Mandell, Douglas, and Bennett's

Principles and Practice
of Infectious Diseases

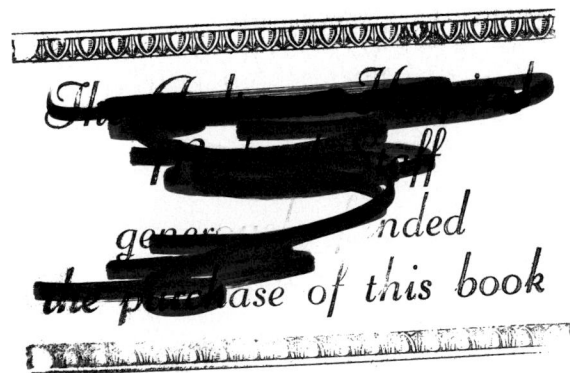

Mandell, Douglas, and Bennett's
Principles and Practice of Infectious Diseases

SIXTH EDITION

Gerald L. Mandell, MD, MACP
Professor of Medicine
Owen R. Cheatham Professor of the Sciences
Division of Infectious Diseases
University of Virginia School of Medicine
Charlottesville, Virginia

John E. Bennett, MD, MACP
Adjunct Professor of Medicine
Uniformed Services University of the Health Sciences
Head, Clinical Mycology Section
Laboratory of Clinical Infectious Diseases
National Institute of Allergy and Infectious Diseases
National Institutes of Health
Bethesda, Maryland

Raphael Dolin, MD
Maxwell Finland Professor of Medicine (Microbiology and Molecular Genetics)
Dean for Academic and Clinical Programs
Harvard Medical School
Boston, Massachusetts

With illustrations by George V. Kelvin

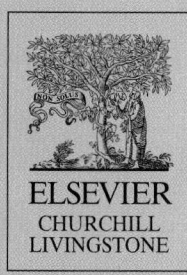

ELSEVIER
CHURCHILL
LIVINGSTONE

162454

ELSEVIER
CHURCHILL
LIVINGSTONE

The Curtis Center
170 S Independence Mall W 300E
Philadelphia, Pennsylvania 19106

MANDELL, DOUGLAS, AND BENNETT'S PRINCIPLES
AND PRACTICE OF INFECTIOUS DISEASES

VOLUME 1: Part no. 9997638247
VOLUME 2: Part no. 9997638239
TWO-VOLUME SET ISBN 0-443-06643-4

NOTICE

Pharmacology is an ever-changing field. Standard safety precautions must be followed, but as new research and clinical experience broaden our knowledge, changes in treatment and drug therapy may become necessary or appropriate. Readers are advised to check the most current product information provided by the maufacturer of each drug to be administered to verify the recommended dose, the method and duration of administration, and contraindications. It is the responsibility of the licensed prescriber, relying on experience and knowledge of the patient, to determine dosages and the best treatment for each individual patient. Neither the publisher nor the author assumes any liability for any injury and/or damage to persons or property arising from this publication.

Previous editions copyrighted 2000, 1995, 1990, 1985, 1979 by Elsevier Inc.

Library of Congress Cataloging-in-Publication Data

Mandell, Douglas, and Bennett's principles and practice of infectious diseases / [edited by]
   Gerald L. Mandell, John E. Bennett, Raphael Dolin.—6th ed.
      p . ; cm.
   Includes bibliographical references and index.
   ISBN 0-443-06643-4
   1. Communicable diseases. I. Title:Principles and practice of infectious diseases. II.
Mandell, Gerald L. III. Douglas, R. Gordon (Robert Gordon) IV. Bennett, John E.
(John Eugene) V. Dolin, Raphael.
   [DNLM: 1. Communicable Diseases. WC 100 M2713 2005]
RC111.M224.2005
616.9—dc22   2004050158

Acquisitions Editor: Tom Hartman
Developmental Editor: Melissa Dudlick
Publishing Services Manager: Frank Polizzano
Design Coordinator: Karen O'Keefe Owens

Printed in the United States of America

Last digit is print number: 9   8   7   6   5   4   3   2   1

CONTRIBUTORS

N. Franklin Adkinson, Jr., MD
Professor of Medicine, Johns Hopkins University School
of Medicine; Johns Hopkins Asthma and Allergy Center,
Baltimore, Maryland
  β-Lactam Allergy

David M. Allen, MD, FAMS
Infectious Diseases Consultant, Medical City Dallas Hospital;
Partner, ID Specialists, P.A., Dallas, Texas
  Acinetobacter Species

Ban M. Allos, MD
Assistant Professor, Departments of Medicine and Preventive
Medicine, Vanderbilt University School of Medicine,
Nashville, Tennessee
  Campylobacter jejuni and Related Species

Harvey J. Alter, MD
Chief, Infectious Diseases Section and Associate Director for
Research, Department of Transfusion Medicine, National Institutes
of Health, Bethesda, Maryland; Clinical Professor of Medicine,
Department of Medicine, Georgetown University Medical School,
Washington, District of Columbia
  Hepatitis G Virus and TT Virus

Guy W. Amsden, PharmD, FCP
Adjunct Assistant Professor, Department of Pharmacology, College
of Physicians and Surgeons of Columbia University, New York;
Attending Pharmacologist in Medicine and Research Scientist,
Department of Adult and Pediatric Medicine and Clinical
Pharmacology Research Center, Bassett Healthcare,
Cooperstown, New York
  Pharmacokinetics and Pharmacodynamics of Anti-infective
  Agents; Tables of Antimicrobial Agent Pharmacology

David A. Anderson, BSc(Hons), PhD
Deputy Director, Macfarlane Burnet Institute for Medical Research
and Public Health, Melbourne, Victoria, Australia
  Hepatitis A Virus

Larry J. Anderson, MD
Chief, Respiratory and Enteric Viruses Branch, Division of Viral
and Rickettsial Diseases, National Center for Infectious Diseases,
Centers for Disease Control and Prevention, Atlanta, Georgia
  Coronaviruses, Including Severe Acute Respiratory Syndrome
  (SARS)—Associated Coronaviruses

David R. Andes, MD
Assistant Professor, Medicine and Microbiology/Immunology,
University of Wisconsin School of Medicine, Madison, Wisconsin
  Cephalosporins

Michael A. Apicella, MD
Professor and Chair, Department of Microbiology, University
of Iowa Roy J. and Lucille A. Carver College of Medicine; Staff
Physician, University of Iowa Hospital and Clinics, Iowa City, Iowa
  Neisseria meningitidis

Gordon L. Archer, MD
Professor, Department of Medicine and Microbiology/Immunology,
Virginia Commonwealth University Medical Center,
Richmond, Virginia
  Staphylococcus epidermidis and Other Coagulase-Negative
  Staphylococci

Michael H. Augenbraun, MD
Associate Professor of Medicine and of Preventive Medicine
and Community Health, State University of New York–Downstate
Medical Center, Brooklyn, New York
  Genital Skin and Mucous Membrane Lesions

Dimitri T. Azar, MD
Professor, Department of Ophthalmology, Harvard Medical School;
Director, Department of Corneal, External Disease, and Refractive
Surgery Services, Massachusetts Eye and Ear Infirmary; Senior
Scientist, Department of Ophthalmology, Schepens Eye Research
Institute, Boston, Massachusetts
  Microbial Conjunctivitis; Microbial Keratitis

Larry M. Baddour, MD
Professor of Medicine, Division of Infectious Diseases, Mayo Clinic
College of Medicine; Consultant, Division of Infectious Diseases,
Mayo Clinic, Rochester, Minnesota
  Infections of Prosthetic Valves and Other Cardiovascular Devices

Lindsey R. Baden, MD
Assistant Professor of Medicine, Harvard Medical School; Clinical
Research Director, Division of Infectious Diseases, Brigham and
Women's Hospital, Boston, Massachusetts
  Vaccines for Human Immunodeficiency Virus-1 Infection

Carol J. Baker, MD
Professor of Pediatrics, Molecular Virology, and Microbiology,
Department of Pediatrics, Section of Infectious Diseases, Baylor
College of Medicine; Attending Physician, Texas Children's
Hospital, Houston, Texas
  Streptococcus agalactiae (Group B Streptococcus)

Ronald C. Ballard, MD
Associate Professor, Department of Clinical Microbiology
and Infectious Diseases, School of Pathology, University of the
Witwatersrand and South African Institute for Medical Research,
Johannesburg, South Africa; Centers for Disease Control
and Prevention, Atlanta, Georgia
  Calymmatobacterium granulomatis (Donovanosis,
  Granuloma Inguinale)

Charles H. Ballow, PharmD, FCCP
Director, Buffalo Clinical Research Center, Buffalo, New York
  Pharmacokinetics and Pharmacodynamics of Anti-infective Agents

Scott D. Barnes, MD
Clinical Fellow in Ophthalmology, Department of Ophthalmology,
Massachusetts Eye and Ear Infirmary, Harvard Medical School,
Boston, Massachusetts
  Microbial Conjunctivitis; Microbial Keratitis

Miriam J. Baron, MD
Instructor, Department of Medicine, Harvard Medical School;
Associate Physician, Department of Medicine, Brigham
and Women's Hospital, Boston, Massachusetts
  Pancreatic Infections

Dan H. Barouch, MD
Instructor in Medicine, Harvard Medical School; Division of Viral
Pathogenesis, Department of Medicine, Beth Israel Deaconess
Medical Center; Division of Infectious Diseases, Department of
Medicine, Brigham and Women's Hospital, Boston, Massachusetts
  Vaccines for Human Immunodeficiency Virus-1 Infection

Kenneth J. Bart, MD, MPH, MSHPM
Director and Professor of Epidemiology and Biostatistics,
Graduate School of Public Health, San Diego State University,
San Diego, California
  Immunization

Byron E. Batteiger, MD
Professor, Department of Medicine and Microbiology
and Immunology, Indiana University School of Medicine,
Indianapolis, Indiana
  Introduction to Chlamydial Diseases; *Chlamydia trachomatis*
  (Trachoma, Perinatal Infections, Lymphogranuloma Venereum,
  and Other Genital Infections)

Gregory J. Bauer, MD
Assistant Professor of Surgery, Department of Surgery, Division of
Burn Surgery, Weill Medical College of Cornell University, New
York, New York
  Burns

Stephen G. Baum, MD
Professor, Department of Medicine, Microbiology and Immunology,
Albert Einstein College of Medicine of Yeshiva University, Bronx,
New York; Chairman, Department of Medicine, Beth Israel Medical
Center, New York, New York
  Adenovirus; Mumps Virus; Introduction to *Mycoplasma* Diseases;
  Mycoplasma pneumoniae and Atypical Pneumonia

Arnold S. Bayer, MD, FACP, FCCP, FIDSA
Professor of Medicine, Department of Internal Medicine, David
Geffen School of Medicine at UCLA, Los Angeles; Associate Chief,
Adult Infectious Diseases, Department of Internal Medicine,
Harbor–UCLA Medical Center; Senior Investigator, St. John's
Cardiovascular Research Center, LA Biomedical Research Institute,
Torrance, California
  Endocarditis and Intravascular Infections

Susan E. Beekmann, RN, MPH
Nurse Epidemiologist, Department of Pathology, University of Iowa
Roy J. and Lucille A. Carver College of Medicine, Iowa City, Iowa
  Infections Caused by Percutaneous Intravascular Devices

Irmgard Behlau, MD
Assistant Professor and Program Director, Infectious Diseases,
Department of Medicine, New Jersey Medical School, University of
Medicine and Dentistry of New Jersey, Newark, New Jersey
  Chronic Meningitis

Beth P. Bell, MD, MPH
Chief, Epidemiology Branch, Division of Viral Hepatitis, National
Center for Infectious Diseases, Centers for Disease Control
and Prevention, Atlanta, Georgia
  Hepatitis A Virus

John E. Bennett, MD, MACP
Adjunct Professor of Medicine, Uniformed Services University of the
Health Sciences; Head, Clinical Mycology Section, Laboratory of
Clinical Infectious Diseases, National Institute of Allergy and
Infectious Diseases, National Institutes of Health, Bethesda, Maryland
  Introduction to Mycoses

Elie F. Berbari, MD
Assistant Professor, Department of Internal Medicine, Division
of Infectious Diseases, Mayo Clinic, Rochester, Minnesota
  Osteomyelitis

Jonathan D. Berman, MD, PhD
Director, Office of Clinical and Regulatory Affairs, National Center
for Complementary and Alternative Medicine, National Institutes
of Health, Bethesda, Maryland
  Complementary and Alternative Medicines for Infectious Diseases

Joseph S. Bertino, Jr., PharmD
Associate Professor of Clinical Pharmacology (in Medicine), College
of Physicians and Surgeons, Columbia University, New York;
Section Chief, Clinical Pharmacology, Department of Medicine,
Bassett Healthcare, Cooperstown, New York
  Pharmacokinetics and Pharmacodynamics of Anti-infective Agents

Holly H. Birdsall, MD, PhD
Associate Professor, Department of Otolaryngology and
Immunology, Baylor College of Medicine; Associate Chief of Staff
for Research, Michael E. DeBakey Veterans Affairs Medical Center,
Houston, Texas
  Antibodies

Alan L. Bisno, MD
Professor, Department of Medicine, University of Miami School of
Medicine; Staff Physician, Miami Veterans Affairs Medical Center,
Miami, Florida
  Pharyngitis; Classification of Streptococci; *Streptococcus
  pyogenes*; Nonsuppurative Poststreptococcal Sequelae:
  Rheumatic Fever and Glomerulonephritis

Martin J. Blaser, MD
Frederick H. King Professor and Chair, Department of Medicine,
New York University School of Medicine; Chief, Medical Services,
Bellevue Hospital Center; Chief, Medical Services, Tisch New York
University Hospital; Staff Physician, Department of Medical
Services, New York Harbor Veterans Affairs Medical Center,
New York, New York
  Introduction to Bacteria and Bacterial Diseases; *Campylobacter
  jejuni* and Related Species; *Helicobacter pylori* and Other Gastric
  Helicobacter Species

William Blattner, MD
Associate Professor and Director of Epidemiology and Prevention
Division, Institute of Human Virology, University of Maryland,
Baltimore, Maryland
  Human T-Cell Lymphotropic Virus Types I and II

Thomas P. Bleck, MD
Louise Nerancy Eminent Scholar in Neurology and Professor of
Neurology, Neurological Surgery, and Internal Medicine, University
of Virginia School of Medicine, Charlottesville, Virginia
  Rhabdoviruses; *Clostridium tetani* (Tetanus); *Clostridium botulinum*
  (Botulism); Botulinum Toxin as a Biological Weapon

David A. Bobak, MD
Associate Professor, Division of Infectious Diseases, Department
of Medicine, Case Western Reserve University School of Medicine;
Director, Traveler's Healthcare Center, and Staff Physician,
University Hospitals of Cleveland/Case Medical Center; Staff
Physician, Department of Hepatitis C Clinic, Louis Stokes Cleveland
Veterans Affairs Medical Center, Cleveland, Ohio
  Nausea, Vomiting, and Noninflammatory Diarrhea

William Bonnez, MD
Associate Professor, Department of Medicine, University
of Rochester School of Medicine and Dentistry; Attending Physician,
Department of Medicine, Strong Memorial Hospital,
Rochester, New York
Papillomaviruses

Luciana L. Borio, MD
Assistant Professor of Medicine, Division of Infectious Diseases,
University of Pittsburgh, Pittsburgh, Pennsylvania; Assistant
Professor of Medicine, Division of Infectious Diseases, Johns
Hopkins Hospital, Baltimore, Maryland
Bioterrorism: An Overview; Plague as an Agent of Bioterrorism

Richard C. Boucher, MD
William Rand Kenan Professor of Medicine, University of North
Carolina at Chapel Hill School of Medicine; Director, Cystic
Fibrosis Center, Chapel Hill, North Carolina
Cystic Fibrosis

Christopher R. Braden, MD
Medical Epidemiologist, Foodborne and Diarrheal Disease Branch,
Division of Bacterial and Mycotic Diseases, National Center for
Infectious Diseases, Centers for Disease Control and Prevention,
Atlanta, Georgia
Foodborne Disease

Barry D. Brause, MD
Clinical Professor of Medicine, Weill Medical College of Cornell
University; Attending Physician, New York Weill Cornell Medical
Center at New York–Presbyterian, Hospital, New York, New York
Infections with Prostheses in Bones and Joints

Kevin E. Brown, MD
Senior Investigator, Hematology Branch, National Heart, Lung, and
Blood Institute, National Institutes of Health, Bethesda, Maryland
Parvovirus

Patricia D. Brown, MD
Associate Professor of Medicine, Division of Infectious Diseases,
Department of Internal Medicine, Wayne State University School
of Medicine, Detroit, Michigan
Infections in Injection Drug Users

Barbara A. Brown-Elliott, MS, MT(ASCP)SM
Senior Research Scientist, Supervisor, Mycobacteria/Nocardia
Laboratory, Department of Microbiology–Biomedical Research,
The University of Texas Health Science Center, Tyler, Texas
Infections Due to Nontuberculous Mycobacteria

Sandra K. Burchett, MD
Assistant Professor, Department of Pediatrics, Harvard Medical
School; Division of Infectious Diseases, Children's Hospital,
Boston, Massachusetts
Pediatric Human Immunodeficiency Virus Infection

James E. Burns, MD, MBA
Clinical Assistant Professor, Department of Pediatrics, University
of Virginia School of Medicine, Charlottesville; Deputy
Commissioner for Public Health Programs, Virginia Department
of Health, Richmond, Virginia
Epiglottitis

Larry M. Bush, MD, FACP
Chief, Infectious Diseases, Department of Medicine, John F.
Kennedy Medical Center; Medical Director, South Florida Clinical
Research, Atlantis Medicine Center, West Palm Beach, Florida
Peritonitis and Intraperitoneal Abscesses

Thomas Butler, MD
Lubbock, Texas
Yersinia Species, Including Plague

David P. Calfee, MD, MS
Assistant Professor, Department of Medicine, Mount Sinai School
of Medicine; Assistant Attending, Mount Sinai Hospital,
New York, New York
Rifamycins

Ellis S. Caplan, MD
Associate Professor of Medicine, University of Maryland School
of Medicine; Section Chief, Infectious Disease, Division of Trauma
Infectious Disease, Shock Trauma Center, University of Maryland
Medical System, Baltimore, Maryland
Hyperbaric Oxygen

Charles C. J. Carpenter, MD, MACP
Professor of Medicine, Department of Medicine, Brown Medical
School; Director, Lifespan/Tufts/Brown Center for AIDS Research,
Providence, Rhode Island
Other Pathogenic Vibrios

Mary T. Caserta, MD
Associate Professor, Department of Pediatrics, University of
Rochester School of Medicine and Dentistry; Attending Physician,
Department of Pediatrics, Golisano Children's Hospital at Strong,
Rochester, New York
Acute Laryngitis

Elio Castagnola, MD
Section for Infections in the Immunocompromised Cancer Patient,
Infectious Diseases Unit, Department of Hematology and Oncology,
G. Gaslini Children's Teaching Hospital, Genoa, Italy
Prophylaxis and Empirical Therapy for Infection
in Cancer Patients

Richard E. Chaisson, MD
Professor of Medicine, Epidemiology, and International Health,
Johns Hopkins University School of Medicine, Baltimore, Maryland
General Clinical Manifestations of Human Immunodeficiency Virus
Infection (Including the Acute Retroviral Syndrome and Oral,
Cutaneous, Renal, Ocular, and Cardiac Diseases); Gastrointestinal
and Hepatobiliary Manifestations of Human Immunodeficiency
Virus Infection

Henry F. Chambers, MD
Professor, Department of Medicine, University of California,
San Francisco, School of Medicine; Chief, Infectious Diseases,
Department of Medicine, San Francisco General Hospital,
San Francisco, California
Penicillins; Other β-Lactam Antibiotics

Stanley W. Chapman, MD
Professor of Medicine and Associate Professor of Microbiology,
University of Mississippi School of Medicine; Division of Infectious
Diseases, University of Mississippi Medical Center, Jackson,
Mississippi
Blastomyces dermatitidis

Manhattan Charurat
Assistant Professor, Institute of Human Virology, University of
Maryland, Baltimore, Maryland
Human T-Cell Lymphotropic Virus Types I and II

Sanjiv Chopra, MD
Faculty Dean for Continuing Education and Professor of Medicine,
Harvard Medical School; Director, Clinical Hepatology, Department
of Medicine, Division of Gastroenterology, Beth Israel Deaconess
Medical Center, Boston, Massachusetts
Acute Viral Hepatitis

Anthony W. Chow, MD, FRCPC, FACP
Professor of Medicine and Director, MD/PhD Program, University of British Columbia Faculty of Medicine; Vancouver Hospital Health Science Center, Vancouver, British Columbia, Canada
    Infections of the Oral Cavity, Neck, and Head

Nicholas P. Cianciotto, PhD
Professor, Department of Microbiology-Immunology, Northwestern University Medical School, Chicago, Illinois
    Legionella

Rebecca A. Clark, MD, PhD
Medicine Department, Louisiana State University Health Sciences Center; HIV Outpatient Program, Medical Center of Louisiana at New Orleans, New Orleans, Louisiana
    Human Immunodeficiency Virus Infection in Women

Robert A. Clark, MD
Professor and Chair, Department of Medicine, University of Texas Health Science Center at San Antonio Medical School; Staff Physician and Chief, Department of Medicine, University Health System; Staff Physician, Medical Service, South Texas Veterans Health Care System, San Antonio, Texas
    Granulocytic Phagocytes

Farley R. Cleghorn, MD, MPH
Adjunct Professor of Medicine, Institute of Human Virology, University of Maryland, Baltimore, Maryland; Director, Center for HIV/AIDS, The Futures Group International, Washington, District of Columbia
    Human Immunodeficiency Viruses

Michael W. Climo, MD
Associate Professor of Medicine and Microbiology/Immunology, Virginia Commonwealth University Medical Center; Hospital Epidemiologist, Infectious Disease Division; Medical Director, HIV/AIDS Program, Hunter Holmes McGuire Veteran Affairs Medical Center, Richmond, Virginia
    Staphylococcus epidermidis and Other Coagulase-Negative Staphylococci

Myron S. Cohen, MD
J. Herbert Bate Distinguished Professor of Medicine, Microbiology, Immunology, and Public Health, University of North Carolina at Chapel Hill School of Medicine, Chapel Hill, North Carolina
    The Acutely Ill Patient with Fever and Rash

Susan E. Cohn, MD, MPH
Associate Professor of Medicine, Department of Medicine, University of Rochester Medical Center, Rochester, New York
    Human Immunodeficiency Virus Infection in Women

Mark Connors, MD
Senior Clinical Investigator, Laboratory of Immunoregulation, National Institutes of Health, Bethesda, Maryland
    The Immunology of Human Immunodeficiency Virus Infection

Joanne Cono, MD, ScM
Senior Medical Officer, Bioterrorism Preparedness and Response Program, National Center for Infectious Diseases, Centers for Disease Control and Prevention, Atlanta, Georgia
    Smallpox and Bioterrorism

Lawrence Corey, MD
Head, Program in Infectious Diseases; Head, Virology Division; and Professor of Laboratory Medicine and Medicine, University of Washington School of Medicine, Seattle, Washington
    Herpes Simplex Virus

William A. Craig, MD
Professor of Medicine and Pharmaceutics, and Consultant, Department of Medicine, University of Wisconsin School of Medicine; Investigator, Department of Research Service, William S. Middleton Memorial Veterans Hospital, Madison, Wisconsin
    Cephalosporins

Kent B. Crossley, MD
Professor, Department of Medicine, University of Minnesota School of Medicine; Veterans Affairs Medical Center, Minneapolis, Minnesota
    Infections in the Elderly

Clyde S. Crumpacker, MD
Professor of Medicine, Harvard Medical School; Physician, Division of Infectious Diseases, Beth Israel Deaconess Medical Center, Boston, Massachusetts
    Cytomegalovirus

James W. Curran, MD, MPH
Dean and Professor, Department of Epidemiology, and Director, Emory Center for AIDS, Rollins School of Public Health, Emory University, Atlanta, Georgia
    Epidemiology and Prevention of Acquired Immunodeficiency Syndrome and Human Immunodeficiency Virus Infection

Bart J. Currie, FRACP, DTM&H
Professor in Medicine, Northern Territory Clinical School, Menzies School of Health Research and Flinders University; Infectious Diseases Physician, Royal Darwin Hospital, Darwin, Northern Territory, Australia
    Burkholderia pseudomallei and *Burkholderia mallei*: Melioidosis and Glanders

Michael P. Curry, MD
Instructor, Department of Medicine, Harvard Medical School; Medical Director, Liver Transplantation, Department of Medicine, Beth Israel Deaconess Medical Center, Boston, Massachusetts
    Acute Viral Hepatitis

Inger Damon, MD, PhD
Chief, Poxvirus Program, Division of Viral and Rickettsial Diseases, National Center for Infectious Diseases, Centers for Disease Control and Prevention, Atlanta, Georgia
    Orthopoxviruses: Vaccinia (Smallpox Vaccine), Variola (Smallpox), Monkeypox, and Cowpox; Other Poxviruses That Infect Humans: Parapoxviruses, Molluscum Contagiosum, and Tanapox; Smallpox and Bioterrorism

Rabih O. Darouiche, MD
Professor, Departments of Medicine and Physical Medicine and Rehabilitation, Infectious Disease Section, Baylor College of Medicine; Director, Center for Prostheses Infection; Staff Physician, Department of Medical (Infectious Disease Section) and Spinal Cord Injury Care Lines, Michael E. Debakey Veterans Affairs Medical Center, Houston, Texas
    Infections in Patients with Spinal Cord Injury

George S. Deepe, Jr., MD
Professor, Department of Internal Medicine, University of Cincinnati College of Medicine; Chief, Division of Infectious Diseases, University Hospital, Cincinnati, Ohio
    Histoplasma capsulatum

Carlos Del Rio, MD
Professor of Medicine (Infectious Diseases), Department of Medicine, Emory University School of Medicine; Chief of Medical Services, Department of Medicine, Grady Memorial Hospital, Atlanta, Georgia
Epidemiology and Prevention of Acquired Immunodeficiency Syndrome and Human Immunodeficiency Virus Infection; Other Gram-Negative and Gram-Variable Bacill

Lisa M. Demeter, MD
Associate Professor, Infectious Diseases Unit, Department of Medicine, University of Rochester School of Medicine and Dentistry, Rochester, New York
JC, BK, and Other Polyomaviruses; Progressive Multifocal Leukoencephalopathy

David T. Dennis, MD, MPH
Faculty Affiliate, Department of Microbiology, Immunology, and Pathology, Colorado State University College of Veterinary Medicine and Biomedical Sciences; Guest Researcher, Division of Vector-Borne Infectious Diseases, Centers for Disease Control and Prevention, Fort Collins, Colorado
Yersinia Species, Including Plague

Peter Densen, MD
Professor, Division of Infectious Diseases, Department of Internal Medicine, University of Iowa Roy J. and Lucille A. Carver College of Medicine, Iowa City, Iowa
Complement

Ben E. De Pauw, MD, PhD
Professor of Medicine, Bloodtransfusion and Transplant Immunology, University Medical Center St. Radboud, Nijmegen, The Netherlands
Infections in the Immunocompromised Host: General Principles; Infections in Patients with Hematologic Malignancies

Terence S. Dermody, MD
Professor, Departments of Pediatrics and Microbiology and Immunology, Vanderbilt University School of Medicine; Director, Elizabeth B. Lamb Center for Pediatric Research; Attending Physician, Pediatric Infectious Diseases, Vanderbilt Children's Hospital, Nashville, Tennessee
Introduction to Viruses and Viral Diseases

Carl W. Dieffenbach, PhD
Director, Basic Science Program, Division of AIDS, National Institute of Allergy and Infectious Diseases, National Institutes of Health, Bethesda, Maryland
Innate (General or Nonspecific) Host Defense Mechanisms

Jules L. Dienstag, MD
Professor of Medicine and Associate Dean for Academic and Clinical Programs, Harvard Medical School; Physician, Gastrointestinal Unit (Medical Services), Massachusetts General Hospital, Boston, Massachusetts
Chronic Viral Hepatitis

William E. Dismukes, MD
Professor of Medicine and Director, Division of Infectious Diseases; Vice-Chairman, Department of Medicine, University of Alabama School of Medicine at Birmingham; Attending Physician, Department of Internal Medicine, University Hospital, UAB Medical Center, Birmingham, Alabama
Chronic Pneumonia

Raphael Dolin, MD
Maxwell Finland Professor of Medicine (Microbiology and Molecular Genetics) and Dean for Academic and Clinical Programs, Harvard Medical School, Boston, Massachusetts
Vaccines for Human Immunodeficiency Virus-1 Infection; Zoonotic Paramyxoviruses: Hendra, Nipah, and Menangle Viruses; Noroviruses and Other Caliciviruses; Astroviruses and Picobirnaviruses

J. Peter Donnelly, PhD
Coordinator, Studies in Supportive Care, Department of Hematology, University Medical Center St. Radboud, Nijmegen University Center for Infectious Diseases, Nijmegen, The Netherlands
Infections in the Immunocompromised Host: General Principles

Michael S. Donnenberg, MD
Professor of Medicine and Professor of Microbiology and Immunology; Head, Division of Infectious Diseases, Department of Medicine, University of Maryland School of Medicine, Baltimore, Maryland
Enterobacteriaceae

Gerald R. Donowitz, MD
Professor of Medicine and Infectious Diseases, Department of Internal Medicine, University of Virginia Health Systems, Charlottesville, Virginia
Oxazolidinones; Acute Pneumonia

Philip R. Dormitzer, MD, PhD
Assistant Professor, Department of Pediatrics, Harvard Medical School; Scientific Associate, Laboratory of Molecular Medicine, Children's Hospital, Boston, Massachusetts
Rotaviruses

J. Stephen Dumler, MD
Professor of Pathology, Division of Medical Microbiology, and Professor, Cellular and Molecular Medicine Program, Johns Hopkins University School of Medicine; Associate Director, Division of Medical Microbiology, Department of Pathology, Johns Hopkins Hospital; Professor, Department of Molecular Microbiology and Immunology, Johns Hopkins University Bloomberg School of Public Health, Baltimore, Maryland
Rickettsia typhi (Murine Typhus); *Ehrlichia chaffeensis* (Human Monocytotropic Ehrlichiosis), *Anaplasma phagocytophilum* (Human Granulocytotropic Anaplasmosis), and Other Ehrlichieae

J. Stephen Dummer, MD
Professor of Medicine, Vanderbilt University School of Medicine; Director, Transplant Infectious Diseases, Vanderbilt Transplant Center, Nashville, Tennessee
Risk Factors and Approaches to Infections in Transplant Recipients; Infections in Solid Organ Transplant Recipients

Herbert L. DuPont, MD
Director, Center for Infectious Diseases, and Professor of Epidemiology, Mary W. Kelsey Chair of Medical Sciences, Department of Medicine, University of Texas-Houston School of Public Health; Chief, Internal Medicine, St. Luke's Episcopal Hospital; H. Irving Schweppe, Jr., MD, Chair in Internal Medicine and Vice Chairman, Department of Medicine, and Clinical Professor, Department of Microbiology and Immunology, Baylor College of Medicine, Houston, Texas
Shigella Species (Bacillary Dysentery)

David T. Durack, MB, PhD
Consulting Professor of Medicine, Duke University School of Medicine, Durham; Becton Dickinson & Co., Research Triangle Park, North Carolina
Fever of Unknown Origin; Prophylaxis of Infective Endocarditis

Marlene L. Durand, MD
Assistant Professor, Department of Medicine, Harvard Medical School; Director, Infectious Disease Service, Massachusetts Eye and Ear Infirmary; Associate Physician, Infectious Disease Unit, Massachusetts General Hospital, Boston, Massachusetts
  Endophthalmitis; Infectious Causes of Uveitis; Periocular Infections

Mark Dybul, MD
Deputy Chief Medical Officer, Office of the U.S. Global AIDS Coordinator, Washington, D.C.
  The Immunology of Human Immunodeficiency Virus Infection

Paul H. Edelstein, MD
Professor, Department of Pathology and Laboratory Medicine, University of Pennsylvania School of Medicine; Director of Clinical Microbiology, Department of Pathology and Laboratory Medicine, University of Pennsylvania Medical System; Attending Physician, Division of Infectious Diseases, University of Pennsylvania Medical Center, Philadelphia, Pennsylvania
  Legionella

Michael B. Edmond, MD, MPH, MPA
Professor and Associate Chair for Education, Department of Internal Medicine, Virginia Commonwealth University School of Medicine; Hospital Epidemiologist and Medical Director of Performance Improvement, Virginia Commonwealth University Medical Center, Richmond, Virginia
  Organization for Infection Control; Isolation

John E. Edwards, Jr., MD
Professor of Medicine, David Geffen School of Medicine at UCLA, Los Angeles; Chief, Division of Infectious Diseases, Harbor/UCLA Medical Center, Torrance, California
  Candida Species

Morven S. Edwards, MD
Professor of Pediatrics, Section of Infectious Diseases, Baylor College of Medicine; Attending Physician, Texas Children's Hospital, Houston, Texas
  Streptococcus agalactiae (Group B Streptococcus)

George M. Eliopoulos, MD
Professor of Medicine, Harvard Medical School; Division of Infectious Diseases, Department of Medicine, Beth Israel Deaconess Medical Center, Boston, Massachusetts
  Principles of Anti-infective Therapy

Jerrold J. Ellner, MD
Professor and Chair, Department of Medicine, New Jersey Medical School, University of Medicine and Dentistry of New Jersey, Newark, New Jersey
  Chronic Meningitis

Suzanne U. Emerson, PhD
Head, Molecular Hepatitis Section, Laboratory of Infectious Diseases, National Institutes of Health, Bethesda, Maryland
  Hepatitis E Virus

N. Cary Engleberg, MD
Professor and Chief, Division of Infectious Diseases, Departments of Internal Medicine and Microbiology and Immunology, University of Michigan Medical School, Ann Arbor, Michigan
  Chronic Fatigue Syndrome

Joel D. Ernst, MD
Director, Division of Infectious Diseases, and Jeffrey Bergstein Professor of Medicine, and Professor of Microbiology, Departments of Medicine and Microbiology, New York University School of Medicine; Attending Physician, Department of Medicine, Bellevue Hospital Center; Attending Physician, Department of Medicine, Tisch Hospital of New York University Medical Center, New York, New York
  Mycobacterium leprae (Leprosy, Hansen's Disease)

Rick M. Fairhurst, MD, PhD
Staff Clinician, Laboratory of Malaria and Vector Research, National Institute of Allergy and Infectious Diseases, National Institutes of Health, Bethesda, Maryland
  Plasmodium Species (Malaria)

Stanley Falkow, PhD
Robert W. and Vivian K. Cahill Professor of Microbiology and Immunology and Professor of Medicine, Departments of Microbiology and Immunology and Medicine, Stanford University School of Medicine, Stanford, California
  A Molecular Perspective of Microbial Pathogenicity

Ann R. Falsey, MD
Associate Professor of Medicine, Department of Medicine, University of Rochester School of Medicine and Dentistry; Attending Physician, Infectious Disease Unit, Rochester General Hospital, Rochester, New York
  Human Metapneumovirus

W. Edmund Farrar, MD
Professor Emeritus of Medicine, Medical University of South Carolina College of Medicine, Charleston, South Carolina
  Erysipelothrix rhusiopathiae

Anthony S. Fauci, MD
Professor, Department of Medicine, University of Maryland School of Medicine, Baltimore; Director, National Institute of Allergy and Infectious Diseases, National Institutes of Health, Bethesda, Maryland
  The Immunology of Human Immunodeficiency Virus Infection

Daniel P. Fedorko, PhD
Staff Scientist, Department of Laboratory Medicine, Warren G. Magnuson Clinical Center, National Institutes of Health, Bethesda, Maryland
  The Clinician and the Microbiology Laboratory

Stephen M. Feinstone, MD
Chief, Laboratory of Hepatitis Viruses, U.S. Food and Drug Administration, Center for Biologics Evaluation and Research, Bethesda, Maryland
  Hepatitis A Virus

Thomas Fekete, MD
Professor of Medicine, Section of Infectious Diseases, Temple University School of Medicine; Professor, Department of Internal Medicine, Temple University Hospital, Philadelphia, Pennsylvania
  Bacillus Species and Related Genera Other than Bacillus anthracis

Steven M. Fine, MD, PhD
Assistant Professor of Medicine, Infectious Diseases Unit, University of Rochester School of Medicine and Dentistry; University of Rochester Medical Center, Rochester, New York
  Vesicular Stomatitis Virus and Related Viruses

Neil O. Fishman, MD
Assistant Professor of Medicine, Division of Infectious Diseases, University of Pennsylvania School of Medicine; Director, Department of Healthcare Epidemiology and Infection Control, Department of Antimicrobial Management Program, University of Pennsylvania Health System, Philadelphia, Pennsylvania
    Antimicrobial Management: Cost and Resistance

Tamara L. Fisk, MD
Assistant Professor, Division of Infectious Diseases, Emory University School of Medicine; Assistant Professor, Department of Infectious Diseases, Emory Crawford Long Hospital, Atlanta, Georgia; Visiting Scientist, International Emerging Infections Program, Thailand Centers for Disease Control and Prevention, Nonthaburi, Thailand
    Cyclospora cayetanensis, Isospora belli, Sarcocystis Species, *Balantidium coli,* and *Blastocystis hominis*

Daniel Fitzgerald, MD
Assistant Professor of Medicine, Division of International Medicine and Infectious Diseases, Department of Medicine, Weill Medical College of Cornell University, New York, New York
    Mycobacterium tuberculosis

Vance G. Fowler, Jr., MD, MHS
Assistant Professor, Department of Medicine, Duke University School of Medicine, Durham, North Carolina
    Endocarditis and Intravascular Infections

David O. Freedman, MD
Professor of Medicine and Epidemiology/International Health, Division of Geographic Medicine, University of Alabama at Birmingham; Director, UAB Travelers Health Clinic, The Kirklin Clinic, University of Alabama Hospital, Birmingham, Alabama; Co-Director, The Gorgas Course in Clinical Tropical Medicine, Tropical Medicine Institute, Cayetano Heredia University, Lima, Peru
    Protection of Travelers; Infections in Returning Travelers

Alicia M. Fry, MD, MPH
Medical Epidemiologist, Foodborne and Diarrhea Diseases Branch, National Center for Infectious Diseases, Centers for Disease Control and Prevention, Atlanta, Georgia
    Foodborne Disease

John Galgiani, MD
Director, Valley Fever Center for Excellence; Professor, Department of Medicine, University of Arizona College of Medicine; Program Director, Department of Infectious Diseases, Southern Arizona Veterans Affairs Health Care System, Tucson, Arizona
    Coccidioides Species

John I. Gallin, MD
Director, Warren G. Magnuson Clinical Center, National Institutes of Health, Bethesda, Maryland
    Evaluation of the Patient with Suspected Immunodeficiency

Robert C. Gallo, MD
Director, Institute of Human Virology and Division of Basic Science, University of Maryland Biotechnology Institute, University of Maryland, Baltimore, Maryland
    Human Immunodeficiency Viruses

Amy Gates, MD
Assistant Clinical Professor in Hematology/Oncology, Positive Health Program, University of California, San Francisco, School of Medicine, San Francisco, California
    Malignancies in Human Immunodeficiency Virus Infection

Jeffrey A. Gelfand, MD
Visiting Professor of Medicine, Harvard Medical School; Professor of Medicine, Tufts University School of Medicine; Physician, Infectious Diseases Division, Department of Medicine, Massachusetts General Hospital; Associate Staff, Department of Medicine, New England Medical Center, Boston, Massachusetts
    Babesia Species

Julie L. Gerberding, MD, MPH
Director, Centers for Disease Control and Prevention; Administrator, Agency for Toxic Substances and Disease Registry, Atlanta, Georgia
    Human Immunodeficiency Virus in Health Care Settings

Anne A. Gershon, MD
Professor, Department of Pediatrics, Columbia University College of Physicians and Surgeons, New York, New York
    Rubella Virus (German Measles); Measles Virus (Rubeola)

David N. Gilbert, MD
Professor of Medicine, Department of Internal Medicine, Oregon Health and Science University School of Medicine; Director of Medical Education and Earle A. Chiles Research Department of Medical Education, Providence Portland Medical Center, Portland, Oregon
    Aminoglycosides

Vee J. Gill, PhD
Microbiology Consultant, Microbiology Laboratory, Department of Pathology, Suburban Hospital Healthcare System, Bethesda, Maryland
    The Clinician and the Microbiology Laboratory; *Capnocytophaga*

Peter H. Gilligan, PhD, D(ABMM), FAAM
Professor, Department of Microbiology-Immunology and Pathology-Laboratory Medicine, University of North Carolina at Chapel Hill School of Medicine; Director, Clinical Microbiology-Immunology Laboratories, University of North Carolina Hospitals, Chapel Hill, North Carolina
    Cystic Fibrosis

Michel P. Glauser, MD
Professor, University of Lausanne; Chief of Service, Service of Infectious Diseases, Department of Medicine, Centre Hospitalier Universitaire Vaudois, Lausanne, Switzerland
    Staphylococcus aureus (Including Staphylococcal Toxic Shock)

Michael S. Glickman, MD
Assistant Professor, Department of Medicine and Immunology, Weill Medical College of Cornell University; Attending Physician, Infectious Diseases Service, Memorial Hospital for Cancer and Allied Diseases; Department Head, Laboratory of Microbial Pathogenesis Immunology Program, Sloan-Kettering Institute, New York, New York
    Cell-Mediated Defense against Infection

Ulf B. Göbel, MD, PhD
Director, Institute for Microbiology and Hygiene, Charité University Hospital, Berlin, Germany
    Stenotrophomonas maltophilia and *Burkholderia cepacia*

Ellie J. C. Goldstein, MD
Clinical Professor, Department of Medicine, David Geffen School of Medicine at UCLA; Chair, Department of Infectious Diseases, Kindred–LA Hospital, Los Angeles; Director, R. M. Alden Research Laboratory, Santa Monica, California
    Bites

Fred M. Gordin, MD
Professor of Medicine, Department of Medicine, George Washington
University School of Medicine; Chief, Infectious Diseases,
Department of Infectious Diseases, Veterans Affairs Medical Center,
Washington, District of Columbia
Mycobacterium avium Complex

Eduardo Gotuzzo, MD, FACP
Professor, Department of Medicine, Cayetano Heredia University;
Director, Alexander von Humboldt Tropical Medicine Institute;
Head, Department of Infectious Diseases and Tropical Medicine,
Hospital Nacional Cayetano Heredia, Lima, Peru
Vibrio cholerae

Paul S. Graman, MD
Professor of Medicine, University of Rochester School of Medicine
and Dentistry; Attending Physician and Clinical Director, Infectious
Diseases Unit, Strong Memorial Hospital, Rochester, New York
Esophagitis

Diane E. Griffin, MD, PhD
Professor and Chair, W. Henry Feinstone Department of Molecular
Microbiology and Immunology, Johns Hopkins University
Bloomberg School of Public Health, Baltimore, Maryland
Encephalitis, Myelitis, and Neuritis

Patricia M. Griffin, MD
Chief, Foodborne Diseases Epidemiology Section, Division
of Bacterial and Mycotic Diseases, National Center for Infectious
Diseases, Centers for Disease Control and Prevention, Atlanta,
Georgia
Foodborne Disease

David E. Griffith, MD
Professor of Medicine, Specialty Care Medicine, University of Texas
Health Center at Tyler, Tyler, Texas
Antimycobacterial Agents

David I. Grove, MD, DSc
Clinical Professor of Infectious Diseases, Department of Medicine,
University of Adelaide Faculty of Medicine; Director, Department of
Clinical Microbiology and Infectious Diseases, Institute of Medical
and Veterinary Science, The Queen Elizabeth Hospital, Adelaide,
South Australia, Australia
Tissue Nematodes, Including Trichinosis, Dracunculiasis,
and the Filariases

Richard L. Guerrant, MD
Thomas H. Hunter Professor of International Medicine; Director,
Center for Global Health, Division of Infectious Diseases and
International Health, University of Virginia School of Medicine,
Charlottesville, Virginia
Principles and Syndromes of Enteric Infection; Nausea, Vomiting,
and Noninflammatory Diarrhea; Inflammatory Enteritides; Enteric
Fever and Other Causes of Abdominal Symptoms with Fever

Jack M. Gwaltney, Jr., MD
Professor Emeritus, Department of Internal Medicine, University
of Virginia School of Medicine; University of Virginia Health
System, Charlottesville, Virginia
The Common Cold; Sinusitis; Acute Bronchitis; Rhinovirus

David W. Haas, MD
Associate Professor, Departments of Medicine, Microbiology,
and Immunology, Vanderbilt University School of Medicine,
Nashville, Tennessee
Mycobacterium tuberculosis

Caroline Breese Hall, MD
Professor of Pediatrics and Medicine, Department of Infectious
Diseases, University of Rochester School of Medicine and Dentistry,
Rochester, New York
Acute Laryngotracheobronchitis (Croup); Bronchiolitis; Respiratory
Syncytial Virus

H. Hunter Handsfield, MD
Professor, Department of Medicine, University of Washington;
Director, STD Control Program, Public Health–Seattle and King
County, Seattle, Washington
Neisseria gonorrhoeae

George J. Hanna, MD
Antiviral Global Project Head, Abbott Laboratories, Abbott Park,
Illinois
Antiretroviral Therapy for Human Immunodeficiency Virus Infection

Barry J. Hartman, MD
Clinical Professor of Medicine, Division of Internal Medicine and
Infectious Diseases, Weill Medical College of Cornell University;
Attending Physician, New York–Presbyterian Hospital–Cornell
Campus, New York, New York
Acinetobacter Species

Roderick J. Hay, MD
Dean and Professor of Dermatology, Faculty of Medicine and Health
Sciences, Queens University Belfast; Attending Physician,
Department of Dermatology, Belfast City Hospital, Belfast, Northern
Ireland, United Kingdom
Dermatophytosis and Other Superficial Mycoses

Frederick G. Hayden, MD
Stuart S. Richardson Professor of Clinical Virology and Professor
of Internal Medicine and Pathology, University of Virginia School
of Medicine, Charlottesville, Virginia
Antiviral Drugs (Other Than Antiretrovirals)

Craig W. Hedberg
Associate Professor, Division of Environmental Health Sciences,
University of Minnesota School of Public Health, Minneapolis,
Minnesota
Epidemiologic Principles

David K. Henderson, MD
Deputy Director for Clinical Care, National Institutes of Health,
Bethesda, Maryland
Hospital Preparedness for Emerging and Highly Contagious
Infectious Diseases: Getting Ready for SARS or Whatever Comes
Next; Infections Caused by Percutaneous Intravascular Devices;
Human Immunodeficiency Virus in Health Care Settings;
Nosocomial Herpesvirus Infections

Donald A. Henderson, MD, MPH
Dean Emeritus, Johns Hopkins University School of Hygiene and
Public Health, Baltimore, Maryland; Professor of Medicine and
Public Health, University of Pittsburgh School of Medicine; Staff,
University of Pittsburgh Center for Biosecurity, Pittsburgh,
Pennsylvania
Bioterrorism: An Overview

J. Owen Hendley, MD
Professor of Pediatrics, University of Virginia School of Medicine;
Attending Physician, Division of Pediatric Infectious Diseases,
University of Virginia Health System, Charlottesville, Virginia
Epiglottitis

Erik L. Hewlett, MD
Professor, Departments of Medicine and Pharmacology,
University of Virginia School of Medicine; Attending Physician,
Department of Internal Medicine, University of Virginia Hospital,
Charlottesville, Virginia
Toxins; *Bordetella* Species

Kevin P. High, MD
Associate Professor of Medicine, Sections of Infectious Diseases
and Hematology/Oncology, Wake Forest University School of
Medicine, Winston-Salem, North Carolina
Nutrition, Immunity, and Infection

Adrian V. S. Hill, MD
Professor of Human Genetics, Wellcome Trust Centre for Human
Genetics, University of Oxford, Oxford, United Kingdom
Human Genetics and Infection

David R. Hill, MD, DTM&H
Honorary Professor, Department of Infectious and Tropical Diseases,
London School of Hygiene and Tropical Medicine; Director,
National Travel Heath Network and Centre, London, United
Kingdom
Giardia lamblia

Alan R. Hinman, MD, MPH
Adjunct Professor, Department of Epidemiology and International
Health, Rollins School of Public Health, Emory University, Atlanta;
Senior Public Health Scientist, Task Force for Child Survival and
Development, Decatur, Georgia
Immunization

Martin S. Hirsch, MD
Professor, Department of Medicine, Harvard Medical School;
Physician, Department of Medicine, Massachusetts General Hospital;
Professor, Infectious Diseases and Immunology, Harvard School
of Public Health, Boston, Massachusetts
Antiretroviral Therapy for Human Immunodeficiency Virus Infection

Steven M. Holland, MD
Chief, Immunopathogenesis Section, Laboratory of Host Defenses,
National Institute of Allergy and Infectious Diseases, National
Institutes of Health, Bethesda, Maryland
Evaluation of the Patient with Suspected Immunodeficiency

Edward W. Hook III, MD
Professor of Medicine and Epidemiology, University of Alabama
School of Medicine, University of Alabama at Birmingham;
Director, STD Control Program for Jefferson County Department of
Health, Birmingham, Alabama
Endemic Treponematoses

David C. Hooper, MD
Chief, Infection Control Unit, Division of Infectious Diseases,
Massachusetts General Hospital, Boston, Massachusetts
Quinolones; Urinary Tract Agents: Nitrofurantoin and Methenamine

C. Robert Horsburgh, Jr., MD, MUS
Professor of Epidemiology, Biostatistics, and Medicine; Chair,
Department of Epidemiology, Boston University School of Public
Health, Boston, Massachusetts
Mycobacterium avium Complex

Duane R. Hospenthal, MD, PhD
Associate Professor of Medicine, F. Edward Hébert School of
Medicine, Uniformed Services University of the Health Sciences,
Bethesda, Maryland; Chief, Infectious Disease Service, Brooke
Army Medical Center, Fort Sam Houston, Texas
Agents of Chromoblastomycosis; Agents of Mycetoma;
Uncommon Fungi

James M. Hughes, MD
Director, National Center for Infectious Diseases, Centers
for Disease Control and Prevention, Atlanta, Georgia
Emerging and Reemerging Infectious Disease Threats;
Foodborne Disease

Molly A. Hughes, MD, PhD
Assistant Professor, Department of Medicine, University of Virginia
School of Medicine; Attending Physician, Department of Internal
Medicine, University of Virginia Hospital, Charlottesville, Virginia
Toxins

Christopher D. Huston, MD
Assistant Professor, Department of Medicine, University of Vermont
College of Medicine; Attending Physician, Department of Medicine,
Division of Infectious Diseases, Fletcher Allen Health Care,
Burlington, Vermont
Microbial Adherence

Jonathon R. Iredell, MD, PhD, FRACP, FRCPA
Senior Lecturer, Department of Medicine, University of Sydney;
Senior Staff Specialist, Centre for Infectious Diseases and
Microbiology, Westmead Hospital, Sydney, New South Wales,
Australia
Nocardia Species

Lisa A. Jackson, MD, MPH
Associate Professor, Department of Epidemiology, School of Public
Health and Community Medicine, University of Washington;
Associate Investigator, Center for Health Studies, Group Health
Cooperative, Seattle, Washington
Chlamydophila (Chlamydia) pneumoniae

Selma M. B. Jeronimo, MD, PhD
Professor, Department of Biochemistry, Federal University of Rio
Grande do Norte, Natal, RN, Brazil
Leishmania Species: Visceral (Kala-Azar), Cutaneous,
and Mucocutaneous Leishmaniasis

Eric C. Johannsen, MD
Instructor, Department of Medicine, Harvard Medical School;
Associate Physician, Division of Infectious Diseases, Brigham
and Women's Hospital, Boston, Massachusetts
Infections of the Liver and Biliary System; Epstein-Barr Virus
(Infectious Mononucleosis)

Caroline C. Johnson, MD
Adjunct Associate Professor, School of Public Health, Drexel
University; Director, Division of Disease Control, Philadelphia
Department of Public Health, Philadelphia, Pennsylvania
Viridans Streptococci, Groups C and G Streptococci,
and *Gemella morbillorum*

Warren D. Johnson, Jr., MD
B.H. Kean Professor of Tropical Medicine; Chief, Division of
International Medicine and Infectious Diseases; Director,
International Health Care Service, Weill Medical College of Cornell
University, New York, New York
Borrelia *Species (Relapsing Fever)*

Robert B. Jones, MD, PhD
Executive Associate Dean for Strategic Planning, Analysis, and
Operations, Indiana University School of Medicine, Indianapolis,
Indiana
Introduction to Chlamydial Diseases; *Chlamydia trachomatis*
(Trachoma, Perinatal Infections, Lymphogranuloma Venereum,
and Other Genital Infections)

Allen B. Kaiser, MD
Chief of Staff, Vanderbilt University Hospital; Vice Chairman for Clinical Affairs, Department of Medicine, Vanderbilt University Medical Center, Nashville, Tennessee
    Postoperative Infections and Antimicrobial Prophylaxis

Angela D. M. Kashuba, PharmD, DABCP
University of North Carolina at Chapel Hill, Chapel Hill, North Carolina
    Pharmacokinetics and Pharmacodynamics of Anti-infective Agents

Dennis L. Kasper, MD
William Ellery Channing Professor of Medicine; Professor of Microbiology and Molecular Genetics, Harvard Medical School; Director, Channing Laboratory, Department of Medicine, Brigham and Women's Hospital, Boston, Massachusetts
    Anaerobic Infections: General Concepts

Bruce A. Kaufman, MD
Professor of Neurosurgery, Medical College of Wisconsin; Chief, Division of Pediatric Neurosurgery Froedtert Hospital, Neurosciences Center, Milwaukee, Wisconsin
    Cerebrospinal Fluid Shunt Infections

Donald Kaye, MD, MACP
Professor of Medicine, Drexel University College of Medicine; Medical Staff, Department of Medicine, Hospital of the Medical College of Pennsylvania, Philadelphia, Pennsylvania
    Polymyxins (Polymyxin B and Colistin); Urinary Tract Infections

Keith S. Kaye, MD, MPH
Assistant Professor of Medicine, Division of Infectious Diseases and International Health, Duke University Medical Center, Durham, North Carolina
    Polymyxins (Polymyxin B and Colistin)

Kenneth M. Kaye, MD
Assistant Professor, Department of Medicine, Harvard Medical School; Staff Physician, Division of Infectious Diseases, Department of Medicine, Brigham and Women's Hospital, Boston, Massachusetts
    Epstein-Barr Virus (Infectious Mononucleosis); Kaposi's Sarcoma-Associated Herpesvirus (Human Herpesvirus Type 8)

George E. Kenny, PhD
Professor Emeritus, Department of Pathobiology, University of Washington School of Medicine, Seattle, Washington
    Genital Mycoplasmas: *Mycoplasma genitalium, Mycoplasma hominis,* and *Ureaplasma* Species

Jay S. Keystone, MD, FRCPC, MSc
Centre for Travel and Tropical Medicine, University of Toronto Faculty of Medicine; Toronto General Hospital, Toronto, Ontario, Canada
    Cyclospora cayetanensis, Isospora belli, Sarcocystis Species, *Balantidium coli,* and *Blastocystis hominis*

Charles H. King, MD
Associate Professor of International Health, Center for Global Health and Diseases, Case Western Reserve University, Cleveland, Ohio
    Cestodes (Tapeworms)

Louis V. Kirchhoff, MD, MPH
Professor, Departments of Internal Medicine and Epidemiology, University of Iowa Roy J. and Lucille A. Carver College of Medicine; Staff Physician, Medical Service, Department of Veterans Affairs Medical Center, Iowa City, Iowa
    Trypanosoma Species (American Trypanosomiasis, Chagas' Disease): Biology of Trypanosomes; Agents of African Trypanosomiasis (Sleeping Sickness)

Jerome O. Klein, MD
Professor, Department of Pediatrics, Boston University School of Medicine and Boston Medical Center, Boston, Massachusetts
    Otitis Externa, Otitis Media, and Mastoiditis

Michael R. Knowles, MD
Professor of Medicine, University of North Carolina at Chapel Hill School of Medicine; Pulmonary/Critical Care Medicine and CF/Pulmonary Research and Treatment Center, Chapel Hill, North Carolina
    Cystic Fibrosis

Igor J. Koralnik, MD
Assistant Professor of Neurology, Harvard Medical School; Director, HIV/Neurology Center, Department of Neurology and Medicine, Beth Israel Deaconess Medical Center, Boston, Massachusetts
    Neurologic Diseases Caused by Human Immunodeficiency Virus-1 and Opportunistic Infections

Joseph A. Kovacs, MD
Head, AIDS Section, Critical Care Medicine Department, Warren G. Magnuson Clinical Center, National Institutes of Health, Bethesda, Maryland
    Toxoplasma gondii

Phyllis Kozarsky, MD
Professor of Medicine, Division of Infectious Diseases, Emory University School of Medicine, Atlanta, Georgia
    Cyclospora cayetanensis, Isospora belli, Sarcocystis Species, *Balantidium coli,* and *Blastocystis hominis*

Margaret James Koziel, MD
Assistant Professor of Medicine, Harvard Medical School, Harvard Institutes of Medicine, Beth Israel Deaconess Medical Center, Boston, Massachusetts
    Hepatitis B Virus and Hepatitis Delta Virus

John N. Krieger, MD
Professor of Urology, University of Washington School of Medicine; Chief of Urology, Veterans Affairs Puget Sound Health Care System; Attending Urologist, Harbor Medical Center and Children's Hospital and Medical Center, Seattle, Washington
    Prostatitis, Epididymitis, and Orchitis

James W. LeDuc, PhD
Director, Division of Viral and Rickettsial Diseases, National Center for Infectious Diseases, Centers for Disease Control and Prevention, Atlanta, Georgia
    Emerging and Reemerging Infectious Disease Threats

Stanley M. Lemon, MD
Dean of Medicine, University of Texas Medical Branch, University of Texas Medical School at Galveston, Galveston, Texas
    Hepatitis C

Paul N. Levett, PhD
Director, WHO Collaborating Center on Leptospirosis, Centers for Disease Control and Prevention, Atlanta, Georgia
    Leptospirosis

Donald P. Levine, MD
Professor of Medicine and Chief, Division of General Internal Medicine, Wayne State University; Vice-Chief of Medicine, Detroit Receiving Hospital, Detroit, Michigan
    Infections in Injection Drug Users

William R. Levis, MD
Attending Physician, Department of Dermatology, New York University School of Medicine; Hansen's Disease Clinic, Bellevue Hospital, New York, New York
Mycobacterium leprae (Leprosy, Hansen's Disease)

Matthew E. Levison, MD
Professor of Medicine and Public Health, Department of Medicine, Drexel University College of Medicine; Attending Staff, Department of Medicine/Infectious Diseases, Medical College of Pennsylvania Hospital, Philadelphia, Pennsylvania
Peritonitis and Intraperitoneal Abscesses

W. Conrad Liles, MD, PhD
Associate Professor of Medicine, Division of Infectious Diseases, and Adjunct Associate Professor, Department of Pathology, University of Washington School of Medicine; Attending Physician, Department of Medicine, University of Washington Medical Center; Attending Physician, Department of Medicine, Harborview Medical Center, Seattle, Washington
Immunomodulators

Aldo A. M. Lima, MD, PhD
Federal University of Ceara, Fortaleza, Brazil
Inflammatory Enteritides

Nathan Litman, MD
Professor, Department of Pediatrics, Albert Einstein College of Medicine of Yeshiva University; Department of Pediatrics, Montefiore Medical Center, Bronx, New York
Mumps Virus

Bennett Lorber, MD, DSc(Hon)
Thomas M. Durant Professor of Medicine and Professor of Microbiology and Immunology, Temple University School of Medicine; Chief, Section of Infectious Diseases, Temple University Hospital, Philadelphia, Pennsylvania
Lung Abscess; *Listeria monocytogenes;* Gas Gangrene and Other *Clostridium*-Associated Diseases; *Bacteroides, Prevotella, Porphyromonas,* and *Fusobacterium* Species (and Other Medically Important Anaerobic Gram-Negative Bacilli)

Daniel Lucey, MD
Professor of Medicine, Uniformed Services University of the Health Sciences, Bethesda, Maryland; Adjunct Professor of Microbiology and Immunology, Georgetown University School of Medicine; Director, Center for Biologic Counterterrorism and Emerging Diseases, Washington Hospital Center, Washington, DC
Bacillus anthracis (Anthrax); Anthrax

Larry I. Lutwick, MD
Professor of Medicine, Division of Infectious Diseases, State University of New York–Downstate School of Medicine; Director, Infectious Diseases, Veterans Affairs New York Harbor Health Care System, Brooklyn Campus, Brooklyn, New York; Bacterial Diseases Moderator, Program for Monitoring Emerging Diseases (ProMED-mail), International Society for Infectious Diseases, New York, New York
Infections in Asplenic Patients

Rob Roy MacGregor, MD
Professor, Department of Medicine, University of Pennsylvania School of Medicine; Attending Physician, Department of Medicine/Infectious Diseases, Hospital of the University of Pennsylvania; Attending Physician, Department of Medicine/Infectious Diseases, Philadelphia Veterans Affairs Medical Center, Philadelphia, Pennsylvania
Corynebacterium diphtheriae

Philip A. Mackowiak, MD, MBA
Professor and Vice Chairman, Department of Medicine, University of Maryland School of Medicine; Chief, Medical Care Clinical Center, Veterans Affairs Maryland Health Care System, Baltimore, Maryland
Temperature Regulation and the Pathogenesis of Fever; Fever of Unknown Origin

Lawrence C. Madoff, MD
Assistant Professor, Department of Medicine, Harvard Medical School; Associate Physician, Department of Medicine, Division of Infectious Diseases and Channing Laboratory, Brigham and Women's Hospital, Boston, Massachusetts
Infections of the Liver and Biliary System; Pancreatic Infections; Splenic Abscess; Appendicitis; Diverticulitis and Typhlitis

James H. Maguire, MD
Chief, Parasitic Diseases Branch, National Center for Infectious Diseases, Centers for Disease Control and Prevention, Atlanta, Georgia
Introduction to Helminth Infections; Intestinal Nematodes (Roundworms); Trematodes (Schistosomes and Other Flukes)

Frank Maldarelli, MD, PhD
Staff Clinician, HIV Drug Resistance Program, National Cancer Institute; Warren G. Magnuson Clinical Center, National Institutes of Health, Bethesda, Maryland
Diagnosis of Human Immunodeficiency Virus Infection

Gerald L. Mandell, MD, MACP
Professor of Medicine, Owen R. Cheatham Professor of the Sciences, Division of Infectious Diseases, University of Virginia School of Medicine, Charlottesville, Virginia
Acute Pneumonia

Lionel A. Mandell, MD, FRCPC, FRCP[Lond]
Professor of Medicine and Chief, Division of Infectious Diseases, McMaster University, Henderson Site, Division of Infectious Diseases, Hamilton, Ontario, Canada
Fusidic Acid

Barbara J. Mann, PhD
Associate Professor, Department of Internal Medicine and Microbiology, University of Virginia School of Medicine, Charlottesville, Virginia
Microbial Adherence

Lewis Markoff, MD
Chief, Laboratory of Vector-Borne Virus Diseases, Division of Viral Products, Center for Biologics Research and Review, U.S. Food and Drug Administration, Bethesda, Maryland
Alphaviruses

Thomas J. Marrie, MD
Professor and Chair, Department of Medicine, University of Alberta Faculty of Medicine; Site Chief for Medicine, University of Alberta Hospital, Edmonton, Alberta, Canada
Coxiella burnetii (Q Fever)

Thomas Marth, Priv.-Doz. DrMed
Chefarzt der Abteilung Innere Medizin mit Schwerpunkten, Gastroenterologie, Onkologie, Diabetologie, und Ernahrungsmedizin, St. Josef-Krankenhaus Zell, Zell/Mosel, Germany
Whipple's Disease

David H. Martin, MD
Harry E. Dascomb, MD, Professor of Medicine and Professor of Microbiology, Immunology, and Parasitology, Louisiana State University School of Medicine; Chief, Section of Infectious Diseases, Department of Medicine, Louisiana State University Health Sciences Center, New Orleans, Louisiana
Trichomonas vaginalis

Georg Maschmeyer, MD
Professor of Internal Medicine, Department of Hematology
and Oncology, Charite University Hospital, Berlin, Germany
Stenotrophomonas maltophilia and *Burkholderia cepacia*

Ellen M. Mascini
Eijkman-Winkler Institute for Microbiology, Infection, and
Inflammation, Utrecht University, Utrecht, The Netherlands
Anaerobic Cocci; Anaerobic Gram-Positive Nonsporulating Bacilli

Henry Masur, MD
Chief, Critical Care Medicine Department, Warren G. Magnuson
Clinical Center, National Institutes of Health, Bethesda, Maryland
Management of Opportunistic Infections Associated with Human
Immunodeficiency Virus Infection

Michael Eric Mathieu, MD
Instructor in Clinical Dermatology, Department of Dermatology,
University of Virginia School of Medicine, Charlottesville; Medical
Staff, Department of Medicine, Winchester Medical Center,
Winchester, Virginia; Medical Staff, Department of Medicine, City
Hospital, Martinsburg, West Virginia
Introduction to Ectoparasitic Diseases; Lice (Pediculosis); Scabies;
Myiasis and Tungiasis; Mites (Including Chiggers); Ticks (Including
Tick Paralysis)

Kenneth H. Mayer, MD
Professor of Medicine and Community Health, Brown Medical
School; Department of Medicine/Infectious Diseases, Miriam
Hospital, Providence, Rhode Island; Director of Medical Research,
Fenway Community Health, Boston, Massachusetts
Sulfonamides and Trimethoprim

John T. McBride, MD
Professor, Department of Pediatrics, Northeast Ohio Universities
College of Medicine, Rootstown; Vice Chair, Department
of Pediatrics, Akron Children's Hospital, Akron, Ohio
Acute Laryngotracheobronchitis (Croup); Bronchiolitis

Carol A. McCarthy, MD
Associate Professor, Department of Pediatrics, University of Vermont
College of Medicine, Burlington, Vermont; Director, Pediatric
Infectious Diseases, Department of Pediatrics, Maine Medical
Center, Portland, Maine
Respiratory Syncytial Virus

William M. McCormack, MD
Chief, Infectious Diseases Division, Department of Medicine,
State University of New York–Downstate Medical Center,
Brooklyn, New York
Urethritis; Vulvovaginitis and Cervicitis

Joseph E. McDade, PhD
Orise Fellow, National Center for Infectious Diseases, Centers
for Disease Control and Prevention, Atlanta, Georgia
Emerging and Reemerging Infectious Disease Threats

Kenneth McIntosh, MD
Professor, Department of Pediatrics, Harvard Medical School; Senior
Associate in Medicine, Division of Infectious Diseases, Children's
Hospital; Professor, Department of Immunology and Infectious
Diseases, Harvard School of Public Health, Boston, Massachusetts
Coronaviruses, Including Severe Acute Respiratory Syndrome
(SARS)–Associated Coronaviruses

Philip B. Mead, MD
Professor and Chair Emeritus, Department of Obstetrics and
Gynecology, University of Vermont College of Medicine; Emeritus
Staff, Department of Obstetrics and Gynecology, Fletcher Allen
Health Care, Burlington, Vermont
Infections of the Female Pelvis

Antone A. Medeiros, MD
Professor, Department of Medicine, Brown Medical School,
Providence, Rhode Island
Molecular Mechanisms of Antibiotic Resistance in Bacteria

Michael H. Merson, MD
Anna M. R. Lauder Professor of Public Health, Dean of Public
Health, and Director, Center for Interdisciplinary Research on AIDS,
Department of Epidemiology and Public Health, Yale University
School of Medicine, New Haven, Connecticut
Global Perspectives on Human Immunodeficiency Virus
Infection and Acquired Immunodeficiency Syndrome

Daniel K. Meyer, MD
Assistant Professor of Medicine, Division of Infectious Diseases,
University of Medicine and Dentistry of New Jersey Robert Wood
Johnson Medical School at Camden; Program Director, Fellowship
Training Program, Division of Infectious Diseases, Cooper
University Hospital, Camden, New Jersey
Other Coryneform Bacteria and *Rhodococcus*

Burt Meyers, MD
Clinical Professor of Medicine, Mount Sinai Hospital, New York,
New York
Tetracyclines and Chloramphenicol; Metronidazole

Samuel I. Miller, MD
Professor, Department of Medicine, Microbiology, and Genome
Sciences, and Professor, Department of Medicine, University
of Washington School of Medicine, Seattle, Washington
Salmonella Species, Including *Salmonella typhi*

Yazdan Mirzanejad, MD, FRCPC, FACP
Clinical Instructor, Division of Infectious Diseases,
Department of Medicine, University of British Columbia Faculty
of Medicine; Clinical Associate, Oak Tree HIV Clinic, Children and
Women Hospital, Vancouver; Consultant, Department of Infectious
Diseases, Surrey Memorial Hospital, Surrey; Consultant, Infectious
Diseases, Department of Infectious Diseases, Royal Columbian
Hospital, New Westminster, British Columbia, Canada
Streptococcus anginosus Group

Candace L. Mitchell, MD
Assistant Professor of Medicine, Section of Infectious Diseases,
Louisiana State University School of Medicine in Shreveport,
Shreveport, Louisiana
Francisella tularensis (Tularemia) as an Agent of Bioterrorism

David H. Mitchell, MBBS, MMedSci (Epi)
Clinical Lecturer, Department of Infectious Diseases, University of
Sydney Faculty of Medicine; Senior Staff Specialist, Centre for
Infectious Diseases and Microbiology, Westmead Hospital,
Westmead, New South Wales, Australia
Nocardia Species

John F. Modlin, MD
Professor and Chair, Department of Pediatrics, Dartmouth Medical
School; Children's Hospital at Dartmouth, Dartmouth-Hitchcock
Medical Center, Lebanon, New Hampshire
Introduction to the Enteroviruses; Poliovirus; Coxsackieviruses,
Echoviruses, and Newer Enteroviruses

Robert C. Moellering, Jr., MD
Herman L. Blumgart Professor of Medicine, Harvard Medical
School; Physician-in-Chief and Chairman, Department of Medicine,
Beth Israel Deaconess Medical Center, Boston, Massachusetts
Principles of Anti-infective Therapy; *Enterococcus* Species,
Streptococcus bovis, and *Leuconostoc Species*

Jose G. Montoya, MD
Associate Professor, Department of Medicine, Division of Infectious Diseases and Geographic Medicine, Stanford University School of Medicine; Attending Physician, Stanford University Medical Center, Stanford; Associate Staff Scientist, Department of Immunology and Infectious Diseases, Research Institute, Palo Alto Medical Foundation, Palo Alto, California
Toxoplasma gondii

Philippe Moreillon, MD
Division of Infectious Diseases, Department of Medicine, University Hospital CHUV, Lausanne, Switzerland
Staphylococcus aureus (Including Staphylococcal Toxic Shock)

J. Glenn Morris, Jr., MD, MPH
Professor and Chairman, Department of Epidemiology and Preventive Medicine, Professor of Medicine (Infectious Diseases), and Professor of Microbiology and Immunology, University of Maryland School of Medicine, Baltimore, Maryland
Human Illness Associated with Harmful Algal Blooms

Caryn Gee Morse, MD
Staff Clinician and Research Fellow, Critical Care Medicine, Warren G. Magnuson Clinical Center, National Institutes of Health, Bethesda, Maryland
Nutrition, Immunity, and Infection

Robert R. Muder, MD
Professor, Department of Medicine, University of Pittsburgh School of Medicine; Hospital Epidemiologist, Infectious Disease Section, Veterans Affairs Pittsburgh Healthcare System, Pittsburgh, Pennsylvania
Other *Legionella* Species

Jean Marie Mulinde, MD
Lead Medical Officer, U.S. Food and Drug Administration, Rockville, Maryland
Hyperbaric Oxygen

Robert S. Munford, MD
Jan and Henri Bromberg Chair in Internal Medicine and Professor, Department of Internal Medicine and Microbiology, University of Texas-Southwestern Medical Center; Parkland Memorial Hospital and Zale-Lipshy University Hospital, Dallas, Texas
Sepsis, Severe Sepsis, and Septic Shock

Timothy F. Murphy, MD
Professor of Medicine and Microbiology, State University of New York at Buffalo School of Medicine and Biomedical Sciences; Chief, Division of Infectious Diseases, Department of Medicine, Veterans Affairs Medical Center, Buffalo, New York
Moraxella (Branhamella) catarrhalis and Other Gram-Negative Cocci; *Haemophilus* Infections

Barbara E. Murray, MD
Professor and Director, Division of Infectious Diseases, Department of Internal Medicine, University of Texas–Houston Medical School; Co-Director, Center for Emerging and Re-emerging Pathogens, University of Texas Health Science Center, Houston, Texas
Glycopeptides (Vancomycin and Teicoplanin), Streptogramins (Quinupristin-Dalfopristin), and Lipopeptides (Daptomycin)

Daniel M. Musher, MD
Professor of Medicine and Microbiology and Immunology, Baylor College of Medicine; Chief, Infectious Diseases Section, Veterans Affairs Medical Center, Houston, Texas
Streptococcus pneumoniae

Esteban C. Nannini, MD
Attending Physician, Department of Infectious Diseases, Sanatorio Parque, Rosario, Santa Fe, Argentina
Glycopeptides (Vancomycin and Teicoplanin), Streptogramins (Quinupristin-Dalfopristin), and Lipopeptides (Daptomycin)

Theodore E. Nash, MD
Head, Gastrointestinal Parasites Section, Laboratory of Parasitic Diseases, National Institute of Allergy and Infectious Disease, National Institutes of Health, Bethesda, Maryland
Visceral Larva Migrans and Other Unusual Helminth Infections

William M. Nauseef, MD
Professor, Inflammation Program and Department of Medicine, University of Iowa Roy J. and Lucille A. Carver College of Medicine; Department of Veterans Affairs, Iowa City, Iowa
Granulocytic Phagocytes

Marguerite A. Neill, MD
Associate Professor, Department of Medicine, Brown Medical School, Providence; Attending Physician, Division of Infectious Disease, Memorial Hospital of Rhode Island, Pawtucket, Rhode Island
Other Pathogenic Vibrios

Judith A. O'Donnell, MD
Associate Professor of Medicine and Public Health, Division of Infectious Disease, Drexel University College of Medicine; Attending Physician and Hospital Epidemiologist, Department of Medicine, Medical College of Pennsylvania Hospital, Philadelphia, Pennsylvania
Topical Antibacterials

Christopher A. Ohl, MD
Associate Professor of Medicine, Section of Infectious Diseases, Wake Forest University School of Medicine; Medical Director, Center for Antimicrobial Utilization, Stewardship, and Epidemiology, North Carolina Baptist Hospital, Winston-Salem, North Carolina
Infectious Arthritis of Native Joints

Michael E. Ohl, MD
Postdoctoral Research Fellow and Clinical Instructor, Departments of Internal Medicine and Family and Community Medicine, University of Missouri School of Medicine, Columbia, Missouri
Salmonella Species, Including *Salmonella typhi*

Pablo C. Okhuysen, MD, FACP
Professor, Department of Medicine, Division of Infectious Diseases, University of Texas–Houston Medical School; Associate Professor, Center for Infectious Diseases, University of Texas Health Science Center–Houston School of Public Health; UTHSC–Houston Director, Memorial Hermann Hospital Clinical Research Center; Staff Physician, Department of Infectious Diseases, Lyndon B. Johnson General Hospital, Houston, Texas
Sporothrix schenckii

Steven M. Opal, MD
Professor, Department of Medicine/Division of Infectious Diseases, Brown Medical School, Providence; Chief, Infectious Disease Division, Department of Medicine/Division of Infectious Diseases, Memorial Hospital of Rhode Island, Pawtucket, Rhode Island
Molecular Mechanisms of Antibiotic Resistance in Bacteria

Walter A. Orenstein, MD
Director, Emory Program for Vaccine Policy and Development, and Associate Director, Emory Vaccine Center, Emory University School of Medicine, Atlanta, Georgia
Immunization

Douglas R. Osmon, MD, MPH
Associate Professor of Medicine, Mayo Clinic College of Medicine
and Mayo Clinic, Rochester, Minnesota
    Osteomyelitis

Michael T. Osterholm, PhD, MPH
Director, Center for Infectious Disease Research and Policy,
and Professor, University of Minnesota School of Public Health,
Minneapolis, Minnesota
    Epidemiologic Principles

Stephen M. Ostroff, MD
Deputy Director, National Center for Infectious Diseases, Centers
for Disease Control and Prevention, Atlanta, Georgia
    Emerging and Reemerging Infectious Disease Threats

Michael N. Oxman, MD
Professor of Medicine and Pathology, University of California,
San Diego, School of Medicine; Veterans Affairs San Diego,
San Diego, California
    Myocarditis and Pericarditis

Eric G. Pamer, MD
Chief, Infectious Diseases Service, Department of Medicine,
Memorial Sloan-Kettering Cancer Center; Head, Laboratory of
Antimicrobial Immunity, Immunology Program, Sloan-Kettering
Institute, New York, New York
    Cell-Mediated Defense against Infection

Peter G. Pappas, MD
Professor, Department of Medicine, University of Alabama School
of Medicine, Birmingham, Alabama
    Chronic Pneumonia

Mark S. Pasternack, MD
Associate Professor of Pediatrics, Harvard Medical School; Chief,
Pediatric Infectious Disease Unit, Massachusets General Hospital
for Children, Massachusetts General Hospital, Boston,
Massachusetts
    Cellulitis and Subcutaneous Tissue Infections; Myositis;
    Lymphadenitis and Lymphangitis

Thomas F. Patterson, MD
Professor, Department of Medicine, Division of Infectious Diseases,
University of Texas Health Science Center at San Antonio, San
Antonio, Texas
    Aspergillus Species

Deborah Pavan-Langston, MD, FACS
Associate Professor, Department of Ophthalmology, Harvard
Medical School; Surgeon, Director of Clinical Virology, Department
of Corneal and External Disease, Massachusetts Eye and Ear
Infirmary, Boston, Massachusetts
    Microbial Conjunctivitis; Microbial Keratitis

Richard D. Pearson, MD
Professor, Departments of Internal Medicine and Pathology,
University of Virginia School of Medicine; Attending Physician,
Department of Internal Medicine, University of Virginia Health
System, Charlottesville, Virginia
    Agents Active against Parasites and Pneumocystis;
    Leishmania Species: Visceral (Kala-Azar), Cutaneous,
    and Mucocutaneous Leishmaniasis

David A. Pegues, MD
Professor of Clinical Medicine, Department of Medicine, David
Geffen School of Medicine at UCLA; Hospital Epidemiologist and
Attending Physician, Division of Infectious Diseases, University
of California, Los Angeles, Medical Center, Los Angeles, California
    Salmonella Species, Including *Salmonella typhi*

Robert L. Penn, MD
Professor of Medicine and Chief, Section of Infectious Diseases,
Louisiana State University School of Medicine in Shreveport; Chief,
Infectious Diseases Section, Louisiana State University Health
Sciences Center, University Hospital, Shreveport, Louisiana
    Francisella tularensis (Tularemia); *Francisella tularensis* (Tularemia)
    as an Agent of Bioterrorism

John R. Perfect, MD
Professor, Department of Medicine, Duke University Medical Center,
Durham, North Carolina
    Cryptococcus neoformans

C. J. Peters, MD
John Sealy Distinguished University Chair in Tropical and Emerging
Virology, Department of Pathology and Microbiology/Immunology,
University of Texas Medical Branch, University of Texas Medical
School at Galveston, Galveston, Texas
    Marburg and Ebola Virus Hemorrhagic Fevers; California
    Encephalitis, Hantavirus Pulmonary Syndrome, and Bunyavirid
    Hemorrhagic Fevers; Lymphocytic Choriomeningitis Virus, Lassa
    Virus, and the South American Hemorrhagic Fevers; Bioterrorism:
    Viral Hemorrhagic Fevers

Phillip K. Peterson, MD
Professor of Medicine, Department of Internal Medicine, University
of Minnesota Medical School-Minneapolis; Director, Infectious
Diseases and International Medicine, Department of Internal
Medicine, Fairview University Medical Center; Director, Infectious
Diseases and International Medicine, Department of Internal
Medicine, Hennepin County Medical Center,
Minneapolis, Minnesota
    Infections in the Elderly

William A. Petri, Jr., MD, PhD
Wade Hampton Frost Professor of Epidemiology and Professor
of Medicine, Microbiology, and Pathology, University of Virginia
School of Medicine; Chief, Division of Infectious Diseases and
International Health, University of Virginia Health System,
Charlottesville, Virginia
    Microbial Adherence

Gerald B. Pier, PhD
Professor of Medicine, Microbiology, and Molecular Genetics,
Harvard Medical School; Microbiologist, Department of Medicine,
Brigham and Women's Hospital, Boston, Massachusetts
    Pseudomonas aeruginosa

Peter Piot, MD, PhD
Executive Director, Joint United Nations Programme on HIV/AIDS
(UNAIDS); Under Secretary-General, United Nations, Geneva,
Switzerland
    Global Perspectives on Human Immunodeficiency Virus Infection
    and Acquired Immunodeficiency Syndrome

Ronald E. Polk, PharmD
Professor and Chairman, Department of Pharmacy, School
of Pharmacy, Virginia Commonwealth University School of
Medicine, Richmond, Virginia
    Antimicrobial Management: Cost and Resistance

Mikulas Popovic, MD, PhD
Professor, Institute of Human Virology, University of Maryland
Biotechnology Institute, Baltimore, Maryland
    Human Immunodeficiency Viruses

John H. Powers, MD, FACP
Infectious Diseases Attending, National Institute of Allergy and Infectious Diseases, National Institutes of Health, Bethesda, Maryland; Clinical Assistant Professor, Department of Medicine, George Washington University School of Medicine, Washington, District of Columbia; Clinical Assistant Professor, Department of Medicine/Infectious Diseases, University of Maryland School of Medicine, Baltimore; Lead Medical Officer, Antimicrobial Drug Development and Resistance Initiatives, Center for Drug Evaluation and Research, U.S. Food and Drug Administration, Rockville, Maryland
Interpreting the Results of Clinical Trials on Antimicrobial Agents

Robert H. Purcell, MD
Co-Chief, Laboratory of Infectious Diseases, and Head, Hepatitis Viruses Section, National Institute of Allergy and Infectious Diseases, National Institutes of Health, Bethesda, Maryland
Hepatitis E Virus

Yok-Ai Que, MD, PhD
Centre Hospitalier Universitaire Vaudois, Medical Critical Care Division, Department of Internal Medicine, Lausanne, Switzerland
Staphylococcus aureus (Including Staphylococcal Toxic Shock)

Anastácio de Queiroz Sousa, MD
Associate Professor of Medicine, Department of Internal Medicine; Director, Nucleo de Medicina Tropical, Federal University of Ceara; Physician and Head, Epidemiology Surveillance Service, Hospital Sao Jose for Infectious Diseases, Fortaleza, Ceara, Brazil
Leishmania Species: Visceral (Kala-Azar), Cutaneous, and Mucocutaneous Leishmaniasis

Ronald Rabinowitz, MD
Assistant Professor of Medicine, Division of Trauma Infectious Disease, University of Maryland School of Medicine; Shock Trauma Center, University of Maryland Health System, Baltimore, Maryland
Hyperbaric Oxygen

Reuben Ramphal, MD
Professor, Department of Medicine, University of Florida College of Medicine, Gainesville, Florida
Pseudomonas aeruginosa

Didier Raoult, MD, PhD
Faculté de Médecine de Marseille, Unité des Rickettsies, Marseille, France
Introduction to Rickettsioses and Ehrlichioses; *Rickettsia rickettsii* and Other Spotted Fever Group Rickettsiae (Rocky Mountain Spotted Fever and Other Spotted Fevers); *Rickettsia akari* (Rickettsialpox); *Coxiella burnetii* (Q Fever); *Rickettsia prowazekii* (Epidemic or Louse-Borne Typhus); Scrub Typhus

Jonathan I. Ravdin, MD
Nesbitt Professor and Chairman, Department of Medicine, University of Minnesota Medical School–Minneapolis; Minneapolis Veterans Affairs Medical Center, Fairview-University Medical Center, Minneapolis, Minnesota
Introduction to Protozoal Diseases; *Entamoeba histolytica* (Amebiasis)

Stuart C. Ray, MD
Associate Professor of Medicine, Division of Infectious Diseases, Department of Medicine, Johns Hopkins University School of Medicine; Active Staff, Department of Medicine, Johns Hopkins Hospital, Baltimore, Maryland
Hepatitis C

Annette C. Reboli, MD
Professor, Department of Medicine, Division of Infectious Diseases, University of Medicine and Dentistry of New Jersey Robert Wood Johnson Medical School, New Brunswick; Hospital Epidemiologist and Head, Infectious Diseases Division, Cooper University Hospital, Camden, New Jersey
Other Coryneform Bacteria and *Rhodococcus; Erysipelothrix rhusiopathiae*

Richard C. Reichman, MD
Professor of Medicine, Microbiology, and Immunology, University of Rochester School of Medicine; Head, Infectious Diseases Unit, University of Rochester Medical Center, Rochester, New York
Papillomaviruses

Michael F. Rein, MD
Professor of Medicine, Department of Infectious Diseases and International Health, University of Virginia School of Medicine; Attending Physician, Department of Internal Medicine, University of Virginia Hospital; Medical Director, Sexually Transmitted Disease Clinic, Thomas Jefferson District Health Department, Charlottesville, Virginia
Urethritis; *Trichomonas vaginalis*

Marvin S. Reitz, Jr., PhD
Professor, Institute of Human Virology; Member, Greenebaum Cancer Center, University of Maryland, Baltimore, Maryland
Human Immunodeficiency Viruses

David A. Relman, MD
Associate Professor, Department of Microbiology and Immunology, Stanford University School of Medicine, Stanford; Chief, Infectious Diseases, Veterans Affairs Palo Alto Health Care System, Palo Alto, California
A Molecular Perspective of Microbial Pathogenicity

Jack S. Remington, MD
Professor, Division of Infectious Diseases, Department of Medicine, Stanford University School of Medicine; Attending Physician, Stanford University Medical Center and Lucille Packard Medical Center, Stanford; Marcus A. Krupp Research Chair and Chairman, Department of Immunology and Infectious Diseases, Research Institute, Palo Alto Medical Foundation, Palo Alto, California
Toxoplasma gondii

Angela Restrepo, MD
Scientific Advisor, Medical and Experimental Mycology Group, Corporación para Investigaciones Biológicas (CIB), Medellin, Antioquia, Colombia, South America
Paracoccidioides brasiliensis

John H. Rex, MD, FACP
Adjunct Professor of Medicine, Department of Internal Medicine, University of Texas–Houston Medical School, Houston, Texas; Vice President and Medical Director for Infection, Astra Zeneca Pharmaceuticals, Macclesfield, Cheshire, United Kingdom
Systemic Antifungal Agents; *Sporothrix schenckii*

Herbert Y. Reynolds, MD
Emeritus Professor of Medicine, Pennsylvania State University College of Medicine; Milton S. Hershey Medical Center, Hershey, Pennsylvania; Medical Officer, Division of Lung Diseases, National Heart, Lung, and Blood Institute, National Institutes of Health, Bethesda, Maryland
Chronic Obstructive Pulmonary Disease, Chronic Bronchitis, and Acute Exacerbations

Kyu Y. Rhee, MD, PhD
Clinical Fellow, Division of International Medicine and Infectious Diseases, Weill Medical College of Cornell University and New York–Presbyterian Hospital–Weill Cornell Medical Center, New York, New York
Borrelia Species (Relapsing Fever)

Lisa D. Rotz, MD
Acting Director, Bioterrorism Preparedness and Response Program, National Center for Infectious Diseases, Centers for Disease Control and Prevention, Atlanta, Georgia
Smallpox and Bioterrorism

Kathryn L. Ruoff, PhD
Department of Pathology, Dartmouth Hitchcock Medical Center, Lebanon, New Hampshire
Classification of Streptococci

Mark E. Rupp, MD
Professor, Department of Internal Medicine, University of Nebraska College of Medicine; Medical Director, Department of Healthcare Epidemiology, Nebraska Medical Center, Omaha, Nebraska
Mediastinitis

Charles E. Rupprecht, VMD, PhD
Chief, Rabies Section, Viral and Rickettsial Zoonoses Branch, Division of Viral and Rickettsial Diseases, Centers for Disease Control and Prevention, Atlanta, Georgia
Rhabdoviruses

Thomas A. Russo, MD, CM
Associate Professor, Department of Medicine, Division of Infectious Diseases, State University of New York at Buffalo School of Medicine and Biomedical Sciences; Staff Physician, Department of Medicine, Division of Infectious Diseases, Veterans Affairs Medical Center; Staff Physician, Department of Medicine, Division of Infectious Diseases, Erie County Medical Center, Buffalo, New York
Agents of Actinomycosis

William A. Rutala, PhD, MPH
Professor, Department of Medicine, University of North Carolina at Chapel Hill School of Medicine; Director, Statewide Program for Infection Control and Epidemiology, and Director, Hospital Epidemiology, Occupational Health, and Safety, University of North Carolina Health Care System, Chapel Hill, North Carolina
The Acutely Ill Patient with Fever and Rash; Disinfection, Sterilization, and Control of Hospital Waste

Mirella Salvatore, MD
Associate, Clinical Fellow, Department of Infectious Diseases, Mount Sinai Medical Center, New York, New York
Tetracyclines and Chloramphenicol; Metronidazole

Frank T. Saulsbury, MD
Professor, Department of Pediatrics, University of Virginia School of Medicine; Head, Division of Immunology and Rheumatology, Department of Pediatrics, University of Virginia Health System, Charlottesville, Virginia
Kawasaki Syndrome

Maria C. Savoia, MD
Vice Dean for Medical Education and Professor, Department of Medicine/Infectious Diseases, University of California, San Diego, School of Medicine; Attending Physician, Department of Medicine/Infectious Diseases, University of California, San Diego, Medical Center, San Diego Veterans Affairs Medical Center, San Diego, California
Myocarditis and Pericarditis

Paul E. Sax, MD
Assistant Professor of Medicine, Harvard Medical School; Clinical Director, Division of Infectious Diseases and HIV Program, Brigham and Women's Hospital, Boston, Massachusetts
Pulmonary Manifestations of Human Immunodeficiency Virus Infection

W. Michael Scheld, MD
Wyeth Professor of Infectious Diseases, Professor of Internal Medicine, and Clinical Professor of Neurosurgery, Department of Internal Medicine, University of Virginia School of Medicine; University of Virginia Health System, Charlottesville, Virginia
Endocarditis and Intravascular Infections; Acute Meningitis

David Schlossberg, MD, FACP
Professor, Department of Medicine, Temple University School of Medicine; Adjunct Professor, Department of Medicine, Jefferson Medical College of Thomas Jefferson University, Philadelphia; Director, Medical Services, Merck & Company, Inc., North Wales, Pennsylvania
Chlamydophila (Chlamydia) psittaci (Psittacosis)

Robert T. Schooley, MD
Tim Gill Professor and Head, Division of Infectious Diseases, University of Colorado Health Sciences Center, Denver; Physician, Department of Medicine, University of Colorado Hospital, Aurora; Physician, Department of Veterans Affairs Medical Center and Denver Department of Health and Hospitals, Denver, Colorado
Epstein-Barr Virus (Infectious Mononucleosis)

Carlos Seas, MD
Associate Professor, Department of Medicine, and Associate Investigator, Alexander von Humboldt Tropical Medicine Institute, Cayetano Heredia University; Attending Physician, Department of Infectious, Tropical, and Dermatological Diseases, Cayetano Heredia National Hospital, Lima, Peru
Vibrio cholerae

Kent A. Sepkowitz, MD
Professor, Department of Medicine, Weill Medical College of Cornell University; Director, Infection Control, Department of Medicine, Memorial Sloan-Kettering Cancer Center, New York, New York
Nosocomial Hepatitis and Other Infections Transmitted by Blood and Blood Products

Edward Septimus, MD
Clinical Professor of Medicine, Department of Infectious Diseases, University of Texas–Houston Medical School; Medical Director, Department of Infectious Diseases and Occupational Health, Memorial Hermann Healthcare System, Houston, Texas
Pleural Effusion and Empyema

Aleem Siddiqui, PhD
Professor, Department of Microbiology, Program in Molecular Biology, University of Colorado Health Sciences Center, Denver, Colorado
Hepatitis B Virus and Hepatitis Delta Virus

Costi D. Sifri, MD
Instructor, Department of Medicine, Harvard Medical School; Clinical Associate, Division of Infectious Diseases, Massachusetts General Hospital, Boston, Massachusetts
Appendicitis; Diverticulitis and Typhlitis

Upinder Singh, MD
Assistant Professor, Departments of Internal Medicine and Microbiology and Immunology, Stanford University School of Medicine, Stanford, California
Free-Living Amebas

Sumathi Sivapalasingam
Instructor, Division of Infectious Diseases, Department of Medicine, New York University School of Medicine, New York, New York
  Macrolides, Clindamycin, and Ketolides

Leonard N. Slater, MD
Professor, Department of Medicine, Infectious Disease Section, University of Oklahoma College of Medicine; Staff Physician and Chairman, Infection Control Committee, Department of Medicine, Oklahoma University Medical Center; Staff Physician and Chairman, Infection Control, Medical Service, Veterans Affairs Medical Center, Oklahoma City, Oklahoma
  Bartonella, Including Cat-Scratch Disease

A. George Smulian, MBBCh
Associate Professor of Medicine, Division of Infectious Diseases, University of Cincinnati College of Medicine; Chief, Infectious Disease Section, Medical Service, Cincinnati Veterans Affairs Medical Center, Cincinnati, Ohio
  Pneumocystis Species

Jack D. Sobel, MD
Professor of Medicine, Division of Infectious Diseases, Wayne State University School of Medicine; Chief, Division of Infectious Diseases, Department of Internal Medicine, Detroit Medical Center, Detroit, Michigan
  Urinary Tract Infections

Tom Solomon, MD, PhD
Lecturer in Neurology, Department of Neurological Science, Clinical Lecturer in Medical Microbiology, University of Liverpool, Liverpool, United Kingdom
  Flaviviruses (Yellow Fever, Dengue, Dengue Hemorrhagic Fever, Japanese Encephalitis, West Nile Encephalitis, St. Louis Encephalitis, Tick-Borne Encephalitis)

David E. Soper, MD
Professor and Vice-Chairman, Department of Obstetrics and Gynecology, Medical University of South Carolina College of Medicine, Charleston, South Carolina
  Infections of the Female Pelvis

Tania C. Sorrell, MB, BS, MD, FRACP
Professor of Clinical Infectious Diseases, Department of Medicine, University of Sydney Faculty of Medicine, Sydney; Director, Department of Infectious Diseases, Westmead Hospital, Westmead, New South Wales, Australia
  Nocardia Species

P. Frederick Sparling, MD
J. Herbert Bate Professor Emeritus, Departments of Medicine and Microbiology and Immunology, University of North Carolina at Chapel Hill School of Medicine; University of North Carolina Hospitals, Chapel Hill, North Carolina
  Neisseria gonorrhoeae

Walter E. Stamm, MD
Professor of Medicine and Head, Division of Allergy and Infectious Diseases, University of Washington School of Medicine, Seattle, Washington
  Introduction to Chlamydial Diseases; *Chlamydia trachomatis* (Trachoma, Perinatal infections, Lymphogranuloma Venereum, and Other Genital Infections)

William M. Stauffer, MD, MSPH, DTM&H
Instructor of Medicine, Department of Internal Medicine, Division of Infectious Disease and International Medicine, University of Minnesota Medical School–Minneapolis, Minneapolis; Clinical Faculty, Center for International Health and International Travel Clinic, Regions Hospital/HealthPartners, St. Paul, Minnesota
  Introduction to Protozoal Diseases; *Entamoeba histolytica* (Amebiasis)

James M. Steckelberg, MD
Professor of Medicine and Chair, Division of Infectious Diseases, Mayo Clinic College of Medicine, Rochester, Minnesota
  Osteomyelitis

Allen C. Steere, MD
Professor, Department of Medicine, Harvard Medical School; Director of Rheumatology, Department of Medicine, Massachusetts General Hospital, Boston, Massachusetts
  Borrelia burgdorferi (Lyme Disease, Lyme Borreliosis)

Neal H. Steigbigel, MD
Professor, Department of Medicine, Division of Infectious Disease and Immunology, New York University School of Medicine; Staff Physician, Medical Service, New York Veterans Affairs Medical Center; Attending Physician, Department of Medicine, Bellevue Hospital Center and New York University Medical Center, New York, New York
  Macrolides, Clindamycin, and Ketolides

James P. Steinberg, MD
Associate Professor of Medicine, Division of Infectious Diseases, Emory University School of Medicine; Hospital Epidemiologist, Chief of Infectious Diseases, and Associate Chief of Medicine, Emory Crawford Long Hospital, Atlanta, Georgia
  Other Gram-Negative and Gram-Variable Bacilli

Theodore S. Steiner, MD
Assistant Professor, Department of Medicine, University of British Columbia Faculty of Medicine; Attending Physician, Vancouver Hospital and Health Sciences Centre, Vancouver, British Columbia, Canada
  Principles and Syndromes of Enteric Infection

Timothy R. Sterling, MD
Associate Professor, Department of Medicine, Division of Infectious Diseases, Vanderbilt University School of Medicine, Nashville, Tennessee
  General Clinical Manifestations of Human Immunodeficiency Virus Infection (Including the Acute Retroviral Syndrome and Oral, Cutaneous, Renal, Ocular, and Cardiac Diseases)

David A. Stevens, MD, FACP
Professor, Department of Medicine, Stanford University School of Medicine, Stanford; Chief, Division of Infectious Diseases, Hospital Epidemiologist, and Co-Director, Clinical Microbiology Laboratory, Santa Clara Valley Medical Center; President, California Institute for Medical Research, San Jose, California
  Systemic Antifungal Agents

Dennis L. Stevens, PhD, MD
Professor, Department of Medicine, University of Washington School of Medicine, Seattle, Washington; Chief, Infectious Diseases, Department of Medicine, Veterans Affairs Medical Center, Boise, Idaho
  Streptococcus pyogenes

Charles W. Stratton, MD
Associate Professor, Departments of Medicine and Pathology, Vanderbilt University School of Medicine; Director, Clinical Microbiology Laboratory, Department of Pathology, Vanderbilt University Medical Center, Nashville, Tennessee
  Streptococcus anginosus Group

Stephen E. Straus, MD
Senior Investigator, Laboratory of Clinical Infectious Diseases, National Institute of Allergy and Infectious Diseases; Director, National Center for Complementary and Alternative Medicine, National Institutes of Health, Bethesda, Maryland
  Complementary and Alternative Medicines for Infectious Diseases; Introduction to Herpesviridae; Human Herpesvirus Types 6 and 7; Herpes B Virus

Larry J. Strausbaugh, MD
Professor, Department of Medicine, Oregon Health and Science University School of Medicine; Hospital Epidemiologist and Staff Physician, Division of Hospital and Specialty Medicine, Portland Veterans Affairs Medical Center, Portland, Oregon
Nosocomial Respiratory Infections

Alan M. Sugar, MD
Professor, Department of Medicine, Boston University School of Medicine, Boston; Director, HIV/AIDS Program and Hepatitis C Virus Program, Director, Infectious Diseases Clinical Services, and Attending Physician, Department of Medicine, Cape Cod Hospital, Hyannis; Attending Physician, Department of Medicine, Boston Medical Center, Boston, Massachusetts
Agents of Mucormycosis and Related Species

Mark S. Sulkowski, MD
Associate Professor, Department of Medicine, Division of Infectious Diseases, Johns Hopkins University School of Medicine; Johns Hopkins Hospital, Baltimore, Maryland
Gastrointestinal and Hepatobiliary Manifestations of Human Immunodeficiency Virus Infection

Morton N. Swartz, MD
Professor, Department of Medicine, Harvard Medical School; Chief, James Jackson Firm, Department of Medicine, Massachusetts General Hospital, Boston, Massachusetts
Cellulitis and Subcutaneous Tissue Infections; Myositis; Lymphadenitis and Lymphangitis

Thomas R. Talbot, MD, MPH
Assistant Professor, Departments of Medicine and Preventive Medicine, Vanderbilt University School of Medicine; Associate Hospital Epidemiologist, Vanderbilt University Medical Center, Nashville, Tennessee
Postoperative Infections and Antimicrobial Prophylaxis

Nathan M. Thielman, MD, MPH
Assistant Professor, Department of Medicine, Division of Infectious Diseases and International Health, Duke University School of Medicine, Durham, North Carolina
Antibiotic-Associated Colitis; Enteric Fever and Other Causes of Abdominal Symptoms with Fever

David L. Thomas, MD
Professor, Johns Hopkins University School of Medicine and Johns Hopkins Hospital, Baltimore, Maryland
Hepatitis C

Anna R. Thorner, MD
Research Fellow, Department of Pathology, Harvard Medical School; Clinical and Research Fellow, Infectious Disease Division, Massachusetts General Hospital and Brigham and Women's Hospital, Boston, Massachusetts
Zoonotic Paramyxoviruses: Hendra, Nipah, and Menangle Viruses

Alan D. Tice, MD, FACP
Associate Professor, Infectious Diseases and Public Health Sciences, University of Hawaii at Mānoa John A. Burns School of Medicine; Active Medical Staff, Department of Internal Medicine, Queen's Medical Center, Honolulu, Hawaii
Outpatient Parenteral Antimicrobial Therapy

Angela María Tobón, MD
Scientific Advisor, Medical and Experimental Mycology Group, Corporación para Investigaciones Biológicas (CIB); Department of Internal Medicine, Hospital La Maria, Medellin, Colombia
Paracoccidioides brasiliensis

Gregory C. Townsend, MD
Associate Professor, Department of Internal Medicine, University of Virginia School of Medicine, Charlottesville, Virginia
The Infectious Diseases Physician and Digital Resources

Edmund C. Tramont, MD
Director, Division of AIDS, National Institute of Allergy and Infectious Diseases, National Institutes of Health, Bethesda, Maryland
Innate (General or Nonspecific) Host Defense Mechanisms; *Treponema pallidum* (Syphilis)

John J. Treanor, MD
Professor of Medicine, Infectious Diseases Unit, University of Rochester School of Medicine and Dentistry; Attending Physician, Department of Medicine, Strong Memorial Hospital, Rochester, New York
Influenza Virus; Noroviruses and Other Caliciviruses; Astroviruses and Picobirnaviruses

Phoebe R. Trubowitz, MD
Oncologist, Department of Hematology/Oncology, Kaiser Permanente Northwest, Portland, Oregon
Malignancies in Human Immunodeficiency Virus Infection

Theodore F. Tsai, MD, MPH
Senior Director, Department of Vaccines, Global Medical Affairs, Wyeth, Collegeville, Pennsylvania
Orthoreoviruses and Orbiviruses; Coltiviruses and Seadornaviruses (Colorado Tick Fever); Flaviviruses (Yellow Fever, Dengue, Dengue Hemorrhagic Fever, Japanese Encephalitis, West Nile Encephalitis, St. Louis Encephalitis, Tick-Borne Encephalitis)

Allan R. Tunkel, MD, PhD
Professor of Medicine and Associate Dean for Admissions, Drexel University College of Medicine, Philadelphia, Pennsylvania
Topical Antibacterials; Approach to the Patient with Central Nervous System Infection; Acute Meningitis; Cerebrospinal Fluid Shunt Infections; Brain Abscess; Subdural Empyema, Epidural Abscess, and Suppurative Intracranial Thrombophlebitis; Viridans Streptococci, Groups C and G Streptococci, and *Gemella morbillorum*

Kenneth L. Tyler, MD
Reuler-Lewin Family Professor of Neurology and Professor of Medicine, Microbiology, and Immunology, University of Colorado School of Medicine; Chief, Neurology Service, Department of Neurology, Denver Veterans Affairs Medical Center, Denver, Colorado
Introduction to Viruses and Viral Diseases; Prions and Prion Diseases of the Central Nervous System (Transmissible Neurodegenerative Diseases)

Arthur O. Tzianabos, PhD
Associate Professor of Medicine, Harvard Medical School; Channing Laboratory, Department of Medicine, Brigham and Women's Hospital, Boston, Massachusetts
Anaerobic Infections: General Concepts

Jo-Anne Van Burik, MD, FACP
Associate Professor, Department of Medicine, University of Minnesota Medical School–Minneapolis, Minneapolis, Minnesota
Infections in Recipients of Hematopoietic Stem Cell Transplantation

Edouard Vannier, PhD
Assistant Professor, Department of Medicine, Tufts University School of Medicine; Attending Physician, Division of Geographic Medicine and Infectious Diseases, Tufts–New England Medical Center, Boston, Massachusetts
Babesia Species

David W. Vaughn, MD, MPH
Director, Military Infectious Diseases Research Program, U.S. Army Medical Research and Materiel Command, Fort Detrick, Maryland
Flaviviruses (Yellow Fever, Dengue, Dengue Hemorrhagic Fever, Japanese Encephalitis, West Nile Encephalitis, St. Louis Encephalitis, Tick-Borne Encephalitis)

Jan Verhoef, MD, PhD
Professor of Clinical Microbiology, Medical Microbiology, Utrecht University; Eijkman-Winkler Institute, University Medical Center, Utrecht, The Netherlands
Anaerobic Cocci; Anaerobic Gram-Positive Nonsporulating Bacilli

Paul E. Verweij, MD, PhD
Professor of Medicine (Medical Microbiology), Department of Medical Microbiology, University Medical Center St. Radboud, Nijmegen, The Netherlands
Infections in Patients with Hematologic Malignancies

Claudio Viscoli, MD
Professor, University of Genoa, Infectious Disease Unit, National Institute of Cancer Research, Genoa, Italy
Prophylaxis and Empirical Therapy for Infection in Cancer Patients

Paul A. Volberding, MD
Professor and Vice Chair, Department of Medicine, and Co-Director, UCSF-GIVI Center for AIDS Research, University of California, San Francisco, School of Medicine; Chief, Medical Service, San Francisco Veterans Affairs Medical Center, San Francisco, California
Malignancies in Human Immunodeficiency Virus Infection

Sanjivini Wadhwa, MD
Fellow in Infectious Disease, Department of Medicine, Harvard Medical School and Beth Israel Deaconess Medical Center, Boston, Massachusetts
Cytomegalovirus

David H. Walker, MD
Professor and Chairman, Department of Pathology; Executive Director, Center for Biodefense and Emerging Infectious Diseases, University of Texas Medical Branch, University of Texas Medical School at Galveston, Galveston, Texas
Rickettsia rickettsii and Other Spotted Fever Group Rickettsiae (Rocky Mountain Spotted Fever and Other Spotted Fevers); Rickettsia prowazekii (Epidemic or Louse-Borne Typhus); Rickettsia typhi (Murine Typhus); Ehrlichia chaffeensis (Human Monocytotropic Ehrlichiosis), Anaplasma phagocytophilum (Human Granulocytotropic Anaplasmosis), and Other Ehrlichieae

Richard J. Wallace, Jr., MD
Chairman, Department of Microbiology, University of Texas Health Center at Tyler, Tyler, Texas
Antimycobacterial Agents; Infections Due to Nontuberculous Mycobacteria

Peter D. Walzer, MD
Professor and Associate Chair for Research, Department of Internal Medicine, University of Cincinnati College of Medicine; Associate Chief of Staff, Department of Research Service, Veterans Affairs Medical Center, Cincinnati, Ohio
Pneumocystis Species

Christine A. Wanke, MD
Associate Professor, Department of Medicine, Tufts University School of Medicine; Director of Clinical HIV Research, Department of Medicine, Tufts–New England Medical Center, Boston, Massachusetts
Tropical Sprue/Enteropathy

John W. Warren, MD
Professor, Department of Medicine, Division of Infectious Diseases, University of Maryland School of Medicine, Baltimore, Maryland
Nosocomial Urinary Tract Infections

Ronald G. Washburn, MD
Professor, Department of Internal Medicine/Infectious Diseases, Louisiana State University School of Medicine in Shreveport; Chief, Department of Infectious Diseases, Shreveport Veterans Affairs Medical Center, Shreveport, Louisiana
Streptobacillus moniliformis (Rat-Bite Fever); Spirillum minus (Rat-Bite Fever)

David J. Weber, MD, MPH
Department of Medicine, Division of Infectious Diseases, University of North Carolina at Chapel Hill School of Medicine, Chapel Hill, North Carolina
The Acutely Ill Patient with Fever and Rash; Disinfection, Sterilization, and Control of Hospital Waste

Arnold N. Weinberg, MD
Professor of Medicine, Harvard Medical School; Physician and Associate Firm Chief, Department of Medicine and Infectious Disease, Massachusetts General Hospital, Boston, Massachusetts
Zoonoses

Geoffrey A. Weinberg, MD
Associate Professor, Department of Pediatrics, University of Rochester School of Medicine and Dentistry; Director, Pediatric HIV Program, Golisano Children's Hospital at Strong and Strong Memorial Hospital, Rochester, New York
Pediatric Human Immunodeficiency Virus Infection

Daniel Weisdorf, MD, FACP
Professor of Medicine and Director, Adult Blood and Marrow Transplant Program, Division of Hematology, Oncology, and Transplantation, Department of Medicine, University of Minnesota, Minneapolis, Minnesota
Infections in Recipients of Hematopoietic Stem Cell Transplantation

Louis M. Weiss, MD, MPH
Professor, Departments of Medicine (Division of Infectious Diseases) and Pathology (Division of Parasitology and Tropical Medicine), Albert Einstein College of Medicine of Yeshiva University; Attending Physician, Department of Medicine, Jack D. Weiler Hospital of the Albert Einstein College of Medicine—Montefiore Medical Center; Attending Physician, Department of Medicine, Jacobi Medical Center, Bronx, New York
Microsporidiosis

Michael E. Weiss, MD
Northwest Asthma and Allergy, Redmond, Washington
β-Lactam Allergy

David F. Welch, PhD
Associate Clinical Professor of Pathology, University of Texas Southwestern Medical Center at Dallas; Medical Microbiologist, Laboratory Corporation of America, Dallas, Texas
Bartonella, Including Cat-Scratch Disease

Thomas E. Wellems, MD, PhD
Head, Malaria Genetics Section, and Acting Chief, Laboratory of Malaria and Vector Research, National Institutes of Allergy and Infectious Diseases, National Institutes of Health, Bethesda, Maryland
Plasmodium Species (Malaria)

Richard P. Wenzel, MD, MSc
Professor and Chairman, Department of Internal Medicine, Virginia Commonwealth University School of Medicine, Richmond, Virginia
Organization for Infection Control; Isolation

Melinda Wharton, MD, MPH
Acting Deputy Director, National Immunization Program, Centers for Disease Control and Prevention, Atlanta, Georgia
Immunization

A. Clinton White, Jr., MD
Professor, Infectious Diseases Section, Department of Medicine, Baylor College of Medicine; Chief, Infectious Diseases Section, Department of Medicine, Ben Taub General Hospital, Houston, Texas
Cryptosporidiosis (Cryptosporidium hominis, Cryptosporidium parvum, and Other Species)

Richard J. Whitley, MD
Professor of Pediatrics, Microbiology, and Medicine; Loeb Scholar in Pediatrics; Director, Division of Pediatric Infectious Diseases; Vice-Chair, Department of Pediatrics; Senior Scientist, Department of Gene Therapy; Senior Scientist, Cancer Research and Training Center; Associate Director for Clinical Studies, Center for AIDS Research; Director, Center for Biodefense and Emerging Infection, University of Alabama School of Medicine, University of Alabama at Birmingham, Birmingham, Alabama
Varicella-Zoster Virus

Barbara Braunstein Wilson, MD
Associate Professor, Department of Dermatology, University of Virginia School of Medicine, Charlottesville, Virginia
Introduction to Ectoparasitic Diseases; Lice (Pediculosis); Scabies; Myiasis and Tungiasis; Mites (Including Chiggers); Ticks (Including Tick Paralysis)

Kenneth H. Wilson, MD
Professor, Department of Medicine, Duke University School of Medicine; Chief, Infectious Diseases Section, Veterans Affairs Medical Center, Durham, North Carolina
Antibiotic-Associated Colitis

Walter R. Wilson, MD
Professor of Medicine, Division of Infectious Diseases, Mayo Clinic College of Medicine; Consultant, Mayo Clinic, Rochester, Minnesota
Infections of Prosthetic Valves and Other Cardiovascular Devices

Frank G. Witebsky, MD
Assistant Chief, Microbiology Service, Department of Laboratory Medicine, Warren G. Magnuson Clinical Center, National Institutes of Health, Bethesda, Maryland
The Clinician and the Microbiology Laboratory

Peter F. Wright, MD
Professor of Pediatrics, Pathology, Microbiology, and Immunology, and Head, Pediatric Infectious Diseases, Vanderbilt University School of Medicine, Nashville, Tennessee
Parainfluenza Viruses

Edward J. Young, MD
Professor, Department of Medicine and Molecular Virology and Microbiology, Baylor College of Medicine; Staff Physician, Section of Infectious Diseases, Veterans Affairs Medical Center, Houston, Texas
Brucella Species

Roger W. Yurt, MD
Johnson & Johnson Distinguished Professor and Vice Chairman, Department of Surgery, Weill Medical College of Cornell University; Director, William Randolph Hearst Burn Center, Department of Surgery, New York–Presbyterian–Weill Cornell Medical Center, New York, New York
Burns

Stephen H. Zinner, MD
Charles S. Davidson Professor of Medicine, Harvard Medical School, Boston; Chair of Medicine, Mount Auburn Hospital, Cambridge, Massachusetts
Sulfonamides and Trimethoprim

John J. Zurlo, MD
Professor, Department of Medicine, Division of Infectious Diseases and Epidemiology, Pennsylvania State University, School of Medicine, Hershey, Pennsylvania
Pasteurella Species

PREFACE TO THE FIRST EDITION

Infectious diseases traverse the usual boundaries established by medical specialists. All organ systems may be involved, and all physicians caring for patients may have to deal with infected patients. The format of this book was chosen with the intent that it would contain the necessary information to aid the practitioner in the understanding, diagnosis, and treatment of infectious diseases. Thus, internists, family or general practitioners, pediatricians, surgeons, obstetrician-gynecologists, urologists, residents and fellows in training, medical students, hospital infection control personnel, and clinical microbiologists should find the book a valuable reference.

In planning this book the editors considered several different patterns of organization. The system adopted allows the reader to approach an infected patient three different ways: (a) by major clinical syndrome, (b) by specific etiologic organisms, and (c) by host characteristics for patients who are compromised.

Principles and Practice of Infectious Diseases consists of four major parts. The book may be perused as whole, or individual chapters may be examined when the reader is concerned with a specific problem. Part I covers the basic principles necessary for a clear understanding of the concepts of diagnosis and management of infectious disease. Chapters dealing with microbial virulence factors, host defense mechanisms, the epidemiology of infectious diseases, and the clinician and microbiology laboratory are included. In addition, there is a comprehensive discussion of anti-infective chemotherapy.

Part II considers major clinical syndromes. The syndromes are described, followed by a discussion of the potential etiologic agents, evaluation of differential diagnostic possibilities, and an outline of presumptive therapy. All major infectious diseases are discussed in this part of the book.

Part III describes all important pathogenic microbes for man and the diseases they cause. The pathogen is classified and described, the epidemiology is discussed, clinical manifestations are listed, and specific information on therapy and prevention is presented. The most comprehensive discussion of a disease entity can be found by reading about both the etiologic agent and the clinical syndrome. Thus, a comprehensive treatment of pneumococcal pneumonia could be found in reading the appropriate sections of the chapters on acute pneumonia and *Streptococcus pneumoniae.* We attempted to make the chapters dealing with etiologic agents and those dealing with syndromes complete. Therefore some repetition was unavoidable.

The final section, Part IV, covers special problems in infectious diseases including nosocomial infections, infections in impaired hosts, immunizations, and protection of travelers.

The editors are grateful to our expert contributors. These physicians are the world's leaders in their fields, and they diligently prepared carefully written, well-referenced "state of the art" chapters. Our secretaries were skillful and meticulous in their attention to the complexities of assembling *Principles and Practice of Infectious Diseases.* John de Carville, executive editor of John Wiley & Sons, encouraged, cajoled, and advised us from the formative steps all the way through to completion. Lastly, and perhaps most important, we are grateful to our wives and children for putting up with interminable editorial work and meetings.

GERALD L. MANDELL, M.D.
R. GORDON DOUGLAS, JR., M.D.
JOHN E. BENNETT, M.D.

PREFACE TO THE SIXTH EDITION

Knowledge about infectious diseases has undergone an extraordinary expansion during the years between publication of the fifth edition of this book, and this, the sixth one. During that time, previously unrecognized infections have emerged, and awareness of the role of microbes as potential agents of terrorism has been heightened. The population of patients whose host defenses are compromised by underlying diseases or by medical treatments continues to increase, and this has resulted in increasingly complex and challenging infections. In those years, important new advancements were made in the development of highly sensitive and specific diagnostic techniques, in antimicrobial therapy, in vaccines, and in appreciation of public health control measures against the spread of infectious diseases.

This new edition has attempted to capture this explosion of new knowledge in an authoritative, complete, yet readable and readily accessible text. Every chapter has been revised, and many new chapters have been added since the last edition. Examples of the latter include chapters on SARS, metapneumovirus, Nipah and Hendra viruses, uncommon fungi, bioterrorism agents, and hospital preparedness for emerging and highly contagious infections. New color figures and revised tables have been added throughout, which will facilitate use of the book.

The continually changing names of microorganisms remains a vexing challenge for infectious disease practitioners and book editors alike. For the sixth edition, we have generally adhered to the names of organisms given in the eighth edition of the *Manual of Clinical Microbiology,* ASM Press, 2003.

As always, a work of this magnitude is impossible without the contributions of our many authors, who brought extraordinary knowledge, experience, and perspective to each of their chapters. Their dedication to the goals of our book is a source of continued inspiration to us, for which we express a most heartfelt gratitude. We also want to express our appreciation for the superb assistance that has been provided by Janet Morgan and Stacy McGrath.

Finally, none of this would have been possible without the encouragement, understanding, and sometimes forbearance of Judy, Shirley, and Kelly, who once again saw their husbands through the process of bringing this book to fruition.

GERALD L. MANDELL, M.D.
JOHN E. BENNETT, M.D.
RAPHAEL DOLIN, M.D.

CONTENTS

VOLUME 1

PART I
BASIC PRINCIPLES IN THE DIAGNOSIS AND MANAGEMENT OF INFECTIOUS DISEASES

SECTION A

Microbial Virulence Factors, 3

1 A Molecular Perspective
of Microbial Pathogenicity, 3
David A. Relman and Stanley Falkow

2 Microbial Adherence, 14
*William A. Petri, Jr., Barbara J. Mann,
and Christopher D. Huston*

3 Toxins, 24
Erik L. Hewlett and Molly A. Hughes

SECTION B

Host Defense Mechanisms, 34

4 Innate (General or Nonspecific) Host Defense
Mechanisms, 34
Carl W. Dieffenbach and Edmund C. Tramont

5 Human Genetics and Infection, 42
Adrian V. S. Hill

6 Antibodies, 52
Holly H. Birdsall

7 Complement, 69
Peter Densen

8 Granulocytic Phagocytes, 93
William M. Nauseef and Robert A. Clark

9 Cell-Mediated Defense against Infection, 117
Michael S. Glickman and Eric G. Pamer

10 Nutrition, Immunity, and Infection, 139
Caryn Gee Morse and Kevin P. High

11 Evaluation of the Patient with Suspected
Immunodeficiency, 149
Steven M. Holland and John I. Gallin

SECTION C

Epidemiology of Infectious Diseases, 161

12 Epidemiologic Principles, 161
Michael T. Osterholm and Craig W. Hedberg

13 Emerging and Reemerging Infectious Disease
Threats, 173
*Stephen M. Ostroff, Joseph E. McDade, James W. LeDuc,
and James M. Hughes*

14 Hospital Preparedness for Emerging and Highly
Contagious Infectious Diseases: Getting Ready
for SARS or Whatever Comes Next, 192
David K. Henderson

SECTION D

Clinical Microbiology, 203

15 The Clinician and the Microbiology
Laboratory, 203
Vee J. Gill, Daniel P. Fedorko, and Frank G. Witebsky

SECTION E

Anti-Infective Therapy, 242

16 Principles of Anti-infective Therapy, 242
Robert C. Moellering, Jr., and George M. Eliopoulos

17 Molecular Mechanisms of Antibiotic Resistance
in Bacteria, 253
Steven M. Opal and Antone A. Medeiros

18 Pharmacokinetics and Pharmacodynamics
of Anti-infective Agents, 271
*Guy W. Amsden, Charles H. Ballow, Joseph S. Bertino, Jr.,
and Angela D. M. Kashuba*

19 Penicillins, 281
Henry F. Chambers

20 Cephalosporins, 294
David R. Andes and William A. Craig

21 Other β-Lactam Antibiotics, 311
Henry F. Chambers

22 β-Lactam Allergy, 318
Michael E. Weiss and N. Franklin Adkinson, Jr.

23 Fusidic Acid, 326
Lionel A. Mandell

24 Aminoglycosides, 328
David N. Gilbert

25 Tetracyclines and Chloramphenicol, 356
Burt Meyers and Mirella Salvatore

26 Rifamycins, 374
David P. Calfee

27 Metronidazole, 388
Mirella Salvatore and Burt Meyers

28 Macrolides, Clindamycin, and Ketolides, 396
Sumathi Sivapalasingam and Neal H. Steigbigel

29 Glycopeptides (Vancomycin and Teicoplanin),
Streptogramins (Quinupristin-Dalfopristin),
and Lipopeptides (Daptomycin), 417
Barbara E. Murray and Esteban C. Nannini

30 Polymyxins (Polymyxin B and Colistin), 435
Keith S. Kaye and Donald Kaye

31 Oxazolidinones, 436
Gerald R. Donowitz

32 Sulfonamides and Trimethoprim, 440
Stephen H. Zinner and Kenneth H. Mayer

33 Quinolones, 451
David C. Hooper

34 Urinary Tract Agents: Nitrofurantoin
and Methenamine, 473
David C. Hooper

35 Topical Antibacterials, 478
Judith A. O'Donnell and Allan R. Tunkel

36 Antimycobacterial Agents, 489
Richard J. Wallace, Jr., and David E. Griffith

37 Systemic Antifungal Agents, 502
John H. Rex and David A. Stevens

38 Antiviral Drugs (Other Than Antiretrovirals), 514
Frederick G. Hayden

39 Immunomodulators, 551
W. Conrad Liles

40 Hyperbaric Oxygen, 563
Ronald Rabinowitz, Jean Marie Mulinde, and Ellis S. Caplan

41 Agents Active against Parasites
and *Pneumocystis*, 568
Richard D. Pearson

42 Complementary and Alternative Medicines
for Infectious Diseases, 603
Jonathan D. Berman and Stephen E. Straus

43 Antimicrobial Management: Cost
and Resistance, 611
Ronald E. Polk and Neil O. Fishman

44 Interpreting the Results of Clinical Trials
on Antimicrobial Agents, 619
John H. Powers

45 Outpatient Parenteral Antimicrobial Therapy, 629
Alan D. Tice

46 Tables of Antimicrobial Agent Pharmacology, 634
Guy W. Amsden

PART II
MAJOR CLINICAL SYNDROMES

SECTION A

Fever, 703

47 Temperature Regulation and the Pathogenesis
of Fever, 703
Philip A. Mackowiak

48 Fever of Unknown Origin, 718
Philip A. Mackowiak and David T. Durack

49 The Acutely Ill Patient with Fever and Rash, 729
David J. Weber, Myron S. Cohen, and William A. Rutala

SECTION B

Upper Respiratory Tract Infections, 747

50 The Common Cold, 747
Jack M. Gwaltney, Jr.

51 Pharyngitis, 752
Alan L. Bisno

52 Acute Laryngitis, 758
Mary T. Caserta

53 Acute Laryngotracheobronchitis (Croup), 760
Caroline Breese Hall and John T. McBride

54 Otitis Externa, Otitis Media, and Mastoiditis, 766
Jerome O. Klein

55 Sinusitis, 772
Jack M. Gwaltney, Jr.

56 Epiglottitis, 784
James E. Burns and J. Owen Hendley

57 Infections of the Oral Cavity, Neck, and Head, 787
Anthony W. Chow

SECTION C

Pleuropulmonary and Bronchial Infections, 803

58 Acute Bronchitis, 803
Jack M. Gwaltney, Jr.

59 Chronic Obstructive Pulmonary Disease, Chronic
Bronchitis, and Acute Exacerbations, 806
Herbert Y. Reynolds

60 Bronchiolitis, 812
Caroline Breese Hall and John T. McBride

61 Acute Pneumonia, 819
Gerald R. Donowitz and Gerald L. Mandell

62 Pleural Effusion and Empyema, 845
Edward Septimus

63 Lung Abscess, 853
Bennett Lorber

64 Chronic Pneumonia, 857
Peter G. Pappas and William E. Dismukes

65 Cystic Fibrosis, 869
Michael R. Knowles, Peter H. Gilligan, and Richard C. Boucher

SECTION D

Urinary Tract Infection, 875

66 Urinary Tract Infections, 875
Jack D. Sobel and Donald Kaye

SECTION E

Sepsis, 906

67 Sepsis, Severe Sepsis, and Septic Shock, 906
Robert S. Munford

SECTION F

Intra-abdominal Infection, 927

68 Peritonitis and Intraperitoneal Abscesses, 927
Matthew E. Levison and Larry M. Bush

69 Infections of the Liver and Biliary System, 951
Eric C. Johannsen and Lawrence C. Madoff

70 Pancreatic Infections, 959
Miriam J. Baron and Lawrence C. Madoff

71 Splenic Abscess, 967
Lawrence C. Madoff

72 Appendicitis, 968
Costi D. Sifri and Lawrence C. Madoff

73 Diverticulitis and Typhlitis, 971
Costi D. Sifri and Lawrence C. Madoff

SECTION G

Cardiovascular Infections, 975

74 Endocarditis and Intravascular Infections, 975
Vance G. Fowler, Jr., W. Michael Scheld, and Arnold S. Bayer

75 Infections of Prosthetic Valves and Other Cardiovascular Devices, 1022
Larry M. Baddour and Walter R. Wilson

76 Prophylaxis of Infective Endocarditis, 1044
David T. Durack

77 Myocarditis and Pericarditis, 1052
Maria C. Savoia and Michael N. Oxman

78 Mediastinitis, 1070
Mark E. Rupp

SECTION H

Central Nervous System Infections, 1079

79 Approach to the Patient with Central Nervous System Infection, 1079
Allan R. Tunkel

80 Acute Meningitis, 1083
Allan R. Tunkel and W. Michael Scheld

81 Cerebrospinal Fluid Shunt Infections, 1126
Allan R. Tunkel and Bruce A. Kaufman

82 Chronic Meningitis, 1132
Irmgard Behlau and Jerrold J. Ellner

83 Encephalitis, Myelitis, and Neuritis, 1143
Diane E. Griffin

84 Brain Abscess, 1150
Allan R. Tunkel

85 Subdural Empyema, Epidural Abscess, and Suppurative Intracranial Thrombophlebitis, 1164
Allan R. Tunkel

SECTION I

Skin and Soft Tissue Infections, 1172

86 Cellulitis and Subcutaneous Tissue Infections, 1172
Morton N. Swartz and Mark S. Pasternack

87 Myositis, 1194
Mark S. Pasternack and Morton N. Swartz

88 Lymphadenitis and Lymphangitis, 1204
Mark S. Pasternack and Morton N. Swartz

SECTION J

Gastrointestinal Infections and Food Poisoning, 1215

89 Principles and Syndromes of Enteric Infection, 1215
Richard L. Guerrant. and Theodore S. Steiner

90 Esophagitis, 1231
Paul S. Graman

91 Nausea, Vomiting, and Noninflammatory Diarrhea, 1236
Richard L. Guerrant and David A. Bobak

92 Antibiotic-Associated Colitis, 1249
Nathan M. Thielman and Kenneth H. Wilson

93 Inflammatory Enteritides, 1263
Richard L. Guerrant and Aldo A. M. Lima

94 Enteric Fever and Other Causes of Abdominal Symptoms with Fever, 1273
Nathan M. Thielman and Richard L. Guerrant

95 Foodborne Disease, 1286
Alicia M. Fry, Christopher R. Braden, Patricia M. Griffin, and James M. Hughes

96 Tropical Sprue/Enteropathy, 1301
Christine A. Wanke

97 Whipple's Disease, 1306
Thomas Marth

SECTION K

Bone and Joint Infections, 1311

98 Infectious Arthritis of Native Joints, 1311
Christopher A. Ohl

99 Osteomyelitis, 1322
Elie F. Berbari, James M. Steckelberg, and Douglas R. Osmon

100 Infections with Prostheses in Bones and Joints, 1332
Barry D. Brause

SECTION L

Diseases of the Reproductive Organs and Sexually Transmitted Diseases, 1338

101 Genital Skin and Mucous Membrane Lesions, 1338
Michael H. Augenbraun

102 Urethritis, 1347
William M. McCormack and Michael F. Rein

103 Vulvovaginitis and Cervicitis, 1357
William M. McCormack

104 Infections of the Female Pelvis, 1372
David E. Soper and Philip B. Mead

105 Prostatitis, Epididymitis, and Orchitis, 1381
John N. Krieger

SECTION M

Eye Infections, 1387

106 Microbial Conjunctivitis, 1387
Scott D. Barnes, Deborah Pavan-Langston, and Dimitri T. Azar

107 Microbial Keratitis, 1395
Scott D. Barnes, Deborah Pavan-Langston, and Dimitri T. Azar

108 Endophthalmitis, 1406
Marlene L. Durand

109 Infectious Causes of Uveitis, 1413
Marlene L. Durand

110 Periocular Infections, 1419
Marlene L. Durand

SECTION N

Hepatitis, 1426

111 Acute Viral Hepatitis, 1426
Michael P. Curry and Sanjiv Chopra

112 Chronic Viral Hepatitis, 1441
Jules L. Dienstag

SECTION O

Acquired Immunodeficiency Syndrome, 1465

113 Global Perspectives on Human Immunodeficiency Virus Infection and Acquired Immunodeficiency Syndrome, 1465
Michael H. Merson and Peter Piot

114 Epidemiology and Prevention of Acquired Immunodeficiency Syndrome and Human Immunodeficiency Virus Infection, 1477
Carlos Del Rio and James W. Curran

115 Diagnosis of Human Immunodeficiency Virus Infection, 1506
Frank Maldarelli

116 The Immunology of Human Immunodeficiency Virus Infection, 1527
Mark Dybul, Mark Connors, and Anthony S. Fauci

117 General Clinical Manifestations of Human Immunodeficiency Virus Infection (Including the Acute Retroviral Syndrome and Oral, Cutaneous, Renal, Ocular, and Cardiac Diseases), 1546
Timothy R. Sterling and Richard E. Chaisson

118 Pulmonary Manifestations of Human Immunodeficiency Virus Infection, 1567
Paul E. Sax

119 Gastrointestinal and Hepatobiliary Manifestations of Human Immunodeficiency Virus Infection, 1575
Mark S. Sulkowski and Richard E. Chaisson

120 Neurologic Diseases Caused by Human Immunodeficiency Virus-1 and Opportunistic Infections, 1583
Igor J. Koralnik

121 Malignancies in Human Immunodeficiency Virus Infection, 1601
Amy Gates, Phoebe R. Trubowitz, and Paul A. Volberding

122 Human Immunodeficiency Virus Infection in Women, 1616
Susan E. Cohn and Rebecca A. Clark

123 Pediatric Human Immunodeficiency Virus Infection, 1638
Geoffrey A. Weinberg and Sandra K. Burchett

124 Antiretroviral Therapy for Human Immunodeficiency Virus Infection, 1655
George J. Hanna and Martin S. Hirsch

125 Management of Opportunistic Infections Associated with Human Immunodeficiency Virus Infection, 1679
Henry Masur

126 Vaccines for Human Immunodeficiency Virus-1 Infection, 1707
Dan H. Barouch, Lindsey R. Baden, and Raphael Dolin

SECTION P

Miscellaneous Syndromes, 1720

127 Chronic Fatigue Syndrome, 1720
N. Cary Engleberg

Index, i

VOLUME 2

PART III
INFECTIOUS DISEASES AND THEIR ETIOLOGIC AGENTS

SECTION A

Viral Diseases, 1729

128 Introduction to Viruses and Viral Diseases, 1729
Terence S. Dermody and Kenneth L. Tyler

DNA Viruses

Poxviridae

129 Orthopoxviruses: Vaccinia (Smallpox Vaccine), Variola (Smallpox), Monkeypox, and Cowpox, 1742
Inger Damon

130 Other Poxviruses That Infect Humans: Parapoxviruses, Molluscum Contagiosum, and Tanapox, 1753
Inger Damon

Herpesviridae

131 Introduction to Herpesviridae, 1756
Stephen E. Straus

132 Herpes Simplex Virus, 1762
Lawrence Corey

133 Varicella-Zoster Virus, 1780
Richard J. Whitley

134 Cytomegalovirus, 1786
Clyde S. Crumpacker and Sanjivini Wadhwa

135 Epstein-Barr Virus (Infectious Mononucleosis), 1801
Eric C. Johannsen, Robert T. Schooley, and Kenneth M. Kaye

136 Human Herpesvirus Types 6 and 7, 1821
Stephen E. Straus

137 Kaposi's Sarcoma–Associated Herpesvirus (Human Herpesvirus Type 8), 1827
Kenneth M. Kaye

138 Herpes B Virus, 1832
Stephen E. Straus

Adenoviridae

139 Adenovirus, 1835
Stephen G. Baum

Papovaviridae

140 Papillomaviruses, 1841
William Bonnez and Richard C. Reichman

141 JC, BK, and Other Polyomaviruses; Progressive Multifocal Leukoencephalopathy, 1856
Lisa M. Demeter

Hepadnaviridae

142 Hepatitis B Virus and Hepatitis Delta Virus, 1864
Margaret James Koziel and Aleem Siddiqui

Parvoviridae

143 Parvovirus B19, 1891
Kevin E. Brown

RNA Viruses

Reoviridae

144 Orthoreoviruses and Orbiviruses, 1899
Theodore F. Tsai

145 Coltiviruses and Seadornaviruses (Colorado Tick Fever), 1900
Theodore F. Tsai

146 Rotaviruses, 1902
Philip R. Dormitzer

Togaviridae

147 Alphaviruses, 1913
Lewis Markoff

148 Rubella Virus (German Measles), 1921
Anne A. Gershon

Flaviviruses

149 Flaviviruses (Yellow Fever, Dengue, Dengue Hemorrhagic Fever, Japanese Encephalitis, West Nile Encephalitis, St. Louis Encephalitis, Tick-Borne Encephalitis), 1926
Theodore F. Tsai, David W. Vaughn, and Tom Solomon

150 Hepatitis C, 1950
David L. Thomas, Stuart C. Ray, and Stanley M. Lemon

151 Hepatitis G Virus and TT Virus, 1981
Harvey J. Alter

Coronaviridae

152 Coronaviruses, Including Severe Acute Respiratory Syndrome (SARS)-Associated Coronavirus, 1990
Kenneth McIntosh and Larry J. Anderson

Paramyxoviridae

153 Parainfluenza Viruses, 1998
Peter F. Wright

154 Mumps Virus, 2003
Nathan Litman and Stephen G. Baum

155 Respiratory Syncytial Virus, 2008
Caroline Breese Hall and Carol A. McCarthy

156 Human Metapneumovirus, 2026
Ann R. Falsey

157 Measles Virus (Rubeola), 2031
Anne A. Gershon

158 Zoonotic Paramyxoviruses: Hendra, Nipah, and Menangle Viruses, 2038
Anna R. Thorner and Raphael Dolin

Rhabdoviridae

159 Vesicular Stomatitis Virus and Related Viruses, 2044
Steven M. Fine

160 Rhabdoviruses, 2047
Thomas P. Bleck and Charles E. Rupprecht

Filoviridae

161 Marburg and Ebola Virus Hemorrhagic Fevers, 2057
C. J. Peters

Orthomyxoviridae

162 Influenza Virus, 2060
John J. Treanor

Bunyaviridae

163 California Encephalitis, Hantavirus Pulmonary Syndrome, and Bunyavirid Hemorrhagic Fevers, 2086
C. J. Peters

Arenaviridae

164 Lymphocytic Choriomeningitis Virus, Lassa Virus, and the South American Hemorrhagic Fevers, 2090
C. J. Peters

Retroviridae

165 Human T-Cell Lymphotropic Virus Types I and II, 2098
William Blattner and Manhattan Charurat

166 Human Immunodeficiency Viruses, 2119
Farley R. Cleghorn, Marvin S. Reitz, Jr., Mikulas Popovic, and Robert C. Gallo

Picornaviridae

167 Introduction to the Enteroviruses, 2133
John F. Modlin

168 Poliovirus, 2141
John F. Modlin

169 Coxsackieviruses, Echoviruses, and Newer Enteroviruses, 2148
John F. Modlin

170 Hepatitis A Virus, 2162
Beth P. Bell, David A. Anderson, and Stephen M. Feinstone

171 Rhinovirus, 2185
Jack M. Gwaltney, Jr.

Caliciviridae and Other Gastrointestinal Viruses

172 Noroviruses and Other Caliciviruses, 2194
John J. Treanor and Raphael Dolin

173 Astroviruses and Picobirnaviruses, 2201
John J. Treanor and Raphael Dolin

Unclassified Viruses

174 Hepatitis E Virus, 2204
Robert H. Purcell and Suzanne U. Emerson

SECTION B

Prion Diseases, 2219

175 Prions and Prion Diseases of the Central Nervous System (Transmissible Neurodegenerative Diseases), 2219
Kenneth L. Tyler

SECTION C

Chlamydial Diseases, 2236

176 Introduction to Chlamydial Diseases, 2236
Walter E. Stamm, Robert B. Jones, and Byron E. Batteiger

177 *Chlamydia trachomatis* (Trachoma, Perinatal Infections, Lymphogranuloma Venereum, and Other Genital Infections), 2239
Walter E. Stamm, Robert B. Jones, and Byron E. Batteiger

178 *Chlamydophila (Chlamydia) psittaci* (Psittacosis), 2256
David Schlossberg

179 *Chlamydophila (Chlamydia) pneumoniae*, 2258
Lisa A. Jackson

SECTION D

Mycoplasma Diseases, 2269

180 Introduction to *Mycoplasma* Diseases, 2269
Stephen G. Baum

181 *Mycoplasma pneumoniae* and Atypical Pneumonia, 2271
Stephen G. Baum

182 Genital Mycoplasmas: *Mycoplasma genitalium, Mycoplasma hominis,* and *Ureaplasma* Species, 2280
George E. Kenney

SECTION E

Rickettsioses and Ehrlichioses, 2284

183 Introduction to Rickettsioses and Ehrlichioses, 2284
Didier Raoult

184 *Rickettsia rickettsii* and Other Spotted Fever Group Rickettsiae (Rocky Mountain Spotted Fever and Other Spotted Fevers), 2287
David H. Walker and Didier Raoult

185 *Rickettsia akari* (Rickettsialpox), 2295
Didier Raoult

186 *Coxiella burnetii* (Q Fever), 2296
Thomas J. Marrie and Didier Raoult

187 *Rickettsia prowazekii* (Epidemic or Louse-Borne Typhus), 2303
Didier Raoult and David H. Walker

188 *Rickettsia typhi* (Murine Typhus), 2306
J. Stephen Dumler and David H. Walker

189 Scrub Typhus, 2309
Didier Raoult

190 *Ehrlichia chaffeensis* (Human Monocytotropic Ehrlichiosis), *Anaplasma phagocytophilum* (Human Granulocytotropic Anaplasmosis), and Other Ehrlichieae, 2310
David H. Walker and J. Stephen Dumler

SECTION F

Bacterial Diseases, 2319

191 Introduction to Bacteria and Bacterial Diseases, 2319
Martin J. Blaser

Gram-Positive Cocci

192 *Staphylococcus aureus* (Including Staphylococcal Toxic Shock), 2321
Philippe Moreillon, Yok-Ai Que, and Michel P. Glauser

193 *Staphylococcus epidermidis* and Other Coagulase-Negative Staphylococci, 2352
Gordon L. Archer and Michael W. Climo

194 Classification of Streptococci, 2360
Alan L. Bisno and Kathryn L. Ruoff

195 *Streptococcus pyogenes*, 2362
Alan L. Bisno and Dennis L. Stevens

196 Nonsuppurative Poststreptococcal Sequelae: Rheumatic Fever and Glomerulonephritis, 2380
Alan L. Bisno

197 *Streptococcus pneumoniae*, 2392
Daniel M. Musher

198 *Enterococcus* Species, *Streptococcus bovis*, and *Leuconostoc* Species, 2411
Robert C. Moellering, Jr.

199 *Streptococcus agalactiae* (Group B Streptococcus), 2423
Morven S. Edwards and Carol J. Baker

200 Viridans Streptococci, Groups C and G Streptococci, and *Gemella morbillorum*, 2434
Caroline C. Johnson and Allan R. Tunkel

201 *Streptococcus anginosus* Group, 2451
Yazdan Mirzanejad and Charles W. Stratton

Gram-Positive Bacilli

202 *Corynebacterium diphtheriae*, 2457
Rob Roy MacGregor

203 Other Coryneform Bacteria and *Rhodococcus*, 2465
Daniel K. Meyer and Annette C. Reboli

204 *Listeria monocytogenes*, 2478
Bennett Lorber

205 *Bacillus anthracis* (Anthrax), 2485
Daniel Lucey

206 *Bacillus* Species and Related Genera Other than *Bacillus anthracis*, 2493
Thomas Fekete

207 *Erysipelothrix rhusiopathiae*, 2496
Annette C. Reboli and W. Edmund Farrar

Gram-Negative Cocci

208 *Neisseria meningitidis*, 2498
Michael A. Apicella

209 *Neisseria gonorrhoeae*, 2514
H. Hunter Handsfield and P. Frederick Sparling

210 *Moraxella (Branhamella) catarrhalis* and Other Gram-Negative Cocci, 2529
Timothy F. Murphy

Gram-Negative Bacilli

211 *Vibrio cholerae*, 2536
Carlos Seas and Eduardo Gotuzzo

212 Other Pathogenic Vibrios, 2544
Marguerite A. Neill and Charles C. J. Carpenter

213 *Campylobacter jejuni* and Related Species, 2548
Martin J. Blaser and Ban M. Allos

214 *Helicobacter pylori* and Other Gastric *Helicobacter* Species, 2557
Martin J. Blaser

215 Enterobacteriaceae, 2567
Michael S. Donnenberg

216 *Pseudomonas aeruginosa*, 2587
Gerald B. Pier and Reuben Ramphal

217 *Stenotrophomonas maltophilia* and *Burkholderia cepacia*, 2615
Georg Maschmeyer and Ulf B. Göbel

218 *Burkholderia pseudomallei* and *Burkholderia mallei*: Melioidosis and Glanders, 2622
Bart J. Currie

219 *Acinetobacter* Species, 2632
David M. Allen and Barry J. Hartman

220 *Salmonella* Species, Including *Salmonella typhi*, 2636
David A. Pegues, Michael E. Ohl, and Samuel I. Miller

221 *Shigella* Species (Bacillary Dysentery), 2655
Herbert L. DuPont

222 *Haemophilus* Infections, 2661
Timothy F. Murphy

223 *Brucella* Species, 2669
Edward J. Young

224 *Francisella tularensis* (Tularemia), 2674
Robert L. Penn

225 *Pasteurella* Species, 2687
John J. Zurlo

226 *Yersinia* Species, Including Plague, 2691
Thomas Butler and David T. Dennis

227 *Bordetella* Species, 2701
Erik L. Hewlett

228 *Streptobacillus moniliformis* (Rat-Bite Fever), 2708
Ronald G. Washburn

229 *Legionella*, 2711
Paul H. Edelstein and Nicholas P. Cianciotto

230 Other *Legionella* Species, 2725
Robert R. Muder

231 *Capnocytophaga*, 2730
Vee J. Gill

232 *Bartonella*, Including Cat-Scratch Disease, 2733
Leonard N. Slater and David F. Welch

233 *Calymmatobacterium granulomatis* (Donovanosis, Granuloma Inguinale), 2748
Ronald C. Ballard

234 Other Gram-Negative and Gram-Variable Bacilli, 2751
James P. Steinberg and Carlos Del Rio

Spirochetes

235 *Treponema pallidum* (Syphilis), 2768
Edmund C. Tramont

236 Endemic Treponematoses, 2785
Edward W. Hook III

237 Leptospirosis, 2789
Paul N. Levett

238 *Borrelia* Species (Relapsing Fever), 2795
Kyu Y. Rhee and Warren D. Johnson, Jr.

239 *Borrelia burgdorferi* (Lyme Disease, Lyme Borreliosis), 2798
Allen C. Steere

240 *Spirillum minus* (Rat-Bite Fever), 2810
Ronald G. Washburn

Anaerobic Bacteria

241 Anaerobic Infections: General Concepts, 2810
Arthur O. Tzianabos and Dennis L. Kasper

242 *Clostridium tetani* (Tetanus), 2817
Thomas P. Bleck

243 *Clostridium botulinum* (Botulism), 2822
Thomas P. Bleck

244 Gas Gangrene and Other *Clostridium*-Associated Diseases, 2828
Bennett Lorber

245 *Bacteroides, Prevotella, Porphyromonas,* and *Fusobacterium* Species (and Other Medically Important Anaerobic Gram-Negative Bacilli), 2838
Bennett Lorber

246 Anaerobic Cocci, 2847
Ellen M. Mascini and Jan Verhoef

247 Anaerobic Gram-Positive Nonsporulating Bacilli, 2849
Ellen M. Mascini and Jan Verhoef

Mycobacterial Diseases

248 *Mycobacterium tuberculosis,* 2852
Daniel Fitzgerald and David W. Haas

249 *Mycobacterium leprae* (Leprosy, Hansen's Disease), 2886
William R. Levis and Joel D. Ernst

250 *Mycobacterium avium* Complex, 2897
Fred M. Gordin and C. Robert Horsburgh, Jr.

251 Infections Caused by Nontuberculous Mycobacteria, 2909
Barbara A. Brown-Elliott and Richard J. Wallace, Jr.

Higher Bacterial Diseases

252 *Nocardia* Species, 2916
Tania C. Sorrell, David H. Mitchell, and Jonathon R. Iredell

253 Agents of Actinomycosis, 2924
Thomas A. Russo

SECTION G

Mycoses, 2935

254 Introduction to Mycoses, 2935
John E. Bennett

255 *Candida* Species, 2938
John E. Edwards, Jr.

256 *Aspergillus* Species, 2958
Thomas F. Patterson

257 Agents of Mucormycosis and Related Species, 2973
Alan M. Sugar

258 *Sporothrix schenckii,* 2984
John H. Rex and Pablo C. Okhuysen

259 Agents of Chromoblastomycosis, 2988
Duane R. Hospenthal

260 Agents of Mycetoma, 2991
Duane R. Hospenthal

261 *Cryptococcus neoformans,* 2997
John R. Perfect

262 *Histoplasma capsulatum,* 3012
George S. Deepe, Jr.

263 *Blastomyces dermatitidis,* 3026
Stanley W. Chapman

264 *Coccidioides* Species, 3040
John Galgiani

265 Dermatophytosis and Other Superficial Mycoses, 3051
Roderick J. Hay

266 *Paracoccidioides brasiliensis,* 3062
Angela Restrepo and Angela María Tobón

267 Uncommon Fungi, 3068
Duane R. Hospenthal

268 *Pneumocystis* Species, 3080
Peter D. Walzer and A. George Smulian

SECTION H

Protozoal Diseases, 3095

269 Introduction to Protozoal Diseases, 3095
Jonathan I. Ravdin and William M. Stauffer

270 *Entamoeba histolytica* (Amebiasis), 3097
Jonathan I. Ravdin and William M. Stauffer

271 Free-Living Amebas, 3111
Upinder Singh

272 *Plasmodium* Species (Malaria), 3121
Rick M. Fairhurst and Thomas E. Wellems

273 *Leishmania* Species: Visceral (Kala-Azar), Cutaneous, and Mucocutaneous Leishmaniasis, 3145
Selma M. B. Jeronimo, Anastácio de Queiroz Sousa, and Richard D. Pearson

274 *Trypanosoma* Species (American Trypanosomiasis, Chagas' Disease): Biology of Trypanosomes, 3156
Louis V. Kirchhoff

275 Agents of African Trypanosomiasis (Sleeping Sickness), 3165
Louis V. Kirchhoff

276 *Toxoplasma gondii,* 3170
Jose G. Montoya, Joseph A. Kovacs, and Jack S. Remington

277 *Giardia lamblia,* 3198
David R. Hill

278 *Trichomonas vaginalis,* 3205
David H. Martin and Michael F. Rein

279 *Babesia* Species, 3209
Jeffrey A. Gelfand and Edouard Vannier

280 Cryptosporidiosis (*Cryptosporidium hominis, Cryptosporidium parvum,* and Other Species), 3215
A. Clinton White, Jr.

281 *Cyclospora cayetanensis, Isospora belli, Sarcocystis* Species, *Balantidium coli,* and *Blastocystis hominis,* 3228
Tamara L. Fisk, Jay S. Keystone, and Phyllis Kozarsky

282 Microsporidiosis, 3237
Louis M. Weiss

SECTION I

Diseases Due to Toxic Algae, 3255

283 **Human Illness Associated with Harmful Algal Blooms, 3255**
J. Glenn Morris, Jr.

SECTION J

Diseases Due to Helminths, 3258

284 **Introduction to Helminth Infections, 3258**
James H. Maguire

285 **Intestinal Nematodes (Roundworms), 3260**
James H. Maguire

286 **Tissue Nematodes, Including Trichinosis, Dracunculiasis, and the Filariases, 3267**
David I. Grove

287 **Trematodes (Schistosomes and Other Flukes), 3276**
James H. Maguire

288 **Cestodes (Tapeworms), 3285**
Charles H. King

289 **Visceral Larva Migrans and Other Unusual Helminth Infections, 3293**
Theodore E. Nash

SECTION K

Ectoparasitic Diseases, 3301

290 **Introduction to Ectoparasitic Diseases, 3301**
Michael Eric Mathieu and Barbara Braunstein Wilson

291 **Lice (Pediculosis), 3302**
Michael Eric Mathieu and Barbara Braunstein Wilson

292 **Scabies, 3304**
Michael Eric Mathieu and Barbara Braunstein Wilson

293 **Myiasis and Tungiasis, 3307**
Michael Eric Mathieu and Barbara Braunstein Wilson

294 **Mites (Including Chiggers), 3310**
Michael Eric Mathieu and Barbara Braunstein Wilson

295 **Ticks (Including Tick Paralysis), 3312**
Michael Eric Mathieu and Barbara Braunstein Wilson

SECTION L

Diseases of Unknown Etiology, 3316

296 **Kawasaki Syndrome, 3316**
Frank T. Saulsbury

PART IV
SPECIAL PROBLEMS

SECTION A

Nosocomial Infections, 3323

297 **Organization for Infection Control, 3323**
Michael B. Edmond and Richard P. Wenzel

298 **Isolation, 3326**
Michael B. Edmond and Richard P. Wenzel

299 **Disinfection, Sterilization, and Control of Hospital Waste, 3331**
William A. Rutala and David J. Weber

300 **Infections Caused by Percutaneous Intravascular Devices, 3347**
Susan E. Beekmann and David K. Henderson

301 **Nosocomial Respiratory Infections, 3362**
Larry J. Strausbaugh

302 **Nosocomial Urinary Tract Infections, 3370**
John W. Warren

303 **Nosocomial Hepatitis and Other Infections Transmitted by Blood and Blood Products, 3381**
Kent A. Sepkowitz

304 **Human Immunodeficiency Virus in Health Care Settings, 3391**
David K. Henderson and Julie L. Gerberding

305 **Nosocomial Herpesvirus Infections, 3409**
David K. Henderson

SECTION B

Infections in Special Hosts, 3421

306 **Infections in the Immunocompromised Host: General Principles, 3421**
J. Peter Donnelly and Ben E. De Pauw

307 **Infections in Patients with Hematologic Malignancies, 3432**
Ben E. De Pauw and Paul E. Verweij

308 **Prophylaxis and Empirical Therapy for Infection in Cancer Patients, 3442**
Claudio Viscoli and Elio Castagnola

309 **Infections in Injection Drug Users, 3462**
Donald P. Levine and Patricia D. Brown

310 **Risk Factors and Approaches to Infections in Transplant Recipients, 3476**
J. Stephen Dummer

311 **Infections in Recipients of Hematopoietic Stem Cell Transplantation, 3486**
Jo-Anne Van Burik and Daniel Weisdorf

312 **Infections in Solid Organ Transplant Recipients, 3501**
J. Stephen Dummer

313 **Infections in Patients with Spinal Cord Injury, 3512**
Rabih O. Darouiche

314 **Infections in the Elderly, 3517**
Kent B. Crossley and Phillip K. Peterson

315 **Infections in Asplenic Patients, 3524**
Larry I. Lutwick

SECTION C

Surgical- and Trauma-Related Infections, 3533

316 **Postoperative Infections and Antimicrobial Prophylaxis, 3533**
Thomas R. Talbot and Allen B. Kaiser

317 Burns, 3547
Gregory J. Bauer and Roger W. Yurt

318 Bites, 3552
Ellie J. C. Goldstein

SECTION D

Immunization, 3557

319 Immunization, 3557
Walter A. Orenstein, Melinda Wharton, Kenneth J. Bart, and Alan R. Hinman

SECTION E

Biodefense, 3591

320 Bioterrorism: An Overview, 3591
Donald A. Henderson and Luciana L. Borio

321 Plague as an Agent of Bioterrorism, 3601
Luciana L. Borio

322 *Francisella tularensis* (Tularemia) as an Agent of Bioterrorism, 3607
Candace L. Mitchell and Robert L. Penn

323 Smallpox and Bioterrorism, 3612
Lisa D. Rotz, Joanne Cono, and Inger Damon

324 Anthrax , 3618
Daniel Lucey

325 *Botulinum* Toxin as a Biological Weapon, 3624
Thomas P. Bleck

326 Bioterrorism: Viral Hemorrhagic Fevers, 3626
C. J. Peters

SECTION F

Zoonoses, 3630

327 Zoonoses, 3630
Arnold N. Weinberg

SECTION G

Protection of Travelers, 3637

328 Protection of Travelers, 3637
David O. Freedman

329 Infections in Returning Travelers, 3646
David O. Freedman

SECTION H

The Internet, 3656

330 The Infectious Diseases Physician and Digital Resources, 3656
Gregory C. Townsend

Index, i

PART I

BASIC PRINCIPLES

IN THE DIAGNOSIS

AND MANAGEMENT

OF INFECTIOUS

DISEASES

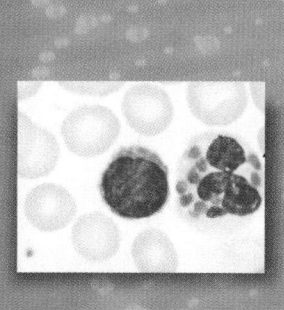

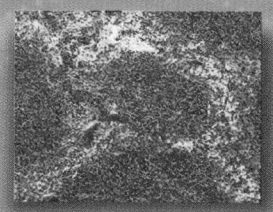

CHAPTER 1

A Molecular Perspective of Microbial Pathogenicity

DAVID A. RELMAN

STANLEY FALKOW

The study of microbial pathogenicity at the genomic and molecular level has altered our view of host-parasite relationships dramatically and has forced the redefinition of some commonly used terms. Thus, after birth, human exposure to myriad microorganisms leads to the establishment (*colonization*) of a complex protective commensal microbial flora. This flora facilitates nutrient acquisition, promotes further differentiation of mucosal structure and function, stimulates the innate and adaptive immune systems, and provides small amounts of human accessory growth factors.[1,2] Composition of the endogenous flora evolves in a generally orderly fashion as diet, hormonal environment, geography, and occasional ecologic disturbances play out their effects on a distinct genetic background. *Infection* is simply the establishment of a microorganism on or within a host; it may be short lived. The human participants in all of these interactions are most often asymptomatic and may exhibit subclinical signs of altered pathophysiology but are generally better off for their encounter with these microorganisms. It is probably fair to say that such is the usual outcome of most host-microbe interactions.

The term *infectious disease* applies when an interaction with a microbe causes damage to the host and the associated damage or altered physiology results in clinical signs and symptoms of disease. Thus, a *pathogen* is usually defined as any microorganism that has the capacity to cause disease. Yet not all pathogens have an equal probability of causing disease in the same host population. *Virulence* provides a quantitative measure of pathogenicity or the likelihood of causing disease. For example, encapsulated pneumococci are more virulent than nonencapsulated pneumococci, and *Escherichia coli* strains that express Shiga-like toxins are more virulent than those that do not express these toxins. *Virulence factors* refer to the properties (i.e., gene products) that enable a microorganism to establish itself on or within a host of a particular species and enhance its potential to cause disease.

It is useful to distinguish "principal" pathogens, which *regularly* cause disease in some proportion of susceptible individuals with apparently *intact* defense systems, from other potentially pathogenic microorganisms. Certain microorganisms with potential for causing disease in humans do not meet this definition. *Pseudomonas aeruginosa* is a good example. This microorganism is not ordinarily a member of the commensal flora of humans and does not usually cause disease in people with intact host defense systems; yet it can clearly cause devastating disease in many hospitalized and immunocompromised patients. Most microorganisms with a capacity for sustained multiplication in humans, including members of the indigenous commensal flora, cause disease more readily in individuals with underlying chronic disease or in those who are otherwise compromised. The common term *opportunist* suits this category of pathogen well. One could extend this argument to say that even for most organisms classified as principal pathogens, for example, *Staphylococcus aureus* and the pneumococcus, some impairment or local breakdown in normal host defense mechanisms must occur for these bacteria to cause disease. Moreover, both of these microorganisms are members of the commensal flora in some individuals for varying periods of time. Thus, it seems clear that the capacity of certain microorganisms to cause disease in seemingly uncompromised human hosts on a regular basis reflects some fundamental difference in their virulence capabilities from those of opportunists and the more numerous commensal species that rarely, if ever, cause disease.

THE ATTRIBUTES OF MICROBIAL PATHOGENS

In simple terms, one can say that to be successful, a pathogen must find an appropriate host niche, multiply there, and repeat this process at some frequency. Actually, a commensal must also meet this test of success. Disease is arguably only an inadvertent outcome of microbial multiplication. What, then, are the distinguishing characteristics that separate pathogens from other microorganisms, including the vast majority of members of the endogenous flora? To cause infection, a microorganism must possess an interactive group of complementary genetic properties, sometimes coregulated, that promote its interaction with a particular host. For a given microorganism, these genetic traits define unique attributes that enable it to follow a common sequence of steps used by organisms that are successful in establishing infection or subsequent disease.[3,4] These traits are reflected as phenotypes for which one or more genes and their gene products may be responsible. Elegant molecular and genetic techniques permit the identification, isolation, and characterization of many of these genes and their products. In complementary fashion, complete genome sequences provide important clues and insight into the potential of a microorganism for causing disease and facilitate genetic approaches.[5] Precise manipulation of the pathogen's genome has led to determination of the roles for some of these putative virulence factors. The availability of the host (e.g., human) genome sequence enables multiple synergistic approaches for understanding virulence, including the identification of host susceptibility traits, genome-wide assessments of host response, and clues about the mechanisms of host defense and pathogen counterdefense.[6]

The results of these analyses lead to the conclusion that the distinguishing characteristic of microorganisms that regularly cause disease is their capacity to breach normal host anatomic, cellular, or biochemical barriers that ordinarily prevent entry by other microorganisms into sterile tissue sites, that is, "to go where others cannot." In addition, many pathogens, particularly those that have the capacity to establish persistent infection in a host, have acquired the capacity to thwart the host's innate and adaptive immune defenses. The distinction, then, between primary pathogen and opportunist is that the pathogen has an *inherent* ability to breach the host barriers that ordinarily restrict other microbes, whereas the opportunist requires some underlying defect or alteration in the host's defenses, whether it be genetic, ecologic (altered microflora), or caused by underlying disease, to establish itself in a usually privileged host niche. Clearly, the state of the host plays an important role in determining outcome.[7,8]

An initial step required of a pathogen is to gain access to the host in sufficient numbers. Such access requires that the microorganism not only make contact with an appropriate surface but also then reach its *unique* niche or microenvironment on or within the host. This requirement is not trivial. Some pathogens must survive for varying periods in the external environment. Others have evolved an effective and suitable means of transmission. To accomplish this goal, the infecting microbe may make use of motility, chemotactic properties, and adhesive structures (or *adhesins*) that mediate binding to specific eukaryotic cell receptors or to other microorganisms (see Chapter 2).[9-12] Pathogens that remain at the surface of skin or mucosa for the duration of infection usually rely upon multiple, redundant adhesins and adherence mechanisms. If the adhesin is immunogenic, expression may be regulated; in addition, antigenic variants may arise (see "Regulation of Bacterial Pathogenicity"). Preexisting microorganisms, the normal flora, provide competition against establishment of the newcomer; furthermore, the latter must adapt, at least temporarily, to the particular nutrient environment in which it now finds itself. As an interesting example of such adaptation, data suggest that intracellular *Neisseria gonorrhoeae* capture enzymatically active host pyruvate kinase using their Opa outer membrane proteins as a means of enhancing local concentrations of pyruvate, which is required for gonococcal intracellular growth.[13]

Normal host defense mechanisms pose the next and most difficult set of obstacles to the arriving pathogen. For any set of specific host defenses, an individual pathogen must have devised a unique and distinctive counterstrategy. Some of the best known mechanisms for countering host defenses include the use of an antiphagocytic capsule and the elaboration of toxins and microbial enzymes that act on host immune cells and destroy anatomic barriers.[14] In addition, microorganisms may use subtle mechanisms to avoid, subvert, or even manipulate host defenses. These strategies include the elaboration of immunoglobulin-specific proteases, iron sequestration mechanisms, coating themselves with host proteins to confuse the immune surveillance system, or causing host cells to signal inappropriately leading to dysregulation of host defenses or even host cell death. Examples of these mechanisms include the production of immunoglobulin A$_1$ protease by *Haemophilus influenzae*, the use of receptors for iron-saturated human transferrin and lactoferrin by *N. gonorrhoeae*, and the coating of *Treponema pallidum* with human soluble fibronectin. *Yersinia*, *Mycobacterium*, and *Bordetella* induce host cell production of interleukin-10, which is a potent immunosuppressive cytokine, thereby downregulating important elements of the innate immune defense. Antigenic variation and intracellular invasion are other common strategies used by successful pathogens to avoid immune detection.[15,16] The intimacy of the relationships between viral pathogens and host is reflected in the frequency with which these pathogens co-opt host molecules and pathways for subverting host defenses (see "Subversion of Host Cellular Processes and Immune Defenses").[17-21]

The ability to multiply is a characteristic of all living organisms. Whether the pathogen's niche in the relevant host be intracellular or extracellular, mucosal or submucosal, within the blood stream or within another privileged anatomic site, pathogens have evolved a distinct set of biochemical tactics to achieve this goal. The success of a pathogen, indeed, of any microorganism, is measured by the degree to which it can multiply on reaching its specific niche and secure its potential transmission to a new susceptible host. The rate of multiplication of the pathogen is, of course, reflected in the duration of the incubation period appreciated by the clinician.

Thus, the outcome of the events just described is determined by the degree to which the pathogen has perpetuated itself and by the nature of the relationship it has established with its host. The result may be altered host physiology and tissue damage, reflected often in clinical manifestations of disease. Infectious disease, in one sense, is simply a by-product of the method and site chosen by pathogens for replication and persistence; disease per se is not a measure of microbial success, and it may reflect the status of the host as much as it does the virulence characteristics of the offending microorganism.[7,8] Death of the host is fortunately a rare event and one that must be viewed with the dispassion of biology as being detrimental to both parties involved! The more usual outcome is sufficient multiplication of the pathogen to ensure its establishment within the host (transient or long-term infection) and to ensure its successful transmission to a new susceptible host.

Why do some pathogens cause disease more readily than others? The strategy used for multiplication on or within the host (i.e., its ability to overcome host barriers) often defines fundamental differences between pathogens that commonly cause acute disease symptoms and those that do not. An organism that can reach and multiply in privileged anatomic sites away from the competitive environment of skin and mucosal surfaces is more likely to disrupt homeostasis in the host and cause disease than one that chooses a different strategy. If a microorganism has evolved a means to nullify or destroy phagocytic cells to multiply successfully, it is more likely to multiply in deeper tissue and cause acute disease. Commensal organisms are content to multiply just enough, in the midst of competing microflora, to persist but not damage the host's self-preserving homeostatic mechanisms. It is important to emphasize that a microorganism exceptionally equipped to multiply in a host may nonetheless be an unexceptional pathogen and only infrequently, if ever, cause clinically manifested disease.

Why are some organisms such as *P. aeruginosa* only opportunists despite their impressive array of virulence factors? An organism has no presupposition about the state of the host defenses when it encounters a human host. For opportunistic pathogens, that state is the main determinant of whether disease is the outcome of their interaction with the host. Many opportunistic infectious agents in compromised hosts are simply transients, "just passing through" in a normal host. This pattern of infection reflects the fact that opportunistic organisms lack an effective means to overcome normal host barriers to infection. Commensals, for example, which are the usual cause of opportunistic infections, may be very adept at colonization, but because of their preferred growth locale (e.g., the mucosal surface) and preferred growth conditions (e.g., a microaerophilic environment), they may have limited growth opportunities outside their restricted niche in an unimpaired individual. As a result, opportunistic infection and disease may be only a rare consequence of their encounter with the compromised host.

Pathogens were once viewed as organisms, largely unadapted to their hosts, that elaborated potent toxins or other powerful aggressive factors that caused the signs and symptoms of disease. The current view is that a microbial pathogen is a highly adapted organism that follows a strategy for survival requiring multiplication on or within another living organism. This survival strategy of necessity produces overt damage to the host. Of course, some infectious diseases occur predominantly in dramatic epidemic form, which argues against the evolution of a balanced host-parasite relationship; however, in many such epidemics, mitigating circumstances involving herd immunity and other underlying social, economic, and political issues impinge on this relationship. Furthermore, some of the most serious infectious diseases occur when humans are infected by microorganisms that prefer and are better adapted to another mammalian host. Then, as seen in many zoonotic diseases, the rules of engagement between both the host and the pathogen are blurred often to the detriment of the host, which serves as an evolutionary dead end for the microbe.

Given the increasingly frequent and unexpected emergence of previously unrecognized pathogens, it is appropriate to question how well we appreciate the true diversity and distribution of extant microorganisms capable of causing human disease. Although most emerging pathogens are zoonotic agents and already adapted to a different host, the question also concerns a more basic uncertainty about how often, in what phylogenetic backgrounds, and through what mechanisms virulence for humans among microbes can arise. Pathogenicity appears to have arisen on multiple occasions throughout the bacterial tree of life but only in a small fraction of the overall phyla; in particular, it is curious that there are currently no known pathogens among the archaea.[22] Three points should be made: (1) pathogen detection and identification remain suboptimal, in part because of continuing dependence on cultivation methods, and therefore a number of novel pathogens may be missed[23]; (2) some potential pathogens may not have had adequate contact with humans to have made themselves known (yet)[24]; and (3) dominant models of microbial disease causation (e.g., introduction of single pathogenic agent into susceptible host is sufficient to cause disease) may be too restrictive, in that some microbial diseases may require a consortium of agents or "pathogenic community structure," thereby creating difficulty for pathogen identification. If we define success for a microbial pathogen without a requirement for long-term survival, a much larger number of organisms may qualify, in being able to cause devastating human disease but only over a limited number of generations. These matters have obvious relevance to the troubling issue of bioterrorism and the potential malevolent use and genetic manipulation of microorganisms.

THE CLONAL NATURE OF BACTERIAL PATHOGENS

Pathogenicity is not a microbial trait that has appeared by chance. Instead, particular microbial strains and species have evolved to carry very specific arrays of virulence-associated genes. By examining the genetic organization of pathogens, opportunists, and nonpathogenic bacteria, one can begin to understand the origins of pathogenicity.

Techniques used in the study of genetic relatedness include primary protein or nucleic acid sequence comparisons and DNA hybridization methods, including DNA microarray-based approaches.[5] Some genetic sequences, such as those of the small- and large-subunit ribosomal RNAs, have been used as reliable evolutionary clocks.[25-27] Comparative analysis of these sequences allows one to infer phylogenetic relationships among all known cellular life. Multilocus enzyme electrophoresis is a method by which chromosomal structure or genotype is deduced from the electrophoretic mobility variations in a number of common metabolic enzymes.[28] The increasing ease with which primary genomic sequence information can be acquired, differences quantified, and these data shared has led to more precise methods of strain characterization such as multilocus sequence typing.[29] These approaches avoid the classic comparisons of phenotypes (i.e., gross observable characteristics of a microbe), which can be unreliable. When these sequence-based techniques are used, a consistent finding emerges concerning the population structure of microorganisms: most natural populations of microorganisms consist of a number of discrete clonal lineages.[30]

The finding of a clonal population structure implies that the rates of recombination of chromosomal genes between different strains of the same species and between different bacterial species are very low. Clonal organization has been substantiated by the concordance between evolutionary trees derived from unrelated chromosomal sequences.[31] At first view, this pattern may seem somewhat unexpected because well-established, naturally occurring mechanisms are in place for horizontal genetic exchange between and within species, including transformation, transduction, and conjugation. However, bacteria are haploid creatures. If horizontal transfer of genetic material and subsequent recombination were frequent occurrences, one would expect to see homogenization of bacterial species and little specialization. In fact, the opposite is true. Bacterial species have remained discrete and distinct taxonomic entities[32] because the bacterial chromosome is a highly integrated and coadapted entity that has resisted rearrangement. Nonetheless, global analysis of bacterial chromosomes reveals chimeric features and significant degrees of lateral gene transfer, with evidence of exogenously acquired segments (approximately 18% of the *E. coli* genome) and subsequent amelioration of base composition and codon usage over millions of years.[33,34]

Analysis of natural populations of microorganisms with pathogenic potential has revealed the prominent representation of a relatively few clones. In fact, most cases of serious disease may be caused by a small proportion of the total number of extant clones that constitute a pathogenic bacterial species. Indeed, in some extreme cases, all members of a species such as *Shigella sonnei* or *Bordetella pertussis* belong to the same clonal type or small group of closely related types. Although it is true of most that have been studied, not all pathogenic bacterial species reveal this pattern of clonal organization. Two notable exceptions are *N. gonorrhoeae* and *Helicobacter pylori*, which appear to use chromosomal recombination to increase their genetic diversity. The genetic variability among gonococcal isolates from discrete geographic locations suggests that this organism is essentially sexual. *Neisseria meningitidis* also demonstrates random chromosomal rearrangement; however, because single clones disseminate rapidly during an epidemic, the population structure of this species may falsely appear to be clonal.[35] *Salmonella* population analysis also suggests that serovars that are most adapted to a specific host species are less genetically diverse than those that infect a wider range of hosts. Indeed, the serovars that are specific to humans form a single, distinct subgroup of related strains.

Clonal analysis has generated other important conclusions concerning the evolution of bacterial species and pathogenic strains in particular. Study of *E. coli* populations in the human intestinal tract indicates that only a small number of clonal lineages persist while numerous unrelated cell lines appear and disappear.[30] *E. coli* urinary tract pathogens causing symptomatic disease in humans are even less genetically diverse than *E. coli* strains found in the intestinal flora or those that cause asymptomatic urinary tract colonization.[36] The nonrandom association of particular versions of different genes within a distinct clone has led to speculation that this species has evolved, not by means of accumulated random recombinational events, but by "random sampling" of clonal populations from the environment with periodic selection and extinction.[33] The evolution of pathogenicity is revealed in part by examination of chromosomal structure and organization.[5,34]

HORIZONTAL EXCHANGE OF VIRULENCE-ASSOCIATED GENES

Study of natural populations of bacteria suggests that the genetic potential for pathogenicity within a bacterial species has arisen among a small number of unrelated clones through means that do not compromise the genetic individuality of the organism or its unique place in nature but nonetheless in a fashion that provides the microbe with genetic and biochemical flexibility for a competitive environment. How might this adaptation have happened? The answer can be approached from two different temporal perspectives: events that take place over months to years and changes that are defined over millions of years (see the next section).

A number of separate observations indicate that microbes frequently carry virulence-associated genes on mobile genetic elements.[3] Bacteriophages and extrachromosomal elements such as bacterial plasmids are supplements to the bacterial genome that allow a microbe to maintain the integrity of its chromosome and still increase its genetic diversity. Some of these mobile elements are able to enter a wide variety of host organisms and may facilitate the transfer of genes that have been selected for their ability to function in diverse genetic backgrounds. These genetic exchanges are observed over the course of infection within a single host or within a population of microorganisms over months to years. Clinicians are painfully aware that genes encoding antibiotic resistance are efficiently disseminated among different microbial species in nature by such means. The presence of virulence factors in pathogenic bacteria is also associated with the presence of plasmids,[37] transposons, and bacteriophages[38,39] to a striking degree, both in gram-positive and in gram-negative species (Table 1-1). For example, cholera toxin is encoded by a vibriophage that is found integrated within the *Vibrio cholerae* chromosome.[40] Expression of the fimbrial receptor for this phage is regulated by the same *V. cholerae* protein, ToxR, that controls expression of the cholera toxin genes (see later). Some transmissible elements such as bacteriophages prefer specific chromosomal sites for integration, for example, transfer RNA genes. This specificity may explain the chromosomal distribution of some virulence genes.

Some bacteria readily exchange random fragments of their cellular DNA with other members of their species through a process known as *transformation*. For some of these species such as *N. gonorrhoeae*, *Streptococcus pneumoniae*, and *H. pylori* transformation in nature may provide an additional means of acquiring genes that are advantageous to their growth and to persistence in the host.

Plasmids, transposons, and phages provide bacteria with the potential for relatively rapid adaptation to an unfavorable, changing, or new environment. Although these mobile genetic elements are often dispensable to the host bacterium, they are typically conserved over substantial periods within diverse cell lineages. This situation is hardly surprising if the mobile element enables the organism to multiply successfully in a host. Often, the mobile element carries multiple virulence-associated genes as a co-adapted block, accompanied by a separate self-regulatory system.

TABLE 1-1 Examples of Plasmid- and Phage-Encoded Virulence Determinants

Organism	Virulence Factor	Biologic Function
Plasmid encoded		
Enterotoxigenic *Escherichia coli*	Heat-labile, heat-stable enterotoxins	Activation of adenylate/guanylate cyclase in the small bowel, which leads to diarrhea
	CFA/I and CFA/II	Adherence/colonization factors
Extraintestinal *E. coli*	Hemolysin	Cytotoxin
Shigella spp. and enteroinvasive *E. coli*	Gene products involved in invasion	Induces internalization by intestinal epithelial cells
Yersinia spp.	Adherence factors and gene products involved in invasion	Attachment/invasion
Bacillus anthracis	Edema factor, lethal factor, and protective antigen	Edema factor has adenylate cyclase activity; lethal factor is a metalloprotease that acts on host signaling molecules
Staphylococcus aureus	Exfoliative toxin	Causes toxic epidermal necrolysis
Clostridium tetani	Tetanus neurotoxin	Blocks the release of inhibitory neurotransmitter, which leads to muscle spasms
Phage encoded		
Corynebacterium diphtheriae	Diphtheria toxin	Inhibition of eukaryotic protein synthesis
Streptococcus pyogenes	Erythrogenic toxin	Rash of scarlet fever
Clostridium botulinum	Botulism neurotoxin	Blocks synaptic acetylcholine release, which leads to flaccid paralysis
Enterohemorrhagic E. coli	Shiga-like toxin	Inhibition of eukaryotic protein synthesis
Vibrio cholerae	Cholera toxin	Stimulates adenylate cyclase in host cells

CFA, colonization factor antigen.
Data from Elwell LP, Shipley PL. Plasmid-mediated factors associated with virulence of bacteria to animals. Annu Rev Microbiol. 1980;34:465-496; and Cheetham BR, Katz ME. A role for bacteriophages in the evolution and transfer of bacterial virulence determinants. Mol Microbiol. 1995;18:201-208.

GENOMICS AND THE EVOLUTION OF PATHOGENICITY

Comparisons of pathogenic and nonpathogenic representatives of a single genus or species usually demonstrate the nonpathogens to be relatively devoid of functional genetic sequences encoding the pathogenic trait or traits. Inactive mutational variants or portions of virulence-associated genes infrequently occur in nonpathogenic strains of the same species. In general, as bacteria evolve from free-living organisms with multiple habitats to obligate pathogens, host-restricted organisms, endosymbionts, or obligate intracellular organisms, their genomes appear to become reduced in size or they accumulate inactive or defective genes (*pseudogenes*), or both.[41] For example, the evolution of *B. pertussis* as a host-specific, human-adapted pathogen from a *Bordetella bronchiseptica*–like ancestor has been accompanied by extensive gene loss and gene inactivation (3816 coding sequences, versus 5007 for *B. bronchiseptica*; 9.4% of coding sequences are pseudogenes, versus 0.4% for *B. bronchiseptica*).[42] In this case, a highly restricted host range has meant loss of genetic diversity. In contrast to *B. bronchiseptica*, which infects multiple animal hosts and can survive in the environment, *B. pertussis* varies little in gene content among different strains isolated over the past 50 years and across several continents.[43] *Bacillus anthracis*, which exists predominantly as an inactive spore, and *Mycobacterium tuberculosis*, which exists primarily in a latent phase in human granulomas, also exhibit limited genomic diversity. *Mycobacterium leprae* displays an extreme degree of gene decay.[44] All three *Bordetella* species share similar complements of virulence-associated genes, although their patterns of expression differ; for example, although all three share genes for pertussis toxin, only *Bordetella pertussis* has a functional promoter.

Not uncommonly, virulence-specific sequences are bounded by repeated DNA segments, some of which represent known insertion elements, which suggests that these virulence genes were once associated with a mobile genetic element or that these genes formerly occupied another chromosomal locale in either the same species or another microorganism altogether. Acquisition of an adhesin, toxin, or serum resistance factor might lead a previously nonpathogenic organism to cause disease in a host that had previously been nonsusceptible.

This concept has been supported by the discovery of "pathogenicity islands."[45,46] The latter are 35- to 200-kilobase segments of chromosomal DNA flanked by insertion or repeat elements, with a nucleotide composition quite unlike that of the surrounding bacterial genome. Pathogenicity islands contain clusters of virulence-associated genes that encode specialized secretion systems, secreted effector molecules, adhesins, and regulatory proteins. *Salmonella typhimurium* is believed to have begun evolving as a pathogen approximately 130 million years ago through the sequential acquisition of at least two pathogenicity islands, one of which mediates internalization within host cells and the other, survival and replication within an intracellular vacuole.[47] The apparent genetic instability of some chromosomal regions, such as the *H. pylori* Cag island, can give rise to an assortment of strains with different virulence capabilities. *Yersinia pestis* provides a dramatic example of evolution through both acquisition and loss of genes. In comparison with the two enteropathogenic *Yersinia* species, the ability of *Y. pestis* to be transmitted by fleas is associated with the acquisition of two unique plasmids and some novel chromosomal genes; conversely, *Y. pestis* appears to be missing or have inactivated a large group of genes that facilitate adaptation to the intestinal tract and invasion through the intestinal epithelial barrier.[48]

Full genome sequencing offers a more complete picture of microbial virulence-associated gene organization, as illustrated in the previous discussions. The first complete genome sequence for a free-living organism, *H. influenzae,* was described in 1995.[49] Since then, more than 150 microbial genome sequences have been completed and released to public databases (see http://www.ncbi.nlm.nih.gov/genomes/Complete.html). Despite the obvious value of a primary genomic blueprint, it is increasingly clear that genetic, genomic, and epidemiologic approaches provide complementary advantages. Each contributes to the search for new chromosomal determinants of virulence.

REGULATION OF BACTERIAL PATHOGENICITY

All bacteria respond to environmental changes with metabolic alterations. A successful host-parasite relationship demands that a pathogen sense its local host environment and distinguish between conditions favorable to rapid growth and those inhospitable and requiring an adaptive or protective response. Consequently, regulating the expression of virulence factors is an additional, yet essential complication of a pathogenic microbe's life.[50] The host presents an array of conditions strikingly distinct from those of the outside environment, conditions that are not easily reproduced in the laboratory. In fact, laboratory culture conditions bias our understanding of microbial adaptation to natural environments. This bias is reflected in the concept of a

TABLE 1-2   Examples of Bacterial Virulence Regulatory Systems

Organism	Regulatory Gene(s)	Environmental Stimuli	Regulated Functions
Escherichia coli	drdX	Temperature	Pyelonephritis-associated pili
	fur	Iron concentration	Shiga-like toxin, siderophores
Bordetella pertussis	bvgAS	Temperature, ionic conditions, nicotinic acid	Pertussis toxin, filamentous hemagglutinin, adenylate cyclase, others
Vibro cholerae	toxR	Temperature, osmolarity, pH, amino acids	Cholera toxin, pili, outer-membrane proteins
Yersinia spp.	lcr loci	Temperature, calcium	Secretion of effector proteins
	virF	Temperature	Adherence, invasiveness
Shigella spp.	virR	Temperature	Invasiveness
Salmonella typhimurium	pag genes	pH	Virulence, macrophage survival
Staphyococcus aureus	agr genes	Cell density	α-, β-Hemolysins; toxic shock syndrome toxin-1, protein A

Data from Miller JF, Mekalanos JJ, Falkow S. Coordinate regulation and sensory transduction in the control of bacterial virulence. Science. 1989;243:916-922; and Mekalanos JJ. Environmental signals controlling the expression of virulence determinants in bacteria. J Bacteriol. 1992;174:1-7.

"viable but nonculturable state" for bacteria in their natural external environment.[51] *V. cholerae*, for example, is thought to persist in this state in brackish estuaries and other saline aquatic environments, sometimes associated with the chitinous exoskeleton of various marine organisms.[52] Transition from this milieu to the contrasting environment of the human small intestinal lumen must be accompanied by substantial genetic regulatory events. The equally dramatic transition for *Borrelia burgdorferi* and *Y. pestis* from arthropod vector to human host is accompanied by significant changes in gene expression.[53]

Changes in temperature, ionic conditions, oxygen concentration, pH, and calcium, iron, and other metal concentrations that might appear more subtle also exert profound effects on the expression of virulence determinants. The environmental regulatory signals that prepare the microbe for its transition from an extracellular to an intracellular state may include some of these parameters. For example, iron is a critical component of many cell metabolic processes; therefore, it is not surprising that animals rely on high-affinity iron-binding and storage proteins to deprive microorganisms from access to this nutrient, especially at the mucosal surface. In turn, most pathogens sense iron availability and induce or repress various iron acquisition systems accordingly.[54] For the gastric pathogen *H. pylori*, pH may be a critical signal. The *H. pylori* response to low pH involves changes in transcript abundance for 7% of its genes and is associated with increased motility, perhaps as a means for penetrating the gastric mucous layer.[55]

Reversible regulation of the expression of virulence genes by temperature is a feature common to many pathogens, including enteropathogenic and uropathogenic *E. coli* (K-88 and K-99 fimbriae, pyelonephritis-associated pilus fimbriae, and K-1 capsular antigen), *Shigella* spp. (invasiveness and Shiga toxin), and *Yersinia* spp. (virulence-associated determinants, including a low-calcium response and outer-membrane proteins). Changes in DNA topology, messenger RNA conformation, and, in the case of the heat shock response, protein stability mediate thermal regulation of these diverse virulence determinants.[56]

The number of well-characterized virulence regulatory systems is rapidly increasing, in part because of the development of rapid methods for screening gene expression on a genome-wide basis (e.g., with the use of DNA microarrays[57]). At the same time, relatively little is known about both the specific environmental signals to which these systems respond and the exact role of these responses in the course of human infection. One common mechanism for bacterial transduction of environmental signals involves two-component regulatory systems that act on gene expression, usually at the transcriptional level.[58] Such systems make use of similar pairs of proteins; one protein of the pair spans the cytoplasmic membrane, contains a transmitter domain, and may act as a sensor of environmental stimuli, whereas the other is a cytoplasmic protein ("response regulator") with a receiver domain and regulates responsive genes or proteins. Sensor proteins are often kinases that phosphorylate themselves at a conserved histidine residue. These high-energy intermediates then transfer their phosphate groups to a conserved aspartate residue within the receiver domain of the response regulator proteins. Competing dephosphorylases determine an overall phosphorylation state of these response regulators and hence their level of activity. Many of these regulators are DNA-binding proteins that regulate transcription of multiple gene targets. Systems of this type control, for example, the permeability properties of the *E. coli* cell envelope in response to osmotic stimuli (EnvZ/OmpR), motor control involved in *E. coli* chemotaxis (CheA/CheY, CheB), the switch from vegetative growth to sporulation by *Bacillus subtilis* (KinA/SpoOF, SpoOA), and even the ability of the soil bacterium *Agrobacterium tumefaciens* to induce tumors in susceptible plant cells in response to phenols found within plant wound exudates (VirA/VirG). *V. cholerae* ToxR and the BvgAS proteins of *B. pertussis* share several features common to these systems, but they also retain significant differences.

The coordinated control of pathogenicity incorporates the important concept of a *regulon*. A regulon is a group of operons or individual genes controlled by a common regulator, usually a protein activator or repressor. This regulator may, in some cases, be the second component of a two-component system. A regulon provides a means by which many genes can respond in concert to a particular stimulus. At other times the same genes may respond independently to other signals. Global regulatory networks are a common feature of microbial virulence as well as basic microbial physiology (Table 1-2). The apparent complexity of virulence regulation in a single microbial pathogen is magnified by the coexistence of multiple interacting ("cross-talking") systems and by regulons within regulons. *P. aeruginosa*, for example, contains genes for 55 sensors and 89 response regulators, whereas *H. pylori* contains genes for 4 and 7, respectively. Perhaps the more restricted number and type of microenvironments occupied by the latter organism reduce the number of cues that it must recognize. Given the limited sensitivity of in vitro models, it appears that some but not all regulatory systems are essential for virulence.

B. pertussis synthesizes a group of surface-associated or extracellular products that are responsible for the pathologic and clinical findings of pertussis. These products include pertussis toxin, filamentous hemagglutinin, adenylate cyclase, dermonecrotic toxin, fimbrial protein, and pertactin. Coordinate expression of these and other virulence factors is orchestrated by the two encoded products of the chromosomal *bvgAS* locus.[59] *Trans*-activation and *trans*-repression are features of the Bvg regulon in which at least 20 unlinked chromosomal *bvg*-activated genes are expressed and a group of other *bvg*-repressed genes silenced, or vice versa, depending on the nature of the immediate environment.

BvgS is a member of the histidine kinase sensor class of bacterial regulatory proteins, but unlike most other members of this class, it also contains a receiver communication module and a regulatory carboxyl-terminal domain. BvgS spans the cytoplasmic membrane; a periplasmic domain responds to temperature and ionic conditions, thereby modulating BvgS activity. At 37° C, BvgS autophosphorylates its transmitter domain, and an ensuing cascade of phosphotransfer events results in phosphorylation of the receiver domain of BvgA, a member of the class of bacterial protein response regulators.[60] BvgA then binds to a DNA recognition sequence located upstream of the *bvgAS* operon itself, the filamentous hemagglutinin structural gene, and other *bvg*-regulated loci and promotes transcription of these genes.[61] Gene repression by *bvg* also occurs at the level of transcription and is mediated by a *bvg*-activated *trans*-acting regulator protein, BvgR, encoded by a locus adjacent to *bvgAS*. Inappropriate expression of repressed gene products during infection may be detrimental. Regulatory cascades allow signal amplification and the possibility of sequential temporal gene expression. For example, with removal of downmodulating conditions, *bvgAS* autoactivation and expression of the crucial adherence factors filamentous hemagglutinin and fimbrial protein precede expression of the other *bvg*-activated genes. With this type of regulatory system, *B. pertussis* can adapt in a measured fashion to the diverse local conditions within the human upper respiratory tract, its natural site of infection.[62] In addition, proteins expressed during an intermediate Bvg phase may be critical for survival of the related pathogen *Bordetella bronchiseptica* outside its animal hosts.[63]

Regulation of the expression of virulence determinants by *V. cholerae* also illustrates the use of a global regulatory protein that in this case serves a dual function. The *toxR* gene product is a transmembrane, DNA-binding protein that regulates expression of cholera toxin, toxin-coregulated pili, and specific outer-membrane proteins.[64] The ToxR protein is thought to sense a variety of environmental regulatory signals, including osmolarity, amino acid concentration, temperature, and pH. ToxR directs expression of these genes indirectly by activating transcription of ToxT, a member of the AraC family of transcriptional regulators.[62] At the level of amino acid sequence, the ToxR protein contains features of both sensor and regulator proteins from the two-component sensory transduction system. The combination of these features into one protein may lead to increased specificity of action. Vibrios in cholera stools may be hyperinfectious and prepared for enhanced transmission.[65] The transcriptional profile of these organisms as they exit patients suggests recent nutrient deprivation, iron limitation, downmodulated toxin expression, and reduced chemotactic activity.[65,66]

Quorum sensing is a means by which bacteria keep track of their cell density and regulate their behavior accordingly.[67] It is inextricably involved in the formation of complex community structures called biofilms by bacteria on environmental surfaces for long-term persistence and resistance to host defenses. Gram-negative organisms secrete and respond to acylated homoserine lactones as a means of cell-cell communication. Production of light by marine vibrios and tissue-degrading enzymes by *P. aeruginosa* is activated by these autoinducing compounds when they reach sufficient concentration.[68] Gram-positive organisms such as *S. aureus* use peptide autoinducers and repressors to sense cell density and regulate toxin expression; these secreted factors might serve as targets for novel immunoprophylactic approaches.[69] *V. cholerae* relies on quorum sensing to regulate biofilm formation on marine plankton and mediate release from these biofilms upon entry into a human host.[70]

Some microbial pathogens (e.g., *N. gonorrhoeae*, *Borrelia recurrentis*, and *Trypanosoma brucei*) periodically vary prominent antigenic components of their surface and, by so doing, may avoid the host immune response. Antigenic variations in *S. typhimurium* and *N. gonorrhoeae* provide examples of alternative molecular mechanisms (i.e., DNA rearrangements) that mediate regulation of the expression of virulence factors. *S. typhimurium* varies an immunodominant antigen by alternating between the expression of two different flagellin genes, H1 and H2. The mechanism for this form of variation involves inversion of a 995-bp chromosomal DNA sequence containing a promoter.[71] By altering expression of flagellin, *S. typhimurium* avoids the host antibody response directed against it.

Pili are essential for virulence of the gonococcus in the human host, probably as a result of their role in adherence to the mucosal target surface.[72] They also elicit a specific local and systemic host antibody response. Intermittent production of pili, as well as variation in the antigenic type of pilus, may be strategies used by the gonococcus to avoid the host immune response. The molecular mechanisms behind these strategies are complex. In general terms, phase and antigenic variation results from DNA rearrangements that move pilin-related sequences scattered around the gonococcal chromosome (in silent *pilS* loci) to the expression site (*pilE* locus). Numerous different pilus types may be expressed by derivatives of a single *N. gonorrhoeae* strain. Gene conversion and other recombination mechanisms may be involved.[16] Among other microbial pathogens, DNA rearrangements account for the antigenic variation of variant surface glycoproteins of *T. brucei*[73] and the antigenic variation of variable major proteins in *Borrelia* spp.[74]

Proper presentation of certain virulence-associated gene products on the microbial surface is now recognized to be as important to pathogenicity as the initial expression of these genes. Presentation entails export pathways, association with other periplasmic or surface factors, and sometimes macromolecular assembly at the surface and is also subject to regulation. Among bacterial pathogens, shared homology is apparent among families of proteins involved in these processes. One family consists of proteins that are known as *chaperones* and *ushers*, concepts first proposed in a model for the assembly of uroepithelium-adherent *E. coli* P pili.[75] Periplasmic chaperones such as PapD escort protein subunits from the cytoplasmic to the outer membrane and assist in their proper folding. Outer-membrane ushers such as PapC target these complexes to a surface assembly site. Folding, transport, and assembly enable a microorganism to present a specific array of surface molecules necessary for eukaryotic cell tropism, intoxication, or entry.[3] A precise configuration of microbial surface molecules might be viewed as an "attack complex," with properties not found in any of the individual components.

MICROBIAL PATHOGENS AS INTRACELLULAR PARASITES

Despite their capacity for an extracellular existence, a wide variety of bacterial and protozoal pathogens have evolved the means to enter, survive, multiply, and even persist within host eukaryotic cells. By so doing, a microorganism avoids host immune defenses and gains access to what are otherwise restricted nutrients. These advantages impose a strong selective evolutionary pressure that is dramatically reflected in the refined strategies developed by microbial pathogens for life within a host cell. These strategies include molecular mimicry, coercion, and intimate adaptation to eukaryotic cellular processes. Collaborative efforts of molecular microbiologists and cell biologists have led to a new discipline called cellular microbiology that has begun to reveal some common themes of these strategies.[3,12,15,76]

To a large degree, the mechanisms used by a microorganism to adhere to a eukaryotic cell dictate whether and how it enters the cell and its subsequent intracellular fate.[12] Most, if not all, intracellular pathogens have multiple means for attachment to a eukaryotic cell surface; the particular combination of microbial attachment factors and cognate host receptors favors selection of one of several entry pathways and predetermines basic features of the intracellular vacuole. However, in a general sense, it is unclear to what extent microbial pathogens accept preprogrammed pathways dictated by phagocytic (e.g., complement and Fc receptors) and nonphagocytic receptors and to what extent they may be able to modify or exploit these pathways. *Toxoplasma gondii* invades and replicates within all types of nucleated mammalian cells. After entry and through unidentified receptors, *T. gondii* resides within a parasitophorous vacuole that is permanently incapable of fusion with other intracellular organelles, including lysosomes. Parasite survival within this vacuole depends on the accompanying lack of acidification, exclusion of lysosomal contents, and specific mechanisms for nutrient acquisition and environmental sensing. However, when this organism is directed to enter eukaryotic cells by means of an alternative pathway (i.e., mediated by receptors for the constant region of immunoglobulin G, Fc), this vacuole fusion block is overcome.[77] Presumably, parasite-directed modifications of the surrounding vacuolar membrane and exclusion of certain host proteins during the earliest stages of entry help create conditions necessary for growth and development of the pathogen.

Some pathogenic microorganisms seem to regulate when and where they enter host cells by using preexistent host signaling pathways.[12] Among the receptors that recognize pathogens and mediate entry are integrins (*Yersinia* spp.), tight junction apparatus cadherins (*Listeria monocytogenes*)[78] and ZO-1 (*H. pylori*),[79] dystroglycans (arenaviruses),[80] and growth factor receptors (*S. typhimurium*). In some of these cases, the pathogens do not depend on only one receptor family for cellular entry. In addition, cell or organ tropism may be determined by recognition of different members of the same family.

Signaling events at the surface of the host cell, between pathogens of the same type, and between pathogen and host cell indicate a complex, highly evolved process of coadaptation and co-optation.[3,15,67] Many of these signals induce rearrangement of host cell cytoskeleton to the advantage of the pathogen. In a particularly dramatic example, enteropathogenic *E. coli* induces the effacement of normal epithelial cell surface architecture and the formation of a specialized structure containing reorganized actin that protrudes from the host cell surface and is called a "pedestal" or pseudopod (Fig. 1-1). Pedestals facilitate intimate attachment but not entry of enteropathogenic *E. coli* to the host cell; attachment is mediated by the bacterial adhesin intimin and a receptor, Tir, that is secreted by enteropathogenic *E. coli* into the host cell and then localized to the host cell membrane at the apical surface of the pedestal.[81] These events require a specialized secretion system (see later) that delivers not only Tir but also effector proteins that direct host cell phosphorylation of Tir and stimulate other signaling pathways. All these factors are encoded by genes found within a pathogenicity island known as the locus for enterocyte effacement; this chromosomal island is also found in some strains of Shiga toxin–producing *E. coli*. Tir from Shiga toxin–producing *E. coli* is immunogenic in humans and exhibits sequence and antigenic diversity among different isolates.[82]

Other forms of cytoskeletal rearrangements are essential to the process by which *Salmonella*, *Shigella*, and other intracellular pathogens enter host cells. *Salmonella* induces "ruffling" of the host cell membrane, which then engulfs the bacterium and leads to internalization through macropinocytosis. This response by nonphagocytic cells is similar to that provoked by growth factors. *Salmonella* Sip proteins and the related *Shigella* Ipa proteins are secreted into host cells after surface contact and are each necessary for the cytoskeletal responses of the host cell and for pathogen entry.

Microbial pathogens that have adapted to an intracellular environment possess diverse and specific strategies for survival and replication. Some pathogens remain within a vacuole (e.g., *Toxoplasma*, *Salmonella*), and some lyse the initial phagosomal membrane and replicate within the host cell cytoplasm (*Shigella*, *Listeria*, *Trypanosoma*, some *Rickettsia* species). Maintenance of specific and favorable vacuolar conditions may entail inhibition of phagolysosomal fusion and acidification (*Toxoplasma*), association of eukaryotic organelles with bacteria-containing vacuoles (*Legionella*, *Salmonella*), and regulation of pH (*Salmonella*). Some of the details of the molecular mechanisms behind these phenomena are now available. For example, *Legionella pneumophila* secretes effectors from its vacuole into the host cytoplasm that lead to redirected trafficking of the bacterial phagosome within the host cell.[76,83] *S. typhimurium* delays and attenuates macrophage phagosomal acidification, during which various regulons (e.g., the PhoP/PhoQ two-component system) mediate bacterial adaptation to a radically changing environment.[84] Some of these regulated *Salmonella* gene products, such as PhoP-activated PagC, are essential for survival within macrophages and recognize pH, magnesium, and manganese ions as transcriptional signals.

Early escape from the vacuole is essential for the growth and virulence of some intracellular pathogens. *L. monocytogenes* relies on several molecules for lysis of the early phagosome, including a pore-forming hemolysin (listeriolysin O) and two forms of phospholipase C. Once in the cytoplasm, *Listeria* replicates and induces its own movement through a remarkable process of host cell actin polymerization and formation of microfilaments within a comet-like tail. *Shigella* also lyses the phagosomal vacuole and induces the formation of similar structures for the purpose of intracytoplasmic movement and cell-cell spread. In both cases, bacterial and host factors involved in actin polymerization have been identified.[85,86] In the same way that microbial pathogens fare differently in their interactions with phagocytic cells, the outcome of intracellular parasitism for the host cell also varies considerably, depending on the specific host cell and pathogen involved.

SUBVERSION OF HOST CELLULAR PROCESSES AND IMMUNE DEFENSES

Pathogens can be distinguished from commensal microorganisms by their ability to subvert host cellular processes for their own advantage.[12,15] Enhanced adherence or internalization of the pathogen, inhibition of host cell antimicrobial activity, altered inflammatory responses, enhanced multiplication, and death are potential outcomes for the host cell and goals for the pathogen. As mentioned earlier, one common mechanism by which bacterial pathogens alter or subvert the host cell involves specialized secretion systems known as the type III or contact-dependent secretion pathway and the type IV secretion pathway.[76,87-89] Type III secretion systems from diverse bacterial pathogens share structural and functional features that suggest an evolutionary relationship with the bacterial flagellar apparatus.[88] These systems are encoded by blocks of genes that are usually located within pathogenicity islands. Using a supramolecular structure that spans the entire cell wall and resembles a hypodermic syringe,[90] pathogens secrete effector molecules directly across host cell membranes. Whereas *Salmonella* and *Shigella* use type III secretion systems (*Salmonella* pathogenicity island 1 [SPI-1] and invasion plasmid systems, respectively) to mediate entry into host cells, *Salmonella* relies on a second type III system (SPI-2) for successful replication within an intracellular vacuole; this second system is expressed only when the organism occupies this privileged niche.

Type III secreted effector molecules mediate diverse tasks. *Salmonella* SopE is secreted by the SPI-1 system and binds directly to members of the Rho small-molecular-weight guanosine triphosphatase

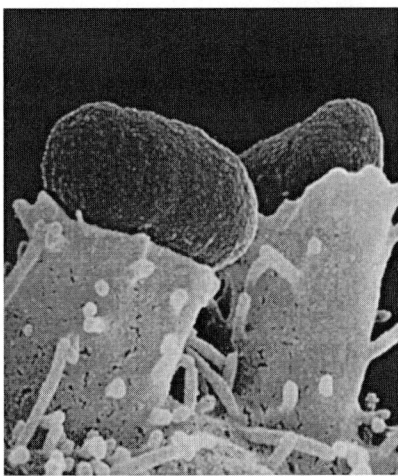

FIGURE 1-1. Scanning electron micrograph depicting pseudopod or "pedestal" formation by enteropathogenic *Escherichia coli* (EPEC) as it interacts with the surface of an epithelial cell. This form of intimate adherence requires a bacterial adhesin, intimin; a receptor of bacterial origin, Tir, that is injected into the host cell; and a series of EPEC-initiated signaling events. Disruption of normal absorptive function results in diarrhea. Other bacterial pathogens are also capable of inducing pedestal formation on intestinal epithelial cells. (From Rosenshine I, Ruschkowski S, Stein M, et al. A pathogenic bacterium triggers epithelial signals to form a functional bacterial receptor that mediates actin pseudopod formation. EMBO J. 1996;15:2613-2624. Courtesy of BB Finlay.)

protein family in the host cell cytoplasm; this action activates membrane ruffling.[91] SopE also stimulates mitogen-activated protein kinases and, thus, nuclear factor κB (NF-κB) and activator protein 1 (AP-1)–mediated nuclear transcriptional responses. The *Yersinia* YopH effector protein is a potent protein tyrosine phosphatase, virulence factor, and antiphagocytic factor. YopJ induces apoptosis in activated macrophages, suppresses tumor necrosis factor-α production, and is critical for *Yersinia* translocation from Peyer's patches to lymphoid tissue and replication in the spleen.[92] A number of pathogens, including *Shigella* and *Salmonella*, are capable of inducing cell death in macrophages and dendritic cells but not epithelial cells. Although the induction of cell death and frank apoptosis is a common shared strategy of many pathogens, each accomplishes this outcome through different mechanisms and with a different precise temporal program.[93]

Manipulation of host cell fate and orchestrated choreography of inflammatory responses are recurrent themes in the strategies of microbial pathogens. Because they establish dependent relationships with host cells, viruses often manipulate host cells in dramatic fashion. Human papillomaviruses and other animal viruses induce expansion of their preferred host niche by interfering with critical cell-cycle controls.[94] In an interesting analogy, *Rickettsia rickettsii* blocks a host cell apoptosis defensive strategy to prolong the life of the infected cell, facilitate rickettsial replication, and then spread to other host cells.[95] Molluscum contagiosum virus protects its host cell from oxidative or ultraviolet-induced damage by expressing a glutathione peroxidase–like selenoprotein that acts as a scavenger of toxic oxygen metabolites.[96] Other opportunistic strategies of viral pathogens include suppression of viral antigen presentation by host cells and interference with host cytokine, complement, and interferon activities.[17-21] Bacteria also modulate local cytokine networks.[15] The scope and sophistication of the means by which pathogens overcome the host barrier to their establishment, replication, persistence, and subsequently exit and transmission to a new host must be seen as one of the most impressive examples of evolutionary diversity and adaptation. We cannot hope to do justice to the topic here, but we do hope to inspire appreciation and respect among clinicians for their microscopic adversaries.

IDENTIFICATION AND CHARACTERIZATION OF VIRULENCE GENES

Characterization of microbial pathogenicity at the molecular level traditionally begins with the identification of a virulence-associated phenotype. Such identification may come from clinical observation, epidemiologic investigation, or the use of a model system that reliably reproduces the microbial phenotype in a manner similar to that seen in natural infection. Traditionally, a virulent strain was compared with a naturally occurring avirulent variant. Such variants, however, may have complex genotypic alterations involving multiple genetic loci. Comparison of strains of naturally occurring virulent and nonvirulent organisms may be even more confounding now that we understand that they may represent entirely different clones of the same species.

Analysis using mutant strains with an identical genetic background is a more desirable approach to the definition of virulence phenotypes. The goal is to identify a single, well-defined genetic lesion that alters a recognizable phenotype and then test the effect of this alteration on the pathogenicity or virulence of the organism in an appropriate model system. The use of insertional elements (e.g., antibiotic-resistant transposons) as mutational agents is an attractive means of accomplishing this aim. Transposons are pieces of DNA that are able to translocate from one genomic site to another. Insertion into a gene usually disrupts its function. Transposons have the advantage of marking the mutagenized genetic locus with a new selectable phenotype, typically antibiotic resistance, but the disadvantage of possible pleiotropic effects on cotranscribed genes or on overall microbial fitness. The development of broad-host-range plasmid vectors carrying well-defined transposons has extended this method of analysis to a number of pathogenic species for which a method of genetic manipulation was not previously available. Once a gene is identified, more precise charac-

terization of the gene product usually follows. By using transposable elements with unique genetic tags, negative selection can be applied to a pool of random mutants in a relevant model of pathogenesis. This approach, known as *signature-tagged mutagenesis*, has identified a number of genes in gram-negative and gram-positive bacteria that are essential for virulence.[97,98]

Genes of interest are usually isolated by screening a "library" of overlapping pieces of a fragmented microbial genome that have been inserted into an appropriate plasmid or bacteriophage vector, which is then introduced into a carrier microorganism. Although *E. coli* K-12 has traditionally served as the carrier, other organisms may be far more useful than *E. coli* if they are easily manipulated genetically and more closely related to the pathogen of interest, for example, use of *B. subtilis* or even *Listeria innocua* to study *L. monocytogenes*. Now, in an era in which there is concern about agents of bioterrorism, such surrogate microbial models become even more urgent. Hence, *Yersinia pseudotuberculosis* can be employed to study many features of the plague bacillus, *Bacillus cereus* for *B. anthracis*, and *Francisella novicida* for *F. tularensis*, thereby providing more safety for the investigator while permitting research on the pathogenic properties of the group. In some instances, only a few hundred carrier organisms bearing such recombinant molecules need to be examined to screen effectively an entire, average-sized bacterial genome.[99] Typical strategies for screening a genomic library may or may not depend on expression of the cloned gene of interest by the carrier organisms. Tools for screening include DNA fragments or oligonucleotides as hybridization probes (e.g., in a high-density format such as a DNA microarray) and antisera for expressed gene products. In some cases, a recombinant host expressing the cloned gene displays a corresponding phenotype that can be exploited for screening purposes: expression of the cloned *inv* locus from *Y. pseudotuberculosis* confers on *E. coli* an ability to invade certain types of cultured eukaryotic cells in vitro.[100] The carrier organisms bearing the recombinant clones, once intracellular, are uniquely resistant to the killing effect of gentamicin, which acts only on extracellular bacteria.

A number of powerful methods have been developed for the identification of virulence-associated genes based on the recognition that they are regulated by the transitions between external and internal host and cellular environments. For example, one can select for mutations that cause a defect in the intracellular growth of certain bacterial pathogens by studying auxotrophic strains that die upon replication in conditions that mimic those found within the host cell. One then imposes a requirement upon a pool of mutagenized auxotrophs that they survive serial passage within host cells under these limiting conditions. This method was the one that first revealed the *Legionella dotA* gene (see earlier). Two more approaches allow one to select for genes and promoters that are preferentially expressed by a microbial pathogen within a host cell or within a host organ. These approaches rely on specially designed vectors into which a complete library of chromosomal genes are cloned such that when the promoters for these genes are activated they turn on the expression of factors that can be easily selected, either by expression of antibiotics, by complementation of an engineered growth-attenuating mutation in the pathogen, or by expression of a fluorescent protein. In the first approach, the application of *in vivo expression technology* to *V. cholerae* and *S. typhimurium* has clarified the conditions encountered by pathogens in vivo as well as their regulatory responses.[101] By using the second approach termed *differential fluorescence induction,* one identifies promoters that are selectively induced within host cells or tissues by fusing random fragments of a pathogen's genome to the gene encoding green fluorescent protein and then applying fluorescence-activated flow cytometry to a pool of recombinant organisms bearing these reporter gene fusions.[102] As an example, differential fluorescence induction has revealed the differential expression of the *Salmonella* SPI-2 pathogenicity island within the phagosomal vacuole.

Broad-based, nonselective approaches for screening an entire genome and its complement of expressed genes are now quite feasible with subtractive hybridization, full genome sequences, and DNA microarray technology. Methods based on subtractive hybridization techniques facilitate the detection of subtle differences between two populations of DNA or RNA. These differences can be amplified by polymerase chain reaction (PCR).[103] An approach of this type was used to identify differences in genomic content among a group of *H. pylori* strains.[104] DNA microarrays are high-density grids of probes displayed on a solid surface; tens or hundreds of thousands of probes can be arrayed in an area of 1 cm². By displaying probes for every gene of a given pathogen on a microarray and hybridizing labeled genomic DNA or complementary DNA, one can obtain a complete gene content or expression profile, respectively, for the pathogen under any desired condition.[5,57] Comparative genomic hybridization analysis of multiple strains of pathogens reveals localized regions of frequent gene gain and loss ("regions of difference," equivalent in many cases to pathogenicity islands) and can provide insight into pathogen evolution as well as novel mechanisms of virulence.[43,105,106] With these approaches, genes and their products are incriminated by their relationship with a disease-associated process. Final proof, however, that a gene is associated with pathogenicity requires that certain criteria be met (see later).

ASSOCIATION OF GENES WITH VIRULENCE: PROOF BY A MOLECULAR FORM OF KOCH'S POSTULATES

Technical advances have brought about a proliferation of reports describing genes thought to be involved in microbial pathogenicity. These advances have dramatized the need for defined criteria by which genes may be assigned a role in pathogenesis. In a manner analogous to Koch's original postulates, these criteria must include return of the putative causal agent (the cloned virulence-associated gene mutated or intact) to the host of origin. Unless one can demonstrate an effect on pathogenicity by this kind of controlled genetic manipulation, causality with respect to virulence has not been proved. Just as the original Henle-Koch postulates have provided a reference point for later revised criteria of microbial causality,[107] the criteria outlined in this section best serve as guidelines, in this case for an experimental approach to the molecular genetic basis of pathogenicity.

A molecular form of Koch's postulates[108] can be stated as follows: (1) The phenotype or property under investigation should be associated significantly more often with pathogenic members of a genus or pathogenic strains of a species than with nonpathogenic members or strains. (2) Specific inactivation of the gene or genes associated with the suspected virulence trait should lead to a measurable decrease in virulence. If inactivation of the gene has taken place in a cloned copy carried by a recombinant host, this mutated gene must be exchanged for the wild-type copy of the gene in the host of origin; the latter must suffer a loss of virulence after the exchange. (3) Restoration of full pathogenicity should accompany replacement of the mutated version of the gene with the wild-type version in the strain of origin.

Technical limitations often face investigators who wish to apply these postulates to an organism poorly characterized from a genetic standpoint. The ability to exchange alleles in the organism under investigation is crucial because it allows a virulence-associated gene to be studied in an isogenic background. Cloned genes carried into the strain of origin on plasmid vectors are exchanged for the analogous chromosomal version of the same genes by means of homologous recombination, an enzyme-catalyzed process by which a segment of DNA replaces an equivalent segment elsewhere that has identical or nearly identical nucleotide sequences. A suicide plasmid cloning vector can be used for this purpose; these vectors are plasmids that can be manipulated in *E. coli*, for example, but are unable to replicate in the organism under investigation. When conjugation is performed in the presence of an antibiotic that selects for the presence of the suicide plasmid, the plasmid becomes recombined into the recipient organism's chromosome because of homology with the cloned gene copy in the plasmid. Subsequent antibiotic selection against the presence of the suicide plasmid allows detection of a second recombinational event that results in excision of the plasmid and replacement of the original chromosomal gene copy with that carried by the plasmid. In this way, chromosomal virulence genes can be modified in a directed fashion.

Another difficulty in the application of a molecular form of Koch's postulates is similar to a problem that faced Koch in his own day: finding an appropriate animal model system. This problem limits the study of microbial pathogenesis as much as any other. It does little good to return a carefully constructed virulence gene mutation to the original strain if its effect on a particular virulence phenotype cannot be evaluated. A model must duplicate relevant pathology commonly observed in the normal host. The animal host must become consistently infected by using a natural route. Clearly, a model of this sort does not exist for many pathogens. At the same time, it should be remembered that exposure to a known human pathogen does not uniformly lead to disease in all humans.

The postulates just outlined are meant to provide principles by which one may study the genes and gene products associated with microbial pathogenesis. This kind of approach can also be used to analyze the internal structure of these genes and the corresponding functional domains of the encoded proteins. These postulates continue to coevolve in conjunction with emerging insights into microbial virulence and rapidly improving experimental approaches and technologies.[109]

MOLECULAR MICROBIOLOGY AT THE BEDSIDE: PATHOGEN DETECTION AND DISCOVERY

As mechanisms of microbial pathogenicity, acquisition of virulence, and drug resistance are revealed, pathogen detection, strain identification, and pathogen discovery assume increasing importance in the practice of clinical infectious diseases.[23] It is already apparent that studies of microbial pathogenicity at the molecular level have made substantial contributions to our understanding of the epidemiology, clinical manifestations, diagnosis, treatment, and immunoprophylaxis of infectious diseases. Even the fundamental issue of disease causation and the possible role of microorganisms in chronic diseases of uncertain etiology must be reexamined in light of newer experimental methods and insight.[110,111]

Infectious disease epidemiology hinges on a clear definition of the clinical problem under study and, moreover, precise identification of the etiologic agent. Molecular techniques provide for the sensitive and specific detection of putative pathogens and supply a means for establishing relationships among multiple isolates of the same species. As a result, seemingly unrelated cases occurring during an outbreak have been connected; similarly, geographically or temporally distinct outbreaks have been linked to the same pathogenic clone. Molecular techniques have been used in other epidemiologic investigations to study transmission mechanisms and the role of avirulent microbial variants in the spread of disease.

Several methods are available with which to define clonal relationships among pathogens in an epidemiologic investigation of disease outbreaks, including restriction endonuclease genomic fingerprinting, pulsed-field gel electrophoresis, plasmid analysis, randomly amplified polymorphic DNA analysis, high-density DNA microarray–based analyses, and primary sequence–based methods such as multilocus sequence typing.[5,29,112,113] Molecular strain typing data sometimes provide the only clue that a group of cases are related, that is, that an outbreak of disease has occurred.[114] Morphologic and metabolic features often fail to indicate the important genetic diversity found within strains; for example, sequence-based typing of *Cryptosporidium parvum* distinguishes animal- from human-adapted isolates, and *H. pylori* population structure can be linked to the historical migration patterns of humans.[115,116]

Nucleic acid amplification techniques have had a far-reaching impact on study of microbial pathogenesis and the diagnosis of infectious diseases. Using PCR, it is possible to detect the presence of a single target DNA or RNA sequence in a sample of 10⁵ cells. This degree of sensitivity is far greater than that achieved by Southern hybridization with a specific DNA probe. Specific PCR assays are available for a long list of microbial pathogens but have failed to penetrate the clinical workplace to a thorough degree.[113,117] The more informative of these assays target microbial genetic sequences that encode specific virulence determinants or antimicrobial-resistance factors. On the other hand, the extraordinary sensitivity of PCR and potential problems with cross-contamination have thus far restricted its use to reference and research laboratories. Suboptimal sample preparation methods and the PCR inhibitors found in many types of clinical specimens pose additional challenges. Other nucleic acid and probe amplification methods include self-sustaining sequence replication, strand displacement amplification, ligase chain reaction, and Q replicase–based probe amplification.[117]

Southern hybridization–DNA probe technology has been applied widely to infectious disease outbreak investigations and field surveillance. Fingerprint patterns have been used to type strains, track isolates, and incriminate particular strains in multiple cases of disease.[118] PCR- and microarray-based methods may eventually supplant Southern hybridization techniques in many of these sorts of investigations. For example, a variety of arthropod-borne microbial pathogens (such as *Y. pestis*, *R. rickettsii*, *Babesia microti*, and some arboviruses) are readily detected in their natural vectors with PCR. *B. burgdorferi* sequences have been amplified from archival tick samples and used to clarify the geographic and temporal origins of Lyme disease in the United States.[119]

Current methods for the identification of microbial pathogens rely heavily on cultivation or propagation in the laboratory. Molecular pathogen discovery methods provide alternative approaches and have spawned new searches for microorganisms that might play important causal roles in a wide variety of poorly explained acute and chronic diseases.[23,111,120,121] The principle behind these methods is reliance on molecular signatures to identify or classify a previously unrecognized pathogen; the most commonly used signature is the genomic sequence, but other small molecules may prove useful. One of these methods targets highly conserved regions of ribosomal DNA sequences by amplifying them directly from digested, infected human tissue.[120] Reliable evolutionary relationships of a putative organism can then be established from these amplified ribosomal DNA sequences. A number of organisms resistant to cultivation or propagation have been identified with non–culture-based methods.[122-124] With the discovery of novel bacterial kingdoms in soil, thermal springs, lakes, and oceans, efforts have begun using the same molecular methods to explore diversity within the commensal microbial communities that populate the skin and mucosal surfaces of the human body.[125-127] With the detection of microbial sequences by highly sensitive methods, new challenges are also posed for clarifying the role of the inferred putative organisms in disease causation.[110]

The application of molecular techniques and theory to infectious disease diagnosis, therapeutics, and prophylaxis has yet to be fully realized. As virulence factors for essential steps in pathogenesis are identified, it should be possible to interfere with their function. As they become better characterized, manipulation of global virulence regulatory systems may have therapeutic value. Patterns of human gene expression associated with the response to infectious disease may serve as signatures, enabling early recognition and classification of patients on the basis of agent or future disease course.[23,128-130] New acellular or recombinant live-attenuated vaccines and vaccine candidates have already resulted from the identification of immunoprotective antigens through molecular and genomic approaches.[131] The increasing availability of microbial full genome sequences will accelerate these efforts. The result should be a more informed and effective approach to the detection, treatment, and prevention of infectious diseases.

REFERENCES

1. Hooper LV, Gordon JI. Commensal host-bacterial relationships in the gut. Science. 2001;292:1115-1158.
2. Hooper LV, Wong MH, Thelin A, et al. Molecular analysis of commensal host-microbial relationships in the intestine. Science. 2001;291:881-884.
3. Finlay BB, Falkow S. Common themes in microbial pathogenicity revisited. Microbiol Mol Biol Rev. 1997;61:136-169.
4. Falkow S. The microbe's view of infection. Ann Intern Med. 1998;129:247-248.
5. Joyce EA, Chan K, Salama NR, Falkow S. Redefining bacterial populations: A post-genomic reformation. Nat Rev Genet. 2002;3:462-473.
6. Relman DA, Falkow S. The meaning and impact of the human genome sequence for microbiology. Trends Microbiol. 2001;9:206-208.
7. Pirofski LA, Casadevall A. The meaning of microbial exposure, infection, colonisation, and disease in clinical practice. Lancet Infect Dis. 2002;2:628-635.
8. Casadevall A, Pirofski LA. Microbial virulence results from the interaction between host and microorganism. Trends Microbiol. 2003;11:157-158; author reply 158-159.
9. Jones GW, Isaacson RE. Proteinaceous bacterial adhesins and their receptors. Crit Rev Microbiol. 1983;10:229-260.
10. Isberg RR, Barnes P. Dancing with the host; flow-dependent bacterial adhesion. Cell. 2002;110:1-4.
11. Kolenbrander PE, Andersen RN, Blehert DS, et al. Communication among oral bacteria. Microbiol Mol Biol Rev. 2002;66:486-505, table of contents.
12. Boyle EC, Finlay BB. Bacterial pathogenesis: Exploiting cellular adherence. Curr Opin Cell Biol. 2003;15:633-639.
13. Williams JM, Chen GC, Zhu L, Rest RF. Using the yeast two-hybrid system to identify human epithelial cell proteins that bind gonococcal Opa proteins: Intracellular gonococci bind pyruvate kinase via their Opa proteins and require host pyruvate for growth. Mol Microbiol. 1998;27:171-186.
14. Rosenberger CM, Finlay BB. Phagocyte sabotage: Disruption of macrophage signalling by bacterial pathogens. Nat Rev Mol Cell Biol. 2003;4:385-396.
15. Hornef MW, Wick MJ, Rhen M, Normark S. Bacterial strategies for overcoming host innate and adaptive immune responses. Nat Immunol. 2002;3:1033-1040.
16. Young D, Hussell T, Dougan G. Chronic bacterial infections: Living with unwanted guests. Nat Immunol. 2002;3:1026-1032.
17. Brander C, Walker BD. Modulation of host immune responses by clinically relevant human DNA and RNA viruses. Curr Opin Microbiol. 2000;3:379-386.
18. Benedict CA, Norris PS, Ware CF. To kill or be killed: Viral evasion of apoptosis. Nat Immunol. 2002;3:1013-1018.
19. Murphy PM. Viral exploitation and subversion of the immune system through chemokine mimicry. Nat Immunol. 2001;2:116-122.
20. Orange JS, Fassett MS, Koopman LA, et al. Viral evasion of natural killer cells. Nat Immunol. 2002;3:1006-1012.
21. Johnston JB, McFadden G. Poxvirus immunomodulatory strategies: Current perspectives. J Virol. 2003;77:6093-6100.
22. Eckburg PB, Lepp PW, Relman DA. Archaea and their potential role in human disease. Infect Immun. 2003;71:591-596.
23. Relman DA. New technologies, human-microbe interactions, and the search for previously unrecognized pathogens. J Infect Dis. 2002;186(Suppl 2):S254-S258.
24. Relman DA. Mining the natural world for new pathogens. Am J Trop Med Hyg. 2002;67:133-134.
25. Pace NR. A molecular view of microbial diversity and the biosphere. Science. 1997;276:734-740.
26. Hugenholtz P, Goebel BM, Pace NR. Impact of culture-independent studies on the emerging phylogenetic view of bacterial diversity. J Bacteriol. 1998;180:4765-4774.
27. Hugenholtz P. Exploring prokaryotic diversity in the genomic era. Genome Biol. 2002;3:REVIEWS0003.
28. Selander RK, Caugant DA, Ochman H, et al. Methods of multilocus enzyme electrophoresis for bacterial population genetics and systematics. Appl Environ Microbiol. 1986;51:873-884.
29. Maiden MC, Bygraves JA, Feil E, et al. Multilocus sequence typing: A portable approach to the identification of clones within populations of pathogenic microorganisms. Proc Natl Acad Sci USA. 1998;95:3140-3145.
30. Whittam TS. Genetic variation and evolutionary processes in natural populations of *Escherichia coli*. In: Neidhardt FC, ed. *Escherichia coli* and *Salmonella typhimurium*. Washington, DC: ASM Press; 1996:2708-2720.
31. Daubin V, Moran NA, Ochman H. Phylogenetics and the cohesion of bacterial genomes. Science. 2003;301:829-832.
32. Falkow S. The evolution of pathogenicity in *Escherichia*, *Shigella*, and *Salmonella*. In: Neidhardt FC, ed. *Escherichia coli* and *Salmonella typhimurium*. Washington, DC: ASM Press; 1996:2723-2729.
33. Lawrence JG, Ochman H. Molecular archaeology of the *Escherichia coli* genome. Proc Natl Acad Sci USA. 1998;95:9413-9417.
34. Ochman H, Moran NA. Genes lost and genes found: Evolution of bacterial pathogenesis and symbiosis. Science. 2001;292:1096-1099.
35. Gupta S, Maiden MC. Exploring the evolution of diversity in pathogen populations. Trends Microbiol. 2001;9:181-185.
36. Johnson JR, Manges AR, O'Bryan TT, Riley LW. A disseminated multidrug-resistant clonal group of uropathogenic *Escherichia coli* in pyelonephritis. Lancet. 2002; 359:2249-2251.
37. Elwell LP, Shipley PL. Plasmid-mediated factors associated with virulence of bacteria to animals. Annu Rev Microbiol. 1980;34:465-496.
38. Cheetham BF, Katz ME. A role for bacteriophages in the evolution and transfer of bacterial virulence determinants. Mol Microbiol. 1995;18:201-208.
39. Boyd EF, Brussow H. Common themes among bacteriophage-encoded virulence factors and diversity among the bacteriophages involved. Trends Microbiol. 2002;10:521-529.
40. Davis BM, Waldor MK. Filamentous phages linked to virulence of *Vibrio cholerae*. Curr Opin Microbiol. 2003;6:35-42.
41. Moran NA. Microbial minimalism: Genome reduction in bacterial pathogens. Cell. 2002;108:583-586.

42. Parkhill J, Sebaihia M, Preston A, et al. Comparative analysis of the genome sequences of *Bordetella pertussis*, *Bordetella parapertussis* and *Bordetella bronchiseptica*. Nat Genet. 2003;35:32-40.

43. Cummings CA, Brinig MM, Lepp PW, et al. *Bordetella* species are distinguished by patterns of substantial gene loss and host adaptation. J Bacteriol. 2004;186: 1484-1492.

44. Cole ST, Eiglmeier K, Parkhill J, et al. Massive gene decay in the leprosy bacillus. Nature. 2001;409:1007-1011.

45. Groisman EA, Ochman H. Pathogenicity islands: Bacterial evolution in quantum leaps. Cell. 1996;87:791-794.

46. Hacker J, Blum-Oehler G, Muhldorfer I, Tschape H. Pathogenicity islands of virulent bacteria: Structure, function and impact on microbial evolution. Mol Microbiol. 1997;23:1089-1097.

47. Groisman EA, Ochman H. How *Salmonella* became a pathogen. Trends Microbiol. 1997;5:343-349.

48. Parkhill J, Wren BW, Thomson NR, et al. Genome sequence of *Yersinia pestis*, the causative agent of plague. Nature. 2001;413:523-527.

49. Fleischmann RD, Adams MD, White O, et al. Whole-genome random sequencing and assembly of *Haemophilus influenzae* Rd. Science. 1995;269:496-512.

50. Guiney DG. Regulation of bacterial virulence gene expression by the host environment. J Clin Invest. 1997;99:565-569.

51. Roszak DB, Colwell RR. Survival strategies of bacteria in the natural environment. Microbiol Rev. 1987;51:365-379.

52. Lipp EK, Huq A, Colwell RR. Effects of global climate on infectious disease: The cholera model. Clin Microbiol Rev. 2002;15:757-770.

53. de Silva AM, Fikrig E. Arthropod- and host-specific gene expression by *Borrelia burgdorferi*. J Clin Invest. 1997;99:377-379.

54. Crosa JH. Signal transduction and transcriptional and posttranscriptional control of iron-regulated genes in bacteria. Microbiol Mol Biol Rev. 1997;61:319-336.

55. Merrell DS, Goodrich ML, Otto G, et al. pH-regulated gene expression of the gastric pathogen *Helicobacter pylori*. Infect Immun. 2003;71:3529-3539.

56. Hurme R, Rhen M. Temperature sensing in bacterial gene regulation—What it all boils down to. Mol Microbiol. 1998;30:1-6.

57. Conway T, Schoolnik GK. Microarray expression profiling: Capturing a genome-wide portrait of the transcriptome. Mol Microbiol. 2003;47:879-889.

58. Parkinson JS. Signal transduction schemes of bacteria. Cell. 1993;73:857-871.

59. Weiss AA, Falkow S. Genetic analysis of phase change in *Bordetella pertussis*. Infect Immun. 1984;43:263-269.

60. Cotter PA, Jones AM. Phosphorelay control of virulence gene expression in *Bordetella*. Trends Microbiol. 2003;11:367-373.

61. Akerley BJ, Miller JF. Understanding signal transduction during bacterial infection. Trends Microbiol. 1996;4:141-146.

62. Cotter PA, Miller JF. In vivo and ex vivo regulation of bacterial virulence gene expression. Curr Opin Microbiol. 1998;1:17-26.

63. Fuchslocher B, Millar LL, Cotter PA. Comparison of *bipA* alleles within and across *Bordetella* species. Infect Immun. 2003;71:3043-3052.

64. Miller VL, Taylor RK, Mekalanos JJ. Cholera toxin transcriptional activator toxR is a transmembrane DNA binding protein. Cell. 1987;48:271-279.

65. Merrell DS, Butler SM, Qadri F, et al. Host-induced epidemic spread of the cholera bacterium. Nature. 2002;417:642-645.

66. Bina J, Zhu J, Dziejman M, et al. ToxR regulon of *Vibrio cholerae* and its expression in vibrios shed by cholera patients. Proc Natl Acad Sci USA. 2003;100:2801-2806.

67. Bassler BL. Small talk. Cell-to-cell communication in bacteria. Cell. 2002;109: 421-424.

68. Donlan RM, Costerton JW. Biofilms: Survival mechanisms of clinically relevant microorganisms. Clin Microbiol Rev. 2002;15:167-193.

69. Camara M, Williams P, Hardman A. Controlling infection by tuning in and turning down the volume of bacterial small-talk. Lancet Infect Dis. 2002;2:667-676.

70. Zhu J, Mekalanos JJ. Quorum sensing–dependent biofilms enhance colonization in *Vibrio cholerae*. Dev Cell. 2003;5:647-656.

71. Simon M, Zieg J, Silverman M, et al. Phase variation: Evolution of a controlling element. Science. 1980;209:1370-1374.

72. McGee ZA, Johnson AP, Taylor-Robinson D. Pathogenic mechanisms of *Neisseria gonorrhoeae*: Observations on damage to human fallopian tubes in organ culture by gonococci of colony type 1 or type 4. J Infect Dis. 1981;143:413-422.

73. Borst P. Antigenic variation and allelic exclusion. Cell. 2002;109:5-8.

74. Meier JT, Simon MI, Barbour AG. Antigenic variation is associated with DNA rearrangements in a relapsing fever *Borrelia*. Cell. 1985;41:403-409.

75. Jones CH, Jacob-Dubuisson F, Dodson K, et al. Adhesin presentation in bacteria requires molecular chaperones and ushers. Infect Immun. 1992;60:4445-4451.

76. Nagai H, Roy CR. Show me the substrates: Modulation of host cell function by type IV secretion systems. Cell Microbiol. 2003;5:373-383.

77. Sinai AP, Joiner KA. Safe haven: The cell biology of nonfusogenic pathogen vacuoles. Annu Rev Microbiol. 1997;51:415-462.

78. Mengaud J, Ohayon H, Gounon P, et al. E-cadherin is the receptor for internalin, a surface protein required for entry of *L. monocytogenes* into epithelial cells. Cell. 1996;84:923-932.

79. Amieva MR, Vogelmann R, Covacci A, et al. Disruption of the epithelial apical-junctional complex by *Helicobacter pylori* CagA. Science. 2003;300:1430-1434.

80. Cao W, Henry MD, Borrow P, et al. Identification of alpha-dystroglycan as a receptor for lymphocytic choriomeningitis virus and Lassa fever virus. Science. 1998;282:2079-2081.

81. Kenny B, DeVinney R, Stein M, et al. Enteropathogenic *E. coli* (EPEC) transfers its receptor for intimate adherence into mammalian cells. Cell. 1997;91:511-520.

82. Paton AW, Manning PA, Woodrow MC, Paton JC. Translocated intimin receptors (Tir) of Shiga-toxigenic *Escherichia coli* isolates belonging to serogroups O26, O111, and O157 react with sera from patients with hemolytic-uremic syndrome and exhibit marked sequence heterogeneity. Infect Immun. 1998;66:5580-5586.

83. Nagai H, Kagan JC, Zhu X, et al. A bacterial guanine nucleotide exchange factor activates ARF on *Legionella* phagosomes. Science. 2002;295:679-682.

84. Waterman SR, Holden DW. Functions and effectors of the *Salmonella* pathogenicity island 2 type III secretion system. Cell Microbiol. 2003;5:501-511.

85. Goldberg MB. Actin-based motility of intracellular microbial pathogens. Microbiol Mol Biol Rev. 2001;65:595-626, table of contents.

86. Cossart P. Actin-based motility of pathogens: The Arp2/3 complex is a central player. Cell Microbiol. 2000;2:195-205.

87. Hueck CJ. Type III protein secretion systems in bacterial pathogens of animals and plants. Microbiol Mol Biol Rev. 1998;62:379-433.

88. Blocker A, Komoriya K, Aizawa S. Type III secretion systems and bacterial flagella: Insights into their function from structural similarities. Proc Natl Acad Sci USA. 2003;100:3027-3030.

89. Pallen MJ, Chaudhuri RR, Henderson IR. Genomic analysis of secretion systems. Curr Opin Microbiol. 2003;6:519-527.

90. Kubori T, Sukhan A, Aizawa SI, Galan JE. Molecular characterization and assembly of the needle complex of the *Salmonella typhimurium* type III protein secretion system. Proc Natl Acad Sci USA. 2000;97:10225-10230.

91. Hardt WD, Chen LM, Schuebel KE, et al. *S. typhimurium* encodes an activator of Rho GTPases that induces membrane ruffling and nuclear responses in host cells. Cell. 1998;93:815-826.

92. Monack DM, Mecsas J, Bouley D, Falkow S. *Yersinia*-induced apoptosis in vivo aids in the establishment of a systemic infection of mice. J Exp Med. 1998;188: 2127-2137.

93. Navarre WW, Zychlinsky A. Pathogen-induced apoptosis of macrophages: A common end for different pathogenic strategies. Cell Microbiol. 2000;2:265-273.

94. Ferenczy A, Franco E. Persistent human papillomavirus infection and cervical neoplasia. Lancet Oncol. 2002;3:11-16.

95. Joshi SG, Francis CW, Silverman DJ, Sahni SK. Nuclear factor kappa B protects against host cell apoptosis during *Rickettsia rickettsii* infection by inhibiting activation of apical and effector caspases and maintaining mitochondrial integrity. Infect Immun. 2003;71:4127-4136.

96. Shisler JL, Senkevich TG, Berry MJ, Moss B. Ultraviolet-induced cell death blocked by a selenoprotein from a human dermatotropic poxvirus. Science. 1998;279: 102-105.

97. Hensel M, Shea JE, Gleeson C, et al. Simultaneous identification of bacterial virulence genes by negative selection. Science. 1995;269:400-403.

98. Chiang SL, Mekalanos JJ, Holden DW. In vivo genetic analysis of bacterial virulence. Annu Rev Microbiol. 1999;53:129-154.

99. Merrell DS, Camilli A. Information overload: Assigning genetic functionality in the age of genomics and large-scale screening. Trends Microbiol. 2002;10:571-574.

100. Isberg RR, Falkow S. A single genetic locus encoded by *Yersinia pseudotuberculosis* permits invasion of cultured animal cells by *Escherichia coli* K-12. Nature. 1985;317:262-264.

101. Angelichio MJ, Camilli A. In vivo expression technology. Infect Immun. 2002; 70:6518-6523.

102. Valdivia RH, Falkow S. Fluorescence-based isolation of bacterial genes expressed within host cells. Science. 1997;277:2007-2011.

103. Lisitsyn N, Wigler M. Cloning the differences between two complex genomes. Science. 1993;259:946-951.

104. Akopyants NS, Fradkov A, Diatchenko L, et al. PCR-based subtractive hybridization and differences in gene content among strains of *Helicobacter pylori*. Proc Natl Acad Sci USA. 1998;95:13108-13113.

105. Salama N, Guillemin K, McDaniel TK, et al. A whole-genome microarray reveals genetic diversity among *Helicobacter pylori* strains. Proc Natl Acad Sci USA. 2000;97:14668-14673.

106. Fitzgerald JR, Reid SD, Ruotsalainen E, et al. Genome diversification in *Staphylococcus aureus*: Molecular evolution of a highly variable chromosomal region encoding the staphylococcal exotoxin-like family of proteins. Infect Immun. 2003;71:2827-2838.

107. Evans AS. Causation and disease: The Henle-Koch postulates revisited. Yale J Biol Med. 1976;49:175-195.

108. Falkow S. Molecular Koch's postulates applied to microbial pathogenicity. Rev Infect Dis. 1988;10(Suppl 2):S274-S276.

109. Falkow S. Molecular Koch's postulates applied to bacterial pathogenicity—A personal recollection 15 years later. Nat Rev Microbiol. 2004;2:67-72.

110. Fredricks DN, Relman DA. Sequence-based identification of microbial pathogens: A reconsideration of Koch's postulates. Clin Microbiol Rev. 1996;9:18-33.

111. Fredricks DN, Relman DA. Infectious agents and the etiology of chronic idiopathic diseases. Curr Clin Top Infect Dis. 1998;18:180-200.

112. Dumler JS, Valsamakis A. Molecular diagnostics for existing and emerging infections. Complementary tools for a new era of clinical microbiology. Am J Clin Pathol. 1999;112:S33-S39.

113. Fredricks DN, Relman DA. Application of polymerase chain reaction to the diagnosis of infectious diseases. Clin Infect Dis. 1999;29:475-486; quiz 487-488.

114. Bender JB, Hedberg CW, Besser JM, et al. Surveillance by molecular subtype for *Escherichia coli* O157:H7 infections in Minnesota by molecular subtyping. N Engl J Med. 1997;337:388-394.

115. Awad-El-Kariem FM, Robinson HA, Petry F, et al. Differentiation between human and animal isolates of *Cryptosporidium parvum* using molecular and biological markers. Parasitol Res. 1998;84:297-301.

116. Covacci A, Telford JL, Del Giudice G, et al. *Helicobacter pylori* virulence and genetic geography. Science. 1999;284:1328-1333.
117. Persing DH, Tenover FC, Versalovic J, et al. Molecular Microbiology: Diagnostic Principles and Practice. Washington, DC: ASM Press; 2004.
118. Verver S, Warren RM, Munch Z, et al. Proportion of tuberculosis transmission that takes place in households in a high-incidence area. Lancet. 2004;363:212-214.
119. Persing DH, Telford SR 3rd, Rys PN, et al. Detection of *Borrelia burgdorferi* DNA in museum specimens of *Ixodes dammini* ticks. Science. 1990;249:1420-1423.
120. Relman DA. The search for unrecognized pathogens. Science. 1999;284:1308-1310.
121. Nikkari S, Lopez FA, Lepp PW, et al. Broad-range bacterial detection and the analysis of unexplained death and critical illness. Emerg Infect Dis. 2002;8:188-194.
122. Relman DA, Loutit JS, Schmidt TM, et al. The agent of bacillary angiomatosis. An approach to the identification of uncultured pathogens. N Engl J Med. 1990;323:1573-1580.
123. Chang Y, Cesarman E, Pessin MS, et al. Identification of herpesvirus-like DNA sequences in AIDS-associated Kaposi's sarcoma. Science. 1994;266:1865-1869.
124. Fredricks DN, Jolley JA, Lepp PW, et al. *Rhinosporidium seeberi*: A human pathogen from a novel group of aquatic protistan parasites. Emerg Infect Dis. 2000;6:273-282.
125. Kroes I, Lepp PW, Relman DA. Bacterial diversity within the human subgingival crevice. Proc Natl Acad Sci USA. 1999;96:14547-14552.
126. Paster BJ, Boches SK, Galvin JL, et al. Bacterial diversity in human subgingival plaque. J Bacteriol. 2001;183:3770-3783.
127. Brinig MM, Lepp PW, Ouverney CC, et al. Prevalence of bacteria of division TM7 in human subgingival plaque and their association with disease. Appl Environ Microbiol. 2003;69:1687-1694.
128. Boldrick JC, Alizadeh AA, Diehn M, et al. Stereotyped and specific gene expression programs in human innate immune responses to bacteria. Proc Natl Acad Sci USA. 2002;99:972-977.
129. Nau GJ, Richmond JF, Schlesinger A, et al. Human macrophage activation programs induced by bacterial pathogens. Proc Natl Acad Sci USA. 2002;99:1503-1508.
130. Whitney AR, Diehn M, Popper SJ, et al. Individuality and variation in gene expression patterns in human blood. Proc Natl Acad Sci USA. 2003;100:1896-1901.
131. Pizza M, Scarlato V, Masignani V, et al. Identification of vaccine candidates against serogroup B meningococcus by whole-genome sequencing. Science. 2000;287:1816-1820.

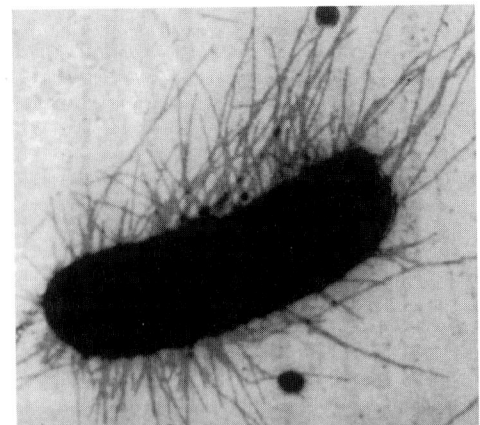

A

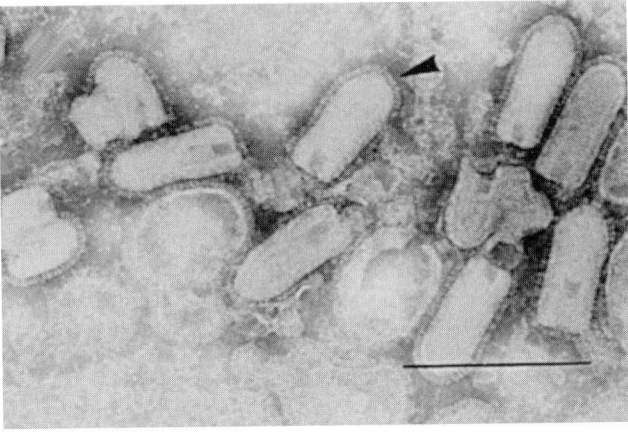

B

FIGURE 2-1. Escherichia coli and vesicular stomatitis virus adhesins. A, Electron micrograph of *E. coli* expressing P fimbriae. **B,** Vesicular stomatitis virus, demonstrating the spikelike protrusions *(arrowhead)* of the viral adherence glycoprotein. Bar = 0.25 μm. (**B** from Klemm P. Fimbrial adhesins of Escherichia coli. *Rev Infect Dis.* 1985;7:321-340.)

CHAPTER **2**

Microbial Adherence

WILLIAM A. PETRI, JR.

BARBARA J. MANN

CHRISTOPHER D. HUSTON

Adherence is the initial interaction of a pathogenic microorganism with its host. It is the route to cellular invasion by intracellular parasites and the first step in host cell killing and toxin delivery by microbial pathogens. Adhesins are microbial molecules that mediate adherence or binding of microbes to the host (Fig. 2-1). Receptors are the host molecules or ligands that microbial adhesins bind to when adherence is initiated. A single adhesin may have more than one receptor, and a single receptor may be recognized by many different adhesins. This chapter will discuss general concepts related to the identification of microbial adhesins and host receptors and provide specific examples of viral, parasite, and bacterial adhesins as illustrations. The central role adhesins play in microbial colonization and pathogenesis makes them ideal targets for preventive and therapeutic interventions. The mechanisms and applications of adherence-inhibitory drugs and molecules in the treatment of human immunodeficiency virus (HIV) infection, picornavirus infections, and urinary tract infections will also be discussed.

EXPERIMENTAL IDENTIFICATION OF AN ADHESIN

Identification of a microbe's adherence mechanism begins with the development of an adherence assay (Table 2-1). Care must be taken that the assay is designed to measure adherence and not motility or invasion. Experiments to measure adherence are often performed at 4° C,

a temperature at which motility and invasion are inhibited. Juxtaposition of microbe and target cell can be accomplished by centrifugation, so motility of the microbe is not required for adherence to take place. Bacterial adherence to cells may also be distinguished from invasion by adding aminoglycosides to the medium after adherence has occurred. Only extracellular bacteria should be killed because aminoglycosides do not penetrate into cells in sufficient quantities to kill intracellular bacteria. Other approaches include mild fixation of target cells to prevent intracellular invasion.

A physiologically relevant substrate is an important component of an adherence assay. Receptors for some microorganisms such as influenza or *Entamoeba histolytica* are ubiquitous, so little, if any, species or tissue restriction to adherence in vitro is noted. However, the adherence of many microorganisms such as polioviruses and rhinoviruses is species specific, and sometimes species and cell type specific as in the case of pathogens such as the Epstein-Barr virus (EBV) and HIV. An adherence assay that measures hepatitis B virus binding to human hepatocytes is more likely to yield information relevant to pathogenesis than one measuring binding to mouse fibroblasts, for example.

Adherence can often be measured visually. The influenza virus adhesin is named *hemagglutinin* (HA) because of the initial observation that purified influenza virions agglutinate erythrocytes. Cell rosetting assays performed with larger microorganisms are a modification of

TABLE 2-1 Approaches to Identifying Adhesins of Pathogenic Microorganisms

Develop an assay that measures adherence to a physiologically relevant substrate.

Inhibit adherence with simple sugars or Fab fragments of monoclonal antibodies directed against the microorganism.

Demonstrate receptor binding activity of the purified putative adhesin, and show that excess adhesin blocks adherence of intact organisms.

Mutate the adhesin gene and demonstrate a change in the adhesive phenotype of the organism.

these hemagglutination assays. Radioactive labeling of the microbe is often used as a means to measure adherence to cells. Care must be taken that the labeling procedure does not kill or significantly alter the microbe; a good test is to show that binding of the radiolabeled microorganism can be inhibited by excess unlabeled microorganism. Likewise, binding of soluble receptors, such as extracellular matrix components, to microorganisms is performed by radiolabeling the receptors, with "specific" binding defined as the amount of radiolabeled receptor bound that is inhibited by excess cold receptor.

Once an assay has been developed to measure the adherence of a pathogen to a cell or substrate, steps can be taken to identify the microbial components participating in adherence. Because the binding of many microbes to host tissues is mediated by microbial lectins, an initial approach is to test whether adherence can be blocked with simple sugars or complex oligosaccharides. Definition of the carbohydrate specificity of adherence can lead to identification of the responsible adhesin via carbohydrate affinity chromatography. Another common approach is to screen monoclonal antibodies produced against the microorganism for their ability to block adherence; inhibitory monoclonal antibodies can be used to identify and purify the putative adhesin.

Antibody inhibition of adherence is most convincing if performed with Fab fragments of antibody (which reduces the likelihood of nonspecific effects of the antibodies from agglutination, steric hindrance, or cross-linking on the microbial surface) or if performed with monoclonal antibodies, where epitope-specific inhibition of adherence can be demonstrated (monoclonal antibodies to some but not all epitopes on an adhesin block its adhesive function, thereby making nonspecific effects of the adherence-inhibitory monoclonal antibody less likely). The purified putative adhesin should be demonstrated to bind to the microbe's receptor, and excess adhesin should be able to inhibit adherence of the intact microbe competitively by preventing binding to the host receptor.

EXPERIMENTAL IDENTIFICATION OF A HOST RECEPTOR

Identification of the receptor for an adhesin is important to understanding the interactions of microbial pathogens with their hosts (Table 2-2). In several pathogens, the species specificity, or tissue or cell tropism, of a microorganism can be explained by the presence or absence of a receptor for the microbial adhesin. Examples include

TABLE 2-2 Approaches to Identifying Host Cell Receptors for Pathogenic Microorganisms

Transfer DNA from a permissive to a nonpermissive cell; identify the transfected DNA that confers permissiveness. This technique exploits the fact that many microorganisms have restricted host ranges (e.g., rhinovirus infects only human and chimpanzee cells) and tissue tropism (e.g., HIV and CD4 cells, Epstein-Barr virus, and B cells).

Produce monoclonal antibodies against host cell surface antigens; screen the antibody for inhibition of binding or infection. Characterize the antigen recognized by the monoclonal antibody.

Identify lectin (carbohydrate recognition) activity of the microorganism's adhesin by blocking the adherence, infectivity, or both of the permissive cell with simple or complex carbohydrates (e.g., sialic acid and influenza hemagglutinin; HIV and galactosylcerebroside).

Affinity-purify the host cell receptor by using microbial adhesin (rarely successful because of the generally low affinity of the adhesin for the solubilized receptor).

TABLE 2-3 Classes of Host Cell Receptors for Microbial Adhesins

Sugars: Sialic acid (orthomyxoviruses and paramyxoviruses, polyomaviruses), galactose *(Entamoeba histolytica),* P blood group antigen (uropathogenic *E. coli*)

Immunoglobulin superfamily: ICAM-1 (rhinoviruses, major group), CD4 (HIV), polioviruses receptor (polio)

Growth factors or growth factor receptors: EGF receptors (vaccinia), erythropoietin receptor (Friend leukemia virus), interleukin-6 (hepatitis B virus)

Integrins: VLA-2 (echovirus)

Extracellular matrix components: Laminin *(Toxoplasma gondii),* fibronectin (streptococci)

Transport proteins: Basic amino acid and phosphate transporter (certain retroviruses)

Complement receptors: CR2 (Epstein-Barr virus)

Antibody-dependent or complement-dependent enhancement of adherence: Antibody-coated dengue virus entry into macrophages via Fcγ1, and IgA-coated Epstein-Barr virus entry via IgA receptor; HIV antibody-dependent enhancement via CR2

EGF, epidermal growth factor; HIV, human immunodeficiency virus; ICAM-1, intercellular adhesion molecule 1.

the B-lymphocyte CR2 receptor for EBV,[1] the T-cell CD4 receptor for HIV,[2,3] and the aminopeptidase N receptor for the pig coronavirus transmissible gastroenteritis virus (TGEV).[4,5] Species specificity of adherence of microbial pathogens has also been demonstrated for poliovirus[6,7] and the major group of rhinoviruses,[8-10] where viral receptors are present on human but not murine cells (Tables 2-3 and 2-4).

Species or tissue specificity for receptors for microbial adhesins suggests an obvious approach to their identification: transfection of DNA from a receptor-positive to a receptor-negative cell line, followed by identification and sequencing of the DNA segment that confers receptor positivity. This approach has been successfully used to identify intercellular adhesion molecule 1 (ICAM-1) as the human receptor for the major group of rhinoviruses[9,10] and to identify the poliovirus receptor, a member of the immunoglobulin gene superfamily.[6,7] The advantage of this approach to receptor identification is that the receptor is cloned and sequenced at the same time that it is identified.

When a restricted host range or tissue tropism cannot be exploited, monoclonal antibodies produced against the host cell have been used to identify the receptor. Monoclonal antibodies that block adherence to or infection of host cells were used to identify ICAM-1 as the receptor for the major group of rhinoviruses,[8] CD4 as the HIV receptor,[2,3] aminopeptidase N as the TGEV coronavirus receptor,[4,5] and "very late antigen" (VLA)-2 as the receptor for echovirus-1.[11]

If the microbial adhesin is a lectin, the carbohydrate structure recognized by the adhesin on host cells can be determined by the effect of different oligosaccharides on inhibition of adherence. In this manner, the detailed structure of the sialic acid–containing oligosaccharide recognized by influenza virus HA has been determined.[12]

TABLE 2-4 Classes of Microbial Adhesins for Host Cell Receptors

Lectins: Sialic acid binding (hemagglutinin envelope glycoproteins of orthomyxoviruses), galactose binding (*Entamoeba histolytica* adherence lectin), P blood group antigen binding (*E. coli* P fimbriae), *trans*-sialidase (*Trypanosoma cruzi*)

Fimbriae (pili): Filamentous bacterial adhesins of *E. coli* (P, S, type 1, K-88, K-99, CFA-1), *Neisseria gonorrhoeae* (type 4), *Salmonella* (type 1), *Vibrio cholerae* (Tcp)

Nonfimbrial bacterial adhesins: Yersinia (Inv and Ail proteins), *Bordetella pertussis* (pertactin), *Mycoplasma pneumoniae* (P1 cytoadhesin), *Treponema pallidum* (fibronectin-binding protein)

Lipid: Streptococcus pyogenes (lipoteichoic acid), *Leishmania* (lipophosphoglycan)

Glycosaminoglycan: Chlamydia trachomatis (heparin sulfate–like glycosaminoglycan)

Viral capsid proteins: Rhinovirus (VP1/VP3); aphthovirus (VP1)

Mechanical: Giardia lamblia (gripping disk)

If the adhesin itself is purified, it can be used to affinity-purify its receptor from the host cell. This approach is not likely to be successful if the interaction of adhesin with receptor is of low affinity, which may be a particular problem when adhesin and receptor have been solubilized during purification. However, this approach successfully identified CR2 as the receptor for EBV.

CENTRAL CONCEPTS IN THE INTERACTIONS BETWEEN ADHESINS AND RECEPTORS

Many adhesins require post-translational processing, especially proteolytic fragmentation, to manifest full biologic activity (Table 2-5). The membrane fusion activity of HA, which is required for viral infectivity, requires processing by a host protease of the intact hemagglutinin (HA_0) into HA_1 and HA_2. This proteolytic fragmentation exposes a highly conserved hydrophobic sequence at the amino terminus of HA_2 that, at acidic pH, is involved in viral entry into the cell by fusion of the viral membrane to the endocytic vacuole cell membrane (Fig. 2-2).[12] Similar processing events are required for the gp160 adhesin of HIV to have functional cell fusion activity, as will be described later. The requirement for host proteases to activate the fusion activity of adhesins may partly explain the tissue tropism of microbial pathogens, inasmuch as the proteases required to activate the adhesins may be present only in certain tissues.

A second important concept is the canyon hypothesis, in which the active site of the adhesin may be inaccessible to antibody because of its location in a "canyon," or depression, in the molecule. This location shields the receptor site from antibody and enables the microbe to conserve the amino acids required for formation of the binding site in the face of antibody-driven variation in the rest of the adhesin sequence. For example, the sialic acid–binding site of influenza HA is formed by the highly conserved amino acids Tyr98, Trp153, His183, Glu190, and Leu194, which are found in an antibody-inaccessible depression at the distal end of the HA; the surface-exposed residues, however, are subject to antigenic variation.[12] In a similar manner, the binding site on the major group of rhinoviruses

for the ICAM-1 receptor is located in a canyon formed by the capsid proteins that is only partially accessible to antibody (Fig. 2-3).[13]

Human adhesins such as *Limax flavus* agglutinin (LFA)-1, complement receptor type 3 (CR3), and integrins require activation in addition to cell surface expression to mediate adherence,[14,15] and microbial adhesins also exist in active and inactive states. One example is the galactose and N-acetyl-D-galactosamine (Gal/GalNAc) specific adherence lectin of *E. histolytica*. Antibodies against different epitopes on this lectin either enhance or inhibit the galactose-binding activity of the lectin, presumably by altering conformations from inactive to active configurations (see later).

Conformational changes in an adhesin may also activate other functions of the adhesin, such as the fusion activities of enveloped virus gly-

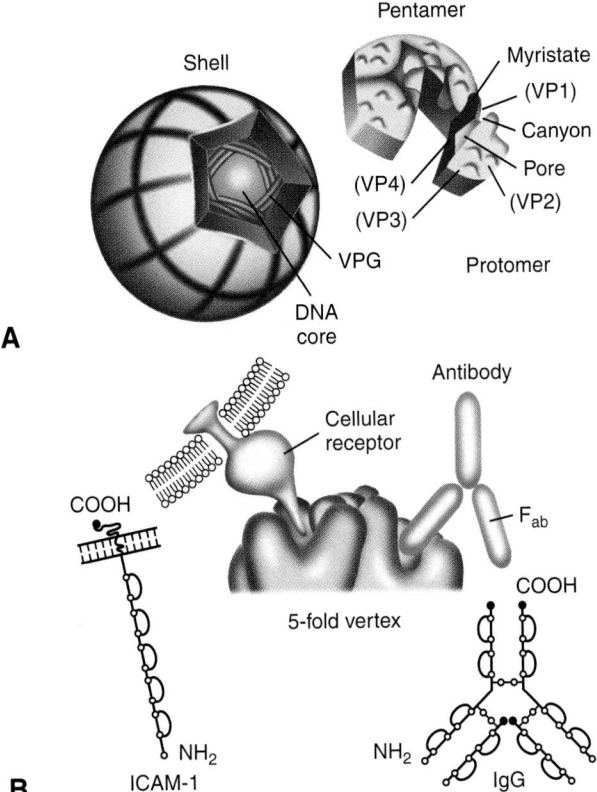

A

B

FIGURE 2-3. Key features in the adherence function of a typical picornavirus. **A,** Exploded diagram showing location of canyon in the middle of the center of the viral capsid protein VP4 pentamer. **B,** Binding of cellular receptor to the floor of the canyon. Note that the binding site of the intercellular adhesion molecule 1 (ICAM-1) molecule, identified as ICAM-1 for major group rhinoviruses, has a diameter roughly half that of an IgG antibody molecule. *(From Rueckert RR. Picornaviridae and their replication. In: Fields BN, Knipe DM, Howley PM, eds. Fields Virology. 3rd ed. Philadelphia: Lippincott-Raven; 1996:623.)*

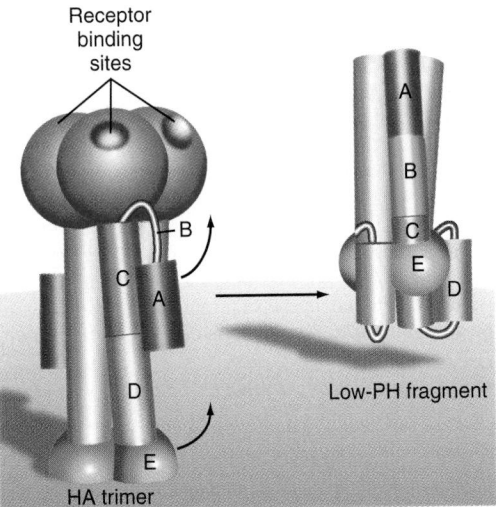

FIGURE 2-2. Schematic representation of the conformation of the influenza hemagglutinin molecule at neutral and acidic pH. The HA trimer is shown protruding from a plane representing the surface of the viral membrane. The main structural units of the low-pH structure (from about residues 40 to 155 of the HA_2 chain) are labeled A to E from the N-terminal end. The fusion peptide, N-terminal to unit A, would protrude well above the heads bearing the receptor binding sites, ideally placed to engage the membrane of the target cell. *(Reprinted by permission from Stuart D. Virus structure: Docking mission accomplished. Nature. 1994;371:19-20, Macmillan Magazines Ltd.)*

coproteins. Some viral adherence glycoproteins, on binding to a receptor or on exposure to low pH in endosomes, undergo conformational changes that expose the hydrophobic fusion domains of the envelope glycoproteins.[16,17]

Single adhesins can have multiple receptors. For example, gp120/41 of HIV binds to CD4 and interacts with membrane-bound chemokine co-receptors (see later) before initiation of viral–host cell membrane fusion.

The immune response to an adhesin (in particular, anti-adhesin antibodies) may enhance adherence, infectivity, or both by facilitating alternative routes of adherence and invasion. Examples of this phenomenon can be found in infections with HIV, *E. histolytica*, dengue virus, and EBV. Enhancement of adherence and infection of Fc receptor–positive monocytes and macrophages by subneutralizing antibodies has been demonstrated for some flaviviruses, including dengue. However, the importance of antibody-dependent enhancement in the pathogenesis of dengue hemorrhagic fever remains controversial.[18] EBV entry into a human epithelial cell line was promoted by polymeric IgA specific for EBV. The virus entered the cells via secretory component–mediated transport when bound to IgA instead of the usual route of entry via the CR2 receptor in B cells and other epithelial cell lines.[19]

The species, tissue, and cell tropism of a microbe is often determined by adhesin–receptor interactions. Examples include EBV and the CR2 receptor on B cells, poliovirus and the poliovirus receptor of human cells, and rhinoviruses and the human ICAM-1 receptor.

SPECIFIC ADHERENCE MECHANISMS AND THEIR ROLES IN PATHOGENESIS

HIV gp120/160

The development of an immune response to the gp120/41 adhesin of HIV to block adherence and invasion by the virus unfortunately leads quickly to the emergence of HIV virions that resist antibody neutralization, as discussed in Chapter 116.[20,21] Understanding the mechanisms of adherence and fusion for HIV thus has more immediate clinical application in the design of fusion and adherence inhibitory drugs (see later). Infection of cells with HIV and other enveloped viruses requires fusion of the viral and cell membranes. The fusion event releases the viral nucleocapsid into the cell cytoplasm and thereby initiates the process of viral infection and replication.[22] This fusion event can occur at the cell surface between the plasma membrane and the viral membrane, as it does for paramyxoviruses, or it can occur between the endosome and viral membranes after phagocytosis of the virus, as in influenza virus infection. The adherence and fusion events are generally mediated by the same viral glycoprotein. In the case of HIV, it appears that the fusion event occurs at the plasma membrane because neutralization of acidic endosomes with weak bases does not interfere with viral entry, and mutation of CD4 to a glycolipid-anchored form that is endocytosed poorly also has no effect on HIV entry.[23,24]

The HIV cell surface glycoprotein is synthesized as a 160-kilodalton glycoprotein. Proteolytic cleavage of gp160 to gp120 and gp41 at a site containing several basic amino acids (arginine and lysine) is required for activation of the glycoprotein and production of infectious virions. Cleavage of gp160 is thought to occur in the trans-Golgi compartment and has been shown in vitro to be mediated by the endoproteinase furin, which cleaves at the consensus sequence Arg-X-Lys/Arg-Arg.[25] Furin also activates the HA protein of the fowl plague influenza virus. In fact, the cleavage sites of the fusion proteins for orthomyxoviruses, paramyxoviruses, and retroviruses are all remarkably conserved. Inhibition of gp160 cleavage with peptide moieties containing the furin consensus sequence or by the ionophore monensin blocks HIV glycoprotein-induced syncytia formation and results in the production of virions with greatly reduced infectivity.[25] Mutation of the carboxyl-terminal amino acid 518 of gp120 from arginine to threonine abolishes both gp160 cleavage and syncytia formation.[26]

Cleavage of gp160 to gp41 and gp120 activates the fusion ability of the viral glycoprotein. The gp41 contains the transmembrane carboxyl terminus of gp160; gp120 remains attached to the virion via noncovalent interactions with gp41. The amino terminus created on gp41 by cleavage of gp160 is hydrophobic and contains the Phe-X-Gly sequence present in the amino termini of the activated fusion proteins of the paramyxoviruses. Mutations in gp160 that affect fusion activity map to the amino terminus of gp41. Thus, the requirement for cleavage of gp160 to gp41 and gp120 is in large part necessary to expose the fusion domain of gp41 for the virion to enter the cell via viral–cell plasma membrane fusion.[23-26]

Binding of HIV to CD4 and chemokine receptors is mediated by gp120.[2,3,27,28] Binding of CD4 by gp120 is a high-affinity interaction and results in the exposure of cryptic epitopes on gp120 and gp41, which indicates that CD4 binding has resulted in a conformational change in the virion glycoproteins.[29] Binding of HIV to CD4 is insufficient for the fusion of viral and cell membranes, as demonstrated by the inability of HIV to enter murine cells engineered to express CD4.[30] The requirement for something in addition to CD4 to allow entry of HIV led to the discovery of chemokine co-receptors for HIV. Macrophage-tropic strains of HIV invade after interaction with the CCR5 chemokine receptor; T-cell–tropic strains require the CXCR4 chemokine receptor.[28,29] CCR5 and CXCR4 consist of seven transmembrane domain G-coupled receptors for chemokines, a group of chemoattractant polypeptides involved in inflammation and infection. Interaction of HIV gp120 with the co-receptor is thought to permit interaction of the fusion domain of gp41 with the host cell (Fig. 2-4). A homozygous deletion mutation in CCR5 is associated with resistance to HIV infection in whites.[29]

Cell tropism (T4 cells versus macrophages) of HIV-1 is determined in part by the interaction of the third variable (V3) loop of gp120 with the macrophage co-receptor CCR5 or the T-cell co-receptor CXCR4. Production of a chimeric gp120 containing the

FIGURE 2-4. Adherence and fusion mechanisms of HIV gp120/gp41. After gp120 binds to CD4 (**A**), a conformational change in gp120 ensues (**B**), allowing it to bind to a co-receptor, CCR5 or CXCR4. The change allows the amino terminus of gp41 to insert into the membrane of the CD4 cell and causes the membrane of the virus and cell to fuse. Membrane fusion thus allows the contents of the virus to enter the cell. *(From Kilby JM, Eron JJ. Novel therapies based on mechanisms of HIV-1 cell entry. N Engl J Med. 2003;348:2228-2238.)*

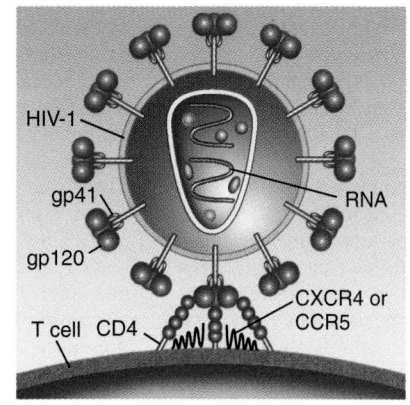

A

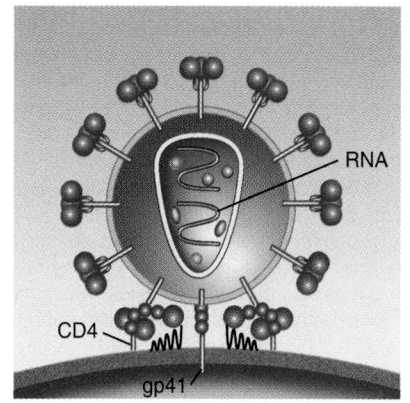

B

V3 loop of the macrophage-tropic BaL isolate of HIV-1 conferred macrophage tropism on the human T-cell leukemia/lymphoma virus IIIB, which is normally a T-cell–tropic virus. The sensitivity of HIV isolates to inhibition by soluble CD4 is also determined by the sequence in the V3 loop.[31-34] Amino acid substitutions in the V3 loop block cell fusion and infectivity without affecting gp160 processing to gp120/gp41 or CD4 binding.[35] Enhancement of HIV infection of cells has also been observed in the presence of anti-gp120/gp41 antibodies. Most of the antibodies enhancing HIV infection have been mapped to the V3 loop; enhancement of infection appears to occur when anti-V3 loop antibodies derived from infection or immunization with gp120 from one strain cross react with, but do not neutralize, the V3 region of another strain. Apparently, V3 hypervariable loops from one isolate may elicit antibodies enhancing infection by another HIV isolate.[36] Antibody-mediated enhancement of HIV infection may be independent of complement or may be mediated by complement and the CR2 receptor; antibodies to the CR2 receptor blocked enhanced infectivity in one experimental system.[37] The biologic significance of antibody-mediated enhancement in HIV infection remains unclear.

Entamoeba histolytica Gal/GalNAc Lectin

Carbohydrate-protein interactions are responsible for the contact-dependent cytotoxicity for which *E. histolytica* was named. A cell surface lectin specific for galactose (Gal) and *N*-acetyl-D-galactosamine (GalNAc) mediates trophozoite adherence to human colonic mucin, colonic epithelium, neutrophils and erythrocytes, certain bacteria, and a variety of cell lines.[38-40] Studies of human neutrophils have confirmed that the Gal/GalNAc lectin (and not fibronectin, vitronectin, CD11/CD18 integrins, complement, or mannose-binding protein) is the only defined adhesin participating in the adherence event.[38-41] Inhibition of contact-dependent killing of Chinese hamster ovary (CHO) cells and other target cells by Gal and GalNAc is greater than 90%. Additionally, CHO cell glycosylation-deficient mutants lacking terminal Gal residues on N- and O-linked sugars are nearly totally resistant to amebic adherence and cytolytic activity.[42,43]

The Gal/GalNAc lectin was identified by carbohydrate affinity chromatography and with adherence-inhibitory monoclonal antibodies (MAbs).[44] The 260-kDa Gal/GalNAc lectin is a heterodimer of transmembrane heavy (170 kDa, Hgl) and glucose-6-phosphate isomerase (GPI)-anchored light (35/31 kDa, Lgl) subunits linked by disulfide bonds (Fig. 2-5). A carbohydrate recognition domain (CRD) has been identified in Hgl.[40] The cytoplasmic tail has homology to the cytoplasmic domain of β_1 and β_2 integrins, including regions implicated in binding of the intracellular signaling molecules Shc and Grb2.[45]

The intermediate subunit of the lectin is noncovalently associated with the 260-kDa heterodimer.[46] Initially identified as a trophozoite surface antigen recognized by MAbs that block trophozoite adherence to mammalian cells in vitro, the 150-kDa lectin has been shown to be associated with the Gal/GalNAc lectin in several different ways. The 150-kDa lectin is present in small amounts in preparations of the Gal/GalNAc lectin that have been purified by either galactose affinity chromatography or anti-Hgl MAb affinity chromatography. Similarly, the 260-kDa lectin is present in small quantities in the immunoaffinity-purified 150-kDa lectin.

Destruction of host cells is contact dependent (via the Gal/GalNAc lectin), extracellular, and apoptotic.[47] Killing requires an intact parasite: amebic filtrates or sonicates are not cytotoxic, and neither is the purified 260-kDa lectin. Pore-forming proteins have historically been implicated in the cytolytic event. A purified 5-kDa amebapore has cytolytic activity for nucleated cells at high concentrations (10 to 100 μM).[38,40] Interestingly, host cell DNA degradation was observed only in cells lysed by the intact parasite, and not in those lysed by the purified amebapore, indicating that the mechanism of cell killing by the purified amebapore is different from that by the intact parasite. Further

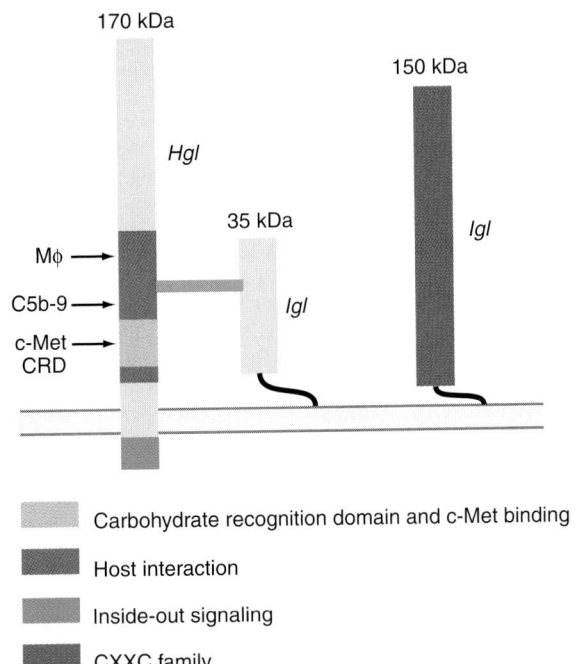

FIGURE 2-5. Gal/GalNAc adherence lectin of *Entamoeba histolytica*. The Gal/GalNAc lectin mediates parasite adherence and is required for contact-dependent killing of host cells. It is present on the plasma membrane of the trophozoite and is composed of three subunits. The integral membrane heavy subunit (Hgl) has a short cytoplasmic tail implicated in intracellular signaling. Located within Hgl is the carbohydrate recognition domain (CRD), which also contains a binding site for the c-Met receptor kinase. Adjacent to the CRD are a complement C5b-9 membrane attack complex inhibitory domain, and sites that stimulate proinflammatory cytokine release by macrophages (Mϕ). Hgl is disulfide bonded to a lipid-anchored light subunit (Lgl). Finally, the lipid-anchored intermediate subunit (Igl) is noncovalently associated with the Hgl-Lgl heterodimer. *(Adapted with permission from Petri WA Jr, Haque R, Mann BJ. The bittersweet interface of parasite and host: Lectin–carbohydrate interactions during human invasion by the parasite* Entamoeba histolytica. *Annu Rev Microbiol. 2002;56:39-64. ©2002 by Annual Reviews www.annualreviews.org.*

demonstrating the importance of an intact parasite for delivery of the cytolytic event, disruption of the cytoskeleton (by expression of dominant negative myosin, by cytochalasin, and by inactivation of Rho) blocked cytotoxicity.[38]

The Gal/GalNAc lectin may also have a role in signaling the initiation of encystation. The formation of the cyst form of *Entamoeba* has been studied in the reptilian parasite *E. invadens*. Coppi and Eichinger have demonstrated that encystation requires the addition of precise amounts of polyvalent galactose-terminated molecules (serum or mucins or *Crithidia fasciculata*).[48] Galactose (but not GalNAc or mannose) blocked encystation of *E. invadens* specifically at the aggregation stage of the encystment process.[48] A homologue of the 260-kDa lectin heavy subunit has been cloned and partially sequenced in *E. invadens* (D. Eichinger, personal communication, February 2004). These studies suggest that Gal/GalNAc lectins are also important in formation of the infectious cyst.

Acquired immunity to amebiasis in humans correlates with an intestinal IgA antibody response against the Gal/GalNAc lectin. Haque and colleagues studied *E. histolytica* infections in children in an urban slum of Dhaka, Bangladesh.[49,50] *E. histolytica* colonization was present in 0% (0/64) of children with, and 13.4% (33/246) without, stool IgA anti-GalNAc lectin antibodies (P = .001). Of these children, 289 were followed for 1 year, and 39% (105/269) had at least one new *E. histolytica* infection, and 3.1% (4/129) of the infections were associated with dysentery. Children who developed a mucosal IgA response against the carbohydrate recognition domain of the lectin during the first year of this study had an 86% reduction in new infections over the second year.[50]

Active immunization of mice with the Gal/GalNAc lectin has recently been shown to prevent intestinal infection. Using a mouse model of intestinal amebiasis, Houpt and colleagues demonstrated that immunization of these mice with the 260-kDa lectin provided nearly 90% protection from intestinal infection.[51] Because the Gal/GalNAc lectin is antigenically conserved and because an anti–lectin IgA is a marker of acquired immunity, an adherence-blocking amebiasis vaccine appears feasible.

Escherichia coli P Fimbriae

Many gram-negative bacteria have adhesive organelles called *fimbriae* or *pili* that mediate attachment to host tissues. Fimbriae are proteinaceous, 2- to 7-nm rodlike structures that are peritrichously arranged on the bacterial cell surface in numbers ranging from 100 to 1000 per cell (see Fig. 2-1).[52,53] They are easily distinguishable from flagella, which are about 20 nm in diameter.[54] There are several different types of fimbriae. They are classified on the basis of common structural features and mechanisms of biogenesis.[52] A single bacterium may produce one or more different types of fimbriae at a time.

Bacteria with specific types of fimbriae have been associated with certain sites of infection. In the case of P or Pap (*p*ili *a*ssociated with *p*yelonephritis) fimbriae on uropathogenic *E. coli*, the presence of P fimbriae has been clearly established as a tropism factor that promotes urinary tract colonization and invasion. Studies of *E. coli* isolates from urinary tract infections (UTIs) have revealed that 60% of cystitis isolates, and 50% to 90% of isolates from adults with pyelonephritis, express P fimbriae.[55-58] In several studies, 100% of isolates from patients with pyelonephritis and bacteremia were positive for P fimbriae.[59-61]

P fimbriae have been shown to bind specifically to uroepithelial cells and P blood group antigens, which are globo-series glycolipids containing the disaccharide α-D-galactopyranosyl-(1,4)-β-D-galactopyranose (Gal-Gal).[62,63] Gal-Gal, which is the minimal receptor moiety, can block the attachment of P fimbriated bacteria to uroepithelial cells.[64] Individuals with high-level expression of P1 blood group antigen are over-represented in populations with recurrent UTIs and pyelonephritis.[65]

The importance of P fimbriae to human UTIs has been demonstrated in human trials.[53] Studies of patients infected by intravesicular inoculation with isogenic strains of *E. coli* 83972, which differed from the parent strain only in their lack of production of P fimbriae, demonstrated that the presence of P fimbriae enhanced the early establishment of *E. coli* in the urinary tract.[66] P fimbriae were also associated with increased levels of interleukin (IL)-6, IL-8, and neutrophils in these patients.[67]

P fimbriae have also been shown to activate cells via the toll-like receptor 4 (TLR-4) pathway.[68] P fimbriated *E. coli* stimulate cytokine responses in TLR-4–positive mice but not in TLR-4 knockout mice. This activation is independent of the lipopolysaccharide (LPS)-CD14 pathway because P fimbriated bacteria with defective LPS are still capable of eliciting cytokine responses.

P fimbriae consist of a rigid helical rod with a thin flexible fibrillar tip and are assembled by the chaperone usher pathway.[52] The adhesin subunit PapG is located at the end of the fibrillar tip.[69-71] A model for fimbrial structure is depicted in Figure 2-6. Each of the three classes or alleles of PapG has a different binding specificity for Gal-Gal globo-series glycolipids and contributes to tissue tropism.[72] Class II PapG is the most common allele in isolates from acute pyelonephritis and first-time cystitis patients. Class II binds to the Gal-Gal globoside GbO₄, which predominates in the upper urinary tract of humans.[73] The saccharides flanking GbO₄ have also been shown to be important for recognition, thus lending further specificity to the interaction.[74] The class III adhesin is frequently found on human cystitis isolates and rarely on pyelonephritis iso-

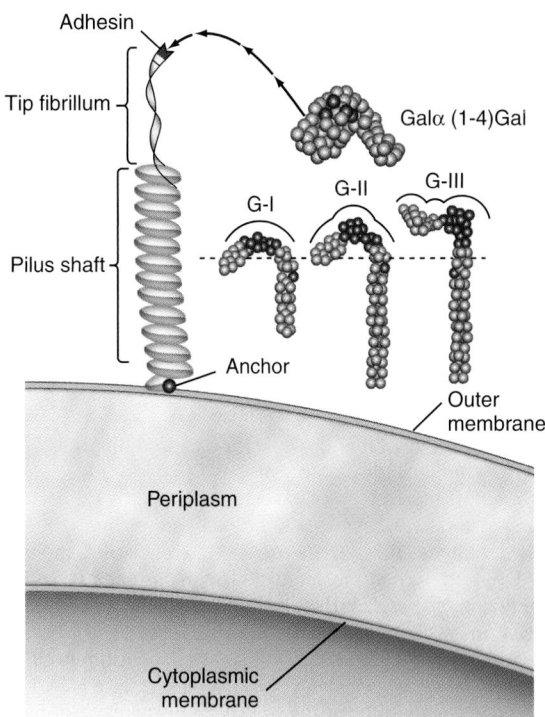

FIGURE 2-6. Model for the organization of P fimbriae subunits. Subunits PapG, F, E, and K constitute the fibrillar tip. The fimbrial rod is composed of *papA* and anchored in the membrane by PapH. See text for details. Subunits are not drawn to scale.

lates. Class III adhesin recognizes GbO₅, or Forssman's antigen, and globoA. Isolates with class III adhesin also frequently occur in secretor-positive individuals who carry globoA on their uroepithelial cells.[75]

P fimbriae undergo a type of phase variation in which an individual bacterium can turn on or off expression of the fimbrial genes. Consequently, within a clonal population, not all bacteria containing the P fimbrial genes will be expressing P fimbriae on their surface. The ability to control the expression of P fimbriae may be advantageous to the bacteria in that it may enable detachment and migration to different sites or provide a mechanism of antigenic variation to avoid recognition by the immune system.[76]

The central role of fimbriae in adherence to host cells makes them logical targets for antimicrobial therapy and vaccine development. Purified fimbriae have served as effective, well-established vaccines for veterinary use for a number of years. One of the first effective fimbrial vaccines was based on K-88 antigen, a fimbriae found on *E. coli* strains that cause diarrheal disease in pigs.[77] Immunization with fimbriae has been achieved using purified fimbriae,[77,78] recombinantly expressed fimbrial adhesin subunit,[79] and live-attenuated strains of *Shigella flexneri* and *Salmonella* that produce heterologous fimbriae or fimbrial subunits.[80,81] Fimbriae have also been engineered to present foreign epitopes. One example is an attenuated *Salmonella* strain engineered to produce a chimeric 987P fimbrial antigen that included epitopes of the transmissible gastroenteritis virus.[82]

Purified P fimbriae have been tested as protective antigens for humans in several animal models. Protection against pyelonephritis in monkeys has been achieved by immunization with purified P fimbriae. Protection was shown to correlate with a high titer of anti-P fimbrial antibodies.[78] Another study reports that PapG-mediated protection is dependent on the presence of a specific cognate receptor.[83] Primates immunized with P fimbriated *E. coli* bearing the class II PapG adhesin were protected against challenge. Immunization with strains of bacteria expressing P fimbriae that lacked PapG or carried a class III PapG allele (whose receptor is not present in the primate bladder) did not result in protective immunity even though these strains produced bladder infections similar to those produced by the wild type. Therefore the antigenic variation of P fimbriae and perhaps the requirement for the appropriate host ligand receptor will have to be considered in development of a broadly effective vaccine.

An alternative to receptor blockage as an antimicrobial treatment is receptor depletion. A glucose analogue and glycosphingolipid biosynthesis inhibitor, N-butyldeoxynojirimycin (NB-DNJ) has been used to deplete human uroepithelial cells and murine urinary tract mucosa of the Gal-Gal glycolipid receptor of P fimbriae.[84] NB-DNJ–treated mice showed reduced susceptibility to experimental UTIs, reduced chemokine secretion, and less neutrophil infiltration than untreated mice.

ADHESINS AND MICROBIAL SYNERGY

It has long been known that one infection can predispose to others. Although a complete discussion of the many possible causes of these microbial interactions is beyond the scope of this chapter, it can be said that altered expression or exposure of microbial receptors on host cells resulting in increased adherence of pathogens appears to be an important mechanism. The occurrence of secondary bacterial pneumonia after influenza infection is one of the most well recognized and well studied examples of microbial synergy, and it is the most common cause of excess mortality during an influenza epidemic.[85]

The usual explanation for the increased occurrence of bacterial pneumonia after influenza is that destruction of the respiratory mucosa exposes basement membrane proteins (e.g., fibrinogen) that bacteria bind. Autopsy studies from patients who died of nosocomial *Staphylococcus aureus* pneumonia during the 1957-1958 influenza pandemic revealed staphylococci adherent to denuded regions of respiratory epithelium.[86] Similarly, pneumococci adhere to exposed portions of basement membrane on tracheas removed from mice after challenge with influenza virus.[87] The inflammatory response to influenza may also alter receptors for bacterial pathogens in the respiratory tract. For example, phosphorylcholine on the surface of virulent pneumococci mediates binding to the platelet-activating factor receptor (PAFr).[88-90] In vitro treatment of endothelial cells with tumor necrosis factor-α or IL-1α increases pneumococcal adherence, an effect blocked by PAFr antagonists.[91] Finally, bacterial neuraminidases have been shown to increase adherence of pneumococci in vitro to tracheal, eustachian tube, and middle ear epithelium using chinchilla tissues.[92-94] Recent studies suggest that influenza viral neuraminidase may similarly degrade sialic acid in the lung, thereby exposing bacterial receptors and increasing bacterial adherence.[95] It remains to be determined if treatment of influenza with neuraminidase inhibitors can prevent secondary bacterial pneumonia, but in limited studies, early treatment of acute influenza has been associated with some reduced bacterial complications and antibiotic use.[96,97]

EXAMPLES OF ADHESINS AS TARGETS FOR THERAPY

Human Immunodeficiency Virus Entry Inhibitors

The critical events leading to attachment and entry of HIV into host cells (see earlier and Fig. 2-4) provide opportunities for preventive and therapeutic interventions, and indeed, HIV entry inhibitors are new classes of antiretroviral agents that have become available or are being developed (Table 2-6). These drugs fall into three classes (attachment inhibitors, chemokine/co-receptor inhibitors, and fusion inhibitors) and are too numerous for inclusive discussion here (see Chapter 124).[98,99] Some examples are briefly outlined here.

Drugs that block viral attachment by inhibiting the initial interaction of viral gp120 with CD4 include soluble CD4, antibody-derived therapies, and small molecule inhibitors that bind to gp120. Soluble CD4, tested in the late 1980s, was first. Despite potent in vitro antiviral activity, efficacy in clinical trials was poor.[100-102] PRO 542 (tetravalent CD4-IgG$_2$ fusion protein) is an antibody-derived HIV entry inhibitor containing four copies of the CD4 virus-binding domain.[103] Compared to monovalent and divalent CD4-based proteins, PRO 542 has as much as 100-fold greater activity against primary HIV-1 isolates and appears more promising in phase 1/2 clinical trials.[104,105] BMS-806, a small molecule that binds to the CD4 interacting region of gp120 and is a potent inhibitor of HIV replication in vitro, is another promising agent currently in clinical trials.[106] Although the peptide-based treatments described previously must be given by injection or infusion, many small molecules are orally bioavailable.

Unlike the attachment inhibitors that directly target the viral gp120 protein, chemokine/co-receptor inhibitors studied to date directly bind the host co-receptors CCR5 or CXCR4. Targeting these host receptors could theoretically result in intolerable toxicity. In addition, in vivo blockade of CCR5, the co-receptor used by most clinical isolates, could drive development of CXCR4-tropic strains that have been associated with more rapid clinical progression to AIDS. Mutants seen in vitro continue to utilize CCR5, suggesting that this may not occur.[107] The small molecule CXCR4 inhibitor AMD-3100 is an early example of drugs in this class. Although active in vitro, this agent caused prolongation of the QT interval in phase 1 trials and was not potent enough to warrant further study.[108] AMD-070, an orally bioavailable small molecule with potent in vitro activity, and others are currently under study. Agents targeting CCR5 include a monoclonal antibody (PRO-140) and the small molecule SCH-C.[109,110] All have potent antiretroviral activity in vitro, but SCH-C was associated with cardiac toxicity in phase 1 clinical trials, reemphasizing the risk of serious side effects with agents that target host receptors.

The greatest success to date has been achieved with agents that block viral fusion. Because the fusion inhibitors remain extracellular and interact with the viral gp41 protein rather than with host receptors, toxicity is limited. As described previously and in Figure 2-4, binding of HIV gp120 to CD4 induces conformational changes that enable interaction with the co-receptor (CCR5/CXCR4). Co-receptor binding results in exposure of the fusion peptide on gp41, which becomes in-

---

TABLE 2-6 Examples of Adhesin-Based Therapies

Organism	Drug	Mechanism/Target
Influenza A and B viruses	Neuraminidase inhibitors	May prevent release of virus and cell-to-cell spread by inhibiting the sialidase activity of viral neuraminidase
Human immunodeficiency virus	Soluble CD4, PRO 542	*Attachment inhibitors:* block initial interaction of viral gp120 with CD4
	AMD-3100, AMD-070, PRO-140, SCH-C	*Chemokine/co-receptor inhibitors:* directly bind CCR5 or CXCR4
	Enfuvirtide (T-20), T-1249, 5-helix	*Fusion inhibitors:* interact with gp41 helical regions; block gp41 folding and viral fusion
Picornaviruses (rhinoviruses, enteroviruses)	WIN compounds (pleconaril)	Bind VP1 protein with resultant conformational change in ICAM-1 binding site
P fimbriated *E. coli*	Cranberry juice (proanthocyanidins)	Inhibit binding to D-Gal-Gal moieties on uroepithelial cells

ICAM-1, intercellular adhesion molecule 1.

serted into the cell membrane. Interaction of two helical regions of gp41 (amino and carboxy) then results in folding of gp41, which pulls the viral and cellular membranes into proximity and enables fusion.[98] Enfuvirtide (T-20), a 36-amino-acid peptide derived from the carboxy-helical region of gp41 that binds to the amino-helical region and blocks folding, is the first clinically available drug in this class.[111] Phase 3 clinical trials in which enfuvirtide was added to an optimized antiviral regimen for heavily treatment-experienced patients demonstrated clinically significant virologic activity (0.932 log_{10} viral copies/mL difference in favor of enfuvirtide-containing treatment arms) after 24 weeks of therapy.[112] T-1249 peptide, which corresponds to a region of the carboxy-helical domain that overlaps T-20, also has potent activity against viral entry and is in phase 1/2 clinical trials. A third peptide inhibitor of HIV fusion, 5-helix, is derived from the amino-helical region and targets the carboxy-helical region of gp41. The use of peptides corresponding to different regions of gp41 should limit cross-resistance to members of this class. Combinations of entry inhibitors to block multiple steps in the attachment/fusion process should further limit development of resistance and may result in synergistic viral suppression. For example, a combination of T-20 and PRO 542 used in vitro resulted in a greater than 10-fold reduction in doses necessary to achieve viral suppression.[113]

Novel Antipicornaviral Drugs

Members of the picornavirus family, specifically the rhinoviruses and enteroviruses, are responsible for a major portion of human viral illnesses. At least 100 distinct rhinovirus serotypes cause the common cold, making development of a preventive vaccine impractical. Understanding the common features of attachment and unsheathing of these viruses on the molecular level, however, has enabled rational development of novel antipicornaviral drugs with broad activity for members of this family (see Table 2-6).[114]

The major receptor binding group of rhinoviruses (90% of isolates) uses the ICAM-1 receptor to attach to host cells.[115-117] As discussed earlier (and see Fig. 2-3), the ICAM-1 binding site is located in a protected canyon formed by the capsid binding proteins. The antiviral WIN compounds, the largest class of antirhinoviral agents studied, all bind to a hydrophobic pocket on the virion capsid protein VP1. Binding in this pocket results in a conformational change that raises the canyon floor and inhibits attachment to ICAM-1.[118] These agents also inhibit uncoating of virion RNA of the minor group rhinoviruses and polioviruses.[119,120] Crystallographic studies of the interaction of a large number of WIN compounds with major and minor group rhinoviruses, polioviruses, and coxsackievirus B3 have led to development of progressively more efficacious drugs.[121] Pleconaril (WIN 63843), an orally available third-generation WIN compound, inhibits replication of approximately 90% of rhinoviruses and enteroviruses and is the first antiviral to show efficacy for treatment of the common cold.[122,123] Pleconaril treatment significantly reduced the duration of cold symptoms (average of 1 day) in two randomized, double-blind, placebo-controlled phase 3 clinical trials.[123] However, a U.S. Food and Drug Administration review panel deemed the effect insufficiently profound and did not recommend approval of the drug. Treatment of adults and older children who have life-threatening enterovirus infections has been associated with reduced severity and duration of symptoms.[124]

Cranberry Juice for Prevention of Urinary Tract Infections

Cranberry juice or cranberry concentrate tablets reduce bacteriuria and recurrent UTIs in women by 12% to 20% compared with placebo.[125-127] Despite the results seen in initial studies, cranberry juice does not inhibit bacterial growth and has no effect on the pH of the urine. Rather, the positive effect of cranberry juice can be attributed to inhibition of bacterial adherence to the urinary tract epithelium. Sobota demonstrated that cranberry juice cocktail inhibited in vitro adherence to uroepithelial cells in greater than 60% of clinical *E. coli* isolates obtained from patients diagnosed with UTIs.[128] This work was extended to include clinical isolates of *E. coli, Proteus, Klebsiella, Enterobacter,* and *Pseudomonas.*[129] Cranberry juice cocktail contains at least two inhibitors of lectin-mediated adherence of uropathogens to uroepithelial cells. It inhibits adherence of *E. coli* isolates expressing type 1 fimbriae (mannose-specific) and P fimbriae (specific for α-D-Gal[1→4]-β-D-Gal).[130] A number of juices inhibit adherence of type 1 fimbriated *E. coli*, but the effect on P fimbriated *E. coli* is only seen with blueberry and cranberry juices.[130,131] Recent studies show that proanthocyanidins (condensed tannins) from cranberries appear to be the compounds in cranberries responsible for preventing uropathogenic P fimbriated *E. coli* from adhering to the urinary tract (see Table 2-6).[132]

MICROBIAL BIOFILMS

Many of the studies of bacterial adherence have been done on free-floating "planktonic" bacteria growing in culture. In nature, however, many bacteria exist in a complex community-like structure known as a biofilm. Biofilms are bacterial populations that are enclosed in a matrix of extracellular polymeric substances.[133] Bacteria form microcolonies with conelike and mushroom-shaped morphologies by adhering to each other and to a surface. Water-filled channels surround the microcolonies and function somewhat like a primitive circulatory system, allowing access to nutrients, elimination of wastes, and interbacterial communication. In industrial settings, biofilms are responsible for fouling storage tanks and clogging water pipes. In the medical arena, biofilms are seen in native valve endocarditis, otitis media, and dental plaque, and they are a problem for cystic fibrosis patients.[133,134] Biofilms also form on synthetic medical implants, including intravascular catheters, artificial valves, pacemakers, orthopedic devices, and contact lenses.[133,134] Table 2-7 lists microorganisms that are commonly associated with indwelling medical devices.

One of the characteristics of biofilms that is of concern to the medical community is increased resistance to antibiotics. Bacterial biofilms have been reported to be up to 500 times more resistant to antibiotics than planktonic cells.[133-135] There are several properties of biofilms that could contribute to increased resistance to antibiotics. The exopolysaccharide matrix, or "slime," that surrounds the cells

---

TABLE 2-7 Biofilm-Associated Microorganisms Isolated from Indwelling Medical Devices

Indwelling Medical Device	*Organisms*
Central venous catheter	Coagulase-negative staphylococci, *Staphylococcus aureus, Enterococcus faecalis, Klebsiella pneumoniae, Pseudomonas aeruginosa, Candida albicans*
Prosthetic heart valve	Viridans streptococci, coagulase-negative staphylococci, enterococci, *S. aureus*
Urinary catheter	*Staphylococcus epidermidis, Escherichia coli, K. pneumoniae, E. faecalis, Proteus mirabilis*
Artificial hip prosthesis	Coagulase-negative staphylococci, hemolytic streptococci, enterococci, *P. mirabilis, Bacteroides* species, *S. aureus*, viridans streptococci, *E. coli, P. aeruginosa*
Artificial valve prosthesis	*C. albicans, Streptococcus mitis, Streptococcus salivarius, Rothia dentrocariosa, Candida tropicalis, Streptococcus sobrinus, S. epidermidis, Stomatococcus mucilaginous*
Intrauterine device	*S. epidermidis, Corynebacterium* species, *S. aureus, Micrococcus* species, *Lactobacillus plantarum*, group B streptococci, *Enterococcus* species, *C. albicans*

Reprinted from Donlan RM. Biofilm formation: A clinically relevant process. Clin Inf Dis. 2001;33:1387-1392, with permission.

may create an exclusion barrier to antimicrobials or directly complex with these agents to inactive them. Bacteria in biofilms grow more slowly, and slower growth may lead to decreased uptake of the drug and other physiologic changes that could affect drug effectiveness.

Biofilms are formed in two phases.[133] The first phase is an initial, reversible adherence to a surface. Several factors are thought to contribute to this initial adherence, including surface hydrophobicity, proteinaceous adhesins, and capsular polysaccharides. The second phase involves intercellular adhesion, which results in microcolony formation and the complex biofilm architecture. In *Pseudomonas aeruginosa*, pili and flagella have been shown to be important in biofilm formations.[136] Strains lacking flagella appear to be unable to establish initial adherence to a substrate, whereas the pili-minus bacteria are defective at the second stage of microcolony formation. Elucidation of the molecular mechanisms of biofilm formation should identify new targets for chemotherapy and provide new approaches to controlling the formation of biofilms.

REFERENCES

1. Fingeroth JD, Weiss JJ, Tedder TF, et al. Epstein-Barr virus receptor of human B lymphocytes is the C3d receptor CR2. Proc Natl Acad Sci U S A. 1984;81:4510-4514.
2. Dalgleish AG, Beverley PC, Clapham PR, et al. The CD4 (T4) antigen is an essential component of the receptor for the AIDS retrovirus. Nature. 1984;312:763-767.
3. Klatzmann D, Champagne E, Chamaret S, et al. T lymphocyte T4 molecule behaves as the receptor for human retrovirus LAV. Nature. 1984;312:767-768.
4. Delmas B, Gelfi J, L'Haridon R, et al. Aminopeptidase N is a major receptor for the enteropathogenic coronavirus TGEV. Nature. 1992;357:417-420.
5. Yeager CL, Ashmun RA, Williams RK, et al. Human aminopeptidase N is a receptor for human coronavirus 229E. Nature. 1992;357:420-422.
6. Mendelsohn CL, Wimmer E, Racaniello VR. Cellular receptor for poliovirus: Molecular cloning, nucleotide sequence, and expression of a new member of the immunoglobulin superfamily. Cell. 1989;56:855-865.
7. Koike S, Horie H, Ise I, et al. The poliovirus receptor protein is produced both as membrane-bound and secreted forms. EMBO J. 1990;9:3217-3224.
8. Tomassini JE, Colonno RJ. Isolation of a receptor protein involved in attachment of human rhinoviruses. J Virol. 1986;58:290-295.
9. Greve JM, Davis G, Meyer AM, et al. The major human rhinovirus receptor is ICAM-1. Cell. 1989;56:839-847.
10. Staunton DE, Merluzzi VJ, Rothlein R, et al. A cell adhesion molecule, ICAM-1, is the major surface receptor for rhinoviruses. Cell. 1989;56:849-853.
11. Bergelson JM, Shepley MP, Chan BMC, et al. Identification of the integrin VLA-2 as a receptor for echovirus 1. Science. 1992;255:1718-1720.
12. Wiley DC, Skehel JJ. The structure and function of the hemagglutinin membrane glycoprotein of influenza virus. Annu Rev Biochem. 1989;56:365.
13. Rossman MG, Arnold E, Erickson JW, et al. The structure of a human common cold virus (rhinovirus 14) and its functional relations to other picornaviruses. Nature. 1985;317:145-153.
14. Altieri DC, Edginton TS. A monoclonal antibody reacting with distinct adhesion molecules defines a transition in the functional state of the receptor CD11b/CD18 (Mac-1). J Immunol. 1988;141:2656.
15. Dustin ML, Springer TA. T cell receptor cross-linking transiently stimulates adhesiveness through LFA-1. Nature. 1989;341:619.
16. Flynn DC, Meyer WJ, MacKenzie JM Jr, et al. A conformational change in Sindbis virus glycoprotein E1 and E2 is detected at the plasma membrane as a consequence of early virus-cell interaction. J Virol. 1990;64:3643-3653.
17. Wahlberg JM, Garoff H. Membrane fusion process of Semliki forest virus I: Low pH-induced rearrangement in spike protein quaternary structure precedes virus penetration into cells. J Cell Biol. 1992;116:339-348.
18. Halstead SB. Pathogenesis of dengue: Challenges to molecular biology. Science. 1988;239:476-481.
19. Sixbey JW, Yao QY. Immunoglobulin A induced shift of Epstein-Barr virus tissue tropism. Science. 1992;255:1578-1580.
20. Wei X, Decker JM, Wang S, et al. Antibody neutralization and escape by HIV-1. Nature. 2003;422:307-313.
21. Kilby JM, Eron JJ. Novel therapies based on mechanisms of HIV-1 cell entry. N Engl J Med. 2003;348:2228-2238.
22. White J, Kielian M, Helenius A. Membrane fusion proteins of enveloped animal viruses. Q Rev Biophys. 1983;16:151-195.
23. Nara PL, Garrity RR, Goudsmit J. Neutralization of HIV-1: A paradox of humoral proportions. FASEB J. 1991;5:2437-2455.
24. Wain-Hobson S. One on one meets two. Nature. 1996;384:117-118.
25. Hallenberger S, Bosch V, Angliker H, et al. Inhibition of furin-mediated cleavage activation of HIV-1 glycoprotein gp160. Nature. 1992;360:358-361.
26. Freed EO, Myers DJ, Risser R. Mutational analysis of the cleavage sequence of the human immunodeficiency virus type 1 envelope glycoprotein precursor gp160. J Virol. 1989;63:4670-4675.
27. Harouse JM, Bhat S, Spitalnik SL, et al. Inhibition of entry of HIV-1 in neural cells by antibodies against galactosyl ceramide. Science. 1991;253:320-323.
28. Feng Y, Broder CC, Kennedy PE, Berger EA. HIV-1 entry co-factor: Functional cDNA cloning of a seven-transmembrane G protein-coupled receptor. Science. 1996;272:872-877.
29. Fauci AS. Host factors and the pathogenesis of HIV-induced disease. Nature. 1996;384:529-534.
30. Maddon PJ, Dalgleish AG, McDougal JS, et al. The T4 gene encodes the AIDS virus receptor and is expressed in the immune system and brain. Cell. 1986;47:333.
31. Safrit JT, Fung MSC, Andrews CA, et al. hu-PBL-SCID mice can be protected from HIV-1 infection by passive transfer of monoclonal antibody to the principal neutralizing determinant of envelope gp120. AIDS. 1993;7:15-21.
32. Hwang SS, Boyle TJ, Lyerly HK, et al. Identification of the envelope V3 loop as the primary determinant of cell tropism in HIV-1. Science. 1991;253:71-74.
33. Hwang SS, Boyle TJ, Lyerly HK, et al. Identification of the envelope V3 loop as the major determinant of CD4 neutralization sensitivity of HIV-1. Science. 1992;257:535-537.
34. Shioda T, Levy JA, Cheng-Mayer C. Macrophage and T cell tropisms of HIV-1 are determined by specific regions of the envelope gp120 gene. Nature. 1991;349:167-169.
35. Page KA, Stearns SM, Littman DR. Analysis of mutations in the V3 domain of gp160 that affect fusion and infectivity. J Virol. 1992;66:524-533.
36. Jiang S, Lin K, Neurath AR. Enhancement of human immunodeficiency virus type 1 infection by antisera to peptides from the envelope glycoproteins gp120/gp41. J Exp Med. 1991;174:1557-1563.
37. Tremblay M, Meloche S, Sekaly RP, et al. Complement receptor 2 mediates enhancement of human immunodeficiency virus 1 infection in Epstein-Barr virus carrying B cells. J Exp Med. 1990;171:1791-1796.
38. Haque R, Huston CD, Hughes M, et al. Current concepts: Amebiasis. N Engl J Med. 2003;348:1565-1573.
39. Ravdin JI, Croft BY, Guerrant RL. Cytopathogenic mechanisms of *Entamoeba histolytica*. J Exp Med. 1980; 152:377-390.
40. Petri WA Jr, Mann BJ, Haque R. The bittersweet interface of parasite and host: Lectin-carbohydrate interactions during human invasion by the parasite *Entamoeba histolytica*. Annu Rev Microbiol. 2002;56:39-64.
41. Chadee K, Petri WA Jr, Innes DJ, Ravdin JI. Rat and human colonic mucins bind to and inhibit the adherence lectin of *Entamoeba histolytica*. J Clin Invest. 1987;80:1245-1254.
42. Li E, Becker A, Stanley SL. Use of Chinese hamster ovary cells with altered glycosylation patterns to define the carbohydrate specificity of *Entamoeba histolytica* adhesion. J Exp Med. 1988;167:1725-1730.
43. Ravdin JI, Stanley P, Murphy CF, Petri WA Jr. Characterization of cell surface carbohydrate receptors for *Entamoeba histolytica* adherence lectin. Infect Immun. 1989;57:2179-2186.
44. Petri WA Jr, Smith RD, Schlesinger PH, et al. Isolation of the galactose binding adherence lectin of *Entamoeba histolytica*. J Clin Invest. 1987;80:1238-1244.
45. Vines RR, Ramakrishnan G, Rogers J, et al. Regulation of adherence and virulence by the *Entamoeba histolytica* lectin cytoplasmic domain, which contains a beta2 integrin motif. Molec Biol Cell. 1998;9:2069-2079.
46. Cheng XJ, Tsukamoto H, Kaneda Y, Tachibana H. Identification of the 150 kDa surface antigen of *Entamoeba histolytica* as a galactose- and *N*-acetyl-D-galactosamine-inhibitable lectin. Parasitol Res. 1998;84:632-639.
47. Huston CD, Miller-Sims V, Petri WA Jr. Apoptotic killing and phagocytosis of host cells by the parasite *Entamoeba histolytica*. Infect Immun. 2003;71:964-972.
48. Coppi A, Eichinger D. Regulation of *Entamoeba invadens* encystation and gene expression with galactose and *N*-acetylglucosamine. Molec Biochem Parasitol. 1999;102:67-77.
49. Beck DL, Tanyuksel M, Mackey A, et al. Sequence conservation of the Gal/GalNAc lectin from clinical isolates. Exp Parasitol. 2002;101:157-163.
50. Haque R, Duggal P, Ali IM, et al. Innate and acquired resistance to amebiasis in Bangladeshi children. J Infect Dis. 2002;186:547-552.
51. Houpt E, Barroso L, Lockhart L, et al. Prevention of intestinal amebiasis by vaccination with the *Entamoeba histolytica* Gal/GalNAc lectin. Vaccine. 2004;22:612-618.
52. Thanassi DG, Hultgren SJ. Assembly of complex organelles: pilus biogenesis in gram-negative bacteria as a model system. Methods. 2000;20:111-126.
53. Wullt B, Bergsten G, Samuelsson M, et al. The role of P fimbriae for *Escherichia coli* establishment and mucosal inflammation in the human urinary tract. Int J Antimicrob Agents. 2002;19:522-538.
54. Silverman M, Simon MI. Bacterial flagella. Annu Rev Microbiol. 1977;31:397-419.
55. Kallenius G, Svenson SB, Hultberg H, et al. Occurrence of P fimbriated *Escherichia coli* in urinary tract infection. Lancet. 1981;2:1369-1372.
56. Latham RH, Stamm WE. Role of fimbriated *Escherichia coli* in urinary tract infections in adult women: Correlation with localization studies. J Infect Dis. 1984;149:835-840.
57. Svanborg-Eden C, Eriksson B, Hanson LA, et al. Adhesion to normal human uroepithelial cells of *Escherichia coli* from children with various forms of urinary tract infection. J Pediatr. 1978;93:398-403.
58. O'Hanley P, Low D, Romero I, et al. Gal-Gal binding and hemolysin phenotypes and genotypes associated with uropathogenic *Escherichia coli*. N Engl J Med. 1985;313:414-420.
59. Brauner A, Leissner M, Wretlind B, et al. Occurrence of P-fimbriated *Escherichia coli* in patients with bacteremia. Eur J Clin Microbiol. 1985;4:566-569.
60. Johnson JR, Roberts PL, Stamm WE. P fimbriae and other virulence factors in *Escherichia coli* urosepsis: Association with patients' characteristics. J Infect Dis. 1987;156:225-229.
61. Otto G, Sandberg T, Marklund BI, et al. Virulence factors and pap genotype in *Escherichia coli* isolates from women with acute pyelonephritis, with or without bacteremia. Clin Infect Dis. 1993;17:448-456.

62. Kallenius G, Mollby R, Svenson SB, et al. The p^k antigen as receptor for the haemagglutinin of pyelonephritic *Escherichia coli* strains. FEMS Microbiol Lett. 1980;7:297-302.

63. Leffler H, Svanborg-Eden C. Chemical identification of glycosphingolipid receptor for *Escherichia coli* attaching to human urinary tract epithelial cells and agglutinating human erythrocytes. FEMS Microbiol Lett. 1980;8:127-134.

64. Svanborg-Eden C, Freter R, Hagberg L, et al. Inhibition of experimental ascending urinary tract infection by an epithelial cell-surface receptor analogue. Nature. 1982;298:560-562.

65. Lomberg H, Eden CS. Influence of P blood group phenotype on susceptibility to urinary tract infection. FEMS Microbiol Immunol. 1989;1:363-370.

66. Wullt B, Bergsten G, Connell H, et al. P fimbriae enhance the early establishment of *Escherichia coli* in the human urinary tract. Mol Microbiol. 2000;38:456-464.

67. Wullt B, Bergsten G, Connell H, et al. P-fimbriae trigger mucosal responses to *Escherichia coli* in the human urinary tract. Cell Microbiol. 2001;3:255-264.

68. Frendeus B, Wachtler C, Hedlund M, et al. *Escherichia coli* P fimbriae utilize the toll-like receptor 4 pathway for cell activation. Mol Microbiol. 2001;40:37-51.

69. Kuehn MJ, Heuser J, Normark S, et al. P pili in uropathogenic *E. coli* are composite fibres with distinct fibrillar adhesive tips. Nature. 1992;356:252-255.

70. Lindberg F, Lund B, Johansson L, et al. Localization of the receptor-binding protein adhesin at the tip of the bacterial pilus. Nature. 1987;328:84-87.

71. Lund B, Lindberg F, Marklund BI, et al. The PapG protein is the α-D-galactopyranosyl-(1-4)-β-D-galactopyranose-binding adhesin of uropathogenic *Escherichia coli*. Proc Natl Acad Sci U S A. 1987;84:5898-5902.

72. Stromberg N, Nyholm P-G, Pashcer I, et al. Saccharide orientation at the cell surface affects glycolipid receptor function. Proc Natl Acad Sci U S A. 1991;88:9340-9344.

73. Johanson I-M, Plos K, Marklund BI, et al. *Pap, papG* and *prsG* DNA sequences in *Escherichia coli* from the fecal flora and the urinary tract. Microb Pathog. 1993;15:121-129.

74. Striker R, Nilsson U, Stonecipher A, et al. Structural requirements for the glycolipid receptor of human uropathogenic *Escherichia coli*. Mol Microbiol. 1995;16:1021-1029.

75. Lindstedt R, Larson G, Falk P, et al. The receptor repertoire defines the host range for attaching *Escherichia coli* strains that recognize globo-A. Infect Immun. 1991;59:1086-1092.

76. van der Woude M, Braaten B, Low D. Epigenetic phase variation of the *pap* operon in *Escherichia coli*. Trends Microbiol. 1996;4:5-9

77. Greenwood PE, Clark SJ, Cahill AD, et al. Development and protective efficacy of a recombinant-DNA derived fimbrial vaccine against enterotoxic colibacillosis in neonatal piglets. Vaccine. 1988;6:389-392.

78. Roberts J, Hardaway K, Kaack B, et al. Prevention of pyelonephritis by immunization with P-fimbriae. J Urol. 1984;131:602-607.

79. Langermann S, Mollby R, Burlein JE, et al. Vaccination with FimH adhesin protects cynomolgus monkeys from colonization and infection by uropathogenic *Escherichia coli*. J Infect Dis. 2000;181:774-778.

80. Ascon MA, Hone DM, Walters N, et al. Oral immunization with a *Salmonella typhimurium* vaccine vector expressing recombinant enterotoxigenic *Escherichia coli* K99 fimbriae elicits elevated antibody titers for protective immunity. Infect Immun. 1998;66:5470-5476.

81. Altboum Z, Barry EM, Losonsky G, et al. Attenuated *Shigella flexneri* 2a Delta guaBA strain CVD 1204 expressing enterotoxigenic *Escherichia coli* (ETEC) CS2 and CS3 fimbriae as a live mucosal vaccine against *Shigella* and ETEC infection. Infect Immun. 2001;69:3150-3158.

82. Chen H, Schifferli DM. Enhanced immune responses to viral epitopes by combining macrophage-inducible expression with multimeric display on a *Salmonella* vector. Vaccine. 2001;19:3009-3018.

83. Soderhill M, Normark S, Ishikawa K, et al. Induction of protective immunity after *Escherichia coli* bladder infection in primates. J Clin Invest. 1997;100:364-372.

84. Svensson M, Frendeus B, Butters T, et al. Glycolipid depletion in antimicrobial therapy. Mol Microbiol. 2003;47:453-461.

85. Glazen WP, Payne AA, Snyder DN, et al. Mortality and influenza. J Infect Dis. 1982;146:313-321.

86. Hers JFP, Masurel N, Mulder J. Bacteriology and histopathology of the respiratory tract and lungs of fatal Asian influenza. Lancet. 1958;2:1164-1165.

87. Plotkowski MC, Puchelle E, Beck G, et al. Adherence of type I *Streptococcus pneumoniae* to tracheal epithelium of mice infected with influenza A/PR8 virus. Am Rev Respir Dis. 1986;134:1040-1044.

88. Cundell DR, Gerard NP, Gerard C, et al. PAF receptor anchors *Streptococcus pneumoniae* to activated human endothelial cells. Adv Exp Med Biol. 1996;416:89-94.

89. Ishizuka S, Yamaya M, Suzuki T, et al. Acid exposure stimulates the adherence of *Streptococcus pneumoniae* to cultured human airway epithelial cells: Effects on platelet-activating factor receptor expression. Am J Respir Cell Mol Biol. 2001;24:459-468.

90. Toumanen EI. The biology of pneumococcal infection. Pediatr Res. 1997;42:253-258.

91. Cundell DR, Gerard NP, Gerard C, et al. *Streptococcus pneumoniae* anchor to activated human cells by the receptor for platelet-activating factor. Nature. 1995;377:435-438.

92. Tong HH, McIver MA, Fisher LM, et al. Effect of lacto-*N*-neotetraose, asialoganglioside-GM1 and neuraminidase on adherence and otitis media-associated serotypes of *Streptococcus pneumoniae* to chinchilla tracheal epithelium. Microb Pathog. 1999;26:111-119.

93. LaMarco KL, Diven WF, Glew RH. Experimental alteration of chinchilla middle ear mucosae by bacterial neuraminidase. Ann Otol Rhinol Laryngol. 1986;95:304-308.

94. Linder TE, Lim DJ, DeMaria TF. Changes in the structure of the cell surface carbohydrates of the chinchilla tubotympanum following *Streptococcus pneumoniae*-induced otitis media. Microb Pathog. 1992;13:293-303.

95. McCullers JA, Bartmess KC. Role of neuraminidase in lethal synergism between influenza virus and *Streptococcus pneumoniae*. J Infect Dis. 2003;187:1000-1009.

96. Treanor JJ, Hayden FG, Vrooman PS, et al. Efficacy and safety of the oral neuraminidase inhibitor oseltamivir in treating acute influenza: A randomized controlled trial. U.S. Oral Neuraminidase Study Group. JAMA. 2000;283:1016-1024.

97. Whitley RJ, Hayden FG, Reisinger KS, et al. Oral oseltamivir treatment of influenza in children. Pediatr Infect Dis J. 2001;20:127-133.

98. Doms RW, Trono D. The plasma membrane as a combat zone in the HIV battlefield. Genes Dev. 2000;14:2677-2688.

99. O'Brien WA. New classes of HIV drugs on the horizon. AIDS Read. 2003;13:s4-s8.

100. Kahn JO, Allan JD, Hodges TL, et al. The safety and pharmacokinetics of recombinant soluble CD4 (rCD4) in subjects with the acquired immunodeficiency syndrome (AIDS) and AIDS-related complex: A phase 1 study. Ann Intern Med. 1990;112:254-261.

101. Schooley RT, Merigan TC, Gaut P, et al. Recombinant soluble CD4 therapy in patients with the acquired immunodeficiency syndrome (AIDS) and AIDS-related complex: A phase I-II escalating dosage trial. Ann Intern Med. 1990;112:247-253.

102. Schacker T, Coombs RW, Collier AC, et al. The effects of high-dose recombinant soluble CD4 on human immunodeficiency virus type 1 viremia. J Infect Dis. 1994;169:37-40.

103. Allaway GP, Davis-Bruno KL, Beaudry GA, et al. Expression and characterization of CD4-IgG2, a novel heterotetramer which neutralizes primary HIV-1 isolates. AIDS Res Hum Retroviruses. 1995;11:533-539.

104. Jacobson JM, Lowy I, Fletcher CV, et al. Single-dose safety, pharmacology, and antiviral activity of the human immunodeficiency virus (HIV) type 1 entry inhibitor PRO 542 in HIV-infected adults. J Infect Dis. 2000;182:326-329.

105. Shearer WT, Israel RJ, Starr S, et al. Recombinant CD4-IgG2 in human immunodeficiency virus type 1-infected children: Phase 1/2 study. J Infect Dis. 2000;182:1774-1779.

106. Stephenson J. Researchers explore new anti-HIV agents. JAMA. 2002;287:1635-1637.

107. Trkola A, Kuhmann SE, Strizki JM, et al. HIV-1 escape from a small molecule, CCR5-specific entry inhibitor does not involve CXCR4 use. Proc Natl Acad Sci U S A. 2002;99:395-400.

108. Hendrix CW, Flexner C, MacFarland RT, et al. Pharmacokinetics and safety of AMD-3100, a novel antagonist of the CXCR-4 chemokine receptor, in human volunteers. Antimicrob Agents Chemother. 2000;44:1667-1673.

109. Trkola A, Ketas TJ, Nagashima KA, et al. Potent, broad-spectrum inhibition of human immunodeficiency virus type 1 by the CCR5 monoclonal antibody PRO 140. J Virol. 2001;75:579-588.

110. Strizki JM, Xu S, Wagner NE, et al. SCH-C (SCH 351125), an orally bioavailable, small molecule antagonist of the chemokine receptor CCR5, is a potent inhibitor of HIV-1 infection in vitro and in vivo. Proc Natl Acad Sci U S A. 2001;98:12718-12723.

111. Wild CT, Shugars DC, Greenwell TK, et al. Peptides corresponding to a predictive alpha-helical domain of human immunodeficiency virus type 1 gp 41 are potent inhibitors of virus infection. Proc Natl Acad Sci U S A. 1994;91:9770-9774.

112. Lalezari JP, Henry K, O'Hearn M, et al. Enfuvirtide, an HIV-1 fusion inhibitor, for drug-resistant HIV infection in North and South America. N Engl J Med. 2003;348:2175-2185.

113. Nagashima KA, Thompson DAD, Rosenfield SI, et al. Human immunodeficiency virus type 1 entry inhibitors PRO 542 and T-20 are potently synergistic in blocking virus-cell and cell-cell fusion. J Infect Dis. 2001;183:1121-1125.

114. McKinlay MA, Pevear DC. Treatment of the picornavirus common cold by inhibitors of viral uncoating and attachment. Annu Rev Microbiol. 1992;46:635-654.

115. Greve JM, Davis G, Meyer AM, et al. The major human rhinovirus receptor is ICAM-1. Cell. 1989;56:839-847.

116. Staunton DE, Merluzzi VJ, Rothlein R, et al. A cell adhesion molecule, ICAM-1, is the major receptor for rhinoviruses. Cell. 1989;56:849-853.

117. Tomassini JE, Graham D, DeWitt CM, et al. cDNA cloning reveals that the major group rhinovirus receptor on HeLa cells is intracellular adhesion molecule-1. Proc Natl Acad Sci U S A. 1989;86:4907-4911.

118. Pevear DC, Fancher MJ, Felock PJ, et al. Conformational change in the floor of the human rhinovirus canyon blocks adsorption to HeLa cell receptors. J Virol. 1989;63:2002-2007.

119. Fox MP, Otto MJ, McKinlay MA. The prevention of rhinovirus and poliovirus uncoating by WIN 51711: A new antiviral drug. Antimicrob Agents Chemother. 1986;30:110-116.

120. Zeichhardt H, Otto MJ, McKinlay MA, et al. Inhibition of poliovirus uncoating by disoxaril (WIN 51711). Virology. 1987;160:281-285.

121. Hadfield AT, Diana GD, Rossmann MG. Analysis of three structurally related antiviral compounds in complex with human rhinovirus 16. Proc Natl Acad Sci U S A. 1999;96:14730-14735.

122. Pevear DC, Tull TM, Seipel ME, et al. Activity of pleconaril against enteroviruses. Antimicrob Agents Chemother. 1999;43:2109-2115.

123. Hayden FG, Herrington DT, Coats TL, et al. Efficacy and safety of oral pleconaril for treatment of colds due to picornaviruses in adults: Results of 2 double-blind, randomized, placebo-controlled trials. Clin Infect Dis. 2003;36:1523-1532.

124. Rotbart HA, Webster AD. Treatment of potentially life-threatening enterovirus infections with pleconaril. Clin Infect Dis. 2001;32:228-235.

125. Avorn J, Monane M, Gurwitz JH, et al. Reduction of bacteriuria and pyuria after ingestion of cranberry juice. JAMA. 1994;271:751-754.

126. Kontiokari T, Sundqvist K, Nuutinen M, et al. Randomised trial of cranberry-lingonberry juice and lactobacillus GG drink for the prevention of urinary tract infections in women. BMJ. 2001;322:1571-1573.

127. Stothers L. A randomized trial to evaluate effectiveness and cost effectiveness of naturopathic cranberry products as prophylaxis against urinary tract infection in women. Can J Urol. 2002;9:1558-1562.

128. Sobota AE. Inhibition of bacterial adherence by cranberry juice: Potential use for the treatment of urinary tract infections. J Urol. 1984;131:1013-1016.

129. Schmidt DR, Sobota AE. An examination of the anti-adherence activity of cranberry juice on urinary and nonurinary bacterial isolates. Microbios. 1988;55:173-181.

130. Zafriri D, Ofek I, Adar R, et al. Inhibitory activity of cranberry juice on adherence of type 1 and type P fimbriated *Escherichia coli* to eucaryotic cells. Antimicrob Agents Chemother. 1989;33:92-98.

131. Ofek I, Goldhar J, Zafriri D. Anti-*Escherichia coli* adhesion activity of cranberry and blueberry juices. N Engl J Med. 1991;324:1599.

132. Howell AB, Vorsa N, Marderosian AD, et al. Inhibition of the adherence of P-fimbriated *Escherichia coli* to uroepithelial-cell surfaces by proanthocyanidin extracts from cranberries. N Engl J Med. 1998;339:1085-1086.

133. Donlan RM, Costerton JW. Biofilms: Survival mechanisms of clinically relevant microorganisms. Clin Microbiol Rev. 2002;15:167-193.

134. Donlan RM. Biofilm formation: A clinically relevant microbiological process. Clin Infect Dis. 2001;33:1387-1392.

135. Gander S. Bacterial biofilms: Resistance to antimicrobial agents. J Antimicrob Chemother. 1996;37:1047-1050.

136. O'Toole GA, Kolter R. Flagellar and twitching motility are necessary for *Pseudomonas aeruginosa* biofilm development. Mol Microbiol. 1998;30:295-304.

CHAPTER **3**

Toxins

ERIK L. HEWLETT

MOLLY A. HUGHES

CLASSIFICATION OF TOXINS

The word *toxin* is derived from the Greek *toxikon*, or "bow poison," and refers to poisonous material placed on arrows by Greek warriors. The implication of this choice of terms for microbial pathogenesis is that the responsible microorganism produces a molecule that it "releases" to affect target cells at a distance. The term was first used by Roux and Yersin to describe a factor released into the culture medium by *Corynebacterium diphtheriae* that caused the death of recipient animals.[1,2] The concept of microbial toxins now requires reexamination, particularly in light of data from the sequencing of the genomes of multiple pathogens and the development of microbial pathogenesis as a discipline. Although in the broadest sense, any material (natural or manufactured) that causes adverse effects to cells or organisms could be considered a toxin, in the present context, this term refers to molecules (predominantly proteins) that are produced by microbes, including bacteria, parasites, fungi, and viruses. This family of microbial products can be categorized in a number of different ways (Table 3-1), including (1) chemical composition (e.g., protein, lipid, lipopolysaccharide), (2) cellular or tissue target of action (i.e., enterotoxins, neurotoxins, leukotoxins), (3) mechanism of action (proteolytic toxins, adenosine diphosphate [ADP]-ribosylating toxins, adenylate cyclase toxins; deamidating toxins), (4) intracellular target molecule (small-molecular-weight G proteins such as Rho or heterotrimeric G proteins, such as G_s or G_i), (5) major biologic effect (dermonecrotic toxin, edema-producing toxin, hemolytic toxin, lymphocytosis-promoting toxin), and (6) the organisms that produce them (pertussis toxin, cholera toxin). Quite clearly, the difficulties associated with describing and classifying these bacterial products reflect limitations in knowledge of their production, target cell interaction, mechanism of action, and clinical significance. The use of powerful investigative techniques provided by genomic and proteomic analyses in combination with cellular and molecular biology has resulted in a dramatic increase in the quantity and quality of information on bacterial toxins. These developments include the discovery of new toxins, determination of the amino acid sequence and crystal structure of many toxins, elucidation of molecular mechanisms of action and identification of new

functions for known toxins, and recognition of family relationships among apparently disparate molecules.[3-6]

It is also clear that the pathogenic process is complex and represents a well-orchestrated sequence of events in which many microbial components play a part, even for diseases that are classically considered to be primarily toxin mediated. These diverse microbial products allow the pathogen access to the appropriate site in the host, provide a means for environmental signals to be transmitted to the bacterium to indicate that the conditions are right for expression of toxins and other virulence determinants, and protect the microbe against clearance by host defenses. The development of microbial pathogenesis as a distinct discipline and the availability of bacterial genome sequences have facilitated the identification of additional virulence factors involved in the activities required for production of infection and disease (see Chapters 1 and 2).[7-11] Many microorganisms produce an additional set of toxins (i.e., colicins) that are directed at other microbes and do not affect eukaryotic cells.[12] Although fascinating in structure and mechanism of action, these molecules are not within the scope of this chapter.

Many of the molecules fitting the definition of toxin are enzymes with very specific intracellular targets within host cells, and a general structural model to which a number of these exotoxins conform has been elaborated. According to the A-B model described by Gill, each of these toxins is composed of a binding (B) domain, component, or subunit and an enzymatic (A or "active") domain or subunit that catalyzes the reaction that is responsible for the effects of the toxin.[13] Isolated A subunits are enzymatically active but lack binding and cell entry capability and thus have no biologic activity (the ability to intoxicate intact cells). Isolated B subunits may bind to target cells and even block the action of holotoxin, but they are, in most instances, nontoxic and biologically inactive. It is now clear, however, that there are exceptions to this model and, although generally applicable and useful as a concept, one should not be limited by this model when investigating a new toxin. For example, isolated B subunits from an increasing number of toxins, such as pertussis toxin, cholera toxin, and heat-labile enterotoxin, and even alpha hemolysin from *Escherichia coli*, elicit biologic effects simply by interacting with receptors on the surface of target cells.[14-16] This phenomenon appears to arise when the molecule to which the toxin binds is a receptor for some hormone or other endogenous signaling agent, and when it is usurped by the toxin for binding and cell entry, the signaling cascade to which it is linked is activated by the foreign ligand or bacterial toxin. Specific examples of B-subunit activities are noted in the discussion of toxins to which this concept is relevant.

Another exception to the A-B model came with discovery of the type III secretion system (see later). Enzymes that seemed similar to isolated A subunits for known toxins were found in the culture medium of gram-negative organisms (such as *Pseudomonas aeruginosa* and *Yersinia pestis*) but were unable to enter target cells or elicit biologic effects because they were lacking a B-subunit domain. The explanation is that these molecules are "injected" into the host cell through the type III secretion apparatus and thus do not require a binding component; apparently, some material is leaked into the medium and is the source of the observed extracellular enzymatic activity.[17]

CONTROL OF SYNTHESIS AND RELEASE OF TOXINS

Molecular biologic approaches have revealed an unanticipated level of complexity in the regulation of microbial virulence, including toxin production and secretion.[7,18] Synthesis of many bacterial toxins and other virulence factors is tightly controlled by regulatory systems that are responsive to environmental conditions (see Chapter 1). For example, the production of diphtheria toxin is virtually eliminated by the presence of iron in the medium, virulence gene expression in *Yersinia* is repressed by calcium, and the expression of cholera toxin and associated virulence factors is controlled by environmental osmolarity.[19-22] In many cases, two-component, environment-sensing systems are responsible for coordinated control of the expression of a group of toxins and virulence factors in a regulon and allow their concurrent production during a particular phase of infection.[18,22-26]

TABLE 3-1 Representative Bacterial Toxins with Enzymatic Mechanisms

Toxin Category	Toxin Name	Organism	Structure	Receptor	Molecular Target(s) and Effect
Adenylate cyclase toxins	Adenylate cyclase toxin	*Bordetella* species	A-B	Direct entry into cell	Activation by calmodulin results in cAMP production in host cell and cAMP-mediated effects, depending on cell type.
	Edema factor, EF (plus protective antigen, PA)	*Bacillus anthracis*	A plus B (two separate proteins)	Anthrax toxin receptor (ATR)	Same as adenylate cyclase toxin.
	ExoY	*Pseudomonas aeruginosa*	A only	Introduced into host cell by type III secretion, eliminating need for B subunit.	Adenylate cyclase activity is calmodulin independent but enhanced by a eukaryotic factor or factors. cAMP-mediated effects are dependent on cell type.
ADP-ribosylating toxins	Cholera toxin (CT)	*Vibrio cholerae*	A-5B	GM1 ganglioside	ADP-ribosylation of $G_{s\alpha}$ activates host cell adenylate cyclase and increases cAMP level and cAMP-mediated fluid secretion.
	Heat-labile toxin (LT-I)	*Escherichia coli*	A-5B	GM1 ganglioside (and weakly binds to surface glycoproteins)	Same as cholera toxin.
	Diphtheria toxin (DT)	*Corynebacterium diphtheriae*	A-B	Heparin-binding EGF-like growth factor–like cell precursor (HB-EGF)	ADP-ribosylation of EF-2 inhibits protein synthesis and causes death.
	Exotoxin A (ETA)	*Pseudomonas aeruginosa*	A-B	α_2-Macroglobulin receptor/low-density lipoprotein receptor–related protein (LRP)	Same as diphtheria toxin.
	Pertussis toxin (PT)	*Bordetella pertussis*	A-5B	Glycoprotein	ADP-ribosylation of several heterotrimeric G proteins results in blockage of signal transduction mediated by those proteins.
	C2 toxin	*Clostridium botulinum*	A-B	Glycoprotein	ADP-ribosylation of G-actin results in inhibition of polymerization and causes cell rounding.
	C3 ADP-ribosyl transferase	*Clostridium botulinum*	A-B	Pinocytosis	ADP-ribosylation of Rho A, B, or C causes their inactivation and cytopathic changes in target cells.
Deamidating toxins	Cytotoxic necrotizing factor (CNF1, CNF2)	*Escherichia coli*	A-B	Unknown	Deamidation of Rho proteins (Rho, Rac, Cdc42) inhibits GTPase activity and results in constitutive activation and an increase in actin stress fibers and focal adhesion.
	Dermonecrotic toxin (DNT)	*Bordetella pertussis*	A-B	Unknown	Deamidation of Rho proteins (as above for CNF1, CNF2); DNT also catalyzes cross-linking of GTPases with polyamines (putrescine, spermidine, spermine), which abrogates GTPase activity and allows Rho to interact with downstream effector molecules.
Glucosylating toxins	Toxins A and B	*Clostridium difficile*	A-B	Glycoprotein for toxin A; unknown for toxin B	Monoglucosylation of Rho proteins (Rho, Rac, Cdc42) at key threonine residues causes their inactivation and subsequent cytopathic changes in target cells and cytokine release.
Metalloprotease toxins	*Bacillus fragilis* enterotoxin	Enterotoxigenic *Bacillus fragilis* protein (ETBF)	(20-kDa protein)	Unknown	Cleavage of E-cadherin (zonula adherens protein) allows disruption of intestinal tight junction and consequently F-actin rearrangement and fluid secretion.
	Botulinum neurotoxin (BoNT)	*Clostridium botulinum*	A-B	GT1b and GD1a gangliosides; probably also synaptotagmin	Cleavage of SNARE protein or proteins blocks ACh secretion and causes flaccid paralysis.
	Tetanus neurotoxin	*Clostridium tetani*	A-B	GD1b gangliosides	Cleavage of protein in SNARE complex results in blocking neurotransmitter secretion and causes spastic paralysis.
	Lethal factor, LF (plus protective antigen, PA)	*Bacillus anthracis*	A plus B (two separate proteins)	Anthrax toxin receptor (ATR)	Cleavage of MAPKKs and potentially other cytoplasmic protein substrates; role of the MAPKK pathway in eliciting host cell death remains unclear.
RNA glycosidase toxins	Shiga toxin	*Shigella dysenteriae*	A-5B	Globotriaosylceramide (Gb3)	Single-site depurination of 28S ribosomal RNA causes inhibition of protein synthesis and cell death.
	Shiga-like toxin	*Escherichia coli*	A-5B	Globotriaosylceramide (Gb3)	Same as Shiga toxin.

ACh, acetylcholine; ADP, adenosine diphosphate; cAMP, cyclic adenosine monophosphate; EF-2, elongation factor 2; EGF, epidermal growth factor; GTPase, guanosine triphosphatase; MAPKK, mitogen-activated protein kinase kinase; SNARE, soluble *N*-ethylmaleimide–sensitive fusion protein–attachment receptor protein complex.

Specific genetic selection systems have been developed to allow detection of bacterial genes activated in vivo, thus providing powerful tools for evaluating putative virulence genes.[4,22,27-29] In *Bordetella pertussis*, induction of the synthesis of different virulence components is staggered so that attachment factors are initially produced to establish the infection and toxins are synthesized and later released to protect against the host response and promote survival.[24,30]

In addition to the regulatory elements within a given toxin operon, there are genes that encode the toxin itself and other genes for proteins involved in activation and export of the toxin after synthesis. Furthermore, the regulatory and structural genes may be chromosomal in location, as is the case for cholera toxin, or plasmid encoded, as is the case for the family of immunologically and functionally homologous heat-labile toxins of *E. coli*.[31] The structural gene for diphtheria toxin is located on a bacteriophage, but the inhibition of toxin synthesis by excess iron is mediated through a metalloregulatory protein, DtxR, that is encoded on the bacterial chromosome. The structural gene for tetanus toxin is located on a large (75-kilobase) plasmid. The pertussis toxin gene is chromosomal and present in three *Bordetella* species and has been detected only in *B. pertussis*, a difference previously attributed to apparent mutations in the promoter region of the gene in *Bordetella parapertussis* and *Bordetella bronchiseptica*. From the *Bordetella* genome sequencing project, however, it now seems that *B. bronchiseptica* is the older species and the promoter in *B. pertussis* may, in fact, contain the mutations, which enhance expression or control thereof.[32] Finally, the gene for staphylococcal enterotoxin may be either chromosomal or plasmid in location, but its production is regulated by genes on a plasmid.[33,34]

Secretion of proteins from bacteria occurs by several different mechanisms and the study of these processes has become an established field of research, which has benefited from the availability of genome sequences of pathogenic organisms.[35] Because the majority of toxins are single- or multiple-component proteins that must be exported, either into the environment or directly into a host cell, to have their effects, protein secretion is a critical element of toxin delivery. The type I to type V secretion systems have been studied in regard to secretion of toxins as well as other proteins and are described in detail in reviews (Table 3-2).[36-38]

Type I secretion is used for export of "repeat-in-toxin" (RTX) toxins, including *E. coli* hemolysin (HlyA), *Pasteurella haemolytica* leukotoxin (LktA) and *B. pertussis* adenylate cyclase toxin (CyaA), and some extracellular proteins, such as enzymes and S-layer protein from *Serratia marcescens*. Secreted proteins are targeted by a carboxyl-terminal signal sequence and are transported directly across cytoplasmic and outer membranes by the three-protein complex.[39] Type II secretion was identified for its role in export of hydrolytic enzymes, such as pullulanase, but has been recognized as the mechanism for secretion of several important toxins, such as cholera toxin and *Pseudomonas* exotoxin A.[40] Expression of the components of the type II pathway is tightly regulated with growth cycle, and distribution of the secretion machinery on the bacterial surface can be polar.[41] The secretion process consists of two steps with a periplasmic intermediate in which toxin assembly occurs.

The type III secretion pathway was discovered in *Yersinia* species but is widely distributed among gram-negative pathogens.[17] The secretory apparatus consists of approximately 25 proteins that form a needle-like structure through which bacterial virulence factors are injected directly into the cytoplasm of target cells.[42] A number of extracellular bacterial proteins, such as ExoS (ADP-ribosyl transferase) and ExoY (adenylate cyclase) from *P. aeruginosa*, appeared to be the A domains of toxins but had no demonstrable toxin activities. With the discovery of the type III system, it became clear that these and many other molecules are effectors that are delivered through that pathway (and thus do not require a B subunit) and are also released at a low level into the medium, even when no target cells are present.

The prototype for type IV secretion is the apparatus in *Agrobacterium tumefaciens* that delivers DNA to target plant cells, result-

TABLE 3-2   Secretion of Bacterial Toxins

Pathway	Organism	Toxin	Protein
Type I	*Escherichia coli*	Hemolysin	HlyA
	Pasteurella haemolytica	Leukotoxin	LktA
	Bordetella pertussis	Adenylate cyclase toxin	CyaA
Type II	*Vibrio cholerae*	Cholera toxin	CtxA
	Pseudomonas aeruginosa	Exotoxin A	ExoA
Type III	*Yersinia* spp.	Yops	Yop E, H, J
	P. aeruginosa	Exoenzyme S	ExoS
	Enteropathogenic *E. coli*	Tir	EspE
Type IV	*B. pertussis*	Pertussis toxin	PtxA
	Helicobacter pylori		CagA
Type V (autotransporters)	*Serratia marcescens*	Hemolysin	
	H. pylori	Vacuolating cytotoxin	VacA
	B. pertussis		BrkA

ing in induction of crown gall tumor formation. Related systems are used by human pathogens, such as *B. pertussis* and *Helicobacter pylori*, for secretion of toxins (pertussis toxin and CagA, respectively).[43] The machinery consists of 11 proteins and catalyzes a process that allows assembly of the holotoxin in the periplasmic space before it is transported into the extracellular medium or, in the case of CagA, injected directly into the host cell.

An additional category of bacterial proteins called "autotransporters" has been identified.[44] Members of this family of proteins are virulence factors, many possessing enzymatic activity, but not all are toxins by the definition used previously. They are novel, however, in that after secretion across the bacterial cytoplasmic membrane they are able to form an amphipathic β-barrel structure and deliver a passenger domain across the outer membrane into the medium. Examples include BrkA, an anticomplement protein from *B. pertussis*, and vacuolating cytotoxin (VacA) from *H. pylori*.[45,46]

ATTACHMENT AND ENTRY OF TOXINS

Most toxins act on intracellular substrates and thus require cell entry to be effective. Most of them conform to the A-B model described earlier and have binding components that interact with specific receptors on target cells, such as the ganglioside GM1 for cholera toxin, GD1b for tetanus toxin, and GD1a and GT1b for botulinum toxin.[13,47,48] The relatively wide distribution of GM1 ganglioside among cell types accounts for the apparent lack of selectivity of cholera toxin in vitro. The specificity of the effect of cholera toxin during infection (secretory diarrhea), however, is due to localization of the organisms and the toxin to the intestinal tract.

The surface receptor to which a toxin binds is also a determinant of the trafficking of the toxin to the site at which the A subunit is ultimately delivered to the cytoplasm. Retrograde transport of cholera toxin to the Golgi complex, where it is finally translocated, is one example of the complex processes used by protein toxins to reach their target substrates.[49] One element of trafficking can involve coupling of toxin-receptor complexes to lipid rafts in the host cell plasma membrane, with that association facilitating entry of the toxin into the host cell. Examples include several pore-forming toxins, cholera toxin, and anthrax toxins.[50-52] The cholera toxin–GM1 ganglioside receptor complex has been shown to couple with lipid raft domains in a cholesterol-dependent fashion.[51] Clustering and internalization of the anthrax toxin receptor (ATR) and the heptameric form of anthrax protective antigen (the B moiety for lethal factor or edema factor) have been shown to be facilitated by a lipid raft–mediated, clathrin-dependent process.[52] Trafficking of toxins has become an important growth area of research at the interface of microbial pathogenesis and cell biology.[6]

Pertussis toxin has been shown to interact with sialic acid–containing glycoproteins, which differ from cell to cell.[14,53,54] Because most cells are sensitive to intoxication by pertussis toxin but often do not contain the same receptors, it appears that a common carbohydrate motif (presumably containing sialic acid) present on different proteins accounts for this "family" of receptor molecules. Diphtheria toxin and *Pseudomonas* exotoxin A catalyze the same reaction intracellularly and are both distributed systemically during infection, yet the resultant disease processes are quite distinct. The differences between the two appear to reside, at least in part, at the level of target cell specificities. For example, diphtheria toxin binds to a complex consisting of a heparin-binding epidermal growth factor–like precursor molecule (HB-EGF) plus CD9, whereas *Pseudomonas* exotoxin A binds to the α_2-macroglobulin/low-density lipoprotein receptor–related protein.[55-57] In light of the reactogenicity of horse serum containing antitoxin, used to treat patients with diphtheria, a modified form of the receptor has been proposed as a possible antidote.[58]

Several different mechanisms can be used by A subunits of A-B toxins to enter the target cell. In each case, however, a large protein molecule must insert into or cross the lipid bilayer.[13] This activity is reflected in the ability of a number of intact A-B toxins or their B subunits to insert into artificial lipid bilayers and create ion-permeable pathways.[59,60] In some cases, such as diphtheria toxin, binding to a surface receptor, uptake into an endocytotic vesicle, and acidification of that vesicle result in a conformational change that enables a part of the toxin molecule to traverse the membrane.[61] The final step in diphtheria toxin translocation is energy requiring and dependent on membrane potential, a proton gradient, and a host cell cytosolic factor.[61] *Pseudomonas* exotoxin A appears to be internalized somewhat differently, with endocytosis into coated pits and routing to the *trans*-Golgi compartment, where proteolytic activation occurs before entry into the cytosol.[62]

Toxins with identical enzymatic mechanisms may enter cells by completely separate and distinct pathways. *B. pertussis* adenylate cyclase toxin, *Bacillus anthracis* edema toxin (edema factor plus protective antigen), and ExoY, an adenylate cyclase from *P. aeruginosa*, each catalyze the production of cyclic adenosine monophosphate (cAMP) from host intracellular adenosine triphosphate stores. Anthrax edema toxin enters the host cell by receptor-mediated endocytosis and requires acidification of the endosome in order to be translocated into the cytosol.[63] Pertussis adenylate cyclase toxin can bind to a receptor, an integrin complex consisting of CD11b/CD18, but how it gains access to its substrate in the cytosol thereafter remains unclear.[64] In cells lacking that receptor, however, this toxin can insert itself directly into the host cell membrane and deliver its catalytic domain by a process that is dependent on extracellular calcium and the target cell membrane potential as a driving force.[65,66] In contrast, *Pseudomonas* ExoY possesses no binding domain but is delivered to the host cell interior by the type III secretion system.[67]

For toxins such as tetanus toxin and botulinum toxin, which have identical substrates, entry and trafficking are critical events in establishment of the clinical manifestations of specific syndromes, which are characterized by spastic and flaccid paralysis, respectively. Putative ganglioside receptors have been identified (primarily GD1b gangliosides for tetanus toxin and GD1a and GT1b gangliosides for botulinum toxin), but the mechanisms for entry and differential intracellular distribution remain unclear. Coreceptors, consisting of a ganglioside and a protein expressed selectively in neuronal tissue, have been proposed for clostridial neurotoxins; synaptotagmin II may represent the protein component for botulinum toxin.[48,68]

MECHANISM OF TOXIN ACTION AND ROLE IN CLINICAL DISEASE

As noted earlier, bacterial toxins do not operate in isolation to cause disease. With the exception of preformed toxins responsible for foodborne illnesses, toxins are produced by organisms during the course of infection of the host, and a complex array of virulence factors is generally involved. In the following sections, several toxins are described along with their mechanisms of action, when known, and their apparent roles in the clinical disease with which they are associated. This list is by no means complete but rather provides some examples of major toxins that are well studied and for which information is more complete. Important toxins that contribute substantially to infectious diseases and are not mentioned here are discussed in the chapters corresponding to the specific organisms or the resulting disease. Several publications provide more comprehensive information on bacterial toxins.[3,6,69]

Toxins of *Bacillus anthracis*

B. anthracis produces three toxin components that are novel in their interaction with cells.[70] None of the three components—edema factor, lethal factor, or protective antigen—has toxin activity alone. Protective antigen is the binding moiety that interacts with target cells to promote the entry of edema factor or lethal factor. Protective antigen binds to a glycoprotein receptor on target cells known as ATR.[71] The ATR shares sequence identity with the extracellular portion of tumor endothelial marker 8 (TEM8), which is found on a number of cell lines and possesses a von Willebrand domain.[71,72] Once protective antigen is bound to the receptor, it is cleaved by a host protease that is furin or furin-like.[71] This process results in the release of a 20-kD fragment and activates the 63-kD portion of protective antigen (PA_{63}) to form a heptamer that binds edema factor or lethal factor.[73] The complex is internalized by receptor-mediated endocytosis and is activated by calmodulin, resulting in increased levels of cAMP.[70] Lethal factor is a zinc-dependent metalloprotease that has been demonstrated to cleave the amino terminus of the mitogen-activated protein kinase kinases, thereby inactivating them.[74-77] Although it remains to be determined what role these substrates play in the rapidly lethal effects of this toxin complex, these data provide convincing evidence of their protease activity in vivo. It is also clear from current studies that these toxins do not act in isolation; their actions are affected by each other as well as other factors from the bacterium and the host.

Toxins of *Bordetella pertussis*

B. pertussis, the causative agent of whooping cough, produces several toxins that have striking effects in experimental systems and are hypothesized to be major contributors to the pathogenesis of the clinical illness.[78,79] Pertussis toxin, also known as lymphocytosis-promoting factor, histamine-sensitizing factor, or islet-activating protein, is expressed by *B. pertussis*. A copy of the operon is present in *B. parapertussis* and *B. bronchiseptica* and is, from all experimental data, transcriptionally silent.[80] Data from the *Bordetella* genome sequencing project have revealed that the differences between the species may have resulted from mutations in *B. pertussis,* leaving open the possibility that low-level expression does occur in these other species.[32] Pertussis toxin acts by ADP-ribosylation of several members of the family of guanine nucleotide–binding (G) proteins involved in signal transduction. The result of this covalent modification is inhibition of G protein function, affecting a variety of effector systems, such as adenylate cyclase, phospholipases, and several types of ion channels. Although pertussis toxin is clearly a virulence factor for *B. pertussis* and a protective antigen present in acellular pertussis vaccines, its target tissue and role in clinical pertussis remain unclear.[78,79,81] Unlike those of tetanus and diphtheria, the clinical manifestations of pertussis cannot be mimicked by experimental administration of pertussis toxin.[82]

Bordetella species also produce other toxins that are significant virulence factors, including adenylate cyclase toxin and tracheal cytotoxin. Adenylate cyclase toxin enters host cells and catalyzes the production of supraphysiologic levels of cAMP, which impair the normal activities of neutrophils and other immune effector cells and may produce fluid and mucous secretion in the respiratory tract.[83] Tracheal cytotoxin is a disaccharide-tetrapeptide that is derived from the bacterial peptidoglycan. It is cytotoxic to respiratory epithelial cells, apparently by eliciting interleukin-1 release and nitric oxide production.[84]

An additional toxin from *Bordetella* species, dermonecrotic toxin, has not been clearly implicated in the pathogenesis of pertussis but has a mechanism of action like that of the cytotoxic necrotizing factors 1 and 2 (CNF1, CNF2) from invasive strains of *E. coli*.[85-87] Dermonecrotic toxin, as its name implies, causes dermonecrosis when injected into the skin of suckling mice. It has significant sequence homology with cytotoxic necrotizing factor, and both toxins alter the cytoskeleton of affected cells, with enhanced actin stress fiber assembly and focal adhesions. These effects are now known to be the result of constitutive activation of Rho by deamidation of glutamine 63 and abolition of its intrinsic guanosine triphosphatase activity.[87,88] This action represents yet another mechanism by which toxins can affect this family of critical signaling proteins.[89]

Diphtheria Toxin

One of the most extensively studied of all bacterial toxins is that produced by bacteriophage-infected *C. diphtheriae*.[2] Diphtheria toxin, the prototype ADP-ribosylating toxin, inhibits protein synthesis in target cells by catalyzing the ADP-ribosylation of a novel amino acid (diphthamide) on elongation factor 2, a host protein required for translocation of ribosomal messenger RNA. Undoubtedly, other products of *C. diphtheriae* are involved in establishment of infection and production and dissemination of the toxin. Nevertheless, the control of clinical diphtheria with the use of diphtheria toxoid attests to the dominant role of this toxin both in the local infection and in the systemic toxicity, morbidity, and mortality of this disease. The crystal structures of multiple forms of diphtheria toxin have been solved, and its receptor on eukaryotic cells has been identified as the extracellular domain of an HB-EGF that also has transmembrane and cytosolic domains.[2,90] An additional host cell component that interacts with the HB-EGF receptor has been identified by Iwamoto and colleagues as a 27-kD diphtheria toxin receptor–associated protein (DRAP27), which is a CD9 antigen homologue.[2,91] It has been shown that CD9 increases the affinity of diphtheria toxin for HB-EGF.[57] Bound diphtheria toxin enters the cell by receptor-mediated endocytosis, with the A subunit being released into the cytosol with the assistance of a complex of host proteins.[92]

As noted in Table 3-1, exotoxin A of *P. aeruginosa* catalyzes a reaction identical to that of diphtheria toxin but is associated with disease processes that are clearly distinct from those of diphtheria. The cellular receptor for exotoxin A has been identified as the α_2-macroglobulin/low-density lipoprotein receptor–related protein.[55] It is likely that the distinct differences between diphtheria and infection with an exotoxin A–producing *P. aeruginosa* are due to different receptors with different cellular distributions. In addition, exotoxin A is only one of a number of virulence factors involved in *Pseudomonas*-induced disease, whereas diphtheria toxin is the major determinant in clinical diphtheria.

Clostridial Neurotoxins

Advances in knowledge of the mechanisms of action of the neurotoxins produced by *Clostridium tetani* and *Clostridium botulinum* have revealed how they cause their respective neurologic diseases and have validated their use as important research probes for cell secretory processes, even beyond the nervous system.[93] These molecules are metalloproteases with remarkable substrate specificities and have as their targets different proteins of the so-called SNARE complex (soluble *N*-ethylmaleimide–sensitive fusion protein–attachment receptor protein complex). The SNARE complex comprises synaptobrevin or vesicle-associated membrane protein (VAMP), 25-kD synaptosome-associated protein (SNAP-25), and syntaxin, which form a complex on vesicles with *N*-ethylmaleimide–sensitive fusion protein. The SNAREs are integral for the fusion of neurotransmitter-containing vesicles with the presynaptic membrane.[94,95] The truly remarkable aspect of these observations is that the serologically distinct botulinum toxins, some of which elicit slightly different clinical manifestations, act on several different proteins in this secretory apparatus. For example, botulinum toxin serotypes B, D, F, and G cleave synaptobrevin-VAMP, each at a different site.[96] In contrast, botulinum toxin serotypes A and E cleave SNAP-25, at distinct sites, and serotype E cleaves both SNAP-25 and syntaxin.[96] Even more striking is the finding that tetanus toxin and botulinum toxin serotype B cleave synaptobrevin-VAMP at the same site and yet, when the toxins are injected into animals, they cause the clinical manifestations of tetanus and botulism, respectively. The latter findings illustrate that the manifestations of the two diseases reflect the different sites of toxin action (i.e., different target cells) rather than different molecular mechanisms.[95,96]

Tetanus Toxin

In contrast to the case of diphtheria, immunization with tetanus toxoid has no effect on the establishment of infection with *C. tetani*. However, the resultant antibody response totally prevents clinical tetanus, a direct consequence of the action of tetanus toxin (tetanospasmin). Tetanus toxin exhibits striking selectivity for neural tissue and is taken up at myoneural junctions for retrograde axonal transport within alpha motor neurons after binding to a receptor, which may be the GD1b gangliosides.[48] The toxin ultimately crosses the synapses in a retrograde direction by an unknown mechanism to reach the axons of inhibitory γ-aminobutyric acid neurons in the spinal cord. It is the toxin-induced inhibition of neurotransmitter release, specifically in the inhibitory neuron, that results in the spastic paralysis characteristic of the disease. However, at high local concentrations, tetanus toxin can cause inhibition of acetylcholine release at the myoneural junction with resultant flaccid paralysis similar to that elicited by botulinum toxin.

Tetanus toxin is a zinc-dependent metalloprotease that appears to act by selective cleavage of a protein component of synaptic vesicles, synaptobrevin II.[97] Toxicity can be prevented by metalloprotease inhibitors, such as the angiotensin-converting enzyme inhibitor captopril, raising the possibility of specific therapeutic intervention that has not been available previously.

Botulinum Toxin

Botulinum toxin is among the most potent toxins known, with a lethal dose (toxin type A) for humans of approximately 1 ng/kg.[98] Botulinum toxin consists of a family of seven immunologically distinct molecules, most of which cause flaccid paralysis by inhibiting myoneural junction acetylcholine release. The mechanism of this neurotoxic activity is the same as that of tetanus toxin, namely, proteolytic cleavage of neuronal proteins involved in vesicle fusion and integral to vesicular trafficking and neurotransmitter release.[48,95] Interestingly, however, some of the substrates and sites of cleavage not only are different from those of tetanus toxin but also differ among the serotypes of botulinum toxin (see Table 3-1).[99]

The classic features of clinical botulism result from the ingestion of preformed toxin in improperly prepared foods, but a subacute intoxication can occur in infants (infant botulism) and adults harboring *C. botulinum* in their gastrointestinal tracts.[100-102] In most cases, the low-level toxin absorption results in listlessness and hypotonia, but the course can be fulminant and infant botulism has been proposed as a cause of sudden infant death syndrome. The ability of botulinum toxin to block muscle contraction at the myoneural junction has led to its use therapeutically in disorders such as blepharospasm, spastic torticollis, and strabismus and more recently other illnesses and conditions, as discussed under "Therapeutic Uses of Bacterial Toxins."

Many strains of *C. botulinum* types C and D also produce a different molecule, C2 toxin, that ADP-ribosylates actin; this action inhibits the polymerization of actin, affects the shape of target cells, and results in enterotoxin activity in vivo.[89,103] C2 toxin represents a family of clostridial ADP-ribosylating toxins that modify actin.

Enterotoxins

The list of bacterial proteins with enterotoxic activities continues to grow, and the heterogeneous molecules included in this group have been discussed extensively in reviews.[104-107] These diverse molecules elicit enterotoxic activity by a variety of mechanisms, including some that remain poorly understood.[104-106] In this section, several representative examples are described briefly, and additional information about individual enterotoxins can be obtained from the appropriate chapter on the enterotoxin-producing organism.

Cholera Toxin

The classic enterotoxin, that produced by *Vibrio cholerae*, is responsible for the voluminous watery diarrhea that is characteristic of clinical cholera.[108] Cholera toxin activates adenylate cyclase of the intestinal epithelial cell by ADP-ribosylation of the B subunit of the stimulatory G protein G_s.[109] Although the resultant elevation in mucosal cell cAMP levels does produce chloride and isotonic intestinal fluid secretion, it is increasingly likely that additional bacterial components and additional regulatory pathways with other mediators are involved.[104,110,111] Prostaglandin, platelet-activating factor, and perhaps 5-hydroxytryptamine have been implicated as potential intermediates in or synergistic components for cholera toxin action.[110,112,113] Furthermore, an intestinal secretory response in volunteers challenged with strains of *V. cholerae* in which the cholera toxin gene had been deleted or disrupted suggests a role for other factors.[114] Subsequent studies have identified accessory cholera enterotoxin, zonula occludens toxin, and an RTX-like molecule in the armamentarium of *V. cholerae*.[104,115,116] The relative roles, if any, of these molecules in diarrhea caused by cholera remain to be determined.

In addition to its well-known action as an enterotoxin, cholera toxin is recognized as an adjuvant for preparations of antigens with which it is administered.[104,117,118] The mechanism for this adjuvant effect is not entirely clear, but it appears that the B subunit of cholera toxin has a modest adjuvant effect and that the enzymatically intact holotoxin is more potent.[119,120]

Escherichia coli Heat-Labile Toxin

The heat-labile toxins produced by *E. coli* share their molecular mechanism of action with cholera toxin but are divided into two categories, heat-labile enterotoxin type 1 (LT-I) and LT-II, which are distinguished immunologically. LT-I toxins are closely related to cholera toxin and have no major structural or functional differences. Organisms producing this toxin infect primarily humans, but the disease is generally milder than that of cholera for reasons that are not well understood. The LT-II heat-labile toxins are associated with diarrheal disease in animals and have an immunologically distinct B subunit and different receptor.[121]

Escherichia coli Heat-Stable Toxin

E. coli organisms can produce toxins other than the heat-labile toxin discussed in the previous section. Heat-stable toxin, known as STa or ST-I, is synthesized as a peptide of 72 amino acids and is cleaved to an active species of 18 or 19 amino acids.[122] It causes diarrhea by binding to and activating endogenous particulate guanylate cyclase, thus eliciting cyclic guanosine monophosphate (cGMP) production.[123,124] Unlike cholera toxin and *E. coli* heat-labile toxin, heat-stable toxin exhibits striking target cell specificity with little activity in extraintestinal tissues. The endogenous ligand for this receptor, called guanylin, has been identified in extracts of rat jejunum and shown to stimulate cGMP production and chloride secretion in intestinal cells.[125] Studies have revealed that phosphorylation of the heat-stable toxin receptor–guanylate cyclase by protein kinase C produces a synergistic activation when heat-stable toxin is added.

Enteropathogenic *E. coli* elicit activation of protein kinase C and an enhanced sensitivity to heat-stable toxin in cells to which they adhere, and that combination may be responsible for the diarrhea occurring in patients infected with those organisms. Other bacterial species such as *Yersinia enterocolitica*, non-01 *V. cholerae*, and *Citrobacter freundii* also produce toxins related to heat-stable toxin, but their roles in diarrheal illnesses are unclear.

Clostridium difficile Toxins A and B

Clostridium difficile, a causative agent of antibiotic-associated pseudomembranous colitis, produces two large protein toxins, toxin A (308 kD) and toxin B (270 kD).[126] Toxin A is classified as an entero-toxin and toxin B as a cytotoxin on the basis of their activities when administered separately, but both have cytotoxic effects, as reflected by cytoskeletal disruption in treated cells. Toxin A appears to be more important in clinical pseudomembranous colitis because of its ability to elicit inflammatory responses by induction of cytokine release.[127] The inflammation and cytokines may be responsible for the decreases in monolayer resistance observed after treatment with toxin A, but it does not alone produce an increase in short-circuit current.[128] The in vivo secretory effects elicited by toxin A apparently involve other mediators because they can be blocked by inhibitors of phospholipase A_2 and platelet-activating factor.[129] At least part of the effects of these toxins appears to result from alterations in tight junction integrity.[130] Toxin A (and probably toxin B) acts by glucosylation of Rho, which disrupts its ability to promote actin polymerization, thus adding another toxin to the growing list of bacterial products that target members of the Rho family.[89]

Bacteroides fragilis Enterotoxin

Diarrhea-associated strains of *B. fragilis* (known as enterotoxigenic *B. fragilis* or ETBF) produce a 20-kD zinc metalloprotease that causes a decrease in monolayer resistance and disruption of the morphology of human intestinal epithelial cells.[131] This toxin elicits fluid secretion in vivo and alters actin cytoskeleton structure in vitro.[132,133] These effects appear to be the result of a new mechanism, namely, proteolytic cleavage of the zonula adherens protein E-cadherin causing loosening of the tight junction in polarized epithelial cells and perhaps signaling some other intracellular events.[134,135]

Shiga and Shiga-like Toxins

Shiga toxin is the prototype of a family of toxins produced by *Shigella dysenteriae* (Shiga toxin), *E. coli*, *C. freundii*, and other organisms (Shiga-like toxins SLT-I and SLT-II, previously known as Vero toxins).[136,137] SLT-I molecules react with antiserum to Shiga toxin, whereas SLT-II molecules do not despite possessing a common mechanism of action. The members of this family conform to the A-B model with a subunit structure similar to that of cholera toxin (A-5B).[138] The binding pentamer interacts with the glycolipid globotriaosylceramide, and the toxin, which is internalized by receptor-mediated endocytosis through clathrin-coated pits, eventually moves to the *trans*-Golgi apparatus.[136,139] Within the cytoplasm, the A subunit causes inhibition of protein synthesis by enzymatic inactivation of the 28S RNA within the 60S ribosomal subunit. This inactivation occurs by enzymatic removal of adenine from a specific adenosine residue, which is the same as the process catalyzed by the plant toxin ricin.

Despite the cytotoxicity elicited in vitro, the role of these toxins in shigellosis and diarrhea associated with infection by Shiga-like toxin–positive, enterohemorrhagic *E. coli* and others remains controversial.[104,136] Shiga toxin, especially in combination with lipopolysaccharide, causes damage to vascular endothelial cells in a fashion that may explain the hemolytic-uremic syndrome known to be associated with infection by *S. dysenteriae* and enterohemorrhagic *E. coli*.[140,141] In this setting, lipopolysaccharide increases expression of the globotriaosylceramide receptor on vascular endothelial cells in a process involving tumor necrosis factor and interleukin-1.[142] Cell damage also appears to depend on endothelial cell production of procoagulant and arachidonic acid metabolites.[143] Even the enterotoxin activity (intestinal fluid accumulation) may represent toxin effects on the villus cells and on the vasculature of the intestinal mucosa.

Pyrogenic Exotoxins

The pyrogenic exotoxins constitute a growing family of molecules that are responsible for a systemic syndrome manifested by fever, shock, and profound immunomodulation.[144,145] Included in this group are toxic shock syndrome toxins, staphylococcal enterotoxins and exfoliative toxins, and pyrogenic exotoxins from *Streptococcus pyogenes* and group B, C, F, and G streptococci.[34,144] In addition to their recognized roles in toxic shock syndrome, scarlet fever, and other streptococcal diseases, evidence now implicates toxic shock syndrome toxin–producing and exfoliative toxin–secreting *Staphylococcus aureus* in Kawasaki syndrome.[146,147] These proteins share the ability to stimulate T-cell proliferation by interaction with the class II major histocompatibility complex on antigen-presenting cells and specific V_β chains of the T-cell receptor and are therefore designated superantigens.[34,148] The important feature of this interaction is that both the T cells and antigen-presenting cells are stimulated to release massive amounts of inflammatory cytokines such as interleukin-1, tumor necrosis factor, macrophage migration inhibition factor, and other monokines and lymphokines, which appear to be the principal mediators of the disease processes associated with these toxins.[34] The crystal structures have been solved for at least some of these superantigens, which allows closer examination of their interaction with the T-cell receptor complex in addition to permitting mutational analysis.[149-151]

At this time, it is not clear whether superantigen activity is the sole mechanism of these illnesses or whether other actions of the toxins may contribute. Staphylococcal enterotoxins elicit emesis in experimental animals, but this activity may occur with other superantigens with different potencies.[144] In addition, toxic shock syndrome toxin 1 has been shown to be cytotoxic for aortic endothelial cells in vitro, a setting in which cytokines should not be present. Thus, it is possible that the various clinical syndromes produced by the organisms that make these toxins reflect the activities of numerous bacterial components directly on host cells as well as the effects of massive mediator release through their function as superantigens.

Other Toxins

The list of toxins discussed in the preceding sections is by no means inclusive. It is merely illustrative of the many different toxin molecules that have been implicated in clinical diseases in humans. Many other toxins have been the subject of basic research investigations concerning structure and molecular mechanisms of action, with little knowledge of their contribution to clinical disease, although notable advances in the understanding of structure and function of these toxins have taken place over the past decade. Some of these other toxins are membrane-damaging toxins, which include pore-forming toxins and cytotoxins. A common feature of these toxins is that they result in disruption or loss of integrity of the phospholipid membrane bilayer of target cells or the formation of a pore in the bilayer, or both.[152] For example, a large number of toxins have the ability to lyse erythrocytes and are thus defined as hemolysins.[153] Some of these hemolysins also have leukotoxic activity or cytolytic activity (cytolysins). Functionally, the membrane-damaging toxins can be categorized into three major classes: (1) toxins that hydrolyze the phospholipids of the membrane bilayer by a variety of enzymatic activities such as phospholipase C activity (as with *C. perfringens* α-toxin), sphingomyelinase activity (e.g., *S. aureus* β-toxin), or phospholipase D activity (e.g., *Vibrio damsela* hemolysin); (2) toxins that act by detergent-like activity causing solubilization of membranes, such as δ-toxins of *S. aureus* and *S. haemolyticus*; and (3) pore-forming toxins, which consist of 75 to 80 cytolysins and are the largest group of the membrane-damaging toxins.

Bacterial pore-forming toxins constitute a large group of proteins produced by gram-negative and gram-positive organisms, some of which can be grouped into families of toxins on the basis of structural or functional characteristics, or both. For example, a large number of pore-forming toxins belong to a family of cholesterol-binding cytolysins that are produced by gram-positive bacteria (including *Clostridium*, *Listeria*, *Streptococcus*, *Bacillus*, and *Arcanobacterium*) and require the presence of cholesterol in the target cell membrane and formation of large oligomeric complexes for their cytolytic activity.[154] The staphylococcal pore-forming toxins include the α-helix γ-hemolysins and the β-barrel pore-forming α-hemolysins and bicomponent leukotoxins, the latter of which are composed of various combinations of S proteins and F proteins.[155,156] Some of the pore-forming toxins produced by gram-negative bacteria (such as *Escherichia*, *Enterobacter*, *Proteus*, and *Bordetella*) have been found, on the basis of amino acid sequence, to contain a glycine-rich repeat region and thus belong to a family of toxins termed RTX that function as hemolysins and leukotoxins.[157,158] Interestingly, some gram-negative bacteria such as *Proteus* and *Serratia* produce bicomponent pore-forming proteins that are inactive individually but become hemolytic or cytolytic, or both, when associated.[159]

Many pore-forming toxins, including *S. aureus* α-hemolysin, *Aeromonas hydrophila* aerolysin, as well as the *B. anthracis* protective antigen, assemble into heptameric channels in the host cell membrane.[160] The *A. hydrophila* pore-forming toxin is released by the organism as an inactive precursor, proaerolysin, that interacts not with a specific receptor protein but with a specific post-translational modification, a glycosyl phosphatidyl inositol (GPI) anchor on the target cell. Proaerolysin is then converted to aerolysin after binding to the GPI by proteolytic cleavage of the toxin. The aerolysin proteins have a complex and unusual mobility pattern on the cell surface, which occurs through involvement of lipid rafts.[50,155,161]

A variety of non–mutually exclusive cellular effects of pore-forming toxins have been described and include (1) release of host cell nutrients leading to cell death (e.g., *A. hydrophila* aerolysin), (2) facilitation of injection of bacterial effector molecules that occur by type III secretion mechanisms (e.g., *S. pyogenes* streptolysin O and perfringolysin O, *H. pylori* VacA), (3) release of an invading bacterium into the host cell cytoplasm by production of the toxin within the phagocytic vacuole and subsequent rupture of the vacuole membrane (e.g., *Listeria monocytogenes* listeriolysin O), and (4) release of an intracellularly replicating bacterium from the host cell (e.g., *Legionella pneumophila* IcmS). Much progress has been made in the past 15 years in elucidation of the structure and function of the pore-forming toxins, and it is anticipated that this field will continue to make rapid advances and provide an understanding of disease processes and pathogenicity related to these toxins.

Therapeutic Uses of Bacterial Toxins

Microbial toxins demonstrate remarkable specificities in their enzymatic activity and target receptor interactions. In addition, the molecules in the host cell that are targeted by these toxins often represent critical elements in signaling pathways. For these reasons, toxins are useful as probes in biomedical research, to elucidate the role of the target molecule or molecules in normal physiology, and as therapeutic reagents for treatment of an increasing number of disease processes. The rapid growth of therapeutic uses for bacterial toxins is illustrated in the literature. In the period 1966 to 1981, less than 1% of citations on botulinum toxin concerned therapeutic applications of this toxin molecule, whereas in 2002, the specific topic of approximately 60% of articles was its use as a treatment modality.

Other than as immunogens in vaccines directed against the toxin, the most extensively developed clinical application for bacterial toxins is in cancer therapy. These engineered therapeutic agents often consist of a fusion protein in which the binding specificity is provided by a monoclonal antibody (immunotoxin) or a natural ligand for a receptor that is limited to the target cell population of interest. Anti-CD22 antibody has been fused with the catalytic domain of *Pseudomonas* exotoxin A to yield recombinant immunotoxin BL22. Because of the restricted distribution of CD22 to B cells and its high level of expression on hairy cell leukemia cells, this construct has activity in this disease and is currently in clinical trials for that purpose.[162] Direct targeting of cells containing a specific receptor was the strategy used with the catalytic and insertion domains of diphtheria toxin fused to interleukin-7.[163]

The paralytic effect of botulinum toxin was first used for control of disorders that involve uncontrolled muscle contractions, such as blepharospasm and torticollis. This agent is now being commonly used for a variety of purposes from temporary reduction of skin wrinkles to treatment of chronic anal fissures and has been evaluated for new applications ranging from vascular headaches to hyperhidrosis.[94,95] Limitations of these uses include infrequent systemic toxicity and development of neutralizing antibodies that reduce effectiveness upon reapplication.[164] Finally, several toxins are being evaluated for their ability to deliver inserted epitopes to the cytoplasm of antigen-presenting cells so that they are handled by the class I major histocompatibility complex pathway and enable the development of cellular responses. Anthrax toxin and pertussis adenylate cyclase toxin have been used in this way, primarily for viral antigens, and several constructs are nearing clinical trials.[165,166]

REFERENCES

1. Roux E, Yersin A. Contribution a l'étude de la diphthérie. Ann Inst Pasteur. 1888;2:629-661.
2. Collier RJ. Understanding the mode of action of diphtheria toxin: A perspective on progress during the 20th century. Toxicon. 2001;39:1793-1803.
3. Freer JH, Alouf JE. The Comprehensive Sourcebook of Bacterial Protein Toxins. 2nd ed. San Diego: Academic Press; 1999.
4. Wren BW. Microbial genome analysis: Insights into virulence, host adaptation and evolution. Nat Rev Genet. 2000;1:30-39.
5. Cossart P. Cellular Microbiology. Washington, DC: ASM Press; 2000.
6. Burns DL. Bacterial Protein Toxins. Washington, DC: ASM Press; 2003.
7. Strauss EJ, Falkow S. Microbial pathogenesis: Genomics and beyond. Science. 1997;276:707-712.
8. Falkow S. Invasion and intracellular sorting of bacteria: Searching for bacterial genes expressed during host/pathogen interactions. J Clin Invest. 1997;100:239-243.
9. Finlay BB, Cossart P. Exploitation of mammalian host cell functions by bacterial pathogens. Science. 1997;276:718-725.
10. Relman DA. Genome-wide responses of a pathogenic bacterium to its host. J Clin Invest. 2002;110:1071-1073.
11. Galan JE. The cell biology of microbial infections: Coming of age. J Cell Biol. 2002;158:387-388.
12. Riley MA, Wertz JE. Bacteriocins: Evolution, ecology, and application. Annu Rev Microbiol. 2002;56:117-137.
13. Gill DM. Seven toxic peptides that cross cell membranes. In: Jeljaszewicz J, Wadstrom T, eds. Bacterial Toxins and Cell Membranes. 1st ed. New York: Academic Press; 1978:291-332.
14. Wong WS, Rosoff PM. Pharmacology of pertussis toxin B-oligomer. Can J Physiol Pharmacol. 1996;74:559-564.
15. Masco D, Van de Walle M, Spiegel S. Interaction of ganglioside GM1 with the B subunit of cholera toxin modulates growth and differentiation of neuroblastoma N18 cells. J Neurosci. 1991;11:2443-2452.
16. Uhlen P, Laestadius A, Jahnukainen T, et al. Alpha-haemolysin of uropathogenic E. coli induces Ca^{2+} oscillations in renal epithelial cells. Nature. 2000;405:694-697.
17. Cornelis GR, Van Gijsegem F. Assembly and function of type III secretory systems. Annu Rev Microbiol. 2000;54:735-774.
18. Cotter PA, DiRita VJ. Bacterial virulence gene regulation: An evolutionary perspective. Annu Rev Microbiol. 2000;54:519-565.
19. Pappenheimer AM Jr. Diphtheria toxin. Annu Rev Biochem. 1977;46:69-94.
20. Straley SC, Plano GV, Skrzypek E, et al. Regulation by Ca^{2+} in the Yersinia low-Ca^{2+} response. Mol Microbiol. 1993;8:1005-1010.
21. Miller VL, Taylor RK, Mekalanos JJ. Cholera toxin transcriptional activator toxR is a transmembrane DNA binding protein. Cell. 1987;48:271-279.
22. Mahan MJ, Heithoff DM, Sinsheimer RL, Low DA. Assessment of bacterial pathogenesis by analysis of gene expression in the host. Annu Rev Genet. 2000;34:139-164.
23. Miller JF, Johnson SA, Black WJ, et al. Constitutive sensory transduction mutations in the Bordetella pertussis bvgS gene. J Bacteriol. 1992;174:970-979.
24. Scarlato V, Arico B, Domenighini M, Rappuoli R. Environmental regulation of virulence factors in Bordetella species. Bioessays. 1993;15:99-104.
25. Merkel TJ, Stibitz S, Keith JM, et al. Contribution of regulation by the bvg locus to respiratory infection of mice by Bordetella pertussis. Infect Immun. 1998;66:4367-4373.
26. Hoch JA, Silhavy TJ. Two-Component Signal Transduction. Washington, DC: ASM Press; 1995.
27. Akerley BJ, Rubin EJ, Camilli A, et al. Systematic identification of essential genes by in vitro mariner mutagenesis. Proc Natl Acad Sci USA. 1998;95:8927-8932.
28. Chiang SL, Mekalanos JJ. Use of signature-tagged transposon mutagenesis to identify Vibrio cholerae genes critical for colonization. Mol Microbiol. 1998;27:797-805.
29. Camilli A, Mekalanos JJ. Use of recombinase gene fusions to identify Vibrio cholerae genes induced during infection. Mol Microbiol. 1995;18:671-683.
30. Uhl MA, Miller JF. Integration of multiple domains in a two-component sensor protein: The Bordetella pertussis BvgAs phosphorelay. EMBO J. 1996;15:1028-1036.
31. Betley MJ, Miller VL, Mekalanos JJ. Genetics of bacterial enterotoxins. Annu Rev Microbiol. 1986;40:577-605.
32. Parkhill J, Sebaihia M, Preston A, et al. Comparative analysis of the genome sequences of Bordetella pertussis, Bordetella parapertussis and Bordetella bronchiseptica. Nat Genet. 2003;35:32-40.
33. Dyer DW, Iandolo JJ. Plasmid-chromosomal transition of genes important in staphylococcal enterotoxin B expression. Infect Immun. 1981;33:450-458.
34. Muller-Alouf H, Carnoy C, Simonet M, Alouf JE. Superantigen bacterial toxins: State of the art. Toxicon. 2001;39:1691-1701.
35. Lee VT, Schneewind O. Protein secretion and the pathogenesis of bacterial infections. Genes Dev. 2001;15:1725-1752.
36. Sandkvist M. Biology of type II secretion. Mol Microbiol. 2001;40:271-283.
37. Plano GV, Day JB, Ferracci F. Type III export: New uses for an old pathway. Mol Microbiol. 2001;40:284-293.
38. Christie PJ. Type IV secretion: Intercellular transfer of macromolecules by systems ancestrally related to conjugation machines. Mol Microbiol. 2001;40:294-305.
39. Koronakis V, Eswaran J, Hughes C. The type I export mechanism. In: Burns D, Barbieri JT, Iglewski BH, Rappuoli R, eds. Bacterial Protein Toxins. Washington, DC: ASM Press; 2003:71-79.
40. Scott ME, Sandkvist M. Toxins and type II secretion systems. In: Burns D, Barbieri JT, Iglewski BH, Rappuoli R, eds. Bacterial Protein Toxins. Washington, DC: ASM Press; 2003:81-94.
41. Scott ME, Dossani ZY, Sandkvist M. Directed polar secretion of protease from single cells of Vibrio cholerae via the type II secretion pathway. Proc Natl Acad Sci USA. 2001;98:13978-13983.
42. Galan JE, Collmer A. Type III secretion machines: Bacterial devices for protein delivery into host cells. Science. 1999;284:1322-1328.
43. Burns D. Type IV secretion systems. In: Burns D, Barbieri JT, Iglewski BH, Rappuoli R, eds. Bacterial Protein Toxins. Washington, DC: ASM Press; 2003:115-127.
44. Henderson IR, Nataro JP. Virulence functions of autotransporter proteins. Infect Immun. 2001;69:1231-1243.
45. Fernandez RC, Weiss AA. Serum resistance in bvg-regulated mutants of Bordetella pertussis. FEMS Microbiol Lett. 1998;163:57-63.
46. Fischer W, Buhrdorf R, Gerland E, Haas R. Outer membrane targeting of passenger proteins by the vacuolating cytotoxin autotransporter of Helicobacter pylori. Infect Immun. 2001;69:6769-6775.
47. Eidels L, Proia RL, Hart DA. Membrane receptors for bacterial toxins. Microbiol Rev. 1983;47:596-620.
48. Bigalke H, Shoer LF. Clostridial neurotoxins. In: Aktories K, Just I, eds. Bacterial Protein Toxins. Berlin: Springer-Verlag; 2000:407-443.
49. Lencer WI. Microbes and microbial toxins: Paradigms for microbial-mucosal toxins. V. Cholera: Invasion of the intestinal epithelial barrier by a stably folded protein toxin. Am J Physiol. 2001;280:G781-G786.
50. Abrami L, Fivaz M, van der Goot FG. Adventures of a pore-forming toxin at the target cell surface. Trends Microbiol. 2000;8:168-172.
51. Wolf AA, Fujinaga Y, Lencer WI. Uncoupling of the cholera toxin–G(M1) ganglioside receptor complex from endocytosis, retrograde Golgi trafficking, and downstream signal transduction by depletion of membrane cholesterol. J Biol Chem. 2002;277:16249-16256.
52. Abrami L, Liu S, Cosson P, et al. Anthrax toxin triggers endocytosis of its receptor via a lipid raft–mediated clathrin-dependent process. J Cell Biol. 2003;160:321-328.
53. Saukkonen K, Burnette WN, Mar VL, et al. Pertussis toxin has eukaryotic-like carbohydrate recognition domains. Proc Natl Acad Sci USA. 1992;89:118-122.
54. Sindt K, Redpath G, Hewlett E, et al. Pertussis toxin activates platelets through an interaction with platelet glycoprotein Ib. Infect Immun. 1994;62:3108-3114.
55. Kounnas MZ, Morris RE, Thompson MR, et al. The alpha 2-macroglobulin receptor–related protein binds and internalizes Pseudomonas exotoxin A. J Biol Chem. 1992;267:12420-12423.
56. Naglich JG, Metherall JE, Russell DW, Eidels L. Expression cloning of a diphtheria toxin receptor: Identity with a heparin-binding EGF-like growth factor precursor. Cell. 1992;69:1051-1061.
57. Cha JH, Brooke JS, Ivey KN, Eidels L. Cell surface monkey CD9 antigen is a coreceptor that increases diphtheria toxin sensitivity and diphtheria toxin receptor affinity. J Biol Chem. 2000;275:6901-6907.
58. Cha JH, Brooke JS, Chang MY, Eidels L. Receptor-based antidote for diphtheria. Infect Immun. 2002;70:2344-2350.
59. Kagan BL, Reich KA, Collier RJ. Orientation of the diphtheria toxin channel in lipid bilayers. Biophys J. 1984;45:102-104.
60. Benson EL, Huynh PD, Finkelstein A, Collier RJ. Identification of residues lining the anthrax protective antigen channel. Biochemistry. 1998;37:3941-3948.
61. Umata T, Sharma KD, Mekada E. Diphtheria toxin and the diphtheria-toxin receptor. In: Aktories K, Just I, eds. Bacterial Protein Toxins. Berlin: Springer-Verlag; 2000:45-66.
62. West SEH. Pseudomonas aeruginosa exotoxin A: Structure/function, production and intoxication of eukaryotic cells. In: Aktories K, Just I, eds. Bacterial Protein Toxins. Berlin: Springer-Verlag; 2000:67-89.
63. Gordon VM, Young WW Jr, Lechler SM, et al. Adenylate cyclase toxins from Bacillus anthracis and Bordetella pertussis. Different processes for interaction with and entry into target cells. J Biol Chem. 1989;264:14792-14796.
64. Guermonprez P, Khelef N, Blouin E, et al. The adenylate cyclase toxin of Bordetella pertussis binds to target cells via the αMβ2 integrin (CD11b/CD18). J Exp Med. 2001;193:1035-1044.
65. Otero AS, Yi XB, Gray MC, et al. Membrane depolarization prevents cell invasion by Bordetella pertussis adenylate cyclase toxin. J Biol Chem. 1995;270:9695-9697.
66. Karimova G, Fayolle C, Gmira S, et al. Charge-dependent translocation of Bordetella pertussis adenylate cyclase toxin into eukaryotic cells: Implication for the in vivo delivery of CD8+ T cell epitopes into antigen-presenting cells. Proc Natl Acad Sci USA. 1998;95:12532-12537.
67. Yahr TL, Vallis AJ, Hancock MK, et al. ExoY, an adenylate cyclase secreted by the Pseudomonas aeruginosa type III system. Proc Natl Acad Sci USA. 1998;95:13899-13904.
68. Nishiki T, Tokuyama Y, Kamata Y, et al. Binding of botulinum type B neurotoxin to Chinese hamster ovary cells transfected with rat synaptotagmin II cDNA. Neurosci Lett. 1996;208:105-108.
69. Aktories K, Jurt I, eds. Bacterial Proteins Toxin. Handbook of Experimental Pharmacology, vol. 145. Berlin: Springer-Verlag; 2000.

70. Leppla SH. Anthrax toxin edema factor: A bacterial adenylate cyclase that increases cyclic AMP concentrations in eukaryotic cells. Proc Natl Acad Sci USA. 1982;79:3162-3166.

71. Bradley KA, Young JA. Anthrax toxin receptor proteins. Biochem Pharmacol. 2003;65:309-314.

72. Liu S, Leppla SH. Cell surface tumor endothelium marker 8 cytoplasmic tail-independent anthrax toxin binding, proteolytic processing, oligomer formation, and internalization. J Biol Chem. 2003;278:5227-5234.

73. Mogridge J, Cunningham K, Collier RJ. Stoichiometry of anthrax toxin complexes. Biochemistry. 2002;41:1079-1082.

74. Duesbery NS, Webb CP, Leppla SH, et al. Proteolytic inactivation of MAP-kinase-kinase by anthrax lethal factor. Science. 1998;280:734-737.

75. Vitale G, Pellizzari R, Recchi C, et al. Anthrax lethal factor cleaves the N-terminus of MAPKKs and induces tyrosine/threonine phosphorylation of MAPKs in cultured macrophages. Biochem Biophys Res Commun. 1998;248:706-711.

76. Chopra AP, Boone SA, Liang X, Duesbery NS. Anthrax lethal factor proteolysis and inactivation of MAPK kinase. J Biol Chem. 2003;278:9402-9406.

77. Park JM, Greten FR, Li ZW, Karin M. Macrophage apoptosis by anthrax lethal factor through p38 MAP kinase inhibition. Science. 2002;297:2048-2051.

78. Locht C, Antoine R, Jacob-Dubuisson F. *Bordetella pertussis*, molecular pathogenesis under multiple aspects. Curr Opin Microbiol. 2001;4:82-89.

79. Mattoo S, Foreman-Wykert AK, Cotter PA, Miller JF. Mechanisms of *Bordetella* pathogenesis. Front Biosci. 2001;6:E168-E186.

80. Arico B, Rappuoli R. *Bordetella parapertussis* and *Bordetella bronchiseptica* contain transcriptionally silent pertussis toxin genes. J Bacteriol. 1987;169:2847-2853.

81. Hewlett EL. Pertussis: Current concepts of pathogenesis and prevention. Pediatr Infect Dis J. 1997;16:S78-S84.

82. Toyota T, Kai Y, Kakizaki M, al. Effects of islet-activating protein (IAP) on blood glucose and plasma insulin in healthy volunteers (phase 1 studies). Tohoku J Exp Med. 1980;130:105-116.

83. Zaretzky FR, Gray MC, Hewlett EL. Direct penetration of bacterial toxins across the plasma membrane. In: Burns D, Barbieri JT, Iglewski BH, Rappuoli R, eds. Bacterial Protein Toxins. Washington, DC: ASM Press; 2003:149-156.

84. Heiss LN, Flak TA, Lancaster JR Jr, et al. Nitric oxide mediates *Bordetella pertussis* tracheal cytotoxin damage to the respiratory epithelium. Infect Agents Dis. 1994;2:173-177.

85. Lacerda HM, Pullinger GD, Lax AJ, Rozengurt E. Cytotoxic necrotizing factor 1 from *Escherichia coli* and dermonecrotic toxin from *Bordetella bronchiseptica* induce p21^rho-dependent tyrosine phosphorylation of focal adhesion kinase and paxillin in Swiss 3T3 cells. J Biol Chem. 1997;272:9587-9596.

86. Masuda M, Betancourt L, Matsuzawa T, et al. Activation of Rho through a cross-link with polyamines catalyzed by *Bordetella* dermonecrotizing toxin. EMBO J. 2000;19:521-530.

87. Horiguchi Y. *Escherichia coli* cytotoxic necrotizing factors and *Bordetella* dermonecrotic toxin: The dermonecrosis-inducing toxins activating Rho small GTPases. Toxicon. 2001;39:1619-1627.

88. Boquet P. Small GTP binding proteins and bacterial virulence. Microbes Infect. 2000;2:837-844.

89. Aktories K. Bacterial toxins that target Rho proteins. J Clin Invest. 1997;99:827-829.

90. Saelinger CB. Receptors for bacterial toxins. In: Burns DL, Barbieri JT, Iglewski BH, Rappuoli R, eds. Bacterial Protein Toxins. Washington, DC: ASM Press; 2003: 131-148.

91. Iwamoto R, Senoh H, Okada Y, et al. An antibody that inhibits the binding of diphtheria toxin to cells revealed the association of a 27-kDa membrane protein with the diphtheria toxin receptor. J Biol Chem. 1991;266:20463-20469.

92. Ratts R, Zeng H, Berg EA, et al. The cytosolic entry of diphtheria toxin catalytic domain requires a host cell cytosolic translocation factor complex. J Cell Biol. 2003;160:1139-1150.

93. Schiavo G, Rossetto O, Tonello F, Montecucco C. Intracellular targets and metalloprotease activity of tetanus and botulism neurotoxins. Curr Top Microbiol Immunol. 1995;195:257-274.

94. Johnson EA. Clostridial toxins as therapeutic agents: Benefits of nature's most toxic proteins. Annu Rev Microbiol. 1999;53:551-575.

95. Turton K, Chaddock JA, Acharya KR. Botulinum and tetanus neurotoxins: Structure, function and therapeutic utility. Trends Biochem Sci. 2002;27:552-558.

96. Rossetto O, Seveso M, Caccin P, et al. Tetanus and botulinum neurotoxins: Turning bad guys into good by research. Toxicon. 2001;39:27-41.

97. Schiavo G, Rossetto O, Benfenati F, et al. Tetanus and botulinum neurotoxins are zinc proteases specific for components of the neuroexocytosis apparatus. Ann NY Acad Sci. 1994;710:65-75.

98. Gill DM. Bacterial toxins: A table of lethal amounts. Microbiol Rev. 1982;46:86-94.

99. Perelle S, Gibert M, Bourlioux P, et al. Production of a complete binary toxin (actin-specific ADP-ribosyltransferase) by *Clostridium difficile* CD196. Infect Immun. 1997;65:1402-1407.

100. Shapiro RL, Hatheway C, Swerdlow DL. Botulism in the United States: A clinical and epidemiologic review. Ann Intern Med. 1998;129:221-228.

101. Cherington M. Clinical spectrum of botulism. Muscle Nerve. 1998;21:701-710.

102. Glatman-Freedman A. Infant botulism. Pediatr Rev. 1996;17:185-186.

103. Boquet P, Munro P, Fiorentini C, Just I. Toxins from anaerobic bacteria: Specificity and molecular mechanisms of action. Curr Opin Microbiol. 1998;1:66-74.

104. Sears CL, Kaper JB. Enteric bacterial toxins: Mechanisms of action and linkage to intestinal secretion. Microbiol Rev. 1996;60:167-215.

105. Ishibashi Y, Arai T. Specific inhibition of phagosome-lysosome fusion in murine macrophages mediated by *Salmonella typhimurium* infection. FEMS Microbiol Immunol. 1990;2:35-43.

106. Popoff MR. Interactions between bacterial toxins and intestinal cells. Toxicon. 1998;36:665-685.

107. Pothoulakis C, LaMont JT. Microbes and microbial toxins: Paradigms for microbial-mucosal interactions II. The integrated response of the intestine to *Clostridium difficile* toxins. Am J Physiol. 2001;280:G178-G183.

108. Carpenter CCJ Jr. Cholera enterotoxin—Recent investigations yield insights into transport processes. Am J Med. 1971;50:1-7.

109. Moss J, Vaughan M. Mechanism of action of choleragen and E. coli heat-labile enterotoxin: Activation of adenylate cyclase by ADP-ribosylation. Mol Cell Biochem. 1981;37:75-90.

110. Thielman NM, Marcinkiewicz M, Sarosiek J, et al. Role of platelet-activating factor in Chinese hamster ovary cell responses to cholera toxin. J Clin Invest. 1997;99:1999-2004.

111. Lundgren O. 5-Hydroxytryptamine, enterotoxins, and intestinal fluid secretion. Gastroenterology. 1998;115:1009-1012.

112. Turvill JL, Mourad FH, Farthing MJ. Crucial role for 5-HT in cholera toxin but not *Escherichia coli* heat-labile enterotoxin-intestinal secretion in rats Gastroenterology. 1998;115:883-890.

113. Peterson JW, Finkelstein RA, Cantu J, et al. Cholera toxin B subunit activates arachidonic acid metabolism. Infect Immun. 1999;67:794-799.

114. Levine MM, Kaper JB. Live oral vaccines against cholera: An update. Vaccine. 1993;11:207-212.

115. Smith PL, Blumberg JB, Stoff JS, Field M. Antisecretory effects of indomethacin on rabbit ileal mucosa in vitro. Gastroenterology. 1981;80:356-365.

116. Baudry B, Fasano A, Ketley J, Kaper JB. Cloning of a gene (*zot*) encoding a new toxin produced by *Vibrio cholerae*. Infect Immun. 1992;60:428-434.

117. Pierce NF, Cray WCJ, Sacci JBJ. Oral immunization of dogs with purified cholera toxin, crude cholera toxin, or B subunit: Evidence for synergistic protection by antitoxic and antibacterial mechanisms. Infect Immun. 1982;37:687-694.

118. Harandi AM, Sanchez J, Eriksson K, Holmgren J. Recent developments in mucosal immunomodulatory adjuvants. Curr Opin Investig Drugs. 2003;4:156-161.

119. Lycke N. The mechanism of cholera toxin adjuvanticity. Res Immunol. 1997;148:504-520.

120. Eriksson K, Holmgren J. Recent advances in mucosal vaccines and adjuvants. Curr Opin Immunol. 2002;14:666-672.

121. Pickett CL, Twiddy EM, Coker C, Holmes RK. Cloning, nucleotide sequence, and hybridization studies of the type IIb heat-labile enterotoxin gene of *Escherichia coli*. J Bacteriol. 1989;171:4945-4952.

122. Rasheed JK, Guzman-Verduzco LM, Kupersztoch YM. Two precursors of the heat-stable enterotoxin of *Escherichia coli*: Evidence of extracellular processing. Mol Microbiol. 1990;4:265-273.

123. Hughes JM, Murad F, Chang B, Guerrant RL. Role of cyclic GMP in the action of heat-stable enterotoxin of *Escherichia coli*. Nature. 1978;271:755-756.

124. Schulz S, Green CK, Yuen PS, Garbers DL. Guanylyl cyclase is a heat-stable enterotoxin receptor. Cell. 1990;63:941-948.

125. Forte LR, Eber SL, Turner JT, et al. Guanylin stimulation of Cl⁻ secretion in human intestinal T84 cells via cyclic guanosine monophosphate. J Clin Invest. 1993;91:2423-2428.

126. Wren BW. Molecular characterisation of *Clostridium difficile* toxins A and B. Rev Med Microbiol. 1992;3:21-27.

127. Rocha MFG, Maia MET, Bezerra LRPS, et al. *Clostridium difficile* toxin A induces the release of neutrophil chemotactic factors from rat peritoneal macrophages: Role of interleukin-1β, tumor necrosis factor alpha, and leukotrienes. Infect Immun. 1997;65:2740-2746.

128. Hecht G, Pothoulakis C, LaMont JT, Madara JL. *Clostridium difficile* toxin A perturbs cytoskeletal structure and tight junction permeability of cultured human intestinal epithelial monolayers. J Clin Invest. 1988;82:1516-1524.

129. Fonteles M, Fang G, Thielman NM, et al. Role of platelet activating factor in the inflammatory and secretory effects of *Clostridium difficile* toxin A. J Lipid Mediat Cell Signal. 1995;11:133-143.

130. Nusrat A, Eichel-Streiber C, Turner JR, et al. *Clostridium difficile* toxins disrupt epithelial barrier function by altering membrane microdomain localization of tight junction proteins. Infect Immun. 2001;69:1329-1336.

131. Chambers FG, Koshy SS, Saidi RF, et al. *Bacteroides fragilis* toxin exhibits polar activity on monolayers of human intestinal epithelial cells (T84 cells) in vitro. Infect Immun. 1997;65:3561-3570.

132. Obiso RJ Jr, Lyerly DM, Van Tassell RL, Wilkins TD. Proteolytic activity of the *Bacteroides fragilis* enterotoxin causes fluid secretion and intestinal damage in vivo. Infect Immun. 1995:3820-3826.

133. Saidi RF, Jaeger K, Montrose MH, et al. *Bacteroides fragilis* toxin rearranges the actin cytoskeleton of HT29/C1 cells without direct proteolysis of actin or decrease in F-actin content. Cell Motil Cytoskeleton. 1997;37:159-165.

134. Wu S, Lim KC, Huang J, et al. *Bacteroides fragilis* enterotoxin cleaves the zonula adherens protein, E-cadherin. Proc Natl Acad Sci USA. 1998;95:14979-14984.

135. Sears CL. The toxins of *Bacteroides fragilis*. Toxicon. 2001;39:1737-1746.

136. O'Brien AD, Tesh VL, Donohue-Rolfe A, et al. Shiga toxin: Biochemistry, genetics, mode of action, and role in pathogenesis. Curr Top Microbiol Immunol. 1992;180:65-94.

137. Schmidt H, Montag M, Bockemuhl J, et al. Shiga-like toxin II–related cytotoxins in *Citrobacter freundii* strains from humans and beef samples. Infect Immun. 1993;61:534-543.

138. Stein PE, Boodhoo A, Tyrrell GJ, et al. Crystal structure of the cell-binding B oligomer of verotoxin-1 from E. coli. Nature. 1992;355:748-750.

139. Sandvig K, Garred O, van Deurs B. Intracellular transport and processing of protein toxins produced by enteric bacteria. In: Paul PS, Francis DH, Benfield D, eds. Mechanisms in the Pathogenesis of Enteric Diseases. New York: Plenum Press; 1997:225-232.

140. Louise CB, Obrig TG. Shiga toxin–associated hemolytic uremic syndrome: Combined cytotoxic effects of Shiga toxin and lipopolysaccharide (endotoxin) on human vascular endothelial cells in vitro. Infect Immun. 1992;60:1536-1543.

141. Kaplan BS. Shiga toxin–induced tubular injury in hemolytic uremic syndrome (Editorial; comment). Kidney Int. 1998;54:648-649.

142. Louise CB, Tran MC, Obrig TG. Sensitization of human umbilical vein endothelial cells to *Shiga* toxin: Involvement of protein kinase C and NF-kappaB. Infect Immun. 1997;65:3337-3344.

143. Adler S, Bollu R. Glomerular endothelial cell injury mediated by Shiga-like toxin-1. Kidney Blood Press Res. 1998;21:13-21.

144. Bohach GA, Stauffacher CV, Ohlendorf DH, et al. The staphylococcal and streptococcal pyrogenic toxin family. Adv Exp Med Biol. 1996;391:131-154.

145. Rago JV, Schlievert PM. Mechanisms of pathogenesis of staphylococcal and streptococcal superantigens. Curr Top Microbiol Immunol. 1998;225:81-97.

146. Leung DY, Meissner C, Fulton D, Schlievert PM. The potential role of bacterial superantigens in the pathogenesis of Kawasaki syndrome. J Clin Immunol. 1995;15 (6 Suppl):11S-17S.

147. Leung DY, Sullivan KE, Brown-Whitehorn TF, et al. Association of toxic shock syndrome toxin–secreting and exfoliative toxin–secreting *Staphylococcus aureus* with Kawasaki syndrome complicated by coronary artery disease. Pediatr Res. 1997; 42:268-272.

148. Marrack P, Kappler J. The staphylococcal enterotoxins and their relatives. Science. 1990;248:705-711.

149. Leder L, Llera A, Lavoie PM, et al. A mutational analysis of the binding of staphylococcal enterotoxins B and C3 to the T cell receptor beta chain and major histocompatibility complex class II. J Exp Med. 1998;187:823-833.

150. Bohach GA. Staphylococcal enterotoxins B and C. Structural requirements for superantigenic and enterotoxigenic activities. Prep Biochem Biotechnol. 1997;27: 79-110.

151. Schlievert PM, Bohach GA, Ohlendorf DH, et al. Molecular structure of *Staphylococcus* and *Streptococcus* superantigens [published erratum appears in J Clin Immunol. 1996;16:126]. J Clin Immunol. 1995;15(6 Suppl):4S-10S.

152. Alouf JE. Pore-forming bacterial protein toxins: An overview. In: Compans RW, Cooper M, Koprowski H, et al, eds. Pore-Forming Toxins. Berlin: Springer-Verlag; 2001:1-14.

153. Menestrina G, Serra MD, Prevost G. Mode of action of β-barrel pore-forming toxins of the staphylococcal α-hemolysin family. Toxicon. 2001;39:1661-1672.

154. Tweten RK, Parker MW, Johnson AE. The cholesterol-dependent cytolysins. Curr Top Microbiol Immunol. 2001;257:15-33.

155. Menestrina G, Serra MD, Prevost G. Staphylococcal pore-forming toxins. Curr Top Microbiol Immunol. 2001;257:53-83.

156. Menestrina G, Serra MD, Prevost G. Mode of action of beta-barrel pore-forming toxins of the staphylococcal alpha-hemolysin family. Toxicon. 2001;39:1661-1672.

157. Welch RA. RTX toxin structure and function: A story of numerous anomalies and few analogies in toxin biology. Curr Top Microbiol Immunol. 2001;257:85-111.

158. Lally ET, Hill RB, Kieba IR, Korostoff J. The interaction between RTX toxins and target cells. Trends Microbiol. 1999;7:356-361.

159. Alouf JE. Pore-forming bacterial protein toxins: An overview. Curr Top Microbiol Immunol. 2001;257:1-14.

160. van der Goot FG. Membrane-damaging toxins: Pore formation. In: Burns D, ed. Bacterial Protein Toxins. Washington, DC: ASM Press; 2003:189-202.

161. Fivaz M, Abrami L, Tsitrin Y, van der Goot FG. Aerolysin from *Aeromonas hydrophila* and related toxins. Curr Top Microbiol Immunol. 2001;257:35-52.

162. Kreitman RJ, Wilson WH, Bergeron K, et al. Efficacy of the anti-CD22 recombinant immunotoxin BL22 in chemotherapy-resistant hairy-cell leukemia. N Engl J Med. 2001;345:241-247.

163. vanderSpek JC, Murphy JR. Fusion protein toxins based on diphtheria toxin: Selective targeting of growth factor receptors of eukaryotic cells. Methods Enzymol. 2000;327:239-249.

164. Klein AW. Complications, adverse reactions, and insights with the use of botulinum toxin. Dermatol Surg. 2003;29:549-556.

165. Lu Y, Friedman R, Kushner N, et al. Genetically modified anthrax lethal toxin safely delivers whole HIV protein antigens into the cytosol to induce T cell immunity. Proc Natl Acad Sci USA. 2000;97:8027-8032.

166. El Azami El Idrissi M, Ladant D, Leclerc C. The adenylate cyclase of *Bordetella pertussis*: A vector to target antigen presenting cells. Toxicon. 2002;40:1661-1665.

CHAPTER **4**

Innate (General or Nonspecific) Host Defense Mechanisms

CARL W. DIEFFENBACH
EDMUND C. TRAMONT

Host defense mechanisms against microbial invasion are a continuum. At one end of the spectrum are the general nonspecific barriers; at the other end, acquired specific immunity (see Chapters 6 through 9); and in between, the steady-state, pattern-recognition immune response known as *innate immunity* (Table 4-1).[1] All of these barriers must be breached for an infection to occur. Understanding of the host/microbe or host/pathogen interaction and the complexity and overlap between general, innate, and adaptive immunity continues to evolve, especially at the molecular level. Additionally the importance of the crosstalk between the various host defense mechanisms has become increasingly apparent, achieving selectivity and specificity, which helps to focus and direct the adaptive response.

The general nonspecific and innate host defense mechanisms represent an effective, broad-based surveillance program that serves as a transitional defense system, holding a foreign invader at bay while setting the stage for the host to develop specific adaptive immunity. These mechanisms provide crucial initial encounters against all microorganisms. The broad nature of the nonspecific and innate host defense mechanisms includes the general nonspecific effects resulting from physical barriers (e.g., intact skin, mucous membranes, microbicidal peptides, mucus, biofilm, cilia, peristalsis, resident microflora, lysozyme, complement). As a pathogen circumvents the general nonspecific defenses, the invading organism is detected or sensed by the host, resulting in the activation of many cell types and synthesis and release of a range of factors, which classically have been described as the *acute-phase response* (see the section on innate immunity and acute-phase response later).[2]

The *acute-phase response* is the term used to describe a range of nonspecific antimicrobial host factors that promote phagocytosis and microbial killing. These factors are produced mainly in the liver as a result of detection and triggering of the innate immune system. Although many of these acute-phase proteins are present at all times,

it is their rapid, quantitative increase that constitutes the acute-phase reaction or response. This response to pathogens results in fever and malaise that typically accompanies the early phases of infection and represents, in broad terms, the events that occur during infection before the establishment or boosting of the specific adaptive immune response. Traditionally, the list of factors that have correlated with acute-phase response include (1) trigger molecules, which constitute signal systems that alert the adaptive immune system, and (2) effector molecules, which are involved in inflammation, antimicrobial scavenging, and promoting and focusing the adaptive immune response.

How does the human host sense a pathogen and trigger this cascade of responses? It has been hypothesized that the host maintains a detection system that, similar to a smoke detector, senses and triggers a response when a microbe has invaded. Insights into how the host detects an invader and what the host detects have come from many unexpected directions.[3] Through many elegant experiments, investigators showed that a set of genes known as the *Toll gene family* was involved in embryonic development and antifungal responses in fruit flies. The importance of this discovery was appreciated fully with the identification of the lipopolysaccharide (LPS) receptor as a Toll-like receptor (TLR) gene.[4] Additional studies have shown that the Toll gene family is conserved in all species from plants to humans and performs similar functions for all multicellular creatures.[5] This effect has been preserved throughout evolution and is referred to as the *innate immune system.* The major gene family that is associated with innate immunity is called the *TLR gene family.*[5,6]

TISSUE TROPISMS AND HEREDITARY FACTORS

The susceptibility, morbidity, and mortality related to virtually every pathogen and to infection in general are influenced significantly by the host's genetic makeup. If a child's parent died from an infectious disease, such as pneumonia, the child may have inherited an increased probability of dying from an infection (Fig. 4-1).[7] The reasons for this increased susceptibility are multifactorial and include defects in innate immunity, such as a Toll receptor gene,[8] complement,[9] cytokine and chemokines or their receptors,[10] degrees of limited human leukocyte antigen (HLA) diversity,[11,12] and cellular receptor specificities.[13] Other factors undoubtedly will be determined in the future.

The microbial ligand and the host receptor vary independently as to their specificity: A receptor may bind to one or many different ligands on microorganisms, and a ligand may bind to one or many different receptors. Most organisms preferentially colonize certain cells (tissues) and spare others. This phenomenon, referred to as *cellular tropism* or *tissue tropism,* is a crucial determinant of host-microorganism relationships. Influenza virus and mycoplasmas preferentially adhere to respiratory epithelial cells; *Escherichia coli* and *Vibrio cholerae* to intestinal cells; and *Streptococcus mutans* to tooth enamel. Gram-positive organisms more readily attach to heart valves than do gram-negative organisms. Also, urinary epithelial cells from persons with recurrent urinary tract infections support the attachment of urinary pathogens more readily than do urinary epithelial cells obtained from

TABLE 4-1 Nonspecific, Innate, and Adaptive Immunity

Property	Nonspecific	Innate	Adaptive
Receptors	None	Fixed in genome Rearrangement not necessary	Encoded in gene segments Rearrangement required
Distribution	Covers every interface with the environment	Cell type or tissue specific	Clonal
Recognition	None, limited	Conserved molecular patterns	Details of molecular structure
Action time	Continuous	Immediate activation of effectors	Delayed activation
Response	Shield holds, provided no breaks in the barrier Acute-phase proteins	Costimulatory molecules cytokines, chemokines Acute-phase proteins	Clonal expansion or anergy, IL-2 Effector cytokines, humoral, cell-mediated immunity

IL-2, interleukin-2.
Modified with permission from Janeway CA, Medzhitov R. Innate immune recognition. Annu Rev Immunol. 2002;20:197-216. ©2002 by Annual Reviews
www.annualreviews.org.

persons not prone to develop these infections.[14] A specific example of cellular tropism is the monocyte-tropic human immunodeficiency virus (HIV-1), which requires the presence of certain chemokine receptors, especially CCR5 or CXCR4, in conjunction with the CD4 molecule, to infect the host cell (see Chapter 116).

Receptors on host cells may change. Evidence suggests that a viral illness can affect tissue tropisms of the oropharynx and tracheobronchial tree to allow easier colonization by bacteria.[15] As the genetics and cellular characteristics of cellular and tissue tropisms become better known, they will offer a new paradigm for the development of treatment modalities and vaccines.

Ligands on microorganisms change more readily. One of the oldest known examples is trypanosomiasis (see Chapter 274). More recently, the switch by HIV-1 from a monocyte-tropic CCR5 or nonsyncytia-inducing phenotype to a T-cell lymphotropic CXCR4 or syncytia-inducing phenotype has been related to selection and disease progression (see Chapter 116).

Infectious diseases represent one of the strongest and most important selection pressures in human evolution (see Chapter 5). Tuberculosis, measles, and smallpox had devastating effects on the native populations of North and South America, presumably because there was no selective pressure on the indigenous populations to evolve "natural immunity" against these pathogens before being exposed through contact with the more urbanized Europeans.

Conversely, the sickle cell trait has a protective effect against falciparum malaria, and the trait benefits inhabitants of areas where this parasite is endemic. Persons homozygous for a mutation in the gene that codes for the CCR5 chemokine receptor ($\Delta32CCR5$) are resistant to contracting HIV-1 through sexual contact.[16] Persons of western European descent, especially persons from the British Isles, are more likely to carry this deletion than are Africans and Asians, who almost never do.[16] A number of genetic changes have been correlated with slow or nonprogression to AIDS, including heterozygosity for $\Delta32CCR5$ or other chemokine polymorphisms, increased secretion of α-defensins, changes in HLA-B*35 subtypes, and upregulation of CD91—the heat-shock protein receptor.[17-20] Although resistance to HIV-1 infection also has been linked to class II HLA-DRB3 discordance, this is more likely due to chance encounter with discordant HLA antigens integrated into the HIV to which the recipient host is exposed.[21] Severity of and susceptibility to tuberculosis have been linked to variations in the *SLS11A1* gene (formerly known as the *NRAMP1* gene), an HLA-DQ allele, and interleukin (IL)-12 deficiency.[22-26] Susceptibility to pneumococcal disease has been linked to defective production of antibody to the pneumococcal capsule,[27] and the congenital absence of a terminal component of complement predisposes to repeated episodes of disseminated neisserial infections (see Chapters 7 and 208).

Other known linkages include HLA-B27 and reactive arthropathy (Reiter's syndrome); HLA-DR4 and chronic Lyme arthritis; the predisposition of persons with blood group O to cholera, which presumably is linked to the expression of glycosphingolipids in the small bowel mucosa; DRB1*01 and DRB1*04 with symptomatic parvovirus B19 infection[28]; HLA-CW*0202 with human papillomavirus–induced cervical cancer[29]; and various polymorphisms with clearance and persistence of cervical human papillomavirus infection,[30] tuberculoid leprosy, acute glomerulonephritis, paralytic poliomyelitis, meningococcal disease,[31] and Dengue hemorrhagic fever.[32] Infections also can affect the susceptibility to allergic and autoimmune diseases. Solid epidemiologic data suggest that the increase in the incidence of these diseases in industrialized countries is a consequence of decreased incidence of infectious diseases.[33] In summary, the outcome of virtually every microbial-host interaction is linked to host genetics.

NATURAL PHYSICAL BARRIERS TO THE ENTRY OF MICROORGANISMS INTO THE BODY

The morphologic integrity of body surfaces is an important and effective first line of defense. The epithelial coverings and linings share many similar properties, such as production of defensins[34] and populations of γδ cells[35] and unique defense molecules, such as lysozyme.[36]

Skin

The intact skin forms an effective mechanical barrier to invasion by microorganisms. The specific antimicrobial properties of skin are principally due to a protective shield consisting of a battery of broad-spectrum defensive chemicals, principally peptides, synthesized as precursors and processed by specific proteases into mature, active forms that target microbial membranes in a manner similar to disinfectants. The two major classes of antimicrobial peptides are cathelicidins and β-defensins.[34,34a] Not only do they function directly to kill microbes, they also act as chemokines to attract migrating phagocytic cells. Four β-defensins—HBD-1, HBD-2, HBD-3, and HBD-4—have been described, and HBD-4 and LL-37 cathelicidin levels are depressed in atopic skin, a condition in which microbial suprainfection is common.[37]

The relative dryness or desiccating effect of skin, its mild acidity (the so-called acid mantle—pH 5 to 6), and the normal skin flora act in concert to form an effective prohibitive environment. Inflamed skin is more permeable to water and is more hospitable to colonization. It has been speculated that oily skin may retard evaporation of water, resulting in increased numbers of colonizing microorganisms. The acidity of the skin results from the breakdown of lipids into fatty acids. Sebum contains few esterified fatty acids, but the normal skin flora partially hydrolyzes the triglycerides, liberating fatty acids. The continual desquamation of skin scales also aids in the elimination of microorganisms. Because few organisms have the ability to penetrate the skin, they usually gain access by some physical means, such as an arthropod vector, trauma, surgical incision, or intravenous catheter.

Mucous Membranes

Because of the inherent moisture with which they are associated, mucous membranes support a broader spectrum and larger number of microorganisms than does skin. Most epithelial cells possess the same peptide shield as skin, however.[38,39] Additionally, body secretions, including saliva, cervical mucus, prostatic fluid, and tears, are endowed with unique antimicrobial properties.[40] Two of the more potent antimicrobial substances are lysozyme and *N*-acetyl muramyl-L-alanine amidase (NAMLAA). Both substances are particularly effective against gram-positive bacteria because they hydrolyze the amino acid backbone of peptidoglycan.[36]

Local secretions also contain immunoglobulins, principally IgG and secretory IgA, which act primarily to agglutinate microorganisms, block competitively the attachment of organisms to receptors on host cells, or both. The body produces more secretory IgA than total IgG. The IgA immunoglobulin is made relatively resistant to proteolysis by complexing with a unique polypeptide known as *secretory piece* and protein, Fv.[41] There is also evidence that mucosal IgA is able to bind intracellular pathogens or products as they are transported to the cell surface.[42]

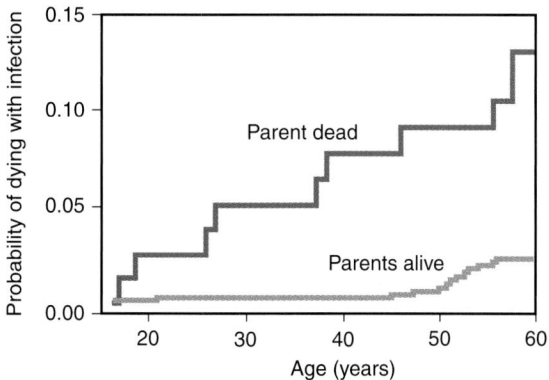

FIGURE 4-1. Probability of dying from an infection before a given age for adoptees with at least one biologic parent who died before age 50 (parent dead) of an infection versus adoptees whose biologic parents were alive at that age (parents alive).

Mucosal secretions also contain significant amounts of iron-binding proteins. The importance of iron for microorganisms is well recognized, and fluids that potentially are exposed to microbes are enriched with iron-binding proteins that act to keep this important factor from the microorganisms. In contrast, microorganisms that routinely colonize skin and mucosal surfaces have evolved mechanisms to acquire iron despite these proteins.[43,44]

Respiratory Tract

The respiratory tract has a formidable array of antimicrobial defense mechanisms.[45,46] The inhaled particles must survive and penetrate the aerodynamic filtration system of the upper airway and tracheobronchial tree. The airflow in these areas is turbulent, causing large particles to come in contact with the mucosal surfaces and face the full array of those defense mechanisms. Humidification also causes hygroscopic organisms to increase in size, aiding trapping.

When a particle is deposited, the mucociliary blanket transports the invading offender away from the lung. Coughing aids this expulsion. This system is amazingly efficient: 90% of deposited material is cleared in less than 1 hour. In addition, the bronchial secretions contain various antimicrobial substances, such as lysozyme, NAMLAA, and β-defensins such as HBD-1 and HBD-2.[47]

After a particle reaches the alveoli, physical expulsion becomes much less effective, and the alveolar macrophages and tissue histiocytes play a more prominent role in protecting the host. These phagocytic cells are assisted in their defense by the collectin surfactants SP-A and SP-D, which bind to and opsonize diverse organisms, including gram-negative bacteria, fungi, and *Pneumocystis carinii*.[48]

Similar to all defense mechanisms, these nonspecific mechanisms can be overcome by the introduction of large numbers of invading organisms (e.g., contaminated respirator), particularly if the host is exposed for an extended period. Their effectiveness is decreased by air pollutants (e.g., cigarette smoke), mechanical respirators, tracheostomy, concomitant infection, allergenic agents, and in some instances genetic defects (e.g., cystic fibrosis).

Intestinal Tract

The acid pH of the stomach and the antibacterial effect of the various pancreatic enzymes, bile, and intestinal secretions are effective first-line antimicrobial defense factors. Paneth cells of the small intestine, located in the crypts of Lieberkühn, secrete antimicrobial substances, such as β-defensins, lysozyme, and type II phospholipase A.[49]

Peristalsis and the normal loss of epithelial cells also act to purge the intestinal tract of harmful microorganisms. Alteration of these parameters can lead to increased susceptibility of the host to infection. *Salmonella* and *Mycobacterium tuberculosis* infections are more common in achlorhydric patients, and slowing peristalsis with belladonna or opium alkaloids prolongs symptomatic disease caused by gastrointestinal pathogens such as *Shigella* species.

The normal bowel microbial flora compete for nutrients (10^{12} organisms per gram of feces), and this plays a crucial protective role. Altering this symbiotic normal intestinal microflora, such as with broad-spectrum antibiotics, can lead to overgrowth of inherently pathogenic organisms (e.g., *Salmonella typhimurium*) or suprainfection with ordinarily commensal organisms (e.g., *Candida albicans*). As always, the interfering competitive capacity of the normal flora can be overcome by the introduction of large numbers of pathogenic organisms. The probability of development of salmonellosis is related directly to the number of *Salmonella* organisms ingested.

Genitourinary Tract

Urine is normally sterile. The factors that contribute to the ability of the urinary tract to resist infection are complex. Urine is bactericidal for some strains of bacteria, mostly because of its pH, although factors such as hypertonicity, urea, and other solutes play a role. Tamm-Horsfall protein is a glycoprotein produced by the kidneys and excreted in large amounts in urine (approximately 50 mg/L). Because many bacteria are avidly bound to it, the protein acts as a sponge and is a natural host defense mechanism against tissue colonization and subsequent infection by preventing these bacteria from gaining a foothold on the cellular lining of the urinary tract.[50]

The lower urinary tract is flushed with urine four to eight times each day, eliminating potential pathogenic organisms, unless they are capable of firmly attaching to epithelial cells of the urinary tract (e.g., *Neisseria gonorrhoeae*, certain strains of *E. coli*). Urinary retention impedes this process.

The length of the male urethra (20 cm in an adult) also provides passive protection, and bacteria seldom gain access to the bladder in men unless introduced by instrumentation. The female urethra is much shorter (5 cm in an adult) and is traversed more readily by microorganisms, which is one reason why urinary tract infections are 14 times more common in women than in men.

The hypotonic state of the kidney medulla presents an unfavorable milieu for most microorganisms. This natural barrier is breached most often by increased glucose levels secondary to hyperglycemia, which accounts for the increased incidence of pyelonephritis in diabetic patients.

The vagina has a unique mechanism of protection. Under hormonal influence, especially estrogen, the vaginal epithelium contains increased amounts of glycogen that *Döderlein's bacilli* and other commensals metabolize into lactic acid. Döderlein's bacilli is an all-encompassing term used to describe acidogenic gram-positive rods, especially lactobacilli, residing in the vagina. Normal vaginal secretions contain 10^8/mL of these bacteria. They establish an acid environment that is unfavorable to most pathogenic microorganisms. The vaginal secretions of women with nonspecific vaginitis or vaginosis, a perturbation of the normally protective vaginal ecosystem, are characterized by an elevated pH.

Eye

Constant bathing of the eye by tears is an effective means of protection. Foreign substances continually are diluted and washed away via the tear ducts into the nasal cavity. Tears also contain large amounts of lysozyme and other antimicrobial substances.

STEADY-STATE COMPONENTS OF NONSPECIFIC IMMUNITY

After microbes breach the integumentary barriers, they encounter additional nonspecific host defenses mediated by soluble factors and cells. Some of these factors are present or circulating at low steady-state physiologic levels but increase twofold to 1000-fold in response to microbial invasion. The level and localization of these humoral and cellular components are regulated primarily by cytokines and chemokines (see Chapter 9).

Complement

Complement refers to a group of 20 or more serum proteins that interact in an orderly fashion that is referred to as the *complement cascade*. Complement can be activated by specific antibody or by the acute-phase reactants, such as C-reactive protein (classic pathway); by the surface components of microorganisms (alternative pathway); and by the collectin mannose-binding protein via interaction with cell surface receptors, such as C1R and C1S.[48,51,52]

Complement activation can lead to direct microbial lysis, but it also plays important roles in phagocytosis, cytokine/chemokine production, and attraction of leukocytes to infected sites. The lytic action of complement is effective: Most intestinal colonizing bacteria are susceptible to complement-mediated lysis. In contrast, strains of enteric bacteria that result in invasive disease typically resist complement-mediated serum bactericidal activity. Most complement components are synthesized by macrophages, with increased production in response to infection (see Chapter 7).

Mannose-Binding Lectin

Mannose-binding lectin is a pluripotent sugar-binding protein found in mammals that discriminates between self and nonself sugar arrays and that, on binding to its targets, activates the complement system. Mannose-binding lectin increases the efficiency of antibody-mediated, complement-dependent immune protection.[53,54] At least three different major human pathogens have hijacked the lectin-binding pathway, however, for the purpose of establishing an infection: HIV,[54] Ebola,[55] and *M. tuberculosis.*[56] In all three diseases, this DC-SIGN-directed pathway is used by the pathogen to avoid direct confrontation with the innate immune system.

Fibronectin

Fibronectin is a high-molecular-weight glycoprotein found in plasma and on cell surfaces that plays a central role in cell-cell adhesion, cell–basement membrane adhesion, clot stabilization, fibroblast migration, and macrophage function. As with all aspects of the host-parasite relationship, a yin-yang phenomenon occurs: Fibronectin covers the receptors of surface cells and blocks the attachment of many microorganisms, such as *Pseudomonas aeruginosa,* but it enhances the binding of other organisms, such as *Staphylococcus aureus,* to host cells.[57]

Phagocytosis

Microorganisms that enter the body are engulfed and killed by a variety of phagocytic cells, such as dendritic cells, polymorphonuclear neutrophils (PMNs), and macrophages. Macrophages are found in all body tissues, whereas PMNs and monocytes circulate in blood and lymph channels. There is the customary crosstalk among all of these sentinel cells, and when a microorganism is sensed or detected, they secrete a variety of chemotactic agents, such as chemokines, which ultimately leads to cellular migration through the tissues resulting in various degrees of inflammation.

When a microbe is internalized into a phagosome, it usually is killed by a variety of lethal microbicidal mechanisms, which include reactive oxygen and nitrogen intermediates and toxic peptides. The dead microorganisms are digested, the microbial peptides bind to major histocompatibility complex (MHC) molecules, and the complex migrates to the cell surface for presentation to its connate T-cell receptor. This process, called *antigen presentation,* results in specific T-cell clonal expansion and is a crucial interface between the innate and the adaptive immune systems.

Opsonin-independent phagocytosis by PMNs is related to the contact angle between the microorganism and the surface on which it rests. As a consequence of this physical relationship, phagocytosis is most efficient when organisms are trapped in small tissue spaces (e.g., alveoli) than when they reside on smooth, open surfaces (e.g., synovium) or float free in the blood.[58]

Mononuclear phagocytes in blood, lymph nodes, spleen, liver, bone marrow, and lung constitute the reticuloendothelial system. These cells recognize microbes, particulate matter, and damaged or senescent host cells by "pattern recognition receptors" on the macrophage surface. The scavenger receptor family (SRAI and SRAII, MACRO, CD36, CD68, and CLA-1)[59] and the mannose receptor[60] detect phospholipid-containing and mannose-containing structures. These structures frequently are present on microbes but are not present on normal host cells. Integrins, notably CD11b/CD18, CD11c/CD18, α_V/β_1, and α_V/β_3, indirectly recognize particulate targets by binding soluble host constituents, including activated complement components, vitronectin, and fibronectin. These soluble molecules interact with fragments of damaged cells, collagen debris, altered platelets, and microbes to enhance their clearance by macrophages.[60,61]

Recognition of collectins (mannose-binding protein, complement component C1q, and the surfactant SP-A) by macrophage receptor C1qRp also enhances phagocytosis of microorganisms coated with these ligands.[62] In addition, CD14 recognizes lipid A from gram-negative bacteria and lipoteichoic acid from gram-positive bacteria. Binding of lipid A to CD14 is facilitated by its attachment to LPS-binding protein. When these receptors are engaged, macrophages become programmed to remove the recognized complexed particles from circulation.

Under resting or steady-state conditions, macrophages and monocytes kill ingested microorganisms by the generation of toxic oxygen and nitrogen metabolites, such as hydrogen peroxide, superoxide, and

nitrous oxide (oxidative killing); nonoxidative killing occurs by defensins, the acidification of phagosomal vacuoles, the deposition of acid hydrolases and other lysosomal enzymes into phagolysosomes, and the production of a variety of granule-associated antimicrobial molecules, including neutrophil peptides 1 through 4, lysozyme, elastase, antileukoproteases, azurocidin, cathepsin G, and bactericidal/permeability–increasing protein.[63-65] These molecules also are released into the plasma and other body fluids during inflammation.[66] Their microbicidal capability is relatively limited, however, compared with that of PMNs and activated macrophages stimulated initially by the acute-phase reactants (proteins) and later by an adaptive immune response.

Persons whose spleens have been surgically removed or functionally impaired dramatically show the importance of the reticuloendothelial system: When encapsulated bacteria, such as pneumococci, are filtered poorly from the blood, they can overwhelm the host more easily by relatively unfettered replication in the blood (see Chapter 315).

INNATE IMMUNITY AND THE ACUTE-PHASE RESPONSE

The human host is armed with a diverse array of sensors to detect an invading pathogen. The best-studied gene family, TLRs, is structurally conserved in all eukaryotes and derives its name from the Toll mutants in *Drosophila.*[5,6] Currently, there are 10 known TLRs in humans (Table 4-2). The TLR gene family functions by detecting specific molecules and patterns of molecules that are unique to pathogens or damaged host tissues. This concept of molecular patterns, or *pathogen-associated molecular patterns* (*PAMPs*), forms the basis for the current view of how the host senses invasion.[5,67-71] Numerous ligands so far have been shown to trigger the 10 different TLRs and include microbial and host cell debris (see Table 4-2).

TABLE 4-2 Toll-like Receptors and Their Ligands[*]

TLR Family	Ligands (Origin)
TLR1	Triacyl lipopeptides (bacteria, mycobacteria)
	Soluble factors (*Neisseria* species)
TLR2	Lipoprotein/lipopeptides (a variety of pathogens)
	Peptidoglycan (gram-positive bacteria)
	Lipoteichoic acid (gram-positive bacteria)
	Lipoarabinomannan (mycobacteria)
	A phenol-soluble modulin (*Staphylococcus* species)
	Glycoinositolphospholipids (*Trypanosoma cruzi*)
	Glycolipids (*Treponema maltophilum*)
	Porins (*Neisseria* species)
	Zymosan (fungi)
	Atypical LPS (*Leptospira interrogans, Porphyromonas gingivalis*)
	HSP70 (host)
TLR3	Double-stranded RNA (virus)
TLR4	LPS (gram-negative bacteria)
	Taxol (plant)
	Fusion protein (RSV)
	Envelope proteins (MMTV)
	HSP60 (*Chlamydia pneumoniae*)
	F-protein (cytomegalovirus)
	HSP60 (host)
	HSP70 (host)
	Type III repeat extra domain A of fibronectin (host)
	Oligosaccharides of hyaluronic acid (host)
	Polysaccharide fragments of heparin sulfate (host)
	Fibrinogen (host)
TLR5	Flagellin (bacteria)
TLR6	Diacyl lipopeptides (*Mycoplasma* species)
TLR7	Imidazoquinoline (synthetic compounds)
	Loxoribine (synthetic compounds)
	Bropirimine (synthetic compounds)
	Guanine nucleoside analogues (synthetic compounds)
TLR8	R848/resiquimod
	Single-stranded RNA
TLR9	CpG DNA (bacteria)
	Chromatin:IgG complexes (host)
TLR10	?

[*]This table shows ligands for mammalian Toll-like receptors (TLRs): pathogen-derived and **host cell–derived ligands (in bold)**.[5,67-69a]

LPS, lipopolysaccharide; MMTV, mouse mammary tumor virus; RSV, respiratory syncytial virus.

Activated TLRs lead to the rapid production of many host cytokines, including IL-1, tumor necrosis factor-α (TNF-α), IL-6, and IL-12, which have redundant, multifactorial effects (Table 4-3). Clinically, this cytokine production results in the full effect of the acute-phase response, including fever (see later). Whether the acute inflammation results from infection or trauma, it is triggered along the same pathway. TLR signaling also activates the adaptive immune response.[71] Adjuvants for all current vaccines function through the activation of the TLR pathways. The most potent adjuvant, Freund's complete adjuvant, is a water-in-oil emulsion containing mycobacterial cell wall components that activates TLR-1, TLR-2, and TLR-4 (see Table 4-2). The simplest adjuvant, alum (aluminum hydroxide), induces molecules involved in antigen presentation in monocytes, MHC class II, CD40, CD54, CD58, CD83, and CD86; drives monocyte differentiation toward a dendritic cell–like morphology; and induces secretion of IL-4, a cytokine with potent antibody production–enhancing properties.[72]

Toll-like Receptors and the Cytokine Cascade

The signaling pathways for some of the TLRs have been defined and are involved in cytokine production (Fig. 4-2).[67] TLR-4, activated by either LPS or the host protein hsp70, activates many signaling pathways through the cytoplasmic tail; the end result is the activation of the transcription factors NF-κB, p38, JNK, and IRF3 (see Fig. 4-2). The NF-κB pathway is the central regulator of cellular transcription in innate and adaptive immunity, and induction of NF-κB is essential for T-cell activation and expansion. The response represents one of the many portals transitioning from innate to adaptive immunity. TLR-4 also triggers many costimulatory molecules, such as CD80/CD86, that aid in the development of antibody-mediated and cell-mediated responses to the pathogen. The IRF-3 pathway activates the interferon response program and is responsible for a profound antiviral state that is effective against all viruses. The result of the signaling and activation of the TLR is that within 4 hours the activated cell is producing the full complement of proinflammatory cytokines, including IL-1, IL-2, IL-6, IL-10, IL-12p40, IL-15, TNF-α, and interferon-α (IFN-α) and interferon-β (see Table 4-3). Through the induction of IL-10 and IL-12, TLR signaling has initiated a cascade that leads to production of interferon-γ and IL-4, which are crucial cytokines for adaptive immune response. As with all other biologic systems, TLR signaling also has a feedback system, which induces signals that attenuate this response, mainly IL-10.

Genetic analysis has allowed precise determination of inherited defects (so-called experiments of nature), and the first genetic deficiency in Toll receptor signaling, *IRAK-4* (interleukin-1 receptor-associated kinase-4), has been described.[8] Children with no detectable IRAK-4 in their cells had recurrent infections and poor inflammatory responses. Further investigation of cells from these patients showed that the cells did not produce TNF-α, IL-1β, IL-12p40, or IL-6 in response to a range of TLR ligands, including LPS. These children were susceptible to only a narrow range of bacterial infections, showing (1) the apparent redundancy built into the innate immune system and (2) the likelihood that this defect will be passed on and potentially expanded in the era of antibiotic therapy, which prolongs their lives into reproducing adults. It is highly likely that similar defects in innate immunity will be elucidated in the future and that this accounts in part for the inherited propensity to die from an infectious disease (see Fig. 4-1).

Cellular Distribution of Toll-like Receptors

Specificity of effects of the innate response are achieved through the distribution of subsets of TLRs on different types of immune effector cells (Table 4-4) and the selective signaling through each receptor (see Fig. 4-2).[5,6,73] TLR-1 and TLR-6 are expressed on all cell subtypes. TLR-2 is highly expressed on monocytes. Plasmacytoid dendritic cells (PDCs) and B cells express strong levels of TLR-7 and TLR-9. B cells express high levels of TLR-10, however, and PDCs show weak expression of this TLR. This is a snapshot of the profile in the resting state, and preliminary data indicate that the regulation of these receptors will be as fluid as the cytokine profile that they trigger.

Toll-like Receptor Signaling and the Initiation and Biasing of Adaptive Immunity

The activation of the innate immune system has several important effects on the adaptive immune response.[74] When stimulated through the

TABLE 4-3 Cytokines and Chemokines* Induced as Part of the Innate Response and Acute-Phase Reaction

IL-1	Inflammatory responses; inducer of acute-phase proteins, edema, and prostaglandin production; production of IL-2; growth of lymphocytes
IL-2	Promotes growth and differentiation of activated T cells and B cells; activates cells of the monocyte/macrophage lineage; induces interferon-γ and TNF-α
IL-4	Promotes B-cell growth and differentiation and Th2-driving cytokine; strong inducer of MHC class II
IL-6	Inducer of acute-phase proteins in hepatocytes; activates PBMCs; B-cell differentiation
IL-8	Enhances inflammation, produced by macrophage and endothelial cells; induces T-cell chemotaxis
IL-10	Attenuator; antagonist to IL-12—downregulates IFN-γ, IL-1, IL-6, and TNF-α; Th2 biasing also activates B cells
IL-12	Antagonist to IL-10; induces IFN-γ, Th1 biasing
IL-13	B-cell growth factor; promotes growth and differentiation of allergic effector cells
IL-15	Promotes growth and differentiation of T cells and B cells; activates cells of the monocyte/macrophage lineage; induces interferon-γ and TNF-α, promotes NK cell toxicity
IL-18	INF-γ inducing (in the presence of IL-12)
IFN-α, IFN-β	Antiviral proteins; induce upregulation of MHC class I
IFN-γ	Activates macrophage; upregulates MHC class I and II; sustains activated T cells; promotes antigen-presenting cell differentiation, Th1 biasing
TNF-α	Major proinflammatory cytokine; inducer of acute-phase response along with IL-1 and IL-6; activates adhesion processes and chemoattraction

*Chemokines as a class mobilize white blood cells to sites of inflammation via transmigration from the vasculature into the tissue to sites of inflammation.

IFN, interferon; IL, interleukin; MHC, major histocompatibility complex; NK, natural killer; PBMCs, peripheral blood mononuclear cells; TNF, tumor necrosis factor.

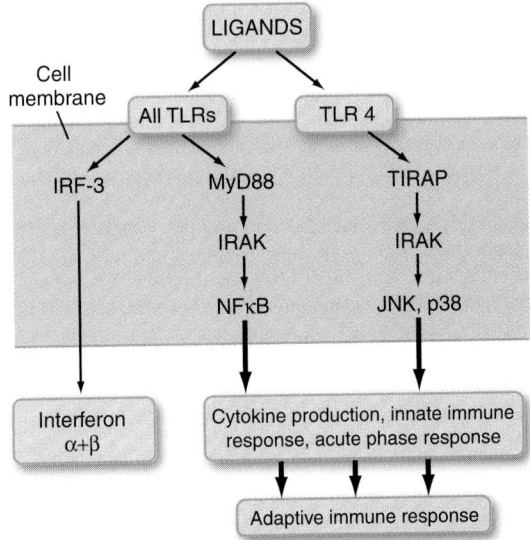

FIGURE 4-2. Toll-like receptor (TLR) signaling pathways. TLR activating molecules, ligands, bind to the TLRs. These molecules are shown graphically within boxes to indicate that this interaction occurs outside of the cell. The TLRs activate three major signaling pathways resulting in the activation of NF-κB, JNK, p38, and IRF-3. A few of the intermediate signaling steps are included, particularly IRAK, because of the genetic defects associated with this step.[8] These steps are shown to occur between two horizontal lines, indicating intracellular action. The effector processes and events are shown at the bottom of the figure in text boxes.

TLR pathways, the PDCs synthesize the costimulatory molecules CD80/CD86 and IL-12. As the PDCs mature and migrate to the draining lymph node, they serve as antigen-presenting cells, driving the adaptive immune response. Additionally, TLRs activate monocytes and macrophages to secrete the regulatory cytokines, IL-10 and IL-12, and liver Kupffer cells to secrete IL-18.[75,76] IL-12 and IL-18 cooperatively promote secretion of IFN-γ by natural killer (NK) cells, driving specific immunity toward type 1 (Th1) T-cell responses characterized by high levels of interferon production, development of delayed-type hypersensitivity, and defense against intracellular microbes. TLR activation of monocytes also produces IL-10, which inhibits IL-12 production, stimulates B-cell proliferation and immunoglobulin synthesis, and drives specific immunity toward Th2 responses, which are characterized by high levels of IL-4 production and synthesis of antibody, particularly IgE. Type 2 (Th2) antibody responses are crucial for the defense against some viruses, encapsulated bacteria, and large extracellular eukaryotes, especially worms.

The pathogen also can have a strong influence on the innate response and the subsequent biasing of the immune response. Helminth infections strongly polarize the immune response toward a Th2 profile because the oligosaccharides lacto-N-fucopentaose and lacto-N-neotetraose of the schistosome egg are Th2 biasing and suppress Th1 responses.[77,78] These sugars also are found in human milk, which may reflect the adaptation of the innate process to increase the likelihood of an antibody response in the neonate to compensate for the loss of maternal antibodies.

Toll-like Receptor Signaling and Acute-Phase Response

Three of the major inflammatory cytokines, IL-1, TNF-α, and IL-6, induced through TLR signaling are largely responsible for triggering the acute-phase response. First, these molecules act as pyrogens, altering the temperature setpoint resulting in a febrile response. These cytokines also induce the synthesis in the liver of many acute-phase proteins, including C-reactive protein[79]; LPS-binding protein[80]; serum amyloid A; haptoglobin; ceruloplasmin; fibrinogen; α₁-acid glycoprotein; complement components C3, C4, C9, factor B, C1 inhibitor, and C4b binding protein; transferrin; procalcitonin; prealbumin; and natural anticoagulants, such as protein C, protein S, antithrombin plasminogen, tissue plasminogen activator, urokinase, vitronectin, plasminogen-activator inhibitor 1, α₁-antitrypsin, α₁-antichymotrypsin, β₂-macroglobulin, pancreatic secretory trypsin inhibitor, granulocyte colony-stimulating factor, fibronectin, ferritin, angiotensinogen, α-fetoprotein, thyroxine-binding globulin, and factor XII.[81] These omnipresent proteins increase the number and function of phagocytic cells and facilitate the delivery of humoral and cellular components to sites of inflammation and constitute a marker of inflammation.[82] The acute-phase response is mediated by a host of cells of the immune system, including

TABLE 4-4 Distribution of Toll-like Receptors (TLRs) in Resting Human Plasmacytoid Dendritic Cells, Monocytes, Natural Killer Cells, B Cells, and T Cells

	PDCs	Monocytes	NK Cells	B Cells	T Cells
TLR-1	+	++	++	++	+
TLR-2	−	++	+	±	±
TLR-3	−	−	+	±	±
TLR-4	−	++	±	±	±
TLR-5	−	+	+	±	+
TLR-6	+	+	+	++	±
TLR-7	+	±	±	+	±
TLR-8	−	+	±	±	±
TLR-9	++	±	±	+	±
TLR-10	±	±	±	+	±

++, greater than 100 mRNA copies per 10³ cells; +, greater than 20 mRNA copies per 10³ cells; ±, detectable mRNA in 10³ cells; −, below limit of detection of the assay.

NK, natural killer; PDCs, plasmacytoid dendritic cells.

From Hornung V Rothenfusser S, Britsch S, et al. Quantitative expression of Toll-like receptor 1-10 mRNA in cellular subsets of human peripheral blood mononuclear cells and sensitivity to CpG oligodeoxynucleotides. J Immunol. 2002;168:4531-4537.

monocytes, Kupffer cells, and T cells[74]; reactions of preexisting humoral defenses; and de novo production of active regulatory molecules (e.g., cytokines/chemokines, prostaglandins, and other eicosanoids) by phagocytes, lymphocytes, and endothelial cells.

Chemokines and Chemotaxis

Two main families of chemokines direct leukocyte migration.[13,83,84] Members of the CXC family, whose first two cysteines are separated by a single amino acid, stimulate chemotaxis of PMNs, eosinophils, monocytes, dendritic cells, NK cells, and T lymphocytes. Members of the CC family, whose first two cysteines adjoin each other, stimulate all these leukocytes except PMNs, which do not express receptors for CC chemokines. More than 45 chemokines, 11 receptors for CC chemokines, and 6 receptors for CXC chemokines have been described. Chemokines upregulate adhesion molecules, stimulate leukocyte migration, and lower the threshold for cell activation. Cytokines, especially TNF-α and IL-1, also increase expression of adhesion molecules on endothelial cells, PMNs, NK cells, and monocytes, which aid in the binding and transmigration of these cells into sites of inflammation.

Although the interactions of chemokines on target cell populations are extraordinarily complex, IL-8 and eotaxin are the predominant chemokine modulators of PMN and eosinophil migration. Resting T cells express few chemokine receptors, but these are strongly upregulated by IL-2 in conjunction with stimulation via the antigen receptor. The most vigorous immigration of T cells to inflammatory sites occurs in conjunction with acquired immunity rather than during the innate response.

Metabolic Changes

Many other metabolic changes reflect mobilization of the host's resources for defense. These include increased production of thyroid-stimulating hormone, vasopressin, insulin, and glucagon. Profound catabolism of muscle protein also can occur as amino acids are used for synthesis of defensive cells and proteins, and resting muscle metabolic activity or shivering increases to raise body temperature.

A decrease in serum iron long has been recognized as a component of the acute-phase response. Many microorganisms must scavenge iron from their environment for optimal growth. Transferrin, an iron-binding protein secreted by hepatocytes under the influence of IL-6, complexes with free iron and limits its availability to microorganisms. Macrophages internalize iron-transferrin complexes, retain the iron, and recycle transferrin, further reducing the availability of free and total serum iron to any potential invader.[85]

Zinc levels decline significantly during acute inflammation. This metal, which has no known tissue stores, enhances lymphocyte responsiveness, aids wound healing, and participates in protein synthesis.[86] Zinc plays a crucial role in regulation of DNA transcription and RNA translation. Its decrease in infection may reflect its increased use by actively metabolizing cells.

IMPAIRMENT AND EXAGGERATION OF GENERAL NONSPECIFIC AND INNATE IMMUNITY

Impaired natural immunity, most conveniently detected by testing for cutaneous delayed hypersensitivity, can occur as a consequence of numerous illnesses. In the United States, end-stage cancer, renal disease, AIDS, liver disease, and alcoholism are the most common underlying illnesses resulting in diminished immune responsiveness. Worldwide, malnutrition is the leading cause of increased susceptibility to and severity of several infections. These include life-threatening bacterial infections of the middle ear, pervasive dental caries, HIV infection, and common childhood infections, especially measles.[87,88] An impaired or dysfunctional immune system is also a crucial determinant of the outcome in sepsis (see Chapter 67).[89]

Nutrition

It is well established that persons with malnutrition, whether preexisting (protein-energy malnutrition) or disease-induced (cytokine-induced malnutrition), have more severe infections. Vitamin A in particular plays a central role.[88,90] Cellular immune dysfunction is affected disproportionately, and nutritional support has a demonstrable beneficial effect on outcome.[91] Before the advent of antibiotics, tuberculosis often was treated successfully by nutrition-based therapies that in some patients included consumption of 20 to 30 eggs per day (see Chapter 10).

Aging

Although the data regarding the effects of aging on immunity and infection are confusing and sometimes conflicting, this process has an impact on the immune system that can be summarized best as immunosenescence. Superimposed and interrelated with this generalized impairment are social isolation and age-related decrements in organ structure and function. Regardless of the setting, there is a higher incidence in elderly persons of pneumonias (twofold), cholecystitis (twofold to eightfold), appendicitis (15-fold to 20-fold), diverticulitis, bacteremia (threefold), asymptomatic bacteriuria, urinary tract infections (fivefold to 10-fold), reactivation of varicella-zoster virus and tuberculosis (10-fold), bacterial meningitis (threefold), and bacterial endocarditis (twofold to threefold). Case-fatality is conspicuously high among patients older than 65 years infected with Severe Acute Respiratory Syndrome (SARS)–associated coronavirus.[91a] The greatest impact of aging is on cell-mediated immunity; there is a lesser but substantial impact on humoral immunity.[92]

Stress

A growing body of evidence has shown an inverse relation between stress and immune function; the end result is an increased susceptibility to infection.[93] The feedback pathways responsible for this effect remain obscure.

Hormones

Increased production of adrenocorticotropic hormone occurs during the acute-phase response and seems to augment the host's survival potential. The depressive effect of excess corticosteroids on inflammation is well known and probably represents an important feedback mechanism to modulate an inflammatory response.

Estrogen affects the lining of the vagina, resulting in increased nonspecific resistance. T-cell function is blunted during pregnancy,[94] which may account for the severity of certain infections, such as those caused by poliomyelitis virus, *Coccidioides immitis*, group A β-hemolytic streptococci, influenza virus, and *N. gonorrhoeae*, particularly in the third trimester.

Dysregulation

The compilation of initial nonspecific response is usually effective in controlling microbial invasion. With overwhelming microbial invasion and release of large amounts of microbial products, however, the failure of feedback control may lead to the catastrophic syndrome of septic shock[89] (see Chapter 67). In addition, if infections are not controlled and become chronic, some metabolic derangements (e.g., decreased serum albumin, iron sequestration, muscle wasting) persist and can become profound.

Normal Indigenous Microbial Flora

The normal commensal flora constitute a crucial ecosystem that plays an important role in protecting the host from microbial invasion by "pathogenic" organisms.[95] Its protective mechanisms include the following: (1) competition for the same nutrients (interference); (2) competition for the same receptors on host cells (tropism); (3) production of secreted products, such as bacteriocins (antibiotics), that are toxic to other organisms, usually of the same species; (4) production of volatile fatty acids or other metabolites that are toxic to competing microbes; (5) continual stimulation of the immune system to maintain low but constant levels of class II histocompatibility (HLA-DR) molecule expression on macrophages and other antigen-presenting cells; and (6) stimulation of cross-protective immune factors, such as "natural" antibodies (see later discussion).

The ultimate effect of the above-listed first three protective mechanisms is to limit the quantity or dominance of any one species. Broad-

spectrum antibiotic therapy decreases the total numbers of bacteria in the gut. This activity results in an increased proportion of normally commensal fungal species and resistant bacterial strains. When the antibiotic therapy is stopped, a natural rebound occurs, and the gut is repopulated. There is a selective advantage, however, to the faster growing aerobic Enterobacteriaceae over the slower replicating anaerobes. This advantage increases the probability of developing a gram-negative bacteremia. Most colonizing organisms are transient, but some persist for life, implying that the biologic cost to the host and microorganism is low.

The microbial flora harbored by the host can be divided into two groups: (1) normal resident flora that are regularly found and, if perturbed, promptly recolonize and (2) a microbial flora that may colonize the host transiently for periods ranging from hours to weeks. Certain organisms characteristically colonize certain body sites (tropism). This fact is taken into consideration when the clinician decides whether a particular organism is behaving in a pathogenic fashion. Bacteria and fungi comprise commensal and symbiotic organisms. Protozoa are less ubiquitous, almost always reside in the gastrointestinal tract, and are more prevalent in developing countries. Mycoplasmas and viruses are much less prevalent members of the host commensal flora.

The species that make up the normal commensal flora are influenced by environmental factors, such as diet, sanitary conditions, air pollution, and hygienic habits.[95,96] Lactobacilli are common intestinal commensals whenever dairy products compose a significant proportion of the dietary intake; protozoa are common intestinal inhabitants of persons living where sanitation is poor; and a patient with underlying chronic bronchitis is more likely than others to harbor *Haemophilus influenzae* in the tracheobronchial tree.

Hormones also may influence the normal commensal flora. Premenarcheal and postmenopausal vaginal flora differ significantly from those present during the childbearing period. The normal commensal flora also are influenced by genetically determined host cell receptors to which microorganisms adhere and which determine or select the microbes that colonize a particular host (see earlier section on tissue tropisms and heredity).

An important beneficial effect of the normal flora on the immune system is to keep it "primed" and more rapid and efficient in its response to invading microorganisms. Antigens normally are presented to the immune system in an ordered and specified way. T cells recognize antigens only after they are displayed on the surface of a macrophage (or other antigen-presenting cell) in physical association with a MHC molecule. Normally, 75% to 85% of circulating monocytes in adults maintain relatively high levels of MHC molecule expression. MHC expression is much lower on the monocytes of human newborns, neonatal mice, and germ-free animals. The constant stimulation by the host's indigenous microbial flora maintains the relatively high level of MHC molecule expression on macrophages and perhaps other antigen-presenting cells, which serves to keep the immune system primed. This modulation results, at least in part, from low-level production of IFN-γ, IL-4, and other cytokines and chemokines by activated T cells (see earlier section on cytokines and Table 4-3) and endothelial cells and represents an important interface between the innate and adaptive immune systems. In contrast to these positive benefits, detrimental consequences of colonization with indigenous microflora include the stimulation of nonfunctional blocking antibodies,[97] cross-reactive responses to host tissues, inappropriate T-cell responses,[98] and chronic low-grade inflammation that is an integral part of chronic degenerative conditions such as cardiovascular disease and cancer.[82,99,100]

Natural Antibodies

Natural antibodies is the term used to designate antibodies that are specific, but not of high affinity, to a microbe found in healthy people without a previous history of infection with the microbe. These antibodies are crucial to the immune defense against many bacteria, especially encapsulated bacteria such as *Neisseria meningitidis* and *H. influenzae* type b.

Some of these antibodies are stimulated as a result of colonization of the oropharynx, gut, or other sites by organisms sharing cross-reactive (cross-protective) antigens. Other antibodies apparently develop independently of antigen stimulation; are "polyreactive" (e.g., react individually with related epitopes); are found in serum and in secretions; and have been observed in newborns, in nude mice, and in germ-free animals.[101] These antibodies are not always beneficial, however. Specific serum IgA antibodies to *N. meningitidis* may predispose an otherwise immune person to become susceptible by preferentially attaching to the organism, blocking the beneficial bactericidal effect of protective IgG and IgM antibodies.[97] The blood group antibodies are a consequence of colonization of the gut by microorganisms bearing cross-reactive antigens. These antibodies are often of low avidity for most cross-reacting microorganisms.

SUMMARY

Pathogens have a formidable task to circumvent and overcome the overlapping, redundant, and integrated host defense mechanisms, from the broad-based general nonspecific defenses, to the pattern-recognizing innate defenses, and, finally, to the specific adaptive immune systems. The most successful pathogens often either hijack crucial components of the immune system (e.g., HIV) or poison crucial components (e.g., cholera). The most susceptible hosts often have a genetic predisposition that increases their susceptibility (e.g., tuberculosis).

REFERENCES

1. Janeway CA, Medzhitov R. Innate immune recognition. Annu Rev Immunol. 2002;20:197-216.
2. Gabay C, Kushner I. Acute-phase proteins and other systemic responses to inflammation. N Engl J Med. 1999;340:448-454.
3. Matzinger P. Tolerance, danger and the extended family. Annu Rev Immunol. 1994;12:991-1045.
4. Poltorak A, He X, Smirnova I, et al. Defective LPS signaling in C3H/HeJ and C57BL/10ScCr mice: Mutations in *Tlr4* gene. Science. 1998;282:2085-2088.
5. Takeda K, Kaisho T, Akira S. Toll-like receptors. Annu Rev Immunol. 2003;21: 335-376.
6. Vasselon T, Detmers PA. Toll receptors: A central element in innate immune responses. Infect Immun. 2002;70:1033-1041.
7. Sorensen TIA, Neilson GG, Anderson PK, et al. Genetic and environmental influences on premature death in adult adoptees. N Engl J Med.1988;318:727-732.
8. Picard C, Puel A, Bonnet M, et al. Pyogenic bacterial infections in humans with IRAK-4 deficiency. Science. 2003;299:2076-2079.
9. Figueroa JE, Densen P. Infectious diseases associated with complement deficiencies. Clin Microbiol Rev. 1991;4:359-395.
10. Dorman SE, Holland SM. Interferon-γ and interleukin-12 pathway defects and human disease. Cytokine Growth Factor Rev. 2000;11:321-333.
11. St Sauver JL, Ovsyannikova IG, Jacobson RM, et al. Associations between human leukocyte antigen homozygosity and antibody levels to measles vaccine. J Infect Dis. 2002;185:1545-1549.
12. Sterling TR, Dorman SE, Chaisson RE, et al. Human immunodeficiency virus-seronegative adults with extrapulmonary tuberculosis have abnormal innate immune responses. Clin Infect Dis. 2001;33:976-982.
13. Luster AD. Chemokines: Chemotactic cytokines that mediate inflammation. N Engl J Med. 1998;338:436-445.
14. Svanburg-Eden C, Jodal V. Attachment of *E. coli* to urinary sediment epithelial cells from urinary tract infection–prone healthy children. Infect Immun. 1979;26:837.
15. Ramirez-Ronda CH, Fuxench-Lopez Z, Nevarez M. Increased pharyngeal bacterial colonization during viral illness. Arch Intern Med. 1981;141:1599.
16. Samson M, Libert F, Doranz BJ, et al. Resistance to HIV-1 infection in caucasian individuals bearing mutant alleles of the CCR-5 chemokine receptor gene. Nature. 1996;382:722-725.
17. Stewart G. Chemokine genes: Beating the odds. Nat Med. 1998;4:275-277.
18. Zhang L, Yu E, Yu T, et al. Contribution of human α-defensin-1, -2 and -3 to the anti-HIV-1 activity of CD8 antiviral factor. Science. 2002;298:995-1000.
18a. Zhang L, Lopez P, He T, et al. Retraction of an interpretation. Science. 2004;303:467.
19. Stebbing J, Gazzard B, Kim L, et al. The heat-shock protein receptor CD91 is up-regulated in monocytes of HIV-1 infected "true" long term non-progressors. Blood. 2003;101:4000-4004.
20. Xiaojiang G, Nelson GW, Karacki P, et al. Effect of a single amino acid change in MHC class I molecules on the rate of progression to AIDS. N Engl J Med. 2001; 344:1668-1675.
20a. Singh KK, Barroga CF, Hughes MD, et al. Genetic influence of CCR5, CCRZ, and SOF-1 variants on human immunodeficiency virus 1 (HIV-1)–related disease progression and neurologic impairment in children with symptomatic HIV-1 infection. J Infect Dis. 2003;188:1461-1472.
21. Hader SL, Hodge TW, Burchacz KA, et al. Discordance at the human leukocyte antigen-DRB3 and protection from human immunodeficiency virus type 1 transmission. J Infect Dis. 2002;185:1729-1733.
22. Bellamy R, Ruwenda C, Corrah T, et al. Variations in the NRAMP1 gene and susceptibility to tuberculosis in West Africans. N Engl J Med. 1998;338:640-643.
23. Goldfeld AE, Delgado JO, Thim S, et al. Association of an HLA-DQ allele with clinical tuberculosis. JAMA. 1998;279:226-228.
24. Altare F, Durandy A, Lammas D, et al. Impairment of mycobacterial immunity in human interleukin-12 receptor deficiency. Science. 1998;280:1432-1438.
25. Awonmyi AA, Marchant A, Howson JMM, et al. Interleukin-10 polymorphism in *SLC11A1* (formerly *NRAMP1*) and susceptibility to tuberculosis. J Infect Dis. 2002; 186:1808-1814.
26. Soborg C, Andersen AB, Madsen HO, et al. Natural resistance-associated macrophage protein 1 polymorphisms are associated with microscopy-positive tuberculosis. J Infect Dis. 2002;186:517-521.
27. Ekdahl K, Braconier HJ, Svanborg C. Impaired antibody response to pneumococcal capsular polysaccharide and phosphorylcholine in adult patients with a history of bacteremic pneumococcal infection. Clin Infect Dis. 1997;5:654-660.
28. Kerr JR, Mattey DL, Thompson W, et al. Association of symptomatic acute human parvovirus B19 infection with human leukocyte antigen class I and II alleles. J Infect Dis. 2002;186:447-452.
29. Wang SW, Hildesheim A, Gao X, et al. Comprehensive analysis of human leukocyte antigen class I allele and cervical neoplasia in 3 epidemiologic studies. J Infect Dis. 2002;186:598-605.
30. Maciag PC, Schlecht NF, Souza PSA, et al. Polymorphisms of the human leukocyte antigen DRB1 and DQB1 genes and the natural history of human papillomavirus infection. J Infect Dis. 2002;186:164-172.
31. van der Pol WL, Huizinga TWJ, Vidarsson G, et al. Relevance of Fcγ receptor and interleukin-10 polymorphisms for meningococcal disease. J Infect Dis. 2001; 184: 1548-1555.
32. Loke H, Bethell DB, Phuong CX, et al. Strong HLA class-restricted T cell responses in dengue hemorrhagic fever: A double-edged sword? J Infect Dis. 2001;184: 1369-1372.
33. Bach JF. The effect of infections on susceptibility to autoimmune and allergic diseases. N Eng J Med. 2002;347:911-920.
34. Zasloff M. Antimicrobial peptides of multicellular organisms. Nature. 2002;415: 389-395.
34a. Zaiou M, Nizet V, Gallo RL, et al. Antimicrobial and protease inhibitory functions of the human cathelicidin (hCAP18/LL-37) prosequence. J Invest Dermatol. 2003;120:810-816.
35. Boismenu R, Havran WL. γδT cells in host defense and epithelial cell biology. Clin Immunol Immunopathol. 1998;86:121-133.
36. Hoijer MA, deGroot R, Lieshout L. Differences in *N*-acetyl muramyl-t-alanine amidase and lysozyme in serum and cerebrospinal fluid of patients with bacterial meningitis. J Infect Dis. 1998;177:102-106.
37. Ong PY, Ohtake T, Brandt C, et al. Endogenous antimicrobial peptides and skin infections in atopic dermatitis. N Engl J Med. 2002;347:185-192.
38. Krisanaprakornkit S, Weinberg A, Perez CN, et al. Expression of the peptide antibiotic human β-defensin 1 in cultured gingival epithelial cells and gingival tissue. Infect Immun. 1988;66:4222-4228.
39. Bals R, Wang X, Wu Z, et al. Human beta-defensin-2 is a salt-sensitive peptide antibiotic expressed in human lung. J Clin Invest. 1998;102:874-880.
40. Jespersgaard C, Hajishengallis H, Russell MW, et al. Identification and characterization of a non-immunoglobulin factor in human saliva that inhibits *Streptococcus mutans* gluconyltransferase. Infect Immun. 2002;70:1136-1142.
41. Bouvet JP, Pries R, Isaki S, et al. Non-immune macromolecular complexes of Ig in the human gut lumen. J Immunol. 1993;151:2562-2571.
42. Mazamec MB, Kaetzel CS, Lamm LE. Intracellular neutralization of virus by immunoglobulin A antibodies. Proc Natl Acad Sci U S A. 1992;89:6901-6905.
43. Singh DK, Parsek MR, Greenberg EP, et al. A component of innate immunity prevents bacterial biofilm development. Nature. 2002;417:552-555.
44. Hill PJ, Cockayne A, Landers P, et al. SirR, a novel iron-dependent repressor in *Staphylococcus epidermidis*. Infect Immun. 1998;66:4123-4129.
45. Tsai H, Raj PA, Bobek LA. Candidacidal activity of recombinant human salivary histadine-5 and variants. Infect Immun. 1996;64:5000-5007.
46. Green GM. In defense of the lung. Am Rev Respir Dis. 1970;102:691-697.
47. Zhao C, Wang I, Lehrer RI. Widespread expression of beta-defensin hBD-1 in human secretory glands and epithelial cells. FEBS Lett. 1996;396:319-322.
48. Epstein J, Eichbaum Q, Sheriff S, et al. The collectins in innate immunity. Curr Opin Immunol. 1996;8:29-35.
49. Ouellette AJ, Selsted ME. Paneth cell defensins: Endogenous peptide components of intestinal host defense. FASEB J. 1996;10:1280-1289.
50. Israde V, Darabi A, McCracken GH. The role of bacterial virulence factors and Tamm-Horsfall protein in the pathogenesis of *E. coli* urinary tract infections in infants. Am J Dis Child. 1987;147:1230-1234.
51. Wolbink GJ, Bossink AW, Groeneveld AB, et al. Complement activation in patients with sepsis is in part mediated by C-reactive protein. J Infect Dis. 1998;177:81-87.
52. Szalai AJ, Arawal A, Greenhough TJ, et al. C-reactive protein: Structural biology, gene expression, and host defense function. Immunol Res. 1997;16:127-126.
53. Jack DL, Jarvis GA, Booth CL, et al. Mannose-binding lectin accelerates complement activation and increases serum killing of *Neisseria meningitidis* serogroup C. J Infect Dis. 2001;184:836-845.
54. Ezekowitz RA. Role of the mannose-binding lectin in innate immunity. J Infect Dis. 2003;187:S335-S339.
55. Baribaud F, Pohlmann S, Leslie G, et al. Quantitative expression and virus transmission analysis of DC-SIGN on monocyte-derived dendritic cells. J Virol. 2002;76:9135-9142.
56. Tailleux L, Schwartz O, Herrmann JL, et al. DC-SIGN is the major *Mycobacterium tuberculosis* receptor on human dendritic cells. J Exp Med. 2003;197:121-127.

57. Mongdolin E, Bajolet O, Cutrona J, et al. Fibronectin-binding proteins of *Staphylococcus aureus* are involved in adherence to human airway epithelium. Infect Immun. 2002;70:620-630.

58. Van Oss CJ, Gillman CF. Phagocytosis as a surface phenomenon: I. Contact angles and phagocytosis of nonopsonized bacteria. J Reticuloendothel Soc. 1972;12:283-292.

59. Yamada Y, Doi T, Hamakubo T, et al. Scavenger receptor family proteins: Roles for atherosclerosis, host defense and disorders of the central nervous system. Cell Mol Life Sci. 1998;54:628-640.

60. Aderem A. Phagocytosis and the inflammatory response. J Infect Dis. 2003;187:S340-345.

61. Hayashi T, Rao SP, Catanzaro A. Binding of the 68-kilodalton protein of *Mycobacterium avium* to alpha (v) beta3 on human monocyte-derived macrophages enhances complement receptor type 3 expression. Infect Immun. 1997;65:1211-1216.

62. Nepomuceno RR, Tenner AJ. C1qRP, the C1q receptor that enhances phagocytosis, is detected specifically in human cells of myeloid lineage, endothelial cells, and platelets. J Immunol. 1998;160:1929-1935.

63. Yagisawa M, Yuo A, Yonemaru M, et al. Superoxide release and NADPH oxidase components in mature human phagocytes: Correlation between functional capacity and amount of functional proteins. Biochem Biophys Res Commun. 1996;228:510-516.

64. Tomee JF, Hiemstra PS, Heinzel WR, et al. Antileukoprotease: An endogenous protein in the innate mucosal defense against fungi. J Infect Dis. 1997;176:740-747.

65. Vaara M. Agents that increase the permeability of the outer membrane. Microbiol Rev. 1992;56:395-411.

66. Ihi T, Nakazato M, Mukae H, et al. Elevated concentrations of human neutrophil peptides in plasma, blood, and body fluids from patients with infections (see comments). Clin Infect Dis. 1997;25:1134-1140.

67. Ozato K, Tsujimura H, Tamura T. Toll-like receptor signaling and regulation of cytokine gene expression in the immune system. BioTechniques. 2002;33:S66-S75.

68. Beg AA. Endogenous ligands of Toll-like receptors: Implications for regulating inflammatory and immune responses. Trends Immunol. 2002;23:509-512.

69. Lee J, Chuang T-H, Redecke V, et al. Molecular basis for immunostimulatory activity of guanine nucleoside analogs: Activation of Toll-like receptor-7. Proc Natl Acad Sci U S A. 2003;100:6646-6651.

69a. Heil F, Hemm H, Hochrein H, et al. Species-specific recognition of single-stranded RNA via toll-like receptor 7 and 8. Science. 2004;303:1526-1529.

70. Janeway CA. Approaching the asymptote? Evolution and revolution in immunology. Cold Spring Harbor Symp Quant Biol. 1989;54:1-13.

71. Schnare M, Barton GM, Holt AC, et al. Toll-like receptors control activation of adaptive immune responses. Nat Immunol. 2001;2:947-950.

72. Ulanova M, Tarkowski A, Hahn-Zoric M, et al. The common vaccine adjuvant aluminum hydroxide up-regulates accessory properties of human monocytes via an interleukin-4-dependent mechanism. Infect Immun. 2001;69:1151-1159.

73. Hornung V, Rothenfusser S, Britsch S, et al. Quantitative expression of Toll-like receptor 1-10 mRNA in cellular subsets of human peripheral blood mononuclear cells and sensitivity to CpG oligodeoxynucleotides. J Immunol. 2002;168:4531-4537.

74. Mak TW, Ferrick DA. The γδ T-cell bridge: Linking innate and acquired immunity. Nat Med. 1998;4:764-765.

75. Trinchieri G. Cytokines acting on or secreted by macrophages during intracelluar infection (IL-10, IL-12, IFN-γ). Curr Opin Immunol. 1997;9:17-23.

76. Kohno K, Kurimoto M. Interleukin 18, a cytokine which resembles IL-1 structurally and IL-12 functionally but exerts its effect independently of both. Clin Immunol Immunopathol. 1998;86:11-15.

77. Okano M, Satoskar AR, Nishizaki K, et al. Lacto-N-fucopentaose III found on *Schistosoma mansoni* egg antigens functions as an adjuvant for proteins by inducing Th2-type response. J Immunol. 2001;167:442-450.

78. Terrazas LI, Walsh KL, Piskorska D, et al. The schistosome oligosaccharide lacto-N-neotetraose expands Gr1+ cells that secrete anti-inflammatory cytokines and inhibit proliferation of naive CD4+ cells: A potential mechanism for immune polarization in helminth infections. J Immunol. 2001;167:5295-5303.

79. Mortensen RF. C-reactive protein, inflammation and innate immunity. Immunol Res. 2001;24:163-176.

80. Dentener MA, Francot GJ, Hiemstra PS, et al. Bactericidal/permeability-increasing protein release in whole blood ex vivo: Strong induction by lipopolysaccharide and tumor necrosis factor-α. J Infect Dis. 1997;175:108-117.

81. Smith OP, White B, Vaughan D, et al. Use of protein C concentrate, heparin, and haemodiafiltration in meningococcus-induced purpura fulminans. Lancet. 1997;350:1590-1593.

82. Ridker PM, Rifai N, Rose L. Comparison of C-reactive protein and low-density lipoprotein cholesterol levels in the prediction of first cardiovascular events. N Engl J Med. 2002;347:1557-1565.

83. Baggiolini M, Dewald B, Moser B. Human chemokines: An update. Annu Rev Immunol. 1997;15:675-705.

84. Baggiolini M. Chemokines and leukocyte traffic. Nature. 1998;392:565-568.

85. Ward CG. Influence of iron on infection. Am J Surg. 1986;151:291-295.

86. Keen CL, Gershwin ME. Zinc deficiency and immune function. Annu Rev Nutr. 1990;10:415-431.

87. Carson WE, Lindemann MJ, Baiocchi R, et al. The functional characterization of interleukin-10 receptor expression on human natural killer cells. Blood. 1995;85:3577-3585.

88. Corman LC. The relationship between nutrition, infection, and immunity. Med Clin North Am. 1985;69:519-531.

89. Hotchkiss RS, Karl IE. The pathophysiology and treatment of sepsis. N Engl J Med. 2003;348:138-150.

90. Semba RD, Graham NM, Caiaffa WT, et al. Increased mortality associated with vitamin A deficiency during human immunodeficiency virus type 1 infection. Arch Intern Med. 1993;153:2149-2154.

91. Souba WW. Nutritional support. N Engl J Med. 1997;336:41-48.

91a. Lians W, Zhu Z, Guo J, et al. Severe Acute Respiratory Syndrome, Beijing, 2003. Emerg Infect Dis. 2004;10:25-31.

92. Yoshikawa TT. Perspective: Aging and infectious diseases—past, present, and future. J Infect Dis. 1997;176:1053-1057.

93. Peterson PK, Chao CC, Molitor T, et al. Stress and pathogenesis of infectious disease. Rev Infect Dis. 1991;13:710-720.

94. Weinberg ED. Pregnancy-associated depression of cell-mediated immunity. Rev Infect Dis. 1984;6:814-831.

95. Mackowiak PA. The normal microbial flora. N Engl J Med. 1982;307:83-86.

96. Moore WEC, Burmeister JA, Brooke CW, et al. Investigation of influences of puberty, genetics and environment on the composition of subgingival periodontal flora. Infect Immun. 1993;61:2891-2898.

97. Griffiss JM. Bactericidal activity by IgA of lytic antibody in human convalescent sera. J Immunol. 1975;114:1779-1784.

98. Looney RJ, Falsey D, Campbell D, et al. Role of cytomegalovirus in the T-cell changes seen in elderly individuals. Clin Immunol. 1999;90:213-219.

99. Wilson M, Seymour R, Henderson B. Bacterial perturbation of cytokine networks. Infect Immun. 1998;66:2401-2409.

100. Mattila KJ, Valtonen VV, Nieminen MS. Role of infection as a risk factor for atherosclerosis, myocardial infarction and stroke. Clin Infect Dis. 1998;26:719-734.

101. Quinn CP, Bernemen A, Pires R, et al. Natural polyreactive secretory immunoglobulin A autoantibodies as a possible barrier to infection in humans. Infect Immun. 1997;65:3997-4004.

CHAPTER **5**

Human Genetics and Infection

ADRIAN V. S. HILL

It is clear that genetic variation in the host has a substantial influence on the course of infectious diseases caused by many microorganisms. Such interactions have been well studied in humans where the pathogens and the host genome are well characterized. In recent years, the methodology and techniques available for analyzing human genetic variation have advanced rapidly, leading to the identification of a large number of genes associated with altered susceptibility to infectious pathogens. The completion in 2003 of the entire human genome sequence provides a very powerful resource for molecular analysis of differential susceptibility. In particular, the availability of millions of new genetic markers with a defined position on the human genome sequence is central to the mapping of susceptibility genes and defining their functional variants. Although many genes have already been associated with susceptibility to various diseases, it is likely that these represent only a small fraction of all the relevant genes. Indeed, susceptibility to most infectious diseases in humans is likely to be highly polygenic, and the identification of susceptibility and resistance genes is providing new insights into disease pathogenesis and resistance mechanisms. Conversely, it appears increasingly likely that a substantial proportion of the functional variation in the human genome has evolved to facilitate defense against infectious pathogens, leading to the observed polygenic variation in susceptibility between individuals and human populations.

MAGNITUDE OF THE HOST GENETIC EFFECT

There are various types of evidence that demonstrate a significant role for host genetics in variable susceptibility to infectious disease. For some infections such as leprosy, disease has long been known to cluster in families,[1] but it is often difficult to assess the relative importance of proximity to an index case and shared genes. Nonetheless, the increased risk of disease in a sibling compared with the general population risk is a useful measure of the extent of the genetic component to a multifactorial disease[2] and appears to be of the order of 1.5 to 5 for several infectious diseases.[3]

Apparent interpopulation and racial differences in susceptibility have also been noted.[4,5] Particularly striking has been the apparent increased susceptibility to viral infections and tuberculosis noted in some previously unexposed populations.[6] In the Qu'Appelle Indians of Saskatchewan, after some decades of exposure to tuberculosis, rates of disease dropped 50-fold.[7] The use of malaria therapy for syphilis in nonimmune individuals[8] and the accidental vaccination of some children with *Mycobacterium tuberculosis* rather than Calmette-Guérin bacillus in Lübeck, Germany, provided direct evidence of variable susceptibility to these pathogens.

In addition to these observational data, two types of study, of adoptees and of twins, have provided more direct quantification of the importance of host genetics in susceptibility to infectious diseases. In a study of more than 900 Scandinavian adoptees, the early death of a biologic, but not an adoptive, parent from an infectious disease was associated with an almost sixfold increase in the risk of an infectious cause of death in the adoptee, consistent with a substantial role for host genetics.[9] Also, several twin studies have found higher concordance rates among monozygotic than among dizygotic twin pairs who share respectively 100% and, on average, 50% of their genes. The diseases studied include tuberculosis, poliomyelitis, leprosy, persistent hepatitis B virus (HBV) infection, *Helicobacter pylori* infection, and malaria[10-15] (Table 5-1). In general, it has been easier to demonstrate a significant role for host genetic factors in infections in which only a proportion of those infected develop disease, in chronic rather than in acute infections, and in the severity of infectious disease rather than in the susceptibility to infection per se.

Approaches

Several different and usually complementary approaches have been taken to identifying genes involved in susceptibility to infectious diseases. By far the most widely adopted strategy in human studies has been the assessment of candidate genes in case-control studies. Here the frequencies of variants of a gene with a possible role in resistance are compared in individuals with and without the disease. In general, large sample sizes are necessary, particularly for rare alleles or multiallelic genes, but such candidate genes have come from a variety of sources. A particular geographic distribution of certain hemoglobin variants suggested that they might play a role in malaria resistance. A few genes have been identified as affecting susceptibility to infection in different strains of mice, leading to assessment of their human homologues. A much larger number of candidate genes have been suggested more recently by studies of the susceptibility of various gene knockout mice to infectious pathogens. Expression analyses of various tissues using microarrays are beginning to provide a new source of candidate genes. Finally, variants of genes known to play roles in immune or innate resistance to infection, such as human leukocyte antigen (HLA) and mannose-binding lectin (MBL), have been evaluated on the basis of their known functions.

A different approach is to search for genetic linkage to, rather than association with, an infectious disease in family studies. Identification of a chromosomal region genetically linked to susceptibility indicates that there is a susceptibility gene (or genes) somewhere in that region.[2] The advantage of this approach is that unknown genes may be mapped and identified without prior information on their function. Although the statistical power of this approach is more limited than that of case-control studies, it does allow a comprehensive screen of the whole genome to be undertaken for major susceptibility genes. A similar approach in mice has led to the mapping of numerous susceptibility genes, and a few of these such as the macrophage gene, *Nramp1*, have then been identified.[16] The human homologue in this case, *NRAMP1* (or *SLC11A1*), has been found to affect susceptibility to tuberculosis,[17] but the human homologue of other murine susceptibility genes, such as the *Mx* influenza resistance gene,[18] is not known to display any functional variation in humans.

A family linkage approach has also been used to map and identify genes that cause rare monogenic susceptibility phenotypes. For example, mutations in the gene for the interferon-γ receptor chain 1 have been found to underlie some rare cases of susceptibility to weakly pathogenic mycobacteria.[19,20] Mutations in various other genes producing more generalized immunodeficiency are described in other chapters, but these are also found at nonpolymorphic frequencies (i.e., at an allele frequency of <1%).

DISEASES

Malaria

More genes have been implicated in differential susceptibility to malaria than to any other disease of humans or other animals (Table 5-2). This in part reflects the early success in identifying the relevance of the sickle hemoglobin polymorphism and the geographic distribution of some malaria resistance alleles.[21] Early evidence of differential susceptibility to malaria in nonimmune subjects came from studies of the use of malaria therapy in the management of syphilis.[8] Marked differences in susceptibility to the same dose and strain of malaria parasite were observed between individuals. Numerous studies of sickle hemoglobin and glucose-6-phosphate dehydrogenase (G6PD) deficiency have provided clear-cut evidence of their protective relevance against *Plasmodium falciparum* malaria,[22,23] and, more recently, compelling evidence has been provided that hemoglobin C,[24,25] which is common in parts of West Africa, and hemoglobin E,[26,27] which is widely distributed in Southeast Asia, are also protective. A few studies have demonstrated protection associated with heterozygosity for β-thalassemia and various α-thalassemia genotypes.[28-30]

There have been relatively few useful interpopulation comparisons of malaria susceptibility. However, a study of different ethnic groups in Mali, West Africa, found significant differences in immune responses to *P. falciparum* and in malaria susceptibility between these that appears to be genetic in origin.[4] The differences could not be explained by the known malaria resistance alleles.

HLA class I and II alleles have both been found to influence malaria susceptibility in Africa in large case-control studies.[31,32] However, it is likely that the particular alleles showing associations differ between populations; there is some evidence that this is so. Such interpopulation heterogeneity can result from many causes, but a prominent one in malaria is likely to be the marked polymorphism of immunodominant malaria antigens. Indeed, HLA has also been found to influence the strain of malaria parasite associated with clinical malaria and complex interaction between parasite strain may lead to further variability in HLA associations.[33] It seems likely that the predominant immune protective mechanisms against malaria vary geographically with transmission patterns.

Malaria parasites vary in their capacity to form rosettes with uninfected erythrocytes and to sequester in capillary beds, and both of these phenotypes have been implicated in increased malaria severity.[34,35] Polymorphic host receptors involved in parasite sequestration, intercellular adhesion molecule-1 (ICAM-1), and CD36 influence susceptibil-

TABLE 5-1 Twin Studies of Some Infectious Diseases

Disease	Population	Concordance		Reference
		MZ	DZ	
Tuberculosis	Germany	65	25	180
	United States	62	18	181
	United Kingdom	32	14	10
Poliomyelitis	United States	36	6	11
Leprosy	India	52	22	12
Hepatitis B	Taiwan	35	4	13
H. pylori	Sweden	81	63	14

All showed significantly higher concordances in monozygotic (MZ) than in dizygotic (DZ) twin pairs.

TABLE 5-2 Some Susceptibility and Resistance Genes Implicated in Parasitic Diseases

Gene	Variant	Disease	Effect
β-Globin	Sickle, thalassemias	Malaria (Pf)	Resistance
α-Globin	Thalassemias	Malaria (Pf)	Resistance
Erythrocyte band 3	27–base pair deletion	Malaria (Pf, Pv)	Resistance
Duffy chemokine receptor	Promoter variant	Malaria (Pv)	Resistance
Glycophorin C	Exon 3 deletion	Malaria (Pf)	Resistance
Glucose-6-phosphate dehydrogenase	Deficiency variants	Malaria (Pf)	Resistance
HLA-B	HLA-B53	Malaria (Pf)	Resistance
HLA-DR	HLA-DRB1*1302	Malaria (Pf)	Resistance
Intracellular adhesion molecule 1	Kilifi variant	Malaria (Pf)	Susceptibility
CD36	Various	Malaria (Pf)	Resistance
Interferon-α receptor	Various	Malaria (Pf)	Resistance
Inducible nitric oxide synthase	Promoter	Malaria (Pf)	Resistance
Tumor necrosis factor	Promoter-308	Malaria (Pf)	Susceptibility
Tumor necrosis factor	Promoter-308	Leishmaniasis	Susceptibility

Pf, *Plasmodium falciparum;* Pv, *Plasmodium vivax.*

ity to severe malaria.[36-39] Thus such host receptors that interact with the surface of the parasitized erythrocyte add to the list of malaria-resistant genes.

Although most genes that influence susceptibility to infectious disease have relatively little effect, a few malaria resistance genes are exceptions. The strength of the protective effect of heterozygosity for hemoglobin S is one, with about 90% reduction in the risk of severe malaria.[31] The protection from *Plasmodium vivax* afforded by the Duffy negative blood group is complete, as this parasite is unable to invade Duffy negative erythrocytes.[40] Finally, Melanesian carriers of a 27–base pair deletion in the erythrocyte band 3 gene appear to be very strongly protected from *P. falciparum*,[41] maintaining the deletion at frequencies of up to 0.35 even though homozygous fetuses do not survive gestation.[42]

The large number of genes implicated in malaria resistance have all been identified by case-control studies or in vitro analyses. Apart from one study showing genetic linkage of malaria to the major histocompatibility complex (MHC),[36] linkage approaches have not been used. However, a thorough genomewide search could reveal many new resistance genes. Malaria provides perhaps the best example of population variation in susceptibility and resistance genes. For example, in West Africa, sickle hemoglobin, the A⁻ allele of G6PD, HLA-B53, and an HLA-DR13 allele are associated with protection, but all of these alleles are either rare or absent in Southeast Asia and Melanesia. In the latter region, hemoglobin E, ovalocytosis, other G6PD alleles, and both α- and β-thalassemia are more prevalent.

Mycobacterial Diseases

Genetic susceptibility studies of mycobacterial diseases have been relatively common for several reasons. Familial clustering of leprosy and tuberculosis was well recognized, and leprosy was regarded by some as a genetic disorder before *Mycobacterium leprae* was identified.[1] An accident in Lübeck, Germany, in which children were immunized with *M. tuberculosis* rather than Calmette-Guérin bacillus provided early evidence for variable susceptibility to tuberculosis. This was substantiated by several large twin studies that found higher concordance rates among monozygotic than among dizygotic twin pairs[10] (see Table 5-1). A large twin study of leprosy in India also reported higher concor-

dance rates for leprosy in monozygotic twins but was inconclusive on the question of genetic susceptibility to leprosy type.[12] Observations on the introduction of tuberculosis to some populations previously free of the infection and disease suggested that the decline in frequency of the disease over time might in part reflect some natural selection for resistance genes.[7] In contrast to malaria, there is evidence that blacks may be more susceptible to infection with *M. tuberculosis* than whites. The clearest data were obtained in a comparison of rates of skin test conversion among socioeconomically matched nursing home residents in the United States.[5] Studies of large pedigrees with multiple cases of leprosy or tuberculosis using complex segregation analysis techniques suggested that just one or two major genes might account for much of the genetic component of susceptibility to these diseases.[43] Analysis of the *M. tuberculosis* genome revealed remarkable sequence conservation between isolates with a lack of single-nucleotide changes, suggesting that host genetic polymorphism might be relatively more important.[44] Finally the chronicity of these diseases and the existence of control programs in many countries have facilitated the recruitment of families as well as unrelated cases.

Several genes have now been associated with susceptibility to particular mycobacterial diseases (Table 5-3). Early studies of HLA variation established the relevance of HLA variation in susceptibility to both tuberculosis and leprosy.[45,46] HLA-DR2 was associated with susceptibility to tuberculoid leprosy in India; more recent data support an association of this HLA type with susceptibility to both tuberculoid and lepromatous forms of leprosy as well as to tuberculosis in several Asian populations.[47-50] Outside of Asia, no clear HLA association has been identified and HLA-DR2 appears not to be associated with susceptibility. Variation in the promoter of the tumor necrosis factor *(TNF)* gene has been associated with susceptibility to lepromatous but not tuberculoid leprosy in Bengal, India, and with altered susceptibility to leprosy per se in Brazil.[51,52]

The natural resistance-associated macrophage protein-1 gene *(NRAMP1)* was suggested as a candidate gene for human mycobacterial disease by identification of its homologue as a susceptibility gene for some intracellular pathogens in mice.[16] Variation in both the 3′-untranslated region and the promoter region of the human *NRAMP1*

TABLE 5-3 Some Susceptibility and Resistance Genes Implicated in Bacterial Diseases

Gene	Variant	Disease	Effect
HLA-DR	HLA-DR2	Tuberculosis	Susceptibility
NRAMP1	5′ and 3′ Variants	Tuberculosis	Susceptibility
Vitamin D receptor	3′ Variant	Tuberculosis	Resistance
Interferon-γ	Intron variant	Tuberculosis	Resistance
HLA-DR	HLA-DR2	Leprosy	Susceptibility
ABO	Blood group O	Cholera	Susceptibility
Mannose-binding lectin	Coding variants	Pneumococcus	Susceptibility
Interferon-γ receptor	Various mutations	Disseminated Calmette-Guérin bacillus	Susceptibility
TLR4	Codon 299	Gram-negative infections	Susceptibility

gene has been associated with susceptibility to pulmonary tuberculosis in West Africans[17] and several other, but not all, populations studied. However, the magnitude of the effect observed in human tuberculosis is relatively modest compared with that suggested by studies of susceptibility to Calmette-Guérin bacillus in mice. Genes with larger effects may be identified by genomewide linkage studies of multicase families, and these have recently suggested that an X-linked gene may influence susceptibility to tuberculosis.[53]

Rare genetic disorders have frequently been informative indicators of disease mechanisms, and this also applies to mycobacterial disease. Children homozygous for mutations in the interferon-γ receptor gene have been found to be remarkably susceptible to weakly pathogenic mycobacteria, including the Calmette-Guérin bacillus vaccine, and have a poor prognosis.[19,20] These children appear to have a limited increase in susceptibility to tuberculosis and a marked susceptibility to salmonellosis. Similarly rare gene "knockout" mutations in interleukin (IL)-12 and IL-12 receptor genes produce this phenotype of marked susceptibility to atypical mycobacterial disease and salmonella, directly implicating this cytokine and pathway in resistance to these pathogens.[54,55] An intronic variant of the interferon-γ gene that may affect binding of the transcription factor nuclear factor (NF)-κB has been associated with resistance to tuberculosis.[56]

Human Immunodeficiency Virus Infection and Acquired Immunodeficiency Syndrome

Studies of cohorts exposed to human immunodeficiency virus (HIV) infection have identified a small proportion of individuals who, despite repeated exposure to infection from infected sexual partners, remain HIV seronegative.[57] Some such resistant sex workers have immunologic evidence of exposure to the virus. There also is clear evidence that individuals vary in the rate of disease progression to acquired immunodeficiency syndrome (AIDS) once infected; several genes have now been found to influence this rate (Table 5-4).

A large number of studies of HLA type and rate of disease progression have been reported. Although there are marked differences between studies, some alleles have now been associated with susceptibility or resistance in more than one population. HLA class I variation is consistently more important than diversity in HLA class II genes. HLA-B35 and the HLA-A1-B8-DR3 haplotype have been associated with more rapid disease progression in several studies.[58-60] Similarly, HLA-B27 and HLA-B57 may be associated with a lower rate of progression.[61,62] Particular combinations of HLA class I and II alleles and variants of the transporter associated with antigen processing (TAP) genes have also been implicated.[63] Evidence of linkage of the MHC to rate of CD4 T-cell decline provides support for the relevance of polymorphism in this region.[64] It is possible to cluster HLA class I types into so-called supertypes based on the types of peptides bound by particular molecules; analysis of supertypes also shows convincing association with rate of disease progression.[65] It has been found that the HLA type of the host appears to influence the pattern of diversity of HIV sequences that emerges during an infection, indicating that HLA variation can directly influence virus evolution.[66]

The discovery of the role of chemokine receptors as co-receptors with CD4 for viral entry into macrophages and lymphocytes has given rise to numerous studies of genetic variants of these receptors and their ligands. The *CCR5* gene associations with resistance to infection and slower disease progression are now well established (see later),[67] and variants in the *CCR2* and *SDF-1* genes have been associated with altered disease progression.[68,69] However, it seems likely that several other relevant genes have yet to be discovered, because the known variants of *CCR5* can account for only a minority of white and none of the African individuals found to be resistant to HIV infection. More limited data support a role for other genes such as *RANTES*,[70] the secretor polymorphism,[71] and macrophage chemoattractant protein-1 (MCP-1)[72] in either susceptibility to infection or disease progression. However, most of the available information on genetic susceptibility comes from studies of susceptibility to clade B virus in North Americans or Europeans, and little is known about genes determining susceptibility in high-prevalence African and Asian populations where other clade types are prevalent.

Persistent Hepatitis

HBV was discovered during population genetic studies, and evidence that carriage of hepatitis B surface antigen tended to run in families was soon noted.[73,74] Some population and family studies suggested the presence of a major autosomal recessive gene. The ability or inability to clear HBV is one of the most striking immunogenetic dichotomies in medicine, with 1% to 12% of infected individuals becoming chronic carriers. One relatively small twin study in Taiwan provided evidence that susceptibility to HBV chronic carriage, but not HBV infection, is genetically determined.[13]

There have been several studies of HLA class I and II genes in HBV infection that initially appeared to show little consistency. A two-stage study of Quatari patients found HLA-DR2 to be associated with viral clearance and HLA-DR7 with viral persistence.[75] A larger study of persistently infected Gambians found a protective association with the *HLA-DRB1*1302* allele as well as a protective effect of heterozygosity in the class II region.[76,77] The same *HLA-DR13* allele may be associated with protection in Europeans.[78] HLA class II antigens have also been associated with the outcome of hepatitis C virus (HCV) infection. In contrast to HBV infection, most individuals fail to clear HCV, and *HLA-DRB1*1101* and the linked *HLA-DQB1*0301* allele have been associated with higher rates of clearance in Europeans.[79]

In single studies, some non-HLA genes, TNF,[80] MBL,[81] and the vitamin D receptor have also been associated with susceptibility to HBV persistence, and haptoglobin genotype may influence clearance of HCV infection.[82] Other genes such as *IL-10*[83] may influence response to antiviral treatment in HBV and HCV infection, and definition of these genetic factors could in the future help identify those most likely to respond to expensive and demanding therapies. The high prevalence of persistent HBV infection in some populations may make it possible to identify major non-MHC genes using family linkage studies. The major complication of these persistent viral infections is chronic liver disease and a high incidence of hepatocellular carcinoma. Other genes may be relevant to these outcomes—in particular, the liver detoxification enzymes, epoxide hydrolase and glutathione *S*-transferase M1, metabolize aflatoxin, a cofactor with persistent HBV infection for risk of hepatocellular carcinoma. A synergistic interaction between these environmental risk factors and genetic variants of the detoxification enzymes has been described.[84]

TABLE 5-4   Some Susceptibility and Resistance Genes Implicated in Viral Diseases

Gene	Variant	Disease	Effect
CCR5	32–Base pair deletion	HIV infection/progression	Resistance
CCR2	Codon 64	HIV progression	Resistance
SDF-1	3′ UTR variant	HIV progression	Resistance
HLA-DR	HLA-DRB1*1302	HBV persistence	Resistance
HLA-DR	HLA-DRB1*11	HCV persistence	Resistance
PRP	Codon 129	Creutzfeldt-Jakob disease	Susceptibility
FUT2	Codon 143 stop	Norwalk virus	Resistance

Other Diseases

Small studies of the FcγRII immunoglobulin receptor, CD32, have been undertaken in recurrent bacterial respiratory infection and in systemic meningococcal infection.[85,86] These suggested that alleles encoding histidine at amino acid position 132, which are associated with greater opsonic activity, may be less frequent in the disease group. Studies of pneumococcal invasive disease revealed an almost threefold higher frequency of individuals homozygous for codon changes in mannose-binding ligand.[87,88] A study of children with a variety of infections also found increased frequencies of MBL-deficiency alleles.[89] In a family study of meningococcal disease, children with first-degree relatives who had low TNF and high IL-10 production were more likely to die, suggesting a role for genes regulating production of these cytokines.[90]

A family linkage study of *Schistosoma mansoni* worm burden in Brazil has found evidence of linkage to a region of the long arm of chromosome 5.[91] This region may also be relevant in Senegalese families and encodes numerous cytokine genes, including IL-4, IL-9, and IL-13. Interestingly, the same region has been genetically linked to various manifestations of atopy and asthma, consistent with the speculation that a gene selected for resistance to helminthic infections might predispose to asthma or atopy. A promoter variant of the *TNF* gene has been associated with mucocutaneous leishmaniasis,[92] and mapping of genes affecting leishmanial infections in mice has suggested candidate genes for the disease in humans.[93,94]

The cystic fibrosis transmembrane regulator, in which mutations produce cystic fibrosis, is the receptor for *Salmonella typhi* raising the possibility that heterozygotes for this disease may be resistant to typhoid.[95] However, studies in humans are required to evaluate this interesting possibility. Little is known of the genetic basis of variable susceptibility to various fungal infections, but polymorphism in the MBL gene and the blood group secretor gene may be relevant. Studies of new-variant Creutzfeldt-Jakob disease (CJD) attributed to infection with the bovine spongiform encephalopathy agent,[96] sporadic CJD,[97] and iatrogenic CJD,[98] as well as kuru,[99,100] have all shown strong associations with variation in the human prion protein *(PPNP)* gene (see later). The maintenance of this genetic variant over long periods of human evolution has been interpreted as evidence for widespread cannibalism in some early human populations.

SPECIFIC SUSCEPTIBILITY AND RESISTANCE GENES

For several human genes, there is compelling evidence that one or more genetic variants affect susceptibility to infectious pathogens (see Tables 5-2 to 5-4). In this section, particular genes are discussed in turn.

Blood Groups

ABO blood groups have been investigated in a large number of infectious diseases in early studies. An association of blood group O with increased severity of cholera symptoms has been found in several studies.[101,102] Blood group O is associated with peptic ulceration, which in turn is associated with *H. pylori* infection. A possible mechanism for this association was suggested by the finding that fucosylation of the Leb receptor for *H. pylori* in the gastric mucosa, found in individuals with A or B blood group, impaired binding of the bacteria.[103] However, *H. pylori* infection is not clearly influenced by ABO blood group type.[104] The ability to secrete blood group substances into saliva and at other mucosal surfaces is genetically determined. Most individuals are secretors, but about 20% of most populations are nonsecretors due to mutation in the fucosyltransferase-2 *(FUT2)* gene.[105] In relatively small studies, nonsecretion has been suggested to be associated with susceptibility to some bacterial and fungal infections and with resistance to certain common viral infections.[106,107] Nonsecretor status is clearly associated with susceptibility to recurrent urinary tract infection,[108] and a possible mechanism for this has been proposed.[109] Nonsecretor status has been found to protect completely against infection with Norwalk virus in volunteer challenge studies.[110]

The most striking blood group association is that relating the Duffy blood group and susceptibility to *P. vivax* malaria. This parasite uses the Duffy blood group antigen as the receptor to invade erythrocytes.[111] The Duffy blood group antigen is a promiscuous chemokine receptor. Most sub-Saharan Africans are Duffy blood group negative due to homozygosity for a mutation in the promoter of this gene. They thus are completely resistant to *P. vivax* infections. Interestingly, such individuals express the Duffy antigen on some other tissues, as the promoter mutation that is in the recognition site for an erythroid-specific enhancer is tissue specific.[112] It is unclear whether the Duffy genotypes prevented *P. vivax* from ever entering Africa or whether an earlier more virulent form of this parasitic infection might have selected the variant in Africa.

Hemoglobin Gene Variants

Based on the distribution of thalassemia in the Mediterranean, Haldane[113] proposed that certain hemoglobin gene variants might have reached high frequencies in malarious regions by providing resistance to this disease. The protective efficacy of sickle hemoglobin in heterozygotes against *P. falciparum* malaria was discovered a few years later.[21] The greatest protection is afforded against death and severe life-threatening malaria, with somewhat less protection against uncomplicated disease and least protection against becoming infected. This pattern of greater protection against disease than infection appears to be found for many resistance genes. Several differences observed in vitro with heterozygous compared with normal red cells have been proposed as the mechanism for this protection; these include impaired invasion and growth of the parasite, decreased rosetting of parasitized cells, decreased expression of a major parasite antigen on the erythrocyte surface, and increased reticuloendothelial clearance. Which of these is of most importance is unclear. The α- and β-thalassemias are extremely common disorders of hemoglobin synthesis leading to imbalanced globin chain production. The mild forms of thalassemia are among the most prevalent single-gene disorders. Both the α- and β-thalassemias have been shown to afford some protection against *P. falciparum* malaria in keeping with their geographical distribution, but the mechanism of protection remains unknown.[24,25] There is no detectable impairment of parasite growth in vitro, and the protection afforded may be less marked than for sickle hemoglobin. Recent studies support a protective role for both hemoglobin C and hemoglobin E against falciparum malaria.[24-27]

Glucose-6-Phosphate Dehydrogenase Deficiency

Erythrocyte G6PD deficiency is found at high frequencies in many tropical and subtropical populations. This is an X-linked disorder that is associated with red cell destruction under certain conditions.[114] A variety of drugs, some infections, and ingestion of fava beans can trigger acute hemolysis, and male G6PD-deficient infants may have neonatal jaundice. More than 100 different mutations of G6PD have been described using molecular analysis, and a small group of uncommon variants is associated with chronic hemolytic anemia in the absence of any environmental agents. The majority of G6PD variants are associated with lesser degrees of enzyme deficiency and are found at higher frequency. Regarding the hemoglobinopathies, the geographic distribution of G6PD deficiency in the "malaria belt" suggested its selective advantage.[7] In several locations, populations with historical malarial exposure had significantly higher frequencies of G6PD deficiency compared with related populations who had not been exposed to malarial selection. As with the hemoglobinopathies, a variety of molecular mutations are associated with this enzyme deficiency: in Africans, G6PD-A−; in the Mediterranean basin, G6PD-Med; and in Asia and Melanesia, several different G6PD variants.[115] In some studies, malaria parasite densities and counts were found to be lower in enzyme-deficient males and sometimes females. However, studies of severe malaria in both East and West Africa have shown that both hemizygous males and heterozygous females are significantly protected.[23] This is in keeping with in vitro studies of erythrocytic cultures of *P. falciparum* that showed impaired growth in G6PD-deficient red cells.[116]

Human Leukocyte Antigens

The pivotal position of HLAs in the initiation and regulation of immune responses together with their well-documented polymorphism has led to numerous studies of their influence on infectious disease susceptibility. The first evidence of HLA effects came from studies of the mycobacterial diseases leprosy and tuberculosis.[44] The HLA class II antigen HLA-DR2 was found to be both associated with and genetically linked to susceptibility to tuberculoid leprosy in India.[44,117] Although initially it appeared that HLA might predominantly influence leprosy type, most studies now indicate that HLA-DR2 in Asian populations predisposes to the development of leprosy per se.[47,49] In several Asian populations, but not in other continents, HLA-DR2 has also been associated with susceptibility to tuberculosis.[48,50,118] The mechanism of these susceptibility associations remains unclear, but it has been speculated that HLA-DR2 may influence the type of immune response developed, leading to stronger humoral but weaker protective cellular responses to mycobacterial antigens.

Studies of malaria susceptibility in African children identified protective associations between particular HLA types and infectious disease. In a large Gambian study, the HLA class I antigen HLA-B53 (now denoted *B*5301*) was associated with resistance to severe malaria.[30] This HLA type is particularly common in Africans, possibly as a result of natural selection by malaria. Cytotoxic T lymphocytes restricted by this HLA class I molecule recognize a peptide epitope from the liver stage of the life cycle of the malaria parasite and may mediate this protective association.[119] In the same study, an HLA class II molecule, HLA-DRB1*1302, a subtype of HLA-DR13 in the older nomenclature, was also associated with resistance to a form of severe malaria, presumably indicating a protective action of CD4+ T cells restricted by this HLA-DR molecule.[30]

In a subsequent study, this same HLA type, *HLA-DRB1*1302,* was associated with resistance to persistent HBV infection in West Africans.[66] In European populations, HLA-DR11 has been associated with resistance to persistent HCV infection.[69] Strong evidence of HLA associations with disease manifestations has also been presented for human papillomavirus infection.[120,121] Numerous studies of HLA and HIV infection have been undertaken. An overview of published studies indicated considerable interpopulation heterogeneity in associations. However, there is compelling evidence of associations between HLA class I types and the rate of disease progression to AIDS, as specified earlier.[59-64] An overall effect of polymorphism in the MHC was elegantly demonstrated in a study of pairs of HIV-infected hemophiliac brothers. Pairs sharing two HLA haplotypes had a more similar rate of CD4 T-cell decline than those sharing only one or zero haplotypes.[64]

The accumulating evidence that particular HLA types are associated with altered susceptibility to infectious disease supports the view that the remarkable diversity of HLA types has been generated and maintained through natural selection by infectious pathogens. The relatively modest magnitude of the reported associations, compared with some HLA associations with autoimmune disease, is in keeping with this possibility. Small selective effects can over time markedly change allele frequencies. The observation that cellular immune responses are restricted by HLA molecules suggested an attractive mechanism whereby heterozygosity for HLA type might be evolutionarily advantageous.[122] Heterozygotes should be able to recognize more peptide epitopes in a foreign pathogen than homozygotes to permit a more protective immune response. A protective effect of heterozygosity has now been observed in relation to HLA class II antigens and clearance of HBV,[123] and for HLA class I antigens and HIV disease progression[60] and human T-cell leukemia/lymphoma virus-1 (HTLV-1) proviral load.[124] Another feature of HLA associations with infectious disease is that associations often vary geographically. In some cases, this may result from geographic strain variation in the infectious pathogen, and an HLA association with the strain of parasite causing infection has been reported in malaria.[33] More detailed analysis of the mechanisms of identified associations should explain further this population diversity and provide insights to immune mechanism of protection and pathogenesis.

Cytokine Genes

Increasing understanding of the pleiotropic regulatory role of various cytokines in immune defense has led to analyses of the role of cytokine genes in several infectious diseases. Studies of the *TNF* gene, located in the class III region of the MHC, have been most rewarding. Several point mutations are found in the promoter of this gene, which may affect the level of TNF production. A variant at position −308 has been associated with susceptibility to cerebral malaria in Africa,[125] to mucocutaneous and visceral leishmaniasis in South America,[92,93] and to lepromatous leprosy in India.[51] Interestingly, serum levels of TNF have been found to be elevated in all of these conditions, and the genetic associations suggest that the elevated *TNF* levels may play a pathogenic role. These genetic associations were identified before there was any in vitro evidence that this promoter variant is associated with increased levels of *TNF* gene expression.[126] Indeed, direct evidence that disease-associated promoter variants have functional effects is only beginning to emerge.[127] Associations have also been described with susceptibility to trachoma,[128] and persistent HBV infection and other promoter variants may also be associated with altered susceptibility to infectious diseases.[62,126] These genetic associations with promoter variants of the *TNF* gene have supported attempts to modulate the severity of various diseases using a variety of anti-TNF reagents. Studies of the families of children with meningococcal disease found that families with low TNF and high IL-10 production in response to endotoxin stimulation in vitro were associated with much higher mortality rates in meningococcal disease,[90] implying a protective role for a proinflammatory cytokine profile.

Searches for infectious disease associations with variants of other cytokine genes have thus far been less fruitful, although variants of IL-1, IL-6, IL-4, and, in particular, IL-10[129] and interferon-γ,[130] have been analyzed in a variety of studies and implicated in a few. However, a susceptibility gene for worm burden in schistosomiasis has been mapped to a region of the long arm of chromosome 5 that encodes a large number of cytokine genes, and it has been suggested that one of these genes may be involved.[91] Also, rare defects in the genes for IL-12p40, IL-12β2 receptor chain, and interferon-γ receptor 1 have been associated with marked susceptibility to some avirulent mycobacteria and salmonella.[19,20,54,55]

Chemokine Receptors

The discovery that certain chemokine receptors act as co-receptors for the invasion of macrophages and lymphocytes by HIV has led to numerous studies of the role of polymorphism in these genes in variable susceptibility to HIV infection and disease progression to AIDS. A 32–base pair deletion in the CCR5 chemokine receptor is found at allele frequencies of up to 10% in European and derived populations.[131] This variant is rare or absent in other populations.[132] CCR5 is the co-receptor for macrophage-tropic strains of HIV-1 involved in viral transmission. Heterozygotes for the 32–base pair deletion progress more slowly to AIDS once infected but are not at reduced risk of HIV infection.[52] In contrast, homozygotes for this variant have very substantial resistance to HIV infection, and only a few infected homozygotes have been identified. Another rarer variant in this gene has been associated with resistance to infection,[133] and haplotypes of several promoter variants are relevant,[134,135] at least in North American cohorts.[136] A particular nucleotide variant of the CCR promoter at position −2459 appears to affect surface CCR receptor levels on monocytes and infectability of Langerhans cells.[137,138] An amino acid change in the linked *CCR2* gene is also associated with slower disease progression to AIDS[68] independent of the *CCR5* variants. Lymphotropic HIV viruses that appear later in the course of infection use the *CXCR4* rather than the *CCR5* receptor. The natural ligand for the *CXCR4* receptor is stromal-derived factor 1 (SDF-1), and variation in the 3′-untranslated region of this gene has also been associated with altered rates of disease progression to AIDS in some, but not all, studies.[67] The effects of these genetic variants underpin current attempts to develop pharmaceutical agents that will block interaction of HIV with these co-receptors.

The high prevalence of the *CCR5* 32–base pair deletion in northern Europeans is intriguing. Analysis of flanking molecular markers has shown that this deletion is found on a rare background haplotype and suggests that it arose less than 3000 years ago.[139,140] This implies that the variant allele has probably been subject to positive selection, but HIV appeared too recently to have been the selective agent. It has been speculated that various other infectious pathogens, including the plague bacillus and the smallpox virus, may have been involved.

Mannose-Binding Lectin

MBL is a serum protein that plays a role in innate immunity. It is a collagenous lectin with at least two important roles in host defense.[141] It binds to sugars, particularly *N*-acetylglucosamine and mannose, on the surface of microorganisms and facilitates their opsonization by macrophages. It also activates complement by means of two MBL-associated serine proteases. Surprisingly, inactivating mutations of this gene are quite prevalent, with frequencies of up to 40% in various populations. Three single amino acid changes are found at codons 52, 54, and 57, each of which leads to a substantial reduction in MBL concentration in heterozygotes. Homozygotes or compound heterozygotes for these variants have absent or extremely low MBL levels in serum. Variation in the promoter of the gene has less marked functional effects.[142] It was originally proposed that MBL might pay a key role in immune defense in late infancy after maternal antibodies had waned and before acquired immunity had been well developed. A cohort study of the rate of acute respiratory infections in young children in Greenland provides some support for this possibility.[143] Case reports and small-scale studies suggested that MBL deficiency might predispose to a variety of infectious diseases,[144] but most initial studies of individual diseases, meningococcal disease, malaria, tuberculosis, and persistent HBV infection failed to show clear associations.[145,146] However, homozygotes for MBL codon changes are susceptible to invasive pneumococcal disease with a 2.5-fold increase in risk.[87,147] MBL deficiency may be associated with an increased risk of exacerbation of chronic obstructive pulmonary disease[148] and an increased duration of febrile neutropenic episodes in children with malignancy.[149] Also, deficiency has been associated with an increased rate of serious infection after chemotherapy,[150] leading to the suggestion that replacement therapy might be beneficial.[151] A small study recently suggested that MBL deficiency may predispose to recurrent vaginal candidiasis, and further study of this condition is warranted.[152]

NATURAL RESISTANCE–ASSOCIATED MACROPHAGE PROTEIN-1

The relevance of natural resistance–associated macrophage protein-1 (*NRAMP1*) to tuberculosis susceptibility was discovered by an unusual route. In studies of mouse strains, susceptibility to species of *Salmonella, Leishmania,* and some mycobacteria was found to be influenced by a single major gene that was mapped and identified by positional cloning.[16] The human homologue of this murine gene *Nramp1* is termed *NRAMP1* or *SLC11A1.* Several sequence changes in *NRAMP1* have been associated with susceptibility to severe pulmonary tuberculosis in West Africa and in Asia.[17,153-155] It is more likely that this gene affects susceptibility to clinical tuberculosis than to infection by *M. tuberculosis,* but this has not been demonstrated. The function of the NRAMP1 gene product remains to be clarified, but it is present only in macrophages and neutrophils and is found on the membrane of the phagolysosome in which *M. tuberculosis* grows.[156] *NRAMP1* is homologous to the more recently described *NRAMP2* gene, which encodes a divalent ion transporter[157]; and the former may influence intraphagosomal iron concentrations and thus affect mycobacterial growth.[158]

Other Genes

Twin studies have indicated that most of the genetic component of variation in cellular and humoral immune responses to some common infectious pathogens appears to map to genes outside of the MHC.[159]

These genes are likely to be numerous and to affect susceptibility to several infectious diseases but have not been identified. One candidate for this type of role is the vitamin D receptor (VDR). The active form of vitamin D (vitamin D_3) has immunoregulatory functions as well as an important role in calcium metabolism.[160] The VDR is expressed in macrophages and activated lymphocytes, and vitamin D_3 leads to increased macrophage activation and a shift in the cytokine secretion profile of lymphocytes to a more Th2-like pattern. Variation in the vitamin D receptor has been associated with resistance to tuberculosis and persistent HBV infection[161] and appears to influence the type of type of leprosy developed,[162] possibly by an influence of the polarization of CD4 T-cell responses. As with vitamin D receptor associations with osteoporosis, gene–environment interactions are likely to be important,[163] so that some population differences in the magnitude of such genetic associations are to be expected.

There has been considerable interest in the possibility that genetic variants of Toll-like receptor (TLR) genes influence susceptibility to infectious diseases. For example, a common variant in the *TLR4* gene has been proposed to influence susceptibility to gram-negative bacterial infections,[164,165] and rare,[166] but uncommon, variants[167] of this gene have been claimed to alter susceptibility to meningococcal disease. A very rare variant of the *TLR2* gene has been implicated in lepromatous leprosy.[168] These early observations suggest that further large-scale genetic studies of these receptors and their signalling pathways may be fruitful.

CJD is caused by infection with *prions,* proteinaceous particles that appear to lack all nucleic acid. Rare familial forms of the disease were initially shown to be due to variation in the host human prion protein (*PRP*) gene.[169,170] In both French and US patients iatrogenically infected with the CJD agent, a marked effect of a very common variation in *PRP* genotype on susceptibility to disease was observed.[98,171] Homozygotes for either of the amino acids, methionine or valine, commonly found at position 129 were markedly more susceptible to disease than heterozygotes. In UK patients with new-variant CJD, caused by infection with the bovine prion that causes bovine spongiform encephalopathy in cattle, only methionine homozygotes have been found among cases.[98]

Cystic fibrosis is the most common life-threatening autosomal recessive disorder in populations of European origin. Causative mutations in the cystic fibrosis transmembrane conductance regulator (CFTR) are found at frequencies of up to 4% in these populations. It is likely, but not certain,[172] that some selective advantage has contributed to the high frequencies of mutations in this gene.[173] Studies in a mouse model of cystic fibrosis led to the suggestion that cholera may have been the selective agent.[174] However, more recent studies have provided stronger support for selection by typhoid rather than by cholera.[95,175] The CFTR molecule was found to be the receptor used by *S. typhi* to enter intestinal epithelial cells.[95] As yet there are no data on CFTR variation and susceptibility to typhoid in humans.

EVOLUTIONARY PERSPECTIVE

From an overview of the information currently available, it seems likely that susceptibility to most infectious diseases will prove to be highly polygenic. The contrary view—that there may be a few major single genes for many infectious diseases—has been suggested by complex segregation analysis of multicase families[43] and may be incorrect.[176] The existence of multiple genes affecting infectious disease susceptibility probably simply reflects the major role that infectious pathogens have played in shaping variation in the human genome through natural selection. Indeed it has been found that genes playing a role in host defense against infectious pathogens evolve at a higher rate than do any other class of genes.[177] Natural selection for resistance to infectious pathogens may also explain why the observed effects of most individual genes are relatively modest in magnitude. In the absence of a counterbalancing selective force, alleles that markedly increased or decreased risk of a major infectious disease would be quickly eliminated or selected to very high frequency, eliminating polymorphism. Such polygenic susceptibility has also been found in extensive analyses of the genetic basis of susceptibility to autoimmune diseases in both humans and mice.[178]

Given the pressure for fixation of selectively advantageous variants, one of the major questions in evolutionary biology has related to the mechanisms maintaining substantial genetic diversity in populations. Some aspects of this question are particularly well addressed in human populations where the host genome and the infectious pathogens have been characterized in most detail. Heterozygote advantage is an attractive mechanism by which two alleles may be maintained in a population and is classically exemplified by the sickle hemoglobin polymorphism and resistance to malaria. However, this appears to be a relatively unusual means of maintaining genetic diversity, and other mechanisms such as frequency-dependent selection and fluctuations in selection may be more generally important. Another factor is likely to be variation in the genome of infectious pathogens. Increasing attention is being paid to specific interactions between variants of the host and the parasite. Particular HLA types have been associated with disease caused by specific serotypes of human papillomavirus,[120] HLA type may also influence the strain of *P. falciparum* causing malaria[33] and HIV may evolve away from prevalent HLA class I types.[66] Furthermore, immunologic mechanisms have been identified that may underlie interaction between competing strains of microorganisms.[33] There may be exquisite specificity in some of these host-parasite interactions leading to co-evolution of genetic variation in the host and pathogen. This implies that individual susceptibility to disease is the result of a variety of genetic factors in both host and pathogen tempered by a constellation of environmental variables. This dynamic evolutionary perspective suggests that the genes affecting susceptibility to an infectious disease may show significant interpopulation heterogeneity due to geographic variation in the pathogen genome, in the environment, and in the frequencies of interacting genes in the host, a prediction well supported by available data on malaria susceptibility.

APPLICATIONS

It is unlikely that most of the genetic component to any infectious disease can be accounted for by the polymorphisms and associations identified to date. The newly available entire human genome sequence and now millions of defined single-nucleotide polymorphisms have greatly enhanced the power of genomic analyses. There are several potential advantages to applying the power of modern molecular genetics to understand genetic susceptibility more fully. An obvious application is in risk prediction. This might influence behavior, the use of prophylactic antimicrobials, or immunization or travel patterns. It is likely that in future it will be possible to offer a genetic profiling test to estimate individual susceptibility to particular pathogens.

Another application is in the understanding of particular pathways used in host resistance to infection. For example, the HLA-B53 association with resistance to malaria[31] supported a protective role for CD8+ T cells in this disease, encouraging efforts to develop vaccines that elicit this immune response.[179] The association of MBL deficiency with susceptibility to pneumococcal invasive disease has revealed a key role for this molecule in innate immunity to this bacterium.

A third application will be the identification of molecules and pathways that are targets for pharmacologic intervention. The demonstration of the almost complete resistance of homozygotes for a deletion in the *CCR5* gene to HIV infection has underpinned attempts to develop pharmacologic blockers of this viral co-receptor. The NRAMP1 gene product may also turn out to be amenable to specific pharmacologic interventions. New techniques of genome-wide analysis offer the prospect of many new target molecules discovered through linkage analysis and positional cloning. The potentially very large number of infectious disease resistance genes and the increasing power of methods available to identify these suggest that there will be much to learn.

REFERENCES

1. Fine PE. Immunogenetics of susceptibility to leprosy, tuberculosis, and leishmaniasis. An epidemiological perspective. Int J Lepr Other Mycobact Dis. 1981;49:437-454.
2. Weeks DE, Lathrop GM. Polygenic disease: Methods for mapping complex disease traits. Trends Genet. 1995;11:513-519.
3. Wallace C, Clayton D, Fine P. Estimating the relative recurrence risk ratio for leprosy in Karonga District, Malawi. Lepr Rev. 2003;74:133-140.
4. Modiano D, Petrarca V, Sirima BS, et al. Different response to *Plasmodium falciparum* malaria in west African sympatric ethnic groups. Proc Natl Acad Sci U S A. 1996;93:13206-13211.
5. Stead WW, Senner JW, Reddick WT, Lofgren JP. Racial differences in susceptibility to infection by *Mycobacterium tuberculosis*. N Engl J Med. 1990;322:422-427.
6. Black FL. Why did they die? Science. 1992;258:1739-1740.
7. Motulsky AG. Metabolic polymorphisms and the role of infectious diseases in human evolution. Hum Biol. 1960;32:28-62.
8. James SP, Nicol WD, Shute PG. A study of induced malignant tertian malaria. Proc R Soc Med. 1932;25:1153-1186.
9. Sorensen TI, Nielsen GG, Andersen PK, Teasdale TW. Genetic and environmental influences on premature death in adult adoptees. N Engl J Med. 1988;318:727-732.
10. Comstock GW. Tuberculosis in twins: A re-analysis of the Prophit survey. Am Rev Respir Dis. 1978;117:621-624.
11. Herndon CN, Jennings RG. A twin-family study of susceptibility to poliomyelitis. Am J Hum Genet. 1951;3:17-46.
12. Chakravarti MR, Vogel F. A twin study on leprosy. Vol. I. Stuttgart: Thieme; 1973 Topics in Human Genetics.
13. Lin TM, Chen CJ, Wu MM, et al. Hepatitis B virus markers in Chinese twins. Anticancer Res. 1989;9:737-741.
14. Malaty HM, Engstrand L, Pedersen NL, Graham DY. *Helicobacter pylori* infection: Genetic and environmental influences. A study of twins. Ann Intern Med. 1994;120:982-986.
15. Jepson AP, Banya WA, Sisay-Joof F, et al. Genetic regulation of fever in *Plasmodium falciparum* malaria in Gambian twin children. J Infect Dis. 1995;172:316-319.
16. Vidal SM, Malo D, Vogan K, et al. Natural resistance to infection with intracellular parasites: Isolation of a candidate for BCG. Cell. 1993;73:469-485.
17. Bellamy R, Ruwende C, Corrah T, et al. Variations in the NRAMP1 gene and susceptibility to tuberculosis in West Africans. N Engl J Med. 1998;338:640-644.
18. Staeheli P, Grob R, Meier E, et al. Influenza virus-susceptible mice carry Mx genes with a large deletion or a nonsense mutation. Mol Cell Biol. 1988;8:4518-4523.
19. Newport MJ, Huxley CM, Huston S, et al. A mutation in the interferon-gamma-receptor gene and susceptibility to mycobacterial infection. N Engl J Med. 1996;335:1941-1949.
20. Jouanguy E, Altare F, Lamhamedi S, et al. Interferon-gamma-receptor deficiency in an infant with fatal bacille Calmette-Guerin infection. N Engl J Med. 1996;335:1956-1961.
21. Allison AC. Protection afforded by sickle-cell trait against subtertian malarial infection. Br Med J. 1954;1:290-294.
22. Allison AC. Polymorphism and natural selection in human populations. Cold Spring Harbor Symp Quant Biol. 1964;29:137-149.
23. Ruwende C, Khoo SC, Snow RW, et al. Natural selection of hemi- and heterozygotes for G6PD deficiency in Africa by resistance to severe malaria. Nature. 1995;376:246-249.
24. Modiano D, Luoni G, Sirima BS, et al. Haemoglobin C protects against clinical *Plasmodium falciparum* malaria. Nature. 2001;414:305-308.
25. Agarwal A, Guindo A, Cissoko Y, et al. Hemoglobin C associated with protection from severe malaria in the Dogon of Mali, a West African population with a low prevalence of hemoglobin S. Blood. 2000;96:2358-2363.
26. Hutagalung R, Wilairatana P, Looareesuwan S, et al. Influence of hemoglobin E trait on the severity of *Falciparum* malaria. J Infect Dis. 1999;179:283-286.
27. Chotivanich K, Udomsangpetch R, Pattanapanyasat K, et al. Hemoglobin E: A balanced polymorphism protective against high parasitemias and thus severe P falciparum malaria. Blood. 2002;100:1172-1176.
28. Willcox M, Bjorkman A, Brohult J, et al. A case-control study in northern Liberia of *Plasmodium falciparum* malaria in haemoglobin S and beta-thalassaemia traits. Ann Trop Med Parasitol. 1983;77:239-246.
29. Allen SJ, O'Donnell A, Alexander ND, et al. alpha+-Thalassemia protects children against disease caused by other infections as well as malaria. Proc Natl Acad Sci U S A. 1997;94:14736-14741.
30. Williams TN, Maitland K, Bennett S, et al. High incidence of malaria in alpha-thalassaemic children. Nature. 1996;383:522-525.
31. Hill AV, Allsopp CE, Kwiatkowski D, et al. Common west African HLA antigens are associated with protection from severe malaria. Nature. 1991;352:595-600.
32. Hill AV, Yates SN, Allsopp CE, et al. Human leukocyte antigens and natural selection by malaria. Philos Trans R Soc Lond B Biol Sci. 1994;346:379-385.
33. Gilbert SC, Plebanski M, Gupta S, et al. Association of malaria parasite population structure, HLA, and immunological antagonism. Science. 1998;279:1173-1177.
34. Carlson J, Helmby H, Hill AV, et al. Human cerebral malaria: Association with erythrocyte rosetting and lack of anti-rosetting antibodies. Lancet. 1990;336:1457-1460.
35. Marsh K, Snow RW. Host-parasite interaction and morbidity in malaria endemic areas. Philos Trans R Soc Lond B Biol Sci. 1997;352:1385-1394.
36. Jepson A, Sisay-Joof F, Banya W, et al. Genetic linkage of mild malaria to the major histocompatibility complex in Gambian children: Study of affected sibling pairs. BMJ. 1997;315:96-97.
37. Fernandez-Reyes D, Craig AG, Kyes SA, et al. A high frequency African coding polymorphism in the N-terminal domain of ICAM-1 predisposing to cerebral malaria in Kenya. Hum Mol Genet. 1997;6:1357-1360.

38. Pain A, Urban BC, Kai O, et al. A non-sense mutation in CD36 gene is associated with protection from severe malaria. Lancet. 2001;357:1502-1503.

39. Omi K, Ohashi J, Patarapotikul J, et al. CD36 polymorphism is associated with protection from cerebral malaria. Am J Hum Genet. 2003;72:364-374.

40. Miller LH, Mason SJ, Dvorak JA, et al. Erythrocyte receptors for *Plasmodium knowlesi* malaria: Duffy blood group determinants. Science. 1975;189:561-563.

41. Genton B, al-Yaman F, Mgone CS, et al. Ovalocytosis and cerebral malaria (Letter). Nature. 1995;378:564-565.

42. Mgone CS, Koki G, Paniu MM, et al. Occurrence of the erythrocyte band 3 (AE1) gene deletion in relation to malaria endemicity in Papua New Guinea. Trans R Soc Trop Med Hyg. 1996;90:228-231.

43. Abel L, Demenais F. Detection of major genes for susceptibility to leprosy and its subtypes in a Caribbean island: Desirade island. Am J Hum Genet. 1988;42:256-266.

44. Sreevatsan S, Pan X, Stockbauer KE, et al. Restricted structural gene polymorphism in the *Mycobacterium tuberculosis* complex indicates evolutionarily recent global dissemination. Proc Natl Acad Sci U S A. 1997;94:9869-9874.

45. de Vries RR, Fat RF, Nijenhuis LE, van Rood JJ. HLA-linked genetic control of host response to *Mycobacterium leprae*. Lancet. 1976;2:1328-1330.

46. Singh SP, Mehra NK, Dingley HB, et al. Human leukocyte antigen (HLA)-linked control of susceptibility to pulmonary tuberculosis and association with HLA-DR types. J Infect Dis. 1983;148:676-681.

47. Rani R, Fernandez Vina MA, Zaheer SA, et al. Study of HLA class II alleles by PCR oligotyping in leprosy patients from north India. Tiss Antigens. 1993;42:133-137.

48. Brahmajothi V, Pitchappan RM, Kakkanaiah VN, et al. Association of pulmonary tuberculosis and HLA in south India. Tubercle. 1991;72:123-132.

49. Todd JR, West BC, McDonald JC. Human leukocyte antigen and leprosy: Study in northern Louisiana and review. Rev Infect Dis. 1990;12:63-74.

50. Bothamley GH, Beck JS, Schreuder GM, et al. Association of tuberculosis and *M. tuberculosis*-specific antibody levels with HLA. J Infect Dis. 1989;159:549-555.

51. Roy S, McGuire W, Mascie-Taylor CG, et al. Tumor necrosis factor promoter polymorphism and susceptibility to lepromatous leprosy. J Infect Dis. 1997;176:530-532.

52. Shaw MA, Donaldson IJ, Collins A, et al. Association and linkage of leprosy phenotypes with HLA class II and tumour necrosis factor genes. Genes Immun. 2001;2:196-204.

53. Bellamy R, Beyers N, McAdam KP, et al. Genetic susceptibility to tuberculosis in Africans: A genome-wide scan. Proc Natl Acad Sci U S A. 2000;97:8005-8009.

54. Fieschi C, Dupuis S, Catherinot E, et al. Low penetrance, broad resistance, and favorable outcome of interleukin 12 receptor beta1 deficiency: Medical and immunological implications. J Exp Med. 2003;197:527-535.

55. Casanova JL, Abel L. Genetic dissection of immunity to mycobacteria: The human model. Annu Rev Immunol. 2002;20:581-620.

56. Rossouw M, Nel HJ, Cooke GS, et al. Association between tuberculosis and a polymorphic NFkappaB binding site in the interferon gamma gene. Lancet. 2003;361:1871-1872.

57. Fowke KR, Nagelkerke NJ, Kimani J, et al. Resistance to HIV-1 infection among persistently seronegative prostitutes in Nairobi, Kenya. Lancet. 1996;348:1347-1351.

58. Scorza Smeraldi R, Fabio G, Lazzarin A, et al. HLA-associated susceptibility to acquired immunodeficiency syndrome in Italian patients with human-immunodeficiency-virus infection. Lancet. 1986;2:1187-1189.

59. Kaslow RA, Duquesnoy R, VanRaden M, et al. A1, Cw7, B8, DR3 HLA antigen combination associated with rapid decline of T-helper lymphocytes in HIV-1 infection. A report from the Multicenter AIDS Cohort Study. Lancet. 1990;335:927-930.

60. Carrington M, Nelson GW, Martin MP, et al. HLA and HIV-1: heterozygote advantage and B*35-Cw*04 disadvantage. Science. 1999; 283:1748-1752.

61. McNeil AJ, Yap PL, Gore SM, et al. Association of HLA types A1-B8-DR3 and B27 with rapid and slow progression of HIV disease. Q J Med. 1996;89:177-185.

62. Migueles SA, Sabbaghian MS, Shupert WL, et al. HLA B*5701 is highly associated with restriction of virus replication in a subgroup of HIV-infected long term nonprogressors. Proc Natl Acad Sci U S A. 2000;97:2709-2714.

63. Kaslow RA, Carrington M, Apple R, et al. Influence of combinations of major histocompatibility genes on the course of HIV-1 infection. Nat Med. 1996;2:405-411.

64. Kroner BL, Goedert JJ, Blattner WA, et al. Concordance of human leukocyte antigen haplotype-sharing, CD4 decline and AIDS in hemophilic siblings. Multicenter Hemophilia Cohort and Hemophilia Growth and Development Studies. AIDS. 1995; 9:275-280.

65. Trachtenberg E, Korber B, Sollars C, et al. Advantage of rare HLA supertype in HIV disease progression. Nat Med. 2003;9:928-935.

66. Moore CB, John M, James IR, et al. Evidence of HIV-1 adaptation to HLA-restricted immune responses at a population level. Science. 2002; 296:1439-1443.

67. Dean M, Carrington M, Winkler C, et al. Genetic restriction of HIV-1 infection and progression to AIDS by a deletion allele of the CKR5 structural gene. Hemophilia Growth and Development Study, Multicenter AIDS Cohort Study, Multicenter Hemophilia Cohort Study, San Francisco City Cohort, ALIVE Study [published erratum appears in Science. 1996;274:1069]. Science. 1996;273:1856-1862.

68. Smith MW, Dean M, Carrington M, et al. Contrasting genetic influence of CCR2 and CCR5 variants on HIV-1 infection and disease progression. Hemophilia Growth and Development Study (HGDS), Multicenter AIDS Cohort Study (MACS), Multicenter Hemophilia Cohort Study (MHCS), San Francisco City Cohort (SFCC), ALIVE Study. Science. 1997;277:959-965.

69. Winkler C, Modi W, Smith MW, et al. Genetic restriction of AIDS pathogenesis by an SDF-1 chemokine gene variant. ALIVE Study, Hemophilia Growth and Development Study (HGDS), Multicenter AIDS Cohort Study (MACS), Multicenter Hemophilia Cohort Study (MHCS), San Francisco City Cohort (SFCC). Science. 1998;279:389-393.

70. An P, Nelson GW, Wang L et al. Modulating influence on HIV/AIDS by interacting RANTES gene variants. Proc Natl Acad Sci U S A. 2002;99:10002-10007.

71. Ali S, Niang MA, N'doye I, et al. Secretor polymorphism and human immunodeficiency virus infection in Senegalese women. J Infect Dis. 2000;181:737-739.

72. Gonzalez E, Rovin BH, Sen L, et al. HIV-1 infection and AIDS dementia are influenced by a mutant MCP-1 allele linked to increased monocyte infiltration of tissues and MCP-1 levels. Proc Natl Acad Sci U S A. 2002;99:13795-13800.

73. Blumberg BS. The nature of Australia antigen: Infectious and genetic characteristics. Prog Liver Dis. 1972;4:367-379.

74. Blumberg BS, Melartin L, Guint RA, Werner B. Family studies of a human serum isoantigen system (Australia antigen). Am J Hum Genet. 1966;18:594-608.

75. Almarri A, Batchelor JR. HLA and hepatitis B infection. Lancet. 1994;344:1194-1195.

76. Thursz MR, Kwiatkowski D, Allsopp CE, et al. Association between an MHC class II allele and clearance of hepatitis B virus in the Gambia. N Engl J Med. 1995; 332:1065-1069.

77. Thursz MR, Thomas HC, Greenwood BM, Hill AV. Heterozygote advantage for HLA class-II type in hepatitis B virus infection (Letter). Nat Genet. 1997;17:11-12.

78. Hohler T, Gerken G, Notghi A, et al. HLA-DRB1*1301 and *1302 protect against chronic hepatitis B. J Hepatol. 1997;26:503-507.

79. Zavaglia C, Bortolon C, Ferrioli G, et al. HLA typing in chronic type B, D and C hepatitis. J Hepatol. 1996;24:658-665.

80. Hohler T, Kruger A, Gerken G, et al. A tumor necrosis factor-alpha (TNF-alpha) promoter polymorphism is associated with chronic hepatitis B infection. Clin Exp Immunol. 1998;111:579-582.

81. Thomas HC, Foster GR, Sumiya M, et al. Mutation of gene of mannose-binding protein associated with chronic hepatitis B viral infection. Lancet. 1996;348:1417-1419.

82. Louagie HK, Brouwer JT, Delanghe JR, et al. Haptoglobin polymorphism and chronic hepatitis C. J Hepatol. 1996;25:10-14.

83. Yee LJ, Tang J, Gibson AW, et al. Interleukin 10 polymorphisms as predictors of sustained response in antiviral therapy for chronic hepatitis C infection. Hepatology. 2001;33:708-712.

84. McGlynn KA, Rosvold EA, Lustbader ED, et al. Susceptibility to hepatocellular carcinoma is associated with genetic variation in the enzymatic detoxification of aflatoxin B1. Proc Natl Acad Sci U S A. 1995;92:2384-2387.

85. Bredius RG, Derkx BH, Fijen CA, et al. Fc gamma receptor IIa (CD32) polymorphism in fulminant meningococcal septic shock in children. J Infect Dis. 1994;170:848-853.

86. Sanders LA, van de Winkel JG, Rijkers GT, et al. Fc gamma receptor IIa (CD32) heterogeneity in patients with recurrent bacterial respiratory tract infections. J Infect Dis. 1994;170:854-861.

87. Roy S, Knox K, Segal S, et al. MBL genotype and risk of invasive pneumococcal disease: A case-control study. Lancet. 2002;359:1569-1573.

88. Kronborg G, Garred P. Mannose-binding lectin genotype as a risk factor for invasive pneumococcal infection. Lancet. 2002;360:1176.

89. Summerfield JA, Sumiya M, Levin M, Turner MW. Association of mutations in mannose binding protein gene with childhood infection in consecutive hospital series. BMJ. 1997;314:1229-1232.

90. Westendorp RG, Langermans JA, Huizinga TW, et al. Genetic influence on cytokine production and fatal meningococcal disease [published erratum appears in Lancet. 1997;349:656]. Lancet. 1997;349:170-173.

91. Marquet S, Abel L, Hillaire D, et al. Genetic localization of a locus controlling the intensity of infection by *Schistosoma mansoni* on chromosome 5q31-q33. Nat Genet. 1996;14:181-184.

92. Cabrera M, Shaw M-A, Sharples C, et al. Polymorphism in tumor necrosis factor genes associated with mucocutaneous leishmaniasis. J Exp Med. 1995;182:1259-1264.

93. Karplus TM, Jeronimo SM, Chang H, et al. Association between the tumor necrosis factor locus and the clinical outcome of *Leishmania chagasi* infection. Infect Immun. 2002;70:6919-6925.

94. Blackwell JM, Black GF, Peacock CS, et al. Immunogenetics of leishmanial and mycobacterial infections: The Belem Family Study. Philos Trans R Soc Lond B Biol Sci. 1997;352:1331-1345.

95. Pier GB, Grout M, Zaidi T, et al. *Salmonella typhi* uses CFTR to enter intestinal epithelial cells. Nature. 1998;393:79-82.

96. Zeidler M, Stewart G, Cousens SN, et al. Codon 129 genotype and new variant CJD (Letter; Comment). Lancet. 1997;350:668.

97. Palmer MS, Dryden AJ, Hughes JT, Collinge J. Homozygous prion protein genotype predisposes to sporadic Creutzfeldt-Jakob disease [published erratum appears in Nature. 1991;352:547]. Nature. 1991;352:340-342.

98. Deslys J-P, Jaeglyy A, d'Aignaux JH, et al. Genotype at codon 129 and susceptibility to Creutzfeldt-Jacob disease. Lancet. 1998;351:1251.

99. Lee HS, Brown P, Cervenakova L, et al. Increased susceptibility to Kuru of carriers of the PRNP 129 methionine/methionine genotype. J Infect Dis. 2001;183:192-196.

100. Mead S, Stumpf MP, Whitfield J, et al. Balancing selection at the prion protein gene consistent with prehistoric kurulike epidemics. Science. 2003;300:640-643.

101. Levine MM, Nalin DR, Rennels MB, et al. Genetic susceptibility to cholera. Ann Hum Biol. 1979;6:369-374.

102. Glass RI, Holmgren J, Haley CE, et al. Predisposition for cholera of individuals with O blood group. Possible evolutionary significance. Am J Epidemiol. 1985;121:791-796.

103. Boren T, Falk P, Roth KA, et al. Attachment of *Helicobacter pylori* to human gastric epithelium mediated by blood group antigens. Science. 1993;262:1892-1895.

104. Umlauft F, Keeffe EB, Offner F, et al. *Helicobacter pylori* infection and blood group antigens: Lack of clinical association. Am J Gastroenterol. 1996;91:2135-2138.

105. Kelly RJ, Rouquier S, Giorgi D, et al. Sequence and expression of a candidate for the human Secretor blood group alpha(1,2)fucosyltransferase gene (FUT2). Homozygosity for an enzyme-inactivating nonsense mutation commonly correlates with the non-secretor phenotype. J Biol Chem. 1995;270:4640-4649.

106. Blackwell CC, Jonsdottir K, Hanson M, et al. Non-secretion of ABO antigens predisposing to infection by *Neisseria meningitidis* and *Streptococcus pneumoniae* (Letter). Lancet. 1986;2:284-285.

107. Raza MW, Blackwell CC, Molyneaux P, et al. Association between secretor status and respiratory viral illness. BMJ. 1991;303:815-818.

108. Sheinfeld J, Schaeffer AJ, Cordon-Cardo C, et al. Association of the Lewis blood-group phenotype with recurrent urinary tract infections in women. N Engl J Med. 1989;320:773-777.

109. Stapleton A, Nudelman E, Clausen H, et al. Binding of uropathogenic *Escherichia coli* R45 to glycolipids extracted from vaginal epithelial cells is dependent on histo-blood group secretor status. J Clin Invest. 1992;90:965-972.

110. Lindesmith L, Moe C, Marionneau S, et al. Human susceptibility and resistance to Norwalk virus infection. Nat Med. 2003;9:548-553.

111. Miller LH, Mason SJ, Clyde DF, McGinniss MH. The resistance factor to *Plasmodium vivax* in blacks. The Duffy blood-group genotype, FyFy. N Engl J Med. 1976;295:302-304.

112. Tournamille C, Colin Y, Cartron JP, Le Van Kim C. Disruption of a GATA motif in the Duffy gene promoter abolishes erythroid gene expression in Duffy-negative individuals. Nat Genet. 1995;10:224-228.

113. Haldane JBS. Disease and evolution. Ricercha Sci. 1949;19(suppl):68-76.

114. Motulsky AG, Stamatoyannopoulos G. Clinical implications of glucose-6-phosphate dehydrogenase deficiency. Ann Intern Med. 1966;65:1329-1334.

115. Vulliamy T, Beutler E, Luzzatto L. Variants of glucose-6-phosphate dehydrogenase are due to missense mutations spread throughout the coding region of the gene. Hum Mutat. 1993;2:159-167.

116. Roth EF Jr, Raventos-Suarez C, Rinaldi A, Nagel RL. Glucose-6-phosphate dehydrogenase deficiency inhibits in vitro growth of *Plasmodium falciparum*. Proc Natl Acad Sci U S A. 1983;80:298-299.

117. de Vries RR, Mehra NK, Vaidya MC, et al. HLA-linked control of susceptibility to tuberculoid leprosy and association with HLA-DR types. Tiss Antigens. 1980;16:294-304.

118. Khomenko AG, Litvinov VI, Chukanova VP, Pospelov LE. Tuberculosis in patients with various HLA phenotypes. Tubercle. 1990;71:1871-1892.

119. Hill AV, Elvin J, Willis AC, et al. Molecular analysis of the association of HLA-B53 and resistance to severe malaria. Nature. 1992;360:434-439.

120. Apple RJ, Erlich HA, Klitz W, et al. HLA DR-DQ associations with cervical carcinoma show papillomavirus-type specificity. Nat Genet. 1994;6:157-162.

121. Wank R, Thomssen C. High risk of squamous cell carcinoma of the cervix for women with HLA-DQw3. Nature. 1991;352:723-725.

122. Doherty PC, Zinkernagel RM. A biological role for the major histocompatibility antigens. Lancet. 1975;1:1406-1409.

123. Thursz MR, Kwiatkowski D, Torok ME, et al. Association of hepatitis B surface antigen carriage with severe malaria in Gambian children. Nat Med. 1995;1:374-375.

124. Jeffery KJ, Siddiqui AA, Bunce M, et al. The influence of HLA class I alleles and heterozygosity on the outcome of human T cell lymphotropic virus type I infection. J Immunol. 2000;165:7278-7284.

125. McGuire W, Hill AV, Allsopp CE, et al. Variation in the TNF-alpha promoter region associated with susceptibility to cerebral malaria. Nature. 1994;371:508-510.

126. Wilson AG, Symons JA, McDowell TL, et al. Effects of a polymorphism in the human tumor necrosis factor alpha promoter on transcriptional activation. Proc Natl Acad Sci U S A. 1997;94:3195-3199.

127. Knight JC, Udalova I, Hill AV, et al. A polymorphism that affects OCT-1 binding to the TNF promoter region is associated with severe malaria. Nat Genet. 1999;22:145-150.

128. Conway DJ, Holland MJ, Bailey RL, et al. Scarring trachoma is associated with polymorphism in the tumor necrosis factor alpha (TNF-alpha) gene promoter and with elevated TNF-alpha levels in tear fluid. Infect Immun. 1997;65:1003-1006.

129. Shin HD, Winkler C, Stephens JC, et al. Genetic restriction of HIV-1 pathogenesis to AIDS by promoter alleles of IL10. Proc Natl Acad Sci U S A. 2000; 97:14467-144672.

130. Rossouw M, Nel HJ, Cooke GS, et al. Association between tuberculosis and a polymorphic NFkappaB binding site in the interferon gamma gene. Lancet. 2003;361:1871-1872.

131. Liu R, Paxton WA, Choe S, et al. Homozygous defect in HIV-1 coreceptor accounts for resistance of some multiply-exposed individuals to HIV-1 infection. Cell. 1996;86:367-377.

132. Martinson JJ, Chapman NH, Rees DC, et al. Global distribution of the CCR5 gene 32-basepair deletion. Nat Genet. 1997;16:100-103.

133. Quillent C, Oberlin E, Braun J, et al. HIV-1-resistance phenotype conferred by combination of two separate inherited mutations of CCR5 gene. Lancet. 1998;351:14-18.

134. McDermott DH, Zimmerman PA, Guignard F, et al. CCR5 promoter polymorphism and HIV-1 disease progression. Multicenter AIDS Cohort Study (MACS). Lancet. 1998;352:866-870.

135. Martin MP, Dean M, Smith MW, et al. Genetic acceleration of AIDS progression by a promoter variant of CCR5. Science. 1998;282:1907-1911.

136. Ramaley PA, French N, Kaleebu P, et al. HIV in Africa (communication arising): Chemokine-receptor genes and AIDS risk. Nature. 2002;417:140.

137. Kawamura T, Gulden FO, Sugaya M, et al. R5 HIV productively infects Langerhans cells, and infection levels are regulated by compound CCR5 polymorphisms. Proc Natl Acad Sci U S A. 2003;100:8401-8406.

138. Salkowitz JR, Bruse SE, Meyerson H, et al. CCR5 promoter polymorphism determines macrophage CCR5 density and magnitude of HIV-1 propagation in vitro. Clin Immunol. 2003;108:234-240.

139. Libert F, Cochaux P, Beckman G, et al. The deltaccr5 mutation conferring protection against HIV-1 has a single and recent origin in Caucasian populations in Northeastern Europe. Hum Mol Genet. 1998;7:399-406.

140. Stephens JC, Reich DE, Goldstein DB, et al. Dating the origin of the CCR5-Delta32 AIDS-resistance allele by the coalescence of haplotypes. Am J Hum Genet. 1998;62:1507-1515.

141. Turner MW. Mannose-binding lectin: The pluripotent molecule of the innate immune system. Immunol Today. 1996;17:532-540.

142. Madsen HO, Garred P, Thiel S, et al. Interplay between promoter and structural gene variants control basal serum level of mannan-binding protein. J Immunol. 1995;155:3013-3020.

143. Koch A, Melbye M, Sorensen P, et al. Acute respiratory tract infections and mannose-binding lectin insufficiency during early childhood. JAMA. 2001;285:1316-1321.

144. Summerfield JA, Ryder S, Sumiya M, et al. Mannose binding protein gene mutations associated with unusual and severe infections in adults. Lancet. 1995;345:886-889.

145. Garred P, Michaelsen TE, Bjune G, et al. A low serum concentration of mannan-binding protein is not associated with serogroup B or C meningococcal disease. Scand J Immunol. 1993;37:468-470.

146. Bellamy R, Ruwende C, McAdam KP, et al. Mannose binding protein deficiency is not associated with malaria, hepatitis B carriage nor tuberculosis in Africans. Q J Med. 1998;91:13-18.

147. Kronborg G, Garred P. Mannose-binding lectin genotype as a risk factor for invasive pneumococcal infection. Lancet. 2002;360:1176.

148. Yang IA, Seeney SL, Wolter JM, et al. Mannose-binding lectin gene polymorphism predicts hospital admissions for COPD infections. Genes Immun. 2003;4:269-274.

149. Neth O, Hann I, Turner MW, Klein NJ. Deficiency of mannose-binding lectin and burden of infection in children with malignancy: A prospective study. Lancet. 2001;358:614-618.

150. Peterslund NA, Koch C, Jensenius JC, Thiel S. Association between deficiency of mannose-binding lectin and severe infections after chemotherapy. Lancet. 2001;358:637-638.

151. Ezekowitz AR. Mannose-binding lectin in prediction of susceptibility to infection. Lancet. 2001;358:598-599.

152. Babula O, Lazdane G, Kroica J, et al. Relation between recurrent vulvovaginal candidiasis, vaginal concentrations of mannose-binding lectin, and a mannose-binding lectin gene polymorphism in Latvian women. Clin Infect Dis. 2003;37:733-737.

153. Ryu S, Park YK, Bai GH, et al. 3′UTR polymorphisms in the NRAMP1 gene are associated with susceptibility to tuberculosis in Koreans. Int J Tuberc Lung Dis. 2000; 4:577-580.

154. Gao PS, Fujishima S, Mao XQ, et al. Genetic variants of NRAMP1 and active tuberculosis in Japanese populations. International Tuberculosis Genetics Team. Clin Genet. 2000;58:74-76.

155. Soborg C, Andersen AB, Madsen HO, et al. Natural resistance-associated macrophage protein 1 polymorphisms are associated with microscopy-positive tuberculosis. J Infect Dis. 2002;186:517-521.

156. Gruenheid S, Pinner E, Desjardins M, Gros P. Natural resistance to infection with intracellular pathogens: The Nramp1 protein is recruited to the membrane of the phagosome. J Exp Med. 1997;185:717-730.

157. Gunshin H, Mackenzie B, Berger UV, et al. Cloning and characterization of a mammalian proton-coupled metal-ion transporter. Nature. 1997;388:482-488.

158. Jabado N, Cuellar-Mata P, Grinstein S, Gros P. Iron chelators modulate the fusogenic properties of *Salmonella*-containing phagosomes. Proc Natl Acad Sci U S A. 2003; 100:6127-6132.

159. Jepson A, Banya W, Sisay-Joof F, et al. Quantification of the relative contribution of major histocompatibility complex (MHC) and non-MHC genes to human immune responses to foreign antigens. Infect Immun. 1997;65:872-876.

160. Tsoukas CD, Provvedini DM, Manolagas SC. 1,25-Dihydroxyvitamin D3: A novel immunoregulatory hormone. Science. 1984;224:1438-1440.

161. Bellamy R, Ruwende C, Corrah T, et al. Tuberculosis and chronic hepatitis B virus infection in Africans and variation in the vitamin D receptor gene. J Infect Dis. 1999;179:721-724.

162. Roy S, Frodsham A, Saha B, et al. Association of vitamin D receptor genotype with leprosy type. J Infect Dis. 1999;179:187-191.

163. Bellamy R. Evidence of gene-environment interaction in development of tuberculosis. Lancet. 2000; 355:588-589.

164. Agnese DM, Calvano JE, Hahm SJ, et al. Human toll-like receptor 4 mutations but not CD14 polymorphisms are associated with an increased risk of gram-negative infections. J Infect Dis. 2002;186:1522-1525.

165. Kiechl S, Lorenz E, Reindl M, et al. Toll-like receptor 4 polymorphisms and atherogenesis. N Engl J Med. 2002;347:185-192.

166. Smirnova I, Mann N, Dols A, et al. Assay of locus-specific genetic load implicates rare Toll-like receptor 4 mutations in meningococcal susceptibility. Proc Natl Acad Sci U S A. 2003;100:6075-6080.

167. Read RC, Pullin J, Gregory S, et al. A functional polymorphism of toll-like receptor 4 is not associated with likelihood or severity of meningococcal disease. J Infect Dis. 2001;184:640-642.

168. Kang TJ, Chae GT. Detection of Toll-like receptor 2 (TLR2) mutation in the lepromatous leprosy patients. FEMS Immunol Med Microbiol. 2001;31:53-58.

169. Goldfarb LG, Brown P, Haltia M, et al. Creutzfeldt-Jakob disease cosegregates with the codon 178Asn PRNP mutation in families of European origin. Ann Neurol. 1992;31:274-281.

170. Chen SG, Parchi P, Brown P, et al. Allelic origin of the abnormal prion protein isoform in familial prion diseases. Nat Med. 1997;3:1009-1015.
171. Brown P, Cervenakova L, Goldfarb LG, et al. Iatrogenic Creutzfeldt-Jakob disease: An example of the interplay between ancient genes and modern medicine. Neurology. 1994;44:291-293.
172. Thompson EA, Neel JV. Allelic disequilibrium and allele frequency distribution as a function of social and demographic history. Am J Hum Genet. 1997;60:197-204.
173. Bertranpetit J, Calafell F. Genetic and geographical variability in cystic fibrosis: Evolutionary considerations. Ciba Found Symp. 1996;197:97-114.
174. Gabriel SE, Brigman KN, Koller BH, et al. Cystic fibrosis heterozygote resistance to cholera toxin in the cystic fibrosis mouse model. Science. 1994;266:107-109.
175. Cuthbert AW, Halstead J, Ratcliff R, et al. The genetic advantage hypothesis in cystic fibrosis heterozygotes: A murine study. J Physiol (Lond). 1995;482:449-454.
176. McGuffin P, Huckle P. Simulation of Mendelism revisited: The recessive gene for attending medical school. Am J Hum Genet. 1990;46:994-999.
177. Murphy PM. Molecular mimicry and the generation of host defense protein diversity (Letter). Cell. 1993;72:823-826.
178. Vyse TJ, Todd JA. Genetic analysis of autoimmune disease. Cell. 1996;85:311-318.
179. McConkey SJ, Reece WH, Moorthy VS, et al. Enhanced T-cell immunogenicity of plasmid DNA vaccines boosted by recombinant modified vaccinia virus Ankara in humans. Nat Med. 2003;9:729-735.

CHAPTER **6**

Antibodies

HOLLY H. BIRDSALL

Those interested in infectious diseases will find the study of antibodies and the B cells that produce them to be useful for many reasons:

- Antibodies are the principal mode of defense against extracellular bacteria and exotoxins, and they can intercept viruses before they enter host cells. Understanding the kinetics of antibody production and the effector functions mediated by antibodies helps predict when and whether patients will recover from infections.
- Understanding the factors that initiate and perpetuate antibody production helps explain how vaccines protect against infectious agents and why some vaccines are less effective for pathogens whose surfaces are dominated by polysaccharide antigens.
- Defects in antibody production are by far the most common of the inherited immunodeficiencies. Moreover, these are also the only type of immunodeficiency that can be treated short of using bone marrow transplantation.
- Detection of a patient's antibody response to a pathogen is often the only means of diagnosing an infection. Knowing the type of antibody response that the patient is currently producing can help ascertain whether the infection is ongoing or resolved.
- Specific antibodies raised in animals are used as reagents to identify antigens, including infectious agents, in tissues. An appreciation of the available assays, their strengths, and their potential pitfalls helps ensure diagnostic accuracy
- Infections sometimes generate copious quantities of antigens that become incorporated into immune complexes with antibodies. Deposition of these immune complexes in blood vessel walls, renal glomeruli, or other vascularized beds causes inflammation that exacerbates the tissue injury caused by the infection.
- Production of autoreactive antibodies that lead to autoimmune disease is often precipitated by infections.

Antibodies are serum proteins that aid in the elimination of pathogens or antigens. Antibodies bind to pathogens and help effector cells recognize, entrap, and eliminate the invaders. Antibodies are produced by B lymphocytes, or B cells. As each B-cell clone matures, it rearranges and mutates its DNA in a manner slightly different from that of other clones. The result is millions of B-cell clones, each producing antibodies with a slightly different configuration at the antigen-binding site. The other end of the antibody molecule has a highly constant structure that allows it to interact with receptors on various cells. Phagocytic cells such as neutrophils and monocytes have receptors that enable them to ingest and kill antibody-coated pathogens. In some cases, antibodies offer protection simply by blocking the attachment of the virus, toxin, or bacterium to host cells. It was recognized in the late 1800s that animals immunized with bacterial toxins produced a circulating substance that could neutralize the toxin's activity. This substance was called an *antitoxin,* and the term was later generalized to *antibody.* In electrophoretic analyses of serum proteins, antibodies migrated in the third, or "gamma," globulin peak, which led to the name *immunoglobulin* (abbreviated Ig).

IMMUNOGLOBULIN STRUCTURE

Basic Antibody Structure

Antibodies look a bit like lobsters, with the two claws serving as antigen-binding clefts (Fig. 6-1). The tail of the lobster-antibody interacts with receptors on neutrophils, monocytes, macrophages, B lymphocytes, dendritic cells, and, in certain cases, mast cells. The carboxyterminal end of certain antibody molecules can also bind to specialized transport receptors that carry them across epithelial barriers into secretions or across the placenta into the fetus. At the insertion point of the claws into the lobster's body is a binding site for C1q, the first protein of the complement cascade, which helps to kill, and clear from the blood, pathogens and other antigens.

The basic antibody monomer is made up of two identical light chains and two identical heavy chains. Structurally, these polypeptide chains can be divided into loops or domains of about 110 amino acids bridged by disulfide bonds. This structural motif is characteristic of all members of the immunoglobulin superfamily, which includes various cell adhesion molecules (CAMs), CD4, CD8, CD28, and members of the B7 family of costimulatory molecules. Light chains have two domains and heavy chains have four or five domains. The domains at the amino ends of heavy and light chains have a highly variable amino acid sequence and are called V domains. The other domains have a relatively constant sequence and are called C domains. Each light chain is paired by disulfide bonds to a heavy chain so that their two V domains come together to form the antigen-binding site. The amino acid sequence variability within the V domains is actually focused in three hypervariable regions. When the protein sequence is folded into a three-dimensional reconstruction, one can see that these hypervariable regions come together to form the walls of the antigen-binding cleft. These stretches of protein sequence are also called complementarity-determining regions (CDRs).

The two heavy chains are linked to each other by disulfide bonds to form the Ig molecule's lobster tail. There are five classes of heavy chains, μ, γ, α, ϵ, and δ, which form the five antibody isotypes IgM, IgG, IgA, IgE, and IgD. Ig isotypes were originally defined by structural homologies and differences recognized by antibodies generated by immunizing phylogenetically distant animal species with human Ig. Allotypes are minor variations in a particular isotype that are found in some, but not all, humans. Allotypic differences were discovered using antibodies generated by immunizing humans (or nonhuman primates) with Ig from other humans. Idiotypes are variations between antibodies from a given donor that are otherwise of the same isotype and allotype. Idiotypic determinants tend to be located in or near the antigen-binding site and would be, for example, the differences between the IgG antibodies specific for measles and the IgG antibodies specific for mumps.

When antigen is first introduced into the host, the initial antibody response is of the IgM class. As the immune response progresses, some B cells begin to make IgG, IgA, or IgE by producing new heavy chains. The antigen-binding specificity is preserved by splicing the heavy chain V domain DNA onto the DNA encoding the C_H domains for the new isotype. Not all isotypes are able to interact with receptors

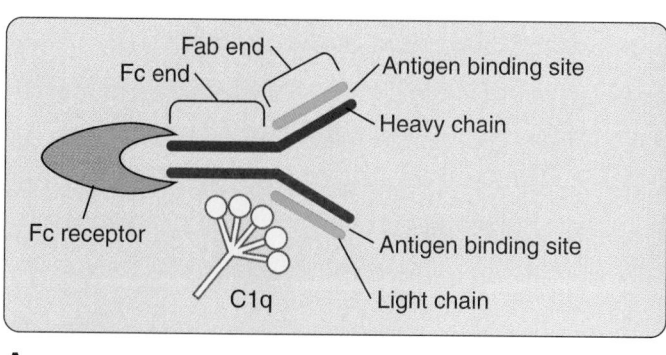
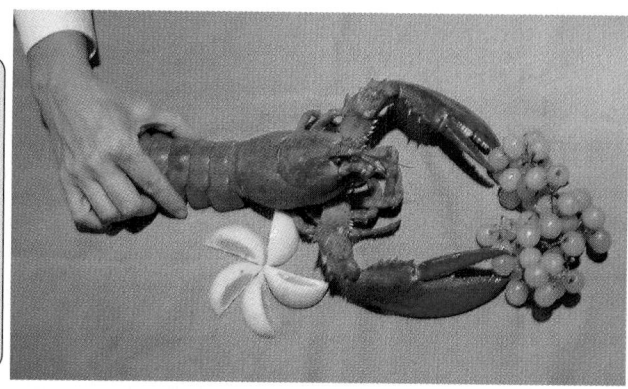

A   B

FIGURE 6-1. **Structure of antibodies.** Antibody molecules are composed of two heavy chains *(red lines)* and two light chains *(blue lines)* held together by disulfide bonds. The two heavy chains join to form a tail (Fc end), which can interact with receptors (FcR) on a variety of cells. The heavy and light chains each contribute to the Fab end. At the 5′ or amino terminal end, these chains form two identical antigen-binding sites, much like the two lobster claws. Near the hinge region of the antibody, there is a binding site for C1q, the first component of the complement cascade.

on immune effector cells or with transport receptors on epithelial cells. As a result, the heavy chain class determines which effector functions can be mediated by an antibody molecule and where it will be found in the body (Table 6-1).

There are only two classes of light chains, kappa (κ) and lambda (λ) and they appear in all five Ig classes. Overall, approximately 60% of antibody molecules use kappa chains and 40% use lambda chains. This information can be useful in the diagnosis of lymphomas. If virtually all of the B cells use the same light chain class (i.e., all κ or all λ), it is likely that they arose by clonal expansion from a single malignant precursor.

F(ab′)₂, Fab, and Fc Pieces

A commonly used nomenclature for antibodies is based on the way the Ig molecule is cleaved by proteases. The fragments are given the name "F" (for fragment) followed by "ab" (for antigen-binding), or "c" for crystallizable. To return to the lobster analogy, the Fab is the head and claws, the Fc is the tail (see Fig. 6-1). The structure of the tail among antibodies of a given isotype is so constant that the Fc fragments can be crystallized—hence the name. Cell receptors for the Fc piece of antibodies are called FcR. A Greek letter indicates their isotype specificity; for example, FcγR binds IgG.

Papain cleaves our imaginary antibody-lobster at approximately mid-thorax, resulting in an Fc tail piece and an F(ab′)₂ piece, with the head and two lobster claws still linked to each other (Fig. 6-2). Under reducing conditions, the disulfide linkage between the two heavy chains is broken, and the lobster-antibody is split in a sagittal direction to generate two Fab′ molecules (note the prime designation). In contrast, pepsin digests the tail into tiny fragments, leaving just the two Fab monomers—claws with no lobster head (see Fig. 6-2).

Proteolytic fragments can be helpful in analyzing how antibodies bind in vitro. For example, to test whether the Fc piece is important for a particular function, you can compare intact antibody with F(ab′)₂ fragments of the same antibody. When using antibodies to stain cells in immunohistochemical or immunofluorescent assays, F(ab′)₂ fragments may be preferable, because this avoids uptake of antibodies via FcR found on many types of cells and tissues. In yet other types of experiments, antibodies are used as surrogate ligands to interact with cell surface receptors. To test whether cross-linking of the cell surface receptor is required for signaling, for example, one can compare the effect of intact or F(ab′)₂ fragments of the antibody, which are dimeric, with Fab or Fab′ fragments, which are monomeric.

Antigen Binding, Affinity, and Avidity

Affinity refers to the strength of the interaction, or the goodness-of-fit between the antigen-binding site and the antigen. Electrostatic, hydrogen-binding, van der Walls, and hydrophobic interactions all contribute to the binding of antibody to antigen. Avidity measures the interaction of the intact antibody molecule with antigen and takes into consideration not only the affinity of the individual binding site but the fact that antibodies, depending on their isotype, have between two and 10 antigen-binding sites. Thus, IgM molecules with low-affinity binding sites can still have relatively high avidity for multivalent antigen, as it is unlikely that all 10 antigen-binding sites, once bound to antigen, will disengage simultaneously.

The portion of the antigen that fits into the antigen-binding cleft is called the *epitope*. The antigen-binding cleft can accommodate as many as six to 12 amino acids. Linear epitopes are composed of contiguous amino acids. Peptide vaccines generate antibodies to linear epitopes. Antibodies can also recognize conformational epitopes formed by amino acids that are brought into apposition with one another by protein folding. Conformational epitopes are not present on denatured antigens or peptides. However, denatured proteins may re-

TABLE 6-1	Characteristics of the Immunoglobulin Classes			
Isotype	*IgM*	*IgG*	*IgA*	*IgE*
Half-life in serum (days)	10	21	6	2
Normal serum level in adults (mg/mL)	0.6-3.5	6.4-13.5	0.7-3.1	.00004
Transported into secretions	±		+	
Crosses placenta to fetus		+		
Blocks binding of pathogens or toxins	+	+	+	
Opsonizes for phagocytosis via FcR		+		
Fixes complement via C1q	+	+		
Mediates ADCC		+		
Binds mast cells				+

ADCC, antibody-dependent cellular cytotoxicity.
Adapted from Stites DP, Stobo JD, Wells JV, eds. Basic and Clinical Immunology. 7th ed. Los Altos, Calif: Appleton & Lange; 1991, with permission.

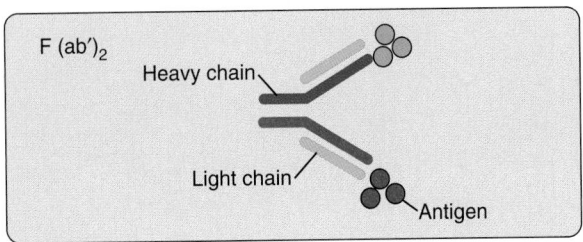
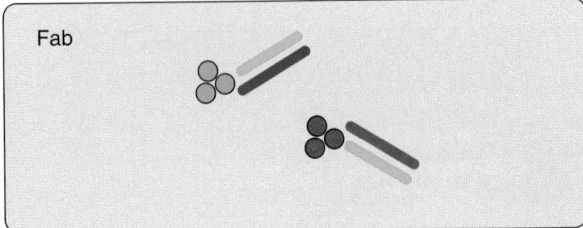

A

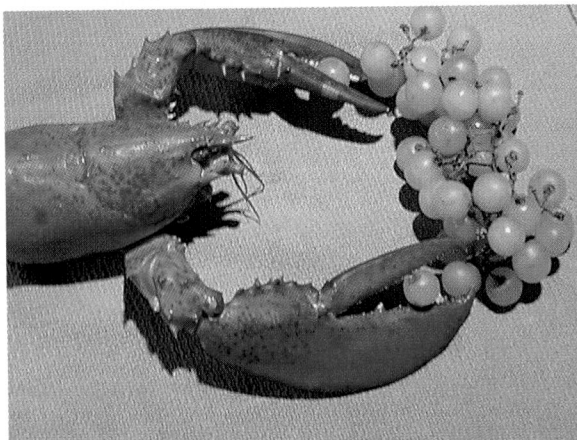
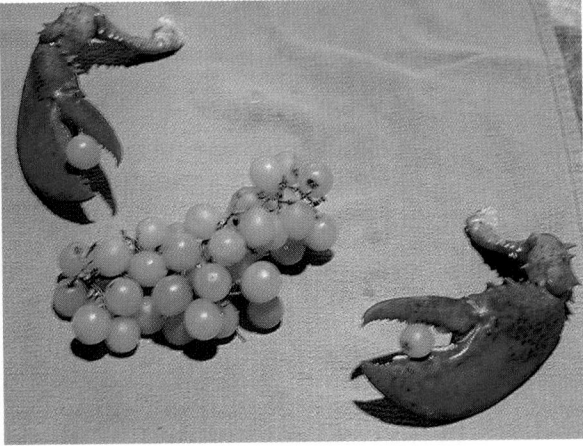

B

FIGURE 6-2.   Cleavage fragments of antibodies. A, Papain digests the immunoglobulin molecule into an F(ab′) fragment. This fragment is still dimeric, but it can no longer interact with FcR. Under reducing conditions, the disulfide bonds holding the two heavy chains together can be broken, leaving two monomeric Fab′ fragments (not shown). **B,** Pepsin digests away all of the Fc piece, leaving two monomeric Fab pieces.

veal novel epitopes that were not accessible on the intact protein. A large antigen may have many epitopes and can react with multiple antibody molecules at the same time.

Immunoglobulin Classes

The concentrations of the five isotypes in serum vary widely, reflecting both different numbers of B cells producing each isotype and different intrinsic half-lives of the Ig classes. The isotype of an antibody dictates where in the body it is likely to be found and what types of effector functions it can mediate (see Table 6-1).

IgM

IgM has the largest molecular weight (900 kilodaltons) of all of the isotypes, which keeps it primarily within the intravascular compartment. It is composed of five immunoglobulin monomers whose μ chains are either covalently linked through disulfide bridges or held noncovalently by a joining, or J, piece. The J piece is produced by the B cell, and it can also hold IgA molecules in multimers. IgM molecules have a total of 10 antigen-binding sites but steric hindrance typically allows only five of the 10 antigen-binding sites to engage antigen simultaneously. Still, this multivalent potential helps to overcome the low affinity for antigen that is characteristic of IgM antibodies. IgM antibodies defend the host by blocking pathogen binding to cells and by aggregating infectious agents, which facilitates their clearance. IgM antibodies are also able to fix (or activate) complement more efficiently than any other isotype. Monomeric IgM is displayed on the surface of B cells. This membrane IgM, or mIgM, allows the B cell to detect when it encounters cognate antigen.

IgG

IgG is by far the most plentiful isotype in the serum because of its high production rate (25 mg/kg/day) and its half-life of 23 days, which is four to 10 times longer than that of the other isotypes. IgG's smaller size allows it to move into tissues, and at any one time, less than 50% of the body burden of IgG is in the circulation. IgG is the only isotype that is carried across the human placenta to the fetus. Beginning at 20 or 21 weeks of gestation,[1] maternal IgG crosses into the fetal circulation by means of a special placental transport receptor, FcRn.[2]

There are four subclasses of the γ heavy chain, IgG$_1$, IgG$_2$, IgG$_3$, and IgG$_4$, and they vary in amino acid composition and degree of glycosylation. IgG$_1$ and IgG$_3$ can fix complement but IgG$_2$ and IgG$_4$ do not. IgG antibodies to proteins tend to be of the IgG$_1$ and IgG$_3$ subclass. Responses to polysaccharides tend to be of the IgG$_2$ subclass,[3] and individuals deficient in IgG$_2$ may show an increased susceptibility to infections with encapsulated organisms.[4] Responses to helminths tend to be of the IgG$_4$ class,[5] but there is no evidence that individuals deficient in IgG$_4$ have a higher susceptibility to these organisms.[3]

IgA

Each day, humans produce about 66 mg of IgA per kilogram of body weight, which is about twice the quantity of IgG produced.[6] However, serum levels of IgA are relatively low because most of the IgA is produced by submucosal plasma cells and immediately transported into secretions. There are two heavy chain subclasses of IgA: IgA$_1$ and IgA$_2$. IgA$_1$ is monomeric and is primarily found in the serum. IgA$_2$ can polymerize into multimers linked by the J piece. IgA$_2$ is transported into the secretions by the cooperative effort of epithelial cells and lymphocytes. Dimeric IgA, produced by submucosal B cells, binds to an epithelial cell membrane protein called secretory component (SC). The IgA is endocytosed and carried through the cytoplasm of the epithelial cells. On the apical side, the SC is cleaved, releasing the IgA into mucosal secretions. A fragment of the SC remains associated with the secretory IgA and protects it from cleavage by proteases in the secretions. IgM can also be carried across epithelium using this process.[7] Some pathogens express ligands that allow them to co-opt this transport system and use it to cross in the reverse direction into the subepithelium.[8] IgA-coated Epstein-Barr virus may gain entry into nasopharyngeal cells by this route.[9]

IgA defends mucosal surfaces against invading pathogens. It cross links pathogens and facilitates their clearance by ciliated epithelium. IgA can block the binding of bacteria, viruses, or toxins to receptors on host mucosal cells. One important role of IgA is to bind food antigens in the intestinal tract and prevent triggering of proinflammatory responses. The relative inability of IgA to initiate inflammatory responses allows food antigens to be sequestered without deleterious consequences.[10] Failure of this process may account for the increased frequency of allergic diseases in IgA-deficient individuals.[11]

IgD

IgD is produced by B cells during some of the early stages of differentiation and is expressed on the cell membrane. Very little is found in the serum. IgD has a role in B-cell signaling but no other apparent effector role in host defense.

IgE

Very little IgE is present in the serum. Mast cells have very high affinity FcεR that scavenges IgE so quickly that its serum half-life is only about 2 days. Once bound to mast cells, IgE persists for a long time, perhaps for the life span of the mast cell. Infused IgE can be detected on murine mast cells up to 7 weeks later.[12] IgE displayed on the mast cell surfaces mediates immediate hypersensitivity or allergic reactions. IgE appears to have a role in defense against parasitic infections. Mast cells are needed to clear intestinal helminthic infections[13] and, when infected, IgE-deficient mice have higher burdens of *Schistosoma mansoni*.[14]

EFFECTOR FUNCTIONS MEDIATED BY ANTIBODIES

Antibodies have no direct microbicidal function but can serve as "transducers" to tag the pathogen and become a physical link between the pathogen and the killing mechanism, typically a leukocyte.

Blocking or Neutralization

Attachment to host cells is a critical step in many infectious processes. Viruses and exotoxins must bind to specific receptors before entering the cell. Bacteria need to adhere to cell surfaces, particularly in locations where the flux of secretions, intestinal contents, or urine tends to dislodge them. Antibodies neutralize or block microbes by binding up or occluding the attachment machinery that allows them to bind to host cells. If they react with the right epitope, antibodies can prevent the binding of viruses,[15] toxins,[16] or bacteria.[17] As an example, antibodies to bacterial endotoxins reduce lethality in animal models[18] and ameliorate gram-negative bacteremia in humans.[19] The challenge for vaccine developers is to identify the epitopes that are integral to the pathogenic process and devise vaccines that generate antibodies that interfere with those critical molecular interactions. Generation of protective immunity may be extremely difficult if, for instance, the key epitope is deep within a cleft in the native protein and is inaccessible to antibodies. Steric hindrance is not the only way that neutralizing antibodies prevent infection. For example, picornavirus has multiple binding sites, but infection can be blocked by a single antibody. This suggests that Ig binding may affect charge characteristics or conformation[20] in the pathogen. Ascertaining that an antibody has "blocking" or "neutralizing" activity must be determined biologically. Antibodies that bind to the pathogen without neutralizing or blocking infection may paradoxically facilitate infection by allowing the pathogen to be taken into the cytoplasm through FcR or other receptors.[21]

Blocking viral and bacterial adherence to mucous membranes is probably the major defensive role of IgA in secretions. Viruses can also be neutralized by IgA within the cytoplasm of epithelial cells in the course of transepithelial transport.[22] Blocking can be accomplished with antibodies of any isotype and even with antibodies from other species. This accounts for the efficacy of equine antitoxin in the early treatment of diseases such as tetanus.[23] Unfortunately, nonhuman Ig is perceived as foreign by the immune system and triggers an antibody response. The complexes of horse Ig and human antibodies to horse Ig caused serum sickness, a condition with considerable morbidity and some mortality.[17] Antisera produced in other animals are rarely used today except in cases such as snake antivenom, where it is not feasible to generate human hyperimmune sera.

Complement Activation

Complement is a series of serum proteins that augment or "complement" the effect of antibodies. Complement proteins attract phagocytic cells and provide "handholds" on the pathogens to facilitate their uptake by the phagocytes. Complement can also lyse pathogens directly by forming pores in the cell wall that permit free flow of water and electrolytes. Many of the complement proteins are proteases that activate the next member in the sequence by cleaving it. Small fragments such as C3a and C5a diffuse away and act as chemoattractants for phagocytes. Larger fragments, such as C3b, remain adherent to the surface of the pathogen and become ligands for receptors on phagocytic cells. The initiation of the cascade and deposition of complement proteins on the surface of a pathogen is greatly accelerated when antibodies participate. Antibodies in this role are said to activate or "fix" complement via the classical pathway. There is an alternative pathway of complement activation in which small amounts of C3 are cleaved spontaneously by hydrolysis and the C3b binds to the surface of the pathogen. This pathway is less efficient than the classical pathway.

IgG and IgM have a site that can bind and activate C1q, the first protein in the cascade. IgG$_4$, IgA, and IgE have no C1q binding sites and do not activate complement by this pathway. For C1q to be activated, at least two of its five arms must interact with Ig. As a pentamer, IgM has five C1q binding sites, so one bound IgM molecule can activate complement by itself. For IgG to activate complement, at least two IgG molecules must bind the pathogen and be sufficiently close together that C1q can interact with both antibodies. Because the C1q binding site is not accessible until the antibody binds to antigen, complement is not activated by soluble Ig in the circulation. Once IgG binds to antigen, a conformational change increases the affinity of its C1q binding site by 10,000-fold.[24] When C1q is engaged by antibodies, it undergoes a conformational change of its own and activates the next member of the cascade. Eventually, C1r, C1s, C4, C2, C3, C5, C6, C7, C8, and C9 are activated. C5, C6, C7, and C8 bind to the surface of the pathogen and form an anchor site for C9. Several C9 molecules polymerize into a tubular structure called the membrane attack complex, which penetrates the wall and lyses the pathogen. Although dramatic to visualize, direct lysis of pathogens by complement seems to have a minor role in host defense. Patients deficient in the terminal components of the complement cascade have few clinical problems besides an increased susceptibility to *Neisseria* infections. The major defensive role of complement is its ability to facilitate the uptake of antigens by phagocytes by a process called opsonization.

Opsonization

Neutrophils, monocytes, and macrophages are collectively referred to as phagocytes on the basis of their ability to ingest antigens. Phagocytes pull pathogens into phagosomes, where the organisms are inundated with toxic agents such as reactive oxygen species, nitric oxide, and enzymes. Phagocytes recognize pathogens using their pattern recognition receptors (PRRs) that recognize endogenous pathogen-associated molecular patterns (PAMPs) on the microbe. However, other ligands can bind to the surface of the pathogen and facilitate phagocytosis. The facilitation is called opsonization, and the ligands, in this role, are called opsonins. Both IgG and C3b can serve as opsonins. FcγR allows phagocytes to bind to IgG-coated targets. This allows phagocytes to recognize infectious agents that may not express any PAMPs. Signaling through the FcγR triggers an oxidative burst that increases the ability of the phagocyte to kill the organism it has just ingested. Complement C3b has a highly reactive thioester bond that al-

TABLE 6-2　Characteristics of Fc Receptors

Receptor	FcγRI	FcγRIIA and B	FcγRIII	FcαRI	FcεRI and RII
CD name	CD64	CD32	CD64	CD89	FcεRII=CD23
Effector function	Phagocytosis	Inhibition	ADCC	Pulmonary phagocytes	Degranulation
			Phagocytosis		
Cell type	Monocytes	B cells	Natural killer cells	Macrophages	Mast cells
	Macrophages	Monocytes	Neutrophils	Neutrophils	Basophils
	Neutrophils	Macrophages	Macrophages	Eosinophils	
		Neutrophils	Eosinophils		
		Eosinophils	Mast cells		
		Platelets			

ADCC, antibody-dependent cellular cytotoxicity.

lows it to bind to substances such as microbes. Accumulation of C3b on the surface of pathogens is greatly accelerated when antibodies bind first, fix C1q, and activate the complement cascade through the classical pathway. As part of the classical pathway, an enzyme is generated that rapidly cleaves C3 to produce large quantities of the reactive C3b fragment. Phagocytes can attach to C3b-coated targets by means of their C3bR. However, to complete the phagocytic process, the leukocyte needs to receive a second stimulus. This can come from the interaction of its FcR with the Fc of IgG bound to the pathogen, or it can come from C5a fragments generated by activated complement. IgM cannot opsonize through an FcR, but a single molecule of IgM is highly effective at fixing complement via C1q, which leads to the deposition of many C3b molecules and the generation of C5a fragments. IgA does not activate complement by the classical C1q pathway. However, IgA can provide a site for deposition of C3b and thereby activate complement through the alternate pathway.[25]

There are four types of receptors for IgG: FcγRI (CD64), FcγRII (CD32), and FcγRIII (CD16) (Table 6-2). Of the three, FcγRI (CD64) has the highest affinity for IgG, and it is the only one that binds monomeric IgG. FcγRI is constitutively expressed on monocytes and macrophages and can be induced on neutrophils. FcγRII and FcγRIII have low intrinsic affinity for monomeric IgG but will bind IgG in immune complexes because the altered conformation of the IgG increases the binding affinity and because the additive effect of many FcRs binding to many IgGs increases the overall avidity of the interaction. Signaling through FcγRIII on natural killer (NK) cells and monocytes triggers antibody-dependent cellular cytotoxicity (ADCC) and production of interferon-γ.[26] IgG$_1$ and IgG$_3$ can interact effectively with FcγRs, but IgG$_2$ and IgG$_4$ do not.

There is an FcR for IgA (CD89) on monocytes, neutrophils, macrophages, and perhaps eosinophils, particularly those in the lungs.[27] There is no FcR for IgM, and antibodies of these classes cannot serve as direct opsonins for phagocytosis. As discussed later, FcγRII is also present on B cells, where it has a negative signaling role that appears to downregulate production when excess quantities of antibody lead to formation of immune complexes.[28]

Antibody-Dependent Cellular Cytotoxicity

ADCC is carried out by monocyte/macrophages, NK cells, and neutrophils. ADCC allows these effector cells to kill targets that are too large to be ingested. Perforins, granzymes, and in some cases reactive oxygen intermediates are involved in this microbicidal activity.[29,30] The role of the IgG antibody in ADCC is to bind to the FcγRIII or FcγRII on the NK cell or monocyte and identify the target cell for killing.

KINETICS OF ANTIBODY PRODUCTION AND DIAGNOSIS OF INFECTIONS

First encounters with an antigen, such as a vaccine, induce a primary antibody response (Fig. 6-3). The primary response can usually be detected about 5 to 7 days after antigen exposure. It is primarily made up of IgM antibodies with a relatively low affinity for antigen. Within several days to weeks, some antibody-producing B cells switch to making antibodies of the same antigen specificity but of an IgG, IgA, or IgE isotype. To switch isotypes, B cells must receive signals from activated T cells. Usually the T cells are activated by the same antigenic stimulus that activated the B cells to produce antibody. However, unrelated agents may also provide the stimuli needed to activate the T cells. T-cell signals also induce the B lymphocytes to generate memory cells. When a second dose of vaccine is administered, several weeks after the first encounter, these memory B cells rapidly divide and begin to produce large quantities of antibody within as little as 1 to 2 days. This is the hallmark of a secondary antibody response. Secondary responses not only occur more rapidly but they generate greater quantities of antibodies and the antibodies are mostly of the IgG isotype, as opposed to IgM. As the B cells divide, they introduce point mutations into the gene sequences encoding the antigen-binding site. Because B-cell survival is dependent on continued antigen stimulation, B cells with mutations that increase the affinity of the antigen-binding site have a competitive advantage at capturing antigen and receiving stimuli that cause them to differentiate and divide. The net effect is to produce IgG antibodies with a higher affinity for the immunizing antigen. The average affinity of antibodies produced in a secondary response is often orders of magnitude higher than that produced during a primary response. As more and more antigen is incorporated in antigen–antibody complexes and metabolized, competition among B cells for antigen stimulation increases. As the antigen stimulus becomes more scarce, this and other regulatory influences act to slow the production of antibody. Only a low level of residual production of IgG persists in response to antigen associated with follicular dendritic cells. However, quiescent memory cells are formed, and these lie in wait for the next challenge with this same antigen. Should antigen reappear, these memory cells can rapidly activate, proliferate, and begin producing antibodies.

When the interval of antigen exposure is well defined, as with vaccines, it is easy to distinguish between the primary and secondary responses. However, with an infection, antigen is released over a prolonged interval and there is no clear border between primary and secondary responses. So long as new clones of B cells are encountering antigen, IgM will be produced. Thus, the presence of IgM antibodies can be taken as indication of an active infection. By contrast, a response that is solely of the IgG isotype is generally considered to be indicative of a resolved infection. During the first few weeks of an infection, responsive B cells proliferate and produce ever-increasing quantities of antibody. Thus, a rising titer of specific antibodies also suggests an active infection. This is typically measured by obtaining a serum sample at presentation (the acute serum) and a second sample one or more weeks later (the convalescent sample). For maximum accuracy, the acute serum should be stored in a freezer and then sent to the laboratory at the same time as the convalescent sample, so that the two samples are assayed at the same time with identical reagents.

LABORATORY MEASUREMENT OF ANTIBODIES

Quantification of Total Immunoglobulin

The amounts of IgG, IgM, and IgA in the serum are readily measurable by most clinical laboratories. In some cases, it may be appropriate to measure individual IgG subclasses as well. Patients missing IgG$_2$, IgG$_3$, or IgG$_4$ may still have normal total IgG levels. As two thirds of IgG is of the IgG$_1$ subclass, a deficiency in this subclass

FIGURE 6-3. **Primary and secondary immune responses.** A first exposure to antigen stimulates production of IgM antibodies *(blue line)*, which become detectable within about a week. The antigen-specific B cells proliferate and some become memory cells. On subsequent exposure to the same antigen, these memory cells are rapidly activated. Antibodies, mainly of the IgG class *(red line)*, appear within about 2 days, and the quantity of antibody produced is much higher than is seen with the primary response. The affinity of the antibodies in the secondary response is also markedly higher than that seen in the primary response.

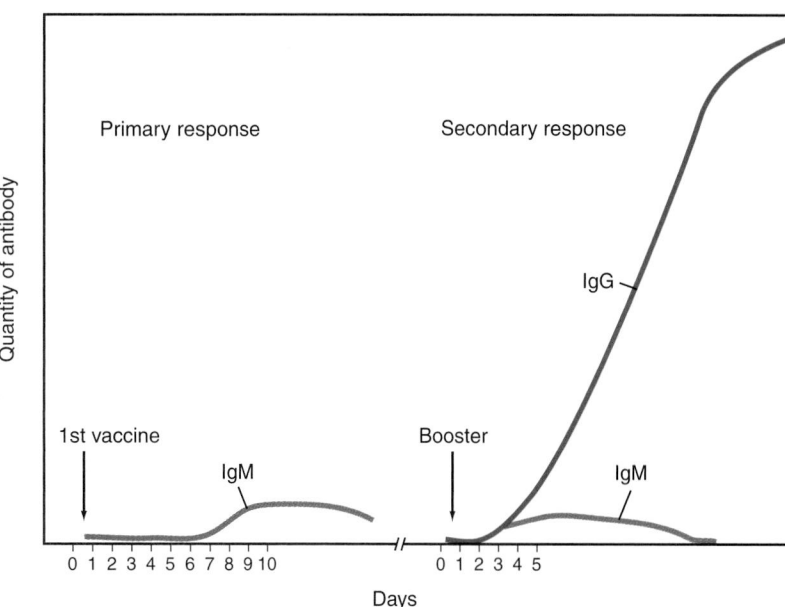

would be apparent when measuring total IgG levels. The most common immunodeficiency is an absence of IgA, often in conjunction with one or more subclasses of IgG. A deficiency of the secretory piece has been described in patients with IgA in their serum but not in their secretions. However, this is a very rare defect and most IgA-deficient patients can be identified by measuring levels of IgA in serum. Measurement of total IgE is not diagnostic of atopy, because serum levels may be normal or only mildly elevated in patients with clinically significant atopic disease (e.g., asthma, allergic rhinitis, urticaria). However, serum IgE may be strikingly elevated in parasitic infections. In evaluating Ig levels in children, the clinician must take great care to use age-specific reference tables, because the normal level varies greatly with age.

Serum Protein Electrophoresis for Monoclonal Gammopathies

Antibody responses are typically polyclonal, meaning that many different types of antibodies are produced that recognize many different epitopes and have many different antigen-binding clefts. In multiple myeloma, or other monoclonal gammopathies, a single B-cell clone proliferates in an unrestricted manner and produces large quantities of a single antibody type. This homogeneous product is referred to as a monoclonal antibody, or M protein. Light chains from this clone may appear in the urine as Bence Jones proteins. On protein electrophoresis, a polyclonal response produces a broad gamma globulin peak because of the variation in electrophoretic mobility, whereas a monoclonal antibody appears as a spike with a single electrophoretic mobility.[31]

Measurement of Functional Antibody

Many times, the only way to diagnose an infection is to demonstrate that the patient is mounting a specific humoral response to the suspected agent. One hallmark of an active infection is the production of increasing quantities of specific antibody. Therefore a good diagnostic test needs to be both specific and quantitative. A second hallmark of an active infection is the presence of IgM antibodies, so a good diagnostic test should be able to identify the isotype of the patient's antibodies.

Today, the most commonly used format is a solid-phase immunosorbent assay. Antigen is immobilized on a plastic surface such as a microtiter plate or beads (Fig. 6-4). The patient's serum is added and allowed to interact with the antigen. Nonspecific, unbound antibody is washed away, and a detection reagent is added to measure the

quantity of patient antibody bound to the antigen. This detection reagent is an antibody to human Ig (anti–human Ig) that has been prepared by immunizing a sheep, rabbit, goat, or other animal. The greater the quantity of patient antibodies adherent to the antigen, the more anti–human Ig there is that binds. The anti–human Ig is typically purified and conjugated with a reagent to facilitate detection. In an enzyme-linked immunosorbent assay (ELISA), the anti-Ig is conjugated with an enzyme, such as a peroxidase or a phosphatase, that converts a substrate to a colored or luminescent product that can be quantified. In a radioimmunoassay (RIA), the anti–human Ig is labeled with a radioisotope, and in a fluorescence-linked immunosorbent assay (FLISA), the anti-Ig is conjugated with a fluorochrome. Class-specific anti-Ig reagents can be prepared by immunizing the animal with a single isotype of human Ig and removing antibodies that cross react with epitopes such as light chain antigens that would be present on other isotypes. Using these, it is possible to determine whether the patient's antibodies are IgM, IgG, IgA, or IgE.

In addition to being isotype specific, solid-phase immunosorbent assays can be made quite sensitive and quantitative. The technology is easily adaptable to processing large numbers of samples in a semi-automated manner. The principal drawback of an immunosorbent assay is false-positive results. There are two possible causes. The only human Ig that is supposed to bind to the antigen-coated plastic is the patient's antigen-specific antibody. However, a patient's Ig molecules can also bind nonspecifically to the plastic well and will be detected by the anti–human Ig. This background binding becomes a particular problem when a patient has abnormally high levels of serum Ig, as may occur in certain chronic infections such as malaria. It is important to run a background determination in which patient serum is added to wells without antigen to measure the nonspecific uptake of Ig. The second cause of false positives involves the nature of the immobilized antigen. In many assays, the antigen is a relatively crude homogenate of the pathogen and contains a complex mixture of biologic products. It is possible that the patient has antibodies that just happen to cross react with an epitope present in the mixture. For this reason, positive results in solid-phase immunosorbent assays such as the human immunodeficiency virus (HIV) ELISA must be verified using more antigen-specific techniques, such as the Western blot.

Western Blot

The Western blot is a way to identify which antigen, within a complex mixture, is recognized by the patient's antibody. The antigen mixture is first separated by molecular size using polyacrylamide gel electrophoresis. The antigens are then transferred, or blotted, onto nitro-cellulose paper. Patient serum is incubated with the paper strip, unbound antibodies are washed away, and bound antibodies are detected with radiolabeled or enzyme-conjugated anti–human Ig. Class-specific anti–human Ig can be used to determine the isotype of the reactive antibodies. Because the antigens are distributed by molecular weight along the strip, one can identify the size, and thus the likely identity, of the antigen recognized by the antibody.

The Western blot is useful in situations where it is suspected that the patient may have cross-reactive antibodies. These are antibodies that just happen to react with something in the antigen mixture, even though the patient has never been exposed to that pathogen. If a patient's antibodies react with only one antigen from a given pathogen, this could be attributed to chance cross-reactivity. However, if the patient has antibodies to multiple antigens from that pathogen, then it is more likely that the infection is due to that pathogen and the patient has mounted a polyclonal antibody response. This is the basis for the interpretation of the Western blot assay for antibodies to HIV. If the patient reacts with a single HIV-associated antigen, this could be just chance cross-reactivity. However, if the patient has antibodies that react with two or more HIV antigens, then the interpretation is that the patient is infected with and is responding to HIV.

Agglutination and Complement Fixation

Some older assay formats that take advantage of the biologic activities of antibodies are still used. For example, agglutination is used to measure antibodies to *Treponema pallidum* in the microhemagglutination (MHA-TP) assay. Agglutination depends on the presence of patient antibodies, which cross link antigen-coated particles. Small antigens can be coated onto the surface of particles such as latex beads or erythrocytes, and then agglutination is apparent on visual inspection. Human IgM antibodies can bind to antigens on two particles, but IgG may be too small to bridge the distance. Therefore anti–human IgG is often added as a "developing reagent" to assist in agglutination.

Agglutination techniques cannot be used to accurately identify the isotype of the patient antibody. However, they are otherwise a useful technique because they can be read within minutes and require only minimal laboratory resources. Results are typically reported as the antibody titer, which is the maximum extent to which a sample can be diluted and still give a positive result. For example, a titer of 1:160 means that one part serum can be mixed with 159 parts of buffer and still produce a positive reaction. Sera are typically tested in serial twofold dilutions, and titer differences between samples are not considered to be statistically different until there is a fourfold or greater difference in the titers of the two samples.

In complement-mediated lysis, red cells are artificially coated with the desired antigen and then mixed with patient serum (as a source of antibodies) and with fresh guinea pig serum (as a source of complement). If the patient serum contains antibodies to the antigen on the red cells, complement will be activated and the red cells will be lysed. The advantage of this assay is the ease of reading the results, which are macroscopically visible. The limitations of this assay involve the difficulty in getting a source of biologically active complement that behaves consistently. Antigen-coated erythrocytes are also unstable and cannot be stored for long periods. As would be predicted from the abilities of different Ig isotypes to activate complement, this format is excellent for measuring IgM, moderately effective for measuring IgG, and not useful for measuring IgA antibodies.

Immunofluorescence and Immunohistochemistry

Immunofluorescence and immunohistochemistry can also be used to measure patient antibodies. The only difference is that the antigen is present in a histologic tissue section or immobilized on a slide. Examples of antigens that might be used are treponemes to look for antibodies to *T. pallidum*. Virus-infected cells can be prepared in the laboratory as a target for virus-specific antibodies. Patient serum is incubated with the slide, unbound antibodies are washed away, and reactive antibodies are detected using a conjugated antibody to human Ig just as in the solid-phase immunosorbent assay. Antibodies conjugated with a fluorochrome are visualized with a fluorescent microscope. Immunohistochemistry uses antibodies conjugated with an enzyme. When exposed to a substrate, the enzyme generates a colored or fluorescent precipitate that deposits in the immediate microenviron-

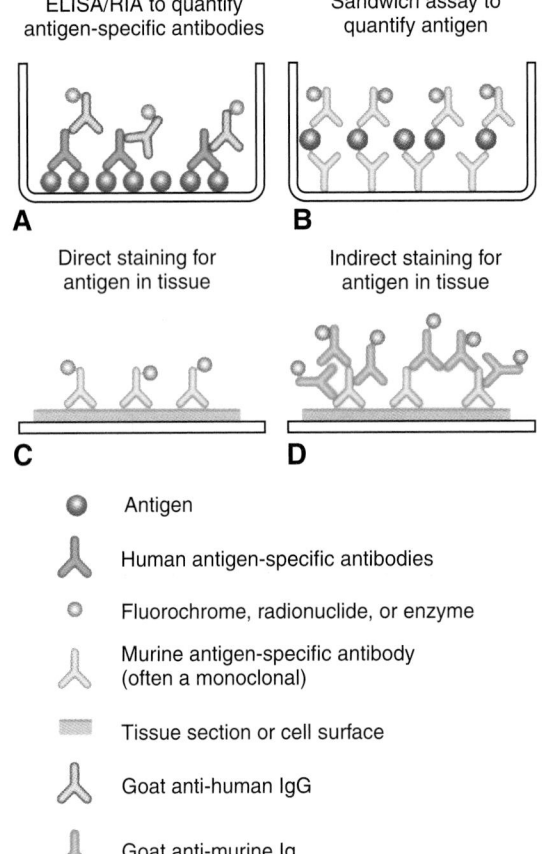

FIGURE 6-4. Structure of antibodies. A, In a solid-phase assay for antigen-specific antibodies, antigen is coated on a surface, typically a plastic well. The patient sample (e.g., serum) is incubated with the antigen, after which unbound antibodies are washed away. Patient antibodies bound to the antigen are detected with an antibody to human Ig produced by immunizing another species (in this case, a goat). The goat anti–human Ig is conjugated with a moiety that allows it to be detected. This could be a radionuclide, a fluorochrome, or an enzyme that converts an added substrate to a colored or luminescent product. **B,** A sandwich format can be used to measure antigen. A capture antibody is immobilized in the plastic well. The source of antigen is added, and then a second antigen-specific antibody is added to detect the bound antigen. This detection antibody is conjugated with a radionuclide, fluorochrome, or enzyme, just as in the previous assay. The two antibody layers in the sandwich assay must recognize different epitopes on the antigen, or the first antibody will occupy all the epitopes and there will be none left for the second antibody to bind. **C,** Direct staining for antigens in tissue or cells uses antigen-specific antibodies (often monoclonal antibodies) that have been purified and conjugated with a detection molecule such as a radionuclide, a fluorochrome, or an enzyme. **D,** Indirect staining for antigens in tissues or cells uses an unconjugated antigen-specific antibody as the first reagent. This antibody is detected with the use of a second antibody (directed against the first antibody) that has been conjugated with a radionuclide, a fluorochrome, or an enzyme. The indirect technique often gives a higher signal than the direct technique, because multiple secondary antibodies (goat anti–mouse Ig in this case) can bind to one primary antibody (mouse monoclonal in this case). However, the background staining for the indirect technique is also considerably higher than is seen with a primary or direct technique.

ment of the conjugated antibody. By using an anti–human Ig selective for a particular Ig class, it is easy to identify the isotype of the patient's antigen-specific antibodies.

Interpretation of immunohistochemistry and immunofluorescence is subjective, or at best semi-quantitative, with results perhaps assignable to a 0 to 4+ scale. It is not possible to determine the exact quantities of antibodies present, although an experienced laboratory may be able to estimate the relative quantity by determining the titer (or extent to which serum can be diluted and still give a positive test). As mentioned before, two samples should not be considered to be statistically different until their titers differ by at least fourfold. It is important to include the appropriate controls. At a minimum, a negative control should be run using the conjugated anti–human Ig alone to evaluate whether it becomes bound to the tissue. It may also be appropriate to run a negative control using human serum in place of the patient's serum to evaluate nonspecific uptake of human Ig. Many cells have Fc receptors, and it is important to verify that neither the patient antibodies nor the anti–human Ig binds to the target cells via their Fc piece. To minimize background signal, it may help to use F(ab′)₂ fragments of the anti–human Ig, and/or to use antibodies produced in goats or sheep as these have a lower affinity for human FcR.

Using Assays to Measure Antigen

Solid-phase immunosorbent assays and immunofluorescence or immunohistochemistry assays can also be used to measure antigens using antibodies prepared by immunizing animals. Monoclonal antibodies are ideal reagents for these assays because these are a reproducible source of antibodies with a well-characterized specificity. The main caveat is that antigen is measured on the basis of its ability to interact with specific antibodies, not by its biologic activity. Unless the antibody measures a conformational epitope, it is very likely that the assay will detect both active and inactive or denatured antigens. Antibodies may also still bind despite the presence of inhibitors that block biologic activity of the antigen in vivo. For example, some cytokines have soluble inhibitors that block their biologic activity. An immunosorbent assay might indicate that a particular serum contained large quantities of cytokine, when, in fact, the presence of inhibitor meant that there was very little cytokine *activity* present.

Solid-phase immunosorbent assays typically use a sandwich format in which a purified antibody to antigen is immobilized on a surface such as a plastic well (see Fig. 6-4). This capture antibody is the bottom layer of the sandwich assay. The patient sample containing antigen is added and allowed to react with the immobilized antibody. Finally, more antigen-specific antibody is added as the top of the sandwich. This second detection antibody is conjugated with a radiolabel, enzyme, or fluorochrome. The more antigen that is captured by the first antibody, the more detection antibody there is that can be captured by the antigen. When using monoclonal antibodies, the capture and detection antibodies must be different clones that recognize different epitopes on the antigen. Otherwise, the capture antibody will react with all of the available epitopes, leaving none for the second antibody.

Immunofluorescent and immunohistochemical techniques are used to locate antigens in patient tissues. For example, to look for virus, sections of patient tissues are probed with antibodies, often monoclonal antibodies, prepared by immunizing animals with viral proteins. The antigen-specific monoclonal antibodies can be directly conjugated with fluorochromes or enzymes and used in a so-called direct, or one-step, detection (see Fig. 6-4).

Alternatively, the antigen-specific antibody, which is typically a mouse monoclonal antibody, is used first, and then bound antibodies are detected with a conjugated anti–mouse IgG prepared in another animal such as rabbit, goat, or sheep. This is a two-step or indirect assay (see Fig. 6-4). Indirect assays often generate a stronger signal, because several conjugated anti–mouse Ig antibodies can bind to each mouse Ig. However, this technique also has a higher background, and appropriate negative controls are critical to the interpretation of the assay. Cells in suspension can be stained with one or more antibodies, each labeled with a different fluorochrome, and analyzed by flow cytometry. The flow cytometer enumerates the cells, measures the fluorescence associated with each, and discriminates between fluorochromes with different emission spectra. Control samples must be analyzed in parallel using fluorochrome-conjugated monoclonal antibodies of the same isotype but specific for irrelevant antigens in order to measure background nonspecific uptake. The signal-to-noise ratio can often be improved by exposing the cells to unconjugated irrelevant IgG from another species, which will help to block the FcR and prevent nonspecific uptake of the fluorochrome-conjugated antibodies.

Immunofluorescence and immunohistochemistry can also be used to detect autoreactive antibodies that bind to antigens in autologous tissues. A direct assay is possible when the involved tissue can be biopsied. Bound autoantibodies are detected by the addition of conjugated antibodies to human Ig. Sometimes, the involved tissue is not accessible and the only option is to look for autoantibodies in the serum. This indirect technique involves incubating patient serum with tissue obtained from surgical samples or autopsies and using conjugated anti–human Ig to detect the patient antibodies that bind.

Measurement of Immune Complexes

Fixed tissue phagocytes in the liver and spleen are responsible for clearing complexes of antigen and antibody. However, if their capacity is exceeded, complexes circulate and deposit in tissues, where they activate complement and incite phagocytes to attempt to ingest the tissues where the antibodies have bound. A diagnosis can be made by demonstrating deposits of immune complexes in the targeted tissues using immunofluorescent or immunohistochemical techniques. A second diagnostic strategy is to measure the quantity of complement components, particularly C3 and C4, in the serum, because their levels will drop when complement is activated by immune complexes. However, interpretation of results can be difficult because C3 is an acute-phase reactant and its level tends to increase during inflammatory conditions.

A third diagnostic strategy is to look for circulating immune complexes in the blood stream. Several approaches can be used.[32,33] Some assays depend on the fact that when IgG or IgM antibodies are engaged with antigen, they also become able to fix C1q. One strategy is to incubate patient serum with immobilized antibodies to C1q and measure how much Ig coprecipitates with the C1q. Another strategy is to add radiolabeled C1q to the serum, precipitate all serum proteins in the size range of immune complexes, and measure the amount of coprecipitating C1q. Another type of assay is based on the fact that circulating immune complexes contain bound C3b. C3b (and the attached complexes) are extracted from the serum using immobilized antibodies to C3b or using the Raji cell line, which has an avid and abundant receptor for C3b. The quantity of human Ig that coprecipitates with the C3b is used as an estimate of the quantity of immune complexes present. The various strategies for measuring immune complexes do not always give concordant results, which suggests that complexes may vary in size, composition, and biologic behavior between patients or at different stages of a disease process.

B-CELL MATURATION AND IMMUNOGLOBULIN PRODUCTION

There is not enough DNA in the human genome to encode each of the millions of antibody specificities that people can produce when appropriately challenged. B cells create antibody diversity by selecting from a series of genes that encode components of the antigen-binding cleft. These are spliced together randomly to produce diverse Ig molecules. The DNA rearrangement process uses enzymes unique to B cells, such as RAG-1 and 2 (named for recombination activating genes), as well as the full array of ubiquitous DNA repair enzymes common to all cells. B cells begin by producing IgM antibodies. With further antigen stimulation and signaling from T cells, progeny of these B cells begin producing IgG, IgA, or IgE antibodies with the same antigen-binding site as the initial IgM. Along with this isotype switch, memory B cells are produced. Memory cells persist for years and are able to rapidly produce large quantities of antibody when appropriately restimulated with antigen.

DNA Rearrangement and Generation of Diverse Antigen-Binding Sites

The bone marrow produces about 10^9 pro-B cells per day. To become B cells, these precursors must undergo a specific series of gene rearrangements (Fig. 6-5 and Table 6-3). The first step is to rearrange the DNA to form a functional μ heavy chain. Four gene segments must be brought together to make a μ chain: the V or variable segment, the D or diversity segment, the J or joining segment, and the μ heavy chain gene. There are 50 functional gene segment choices for V, 27 choices for D, six choices for J, and one μ gene. Through random selection of these segments, 8100 ($50 \times 27 \times 6$) different IgM specificities can be generated using a mechanism called combinatorial diversity. The genes are brought together in a specific order. One of the D genes is spliced to one of the J genes, and then this DJ gene is spliced to one of the V genes. Note the overlapping nomenclature: "V" is used to designate the V gene segment and also to designate the V domains at the 5' ends of the heavy and light chains.

The antigen-binding cleft is formed by the pairing of the V domain from the heavy and light chain. Each of these V domains has three hypervariable regions or CDRs. Two CDRs are encoded in the V gene, and the third CDR is encoded by DNA that spans the splice junction between the V and J segments. Sloppiness or wobble in the splicing of these genes inserts more variability through junctional diversity. To splice the gene segments, the B cell must cleave its DNA. However, the cut ends are not immediately joined to the next gene. Instead, the end is sealed back on itself to form a hairpin loop. The loop is cut open again, but not necessarily at the same place. Shift in the exact location of the opening cut introduces variability into the gene sequence. Furthermore, additional nucleotides can be introduced to (or removed from) the cut end before it is spliced to the next gene.

These DNA rearrangements are a risky process for the B cell. Stop codons can be inadvertently introduced. In approximately two thirds of the cases, the reading frame is moved out of sequence and the gene no longer encodes a functional protein. Therefore, before it proceeds further, the B cell must verify that the rearranged VDJ gene encodes a functional μ chain gene. To test for functionality, the B cell attempts to pair the μ chain with a surrogate light chain and express the product on the cell membrane. It is not known how the B cell confirms that these two proteins are successfully displayed. However, if the criteria for success are met, the heavy chain gene on the other chromosome is prevented from rearranging by a process called allelic exclusion. If the μ chain does not display properly, the pro-B cell attempts to rearrange the other heavy chain allele.

Once rearrangement at the heavy chain locus is closed, the pro-B cell divides, it becomes a pre-B cell, and the light chain locus is open for rearrangement (see Table 6-3). The rearrangement process for light chains is the same as for heavy chains, with the exception that light chain genes have only V, J, and constant region segments—they do not have a D segment. However, the odds of success are better than for μ chains, because there are four potential light chain alleles with which to attempt a productive rearrangement. The B cell tries to rearrange one of the kappa light chains first. If that fails, it tries the other kappa allele and then the lambda chain alleles.

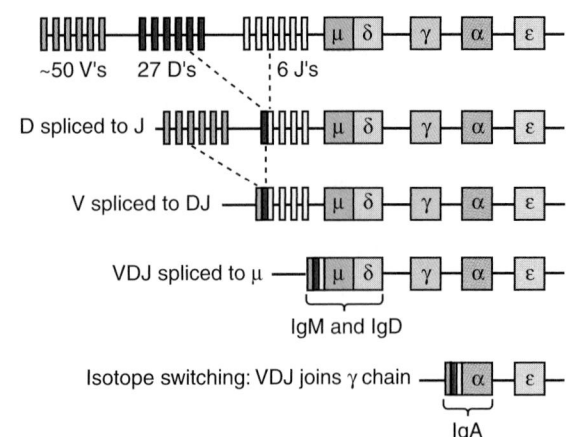

FIGURE 6-5. DNA rearrangement. The scheme for rearranging heavy CD4+ chain genes begins with splicing one of the D gene segments to one of the J gene segments. The DJ product is spliced to the V segment, and this is spliced to the μ chain gene. DNA encoding μ and δ chains are adjacent to each other, and the B cell can produce a single mRNA spanning both. Through alternative splicing in post-translational steps, the B cell produces both IgM and IgD, which are expressed on the B-cell surface. The B cell also produces secreted IgM. After it receives signals from activated T cells, the B cell can switch from production of IgM to production of IgG, IgA, or IgE. The VDJ segment is spliced onto the new heavy chain genes, thereby preserving the antigen specificity of the antibodies produced.

Because both light and heavy chains contribute to the antigen-binding site, the range of diversity is further expanded by the multiple possibilities for the light chain. Once both light and heavy chains are successfully rearranged to form functional membrane IgM (mIgM), the cell officially becomes an immature B cell, ready to encounter antigen (see Table 6-3).

Deletion of Autoreactive Clones

The next step is to eliminate any B cells producing autoreactive antibodies that might injure the host. Immature B cells at this stage express IgM but no IgD on their surface. They are still in the bone marrow, and any antigens they encounter in this environment are likely to be self antigens, or autoantigens. If their mIgM is cross-linked by antigen, the B cell clone is removed from the repertoire. These B cells are induced to undergo apoptosis in a process called clonal deletion, or they may become anergic or unresponsive to antigen. There is one potential rescue for the autoreactive B cell. If sufficient levels of the enzyme RAG remain in the cytoplasm, the autoreactive B cell can try to rearrange a new light chain gene in the hope that the new IgM will no longer react with self antigens. This process is called receptor editing.

Antigen Stimulation—First Signal

As the B cells leave the bone marrow, they begin to express both IgD and IgM on their membrane. To produce both isotypes simultaneously,

TABLE 6-3 Stages of B Cell Development				
Cell Stage	*Pro-B*	*Pre-B*	*Immature B*	*Mature B*
DNA rearrangement for immunoglobulin	μ Chain being rearranged	Heavy chain complete; light chain being rearranged	Heavy and light chains complete	Isotype switch; Somatic hypermutation in germinal center
Membrane immunoglobulin	None	μ Chain with surrogate light chain	IgM	IgM and IgD
Response to interaction with antigen	None	None	Receptor editing or deletion of autoreactive clones	Survival dependent on antigen stimulation

Ig, immunoglobulin.

the B cell generates a long messenger RNA (mRNA) molecule that includes the rearranged VDJ region, the μ gene, and the δ gene. By alternative splicing, the B cell can use this mRNA to produce IgM or IgD. This is a very different process from that used for isotype switching. The class switch from IgM to IgG, IgA, or IgE is irreversible because the B cell splices the VDJ sequence to a new heavy chain gene (γ, α, or ε) and discards the intervening DNA (see Fig. 6-5).

Production of IgD is an important threshold in the life of a B cell. From here forward, not only will interaction with antigen have a stimulatory effect but the B cell's survival will be dependent on repeated stimulation by antigen. Naive B cells leaving the bone marrow have about 1 week in which to locate their cognate antigen. Eighty percent of B cells fail to do so and die.[34] B cells induced to become anergic by premature exposure to antigen are also unable to respond to antigen and also die.

Membrane IgM is also called the B-cell (antigen) receptor, or BCR. When it interacts with cognate antigen, mIgM reorganizes into lipid rafts in the B-cell membrane. However, the cytoplasmic tail of mIgM has no signaling capability on its own. Signaling is carried out instead by two other cytoplasmic proteins, Igα and Igβ, which associate with the IgM in the lipid raft. These function much like the T cell's co-receptors, CD3 and ζ chain. Like CD3 and the ζ, Igα and Igβ have immunoreceptor tyrosine-based activation motifs (ITAMs). When IgM is cross-linked, these ITAMS are phosphorylated, which allows docking of the tyrosine kinase Syk. Syk is the B-cell equivalent of ZAP-70 in T cells. Syk and other tyrosine kinases activate the Ras–mitogen-activated protein (MAP) kinase pathway and the phosphatidylinositol-specific phospholipase C pathway, leading to increased cytosolic calcium and diacylglycerol (DAG). Ultimately, transcription factors such as nuclear factor of activated T cells (NFAT), nuclear factor of kB cells (NFkB), and activator protein (AP)-1 are produced.[35,36] Antigen-mediated signaling can be greatly enhanced by the participation of several B-cell co-receptors.

Co-receptors Amplify or Suppress Antigen Signaling

CD21, CD19, and CD81 form the B-cell co-receptor complex. CD21, also known as complement receptor 2 (CR2), binds C3d. C3d is a degradation product of C3b, which accumulates on the surface of pathogens when complement is activated. While antigen on the pathogen interacts with mIgM, the C3d can cross link the CD21 on the B cells. This brings the cytoplasmic tail of CD19 into proximity with the BCR, where it can be phosphorylated by Syk and bound to Igα or Igβ. The phosphorylated CD19 ultimately activates phosphatidylinositol-3 (PI3)-kinase. Src family kinases linked to CD21 can also phosphorylate ITAMs in the Igα and Igβ.[37] The net effect of co-receptor involvement is to increase the concentration of signaling molecules. In a murine model, involvement of the co-receptor complex, modeled by cross linking CD21 with antibodies, reduced the quantity of antigen needed to induce an immune response by 1000-fold.[38]

Other receptors, such as FcγRIIB, have an opposite effect and downregulate mIgM signaling. The cytoplasmic tail of FcγRIIB has an immunoreceptor tyrosine-based *inhibitory* motif (ITIM) that inhibits the activity of ITAMs. ITIM activates a phosphatase that dephosphorylates the ITAM and interrupts the signaling pathway. As a result, when immune complexes containing antigen and IgG interact with the B cell, the enhancing signal delivered by the interaction of mIgM with antigen is countered by an inhibitory signal arising from the interaction of IgG with the FcγRIIB.[28] This regulatory role for FcγRIIB was demonstrated by cross linking mIgM with IgG anti-IgM, as a surrogate for antigen. Intact IgG anti-IgM, which interacted with both mIgM and FcγRIIB, suppressed antibody responses. Treatment with F(ab')$_2$ fragments of the same anti-IgM, which could cross link mIgM but could not interact with FcR, stimulated antibody production.[39]

Second Signals and B–T Interactions

Before they can switch from production of IgM to production of IgG, IgA, or IgE, B cells need to receive a second signal from activated

CD4$^+$ helper T cells (Fig. 6-6). Activated T cells express CD40 ligand (CD40L, or CD154) that binds to CD40 on B cells and activates the B cell.[40] The critical role of CD40–CD40L interactions is best illustrated by the defects seen in individuals with a congenital deficiency of CD40L and a condition called hyper-IgM syndrome, or Omen's syndrome. Without CD40L, the T cells cannot stimulate CD40 on B cells. These patients' B cells produce greater than normal quantities of IgM, but they are unable to switch to production of other isotypes or to form germinal centers in lymph nodes.

Adhesion molecules such as intercellular adhesion molecule 1 (ICAM-1; CD54) and lymphocyte function–associated molecule 1 (LFA-1; CD11a/CD18) stabilize the B and T cell as a conjugate pair. The two may remain in contact for many hours as the T cell secretes cytokines in a polarized direction into the space between them. B cells can respond to numerous T-cell–derived cytokines, including interleukin (IL)-2, IL-4, IL-5, IL-6, and transforming growth factor β (TGFβ). IL-10 and TGFβ drive the B cell to switch to the IgA isotype, whereas IL-6 induces it to become a high-rate IgA-producing plasma cell.[41] IL-4 and IL-5 promote switching to the IgE isotype.

After the B cell is stimulated by the T cell, it begins to divide every 6 to 7 hours and generates several thousand daughter cells. At this point, nature raises the stakes for the B cell. The cell is set up to die by apoptosis through a decrease in the level of Bcl-2 and an increase in Fas. If, however, the B cell finds antigen that interacts with its surface immunoglobulin, levels of Bcl-X$_L$ increase and the B cell survives. If this does not occur, the B cell dies through Fas-mediated pathways of apoptosis. To make it even more challenging for itself, the B cell ceases expression of surface IgD and expresses only low quantities of IgM. To enhance their ability to bind antigen, B cells undergo somatic hypermutation of the antibody gene. In somatic hypermutation, B cells introduce one mutation per 10^3 base pairs within the gene that encodes antigen-binding clefts. This is a 10 million–fold increase over the baseline mutation rate for other somatic cells. Because continued stimulation by antigen is a prerequisite for survival, when antigen becomes scarce, B cells must compete by modifying their antigen-binding sites in the hope of generating a sequence with a higher affinity for antigen. As antigen is cleared, only B cells making antibodies with the highest binding affinity will be able to compete for the critical survival signal provided by antigen. As a result, the average affinity of the antibody response becomes higher and higher. Somatic hypermutation takes place within the follicular region of the lymph node or spleen in germinal centers.[42] B cells move through the basal light zone, competing for antigen expressed on follicular dendritic cells. Survivors become memory cells and plasma cell precursors.[43] Plasma cells can produce antibodies at a highly accelerated rate for a period of days, or perhaps even longer. Other B-cell progeny become memory cells and appear to survive for years.[44,45]

How B Cells Find and Activate T Cells

How does a B cell find the one-in-a-million T cell that is specific for a peptide from the same antigen? After B cells leave the marrow, they circulate through the blood stream and pass through the lymph nodes or spleen looking for cognate antigens brought in from the periphery by dendritic cells. B cells that do not find their antigen pass on to the next node. B cells that are activated by antigen express chemokine receptor CCR7, which makes them responsive to chemokines produced by stromal cells in the T-cell zone.[46,47] Activated T cells, in turn, are drawn toward the chemokines produced in the B-cell zone.[48]

B cells can also increase their odds of contacting activated T cells specific for the same antigen by becoming antigen-presenting cells (APCs). B cells ingest antigen and present relevant peptides to activate the very T cells they need. Unlike monocytes or dendritic cells, which pick up antigens on a random basis, B cells have an antigen-specific capture mechanism—their mIgM. The B cell internalizes the mIgM–antigen complex and incorporates these complexes into an endosomal compartment. The antigen is degraded into peptides and displayed at the cell surface in major histocompatibility complex (MHC) class II molecules. When mIgM is cross linked by antigen, the B cell is activated to display even more MHC class II antigen, and these pref-

FIGURE 6-6. B cells and T cells each need two signals. **Top,** The first signal for B cells comes when antigen cross links membrane Ig. If this occurs when the immature B cell is expressing only IgM, the signal is inhibitory. However, once the B cell is expressing both IgM and IgD, encounter with antigen is stimulatory. **Middle,** T cells are activated by encounter with antigen-presenting cells (APCs) such as dendritic cells. T cells need to recognize their cognate antigenic peptide expressed in a major histocompatibility complex (MHC) class II molecule and they need a signal through their CD28 receptor. The ligand for CD28 is one of the members of the B7 family (CD80 and CD86). APCs upregulate their expression of B7 molecules when they encounter proinflammatory stimuli such as PAMPs on the antigen. This second APC signal confirms to the T cell that the antigen is "dangerous" and an immune response is needed. **Bottom,** To switch from IgM to other isotypes and to form memory cells, B cells need signal(s) from activated T cells. These second signals include the interaction of CD40 on B cells with CD40L (CD154) on activated T cells and various T-cell–derived cytokines.

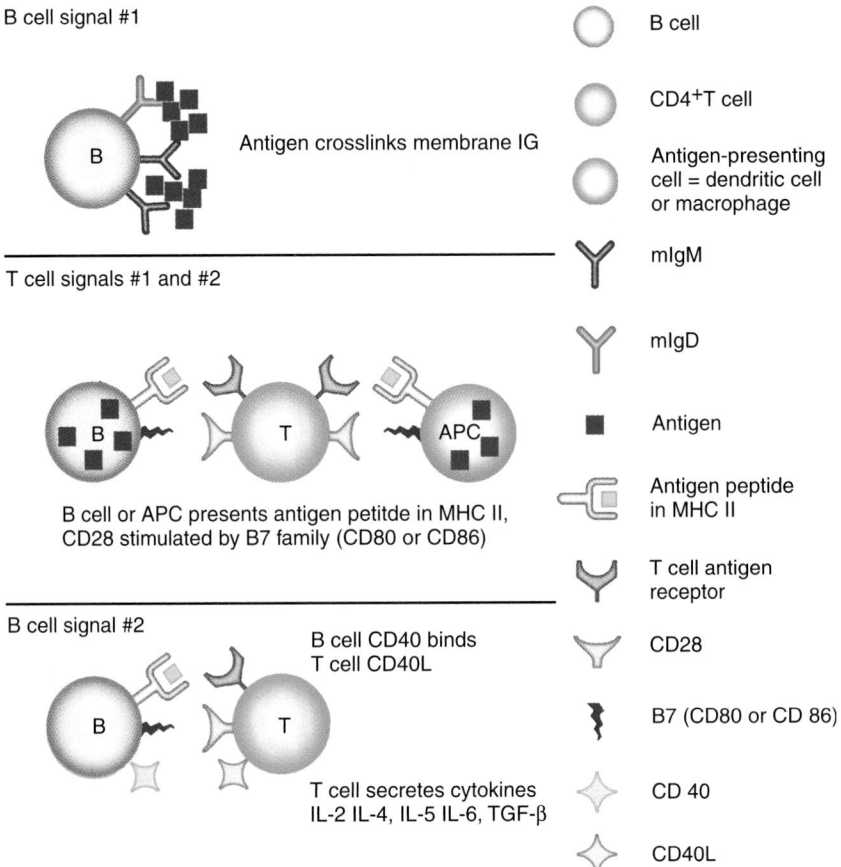

erentially display peptides from antigens that were bound by the mIgM. The peptides in the MHC class II molecules are then presented to CD4+ T cells. Because the antigen was picked up with the B cell's mIgM, the B cell is presenting just the right peptides to engage T cells with the appropriate antigen specificity.

In addition to their ability to select the right T cells, antigen-activated B cells can also provide the necessary costimulatory molecules required to activate the T cell's CD28 receptor.[49] T cells require two signals to be activated. The first signal comes through their antigen receptor, and the second signal comes through CD28. The two-signal requirement ensures that T cells do not mount an immune response to self antigens. T cells have no way to discriminate pathogens from harmless antigens. If T cells were activatable with just one signal, they would respond to every peptide that fit their antigen receptors, and the host could be overwhelmed by inflammatory processes. It is the role of the APC to tell the T cell when antigen is "dangerous" and merits an immune response. APCs do this by expressing members of the B7 family whenever they encounter danger. There are two homologous members of the B7 family: B7-1 (CD80) and B7-2 (CD86). The B7 molecules bind to CD28 and deliver the critical second signal that activates T cells and keeps them alive. T cells stimulated by antigen but not CD28 undergo apoptosis.

How do the APCs identify danger? These cells identify pathogens by using an assortment of receptors collectively called PRRs.[50] PRRs bind to PAMPs such as lipopolysaccharide, peptidoglycans, lipoteichoic acids, mannans, bacterial DNA, and double-stranded RNA. When the PRR is engaged by a PAMP, the APC recognizes this as a pathogen and begins to display the B7 costimulatory molecules. Cross-linking of mIgM, MHC class II molecules, or CD40 upregulates B7 molecules on B cells and transforms them into effective APCs.[51]

Conjugated polysaccharide vaccines depend on the ability of B cells to serve as their own APCs to present antigen to T cells (Fig. 6-7). Polysaccharides make poor vaccines because they cannot stimulate the

production of specific IgG antibodies. B cells producing antibodies to polysaccharides cannot make the switch from IgM to IgG and cannot generate memory cells because there are no specific T cells to provide the necessary second signals. There are no polysaccharide-specific T cells, because T cells recognize peptides displayed in MHC molecules and polysaccharides do not generate peptides. Conjugate vaccines are designed to fool T cells specific for other antigens into providing help to polysaccharide-specific B cells. A conjugate vaccine links the polysaccharide (PS) antigen to a protein, such as tetanus toxoid, for which the host already has specific T cells. PS-specific B cells internalize the conjugate using their mIgM. The conjugate is degraded, and peptides from the tetanus toxoid are displayed in the B cell's MHC class II molecule. T cells specific for tetanus toxoid peptides will pair up with this PS-specific B cell and provide the necessary help to drive isotype switching and formation of memory cells.

T-Cell–Independent Antigens

Some antigens can provide a type of second signal to the B cell without the participation of T cells. Examples of T-cell–independent (TI) antigens include the polysaccharides of *Haemophilus influenzae* type b, peptidoglycans, *Staphylococcus* protein A, and many viruses. TI antigens typically have highly repetitive motifs and a flexible structure. Their repetitive structure and flexible backbone allow them to interact with large numbers of mIgM molecules that aggregate into a single focus and deliver a potent signal to the B cell. Many TI antigens are pathogens that also become coated with C3d. This allows them to cross link CD21, which shares a lipid raft with mIgM in the B cell membrane, and this further amplifies the signaling pathways within the cytoplasm. B cells activated by TI antigens are still dependent on cytokines, but they may receive these from non–T-cell sources such as macrophages.

B cells in the marginal zone of secondary lymphoid tissue have a preselected set of BCRs that are biased toward TI antigens, particularly

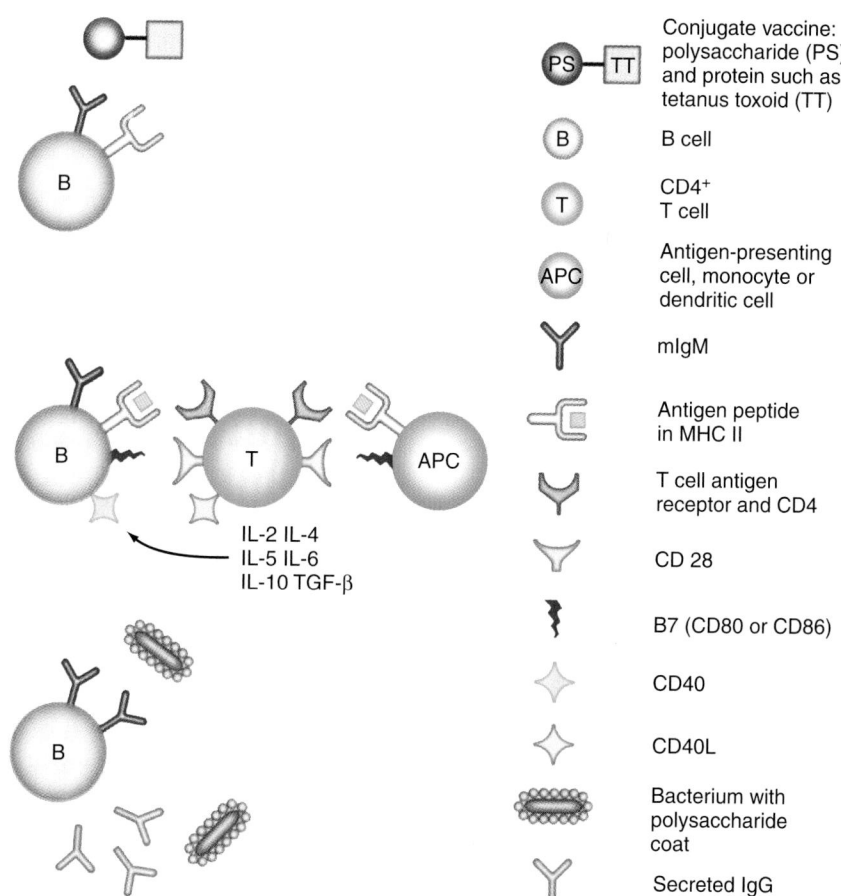

FIGURE 6-7. Conjugate vaccines. The conjugate vaccine is designed to induce production of IgG antibodies to polysaccharide (PS) antigens, which would normally be unable to induce IgG antibodies. Polysaccharides do not induce IgG antibodies because antigen-presenting cells (APCs) cannot degrade them into the peptides that must be presented in major histocompatibility complex (MHC) class II molecules in order to stimulate antigen-specific T cells. The vaccine consists of the PS antigen linked to a protein antigen, such as tetanus toxoid (TT), to which the host has primed antigen-specific T cells. B cells able to make PS-specific antibodies ingest the vaccine through their PS-specific membrane IgM (mIgM). The B cells degrade the vaccine molecule and present the TT peptides in their MHC class II molecules to a TT-specific activated CD4+ T cell. The T cell can be activated by the B cell, or by prior interaction with a dendritic cell displaying TT peptides. The activated TT-specific T cell provides PS-specific B cells (displaying peptides from TT) with the necessary help in the form of CD40–CD40L interactions and cytokines. Having received the necessary signals from a T cell, the PS-specific B cell can switch to production of IgG and can generate long-lived memory cells.

carbohydrate antigens. These B cells respond to blood-borne pathogens such as bacteria that are trapped by macrophages located around the marginal zone. Because they do not require the participation of T cells, marginal zone B cells provide a pseudo-innate response to bacteremia by quickly releasing IgM antibodies.

Downregulation of Antibody Production

Once the antigen is cleared, antibody responses decline. There are several mechanisms that cause this to happen. Immune complexes formed between antigen and excess IgG antibody deliver inhibitory signals to the B cell by interacting with FcγRIIB, as described previously.[52] Anti-idiotypic antibodies spontaneously arise during an immune response and may have a role in both upregulating and downregulating immune responses.[53] Anti-idiotypic antibodies are autoantibodies that react with epitopes in or near the antigen-binding site of an antibody. Because they recognize epitopes unique to a particular clone, they can modulate B cells in a highly selective manner. Anti-idiotypes interacting with mIgM before the immature B cell expresses IgD can suppress antibody production. T-cell help also declines. Repetitively activated T cells begin to express both Fas and its ligand, FasL. Reciprocal interactions be-

tween activated cells expressing both Fas and FasL lead to mutual apoptotic death.[54] Late in an immune response, activated T cells also begin to express CTLA-4. CTLA-4 binds the B7 costimulatory molecules with a much higher affinity than does CD28.[55] Whereas CD28 sends a stimulatory signal, CTLA-4 sends an inhibitory signal to the T cell. Finally, as antigen becomes scarce, fewer T cells and B cells receive the antigen signals necessary for continued activation and survival.

B1 Cells

The "usual" B cells discussed until now are called B2 cells to distinguish them from B1 cells. B1 cells are located primarily in the peritoneal and pleural spaces,[56] and they have a unique surface marker, CD5. B1 cells appear to regenerate continuously in the periphery rather than in the bone marrow. They produce only IgM, which suggests that they do not receive help from T cells. Their antigen-binding clefts are encoded directly by germline sequences, and the antigens they recognize tend to be microbial polysaccharides and effete or denatured host proteins. They may serve a housekeeping function by facilitating the clearance of cellular debris.[57] B1 cells are thought to be the source of the many "natural" antibodies to microbial antigens, particularly those found on normal gut flora. These antibodies are present in low levels even in individuals who have not been deliberately immunized. Even animals that have been raised in "germ-free" environments have low levels of circulating natural antibodies that react with a variety of commensal organisms.

ANTIBODY-MEDIATED PATHOLOGY

Gell and Coombs Classification of Hypersensitivity Responses

Hypersensitivity reactions are immune responses that cause tissue injury and thus morbidity for the host. In some cases, an aberrant autoimmune response is specifically directed to host antigens and host cells. In many other cases, host cells are merely innocent bystanders injured in the course of an exuberant immune response. The Gell and Coombs classification divides hypersensitivity reactions into four types based on their underlying mechanism of action. Types I, II, and III are mediated by antibodies and will be discussed here. Although few diseases can be uniquely attributed to a single Gell and Coombs class, the classification scheme is a useful foundation for understanding pathogenetic mechanisms. It should also be noted that the term *hypersensitivity reaction* is often used, in a potentially paradoxical manner, to describe defense mechanisms that are actually beneficial to the host. For example, granulomas formed in response to tuberculous organisms help to contain the bacillus, yet we refer to them as being formed by a type IV hypersensitivity mechanism.

Type I Hypersensitivity

Type I reactions involve the degranulation of mast cells and the release of pre-formed stores of histamine and heparin. The degranulated mast cell also begins to produce leukotrienes, prostaglandins, cytokines such as tumor necrosis factor (TNF)-α, and proteases. Local release of mast cell contents causes wheal-and-flare reactions, urticaria, and hives. Massive simultaneous degranulation of large numbers of mast cells throughout the body causes anaphylaxis, with a reduction in blood pressure, a loss of fluids through permeable vessel walls, and constriction of smooth muscle. Mast cells can be degranulated by cross-linking of IgE antibodies held in FcϵR on the mast cell surface. Opioids and contrast dyes can also degranulate mast cells but do not act through IgE or FcϵR. As a result, the responses they trigger are referred to as anaphylactoid reactions. Fragments from the third and fifth complement proteins (C3a and C5a) can also degranulate mast cells, and these molecules are referred to as anaphylatoxins. As they respond to intrinsically harmless substances such as penicillin or ragweed, type I hypersensitivity reactions seem to have no role except to make the host miserable. However, this same fundamental process is critical for defense against intestinal parasites. Degranulation of mast cells in the gastrointestinal tract increases motility and aids in the expulsion of helminths.

Type II Hypersensitivity

Type II reactions involve antibodies reacting with antigens on the surface of host cells. Cells decorated with antibodies may be lysed by activated complement or phagocytosed by neutrophils or monocyte-macrophages. Antibodies may bind to host cells because they are self-reactive, or autoantibodies. For example, autoimmune hemolytic anemia is caused by antibodies to red cells. Antibodies can also target external antigens that have bound to host cells. For example, patients with antibodies to penicillin can develop hemolytic anemia when penicillin binds to their red cells.

The Origin of Autoreactive Antibodies

It may be helpful, at this point, to review the mechanisms that prevent the development of autoimmunity and discuss how these processes might be circumvented. The immune system makes an attempt to remove B cells that are making autoantibodies. If B cells encounter their cognate antigen early in differentiation, they are induced to undergo apoptosis or become unresponsive. This window of vulnerability occurs when immature B cells first express IgM and before they express IgD. Geographically, these B cells are likely to be in the bone marrow, or in early transition into the periphery, and any antigens they encounter are likely to be self antigens. The nature of the antigen signaling also appears to dictate whether a B cell will become responsive or anergic. Stimuli that tend to induce anergy include chronic stimuli, oligovalent antigens, low-affinity interactions, and immune complexes that can interact simultaneously with ITIM-containing FcγRIIb on the B cell. Central induction of tolerance appears to be only partially effective, as virtually all individuals have circulating B cells that can be driven, in vitro, to produce antibodies reactive with autoantigens. Furthermore, mature B cells in germinal centers undergo somatic hypermutation and introduce new mutations into the DNA that codes for the antigen-binding site. Thus, it is possible that germinal center B cells could begin to make autoantibodies after they have passed the screening at their exit from the bone marrow.

As the control from the B-cell side is leaky, much of the responsibility for preventing autoimmune reactions falls on the T cell.[58] As T cells mature in the thymus, they are carefully examined for their ability to bind to autologous antigens. A unique system allows thymic epithelium to express a variety of proteins normally only found in extrathymic tissues. Thus, the T cell can be tested against a surprisingly wide repertoire of self antigens while still within the thymus. Immature T cells that bind with high affinity to autologous antigens are deleted by a process called negative selection. After they leave the thymus, T cells cannot be activated by cognate antigen alone—they require a second signal transmitted through CD28. T cells that receive a signal through their antigen receptor without an accompanying signal through CD28 are induced to undergo apoptosis. CD28 signaling is accomplished by B7 costimulatory molecules displayed on APCs. APCs upregulate the expression of B7 molecules when they recognize danger signals or PAMPs on the pathogen. APCs displaying peptides from host antigens generally do not express B7 molecules. However, in the course of an infection, an APC could display autologous peptides at a time when it has also been stimulated by proinflammatory cytokines to express B7 costimulatory molecules. Thus, during an infection or other inflammatory conditions, T cells recognizing peptides from self antigens may be activated and may, in turn, provide help to autoreactive B cells.

Another mechanism leading to autoimmunity is molecular mimicry, which involves pathogen-derived antigens that closely resemble host antigens. Examples of molecular mimicry include cross-reactive epitopes found on the M protein of *Streptococcus pyogenes* and proteins in the myocardial sarcolemma,[59] and cross-reactive peptides found in both *Trypanosoma cruzi* and human neurons.[60] Although the first peptide recognized as a result of molecular mimicry may not trigger an autoimmune disease, the immune response tends to expand to other epitopes on the same protein in a process called epitope spreading.[61] B cells produce antibodies to one epitope on a protein. Through their mIgM, these B cells take up the protein, process it to antigenic peptides, and display these, in large numbers, along with costimulatory signals that were presumably induced by a coexistent inflammatory stimulus. The activated B cell, in its role as an APC, activates T cells that recognize other epitopes from the same protein. This expands the repertoire of CD4 cells that are activated and allows them to help a still wider array of B cells.[62] Eventually, this expanding repertoire can include autoreactive T cells and B cells whose specificity leads them to injure host tissues.

Type III Hypersensitivity

Type III hypersensitivity reactions are inflammatory responses triggered by immune complexes deposited in various tissues. Phagocytes try to ingest the immune complexes bound to tissues. Although tissues decorated with complexes are too large to be ingested, the phagocytes nonetheless try, and in the process release injurious proteolytic enzymes and proinflammatory cytokines. The immune complexes can also activate complement, which deposits on the cell surface. Host cells generally protect themselves from complement attack with proteins that block formation of the membrane attack complex and accelerate the inactivation of complement components. However, when immune complexes activate complement through the classical pathway, the host may be unable to produce inactivator proteins at a sufficient rate. In type III hypersensitivity reactions, the tissue involved depends solely on where the immune complexes deposit; the antigenic specificity of the antibodies is irrelevant. For example, complexes of antibodies and hepatitis antigens cause vasculitis if they deposit in blood vessel walls or glomerulonephritis if they deposit in the kidney.

Infectious diseases are commonly associated with type III hypersensitivity reactions because the pathogen provides a continuous source of large quantities of antigen to be incorporated into immune complexes.[63,64] The formation of immune complexes depends on the relative quantities of antigen and antibody. In the presence of excess quantities of antigen, each antibody can bind its own antigen, and the complexes remain small. In the presence of excess antibody, antigen is covered with antibody, and again the complexes are small. However, when the antigen and antibody are present in near equivalence, antibodies will cross link contiguous antigen molecules and the ensuing lattice forms a large immune complex. Antibodies with low affinities release antigen quickly and tend to form small complexes regardless of their relative abundance.

Rheumatoid factors are antibodies that react with human (autologous) IgG and are a frequent component of immune complexes. These naturally occurring autoantibodies are found in virtually all people. The sequences coding for many of these specificities are in the germ line and are expressed with little DNA rearrangement.[65,66] Their preservation in the germline DNA sequence suggests that these antibodies may have an immunoregulatory role.[67] Anti-immunoglobulins that react with epitopes in or near the antigen-binding site may emulate antigen signaling and have either positive or negative effects on antibody production by B cells.[68,69] They may also facilitate the clearance of effete molecules of Ig.[70] In cases of chronic infection or inflammation, levels of rheumatoid factors can become quite elevated and contribute significantly to immune complexes that cause tissue injury. Cryoglobulinemia is a vasculitis triggered by complexes of rheumatoid factors and IgG that deposit preferentially in sites of reduced body temperature.

Hypergammaglobulinemia

Chronic infections such as malaria, endocarditis,[71] trypanosomiasis,[72] and infections associated with cystic fibrosis[73] increase circulating Ig levels well above the normal range. The mechanism is thought to be bystander activation of B cells, as few of the antibodies produced are specific for antigens associated with the infectious agent. Epstein-Barr virus (EBV) is also associated with elevated Ig levels, because the virus infects and activates a wide array of B cells, which then produce antibodies of diverse (polyclonal) specificities.[74] Sera with very high Ig levels have higher levels of nonspecific binding in assays for specific antibodies. This high background can lead to a false-positive reading if the appropriate background subtractions are not done. Hypergammaglobulinemias are not associated with any defined pathology, with the exception of hyperimmunoglobulinemia D and the inherited periodic fever syndrome, in which overproduction of IgD may trigger chronic inflammation.[75]

IMMUNODEFICIENCIES

IgA Deficiency

Among the inherited immunodeficiencies, defects involving B cells are far more common than those involving T cells or phagocytes. The most common inherited immunodeficiency is selective IgA deficiency, which affects about one in 300 to 700 individuals. There appear to be both incompletely penetrant autosomal dominant and recessive modes of inheritance. Many of these patients appear to remain relatively healthy and asymptomatic. The true prevalence of this disease became apparent only

when serum Ig levels were systematically measured in blood donors. Symptoms may be minimized because of compensatory transport of IgM into secretions.[7] A few IgA-deficient individuals develop recurrent sinopulmonary infections, atopy, autoimmune disorders, and malignancies. Their allergies are often directed toward dietary antigens, and it is postulated that the atopy occurs because they are unable to block absorption of environmental antigens from their gastrointestinal (GI) surfaces. Individuals with the most morbidity often have a combined deficiency of both IgA and one or more of the IgG subclasses, particularly IgG_2 or IgG_4. Some of these persons go on to develop common variable immunodeficiency syndrome (CVID). Ig replacement does not benefit patients with IgA deficiency for two reasons. First, the Ig preparations do not contain much IgA. Second, IgA_1 delivered into the blood is not transported across mucosal surfaces; only IgA_2 antibodies produced in the submucosal lymphoid tissue are transported across epithelial barriers into the secretions. Persons with congenital IgA deficiency are potentially at risk for anaphylactic reactions to IgA in intravenously administered preparations of immunoglobulins or in unwashed packed red cells.[76]

Agammaglobulinemias

Children with inherited profound antibody deficiencies remain well for the first 6 to 9 months of life because of maternal IgG antibodies acquired transplacentally. The half-life of IgG is approximately 3 weeks, and after six to nine half-lives, the maternal IgG levels have fallen below protective levels. Thereafter, these children begin to develop infections such as sinusitis, otitis media, and pneumonias. *Streptococcus pneumoniae, Haemophilus influenzae,* meningococci, and *Mycoplasma* species are particularly common infectious agents.[77] By the time the underlying etiology is recognized and treated, these children may have already developed irreversible bronchiectasis. Intestinal infections with *Salmonella, Shigella, Campylobacter, Giardia,* and rotavirus are also common.[78,79] Rheumatologic symptoms occur in 10% to 30%.[79] They are prone to septic arthritis from both common bacterial agents and unusual organisms such as *Mycoplasma* and *Ureaplasma* species.[78,80] They may also develop synovitis in the absence of infectious agents. These patients are also uniquely vulnerable to a chronic meningitis with enterovirus that often proves fatal.[81] Vaccination with inactivated agents is futile because they cannot produce the desired antibodies. Live vaccines are to be avoided, as vaccine-induced poliomyelitis has occurred in patients with agammaglobulinemia.[82]

Many of the conditions that affect B cell maturation and antibody production are X-linked. The most severe is X-linked agammaglobulinemia, which is caused by a defect in one of the cytoplasmic signal-transducing kinases in B cells.[83] The defective protein is Bruton tyrosine kinase (btk), and the condition is also called Bruton's agammaglobulinemia. Without btk, B cells are arrested at the pre-B stage and cannot develop into surface-immunoglobulin–expressing cells.[84] Many types of mutations of this gene have been described, but there is no apparent correlation between the specific mutation and the severity of the disease. Affected boys have less than 100 mg/dL of IgG and no serum IgM or IgA. B cells are virtually absent from bone marrow or periphery, but T cells are normal.

Hyper-IgM Syndrome

Hyper-IgM syndrome is usually X-linked, although there is a form that affects girls. These children have the same recurrent pyogenic infections seen in boys with X-linked agammaglobulinemia. However, patients with hyper-IgM syndrome are also uniquely susceptible to *Pneumocystis* pneumonia. They have normal numbers of circulating B cells, low levels of IgG and IgA, and greater than normal levels of IgM. The defect is in their T cells, not B cells. They lack the CD40 ligand (CD154) that is typically expressed on the surfaces of activated T cells. Without this molecule, activated T cells cannot bind to CD40 on B cells and induce isotype switching. Thus, the B cells continue to produce IgM, but they do not switch to IgG or IgA and do not exhibit the affinity maturation that is characteristic of a secondary response. As might be predicted, their lymph nodes are populated with cells, but they have no organized germinal centers. Their susceptibility to *Pneumocystis* pneumonia may reflect the inability of their T cells to interact with CD40 on monocytes and activate their full microbicidal potential. The patients are also prone to autoimmune hemolytic anemia, thrombocytopenic purpura, and recurrent neutropenia.[77]

Common Variable Immunodeficiency

The onset of CVID is typically between ages 15 and 25 years of age,[85,86] which is strikingly later than the congenital agammaglobulinemias. Although the late onset suggests an acquired etiology, there is a familial pattern that supports a genetic predisposition. These patients often, but not always, have normal numbers of B cells, which express surface immunoglobulins but produce only very small quantities of circulating secreted Ig.[87] The underlying cause or causes are not yet well defined, but the defect may actually lie with the T cell.[88] Patients with CVID are prone to malabsorption syndromes and autoimmune disorders. Some develop a sarcoid-like picture.[89] They are also at increased risk for GI malignancies and lymphomas.[90] Relatives of patients with CVID have a higher than normal incidence of IgA deficiency,[91] autoimmune disorders, and malignancies.[92]

IgG Subclass Deficiencies

Subclass deficiencies are an uncommon cause of susceptibility to infection. Isolated deficiency of IgG_1 would lead to significant morbidity because this subclass dominates the IgG response, but this condition is rare. IgG_2 subclass deficiencies are often seen in combination with defects in IgG4, IgE, or IgA. Patients deficient in IgG_2, IgG_3, or IgG_4 sometimes have recurrent bacterial infections,[4,93] but usually they do not.[94] When an IgG subclass deficiency is suspected, it should be verified that the patient is deficient in the ability to produce functional antibody before Ig replacement is proposed. This can be done by measuring the quantities of antibody before and after a booster vaccine for antigens such as diphtheria or tetanus.

Selective Immunodeficiencies

A few immunodeficiencies affect just the response to particular pathogens. Individuals with X-linked lymphoproliferative disease (Duncan's disease) are unable to mount an adequate response to EBV. Their B cells remain infected with the EBV and continue to proliferate. Another example of a pathogen-specific immunodeficiency involves people who are missing the VκA2 gene segment. This gene is often involved in the production of antibodies to *H. influenzae*. Presumably, the sequence of this V gene codes for an antigen-binding site that closely matches epitopes on this bacteria. Many members of the Navajo tribe are missing this V segment, and those individuals without it are more prone to infections with *H. influenzae*.[95]

Combined T-Cell and B-Cell Defects

Children with severe combined immunodeficiency are unable to generate mature B cells or T cells. They are susceptible to all types of pathogens, including pyogenic bacteria, viruses, fungi, and assorted opportunistic infections. Wiskott-Aldrich is an X-linked disease characterized by thrombocytopenia, severe eczematoid dermatitis, and deficient T- and B-cell responses.[96] Patients have normal numbers of T and B cells, but a defect in signal transduction impairs their ability to mount antigen-directed antibody responses.[97] IgM and IgG levels are low, but IgE and IgA levels are high.[77] These children are vulnerable to infections with *S. pneumoniae* and *H. influenzae* and may need immune globulin, intravenous (IGIV) prophylaxis.[96] Children with ataxia telangiectasia have defects in DNA repair mechanisms that may ultimately affect their immunoglobulin genes. IGIV should be given to children with demonstrable defects in their ability to generate antibodies to childhood vaccines.[77,98]

Malignancy

Antibody deficiencies may be seen with chronic lymphocytic leukemia, multiple myeloma, and Waldenström's macroglobuline-

mia.[99] This may be caused by decreased numbers of B cells and suppression of normal antibody production by cellular elements of the tumor or by their products.[100]

Clinical Evaluation of Suspected Humoral Immunodeficiency

The community-based physician should be able to initiate an evaluation for humoral immunodeficiency by looking for total Ig levels and the presence of functional antibody. Levels of total Ig, including IgG subclasses, are readily available from community clinical labs. The normal range varies widely with age, and it is critical to use age-matched reference tables when evaluating children. A simple test for functional antibodies is to test for antibodies to blood group antigens, because these are formed spontaneously to the A or B blood group antigens that a person does not possess. Community clinical labs can also evaluate whether a patient has antibodies to various infectious agents for which there is documented evidence of prior immunization—for example, mumps, hepatitis, and rubella. More extensive evaluations can be carried out, when indicated, by a specialist—for example, enumeration of B cells and T cells in the circulation, and an estimate of the ability of a patient's lymphocytes to respond to stimuli that normally cause leukocytes to proliferate and produce Ig in vitro. Patients can be immunized with a novel antigen not encountered in nature, such as the bacteriophage ΦX174, to evaluate their ability to mount a specific humoral immune response in vivo. Additional testing, including the evaluation of phagocyte function and the signaling pathways that endow APCs with the ability to stimulate host B and T cells, may be needed to fully evaluate immunodeficient patients.

THERAPEUTIC USES OF ANTIBODIES

Passive Immunization

Antibodies prepared from one person are effective when injected into another individual. Passive immunization is the administration of Ig prepared from individuals known to have high levels of antibodies to the infectious agent in question. It can be used for an immunocompromised host when the ability to generate a sufficient immune response to vaccination is in doubt. For example, immunosuppressed allograft recipients may need cytomegalovirus (CMV) immune serum after inadvertent exposure to CMV.

Passive vaccination is also used when a patient cannot make antibodies in sufficient time to protect against disease. For example, *Clostridium tetani* in a contaminated wound can produce lethal quantities of toxin long before an unvaccinated host could make neutralizing antibodies to the toxin. In such a case, the patient should receive tetanus immune globulin. The patient should also be vaccinated to protect against tetanus in the event of future injuries. Simultaneous administration of antibodies (hyperimmune serum) and antigen (toxoid vaccine) will not prevent the development of an adequate immune response. In fact, dendritic cells may store immune complexes and use them to stimulate B cells over long periods. The patient who has been previously vaccinated for tetanus should have some circulating antibodies to tetanus toxin, and a booster tetanus toxoid vaccine will trigger the rapid production of large quantities of additional toxoid-specific antibodies as a secondary response.

Another indication for passive vaccination is snake bite, which requires the use of antivenin. It is not practical, and indeed may be dangerous, to immunize human volunteers with the antigen. Because individuals immune through natural exposure are rarely available, it is necessary to use antisera prepared from immunized animals. Antibodies from other species are perfectly adequate, as their major role, in this case, is to block the binding of toxins to cell receptors. The great disadvantage is that the antibodies from other species can trigger an immune response and a type III hypersensitivity reaction, particularly with repeat administration.

Immune Globulin, Intravenous Replacement

Individuals with agammaglobulinemia or hypogammaglobulinemia need lifelong replacement with antibodies that can protect them against the diverse infectious agents they will encounter in ordinary life activities. Ig replacement is unlikely to be necessary until IgG levels fall below 200 mg/dL. Even with low overall levels of IgG, some patients may still make adequate levels of specific antibodies. This can be readily assessed using clinically available tests that measure response to vaccines such as tetanus toxoid, *H. influenza* type b toxoid conjugate, or hepatitis B. Patients with agammaglobulinemia typically require 100 to 500 mg/kg of immunoglobulin every 3 to 4 weeks. Preparations specifically designed for IV administration are available. IGIV must be free of aggregated Ig, which can act like an immune complex and trigger type III hypersensitivity reactions. The life span of infused IgG is about 21 days. With repeated infusions at 3- to 4-week intervals, the trough levels slowly rise. The goal is to ensure that levels do not drop below 400 to 500 mg/dL. Infusions may be accompanied by fever, chills, myalgias, headache, and nausea, but these tend to become less frequent after repeated infusions.[98,101]

Because of its success in treating infectious diseases, clinicians began administering IGIV for inflammatory conditions whose etiology was unknown but was speculated to be of infectious origin. IGIV is currently approved by the U.S. Food and Drug Administration for the treatment of idiopathic thrombocytopenic purpura[102] and Kawasaki syndrome.[103] However, IGIV is beneficial in a wide variety of other conditions, such as Guillain-Barré syndrome,[104] myasthenia gravis,[105] and a variety of inflammatory myopathies.[106] It may also be beneficial in toxic shock syndrome.[107]

The mechanisms by which IGIV ameliorates these conditions are not known and may well vary with the disease. IGIV should contain antibodies that neutralize bacteria, toxins, or superantigens that might be responsible for the disease.[108] The IGIV preparations are made from the plasma of at least 1000 and sometimes up to 100,000 donors. Thus, the array of antigen-binding sites represents essentially the entire human repertoire. Within this repertoire, there may be anti-idiotypic antibodies that can downregulate pathologic autoimmune responses in certain patients.[109] IGIV infusions also appear to downregulate production of inflammatory cytokines, possibly because of cytokine-specific antibodies.[110,111] In cases where antibody-coated host cells are attacked by the immune system, IGIV may slow the process by blockading the reticuloendothelial system.[112] Because the half-life of IgG is influenced by the serum concentration, raising the serum level of IgG with IGIV may accelerate the clearance of autoantibodies. It is even possible that some of the effects of IgG are not caused by antibodies at all but rather by other serum proteins that are present in trace quantities. For example, CD4, CD9, HLA molecules, and cytokines are all present in low levels.[113,114]

Monoclonal Antibodies

Uniform and reproducible preparations of antibodies are also used as therapeutic drugs in vivo and as reagents in vitro. The availability of monoclonal antibodies has greatly enhanced this field. To produce monoclonal antibodies, an animal, typically a mouse or rat, is immunized with the desired antigen. B cells from the immunized animal are fused with malignant B cells that do not produce their own Ig, with the goal of producing a hybridoma that proliferates indefinitely and produces IgG at a high rate. The fused cells are distributed, one to a well, and allowed to proliferate. The supernate is assayed for specific antibody, and clones producing high levels of desirable antibody are selected and propagated indefinitely.

The therapeutic use of monoclonal antibodies is expanding rapidly. Monoclonal antibodies to T cells are used to suppress graft rejections.[115] Monoclonal antibodies to lymphomas and antigens in solid tumors are used as part of chemotherapeutic regimens. Antibodies to cytokines or to their receptors are used to interfere with the activity of proinflammatory mediators such as TNF-α.[116] Because they are of murine origin, monoclonal antibodies are seen as foreign proteins and the patient eventually develops antibodies to them. Once complexed with human anti–mouse antibodies, the monoclonal antibodies are cleared more rapidly and thus become less effective.[117] To circumvent this, techniques have been developed for humanizing the monoclonal antibody. For example, the variable region of the murine

antibody is spliced onto the constant region of a human antibody.[118] Similar technology has been used to develop bifunctional molecules. For example, the Fc of IgG has been fused with CD4 to make a protein that might help to clear HIV by using the aminoterminal CD4 analogue to bind HIV and the Fc piece to bind to phagocytic cells. Chemical linkages have also been used to try to broaden the effector functions of IgG. Toxins have been conjugated to antibodies in the hope that the antibody will lead the toxin to the desired cellular target. Radionuclides have been conjugated to antibodies and used to localize tumor cells.

REFERENCES

1. Kohler PF, Farr RS. Elevation of cord over maternal IgG immunoglobulin: Evidence for an active placental IgG transport. Nature. 1966;210:1070-1071.
2. Ravetch JV, Margulies DH. Immunology: New tricks for old molecules. Nature. 1994;372:323-324.
3. Preud'homme JL, Hanson LA. IgG subclass deficiency. Immunodefic Rev. 1990; 2:129-149.
4. Oxelius VA, Laurell AB, Lindquist B, et al. IgG subclasses in selective IgA deficiency: Importance of IgG2-IgA deficiency. N Engl J Med. 1981;304:1476-1477.
5. Ottesen EA, Skvaril F, Tripathy SP, et al. Prominence of IgG4 in the IgG antibody response to human filariasis. J Immunol. 1985;134:2707-2712.
6. Mestecky J, McGhee JR. Immunoglobulin A (IgA): Molecular and cellular interactions involved in IgA biosynthesis and immune response. Adv Immunol. 1987; 40:153-245.
7. Mellander L, Bjorkander J, Carlsson B, Hanson LA. Secretory antibodies in IgA-deficient and immunosuppressed individuals. J Clin Immunol. 1986;6:284-291.
8. Phalipon A, Corthesy B. Novel functions of the polymeric Ig receptor: Well beyond transport of immunoglobulins. Trends Immunol. 2003;24:55-58.
9. Sixbey JW, Yao QY. Immunoglobulin A-induced shift of Epstein-Barr virus tissue tropism. Science. 1992;255:1578-1580.
10. Stokes CR, Soothill JF, Turner MW. Immune exclusion is a function of IgA. Nature. 1975;255:745-746.
11. Burks AW, Steele RW. Selective IgA deficiency. Ann Allergy. 1986;57:3-13.
12. Kubo S, Nakayama T, Matsuoka K, et al. Long term maintenance of IgE-mediated memory in mast cells in the absence of detectable serum IgE. J Immunol. 2003; 170:775-780.
13. Lantz CS, Boesiger J, Song CH, et al. Role for interleukin-3 in mast-cell and basophil development and in immunity to parasites. Nature. 1998;392:90-93.
14. King CL, Xianli J, Malhotra I, et al. Mice with a targeted deletion of the IgE gene have increased worm burdens and reduced granulomatous inflammation following primary infection with *Schistosoma mansoni*. J Immunol. 1997;158:294-300.
15. Mandel B. Neutralization of animal viruses. Adv Virus Res. 1978;23:205-268.
16. Metzger JF, Lewis GE Jr. Human-derived immune globulins for the treatment of botulism. Rev Infect Dis. 1979;1:689-692.
17. Kauppi-Korkeila M, van Alphen L, Madore D, et al. Mechanism of antibody-mediated reduction of nasopharyngeal colonization by *Haemophilus influenzae* type b studied in an infant rat model. J Infect Dis. 1996;174:1337-1340.
18. Johns M, Skehill A, McCabe WR. Immunization with rough mutants of *Salmonella minnesota*: IV. Protection by antisera to O and rough antigens against endotoxin. J Infect Dis. 1983;147:57-67.
19. Ziegler EJ, McCutchan JA, Fierer J, et al. Treatment of gram-negative bacteremia and shock with human antiserum to a mutant *Escherichia coli*. N Engl J Med. 1982; 307:1225-1230.
20. Rossmann MG. Neutralization of small RNA viruses by antibodies and antiviral agents. FASEB J. 1989;3:2335-2343.
21. Halstead SB, O'Rourke EJ. Antibody-enhanced dengue virus infection in primate leukocytes. Nature. 1977;265:739-741.
22. Mazanec MB, Kaetzel CS, Lamm ME, et al. Intracellular neutralization of virus by immunoglobulin A antibodies. Proc Natl Acad Sci U S A. 1992;89:6901-6905.
23. Blake PA, Feldman RA, Buchanan TM, et al. Serologic therapy of tetanus in the United States, 1965-1971. JAMA. 1976;235:42-44.
24. Burton DR. Immunoglobulin G: Functional sites. Mol Immunol. 1985;22:161-206.
25. Pfaffenbach G, Lamm ME, Gigli I. Activation of the guinea pig alternative complement pathway by mouse IgA immune complexes. J Exp Med. 1982;155:231-247.
26. Cassatella MA, Anegon I, Cuturi MC, et al. Fc gamma R(CD16) interaction with ligand induces Ca2+ mobilization and phosphoinositide turnover in human natural killer cells. Role of Ca2+ in Fc gamma R(CD16)-induced transcription and expression of lymphokine genes. J Exp Med. 1989;169:549-567.
27. Hostoffer RW, Krukovets I, Berger M. Increased Fc alpha R expression and IgA-mediated function on neutrophils induced by chemoattractants. J Immunol. 1993;150:4532-4540.
28. Bich-Thuy LT, Revillard JP. Selective suppression of human B lymphocyte differentiation into IgG-producing cells by soluble Fc gamma receptors. J Immunol. 1982;129:150-152.
29. Trinchieri G. Biology of natural killer cells. Adv Immunol. 1989;47:187-376.
30. Cao D, Boxer L, Peety H. Deposition of reactive oxygen metabolites onto and within living tumor cells during neutrophil-mediated antibody-dependent cellular cytotoxicity. J Cell Physiol. 1993;156:428-436.
31. Kyle RA. Sequence of testing for monoclonal gammopathies. Arch Pathol Lab Med. 1999;123:114-118.
32. Agnello V. Immune complex assays in rheumatic diseases. Hum Pathol. 1983;14:343-349.

33. Theofilopoulos AN, Dixon FJ. The biology and detection of immune complexes. Adv Immunol. 1979;28:89-220.

34. Allman DM, Ferguson SE, Lentz VM, Cancro MP. Peripheral B cell maturation: II. Heat-stable antigen(hi) splenic B cells are an immature developmental intermediate in the production of long-lived marrow-derived B cells. J Immunol. 1993;151:4431-4444.

35. Niiro H, Clark EA. Regulation of B-cell fate by antigen-receptor signals. Nat Rev Immunol. 2002;2:945-956.

36. Kurosaki T. Regulation of B-cell signal transduction by adaptor proteins. Nat Rev Immunol. 2002;2:354-363.

37. Carter RH, Fearon DT. CD19: Lowering the threshold for antigen receptor stimulation of B lymphocytes. Science. 1992;256:105-107.

38. Dempsey PW, Allison ME, Akkaraju S, et al. C3d of complement as a molecular adjuvant: Bridging innate and acquired immunity. Science. 1996;271:348-350.

39. Phillips NE, Parker DC. Cross-linking of B lymphocyte Fc gamma receptors and membrane immunoglobulin inhibits anti-immunoglobulin-induced blastogenesis. J Immunol. 1984;132:627-632.

40. Clark EA, Ledbetter JA. How B and T cells talk to each other. Nature. 1994;367:425-428.

41. Fujihashi K, McGhee JR, Lue C, et al. Human appendix B cells naturally express receptors for and respond to interleukin 6 with selective IgA1 and IgA2 synthesis. J Clin Invest. 1991;88:248-252.

42. Kelsoe G. The germinal center: A crucible for lymphocyte selection. Semin Immunol. 1996;8:179-184.

43. Calame KL. Plasma cells: Finding new light at the end of B cell development. Nat Immunol. 2001;2:1103-1108.

44. Slifka MK, Ahmed R. Long-lived plasma cells: A mechanism for maintaining persistent antibody production. Curr Opin Immunol. 1998;10:252-258.

45. Sprent J. T, B memory cells. Cell. 1994;76:315-322.

46. Reif K, Ekland EH, Ohl L, et al. Balanced responsiveness to chemoattractants from adjacent zones determines B-cell position. Nature. 2002;416:94-99.

47. Zlotnik A, Yoshie O. Chemokines: A new classification system and their role in immunity. Immunity. 2000;12:121-127.

48. Randolph DA, Huang G, Carruthers CJ, et al. The role of CCR7 in TH1 and TH2 cell localization and delivery of B cell help in vivo. Science. 1999;286:2159-2162.

49. Lenschow DJ, Sperling AI, Cooke MP, et al. Differential up-regulation of the B7-1 and B7-2 costimulatory molecules after Ig receptor engagement by antigen. J Immunol. 1994;153:1990-1997.

50. Medzhitov R, Janeway C Jr. Innate immunity. N Engl J Med. 2000;343:338-344.

51. Lenschow DJ, Walunas TL, Bluestone JA. CD28/B7 system of T cell costimulation. Annu Rev Immunol. 1996;14:233-258.

52. Heyman B. Regulation of antibody responses via antibodies, complement, and Fc receptors. Annu Rev Immunol. 2000;18:709-737.

53. Jerne NK. Idiotypic networks and other preconceived ideas. Immunol Rev. 1984;79:5-24.

54. Nagata S, Suda T. Fas and Fas ligand: lpr and gld mutations. Immunol Today. 1995;16:39-43.

55. Egen JG, Kuhns MS, Allison JP. CTLA-4: New insights into its biological function and use in tumor immunotherapy. Nat Immunol. 2002;3:611-618.

56. Kearney JF. CD5+ B-cell networks. Curr Opin Immunol. 1993;5:223-226.

57. Pisetsky DS. DNA and the immune system. Ann Intern Med. 1997;126:169-171.

58. Kamradt T, Mitchison NA. Tolerance and autoimmunity. N Engl J Med. 2001;344:655-664.

59. Dale JB, Beachey EH. Epitopes of streptococcal M proteins shared with cardiac myosin. J Exp Med. 1985;162:583-591.

60. Van Voorhis WC, Schlekewy L, Trong HL. Molecular mimicry by Trypanosoma cruzi: The F1-160 epitope that mimics mammalian nerve can be mapped to a 12-amino acid peptide. Proc Natl Acad Sci U S A. 1991;88:5993-5997.

61. Davidson A, Diamond B. Autoimmune diseases. N Engl J Med. 2001;345:340-350.

62. Liang B, Mamula MJ. Molecular mimicry and the role of B lymphocytes in the processing of autoantigens. Cell Mol Life Sci. 2000;57:561-568.

63. Carson CW, Conn DL, Czaja AJ, et al. Frequency and significance of antibodies to hepatitis C virus in polyarteritis nodosa. J Rheumatol. 1993;20:304-309.

64. Agnello V, Chung RT, Kaplan LM. A role for hepatitis C virus infection in type II cryoglobulinemia. N Engl J Med. 1992;327:1490-1495.

65. Radoux V, Chen PP, Sorge JA, Carson DA. A conserved human germline V kappa gene directly encodes rheumatoid factor light chains. J Exp Med. 1986;164:2119-2124.

66. Pascual V, Randen I, Thompson K, et al. The complete nucleotide sequences of the heavy chain variable regions of six monospecific rheumatoid factors derived from Epstein-Barr virus-transformed B cells isolated from the synovial tissue of patients with rheumatoid arthritis: Further evidence that some autoantibodies are unmutated copies of germ line genes. J Clin Invest. 1990;86:1320-1328.

67. Birdsall HH, Rossen RD. Regulation of antibody release by naturally occurring anti-immunoglobulins in cultures of pokeweed mitogen-stimulated human peripheral blood lymphocytes. J Immunol. 1984;133:1257-1264.

68. Nisonoff A. Idiotypes: Concepts and applications. J Immunol. 1991;147:2429-2438.

69. Jerne NK. Towards a network theory of the immune system. Ann Immunol (Paris). 1974;125C:373-389.

70. Pascual V, Victor K, Randen I, et al. IgM rheumatoid factors in patients with rheumatoid arthritis derive from a diverse array of germline immunoglobulin genes and display little evidence of somatic variation. J Rheumatol Suppl. 1992;32:50-53.

71. Phair JP, Clarke J. Immunology of infective endocarditis. Prog Cardiovasc Dis. 1979;22:137-144.

72. Kobayakawa T, Louis J, Izui S, Lambert PH. Autoimmune response to DNA, red blood cells, and thymocyte antigens in association with polyclonal antibody synthesis during experimental African trypanosomiasis. J Immunol. 1979;122:296-301.

73. Moss RB. Hypergammaglobulinemia in cystic fibrosis: Role of Pseudomonas endobronchial infection. Chest. 1987;91:522-526.

74. Carter RL. Antibody formation in infectious mononucleosis: II. Other 19S antibodies and false-positive serology. Br J Haematol. 1966;12:268-275.

75. Drenth JP, Haagsma CJ, van der Meer JW. Hyperimmunoglobulinemia D and periodic fever syndrome: The clinical spectrum in a series of 50 patients. International Hyper-IgD Study Group. Medicine (Baltimore). 1994;73:133-144.

76. Burks AW, Sampson HA, Buckley RH. Anaphylactic reactions after gamma globulin administration in patients with hypogammaglobulinemia: Detection of IgE antibodies to IgA. N Engl J Med. 1986;314:560-564.

77. Rosen FS, Cooper MD, Wedgwood RJ. The primary immunodeficiencies. N Engl J Med. 1995;333:143-440.

78. Hermaszewski RA, Webster AD. Primary hypogammaglobulinaemia: A survey of clinical manifestations and complications. Q J Med. 1993;86:31-42.

79. Saulsbury FT, Winkelstein JA, Yolken RH. Chronic rotavirus infection in immunodeficiency. J Pediatr. 1980;97:61-65.

80. Forgacs P, Kundsin RB, Margles SW, et al. A case of Ureaplasma urealyticum septic arthritis in a patient with hypogammaglobulinemia. Clin Infect Dis. 1993;16:293-294.

81. McKinney RE, Katz SL, Wilfert CM. Chronic enteroviral meningoencephalitis in agammaglobulinemic patients. Rev Infect Dis. 1987;9:334-356.

82. Buckley RH. Immunodeficiency diseases. JAMA. 1992;268:2797-2806.

83. Conley ME, Cooper MD. Genetic basis of abnormal B cell development. Curr Opin Immunol. 1998;10:399-406.

84. Clark JA, Callicoat PA, Brenner NA, et al. Selective IgA deficiency in blood donors. Am J Clin Pathol. 1983;80:210-213.

85. Sicherer SH, Winkelstein JA. Primary immunodeficiency diseases in adults. JAMA. 1998;279:58-61.

86. Hermans PE, Diaz-Buxo JA, Stobo JD. Idiopathic late-onset immunoglobulin deficiency: Clinical observations in 50 patients. Am J Med. 1976;61:221-237.

87. Spickett GP, Webster AD, Farrant J. Cellular abnormalities in common variable immunodeficiency. Immunodefic Rev. 1990;2:199-219.

88. Jaffe JS, Eisenstein E, Sneller MC, Strober W. T-cell abnormalities in common variable immunodeficiency. Pediatr Res. 1993;33(Suppl 1):S24-27; discussion S27-28.

89. Fasano MB, Sullivan KE, Sarpong SB, et al. Sarcoidosis and common variable immunodeficiency: Report of 8 cases and review of the literature. Medicine (Baltimore). 1996;75:251-261.

90. Sneller MC, Strober W, Eisenstein E, et al. NIH conference: New insights into common variable immunodeficiency. Ann Intern Med. 1993;118:720-730.

91. Wilton AN, Cobain TJ, Dawkins RL. Family studies of IgA deficiency. Immunogenetics. 1985;21:333-342.

92. Friedman JM, Fialkow PJ, Davis SD, et al. Autoimmunity in the relatives of patients with immunodeficiency diseases. Clin Exp Immunol. 1977;28:375-388.

93. Bjorkander J, Bake B, Oxelius VA, Hanson LA. Impaired lung function in patients with IgA deficiency and low levels of IgG2 or IgG3. N Engl J Med. 1985;313:720-724.

94. Lefranc MP, Hammarstrom L, Smith CI, Lefranc G. Gene deletions in the human immunoglobulin heavy chain constant region locus: Molecular and immunological analysis. Immunodefic Rev. 1991;2:265-281.

95. Feeney AJ, Atkinson MJ, Cowan MJ, et al. A defective Vkappa A2 allele in Navajos which may play a role in increased susceptibility to Haemophilus influenzae type b disease. J Clin Invest. 1996;97:2277-2282.

96. Standen GR. Wiskott-Aldrich syndrome: A multidisciplinary disease. J Clin Pathol. 1991;44:979-982.

97. Derry JM, Ochs HD, Francke U. Isolation of a novel gene mutated in Wiskott-Aldrich syndrome. Cell. 1994;78:635-644. Erratum, Cell. 79:following 922.

98. Buckley RH, Schiff RI. The use of intravenous immune globulin in immunodeficiency diseases. N Engl J Med. 1991;325:110-117.

99. Meyers BR, Hirschman SZ, Axelrod JA. Current patterns of infection in multiple myeloma. Am J Med. 1972;52:87-92.

100. Pilarski LM, Andrews EJ, Mant MJ, Ruether BA. Humoral immune deficiency in multiple myeloma patients due to compromised B-cell function. J Clin Immunol. 1986;6:491-501.

101. Berkman SA, Lee ML, Gale RP. Clinical uses of intravenous immunoglobulins. Ann Intern Med. 1990;112:278-292.

102. Blanchette V, Imbach P, Andrew M, et al. Randomised trial of intravenous immunoglobulin G, intravenous anti-D, and oral prednisone in childhood acute immune thrombocytopenic purpura. Lancet. 1994;344:703-707.

103. Laupland KB, Dele Davies H. Epidemiology, etiology, and management of Kawasaki disease: State of the art. Pediatr Cardiol. 1999;20:177-183.

104. Bril V, Allenby K, Midroni G, et al. IGIV in neurology: Evidence and recommendations. Can J Neurol Sci. 1999;26:139-152.

105. Gajdos P, Chevret S, Clair B, et al. Plasma exchange and intravenous immunoglobulin in autoimmune myasthenia gravis. Ann N Y Acad Sci. 1998;841:720-726.

106. Dalakas MC, Quarles RH, Farrer RG, et al. A controlled study of intravenous immunoglobulin in demyelinating neuropathy with IgM gammopathy. Ann Neurol. 1996;40:792-795.

107. Barry W, Hudgins L, Donta ST, Pesanti EL. Intravenous immunoglobulin therapy for toxic shock syndrome. JAMA. 1992;267:3315-3316.

108. Kazatchkine MD, Kaveri SV. Immunomodulation of autoimmune and inflammatory diseases with intravenous immune globulin. N Engl J Med. 2001;345:747-755.

109. Malik U, Oleksowicz L, Latov N, Cardo LJ. Intravenous gamma-globulin inhibits binding of anti-GM1 to its target antigen. Ann Neurol. 1996;39:136-139.

110. Ross C, Svenson M, Hansen MB, et al. High avidity IFN-neutralizing antibodies in pharmaceutically prepared human IgG. J Clin Invest. 1995;95:1974-1978.

111. Campbell DE, Georgiou GM, Kemp AS. Pooled human immunoglobulin inhibits IL-4 but not IFN-gamma or TNF-alpha secretion following in vitro stimulation of mononuclear cells with staphylococcal superantigen. Cytokine. 1999;11:359-365.

112. Fehr J, Hofmann V, Kappeler U. Transient reversal of thrombocytopenia in idiopathic thrombocytopenic purpura by high-dose intravenous gamma globulin. N Engl J Med. 1982;306:1254-1258.

113. Lam L, Whitsett CF, McNicholl JM, et al. Immunologically active proteins in intravenous immunoglobulin. Lancet. 1993;342:678.

114. Blasczyk R, Westhoff U, Grosse-Wilde H. Soluble CD4, CD8, and HLA molecules in commercial immunoglobulin preparations. Lancet. 1993;341:789-790.

115. A randomized clinical trial of OKT3 monoclonal antibody for acute rejection of cadaveric renal transplants. Ortho Multicenter Transplant Study Group. N Engl J Med. 1985;313:337-342.

116. Feldmann M, Maini RN, Bondeson J, et al. Cytokine blockade in rheumatoid arthritis. Adv Exp Med Biol. 2001;490:119-127.

117. Baert F, Noman M, Vermeire S, et al. Influence of immunogenicity on the long-term efficacy of infliximab in Crohn's disease. N Engl J Med. 2003;348:601-608.

118. Winter G, Milstein C. Man-made antibodies. Nature. 1991;349:293-299.

CHAPTER **7**

Complement

PETER DENSEN

Functional activity attributable to the complement system was first described between 1888 and 1894 when a series of studies demonstrated that fresh serum contained a heat-labile bactericidal factor called *alexin.*[1] Subsequently, it was shown that a heat-stable factor present in convalescent serum also contributed to bactericidal activity. At the turn of the century, Paul Erlich used the term *complement* to describe the heat-labile factor and *ambocepto* (antibody) to describe the heat-stable factor. With the 20th century came the recognition that complement was composed of more than one component. However, it was not until 1941 that Louis Pillemer was able to separate functionally distinct components of the classic pathway from various serum fractions. In the early 1950s, Pillemer also described an antibody-independent mechanism for complement activation that he referred to as the *properdin pathway.*[1-3] However, the protein purification techniques of the time were unable to provide complement components of sufficient purity to convince others of the existence of this pathway.

With the 1960s and 1970s came the development of a mathematical model capable of describing the sequential activation of complement, as well as new techniques for purification of individual complement components. The latter development led to the rediscovery of Pillemer's work, characterization of these proteins, and delineation of mechanisms that control their activity. The 1980s brought the recognition that the complement system also consists of membrane proteins—both receptors and inhibitors—that respectively mediate the cellular consequences of complement action and protect host cells from the detrimental effects of complement activation. With this advance came the appreciation that the complement functions optimally at the interface between the fluid phase and the cell surface. Toward the end of the 20th century, an explosion in molecular biology led to the cloning and structural characterization of all the complement proteins and an understanding of the molecular basis for their deficiency states; the characterization of a third pathway of complement activation—the mannose-binding lectin pathway; and the use of genetically engineered mice to dissect the molecular details of complement function. Through this process, the roles and implications of complement, both as a bridge between the innate and acquired immune systems and in the disposal of immune complexes and apoptotic cells, have been more clearly delineated. As a consequence of these revelations, the view of the complement system as a host defense system by virtue of its ability to promote inflammation has been replaced by a more global one in which it serves as a host defense mechanism by virtue of both inflammatory and anti-inflammatory actions.[4]

The complement system comprises more than 30 proteins (Table 7-1). Sequential activation of the pathway proteins mediates the beneficial consequences of complement activation, which include distinction between self and nonself, the development of an inflammatory response, elimination of microbial pathogens, enhancement of the adaptive immune response, and limitation of the potential for an inflammatory response through the disposal of immune complexes and apoptotic cells

TABLE 7-1 Complement Plasma Proteins

Component	Approximate Serum Concentration (μg/mL)	Molecular Weight	Chain Structure*	Number of Genetic Loci	Chromosomal Assignment†
Classic pathway					
C1q	70	410,000	(A, B, C) X 6	3 (A, B, C)	1p
C1r	34	170,000	Dimer of two identical chains	1	12p
C1s	31	85,000	Dimer of two identical chains	1	12p
C14	600	206,000	β-α-γ	2 (C4A, C4B)	6p
C2	25	117,000	One chain	1	6p
Lectin (mannose-binding) pathway					
MBP	1–2	40,000	Homo-oligomers	1	10q
MASPs	ND	74–94,000	A–B	1 per MASP	3q
Alternative pathway					
D (adipsin)	1	24,000	One chain	1	ND
C3	1300	195,000	β-α	1	19q
B	200	95,000	One chain	1	6p
Membrane attack complex					
C5	80	180,000	β-α	1	9q
C6	60	128,000	One chain	1	5p
C7	55	97,000	One chain	1	5p
C8	65	150,000	Three nonidentical chains α-γ, β	3 (A, B, G)	α,β,1p γ 9q
C9	60	79,000	One chain	1	5p

*For multichain components, parentheses indicate subunit structure; commas indicate noncovalent linkage of chains arising from separate genes; solid lines indicate covalent linkage of chains arising from posttranslational cleavage of a proenzyme molecule, with chains listed in order beginning at the amino terminus of the proenzyme molecule; dashed line indicates covalent linkage of chains arising from separate genes.

†p indicates the short arm and q the long arm of the chromosome.

BP, binding protein; C1-INH, C1 inhibitor; H, heavy chain; L, light chain; MBP, mannose-binding protein; MASP, mannose-binding lectin–associated serine protease; ND, not determined.

Continued

TABLE 7-1 Complement Plasma Proteins—cont'd

Component	Approximate Serum Concentration (μg/mL)	Molecular Weight	Chain Structure*	Number of Genetic Loci	Chromosomal Assignment
Control proteins					
Positive regulation					
Properdin	25	220,000	Cyclic polymers of a single 57-kD chain	1	Xp
Negative regulation					
C1-INH	200	105,000	One chain	1	11q
C4bBP	250	550,000	Seven identical chains	1	1q
Factor H	500	150,000	One chain	1	1q
Factor I	34	90,000	β-γ	1	4q
Anaphylatoxin inactivator (carboxypeptidase N)	35	310,000	Dimer of two nonidentical chains (H, L) × 2	ND	ND
S protein (vitronectin)	350	80,000	1 chain	1	ND
SP-40,40 (clusterin)	50	80,000	α-β	1	8p

*For multichain components, parentheses indicate subunit structure; commas indicate noncovalent linkage of chains arising from separate genes; solid lines indicate covalent linkage of chains arising from posttranslational cleavage of a proenzyme molecule, with chains listed in order beginning at the amino terminus of the proenzyme molecule; dashed line indicates covalent linkage of chains arising from separate genes.

†p indicates the short arm and q the long arm of the chromosome.

BP, binding protein; C1-INH, C1 inhibitor; H, heavy chain; L, light chain; MBP, mannose-binding protein; MASP, mannose-binding lectin–associated serine protease; ND, not determined.

(Fig. 7-1).[4] The complement system is activated by a wide variety of chemically diverse substances, even in the absence of antibody. Consequently, the multiplicity of its physiologic effects is felt early in the course of infection. In many instances, antibody and complement are synergistic in providing effective host defense. Specific antibody or binding by mannose-binding protein (MBP) leads to more rapid and efficient complement activation and serves to direct complement deposition to nearby sites on the surfaces of invading pathogens. Opsonization of infectious agents with both antibody and complement leads to more efficient ingestion and killing of these microbes than does opsonization with either substance alone. Similarly, the presence of receptors on lymphocytes for immunoglobulin and complement supports a cooperative role for these substances in both affector and effector pathways of the immune response. "In such a way, a highly specific response mediated by the tertiary structure of an antibody molecule can be coupled with the more general cellular or humoral responses of the phagocytic and complement system to eradicate attacking organisms."[5]

FIGURE 7-1. The complement cascade. Within each pathway, the components are arranged in order of their activation and aligned opposite their functional and structural analogues in the other pathways. Rounded boxes relate to activation of the pathways; squared boxes reflect complement functions; asterisks indicate sites of downregulation of complement activity (see Table 7-2).

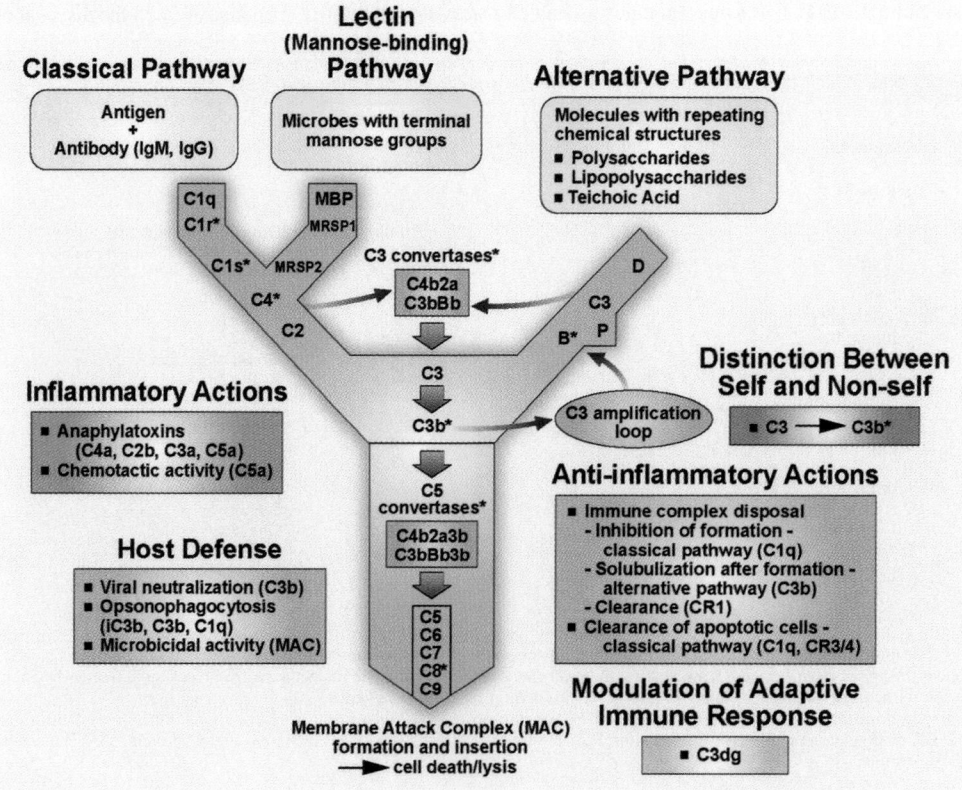

COMPLEMENT SYNTHESIS, CATABOLISM, AND DISTRIBUTION

Studies using cultured hepatocytes coupled with an examination of complement component polymorphisms in patients before and after orthotopic liver transplantation have established the liver as the major site of synthesis for most complement components.[6-8] The fractional catabolic rate for several complement components indicates that they are among the most rapidly metabolized of all plasma proteins. The catabolic rates of these proteins are independent of their serum concentrations, whereas synthetic rates correlate with these concentrations, indicating that the rate of synthesis is the major determinant of plasma concentration.[9]

The concentrations of individual complement components fluctuate over time. In part, this fluctuation reflects the fact that many of these proteins are acute-phase reactants, the synthesis of which can be modulated twofold to fivefold by a variety of immune mediators, including interleukin-1 (IL-1), IL-6, tumor necrosis factor (TNF), interferon-γ (IFN-γ), and endotoxin.[10,11] In most cases, enhanced synthesis is mediated at the transcriptional level.

A variety of other cells also synthesize and secrete a number of complement proteins. Most notable among these are monocytes, macrophages, and adipocytes, but microglia, astrocytes, fibroblasts, and endothelial cells are also important sites of local complement production.[12] Complement synthesis by monocytes can be modulated by IFN-γ, endotoxin, IL-1, and TNF.[13,14] Local synthesis is an important aspect of complement-mediated host defense, as evidenced by the observation that monocytes and macrophages can synthesize sufficient amounts of complement to promote opsonization, ingestion, and killing of bacteria.[15]

In healthy persons, most complement is found in plasma. Concentrations of complement proteins in normal mucosal secretions are approximately 5% to 10% of serum levels, and in normal spinal fluid, they are even lower, perhaps 1% or less. In the presence of local inflammation, complement concentrations in mucosal secretions and in cerebrospinal fluid increase, most likely as a result of altered vascular permeability barriers but also as a consequence of enhanced synthesis and secretion by local mononuclear cells.

Serum complement activity is reduced in preterm infants in proportion to the magnitude of their immaturity.[16] In contrast, complement levels in healthy full-term infants range from 60% to 100% of those in healthy adults. Despite these almost normal levels, defective complement activation via either the classic or the alternative pathway has been noted in as many as 40% of such infants.[17-19]

COMPLEMENT ACTIVATION

Generation of the Classic Pathway C3 Convertase

The classic pathway can be activated either by antibody or via mannose-binding protein (see Fig. 7-1). In the former case, activation occurs through the formation of an immune complex as a consequence of antigen recognition by immunoglobulin (Ig)M or IgG, C1 binding, and sequential enzymatic activation of downstream complement components.[20] The third constant domain (C_H3) of the heavy chain of IgM, especially glycosylation at Asn 402, and the C_H2 and C_H3 regions of IgG play particularly important roles in the binding of C1 by antibody.[21,22] Amino acid sequence differences in the C_H2 region contribute to the different complement-activating potentials among the IgG subclasses (IgG$_3$ > IgG$_1$ > IgG$_2$).[23]

C1 is a trimolecular complex containing one molecule of C1q and two molecules each of C1r and C1s. C1q consists of a central core with six radiating, collagen-like fibrillar strands that terminate in globular heads, which contain the antibody-binding sites.[19,23] Although C1q can bind directly to negatively charged surfaces and in doing so exert functionally important effects (e.g., elimination of apoptotic cells),[24] C1q binding is classically initiated as a consequence of the recognition of antigen by antibody. In the case of IgM, functionally important C1q binding occurs after the change in configuration that accompanies binding of a single IgM molecule to multiple sites on the target particle. In contrast, functionally effective C1q binding to IgG

requires that two IgG molecules be cross linked via the globular heads on C1q. This topographic stipulation dictates that many IgG molecules be bound to a target particle to ensure sufficient density for doublet formation. Functionally this requirement means that complement activation by IgG is less efficient than that by IgM.[20,25]

C1 binding by antibody results in a change in the structural configuration of the C1q molecule such that the C1r and C1s tetramer contained within the cagelike structure formed by the radiating pods of C1q becomes autocatalytically active. This structural alteration may involve the release of C1 inhibitor, which binds reversibly to proenzyme C1. C1r and C1s are structurally related molecules that consist of a head (bearing the serine esterase enzymatic site) and a tail (bearing the binding site). The subunits are aligned linearly such that the central portion of the tetramer is formed by two C1r subunits linked through their catalytic domains. Each C1r molecule is joined to a C1s molecule via binding sites in the tail regions of respective subunits. This linear arrangement allows the tetramer to assume a figure-eight configuration so that all four catalytic domains are in close proximity. In this configuration, each C1r molecule is believed to activate the other C1r molecule, which in turn activates C1s.[26-28]

Expression of enzymatic activity by C1r and C1s represents the initial activation and amplification step in the classic pathway. Many molecules of substrate are cleaved by a given enzyme complex, resulting in the fixation of subsequent complement components in the cascade in close proximity to the antibody-binding site. Therefore, antibody serves not only to activate complement in a kinetically efficient manner but also to deposit it nearby on the target surface, which includes the antibody itself (see later).

Activated C1s cleaves a 9-kD fragment, C4a, from the amino terminus of the α-chain of C4. This results in exposure of an internal thioester bond that links the SH group of a cysteine residue with the carboxyl-terminal group of glutamic acid. This bond is subject to nucleophilic attack by hydroxyl or amino groups, leading to the formation of covalent ester or amide linkages.[29-31] Through this reaction, along with the analogous one involving C3 (Fig. 7-2), the complement system acquires a chemically stable association with the target surface. Because of gene duplication, two slightly different C4 genes are formed—C4A and C4B. The product of the C4A gene preferentially forms amide bonds with target surfaces and is hemolytically less active than the product of the C4B gene, which preferentially forms ester bonds.[32-34] Consequently, C4A binds more effectively to proteins (e.g., antigen-antibody complexes) than does C4B.[33,35,36] The molecular basis for this difference is associated with an aspartic acid residue in the C4A molecule and a histidine residue in the C4B molecule, both of which influence the susceptibility of the thioester bond to nucleophilic attack by reactive groups on the target surface. This difference may play a role in the clinical presentation of patients with inherited deficiencies of C4A and C4B molecules.[35,36]

Activated C1s also cleaves C2 to produce a small fragment, C2b, which is released into the environment, and a larger fragment, C2a, which binds to C4b on the surface of the target particle. This complex, C4b2a, is the classic pathway C3 convertase (see Fig. 7-1). It is inherently labile, but unless C4b is inactivated following dissociation, it can bind newly generated C2a derived from further cleavage of C2 by C1s.[20,30]

Although recognition of antigen by antibody is the historically preeminent initiator of classic pathway activation, recent studies have confirmed a vital clinical role for complement activation via the mannose-binding lectin pathway (see Fig. 7-1). MBP is a collagenous lectin (collectin) that is composed of three identical subunits, each terminating in a calcium-dependent carbohydrate recognition domain. MBP is structurally and functionally homologous to C1q.[37,38] Like C1q, it exists in serum as a complex with serine proteases—MBP-associated serine proteases (MASPs). Four such molecules—MASP 1 to 3 and MAP 19—are the product of two genes that appear to have arisen from a common ancestor shared with C1r and C1s.[39] The exact function of each of the MASPs is unclear at this time, but MASP 2 plays a particular role in cleaving C4 and C2 and generating the classic pathway C3 convertase, as described previously.[37-39]

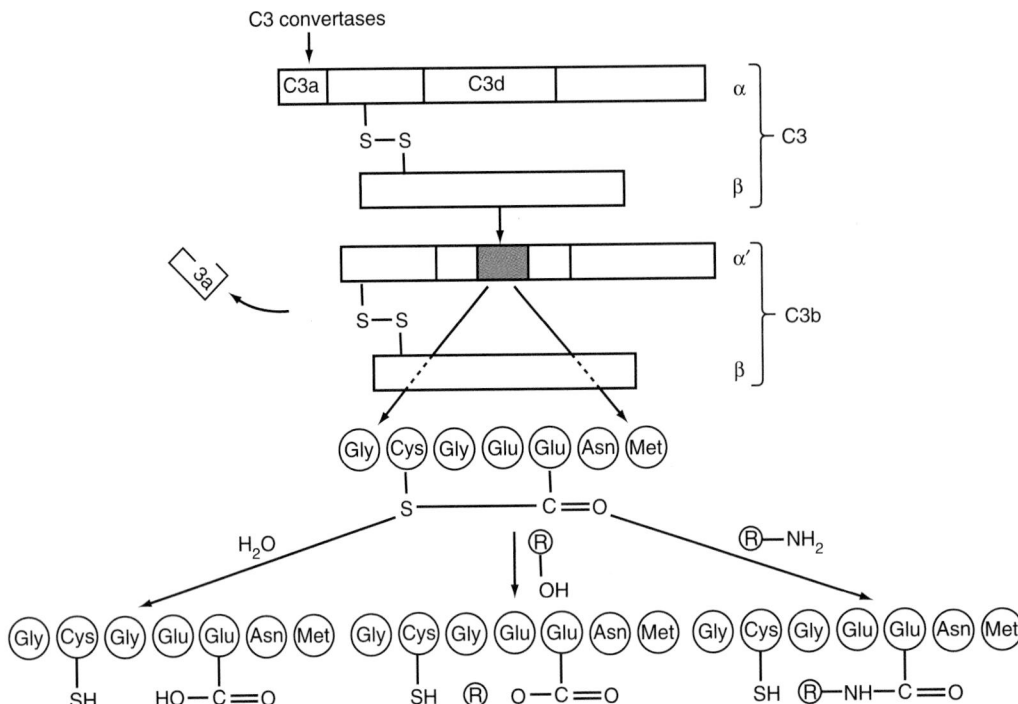

FIGURE 7-2. C3 Activation and fate of the internal thioester bond. During activation, C3a is released from the amino terminus of the α-chain of C3. The exposed internal thioester bond becomes accessible to nucleophilic attack and can react with water or available hydroxyl or amine groups on cell surfaces. Analogous reactions occur with C4. Together, these reactions involving C3 and C4 are responsible for covalently linking complement deposition to the cell surface. *(From Gordon DL, Hostetter MK. Complement and host defense against microorganisms. Pathology. 1986;18:365-375. www.tandf.co.uk/journals)*

The carbohydrate recognition domains on MBP bind to a variety of terminal monosaccharides, including mannose, *N*-acetyl-mannosamine, *N*-acetyl-D-glucosamine, fucose, and glucose. Hence, this activation sequence is probably more properly referred to as the *lectin-binding pathway*. These sugars frequently decorate microbial surfaces, but they only rarely appear as the terminal unit on oligosaccharides or glycoconjugates of human cells. Its ability to bind to a variety of sugars establishes MBP as a pattern recognition receptor. This feature has immense implications for host defense because it provides a mechanism for differentiating nonself from self and for rapidly activating the complement cascade. In these respects, MBP shares several critical features with IgM or "natural antibody": Both are polyreactive and bind to surface carbohydrates, and for both, binding of a single molecule is sufficient for complement activation. Equally important, unlike IgG, recognition is not delayed by the need for clonal expansion of a specific population of lymphocytes.[4,37,38]

Generation of the Alternative-Pathway C3 Convertase

Activation of complement by the alternative pathway displays several unique features. First, antibody is not required, although it can facilitate the activation process. Second, activation proceeds both in the fluid phase and on cell surfaces. Fluid-phase activation occurs continuously at a low rate that is tightly controlled by plasma regulatory proteins. Spillover from the fluid phase results in complement deposition both on cells of the host and on intruding microorganisms. Therefore, host cells must possess a mechanism by which to limit the effects of complement fixation (i.e., they are "nonactivators"), whereas intruding microorganisms must provide a surface that allows complement activation to proceed further (i.e., they are "activators").[30,40,41] Third, a component of the activation process, C3b, is also a product of the reaction, so that a positive-feedback loop is generated that amplifies the activation process. Consequently, C3b deposition resulting from C3 cleavage by either the alternative- or classic pathway C3 convertase can initiate the alternative-pathway amplification loop (see Fig. 7-1).[30,40,41] The time required until amplification occurs makes complement

activation via the alternative pathway three to five times less efficient kinetically than activation via the classic pathway on the same target.[42] This delay is characteristic for a given target but differs among different target particles.[41] Fourth, in contrast to the classic pathway, in which antibody or MBP directs covalent C4b binding in clusters about the respective binding sites, covalent C3b binding mediated by the alternative pathway occurs randomly over the surface of the target particle.[40,41] The random nature of this process contributes in part to the delay in complement activation that occurs via this pathway.

C3 is the critical reactant of the alternative pathway. It is structurally and functionally analogous to C4 (see Fig. 7-2) and contains an internal thioester bond within its α-chain.[43] This internal thioester bond undergoes spontaneous low-rate hydrolysis to form C3(H₂O), as is shown in Figure 7-2. For a brief moment before its inactivation by the control protein factors H and I, C3(H₂O) can form a complex with factor B. Once bound to C3, factor B can be cleaved by factor D, the rate-limiting enzyme in the alternative pathway, to yield C3(H₂O)Bb—a fluid-phase C3 convertase. C3(H₂O)Bb reacts with intact C3 to cleave a 9-kD peptide fragment, C3a, from the amino terminus of the α-chain.[40,41] Analogous to the situation with C4, this process results in exposure of the internal thioester in the α-chain. The resulting metastable C3b can form covalent ester or amide linkages with appropriate chemical constituents on the surfaces of nearby cells. Surface-bound C3b can bind additional factor B, which in turn can be cleaved by factor D to produce C3bBb. This complex is the alternative-pathway C3 convertase, which is capable of cleaving additional C3, thereby initiating the amplification phase of the alternative pathway. Like its classic pathway analogue, this convertase is inherently labile with a half-life of approximately 90 seconds. Properdin binding to C3bBb stabilizes the complex and prolongs its half-life 5- to 10-fold,[44,45] thereby providing reaction conditions sufficient for further C3 cleavage and signaling initiation of the amplification phase of alternative-pathway activation.

Although antibody is not required for activation of the alternative pathway, it acts synergistically with properdin to facilitate the activation process.[46-48] Facilitation depends on the Fab portion of the antibody molecule rather than the Fc fragment responsible for classic pathway activation,[48-52] but not all antibodies can enhance activation. For example, guinea pig IgG$_1$ but not IgG$_2$ can augment alternative-pathway activation.[53] The molecular basis for facilitation is uncertain but may depend on the identity of the carbohydrate moieties present on IgG.[54] The hydroxyl groups in these moieties can serve as sites for ester bond formation with C3.[49] Moreover, the alternative-pathway C3 convertase generated on IgG is relatively resistant to the action of the regulatory proteins.[55,56] This property may contribute to the ability of antibody to facilitate alternative-pathway activation.

C3—The Linchpin of the Complement System

The critical importance of C3 in the complement cascade is evident from its position at the convergence of the classic and alternative pathways, its role in activating and amplifying alternative-pathway activation, the multitude of functional activities associated with its various cleavage products, the fact that it is a major point of regulation of complement activity (see Fig. 7-1), and the fact that its concentration in plasma (1.6 mg/mL) exceeds by 2- to 10-fold the concentration of all other complement components (see Table 7-1).[57] The α-chain of C3b is subject to proteolytic cleavage by factor I to yield C3bi and by less well-defined proteases to yield C3dg and C3d. Each of these progressively smaller C3 fragments remains linked to the cell surface via the original covalent bond, and each can react with specific receptors on phagocytic and lymphocytic cells. However, *only* C3b can perpetuate complement activation. C3b binding to the C3 convertases generates new complexes—C4bC2aC3b and C3bBbC3b—the C5 convertases, which are responsible for cleaving C5 and initiating assembly of the membrane attack complex (MAC).

Assembly of the Membrane Attack Complex

C5 is the structural homologue of C4 and C3, except that its α-chain does not contain an internal thioester bond. Instead, the amino acids cysteine and glutamine, which form the internal thioester in C4 and C3, have been replaced by serine and alanine.[58,59] The enzymes responsible for C5 cleavage—C5 convertases—are formed from the C3 convertases as more C3 is cleaved and additional C3b binds covalently to the convertase complex. The additional C3b in these complexes increases their affinity for C5, converting the C3 convertases to C5 convertases—C4bC2aC4bn and C3bBbC3bn.[60] Analogous to C4 and C3, activation of C5 proceeds via cleavage of an 11.2-kD fragment—C5a—from the amino terminus of its α-chain. The remaining C5b binds noncovalently to the surface of the target particle.[61] The other terminal complement components—C6, C7, C8β, C8α-γ, and C9—share a high level of structural organization at both DNA and protein levels.[62-64] Unlike the early components of the classic and alternative pathways, these proteins lack enzymatic activity but as a group are characterized by their amphipathic properties. They circulate in plasma in hydrophilic form, undergoing hydrophobic transformation on binding to the nascent MAC.[61] Assembly of the MAC begins when C5b binds to hydrophobic sites on the cell surface and expresses a metastable binding site for C6. Both C6 and C7 bind to the α-chains of C5b through binding domains in their carboxyl termini to form a stable trimolecular complex—C5b-7.[61] Subsequently, C8 binds to C5b via a site on its β-chain.[65,66] In the final step, C8 initiates polymerization of C9 through a binding site on C8α-γ.[67] A current model of this process suggests that the function of C5b-8 is to create a discontinuity in the membrane lipid bilayer, thereby establishing an environment for the stepwise unfolding, insertion, and polymerization of monomeric C9.[68] In its completely assembled state, the MAC consists of a single molecule each of C5b, C6, C7, and C8 and multiple (1 to 18) molecules of C9.[61]

Fully inserted and polymerized C9 has a tubular shape and the properties of an integral membrane protein.[61,68] It is responsible for the characteristic electron microscopic appearance of membrane holes that appear during effective complement activation. The inner aspect of this tubular structure is hydrophilic and allows the passage of water and ions, whereas the outer surface of the structure is hydrophobic and causes varying degrees of membrane disorganization during insertion.[61,68] Both of these effects are thought to contribute to the microbicidal and cytolytic properties of the MAC.

REGULATION OF COMPLEMENT ACTIVATION

A major feature of the complement cascade is its controlled production of an inflammatory reaction sufficient to enhance host defense and the immune response, yet not so potent as to lead to host injury. Upregulation of this process is achieved by the inherent property of enzymes to turn over multiple substrate molecules rapidly and by stabilization of enzyme complexes (e.g., by properdin). Downregulation is achieved in a temporal fashion by the short half-lives of the enzymatic complexes and the anaphylatoxins and in a spatial manner by direction of complement activation to the target surface (e.g., by antibody). Modulation of the potentially injurious effects of indiscriminate complement activation is achieved by specific regulatory proteins that act at three major levels: activation (C1), effector initiation (C3), and cytolysis (MAC). Unique disease entities that result from a deficiency of these control proteins are testimony to the importance of complement regulation.

Regulation of C1 Activation

As described previously, C1 esterase inhibitor (C1-INH) binds reversibly to pro-C1, thereby preventing its spontaneous activation.[25] Binding of C1q to antibody subverts this control by causing dissociation of C1-INH from pro-C1 and allowing autocatalytic cleavage to proceed. At some point after C1 activation, C1-INH binds covalently to the active sites on C1r and C1s, inactivating their catalytic function and dissociating them from C1q. C1-INH neither prevents nor inhibits initial activation; rather, its roles are to prevent amplification of fluid-phase C1 activation and to limit excessive activation on the target cell. Complete C1 inactivation requires the binding of four molecules of C1-INH, one per catalytic site. In contrast to its binding to pro-C1, C1-INH binding to C1r and C1s is irreversible and thereby prevents cleavage of C4 and controls the initial amplification step of classic pathway activation.[25,69]

Regulation of the C3 Convertases

As indicated in Figure 7-1, the classic and alternative-pathway C3 convertases are functionally analogous molecules. Control of their activity occurs via three basic mechanisms that use functionally identical or shared regulator proteins (Table 7-2).[30,41,46] First, both convertases are inherently labile and undergo spontaneous decay, with the loss of C2a or Bb from their respective complexes. Second, the rate of spontaneous decay can be accelerated by regulatory proteins, C4b binding protein (C4b BP), and factor H. These proteins compete with C2a and Bb for binding sites on C4b and C3b, thereby inhibiting new convertase formation and enhancing the rate of dissociation of already formed convertases. Third, exposure of C3b and C4b makes them highly susceptible to cleavage by factor I, thereby eliminating their ability to reform the respective C3 convertases.[46,69a,70,71] Under typical circumstances, the functional half-life of C3b is just 90 seconds, whereas its cleavage product, iC3b, has a half-life of approximately 35 minutes.

Several additional points have emerged from the many studies on C3 convertase regulation. First, control of C3 convertase activity is expressed both in the fluid phase and on host cell surfaces. C4b BP and factor H modulate convertase activity both in the fluid phase and on surfaces, whereas membrane-bound proteins (complement receptor 1 [CR1], membrane cofactor protein [MCP], and decay-accelerating factor [DAF]) primarily control convertase activity on cell surfaces. Second, control proteins accelerate the decay of the C3 convertases (decay factors [DAF]) or promote factor I–mediated cleavage of C3b or C4b (cofactor activity [MCP]), or both (CR1, C4b BP, factor H). Third, C4b BP and factor H, unlike their membrane-bound counterparts, exhibit relative specificity for the classic and alternative-pathway C3 convertases, respectively.[70-72] Of these two serum proteins, it is clear that factor H plays the dominant regulating role, a feature supported by its greater serum concentration.

TABLE 7-2 Plasma and Membrane Proteins That Regulate or Mediate Complement Activity

Location, Protein	Specificity	Functions
Plasma		
C1-INH	C1r, C1s	Binds to and inactivates C1r and C1s in the C1 complex
C4bBP	C4b	Inhibits assembly and accelerates decay of C4b2a; cofactor for C4b cleavage by factor I
Factor H	C3b	Inhibits assembly and accelerates decay of C3bBb; cofactor for C3b cleavage by factor I
Factor I	C4b, C3b	Proteolytic inactivation of C4b and C3b
Properdin	C3bBb	Stabilizes alternative-pathway C3 convertase
S protein (vitronectin), (clusterin)	C5b-7	Binds fluid-phase C5b-7; prevents attachment of SP-40,40 C5b-7 and C5b-9 to membranes
Carboxypeptidase N	C4a, C3a, C5a	Inactivates these anaphylatoxins by removal of carboxy-terminal arginine
Cell Membranes		
CR1 (CD35)	C3b, C4b, iC3b	Inhibits assembly and accelerates decay of C3 convertases; binds immune complexes to erythrocytes; phagocytosis
Membrane cofactor protein	(CD46) C3b, C4b	Cofactor for cleavage of C4b/C3b by factor I
Decay-accelerating factor (CD55)	C4b2a, C3bBb	Promotes decay of C3 convertases
CR2 (CD21)	C3d, C3dg	Phagocytosis; modulates B-cell responses; Epstein-Barr virus receptor
CR3 (CD11b/CD18)	iC3b	Phagocytosis
CR4 (CD11c/CD18)	C3dg, C3d	Phagocytosis
CD59	C8 in C5b-8	Binds to C8; inhibits polymerization of C9
C3a/C4aR	C3a, C4a	Vasodilation
C5aR	C5a, C5a des Arg	Chemotaxis, cell activation, cytokine secretion
C1qR	C1q	Phagocytosis

CR, complement receptor.

The combined actions of these membrane-bound and serum proteins serve to confine the spread of complement activation and, by inactivating cell-bound C4 and C3, to protect host cells. In so doing, they distinguish self from nonself with respect to the deleterious effects of complement activation (see later).[73]

Regulation of the Membrane Attack Complex

Assembly of the MAC is controlled in two ways: by proteins that bind to the C5b-7 complex and by those that inhibit C9 incorporation and polymerization within the MAC. Nascent C5b-7 molecules have the potential to insert into any cell membrane and are not restricted to the surface on which complement is activated. By binding to this trimolecular complex, S protein (vitronectin) and clusterin abrogate its ability to insert into cell membranes and consequently its hemolytic potential. These proteins, by binding to C8, C9, or both, can also inhibit the incorporation of these components into the nascent MAC, but they act much more potently at the level of C5b-7.

Although several proteins inhibit C9 incorporation and polymerization within the MAC, by far the most potent is CD59. CD59 is very widely distributed. Its presence as a membrane protein probably accounts for homologous restriction,[74] a phenomenon whereby cells are not lysed by complement from the same species but can be (although are not always) lysed by complement from a different species. Although it is clear that CD59 binds to C9, the site of binding and the mechanism by which it prevents C9 incorporation and polymerization within the MAC are unclear.[70]

Nucleated eukaryotic cells are resistant to complement-mediated cytolysis, even in the face of a nonhomologous complement source. Resistance is associated with the capacity of the cell to maintain high synthetic rates of membrane lipids and the ability to shed MAC from the cell surface.[75-77] Insertion of the MAC in eukaryotic cell membranes is accompanied by a rapid influx of calcium, generation of multiple signals, and stimulation of arachidonic acid metabolism.[78-80] These events probably promote normal physiologic functions and contribute to host cell injury.

Basis for Discriminating between Host and Microbial Cell Surfaces

The potential of C4 and C3 to form covalent bonds with reactive groups on cell surfaces makes them inherently incapable of distinguishing between host and microbial cells. Consequently, additional factors must determine discrimination between self and nonself, if the outcome of complement activation is to be expressed beneficially for host defense.[73] These factors must inhibit activation of complement amplification on

host cells ("nonactivators") yet permit amplification on the surfaces of microbial organisms ("activators"). One element of this discriminatory process is the presence of complement regulatory proteins in the membranes of host cells but not on the cells of microbial organisms (see earlier).[73] Another determinant is the chemical composition of the cell surface. Because covalent bond formation is nondiscriminatory, the basis for discrimination must lie in the capacity for chemical differences on the cell surface to affect the outcome of the competition between factor B and factor H for the binding site on C3b, which in turn determines C3 convertase formation or decay and whether a particular cell surface will activate the alternative pathway. For example, C3b bound to the surface of a nonactivating particle binds factor H with about 100-fold greater affinity than does C3b that is bound to an activator particle. Consequently, factor B binding and subsequent amplification of complement activation are favored on the latter particle.[30,41,46]

Chemical constituents that influence the microenvironment in which the competition between factor B and factor H for C3b occurs include sialic acid and sulfated acid mucopolysaccharides (e.g., heparan sulfate). These molecules, present on most human cells, act through an anion-binding site on factor H to enhance its affinity for C3b, thereby contributing to the nonactivator status of host cells.[81-84] Sialic acid is also a prominent chemical constituent of capsular polysaccharides on type 3 group B streptococci, K1 *Escherichia coli*, and groups B and C meningococci.[46] Consequently, the capsules of these organisms are nonactivators of the alternative pathway and are poor stimuli for antibody production. In this context, it is noteworthy that K1 *E. coli*, group B streptococci, and group B meningococci are prominent causes of neonatal and infant sepsis and meningitis. The frequent absence in these patients of specific antibody to activate the classic pathway, coupled with bacterial sialic acid–mediated inhibition of alternative-pathway activity, may provide the ideal clinical setting for infection by these organisms.

Chemical constituents other than sialic acid also affect the outcome of the competition between factors B and H for C3b. For example, sheep and human erythrocytes contain an extensive amount of sialic acid on their surfaces and are normally nonactivators of the alternative pathway.[82-85] Enzymatic removal of sialic acid from these cells converts sheep but not human erythrocytes into activating particles. Moreover, the chemical introduction of lipopolysaccharide molecules capable of activating the alternative pathway into the membrane of sheep erythrocytes converts them from nonactivating to activating particles despite the presence of sialic acid.[85]

In summary, the C3 convertases represent the major site of both complement amplification and complement regulation. The membranes of host cells contain specific proteins that act to downregulate the C3 convertases and other chemical constituents that enhance the affinity of fluid-phase factor H for surface-bound C3b and promote its regulatory activity. In contrast, the chemical microenvironment on microbial surfaces is the major determinant of the outcome of the competition between C3b- and C4b BP with C4b in formation of the classic pathway convertase, and between Bb and factor H with C3b in formation of the alternative-pathway convertase. Nonpathogenic microbes typically possess an activating surface environment, whereas pathogenic microbes usually manifest a nonactivating environment.

COMPLEMENT RECEPTORS

Complement receptors have been described primarily on peripheral blood cells, including erythrocytes, neutrophils, monocytes, B and T lymphocytes, and platelets. They fall into two broad categories: those that bind diffusible complement fragments released during activation of the complement cascade and those that bind complement components deposited on cell surfaces such that the component serves as a bifunctional ligand, or bridge, linking the target cell to the receptor (see Table 7-2).

The former receptors mediate many of the clinical manifestations of the inflammatory response in that they bind C4a, C3a, and C5a, the complement-derived inflammatory mediators. Of these, the high-affinity C5a receptor has been best studied. It is present on neutrophils and monocytes, and its perturbation causes migration (chemotaxis) of these cells in the direction of increasing C5a concentration. Experimental evidence has confirmed the presence of receptors for C3a on B lymphocytes, guinea pig ileum, vascular endothelium, adipocytes, and mast cells.[86]

The latter category of receptors includes C1qR, CR1, CR2, CR3, and CR4. C1qR is a carbohydrate-rich protein expressed on phagocytic cells and lymphocytes that modulates phagocytosis, cytokine release, cytotoxicity, and interactions with endothelial cells. Functional ligands in addition to C1q that are recognized by C1qR include MBP, surfactant protein A, and conglutinin, all of which exhibit structural homology with C1q.[26]

Receptors for the cleavage products of C3 and C4 (CR1, CR2, CR3, and CR4) have been studied more extensively. Although they recognize closely related ligands, each of these receptors is structurally distinct and exhibits a unique pattern of distribution across peripheral blood cells.[87,88] A portion of these receptors are linked to the cellular cytoskeleton, an association important for signal transduction.[89]

CR1, the C3b/C4b receptor, is present on erythrocytes, neutrophils, monocytes, B cells, subpopulations of T cells, follicular dendritic cells, and glomerular podocytes. Four polymorphic variants vary in size (190 to 280 kD) and in the number of C3b/C4b binding sites.[90] The number of CR1 molecules per cell is determined genetically but varies with cell type and disease activity. CR1 mediates immune complex binding and clearance, promotes ingestion of C3b/C4b-bearing particles, modulates certain lymphocyte functions,[87,88] and carries certain blood group antigens.[91]

CR3 and CR4 are members of the integrin family of heterodimeric proteins.[92] They recognize iC3b as the major binding ligand. CR3 also binds to C3b and C3dg and bears a lectin-like domain that recognizes specific carbohydrates on microbial surfaces.[93] The three-amino-acid sequence arginine-glycine-aspartic acid (Arg-Gly-Asp), which is present in C3 and other ligands, represents an important binding motif for CR3.[93-95] Together CR3 and CR4, particularly the former, recognize the various combinations of C3b, iC3b, and C3dg present on the surfaces of microbial cells and play a major role in their elimination by all types of phagocytic cells.[96] In addition, CR3 plays an important role in adherence-related functions of neutrophils (see Chapter 8).

CR2 is present on B lymphocytes and follicular dendritic cells and serves to recognize C3d and C3dg. The association of CR2 and CD19 in the B-cell membrane constitutes an important mechanism for B-cell activation.[97] CR2 acts to target C3dg-bearing particles or immune complexes to lymphocyte-rich areas in the spleen and lymph nodes, thereby driving antigen activation of these cells and promoting long-term immunologic memory.

FAMILIES OF COMPLEMENT PROTEINS

The preceding material and the representation of the complement cascade presented in Figure 7-1 emphasize features shared by both pathways with respect to their activation and regulation. It is apparent from these similarities that a number of complement components belong to several different protein families. These include the serine protease family (C1r, C1s, MASPs 1 to 3, MAP 19, C2, factor D, factor B, and factor I); disulfide-linked, multichained molecules with homology to an ancestral protein that contained an internal thioester bond (C4, C3, and C5); proteins that are the products of class III major histocompatibility complex (MHC) genes located on chromosome 6 (C2, factor B, C4A, and C4B); proteins that bind C3 and C4 fragments and belong to a closely clustered supergene family located on the long arm of chromosome 1 (C4b BP, factor H, DAF, MCP, CR1, and CR2); and proteins that share homology with the low-density lipoprotein (LDL) receptors (C6, C7, C8α, C8β, and C9).[98]

Among these families, interest has focused on those components that are the products of class III MHC genes, the regulatory protein supergene family on chromosome 1, and the proteins with homology to the LDL receptor. MHC III genes are located between the class I and class II loci on the short arm of chromosome 6.[99] The genetic material in this region appears to have undergone two duplication events, resulting in the one hand in the structurally and functionally related proteins C2 and factor B, and on the other in the C4 and 21-hydroxylase A and B variants.[98-100] Recombinant events in this region of the chromosome tend to be suppressed, thereby leading to the usual inheritance of the entire region intact from each parent.[101] The polymorphic variants of the complement components encoded by these genes in a given individual are referred to as *complotypes*.[102] The association of specific complotypes with specific products of the MHC I and II genes probably contributes to the association of specific complotypes with certain disease states (e.g., systemic lupus erythematosus [SLE]).[103]

Proteins encoded by the complement regulatory protein loci on the long arm of chromosome 1 share a common structural organization with each other, with other complement components that bind to C3 and C4 (e.g., C2, factor B), and with some other complement and noncomplement proteins that do not bind these two components.[104,105] These molecules contain a structural motif called *short consensus repeats (SCRs)*.[105] SCRs are tandem repeats of approximately 60 amino acids that share a conserved consensus sequence in which paired cysteine residues are linked to form a double-loop structure. The number of repeats varies considerably among the control proteins: MCP and DAF contain 4, CR2 has 16, factor H has 20, CR1 has 30, and C4b BP has 59. SCRs constitute the binding domain for C3b and for other molecules. Two to four SCRs are typically required to form a complete binding site, but the number of SCRs and which ones in a sequence form a specific binding site differ among the proteins.[105,106] The binding specificity of these sites and their functional consequences have become increasingly evident with the identification of associations of distinctive disease pathology with specific complement-deficient states (e.g., hemolytic-uremic syndrome and factor H deficiency; see later).

The LDL receptor–related complement proteins are cysteine-rich molecules. Each molecule (except C8α) contains an even number of cysteine residues, which are clustered at the amino and carboxyl ends of the protein and participate in disulfide bond formation. Those clustered at the amino terminus of the molecule share homology with the LDL receptor, whereas those at the carboxyl terminus share homology with epidermal growth factor. The large number of disulfide bonds in these molecules is thought to convey a tertiary structure that facilitates the hydrophilic-hydrophobic transition that occurs on their interaction with lipid membranes during the assembly of the MAC.[62,63]

COMPLEMENT-MEDIATED FUNCTIONS

Complement plays a major role in distinction between self and nonself, development of an inflammatory response, elimination of microbial pathogens, modulation of the adaptive immune response, and, through the disposal of immune complexes and apoptotic cells, limitation of the potential for an injurious inflammatory response (see Fig. 7-1).[4]

Whether initial formation of a C3 convertase is followed by its enhanced decay or by its amplification is the event that distinguishes self from nonself, respectively, as has been described earlier.[4]

Small, diffusible peptide fragments released from C4, C3, C5, and probably C2 during their activation initiate and modulate the inflammatory response.[86] Collectively, C4a, C3a, and C5a are referred to as *anaphylatoxins*, and together, they stimulate histamine release from mast cells (C3a), promote vascular dilation (C3a, C4a), increase endothelial permeability (C3a), and stimulate neutrophil responses (C5a). In addition to these proinflammatory activities, C3a acts via its receptor on B cells to downregulate cytokine synthesis and antibody production.[107] Carboxypeptidase N–mediated removal of the carboxyl-terminal arginine from the anaphylatoxins abrogates their functional activity by preventing their interaction with specific receptors.[97] In the case of C5a des Arg (the inactivated form of C5a), chemotactic activity is restored by association with vitamin D–binding protein.[108,109] The activity of this complex is inhibited by free Bb, which is often present in the sera of patients with active SLE.[110]

Complement activation promotes the elimination of microorganisms in conjunction with phagocytic cells via opsonophagocytosis or, in the case of certain gram-negative pathogens, by direct bactericidal attack. Complement-mediated opsonophagocytosis promotes uptake via complement receptors, predominantly CR1 and CR3, that recognize C3b and iC3b as described previously (see Table 7-2). In the case of bacteria, opsonization with C3b or iC3b, especially in conjunction with IgG, promotes ingestion of the organism and triggers the microbicidal mechanisms of phagocytic cells (see Chapter 8). Ingestion appears to be more efficient when the organism is opsonized with iC3b than with C3b.[111,112] Complete activation of the complement cascade, with assembly of the MAC and its effective insertion into cell membranes, results in the death and eventual lysis of the cell. Death and lysis are independent events, and in the case of prokaryotes, evidence suggests that a metabolic response is required by the organism before the lethal effects of the MAC can be expressed.[113] For some organisms, the assembly of the MAC through C8 is sufficient for killing[114]; however, in all cases, the incorporation of C9 accelerates this process. Complement-mediated virucidal activity has also been well described and in some cases seems to require deposition of only the early components of the classic pathway.[115]

Substantial data indicate that C3 modulates the adaptive immune response.[116] This evidence includes (1) the absolute requirement for C3 binding for antigen localization within splenic and lymphoid germinal centers; (2) the presence of complement receptors, especially CR2, on B lymphocytes, follicular dendritic cells, and other antigen-presenting cells; (3) impaired antibody responses in animals or humans who lack one of the complement components (C1, C2, C4, C3) required for classic pathway C3 convertase formation, and restoration of the immune response by replacement of the missing component; and (4) the association of these deficiencies in humans with depressed concentrations of IgG_4 and IgG_2.[29,116-120] In general, these studies demonstrate that soluble C3 fragments (especially C3a) inhibit adaptive immune responses, whereas C3 fragments (especially C3d) covalently linked to target particles enhance these responses. In particular, ligation of C3d to its receptor, CR2, leads to its association with CD19 in the B-cell membrane and constitutes an important signal for the activation of these cells.[97] It is important to note that C3d acts as an immune adjuvant when bound to antigen, as is demonstrated by a 100- to 1000-fold reduction in concentration of the antigen necessary to activate B cells. This adjuvant role is most critical in enhancing response to antigens with a low affinity for the B-cell receptor.[118,121,122] The clinical importance of this adjuvant role is evident in the inverse correlation

that exists between the extent of C3b degradation on a given pneumococcal polysaccharide and the ability of that polysaccharide to elicit an immune response when administered as part of the polyvalent vaccine.[123] In addition to its adjuvant role, C3d facilitates isotype switching, anamnestic responses after secondary antigenic exposure, and B-cell survival and long-term immunologic memory.[116] In summary, although an absolute complement requirement does not exist for generation of the humoral immune response, C3 facilitates antigen localization and presentation, acts as an immune adjuvant to reduce the amount of antigen required to evoke an optimal immune response, and participates both directly in the activation of B cells and indirectly by promoting cytokine synthesis. In addition, recent studies show that C3 fragments promote the expansion of CD8 T cells after viral infection, indicating a role for complement in the development of both B- and T-cell acquired immune responses.[124]

The incorporation of complement in immune complexes enhances clearance and helps to minimize the potential for tissue damage.[125,126] This process includes inhibition of immune complex precipitation, solubilization of immune complexes, and clearance of C3b-bearing immune complexes via the CR1 receptor. Under conditions of antibody excess or antibody-antigen equivalence, the probability that both antigen-binding sites on a single antibody will bind to epitopes on a single antigen and the probability that multiple antibody molecules will bind to a given molecule of antigen are increased. This situation promotes antibody-antibody interactions via Fc fragments and subsequent immune complex precipitation.[125] C1q binding to the Fc portion of antibody inhibits Fc–Fc interactions and leads to covalent binding of C3b to the immune complex. Subsequent recruitment of the alternative pathway via the C3b amplification loop promotes further C3b deposition within the immune complex lattice, thereby reducing the forces that hold the lattice together and causing separation (solubilization) of smaller complexes from the lattice network. Thus, classic pathway activation inhibits immune complex precipitation, whereas the alternative pathway promotes immune complex solubilization.[125,126] However, in the context of disease pathogenesis, it must be stressed that complement is 10 times more efficient in inhibiting immune complex precipitation than in solubilizing precipitated complexes. This property probably contributes greatly to the close association of classic pathway component deficiencies with immune complex disease formation (e.g., SLE).

In healthy persons, most immune complexes bearing C3b are bound to cells bearing C3b receptors (CR1). The number of these receptors per cell varies from a low of 950 for erythrocytes to a high of 57,000 for neutrophils.[127] However, because there are 1000 times more erythrocytes than leukocytes, 95% of the CR1 receptors in the peripheral circulation are located on erythrocytes. Consequently, immune complexes bearing C3b are 500 to 1000 times more likely to be cleared from the circulation by erythrocytes than by leukocytes.[127] These complexes are removed from the erythrocyte, along with the CR1, during passage through the liver and the spleen. This extraction probably involves fixed macrophages that line the sinusoids of these organs.[128]

Recent studies have extended our understanding of the anti-inflammatory role played by complement in promoting the clearance of apoptotic cells. Under steady-state conditions, the billions of host cells that die every day are eliminated with minimum induction of inflammation or an immune response. Despite the number of cells involved and completion of the apoptotic cycle over a period of several hours, few apoptotic cells are identified in tissues or in the circulation. Rapid complement-dependent phagocytic removal of apoptotic cells by macrophages appears to account for this apparent paradox. During apoptosis, the cell membrane bulges to form blebs that contain macromolecular complexes of proteins and nucleic acids, a finding that may be a significant contributing factor in the development of SLE (see later). The exposed surface of the bleb contains several unique phospholipids that have been translocated from the inner to the outer leaflet of the lipid bilayer of normal cell membranes. Some of these phospholipids, especially phosphatidylserine, bind C1q directly to activate the classic pathway. An analogous process occurs on ischemic cells upon reperfusion. Unlike viable eukaryotic cells, apoptotic cells and ischemic cells "permit" both C3 convertase formation and amplification. These cells can then be eliminated via C1qR, CR3, and CR4 on mononuclear cells, fixed macrophages, and dendritic cells. Elimination in this fashion minimizes the inflammatory potential of injured cells. Disruption of this process may be critical to the development of SLE (see later).[129,130]

MICROBIAL INTERACTIONS WITHIN THE COMPLEMENT SYSTEM

The demonstration by Roantree and Rantz[131] that gram-negative bacteria isolated from blood were almost always resistant to complement-mediated killing, whereas two thirds of those isolated from mucosal surfaces were serum sensitive, was one of the first to suggest an important clinical role for complement-mediated bactericidal activity in host defense. This suggestion was borne out by subsequent studies of complement-deficient persons (see later) and by elucidation of the strategies and extent to which microorganisms go to escape host defense mechanisms. In the case of complement, these strategies parallel those employed by host cells to circumvent injury during the inflammatory response, that is, they are focused on decreasing complement activation, accelerating convertase decay, and inhibiting the formation or insertion of the MAC.[132,133] In many instances, the microbial proteins responsible for these effects share molecular, structural, immunologic, and functional homology with their human counterparts.

Elegant experiments correlating virulence with lipopolysaccharide composition and complement activation in three isogenic *Salmonella typhimurium* variants, which differ only in the chemical structure of their lipopolysaccharide side chains, demonstrated the importance of limited complement deposition on the surfaces of bacteria. The ability of these variants to activate complement via the alternative pathway varied inversely with their relative in vivo virulence. The greatest rate of C3 consumption and extent of C3b deposition were initiated by the least virulent strains. Subsequent experiments demonstrated that discrete differences in O-antigen structure were expressed at the level of alternative-pathway amplification, as manifested in the greater affinity of factor B for C3b on the surface of the least virulent compared with the most virulent strains. In contrast, the affinity of factor H for C3b was the same in all strains.[134-139]

To date, molecules analogous to the complement regulatory proteins that accelerate the decay of C3 convertases have not been identified in bacteria, although they are well described in multicellular parasites and viruses. The striking metamorphosis that protozoa undergo during transformation from insect- to human-infective forms is accompanied by the acquisition of resistance to complement-dependent killing. This phenomenon has been studied most extensively in *Trypanosoma cruzi,* in which the surface proteins gp72 and gp160 have been identified that block assembly and promote decay of the alternative-pathway C3 convertase.[132,133,140] These proteins function in a manner identical to human CR1 and DAF (see Table 7-2). In the case of gp160, structural homology to DAF appears to underlie functional homology.

Appropriation of complement regulatory proteins is a strategy employed by a wide range of microbial pathogens, including *Streptococcus pyogenes, Streptococcus pneumoniae, Neisseria gonorrhoeae, Neisseria meningitidis, Yersinia enterocolitica, Borrelia burgdorferi, Candida albicans, Echinococcus granulosus,* and *Onchocerca volvulus* group A streptococci. These organisms express any of a number of complement regulatory-acquiring proteins (CRASPs 1–5) on their surfaces. A chief binding target of these proteins is factor H, although the site on which factor H binds varies slightly among the CRASPs.[141] M protein in group A streptococci functions as a CRASP. Its C repeats promote binding not just of factor H but also of C4b BP, factor H, and MCP. That group A streptococci bind multiple proteins that regulate complement at the level of C3 attests to the critical importance

of C3 activity for survival of the organism and likewise for host defense against the organism. Through these interactions, M protein not only limits complement deposition on the streptococcal surface but also promotes adhesion to the surfaces of keratinocytes in the skin.[141,142]

Other organisms employ different but related strategies. The envelope of type 1 herpes simplex virus contains a virus-specific protein, gC-1, that interferes with properdin-dependent stabilization of the alternative-pathway C3 convertase, thereby limiting complement-mediated effects. Deletion mutants lacking gC-1 are exquisitely sensitive to complement-mediated lysis. Natural mutants have not been isolated with any frequency in surveys of clinical specimens, attesting to the importance of this protein and perhaps this mechanism in the pathogenesis of infection. Vaccinia virus bears a C4b BP structural and functional homologue that accelerates the decay of the classic pathway convertase.[133,143-145]

A variation on this theme occurs in serum-sensitive gonococci isolated from patients with symptomatic local genital disease. These organisms possess a sialyl transferase but lack the ability to synthesize cytidine monophospho-*N*-acetyl neuraminic acid (CMP-NANA). Consequently, they are incapable of endogenous sialylation of their lipopolysaccharide; rather, they appropriate host CMP-NANA for this purpose. Exogenous sialylation (1) confers serum resistance to these gonococci by reducing the binding of bactericidal antibody,[146] (2) reduces phagocytic uptake, and (3) may alter C3 cleavage and intracellular survival. T. cruzi accomplishes the same effect via a *trans*-sialidase that removes terminal sialic acid residues from host glycoconjugates and transfers them to acceptor molecules on the parasite surface.[140]

The increasing availability of DNA sequence data banks and investigations into molecular pathogenesis have served to focus attention on virus–complement interactions and the mechanisms by which these organisms elude complement-mediated attack. Studies of the human immunodeficiency virus (HIV) are particularly illustrative. During viral replication, the virus is assembled and released from the infected cell by budding—a process that incorporates host cell membrane proteins into the viral envelope. Host cell DAF and CD59 incorporated into the viral envelope in this manner function efficiently to limit amplified complement deposition on HIV and its subsequent lysis. In addition, the HIV-specific envelope proteins gp120 and gp41 both contain factor H binding domains, which, in the case of the latter protein, demonstrate significant homology with C3. Factor H passively absorbed from serum and secretions serves to further limit complement deposition on the virus.[143,147]

Other organisms owe their serum resistance to functional homologues of CD59, the protein that interferes with MAC assembly on host cell membranes. For example, the galactose-specific adhesin of *Entamoeba histolytica* not only functions in this manner but also shares DNA sequence homology and antigenic cross-reactivity with CD59.[148] Plasmids in *S. typhimurium* and *Y. enterocolitica* contain the *rck* and *Ail* genes, respectively, which encode products of a family of virulence-associated outer membrane proteins. By preventing C9 polymerization, these proteins mediate serum resistance and therefore function similarly to CD59.[149,150]

Capsular polysaccharides are another example of microbial surface structures that modulate the effects of complement deposition on the organism and interaction of the organism with the host. In the absence of specific antibody, these polysaccharides—especially those on serogroup B and Y meningococci and type III group B streptococci—contain sialic acid and are poor activators of complement. The capsule, by masking C3 deposited on subcapsular structures, serves to block its interaction with appropriate complement receptors on phagocytic cells. These effects account in large measure for the antiphagocytic properties of these structures. In addition, capsular polysaccharides and outer membrane blebs are shed during organism growth and complement attack. Shedding serves to abort complement attack at the organism surface and may act to decoy complement activation away from the intact organism.[132] The ability of capsular-specific antibody to reverse these effects is testimony to the importance of antibody in redirecting complement deposition to a relevant site on the surface of the organism.[151] In an analogous manner, the long lipopolysaccharide O-antigen side chains on gram-negative bacilli restrict complement activation to sites distant from the outer membrane and hinder access of C5b-9 complexes to it. The failure of these complexes to localize to hydrophobic domains in the outer membrane results in their shedding and the survival of the organism and contributes to serum resistance.[132,152]

Gram-negative bacteria possessing truncated lipopolysaccharide molecules (e.g., *Haemophilus influenzae,* meningococci, gonococci) are not innately resistant to the bactericidal effects of the complement system but do require antibody for effective sensitization and complement deposition. The absence of bactericidal antibody renders these organisms serum resistant and contributes to greater frequency of *H. influenzae* and meningococcal disease during the first several years of life.

Gonococci isolated from patients with disseminated gonococcal infection are resistant to the bactericidal activity of normal human serum.[153] The serum resistance of these strains is multifactorial. In the absence of bactericidal antibody, the MAC is assembled on the organism surface but fails to insert properly into the outer membrane.[154,155] MAC insertion and killing occur normally in the presence of antilipopolysaccharide IgG found in the convalescent serum of some patients with this infection.[156,157] However, some sera also contain IgG specific for gonococcal outer membrane protein 3.[158,159] This antibody competes with bactericidal antibody for binding sites on the surface of the organism, thereby blocking its bactericidal effect. Although the blocking antibody promotes complement deposition on the organism, it apparently does so at sites that do not lead to the killing of the organism.[160] Blocking antibody also appears to account for the resistance of meningococci to killing by the serum of some adults who acquire this infection.[161,162] These findings illustrate the influence of the composition of the outer membrane of gram-negative bacteria in determining sensitivity to complement-mediated killing and the importance to the host of specific antibody in overcoming the resistance of these organisms to killing.[163]

Appreciation has been growing of the number of intracellular pathogens that use complement receptors to gain entry into cells.[106] Entry in this fashion varies as to whether it initiates an appropriate signal transduction response, and whether it is sufficient to establish effective intracellular infection. For example, gp350 on Epstein-Barr virus serves as a ligand for CR2 to initiate viral entry into B cells. The resulting cellular transformation probably contributes to the polyclonal gammopathy observed early in infectious mononucleosis.[164-166] In addition to its factor H binding domain, HIV gp120 contains several C3b binding regions. Cells harboring latent HIV can be activated by the uptake of additional HIV or other particles via CR3. Interactions via this receptor can induce the cellular transcription factor NFκB, which in turn binds to promoter regions in the virus to stimulate generation of progeny virus. *Leishmania* species, *Legionella pneumophila,* and various *Mycobacteria* and *Babesia* spp. also use CR1 and CR3, alone or in combination, to gain intracellular access. The effects of these modes of entry on cellular activation and organism replication have not been well elucidated. However, recent clinical data support a striking association of MBP gene polymorphisms with susceptibility to mycobacterial infections: Individuals with a polymorphism that results in low serum MBP concentrations had a lower incidence of infection than those with a polymorphism that results in high MBP serum concentrations. These data are supportive of a clinically important role for complement and its receptors in promoting intracellular access to these organisms.[4,37]

Over the past decade, our concept of extracellular organisms has been modified by the recognition that many of these organisms can enter and survive in epithelial cells. Both meningococcus and gonococcus, like measles virus, use CD46 (see Table 7-2) to gain entry to such cells to activate intracellular signaling cascades that are important for their infectivity.[167,168]

COMPLEMENT DEFICIENCY STATES

Frequency

Complement deficiency states can be either acquired or inherited. Acquired deficiency states can occur acutely, as part of an abrupt insult such as infection, or in conjunction with chronic rheumatologic or autoimmune disease. The frequency of inherited complement deficiencies in the general population is about 0.03%. Because these states are rare, the usefulness of screening tests is greatest in populations that bear the clinical correlates of abnormal complement inheritance, that is, persons with rheumatologic disease or recurrent bacterial infection.[169,170] The frequency of complement deficiencies reported among persons with these disorders is affected by both methodologic and biologic factors.[171] The most important methodologic variables include sample size and degree of ascertainment. The most important biologic considerations are the ethnic makeup of the population and the incidence of the target disease in that population.

One such study, employing immunologic and functional assays, detected a single individual with homozygous C2 deficiency among 545 patients with rheumatologic disease.[171] This frequency (0.2%) is approximately 10-fold greater than that in the general population. Studies that used DNA typing methodologies have found the frequency of homozygous C2 deficiency in whites with SLE to be about 1.7%.[172,173] These studies provide clear support for the association of complement deficiency states with certain rheumatologic disorders, in particular, SLE.[174]

Reports of an association between systemic meningococcal and gonococcal infections and inherited deficiency of C5, C6, C7, or C8 have led to several studies of the frequency of such deficiencies among patients with these infections. These studies have found as few as 0 of 47 (<2%) and as many as 8 of 16 (50%) complement-deficient individuals who presented with a first episode of documented meningococcal disease.[170,171] Analysis of these studies demonstrates an inverse relationship between the prevalence of complement deficiency in persons with meningococcal disease and the incidence of disease in the general population, that is, high prevalence in populations with hypoendemic disease and low prevalence in populations with epidemic disease (Fig. 7-3). This finding suggests that the overall prevalence of complement deficiencies is relatively constant (0.03% to 0.11%) but that, among populations in which the level of protective antibody is low and meningococcal disease is epidemic, a greater number of

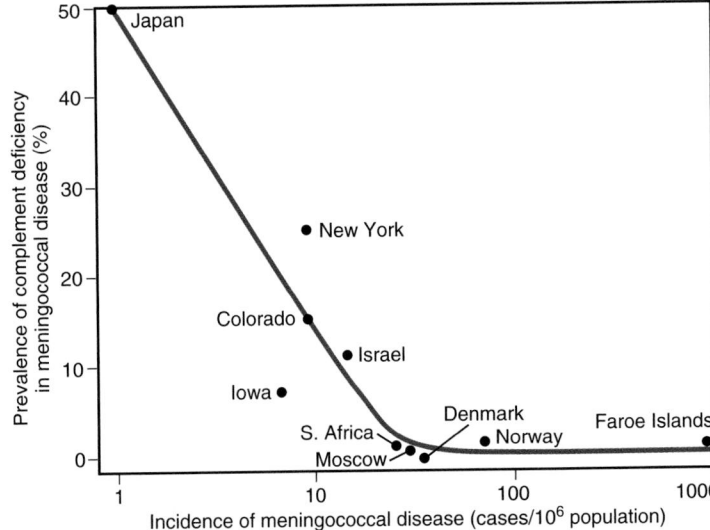

FIGURE 7-3. Relationship between the prevalence of complement deficiency and the incidence of meningococcal disease. *(From Figueroa JE, Densen P. Infectious diseases associated with complement deficiencies. Clin Microbiol Rev. 1991;4:359-395.)*

healthy than complement-deficient persons will be infected because the numbers of healthy persons who lack specific antibody are significantly greater than the numbers of those who are complement deficient. As the level of immunity in the population increases, the incidence of meningococcal disease falls; however, because the prevalence of complement deficiency in the general population is relatively stable, the frequency of infectious states among persons with meningococcal disease increases, that is, complement deficiency becomes a proportionately greater determinant of the risk of infection.[171] The best estimate of inherited complement deficiency states among patients with *endemic* neisserial disease (approximately 10 cases/million population; see Fig. 7-3) is about 5% to 10%. However, the likelihood of complement deficiency is increased dramatically (31%) among patients who have had more than one episode of meningococcal infection, or who have a family history of meningococcal disease.

Although the numbers of infections caused *by S. pneumoniae* and *H. influenzae* appear to be increased in patients with complement deficiencies, the prevalence of complement deficiency among persons with systemic infection caused by these organisms does not appear to be markedly different from that in the population at large.[175] The basis for this apparent paradox, especially for *H. influenzae,* which shares many features with meningococci, is unknown.

Classic Pathway Deficiencies

Patients who lack one of the classic pathway components or who exhibit specific polymorphisms for these proteins exhibit marked susceptibility to autoimmune disease, as well as some increase in the risk of infection. For the purposes of discussion, this section first touches upon methodologic issues in and outcomes of association studies; then, specific pathophysiologic points are addressed that relate these complement deficiencies to SLE and infection.

Disease Association Studies

The association of immune disorders, in particular SLE, with complement deficiency states is most evident in persons lacking C1, C4, C2, or C3 (Table 7-3). Even though these inherited deficiencies are present in a small minority of patients with SLE, their association with this disorder is convincingly underscored by the very high penetrance of the disease in these patients, for example, 87% in patients with C1q deficiency (see later). However, uncertainty exists as to whether both homozygous and heterozygous complement deficiencies constitute a risk factor for SLE, or if only the former states constitute such a risk. Early studies that employed immunologic and functional assays suggested an association in both homozygous and heterozygous deficient persons. More recent studies that used DNA-typing techniques strongly suggest that, at least in C1q and C2 deficiency, the association exists only for the homozygous state.[173,174] Analysis of this issue in patients with partial C4 deficiency is complicated by two factors: the existence of two C4 genes, and the inclusion of null genes among an extended haplotype that contains multiple genes, many of which have been associated with autoimmune disorders.

The existence of two separate C4 genes, C4A and C4B, dictates that complete C4 deficiency (i.e., the absence of the products of all four C4 genetic loci) is extremely rare. Conversely, heterozygous C4 deficiency is very common, occurring in approximately 25% of the general population.[176]

As a result of linkage disequilibrium, the C2 and C4 null genes occur predominantly as part of distinct, extended haplotypes. These haplotypes include MHC I, MHC II, complement, and TNF genes, all of which are candidate disease susceptibility genes. The specific haplotype associated with C2 deficiency—DR2, C4A4, C4B4, BFS, C2Q0, B18, A25, DQB1*0201, DQA1*0501, DRB1*0103, C4B1, C4AQ0, BfS, TNFA*1, TNFB*2, B8, A1—occurs in about 93% of affected persons.[177] For C4 deficiency, this haplotype is HLA-A1, B8, DRB1*0103, DQA1*0501, DQB1*0201, Bf*s, C2*C, C4AQ0, C4B1, TNFA*1, TNFB*2.[178,179] Multivariate analysis of DR and C4 gene types has confirmed an independent contribution of C4AQ0 and DR antigens to the development of SLE. The C4B null gene (C4BQ0) was

not associated with SLE.[180] The chemical preference of the internal thioester in C4A to form amide bonds and to react with immune complexes may contribute to the effect that the C4A null gene has on the development of SLE.[31-33]

Association with Systemic Lupus Erythematosus. The pathophysiologic basis for the association between these complement deficiencies and SLE is incompletely understood, but our emerging understanding of the role of the classic pathway in the clearance of apoptotic cells (see earlier) has provided additional insight and an increasingly compelling logic for this association.[129,130] Despite the insights afforded by studies of these individuals and of genetically engineered complement-deficient mice, it is clear that predisposition to SLE in toto remains genetically multifactorial.[181]

The key clinical features of SLE in complement-deficient persons include its early age of onset (median age, 7 years), increased severity (often with impressive photosensitivity), central nervous system involvement, and increased frequency of glomerulonephritis.[182,183] A striking hierarchy of decreasing penetrance of SLE is seen among classic pathway deficiencies: 93%, 57%, 57%, 75%, and 10% for C1q, C1r, C1s, C4, and C2 deficiencies, respectively. This hierarchical relationship is also generally evident in the severity of SLE and in the frequency and type of autoantibodies present in the sera of these patients. SLE is more severe in patients with C1q, C1r, C1s, or C4 deficiency.[182-186] In persons with C2 deficiency, the severity of SLE appears to be similar to that in the general population, whereas in C3-deficient persons, SLE may be less severe.[175,179]

Additional evidence of the importance of complement deficiency as a predisposing factor for SLE comes from studies of the occurrence of SLE in some patients with acquired hypocomplementemia. Among these studies, C1 inhibitor deficiency is especially interesting because the absence of this regulatory protein is associated with uncontrolled consumption of the classic pathway complement components, which is particularly severe and prolonged in a small number of patients. It appears that it is these patients who are at risk for development of SLE.[183]

The unique functional roles played by the classic pathway, impairment of which seems to play a role in the development of SLE, are (1) elimination of apoptotic cells and (2) clearance of immune complexes.

As noted previously, membrane blebs on apoptotic cells express phosphatidylserine to which C1q can bind, thereby activating the classic pathway and promoting opsonophagocytic elimination by complement receptors on macrophages and mononuclear cells. Engulfment of apoptotic cells via these receptors appears not to initiate a prominent inflammatory response.[129,130] It is interesting to note that sunlight is very effective in inducing apoptosis of cells in the dermis.[24] This observation probably helps explain the photosensitivity rash that is a hallmark of SLE, as well as the positive lupus band test that is demonstrated in skin biopsy specimens of people with SLE regardless of disease activity. The inability of macrophages to clear apoptotic cells effectively is associated with an increased display of apoptotic cell debris on the surfaces of dendritic cells, where it may be presented to autoreactive lymphocytes as an early step in the development of autoantibodies and autoreactive T cells. Particularly intriguing is the observation that membrane blebs on apoptotic cells contain the very macromolecular complexes of ribonucleic proteins to which the autoantibodies observed in SLE are directed, and that the relevant epitopes on these complexes become exposed during incorporation into these blebs.[4,129,130]

Approximately one third of all patients with SLE develop autoantibodies to C1q. The critical role played by C1q in binding to apoptotic blebs places it in proximity to the molecular complexes to which autoantibodies are formed. Perhaps this location contributes to the propensity for autoantibody formation to C1q. Antibody to C1q effectively promotes complement consumption via the classic pathway. The greater the depression in classic pathway components, the greater the potential impairment in the clearance of apoptotic cells—a situation that presumably further impairs apoptotic cell clearance.[187]

TABLE 7-3 Complement Deficiency States

Component	No. of Reported Patients	Mode of Inheritance	Functional Defects	Disease Associations
Classic Pathway				
C1qrs	31	ACD	Impaired IC handling, delayed C′ activation, impaired immune response	CVD, 48%; infection (encaps bact), 22%; both, 18%; healthy, 12%
C4	21	ACD		
C2	109	ACD		
Lectin (mannose-binding) pathway		MBP	Many	
MBP	Many	ACD	Impaired complement activation	Pyogenic infection; meningococcal disease
		ACD	Defective association with MBP	Ulcerative colitis, CVD, pneumococcal disease
MASP-2	1			
Alternative pathway				
D	3	ACD	Impaired C′ activation in absence of specific antibody	Infection (meningococcal), 74%; healthy, 26%
P	70	XL		
Junction of classic and alternative pathways				
C3	19	ACD	Impaired IC handling, opson/phag; granulocytosis, CTX, immune response, and absent SBA	CVD, 79%; recurrent infection (encaps bact), 71%
Terminal components				
C5	27	ACD	Impaired CTX; absent SBA	Infection (*Neisseria*, primarily meningococcal), 58%; CVD, 4%
C6	77	ACD	Absent SBA	Both, 1%
C7	73	ACD		Healthy, 25%
C8	73	ACD		
C9	165	ACD	Impaired SBA	Healthy, 91%; infection, 9%
Plasma proteins regulating C′ activation				
C1-INH	Many	AD; Acq	Uncontrolled generation of an inflammatory mediator on C′ activation	Hereditary angioedema
H	13	ACD	Uncontrolled AP activation→low C3	CVD, 40%; CVD plus infection (encaps bact), 40%; MPGN; aHUS, healthy, 20%
I	14	ACD	Uncontrolled AP activation→low C3	Infection (encaps bact), 100%
Membrane proteins regulating C′ activation				
Membrane cofactor protein	9	ACD/AD	Uncontrolled AP amplification on mast cells	aHUS
Decay-accelerating factor Homologous restriction factor CD59	Many	Acq	Impaired regulation of C3b and C8 deposited on host RBC; PMN, platelets→cell lysis	Paroxysmal nocturnal hemoglobinuria
CR3	>20	ACD	Impaired PMN adhesive functions (i.e., margination), CTX, C3bi-mediated opson/phag	Infection (*Staphylococcus aureus*, *Pseudomonas* spp.), 100%
Autoantibodies				
C3 nephritic factors	>59	Acq	Stabilize AP, convertase→low C3	MPGN, 41%; PLD, 25%; infection (encaps bact), 16%; MPGN plus PLD, 10%; PLD plus infection, 5%; MPGN plus PLD plus infection, 3%; MPGN plus infection, 2%
C4 nephritic factor		Acq	Stabilize CP, C3 convertase→low C3	Glomerulonephritis, 50%; CVD, 50%

ACD, autosomal codominant; Acq, acquired; AD, autosomal dominant; aHUS, atypical hemolytic uremic syndrome; AP, alternative pathway; C′, complement; CP, classic pathway; CTX, chemotaxis; CVD, collagen vascular disease; encaps bact, encapsulated bacteria; IC, immune complex; MBP, mannose-binding protein; MASP, mannose-binding protein–associated serine protease; MPGN, membranoproliferative glomerulonephritis; opson/phag, opsonophagocytosis; PLD, partial lipodystrophy; PMN, polymorphonuclear neutrophil; RBC, red blood cell; SBA, serum bactericidal activity; XL, X-linked.
Data from refs. 163 and 164.

Patients with high concentrations of antibody to C1q may also develop hypocomplementemic urticarial vasculitis. Clinically, these patients present with chronic urticaria and associated leukocytoclastic vasculitis. They may also develop angioedema, airways obstruction, glomerulonephritis, and neuropathy. Their laboratory findings are characterized by profound hypocomplementemia (as measured by total hemolytic complement [CH50]) and marked depression of C1q, C4, and C2 concentrations, as well as a moderate reduction in C3.[187]

Approximately one third of patients with SLE develop antibodies to phospholipids, again presumably as a result of the exposure of these molecules in apoptotic cell blebs. These patients may present with recurrent thrombotic events or spontaneous abortion—the clinical hallmarks of the antiphospholipid syndrome. Recently, fetal wastage in these patients has been shown to be causally related to both placental infarction and massive complement consumption in the fetus. The factors that determine which patients with SLE develop which autoantibodies (e.g., to C1q or phospholipids) are unknown.[187,188]

In addition to altered apoptotic cell elimination, complement-deficient patients with SLE display several distinct abnormalities in immune complex clearance that have been documented by elegant in vivo experiments.[189-192] These abnormalities include (1) increased size of immune complexes, consistent with the key role of C1q in inhibiting complex formation (see earlier); (2) decreased numbers of CR1 on erythrocytes, consistent with their increased removal in association with immune complexes during passage through the spleen[191A] (see earlier); (3) an increased proportion of immune complexes circulating unbound in plasma rather than bound to red blood cells, consistent with both less C3 bound to the complexes and fewer CR1 on erythrocytes; and (4) altered rate and pattern of immune complex clearance by the liver and spleen—a greater number of complexes being removed more rapidly by the liver, with a portion of these being released back into the circulation after a short delay.[127,128,182] The altered clearance reflects the greater proportion of complexes circulating in an unbound state and their uptake by IgG receptors on hepatic macrophages. A portion of these receptors exhibit relatively low affinity for IgG and release the complexes over time. In contrast, splenic removal of immune complexes is almost totally C3 and CR1 dependent. It is important to note that each of these abnormalities, with the exception of CR1 number, is reversed by replacement of the missing complement component,[191] and reduction in the number of circulating immune complexes as a consequence of effective treatment for SLE is associated with an increase in the number of CR1 on circulating erythrocytes. The view of the role of immune complexes and complement in producing tissue injury is changing. Studies in genetically engineered mice suggest that tissue injury reflects a greater role for events consequent to the engagement of immune globulin receptors and also for the phlogistic activities of complement anaphylatoxins, especially C5a.[187]

Association with Infection. The relatively low frequency of infection (20%) in persons with a deficiency of C1, C4, or C2, compared with other component deficiencies (see Table 7-3), has been attributed to the presence of an intact alternative pathway in these patients. Bacterial infection, when it occurs, is usually caused by encapsulated bacteria, especially *S. pneumoniae*, and may be recurrent. The most common sites of infection are the sinopulmonary tree, meninges, and blood.[169,170]

Mannose-Binding Lectin Pathway Deficiencies

MBP Deficiency

In 1976, a group of children with recurrent infection and failure to thrive were described whose serum failed to opsonize *Saccharomyces cerevisiae*. This defect was subsequently found in 5% to 7% of the general population. In 1989, MBP deficiency was identified in a substantial proportion of these patients.[193] Although the association with infection has been best documented in children, it spans the entire age range and has been confirmed in multiple ethnic populations. One study that used genetic techniques found MBP deficiency in 42% of 345 children admitted with infection to a single hospital compared with 24% of 272 children admitted to the same hospital for other reasons. The prevalence of an abnormal MBP gene among infected children was nearly twice that in uninfected children (23% versus 13%), and homozygous deficiency was strikingly prevalent (3%) in the entire group of hospitalized children. In this study, affected patients with MBP deficiency presented with a wide variety of infections caused by a broad range of organisms. Common diagnoses included sinopulmonary infection (31%), meningococcal disease (13%), and fever of unknown origin (10%). The basis for the incomplete penetrance of infection among affected individuals with MBP deficiency is unknown but likely reflects polymorphisms in other genes, as well as environmental effects.[194,195]

MBP is encoded by a single gene that contains four exons. The first exon encodes the signal peptide and the collagen-like region, the second exon encodes the remainder of the collagen region, the third encodes the "neck" region, and the fourth encodes the carbohydrate recognition domain. All three of the known MBP deficiencies that cause mutations are clustered closely in the first exon. Each of these point mutations results in an amino acid substitution that interferes with oligomerization of three single chains to form the mature protein, and each is associated with reduced serum concentrations of MBP.[4,39]

In addition to mutations in the coding portion of the gene, three polymorphic sites are found in the promoter region of the gene: H/L, X/Y, and P/Q. Four of the total possible polymorphic combinations (LXP, LYP, LYQ, and HYP) account for most of the observed promoter haplotypes. These polymorphisms affect transcription of the gene through alterations in the binding of transcriptional factors, with LXP being associated with the lowest MBP serum concentration and

HYP with the highest. These polymorphisms also exist in linkage disequilibrium with the three structural mutations in exon 1 to create haplotypes that differ markedly in their frequency among various populations. Thus, MBP serum concentrations reflect the aggregate effects of promoter polymorphisms, structural gene mutations, and interaction between these two. Low MBP concentrations are associated with an increased risk of pyogenic infection, as noted earlier; however, they may protect against mycobacterial infection. Conversely, high MBP serum concentrations may increase the risk of mycobacterial infection.[4,39]

MASP 2 Deficiency

A single patient with MASP 2 deficiency has recently been described. This patient manifested ulcerative colitis at age 13, erythema multiforme bullosum at age 29, and three episodes of severe pneumococcal infection between ages 28 and 30. Severe hypocomplementemia and antibodies to C1q were documented at age 35, along with low concentrations of MASP 2 and defective association between MBP and MASP 2. MASP deficiency in this patient was shown to be due to a point mutation that resulted in the replacement of an aspartic acid residue by glycine. The substitution of a neutral for an acidic amino acid was postulated to alter tertiary structure and binding function. Recombinant MASP 2 protein bearing this amino acid substitution displayed altered binding to MBP that mirrored that observed in the patient's serum.[196]

Alternative-Pathway Deficiencies

Inherited deficiencies of components of the alternative pathway are less common than those of other complement proteins. To date, no individuals with homozygous factor B deficiency have been identified (see Table 7-3). In the presence of specific antibody, persons with alternative-pathway defects activate the classic pathway normally, but in the absence of specific antibody, a defect in alternative-pathway activation leads to a profound abnormality in complement activation and serum bactericidal activity. Infection in such persons may therefore be expected to have dire consequences, a prediction borne out in patients with properdin deficiency (Table 7-4). However, this prediction is not borne out in factor B knockout mice. These mice breed, develop, and survive normally when reared in conventional housing. They also demonstrate normal lymphoid maturation and antibody production and are no more susceptible to endotoxin challenge than are control mice.[197,198] Resolution of this apparent discrepancy awaits identification of humans with this deficiency.

Properdin deficiency is an X-linked trait that predisposes three quarters of affected persons to meningococcal infection. Such infection is frequently characterized by a fulminant course and a high mortality rate; consequently, recurrent infections are uncommon.[199,200] Three properdin-deficient variants have been described: type 1, characterized by extremely low concentrations (<0.1 μg/mL) of properdin and absent properdin function[199,200]; type 2, characterized by a low concentration (~2 μg/mL) of antigenically detectable but functionally altered properdin; and type 3, characterized by a normal concentration (~25 μg/mL) of antigenically detectable properdin but absent function.[201,202]

C3 Deficiency

Primary C3 Deficiency

Primary C3 deficiency is uncommon (see Table 7-3). As might be expected from its position and function as the linchpin of the complement cascade, virtually all persons with this defect are seriously ill.[169,170] Approximately three quarters develop SLE or a related rheumatologic syndrome. Moreover, the inability to use either the classic or the alternative pathway results in a multitude of severe defects in host defense, including impairments in opsonization, immune response, neutrophil chemotaxis, and the ability to generate serum bactericidal activity. Consequently, severe and recurrent pneumococcal, *H. influenzae,* and meningococcal infections involving the sinopulmonary tree, meninges, and blood stream are common, occurring in about 70% of such patients.[169,170]

TABLE 7-4 Comparison of Meningococcal Disease in Normal and Late Complement Component- and Properdin-Deficient Patients

Characteristics	Normal	Deficient in C5, C6, C7, or C8	Deficient in C9	Properdin Deficient*
No. of homozygotes	—	250	165	54–70
No. with meningococcal disease	—	146	15	25–37
Frequency of infection (%)	0.0072	58	9.1	46–53
Median age at first episode (yr)	3	17	16	14–11.5
Recurrence rate (%)	0.34	44	0	2–1.4
Relapse rate (%)	0.6	7.9	0	0
Mortality per 100 episodes (%)	19	1.5	0	12–51.4
Infecting serogroup				
No. of isolated	3184	67	2	16
B (%)	50	19.4	50	18.7
Y (%)	4.4	32.8	0	37.5

*Where a range is given, the first number refers to documented cases and the second number refers to documented plus probable and possible cases.
From Densen P. Human complement deficiency states and infection. In: Whaley K, Loos M, Weiler JM, eds. Complement in Health and Disease. Dordrecht, The Netherlands: Kluwer Academic Publishers; 1993;173–197, with permission.

Secondary C3 Deficiency

Secondary C3 deficiency is observed in patients with an inherited absence of either factor H or factor I as a result of uncontrolled alternative-pathway activation that leads to C3 consumption and low serum C3 concentrations (<10%). Autoantibodies to either C3 (C3 nephritic factor [C3 nef]) or factor H lead to low C3 concentrations via a similar mechanism. All such patients exhibit varying degrees of susceptibility to infection, especially to meningococcal disease, as a consequence of impaired host defense mechanisms. In addition, patients with factor H deficiency or C3 nef exhibit an increased incidence of type II membranoproliferative glomerulonephritis (see later), and some patients with C3 nef develop partial lipodystrophy (see Table 7-3).[203,204]

Factor H Deficiency

Recent studies have added measurably to our understanding of the role of factor H in normal vascular homeostasis. Factor H is a member of the family of proteins that bind to C3 and C4. These proteins are characterized by SCRs that are responsible for binding specificity (see earlier). As a multifunctional, multiligand binding protein, factor H contains 20 SCRs. SCR 1 to 4 are required for expression of C3 convertase decay and factor I cofactor activity; SCR 1 to 4, 12 to 14, and 19 to 20 play a role in C3b binding; SCR 7, 12 to 14, and 20 mediate binding to heparin and other polyanions, and SCR 7 to 11 are responsible for C-reactive protein (CRP) binding. In its native configuration, the two ends of the factor H molecule are in close proximity, with SCR 20 being directly exposed for binding to its respective ligands. That factor H is the most abundant complement control protein and the third most abundant component overall (see Table 7-1) further attests to its functional importance.[141]

Quantitative Factor H Deficiency—Membranoproliferative Glomerulonephritis

Primary factor H deficiency is an autosomal recessive disorder characterized by low or absent factor H concentrations and low concentrations of C3. As noted earlier, the secondary consumption of C3 that occurs in these individuals is associated with increased risk of infection. A number of these patients also develop type II membranoproliferative glomerulonephritis (MPGN II) at an early age. This disorder is characterized by the deposition of substantial quantities of C3 in glomerular capillary walls and an associated thickening of the glomerular basement membrane with consequent impaired function. Because MPGN II is not a feature of patients with primary C3 deficiency, C3 deposition appears to be a critical pathologic event. The importance of C3 deposition in this pathophysiologic process is supported by the development of histologically typical MPGN II in factor H–deficient pigs and its prevention by infusion of factor H.[205,206]

Qualitative Factor H Deficiency—Atypical Hemolytic-Uremic Syndrome

Hemolytic-uremic syndrome (HUS) is characterized by microangiopathic hemolytic anemia, thrombocytopenia, and acute renal failure. Most cases occur in young people who present with fever and Shiga toxin–positive diarrhea caused by *E. coli* O157-H7. A small percentage of HUS cases occur in patients without diarrhea, and some of these exhibit familial clustering consistent with an autosomal dominant pattern of inheritance.[207,208] Investigation of these patients has led to the identification of persons with normal complement and factor H levels, but whose factor H bears mutations that affect its function. A striking majority of these mutations are clustered in SCR 20, which is exposed and mediates binding to C3b and heparin.[209,210] Factor H from these individuals is fully capable of regulating C3 convertase formation and expressing cofactor activity in the fluid phase, consistent with normal SCR 1 to 4 integrity. However, it binds poorly to C3b or heparin-coated surfaces, as well as to cultured endothelial cells.[211,212]

Hypothesis—C3, Factor H, MCP, and Vascular Disease

The striking deposition of C3 on glomerular capillary endothelial cells in MPGN II and the association of factor H deficiency with MPGN II, as well as its amelioration by factor H replacement, confirm that the loss of normal control of C3 activation and deposition via the alternative pathway plays a key role in the pathogenesis of MPGN II. The basis for preferential C3 activation and deposition in the glomerular vascular bed is unclear but may well be related to the enhanced spontaneous C3 activation that occurs via the alternative pathway in a relatively low pH environment. In the absence of factor H, local C3 activation and amplification lead to unrestrained C3 deposition on glomerular endothelial cells and subsequent MPGN II. The situation in factor H–associated HUS contrasts with MPGN II in that fluid phase activation of the alternative pathway remains regulated under normal conditions. However, a systemic insult that leads to widespread complement activation and C3b deposition on endothelial surfaces provides a nidus for C3 convertase formation that cannot be regulated by the dysfunctional factor H and rapidly exceeds the capacity of factor H that is encoded by the normal allele to control amplification and further C3b deposition. This sequence of events appears critical to the development of HUS in these individuals and provides general insight into the pathophysiology of typical HUS.[211-213]

Further support for these conclusions stems from two very recent reports of atypical hemolytic uremic syndrome in individuals with mutations in the gene encoding membrane cofactor protein (MCP or CD46). CD46 functions in the membrane as a factor H homologue to limit the amount of C3 deposition and amplification of the alternative pathway on host cells. CD46 expression is particularly robust in glomerular capillary endothelial cells. Thus, in the presence of enhanced alternative pathway activation, reduced concentrations of either plasma factor H or membrane CD46 provides an ideal setting for C3 deposition on cell membranes and resultant impairment in cell function as exemplified by both MPGN II and atypical hemolytic uremic syndrome.[213a-c]

Late Complement Component Deficiencies

Persons with a deficiency of one of the terminal complement components exhibit a striking susceptibility to systemic neisserial infections, especially meningococcal disease. Despite the chemotactic defect associated with C5 deficiency, the clinical manifestations of meningococcal disease in persons with this defect and in those with other terminal component deficiencies are remarkably similar.[171] Therefore, the basis for the occurrence of meningococcal disease in these persons appears to be their inability to assemble the MAC and express complement-dependent bactericidal activity.

This conclusion is supported by detailed population-based epidemiologic studies that demonstrate an approximate 5000-fold increase in risk of meningococcal disease in C7-deficient compared with complement-sufficient Japanese patients. In contrast, C9-deficient Japanese patients experienced an approximate 700-fold increase in risk.[214] The increased risk of meningococcal disease in persons deficient in C5, C6, C7, or C8, compared with those deficient in C9, is consistent with in vitro studies demonstrating that C9-deficient sera can kill meningococci, albeit at a slower rate.[114] This dose-response relationship, coupled with the fact that the structural genes that encode these proteins are located on multiple chromosomes, provides strong evidence for a cause-and-effect relationship between the absence of complement-dependent bactericidal activity and the increased susceptibility of these persons to meningococcal disease.

Molecular Basis for Inherited Complement Deficiencies

As with most other inherited conditions, the basis for complement deficiency states exhibits substantial heterogeneity, especially among persons who represent different ethnic or racial ancestries. Within a defined ethnic or racial population, the probability that a single molecular defect will predominate is substantially increased. A corollary of this principle is that the same deficiency occurring among persons of different backgrounds is likely to exhibit molecular heterogeneity. The latter generalization is useful in the selection of patients whose deficiencies, when characterized at the molecular level, are likely to yield new information. Future studies may focus on the possible association of various component polymorphisms with different disease states.

Classic Pathway Deficiencies

C1q is the product of three separate genes (A, B, and C; see Table 7-1). Mutations in each of these genes have been associated with C1q deficiency. A predominant mutation has not yet emerged from the few patients whose defect has been characterized, nor is there any apparent difference in the clinical picture among persons with these various defects.[215]

C2 deficiency is probably the most common of all the complement deficiencies. It occurs predominantly in white persons of northern European extraction and is inherited in association with a distinct haplotype. The molecular basis for this defect in 93% of cases is a 28-bp gene deletion that causes skipping of exon 6 during messenger RNA (mRNA) splicing. Exon skipping in turn results in the generation of a premature stop codon and the synthesis of a nonfunctional protein.[216,217]

The predominant molecular basis for C4A and C4B deficiencies involves large deletions that encompass both the respective C4 and associated 21-hydroxylase genes.[178] A 2-bp insertion in exon 29 of the C4A gene has been reported in association with the haplotype HLA-B60 DR6.[218]

Mannose-Binding Lectin Pathway Deficiencies

MBP and MASP 2 deficiencies that have been characterized are due to point mutations that interfere with secretion of the protein.[37,196] As noted earlier, the serum concentration of MBP also reflects polymor-phisms in the promoter portion of the gene that exist in linkage disequilibrium with the mutations in the structural portion of the gene.[37]

Alternative-Pathway Deficiencies

Factor H deficiency in both humans and pigs is due to point mutations that disrupt disulfide pairing within the SCR modules, which results in their retention in the endoplasmic reticulum and failed secretion of the altered factor H.[219] Functional factor H deficiency is due largely to point mutations in SCR 20 that impair binding of the molecule to C3b, heparin, and endothelial cells, as described earlier.[209-212] The molecular basis for factor I deficiency has been established in two kindred. Three of the four null alleles were identical and led to the substitution of a leucine for a histidine. The altered protein was secreted in vitro, but no factor I was detected in the patients' sera, suggesting that the secreted molecules were catabolized extracellularly.[220]

As noted previously, three phenotypic forms of properdin deficiency have been described based on the concentration and residual function of properdin in patient sera. The molecular basis of this deficiency has been delineated in four families with type 1 deficiency (no detectable properdin), two with type 2 deficiency (low levels of functional properdin), and one with type 3 deficiency (normal levels of a dysfunctional molecule) and has proved to be highly heterogeneous.[221] Type 1 deficiency stems from different mutations, all of which result in premature stop codon formation and the production of truncated proteins, which are presumably neither functional nor secreted.[222] Type 2 deficiency arises from separate mutations that lead to amino acid substitutions that could affect molecular charge. The altered molecules are secreted normally but appear to have an accelerated rate of extracellular catabolism.[222] Type 3 deficiency results from an amino acid substitution that affects neither the secretion of the molecule nor its extracellular catabolism. Instead, folding of the molecule seems to be altered and appears to lead indirectly to a decreased affinity of properdin for C3b.[223]

C3 Deficiency

Primary C3 deficiency is uncommon; when recognized, it has occurred in ethnically diverse populations. The molecular basis for this deficiency, which has been characterized in four patients, has revealed two different splicing defects—a substantial deletion and a single-base-pair change that leads to a defect in C3 secretion.[224]

Late Complement Component Deficiencies

The basis for C5 deficiency is molecularly heterogeneous, with multiple but different defects in whites and African Americans. In one study, all of the African American patients were compound heterozygotes who possessed nonsense mutations in exons 1 and 36.[225]

Several distinct types of C6 deficiency have been described, including complete deficiency and two different subtotal deficiencies, one of which occurs in association with subtotal C7 deficiency. Worldwide, complete C6 deficiency is molecularly diffuse. This deficiency is particularly common among native Africans from the Western Cape in South Africa. Three separate single-base-pair deletions have been described in this population. Of these, the 879delG is most common. Together with an 1195delG null allele, it accounts for a characteristic set of C6/C7 DNA haplotypes. The 1195delG and 1936delG alleles have also been reported in African Americans.[226,227] Isolated subtotal C6 deficiency is caused by an abnormal 5′ splice donor site in intron 15, which results in the reduced secretion of a C6 molecule that is 13.5% shorter than normal but retains functional activity.[228]

A missense mutation in exon 9 appears to account for most cases of C7 deficiency among Israeli families of Moroccan Sephardic Jewish descent.[229] In contrast, deletion of exons 7 and 8 appears to be the predominant cause of this deficiency in the Irish population.[230]

The structural genes for C6 and C7 are tightly linked on chromosome 5 (see Table 7-1). Combined subtotal C6/C7 deficiency (SD) states represent novel combinations of the C6 SD allele with a C7 SD allele and various C6 and C7 null alleles. These partial deficiencies typically come to clinical attention when some initiating event generates production of the C5b6 complex, which in turn converts a partial deficiency to a total one. Persons in whom the two SD alleles are shared in combination with a C6 null allele are functionally C6 SD. Their serum contains a near-normal concentration of C7, despite the presence of the C7 SD allele, because the markedly reduced C6 activity is insufficient to lead to consumption of the existing C7. Complement consumption converts the subtotal state to complete C6 deficiency. In contrast, persons in whom the C6 SD allele is paired with two different C7 SD alleles are functionally C7 deficient, despite the expression, albeit reduced, of functional C7, because the C5b6 complex consumes the C7.[231,232]

Three genes (see Table 7-1) encode the C8 molecule, but defects have been reported in only the A and B genes. C8β deficiency occurs predominantly in white persons, especially those of Russian descent. About 85% of the C8β null alleles described to date have been caused by a C→T transition in exon 9, and 95% of all the C8β null alleles characterized to date have been caused by C→T transitions. It is unclear why C→T transitions should be such a common underlying mechanism for this deficiency.[233] A splicing defect in the C8A gene that results in a 10-bp insertion in the associated RNA has been described as the basis for C8α deficiency in several African Americans with C8α-γ deficiency.[234] In contrast, a point mutation that disrupts the universally conserved 5′ splice site sequence at the boundary between the second exon and intron appears common in the Japanese.[235]

C9 deficiency is particularly common in the Japanese population. In this population, a C→T transition in exon 4 that converts an arginine codon to a stop codon is the dominant mutation associated with this deficiency.[236] The basis for C9 deficiency among white populations is molecularly diverse.[236,237]

Meningococcal Infection in Complement Deficiency States

Meningococcal disease is the single most common infection sustained by persons with complement deficiency, accounting for 75% to 85% of etiologically identified infections.[169,170] Although meningococcal disease has been reported in persons with a deficiency of any of the plasma complement proteins, it is most common in those with a deficiency of properdin, C5, C6, C7, or C8, of whom 50% to 60% experience at least one episode during their lifetime. This striking association confirms the importance of the complement system in host defense against meningococci.

Meningococcal disease in patients with these complement deficiencies exhibits several unique features that help to distinguish it from that in complement-sufficient persons (see Table 7-4). These features provide important clinical clues that should suggest to the clinician the underlying presence of a deficiency and the need to screen for a complement deficiency state. These features are unlikely to result solely from ascertainment bias for the following reasons. First, they have been confirmed in multiple studies in varied populations around the world. Second, each feature has been borne out by investigations of complement-deficient families after exclusion of the proband from the analysis. Third, at least in the case of the late complement component deficiencies, family studies have failed to reveal undiagnosed infection or unexplained or premature death.

Data compiled from the literature and from a detailed population-based study suggest that these complement deficiency states increase the risk of meningococcal disease by 5000- to 10,000-fold. In the general population, the median age at onset of meningococcal infection is 3 years, and 56% of infections occur before 5 years of age; in contrast, the median age of first infection in complement-deficient patients is 17 years, and only 10% of infections occur before 5 years of age. Therefore, most deficient persons pass through the age of life when the deficiency might be expected to increase maximally their susceptibility to meningococcal disease without evidence of that susceptibility. The basis for this observation is unknown, but it suggests that unidentified factors may modulate the susceptibility of deficient persons to infection later in life.

Meningococcal disease in complement-deficient patients is caused by uncommon serogroups—particularly groups Y, W135, and X—more often than in persons without complement deficiencies.[169,170,238]

Conversely, the prevalence of these deficiencies is increased among patients with meningococcal disease caused by these serogroups.[239] The physiologic basis for this observation is not known with certainty, but factors that may be important include (1) the critical requirement for anticapsular antibody for prevention of disease in deficient compared with normal persons; (2) better elimination of group B isolates by phagocytic cells in the absence of capsular antibody[240]; and (3) the propensity for uncommon meningococcal serogroup organisms to cause disease in older persons.[241] Nevertheless, meningococci and gonococci isolated from complement-deficient patients with systemic neisserial infection do not differ significantly in their biologic properties from the same organisms isolated from complement-sufficient patients.[242] Therefore, the absence of complement-dependent bactericidal activity does not automatically provide access to the blood stream to less virulent, serum-sensitive organisms.

Recurrent meningococcal disease, defined as a new infection that occurs more than 1 month after a previous episode, occurs in about 40% to 45% of persons deficient in C5, C6, C7, or C8. This recurrence rate is approximately 100 to 150 times greater than that in the general population. Results of statistical analysis of the number of patients with a specified number of episodes of meningococcal disease are consistent with the interpretation that the risk of meningococcal disease in complement-deficient persons is independent of previous infection,[170] that is, previous disease does not reduce the risk of subsequent meningococcal infection in these patients. In that study, the estimated probability of each infection was 0.39.[170] A similar analysis, using a slightly different statistical approach, led to an identical conclusion and produced an estimated probability of infection of 0.6.[243,244] The latter analysis also demonstrated that the interval between infections (4 to 5 years) did not differ, again suggesting that previous disease does not reduce the risk of subsequent meningococcal infection. The explanation for the failure of previous infection to reduce the risk of subsequent episodes of meningococcal disease in these complement-deficient persons appears to lie in their critical dependence on capsular antibodies for protection and the fact that infection constitutes a relatively poor stimulus for production of these antibodies. These antibodies are highly efficient in promoting opsonophagocytic elimination of meningococci. In contrast, antibodies to subcapsular antigens, although bactericidal and protective in the normal host, are poor opsonins and afford little protection in complement-deficient patients who lack the effector proteins necessary for the expression of bactericidal activity.[245]

Relapse of meningococcal disease, defined as infection with the same serogroup that occurs less than 1 month after the initial infection, is noted in 7.6% of patients deficient in C5 through C8 with meningococcal disease reported in the literature. This frequency, which is approximately 10 times greater than that in the general population, suggests that meningococci may be sequestered intracellularly, where they are relatively protected from antibiotics.[170]

One of the most striking aspects of meningococcal disease in persons with late complement component deficiencies is that, despite a several thousand–fold increase in the risk of infection, they experience a 5- to 10-fold reduction in the chance of dying from the disease, compared with healthy persons.[170] Therefore, the same defect that predisposes to infection appears to provide protection from the lethal consequences of the disease. This remarkable observation suggests that the host's exuberant response to the organism is as much responsible for the clinical manifestations and outcome as is the organism itself. This deduction is supported by the report of Brandtzaeg and colleagues[246] of a close correlation between the extent of complement activation and mortality in meningococcal disease and suggests that the latter is in part dependent on the assembly of the MAC.

The basis for the lower mortality from meningococcal disease observed in persons deficient in late complement components is unknown, but variables that may be relevant include milder disease,[243] the possibility that fewer organisms are required to initiate infection, an ability to better tolerate a given endotoxin load,[247] and less host cell injury.

The possibility that fewer organisms may be required to establish systemic meningococcal disease in deficient than in normal persons is attractive, but data that address this point are conspicuously absent in the literature. Such an effect would account for the increased number of infections and also for the milder disease and the decreased case fatality rate, in that mortality is directly related to the number of organisms in the blood stream.[248,249] A reduction in the organism load might translate into a lower concentration of circulating endotoxin and less systemic inflammation. Alternatively, because insertion of the MAC into the outer membrane of gram-negative organisms results in the release of free endotoxin, the inability of persons with late complement component deficiencies to assemble the MAC may be associated with a reduction in the quantity of circulating endotoxin for a given load of organisms. This reduction in turn might lessen ongoing complement activation and decrease secretion of various cytokines linked to the development of septic shock in meningococcal disease.[246,250-254] Finally, insertion of the MAC into host cell membranes might occur in vivo as a consequence of exuberant complement activation in the vicinity of innocent bystander cells, or as a consequence of endotoxin binding to these cells and subsequent complement activation on their surfaces. For example, MAC insertion activates leukocytes, stimulating release of a plethora of potentially noxious mediators[255-257] and increased expression of procoagulant molecules on endothelial cells.[258] Interruption of these processes in the patient with a late complement component deficiency would result in an improved ability to tolerate a given load of organisms and endotoxin.

Attention has been drawn to functional differences among the various polymorphic forms of the FcγRIIa receptor on phagocytic cells and the possible linkage of a poor IgG$_2$ binding allotype to meningococcal disease in the general population.[259] Characterization of these polymorphisms in patients with late complement component deficiency revealed a significant association of the FcγRIIa allotype with infection, whereas neutrophils from persons with late complement component deficiency without infection were more likely to bear FcγRIIIb and to phagocytose and kill meningococci effectively. These observations suggest a possible explanation for the fact that not all patients with late complement component deficiency become infected with meningococci.[260-262]

Other Complement Deficiency States

Hereditary Angioedema—C1 Inhibitor Deficiency

Persons lacking C1-INH present with a distinctive clinical picture historically referred to as hereditary angioneurotic edema (HANE or HAE).[263] The hereditary form of this disease was recognized more than 100 years ago, and an acquired variant was identified more recently as a distinct entity. HAE is an autosomal dominant disorder, but about 20% of newly identified patients lack a positive family history and reflect spontaneous mutations. Type 1 HAE accounts for 75% to 85% of cases and is characterized by the presence of low (5% to 30%) levels of normal C1-INH protein arising from the intact allele. Type 2 HAE is characterized by the presence of normal to increased levels of antigenic C1-INH, representing a mixture of functional and dysfunctional gene products.[69,263-265]

The acquired forms of this disorder (AAE) are considerably less common. Historically, two variants have been recognized: one occurs in association with B-lymphocyte disorders and the other because of the presence of an autoantibody to C1-INH. However, studies suggest that this distinction may be inaccurate and that autoantibodies account for both types of AAE. Antibody binding does not interfere with cleavage of C1-INH by C1s but rather prevents the formation of a covalent linkage between the enzyme and the cleaved inhibitor. This alteration effectively converts C1-INH from an inhibitor to a substrate and permits C1s action to continue unchecked. In turn, this leads to complement consumption in the fluid phase and associated low levels of C1s, C1r, C4, and C2 that are the hallmark of the disease.[265-267]

Because the hereditary form of this disorder is inherited as an autosomal dominant trait, the serum from all of these patients contains some normally functioning C1-INH.[69] In contrast, persons with the acquired variants have markedly reduced or absent functional C1-INH activity in their serum. As a consequence of this basic difference, the serum from patients with the hereditary form of this disorder contains normal amounts of C1 and C1q but reduced levels of C4 and C2, whereas serum from those with the acquired variants contains strikingly reduced amounts of C1, C1q, C4, and C2.[69,263-265]

The health of patients with this disorder is punctuated by attacks of nonpitting, nonpruritic, and nonpainful edema of the extremities, face, or larynx. Angioedema of the larynx is the most severe complication of the disorder and is a common cause of death in these patients. The gastrointestinal tract may also be affected, and such attacks manifest as episodes of acute, crampy abdominal pain frequently associated with nausea, vomiting, and occasionally diarrhea. In the inherited form of the disorder, attacks generally begin in childhood, increase in frequency and worsen in severity during adolescence, increase during menstruation, are markedly reduced during pregnancy, and diminish gradually in the fifth and sixth decades of life. A typical attack lasts 2 to 3 days. Acute, life-threatening attacks should be treated with C1-INH concentrate. Administration of impeded androgens to increase the biosynthesis of C1-INH has been employed successfully for long-term management of the hereditary form of the disease.[69,263]

The mechanism whereby C1-INH deficiency produces the clinical syndrome of angioedema is incompletely understood. Evidence exists to support a role for both complement-derived and contact system mediators. Intradermal injection of activated C1s leads to nonpainful, nonpruritic swelling in both humans and guinea pigs. This response does not occur if activated C1 is injected into C2-deficient humans or guinea pigs but is observed after injection into C3-deficient patients.[268] These data provide support for a C2-derived anaphylatoxin in the clinical picture of angioedema. However, in addition to its role as the sole inhibitor of C1 esterase, C1-INH is an important inhibitor, if not the major inhibitor, of factor XII and kallikrein. Plasma from patients with HAE exhibits an impaired ability to inactivate these mediators. Detailed studies of a particular family with dysfunctional C1-INH demonstrated that the molecule was defective in its ability to inhibit C1r and C1s but retained full ability to complex and inhibit kallikrein and factor XIIa. None of the 10 family members whose sera possessed this dysfunctional C1-INH had ever experienced an attack of angioedema.[269] These data support an important role for the contact system in the clinical picture of HAE. Together, these separate lines of inquiry suggest that symptoms probably result from the interaction of several factors within these cascade systems.[69,270]

As expected from the different C1-INH protein phenotypes, the genetic basis for HAE is heterogeneous. A substantial proportion of the type 1 HAE defects are associated with mutations within short, interspersed nucleotide elements called *Alu* clusters. These mutations cause a variety of rearrangements that lead to deletions or duplications within the gene, impaired transcription, and reduced levels of specific mRNA and plasma concentrations of C1-INH. In contrast, type 2 HAE, which is generally associated with normal concentrations of a dysfunctional protein, is typically caused by point mutations. These mutations usually affect the arginine at the reactive center of the molecule or amino acids in its immediate vicinity. Occasionally, mutations affect C1-INH glycosylation. In all instances, the mutation leads to the synthesis of a protein with an altered ability to react with its substrates. The resulting altered catabolism is responsible for the normal or elevated concentration of plasma C1-INH.[271-273]

Paroxysmal Nocturnal Hemoglobinuria

Paroxysmal nocturnal hemoglobinuria (PNH) is an uncommon syndrome that typically occurs in adults during their thirties to their fifties. Classically, affected persons present with bouts of intravascular hemolysis that are worse at night and last for several days to weeks. The events precipitating hemolysis are usually inapparent. The basis for the increased hemolysis at night is unclear but may relate to a lower pH in the small vessels of the peripheral venous circulation. In contrast, the more common presentation, which occurs in about half of patients, is one of chronic hemolysis. Patients may have back pain, cramping abdominal pain, and headaches. Although the major clinical features of the disease relate to intravascular hemolysis, the full syndrome includes a propensity to venous thrombosis and diminished hematopoiesis. The thrombosis is unusual in that it typically involves major intra-abdominal and hepatic veins and is often precipitated by surgery.[274-276]

The basic problem in patients with PNH is an increased susceptibility of their erythrocytes to hemolysis. The peripheral blood of these patients contains varying proportions of three populations of erythrocytes. PNH type 1 cells are normal, whereas type 2 and type 3 PNH cells exhibit, respectively, three- to sixfold and 15- to 25-fold increased sensitivity to complement-mediated lysis. The severity of the clinical picture correlates best with the proportion of type 3 cells present in the peripheral circulation.[277]

PNH cells lack more than 20 different surface proteins. The presence of these molecules in normal amounts on endothelial cells in persons with PNH supports the clonal origin of this disorder within bone marrow precursor cells. The feature shared by these proteins is their linkage to the cell membrane through a carboxyl-terminal glycosylphosphatidylinositol (GPI) anchor.[278] PNH arises as a result of a defect in the first step of the synthesis of the GPI anchor responsible for linking the missing surface proteins to the cell membrane. This step is catalyzed by an enzyme that transfers activated *N*-acetyl glucose to the phosphatidylinositol acceptor.[279] This enzyme is the presumed product of the *PIGA* gene, and multiple mutations in this gene have been reported in association with PNH. Unlike most defects that affect synthetic pathways, these genetic abnormalities are expressed in dominant fashion in progeny cells. This unusual event arises because the *PIGA* gene is located on the X chromosome, and the somatic mutations in this gene arise after inactivation of one of the X chromosomes.[276,278]

Two of the proteins that are missing from the membranes of PNH cells are the complement regulatory proteins DAF and CD59.[280,281] The inability to regulate complement deposition on PNH cells explains the underlying pathophysiology of this disorder. It is interesting to note that persons with an inherited defect that affects expression of only DAF on their erythrocyte membranes do not exhibit the PNH phenotype, whereas those lacking solely the CD59 molecule account directly for the increased susceptibility of PNH cells to intravascular hemolysis.

In the absence of CD59, many MACs are inserted into the platelet membrane, cause vesiculation, and provide sites at which prothrombinase is generated with resultant thrombin formation. These alterations may contribute to the susceptibility of patients with PNH to thrombosis. In addition, the absence of the GPI-linked urokinase receptor from PNH cells may render clots more resistant to dissolution, although neither of these abnormalities explains the propensity for intra-abdominal thrombus formation. Similarly, the absence of the GPI-linked FcγRIII receptor from phagocytic cells may contribute to the slightly increased susceptibility of these patients to infection. Studies on the diminished hematopoiesis that occurs in patients with PNH suggest that PNH cells do not possess a proliferative advantage within the marrow. However, in an abnormal marrow in which normal cells are at a survival disadvantage, PNH cells appear to be resistant to abnormal influences and emerge as the predominant cell type. The absence of a GPI-linked receptor (e.g., for a growth factor) has been postulated as the basis for this effect. Whether the factors that contribute to the development of an abnormal marrow environment are the same as those giving rise to the somatic mutation responsible for PNH is unknown.[275,276,278,284]

COMPLEMENT IN DISEASE STATES

The increasing availability of genetically engineered mice coupled with modern molecular techniques is leading to a progressively sophisticated understanding of the role of complement in different types of inflammation and in the pathogenesis of tissue injury and repair. Mediators released during complement activation may play a role in the development of symptoms or in the outcome of these disorders. Evidence that supports this suggestion includes (1) the observation that the extent of complement activation often parallels disease activity, (2) complement deposition at the site of tissue injury, and (3) in animal models of these disorders, the observation that specific manipulation of complement activation modulates the course of disease. The role of complement has been studied most extensively in infectious diseases, rheumatologic disorders, and glomerulonephritis characterized by obvious inflammation. However, it has become increasingly clear that complement activation and mediator generation play important roles in such diverse entities as atherosclerosis,[285] restenosis, postperfusion injury,[286] demyelination disorders,[287-289] a variety of dermatoses,[290] and hyperacute graft rejection in xenogeneic transplantation.[291,292] Damage in these disorders is complement dependent, that is, it can be prevented by complement depletion or by infusion of proteins that regulate complement activation, such as soluble CR1 and CD46,[293-295] or, in the case of xenotransplantation, rejection can be prevented by the development of transgenic animals whose organs express the genes for human complement regulatory molecules.[296]

Infectious Diseases

Complement activation during infection is particularly impressive in diseases like dengue fever, bacterial endocarditis, and sepsis, in which the organisms or their products react with antibodies to form circulating immune complexes and initiate complement consumption. It is especially striking in meningococcal disease, although less so in other forms of gram-negative sepsis and septic shock. Studies have convincingly demonstrated a protective role for complement in endotoxic shock. Genetically engineered C3- and C4-deficient mice did not clear endotoxin as efficiently, had higher levels of TNF and IL-1, and had much higher mortality rates than did wild-type mice. C1-INH and fibrinogen levels were also lower in the deficient mice. Reconstitution of the deficient mice with C1-INH significantly reduced mortality and restored fibrinogen concentrations to normal, despite the persistent deficiency of C3 or C4. Together, these findings indicate that endotoxin-containing immune complexes initiate complement consumption via the classic pathway, and that failure to incorporate C3 into the immune complexes leads to deficient endotoxin clearance, ongoing complement consumption, and C1-INH depletion. The absence of C1-INH permits contact system activation, as manifested by fibrinogen consumption (a potential counterpart of disseminated intravascular coagulation in humans). The fact that C1-INH replacement protected the deficient animals and restored fibrinogen levels to normal strongly implicates the direct involvement of the contact system in endotoxic shock and death.[297] Subsequent experiments have demonstrated that the immune complexes that initiated this sequence of events were composed of IgM natural antibody with specificity for the endotoxin O-antigen.[298] In this respect, these results are reminiscent of those implicating natural antibody and complement consumption via the classic pathway in reperfusion injury.[286]

Studies strongly implicate C5a as a key mediator in the development of septic shock and the acute respiratory distress syndrome in humans,[299,300] as well as in a monkey model of gram-negative shock[301] and in the cecal ligation puncture (CLP) model of sepsis in the rat. Of the two animal models, CLP most closely mimics sepsis in humans; affected rats, left untreated, die in 4 to 5 days.[302] Investigators who have used this model have demonstrated substantial C5a bound to neutrophils, which in turn exhibit a markedly suppressed oxidative burst. Treatment of the animals with anti-C5a antibody at the time of CLP reduces rat mortality by 50%, prevents neutrophil dysfunction, and is associated with a marked reduction in bacterial counts in the blood, liver, and spleen.[302] These studies also show that C5aR expression is upregulated in the lung, liver, kidney, and heart early in the course of sepsis, and that blockade of this receptor with specific antibody not only improves survival but also reduces the serum concentrations of IL-6 and TNF-α.[303] Immune suppression is a newly recognized hallmark of sepsis in humans, as is evidenced by the depletion of lymphocytes in the white pulp of the spleen and by peripheral lymphocytopenia that is temporally associated with the multiorgan failure syndrome.[304] In the CLP model, immunodysregulation occurs as a result of caspase-dependent, NFκB-independent apoptosis of T lymphocytes in the context of decreased expression of Bcl-X$_L$. Lymphocyte apoptosis can be blocked by anti-C5a administration.[305] Whether this apoptosis-sparing effect is due to direct inhibition of events downstream from the ligation of T-cell lymphocyte C5aR or is a consequence of decreased cytokine levels (e.g., IL-6) is currently unknown.[306]

Complement, in conjunction with the reticuloendothelial system, plays a critical role in the removal of encapsulated bacteria from the blood stream.[307] Delineation of the contribution of these variables to the clearance process, which has been accomplished in an animal model of pneumococcal bacteremia, has demonstrated that the more virulent the organism, the greater the role of the spleen in performing this clearance function.[308,309] Complement depletion led to a significant decrease in the number of pneumococci needed to kill 50% of the animals, demonstrating an important role for complement in the clearance function. In addition, clearance of pneumococci was similar in healthy and in C4-deficient animals, indicating that complement activation and fixation to bacteria via the alternative pathway were particularly relevant in this process. Moreover, the presence of immune antibody shifted the burden of clearance from the spleen to the liver, and this effect was absolutely dependent on a functional alternative-complement pathway.[310]

Rheumatologic Disorders

Substantial clinical and experimental evidence links complement deficiency syndromes and complement activation to a variety of rheumatologic diseases, most notably SLE.[311] Additional support for this relation is the finding that pharmacologic agents (e.g., hydralazine, isoniazid) associated with medication-induced SLE inactivate C4 by nucleophilic attack on its internal thioester and formation of amide bonds.[312] Evidence that complement activation may be associated with manifestations of the disease and with tissue injury includes the demonstration of C3 and immune complex deposition at the dermal-epidermal junction in cutaneous lesions from patients with either SLE or discoid lupus erythematosus. Similar immunohistochemical alterations have been demonstrated in biopsy specimens of healthy skin from the same patients. However, the finding of MAC in areas of affected but not unaffected skin from these patients strengthens the hypothesis that complement activation may partially mediate tissue injury in these disorders.[290]

Incorporation of C3 into immune complexes promotes their binding to C3b receptors (CR1) on erythrocytes, as has been noted earlier. Erythrocyte CR1 are removed along with immune complexes during passage through the liver and spleen. The number of erythrocyte CR1 molecules is reduced in persons with disorders such as SLE that are characterized by circulating immune complexes.[191A] The degree of CR1 reduction correlates well with disease activity and with the extent of complement activation. The decrease in CR1, coupled with the inability of circulating erythrocytes to resynthesize them, further exacerbates the defect in immune complex clearance, thereby promoting their deposition in the tissues, with resultant damage to the host. The number of erythrocyte CR1 molecules returns to the genetically prescribed level once the disease is controlled and erythrocyte numbers have returned to normal.

Renal Disorders

Complement deposition in renal diseases that are associated with immune disorders is related to the deposition of immune complexes within the kidney,[313-319] whereas complement deposition in the absence of immune complexes is postulated to occur through activation of the alternative pathway.[320] In a rat model of chronic tubulointerstitial disease, loss of renal mass and function was correlated with increased ammonia production and systemic acidosis. Under these conditions, peritubular deposition of C3 and the MAC was readily demonstrated. However, deposition of these components and evidence of tubulointerstitial inflammation were markedly decreased in diseased animals treated with sodium bicarbonate. These and other findings indicate that ammonia attacks the C3 internal thioester to form amidated C3. Amidated C3 serves to activate the alternative-complement pathway in the fluid phase, leads to C3 and C5b-9 deposition in the tissue, and

elicits an inflammatory response and tissue injury.[320,321] The resulting intrarenal complement depletion may also contribute to the development of chronic bacterial pyelonephritis.[322]

Experiments using C6-sufficient and -deficient rabbits and the infusion of C8-deficient serum into rats have clearly demonstrated that the development of proteinuria in membranous glomerulonephritis depends on the assembly and deposition of a complete MAC on the glomerular epithelial cells.[315,318] A substantial portion of this injury results from MAC-mediated stimulation of prostaglandin and thromboxane synthesis because development of proteinuria was reduced by treatment with indomethacin, an inhibitor of cyclooxygenase.[323]

Many patients with chronic renal disease ultimately require hemodialysis. Exposure of plasma to first-use filter membranes during dialysis results in complement activation.[324] Anaphylatoxins released during this process (e.g., C5a) have been associated in a concentration-dependent and temporal fashion with the onset of respiratory distress in some dialysis patients.[300,324,325] This association is believed to relate in part to C5a-dependent neutrophil aggregation and stimulation and the formation of microemboli and their deposition in the lung (see Chapter 8).[300]

EVALUATION AND TREATMENT OF COMPLEMENT DISORDERS

Evaluation

Evaluation of the complement system is indicated when the diagnosis of a complement deficiency state is being considered, or when specific measures of complement proteins are being used to assess disease activity or response to therapy. As has been pointed out previously, several clinical clues should lead the clinician to suspect a complement deficiency state.[169,170] Foremost among these is a medical or family history of recurrent systemic infection caused by encapsulated bacteria, especially meningococci. A family history of fulminant meningococcal disease occurring in males in alternate generations should suggest the possibility of X-linked properdin deficiency. Meningococcal disease occurring in persons older than 10 years of age, especially when caused by non–group B meningococci, warrants evaluation of the complement system, because 5% to 10% of these patients have a complement deficiency state, even in the absence of recurrent disease. Likewise, a history of SLE in family members or the occurrence of atypical features of SLE should also suggest the need for evaluation of the complement system. Specific syndromes, including HUS, partial lipodystrophy, angioedema, and PNH, are other indications for assessment of complement function.

Any of a number of specific complement deficiencies can produce one of the typical clinical syndromes associated with these disorders; hence, it is important in the initial evaluation of such patients that a test be used that measures the function of the entire complement cascade. For the purposes of diagnosing a complement deficiency, complement assessment should be done when the patient has recovered from any acute illness, or after the disease has been controlled by treatment. The most common of these tests is the CH_{50}, which measures the function of the classic and terminal complement pathways. When defects in the alternative pathway are being considered, an analogous test that evaluates alternative-pathway function should be requested. Many hospital laboratories do not perform the latter test, so it may be necessary to contact a research or commercial laboratory with specific expertise in this area. A negative or extremely low result in either of these two assays warrants further diagnostic evaluation. The combined results of the tests of classic and alternative-pathway functions should suggest which additional tests need to be performed. If both the classic and alternative-pathway CH_{50} values are extremely low, the defect must lie in one of the components shared by both pathways: C3 through C9 (see Fig. 7-1). If the alternative pathway is normal but the classic pathway is not, the deficient component must be C1, C2, or C4. Conversely, a normal classic but a defective alternative pathway suggests a defect in factor D, factor B, or properdin. Diagnosis of these specific defects can frequently be accomplished by the use of immunochemical methods to demonstrate an absence of the relevant antigen. However, several complement deficiency states involve absent function in the presence of normal amounts of antigenic protein. Hence, confirmation of the diagnosis of a specific component deficiency should be documented by specific functional assays for the protein under consideration and by demonstration that replacement of the missing component restores both specific and total complement activity. Such assays usually require the expertise of a laboratory that specializes in complement function.

Treatment

Two major aspects characterize the treatment of patients with complement deficiency states: replacement of the missing protein and prevention of infection. Although advances in our knowledge of the molecular basis of the various complement deficiency states may provide an alternative means of therapy in the future, replacement of a deficient component at the present time usually requires infusion of fresh-frozen plasma. This approach has been successfully employed in therapy for acute attacks of angioedema,[69,263] in restoration of C3 levels toward normal in patients with C3 deficiency, and in treatment of a C2-deficient patient with SLE unresponsive to conventional therapy.[326,327] It has also been recommended as a possible therapeutic option for patients with atypical HUS and dysfunctional factor H. In consideration of this approach, several potential limitations should be considered. First, the half-life of most complement proteins in vivo is short,[9] although a notable exception occurs in patients with low C3 levels caused by factor I deficiency. In these patients, replacement therapy restores factor I activity, thereby markedly reducing the accelerated breakdown of C3 that is observed in this disorder.[328] Second, replacement of a genetically absent protein may stimulate the production of antibody to the missing component, thereby limiting the value of subsequent therapy. This consideration is of limited concern in persons with autosomally inherited disorders such as hereditary angioedema, whose serum contains some normal protein, or in persons with other complement deficiency disorders characterized by the presence of antigenically normal amounts of a dysfunctional protein (e.g., qualitative factor H deficiency). Third, the relative infrequency of infection in most of these patients must be balanced against the potential risk of acquisition of a variety of bloodborne infections during plasma infusion, especially because alternative modes of therapy are available. Whether the short-term infusion of fresh-frozen plasma might be beneficial in the treatment of life-threatening infection,[329] especially in properdin-deficient patients, remains untested. The use of impeded androgens to enhance the in vivo biosynthesis of C1-INH provides a long-term alternative approach to replacement of this protein.[69,263,330]

The development of humanized monoclonal antibodies has opened the door in a highly specific manner to blockade of the complement cascade and its effector functions. For example, anti-C5 is being evaluated for its ability to limit MAC formation and insertion in the red cells of patients with PNH. Monoclonal antibodies to C5a may undergo evaluation for the prevention of sepsis in high-risk patients in the intensive care unit setting.

Prevention of infection in complement-deficient patients is best achieved through vaccination. All deficient persons should be vaccinated with the tetravalent meningococcal vaccine. Those with classic pathway deficiencies should also receive the polyvalent pneumococcal and conjugated *H. influenzae* vaccines. Given the low cost and high potential benefit of these vaccines, all three vaccines should probably be administered to any individual with complement deficiency. Conjugate vaccines, such as that for *H. influenzae*, which initiate a T-cell–dependent response, stimulate the production of higher antibody concentrations and their longer persistence, and induce immunologic memory. The elicitation of T-cell help by such vaccines circumvents the qualitative defect in antibody production observed in these patients[331]; thus, when available, these vaccines are preferred.

Successful vaccination leads to the production of anticapsular antibodies that promote utilization of the classic pathway in patients with an alternative-pathway defect and facilitate alternative-pathway utilization in patients who lack one of the classic pathway components.[47,200] In such patients, these antibodies may promote bactericidal activity, as well as microbial elimination, by enhancing opsonophagocytosis.

Neither clinical nor in vitro studies have explored the potential for vaccination to help protect C3-deficient persons from infection. The theoretical basis for this approach lies in the ability of antibody alone to facilitate phagocytic elimination of organisms, albeit at a reduced rate of killing. This property is most relevant to the clearance of organisms from the blood stream via the reticuloendothelial system, in which the structural architecture and lining of the sinusoids with tissue macrophages contribute greatly to surface phagocytosis.[307,308] In view of the suboptimal response to protein and polysaccharide antigens in C1-, C2-, C4-, and C3-deficient humans and animals, documentation of the patient's response to vaccination with these antigens seems prudent.

Although anticapsular antibody cannot enhance serum bactericidal activity in persons with a deficiency of one of the terminal complement proteins, it promotes opsonization and killing of these organisms by phagocytic cells.[240] In vitro studies of prevaccination and postvaccination sera have documented the ability of these patients to respond to the tetravalent meningococcal vaccine and the likelihood that that response will facilitate phagocytic killing of the corresponding meningococci.[245,332,333] In addition, clinical investigations have documented that vaccination reduces the frequency of infection from 0.15 to 0.04 episode per year and prolongs the interval between infections from 3.6 to more than 6 years.[334,335] These studies, like those in other groups of complement-deficient individuals, attest to the usefulness of vaccination as an immunologic means to circumvent the major clinical manifestations of these deficiencies.

An alternative strategy for the prevention of meningococcal disease is the use of prophylactic antibiotics.[336] This approach significantly reduces the frequency of infection in C6-deficient persons and has its greatest use in populations in whom group B disease is highly prevalent.[337] It is unclear whether prophylaxis should be lifelong, or whether the development of antibiotic resistance will limit the efficacy of this approach.

REFERENCES

1. Ross GD. Introduction and history of complement research. In: Ross GD, ed. Immunobiology of the Complement System. Orlando, Fla: Academic Press; 1986:1-20.
2. Ratnoff WD. A war with the molecules: Louis Pillemer and the history of properdin. Perspect Biol Med. 1980;23:638-657.
3. Lepow IH. Louis Pillemer, properdin, and scientific controversy. J Immunol. 1980; 125:471-478.
4. Walport MJ. Complement (two parts). N Engl J Med. 2001;344:1058-1066, 1140-1144.
5. Root RK, Ryan JL. Humoral immunity and complement. In: Mandell GL, Douglas RG Jr, Bennett JE, eds. Principles and Practice of Infectious Diseases. 2nd ed. New York: Churchill Livingstone; 1985:31-56.
6. Morris KM, Aden DP, Knowles BB, et al. Complement biosynthesis by the human hepatoma-derived cell line HepG2. J Clin Invest. 1982;70:906-913.
7. Perlmutter DH, Colten HR. Molecular immunobiology of complement biosynthesis: A model of single-cell control of effector-inhibitor balance. Annu Rev Immunol. 1986;4:231-251.
8. Alper CA, Raum D, Awdeh ZL, et al. Studies of hepatic synthesis in vivo of plasma proteins, including orosomucoid, transferrin, α₁-antitrypsin, C8, and factor B. Clin Immunol Immunopathol. 1980;16:84-89.
9. Ruddy S, Carpenter CB, Chin KW, et al. Human complement metabolism: An analysis of 144 studies. Medicine (Baltimore). 1975;54:165-178.
10. Mier JW, Dinarello CA, Atkins MB, et al. Regulation of hepatic acute phase protein synthesis by products of interleukin 2 (IL-2)-stimulated human peripheral blood mononuclear cells. J Immunol. 1987;139:1268-1272.
11. Baumann H, Richards C, Gauldie J. Interaction among hepatocyte-stimulating factors, interleukin 1, and glucocorticoids for regulation of acute phase plasma proteins in human hepatoma (HepG2) cells. J Immunol. 1987;139:4122-4128.
12. Morgan BP, Gasque P. Extrahepatic complement biosynthesis: Where, when and why? Clin Exp Immunol. 1997;107:1-7.
13. Strunk RC, Cole FS. γ-Interferon increases expression of class III complement genes C2 and factor B in human monocytes and in murine fibroblasts transfected with human C2 and factor B genes. J Biol Chem. 1985;260:15280-15285.
14. Strunk RC, Whitehead AS, Cole FS. Pretranslational regulation of the synthesis of the third component of complement in human mononuclear phagocytes by the lipid A portion of lipopolysaccharide. J Clin Invest. 1985;76:985-990.

15. Hetland G, Eskeland T. Formation of the functional alternative pathway of complement by human monocytes in vitro as demonstrated by phagocytosis of agarose beads. Scand J Immunol. 1986;23:301-308.

16. Notarangelo LD, Chirico G, Chaira A, et al. Activity of classical and alternative pathways of complement in preterm and small for gestational age infants. Pediatr Res. 1984;18:281-285.

17. Johnston RB Jr, Altenburger KM, Atkinson AW Jr, et al. Complement in the newborn infant. Pediatrics. 1979;64(Suppl):781-786.

18. Mills EL, Björksten B, Quie PG. Deficient alternative complement pathway activity in newborn sera. Pediatr Res. 1979;13:1341-1344.

19. Edwards MS, Buffone GJ, Fuselier PA, et al. Deficient classical complement pathway activity in newborn sera. Pediatr Res. 1983;17:685-688.

20. Lachmann PJ, Hughes-Jones NC. Initiation of complement activation. Springer Semin Immunopathol. 1984;7:143-162.

21. Muraoka S, Shulman MJ. Structural requirements for IgM assembly and cytolytic activity: Effects of mutations in the oligosaccharide acceptor site at Asn402. J Immunol. 1989;142:695-701.

22. Wright JF, Shulman MJ, Isenman DE, et al. C1 binding by mouse IgM. The effect of abnormal glycosylation at position 402 resulting from a serine to asparagine exchange at residue 406 of the μ-chain. J Biol Chem. 1990;265:10506-10513.

23. Tao M-H, Canfield SM, Morrison SL. The differential ability of human IgG1 and IgG4 to activate complement is determined by the COOH-terminal sequence of the C_H2 domain. J Exp Med. 1991;173:1025-1028.

24. Korb LC, Ahearn JM. C1q binds directly and specifically to surface blebs of apoptotic human keratinocytes: Complement deficiency and systemic lupus erythematosus revisited. J Immunol. 1997;158(10):4525-4528.

25. Cooper NR. The classical complement pathway: Activation and regulation of the first complement component. Adv Immunol. 1985;37:151-216.

26. Malhotra R, Sim RB, Reid KBM. Interaction of C1q, and other proteins containing collagen-like domains, with the C1q receptor. Biochem Soc Trans. 1990;18:1145-1148.

27. Arlaud GJ, Colomb MG, Gagnon J. A functional model of the human C1 complex. Immunol Today. 1987;8:106-111.

28. Schumaker VN, Zavodszky P, Poon RH. Activation of the first component of complement. Annu Rev Immunol. 1987;5:21-42.

29. Fearon DT. Complement. J Allergy Clin Immunol. 1983;71:520-529.

30. Müller-Eberhard HJ. Molecular organization and function of the complement system. Annu Rev Biochem. 1988;57:321-347.

31. Isenman DE, Young JR. The molecular basis for the difference in immune hemolysis activity of the Chido and Rodgers isotypes of human complement component C4. J Immunol. 1984;132:3019-3027.

32. Law SKA, Dodds AW, Porter RR. A comparison of the properties of two classes, C4A and C4B, of the human complement component C4. EMBO J. 1984;3:1819-1823.

33. Dodds AW, Law SK, Porter RR. The origin of the very variable haemolytic activities of the common human complement component C4 allotypes including C4-A6. EMBO J. 1985;4:2239-2244.

34. Schifferli JA, Steiger G, Paccaud J-P, et al. Difference in the biological properties of the two forms of the fourth component of human complement (C4). Clin Exp Immunol. 1986;63:473-477.

35. Schifferli JA, Hauptmann G, Paccaud J-P. Complement-mediated adherence of immune complexes to human erythrocytes. FEBS Lett. 1987;213:415-418.

36. Naama JK, Niven IP, Zoma A, et al. Complement, antigen-antibody complexes and immune complex disease. J Clin Lab Immunol. 1985;17:59-67.

37. Jack DL, Klein NJ, Turner MW. Mannose-binding lectin: Targeting the microbial world for complement attack and opsonophagocytosis. Immunol Rev. 2001;180:86-99.

38. Wallis R. The lectin-pathway of complement activation: MBL, other collectins and ficolins. Immunobiology. 2002;204:433-445.

39. Schwaeble W, Dahl MR, Thiel S, et al. The mannan-binding lectin-associated serine proteases (MASPs) and MAp19: Four components of the lectin pathway activation complex encoded by two genes. Immunobiology. 2002;205:455-466.

40. Pangburn MK, Müller-Eberhard HJ. The alternative pathway of complement. Springer Semin Immunopathol. 1984;7:163-192.

41. Pangburn MK. The alternative pathway. In: Ross GD, ed. Immunobiology of the Complement System. Orlando, Fla: Academic Press; 1986:45-62.

42. Densen P, McRill C, Ross SC. The contribution of the alternative and classical complement pathways to gonococcal killing and C3 fixation. In: Poolman JT, Zanen HC, Meyer TF, et al, eds. Gonococci and Meningococci. Dordrecht: Kluwer Academic Publishers; 1988:693-697.

43. Gordon DL, Hostetter MK. Complement and host defense against microorganisms. Pathology. 1986;18:365-375.

44. Fearon DT, Austen KF. Properdin: Initiation of alternative complement pathway. Immunology. 1975;72:3220-3224.

45. Fearon DT, Austen KF. Properdin: Binding to C3b and stabilization of the C3b-dependent C3 convertase. J Exp Med. 1975;142:856-863.

46. Fearon DT, Austen KF. The alternative pathway of complement: A system for host resistance to microbial infection. N Engl J Med. 1980;303:259-263.

47. Söderström C, Braconier JH, Danielsson D, et al. Bactericidal activity for *Neisseria meningitidis* in properdin-deficient sera. J Infect Dis. 1987;156:107-112.

48. Schenkein HA, Ruddy S. The role of immunoglobulins in alternative complement pathway activation by zymosan: II. The effect of IgG on the kinetics of the alternative pathway. J Immunol. 1981;126:11-15.

49. Ratnoff WD, Fearon DT, Austen KF. The role of antibody in the activation of the alternative complement pathway. Springer Semin Immunopathol. 1983;6:361-371.

50. Winkelstein JA, Shin HS. The role of immunoglobulin in the interaction of pneumococci and the properdin pathway: Evidence for its specificity and lack of requirement for the Fc portion of the molecule. J Immunol. 1974;112:1635-1642.

51. Nelson B, Ruddy S. Enhancing role of IgG in lysis of rabbit erythrocytes by the alternative pathway of human complement. J Immunol. 1979;122:1994-1999.

52. Schenkein HA, Ruddy S. The role of immunoglobulins in alternative complement pathway activation by zymosan: I. Human IgG with specificity for zymosan enhances alternative pathway activation by zymosan. J Immunol. 1981;126:7-10.

53. Nicholson-Weller A, Daha MR, Austen KF. Different functions for specific guinea pig IgG1 and IgG2 in the lysis of sheep erythrocytes by C4-deficient guinea pig serum. J Immunol. 1981;126:1800-1804.

54. Capel PJA, Groeneboer O, Grosveld G, et al. The binding of activated C3 to polysaccharides and immunoglobulins. J Immunol. 1978;121:2566-2572.

55. Fries LF, Gaither TA, Hammer CH, et al. C3b covalently bound to IgG demonstrates a reduced rate of inactivation by factors H and I. J Exp Med. 1984;160:1640-1655.

56. Joiner KA, Fries LF, Schmetz MA, et al. IgG bearing covalently bound C3b has enhanced bactericidal activity for *Escherichia coli* O111. J Exp Med. 1985;162:877-889.

57. Lambris JD, Müller-Eberhard HJ. The multifunctional role of C3: Structural analysis of its interactions with physiological ligands. Mol Immunol. 1986;23:1237-1242.

58. Wetsel RA, Lemons RS, Le Beau MM, et al. Molecular analysis of human complement component C5: Localization of the structural gene to chromosome 9. Biochemistry. 1988;27:1474-1482.

59. Lundwall AB, Wetsel RA, Kristenson T, et al. Isolation and sequence analysis of a cDNA clone encoding the fifth complement component. J Biol Chem. 1985;260:2108-2112.

60. Pangburn MK, Rawal N. Structure and function of complement C5 convertase enzymes. Biochem Soc Trans. 2002;30:1006-1010.

61. Müller-Eberhard HJ. The membrane attack complex of complement. Annu Rev Immunol. 1986;4:503-528.

62. Stanley K, Luzio P. A family of killer proteins. Nature. 1988;334:475-476.

63. Tschopp J, Mollnes T-E. Antigenic crossreactivity of the α subunit of complement component C8 with the cysteine-rich domain shared by complement component C9 and low density lipoprotein receptor. Proc Natl Acad Sci U S A. 1986;83:4223-4227.

64. Haefliger J-A, Tschopp J, Nardelli D, et al. Complementary DNA cloning of complement C8β and its sequence homology to C9. Biochemistry. 1987;26:3551-3556.

65. Monahan JB, Sodetz JM. Binding of the eighth component of human complement to the soluble cytolytic complex is mediated by its β subunit. J Biol Chem. 1980;255:10579-10582.

66. Stewart JL, Kolb WP, Sodetz JM. Evidence that C5b recognizes and mediates C8 incorporation into the cytolytic complex of complement. J Immunol. 1987;139:1960-1964.

67. Stewart JL, Sodetz JM. Analysis of the specific association of the eighth and ninth components of human complement: Identification of a direct role for the α subunit of C8. Biochemistry. 1985;24:4598-4602.

68. Stanley KK, Page M, Campbell AK, et al. A mechanism for the insertion of complement component C9 into target membranes. Mol Immunol. 1986;23:451-458.

69. Davis AE III. C1 inhibitor and hereditary angioneurotic edema. Annu Rev Immunol. 1988;6:595-628.

69a. Fearon DT, Austen KF. The alternative pathway of complement: A system for host resistance to microbial infection. N Engl J Med. 1980;303:259-263.

70. Liszewski MK, Farries TC, Lublin DM, et al. Control of the complement system. Adv Immunol. 1996;61:201-283.

71. Holers VM, Cole JL, Lublin DM, et al. Human C3b- and C4b-regulatory proteins: A new multi-gene family. Immunol Today. 1985;6:188-192.

72. Davies A. Policing the membrane: Cell surface proteins which regulate complement. Res Immunol. 1997;147:82-87.

73. Atkinson JP, Farries T. Separation of self from non-self in the complement system. Immunol Today. 1987;8:212-215.

74. Rollins SA, Zhao J, Ninomiya H, et al. Inhibition of homologous complement by CD59 is mediated by a species-selective recognition conferred through binding to C8 within C5b-8 or C9 within C5b-9. J Immunol. 1991;146:2345-2351.

75. Carney DF, Koski CL, Shin ML. Elimination of terminal complement intermediates from the plasma membrane of nucleated cells: The rate of disappearance differs for cells carrying C5b-7 or C5b-8 or a mixture of C5b-8 with a limited number of C5b-9. J Immunol. 1985;134:1804-1809.

76. Ramm LE, Whitlow MB, Koski CL, et al. Elimination of complement channels from the plasma membranes of U937, a nucleated mammalian cell line: Temperature dependence of the elimination rate. J Immunol. 1983;131:1411-1415.

77. Schlager SI, Ohanian SH, Borsos T. Correlations between the ability of tumor cells to resist humoral immune attack and their ability to synthesize lipid. J Immunol. 1978;120:463-471.

78. Imagawa DK, Osifchin NE, Paznekas WA, et al. Consequences of cell membrane attack by complement: Release of arachidonate and formation of inflammatory derivatives. Proc Natl Acad Sci U S A. 1983;80:6647-6651.

79. Betz M, Hansch GM. Release of arachidonic acid: A new function of the late complement components. Immunobiology. 1984;166:473-483.

80. Carney DF, Lang TJ, Shin ML. Multiple signal messengers generated by terminal complement complexes and their role in terminal complement complex elimination. J Immunol. 1990;145:623-629.

81. Gordon DL, Kaufman RM, Blackmore TK, et al. Identification of complement regulatory domains in human factor H. J Immunol. 1995;155:348-356.

82. Fearon DT, Austen KF. Activation of the alternative complement pathway with rabbit erythrocytes by circumvention of the regulatory action of endogenous control proteins. J Exp Med. 1977;146:22-33.

83. Fearon DT. Regulation by membrane sialic acid of β1H-dependent decay-dissociation of amplification C3 convertase of the alternative complement pathway. Proc Natl Acad Sci U S A. 1978;75:1971-1975.

84. Kazatchkine MD, Fearon DT, Austen KF. Human alternative complement pathway: Membrane-associated sialic acid regulates the competition between B and β1H for cell-bound C3b. J Immunol. 1979;122:75-81.

85. Pangburn MK, Morrison DC, Schreiber RD, et al. Activation of the alternative complement pathway: Recognition of surface structures on activators by bound C3b. J Immunol. 1980;124:977-982.

86. Hugli TE. Biological activities of fragments derived from human complement components. Prog Immunol. 1983:419-426.

87. Ross GD, Medof ME. Membrane complement receptors specific for bound fragments of C3. Adv Immunol. 1985;37:217-267.

88. Wilson JG, Andriopoulos NA, Fearon DT. CR1 and the cell membrane proteins that bind C3 and C4: A basic and clinical review. Immunol Res. 1987;6:192-209.

89. Jack RM, Ezzell RM, Hartwig J, et al. Differential interaction of the C3b/C4b receptor and MHC class I with the cytoskeleton of human neutrophils. J Immunol. 1986; 137:3996-4003.

90. Krych M, Hourcade D, Atkinson JP. Sites within the complement C3b/C4b receptor important for the specificity of ligand binding. Proc Natl Acad Sci U S A. 1991;88:4353-4357.

91. Moulds JM, Nickells MW, Moulds JJ, et al. The C3b/C4b receptor is recognized by the Knops, McCoy, Swain-Langley, and York blood group antisera. J Exp Med. 1991;173:1159-1163.

92. Hynes RO. Integrins: A family of cell surface receptors. Cell. 1987;48:549-554.

93. Wright SD, Levin SM, Jong MTC, et al. CR3 (CD11b/CD18) expresses one binding site for Arg-Gly-Asp-containing peptides and a second site for bacterial lipopolysaccharide. J Exp Med. 1989;169:175-183.

94. Wright SD, Reddy A, Jong MTC, et al. C3bi receptor (complement receptor type 3) recognizes a region of complement protein C3 containing the sequence Arg-Gly-Asp. Proc Natl Acad Sci U S A. 1987;84:1965-1968.

95. Ruoslahti E, Pierschbacher MD. Arg-Gly-Asp: A versatile cell recognition signal. Cell. 1986;44:517-518.

96. Myones BL, Dalzell JG, Hogg N, et al. Neutrophil and monocyte cell surface p150,95 has iC3b-receptor (CR4) activity resembling CR3. J Clin Invest. 1988;81:64-51.

97. Matsumoto AK, Kopicky-Burd J, Carter RH, et al. Intersection of the complement and immune systems: A signal transduction complex of the B lymphocyte-containing complement receptor type 2 and CD19. J Exp Med. 1991;173:55-64.

98. Perlmutter DH, Colten HR. Complement molecular genetics. In: Gallin JI, Goldstein IM, Snyderman R, eds. Inflammation: Basic Principles and Clinical Correlates. New York: Raven; 1988:75-88.

99. Campbell RD. The molecular genetics and polymorphism of C2 and factor B. Br Med Bull. 1987;43:37-49.

100. Campbell RD, Law SKA, Reid KBM, et al. Structure, organization, and regulation of the complement genes. Annu Rev Immunol. 1988;6:161-195.

101. Awdeh ZL, Raum D, Yunis EJ, et al. Extended HLA/complement allele haplotypes: Evidence for T/t-like complex in man. Proc Natl Acad Sci U S A. 1983;80:259-263.

102. Alper CA, Raum D, Karp S, et al. Serum complement "supergenes" of the major histocompatibility complex in man (complotypes). Vox Sang. 1983;45:62-67.

103. Porter RR. Complement polymorphism, the major histocompatibility complex and associated diseases: A speculation. Mol Biol Med. 1983;1:161-168.

104. Kristensen T, D'Eustachio P, Ogata RT, et al. The superfamily of C3b/C4b-binding proteins. FASEB J. 1987;46:2463-2469.

105. Reid KBM, Bentley DR, Campbell RD, et al. Complement system proteins which interact with C3b or C4b: A superfamily of structurally related proteins. Immunol Today. 1986;7:230-234.

106. Seya T. Human regulator of complement activation (RCA) gene family proteins and their relationship to microbial infection. Microbiol Immunol. 1995;39:295-305.

107. Fischer WH, Hugli TE. Regulation of B cell functions by C3a and C3a^{desArg}: Suppression of TNF-α, IL-6, and the polyclonal immune response. J Immunol. 1997; 159:4279-4286.

108. Perez HD, Kelly E, Chenoweth D, et al. Identification of the C5a des Arg cochemotaxin: Homology with vitamin D-binding protein (group-specific component globulin). J Clin Invest. 1988;82:360-363.

109. Kew RR, Webster RO. Ge-globulin (vitamin D-binding protein) enhances the neutrophil chemotactic activity of C5a and C5a des Arg. J Clin Invest. 1988;82:364-369.

110. Perez HD, Hooper C, Volanakis J, et al. Specific inhibitor of complement (C5)-derived chemotactic activity in systemic lupus erythematosus related antigenically to the Bb fragment of human factor B. J Immunol. 1987;139:484-489.

111. Gordon DL, Hostetter MK. Complement and host defense against microorganisms. Pathology. 1986;18:365-375.

112. Hostetter MK, Krueger RA, Schmeling DJ. The biochemistry of opsonization: Central role of the reactive thiolester of the third component of complement. J Infect Dis. 1984;150:653-661.

113. Taylor PW. Bactericidal and bacteriolytic activity of serum against gram-negative bacteria. Microbiol Rev. 1983;47:46-83.

114. Harriman GR, Esser AF, Podack ER, et al. The role of C9 in complement-mediated killing of Neisseria. J Immunol. 1981;127:2386-2390.

115. Cooper NR, Nemerow GR. Complement-dependent mechanisms of virus neutralization. In: Ross GD, ed. Immunobiology of the Complement System. Orlando, Fla: Academic Press; 1986:139-162.

116. Erdei A, Fust G, Gergely J. The role of C3 in the immune response. Immunol Today. 1991;12:332-337.

117. Papamichail M, Gutierrez C, Embling P, et al. Complement dependence of localisation of aggregated IgG in germinal centres. Scand J Immunol. 1975;4:343-347.

118. Bird P, Lachmann PJ. The regulation of IgG subclass production in man: Low serum IgG4 in inherited deficiencies of the classical pathway of C3 activation. J Immunol. 1988;18:1217-1222.

119. Dempsey PW, Allison MED, Akkaraju S, et al. C3d of complement as a molecular adjuvant: Bridging innate and acquired immunity. Science. 1996;271:348-350.

120. Böttger EC, Bitter-Suermann D. Complement and the regulation of humoral immune responses. Immunol Today. 1987;8:261-264.

121. Carroll M. The role of complement in B cell activation and tolerance. Adv Immunol. 2000;74:61-88.

122. Barrington R, Zhang M, Fischer M, et al. The role of complement in inflammation and adaptive immunity. Immunol Rev. 2001;80:5-15.

123. Hostetter MK. Serotypic variations among virulent pneumococci in deposition and degradation of covalently bound C3b: Implications for phagocytosis and antibody production. J Infect Dis. 1986;153:682-693.

124. Suresh M, Molina H, Salvato MS, et al. Complement component 3 is required for optimal expansion of CD8 T cells during a systemic viral infection. J Immunol. 2003; 170:788-794.

125. Miller GW, Nusenzweig V. A new complement function: Solubilization of antigen-antibody aggregates. Proc Natl Acad Sci U S A. 1975;72:418-422.

126. Schifferli JA, Ng YC, Peters DK. The role of complement and its receptor in the elimination of immune complexes. N Engl J Med. 1986;315:488-495.

127. Siegel I, Liu TL, Gleicher N. The red-cell immune system. Lancet. 1981;2:556-559.

128. Cornacoff JB, Hebert LA, Smead WL, et al. Primate erythrocyte-immune complex-clearing mechanism. J Clin Invest. 1983;71:236-247.

129. Mevorach D, Mascarenhas J, Gershov D, et al. Complement-dependent clearance of apoptotic cells by human macrophages. J Exp Med. 1998;188:2313-2320.

130. Taylor PR, Carugati A, Fadok V, et al. A hierarchical role for classical pathway complement proteins in the clearance of apoptotic cells in vivo. J Exp Med. 2000; 192:359-366.

131. Roantree RJ, Rantz LA. A study of the relationship of the normal bactericidal activity of human serum to bacterial infection. J Clin Invest. 1960;39:72-81.

132. Joiner K. Complement evasion by bacteria and parasites. Annu Rev Microbiol. 1988;42:201-230.

133. Cooper NR. Complement evasion strategies of microorganisms. Immunol Today. 1991;12:327-332.

134. Leive LL, Jimenez-Lucho VE. Lipopolysaccharide O-antigen structure controls alternative pathway activation of complement: Effects on phagocytosis and virulence of Salmonella. In: Leive L, ed. Microbiology. Washington, DC: American Society for Microbiology; 1986:14-17.

135. Liang-Takasaki C-J, Mäkelä PH, Leive L. Phagocytosis of bacteria by macrophages: Changing the carbohydrate of lipopolysaccharide alters interaction with complement and macrophages. J Immunol. 1982;128:1229-1235.

136. Liang-Takasaki C-J, Saxén H, Mäkelä PH, et al. Complement activation by polysaccharide of lipopolysaccharide: An important virulence determinant of Salmonella. Infect Immun. 1983;41:563-569.

137. Grossman N, Leive L. Complement activation via the alternative pathway by purified Salmonella lipopolysaccharide is affected by its structure but not its O-antigen length. J Immunol. 1984;132:376-385.

138. Grossman N, Joiner KA, Frank MM, et al. C3b binding, but not its breakdown, is affected by the structure of the O-antigen polysaccharide in lipopolysaccharide from Salmonella. J Immunol. 1986;136:2208-2215.

139. Jimenez-Lucho VE, Joiner KA, Foulds J, et al. C3b generation is affected by the structure of the O-antigen polysaccharide in lipopolysaccharide from Salmonella. J Immunol. 1987;139:1253-1259.

140. Hall BF, Joiner KA. Developmentally regulated virulence factors of Trypanosoma cruzi and their relationship to evasion of host defences. J Eukaryot Microbiol. 1993; 40:207-213.

141. Zipfel PF, Skerka C, Hellwage J, et al. Factor H family proteins: On complement, microbes and human diseases. Biochem Soc Trans. 2002;30:971-978.

142. Thern A, Stenberg L, Dahlbäck B, et al. Ig-binding surface proteins of Streptococcus pyogenes also bind human C4b-binding protein (C4BP), a regulatory component of the complement system. J Immunol. 1995;154:375-386.

143. Lachmann PJ, Davies A. Complement and immunity to viruses. Immunol Rev. 1997;159:69-77.

144. Kotwal GJ, Moss B. Vaccinia virus encodes a secretory polypeptide structurally related to complement control proteins. Nature. 1988;335:176-178.

145. Kotwal GJ, Isaacs SN, McKenzie R, et al. Inhibition of the complement cascade by the major secretory protein of vaccinia virus. Science. 1990;250:827-830.

146. Smith H, Cole JA, Parsons NJ. The sialylation of gonococcal lipopolysaccharide by host factors: A major impact on pathogenicity. FEMS Microbiol Lett. 1992;100: 287-292.

147. Stoiber H, Clivio A, Dierich MP. Role of complement in HIV infection. Ann Rev Immunol. 1997;15:649-674.

148. Braga LL, Ninomiya H, McCoy JJ, et al. Inhibition of the complement membrane attack complex by the galactose-specific adhesin of Entamoeba histolytica. J Clin Invest. 1992;90:1131-1137.

149. Heffernan EJ, Reed S, Hackett J, et al. Mechanism of resistance to complement-mediated killing of bacteria encoded by the Salmonella typhimurium virulence plasmid gene rck. J Clin Invest. 1992;90:953-964.

150. Bliska JB, Falkow S. Bacterial resistance to complement killing mediated by the Ail protein of Yersinia enterocolitica. Proc Natl Acad Sci U S A. 1992;89:3561-3565.

151. Brown EJ. Interaction of gram-positive microorganisms with complement. Curr Top Microbiol Immunol. 1985;121:159-197.

152. Joiner KA, Grossman N, Schmetz M, et al. C3 binds preferentially to long-chain lipopolysaccharide during alternative pathway activation by Salmonella montevideo. J Immunol. 1986;136:710-715.

153. Schoolnik GK, Buchman TM, Holmes KK. Gonococci causing disseminated gonococcal infection are resistant to the bactericidal action of normal human sera. J Clin Invest. 1976;58:1163-1173.

154. Joiner KA, Warren KA, Brown EJ, et al. Studies on the mechanism of bacterial resistance to complement-mediated killing: IV. C5b-9 forms high molecular weight complexes with bacterial outer membrane constituents on serum-resistant but not on serum-sensitive *Neisseria gonorrhoeae*. J Immunol. 1983;131:1443-1451.

155. Harriman GR, Podack ER, Braude AI, et al. Activation of complement by serum-resistant *Neisseria gonorrhoeae*. J Exp Med. 1982;156:1235-1249.

156. Rice PA, Kasper DL. Characterization of gonococcal antigens responsible for induction of bactericidal antibody in disseminated infection. J Clin Invest. 1977;60:1149-1158.

157. Densen P, Gulati S, Rice PA. Specificity of antibodies against *Neisseria gonorrhoeae* that stimulate neutrophil chemotaxis: Role of antibodies directed against lipooligosaccharides. J Clin Invest. 1987;80:78-87.

158. Rice PA, Kasper KL. Characterization of serum resistance of *Neisseria gonorrhoeae* that disseminate: Roles of blocking antibody and gonococcal outer membrane proteins. J Clin Invest. 1982;70:157-167.

159. Rice PA, Vayo HE, Tam MR, et al. Immunoglobulin G antibodies directed against protein III block killing of serum-resistant *Neisseria gonorrhoeae* by immune serum. J Exp Med. 1986;164:1735-1748.

160. Joiner KA, Scales R, Warren KA, et al. Mechanism of action of blocking immunoglobulin G for *Neisseria gonorrhoeae*. J Clin Invest. 1985;76:1765-1772.

161. Griffiss MJ, Bertram MA. Immunoepidemiology of meningococcal disease in military recruits: II. Blocking of serum bactericidal activity by circulating IgA early in the course of invasive disease. J Infect Dis. 1977;136:733-739.

162. Griffiss JM. Epidemic meningococcal disease: Synthesis of a hypothetical immunoepidemiologic model. Rev Infect Dis. 1982;4:159-172.

163. Frank MM, Joiner K, Hammer C. The function of antibody and complement in the lysis of bacteria. Rev Infect Dis. 1987;9(Suppl 5):537-545.

164. Cooper NR, Moore MD, Nemerow GR. Immunobiology of CR2, the B lymphocyte receptor for Epstein-Barr virus and the C3d complement fragment. Annu Rev Immunol. 1988;6:85-113.

165. Fingeroth JD, Weis JJ, Tedder TF, et al. Epstein-Barr virus receptor of human B lymphocytes is the C3d receptor CR2. Proc Natl Acad Sci U S A. 1984;81:4510-4514.

166. Montefiori DC, Stewart K, Ahearn JM, et al. Complement-mediated binding of naturally glycosylated and glycosylation-modified human immunodeficiency virus type 1 to human CR2 (CD21). J Virol. 1993;67:2699-2706.

167. Lee SW, Bonnah RA, Higashi DL, et al. CD46 is phosphorylated at tyrosine 354 upon infection of epithelial cells by *Neisseria gonorrhoeae*. J Cell Biol. 2002;156:951-957.

168. Johansson L, Rytkönen A, Bergman P, et al. CD46 in meningococcal disease. Science. 2003;301:373-375.

169. Ross SC, Densen P. Complement deficiency states and infection: Epidemiology, pathogenesis and consequences of neisserial and other infections in an immune deficiency. Medicine (Baltimore). 1984;63:243-273.

170. Figueroa JE, Densen P. Infectious diseases associated with complement deficiencies. Clin Microbiol Rev. 1991;4:359-395.

171. Densen P. Human complement deficiency states and infection. In: Whaley K, Loos M, Weiler JM, eds. Complement in Health and Disease. Dordrecht, The Netherlands: Kluwer Academic Publishers; 1993:173-197.

172. Glass D, Raum D, Gibson D, et al. Inherited deficiency of the second component of complement. J Clin Invest. 1976;58:853-861.

173. Truedsson L, Sturfelt G, Nived O. Prevalence of the type I complement C2 deficiency gene in Swedish systemic lupus erythematosus patients. Lupus. 1993;2:325-327.

174. Sullivan KE, Petri MA, Schmeckpeper BJ, et al. Prevalence of a mutation causing C2 deficiency in systemic lupus erythematosus. J Rheumatol. 1994;21:1128-1133.

175. Ekdahl K, Truedsson L, Sjöholm AG, et al. Complement analysis in adult patients with a history of bacteremic pneumococcal infections or recurrent pneumonia. Scand J Infect Dis. 1995;27:111-117.

176. Agnello V. Lupus diseases associated with hereditary and acquired deficiencies of complement. Springer Semin Immunopathol. 1986;9:161-178.

177. Hauptmann G, Goetz J, Uring-Lambert B, et al. Component deficiencies: 2. The fourth component. Prog Allergy. 1986;39:1232-1249.

178. Awdeh ZL, Raum DD, Glass D, et al. Complement-human histocompatibility antigen haplotypes in C2 deficiency. J Clin Invest. 1981;67:581-583.

179. Kemp ME, Atkinson JP, Skanes VM, et al. Deletion of C4A genes in patients with systemic lupus erythematosus. Arthritis Rheum. 1987;30:1015-1022.

180. Walport MJ, Davies KA, Morley BJ, et al. Complement deficiency and autoimmunity. Ann N Y Acad Sci. 1997;815:267-281.

181. Howard PF, Hochberg MC, Bias WB, et al. Relationship between C4 null genes, HLA-D region antigens, and genetic susceptibility to systemic lupus erythematosus in Caucasian and Black Americans. Am J Med. 1986;81:187-193.

182. Sullivan KE, Jawad AF, Piliero LM, et al. Analysis of polymorphisms affecting immune complex handling in systemic lupus erythematosus. Rheumatology. 2003;42:446-452.

183. Agnello V. Lupus diseases associated with hereditary and acquired deficiencies of complement. Springer Semin Immunopathol. 1986;9:161-178.

184. Davies KA, Schifferli JA, Walport MJ. Complement deficiency and immune complex disease. Springer Semin Immunopathol. 1994;15:397-416.

185. Bowness P, Davies KA, Norsworthy PJ, et al. Hereditary C1q deficiency and systemic lupus erythematosus. QJM. 1994;87:455-464.

186. Provost TT, Arnett FC, Reichlin M. Homozygous C2 deficiency, lupus erythematosus, and anti-Ro (SSA) antibodies. Arthritis Rheum. 1983;26:1279-1282.

187. Walport MJ. Complement and systemic lupus erythematosus. Arthritis. 2002;4(Suppl 3):S279-S293.

188. Salmon JE, Girardi G, Holers VM. Complement activation as a mediator of antiphospholipid antibody induced pregnancy loss and thrombosis. Ann Rheum Dis. 2002;61(Suppl 2):ii46-ii50.

189. Schifferli JA, Peters DK. Complement, the immune-complex lattice, and the pathophysiology of complement-deficiency syndromes. Lancet. 1983;2:957-959.

190. Schifferli JA, Steiger G, Hauptmann G, et al. Formation of soluble immune complexes by complement in sera of patients with various hypocomplementemic states. J Clin Invest. 1985;76:2127-2133.

191. Davies KA, Peters AM, Beynon HL, et al. Immune complex processing in patients with systemic lupus erythematosus: In vivo imaging and clearance studies. J Clin Invest. 1992;90:2075-2083.

191A. Ross GD, Yount WJ, Walport MJ, et al. Disease-associated loss of erythrocyte complement receptors (CR1, C3b receptors) in patients with systemic lupus erythematosus and other diseases involving autoantibodies and/or complement activation. J Immunol. 1985;135:2005-2014.

192. Davies KA, Erlendsson K, Beynon HL, et al. Splenic uptake of immune complexes in man is complement-dependent. J Immunol. 1993;151:3866-3873.

193. Super M, Thiel S, Lu J, et al. Association of low levels of mannan-binding protein with a common defect of opsonisation. Lancet. 1989;2:1236-1239.

194. Summerfield JA, Sumiya M, Levin M, et al. Association of mutations in mannose binding protein gene with childhood infection in consecutive hospital series. Brit Med J. 1997;314:1229-1232.

195. Hibberd ML, Sumiya M, Summerfield JA, et al. Association of variants of the gene for mannose-binding lectin with susceptibility to meningococcal disease. Lancet. 1999;353:1049-1053.

196. Stengaard-Pedersen K, Thiel S, Gadjeva M, et al. Inherited deficiency of mannan-binding lectin-associated serine protease 2. N Engl J Med. 2003;349:554-560..

197. Matsumoto M, Fukuda W, Circolo A, et al. Abrogation of the alternative complement pathway by targeted deletion of murine factor B. Proc Natl Acad Sci U S A. 1997;94:8720-8725.

198. Pekna M, Hietala MA, Landin A, et al. Mice deficient for the complement factor B develop and reproduce normally. Scand J Immunol. 1998;47:375-380.

199. Sjöholm AG, Braconier J-H, Söderström C. Properdin deficiency in a family with fulminant meningococcal infections. Clin Exp Immunol. 1982;50:291-297.

200. Densen P, Weiler JM, Griffiss JM, et al. Familial properdin deficiency and fatal meningococcemia: Correction of the bactericidal defect by vaccination. N Engl J Med. 1987;316:922-926.

201. Sjöholm AG, Söderström C, Nilsson L-A. A second variant of properdin deficiency: The detection of properdin at low concentration in affected males. Complement. 1988;5:130-140.

202. Sjöholm AG, Kuijper EJ, Tijssen CC, et al. Dysfunctional properdin in a Dutch family with meningococcal disease. N Engl J Med. 1988;319:33-37.

203. Sissons JGP, West RJ, Fallow J, et al. The complement abnormalities of lipodystrophy. N Engl J Med. 1976;294:461-465.

204. Ipp MM, Minta JO, Gelfand EW. Disorders of the complement system in lipodystrophy. Clin Immunol Immunopathol. 1977;7:281-287.

205. Zipfel PF. Complement factor H: Physiology and pathophysiology. Semin Thromb Hemost. 2001;27:191-199.

206. Hegasy GA, Manuelian T, Hogasen K, et al. The molecular basis for hereditary porcine membranoproliferative glomerulonephritis type II. Am J Pathol. 2002;161:2027-2034.

207. Taylor CM. Hemolytic-uremic syndrome and complement factor H deficiency: Clinical aspects. Semin Thromb Hemost. 2001;27:185-190.

208. Neumann HPH, Salzmann M, Bohnert-Iwan B, et al. Haemolytic uraemic syndrome and mutations of the factor H gene: A registry-based study of German speaking countries. J Med Genet. 2003;40:676-681.

209. Richards A, Buddles MR, Donne RL, et al. Factor H mutations in hemolytic uremic syndrome cluster in exons 18-20, a domain important for host cell recognition. Am J Hum Genet. 2001;68:485-490.

210. Pérez-Caballero D, González-Rubio C, Gallardo ME, et al. Clustering of missense mutations in the c-terminal region of factor H in atypical hemolytic uremic syndrome. Am J Hum Genet. 2001;68:478-484.

211. Manuelian T, Hellwage J, Meri S, et al. Mutations in factor H reduce binding affinity to C3b and heparin and surface attachment to endothelial cells in hemolytic uremic syndrome. J Clin Invest. 2003;111:1181-1190.

212. Sánchez-Corral P, Pérez-Caballero D, Huarte O, et al. Structural and functional characterization of factor H mutations associated with atypical hemolytic uremic syndrome. Am J Hum Genet. 2002;71:1285-1295.

213. Hindmarsh EJ, Marks RM. Complement activation occurs on subendothelial extracellular matrix in vitro and is initiated by retraction or removal of overlying endothelial cells. J Immunol. 1998;160:6128-6136.

213a. Richards A, Kemp EJ, Liszewski MK, et al. Mutations in human complement regulator, membrane cofactor protein (CD46), predispose to development of familial hemolytic uremic syndrome. Proc Natl Acad Sci U S A. 2003;100:12966-12971.

213b. Noris M, Brioschi S, Caprioli J, et al. Familial haemolytic uraemic syndrome and an MCP mutation. Lancet. 2003;362:1542-1547.

213c. Bonnardeaux A, Pichette V. Complement dysregulation in haemolytic uraemic syndrome. Lancet. 2003;362:1514-1515.

214. Nagata M, Hara T, Aoki T, et al. Inherited deficiency of ninth component of complement: An increased risk of meningococcal meningitis. J Pediatr. 1989;114:260-264.

215. Slingsby JH, Norsworthy P, Pearce G, et al. Homozygous hereditary C1q deficiency and systemic lupus erythematosus: A new family and the molecular basis of C1q deficiency in three families. Arthritis Rheum. 1996;39:663-670.

216. Johnson C, Densen P, Cole FS, et al. Molecular heterogeneity of human C2 deficiency. N Engl J Med. 1992;326:871-874.

217. Johnson CA, Densen P, Hurford R, et al. Type I human complement C2 deficiency: A 28-base pair gene deletion causes skipping of exon 6 during RNA splicing. J Biol Chem. 1992;267:9347-9353.

218. Barba G, Rittner C, Schneider PM. Genetic basis of human complement C4a deficiency. J Clin Invest. 1993;91:1681-1686.
219. Ault BH, Schmidt BZ, Fowler NL, et al. Human factor H deficiency: Mutations in framework cysteine residues and block in H protein secretion and intracellular catabolism. J Biol Chem. 1997;272:25168-25175.
220. Vyse TJ, Morley BJ, Bartok I, et al. The molecular basis of hereditary complement factor I deficiency. J Clin Invest. 1996;97:925-933.
221. Truedsson L, Westberg J, Fredrikson GN, et al. Human properdin deficiency has a heterogeneous genetic background. Immunopharmacology. 1997;38:203-206.
222. Westberg J, Fredrikson GN, Truedsson L, et al. Sequence-based analysis of properdin deficiency: Identification of point mutations in two phenotypic forms of an X-linked immunodeficiency. Genomics. 1995;29:1-8.
223. Fredrikson GN, Westberg J, Kuijper EJ, et al. Molecular characterization of properdin deficiency type III: Dysfunction produced by a single point mutation in exon 9 of the structural gene causing a tyrosine to aspartic acid interchange. J Immunol. 1996; 157:3666-3671.
224. Singer L, Colten HR, Wetsel RA. Complement C3 deficiency: Human, animal and experimental models. Pathobiology. 1994;62:14-28.
225. Wang X, Fleischer DT, Whitehead WT, et al. Inherited human complement C5 deficiency: Nonsense mutations in exons 1 (Gln1 to Stop) and 36 (Arg1458 to Stop) and compound heterozygosity in three African-American families. J Immunol. 1995;154: 5464-5471.
226. Hobart MJ, Fernie BA, Fijen KA, et al. The molecular bases of C6 deficiency in the Western Cape, South Africa. Hum Genet. 1998;103:506-512.
227. Nishizaka T, Horiuchi T, Zhu ZB, et al. Molecular bases for inherited human complement component C6 deficiency in two unrelated individuals. J Immunol. 1996; 156:2309-2315.
228. Würzner R, Hobart MJ, Fernie BA, et al. Molecular basis of subtotal complement C6 deficiency: A carboxy-terminally truncated but functionally active C6. J Clin Invest. 1995;95:1877-1883.
229. Fernie BA, Orren A, Sheehan G, et al. Molecular bases of C7 deficiency: Three different defects. J Immunol. 1997;159:1019-1026.
230. O'Hara AM, Fernie BA, Moran AP, et al. C7 deficiency in an Irish family: A deletion defect which is predominant in the Irish. Clin Exp Immunol. 1998;114(3):355-361.
231. Fernie BA, Würzner R, Orren A, et al. Molecular bases of combined subtotal deficiencies of C6 and C7: Their effects in combination with other C6 and C7 deficiencies. J Immunol. 1996;157:3648-3657.
232. Würzner R, Platonov AE, Beloborodov VB, et al. How partial C7 deficiency with chronic and recurrent bacterial infections can mimic total C7 deficiency: Temporary restoration of host C7 levels following plasma transfusion. Immunology. 1996;88:407-411.
233. Saucedo L, Ackermann L, Platonov AE, et al. Delineation of additional genetic bases for C8β deficiency: Prevalence of null alleles and predominance of C→T transition in their genesis. J Immunol. 1995;155:5022-5028.
234. Densen P, Ackermann L, Saucedo L, et al. The genetic basis for human C8α-γ deficiency (Abstract). Boston: XVI International Complement Workshop; 1996.
235. Kojima T, Horiuchi T, Nishizaki H, et al. Genetic basis of human complement C8α-γ deficiency. J Immunol. 1998;161:3762-3766.
236. Witzel-Schlömp K, Späth PJ, Hobart MJ, et al. Identification of two mutations causing deficiency and revision of the gene structure. J Immunol. 1997;158:5043-5049.
237. Witzel-Schlömp K, Hobart MJ, Fernie BA, et al. Heterogeneity in the genetic basis of human complement C9 deficiency. Immunogenetics. 1998;48:144-147.
238. Fijen CAP, Kuijper EJ, Tjia HG, et al. Complement deficiency predisposes for meningitis due to nongroupable meningococci and Neisseria-related bacteria. Clin Infect Dis. 1994;18:780-784.
239. Fijen CA, Kuijper EJ, Hannema AJ, et al. Complement deficiencies in patients over ten years old with meningococcal disease due to uncommon serogroups. Lancet. 1989;2:585-588.
240. Ross SC, Rosenthal PJ, Berberich HM, et al. Killing of Neisseria meningitidis by human neutrophils: Implications for normal and complement-deficient individuals. J Infect Dis. 1987;155:1266-1275.
241. Anonymous. Analysis of endemic meningococcal disease by serogroup and evaluation of chemoprophylaxis. J Infect Dis. 1976;134:201-204.
242. Ross SC, Berberich HM, Densen P. Natural serum bactericidal activity against Neisseria meningitidis isolates from disseminated infections in normal and complement-deficient hosts. J Infect Dis. 1985;152:1332-1335.
243. Beloborodov VB, Platonov AE. Meningococcal disease in the USSR in patients with deficiencies in late complement components. In: Achtman M, Kohl P, Marchal C, et al, eds. Neisseriae 1990. Berlin: Walter de Gruyter; 1991:659-663.
244. Platonov AE, Beloborodov VB, Vershinina IV. Meningococcal disease in patients with late complement deficiency: Studies in the U.S.S.R. Medicine (Baltimore). 1993;72:374-392.
245. Andreoni J, Kayhty H, Densen P. Vaccination and the role of capsular polysaccharide antibody in prevention of recurrent meningococcal disease in late complement component-deficient individuals. J Infect Dis. 1993;168:227-231.
246. Brandtzaeg P, Mollnes TE, Kierulf P. Complement activation and endotoxin levels in systemic meningococcal disease. J Infect Dis. 1989;160:58-65.
247. Brown DL, Lachmann PJ. The behaviour of complement and platelets in lethal endotoxin shock in rabbits. Int Arch Allergy Immunol. 1973;45:193-205.
248. Zwahlen A, Waldvogel FA. Magnitude of bacteremia and complement activation during Neisseria meningitidis infection: Study of two co-primary cases with different clinical presentations. Eur J Clin Microbiol. 1984;3:439-441.
249. Sullivan TD, LaScolea LJ Jr. Neisseria meningitidis bacteremia in children: Quantitation of bacteremia and spontaneous clinical recovery without antibiotic therapy. Pediatrics. 1987;80:63-67.
250. Brandtzaeg P, Kierulf P, Gaustad P, et al. Plasma endotoxin as a predictor of multiple organ failure and death in systemic meningococcal disease. J Infect Dis. 1989; 159:195-204.
251. Waage A, Brandtzaeg P, Halstensen A, et al. The complex pattern of cytokines in serum from patients with meningococcal septic shock: Association between interleukin 6, interleukin 1, and fatal outcome. J Exp Med. 1989;169:333-338.
252. Girardin E, Grau GE, Dayer JM, et al. Tumor necrosis factor and interleukin-1 in the serum of children with severe infectious purpura. N Engl J Med. 1988;319:397-400.
253. Waage A, Halstensen A, Espevik T. Association between tumour necrosis factor in serum and fatal outcome in patients with meningococcal disease. Lancet. 1987;1:355-357.
254. Waage A, Halstensen A, Shalaby R, et al. Local production of tumor necrosis factor α, interleukin 1, and interleukin 6 in meningococcal meningitis: Relation to the inflammatory response. J Exp Med. 1989;170:1859-1867.
255. Morgan BP. Mechanisms of tissue damage by the membrane attack complex of complement. Complement Inflamm. 1989;6:104-111.
256. Sims PJ, Wiedmer T. The response of human platelets to activated components of the complement system. Immunol Today. 1991;12:338-342.
257. Platonov AE, Gracheva AM. Effects of lipopolysaccharide from N. meningitidis on human granulocyte lysis and chemiluminescence. In: Achtman M, Kohl P, Marchal C, et al, eds. Neisseriae 1990. Berlin: Walter de Gruyter; 1991:627-631.
258. Hamilton KK, Hattori R, Esmon CT, et al. Complement proteins C5b-9 induce vesiculation of the endothelial plasma membrane and expose catalytic surface for assembly of the prothrombinase enzyme complex. J Biol Chem. 1990;265:3809-3814.
259. Bredius RGM, Derkx BHF, Fijen CAP, et al. Fc receptor IIa (CD32) polymorphism in fulminant meningococcal septic shock in children. J Infect Dis. 1994;170:848-853.
260. Fijen CAP, Bredius RGM, Kuijper EJ. Polymorphism of IgG Fc receptors in meningococcal disease (Letter). Ann Intern Med. 1993;119:636.
261. Fijen CAP, et al. Complement deficiency and the role of Fc receptors, properdin and C3 in phagocytosis of meningococci. In: Fijen CAP, ed. Meningococcal Disease and Complement Deficiencies in the Netherlands. Amsterdam: University of Amsterdam; 1995:157-175.
262. Platonov AE, Kuijper EJ, Vershinina IV, et al. Meningococcal disease and polymorphism of FcγRIIa (CD32) in late complement component-deficient individuals. Clin Exp Immunol. 1998;111:97-101.
263. Frank MM, Gelfand JA, Atkinson JP. Hereditary angioedema: The clinical syndrome and its management. Ann Intern Med. 1976;84:580-593.
264. Frank MM. C1 esterase inhibitor: Clinical clues to the pathophysiology of angioedema. J Allergy Clin Immunol. 1986;78:848-850.
265. Cicardi M, Agostoni A. Hereditary angioedema. N Engl J Med. 1996;334:1666-1667.
266. Whaley K, Sim RB, He S. Autoimmune C1-inhibitor deficiency. Clin Exp Immunol. 1996;106:423-426.
267. Cicardi M, Beretta A, Colombo M, et al. Relevance of lymphoproliferative disorders and of anti-C1-inhibitor autoantibodies in acquired angioedema. Clin Exp Immunol. 1996;106:475-480.
268. Strang CJ, Auerbach HS, Rosen FS. C1s-induced vascular permeability in C2-deficient guinea pigs. J Immunol. 1986;137:631-635.
269. Zahedi R, Bissler JJ, Davis AE, et al. Unique C1 inhibitor dysfunction in a kindred without angioedema: II. Identification of an Ala443Val substitution and functional analysis of the recombinant mutant protein. J Clin Invest. 1995;95:1299-1305.
270. Zahedi R, Wisnieski J, Davis AE. Role of the P2 residue of complement 1 inhibitor (Ala443) in determination of target protease specificity: Inhibition of complement and contact system proteases. J Immunol. 1997;159:983-988.
271. Davis AE. C1 inhibitor: Functional analysis of naturally-occurring mutant proteins. In: Church FC, Cunningham DD, Ginsburg D, et al, eds. Chemistry and Biology of Serpins. New York: Plenum; 1997:185-194.
272. Agostini A, Cicardi M. Hereditary and acquired C1-inhibitor deficiency: Biological and clinical characteristics in 235 patients. Medicine (Baltimore). 1992;71:206-215.
273. Donaldson VH, Bissler JJ. C1 inhibitors and their genes: An update. J Lab Clin Med. 1993;119:330-333.
274. Rosse WF, Parker CJ. Paroxysmal nocturnal haemoglobinuria. Clin Haematol. 1985;14:105-125.
275. Rosse WF. Hematopoiesis and the defect in paroxysmal nocturnal hemoglobinuria (Editorial). J Clin Invest. 1997;100:953-954.
276. Luzzatto L, Bessler M, Rotoli B. Somatic mutations in paroxysmal nocturnal hemoglobinuria: A blessing in disguise? Cell. 1997;88:1-4.
277. Rosse WF. The control of complement activation by the blood cells in paroxysmal nocturnal hemoglobinuria. Blood. 1986;67:268-269.
278. Rosse WF, Ware RE. The molecular basis of paroxysmal nocturnal hemoglobinuria. Blood. 1995;86:3277-3286.
279. Armstrong C, Schubert J, Ueda E, et al. Affected paroxysmal nocturnal hemoglobinuria T lymphocytes harbor a common defect in assembly of N-acetyl-D-glucosamine inositol phospholipid corresponding to that in class A thy-1-murine lymphoma mutants. J Biol Chem. 1992;267:25347-25351.
280. Nicholson-Weller A, March JP, Rosenfeld SI, et al. Affected erythrocytes of patients with paroxysmal nocturnal hemoglobinuria are deficient in the complement regulatory protein, decay accelerating factor. Proc Natl Acad Sci U S A. 1983;80:5066-5070.
281. Holguin MH, Fredrick LR, Bernshaw NJ, et al. Isolation and characterization of a membrane protein from normal human erythrocytes that inhibits reactive lysis of the erythrocytes of paroxysmal nocturnal hemoglobinuria. J Clin Invest. 1989;84:7-17.
282. Holguin MH, Wilcox LA, Bernshaw NJ, et al. Relationship between the membrane inhibitor of reactive lysis and the erythrocyte phenotypes of paroxysmal nocturnal hemoglobinuria. J Clin Invest. 1989;84:1387-1394.

283. Yamashina M, Ueda E, Kinoshita T, et al. Inherited complete deficiency of 20-kilodalton homologous restriction factor (CD59) as a cause of paroxysmal nocturnal hemoglobinuria. N Engl J Med. 1990;323:1184-1189.

284. Devetten MP, Liu JM, Ling V, et al. Paroxysmal nocturnal hemoglobinuria: New insights from murine Pig-a-deficient hematopoiesis. Proc Assoc Am Physicians. 1997;109:99-110.

285. Torzewski J, Bowyer DE, Waltenberger J, et al. Processes in atherogenesis: Complement activation. Atherosclerosis. 1997;132:131-138.

286. Weiser MR, Williams JP, Moore FD, et al. Reperfusion injury of ischemic skeletal muscle is mediated by natural antibody and complement. J Exp Med. 1996;183:2343-2348.

287. Koski CL, Sanders ME, Swoveland PT, et al. Activation of terminal components of complement in patients with Guillain-Barré syndrome and other demyelinating neuropathies. J Clin Invest. 1987;80:1492-1497.

288. Cammer W, Brosnan CF, Basile C, et al. Complement potentiates the degradation of myelin proteins by plasmin: Implications for a mechanism of inflammatory demyelination. Brain Res. 1986;364:91-101.

289. Mollnes TE, Vandvik B, Lea T, et al. Intrathecal complement activation in neurological diseases evaluated by analysis of the terminal complement complex. J Neurol Sci. 1987;78:17-28.

290. Biesecker G, Lavin L, Ziskind M, et al. Cutaneous localization of the membrane attack complex in discoid and systemic lupus erythematosus. N Engl J Med. 1982;306:264-270.

291. Platt JL, Vercellotti GM, Dalmasso AP, et al. Transplantation of discordant xenografts: A review of progress. Immunol Today. 1990;11:450-455.

292. Dalmasso AP, Vercellotti GM, Fischel RJ, et al. Mechanism of complement activation in the hyperacute rejection of porcine organs transplanted into primate recipients. Am J Pathol. 1992;140:1157-1166.

293. Xia W, Fearon DT, Kirkman RL. Effect of repetitive doses of soluble human complement receptor type 1 on survival of discordant cardiac xenografts. Transplant Proc. 1993;25:410-411.

294. Loveland BE, Johnstone RW, Russell SM, et al. Increased susceptibility to endotoxin shock in complement C3- and C4-deficient mice is corrected by C1 inhibitor replacement. Transplant Proc. 1993;25:396-397.

295. Weisman HF, Bartow T, Leppo MK, et al. Soluble human complement receptor type 1: In vivo inhibitor of complement suppressing post-ischemic myocardial inflammation and necrosis. Science. 1990;249:146-151.

296. White DJG, Yannoutsos N. Production of pigs transgenic for human DAF to overcome complement-mediated hyperacute xenograft rejection in man. Res Immunol. 1996;147:88-94.

297. Fischer MB, Prodeus AP, Nicholson-Weller A, et al. Increased susceptibility to endotoxin shock in complement C3- and C4-deficient mice is corrected by C1 inhibitor replacement. J Immunol. 1997;159:976-982.

298. Reid RR, Prodeus AP, Khan W, et al. Endotoxin shock in antibody-deficient mice. J Immunol. 1997;159:970-975.

299. Weaver LJ, Craddock PR, Jacob HS. Association of complement activation and elevated plasma-C5a with adult respiratory distress syndrome: Pathophysiological relevance and possible prognostic value. Lancet. 1980;1:947-949.

300. Jacob HS, Craddock PR, Hammerschmidt DE, et al. Complement-induced granulocyte aggregation: An unsuspected mechanism of disease. N Engl J Med. 1980;302:789-794.

301. Stevens JH, O'Hanley P, Shapiro JM, et al. Effect of anti-C5a antibodies on the adult respiratory distress syndrome in septic primates. J Clin Invest. 1986;77:1812-1816.

302. Czermak BJ, Sarma V, Pierson CL, et al. Protective effects of C5a blockade in sepsis. Nature Medicine. 1999;5:788-792.

303. Riedemann NC, Guo RF, Neff TA, et al. Increased C5a receptor expression in sepsis. J Clin Invest. 2002;110:101-108.

304. Hotchkiss R, Karl IE. The pathophysiology and treatment of sepsis. N Engl J Med. 2003;348:138-150.

305. Guo RF, Huber-Lang M, Wang X, et al. Protective effects of anti-C5a in sepsis-induced thymocyte apoptosis. J Clin Invest. 2000;106:1271-1280.

306. Riedemann NC, Neff TA, Guo RF, et al. Protective effects of Il-6 blockade in sepsis are linked to reduced C5a receptor expression. J Immunol. 2003;170:503-507.

307. Hosea SW, Brown EJ, Frank MM. The critical role of complement in experimental pneumococcal sepsis. J Infect Dis. 1980;142:903-909.

308. Brown EJ, Hosea SW, Frank MM. The role of the spleen in experimental pneumococcal bacteremia. J Clin Invest. 1981;67:975-982.

309. Bohnsack JF, Brown EJ. The role of the spleen in resistance to infection. Annu Rev Med. 1986;37:49-59.

310. Brown EJ, Hosea SW, Frank MM. The role of antibody and complement in the reticuloendothelial clearance of pneumococci from the bloodstream. Rev Infect Dis. 1985;5(Suppl):797-805.

311. Atkinson JP. Complement activation and complement receptors in systemic lupus erythematosus. Springer Semin Immunopathol. 1986;9:179-194.

312. Sim E, Gill EW, Sim RB. Drugs that induce systemic lupus erythematosus inhibit complement component C4. Lancet. 1984;2:422-424.

313. Biesecker G, Katz S, Koffler D. Renal localization of the membrane attack complex in systemic lupus erythematosus nephritis. J Exp Med. 1981;151:1790-1791.

314. Falk RJ, Dalmasso AP, Kim Y, et al. Neoantigen of the polymerized ninth component of complement: Characterization of a monoclonal antibody and immunohistochemical localization in renal disease. J Clin Invest. 1983;72:560-573.

315. Groggel GC, Adler S, Rennke HG, et al. Role of the terminal complement pathway in experimental membranous nephropathy in the rabbit. J Clin Invest. 1983;72:1948-1957.

316. Adler S, Baker PJ, Pritzl P, et al. Detection of terminal complement components in experimental immune glomerular injury. Kidney Int. 1984;26:830-837.

317. Cybulsky AV, Rennke HG, Feintzeig ID, et al. Complement-induced glomerular epithelial cell injury: Role of the membrane attack complex in rat membranous nephropathy. J Clin Invest. 1986;77:1096-1107.

318. Cybulsky AV, Quigg RJ, Salant DJ. The membrane attack complex in complement-mediated glomerular epithelial cell injury: Formation and stability of C5b-9 and C5b-7 in rat membranous nephropathy. J Immunol. 1986;137:1511-1516.

319. Rus HG, Niculescu F, Nanulescu M, et al. Immunohistochemical detection of the terminal C5b-9 complement complex in children with glomerular diseases. Clin Exp Immunol. 1986;65:66-72.

320. Nath KA, Hostetter MK, Hostetter TH. Pathophysiology of chronic tubulointerstitial disease in rats: Interactions of dietary acid load, ammonia, and complement component C3. J Clin Invest. 1985;76:667-675.

321. Gordon DL, Krueger RA, Quie PG, et al. Amidation of C3 at the thiolester site: Stimulation of chemiluminescence and phagocytosis by a new inflammatory mediator. J Immunol. 1985;134:3339-3345.

322. Beeson PB, Rowley D. The anticomplementary effect of kidney tissue: Its association with ammonia production. J Exp Med. 1959;110:685-698.

323. Cybulsky AV, Lieberthal W, Quigg RJ, et al. A role for thromboxane in complement-mediated glomerular injury. Am J Pathol. 1987;128:45-51.

324. Hakim RM, Breillatt J, Lazarus MJ, et al. Complement activation and hypersensitivity reactions to dialysis membranes. N Engl J Med. 1984;311:878-882.

325. Craddock PR. Complement and granulocyte activation and deactivation during hemodialysis. In: Lysaght MJ, Gurland JG, eds. Plasma Separation and Plasma Fractionation. Basel: S Karger AG; 1983:14-21.

326. Steinsson K, Erlendsson K, Valdimarsson H. Successful treatment with plasma infusions in a patient with deficiency of the second component of complement and systemic lupus erythematosus: Clinical experience over a 45 month period. Arthritis Rheum. 1989;32:906.

327. Erlendsson K, Traustadóttir K, Freysdóttir J, et al. Reciprocal changes in complement activity and immune-complex levels during plasma infusion in a C2-deficient SLE patient. Lupus. 1993;2:161-165.

328. Barrett DJ, Boyle MDP. Restoration of complement function in vivo by plasma infusion in factor I (C3b inactivator) deficiency. J Pediatr. 1984;104:76-81.

329. Rao CP, Minta JO, Laski B, et al. Inherited C8β subunit deficiency in a patient with recurrent meningococcal infections: In vivo functional kinetic analysis of C8. Clin Exp Immunol. 1985;60:183-190.

330. Pitts JS, Donaldson VH, Forristal J, et al. Remissions induced in hereditary angioneurotic edema with an attenuated androgen (danazol): Correlation between concentrations of C1-inhibitor and the fourth and second components of complement. J Lab Clin Med. 1978;92:501-507.

331. Ada G. Vaccines and vaccination. N Engl J Med. 2001;345:1042-1053.

332. Platonov AE, Beloborodov VB, Pavlova LI, et al. Vaccination of patients deficient in a late complement component with tetravalent meningococcal capsular polysaccharide vaccine. Clin Exp Immunol. 1995;100:32-39.

333. Biselli R, Casapollo I, D'Amelio R, et al. Antibody response to meningococcal polysaccharides A and C in patients with complement defects. Scand J Immunol. 1993;37:644-650.

334. Fijen CAP, Kuijper EJ, van Leeuwen Y, et al. Antibody response of complement deficient patients to tetravalent meningococcal polysaccharide vaccine (Abstract). Proceedings of the Ninth International Pathogenic *Neisseria* Conference, Winchester, England, September 26-30, 1994:440.

335. Platonov AE, Vershinina IV, Dankert J, et al. Long-term follow-up of late complement component deficient patients vaccinated with meningococcal polysaccharide vaccine: Antibody persistence and efficacy of vaccination (Abstract). Abstracts of the Tenth International Pathogenic Neisseria Conference, Baltimore, Maryland, September 8-13, 1996:235.

336. Densen P, Brown EJ, O'Neill GJ. Inherited deficiency of C8 in a patient with recurrent meningococcal infections: Further evidence for a dysfunctional C8 molecule and nonlinkage to the HLA system. J Clin Immunol. 1983;3:90-99.

337. Potter PC, Frasch CE, van der Sande WJ, et al. Prophylaxis against *Neisseria meningitidis* infections and antibody responses in patients with deficiency of the sixth component of complement. J Infect Dis. 1990;161:932-937.

Granulocytic Phagocytes

WILLIAM M. NAUSEEF

ROBERT A. CLARK

Vertebrate immunity represents the integration of two systems, the innate and the acquired immune systems, that together respond to a variety of threats, including those posed by microbial nonself in the context of infection.[1,2] Innate (natural) immunity is the ability to respond immediately to an infectious challenge regardless of previous exposure of the host to the invading agent and represents mechanisms encoded in germline genes. Elements of the innate system include phagocytic cells, namely polymorphonuclear leukocytes (PMNs) and mononuclear phagocytes, and circulating soluble proteins, including components of the complement system (see Chapters 4 and 7). This relatively nonspecific pattern recognition system has functional analogues in the immune systems of a wide variety of multicellular organisms, including plants and insects. As such, this evolutionarily ancient system represents a rapid and sensitive surveillance mechanism of host defense when the organism is challenged with an invading microorganism previously unseen by the host's immune system. In contrast, acquired (adaptive) immunity (see Chapters 6 and 9) is the product of somatic gene rearrangement and has remarkable capacity to recognize and respond to a wide diversity of structures and to discriminate precisely among them. Lymphocytes (both B and T cells) and antibodies represent the cellular and circulating protein elements, respectively, of adaptive immunity. In contrast to the innate system, adaptive immunity is restricted to vertebrates and represents a precisely tuned means by which host cells define specifically the nature of the invading pathogen or tumor cell. Such precision, however, requires time for antigens to be processed and specific antibodies to be generated. Therefore, the adaptive system is slower to respond to new challenges than is the innate system, although the latter lacks specificity. Granulocytes, the most numerous leukocytes in the peripheral circulation, include neutrophils, eosinophils, and basophils. Structurally, these cells share a multilobed nucleus and the presence of numerous membrane-bound, characteristically staining cytoplasmic granules, but functionally they differ significantly.

NEUTROPHILS

Development

Neutrophils arise from pluripotent stem cells located in the bone marrow. The processes of proliferation and differentiation are precisely orchestrated by the coordinated activity of colony-stimulating factors (CSFs) for myeloid cells.[3,4] These molecules influence the survival and direct the maturation and proliferation of myeloid cells. Each factor is named for the colony produced under its influence: GM-CSF, for granulocytes and macrophages; G-CSF, for granulocytes; M-CSF, for monocytes and macrophages; and multi-CSF (or interleukin-3 [IL-3]), for a variety of colonies including neutrophils, macrophages, eosinophils, megakaryocytes, and erythroid cells. Although lineage-specific cytokines mediate acquisition of granulocytic features, precise details of their regulation are not understood.[5-7] In addition, cytokines, including GM-CSF and G-CSF, may enhance function and prolong neutrophil survival by delaying the apoptosis these cells usually undergo.[8]

Granulocyte development in the bone marrow can be divided into a mitotic phase and a postmitotic phase, each lasting approximately 1 week. During the mitotic phase, cells mature sequentially from myeloblasts into promyelocytes and myelocytes.[9] Maturation is associated with the appearance of the cytoplasmic granules characteristic of neutrophils, basophils, and eosinophils. The postmitotic phase of development includes metamyelocytes, band (or immature) neutrophils, and mature neutrophils.

Coincident with the morphologic changes, cells acquire the specific surface markers and functional properties of more mature cells.[10] For example, Fc receptors appear as the cells develop into promyelocytes, cells become competent for phagocytosis in the early myelocyte stage, and complement receptors appear in the late myelocyte and metamyelocyte stages. Oxygen-dependent microbicidal activity appears in the early metamyelocyte stage, and cells in the late metamyelocyte–band stage demonstrate increased adhesiveness, cell motility, and chemotactic responses.[10] In addition, coordinated expression of genes encoding the granule proteins is synchronized with early stages of myeloid development, and normal granulocytic differentiation is intimately linked with expression of proteins localized in specific granules.[11] Although they are incompletely understood at this time, the

hematopoietic growth factors direct myeloid differentiation by modulating transcription factors that regulate genes responsible for a specific myeloid phenotype.[7,11]

Morphologic and Structural Characteristics

The earliest histochemical studies of neutrophils classified the membrane-bound intracellular granules by their staining characteristics. Two populations of granules were distinguished based on staining with azure A: the positively staining azurophilic granules and the unstained specific granules. Sophisticated subcellular fractionation and analysis of neutrophil organelles have refined significantly our appreciation of the complexity and heterogeneity of neutrophil granules.[12] In addition to insights into the biologic roles of the various proteins in the matrix of the granules, studies have identified functionally important proteins within the membranes of particular granule subsets.

At a first approximation, neutrophil granules can be categorized based on peroxidase staining. The peroxidase-positive granules are also known as *primary granules*, because they arise first in granulopoiesis, and as *azurophilic granules*, based on histochemical staining. Azurophilic granules contain myeloperoxidase (MPO)[13]; a variety of proteolytic enzymes, including cathepsins, proteinase-3,[14] and elastase[15]; and the antimicrobial defensins[16] and bactericidal permeability-increasing protein (BPI) (Table 8-1).[17] Because of the acid hydrolase activity of the azurophilic granule contents, this compartment has been considered lysosomal in nature. However, azurophilic granules lack lysosome-associated membrane protein, an identifying marker for lysosomes. Moreover, proteins such as MPO[18] and the defensins[19] do not segregate into the azurophilic granule by means of the mannose-6-phosphate receptor, a targeting system characteristic of lysosomal proteins. Taken together, these observations suggest that the azurophilic granule may be a specialized organelle that is distinctly different from conventional primary lysosomes.

Based in large part on studies by Borregaard and colleagues,[12,20] the peroxidase-negative granules can be categorized as *specific granules, gelatinase granules,* and *secretory vesicles*. The contents of the specific and gelatinase granules overlap to a significant extent (see Table 8-1)[21] but differ from those of azurophilic granules and secretory vesicles. More striking, however, is the distribution of functionally important plasma membrane proteins in the membranes of peroxidase-negative granules.[22] These membranes contain cytochrome-b_{558},[23,24] an essential component of the nicotinamide adenine dinucleotide phosphate

TABLE 8-1 Characteristics of Neutrophil Granules

Characteristics	Primary (Azurophil)	Specific (Secondary)
Contents	Acid hydrolases	Lactoferrin
	β-Glucuronidase	Lysozyme
	α-Mannosidase	Vitamin B$_{12}$–binding protein
	Arylsulfatase	Collagenase (?)
	5′-Nucleotidase	Monocyte chemotactic factor
	Acid protease (cathepsin)	C3 and C5 cleaving proteases
	Neutral proteases	Membrane-bound receptors
	Cathepsin G	CR3
	Elastase	CR4
	Collagenase (?)	C5a
	Myeloperoxidase	fMLP receptor
	Cationic proteins	Laminin
	Defensins	Membrane bound
	Lysozyme	Components of NADPH
	Acid mucopolysaccharide	Oxidase system
pH Optimum	5.5-6.5	Cytochrome-b_{558}
Degranulation	Degranulation delayed > 50% into phagosome	7-7.5
		Degranulates first >90%
Function	Microbial killing	Exocytosis
	Digestion	Inflammatory process

fMLP, formyl-methionyl-leucyl-phenylalanine; NADPH, nicotinamide adenine dinucleotide phosphate.

(NADPH)–dependent oxidase (discussed later); receptors for chemotactic peptides[25]; extracellular matrix proteins[26]; cytokines[27]; opsonins[28]; and adhesion proteins.[29,30] They therefore represent an intracellular reservoir of functionally important membrane proteins that can be quickly recruited to the cell surface during neutrophil activation. The presence of such compartments is ideally suited to the central role of neutrophils as the major circulating cell in the innate immune system; a reservoir of readily accessible functional proteins allows a rapid response without the delays that would be incurred by requirements for new protein synthesis. The functional consequences of this compartmentalization of proteins in the matrix and in the membrane of granules are discussed later.

During maturation the nucleus becomes segmented and the cytoskeletal elements, microfilaments and microtubules, appear in the cytoplasm. A meshwork of microfilaments makes up the clear cortical veil that surrounds the cell and forms the lamellipodium of an advancing cell (Fig. 8-1). These structures are polymers of actin, a protein representing 5% to 10% of the total cellular protein. Actin, together with a number of other interacting proteins, constitutes the contractile machinery of the cell that generates locomotion.[31] Actin monomers (G-actin), in the presence of actin-binding protein, polymerize to form cross-linked actin filaments (F-actin). Regulation of the length of the filaments and the degree of cross-linking provides for the physicochemical dynamics of actin flux between the gel and sol states. Filament length is controlled by several different proteins. Profilin serves to sequester G-actin and may provide a mechanism for rapid transport of actin to sites of polymerization. Acumentin, by initiating multiple sites of filament formation (nucleation) and preferentially inhibiting actin monomer exchange from the "slow-growing" end of elongating filaments, maintains actin in short filaments. Gelsolin, a calcium-modulated protein that initiates filament nucleation, binds to the "fast-growing" end of the filaments and can split preformed actin filaments. In the presence of adenosine triphosphate (ATP), myosin repetitively dissociates and binds to cross-linked actin. Myosin binding changes the cross-linking angle between actin filaments from 90 to 45 degrees, which results in movement of the filaments. In this way myosin serves to harness the changes in the physicochemical state of actin so as to give directionality to cell movement. Changes in calcium concentration that occur with membrane perturbation, directly and in concert with calmodulin, exert control over the contractile process by regulating myosin kinase and gelsolin. As a result, intracellular calcium gradients provide for an increase in polymerized actin in regions of high calcium concentration.

Actin filaments are associated with the cytoskeleton or with the plasma membrane via membrane skeletal proteins. Stimulation of the cell with chemotactic factors causes an abrupt increase in the amount of actin associated with the cytoskeleton[32] and a shift in microfilament organization from a parallel strand to a cross-hatched meshwork most evident at the leading edge of the directionally polarized cell.[33]

Microtubules are hollow structures composed of dimers of tubulin. In contrast to the role of microfilaments in directed locomotion and changes in cell shape, microtubules appear to be necessary for the initial orientation of the cell in a chemotactic gradient and for the spatial organization of structures within the cell during locomotion. They also may be involved in vesicle transport, degranulation, and the regulation of cell surface microviscosity during phagocytosis.

Mature neutrophils (Fig. 8-2; see also Fig. 8-1) are characterized by a paucity of ribosomal material and mitochondria, in keeping with the low levels of synthetic processes in these cells. However, neutrophils actively synthesize a selected group of proteins, including major histocompatibility complex (MHC) class I molecules,[34] complement receptors,[35] IL-8,[36] tumor necrosis factor-α (TNF-α), G-CSF, M-CSF, IL-1, IL-6, and interferon-α (IFN-α).[37] Recent studies using sensitive assays to measure transcripts indicate an even broader array of actively transcribed genes in neutrophils, both at rest and during phagocytosis.[38-41] Glycogen granules fill the cytoplasm and serve as a source of energy for neutrophil function.

Receptors with specificity for a number of humoral substances, including immunoglobulin G (IgG),[42] IgA, the complement fragments C3b and iC3b,[43] and several chemotactic factors (most notably the formyl-methionyl peptide receptor family[44]) have been identified and characterized both functionally and structurally.[45] These receptors are homogeneously distributed over the surface of the resting cell but undergo an asymmetric clustering at the front of the cell when it becomes polarized in response to a chemotactic stimulus. The distribution of receptors with different ligand specificities can be independently regulated even though stimulation via these receptors may result in similar functional effects.[46] Moreover, the various neutrophil functional responses exhibit differential requirements for receptor occupancy. For example, maximal degranulation requires brief receptor occupancy, whereas sustained oxidative responses depend on continuous ligand binding to the receptor.[47]

Neutrophil Kinetics

The daily production of mature PMNs in a healthy adult is on the order of 10^{11} cells. During acute infection or other inflammatory stresses, neutrophils are mobilized from the marrow reserve, which contains up to 10 times the normal daily neutrophil requirement. In the face of a persistent stimulus this reserve may be depleted, but only if there is nutritional deficiency or other disorder (e.g., ethanol abuse) that compromises mechanisms for augmenting delivery to meet demands. Increased stem cell input, increased mitoses during the mitotic stage

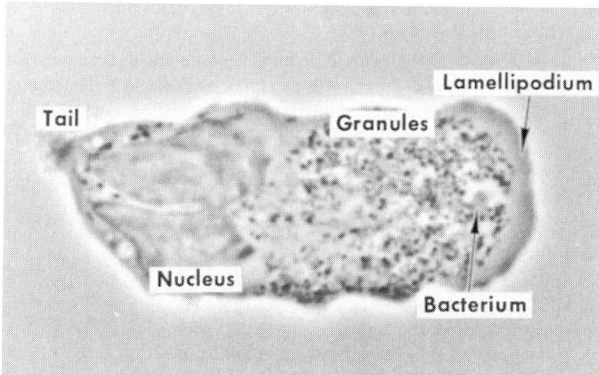

FIGURE 8-1. Phase-contrast photomicrograph of a human neutrophil.

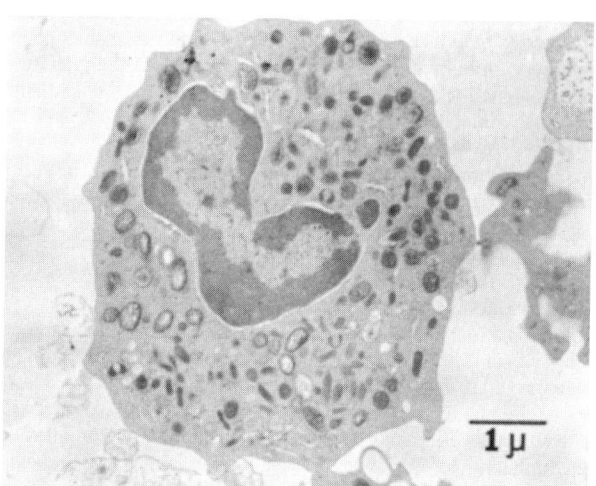

FIGURE 8-2. Electron micrograph of a human neutrophil. Note the granules *(large oval structures)*, glycogen particles *(small dark particles)*, but few other visible organelles.

of development, use of a store of cells whose maturation had been inhibited (so-called hiatal cells), and shortening of the maturation time within the marrow may all occur.[48] Multiplication and differentiation of stem cells is stimulated by the CSF produced by peripheral blood monocytes, tissue macrophages, and stimulated lymphocytes.[48,49]

Approximately 5% (about 4×10^8 cells per kilogram of body weight) of the total granulocyte pool is located in two compartments of similar size: the intravascular circulating cells and the marginating cells. A dynamic equilibrium exists between these two compartments, as cells exhibit transient endothelial interactions (margination) and then resume rapid flow, reflecting the balance between intercellular adherence and shear forces. The intravascular half-life of these cells is 6 to 8 hours, whereas their persistence in extravascular sites ranges from a few hours to several days. Granulocytosis, a hallmark of acute inflammation, is a consequence of certain physiologic and pharmacologic stimuli that typically alter the distribution of neutrophils among the various granulocyte pools rather than increase cell production. For example, the acute administration of corticosteroids or endotoxin, perhaps mimicking pathophysiologic events that occur in severe infection, promotes granulocyte release from the marrow reserve. Long-term steroid administration produces granulocytosis primarily by decreasing neutrophil adherence and shifting cells from the marginating to the circulating pool. Similarly, exercise, stress, epinephrine, hypoxia, aspirin, and alcohol cause granulocytosis by mobilizing marginating cells.

The Inflammatory Response

Inflammation represents a remarkably integrated cascade of events involving both cellular and soluble factors that are precisely orchestrated, both spatially and temporally. As such, it is best conceptualized as a complex network of interdigitated signals that modulate the responses of different cells and circulating molecules that in turn interact and are subject to a variety of regulatory checkpoints that operate by local, systemic, and neural mechanisms.[50,51] Within the context of host response to microbial nonself, the innate immune system sits poised to respond rapidly to perceived threats and in a stepwise fashion to recognize, contain, kill, and destroy potential pathogens. As all successful biologic systems represent a balance among competing forces, the return of the host to homeostasis after an acute inflammatory response requires initiation of a properly timed and appropriately proportioned anti-inflammatory cascade. Thus the acute response of neutrophils requires systemic recognition of a local threat with delivery of effector cells to the noxious site to contain, kill, and degrade potential pathogens before anti-inflammatory events supervene to trigger neutrophil apoptosis en route to resolution of the inflammatory reaction. Furthermore, recent studies emphasize that the noninflammatory homeostatic state represents the result of active modulation of proinflammatory surveillance systems rather than simply the absence of inflammatory stimuli, lending an additional layer of complexity and feedback signaling to an already intricate system.

Prologue

Circulating neutrophils are functionally heterogeneous, with the majority (80%) having the capacity to form IgG rosettes.[52] Because release from the bone marrow is not synchronized, this heterogeneity probably reflects maturational differences within a single cell line, although its biologic significance is uncertain. In contrast, tissue neutrophils are homogeneous, and more than 96% are capable of IgG rosette formation.[52] They contain fewer lysosomal granules and more glycogen than do their circulating counterparts because anaerobic glycolysis provides the energy for cell movement through the tissues.[53] The phenotypic difference between circulating and tissue neutrophils could reflect determinants needed for neutrophils to immigrate into tissue, influences of transmigration per se, elements in the tissue compartment, or other factors. In any case, the tissue neutrophil exhibits a phenotype different from that of the circulating, unstimulated neutrophil. For example, exudative neutrophils synthesize significantly more IL-8 than do neutrophils in circulation.[54] Furthermore, neutrophils exposed to concentrations of mediators that are too low to directly stimulate nevertheless prepare the cell for an enhanced response to a second, unrelated stimulus, in a phenomenon known as *priming*.[55] A broad array of inflammatory mediators, including chemotactic factors, endotoxin, cytokines, and certain lipids, can prime the neutrophil, as can transmigration across the endothelium. The primed state exists with respect to each of the major aspects of neutrophil function, persists for an extended period (longer than 20 minutes) in relation to the response elicited by direct stimulation of the cell, and is reversible. Although the molecular basis for priming of neutrophils is not understood, one study of the effects of endotoxin on neutrophil oxidase activity suggests that partial assembly of the oxidase at the plasma membrane may be responsible in part for the altered activation state of the cell.[56] Given the broad phenotypic features of the primed state, it is likely that alterations in proximal elements of the cellular response system, such as the organization of the plasma membrane and distribution of receptors and components of signal transduction machinery,[57] contribute to the more responsive state of the cell.

Step 1—Recruitment to the Inflammatory Site

To combat invading microorganisms, neutrophils must emigrate from the circulation and into the extravascular tissue space. Extravascular recruitment of neutrophils represents the summation of coordinated interactions of cells, specific receptors, and soluble mediators. The process involves at least four discrete steps: rolling adhesion, integrin activation, firm adhesion, and transmigration (Fig. 8-3).[58] These events are mediated in turn by four classes of adhesion proteins: selectins, integrins, immunoglobulin-like proteins, and mucin-like selectin ligands. In addition to neutrophils and endothelial cells, platelets figure prominently in the initiation of the inflammatory response, colocalizing with neutrophils and participating in P-selectin–dependent leukocyte binding.[59] Taken together, the cooperation of several cell types and their secreted products culminates in events necessary to recruit circulating neutrophils to the site of inflammation, and the activation of autocrine and paracrine feedback loops modulates the extent of the host response.[60]

Through a process of repetitive ligand-receptor binding and release, marginating granulocytes become lightly adherent to endothelial cells and, under the influence of the physiologic shear forces of blood flow, tumble or roll slowly along the vessel wall (see Fig. 8-3). The molecules mediating rolling adhesion are called *selectins* to indicate that the amino terminal lectin domain mediates their selective function and cellular expression. These molecules are homologous to C-type lectins, requiring calcium for expression of binding activity. Individual members of this family are named for the cell type on which they were originally identified (E, endothelia; L, lymphocytes; P, platelets). Although attention has focused on binding to sialylated Lewis X and A (sLe^X, sLe^A) glycoproteins, selectins also interact with sulfated and phosphorylated polysaccharides such as heparin and mannose-6-phosphate. Individual selectins exhibit different but overlapping binding specificities, the bases for which largely remain to be determined.[61]

The presence of unique selectins on endothelial cells and neutrophils means that rolling adhesion can be modulated bidirectionally. For example, L-selectin is constitutively expressed on neutrophils and appears to be shed after cell activation. In contrast, little or no E-selectin is present on resting endothelial cells, either in vitro or in vivo. Stimulation of these cells leads to inducible and transient E-selectin expression, which peaks about 4 hours after stimulation and dissipates over 24 hours.

When neutrophils tumbling along the venule wall encounter inflammatory mediators and stimulated endothelial cells, adhesion between the two cell types rapidly shifts to a high-affinity state. This second step in transendothelial migration reflects activation of β_2-integrins. The β_2- or leukocyte integrins are members of a large family of heterodimeric molecules that mediate cell-cell and cell-matrix interactions.[62] This family is subdivided on the basis of eight different β-chains, any one of which can associate with multiple α-chains to

FIGURE 8-3. Steps in the emigration of neutrophils from the vascular space. Neutrophils are depicted entering the marginating pool in a postcapillary venule. Initial adhesion is mediated by neutrophil (L) and endothelial (E, P) selectins and by their respective carbohydrate ligands on the opposing cell surface. Blood flow shear forces propel the lightly adherent neutrophils forward with a rolling or tumbling motion. Inflammatory mediators diffusing into the blood stream from sites of microbial invasion in the tissues bind to specific receptors and upregulate the functional expression of β_2-integrins (LFA-1; Mo-1; p150,95) on neutrophils as well as intercellular adhesion molecules (ICAM) on epithelial cells. These alterations promote a change in neutrophil shape and the firm adhesion of these cells to the vessel wall. Platelet-endothelial cell adhesion molecules (PECAM) localized to interendothelial cell junctions interact with PECAM on the neutrophil surface to permit neutrophil migration between endothelial cells. Once in the tissues, the polarized neutrophils move up the mediator concentration gradient to reach the site of microbial invasion. Type 2 leukocyte adhesion deficiency (†) is caused by the absence on neutrophil glycoproteins of the primary carbohydrate ligand (small dots in diagram), sLe^x, for E-selectin. Type 1 leukocyte adhesion deficiency (*) is caused by the lack of β_2-integrin expression on the neutrophil surface.

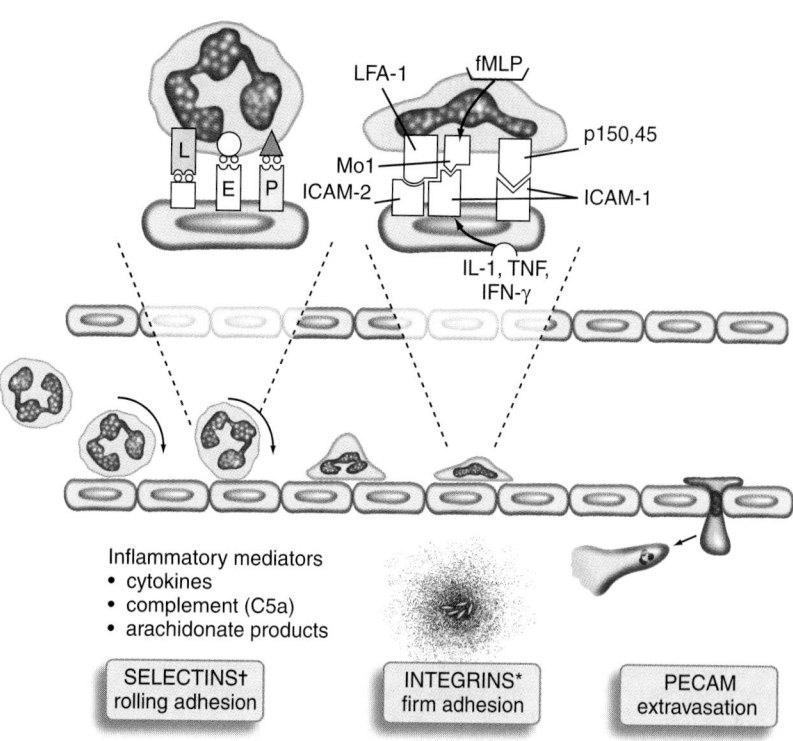

form a unique $\alpha\beta$ pair. Both the α- and β-chains are transmembrane molecules with short cytoplasmic tails and large extracellular globular heads that interact to form the ligand-binding site. The three neutrophil integrins have a common 95-kDa β-chain, CD18, and distinct α-chains. These molecular complexes are also referred to as leukocyte function-associated antigen-1, or LFA-1 ($\alpha_L\beta_2$, CD11a/CD18), Mo-1 or Mac-1 ($\alpha_M\beta_2$, CD11b/CD18), and p150,95 ($\alpha_X\beta_2$, CD11c/CD18).[63] Mo-1 and p150,95 also function as receptors (CR3 and CR4, respectively) for the opsonic C3 fragments iC3b and C3d. Endothelial counter-receptors for the β_2-integrins include intercellular adhesion molecule-1 (ICAM-1) and ICAM-2. LFA-1 binds to both ICAM-1 and ICAM-2, whereas Mo-1 and p150,95 bind only to ICAM-1 but at different sites from that for LFA-1. An additional LFA-1 counter-receptor, ICAM-3, is not present on endothelium but is expressed on all hematopoietic cells, where it may be involved in leukocyte-leukocyte interactions.[64,65] In addition to the β_2-integrins, PMNs possess on their surface the leukocyte response integrin,[66] which, together with integrin-associated protein, modulates cellular responses, particularly those induced by extracellular matrix proteins.[67-69] Although the precise details of the interactions of these various proteins are unknown, their importance is inferred from the observation that mice deficient in integrin-associated protein are unable to mount an inflammatory response after intraperitoneal challenge.

Integrin function requires calcium, a specific membrane environment, and appropriate stimuli such as chemoattractant peptides.[63] These stimuli appear to modulate integrin binding affinity by altering the interaction of the intracytoplasmic tails with each other and with the cytoskeleton. Integrin activation results in increased number and avidity of β_2-integrins as well as clustering of receptors and cytoskeletal rearrangement. Neutrophils change from spherical granulocytes with relatively little surface area involved in cell-cell contact to flattened cells with a broad surface area for cellular interactions (see Fig. 8-3). Blood flow shear forces are no longer able to propel them forward along the vessel wall. This firm adhesion, the third step in transmigration, is mediated through interactions between β_2-integrins on neutrophils and ICAM-1 and ICAM-2 on endothelial cells.[70]

ICAM-2 is constitutively expressed on endothelial cells and therefore may provide the initial endothelial ligand underlying the rapid development of firm adhesion. In contrast, ICAM-1, like E-selectin, undergoes marked upregulation when endothelium is exposed to IL-1 or TNF. It differs from E-selectin in that low-level expression is present on unstimulated cells, peak expression occurs over 12 to 24 hours and is sustained, and expression is also induced by IFN-γ. The ability of corticosteroids to inhibit E-selectin and ICAM-1 upregulation in the face of endotoxin, a potent stimulus for their expression, attests to the feasibility of anti-inflammatory strategies directed at adhesion molecules.

Endothelial cells play an active role in upregulating adherence events. For example, stimulated endothelial cells secrete IL-8, which both attracts and directly activates neutrophils, and upregulates expression of platelet-activating factor, which can engage its receptor on neutrophils. Transmigration, the final step in neutrophil immigration into tissue (see Fig. 8-3), involves at least two specific proteins: platelet-endothelial cell adhesion molecule (PECAM or CD31) and integrin-associated protein (IAP or CD47). Both proteins are localized at the intercellular junctions between endothelial cells, and antibodies to each block transmigration.[70] Current dogma dictates that transmigration occurs between endothelial cells, perhaps by neutrophil-dependent transient disorganization of adherens junctions at cell-cell interfaces,[71] although one study indicates that neutrophil extravasation may also occur by transcellular pathways.[72]

Transmigration is rapid, occurring in less than 2 minutes after leukocyte-endothelial contact is established, and remarkably efficient in that the event transpires without compromise to the integrity of the endothelial monolayer.[73] Recent studies have identified a novel sub-plasmalemmal membrane network in endothelial cells that directly associates with the junctional surface.[74] PECAM-1 recycles between this compartment and the sites of the endothelial junction where leukocytes migrate, presumably supplying critical PECAM-1, membrane, or both to facilitate diapedesis. Interactions between neutrophils and endothelial cells may negatively feed back on endothelial cell function, as transmigrating neutrophils decrease nuclear NF-κB in IL-1β-stimulated endothelial monolayers in a PECAM-1–dependent fashion.[75]

Although this paradigm applies to neutrophil extravasation from the vascular lumen into tissue, transmigration of neutrophils across epithelial barriers from tissue into visceral lumina, which is necessary in infections involving the gastrointestinal, genitourinary, and respiratory tracts, deviates significantly from this theme. Major insights into the mechanisms of neutrophil interaction with polarized epithelial cells have been derived from studies with human cell lines such as T84 and HT29.[76] Neutrophils can bind to either surface of these cells, and transmigration can occur in either direction. Binding to the basolateral surface of T84 cells is mediated by neutrophil β_2-integrins and an unidentified counterligand on the epithelial cell that is neither ICAM-1 nor a known selectin. In contrast, neutrophil binding to the apical surface of intestinal epithelial cells is dependent on ICAM-1.[76,77] Basolateral-to-apical migration of neutrophils across T84 cells requires expression of CD47,[78,79] but the determinants of apical-to-basolateral migration have not been identified. Evidence suggests that the mechanism for transmigration in each direction is distinct, because immunomodulators such as lipoxin A_4[80] and IFN-γ[81] stimulate movement toward the basolateral surface but inhibit luminal migration. The interactions between epithelial cells and migrating neutrophils are remarkably coordinated, as evidenced by reciprocal secretion of adenosine and IL-6 by monolayers of T84 cells.[82] The primed or activated neutrophil recruited to the luminal surface of the epithelial monolayer releases 5' AMP (adenosine monophosphate), a substrate for conversion to adenosine by the action of 5' ectonucleotidase present on the apical membrane of intestinal epithelium. In response to the adenosine, the epithelial cells release IL-6 from the surface that in turn stimulates neutrophils. Furthermore, transmigration across intestinal epithelium triggers neutrophil release of elastase, which then disrupts the apical junctions in a very localized fashion, perhaps contributing to the loss of epithelial cell integrity during colitis.[83]

Eventual characterization of regulated neutrophil movement across epithelium and the interactions between epithelial cells and migrated neutrophils will provide important insights into the pathophysiology of infectious diseases at such epithelial surfaces.

Neutrophil migration through tissue is likewise the consequence of a carefully regulated process involving the sequential release and compartmentalization of a wide variety of inflammatory mediators. Early (0 to 5 hours) neutrophil influx into an area of induced injury appears predominantly to reflect the effects of IFN-γ, C5a, and leukotriene B_4. IL-8 and IL-6 appear in a second wave of mediator activity (at 5 to 24 hours) and IL-1α, GM-CSF, and TNF-α in a third wave of activity (8 to 24 hours), whereas concentrations of IL-1, IL-2, and IL-4 remain unchanged. C5a, leukotriene B_4, and IL-8 are potent neutrophil chemoattractants, as are hydroxyeicosatetraenoic (HETE) acids and microbial oligopeptides analogous to N-formyl-methionyl-leucyl-phenylalanine (fMLP).

Tissue migration of neutrophils also reflects remarkable temporal regulation, well illustrated by the shift in the biosynthesis of lipid mediators during inflammation.[84] Proinflammatory molecules such as leukotrienes and prostaglandins are generated endogenously at inflammatory sites and stimulate neutrophil degranulation and chemotaxis. Whereas the arachidonate released by activated neutrophils is converted to leukotriene B_4 (LTB$_4$) by neutrophil 5'-lipoxygenase, the arachidonate in the exudate likewise becomes a substrate for the 15'-lipoxygenase expressed by tissue macrophages recruited to the site. The latter reaction generates lipoxin A_4 (LXA$_4$), which inhibits neutrophil activation in a receptor-dependent fashion and blocks inflammation. Taken together, the shift from proinflammatory leukotrienes and prostaglandins early to anti-inflammatory lipoxins late provides a mechanism for the sequential promotion of exudate formation followed by resolution mediated by transcellular metabolism of lipid mediators generated in situ.

Among the soluble mediators that can recruit leukocytes, the chemokines represent a diverse and biologically important class of proteins. Chemokines are a family of structurally related, pluripotent proteins that trigger leukocyte activation,[85] including adherence, chemotaxis, degranulation, and priming of the neutrophil oxidase; participate in angiogenesis; and figure prominently in host response to infection with human immunodeficiency virus (HIV).[86] Chemokines are classified into two major families, CXC and CC, distinguished by the presence or absence of an amino acid between the first two cysteines

in the protein. All chemokines targeted for neutrophils are in the CXC family, the most important of which is IL-8. Secreted by leukocytes, platelets, fibroblasts, epithelial cells, and activated endothelium, IL-8 triggers the full range of cellular responses in neutrophils. IL-8 activation of neutrophils is mediated by engagement of one of two G-protein–coupled membrane receptors that specifically recognize the chemokine.

Of importance from the point of view of pathogenesis of infection, several organisms have mimicked chemokine receptors as a means by which to enter cells. For example, US28, a gene product of human cytomegalovirus,[44] and ECRF3, a protein of *Herpesvirus saimiri*,[87] represent virally encoded proteins with significant structural homology to chemokine receptors. In addition, HIV enters target cells by utilizing CD4 and specific chemokine receptors.[88,89] Moreover, genetic polymorphisms in certain of these chemokine receptors have significant effects on susceptibility to or rate of progression of HIV-1 infection.[90] It is clear that chemokines and their receptors have a pivotal place in the inflammatory response and in the pathogenesis of certain infectious diseases.

Chemotactic stimuli bind to high-affinity receptors on the leukocyte surface. Receptors for IL-8, fMLP, and C5a are members of a large family of proteins characterized by an external ligand-binding domain, seven membrane-spanning segments, and cytoplasmic regions that couple to G proteins.[44] In the presence of chemoattractant gradients across the cell as small as 0.1% to 1.0% (e.g., as the attractant diffuses from a focus of infection), ligand-linked receptors distribute asymmetrically and trigger the directed movement (chemotaxis) and net accumulation of neutrophils at sites of increasing concentrations of attractant (Fig. 8-4). How the chemoattractant signal is transduced to cell movement is not precisely understood, but calcium fluxes, actin, and a number of actin-binding and regulatory proteins of the cytoskeleton are centrally involved,[91] as are leukocyte-adherence molecules and the extracellular matrix. Just as mystifying is how the migrating neutrophil deciphers and prioritizes competing signals that drive chemotaxis. For example, within the inflammatory site the advancing neutrophil encounters host chemoattractants such as IL-8 and LTB$_4$ as well as bacterially derived or generated factors such as fMLP or C5a, respectively. Recent data suggest that an intracellular signaling hierarchy exists that favors neutrophil responses to targets derived from or by bacteria in preference to host chemokines.[92] The binding of chemoattractants to their receptors also initiates elements of the microbicidal response, namely, degranulation and the respiratory burst, although these responses generally require higher concentrations of the stimulus than does chemotaxis. For this reason, activation of these distal events may be delayed until the cell is in proximity to the infected tissue site.

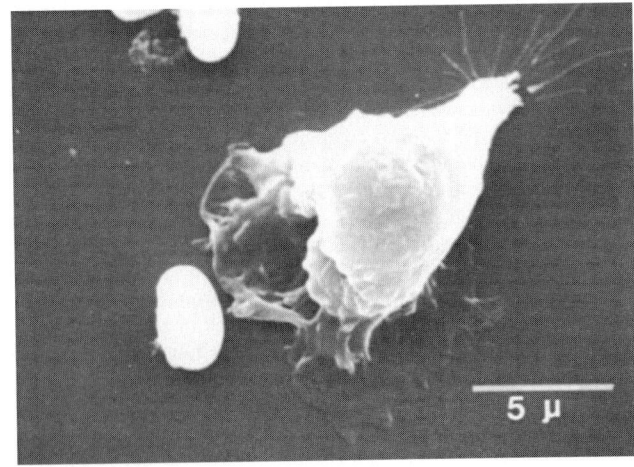

FIGURE 8-4. Scanning electron micrograph of a neutrophil extending a pseudopod toward *Candida albicans*.

Step 2—Ingestion

Phagocytosis is the intracellular uptake of particles greater than 0.5 mm by a mechanism independent of clathrin but dependent on the polymerization of actin. After attachment to the cell surface, the phagocytic particle is internalized, with subsequent phagosome maturation (described later) and eventual delivery to and fusion with the lysosome to form a phagolysosome.[93,94] Neutrophils may ingest some microorganisms in the absence of serum factors by a process known as lectinophagocytosis, wherein surface proteins on one or both cells recognize specific carbohydrates on the other cell. However, most bacteria must be opsonized for attachment to and ingestion by neutrophils to occur efficiently.

Specific IgG and complement are the major opsonic factors promoting recognition and ingestion of most microorganisms by neutrophils. Antibody promotes phagocytic uptake by neutralizing antiphagocytic molecules on the bacterial surface (e.g., capsular polysaccharide), efficiently activating the classic pathway of complement and promoting deposition of opsonic fragments of C3 on the bacterial surface, physically linking the organism to the neutrophils and engaging the IgG receptor in the neutrophil membrane. Activation of complement via either the alternative or the classic pathway leads to C3b and iC3b deposition on the microbial surface (see Chapter 7), and C1q deposition enhances Fc receptor–dependent ingestion.[95] Opsonization directly alters the organism by making the relatively hydrophilic microbial surface more hydrophobic and therefore more readily ingested.

Distinct receptors for IgG (FcγRI through RIII), but not other immunoglobulins, and for C3b (CR1) and iC3b (CR3) are present in the neutrophil membrane.[42,43] In addition to its iC3b-binding site, CR3 also bears a carbohydrate recognition domain that may play a role in lectinophagocytosis. Data suggest that Fcγ receptors mediate phagocytosis via calcium-dependent pathways, whereas CR1 and CR3 use calcium-independent pathways.[96] FcγRII and RIII are low- to moderate-affinity receptors that are constitutively expressed, whereas the high-affinity FcγRI is present only after cell stimulation (e.g., by IFN-γ).[97] Intracellular pools of Fc receptors have not been identified, but reserves have been described for both CR1 and CR3.[43] These receptor pools are rapidly mobilized to the surface after stimulation of the cell by a variety of inflammatory mediators.

Binding of either IgG or C3 increases the rate of phagocytosis of appropriately sensitized erythrocytes. However, Fc receptor-dependent interactions with this target initiate microfilament polymerization and ingestion only in unprimed cells. In contrast, complement deposition alone is sufficient to promote ingestion of a number of bacteria, a finding that emphasizes the heterogeneity among opsonic requirements for different particles. In most cases, phagocytosis is most efficient when organisms are coated with both IgG and C3, thereby allowing cooperative interaction of the two types of receptors.

Ingestion is the result of the sequential interaction between opsonic ligands distributed over the particle surface and their receptors on the phagocyte membrane.[98] The sequential interaction of these opsonic ligands with their receptors in the phagocytic membrane initiates polymerization of actin microfilaments in the cytoplasm underlying the site of particle attachment and results in circumferential flow of the cell membrane about the opsonized particle and its enclosure within a phagosome (Fig. 8-5; see also Fig. 8-4).[99,100]

Increased attention has been paid to the important phagocytic role played by receptors that do not bind to opsonins, especially in soft tissues where neutrophil function is most critical. Receptors for fibronectin and laminin, proteins that constitute part of the extracellular matrix secreted by endothelial cells, recognize the Arg-Gly-Asp (RGD) amino acid sequence in these extracellular matrix proteins.[101] Although these proteins in solution fail to promote ingestion of target particles, neutrophils adherent to surfaces coated with proteins containing this sequence display enhanced capacity to ingest C3-coated particles when stimulated with a variety of chemotactic factors. This enhancement requires neutrophil adherence to the matrix protein but not interaction of the matrix protein with the target particles or an increase in FcγR or C3 receptor number. Hence these proteins are not opsonins but rather enhance phagocytosis by converting C3 receptors from a binding mode to one mediating ingestion. Studies have assigned an important role for the vitronectin receptor ($\alpha_V\beta_3$) in modulating phagocytosis via the $\alpha_{5\beta1}$ receptor on mononuclear phagocytes.[102] Such findings reinforce the notion that migrating phagocytes modulate their phagocytic capacity according to the tissue context in which they function.

Step 3—Intracellular Disposition of the Ingested Microbe

Once internalization has begun, actin polymerization in the cytoplasm immediately adjacent to the nascent phagosome occurs and actin-binding proteins are recruited to the periphagosomal space. In an orderly fashion, cytosolic proteins associate with and disassociate from the phagosome sequentially, with eventual fusion of the phagosome with the neutrophil granules. In the mature phagosome, optimal microbicidal activity represents the coordinated generation of oxygen-derived species by activation of the NADPH-dependent oxidase and release of granule components. As discussed later, the successful survival of several intracellular pathogens reflects their ability to elude or undermine events critical for normal phagosomal maturation and complete recruitment of the elements essential for microbicidal action.

Oxidative Burst. The oxidative or respiratory burst is mediated by a multicomponent system present as an enzymatically active complex in the plasma membrane and phagosomal membrane of stimulated neutrophils.[103,104] Such enzymatic activity is not detected in resting, nonstimulated neutrophils. A similar, if not identical, enzyme system is found in stimulated eosinophils, monocytes, and macrophages. The respiratory burst enzyme transports electrons from cytosolic NADPH to molecular oxygen to generate superoxide anion ($O\bullet_2^-$), the one-electron reduction product of oxygen, as the immediate product:

$$2O_2 + NADPH \rightarrow 2O\bullet_2^- + H^+ + NADP^+$$

Important features of the oxidase include the 1:1 stoichiometry between oxygen consumption and superoxide formation, the two-electron oxidation of the pyridine nucleotide compared with the one-electron reduction of oxygen, the formation of protons, and the generation of NADP$^+$, which must be reduced back to NADPH to sustain the reaction.

Most of the superoxide formed readily undergoes dismutation to hydrogen peroxide and oxygen:

$$2O\bullet_2^- + 2H^+ \rightarrow H_2O_2 + O_2$$

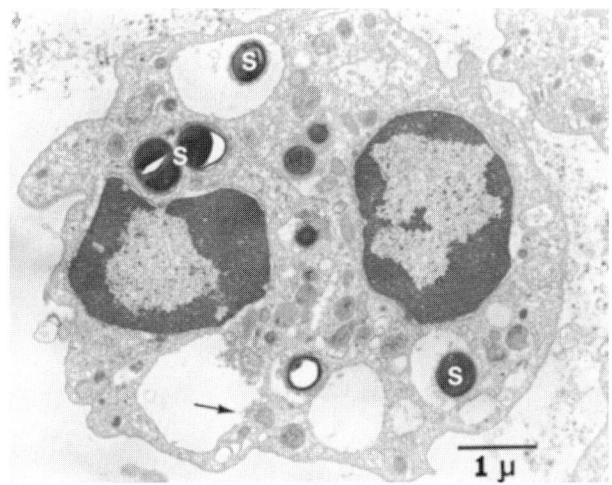

FIGURE 8-5. Electron micrograph of a neutrophil that has ingested *Staphylococcus aureus* (S). Bacteria are in phagocytic vacuoles formed by invagination of the external cell membrane. Degranulation into a phagocytic vacuole can be seen at the lower left (*arrow*).

This reaction is catalyzed by superoxide dismutase, but also occurs spontaneously with rapid kinetics at acidic pH, where a significant portion of the superoxide exists in its protonated form, the perhydroxy radical ($HO•_2^-$). This is a result of the high rate constant for the reaction between $O•_2^-$ and $HO•_2^-$. In the acidic environment of the phagocytic vacuole, superoxide is converted quantitatively to hydrogen peroxide. Because 1 mole of oxygen is regenerated for each mole of hydrogen peroxide formed, there is a net 1:1 stoichiometry between oxygen consumption and hydrogen peroxide formation, but a 2:1 relation between $O•_2^-$ and H_2O_2.

Detoxification of $O•_2^-$ and H_2O_2 is carried out by cellular enzyme systems. At neutral or basic pH, superoxide dismutase markedly accelerates the dismutation reaction. H_2O_2 is metabolized both by catalase and through the glutathione system. Catalase converts H_2O_2 directly to water and oxygen, whereas glutathione peroxidase utilizes reduced glutathione (GSH) to reduce H_2O_2 to water. NADPH provides the reducing equivalents for the glutathione reductase–catalyzed regeneration of GSH from glutathione (GSSG). NADPH levels must be maintained in order to support both the superoxide-forming oxidase and the glutathione cycle. The reduced pyridine nucleotide is regenerated by the activity of the hexose monophosphate shunt, which is enhanced 15- to 30-fold during phagocytosis.

The dormant respiratory burst oxidase of the resting neutrophil is activated as the cell is stimulated (e.g., during phagocytosis). The lag period between stimulus exposure and expression of NADPH oxidase activity varies from 10 or 20 seconds to 1 or 2 minutes, depending on the stimulus. It appears that the lag time reflects the period required for assembly of the multiple components of the oxidase at the cytoplasmic face of the plasma membrane or phagosomal membrane. On the basis of studies in both intact neutrophils and in vitro cell-free systems, the components of the NADPH oxidase comprise integral membrane proteins as well as soluble cytosolic proteins (Fig. 8-6).[104,105]

Within the membrane is cytochrome-b_{558}, so designated because of a characteristic 558-nm peak in its redox difference spectrum.[106-108] It is a heterodimer composed of large and small subunits, gp91phox and p22phox (phox stands for phagocyte oxidase), respectively, which are firmly but noncovalently associated. This protein has two different types of redox centers: a flavin adenine dinucleotide (FAD) domain and two heme prosthetic groups.[109,110] Cytochrome-b_{558} appears to be the sole catalytic subunit of the oxidase. The substrate, NADPH, binds to a domain within the flavoprotein portion of the molecule and is oxidized by the transfer of two electrons to FAD. Then follow two single-electron reductions of the heme groups ($Fe^{3+} \rightarrow Fe^{2+}$). The very low midpoint potential of the reduced hemes allows them to react directly with molecular oxygen, reoxidizing the iron moieties and forming two molecules of superoxide, $O•_2^-$.

Although cytochrome-b_{558} appears to mediate the catalytic functions of the respiratory burst oxidase, other proteins are required for enzyme activation and activity. Two necessary proteins, p47phox and p67phox, are present in neutrophil cytosol,[111-115] existing, at least in part, as a complex with one another.[104,116,117] The primary structure of p47phox includes a very cationic carboxyl-terminal domain containing several serine residues that serve as substrates for phosphorylation by several kinases including protein kinase C (PKC) or related enzymes.[114] In the stimulated neutrophil, some sites on p47phox are phosphorylated and the partially phosphorylated protein then translocates to the plasma membrane, where additional sites are phosphorylated.[118-122] There is also evidence for phosphorylation-independent determinants of p47phox translocation.[123]

The functioning oxidase assembles at the plasma membrane, and cytochrome-b_{558} appears to be the membrane docking site for p47phox.[105] Specific sites of gp91phox and p22phox have been implicated as mediating interactions with the cytosolic components.[124-126] Neutrophil stimulation also results in membrane translocation of p67phox, probably as a result of its association with p47phox; p67phox fails to translocate in the absence of p47phox, although p47phox is competent for translocation by itself.[121]

Both p47phox and p67phox contain two copies of a 50–amino acid domain related to a region of the Src oncoprotein designated SH3 (src homology region 3).[113,115] Proline-rich motifs similar to those that bind to SH3 domains in other proteins[127] are present in p47phox, p67phox, and p22phox. In general, SH3 domains are thought to mediate binding to cytoskeletal and membrane elements. Both SH3 and proline-rich segments of the oxidase proteins are involved in the protein-protein

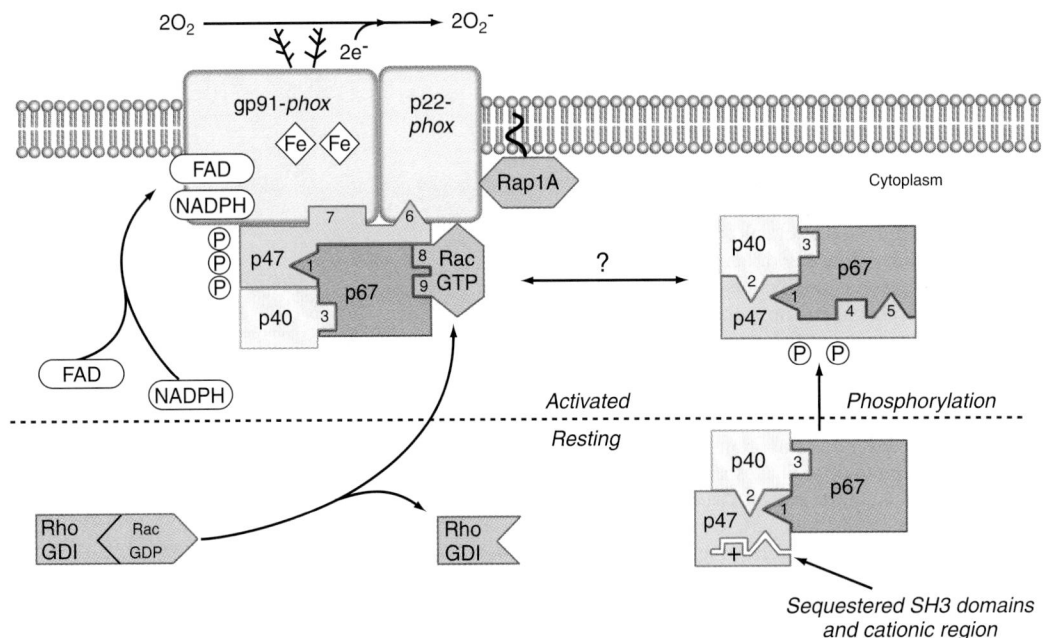

FIGURE 8-6. Model of the agonist-dependent assembly of the neutrophil respiratory burst oxidase. Numbers 1 through 7 represent associations mediated by interactions between SH3 domains and proline-rich regions *(triangular shapes)* or by other protein-protein binding motifs *(square shapes)*. *(Modified from DeLeo FR, Quinn MT. Assembly of the phagocyte NADPH oxidase: Molecular interactions of oxidase proteins. J Leukoc Biol. 1996;60:677-691.)*

interactions required for oxidase activation and function.[128,129] The net effect of phosphorylation and translocation of cytosolic components is the assembly on the membrane of the active oxidase complex, composed of the cytochrome-b_{558} subunits, p47phox, p67phox, and perhaps other constituents including RAC2 and p40phox.

In cell-free model systems, requirements for additional proteins have been demonstrated. In keeping with the enhancement of oxidase activation in these systems by guanosine triphosphate (GTP) or nonhydrolyzable GTP analogues, the low-molecular-weight GTP-binding proteins RAC1 or RAC2, depending on species and type of phagocytic cell,[130-132] have been implicated as essential elements of the oxidase. The RAC proteins are isolated together with another protein, rhoGDI (the guanoside diphosphatase dissociation inhibitor of p21rho), which may also be involved in the oxidase system. Modification of the carboxyl terminus of RAC by isoprenylation with a 20-carbon (geranylgeranyl) fatty acid and carboxymethylation promotes association with rhoGDI and with membranes and is required for optimal activity.[133,134] During neutrophil stimulation, RAC translocates to the plasma membrane but in a fashion independent of the redistribution of p47phox and p67phox.[135-137] Another small GTP-binding protein, RAP1A, is closely associated with cytochrome-b_{558}, but whether it is involved in NADPH oxidase assembly or function is unknown.[138] An additional oxidase-related cytosolic protein, p40phox, exhibits homology to p47phox,[138] including the presence of an SH3 domain, and may serve as a regulator of enzyme activation.[139-141]

The active respiratory burst oxidase is topographically oriented in the membrane to promote the delivery of toxic products of oxygen reduction to the ingested microorganism. The binding site for NADPH is on the cytoplasmic face of the membrane, whereas the reaction product superoxide is formed at the vacuolar side. Oxidase activation on the external plasma membrane results in extracellular release of superoxide, a process important in the oxidative attack on attached but uningested organisms (e.g., protozoa) and on adjacent host cells. Despite indirect evidence that reactive products of the oxidase inactivate the enzyme,[142] the precise mechanisms by which oxidase activity is regulated and terminated are unknown.

Several homologues of the phagocyte NADPH oxidase have been recently discovered. The NOX gene family comprises to date five members with homology to gp91phox (also now designated as NOX2) plus two others known as dual oxidases (DUOX subfamily). Each member of the NOX family is expressed in a restricted range of tissues. For example, NOX1 is found primarily in colon epithelium, whereas NOX4 is detected mostly in the kidney.[143-145] In the case of NOX1, cytosolic cofactors homologous to p47phox and p67phox have been identified.[146-148] Whether any of the nonphagocyte NADPH oxidase systems are important in the host defense against infection remains to be determined.

Degranulation. In parallel with activation of the oxidative burst, stimulated neutrophils undergo exocytosis and release their granule contents.[149] This process is remarkably selective in its regulation of distinct granule subpopulations for fusion with different membranes. For example, fusion of granule membranes with the phagosome, with subsequent exocytosis into the phagolysosome, involves different fusogenic proteins and different granule populations than does extracellular release of granule contents.[149] Most extensively studied have been the differential calcium requirements for exocytosis of neutrophil granules.[150,151] In addition, the release of given granule populations depends on the specific stimulus and the particular opsonin used.[152]

Stimulated exocytosis requires cytoskeletal rearrangement[153,154] with redistribution of actin-binding proteins such as myristoylated alanine-rich C-kinase substrates (MARCKS).[155,156] Fusogenic proteins on the granules, including annexins,[157] syntaxin 4, vesicle-associated membrane protein-2 (VAMP-2), and other cytosolic soluble N-ethylmaleimide-sensitive attachment proteins (SNAPs),[158,159] mediate association at the target membranes with specific receptors, including various target SNAP receptors (t-SNAREs).[158,160] Lipid modification probably contributes critically to fusion of the granule membrane with the plasma or phagosomal membrane, and such remodeling depends on the redistribution and activation of cytosolic phospholipases.[161,162] The

intraphagosomal pH must be modified for optimal activation of some of the granule contents. To that end, activation recruits to the phagosomal membrane Na$^+$/H$^+$ exchangers, Na$^+$, K$^+$-ATPases, and vacuolar-type proton ATPases from membrane-bound granule intracellularly.[163,164]

As discussed previously, the granules of neutrophils differ not only in the luminal contents but also in the proteins inserted in their membranes. Azurophilic granules fuse predominantly with the phagosome, thereby delivering to the ingested organism microbicidal and hydrolytic proteins at high concentration. On the other hand, specific granules and secretory vesicles fuse preferentially with the plasma membrane, releasing contents extracellularly and bringing to the cell surface a variety of functionally important membrane proteins, including integrins, cytochrome-b_{558}, and receptors for chemotactic agents and opsonins. Taken together, the process of degranulation affords concurrent recruitment of critical membrane proteins (e.g., cytochrome-b_{558}) to the cell surface, release of essential elements of the oxygen-dependent microbicidal system (e.g., MPO), and discharge of proteins that possess direct antimicrobial activity (e.g., defensins, BPI).

Step 4—Resolution of the Inflammatory Response

Neutrophils have a relatively short half-life, approximately in circulation but longer in tissue, and constitutively undergo apoptosis before being cleared by tissue macrophages.[165,166] This fate, rather than undergoing necrotic cell death, avoids the release of granule proteins and other cytotoxic agents that might promote tissue damage. Neutrophils express members of the Bcl-2 family of apoptotic proteins, notably the pro-apoptotic proteins Bax, Bid, Bak, and Bad but not the anti-apoptotic Bcl-2.[167,168] Neutrophil apoptosis is caspase mediated, reflecting the involvement of mitochondria and complex cross-talk among several signaling pathways including the caspases, reactive oxygen species, and mitogen-activated protein (MAP) kinases.[169-171] Several molecules on the neutrophil surface have been implicated as participants in receptor-mediated uptake of apoptotic neutrophils by tissue macrophages, including phosphatidylserine exposed from the inner leaflet of the plasma membrane, altered membrane carbohydrates, and oxidized membrane phospholipids.[172] Likewise, a variety of receptors have been proposed to mediate uptake, including a phosphatidylserine receptor, scavenger receptors, and the coordinated activity of CD36 and the integrin $\alpha_{v\beta3}$.[172]

Within the context of the acute inflammatory response, cytokines released at the site delay apoptosis, thereby extending the neutrophil life span and permitting their participation in host defense. Cytokines modulate pro- and anti-apoptotic pathways in a variety of ways and the initiation of phagocytosis by neutrophils accelerates apoptosis with an associated downregulation of their proinflammatory capacity.[173-175] Thus the stimulated neutrophil, at the peak of its response to an invading microbe, initiates pathways leading to decreased proinflammatory activity and to apoptosis, en route to resolution of the acute phase of the inflammatory response.[176] Evidence supporting this interpretation comes from a consideration of the local consequences when accelerated apoptosis is not triggered by neutrophil stimulation. Neutrophils from individuals with chronic granulomatous disease (vide infra) undergo delayed apoptosis after stimulation[174,175] and produce less prostaglandin D_2, an anti-inflammatory mediator, deficiencies that may contribute to the chronic inflammation and granuloma formation that are hallmarks of this disease.

Microbicidal Mechanisms

Postphagocytic events deliver the products of degranulation and the respiratory burst to the phagocytic vacuole, a closed space in which an ingested microbe is exposed to high concentrations of toxic substances while the exposure of the phagocyte and other cells to these potentially injurious agents is limited (see Fig. 8-5). Antimicrobial mechanisms are classified by their dependence or lack of dependence on the products of the oxidative burst.

Oxygen-dependent bactericidal mechanisms can be divided into MPO-dependent and MPO-independent reactions. The essential requirements for the MPO-mediated bactericidal mechanisms, as first described by Klebanoff,[177,178] are MPO (released from the primary granule), hydrogen peroxide (generated by the respiratory burst), and a halide ion. In addition, the low pH present in the phagocytic vacuole enhances the enzymatic and microbicidal activity of MPO. Hydrogen peroxide by itself has bactericidal properties, but in the presence of MPO the microbicidal potency of this system is enhanced 50-fold. The particular halide cofactor used in the MPO–hydrogen peroxide reaction affects potency, the effect of iodide being greater than that of bromide, which is greater than that of chloride. However, at physiologic concentrations, chloride appears to be the predominant cofactor for this reaction in the cell.[177]

Hypochlorous acid, formed by the neutrophil when chloride serves as the cofactor, is a potent oxidizing and microbicidal agent.[178,179] Other products, including chlorine gas, chlorinated sterols, tyrosyl radicals, and nitric oxide–derived reactants, are generated by neutrophils via MPO-catalyzed reactions.[180-184] The precise events responsible for the microbicidal activity of the MPO system are incompletely characterized. Candidate target sites in bacteria include components of the electron transport chain, iron-sulfur centers, penicillin-binding proteins, and sites in bacterial membranes that are necessary for initiation of chromosomal replication.[185-188] Oxidation of some of these molecules may lead to the release of free iron, which can then participate in the formation of the highly reactive hydroxyl radical.[189] In addition to these effects, the MPO–hydrogen peroxide–halide system promotes the formation of singlet oxygen, decarboxylation of amino acids to form toxic aldehydes, and generation of chloramines,[190] agents that may contribute to neutrophil microbicidal activity.[191] Studies have implicated the MPO–hydrogen peroxide–halide system in tissue injury, oxidation of lipids, and possibly in atherogenesis, extending the biologic importance of this system beyond its microbicidal activity.[192-194]

Metabolites of oxygen for which a role in neutrophil bactericidal activity has been suggested include hydrogen peroxide, superoxide anion, singlet oxygen, and hydroxyl radical. The fact that catalase, which degrades hydrogen peroxide, protects bacteria from the bactericidal effects of neutrophils[195] supports a direct germicidal effect of hydrogen peroxide. Superoxide, by itself, is thought to play little role in the killing of microorganisms because, for example, bacteria incubated in a cell-free, superoxide-generating system survive normally. However, under appropriate conditions superoxide can react with other products of oxygen metabolism to generate hydroxyl radical and singlet oxygen. The bactericidal effect of these oxygen-derived free radicals may result from the initiation of a chain of oxidizing events in the bacterial cell wall.[191]

Hydroxyl radical is a potent bactericidal agent that can be formed by the direct reaction of superoxide with hydrogen peroxide, a reaction that occurs slowly on its own, but is catalyzed by ferric ion.[196] Sensitive analytical systems indicate that activated neutrophils produce hydroxyl radical by two different mechanisms, one dependent on the catalytic activity of MPO,[197] and the other requiring transition metals in the Haber-Weiss reaction.[198] The relative contribution of each mechanism to the overall production of hydroxyl radical in vivo depends on the availability of exogenous transition metals, usually iron. In the presence of supplemental iron, hydroxyl radical generation occurs through the Haber-Weiss reaction. However, lactoferrin and transferrin can interfere with this reaction by binding iron in a noncatalytic form. Therefore, under physiologic conditions it appears that the small amounts of hydroxyl radical generated by stimulated neutrophils are derived from the MPO-dependent pathway.

Underemphasized in the past has been the importance of oxygen-independent antimicrobial systems in overall innate immunity and neutrophil-dependent host defense.[199-201] The involvement of these mechanisms is clearly demonstrated by the ability of neutrophils to kill some organisms under anaerobic conditions. Agents contributing to oxygen-independent microbicidal activity include acid, defensins, BPI, lactoferrin, lysozyme, and a variety of cationic proteins. In human neutrophils, the pH in the phagosome decreases to about 6.0.[202] Although some microorganisms (e.g., pneumococci) are killed by the effects of acid alone, most bacteria are resistant to the acid environment per se. The main effect of the low pH in the phagocytic vacuole is to potentiate the microbicidal and degradative activity of the granule enzymes.

Defensins are potent antimicrobial peptides in the primary granules of neutrophils[203,204] and in epithelial cells of the gut and the genitourinary tract.[205,206] Defensins and closely related proteins are widely distributed in nature (e.g., the hemolymph of insects[207]) and probably represent an ancient mechanism for host defense. In general, defensins are small molecules (3 to 4 kDa) rich in arginine and containing a characteristic disulfide motif. Elegant studies have defined many of the physical properties of purified defensins[208-210] and provided insight into their mechanism of action, which involves insertion into microbial membranes resulting in the formation of pores that allow efflux of cytoplasmic components. The spectrum of organisms against which defensins are active is extremely broad, including gram-positive and gram-negative bacteria, fungi, and enveloped viruses.

BPI is a 59-kDa protein located in the primary granule of neutrophils. Its antimicrobial activity resides in a 25-kDa amino-terminal fragment.[211,212] In addition, BPI binds to lipopolysaccharide[213] and blocks the release of TNF elicited by bacteria,[214] properties that suggest the clinical utility of recombinant BPI, or a fragment thereof, in the treatment or prevention of lipopolysaccharide-dependent sequelae of acute bacterial infection. Clinical trials with recombinant amino-terminal BPI have demonstrated efficacy in ameliorating morbidity and mortality in disseminated meningococcal disease in children.[215]

Lactoferrin is an iron-binding protein found in secretions bathing mucosal membranes and in the specific granules of neutrophils.[216] Lactoferrin's bacteriostatic properties reflect its ability to deprive bacteria of the iron required for growth, an effect eliminated by saturation of its iron-binding sites.[216] Lactoferrin plays a role in the alteration of the physicochemical properties of the neutrophil membrane that occurs during degranulation,[217] in the modulation of hydroxyl radical production,[196] in the regulation of granulopoiesis,[218] and in the modulation of complement function.[219]

Lysozyme, found mainly in the specific granules but also present in the primary granules, hydrolyzes the glycoside bond between N-acetylmuramic acid and N-acetylglucosamine, a component of the peptidoglycan in bacterial cell walls. Although the bactericidal properties of lysozyme reflect this activity, peptide substitutions on the N-acetylmuramic acid residue in most bacteria make this bond inaccessible to lysozyme, thereby limiting its bacteriolytic properties. However, in the context of the complex environment of an inflammatory reaction, a bacterial cell wall already damaged by complement or granule proteins may allow access of lysozyme to its site of action.

Additional cationic proteins isolated from neutrophil primary granules[199,211] demonstrate preferential activity against specific bacterial species. These proteins include a 37-kDa cationic antimicrobial protein, the activity of which is favored by the intraphagosomal acid pH[220,221]; p15s[222]; azuricidin[223]; indolicin[224]; and cathelicidins.[225] Understanding of the principles of antimicrobial activity of these proteins is incomplete at this time. In some cases it involves temperature-independent binding to the organism via ionic interactions followed by temperature-dependent insertion into the outer membrane via hydrophobic interactions.[211] These sequential events result in increased permeability of the bacterial outer membrane and the subsequent death of the organism.

Microbial Defenses against Phagocytes

Ongoing investigation in microbial pathogenesis reflects the scientific advances in molecular microbiology and eukaryotic cell biology. In many ways, results from using these newer analytical approaches challenge our conventional understanding of microbial pathogenesis and the biologic meaning of colonization, commensalism, infection, and disease.[226] The application of genetic arrays to the host-microbe interaction has revealed the remarkably dynamic and interactive nature both of the invading microorganism and of the responsive host cell. Neutrophil phagocytosis elicits transcription of an array of genes[227] and group A streptococci undergo complex transcriptional response to evade the activities of neutrophils.[228,229] The ingested microbe responds to its immediate environment rapidly and specifically. For example, among the many genes expressed by *Escherichia coli* 7 minutes after being ingested by normal neutrophils are those regulated by OxyR, an oxygen-sensing transcription factor.[230] However the same strain of *E. coli* does not express OxyR-regulated genes when ingested by chronic granulomatous disease (CGD) neutrophils, cells lacking the capacity to generate reactive oxygen species and thereby to create an oxidant stress with the phagosome.

Within the complex context of the interactive cell biology between host and microbe, it is clear that pathogens have evolved molecular strategies for neutralizing one or more of the discrete steps in normal host defense.[231,232] To that end, the invading microorganism may exploit specific aspects of normal mammalian cell biology, including adhesive properties, signal transduction pathways, cytoskeletal rearrangements, and vacuolar trafficking,[233] or, as with *Chlamydia*, alter genes involved in multiple cellular pathways.[234] In some cases these properties are manifest only when microbes are in the appropriate host, demonstrating the exquisitely precise manner in which the invading microorganism has adapted to the context of the mammalian host.[235,236]

In some cases bacteria adhere to surface proteins on target phagocytes, as with certain *Neisseria* and CD66 on the neutrophil surface.[237] In other situations, bacterial proteins secreted into target cells may modify the host cell response, as is the case with the Yop proteins of *Yersinia*. Once secreted into the host cell, the various members of the Yop family of proteins impair phagocytosis, induce apoptosis, paralyze cellular actin, and, in the case of the tyrosine phosphatase YopH, block Fc receptor–mediated activation of the respiratory burst oxidase.[238,239] In other settings, multiple mammalian cell types are targeted. For example, a glycoprotein of Ebola virus, in its secreted form, engages the neutrophil Fc receptor and inhibits cell activation and, in its transmembrane form, interacts with endothelial cells. In this way the virus simultaneously inhibits the neutrophil-dependent early inflammatory response and induces endothelial cell damage, the clinical hallmark of Ebola virus infection.[240]

Even within the phagocyte microbes have devised ways to subvert or avoid host defenses and survive. For example, within mononuclear phagocytes, mycobacteria block the fusion of lysosomes with phagosomes and inhibit recruitment of the endosomal vacuolar proton ATPase that mediates phagosomal acidification. The aberrant compartmentalization of mycobacteria depends on the viability of the organism, assigning the organism an active role in the subversion of fusion, and results in the avoidance by the organism of the microbicidal and hydrolytic contents of the phagocyte's lysosomes. In an analogous fashion, *Chlamydia* remain in an intracellular vacuole dissociated from the endosomal pathway of the host cell.[241] *Salmonella* evades the consequences of the phagocyte's reactive oxygen species by entering macrophages into a compartment free of the components of the NADPH oxidase.[242-244] Success of the process depends on a functional type III secretion system in *Salmonella*, although it is not known if bacterial products actively exclude flavocytochrome-b_{558} from the nascent phagosome or inhibit normal macrophage responses that recruit the membrane elements necessary for organization and assembly of a functional NADPH oxidase. On the other hand, in the case of intraphagocytic *Leishmania* spp., the phagosomes acquire markers from the lysosomal compartment and the intraphagolysosomal pH is appropriately acidic, although organisms survive.[245,246] Other organisms escape the vacuole and invade the cytoplasm of the host cell, targeting a variety of host proteins or organellar systems. Even with the limited details available, it is clear that there is as broad a range of microbial tactics for pathogenesis as there are host cell targets and their elucidation will provide insights into the biology of both the host and the pathogen.

DEFECTS IN NEUTROPHIL FUNCTION

Defects in neutrophil function can result from decreased numbers of mature neutrophils or abnormalities in chemotaxis, ingestion, or bactericidal mechanisms.[247] Table 8-2 summarizes these defects. Infections resulting from quantitative or qualitative defects in neutrophil function

TABLE 8-2 Defects in Neutrophil Function

Neutropenia
  Acquired
    Drug induced
    Autoimmune
    Cancer related
  Hereditary
    Infantile genetic agranulocytosis
    Familial neutropenia
    Cyclic neutropenia
Qualitative defects
  Adhesion defects
    Leukocyte adhesion deficiency
      Type 1, integrin deficiency
      Type 2, E-selectin ligand deficiency
  Chemotactic defects
    Humoral
      Complement deficiency
      Inhibitors
      Immune complexes
      Hyperimmunoglobulinemia E (Job's) syndrome
    Cellular
      Chédiak-Higashi syndrome
      Hypophosphatemia
      Lazy leukocyte syndrome
  Opsonic defects
    Complement deficiency
    Antibody deficiency
  Defects in intracellular killing
    Abnormal respiratory burst
      Chronic granulomatous disease
      Glucose-6-phosphate dehydrogenase deficiency
    Granule abnormalities
      Myeloperoxidase deficiency
      Specific granule deficiency
      Chédiak-Higashi syndrome

share a tendency to be prolonged, slowly responsive to antibiotics, and recurrent. Qualitative defects may be intrinsic or extrinsic to the neutrophil. In general, the intrinsic defects of qualitative neutrophil function are more severe than are the extrinsic defects. Staphylococci, gram-negative organisms, and fungi are the usual pathogens responsible for these infections. Encapsulated bacteria frequently cause infection in patients with defective serum opsonic activity. Essentially any organ system may be the site of infections associated with neutrophil defects. Patients with severe neutropenia tend to experience bacteremia with a septic clinical picture, whereas those with qualitative functional defects most commonly develop localized infection, especially cutaneous infections with associated adenitis. However, defects in microbicidal activity are associated with such complications as liver abscess, osteomyelitis, sinopulmonary infections, and central nervous system infections. Inflammatory periodontal disease is commonly encountered in patients with neutrophil dysfunction and may be a useful early marker of impaired host defenses.

Neutropenia

The most common granulocyte defect encountered is the absolute reduction of circulating neutrophils. The lower limit of normal for circulating neutrophils is 1500 to 2000 cells/mm³. The risk of acquiring an infection increases progressively with both the duration and the magnitude of the granulocytopenia at fewer than 1500 cells/mm³. At fewer than 500 cells/mm³, there is a dramatic increase in the incidence of infection.[248]

The acquired neutropenias are most often related to drug therapy and may be either a predictable result of cytotoxic therapy or an idiosyncratic reaction. The former is frequently encountered during chemotherapy for various neoplastic and immunologic disorders. Neutropenia caused by idiosyncratic drug reactions is observed with phenothiazines, sulfonamides, penicillins, cephalosporins, and vancomycin. Chloramphenicol can cause both a predictable and an idiosyncratic neutropenia. The latter is rare, but when it occurs is frequently fatal. Increased granulocyte destruction may occur as a result of splenic sequestration, which may be immunologically mediated by antibody[249] or secondary to any of the causes of hypersplenism. Splenectomy may be beneficial in restoring neutrophil counts toward normal.

The availability of recombinant CSFs has afforded clinicians a therapeutic option for treatment of acquired cytopenias.[4,248] Most clinical experience has been with G-CSF and GM-CSF, primarily for treatment of the granulocytopenia associated with cancer chemotherapy and bone marrow transplantation (reviewed in reference 250). These agents have been used to stimulate hematopoiesis in myelodysplastic syndromes, aplastic anemia, and cytopenias resulting from chemotherapy. Likewise, GM-CSF has been used to overcome HIV-mediated leukopenias and, in some cases, to permit use of myelosuppressive antiviral agents. Not only is the number of circulating cells increased, but the biologic function and bactericidal activity of the recruited cells are normal.[251] However, current data do not support the use of these agents as an adjunct to antibiotics in infected patients with normal neutrophil production.[252]

Hereditary neutropenia is observed either as a solitary defect or in association with other defects. The neutropenia can be severe as in infantile genetic agranulocytosis, moderate as in familial (benign) neutropenia, or cyclic. Infantile genetic agranulocytosis (Kostmann's syndrome) is an autosomal recessive disorder characterized by granulocyte maturation arrest and severe infection with death in infancy. Progenitor cells from some patients with Kostmann's syndrome are hyporesponsive to G-CSF, and a subset of these individuals have a somatic point mutation in the gene encoding the G-CSF receptor.[253] Some hereditary neutropenias are accompanied by an apparent compensatory monocytosis. Cyclic neutropenia is a rare autosomal dominant defect of myelopoiesis characterized by the periodic disappearance of neutrophils and other blood elements from the circulation. Early granulocyte precursors are present in the marrow during the neutropenia, suggesting a transient maturation arrest. The duration of neutropenia ranges from 5 to 8 days, followed by a 2- to 5-week period with normal numbers of circulating neutrophils. In any given patient, the periodic oscillations are highly predictable. During the neutropenic state, the patient experiences aphthous stomatitis, fever, malaise, and cutaneous infections. The disease is usually recognized during childhood, and there is no amelioration with age. Treatment with either recombinant G-CSF[254] or alternate-day prednisolone[255] attenuates the oscillations in neutrophil maturation.

Leukocyte Adhesion Deficiency Syndromes

The hallmark of the leukocyte adhesion deficiency (LAD) syndromes is severe, prolonged, and recurrent infection in the face of a marked granulocytosis. Blood neutrophil counts are often 2 to 20 times higher than normal, even in the absence of infection. Despite this impressive granulocytosis, pus formation (the accumulation of neutrophils in tissues) is limited, and patients develop abscesses that manifest relatively few of the classic signs of infection. This abnormality reflects impaired adhesion of affected cells within the vasculature and their inability to immigrate into the tissue. Two types of LAD have been described: LAD-1,[256] in which integrin expression is abnormal, and LAD-2,[257] in which expression of the primary selectin ligand sLe^x on granulocytes is essentially absent (see Fig. 8-3). In vivo, cells from patients with type 1 deficiency display normal rolling adhesion, but are unable to adhere firmly to the venule walls or to emigrate from the vasculature.[258] In contrast, cells from those with type 2 deficiency fail to adhere to stimulated venules exposed to normal shear forces, and they do not exhibit rolling adhesion. Because integrin function is intact, these cells can adhere to the vessel wall and can immigrate into the tissues if shear forces are absent.

LAD-1 results from mutations in the gene encoding the β_2-integrin subunit CD18 and is inherited in an autosomal recessive manner. Nearly 40 different mutations in *INTG2* gene have been associated with LAD-1.[259] There is frequently a history of consanguinity, and both severe and moderate phenotypes are recognized. Patients with

this syndrome typically present with prolonged and/or recurrent staphylococcal and *Pseudomonas* infections beginning in infancy, often in the perinatal period. Patients with the severe phenotype exhibit poor wound healing. As a consequence, they often have delayed separation of the umbilical cord, a useful clinical diagnostic clue, and may develop omphalitis. Infections involving the soft tissues, mucosal surfaces, and the intestinal tract are common. Cutaneous infections frequently become necrotic. Initially these lesions may resemble ecthyma gangrenosum, whereas later they may assume an appearance more akin to pyoderma gangrenosum. Affected persons who survive infancy universally develop acute gingivitis with eruption of primary dentition. The gingivitis persists and results in progressive gingival hypertrophy and alveolar bone loss. Although survival into adulthood is not unusual, particularly in patients with the moderate phenotype, 41% of affected individuals die before the age of 2 years.[256,260]

Evaluation of neutrophil function demonstrates impaired adherence to artificial substrates, impaired chemotaxis in vivo and in vitro, and impaired respiratory burst in response to the ingestion of particles coated with iC3b but not IgG.[247,256] Affected neutrophils exhibit an abnormal burst in oxidative metabolism after stimulation with soluble stimuli, depending on which stimulus is used and the nature of the association between its receptor and the cytoskeleton.[261]

Leukocytes from patients with the severe phenotypic expression of LAD-1 bear less than 0.3% of the normal quantity of all three β_2-integrins, whereas moderately affected patients have 2.5% to 6% of the integrin expression level of healthy people.[260] In affected individuals, the surface expression of both the α- and β-chains is abnormal. However, the α-chain is present in normal amounts within the cell. The predominant basis for this syndrome is abnormal β-chain synthesis, which impairs intracellular assembly of the αβ-heterodimer for transport of the molecular complex to the cell surface.[262] Molecular analysis has demonstrated a spectrum of β-gene mutations that cause abnormalities ranging from failure to produce messenger RNA (mRNA) in some persons with the severe disease phenotype, to production of an abnormally sized precursor β-protein, to absence of any readily apparent defect.[263]

LAD-2 is an autosomal recessive disorder that has been described in three Arab-Israeli families from the vicinity of Nazareth and one Turkish child.[264-267] In addition to the infectious complications seen in patients with LAD-1, these people have a distinct facial appearance, short stature, microcephaly, mental retardation,[257,265] and the rare Bombay blood phenotype (hh). They develop recurrent bacterial infections, primarily pneumonia, beginning early in life. Periodontal infections, otitis media, and focal cellulitis have also been reported, but infection caused by a predominant organism has not been striking.[265] Patients with LAD-2 lack fucosylated glycoconjugates, and their underlying defect appears to be defective GDP-fucose biosynthesis secondary to a mutation in the gene encoding the GDP-fucose transporter.[266] Although the clinical phenotypes of the four patients are similar, only the Turkish child responded to oral fucose therapy with a decrease in the rate of infection, reduced leukocytosis, and appearance of fucosylated glycoconjugates on his neutrophils.[267] Whereas all three Arab patients have the same missense mutation, whereby arginine replaces threonine at codon 308 (T308R), the Turkish child has cysteine substituted for arginine at codon 147 (R147C), providing a genetic correlate for the different clinical and biochemical features. Despite the generalized nature of the defect, endothelial cells from LAD-2 patients support neutrophil rolling in vitro, demonstrating that the fucose is not essential for function of L-selectin ligands on vascular endothelium.[266]

In vivo assessment of neutrophil function reveals a marked impairment of both random motility and directed migration. Oxidative response to a particulate stimulus is within the normal range, although lower than that from simultaneously evaluated normal cells. Phorbol myristate acetate, a soluble stimulus, also evokes a normal, although somewhat greater than average, oxidative response from these cells. Lymphocyte number, subset distribution, and mitogenic responses are normal, as is natural killer cell activity.[257]

Chemotactic Defects

Defective neutrophil chemotaxis has been described in a number of pathologic conditions, in some cases as an apparently isolated abnormality, but also associated with impairment of other neutrophil functions. Some defects (extrinsic) are secondary to humoral factors, either decreases in chemoattractants or the presence of inhibitors, whereas others are due to intrinsic cellular abnormalities of the neutrophil.

Extrinsic Abnormalities

Neutrophil chemotactic defects resulting from extrinsic factors may be caused by abnormalities involving the complement cascade. These include genetic deficiencies (C3, C5) and decreased synthesis (cirrhosis, kwashiorkor, premature birth), hypercatabolism, and increased loss of serum proteins, as for example in patients with severe burns. Some investigators have noted a depression in neutrophil chemotactic responses in patients with diabetes mellitus that is independent of serum osmolality. The defect is mild and is most readily demonstrated in juvenile-onset diabetic patients. Chemotactic responsiveness of diabetic neutrophils can be restored in vitro by incubation with insulin.[268]

Inhibitors of chemotaxis may express their effect either directly on the phagocyte or indirectly by neutralizing the chemoattractant properties of complement. Polymeric IgA is cytophilic for neutrophils and can markedly depress chemotaxis.[269] Defective chemotaxis has been described in a number of diseases characterized by circulating immune complexes, including rheumatoid arthritis, systemic lupus erythematosus, and subacute bacterial endocarditis. The sera from about 40% of patients with systemic lupus erythematosus contain an inhibitor that is specific for C5-derived chemotactic activity, but does not interfere with the expression of other C5-mediated functions. Its presence correlates with disease activity and the resultant chemotactic defect with the enhanced susceptibility of these patients to infection.[270] The inhibitor has been identified as the Bb fragment of complement factor B, and it exerts its effect by inhibiting the interaction of C5a des Arg with co-chemotaxin in serum.[271]

A defect in neutrophil chemotaxis has been described in patients with juvenile periodontitis, a familial disorder characterized by periodontitis occurring in the absence of severe dental disease. Serum from some of these patients contains an inhibitor of chemotaxis, and the resultant defect in chemotaxis has been postulated to play a role in the pathogenesis of this disease.[272] In addition, neutrophils from some of these patients bear fewer chemoattractant receptors than do cells from unaffected persons, and an apparent structural abnormality of certain isoforms of the formyl peptide chemoattractant receptor has been reported.[273,274] Of particular note is the report of an acquired neutrophil chemotaxis defect in two adults with gingival infection caused by *Capnocytophaga* spp. Eradication of infection resulted in a return to normal of neutrophil function. Sonicates of *Capnocytophaga* and filtrates of broth in which the organism had been grown inhibited the chemotactic response of normal neutrophils. These findings suggest that the impaired chemotaxis associated with some forms of periodontal disease may be caused by the presence of bacterial products in the circulation.[275]

Chemotactic inhibitors whose mode of action appears to be the inactivation of chemotactic substances have been described in Hodgkin's disease, sarcoidosis, leprosy, and cirrhosis. These inhibitors are usually present at low levels in normal serum and significantly affect chemotaxis only when present in high concentrations. Recurrent skin infections and abnormal neutrophil chemotaxis have also been associated with an IgG antineutrophil antibody.[276]

Intrinsic Abnormalities

Chédiak-Higashi Syndrome. Chédiak-Higashi syndrome (CHS) is a rare autosomal recessive trait caused by mutations of the *LYST* gene at chromosome 1q42-43.[277] The disease affects lysosomes in melanocytes, Schwann cells, renal tubular cells, thyroid cells, and all types of leukocytes (Fig. 8-7). The giant and dysmorphic lysosomes account for the physical findings of partial oculocutaneous albinism, rotatory nystagmus, peripheral neuropathy, and recurrent in-

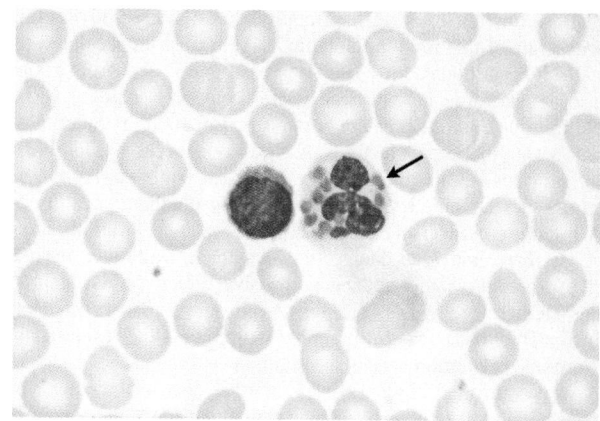

FIGURE 8-7. Neutrophil and lymphocyte from a patient with Chédiak-Higashi syndrome. Note the large abnormal growth granules *(arrow)*.

fections. Laboratory abnormalities include anemia, leukopenia, thrombocytopenia, and intramedullary destruction of blood elements with secondary elevations in serum lysozyme and deficiencies in iron and folate. In some patients there is an unpredictable transformation of the disease to a lymphoma-like accelerated phase with associated hepatosplenomegaly, lymphadenopathy, and lymphocytic infiltration of organs. Both T-cell– and natural killer cell–mediated cytotoxicity are depressed, and studies have identified defective MHC class II peptide loading and antigen presentation in cells derived from patients with CHS.[278]

Neutrophils from patients with CHS exhibit defective chemotactic responses[279] and, although microbial ingestion occurs normally, intracellular survival of bacteria is generally prolonged. Bacterial killing rates are most abnormal during the first 20 minutes of contact in vitro, but approach normal levels at 2 hours, apparently reflecting the delayed release of lysosomal enzymes into phagocytic vacuoles. Because the metabolic burst is normal,[280] the intracellular killing defect appears to result primarily from delayed degranulation into the developing phagolysosome.

Although infections are common in patients with this syndrome, significant morbidity also results from the progressive peripheral neuropathy caused by axonal dysfunction.[281] The primary cellular defect in CHS is the function of a lysosomal trafficking regulator, the product of the *LYST* gene,[282,283] which is essential for normal vesicle sorting in the endosomal pathway.

Current management of patients with CHS is limited to prophylactic use of antibiotics such as trimethoprim-sulfamethoxazole and supportive care. Bone marrow transplantation is effective therapy for the chronic progressive symptoms and the accelerated phase of the disease, but has no impact on the peripheral neuropathy.[284]

Hyperimmunoglobulinemia E with Impaired Chemotaxis (Job's Syndrome). Job's syndrome, as originally described, is an affliction of fair-skinned, red-haired women that is characterized by eczema, recurrent "cold" staphylococcal skin abscesses, sinusitis, and otitis media.[285,286] However, the disorder also occurs in men and in African Americans.[287] Many of the patients have coarse facial features and a broad nasal bridge. In addition to cutaneous staphylococcal infection, recurrent pneumonia and mucocutaneous candidiasis are common. Patients may have mild eosinophilia, and the neutrophils of most patients exhibit impaired chemotaxis, although this feature is variable. Defective chemotaxis appears to correlate best with the severity of the eczema, and in some patients is detectable only during relapses of their dermatitis. Mononuclear cells from these patients, but not from normal persons or atopic patients, spontaneously produce a factor that inhibits the chemotactic responses of normal neutrophils and monocytes.[288] All patients have markedly elevated (more than 10 times normal) serum levels of IgE, primarily due a decreased fractional catabolic rate of this immunoglobulin.[289] Antistaphylococcal and anti-*Candida* IgE antibodies have been demonstrated in sera from patients with Job's syndrome, but not from healthy controls or patients with elevated IgE due to atopic disease or parasitic infection, or patients with chronic staphylococcal infections. Antistaphylococcal antibody of the IgM class is also elevated in the sera from these patients, whereas specific IgA is low and the IgG level no different from that in healthy controls. Infection is inversely correlated with the concentrations of specific IgE, IgA, and IgM, suggesting that these antibodies normally exert a protective rather than a permissive effect against staphylococci.[290] It therefore appears that Job's syndrome does not represent an intrinsic defect of neutrophil function, but rather is the result of aberrant immune regulation.

A well-controlled clinical trial established that levamisole, which had been reported to improve neutrophil function in a few patients with Job's syndrome, was not efficacious and was actually associated with an increase in the number of infections.[291] Therefore, management should be directed toward early detection of infection, prolonged treatment with appropriate antibiotics, and early surgical drainage of abscesses, keeping in mind their tendency to lack the usual features of inflammatory reactions.[286,287]

Other Disorders. A mild and variable defect in neutrophil chemotaxis has been described in patients with Kartagener's (immotile cilia) syndrome, in which there is an abnormality in the linkage between microtubules and cilia.[292] An acquired but reversible defect in neutrophil function has been described with severe hypophosphatemia (<1 mg/dL) caused by phosphate-free hyperalimentation. The defect in these cells is thought to result from an inability to generate ATP from anaerobic glycolysis.[293]

Abnormal Phagocytosis

Defective opsonization occurs with inherited or acquired deficiencies of the early complement components (especially C3) or immunoglobulin. Similar derangements accompany the paraproteinemias and a number of other neoplastic and non-neoplastic disorders characterized by hypoglobulinemia or hypocomplementemia. Patients with these types of opsonic disorders frequently have recurrent infections with encapsulated bacteria, particularly pneumococci and *Haemophilus influenzae*. Infection with these organisms in the splenectomized person can manifest as fulminant bacteremia or meningitis accompanied by disseminated intravascular coagulation.[294]

In 1968, Miller and colleagues[295] reported that sera from 5% to 7% of the population were defective in opsonizing baker's yeast. A number of these individuals suffered recurrent upper respiratory tract infections, and some had diarrhea with associated failure to thrive. The basis for this defect remained obscure until Turner and co-workers[296] discovered that the concentration of mannan-binding protein (MBP) was low in affected subjects. MBP acts to enhance complement activation and deposition on mannose-rich surfaces. The usual molecular basis for this defect is a point mutation resulting in the replacement in exon 1 of a glycine residue with aspartic acid, a change postulated to interfere with MBP triple helix formation, with consequent retention of the protein and intracellular degradation.[297]

Defects in Intracellular Killing

Impaired neutrophil intracellular microbicidal activity may be a consequence of either an abnormal respiratory burst oxidase or the failure to deliver active granule enzymes. Those diseases in which microbicidal defects have been well characterized represent inherited disorders.[298,299] Although functional decreases in microbial killing have been described in patients with certain acquired inflammatory, metabolic, and malignant diseases, these observations have been neither widely confirmed nor characterized at a biochemical level.

Abnormal Respiratory Burst

Chronic Granulomatous Disease. Patients with the hereditary disorder known as CGD characteristically experience recurrent and often severe pyogenic infections, a granulomatous tissue response, and impaired phagocyte microbicidal activity due to the absence of respiratory burst oxidase activity.[300-303] Although initially described as an X-linked disorder, with males affected and mothers and sisters serving as heterozygous carriers, CGD can be transmitted with the inheritance pattern of either an autosomal or an X-linked disease, depending on the molecular defect.[304] The remarkable insights into the components and regulation of the NADPH-dependent oxidase made possible by the development of the broken cell assay[305,306] also provided investigators with a means by which to classify the various forms of CGD (Table 8-3).

The membrane component of the NADPH oxidase is the heterodimeric cytochrome-b_{558}. The gene for the large subunit (gp91*phox*) is located on the X chromosome and is the site of mutation in all patients with X-linked CGD.[106,304,307-309] Rarely (in less than 5% of CGD patients), mutations occur in the gene for the small subunit (p22*phox*), which is on chromosome 16. In most cases deletion or frameshift mutations result in a failure to synthesize the affected subunit of the cytochrome. When one subunit is absent, neither is inserted into the membrane, and the characteristic heme spectrum featuring a 558-nm peak is not present.[310] In rare kindreds single point mutations result in synthesis of nonfunctional flavocytochrome,[311] especially when defects are present in critical functional domains such as the binding site for NADPH or flavin. Mutations also include alterations in the site on the cytochrome for docking p47*phox*, leaving affected cells unable to assemble a functional oxidase.[312]

In most patients with autosomally inherited CGD, the neutrophils lack the cytosolic oxidase component p47*phox*.[301,313] Mutations in the p47*phox* gene account for approximately one third of all cases of CGD. Unlike the cytochrome-*b* mutations, which comprise many different lesions, most examples of p47*phox* deficiency[104,314,315] are caused by a two-base deletion at an exon splice site that results in a frameshift and early termination of translation. Most of the patients studied to date appear to be homozygous for this deletion, although examples have been described of patients who are compound heterozygotes for this mutation and either a single-base frameshift deletion at another site or missense mutations.[104,315] The high prevalence of this deletion of guanine and thymine, also present in a homologous pseudogene on chromosome 7, may reflect recombination of normal and pseudogene sequences.[316] Mutations in the gene for p67*phox* are less common, accounting for perhaps 5% of CGD cases.[313] The

TABLE 8-3	Genetic Types of Chronic Granulomatous Disease					
Defective Component	**Relative Frequency (%)***	**Gene Locus**	**Mutations**	**Biochemical Features**		
				Membranes	**Cytosol**	
gp91*phox*	55-60	Xp21.1	Large deletion/ frameshift, missense	Cytochrome-*b* absent in most, but present in missense mutations	Normal	
p22*phox*	<5	16q24	Deletion/frameshift, missense	Same as for gp91*phox*	Normal	
p47*phox*	30-35	7q11.23	Deletion/frameshift, missense	Normal	p47*phox* absent	
p67*phox*	<5	1q25	Unknown	Normal	p67*phox* absent	

*Percentage of all chronic granulomatous disease patients.[239,421]

p67*phox* protein is usually absent, and several specific mutations have been defined.[303,317] In one kindred, a p67*phox* allele with a triplet nucleotide deletion resulted in an in-frame loss of a lysine residue that was shown in vitro to disrupt p67*phox*-RAC binding.[318]

In all thoroughly characterized cases to date, the CGD phenotype is explained by a defect in a gene for one of the four peptide oxidase components—the two cytochrome-*b* subunits and the cytosolic proteins p47*phox* and p67*phox*. These findings underscore the critical roles that each of these proteins plays in oxidase function. A single family with a genetic abnormality in RAC2 has recently been described.[319-321] The missense mutation observed in this kindred results in the formation of an inhibitory form of the RAC2 protein. The clinical phenotype includes recurrent infections and an abnormal respiratory burst, but is considerably more complex than classical CGD.

In spite of genetic heterogeneity, the biochemical phenotype common to all forms of CGD is the failure of phagocytic cells to generate a respiratory burst in response to phagocytic or soluble stimuli. Because no oxygen-derived microbicidal agents (e.g., superoxide, hydrogen peroxide, hydroxyl radical, hypochlorous acid) are formed, there is a severe defect in intracellular killing of phagocytized microorganisms. Catalase-negative organisms such as the pneumococcus and other streptococci are killed normally because microbial hydrogen peroxide accumulates within the phagocytic vacuole and essentially reconstitutes the defective MPO–hydrogen peroxide–halide system. The basis for this is twofold: (1) microbes that do not produce catalase are also incapable of synthesizing other heme enzymes and therefore utilize flavoprotein pathways that produce peroxide as a byproduct of oxidative metabolism; (2) the peroxide generated can accumulate because it is not degraded by catalase. The preservation of microbicidal activity of CGD cells against catalase-negative microorganisms translates into an absence of major clinical infections caused by these species in patients with CGD.

In general, the clinical manifestations of the different genetic forms of CGD are quite similar, notwithstanding some evidence for a more severe course in X-linked compared with autosomally inherited disease. Infectious complications often begin in infancy and recur throughout childhood and adolescence. In patients who survive into adulthood, there may be a lessening of clinical severity. Occasionally, there is a relatively mild clinical course during childhood, and some patients may not come to medical attention until they are adolescents or even adults.[322,323] Infections may affect virtually any organ system, but the most common manifestations are suppurative lymphadenitis, subcutaneous abscesses, pneumonia, lung abscess, liver abscess, and osteomyelitis. Stomatitis, blepharitis, and pyogenic dermatitis frequently are recurring problems. The most characteristic pathogens are *Staphylococcus aureus, Serratia marcescens, Burkholderia cepacia,* and *Aspergillus* spp., although a wide variety of other catalase-positive bacteria and fungi may cause disease as well. Certain infections, for example *Serratia* osteomyelitis, are particularly suggestive of the diagnosis of CGD. A study of *Aspergillus nidulans* infection in a p47*phox* knockout mouse model suggested that catalase may not represent a significant fungal virulence factor in hosts with impaired oxidase function,[324] but this observation likely reflects the lack of hydrogen peroxide generation by *Aspergillus*. The presence of catalase represents a determinant virulence only when the pathogen has the potential to generate hydrogen peroxide.

Infections in CGD patients can follow an acute course, but more often one observes subacute or chronic progression with poor wound healing, a mixed acute and chronic inflammatory response, and granuloma formation. The basis for the granulomatous inflammation is not clear, but it is thought to relate to the persistence of viable intracellular microorganisms. In certain tissue sites obstructive lesions may develop, as in xanthogranulomatous urinary tract disease[325] or granulomatous bowel involvement that resembles Crohn's disease.[326] Perirectal involvement with fissures or inflammatory masses is a rather common manifestation. The physical examination of CGD patients often reveals dermatitis, lymphadenitis, enlargement of liver and spleen, and retardation of normal rates of growth and development. Routine

laboratory studies may indicate an anemia associated with chronic inflammation, leukocytosis to a moderate level (generally <15,000 to 20,000 cells/mm³), hyperglobulinemia, and an elevated erythrocyte sedimentation rate. Pathologic examination of infected tissues usually demonstrates inflammatory masses with granulomata that may or may not progress to areas of frank necrosis, sometimes with well-defined abscesses. Lipid-filled histiocytes are found in liver, spleen, lymph nodes, gut, and other tissues of some CGD patients.

The diagnosis of CGD can be established using assays for any of the products of the neutrophil respiratory burst. The most used method is the nitroblue tetrazolium (NBT) slide test. Neutrophils adherent to a microscope coverslip are stimulated in the presence of NBT, a soluble yellow dye that is reduced by superoxide to formazan, an insoluble precipitate that stains the cells dark blue or black. In normal control subjects, essentially 100% of the neutrophils stain with NBT. In contrast, neutrophils from CGD patients are uniformly NBT negative, whereas female carriers of X-linked CGD exhibit a mixture of NBT-positive and NBT-negative cells owing to the expression of only one of the X chromosomes in any somatic female cell (lyonization). Although the average distribution of the two cell types in female carriers is 50:50, skewing toward a higher proportion of either defective (CGD) or normal cells occurs. Most female carriers of CGD maintain good health and normal host defenses, but some develop a cutaneous syndrome similar to discoid lupus, full-blown systemic lupus erythematosus, or recurring infections.[327] Clinical manifestations in carriers are more likely when lyonization is skewed toward predominantly CGD-like neutrophils.

In the past decade sensitive fluorometric assays have been applied to identify patients with CGD and carriers of the X-linked form of the disease. The most sensitive system utilizes the fluorescent probe dihydrorhodamine 123 (DHR) in a flow cytometric assay.[328] The DHR assay is sufficiently sensitive to detect populations of normal cells as low as 0.1% and has been applied to quantitate and monitor the subpopulation of normally functioning cells after gene therapy. Carriers of X-linked CGD can be easily identified and their degree of lyonization quantitated using the DHR assay. However, in the diagnosis of CGD, all abnormal DHR assays should be confirmed by the NBT slide test because the DHR assay depends on a variety of variables, including the amount of MPO in neutrophils,[329] allowing completely MPO-deficient subjects to be incorrectly identified as having CGD.

The management of patients with CGD is based largely on the early recognition and aggressive treatment of infections.[330] Specific microbiologic diagnosis should be established whenever possible and, if necessary, empiric therapy should be directed against the pathogens characteristically encountered in such patients (i.e., *S. aureus*, certain gram-negative bacilli, *Aspergillus*). Surgical incision and drainage are often required, although the surgeon may encounter an inflammatory granulomatous mass rather than a discrete abscess. Obstructive lesions are occasionally responsive to steroids, which when used in a limited fashion do not increase substantially the risk of secondary infection. Because the utility of granulocyte transfusions has not been established, they are not generally recommended, although their use in severe infections unresponsive to standard treatment may be worth considering. Prophylactic use of antibacterial agents is of well-established benefit in patients with CGD. The preferred agent is trimethoprim-sulfamethoxazole, although antistaphylococcal semisynthetic penicillins or cephalosporins are considered good alternatives in sulfonamide-intolerant patients. A recent study suggested that prophylactic itraconazole is effective in decreasing the incidence of fungal infections in CGD patients.[331] In patients who experience morbidity from infections despite the use of prophylactic antimicrobial agents, the use of recombinant IFN-γ should be considered. In a randomized controlled trial, this agent, given in a dose of 50 μg/m² three times weekly by the subcutaneous route, reduced by 72% the incidence of serious infections, regardless of the genetic form of the disease and with relatively few side effects.[332] Notwithstanding the reported effects of IFN-γ on oxidative metabolism and microbicidal activity of CGD phagocytes,[333-335] its mechanism of action in patients is not clear.[336] In a rare kindred with a defect in the regulatory domain of the gp91*phox* subunit of cytochrome-b_{558}, the cytokine appears to upregulate gene expression and restore cytochrome synthesis and function to normal,[337] although clearly this is not the mechanism of action in most patients.

Long-term reconstitution of normal phagocyte function in patients with CGD might be achieved by bone marrow transplantation.[338] However, the morbidity and mortality of this mode of treatment are high, and results in a few CGD patients have been variable. Gene transfer may ultimately prove to be the preferred means of definitive treatment. In vitro reconstitution of oxidase function in CGD cells has been achieved in several systems, including peripheral blood CD34+ progenitor cells from subjects with p47*phox* or p67*phox* deficiency.[339,340] Very promising is the report of studies by Malech in which five patients with p47*phox* deficiency achieved extended, albeit low-level, reconstitution of oxidase function in vivo.[341,342] Better targeting vectors and specialized conditioning regimens for patients offer the promise of a durable correction of oxidase dysfunction by genetic therapy in the future.[304,343] The prognosis in CGD patients has improved considerably over the last 20 years, based on increased recognition, aggressive treatment of infections, and prophylactic approaches to preventing infectious complications.

Glucose-6-Phosphate Dehydrogenase Deficiency. Although erythrocyte and leukocyte glucose-6-phosphate dehydrogenase (G6PD) are products of the same gene, the common form of G6PD deficiency that manifests as a hemolytic anemia in African Americans is not associated with neutrophil dysfunction. This discrepancy reflects the fact that the deficiency is caused by an unstable enzyme, the activity of which diminishes over a period that exceeds the life expectancy of the neutrophil. Neutrophil dysfunction does occur in rare cases of G6PD deficiency in whites who are missing or have less than 5% of the normal levels of G6PD. Neutrophil function is abnormal in this disorder because, in the absence of G6PD, glucose cannot be metabolized via the hexose monophosphate shunt, and as a consequence NADPH cannot be regenerated from NADP to support oxidase activity. Aside from the presence of a hemolytic anemia, the clinical, laboratory, and genetic (X-linked) presentation can be quite similar to that of CGD. The NBT test is abnormal, as are other parameters of the respiratory burst. The failure of methylene blue to stimulate hexose monophosphate shunt activity and the low level of G6PD distinguish this defect from classic CGD.[344]

Myeloperoxidase Deficiency

Once thought to be a rare disorder, neutrophil MPO deficiency is now recognized as the most common of all neutrophil functional disorders, with a frequency of 1 per 2000 to 4000 people for whom leukocyte counts are performed. This discrepancy is explained by the facts that the overwhelming majority of such persons are healthy and that detection of this condition has been greatly facilitated by the widespread use of flow cytometry techniques that use peroxidase staining for leukocyte differential counts.[345] Eosinophil peroxidase is normal in this disorder. An autosomal recessive manner of inheritance has been reported, but the inheritance pattern is much more complex, probably reflecting the heterogeneity of the responsible genotypes.[346] Of all the patients recognized with this disorder, only six have had serious infections. Systemic candidiasis occurred in four of these patients, three of whom also had diabetes mellitus.[298,299]

Because the cell is devoid of MPO-dependent but not other oxidative killing mechanisms, there is delayed but not absent intracellular killing in MPO-deficient neutrophils. Delayed killing is more pronounced for fungi than for bacteria,[347] which suggests an explanation for the clinical findings in this disorder. Chemotaxis, phagocytosis, and degranulation are normal, but the respiratory burst is enhanced. The supranormal oxidative metabolism may be caused by absent MPO-dependent inactivation of the oxidase system[142] and may help explain the lack of clinical expression of this defect in most patients.

Normal MPO is the product of a single gene on chromosome 17. Post-translational processing of a glycosylated (89-kDa) primary gene product results in a mature molecule containing heavy (59-kDa)

α-chain and light (13.5-kDa) β-chains.[299,348,349] The current structural model suggests that the chain content of mature MPO is an $(\alpha\beta)_2$ molecule and that processing and lysosomal targeting are independent of the mannose-6-phosphate receptor system.[350] Most patients with MPO deficiency have a defect in post-translational processing such that their neutrophils have immunochemical evidence of an MPO precursor but no mature protein.[351,352] However, one report described a patient with a pretranslational defect causing MPO deficiency,[353] highlighting the heterogeneity of the molecular defects causing this disorder. To date, three mutations in the coding sequence of MPO have been identified in persons with inherited deficiency,[352,354,355] but it is probable that many different mutations underlie this common disorder.[346,356]

MPO deficiency has also been recognized as an acquired defect accompanying some myeloproliferative disorders, particularly acute myelogenous leukemia. In the leukemic but not the preleukemic state, this deficiency is associated with an increased risk of infection. However, large population studies suggest that MPO deficiency may predispose to infection and influence risk for malignant disease[357,358] and murine models of MPO deficiency have implicated its impact on the risk for candidiasis,[359] atherosclerosis,[360] central nervous system disease,[361] and vasculitis.[362-364] Polymorphisms in the promoter region of the MPO gene may influence the relative risk for diseases in the cardiovascular system,[365] gastrointestinal tract,[366] and central nervous system[367-371] and for cancer.[372-376]

Specific Granule Deficiency

The absence of specific granules has been recognized in five patients with recurrent infection.[377] The peripheral leukocyte count in such patients is normal when they are uninfected, and the diagnosis is established by the apparent absence of intracellular granules on routine Wright stain (primary granules do not take up Wright stain). Close examination reveals a bilobed nuclear morphology with nuclear blocks and clefts. In addition, eosinophils are affected in this disorder.[378] Specific granule contents (e.g., lactoferrin, vitamin B_{12}–binding protein) are absent, as is membrane alkaline phosphatase.[377] Unexpectedly, the neutrophils of affected patients are almost completely devoid of defensins, proteins that normally constitute one third of the azurophilic granule contents.[379] Only myeloid cells are affected, because the lactoferrin content of nasal secretions and tears is normal.[380]

The molecular basis of specific granule deficiency has been identified and logically explains the biochemical phenotype involving more than a single gene product. CCAAT/enhancer binding protein epsilon (C/EBPϵ), the member of the protein family of transcription factors that is expressed in myeloid and T cells,[381] is defective in patients with specific granule deficiency.[382] A small deletion in the second exon of the C/EBPϵ gene results in a frame shift and production of a truncated protein lacking the essential dimerization domain.[382] As a result of these changes, there is defective myelopoiesis at the level of promyelocyte transition. Defects in C/EBPϵ affect expression of secondary granule proteins in eosinophils as well as neutrophils[383] and result in a range of functional defects, including the absence of tertiary granule expression and aberrant chemotaxis, in both affected human and murine knockout models.[384-386]

Therapy for Neutrophil Defects

Antimicrobial Prophylaxis

The recurrent and severe infections that occur in many patients with abnormal neutrophil function have made the administration of prophylactic antibiotics common despite concerns about colonization and infection with resistant microorganisms. The low prevalence of these disorders has made controlled trials of prophylactic antibiotics difficult. Nonetheless, the broad antimicrobial spectrum of trimethoprim-sulfamethoxazole against both gram-positive and gram-negative bacteria, coupled with its penetration and concentration within neutrophils, probably explains its apparent effectiveness in reducing infections in patients with CGD. Prophylactic antibiotic therapy in patients with CGD has been associated with an increase in the average infection-free interval from 9.6 to 40 months.[330] The effect of antibiotics on intracellular killing mechanisms received attention with the demonstration that staphylococci exposed to sublethal concentrations of cell wall–active antibiotics for a short time were more readily killed by neutrophils than were staphylococci grown in the absence of antibiotics. Improved killing resulted from an enhancement in nonoxidative bactericidal mechanisms and was both organism and antibiotic specific. The significance of these findings for patient management is unknown. A randomized controlled trial with alternating drug and placebo cycles administered to 39 CGD patients found an incidence of one serious and no superficial fungal infections during itraconazole treatment cycles, versus seven serious and five superficial fungal infections during placebo cycles.[331]

Granulocyte Transfusions

Granulocyte transfusions have been used therapeutically in febrile granulocytopenic patients. Theoretically, to achieve a blood neutrophil count of 1000 cells/mm^3 after transfusion, approximately 1×10^{10} neutrophils (all the neutrophils in 2 to 3 L of blood) are required daily for the average adult. However, many patients show no significant rise in the peripheral leukocyte count after transfusion of this number of cells.[387,388] Two basic methods of procurement have been devised: centrifugation and filtration leukapheresis. The former method uses differences in density among blood cells to achieve separation. Filtration makes use of the ability of neutrophils to adhere to nylon wool to achieve separation from other cells. Cells obtained by both procedures are functional both in vitro and in vivo, but those obtained by filtration leukapheresis exhibit cytoplasmic vacuolization and surface distortion, as well as a loss of granule contents and reduced bactericidal capacity. In addition, up to 75% of the recipients of cells obtained by leukapheresis have transfusion reactions, predominantly fever and chills, compared with 15% of the recipients of cells obtained by centrifugation.[388] These differences aside, administration of cells obtained by either method to granulocytopenic patients with infection has been beneficial in some but not all controlled trials.[387,388] Granulocytopenic patients with proven bacterial infection who received daily granulocyte transfusions for the duration of their infection survived longer than did infected nontransfused control patients. All patients received therapy appropriate for their infections.[388,389] Leukocyte transfusions have appeared to be therapeutically successful in a limited number of patients with neutrophil bactericidal defects and progressive infection. By using a positive NBT test as a marker, delivery to and persistence of transfused normal leukocytes at the site of infection were documented in a patient with CGD.[390]

Although leukocyte transfusion may be beneficial for certain infected granulocytopenic patients, associated complications have limited their use. These complications include (1) transfusion-associated cytomegalovirus infection, (2) allosensitization to human leukocyte antigens, (3) difficulties in locating adequate numbers of suitable donors, (4) risks to the donor, (5) high cost of the procedure, and (6) an increased incidence of acute pulmonary reactions when transfusions are given in conjunction with amphotericin B administration.[391] This reaction most commonly occurs when amphotericin B treatment is initiated simultaneously with or after transfusion and is characterized by the acute onset of respiratory decompensation, pulmonary infiltrates, and intra-alveolar hemorrhage.[391]

A potentially serious complication of red cell or white cell transfusions in patients with CGD may occur because of abnormalities of the Kell antigen system and the Kell-related antigen K_x. This antigen is present on the surface of red and white blood cells from healthy people and from patients with autosomally transmitted CGD. K_x is absent from the neutrophils of most patients with the X-linked form of the disease because of the close linkage of the CGD and X_k genes on the X chromosome. In addition, some patients with X-linked CGD exhibit the rare McLeod phenotype, in which K_x and the standard Kell antigens are absent from erythrocytes and leukocytes and a mild hemolytic anemia occurs. Failure to recognize this antigenic abnormality can result in severe transfusion reactions. As a consequence of

these complicating aspects, leukocyte transfusion seems best reserved for the patient with severe granulocytopenia or functionally defective neutrophils who has a serious bacterial or fungal infection that has not responded to appropriate antimicrobial therapy. Donors should preferably be seronegative for cytomegalovirus.

Bone Marrow Transplantation

There are published reports of several patients, one with LAD and three with CGD, undergoing successful bone marrow engraftment with subsequent clinical improvement. Two of the patients with CGD ultimately rejected their transplant, but continued to enjoy clinical improvement. This result illustrates the difficulty in meaningfully evaluating this procedure in these types of patients. Moreover, given the increased infection-free interval and survival rates observed with the use of prophylactic antibiotics and IFN-γ in patients with CGD,[332] it seems reasonable to reserve such aggressive therapy for unusual situations.

Although allogeneic hematopoietic stem-cell transplantation has succeeded in selected cases in restoring granulocyte function to patients with CGD, the associated morbidity and mortality represent significant obstacles to widespread application of this intervention, except for patients most devastated by their underlying illness. Efforts to moderate the extent of myeloablation during conditioning of the recipient result in less toxicity but still incur significant graft-versus-host disease due to the presence of active T cells in the donor graft. Recently the use of nonmyeloablative conditioning of the recipient coupled with T-cell depletion of the donor and transplantation of stem cells from an HLA-identical sibling has demonstrated promising results in a study of 10 patients with CGD.[392]

Gene Therapy

Indirect evidence suggests that CGD may be an inherited disease amenable to gene therapy. Given that the most common form of CGD is due to mutation of *CYBB*, the X-chromosome gene encoding gp91*phox*, maternal carriers of X-CGD have a chimeric population of circulating granulocytes, reflecting the inactivation of a single X-chromosome in somatic cells. In most cases there is a nearly equal number of normal and mutant neutrophils, and carriers experience no increase in the number or severity of clinical infections. However, skewed inactivation can result in a clinical phenotype indistinguishable from that of CGD, generally seen when the percentage of normal neutrophils falls below 10%.[393-397] Based on such observations, it is possible that correction of only 10% of circulating neutrophils will provide the recipient with sufficient phagocyte oxidase function to be protective. Ongoing studies in murine models[398-400] focus on the conditioning protocols and specific vectors that optimize both efficiency of gene transfer and durability of functional expression. For example, a clinical trial using p47*phox* succeeded in reconstituting function in the recipients but at 1 year, less than 0.1% of the circulating neutrophils were still functional.[401] Recent advances in the retroviral and lentiviral vectors and application of the NOD/SCID mouse system to assess success of transduced CD34$^+$ stem cells have shown promise, in some cases resulting in ex vivo transduction of more than 95% of the cells and 14% to 77% transgene expression in vivo in engrafted human cells.[402]

Evaluating Phagocyte Function

The most important step in the evaluation of possible abnormalities of neutrophil function is to obtain a good clinical history and a leukocyte count with a stained blood smear. Serum immunoglobulin and complement levels should be determined. An NBT test, requiring only a drop or two of blood, is simple and fast and definitively rules in or out CGD. Further evaluation depends on the results of these simple screening tests (Table 8-4) (see Chapter 11).

EOSINOPHILS

Eosinophils are bone marrow–derived, tissue-based granulocytes located subjacent to the skin and mucosal lining of the respiratory and gastrointestinal tracts.[403,404] In these locations they play a role in host

TABLE 8-4 Evaluation of Neutrophil Function[422,423]

Phagocytosis and bactericidal activity[303]
Leukocyte and differential count
Adherence
Migration to site
Chemotaxis
Phagocytosis and bactericidal activity[424]
Postphagocytic activity
    Oxygen consumption
    Hexose monophosphate shunt
    Iodination
    Nitroblue tetrazolium[425,426]
    Degranulation
    Chemiluminescence[427]

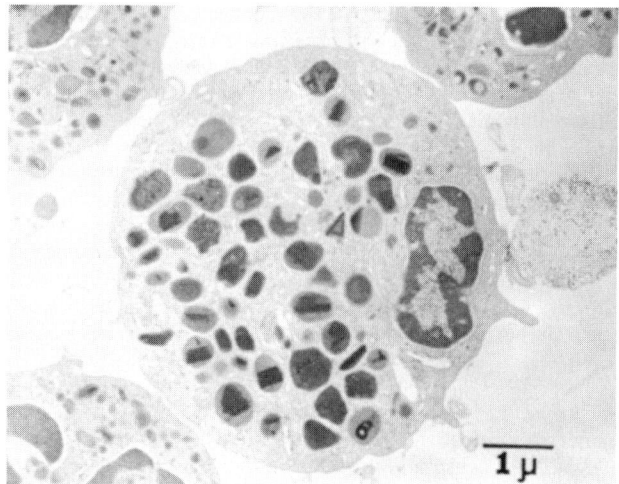

FIGURE 8-8. Electron micrograph of a human eosinophil. Note the prominent granules with crystalloid cores.

defense against helminthic infection; hypersensitivity diseases, especially bronchial asthma; and certain dermatologic conditions. In general, eosinophils have a functional repertoire similar to that of neutrophils,[403,405] although there are several significant differences in the activities of these two phagocytic granulocytes.

Eosinophils develop from marrow stem cells over a 5- to 6-day period.[406] Eosinophilopoiesis in humans appears to be uniquely dependent on IL-5, with IL-3 and GM-CSF also contributing to a lesser degree. IL-5 concentrations correlate with the appearance and magnitude of eosinophilia in vivo.[407] Eosinophil maturation is accompanied by the appearance of three characteristic granule populations: primary, secondary, and small granules (Fig. 8-8). Primary granules are electron dense and appear during the promyelocyte stage of development. Secondary granules are distinguished by their larger size, an electron-dense crystalloid core containing MBP, and an electron-lucent matrix containing eosinophil cationic protein, eosinophil-derived neurotoxin, and eosinophil peroxidase. Small granules contain acid phosphatase and arylsulfatase B. Mature eosinophils also possess secretory IgA receptors as well as low-affinity IgG (FcγRII) and IgE receptors. Receptors for complement (CR1, CR3, ClqR, C5a), cytokines (IL-5, IL-3, GM-CSF, IFN-γ, TNF), platelet-activating factor, and leukotriene B$_4$ have also been reported.[408] The number and functional competence of these receptors are presumably regulated in a manner analogous to that documented for neutrophils.

Circulating eosinophils can be separated into two populations based on their buoyant density. Most of the eosinophils in normal persons are characterized as dense or normodense. Hypodense eosinophils are cells that have been activated: They express a greater number of functionally competent receptors, exhibit a higher resting level of oxidative metabolism, and predominate in the blood and tissues of persons with eosinophilia.

The intravascular half-life of eosinophils is about 2 hours. Eosinophil migration involves different adhesion molecules than does neutrophil transmigration.[409,410] In addition to the β$_2$-integrins also expressed by neutrophils, eosinophils express α$_4$β$_1$, α$_4$β$_7$, and α$_6$β$_1$[411] integrins and display a form of P-selectin glycoprotein ligand 1 (PSGL-1) that binds more avidly to endothelial P-selectin than does the form expressed by neutrophils.[412-414] That eosinophil transmigration is normal in LAD-1 provides evidence that β$_2$-integrins are not required for this process. Association with endothelium appears to be mediated by IL-5–dependent upregulation of α$_4$β$_1$ on eosinophils and its counter-receptor, vascular cell adhesion molecule-1, on endothelial cells.[415]

In murine models of helminthic infection, the major source of IL-5 is the T-helper cell subset, Th2. The outcome of the infection appears to depend on whether Th1 or Th2 cell responses predominate and on the identity of the parasites. Because IL-5 is intimately involved in eosinophil production, activation, and transmigration in humans, its modulation is an attractive therapeutic strategy for affecting this type of eosinophil-dependent event.[407]

Substantial evidence supports a role for eosinophils in immunity to helminthic parasites, as demonstrated by the greater worm burden and tissue damage in animals treated with antieosinophil serum and by the finding that the transfer of passive immunity requires the presence of these cells. This conclusion is buttressed by the demonstration of eosinophils on and around degenerating parasites in vivo and by the ability of eosinophils to kill these organisms in vitro.[416,417]

Killing of parasites is related to exocytosis of eosinophil granule contents onto the parasite surface while it is in close apposition to the eosinophils.[418,419] The eosinophil peroxidase–hydrogen peroxide–halide oxidation system plays a minor role in anthelminthic activity.[420] Rather, the cationic granule proteins are responsible for the bulk of this activity. On a molar, basis eosinophil cationic protein exerts a more potent anthelminthic effect than does MBP, but the greater quantity of the latter in the eosinophil makes its contribution more significant. The effect of these proteins is also specific for different stages in the life cycle of the parasite.

Recognition that eosinophil granules contain a number of substances capable of inactivating the chemical mediators of anaphylaxis has led to the suggestion that the eosinophil may modulate the severity of type I hypersensitivity reactions.[421] In this scenario, stimulation of basophils and mast cells by the interaction of surface IgE with specific antigen results in the release of substances important in type I hypersensitivity reactions. These include vasoactive amines, slow-reacting substances of anaphylaxis (leukotrienes C, D, and E), platelet-activating factor, and eosinophil chemotactic factor of anaphylaxis (ECF-A). Histamine and ECF-A attract eosinophils to the site of antigen reaction with basophils and mast cells. ECF-A can also stimulate eosinophil degranulation, as can immune complexes that the eosinophil phagocytizes. Histaminase secreted by the eosinophil may inactivate local histamine, and a substance present in eosinophils may inhibit further histamine secretion by basophils. Arylsulfatase and phospholipase present in the smaller eosinophil granules are capable of inactivating leukotrienes C, D, and E and platelet-activating factor. Therefore, eosinophils may modulate immediate hypersensitivity reactions by inhibiting the release of mediators of the type I reaction as well as by destroying mediators that have already been released.[420]

The association of eosinophilia of several weeks' duration with the development of endocardial lesions and the isolation of an eosinophil-derived neurotoxin capable of reproducing the neurologic picture observed in patients with cerebrospinal fluid eosinophilia strongly support a role for the eosinophil in the pathogenesis of tissue injury in certain disorders, most prominent of which is bronchial asthma. Substantial evidence indicates that eosinophil MBP is an important mediator of tissue injury. For example, increased quantities of MBP are detectable in the bronchial washings from patients with asthma but not from those with other pulmonary disorders. Nanomolar concentrations of MBP but not other cationic proteins cause exfoliation of epithelial cells, impaired ciliary function, net chloride secretion, and bronchial hyperreactivity. Immunofluorescent staining of bronchial epithelium in autopsy specimens from patients who died from asthma revealed extensive deposition of MBP in the peribronchial areas and overlying regions of bronchial epithelial denudation. These findings were not observed in autopsy material obtained from patients whose deaths were related to other pulmonary diseases. The importance of epithelial denudation lies in the resultant enhanced responsiveness of the underlying bronchial smooth muscle to contractile agonists, including acetylcholine and histamine, as well as to leukotriene C$_4$ produced by eosinophils.[408]

REFERENCES

1. Janeway, C. How the immune system works to protect the host from infection: A personal view. Proc Natl Acad Sci U S A. 2001;98:7461-7468.
2. Medzhitov R, Janeway C. Innate immunity. N Engl J Med. 2000;343:338-344.
3. Dale DC. Colony-stimulating factors for the management of neutropenia in cancer patients. Drugs. 2002;62:1-15.
4. Nemuaitis J. A comparative review of colony-stimulating factors. Drugs. 1997;54:709-729.
5. Kehrl JH. Hematopoietic lineage commitment: Role of transcription factors. Stem Cells. 1995;13:223-241.
6. Metcalf D. Hematopoietic regulation: Redundancy or subtlety? Blood. 1993;82:3515-3523.
7. Tenen DG, Hromas R, Licht JD, et al. Transcription factors, normal myeloid development, and leukemia. Blood. 1997;90:489-519.
8. Colotta F, Re F, Polentarutti N, et al. Modulation of granulocyte survival and programmed cell death by cytokines and bacterial products. Blood. 1992; 80:2012-2020.
9. Bainton DF. Differentiation of human neutrophilic granulocytes: Normal and abnormal. Prog Clin Biol Res. 1977;13:1.
10. Glasser L, Fiederlein RL. Functional differentiation of normal human neutrophils. Blood. 1987;69:937-944.
11. Sigurdsson F, Khanna-Gupta A, Lawson N, et al. Control of late neutrophil-specific gene expression: Insights into regulation of myeloid differentiation. Semin Hematol. 1990;34:303-310.
12. Borregaard N, Cowland JB. Granules of the human neutrophilic polymorphonuclear leukocyte. Blood. 1997;89:3503-3521.
13. Cramer E, Pryzwansky KB, Villeval J-C, et al. Ultrastructural localization of lactoferrin and myeloperoxidase in human neutrophils by immunogold. Blood. 1985;65:423-432.
14. Csernok E, Ludemann J, Gross WL, et al. Ultrastructural localization of proteinase 3, the target antigen of anti-cytoplasmic antibodies circulating in Wegener's granulomatosis. Am J Pathol. 1990;137:1113-1120.
15. Ohlsson K, Olsson I. The neutral proteases of human granulocytes: Isolation and partial characterization of granulocyte elastase. Eur J Biochem. 1974;42:519-527.
16. Rice WG, Ganz T, Kinkade JM, et al. Defensin-rich dense granules of human neutrophils. Blood. 1987;70:757-765.
17. Weiss J, Olsson I. Cellular and subcellular localization of the bactericidal/permeability-increasing protein of neutrophils. Blood. 1987;69:652-659.
18. Nauseef WM, McCormick S, Yi H. Roles of heme insertion and the mannose-6-phosphate receptor in processing of the human myeloid lysosomal enzyme, myeloperoxidase. Blood. 1992;80:2622-2633.
19. Valore EV, Ganz T. Posttranslational processing of defensin precursors in immature human myeloid cells. Blood. 1992;79:1538-1544.
20. Sengelov H, Nielsen MH, Borregaard N. Separation of human neutrophil plasma membrane from intracellular vesicles containing alkaline phosphatase and NADPH oxidase activity by free flow electrophoresis. J Biol Chem. 1992;267:14912-14917.
21. Kjeldsen L, Bainton DF, Sengelov H, et al. Structural and functional heterogeneity among peroxidase-negative granules in human neutrophils: Identification of a distinct gelatinase-containing granule subset by combined immunocytochemistry and subcellular fractionation. Blood. 1993;82:3183-3191.
22. Borregaard N, Kjeldsen L, Lollike K. Granules and vesicles of human neutrophils: The role of endomembranes as source of plasma membrane proteins. Eur J Haematol. 1993;51:318-322.
23. Calafat J, Kuijpers TW, Janssen H, et al. Evidence for small intracellular vesicles in human blood phagocytes containing cytochrome b558 and the adhesion molecule CD11b/CD18. Blood. 1993;81:3122-3129.
24. Borregaard N, Heiple JM, Simons ER, et al. Subcellular localization of the b-cytochrome component of the human neutrophil microbicidal oxidase: Translocation during activation. J Cell Biol. 1983;97:52-61.
25. Sengelov H, Boulay F, Kjeldsen L, et al. Subcellular localization and translocation of the receptor for N-formylmethionyl-leucyl-phenylalanine in human neutrophils. Biochem J. 1994;299:473-479.
26. Singer II, Scott S, Kawka DW, et al. Adhesomes: Specific granules containing receptors for laminin, C3bi/fibrinogen, fibronectin, and vitronectin in human polymorphonuclear leukocytes and monocytes. J Cell Biol. 1989;109:3169-3182.
27. Porteu F, Nathan CF. Mobilizable intracellular pool of p55 (type I) tumor necrosis factor receptors in human neutrophils. J Leukoc Biol. 1992;52:122-124.
28. Sengelov H, Kjeldsen L, Kroeze W, et al. Secretory vesicles are the intracellular reservoir of complement receptor 1 in human neutrophils. J Immunol. 1994;153:804-810.
29. Borregaard N, Kjeldsen L, Sengelov H, et al. Changes in subcellular localization and surface expression of L-selectin, alkaline phosphatase, and Mac-1 in human neutrophils during stimulation with inflammatory mediators. J Leukoc Biol. 1994;56:80-87.
30. Sengelov H, Kjeldsen L, Diamond MS, et al. Subcellular localization and dynamics of Mac-1 ($\alpha_{m\beta2}$) in human neutrophils. J Clin Invest. 1993;92:1467-1476.
31. Stossel TP. On the crawling of animal cells. Science. 1993;260:1086-1094.
32. White JR, Naccache PH, Sha'afi RI. Stimulation by chemotactic factor of actin association with the cytoskeleton in rabbit neutrophils. J Biol Chem. 1983; 258:14041-14047.
33. Ryder MI, Weinreb RN, Niederman R. The organization of actin filaments in human polymorphonuclear leukocytes. Anat Rec. 1984;209:7-20.
34. Neuman E, Huleatt JW, Vargas H, et al. Regulation of MHC class I synthesis and expression by human neutrophils. J Immunol. 1992;148:3520-3527.
35. Neuman E, Huleatt JW, Jack RM. Granulocyte-macrophage colony-stimulating factor increases synthesis and expression of CR1 and CR3 by human peripheral blood neutrophils. J Immunol. 1990;145:3325-3332.
36. Cassatella MA, Bazzoni F, Ceska M, et al. IL-8 production by human polymorphonuclear leukocytes: The chemoattractant formyl-methionyl-leucyl-phenylalanine induces the gene expression and release of IL-8 through a pertussis toxin-sensitive pathway. J Immunol. 1992;148:3216-3220.
37. Jack RM, Fearon DT. Selective synthesis of mRNA and proteins by human peripheral blood neutrophils. J Immunol. 1988;140:4286-4293.
38. Lian ZY, Kluger DS, Greenbaum D, et al. Genomic and proteomic analysis of the myeloid differentiation program: Global analysis of gene expression during induced differentiation in the MPRO cell line. Blood. 2002;100:3209-3220.
39. Kobayashi SD, Braughton KR, Whitney AR, et al. Bacterial pathogens modulate an apoptosis differentiation program in human neutrophils. Proc Natl Acad Sci U S A. 2003;100:10948-10953.
40. Kobayashi SD, Voyich JM, Buhl CL, et al. Global changes in gene expression by human polymorphonuclear leukocytes during receptor-mediated phagocytosis: Cell fate is regulated at the level of gene expression. Proc Natl Acad Sci U S A. 2002;99:6901-6906.
41. Voyich JM, Sturdevant DE, Braughton KR, et al. Genome-wide protective response used by group A streptococcus to evade destruction by human polymorphonuclear leukocytes. Proc Natl Acad Sci U S A. 2003;100:1996-2001.
42. McKenzie SE, Schreiber AD. Fc gamma receptors in phagocytes. Curr Opin Hematol. 1998;5:16-21.
43. Sengelov H. Complement receptors in neutrophils. Crit Rev Immunol. 1995;15:107-131.
44. Murphy PM. The molecular biology of leukocyte chemoattractant receptors. Annu Rev Immunol. 1994;12:593-633.
45. Daeron M. Fc receptor biology. Ann Rev Immunol. 1997;15:203-234.
46. Bender JG, Van Epps DE, Chenoweth DE. Independent regulation of human neutrophil chemotactic receptors after activation. J Immunol. 1987;139:3028-3033.
47. Korchak HM, Wildenfeld C, Rich AM, et al. Stimulus response coupling in the human neutrophil. J Biol Chem. 1984;259:7439-7445.
48. Walker RI, Willemze R. Neutrophil kinetics and regulation of granulopoiesis. Rev Infect Dis. 1980;2:282-292.
49. Sachs L. The molecular control of blood cell development. Science. 1987;238:1374-1379.
50. Nathan C. Points of control in inflammation. Nature. 2000;420:846-852.
51. Tracey KJ. The inflammatory reflex. Nature. 2002;420:853-859.
52. Gallin JI. Human neutrophil heterogeneity exists, but is it meaningful? Blood. 1984;63:977-983.
53. Robinson JM, Karnovsky ML, Karnovsky MJ. Glycogen accumulation in polymorphonuclear leukocytes, and other intracellular alterations that occur during inflammation. J Cell Biol. 1982;95:933.
54. Kuhns DB, Gallin JI. Increased cell-associated IL-8 in human exudative and A23187-treated peripheral blood neutrophils. J Immunol. 1995;154:6556-6562.
55. Bender JG, McPhail LC, Van Epps DE. Exposure of human neutrophils to chemotactic factors potentiates activation of the respiratory burst enzyme. J Immunol. 1983;130:2316-2323.
56. DeLeo FR, Renee J, McCormick S, et al. Neutrophils exposed to bacterial lipopolysaccharide up-regulate NADPH oxidase assembly. J Clin Invest. 1998; 101:455-463.
57. Keil ML, Solomon NL, Lodhi IJ, et al. Priming-induced localization of G$_{io2}$ in high density membrane microdomains. Biochem Biophys Res Commun. 2003;301:862-872.
58. Muller WA. Leukocyte-endothelial-cell interactions in leukocyte transmigration and the inflammatory response. Trends Immunol. 2003;24:327-334.
59. Frenette PS, Moyna C, Hartwell DW, et al. Platelet-endothelial interactions in inflamed mesenteric venules. Blood. 1998;91:1318-1324.
60. Celi A, Lorenzet R, Furie B, et al. Platelet-leukocyte-endothelial cell interaction on the blood vessel wall. Semin Hematol. 1997;34:327-335.
61. Nelson RM, Venot A, Bevilacqua MP, et al. Carbohydrate-protein interactions in vascular biology. Annu Rev Cell Dev Biol. 1995;11:601-631.
62. Gahmberg CG, Tovanen M, Kotovuori P. Leukocyte adhesion: Structure and function of human leukocyte 2 integrins and their cellular ligands. Eur J Biochem. 1997;245:215-232.
63. Smyth SS, Joneckis CC, Parise LV. Regulation of vascular integrins. Blood. 1993;81:2827-2843.
64. De Fougerolles AR, Klickstein LB, Springer TA. Cloning and expression of intercellular adhesion molecule 3 reveals strong homology to the immunoglobulin family counter-receptors for lymphocyte function-associated antigen 1. J Exp Med. 1993;177:1187-1192.
65. De Fougerolles AR, Diamond MS, Springer TA. Heterogeneous glycosylation of ICAM-3 and lack of interaction with Mac-1 and p150,95. Eur J Immunol. 1995;25:1008-1012.
66. Gresham HD, Goodwin JL, Allen PM, et al. A novel member of the integrin receptor family mediates Arg-Gly-Asp-stimulated neutrophil phagocytosis. J Cell Biol. 1989;108:1935-1943.
67. Gresham HD, Graham IL, Griffin GL, et al. Domain-specific interactions between entactin and neutrophil integrins. J Biol Chem. 1996;271:30587-30594.
68. Lindberg FP, Gresham HD, Reinhold MI, et al. Integrin-associated protein immunoglobulin domain is necessary for efficient vitronectin bead binding. J Cell Biol. 1996;134:1313-1322.
69. Zhou M, Brown EJ. Leukocyte response integrin and integrin-associated protein act as a signal transduction unit in generation of a phagocyte respiratory burst. J Exp Med. 1993;178:1165-1174.

70. Brown E. Neutrophil adhesion and the therapy of inflammation. Semin Hematol. 1997;34:319-326.
71. Del Maschio A, Zanetti A, Corada M, et al. Polymorphonuclear leukocyte adhesion triggers the disorganization of endothelial cell-to-cell adherens junctions. J Cell Biol. 1996;135:497-510.
72. Feng D, Nagy JA, Pyne K, et al. Neutrophils emigrate from venules by a transendothelial cell pathway in response to FMLP. J Exp Med. 1998;187:903-915.
73. Muller WA. Leukocyte-endothelial cell interactions in the inflammatory response. Lab Invest. 2002;82:521-524.
74. Mamdouh Z, Chen X, Pierini LM, et al. Targeted recycling of PECAM from endothelial surface-connected compartments during diapedesis. Nature. 2003;421:748-753.
75. Cepinskas G, Savickiene J, Ionescu CV, Kvietys PR. PMN transendothelial migration decreases nuclear NF-κB in IL-β-activated endothelial cells: role of PECAM-1. J Cell Biol. 2003;161:641-651.
76. Parkos CA, Colgan SP, Madara JL. Interactions of neutrophils with epithelial cells: Lessons from the intestine. J Am Soc Nephrol. 1994;5:138-152.
77. Parkos CA, Colgan SP, Bacarra AE, et al. Intestinal epithelia (T84) possess basolateral ligands for CD11b/CD18-mediated neutrophil adherence. Am J Physiol. 1995; 268:C472-C479.
78. Parkos CA, Colgan SP, Liang TW, et al. CD47 mediates post-adhesive events required for neutrophil migration across polarized intestinal epithelia. J Cell Biol. 1996; 132:437-450.
79. Lindberg FP, Bullard DC, Caver DE, et al. Decreased resistance to bacterial infection and granulocyte defects in IAP-deficient mice. Science. 1996;274:795-798.
80. Colgan SP, Serhan CN, Parkos CA, et al. Lipoxin A4 modulates transmigration of human neutrophils across intestinal epithelial monolayers. J Clin Invest. 1993;92:75-82.
81. Colgan SP, Parkos CA, Delp C, et al. Neutrophil migration across cultured intestinal epithelial monolayers is modulated by epithelial exposure to IFN-gamma in a highly polarized fashion. J Cell Biol. 1993;120:785-798.
82. Sitaraman S, Merlin D, Wang L, et al. Neutrophil-epithelial crosstalk at the intestinal lumenal surface mediated by reciprocal secretion of adenosine and IL-6. J Clin Invest. 2001;107:861-869.
83. Ginzberg HH, Cherapanov V, Dong Q, et al. Neutrophil-mediated epithelial injury during transmigration: Role of elastase. Am J Physiol Gastrointest Liver Physiol. 2001;281:G705-G717.
84. Levy BD, Clish CB, Schmidt B, et al. Lipid mediator class switching during acute inflammation: Signals in resolution. Nat Immunol. 2001;2:612-619.
85. Baggiolini M. Chemokines and leukocyte traffic. Nature. 1998;392:565-568.
86. Adams DH, Lloyd AR. Chemokines: Leucocyte recruitment and activation cytokines. Lancet. 1997;349:490-495.
87. Ahuja SK, Murphy PM. Molecular piracy of mammalian interleukin-8 receptor type B by *Herpesvirus saimiri*. J Biol Chem. 1993;268:20961-20964.
88. Dragic T, Litwin V, Allaway GP, et al. HIV-1 entry into CD4+ cells is mediated by the chemokine receptor CC-CKR-5. Nature. 1996;381:667-673.
89. Deng HK, Liu R, Ellemeirer W, et al. Identification of a major co-receptor for primary isolates of HIV. Nature. 1996;381:661-666.
90. Mummidi S, Gonzalez E, Ahuja SS, et al. Genealogy of the CCR5 locus and chemokine system gene variants associated with altered rates of HIV-1 disease progression. Nat Med. 1998;4:786-793.
91. Hallett MB. Controlling the molecular motor of neutrophil chemotaxis. Bioessays. 1997;19:615-621.
92. Heit B, Tavener S, Raharjo E, Kubes P. An intracellular signaling hierarchy determines direction of migration in opposing chemotactic gradients. J Cell Biol. 2002; 159:91-102.
93. Aderem A. How to eat something bigger than your head. Cell. 2002;110:5-8.
94. Greenberg S, Grinstein S. Phagocytosis and innate immunity. Curr Opin Immunol. 2002;14:136-145.
95. Bobak DA, Gaither TA, Frank MM, et al. Modulation of FcR function by complement: Subcomponent Clq enhances the phagocytosis of IgG-opsonized targets by human monocytes and culture-derived macrophages. J Immunol. 1987;138:1150-1156.
96. Lew DP, Andersson T, Hed J, et al. Ca^{2+}-dependent and Ca^{2+}-independent phagocytosis in human neutrophils. Nature. 1985;315:509-511.
97. Petroni KC, Shen L, Guyre PM. Modulation of human polymorphonuclear leukocyte IgG Fc receptors and Fc receptor-mediated functions by IFN-γ and glucocorticoids. J Immunol. 1988;140:3467-3472.
98. Swanson JA, Baer SC. Phagocytosis by zippers and triggers. Trends Cell Biol. 1995;5:89-93.
99. Griffin FM, Griffin JH, Leider JE, et al. Studies on the mechanism of phagocytosis: I. Requirements for circumferential attachment of particle bound ligands to specific receptors on the macrophage plasma membrane. J Exp Med. 1975;142:1263.
100. Griffin FM, Griffin JA, Silverstein SC. Studies on the mechanism of phagocytosis: II. The interaction of macrophages with anti-immunoglobulin IgG-coated bone marrow derived lymphocytes. J Exp Med. 1976;144:788.
101. Ruoslahti E, Pierschbacher MD. Arg-Gly-Asp: A versatile cell recognition signal. Cell. 1986;44:517-518.
102. Blystone SD, Graham IL, Lindberg FP, et al. Integrin avβ3 differentially regulates adhesion and phagocytic functions of the fibronectin receptor, a5β1. J Cell Biol. 1994;127:1129-1137.
103. Babior BM, Lambeth JD, Nauseef W. The neutrophil NADPH oxidase. Arch Biochem Biophys. 2002;397:342-344.
104. Clark RA. Activation of the neutrophil respiratory burst oxidase. J Infect Dis.1999; 179:S309-S317.
105. DeLeo FR, Quinn MT. Assembly of the phagocyte NADPH oxidase: Molecular interactions of oxidase proteins. J Leukoc Biol. 1996;60:677-691.
106. Teahan C, Rowe P, Parker P, et al. The X-linked chronic granulomatous disease gene codes for the b-chain of cytochrome b-245. Nature. 1987;327:720-721.
107. Parkos CA, Allen RA, Cochrane CG, et al. Purified cytochrome b from human granulocyte plasma membrane is comprised of two polypeptides with relative molecular weights of 91,000 and 22,000. J Clin Invest. 1987;80:732-742.
108. Dinauer MC, Orkin SH, Brown R, et al. The glycoprotein encoded by the X-linked chronic granulomatous disease locus is a component of the neutrophil cytochrome b complex. Nature. 1987;327:717-720.
109. Rotrosen D, Yeung CL, Leto TL, et al. Cytochrome b_{558}: The flavin-binding component of the phagocyte NADPH oxidase. Science. 1992;256:1459-1462.
110. Segal AW, West I, Wientjes F, et al. Cytochrome b_{-245} is a flavocytochrome containing FAD and the NADPH-binding site of the microbicidal oxidase of phagocytes. Biochem J. 1992;284:781-788.
111. Volpp BD, Nauseef WM, Clark RA. Two cytosolic neutrophil oxidase components absent in autosomal chronic granulomatous disease. Science. 1988;242:1295-1297.
112. Nunoi H, Rotrosen D, Gallin JI, et al. Two forms of autosomal chronic granulomatous disease lack distinct neutrophil cytosol factors. Science. 1988;242:1298-1301.
113. Volpp BD, Nauseef WM, Donelson JE, et al. Cloning of the cDNA and functional expression of the 47 kilodalton cytosolic component of the human neutrophil respiratory burst oxidase. Proc Natl Acad Sci U S A. 1989;86:7195-7199.
114. Lomax KJ, Leto TL, Nunoi H, et al. Recombinant 47-kilodalton cytosol factor restores NADPH oxidase in chronic granulomatous disease. Science. 1989;245:409-412.
115. Leto TL, Lomax KJ, Volpp BD, et al. Cloning of a 67-kD neutrophil oxidase factor with similarity to a noncatalytic region of $p60^{c\text{-}src}$. Science. 1990;248:727-730.
116. Park J-W, Ma M, Ruedi JM, et al. The cytosolic components of the respiratory burst oxidase exist as a M_r (approx.) 240,00 complex that acquires a membrane-binding site during activation of the oxidase in a cell-free system. J Biol Chem. 1992;267:17327-17332.
117. Iyer SS, Pearson DW, Nauseef WM, Clark RA. Evidence for a readily dissociable complex of p47phox and p67phox in cytosol of unstimulated human neutrophils J Biol Chem. 1994;269:22405-22411.
118. Heyworth PG, Shrimpton CF, Segal AW. Localization of the 47 kDa phosphoprotein involved in the respiratory-burst NADPH oxidase of phagocytic cells. Biochem J. 1989;260:243-248.
119. Rotrosen D, Leto TL. Phosphorylation of neutrophil 47-kDa cytosolic oxidase factor: Translocation to membrane is associated with distinct phosphorylation events. J Biol Chem. 1990;265:19910-19915.
120. Clark RA, Volpp BD, Leidal KG, et al. Two cytosolic components of the human neutrophil respiratory burst oxidase translocate to the plasma membrane during cell activation. J Clin Invest. 1990;85:714-721.
121. Heyworth PG, Curnutte JT, Nauseef WM, et al. Neutrophil nicotinamide adenine dinucleotide phosphate oxidase assembly: Translocation of *p47-phox* and *p67-phox* requires interaction between *p47-phox* and cytochrome b_{558}. J Clin Invest. 1991;87:352-356.
122. Nauseef WM, Volpp BD, McCormick S, et al. Assembly of the neutrophil respiratory burst oxidase: Protein kinase C promotes cytoskeletal and membrane association of cytosolic oxidase components. J Biol Chem. 1991:266:5911-5917.
123. Nauseef WM, McCormick S, Renee J, et al. Functional domain in an arginine-rich carboxyl-terminal region of p47phox. J Biol Chem. 1993;268:23646-23651.
124. Rotrosen D, Kleinberg ME, Nunoi H, et al. Evidence for a functional cytoplasmic domain of phagocyte oxidase cytochrome b558. J Biol Chem. 1990:265:8745-8750.
125. Kleinberg ME, Mital D, Rotrosen D, et al. Characterization of a phagocyte cytochrome b_{558} 91-kilodalton subunit functional domain: Identification of peptide sequence and amino acids essential for activity. Biochemistry. 1992:31:2686-2690.
126. DeLeo FR, Yu L, Burritt JB, et al. Mapping sites of interaction of p47-phox and flavocytochrome *b* with random-sequence peptide phage display libraries. Proc Natl Acad Sci U S A. 1995;92:7110-7114.
127. Pawson T, Schlessinger J. SH2 and SH3 domains. Curr Biol. 1993;3:434-442.
128. McPhail LC. SH3-dependent assembly of the phagocyte NADPH oxidase. J Exp Med. 1994;180:2011-2015.
129. Leto TL, Adams AG, de Mendez I. Assembly of the phagocyte NADPH oxidase: Binding of Src homology 3 domains to proline-rich targets. Proc Natl Acad Sci U S A. 1994;91:10650-10654.
130. Abo A, Pick E, Hall A, et al. Activation of the NADPH oxidase involves the small GTP-binding protein $p21^{rac1}$. Nature. 1991;353:668-670.
131. Knaus UG, Heyworth PG, Evans T, et al. Regulation of phagocyte oxygen radical production by the GTP-binding protein Rac 2. Science. 1991;254:1512-1515.
132. Bokoch GM, Diebold BA. Current molecular models for NADPH oxidase regulation by Rac GTPase. Blood. 2002;100:2692-2696.
133. Philips MR, Pillinger MH, Staud R, et al. Carboxyl methylation of Ras-related proteins during signal transduction in neutrophils. Science. 1993;259:977-980.
134. Ando S, Kaibuchi K, Sasaki T, et al. Post-translational processing of *rac* p21s is important both for their interaction with the GDP/GTP exchange proteins and for their activation of NADPH oxidase. J Biol Chem. 1992;267:25709-25713.
135. Quinn MT, Evans T, Loetterle LR, et al. Translocation of Rac correlates with NADPH oxidase activation: Evidence for equimolar translocation of oxidase components. J Biol Chem. 1993;268:20983-20987.
136. Abo A, Webb MR, Grogan A, et al. Activation of NADPH oxidase involves the dissociation of $p21^{rac}$ from its inhibitory GDP/GTP exchange protein (rhoGDI) followed by its translocation to the plasma membrane. Biochem J. 1994;298:585-591.
137. Heyworth PG, Bohl BP, Bokoch GM, et al. Rac translocates independently of the neutrophil NADPH oxidase components $p47^{phox}$ and $p67^{phox}$: Evidence for its interaction with flavocytochrome b_{558}. J Biol Chem. 1994;269:30749-30752.
138. Quinn MT, Mullen ML, Jesaitis AJ, et al. Subcellular distribution of the Rap 1A protein in human neutrophils: Colocalization and cotranslocation with cytochrome b_{559}. Blood. 1992;79:1563-1573.
139. Wientjes FB, Hsuan JJ, Totty NF, et al. p40phox, A third cytosolic component of the activation complex of the NADPH oxidase to contain src homology 3 domains. Biochem J. 1993;296:557-561.

140. Wientjes FB, Panayotou G, Reeves E, et al. Interactions between cytosolic components of the NADPH oxidase: p40*phox* interacts with both p67*phox* and p47*phox*. Biochem J. 1996;317:919-924.

141. Sathyamoorthy M, de Mendez I, Adams AG, et al. p40*phox* Down-regulates NADPH oxidase activity through interactions with its SH3 domain. J Biol Chem. 1997; 272:9141-9146.

142. Jandl RC, Andre-Schwartz J, Borges-Dubois L, et al. Termination of the respiratory burst in human neutrophils. J Clin Invest. 1978;61:1176.

143. Suh Y-A, Arnold RS, Lassegue B, et al. Cell transformation by the superoxide-generating oxidase Mox1. Nature. 1999;401:79-82.

144. Banfi B, Maturana A, Jaconi S, et al. Mammalian H⁺ channel generated through alternative splicing of the NADPH oxidase homologue NOH-1. Science. 2000; 287:138-142.

145. Lambeth JD, Cheng GJ, Arnold RS, Edens WA. Novel homologs of gp91*phox*. Trends Biochem Sci. 2000;25:459-461.

146. Bánfi B, Clark RA, Steger K, Krause KH. Two novel proteins activate superoxide generation by the NADPH oxidase NOX1. J Biol Chem. 2003;278:3510-3513.

147. Geiszt M, Lekstrom K, Witta J, Leto TL. Proteins homologous to p47*phox* and p67*phox* support superoxide production by NAD(P)H oxidase 1 in colon epithelial cells. J Biol Chem. 2003;278:20006-20012.

148. Takeya R, Ueno N, Kami K, et al. Novel human homologues of p47*phox* and p67*phox* participate in activation of superoxide-producing NADPH oxidases J Biol Chem. 2003;278:25234-25246.

149. Tapper H. The secretion of preformed granules by macrophages and neutrophils. J Leukoc Biol. 1996;59:613-622.

150. Nüsse O, Serrander L, Lew DP, et al. KH. Ca⁺⁺ -induced exocytosis in individual human neutrophils: High- and low-affinity granule populations and submaximal responses. EMBO J. 1998;17:1279-1288.

151. Nüsse O, Serrander L, Foyouzi-Youssefi R, et al. Store-operated Ca⁺⁺ influx and stimulation of exocytosis in HL-60 granulocytes. J Biol Chem. 1997;272:28360-28363.

152. Tapper H, Grinstein S. Fc receptor-triggered insertion of secretory granules into the plasma membrane of human neutrophils: Selective retrieval during phagocytosis. J Immunol. 1997;159:409-418.

153. Aunis D, Bader M-F. The cytoskeleton as a barrier to exocytosis in secretory cells. J Exp Biol. 1988;139:253-266.

154. Boyles J, Bainton DF. Changes in plasma-membrane-associated filaments during endocytosis and exocytosis in polymorphonuclear leukocytes. Cell. 1981;24:905-914.

155. Allen L-AH, Aderem A. Protein kinase C regulates MARCKS cycling between the plasma membrane and lysosomes in fibroblasts. EMBO J. 1995;14:1109-1120.

156. Allen L-AH, Aderem A. A role for MARCKS, the isozyme of protein kinase C and myosin I in zymosan phagocytosis by macrophages. J Exp Med. 1995;182:829-840.

157. Rosales JL, Ernst JD. Calcium-dependent neutrophil secretion: Characterization and regulation by annexins. J Immunol. 1997;159:6195-6202.

158. Whiteheart SW, Kubalek EW. SNAPs and NSF: General members of the fusion apparatus. Trends Cell Biol. 1995;5:64-68.

159. Brumell JH, Volchuk A, Sengelov H, et al. Subcellular distribution of docking/fusion proteins in neutrophils, secretory cells with multiple exocytic compartments. J Immunol. 1995;155:5750-5759.

160. Hackam DJ, Rotstein OD, Bennett MK, et al. Characterization and subcellular localization of target membrane soluble NSF attachment protein receptors (t-SNAREs) in macrophages: Syntaxins 2, 3, and 4 are present on phagosomal membranes. J Immunol. 1996;156:4377-4383.

161. Blackwood RA, Smolen JE, Tranoue A, et al. Phospholipase D activity facilitates Ca⁺⁺-induced aggregation and fusion of complex liposomes. Am J Physiol. 1997; 242:C1285.

162. Hessler RJ, Blackwood RA, Brock TG, et al. Identification of glyceraldehyde-3-phosphate dehydrogenase as a Ca⁺⁺-dependent fusogen in human neutrophil cytosol. J Leukoc Biol. 1998;63:331-336.

163. Hackam DJ, Rotstein OD, Zheng WJ, et al. Regulation of phagosomal acidification. Differential targeting of Na⁺/H⁺ exchangers, Na⁺K⁺-ATPases, and vacuolar-type H⁺-ATPases. J Biol Chem. 1997;272:29810-29820.

164. Nanda A, Brumell JH, Nordström T, et al. Activation of proton pumping in human neutrophils occurs by exocytosis of vesicles bearing vacuolar-type H⁺-ATPases. J Biol Chem. 1996;271:15963-15970.

165. Akgul C, Moulding DA, Edwards SW. Molecular control of neutrophil apoptosis. FEBS Lett. 2001;487:318-322.

166. Weinmann P, Scharffetter-Kochanek K, Forlow SB, et al. A role for apoptosis in the control of neutrophil homeostasis in the circulation: Insights from CD18-deficient mice. Blood. 2003;101:739-746.

167. Villunger A, Scott C, Bouillet P, Strasser A. Essential role for the BH3-only protein bim but redundant roles for bax, bcl-2, and bcl-w in the control of granulocyte survival. Blood. 2003;101:2393-2400.

168. Moulding DA, Akgul C, Derouet M, et al. BCL-2 family expression in human neutrophils during delayed and accelerated apoptosis. J Leukoc Biol. 2001;70:783-792.

169. Yamamoto A, Taniuchi S, Tsuji S, et al. Role of reactive oxygen species in neutrophil apoptosis following ingestion of heat-killed *Staphylococcus aureus*. Clin Exp Immunol. 2002;129:479-484.

170. Ottonello L, Frumento G, Arduino N, et al. Differential regulation of spontaneous and immune complex-induced neutrophil apoptosis by proinflammatory cytokines. Role of oxidants, bax and caspase-3. J Leukoc Biol. 2002;72:125-132.

171. Fossati G, Moulding DA, Spiller DG, et al. The mitochondrial network of human neutrophils: Role in chemotaxis, phagocytosis, respiratory burst activation, and commitment to apoptosis. J Immunol. 2003;170:1964-1972.

172. Fadok VA, Bratton DL, Henson PM. Phagocyte receptors for apoptotic cells: Recognition, uptake, and consequences. J Clin Invest. 2001;108:957-962.

173. Coussens LM, Werb Z. Inflammation and cancer. Nature. 2002;420:860-867.

174. Kobayashi SD, Voyich JM, Braughton KR, DeLeo FR. Down-regulation of proinflammatory capacity during apoptosis in human polymorphonuclear leukocytes. J Immunol. 2003;170:3357-3368.

175. Brown JR, Goldblatt D, Buddle J, Morton L, Thrasher AJ. Diminished production of anti-inflammatory mediators during neutrophil apoptosis and macrophage phagocytosis in chronic granulomatous disease (CGD). J Leukoc Biol. 2003;73:591-599.

176. Coxon A, Rieu P, Barkalow FJ, et al. A novel role for the β2 integrin CD11b/CD18 in neutrophil apoptosis: A homeostatic mechanism in inflammation. Immunity. 1996;5:653-666.

177. Klebanoff SJ. Myeloperoxidase: Occurrence and biological function. In: Everse J, Everse K, Grisham M, eds. Peroxidases in Chemistry and Biology. Boca Raton, Fla: CRC Press; 1991:1-36.

178. Klebanoff SJ. Antimicrobial mechanisms in neutrophilic PMN leukocytes. Semin Hematol. 1975;12:117.

179. Hurst JK. Myeloperoxidase: Active site structure and catalytic mechanisms. In: Everse J, Everse KE, Grisham MB, eds. Peroxidases in Chemistry and Biology. Boca Raton, Fla: CRC Press; 1991:37-62.

180. Jiang Q, Griffin DA, Barofsky DF, et al. Intraphagosomal chlorination dynamics and yields determined using unique fluorescent bacterial mimics. Chem Res Toxicol. 1997;10:1080-1089.

181. Hazen SL, Hsu FF, Mueller DM, et al. Human neutrophils employ chlorine gas as an oxidant during phagocytosis. J Clin Invest. 1996;98:1283-1289.

182. Hazen SL, Hsu FF, Duffin K, et al. Molecular chlorine generated by the myeloperoxidase-hydrogen peroxide-chloride system of phagocytes converts low density lipoprotein cholesterol into a family of chlorinated sterols. J Biol Chem. 1996;271:23080-23088.

183. Jacob JS, Cistola DP, Hsu FF, et al. Human phagocytes employ the myeloperoxidase-hydrogen peroxide system to synthesize dityrosine, trityrosine, pulcherosine, and isodityrosine by a tyrosyl radical-dependent pathway. J Biol Chem. 1996;271:19950-19956.

184. Eiserich JP, Hristova M, Cross CE, et al. Formation of nitric oxide-derived inflammatory oxidants by myeloperoxidase in neutrophils. Nature. 1998;391:393-397.

185. Rosen H, Michel BR, VanDevanter DR, et al. Differential effects of myeloperoxidase-derived oxidants on *Escherichia coli* DNA replication. Infect Immun. 1998;66:2655-2659.

186. Rosen H, Orman J, Rakita RM, et al. Loss of DNA-membrane interactions and cessation of DNA synthesis in myeloperoxidase-treated *Escherichia coli*. Proc Natl Acad Sci U S A. 1990;87:10048-10052.

187. Rakita RM, Rosen H. Penicillin-binding protein inactivation by human neutrophil myeloperoxidase. J Clin Invest. 1991;88:750-754.

188. Hurst JK, Barrette WC Jr, Michel BR, et al. Hypochlorous acid and myeloperoxidase-catalyzed oxidation of iron-sulfur clusters in bacterial respiratory dehydrogenases. Eur J Biochem. 1991;202:1275-1282.

189. Rosen H, Klebanoff SJ. Oxidation of microbial iron-sulfur centers by the myeloperoxidase-H₂O₂-halide antimicrobial system. Infect Immun. 1985;47:613-618.

190. Thomas EL, Jefferson MM, Grisham MB. Myeloperoxidase-catalyzed incorporation of amines into proteins: Role of hypochlorous acid and dichloramines. Biochemistry. 1982;24:6299-6308.

191. Klebanoff SJ. Oxygen-dependent cytotoxic mechanisms of phagocytes. Adv Host Defense Mech. 1982;1:111.

192. Berliner JA, Heinecke JW. The role of oxidized lipoproteins in atherogenesis. Free Radic Biol Med. 1996;20:707-727.

193. Hazen SL, Heinecke JW. 3-Chlorotyrosine, a specific marker of myeloperoxidase-catalyzed oxidation, is markedly elevated in low density lipoprotein isolated from human atherosclerotic intima. J Clin Invest. 1997;99:2075-2081.

194. Daugherty A, Dunn JL, Rateri DL, et al. Myeloperoxidase, a catalyst for lipoprotein oxidation, is expressed in human atherosclerotic lesions. J Clin Invest. 1994;94:437-444.

195. Mandell GL. Catalase, superoxide dismutase, and virulence of *S. aureus*. J Clin Invest. 1975;55:561.

196. Cohen MS, Britigan BE, Hassett DJ, et al. Phagocytes, O₂ reduction, and hydroxyl radical. Rev Infect Dis. 1988;10:1088.

197. Ramos CL, Pou S, Britigan BE, et al. Spin trapping evidence for myeloperoxidase-dependent hydroxyl radical formation by human neutrophils and monocytes. J Biol Chem. 1992;267:8307-8312.

198. Pou S, Cohen MS, Britigan BE, et al. Spin trapping and human neutrophils: Limits of detection of hydroxyl radical. J Biol Chem. 1989;264:12299-12302.

199. Levy O. Antibiotic proteins of polymorphonuclear leukocytes. Eur J Haematol. 1996; 56:263-277.

200. Ganz T, Weiss J. Antimicrobial peptides of phagocytes and epithelia. Semin Hematol. 1997;34:343-354.

201. Lehrer RI, Ganz T. Defensins of vertebrate animals. Curr Opin Immunol. 2002;14:96-102.

202. Mandell GL. Intraphagosomal pH of human polymorphonuclear neutrophils. Proc Soc Exp Biol Med. 1970;134:447.

203. Lehrer RI, Ganz T, Selsted ME. Defensins: Endogenous antibiotic peptides of animal cells. Cell. 1991;64:229-230.

204. Lehrer RI, Lichtenstein AK, Ganz T. Defensins: Antimicrobial and cytotoxic peptides of mammalian cells. Annu Rev Immunol. 1993;11:105-128.

205. Ganz T. Microbiology—Gut defence. Nature. 2003;422:478-479.

206. Valore EV, Park CH, Quayle AJ, et al. Human β-defensin-1: An antimicrobial peptide of urogenital tissues. J Clin Invest. 1998;101:1633-1642.

207. Hoffmann JA, Hetru C. Insect defensins: Inducible antibacterial peptides. Immunol Today. 1992;13:411-415.

208. Hill CP, Yee J, Selsted ME, et al. Crystal structure of defensin HNP-3, an amphiphilic dimer: Mechanisms of membrane permeabilization. Science. 1991;251:1481-1485.

209. Zhang X-L, Selsted ME, Pardi A. NMR studies of defensin antimicrobial peptides: 1. Resonance assignment and secondary structure determination of rabbit NP-2 and human HNP-1. Biochemistry. 1992;31:11348-11356.

210. Pardi A, Zhang X-L, Selsted ME, et al. NMR studies of defensin antimicrobial peptides: 2. Three-dimensional structures of rabbit NP-2 and human HNP-I. Biochemistry. 1992;31:11357-11364.

211. Elsbach P, Weiss J. Oxygen-independent bactericidal systems of polymorphonuclear leukocytes. In: Weissmann G, ed. Advances in Inflammation Research, v. 2. New York: Raven; 1981:95.

212. Ooi CE, Weiss J, Elsbach P, et al. A 25-kD NH2-terminal fragment carries all the antibacterial activities of the human neutrophil 60-kD bactericidal/permeability-increasing protein. J Biol Chem. 1987;262:14891.

213. Tobias PS, Soldau K, Iovine NM, et al. Lipopolysaccharide (LPS)-binding proteins BPI and LBP form different types of complexes with LPS. J Biol Chem. 1997; 272:18682-18685.

214. Weiss J, Elsbach P, Shu C, et al. Human bactericidal/permeability-increasing protein and a recombinant NH-terminal fragment cause killing of serum-resistant gram-negative bacteria in whole blood and inhibit tumor necrosis factor release induced by the bacteria. J Clin Invest. 1992;90:1122-1130.

215. Giroir BP, Quint PA, Barton P, et al. Preliminary evaluation of recombinant amino-terminal fragment of human bactericidal/permeability-increasing protein in children with severe meningococcal sepsis. Lancet. 1997;350:1439-1443.

216. Oram JD, Reiter B. Inhibition of bacteria by lactoferrin and other iron-chelating agents. Biochem Biophys Acta. 1968;170:351.

217. Boxer LA, Coates TD, Haak RA, et al. Lactoferrin deficiency associated with altered granulocyte function. N Engl J Med. 1982;387:404.

218. Broxmeyer HE, Smithyman A, Eger RR, et al. Identification of lactoferrin as the granulocyte-derived inhibitor of colony-stimulating activity production. J Exp Med. 1978;148:1052.

219. Kijlstra A, Jeurissen HM. Modulation of classical C3 convertase of complement by tear lactoferrin. Immunology. 1982;47:263.

220. Shafer WM, Martin LE, Spitznagel JK. Cationic antimicrobial proteins isolated from human neutrophil granulocytes in the presence of diisopropyl flurophosphate. Infect Immun. 1984;45:29.

221. Shafer WM, Martin LE, Spitznagel JK. Late intraphagosomal hydrogen ion concentration favors the in vitro antimicrobial capacity of a 37-kilodalton cationic granule protein of human neutrophil granulocytes. Infect Immun. 1986;53:651.

222. Levy O, Weiss J, Zarember K, et al. Antibacterial 15-kDa protein isoforms (p15s) are members of a novel family of leukocyte proteins. J Biol Chem. 1993;268:6058-6063.

223. Campanelli D, Detmers PA, Nathan CF, et al. Azurocidin and a homologous serine protease from neutrophils: Differential antimicrobial and proteolytic properties. J Clin Invest. 1990;85:904-915.

224. Selsted ME, Novotny MJ, Morris WL, et al. Indolicidin, a novel bactericidal tridecapeptide amide from neutrophils. J Biol Chem. 1992;267:4292-4295.

225. Zanetti M, Gennaro R, Romeo D. Cathelicidins: A novel protein family with a common proregion and a variable C-terminal antimicrobial domain. FEBS Lett. 1996; 374:1-5.

226. Casadevall A, Pirofski L. Host-pathogen interactions: Basic concepts of microbial commensalism, colonization, infection, and disease. Infect Immun. 2000;68:6511-6518.

227. Kobayashi SD, Voyich JM, Buhl CL, et al. Global changes in gene expression by human polymorphonuclear leukocytes during receptor-mediated phagocytosis: Cell fate is regulated at the level of gene expression. Proc Natl Acad Sci U S A. 2002;99:6901-6906.

228. Voyich JM, Sturdevant DE, Braughton KR, et al. Genome-wide protective response used by group A streptococcus to evade destruction by human polymorphonuclear leukocytes. Proc Natl Acad Sci U S A. 2003;100:1996-2001.

229. Kobayashi SD, Braughton KR, Whitney AR, et al. Bacterial pathogens modulate an apoptosis differentiation program in human neutrophils. Proc Natl Acad Sci U S A. 2003;100:10948-10953.

230. Staudinger BJ, Oberdoerster MA, Lewis PJ, Rosen H. mRNA expression profiles for Escherichia coli ingested by normal and phagocyte oxidase-deficient human neutrophils. J Clin Invest. 2002;110:1151-1163.

231. Finlay BB, Cossart P. Exploitation of mammalian host cell functions by bacterial pathogens. Science. 1997;276:718-725.

232. Theriot JA. The cell biology of infection by intracellular bacterial pathogens. Annu Rev Cell Dev Biol. 1995;11:213-239.

233. Rosenberger CM, Finlay BB. Phagocyte sabotage: Disruption of macrophage signalling by bacterial pathogens. Mol Cell Biol. 2003;4:385-396.

234. Dezube BJ, Zambela M, Sage DR, et al. Characterization of Kaposi sarcoma-associated herpesvirus/human herpesvirus-8 infection of human vascular endothelial cells: Early events. Blood. 2002;100:888-896.

235. Vlavidia RH, Falkow S. Probing bacterial gene expression within host cells. Trends Microbiol. 1997;5:360-363.

236. Guiney DG. Regulation of bacterial virulence gene expression by the host environment. J Clin Invest. 1998;99:565-569.

237. Virgi M, Makepeace K, Ferguson DJ, et al. Carcinoembryonic antigens (CD66) on epithelial cells and neutrophils and receptor for Opa proteins of pathogenic neisseriae. Mol Microbiol. 1996;22:941-950.

238. Monack DM, Mecsas J, Ghori J, et al. Yersinia signals macrophages to undergo apoptosis and YopJ is necessary for this cell death. Proc Natl Acad Sci U S A. 1997;94:10385-10390.

239. Sory MP, Boland A, Lambermont I, et al. Identification of the YopE and YopH domains required for secretion and internalization into the cytosol of macrophages, using cyaA gene fusion approach. Proc Natl Acad Sci U S A. 1995;92:11198-12002.

240. Yang Z, Delgado R, Xu L, et al. Distinct cellular interactions of secreted and transmembrane Ebola virus glycoproteins. Science. 1998;279:1034-1037.

241. Hackstadt T, Scidmore MA, Rockey DD. Lipid metabolism in Chlamydia trachomatis-infected cells: Directed trafficking of Golgi-derived sphingolipids to the chlamydial inclusion. Proc Natl Acad Sci U S A. 1995;92:4877-4881.

242. Vazquez-Torres A, Xu Y, Jones-Carson J, et al. Salmonella pathogenicity island 2-dependent evasion of the phagocyte NADPH oxidase. Science. 2000;287:1655-1658.

243. Vazquez-Torres A, Fang FC. Salmonella evasion of the NADPH phagocyte oxidase. Microb Infect. 2001;3:1313-1320.

244. Gallois A, Klein J, Allen L-AH, et al. Salmonella pathogenicity island 2-encoded type III secretion system mediates exclusion of NADPH oxidase assembly from the phagosomal membrane. J Immunol. 2001;166:5741-5748.

245. Russell DG, Xu S, Chakraborty P. Intracellular trafficking and the parasitophorous vacuole of Leishmania mexicana-infected macrophages. J Cell Sci. 1992;103:1193-1210.

246. Antoine JC, Prina E, Jovanne C, et al. Parasitophorous vacuoles of Leishmania amazonensis-infected macrophages maintain an acidic pH. Infect Immun. 1990;58:779-787.

247. Malech HL, Gallin JI. Neutrophils in human diseases. N Engl J Med. 1987;317:687.

248. Bodey GP, Buckley M, Sathe YS, et al. Quantitative relationship between circulating leukocytes and infection in patients with acute leukemia. Ann Intern Med. 1966; 64:328.

249. Dale DC. Immune and idiopathic neutropenia. Curr Opin Hematol. 1998;5:33-36.

250. Hübel K, Engert A. Clinical applications of granulocyte colony-stimulating factor: An update and summary. Ann Hematol. 2003;82:207-213.

251. Allen RC, Stevens PR, Price TH, et al. In vivo effects of recombinant human granulocyte colony-stimulating factor on neutrophil oxidative functions in normal human volunteers. J Infect Dis. 1997;175:1184-1192.

252. Root RK, Ladato RF, Patrick W, et al. Multicenter, double-blind, placebo-controlled study of the use of filgrastim in patients hospitalized with pneumonia and severe sepsis. Crit Care Med. 2003;31:367-373.

253. Dong F, Hoefsloot LH, Schelen AM, et al. Identification of a nonsense mutation in the granulocyte-colony-stimulating factor receptor in severe congenital neutropenia. Proc Natl Acad Sci U S A. 1994;91:4480-4484.

254. Hammond WP, Price TH, Souza LM, et al. Treatment of cyclic neutropenia with granulocyte colony-stimulating factor. N Engl J Med. 1989;320:1306-1311.

255. Wright DG, Fauci AS, Dale DC, et al. Correction of human cyclic neutropenia with prednisolone. N Engl J Med. 1978;298:295.

256. Anderson DC, Springer TA. Leukocyte adhesion deficiency: An inherited defect in the Mac-l, LFA-1, and p150,95 glycoproteins. Annu Rev Med. 1987;38:1975-1994.

257. Etzioni A, Frydman M, Pollack S, et al. Recurrent severe infections caused by a novel leukocyte adhesion deficiency. N Engl J Med. 1992;327:1789-1792.

258. von Andrian UH, Berger EM, Ramezani L, et al. In vivo behavior of neutrophils from two patients with distinct inherited leukocyte adhesion deficiency syndromes. J Clin Invest. 1993;91:2893-2897.

259. Roos D, Law SKA. Hematologically important mutations: Leukocyte adhesion deficiency. Blood Cells Mol Dis. 2001;27:1000-1004.

260. Anderson DC, Schmalsteig FC, Finegold MJ, et al. The severe and moderate phenotypes of heritable Mac-l, LFA-I deficiency: Their quantitative definition and relation to leukocyte dysfunction and clinical features. J Infect Dis. 1985;152:668.

261. Nauseef WM, de Alarcon P, Bale JF, et al. Aberrant activation and regulation of the oxidative burst in neutrophils with Mo-1 glycoprotein deficiency. J Immunol. 1986;137:636.

262. Springer TA, Thompson WS, Miller LJ, et al. Inherited deficiency of the Mac-l, LFA-1, p150,95 glycoprotein family and its molecular basis. J Exp Med. 1984;160:1901.

263. Roos D, Law SKA. Hematologically important mutations: Leukocyte adhesion deficiency. Blood Cells Mol Dis. 2001;27:1000-1004.

264. Hidalgo A, Ma S, Peired AJ, et al. Insights into leukocyte adhesion deficiency type 2 from a novel mutation in the GDP-fucose transporter gene. Blood. 2003;101:1705-1712.

265. Frydman M, Etzioni A, Eidlitz-Markus T, et al. Rambam-Hasharon syndrome of psychomotor retardation, short stature, defective neutrophil motility, and Bombay phenotype. Am J Med Genet. 1992;44:297-302.

266. Karsan A, Cornejo CJ, Winn RK, et al. Leukocyte adhesion deficiency type II is a generalized defect of de novo GDP-fucose biosynthesis. J Clin Invest. 1998; 101:2438-2445.

267. Etzioni A, Sturla L, Antonellis A, et al. Leukocyte adhesion deficiency (LAD) type II/carbohydrate deficient glycoprotein (CDG) IIc founder effect and genotype/phenotype correlation. Am J Med Genet. 2002;110:131-135.

268. Gallin JI. Abnormal phagocyte chemotaxis: Pathophysiology, clinical manifestations, and management of patients. Rev Infect Dis. 1981;3:1196.

269. Van Epps DE, Williams RC. Suppression of leukocyte chemotaxis by human IgA myeloma components. J Exp Med. 1976;144:1227.

270. Perez HD, Lipton M, Goldstein IM. A specific inhibitor of complement (C5)-derived chemotactic activity in serum from patients with systemic lupus erythematosus. J Clin Invest. 1978;62:29.

271. Perez HD, Hooper C, Volanakis J, et al. Specific inhibitor of complement derived chemotactic activity in systemic lupus erythematosus related antigenically to the Bb fragment of human factor B. J Immunol. 1987;139:484.

272. Clark RA, Page RC, Wilde G. Defective neutrophil chemotaxis in juvenile periodontitis. Infect Immun. 1977;18:694.

273. Van Dyke TE. Role of the neutrophil in oral disease: Receptor deficiency in leukocytes from patients with juvenile periodontitis. Rev Infect Dis. 1985;7:419.

274. Perez HD, Kelly E, Elfman F, et al. Defective polymorphonuclear leukocyte formyl peptide receptor(s) in juvenile periodontitis. J Clin Invest. 1991;87:971-976.

275. Shurin SB, Socransky SS, Sweeney E, et al. A neutrophil disorder induced by Capnocytophaga: A dental micro-organism. N Engl J Med. 1979;301:849.

276. Kramer N, Perez HD, Goldstein IM. An immunoglobulin (IgG) inhibitor of polymorphonuclear leukocyte motility in a patient with recurrent infection. N Engl J Med. 1980;303:1253.

277. Barrat FJ, Auloge L, Pastural E, et al. Genetic and physical mapping of the Chédiak-Higashi syndrome on chromosome 1q42-43. Am J Hum Genet. 1996;59:625-632.

278. Faigle W, Raposo G, Tenza D, et al. Deficient peptide loading and MHC class II endosomal sorting in a human genetic immunodeficiency disease: The Chédiak-Higashi syndrome. J Cell Biol. 1998;141:1121-1134.

279. Clark RA, Kimball HR. Defective granulocyte chemotaxis in the Chédiak-Higashi syndrome. J Clin Invest. 1971;50:2645.

280. Root RK, Rosenthal AS, Balestra DJ. Abnormal bactericidal, metabolic, and lysosomal functions of Chédiak-Higashi syndrome leukocytes. J Clin Invest. 1972;51:649.

281. Spritz RA. Genetic defects in Chédiak-Higashi syndrome and the beige mouse. J Clin Immunol. 1998;18:97-105.

282. Barbosa MDFS, Nguyen QA, Tchernev VT, et al. Identification of the homologous beige and Chédiak-Higashi syndrome genes. Nature. 1996;382:262-265.

283. Nagle DL, Karim MA, Woolf EA, et al. Identification and mutation analysis of the complete gene for Chédiak-Higashi syndrome. Nat Genet. 1996;14:307-311.

284. Haddad E, Le Deist F, Blanche S, et al. Treatment of Chédiak-Higashi syndrome by allogenic bone marrow transplantation: Report of 10 cases. Blood. 1995;85:3328-3333.

285. Davis SD, Schaller J, Wedgwood RJ. Job's syndrome: Recurrent "cold" staphylococcal abscesses. Lancet. 1966;1:1013.

286. Grimbacher B, Holland SM, Gallin JI, et al. Hyper-IgE syndrome with recurrent infections—An autosomal dominant multisystem disorder. N Engl J Med. 1999; 340:692-702.

287. Donabedian H, Gallin JI. The hyperimmunoglobulinemia E recurrent-infection (Job's) syndrome. Medicine (Baltimore). 1983;62:195.

288. Donabedian H, Gallin JI. Mononuclear cells from patients with the hyperimmunoglobulinemia E recurrent infection syndrome produce an inhibitor of leukocyte chemotaxis. J Clin Invest. 1982;69:1155.

289. Dreskin SC, Goldsmith PK, Strober W, et al. Metabolism of immunoglobulin E in patients with markedly elevated serum immunoglobulin E levels. J Clin Invest. 1987;79:1764.

290. Dreskin SC, Goldsmith PK, Gallin JI. Immunoglobulins in the hyperimmunoglobulin E and recurrent infection (Job's) syndrome. J Clin Invest. 1985;75:26.

291. Donabedian H, Alling DW, Gallin JI. Levamisole is inferior to placebo in the hyperimmunoglobulin E recurrent-infection (Job's) syndrome. N Engl J Med. 1982; 307:290.

292. Ottonello L, Daprio P, Pastorino G, et al. Neutrophil dysfunction and increased susceptibility to infection. Eur J Clin Invest. 1998;19:434.

293. Craddock PR, Yawata P, Van Santen L, et al. Acquired phagocyte dysfunction: A complication of the hypophosphatemia of parenteral hyperalimentation. N Engl J Med. 1974;290:1403.

294. Bisno AL, Freeman JC. The syndrome of asplenia, pneumococcal sepsis, and disseminated intravascular coagulation. Ann Intern Med. 1970;72:389.

295. Miller ME, Seals J, Kaye R, et al. A familial, plasma associated defect of phagocytosis: A new cause of recurrent bacterial infections. Lancet. 1968;2:60-63.

296. Super M, Thiel S, Lu J, et al. Association of low levels of mannan-binding protein with a common defect of opsonisation. Lancet. 1989;1236-1239.

297. Turner MW, Hamvas RM. Mannose-binding lectin: Structure, function, genetics and disease associations. Rev Immunogenet. 2000;2:305-322.

298. Malech HL, Nauseef WM. Primary inherited defects in neutrophil function: Etiology and treatment. Semin Hematol. 1997;34:279-290.

299. Dinauer MC, Nauseef WM, Newburger PE. Inherited disorders of phagocyte killing. The Metabolic and Molecular Bases of Inherited Diseases. New York: McGraw-Hill; 2001:4857-4887.

300. Curnutte JT. Chronic granulomatous disease: The solving of a clinical riddle at the molecular level. Clin Immunol Immunopathol. 1993;67:S2-S15.

301. Winkelstein JA, Marino MC, Johnston RB Jr, et al. Chronic granulomatous disease—Report on a national registry of 368 patients. Medicine. 2000;79:155-169.

302. Dinauer MC, Orkin SH. Chronic granulomatous disease. Annu Rev Med.1992;43: 117-124.

303. Meischl C, Roos D. The molecular basis for chronic granulomatous disease. Springer Semin Immunopathol. 1998;19:417-434.

304. Heyworth PG, Curnutte JT, Rae J, et al. Hematologically important mutations: X-linked chronic granulomatous disease (second update). Blood Cells Mol Dis. 2001;27:16-26.

305. Bromberg Y, Pick E. Activation of NADPH-dependent superoxide production in a cell-free system by sodium dodecyl sulfate. J Biol Chem. 1985;260:13539-13545.

306. Heyneman RA, Vercauteren RE. Activation of a NADPH-dependent oxidase from horse polymorphonuclear leukocytes in a cell-free system. J Leukoc Biol. 1984;36:751-759.

307. Royer-Pokora B, Kunkel LM, Monaco AP, et al. Cloning the gene for an inherited human disorder—chronic granulomatous disease—on the basis of its chromosomal location. Nature. 1986;322:32-38.

308. Rae J, Newburger PE, Dinauer MC, et al. X-linked chronic granulomatous disease: Mutations in the CYBB gene encoding the gp91-phox component of the respiratory burst oxidase. Am J Hum Genet. 1998;62:1320-1331.

309. Heyworth PG, Curnutte JT, Noack D, et al. Hematologically important mutations: X-linked chronic granulomatous disease, an update. Blood Cells Mol Dis. 1997;23:443-450.

310. Parkos CA, Dinauer MC, Jesaitis AJ, et al. Absence of both the 91 kD and 22 kD subunits of human neutrophil cytochrome b in two genetic forms of chronic granulomatous disease. Blood. 1989;73:1416-1420.

311. Dinauer MC, Curnutte JT, Rosen H, et al. A missense mutation in the cytochrome b heavy chain in cytochrome-positive X-linked chronic granulomatous disease. J Clin Invest. 1989;84:2012-2016.

312. Dinauer MC, Pierce EA, Erickson RW, et al. Point mutation in the cytoplasmic domain of the neutrophil p22-phox cytochrome b subunit is associated with a nonfunctional NADPH oxidase and chronic granulomatous disease. Proc Natl Acad Sci U S A. 1991;88:11231-11235.

313. Clark RA, Malech HL, Gallin JI, et al. Genetic variants of chronic granulomatous disease: Prevalence of deficiencies of two cytosolic components of the NADPH oxidase system. N Engl J Med. 1989;321:647-652.

314. Casimir CM, Bu-Ghanim HN, Rodaway ARF, et al. Autosomal recessive chronic granulomatous disease caused by deletion at a dinucleotide repeat. Proc Natl Acad Sci U S A. 1991;88:2753-2757.

315. Volpp BD, Lin Y. In vitro molecular reconstitution of the respiratory burst in B lymphoblasts from p47-phox-deficient chronic granulomatous disease. J Clin Invest. 1993;91:201-207.

316. Gorlach A, Lee PL, Roesler J, et al. A p47-phox pseudogene carries the most common mutation causing p47-phox-deficient chronic granulomatous disease. J Clin Invest. 1997;100:1907-1918.

317. Bonnizzato A, Russo MP, Donini M, et al. Identification of a double mutation (D160V-K161E) in the p67phox gene of a chronic granulomatous disease patient. Biochem Biophys Res Commun. 1997;231:861-863.

318. Leusen JHW, De Klein A, Hilarius PM, et al. Disturbed interaction of p21-rac with mutated p67-phox causes chronic granulomatous disease. J Exp Med. 1996; 184:1243-1249.

319. Ambruso DR, Knall C, Abell AN, et al. Human neutrophil immunodeficiency syndrome is associated with an inhibitory Rac2 mutation. Proc Natl Acad Sci U S A. 2000;97:4654-4659.

320. Williams DA, Tao W, Yang FC, et al. Dominant negative mutation of the hematopoietic-specific Rho GTPase, Rac2, is associated with a human phagocyte immunodeficiency. Blood. 2000;96:1646-1654.

321. Kurkchubasche AG, Panepinto JA, Tracy TF Jr, et al. Clinical features of a human Rac2 mutation: A complex neutrophil dysfunction disease. J Pediatr. 2001;139:141-147.

322. Clark RA, Klebanoff SJ. Chronic granulomatous disease: Studies of a family with impaired neutrophil chemotactic, metabolic and bactericidal function. Am J Med. 1978;65:941-948.

323. Schapiro BL, Newburger PE, Klempner MS, et al. Chronic granulomatous disease presenting in a 69-year-old man. N Engl J Med. 1991;325:1786-1790.

324. Chang YC, Segal BH, Holland SM, et al. Virulence of catalase-deficient Aspergillus nidulans in p47phox-1-mice. J Clin Invest. 1998;101:1843-1850.

325. Aliabadi H, Gonzalez R, Quie PG. Urinary tract disorders in patients with chronic granulomatous disease. N Engl J Med. 1989;321:706-708.

326. Ament ME, Ochs HD. Gastrointestinal manifestations of chronic granulomatous disease. N Engl J Med. 1973;288:382-387.

327. Sillevis Smitt JH, Weening RS, Krieg SR, et al. Discoid lupus erythematosus-like lesions in carriers of X-linked chronic granulomatous disease. Br J Dermatol. 1990; 122:643-650.

328. Vowells SJ, Sekhsaria S, Malech HL, et al. Flow cytometric analysis of the granulocyte respiratory burst: A comparison study of fluorescent probes. J Immunol Methods. 1995;178:89-97.

329. van Pelt LJ, van Zwieten R, Weening RS, et al. Limitations in the use of dihydrorhodamine 123 for flow cytometric analysis of the neutrophil respiratory burst. J Immunol Methods. 1996;191:187-196.

330. Segal BH, Leto TL, Gallin JI, et al. Genetic, biochemical, and clinical features of chronic granulomatous disease. Medicine. 2000;79:170-200.

331. Gallin JI, Alling DW, Malech HL, et al. Itraconazole to prevent fungal infections in chronic granulomatous disease. N Engl J Med. 2003;348:2416-2422.

332. International Chronic Granulomatous Disease Study Group. A controlled trial of interferon gamma to prevent infection in chronic granulomatous disease. N Engl J Med. 1991;324:509-516.

333. Sechler JMG, Malech HL, White CJ, et al. Recombinant human interferon reconstitutes defective phagocyte function in chronic granulomatous disease of childhood. Proc Natl Acad Sci U S A. 1988;85:4874-4878.

334. Ezekowitz RAB, Orkin SH, Newburger PE. Recombinant interferon gamma augments phagocyte superoxide production and X-chronic granulomatous disease gene expression in X-linked variant chronic granulomatous disease. J Clin Invest. 1987; 80:1009-1016.

335. Ezekowitz RAB, Dinauer MC, Jaffee HS, et al. Partial correction of the phagocyte defect in patients with X-linked chronic granulomatous disease by subcutaneous interferon gamma. N Engl J Med. 1988;319:146-151.

336. Woodman RC, Erickson RW, Rae J, et al. Prolonged recombinant interferon-gamma therapy in chronic granulomatous disease: Evidence against enhanced neutrophil oxidase activity. Blood. 1992;79:1558-1562.

337. Newburger PE, Ezekowitz RAB. Cellular and molecular effects of recombinant interferon gamma in chronic granulomatous disease. Hematol Oncol Clin North Am. 1988;2:267-276.

338. Calvino MC, Maldonado MS, Otheo E, et al. Bone marrow transplantation in chronic granulomatous disease. Eur J Pediatr. 1996;155:877-879.

339. Sekhsaria S, Gallin JI, Linton GF, et al. Peripheral blood progenitors as a target for genetic correction of p47phox-deficient chronic granulomatous disease. Proc Natl Acad Sci U S A. 1993;90:7446-7450.

340. Weil WM, Linton GF, Whiting-Theobald N, et al. Genetic correction of p67phox deficient chronic granulomatous disease using peripheral blood progenitor cells as a target for retrovirus mediated gene transfer. Blood. 1997;89:1754-1761.

341. Malech HL, Maples PB, Whiting-Theobald N, et al. Prolonged production of NADPH oxidase-corrected granulocytes after gene therapy of chronic granulomatous disease. Proc Natl Acad Sci U S A. 1997;94:12133-12138.

342. Grez M, Becker S, Saulnier S, et al. Gene therapy of chronic granulomatous disease. Bone Marrow Transplant. 2000;25:S99-S104.

343. Malech HL, Bauer TR Jr, Hickstein DD. Prospects for gene therapy for neutrophil defects. Semin Hematol. 1997;34:355-361.

344. Babior GL, Crowley CA. Chronic granulomatous disease and other disorders of killing by phagocytes. In: Steinbury JB, Wyngaarden JB, Frederickson DS, et al, eds. The Metabolic Basis of Inherited Disease. 5th ed. New York: McGraw-Hill; 1983;1969.

345. Parry MF, Root RK, Metcalf JA, et al. Myeloperoxidase deficiency: Prevalance and clinical significance. Ann Intern Med. 1981;95:293.

346. Nauseef WM, Cogley M, Bock S, et al. Pattern of inheritance in hereditary myeloperoxidase deficiency associated with the R569W missense mutation. J Leukoc Biol. 1998;63:264-269.

347. Lehrer RJ, Cline MJ. Leukocyte myeloperoxidase deficiency and disseminated candidiasis: The role of myeloperoxidase in resistance to Candida infection. J Clin Invest. 1969;48:1478.

348. Nauseef WM. Insights into myeloperoxidase biosynthesis gained from cases of inherited deficiency. J Mol Med. 1998;76:661-668.

349. Nauseef WM. Posttranslational processing of a human myeloid lysosomal protein, myeloperoxidase. Blood. 1987;70:1143-1150.

350. Nauseef WM, McCormick S, Yi H. Roles of heme insertion and the mannose-6-phosphate receptor in processing of the human myeloid lysosomal enzyme, myeloperoxidase. Blood. 1992;80:2622-2633.

351. Nauseef WM, Root RK, Malech HL. Biochemical and immunologic analysis of hereditary myeloperoxidase deficiency. J Clin Invest. 1983;71:1297.

352. Nauseef WM, Brigham S, Cogley M. Hereditary myeloperoxidase deficiency due to a missense mutation of arginine to tryptophan. J Biol Chem. 1994;369:1212-1216.

353. Tobler A, Selsted ME, Miller CW, et al. Evidence for a pretranslational defect in hereditary and acquired myeloperoxidase deficiency. Blood. 1989;73:1980-1986.

354. DeLeo FR, Goedken M, McCormick SJ, et al. A novel form of hereditary myeloperoxidase deficiency linked to endoplasmic reticulum/proteasome degradation. J Clin Invest. 1998;101:2900-2909.

355. Romano M, Dri P, Dadalt L, et al. Biochemical and molecular characterization of hereditary myeloperoxidase deficiency. Blood. 1997;90:4126-4134.

356. Petrides PE. Molecular genetics of peroxidase deficiency. J Mol Med. 1998;76:688-698.

357. Lanza F. Pathology of myeloperoxidase deficiency. J Mol Med. 1998;76:676-681.

358. Kutter D. Recent developments in myeloperoxidase deficiency. J Mol Med. 1998; 76:669-675.

359. Aratani Y, Kura F, Watanabe H, et al. Critical role of myeloperoxidase and nicotinamide adenine dinucleotide phosphate-oxidase in high-burden systemic infection of mice with Candida albicans. J Infect Dis. 2002;185:1833-1837.

360. Brennan ML, Anderson MM, Shih DM, et al. Increased atherosclerosis in myeloperoxidase-deficient mice. J Clin Invest. 2001;107:419-430.

361. Brennan ML, Gaur A, Pahuja A, et al. Mice lacking myeloperoxidase are more susceptible to experimental autoimmune encephalomyelitis. J Neuroimmunol. 2001; 112:97-105.

362. Xiao H, Heeringa P, Hu P, et al. Antineutrophil cytoplasmic autoantibodies specific for myeloperoxidase cause glomerulonephritis and vasculitis in mice. J Clin Invest. 2002;110:955.

363. Ishida-Okawara A, Ohareseki T, Takahashi K, et al. Contribution of myeloperoxidase to coronary artery vasculitis associated with MPO-ANCA production. Inflammation. 2001;25:381-387.

364. Reynolds WF, Stegeman CA, Tervaert JWC. -463 G/A myeloperoxidase promoter polymorphism is associated with clinical manifestations and the course of disease in MPO-ANCA-associated vasculitis. Clin Immunol. 2002;103:154-160.

365. Zhang R, Brennan M-L, Fu X, et al. Association between myeloperoxidase levels and risk of coronary artery disease. JAMA. 2001;286:2136-2142.

366. Hamajima N, Matsuo K, Suzuki T, et al. Low expression myeloperoxidase genotype negatively associated with Helicobacter pylori infection. Jpn J Cancer Res. 2001; 92:488-493.

367. Combarros O, Infante J, Llorca J, et al. The myeloperoxidase gene in Alzheimer's disease: A case-control study and meta-analysis. Neurosci Lett. 2002;326:33-36.

368. Nelissen I, Fiten P, Vandenbroeck K, et al. PECAM1, MPO and PRKAR1A at chromosome 17q21-q24 and susceptibility for multiple sclerosis in Sweden and Sardinia. J Neuroimmunol. 2000;108:153-159.

369. Reynolds WF. The role of myeloperoxidase in myeloid leukemia and multiple sclerosis. In Nauseef WM, Petrides PE, eds. The Peroxidase Multigene Family of Enzymes. Berlin, Heidelberg, New York: Springer-Verlag; 2000:93-101.

370. Reynolds WF, Hiltunen M, Pirskanen M, et al. MPO and APOe4 polymorphisms interact to increase risk for AD in Finnish males. Neurology. 2000;55:1284-1290.

371. Reynolds WF, Rhees J, Maciejewski D, et al. Myeloperoxidase polymorphism is associated with gender specific risk for Alzheimer's disease. Exp Neurol. 1999;155:31-41.

372. Cascorbi I, Henning S, Brockmöller J, et al. Substantially reduced risk of cancer of the aerodigestive tract in subjects with variant-463A of the myeloperoxidase gene. Cancer Res. 2000;60:644-649.

373. Kantarci OH, Lesnick TG, Yang P, et al. Myeloperoxidase-463 (G→A) polymorphism associated with lower risk of lung cancer. Mayo Clin Proc. 2002;77:17-22.

374. Lu W, Xing D, Qi J, et al. Genetic polymorphism in myeloperoxidase but not GSTM1 is associated with risk of lung squamous cell carcinoma in a Chinese population. Int J Cancer. 2002;102:275-279.

375. London SJ, Lehman TA, Taylor JA. Myeloperoxidase genetic polymorphism and lung cancer risk. Cancer Res. 1997;57:5001-5003.

376. Schabath MB, Spitz MR, Hong WK, et al. A myeloperoxidase polymorphism associated with reduced risk of lung cancer. Lung Cancer. 2002;37:35-40.

377. Gallin JI. Neutrophil specific granule deficiency. Annu Rev Med. 1985;36:263.

378. Rosenberg HF, Gallin JI. Neutrophil-specific granule deficiency includes eosinophils. Blood. 1993;82:268-273.

379. Ganz T, Metcalf JA, Gallin JI, et al. Microbicidal/cytotoxic proteins of neutrophils are deficient in two disorders: Chediak-Higashi syndrome and "specific" granule deficiency. J Clin Invest. 1988;82:552-556.

380. Lomax KJ, Gallin JI, Rotrosen D, et al. Selective defect in myeloid cell lactoferrin gene expression in neutrophil specific granule deficiency. J Clin Invest. 1989;83:514-519.

381. Lekstrom-Himes J, Xanthopoulos KG. Biological role of the CCAAT/enhancer-binding protein family of transcription factors. J Biol Chem. 1998;273:28545-28548.

382. Lekstrom-Himes JA, Dorman SE, Lopar P, et al. Neutrophil-specific granule deficiency results from a novel mutation with loss of function of the transcription factor CCAAT/enhancer binding protein. J Exp Med. 1999;189:1847-1852.

383. Gombart AF, Kwok SH, Anderson KL, et al. Regulation of neutrophil and eosinophil secondary granule gene expression by transcription factors C/EBPε and PU.1. Blood. 2003;101:3265-3273.

384. Gallin JI, Fletcher MP, Seligmann BE, et al. Human neutrophil-specific granule deficiency: A model to assess the role of neutrophil-specific granules in the evolution of the inflammatory response. Blood. 1983;59:1317-1329.

385. Lekstrom-Himes J, Xanthopoulos KG. CCAAT/Enhancer binding protein E is critical for effective neutrophil-mediated response to inflammatory challenge. Blood. 1999;93:3096-3105.

386. Gombart AF, Koeffler HP. Neutrophil specific granule deficiency and mutations in the gene encoding transcription factor C/EBP(epsilon). Curr Opin Hematol. 2002;9:36-42.

387. Yeghen T, Devereux S. Granulocyte transfusion: A review. Vox Sanguinis. 2001;81:87-92.

388. Herzig RH, Herzig GP, Grano RG, et al. Successful granulocyte transfusion therapy for gram-negative septicemia. N Engl J Med. 1977;296:701.

389. Alavi JB, Root RK, Djerassi I, et al. A randomized clinical trial of granulocyte transfusions for infections in acute leukemia. N Engl J Med. 1977;296:706.

390. Buescher ES, Gallin JI. Leukocyte transfusion in chronic granulomatous disease. N Engl J Med. 1982;307:800.

391. Wright DG, Robichaud KJ, Pizzo PA, et al. Lethal pulmonary reactions associated with the combined use of amphotericin B and leukocyte transfusions. N Engl J Med. 1981;304:1185.

392. Horwitz M, Barrett J, Brown M, et al. Treatment of chronic granulomatous disease with nonmyeloablative conditioning and a T-cell-depleted hematopoietic allograft. N Engl J Med. 2001;344:881-888.

393. Miyazaki S, Shin H, Goya N, Nakagawara A. Identification of a carrier mother of a female patient with chronic granulomatous disease. J Pediatr. 1976;89:784-786.

394. Mills EL, Rholl KS, Quie PG. X-linked inheritance in females with chronic granulomatous disease. J Clin Invest. 1980;66:332-340.

395. Johnston RB III, Harbeck RJ, Johnston RB Jr. Recurrent severe infections in a girl with apparently variable expression of mosaicism for chronic granulomatous disease. J Pediatr. 1985;106:50-55.

396. Oez S, Welte K, Platzer E, Kalden JR. A simple assay for quantifying the inducible adherence of neutrophils. Immunobiology. 1990;180:308-315.

397. Bolscher BGJM, De Boer M, De Klein A, et al. Point mutations in the β-subunit of cytochrome b_{558} leading to X-linked chronic granulomatous disease. Blood. 1991;77:2482-2487.

398. Kume A, Dinauer MC. Gene therapy for chronic granulomatous disease. J Lab Clin Med. 2000;135:122-128.

399. Björgvinsdóttir H, Ding CJ, Pech N, et al. Retroviral-mediated gene transfer of gp91^{phox} into bone marrow cells rescues defect in host defense against Aspergillus fumigatus in murine X-linked chronic granulomatous disease. Blood. 1997;89:41-48.

400. Dinauer MC, Li LL, Björgvinsdóttir H, et al. Long-term correction of phagocyte NADPH oxidase activity by retroviral-mediated gene transfer in murine X-linked chronic granulomatous disease. Blood. 1999;94:914-922.

401. Malech HL, Maples PB, Whiting-Theobald N, et al. Prolonged production of NADPH oxidase-corrected granulocytes after gene therapy of chronic granulomatous disease. Proc Natl Acad Sci U S A. 1997;94:12133-12138.

402. Brenner S, Whiting-Theobald NL, Linton GF, et al. Concentrated RD114-pseudotyped MFGS-gp91^{phox} vector achieves high levels of functional correction of the chronic granulomatous disease oxidase defect in NOD/SCID/β2m $^{-/-}$ repopulating mobilized human peripheral blood CD34^{+} cells. Blood. 2003;102:2789-2797.

403. Weller PF. Human eosinophils. J Allergy Clin Immunol. 1997;100:283-287.

404. Hirai K, Miyamasu M, Takaishi T, et al. Regulation of the function of eosinophils and basophils. Crit Rev Immunol. 1997;17:325-352.

405. Boyce JA. The pathology of eosinophilic inflammation. Allergy Asthma Proc. 1997;18:293-300.

406. Spry CJE. Mechanisms of eosinophilia: V. Kinetics of normal and accelerated eosinophilopoiesis. Cell Tissue Kinet. 1971;4:351.

407. Sanderson CJ. Interleukin-5, eosinophils, and disease. Blood. 1992;79:3101-3109.

408. Gleich GJ, Adolphson CR, Leiferman KM. The biology of eosinophilic leukocyte. Annu Rev Med. 1993;44:85-101.

409. Kitayama J, Mackay CR, Ponath PD, et al. The C-C chemokine receptor CCR3 participates in stimulation of eosinophil arrest on inflammatory endothelium in shear flow. J Clin Invest. 1998;101:2017-2024.

410. Henderson WR, Chi EY, Albert RK, et al. Blockade of CD49d (α₄ integrin) on intrapulmonary but not circulating leukocytes inhibits airway inflammation and hyperresponsiveness in a mouse model of asthma. J Clin Invest. 1997;100:3083-3092.

411. Sriramarao P, Von Andrian UH, Butcher EC, et al. L-Selectin and very late antigen-4 integrin promote eosinophil rolling at physiological shear rates in vivo. J Immunol. 1994;153:4238-4246.

412. Henriques GMO, Miotla JM, Cordeiro RSB, et al. Selectins mediate eosinophil recruitment in vivo: A comparison with their role in neutrophil influx. Blood. 1996; 87:5297-5304.

413. Noursharrgh S. Mechanisms of neutrophil and eosinophil accumulation in vivo. Am Rev Respir Dis. 1993;148:S60-S64.

414. Wardlaw AJ, Walsh GM, Symon FA. Adhesion interactions involved in eosinophil migration through vascular endothelium. Ann N Y Acad Sci. 1996;796:124-137.

415. Dobrina A, Menegazzi R, Carlos TM, et al. Mechanisms of eosinophil adherence to cultured vascular endothelial cells: Eosinophils bind to the cytokine-induced endothelial ligand vascular cell adhesion molecule-1 via the very late activation antigen-4 integrin receptor. J Clin Invest. 1991;88:20-26.

416. David JR, Vadas MA, Butterworth AE, et al. Enhanced helminthotoxic capacity of eosinophils from patients with eosinophilia. N Engl J Med. 1980;303:1147.
417. Mahmoud AAF, Warren KS, Peters PA. A role for the eosinophil in acquired resistance to *Schistosoma mansoni* infection as determined by antieosinophil serum. J Exp Med. 1975;142:805.
418. McLaren DJ, MacKenzie CD, Ramalho-Pinto FJ. Ultrastructural observations on the in vitro interaction between rat eosinophils and some parasitic helminths (*Schistosoma mansoni, Trichinella spiralis* and *Nippostrongylus brasiliensis*). Clin Exp Immunol. 1977;30:105.
419. Densen P, Mahmoud AAF, Sullivan J, et al. Demonstration of eosinophil degranulation on the surface of opsonized schistosomules by phase-contrast cinemicrography. Infect Immun. 1978;22:282.
420. Weller PF, Goetzl EJ. The human eosinophil: Roles in host defense and tissue injury. Am J Pathol. 1980;100:790.
421. Buttersworth AE, David JR. Eosinophil function. N Engl J Med. 1981;304:154.
422. Metcalf JA, Gallin JI, Nauseef WM, et al. Laboratory of Neutrophil Function. New York: Raven; 1985.
422. Carulli G. Applications of flow cytometry in the study of human neutrophil biology and pathology. Hematopathol Mol Hematol. 1996;10:39-61.
424. Rest RF. Measurement of human neutrophil respiratory burst activity during phagocytosis of bacteria. Methods Enzymol. 1994;236:119-136.
425. Ochs HD, Igo RP. The nitroblue tetrazolium slide test: A simple screening method for detecting chronic granulomatous disease and female carriers. J Pediatr. 1973;83:77-82.
426. Baehner RL, Nathan DG. Quantitative nitroblue tetrazolium dye test in chronic granulomatous disease. N Engl J Med. 1968;278:971.
427. Allen RC. Phagocytic leukocyte oxygenation activities and chemiluminescence: A kinetic approach to analysis. Methods Enzymol. 1986;133:449-493.

CHAPTER **9**

Cell-Mediated Defense against Infection

MICHAEL S. GLICKMAN
ERIC G. PAMER

The principal function of the mammalian immune system is to control infectious diseases. The existence of an immune system first was suspected when individuals surviving a bout with plague were noted to be resistant to reinfection. Long before any detailed understanding of its function, the immune system was exploited for therapeutic benefit. One of the earliest examples of vaccination occurred in China to prevent outbreaks of smallpox, later in Turkey, and later still, but to greater acclaim, in England by Jenner's immunization strategy with vaccinia.[1,2] The demonstration that passive transfer of serum from immune individuals conferred specific protection against some pathogens led to the conclusion that immunity is conferred exclusively by serum factors, such as antibodies.[3] Half a century later, the original studies of Metchnikoff showing cell-mediated killing of microbes were resurrected by the demonstration that cells obtained from immune animals, on transfer into naive animals, provided pathogen-specific protective immunity.[4-6]

Early studies of cell-mediated immunity were difficult. First, cells that we now appreciate as distinct, such as B cells and T cells, are morphologically similar and impossible to distinguish by microscopic appearance. To characterize these cells required the development of methods to identify them directly on the basis of cell surface markers. Second, the demonstration of cell-mediated immunity required experiments with inbred mice because cell transfer between outbred animals generally results in rapid rejection of transferred cells. Were it not for the curiosity of immunologists trying to decipher the rules of tissue transplantation, in the process identifying and characterizing the major histocompatibility complex (MHC), we still might be mystified by the role of T lymphocytes in antimicrobial defense. The concept of MHC restriction, an axiom of T-cell biology, is relatively new to immunology, having been shown definitively by Zinkernagel and Doherty[7] in the 1970s.

PRIMER ON BASIC IMMUNOLOGIC TECHNIQUES: FOUNDATION OF IMMUNOLOGIC MODELS

Rapid evolution of immunologic techniques has facilitated the increasingly sophisticated view of the mammalian immune system. Understanding current immunologic techniques is important for the practicing infectious diseases specialist for two reasons. First, these techniques form the basis on which we formulate our understanding of protective immunity. Second, immunologic techniques, such as flow cytometry, intracellular cytokine and MHC tetramer staining, and ELISPOT assays, increasingly are used in the clinical setting to evaluate immunologic function. We briefly review some of the more recently developed immunologic techniques that are increasingly evident in the clinical literature.

Characterizing and Measuring Pathogen-Specific Immunity

Advances in immunology often have resulted from the development of tools that enable investigators to visualize previously unapparent physical distinctions or processes. The generation of monoclonal antibodies revolutionized cellular immunology by distinguishing morphologically similar cell populations, such as B cells and CD4+ and CD8+ T cells. Flow cytometry, now a routine tool in the immunologist's laboratory, radically transformed immunologic analysis by allowing rapid and efficient analysis of complex lymphoid cell populations.[8] A flow cytometer analyzes single cells for the presence of multiple, fluorescently labeled monoclonal antibodies or dyes and allows each cell in a complex population to be scored for multiple cellular markers. This powerful technique provides a detailed picture of mixed cell populations, such as lymph node, spleen, or peripheral blood cells (Fig. 9-1). With the steady introduction of new monoclonal antibodies specific for novel surface or intracellular proteins, flow cytometry continues to uncover increasingly greater complexity among cell populations that previously were assumed to be homogeneous. A recurring theme in immunologic studies is the discovery that a cell subset, on the basis of a new marker, can be divided into two or three distinct cell populations. Although flow cytometry is used routinely in the clinical arena for CD4/CD8 T-cell quantitation in human immunodeficiency virus (HIV)–infected and other immunocompromised patients, it is likely that this technique will play an increasing role in the management of patients with infectious diseases.

More recent technical innovations that have affected cellular immunology studies involve the precise quantitation of antigen-specific T lymphocytes. Three methods—ELISPOT assays, intracellular cytokine staining, and MHC tetramers—have revolutionized the study of pathogen-specific T-cell responses. Before these techniques were available, the frequency of antigen-specific lymphocytes could be estimated only by very labor-intensive and time-consuming methods. The ELISPOT assay is relatively simple and does not require a flow cytometer, an attractive feature if a flow cytometer is not available. Nevertheless, ELISPOT assays provide accurate, quantitative data and can be performed with complex mixtures of cells, such as peripheral blood mononuclear cells or lymph node or spleen cells.[9] To perform this assay, complex mixtures of cells are stimulated with antigen on a membrane coated with a monoclonal antibody specific for a cytokine, such as interferon (IFN)-γ, tumor necrosis factor (TNF), or interleukin (IL)-4. Antigen-specific T cells in the mixture, on stimulation, release cytokines that are captured by membrane-bound antibodies directly adjacent to the stimulated cell. Bound cytokines are detected with a secondary, enzyme-conjugated monoclonal antibody in a fashion identical to a standard sandwich enzyme-linked immunosorbent assay. Each stimulated cell leaves a "spot" on the membrane, and the number of spots is quantified by direct visualization through a dissecting microscope (Fig. 9-2). ELISPOT assays provided the first technique to quantitate the presence of antigen-specific T cells, based on their ability to respond to antigen by cytokine secretion.

Intracellular cytokine staining is similar to the ELISPOT, in that complex cell populations are stimulated with an antigen, but in the

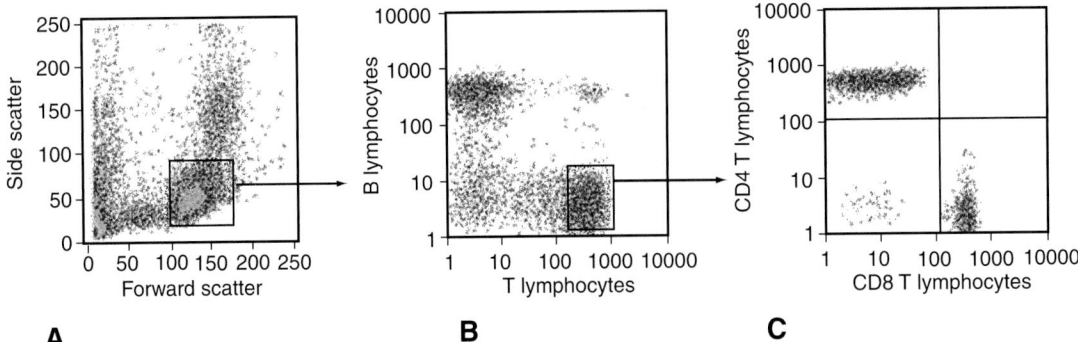

FIGURE 9-1.   Flow cytometry can be used to identify distinct immune cell populations within a complex mixture of cells. **A,** The forward light scatter versus the side scatter of individual cells, which is a measure of the cell's relative size and granularity. Cells within the enclosed box are selected (gated) and consist of monocytes and lymphocytes. **B,** The gated cells are divided further into B cells and T cells on the basis of staining with specific monoclonal antibodies with differing fluorescent emissions. The box surrounds the T-cell population. **C,** Staining of the gated T-cell population for surface expression of CD4+ or CD8+, using monoclonal antibodies that are fluorescent at two additional wavelengths.

presence of either Brefeldin A or monensin, drugs that inhibit cellular secretion of cytokines.[10] During this incubation, cytokines are produced by antigen-specific T cells, but instead of being secreted, they accumulate within the cell. After stimulation, cells are fixed and permeabilized, then stained with cytokine-specific, fluorescently tagged antibodies. Permeabilization with a dilute detergent is necessary to provide antibody access to the accumulated intracellular cytokine. Stained cells are examined by flow cytometry (Fig. 9-3), and antigen-specific T cells are identified and quantified on the basis of cytokine production, but also can be scored for other characteristics (size, granularity, activation and differentiation markers, antigen receptor expression). Although technically more demanding, intracellular cytokine staining is more informative than the ELISPOT assay.

A newer and more direct method for quantifying antigen-specific T cells involves the use of MHC tetramers.[11] Because the interaction between T-cell receptors (TCRs) and MHC peptide complexes is of low affinity, attempts to identify antigen-specific T cells with soluble MHC/peptide complexes routinely failed (see later). Generation of tetrameric forms of MHC/peptide complexed with a fluorophore readily enabled antigen-specific T cells to be stained and identified with flow cytometry (Fig. 9-4). In addition, tetramer staining can be used to isolate viable, pathogen-specific T lymphocytes.[12] An advantage of MHC tetramer staining over either intracellular cytokine staining or ELISPOT assays is that T-cell detection does not depend on cytokine production, which depends on the T-cell phenotype. In some circumstances, T cells may be anergized, in which case they do not produce cytokines on antigen stimulation. Although intracellular cytokine

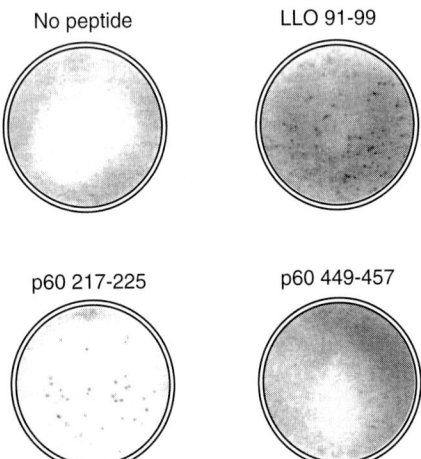

FIGURE 9-2.   The ELISPOT assay quantifies T-cell responses to distinct peptides after infection. The four panels show interferon-γ production by spleen cells derived from mice infected with *Listeria monocytogenes* on stimulation with either no peptide or three defined, MHC class I–restricted peptide epitopes. Each spot represents the activation of an individual cell by a specific peptide. The frequency of antigen-specific T cells can be calculated by counting the number of spots on the filter and dividing by the number of cells placed in the well. *(Redrawn from Vijh S, Pamer EG. Immunodominant and subdominant CTL responses to* Listeria monocytogenes *infection. J Immunol. 1997;158:3366.)*

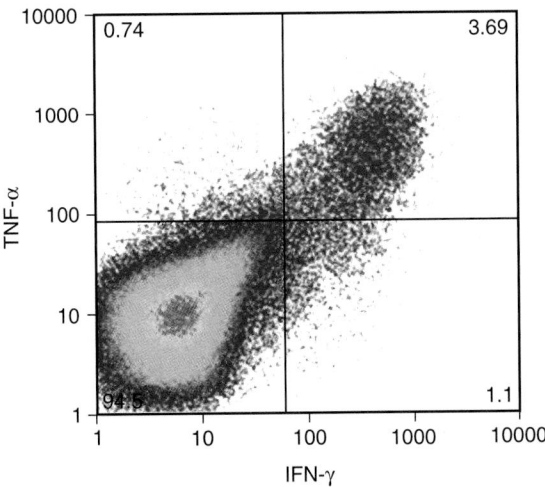

FIGURE 9-3.   Intracellular cytokine staining is another method for quantifying antigen-specific T lymphocytes in complex mixtures of cells. Using this method, spleen cells or peripheral blood cells are stimulated transiently with antigenic peptides, then stained with monoclonal antibodies for the production of cytokines. The dot plot shows interferon (IFN)-γ and tumor necrosis factor (TNF)-α production by peripheral blood lymphocytes on stimulation with an antigenic bacterial peptide. The peptide-specific T-cell population shows concurrent production of both cytokines, a common finding for pathogen-specific CD8+ T lymphocytes. The percentage of cells producing TNF-α, IFN-γ, or both is indicated in the plot quadrants.

staining and MHC tetramer staining are considered methods for quantifying T cells, they are complementary methods that together provide more information than either assay alone.

In many cases, the above-described quantitative assays radically revised prior estimates of pathogen-specific T-cell frequencies.[13-15] The previous gold standard method for quantifying antigen-specific T cells, limiting dilution analysis, underestimated pathogen-specific T cell-frequencies by a factor of 100 to 1000.[16] The fact that in some infections, such as primary Epstein-Barr virus (EBV) infection, the frequency of virus-specific CD8+ T cells approaches 70% continues to amaze immunologists.[17,18] Although EBV is arguably an extreme example, in other infections, such as those caused by HIV, herpes simplex virus, influenza virus, and *Listeria monocytogenes,* pathogen-specific T-cell frequencies are astonishingly large, generally ranging from 2% to 25%.[14,15,19,20] The immunologic techniques described here are now fundamental to the investigations of pathogen-specific cellular immunity and have made the diagnostic and therapeutic use of antigen-specific T cells a reality.

Lymphoid Anatomy

Studies of the human immune system to a large extent have been restricted to circulating blood cells and, much less frequently, have focused on lymphocytes derived from lymph nodes, spleen, or other tissues. Studies in mice largely have focused on lymphocytes derived from spleen and lymph nodes and, more recently, mucosal tissues such as gut. In aggregate, however, studies with humans and mice have provided a fairly detailed picture of immune system compartmentalization. Understanding of immune cell populations in various lymphoid and nonlymphoid tissues has increased dramatically,[21] as has understanding of the signals that direct the trafficking of lymphocytes in vivo.[22] Although exceptions to this rule may exist, T-cell–mediated immune responses generally are initiated in secondary lymphoid tissues, specifically lymph nodes and spleen.[23] Subsequently, activated lymphocytes traffic to nonlymphoid sites of infection. Even after infection with microbial pathogens that do not infect lymphoid tissues directly, naive, specific T cells are activated in secondary lymphoid tissues, then traffic to the actual site of infection. Because lymphoid tissues play this vital role in adaptive immunity, understanding the anatomy of the lymph node and spleen is essential to understanding the commingling of antigen with its cognate immune cell.

Lymph Nodes

Lymph nodes serve as a nexus for lymphocyte interaction with antigen-presenting cells, overcoming the difficult problem of bringing together rare, antigen-specific lymphocytes with small quantities of antigen.[24] Lymph nodes receive blood flow through arteries that enter the hilum of the node and receive lymphatic drainage from peripheral tissues

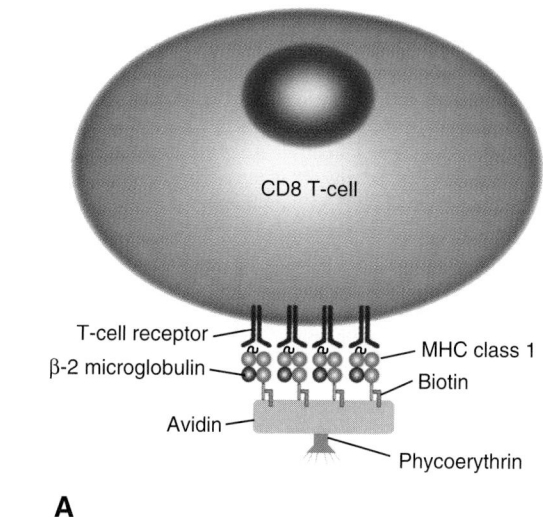

A

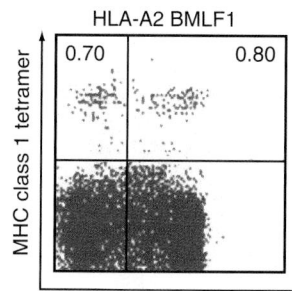 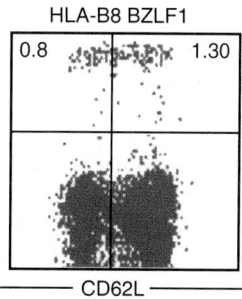 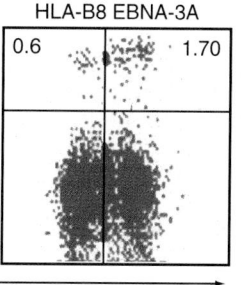

B

FIGURE 9-4. Major histocompatibility complex (MHC) tetramers are able to stain antigen-specific T lymphocytes because they simultaneously can interact with multiple antigen-specific T-cell receptors. Although the association of individual T-cell receptors with MHC complexes is transient, in the setting of multiple simultaneous interactions, binding becomes stable. In most studies, MHC tetramers are generated by biotinylating the C-terminus of soluble MHC molecules that contain a specific antigenic peptide, followed by complex formation with a fluorescently labeled avidin molecule, which contains four biotin-binding sites. **A,** MHC tetramer complex associated with an antigen-specific T lymphocyte. **B,** MHC tetramer staining of human peripheral blood mononuclear cells using tetramers complexed with three different Epstein-Barr virus–derived peptides. The percentage of CD8+ T cells specific for each of these peptides is indicated in the plots. (*A, Courtesy of Dirk H. Busch, Technical University, Munich.*)

through the subcapsular space. Although highly investigated, the mechanics of fluid and cellular movement through lymph nodes have been elucidated only recently. Nevertheless, because T-cell responses to infectious pathogens begin in lymph nodes, inflammatory cytokines induced at the site of infection, pathogen-derived antigens, and specific T cells all travel these recently defined avenues.

Figure 9-5 provides a schematic view of a lymph node. Lymph draining from peripheral tissues enters the subcapsular space of a lymph node, then flows through the capsular sinus to the medullary sinus.[25] Dendritic cells, potentially carrying pathogen-derived antigens from the site of infection, enter the subcapsular sinus and the lymph node cortex, directly contacting naive lymphocytes in the paracortical cords.[26] Although dendritic cells have direct access to the paracortical cords, small protein molecules, such as cytokines and chemokines, and small microbe-derived molecules, do not enter the paracortical cords directly.[25] Instead the small molecules are channeled into conduits defined by a tight network of fibroblastic reticular cells surrounding an extracellular matrix consisting of collagen bundles. The collagen fibers provide structural support to the lymph node and define its architecture. The lymphatic conduits associated with these collagen fibers provide connections between the subcapsular and cortical sinuses and the high endothelial venules (HEVs), enabling fluid flow and substrate transport from peripheral tissues, via the subcapsular sinuses to the HEV, the site of cellular entry into the lymph node from the blood stream.[25] The utility of this complicated system of lymphatic channels will become apparent.

Blood flow to the lymph node, after entering the lymph node hilum, is channeled through the HEV, where circulating lymphoid cells can adhere and traverse from the lumen into the paracortical cords of the lymph node. On traversing the HEV, lymphocytes enter the perivenular channel, a narrow space bounded by fibroblastic reticular cells, that provides entry into the corridors of the paracortical cord. The paracortical cord is a labyrinthine structure that accommodates many T cells that are presumed to roam the corridors, eventually exiting by moving either toward a B-cell follicle or toward a cortical or medullary sinus.[27] As lymphocytes move, side by side, through this labyrinth, they have extensive opportunities to contact antigen-bearing dendritic cells that have entered the cord from the subcapsular sinus. If lymphocytes recognize an antigen presented by a dendritic cell, the T-cell activation process is initiated.

The flow of antigen-presenting cells, lymphocytes, and messenger molecules into and through lymph nodes in response to infection is a masterpiece of systems engineering. The flow of cells and inflammatory mediators to the lymph node from distant sites of infection is directed precisely to optimize the opportunity for pathogen-specific lymphocyte activation. Beginning with a peripheral site of infection, microbial antigens are taken up by tissue dendritic cells that, after receiving signals through innate immune receptors, mature and travel through lymphatic channels to a draining lymph node.[28] Concurrent with dendritic cell migration, inflammatory cytokines and chemokines produced at the site of infection also travel in lymph to the draining lymph node.[29] This cellular and cytokine cocktail enters the subcapsular space of the draining lymph node. Here the molecular and cellular immigrants follow different paths. Antigen-bearing dendritic cells directly move into the collection of lymphocytes in the paracortical cords, traversing a cellular barrier that, paradoxically, permits cells, but not much smaller molecules, to cross. Inflammatory cytokines and chemokines enter the fibroblastic, reticular cell–bounded conduits that lead to the HEV, where they relay the message to circulating lymphocytes to adhere and traverse the endothelium. The recruitment of lymphocytes into the paracortical cords is rapid and efficient, and the labyrinths can become engorged with lymphocytes within a few hours of an inflammatory stimulus.

SPLEEN

The spleen is a large secondary lymphoid organ that also serves as an important filtration site for clearance of microbial pathogens from the blood stream.[30] Although spleen and lymph nodes share many T-cell, B-cell, and dendritic-cell subsets and are similarly complex at the microanatomic level, they also differ in some important respects (Fig. 9-6). The spleen is not a site for lymphatic drainage. Instead, antigens, pathogens, and circulating cells enter the spleen through the splenic artery. The splenic artery branches into central arterioles, which course through the splenic cortex and are surrounded by lymphocytes in a structure called the *periarteriolar sheath*.[31] T lymphocytes are most proximal to the central arteriole and are surrounded by aggregates of B lymphocytes in regions called *B-cell follicles* (see Fig. 9-6B). The densely packed B and T lymphocytes constitute the splenic white pulp and are surrounded by the marginal zone (see Fig. 9-6C), which separates white pulp from red pulp.[32] The splenic red pulp is rich in macrophages and contains many red blood cells, resulting from the percolating blood flow delivered by the termini of the splenic arterioles. The blood flow to the spleen predominantly ter-

FIGURE 9-5. The microanatomy of lymph nodes is highly complex. This schematic provides an outline of lymph node anatomy at a level that cannot be visualized by light microscopy, but that has been deduced by trafficking analyses of low-molecular-weight markers that were introduced experimentally into lymph and blood circulating into intact lymph nodes. Low-molecular-weight proteins, such as chemokines, can flow from the lymph node sinus through the conduit system to the high endothelial venules (HEV), through which the blood supply of the lymph node circulates, where they can influence the recruitment of circulating lymphocytes. CF, collagen fibers, which provide structural support to the conduits and the lymph node; FC, fibroblastic conduit; FRC, fibroblastic reticular cells, which surround the conduits; IDC, interdigitating dendritic cells, which can present antigens to T lymphocytes entering the paracortex through the HEV; JC, junctional complexes, which provide a tight barrier to the contents of the conduit; SLC, sinus-lining cells. (*Courtesy of Stephen Shaw, National Institutes of Health, Bethesda, Md.*)

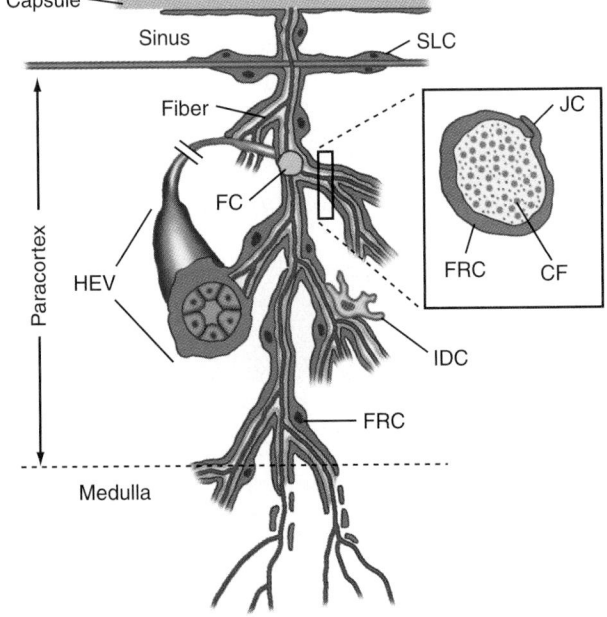

minates in the red pulp and the marginal zone. Most pathogens, on clearance from the blood stream, first are localized to the marginal zone and red pulp of the spleen.[33] With respect to cellular trafficking into the spleen, it seems that the major entry point into the white pulp is from the marginal zone.[34] From here, activated antigen-presenting cells can enter the white pulp areas, most likely by traversing the marginal zone sinus and the metallophilic macrophage layer that forms a boundary between white pulp and marginal zone. Access of protein antigens and other molecules into the splenic white pulp is highly restricted and, in many ways, similar to the system identified in lymph nodes. Specifically, small channels that surround collagen fibers and are formed by fibroblastic reticular cells enter the T-cell and the B-cell zones of the spleen and deliver small molecules (i.e., generally <60 kD) into the white pulp. The channels found in B-cell follicles bind chemokines associated with the recruitment of B cells, whereas the channels identified in T-cell zones bind chemokines associated with T-cell recruitment.[35]

Chemokine-Mediated and Integrin-Mediated Trafficking to Lymphoid Tissues

The mechanism of entry of T and B lymphocytes into lymph nodes has been investigated in great detail, and the sequence of events is well characterized. First, lymphocytes passing through HEVs roll along the surface of the endothelium in a process that involves selectins on lymphocytes and counterreceptors on the endothelial surface.[36-38] The next step, which is crucial for entry into the lymph node, involves recognition of chemokines on the endothelial surface by chemokine receptors on the lymphocyte surface, which triggers a G_i-protein–mediated activation process that induces integrin-mediated adhesion and movement across the endothelium.[22,39] In recent years, many of the components of this process have been delineated. The chemokine receptors CXCR4 and CCR7 are activated by the chemokine CXCL12, promoting the entry of B lymphocytes into peripheral lymph nodes. B-cell entry into Peyer's patches is mediated by CXCL13 and CXCR5.[40] LFA-1/ICAM-1 and $\alpha4\beta1$/VCAM interactions are required for B-cell retention in the marginal zone of the spleen.[41] Antibody-blocking studies showed that B-cell entry into follicles requires interaction between LFA-1 on lymphocytes and ICAM-1 on spleen cells. The interaction between $\alpha4\beta1$ integrin molecules and VCAM also contributes to B-cell entry into splenic follicles.[42] When lymphocytes have entered the splenic white pulp, their movement between T-cell and B-cell zones is dictated in large part by chemokines and their respective receptors. B lymphocytes, on activation by antigen, upregulate the expression of CCR7, a chemokine receptor that responds to CCL19 and CCL21 chemokines.[43] Naive T lymphocytes express CCR7, allowing them to respond to CCL19 and CCL21 and directing them to T-cell zones of lymph nodes. When activated by antigen, the upregulation of CCR7 on B cells directs them to the T-cell zone, enabling their direct interaction with T cells and enabling B-cell antigen presentation to T cells and T-cell–mediated maturation of B cells.[43]

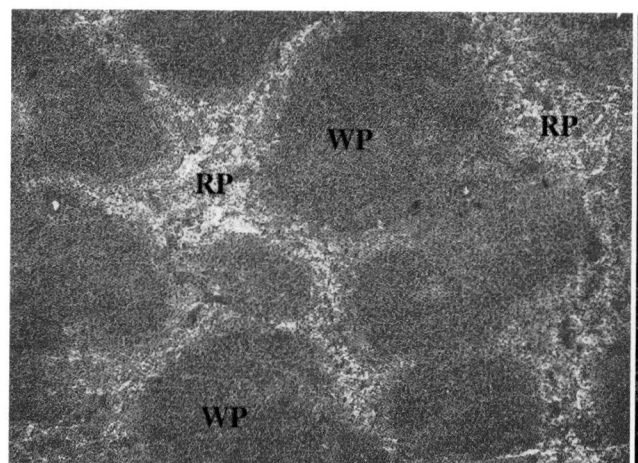

A

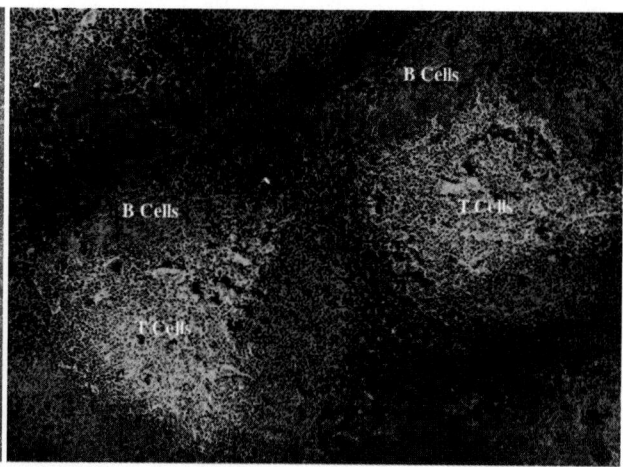

B

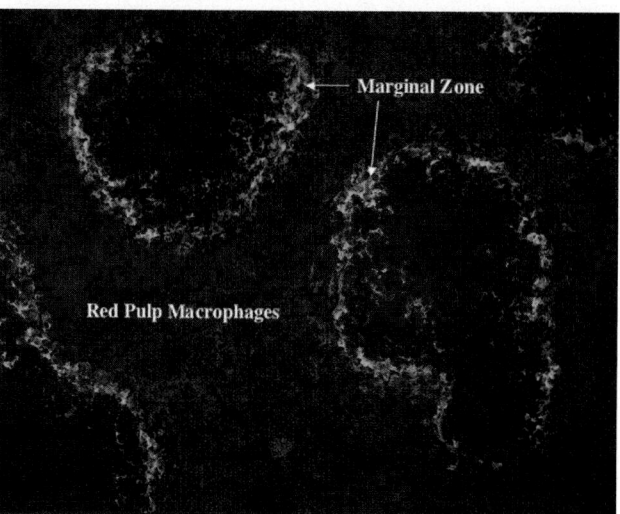

C

FIGURE 9-6.   The spleen is a complex secondary lymphoid organ with compartmentalized cell populations. **A,** Spleen section stained with hematoxylin and eosin shows areas of densely packed cells, referred to as the *white pulp* (WP), separated by areas with more dispersed cell populations, referred to as the *red pulp* (RP). **B,** Spleen section that has been stained with fluorescently labeled antibodies specific for B cells (orange) and T cells (green) shows the distinct localization of B cells and T cells within the white pulp. **C,** Staining for macrophages (orange) and the splenic marginal zone (green) shows the density of macrophages and phagocytic cells in the red pulp and marginal zone.

Immune Tissues Associated with Mucosal Surfaces

One of the challenges faced by the immune system is to distinguish pathogens from innocuous microbes. This issue is of particular relevance in the intestine, a location that is teeming with microbes that, under most circumstances, pose little threat to healthy individuals. Aberrant inflammatory and T-cell–mediated responses to commensal microbes are postulated to underlie the pathogenesis of various inflammatory bowel syndromes.[44] The intestine also is one of the most important portals of entry for viral, bacterial, protozoal, and helminth pathogens.[45]

T lymphocytes are prevalent in the intestinal mucosa and can be found within the epithelial layer, in the lamina propria, and within lymphoid tissues such as Peyer's patches and mesenteric lymph nodes.[46] T lymphocytes in the epithelial layer are a diverse population that in aggregate are called *intraepithelial lymphocytes*. Some intraepithelial lymphocytes express CD8$^+$ α/β chains, some express exclusively CD8$^+$ α chains, and some do not express CD8$^+$.[47] With respect to TCRs, some express $\alpha\beta$ TCRs, whereas others express $\gamma\delta$ TCRs.[48-50] Nearly all intraepithelial lymphocytes express adhesion molecules associated with an activated phenotype and readily express effector functions, such as cytolytic activity and cytokine secretion. The intestinal lamina propria also is populated with T lymphocytes, but in this site conventional CD8$^+$ α/β-expressing T cells with $\alpha\beta$ TCRs predominate.[51,52] Despite the likely importance of T lymphocytes in intestinal immune defense, little is known about their mechanism of antimicrobial activity in mucosal surfaces. Although intestinal epithelial cells are postulated to present antigen to T lymphocytes,[53-55] dendritic cells also have been shown in intestinal tissues. Two reports have shown that dendritic cells sample intestinal contents by transiently traversing the tight junctions of the intestinal epithelial cell layer.[56,57] After engulfing bacterial pathogens, such as *Salmonella typhimurium,* dendritic cells migrate to secondary lymphoid tissues to activate naive T lymphocytes.

Studies in mouse models have shown that intestinal infection with viral or bacterial pathogens induces robust expansion of pathogen-specific T lymphocytes in the small intestinal epithelium and lamina propria.[51,52,58] Systemic infection with viruses, such as vesicular stomatitis virus, or the intracellular bacterium *L. monocytogenes* also induces marked increases in the frequency of pathogen-specific CD8$^+$ T cells in the gut, suggesting that these T cells traffic to the intestine during systemic immune responses. The concept that immune responses to infectious pathogens result in the distribution of pathogen-specific T lymphocytes throughout the body is supported by two studies that measured whole-animal immunity.[59,60] In both studies, although T-cell priming occurred in secondary lymphoid tissues, after priming, antigen-specific T lymphocytes were found at higher frequencies in nonlymphoid tissues, such as liver, lamina propria, and adipose tissues.

Influenza virus infection has been used in animal models to characterize pulmonary CD8$^+$ T-cell responses. During acute infection, influenza-specific T cells in the lungs are highly cytolytic, and most produce IFN-γ on peptide stimulation.[61] The kinetics of influenza virus–specific CD8$^+$ T-cell expansion, differentiation, and contraction are distinct in different tissues.[62] Virus-specific CD8$^+$ T cells persist at very high frequencies in airways and lung parenchyma after infection and, in contrast to splenic and lymph node memory T cells, rapidly express effector functions on reexposure to antigen.[63] Rapidly responsive, virus-specific T cells also persist in the nasal mucosa.[64] Activated and memory T cells are superior at trafficking to influenza virus–infected lungs,[65] a process that is not driven by antigen because even non–virus-specific, activated T cells traffic to infected lungs.[66]

The dynamics of T-cell trafficking and expansion in nonlymphoid tissues during infection is just starting to be explored. Although it is unclear how high frequencies of antigen-specific T cells are maintained in peripheral tissues, one likely explanation is that tissue expression of cytokines, such as IL-7 and IL-15, support the survival and perhaps replication of memory T cells.[67]

Microbial Pathogenesis and the Cellular Immune System

The diverse properties of microbial pathogens provide a daunting challenge for the cellular immune system, and the relationship between individual classes of microbial pathogens and specific arms of the cellular immune system is instructive and fascinating. Although the details of cellular immune responses vary substantially among pathogens, broad generalizations are useful to understand the general themes of cellular immune responses in antimicrobial defense. In most cases, the subcellular anatomic location of a pathogen predicts the arm of the cellular immune response that is necessary for the control of that particular pathogen. In many cases, the most definitive information about the important arms of antimicrobial defense for a particular pathogen has come from natural or acquired deficiency states, in particular, defects in immune receptors or signaling molecules. In addition, although different classes of pathogens are associated with a particular type of cellular immune response, many pathogens have developed sophisticated molecular countermeasures to avoid elimination.

Viral Infections

In general, cellular immune responses against viral infections involve MHC class I presentation of virally derived peptide antigens to CD8$^+$ T cells. Because viral pathogens replicate within their host cell, their elimination by the cellular immune system involves either cytolytic destruction of the infected host cell by virus-specific lymphocytes or inhibition of viral replication in host cells.[68] Because viruses, by necessity, use the host cell for protein synthesis, viral proteins are ready substrates for the MHC class I antigen-processing pathway.

There are several reports of congenital deficiency of CD8$^+$ T cells or MHC class I function. Deficiency in TAP, the antigen transporter necessary for MHC class I peptide loading, was documented in several families.[69,70] These patients express dramatically reduced levels of MHC class I surface expression and CD8$^+$ T cells. In contrast to the canonical function presented for CD8$^+$ T cells in antiviral defense, these TAP1-deficient patients and a patient deficient in CD8$^+$ α chain did not manifest increased susceptibility to viral infection and instead presented with recurrent pulmonary bacterial infections leading to bronchiectasis. One of these patients had adequate titers to cytomegalovirus (CMV), rubella, and other viruses, confirming prior exposure and successful protective immunity.[71] Although the clinical manifestations of deficient CD8$^+$ T-cell function and understanding from animal models are not reconciled easily, studies of MHC class I polymorphisms and susceptibility to HIV infection support a role for CD8$^+$ T cells in control of viral infections.[72,73]

Some viruses become transcriptionally inactive after host cell infection and represent a particular challenge for the cellular immune system. Although transcriptionally inactive, these viruses cannot be detected by antigen-specific T lymphocytes because viral proteins are unavailable for processing and presentation by MHC class I molecules. The human herpesviruses belong to this class of viral pathogens. Although primary active infection with these viruses is controlled, herpesviruses establish clinical latency and can cause intermittent disease or disease in the setting of impaired immunity. As might be predicted, many viruses employ strategies to avoid detection or elimination by CD8$^+$ T cells using a variety of clever mechanisms, which are described in greater detail in the antigen-processing section.

In addition to directly interfering with antigen presentation, many viral pathogens encode proteins that can interfere with cytokine signaling or chemokine-mediated cell recruitment. EBV contains a gene for an IL-10 homologue that shares 87% sequence identity with human IL-10. The EBV IL-10, on binding the IL-10 receptor, induces predominantly the immunosuppressive effects of this pleiotropic cytokine. Poxviruses express an IL-18–binding protein that can bind IL-18 with high affinity, interfering with early IFN-γ–mediated inflammatory responses. Poxviruses also express proteins that bind CC chemokines with high affinity, preventing their association with chemokine receptors on the surface of inflammatory cells. This latter strategy likely interferes with the recruitment of monocytes, natural killer (NK) cells and activated T lymphocytes to sites of viral infection.

Intracellular Bacteria

Many important human pathogens have evolved mechanisms to escape antibody-mediated, complement-mediated, and neutrophil-mediated immune defense. One of the most effective escape mechanisms involves entering host cells, often phagocytic cells. In this circumstance, the host cell becomes a protective barrier from extracellular microbicidal defenses. Bacterial pathogens have used many clever strategies to exploit the interior of host cells to their benefit, by manipulating intracellular trafficking pathways or targeting specific intracellular niches. The challenge facing the cell-mediated immune system is to detect and eliminate these pathogens.

Phagosomal Pathogens

Multiple bacterial pathogens that parasitize phagocytic cells, such as macrophages, reside within the endosomal-phagosomal network. These pathogens often are accessible to the MHC class II antigen presentation network and can colocalize with the antimicrobial effector molecules of macrophages that are delivered to the phagolysosome. Prototypical pathogens of this type include *Mycobacterium* and *Salmonella* spp. Control of these pathogens depends most on CD4$^+$ T-cell activation of antimicrobial killing through IFN-γ. IFN-γ secreted by T cells activates macrophages to kill pathogens through nitric oxide, reactive oxygen intermediates, and lysosomal enzymes. Strong evidence for the importance of these pathways of intracellular killing comes from clinical observation and mouse studies.

In many parts of the world, infants are exposed parenterally to live mycobacteria in the form of bacille Calmette-Guérin (BCG) vaccination. Although highly attenuated compared with its parent *Mycobacterium bovis* strain, BCG can replicate within human hosts in impaired host immunity. This massive cohort of mycobacteria-exposed infants has revealed several inherited defects in antimycobacterial immunity. The clinical syndrome has been called *mendelian susceptibility to mycobacterial disease*[74] and includes patients with disseminated BCG infection and progressive infection with low-pathogenicity mycobacteria. These patients also show increased susceptibility to *Salmonella* infections. All of the mutations that cause this mendelian susceptibility to mycobacterial disease are in the IFN-γ pathway, including IFN-γ receptor mutations, Stat1 mutations, and IL-12 cytokine/receptor.[75-77] Mice rendered deficient in IFN-γ are highly susceptible to intracellular bacterial pathogens, including *Mycobacterium tuberculosis* and *Salmonella,* providing support for the importance of the Th1-mediated stimulation of antimicrobial killing of phagosomal pathogens.

The data presented here document the central role of the Th1 immunity in protection from and control of phagosomal pathogens. As such, it is logical to assume that pathogens of this type have evolved countermeasures to dampen or subvert effective host immunity. *M. tuberculosis* infection of macrophages renders these cells resistant to activation with IFN-γ,[78] limiting the bacteriostatic actions of the host cell that depend on this cytokine. *M. tuberculosis* also prevents acidification of vacuoles by excluding the proton–adenosine triphosphatase (ATPase) from the endosomes it occupies. One possible outcome of diminished vacuolar acidification is decreased antigen degradation resulting in diminished presentation of mycobacterial peptides by MHC class II molecules. Other pathogens, such as *Legionella pneumophila,* segregate themselves in an endosomal compartment that does not communicate with the MHC class II antigen-processing pathway.[79]

Cytoplasmic Pathogens

Some bacterial pathogens have evolved a different intracellular survival strategy. These pathogens, which include *L. monocytogenes, Shigella flexneri,* and various *Rickettsia* spp., escape the phagocytic vacuole and replicate in the cytoplasm of host cells. These pathogens secrete proteins that are essential for virulence and that destroy the vacuolar membrane, providing direct access to the host cell cytosol. In terms of the cellular immune response, these pathogens are thematically similar to viruses because defense against these agents predominantly depends on the MHC class I/CD8$^+$ T-cell axis. Because of their cytoplasmic location, the antimicrobial effector mechanisms of phagocytic cells cannot be localized spatially to the cytoplasmic site of infection, necessitating killing of the infected cell by cytolytic T cells to eliminate the infection. Extensive evidence from animal models of *L. monocytogenes*

supports the role of CD8$^+$ T cells in protective immunity against cytoplasmic bacterial pathogens.

Extracellular Bacteria

Bacteria that replicate extracellularly are accessible to antibody-mediated neutralization or killing by externalized microbial products of phagocytic cells. Defense against pyogenic bacteria, such as *Staphylococcus aureus* and pneumococcus, depends on adequate humoral immunity and intact neutrophil function. To the extent that adequate specific and high-affinity antibody production depends on CD4$^+$ T-cell–helper function, patients with impaired CD4$^+$ T-cell function are susceptible to these pathogens. A role for CD8$^+$ T-cell responses in defense against extracellular bacteria has been postulated in anaerobic abscesses. In this setting, CD8$^+$ T cells have been shown to recognize the carbohydrates of *Bacteroides fragilis.*

INNATE IMMUNE RECOGNITION: SETTING THE STAGE FOR T-CELL RESPONSES

It is conventional to divide the mammalian immune system into the adaptive system, which consists of B cells and T cells expressing distinct, genetically recombined receptors that are exquisitely specific but infrequent, and the innate system, consisting of prevalent cells that express common receptors that bind to molecular patterns unique to microbes. The discovery of an extensive family of innate immune receptors that recognize microbial molecules ranging from lipopolysaccharide to flagellin to CpG DNA has opened up the most exciting new area of investigation in infectious disease immunology. Although this area falls into the realm of innate immunity, it is clear from investigations in this field that recognition of microbial molecules forms the foundation for the adaptive immune response. Although studies have identified and characterized "bridges" between the innate and adaptive immune systems, it is increasingly apparent that these two arms of the immune system are associated so intricately with each other as to be inseparable. With so many experiments showing the connections between the innate and the adaptive immune systems, it is unrealistic to think of adaptive immune responses to infection without considering the innate inflammatory responses induced by the pathogen.

As detailed in this chapter, the molecular basis for antigen-specific immune responses derives from combinatorial receptors (αβ TCRs) that have almost infinitely diverse specificity. This system ensures that a great diversity of pathogenic antigens can be recognized, but because pathogen-specific cells are infrequent, it requires time for expansion of these cells to relevant numbers. In the hours after pathogen breach of an anatomic barrier, the most rapid pathogen recognition events are mediated by cells bearing innate immune receptors. These receptors are not combinatorial, but recognize broad classes of microbial molecules that serve as a general signal of infection. This recognition event, rapid but relatively nonspecific, plays an essential role in the generation of pathogen-specific immunity through the generation of cytokines and chemokines that recruit antigen-specific cells to the site of infection. This section briefly details the major known receptors of the innate immune system and links the function of these receptors to antigen-specific cellular immunity.

Molecular Recognition of Microbial Products

Although the concept that microbial products are recognized by specific receptors of the innate immune system is not new, more recent investigation has expanded dramatically understanding of the receptors involved in this process.

Toll-like Receptors

Toll-like receptors (TLRs) are a family of at least 10 distinct transmembrane proteins that mediate recognition of microbial products. In general, recognition of extracellular microbial products by TLRs results in the activation of NFκB, a transcription factor that promotes the expression of genes associated with immune defense. TLR-mediated signals induce the secretion of proinflammatory cytokines, such as TNF and IL-12, and induce the maturation of dendritic cells, enabling them to activate naive, pathogen-specific T lymphocytes. In addition, stimulation of TLRs can stimulate directly antimicrobial effector mechanisms of the host cell, limiting pathogen replication until adaptive immune cells are recruited to the site of infection.[80] Individual TLRs recognize specific microbial products that have been termed *pathogen-associated molecular patterns*. This model of TLR-mediated recognition reflects the noncombinatorial nature of TLRs and their recognition of bacterial products that are essential for viability, limiting the ability of the pathogen to escape detection by innate immunity.

Although the field of TLR-mediated recognition of microbial products is at an early stage, the specificity of many TLRs already has been determined. TLR-4 is associated with lipopolysaccharide (LPS) recognition; TLR-5, with bacterial flagellin; TLR-9, with CpG DNA; TLR-3, with dsRNA; and TLR-2 with bacterial lipoprotein recognition.[81] The potential specificity of the TLR family is broader than initially anticipated because heterodimerization of TLRs can mediate novel antigen-binding specificities. In addition, although TLRs are crucial to recognition of distinct microbial products, in most cases it is unknown whether the TLR binds the microbial product directly or recognizes a complex of microbial product with an associated host molecule, such as occurs with TLR-4 and CD14/LPS. Although the spectrum of microbial products recognized by TLRs is large and expanding, it is becoming clear that this system alone does not serve as the sole pattern recognition system in innate immunity.

The availability of TLR-deficient and MyD88-deficient mice has revealed substantial variability in the importance of these molecules in defense against different microbial pathogens. MyD88-deficient mice are highly susceptible to *Toxoplasma gondii* infection,[82,83] but TLR-2 and TLR-4 are dispensable for anti-*Toxoplasma* immunity. In contrast, MyD88 and TLR-2 are important for defense against *S. aureus* infection.[84] Neither TLR-2 nor TLR-4 is important for host defense in a murine polymicrobial infection model, whereas MyD88 deficiency favors host survival.[85] Similarly, TLR-2–deficient and TLR-4–deficient mice are not altered dramatically in their susceptibility to *M. tuberculosis* infection, although TLR-4 may have some role in antimycobacterial immunity.[86,87] These data suggest a role for TLR-mediated antimicrobial defense in some infections but not others, suggesting that other innate immune recognition systems also must be important.

Nods

Toll receptors are expressed at the cell surface as transmembrane proteins. As such, they recognize extracellular microbial products or products in phagocytic vacuoles. They are not known to recognize intracellular microbial products, however, suggesting that a distinct system of intracellular innate immune receptors may exist. The Nod family of receptors may serve this function. The biologic functions of the Nod family of proteins are poorly understood, but early investigations suggest that they function as intracellular sensors of specific microbial products, including LPS and muramyl dipeptide.[88-90] A polymorphism of Nod2 is linked to inflammatory bowel disease in a subset of patients.[91,92] Although Nod1 and Nod2 are the most intensely studied proteins of this family, the family is large, suggesting that the full spectrum of intracellular innate immune recognition has yet to be discovered.[88]

Other Receptors Implicated in Innate Immune Recognition

Before the discovery of TLRs and Nod proteins, many host proteins were implicated in the binding of microbial products. The scavenger receptor, a protein expressed on macrophages, has been shown to bind gram-positive bacteria via interactions with lipoteichoic acid.[93] The mannose receptor is a lectin expressed on phagocytic cells that binds a wide variety of microbial-derived carbohydrates. In vitro, the mannose receptor mediates phagocytosis of many microbes and microbial products, including *Candida*, *M. tuberculosis*, and Lipoarabinomannan.[94]

The exact role of the mannose receptor in mediating host defense through innate immune recognition still is being clarified, however, through the use of mouse strains deficient in this receptor. Early investigations of this type have not documented a clear role for the mannose receptor and defense against *Candida albicans* infection.[95] The exact in vivo role of the mannose receptor in host defense against other pathogens is undefined.

Links between Innate Immune Recognition and Adaptive Immune Response

Although it is logical to postulate that innate immune recognition of microbes is essential to adaptive antigen-specific immunity, the details of this relationship are incompletely defined. More recent studies have begun to examine the relationship between specific innate immune recognition events and later adaptive responses. Immunization with model antigens and Freund's adjuvant in MyD88-deficient mice leads to impaired T-cell responses and abnormal isotype-specific antibody production,[96] suggesting that TLR recognition is essential for proper Th1 adjuvant effects. Clinical evidence from leprosy has linked a polymorphism in TLR-2 to lepromatous leprosy in Korean patients,[97] and the presence of this polymorphism prevents proinflammatory responses on recognition of *Mycobacterium leprae* in vitro.[98,99] These data support the general idea that early recognition of microbial products is essential for the presence and quality of the later immune response. Investigation into the detailed relationship between innate and adaptive immunity is forthcoming in the near future.

T-Lymphocyte–Mediated Antimicrobial Responses

Introduction to T-Cell–Mediated Immune Defense

T lymphocytes orchestrate and mediate cellular defenses against infection by microbial pathogens.[100,101] T lymphocytes confer long-term, pathogen-specific protective immunity against reinfection. After the discovery that T cells play an essential role in antimicrobial defense, great effort and ingenuity was expended to unravel the molecular mechanisms underlying pathogen specificity and long-term memory. The complexity of this process, the arcane nomenclature, and the perpetual new discoveries of cytokines and cell subsets make the area of T-cell–mediated immune defense challenging, if not daunting, to the clinician. Nevertheless, to understand infectious diseases fully and to understand the genesis of immunity fully, it is necessary to become familiar with the role T lymphocytes play in modulating inflammatory responses and microbial clearance.

Presentation of Antigens to T Lymphocytes

Several aspects of T-lymphocyte recognition of antigens distinguish this process from antibody-mediated antigen recognition. First, T lymphocytes recognize antigens only in the context of MHC haplotype-matched, antigen-presenting cells.[7] Early studies also indicated that antigen-presenting cells degrade pathogen-derived proteins in a time-dependent process that requires antigen internalization followed by transport to the cell surface.[102] Further characterization of this process revealed that T cells detect peptide fragments of pathogen-derived proteins and that short synthetic peptides representing short fragments of pathogen-derived proteins could stimulate T lymphocytes.[103,104]

Another complicating aspect of T-cell–mediated recognition of pathogen-derived antigens was the requirement for MHC molecules in this process. The precise nature of MHC involvement in antigen presentation became clear only with the crystallization of HLA-A2, which showed a globular protein with a central groove that precisely accommodates a solitary peptide.[105,106] The other important development that allowed a complete picture of the T-cell recognition process was the identification of the TCR.[107] This heterodimeric protein, consisting of two transmembrane chains, provides diversity and specificity by a gene recombination process that is mechanistically similar to the generation of antibody diversity in B cells.[108]

FIGURE 9-7. Major histocompatibility complex (MHC) class I molecules bind short antigenic peptides in a central groove formed by two α helices of the heavy chain. The T-cell receptor binds the peptide, but also associates with the MHC class I molecule to transmit an activation signal to the T lymphocyte. The structures that are depicted represent the murine H2-K^b MHC class I molecule (shown in purple) binding a peptide derived from vesicular stomatitis virus (shown in green). β$_2$-Microglobulin is shown in pink. The left panel shows a side view of the structure, whereas the right view of the complex is from the top, as it would be detected by the T-cell receptor on a CD8$^+$ T cell. (Courtesy of Dr. Chris Garcia, Stanford University, Palo Alto, CA.)

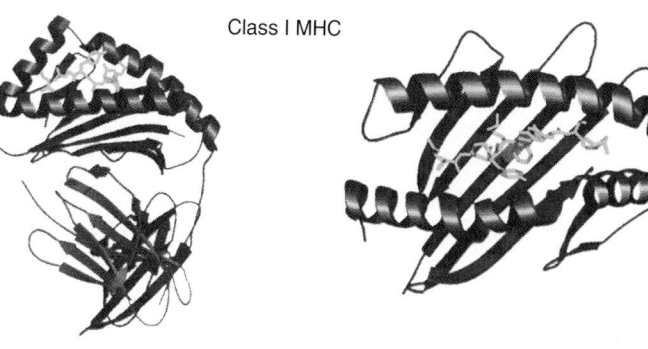

Class I MHC

Major Histocompatibility Complex Structure and Peptide Binding

Major Histocompatibility Complex Class I Structure

MHC class I molecules present peptide antigens to CD8$^+$ T lymphocytes. Most nucleated cells express MHC class I molecules, although the amount on the cell surface varies dramatically among different cell types and under different inflammatory conditions.[109] Most MHC class I molecules are transmembrane proteins and require association with β$_2$-microglobulin for proper folding and trafficking to the cell surface. The characteristic structural features of MHC class I molecules are α1, α2, and α3 domains, which form a globular protein with a β-pleated sheet forming the floor of the peptide binding groove, bounded by two helical regions that form the sides of the groove.[105,106,110] An important feature of MHC class I grooves that distinguishes them from MHC class II grooves is the restricted size of the peptides that can be accommodated. MHC class I molecules typically bind peptides that are 9 amino acids in length because the groove is closed at both ends.[111] The structure of an MHC class I molecule binding a virally derived peptide is shown in Figure 9-7.

MHC class I molecules are highly polymorphic. Although different allomorphs of MHC class I are structurally similar and can bind many different peptides, the peptides that different allelic forms of MHC class I bind are distinct.[111] Each allomorph of MHC class I binds a distinct subset of peptides because of structural differences between the peptide binding grooves. Most MHC class I molecules have a groove with two or three deeper pockets that provide space for bulky amino acid side chains. The peptide sequences that a particular MHC class I molecule can bind is determined by the shape, depth, and charge of the groove and its binding pockets. Because most individuals express six different MHC class I alleles (two each of HLA-A, HLA-B, and HLA-C), a diversity of pathogen-derived peptide sequences can be presented to T lymphocytes. Elution of peptides from the HLA-A2 MHC class I molecule and analysis by mass spectrometry revealed that HLA-A2

can bind thousands of distinct peptides that share a common motif but derive from a plethora of cellular proteins.[112]

Although binding of peptides and interaction with TCRs is mediated entirely by the MHC class I protein, stable surface expression of peptide/MHC class I complexes requires the association with β$_2$-microglobulin. This 12-kD protein is not membrane bound but binds to membrane-bound MHC class I molecules, providing structural stability. In the absence of β$_2$-microglobulin, most MHC class I molecules fold improperly and are destroyed before leaving the endoplasmic reticulum.[113]

Major Histocompatibility Complex Class II Structure

MHC class II molecules present peptides to CD4$^+$ T cells.[114] In contrast to MHC class I molecules, expression of MHC class II molecules is restricted to only a few cell types: macrophages, dendritic cells, and B lymphocytes. On activation, endothelial cells also can express MHC class II molecules.[115] Regulation of MHC class II expression is mediated in part by the class II transactivator protein (CIITA), which enhances expression of not only MHC class II molecules, but also the associated invariant chain and other molecules associated with MHC class II antigen processing.[116] An important human primary immunodeficiency syndrome associated with profound immunosuppression is the bare lymphocyte syndrome, so named because circulating peripheral blood mononuclear cells do not express surface MHC class II molecules. This disease is associated with mutation in the gene for CIITA, a transcription factor that regulates MHC class II gene expression.[117,118]

Although MHC class II molecules share many features with MHC class I molecules, there are some important distinctions (Fig. 9-8). First, the folded MHC class II molecule consists of two transmembrane proteins, an α chain and a β chain, which together form a protein with an open-ended peptide binding groove.[119] The open-endedness of the MHC class II groove accounts for the binding of substantially longer

FIGURE 9-8. Major histocompatibility complex (MHC) class II molecules also bind antigenic peptides in a groove formed by the α and β chains. In contrast to peptides bound by MHC class I molecules, which are of defined length, the MHC class II structure accommodates peptides of various lengths. The MHC class II α and β chains are shown in pink and purple, while the antigenic peptide is shown in green. The left panel shows a view of the complex from the side, whereas the right panel shows a view from the top, as it would be detected by a T-cell receptor on a CD4 T cell. (Courtesy of Dr. Chris Garcia, Stanford University, Palo Alto, CA.)

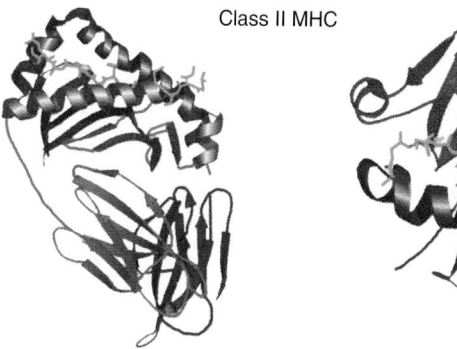 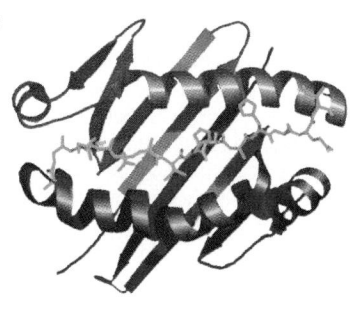

Class II MHC

peptides than seen with MHC class I molecules.[120] Peptides bound by MHC class II molecules typically are longer than 10 amino acids, occasionally more than 20 amino acids in length. In the case of MHC class II molecules, the base of the groove is a β-pleated sheet that is formed by both chains of the heterodimer.[119] The structure of an MHC class II molecule binding an antigenic peptide is shown in Figure 9-8.

Mechanisms of Antigen Processing: Major Histocompatibility Complex Class I Antigen Processing Pathway

Long before the details of the antigen processing pathways were defined, it was shown that the antigens presented by MHC class I and MHC class II molecules derived from different cellular compartments.[121,122] Because peptides bound by MHC class I molecules frequently are derived from cytosolic proteins, either endogenous proteins or viral antigens synthesized in the cytosol, it became a challenge to define the mechanism of peptide generation in the cytosol and the route of peptide transport to the MHC class I binding groove. After the serendipitous discovery of an MHC-encoded peptide transporter,[123] the pathway for peptide presentation by MHC class I molecules gradually was deciphered. The MHC class I antigen processing pathway begins in the cytosol with the degradation of a protein that, most often, is an endogenous self-protein, but in the setting of viral infection can be a virally encoded protein.[109,124] Protein degradation is mediated by proteasomes, which are multicomponent, multicatalytic proteases that consist of four stacked rings that each consist of seven proteins that, in aggregate, form a barrel shape.[125] In activated cells or after exposure to IFN-γ, the composition of proteasomes can change, with some components replaced by subunits that enhance the generation of antigenic peptides and other components added to the ends of the barrel to alter the efficiency and perhaps specificity of protein degradation.[126,127] Proteasomes target proteins for degradation by a variety of distinct mechanisms. Misfolded proteins may reveal peptide sequences that are recognized by proteasomes, leading to their degradation.[124] Alternatively, many proteins targeted by proteasomes are conjugated to ubiquitin by enzymes that recognize the phosphorylation of specific amino acids. Addition of multiple ubiquitin moieties to a protein is a signal for rapid, proteasome-mediated degradation.[124]

In the setting of infection, it is unclear whether pathogen-derived proteins are degraded selectively and targeted for presentation by MHC class I molecules. Bacterial proteins that find their way into the cytosol are degraded rapidly because they express unique amino terminal amino acids[128] or because they contain internal amino acid sequences that promote rapid degradation.[129] In most circumstances, however, pathogen-derived antigens probably are degraded nonselectively along with endogenous proteins. Pathogen-derived peptides must compete with far more prevalent endogenous peptides for a place in an MHC class I peptide binding groove.

Proteasomes do not degrade antigens into amino acids. Rather, they generate peptides that, by virtue of the length of the proteasome channel, are 9 to 12 amino acids in length.[130] Somehow, by mysterious mechanisms, proteasome-generated peptides are bound to the peptide transporter named *transporter associated with antigen processing* (TAP). This heterodimeric, ATP-dependent transporter efficiently moves peptides from the cytosol into the lumen of the endoplasmic reticulum. TAP is not a selective peptide transporter (i.e., most peptide sequences are well transported by TAP), although certain residues decrease the efficiency of transport.[131,132] Peptide length also influences the efficiency of peptide transport, with peptides shorter than 6 amino acids or longer than 14 amino acids being poorly transported. TAP is the major peptide transporter involved in the generation of peptide/MHC class I complexes; mice with genetic deletions of TAP have markedly decreased levels of surface MHC class I and markedly diminished numbers of CD8+ T cells.[133] TAP deficiency has been identified rarely in humans and is associated with markedly decreased numbers of circulating CD8+ T cells and modest immunodeficiency.[69,70]

The TAP1 and TAP2 molecules each contain seven transmembrane regions and an ATP binding site and together, by mechanisms that remain poorly defined, transport peptides from the cytosol into the endoplasmic reticulum lumen.[134] Newly synthesized MHC class I molecules associate with TAP in the endoplasmic reticulum, along with several other endoplasmic reticulum resident proteins and chaperones.[135] Among these proteins, tapasin is a protein 428 amino acids long that plays an important accessory role in MHC class I/peptide complex formation.[136] Other chaperone molecules, such as calnexin and calreticulin,[137] and the thiol reductase ERp57[138,139] also associate with MHC class I/β2-microglobulin/peptide complexes. In the case of MHC class I, peptide length is an important parameter, and mechanisms to ensure proper peptide length have been discovered only recently with the identification of endoplasmic reticulum proteases that trim peptides before their final integration into the class I groove.[140-143]

Only after the MHC class I molecule has bound an appropriate peptide is the MHC class I/β2-microglobulin/peptide complex released from TAP, allowing the complex to traffic via the Golgi complex to the cell surface. On the way to the cell surface, N-linked glycans are added and modified on the MHC class I molecule. The MHC class I antigen processing pathway is regulated by inflammation. IFN-γ, in particular, is a cytokine that impacts the MHC class I pathway at multiple levels.[143] First, transcription of many components of the MHC class I pathway is upregulated by IFN-γ, including MHC class I molecules, TAP, tapasin, and several components of the proteasome. Specifically, three subunits of the proteasome, LMP-2, LMP-7, and MECL, are induced and replace three subunits of the core proteasome complex.[144-146] Additional accessory proteins that modify proteasome efficiency and specificity also are induced by IFN-γ. Prominent among these is PA28, an activator that consists of six subunits that form rings that can cap the ends of the proteasome.[147] The PA28 activator can increase the efficiency with which virus-derived, MHC class I–restricted epitopes are presented to CD8+ T cells.[148] In the setting of infection, the MHC class I antigen processing pathway is enhanced, allowing more efficient presentation of pathogen-derived peptides to CD8+ T lymphocytes. The MHC class I antigen processing pathway is outlined in Figure 9-9.

Viral Intervention with the Major Histocompatibility Complex Class I Antigen Processing Pathway

CD8+ T lymphocytes and the MHC class I antigen processing pathway are involved principally in defense against viral infection. The length to which viral pathogens have gone to subvert the MHC class I antigen processing pathway is fascinating and indicates the importance of this process in antiviral defense. It was an early observation that cells infected with herpes family viruses downregulate MHC class I expression. Exploration of the mechanism behind this observation uncovered many viral proteins that block distinct steps along the MHC class I antigen processing pathway.[149] ICP47 is encoded by herpes simplex virus and blocks human TAP by plugging the peptide transport channel from the cytosolic side.[150,151] Using a similar strategy, but with a completely distinct protein, the human CMV-encoded protein US6 blocks TAP transport by obstructing the peptide transporter from the endoplasmic reticulum luminal side.[152,153] Human CMV also uses several other mechanisms to prevent MHC class I molecules from appearing on the cell surface. The US3 protein binds MHC class I molecules in the endoplasmic reticulum and prevents their trafficking to the cell surface.[154,155] A similar strategy also is used by adenoviruses, which encode the type I membrane protein E3-19K.[156,157] This protein binds MHC class I molecules in the endoplasmic reticulum lumen and prevents their egress from endoplasmic reticulum by expressing an endoplasmic reticulum retention motif on its cytoplasmic tail. Another strategy for downregulating surface MHC class I retention is to displace endoplasmic reticulum luminal MHC class I molecules into the cell's cytoplasm, where they are ubiquitinated rapidly and degraded by proteasomes. Human CMV encoded two proteins, US2 and US11,

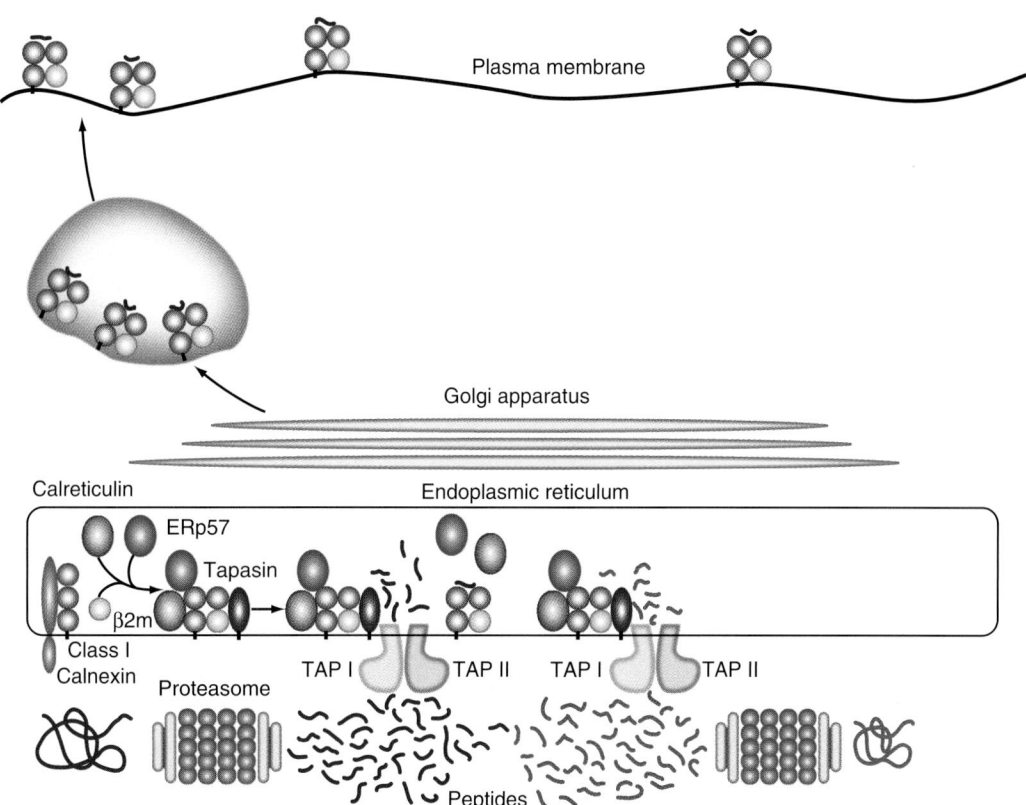

FIGURE 9-9. Major histocompatibility complex (MHC) class I antigen processing pathway begins in the cytoplasm with the degradation of proteins by proteasomes. Peptides are transported into the lumen of the endoplasmic reticulum, where they are bound by MHC class I molecules and transported to the cell surface. *(Courtesy of Anne Ackerman and Peter Cresswell, Yale University, New Haven, CT.)*

which mediate this process.[157,158] Remarkably, transport of proteins from the endoplasmic reticulum lumen back to the cytosol via the Sec61 translocon is a normal process that usually is restricted to misfolded or otherwise nonfunctional proteins. US2 and US11 seem to accelerate this process selectively for MHC class I molecules. Crystallographic studies have characterized the binding of US2 to MHC class I molecules.[159]

The Kaposi's sarcoma herpesvirus also downregulates surface MHC class I expression, but by another mechanism. Two Kaposi's sarcoma herpesvirus–encoded proteins, K3 and K5, function as ubiquitin ligases that selectively conjugate ubiquitin to the cytoplasmic tail of MHC class I molecules and B7.2 costimulatory molecules.[160,161] On ubiquitination, surface MHC class I molecules are internalized rapidly and targeted for lysosomal degradation. HIV also has evolved mechanisms to downregulate surface expression of MHC class I molecules.[162-164] In this case, the retrovirally encoded Nef protein selectively downregulates the expression of HLA-A and HLA-B molecules by associating with the clathrin adaptor complex.

An important consequence of MHC class I downregulation is that affected cells become susceptible to NK cell–mediated lysis. NK cells express receptors that inhibit NK cell activation on contact with MHC class I molecules. To prevent NK cell–mediated lysis of virally infected cells, human CMV encodes an MHC class I–like molecule, UL18,[165,166] which acts as a decoy for the NK cell inhibitory receptor, LIR-1,[167] providing yet another level of camouflage to the viral pathogen.

Major Histocompatibility Complex Class I Cross-Priming

The MHC class I antigen processing pathway performs two principal functions. First, it presents antigens to naive CD8+ T cells in a manner

that promotes their activation, proliferation, and differentiation. Second, it must present antigens to activated CD8+ T cells as a signal of cellular infection. From extensive work in the 1990s, it now is clear that the first function is predominantly, if not exclusively, mediated by dendritic cells that, most often, are not infected directly with the pathogen.[168,169] Any MHC class I–expressing cell that becomes infected can perform the second function. The rules of antigen processing differ in these two circumstances. The conventional MHC class I antigen processing pathway, as described in the preceding sections, applies to the second function. When cells become directly infected, pathogen-derived antigens are degraded by the infected cell and presented on the cell surface in the context of MHC class I molecules.[170] MHC class I antigen presentation by dendritic cells is more complex and is not restricted to endogenous cytosolic proteins. Because they are not infected directly, the major route for CD8+ T-cell priming involves uptake of debris from infected cells by dendritic cells, and re-presentation of pathogen-derived peptides[171] by an as yet incompletely defined antigen processing pathway that involves endocytosis and TAP-mediated transport of antigen into the endoplasmic reticulum.[172] This cumbersome route for CD8+ T-cell priming ensures that CD8+ T-cell priming occurs in a regulated fashion and likely represents an essential hurdle to prevent overly robust CD8+ T-cell responses to systemic viral infections.

Major Histocompatibility Complex Class II Antigen Processing Pathway

The MHC class II antigen processing pathway presents peptides to CD4+ T lymphocytes. Although there is some similarity to the MHC class I antigen processing pathway, there are some crucial distinctions. First, most of the peptides presented by MHC class II molecules de-

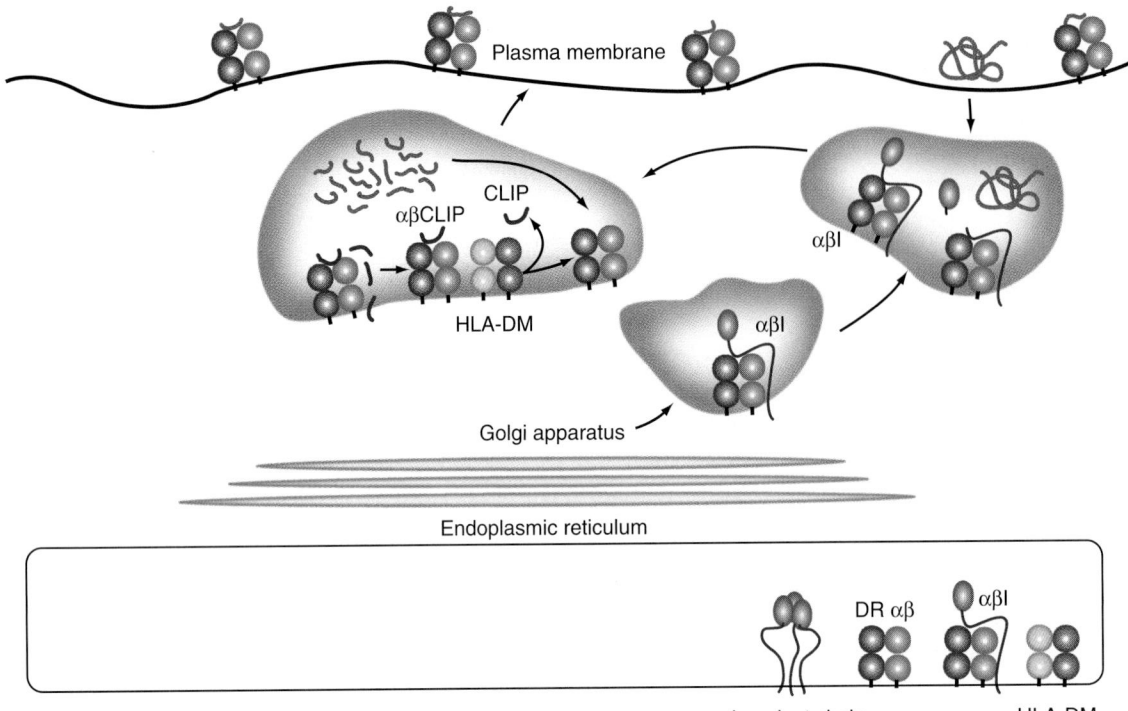

FIGURE 9-10. MHC class II antigen processing pathway presents peptides derived from extracellular proteins to CD4⁺ T lymphocytes. Peptides are generated in an endosomal compartment and associate with MHC class II molecules, then are carried to the cell surface. *(Courtesy of Anne Ackerman and Peter Cresswell, Yale University, New Haven, CT.)*

rive from extracellular proteins that have been endocytosed by MHC class II–bearing cells.[120] Additional peptides are derived from membrane or secretory proteins that are degraded in endosomal compartments during transport to the cell surface. With respect to antimicrobial responses, the MHC class II antigen processing pathway has been implicated principally in the response to extracellular pathogens and pathogens that reside within vacuolar compartments, such as *S. typhimurium* and *M. tuberculosis*.[173,174] Because CD4⁺ T-cell responses also are essential for complete priming, activation, and differentiation of CD8⁺ T-cell responses, however, it is difficult to attribute immune susceptibility directly to CD4⁺ T-cell deficiency.[175] The implications and complexities of CD4⁺ T-cell deficiency have been made clear by the HIV epidemic.[176,177]

The first step in the MHC class II antigen processing pathway is the synthesis of MHC class α and β chains into the endoplasmic reticulum lumen and the synthesis of invariant chain. By and large, MHC class II molecules do not bind antigenic peptides in the endoplasmic reticulum. The α and β chains fold, using the invariant chain, which is a copious, membrane-bound protein, as a substitute for peptide.[178] A portion of the invariant chain occupies the MHC class II groove as the complex exits the endoplasmic reticulum, traverses the Golgi complex, and traffics to the endosomal compartments.[179,180] On acidification of the endosomal compartment, proteases, such as cathepsin D and cathepsin B, are activated and degrade all parts of the invariant chain except for the portion that is protected by the MHC class II groove.[181,182] It is in the acidified endosome, in a compartment called *MIIC*, that MHC class II molecules can intersect with endocytosed antigens in the process of degradation.[183,184] In a complex, topologically challenging series of events, the invariant chain fragment is replaced by a proteolytically generated peptide. Although MHC class II molecules, similar to MHC class I mole-

cules, are selective with respect to peptide binding, because the groove is open and can accommodate peptides in various registers, the range of peptides that are bound is greater and the binding stringency relaxed. The mechanics of MHC class II peptide binding still are mysterious but are known to be accelerated by the presence of another MHC-encoded, MHC class II–like molecule that resides in MIICs.[185] This protein, HLA-DM, is believed to participate in the extraction of the invariant chain peptide fragment from the MHC class II molecule, enhancing the binding of other, potentially antigen-derived peptides. In addition to proteases, a thiol-reductase called *GILT* also is involved in the denaturation of some antigens before their degradation and presentation by MHC class II molecules.[186]

On peptide binding in the MIIC, MHC class II molecules traffic to the cell surface, where the MHC class II/peptide complex can be detected by CD4⁺ T cells. MHC class II molecules are reinternalized, and it is possible that these complexes return to the endosomal compartments, acquiring new peptides before returning to the cell surface. The extent to which this pathway contributes to the MHC class II antigen processing pathway during immune responses to infection is incompletely defined.[187] Figure 9-10 outlines the MHC class II antigen processing pathway.

CD1

The CD1 family comprises antigen-presenting molecules that resemble MHC class I molecules in general structure and in their association with β₂-microglobulin. The human CD1 locus on chromosome 1 contains five distinct genes that encode for proteins termed *CD1a* through *CD1e*. Consistent with their structural similarity to MHC class I, CD1 molecules generally are highly expressed on antigen-presenting cells, present antigens for recognition by the TCR, and interact with T lym-

FIGURE 9-11.   The structure of CD1 molecules differs from the structure of major histocompatibility complex (MHC) class I molecules, but also shares substantial similarities. This figure shows the structure of the human CD1b molecule binding the lipid ganglioside G_{M2}. The CD1 chain is shown in blue, and β_2-microglobulin is shown in pink. The lipid is shown in green. The left panel is a side view of the complex, whereas the right panel shows a view from the top, as it would be detected by a T-cell receptor. *(Courtesy of Dr. Chris Garcia, Stanford University, Palo Alto, CA.)*

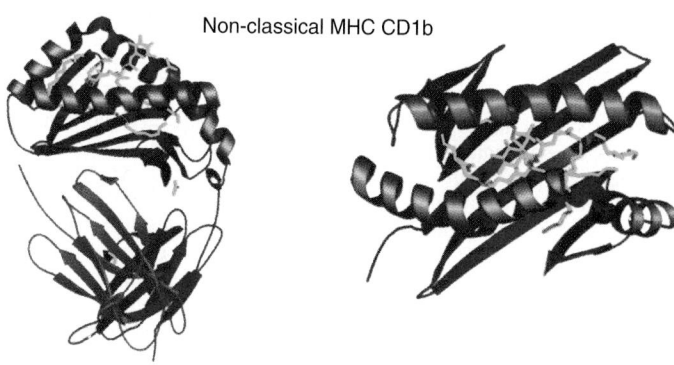

Non-classical MHC CD1b

phocytes. CD1 molecules differ dramatically from the MHC in the class of antigens presented, however. In contrast to the peptide antigens presented by the MHC, CD1 proteins present lipid and glycolipid antigens to T cells, a discovery that radically expanded the universe of antigens recognized by T lymphocytes. Figure 9-11 shows the structure of the human CD1b molecule presenting the ganglioside G_{M2}.[188] This section reviews the antigens presented by CD1, the lymphocytes that recognize these antigens, and the importance of this antigen-presenting system in host defense against specific infectious diseases.

CD1 Protein Structure

CD1 proteins are single-pass transmembrane proteins that have a short intracellular domain. The extracellular portion of CD1 is composed of three domains that mediate antigen binding, whereas specific motifs in the intracellular domain control CD1 trafficking to intracellular compartments (discussed further later). The extracellular domains of CD1 molecules form an antigen binding groove that is structurally analogous to the peptide binding groove of the MHC. Consistent with the lipid presentation function of CD1, the antigen binding groove contains multiple hydrophobic pockets that can accommodate the aliphatic chains of lipid antigens. The three-dimensional structure of mouse CD1[189] and human CD1b[188] reveals a complicated network of hydrophobic channels that can accommodate diverse lipids of varying aliphatic chain length (see Fig. 9-11). All CD1 proteins associate with β_2-microglobulin, which is required for the proper cell surface expression and function of CD1 antigen presentation.[190,191] In contrast to the five CD1 isoforms found in humans, mice lack CD1a, CD1b, and CD1c and have a duplicated CD1d gene. This important difference between mice and human CD1 complicates the experimental analysis of CD1 function because the powerful tools of genetically altered mice are not available to analyze the function of CD1a, CD1b, or CD1c.

Antigens Presented by CD1

Mycobacterial lipids were the first antigens found to be presented by CD1 to T cells.[192,193] CD1b presents glycosylated and free mycolic acids and Lipoarabinomannan, two major lipid and glycolipid components of the *M. tuberculosis* cell envelope. Further analyses of the structure of CD1-presented lipids revealed that T-cell recognition of CD1b-presented glycolipids was exquisitely sensitive to the fine structure of the carbohydrate head group but relatively insensitive to alterations in the structure of the lipid tail.[194] These observations, along with later characterization of CD1c-presented mycobacterial isoprenoid glycolipids,[194] have led to a model of CD1 lipid antigen presentation in which the hydrophilic head group is exposed and available for TCR interactions, whereas the hydrophobic lipid tails of the antigen are bound within the hydrophobic pockets of the CD1 protein.

Since this initial identification of mycobacterial antigens, CD1-presented antigens have expanded to include other microbial products, self-derived glycolipids, and other natural products. One important natural product that is presented by mouse CD1 is α-galactosyl ceramide, which is derived from marine sponges. α-Galactosyl ceramide, which presumably resembles a physiologically relevant glycolipid, is presented to a limited subpopulation of T cells generally termed *NK-T cells* owing to their dual expression of NK cell markers and the TCR. α-Galactosyl ceramide is a strong activator of these T cells and has been used extensively to study the effect of CD1d-mediated NK-T cell activation on host defense against infections and tumors.

Cell Biology of CD1 Antigen Processing and Loading

Individual CD1 isoforms are differentially enriched in different intracellular compartments, suggesting that each isoform of CD1 has evolved to survey the microbial antigens that appear in distinct parts of the endosomal-lysosomal network.[195] All CD1 isoforms are found at the cell surface and are internalized during endocytosis. CD1a is found predominantly in early endosomes, CD1c in late endosomes, and CD1b/d in late endosomes and lysosomes. Specific amino acid residues in their short intracellular tails target CD1 isoforms to these various compartments by binding cytosolic adaptor molecules that mediate organelle trafficking.[196-198] Although the precise functional implications of this trafficking pattern for the immune response are still being elucidated, each CD1 isoform may survey a distinct intracellular compartment for distinct lipid structures from distinct pathogens. Figure 9-12 summarizes recently deduced CD1 trafficking pathways.

NK-T Cells

As discussed earlier, T lymphocytes bear a combinatorial diversity of TCRs that determine antigen binding specificity. A small subset of T lymphocytes, generally termed *NK-T cells,* expresses a limited repertoire of TCRs that includes a single TCR α chain (Vα14) and a limited number of Vβ chains. In addition to the TCR, these cells also express NK cell markers and are either CD4$^+$ or double negative (CD4$^-$/CD8$^-$). NK-T cells are of particular interest because they respond to lipid antigens presented on CD1d, and a defined glycolipid (α-galactosyl ceramide) strongly activates these cells. The close functional association between CD1d and NK-T cells has major implications for understanding the animal models of CD1 deficiency. Because NK-T cells are positively selected in the thymus by CD1, CD1-deficient mice lack NK-T cells. NK-T cells seem to play a role in immune defense against *Borrelia burgdorferi* infections[199] and participate in defense against viral hepatitis.[200]

CD1 Antigen Presentation and Host Defense against Infectious Diseases

Mycobacteria

Mycobacterial lipids, specifically mycolic acids, were the first CD1-presented antigens.[192] Several other mycobacterial lipid antigens are presented by CD1, including Lipoarabinomannan[193] and glycosylated isoprenoids.[201] Although it is clear that CD1 presents mycobacterial lipid antigens to cloned T-cell lines, the exact role of CD1 in antimicrobial defense still is being elucidated. Possibly because of the noted differences between mouse and human CD1 loci, the mouse model has not been informative in defining an important role for CD1 in immune defense against mycobacterial infection. Mice deficient in CD1 are unaffected in their sensitivity to *M. tuberculosis* infection,[202,203] although neutralization of CD1 with monoclonal antibodies had some deleterious effect on murine defense against tuberculosis infection.[204] The importance of CD1 antigen presentation in human resistance to tuberculosis is more difficult to examine directly, however. Recent purified protein derivative converters have CD1-restricted T cells that react to mycobacterial isoprenoid glycolipids, showing that CD1-restricted antigen presentation does occur in the context of human infection. In addition, CD1a through CD1c are expressed strongly on dendritic cells in tuberculoid leprosy lesions and reversal reactions, but not in lepromatous lesions, suggesting the CD1 expression is correlated with effective antimycobacterial immunity.[205] The emerging role of CD1 antigen presentation has been linked closely with mycobacterial lipid antigens. Although this system surely does not exist solely for the purpose of defense against mycobacterial infections, it is widely accepted that CD1 molecules likely play an important role in antimycobacterial immunity.

Other Infections

Several other studies using mouse models or α-galactosyl ceramide–activated NK-T cells have shown roles for CD1 and NK-T cells in antimicrobial defense against tuberculosis,[206] *Cryptococcus neoformans,*[207] malaria, trypanosomiasis,[208] and others.[209] The precise roles of CD1 versus NK-T cells and the full spectrum of CD1-presented antigens would be an active area of ongoing investigation.

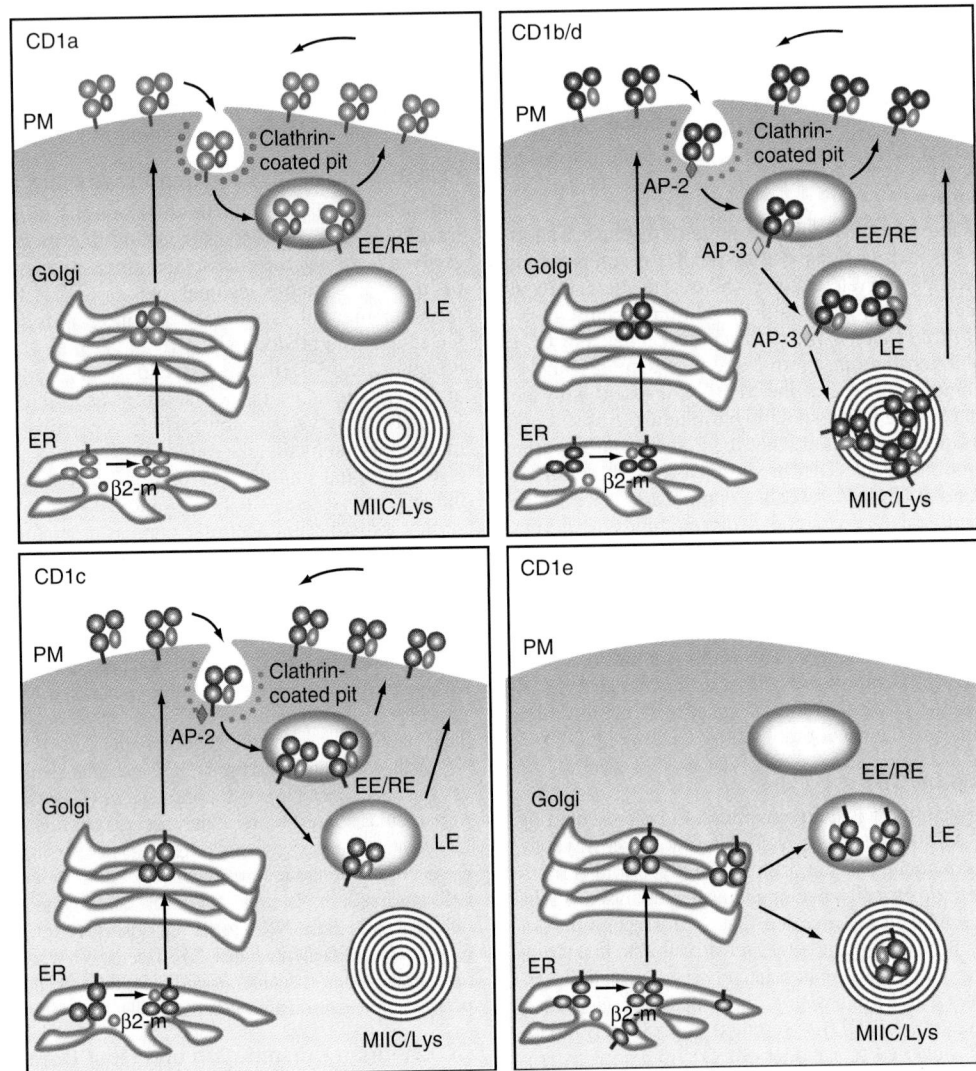

FIGURE 9-12. Intracellular trafficking of CD1 isoforms. Each panel depicts a distinct pattern of CD1 trafficking. All CD1 isoforms associate with β₂-microglobulin, and all isoforms except CD1e are targeted to the cell surface via the secretory pathway. CD1 is internalized and targeted to distinct locations in the lysosomal endosomal network based on the interaction of the CD1 cytoplasmic tails with adapter proteins (AP2, AP3). The varying compartments in the endosomal/lysosomal network are early endosomes/recycling endosomes (EE/RE, CD1a), late endosomes (LE, CD1c), and MHC class II compartment/lysosomes (MIIC/Ly, Cd1b/d). The differing subcellular distributions of CD1 isoforms may reflect surveillance of these compartments for distinct lipid antigens. *(Courtesy of Steven Porcelli, Albert Einstein Medical College, Bronx, NY.)*

MAJOR HISTOCOMPATIBILITY COMPLEX IMMUNOGENETICS

The MHC, so named because its discovery resulted from studies of tissue transplant rejection, contains many of the genes associated with cell-mediated immune defenses. The MHC class I molecules HLA-A, HLA-B, and HLA-C are encoded in the MHC, as are the α and β chains of MHC class II molecules HLA-DR, HLA-DP, and HLA-DQ. In addition to these genes, genes associated with the antigen processing pathways are found in the MHC. Several proteasome subunits, LMP-2, LMP-7, and MECL-1; the peptide transporter TAP1 and TAP2 proteins; and the MHC class II processing–associated HLA-DM and HLA-DO proteins are encoded in the MHC.[126] TNF and its receptor also are encoded in the MHC. A map of the human MHC is shown in Figure 9-13.

An important feature of the MHC, which led to its discovery, is the polymorphism of some of its genes, particularly the MHC class I and class II genes.[210] For the MHC class I HLA-A gene, there are more than 100 known alleles. Although some of these alleles bind similar peptides, most, by virtue of their morphologically distinct peptide binding grooves, bind distinct families of peptides. The evolutionary force driving the diversity of MHC alleles comes from the microbial world and its ability to undergo antigenic variation.[211,212] It is clear from studies of African populations where malaria is endemic that certain HLA alleles are associated with a greater ability to survive malaria infection.[213,214] Conversely, malaria has a confounding ability to alter protein sequences that are bound by HLA molecules, allowing parasite populations to evolve that are invisible to individuals with certain HLA molecules.[215] This type of escape strategy also has been described for viral pathogens,[216,217] including HIV,[218] where cytotoxic T-lymphocyte viral escape mutants are complicating efforts for an effective vaccine.

The HLA locus also encodes proteins for MHC class I molecules that are not highly polymorphic. These molecules also are called *MHC class Ib* molecules and in humans consist of HLA-E, HLA-F, and HLA-G. HLA-G is highly expressed in the placenta, and it has been suggested that it plays a role in protecting cells from NK cell–mediated lysis.[219] HLA-E is another MHC class Ib molecule that plays a role in NK cell–mediated cytolysis. HLA-E binds the signal sequences of conventional MHC class I molecules, providing a readout of the cell's synthesis of MHC class I molecules. HLA-E also binds to NK cell receptors, CD94/NKG2B and CD94/NKG2C, which inhibits NK cell–mediated cytolysis.[220] The role of these proteins in antimicrobial immunity is unclear, although there is evidence that HLA-E can present antigens derived from *M. tuberculosis* to T lymphocytes.[221] Because MHC class Ib molecules generally are highly conserved among individuals (i.e., they are not highly polymorphic, similar to the HLA-A, HLA-B, and HLA-C molecules), there has been interest in exploiting them for pathogen-specific vaccine development.[221] Mice have many MHC class Ib molecules that are encoded within the Q, T, and M regions of the murine MHC.[222,223] One molecule, referred to as *H2-M3*, has been shown to play a role in defense against infection.[224,225] H2-M3 is structurally similar to conventional MHC class I molecules except that the peptide binding groove specifically accommodates peptides that contain *N*-formyl methionine at the amino terminus.[226] Because bacterial, but not eukaryotic, protein synthesis initiates with *N*-formyl methionine, H2-M3 molecules selectively bind peptide of bacterial origin.[227] During murine infection with the intracellular bacterium *L. monocytogenes,* a substantial fraction of CD8+ T cells are specific for bacterially derived, *N*-formyl methionine–containing peptides presented by H2-M3.[228] H2-M3–restricted CD8+ T cells expand more rapidly during bacterial infection than conventional CD8+ T cells and make a relatively minor contribution to memory T-cell responses. Qa-1 is another murine MHC class Ib molecule that has been implicated in antimicrobial defense. Mice infected with *S. typhimurium* mount CD8+ T-cell responses that are specific for a bacterial GroEL-derived peptide in the context of Qa-1.[229-231]

Thymic Selection of CD4+ and CD8+ T Cells

Mature CD4+ and CD8+ T cells are generated in the thymus by a complex process of positive and negative selection.[232] As mentioned earlier, T cells detect peptide antigen in the context of MHC molecules and express receptors that bind the foreign antigen and the MHC molecule. Thymic selection has evolved to ensure that peripheral T cells are able to interact with self-MHC molecules, through the process of positive selection, but not to respond to self-peptides, through the process of negative selection. Progenitors for T lymphocytes originate in the bone marrow and travel to the thymus, where they enter the cortex at the double-negative stage, as defined by the absence of CD4+ and CD8+ on the cell surface. In the thymic cortex, the TCR β chain gene undergoes VDJ recombination, which, if successful, gives rise to the TCR β chain protein. This gene recombination event is catalyzed by the *RAG1* and *RAG2* genes.[233] The newly recombined TCR β chain first forms a complex with the invariant pre-TCR α chain and travels to the cell surface.[234,235] If this process is successful, the endogenous α chain locus undergoes VJ recombination and in subsequent TCR complexes replaces the pre-TCR α. At this stage, the cell upregulates the expression of CD4+ and CD8+ on its cell surface and is referred to as a *double-positive thymocyte*. Positive selection occurs first through a process in which the double-positive thymocyte interacts with a thymic epithelial cell. Although the precise requirements for positive selection are controversial, the consensus is that low avidity interactions between the TCR on the double-positive thymocyte and MHC/peptide complexes on the thymic epithelial cell drive the cell proliferation and survival, whereas high-affinity interactions or no interaction results in cell demise.[236,237] On completion of positive selection, the double-positive thymocyte downregulates either CD4+ or CD8+, depending on whether positive selection occurred on MHC class II or class I. At this stage, thymocytes enter the thymic medulla, where they come into contact with bone marrow–derived dendritic cells and medullary epithelial cells expressing a range of self-antigens. High-affinity interaction with self-antigens results in deletion of the single positive thymocyte, providing a second opportunity to eliminate potentially autoreactive T lymphocytes. Studies have identified a transcription factor, AIRE, which promotes the ectopic expression of peripheral antigens in the thymus.[238] Individuals lacking AIRE develop severe autoimmune diseases.

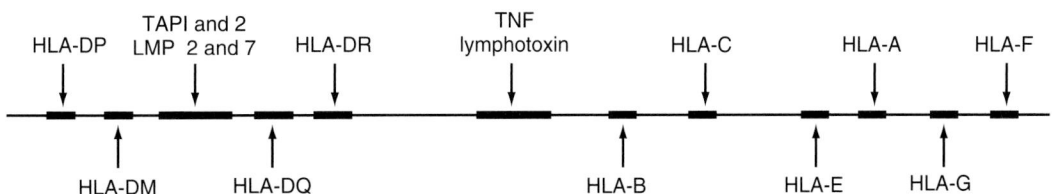

FIGURE 9-13. The major histocompatibility complex (MHC) contains genes for many proteins involved in adaptive immune defense against infectious diseases. In addition to MHC class I and class II genes, the MHC also contains genes for tumor necrosis factor (TNF), lymphotoxin, and many of the genes associated with antigen processing.

On completion of positive and negative selection, thymocytes exit the thymus and become part of the peripheral T-cell compartment. Naive T cells generally express high levels of CD62L (also called *L-selectin*) and the chemokine receptor CCR7,[239] a combination of adhesion molecule and chemokine receptor that targets cells for the T-cell zone of lymph nodes and spleen. The diversity of T cells in the peripheral compartment is enormous; it is estimated that naive T cells of an immunologically normal mouse express approximately 25 million distinct TCRs.[240]

Thymic selection is crucial for the development of peripheral T lymphocytes. In patients with DiGeorge's syndrome, there is a congenital absence of thymic tissue and a corresponding absence of peripheral T lymphocytes.[241] Transplantation of thymic tissue into these patients corrects this problem.[242]

Thymic function dramatically diminishes in humans on aging. Young children have active thymic function and produce large numbers of naive T lymphocytes, whereas older adults have a markedly smaller thymus that produces few new T lymphocytes. Even adults in their 50s continue to have active thymic tissue in the mediastinum, however.[243] Analysis of peripheral blood T lymphocytes from these older individuals indicates that some are recent thymic emigrants, suggesting the thymus continues to function despite its relatively small size. Many factors and circumstances can decrease thymic function, however. Administration of steroids results in thymic involution and decreased output of naive T lymphocytes. Along similar lines, many forms of chemotherapy also are toxic to the thymus and result in thymic atrophy and diminished output of T lymphocytes. This issue is of particular importance in bone marrow transplantation, where long-term survival depends on the reconstitution of the peripheral T-cell compartment. Studies that measured TCR excision circles, an indication of recent emigration from the thymus, have shown that thymic function does return in the transplant setting.[244]

Thymic function also is relevant in HIV infection,[245] particularly in patients with advanced HIV disease initiated on highly active antiviral therapy. In this setting, viral replication often is halted, but increases in the peripheral CD4+ T-cell count depend on thymic production of new, naive T cells or expansion of the residual peripheral T-cell compartment or both.[246] The extent to which thymic function contributes to the redevelopment of the T-cell population in HIV-infected patients has been investigated by TCR excision circle analysis.[247]

T-Cell Activation

T-lymphocyte activation is a remarkably complex process.[248] Although specificity is provided by interaction of TCRs with cognate MHC peptide complexes, many other concurrent processes are necessary for the induction of T-cell proliferation and differentiation. The most important signal after engagement of the TCR with the MHC/peptide complex is mediated by CD28 on the T cell and B7.1 and B7.2 on the antigen-presenting cell.[249] This interaction induces IL-2 production by T lymphocytes, which promotes their proliferation. On activation, T lymphocytes express CTLA-4, which also binds B7.1 and B7.2, but instead of stimulating proliferation, this signaling molecule inhibits proliferation and acts as a brake on expansion. Studies have identified many other related B7 molecules that seem to play a role in the activation of T lymphocytes in peripheral tissues.[250] One of these molecules, B7h, interacts with the inducible molecule ICOS on the surface of activated T cells and promotes their differentiation toward the Th2 phenotype.[251-253]

Many receptors that belong in the TNF receptor superfamily also play a role in the activation and differentiation of T lymphocytes.[254] Among these, CD40 and CD40L are perhaps the most completely investigated. The role of CD40L in T-cell and B-cell immunity first became apparent with the discovery that individuals with the hyper-IgM syndrome had genetic defects in the gene encoding CD40L.[255-257] Not only do individuals with this disease have difficulty with antibody isotype switching, accounting for the high circulating IgM levels, but they are also susceptible to infections with *Pneumocystis carinii*, suggesting defective T-cell–mediated immunity. In mice deficient for CD40 or CD40L, T-cell activa-

tion and maintenance of memory T-cell populations are defective, accounting for increased susceptibility to some infections.[258] Other receptors, such as 4-1BB and OX40, also have been implicated as playing a positive role in the generation of pathogen-specific T-cell responses.[259-261]

The interface between T lymphocytes and antigen-presenting cells is a highly organized structure called the *immunologic synapse*.[262] In this structure, TCRs occupy center stage, forming a bull's eye that is surrounded by adhesion molecules, such as ICAM and LFA-1.[263] Costimulatory molecules, such as CD28, also are present in the synapse, as are essential signaling molecules, such as PKC-θ.[264] Synapse formation occurs when an antigen-specific T cell encounters an antigen-presenting cell, enabling these cells to engage each other for several hours, a process that is likely essential for T-cell activation.

Antigen-Presenting Cells

Priming of naive T lymphocytes is mediated predominantly by dendritic cells.[265] As dendritic cells are characterized in greater detail, it is becoming increasingly apparent that they are a complex, heterogeneous population.[266] One of the major functions of dendritic cells is to present antigens to T lymphocytes and promote their proliferation and differentation. The high levels of surface MHC class I and class II and the expression of an array of costimulatory molecules enable dendritic cells to stimulate naive T cells effectively. The role of dendritic cells in antimicrobial defense extends, however, beyond stimulation of T cells. Dendritic cells derived from monocytes express a range of TLRs that induce dendritic cell activation and the expression of cytokines that can orchestrate the innate inflammatory response.[267,268] Some dendritic cells, such as plasmacytoid dendritic cells,[269,270] express high levels of TLR7 and TLR9 and, on stimulation, secrete very high levels of type I IFNs. Monocyte-derived dendritic cells express TLR1, TLR2, TLR4, TLR5, and TLR8 and respond to a range of bacterial molecules.[267] Some dendritic cells express TNF on stimulation,[271] whereas others, predominantly cells expressing CD8α, secrete IL-12 on stimulation.[267,268] A receptor that recognizes fungal-derived β-glucans named *Dectin-1* was found to induce dendritic cell activation in conjunction with TLR signaling.[94,272,273]

Dendritic cells are postulated to pick up antigens in peripheral tissues, and to transport antigens to draining lymph nodes.[28] Peripheral tissues, such as skin, contain resident dendritic cells that, after inflammatory stimuli, traffic to the T-cell regions of draining lymph nodes. The precise role of different dendritic cell populations in tissues is incompletely defined. Although skin Langerhans dendritic cells were assumed to transport antigens from inflamed skin, more recent studies have shown that particulate antigens injected into skin are taken up by monocytes that are recruited from the blood stream to the site of injection.[28] These monocytes enter the skin's lymphatics and traffic to the lymph node, where they differentiate into dendritic cells that are capable of priming naive T lymphocytes. Trafficking of activated dendritic cells into lymph nodes involves the upregulation of CCR7 on dendritic cells, enabling them to respond to CCL19 and CCL21, which are expressed in the lymph node paracortex.[274] Dendritic cells, when migrating to lymph nodes, secrete cysteinyl leukotrienes, in a process that depends on multidrug resistance–associated protein 1 (MRP-1). The cysteinyl leukotriene LTC$_4$ enhances dendritic cell responsiveness to CCL19.

Dendritic cells, although they play an essential role in T-cell priming, also participate in the innate inflammatory response, setting the stage for the T-cell response. One of the first in vivo demonstrations of this role for dendritic cells came from studies of the cytokine response to injected *T. gondii* antigens.[275] CD8+ dendritic cells were the major source of IL-12 production that occurred within hours of antigen injection. Induction of IL-12 is transient, and *T. gondii*–stimulated dendritic cells quit making IL-12 within 24 hours and do not respond to further simulation for 1 week.[276] CD8+ dendritic cells stimulated with *T. gondii* extracts eventually downregulate IL-12 production in a process that is mediated by lipoxin A4, an eicosanoid inhibitor of acute inflammation.[277] Although chemokine receptors typically are implicated in chemotactic recruitment of cells, they have been shown to enhance cytokine secretion. CCR5 stimulation on CD8$^+$ dendritic cells induces the production of IL-12.[278] *T. gondii* produces a protein that binds to CCR5, enhancing the production of IL-12.[279]

T-Cell Expansion and Differentiation

CD8$^+$ T Cells

The development of methods that precisely quantify antigen-specific T-cell responses has added an important dimension to the understanding of pathogen-specific immunity. Studies in animal models have provided the clearest picture of pathogen-specific T-cell responses. CD8$^+$ T-cell responses are induced rapidly after infection with viruses, such as lymphocytic choriomeningitis virus, and bacteria, such as *L. monocytogenes*.[13,15] Using MHC class I tetramers or intracellular cytokine staining, pathogen-specific T cells are detectable 5 days after infection and expand rapidly to peak frequencies approximately 8 days after infection. Studies using adoptively transferred T cells of defined specificity, labeled with a fluorescent dye, have shown that antigen-specific T cells undergo rapid proliferation during this phase of the immune response, dividing at a rate of approximately once every 6 hours.[280] In a matter of a few days, the frequency of antigen-specific T cells can increase from 1 in 100,000 CD8$^+$ T cells to 1 in 2 CD8$^+$ T cells in some viral infections.

During the early immune response, CD8$^+$ T cells differentiate into effector T cells by acquiring effector functions that typically include production of cytokines, such as IFN-γ and TNF, and molecules associated with cytolytic killing, such as perforin, granzyme B, and granulysin.[281] In addition, some cytokine receptors, such as the IL-7 receptor, which transmits homeostatic signals to naive T cells, are downregulated, whereas other receptors, such as the high-affinity IL-2 receptor, are upregulated.[282] The mechanisms that drive CD8$^+$ T-cell proliferation and differentiation during immune responses to infection remain incompletely defined. Studies indicate, however, that T cells acquire a program during early encounters with antigens, then undergo proliferation and differentiation independent of further encounters with antigens or with the inflammation associated with infection.[283,284] Although innate inflammation and T-cell priming are intricately interwoven processes, when primed, T cells follow a pathway that is remarkably independent of inflammation.

When CD8$^+$ T cells complete the expansion phase, the frequency of pathogen-specific CD8$^+$ T cells decreases, ultimately giving rise to a residual memory T-cell population. Similar to the expansion phase, the contraction phase of CD8$^+$ T-cell responses is antigen and inflammation independent.[285] Characterization of gene expression by CD8$^+$ T cells during an immune response to infection showed that molecules associated with cell survival, prominently BCL-2, are regulated in a fashion that leaves effector T cells vulnerable to apoptosis.[286] Downregulation of BCL-2 expression along with upregulation of cell surface Fas enhances CD8$^+$ T-cell death.

CD4$^+$ T Cells

CD4$^+$ T cells also respond to microbial infection. Although the kinetics of their responses are less well defined, increasingly investigators are characterizing CD4$^+$ T-cell differentiation and expansion after infection.[287,288] In infections associated with robust and rapid CD8$^+$ T-cell responses, the CD4$^+$ T-cell response generally follows parallel kinetics. Long-term survival of CD4$^+$ memory T cells seems to differ, however, from CD8$^+$ memory T-cell survival.[289] In virally infected mice, memory CD4$^+$ T cells decrease in frequency, whereas memory CD8$^+$ T-cell frequencies are maintained at stable levels. In other scenarios, however, such as *S. typhimurium* or *M. tuberculosis* infection, the kinetics of CD4$^+$ T-cell responses seem to be delayed, with peak CD4$^+$ T-cell populations occurring only after 3 weeks of infection.[290]

At the time of priming, responding CD4$^+$ T cells can choose one of two pathways of differentiation.[291] If they choose to become Th1 cells, they upregulate the expression of IFN-γ and participate in the activation of cellular defenses against a range of intracellular bacterial and protozoal pathogens. If they differentiate into Th2 cells, they express high levels of IL-4 and potentially IL-13 and IL-5; induce mucus secretion, IgE production, and eosinophil recruitment; and participate in the elimination of intestinal pathogens and infections by large, multicellular pathogens, such as helminths.[292] Although the differentiation of CD4$^+$ T cells is of great relevance to antimicrobial defense, the aberrant differentiation of CD4$^+$ T cells into Th2 cells is also the root cause of allergic diseases, such as asthma and anaphylactic reactions to various substances ranging from antibiotics to peanuts.

Identifying the mechanisms that drive primed T cells down the Th1 or Th2 pathway has been an intense area of research since the 1980s. One of the earliest steps in the differentiation process is the induction of either GATA-3, in the case of Th2 differentiation,[293] or T-bet, in the case of Th1 differentiation.[294] Expression of T-bet in T cells activates the expression of Th1 cytokines and downregulates the expression of Th2 cytokines. The precise stimuli driving the induction of one factor or the other are controversial, although there is consensus that the nature of the innate inflammatory response plays a role. Early production of IL-4, perhaps by mast cells or NK-T cells, drives CD4$^+$ T cells in the direction of the Th2 phenotype, whereas early production of IFN-γ drives the development of Th1 CD4$^+$ T cells.[291] IL-12 is believed to play an important role in the expansion of Th1 CD4$^+$ T cells.[295] In the absence of MyD88, an adaptor molecule that is essential for most TLR-mediated signaling, including the induction of IL-12, CD4$^+$ T cells differentiate into Th2 T cells, whereas in the presence of intact TLR signaling, they differentiate into Th1 T cells.[296]

When CD4$^+$ T cells have differentiated into Th1 or Th2 cells, they are committed to their phenotype. Analysis of DNA methylation and histone acetylation showed that the IL-4 locus in the case of Th2 cells, or the IFN-γ locus in the case of Th1 cells, becomes epigenetically remodeled.[297,298] This process ensures that T cells, on reencountering the pathogen, rapidly express the same cytokine profile that was induced during T-cell priming.

Differentiation of CD4$^+$ T cells during immune responses has profound implications for the outcome of infection. Murine infection with the protozoan pathogen *Leishmania major* results in a CD4$^+$ T-cell response that, depending on the mouse strain, can be either Th1 or Th2.[299] Because *L. major* survives within macrophage vacuoles, a Th1 response is beneficial and results in parasite killing. In mice mounting a Th2 response, infection with *L. major* is progressive and ultimately lethal. The mechanisms that determine whether an *L. major*–specific T-cell response will be Th1 or Th2 are complex and incompletely understood. Early expression of IL-4 induces Th2 responses, whereas early expression of IFN-γ induces Th1 differentiation. Genetic studies suggest that the process of CD4$^+$ T-cell differentiation after *L. major* infection is multifactorial, involving more than five different loci.[299] In some mouse strains, Th2 responses occur because of T-cell responses to one dominant antigen called *LACK*.[300] In the absence of a T-cell response to this specific antigen, the responding CD4$^+$ T cells differentiate into Th1 cells.

As has been described for CD8$^+$ T cells, CD4$^+$ T-cell expansion during immune responses does not require continuous exposure to antigen.[301] The dose of antigen that naive CD4$^+$ T cells encounter during priming influences their differentiation into Th1 or Th2 cells. Higher doses of antigen are associated with differentiation into Th1 cells, whereas low-dose antigen exposure induces Th2 differentiation.[302]

CD8$^+$ T-Lymphocyte Effector Functions

As a rule, T lymphocytes orchestrate antimicrobial defense but do not participate directly in microbial killing. One strategy that T cells use to disable microbes is to secrete cytokines and chemokines that can activate other cells (e.g., macrophages and B cells) or recruit other cells (e.g., monocytes and neutrophils) to sites of infection. The other strategy used by T lymphocytes is to lyse and destroy microbially infected cells, depriving the pathogen of an environment that is suitable for its replication or long-term survival or both. These functions, collectively called *T-lymphocyte effector functions*, are expressed selectively by different T-cell subsets, providing a diversity of antimicrobial mechanisms.[281]

One of the principal effector functions of CD8$^+$ T cells is the ability to lyse pathogen-infected cells. This function is particularly effective in defense against some viral infections, in which lysis of the host cell prevents further viral replication.[303] The most rapid cytolytic mechanism involves release of perforin granules by antigen-activated CD8+ T lymphocytes. Perforin lyses the target cell membrane and enables granzymes, which also are released by cytolytic T cells, to enter the target cell and initiate the apoptotic pathway.[304] In addition to perforin/granzyme–mediated lysis, CD8+ T cells also can mediate target cell death by expressing Fas ligand, which can engage Fas on the target cell surface, resulting in Fas-mediated death. Cytolysis mediated by CD8+ T cells generally targets a host cell and not the microbe. Studies have shown, however, that human T cells produce a cytolytic protein called *granulysin* that can kill bacteria directly, including *M. tuberculosis*.[305] Granulysin is produced by CD8+ and CD4+ T cells and has been implicated in defense against *M. leprae*.[306]

In addition to being cytolytic, CD8+ T cells produce cytokines. In the setting of most infections, pathogen-specific CD8+ T cells secrete IFN-γ and TNF, which enhances macrophage-mediated and neutrophil-mediated microbial killing.[281] In addition to cytokines, CD8+ T cells produce chemokines, such as RANTES, Mip-1α, and Mip-1β. Expression of these chemokines by CD8+ T cells has been suggested as playing a role in reducing HIV infectivity.[307] A more likely role for chemokine secretion by T cells is to recruit inflammatory cells to sites of T-cell activation.

T-Lymphocyte Memory

A hallmark of the adaptive T-lymphocyte response is its capacity for antigen-specific memory.[308] It is well established that T lymphocytes with specificity for a particular pathogen can persist in the host for many years after the pathogen has been eliminated. It also is clear that T lymphocytes can persist in the host without reexposure to antigen, either from exogenous sources or from antigen depots that might be maintained after the resolution of primary infection. The mechanism of memory T-cell maintenance has been difficult to discern, but in recent years substantial progress has been made. One important finding came from studies of naive and memory T lymphocytes transferred into mice that lack MHC molecules. Naive T cells were found to depend on the presence of MHC molecules for long-term survival, whereas memory T cells could survive and undergo homeostatic proliferation in the absence of any MHC molecules.[309] This result indicated that maintenance of naive and memory T cells is fundamentally different. Further studies determined that memory CD8+ T lymphocytes specific for a viral pathogen diminished in frequency in the absence of IL-15 or if they did not express the IL-15 receptor.[310-312] In murine CD8+ T cells, IL-15 seems to be the essential cytokine that maintains memory T-cell populations. Although CD4+ and CD8+ T lymphocytes share many features, there also are some important distinctions. Although viral infection induces CD8+ memory T-cell populations that persist at relatively constant levels over time, virus-specific CD4+ memory T cells decrease in frequency.[289] CD4+ memory T cells also are not affected by the presence or absence of IL-15, suggesting that their maintenance may depend on other, yet to be discovered factors.

The molecular mechanisms for memory T-cell generation have been areas of intense investigation and speculation. Several models of memory T-cell generation have been proposed, including the idea that memory T cells rapidly distinguish themselves from conventional effector T cells during the primary immune response.[308] Most data support an alternate model, however, of naive T cells differentiating into effector T cells, then further differentiating into memory T cells.[286] Comparison of the TCR repertoire of pathogen-specific effector and memory T cells suggested that these two populations shared a common ancestry.[313] A more direct analysis of memory T cells, using a clever genetic marking strategy, showed that memory T cells had expressed genes associated with the acquisition of effector functions, further supporting the notion that memory T cells derive from effector T cells.[314] A remaining controversy concerns the amount of time required for the generation of memory CD8+ T lymphocytes. A study suggests that memory T lymphocytes require 3 to 4 weeks to differentiate

fully,[286] whereas earlier studies suggested that memory responses could be elicited at earlier time points.[315] Although this issue may seem to be a concern only to CD8+ T-cell aficionados, it has significance for the design of prime-boost immunization strategies.

The interaction between CD4+ and CD8+ T cells during immune responses to infection also has been elucidated in recent years. The old notion that CD4+ T cells produce IL-2 to enhance CD8+ T-cell proliferation and differentiation has been supplanted by a more complicated model. During immunization in the absence of inflammation, CD8+ T-cell priming depends on the presence of CD4+ T-cell help. CD4+ T cells can provide help through two mechanisms. First, they can activate antigen-presenting dendritic cells through CD40/CD40L interactions, upregulating the expression of costimulatory molecules on the surface of the antigen-presenting cell.[316-318] Second, a more recent study showed that CD4+ T cells could interact directly with CD8+ T cells through CD40/CD40L interactions.[258] Under priming conditions associated with greater innate inflammation, CD8+ T-cell priming and expansion can occur without CD4+ T-cell help. Several studies have shown, however, that long-term memory responses of CD8+ T cells primed in the absence of CD4+ T cells are compromised. These studies indicate that CD8+ T-cell memory is programmed during the priming process through CD4+ T-cell–mediated stimuli that are distinct from the stimuli required for proliferation and effector differentiation.[319-321] Much more work is required to work out the mechanisms of CD8+ T-cell memory generation, but the results will be of great relevance for the development of vaccines against pathogens such as HIV, hepatitis C virus, malaria, and tuberculosis.

Detailed characterization of memory T lymphocytes has uncovered a level of diversity that is likely relevant for antimicrobial defense. This discovery has led to the division of memory T lymphocytes into two populations: effector memory T cells and central memory T cells.[322] The former population expresses low levels of CD62L and CCR7, actively expresses effector functions (e.g., cytokine synthesis and cytolytic activity), and traffics to peripheral rather than secondary lymphoid tissues. Central memory T cells express high levels of CD62L and CCR7, do not actively express effector functions, and traffic preferentially to secondary lymphoid tissues. These two populations of memory T cells are postulated to play different roles in providing protective immunity. Effector memory T cells are present in tissues and are ready to engage the pathogen, should invasion occur. Central memory T cells are believed to provide a source of effector memory cells and, although they would be anticipated to require more time for activation, can play a role in protective immunity. Studies of patients enduring chronic viral infections show an even greater level of diversity among memory T lymphocytes.[323]

T Regulatory Cells

The rapid proliferation of pathogen-specific T lymphocytes, although essential for pathogen clearance and the establishment of long-term protective immunity, poses a significant problem for the mammalian host. First, if the proliferative phase of the T-cell response lasts too long, the immune compartment could be overwhelmed easily by pathogen-specific T lymphocytes. In addition, because of the potential for T-cell cross-reactivity with self-antigens, there is a risk that overly robust T-cell expansion in response to infection could give rise to autoreactive T lymphocytes that could result in autoimmunity. The notion that a specialized T-lymphocyte population might control or suppress T-lymphocyte responses is not new.[324] The identity of the suppressor T cell, which is referred to more commonly as a *T regulatory cell,* was determined only recently, however.[325] T regulatory cells first were identified as a CD4+/CD25+ T-cell subset that could be found in normal mice and constituted roughly 10% of the CD4+ T-cell population.[326] This T-cell population had the remarkable ability to prevent autoimmune inflammatory bowel disease when transferred into mice with a predilection for inflammatory bowel disease. Further studies have shown that CD4+/CD25+ T regulatory cells suppress the activation of autoimmune T lymphocytes, although the precise mechanisms that are involved in suppression need to be elucidated.[325]

Although transforming growth factor-β and IL-10 have been implicated in this process, they are dispensable for in vivo suppression by T regulatory cells. Similar to conventional CD4+ and CD8+ T lymphocytes, T regulatory cells are selected in the thymus on thymic epithelial cells.[327] Thymic selection of T regulatory cells is distinguishable from the selection of conventional T cells by the requirement for Foxp3. Foxp3-deficient mice develop CD4+ T-cell–mediated, lethal, multiorgan autoimmune disease because they are deficient in CD4+/CD25+ T regulatory cells.

In contrast to NK-T cells, CD4+/CD25+ T regulatory cells express a broad range of TCRs, suggesting that they likely respond specifically to microbial antigens. Although T regulatory cells restrain specific T-cell responses, mechanisms are in place to limit T regulatory cell–mediated inhibition of antimicrobial T-cell responses. TLR-mediated microbial stimuli induce the production of IL-6 by dendritic cells, which blocks T regulatory cell–mediated suppression of antigen-specific CD4+ T-cell proliferation.[96]

Natural Killer Cells

NK cells are lymphocytes that do not express TCRs, but express a family of receptors responsible for their activation and inhibition. Several extensive reviews on this topic have been published.[328-330] These cells are active in defense against tumors and infectious organisms, particularly viruses. Their importance in antiviral defense is emphasized by the report of a patient with severe herpesvirus infections who lacked NK cells.[331] The activation of NK cells against a malignant or parasitized target cell or their ignorance of normal cells is mediated by a family of NK-cell receptors. Because these receptors are non-combinatorial, the molecules they recognize on target cells are relatively conserved, analogous to the recognition of conserved molecular patterns by other receptors in the innate immune system. The best studied of the inhibitory receptors is Ly49a (mouse)/CD94 (human). These molecules recognize MHC class I molecules on the surface of potential target cells and transduce an inhibitory signal that prevents NK-cell cytolysis, preventing killing of normal cells. In contrast, activating NK-cell receptors recognize more diverse ligands, including host MHC and direct recognition of viral proteins expressed on infected cells.[332] A direct role of NK cells in antimicrobial defense is best established for CMV infections.[333,334]

REFERENCES

1. Halsband RE. The Complete Letters of Lady Mary Wortley Montagu. Oxford: Clarendon Press; 1966.
2. Jenner E. An inquiry into the causes and effects of the variolae vaccinae, a disease discovered in some of the western counties of England, particularly Gloucestershire, and known by the name of the cow pox. 1st ed. London: Low, Sampson; 1798.
3. Silverstein AM. A history of immunology. 1st ed. San Diego, Calif: Academic Press; 1989.
4. Landsteiner K, Chase MW. Experiments on transfer of cutaneous sensitivity to simple compounds. Proc Soc Exp Biol Med 1942;49:688-689.
5. Chase MW. The cellular transfer of cutaneous hypersensitivity to tuberculin. Proc Soc Exp Biol Med 1945;59:134-135.
6. Mackaness GB, Blanden RV. Cellular immunity. Prog Allergy 1967;11:89-140.
7. Zinkernagel RM, Doherty PC. Restriction of in vitro T cell-mediated cytotoxicity in lymphocytic choriomeningitis within a syngeneic or semiallogeneic system. Nature 1974;248:701-702.
8. Herzenberg LA, De Rosa SC. Monoclonal antibodies and the FACS: Complementary tools for immunobiology and medicine. Immunol Today 2000;21:383-390.
9. Miyahira Y, Murata K, Rodriguez D, et al. Quantification of antigen specific CD8+ T cells using an ELISPOT assay. J Immunol Methods 1995;181:45-54.
10. Suni MA, Picker LJ, Maino VC. Detection of antigen-specific T cell cytokine expression in whole blood by flow cytometry. J Immunol Methods 1998;212:89-98.
11. Altman JD, Moss PA, Goulder PJ, et al. Phenotypic analysis of antigen-specific T lymphocytes. Science 1996;274:94-96.
12. Knabel M, Franz TJ, Schiemann M, et al. Reversible MHC multimer staining for functional isolation of T-cell populations and effective adoptive transfer. Nat Med 2002;8:631-637.
13. Murali-Krishna K, Altman JD, Suresh M, et al. Counting antigen-specific CD8 T cells: A reevaluation of bystander activation during viral infection. Immunity 1998;8:177-187.
14. Flynn KJ, Belz GT, Altman JD, et al. Virus-specific CD8+ T cells in primary and secondary influenza pneumonia. Immunity 1998;8:683-691.
15. Busch DH, Pilip IM, Vijh S, Pamer EG. Coordinate regulation of complex T cell populations responding to bacterial infection. Immunity 1998;8:353-362.
16. Doherty PC, Christensen JP. Accessing complexity: The dynamics of virus-specific T cell responses. Annu Rev Immunol 2000;18:561-592.
17. Tan LC, Gudgeon N, Annels NE, et al. A re-evaluation of the frequency of CD8+ T cells specific for EBV in healthy virus carriers. J Immunol 1999;162:1827-1835.
18. Callan MF, Tan L, Annels N, et al. Direct visualization of antigen-specific CD8+ T cells during the primary immune response to Epstein-Barr virus in vivo. J Exp Med 1998;187:1395-1402.
19. Waldrop SL, Pitcher CJ, Peterson DM, et al. Determination of antigen-specific memory/effector CD4+ T cell frequencies by flow cytometry: Evidence for a novel, antigen-specific homeostatic mechanism in HIV-associated immunodeficiency. J Clin Invest 1997;99:1739-1750.
20. Wallace ME, Keating R, Heath WR, Carbone FR. The cytotoxic T-cell response to herpes simplex virus type 1 infection of C57BL/6 mice is almost entirely directed against a single immunodominant determinant. J Virol 1999;73:7619-7626.
21. Lefrancois L, Masopust D. T cell immunity in lymphoid and non-lymphoid tissues. Curr Opin Immunol 2002;14:503-508.
22. Cyster JG. Chemokines and cell migration in secondary lymphoid organs. Science 1999;286:2098-2102.
23. Weninger W, Manjunath N, von Andrian UH. Migration and differentiation of CD8+ T cells. Immunol Rev 2002;186:221-233.
24. Gretz JE, Anderson AO, Shaw S. Cords, channels, corridors and conduits: Critical architectural elements facilitating cell interactions in the lymph node cortex. Immunol Rev 1997;156:11-24.
25. Gretz JE, Norbury CC, Anderson AO, et al. Lymph-borne chemokines and other low molecular weight molecules reach high endothelial venules via specialized conduits while a functional barrier limits access to the lymphocyte microenvironments in lymph node cortex. J Exp Med 2000;192:1425-1440.
26. Norbury CC, Malide D, Gibbs JS, et al. Visualizing priming of virus-specific CD8+ T cells by infected dendritic cells in vivo. Nat Immunol 2002;3:265-271.
27. Kaldjian EP, Gretz JE, Anderson AO, et al. Spatial and molecular organization of lymph node T cell cortex: A labyrinthine cavity bounded by an epithelium-like monolayer of fibroblastic reticular cells anchored to basement membrane-like extracellular matrix. Int Immunol 2001;13:1243-1253.
28. Randolph GJ, Inaba K, Robbiani DF, et al. Differentiation of phagocytic monocytes into lymph node dendritic cells in vivo. Immunity 1999;11:753-761.
29. Palframan RT, Jung S, Cheng G, et al. Inflammatory chemokine transport and presentation in HEV: A remote control mechanism for monocyte recruitment to lymph nodes in inflamed tissues. J Exp Med 2001;194:1361-1373.
30. Kraal G. Cells in the marginal zone of the spleen. Int Rev Cytol 1992;132:31-74.
31. Van den Eertwegh AJ, Boersma WJ, Claassen E. Immunological functions and in vivo cell-cell interactions of T cells in the spleen. Crit Rev Immunol 1992;11:337-380.
32. Nolte MA, Hoen EN, van Stijn A, et al. Isolation of the intact white pulp: Quantitative and qualitative analysis of the cellular composition of the splenic compartments. Eur J Immunol 2000;30:626-634.
33. Geijtenbeek TB, Groot PC, Nolte MA, et al. Marginal zone macrophages express a murine homologue of DC-SIGN that captures blood-borne antigens in vivo. Blood 2002;100:2908-2916.
34. Balazs M, Martin F, Zhou T, Kearney J. Blood dendritic cells interact with splenic marginal zone B cells to initiate T-independent immune responses. Immunity 2002;17:341-352.
35. Nolte MA, Belien JA, Schadee-Eestermans I, et al. A conduit system distributes chemokines and small blood-borne molecules through the splenic white pulp. J Exp Med 2003;198:505-512.
36. Springer TA. Traffic signals on endothelium for lymphocyte recirculation and leukocyte emigration. Annu Rev Physiol 1995;57:827-872.
37. Girard JP, Springer TA. High endothelial venules (HEVs): Specialized endothelium for lymphocyte migration. Immunol Today 1995;16:449-457.
38. Takagi J, Springer TA. Integrin activation and structural rearrangement. Immunol Rev 2002;186:141-163.
39. Ansel KM, Cyster JG. Chemokines in lymphopoiesis and lymphoid organ development. Curr Opin Immunol 2001;13:172-179.
40. Okada T, Ngo VN, Ekland EH, et al. Chemokine requirements for B cell entry to lymph nodes and Peyer's patches. J Exp Med 2002;196:65-75.
41. Lu TT, Cyster JG. Integrin-mediated long-term B cell retention in the splenic marginal zone. Science 2002;297:409-412.
42. Lo CG, Lu TT, Cyster JG. Integrin-dependence of lymphocyte entry into the splenic white pulp. J Exp Med 2003;197:353-361.
43. Reif K, Ekland EH, Ohl L, et al. Balanced responsiveness to chemoattractants from adjacent zones determines B-cell position. Nature 2002;416:94-99.
44. Mayer L. Mucosal immunity. Pediatrics 2003;111(6 Pt 3):1595-1600.
45. Mayer L. Innate and acquired immunity at mucosal surfaces. Viral Immunol 2000;13:477-480.
46. Lefrancois L, Fuller B, Huleatt JW, et al. On the front lines: Intraepithelial lymphocytes as primary effectors of intestinal immunity. Springer Semin Immunopathol 1997;18:463-475.
47. Huleatt JW, Lefrancois L. Antigen-driven induction of CD11c on intestinal intraepithelial lymphocytes and CD8+ T cells in vivo. J Immunol 1995;154:5684-5693.
48. Lefrancois L. Intraepithelial lymphocytes of the intestinal mucosa: Curiouser and curiouser. Semin Immunol 1991;3:99-108.
49. Lefrancois L. Extrathymic differentiation of intraepithelial lymphocytes: Generation of a separate and unequal T-cell repertoire? Immunol Today 1991;12:436-438.
50. Lefrancois L. Maturation, selection and specificity of Tcr gamma delta T cells. Immunol Res 1992;11:54-65.
51. Pope C, Kim SK, Marzo A, et al. Organ-specific regulation of the CD8 T cell response to Listeria monocytogenes infection. J Immunol 2001;166:3402-3409.
52. Huleatt JW, Pilip I, Kerksiek K, Pamer EG. Intestinal and splenic T cell responses to enteric Listeria monocytogenes infection: Distinct repertoires of responding CD8 T lymphocytes. J Immunol 2001;166:4065-4073.
53. Hershberg RM, Mayer LF. Antigen processing and presentation by intestinal epithelial cells—polarity and complexity. Immunol Today 2000;21:123-128.

54. Blumberg RS, Lencer WI, Zhu X, et al. Antigen presentation by intestinal epithelial cells. Immunol Lett 1999;69:7-11.

55. Mayer L. Current concepts in mucosal immunity: I. Antigen presentation in the intestine: New rules and regulations. Am J Physiol 1998;274(1 Pt 1):G7-9.

56. Vazquez-Torres A, Jones-Carson J, Baumler AJ, et al. Extraintestinal dissemination of *Salmonella* by CD18-expressing phagocytes. Nature 1999;401:804-808.

57. Rescigno M, Urbano M, Valzasina B, et al. Dendritic cells express tight junction proteins and penetrate gut epithelial monolayers to sample bacteria. Nat Immunol 2001;2:361-367.

58. Masopust D, Jiang J, Shen H, et al. Direct analysis of the dynamics of the intestinal mucosa CD8 T cell response to systemic virus infection. J Immunol 2001;166:2348-2356.

59. Masopust D, Vezys V, Marzo AL, et al. Preferential localization of effector memory cells in nonlymphoid tissue. Science 2001;291:2413-2417.

60. Reinhardt RL, Khoruts A, Merica R, et al. Visualizing the generation of memory CD4 T cells in the whole body. Nature 2001;410:101-105.

61. Belz GT, Altman JD, Doherty PC. Characteristics of virus-specific CD8(+) T cells in the liver during the control and resolution phases of influenza pneumonia. Proc Natl Acad Sci U S A 1998;95:13812-13817.

62. Marshall DR, Turner SJ, Belz GT, et al. Measuring the diaspora for virus-specific CD8+ T cells. Proc Natl Acad Sci U S A 2001;98:6313-6318.

63. Hogan RJ, Usherwood EJ, Zhong W, et al. Activated antigen-specific CD8+ T cells persist in the lungs following recovery from respiratory virus infections. J Immunol 2001;166:1813-1822.

64. Wiley JA, Hogan RJ, Woodland DL, et al. Antigen-specific CD8(+) T cells persist in the upper respiratory tract following influenza virus infection. J Immunol 2001; 167:3293-3299.

65. Cerwenka A, Morgan TM, Dutton RW. Naive, effector, and memory CD8 T cells in protection against pulmonary influenza virus infection. Homing properties rather than initial frequencies are crucial. J Immunol 1999;163:5535-5543.

66. Topham DJ, Castrucci MR, Wingo FS, et al. The role of antigen in the localization of naive, acutely activated, and memory CD8(+) T cells to the lung during influenza pneumonia. J Immunol 2001;167:6983-6990.

67. Jameson SC. Maintaining the norm: T-cell homeostasis. Nat Rev Immunol 2002;2: 547-556.

68. Guidotti LG, Ishikawa T, Hobbs MV, et al. Intracellular inactivation of the hepatitis B virus by cytotoxic T lymphocytes. Immunity 1996;4:25-36.

69. de la Salle H, Zimmer J, Fricker D, et al. HLA class I deficiencies due to mutations in subunit 1 of the peptide transporter TAP1. J Clin Invest 1999;103:R9-R13.

70. de la Salle H, Hanau D, Fricker D, et al. Homozygous human TAP peptide transporter mutation in HLA class I deficiency. Science 1994;265:237-241.

71. de la Calle-Martin O, Hernandez M, Ordi J, et al. Familial CD8 deficiency due to a mutation in the CD8 alpha gene. J Clin Invest 2001;108:117-123.

72. Carrington M, Nelson GW, Martin MP, et al. HLA and HIV-1: Heterozygote advantage and B*35-Cw*04 disadvantage. Science 1999;283:1748-1752.

73. Kaslow RA, Carrington M, Apple R, et al. Influence of combinations of human major histocompatibility complex genes on the course of HIV-1 infection. Nat Med 1996;2:405-411.

74. Doffinger R, Dupuis S, Picard C, et al. Inherited disorders of IL-12- and IFNgamma-mediated immunity: A molecular genetics update. Mol Immunol 2002;38:903-909.

75. de Jong R, Altare F, Haagen IA, et al. Severe mycobacterial and *Salmonella* infections in interleukin-12 receptor-deficient patients. Science 1998;280:1435-1438.

76. Jouanguy E, Altare F, Lamhamedi S, et al. Interferon-gamma-receptor deficiency in an infant with fatal bacille Calmette-Guerin infection. N Engl J Med 1996;335:1956-1961.

77. Doffinger R, Jouanguy E, Dupuis S, et al. Partial interferon-gamma receptor signaling chain deficiency in a patient with bacille Calmette-Guerin and *Mycobacterium abscessus* infection. J Infect Dis 2000;181:379-384.

78. Ting LM, Kim AC, Cattamanchi A, et al. *Mycobacterium tuberculosis* inhibits IFN-gamma transcriptional responses without inhibiting activation of STAT1. J Immunol 1999;163:3898-3906.

79. Clemens DL, Horwitz MA. Membrane sorting during phagocytosis: Selective exclusion of major histocompatibility complex molecules but not complement receptor CR3 during conventional and coiling phagocytosis. J Exp Med 1992;175:1317-1326.

80. Thoma-Uszynski S, Stenger S, Takeuchi O, et al. Induction of direct antimicrobial activity through mammalian toll-like receptors. Science 2001;291:1544-1547.

81. Takeda K, Kaisho T, Akira S. Toll-like receptors. Annu Rev Immunol 2003;21:335-376.

82. Scanga CA, Aliberti J, Jankovic D, et al. Cutting edge: MyD88 is required for resistance to *Toxoplasma gondii* infection and regulates parasite-induced IL-12 production by dendritic cells. J Immunol 2002;168:5997-6001.

83. Chen M, Aosai F, Norose K, et al. Involvement of MyD88 in host defense and the down-regulation of anti-heat shock protein 70 autoantibody formation by MyD88 in *Toxoplasma gondii*-infected mice. J Parasitol 2002;88:1017-1019.

84. Takeuchi O, Hoshino K, Akira S. Cutting edge: TLR2-deficient and MyD88-deficient mice are highly susceptible to *Staphylococcus aureus* infection. J Immunol 2000;165: 5392-5396.

85. Weighardt H, Kaiser-Moore S, Vabulas RM, et al. Cutting edge: Myeloid differentiation factor 88 deficiency improves resistance against sepsis caused by polymicrobial infection. J Immunol 2002;169:2823-2827.

86. Abel B, Thieblemont N, Quesniaux VJ, et al. Toll-like receptor 4 expression is required to control chronic *Mycobacterium tuberculosis* infection in mice. J Immunol 2002;169:3155-3162.

87. Reiling N, Holscher C, Fehrenbach A, et al. Cutting edge: Toll-like receptor (TLR)2- and TLR4-mediated pathogen recognition in resistance to airborne infection with *Mycobacterium tuberculosis*. J Immunol 2002;169:3480-3484.

88. Inohara N, Nunez G. NODs: Intracellular proteins involved in inflammation and apoptosis. Nat Rev Immunol 2003;3:371-382.

89. Girardin SE, Boneca IG, Carneiro LA, et al. Nod1 detects a unique muropeptide from gram-negative bacterial peptidoglycan. Science 2003;300:1584-1587.

90. Ogura Y, Inohara N, Benito A, et al. Nod2, a Nod1/Apaf-1 family member that is restricted to monocytes and activates NF-kappaB. J Biol Chem 2001;276:4812-4818.

91. Ogura Y, Bonen DK, Inohara N, et al. A frameshift mutation in NOD2 associated with susceptibility to Crohn's disease. Nature 2001;411:603-606.

92. Hugot JP, Chamaillard M, Zouali H, et al. Association of NOD2 leucine-rich repeat variants with susceptibility to Crohn's disease. Nature 2001;411:599-603.

93. Dunne DW, Resnick D, Greenberg J, et al. The type I macrophage scavenger receptor binds to gram-positive bacteria and recognizes lipoteichoic acid. Proc Natl Acad Sci U S A 1994;91:1863-1867.

94. Gordon S. Pattern recognition receptors: Doubling up for the innate immune response. Cell 2002;111:927-930.

95. Lee SJ, Zheng NY, Clavijo M, et al. Normal host defense during systemic candidiasis in mannose receptor-deficient mice. Infect Immun 2003;71:437-445.

96. Pasare C, Medzhitov R. Toll pathway-dependent blockade of CD4+CD25+ T cell-mediated suppression by dendritic cells. Science 2003;299:1033-1036.

97. Kang TJ, Chae GT. Detection of Toll-like receptor 2 (TLR2) mutation in the lepromatous leprosy patients. FEMS Immunol Med Microbiol 2001;31:53-58.

98. Bochud PY, Hawn TR, Aderem A. Cutting edge: A toll-like receptor 2 polymorphism that is associated with lepromatous leprosy is unable to mediate mycobacterial signaling. J Immunol 2003;170:3451-3454.

99. Kang TJ, Lee SB, Chae GT. A polymorphism in the toll-like receptor 2 is associated with IL-12 production from monocyte in lepromatous leprosy. Cytokine 2002;20:56-62.

100. Wong P, Pamer EG. CD8 T cell responses to infectious pathogens. Annu Rev Immunol 2003;21:29-70.

101. Raupach B, Kaufmann SH. Immune responses to intracellular bacteria. Curr Opin Immunol 2001;13:417-428.

102. Allen PM, Unanue ER. Antigen processing and presentation at a molecular level. Adv Exp Med Biol 1987;225:147-154.

103. Bastin J, Rothbard J, Davey J, et al. Use of synthetic peptides of influenza nucleoprotein to define epitopes recognized by class I-restricted cytotoxic T lymphocytes. J Exp Med 1987;165:1508-1523.

104. Townsend AR, Rothbard J, Gotch FM, et al. The epitopes of influenza nucleoprotein recognized by cytotoxic T lymphocytes can be defined with short synthetic peptides. Cell 1986;44:959-968.

105. Bjorkman PJ, Strominger JL, Wiley DC. Crystallization and X-ray diffraction studies on the histocompatibility antigens HLA-A2 and HLA-A28 from human cell membranes. J Mol Biol 1985;186:205-210.

106. Bjorkman PJ, Saper MA, Samraoui B, et al. The foreign antigen binding site and T cell recognition regions of class I histocompatibility antigens. Nature 1987;329:512-518.

107. Davis MM, Bjorkman PJ. T-cell antigen receptor genes and T-cell recognition. Nature 1988;334:395-402.

108. Gellert M. V(D)J recombination: RAG proteins, repair factors, and regulation. Annu Rev Biochem 2002;71:101-132.

109. Pamer E, Cresswell P. Mechanisms of MHC class I-restricted antigen processing. Annu Rev Immunol 1998;16:323-358.

110. Wilson IA, Fremont DH. Structural analysis of MHC class I molecules with bound peptide antigens. Semin Immunol 1993;5:75-80.

111. Falk K, Rotzschke O, Stevanovic S, et al. Allele-specific motifs revealed by sequencing of self-peptides eluted from MHC molecules. Nature 1991;351:290-296.

112. Hunt DF, Henderson RA, Shabanowitz J, et al. Characterization of peptides bound to the class I MHC molecule HLA-A2.1 by mass spectrometry. Science 1992;255:1261-1263.

113. Song ES, Yang Y, Jackson MR, Peterson PA. In vivo regulation of the assembly and intracellular transport of class I major histocompatibility complex molecules. J Biol Chem 1994;269:7024-7029.

114. Cresswell P. Assembly, transport, and function of MHC class II molecules. Annu Rev Immunol 1994;12:259-293.

115. Pober JS, Kluger MS, Schechner JS. Human endothelial cell presentation of antigen and the homing of memory/effector T cells to skin. Ann N Y Acad Sci 2001;941:12-25.

116. Ting JP, Trowsdale J. Genetic control of MHC class II expression. Cell 2002;109(Suppl):S21-33.

117. Steimle V, Reith W, Mach B. Major histocompatibility complex class II deficiency: A disease of gene regulation. Adv Immunol 1996;61:327-340.

118. Steimle V, Otten LA, Zufferey M, et al. Complementation cloning of an MHC class II transactivator mutated in hereditary MHC class II deficiency (or bare lymphocyte syndrome). Cell 1993;75:135-146.

119. Stern LJ, Brown JH, Jardetzky TS, et al. Crystal structure of the human class II MHC protein HLA-DR1 complexed with an influenza virus peptide. Nature 1994;368:215-221.

120. Rudensky A, Preston-Hurlburt P, Hong SC, et al. Sequence analysis of peptides bound to MHC class II molecules. Nature 1991;353:622-627.

121. Moore MW, Carbone FR, Bevan MJ. Introduction of soluble protein into the class I pathway of antigen processing and presentation. Cell 1988;54:777-785.

122. Morrison LA, Lukacher AE, Braciale VL, et al. Differences in antigen presentation to MHC class I- and class II-restricted influenza virus-specific cytolytic T lymphocyte clones. J Exp Med 1986;163:903-921.

123. Monaco JJ. A molecular model of MHC class-I-restricted antigen processing. Immunol Today 1992;13:173-179.

124. Goldberg AL, Cascio P, Saric T, et al. The importance of the proteasome and subsequent proteolytic steps in the generation of antigenic peptides. Mol Immunol 2002; 39:147-164.

125. Kloetzel PM. Antigen processing by the proteasome. Nat Rev Mol Cell Biol 2001;2: 179-187.

126. Monaco JJ, Nandi D. The genetics of proteasomes and antigen processing. Annu Rev Genet 1995;29:729-754.

127. Griffin TA, Nandi D, Cruz M, et al. Immunoproteasome assembly: Cooperative incorporation of interferon gamma (IFN-gamma)-inducible subunits. J Exp Med 1998; 187:97-104.

128. Sijts AJ, Pilip I, Pamer EG. The *Listeria monocytogenes*-secreted p60 protein is an N-end rule substrate in the cytosol of infected cells: Implications for major histocompatibility complex class I antigen processing of bacterial proteins. J Biol Chem 1997;272:19261-19268.

129. Decatur AL, Portnoy DA. A PEST-like sequence in listeriolysin O essential for *Listeria monocytogenes* pathogenicity. Science 2000;290:992-995.

130. Dick TP, Ruppert T, Groettrup M, et al. Coordinated dual cleavages induced by the proteasome regulator PA28 lead to dominant MHC ligands. Cell 1996;86:253-262.

131. Androlewicz MJ, Cresswell P. How selective is the transporter associated with antigen processing? Immunity 1996;5:1-5.

132. Androlewicz MJ, Cresswell P. Human transporters associated with antigen processing possess a promiscuous peptide-binding site. Immunity 1994;1:7-14.

133. Van Kaer L, Ashton-Rickardt PG, Ploegh HL, et al. TAP1 mutant mice are deficient in antigen presentation, surface class I molecules, and CD4-8+ T cells. Cell 1992;71:1205-1214.

134. Karttunen JT, Lehner PJ, Gupta SS, et al. Distinct functions and cooperative interaction of the subunits of the transporter associated with antigen processing (TAP). Proc Natl Acad Sci U S A 2001;98:7431-7436.

135. Ortmann B, Androlewicz MJ, Cresswell P. MHC class I/beta 2-microglobulin complexes associate with TAP transporters before peptide binding. Nature 1994;368:864-867.

136. Ortmann B, Copeman J, Lehner PJ, et al. A critical role for tapasin in the assembly and function of multimeric MHC class I-TAP complexes. Science 1997;277:1306-1309.

137. Sadasivan B, Lehner PJ, Ortmann B, et al. Roles for calreticulin and a novel glycoprotein, tapasin, in the interaction of MHC class I molecules with TAP. Immunity 1996;5:103-114.

138. Hughes EA, Cresswell P. The thiol oxidoreductase ERp57 is a component of the MHC class I peptide-loading complex. Curr Biol 1998;8:709-712.

139. Diedrich G, Bangia N, Pan M, et al. A role for calnexin in the assembly of the MHC class I loading complex in the endoplasmic reticulum. J Immunol 2001;166:1703-1709.

140. Shastri N, Schwab S, Serwold T. Producing nature's gene-chips: The generation of peptides for display by MHC class I molecules. Annu Rev Immunol 2002;20:463-493.

141. Serwold T, Gaw S, Shastri N. ER aminopeptidases generate a unique pool of peptides for MHC class I molecules. Nat Immunol 2001;2:644-651.

142. Serwold T, Gonzalez F, Kim J, et al. ERAAP customizes peptides for MHC class I molecules in the endoplasmic reticulum. Nature 2002;419:480-483.

143. Fruh K, Yang Y. Antigen presentation by MHC class I and its regulation by interferon gamma. Curr Opin Immunol 1999;11:76-81.

144. Ustrell V, Realini C, Pratt G, et al. Human lymphoblast and erythrocyte multicatalytic proteases: Differential peptidase activities and responses to the 11S regulator. FEBS Lett 1995;376:155-158.

145. Van Kaer L, Ashton-Rickardt PG, Eichelberger M, et al. Altered peptidase and viral-specific T cell response in LMP2 mutant mice. Immunity 1994;1:533-541.

146. Fehling HJ, Swat W, Laplace C, et al. MHC class I expression in mice lacking the proteasome subunit LMP-7. Science 1994;265:1234-1237.

147. Gray CW, Slaughter CA, DeMartino GN. PA28 activator protein forms regulatory caps on proteasome stacked rings. J Mol Biol 1994;236:7-15.

148. Groettrup M, Soza A, Eggers M, et al. A role for the proteasome regulator PA28alpha in antigen presentation. Nature 1996;381:166-168.

149. Ploegh HL. Viral strategies of immune evasion. Science 1998;280:248-253.

150. York IA, Roop C, Andrews DW, et al. A cytosolic herpes simplex virus protein inhibits antigen presentation to CD8+ T lymphocytes. Cell 1994;77:525-535.

151. Hill A, Jugovic P, York I, et al. Herpes simplex virus turns off the TAP to evade host immunity. Nature 1995;375:411-415.

152. Hengel H, Koopmann JO, Flohr T, et al. A viral ER-resident glycoprotein inactivates the MHC-encoded peptide transporter. Immunity 1997;6:623-632.

153. Ahn K, Gruhler A, Galocha B, et al. The ER-luminal domain of the HCMV glycoprotein US6 inhibits peptide translocation by TAP. Immunity 1997;6:613-621.

154. Ahn K, Angulo A, Ghazal P, et al. Human cytomegalovirus inhibits antigen presentation by a sequential multistep process. Proc Natl Acad Sci U S A 1996;93:10990-10995.

155. Jones TR, Wiertz EJ, Sun L, et al. Human cytomegalovirus US3 impairs transport and maturation of major histocompatibility complex class I heavy chains. Proc Natl Acad Sci U S A 1996;93:11327-11333.

156. Paabo S, Severinsson L, Andersson M, et al. Adenovirus proteins and MHC expression. Adv Cancer Res 1989;52:151-163.

157. Wiertz EJ, Jones TR, Sun L, et al. The human cytomegalovirus US11 gene product dislocates MHC class I heavy chains from the endoplasmic reticulum to the cytosol. Cell 1996;84:769-779.

158. Wiertz EJ, Tortorella D, Bogyo M, et al. Sec61-mediated transfer of a membrane protein from the endoplasmic reticulum to the proteasome for destruction. Nature 1996;384:432-438.

159. Gewurz BE, Gaudet R, Tortorella D, et al. Antigen presentation subverted: Structure of the human cytomegalovirus protein US2 bound to the class I molecule HLA-A2. Proc Natl Acad Sci U S A 2001;98:6794-6799.

160. Coscoy L, Ganem D. Kaposi's sarcoma-associated herpesvirus encodes two proteins that block cell surface display of MHC class I chains by enhancing their endocytosis. Proc Natl Acad Sci U S A 2000;97:8051-8056.

161. Coscoy L, Ganem D. A viral protein that selectively downregulates ICAM-1 and B7-2 and modulates T cell costimulation. J Clin Invest 2001;107:1599-1606.

162. Le Gall S, Erdtmann L, Benichou S, et al. Nef interacts with the mu subunit of clathrin adaptor complexes and reveals a cryptic sorting signal in MHC I molecules. Immunity 1998;8:483-495.

163. Piguet V, Wan L, Borel C, et al. HIV-1 Nef protein binds to the cellular protein PACS-1 to downregulate class I major histocompatibility complexes. Nat Cell Biol 2000;2:163-167.

164. Cohen GB, Gandhi RT, Davis DM, et al. The selective downregulation of class I major histocompatibility complex proteins by HIV-1 protects HIV-infected cells from NK cells. Immunity 1999;10:661-671.

165. Reyburn HT, Mandelboim O, Vales-Gomez M, et al. The class I MHC homologue of human cytomegalovirus inhibits attack by natural killer cells. Nature 1997;386:514-517.

166. Farrell HE, Vally H, Lynch DM, et al. Inhibition of natural killer cells by a cytomegalovirus MHC class I homologue in vivo. Nature 1997;386:510-514.

167. Chapman TL, Heikema AP, West AP Jr, et al. Crystal structure and ligand binding properties of the D1D2 region of the inhibitory receptor LIR-1 (ILT2). Immunity 2000;13:727-736.

168. Sigal LJ, Crotty S, Andino R, et al. Cytotoxic T-cell immunity to virus-infected non-haematopoietic cells requires presentation of exogenous antigen. Nature 1999;398:77-80.

169. Jung S, Unutmaz D, Wong P, et al. In vivo depletion of CD11c(+) dendritic cells abrogates priming of CD8(+) T cells by exogenous cell-associated antigens. Immunity 2002;17:211-220.

170. Shen H, Miller JF, Fan X, et al. Compartmentalization of bacterial antigens: Differential effects on priming of CD8 T cells and protective immunity. Cell 1998;92:535-545.

171. Carbone FR, Bevan MJ. Class I-restricted processing and presentation of exogenous cell-associated antigen in vivo. J Exp Med 1990;171:377-387.

172. Kovacsovics-Bankowski M, Rock KL. A phagosome-to-cytosol pathway for exogenous antigens presented on MHC class I molecules. Science 1995;267:243-246.

173. Hess J, Ladel C, Miko D, et al. *Salmonella typhimurium* aroA-infection in gene-targeted immunodeficient mice: Major role of CD4+ TCR-alpha beta cells and IFN-gamma in bacterial clearance independent of intracellular location. J Immunol 1996;156:3321-3326.

174. Caruso AM, Serbina N, Klein E, et al. Mice deficient in CD4 T cells have only transiently diminished levels of IFN-gamma, yet succumb to tuberculosis. J Immunol 1999;162:5407-5416.

175. Zajac AJ, Blattman JN, Murali-Krishna K, et al. Viral immune evasion due to persistence of activated T cells without effector function. J Exp Med 1998;188:2205-2213.

176. Sepkowitz KA. AIDS—the first 20 years. N Engl J Med 2001;344:1764-1772.

177. Sepkowitz KA. Opportunistic infections in patients with and patients without acquired immunodeficiency syndrome. Clin Infect Dis 2002;34:1098-1107.

178. Bryant PW, Lennon-Dumenil AM, Fiebiger E, et al. Proteolysis and antigen presentation by MHC class II molecules. Adv Immunol 2002;80:71-114.

179. Cresswell P. Invariant chain structure and MHC class II function. Cell 1996;84:505-507.

180. Arunachalam B, Cresswell P. Molecular requirements for the interaction of class II major histocompatibility complex molecules and invariant chain with calnexin. J Biol Chem 1995;270:2784-2790.

181. Nakagawa T, Roth W, Wong P, et al. Cathepsin L: Critical role in Ii degradation and CD4 T cell selection in the thymus. Science 1998;280:450-453.

182. Villadangos JA, Ploegh HL. Proteolysis in MHC class II antigen presentation: Who's in charge? Immunity 2000;12:233-239.

183. Peters PJ, Raposo G, Neefjes JJ, et al. Major histocompatibility complex class II compartments in human B lymphoblastoid cells are distinct from early endosomes. J Exp Med 1995;182:325-334.

184. Pierre P, Denzin LK, Hammond C, et al. HLA-DM is localized to conventional and unconventional MHC class II-containing endocytic compartments. Immunity 1996;4:229-239.

185. Denzin LK, Cresswell P. HLA-DM induces CLIP dissociation from MHC class II alpha beta dimers and facilitates peptide loading. Cell 1995;82:155-165.

186. Maric M, Arunachalam B, Phan UT, et al. Defective antigen processing in GILT-free mice. Science 2001;294:1361-1365.

187. Watts C. Capture and processing of exogenous antigens for presentation on MHC molecules. Annu Rev Immunol 1997;15:821-850.

188. Gadola SD, Zaccai NR, Harlos K, et al. Structure of human CD1b with bound ligands at 2.3 A, a maze for alkyl chains. Nat Immunol 2002;3:721-726.

189. Zeng Z, Castano AR, Segelke BW, et al. Crystal structure of mouse CD1: An MHC-like fold with a large hydrophobic binding groove. Science 1997;277:339-345.

190. Bauer A, Huttinger R, Staffler G, et al. Analysis of the requirement for beta 2-microglobulin for expression and formation of human CD1 antigens. Eur J Immunol 1997;27:1366-1373.

191. Brutkiewicz RR, Bennink JR, Yewdell JW, et al. TAP-independent, beta 2-microglobulin-dependent surface expression of functional mouse CD1.1. J Exp Med 1995;182:1913-1919.

192. Beckman EM, Porcelli SA, Morita CT, et al. Recognition of a lipid antigen by CD1-restricted alpha beta+ T cells. Nature 1994;372:691-694.

193. Sieling PA, Chatterjee D, Porcelli SA, et al. CD1-restricted T cell recognition of microbial lipoglycan antigens. Science 1995;269:227-230.

194. Moody DB, Reinhold BB, Guy MR, et al. Structural requirements for glycolipid antigen recognition by CD1b-restricted T cells. Science 1997;278:283-286.

195. Moody DB, Porcelli SA. Intracellular pathways of CD1 antigen presentation. Nat Rev Immunol 2003;3:11-22.

196. Sugita M, Cao X, Watts GF, et al. Failure of trafficking and antigen presentation by CD1 in AP-3-deficient cells. Immunity 2002;16:697-706.

197. Briken V, Jackman RM, Dasgupta S, et al. Intracellular trafficking pathway of newly synthesized CD1b molecules. EMBO J 2002;21:825-834.

198. Briken V, Jackman RM, Watts GF, et al. Human CD1b and CD1c isoforms survey different intracellular compartments for the presentation of microbial lipid antigens. J Exp Med 2000;192:281-288.

199. Kumar H, Belperron A, Barthold SW, et al. Cutting edge: CD1d deficiency impairs murine host defense against the spirochete, *Borrelia burgdorferi*. J Immunol 2000;165:4797-4801.

200. Baron JL, Gardiner L, Nishimura S, et al. Activation of a nonclassical NKT cell subset in a transgenic mouse model of hepatitis B virus infection. Immunity 2002;16:583-594.

201. Moody DB, Ulrichs T, Muhlecker W, et al. CD1c-mediated T-cell recognition of iso-prenoid glycolipids in *Mycobacterium tuberculosis* infection. Nature 2000;404: 884-888.

202. Sousa AO, Mazzaccaro RJ, Russell RG, et al. Relative contributions of distinct MHC class I-dependent cell populations in protection to tuberculosis infection in mice. Proc Natl Acad Sci U S A 2000;97:4204-4208.

203. Behar SM, Dascher CC, Grusby MJ, et al. Susceptibility of mice deficient in CD1D or TAP1 to infection with *Mycobacterium tuberculosis*. J Exp Med 1999;189: 1973-1980.

204. Szalay G, Zugel U, Ladel CH, et al. Participation of group 2 CD1 molecules in the control of murine tuberculosis. Microbes Infect 1999;1:1153-1157.

205. Sieling PA, Jullien D, Dahlem M, et al. CD1 expression by dendritic cells in human lep-rosy lesions: Correlation with effective host immunity. J Immunol 1999;162:1851-1858.

206. Chackerian A, Alt J, Perera V, et al. Activation of NKT cells protects mice from tu-berculosis. Infect Immun 2002;70:6302-6309.

207. Kawakami K, Kinjo Y, Yara S, et al. Activation of Valpha14(+) natural killer T cells by alpha-galactosylceramide results in development of Th1 response and local host resistance in mice infected with *Cryptococcus neoformans*. Infect Immun 2001;69:213-220.

208. Duthie MS, Wleklinski-Lee M, Smith S, et al. During *Trypanosoma cruzi* infection CD1d-restricted NK T cells limit parasitemia and augment the antibody response to a glycophosphoinositol-modified surface protein. Infect Immun 2002;70:36-48.

209. Kronenberg M, Gapin L. The unconventional lifestyle of NKT cells. Nat Rev Immunol 2002;2:557-568.

210. Little AM, Parham P. Polymorphism and evolution of HLA class I and II genes and molecules. Rev Immunogenet 1999;1:105-123.

211. Parham P, Adams EJ, Arnett KL. The origins of HLA-A,B,C polymorphism. Immunol Rev 1995;143:141-180.

212. Adams EJ, Parham P. Species-specific evolution of MHC class I genes in the higher primates. Immunol Rev 2001;183:41-64.

213. Cooke GS, Hill AV. Genetics of susceptibility to human infectious disease. Nat Rev Genet 2001;2:967-977.

214. Hill AV, Allsopp CE, Kwiatkowski D, et al. Common west African HLA antigens are associated with protection from severe malaria. Nature 1991;352:595-600.

215. Plebanski M, Lee EA, Hannan CM, et al. Altered peptide ligands narrow the reper-toire of cellular immune responses by interfering with T-cell priming. Nat Med 1999;5:565-571.

216. Pircher H, Moskophidis D, Rohrer U, et al. Viral escape by selection of cytotoxic T cell-resistant virus variants in vivo. Nature 1990;346:629-633.

217. Ciurea A, Hunziker L, Martinic MM, et al. CD4+ T-cell-epitope escape mutant virus selected in vivo. Nat Med 2001;7:795-800.

218. Goulder PJ, Brander C, Tang Y, et al. Evolution and transmission of stable CTL es-cape mutations in HIV infection. Nature 2001;412:334-338.

219. Hunt JS, Petroff MG, Morales P, et al. HLA-G in reproduction: Studies on the maternal-fetal interface. Hum Immunol 2000;61:1113-1117.

220. Braud VM, Allan DS, O'Callaghan CA, et al. HLA-E binds to natural killer cell re-ceptors CD94/NKG2A, B and C. Nature 1998;391:795-799.

221. Heinzel AS, Grotzke JE, Lines RA, et al. HLA-E-dependent presentation of Mtb-derived antigen to human CD8+ T cells. J Exp Med 2002;196:1473-1481.

222. Weiss EH, Golden L, Fahrner K, et al. Organization and evolution of the class I gene family in the major histocompatibility complex of the C57BL/10 mouse. Nature 1984;310:650-655.

223. Steinmetz M, Minard K, Horvath S, et al. A molecular map of the immune response re-gion from the major histocompatibility complex of the mouse. Nature 1982;300:35-42.

224. Pamer EG, Wang CR, Flaherty L, et al. H-2M3 presents a *Listeria monocytogenes* peptide to cytotoxic T lymphocytes. Cell 1992;70:215-223.

225. Kurlander RJ, Shawar SM, Brown ML, et al. Specialized role for a murine class I-b MHC molecule in prokaryotic host defenses. Science 1992;257:678-679.

226. Wang CR, Castano AR, Peterson PA, et al. Nonclassical binding of formylated pep-tide in crystal structure of the MHC class Ib molecule H2-M3. Cell 1995;82:655-664.

227. Shawar SM, Cook RG, Rodgers JR, et al. Specialized functions of MHC class I mol-ecules: I. An N-formyl peptide receptor is required for construction of the class I anti-gen Mta. J Exp Med 1990;171:897-912.

228. Kerksiek KM, Busch DH, Pilip IM, et al. H2-M3-restricted T cells in bacterial infec-tion: Rapid primary but diminished memory responses. J Exp Med 1999;190:195-204.

229. Lo WF, Ong H, Metcalf ES, et al. T cell responses to Gram-negative intracellular bac-terial pathogens: A role for CD8+ T cells in immunity to *Salmonella* infection and the involvement of MHC class Ib molecules. J Immunol 1999;162:5398-5406.

230. Lo WF, Woods AS, DeCloux A, et al. Molecular mimicry mediated by MHC class Ib molecules after infection with gram-negative pathogens. Nat Med 2000;6:215-218.

231. Soloski MJ, Metcalf ES. The involvement of class Ib molecules in the host response to infection with *Salmonella* and its relevance to autoimmunity. Microbes Infect 2001;3:1249-1259.

232. Starr TK, Jameson SC, Hogquist KA. Positive and negative selection of T cells. Annu Rev Immunol 2003;21:139-176.

233. Fugmann SD, Lee AI, Shockett PE, et al. The RAG proteins and V(D)J recombina-tion: Complexes, ends, and transposition. Annu Rev Immunol 2000;18:495-527.

234. von Boehmer H, Aifantis I, Azogui O, et al. The impact of pre-T-cell receptor signals on gene expression in developing T cells. Cold Spring Harb Symp Quant Biol 1999;64:283-289.

235. Aifantis I, Azogui O, Feinberg J, et al. On the role of the pre-T cell receptor in al-phabeta versus gammadelta T lineage commitment. Immunity 1998;9:649-655.

236. Goldrath AW, Bevan MJ. Selecting and maintaining a diverse T-cell repertoire. Nature 1999;402:255-262.

237. Hogquist KA, Jameson SC, Heath WR, et al. T cell receptor antagonist peptides in-duce positive selection. Cell 1994;76:17-27.

238. Anderson MS, Venanzi ES, Klein L, et al. Projection of an immunological self shadow within the thymus by the aire protein. Science 2002;298:1395-1401.

239. Sallusto F, Lenig D, Mackay CR, et al. Flexible programs of chemokine receptor ex-pression on human polarized T helper 1 and 2 lymphocytes. J Exp Med 1998;187:875-883.

240. Arstila TP, Casrouge A, Baron V, et al. A direct estimate of the human alphabeta T cell receptor diversity. Science 1999;286:958-961.

241. Perez E, Sullivan KE. Chromosome 22q11.2 deletion syndrome (DiGeorge and velo-cardiofacial syndromes). Curr Opin Pediatr 2002;14:678-683.

242. Bonilla FA, Geha RS. 12. Primary immunodeficiency diseases. J Allergy Clin Immunol 2003;111(2 Suppl):S571-581.

243. Jamieson BD, Douek DC, Killian S, et al. Generation of functional thymocytes in the human adult. Immunity 1999;10:569-575.

244. Lewin SR, Heller G, Zhang L, et al. Direct evidence for new T-cell generation by pa-tients after either T-cell-depleted or unmodified allogeneic hematopoietic stem cell transplantations. Blood 2002;100:2235-2242.

245. Su L, Kaneshima H, Bonyhadi M, et al. HIV-1-induced thymocyte depletion is asso-ciated with indirect cytopathogenicity and infection of progenitor cells in vivo. Immunity 1995;2:25-36.

246. Sempowski GD, Haynes BF. Immune reconstitution in patients with HIV infection. Annu Rev Med 2002;53:269-284.

247. Diaz M, Douek DC, Valdez H, et al. T cells containing T cell receptor excision cir-cles are inversely related to HIV replication and are selectively and rapidly released into circulation with antiretroviral treatment. AIDS 2003;17:1145-1149.

248. Chambers CA, Allison JP. Costimulatory regulation of T cell function. Curr Opin Cell Biol 1999;11:203-210.

249. Lenschow DJ, Walunas TL, Bluestone JA. CD28/B7 system of T cell costimulation. Annu Rev Immunol 1996;14:233-258.

250. Liang L, Sha WC. The right place at the right time: Novel B7 family members regu-late effector T cell responses. Curr Opin Immunol 2002;14:384-390.

251. Tafuri A, Shahinian A, Bladt F, et al. ICOS is essential for effective T-helper-cell re-sponses. Nature 2001;409:105-109.

252. McAdam AJ, Greenwald RJ, Levin MA, et al. ICOS is critical for CD40-mediated an-tibody class switching. Nature 2001;409:102-105.

253. Dong C, Temann UA, Flavell RA. Cutting edge: Critical role of inducible costimula-tor in germinal center reactions. J Immunol 2001;166:3659-3662.

254. Locksley RM, Killeen N, Lenardo MJ. The TNF and TNF receptor superfamilies: Integrating mammalian biology. Cell 2001;104:487-501.

255. Allen RC, Armitage RJ, Conley ME, et al. CD40 ligand gene defects responsible for X-linked hyper-IgM syndrome. Science 1993;259:990-993.

256. DiSanto JP, Bonnefoy JY, Gauchat JF, et al. CD40 ligand mutations in x-linked im-munodeficiency with hyper-IgM. Nature 1993;361:541-543.

257. Aruffo A, Farrington M, Hollenbaugh D, et al. The CD40 ligand, gp39, is defective in activated T cells from patients with X-linked hyper-IgM syndrome. Cell 1993;72:291-300.

258. Bourgeois C, Rocha B, Tanchot C. A role for CD40 expression on CD8+ T cells in the generation of CD8+ T cell memory. Science 2002;297:2060-2063.

259. Bertram EM, Lau P, Watts TH. Temporal segregation of 4-1BB versus CD28-mediated costimulation: 4-1BB ligand influences T cell numbers late in the primary response and regulates the size of the T cell memory response following influenza infection. J Immunol 2002;168:3777-3785.

260. Halstead ES, Mueller YM, Altman JD, et al. In vivo stimulation of CD137 broadens primary antiviral CD8+ T cell responses. Nat Immunol 2002;3:536-541.

261. Weinberg AD, Vella AT, Croft M. OX-40: Life beyond the effector T cell stage. Semin Immunol 1998;10:471-480.

262. Dustin ML. Coordination of T cell activation and migration through formation of the immunological synapse. Ann N Y Acad Sci 2003;987:51-59.

263. Dustin ML, Colman DR. Neural and immunological synaptic relations. Science 2002;298:785-789.

264. Arendt CW, Albrecht B, Soos TJ, et al. Protein kinase C-theta: Signaling from the center of the T-cell synapse. Curr Opin Immunol 2002;14:323-330.

265. Mellman I, Steinman RM. Dendritic cells: Specialized and regulated antigen pro-cessing machines. Cell 2001;106:255-258.

266. Shortman K, Liu YJ. Mouse and human dendritic cell subtypes. Nat Rev Immunol 2002;2:151-161.

267. Kadowaki N, Ho S, Antonenko S, et al. Subsets of human dendritic cell precursors express different toll-like receptors and respond to different microbial antigens. J Exp Med 2001;194:863-869.

268. Jarrossay D, Napolitani G, Colonna M, et al. Specialization and complementarity in microbial molecule recognition by human myeloid and plasmacytoid dendritic cells. Eur J Immunol 2001;31:3388-3393.

269. O'Keeffe M, Hochrein H, Vremec D, et al. Mouse plasmacytoid cells: Long-lived cells, heterogeneous in surface phenotype and function, that differentiate into CD8(+) dendritic cells only after microbial stimulus. J Exp Med 2002;196:1307-1319.

270. Cella M, Facchetti F, Lanzavecchia A, et al. Plasmacytoid dendritic cells activated by influenza virus and CD40L drive a potent TH1 polarization. Nat Immunol 2000;1: 305-310.

271. Schakel K, Kannagi R, Kniep B, et al. 6-Sulfo LacNAc, a novel carbohydrate modi-fication of PSGL-1, defines an inflammatory type of human dendritic cells. Immunity 2002;17:289-301.

272. Gantner BN, Simmons RM, Canavera SJ, et al. Collaborative induction of inflamma-tory responses by dectin-1 and Toll-like receptor 2. J Exp Med 2003;197:1107-1117.

273. Brown GD, Herre J, Williams DL, et al. Dectin-1 mediates the biological effects of beta-glucans. J Exp Med 2003;197:1119-1124.

274. Robbiani DF, Finch RA, Jager D, et al. The leukotriene C(4) transporter MRP1 regulates CCL19 (MIP-3beta, ELC)-dependent mobilization of dendritic cells to lymph nodes. Cell 2000;103:757-768.

275. Reis e Sousa C, Hieny S, Scharton-Kersten T, et al. In vivo microbial stimulation induces rapid CD40 ligand-independent production of interleukin 12 by dendritic cells and their redistribution to T cell areas. J Exp Med 1997;186:1819-1829.

276. Reis e Sousa C, Yap G, Schulz O, et al. Paralysis of dendritic cell IL-12 production by microbial products prevents infection-induced immunopathology. Immunity 1999;11:637-647.

277. Aliberti J, Hieny S, Reis e Sousa C, et al. Lipoxin-mediated inhibition of IL-12 production by DCs: A mechanism for regulation of microbial immunity. Nat Immunol 2002;3:76-82.

278. Aliberti J, Reis e Sousa C, Schito M, et al. CCR5 provides a signal for microbial induced production of IL-12 by CD8 alpha+ dendritic cells. Nat Immunol 2000;1:83-87.

279. Aliberti J, Valenzuela JG, Carruthers VB, et al. Molecular mimicry of a CCR5 binding-domain in the microbial activation of dendritic cells. Nat Immunol 2003;4:485-490.

280. Blattman JN, Antia R, Sourdive DJ, et al. Estimating the precursor frequency of naive antigen-specific CD8 T cells. J Exp Med 2002;195:657-664.

281. Harty JT, Tvinnereim AR, White DW. CD8+ T cell effector mechanisms in resistance to infection. Annu Rev Immunol 2000;18:275-308.

282. Schluns KS, Kieper WC, Jameson SC, et al. Interleukin-7 mediates the homeostasis of naive and memory CD8 T cells in vivo. Nat Immunol 2000;1:426-432.

283. Mercado R, Vijh S, Allen SE, et al. Early programming of T cell populations responding to bacterial infection. J Immunol 2000;165:6833-6839.

284. Kaech SM, Ahmed R. Memory CD8+ T cell differentiation: Initial antigen encounter triggers a developmental program in naive cells. Nat Immunol 2001;2:415-422.

285. Badovinac VP, Porter BB, Harty JT. Programmed contraction of CD8(+) T cells after infection. Nat Immunol 2002;3:619-626.

286. Kaech SM, Hemby S, Kersh E, et al. Molecular and functional profiling of memory CD8 T cell differentiation. Cell 2002;111:837-851.

287. Roman E, Miller E, Harmsen A, et al. CD4 effector T cell subsets in the response to influenza: Heterogeneity, migration, and function. J Exp Med 2002;196:957-968.

288. Stetson DB, Mohrs M, Mallet-Designe V, et al. Rapid expansion and IL-4 expression by *Leishmania*-specific naive helper T cells in vivo. Immunity 2002;17:191-200.

289. Homann D, Teyton L, Oldstone MB. Differential regulation of antiviral T-cell immunity results in stable CD8+ but declining CD4+ T-cell memory. Nat Med 2001;7:913-919.

290. Kaufmann SH. Immunity to intracellular microbial pathogens. Immunol Today 1995;16:338-342.

291. Szabo SJ, Sullivan BM, Peng SL, et al. Molecular mechanisms regulating Th1 immune responses. Annu Rev Immunol 2003;21:713-758.

292. Finkelman FD, Wynn TA, Donaldson DD, et al. The role of IL-13 in helminth-induced inflammation and protective immunity against nematode infections. Curr Opin Immunol 1999;11:420-426.

293. Zheng W, Flavell RA. The transcription factor GATA-3 is necessary and sufficient for Th2 cytokine gene expression in CD4 T cells. Cell 1997;89:587-596.

294. Finotto S, Neurath MF, Glickman JN, et al. Development of spontaneous airway changes consistent with human asthma in mice lacking T-bet. Science 2002;295:336-338.

295. Murphy KM, Reiner SL. The lineage decisions of helper T cells. Nat Rev Immunol 2002;2:933-944.

296. Barton GM, Medzhitov R. Control of adaptive immune responses by Toll-like receptors. Curr Opin Immunol 2002;14:380-383.

297. Bird JJ, Brown DR, Mullen AC, et al. Helper T cell differentiation is controlled by the cell cycle. Immunity 1998;9:229-237.

298. Lee DU, Agarwal S, Rao A. Th2 lineage commitment and efficient IL-4 production involves extended demethylation of the IL-4 gene. Immunity 2002;16:649-660.

299. Sacks D, Noben-Trauth N. The immunology of susceptibility and resistance to *Leishmania major* in mice. Nat Rev Immunol 2002;2:845-858.

300. Julia V, Rassoulzadegan M, Glaichenhaus N. Resistance to *Leishmania major* induced by tolerance to a single antigen. Science 1996;274:421-423.

301. Swain SL, Hu H, Huston G. Class II-independent generation of CD4 memory T cells from effectors. Science 1999;286:1381-1383.

302. Constant S, Pfeiffer C, Woodard A, et al. Extent of T cell receptor ligation can determine the functional differentiation of naive CD4+ T cells. J Exp Med 1995;182:1591-1596.

303. Kagi D, Seiler P, Pavlovic J, et al. The roles of perforin- and Fas-dependent cytotoxicity in protection against cytopathic and noncytopathic viruses. Eur J Immunol 1995;25:3256-3262.

304. Lowin B, Peitsch MC, Tschopp J. Perforin and granzymes: Crucial effector molecules in cytolytic T lymphocyte and natural killer cell-mediated cytotoxicity. Curr Top Microbiol Immunol 1995;198:1-24.

305. Stenger S, Hanson DA, Teitelbaum R, et al. An antimicrobial activity of cytolytic T cells mediated by granulysin. Science 1998;282:121-125.

306. Ochoa MT, Stenger S, Sieling PA, et al. T-cell release of granulysin contributes to host defense in leprosy. Nat Med 2001;7:174-179.

307. Wagner L, Yang OO, Garcia-Zepeda EA, et al. Beta-chemokines are released from HIV-1-specific cytolytic T-cell granules complexed to proteoglycans. Nature 1998;391:908-911.

308. Ahmed R, Gray D. Immunological memory and protective immunity: Understanding their relation. Science 1996;272:54-60.

309. Murali-Krishna K, Lau LL, Sambhara S, et al. Persistence of memory CD8 T cells in MHC class I-deficient mice. Science 1999;286:1377-1381.

310. Becker TC, Wherry EJ, Boone D, et al. Interleukin 15 is required for proliferative renewal of virus-specific memory CD8 T cells. J Exp Med 2002;195:1541-1548.

311. Goldrath AW, Sivakumar PV, Glaccum M, et al. Cytokine requirements for acute and basal homeostatic proliferation of naive and memory CD8+ T cells. J Exp Med 2002;195:1515-1522.

312. Schluns KS, Williams K, Ma A, et al. Cutting edge: Requirement for IL-15 in the generation of primary and memory antigen-specific CD8 T cells. J Immunol 2002;168:4827-4831.

313. Busch DH, Pilip I, Pamer EG. Evolution of a complex T cell receptor repertoire during primary and recall bacterial infection. J Exp Med 1998;188:61-70.

314. Jacob J, Baltimore D. Modelling T-cell memory by genetic marking of memory T cells in vivo. Nature 1999;399:593-597.

315. Busch DH, Kerksiek KM, Pamer EG. Differing roles of inflammation and antigen in T cell proliferation and memory generation. J Immunol 2000;164:4063-4070.

316. Bennett SR, Carbone FR, Karamalis F, et al. Help for cytotoxic-T-cell responses is mediated by CD40 signalling. Nature 1998;393:478-480.

317. Schoenberger SP, Toes RE, van der Voort EI, et al. T-cell help for cytotoxic T lymphocytes is mediated by CD40-CD40L interactions. Nature 1998;393:480-483.

318. Ridge JP, Di Rosa F, Matzinger P. A conditioned dendritic cell can be a temporal bridge between a CD4+ T-helper and a T-killer cell. Nature 1998;393:474-478.

319. Sun JC, Bevan MJ. Defective CD8 T cell memory following acute infection without CD4 T cell help. Science 2003;300:339-342.

320. Shedlock DJ, Shen H. Requirement for CD4 T cell help in generating functional CD8 T cell memory. Science 2003;300:337-339.

321. Janssen EM, Lemmens EE, Wolfe T, et al. CD4+ T cells are required for secondary expansion and memory in CD8+ T lymphocytes. Nature 2003;421:852-856.

322. Sallusto F, Lenig D, Forster R, et al. Two subsets of memory T lymphocytes with distinct homing potentials and effector functions. Nature 1999;401:708-712.

323. Appay V, Dunbar PR, Callan M, et al. Memory CD8+ T cells vary in differentiation phenotype in different persistent virus infections. Nat Med 2002;8:379-385.

324. Gershon RK, Kondo K. Cell interactions in the induction of tolerance: The role of thymic lymphocytes. Immunology 1970;18:723-737.

325. Shevach EM. CD4+ CD25+ suppressor T cells: More questions than answers. Nat Rev Immunol 2002;2:389-400.

326. Sakaguchi S, Sakaguchi N, Asano M, et al. Immunologic self-tolerance maintained by activated T cells expressing IL-2 receptor alpha-chains (CD25): Breakdown of a single mechanism of self-tolerance causes various autoimmune diseases. J Immunol 1995;155:1151-1164.

327. Fontenot JD, Gavin MA, Rudensky AY. Foxp3 programs the development and function of CD4+CD25+ regulatory T cells. Nat Immunol 2003;4:330-336.

328. Yokoyama WM, Plougastel BF. Immune functions encoded by the natural killer gene complex. Nat Rev Immunol 2003;3:304-316.

329. Cerwenka A, Lanier LL. Ligands for natural killer cell receptors: Redundancy or specificity. Immunol Rev 2001;181:158-169.

330. Natarajan K, Dimasi N, Wang J, et al. Structure and function of natural killer cell receptors: Multiple molecular solutions to self, nonself discrimination. Annu Rev Immunol 2002;20:853-885.

331. Biron CA, Byron KS, Sullivan JL. Severe herpesvirus infections in an adolescent without natural killer cells. N Engl J Med 1989;320:1731-1735.

332. Arase H, Mocarski ES, Campbell AE, et al. Direct recognition of cytomegalovirus by activating and inhibitory NK cell receptors. Science 2002;296:1323-1326.

333. Brown MG, Dokun AO, Heusel JW, et al. Vital involvement of a natural killer cell activation receptor in resistance to viral infection. Science 2001;292:934-937.

334. Biron CA, Brossay L. NK cells and NKT cells in innate defense against viral infections. Curr Opin Immunol 2001;13:458-464.

CHAPTER **10**

Nutrition, Immunity, and Infection

CARYN GEE MORSE

KEVIN P. HIGH

Although the effects of malnutrition are recorded throughout human history, the links between nutrition, immunity, and resistance to infection have only begun to be explored in a scientific fashion during the past half-century.[1] This relationship was first identified in the developing world, where great obstacles may exist in merely obtaining sufficient calories or protein. As understanding of the influence of specific micronutrients on immune responses has evolved, it has become clear that specific populations are at risk for malnutrition-induced immune dysfunction, even in industrialized nations where protein-calorie malnutrition is rare. Recent studies even suggest that malnutrition influences not only immune function but also virulence of infectious agents, progression of chronic infections such as human immunodeficiency virus

(HIV), and transcriptional regulation of inflammatory genes that may determine the outcome of sepsis.[1] This chapter explores these relationships pertinent to the understanding and practice of infectious diseases.

EPIDEMIOLOGY OF MALNUTRITION AND CLINICAL RELEVANCE

The World Health Organization (WHO) estimates that more than 30% of residents in developing nations are affected by hunger and malnutrition. Protein-energy malnutrition (PEM) is cited as the primary cause of immunodeficiency worldwide, with infants, children, adolescents, and elderly people being most affected. According to WHO, in 1995 nearly 50% of the 10.7 million deaths among children younger than the age of 5 were associated with malnutrition. PEM affects more than 25% of children worldwide, with an estimated 150 million children considered underweight and 182 million experiencing growth retardation. Geographically, 70% of children with PEM reside in Asia, another 26% in Africa, and approximately 4% in Latin America and the Caribbean.

Whereas the incidence of overt hunger and malnutrition is highest in developing nations, vulnerable populations in more affluent societies are also affected by malnutrition. At-risk populations include children, the elderly, pregnant women, homeless people, alcohol abusers, persons affected by acute and chronic illnesses including HIV/acquired immunodeficiency syndrome (AIDS) and end-stage renal disease, and those under self-imposed dietary restriction such as persons with anorexia nervosa or bulimia and consumers of vegetarian diets.

Malnutrition can be broadly defined as a decrease in nutrient reserve. Under this definition undernutrition is prevalent even in the United States, affecting up to 15% of ambulatory outpatients,[2] 25% to 60% of long-term care patients,[3] and 35% to 65% of hospitalized patients.[4,5] Malnutrition is associated with an increased risk of infection,[6] respiratory and cardiac illness,[7,8] venous thromboembolic disease, pressure ulcers,[9] perioperative mortality, and multisystem organ failure.[7,8]

In contrast with the extensive morbidity and mortality associations documented with undernutrition, the epidemic of obesity now affecting children, adolescents, and up to half of adults residing in some industrialized nations is poorly studied with regard to infection. Diet and obesity have been linked to increasing rates of diabetes mellitus; cardiovascular diseases, including coronary artery disease; stroke; gastrointestinal (GI) disorders; cancer; and arthritis. Obesity and the increase in chronic diseases are not limited to the developed world. In five out of six WHO regions, deaths caused by chronic diseases dominate mortality statistics, and nearly 80% of all deaths worldwide attributable to chronic diseases occur in the developing world.[10]

The National Research Council (NRC) recommends daily allowances for protein, vitamins, and minerals for healthy adults, specifying ranges for both men and women.[11]

NUTRITIONAL ASSESSMENT AND DIAGNOSIS OF MALNUTRITION

Whereas no integrated standard exists to diagnose malnutrition, a number of different approaches to nutritional screening and assessment have been described. The nutritional evaluation begins with a

TABLE 10-1 Classification of Overall Nutritional Status by Body Mass Index

Body Mass Index (kg/m²)	Overall Nutritional Status
<16	Severely malnourished
16-16.9	Moderately malnourished
17-18.4	Mildly malnourished
18.5-24.9	Normal nutritional status
25-29.9	Overweight
30-34.9	Obese (class I)
35-39.9	Obese (class II)
≥40	Obese (class III)

Adapted with permission from Feldman M, Friedman LS, Sleisenger MH. Sleisenger & Fordtran's Gastrointestinal and Liver Disease. 7th ed. Philadelphia: Elsevier; 2002:123.

TABLE 10-2 Visceral and Somatic Protein Assays in Clinical Use for Nutritional Assessment

Nutritional Level	Albumin (g/dL)	Prealbumin (mg/dL)	Transferrin (mg/dL)	Urinary Creatinine Excretion (%)
Half-life in serum	20 days	2 days	8-10 days	NA
Normal	3.5-5.5	15.7-29.6	250-300	>90
Mild depletion	2.8-3.5	10-15	150-250	80-90
Moderate depletion	2.1-2.7	5-10	100-150	60-80
Severe depletion	<2.1	<100	<5	<60

Adapted with permission from Katz DL. Malnutrition and cachexia. In: Katz DL, ed. Nutrition in Clinical Practice. Philadelphia: Lippincott Williams & Wilkins; 2001:188.

comprehensive history and physical examination followed by an evaluation of dietary intake, measurements of body composition, and a metabolic assessment that includes laboratory parameters and markers of immune function (Table 10-1).

Several biochemical markers of nutritional status can give a general indication of nutritional reserve.[12] Assessment of visceral proteins includes albumin, prealbumin, and transferrin. Albumin is most commonly used to assess visceral protein status, although its use in the assessment of acute malnutrition is limited by its prolonged half-life. Albumin levels are also subject to rapid declines in times of physiologic stress, including septic shock and other acute illness states. Prealbumin has a shorter half-life and is used more commonly to assess acute nutritional deficiencies. Like albumin, prealbumin is also subject to rapid drops in acute illness. Transferrin has an intermediate half-life and can be used instead of albumin when acute malnutrition is being assessed. Decreases in markers of visceral protein status are not specific and may have other etiologies, including hepatic disease and increased capillary permeability. Somatic protein status, indicating muscle mass and condition, can be measured using 24-hour urinary creatinine excretion (Table 10-2).[13]

Global indicators of cell-mediated immune function are commonly employed to assess malnutrition and can be estimated by total lymphocyte count (TLC) and delayed-type hypersensitivity testing with a series of common antigens. Compromise of cell-mediated immunity (CMI) due to malnutrition is suggested by a TLC of 1000/mm³ or the lack of skin test induration greater than 5 mm above glycerin control at 48 hours, unless another cause of lymphocyte dysfunction is present.[12] However, these tests should be interpreted cautiously during an acute illness that may depress CMI in the absence of malnutrition.

PROTEIN-ENERGY MALNUTRITION AND IMMUNE FUNCTION

Normal nutritional status represents a balance between nutrient requirements and nutrient intake. Malnutrition can be caused by specific nutrient deficiencies or more commonly overall deficiency of protein and energy. PEM has been used to describe nutritional macrodeficiency syndromes, including marasmus (deficiency of calories), kwashiorkor (deficiency of protein), nutritional dwarfism in children, and wasting syndromes in adults.

Primary PEM is caused by inadequate nutrient intake and typically affects children and elderly people. The functional and structural abnormalities associated with primary PEM are often reversible with nutritional therapy. However, prolonged primary PEM can result in serious and irreversible changes in organ function and growth. Secondary PEM is the result of illnesses, injuries, or treatments that alter appetite, digestion, absorption, or metabolism. The major causes of secondary PEM include disorders that affect GI tract function, wasting disorders, and critical illness. Although the nutritional deficits of patients with PEM due to GI tract dysfunction often can be restored to normal if adequate nutritional support can be provided by dietary supplements, enteral tube feeding, or parenteral nutrition, wasting disorders such as cancer or AIDS are characterized by involuntary weight loss often despite increased caloric intake. In wasting diseases, alterations in metabolism are responsible for a greater loss of muscle tissue than would be expected from reductions of caloric intake alone, and restoration of muscle mass by nutritional supplementation is unlikely unless the underlying inflammatory disease is treated. In addition, weight gain that occurs as a result of nutritional support in those syndromes is usually caused by increases in fat mass and body water without significant changes in lean tissue.

PEM has been associated with a number of impairments in the immune response.[14] Documented abnormalities of innate immunity include reduced production of cytokines, reduced phagocytosis, interruptions in the integrity of physical barriers and diminished quality of mucus, and reductions in complement (C3 and C5).[15-17] Alterations in adaptive immunity include reduced or delayed cutaneous hypersensitivity to recall and new antigens, reductions in CD4+ and CD8+ T-cell subsets, CD4+/CD8+ ratio, lymphocyte proliferative capacity, and reductions in immunoglobulin G (IgG) and secretory IgA.[15,18] In addition, malnourished children and elderly adults demonstrate elevated baseline biomarkers of inflammation such as interleukin-6 (IL-6).[18,19]

SPECIFIC NUTRIENTS AND THEIR ROLE IN IMMUNITY

Fat-Soluble Vitamins

Vitamin A. Vitamin A deficiency is the leading cause of preventable blindness in children and raises the risk of disease and death from severe infections. WHO estimates that 100 to 140 million children are vitamin A deficient.[20]

Vitamin A is a subclass of the retinoic acids, a family of lipid-soluble compounds that include retinols, β-carotenes, and other carotenoids. Retinol, or preformed vitamin A, is the most active form and is mostly found in animal food sources or can be synthesized from carotenoids. The major functions of vitamin A are in vision, cell differentiation, and tissue growth. The important role of vitamin A in immune system function is well established, and several excellent and comprehensive reviews are available.[21,22] Vitamin A deficiency can affect host immunity through direct actions on immune cell function and indirect effects on epithelial cell differentiation and thereby host barrier defenses. Vitamin A plays a pivotal role in the differentiation and maturation of epithelial cells through the regulation of keratin synthesis.[23] Vitamin A deficiency results in squamous metaplasia and reductions in the number of mucus secreting cells. Rapidly dividing epithelial cells on the mucosal surfaces of the lung and gut are especially susceptible to the effects of vitamin A deficiency, and interruptions in the integrity of these surfaces allow increased bacterial translocation and may increase risk of infection.[24]

Vitamin A deficiency results in reduced mitogen-stimulated T-cell proliferation and antigen-specific IgA and IgG production, impairs the ability of CD4+ T lymphocytes to stimulate Th2 responses (B-cell antigen-specific IgG1 responses), and limits the ability of neutrophils to phagocytose bacterial pathogens.[21,22,25]

The effect of vitamin A supplementation on human immune responses has been examined in a number of randomized, double-blind placebo-controlled trials of undernourished and malnourished children in developing nations. Antibody-mediated responses are impaired in individuals with vitamin A deficiency,[26] and supplementation has been demonstrated to improve antibody titer responses to measles vaccine, sustain gut integrity,[24] and lower the incidence of respiratory tract infections in some studies but not in others.[27-29] Supplemental vitamin A has also been associated with reduced mortality from measles and diarrhea[27,29,30] but not pneumonia.[28,30] Additional studies in HIV-positive persons has suggested an association between vitamin A deficiency and increased mortality, disease progression,[31] and vertical transmission of HIV.[32,33]

In light of these trials and others demonstrating beneficial effects of vitamin A supplementation on immune function and its efficacy in preventing infection, WHO recommends vitamin A supplementation be provided to all at-risk people, primarily children and women of childbearing age residing in developing nations, even in the absence of signs and symptoms of deficiency. Implementation of this program has been one of the great WHO success stories.[20,30,34]

Vitamin A can also be used therapeutically after the onset of some viral illnesses. The prototypical example here is that of measles virus. Epidemiologic studies suggest more than half of well-nourished measles victims in developed countries will have low serum vitamin A levels despite adequate body stores.[35] Brief, high-dose vitamin A supplementation has been shown in several trials to reduce morbidity and mortality in measles.[30,36,37] Although there is little debate regarding the efficacy of vitamin A in populations at high risk for vitamin A deficiency, some have questioned whether vitamin A therapy offers any advantage in developed countries where retinol deficiency is uncommon. The rarity of rubeola infection in the developed world suggests this debate will not be settled soon. However, similar trials in related Paramyxoviridae infections (e.g., respiratory syncytial virus [RSV]) have provided mixed results. Some demonstrate benefit, particularly in those with severe disease,[38,39] whereas others found no benefit or even potential harm.[40] Further, excess of vitamin A may produce acute toxic manifestations (headache, vomiting, stupor, and papilledema). Chronic toxicity is associated with weight loss, nausea, and vomiting; dryness of the mucosa of the lips; bone and joint pain; hyperostosis; and hepatomegaly with parenchymal damage and fibrosis. Additionally, in the 1990s two large trials evaluating the role of β-carotene in lung cancer prevention observed an increased risk of lung cancer in subjects receiving β-carotene.[41,42] While the increased cancer risk occurred in smokers receiving β-carotene, the reasons for these findings remain unclear and emphasize the need for further study on the role of retinoids in human health and immunity, before widespread supplementation with retinoid precursors can be recommended in well-nourished populations.

Vitamin E. A group of eight closely related fat-soluble compounds—four tocopherols and four tocotrienols—all exhibit vitamin E biologic activity, but α-tocopherol is the most active, abundant in many foods and most widely available as a supplement. An essential nutrient, vitamin E is one of a group of antioxidants that serve to scavenge free radicals formed in redox reactions throughout the body.[43] Vitamin E plays a role in termination of free radical–generated lipid peroxidation chain reactions, particularly in cellular and subcellular membranes that are rich in polyunsaturated lipids. Vitamin E activity is complemented by that of selenium, which, as a constituent of glutathione peroxidase, also metabolizes peroxides before they cause membrane damage.

Hypovitaminosis E resulting from a deficient diet is uncommon in the Western world and occurs almost exclusively in association with severe fat malabsorption, low-birth-weight infants, and with rare genetic disorders such as abetalipoproteinemia. Vitamin E supplementation has multiple immunologic effects, including enhanced T-cell proliferation perhaps mediated by suppression of prostaglandin E_2 (PGE_2) production (a T-cell–suppressive compound) and enhancing delayed-type hypersensitivity (DTH) responses.[43-45] Clinical effects of vitamin E supplementation have primarily been studied in the elderly (see "Special Populations" below).

Water-Soluble Vitamins

Vitamin C. Vitamin C (ascorbic acid) is the most powerful biologic reductant available to cells and provides reducing equivalents for a number of biochemical reactions involving iron and copper. As a reducing agent ascorbic acid plays a crucial role as an enzymatic cofactor and antioxidant in a number of physiologically important processes including fatty acid transport, collagen synthesis, and neurotransmitter formation.[44] Vitamin C plays a role in prostaglandin metabolism and may attenuate the inflammatory response and sepsis syndrome.[45]

In humans vitamin C deficiency is manifested as scurvy, the principal feature of which is impaired collagen synthesis with signs including capillary fragility, bleeding gums, delayed wound healing, and impaired bone formation. Human trials demonstrate increases in lymphoproliferative capacity and phagocytic functions of peripheral blood neutrophils and a decrease in serum levels of lipid peroxides and cortisol with vitamin C supplementation. Animal studies and a limited number of human studies have suggested an immunomodulatory role for ascorbic acid with increased resistance to viral illness and some anticarcinogenic effects, perhaps via reducing T-cell apoptosis.[45]

More than 30 trials have been performed to determine whether vitamin C might prevent or treat the common cold. A recent comprehensive review concluded that vitamin C had no beneficial effects on the incidence of common colds, but a consistent reduction in the duration of cold symptoms was seen (range: 0.07% to 39% reduction in symptom days) and larger doses demonstrated a trend toward greater benefit.[46]

In contrast with most other dietary antioxidants, vitamin C appears to be safe even at very high levels of consumption. However, in vitro studies have demonstrated suppression of T-cell proliferation and adhesion and reduced neutrophil phagocytosis of *Candida albicans* at high levels of vitamin C concentrations,[45] suggesting extremely high doses should be avoided.

Trace Metals

Zinc. Zinc (Zn^{2+}) is a dietary trace mineral that plays a critical role in the structure of cell membranes and in the function of cells of the immune system. Zinc is required for the activity of more than 300 enzymes associated with carbohydrate and energy metabolism, protein synthesis and degradation, nucleic acid synthesis, heme biosynthesis, and carbon dioxide transport.

Zinc deficiency occurs most commonly in association with starvation, PEM, and malabsorption syndromes. In the developed world zinc deficiency is seen primarily in children and the elderly though it is estimated that a larger proportion of North Americans may be at risk.[47] Zinc deficiency has been documented in association with numerous conditions of relative immunocompromise, including pregnancy, alcoholism, kidney disease, burns, inflammatory bowel disease, and HIV.

Clinical manifestations of zinc deficiency include growth impairment, delayed sexual maturation, hypogonadism, impotence, oligospermia, alopecia, dysgeusia, night blindness, impaired wound healing, skin abnormalities and impaired immunity. In animals, zinc deficiency results in atrophy of lymphoid tissue, depressed responses to T-lymphocyte–dependent and T-lymphocyte–independent antigens and decreased primary and secondary antibody responses. Decreases have also been observed in natural killer cell activity and responses to cutaneous sensitization in zinc-deficient mice. Diminished in vivo cytotoxic T-killer activity against allogeneic tumor cells has been described.[48] Challenging zinc-deficient mice with infectious agents such as *Trypanosoma cruzi* or nematodes results in increased mortality versus zinc-replete animals due to impaired defenses.[49] In normal human subjects in whom zinc deficiency is induced by dietary restriction, abnormalities were noted in serum thymulin activity, T-cell recruitment, cytolytic T-cell percentage, and natural killer (NK) cell activity.[50]

Clinical trials have examined the role of zinc in immune system modulation during infection and other illnesses. For children living in developing nations, zinc supplementation reduced the duration and intensity of diarrheal illness, acute lower respiratory tract infections, and pneumonia.[51] Further, zinc supplementation has been shown to limit growth stunting in children affected by acute diarrheal illness in underdeveloped areas. Children receiving zinc supplements had higher $CD3^+$ and $CD4^+$ lymphocyte counts and $CD4^+/CD8^+$ ratios in peripheral blood and improved cell-mediated immunity when compared with controls. Zinc supplementation also reduces the incidence of clinical disease caused by *Plasmodium falciparum*.[45,51] In patients with sickle cell disease, zinc supplementation increased IL-2 production and decreased microbiologically confirmed infections and hospitalizations.[52]

A number of studies have evaluated the role of zinc in protection against the common cold. In vitro, zinc salts have been found to inhibit rhinovirus replication. Postulated mechanisms include interference in rhinoviral protein cleavage and assembly of viral particles and protection of plasma membranes against lysis by cytotoxic agents, such as microbial toxins and complement.[45] Transient elevations in zinc concentration in and around the nasal cavity may promote the attachment of zinc complexes to known intercellular adhesion molecule binding sites on rhinovirus surfaces, preventing rhinovirus binding to mucosal cells and interrupting infection.[53] It has also been suggested that common cold symptoms, sneezing and nasal discharge, may be reduced in

intensity by elevations in intranasal zinc salts through production of a "chemical clamp" on trigeminal and facial nerve endings.[53] Some beneficial effects of zinc supplementation may simply be due to correction of a subclinical zinc deficiency.[45]

However, other studies and trials have cast doubt on the validity of these findings. The in vitro inhibitory effect of zinc on rhinovirus replication has been found to be weak, and human trials measuring the effect of zinc on viral shedding found no effect on duration or magnitude of shedding.[54] Additionally, serum zinc concentrations are well below those required for a direct antiviral effect,[54] and although concentrations in oral saliva reach sufficient levels, there is no evidence that this zinc-saliva mixture reaches the nasal mucosa, the site of viral infection. A meta-analysis of eight published randomized trials found no clear benefit for the use of zinc lozenges in the treatment of the common cold.[55]

Selenium. Selenium is essential for the function of selenium-dependent proteins, which play critical roles in the redox regulation of key enzymes, transcription factors, and receptors. Beyond its role as an antioxidant, selenium may have additional immune properties that contribute to the maintenance of normal immune function and cancer prevention. To date, approximately 35 selenoproteins have been identified. The significance of many of these proteins remains to be clarified.

Selenium is ubiquitous in the soil and enters the diet through both plant and animal sources. Dietary intake varies depending on geographic region. Overt selenium deficiency is rare and is limited to certain regions of China. However, the effects of relative selenium deficiency on disease susceptibility and disease progression remain only partially characterized and are a subject of intense ongoing study.

Selenium deficiency has been shown to decrease the production of free radicals and killing by neutrophils, IL-2 receptor affinity and expression on T cells, T-cell proliferation and differentiation, and lymphocyte cytotoxicity. In vitro, selenium deficiency results in enhanced neutrophil adherence to endothelial cells, an early event in the inflammatory response.[45,56] In both mice and humans, supplementation with selenium has been shown to increase lymphocyte proliferative responses, IL-2 receptor expression, and macrophage and cytolytic T-lymphocyte–dependent tumor cytotoxicity.[45,57] Even at plasma selenium levels associated with normal dietary intake in the United States, supplementation with 200 µg selenium per day has considerable immunoenhancing effects, though an upper limit is likely as "megadose" therapy may be associated with reduced immunity.[56]

Selenium deficiency has not only been linked to poor immune responses against viral infections but to enhancement of organism *virulence* itself. Data in selenium-deficient mice infected with either coxsackievirus B or influenza virus demonstrate that viral replication within nutritionally deficient hosts can lead to marked mutations in the viral genome, in the case of influenza specifically the matrix (M) proteins M1 and M2.[57] These mutations alter the virulence of influenza, increasing the severity of illness in subsequent hosts even if the hosts are adequately nourished (Fig. 10-1).[57,58] Thus nutritionally deficient hosts may contribute to mutations in the viral genome during replication within the host and produce viruses with enhanced virulence, although human data are lacking.

Iron. Iron deficiency is the most common trace element deficiency worldwide. It is estimated to affect 20% to 50% of the world's population, including infants, children, and women of childbearing age in tropical regions.[59] The effects of iron deficiency are seen in multiple systems of the human body, including the immune system.[60] In animal and human studies iron deficiency has been associated with impairments in cell-mediated immunity, reductions in neutrophil activity with decreased myeloperoxidase activity and bactericidal activity, and diminished NK-cell activity.[60] Iron deficiency has been shown to impair lymphocyte and neutrophil functions in children, though no resultant increase in susceptibility to infection has been described.[61] Whereas iron deficiency and infection often coexist in developing nations, except in the well-documented association between GI blood loss and heavy infestations of hookworm, a cause-and-effect relationship has not been established.

Many of the immune abnormalities associated with iron deficiency appear to be reversible with iron replacement, but this has

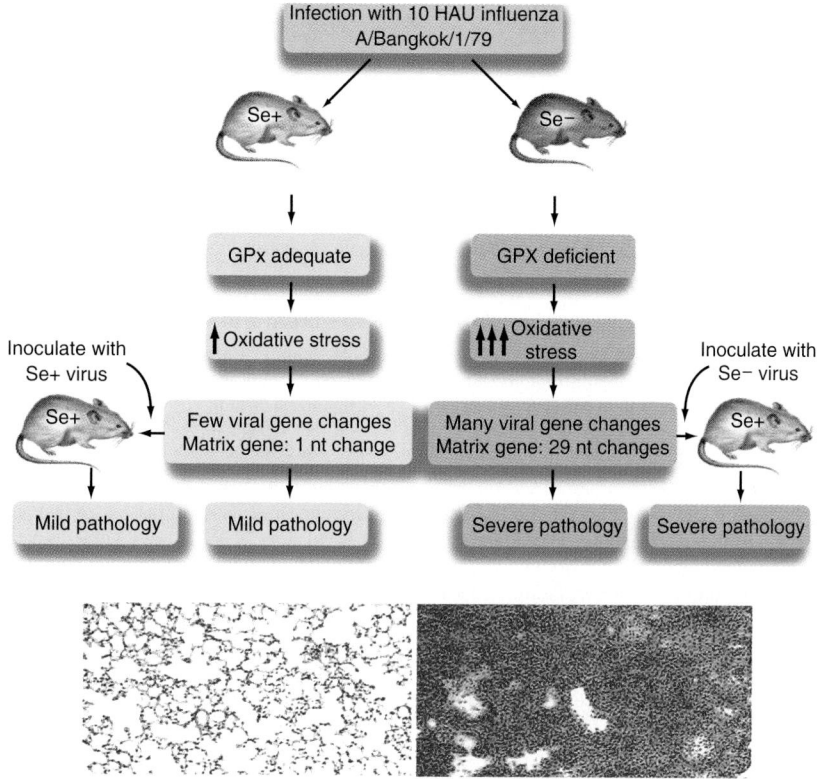

FIGURE 10-1. Enhanced virulence of influenza virus after passage in selenium-deficient mice. GPx, glutathione peroxidase; nt, nucleotide; Se, selenium; +, nondeficient; −, deficient. *(Reprinted with permission from Nelson HK, Shi Q, Van Dael P, et al. Host nutritional selenium status as a driving force for influenza virus mutations. FASEB J. 2001;15:18468.)*

been difficult to demonstrate in human studies.[60] Studies in laboratory animals have been more consistent, demonstrating reversible, deleterious effects of iron deficiency on measures of functional immunity,[60] even in mildly iron-deficient animals.

Most clinicians routinely replace iron in documented iron deficiency to avoid anemia. However, controversy exists over possible deleterious effects of iron supplementation in some settings. Many microorganisms require trace elements like iron and zinc for survival and replication in the host and may increase in pathogenicity with supplementation. Indeed microbiology studies have shown a relationship between the availability of iron and bacterial virulence.[45,60] Further, parenteral iron supplementation has been shown in human and animal studies to be harmful when administered during infection.[60] Thus administration of iron, particularly intravenous iron, or iron-chelating agents such as deferoxamine should be delayed in subjects with active infection.

Fatty Acids

Three major groups of dietary fatty acids, oleic acid, linoleic acid, and linolenic acid, serve as precursors for the biosynthesis of polyunsaturated fatty acids (PUFAs). Metabolic competition exists among these groups of fatty acids, and modification of dietary fatty acid intake can lead to alterations in the fatty acid composition of tissue lipids and in turn changes in cellular responses.

Twenty carbon PUFAs, including arachidonic acid and eicosapentaenoic acid (EPA), can be enzymatically converted to eicosanoids, as shown in Figure 10-2. Extensive data suggest a strong modulatory role for fatty acids in various cellular responses, including inflammation and immune function.[45,62] Growing evidence now suggests that fatty acids also act as second messengers or regulators of signal-transducing molecules.[63]

Among the fatty acids, it is the omega-3 PUFAs that possess the most potent immunomodulatory activities, and among the omega-3 PUFAs, those found concentrated in fish oil, EPA, and docosa-hexaenoic acid (DHA), are more biologically potent than α-linolenic acid (ALA).[64]

Ex vivo studies of human cells have demonstrated a correlation between consumption of fish oil and inhibition of prostaglandin (PG) and leukotriene synthesis leading to reductions in PGE$_2$, thromboxane A$_2$, and leukotriene B$_4$ and increases in thromboxane A$_3$, prostacyclin

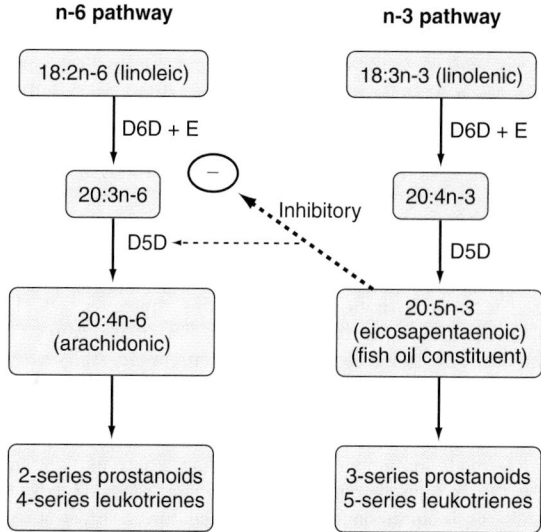

FIGURE 10-2. Production of biologically active metabolites of arachidonic acid is inhibited by n-3 eicosanoids. Abbreviations: D6D, Δ-6 desaturase; E, elongase; D5D, Δ-5 desaturase. *(From McCowen KC, Bistrian BR. Immunonutrition: Problematic or problem solving? Am J Clin Nutr. 2003 Apr;77[4]:764-770. ©American Journal of Clinical Nutrition. American Society for Clinical Nutrition.)*

PGI$_3$, and leukotriene B$_5$.[64] There have been a number of clinical trials assessing the benefits of dietary supplementation with fish oils in several inflammatory and autoimmune diseases in humans, including rheumatoid arthritis, Crohn's disease, ulcerative colitis, psoriasis, lupus erythematosus, multiple sclerosis, and migraine headaches. Many of the placebo-controlled trials of fish oil in chronic inflammatory diseases reveal benefit, including decreased disease activity and reduced use of anti-inflammatory drugs. Samples of peripheral blood mononuclear cells from these patients show suppressed synthesis of two principal mediators of inflammation, IL-1 and tumor necrosis factor-α (TNF-α), as compared with patients receiving placebo.[45]

Reduction of T-cell–derived IL-2 production by the intake of omega-3 PUFAs has also been demonstrated in humans and mice. In addition, consuming diets supplemented with fish oil leads to the suppression of mitogen-induced proliferation of T cells and delayed-type hypersensitivity skin responses, which suggests a generalized decrease in T-cell–mediated immune responses.[45,62]

Recent studies in animal models of acute respiratory distress syndrome (ARDS) have suggested a high-fat diet containing EPA (fish oil), gamma-linolenic acid (GLA; borage oil) (EPA plus GLA), and antioxidants can improve lung microvascular permeability, oxygenation, and cardiopulmonary function and reduce proinflammatory eicosanoid synthesis and lung inflammation.[65] In one prospective, double-blind randomized controlled trial of seriously ill patients, those receiving enteral feed supplemented with EPA plus GLA required significantly fewer days of ventilatory support and had a decreased length of stay in the intensive care unit compared with controls. Beneficial effects of the EPA-plus-GLA diet on pulmonary neutrophil recruitment and gas exchange were also observed.[66]

NUTRITIONAL SUPPLEMENTATION

Anorexia occurs both in patients with current nutritional deficiencies and in those at risk for malnutrition. Simple strategies to combat anorexia include modifications of meal size, timing and content, and prioritizing calorically dense foods. When efforts to modify diet fail to provide adequate nutrition, options include the use of diet supplements, appetite stimulants, or direct delivery of nutrients via enteral or parenteral means.

Strategies to maximize the nutritional status of hospitalized or severely ill patients have undergone significant change in the past 35 years. Improvements in intravenous catheters, catheter care, nutrient formulations, and laboratory monitoring facilitated a rise in the use of total parenteral nutrition (TPN) during the 1970s and 1980s. Enteral nutrition was perceived to be labor intensive and associated with multiple complications, and parenteral nutrition became the preferred route of nutritional support in many patients. In the past decade, however, a growing body of evidence has demonstrated that enteral feeding has significant advantages over TPN, including cost, safety, and enhancement of gut integrity and immune system responses.

Enteral Feeding and "Immunonutrition"

Most studies in burn victims and surgical patients have demonstrated clinical benefits of early enteral feeding (within 24 to 48 hours) when compared with IV hydration alone, and this strategy is widely employed, though contradictory data exist.[67,68] Formulas designed to improve immune function through the use of immunologically active micronutrients including glutamine, arginine, omega-3 fatty acids, nucleotides, and β-carotene have shown significant promise in laboratory experiments and in several small clinical studies. This approach has been termed "immunonutrition."[69] Pediatric burn unit patients administered a diet supplemented with arginine, omega-3 fatty acids, zinc, and other immunonutrients sustained fewer infections and a shorter length of stay per percent body burn than patients fed conventional enteral diets.[70] General surgical patients receiving a diet supplemented with arginine, nucleotides, and fish oil may have a significantly lower incidence of bacteremia and shorter length of stay if able to tolerate at least 800 mL/day of an immune-enhancing diet.[69] Patients undergoing surgery for upper GI malignancy most clearly

benefit from similar immune-enhancing formulations and experience fewer infections and shorter lengths of stay,[69] and similar findings were reported in two prospective studies of patients sustaining blunt or penetrating trauma.[69] One of these studies found that patients randomized to the immune-enhancing diet required fewer days of antibiotics than patients randomized to the control diet.[71] Because the diet formulations include multiple immunologically active nutrients, discerning the clinically active and relevant component or components is difficult. Current animal and human studies seek to better define the role of these micronutrients in immune responses; most important will be larger, adequately powered studies.[69]

Total Parenteral Nutrition

The Veteran Affairs (VA) TPN Cooperative Study,[72] a multicenter prospective randomized controlled trial, evaluated the effectiveness of perioperative TPN in surgical patients stratified by nutritional status. No significant differences in 30-day postoperative mortality and 90-day complication rates and mortality were found between the TPN and control groups. Subgroup analysis revealed a slight increase in infectious complications in patients classified as borderline or mildly malnourished in the TPN group when compared with controls. The increase in infectious complications in the TPN group was compensated for by a decrease in noninfectious complications, however. The overall complication rate in severely malnourished patients given TPN was lower, though this difference failed to meet statistical significance. The authors concluded that perioperative TPN was not beneficial in borderline or mildly malnourished patients and that TPN may actually be harmful in this group because of increased risk of infection. Subsequent trials have substantiated the findings of the VA TPN Cooperative Study though concern exists over the clinical application of the VA and other early studies in light of advances made in TPN solutions since the trials were conducted.

Total Parenteral Nutrition versus Total Enteral Nutrition

Although numerous studies in animals and humans have compared the effects of enteral and parenteral feeds on markers of nutrition and immunologic status, only a few randomized clinical trials exist. Data from several of these studies were included in a meta-analysis of eight trials of trauma and general surgery patients that concluded patients receiving total enteral nutrition (TEN) developed fewer septic complications suggesting a benefit over TPN in critically ill patients.[73]

The increased incidence of infection in people receiving parenteral nutrition cannot be explained by catheter-related complications alone. The mechanisms underlying the reduced septic complications with enteral nutrition versus parenteral nutrition are currently not known, but do not appear to be due to differences in restoration of nutritional status. One hypothesis to explain the increased rate of infection in parenterally fed patients is that intravenous nutrition induces immunosuppression. In animals, TPN has been shown to impair white blood cell function, including locomotion and phagocytosis, decrease CD4$^+$ and CD8$^+$ lymphocyte count, and alter cytokine release. TPN has been associated with intestinal mucosal atrophy, decreased microvillous height, and decreases in brush-border hydrolase and nutrient transporter activity. These changes and associated bacterial overgrowth likely result in the increased bacterial translocation from the intestinal lumen to local lymph nodes demonstrated in animals receiving TPN, whereas enteral nutrition has been shown to support the gut barrier and gut-associated lymphoid tissue.[74,75]

SPECIAL POPULATIONS

Nutritional concerns plague many special populations commonly seen by infectious disease practitioners. These include patients with cancer, diabetes, end-stage renal disease, transplant recipients, and others. However, to note specific concerns in each of these populations is beyond the scope of this chapter. To illustrate many of the general issues discussed above, two clinical populations of specific interest are highlighted: patients afflicted with HIV/AIDS and older adults. Research in these two groups is of particularly high quality with a plethora of well-designed epidemiologic and interventional studies.

Human Immunodeficiency Virus/Acquired Immunodeficiency Syndrome

Recognition of malnutrition and principles of nutritional management are important aspects of the primary care of HIV-infected patients.[76,77] Severe malnutrition in HIV-infected persons is recognized as the "wasting syndrome," defined by the Centers for Disease Control and Prevention (CDC) as a body weight loss of greater than or equal to 10% with associated fatigue, fever, and diarrhea unexplained by another cause, but any weight loss of more than 5% is associated with accelerated disease progression, impaired functional status, and increased mortality.[78] Early in the HIV epidemic, studies reported wasting in up to 20% of patients at the time of AIDS diagnosis in the United States. Despite advances in the management and therapy of HIV infection, the wasting syndrome and other forms of malnutrition remain highly prevalent in HIV-infected persons.[79] Wasting is associated with increased mortality and remains a significant prognostic factor in advanced HIV disease.

The etiology of AIDS-associated wasting is multifactorial. Wasting has been associated with decreased oral intake, malabsorption syndromes, endocrine dysfunction, and increased cytokine production. Reductions in food intake may be caused by disease or drug-associated anorexia, central nervous system dysfunction, dysphagia, and odynophagia. Absorption may be impaired by infectious or drug-associated intestinal inflammation, dysfunction, and diarrhea. Endocrine abnormalities include alterations in thyroid and adrenal function and fluctuations in growth hormone levels. Production of proinflammatory cytokines leads to accelerated metabolic degradation of essential micronutrients, further compromising the HIV-infected host. The use of nutritional therapy throughout the course of HIV infection, and with increased intensity during symptomatic infection, can slow and perhaps reverse the compounding effects of nutritionally associated immunodeficiency.

PEM is the most common form of malnutrition seen in HIV disease worldwide, but alterations in the stores of fat- and water-soluble vitamins and trace elements are also seen.[80-82] Vitamin A deficiency has been associated with the progression of HIV disease, development of secondary infections, increased HIV-associated mortality, and increased maternal-fetal transmission.[32,83-85] Deficiencies in water-soluble vitamins appear to occur less frequently than with fat-soluble vitamins and only cobalamin (B_{12}) is associated with HIV disease progression.[86] Of the trace elements, deficiencies in iron, zinc, and selenium have been described. Zinc levels decline as HIV disease progresses, and zinc supplementation in HIV infection has been shown to improve immune responses though clinical benefits have not been documented.[87]

Selenium deficiency occurs more commonly in HIV-infected persons as documented by low plasma and red blood cell levels of selenium, diminished activity of glutathione peroxidase, and low selenium levels in cardiac muscle of AIDS patients. Plasma selenium concentrations may be reduced by up to 50% in AIDS patients with relative selenium deficiency described in more than 60% of HIV-positive persons.[88] The mechanism of selenium depletion in HIV-infected individuals is poorly understood, and is likely multifactorial. Declines in selenium levels have been documented even in the earliest stages of HIV infection,[89] and accelerated progression of HIV disease has been described in patients with selenium deficiency.[90,91] However, selenium supplementation trials in HIV-infected individuals have failed to demonstrate improvements in CD4+ cell count, rates of opportunistic infections, or mortality despite improvements in markers of oxidative stress.[91]

Strategies to Combat Weight Loss and Wasting Associated with Human Immunodeficiency Virus

Enhanced dietary protein or total caloric intake can be effective for increasing total body protein and muscle mass in patients with known weight loss and should be encouraged as the initial approach to weight loss in HIV-positive persons. Many other therapies for wasting in HIV infection have been employed and are briefly reviewed below.

Appetite Stimulants. Dronabinol is a cannabinol derivative approved to increase appetite in patients with AIDS-related anorexia and weight loss. Dronabinol has been shown to result in significantly increased appetite, but no change in weight and at the cost of significant side effects.[92]

Exercise. Trials of resistance exercise in HIV-infected men have demonstrated conflicting results with regard to gains in muscle mass. In one randomized, placebo-controlled 16-week trial in 61 men with AIDS, weight loss, and *low* serum testosterone levels, resistance exercise resulted in a significant increase in body weight and muscle strength.[93] In a similar 12-week trial of 54 men with AIDS and weight loss but *normal* testosterone levels, exercise alone failed to result in increases in either body weight or muscle strength, although there was an increase in muscle mass.[94]

Steroids. Steroid hormones commonly used to treat HIV-induced tissue wasting include testosterone, megestrol acetate, and dehydroepiandrosterone (DHEA).

Whereas testosterone therapy may offer the most benefit to men with proven hypogonadism, testosterone can also be effective in men who are eugonadal.[95] Intramuscular (IM) testosterone can lead to increases in lean body mass and significantly improve quality of life.[81,95,96] In contrast, randomized trials of transscrotal or transcutaneous testosterone have shown no or nonsignificant changes in muscle mass and no benefit on self-reported quality of life.[97,98]

Smaller doses of transdermal testosterone may be effective in women with HIV infection. In one study, weight gain and social functioning improved in women who received 0.15 mg/day of testosterone, but not in those who received 0.3 mg/day, as compared with the placebo group.[99]

Anabolic steroids other than testosterone may have utility in treating weight loss in HIV-positive persons. In two trials in HIV-infected men with normal serum testosterone levels, oxandrolone therapy resulted in small increases in weight, strength, and lean body mass, especially when combined with an exercise program.[100] Megestrol acetate (Megace), given orally in a dose of 400 to 800 mg/day, has been shown to increase both appetite and weight when compared with placebo. The increase in weight, however, is largely fat not muscle.[101] Transient adrenal insufficiency and glucose intolerance may occur during and following use. DHEA may have some beneficial effects on reducing fatigue and elevating mood,[102] but there are no convincing data from controlled trials to support the use of DHEA for the prevention or treatment of HIV-associated weight loss.

Growth Hormone. A number of peptide hormones are being used in an attempt to reverse tissue wasting in HIV disease. The best studied is recombinant human growth hormone (GH). Although GH secretion is rarely deficient in HIV-infected patients, it is theorized that possible GH resistance in HIV may be overcome by the administration of GH and that this may result in benefits in muscle mass. Pharmacologic use of growth hormone has been shown to improve nitrogen balance and increase lean body mass in HIV-infected patients with wasting and to promote lean tissue retention in those with secondary infections.[94] Other trials have suggested no sustainable benefit to therapy or that modest benefits were outweighed by adverse effects and high costs.[103,104]

Anticytokine Therapies. Many studies have suggested that proinflammatory cytokines contribute to the metabolic abnormalities and weight loss associated with HIV disease. As a result, cytokine suppressors have been evaluated as potential treatments for wasting. Placebo-controlled trials in patients with HIV have shown that thalidomide, a suppressor of TNF-α production, produces weight gain.[105,106] However, some trials demonstrated modest but significant elevations in viral load.[106]

Overall Conclusions Regarding Therapy for Wasting Associated with Human Immunodeficiency Virus. Though a number of agents appear promising in the treatment of HIV-related weight loss and have shown *statistically* significant increases in body weight, no currently available therapy offers *clinically* significant and sustained increases in lean body mass. Increasing calorie and protein intake from

TABLE 10-3 The Prevalence of Nutritional Deficiencies in Older Adults Residing in Various Settings

Nutrient	Long-Term Care or Hospitalized	Community-Dwelling
Protein-calorie	17%-85%	10%-25%
Vitamin A	2%-20%	2%-8%
Vitamin B_{12}	ND	7%-15%
Vitamin E	5%-15%	ND
Zinc	ND	15%-25%

ND, no data.
Data are pooled from multiple studies.

diet and engaging in regular resistance exercise do appear to result in weight gain and seem to be prudent recommendations. Treatment with anabolic steroids, particularly IM testosterone in testosterone-deficient men, may offer sustainable gains in muscle mass and improvements in mood and quality of life.

Older Adults

The elderly represent a population at significant risk for malnutrition and its related health problems. Malnutrition and decreased oral intake in older adults is often multifactorial. In the inpatient setting, "nothing by mouth" orders, inability to feed oneself, and increased caloric needs head the list. In the outpatient setting, depression, medications, dental/swallowing problems, and social issues (e.g., choices between food and medicine) are paramount. Special focus should be applied to residents of long-term care, as they represent a population at further increased risk for nutritional deficiencies and infection. Age-related immune dysfunction is likely influenced by nutritional status.[107] Morley has reviewed the biology of anorexia in older adults and suggested the mnemonic Meals on Wheels to highlight the causes of malnutrition in older adults.[108]

Studies of hospitalized older adults, using anthropometric measures and laboratory values such as serum albumin, have shown an estimated 40% to 60% to be malnourished.[109,110] A prospective study of nonterminally ill elderly patients discharged from an acute care hospital

found a body mass index (BMI) equal to 20 kg/m² to be associated with a markedly increased risk of mortality within 1 year.[111] Among long-term and subacute care residents the prevalence of malnutrition is 15% to 66%.[112] In outpatient elderly patients, the incidence of malnutrition has been identified primarily by determining weight loss. Data from the Nutritional Screening Initiative suggested loss of body weight greater than 5% in 1 month, greater than 7.5% in 3 months, or greater than 10% in 6 months to be clinically significant.[113] The National Health and Nutrition Examination Survey Follow-up Study found that over 10 years of follow-up 50% of people ages 65 to 74 lost at least 5% of their body weight, whereas 26% of women and 14% of men lost at least 15% of their body weight.[114] Micronutrient deficiencies are also prevalent among older adults, with 10% to 30% having subnormal levels of some vitamins or minerals (Table 10-3).

Nutritional Supplements in Older Adults: Effects on Immunity and Clinical Outcomes

Although malnutrition in the elderly is clearly associated with impaired immunity and poor clinical outcomes, nutritional supplementation has not definitively been shown to reverse this trend. Many studies examining only immune response variables rather than clinical end points have been performed and recently reviewed.[115] Studies specifically addressing clinical end points are emphasized below.

Multivitamin and Trace Mineral Supplements. Studies of multivitamin-mineral supplementation for the prevention of infection have been performed in both outpatient healthy elderly and long-term care residents and are summarized in Table 10-4.[116,117] Overall, nutritionally at-risk older adults in the community experience fewer days of illness and antibiotic use compared with placebo-treated patients.[115,118] Trace minerals (zinc and selenium) appear to be more effective than multivitamins (MVIs) in residents of long-term care for reducing the incidence of respiratory tract infection but have little effect on urinary tract infection or pressure ulcers.[9,119,120]

Vitamin E. Vitamin E has been shown to enhance both humoral and cell-mediated immune responses in elderly individuals. Supplementation with daily vitamin E at 200 or 800 mg/day in healthy older adults improved delayed-type hypersensitivity responses and immunization responses to hepatitis B, but not pneumococcal polysaccharide

TABLE 10-4 Recent Randomized, Placebo-Controlled Nutrient Supplementation Trials in Older Adults

Reference, Year	Sample Size/Population	Time (mo)	Randomized Groups	Outcome Measured	Comment
125 (1992)	N = 296, community-dwelling	12	1. Daily MVI plus Zn^{2+} and Se 2. Placebo	MD-confirmed infection, antibiotic use	Lower incidence of infection and antibiotic use in the supplemented group
126 (1997)	N = 81, nursing home	24	1. Daily MVI 2. Daily Zn^{2+} and Se 3. Both daily 4. Placebo	MD-confirmed respiratory/urogenital infection, mortality	No mortality difference, lower infection with trace minerals or TM + MVI, but not MVI alone group
129 (1997)	N = 88, community-dwelling	8	1. Daily vitamin E 60 2. Daily vitamin E 200 3. Daily vitamin E 800 4. Placebo	Self-reported illness, immune responses	Borderline reduction in illness ($P = 0.10$), improved DTH and primary antibody responses
127 (1999)	N = 725, nursing home	24	1. Daily MVI 2. Daily Zn^{2+} and Se 3. Both daily 4. Placebo	MD-confirmed respiratory/urogenital infection, mortality	No mortality difference, borderline reduction in infection ($P = 0.06$) and improved influenza vaccine responses in trace mineral, but not MVI alone group
130 (2002)	N = 652, community-dwelling	15	1. Daily MVI plus Zn^{2+} and Se 2. Daily MVI plus Zn^{2+} and SE plus vitamin E 3. Vitamin E 4. Placebo	Self-reported respiratory infection	No difference in incidence of infection; significantly *worse* symptom severity in vitamin E recipients
123 (2003)	N = 130 (only 33 >age 65 y; others were diabetic patients), community-dwelling	12	1. Daily MVI plus Zn^{2+} and Se 2. Placebo	Self-reported infection confirmed by MD	Lower incidence of infection overall ($P < 0.001$) and in subset with type 2 DM ($P < 0.001$), but not in elderly subset $P > 0.2$)

DM, diabetes mellitus; DTH, delayed-type hypersensitivity; MD, medical doctor; MVI, multivitamin; Se, selenium; TM, Zn^{2+} + Se; Zn^{2+}, zinc.

or tetanus.[121,122] However, another study showed the severity of symptoms due to infection was significantly *worse* in the vitamin E group (versus placebo) with higher total illness duration and number of symptoms, and more frequent fever and activity restriction compared with those not receiving vitamin E[123] (due to enhanced immune responses in the vitamin E recipients?). Therefore, although there is currently no evidence to support the use of vitamin E supplementation for reducing the incidence of infection, there may be measurable effects on immune responses, and determination of its overall role in nutritional supplementation of older adults requires further study.

Overall Conclusions Regarding Nutritional Supplementation in Older Adults. Nutrient factors likely play a role in the immunosuppressed state prevalent in older adults. Limited studies demonstrating improvement in immune function are promising. Of studies examining clinical end points, nutritional status of the study population appears to be important and may explain variations in study findings. At-risk populations with higher rates of subclinical nutrient deficiency appear to derive greatest benefit. Thus far, studies indicate that use of multivitamin and trace mineral supplementation may be most beneficial, particularly trace mineral supplementation in the long-term care population. Further study is needed regarding the use of vitamin E in the prevention of infection in older adults; current studies are inconclusive with some demonstrating benefits, others suggesting increased severity of infectious symptoms. Early recognition and investigation of malnutrition in the elderly remain the most important factors in prevention.

REFERENCES

1. Keustch GT. The history of nutrition: Malnutrition, infection and immunity. J Nutr. 2003 Jan;133(1):336S-340S.
2. Wilson MG, Vaswani S, Liu D. Prevalence and causes of undernutrition in medical outpatients. Am J Med. 1998;104:56-63.
3. Kerstetter JE, Holthausen BA, Fitz PA. Malnutrition in the institutionalized older adult. J Am Diet Assoc. 1992 Sep;92(9):1109-1116.
4. Guigoz Y, Lauque S, Vellas BJ. Identifying the elderly at risk for malnutrition. The Mini Nutritional Assessment. Clin Geriatr Med. 2002 Nov;18(4):737-757.
5. Sullivan DH. The role of nutrition in increased morbidity and mortality. Clin Geriatr Med. 1995 Nov;11(4):661-674.
6. Bistrian BR, Sherman M, Blackburn GL, et al. Cellular immunity in adult marasmus. Arch Intern Med. 1977;137(10):1408-1411.
7. Windsor JA, Hill GL. Weight loss with physiologic impairment. A basic indicator of surgical risk. Ann Surg. 1988 Mar;207(3):290-296.
8. Windsor JA, Hill GL. Risk factors for post-operative pneumonia: The importance of protein depletion. Ann Surg 1988; 208(2):209-214.
9. Thomas DR. Improving outcome of pressure ulcers with nutritional interventions: A review of the evidence. Nutrition. 2001 Feb;17(2):121-125.
10. The World Health Report 2002: Reducing risks, promoting healthy life. Geneva:World Health Organization; 2002.
11. www.nationalacademies.org
12. Omran ML, Morley JE. Assessment of protein energy malnutrition in older persons, part II: Laboratory evaluation. Nutrition. 2000 Feb;16(2):131-140.
13. Katz DL. Malnutrition and cachexia. In: Katz DL, ed. Nutrition in Clinical Practice. Philadelphia: Lippincott Williams & Wilkins; 2001:188.
14. Woodward B. Protein, calories, and immune defenses. Nutr Rev. Jan 1998;56(1 Pt 2):S84-S92.
15. Chandra RK, Wadhwa M. Nutritional modulation of intestinal mucosal immunity. Immunol Invest. 1989 Jan-May;18(1-4):119-126.
16. Erickson KL, Medina EA, Hubbard NE. Micronutrients and innate immunity. J Infect Dis. 2000;182(Suppl 1):S5-S10.
17. Sakamoto M, Fujisawa Y, Nishioka K. Physiologic role of the complement system in host defense, disease, and malnutrition. Nutrition. 1998;14:391-398.
18. Sauerwein RW, Mulder JA, Mulder L, et al. Inflammatory mediators in children with protein-energy malnutrition. Am J Clin Nutr. 1997 May; 65(5):1534-1539.
19. Lipshitz DA. Nutrition, aging, and the immunohematopoietic system. Clin Geriatr Med. 1987 May; 3(2):319-328.
20. WHO/UNICEF/IVACG. Vitamin A supplements: A guide to their use in the treatment and prevention of vitamin A deficiency and xerophthalmia. 2nd ed. Geneva: World Health Organization; 1997.
21. Semba RD. The role of vitamin A and related retinoids in immune function. Nutr Rev 1998;56:S38-S48.
22. Stephensen CB. Vitamin A, infection and immune function. Annu Rev Nutr. 2001;21:167-192.
23. Rosenthal D, Lancillotti F, Darwiche N, et al. Regulation of epithelial differentiation by retinoids. In: Blumhoff R, ed. Vitamin A in Health and Disease. New York: Marcel Dekker; 1994:425-450.
24. Thurnam DI, Northrop-Clewes CA, McCullough FSW, et al. Innate immunity, gut integrity and vitamin A in Gambian and Indian infants. J Infect Dis. 2000;182:S23-S38.
25. Blomhoff HK, Smeland EB. Role of retinoids in normal hematopoiesis and the immune system. In: Blumhoff R, ed. Vitamin A in Health and Disease. New York: Marcel Dekker; 1994:45184.
26. Cantorna MT, Nashold FE, Chun TY, Hayes CE. In vitamin A deficiency multiple mechanisms establish a regulatory T helper cell imbalance with excess Th1 and insufficient Th2 function. J Immunol. 1994;152:1515-1522.
27. Barreto ML, Santos LM, Assis AM, et al. Effect of vitamin A supplementation on diarrhea and acute lower respiratory tract infections in young children in Brazil. Lancet. 1994;344:228-231.
28. Dibley MJ, Sadjimin T, Kjolhede CL, Moulton LH. Vitamin A supplementation fails to reduce incidence of acute respiratory illness and diarrhea in preschool-age Indonesian children. J Nutr. 1996;126:434-442.
29. Fawzi WW, Chalmers TC, Herrera MG, Moesteller F. Vitamin A supplementation and child mortality. JAMA. 1993;269:898-903.
30. The Vitamin A and Pneumonia Working Group. Potential interventions for the prevention of childhood pneumonia in developing countries: A meta-analysis of data from field trials to assess the impact of vitamin A supplementation on pneumonia morbidity and mortality. Bulletin WHO. 1995;73:609-619.
31. Semba D, Graham NM, Caiaffa WT, et al. Increased mortality associated with vitamin A deficiency during human immunodeficiency virus type 1 infection. Arch Intern Med. 1993;153:2149-2154.
32. Greenberg BL, Semba RD, Vink PE, et al. Vitamin A deficiency and maternal-infant transmissions of HIV in two metropolitan areas of the United States. AIDS. 1997;11:325-332.
33. Semba RD. Overview of the potential role of vitamin A in mother-to-child transmission of HIV-1. Acta Paediatr. 1997;(Suppl 421):107-112.
34. www.who.int/vaccines-documents/DocsPDF/www9837.pdf.
35. Butler JC, Havens PL, Sowell AL, et al. Measles severity and serum retinol (vitamin A) concentration among children in the United States. Pediatrics. 1993 June; 91(6):1176-1181.
36. Hussey GD, Klein M. A randomized, controlled trial of vitamin A in children with severe measles. N Engl J Med. 1990 July 19;323(3):160-164.
37. Coutsoudis A, Kiepiela P, Coovadia HM, Broughton M. Vitamin A supplementation enhances specific IgG antibody levels and total lymphocyte numbers while improving morbidity in measles. Pediatr Infect Dis J. 1992 Mar;11(3):203-209.
38. Kawasaki Y, Hosoya M, Katayose M, Suzuki H. The efficacy of oral vitamin A supplementation for measles and respiratory syncytial virus (RSV) infection. Kansenshogaku Zasshi. 1999 Feb;73(2):104-109.
39. Dowell SF, Papic Z, Bresee JS, et al. Treatment of respiratory syncytial virus infection with vitamin A: A randomized, placebo-controlled trial in Santiago, Chile. Pediatr Infect Dis J. 1996 Sep;15(9):782-786.
40. Bresee JS, Fisher M, Dowell SF, et al. Vitamin A therapy for children with respiratory syncytial virus infection: A multicenter trial in the United States. Pediatr Infect Dis J. 1996 Sep;15(9):777-782.
41. The Alpha-Tocopherol, Beta Carotene Cancer Prevention Study Group. The effect of vitamin E and beta carotene on the incidence of lung cancer and other cancers in male smokers. N Engl J Med. 1994 Apr 14;330(15):1029-1035.
42. Omenn GS, Goodman GE, Thornquist MD, et al. Effects of a combination of beta carotene and vitamin A on lung cancer and cardiovascular disease. N Engl J Med. 1996 May 2;34(18):1150-1155.
43. Meydani M. Vitamin E. Lancet. 1995 Jan 21;345(8943):170-175.
44. Rucker R. Vitamins: Overview and metabolic functions. In: Gershwin ME, German JB, Keen CL, eds. Nutrition and Immunology. Totowa, NJ: Humana; 2000:75-96.
45. Field CJ, Johnson IR, Schley PD. Nutrients and their role in host resistance to infection. J Leukoc Biol. 2002 Jan;71:16-32.
46. Douglas RM, Chalker EB, Treacy B. Vitamin C for prevention and treating the common cold. Cochrane Database Syst Rev. 2000;(2):CD000980.
47. Prasad AS. Zinc: An overview. Nutrition 1995 Jan-Feb;11(Suppl 1):93-99.
48. Keen C, Gershwin M. Zinc deficiency and immune function. Annu Rev Nutr. 1990;10:415-431.
49. Dardenne M. Zinc and immune function. Eur J Clin Nutr. 2002 Aug;56 (Suppl 3): S20-S23.
50. Shi HN, Scott ME, Stevenson MM, Koski KG. Energy restriction and zinc deficiency impair the functions of murine T cells and antigen-presenting cells during gastrointestinal nematode infection. J Nutr. 1998 Jan;128(1):20-27.
51. Black RE. Zinc deficiency, infectious disease and mortality in the developing world. J Nutr. 2003 May;133(5 Suppl 1):1485S-1489S.
52. Prasad AS, Beck FW, Kaplan J, et al. Effect of zinc supplementation on incidence of infections and hospital admissions in sickle cell disease. Am J Hematol 1999;61:194-202.
53. Novick SG, Godfrey JC, Godfrey NJ, Wilder HR. How does zinc modify the common cold? Med Hypoth. 1996;46:295-302.
54. Farr BM, Conner EM, Betts RF, et al. Two randomized controlled trials of zinc gluconate lozenge therapy of experimentally induced rhinovirus colds. Antimicrob Agents Chemother. 1987;31:1183-1187.
55. Jackson JL, Lesho E, Peterson C. Zinc and the common cold: A meta-analysis revisited. J Nutr. 2000;130:1512S-1515S.
56. McKenzie RC, Rafferty TS, Beckett GJ. Selenium: An essential element for immune function. Immunol Today. 1998 Aug;19(8):342-345.
57. Nelson HK, Shi Q, Van Dael P, et al. Host nutritional selenium status as a driving force for influenza virus mutations. FASEB J. 2001;15:18468.
58. Beck MA, Shi Q, Morris VC, Levander OA. Rapid genomic evolution of a non-virulent coxsackievirus B3 in selenium-deficient mice results in selection of identical virulent isolates. Nat Med. 1995;1:433.
59. Ramakrishnan U. Prevalence of micronutrient malnutrition worldwide. Nutr Rev. 2002 May; 60(5 Pt 2):S46-S52.

60. Oppenheimer SJ. Iron and its relation to immunity and infectious disease. J Nutr. 2001 Feb; 131(S-2):616S-635S.

61. Dallman PR. Manifestations of iron deficiency. Semin Hematol. 1982 Jan;19(1):19-30.

62. Calder PC, Grimble RF. Polyunsaturated fatty acids, inflammation and immunity. Eur J Clin Nutr. 2002 Aug;56(Suppl 3):S14-S19.

63. Hwang D. Fatty acids and immune responses—A new perspective in searching for clues to mechanisms. Annu Rev Nutr. 2000;20:431-456.

64. Simopoulos AP. Omega-3 fatty acids in inflammation and autoimune diseases. J Am Coll Nutr. 2002 Dec;21(6):495-505.

65. Pacht ER, DeMichele SJ, Nelson JL, et al. Enteral nutrition with eicosapentaenoic acid, gamma-linolenic acid, and antioxidants reduces alveolar inflammatory mediators and protein influx in patients with acute respiratory distress syndrome. Crit Care Med. 2003 Feb; 31(2):491-500.

66. Gadek JE, DeMichele SJ, Karlstad MD, et al. Effect of enteral feeding with eicosapentaenoic acid, gamma-linolenic acid, and antioxidants in patients with acute respiratory distress syndrome. Enteral Nutrition in ARDS Study Group. Crit Care Med. 1999 Aug;27(8):1409-1420.

67. Carr C, Ling EK, Boulos P, Singer M. Randomized trial of safety and efficacy of immediate postoperative enteral feeding in patients undergoing gastrointestinal resection. BMJ. 1996;312:869-871.

68. Heslin MJ, Latkany L, Leung D, et al. A prospective, randomized trial of early enteral feeding after resection of upper gastrointestinal malignancy. Ann Surg 1997; 226:567-580.

69. McCowen KC, Bistrian BR. Immunonutrition: Problematic or problem solving? Am J Clin Nutr. 2003 Apr;77(4):764-770.

70. Gottschlich MM, Jenkins M, Warden GD, et al. Differential effects of three enteral dietary regimens on selected outcome variables in burn patients. JPEN. 1990;14:225-236.

71. Kudsk KA, Minard G, Croce MA, et al. A randomized trial of isonitrogenous enteral diets after severe trauma. An immune-enhancing diet reduces septic complications. Ann Surg. 1996 Oct;224(4):531-540; discussion 540-543.

72. The Veterans Affairs Total Parenteral Nutrition Cooperative Study Group. Perioperative total parenteral nutrition in surgical patients. N Engl J Med. 1991 Aug 22;325(8):525-532.

73. Moore FA, Feliciano DV, Andrassy RJ, et al. Early enteral feeding, compared with parenteral, reduced postoperative septic complications—The results of a meta-analysis. Ann Surg. 1992;216:172-183.

74. Shou J, Lappin J, Minnard EA, Daly JM. Total parenteral nutrition, bacterial translocation, and host immune function. Am J Surg. 1994;167:145-150.

75. Alverdy JC, Aoys E, Moss G. Total parenteral nutrition promotes bacterial translocation from the gut. Surgery 1988;104:185-190.

76. Knox T, Zafonte-Sanders M, Fields-Gardner C, et al. Assessment of nutritional status, body composition, and human immunodeficiency virus–associated morphologic changes. Clin Infect Dis. 2003 Apr(Suppl 2):36:S63-S68.

77. Nerad J, Romeyn M, Silverman E, et al. General nutrition management in patients infected with human immunodeficiency virus. Clin Infect Dis. 2003 Apr(Suppl 2):36:S52-S62.

78. Wheeler DA. Weight loss and disease progression in HIV infection. AIDS Read. 1999 Aug; 9(5):347-353.

79. Wanke CA, Silva M, Knox TA, et al. Weight loss and wasting remain common complications in individuals infected with human immunodeficiency virus in the era of highly active antiretroviral therapy. Clin Infect Dis. 2000 Sep;31(3):803-805.

80. Beach RS, Mantero-Atienza E, Shor-Posner G, et al. Specific nutrient abnormalities in asymptomatic HIV-1 infection. AIDS. 1992 July;6(7):701-708.

81. Coodley, GO, Goodley MK. A trial of testosterone therapy for HIV-associated weight loss. AIDS. 1997 Sep;11(1):1347-1352.

82. Baum MK, Shor-Posner G, Lu Y, et al. Micronutrients and HIV-1 disease progression. AIDS. 1995 Sep;9(9):1051-1056.

83. Semba RD, Miotti PG, Chiphangwi JD, et al. Infant mortality and maternal vitamin A deficiency during human immunodeficiency virus infection. Clin Infect Dis. 1995; 21:966-972.

84. Coutsoudis A, Bobat RA, Coovadia HM, et al. The effects of vitamin A supplementation on the morbidity of children born to HIV-infected women. Am J Public Health. 1995 Aug;85(8 Pt 1):1076-1081.

85. Fawzi WW, Mbise RL, Hertzmark E, et al. A randomized trial of vitamin A supplements in relation to mortality among human immunodeficiency virus–infected and uninfected children in Tanzania. Pediatr Infect Dis J. 1999 Feb;18(2):127-133.

86. Tang AM, Graham NM, Chandra RK, Saah AJ. Low serum vitamin B-12 concentrations are associated with faster human immunodeficiency virus type 1 (HIV-1) disease progression. J Nutr. 1997 Feb;127(2):345-351.

87. Baum MK, Shor-Posner G, Campa A. Zinc status in human immunodeficiency virus infection. J Nutr. 2000 May;130(Suppl 5S):1421S-1423S.

88. Constans J, Peuchant E, Pellegrin JL, et al. Fatty acids and plasma antioxidants in HIV-positive patients, correlation with nutritional and immunological status. Clin Biochem. 1995 Aug;28(6):421-426.

89. Look MP, Rockstroh JK, Rao GS, et al. Serum selenium versus lymphocyte subsets and markers of disease progression and inflammatory response in human immunodeficiency virus-1 infection. Biol Trace Elem Res. 1997 Jan;56(1):31-41.

90. Baum MK, Shor-Posner G, Lai S. High risk of HIV-related mortality is associated with selenium deficiency. J Acquir Immune Defic Syndr. 1997;15:370-374.

91. Campa A, Shor-Posner G, Indacochea F, et al. Mortality risk in selenium-deficient HIV-positive children. J Acquir Immune Defic Syndr. 1999;20:508-513.

92. Struwe M, Kaempfer SH, Geiger CJ, et al. Effect of dronabinol on nutritional status in HIV infection. Ann Pharmacother. 1993 Jul-Aug;27(7-8):827-831.

93. Bhasin S, Storer TW, Javanbakht M, et al. Testosterone replacement and resistance exercise in HIV-infected men with weight loss and low testosterone levels. JAMA. 2000;283:763.

94. Grinspoon S, Mulligan K, Department of Health and Human Services Working Group on the Prevention and Treatment of Wasting and Weight Loss. Weight loss and wasting in patients infected with human immunodeficiency virus. Clin Infect Dis. 2003 Apr 1;36(Suppl 2):S69-S78.

95. Rabkin JG, Wagner GJ, Rabkin R. Testosterone therapy for human immunodeficiency virus–positive men with and without hypogonadism. J Clin Psychopharmacol. 1999;19:19.

96. Grinspoon S, Corcoran C, Parlman K, et al. Effects of testosterone and progressive resistance training in eugonadal men with AIDS wasting. A randomized, controlled trial. Ann Intern Med. 2000;133:348.

97. Bhasin S, Storer TW, Asbel-Sethi N, et al. Effects of testosterone replacement with a nongenital, transdermal system, Androderm, in human immunodeficiency virus–infected men with low testosterone levels. J Clin Endocrinol Metab. 1998;83:3155.

98. Dobs AS, Cofrancesco J, Nolten WE, et al. The use of a transscrotal testosterone delivery system in the treatment of patients with weight loss related to human immunodeficiency virus infection. Am J Med. 1999;107:126.

99. Miller K, Corcoran C, Armstrong C, et al. Transdermal testosterone administration in women with acquired immunodeficiency syndrome wasting: A pilot study. J Clin Endocrinol Metab. 1998;83:2717.

100. Strawford A, Barbieri T, Van Loan M, et al. Resistance exercise and supraphysiologic androgen therapy in eugonadal men with HIV-related weight loss: A randomized controlled trial. JAMA. 1999;281:1282.

101. Strang P. The effect of megestrol acetate on anorexia, weight loss and cachexia in cancer and AIDS patients. Anticancer Res. 1997;17(1B):657-662.

102. Rabkin JG, Ferrando SJ, Wagner GJ, Rabkin R. DHEA treatment for HIV+ patients: Effects on mood, androgenic and anabolic parameters. Psychoneuroendocrinology. 2000;57:141.

103. Lee PDK, Pivarnik JM, Bukar JG, et al. A randomized, placebo-controlled trial of combined insulin-like growth factor I and low dose growth hormone therapy for wasting associated with human immunodeficiency virus infection. J Clin Endocrinol Metab. 1996; 81:2968.

104. McNurlan MA, Garlick PJ, Steigbigel RT, et al. Responsiveness of muscle protein synthesis to growth hormone administration in HIV-infected individuals declines with severity of disease. J Clin Invest. 1997;100:2125.

105. Reyes-Teran G, Sierra-Madero JG, del Cerro VM, et al. Effects of thalidomide on HIV-associated wasting syndrome: A randomized, double-blind, placebo-controlled clinical trial. AIDS. 1996;10:15017.

106. Kaplan G, Thomas S, Fierer DS, et al. Thalidomide for the treatment of AIDS-associated wasting. AIDS Res Hum Retroviruses. 2000;16:134555.

107. High KP. Micronutrient supplementation and immune function in the elderly. Clin Infect Dis. 1999;28:717-722.

108. Morley JE. Anorexia and weight loss in older persons. J Gerontol A Biol Sci Med Sci. 2003 Feb;58(2):131-137.

109. Mowe M, Bohmer T. The prevalence of undiagnosed protein-calorie undernutrition in a population of hospitalized elderly patients. J Am Geriatr Soc. 1991;39:1089-1092.

110. Constans T, Bacq Y, Brechot JF, et al. Protein-energy malnutrition in elderly medical patients. J Am Geriatr Soc. 1992;40:263-268.

111. Liu L, Bopp MM, Roberson PK, Sullivan DH. Undernutrition and risk of mortality in elderly patients within 1 year of hospital discharge. J Gerontol A Biol Sci Med Sci. 2002 Nov; 57(11):M741-M746.

112. Thomas DR, Zdrowski CD, Wilson M, et al. Malnutrition in subacute care. Am J Clin Nutr. 2002;75:308-313.

113. Ham RJ. Indicators of poor nutritional status in older Americans. Report of nutrition screening 1: Towards a common view. A consensus conference sponsored by the Nutrition Screening Initiative. Washington, DC: Nutrition Screening Initiative; 1991.

114. Williamson DF. Descriptive epidemiology of body weight and weight change in U.S. adults. Ann Intern Med. 1993;119:646-649.

115. High KP. Nutritional strategies to boost immunity and prevent infection in the elderly. Clin Infect Dis. 2001;33:1892-1900.

116. Barringer TA, Kirk JK, Santaniello AC, et al. Effect of multivitamin and mineral supplement on infection and quality of life. Ann Intern Med. 2003;138:365-371.

117. Buchanan CK, High KP. Nutrition, aging, and infection. Clin Geriatr. 2003;12:44-53.

118. Chandra RK. Effect of vitamin and trace-element supplementation on immune responses and infection in elderly subjects. Lancet. 1992;340:1124-1127.

119. Girodon F, Lombard M, Galan P, et al. Effect of micronutrient supplementation on infection in institutionalized elderly subjects: A controlled trial. Ann Nutr Metab. 1997;41:98-107.

120. Girodon F, Galan P, Monget A, et al. Impact of trace elements and vitamin supplementation on immunity and infections in institutionalized elderly patients: A randomized controlled trial. Arch Intern Med. 1999;159:748-754.

121. Meydani SN, Barklund MP, Liu S, et al. Vitamin E enhances cell-mediated immunity in healthy elderly subjects. Am J Clin Nutr. 1990;52:557-563.

122. Meydani SN, Meydani M, Blumberg JB, et al. Vitamin E supplementation and in vivo immune response in healthy subjects. JAMA. 1997;277:1380-1386.

123. Graat JM, Schouten EG, Kok FJ. Effect of daily vitamin E and multivitamin-mineral supplementation on acute respiratory tract infections in elderly persons: A randomized controlled trial. JAMA. 2002; 288(6):715-721.

CHAPTER **11**

Evaluation of the Patient with Suspected Immunodeficiency

STEVEN M. HOLLAND

JOHN I. GALLIN

The most common causes of immunodeficiency are iatrogenic and are a result of the widespread use of therapies that modulate the immune system either by design or incidentally. With the expanding recognition, characterization, and—in an increasing number of cases—correction of immune abnormalities, making the correct diagnosis is no longer of only academic interest. Identification and cloning of disease-related genes have now made precise antenatal diagnosis and genetic counseling a reality. The promise of the emerging field of gene transfer technology makes it essential to use a sensible, problem-oriented approach to the patient in whom these issues are raised. Following are some general principles involved in the consideration of whether a patient may have an immunodeficiency and how to proceed with a diagnostic evaluation before, or as an adjunct to, referral or discussion with a specialist.

THE INDEX OF SUSPICION

Concern about the immune status of a patient is usually raised on the basis of the frequency or severity of infections or the finding of an unusual infectious agent. Table 11-1 lists some infectious organisms and the affected limb of host defense implied by their isolation. Clearly, not every isolation of a herpesvirus or *Staphylococcus* implies an immunodeficiency in a specific patient. However, in the setting of abnormally frequent infections or failure to thrive, isolation of these organisms from patient samples should make one consider possible underlying diagnoses. In contrast, identification of *Pneumocystis, Burkholderia (Pseudomonas) cepacia, Aspergillus,* or *Nocardia* from a patient without a known immunodeficiency is sufficient grounds for pursuing the probability of an underlying defect.

Recurrent hematogenous neisserial infections indicate deficiencies in the late components of complement.[1] *Pneumocystis carinii* pneumonia indicates T-cell abnormalities.[2] *B. cepacia* bacteremia strongly suggests chronic granulomatous disease.[3] Some specific immunodeficiencies are listed in Table 11-2, along with the gene defect, if known,

and some pertinent findings. Recognition and appreciation of the genetic basis of these disorders have been critical to the development of therapy for them and are fundamental to the curative approaches that are now being implemented.

INITIAL EVALUATION

The screening approach to a patient with suspected immunodeficiency is listed in Table 11-3. Careful attention to historical detail is critical. Age of onset of the illness is helpful; Job's syndrome often has an onset within the first days to weeks of life, whereas antibody deficiency states appear only after several months of life when maternal immunoglobulin levels have fallen.[4] Failure to thrive and diarrhea are important points in favor of a substantial problem but are not specific in terms of etiology. Birth history should include the condition and time of separation of the umbilical stump, because stump separation is abnormally delayed in leukocyte adhesion deficiency (LAD).[5] The past medical history should note the administration of vaccines, especially for measles, mumps, and rubella, and Calmette-Guérin bacillus (BCG), difficulties with which are suggestive of dysfunctional T-cell or monocyte immunity. A dental history can be quite informative because patients with abnormalities of phagocytic defense often have gingivitis with periodontal disease[6] (Fig. 11-1), and patients with Job's syndrome usually have severely delayed deciduation of the primary teeth.[7] Specific questioning regarding parental consanguinity is critical.

Physical examination can yield findings diagnostic or highly suggestive of lesions in specific arms of the immune system. Facial anomalies, including hypertelorism, a shortened philtrum, and down-slanting palpebral fissures, are encountered in DiGeorge's syndrome,[8] whereas characteristic facies with a broad nose and a triangular mandible are seen in the syndrome of extremely elevated IgE and recurrent infections (Job's syndrome).[7,9] Hair with a silvery sheen and irregular melanin production is seen in Chédiak-Higashi syndrome.[10] In general, poor dentition, gingivitis, aphthous ulcers, and tooth loss are seen in phagocytic defects such as chronic granulomatous disease (CGD) and LAD,[6] whereas retained primary teeth are encountered in Job's syndrome.[7] Cutaneous signs of immune defects include telangiectases over the bulbar conjunctivae and skin in ataxia-telangiectasia, the severe eczema that accompanies Job's syndrome, or the dystrophic scarring seen in LAD.

The initial laboratory examination should consist of a complete blood count with differential, platelet count, examination of the peripheral blood smear, and erythrocyte sedimentation rate. Chédiak-Higashi syndrome and neutrophil-specific granule deficiency can be detected on peripheral smear, whereas Kostmann's syndrome (congenital agranulocytosis) and Wiskott-Aldrich syndrome can be largely excluded by normal neutrophil or platelet counts, respectively. An immunoglobulin (Ig) profile with total IgA, IgM, and IgG levels

---

TABLE 11-1 Selected Pathogens Associated with Immunodeficiency Diseases

Pathogen	History	Host Defense Affected	Clinical Examples
Pneumocystis carinii, Cryptococcus neoformans, herpesviruses	Disseminated infections, opportunistic infections, persistent viral infections	T cells	Severe combined immunodeficiency, acquired immunodeficiency syndrome
Haemophilus influenzae, Streptococcus pneumoniae, Giardia lamblia, Campylobacter spp., enteroviruses	Recurrent respiratory infections with encapsulated organisms, chronic diarrhea, aseptic meningitis	B cells	Common variable immunodeficiency, X-linked agammaglobulinemia
Staphylococcus aureus, Burkholderia cepacia, Serratia marcescens, Aspergillus spp., *Nocardia* spp.	Gingivitis, aphthous ulcers, recurrent pyogenic infections, delayed umbilical stump separation	Phagocytes	Chronic granulomatous disease, Chédiak-Higashi syndrome, leukocyte adhesion deficiency
Neisseria spp.	Recurrent bacteremia, recurrent meningitis	Complement	Late complement component deficiency
Staphylococcus aureus, H. influenzae, S. pneumoniae, Candida albicans	Eczema, kyphoscoliosis, pathologic fractures, pulmonary and cutaneous infections, mucocutaneous candidiasis	T cells, phagocytes	Hyperimmunoglobulin E–recurrent infections (Job's syndrome)

TABLE 11-2 Congenital Immunodeficiencies

Clinical Disease	Affected Gene Product*	Chromosomal Location	Inheritance	Functional Defect	Important Findings	References
T Cells						
Severe combined immunodeficiency (SCID)						2, 16
X-linked SCID	Interleukin (IL)-2 receptor gamma common chain	Xq13–21.1	X	T-cell proliferation, antibody production	Lymphopenia, hypo-gammaglobulinemia	2, 16
Adenosine deaminase (ADA) deficiency	Adenosine deaminase	20q13–ter	AR	T-cell functions, antibody production	Absent ADA activity, lymphopenia, hypo-gammaglobulinemia	14
Purine nucleoside phosphorylase (PNP) deficiency	Purine nucleoside phosphorylase	14q13.1	AR	T-cell functions	Absent PNP activity, low CD3$^+$ cells, increased NK cells, low uric acid	15
Defective major histocompatibility complex (MHC) molecules	RF-X	19q13	AR	Cell-mediated immunity	B cells normal, Ig normal or low, absent MHC molecules	24
IL-2 deficiency	Nuclear factor–activated T cells (NFAT)	?	AR	Cell-mediated immunity, antibody production	Lymphopenia, hypo-gammaglobulinemia	20-23
Reticular dysgenesis	?	?	AR	Pancytopenia	Pancytopenia	11-13, 16, 17
DiGeorge's syndrome, velocardiofacial syndrome, CATCH 22	Many candidates in the deleted region; TBX1	22q11.21–q11.23	AD	Anomalous development of 3rd and 4th pharyngeal pouches	Thymic aplasia, parathyroid aplasia, cardiac anomalies, abnormal facies	8, 26
Ataxia-telangiectasia	Ataxia-telangiectasia mutated (ATM)	11q22.3	AR	DNA repair, T cells	Low IgA, Low CD3 and CD4 cells, malignancies	27
Wiskott-Aldrich syndrome	Wiskott-Aldrich syndrome protein (WASP)	Xq11–11.3	X	T cells and platelets	Eczema, thrombocytopenia, low platelet volume, low IgM, high IgA, IgE	28-33
B Cells						
X-linked agamma-globulinemia	B-cell progenitor kinase (BPK)	Xq22	X	B cells	Very low antibody levels	2, 34, 35
Immunodeficiencies with hyper-IgM	CD40 ligand (CD40L, gp39)	Xq26	X	B cells, T cells B cells, monocytes	High IgM, low IgG, IgA, poor T-cell responses	36, 37
	NFκB essential modulator (NEMO)	Xq28	X	Neutrophils	High or normal IgM, low IgG, broad spectrum of infections	38-91
	CD40	20q12	AR	Monocytes	High or normal IgM, low IgG, poor T-cell function	39
	Activation-induced cytidine deaminase (AID)	12p13	AR	B cells	Lymph nodes present, normal to high IgM, low IgG	40
X-linked lympho-proliferative syndrome (Duncan's syndrome)	SLAM-associated protein (SAP)	Xq25	X	EBV response	Low EBNA antibody, uncontrolled cellular activation	41-43
Common variable immunodeficiency	ICOS and others	2q33 and others	AR	Antibody synthesis, T-cell function	Low IgG, poor antibody response, low IgA common	44, 121
IgA deficiency	IgA	?6p21.3	AR	IgA	Associated with other immunodeficiencies	44, 45
Phagocytes						
Chronic granulomatous disease (CGD)				Bacterial and fungal killing defective in all forms of CGD	Infections with catalase+ microbes, granulomas, and reduced superoxide generation	70, 72
X-linked CGD	gp91phox	Xp21.1	X 70% of CGD			
Autosomal recessive CGD	p22phox	16q24	AR <5% of CGD	—	—	
	p47phox	7q11.23	AR 25% of CGD	—	—	
	p67phox	1q25	AR <5% of CGD	—	—	

*The affected gene product is not always the gene in which the lesion has occurred. The genetic lesion may disable a regulatory gene required for expression or function of the affected gene product.

AD, autosomal dominant; AR, autosomal recessive; BCG, bacille Calmette-Guérin; EBNA, Epstein-Barr virus nuclear antigen; EBV, Epstein-Barr virus; GDP, guanosine diphosphate; ICOS, inducible costimulator; Ig, immunoglobulin; NFκB, nuclear factor κB; NK, natural killer; RF, regulatory factor; SLAM, signaling lymphocyte activation molecule; X, X-linked inheritance.

TABLE 11-2   Congenital Immunodeficiencies—cont'd

Clinical Disease	Affected Gene Product*	Chromosomal Location	Inheritance	Functional Defect	Important Findings	References
Severe chronic neutropenia and cyclic neutropenia	Neutrophil elastase (ELA2)	19p13	AD	Neutropenia	Cyclic hematopoiesis, cycle ~21 days; some cases constant	47, 48, 51
	Growth factor independent 1(GFI1)	1p22	AD	Neutropenia	Severe neutropenia	49
Warts, hypogamma-globulinemia, infections, and myelokathexis	CXCR4	2q21	AD	Impaired chemokine receptor activity	Impaired neutrophil exit from the marrow (myelokathexis), low IgG, warts	122
Chédiak-Higashi syndrome	Lysosomal transport protein (LYST)	1q43	AR	Chemotactic defect, neutropenia	Giant granules in neutrophils, oculo-cutaneous albinism	54-56
Leukocyte adhesion deficiency type 1	CD18	21q22.3	AR	Absent leukocyte integrins	Chronic leukocytosis, delayed umbilical cord separation, recurrent infections	5, 59, 60
Leukocyte adhesion deficiency type 2	Sialyl-Lewis X [due to mutations in GDP-fucose transporter-1 (FUCT1)]	11	AR	E-selectin ligand, fucose metabolism	Short stature, mental retardation, Bombay blood type	58, 61
Neutrophil specific granule deficiency	CCAAT enhancer binding protein (C/EBPε)	3q21	AR	Neutrophil granule products	Absent neutrophil-specific granules, absent defensins (primary granules)	62-67
IL-1 receptor–associated kinase-4 (IRAK 4) deficiency	IRAK 4	12q12	AR	Signal transduction through the Toll-like receptors, the IL-1 receptor, and others	Severe pyogenic infections in childhood	89, 90
Myeloperoxidase deficiency	Myeloperoxidase (MPO)	17q21–q23	AR	Catalysis of superoxide to hydrogen peroxide	Absent MPO, usually unassociated with infections	68
Interferon (IFN)-γ receptor 1 deficiency	IFN γR1	6q23-q24	AR	Absence of IFN-γ binding	Recurrent nontuberculous mycobacterial and Salmonella infections	93-95
			AD	Overaccumulation of defective receptor	Nontuberculous mycobacterial osteomyelitis	97, 98
IFN-γ receptor 2 deficiency	IFN γR2	21q22.1-q22.2	AR	Absence of IFN-γ signaling	Recurrent nontuberculous mycobacteria	96
Interleukin (IL)-12 receptor β1 deficiency	IL-12RB1	19p13.1	AR	Absence of IL-12 signaling	Recurrent nontuberculous mycobacterial and Salmonella infections	99, 100, 102
IL-12 p40 deficiency (IL-12p40)	IL-12p40	5q31	AR	Lack of IL-12 leading to low production of IFN-γ	Recurrent nontuberculous mycobacterial and Salmonella infections	101
Signal transducer and activator of transcription 1 (STAT1)	STAT1	2q32.2	AD	Reduced IFN-γ receptor signaling	Severe disseminated nontuberculous myco-bacteria and BCG	103
			AR	Absent IFN-γ and IFN alfa/beta receptor signaling	Disseminated fatal mycobacterial and viral infections	104
Hyper IgE–recurrent infection syndrome (Job's syndrome)	?	?4q	AD	Intermittently poor chemotaxis, ?CD8 T-cell dysfunction	Extremely high IgE, eczema, facial, dental and bony abnormal-ities, pneumatocele formations	7, 105, 112

Complement

Classical Pathway

Clinical Disease	Affected Gene Product*	Chromosomal Location	Inheritance	Functional Defect	Important Findings	References
C1q deficiency	C1q	1p36.3	AR	Antibody-dependent complement lysis is depressed in all forms of classic complement component deficiencies	Low CH$_{50}$ is seen with all forms of classic complement component deficiency. Individual components are very low or absent	1
C1r deficiency	C1r	12p13	AR			
C1s deficiency	C1s	12p13	AR			
C2 deficiency	C2	6p21.3	AR			
C3 deficiency	C3	19p13.3	AR			
C4A deficiency	C4A	6p21.3	AR			
C4B deficiency	C4B	6p21.3	AR		Autoimmune disease is common in early-component deficiencies (C1–C4)	
C5 deficiency	C5	9q34.1	AR			
C6 deficiency	C6	5p13	AR			
C7 deficiency	C7	5p13	AR			
C8 deficiency	C8	1p32	AR		Bacteremia and meningitis are common in all types of complement deficiency	
C9 deficiency	C9	5p13	AR			

Alternative Pathway

Clinical Disease	Affected Gene Product*	Chromosomal Location	Inheritance	Functional Defect	Important Findings	References
Properdin deficiency	Properdin	Xp11.4-23	X	Antibody-independent complement lysis is depressed in alternative complement component deficiencies	More severe susceptibility to infection than classic component deficiencies	
Factor H deficiency	Factor H	1q32	AR			
Factor I deficiency	Factor I	4q25	AR			

TABLE 11-3   Screening Evaluations for Immune Defects

History
  Medications and treatments
  Relatedness of parents, umbilical stump separation, age of onset, dental history
  Frequency, severity, distribution, types of infections
  Vaccination history, especially live vaccines
  Causative infectious agents
Physical
  Weight and height
  Hair: sheen, pigmentation
  Abdomen: organomegaly
  Skin: dystrophic scars, telangiectases, eczema, warts
  Oropharynx: thrush, ulcers, gingivitis, secondary tooth eruption
  Facies: hypertelorism, eye slant, philtrum
  Skeleton: kyphoscoliosis, fractures
Routine laboratory values
  Complete blood count
    Differential: lymphopenia, neutropenia, eosinophilia
    Peripheral smear: giant granules, specific (secondary) granules
    Platelet count: thrombocytopenia
    Erythrocyte sedimentation rate: usually elevated in infection
  Chemistries
    Serum calcium
    Serum uric acid
    Liver functions
  Immunoglobulins
    IgA, IgM, IgG, IgE
    Isohemagglutinins
    Antibody titers (tetanus, pneumococcus, etc.)
  Complement
    Total hemolytic complement (CH_{50})
Radiography
  Plain chest films: kyphoscoliosis, pneumatoceles, scarring

will help detect cases of IgA deficiency as well as hypogamma-globulinemia. In cases in which eczema is a prominent feature or Job's syndrome is suspected, measurement of IgE levels is indicated. A functional challenge of the humoral immune system, such as preimmunization and postimmunization antibody levels, may be informative. Testing of total hemolytic complement (CH_{50}) gives a quick assessment of the functional integrity of the classic component of the complement cascade from C1 through the membrane attack complex (C5-C9). Plain radiographs of the chest can demonstrate pulmonary scarring, pneumatoceles, and destruction, often encountered in phagocyte defects and Job's syndrome. Scoliosis, osteoporosis, rib and long bone fractures, and their sequelae are frequently seen in Job's syndrome.[7,9]

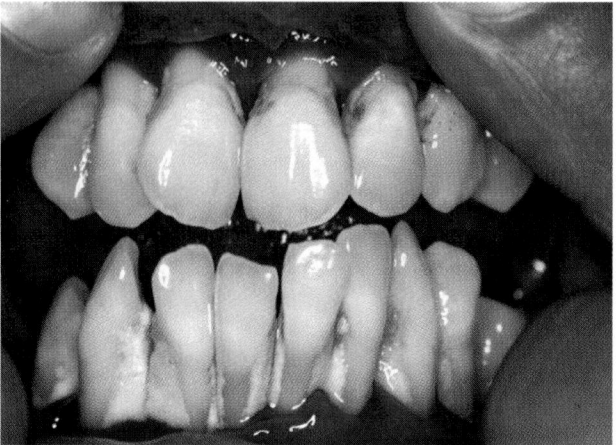

FIGURE 11-1.   Severe periodontal disease in leukocyte adhesion deficiency (LAD)-1 as shown by gum recession.

LYMPHOCYTE IMMUNE DEFECTS

T Cells and Cell-Mediated Immunity

The initial manifestation of congenital T-cell defects usually, but not always, occurs within the first few months of life and includes severe mucocutaneous candidiasis, recurrent persistent respiratory infections, diarrhea, and failure to thrive. A broad spectrum of onset and severity is seen. Reticular dysgenesis occurs within the first weeks of life and is characterized by pancytopenia, infection, and early demise.[11-13] The lymphocyte enzymopathies (adenosine deaminase deficiency and purine nucleoside phosphorylase deficiency) tend to occur after several months of life when lymphocyte counts begin to fall because of accumulation of the toxic metabolites deoxyadenosine triphosphate and deoxyguanosine triphosphate, respectively.[14,15] The occurrence of *P. carinii* pneumonia, disseminated Calmette-Guérin bacillus infection after vaccination, persistent poliovirus infection after oral polio vaccination, or persistent respiratory virus infection should initiate consideration of a defect in lymphocyte function.[16] Graft-versus-host disease, either acquired from in utero transfer of maternal lymphocytes or through transfusion of unirradiated blood, may be the underlying cause of cutaneous eruptions, transaminase elevations, or malabsorption and diarrhea and is a strong indicator of defective T-cell immunity.[16]

In many forms of T-cell abnormality, B-cell function is also compromised, and both cell-mediated and humoral deficiencies occur, a state referred to as severe combined immunodeficiency.[16] This syndrome tends to be recognized after maternal antibody levels wane and recurrent bacterial infections begin. The finding of low immunoglobulin levels in association with marked lymphopenia in the appropriate setting should lead to the consideration of severe combined immunodeficiency.[2]

The most direct and simplest assessment of T-cell immune status is the determination of lymphocyte number, which is obtained in the screening differential count. Circulating lymphocyte numbers range from about 7000 cells/µL in infants to 4000 cells/µL in children and about 2000 cells/µL in adolescents and adults through old age.[17] Of these lymphocytes, roughly half are T cells, with the remainder split between B cells and natural killer cells. Severe quantitative abnormalities of lymphocytes are relatively uncommon; low absolute lymphocyte numbers are encountered in the great majority of cases of severe combined immunodeficiency as well as in several other congenital immunodeficiencies (see Table 11-2). Acquired immunodeficiency syndrome (AIDS), high plasma corticosteroid levels (iatrogenic or endogenous), obstructed lymphatic circulation (e.g., intestinal lymphangiectasia), severe systemic illness (e.g., carcinomatosis, miliary tuberculosis), systemic lupus erythematosus, sarcoid, cytotoxic or immunosuppressive therapy, and severe right-sided congestive heart failure can also cause lymphocytopenia.

T-lymphocyte function is initially and most easily assayed in vivo by testing of type IV cell-mediated immunity, or delayed-type hypersensitivity (DTH) (Table 11-4). DTH is elicited by the intradermal injection of an antigen to which the patient has been exposed. Antigen-specific CD4+ T cells are recruited, and in turn, these T cells recruit macrophages with resulting interstitial fibrin deposition and induration. Erythema and edema are seen early after the injection but are not indicative of DTH. Frank induration is best appreciated between 24 and 48 hours and then gradually falls off. Effective DTH is indicated by induration.

In the screening evaluation for immune defects, it is important to consider the patient's antigenic experience, such as immunizations, previous infections, and regional exposures in the selection of antigens. It is critical to test several different antigens simultaneously for the determination of T-cell responsiveness, such as mumps, *Candida, Trichophyton,* streptococcal antigens, and tetanus. The demonstration of intact DTH confirms the presence of functional CD4+ T cells and excludes most of the congenital defects in cell-mediated immunity. Importantly, DTH can be preserved until relatively late into human immunodeficiency virus (HIV) infection. Therefore, the presence of DTH should not be considered evidence against HIV infection per se.

TABLE 11-4   Directed Tests of Immune Function

T cells
    Fluorescence-activated cell sorting (FACS) (lymphocyte subsets,
        cytokine receptors)
    Delayed-type hypersensitivity: mumps, *Candida*, tetanus, *Trichophyton*
    Lymphocyte enzymes (adenosine deaminase and purine nucleoside
        phosphorylase)
    Cytokine production and response
    In vitro proliferation: stimulation with antigen, lectin, antibody,
        allogeneic cells, phosphokinase C stimulants, and calcium
        ionophores
B cells
    FACS
    Antigen challenge, recall or new
    In vitro antibody production
Phagocytes
    FACS for leukocyte adhesion molecules
    Dihydrorhodamine oxidation, nitroblue tetrazolium reduction
    Superoxide generation, hydrogen peroxide generation
    Adherence
    Staphylococcicidal activity
    Chemotaxis
    Phagocytosis
Complement
    Assay of individual complement components, functional or quantitative

Selective anergy to the antigens of the offending organism has been observed in active visceral leishmaniasis and lepromatous leprosy. These specific defects have reversed after successful treatment of the underlying infection.[18] Complete anergy to a battery of antigens is a relatively nonspecific finding in terms of etiology insofar as the differential diagnosis includes all the entities that cause lymphopenia. However, anergy makes further evaluation of the cell-mediated immune system reasonable.

Fluorescence-activated cell sorting (FACS) analysis now allows rapid enumeration and characterization of lymphocyte, monocyte, and neutrophil subsets.[19] Access to FACS analysis is widely available. Lymphocyte subset determination, specifically for CD4$^+$ T cells, is standard in the management of HIV infection to provide guideposts for initiation of antiviral and prophylactic therapy. With the recent identification and cloning of certain immunodeficiency-related genes, FACS is able to confirm or exclude specific diagnoses.

Evaluation of T-cell function in vitro requires laboratory personnel skilled in the isolation, preparation, and stimulation of peripheral blood mononuclear cells. Stimulation is typically done on unseparated peripheral blood mononuclear cells and therefore represents the product of both lymphocyte and monocyte contributions. Proliferation is usually measured as triffiated (^{3}H)-thymidine incorporation into the DNA of dividing lymphocytes after stimulation with cell membrane–binding lectins (phytohemagglutinin, concanavalin A, pokeweed mitogen), direct stimulants of cellular signaling pathways that bypass the need for membrane components (phorbol myristate acetate and calcium ionophore), antigens (purified protein derivative, *Candida*, tetanus), cytokines (interleukin-2 [IL-2]), or allogeneic cells (mixed lymphocyte reaction).[19] Significantly low proliferation in vitro can result from absent cell surface receptors such as the CD3 complex,[20] antigen-specific anergy as in leishmaniasis,[18] IL-2 deficiencies,[21-23] or major histocompatibility complex abnormalities.[24] Two important CD4$^+$ T-cell subsets are distinguished. Th1 cells produce interferon-γ and IL-2 and are the predominant cells in the DTH response. Th2 cells produce IL-4, IL-5, and IL-10 and can regulate the differentiation of B cells and eosinophils. Both of these cell types regulate each other and therefore open new areas for the likely discovery of immune defects and new therapeutic manipulations of their relationship.[25] Cytokine levels in the supernates of stimulated and unstimulated cells can be readily determined and may demonstrate states of either deficiency[21-23] or excess.

DiGeorge's syndrome is caused by anomalous development of the third and fourth pharyngeal pouches with agenesis of the thymus and parathyroids and subsequent immunodeficiency and hypocalcemia.

Neonatal tetany is an expected manifestation.[26] The defect in DiGeorge's syndrome is due to interstitial deletions in chromosome 21, but specific genes have not yet been identified.[8] Ataxia-telangiectasia is associated with low IgA and low CD3$^+$ and CD4$^+$ T-cell levels, progressive ataxia, and oculocutaneous telangiectases. These patients usually experience recurrent bacterial respiratory infections and are at increased risk of malignancy because of abnormalities in DNA repair.[2,27] Wiskott-Aldrich syndrome is characterized by eczema, elevated IgE, thrombocytopenia with small platelets, and recurrent opportunistic infections.[28] The gene product defective in Wiskott-Aldrich syndrome has been identified as Wiskott-Aldrich syndrome protein (WASP).[29-31] Mutations in WASP also have been found to cause X-linked thrombocytopenia[32] and X-linked neutropenia.[33]

B Cells and Humoral Immunity

Almost 50 years have elapsed since the first description of an immunodeficiency syndrome, X-linked agammaglobulinemia (XLA), by Colonel Bruton.[34] The clinical features of immunoglobulin defects are distinct from those of T-cell or combined defects. The age of onset for congenital deficiencies is between 6 months and 2 years, and the initial infections are predominantly with encapsulated bacteria. The thymus gland is present and apparently normal in XLA, but peripheral lymphoid tissues such as tonsils and lymph nodes are essentially absent.[35] B cells and plasma cells in the circulation and the periphery are rare despite normal numbers of pre-B cells in the bone marrow. These patients have elevated T-cell numbers, normal T-cell subsets, and intact T-cell functions. Although they have significant problems with bacterial infections, patients with XLA also have severe difficulty with persistent, disseminated echovirus infections, especially in the central nervous system. Immunoglobulin G (IgG), IgA, and IgM levels are extremely low, as are those of isohemagglutinins. No antibody to either new or previously administered antigens is detectable. In contrast, patients with any of the syndromes that can give rise to the hyperimmunoglobulin M syndrome (the X-linked deficiency of CD40 ligand [CD40L or CD154][36,37]; X-linked ectodermal dysplasia with immunodeficiency[38]; autosomal recessive CD40 deficiency[39]; and autosomal recessive activation-induced cytidine deaminase deficiency[40]) may have preserved lymphoid tissue mass, hepatosplenomegaly, normal numbers of B cells and T cells, and variable neutropenia. Autoimmune phenomena such as Coombs-positive hemolytic anemia and thrombocytopenia are common. IgM is often normal to elevated, and IgG and IgA are usually quite low; isohemagglutinins may be elevated.[35] The X-linked lymphoproliferative disorder, Duncan's syndrome, occurs in males only after infection with Epstein-Barr virus and results in a full-blown immunodeficiency syndrome that can be fatal.[41] The gene has been identified as a protein that is associated with the signaling lymphocyte-activation molecule (SLAM); the SLAM-associated protein is called SAP and is a critical T-cell–signaling molecule.[42,43]

The initial test for the integrity of the humoral arm of immunity is a determination of levels of isohemagglutinins (see later) and levels of IgG, IgA, and IgM. Normal immunoglobulin levels are relatively low in infancy and childhood and increase with age. If immunoglobulin levels are appropriate, XLA can be excluded. Low immunoglobulin levels may be seen in the first year of life in the transient hypogammaglobulinemia of infancy.[2,35] However, these infants usually have detectable isohemagglutinins and can mount antibody responses to new antigenic challenges. Despite family histories notable for relatives with immunodeficiencies, patients with transient hypogammaglobulinemia of infancy tend to normalize their immunoglobulin levels over the first 2 years of life. The finding of depressed levels of immunoglobulin, especially in an adult with recurrent bacterial sinopulmonary infections, raises the possibility of common variable immunodeficiency.[44] Common variable immunodeficiency is a heterogeneous group of diseases that share the features of hypogammaglobulinemia and an increased susceptibility to chronic enteric infections with *Giardia lamblia, Campylobacter,* and disseminated echovirus infections, in addition to sinopulmonary bacterial infections. Patients with common variable immunodeficiency often have low isohemagglutinin levels and abnormal DTH and fail to make antibody to new antigens. IgG subclass analysis may show selective defects in IgG_1 and IgG_3 or in IgG_2 and IgG_4, in addition to defects in IgA.[44] However, the value of checking IgG subclasses is debated.[45]

Isohemagglutinins are IgM antibodies directed against blood group A and B antigens, which occur in all healthy people except those with blood group AB. By the age of 3 years, 98% of patients with blood groups A, B, or O have isohemagglutinins with a titer of at least 1:16.[44] Isohemagglutinin levels are determined in blood banks as a prerequisite to transfusion. Challenge with antigen is probably the simplest and most effective method for determining the functional integrity of the humoral immune system. Use of a recall antigen allows testing of anamnestic responses. Novel antigens such as bacteriophage ΦX174 or keyhole limpet hemocyanin make possible the testing of antibody responses during immunoglobulin administration. Polysaccharide pneumococcal vaccinations examine the response to polysaccharide antigen, whereas tetanus challenge is more specific for peptide responses. Serum titers should be checked before and 2 weeks after immunization.

PHAGOCYTE IMMUNE DEFECTS: NEUTROPHILS

The clinical findings of patients with neutrophil disorders often share common features: gingivitis, periodontal disease, and oral ulceration.[6] Cutaneous infections with *Staphylococcus aureus* are recurrent and can be severe. In neutrophil disorders characterized by inadequate inflammation (neutropenia, LAD, Chédiak-Higashi syndrome, neutrophil-specific granule deficiency), infections can extend locally and subcutaneously with little reaction until marked destruction has taken place. Visceral and especially sinopulmonary involvement is a feature that helps distinguish neutrophil defects from other syndromes in the differential diagnosis. Hepatic abscess is a frequent manifestation of CGD and is most often caused by *S. aureus,* an organism rarely encountered at that anatomic site in patients with normal neutrophils.

Neutropenia

A neutrophil count below 500 cells/μL carries a profound risk of bacterial and fungal infection.[46] Although this principle was first extensively documented and is still most frequently displayed in cancer and leukemia patients undergoing combination chemotherapy, its importance has been confirmed in patients with genetic disorders that affect neutrophil number. Cyclic neutropenia or cyclic hematopoiesis is a rare disease occurring in autosomal dominant, spontaneous, and acquired forms characterized by relatively regular 21-day oscillations in the levels of blood neutrophils, monocytes, eosinophils, lymphocytes, platelets, and reticulocytes.[47] The defects, now known to be multiple and at the level of the hematopoietic stem cell, are the result of mutations in neutrophil elastase[48] or growth factor–independent 1 (GFI1).[49] Patients are usually first seen in childhood and have recurrent episodes of fever, malaise, mucosal ulcers, and, occasionally, life-threatening infections associated with periods of profound neutropenia (<200/μL).[47] Adult-onset cases have been described with an associated clonal proliferation of large granular lymphocytes (CD8$^+$/CD57$^+$) as well. Neutrophil number is transiently impaired, but function is normal. The diagnosis is suspected in children with recurrent stomatitis, gingivitis, cutaneous infections, lymphadenopathy, and fever. The diagnosis should be entertained in patients with intermittent neutropenia, especially if a periodicity around 21 days can be documented on serial blood draws. Molecular diagnostics should be pursued to confirm the specific gene involved. In congenital agranulocytosis (severe congenital neutropenia or Kostmann's syndrome[50]), neutrophil counts are consistently low from birth and show no periodicity. Interestingly, congenital agranulocytosis is also caused by mutations in neutrophil elastase, but these cluster in a different part of the molecule from those that cause cyclic neutropenia.[51] Neutropenic syndromes are successfully treated with recombinant granulocyte colony-stimulating factor, but myeloid malignancies are increased in this population.[52,53]

Chédiak-Higashi Syndrome

Chédiak-Higashi syndrome is a rare autosomal recessive disorder caused by defects in the lysosomal transport protein (Lyst).[54,55] It is characterized by recurrent bacterial infections, partial oculocutaneous albinism, photophobia, nystagmus, and peripheral neuropathy.[10] Many patients die in childhood from infection. An aggressive "lymphoproliferative" phase with diffuse organ infiltration and death develops in about half of the patients who survive into adolescence. Several patients have lived into adulthood, at which time an aggressive, severe, debilitating peripheral neuropathy is a common feature.[10] Pathologically, giant abnormal granules are found in neutrophils, melanocytes, hair, Schwann cells, the central nervous system, peripheral ganglia, capillary epithelium, renal tubular epithelium, erythroid precursors, fibroblasts, and other granule-containing cells.[10] In neutrophils, the granules are formed mainly by fusion of azurophilic or primary granules to each other, and to a lesser extent by fusion to specific or secondary granules.[56]

Features of Chédiak-Higashi syndrome include central and peripheral nervous system involvement with peripheral neuropathy, myopathy, autonomic dysfunction, and leptomeningeal involvement.[10] Lymphohistiocytic infiltration of axons and myelin sheaths occurs in patients with peripheral neuropathy and in ganglia in patients with autonomic neuropathy. Melanin granules seen in the neurons of the substantia nigra are large, irregular, and clumped. These aggregates of melanosomes seem to increase in size and number with age. Low intelligence has been noted in some series.[10] The diagnosis of Chédiak-Higashi syndrome is easily made by inspection of the peripheral smear for giant lysosomes or microscopic examination of hair for characteristic melanin clumps.

Leukocyte Adhesion Deficiency

Leukocyte adhesion to endothelium and other leukocytes is mediated by several sets of molecules, among which are the integrins and the selectins. It is now recognized that defects in either of these two intercellular adhesion pathways can lead to overlapping clinical phenotypes. LAD type 1 is a rare autosomal recessive disorder involving one set of the leukocyte integrins—the molecules required for leukocyte adherence to endothelium, other leukocytes, and bacteria.[5,57] Deficiency of the integrin component CD18 leads to a corresponding deficiency of the complexes leukocyte function–associated antigen (LFA)-1, Mac-1, and p150,95, and to the resulting abnormalities of cellular adhesion. These abnormalities are predictable from the basic defect. The absence of a marginated pool of neutrophils leads to chronic leukocytosis, whereas the poor inflammatory response leads to recurrent infections.

LAD-1 encompasses two broad categories, severe and moderate, depending on the degree of CD18 deficiency.[5] Patients with severe deficiency (<0.5%) of normal protein expression are characterized by delayed umbilical stump separation, umbilical stump infection, persistent leukocytosis in the absence of active infection (>15,000/μL), and severe destructive periodontitis with associated loss of dentition and alveolar bone. Recurrent infections of the skin, upper and lower airways, bowel, and perirectal area and septicemia are common and usually due to *S. aureus* or gram-negative rods, most notably *Pseudomonas* species. Infections tend to be necrotizing and may progress to ulceration but demonstrate an almost complete absence of neutrophil invasion on histopathologic analysis. Patients with a moderate form of the disease (3% to 30% of normal expression) tend to have normal umbilical stump separation, have LAD diagnosed later in life, and less commonly have life-threatening infections. Leukocytosis is still the rule, as is delayed wound healing and periodontal disease. Although patients with a moderate form of the disease are less ill and tend to live past childhood, deaths from infection have been reported in young adults.[5]

Laboratory findings in general reflect the clinical differences between severe and moderate phenotypes of the disease, with the severe form showing more profound deficiencies than the moderate form. Abnormalities include grossly defective granulocyte and mononuclear cell mobilization into Rebuck skin windows in vivo and diminished neutrophil migration in response to the bacterial chemoattractant f-Met-Leu-Phe in vitro despite normal numbers of receptors.[5] These laboratory abnormalities are demonstrated in vivo in histologic sections of infected tissues, which show the presence of some mononuclear cells but very low numbers of neutrophils. Granulocyte adherence to glass, plastic, nylon, wool, and other LAD granulocytes is greatly reduced and not stimulated by exposure to f-Met-Leu-Phe or phorbol myristate acetate. The absence of CD18 leads to the absence of Mac-1 and the iC3b receptor CR3. Therefore, complement-mediated phagocytosis is severely impaired, whereas IgG-mediated phagocytosis is normal. Although viral infections are not usually special problems in LAD, antibody-dependent cellular cytotoxicity by patient cells is also diminished. Oxidative metabolism in response to phorbol myristate acetate or calcium ionophore is normal in patient granulocytes as measured by nitroblue tetrazolium reduction or chemiluminescence. Neutrophil primary and secondary granule release in response to phorbol myristate acetate or chemoattractants is normal in LAD cells, whereas the response after zymosan particle ingestion is depressed.

The diagnosis is established by eliciting a thorough history, with special attention directed to consanguinity, evidence of depressed inflammation in the neonatal period, delayed umbilical stump separation, and recurrent infections. A dental history is helpful inasmuch as most of these patients have severe problems with gingivitis, periodontal disease, tooth loss, and alveolar bone erosion. Wounds often heal abnormally, with dystrophic, paper-thin scars remaining. The diagnosis is confirmed by FACS, which shows reduction or absence of the components of the leukocyte adhesion molecules CD18, CD11a, CD11b, and CD11c.

In LAD-2, neutrophil adherence to endothelial cells is defective because of absence of the sialyl-Lewis X antigen on the neutrophil surface, which is the binding site for E-selectin.[58-60] The patients have neutrophilia, recurrent pulmonary, periodontal, and cutaneous infections, abnormal chemotaxis, mental retardation, short stature, distinctive facies, and the Bombay (hh) blood phenotype. The underlying defect is autosomal recessive and caused by mutations in guanosine diphosphate (GDP)-fucose transporter-1.[58,61] This disease is now known as congenital disorder of glycosylation IIc.

Neutrophil-Specific Granule Deficiency

Neutrophil-specific (secondary) granule deficiency is a rare (eight cases identified), heterogeneous disease characterized by a profound reduction or absence of neutrophil-specific granules and their contents.[62] Associated abnormalities in the few patients reported include bilobed or trilobed neutrophil nuclei, absence of some neutrophil primary (azurophil) granule proteins, mononuclear eosinophils without eosinophilic granules, and dysfunction of platelet α-granules. The neutrophil-specific granule protein lactoferrin has been shown to be diminished or absent in these patients' neutrophils, and the defective production of lactoferrin is relatively tissue specific, with normal production by lacrimal glands but no production in neutrophils or eosinophils.[62-64] Sibling deaths at early ages, consanguineous marriages in the parents of patients, and occurrence of the syndrome in females lead to the assumption of an autosomal recessive pattern of inheritance for neutrophil-specific granule deficiency. The development of a mouse model that displays clinical features of neutrophil-specific granule deficiency by deletion of the gene *C/EBP*ε, a regulator of myeloid development, focused attention on this regulatory gene family in this disease.[65] One of the cases of neutrophil-specific granule deficiency has been shown to result from mutation in the transcriptional regulator c/EBPε.[66,67]

Myeloperoxidase Deficiency

Myeloperoxidase (MPO, also called verdoperoxidase), the heme-binding protein that makes pus green, catalyzes the conversion of hydrogen peroxide to hypochlorous acid (bleach). MPO deficiency, the most common neutrophil disorder, affects about 1 in 2000 persons but is quite silent in most cases. Neutrophil function is affected by MPO deficiency in a variety of ways. The respiratory burst in MPO-deficient neutrophils is prolonged, and as a result, exaggerated amounts of hydrogen

peroxide are produced.[68] The increased hydrogen peroxide production probably compensates functionally for the defect in hypochlorous acid production. Phagocytosis is normal to increased in MPO-deficient neutrophils, whereas bactericidal activity is somewhat slower than normal. Killing of *Aspergillus* conidia by MPO-deficient neutrophils is retarded, whereas the combination of MPO-deficient neutrophils with CGD neutrophils (see "Chronic Granulomatous Disease," next), which are unable to generate hydrogen peroxide but do produce MPO, results in normal killing of *Aspergillus* conidia.[69] Pathologic sequelae of MPO deficiency are brought out only in the presence of other impairments of host defense such as diabetes mellitus. A very few MPO-deficient diabetic patients have had severe yeast infections.

Chronic Granulomatous Disease

CGD is a genetically heterogeneous group of disorders of phagocytic cell oxidative metabolism characterized by recurrent life-threatening infections with bacteria and fungi and dysregulated granuloma formation.[70] The frequency is greater than 1 in 200,000 persons.[71] CGD is caused by a defect in the reduced nicotinamide-adenine dinucleotide phosphate oxidase, which is responsible for the respiratory burst and the generation of phagocyte hydrogen peroxide (Fig. 11-2). Clinically, CGD is quite variable; the time of onset may occur from infancy to late adulthood, although it is diagnosed in most patients while toddlers and young children. However, CGD is diagnosed in a significant number of patients later in life.[70-72] Children with CGD tend to be short and small for their age but eventually achieve the height predicted by their parents' height.[73]

Pulmonary, cutaneous, lymphatic, and hepatic infections are frequent. Osteomyelitis, perianal abscess, and gingivitis are also common.[70-72] The microbiology of infections associated with CGD is remarkable for its relative specificity: *S. aureus, B. cepacia, Serratia marcescens, Nocardia* species, and *Aspergillus* species account for the overwhelming majority of infections (Fig. 11-3). As in other neutrophil abnormalities, the most common offender in CGD is *S. aureus*. Whereas the typical case of liver abscess in an immunologically normal patient involves enteric organisms and is liquid and easily drained, the liver abscesses encountered in patients with CGD are dense, caseous, and staphylococcal (Fig. 11-4). In the absence of antibiotic prophylaxis, lung, skin, and bone infections are also usually staphylococcal. However, *Aspergillus* species and some of the rarer fungi such as *Exophiala dermatitidis*[74] and *Paecilomyces* species[75] are encountered in CGD. Infections with *Nocardia* species, *Chromobacterium*

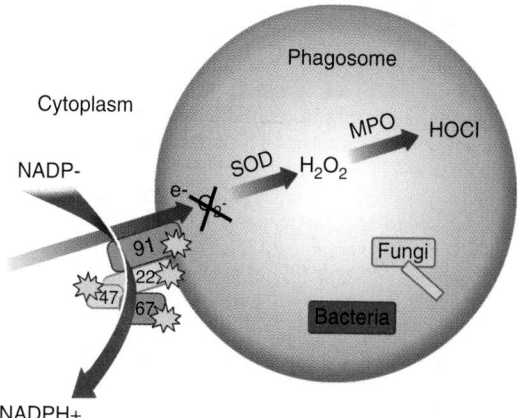

FIGURE 11-2. The neutrophil oxidative burst is mediated by the structural components of the NADPH oxidase: the membrane-bound components gp91*phox* and p22*phox* and the cytosolic factors p47*phox* and p67*phox*. In the setting of cellular activation, these factors coalesce on the phagosome membrane and catalyze the transfer of an electron from NADPH to molecular oxygen. This in turn creates superoxide, which is converted to hydrogen peroxide and then to hypochlorous acid (bleach). The genetic absence of any of these structural components causes chronic granulomatous disease (CGD).

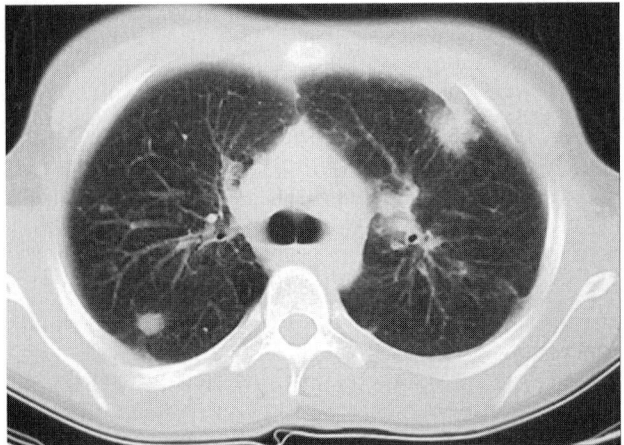

FIGURE 11-3. Multifocal asymptomatic *Aspergillus fumigatus* pneumonia in a patient with chronic granulomatous disease.

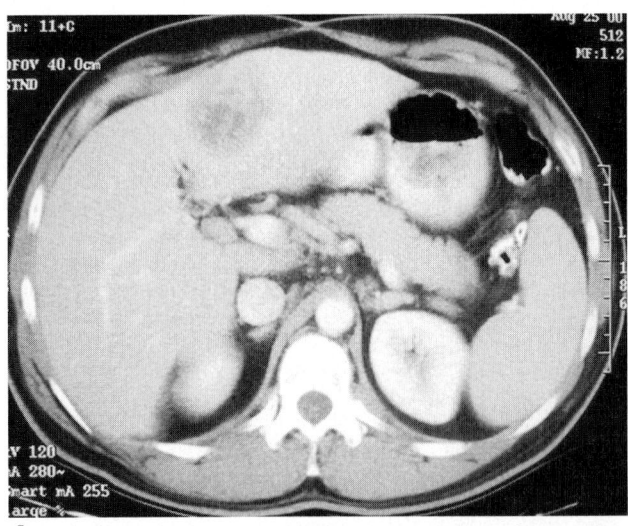

A

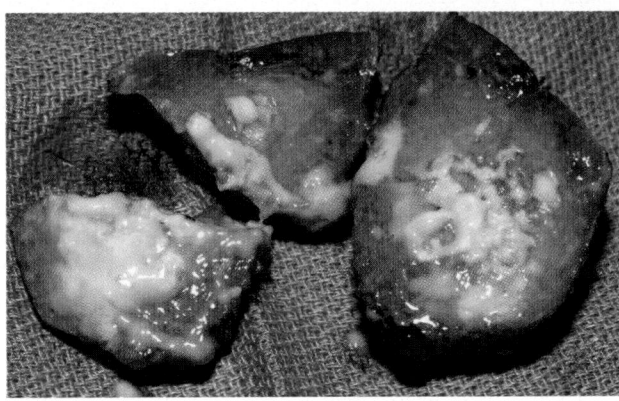

B

FIGURE 11-4. **A,** Staphylococcal liver abscess in a patient with chronic granulomatous disease. It is large, diffuse, and multiloculated. **B,** The excised abscess shows a dense fibrocaseous mass that is typically not amenable to catheter drainage and requires surgical removal.

violaceum, S. marcescens, and *B. cepacia* are seen frequently in patients with CGD and strongly suggest the diagnosis.[3,70-72,76] Bony involvement can occur by direct extension in the case of *Aspergillus* or hematogenously, as in the case of *Staphylococcus* and *Nocardia.*[77] Infection with *Aspergillus nidulans* is especially aggressive and requires more intensive therapy than does infection with *Aspergillus fumigatus.*[78] The advent of antibiotic prophylaxis has altered the frequency of infections in CGD and has reduced the frequency of staphylococcal infections in particular.[3,73] Therefore, infections outside the liver or lymph nodes occurring in CGD patients who have been taking antibacterial prophylaxis should not be presumed to be staphylococcal. The rate of fungal infections in CGD is lower than that for bacterial infections and has apparently not changed in the setting of prophylactic antibiotics.[79] The recent introduction of itraconazole prophylaxis for prevention of fungal infections in CGD should further reduce infection frequency and severity.[80]

The granulomas that occur in CGD are presumed to originate from an inflammatory response to infectious or irritative foci (e.g., sutures) that fails to eradicate the infection or irritation. This may be because hydrogen peroxide, a moiety missing in CGD phagocytes, is involved in the degradation of inflammatory mediators such as leukotrienes and complement factors.[81,82] This persistent inflammatory reaction may lead to exuberant and often obstructive granulomatous lesions. The gastrointestinal and genitourinary tracts are frequently involved by granulomatous lesions in CGD, sometimes as the site of the initial complaint, sometimes asymptomatically. Ament and Ochs noted frequent malabsorption, intrinsic factor–unresponsive vitamin B_{12} deficiency, abundant lipid-pigmented histiocytes in small bowel biopsy specimens, and pigmented histiocytes and granulomas in rectal biopsy material.[83] These findings were present in patients with both autosomal and X-linked disorders. Esophageal, jejunal, ileal, cecal, rectal, and perirectal involvement with granulomas, often mimicking Crohn's disease, occur in 30% of patients with CGD, affecting patients with X-linked more than autosomal disorders.[84] Gastric outlet obstruction is an especially common manifestation and may be the initial feature of CGD. In a comprehensive review of genitourinary manifestations, Walther and colleagues found that 38% of patients with CGD had some kind of urologic event, including bladder granulomas, ureteral obstruction, and urinary tract infection.[85] The diagnosis of CGD is made by assays of superoxide or hydrogen peroxide production, such as nitroblue tetrazolium reduction, or of dihydrorhodamine oxidation. Mothers of boys with the X-linked form of CGD are obligate carriers of a defective X chromosome. Therefore, by lyonization, a certain proportion of the mother's cells will fail to oxidize dihydrorhodamine and thus give a characteristic mosaic pattern. By performing a dihydrorhodamine test on the mother's blood, one can determine the broad lines of inheritance of CGD in a given male.

An important adjunct to therapy is interferon-γ, a cytokine with neutrophil and monocyte-macrophage–stimulating properties that has reduced the frequency and severity of infections in patients with CGD.[86] Although granulocyte transfusions supply only a small portion of the body's normal neutrophil output in a day, they may be effective in helping to clear severe infections. Transfused granulocytes produce superoxide, which can be used by the intact MPO system in CGD neutrophils, thereby allowing the biochemical defect to be bypassed.[87] The granulomatous complications of CGD pose a special problem in management. Although these patients are already somewhat immunocompromised, the judicious use of corticosteroids in conjunction with antibiotics has been successful in opening and maintaining the patency of hollow viscera in patients with CGD.[88]

DEFECTS AFFECTING PHAGOCYTE SIGNALING

Defects in the molecule necessary for signaling from the IL-1 receptor and the Toll-like receptors, the IL-1 receptor–associated kinase-4 (IRAK-4), lead to severe, recurrent pyogenic infections in infancy and childhood.[89,90] Interestingly, the clinical phenotype in this defect seems to ameliorate with age. The nuclear factor kappa B (NFκB) essential modulator (NEMO) is required to transduce signal farther downstream from IRAK-4.[38,91] Therefore, patients with defects in NEMO have a more profound defect that encompasses pyogenic as well as mycobacterial, viral, and *Pneumocystis* infections. Many of these patients also have mild to moderate forms of ectodermal dysplasia, reflecting the fact that this morphogenic pathway also signals through NFκB.

PHAGOCYTE AND LYMPHOCYTE DEFECTS AFFECTING MONONUCLEAR CELLS

Although tuberculosis is highly virulent in humans and infects more than one third of the globe's population, infections with nontuberculous mycobacteria are much less common, and when these infections are disseminated, they bespeak substantial immunocompromise. If HIV infection and iatrogenic causes are excluded, one is left with patients with intrinsic immune defects, some of which have recently been characterized at a genetic level.

Interferon-γ is an absolutely critical cytokine in the control of mycobacteria.[92] It is produced by lymphocytes and acts through its cognate receptor on monocyte-macrophages to facilitate the killing of intracellular parasites such as mycobacteria (Fig. 11-5). Therefore, it is expected and observed that severe, disseminated infections with nontuberculous mycobacteria such as *Mycobacterium avium* complex develop in humans with defects in either the ligand binding (interferon-γ receptor 1) or the signal transducing (interferon-γ receptor 2) chains of the interferon-γ receptor.[93-96] These infections often have their onset in childhood, and if BCG is given to these infants, it often disseminates. Patients with complete defects of the interferon-γ receptors have autosomal recessive defects and characteristically fail to form granulomas and have very high mortality from their *M. avium* complex infections. They are also susceptible to recurrent disseminated infections with the intracellular pathogen *Salmonella*. Rare patients have partial defects in interferon-γ receptor 1, resulting in an intermediate phenotype with severe but curable mycobacterial infections and retained ability to form granulomas.[97] The autosomal dominant form of interferon-γ receptor deficiency is the most common: patients present in childhood and later, typically with treatable nontuberculous mycobacterial infections involving bone. In these patients, the interferon-γ receptor 1 is overaccumulated on the cell surface due to a common mutation in the intracellular domain.[98] The diagnosis of complete recessive (receptor absent) or partial dominant (receptor increased) interferon-γ receptor 1 deficiency is most easily accomplished by examination of the cell surface for interferon-γ receptor 1 expression by flow cytometry. However,

demonstration of protein-positive interferon-γ receptor 1 deficiency and all cases of interferon-γ receptor 2 deficiency must still be performed by functional and molecular assays.

IL-12 is a monocyte-macrophage product that acts on lymphocytes to drive the production of interferon-γ. As expected, in the absence of IL-12 signal transduction as a result of defects in the IL-12 receptor or the absence of IL-12p40, disseminated infections with nontuberculous mycobacteria and *Salmonella* occur.[99,100] However, because patients with IL-12 or IL-12 receptor defects have some residual interferon-γ production, granuloma formation is preserved and these patients tend to be less severely affected than those with complete interferon-γ receptor defects.[101,102] Treatment of IL-12 or IL-12 receptor–deficient patients with disseminated mycobacterial infections can be greatly aided by the use of interferon-γ. The diagnosis of IL-12 receptor deficiency currently requires functional or molecular assays.

The signal transducer and activator of transcription 1 (STAT1) transduces most signals from the interferon-γ and interferon-α receptors. Autosomal dominant mutations in STAT1 affect only the interferon-γ receptor signaling, and they result in disseminated nontuberculous mycobacterial infections in childhood.[103] However, more severe complete recessive defects impair the interferon-α signaling as well and lead to severe mycobacterial and viral infections.[104]

Hyperimmunoglobulin E–Recurrent Infection Syndrome (Job's Syndrome)

Job's syndrome is a rare disorder characterized by recurrent infections (typically of the lower respiratory system and skin), eczema, extremely elevated levels of IgE, and eosinophilia. Most patients have facial abnormalities, including ocular hypertelorism, a prominent, protruding, triangular mandible, and a broad, somewhat bulbous nose.[4,7,9,105] Failure of primary teeth to exfoliate is common and results in a frequent need for dental extractions to allow eruption of normal secondary teeth.[7,106] Moderate scoliosis develops in most patients. Many also have abnormalities of bone formation and metabolism, which may result in fractures.[107,108] Craniosynostosis has been reported in several patients.[7,9,105] Job's syndrome appears to occur spontaneously in all racial and ethnic groups and seems to be transmitted as an autosomal dominant trait with variable penetrance.[4,7]

Patients are usually noted within the first days to months of life to have severe eczema, mucocutaneous candidiasis, and cutaneous, sinus, or pulmonary infections, predominantly with *S. aureus* or *Haemophilus influenzae*. Pneumatoceles are often noted by adolescence, and these in turn provide a hospitable site for subsequent infections with *Aspergillus* and *Pseudomonas aeruginosa* (Fig. 11-6). Otitis media and externa are relatively common, as are intertriginous infections and breast abscesses. Infections occur less frequently in bones and joints and very infrequently in the liver, kidneys, and gastrointestinal tract. Documented sepsis is rare. Recurrent "cold" abscesses of the skin are commonly due to staphylococci. The lack of robust inflammation is a manifestation of the impaired inflammatory response in these patients

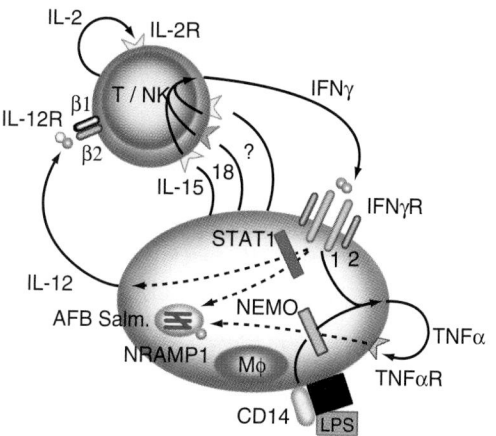

FIGURE 11-5. **The interacting cytokine and receptor pathways that regulate the resistance to and killing of mycobacteria and *Salmonella*.** Lesions resulting in severe disseminated mycobacterial disease have been described in the interferon (IFN)-γ receptors, signal transducer and activator of transcription 1 (STAT1), interleukin (IL)-12 p40, IL-12 receptor (R) β1, and the signal transducing molecule, nuclear factor (NF)κB essential modulator (NEMO). AFB, acid-fast bacilli; LPS, lipopolysaccharide; NRAMP, natural resistance-associated macrophage protein; TNF, tumor necrosis factor.

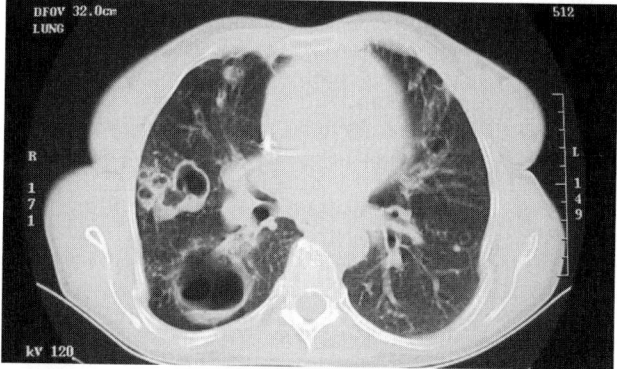

FIGURE 11-6. Multifocal postinflammatory pneumatoceles in a patient with hyper-IgE–recurrent infection (Job's) syndrome.

insofar as substantial infection may elicit only modest reaction and is often unassociated with a sense of illness on the part of the patient. Pathogens that have been recovered from patients with Job's syndrome include *S. aureus, H. influenzae, Aspergillus* species, *P. aeruginosa, Streptococcus pneumoniae,* group A streptococci, *P. (carinii) jirovecii, Cryptococcus neoformans,* and *Candida albicans.*[4,7,9,105]

The syndrome is defined by marked elevations of IgE (>2000 IU/mL), with levels of more than 50,000 IU/mL reported.[4,7,9] Levels may start out elevated in cord blood and then climb through infancy and childhood.[109] In addition, levels may decline into the normal range over time.[7] Therefore, although a high IgE level is one of the diagnostic criteria for Job's syndrome, authentic cases do at times lack this particular feature. Catabolism of IgE is abnormally reduced in both Job's syndrome and atopic dermatitis, thus further contributing to the elevated levels of IgE seen in these syndromes.[110] A high proportion of the IgE in Job's syndrome binds to *S. aureus* and *C. albicans.*[111] White blood cell counts are typically normal but have been reported to range from 1700 to 60,000/µL.[4,7,9] Chronic leukopenia with borderline neutropenia has been observed in several patients.[9] Mild to moderate eosinophilia is the rule, although exceptions do occur.[7] No correlation between IgE levels and the degree of eosinophilia or clinical disease has been made.[7,9] Chemotaxis is abnormal in this syndrome, at least some of the time in most of the patients.[9] However, until the disease gene is found and its functions clearly defined, clinical criteria requiring both immunologic and somatic features are the basis for making the accurate diagnosis of hyperimmunoglobulin E–recurrent infection syndrome: extremely elevated IgE, eczema, recurrent sinopulmonary infections, recurrent skin abscesses, failure of primary dental deciduation, scoliosis, characteristic facies, and a positive family history.[112]

Complement-Mediated Immunity

Deficiencies in complement components are clinically manifested as recurrent systemic bacterial infections. Bacteremia and meningitis are common in all the complement deficiencies.[1] Pneumonia is common in the early classic pathway (C1, C4, C2) and alternative pathway (factors I and H, properdin, C3) defects. Late-component defects (C5-C9) are associated with recurrent *Neisseria* bacteremia and meningitis. Surprisingly, the bacteremias associated with late-component defects occur at a much later age (average, 17 years) than does meningococcal bacteremia in the healthy population. Although these patients also have much higher rates of relapse and reinfection than healthy people have, their mortality from the infection is lower than normal. Patients with deficiencies of the early components of complement, C1, C4, C2, and C3, tend to have considerably higher rates of collagen-vascular disease such as systemic and discoid lupus erythematosus than do either healthy populations or patients with late-component defects.

Except for properdin deficiency, which is X-linked, complement deficiency states are inherited as autosomal recessive disorders. Heterozygotes have 50% of normal levels, whereas homozygous defective persons tend to have very low levels, if any, of the affected component. Screening for the presence of complement deficiencies is best accomplished by use of the test for total hemolytic complement (the CH$_{50}$ assay). This test examines the integrity of the classic pathway of the complement system by determining the ability of complement in patient serum to lyse antibody-coated sheep erythrocytes in vitro. Cell lysis leads to the release of hemoglobin, which can be determined spectrophotometrically. Specific classic complement component defects can be detected by a modified CH$_{50}$ assay that uses purified proteins and selectively omits the one to be assayed so that patient serum must supply the missing factor.[19] Direct determinations of immunologically reactive protein, including members of the alternative pathway, can be performed with enzyme-linked immunosorbent assays or diffusion assays. These types of direct assay systems do not offer functional data but can help quantify apparent functional defects.

Acquired Immune Deficiencies

The most common forms of immunodeficiency encountered are acquired after birth and are not clearly traceable to an immune genetic basis. Like other immunodeficiencies, they are best approached by a thorough history and physical examination to search for associated findings and to guide diagnostic testing. Special attention to the infecting organisms can point to underlying abnormalities in host defense. AIDS is caused by HIV, which induces progressive CD4$^+$ T-cell depletion.[113] A syndrome that is manifested, like AIDS, by opportunistic infections but is unassociated with HIV infection is idiopathic CD4$^+$ lymphopenia.[114] The diagnosis is made by excluding all other known causes of immunodeficiency, including HIV, and determining that the CD4$^+$ T-cell count is 300/µL or less. Certain malignancies, particularly hematopoietic and lymphoid malignancies, result in immune dysfunction by causing a deficiency in immune effector cells or dysregulation of such activities as antibody synthesis, and are associated with severe or opportunistic infections. Drug therapy can be complicated by rare or idiosyncratic reactions such as aplastic anemia with chloramphenicol or drug-induced neutropenia.[115] Iron overload and chelation therapy with deferoxamine provide a hospitable environment for certain bacteria, notably *Yersinia enterocolitica.*[116-118] Splenectomy, especially posttraumatic splenectomy, predisposes to overwhelming infection with encapsulated organisms such as *S. pneumoniae* and *Capnocytophaga canimorsus* (DF-2) and parasites such as *Babesia microti* and *Plasmodium* species.[119] Severe thermal injury is associated with selective degranulation of neutrophil-specific granules, decreased chemotaxis, and profound susceptibility to infection.[120]

REFERENCES

1. Ross SC, Denson P. Complement deficiency states and infection: Epidemiology, pathogenesis and consequences of neisserial and other infections in an immune deficiency. Medicine (Baltimore). 1984;63:243-273.
2. Buckley RH. Primary immunodeficiency diseases due to defects in lymphocytes. N Engl J Med. 2000;343:1313-1324.
3. O'Neil KM, Herman JH, Modlin JF, et al. *Pseudomonas cepacia:* An emerging pathogen in chronic granulomatous disease. J Pediatr. 1986;108:940-942.
4. Buckley RH, Becker WG. Abnormalities in the regulation of human IgE synthesis. Immunol Rev. 1978;41:288-314.
5. Anderson DC, Schmalsteig FC, Finegold MJ, et al. The severe and moderate phenotypes of heritable Mac-1, LFA-1 deficiency: Their quantitative definition and relation to leukocyte dysfunction and clinical features. J Infect Dis. 1985;152:668-689.
6. Charon JA, Mergenhagen SE, Gallin JI. Gingivitis and oral ulceration in patients with neutrophil dysfunction. J Oral Pathol. 1985;14:150-155.
7. Grimbacher B, Holland SM, Gallin JI, et al. Hyper IgE syndrome with recurrent infections: An autosomal dominant multisystem disorder. N Engl J Med. 1999;340:692-702.
8. Perez E, Sullivan KE. Chromosome 22q11.2 deletion syndrome (DiGeorge and velocardiofacial syndromes). Curr Opin Pediatr. 2002;14:678-683.
9. Donabedian H, Gallin JI. The hyperimmunoglobulin E recurrent infection (Job's) syndrome: A review of the NIH experience and the literature. Medicine (Baltimore). 1983;62:195-208.
10. Blume RS, Wolff SM. The Chédiak-Higashi syndrome: Studies in four patients and a review of the literature. Medicine (Baltimore). 1972;51:247-280.
11. Ownby DR, Pizzo SV, Blackmon L, et al. Severe combined immunodeficiency with leukopenia (reticular dysgenesis) in siblings: Immunologic and histopathologic findings. J Pediatr. 1976;89:382-387.
12. Roper M, Parmley RT, Crist WM, et al. Severe congenital leukopenia (reticular dysgenesis): Immunologic and morphologic characterizations of leukocytes. Am J Dis Child. 1985;139:832-835.
13. Cham B, Bonilla MA, Winkelstein J. Neutropenia associated with primary immunodeficiency syndromes. Semin Hematol. 2002;39:107-112
14. Hirschhorn R. Adenosine deaminase deficiency. Immunodefic Rev. 1990;2:175-198.
15. Markert ML. Purine nucleoside phosphorylase deficiency. Immunodefic Rev. 1991;3:45-81.
16. Fischer A. Primary T-lymphocyte immunodeficiencies. Clin Rev Allergy Immunol. 2001;20:3-26[AU8].
17. Williams WJ, Nelson DA, Morris MW. Examination of the blood. In: Williams WA, Beutler E, Erslev AJ, et al, eds. Hematology. 4th ed. New York: McGraw-Hill; 1990:9-24.
18. Carvalho EM, Bacellaro O, Barral A, et al. Antigen specific immunosuppression in visceral leishmaniasis is cell mediated. J Clin Invest. 1989;83:860-864.
19. Marti GE, Stetler-Stevenson M, Bleesing JJ, Fleisher TA. Introduction to flow cytometry. Semin Hematol. 2001;38:93-99.
20. Alarcon B, Regueiro JR, Arnaiz-Villena A, et al. Familial defect in the surface expression of the T cell receptor-CD3 complex. N Engl J Med. 1988;319:1203-1208.
21. Pahwa R, Chatila T, Pahwa S, et al. Recombinant interleukin 2 therapy in severe combined immunodeficiency disease. Proc Natl Acad Sci U S A. 1989;86:5069-5073.

22. Weinberg K, Parkman R. Severe combined immunodeficiency due to a specific defect in the production of interleukin 2. N Engl J Med. 1990;322:1718-1723.

23. Chatila T, Castigli E, Pahwa R, et al. Primary combined immunodeficiency resulting from defective transcription of multiple T-cell lymphokine genes. Proc Natl Acad Sci U S A. 1990;87:10033-10037.

24. Griscelli C, Lisowska-Grospierre B, Mach B. Combined immunodeficiency with defective expression in MHC class II genes. Immunodefic Rev. 1989;1:135-153.

25. Mossmann TR, Moore KW. The role of IL10 in cross regulation of Th1 and Th2 responses. Immunol Today. 1991;12:48-53.

26. Muller W, Peter HH, Wilken M, et al. The DiGeorge syndrome: I. Clinical evaluation and course of partial and complete forms of the syndrome. Eur J Pediatr. 1988;147:496-502.

27. Gatti RA, Becker-Catania S, Chun HH, et al. The pathogenesis of ataxia-telangiectasia: Learning from a Rosetta Stone. Clin Rev Allergy Immunol. 2001;20:87-108.

28. Aldrich RA, Steinberg AG, Campbell DC. Pedigree demonstrating a sex-linked recessive condition characterized by draining ears, eczematoid dermatitis, and bloody diarrhea. Pediatrics. 1954;13:133-139.

29. Derry JM, Ochs HD, Francke U. Isolation of a novel gene mutated in Wiskott-Aldrich syndrome. Cell. 1994;78:635-644.

30. Symons M, Derry JM, Karlak B, et al. Wiskott-Aldrich syndrome protein, a novel effector for the GTPase CDC42Hs, is implicated in actin polymerization. Cell. 1996;84:723-734.

31. Thrasher AJ. WASp in immune-system organization and function. Nat Rev Immunol. 2002;2:635-646.

32. Villa A, Notarangelo L, Macchi P, et al. X-linked thrombocytopenia and Wiskott-Aldrich syndrome are allelic diseases with mutations in the WASP gene. Nat Genet. 1995;9:414-417.

33. Devriendt K, Kim AS, Mathijs G, et al. Constitutively activating mutation in WASP causes X-linked severe congenital neutropenia. Nat Genet. 2001;27:313-317.

34. Bruton OC. Agammaglobulinemia. Pediatrics. 1952;9:722-728.

35. Waldmann TA. Immunodeficiency diseases: Primary and acquired. In: Samter M, ed. Immunological Diseases. 4th ed. New York: Little Brown; 1988:411-465.

36. Allen RC, Armitage RJ, Conley ME, et al. CD40 ligand gene defects responsible for X-linked hyper-IgM syndrome. Science. 1993;259:990-993.

37. Aruffo A, Farrington M, Hollenbaugh D, et al. The CD40 ligand, gp39, is defective in activated T cells from patients with X-linked hyper-IgM syndrome. Cell. 1993;72:291-300.

38. Doffinger R, Smahi A, Bessia C, et al. X-linked anhidrotic ectodermal dysplasia with immunodeficiency is caused by impaired NF-kappaB signaling. Nat Genet. 2001;27:277-285.

39. Ferrari S, Giliani S, Insalaco A, et al. Mutations of CD40 gene cause an autosomal recessive form of immunodeficiency with hyper IgM. Proc Nat Acad Sci U S A. 2001;98:12614-12619.

40. Revy P, Muto T, Levy Y, et al. Activation-induced cytidine deaminase (AID) deficiency causes the autosomal recessive form of the hyper-IgM syndrome (HIGM2). Cell. 2000;102:565-575.

41. Sullivan JL, Woda BA. X-linked lymphoproliferative syndrome. Immunodefic Rev. 1989;1:325-347.

42. Coffey AJ, Brooksbank RA, Brandau O, et al. Host response to EBV infection in X-linked lymphoproliferative disease results from mutations in an SH2-domain encoding gene. Nat Genet. 1998;20:129-135.

43. Crotty S, Kersh EN, Cannons J, et al. SAP is required for generating long-term humoral immunity. Nature. 2003;421:282-287.

44. Cunningham-Rundles C. Common variable immunodeficiency. Curr Allergy Asthma Rep. 2001;1:421-429.

45. Buckley RH. Immunoglobulin G subclass deficiency: Fact or fancy? Curr Allergy Asthma Rep. 2002;2:356-360.

46. Bodey GP, Buckley M, Sathe YS, et al. Quantitative relationships between circulating leukocytes and infection in patients with acute leukemia. Ann Intern Med. 1966;64:328-340.

47. Wright DG, Dale DC, Fauci AS, et al. Human cyclic neutropenia: Clinical review and long term follow up of patients. Medicine (Baltimore). 1981;60:1-13.

48. Horwitz M, Benson KF, Person RE, et al. Mutations in ELA2, encoding neutrophil elastase, define a 21-day biological clock in cyclic haematopoiesis. Nat Genet. 1999;23:433-436.

49. Person RE, Li F-Q, Duan Z, et al. Mutations in proto-oncogene GFI1 cause human neutropenia and target ELA2. Nat Genet. 2003;34:308-312.

50. Kostmann R. Infantile genetic agranulocytosis: A review with presentation of ten new cases. Acta Paediatr Scand. 1975;64:362-368.

51. Dale DC, Person RE, Bolyard AA, et al. Mutations in the gene encoding neutrophil elastase in congenital and cyclic neutropenia. Blood. 2000;96:2317-2322.

52. Bonilla MA, Gillio AP, Ruggiero M, et al. Effects of recombinant human granulocyte colony-stimulating factor on neutropenia in patients with congenital agranulocytosis. N Engl J Med. 1989;320:1574-1580.

53. Dale DC, Cottle TE, Fier CJ, et al. Severe chronic neutropenia: Treatment and follow-up of patients in the Severe Chronic Neutropenia International Registry. Am J Hematol. 2003;72:82-93.

54. Barbosa MD, Nguyen QA, Tchernev VT, et al. Identification of the homologous beige and Chédiak-Higashi syndrome genes. Nature. 1996;382:262-265.

55. Nagle DL, Karim MA, Woolf EA, et al. Identification and mutation analysis of the complete gene for Chédiak-Higashi syndrome. Nat Genet. 1996;14:307-311.

56. Rausch PG, Pryzwansky KB, Spitznagel JK. Immunocytochemical identification of azurophilic and specific granule markers in the giant granules of Chédiak-Higashi neutrophils. N Engl J Med. 1978;298:693-698.

57. Kishimoto TK, Larson RS, Corbi AL, et al. The leukocyte integrins. Adv Immunol. 1989;46:149-182.

58. Etzioni A, Frydman M, Pollack S, et al. Brief report: Recurrent severe infections caused by a novel leukocyte adhesion deficiency. N Engl J Med. 1992;327:1789-1792.

59. Springer TA. Adhesion receptors of the immune system. Nature. 1990;346:425-434.

60. Butcher EC. Leukocyte-endothelial cell recognition: 3 (or more) steps to specificity and diversity. Cell. 1991;67:1033-1036.

61. Lubke T, Marquardt T, Etzioni A, et al. Complementation cloning identifies CDG-IIc, a new type of congenital disorder of glycosylation, as a GDP-fucose transporter deficiency. Nat Genet. 2001;28:73-76.

62. Gallin JI, Fletcher MP, Seligmann BE, et al. Human neutrophil specific granule deficiency: A model to assess the role of the neutrophil specific granules in the evolution of the inflammatory response. Blood. 1982;59:1317-1329.

63. Lomax KJ, Gallin JI, Rotrosen D, et al. Selective defect in myeloid cell lactoferrin gene expression in neutrophil specific granule deficiency. J Clin Invest. 1989;83:514-519.

64. Rosenberg HF, Gallin JI. Neutrophil specific granule deficiency includes eosinophils. Blood. 1993;82:268-273.

65. Yamanaka R, Barlow C, Lekstrom-Himes J, et al. Impaired granulopoiesis, myelodysplasia, and early lethality in CCAAT/enhancer binding protein epsilon-deficient mice. Proc Natl Acad Sci U S A. 1997;94:13187-13192.

66. Lekstrom-Himes J, Dorman SE, Kapar P, et al. Neutrophil-specific granule deficiency results from a novel mutation with loss of function of the transcription factor CCAAT/enhancer binding protein ε. J Exp Med. 1999;189:1842-1852.

67. Gombart AF, Koeffler HP. Neutrophil specific granule deficiency and mutations in the gene encoding transcription factor C/EBP(epsilon). Curr Opin Hematol. 2002;9:36-42.

68. Nauseef WM. Myeloperoxidase deficiency. Hematol Oncol Clin North Am. 1988;2:135-158.

69. Rex JH, Bennett JE, Gallin JI, et al. Normal and deficient neutrophils can cooperate to damage *Aspergillus fumigatus* hyphae. J Infect Dis. 1990;162:523-528.

70. Segal BH, Leto TL, Gallin JI, et al. Genetic, biochemical, and clinical features of chronic granulomatous disease. Medicine (Baltimore). 2000;79:170-200.

71. Winkelstein JA, Marino MC, Johnston RB Jr, et al. Chronic granulomatous disease: Report on a national registry of 368 patients. Medicine (Baltimore). 2000;79:155-169.

72. Muoy R, Fisher A, Vilmer E, et al. Incidence, severity and prevention of infections in chronic granulomatous disease. J Pediatr. 1989;114:555-560.

73. Buescher ES, Gallin JI. Stature and weight in chronic granulomatous disease. J Pediatr. 1984;104:911-913.

74. Kenney RT, Kwon-Chung KJ, Waytes AT, et al. Successful treatment of systemic *Exophiala dermatitidis* infection in a patient with chronic granulomatous disease. Clin Infect Dis. 1992;1:235-242.

75. Williamson PR, Kwon-Chung KJ, Gallin JI. Successful treatment of *Paecilomyces varioti* infection in a patient with chronic granulomatous disease and a review of *Paecilomyces* species infections. Clin Infect Dis. 1992;5:1023-1026.

76. Gallin JI, Buescher ES, Seligmann BE, et al. Recent advances in chronic granulomatous disease. Ann Intern Med. 1983;99:657-674.

77. Sponseller PD, Malech HL, McCarthy EF, et al. Skeletal involvement in chronic granulomatous disease of childhood. J Bone Joint Surg Am. 1991;73:37-51.

78. Segal BH, DeCarlo ES, Kwon-Chung KJ, et al. *Aspergillus nidulans* infection in chronic granulomatous disease. Medicine (Baltimore). 1998;77:345-354.

79. Margolis DM, Melnick DA, Alling DW, et al. Trimethoprim-sulfamethoxazole prophylaxis in the management of chronic granulomatous disease. J Infect Dis. 1990;162:723-726.

80. Gallin JI, Alling DW, Malech HL, et al. Itraconazole to prevent fungal infections in chronic granulomatous disease. N Engl J Med. 2003;348:2416-2422.

81. Henderson WR, Klebanoff SJ. Leukotriene production and inactivation by normal, chronic granulomatous disease and myeloperoxidase-deficient neutrophils. J Biol Chem. 1983;258:13522-13527.

82. Segal BH, Kuhns DB, Ding L, et al. Thioglycolate peritonitis in mice lacking C5, 5-lipoxygenase, or p47(phox): Complement, leukotrienes, and reactive oxidants in acute inflammation. J Leukoc Biol. 2002;71:410-416.

83. Ament ME, Ochs HD. Gastrointestinal manifestations of chronic granulomatous disease. N Engl J Med. 1973;288:382-387.

84. Marciano BE, Rosenzweig SD, Kleiner DE, et al. Gastrointestinal involvement in chronic granulomatous disease. Pediatrics. In press.

85. Walther MM, Malech H, Berman A, et al. The urologic manifestations of chronic granulomatous disease. J Urol. 1992;147:1314-1318.

86. International Chronic Granulomatous Disease Cooperative Study. A controlled trial of interferon gamma to prevent infection in chronic granulomatous disease. N Engl J Med. 1991;324:509-516.

87. Buescher ES, Gallin JI. Leukocyte transfusions in chronic granulomatous disease: Persistence of transfused leukocytes in sputum. N Engl J Med. 1982;307:800-803.

88. Chin TW, Stiehm ER, Falloon J, et al. Corticosteroids in treatment of obstructive lesions of chronic granulomatous disease. J Pediatr. 1987;111:349-352.

89. Picard C, Puel A, Bonnet M, et al. Pyogenic bacterial infections in humans with IRAK-4 deficiency. Science. 2003;299:2076-2079.

90. Medvedev AE, Lentschat A, Kuhns DB, et al. Distinct mutations in IRAK-4 confer hyporesponsiveness to lipopolysaccharide and interleukin-1 in a patient with recurrent bacterial infections. J Exp Med. 2003;198:521-531.

91. Jain A, Ma CA, Liu S, et al. Specific missense mutations in NEMO result in hyper-IgM syndrome with hypohydrotic ectodermal dysplasia. Nat Immun. 2001;2:223-228.

92. Dorman SE, Holland SM. Interferon-gamma and interleukin-12 pathway defects and human disease. Cytokine Growth Factor Rev. 2000;11:321-333.

93. Newport MJ, Huxley CM, Huston S, et al. A mutation in the interferon-gamma-receptor gene and susceptibility to mycobacterial infection. N Engl J Med. 1996;335:1941-1949.

94. Jouanguy E, Altare F, Lamhamedi S, et al. Interferon-gamma-receptor deficiency in an infant with fatal bacille Calmette-Guérin infection. N Engl J Med. 1996;335: 1956-1961.

95. Holland SM, Dorman SE, Kwon A, et al. Abnormal regulation of interferon-gamma, interleukin-12, and tumor necrosis factor-alpha, in human interferon-gamma receptor 1 deficiency. J Infect Dis. 1998;178:1095-1104.

96. Dorman SE, Holland SM. Mutation in the signal-transducing chain of the interferon-gamma receptor and susceptibility to mycobacterial infection. J Clin Invest. 1998;101:2364-2369.

97. Jouanguy E, Lamhamedi-Cherradi S, Altare F, et al. Partial interferon gamma receptor 1 deficiency in a child with tuberculoid bacillus Calmette-Guérin infection and a sibling with clinical tuberculosis. J Clin Invest. 1997;100:2658-2664.

98. Jouanguy E, Lamhamedi-Cherradi S, Lammas D, et al. A human IFNGR1 small deletion hotspot associated with dominant susceptibility to mycobacterial infection. Nat Genet. 1999;21:370-378.

99. de Jong R, Altare F, Haagen IA, et al. Severe mycobacterial and *Salmonella* infections in interleukin-12 receptor-deficient patients. Science. 1998;280:1435-1438.

100. Altare F, Durandy A, Lammas D, et al. Impairment of mycobacterial immunity in human interleukin-12 receptor deficiency. Science. 1998;280:1432-1435.

101. Picard C, Fieschi C, Altare F, et al. Inherited interleukin-12 deficiency: IL12B genotype and clinical phenotype of 13 patients from six kindreds. Am J Hum Genet. 2002;70:336-348.

102. Fieschi C, Dupuis S, Catherinot E, et al. Low penetrance, broad resistance, and favorable outcome of interleukin 12 receptor beta1 deficiency: Medical and immunological implications. J Exp Med. 2003;197:527-535.

103. Dupuis S, Dargemont C, Fieschi C, et al. Impairment of mycobacterial but not viral immunity by a germline human STAT1 mutation. Science. 2001;293:300-303.

104. Dupuis S, Jouanguy E, Al-Hajjar S, et al. Impaired response to interferon-gamma/beta and lethal viral disease in human STAT1 deficiency. Nat Genet. 2003; 33:388-391.

105. Geha RS, Leung DYM. Hyper immunoglobulin E syndrome. Immunodefic Rev. 1989;1:155-172.

106. O'Connell AC, Puck JM, Grimbacher B, et al. Delayed eruption of permanent teeth in hyperimmunoglobulinemia E recurrent infection syndrome. Oral Surg Oral Med Oral Pathol Oral Radiol Endod. 2000;89:177-185.

107. Lallemand D, Kalifa G, Buriot D, et al. Constitutional bone anomalies in congenital immune deficiencies. Ann Radiol. 1978;22:108-118.

108. Leung DYM, Key L, Steinberg JJ, et al. Increased in vitro bone resorption by monocytes in the hyperimmunoglobulin E syndrome. J Immunol. 1988;140:84-88.

109. Dreskin SC, Gallin JI. Evolution of the hyper immunoglobulin E and infection (HIE, Job's) syndrome in a young girl. J Allergy Clin Immunol. 1987;80:746-751.

110. Dreskin SC, Goldsmith PK, Strober W, et al. Metabolism of immunoglobulin E in patients with markedly elevated serum immunoglobulin E levels. J Clin Invest. 1987;79:1764-1772.

111. Berger M, Kirkpatrick CH, Goldsmith PK, et al. IgE antibodies to *Staphylococcus aureus* and *Candida albicans* in patients with the syndrome of hyperimmunoglobulin E and recurrent infections. J Immunol. 1980;125:2437-2443.

112. Grimbacher B, Schaffer AA, Holland SM, et al. Genetic linkage of hyper-IgE syndrome to chromosome 4. Am J Hum Genet. 1999;65:735-744.

113. Letvin NL, Walker BD. Immunopathogenesis and immunotherapy in AIDS virus infections. Nat Med. 2003;9:861-866.

114. Smith DK, Neal JJ, Holmberg SD, Centers for Disease Control Idiopathic CD4+ T-Lymphocytopenia Task Force. Unexplained opportunistic infections and CD4+ T-lymphocytopenia without HIV infection: An investigation of cases in the United States. N Engl J Med. 1993;328:373-379.

115. Singh N, Yu VL, Mielles LA, et al. Beta-lactam antibiotic induced leukopenia in severe hepatic dysfunction: Risk factors and implications for dosing in patients with liver disease. Am J Med. 1993;94:251-256.

116. Leighton PM, MacSween HM. *Yersinia* hepatic abscesses subsequent to long term iron therapy. JAMA. 1987;257:964-965.

117. Gallant T, Freedman MH, Vellend H, et al. *Yersinia* sepsis in patients with iron overload treated with desferrioxamine (Letter). N Engl J Med. 1986;314:1643.

118. Mofenson HC, Caraccio TR, Sharieff N. Iron sepsis: *Yersinia enterocolitica* septicemia possibly caused by an overdose of iron (Letter). N Engl J Med. 1987;316:1092-1093.

119. Case 29-1986: DF-2 sepsis in a splenectomized patient. N Engl J Med. 1986;315: 241-249.

120. Davis JM, Dineen P, Galin JI. Neutrophil degranulation and abnormal chemotaxis after thermal injury. J Immunol. 1990;124:1467-1471.

121. Grimbacher B, Hutloff A, Schlesier M, et al. Homozygous loss of ICOS is associated with adult-onset common variable immunodeficiency. Nat Immunol. 2003;4: 261-268.

122. Hernandez PA, Gorlin RJ, Lukens JN, et al. Mutations in the chemokine receptor gene CXCR4 are associated with WHIM syndrome, a combined immunodeficiency disease. Nat Genet. 2003;34:7074.

CHAPTER **12**

Epidemiologic
Principles

MICHAEL T. OSTERHOLM
CRAIG W. HEDBERG

EPIDEMIOLOGIC STUDIES

Epidemiology is the study of health-related events in defined populations. These include specific diseases and conditions and the exposures and host factors that contribute to their occurrence. The science of epidemiology was originally derived from the study of epidemics and has now been broadened to encompass all phenomena related to health in populations.[1] Simply stated, epidemiology involves the careful description of events within populations and the comparison of rates at which these events occur between groups within those populations. Similar concepts and methods of epidemiology apply to both infectious and noninfectious diseases.[2] The strength and adaptability of epidemiologic methods lie in their underlying simplicity. For example, John Snow's application of epidemiologic study methods led to the classic intervention of pulling the handle from the Broad Street pump during an outbreak of cholera in London in 1851. His work was based on a careful description of his observations and his quantitative approach in analyzing the occurrence of cholera among the citizens of London. The influence of his work led to legislation mandating that all the water companies in London filter their water. Of note, it was not until 1883 that Robert Koch discovered *Vibrio cholerae.*[3]

Goals of Epidemiologic Analysis

As applied to infectious diseases, at least 10 goals of epidemiologic analysis can be listed: (1) Describe patterns of infection and disease occurrence in populations; (2) identify outbreaks or unusual rates of disease occurrence; (3) facilitate laboratory-based efforts to identify infectious agents; (4) describe the occurrence of asymptomatic infection and the spectrum of disease associated with specific agents; (5) provide population-based descriptions of clinical illness to improve the specificity of diagnosis for individual diseases; (6) assist in the understanding of disease pathogenesis; (7) identify and characterize factors in the chain of infection that contribute to agent transmission and the development of disease; (8) develop and evaluate treatment protocols through clinical trials; (9) develop and evaluate primary, secondary, and tertiary prevention and control measures for individuals; and (10) describe and assess the use of prevention measures on a community-wide basis. These comprehensive goals far exceed what is often considered to be the goal of epidemiologic analysis, that is, to investigate and control epidemics or outbreaks.

These goals can be illustrated by a historical review of the unfolding of the human immunodeficiency virus (HIV) epidemic. After the acquired immunodeficiency syndrome (AIDS) was initially described in 1981, a national epidemiologic surveillance case definition was developed. Subsequent disease surveillance was initiated to characterize the cases by standard measures of time, place, and person and to identify population groups at risk. Based on these efforts, an infectious etiology was hypothesized early in the epidemic, before the first laboratory evidence of an etiologic agent was presented. Combined clinical, epidemiologic, and laboratory studies led to identification of HIV as the cause of AIDS and to the development of sensitive and specific serologic tests for infection. This progress in turn led to studies that characterized the spectrum of illness associated with HIV infection. Epidemiologic studies of persons infected with HIV (with or without AIDS) have characterized the routes of HIV transmission, have shown that the occurrence of other sexually transmitted diseases can increase the risk of HIV transmission, and have demonstrated that HIV infection can enhance the transmission of other agents such as *Mycobacterium tuberculosis.* Clinical trials were conducted to assess the efficacy of antiretroviral agents and combinations of drugs for the purposes of increasing the effectiveness of therapy and reducing the rate of resistance to individual drugs. Development of potential HIV vaccines is progressing through animal trials and phase I human trials. Multiple other trials have also been conducted to assess the efficacy of a range of antimicrobial agents aimed at preventing a variety of opportunistic infections. Finally, community-based programs developed on the basis of epidemiologic data have worked to promote behavior change aimed at reducing the risk of HIV transmission. Epidemiologic methods have also been applied to the evaluation of these community-based programs. These examples illustrate the broad role that epidemiologic methods have played in our understanding and control of the HIV epidemic.

During 2003, the global application of combined clinical, epidemiologic, and laboratory studies led to the rapid detection, characterization, and ultimately control of an epidemic of severe acute respiratory syndrome (SARS) caused by a novel coronavirus.[4-6] Although questions remain about the reservoir of SARS coronavirus, the global response to SARS serves as a model for the usefulness of epidemiologic methods.

Defining Infections, Diseases, and Populations

An essential aspect of any epidemiologic study is careful definition of the infection, disease, condition, or factor that is being studied. Specificity and sensitivity are concepts that are frequently used in reference to laboratory test performance, particularly when tests are used for screening purposes.[1] However, in the epidemiologic study of infectious diseases, it is important that the concepts of specificity and sensitivity be applied more broadly in terms of diagnosis of infection and disease. For example, the diagnosis of smallpox was both highly specific and sensitive. Few other diseases could be confused with smallpox (i.e., the diagnosis was specific), and clinical disease developed in most people who became infected with smallpox virus (i.e., the diagnosis was sensitive). Because of these qualities of smallpox, along with the fact that humans were the only important reservoir for the smallpox virus and the development of highly immunogenic vaccines, smallpox was successfully eradicated.[7] In contrast, many clinical conditions and syndromes, such as diarrhea, are caused by more than one etiologic agent. Thus, epidemiologic studies of diarrheogenic *Escherichia coli* are complicated because (1) diarrhea is not specific for *E. coli* and (2) the sensitivity of *E. coli* detection is limited owing to an array of virulence factors that can result in disease and yet are not detected by standard biochemical tests.[8]

Conversely, *E. coli* O157-H7 infections may lead to a broad spectrum of clinical illnesses, including uncomplicated diarrhea, hemorrhagic colitis, and hemolytic-uremic syndrome (HUS). Depending on whether the goals of a particular study focus on the clinical illness or the specific agent, investigators may choose a case definition that casts a wide net, or they may choose a more narrow case definition. The type of definition can have a substantial impact on study results and should be carefully considered before a specific study is undertaken.

Epidemiologic studies may be designed to evaluate outcome variables other than infection or disease occurrence. In these situations, how the outcome variables and study population are defined and measured can affect interpretation of the results and validity of the conclusions. For example, in the development of recombinant vaccines for hepatitis B virus, two vaccine formulations containing either 10 μg or 20 μg of hepatitis B surface antigen (HBsAg) in each dose were evaluated in clinical trials. Higher antibody titers developed in subjects who were administered vaccine with 20 μg HBsAg per dose than in those who were provided vaccine with 10 μg HBsAg per dose. Both doses produced sufficient levels of antibody to be considered protective against infection, and both vaccines were licensed by the U.S. Food and Drug Administration. However, when the vaccines were more broadly administered to Minnesota hospital employees, those who received vaccine with 20 μg HBsAg per dose were more likely than persons given the 10 μg dose vaccine to have detectable antibody when tested within 6 months after completion of the three-dose series.[9] The results of this investigation suggested that sociodemographic factors of the community-vaccinated population, such as age, sex, weight, and smoking, affected the outcome of vaccination programs in ways that were not predicted by the clinical trials.[10]

Establishing specific enrollment criteria for cases of infection or disease in epidemiologic studies is critical to obtaining valid and biologically meaningful results. For example, large multistate outbreaks of *E. coli* O157-H7 have been documented with increasing frequency. However, without molecular subtyping of *E. coli* O157-H7 strains, population-based surveillance is limited in its ability to detect and determine when an unexpected number or temporal clustering of cases actually documents a common vehicle-associated outbreak. In Minnesota during 1994 and 1995, of 317 reported cases of *E. coli* O157-H7 infection for which isolates were available for pulsed-field gel electrophoresis (PFGE), 143 distinct PFGE patterns were identified.[11] Ten outbreaks of *E. coli* O157-H7 were identified during that time; these accounted for only 56 (18%) of the cases. Most cases represented sporadic infections not related to a single food vehicle. Because of its discriminatory ability, the Centers for Disease Control and Prevention (CDC) adopted PFGE as the standardized molecular subtyping for national surveillance (PulseNet).[12] PulseNet has played an important role in the identification and investigation of several multistate outbreaks of foodborne disease.

A similar issue regarding the definition of cases and the population in which they occur confronts public health officials when they must consider intervention activities because of a possible outbreak of some selected infectious disease. It is common practice to define outbreaks as the occurrence of cases of disease at a frequency greater than that expected.[1] When an outbreak occurs, it is necessary to define the population at risk (i.e., the denominator) if an accurate measure of the rate of disease is to be calculated. For example, it is not unusual to recognize a cluster of cases of *Neisseria meningitidis* disease in the community. Because outbreaks of invasive *N. meningitidis* disease are known to occur in closed populations, such as persons living in dormitories and barracks, and because a vaccine and antibiotic chemoprophylaxis are available to prevent or control these outbreaks, the occurrence of multiple cases of meningococcal disease inevitably prompts a rapid public health assessment.[13] Cases of meningococcal disease tend to occur during well-described seasonal peak periods, so it is possible that a cluster of unrelated cases may occur in a defined population. The need for public health intervention is quite different for a cluster of cases related to a single outbreak-associated strain versus a cluster of cases in which each is caused by a different group or strain of *N. meningitidis*.[14] However, in many situations, strains are not available for further subtyping because laboratory capacity to distinguish strains is limited.

A companion problem to defining cases is specifying the definition of the population at risk. To determine whether cases of disease are occurring at a frequency greater than that expected, it is necessary to consider baseline incidence rates of disease. For example, in the United States, *N. meningitidis* invasive disease occurs at a rate of approximately 1 to 2 cases per 100,000 persons per year.[15] Many of these cases occur seasonally (i.e., in the winter months) and among young children. Thus, expected temporal clustering in the winter months could make a short-term observed rate of occurrence appear excessive when compared with the annual rate of disease. A similar issue is the fact that cases often occur in one or more identified populations (i.e., school, workplace, church group) that are of limited size; therefore, rate comparisons may be meaningless. For example, 1 case of meningococcal disease in a school of 1000 students could be represented as a rate of 100 per 100,000 persons per year. Although this figure is 50 times the expected annual population rate, it cannot reason-

ably be interpreted as defining an outbreak. Thus, timely decisions regarding major community-based interventions after the observation of a cluster of meningococcal cases will often be made without adequate information regarding the status of a possible outbreak. Similar situations occur with other pathogens as well.

Two common measures of the occurrence of disease in populations are incidence and prevalence.[1] *Incidence* represents the occurrence of new cases of infection or disease per unit of population per time period. It is common to express incidence rates in terms of person-years of exposure. *Prevalence* describes the number of current cases of disease per population unit at the time of observation. The relationship between incidence and prevalence depends on the duration of infection or disease. For example, the incidence of measles over the period of a year is always greater than its prevalence at a given point because the disease has a very short duration. In contrast, the prevalence of HIV infection is always greater than its incidence because the infection is chronic and infected persons may live for years after onset of the initial infection.

Biology and Statistics

The results of epidemiologic studies to compare the risk of infection or disease and the presence or absence of specific risk factors are presented in terms of relative risk and odds ratios. *Relative risk* is the ratio of the rate of illness or infection among persons who were exposed to the rate of illness or infection in persons who were not exposed (Fig. 12-1). Relative risks may also be called rate ratios and are the products of cohort studies. In case-control studies, *odds ratios* are determined and approximate the relative risk. Odds ratios provide a valid estimate of the relative risk under conditions that prevail in most case-control studies, that is, the cases of disease are newly diagnosed, prevalent cases are not included in the control group, and the selection of cases and controls is not based on exposure status.[16]

An increased relative risk or odds ratio (i.e., >1.0) for an exposure variable indicates that the exposure is related to an increased risk of disease. Similarly, a decreased relative risk or odds ratio (i.e., <1.0) indicates that the exposure variable is related to a decreased risk of

	Disease present	Disease absent
Exposure present	a	b
Exposure absent	c	d

A. The relative risk is calculated as: $\dfrac{[a/(a+b)]}{[c/(c+d)]}$

The odds ratio is calculated as: $\dfrac{ad}{bc}$

B. Calculation of population-attributable risk percent:

$$\frac{(\text{prevalence of exposure})(\text{relative risk}-1)}{1+(\text{prevalence of exposure})(\text{relative risk}-1)} \times 100$$

FIGURE 12-1. The Calculation of and Relationship Among Relative Risks, Odds Ratios, and Attributable Risks. A, The calculation of relative risks and odds ratios from a two-by-two table. The odds ratio provides a valid estimate of the relative risk under conditions that prevail in most case-control studies, including (1) that the cases of disease are newly diagnosed, (2) that prevalent cases are not included in the control group, and (3) that the selection of cases and controls is not based on exposure status. **B,** The calculation of population-attributable risk percent. In a case-control study, attributable risk can be estimated from the prevalence of exposure among controls (b/b + d) and the odds ratio. The validity of this approach is limited by how representative controls of the population are and how well the odds ratio estimates the relative risk.

disease. For example, the consumption of undercooked eggs has been associated with an increased risk for *Salmonella enterica* serotype Enteritidis infection in outbreak settings and for sporadic *S. enteritidis* infections in the community.[17] Although relative risks and odds ratios do provide a measure of the risk of disease associated with a specific factor, they do not directly describe how much disease in the community can be attributed to that factor. Rather, the *attributable risk* or *fraction* considers both the relative risk for an exposure variable and the proportion of the population exposed to that variable. In Minnesota, persons who consumed undercooked eggs had approximately a fourfold greater risk of *S*. Enteritidis infection than those who did not eat undercooked eggs. Based on an estimate of the frequency of eating undercooked eggs among the general population, investigators determined that 37% of sporadic *S*. Enteritidis infections in Minnesota adults could be attributed to the consumption of undercooked eggs.[18] Thus, both relative risk and attributable risk are important measures for describing the epidemiology of infectious diseases and for determining public health priorities.

In the process of studying the epidemiology of infectious diseases, many factors are evaluated to determine their relationship or association with a specific disease. Statistical associations, both positive and negative, may represent a true causal relationship, a confounding relationship with another factor, or a chance occurrence. When more than one factor is statistically associated with infection or disease status in univariate, or single-variable, analyses, the relationship between individual factors and infection or disease status can be evaluated by multivariate regression analysis.[19] These procedures allow the investigator simultaneously to control for a combination of factors in the analysis and to determine whether any of the risk factors are associated with infection or disease status independent of other factors. Another critical way of distinguishing among causation, confounding, and chance is to assess the biologic plausibility of the association. An unexpected statistical association found in conjunction with an epidemiologic study may result in a new understanding of how agent transmission or disease occurs. The temptation to stretch the plausibility of biology to provide meaning to statistical results is a constant danger. However, such results may be a useful guide in the evaluation of new hypotheses in future studies.

Furthermore, "statistically significant results" may be unimportant from a disease control or a practical perspective. Statistical significance, which historically has been considered to be an event that happens less than once every 20 times by chance alone (i.e., $P < .05$), is a combination of both the sample size and the strength or degree of association. Studies with a large number of persons enrolled can produce statistically significant results of weak associations (i.e., relative risks or odds ratios greater than 1 but less than 2), whereas studies with a limited number of persons enrolled may not be able to produce statistically significant results even with moderately strong or increased associations (i.e., relative risks or odds ratios greater than 5).

Determining Epidemiologic Methods Appropriate to the Study Setting

The clinical trial is cited as the gold standard of epidemiologic research. However, many epidemiologic studies cannot take place under such rigorously controlled conditions. Taking advantage of opportunities to study diseases in clinical and community settings is one of the strengths of epidemiology. In the setting of a clinical practice, epidemiology may involve studying a series of patients, participating in multicenter trials, or being a source for reporting cases of disease to public health officials. This last aspect of epidemiologic study may be a legal obligation, but it should also be viewed as an opportunity for all practicing clinicians to participate in the practice of community-based epidemiology. Academically based research centers are often settings for clinical trials, studies requiring newly developed laboratory methods, or studies derived from referrals to clinical specialty groups. Public health departments typically do not have direct access to or contact with patients for clinical trials, but they are responsible for surveillance of reportable diseases and the investigation of outbreaks. Recently, a subject for debate has been how to distinguish public health surveillance from research and

how to address the ethical considerations of that distinction.[20] Each of the settings described previously provides opportunities for epidemiologic studies that have made major contributions to the understanding, prevention, and control of infectious diseases.

Several major constraints are confronted in the design of epidemiologic studies of infectious diseases. Time is frequently a problem in the investigation of outbreaks. The need to quickly design and conduct outbreak investigations has grown with both the increased frequency of widespread foodborne outbreaks and concerns over the potential for intentional contamination of the food supply. This necessarily limits the investigator's ability to fully explore the outbreak setting and can result in the loss of information. In any study that involves the retrospective collection of data, information may be lost because of difficulty in recalling exposure or in verifying information about the exposure.

For many infectious diseases, it may be difficult to identify sufficient numbers of cases in clinical settings for meaningful epidemiologic studies to be conducted. In such situations, multisite collaborative projects are often needed. For example, a CDC work group on prevention of invasive group A streptococcal disease among household contacts concluded in 1995 that the data gleaned from a single study conducted in Ontario, Canada, were inadequate to recommend chemoprophylaxis to household contacts.[21,22] Although the Canadian study suggested an increased risk of invasive disease among household contacts, this assessment was based on only four subsequent cases in households. Based on the recommendations of the work group, a multisite study coordinated by the CDC was initiated in several states and areas with active surveillance of invasive group A streptococcal disease. Results of this ongoing surveillance continue to suggest that outbreaks of invasive disease among household contacts are rare and that recommendations for chemoprophylaxis need to be made on an individual basis.[23,24]

Types of Epidemiologic Studies

Several schemes can be used to classify or define types of epidemiologic studies (Table 12-1). Studies can be classified as *descriptive* or *analytic* and *observational* or *experimental*. A descriptive study is designed to describe only the existing distribution of case characteristics without regard to causal or other hypotheses.[25] For example, the results of community-based surveillance for *Campylobacter* infection may include a summary of all cases reported in a given year by the date of onset, county of residence, age, sex, and race. An analytic study is one designed to examine associations, particularly hypothesized causal relationships.[25] A case-control study could be designed to examine whether consumption of ready-to-eat meat and poultry products is a risk factor for cases of invasive listeriosis infections identified through surveillance activities. In addition to case-control studies, cohort studies, clinical trials, and cross-sectional surveys are common types of analytic studies. In practice, most epidemiologic studies involve both descriptive and analytic elements.

A more relevant distinction can be made between observational and experimental studies. Observational studies are conducted in natural settings in which changes in one characteristic are studied in relation to others without the intervention of the investigator.[26] Observational studies represent the bulk of epidemiologic research because they focus on events, exposures, and diseases that occur in the population during the course of routine living conditions. In contrast, experimental studies are those in which the study conditions are under

TABLE 12-1 Classification Schemes for Epidemiologic Studies

	Observational	Experimental
Descriptive	Surveillance	—
	Case series	
Analytic	Outbreak investigations	Clinical trials
	Cross-sectional surveys	Community interventions
	Seroprevalence surveys	
	Case-control studies	
	Cohort studies	
	Seroincidence studies	

the direct control of the investigator.[26] Such studies may include randomization of subjects to treatment or placebo groups and blinding of subject and investigator to placement status. Clinical trials are the prototypic experimental study. On a broader scale, community intervention trials can also be conducted.

OBSERVATIONAL STUDIES

Disease Surveillance

Disease surveillance is an ongoing process that involves the systematic collection, analysis, interpretation, and dissemination of information regarding the occurrence of diseases in defined populations so that public health action can take steps to reduce morbidity and mortality.[27] Surveillance can be conducted in the community and in institutional settings, where it may form the basis for an infection-control program. For most infectious diseases, community-based surveillance is the domain of public health departments at the local or state level. All jurisdictions require licensed physicians to report the occurrence of selected diseases to the health department.[28] Typically, such diseases include sexually transmitted diseases, vaccine-preventable diseases, blood-borne pathogens, tuberculosis, certain invasive bacterial diseases, and enteric infections caused by *Salmonella, Shigella,* and *Campylobacter.* In addition to categoric reporting, most states require reporting of disease outbreaks, regardless of the cause, and have some provision for soliciting reports of new and emerging diseases. In some situations, syndromal surveillance may be appropriate, as opposed to surveillance based on isolation of a specific infectious agent. Surveillance of influenza-like illness in sentinel physician practices, nursing homes, or schools is a way of monitoring influenza activity each influenza season. Surveillance for chronic liver disease may be a way to measure the burden of disease caused by hepatitis C in the United States.[29] Surveillance for unexplained deaths from possible infectious causes with characterization of such deaths according to the clinical syndrome at the initial evaluation is a way to monitor the emergence of potential new infectious disease threats.[30] Finally, syndromal surveillance has been established in several large cities to serve as an early-warning system for the detection of bioterrorist events.[31,32]

Over the past 10 years, surveillance for certain pathogens has evolved to include surveillance for antimicrobial resistance. Surveillance for drug-resistant tuberculosis is now essentially routine in all jurisdictions.[33] Successive waves of emergence and clonal dispersion of multidrug-resistant *Salmonella* Typhimurium DT104 and multidrug-resistant *Salmonella* Newport among food animals and humans in the United States were recently detected through national surveillance undertaken to monitor resistant enteric infections.[34,35] Several state health departments now monitor the occurrence of drug-resistant pneumococcal infections in their jurisdictions, and national data have been developed as well.[36] The importance of surveillance for drug-resistant infections will continue to grow in the 21st century; data collected through public health surveillance can be extremely useful to clinical care providers.

Case reports for use in surveillance can be collected in an active or passive manner. *Active surveillance* involves a regular, systematic effort to contact reporting sources or to review records within an institution to ascertain information on the occurrence of newly diagnosed diseases or infections. An example of an active surveillance system for foodborne illnesses is the Foodborne Diseases Active Surveillance Network (FoodNet), which operates as part of the CDC's Emerging Infections Program.[37] Active laboratory-based surveillance for confirmed cases of *Campylobacter, Cryptosporidium, Cyclospora, E. coli* O157-H7, *Listeria, Salmonella, Shigella,* and *Vibrio* was initiated in five Emerging Infections Program sites in 1996 and was expanded to 10 sites in 2003. Each clinical laboratory in each surveillance catchment area is contacted weekly or monthly to ensure that all confirmed infections under surveillance have been reported. *Passive surveillance* relies on the individual clinician or laboratory to initiate the report. Although surveillance systems are labeled as active or passive according to how cases are reported, all surveillance systems require an active review and analysis of reported cases, with dissemination of results to key stakeholders.[27]

Two key qualities of community-based surveillance for infectious diseases that must be considered when surveillance data are interpreted include representativeness and timeliness. These qualities vary by disease according to multiple factors. The first factor of importance is that the patient must seek medical attention. It is not common for persons with mild or limited illness to seek medical attention. Second, the physician must seek laboratory testing of appropriate clinical specimens to confirm the diagnosis. Third, the laboratory must have the capability to identify the agent. Fourth, the physician and laboratory must report the clinical and laboratory findings to public health officials in a timely manner. Fifth, the availability of molecular subtyping techniques such as PFGE and the ability to electronically compare PFGE patterns through the national computer network PulseNet can greatly increase both the sensitivity and the specificity of pathogen-specific surveillance. Even in states in which laboratory-based infectious disease reporting is required, confusion over who has responsibility for reporting may be noted among physicians and laboratory officials. Finally, public health agencies must have the resources to conduct timely and routine follow-up of such reports to ascertain basic case demographic and other relevant data. Failure at any step of this process will result in loss of information by the community-based surveillance system.

The efficiency of community-based surveillance systems varies greatly, depending on the disease that needs to be identified, how the diagnosis is made, and what resources are targeted toward the surveillance effort.[27] Diseases that require a diagnosis based on clinical findings, such as Lyme disease, present difficulties because many patients may not be seen when the typical clinical manifestations of the disease are present, and laboratory testing is not adequate for establishing the diagnosis. In contrast, the diagnosis of measles can be confirmed by specific serologic testing regardless of whether or not the physician sees the patient when the pathognomonic clinical features of the disease are present. Surveillance for invasive bacterial diseases such as those caused by *Haemophilus influenzae* type B and *N. meningitidis* is facilitated by the need for medical treatment because of the relative severity of the disease and the laboratory-supported diagnosis. For diseases such as these, active case ascertainment can greatly enhance the effectiveness of surveillance activities. However, active surveillance requires the commitment of personnel and other resources that are limited for many reportable diseases. Typically, active surveillance may be conducted for a limited period when complete data are most critical. Examples include the characterization of emerging diseases such as AIDS or SARS or special surveillance projects aimed at assessing an intervention, such as evaluating whether the occurrence of intussusception was causally related to the use of rotavirus vaccine.[38] Most infectious disease surveillance conducted by public health departments in the United States is passive in that it relies on the physician or the laboratory to initiate the report. Passive surveillance systems are subject to selection bias because disease reports are likely to come from a nonrepresentative sample of practicing physicians who may report specific diseases because of personal interest.[27] In addition, some data (i.e., age and sex versus clinical and pathologic information) may be more readily reported because of ease of ascertainment.[27]

Active surveillance is relatively more common in the hospital setting. For example, surveillance of nosocomial infections is an important hospital infection-control activity.[39] This highly specialized surveillance system has the operational advantage of a defined population, routine clinical observation of the patient population, and direct access to the laboratory. Hospital-based surveillance has been a primary epidemiologic tool in the study of drug-resistant organisms.[40]

Case Series

A common type of descriptive study that is conducted in clinical settings is the case series. A case series describes the clinical features of a disease and the demographic profiles and other interesting features of patients with the disease. Case series are typically the domain of practicing clinicians and serve as a way of communicating significant clinical observations. For example, the SARS epidemic was first recognized outside of

China as an unusual series of cases of patients with atypical pneumonia.[41] As the case series grew, with evidence of transmission to hospital staff, it became apparent that an unusual outbreak was occurring.

Case-Control Studies

In case-control studies, persons with infection or disease are compared with controls (i.e., persons without the infection or disease under study) with respect to previous exposures likely to be related to agent transmission.[1] Case-control studies by nature are retrospective because the outcome (i.e., case status) is known at the outset of the study. Case-control studies are the most widely conducted type of epidemiologic study because they are relatively cheap, powerful, and adaptable to many settings.[19] For example, in a nationwide outbreak of *S.* Enteritidis infection, the results of a case-control study identified the ice cream made by a large national producer as the source of the outbreak 10 days before *S.* Enteritidis could be isolated from samples of the implicated ice cream.[42] When *S.* Enteritidis was isolated from the ice cream, it was shown to be present at levels lower than one to six organisms per half-cup serving—levels that rendered insensitive the microbiologic surveillance of ice cream. Furthermore, the case-control study identified contamination of pasteurized ice cream premix during transport in tanker trailers that had previously carried nonpasteurized liquid eggs, even though regulatory officials were not able to isolate *S.* Enteritidis from any environmental samples.

The primary considerations for design of case-control studies include defining cases, establishing enrollment criteria, identifying suitable controls, and developing interview or other data collection processes that do not systematically result in different standards of data collection for cases versus controls. In the community setting, it is customary for controls to be selected from the same area of residence as the cases. It is desirable for controls to resemble cases with respect to variables that are not being studied. Controls may also be matched by age, sex, or any other factor that the investigator considers important. For example, in the study of risk factors for listeriosis, it has been important for investigators to select or match controls with a similar risk of illness based on the presence of an immuno-compromising condition or treatment. This is necessary because healthy community controls who have exactly the same exposures are still less likely to develop disease. Thus, a case-control study of listeriosis that includes healthy community-based controls would require simultaneous attempts to assess risk for exposure, as well as risk for illness given exposure. However, overmatching, such as that requiring controls to have the same birthdays as the cases, may make it difficult for investigators to identify and recruit controls. Also, once a variable has been used as a matching criterion, it is no longer available for evaluation. In hospital settings, controls are frequently selected from patients with unrelated diagnoses who might otherwise be comparable to the case patients.

Analysis of case-control studies involves comparing exposure differences between cases and controls. Such comparison allows for the study of associations between exposure and disease even when the disease is a rare outcome of the exposure. For example, a case-control study of Guillain-Barré syndrome demonstrated an association between *Campylobacter* infection and Guillain-Barré syndrome.[43] This association could not have been evaluated easily in a prospective cohort study because of the large population size necessary for identification of a similar number of Guillain-Barré syndrome cases. The power of case-control methodology stems from the fact that although illness may be an uncommon outcome of a given exposure, the common history of exposure among cases may stand in stark contrast to the exposure history of controls.

Cohort Studies

In cohort studies, the development of infection or disease is observed in groups who are either exposed or not exposed to the previously defined risk factors.[1] Cohort studies are traditionally considered prospective studies. However, this nomenclature is misleading because in reality, cohort studies can be prospective or retrospective, depending on how the exposed and comparison groups have been identified and monitored. Cohort studies provide the advantage of enabling a direct measurement of illness rates by exposure status, which allows direct measurement of relative risk. Furthermore, when conducted prospectively, cohort studies allow the investigator to maintain better control over data collection and identification of potentially confounding variables. The use of cohort studies is limited to groups in which exposures can be defined and measured.

Cohort studies of homosexual men have helped in the evaluation of risk factors for transmission of HIV, hepatitis B virus, and hepatitis C virus.[44,45] These studies are also examples of *seroincidence surveys,* in which the appearance of antibody to an agent in the second of two sequentially collected specimens indicates infection with that agent somewhere between the two times of collection.[35] Seroincidence surveys allow the investigator to (1) define total infection rates, (2) relate infection rates to previous antibody levels, and (3) identify risk factors for infection.[46] Prospective cohort studies are limited because of the enrollment size and observation period requirements for diseases of low incidence. Retrospective cohort studies in which previous exposures can be identified offer the advantage that no additional observation periods are required. However, they may be limited by the recall of study subjects or the inadequacy of available medical records.

Cross-sectional Surveys

Cross-sectional surveys provide a point-in-time assessment of a particular population or study group. These surveys may be conducted to determine the prevalence of a disease in the community, but a more common use is to establish the prevalence of risk factors or serologic markers of infection.[16] For example, a cross-sectional survey of patients attending a sexually transmitted disease clinic demonstrated that hepatitis C virus infection occurred infrequently; however, patients with a history of intravenous drug use had a significantly higher rate of serologic markers for hepatitis C virus infection.[47]

An important type of cross-sectional survey is the *seroprevalence survey.* Serologic prevalence data reflect total infection rates and thereby represent both clinical and subclinical (or asymptomatic) infections. Seroprevalence surveys can therefore provide information on patterns of infection or immunity to agents that could not be obtained by ordinary surveillance methods based on the reporting of clinical cases.[46] For example, seroprevalence surveys have demonstrated that <1% of human West Nile virus infections result in serious neurologic illness, and about 20% cause systemic febrile illness.[48]

Outbreak Investigations

A final category of observational study that integrates multiple epidemiologic methods is the outbreak investigation. A special feature of outbreak investigations is that they are frequently conducted with a sense of urgency because of the ongoing occurrence of cases, the need to rapidly implement control measures, or intense public and media interest in the outbreak. Investigations of the first documented outbreak of legionnaires' disease, the 1993 outbreak of hantavirus-associated respiratory illness in the southwestern United States, and the posting of anthrax-contaminated letters were lead stories for national news media. The importance of rapid investigation of outbreaks has increased as perceptions of the threats posed by such events have been enhanced, whether naturally emerging or intentional. Although standard methods for conducting outbreak investigations have been published,[26] strict adherence to a sequential approach to outbreak investigations, frequently implied by such publications, can be a barrier to the timely identification of the source.

Specific surveillance systems have been established for outbreaks of foodborne and waterborne diseases, influenza, and a range of infections in institutional settings. At the local or state level, outbreaks may be reported because a physician or the public is aware of the health department's existence and desires some intervention. Once an outbreak has been recognized, it is necessary that the extent of the outbreak be determined in terms of person, place, and time. For example, the nationwide outbreak associated with Schwan's ice cream initially appeared as an increased occurrence of cases in southeastern Minnesota.[42] These cases served to index the larger outbreak occurring throughout the distribution area for the implicated product. Similarly, the increased occurrence of *Salmonella* Agona infection in several states during April and May of 1998 led to the identification of a nationwide outbreak associated with toasted oats cereal, a previously unrecognized vehicle for salmonellosis. Molecular subtyping by PFGE was critical in (1) identification of the outbreak-associated strain of *S.* Agona, (2) exclusion of sporadic *S.* Agona infections identified through surveillance, and (3) provision of a specific case definition for use in the case-control study that implicated the cereal.[49]

Molecular subtyping by PFGE and comparison of subtype patterns through PulseNet facilitated identification of a multistate outbreak of listeriosis that occurred from August to December of 1998.[50] The use of molecular subtyping allowed this investigation to compare outbreak-associated *Listeria* cases with sporadic cases unrelated to the outbreak. The outbreak was associated with the consumption of hot dogs and luncheon meat manufactured at a single plant. Although subtype results enabled the identification of cases with a high degree of specificity, preliminary results of epidemiologic investigations that identified the likely source did not lead to appropriate public health interventions, and product recall and public notification were delayed until after the outbreak strain of *Listeria monocytogenes* had been isolated from the implicated hot dogs. Although the prolonged incubation period for *Listeria* complicates the process of identifying potential sources, routine use of subtyping and interviews of patients as they are identified could lead to quicker and more successful investigations. In addition, the use of case-case comparisons should be advantageous in any outbreak setting in which results of subtyping can distinguish outbreak from unrelated cases.[51] Such methods should be applicable to any of the agents tracked by PulseNet.

The second major category of foodborne outbreaks consists of those that are recognized because of the occurrence of a similar illness among persons with a common exposure, such as eating at a restaurant or attending a banquet. Although many of these outbreaks seem to be self-limited events unique to the establishment, they may serve to index much larger outbreaks. They also provide opportunities for identification of emerging foodborne pathogens. For example, in both 1996 and 1997, nationwide outbreaks of cyclosporiasis associated with raspberries imported from Guatemala were manifested as a large series of otherwise unrelated outbreaks associated with restaurants, banquets, and parties.[52,53] It was only through collective investigation and tracing of the product back from these individual events that the nature of the outbreak was recognized. Similarly, the investigation of an outbreak of gastrointestinal illness with clinical and epidemiologic features of enterotoxigenic *E. coli* at a restaurant led to the identification of a novel strain of atypical enteropathogenic *E. coli*.[8] Nationwide surveillance efforts conducted by individual states, coordinated by the CDC, and facilitated by activities such as FoodNet and PulseNet offer great promise for enhancing our understanding of foodborne diseases over the coming years. For example, FoodNet data formed much of the basis for the CDC's estimate that 76 million foodborne illnesses occur each year.[54] In addition, FoodNet's population survey *Atlas of Exposures* provides a reasonable starting point for a priori hypothesis testing of exposures reported by patients interviewed during the early stages of outbreak investigation.

EXPERIMENTAL STUDIES

Clinical Trials

Clinical trials are research activities that involve the administration of a treatment or prevention regimen to humans to evaluate its safety and efficacy.[1] In general, these trials involve a comparison of clinical outcomes in patients receiving treatment with the outcomes of a comparable control group. Most clinical trials of interest in infectious disease epidemiology involve antimicrobial agents and vaccines. An early forerunner to the modern clinical trial was a U.S.-based smallpox trial conducted in 1800.[55] During the 1950s, several multicenter trials were developed to evaluate chemotherapy in the treatment of tuberculosis.[56] In 1953, the U.S. poliomyelitis vaccine trials were conducted in collaboration with the U.S. Public Health Service and state health departments.[57]

Many considerations are involved in the design of a clinical trial. First, should the trial be conducted at all? Is enough known about the safety and biologic activity of the treatment or vaccine to allow it to be administered to patients? This consideration requires some knowledge of the immunogenicity of candidate vaccines or the in vitro activity of an antibiotic against specific pathogens. Second, would patients be harmed if the treatment or vaccine were withheld? These issues have gained particular attention in trials of drugs for the treatment of HIV infection. Concern expressed by AIDS activists and some clinicians about withholding potentially life-extending treatments has forced the U.S. Food and Drug Administration to sanction the use of a secondary and less rigorous treatment and evaluation protocol in designated AIDS clinics.[58] Recently, concern has been expressed regarding the enrollment of individuals at risk for HIV infection in HIV vaccine trials. The need to maintain behavior-related education intervention for participants in clinical trials reduces the likelihood that vaccine efficacy will be demonstrated because of the lack of new infections among placebo recipients; however, to withhold such education would be unethical.

Other considerations include the specification of both test and control treatments, an outcome measure for evaluating the treatments, a bias-free method for assigning patients to treatment groups, and calculation of the necessary sample size.[59] Sample size calculations are affected by the number of treatment groups to be studied, the desired significance level for rejecting the null hypothesis, the statistical power for detecting a difference, and the desired detectable treatment difference.

Limitations of clinical trials relate largely to the size of the trial and how well the treatment groups reflect the larger target population for the vaccine or treatment.[10] As has been noted earlier, the results of hepatitis B virus (HBV) vaccine trials did not adequately predict the performance of vaccines among health care workers. In addition, sample size limitations may not allow for the full characterization of potentially rare complications, such as intussusception that occurs after administration of rotavirus vaccine.[38] In these situations, postlicensure surveillance becomes a critical measure of the safety and effectiveness of a particular vaccine or treatment.

Community Intervention Trials

Community intervention trials are related to the clinical trial but are carried out on a larger scale. In these experiments, large groups or communities are selected to receive a therapeutic or preventive regimen.[59] For example, the efficacy of normal human immune globulin prophylaxis to control hepatitis A outbreaks in child care facilities was demonstrated in a community trial in Phoenix.[60] Community trials are particularly well suited to broad-based interventions such as changing physician antibiotic prescribing practices through the promotion of judicious antibiotic use.[61]

THE HOST-AGENT RELATIONSHIP

Although advances in medical science have made us less vulnerable to some infectious disease epidemics and pandemics, these diseases continue to occur as they have throughout human history. As recently as the late 1960s, it was suggested by leading medical authorities in this country, including the surgeon general, that it was time "to close the book on infectious diseases."[62] However, infectious diseases remain the leading cause of death worldwide. The world's human and animal populations continue to struggle against an increasingly recognized number of viral, bacterial, protozoal, helminthic, and fungal agents.

A recent National Academy of Sciences Institute of Medicine report suggested that because of the combination of emerging social, political, and economic factors favoring infectious agents in humans and animals, "a transcendent moment nears upon the world for a microbial perfect storm."[63] Thirteen factors identified in the report favor the emergence of infectious agents. They include microbial adaptation and change, human susceptibility to infection, climate and weather, changing ecosystems, human demographics and behavior, economic development and land use, international travel and commerce, technology and industry, breakdown of public health measures, poverty and social inequality, war and famine, lack of political will, and intent to harm.

For the study of infectious disease epidemiology, it is important that both infection and disease be considered, for these may be different.

Infection results from an encounter with a potentially pathogenic agent with a susceptible human host in conjunction with a suitable portal of entry. The source of most human infections lies outside the individual human host; thus, exposure to the environment or other infected hosts is a key factor. *Disease* is one of the possible outcomes of infection, and its development is related to factors of both the host and the agent.

Whereas the clinician is primarily concerned with disease, the epidemiologist is interested in both infection and disease. Because infection without disease occurs frequently for many agents, a study of only clinical illness may provide a misleading understanding of the epidemiology of a specific infectious disease in the community. For example, adults infected with the hepatitis A virus (HAV) frequently experience clinical hepatitis, whereas infants and toddlers with HAV infection are usually asymptomatic.[64] Thus, to determine the incidence of hepatitis A associated with child care facilities and subsequent transmission to family members and child care providers, investigators need to assess both the diagnosis of asymptomatic HAV infection and the level of HAV-related disease.

If the balance between agent and host favors the agent, infection (and in some instances disease) will occur. This relationship among the agent, the route or mechanism of transmission, and the host is referred to as the *chain of infection.* Control and prevention of infection depend on sufficient understanding of the dynamics of these interrelated factors.

Frequently, characteristics of the agent or host are seen as independent factors. However, it is necessary that both the host and the agent be considered together in any discussion of the relationship that results in infection and disease. For example, smallpox was a disease of dramatic human suffering; historically, it has been one of the most feared of all infectious diseases. Yet the ability of the smallpox virus (variola virus) to infect and cause disease only in humans and subhuman primates was an important consideration in approaches to control and prevention (i.e., vaccination of the human population).[65] Consideration of the smallpox virus as highly virulent must be tempered by the fact that inoculation studies of this virus into many animal species did not result in infection. In contrast, most *Salmonella* serotypes may cause mild to severe infection in humans and a variety of animal species. A notable exception is *Salmonella* Typhi, which causes infection only in humans. Thus, any description of the characteristics of either the agent or the host must be understood in the context of their interrelationships.

AGENT

Any agent or microorganism is of epidemiologic importance if it can be transmitted through the environment, causes infection in a host (either human or animal), and produces clinical disease. Such agents, regardless of their classification as bacterial, viral, protozoal, helminthic, or fungal, are considered the first necessary component of the chain of infection. Three characteristics of agents must be considered in terms of their epidemiologic importance[66]: (1) Those characteristics of agents that are involved in their spread or transport through the environment, (2) characteristics that are involved in the production of infection, and (3) characteristics that are involved in the production of disease.

The characteristics of agents involved in spread through the environment vary with the method of transmission. However, regardless of the method of transmission, it is necessary for a minimum number of organisms to survive transport through the environment if they are to reach and enter a susceptible host. For agents that are transmitted by direct person-to-person contact, their ability to survive stressful environmental conditions (such as changes in temperature, humidity, or pH) tends to be minimal. In contrast, agents that are capable of actual multiplication within the environment (i.e., in food products, water, soil, and plants) have a unique advantage for survival. Some agents such as *Legionella pneumophila* or *Bacillus anthracis* do not necessarily multiply within the environment; however, they can survive for months in relatively hostile conditions, including distilled water or soil.[67,68] For those agents for which humans are the only known reservoir, the longer the time between the likelihood of contact between two susceptible hosts, the greater the resistance that the agent must have to environmental conditions such as heat, drying, ultraviolet light, or dilution by airflow.

Finally, some agents have the capacity to infect a nonhuman host such as animals, birds, or an insect vector. Such nonhuman hosts may play an important role in maintenance of the agent in the environment.

The ability of an agent to cause infection or disease has to be considered in the context of host characteristics. For example, an agent is considered to *colonize* a host when its presence in that host does not cause a specific immune response or infection. However, should the relationship between the agent and the host change, such as when *E. coli* is introduced from the gastrointestinal tract into the blood stream, infection can result. These types of infection are known as *endogenous.* If the agent is transported from an external source to the host (*exogenous infection*) and the balance between the agent and the host favors the agent, infection usually develops.

Several aspects of the agent-host relationship can be related to the agent. Other aspects must be considered only in the context of both agent and host characteristics. For example, *infectiousness* is a characteristic of an agent that is concerned with the relative ease with which it is transmitted to other hosts. A droplet-spread infection, such as a respiratory virus, tends to be more infectious than an infection transmitted by direct contact, such as a sexually transmitted disease. Characteristics of the portals of exit and entry are thus determinants of infectiousness, as is the agent's ability to survive away from the host. Some factors that are often ascribed to an agent are actually the result of both agent and host characteristics. These factors include infectivity, pathogenicity, virulence, and antigenicity or immunogenicity.

Infectivity is typically defined as the characteristic of the infectious agent that embodies its capability to enter, survive, and multiply in the host. A measure of infectivity is the *secondary attack rate.* Infectivity is often expressed as the number infected divided by the number susceptible and exposed. In a population with an increased number of individuals with compromised specific or nonspecific immune responses, a higher proportion of exposed individuals actually become infected. For example, individuals who have decreased gastric acidity because of antacid use are at higher risk for the development of salmonellosis at a lower infectious dose than those with normal gastric pH.[69]

Pathogenicity is the property of an agent that determines the extent to which overt disease is produced in an infected population.[1] The pathogenicity of an agent is measured by the ratio of the number of persons in whom clinical disease develops to the number of infections. Again, pathogenicity is frequently considered a property of the agent alone; however, host characteristics play an important role in defining pathogenicity. For example, as has been noted earlier, the ratio of disease to total infections related to HAV varies widely according to host age.[64] In general, those agents with the highest levels of pathogenicity possess characteristics that protect them against nonspecific host defenses. In addition, they may elaborate a number of enzymes or toxins or may induce host-mediated disease associated with the immune response to infection.

The *gradient of infection,* or *biologic gradient,* is the range of manifestations of illness in the host that result from infection with an agent. It extends from death at one extreme to inapparent or subclinical illness at the other. In this regard, *virulence* is frequently used as a quantitative expression for the disease-producing potential of a pathogenic agent. It is defined as the rate of the number of cases of serious or disability-producing infections to the total number of people infected.[1] When death is the only criterion used to determine severity, it is referred to as the *case-fatality rate.*

From an epidemiologic perspective, the *virulence* of an organism must be viewed in light of the host. For example, the clinical outcome of HBV infection, which ranges from limited, subclinical infection to the development of acute fulminant hepatitis, is related to immune-mediated disease and important genetic factors of the host.[70] Similarly, the severity of tuberculosis is increased among blacks with host characteristics similar to those of patients of other races.[71] The development of drug resistance among organisms (regardless of the mechanism) is an important consideration related to virulence. Infection that is caused by agents that are sensitive to a variety of antimicrobial drugs is less likely to cause serious disease if it is treated in a timely and appropriate manner than infection caused by a highly resistant organism. With rapidly increasing drug resistance among all groups of infectious agents, this virulence characteristic will become even more important in the future.[72,73]

Finally, the last characteristic usually ascribed to an agent is *antigenicity* or *immunogenicity*. It is defined as the ability of an agent to produce a systemic or local immunologic reaction in the host.[1] However, this characteristic must also be considered in the context of both agent and host. The antigenicity of an agent is important from a clinical perspective because it is a primary determinant of the host's ability to mount an initial immune response to infection, thus affecting both pathogenicity and virulence. It also affects the host's development of long-term immunity to a specific agent. Thus, it is a critical factor in the assessment and development of vaccines for human and animal use.

In general, the host immune system includes all physiologic mechanisms with the capacity to recognize materials foreign to themselves and to neutralize, eliminate, or metabolize them with or without injury to their own tissues.[74] The immune response may be classified into two categories: specific and nonspecific. Specific immune responses are observed upon exposure to a foreign configuration, including infectious agents, and subsequent recognition of and reaction to that agent. An example of this type of response is the development of both humoral and cell-mediated immunity related to a specific agent.[75] A nonspecific response occurs after initial and subsequent exposure to a foreign antigen, and although it is selective in differentiating "self" from "nonself," it is not dependent on selective recognition. A number of factors modify the host immune mechanisms, including genetic, age-related, metabolic, environmental, anatomic, physiologic, and microbial factors.

The complex nature of the interaction between an agent and a host can be demonstrated by the relationship between *H. influenzae* type b and the age of the host. Children younger than 2 years do not mount an effective immune response to agents with capsular polysaccharide (i.e., *H. influenzae* type b, *N. meningitidis, Streptococcus pneumoniae*).[76] Polysaccharide antigens are T-cell–independent antigens, in contrast to protein antigens, which induce a T-cell effect. T-cell–independent antigens are poorly handled by children younger than 2 years of age because of the lack of maturation of their immune system. Thus, efforts were undertaken to develop vaccines for *H. influenzae* in younger children. This approach required that the *H. influenzae* type b polysaccharide be conjugated to various carrier proteins.[76] This combination of polysaccharide and protein has resulted in vaccines with enhanced immunogenicity, which is caused by induction of a T-cell response in infants. Use of the second-generation *H. influenzae* conjugate vaccines in infants in the United States has resulted in a dramatic decrease in the occurrence of invasive *H. influenzae* type b disease in children under 2 years of age.[77] Similar efforts are under way to develop conjugated polysaccharide vaccines for *N. meningitidis* and *S. pneumoniae*. Because vaccines have proved to be one of the most cost-effective methods of preventing infectious diseases, the need to understand antigenicity in terms of both the agent and the host is a high priority.

HOST

As was noted in the previous section regarding the agent, the characteristics of the host also play an important role in the eventual outcome of an agent-host interaction. Host factors that influence exposure, infection, and disease are summarized in Table 12-2. Factors can be classified into two categories: Those that influence exposure and those that influence the likelihood of infection and the occurrence and severity of disease.

All factors that influence human exposure to an infectious agent depend on contact with sources of infection within the environment or the promotion of person-to-person transmission.[66] The importance of factors that influence exposure tends to change by host age, culture, geographic residence, season, and family status.

Although most factors that influence infection and the occurrence and severity of disease are related to the host, the characteristics of both the agent and the host, as described by pathogenicity, virulence, and antigenicity, are important. Also, infectious dose of the agent, mechanisms of disease production, antibiotic resistance of the infecting agent, and portal of entry contribute to infection and disease status.[66] For most infections, two host factors play a key role in determining the likelihood of clinical illness and the severity of that illness: The immune status of the host and patient age at the time of infection. The highest levels of pathogenicity and virulence associated with the agent-host relationship tend to occur very early in life, when immune disease mechanisms are immature, or at an old age, when they may be deteriorating. Finally, genetic factors tend to influence both susceptibility and disease outcome, although they are primarily related to the host immune response to infection.

ROUTES OF TRANSMISSION

Transmission of infectious agents is defined as any mechanism by which an infectious agent is spread through the environment or to another person.[1,78] These mechanisms can be classified as either direct or indirect.

Of the three different modes of direct agent transmission, the most common is associated with direct and immediate transfer of an infectious agent to a receptive portal of entry through which the human infection is established. This type of direct-contact transmission occurs in association with touching, kissing, or sexual intercourse or by the direct projection (droplet spread) of droplet spray from an infected host onto the conjunctiva or the mucous membranes of the nose or mouth. Typically, droplet spread is limited to a distance of approximately 1 m. The second type of direct transmission occurs when susceptible tissue of the host is exposed to the agent, such as by the bite of a rabid ani-

TABLE 12-2 Host Factors That Influence Exposure, Infection, and Disease

Factors That Influence Exposure

Animal exposure, including pets
Behavioral factors related to age, drug usage, alcohol consumption
Blood or blood product receipt
Child daycare attendance
Closed living quarters: military barracks, dormitories, homeless shelters, facilities for the elderly and mentally handicapped, prisons
Food and water consumption
Familial exposure
Gender
Hospitalization or outpatient medical care
Hygiene practices, including toilet training and hand washing
Occupation
Recreational activities, including sports and recreational injecting drug use
Sexual activity: heterosexual and homosexual, type and number of partners
School attendance
Socioeconomic status
Travel, especially to developing countries
Vector exposure

Factors That Influence Infection and the Occurrence and Severity of Disease

Age at the time of infection
Alcoholism
Anatomic defect
Antibiotic resistance (agent)
Antibiotic use (host)
Coexisting noninfectious diseases, especially chronic
Coexisting infections
Dosage: amount and virulence of the organism to which the host is exposed
Duration of exposure to the organism
Entry portal of the organism and presence of trauma at the site of implantation
Gender
Genetic makeup, especially influences on the immune response
Immune state at the time of infection, including immunization status
Immunodeficiency (specific or nonspecific): natural, drug induced, or viral (HIV)
Mechanism of disease production: inflammatory, immunopathologic, or toxic
Nutritional status
Receptors for organism on cells needed for attachment or entry of the organism

Adapted from Evans AS, Brachman PS. Bacterial Infections of Humans: Epidemiology and Control. 3rd ed. New York: Plenum; 1998.

mal, or when it comes in contact with soil or decaying matter, in which the agent usually leads a saprophytic existence (e.g., systemic mycosis). Recently, direct human contact with infected pet prairie dogs led to an outbreak of monkeypox in the United States.[79] Finally, transplacental transmission is another form of direct transmission.

The three primary mechanisms of indirect agent transmission are vehicle borne, vector borne, and airborne. Vehicle-borne transmission occurs when any material serves as an intermediate means by which an infectious agent is transported or introduced into the susceptible host through a suitable portal of entry. These materials may include water; food; biologic products such as blood, serum, plasma, tissues, and organs; and objects (fomites) such as toys, soiled clothing, bedding, or surgical instruments. It is not necessary for the agent to multiply or develop in or on the vehicle before it is transmitted.

The second method of indirect transmission is vector borne. The two different types of vector-borne transmission are mechanical and biologic. Mechanical transmission occurs when an insect carries an infectious agent through the soiling of its feet or proboscis or through carriage in its gastrointestinal tract. Mechanical transmission does not require multiplication or development of the organism. In contrast, biologic vector-borne transmission occurs when propagation (multiplication), cyclic development, or a combination of these events (cyclopropagative) is required before the arthropod can transmit the infected form of the agent to humans.

The third type of indirect transmission is airborne, which involves the dissemination of aerosols with infectious agents to a suitable portal of entry in a host, usually the respiratory tract. These aerosols are suspensions of particles in the air that consist partially or wholly of infectious agents. The particles are in the range of 1 to 5 μm. (Note that airborne transmission does not include droplets and other large particles that promptly settle out. As has been noted earlier, these agents are included under direct transmission.) Some infections transmitted by the airborne route may be carried great distances from their sources, as has been documented by outbreaks of measles, legionnaires' disease, and anthrax.[80,81] For this reason, concern is great that agents such as *B. anthracis* and *Yersinia pestis* will be used as weapons of mass destruction in a civilian bioterrorism event.[82,83]

DISEASE PREVENTION AND CONTROL

Individual-, Institution-, Community-, and World-Based Strategies

Disease prevention and control activities for infectious agents occur at four levels. The first level is targeted to the individual and is predominantly the domain of the clinician. A variety of prevention activities can be targeted to individuals through their primary care provider. Use of chemoprophylaxis to prevent surgical wound infection is an example of a control measure targeted to the individual. The second level is that of the institution, which is predominantly the domain of the infection-control practitioner or the school health official. This level includes health care facilities, nursing homes, other residential facilities, and schools. Programs to prevent the spread of blood-borne pathogens or tuberculosis to health care workers in hospitals are examples of control strategies targeted at the institutional level. The third level is targeted to the community in general and is predominantly the domain of public health agencies (at the local, state, and national levels). Removal of a contaminated food product from the market is an example of a control measure targeted to the community. Finally, the fourth level is related to global strategies. For a number of important pathogens, it has become clear that global control strategies are critical if disease occurrence within the United States is to be changed. The growing proportion of tuberculosis cases among refugees and immigrants to the United States and ongoing episodes of importation of measles from abroad are two examples pertinent to U.S. disease control in the late 1990s and early 21st century.

Although some control measures are specific to these different levels, a substantial amount of overlap can occur. For example, immuniza-

tion programs operate at all four levels. Clinicians play an important role in the health maintenance of individual patients by providing immunizations against a variety of pathogens. Immunization programs are also an important activity at the institutional level, such as routine annual immunization against influenza in nursing homes and immunization of health care workers against HBV. Public health agencies monitor vaccination levels in the community and provide vaccination clinics that are open to the public. Finally, ensuring that foreign travelers from countries with selected endemic vaccine-preventable diseases are adequately vaccinated before they travel is a critical control measure for the prevention of diseases such as measles.

During assessment or development of disease prevention and control activities targeted to infectious diseases, the weakest link in the chain of infection (agent, transmission, host) also needs to be considered for each specific pathogen. In some situations, control of the agent in a specific reservoir may be the best way to reduce disease occurrence. Chlorination of water and pasteurization of milk are examples of destroying an agent in its reservoir or eliminating a possible mode of transmission.

Strategies aimed at the level of transmission need to be tailored to the type of transmission involved. For example, the use of condoms in the prevention of sexually transmitted diseases is a control strategy targeted at preventing contact transmission. Transmission through common vehicles frequently involves food and water and may involve other vehicles such as blood in the case of transfusions. Irradiation of food and screening of blood for infectious agents are control activities targeted to a common vehicle. An example of a control activity targeted to airborne transmission is the use of respirators to prevent transmission of tuberculosis in the health care setting. Control of vector-borne transmission can be targeted toward destroying the vector or its breeding sites or toward the use of protective clothing and repellents.

Finally, methods to limit population mixing between infected and infectious patients and uninfected individuals can result in the application of isolation or quarantine. Often referred to as "police powers," federal, state, and local governments, depending on specific legal authorities, can control the movement of individuals or populations to protect the general public from communicable diseases.[84,85] Isolation is the process and procedure whereby an infected individual is prevented from potentially transmitting a communicable disease to others. Traditionally, it has been applied to individuals with serious, life-threatening infections that have not or cannot be treated so as to render the patient noninfectious. Recently, the potential for bioterrorism-related illnesses such as smallpox and pneumonic plague and the occurrence of SARS have highlighted this issue. Quarantine, that is, the separation and/or restriction of movement of persons who are not ill but are believed to have been exposed to infection to prevent transmission of diseases, was developed in the 14th century but has been implemented rarely on a large scale during the past century. The SARS pandemic has demonstrated that governments might use quarantine as a public health tool to control infectious diseases, particularly when other preventive interventions (e.g., vaccines and antibiotics) are unavailable.[85,86]

In some instances, the best mechanism for preventing disease occurrence is modification of the host, such as that which occurs by developing or boosting immunity through active or passive immunization. Other examples of control activities targeted to the host include improving nutritional status and providing chemoprophylaxis against a variety of agents.

Assessment of Risk, Feasibility, Cost, and Effectiveness

When disease prevention and control strategies are being developed, several issues need to be considered, including risk, feasibility, cost, and effectiveness. Risk can be defined by the potential for exposure. Epidemiologic studies or analysis of surveillance data can serve to define persons or populations at risk and can quantify risk within different populations. At the individual level, risk can be evaluated by assessment of host characteristics, such as the need for prophylaxis against *Pneumocystis jirovecii* pneumonia for persons with HIV infection and T-cell depletion.[87] An example of evaluating risk at the institutional level is assessment of occupational exposure to infectious agents such as blood-borne pathogens. At the community level, groups at risk for a variety of conditions can be defined by demographic features (such as age, race, country of origin, socioeconomic status, and geographic location). For example, persons born outside the United States are at increased risk for infectious diseases such as tuberculosis or for being chronic carriers of infection such as hepatitis B. Screening programs targeted to these populations with subsequent interventions (such as isoniazid prophylaxis for persons with *M. tuberculosis* infection or immunization of susceptible household contacts of HBV carriers) can serve as important community-based strategies for prevention of infectious disease occurrence.[88,89] Another example of defining risk at the community level is assessment of behavior that increases the risk for specific diseases, such as injecting drug use as a risk behavior for acquiring HIV or hepatitis C virus (HCV) infection. Education and drug treatment programs targeted to this population can serve as important disease prevention and control strategies. Finally, assessing the population of species-specific mosquitoes and the viability of local breeding sites can provide a risk assessment of the likelihood of vector-borne disease transmission such as that which occurs with West Nile virus infection.[90,91]

In the development of control programs, the feasibility of a strategy also needs to be assessed. Feasibility is dependent on the sociodemographic factors of the population involved. For example, high immunization rates can clearly prevent the occurrence of infectious diseases. In the United States, immunizations should be readily available; however, in the late 1980s, numerous large outbreaks of measles occurred in U.S. inner city populations because of low immunization rates.[92] A variety of sociodemographic factors contributed to these low rates, such as inadequate access to medical care and other barriers to immunization. Until such barriers are removed and control strategies are developed to specifically target such populations, adequate control of vaccine-preventable diseases in the United States cannot be accomplished.[93]

Cost and availability of resources also need to be considered when control strategies are developed. Adequate water treatment facilities and distribution systems in developing countries would do much to eliminate the spread of cholera. However, in many countries, resources to build and develop such facilities are not available. Consequently, control strategies need to be focused on simpler, less expensive methods such as boiling water or improving water storage in the home.

Finally, control strategies need to be evaluated for their effectiveness. For example, the effectiveness of the control strategy is a critical issue in the evaluation of ways to curb the HIV epidemic in the absence of vaccination. Evaluation of HIV prevention educational programs or HIV counseling and testing programs is essential in assessing the effectiveness of currently available strategies. Cost-effectiveness models are often used in the development of recommendations for population-based vaccination programs.[94,95]

Primary, Secondary, or Tertiary Prevention

Prevention strategies for infectious disease can be characterized by the traditional concepts of primary, secondary, and tertiary prevention.[1] *Primary prevention* can be defined as the prevention of infection by personal and community-wide efforts. *Secondary prevention* includes measures available to individuals and the population for the detection of early infection and effective intervention. *Tertiary prevention* consists of measures available to reduce or eliminate the long-term impairment and disabilities caused by infectious disease.

Primary Prevention

A key example of primary prevention is immunoprophylaxis, which can be active or passive. Active immunoprophylaxis involves the administration of all or part of a microorganism (live or inactivated) or a product of that microorganism (such as a toxoid) to alter the host by stimulating an immunologic response aimed at protecting against infection. Live vaccines are often more immunogenic than inactivated vaccines and may require fewer booster doses. Live-attenuated vaccines contain weakened or avirulent viruses or bacteria. They are generally contraindicated in immunocompromised persons. Examples of live-attenuated vaccines include vaccines against measles, mumps, rubella, and yellow fever; oral polio vaccine; oral typhoid vaccine; and Calmette-Guérin bacillus vaccine.[78] Examples of vaccines created from inactivated organisms include inactivated polio vaccine and vaccines against anthrax, influenza, hepatitis B, cholera, pertussis, and rabies.[78] Examples of polysaccharide vaccines include pneumococcal and meningococcal vaccines; *H. influenzae* type b conjugate vaccine is a polysaccharide-protein conjugate.[64] Examples of toxoid vaccines include tetanus, diphtheria, and botulinal toxoids.[78]

Currently, at least four types of active immunization programs are being conducted. The first is routine childhood immunization. Current practices include routine childhood immunization against measles, mumps, rubella, tetanus, diphtheria, pertussis, *H. influenzae* type b, and hepatitis B.[96,97] In many parts of the world, Calmette-Guérin bacillus vaccine is also given routinely in early childhood. Recently, childhood vaccines have become available to prevent infections caused by HAV and by varicella-zoster virus. As the routine childhood immunization schedule becomes increasingly complex, new methods of vaccine delivery need to be developed. Of particular interest is the development of new multiple-antigen vaccines to simplify the routine schedule and maximize efficiency of vaccine delivery. The goals of routine childhood immunization are twofold: First, to protect the individual and second to provide herd immunity, which can be effective in controlling certain diseases at the population level (such as measles, mumps, rubella, and *H. influenzae*).[98] Ongoing adequate surveillance for these diseases is essential for monitoring the effectiveness of population-based immunization programs so that strategies can be adapted as needed. The expansion of measles immunization to a two-dose schedule in the United States in 1989 is an example of the use of surveillance data to revise immunization practices.[99]

A second type of immunization program is travel-related immunization. Examples include the administration of typhoid, yellow fever, Japanese encephalitis, and meningococcal vaccines for travel to areas endemic for these conditions. The third type of program is immunization of selected at-risk populations. For example, influenza vaccine is currently recommended in the United States annually for persons who are at increased risk for complications (persons 50 years of age and older, residents of nursing homes, adults with certain chronic diseases, children who are receiving long-term aspirin therapy and may be at risk for Reye's syndrome, and women who will be in the second or third trimester of pregnancy during the influenza season) and for persons who can transmit influenza to those at high risk.[100] Pneumococcal vaccine is also recommended for selected high-risk populations, including persons 65 years of age or older, persons with certain chronic diseases, and persons with certain immunosuppressive conditions. In outbreak settings, community-wide vaccination may be used to protect those at risk of exposure, such as that during community outbreaks of serogroup C meningococcal disease.[99]

The final type of immunization program is based on occupational exposure. Recommendations for the immunization of health care workers have been made because of their special risk of exposure to a variety of vaccine-preventable diseases. Examples include immunization of laboratory workers against anthrax, rabies, smallpox, and botulism in settings in which these organisms are, or may be, handled; immunization of health care workers against measles or smallpox and hepatitis B based on exposure to blood-borne pathogens; and immunization of those who respond to bioterrorism-related anthrax or smallpox.[99,101,102]

Active immunization is also used in certain postexposure situations, including immunization after exposure to *N. meningitidis*, HBV, measles, pertussis, and rabies. Some of these vaccines are given in conjunction with various types of immune globulin in the postexposure setting.

Passive immunization involves the administration of preformed antibodies, often to specific agents, after exposure. The broadest form of passive immunization is the use of normal human immune globulin (also referred to as *gamma globulin*). It is most often used after exposure to HAV and may be effective if given within 14 days after exposure.[89] Normal human immune globulin is also recommended before travel to countries endemic for hepatitis A. It may be effective in reducing clinical disease in persons exposed to measles if provided within 6 days after exposure.[99] For persons with hypogammaglobulinemia or agammaglobulinemia, it may be given as immunoglobulin (Ig) G replacement therapy. Multiple specific types of immune globulin are used in postexposure settings to prevent infection. Examples include immune globulin specific to HBV, cytomegalovirus, rabies, varicella-zoster virus, and tetanus.

A second type of primary prevention is antimicrobial prophylaxis, often referred to as chemoprophylaxis. Use of effective chemoprophylaxis requires that the infectious agent be susceptible to the antimicrobial used. As a primary prevention strategy, it may be used before or after exposure to prevent infection. Examples of chemoprophylaxis in the postexposure setting include exposure to pertussis (e.g., erythromycin), *N. meningitidis* (e.g., rifampin), influenza A virus (e.g., amantadine, rimantadine), influenza A or B virus (zanamivir or oseltamivir), and HIV (e.g., zidovudine). Use of antiretroviral drugs by HIV-infected pregnant women has been shown to substantially reduce the risk of perinatal HIV infection.[103] Prophylaxis against surgical wound infection with broad-spectrum coverage before surgery and prophylaxis of neonates against ophthalmia neonatorum are examples of chemoprophylaxis used in the hospital setting. In such situations, chemoprophylaxis is used because a likelihood of exposure to pathogenic organisms is present, even though exposure is not clearly documented. Chemoprophylaxis is also used in anticipation of exposure during travel (such as that for the prevention of malaria through the use of chloroquine or mefloquine); antimicrobials against enteric pathogens can be used to prevent traveler's diarrhea.

In addition to immunoprophylaxis and chemoprophylaxis, other important primary prevention activities are aimed at individual, institutional, and community levels. Examples have been discussed in earlier sections of this chapter.

Secondary Prevention

Secondary prevention activities traditionally entail chemoprophylaxis and involve the identification of early or asymptomatic infection with subsequent treatment so that such infections are eradicated and sequelae are prevented. Although most secondary prevention programs involve intervention at the individual level through the use of chemoprophylaxis, such programs often operate within the context of a population-based or institution-based screening effort. Routine screening programs for sexually transmitted diseases such as *Chlamydia* infection are examples of secondary prevention strategies.[104,105] Contact investigations for partners of persons with sexually transmitted diseases are also part of a secondary prevention strategy focused on those at the highest risk of infection (i.e., those with known exposure).[104] Another example of a secondary prevention program that uses chemoprophylaxis is the screening of high-risk populations for tuberculosis infection and subsequent therapy with an antimicrobial such as isoniazid to prevent active disease.

Although most secondary prevention strategies involve chemoprophylaxis (and rarely immunoprophylaxis), the concept can be broadened to other prevention efforts aimed at intervention and correction of a recognized specific health hazard. Most such efforts occur at the community level. Examples of community-based secondary prevention efforts include the early identification of contaminated products through outbreak investigations and the subsequent removal of such products from the market to prevent additional illnesses and restore "the community's health." A boil-water order for a waterborne disease outbreak of cryptosporidiosis is another example of a secondary prevention strategy aimed at correcting an existing community-wide problem.

Tertiary Prevention

Tertiary prevention efforts are measures to eliminate long-term impairment and disability that may result from an existing condition. Because most infectious diseases are treatable, tertiary prevention activities are less common than those used with chronic diseases such as hypertension, diabetes, and coronary artery disease. However, this concept is still applicable to the control of infectious diseases inasmuch as some viral infections are chronic and cannot be eradicated. Current treatment of HIV infection, including prophylaxis against other opportunistic agents, is an example of a tertiary prevention activity.

REFERENCES

1. Last JM, ed. A Dictionary of Epidemiology. 2nd ed. New York: Oxford; 1988.
2. Barrett-Connor E. Infectious and chronic disease epidemiology: Separate and unequal? Am J Epidemiol. 1979;109:245-249.
3. Snow J. On the Mode of Communication of Cholera. London: 1855. Reprinted in Frost WH, ed. Snow on Cholera. New York: Commonwealth Fund; 1936.
4. Lee N, Hui D, Wu A, et al. A major outbreak of severe acute respiratory syndrome in Hong Kong. N Engl J Med. 2003;348:1977-1985.
5. Ksiazek TG, Erdman D, Goldsmith C, et al. A novel coronavirus associated with severe acute respiratory syndrome. N Engl J Med. 2003;348:1953-1966.
6. Lipsitch M, Cohen T, Cooper B, et al. Transmission dynamics and control of severe acute respiratory syndrome. Science. 2003;300:1966-1970.
7. World Health Organization. Global eradication of smallpox. Bull World Health Org. 1980;58:161-163.
8. Hedberg CW, Savarino SJ, Besser JM, et al. An outbreak of foodborne illness caused by *Escherichia coli* O39:NM, an agent not fitting into the existing scheme for classifying diarrheogenic *E. coli*. J Infect Dis. 1997;176:1625-1628.
9. Wood RC, MacDonald KL, White KE, et al. Risk factors for lack of detectable antibody following hepatitis B vaccination of Minnesota health care workers. JAMA. 1993;270:2935-2939.
10. Maldonado G, Greenland S. Estimating causal effects. Int J Epidemiol. 2002;31:422-429.
11. Bender JB, Hedberg CW, Besser JM, et al. Surveillance for *Escherichia coli* O157:H7 infections in Minnesota by molecular subtyping. N Engl J Med. 1997;337:388-394.
12. Swaminathan B, Barrett TJ, Hunter SB, et al. PulseNet: The molecular subtyping network for foodborne bacterial disease surveillance, United States. Emerg Infect Dis. 2001;7:382-389.
13. Centers for Disease Control and Prevention. Prevention and control of meningococcal disease: Recommendations of the Advisory Committee on Immunization Practices (ACIP). MMWR Morb Mortal Wkly Rep. 2000;49(RR-07):1-10.
14. Popovic T, Schmink S, Rosenstein N, et al. Evaluation of pulsed-field gel electrophoresis in epidemiological investigations of meningococcal disease outbreaks caused by *Neisseria meningitides* serogroup C. J Clin Microbiol. 2001;39:75-85.
15. Rosenstein NE, Perkins BA, Stephens DS, et al: The changing epidemiology of meningococcal disease in the United States, 1992-1996. J Infect Dis. 1999;180:1894-1901.
16. Hennekens CH, Burning JE. Epidemiology in Medicine. Boston: Little, Brown; 1987.
17. St Louis ME, Morse DL, Potter ME, et al. The emergence of grade A eggs as a major source of *Salmonella enteritidis* infections. New implications of the control of salmonellosis. JAMA. 1988;259:2103-2107.
18. Hedberg CW, David MJ, White KE, et al. Role of egg consumption in sporadic *Salmonella enteritidis* and *Salmonella typhimurium* infections in Minnesota. J Infect Dis. 1993;167:107-111.
19. Schlesselman JJ, Stolley PD. Case-Control Studies. Design, Conduct, Analysis. New York: Oxford; 1982.
20. Fairchild AL, Bayer R. Ethics and the conduct of public health surveillance. Science. 2004;303:631-632.
21. Centers for Disease Control and Prevention. Prevention of invasive group A streptococcal disease among household contacts of case-patients and among postpartum postsurgical patients. Clin Infect Dis. 2002;35:950-959.
22. Davies HD, McGeer A, Schwartz B, et al. A prospective, population-based study of invasive group A streptococcal infections, including toxic shock syndrome and the risk of secondary invasive disease. N Engl J Med. 1996;335:547-554.
23. Centers for Disease Control and Prevention. Prevention of invasive group A streptococcal disease among household contacts of case patients and among postpartum and postsurgical patients. Clin Infect Dis. 2002;35:950-959.
24. Robinson KA, Rothrock G, Phan Q, et al. Risk for severe group A streptococcal disease among patients' household contacts. Emerg Infect Dis. 2003;9:443-447.
25. Lilienfeld AM, Lilienfeld DE. Foundations of Epidemiology. 2nd ed. New York: Oxford; 1980.
26. Kelsey JL, Thompson WD, Evans AS. Methods in Observational Epidemiology, v. 10. Monographs in Epidemiology and Biostatistics. New York: Oxford; 1986.
27. Centers for Disease Control and Prevention. Updated guidelines for evaluating public health surveillance systems: Recommendations from the Guidelines Working Group. MMWR Morb Mortal Wkly Rep. 2001;50:RR-13.
28. Chorba TL, Berkelman RL, Saffor SK, et al. Mandatory reporting of infectious diseases by clinicians. JAMA. 1989;262:3018-3026.
29. Centers for Disease Control and Prevention. Recommendations for prevention and control of hepatitis C virus (HCV) infection and HCV-related chronic disease. MMWR Morb Mortal Wkly Rep. 1998;47(RR-19):1-39.
30. Perkins BA, Flood JM, Danila R, et al. Unexplained deaths due to possibly infectious causes in the United States: Defining the problem and designing surveillance and laboratory approaches. Emerg Infect Dis. 1996;2:47-53.
31. Buehler JS, Berkelman RL, Hartley DM, et al. Syndromic surveillance and bioterrorism-related epidemics. Emerg Infect Dis. 2003;9:1197-1204.

32. Centers for Disease Control and Prevention. Syndromic surveillance for bioterrorism following the attacks on the World Trade Center—New York City, 2001. MMWR Morb Mortal Wkly Rep. 2002;51:13-15.

33. Moore M, Onorato IM, McCray E, et al. Trends in drug-resistant tuberculosis in the United States, 1993-1996. JAMA. 1997;278:833-837.

34. Glynn MK, Bopp C, Dewitt W, et al. Emergence of multidrug-resistant *Salmonella enterica* serotype *typhimurium* DT104 infections in the United States. N Engl J Med. 1998;338:1333-1338.

35. Gupta A, Fontana J, Crowe C, et al. Emergence of multi-drug resistant *Salmonella enterica* serotype *newport* infections resistant to expanded spectrum cephalosporins in the United States. J Infect Dis. 2003;188:1707-1716.

36. Breiman RF, Butler JC, Tenover FC, et al. Emergence of drug-resistant pneumococcal infections in the United States. JAMA. 1994;271:1831-1835.

37. Centers for Disease Control and Prevention. The Foodborne Diseases Active Surveillance Network, 1996. MMWR Morb Mortal Wkly Rep. 1997;46:258-261.

38. Murphy TV, Smith PJ, Gargiullo PM, Schwartz B. The first rotavirus vaccine and intussusception: epidemiological studies and policy decisions. J Infect Dis. 2003; 187:1309-1313.

39. Centers for Disease Control and Prevention. Public health: Surveillance, prevention and control of nosocomial infections. MMWR Morb Mortal Wkly Rep. 1992;41:783-787.

40. Williams REO. Changing perspectives in hospital infection. In: Proceedings of the International Conference on Nosocomial Infections. Atlanta: Centers for Disease Control; 1970:1-10.

41. Tsang KW, Ho PL, Ooi GC, et al. A cluster of cases of severe acute respiratory syndrome in Hong Kong. N Engl J Med. 2003;348:1977-1985.

42. Hennessey TW, Hedberg CW, Slutsker L, et al. A national outbreak of *Salmonella enteritidis* infections from ice cream. N Engl J Med. 1996;334:1281-1286.

43. Mishu B, Blaser MJ. Role of infection due to *Campylobacter jejuni* in the initiation of Guillain-Barré syndrome. Clin Infect Dis. 1993;17:104-108.

44. Moss AR, Osmond D, Bacchetti P, et al. Risk factors for AIDS and HIV seropositivity in homosexual men. Am J Epidemiol. 1987;125:1035-1047.

45. Osmond DH, Charlebois E, Sheppard HW, et al. Comparison of risk factors for hepatitis C and hepatitis B infection in homosexual men. J Infect Dis. 1993;167:66-71.

46. Evans AS, ed. Viral Infections of Humans. Epidemiology and Control. 2nd ed. New York: Plenum; 1982.

47. Weinstock HS, Bolar G, Reingold AL, Polish LB. Hepatitis C virus infection among patients attending a clinic for sexually transmitted diseases. JAMA. 1993;269:392-394.

48. Centers for Disease Control and Prevention. Serosurveys of West Nile virus infection—New York and Connecticut counties, 2000. MMWR Morb Mortal Wkly Rep. 2001;50:31-39.

49. Centers for Disease Control and Prevention. Multistate outbreak of *Salmonella* serotype *agona* infections linked to toasted oats cereal—United States, April-May 1998. MMWR Morb Mortal Wkly Rep. 1998;47:402-464.

50. Centers for Disease Control and Prevention. Multistate outbreak of listeriosis—United States, 1998. MMWR Morb Mortal Wkly Rep. 1998;47:1085-1086.

51. McCarthy N, Giesecke J. Case-case comparisons to study causation of common infectious diseases. Int J Epidemiol. 1999;28:764-768.

52. Herwaldt BL, Ackers ML. An outbreak in 1996 of cyclosporiasis associated with imported raspberries. The Cyclospora Working Group. N Engl J Med. 1997;336:1548-1556.

53. Herwaldt BL, Beach MJ. The return of *Cyclospora* in 1997: Another outbreak of cyclosporiasis in North America associated with imported raspberries. The Cyclospora Working Group. Ann Intern Med. 1999;130:210-220.

54. Mead PS, Slutsker L, Dietz V, et al. Food-related illness and death in the United States. Emerg Infect Dis. 1999;5:607-625.

55. Waterhouse B. A Prospect for Exterminating the Smallpox. Cambridge, England: Cambridge; 1800.

56. Tucker WB. The evolution of the cooperative studies in the chemotherapy of tuberculosis of the Veteran's Administration and Armed Forces of the USA: An account of the evolving education of the physician in clinical pharmacology. Adv Tuber Res. 1960;10:1-68.

57. Francis T, Karns RF, Voight RB, et al. An evaluation of the 1954 poliomyelitis vaccine trial: Summary report. Am J Pub Health. 1955;45(Suppl):S1-S51.

58. Austin SC, Stolley PD, Lasky T. The history of malariotherapy for neurosyphilis. Modern parallels. JAMA. 1992;268:516-519.

59. Meinert CL. Clinical Trials. Design, Conduct and Analysis, v. 8. Monographs in Epidemiology and Biostatistics. New York: Oxford; 1986.

60. Hadler SC, Erben JJ, Matthews D, et al. Effect of immunoglobulin on hepatitis A in day-care centers. JAMA. 1983;249:48-53.

61. Schwartz B. Preventing the spread of antimicrobial resistance among bacterial respiratory pathogens in industrialized countries: The case for judicious antimicrobial use. Clin Infect Dis. 1999;28:211-213.

62. Berkelman RL, Hughes JM. The conquest of infectious diseases: Who are we kidding? Ann Intern Med. 1993;119:426-428.

63. Smolinski MS, Hamburg MA, Lederberg J, eds. Microbial Threats to Health: Emergence, Detection, and Response. Washington, DC: National Academies Press; 2003.

64. Hadler SC, Webster HM, Erben JJ, et al. Hepatitis A in day care centers—a communitywide assessment. N Engl J Med. 1980;302:1222-1227.

65. Benenson AS. Smallpox. In: Evans AS, ed. Viral Infections of Humans: Epidemiology and Control. New York: Plenum; 1982:541-568.

66. Evans AS, Brachman PS, eds. Bacterial Infections of Humans: Epidemiology and Control. 3rd ed. New York: Plenum; 1998.

67. Fox M, Kaufmann AF, Zendel SA, et al. Anthrax in Louisiana, 1971: Epizootiologic study. J Am Vet Med Assoc. 1973;163:446-451.

68. Skaliy P, McEachern HV. Survival of the legionnaires' disease bacterium in water. Ann Intern Med. 1979;90:577-580.

69. Black PH, Kunz LJ, Swartz MN. Salmonellosis—a review of some unusual aspects. N Engl J Med. 1960;262:811-816, 846-870, 921-927.

70. Lau JYN, Wright TL. Molecular virology and pathogenesis of hepatitis B. Lancet. 1993;342:1335-1339.

71. Stead WW, Senner JW, Reddick WT, Lofgren JP. Racial differences in susceptibility to infection by *Mycobacterium tuberculosis*. N Engl J Med. 1990;322:422-427.

72. Cohen ML. Epidemiology of drug resistance: Implications for a post-antimicrobial era. Science. 1992;257:1050-1055.

73. Levy SB. Confronting multidrug resistance: A role for each of us. JAMA. 1993; 269:1840-1842.

74. Bellanti JA. Immunology II. Philadelphia: WB Saunders; 1978.

75. Nossal GJV. Current concepts: Immunology: The basic components of the immune system. N Engl J Med. 1987;316:1320-1325.

76. Granoff DM, Munson RS Jr. Prospects for prevention of *Haemophilus influenzae* type b disease by immunization. J Infect Dis. 1986;153:448-461.

77. Murphy TV, White KE, Pastor P, et al. Declining incidence of *Haemophilus influenzae* type b since introduction of vaccination. JAMA. 1993;269:246-248.

78. Chin James E, ed. Control of Communicable Diseases Manual. 17th ed. Washington, DC: American Public Health Association; 2000.

79. Reed KD, Melski JW, Graham MB, et al. The detection of monkeypox in humans in the western hemisphere. N Engl J Med. 2004;350:342-350.

80. Ehresmann KR, Hedberg CW, Grimm MB, et al. An outbreak of measles at an international sporting event with airborne transmission in a domed stadium. J Infect Dis. 1995;171:679-683.

81. Meselson M, Guillemin J, Hugh-Jones M, et al. The Sverdlovsk anthrax outbreak of 1979. Science. 1994;266:1202-1208.

82. Inglesby TV, O'Toole T, Henderson DA, et al. Anthrax as a biological weapon, 2002. JAMA. 2002;287:2236-2252.

83. Inglesby TV, Dennis DT, Henderson DA, et al. Plague as a biological weapon: Medical and public health management. JAMA. 2000;283:2281-2290.

84. Barbera J, Macintyre A, Gostin L, et al. Large-scale quarantine following biological terrorism in the United States: Scientific examination, logistic and legal limits, and possible consequences. JAMA. 2001;286:2711-2717.

85. Centers for Disease Control and Prevention. Use of quarantine to prevent transmission of severe acute respiratory syndrome—Taiwan, 2003. MMWR Morb Mortal Wkly Rep. 2003;52:680-683.

86. Misrahi JJ, Foster JA, Shaw FE, et al. HHS/CDC legal response to SARS outbreak. Emerg Infect Dis. 2004;10:353-355.

87. Centers for Disease Control. Recommendations for prophylaxis against *Pneumocystis carinii* pneumonia for adults and adolescents infected with human immunodeficiency virus. MMWR Morb Mortal Wkly Rep. 1992;41(RR-4):1-11.

88. American Thoracic Society. Control of tuberculosis in the United States. Am Rev Respir Dis. 1992;146:1623-1633.

89. Centers for Disease Control. Protection against viral hepatitis: Recommendations of the Immunization Practices Advisory Committee. MMWR Morb Mortal Wkly Rep. 1990;39(RR-2):1-26.

90. Centers for Disease Control and Prevention. Epidemic/Epizootic West Nile Virus in the United States: Guidelines for Surveillance, Prevention, and Control. 3rd rev. Atlanta: CDC; 2003.

91. Nash D, Mostashari F, Fine A, et al. The outbreak of West Nile Virus infection in the New York City area in 1999. N Engl J Med. 2001;344:1807-1814.

92. The National Vaccine Advisory Committee. The measles epidemic: The problems, barriers, and recommendations. JAMA. 1991;266:1547-1552.

93. Shalala DE. Giving pediatric immunizations the priority they deserve. JAMA. 1993;269:1844-1845.

94. Tucker AW, Haddix AC, Bresee JS, et al. Cost-effectiveness analysis of a rotavirus immunization program for the United States. JAMA. 1998;279:1371-1376.

95. Sisk JE, Moskowitz AJ, Whang W, et al. Cost-effectiveness of vaccination against pneumococcal bacteremia among elderly people. JAMA. 1997;278:1333-1339.

96. Pickering LK, ed. Red Book: 2003 Report of the Committee on Infectious Diseases. 26th ed. Elk Grove Village, IL: American Academy of Pediatrics: 2003.

97. Atkinson WL, Pickering LK, Schwartz B, et al. General recommendations on immunization: Recommendations of the Advisory Committee on Immunization Practices (ACIP) and the American Academy of Family Physicians (AAFP). MMWR Morb Mortal Wkly Rep. 2002;51:1-36.

98. Fine PE. Herd immunity: History, theory, practice. Epidemiol Rev. 1993;15:265-302.

99. Centers for Disease Control. Measles prevention: Recommendations of the Immunization Practices Advisory Committee. MMWR Morb Mortal Wkly Rep. 1989;38:1-13.

100. Bridges CB, Harper SA, Fukuda K, et al. Prevention and Control of Influenza: Recommendations of the Advisory Committee on Immunization Practices (ACIP). MMWR Morb Mortal Wkly Rep. 2003;52:1-36.

101. Centers for Disease Control and Prevention. Notice to readers: Use of anthrax vaccine in response to terrorism: Supplemental recommendations of the Advisory Committee on Immunization Practices. MMWR Morb Mortal Wkly Rep. 2002;51:1024-1026.

102. Wharton M, Strikas RA, Harpaz R, et al. Recommendations for using smallpox vaccine in a pre-event vaccination program: Supplemental recommendations of the Advisory Committee on Immunization Practices (ACIP) and the Healthcare Infection Control Practices Advisory Committee (HICPAC). MMWR Morb Mortal Wkly Rep. 2003;52:1-16.

103. Centers for Disease Control and Prevention. Public health services task force recommendations for the use of antiretroviral drugs in pregnant women infected with HIV-1 for maternal health and for reducing perinatal HIV-1 transmission in the United States. MMWR Morb Mortal Wkly Rep. 1998;47:1-30.

Chapter 13   Emerging and Reemerging Infectious Disease Threats   173

104. Centers for Disease Control. 1993 sexually transmitted diseases treatment guidelines. MMWR Morb Mortal Wkly Rep. 1993;42:1-102.

105. Centers for Disease Control and Prevention. Recommendations for the prevention and management of *Chlamydia trachomatis* infections, 1993. MMWR Morb Mortal Wkly Rep. 1993;42:1-39.

CHAPTER **13**

Emerging and Reemerging Infectious Disease Threats

STEPHEN M. OSTROFF

JOSEPH E. McDADE

JAMES W. LeDUC

JAMES M. HUGHES

Throughout history, outbreaks of infectious disease have periodically spread across different populations and regions, affected largely by movement of people, animals, and commercial goods into new areas. In the 16th century, Spanish explorers reportedly brought smallpox to the New World and returned with syphilis.[1,2] The 1918 influenza outbreak killed more than 25 million persons throughout the world in a little over 1 year. The epidemic of human immunodeficiency virus/ acquired immunodeficiency syndrome (HIV/AIDS) had spread globally by the time the disease, now an unremitting pandemic claiming millions of lives each year,[3] was recognized. In early 2003, the emergence of severe acute respiratory syndrome (SARS) reminded the world that new infectious agents can spread globally in a matter of weeks, impacting national security and the global economy and requiring international collaboration to stop their spread.

During the early and mid 20th century, advances in medicine and science brought new optimism to the struggle against infectious disease. Improvements in sanitation and overall living conditions led to safer food and drinking water and improved waste management and disposal. The development and widespread delivery of effective vac-

cines and the production of safe and effective antimicrobial agents further reduced morbidity and mortality from many previously widespread infectious threats. As a result, a major increase in overall life expectancy has occurred over the second half of the 20th century— from 46.5 years in 1950-1955 to 65.2 years in 2002.[3]

These successes, however, do not apply to the poorest countries. In the 48 least developed countries, life expectancy is just 51 years, compared with 78 years in high-income countries.[4] Gains in life expectancy have been reversed in many developing countries, especially in sub-Saharan Africa, where adult mortality is now higher than it was 30 years ago, primarily because of HIV/AIDS.[5] Among children, health disparities between the developed and the developing world are further magnified. According to the World Health Organization (WHO), of 10.5 million deaths reported in 2002 among children younger than 5 years of age, 98% occurred in developing countries.[3]

Infectious diseases contribute disproportionately to these figures (Fig. 13-1). Of the estimated 57 million deaths that occurred throughout the world in 2002, nearly 15 million (26%) were infectious disease related (Table 13-1), the vast majority of which occurred among persons from developing countries. These statistics, however, do not reflect the true burden of death from infectious diseases because underreporting remains a major factor, particularly in the developing world, and because many deaths with infectious causes are not categorized as infection related. Examples include deaths from cancer secondary to infectious causes, cardiovascular deaths resulting from poststreptococcal rheumatic heart disease, and maternal deaths due to puerperal sepsis.

In 1992, the Institute of Medicine (IOM) published a report[6] that described the increasing public health challenges created by emerging infections. The report sought to highlight the need for improvements in public health to address the risks posed by "new, reemerging, or drug-resistant infections whose incidence in humans has increased within the past two decades." The report identified the following six factors that underlie infectious disease emergence: (1) changes in human demographics and behavior; (2) the impact of new technologies and industries; (3) economic development and changes in land use; (4) increased international travel and commerce; (5) microbial adaptation and change; and (6) the breakdown of public health measures. In March of 2003, the IOM published an update[7] to this report, expanding on both the threats of emerging infectious diseases and the need for increased global recognition and response to address them. In addition to the six underlying factors listed here, the new report cites seven other factors that can contribute to the emergence of global

FIGURE 13-1. Global Causes of Death, 2002. Distribution of global causes of death based on an estimated 57,027,000 deaths in 2002. *(Source: World Health Organization. The World Health Report 2003. Geneva: World Health Organization; 2003.)*

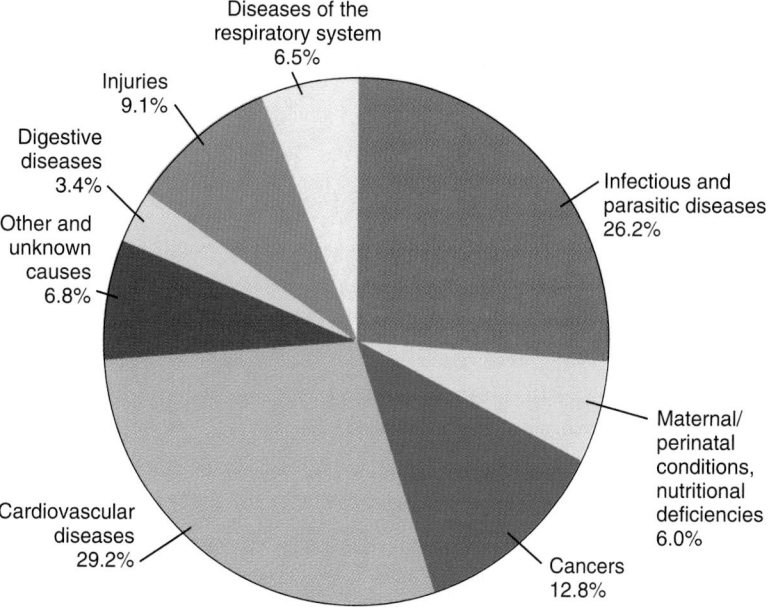

TABLE 13-1   Leading Infectious and Parasitic Causes of Death Worldwide, 2002*

Diseases	No. of Deaths	Percentage of All Deaths
Acute lower respiratory tract infection	3,766,000	6.6
HIV/AIDS	2,821,000	4.9
Diarrheal disease	1,767,000	3.1
Tuberculosis	1,605,000	2.8
Malaria	1,222,000	2.1
Measles	760,000	1.3
Pertussis	301,000	0.5
Tetanus	292,000	0.5
Sexually transmitted infections, excluding HIV	180,000	0.3
Meningitis	173,000	0.3

*Based on 57 million estimated deaths.
AIDS, acquired immunodeficiency syndrome; HIV, human immunodeficiency virus.
From World Health Organization. The World Health Report 2003. Geneva: World Health Organization; 2003.

TABLE 13-2   Examples of Newly Identified Agents/Diseases, 1993–2003

Year	Microbe	Disease
1993	Sin Nombre virus	Hantavirus pulmonary syndrome
1994	Sabia virus	Brazilian hemorrhagic fever
1994	Hendra virus	Encephalitic disease transmitted from horses to humans
1995	Human herpesvirus 8 (HHV-8)	Associated with Kaposi's sarcoma in AIDS patients
1996	New-variant Creutzfeldt-Jakob disease agent	Progressive, degenerative neurologic disease
1997	H5N1 strain of avian influenza	Severe, often fatal influenza transmitted from chickens to humans
1999	Nipah virus	Encephalitic disease transmitted from pigs to humans
2001	Human metapneumovirus	Acute respiratory infections
2003	SARS-associated coronavirus	Severe acute respiratory syndrome (SARS)

microbial threats. Combined, these 13 factors can be broadly categorized into four domains: genetic and biologic factors; physical environmental factors; ecologic factors; and social, political, and economic factors. These domains can work singly or in combination to affect the interaction of humans and microbes and to produce an emerging microbial threat (Fig. 13-2).

Today's highly globalized and interconnected world enhances these factors, allowing infectious pathogens rapid and easy access to new environments and populations and increasing the spread of antimicrobial resistance. Over the past decade, new infectious agents

have surfaced at an alarming rate (Table 13-2). Examples include hantavirus, Hendra and Nipah viruses, the agent responsible for new-variant Creutzfelt-Jakob disease, and the newly recognized coronavirus that causes SARS. In addition, previously recognized diseases such as West Nile virus infection and Rift Valley fever have emerged on new continents, and others such as epidemic cholera and dengue in Central and South America and pertussis in The Netherlands have reemerged with renewed intensity. Moreover, incidents such as the 2001 anthrax attacks in the United States have heightened concerns regarding the intentional use of infectious agents for harm.

This chapter examines the epidemiology of several of the leading infectious causes of global morbidity and mortality (see Table 13-1). The increasing problem of antimicrobial resistance—a major factor contributing to the impact of these diseases—is also discussed. In addition, several infectious diseases that have emerged or reemerged over the past decade are mentioned. Some of these are discussed in further detail elsewhere in this book. All of them are a cause for concern.

ACUTE RESPIRATORY INFECTION

Acute respiratory infection is the leading cause of mortality from infectious diseases in the world. Each year, almost 4 million persons die as a result of acute infection of the respiratory tract.[3] Acute respiratory infection constitutes a broad category of diseases that include infections of both the upper and lower respiratory tract, such as acute pharyngitis, epiglottitis, bronchitis, pneumonia, and influenza. Although upper respiratory tract infection can cause severe illness (e.g., poststreptococcal rheumatic fever and streptococcal toxic shock syndrome), about 98% of all respiratory disease–related deaths result from infection of the lower respiratory tract.[3] Mortality rates are especially high among young children.[8] Significant influenza and pneumonia–associated mortality rates also occur in persons older than 65 years of age and in individuals with chronic underlying pulmonary disease. In the United States, influenza and pneumonia are the leading cause of infectious disease–related mortality and the seventh leading overall cause of death.[9] Pneumonia is also an important nosocomial problem. It is the second most common infectious complication of hospitalization, the most frequent infection in the critical care setting, and the infectious complication that most often produces a fatal outcome.[10-13]

Infants and young children (younger than 5 years of age) throughout the world have been estimated to have from 3 to 11 episodes of acute respiratory infection per year, with the highest incidence occurring during the first year of life.[14-25] Studies examining the frequency of respiratory infection in children suggest that incidence has re-

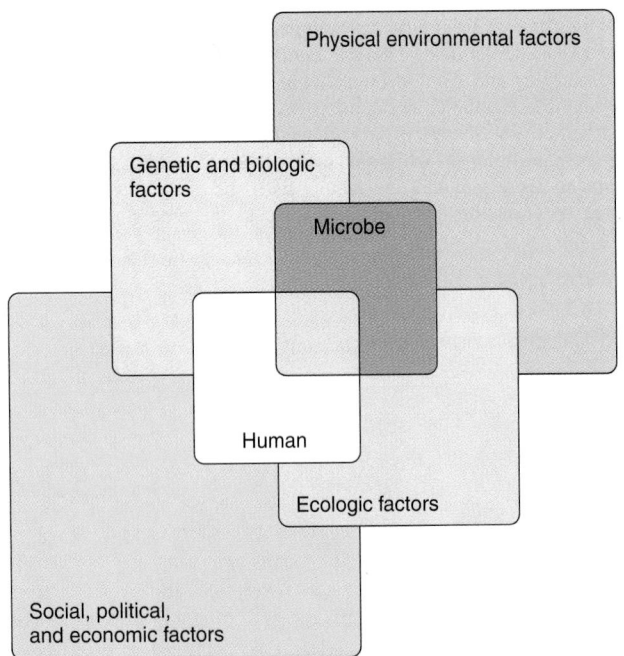

FIGURE 13-2. The Convergence Model. The microbe–host interaction is influenced by the interlocking domains of the determinants of the emergence of infection: genetic and biologic factors; physical environmental factors; ecologic factors; and social, political, and economic factors. (*From Smolinski MS, Hamburg MA, Lederberg J, eds, for the Committee on Emerging Microbial Threats to Health in the 21st Century, Board on Global Health, Institute of Medicine. Microbial Threats to Health: Emergence, Detection, and Response. Washington, DC: National Academy Press; 2003.*)

mained stable over time and is similar among children in developed and developing countries and among those residing in temperate and tropical climates.[14-23] Despite these similarities, children in developing countries are at far greater risk of having a fatal outcome from respiratory infection compared with children in developed countries. Estimates reveal a greater than 30-fold higher risk of a fatal outcome among such children; more than 95% of childhood deaths from respiratory infection occur in less developed parts of the world.[8,14]

Regardless of geographic location, the agents most often responsible for acute respiratory infection are viruses.[8,26] Among these, respiratory syncytial virus, parainfluenza, adenovirus, and influenza have been most frequently linked to childhood respiratory infection.[8,27] These agents most commonly produce self-limited illness but can be an important cause of pneumonia and death.[28-32] Bacterial agents play a major role in the etiology of acute lower respiratory tract infection and are considered the major reason for high mortality rates among children with pneumonia in the developing world. In this setting, lung puncture studies of clinically and radiologically diagnosed childhood pneumonia have consistently demonstrated *Streptococcus pneumoniae*, *Haemophilus influenzae*, and *Staphylococcus aureus* to be the three most commonly isolated bacterial agents.[33] Analysis of nine lung puncture studies of children with pneumonia showed that 63% (range, 21% to 78%) of specimens yielded a bacterial pathogen.[33] The number of children enrolled in these studies ranged from 18 to 233. Among specimens positive for bacterial growth, 38% yielded *S. pneumoniae* (range, 18% to 83%), 37% yielded *H. influenzae* (range, 13% to 85%), and 23% yielded *S. aureus* (range, 0% to 37%). Observed differences between the studies, which were conducted at different times over a 4-decade period, may reflect varying study designs, sampling methods, diagnostic criteria, or culture techniques. The role of other bacterial agents known to be major causes of pneumonia in developed countries (such as *Chlamydophila pneumoniae* and *Mycoplasma pneumoniae*)[34-37] as causes of childhood pneumonia in the developing world has not been well defined.

A number of factors have been proposed to explain (1) the increased likelihood that an episode of acute respiratory infection will be complicated by pneumonia and (2) the high mortality rate from respiratory infection among children in developing countries. Factors associated with the host and with the environment are both considered to be important. Low birth weight resulting from prematurity, intrauterine growth retardation,[38] and malnutrition[39-41] are host risk factors that have been strongly associated with an increased risk of both pneumonia and fatal outcome from respiratory infection; breast-feeding has been shown to be protective.[42] Vitamin A deficiency has been identified as a risk factor for pneumonia in children.[43] However, a placebo-controlled study in Haiti suggested an increased risk of symptoms of respiratory infection after routine vitamin A supplementation.[44] Environmental determinants linked to childhood respiratory infection and pneumonia include household crowding,[18] smoking within the household,[45-47] attendance in child care settings,[45,48] and environmental pollution,[49-52] particularly the use of biomass smoke-producing fuels in the household (although studies of the latter have yielded inconsistent results). It is also possible that such environmental risks simply represent markers for other yet to be identified factors.

It is also important that the serotype distribution among disease-causing *S. pneumoniae* and *H. influenzae* be defined so that the potential usefulness of vaccines as a prevention strategy for childhood pneumonia and development of antimicrobial resistance can be delineated. Between 34% and 94% of *H. influenzae* organisms isolated from cultures taken from children with pneumonia were found to be non–type b, and a significant proportion were nontypable, which suggests a limited potential for *H. influenzae* type b vaccine to prevent childhood pneumonia;[8] additional studies to address this issue are clearly needed.

Polyvalent polysaccharide pneumococcal vaccines are poorly immunogenic in children younger than the age of 2 years—the age group at highest risk for pneumonia-related mortality. However, in early 2000, a heptavalent protein-polysaccharide conjugate vaccine was licensed in the United States for use in young children.[53,54] In clinical trials, this vaccine was demonstrated to have 97.4% efficacy in the prevention of invasive pneumococcal disease caused by vaccine-associated serotypes.[55] It was also shown to reduce the incidence of radiographically confirmed pneumonia in children younger than 2 years of age[56] and to slightly reduce the incidence of acute otitis media.[57,58] Postlicensure studies have demonstrated that this vaccine has had a profound impact on the incidence of pneumococcal disease in children in the United States.[59,60] In one study, the incidence of invasive pneumococcal disease in children younger than 1 year of age fell from between 51.5 and 98.2 cases per 100,000 person-years before licensure to 9.4 cases per 100,000 person-years after introduction of the vaccine.[59] National surveillance data demonstrated a 69% decline in rates of invasive pneumococcal disease in children younger than 2 years of age in 2001 (after licensure) compared with the rates in 1998-1999.[60] Other data suggest that pneumococcal conjugate vaccine is having an indirect beneficial impact on antimicrobial resistance among pneumococci.

The role of the currently licensed conjugate pneumococcal vaccine in developing countries needs to be defined. Pneumococcal serotype distributions are known to vary geographically and temporally,[61] and vaccine immunogenicity may be suboptimal in malnourished children. Because the number of serotypes that can be included in the vaccine is limited, reductions in invasive disease incidence may not be equivalent to those in the United States. In addition, vaccine formulations tailored to maximally cover prevailing serotypes may need to be developed for specific locations. The current cost of the vaccine also makes widespread use in developing countries prohibitive. However, if current barriers can be overcome, this vaccine holds the promise of substantially reducing the high burden of illness from acute respiratory infection in the developing world.[62]

Our understanding of the causes of acute respiratory infection continues to evolve. Several newly identified agents of acute respiratory disease have recently been reported.

Human Metapneumovirus

In 2001, human metapneumovirus (HMPV), a member of the paramyxovirus family, was first reported as the cause of acute respiratory infection in hospitalized children.[63] In the initial case series from The Netherlands, the virus was identified in 28 children with upper and lower respiratory tract illnesses similar to those produced by respiratory syncytial virus. Accompanying serologic studies found that virtually all persons tested had evidence of past exposure to metapneumovirus.[63] Although the epidemiology and clinical spectrum of human metapneumovirus infection remain undefined, a number of subsequent reports have documented that such infection occurs throughout the world as a common, seasonal cause of community-acquired respiratory disease, accounting for up to 10% of acute upper respiratory infection for which another etiologic agent has not been identified.[64-71] HMPV-associated respiratory disease (upper and lower respiratory tract) occurs in both children and adults, can cause severe disease in persons with underlying health conditions, and can precipitate wheezing episodes and exacerbate asthma.

Severe Acute Respiratory Syndrome (SARS)

Early in the year 2003, an explosive outbreak of adult respiratory distress syndrome was first reported in residents and persons who had recently visited Hong Kong.[72,73] A similar illness was reported in the adjacent southern Chinese province of Guangdong, with the first cases recognized in November of 2002.[74] This disease appeared readily transmitted to health care workers and household members in close contact with ill patients. Initial hypotheses for the cause of the illness, which was designated severe acute respiratory syndrome (SARS) by the World Health Organization (WHO), focused on agents such as avian influenza virus, HMPV, and *C. pneumoniae*. However, subsequent testing among a network of collaborating laboratories in affected locations identified a previously unrecognized coronavirus as the causative agent.[75-78]

With the use of a case definition that included (1) the presence of respiratory symptoms, (2) radiographic evidence of infiltrates or of acute respiratory distress syndrome, and (3) presence in or travel to an affected area (or contact with an individual who had been in an affected area), a total of 8096 probable cases of SARS were reported to WHO from nearly 30 countries as occurring between November of 2002 and July of 2003 (when person-to-person transmission was declared to have been interrupted) (Table 13-3).[79] Locations with sustained local transmission accounted for 98% of all cases and included mainland China (5327 probable cases—66%), Hong Kong (1755—22%), Taiwan (346—4%), Canada (251—3%), and Singapore (238—3%). For all locations, the case-fatality rate for probable cases was 10%. In the five most greatly affected locations, mortality ranged from 7% to 17% of probable cases, with the lowest proportion in mainland China and the highest in Canada and Hong Kong.[79] Poor outcomes appeared to be age related, with estimated mortality rates from SARS approaching 50% in persons older than 60 years of age.[80] Mortality was also more common in persons with preexistent conditions such as diabetes mellitus and cardiac disease.[81,82]

The 2002-2003 SARS epidemic was unusual in several respects. First, few cases of illness were recognized or reported in children.[83-85] Second, a high proportion of cases occurred in health care workers.[86,87] In the five most affected locations, 20% of all cases were observed in health care workers (range, 19% [China] to 43% [Canada]).[79] Third, the transmission dynamics were highly variable. Most individuals appeared not to transmit the disease to other persons.[88,89] However, in certain situations, referred to as "super-spreading" events, infected individuals were linked to a large number of subsequent cases (Fig. 13-3).[72,90-92] The basis for the super-spreading phenomenon is unknown. Possible hypotheses include host or environmental factors, virus burden, coinfection, and medical interventions that may have widely aerosolized the virus.

SARS transmission was documented in a number of settings. These included inpatient and outpatient health care settings, hotels, an apartment complex, conveyances (airplanes, trains, taxicabs), religious gatherings, and the community.[73,80,82,92-97] In most of these settings, close, direct contact appeared to be the most important factor associated with disease transmission, suggesting that droplet or fomite transmission was the predominant mode of spread.[98] The role of alternative modes of transmission, particularly aerosols and environmental contamination, is less clear but best fits disease patterns in certain settings.[99,100] No evidence supports foodborne or blood-borne transmission of SARS coronavirus.

Genetic analysis of the SARS coronavirus determined that it was unlike other known members of the coronavirus family, including those previously associated with upper respiratory infection in humans.[101-104] Retrospective analyses of banked respiratory and serologic specimens detected no evidence of human disease before the late 2002 outbreak was recognized in China. Surveys in South China detected potential zoonotic reservoirs for the virus in exotic live animals sold in markets for human consumption, as well as serologic evidence of human infection in persons who worked in these markets.[104,105] The implications of these findings for control of SARS are uncertain.

Although longer incubation periods may have occasionally occurred, the generally accepted upper limit for the incubation period for SARS is 10 days.[73,80] Infected persons experience a nonspecific febrile prodromal illness followed by abrupt or gradual respiratory compromise, often requiring mechanical ventilation and characterized by various clinical, laboratory, and radiographic features (Table 13-4).[106] A variety of antiviral, immunomodulatory, and immunosuppressive agents were used alone and in combination to treat SARS-affected persons, with systemic steroids showing the most consistent beneficial results.[107-112] However, persons treated with high-dose steroids often experienced significant secondary complications and superinfections,[113] and cases of aseptic necrosis of the femoral head have been reported in the lay media. If disease recurs, controlled clinical trials of interventions will be needed to determine optimal therapies. Among survivors, prolonged (weeks to months) shedding of SARS coronavirus nucleic acid in the respiratory, urinary, and gastrointestinal tracts has been documented, even after recovery.[114] The long-term sequelae of SARS infection among survivors are unknown.

A variety of measures were instituted to control the unprecedented rapid global spread of SARS. These included isolation and other infection-control measures in the health care setting; institutional, household, and community quarantine and isolation; temperature screening and thermal scanning; environmental decontamination; and the use of personal protective measures such as masks and hand washing.[115] Most of these interventions did not undergo rigorous efficacy or cost-effectiveness evaluations. However, in one retrospective hospital-based study, the use of personal protective measures such as hand washing, gloves, masks, and respirators was found to significantly reduce the risk of infection.[98] Another study showed that the most important factor associated with SARS control was rapid identification and isolation of persons suspected of having the disease.[80]

DIARRHEAL DISEASE

Diarrheal disease remains a leading global cause of infectious disease morbidity and death, resulting in approximately 2.5 million deaths per year.[116] Although diarrheal disease affects persons in all geographic lo-

TABLE 13-3 Summary of Probable Cases of Severe Acute Respiratory Syndrome (SARS) with Onset of Illness from November 1, 2002, to July 31, 2003

Area of Report	No. of Cases	Percentage of Cases in Health Care Workers	Deaths (CFR)
China	5327	19%	349 (7)
Hong Kong	1755	22%	299 (17)
Taiwan	346	20%	37 (11)
Canada	251	43%	43 (17)
Singapore	238	41%	33 (14)
Other	182	25%	13 (7)
Total	**8096**	**21%**	**774 (10)**

CFR, case-fatality ratio.
Source: World Health Organization. Data through September 26, 2003.

TABLE 13-4 Common Clinical Features of Severe Acute Respiratory Syndrome (SARS)

Clinical Feature	Common Findings with SARS-Associated Coronavirus Infection
Initial symptoms	Nonrespiratory prodrome lasting 2 to 7 days characterized by one or more of the following:
	Fever
	Rigors
	Headache
	Malaise
	Myalgia
	Diarrhea
	Respiratory phase beginning 2 to 7 days after onset, characterized by:
	Nonproductive cough
	Dyspnea
	Absence of upper respiratory symptoms
Laboratory findings	Normal or low total leukocyte cell count
	Lymphopenia
	Mildly depressed platelet count
	Elevated lactate dehydrogenase levels
	Elevated creatine phosphokinase levels
	Elevated transaminase levels
	Prolonged activated partial thromboplastin time
Radiographic findings	Abnormal chest radiograph results in almost all patients by the second week of illness

From Jernigan JA, Low DE, Helfand RF. Combining clinical and epidemiologic features for early recognition of SARS. Emerg Infect Dis. 2004;10:327-333.

cations and age groups, the greatest burden of severe illness and death falls disproportionately on infants and young children in developing nations. Estimates suggest that more than 80% of all diarrheal disease deaths occur in children younger than 5 years of age in developing countries, accounting for 21% of all deaths in these areas.[3,116] Diarrheal disease also produces substantial morbidity, with 4 billion acute episodes estimated to occur on an annual basis, affecting growth and cognitive development[117] and resulting in persistent illness (of longer than 2 weeks) in 10% of cases.[118] Studies among children in developing countries have found a range of one to ten episodes of diarrhea per year; most have reported three to five episodes per year.[118-124] A survey among the general population in the United States reported a rate of 1.4 episodes of diarrhea per year, translating to 200 million to 375 million episodes annually.[125]

The pathogens that produce diarrhea are transmitted in three main ways. These are foodborne transmission, waterborne transmission, and person-to-person transmission. Although systematic studies are difficult to perform, it is likely that the relative importance of these transmission patterns varies in different settings. Estimates in the United States suggest that 76 million episodes of foodborne illness occur per annum, resulting in 325,000 hospitalizations and 5000 fatalities.[126]

The pathogens that cause diarrheal illness also differ in their modes of transmission. For example, nontyphoidal *Salmonella* species are transmitted principally through food, *Shigella* species are transmitted mainly from person to person, and *Cryptosporidium parvum* is principally waterborne. Determination of the patterns of pathogen distribution provides a sound surrogate marker for the relative importance of different modes of transmission in a given location.

The causes of diarrheal disease do not remain static over time, even in a single location. Fluctuations may result from the introduction of

an organism not previously present, the recognition of a new agent, changing levels of sanitation from man-made or natural disasters, or climatic variations. The introduction of classic cholera into Latin America is one example. This illness had not been recognized in South America during the 20th century, but in January of 1991, cases were identified in coastal Peru.[127] Within weeks, thousands of cases were occurring, and cholera quickly became the most commonly diagnosed cause of diarrheal illness in many parts of Peru.[128-130] Over the next 3 years, the disease spread throughout mainland South and Central America, significantly altering the distribution of etiologic agents of diarrheal disease.[129] *Vibrio cholerae* O139 is an example of a newly recognized pathogen that had a significant impact on the distribution of agents that produce diarrheal disease. This organism was first detected in South Asia in 1992, and it quickly spread to many regions of India and Bangladesh.[131-135] Studies conducted in Bangladesh suggested that shortly after its introduction, *Vibrio cholerae* O139 became the agent most commonly linked to cholera in that country. Since then, its impact has fluctuated in place and time throughout areas of South Asia.[134,136]

The international movement of foods can also alter the spectrum of diarrheal pathogens.[137] In 1996, thousands of cases of cyclosporiasis due to the parasitic agent *Cyclospora cayetanensis* occurred in the United States and Canada among persons who consumed fresh raspberries imported from Guatemala.[138] Before this episode, only small numbers of persons with cyclosporiasis had been recognized in North America, and these cases were mainly associated with travel to developing countries.[139] *Escherichia coli* O157-H7 significantly affected pathogen distribution patterns in the developed parts of the world after the agent was first recognized.[140] After its recognition in the United States in 1982, this foodborne agent rapidly became the most common

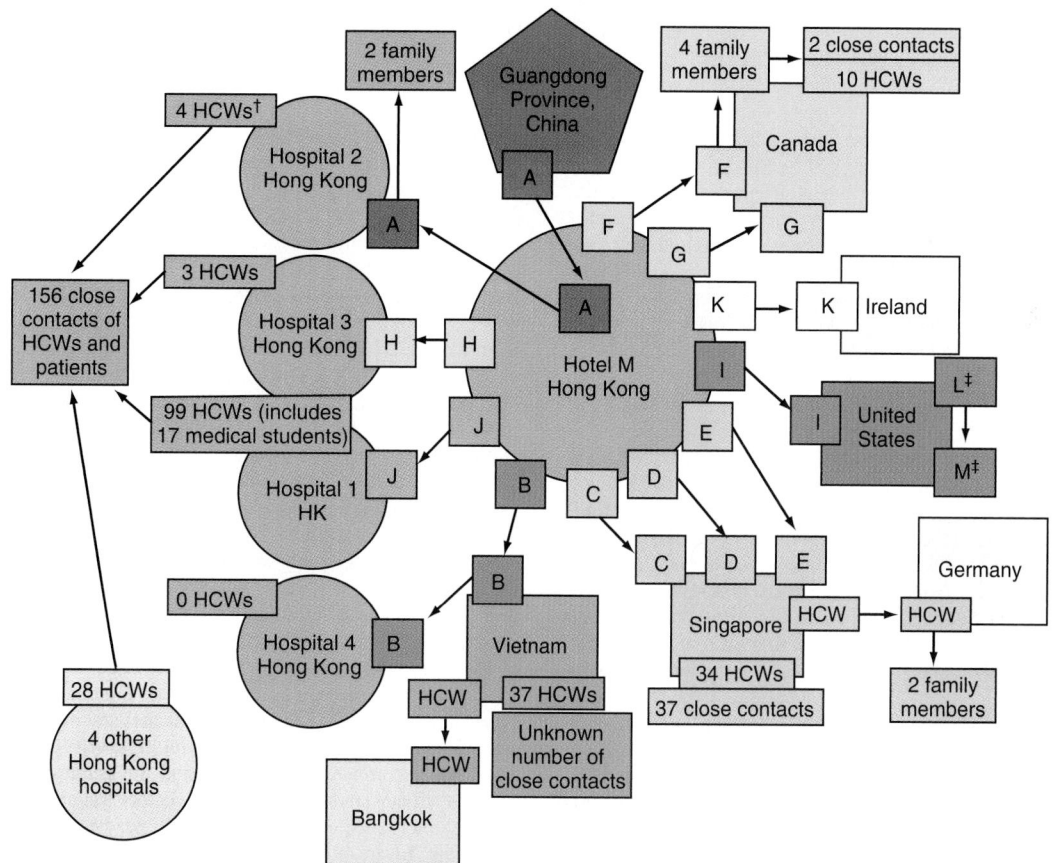

FIGURE 13-3. **Chain of Transmission Among Guests at Hotel M—Hong Kong, 2003.**[*]
[*]Data as of March 28, 2003.
[†]Health care workers.
[‡]Guests L and M (spouses) were not at Hotel M during the same time as index Guest A but were at the hotel during the same times as Guests G, H, and I, who were ill during this period.

cause of bloody diarrhea in many locations in North America.[141] Recent surveys have found that it is the fourth most commonly isolated bacterial agent of diarrheal disease in the United States.[141] In 1996, it produced massive outbreaks of diarrheal disease and the hemolytic-uremic syndrome in Japan,[142] and more recently, it has produced major waterborne outbreaks in North America.[143,144] Shigellosis is an example of a disease with rapid emergence in areas with disrupted sanitation. Along with cholera, it has been a common problem in areas with social disruption as a result of war, especially when large numbers of refugees have lacked access to water and sanitation services.[145-147]

Viruses are an increasingly recognized cause of sporadic and outbreak-associated diarrheal diseases.[148] Noroviruses (previously called Norwalk-like viruses) are transmitted not only from person to person but also by food and water. They have become an increasing source of diarrheal illness outbreaks among cruise ship passengers and in military settings.[149-151]

Because the pathogens responsible for diarrheal disease vary over time, even in the same location, longitudinal studies are important for defining the etiology of diarrheal disease. Data from studies of the causes of acute diarrheal illness in young children in developing countries suggest that the most common etiologic agents are rotavirus, enterotoxigenic E. coli, and Shigella species.[118] Their relative importance is difficult to determine because findings have varied depending on the population studied, the types of specimens collected, the pathogens sought, and the detection methods used. Rotavirus infections affect all age groups, but most severe illness and hospitalization occurs in children younger than age 2 years, who often develop dehydrating diarrhea from the infection.[152-154] Because infants are vulnerable to the complications of diarrhea, particularly dehydration, rotavirus has been estimated to cause up to 30% of acute diarrheal deaths.[153] In two recent studies in the developing world, this agent was found in less than 20% of acute diarrheal episodes among children younger than 5 years of age.[155,156] In these same studies, pathogenic forms of E. coli were found in less than 15% of episodes, and Shigella species accounted for between 6% and 13% of episodes. Because bacterial dysentery produced by Shigella species is severe and can be accompanied by the complication of hemolytic-uremic syndrome in children infected with Shigella dysenteriae type 1, the impact of shigellosis as a cause of diarrheal morbidity and mortality among persons in developing countries is substantial.[157,158] Other agents that are increasingly appreciated as important causes of diarrheal disease among children in developing countries include Campylobacter jejuni/coli and C. parvum, although these agents have not been as well studied.[159-163]

Rotavirus is also an important cause of childhood diarrhea and hospitalization in developed countries, with four out of five children in the United States experiencing this infection by age 5 years and with an estimated 55,000 annual hospitalizations.[153] In the early 1990s, it was estimated that 5.2 per 1000 children younger than 5 years of age in England and Wales were hospitalized with rotavirus-associated illness during a 1-year period.[164] Among both children and adults in developed countries, viral agents, particularly small, round viruses (including noroviruses), are among the most common causes of diarrhea.[165,166] Systematic studies in the United States indicate that among the bacterial diarrheal pathogens, C. jejuni/coli is the most common agent, followed by nontyphoidal Salmonella species, shigellosis, and E. coli O157-H7.[141] Although this distribution is similar in other developed countries, serotypes other than O157-H7 can be the predominant form of Shiga toxin–producing E. coli in other locations.[167,168] These findings suggest that foodborne sources are an important cause of diarrheal disease in the developed world in that all but Shigella species are transmitted principally through foods. Notifiable disease data demonstrate trends in the occurrence of these pathogens but severely underestimate their incidence. As an example, 45,970 cases of salmonellosis were reported in the United States in 1995, but calculations suggest that almost 2 million cases of this infection occur each year.[169,170] The role of waterborne parasites, particularly C. parvum, is underrecognized in developed countries.[171]

The global patterns of diarrheal disease are likely to continue to evolve. Efforts continue toward the development of vaccines against

agents of diarrheal disease, especially rotavirus and enterotoxigenic E. coli.[172] New formulations of rotavirus vaccine have been developed after a tetravalent rhesus–human reassortant rotavirus vaccine was linked to intussusception in infants and was withdrawn from the market.[173-175] These vaccines have the potential to decrease the burden of diarrheal disease among persons in the developing world. In addition, food production practices are changing, with greater volumes of fresh fruits and vegetables grown in the developing world for export to developed countries.[137] This practice has resulted in the transfer of agents like C. cayetanensis and V. cholerae in exported products—a situation that is likely to continue.[138,176] Changes in food distribution practices increase the potential for widespread, multinational disease outbreaks.[177] Climate change, which has been reported to affect the spread of cholera; the increasing populations of immunocompromised individuals who have a different spectrum of pathogens responsible for diarrheal illness; and increasing global travel can all influence future trends in diarrheal disease in ways that may be difficult to predict.

VECTOR-BORNE AND ZOONOTIC DISEASES

Most of the emerging infections recognized during the past decade have been zoonoses (see Table 13-2), with the proportion of all emerging infections that are zoonotic estimated at approximately 75%.[178] Diseases transmitted by vectors have posed particular challenges, both in tropical areas, where many previously controlled diseases have resurged, and throughout the world, as diseases such as Japanese encephalitis, West Nile meningoencephalitis, and Rift Valley fever have emerged in new areas. Changes in ecologic and environmental conditions, along with international travel and commerce, play key roles in the persistence, resurgence, and emergence of these diseases.[7]

Dengue

Dengue is the most important mosquito-borne viral disease that affects humans. Its global distribution is comparable to that of malaria, and an estimated 2.5 billion people live in areas at risk for epidemic transmission.[179] The disease is endemic in Africa, the Americas, and parts of the Middle East, Asia, and the Western Pacific. The frequency of dengue and its more severe complications—dengue hemorrhagic fever (DHF) and dengue shock syndrome—has been increasing dramatically since 1980; an estimated 50 million infections occur annually.[179] Dengue is a mosquito-borne viral disease caused by any of four antigenically distinct virus serotypes (DEN-1, -2, -3, -4) of the genus Flavivirus. Infection with one of these serotypes is not cross-protective. Infection with dengue viruses produces a spectrum of clinical illness that ranges from a nonspecific viral syndrome to severe and fatal hemorrhagic disease.[180-182] DHF is a life-threatening condition characterized by capillary permeability that may lead to hypovolemic shock and death. Important risk factors for DHF include the strain and serotype of the infecting virus, as well as the age, immune status, and genetic predisposition of the patient. In endemic areas, most deaths from dengue infection occur in children younger than 15 years of age.[180]

Dengue is transmitted by Aedes aegypti, a domestic, day-biting mosquito. This mosquito was historically found in Africa but spread throughout the tropical regions of the world during the past 2 centuries through international commerce. A. aegypti is well adapted to the urban environment, feeding on humans and breeding in containers found in areas where water is stored or allowed to accumulate, such as discarded cans, bottles, plastic containers, and tires. A global pandemic of dengue began in Southeast Asia after World War II and has intensified over the past 15 years. Epidemics caused by multiple serotypes (hyperendemicity) have become more frequent, and the geographic distribution of both the viruses and their mosquito vectors has expanded.

The emergence of dengue and DHF has been most dramatic in the Americas. In an effort to prevent urban yellow fever, which is also transmitted by A. aegypti, the Pan American Health Organization established a program in the 1950s and 1960s to eradicate the species from most of Central and South America.[179,183] As a result, epidemic dengue occurred only sporadically in some Caribbean islands during this period. The success of the program, however, led to its gradual discontinuation beginning in 1970. Since that time, *A. aegypti* has reestablished itself firmly in the region, now exceeding the extent of distribution that was seen before the eradication program began (Fig. 13-4). Epidemics of dengue fever are now routinely seen in Venezuela, Colombia, Brazil, and other locations in Latin America and the Caribbean.[184,185]

No therapy is effective for dengue infection, and treatment is symptomatic.[179] Recently, attenuated candidate vaccines have been developed, and research is under way to develop second-generation recombinant vaccine viruses. However, it is unlikely that an effective dengue vaccine will be available for public use in the near future.

Efforts to reverse the recent trend of increased epidemic activity and geographic expansion of dengue are not promising. New dengue virus strains and serotypes will likely continue to be introduced into many areas with high population levels of *A. aegypti*. In the absence of new mosquito control technology, public health authorities have emphasized disease prevention and insect control through community efforts to reduce larval breeding sources. Improved laboratory-based surveillance systems that can provide early warning of a potential dengue epidemic are also needed to alert the public to take protective action and physicians to diagnose and properly treat cases.

West Nile Virus

West Nile virus (WNV) provides a clear example of the ability of vector-borne diseases to emerge and spread rapidly in new areas. The virus was first isolated in 1937 from an apparently well individual from the West Nile district of Uganda.[186] For decades, WNV has been recognized as an important endemic and occasionally epidemic disease in Africa and the Middle East, causing primarily minor febrile illness.[187,188] Recently, major outbreaks associated with severe neurologic disease have been reported in Romania,[188,189] Russia,[190] Israel,[191,192] the United States,[193] and Canada.[194] The disease was first reported in North America in 1999 when the virus caused an outbreak of severe neuroinvasive disease that resulted in seven deaths in New York City.[195] Despite its extensive spread in nature, the virus showed limited spread to humans in the United States until 2002, when more than 4100 cases, including nearly 3000 (75%) cases of severe neuroinvasive disease and 284 deaths, were reported (Fig. 13-5).[196] In addi-

tion to an unusual proportion of severe cases, the 2002 U.S. epidemic revealed several new clinical syndromes and five new modes of transmission, including transmission to recipients of transplanted organs and transfused blood.[196-198] The virus has spread to both Canada and Mexico, and evidence of transmission has been documented in the Caribbean and Central America.[199] In the 2003 U.S. outbreak, more than 9800 cases and more than 260 deaths were reported; compared with 2002 events, a lower proportion of patients (30%) were reported with severe neuroinvasive disease likely reflecting improved diagnosis of these conditions in persons with WNV fever because of the availability of new diagnostic tests.

WNV is a single-stranded RNA virus of the family Flaviviridae (genus *Flavivirus*), which is part of the Japanese encephalitis virus antigenic complex. In addition to Japanese encephalitis, this complex includes St. Louis encephalitis virus, Murray Valley encephalitis virus, and Kunjin virus, a subtype of WNV.[187] The virus is maintained in a bird-mosquito-bird cycle, with birds developing high levels of viremia and serving as amplifying hosts. Mosquitoes primarily of the genus *Culex* transmit WNV, although the virus has been isolated from many genera and species of mosquitoes. Although most species of birds generally remain asymptomatic, WNV-related mortality has been noted in more than 160 avian species in the United States and Canada.[200] Crows and related birds of the family Corvidae are especially susceptible to mortality from WNV infection, and die-offs of these birds have been used as one indicator of active WNV transmission.[200]

Most WNV infections in humans are asymptomatic; however, severe and sometimes fatal complications occur, especially among older individuals. The incubation period is normally 2 to 14 days,[186,187,196] although incubation periods of up to 21 days have been documented in patients infected through organ transplantation.[198] West Nile virus usually produces a mild illness that lasts from 3 to 6 days. In addition to fever, symptoms include malaise, headache, myalgia, eye pain, and in some pharyngitis, nausea, vomiting, diarrhea, abdominal pain, and rash.[186,187,196,201,202] Less than 1% of persons with WNV infection develop severe illness characterized by acute neurologic manifestations, usually encephalitis or meningoencephalitis, occasionally with fatal outcome.[189,196] More than 90% of persons with severe disease have fever, often accompanied by severe weakness, gastrointestinal tract symptoms, and headache.[192,195] Movement disorders and a polio-like

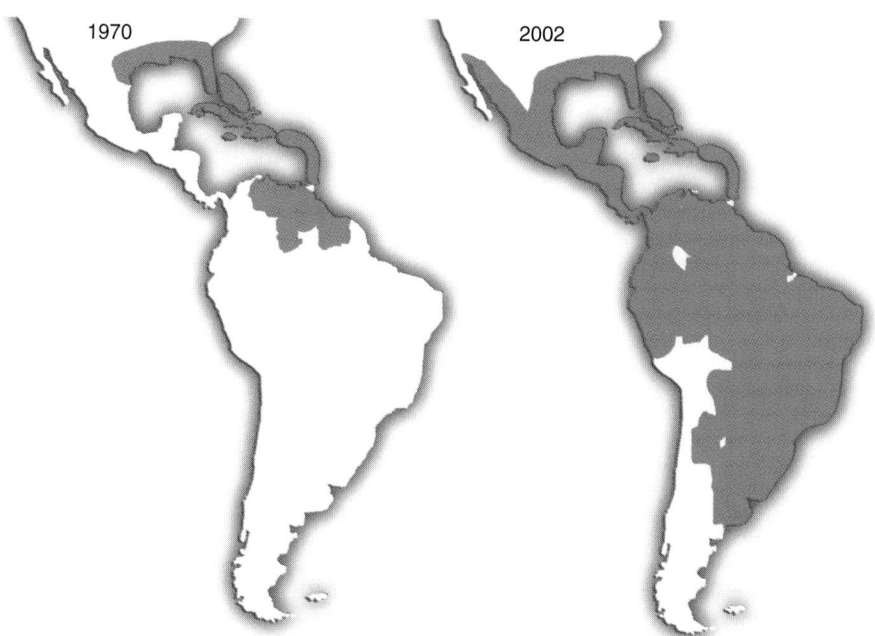

1970   2002

FIGURE 13-4. Distribution of *Aedes aegypti* in the Americas in 1970 (at the end of the mosquito eradication program) and in 2002. (*Source: CDC and PAHO.*)

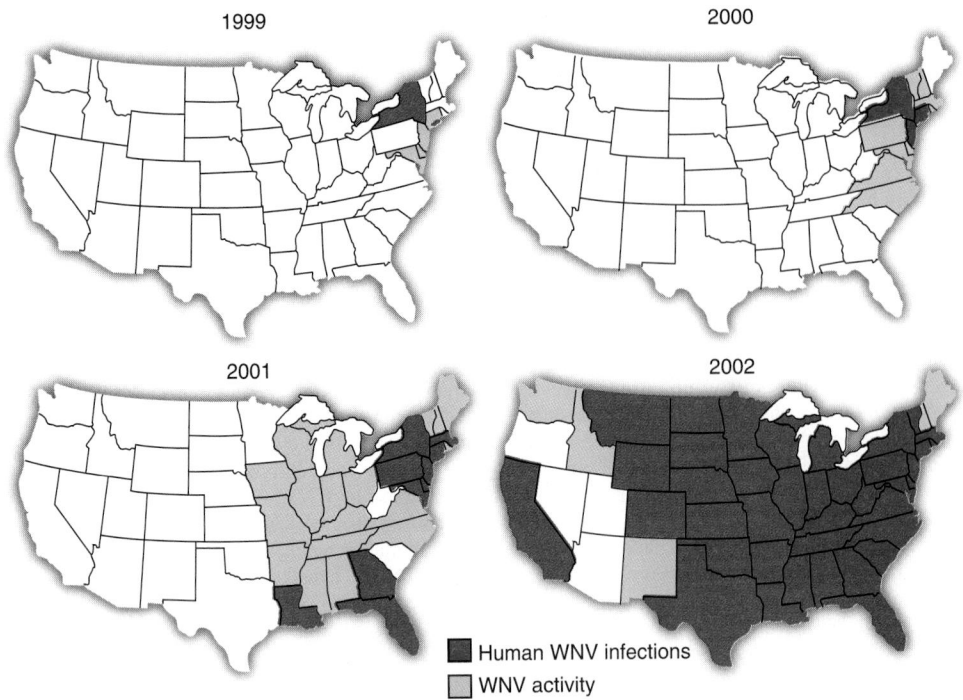

FIGURE 13-5. West Nile Virus Activity, United States, 1999-2002.

acute flaccid paralysis have also been reported.[203] Those suffering polio-like paralysis have a poor long-term outcome.[203]

West Nile virus has clearly established itself in North America, and every indication is that it will continue to expand its range southward to include much of Central and South America. Prevention of WNV infection currently relies on mosquito control, the use of personal protective measures, and screening of the blood supply. Candidate vaccines for human use are in development; however, it may be several years before a safe and effective vaccine is available for those at risk.[204]

Hendra and Nipah Viruses

Hendra and Nipah are two closely related novel viruses discovered during the past decade. Both are members of the virus family Paramyxoviridae; together, they make up a newly proposed genus, *Henipavirus*. Hendra virus was first recognized in a suburb of Brisbane, Australia, in 1994 during an outbreak of acute respiratory disease that occurred among horses and their trainer; a total of 13 horses and the trainer died during the outbreak.[205] Additional isolated cases or small clusters of fatal equine and human infections of the Hendra virus have subsequently been identified elsewhere in northern Australia. Investigations into the origin of Hendra found anti-Hendra antibodies in serum collected from various species of fruit bats (flying foxes); further studies were able to successfully isolate Hendra virus from individual fruit bats, although infected individuals do not appear to suffer clinical illness from the infection.[206,207] No evidence suggests person-to-person spread of the Hendra virus; however, horses appear to shed infectious virus in nasal secretions and urine, which may lead to transmission between animals.

Shortly after recognition of the Hendra virus, an outbreak of acute illness in pigs and humans was discovered in peninsular Malaysia and Singapore. A novel virus, named Nipah virus (after the site where it was first isolated), was found to be the cause of the outbreak. Between September of 1998 and April of 1999, the outbreak devastated pig farms in central and southern Malaysia, subsequently spreading into Singapore with the importation of sick animals. The disease in pigs was characterized by acute onset of a febrile illness with respiratory symptoms. Although the mortality rate among pigs was only about 5% to 15%, the disease was highly contagious and

rapidly spread among pigs and to humans associated with pig rearing and processing. Illness in humans was more severe and was characterized by fever, headache, myalgia, and rapidly progressing neurologic involvement, often leading to coma and death. Of 265 persons infected, 105 (40%) died during their illness; among those recovering, a few have subsequently suffered relapses, some fatal.[208] The outbreak was finally controlled when all transport of pigs was halted and about 1.1 million pigs were destroyed, causing enormous economic hardship for this sector of the economy.[208]

Nipah virus was isolated and characterized during the outbreak and was shown to be similar to, although clearly distinct from, Hendra virus. Based on these similarities, the search for reservoir hosts of Nipah focused on fruit bats; as with Hendra virus, anti-Nipah antibodies have now been detected in several species of bats, primarily fruit-eating flying foxes, and in some insectivorous bats.[209]

Recognition of these viruses has been limited to outbreaks that occurred in northern Australia, the Malay Peninsula, and, more recently, Bangladesh; however, the range of pteropid fruit bats is much wider, and it is clearly possible that other locations are at risk for infection by these viruses or others yet to be discovered. Indeed, serologic surveys of bats captured in Cambodia found evidence of antibodies reactive with Nipah virus.[210]

Monkeypox

Several other zoonotic diseases have recently emerged in new areas. In 2003, monkeypox, a rare viral disease that occurs mainly in the rainforest countries of central and West Africa, was reported among prairie dogs and humans in the United States.[211,212] Traceback investigations implicated a shipment of animals from Ghana as the probable source of introduction of monkeypox virus into the United States. The shipment contained approximately 800 small mammals of nine different species, including six genera of African rodents. These rodents included rope squirrels (*Funisciurus* sp.), tree squirrels (*Heliosciurus* sp.), Gambian giant rats (*Cricetomys* sp.), brush-tailed porcupines (*Atherurus* sp.), dormice (*Graphiurus* sp.), and striped mice (*Hybomys* sp.). Laboratory testing of available animals from this shipment found evidence of monkeypox virus in several species, including one Gambian giant rat, three dormice, and two rope squirrels. Prairie dogs became infected by con-

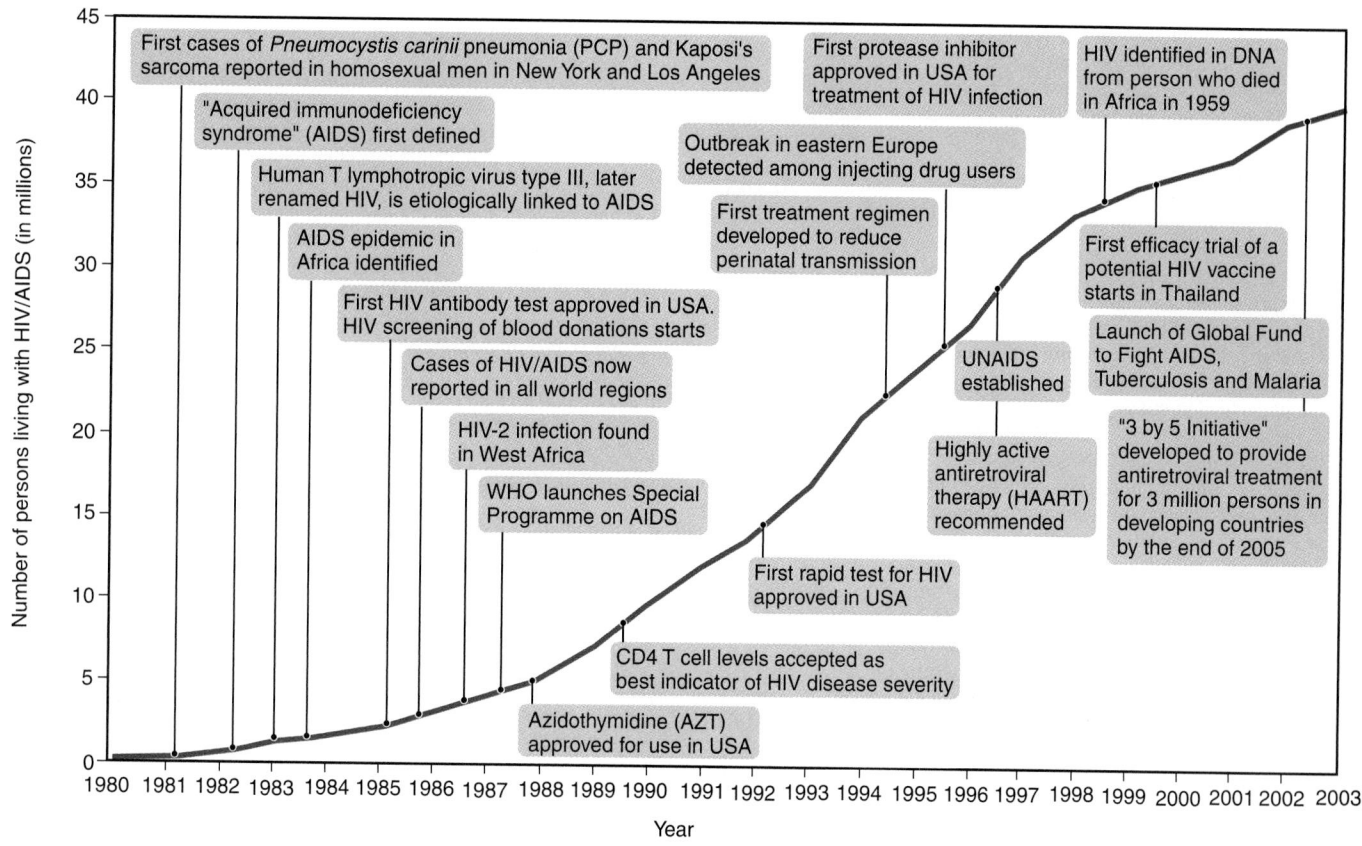

FIGURE 13-6. The HIV/AIDS Epidemic. *(Source: Adapted from WHO/UNAIDS.)*

tact with Gambian rats from this shipment as part of transport and holding of exotic animals for sale as pets. Human infection occurred from contact with infected prairie dogs. In total, 72 cases, of which 37 were laboratory confirmed, were reported from 6 Midwestern states.

Human monkeypox was first identified in 1970 in a region of the Democratic Republic of Congo, from which smallpox had been eradicated 2 years earlier.[213] Monkeypox is caused by an orthopoxvirus and has clinical similarities to smallpox virus but with distinct epidemiologic and biologic differences.[214-217] The incubation period, which usually lasts 7 to 17 days, is followed by the onset of a prodrome of fever, headache, backache, and fatigue. Similar to smallpox, a rash develops that involves macules, papules, vesicles, pustules, and crusts that evolve over 14 to 21 days.[218] Most patients with monkeypox develop pronounced lymphadenopathy—a major clinical difference from smallpox.[218] Low rates of person-to-person transmission of monkeypox have been reported, with case-fatality rates ranging from 1% to 10% in Africa and with higher death rates among young children.[214,218]

The 2003 U.S. outbreak illustrates the serious public health threat that can result from the introduction of nonindigenous pathogens from exotic species of animals. Infections transmitted directly or secondarily to humans by rodents have all occurred in recent years. Compounding the severity of this situation is the potential for many of these infections to be used as biologic weapons. To address these threats—both naturally occurring and intentional—efforts are needed to reexamine and strengthen public health laws that address the importation of exotic animals in the context of control of infectious disease. Toward this end, the U.S. Centers for Disease Control and Prevention (CDC) and the U.S. Food and Drug Administration (FDA) issued a joint order in 2003 that prohibited the importation of any African rodent, along with the sale and transport within the United States and the release into the wild of prairie dogs and certain African rodents. An interim final rule has been issued and is available for public comment.[219]

HUMAN IMMUNODEFICIENCY VIRUS, TUBERCULOSIS, AND MALARIA

Each year, more than half of the deaths associated with infectious disease continue to be attributed to three illnesses—HIV/AIDS, tuberculosis, and malaria. These diseases, especially tuberculosis and HIV/AIDS, involve interconnected epidemics, profoundly affecting health and serving as major obstacles to economic growth and development in many of the poorest countries in the world. Although fueled within impoverished areas, these diseases also continue to affect developed countries, in part owing to immigration and international travel but also resulting from domestic factors such as homelessness and drug abuse.

Human Immunodeficiency Virus

Recognition of the first cases of AIDS in 1981 among previously healthy homosexual men in the United States was the first indication of a new pathogen that would become the most destructive infectious agent of the 20th century. Despite increasing information on the virus and the disease, as well as tremendous strides in prevention and treatment (Fig. 13-6), the numbers are staggering. Current estimates include approximately 28 million deaths from HIV/AIDS, approximately 40 million persons living with the disease, and more than 14 million children orphaned by the disease.[3] In 2003 alone, it is estimated that approximately 3 million people died from AIDS and 5 million people, including 700,000 children, became newly infected.[220] Compounding the problem is the fact that most HIV-infected individuals do not know they are infected. Worldwide, HIV/AIDS is the leading cause of death and morbidity among adults 15 to 59 years of age.[5]

Recent studies on the origin of AIDS suggest that humans first became infected with HIV in the early to mid 20th century by nonhuman primates infected with simian immunodeficiency virus (SIV).[221,222]

This hypothesis is based on several findings such as similarities in the genetic organization of the viruses and in the geographic location of both the natural host and the earliest reported cases of human infection. HIV infections have been classified as types 1 and 2 (HIV-1 and HIV-2), with HIV-1 primarily responsible for the global pandemic. HIV-1 is most closely related to SIVcpz, a virus isolated from the chimpanzee *Pan troglodytes troglodytes*.[221,222] Based on genetic diversity, HIV-1 is divided into three groups—the main group (group M), found throughout the world; the outlier group (group O), found primarily in western equatorial Africa; and the non-M, non-O group (group N), found among some individuals from Cameroon.[223,224] HIV-1 group M viruses have been further divided into at least nine different subtypes and multiple recombinant forms, with subtypes A, B, and C accounting for nearly 90% of the world's infections.[223,225] These findings have particular relevance for efforts to develop an effective vaccine against a highly adaptable virus.

Although the HIV/AIDS epidemic has had tremendous medical, social, and economic impact on virtually all areas of the world, countries in Africa, especially sub-Saharan Africa, continue to be the most severely affected. In 2003, more than 26 million people in this region were living with HIV and 3.2 million became infected, primarily through sexual contact.[220] More than two thirds of all AIDS deaths have occurred in this region.[220] In some sub-Saharan countries, the epidemic has reduced life expectancy by almost half.[5]

Although the epidemic continues to be most profound in Africa, increasing rates of HIV transmission are reported in other parts of the world—primarily Eastern Europe and Asia. With 7.2 million infections already reported, China and India are feared to be in the beginning of explosive outbreaks.[220] In some parts of China, HIV infection rates of 35% to 80% have been found among injecting drug users.[220] In Eastern Europe and central Asia, an estimated 180,000 to 280,000 new infections occurred in 2003, bringing the total number of HIV-infected persons in this region to approximately 1.5 million.[220] Many infections in these regions have been attributed to injecting drug use, but heterosexual contact has now become the primary mode of transmission in these countries. The epidemic appears to have leveled off or decreased in many areas initially affected by the disease such as the United States and Western Europe; however, increasing rates have been observed in some populations, including men who have sex with men and racial and ethnic minority groups in the United States.[226-228]

Despite a death rate of almost 100% for untreated persons, tremendous progress has been made in the clinical treatment of infected persons. The use of combination antiretroviral therapy offers many infected individuals the potential for management of the disease as a chronic condition. However, access to such treatment is limited and is restricted primarily to persons in high-income countries, leaving behind the most vulnerable populations (Table 13-5). As an example, it is estimated that approximately 4.1 million persons in sub-Saharan Africa are in need of such therapy, but less than 2% have access to the drugs.[5]

Containing this pandemic will require new strategies in prevention and treatment, as well as a commitment to confronting many of the issues that contribute greatly to its spread, such as poverty, social inequality, and stigmatization. Toward this end, the WHO and the Joint United Nations Programme on HIV/AIDS (UNAIDS) have developed a detailed plan to provide antiretroviral treatment to 3 million HIV-infected persons in developing countries by the end of 2005.[229] The strategy, called "The 3 by 5 Initiative," is a collaborative effort among many countries, organizations, and individuals designed to treat existing and prevent new infections among persons living in the poorest countries affected. To lessen the development of antimicrobial resistance against the treatment regimens—an increasing problem with HIV infection—the protocol involves the use of four simplified but effective treatment regimens, as well as easy-to-use diagnostic and monitoring tests. Although the main goal of the initiative is to provide access to effective treatment, additional benefits are anticipated, including increased testing for and awareness of infection and reduced stigmatization about the disease. Moreover, in addition to improved health, persons who receive such treatment will have lower viral loads, causing them to be less likely to transmit infection to others.

Tuberculosis

Unlike HIV, *Mycobacterium tuberculosis* emerged as a major disease threat more than 15,000 years ago.[230] Its impact continues today, however, with nearly 1.9 billion persons infected.[231] Although not all of these individuals will become ill, those who develop active tuberculosis (TB) will infect an estimated 10 to 15 other persons each year.[232] Annually, approximately 2 million people, most (98%) from developing countries, die from tuberculosis.[232,233] These fatalities occur mostly from a pool of more than 8 million new cases of tuberculosis per year, many of which are caused by strains resistant to antituberculosis drugs.[232]

In the developed countries of the world, illness and death from tuberculosis declined dramatically throughout much of the 20th century. These declines, which predated the availability of antituberculosis drugs (beginning in the 1940s with streptomycin), were probably due to improved living conditions and decreasing opportunities for exposure.[234] In 1953, based on information from a newly established tuberculosis reporting system, tuberculosis incidence in the United States was 53 cases per 100,000 population.[235] From 1953 to 1984, tuberculosis rates steadily declined at an average rate of 5.8% per year to 9.4 cases per 100,000 population.[236]

Beginning in 1985, however, this downward trend was reversed, primarily owing to the emerging HIV/AIDS epidemic, widespread immigration of individuals from countries heavily affected by tuberculosis, and the dismantling of the tuberculosis control infrastructure. By 1992, the number of new cases had increased by 20% to 26,673 persons.[236] Similar trends were observed in western European countries (Spain—28% increase between 1990 and 1992; Italy—27% increase between 1988 and 1992; and The Netherlands—19% increase between 1987 and 1992).[237] Implementation of directly observed therapy has substantially improved therapeutic compliance and has reduced disease transmission. From 1992 to 2000, the prevalence of TB in the United States decreased by 39%.[238] However, the rate of decline has slowed, and from 2000 to 2001, reported cases declined by only 2%, with 50% of the 15,989 annual cases occurring in foreign-born individuals.[236]

Despite decreases in tuberculosis rates observed in many areas, overall incidence has been increasing by approximately 0.4% to 3% per year in most countries.[7,239] However, much higher rates of increase have been reported in many areas, including Eastern Europe and Africa, and the largest numbers of cases are reported in Southeast Asia.[232] In some areas, one third or more of the population is infected with *M. tuberculosis* (compared with 6% in the United States).[237]

HIV infection is known to be the strongest risk factor for the progression of tuberculosis infection to active disease. For non–HIV-infected persons infected with tuberculosis, the cumulative lifetime risk of active disease ranges between 5% and 10%.[240] In contrast, HIV-infected persons have a 10% annual risk of progression to active tuberculosis.[241] In areas of the world with rapidly escalating HIV prevalence, the impact on

TABLE 13-5 Antiretroviral Therapy Coverage of Adults in Developing Countries by WHO Region, December 2002

Region	Number of People	Estimated Need	Coverage
Africa	50,000	4,100,000	1%
Americas	196,000	370,000	53%
Europe	7000	80,000	9%
Eastern Mediterranean	3000	9000	29%
Southeast Asia and western Pacific	43,000	1,000,000	4%
All WHO regions	300,000	5,500,000	5%

From World Health Organization. The World Health Report 2003. Geneva: World Health Organization; 2003.

the occurrence of active tuberculosis has been dramatic. One study of data from sub-Saharan Africa demonstrated that tuberculosis rates were declining by 1.6% per year before 1985 but since then have increased by 7.7% annually.[242] In one city in Thailand, the proportion of tuberculosis patients who were HIV-positive increased from 1.5% to 45.5% in only 4 years.[243] Worldwide, tuberculosis is a leading cause of morbidity and mortality among both HIV-infected persons and their family members and close contacts. In the absence of strengthened control measures, the WHO estimates that between 2002 and 2020, nearly 1 billion people will be newly infected, more than 150 million will become sick from the disease, and more than 36 million will die.[232]

As with HIV/AIDS, stopping the spread of tuberculosis will require a global response. In collaboration with international partners, the WHO has recommended an international strategy for detecting and treating tuberculosis, especially in low- and middle-income countries.[239] The strategy, called *DOTS* for directly observed therapy, includes the following five key elements: (1) political commitment, (2) microscopy services, (3) drug supplies, (4) surveillance and monitoring systems, and (5) the use of highly efficacious regimens with direct observation of treatment—an important step in helping to reduce the development of antimicrobial resistance. A supplement to this strategy, called *DOTS-Plus*, has also been developed to address issues such as the use of second-line antituberculosis drugs in areas with a high prevalence of multidrug-resistant tuberculosis (MDR-TB). Since 1995, more than 10 million persons infected with tuberculosis throughout the world have received effective treatment through these programs.[239]

Malaria

In addition to HIV and tuberculosis, malaria has remained a major global health threat, causing an estimated 300 to 500 million cases and 1.5 to 2.7 million deaths each year, more than 90% of which occur among young children in Africa.[244-246] Although it was considered a target for eradication as recently as the 1960s,[247] the disease is endemic in more than 90 countries, placing approximately 40% of the world's population at risk (Fig. 13-7).[246,248] A mosquito-borne disease primarily transmitted in tropical areas, malaria disproportionately affects children younger than 5 years of age and pregnant women. These groups, along with nonimmune persons who visit malarious areas, are at greatest risk of severe disease or death from malaria.[249] Significant morbidity and mortality also occur among pregnant women, especially during the first pregnancy.[250,251] These patterns reflect the role of partial immunity, which develops from repeated exposure to the parasite in areas of intense disease transmission.[252,253] In areas of less intense, or intermittent, exposure to malaria, partial immunity either does not develop or is not sustained, and all age groups can be affected by the disease.

Malaria is transmitted primarily in tropical and subtropical regions in sub-Saharan Africa, Central and South America, Hispaniola, the Middle East, India, Southeast Asia, and Oceania.[249] Within these areas, the risk of transmission is highly variable and is affected largely by climate. Although most transmission of malaria occurs in rural areas, explosive population growth has contributed to increased transmission in many urban areas. Developed countries also continue to be affected by malaria because of international travel, commerce, and migration.[254] In the United States, between 1000 and 1500 cases have been reported annually in recent years, most often among individuals who acquired their infections during travel to malarious areas.[255] Information collected from ill persons suggests that many cases occurred in foreign-born persons who have resided in the United States and returned to their country of origin for visits. In such individuals, existing immunity may have waned during the interval since they relocated to the United States. In addition, several cases of autochthonous (i.e., locally acquired) mosquito-borne malaria have been reported in the United States in recent years.[254,256-258] Although none of these incidents has resulted in sustained transmission, increases in international travel and commerce, along with the presence of competent vectors and favorable environmental conditions, have caused continued concern about transmission of the disease in nonendemic areas.

Four species of *Plasmodium* are capable of producing malaria in humans: *P. falciparum*, *P. vivax*, *P. malariae*, and *P. ovale*. All are transmitted to humans by *Anopheles* species mosquitoes, with *Anopheles gambiae* the most efficient vector.[259] *P. falciparum* and *P. vivax* cause most cases of malaria in humans; however, *falciparum* malaria is considered the greater public health concern because of its more severe clinical manifestations and higher mortality. *P. falciparum* causes more than 90% of all the malaria infections in sub-Saharan Africa and Haiti and more than two thirds of infections in Southeast Asia. *P. vivax* infections predominate in Central America, most malarious areas of South America, and the Indian subcontinent, but are rare in Africa owing to genetic factors that inhibit red blood cell invasion by the parasite.[260] *P. ovale* infection is limited to small foci in sub-Saharan Africa and Papua New Guinea, and *P. malariae* occurs at low frequencies in many areas with endemic malaria transmission.

As a result of eradication efforts during the 1950s and 1960s, which consisted largely of vector control and chemotherapy, the incidence of malaria fell, particularly in temperate zones and some island nations, and the disease was eliminated in Europe, the Asian former Soviet Union, the United States, and most of the Caribbean.[261] Upon cessation of eradication efforts, the disease began to increase, especially in parts

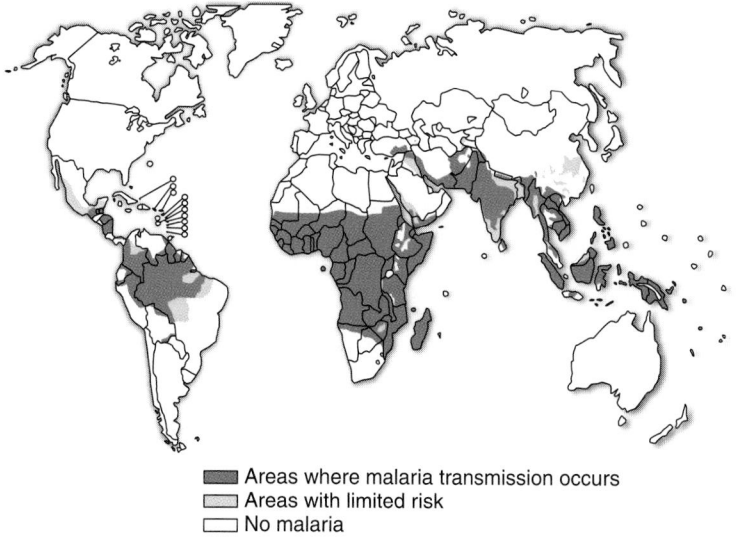

   ■ Areas where malaria transmission occurs
   □ Areas with limited risk
   □ No malaria

FIGURE 13-7. World Malaria Situation. Malaria is endemic to tropical and subtropical regions. *(Source: Geneva: World Health Organization; 2003.* *http://www.who.int/ith/chapter05_m08_malaria.html.)*

of Asia and South America.[245] In Africa, however, the global eradication program was not implemented, and the incidence of disease is increasing at alarming rates.[245] The reemergence of malaria has several explanations, including expanding human populations in tropical locations and ineffective or absent vector-control programs.[248,261] Climate change, natural disasters, and displacement may also play a role.[248,262] However, the evolution of drug resistance is probably the most critical problem in the treatment and control of malaria, especially in Africa. Both *P. falciparum* and *P. vivax* have been shown to be resistant to antimalarial drugs.[249] *P. falciparum* is resistant to most currently used antimalarial drugs, although resistance varies widely by geographic area.[249] Resistance to chloroquine and/or primaquine has been found for some *P. vivax* infections.[263,264] In many parts of Africa, both chloroquine and sulfadoxine-pyrimethamine are ineffective against the disease.[265,266]

Because the malaria parasite has consistently demonstrated its ability to develop drug resistance and the vectors to develop insecticide resistance,[267] efforts to find new control strategies have been undertaken. In the 1990s, randomized trials conducted in areas of stable malaria transmission found that use of insecticide-treated bed nets (ITNs) dramatically improved the health of young children, reducing overall child mortality by approximately one fifth.[259,268-271] More recently, ITNs have been shown to provide significant health benefits in areas of intense, perennial malaria transmission.[259,272,273] In addition, artemisinin-class combination therapies have shown promising results in reducing treatment failure, the presence of infectious mosquitoes, and the development of resistance.[265]

Despite the success of these strategies, lack of education and resources has restricted their use among many at-risk populations. To address this issue and to strengthen overall malaria treatment and control efforts, several global initiatives have been developed that involve local, national, regional, and international organizations. One of these programs, the "Roll Back Malaria" campaign, was begun in 1998 by the WHO to develop new and strengthen existing malaria-related activities, enabling widespread access to effective treatment and prevention. The overall goal of the campaign is to halve the number of malaria deaths by 2010 and again by 2015.[274]

An additional step toward reducing the severe health and economic consequences of these three interconnected diseases is the Global Fund to Fight AIDS, Tuberculosis, and Malaria. A partnership between the WHO and public and private organizations in both high- and low-income countries, the Global Fund is designed to enable substantial allocation of resources to address these diseases in countries most in need. Through these efforts, more than $600 million was provided to 40 countries in 2002.

ANTIMICROBIAL DRUG RESISTANCE

Resistance to antimicrobal drugs is a pervasive public health problem. Drug resistance increases mortality, prolongs morbidity, and, by extending the period of infectivity, enhances disease transmission. Resistance also extends the length of hospital stays and adds considerably to health care costs.

Tuberculosis

Drug resistance in tuberculosis, particularly resistance to the first-line bactericidal agents isoniazid and rifampin, has become a major concern throughout the world.[275-277] In 1998, the WHO's Global Tuberculosis Program summarized published data on patterns of drug resistance.[278] In general, levels of acquired drug resistance (i.e., resistance in cases of previously diagnosed and treated disease) were higher than those of primary drug resistance. Rates of primary MDR-TB (resistance to at least isoniazid and rifampin) around the world ranged from 0% to 11% (median, 0.5%), but high rates of acquired multidrug-resistant disease were found in several areas (Nepal, 48%; Gujarat, India, 33%; New York City, 30%). However, the levels of drug resistance in New York City subsequently declined, a finding that probably reflects strengthened control programs and wider use of directly observed therapy.[279]

Worldwide, an estimated 273,000 new cases of MDR-TB occurred in the year 2000.[280] In 2002, rates of MDR-TB among new cases were 3% or higher in 12 major geographic regions, although rates varied from 0% to 14.1% throughout the different regions.[281] Globally, an estimated 50 million people may be infected with drug-resistant tuberculosis.[282] Antimicrobial drug resistance is particularly problematic in countries with limited laboratory capability for determining drug resistance; in such countries, inappropriate regimens contribute to the development of acquired resistance.

Staphylococcus aureus

Treatment of *Staphylococcus aureus* infections is complicated by the increasing incidence of methicillin-resistant *S. aureus* (MRSA) in both community- and health care–associated settings.[283-288] MRSA emerged in the hospital environment in England in 1961, shortly after methicillin was introduced, and the incidence of MRSA has increased steadily since that time.[289,290] For example, in 1990, 22% of all nosocomial *S. aureus* isolates were methicillin resistant,[291] but by 2000, the rate had increased to more than 55%.[284] Initially, health care–associated MRSA infections occurred most often in large hospitals, but now these infections are common in small and medium-sized hospitals and in long-term care facilities. MRSA actually refers to resistance to oxacillin and nafcillin because methicillin is no longer available commercially.

Community-associated MRSA infections may occur among persons with none of the expected risk factors, such as recent hospitalization, recent drug therapy, or exposure to a previously hospitalized patient.[285-287] Infections with MRSA have been reported among children,[285,286] inmates of correctional facilities,[292] athletic teams, and men who have sex with men.[293] Available data suggest that community-associated strains are more likely to cause skin or soft tissue infection and are more likely to occur in younger persons than are strains associated with health care facilities. At least four pediatric cases have resulted in fatalities.[285] A foodborne outbreak of MRSA has also been reported, presumably caused by a food handler who became infected while visiting a nursing home.[294]

Analysis of MRSA isolates from persons with community- or hospital-associated MRSA infection has provided valuable insight into the pathogenic potential of community-associated strains. In one study, 31 of 32 community-associated MRSA isolates proved highly related when analyzed by several subtyping methods. These 31 isolates also produced high levels of staphylococcal enterotoxin B or C (but not toxic shock syndrome [TSS] toxin-1)—superantigens that may induce nonmenstrual TSS. In contrast, none of 32 hospital-associated MRSA isolates produced any of the three superantigens.[295] Thus, community-associated MRSA infection may pose a significant public health threat, not only because of antibiotic resistance but also because of considerable pathogenic potential. Fortunately, community-associated strains of MRSA remain susceptible to some non–β-lactam drugs.

The origin of community-associated MRSA is a subject of active investigation. Initially thought to have "escaped" from health care settings, community-associated MRSA strains apparently arose independently, acquiring a mobile genetic element that contains a novel gene for methicillin resistance (i.e., the staphylococcal cassette chromosome *mec* [SCC*mec*] gene), which became incorporated into previously susceptible strains of *S. aureus* capable of causing nonmenstrual TSS.[295] Detailed genomic sequencing identified a unique resistance determinant (called type IV SCC*mec*) in community-associated MRSA strains.[296] The novel element is much smaller than SCC*mec* found in hospital-associated MRSA strains, contains novel genes for excision and integration into the *S. aureus* chromosome, and does not include other antibiotic resistance genes.[296,297] The type IV SCC*mec* element has been found in strains widely separated temporally and geographically (e.g., from the United States to Australia).[298]

Vancomycin is currently considered the treatment of last resort for MRSA infection, but strains of *S. aureus* with reduced susceptibility to vancomycin have been reported, first in Japan in 1996[299,300] and subsequently in the United States,[301-303] France,[304] the United Kingdom,[305] and Germany.[306] The National Committee for Clinical Laboratory Standards (NCCLS) has defined susceptible strains as those in which concentrations of vancomycin ≤ 4 µg/mL inhibit growth; isolates of vancomycin-intermediate *S. aureus* (VISA) require concentrations of 8 to 16 µg/mL for inhibition; and vancomycin-resistant *S. aureus* (VRSA) require >32 µg/mL to inhibit growth.[307] As of June 2003, eight VISA and two VRSA infections had been confirmed in the United States.[301,308-311] Both VRSA isolates contained the vanA resistance determinant commonly seen in enterococci.

Some automated methods do not readily distinguish VISA isolates from vancomycin-susceptible isolates, nor did automated methods detect the VRSA isolate from Pennsylvania.[310] Disk diffusion methods are not accurate for identifying isolates with reduced susceptibility to vancomycin. The CDC uses three criteria to identify VISA and VRSA strains—broth microdilution, E-test, and growth on commercial Brain Heart infusion agar containing 6 µg/mL of vancomycin.[307] Isolates of *S. aureus* with reduced susceptibility to vancomycin remain susceptible to several antimicrobial agents (e.g., trimethoprim-sulfamethoxazole) and to new drugs, such as linezolid, streptogramins (quinupristin-dalfopristin), and daptomycin.[307,312] Although no clear consensus has been reached on the best approaches for containing the spread of VISA or VRSA infections, interim guidelines have been published by the CDC (available online at www.cdc.gov/ncid/hip/ARESIST/visa_vrsa_guide.pdf);[313] preliminary guidelines for the judicial use of vancomycin are also available.[314]

Enterococci

The emergence of vancomycin-resistant enterococci (VRE) is another issue of concern. *Enterococcus faecalis* and *E. faecium*, natural inhabitants of the gastrointestinal tract, are serious opportunistic pathogens, especially in intensive care units (ICUs). Both species can cause surgical site infections, urinary tract infections, and bacteremias, although *E. faecalis* is more commonly the responsible agent.

Vancomycin-resistant enterococci were first observed in Europe in 1986[315] and in the United States in 1987[316] and are now found with increasing frequency. For example, of more than 2500 isolates of enterococci obtained from ICUs during the year 2000, 26% were resistant to vancomycin.[317,318] Although *E. faecium* is isolated less frequently than *E. faecalis* in the United States, an overwhelming majority of VRE isolates are *E. faecium*.[319] The intrinsic resistance of VRE to other antimicrobial drugs severely limits therapeutic options. For example, among 185 isolates of *E. faecium* tested in one study for susceptibility to 17 drugs, a vast majority were fully resistant or had diminished susceptibility to 13 drugs. All isolates were susceptible to linezolid, most (75%) were also susceptible to chloramphenicol, and 66% were susceptible to rifampin.[318] Other studies have reported similar results.[320] However, resistance to linezolid[321] and quinupristin-dalfopristin[322] has been reported.

The increased frequency of VRE has been attributed largely to clonal spread, and the number of individual clones of VRE in a given locus appears to increase over time as VRE becomes endemic in a particular site. For example, when the 185 VRE isolates described previously were analyzed by pulsed-field gel electrophoresis (PFGE), 65 strains could be identified by unique PFGE patterns: 34 distinct clones were identified among the remaining 120 isolates. These results, in conjunction with corresponding epidemiologic data, suggest the transfer of VRE strains between and within two adjacent health institutions.[318] The ability of enterococci to withstand extreme environmental stress is a major factor in their stability once they have been introduced into the hospital environment.

Mobile DNA is the principal mechanism for the acquisition of vancomycin resistance in enterococci. Genomic sequencing of *E. faecalis* strain V583 revealed that more than 25% of the genome is composed of mobile or foreign DNA, including integrated phage regions, insertion elements, conjugative and composite transposons, and integrated plasmid genes. Resistance in this strain is encoded by a newly recognized mobile element similar to the *E. faecalis* vanB (vancomycin resistance) conjugative transposon Tn*1549*. Presumably, the propensity of enterococci to incorporate mobile genetic elements contributes to their unique ability to acquire and disseminate antimicrobial resistance genes.[323]

Streptococcus pneumoniae

Streptococcus pneumoniae remains the leading cause of community-acquired pneumonia, acute otitis media, and meningitis. In the United States, seven serotypes (4, 6B, 9V, 14, 18C, 19F, 23F) are responsible for 80% of infections among children younger than 6 years of age and for 50% of infections among persons of other ages.[324] Drug resistance among *S. pneumoniae* infections, first described in the 1960s in Australia, has now been reported throughout the world.[325] In many geographic areas, the frequency of resistance among pneumococci rose rapidly during the 1990s.[326-329] In the United States during the 1980s, only 1 (0.02%) of 5459 isolates of pneumococci from normally sterile sites exhibited high-level penicillin resistance.[330] By 1998, 24% of isolates obtained from patients with invasive pneumococcal disease had either high or intermediate levels of resistance.[327] Penicillin-resistant isolates also were more likely than susceptible isolates to be resistant to other antimicrobial drugs. For example, between 1995 and 1998, resistance to three or more classes of drugs increased from 9% to 14%.[327] The clinical significance of intermediate levels of resistance to penicillin among persons with pneumonia is uncertain.[331,332] High-level resistance associated with treatment failure has been reported,[333] but even this finding has been inconsistent,[331] and prospective studies are difficult to perform because of delays in laboratory confirmation of resistance patterns. Data from Europe in the 1990s indicated that penicillin nonsusceptibility (intermediate and high-level resistance) varied from 45% in Spain to a range of 4% to 7% in the United Kingdom.[334-336] In one Hong Kong hospital, penicillin nonsusceptibility increased from 6.6% to 55.8% of isolates in only 2 years.[337] In Mexico City, 22% of pneumococcal isolates from children with invasive disease were found to have high-level resistance.[338] In other locations, low frequencies of penicillin resistance were found. For example, one survey in Ethiopia in the early 1990s identified no penicillin-resistant strains.[339] As demonstrated in these examples, resistance patterns may be highly variable, possibly reflecting different patterns of antimicrobial use and other undefined factors. Local patterns of resistance must be understood for proper selection of therapy.

Fluoroquinolones are frequently recommended for the treatment of older adults with pneumococcal pneumonia, especially if resistance to β-lactam antibiotics is suspected. However, fluoroquinolone-resistant pneumococci have also been reported in the United States.[340-342] Some isolates, especially those with reduced susceptibility to levofloxacin, also have reduced susceptibilities to other antimicrobial drugs used for treating pneumococcal pneumonia, such as penicillin, trimethoprim-sulfamethoxazole, cefotaxime, and erythromycin, leaving few therapeutic options for patients with invasive pneumococcal disease.[342] A seven-valent pneumococcal conjugate vaccine (PCV7), comprising the seven serotypes listed earlier and licensed for use in infants and young children, prevents disease. In initial evaluations, efficacies for prevention of otitis media and invasive pneumococcal disease by the same serotypes were 57% and 94%, respectively.[343,344] In the United States, 1 year after the vaccine was introduced, the overall rate of invasive pneumococcal disease decreased by nearly 70% among children younger than 2 years old and was 32% lower among adults 20 to 39 years of age; disease attributable to strains nonsusceptible to penicillin was 35% lower in 2001 than in 1999.[345] Reduced nasopharyngeal carriage of certain strains of pneumococci, a likely consequence of vaccination, could affect the epidemiology of pneumococcal disease.

Diarrheal Bacterial Pathogens

Antimicrobial resistance has developed among many of the major diarrheal bacterial pathogens. In sub-Saharan Africa, *Shigella dysenteriae* has become resistant to multiple drugs, and multidrug-resistant strains have caused major disease outbreaks with high mortality in refugee settings.[346] In the United States, sequential surveys and the National Antimicrobial Resistance Monitoring System (NARMS) have documented increasing levels of resistance among *Salmonella* isolates from humans. In 1979/1980, a total of 17% of *Salmonella* isolates exhibited antimicrobial resistance.[347] By 1989/1990, this proportion had risen to 31%, with 25% of strains demonstrating multiple-drug resistance.[348] In a 1997 NARMS survey that used a different methodology, a total of 34% of *Salmonella* strains were drug resistant, including 27% that were resistant to multiple drugs.[349] *Salmonella* Typhimurium DT104 was first recognized in Great Britain in 1984 and quickly became the second most commonly isolated *Salmonella* strain from humans in that country.[350] First recognized in the United States in 1985, the strain did not appear widespread until the late 1990s but is now thought to produce more than 25% of all *S.* Typhimurium infections.[351] Now distributed virtually worldwide, *Salmonella* Typhimurium DT104 is invariably resistant to five antimicrobial agents; resistance to other drugs, including fluoroquinolones, has also been reported.[352-355] The use of antimicrobial agents as growth promoters in animals is thought to contribute to the rising levels of resistance among foodborne zoonotic pathogens, but other factors are also likely to be responsible.[356-358] Infections with *Salmonella* Newport have also risen dramatically in the United States in recent years, from 5% of all cases of salmonellosis in 1997 to 10% in 2001. In another disturbing trend, the increased frequency of *Salmonella* Newport infections is occurring at the same time that multidrug-resistant strains of the organism are becoming widely disseminated.[359] It is important to note that multidrug-resistant *Salmonella* Newport is commonly resistant to third-generation cephalosporins.[360]

Neisseria gonorrhoeae

Drug-resistant *Neisseria gonorrhoeae* has become a serious problem that threatens the control of gonorrhea. For example, during the late 1980s and early 1990s, resistance of gonococci to penicillin and tetracycline had emerged worldwide. In the United States in 1992, 43.6% of isolates were resistant to penicillin, tetracycline, or both drugs.[361] Fluoroquinolones and cephalosporins were then recommended as treatments for patients with uncomplicated gonococcal urethritis. As the proportion of patients treated with quinolones increased, fluoroquinolone-resistant gonococci emerged dramatically, especially in the Far East. For example, in Hong Kong, the proportion of fluoroquinolone-resistant gonococci increased from 0.5% in 1992 to 10.4% in 1994.[362,363] From 1994 to 1995, 36% of strains in Hong Kong, 54% of strains in the Philippines, and 22% of isolates in Thailand had acquired decreased susceptibility to ciprofloxacin and ofloxacin.[362] In Japan, resistance to ciprofloxacin increased from 6.6% in 1993/1994 to 24.4% in 1997/1998.[364] Fluoroquinolone resistance among isolates of *N. gonorrhoeae* obtained from sexually transmitted disease patients now exceeds 40% in parts of Asia and the western Pacific.[365-367] Well-established foci also exist elsewhere, for example, in Greece,[368] Denmark,[369] The Netherlands,[370] and Israel.[371,372]

In Israel, multidrug-resistant gonococci, including strains with high-level ciprofloxacin resistance, emerged rapidly. Fluoroquinolone-resistant gonococci, which also had decreased susceptibility to penicillin and tetracycline, were first identified in Israel in 1999; the following year, 54% of isolates from patients in Jerusalem and 51% of isolates from patients in the Tel Aviv area were resistant to fluoroquinolones.[371,372] When isolates of ciprofloxacin-resistant gonococci from different parts of Israel were subtyped by PFGE, all were found to be identical or closely related strains, suggesting that a single resistant clone became widely disseminated once it had been introduced into the country.[372] A dramatic increase in the incidence of male gonococcal urethritis occurred at the same time. Similarly, genotypic analyses of ciprofloxacin-resistant strains in Denmark suggested that most isolates, although they had originated in different geographic areas, had come from a single drug-resistant clone that apparently had been spread worldwide.[369] In contrast, multiple subtypes of drug-resistant *N. gonorrhoeae* emerged in Thailand in 1998/1999, suggesting the proliferation of endemic strains as well as the importation of others.[373]

Foci of fluoroquinolone-resistant gonococci have been identified in the United States since the early 1990s.[374,375] Fluoroquinolone resistance appears to be well established (i.e., has a sustained prevalence >1%) in Hawaii and California but occurs with less frequency in other states.[361,366] From 1991 through 1997, few resistant strains of *N. gonorrhoeae* were identified in Hawaii, and genotypic and phenotypic analyses of fluoroquinolone resistance indicated that most isolates were distinct and had been imported; few cases of secondary transmission had occurred, and no particular strains had become established. Beginning in 1998, however, clonal spread of certain strains occurred, suggesting an increased frequency of endemic spread.[376] In the United States, most strains of *N. gonorrhoeae* remain susceptible to cefixime, ceftriaxone, or spectinomycin,[361] all of which are recommended for patients who acquire infection in areas where resistance to fluoroquinolones is >1%. Use of fluoroquinolones remains an option for patients who have become infected in areas with lower prevalence rates.[366] Continued susceptibility testing of local isolates is also highly recommended to ensure appropriate treatment of patients.

FUTURE CHALLENGES

In addition to the emerging and reemerging diseases that have been discussed, many other infectious agents continue to present significant challenges to global health. A major concern is the threat of another influenza pandemic, a seemingly increasing inevitability as highly pathogenic and rapidly mutating strains such as H5N1 become further established in avian populations and cocirculate with human influenza viruses in some Asian countries (Fig. 13-8).[377,378] In early 2004, millions of chickens in Asia were infected with H5N1 strains of influenza A, and a number of cases in humans were reported with limited person-to-person spread. Other infectious threats include the risk of international foodborne disease outbreaks and the resurgence of urban yellow fever in Latin America and its possible introduction into Asia. In addition, associations between infectious agents and many chronic conditions continue to be demonstrated, including the roles of hepatitis B and C

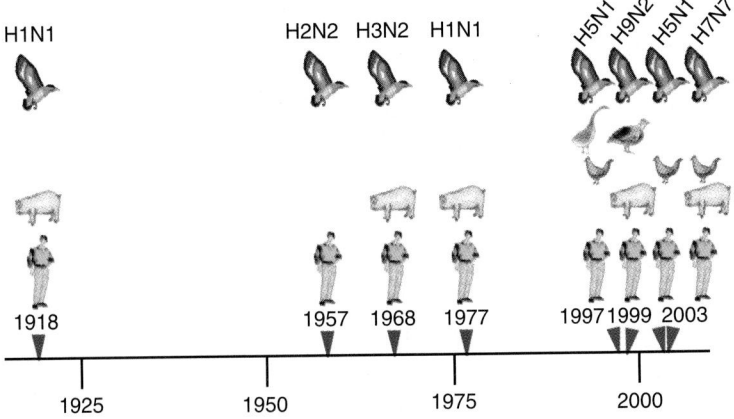

FIGURE 13-8. Influenza A Outbreaks, 1918-2003. Documented human influenza A infections characterized by multiple cases and the species of animals implicated in the outbreaks. *(Reprinted with permission from Webby RJ, Webster RG. Are we ready for pandemic influenza? Science. 2003;302:1519-1522. Copyright 2003 AAAS.)*

viruses in chronic liver disease and hepatocellular carcinoma, of human papillomaviruses in cervical cancer, and of *Helicobacter pylori* infection in peptic ulcer disease and gastric cancer. Additional associations will likely be discovered, presenting new challenges as well as new opportunities for treatment and prevention. Moreover, acts of bioterrorism, such as the anthrax attacks in the United States in 2001, remain a significant concern for much of the world. However, as the past decade has clearly indicated, that new infectious agents will continue to be recognized, underscoring the need to expect the unexpected.

Addressing the threat of infectious diseases will require efforts to confront many of the conditions that contribute to their spread.[7] Moreover, policymakers and public health officials must recognize that diseases and conditions in one country affect the health and stability of the rest of the world. As part of these efforts, in the year 2000, at the United Nations Millennium Summit, representatives from a large number of nations resolved to help reduce human poverty and its ramifications. Called the "Millennium Development Goals," this agreement requires countries to enhance their efforts to address inadequate incomes; lack of food, clean water, and health care; substandard education; gender inequality; and environmental deterioration. Target areas within the goals provide measurable steps by which development can be advanced and poverty reduced throughout the world by the year 2015.

Preparing for and successfully responding to infectious disease threats will require sound and effective national and international health systems; strong multidisciplinary partnerships among clinical, public health, research, and veterinary specialists worldwide; and innovative and consistent efforts to communicate essential and timely health information to persons at risk.[379,380] Finally, as experience continues to demonstrate, avoiding complacency in these efforts and maintaining vigilance for unusual signs and symptoms will remain critical first steps in recognition of and response to new and reemerging threats from infectious diseases.

REFERENCES

1. McNeill WH. Plagues and Peoples. Garden City, NY: Anchor Press, Doubleday; 1976.
2. Burnet M, White DO. Natural History of Infectious Disease. London: Cambridge University Press; 1972.
3. World Health Organization. World Health Report 2003—Shaping the Future. Geneva: World Health Organization; 2003.
4. World Health Organization. Macroeconomics and Health: Investing in Health for Economic Development. Report of the Commission on Macroeconomics and Health. Geneva: World Health Organization; 2001.
5. Jong-wook L. Global health improvement and WHO: Shaping the future. Lancet. 2003;362:2083-2088.
6. Lederberg J, Shope RE, Oaks SC Jr, eds, for the Committee on Emerging Microbial Threats to Health, Division of Health Sciences Policy, Division of International Health, Institute of Medicine. Emerging Infections: Microbial Threats to Health in the United States. Washington, DC: National Academy Press; 1992.
7. Smolinski MS, Hamburg MA, Lederberg J, eds, for the Committee on Emerging Microbial Threats to Health in the 21st Century, Board on Global Health, Institute of Medicine. Microbial Threats to Health: Emergence, Detection, and Response. Washington, DC: National Academy Press; 2003.
8. Berman S. Epidemiology of acute respiratory infections in children of developing countries. Rev Infect Dis. 1991;13:S454-S462.
9. Centers for Disease Control and Prevention. Deaths: Preliminary data for 2002. National Vital Statistics Reports. 2001;49:1-40.
10. Craven DE, Steger KA. Hospital-acquired pneumonia: Perspectives for the healthcare epidemiologist. Infect Control Hosp Epidemiol. 1997;18:783-795.
11. Greenaway CA, Embil J, Orr PH, McLeod J, Dyck B, Nicolle LE. Nosocomial pneumonia on general medical and surgical wards in a tertiary-care hospital. Infect Control Hosp Epidemiol. 1997;18:749-756.
12. Gerberding JL. Hospital-onset infections: A patient safety issue. Ann Intern Med. 2002;137:665-670.
13. Richards MJ, Edwards JR, Culver DH, Gaynes RP. Nosocomial infections in combined medical-surgical intensive care units in the United States. Infect Control Hosp Epidemiol. 2000;21:510-515.
14. Graham NMH. The epidemiology of acute respiratory infections in children and adults: A global perspective. Epidemiol Rev. 1990;12:149-178.
15. Vathanophas K, Sangchai R, Raktham S, et al. A community-based study of acute respiratory tract infection in Thai children. Rev Infect Dis. 1990;12:S957-S965.

16. Borrero I, Fajardo L, Bedoya A, Zea A, Carmona F, de Borrero MF. Acute respiratory tract infections among a cohort of children from Cali, Columbia. Rev Infect Dis. 1990;12:S950-S956.
17. Tupasi TE, de Leon LE, Lupisan S, et al. Patterns of acute respiratory tract infection in children: A longitudinal study in a depressed community in Metro Manila. Rev Infect Dis. 1990;12:S940-S949.
18. Selwyn BJ. The epidemiology of acute respiratory tract infection in young children: Comparison of findings from several developing countries. Coordinated Data Group of BOSTID Researchers. Rev Infect Dis. 1990;12:S870-S888.
19. Zaman K, Baqui AH, Yunus M, et al. Acute respiratory infections in children: A community-based longitudinal study in rural Bangladesh. J Trop Pediatr. 1997;43:133-137.
20. Singh MP, Nayar S. Magnitude of acute respiratory infections in under five children. J Commun Dis. 1996;28:273-278.
21. Fagbule D, Parakoyi DB, Spiegel R. Acute respiratory infections in Nigerian children: Prospective cohort study of incidence and case management. J Trop Pediatr. 1994;40:279-284.
22. Hortal M, Contera M, Mogdasy C, Russi JC. Acute respiratory infections in children from a deprived urban population from Uruguay. Rev Inst Med Trop Sao Paulo. 1994;36:51-57.
23. Monto AS, Sullivan KM. Acute respiratory illness in the community. Frequency of illness and the agents involved. Epidemiol Infect. 1993;110:145-160.
24. Enarson DA, Chretien J. Epidemiology of respiratory infectious diseases. Curr Opin Pulm Med. 1999;5:128-135.
25. Koch A, Sorensen P, Homoe P, et al. Population-based study of acute respiratory infections in children, Greenland. Emerg Infect Dis. 2002;8:586-593.
26. Monto AS. Epidemiology of viral respiratory infections. Am J Med. 2002;112(suppl 6A):4s-12s.
27. Weigl JA, Puppe W, Grondahl B, Schmitt HJ. Epidemiological investigation of nine respiratory pathogens in hospitalized children in Germany using multiplex reverse-transcriptase polymerase chain reaction. Eur J Clin Microbiol Infect Dis. 2000;19:336-343.
28. Ruuskanen O, Ogra PL. Respiratory syncytial virus. Curr Probl Pediatr. 1993;23:50-79.
29. Weber MW, Mulholland EK, Greenwood BM. Respiratory syncytial virus infection in tropical and developing countries. Trop Med Int Health. 1998;3:268-280.
30. Siritantikorn S, Puthavathana P, Suwanjutha S, et al. Acute viral lower respiratory infections in children in a rural community in Thailand. J Med Assoc Thai. 2002;85(suppl 4):S1167-S1175.
31. Crowcroft NS, Cutts F, Zambon MC. Respiratory syncytial virus: An underestimated cause of respiratory infection, with prospects for a vaccine. Commun Dis Public Health 1999;2:234-241.
32. Muller-Pebody B, Edmunds WJ, Zambon MC, Gay NJ, Crowcroft NS. Contribution of RSV to bronchiolitis and pneumonia-associated hospitalizations in English children, April 1995-March 1998. Epidemiol Infect. 2002;129:99-106.
33. Shann F. Etiology of severe pneumonia in children in developing countries. Pediatr Infect Dis J 1986;5:247-252.
34. Heiskanen-Kosma T, Korppi M, Laurila A, Jokinen C, Kleemola M, Saikku P. *Chlamydia pneumoniae* is an important cause of community-acquired pneumonia in school-aged children: Serological results of a prospective, population-based study. Scand J Infect Dis. 1999;31:255-259.
35. Principi N, Esposito S, Blasi F, Allegra L, Mowgli Study Group. Role of *Mycoplasma pneumoniae* and *Chlamydia pneumoniae* in children with community-acquired lower respiratory tract infections. Clin Infect Dis. 2001;32:1281-1289.
36. Schmidt SM, Muller CE, Mahner B, Wiersbitzky SK. Prevalence, rate of persistence and respiratory tract symptoms of *Chlamydia pneumoniae* infection in 1211 kindergarten and school age children. Pediatr Infect Dis J. 2002;21:758-762.
37. Nelson CT. *Mycoplasma* and *Chlamydia pneumoniae* in pediatrics. Semin Respir Infect. 2002;17:10-14.
38. Datta N, Kumar V, Kumar L, Singhi S. Application of case management to the control of acute respiratory infections in low-birth-weight infants: A feasibility study. Bull World Health Organ. 1987;65:77-82.
39. Tupasi TE, Velmonte MA, Sanvictores MEG, et al. Determinants of morbidity and mortality due to acute respiratory infections: Implications for intervention. J Infect Dis. 1988;157:615-623.
40. Keusch GT. Nutritional effects on response of children in developing countries to respiratory tract pathogens: Implications for vaccine development. Rev Infect Dis. 1991;13:S486-S491.
41. Victora CG, Smith PG, Barros FC, et al. Risk factors for deaths due to respiratory infections among Brazilian infants. Int J Epidemiol. 1989;18:918-925.
42. Watkins CJ, Leeder SR, Corkhill RT. The relationship between breast and bottle feeding and respiratory illness in the first year of life. J Epidemiol Commun Health. 1979;33:180-182.
43. Sommer A, Katz J, Tarwotjo I. Increased risk of respiratory disease and diarrhea in children with preexisting mild vitamin A deficiency. Am J Clin Nutr. 1984;40:1090-1095.
44. Stansfield SK, Pierre-Louis M, Lerebours G, Augustin A. Vitamin A supplementation and increased prevalence of childhood diarrhoea and acute respiratory infections. Lancet. 1993;342:578-582.
45. Forastiere F, Corbo GM, Michelozzi P, et al. Effects of environment and passive smoking on the respiratory health of children. Int J Epidemiol. 1992;21:66-73.
46. Holberg CJ, Wright AL, Martinez FD, Morgan WJ, Taussig LM, Group Health Medical Associates. Child day care, smoking by caregivers, and lower respiratory tract illness in the first 3 years of life. Pediatrics. 1993;91:885-892.

47. Peat JK, Keena V, Harakeh Z, Marks G. Parental smoking and respiratory tract infections in children. Paediatr Respir Rev. 2001;2:207-213.

48. Woodward A, Douglas RM, Graham NMH, Miles H. Acute respiratory illness in Adelaide children—the influence of child care. Med J Aust. 1991;154:805-808.

49. Frampton MW, Samet JM, Utell MJ. Environmental factors and atmospheric pollutants. Semin Respir Infect. 1991;6:185-193.

50. Armstrong JRM, Campbell H. Indoor air pollution and lower respiratory tract infections in young Gambian children. Int J Epidemiol. 1991;20:424-429.

51. Anonymous. Indoor air pollution and acute respiratory infections in children. Lancet. 1992;339:396-398.

52. Smith KR, Samet JM, Romieu I, Bruce N. Indoor air pollution and acute lower respiratory infections in children. Thorax. 2000;55:518-532.

53. Darkes MJ, Plosker GL. Pneumococcal conjugate vaccine (Prevnar; PNCRM7): A review of its use in the prevention of Streptococcus pneumoniae infection. Paediatr Drugs. 2002;4:609-630.

54. Pelton SI, Klein JO. The future of pneumococcal conjugate vaccines for prevention of pneumococcal diseases in infants and children. Pediatrics. 2002;110:805-814.

55. Black S, Shinefield H, Fireman B, et al. Efficacy, safety, and immunogenicity of heptavalent pneumococcal conjugate vaccine in children. Pediatr Infect Dis J. 2000;19:187-195.

56. Black SB, Shinefield HR, Ling S, et al. Effectiveness of heptavalent pneumococcal conjugate vaccine in children younger than five years of age for prevention of pneumonia. Pediatr Infect Dis J. 2002;21:810-815.

57. Straetemans M, Sanders EA, Veenhoven RH, Schilder AG, Damoiseaux RA, Zielhuis GA. Review of randomized controlled trials on pneumococcal vaccination for prevention of otitis media. Pediatr Infect Dis J. 2003;22:515-524.

58. Fireman B, Black SB, Shinefield HR, Lee J, Lewis E, Ray P. Impact of the pneumococcal conjugate vaccine on otitis media. Pediatr Infect Dis J. 2003;22:10-16.

58. Black SB, Shinefield HR, Hansen J, Elvin L, Laufer D, Malinoski F. Postlicensure evaluation of the effectiveness of seven valent pneumococcal conjugate vaccine. Pediatr Infect Dis J. 2001;20:1105-1107.

60. Whitney CG, Farley MM, Hadler J, et al. Decline in invasive pneumococcal disease after the introduction of protein-polysaccharide conjugate vaccine. N Engl J Med. 2003;348:1737-1746.

61. Sniadack DH, Schwartz B, Lipman H, et al. Potential interventions for the prevention of childhood pneumonia: Geographic and temporal differences in serotype and serogroup distribution of sterile site pneumococcal isolates from children—implications for vaccine strategies. Pediatr Infect Dis J. 1995;14:503-510.

62. Whitney CG, Pickering LK. The potential of pneumococcal conjugate vaccines for children. Pediatr Infect Dis J. 2002;21:961-970.

63. Van den Hoogen BG, De Jong JC, Groen J, et al. A newly discovered human pneumovirus isolated from young children with respiratory tract disease. Nat Med. 2001;7:719-724.

64. Nissen MD, Siebert DJ, Mackay IM, Sloots TP, Withers SJ. Evidence of human metapneumovirus in Australian children. Med J Aust. 2002;176:188.

65. Stockton J, Stephenson I, Fleming D, Zambon M. Human metapneumovirus as a cause of community-acquired respiratory illness. Emerg Infect Dis. 2002;8:897-901.

66. Boivin G, Abed Y, Pelletier G, et al. Virological features and clinical manifestations associated with human metapneumovirus: A new paramyxovirus responsible for acute respiratory-tract infections in all age groups. J Infect Dis. 2002;186:1330-1334.

67. Jartti T, van den Hoogen B, Garofalo RP, Osterhaus AD, Ruuskanen O. Metapneumovirus and acute wheezing in children. Lancet. 2002;360:1393-1394.

68. Freymouth F, Vabret A, Legrand L, et al. Presence of the new human metapneumovirus in French children with bronchiolitis. Pediatr Infect Dis J. 2003;22:92-94.

69. Falsey AR, Erdman D, Anderson LJ, Walsh EE. Human metapneumovirus infections in young and elderly adults. J Infect Dis. 2003;187:785-790.

70. Kahn JS. Human metapneumovirus: A newly emerging respiratory pathogen. Curr Opin Infect Dis. 2003;16:255-258.

71. Esper F, Boucher D, Weibel C, Martinello RA, Kahn JS. Human metapneumovirus infection in the United States: Clinical manifestations associated with a newly emerging respiratory pathogen in children. Pediatrics. 2003;111:1407-1410.

72. Tsang KW, Ho Pl, Ooi GC, et al. A cluster of cases of severe acute respiratory syndrome in Hong Kong. N Engl J Med. 2003;348:1977-1985.

73. Lee N, Hui D, Wu A, et al. A major outbreak of severe acute respiratory syndrome in Hong Kong. N Engl J Med. 2003;348:1986-1994.

74. Wu W, Wang J, Liu P, et al. A major outbreak of severe acute respiratory syndrome in Guangzhou, China. Chin Med J. 2003;116:811-818.

75. Peiris JSM, Lai ST, Poon LLM, et al. Coronavirus as a possible cause of severe acute respiratory syndrome. Lancet. 2003;361:1319-1325.

76. Ksaizek TG, Erdman D, Goldsmith C, et al. A novel coronavirus associated with severe acute respiratory syndrome. N Engl J Med. 2003;348:1953-1966.

77. Drosten C, Gunther S, Preiser W, et al. Identification of a novel coronavirus in patients with severe acute respiratory syndrome. N Engl J Med. 2003;348:1967-1976.

78. Kuiken T, Fouchier RAM, Schutten M, et al. Newly discovered coronavirus as the primary cause of severe acute respiratory syndrome. Lancet. 2003;362:263-270.

79. World Health Organization. Cumulative number of reported cases of severe acute respiratory syndrome (SARS). Geneva: World Health Organization; 2003. Available at http://www.who.int/csr/sarscountry/en/

80. Donnelly CA, Ghani AC, Leung GM, et al. Epidemiological determinants of spread of causal agent of severe acute respiratory syndrome in Hong Kong. Lancet. 2003;361:1761-1766.

81. Chan JW, Ng CK, Chan YH, et al. Short term outcome and risk factors for adverse clinical outcomes in adults with severe acute respiratory syndrome (SARS). Thorax. 2003;58:686-689.

82. Booth CM, Matukas LM, Tomlinson GA, et al. Clinical features and short-term outcomes of 144 patients with SARS in the Greater Toronto area. JAMA. 2003;289:2801-2809.

83. Hon KLE, Leung CW, Cheng WTF, et al. Clinical presentation and outcome of severe acute respiratory syndrome in children. Lancet. 2003;361:1701-1703.

84. Chiu WK, Cheung PCH, Ng KL, et al. Severe acute respiratory syndrome in children: Experience in a regional hospital in Hong Kong. Pediatr Crit Care Med. 2003;4:279-283.

85. Van Bever H, Hia C, Chye QS. Childhood SARS in Singapore. Arch Dis Child. 2003;88:742.

86. Avendano M, Derkach P, Swan S. Clinical course and management of SARS in health care workers in Toronto: A case series. Can Med Assoc J. 2003;168:1649-1660.

87. Centers for Disease Control and Prevention. Cluster of severe acute respiratory syndrome cases among protected health-care workers. Toronto, Canada, April 2003. MMWR CDC Surveill Sum. 2003;52:433-436.

88. Centers for Disease Control and Prevention. Severe acute respiratory syndrome—Singapore, 2003. MMWR CDC Surveill Sum. 2003;52:405-411.

89. Schrag SJ. SARS surveillance during emergency public health response, United States, March-July 2003. Emerg Infect Dis. 2004;10:185-194.

90. Lipsitch M, Cohen T, Cooper B, et al. Transmission dynamics and control of severe acute respiratory syndrome. Science. 2003;300:1966-1970.

91. Shen Z. Superspreading SARS events, Beijing, 2003. Emerg Infect Dis. 2004;10:256-260.

92. Poutanen SM, Low DE, Henry B, et al. Identification of severe acute respiratory syndrome in Canada. N Engl J Med. 2003;348:1995-2005.

93. Dwosh HA, Hong H, Austgarden D, et al. Identification and containment of an outbreak of SARS in a community hospital. Can Med Assoc J. 2003;168:1415-1420.

94. Fisher DA, Chew MH, Lim YT, Tambyah PA. Preventing local transmission of SARS: Lessons from Singapore. Med J Aust. 2003;178:555-558.

95. Flint J, Burton S, Macey JF, et al. Assessment of in-flight transmission of SARS—results of contact tracing, Canada. Can Commun Dis Rep. 2003;29:105-110.

96. Olsen SJ, Chang HL, Cheung TYY, et al. Transmission of severe acute respiratory syndrome on aircraft. N Engl J Med. 2003;349:2416-2422.

97. Ho AS, Sung JJY, Chan-Yeung M. An outbreak of severe acute respiratory syndrome among hospital workers in a community hospital in Hong Kong. Ann Intern Med. 2003;139:564-567.

98. Seto WH, Tsang D, Yung RWH, et al. Effectiveness of precautions against droplets and contact in prevention of nosocomial transmission of severe acute respiratory syndrome (SARS). Lancet. 2003;361:1519-1520.

99. Department of Health, Hong Kong Special Administrative Region. Outbreak of severe acute respiratory syndrome (SARS) at Amoy Gardens, Kowloon Bay, Hong Kong. Main findings of the investigation, April 17, 2003. Available at www.info.gov.hk/info/ap/pdf/amoy_e.pdf

100. Ng SKC. Possible role of an animal vector in the SARS outbreak at Amoy Gardens. Lancet. 2003;362:570-572.

101. Holmes KV. SARS-associated coronavirus. N Engl J Med. 2003;348:1948-1951.

102. Marra MA, Jones SJM, Astell CR, et al. The genome-sequence of the SARS-associated coronavirus. Science. 2003;300:1399-1404.

103. Rota PA, Oberste MS, Monroe SS, et al. Characterization of a novel coronavirus associated with severe acute respiratory syndrome. Science. 2003;300:1394-1399.

104. Ruan YJ, Wei CL, Ee LA, et al. Comparative full-length genome sequence analysis of 14 SARS coronavirus isolates and common mutations associated with putative origins of infection. Lancet. 2003;361:1779-1785.

105. Guan Y, Zheng BJ, He YQ, et al. Isolation and characterization of viruses related to the SARS coronavirus from animals in Southern China. Science. 2003;300:276-278.

106. Jernigan JA. Combining clinical and epidemiologic features for early recognition of SARS. Emerg Infect Dis. 2004;10:327-333.

107. Cinatl J, Morganstern B, Bauer G, Chandra P, Rabenau H, Doerr HW. Treatment of SARS with human interferons. Lancet. 2003;362:293-294.

108. Fowler RA, Lapinsky SE, Hallett D, et al. Critically ill patients with severe acute respiratory syndrome. JAMA. 2003;290:367-373.

109. Lew TW, Kwek TK, Tai D, et al. Acute respiratory distress syndrome in critically ill patients with severe acute respiratory syndrome. JAMA. 2003;290:374-380.

110. Oba Y. The use of corticosteroids in SARS. N Engl J Med. 2003;348:2034-2035.

111. So LK, Lau AC, Yam LY, et al. Development of a standard treatment protocol for severe acute respiratory syndrome. Lancet. 2003;361:1730-1733.

112. Tsang KW, Lam WK. Management of severe acute respiratory syndrome: The Hong Kong University experience. Am J Respir Crit Care Med. 2003;168:417-424.

113. Wang H, Ding Y, Li X, et al. Fatal aspergillosis in a patient with SARS who was treated with corticosteroids. N Engl J Med. 2003;349:507-508.

114. Peiris JSM, Chu CM, Cheng VCC, et al. Clinical progression and viral load in a community outbreak of coronavirus-associated SARS pneumonia: A prospective study. Lancet. 2003;361:1767-1772.

115. Pang X, Zhu Z, Xu F, et al. Evaluation of control measures implemented in the severe acute respiratory syndrome outbreak in Beijing, 2003. JAMA. 2003;290:3215-3221.

116. Kosek M, Bern C, Guerrant RL. The global burden of diarrhoeal disease, as estimated from studies published between 1992 and 2000. Bull World Health Organ. 2003;81:197-204.

117. Moore SR, Lima AAM, Conaway MR, et al. Early childhood diarrhoea and helminthiases associated with long-term linear growth faltering. Int J Epidemiol. 2001;30:1457-1464.

118. DuPont HL. Diarrheal diseases in the developing world. Infect Dis Clin North Am. 1995;2:313-324.

119. Muhe L, Byass P, Friej L, Sandstrom A, Wall S. A one-year community study of under-fives in rural Ethiopia: Patterns of morbidity and mortality. Public Health. 1995;109:99-109.

120. Gupta DN, Sircar BK, Sengupta PG, et al. Epidemiological and clinical profiles of acute invasive diarrhoea with special reference to mucoid episodes: A rural community-based longitudinal study. Trans R Soc Trop Med Hyg. 1997;90:544-547.
121. Jousilahti P, Madkour SM, Lambrechts T, Sherwin E. Diarrhoeal disease morbidity and home treatment practices in Egypt. Public Health. 1997;111:5-10.
122. Mirza NM, Caulfield LE, Black RE, Macharia WM. Risk factors for diarrheal duration. Am J Epidemiol. 1997;146:776-785.
123. Isenbarger DW, Hien BT, Ha HT, et al. Prospective study of the incidence of diarrhoea and prevalence of bacterial pathogens in a cohort of Vietnamese children along the Red River. Epidemiol Infect. 2001;127:229-236.
124. Aranda-Michel J, Giannella RA. Acute diarrhea: A practical review. Am J Med. 1999;106:670-676.
125. Herikstad H, Yang S, Van Gilder TJ, et al. A population-based estimate of the burden of diarrhoeal illness in the United States: FoodNet, 1996-7. Epidemiol Infect. 2002;129:9-17.
126. Mead PS, Slutsker L, Dietz V, et al. Food-related illness and death in the United States. Emerg Infect Dis. 1999;5:607-625.
127. Morris JG Jr. Cholera and other types of vibriosis: A story of human pandemics and oysters on the half shell. Clin Infect Dis. 2003;37:272-280.
128. Ries AA, Vugia DJ, Beingolea L, et al. Cholera in Piura, Peru: A modern urban epidemic. J Infect Dis. 1992;166:1429-1433.
129. Begue RE, Castellares G, Hayashi KE, et al. Diarrheal disease in Peru, after the introduction of cholera. Am J Trop Med Hyg. 1994;51:585-589.
130. Vugia DJ, Rodriguez M, Vargas R, et al. Epidemic cholera in Trujillo, Peru, 1992: Utility of a clinical case definition and shift in *Vibrio cholerae* O1 serotype. Am J Trop Med Hyg. 1994;50:566-569.
131. Nair GB, Ramamurthy T, Bhattacharya SK, et al. Spread of *Vibrio cholerae* O139 Bengal in India. J Infect Dis. 1994;169:1029-1034.
132. Siddique AK, Zaman K, Akram K, Mutsuddy P, Eusof A, Sack RB. Emergence of a new epidemic strain of *Vibrio cholerae* in Bangladesh. An epidemiological study. Trop Geographical Med. 1994;46:147-150.
133. Anonymous. Large epidemic of cholera-like disease in Bangladesh caused by *Vibrio cholerae* O139 synonym Bengal. Lancet. 1993;342:387-390.
134. Faruque SM, Sack DA, Sack RB, Colwell RR, Takeda Y, Nair GB. Emergence and evolution of *Vibrio cholerae* O139. Proc Natl Acad Sci U S A. 2003;100:1304-1309.
135. Ramamurthy T, Yamasaki S, Takeda Y, Nair GB. *Vibrio cholerae* O139 Bengal: Odyssey of a fortuitous variant. Microb Infect. 2003;5:329-344.
136. Sinha S, Chakraborty R, De K, et al. Escalating association of *Vibrio cholerae* O139 with cholera outbreaks in India. J Clin Microbiol. 2002;40:2635-2637.
137. Tauxe RV. Emerging foodborne pathogens. Int J Food Microbiol. 2002;78:31-41.
138. Herwaldt BL, Ackers ML, Cyclospora Working Group. An outbreak in 1996 of cyclosporiasis associated with imported raspberries. N Engl J Med. 1997;336:1548-1556.
139. Soave R. *Cyclospora*: An overview. Clin Infect Dis. 1996;23:429-437.
140. Armstrong GL, Hollingsworth J, Morris JG Jr. Emerging foodborne pathogens: *Escherichia coli* O157:H7 as a model of entry of a new pathogen into the food supply of the developed world. Epidemiol Rev. 1996;18:29-51.
141. Slutsker L, Ries AA, Greene KD, Wells JG, Hutwagner L, Griffin PM. *Escherichia coli* O157:H7 diarrhea in the United States: Clinical and epidemiologic features. Ann Intern Med. 1997;126:505-513.
142. Michino H, Araki K, Minami S, et al. Massive outbreak of *Escherichia coli* O157:H7 infection in schoolchildren in Sakai City, Japan, associated with consumption of white radish sprouts. Am J Epidemiol. 1999;150:787-796.
143. Hrudey SE, Payment P, Huck PM, Gillham RW, Hrudey EJ. A fatal waterborne disease epidemic in Walkerton, Ontario: Comparison with other waterborne outbreaks in the developed world. Water Sci Technol. 2003;47:7-14.
144. Bopp DJ, Saunders BD, Waring AL, et al. Detection, isolation, and molecular subtyping of *Escherichia coli* O157:H7 and *Campylobacter jejuni* associated with a large waterborne outbreak. J Clin Microbiol. 2003;41:174-180.
145. Hatch DL, Waldman RJ, Lungu GW, Piri C. Epidemic cholera during refugee resettlement in Malawi. Int J Epidemiol. 1994;23:1292-1299.
146. Engels D, Madaras T, Nyandwi S, Murray J. Epidemic dysentery caused by *Shigella dysenteriae* type 1: A sentinel site surveillance of antimicrobial resistance patterns in Burundi. Bull World Health Organ. 1995;73:787-791.
147. Shears P. *Shigella* infections. Ann Trop Med Parasitol. 1996;90:105-114.
148. Bresee JS, Widdowson MA, Monroe SS, Glass RI. Foodborne viral gastroenteritis: Challenges and opportunities. Clin Infect Dis. 2002;35:748-753.
149. Centers for Disease Control and Prevention. Norovirus activity—United States, 2002. MMWR Morb Mortal Wkly Rep. 2003;52:41-45.
150. Bohnker BK, Thornton S. Explosive outbreaks of gastroenteritis in the shipboard environment attributed to norovirus. Military Med. 2003;168:iv.
151. Centers for Disease Control and Prevention. Outbreak of acute gastroenteritis associated with Norwalk-like viruses among British military personnel——Afghanistan, May 2002. MMWR Morb Mortal Wkly Rep. 2002;51:477-479.
152. Bishop RF. Natural history of human rotavirus infection. Arch Virol Suppl. 1996;12:119-128.
153. Glass RI, Kilgore PE, Holman RC, et al. The epidemiology of rotavirus diarrhea in the United States: Surveillance and estimates of disease burden. J Infect Dis. 1996;174(Suppl):S5-S11.
154. Unicomb LE, Kilgore PE, Faruque SG, et al. Anticipating rotavirus vaccines: Hospital-based surveillance for rotavirus diarrhea and estimates of disease burden in Bangladesh. Pediatr Infect Dis J. 1997;16:947-951.
155. Suwatano O. Acute diarrhea in under five-year-old children admitted to King Mongkut Prachomklao Hospital, Phetchaburi province. J Med Assoc Thai. 1997; 80:26-33.
156. Saida SM, Iijima Y, Sang WK, et al. Epidemiological study on infectious diarrheal diseases in children in a coastal rural area of Kenya. Microbiol Immunol. 1997; 41:773-778.
157. Townes JM, Quick R, Gonzales OY, et al. Etiology of bloody diarrhea in Bolivian children: Implications for empiric therapy. J Infect Dis. 1997;175:1527-1530.
158. Bhimma R, Rollins NC, Coovadia HM, Adhikari M. Post-dysenteric hemolytic uremic syndrome in children during an epidemic of *Shigella* dysentery in Kwazulu/Natal. Pediatr Nephrol. 1997;11:560-564.
159. Lindblood GB, Ahren C, Changalucha J, et al. *Campylobacter jejuni/coli* and enterotoxigenic *Escherichia coli* (ETEC) in faeces from children and adults in Tanzania. Scand J Infect Dis. 1995;27:589-593.
160. Blaser MJ. Epidemiologic and clinical features of *Campylobacter jejuni* infections. J Infect Dis. 1997;176(Suppl):S103-S105.
161. Bhattacharya MK, Teka T, Faruque AS, Fuchs GJ. *Cryptosporidium* infection in children in urban Bangladesh. J Trop Pediatr. 1997;43:282-286.
162. Agnew DG, Lima AA, Newman RD, et al. Cryptosporidiosis in northeastern Brazilian children: Association with increased diarrhea morbidity. J Infect Dis. 1998; 177:754-760.
163. Isenbarger DW, Hien BT, Ha HT, et al. Prospective study of the incidence of diarrhoea and prevalence of bacterial pathogens in a cohort of Vietnamese children along the Red River. Epidemiol Infect. 2001;127:229-236.
164. Ryan MJ, Ramsay M, Brown D, Gay NJ, Farrington CP, Wall PG. Hospital admissions attributable to rotavirus infection in England and Wales. J Infect Dis. 1996; 174:S12-S18.
165. Blacklow NR, Greenberg HB. Viral gastroenteritis. N Engl J Med. 1991;325:252-264.
166. Kapikian AZ. Overview of viral gastroenteritis. Arch Virol Suppl. 1996;12:7-19.
167. Goldwater PN, Bettelheim KA. The role of enterohemorrhagic *Escherichia coli* serotypes other than O157:H7 as causes of disease. Commun Dis Intelligence. 1995;19:2-4.
168. Huppertz HI, Busch D, Schmidt H, Aleksic S, Karch H. Diarrhea in young children associated with *Escherichia coli* non-O157 organisms that produce Shiga-like toxin. J Pediatr. 1996;128:341-346.
169. Centers for Disease Control and Prevention. Summary of notifiable diseases, United States, 1995. MMWR CDC Surveill Sum. 1995;44:1-87.
170. Chalker RB, Blaser MJ. A review of human salmonellosis III. Magnitude of *Salmonella* infection in the United States. Rev Infect Dis. 1988;10:111-124.
171. Meinhardt PL, Casemore DP, Miller KB. Epidemiologic aspects of human cryptosporidiosis and the role of waterborne transmission. Epidemiol Rev. 1996;18: 118-136.
172. Cohen D, Orr N, Haim M, et al. Safety and immunogenicity of two different lots of the oral, killed enterotoxigenic *Escherichia coli*–cholera toxin B subunit vaccine in Israeli young adults. Infect Immun. 2000;68:4492-4497.
173. Murphy TV, Gargiullo PM, Massoudi MS, et al. Intussusception among infants given an oral rotavirus vaccine. N Engl J Med. 2001;344:564-572.
174. Offit PA. The future of rotavirus vaccines. Semin Pediatr Infect Dis. 2002;13: 190-195.
175. Cunliffe NA, Bresee JS, Hart CA. Rotavirus vaccines: Development, current issues, and future prospects. J Infect. 2002;45:1-9.
176. Taylor JL, Tuttle J, Pramukul T, et al. An outbreak of cholera in Maryland associated with imported commercial frozen fresh coconut milk. J Infect Dis. 1993;167: 1330-1335.
177. Threlfall EJ, Hampton MD, Ward LR, Rowe B. Application of pulsed-field gel electrophoresis to an international outbreak of *Salmonella agona*. Emerg Infect Dis. 1996;2:130-132.
178. Taylor LN, Ltham SM, Woolhouse ME. Risk factors for human disease emergence. Philos Trans R Soc Lond B Biol Sci. 2001;356:983-989.
179. Gubler DJ. Epidemic dengue/dengue hemorrhagic fever as a public health, social, and economic problem in the 21st century. Trends Microbiol. 2002;10:100-103.
180. Kautner I, Robinson MJ, Kuhnle U. Dengue virus infection: Epidemiology, pathogenesis, clinical presentation, diagnosis, and prevention. J Pediatr. 1997;131:516-524.
181. Hayes EB, Gubler DJ. Dengue and dengue hemorrhagic fever. Pediatr Infect Dis J. 1992;11:311-317.
182. Kalayanarooj S, Vaughn DW, Nimmannitya S, et al. Early clinical and laboratory indicators of acute dengue illness. J Infect Dis. 1997;176:313-321.
183. Gratz NG. Emerging and resurging vector-borne diseases. Annu Rev Entomol. 1999;44:51-75.
184. Pinhiero FP, Corber SJ. Global situation of dengue and dengue haemorrhagic fever, and its emergence in the Americas. World Health Stat Q. 1997;50:161-169.
185. Kouri G, Guzman MG, Valdes L, et al. Reemergence of dengue in Cuba: A 1997 epidemic in Santiago de Cuba. Emerg Infect Dis. 1998;4:89-92.
186. Petersen LR, Marfin AA. West Nile virus: A primer for the clinician. Ann Intern Med. 2002;137:173-179.
187. Campbell GL, Marfin AA, Lanciotti RS, Gubler DJ. West Nile virus. Lancet Infect Dis. 2002;2:519-529.
188. Savage HM, Ceianu C, Nicolescu G, et al. Entomologic and avian investigations of an epidemic of West Nile fever in Romania in 1996, with serologic and molecular characterization of a virus isolate from mosquitoes. Am J Trop Med Hyg. 1999;61:600-611.
189. Tsai TF, Popovici F, Cernescu C, Campbell GL, Nedelcu NI. West Nile encephalitis epidemic in southeastern Romania. Lancet. 1998;352:767-771.
190. Platonov AE, Shipulin GA, Shipulina OY, et al. Outbreak of West Nile virus infection, Volgograd Region, Russia, 1999. Emerg Infect Dis. 2001;7:128-132.
191. Weinburger M, Pitlik SD, Gandacu D, et al. West Nile fever outbreak, Israel, 2000: Epidemiologic aspects. Emerg Infect Dis. 2001;7:686-691.

192. Chowers M, Lang, R, Nassar F, et al. Clinical characteristics of the West Nile fever outbreak, Israel, 2000. Emerg Infect Dis. 2001;7:675-678.

193. Centers for Disease Control and Prevention. Provisional surveillance summary of the West Nile virus epidemic—United States, January-November 2002. MMWR CDC Surveill Sum. 2002;51:1129-1133.

194. Drebot MA, Lindsay R, Barker IK, et al. West Nile virus surveillance and diagnostics: A Canadian perspective. Can J Infect Dis. 2003;14:114.

195. Nash D, Mostashari F, Fine A, et al. The outbreak of West Nile virus infection in the New York City area, 1999. N Engl J Med. 2001;344:1807-1814.

196. Petersen LR, Marfin AA, Gubler DJ. West Nile virus. JAMA. 2003;290;524-528.

197. Pealer LN, Marfin AA, Petersen LR, et al. Transmission of West Nile virus through blood transfusion in the United States in 2002. N Engl J Med. 2003;349:1236-1245.

198. Iwamoto M, Jernigan DB, Guasch A, et al. Transmission of West Nile virus from an organ donor to four transplant recipients. N Engl J Med. 2003;348:2196-2203.

199. Centers for Disease Control and Prevention. Epidemic/epizootic West Nile virus in the United States: Guidelines for surveillance, prevention, and control of West Nile virus infection. Available at http://www.cdc.gov/ncidod/dvbid/westnile/resources/wnv-guidelines-aug-2003.pdf

200. Komar N, Langevin S, Hinten S, et al. Experimental infection of North American birds with the New York 1999 strain of West Nile virus. Emerg Infect Dis. 2003;9:311-322.

201. Marberg K, Goldblum N, Sterk VV, Jasinska-Klingberg W, Klingberg MA. The natural history of West Nile fever. I: Clinical observations during an epidemic in Israel. Am J Hyg. 1956;64:259-269.

202. Hubálek Z. Comparative symptomatology of West Nile fever. Lancet. 2001;358: 254-255.

203. Sejvar JJ, Haddad MB, Tierney BC, et al. Neurologic manifestations and outcome of West Nile virus infection. JAMA. 2003;290:511-515.

204. Monath TP. Prospects for development of a vaccine against the West Nile virus. Ann N Y Acad Sci. 2001;951:1-12.

205. Murray K, Selleck P, Hooper P, et al. A morbillivirus that caused fatal disease in horses and humans. Science. 1995;268:94-97.

206. Halpin K, Young P, Field H, Mackenzie J. Isolation of Hendra virus from pteropid bats: A natural reservoir of Hendra virus. J Gen Virol. 2000;81:1927-1932.

207. Mackenzie JS, Chua KB, Daniels PW, et al. Emerging viral diseases of southeast Asia and the Western Pacific. Emerg Infect Dis. 2001;7:497-504.

208. Chua KB. Nipah virus outbreak in Malaysia. J Clin Virol. 2003;26:265-275.

209. Chua KB, Koh CL, Hooi PS, et al. Isolation of Nipah virus from Malaysian Island flying foxes. Microb Infect. 2002;4:145-151.

210. Olson JG, Rupprecht C, Rollin PE, et al. Antibodies to Nipah-like virus in bats (*Pteropus lylei*), Cambodia. Emerg Infect Dis. 2002;8:987-988.

211. Centers for Disease Control and Prevention. Multistate outbreak of monkeypox—Illinois, Indiana, and Wisconsin, 2003. MMWR CDC Surveill Sum. 2003;52: 537-540.

212. Reed KD, Melski JW, Graham MB, et al. The detection of monkeypox in humans in the western hemisphere. N Engl J Med. 2004;350:342-350.

213. Landyl ID, Ziegler P, Kima A. A human infection caused by monkeypox virus in Basankusu Territory, Democratic Republic of the Congo (DRC). Bull World Health Organ. 1972;46:593-597.

214. Breman JG. Monkeypox: An emerging infection for humans? In: Scheld WM, Craig WA, Hughes JM, eds. Emerging Infections 4. Washington, DC: ASM Press; 2000: 45-76.

215. Shchelkunov SN, Totmenin AV, Babkin IV, et al. Human monkeypox and smallpox viruses: Genomic comparison. FEBS Lett. 2001;509:66-70.

216. Shchelkunov SN, Totmenin AV, Safronov PF, et al. Analysis of the monkeypox genome. Virology. 2002;297:172-194.

217. Technical Advisory Group on Human Monkeypox: Report of a WHO meeting. Geneva, Switzerland: World Health Organization; January 11-12, 1999.

218. Jezek ZM, Sczeniowski KM, Paluku M, et al. Human monkeypox: Clinical features of 282 patients. J Infect Dis. 1987;156:293-298.

219. Control of Communicable Diseases; Restrictions on African Rodents, Prairie Dogs, and Certain Other Animals. Interim Final Rule by the Food and Drug Administration and Centers for Disease Control and Prevention. Available at http://edocket.access.gpo.gov/2003/03-27557.htm

220. Joint United Nations Programme on HIV/AIDS (UNAIDS) and World Health Organization (WHO). AIDS Epidemic Update. Geneva: UNAIDS; 2003.

221. Gao F, Bailes E, Robertson EL. Origin of HIV-1 in the chimpanzee *Pan troglodytes troglodytes*. Nature. 1999;397:436-441.

222. Hahn BH, Shaw GM, DeCock KM. AIDS as a zoonosis: Scientific and public health implications. Science. 2000;287:607-614.

223. Quinn TC. The global epidemiology of AIDS. In: Scheld WM, Murray BE, Hughes JM, eds. Emerging Infections 6. Washington, DC: ASM Press; 2004:59-82.

224. Korber B, Muldoon M, Theiler J, et al. Timing the ancestor of the HIV-1 pandemic strains. Science. 2000;288:1786-1789.

225. Osamanov S, Pattou N, Walker N, Schwardlander B, Esparza J. Estimated global distribution and regional spread of HIV-1 genetic subtypes in the year 2000. J Acquir Immune Defic Syndr Hum Retrovirol. 2002;29:184-190.

226. Karon JM, Fleming PL, Steketee RW, DeCock KM. HIV in the United States at the turn of the century: An epidemic in transition. Am J Public Health. 2001;91: 1060-1068.

227. Wolitski RJ, Valdiserri RO, Denning PH, Levine WC. Are we headed for a resurgence of the HIV epidemic among men who have sex with men? Am J Public Health. 2001;91:883-888.

228. Centers for Disease Control and Prevention. Increases in HIV diagnoses: 29 states, 1999-2002. MMWR CDC Surveill Sum. 2003;52:1145-1148.

229. World Health Organization. Treating 3 million by 2005: Making it happen: The WHO strategy: The WHO and UNAIDS global initiative to provide antiretroviral therapy to 3 million people with HIV/AIDS by the end of 2005. Geneva: World Health Organization; 2003. Available at http://www.who.int/3by5/publications/documents/isbn9241591129/en/

230. Kapur V, Wittam TS, Musser JM. Is *Mycobacterium tuberculosis* 15,000 years old? J Infect Dis. 1994;170:1348-1349.

231. Dye C, Scheel S, Dolan P, Pathania V, Raviglione MC, for the WHO Global Surveillance and Monitoring Project. Global burden of tuberculosis: Estimated incidence, prevalence, and mortality by country. JAMA. 1999;282:677-686.

232. World Health Organization. Tuberculosis. Fact Sheet No. 104. Geneva: World Health Organization; 2002. Available at http://www.who.int/mediacentre/factsheets/who104/en/

233. Mukadi YD, Maher D, Harries A. Tuberculosis case fatality rates in high HIV prevalence populations in sub-Saharan Africa. AIDS. 2001;15:143-152.

234. Wilson LG. The historical decline of tuberculosis in Europe and America: Its causes and significance. J History Med Allied Sci. 1990;45:366-396.

235. Centers for Disease Control and Prevention. Reported tuberculosis in the United States, 2001. Atlanta: U.S. Department of Health and Human Services, Centers for Disease Control and Prevention; September 2002.

236. Navin TR, McNabb SJN, Crawford JT. The continued threat of tuberculosis. Emerg Infect Dis. 2002;8:1187.

237. World Health Organization. TB, A Global Health Emergency. WHO Report on the TB Epidemic. World Health Organization, 1994, Document No. WHO/TB/94.177.

238. Bloom BR. Tuberculosis—the global view. N Engl J Med. 2002;346:1434-1435.

239. World Health Organization. WHO Report 2003. Global Tuberculosis Control: Surveillance, Planning, Financing. Geneva: World Health Organization; 2003. Available at http://www.who.int/gtb/publications/globrep/

240. Rieder HL, Cauthen GM, Comstock GW, Snider DE Jr. Epidemiology of tuberculosis in the United States. Epidemiol Rev. 1989;11:79-98.

241. Shafer RW, Edlin BR. Tuberculosis in patients with human immunodeficiency virus: Perspective on the past decade. Clin Infect Dis. 1996;22:683-704.

242. Cantwell MF, Binkin NJ. Tuberculosis in sub-Saharan Africa: A regional assessment of the impact of the human immunodeficiency virus and National Tuberculosis Control Program quality. Tuber Lung Dis. 1996;77:220-225.

243. Yanai CM, Uthaivoravit W, Panich V, et al. Rapid increase in HIV-related tuberculosis, Chiang Rai, Thailand, 1990-1994. AIDS. 1996;10:527-531.

244. World Health Organization. WHO Expert Committee on Malaria: Twentieth Report. Geneva: World Health Organization; 2000.

245. Nchinda TC. Malaria: A reemerging disease in Africa. Emerg Infect Dis. 1998;4: 398-403.

246. World Health Organization. Malaria. Fact Sheet No. 94. Geneva: World Health Organization; 2003. Available at http://www.who.int/inf-fs/en/fact094.html

247. Pampana EJ. A Textbook of Malaria Eradication. London: Oxford University Press; 1963.

248. Martens P, Hall L. Malaria on the move: Human population movement and malaria transmission. Emerg Infect Dis. 2000;6:103-108.

249. Bloland PB. Drug Resistance in Malaria. Geneva: World Health Organization; 2001.

250. Silver HM. Malarial infection during pregnancy. Infect Dis Clin North Am. 1997;11:99-107.

251. Steele RW. Malaria in children. Adv Pediatr Infect Dis. 1996;12:325-349.

252. Marsh K, Snow RW. Host-parasite interaction and morbidity in malaria endemic areas. Philos Trans R Soc Lond B Biol Sci. 1997;352:1385-1394.

253. Warsame M, Wernsdorfer WH, Perlmann H, et al. A malariometric survey in a rural community in the Muheza district, Tanzania: Age profiles in the development of humoral immune responses. Acta Trop 1997;68:239-253.

254. Zucker JR. Changing patterns of autochthonous malaria transmission in the United States: A review of recent outbreaks. Emerg Infect Dis. 1996;2:37-43.

255. Centers for Disease Control and Prevention. Malaria surveillance—United States, 2001. MMWR CDC Surveill Sum. 2003;52:1-14.

256. Centers for Disease Control and Prevention. Probable locally acquired mosquito-transmitted *Plasmodium vivax* infection—Suffolk County, New York, 1999. MMWR CDC Surveill Sum. 2000;49:495-498.

257. Centers for Disease Control and Prevention. Local transmission of *Plasmodium vivax* malaria—Virginia, 2002. MMWR CDC Surveill Sum. 2002;51:921-923.

258. Centers for Disease Control and Prevention. Local transmission of *Plasmodium vivax* malaria—Palm Beach County, Florida, 2003. MMWR CDC Surveill Sum. 2003; 52:908-911.

259. Nahlen BL, Clark JP, Alnwick D. Insecticide-treated bed nets. Am J Trop Med Hyg. 2003;68:1-2.

260. Miller LH, McAuliffe FM, Mason SJ. Erythrocyte receptors for malaria merozoites. Am J Trop Med Hyg. 1977;26:204-208.

261. Krogstad DJ. Malaria as a reemerging disease. Epidemiol Rev. 1996;18:77-89.

262. Bourma MJ, Dye C. Cycles of malaria associated with El Nino in Venezuela. JAMA. 1997;278:1772-1774.

263. Murphy GS, Basri H, Andersen M, et al. *Vivax* malaria resistant to treatment and prophylaxis with chloroquine. Lancet. 1993;341:96-100.

264. Looareesuwan S, Buchachart K, Wilairatana P, et al. Primaquine-tolerant *Vivax* malaria in Thailand. Ann Trop Med Parasitol. 1997;91:939-943.

265. Attaran A, Barnes KI, Curtis C, et al. WHO, the Global Fund, and medical malpractice in malaria treatment. Lancet. 2004;363:237-240.

266. World Health Organization. Position of WHO's Roll Back Malaria Department on Malaria Treatment Policy. November, 2003. Available at http://www.emro.who.int/rbm/

267. Roberts DR, Andre RG. Insecticide resistance issues in vector-borne disease control. Am J Trop Med Hyg. 1994;50:21-34.

268. D'Alessandro U, Olaleye BO, McGuire W, et al. Mortality and morbidity from malaria in Gambian children after introduction of an impregnated bed-net programme. Lancet. 1995;345:479-483.
269. Binka F, Kubaje A, Adjuik M, et al. Impact of permethrin impregnated bednets on child mortality in Kassena-Nankana district, Ghana: A randomized controlled trial. Trop Med Int Health. 1996;1:147-154.
270. Habluetzel A, Diallo DA, Esposito F, et al. Do insecticide-treated curtains reduce all-cause child mortality in Burkina Faso? Trop Med Int Health. 1997;2:855-862.
271. Nevill C, Some E, Mung'ala V, et al. Insecticide-treated bednets reduce mortality and severe morbidity from malaria among children on the Kenyan coast. Trop Med Int Health. 1996;1:139-146.
272. Phillips-Howard PA, Nahlen BL, Kolczak MS, et al. Efficacy of permethrin-treated bed nets in the prevention of mortality in young children in an area of high perennial malaria transmission in Western Kenya. Am J Trop Med Hyg. 2003;68:23-29.
273. ter Kuile FO, Terlouw DJ, Phillips-Howard PA, et al. Impact of permethrin-treated bed nets on malaria and all-cause morbidity in young children in an area of intense perennial malaria transmission in Western Kenya: Cross-sectional survey. Am J Trop Med Hyg. 2003;68:100-107.
274. Nabarro DN, Talyer EM. The "Roll Back Malaria" campaign. Science. 1998; 280:2067-2068.
275. Parsons LM, Driscoll JR, Taber HW, et al. Drug resistance in tuberculosis. Infect Dis Clin North Am. 1997;11:905-928.
276. Bradford WZ, Daley CL. Multiple drug-resistant tuberculosis. Infect Dis Clin North Am. 1998;12:157-172.
277. Snider DE Jr, Castro KG. The global threat of drug-resistant tuberculosis. N Engl J Med. 1998;338:1689-1690.
278. Pablos-Mendez A, Raviglione MC, Laszlo A, et al. Global surveillance for antituberculosis-drug resistance, 1994-1997. N Engl J Med. 1998;338:1641-1649.
279. Fujiwara PI, Cook SV, Rutherford CM, et al. A continuing survey of drug-resistant tuberculosis, New York City, April 1994. Arch Intern Med. 1997;157:531-536.
280. Dye C, Espinal MA, Watt CJ, et al. Worldwide incidence of multidrug-resistant tuberculosis. J Infect Dis. 2002;185:1197-1202.
281. Kim SJ. Current problems of drug-resistant tuberculosis and its control. Kekkaku. 2002;77:735-740.
282. Kremer LS, Bestra GS. Current status and future development of antitubercular chemotherapy. Expert Opin Invest Drugs. 2002;11:1033-1049.
283. Lowy FD. Staphylococcus aureus infections. N Engl J Med. 1998;339:520-532.
284. Centers for Disease Control and Prevention. National Nosocomial Infections Surveillance (NNIS) system report, data summary from January 1992-June 2001. Am J Infect Control. 2001;29:404-421.
285. Centers for Disease Control and Prevention. Four pediatric deaths from community-acquired methicillin-resistant Staphylococcus aureus—Minnesota and North Dakota, 1997-1999. MMWR Morb Mortal Wkly Rep. 1999;48:707-710.
286. Herold BC, Immergluck LC, Maranan MC, et al. Community-acquired methicillin-resistant Staphylococcus aureus in children with no identified predisposing risk. JAMA. 1998;279:593-598.
287. Chambers HF. The changing epidemiology of Staphylococcus aureus. Emerg Infect Dis. 2001;7:178-182.
288. O'Brien FG, Pearman JW, Gracey M, et al. Community strain of methicillin-resistant Staphylococcus aureus involved in a hospital outbreak. J Clin Microbiol. 1999;37:2858-2862.
289. Simor AE, Ofner-Agostini M, Bryce E, et al. The evolution of methicillin-resistant Staphylococcus aureus in Canadian hospitals: 5 years of national surveillance. CMAJ 2001;165:21-26.
290. van Belkum A, Verbrugh H. 40 years of methicillin resistant Staphylococcus aureus. BMJ. 2001;323:644-645.
291. Wenzel RP, Nettleman MD, Jones RN, et al. Methicillin-resistant Staphylococcus aureus: Implications for the 1990s and effective control measures. Am J Med. 1991;91(Suppl):221S-227S.
292. Centers for Disease Control and Prevention. Methicillin-resistant Staphylococcus aureus skin or soft tissue infections in a state prison—Mississippi, 2000. MMWR Morb Mortal Wkly Rep. 2001;50:919-922.
293. Centers for Disease Control and Prevention. Public Health Dispatch: Outbreaks of community-associated methicillin-resistant Staphylococcus aureus skin infection—Los Angeles County, California, 2002-2003. MMWR Morb Mortal Wkly Rep. 2003;52:88.
294. Groom AV, Wolsey DH, Naimi TS, et al. Community-acquired methicillin-resistant Staphylococcus aureus in a rural American Indian community. JAMA. 2001;286:1201-1205.
295. Fey PD, Saïd-Salim B, Rupp ME, et al. Comparative molecular analysis of community- or hospital-acquired methicillin-resistant Staphylococcus aureus. Antimicrob Agents Chemother. 2003;47:196-203.
296. Ma XX, Ito T, Tiensasitorn C, et al. Novel type of staphylococcal cassette chromosome mec identified in community-acquired methicillin-resistant Staphylococcus aureus strains. Antimicrob Agents Chemother. 2002;46:1147-1152.
297. Katayama Y, Ito T, Hiramatsu K. A new class of genetic element, staphylococcus cassette chromosome mec, encodes methicillin resistance in Staphylococcus aureus. Antimicrob Agents Chemother. 2000;44:1549-1555.
298. Okuma K, Iwakawa K, Turnidge JD, et al. Dissemination of new methicillin-resistant Staphylococcus aureus clones in the community. J Clin Microbiol. 2002;40: 4289-4294.
299. Hiramatsu K, Hanaki H, Ino T, et al. Methicillin-resistant Staphylococcus aureus clinical strain with reduced vancomycin susceptibility. J Antimicrob Chemother. 1997; 40:135-136.
300. Hiramatsu K, Aritaka N, Hanaki H, et al. Dissemination in Japanese hospitals of strains of Staphylococcus aureus heterogeneously resistant to vancomycin. Lancet. 1997;350:1670-1673.
301. Smith TL, Pearson ML, Wilcox KR, et al, for the Glycopeptide-Intermediate Staphylococcus aureus Working Group. Emergence of vancomycin resistance in Staphylococcus aureus. N Engl J Med. 1999;340:493-501.
302. Rotun SS, McMath V, Schoonmaker DJ, et al. Staphylococcus aureus with reduced susceptibility to vancomycin isolated from a patient with fatal bacteremia. Emerg Infect Dis. 1999;5:147-149.
303. Centers for Disease Control and Prevention. Staphylococcus aureus with reduced susceptibility to vancomycin—Illinois, 1999. MMWR Morb Mortal Wkly Rep. 2000; 48:1165-1167.
304. Ploy MC, Grélaud C, Martin C, et al. First clinical isolate of vancomycin-intermediate Staphylococcus aureus in a French hospital. Lancet. 1998;351:1212.
305. Howe RA, Bowker KE, Walsh TR, et al. Vancomycin-resistant Staphylococcus aureus. Lancet. 1998;351:602.
306. Bierbaum G, Fuchs K, Lenz W, et al. Presence of Staphylococcus aureus with reduced susceptibility to vancomycin in Germany. Eur J Clin Microbiol Infect Dis. 1999;18:691-696.
307. Tenover FC, Biddle JW, Lancaster MV. Increasing resistance to vancomycin and other glycopeptides in Staphylococcus aureus. Emerg Infect Dis. 2001;7:327-331.
308. Fridkin SK. Vancomycin-intermediate and -resistant Staphylococcus aureus: What the infectious disease specialist needs to know. Clin Infect Dis. 2001;32:108-115.
309. Chang S, Sievert DM, Hageman JC, et al. Infection with vancomycin-resistant Staphylococcus aureus containing the vanA resistance gene. N Engl J Med. 2003; 348:1342-1347.
310. Centers for Disease Control and Prevention. Public Health Dispatch: Vancomycin-resistant Staphylococcus aureus—Pennsylvania, 2002. MMWR Morb Mortal Wkly Rep. 2002;51:902.
311. Centers for Disease Control and Prevention. Staphylococcus aureus resistant to vancomycin—United States, 2002. MMWR Morb Mortal Wkly Rep. 2002;51:565-567.
312. Tenover FC, Lancaster MV, Hill BC, et al. Characterization of staphylococci with reduced susceptibilities to vancomycin and other glycopeptides. J Clin Microbiol. 1998;36:1020-1027.
313. Centers for Disease Control and Prevention. Interim guidelines for prevention and control of staphylococcal infection associated with reduced susceptibility to vancomycin. MMWR Morb Mortal Wkly Rep. 1997;46:626-628, 635-636.
314. Centers for Disease Control and Prevention. Recommendations for preventing the spread of vancomycin resistance: Recommendations of the Hospital Infection Control Practices Advisory Committee (HICPAC). MMWR Morb Mortal Wkly Rep. 1995;44(no. RR-12).
315. Leclercq R, Derlot E, Duval J, et al. Plasmid-mediated resistance to vancomycin and teicoplanin in Enterococcus faecium. N Engl J Med. 1988;319:157-161.
316. Kaplan AH, Gilligan PH, Facklam RR. Recovery of resistant enterococci during vancomycin prophylaxis. J Clin Microbiol. 1988;26:1216-1218.
317. National Nosocomial Infections Surveillance (NNIS) System Report, Data Summary from January 1992-June 2001, issued August 2001. Am J Infect Control. 2001;29:404-421.
318. Chavers LS, Moser SA, Benjamin WH, et al. Vancomycin-resistant enterococci: 15 years and counting. J Hosp Infect. 2003;53:159-171.
319. Rice LB. Emergence of vancomycin-resistant enterococci. Emerg Infect Dis. 2001;7:183-187.
320. Low DE, Keller N, Barth A, et al. Clinical prevalence, antimicrobial susceptibility, and geographic resistance patterns of enterococci: Results from the Sentry Antimicrobial Surveillance Program, 1997-1999. Clin Infect Dis. 2001;15(Suppl): S133-S145.
321. Prystowsky J, Siddiqui F, Chosay J, et al. Resistance to linezolid: Characterization of their occurrences in vancomycin-resistant enterococci. Antimicrob Agents Chemother. 2001;45:2154-2156.
322. Karlowsky JA, Zhanel GG, Hoban DJ. Vancomycin-resistant enterococci (VRE) colonization of high-risk patients in tertiary care Canadian hospitals. Canadian VRE Surveillance Group. Diagn Microbiol Infect Dis. 1999;35:1-7.
323. Paulsen IT, Eanerjei L, Mysers GSA, et al. Role of mobile DNA in the evolution of vancomycin-resistant Enterococcus faecalis. Science. 2003;299:2071-2074.
324. Centers for Disease Control and Prevention. Preventing pneumococcal disease among infants and young children: Recommendations of the Advisory Committee on Immunization Practices (ACIP). MMWR Morb Mortal Wkly Rep. 2000;49(RR09): 1-38.
325. Campbell GD Jr, Silberman R. Drug-resistant Streptococcus pneumoniae. Clin Infect Dis. 1998;26:1188-1195.
326. Breiman RF, Butler JC, Tenover FC, et al. Emergence of drug-resistant pneumococcal infections in the United States. JAMA. 1994;271:1831-1835.
327. Whitney CG, Farley MM, Hadler J, et al. Increasing prevalence of multidrug-resistant Streptococcus pneumoniae in the United States. N Engl J Med. 2000;343:1917-1924.
328. Forward KR. The epidemiology of penicillin resistance in Streptococcus pneumoniae. Semin Respir Infect. 1999;14:243-254.
329. Collignon PJ, Turnidge JD. Antibiotic resistance in Streptococcus pneumoniae. Med J Aust. 2000;173(Suppl):S58-S64.
330. Spika JS, Facklam RR, Plikaytis BD, et al. Antimicrobial resistance of Streptococcus pneumoniae in the United States, 1979-1987. J Infect Dis. 1991;163:1273-1278.
331. Palleres R, Liñares J, Vadillo M, et al. Resistance to penicillin and cephalosporin and mortality from severe pneumococcal pneumonia in Barcelona, Spain. N Engl J Med. 1995;333:474-480.
332. Friedland IR. Comparison of response to antimicrobial therapy of penicillin-resistant and penicillin-susceptible pneumococcal disease. Pediatr Infect Dis J. 1995;14: 885-890.

333. Friedland IR, McCracken GH Jr. Management of infections caused by antibiotic-resistant *Streptococcus pneumoniae*. N Engl J Med. 1994;331:377-382.

334. Pradier C, Dunais B, Carsenti-Etesse H, et al. Pneumococcal resistance patterns in Europe. Eur J Clin Microbiol Infect Dis. 1997;16:644-647.

335. Miller E, Waight P, Efstratiou A, et al. Epidemiology of invasive and other pneumococcal disease in children in England and Wales, 1996-1998. Acta Paediatr Suppl. 2000;89:11-16.

336. Reacher MH, Shah A, Livermore DM, et al. Bacteraemia and antibiotic resistance of its pathogens reported in England and Wales between 1990 and 1998: Trend analysis. BMJ. 2000;320:213-216.

337. Lyon DJ, Scheel O, Fung KS, et al. Rapid emergence of penicillin-resistant pneumococci in Hong Kong. Scand J Infect Dis. 1996;28:375-376.

338. Echaniz-Aviles G, Velazquez-Meza ME, Carnalla-Barajas MN, et al. Antimicrobial susceptibilities and capsular types of invasive *Streptococcus pneumoniae* isolated in children in Mexico City. Microb Drug Resist. 1997;3:153-157.

339. Ringertz S, Muhe L, Krantz I, et al. Prevalence of potential respiratory disease bacteria in children in Ethiopia: Antimicrobial susceptibility of the pathogens and use of antibiotics among the children. Acta Paediatr. 1993;82:843-848.

340. Doern GV, Pfaller MA, Erwin ME, et al. The prevalence of fluoroquinolone resistance among clinically significant respiratory tract isolates of *Streptococcus pneumoniae* in the United States and Canada—1997 results from the SENTRY Antimicrobial Surveillance Program. Diagn Microbiol Infect Dis. 1998;32:313-316.

341. Chen DK, McGeer A, de Azavedo JC, et al. Decreased susceptibility of *Streptococcus pneumoniae* to fluoroquinolones in Canada. Canadian Bacterial Surveillance Network. N Engl J Med. 1999;341:233-239.

342. Centers for Disease Control and Prevention. Resistance of *Streptococcus pneumoniae* to fluoroquinolones—United States, 1995-1999. MMWR Morb Mortal Wkly Rep. 2001;50:800-804.

343. Eskola J, Kilpi T, Palmu A, et al. Efficacy of a pneumococcal conjugate vaccine against acute otitis media. N Engl J Med. 2001;344:403-409.

344. Black S, Shinefield H, Fireman B, et al. Efficacy, safety, and immunogenicity of heptavalent pneumococcal conjugate vaccine in children. Pediatr Infect Dis J. 2000;19:187-195.

345. Whitney CG, Farley MM, Hadler J. Decline in invasive pneumococcal disease after the introduction of protein-polysaccharide conjugate vaccine. N Engl J Med. 2003;348:1737-1746.

346. Engels D, Madaras T, Nyandwi S, et al. Epidemic dysentery caused by *Shigella dysenteriae* type 1: A sentinel site surveillance of antimicrobial resistance patterns in Burundi. Bull World Health Organ. 1995;73:787-791.

347. Riley LW, Cohen ML, Seals JE, et al. Importance of host factors in human salmonellosis caused by multiresistant strains of *Salmonella*. J Infect Dis. 1984;149:878-883.

348. Lee LA, Puhr ND, Maloney EK, et al. Increase in antimicrobial-resistant *Salmonella* infections in the United States, 1989-1990. J Infect Dis. 1994;170:128-134.

349. National Antimicrobial Resistance Monitoring System: 1997 Annual Report. Atlanta: Centers for Disease Control and Prevention; 1998.

350. Threlfall EJ, Frost JA, Ward LR, et al. Increasing spectrum of resistance in multiresistant *Salmonella typhimurium*. Lancet. 1996;347:1053-1054.

351. Glynn MK, Bopp C, Dewitt W, et al. Emergence of multidrug-resistant *Salmonella enterica* serotype Typhimurium DT104 infections in the United States. N Engl J Med. 1998;338:1333-1338.

352. Threlfall EJ, Ward LR, Rowe B. Increasing incidence of resistance to trimethoprim and ciprofloxacin in epidemic *Salmonella typhimurium* DT104 in England and Wales. Eurosurveillance. 1997;2:81-84.

353. Molbak K, Baggesen DL, Aarestrup FM, et al. An outbreak of multi-drug-resistant, quinolone-resistant *Salmonella enterica* serotype typhimurium DT104. N Engl J Med. 1999;341:1420-1425.

354. Hakanen A, Kotilainen P, Jalava J, et al. Detection of decreased fluoroquinolone susceptibility in *Salmonella* and validation of nalidixic acid screening test. J Clin Microbiol. 1999;37:3572-3577.

355. Helms M, Vastrup P, Gerner-Smidt P, et al. Excess mortality associated with antimicrobial drug-resistant *Salmonella typhimurium*. Emerg Infect Dis. 2002;8:490-495.

356. Witte W. Medical consequences of antibiotic use in agriculture. Science. 1998;279:996-997.

357. Angulo FJ, Johnson KR, Tauxe RV, et al. Origins and consequences of antimicrobial-resistant nontyphoidal *Salmonella*: Implications for the use of fluoroquinolones in food animals. Microb Drug Resist. 2000;6:77-83.

358. Threlfall EJ, Ward LR, Frost JA, et al. The emergence and spread of antibiotic resistance in food-borne bacteria. Int J Food Microbiol. 2000;62:1-5.

359. Centers for Disease Control and Prevention. Outbreak of multidrug-resistant *Salmonella* Newport—United States, January-April 2002. MMWR Morb Mortal Wkly Rep. 2002;51:545-548.

360. Gupta A, Fontana J, Crowe C, et al. Emergence of multidrug-resistant *Salmonella enterica* serotype Newport infections resistant to expanded-spectrum cephalosporins in the United States. J Infect Dis. 2003;188:1707-1716.

361. Centers for Disease Control and Prevention. Sexually Transmitted Disease Surveillance 2001 Supplement: Gonococcal Isolate Surveillance Project (GISP) Annual Report 2001. Atlanta: U.S. Department of Health and Human Services; October 2002.

362. Knapp JS, Fox KK, Trees D, et al. Fluoroquinolone resistance in *Neisseria gonorrhoeae*. Emerg Infect Dis. 1997;3:33-39.

363. Kam KM, Lo K-K, Ng K-Y-H, et al. Rapid decline in penicillinase-producing *Neisseria gonorrhoeae* in Hong Kong associated with emerging 4-fluoroquinolone resistance. Genitourin Med. 1995;71:141-144.

364. Tanaka M, Nakayama H, Haraoka M, et al. Antimicrobial resistance of *Neisseria gonorrhoeae* and high prevalence of ciprofloxacin-resistant isolates in Japan, 1993 to 1998. J Clin Microbiol. 2000;38:521-525.

365. WHO Western Pacific Gonococcal Antimicrobial Surveillance Programme. Surveillance of antibiotic resistance in *Neisseria gonorrhoeae* in the WHO Western Pacific Region, 2000. Commun Dis Intelligence. 2001;25:274-277.

366. Centers for Disease Control and Prevention. Increases in fluoroquinolone-resistant *Neisseria gonorrhoeae*—Hawaii and California, 2001. MMWR Morb Mortal Wkly Rep. 2002;51:1041-1044.

367. Ye S, Su X, Wang Q, et al. Surveillance of antibiotic resistance of *Neisseria gonorrhoeae* isolates in China, 1993-1998. Sex Transm Dis. 2002;29:242-245.

368. Mavroidi A, Tzouvelekis LS, Tassios PT, et al. Characterization of *Neisseria gonorrhoeae* strains with decreased susceptibility to fluoroquinolones isolated in Greece from 1996 to 1999. J Clin Microbiol. 2000;38:3489-3491.

369. Su X, Lind I. Molecular basis of high-level ciprofloxacin resistance in *Neisseria gonorrhoeae* strains isolated in Denmark from 1995 to 1998. Antimicrob Agents Chemother. 2001;45:117-123.

370. deNeeling AJ, van Santen-Verheuvel M, Spaargaren J, et al. Antimicrobial resistance of *Neisseria gonorrhoeae* and emerging ciprofloxacin resistance in the Netherlands, 1991 to 1998. Antimicrob Agents Chemother. 2000;44:3184-3185.

371. Dan M, Poch F, Sheinberg B. High prevalence of high-level ciprofloxacin resistance in *Neisseria gonorrhoeae* in Tel Aviv, Israel: Correlation with response to therapy. Antimicrob Agents Chemother. 2002;46:1671-1673.

372. Yagupsky P, Schahar A, Peled N, et al. Increasing incidence of gonorrhea in Israel associated with countrywide dissemination of a ciprofloxacin-resistant strain. Eur J Clin Microbiol Infect Dis. 2002;21:368-372.

373. Trees DL, Sirivongrangson P, Schultz AJ, et al. Multiclonal increase in ciprofloxacin-resistant *Neisseria gonorrhoeae*, Thailand, 1998-1999. Sex Transm Dis. 2002;29:668-673.

374. Knapp JS, Washington JA, Doyle LJ, et al. Persistence of *Neisseria gonorrhoeae* strains with decreased susceptibilities to ciprofloxacin and ofloxacin in Cleveland, Ohio, from 1992 through 1993. Antimicrob Agents Chemother. 1994;38:2194-2196.

375. Gordon SM, Carlyn CJ, Doyle LJ, et al. The emergence of *Neisseria gonorrhoeae* with decreased susceptibility to ciprofloxacin in Cleveland, Ohio: Epidemiology and risk factors. Ann Intern Med. 1996;125:465-470.

376. Trees DL, Sandul AL, Neal SW, et al. Molecular epidemiology of *Neisseria gonorrhoeae* exhibiting decreased susceptibility and resistance to ciprofloxacin in Hawaii, 1991-1999. Sex Transm Dis. 2001;28:309-314.

377. Webby RJ, Webster RG. Are we ready for pandemic influenza? Science. 2003;302:1519-1522.

378. World Health Organization. Avian influenza A(H5N1) in humans in Viet Nam and in poultry in Asian countries—update 2, January 16, 2003. Available at http://www.who.int/csr/don/2004_01_16/en/

379. Gerberding JL, Hughes JM, Koplan JP. Bioterrorism preparedness and response: Clinicians and public health agencies as essential partners. JAMA. 2002;287:898-900.

380. Hughes JM. The SARS response-building and assessing an evidence-based approach to future global microbial threats. JAMA. 2003;290:3251-3253.

CHAPTER **14**

Hospital Preparedness for Emerging and Highly Contagious Infectious Diseases

Getting Ready for SARS or Whatever Comes Next

DAVID K. HENDERSON

The events of the past 5 years have made it clear that health care institutions have an unprecedented need to be prepared for a variety of problems that would have been considered unimaginable only 10 years ago.[1] The horrifying events of September 11, 2001, the intentional release of anthrax as a weapon of bioterrorism, the emergence of West Nile virus as a pathogen in the United States, the epidemic of severe acute respiratory syndrome (SARS), the zoonotic spread of monkeypox in the United States, and the effort to vaccinate health care workers against smallpox because of concerns about its potential release as an agent of bioterrorism—each underscores the necessity for a new level of preparedness for health care institutions. The purpose of this chapter is to assess what we have learned from these and other recent events in terms of preparing our institutions for biologic, hospital, and public health emergencies and to outline some basic principles to use in preparing health care institutions for managing patients infected with highly contagious pathogens.

GENERAL EMERGENCY PREPAREDNESS

Every health care institution should develop a general emergency preparedness plan. Details of such plans are well beyond the scope of this chapter; however, general guidelines for the development of preparedness plans can be found on the Internet at a variety of reliable publicly and privately sponsored sites. Ferguson and her colleagues have recently identified 43 websites that are highly relevant to bioterrorism preparedness for infectious disease clinicians and epidemiologists.[2] They classify these websites into several categories, including general purpose sites, biologic agent information, laboratory information, infection control reference materials, epidemiology information, mental health information, preparedness resources, clinical and public education materials, and research resources.[2]

At my own institution, the Clinical Center of the National Institutes of Health (NIH), we have found it useful to develop both a detailed emergency management plan and a quick-reference flipchart (Fig. 14-1) that is readily available to staff throughout the institution. The flipchart contains important information about plan activation, appropriate first responses, hospital evacuation routes, and information germane to specific types of emergencies (e.g., fire, biologic, radiologic, chemical, and explosive). These flipcharts hang on the walls on each of our inpatient and outpatient care sites in highly conspicuous places. Although these charts are not all-encompassing, they do contain easily accessible core information that staff can use for both education and emergent direction.

To be able to respond appropriately to emergency situations, institutions need to create teams that can respond quickly and decisively when events require emergency or immediate action. These teams should be strategically constructed to include individuals who possess a broad range of competencies, including safety, hospital epidemiology, building management, information systems, nursing, medicine, law enforcement, fire safety, hospital administration, finance, human resources, pharmacy, material handling, and communication. Although institutions cannot plan for every possible contingency, they can develop systems and processes that have sufficient flexibility to allow the institution to be able to respond quickly to a variety of different types of emergencies. Once the team is in place, the institution must practice implementing and managing responses to a variety of different kinds of emergencies. In this so-called pre-event planning, both tabletop and full disaster drills are critical components of emergency preparedness. Practicing responses will provide remarkably useful insight into what works and what does not, and what systems and processes need to be redesigned, reconfigured, or restructured to optimize the responsiveness of the institution.

Surge Capacity

An issue that must be addressed by emergency departments and by an institution's administration in the emergency preparedness planning process is characterization of the institution's and the community's surge capacity.[3-5] Communities and community-based health care institutions need to develop strategies for managing large numbers of patients who have epidemic infections or other types of casualties. In addition, as part of its planning for emergency preparedness, each institution should develop plans for creating as much surge capacity as it can by developing plans to transfer patients, by

discharging patients who can be discharged, by canceling elective admissions and procedures, by commissioning units that have been decommissioned, and by studying institutional air-handling and infrastructure to see how large numbers of patients who have highly contagious diseases can be cared for (see later). The importance of understanding the flow of patients into the institution during an acute emergency—either infectious or noninfectious—cannot be overstressed. Developing the capacity to provide emergency care to the patients who arrive in the second or third wave of an epidemic or catastrophe, who are frequently more ill than those in the first wave, is a key part of emergency preparedness. Similarly, the institution must work closely with the other health care organizations as well as with the public health authorities in the local community and in the geographic region to develop a community-wide or region-wide approach to the management of mass casualties.

Communication

Finally, a critical part of general emergency preparedness is communication. Effective communication strategies are essential not only within your own institution but also with other institutions in your community, as well as with local and regional public health authorities. A detailed communications plan, including the creation of an institutional communications core or command/control center, and a highly functioning local and regional communications network are integral parts of every emergency preparedness plan. Figure 14-2 is a schematic diagram of the structural elements of the communications plan for the NIH Clinical Center.

INFECTION CONTROL PREPAREDNESS FOR HIGHLY CONTAGIOUS MICROORGANISMS

Rapid Diagnosis and Detection

Perhaps the single most important approach to managing highly contagious diseases in the health care setting is maintaining a high index of suspicion for these diagnoses. Highly contagious emerging infections and other organisms that have the potential for epidemic spread (either as a result of natural infection or as a result of acts of bioterrorism) are listed in Table 14-1. Space does not permit a detailed discussion of management/response issues relevant to each of these agents; however, each is discussed in the relevant chapters of this textbook and, in addition, specific public health management responses for smallpox, plague, anthrax, tularemia, botulism, poliomyelitis, and hemorrhagic fever virus infections have been recently discussed in detail in the medical literature.[6-16]

For all of these infectious diseases, maintaining a high index of suspicion (especially in epidemic settings) will facilitate the immediate and appropriate use of isolation and containment strategies when these patients present to the hospital. Emergency room staff must be particularly attuned to these diagnoses, as they represent the first line of institutional defense. Clearly, the greatest risks for nosocomial and occupational transmission of these epidemic infectious disease agents arise when the diagnosis is not suspected and the index patient is neither diagnosed nor isolated appropriately. One of the most important lessons learned from the SARS epidemic is that spread to health care providers occurred primarily when the diagnosis of the index case was not appreciated, the patient was not isolated appropriately, and health care providers were not using appropriate isolation procedures, including the appropriate personal protective devices (discussed later). Although rapid diagnosis remains a formidable problem in many epidemic settings, advancing technology has made new, rapid diagnostic tests for many of these pathogens a reality,[17-23] including the recent development of a TaqMan 5′ hydrolysis fluorogenic polymerase chain reaction (PCR) that is able to detect potential pathogens (e.g., *Francisella tularensis* in tissues of infected mice)[18] using a hand-held portable fluorescence thermocycler designed for use in the field. In any event, maintaining vigilance and a high index of suspicion for contagious infectious diseases simply

FIGURE 14-1. Emergency management flipchart used at the NIH Clinical Center.

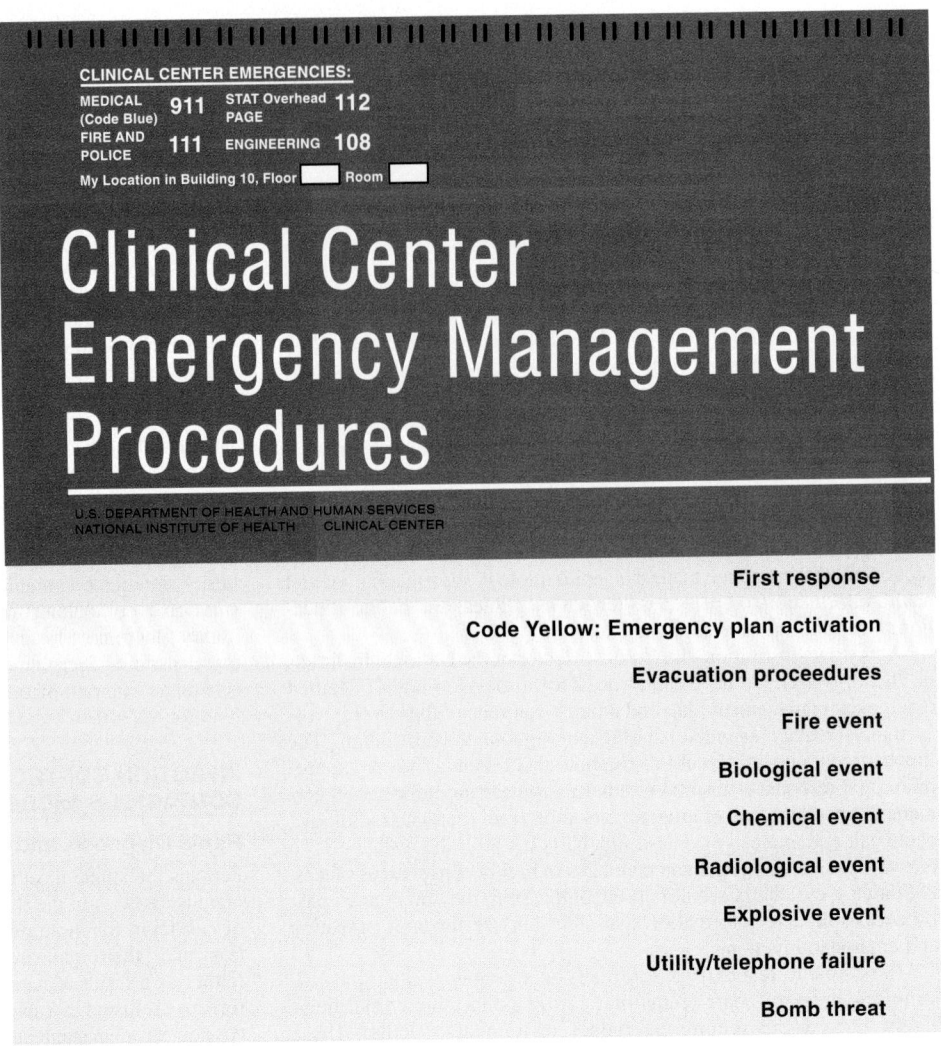

CLINICAL CENTER EMERGENCIES:

MEDICAL (Code Blue)	911	STAT Overhead PAGE	112
FIRE AND POLICE	111	ENGINEERING	108

My Location in Building 10, Floor ▢   Room ▢

Clinical Center Emergency Management Procedures

U.S. DEPARTMENT OF HEALTH AND HUMAN SERVICES
NATIONAL INSTITUTE OF HEALTH   CLINICAL CENTER

First response

Code Yellow: Emergency plan activation

Evacuation proceedures

Fire event

Biological event

Chemical event

Radiological event

Explosive event

Utility/telephone failure

Bomb threat

---

must become a high priority for health care institutions in the United States, as this practice will afford by far the most effective first-line defense against the nosocomial spread of these organisms.

Syndromic Surveillance for Outbreak Detection

In addition to rapid laboratory tests to detect suspected pathogens, institutions across the United States have set up syndromic surveillance techniques that can detect clusters of these types of infections and rapidly notify emergency departments in hospitals that an epidemic may be occurring, with the result that this can be accomplished much sooner than would have been possible in the past.[24-30] A number of different approaches have been used to conduct syndromic surveillance, but one of these systems, established jointly by several health plans and the Centers for Disease Control and Prevention (CDC), provides national coverage that includes more than 20 million subscribers of the plans. This system can be "set" to assess daily counts of individuals who have specific syndromes in defined geographic regions. The system protects the medical privacy of the affected individuals and is less labor-intense than similar reporting systems.[30] Use of these syndromic surveillance systems will very likely make it possible for institutions to share information about potential epidemics far faster than has ever been possible, thereby decreasing the window of opportunity for control of transmission of these infections.

Policies, Procedures, and Administrative Controls

The major concern about managing patients who have highly contagious diseases in the hospital is the concern for spread to staff, to other patients, to visitors, and to the families of individuals who have nosocomial or occupational exposures. Although the early days of the human immunodeficiency virus/acquired immunodeficiency syndrome (HIV/AIDS) epidemic in the 1980s taught us a great deal about managing unknown transmission risks in the hospital, the SARS epidemic of 2002/2003 was perhaps even more instructive. By the time most institutions were aware that they were hospitalizing patients with AIDS, the CDC had provided institutions and providers with reasonably clear indications about the epidemiology and routes of transmission for this disease, and at least some early suggestion about the magnitude of risk for occupational/nosocomial transmission. HIV/AIDS—from its earliest identification—appeared to be a blood-borne and sexually transmitted disease. Early evaluation of HIV epidemiology suggested that risk for occupational/nosocomial transmission was likely to be present; however, the risks and routes of transmission appeared to be similar to (or perhaps even substantially smaller than) the known risk for occupational infection with other blood-borne pathogens. Although the management of HIV-infected patients was initially associated with considerable angst and turmoil among staff in our own hospital, educating staff members about the

FIGURE 14-2. Schematic diagram illustrating an organizational communication plan for emergencies.

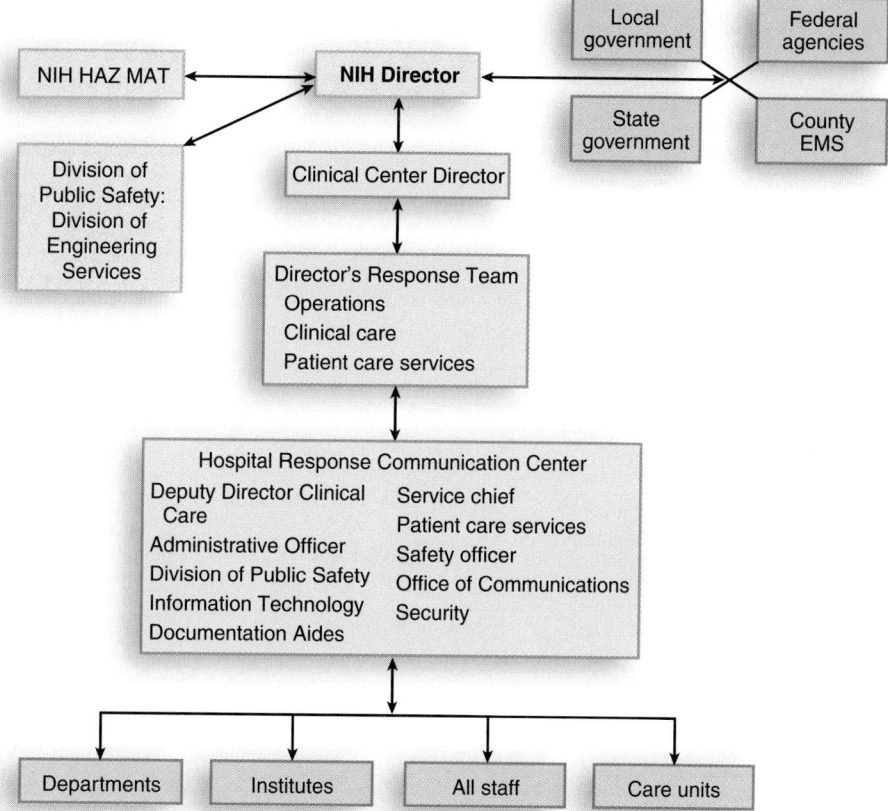

risks as we learned about them and ensuring that staff members understood the epidemiologic similarities of the new disease to other blood-borne pathogens that had long been prevalent (and presenting substantial risk) in the health care setting provided a convenient framework for thinking about the new disease.

On the other hand, the SARS epidemic presented institutions with a disease that had a less clear (and, at some level, perhaps even more frightening) epidemiology. The majority of cases appeared to be transmitted by close personal contact (i.e., in a manner like that of known human coronavirus or rhinovirus infections); however, instances also occurred in which numbers of exposed individuals were infected by so-called supershedders or superspreaders.[31,32] In China, Hanoi, Hong Kong, and Toronto, many, if not most, of the individuals infected by these superspreading patients were health care workers.[32-41] Because of the less-than-clear epidemiology, the potential for droplet or airborne spread, and the apparent risks for hospital staff, health care providers,[42,43] and of course the public,[44] substantial concern was generated about the potential for uncontrollable spread of SARS in health care institutions and in the community.

Intentional release of certain diseases thought to represent a threat for bioterrorism (e.g., plague, smallpox, tularemia, and perhaps the viral hemorrhagic fevers [see Table 14-1]) would almost certainly provoke similar (if not more substantial) community and institutional responses. Because of the potential for chaos associated with the presence of patients infected with any of these types of pathogens in health care institutions, all institutions should develop policies and procedures to manage patients who have highly contagious diseases in the hospital. Examples of policies developed specifically for managing

patients who have highly contagious diseases at the Clinical Center are listed in Table 14-2.

In the setting of an epidemic (for example, a SARS epidemic), institutions in areas experiencing the epidemic should have in place strategies for monitoring fever and respiratory symptoms in hospitalized patients and visitors and should maintain a high level of vigilance and continued surveillance—even after the epidemic appears to be receding. This very high index of suspicion should be applied consistently, not only to all patients (including those admitted for reasons other than those directly linked to the epidemic) but also to all staff members who develop any signs or symptoms consistent with the disease. Failure to do so very likely contributed to the spread of infection in the second wave of the SARS epidemic in Toronto in 2003.[34]

ISOLATION TECHNIQUE AND PERSONAL PROTECTIVE EQUIPMENT

Certain of the specific issues, policies, and procedures outlined in Table 14-2 are worthy of additional discussion and emphasis. Perhaps paramount among these issues is the appropriate use of isolation precautions.

Experience from the SARS epidemic of 2002/2003 demonstrated that use of appropriate isolation techniques for these patients could result in the successful containment of the infection in the hospital—even in countries that had extremely limited infection control resources. In the 2002/2003 epidemic, SARS appeared to be transmitted primarily by close personal contact, with occasional instances of (presumably) droplet or airborne spread associated with the superspreaders. Developing strategies that limited opportunities for nosocomial

TABLE 14-1 Highly Contagious Agents and Agents of Known Bioterrorism Potential

Agents/Diseases in Category A
Anthrax—*Bacillus anthracis*
Botulism—*Clostridium botulinum* (toxin)
Plague—*Yersinia pestis*
Smallpox—*Variola major*
Tularemia—*Francisella tularensis*
Viral hemorrhagic fevers (filoviruses [e.g., Ebola, Marburg] and arenaviruses [e.g., Lassa, Machupo])

Agents/Diseases in Category B
Brucellosis (*Brucella* spp.)
Clostridium perfringens (Epsilon toxin)
Food safety threats
 Salmonella species
 Escherichia coli O157:H7
 Shigella spp.
Glanders—*Burkholderia mallei*
Melioidosis—*Burkholderia pseudomallei*
Psittacosis—*Chlamydia psittaci*
Q fever—*Coxiella burnetii*
Ricinus communis (castor beans) (ricin toxin)
Staphylococcal enterotoxin B
Typhus fever—*Rickettsia prowazekii*
Viral encephalitis (alphaviruses [e.g., Venezuelan equine encephalitis, eastern equine encephalitis, western equine encephalitis])
Water safety threats
 Vibrio cholerae
 Cryptosporidium parvum

Agents/Diseases in Category C
Nipah virus
Hantavirus

Agents/Diseases Not Listed in CDC Categories but Having Substantial Epidemic Potential
Pandemic influenza
Severe acute respiratory syndrome (SARS) coronavirus
Orthopoxviruses other than Variola (e.g., monkeypox)

Definitions

Category A
Could be easily disseminated or transmitted from person to person
May result in high mortality rates and have the potential for major public health impact
Might cause public panic and social disruption
Requires special action for public health preparedness

Category B
Are moderately easily disseminated
May result in moderate morbidity rates and relatively low mortality rates
Requires enhancements of diagnostic capacity and enhanced disease surveillance

Category C
Includes emerging pathogens that could be engineered for mass dissemination
Broadly available
Easily produced and disseminated
Potential for high morbidity and mortality rates and major health impact

Modified from Centers for Disease Control and Prevention. Biological agents/diseases, by category: Public health emergency preparedness and response. Available at http://www.bt.cdc.gov/agent/agentlist-category.asp#a.

TABLE 14-2 Issues, Policies, and Procedures for Management of Hospital Patients Who Have Highly Contagious Diseases

1. Strict isolation procedures (or, alternatively, special categories of isolation that address unique features of a disease—e.g., "special respiratory precautions" for patients with SARS); for SARS, the CDC recommends a combination of "standard precautions," "contact precautions," and "airborne precautions."[56]
2. Procedure for patient arrival (preferably a flow sheet), including information about interhospital transfer
3. Procedure for cohorting the care of individuals infected with highly contagious infections
4. Admitting procedures
5. Procedure for patient intrahospital transport
6. Procedure identifying appropriate personal protective equipment and techniques for using it (i.e., donning, using, and removing) appropriate to the disease, including procedures for fit-testing of respirators, as appropriate[36,53]
7. Procedure for provision of safe consultative care—that is, for individuals not on the immediate care team (e.g., needed consultants) to enter the isolation room
8. Procedure for the use of a monitor to ensure compliance with infection control procedures and to identify potential breaks in technique that might result in opportunities for nosocomial spread
9. Emergency resuscitative (i.e., code blue) infection control procedures
10. Safe laboratory processing and specimen handling procedures[57,58]
11. Procedures for appropriate transport of laboratory (i.e., microbiology, chemistry, hematology, immunology, and transfusion medicine) specimens
12. Special sterilization and disinfection procedures, including procedures for cleaning and disinfecting endoscopes and bronchoscopes
13. Procedure for endotracheal intubation, sputum induction, nasopharyngeal wash, and other procedures that have substantial potential for aerosolization[54]
14. Procedure for essential radiologic (or other imaging) studies, including techniques for decontamination of films and equipment
15. Ambulatory care procedures for patients not requiring hospitalization or those requiring follow-up visits
16. Procedures for field visits, when appropriate
17. Anatomic and surgical pathology procedures (including autopsy procedures[59])
18. Procedures for managing infrastructure (i.e., to optimize isolation and air handling)
19. Procedures for limiting visitors and procedures for monitoring fever and respiratory symptoms among hospitalized patients and visitors
20. Procedures for working with public health authorities and with surrounding institutions to address the conjoint management of large numbers of patients in an epidemic setting
21. Special surgical infection-control procedures (see text)
22. Procedures for screening and triage of staff and visitors for signs and symptoms of the epidemic disease[61]
23. Procedure for surveillance and detection of exposures and infections among staff participating in the care of patients with the epidemic infectious disease[60]
24. Procedure for managing health care workers who have had exposures to patients with the epidemic disease, including the use of administrative leave and quarantine, if necessary
25. Procedure for isolating a building, floor, or significant geographic area in the institution to be able to provide safe care for large numbers of infected patients while not placing other patients and staff at risk

spread and that emphasized the *control* aspect of infection control became the primary operative strategy for institutions dealing directly with the epidemic. Designing and implementing appropriate isolation procedures for highly contagious diseases are crucial for institutional containment of these infections. In the setting of a putative epidemic, isolation strategies should be tailored specifically to the disease or epidemic circumstances.

As a general rule, the approach that we have taken at the NIH Clinical Center is to begin with conservative guidelines and then to relax the guidelines as reliable information suggests it is safe to do so. For example, our first patients with AIDS were hospitalized in April of 1981, well in advance of the identification of the syndrome. When we

learned that this syndrome appeared to represent an epidemic of a transmissible infectious disease, we developed conservative isolation guidelines for the management of these patients. As the blood-borne and sexually transmitted epidemiology of the disease became increasingly apparent, we modulated and reformatted the guidelines to reflect the new information.

Similarly, at the beginning of the 2002/2003 SARS epidemic, while preparing for SARS patients to be admitted to the NIH Clinical Center and anticipating our participation in clinical research protocols studying the pathogenesis, immunopathogenesis, and natural history of SARS, our staff was expressing substantial anxiety about the risks that patients with this potentially highly contagious disease presented to the often severely immunocompromised patients at the Clinical

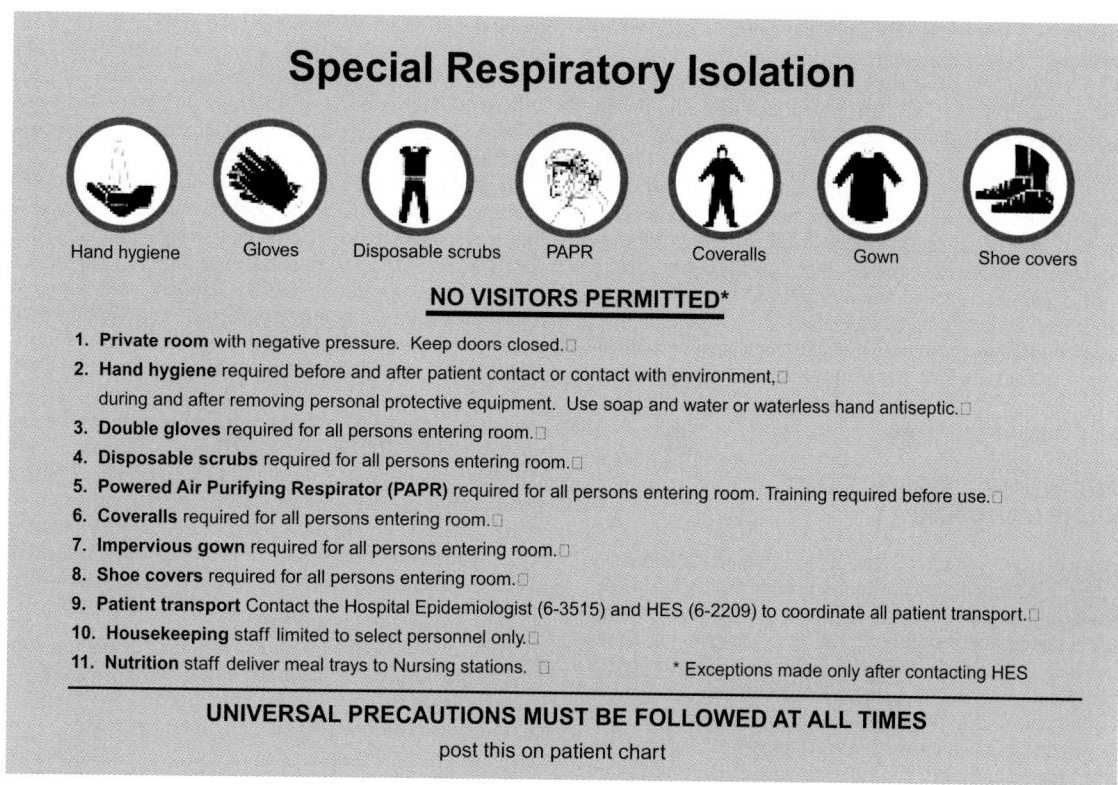

FIGURE 14-3. Isolation placard used at the NIH Clinical Center for patients requiring special respiratory isolation precautions.

Center. We developed a new category of isolation, called *special respiratory precautions* (Fig. 14-3), to use when caring for these patients (and others infected with pathogens transmitted in a similar fashion) and extensively trained our staff about the epidemiology, transmissibility, and effective prevention strategies for this new syndrome.

Because of the remarkable over-representation of health care workers among patients infected with the SARS virus,[34,36,40,45-50] we also developed a policy requiring cohorting of primary care personnel. We designed a small area on two units where these protocol patients would be safely housed, and we developed immediately proximate staging areas for staff, so that staff providing care for the SARS patients would have extremely limited, if any, interaction with staff providing care for other patients (e.g., at the nurses' station).

Use of appropriate personal protective devices is another important aspect of any successful approach to containing infectious diseases in health care institutions. General guidelines for the use of personal protective devices are included in the overall CDC infection control guidelines.[51,52] Specific approaches to the use of personal protective equipment should be tailored to what is known about the risks and routes of transmission of the disease in question. Because of the early concern about the potential for airborne and droplet transmission of the SARS coronavirus, we initially elected to recommend the use of extremely conservative respiratory protection (i.e., the routine use of powered, air-purifying respirators [PAPRs] for the care of these patients). The CDC initially recommended the use of N-95 (or N-99 or N-100) respirators for the care of SARS patients[53] but subsequently also commented that, for certain procedures associated with a high risk for aerosol formation (e.g., endotracheal intubation, bronchoscopy), the use of higher levels of protection (e.g., PAPRs) may be advisable.[54]

One important component of any respiratory protection program in a health care institution is ensuring that staff members are both familiar with the respiratory protection devices in use and are comfortable with their use. For all respirators, a fit-testing program is essential to ensure that the staff members are entirely aware of how the devices work and how they can ensure maximal safety.[53] In the case of N-95, N-99, and N-100 masks, attaining a facial seal is a crucial component of safe and effective use. In the Toronto SARS epidemic, some infections occurred in health care providers as a result of the inappropriate or ineffective use of "N-95-equivalent" respirators.[36] It was believed that some instances of nosocomial SARS virus transmission in the Toronto epidemic were most likely to be due to failure of the health care worker to protect the ocular mucous membranes from droplet contamination (even though an N-95 equivalent mask was worn).[36] Thus, if an N-95 mask is chosen for this type of isolation, protective eyewear or face shields should also be used. If and when information becomes available that clarifies the nosocomial epidemiology and that identifies risks for superspreader status, we may be able to relax our initial guidelines. Although in the earliest experience with this agent, primary risk for spread appeared to be by direct or close personal contact, some infections occurred (both in the Metropole Hotel in Hong Kong[55] and at health care institutions in Toronto)[36,45] in the absence of close contact. Again, airborne transmission could not be excluded for these cases, and for this reason, we decided that initially maintaining a conservative approach was most prudent.

Because of the risk for environmental spread of the SARS coronavirus (suggested in some nosocomial cases and at the Amoy Gardens apartment complex in Hong Kong),[55] the use of closely monitored contact precautions was also felt to be necessary. Gloves and gowns should be used routinely for care of these patients and should be managed carefully to minimize the risk for contamination as they are removed. Because of concern about the potential for inadvertent, unnoticed contamination, we also designed and implemented a nurse-monitor position for patients requiring this level of isolation precaution. This individual is positioned in the hall, retrieves supplies or other necessary items for the staff in the room, monitors compliance with infection control procedures, keeps a record of all individuals entering the room and the times of entry, and notifies staff when breaks in technique or potential for contamination may have occurred. The SARS coronavirus has been shown to be reasonably stable in the environment[55]; hence, the clear potential for fomite or environmental spread exists. Although the SARS virus appears to be relatively stable (for an RNA virus) in the environment, it is highly susceptible to most commercially available disinfectants or sterilants.[55] Because of the risk for environmental or fomite spread, disposable equipment and supplies should be used for these patients whenever possible. If patient care devices (e.g., stethoscopes) are to be reused on other patients, special attention should be paid to their disinfection after use on the epidemic cases.[56]

Other aspects of infection control that need to be carefully considered in epidemic settings include handling of laboratory specimens and specimen processing[57,58] and anatomic pathologic procedures (i.e., for autopsies and surgical specimens).[59]

HEALTH CARE WORKER SURVEILLANCE AND EXPOSURE MANAGEMENT

Institutions, particularly those directly involved in the management of infected patients during an epidemic, should develop strategies for detecting and managing staff who participate in the care of these patients as well as those who are inadvertently exposed to patients with the infection.[60] Surveillance of health care workers who are caring for SARS patients, working with specimens from these patients, or working in the same environment of care is essential for two reasons. First, surveillance will provide a mechanism to ensure that workers who become ill receive appropriate care. Second, individuals identified as infected can be placed in isolation to prevent transmission to family, patients, other employees, and visitors. Institutions should develop strategies that ensure that they can identify all personnel who enter the rooms of SARS patients or who participate in the care of these patients in other parts of the hospital. Personnel caring for SARS patients, working with specimens from these patients, or working in the immediate vicinity of the patients should be instructed to notify their occupational medicine program or the hospital epidemiology staff if they develop signs or symptoms consistent with infection. Institutions should also monitor the health care workforce for absenteeism increases. Finally, as noted earlier, institutions should promptly report clusters of respiratory infections to local and state health authorities.

In the SARS epidemics in Hong Kong, Singapore, Hanoi, Peking, and Toronto, health care workers who developed SARS transmitted infection to patients and staff within health care facilities, especially before the presence of the institutional epidemic was recognized. For this reason, staff members who sustain exposures to SARS patients should be placed on administrative leave for at least 10 days. The CDC recommends that exposed health care workers need not limit their activities outside of the health care setting but should undergo active surveillance for symptoms, including measurement of body temperature twice daily and monitoring for respiratory symptoms for 10 days after the exposure.[60] In light of the fact that infections occurred despite the attempted use of appropriate infection control procedures,[36] health care workers participating in the care of SARS patients should, in addition to following appropriate precautions, be instructed to monitor body temperature at least twice daily concurrently and for 10 days after the last exposure to a SARS patient. Institutions' occupational medicine or hospital epidemiology staff should regularly discuss the health status of each of these employees during her or his participation in care and for 10 days after the last contact with a SARS patient, specifically inquiring during each interaction about fever and respiratory symptoms.[60] Any health care worker being monitored in this fashion who develops fever or respiratory symptoms or both within 10 days after exposure should be instructed not to report for duty but rather to stay home and report the clinical status to the occupational medicine staff (or equivalent) immediately. If the health care worker requires clinical evaluation, arrangements should be made in advance with hospital staff to ensure that patients, staff, and visitors do not sustain exposures as a result of the health care worker's visit. Individuals who meet the SARS case definition should be placed into quarantine until at least 10 days after the resolution of all signs and symptoms. Every effort should be expended to ensure that the infected health care provider receives the best available care.

Instances in which the outcomes are less straightforward (e.g., the health care worker does not meet the surveillance case definition, the illness resolves rapidly) should be managed with an eye to minimizing risk. Current CDC recommendations suggest that workers whose illnesses improve or resolve within 72 hours after symptom onset be allowed to return to duty after appropriate consultation with both institutional hospital epidemiology staff and local public health authorities.[60] If the health care worker's illness does not meet the CDC case definition, but the individual has persistent symptoms, care should be individualized. The CDC recommends that precautions be continued for at least an additional 72 hours.[60] Although definitive laboratory studies for the diagnosis of SARS do not yet exist, SARS coronavirus serology tests or PCR detection of viral RNA for this virus may assist in clarifying cases that do not meet the surveillance case definition.[36]

A special case arises when a health care worker's symptoms begin while at work. Such individuals should do the following:

1. Immediately don a surgical mask
2. Immediately notify the supervisor, the occupational medicine staff, and the hospital epidemiology staff (so they can begin an outbreak investigation)
3. Immediately leave patient care areas

EDUCATION

Education of staff, patients, and visitors is crucial to being able to provide safe care for patients infected with highly contagious pathogens. Especially in situations in which the epidemiology, transmission routes, and transmissibility are incompletely understood, the role of candid, ongoing educational sessions for staff—underscoring what is known and what is not known about the disease, as well as what measures are being instituted to maximize safety and minimize risk—cannot be overemphasized. Patients admitted to the hospital for other reasons may also have substantial anxieties about risks for themselves and their families. Educational strategies, including the development of educational materials, lists of frequently asked questions and answers, flyers, videotapes, and even short didactic presentations designed for the lay public (providing ample time for discussion), are all strategies that may be useful in explaining how risks are being managed.

Communication of new findings and developments with institutional staff is a sine qua non for being able to continue to provide high-quality care in the hospital setting. As was the case with the HIV epidemic in the 1980s, staff members will be more at ease if they have confidence that the institution will share all new developments as soon as the institution becomes aware of them—even if the news is not all good. If staff members lack confidence in the institutional leadership, providing effective, safe care for patients who have highly contagious diseases, or for patients who have infectious diseases for which the epidemiology and transmissibility are not fully delineated, is likely to be extremely problematic if not impossible.

ENLISTING THE ASSISTANCE OF PATIENTS AND VISITORS—SCREENING

When concern exists about the potential for epidemic spread of infection (as occurred during the SARS epidemic), institutions should develop screening procedures for all individuals entering the hospital.[61] No one strategy for screening has been identified as being more effective than any other. In some countries, all individuals entering the country were aggressively screened for elevated temperatures, for res-

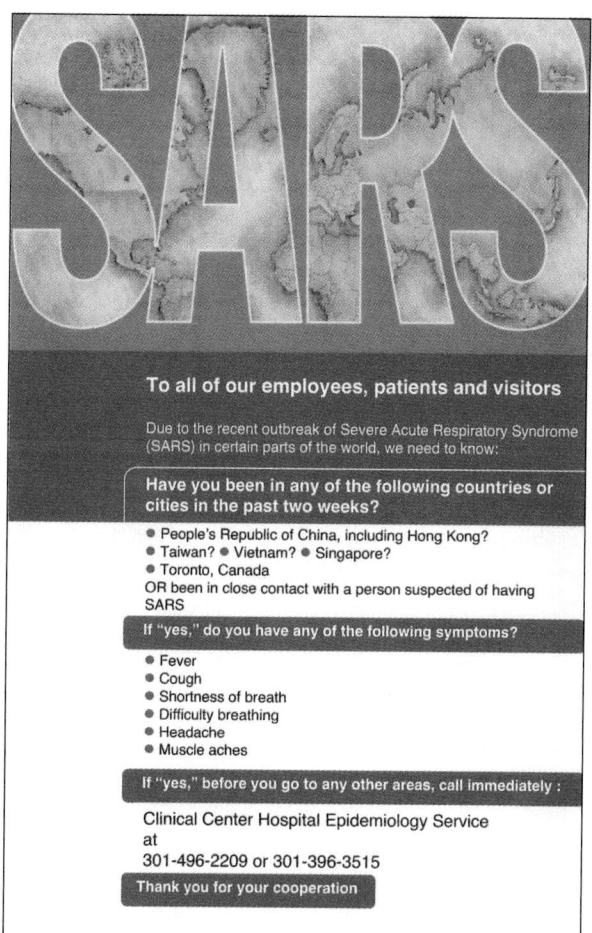

FIGURE 14-4. Self-screening poster used at the NIH Clinical Center to assist in identification of patients at risk for SARS coronavirus infection. *(Modified from a similar poster used at Johns Hopkins Hospital, courtesy of Johns Hopkins Medicine/Max Boam and Trish Perl, M.D., and used with permission.)*

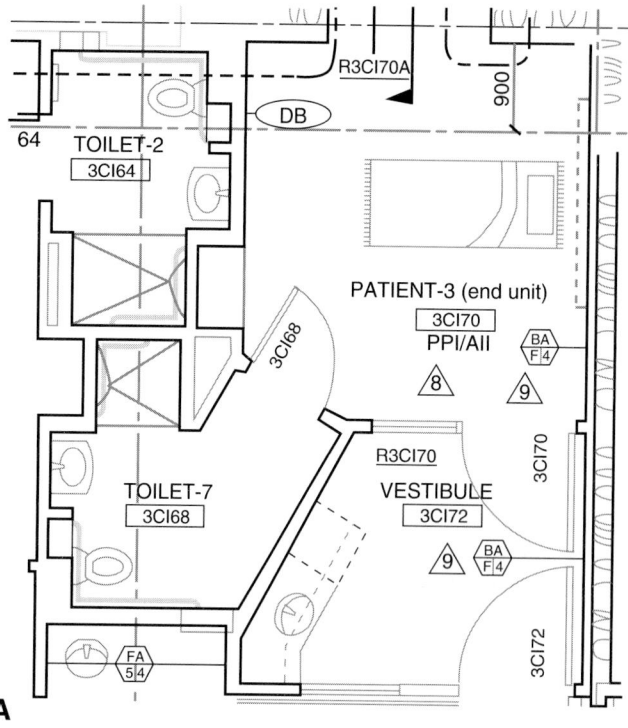

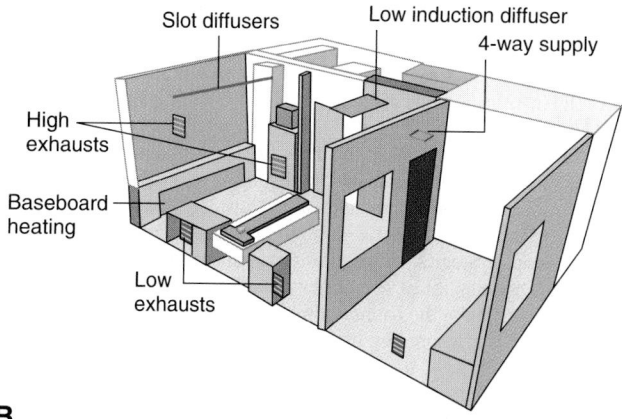

FIGURE 14-5. A, Schematic diagram of an isolation room at the new Mark O. Hatfield Clinical Research Center, NIH, illustrating anteroom/vestibule. **B,** Artist's rendition of the ventilation plan for the new NIH Clinical Research Center isolation room.

piratory symptoms, and for recent travel to areas known to have epidemic spread of SARS. Other countries simply gave people entering the country from an area known to have epidemic spread a card that delineated how they should monitor themselves and what to do if they developed symptoms consistent with SARS.

Some health care institutions (particularly those in areas experiencing the full brunt of the epidemic) took an aggressive approach to health care providers who were caring for SARS patients, monitoring them for fever and respiratory symptoms. Other institutions relied on self-screening and self-reporting. An example of a self-screening poster developed at Johns Hopkins University Hospital that was modified for use at the NIH Clinical Center is depicted in Figure 14-4. At the very least, institutions need to develop policies and procedures for the conduct of such screening, as well as an algorithm or flowchart for the management of individuals who present with a positive screen.[61]

INFRASTRUCTURAL PREPAREDNESS

Safe management of patients infected with highly contagious pathogens depends in part on the integrity of an institution's infection control infrastructure. Optimally, institutions should have negative-pressure isolation rooms in which such patients can be housed. Figure 14-5 depicts both a schematic diagram of an isolation room in the new Mark O. Hatfield Clinical Research Center and an artist's rendition of

the air supply. The important characteristics of an ideal isolation room are delineated in Table 14-3. Not all institutions have isolation facilities that meet this ideal. Particularly in institutions that lack ideal negative-pressure isolation rooms, hospital epidemiology program staff members must be knowledgeable about the unique air handling characteristics of their own institutions. Specifically, hospital epidemiology program personnel must be aware whether their institutions have single-pass or recirculated air. If the air is recirculated, is it filtered, and if so, by what technique? Furthermore, epidemiology program staff members need to be aware of what they can do to optimize the infrastructural characteristics of their own institutions. If patient care rooms are positive with respect to air pressure to the corridor, can

TABLE 14-3   Hospital Infrastructure Issues Related to Managing Aerosolized or Airborne Contagious Infections

Optimal characteristics of isolation rooms for patients who have infectious diseases that can be airborne or aerosolized:
1. Each patient isolation room should have an anteroom (see Fig. 14-5).
2. These rooms should have consistently negative pressure (i.e., patient room is negative to anteroom; anteroom is negative to corridor).
3. Pressure gradients from corridor to anteroom and from anteroom to patient room should be constantly monitored (optimally with both auditory alarms and visual documentation of gradient).
4. Single-pass air handling (i.e., no recirculation)*
5. At least 12 air changes per hour
6. Optimally, air enters near the top of the room and exhausts through unobstructed grates near the floor.
7. Negative pressure procedure space
8. Negative pressure (or otherwise safe) area for operations (if necessary)

*If air is recirculated, it should be HEPA-filtered before its return.

these rooms be made negative by putting a window fan in the room, by regulating air flow into the room, or by increasing the exhaust rates?[62] Epidemiology program staff should determine the direction of air flow into or from patient care units and individual patient care rooms. (For example, in my own older institution, the air generally flows up the elevator shafts, is swept down the patient care units from the central elevator lobby in both directions, and then exits from the distal end of the units through large exhaust grates.) Staff should plan responses and isolation strategies on the basis of the unique characteristics of their own institutions. In the event of a bioterrorism attack or a rapidly spreading epidemic, institutions may be required to deal with a significant number of patients who have contagious diseases. To deal with this type of problem, institutional staff members need to be aware of which components of the institution (e.g., separate buildings, floors, specific geographic areas) can be effectively isolated from the remainder of the institution to be able to provide care for large numbers of infected patients.

Institutions also must plan for some unexpected contingencies. For example, some patients infected with highly contagious pathogens may require emergency operative procedures. As operating theaters are positive in pressure to the surrounding environment, institutions must develop strategies to provide emergency care without putting other patients and staff at risk. Creative solutions include developing the capacity to make the rooms immediately adjacent to the positive-pressure operating room negative to the outside environment. When the adjacent rooms are negative to the external environment, the potentially contaminated air can be exhausted directly outside. Staff should be precluded from entering these adjacent areas unless they have an absolute need to enter, and then they should enter only when wearing appropriate personal protective equipment.

Ambulatory care facilities, clinics, and emergency departments have unique problems with respect to isolation facilities (see "Special Problems," later).

PATIENT TRANSPORT

Another issue that has to be carefully considered and planned for is the movement of patients who have highly contagious diseases, into and, when necessary, around and through the health care institution. As a risk-reduction strategy, movement of these patients should be as limited as is possible. When patients must leave their isolation rooms for procedures or examinations, their movement must be strictly controlled and isolation must be optimally maintained. In our own hospital, we have generated flowcharts for patient transport (e.g., to the imaging sciences area or to the operating theater) should a clinical circumstance arise absolutely necessitating transport. The key to successful transportation of such patients is effective communication among members of our staff. Clinical Center staff have developed procedures to use a mobile, high-efficiency particulate air (HEPA)-filtered isolation device (the Demistifier, Peace Medical Inc., Orange, N.J.) (Fig. 14-6) for transporting patients infected or potentially infected with highly contagious pathogens that have the potential for airborne or efficient droplet spread. Although the efficacy of such devices in reducing risk for airborne transmission of airborne pathogens remains to be demonstrated, these devices do appear to provide an extra measure of containment for highly contagious organisms.

VISITORS

Decisions about an institutional approach to visitors have to be made on an event-by-event basis. Among the factors that must be considered in setting institutional policy are the psychological impact of limiting visitors for the patient and family, the ease of spread of the infection, the risks to other patients in the institution, the risks to health care workers who might be inadvertently exposed, and the risks for accelerating community spread of the disease. On the basis of these and other factors, the Clinical Center has proposed a "no visitors" policy for patients infected with the SARS coronavirus, at least during the time when these individuals are known to be infected and potentially infectious. Others have taken a similar approach and found it to be effective.[34] Nonetheless, the psychological effects of such a policy for patients; the psychological effects of having an epidemic, highly contagious disease; and the psychological effects of having a disease with few options for care, not to mention a frighteningly high mortality, cannot be understated for these patients. Every effort should be made to provide psychological support for both the patients and the staff involved in the care of the patients in such a setting. Experience from the SARS epidemic has taught us that the psychological impact of such an illness—including fear, depression, loneliness, boredom, remorse, resentment, and concern about the effects of quarantine and contagion on family members and friends—can be devastating.[43,63]

If institutions decide to allow visitors during an ongoing epidemic, careful screening and triage of visitors must take place at the time of their arrival at the institutions.[61,62]

SPECIAL PROBLEMS

A few issues relating to the provision of care in the setting of an epidemic of contagious infectious disease are worthy of additional emphasis, including issues directly related to ambulatory care or the

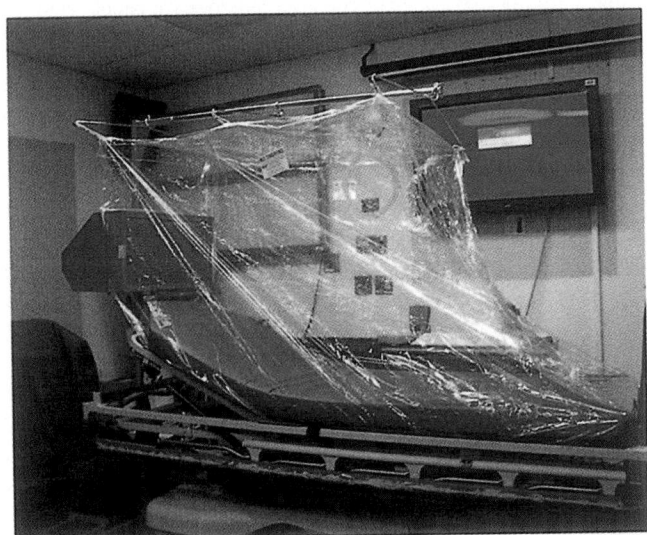

FIGURE 14-6. A HEPA-filtered mobile isolation device (Demistifier, Peace Medical Inc., Orange, N.J.), designed for transport of patients with contagious diseases.

emergency department, and issues relating to the organization's approach to the media when an epidemic is occurring.

Emergency Department and Ambulatory Care Issues

Because of difficulty in exerting tight control over their respective environments, emergency departments and ambulatory care facilities have unique problems with respect to the containment of infectious diseases spread through the air or by efficient droplet spread. For this reason institutions need to develop sensitive screening criteria for epidemic infectious diseases when the risk for transmission is present.[61,62] In the setting of an ongoing epidemic, all individuals entering the institution should be asked to self-screen (see Fig. 14-3), but staff should also rigorously screen each new patient or visitor who enters the building.[61,62]

During the SARS epidemic, many hospitals around the world posted large signs outside emergency departments and ambulatory care areas notifying patients about the epidemic, listing screening criteria, and encouraging individuals who have positive screening criteria (e.g., fevers or respiratory symptoms) to don a surgical mask before entering the institution. Some institutions provided a supply of masks outside the entrance to the facility in an attempt to increase the efficacy of this strategy. Screening criteria that are as sensitive as possible should be developed for the screening process.[61,62] A high index of suspicion for epidemic diseases is the best defense against spread. Containment depends heavily on early identification and implementation of appropriate infection control measures.

Many emergency departments and ambulatory care settings do not have adequate (or sometimes any) isolation facilities. Emergency room and ambulatory care staff need to work with the institution's hospital epidemiology program and building safety staff to delineate airflow patterns in their respective departments. Once the airflow patterns are known, the best available isolation area should be designated and staff should be trained about placing patients who meet screening criteria into isolation. During the SARS epidemic of 2002/2003—even where the infrastructure was less than ideal—initiation of isolation and use of appropriate infection control strategies and procedures ultimately resulted in containment of the infection in hospitals around the world.

Institutions also need to develop processes for the safe management of individuals who have positive screens and are then placed into isolation. Health care workers should immediately don protective gear appropriate to the infection for which containment is being attempted. Procedures need to be developed that address the management of such patients, whether they are discharged to home to be followed remotely, managed briefly in the emergency department or ambulatory care area, transferred to another facility, or admitted to an isolation room in the institution.

Media Management

Dealing with the mass media is a major challenge for institutional staff when the institution is participating in the care of patients who have highly transmissible or poorly defined infectious diseases. Important aspects of media management include (1) deciding what the two or three most important components of the institution's primary message for the public should be—that is, deciding what pieces of data consistently transmit the most important information to the public; (2) crafting a media management plan that ensures that a limited number of spokespersons (preferably one) present the institution's message in the most consistent and constructive way possible; and (3) ensuring that when difficult issues and questions arise, the spokesperson returns to the *message* after delivering the most balanced response possible to the challenging or difficult inquiry. The individual interacting with the media should keep answers short and straight to the point, should be as candid as possible, should attempt to frame risk in a perspective that the public can understand, and should be able to identify other experts who can corroborate her or his account of the issues.[64] Developing an adversarial relationship with the media or ignoring the media will be of no value—either to the media or to the institution.

REFERENCES

1. Franz DR, Zajtchuk R. Biological terrorism: Understanding the threat, preparation, and medical response. Dis Mon. 2002;48:493.
2. Ferguson NE, Steele L, Crawford CY, et al. Bioterrorism web site resources for infectious disease clinicians and epidemiologists. Clin Infect Dis. 2003;36:1458.
3. Wein LM, Craft DL, Kaplan EH. Emergency response to an anthrax attack. Proc Natl Acad Sci U S A. 2003;100:4346.
4. Hupert N, Mushlin AI, Callahan MA. Modeling the public health response to bioterrorism: Using discrete event simulation to design antibiotic distribution centers. Med Decis Making. 2002;22:S17.
5. Burkle FM Jr. Mass casualty management of a large-scale bioterrorist event: An epidemiological approach that shapes triage decisions. Emerg Med Clin North Am. 2002;20:409.
6. Inglesby TV, Henderson DA, Bartlett JG, et al. Anthrax as a biological weapon: Medical and public health management. Working Group on Civilian Biodefense. JAMA. 1999;281:1735.
7. Henderson DA, Inglesby TV, Bartlett JG, et al. Smallpox as a biological weapon: Medical and public health management. Working Group on Civilian Biodefense. JAMA. 1999;281:2127.
8. Inglesby TV, Dennis DT, Henderson DA, et al. Plague as a biological weapon: Medical and public health management. Working Group on Civilian Biodefense. JAMA. 2000;283:2281.
9. Dennis DT, Inglesby TV, Henderson DA, et al. Tularemia as a biological weapon: Medical and public health management. JAMA. 2001;285:2763.
10. Arnon SS, Schechter R, Inglesby TV, et al. Botulinum toxin as a biological weapon: Medical and public health management. JAMA. 2001;285:1059.
11. Inglesby TV, O'Toole T, Henderson DA, et al. Anthrax as a biological weapon, 2002: Updated recommendations for management. JAMA. 2002;287:2236.
12. Henderson DA. Countering the posteradication threat of smallpox and polio. Clin Infect Dis. 2002;34:79.
13. Borio L, Inglesby T, Peters CJ, et al. Hemorrhagic fever viruses as biological weapons: Medical and public health management. JAMA. 2002;287:2391.
14. Brocato CE, Miller GT: The next agent of terror? Understanding smallpox & its implications for prehospital crews. JEMS. 2002;27:44.
15. Kraut A, Mullan F, Riegelman R, et al. Public health in the age of bioterrorism. Responsive Community. 2002;12:59.
16. Veenema TG. Diagnosis, management, and containment of smallpox infections. Disaster Manag Response. 2003;1:8.
17. Karhukorpi EK, Karhukorpi J. Rapid laboratory diagnosis of ulceroglandular tularemia with polymerase chain reaction. Scand J Infect Dis. 2001;33:383.
18. Emanuel PA, Bell R, Dang JL, et al. Detection of *Francisella tularensis* within infected mouse tissues by using a hand-held PCR thermocycler. J Clin Microbiol. 2003;41:689.
19. Drosten C, Gottig S, Schilling S, et al. Rapid detection and quantification of RNA of Ebola and Marburg viruses, Lassa virus, Crimean-Congo hemorrhagic fever virus, Rift Valley fever virus, dengue virus, and yellow fever virus by real-time reverse transcription–PCR. J Clin Microbiol. 2002;40:2323.
20. De Paula SO, Pires Neto RJ, Correa JA, et al. The use of reverse transcription–polymerase chain reaction (RT-PCR) for the rapid detection and identification of dengue virus in an endemic region: A validation study. Trans R Soc Trop Med Hyg. 2002;96:266.
21. Espach A, Romito M, Nel LH, et al. Development of a diagnostic one-tube RT-PCR for the detection of Rift Valley fever virus. Onderstepoort J Vet Res. 2002;69:247.
22. Ellerbrok H, Nattermann H, Ozel M, et al. Rapid and sensitive identification of pathogenic and apathogenic *Bacillus anthracis* by real-time PCR. FEMS Microbiol Lett. 2002;214:51.
23. Espy MJ, Uhl JR, Sloan LM, et al. Detection of vaccinia virus, herpes simplex virus, varicella-zoster virus, and *Bacillus anthracis* DNA by LightCycler polymerase chain reaction after autoclaving: Implications for biosafety of bioterrorism agents. Mayo Clin Proc. 2002;77:624.
24. Section II: Event-based syndromic surveillance systems. J Urban Health. 2003;80 (Suppl 1):i123-i126.
25. Section I: Syndromic surveillance using emergency department data. J Urban Health. 2003;80(Suppl 1):i117.
26. Duchin JS. Epidemiological response to syndromic surveillance signals. J Urban Health. 2003;80(Suppl 1):i115.
27. Pavlin JA. Investigation of disease outbreaks detected by "syndromic" surveillance systems. J Urban Health. 2003;80(Suppl 1):i107.
28. Lober WB, Trigg LJ, Karras BT, et al. Syndromic surveillance using automated collection of computerized discharge diagnoses. J Urban Health. 2003;80(Suppl 1):i97.
29. Lombardo J, Burkom H, Elbert E, et al. A systems overview of the electronic surveillance system for the early notification of community-based epidemics (ESSENCE II). J Urban Health. 2003;80(Suppl 1):i32.
30. Platt R, Bocchino C, Caldwell B, et al. Syndromic surveillance using minimum transfer of identifiable data: The example of the national bioterrorism syndromic surveillance demonstration program. J Urban Health. 2003;80(Suppl 1):i25.
31. Riley S, Fraser C, Donnelly CA, et al. Transmission dynamics of the etiological agent of SARS in Hong Kong: Impact of public health interventions. Science. 2003;300:1961.
32. Centers for Disease Control and Prevention. Severe acute respiratory syndrome: Singapore, 2003. MMWR Morb Mortal Wkly Rep. 2003;52:405.
33. Centers for Disease Control and Prevention. Severe acute respiratory syndrome: Taiwan, 2003. MMWR Morb Mortal Wkly Rep. 2003;52:461.

34. Centers for Disease Control and Prevention. Update: Severe acute respiratory syndrome: Toronto, Canada, 2003. MMWR Morb Mortal Wkly Rep. 2003;52:547.

35. Centers for Disease Control and Prevention. Outbreak of severe acute respiratory syndrome: Worldwide, 2003. MMWR Morb Mortal Wkly Rep. 2003;52:226.

36. Centers for Disease Control and Prevention. Cluster of severe acute respiratory syndrome cases among protected health-care workers: Toronto, Canada, April 2003. MMWR Morb Mortal Wkly Rep. 2003;52:433.

37. Centers for Disease Control and Prevention. Update: Outbreak of severe acute respiratory syndrome: Worldwide, 2003. MMWR Morb Mortal Wkly Rep. 2003;52:269.

38. Avendano M, Derkach P, Swan S. Clinical course and management of SARS in health care workers in Toronto: A case series. CMAJ. 2003;168:1649.

39. Peng GW, He JF, Lin JY, et al. Epidemiological study on severe acute respiratory syndrome in Guangdong province. Zhonghua Liu Xing Bing Xue Za Zhi. 2003;24:350.

40. Seto WH, Tsang D, Yung RW, et al. Effectiveness of precautions against droplets and contact in prevention of nosocomial transmission of severe acute respiratory syndrome (SARS). Lancet. 2003;361:1519.

41. Vu TH, Cabau JF, Nguyen NT, et al. SARS in northern Vietnam. N Engl J Med. 2003;348:2035.

42. Clark J. Fear of SARS thwarts medical education in Toronto. BMJ. 2003;326:784.

43. Maunder R, Hunter J, Vincent L, et al. The immediate psychological and occupational impact of the 2003 SARS outbreak in a teaching hospital. CMAJ. 2003;168:1245.

44. Razum O, Becher H, Kapaun A, et al. SARS, lay epidemiology, and fear. Lancet. 2003;361:1739.

45. Dwosh HA, Hong HH, Austgarden D, et al. Identification and containment of an outbreak of SARS in a community hospital. CMAJ. 2003;168:1415.

46. Lee N, Hui D, Wu A, et al. A major outbreak of severe acute respiratory syndrome in Hong Kong. N Engl J Med. 2003;348:1986.

47. Peiris JS, Chu CM, Cheng VC, et al. Clinical progression and viral load in a community outbreak of coronavirus-associated SARS pneumonia: A prospective study. Lancet. 2003;361:1767.

48. Tan YM, Chow PK, Soo KC. Severe acute respiratory syndrome: Clinical outcome after inpatient outbreak of SARS in Singapore. BMJ. 2003;326:1394.

49. Tomlinson B, Cockram C. SARS: Experience at Prince of Wales Hospital, Hong Kong. Lancet. 2003;361:1486.

50. Wong TW. An outbreak of SARS among healthcare workers. Occup Environ Med. 2003;60:528.

51. Garner JS. Guideline for isolation precautions in hospitals. The Hospital Infection Control Practices Advisory Committee. Infect Control Hosp Epidemiol. 1996;17:53.

52. Bolyard EA, Tablan OC, Williams WW, et al. Guideline for infection control in healthcare personnel, 1998. Hospital Infection Control Practices Advisory Committee. Infect Control Hosp Epidemiol. 1998;19:407.

53. Centers for Disease Control and Prevention. Interim domestic guidance on the use of respirators to prevent transmission of SARS. May 6, 2003. Available at http://www.cdc.gov/ncidod/sars/respirators.html. (Accessed July 16, 2003.)

54. Centers for Disease Control and Prevention. Interim domestic infection control precautions for aerosol-generating procedures on patients with severe acute respiratory syndrome (SARS). May 20, 2003. Available at http://www.cdc.gov/ncidod/sars/aerosolinfectioncontrol.html. (Accessed July 16, 2003.)

55. Tsang T. SARS: Environmental issues. June 18, 2003. Available at http://www.who.int/csr/sars/conference/june_2003/materials/presentations/en. (Accessed July 15, 2003.)

56. Centers for Disease Control and Prevention. Updated interim domestic infection control guidance in the health-care and community setting for patients with suspected SARS. May 1, 2003. Available at http://www.cdc.gov/ncidod/sars/infectioncontrol.html. (Accessed July 15, 2003.)

57. Centers for Disease Control and Prevention. Interim laboratory biosafety guidelines for handling and processing specimens associated with severe acute respiratory syndrome (SARS). April 16, 2003. Available at http://www.cdc.gov/ncidod/sars/s arslabguide.html. (Accessed July 16, 2003.)

58. World Health Organization. WHO biosafety guidelines for handling of SARS specimens. April 25, 2003. Available at http://www.who.int/csr/sars/biosafety 2003_04_25/en/. (Accessed July 15, 2003.)

59. Centers for Disease Control and Prevention. Safe handling of human remains of severe acute respiratory syndrome (SARS) patients: Interim domestic guidance. May 15, 2003. Available at http://www.cdc.gov/ncidod/sars/autopsy.html. (Accessed July 16, 2003.)

60. Centers for Disease Control and Prevention. Interim domestic guidance for management of exposures to severe acute respiratory syndrome (SARS) for health-care settings. June 24, 2003. Available at http://www.cdc.gov/ncidod/sars/exposureguidance.htm. (Accessed July 15, 2003.)

61. Centers for Disease Control and Prevention. Updated interim domestic guidelines for triage and disposition of patients who may have severe acute respiratory syndrome (SARS). April 25, 2003. Available at http://www.cdc.gov/ncidod/sars/triage_interim_guidance.html. (Accessed July 15, 2003.)

62. World Health Organization. Hospital infection control guidance for severe acute respiratory syndrome (SARS). April 24, 2003. Available at http://www.who.int/csr/sars/infectioncontrol/en. (Accessed July 15, 2003.)

63. Huang Y. Psychosocial aspects of SARS in China. June 18, 2003. Available at http://www.who.int/csr/sars/conference/june_2003/materials/presentations/en/. (Accessed July 15, 2003.)

64. Stamm K, Williams JW Jr, Noel PH, et al. Helping journalists get it right: A physician's guide to improving health care reporting. J Gen Intern Med. 2003;18:138.

CHAPTER **15**

The Clinician and the Microbiology Laboratory

VEE J. GILL

DANIEL P. FEDORKO

FRANK G. WITEBSKY

The clinician and the microbiology laboratory are partners in determining the etiology of infection; as part of this process, it is essential that they actively communicate with each other. Unfortunately, the current trend to consolidate laboratory services and to move them off-site has made timely communication between laboratory personnel and patient care providers more difficult to attain.[1] These changes, along with other cost-cutting measures, make it even more imperative that the infectious diseases physician and the microbiology laboratory work together to facilitate effective patient care and management. The following expectations regarding the laboratory's and the clinician's responsibilities should be recognized and addressed.

The laboratory must ensure that its operation meets all current regulatory requirements (Clinical Laboratory Improvement Amendments [CLIA]), including initial verification and ongoing validation of procedures that are used by the laboratory.[2-4] It should have a responsible program of quality control, as well as quality assurance benchmarks by which it can gauge its performance. Minimizing costs is essential but must be done without significant compromise of the quality of results. As part of an ongoing process, the laboratory director should be looking for state-of-the-art methodology that improves performance and is relevant to the specific hospital population for which services are provided. Through the hospital informational network, the laboratory should provide clinicians with easy access to specific guidelines for optimal collection and transport of specimens, as well as guidelines for common laboratory policies, for example, policies limiting the number of specimens that can be submitted per day or per week. These policies should be included on the ordering screens, which should also display practical information about specific tests, such as what pathogens are screened for when a routine bacterial stool culture is ordered. Reporting of urgent and significant results such as positive blood cultures is mandatory, but preliminary or interim "significant" reports should also be provided to aid the clinician in patient management. Critical to optimal functioning of a laboratory are its interactions with other hospital personnel, including patient care staff, hospital infection-control officers, and pharmacists, as well as the infectious diseases physicians with whom the laboratory should be interacting on a daily basis. The use of good notification and informational guidelines with each of these groups is important (1) for maintenance of effective hospital infection control, and (2) to deter the emergence of resistant organisms through the indiscriminate or inappropriate use of antibiotics.

The responsibilities of the clinician, particularly of the infectious diseases physician, include acquiring a substantive understanding of the laboratory's policies and methods used for commonly ordered cultures so that the infectious diseases physician can provide meaningful feedback to the patient's primary physician, who may be awaiting the test results. The laboratory expects that the infectious diseases physician will recommend the best specimen type, will request the most appropriate test from the laboratory's menu, and will contact the laboratory if further information or clarification is needed. The clinician should also alert the laboratory when a particular organism is sought that may be unusual or that may require a special setup (e.g., *Corynebacterium diphtheriae, Bartonella* spp.), or when a potentially hazardous organism is expected (e.g., *Francisella tularensis,* multidrug-resistant *Mycobacterium tuberculosis, Coccidioides immitis*). On a similar note, discussion with laboratory personnel would be beneficial in explaining out-of-the-ordinary situations in which deviation from normal laboratory policy would best serve the patient's interests (e.g., extended incubation, additional antibiotic susceptibility tests). In the provision of care to immunocompromised patients or when difficult diagnostic problems arise, numerous cultures or tests are often requested on a specimen for which there may be inadequate quantity; the clinician should prioritize the test requests for the laboratory based on the highest clinical suspicions because the laboratory staff cannot objectively assess test prioritization. The infectious diseases physician should bring to laboratory management's attention policies or procedures that are recurrent problems for which solutions should be sought.

Both the microbiology laboratory and the infectious diseases physician need to regularly update their knowledge of organism nomenclature, which seems to be constantly changing. It is as difficult for laboratorians as it is for physicians to stay current with taxonomic changes and the discovery of new organisms. The laboratory must change and add names in a timely yet appropriate fashion, and the infectious diseases physician must be aware of significant changes or additions and must be ready to discuss them with primary patient care physicians. Much of the taxonomic reorganization now under way is driven by our increased capability for grouping organisms according to genetic relatedness, which was shown initially by DNA hybridization but has been refined by advanced molecular evolutionary genetic studies.[5,6] These analyses will lead us to taxonomic schemes that are more objective and, one hopes, more accurate in portraying the phylogenetic relationships of organisms.

Hospital epidemiology is another area of shared concern for the microbiology service and for hospital infection-control officers who must have a surveillance program that leads to rapid detection of potential infectious outbreaks. In such situations, the appropriate organisms must be stored so that typing can be done if needed. Molecular techniques can rapidly and reliably identify whether a single strain is causing an outbreak. Timely receipt of this information leads to more effective use of control measures throughout the hospital and helps to identify sources, carriers, and patterns of spread. Although strain typing is ideally done in the hospital laboratory, this is beyond the capability of most community hospital laboratories, which instead must rely on either county or state laboratories to analyze organisms for them.

Figure 15-1 provides a general scheme of the types of methods used in the diagnosis of infectious agents. The specific methods and the relative usefulness of the tests used vary according to the microorganism being sought. In the following section, we summarize guidelines for specimen selection, collection, and transport; we then briefly describe the detection and identification methods that are currently available. Molecular techniques to aid in the laboratory diagnosis of infectious diseases have added another dimension to the traditional stain, culture, and serology repertoire of the microbiology laboratory. Although such testing is currently limited in its availability and proven usefulness, molecular testing by the clinical laboratory will likely play an increasingly prominent role in infectious disease diagnosis.

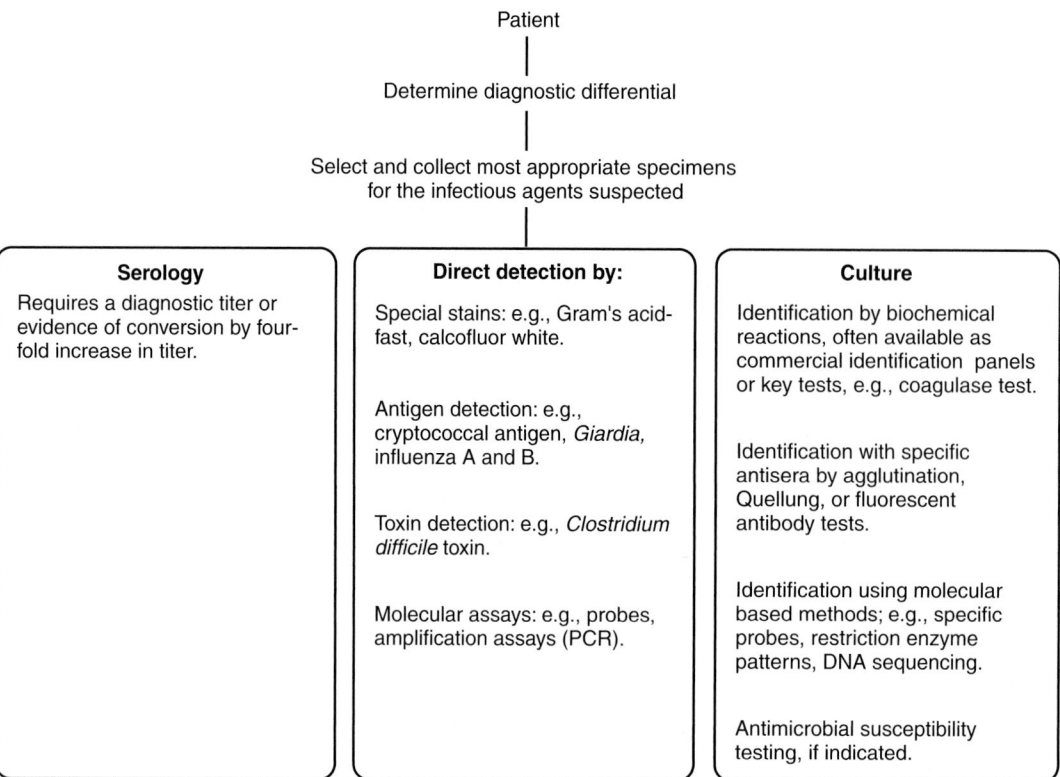

FIGURE 15-1.   Methodologies used in the diagnosis of infectious agents. PCR, polymerase chain reaction.

SPECIMEN SELECTION, COLLECTION, AND PROCESSING

Submission of the best specimen type for a particular test or for recovery of a specific microorganism is of paramount importance for a successful outcome. It is obvious, however, that such a specimen, if placed in the wrong container, obtained incorrectly, or left undelivered for a prolonged period, will lead to less reliable, if not falsely negative, results. Clear guidelines for specimen submission must be readily available to doctors, nurses, and other personnel who are involved in the collection and transport of specimens.

General Criteria for Specimen Selection

Selection of the type of specimen that one should send for testing depends on multiple factors. Although it seems intuitively obvious that the best specimen is one that probably contains the infecting organism, a direct correlation is not always found between the apparently infected site and successful detection. Specimen selection must also be based on the known characteristics of certain infectious processes or infectious agents. For example, pneumonia caused by *Legionella pneumophila* is only poorly diagnosed from expectorated sputum, whereas urine from the patient might yield a positive *Legionella* urinary antigen test. If, however, the patient has been infected with *Legionella* spp. other than *L. pneumophila* serotype 1, the optimal specimen for diagnosis would be either bronchoalveolar lavage or lung biopsy because the urinary antigen test detects only serotype 1. Thus, selection of the most appropriate specimen must be made with knowledge of the relative yields of different specimens for different organisms and different tests. Here again, the laboratorian and the infectious diseases physician must work to educate primary care physicians about this information. Selection of the best array of tests for specific types of infections or for specific microorganisms is not always obvious; in addition, patient tolerance of diagnostic procedures may limit the potential for obtaining the most definitive specimen type.

General Criteria for Specimen Collection and Transport

Proper specimen collection ideally should start before the administration of chemotherapeutic agents (e.g., antibiotic, antiviral, antifungal) so that the recovery of microorganisms will not be compromised. Collection must then proceed with care to prevent contamination of the specimen with normal flora that may be encountered during the collection process, although such contamination may sometimes be unavoidable.

Amounts of material that are adequate for needed tests must be obtained. This information needs to be relayed by the infectious diseases physician to the individual obtaining the specimen, often a surgeon, dermatologist, or other specialist, who may not be aware of all the tests that will be ordered. Too often, laboratories are hampered by inadequate amounts of sterile body fluids (such as cerebrospinal fluid [CSF] or pleural fluid) that must be cultured or directly tested for multiple agents. This shortage of material is particularly significant when an invasive procedure is used to obtain the specimen because the procedure is unlikely to be repeated in the event of insufficient quantities. Even material taken with a swab must be examined so that adequacy of the sampled material can be determined for the various tests that are to be requested. In general, swab cultures should be reserved for superficial skin lesions or throat swabs. Two sets of swabs may be needed if multiple test requests will be made, particularly if both direct smears and cultures are intended. When a collection of fluid or pus is to be sampled, aspirated material is preferable to the use of swabs. A particularly important culture type that is dependent on adequate volume for maximal sensitivity is the blood culture. Although a sufficient volume of blood may be difficult to obtain from some patients, good effort should be made to obtain the recommended amount of blood to increase the likelihood of successful culture.

Complete instructions should be provided to those who will be collecting specimens that require special handling. Common questions, such as what to put the biopsy in for transport to the laboratory, how to culture for anaerobes, how to collect and transport material for direct tests such as a fluorescent antibody test on skin lesions for varicella-zoster virus (VZV), what to use for *Chlamydia* cultures, and so forth, should be anticipated. Clear answers to these and similar questions could prevent discarding of specimens because of improper collection or having valuable specimens placed in bacteriostatic saline or formalin. All of this information should be readily available and easily accessible to physicians and nurses through the hospital or laboratory computer system or in a widely distributed laboratory guide.

Transport of specimens to the microbiology laboratory must be done in a timely fashion, which is particularly important in the handling of urgent requests. The laboratory should determine in what manner and how often specimens should be delivered and should periodically monitor this process to make sure that delivery to the laboratory is occurring as expected. Specimens should not be allowed to sit

for hours; even if the specimen may remain perfectly suitable for culture, such as urine in buffered tubes, delay in transport results in later processing and a shorter "overnight" incubation period. For some lengthy tests that may take 4 to 6 hours for completion, such as certain immunoassays, late arrival may mean postponing performance of the test until the following day. Laboratories often have daily cutoff times for certain tests if the test is to be completed on the same day that the specimen is received.

Table 15-1 summarizes generally accepted guidelines for specimen collection and transport of common specimen types. Although different laboratories have similar policies, little absolute uniformity in the practice of microbiology is seen from laboratory to laboratory, so the clinician must be sure to understand the guidelines for each specific laboratory. Not all situations can be covered under general guidelines.

TABLE 15-1 Collection and Transport* Guidelines for Commonly Submitted Specimens

Specimen	Collection Guidelines	Other Comments
Abscess	Aspirate of pus or fluid in anaerobic transport vial is preferred. Swabs usually have insufficient material for Gram stain and culture. Specify location of abscess for optimal plating. Aspirate is appropriate for routine, anaerobic, fungal, and mycobacterial culture.	Specimen sent immediately in syringe is also acceptable, but without a needle attached. Provide additional pertinent information (e.g., cat-bite, needle aspirate of liver).
Biopsies	Keep specimen moist and transport rapidly to lab. Do not use bacteriostatic saline or formalin. Biopsies are suitable specimens for routine, fungal, mycobacterial, viral, and anaerobic cultures, depending on site of biopsy.	Always specify the type of tissue, and indicate the specific pathogen sought, if other than routine bacteria, (e.g., *Nocardia, Bartonella, Histoplasma*).
Blood for Culture	Prepare site with 70% alcohol, then with tincture of iodine or an iodophor. Cleanse top of culture bottles/tubes with 70% alcohol; do not change needles to inoculate.	All blood cultures should be transported ASAP to start incubation or processing. (Differing skin preparation methods have been proposed; follow specific hospital recommendations.)
Routine Bacteria	20–30 mL/adults and 1–3 mL/child are *minimum* amounts for each episode; peripheral draws are preferred. 3 culture sets/day maximum, 2 sets/episode minimum.	Do not use smaller blood volumes in pediatric bottles **for adults** because this decreases culture sensitivity. SPS may inhibit some organisms (see text).
Anaerobes	If anaerobic bottle is not part of the laboratory's routine culture set, contact laboratory for instructions.	
Bartonella	10 mL in lysis-centrifugation tube is preferred method. Bottle systems may be much slower; contact laboratory.	
Brucella	Routine broth culture systems, biphasic systems, and lysis-centrifugation are used; contact laboratory.	
Leptospira	One to three drops of fresh or SPS blood is needed to inoculate special media; collect within first week of illness.	Contact laboratory in advance.
Fungi	Use routine blood culture system for *Candida/Cryptococcus* or 10 mL in lysis-centrifugation tube, or 3–5 mL in fungal blood culture bottle or biphasic system.	Specify if culture for *Malassezia* is needed. (Histoplasma or cryptococcal antigen tests require serum tubes.)
Mycobacteria	10 mL in lysis-centrifugation tube; amount of blood or lysed sediment needed for bottle systems for mycobacteria depends on system used.	
Blood for Parasites		
Malaria or Babesia	Prepare thick and thin smears from fingerstick or EDTA blood; examine multiple specimens over 48–72 hr.	Transport ASAP for smear preparation.
Trypanosomes	Prepare multiple thick and thin smears from fingerstick or EDTA blood during febrile episodes. Culture is possible but is not generally available.	Transport ASAP for wet mount or smear preparation.
Microfilariae	Obtain blood according to observed periodicity; concentration techniques such as thick smears can be used; contact laboratory.	Transport ASAP for smear preparation.
Bone Marrow	Obtain 1–2 mL of marrow for diagnosis of histoplasmosis, miliary tuberculosis, brucellosis, or *Salmonella typhi*. Also good for diagnosis of leishmaniasis.	Aspirating more than 2 mL will dilute marrow with peripheral blood.
Catheter		
Intravenous	Remove aseptically, cut at least a 2-inch segment from tip, and place segment in sterile container.	Transport ASAP to prevent drying out.
Foley	Not acceptable for culture.	
Drainage	Not recommended for culture; needle aspirate of fluid or abscess preferred.	Drainage tubes may be superficially contaminated, making culture interpretation difficult.

Continued

*It is assumed that appropriate transport media will be provided and used.
ASAP, as soon as possible; CSF, cerebrospinal fluid; EDTA, ethylenediamine tetraacetic acid; KOH, potassium hydroxide, LCR, ligase chain reaction; MRSA, methicillin-resistant *Staphylococcus aureus;* NP, nasopharynx; PCR, polymerase chain reaction; R/O, rule out; RT, room temperature; SDA, strand displacement amplification; SPS, sodium polyanethole sulfonate anticoagulant; TMA, transcription-mediated amplification.

TABLE 15-1   Collection and Transport* Guidelines for Commonly Submitted Specimens—cont'd

Specimen	Collection Guidelines	Other Comments
Eye (Lid, Conjunctiva, Corneal Scrapings)	Bacterial, fungal, chlamydial, mycobacterial, or viral cultures may be requested from these sites.	Notify laboratory if you are looking for *Acanthamoeba* or microsporidia.
Fluids (Body Fluids Other Than Blood, Urine)		
Pleural Peritoneal Synovial Cardiac, etc.	Send at least 2–5 mL for bacteria, >10 mL for fungi and/or mycobacteria. Use anaerobic transport media if indicated. Viral etiology may be considered for pericardial fluids.	Excess peritoneal fluid inoculated into blood culture bottles may increase sensitivity of culture for routine bacteria. Send ASAP.
CSF for Culture	1–2 mL for bacteria, viruses 5–10 mL for mycobacteria or fungi	Send immediately. Alert laboratory if anaerobic culture is indicated because anaerobes may not be detected by the laboratory's routine culture, or for diagnosis of primary amebic meningoencephalitis.
CSF for Antigen	1–2 mL for cryptococcal antigen	Cross-reaction with *Trichosporon* spp. may occur.
Genital Tract (Commonly Submitted Specimens)		
Cervical Urethral Vaginal or Penile	Use transport media/containers appropriate for organisms sought (*Neisseria gonorrhoeae, Chlamydia, Ureaplasma*, etc)	Transport quickly. Laboratory may want specimen planted directly; swabs or plates need to be transported to lab ASAP.
Ulcer or Discharge	Follow laboratory guidelines for syphilis, soft chancre, herpes, yeast, *Trichomonas, Gardnerella, N. gonorrhoeae.*	Check with laboratory to determine which tests are available because some organisms are difficult to detect by culture. Anaerobic cultures are not performed.
Respiratory, Upper		
Nose	Anterior nares swabs usually submitted only for detection of staphylococcal or streptococcal carriers.	Use bacterial transport media; specify organism (e.g., R/O MRSA).
Nasopharynx	NP specimen appropriate for *Bordetella pertussis, Corynebacterium diphtheriae, N. gonorrhoeae, Neisseria meningitidis.* Alert laboratory before sending.	Cough plates for pertussis are not recommended; use calcium alginate swabs and plate directly or send to laboratory ASAP.
Oral Cavity	(e.g., swabs or scrapings taken from oral lesions)	
Bacteria	Not usually cultured, but direct smears may be used to demonstrate fusospirochetal disease.	
Fungi	Gram stain, calcofluor white stain, or KOH preparation can be used for direct detection of yeast. Culture not generally done unless identification or susceptibilities of yeast are wanted.	Follow laboratory guidelines for submission of samples for direct smears.
Sinus Aspirate	Submit in anaerobic transport if anaerobes are suspected. Bacterial and fungal smears and cultures may be indicated.	
Throat	Swab areas of purulence or ulceration. Notify laboratory if you are looking for organism other than group A streptococci.	Use transport media. Be sure to specify when you are looking for diphtheria or pertussis.
Respiratory, Lower		
All Specimens of Lower Respiratory Secretions	Specimens should be refrigerated if transport will be delayed, to prevent overgrowth with commensals.	For multiple test requests, be sure that specimen volume is adequate.
Sputum Bacteria	Sputa are screened for acceptability by absence or low numbers of squamous epithelial cells in the presence of neutrophils. Not suitable for anaerobic culture. Not recommended for *Legionella* culture.	Expectorated sputa may not be best specimen for diagnosis of bacterial pneumonia. Lavages or biopsies are more definitive. Concomitant blood cultures are recommended.
Mycobacteria	First, early morning specimen is preferred, not pooled. Should not be screened for adequacy. Send 3 consecutive first morning specimens for optimal diagnosis.	
Fungi	Should not be screened for adequacy. Send 3 consecutive first morning specimens for optimal diagnosis. **Induced** sputum recommended for *Pneumocystis.*	If known, specify particular agent of concern (e.g., *Cryptococcus, Histoplasma, Nocardia*). Isolation of *Candida* sp. from sputum is not diagnostic of *Candida* pneumonia.
Parasites	Acceptable for parasite detection (e.g., *Strongyloides, Ascaris* larvae)	
Sputum, Induced	Induction with nebulized saline is used primarily to obtain specimens suitable for either mycobacterial or *Pneumocystis* diagnosis.	Quantity of specimen is generally limited (<2 mL), so tests requested should be prioritized. Substantial contamination with oral flora makes this specimen unsuitable for culture of routine bacteria.
Tracheal Aspirate	Acceptable for same tests as sputum; not screened for acceptability like sputa.	Significance of potential pathogens such as Gram-negative rods cannot be determined owing to rapid, heavy colonization of these sites with organisms.
Transtracheal Aspirate	Acceptable for same tests as sputum; this procedure bypasses the oral cavity, so anaerobic cultures are also acceptable.	This procedure is only infrequently performed.

*It is assumed that appropriate transport media will be provided and used.

ASAP, as soon as possible; CSF, cerebrospinal fluid; EDTA, ethylenediamine tetraacetic acid; KOH, potassium hydroxide, LCR, ligase chain reaction; MRSA, methicillin-resistant *Staphylococcus aureus;* NP, nasopharynx; PCR, polymerase chain reaction; R/O, rule out; RT, room temperature; SDA, strand displacement amplification; SPS, sodium polyanethole sulfonate anticoagulant; TMA, transcription-mediated amplification.

TABLE 15-1 Collection and Transport* Guidelines for Commonly Submitted Specimens—cont'd

Specimen	*Collection Guidelines*	*Other Comments*
Bronchial Wash/Brush	These specimens are usually not screened for acceptability like sputa.	For detection of all pathogens, bronchoalveolar lavage (see later) is considered better than bronchial wash.
Bacteria	Suitable for culture of common bacterial pathogens, but only sheathed brush specimens are acceptable for anaerobic cultures.	Specimens are contaminated with oral flora so that assessment of the significance of routine bacteria is still problematic.
Legionella	Process ASAP for *Legionella* because saline may be detrimental.	
Mycobacteria	May be preferable to expectorated sputum.	
Fungi	Preferable to expectorated sputum. Also acceptable for detection of *Pneumocystis*.	Growth of *Candida* and other opportunistic fungi does not necessarily predict significance.
Parasites	Suitable for detection of *Strongyloides,* cryptosporidia, microsporidia, *Toxoplasma*.	
Bronchoalveolar Lavage	Can be used for same tests as bronchial wash/brush. Particularly better than bronchial wash for *Pneumocystis*.	Although properly obtained lavages have minimal contamination with oral flora, significance of *Candida*, molds, and opportunistic bacteria may still be unclear. Some laboratories use quantitation of bacteria to help assess significance.
Skin Scrapings for Dermatophytes	Scrape skin at active edge of lesion; avoid blood. Place in sterile petri dish.	
Skin Lesion	Specimen taken from advancing edge is recommended. Biopsy may be more definitive than swabs of lesion. Appropriate for routine, fungal, and mycobacterial culture, *Leishmania* by smear or culture.	Transport swabs in transport media to prevent drying out. Specifying species of fungus or *Mycobacterium* sought is helpful.
Rectal Swabs (see Stool)	Only rarely acceptable when one is looking for diarrheal pathogens. Send fresh stool instead (see stool guidelines later). Avoid fecal material on anal swabs for *N. gonorrhoeae* culture. Perianal samples used for detection of pinworm.	Occasionally, an infant or very ill patient with diarrhea may require use of rectal swab. For pinworm, use scotch tape preparation or swube device.
Stool Bacteria	Send up to three specimens (1/day). Notify laboratory if *Vibrio, Yersinia, Aeromonas,* or enterohemorrhagic *Escherichia coli* is being looked for. Transport immediately or hold in refrigerator (less desirable).	Be aware of what pathogens are "routinely" screened for by laboratory, in particular *Campylobacter* should be routine. Stool from patients in hospital for >3 days is not accepted by some laboratories.
Ova and Parasites	Transport fresh specimen to laboratory quickly. Preservatives for transport may be supplied by laboratories. Three specimens on 3 separate days is sufficient for screening.	Alert laboratory when specific pathogens are suspected (e.g., *Strongyloides,* cryptosporidia, microsporidia, *Isospora*). *Giardia* enzyme immunoassays may need to be specifically requested.
C. difficile Toxin	No more than 1 per day or 3 specimens for initial screening is acceptable. Deliver ASAP, or refrigerate or freeze specimen. Isolation of organism is not generally done. Assays are usually done for toxin.	Find out what kind of assay is used, turnaround time, sensitivity, and specificity of assay.
Urine Cultures	Keep refrigerated and transport to laboratory promptly, or submit in urine tube with preservative.	Proper instruction for midstream collection should be routinely provided. Straight catheter collection provides specimen with less or no external contamination.
Bacteria	Most commonly clean voided. Only suprapubic aspirate is acceptable for anaerobic culture.	*Candida* sp. will also be detected by routine bacterial cultures.
Leptospira	Culture within 2 hr or neutralize to pH 7.0; collect **after** first week of illness.	Contact laboratory in advance.
Mycobacteria	Send >20 mL, use first morning urine.	DO NOT SEND 24-hr specimens.
Fungi	Send >20 mL, specify fungus being sought.	Check with laboratory on policy for *Candida* culture.
Urine–Other Tests		
N. gonorrhoeae	Amount of urine and storage conditions depend on method used; follow guidelines.	Nucleic acid amplification assays (PCR, LCR, SDA) can detect *Chlamydia* also.
Chlamydia	Amount of urine and storage conditions depend on method used; follow guidelines.	Nucleic acid amplification assays (PCR, LCR, SDA, TMA). PCR, LCR, SDA can be used for simultaneous detection of *N. gonorrhoeae*.
Legionella Antigen	Submit 1–2 mL in suspected cases of *Legionella* pneumonia.	Will detect only *Legionella pneumophila*, serotype 1.
Histoplasma Antigen	Send 1–2 mL for *Histoplasma* antigen.	May aid in diagnosis of systemic infections, but cross-reaction with other fungi occurs.
Schistosoma haematobium	Collect midday urine, particularly that containing mucus and blood.	
Trichomonas	Collect first-voided urine, and transport quickly. DO NOT REFRIGERATE.	For males, prostatic massage may promote detection.
Wound (See abscess, skin lesion)	Decontaminate open lesion first. Aspirate if possible; if swabs must be used, be sure that quantity is sufficient for stains and cultures. Open, superficial wounds are not suitable for anaerobic culturing. Identify type/location of wound.	Transport in anaerobic transport media ASAP if anaerobes suspected. Use transport media for all swabs.

For these instances, the physician should contact laboratory personnel to discuss the best procedures for ensuring optimal handling of the specimen. For more extensive guidelines or for recommendations that are beyond the scope of this chapter, other sources are available.[7,8]

SPECIFIC GUIDELINES AND RECOMMENDATIONS FOR MAJOR CATEGORIES OF INFECTION

This section summarizes pertinent laboratory information, predominantly that related to bacterial infection. Viral, fungal, and mycobacterial infections are only briefly mentioned here but are covered more specifically in separate sections to follow. Likewise, common parasitic test requests are included here, but more extensive discussion can be found in relevant parasitology chapters.

Respiratory Tract Infection

Laboratories typically subdivide respiratory specimens into two major categories—upper respiratory and lower respiratory. Common upper respiratory specimens include throat swabs, nasopharyngeal swabs or washes, and mouth or oral cavity swabs or scrapings. Sinus aspiration and culture for otitis media is submitted only occasionally for specific problematic cases because empirical therapy without culture is generally effective.

In throat swabs, laboratories look for the presence or absence of group A streptococci (*Streptococcus pyogenes*) only, unless a specific request is submitted to look for other agents. Although it is recognized that groups C and G β-hemolytic streptococci may also cause pharyngitis, the lack of proven rheumatic fever sequelae, as well as only rare reports of associated poststreptococcal glomerulonephritis, has deterred laboratories from screening for and reporting these isolates. Rapid antigen tests (enzyme immunoassays [EIAs]) for detection of group A streptococci are widely used because they give results within 15 to 20 minutes that, if positive, can justify the immediate initiation of antibiotic therapy. Although they are highly specific, these tests vary in their sensitivity, especially for detecting very low numbers of organisms.[9] The quality of the specimen varies according to the effectiveness of the sampling process; therefore, very low numbers of organisms may still be significant. Although recommendations vary for the diagnosis of group A streptococcal pharyngitis,[10,11] its higher incidence in children and adolescents make it prudent for the clinician to follow any negative rapid test with a traditional culture both for these patients and for adults who have highly suggestive clinical presentations. Antibiotic susceptibility testing is not routinely done on *S. pyogenes* because all isolates remain universally susceptible to penicillin.

If other agents of pharyngitis are sought, such as *Neisseria gonorrhoeae*, the laboratory must be notified because cultures for agents other than *S. pyogenes* are not routinely done. Throat swabs or nasopharyngeal specimens may also be submitted when diphtheria is suspected, but special smears and isolation media should be used, and *C. diphtheriae* isolates must be tested for toxigenicity. For *Bordetella pertussis* culture, either nasopharyngeal swabs or aspirates are recommended rather than throat swabs or "cough plates." Dacron, rayon, or calcium alginate swabs should be used for culture, and because special media are required for optimal growth of *B. pertussis*, the laboratory should be notified in advance. If a polymerase chain reaction (PCR)-based method is to be applied, calcium alginate swabs should not be used because these have been found to inhibit the PCR reaction.[12]

Lower respiratory tract infections, primarily pneumonia, most often are initially cultured with the use of expectorated sputa or tracheal aspirates because these specimens can be obtained with minimal patient discomfort. More aggressive culturing is attained by way of sputum induction for patients who produce only scant sputum or by bronchoscopic procedures, including bronchial washes, bronchial brushes, transbronchial biopsies, and bronchoalveolar lavages. In select situations, lung biopsies are performed, particularly when less invasive specimens have yielded no diagnosis. Although sputa and tracheal aspirates are readily obtained, the significance of the potential pathogens that are isolated is sometimes difficult to assess.[13] Also important is that expectorated sputum is insensitive for the detection of *Legionella* or *Pneumocystis*. To eliminate unnecessary and potentially misleading culture results, laboratories use microscopy screening guidelines to reject sputum specimens that are poor in quality. Rejection is usually based on the observation of many squamous epithelial cells, which generally correlates with significant oropharyngeal contamination. The presence of polymorphonuclear leukocytes usually indicates good specimen quality, but this criterion should not be required in a granulocytopenic patient. Although sputa should be screened upon submission for routine bacterial culture, rejection criteria based on specimen quality have not been validated for *Legionella*, fungal, and mycobacterial cultures.

Lower respiratory specimens obtained by bronchoscopic procedures or by lung biopsy should always be regarded as important specimens that require prompt laboratory attention. Diagnoses obtained by the use of bronchoalveolar lavage and transbronchial biopsy have significantly decreased the need for open lung biopsies. The range of microorganisms that cause lower respiratory tract infection is broad, and selection of appropriate tests relies on whether the infection is thought to be community acquired or nosocomial in origin, as well as on other relevant clinical information, including the type of infiltrate, the immunologic status and underlying disease of the patient, the history of exposure to known pathogens, travel or occupational exposure, and so forth. Table 15-2 summarizes the microorganisms that often enter into the differential diagnosis and the types of tests that can be used to establish an infectious etiology. To help determine the significance of potential pathogens that could instead be mere colonizers, some laboratories use a quantitative procedure with suggested significance cutoffs to analyze the culture results from bronchoalveolar lavage fluids.[14] The guidelines used by a laboratory should be known to the infectious diseases physician, and the appropriateness of the interpretation should be assessed in light of the type of patient tested and any clinical concerns.

Because the diagnosis of pneumonia in an immunocompromised host has become a frequent and often urgent problem, laboratories have made significant strides in establishing some of these diagnoses more expeditiously than they did in the past. The diagnosis of *Pneumocystis* pneumonia can be made from either induced sputum or bronchoalveolar lavage fluid with stains that can be done within a few hours.[15] Microbiology laboratories should make an effort to offer this service because in many situations they can provide results sooner than the cytopathology laboratory, and these results may have a significant impact on patient management. Improved fungal stains with calcofluor white rather than traditional wet mount have greatly improved direct detection of fungi. Likewise, the use of fluorochrome smears for acid-fast bacilli rather than the older Ziehl-Neelsen or Kinyoun stain has improved the sensitivity of direct detection of mycobacteria. Radiometric culture methods, as well as other new culture systems for mycobacteria, have reduced time to detection. Despite these improvements, more sensitive and specific methods are still needed for detection of *Legionella*, *Chlamydia*, *Mycoplasma*, and fungi, particularly *Histoplasma* and *Cryptococcus*, in lower respiratory specimens. For these and other organisms, molecular amplification assays may be the best approach to improving our diagnostic capabilities.[16,17]

Diagnosis of pneumonias caused by *L. pneumophila* serogroup 1 and *Streptoccus pneumoniae* may be facilitated by the use of urinary antigen assays. Rapid EIA tests, which are now available for detecting antigens of these organisms in patients' urine, have been found to be relatively sensitive. In the case of *Legionella*, only serogroup 1 will be detected in this way, so that culture must still be used to detect other serogroups and species of *Legionella*. A recent review of trends, however, has shown a decrease in diagnosis of legionellosis by culture and a notable increase in the use of urinary EIA instead.[18] Routine cultures are also recommended for *S. pneumoniae* even if urine EIA testing is done. The actual advantage afforded by this assay for diagnosis of pneumococcal infection is yet to be determined.

TABLE 15-2   **Diagnosis of Lower Respiratory Tract Pathogens**

Organism	Acceptable Specimens	Tests Available	Comments
Common bacteria*	S, B, L	Gram stain, culture	1–5 days for isolation and identification
	Urine	Antigen assay	EIA for pneumococcal antigen
Legionella	B, L	FA	Poor test, not recommended
		Culture	Requires special media, incubation for 10–12 days
	Urine	Antigen assay	EIA for *Legionella pneumophila* serotype 1 only
Mycobacteria	S, IS, B, L	Acid-fast stains	Fluorochrome stains preferred
		Nucleic acid amplification	Higher sensitivity for smear-positive specimens; direct test for *Mycobacterium tuberculosis* only
		Culture	Rapid methods preferred (e.g., radiometric, newer automated systems). 4–6 week incubation is standard
Nocardia	S, IS, B, L	Modified acid-fast stain	Include positive and negative controls when staining
		Culture	Incubate up to 4 weeks
Fungi	S, IS, B, L	Calcofluor white stain	Superior to unstained wet mounts
		Culture	Specify if *Histoplasma* or *Coccidioides* is suspected. Incubate 6 weeks
	Serum and CSF	Cryptococcal antigen	By latex agglutination or EIA
	Serum and urine	*Histoplasma* antigen	Must be sent to commercial laboratory
Pneumocystis	IS, B, L	*Pneumocystis* stains (nonculturable agent)	FA, Giemsa, Toluidine blue O, silver stains, etc
Mycoplasma pneumoniae	S, NP, B, L	No direct stains	
		Culture	Not done routinely, requires 7–10 days.
	Serum	Serology (CF)	4–9 week conversion time
		Cold agglutinins	CA titers are nonspecific
Chlamydia pneumoniae	NP, ?B, ?L	No direct stains	
		Culture	Fastidious, difficult to grow; not readily available
	Serum	Serology, CF	Cross-reacts within the genus, 4–6 week conversion time
		Serology, microimmuno-fluorescence	Not widely available
Viruses	NP, B, L	FA, enzyme immunoassay	Available only for certain viruses
		Culture	Rapid shell vials, hold 2–5 days Standard tubes, hold 4–6 weeks

*Common bacteria including staphylococci, streptococci, Enterobacteriaceae, *Pseudomonas*, etc.

B, bronchial washes, brushes, biopsies, bronchoalveolar lavage; CA, cold agglutinins; CF, complement fixation; CSF, cerebrospinal fluid; EIA, enzyme immunoassay; FA, fluorescent antibody; IS, induced sputum; L, lung biopsy; NP, nasopharyngeal suction or swab; S, sputum, tracheal aspirates.

Blood-Stream Infections

Blood cultures are considered one of the most significant specimen types processed by the microbiology laboratory. Every laboratory has strict notification policies to ensure that positive blood cultures are promptly reported to the physician. Automated blood culture systems now provide us with the capability of "continuous monitoring," by which a growth reading is automatically taken every 10 to 20 minutes throughout the day to detect positive cultures as quickly as possible. Monitoring does not require entry into bottles, so contamination rates remain low. Nonbottle systems such as the lysis-centrifugation system (Isolator, Wampole Laboratories, Cranbury, NJ) are used in some hospitals for routine bacteria, fungi, or mycobacteria, or for fastidious organisms such as *Bartonella* or *Brucella*. Although lysis-centrifugation offers advantages such as colony counts and isolated colonies for rapid identification, it remains a fairly labor-intensive method that has rates of contamination higher than those of bottle systems and therefore is not widely used.

For most common, nonfastidious pathogens, the type of blood culture system used is probably not as significant a factor in the reliable detection of septicemia as are other important considerations, such as collection before the start of antibiotics, drawing of a sufficient volume of blood, and use of a phlebotomy team for drawing cultures. Optimal blood culturing starts with proper skin preparation for venipuncture: The skin surface is first cleansed with 70% alcohol, followed by tincture of iodine (1 minute) or povidone iodine (2 minutes). The septum of the culture bottle or tube needs only to be wiped with 70% alcohol, and the blood must be immediately injected without a needle change. Blood cultures should be transported to the laboratory promptly so that processing and incubation can be started without delay. The volume of blood cultured and the number of sets drawn are particularly important factors that determine the success of detection. Often, the number of organisms per milliliter of blood is low, or the circulation of organisms may be intermittent, so the current recommendation for adult patients is that the clinician should draw at least two separate blood cultures that total 30 to 40 mL of blood. Separate venipunctures should be performed to help in the interpretation of cultures that contain skin flora such as *Staphylococcus epidermidis* and *Corynebacterium* species. In cases of fever of unknown origin, subsequent sets at later times in the day may be indicated. For children, the maximum amount of blood that can be taken depends on the weight and clinical status of the child; usually, 1 to 3 mL may be obtained from a child younger than 6 years of age, whereas neonates may be able to afford only 0.5 to 1 mL. When the volume drawn is 2 mL or less, pediatric blood culture systems should be used to achieve the optimal blood-to-broth dilution ratio. The use of pediatric bottles for adult patients or for older children results in less blood cultured; this should be discouraged except in the most unusual circumstances because smaller volumes significantly compromise the effectiveness of blood cultures. For both children and adults, blood cultures should be obtained before the start of antibiotic therapy to prevent inhibition of organism growth.

In recent years, many bacteremias have been associated with the increased use of catheters for intravenous access, including long-term percutaneous catheters and subcutaneous implanted devices and short-term catheters used for a variety of limited vascular access needs. Hospitals in which the use of indwelling intravenous lines is commonplace have seen an increase in organisms such as coagulase-negative staphylococci, corynebacteria, *Bacillus*, yeast, and even a variety of uncommon but opportunistic gram-negative rods. Microbiologists have long recommended that blood for cultures should not be drawn through catheters because a positive culture may represent not true septicemia, but rather colonization or localized infection of the catheter site. Some laboratories perform semiquantitative catheter tip cultures according to the guidelines of Maki and colleagues[19] to help determine the likelihood of catheter-related infection. Despite laboratory recommendations that blood for cultures should not be drawn through intravenous catheters, the ease of drawing blood through these catheters with little discomfort to the patient has made this practice common. In addition, physicians may have clinically significant concerns about keeping the catheter in place and treating with antibiotics without removal of the catheter. For these reasons, the use of catheter-drawn blood cultures continues to be on the rise. For laboratories that use quantitative blood culture systems (e.g., Isolator), a substantially higher colony count from cultures on catheter-drawn blood versus peripheral blood cultures is commonly used to identify a catheter-related focus for the bacteremia.

In most hospitals, the most common blood culture isolates are *S. epidermidis* and other coagulase-negative staphylococci.[20] The frequent occurrence of these organisms as contaminants that originate from the patient's skin or as true infecting agents from colonized or infected catheters in immunocompromised hosts has led laboratories to establish various reporting policies to lessen unnecessary additional work. In many hospitals, algorithms are used to suggest that certain positive cultures are "contaminants," and further workup such as species identification and antibiotic susceptibility testing will not be pursued unless the physician so directs.[21]

Standard blood culture protocols usually provide one aerobic and one anaerobic bottle for each blood culture set. Examination of the usefulness and cost-effectiveness of routine inclusion of an anaerobic bottle for all blood cultures has led to the suggestion that anaerobic blood cultures should be done only by specific request, and that the second bottle instead should be an additional aerobic bottle.[22] This practice would increase the overall sensitivity of the culture for aerobic and facultatively anaerobic bacteria and fungi. However, unanticipated sepsis with anaerobes would place patients at high risk for serious, potentially life-threatening infection.[23] At present, each hospital should determine the combination of bottles that would be most desirable for its patient population. In addition to an aerobic/anaerobic or aerobic/aerobic two-bottle set, the use of resin-containing bottles, different broth media, or fungal broth media can be considered.

Blood cultures are usually incubated for 5 to 7 days, except for specific situations, for example, when fastidious organisms are anticipated such as *Brucella* and *Bartonella*, or in cases of suspected subacute bacterial endocarditis or prolonged fever of unknown origin. Laboratory policies on extended incubation (e.g., from 2 to 4 weeks) vary according to the type of blood culture system used. For some bottle systems, weekly subcultures, acridine orange staining, or both are recommended for reliable detection of organisms such as *Brucella, Bartonella, Campylobacter,* or *Helicobacter.* Organisms such as *N. gonorrhoeae, Neisseria meningitidis, Gardnerella vaginalis, Streptobacillus moniliformis,* and *Peptostreptococcus anaerobius* may be inhibited by the anticoagulant used in most blood culture systems—sodium polyanethole sulfonate—so culture for these agents requires media without this anticoagulant. Optimal methods should be used whenever possible for the growth of *Brucella, Bartonella, Campylobacter, Helicobacter, Abiotrophia, Legionella, Nocardia,* and *Malassezia.* Table 15-3 provides a general overview of the usefulness of specific blood culture methods for various organisms. Further discussion of blood cultures for mycobacteria, fungi, and viruses is provided later in this chapter.

Intravenous Catheter Tip Cultures

As has been mentioned earlier, semiquantitative culture of catheter tips obtained by rolling the tip across a blood-agar plate is the method used most commonly. A breakpoint of 15 or more colonies suggests that these organisms are indicative of catheter infection,[19] although other investigators suggest that a lower breakpoint such as 5 colonies more accurately identifies infection.[24] Other methods include simple qualitative cultures done by incubation of the tip immersed in broth, by culture of sonicates of segments or tips, or by intraluminal flushing of the catheter tip with broth to culture the inside of the catheter segment. Quantitative culture performed by flushing, sonicating, or vortexing the catheter segment and then preparing and plating a set of dilutions for colony counts is more labor intensive but may be a more accurate predictor of catheter-related sepsis.[25] Guidelines have been established for the prevention of catheter-related infection; these include definitions for different types of catheter-related infections.[26] Use of these definitions should help in the standardization and improvement of future analyses of catheter-related infections.

Central Nervous System Infections

CSF is another type of specimen that requires immediate processing, as well as prompt reporting of results of Gram stain or other direct tests such as cryptococcal antigen assays or acid-fast stains. These specimens must be transported to the laboratory quickly because fastidious organisms such as *N. meningitidis* may become nonviable if the specimen is allowed to sit at room temperature or in a refrigerator. Because multiple tubes are sent for microbiologic, hematologic, and chemistry analyses, it is important that the most turbid specimen be used for microbiology and that enough fluid be allocated for adequate coverage of the culture requests. Gram stain and routine culture may require only 1 to 2 mL of CSF; however, if fungal or mycobacterial infection is suspected, larger volumes of CSF, preferably more than 2 mL for each test, increase the likelihood of successful culture.

Gram stains should be done on all spinal fluids with the use of a concentrated sediment smear prepared by centrifugation or by means of a cytocentrifuge. Because the number of organisms present may be low but the nature of the organisms seen on direct Gram stain could be of immediate critical assistance in the initiation of optimal antibiotic coverage, it is particularly important that these stains be done on well-concentrated smears, and that results be reported to the physician immediately. If properly done and read by someone with microscopic expertise, the direct Gram stain can provide a preliminary answer in 60% to 80% of untreated cases; it is most sensitive for *Haemophilus influenzae* and less sensitive for *N. meningitidis* and *S. pneumoniae.*

TABLE 15-3 Special Blood Culture Methods[*]

Organism	Method	Comments
Abiotrophia and *Granulicatella*	Bottle systems	Subculture to blood agar with pyridoxal or place staphylococcal streak for satelliting growth
Bartonella	Lysis-centrifugation	More sensitive and faster than bottle systems. Use fresh blood agar; incubate 12–14 days
Brucella	Lysis-centrifugation (5%–10% CO_2)	LC may be most sensitive with earliest detection (3–5 days)
	Bi-phasic systems (5%–10% CO_2)	Regularly flood agar with broth phase
	Bottle systems (5%–10% CO_2)	Do weekly blind subcultures. No growth in anaerobic bottles
Campylobacter and *Helicobacter*	Bottle systems	Stain with acridine orange; may have minimal growth indices, slow growth
	Lysis-centrifugation	Blood plates must be incubated in reduced O_2 atmosphere
Legionella	Lysis centrifugation	Plate LC concentrate onto BCYE plates
Leptospira	Fletcher's semisolid or EMJH[†] medium	Only during 1st week of illness; incubate in dark, in air, 28–29°C, 4–6 weeks. Use darkfield or phase-contrast microscopy
Nocardia	Lysis-centrifugation or bottle system	Extend incubation of primary blood agar plates or of bottles

[*]Blood cultures for mycobacteria and fungi are discussed in subsequent sections.
[†]Elinghausen, McCullough, Johnson, and Harris medium for leptospires.
BCYE, buffered charcoal yeast extract agar; LC, lysis centrifugation.

Bacterial antigen tests for *S. pneumoniae, H. influenzae, N. meningitidis,* group B streptococci (*Streptococcus agalactiae*), and *Escherichia coli* K1 are offered by few laboratories. Their overall cost-effectiveness has been decreased because of the dramatic reduction in *H. influenzae* meningitis that occurred after the introduction of *H. influenzae* type b vaccine. Laboratories need to determine the real benefit, if any, of maintaining these tests in their hospital setting because they rarely affect patient management for acute bacterial meningitis.[27] If the direct Gram stain is negative, initiation of antibiotic therapy based on the most appropriate empirical coverage rather than in response to antigen testing is a safer course of action in life-threatening situations. Culture yields the definitive diagnosis and should determine whether modification of antibiotic coverage is warranted. Bacterial antigen test results should not be used to modify initial empirical therapy. Antigen testing for *Cryptococcus neoformans,* however, is both a sensitive and a specific way of establishing the diagnosis of cryptococcal meningitis. Such testing, which can be done either by latex agglutination assays or by EIAs, has replaced the India ink wet preparation as the direct test of choice.

Most bacteria that cause acute meningitis grow well on chocolate agar, unless they have been damaged by antibiotic intervention. This medium allows for good growth of the primary pathogens, including *E. coli* and group B streptococci in neonates and infants; *Listeria* in neonates, infants, immunosuppressed patients, and the elderly; *H. influenzae* predominantly in children; *N. meningitidis* either in children or in adults; and *S. pneumoniae* in children, adults, and the elderly. As has been previously mentioned, since the introduction of *H. influenzae* type b vaccine, a notable drop has occurred in meningitis caused by this organism; therefore, *S. pneumoniae, N. meningitidis,* and *Listeria monocytogenes* are currently the most common agents of bacterial meningitis.[28] The use of multitarget PCR techniques to increase the sensitivity of detection of these bacterial pathogens is ideal for rapid, specific diagnosis of critical infections that are usually caused by only a few species of bacteria.[29] *C. neoformans,* which is of particular concern in immunocompromised patients, also grows well on chocolate or blood-agar plates, and colonies can be detected within a few days. Detection of mycobacteria and viruses from central nervous system specimens is discussed later in this chapter. Spinal fluid specimens are not generally cultured for anaerobic bacteria unless a specific request is made.

Sterile Body Fluid Infections Other Than Blood, Urine, and Cerebrospinal Fluid (Peritoneal Fluid/Dialysate; Pleural, Synovial, Pericardial Fluids)

Normal sterile body fluids are concentrated by either centrifugation or filtration if the volume of specimen is sufficient because the number of organisms may be low. To improve culture sensitivity, culturing of larger volumes of fluid in blood culture bottles has been recommended, particularly for peritoneal and dialysate fluids.[30] This concept may be expanded to improve the recovery of organisms from all types of sterile fluid because some automated blood culture systems have been approved for use with these specimens. Although the use of blood culture bottles that are read by automated instrumentation streamlines work for laboratories, undiluted specimen should also be sent along with the bottles so that direct Gram stains can be made and agar media inoculated. The types of organisms seen on direct Gram stain of the fluid can give initial guidance regarding antibiotic coverage; the ability to work with isolated colonies from agar plates provides more rapid organism identification and susceptibility testing than can be achieved with broth media. Direct plating of the fluids allows detection of mixed infections, whereas growth in broth may initially reveal only the most rapidly growing organism. Unlike the narrow spectrum of organisms isolated from CSF, other body fluids can be infected with a wide range of bacteria, fungi, mycobacteria, and viruses. When fluid is limited in quantity, the clinician must prioritize and select the most appropriate array of tests to request. Although any growth from these fluids must be considered significant and reported immediately, clinical judgment is required in assessing real significance because contamination during collection and processing of the specimen occasionally occurs.

Urinary Tract Infection

Urine culture, primarily with clean-voided midstream urine samples, remains one of the microbiology laboratory's most requested tests. The accuracy and therefore the usefulness of the culture results, however, are dependent on how well the specimen is collected and how promptly it arrives at the laboratory. Specific, detailed instructions should be given to each patient at the time of urine collection to minimize contamination with genital bacteria. Laboratories should ensure that specimen delivery occurs within 2 hours of collection or, if this is not possible, that refrigeration is provided until the time of pickup, or that urine transport tubes that contain preservatives are supplied. Laboratories will not culture Foley catheter tips. Suprapubic aspirates, done primarily in infants or other patients in whom assessment of clean-voided urine is difficult, should be clearly labeled as such so that all growth is identified and reported. This recommendation also holds for specimens obtained at cystoscopy or by other invasive procedures. Anaerobic cultures are not performed unless specifically requested, and these must be done on suprapubically aspirated urine.

Rapid screening techniques for urinary tract infection include direct Gram stains and a variety of commercially available products such as dipstick methods, bioluminescence, and filtration devices. A Gram stain is prepared by placing a drop of well-mixed, uncentrifuged urine onto a slide, air-drying, and then staining. The slide is read with the oil immersion lens; 1 or more organisms per oil immersion field is equivalent to 10^5 or more colony-forming units per milliliter. If the Gram stain is read by a well-trained microscopist, correlation of stain with culture results should be quite good for colony counts of 10^5 or greater. The presence of mixed bacterial types or a moderate amount of squamous epithelial cells usually indicates contamination with normal genital flora. Also, direct Gram stains cannot be used to detect situations in which 10^4 colony-forming units per milliliter or fewer might be considered significant. Use of other rapid screening methods may provide some efficiency if the method has a high negative predictive value and is used to screen out specimens that would be culture negative. If detection of lower colony counts (10^4 to 10^5) is desired, however, care should be taken to ensure that these specimens are not eliminated through the screening procedure. In addition, the reliability of the screening system should be determined, particularly for patients who are neutropenic.

Fortunately, the most common urinary tract pathogens are easy to grow, and grow quickly. These organisms include *Escherichia, Klebsiella, Enterobacter, Proteus, Pseudomonas, Enterococcus,* and *Staphylococcus* spp. Contaminants that are generally disregarded include lactobacilli, diphtheroids, nonenterococcal α-hemolytic streptococci, and coagulase-negative staphylococci other than *Staphylococcus saprophyticus.* In some patient populations, high colony counts of *S. epidermidis* may also be considered significant. Yeast, particularly *Candida* species, may be isolated from routine midstream urine cultures, often in quantities deemed significant for bacteria. Determination of true urinary tract infection with yeast, however, may require more invasively obtained specimens because heavy genital colonization, long-term urinary catheterization, or both may make this distinction difficult. The value of colony counts in the prediction of true yeast urinary infection has not been well documented or substantiated, particularly in recent years.

Urine specimens are also used for the detection of other fungi, mycobacteria, *Leptospira,* viruses, and *Chlamydia.* Further discussion of their use with these organisms is found later in this chapter and in the specific chapters related to these organisms. For culture of fungi and mycobacteria, first morning specimens are recommended.

Gastrointestinal Infection

Gastritis

The discovery of *Helicobacter pylori* and its association with gastritis has resulted in the need for diagnostic verification of the presence or absence of this organism. Detection of serum antibody to *H. pylori* is widely used to provide evidence of past or recent infection. The urea breath test is another noninvasive test procedure that can be used.

Culture of this organism requires gastric tissue that must be inoculated onto enriched media under microaerophilic conditions; growth is generally not visible before 3 days of incubation. Growth of the organism may be desired when it is believed that treatment failure is related to antibiotic resistance, which requires in vitro antibiotic susceptibility testing for confirmation. Gastric tissue can also be used to demonstrate the organism by Gram stain or by special histologic stains, or to perform rapid presumptive tests to detect the hydrolysis of urea caused by *H. pylori*. These rapid tests generally rely on an obvious color (pH) change caused by the presence of a potent urease in the gastric biopsy tissue. A less invasive alternative involves testing the patient's stool for the presence of *H. pylori* antigen with the use of commercially available EIA products. These assays provide greater than 90% sensitivity and specificity.[9,31]

Diarrheal Disease

Acute diarrhea can have a wide variety of etiologies, including bacteria, viruses, and parasites. Stool specimens are preferred to rectal swabs and should be transported to the laboratory quickly. Recommendations for minimizing unnecessary stool cultures include rejection of routine bacterial stool cultures in patients who have been hospitalized for 3 days or longer.[32] Most laboratories also have guidelines that limit specimen submissions to one per day and no more than three specimens (on successive days) for initial screening of acute gastroenteritis.

The spectrum of bacterial diarrheal pathogens is relatively well defined, and all laboratories have a "routine" setup to look for the common agents, which should include at a minimum *Campylobacter, Salmonella,* and *Shigella*. The presence of white blood cells suggests invasive infection with *Campylobacter, Shigella,* or enteroinvasive *E. coli,* so direct Gram stains are sometimes requested in the search for leukocytes. Enrichment broths to detect small numbers of organisms may or may not be performed, depending on each hospital's experience in terms of their overall usefulness. When stool specimens are submitted for bacterial culture, certain pathogens such as *Vibrio* or *Aeromonas* may need to be specifically requested.

Although enterohemorrhagic *E. coli* (also referred to as Shiga-like toxin– or Vero toxin–producing *E. coli,* including O157-H7) is a significant pathogen, recovery of this organism, even with selective media, is often low except in an outbreak situation or with bloody stool specimens. For this reason, many laboratories screen for enterohemorrhagic *E. coli* only when specifically requested. All laboratories must have this capability because serious infections such as hemolytic-uremic syndrome and severe hemorrhagic colitis can be caused by enterohemorrhagic *E. coli*. Commercially available enzyme-linked immunosorbent assays (ELISAs) that can be used directly on stool specimens or on culture isolates provide simple tests with acceptable sensitivities and specificities compared with culture, although at an added cost. Other known pathogens, particularly the various types of diarrhea-producing *E. coli,* *Vibrio* spp. (*Vibrio cholerae* and halophilic vibrios), *Yersinia,* and *Aeromonas* spp., may need to be specifically requested because they may not be detected by the laboratory's routine screening procedures. Additional specific selective media would need to be included for optimal sensitivity. These include thiosulfate-citrate–bile salts–sucrose agar for *Vibrio,* and cefsulodin-irgasan-novobiocin agar for *Aeromonas* and *Yersinia*.

For *Clostridium difficile,* toxin detection rather than organism culture is recommended. When culture is needed for epidemiologic or comparative study purposes, a specific request and a selective medium (cycloserine cefoxitin egg yolk–fructose agar) that has been incubated anaerobically are required. Toxin assays vary in sensitivity and specificity, with the labor-intensive, time-consuming tissue culture assay being the most specific. Rapid latex agglutination assays and the early versions of EIAs proved to be insufficiently sensitive and specific, but the newer-generation EIAs that detect toxins A and B provide acceptable performance.[33] Wide variation in sensitivities, specificities, and positive and negative predictive values of these assays has been observed. However, these simpler, more rapid assays can have an immediate impact on patient care decisions since results are available in a matter of hours rather than days. It should be mentioned that some laboratories use an EIA that detects glutamate dehydrogenase as a rapid screening assay to rule out *C. difficile* disease. This assay cannot distinguish between toxigenic and nontoxigenic strains; thus, although it may have reasonable sensitivity, the positive predictive value is lower than desirable and requires that a specific toxin assay be used for confirmation. In the evaluation of new methods such as EIAs, difficulty is always encountered in establishing what constitutes a "true" positive because even the tissue culture assay that is treated as the gold standard may not be an adequately sensitive standard.

Parasitic etiologies have become more common, particularly with greater recognition of cryptosporidial infection. Receipt of fresh specimens is important, and if delay is expected, the specimen should be placed in an appropriate fixative generally supplied by the laboratory. When *Cryptosporidium, Cyclospora,* or microsporidia are sought, the request must be specified because special techniques are needed to detect these organisms. Detection of *Giardia* infection has been improved by the development of immunoassays. As has been suggested for the submission of stool for routine cultures, it is similarly recommended that stool for parasitic evaluation be limited to the first 3 days of hospitalization.[34]

Genital Infections, Including Sexually Transmitted Diseases

The genital tract normally contains many organisms that reside as colonizing flora, including coagulase-negative staphylococci, lactobacilli, corynebacteria, streptococci, anaerobes, and yeast. On occasion, genital tract infection may be caused by members of this endogenous population, for example, by *G. vaginalis* or *S. agalactiae*. In addition, specific pathogens, particularly those involved in sexually transmitted diseases, must be considered when infectious etiologies are determined. Commonly submitted specimens include vaginal or penile discharge, genital ulcers, and urethral, cervical, and anorectal swabs. Genital infections can be caused by many different bacteria, including actinomycetes, *Haemophilus* spp., *Staphylococcus aureus,* Enterobacteriaceae, *N. gonorrhoeae,* group A and group B streptococci, and anaerobes, to name a few. In addition to bacteria, *Ureaplasma urealyticum, Chlamydia trachomatis, Trichomonas,* and viruses may need to be included in the infectious differential. Certain pathogens are known to be associated with specific types of genital infection; thus, the physician bases the selection of culture requests on the suspected type or location of infection.

Vaginitis with accompanying discharge can be caused by *Trichomonas vaginalis, Candida,* or bacteria, as in the case of bacterial vaginosis. *T. vaginalis* is often diagnosed microscopically in wet mounts of vaginal secretions, although culture of this organism has been shown to be more sensitive. More recently, monoclonal fluorescent antibody stains have become available; they are more costly than traditional wet mounts but may be more sensitive. Vaginal candidiasis is most frequently diagnosed by direct smears that show many budding yeast and pseudohyphae. Although culture of *Candida* can be accomplished rapidly and easily, growth of *Candida* is not necessarily diagnostic of candidal infection because many asymptomatic women harbor *Candida* spp. The etiology of nonspecific vaginitis or bacterial vaginosis is controversial, with organisms such as *G. vaginalis, Mobiluncus, Mycoplasma hominis,* and anaerobic gram-negative rods thought to play a role, most likely through coinfection or overgrowth with these organisms. The diagnosis of bacterial vaginosis is not based on bacterial culture because growth and identification of these presumed pathogens is difficult, slow, and therefore expensive. Gram stain of vaginal secretions suggests bacterial vaginosis when evidence of *Gardnerella* is detected by the presence of "clue cells," or when a prevalence of delicate gram-negative and gram-variable curved or fusiform bacteria, along with a reduction or absence of typical lactobacillary forms, is noted. The watery character of the discharge, a pH greater than 4.5, and the characteristic fishy amine odor are also used to support this diagnosis.[35]

N. gonorrhoeae is a major pathogen in genital infections such as cervicitis, salpingitis, urethritis, and epididymitis. Because this organism is delicate, specimens should be sent in appropriate transport media, should be transported promptly, and should never be refrigerated. The specimen type will depend on the site of infection, but anorectal or oropharyngeal specimens may also be sent with a specific request to look for *N. gonorrhoeae*. Gram stain and culture are still indicated, although newer nonculture methods, particularly DNA hybridization (probe) or amplification assays, are increasingly used because of their speed and accuracy. Isolation of *N. gonorrhoeae* would still be needed if antibiotic susceptibility testing were required. The direct Gram stain is the most rapid and inexpensive way of making a presumptive diagnosis of gonococcal infection in symptomatic men. The sensitivity and specificity of urethral smears in these instances, when read by trained microscopists, are as high as 95%. The sensitivity decreases when urethral specimens from asymptomatic men are examined, although the specificity remains good. Gram stains of cervical discharge are thought to be less reliable because of the presence of other organisms, which can make interpretation error prone; these stains are done by some laboratories but may be discouraged by others because of concerns about accuracy.

Infections caused by *N. gonorrhoeae* and *C. trachomatis* are often clinically difficult to distinguish and coinfection is common, so diagnostic testing should include methods that will detect both agents. Although cell culture methods and rapid shell vial cultures are available for the growth of *C. trachomatis,* they are done only by a limited number of laboratories. Instead of cultures, direct immunofluorescence with specific monoclonal antibodies or commercially available EIA assays has been used. The commercial development of specific DNA probes for *C. trachomatis* has further advanced sensitive and specific detection in urethral and endocervical specimens. Alternative molecular methods, which rely on nucleic acid amplification techniques (PCR, ligase chain reaction, and transcription-mediated amplification), have been designed to detect both *N. gonorrhoeae* and *C. trachomatis*. Amplification methods can be used on urine samples with excellent sensitivity, which is a decided benefit. The rapidity and increased sensitivity of these assays are attractive, although the increased cost of amplification tests must also be considered.

Other pathogens that cause genital infection include *Treponema pallidum, Haemophilus ducreyi, Ureaplasma,* and herpes simplex virus (HSV). Diagnostic recommendations for these and other organisms are beyond the scope of this section and can be found in the relevant chapters devoted to these organisms.

Skin, Skeletal, and Soft Tissue Infections

These infections most frequently involve bacteria and less commonly are caused by mycobacteria and fungi. Specimens sent to the laboratory include tissue biopsy specimens, aspirates or swabs of abscesses, wound swabs, material obtained by surgical débridement, and drainage samples. The usefulness of these cultures may be limited by the character of the lesion being cultured because lesions that connect with skin, mucosal surfaces, or gastrointestinal contents are encumbered by the presence of indigenous microflora. For meaningful culture results, laboratories prefer surgically obtained tissue samples, aspirates of closed abscesses, and an aliquot of pus or fluid rather than swab samples. When anaerobic bacteria are expected, the specimen should be inoculated into an anaerobic transport container and delivered promptly. Swabs of superficial skin ulcers, from the skin surface of a sinus tract, or from open abscesses commonly yield mixed bacterial flora and often do not reflect the organisms of true infectious significance. For these infections, every effort should be made to sample from the deeper aspects of the lesion with careful avoidance of the contaminated tissue surface so that the best possible specimen is obtained.

Wound infections and abscesses are caused by many different organisms, including routine bacteria, anaerobic bacteria, mycobacteria, and fungi. A long list of these organisms is not helpful, but it is important for the clinician and the laboratory technician to recognize that certain organisms are often associated with particular types of wounds or abscesses. An infected animal bite may yield *Pasteurella multocida* or *Capnocytophaga cynodegmi*; a post-traumatic hand infection may yield *S. aureus, Mycobacterium marinum,* or *Sporothrix schenckii,* depending on the source of trauma; a postoperative wound infection might yield *Pseudomonas* or *Acinetobacter* spp., among others. Laboratory guidelines include media and methods suitable for the isolation of most rapidly growing bacteria. Fungal, mycobacterial, and anaerobic cultures must be specifically requested if these organisms are suspected. When fastidious organisms such as *Francisella, Brucella,* or *Bartonella* are sought, the laboratory should be notified so that cultures can be set up appropriately and held for prolonged incubation as needed. Providing the laboratory with the location or type of wound, abscess, or tissue is often useful because it may hasten the recognition of specific pathogens known to be associated with that particular type of infection (e.g., cat bite, brain abscess).

Whenever an ample amount of specimen is available, a direct Gram stain should be performed to obtain some preliminary indication of the infecting organism(s). In some instances, if antibiotic therapy has been initiated, direct smear may be the only available guide to the etiology because growth may be inhibited. On tissue specimens, impression smears made by gentle pressing of a freshly cut surface of the tissue onto a slide should be examined in place of or in addition to ground tissue smears. Impression smears are easier to read and interpret than those made from material that has been ground or macerated. In addition to Gram stains, calcofluor white stains for fungi and acid-fast stains for mycobacteria can be done on impression smears. Direct Gram stains are of significant value not only for providing the physician with preliminary information about the type of organism(s) present but also as a guide for the microbiologist who is examining the culture. The presence of many epithelial cells, for example, indicates skin contamination, whereas observation of many polymorphonuclear leukocytes suggests a good-quality specimen. The types of organisms seen should be correlated with culture results because such correlation may sometimes help in the recognition of organisms that do not grow well under routine aerobic culture conditions. For example, faintly staining gram-negative rods that do not grow on routine aerobic plates should suggest the possibility of an anaerobic organism such as *Bacteroides.*

In some hospital settings, quantitative wound or tissue biopsy specimen cultures have been used to help predict the likelihood of wound sepsis and for the performance of skin grafts. Quantitative culture requires weighing and careful preparation of the specimen for serial dilutions to determine whether the colony count is greater than 10^5 colony-forming units per gram of tissue. Such colony counts are correlated with a greater likelihood of infection associated with wound closure. Direct Gram smears of known quantities of specimen can also be used to give an immediate assessment of organism load. Because quantitative cultures are time consuming and labor intensive, not all laboratories have procedures in place for performing these assays; the availability of quantitative wound cultures should be checked through consultation with the laboratory before tests are ordered.

INFECTIONS CAUSED BY AGENTS OF BIOTERRORISM

Bacillus anthracis, Francisella tularensis, Yersinia pestis, and *Brucella* spp. are the bacterial agents considered most likely to be used for bioterrorism. When such an event is suspected, the laboratory should be notified to put its bioterrorism protocol in place. Past experience with *B. anthracis* spread by intentionally contaminated mail has led to the development of better methods of screening for and confirming identification of *B. anthracis*. Once the laboratory identifies a nonhemolytic, nonmotile *Bacillus*, confirmation of *B. anthracis* can be provided rapidly by reference laboratories with the use of either PCR or fluorescent antibody assays specific for the pathogen. *F. tularensis* and *Brucella* require biosafety level (BSL) 3 precautions because they are known laboratory hazards. Although *Y. pestis* can be worked with caution at the BSL 2 level, most laboratories would likely choose to use BSL 3 precautions owing to the risk of unintended aerosolization. Promising results with rapid dipstick methods for detecting IgM for brucellosis and typhoid fever may improve rapid and specific diagnosis.[36] For more detailed information on these and other potential agents, consult the chapter on bioterrorism or chapters on specific agents of bioterrorism.

DETECTION AND IDENTIFICATION METHODS

As was shown in Figure 15-1, microorganisms can be identified in patient materials either by direct detection, which is commonly accomplished by special stains, or by culture methods that rely on growth of the organisms. In this section, bacterial detection and identification are discussed, with only superficial mention of methods used for mycobacteria, fungi, and viruses, each of which is discussed in greater detail in later sections of this chapter. Parasitology methods are covered more extensively in a separate chapter.

Direct Detection of Microorganisms in Patient Specimens

Microscopic Observation

Table 15-4 shows the stains most commonly used directly on patient specimens and the types of organisms that they detect. The Gram stain is a simple, yet reliable stain that can provide important preliminary information on whether a bacterial infection has been caused by a gram-negative or a gram-positive organism and whether the organism is a rod or a coccus. When read by an individual with microscopy expertise, the Gram stain gives an indication of the quality of the specimen; in addition to routine bacteria, it may reveal yeast and molds, and occasionally, parasites, mycobacteria, and *Nocardia*. As with all other direct stains, detection sensitivity is limited by the amount of material that can be reviewed on a slide, and if the number of organisms is low, they may not be seen.

Although the Gram stain provides a category of organism as a preliminary guide, it is a nonspecific stain. Specific stains that use antiserum conjugated to a fluorescent label are not used widely for direct detection of bacteria in patient specimens. At present, fluorescent antibody (FA) stains for *Legionella* and *B. pertussis* are the only ones still offered by some laboratories. Both of these commercially available stains are not considered to be effective for use in direct detection because the *Legionella* FA stain has low sensitivity, and *B. pertussis* FA has low specificity. The results of FA staining should be used with caution because false positives may occur from cross-reactivity with other organisms, and false negatives may result from poor quality of the antiserum or too few organisms. FA stains are always subject to technical concerns, primarily in reading and interpretation, which should be done only by trained individuals. FA stains have been used successfully for other organisms, including *Chlamydia*, some viruses, and some parasites (see specific chapters).

Wet mounts have traditionally been used for detection of fungi and parasites. The addition of potassium hydroxide to a wet preparation helps clarify the background of tissue cells, mucus, or proteinaceous materials and allows for better visualization of yeast or hyphal structures. Further discussion on direct detection by stains specific for fungi (including *Pneumocystis*), mycobacteria, and aerobic actinomycetes, as well as other methods of detection such as fungal antigen assays, can be found in later sections of this chapter.

Antigen Detection by Agglutination or Enzyme Immunoassays

Direct testing of patient specimens with simplified antigen assays has become more common and has been used for a variety of microorganisms. These assays are usually simple and rapid for laboratories to perform, and if reasonably sensitive and specific, they are adopted fairly rapidly into laboratory routine. Table 15-5 shows some of the assays that are currently being used. Commonly used EIA kits include either microtitration plate assays that require 2 to 4 hours for completion, or membrane immunoassays that take less than 15 minutes to complete. Depending on the organism being sought, tests are designed and approved for use with serum, CSF, stool, respiratory secretions, or urine. Antigenic assays for *C. difficile* and enterohemorrhagic *E. coli* are based on detection of the toxins rather than the organism. On request, or preferably as part of the laboratory report, performance characteristics of the assays should be supplied so that an educated assessment of

TABLE 15-4 Commonly Used Direct Stains for Microorganisms

Type of Stain	Comments
Gram stain	Determines Gram-positive versus Gram-negative bacteria, and provides general morphology (rods or cocci); also stains yeast. Filamentous fungi stain poorly; *Nocardia* and mycobacteria stain variably, often with a beaded appearance.
Acridine orange (AO)	AO stains are useful for viewing bacteria that are difficult to see on Gram stain, particularly in blood culture bottles (*Campylobacter*, *Helicobacter*, anaerobes, etc). Requires a fluorescent microscope.
Mycobacterial stains	Ziehl-Neelsen and Kinyoun stains are carbolfuchsin-based stains widely used for mycobacteria. Fluorochrome stains using auramine and rhodamine dyes that bind to the cell wall mycolic acids are more sensitive and easier to screen.
Nocardial stains	Often referred to as modified acid-fast stains, these have weaker or shorter decolorization steps than do traditional AFB stains, to demonstrate the acid-fastness of *Nocardia*. Also can be used for *Cryptosporidium*, *Cyclospora*, and *Isospora*.
Calcofluor white (CF)	CF is a whitening agent that binds to cellulose and chitin and is useful for staining fungi. Yeast and molds fluoresce brightly, making this a more sensitive stain than traditional wet mounts, but it requires a fluorescent microscope.
Fluorescent antibody stains (FA)	FA stains use monoclonal or polyclonal antibodies against specific organisms. The assays can be either direct FA or indirect FA, but most commonly use fluorescein isothiocyanate (FITC) as the fluorochrome.

AFB, acid-fast bacillus.

TABLE 15-5 Direct Antigen Detection Tests by Agglutination Assays or by Enzyme Immunoassays

Latex Agglutination	Enzyme Immunoassays
Bacterial antigens (used primarily for CSF specimens)	Bacterial antigens
Group B *Streptococcus*	Group A *Streptococcus*
Haemophilus influenzae, type b	*Legionella pneumophila*, serotype 1
Streptococcus pneumoniae	*Helicobacter pylori*
Neisseria meningitidis	*Streptococcus pneumoniae*
	Bacterial toxins
	Clostridium difficile
	Shiga-like toxins of *Escherichia coli*
Fungal antigen	Fungal antigen
Cryptococcus neoformans	*Cryptococcus neoformans*
	Parasitic antigens
	Giardia lamblia
	Cryptosporidium parvum
	Entamoeba dispar/histolytica
	Viral antigens
	Adenovirus 40/41
	Herpes simplex
	Influenza A and B
	Respiratory syncytial virus
	Rotavirus
	Chlamydial antigen
	Chlamydia trachomatis

CSF, cerebrospinal fluid.

the assessment of a positive or negative test can be made. The sensitivities and specificities of different commercial products may vary, even when testing is done for the same organism. Some EIA assays are best used in conjunction with, rather than in place of, cultures for improved detection of specific pathogens.

Molecular Assays

Development of molecular assays for the direct detection of microorganisms is an actively growing specialty. A comprehensive overview of diagnostic molecular microbiology has been provided by Hayden and Persing.[37] The first commercially offered assays for bacteria were based on DNA probe technology that detected specific ribosomal RNA sequences (Gen-Probe, San Diego, CA). This system currently uses acridinium ester–labeled, single-stranded DNA probes to detect complementary ribosomal RNA sequences of the target organism; this reaction is measured by chemiluminescence read on a luminometer. The method has been used as a direct test for only a few bacteria, mainly *N. gonorrhoeae* and *C. trachomatis,* but it is more widely used for culture confirmation of dimorphic fungi and mycobacterial species once colony or broth growth has become available.

Amplification techniques such as those using PCR or the ligase chain reaction provide increased sensitivity because of the extensive amplification of target nucleic acid. Various commercial amplification systems for the clinical laboratory that have been approved by the US Food and Drug Administration (FDA) are increasingly available, although in-house development of PCR assays has been under way for years. PCR assays developed in-house, as well as prospective commercial amplification systems that are under development, have been tested in many university- or research-affiliated institutions to validate the performance of these assays. Results from these investigations have been most encouraging and suggest that molecular diagnostics will usefully expand the ability of laboratories to detect organisms present in very low quantities, those that are difficult or slow to grow, and agents that are yet "undiscovered."[38] The potential power of these tools is substantial, and simplification of technology will eventually bring molecular methods more into the realm of possibility for the average clinical laboratory. The spectrum of validated assays, particularly for bacteria, is limited, and performance of these assays is technically complex and requires well-trained and knowledgeable personnel.

The experience of laboratories that offer molecular amplification assays has highlighted problems about which both the physician and the microbiologist need to be aware. The first critical issue is that of false-positive reactions because of amplicon (PCR product) contamination of the work area. False positives can lead to serious consequences in patient care, so laboratories must be particularly diligent about avoiding amplicon carryover. Control over this contamination can be exerted by allocation of separate work areas, pipettes, and reagents for the various components of the assay, as well as by the use of methods designed to inactivate the product from further amplification. A second source of error is false-negative results caused by inhibitors of the PCR reaction that are present in the patient's specimen, in the specimen transport medium, or in materials such as calcium alginate swabs. Although most assays use positive controls that contain known target, as well as external amplification controls, to detect inhibition as part of the quality control process, the best index of inhibition uses internal controls that mimic the target primers. Use of internal controls that are included in the test reaction mixture gives the most accurate assessment of inhibition.[39]

In addition to these important technical considerations, clinical assessment of amplification assays has yet to be accomplished for most microorganisms. For agents that are considered pathogens that need treatment or intervention regardless of the quantity, source, or medical status of the host, a positive amplification result may be interpreted in the same manner as a positive culture or other currently accepted measures of diagnosis (e.g., FA, EIA for antigen). For most other agents, however, amplification baseline information must be accumulated for various patient populations and correlated not only with traditional

detection methods but also with usefulness for patient care purposes. Because it is likely that PCR assays will be much more sensitive than the current traditional test for a particular organism, a higher rate of detection of "asymptomatic carriers" may occur, so the threshold for infection with the use of amplification techniques would be different from an assessment based on culture positivity. At this stage of molecular diagnostics in microbiology, it is prudent for the infectious diseases physician and the laboratory director to be critical in their acceptance and interpretation of results. The transition from research-based testing to clinical laboratory routine testing has been aided by the development of CLIA regulations and National Committee for Clinical Laboratory Standards (NCCLS) guidelines[40] that cover molecular laboratory requirements, along with the necessary validation of assays that must be provided by either commercial vendors or those offering tests that have been developed in-house.

Recent advances in molecular amplification include "real-time PCR," an exciting technology that significantly improves on traditional amplification-based techniques, which generally require postamplification inverventions to detect and measure the products of amplification. In real-time PCR systems, amplification and detection are carried out in a single, closed vessel, thereby eliminating cross-contamination risks due to carryover of amplicons. Multiple genes can be amplified and recognized in one reaction mixture with the use of dye-labeled probes (fluorophores) that are spectrally distinct. A full description of these methods can be found elsewhere.[41] Real-time PCR provides rapid automated quantitation of PCR products (<4 hr) and allows simultaneous detection and discrimination of multiple targets in one assay, with little risk of crossover contamination. These qualities make real-time PCR ideal for clinical situations in which a specific set of pathogens can be anticipated (e.g., bacterial meningitis, community-acquired pneumonias).

Detection by Culture

Much of diagnostic bacteriology has long relied on the growth of organisms on appropriate culture media and has traditionally based identification on biochemical characteristics. Clinical microbiology textbooks are available to help a laboratory determine the "standard" culture setups for various organisms.[7,8] Culture and identification methods for the subspecialties of mycology, mycobacteriology, and virology are discussed in later sections of this chapter; here, we focus mainly on culture of routine bacteria.

For common specimen types, laboratories use enriched all-purpose media, such as blood or chocolate agar, which grow most of the ordinary bacterial pathogens. For specimens that might contain mixed microbial flora, additional plates such as MacConkey or eosin-methylene blue agar for gram-negative bacteria and phenylethyl alcohol agar for gram-positive bacteria would also be inoculated. A broth medium into which a larger aliquot of specimen can be inoculated may be used to help in the detection of small numbers of organisms. Table 15-6 lists some of the organisms for which special enriched or selective media are required for optimal recovery. In addition to the selection of appropriate media, use of the optimal atmosphere (aerobic, aerobic with CO_2, microaerophilic, anaerobic) and temperature (25° C, 37° C, 42° C) is important.

Identification by Biochemical Methods

Once colony growth is evident on agar media, Gram stain morphology and characteristics such as colony size, color, and shape, and the presence or absence of hemolytic activity are used by the microbiologist in selection of the appropriate identification procedure. An experienced microbiologist often is able to provide reliable preliminary information on a culture on the basis of these early characteristics. For most common bacterial pathogens, identification can be done fairly simply and rapidly because of the availability of rapid key tests and miniaturized identification panels. For example, an opaque white, gray, or light yellow colony that on Gram stain appears as gram-positive cocci found predominantly in clusters will be tested promptly with a latex agglutination reagent for coagulase/protein A detection to determine

TABLE 15-6   Special Media Used for Specific Pathogens*

Organism	Media	Comments
Bordetella pertussis	Bordet-Gengou (BG) + methicillin or cephalexin Regan-Lowe cephalexin agar Horse blood charcoal agar	NP swabs rather than cough plates are recommended. *B. pertussis* will also grow on BCYE.
Burkholderia cepacia	PC agar OFPBL agar BCSA agar	Highly selective for *B. cepacia*; particularly useful for sputum cultures from cystic fibrosis patients.
Corynebacterium diphtheriae	Tinsdale agar (Tins) Cystine-tellurite blood agar Loeffler's slant	Brown halo around colonies on Tins is presumptive for *C. diphtheriae*. Use Loeffler's for "Chinese letter" forms.
Francisella tularensis	Blood- or chocolate-cystine agar	*Francisella* will also grow on most chocolate and Thayer-Martin agars, as well as on BCYE agar.
Legionella	Buffered charcoal yeast extract agar (BCYE)	BCYE formula that includes antibiotics can be used to inhibit growth of other organisms.
Leptospira	Fletcher's or Stuart's medium with rabbit serum, or *Leptospira* medium with BSA-Tween-80	Incubate cultures in the dark at 28–30° C for up to 6 weeks, and examine by darkfield microscopy.
Neisseria gonorrhoeae, meningitidis	Modified Thayer-Martin agar (MTM) New York City agar (NYC)	Both media inhibit growth of other bacteria and yeast.

*Not including gastrointestinal pathogens.
BCSA, *Burkholderia cepacia*–selective agar; BSA, bovine serum albumin; NP, nasopharyngeal; PC, *Pseudomonas cepacia*; OFPBL, "oxidative-fermentative base, polymyxin B, bacitracin, lactose."

whether it is *S. aureus* or a coagulase-negative *Staphylococcus* species. Specific laboratory procedures used for identification of organisms are not uniform from laboratory to laboratory because of the multiple choices of commercial products available for identification of each bacterial species. Table 15-7 describes key tests that are commonly used, along with colony and Gram stain morphology, to identify certain species of bacteria.

Biochemical differentiation of organisms used to be generally simple, inexpensive, and often rapid. Over the past 5 years, this process has become complicated by the explosion of newly recognized organisms and associated name changes brought about by more accurate taxonomic classification of organisms through molecular techniques such as 16S rRNA gene sequencing and DNA hybridization. Simplified schemes that were formerly based on a few key reactions or dichotomous flow charts can no longer be "simple" owing to the increased number of genera and species that must be included for error-free identification. Attempts to construct algorithms or flow charts result in highly complicated charts or diagrams[7] that are impractical for routine laboratory usage. Our improved ability to analyze organisms has revealed that only subtle phenotypic differences may exist among closely related species, making it necessary for laboratories to rely on commercial multitest identification panels to accurately identify isolates

to genus and species. Fortunately for the laboratory and clinicians, those pathogens that were common and significant in the past have remained common and significant, and most can be identified simply and rapidly (e.g., *S. aureus, E. coli, Pseudomonas aeruginosa*). With this approach, the NCCLS has provided guidelines for reliable, abbreviated identification of certain bacterial and yeast species.[42] It is generally the less commonly encountered organisms that require more extensive evaluation, and such unusual organisms may not be included in the database of identification panels. The laboratory must be aware of the robustness of the systems that it uses and must check to ensure that name changes are updated regularly. Table 15-8 shows some recent taxonomic changes of note. For organisms that are metabolically inactive or those that are difficult or slow to grow, molecular rather than biochemical identification may be more accurate and eventually may even be more rapid.

Gram-Positive Cocci

Gram-positive cocci can be subdivided into several important categories. Aerobic or facultatively anaerobic gram-positive cocci are regarded as staphylococcal-like by virtue of microscopic morphology that shows cocci in groups, clusters, or tetrads, and as streptococcal-like by the appearance of cocci in pairs and chains in broth media. In

TABLE 15-7   Common Biochemical Reactions Used to Identify Bacteria

Biochemical Test	Primary Use of Test
ALA test (δ-aminolevulinic acid)	Rapid presumptive differentiation of *Haemophilus influenzae* from *Haemophilus parainfluenzae* isolated from upper respiratory specimens.
Bacitracin (A) disk (0.04 U bacitracin)	For presumptive identification of group A β-hemolytic streptococci, which are all sensitive to low concentrations of bacitracin.
Bile solubility	For rapid differentiation of pneumococci (which are bile soluble) from other α-hemolytic streptococci.
Catalase	An important characteristic that defines significant major groups of bacteria, (e.g., staphylococci [catalase +], streptococci [catalase −]).
Coagulase	A positive coagulase test is the key criterion for identification of *Staphylococcus aureus*.
Hippurate hydrolysis	A positive test is used for presumptive identification of group B streptococci, and also for *Campylobacter jejuni*.
Indole	A rapid test is used for presumptive identification of *Escherichia coli* from urine specimens, but indole production is used for the identification of many different Gram-negative rods.
Optochin (Ethylhydrocupreine hydrochloride)	Susceptibility to optochin is presumptive identification of *Streptococcus pneumoniae*.
Oxidase	This is a key reaction to help differentiate Gram-negative rods (e.g., Enterobacteriaceae are oxidase negative; *Pseudomonas* are positive).
PYR hydrolysis (L-pyrrolidonyl-β-naphthylamide)	Used primarily for Gram-positive cocci in chains; a positive test suggests *Streptococcus pyogenes*, *Enterococcus* sp., or *Abiotrophia/Granulicatella* sp.
X and V factor requirements	Factor requirements are used to help identify the different species of *Haemophilus*; *H. influenzae* requires both X and V for growth; *H. parainfluenzae* requires only V factor.

TABLE 15-8 Recent Taxonomic Changes

Old Designation	New Name
Gram-Positive Cocci	
Abiotrophia adiacens, elegans	Granulicatella adiacens, elegans
Leuconostoc paramesenteroides	Weisella paramesenteroides
Staphylococcus caseolyticus	Macrococcus caseolyticus
Stomatococcus mucilaginosus	Rothia mucilaginosa
Gram-Positive Bacilli	
"Corynebacterium aquaticum"	Leifsonia aquatica
Gram-Negative Bacilli	
Achromobacter CDC group Vd	Ochrobactrum anthropi
Agrobacterium radiobacter	Rhizobium radiobacter
CDC Group DF3	Dysgonomonas capnocytophagoides
CDC Group DF3-like	Dysgonomonas gadei
CDC Group IVc-2	Ralstonia paucula
CDC Group IVe	Oligella urealytica
Flavobacterium gleum, indologenes, meningosepticum	Chryseobacterium gleum, indologenes, meningosepticum
Flavobacterium breve	Empedobacter brevis
Flavobacterium odoratum	Myroides odoratus/odoratimimus
Flavobacterium multivorans, spiritivorum	Sphingobacterium multivorans, spiritivorum
Moraxella phenylpyruvica	Psychrobacter phenylpyruvicus
Moraxella urethralis	Oligella urethralis
Pasteurella ureae	Actinobacillus ureae
Pseudomonas (Comamonas) acidovorans	Delftia acidovorans
Pseudomonas diminuta, vesicularis	Brevundimonas diminuta, vesicularis
Pseudomonas paucimobilis	Sphingomonas paucimobilis
Pseudomonas (Burkholderia) pickettii	Ralstonia pickettii
pickettii biovar 3	Ralstonia mannitolilytica
Weeksella zoohelcum	Bergeyella zoohelcum

recent years, additional genera and species of gram-positive cocci have become clinically significant and have complicated earlier simplified schemes, particularly those cocci that appear staphylococcal in morphology but are catalase negative. Although any of these organisms can be encountered as true pathogens on occasion, most of the less common species are infrequent agents of serious infection. Table 15-9 briefly summarizes the many different genera and species of clinically encountered aerobic and facultatively anaerobic gram-positive

cocci on the basis of a few important phenotypic characteristics. Strictly anaerobic gram-positive cocci occur either in clusters or in chains; nomenclature and identification for this group can be found in the chapter devoted to anaerobic cocci (Chapter 246).

The catalase test distinguishes common catalase-producing organisms such as *Staphylococcus* and *Micrococcus* from noncatalase producers such as *Streptococcus* and *Enterococcus*. For gram-positive cocci that appear staphylococcal according to colony morphology and color, a coagulase test is used to separate coagulase-positive *S. aureus* from coagulase-negative staphylococci, most commonly *S. epidermidis*, and other similar-appearing organisms. Methods include a standard tube coagulase test that is used to look for fibrin clot formation in plasma, a rapid slide coagulase test that requires a subsequent tube coagulase test for all negative reactions, and a rapid latex agglutination test that detects both clumping factor and protein A of *S. aureus*. Latex agglutination tests take only a few minutes to perform, and unlike with the slide coagulase test, negative reactions do not have to be confirmed with a tube coagulase test. The reliability of these tests is high, although both false-positive and false-negative reactions may occur. Some have reported that particular latex agglutination tests may not be reliable for the identification of methicillin-resistant *S. aureus,* although this experience does not appear to be generalized. Because the various commercial products vary in their performance, it is important for the microbiologist and the infectious diseases physician to know the characteristics of the particular assay used. Newer latex agglutination products with increased sensitivity have decreased false-negative reactions but may result in a higher false-positive rate. In most laboratories, an organism that yields a positive latex agglutination test would be identified as *S. aureus,* whereas organisms that are negative would be classified as "coagulase-negative staphylococci." For coagulase-negative staphylococci, species determinations are not routinely done, although some laboratories identify species from cases of significant bacteremia or other significant infections, as well as from urine cultures with high colony counts. The latter identification commonly uses resistance to novobiocin to detect *S. saprophyticus,* a known urinary tract pathogen found predominantly in young women. Species identification may be obtained from commercially available staphylococcal identification panels. Such identification is reasonably reliable, particularly for the most common species—*S. epidermidis;* newer species may be missing from commercial panel databases and either will not be identified or will be identified incorrectly.

TABLE 15-9 Clinically Encountered Aerobic and Facultatively Anaerobic Gram-Positive Cocci: A Simplified Recognition Scheme

		Microscopic Arrangement: Groups, Clusters, or Tetrads	
Catalase +			
	Coagulase +		Staphylococcus aureus (rarely, Staphylococcus intermedius)
	Coagulase −		
		Bacitracin R (0.04-μg disk)	Staphylococcus species (coagulase-negative), Macrococcus
		Bacitracin S (0.04-μg disk)	Alloiococcus, Kocuria, Micrococcus, Rothia mucilaginosa
Catalase−			
	Vancomycin-resistant		Pediococcus
	Vancomycin-sensitive		Aerococcus, Dolosigranulum, Facklamia languida, Gemella haemolysans, Helcococcus, Rothia
		Microscopic Arrangement: Pairs and Chains (all are catalase negative)	
β-Hemolytic			
	*PYR+		Streptoccous pyogenes (occasional Enterococcus)
	PYR −		β-hemolytic Streptococcus group B, C, F, or G
Nonhemolytic or α-hemolytic			
	PYR+		
		†Bile esculin +	Enterococcus (less commonly, Lactococcus, Vagococcus)
		Bile esculin −	Occasional Streptococcus pneumoniae‡
			Abiotrophia, Dolosicoccus, Facklamia, Gemella, Globicatella, Granulicatella, Ignavigranum
	PYR −		
		Vancomycin-resistant	Leuconostoc
		Vancomycin-sensitive	Streptococcus bovis group, viridans streptococci (includes Mitis, Anginosus, Mutans, and Salivarius groups), Streptococcus group B, Lactococcus, Streptococcus pneumoniae‡

*PYR, L-pyrrolidonyl-β-naphthylamide hydrolysis.
†Bile esculin, ability to tolerate bile and hydrolyze esculin.
‡S. pneumoniae readily identified by specific antisera, bile solubility +, or susceptibility to optochin.

In addition to *Staphylococcus* and *Micrococcus,* other gram-positive cocci arranged in groups, tetrads, or clusters have been described. These include those that are catalase positive (*Rothia mucilaginosa* [formerly *Stomatococcus mucilaginosus*], *Alloiococcus*) and those that are catalase negative (*Pediococcus, Aerococcus, Facklamia languida, Gemella haemolysans, Dolosigranulum, Helcococcus*). Most reside as normal human flora, so identification of these organisms would be pursued only when they have been isolated from a critical site such as blood and are assumed to be pathogens. Although five species of *Pediococcus* have been identified, *P. acidilactici* and *P. pentosaceus* are the species most commonly isolated from human clinical specimens.[43] Unlike the other genera, pediococci can be found in fermented vegetables, dairy products, and meat. *Pediococcus* is usually vancomycin resistant and should be suspected by virtue of this feature, although these organisms are only rarely opportunistic pathogens. *R. mucilaginosa* has been isolated from blood cultures in association with intravenous line sepsis and may initially look like coagulase-negative staphylococci until its colonies become adherent, gummy, and difficult to lift from the agar surface. The genus *Aerococcus* comprises five species and may be confused with α-hemolytic enterococci because both genera are catalase negative and PYR positive (i.e., they produce pyrrolidonyl arylamidase). Laboratories have limited experience with these "other" genera and species because they are not encountered frequently, especially as significant pathogens, and may escape identification if simplified tests that employ only a few key reactions are used.

Initial identification of streptococci and enterococci relies on the type of hemolysis observed on blood agar, as well as on colony size and morphology. For β-hemolytic streptococci, rapid testing to identify group A *Streptococcus* (*S. pyogenes*) is done by means of either the positive PYR test of this species or the presence of group A antigen as detected by latex agglutination with specific antisera. Both of these tests take less than 30 minutes to perform and can thus be done on the same day that colonies are observed, whereas the traditional method, which uses susceptibility to low-content bacitracin disks (A disk), requires overnight incubation and may yield false-positive reactions owing to bacitracin-susceptible strains of group C and G streptococci. β-Hemolytic streptococci from throat cultures are usually identified as group A or non–group A. When β-hemolytic streptococci are isolated from other significant sources such as blood, group identification is readily determined by latex agglutination, which is available for groups A, B, C, D, F, and G, or by commercial biochemical panels for identification of streptococcal species. Group B *Streptococcus* (*S. agalactiae*) is an important pathogen that in the past was identified either by its ability to hydrolyze hippurate or by a positive CAMP (Christie, Atkins, and Munch-Peterson) test to demonstrate synergistic hemolysis with *S. aureus.* These tests are inexpensive and reliably accurate; latex agglutination with group B antisera is fast, simple, and accurate but more expensive.

The extent of identification of *Enterococcus* spp. is dependent on individual laboratory policies. A key reaction that rapidly suggests a presumptive identification of *Enterococcus* is a positive PYR test, as has just been described for *S. pyogenes.* As is shown in Table 15-9, however, a positive PYR test is only presumptive because of the host of other species that are also PYR positive. Nonetheless, for a non-hemolytic or an α-hemolytic streptococcal organism, a positive PYR test is regarded as presumptive evidence of *Enterococcus.* Enterococcal isolates from blood and other sterile fluid sites are almost always identified to the species level, as are strains that are vancomycin resistant. Urinary or wound isolates, however, are often identified as *Enterococcus* without further species identification. Enterococcal species can be identified well with commercially available panels, and species identification has become a matter of greater interest and concern because of the emergence of vancomycin-resistant strains. *Enterococcus faecalis* is the most common species of *Enterococcus* encountered, and although *E. faecium* is second in frequency, it is often more difficult to treat because of multiple antibiotic resistances.

S. pneumoniae produces α-hemolytic colonies that have a coin- or a "checker"-shaped flat colony or a wet mucoid colony. Rapid presumptive identification can be obtained by placement of a drop of desoxycholate onto the colonies and observation of the disappearance of colonies (bile solubility), or by latex agglutination methods that use polyvalent (omni) pneumococcal antiserum. Presumptive identification of pneumococci can also be based on susceptibility to optochin (ethylhydrocupreine hydrochloride), which differentiates *S. pneumoniae* from other α-hemolytic streptococci, although this test requires overnight incubation.

α-Hemolytic and nonhemolytic streptococci that are nongroupable and are not pneumococci or enterococci are commonly found as human oral or gastrointestinal flora. These organisms have been called "viridans" or "green" streptococci and are not generally identified unless they are clearly significant, as in cases of bacteremia in an immunocompromised host or subacute bacterial endocarditis. These species of streptococci are difficult to identify accurately, although some commercial identification panels are available. Taxonomic modifications made for clinical reporting purposes have simplified the identification of these organisms by putting them into related subgroups rather than species.[44] These include *Streptococcus anginosus* group, *Streptococcus bovis* group, *Streptococcus mutans* group, *Streptococcus mitis* group, *Streptococcus salivarius group,* and *Streptococcus sanguis* group. These streptococci are no longer uniformly susceptible to penicillin in that intermediate as well as outright resistance has been seen, so in vitro susceptibility testing is warranted in patients with serious infection.[45] Similar in morphology to α-hemolytic streptococci are nutritionally deficient streptococci or "satelliting" streptococci, now designated as *Abiotrophia* and *Granulicatella* species. Members of these genera cannot grow on blood or chocolate agar unless the agar has been supplemented with pyridoxal. Although they do grow in broth blood cultures, they fail to grow upon subculture onto unsupplemented blood or chocolate agar. These organisms are also PYR positive, similar to enterococci and *S. pyogenes,* but PYR reactions may be delayed and weak.

Other more recently described species that appear as gram-positive cocci or coccobacilli in chains belong to the genera *Dolosicoccus, Facklamia, Globicatella, Ignavigranum, Lactococcus, Leuconostoc,* and *Vagococcus.* Of these, *Leuconostoc* is notable because of its inherent vancomycin resistance. It is often initially thought to be a streptococcus until antibiotic susceptibility testing reveals vancomycin resistance. Additional tests are then needed to firmly identify the isolate as *Leuconostoc.* The other genera mentioned here are unusual isolates that may be difficult to recognize and identify unless more extensive biochemical reactions are evaluated or molecular identification techniques are used. Almost all have been reported from clinically significant sites such as blood, urine, and wounds, but the clinical role of each must be evaluated on a case-by-case basis, according to the specific infectious presentation.

Gram-Positive Rods. In this section, only the aerobic and facultatively anaerobic gram-positive rods are discussed (Table 15-10); mycobacteria and *Nocardia* are described later in the chapter. The first major distinction made in this group of bacteria is whether they are capable of forming spores. Demonstration of spores in an organism that is growing aerobically is considered presumptive identification of *Bacillus,* although occasional species of *Paenibacillus* or *Brevibacillus* might be encountered. Aerotolerant clostridial species such as *Clostridium tertium* do not sporulate under aerobic conditions. Identification of the different species of *Bacillus* is labor intensive and time consuming because of the lack of commercially available identification panels for *Bacillus.* Most isolates of *Bacillus* are laboratory contaminants; on occasion, *Bacillus* causes bacteremia in an immunocompromised host, usually in association with intravenous catheters and most commonly caused by strains of *Bacillus subtilis, Bacillus cereus,* and *Bacillus licheniformis.* Because of past and potential future use of *B. anthracis* for bioterrorism, however, all laboratories must be able to culture, recognize, and presumptively identify this agent, and then must submit the organism to proper agencies for confirmation.

TABLE 15-10 Clinically Encountered Aerobic and Facultatively Anaerobic Gram-Positive Bacilli: A Simplified Recognition Scheme

Spores Formed on Aerobic Media, and Catalase +	*Bacillus* (occasionally, *Paenibacillus, Brevibacillus*)
Non–Spore Forming	
Catalase +, yellow pigmented	*Cellulomonas, Cellulosimicrobium, Curtobacterium, Exiguobacterium, Leifsonia aquatica ("Corynebacterium aquaticum"), Microbacterium, Oerskovia, Corynebacterium* (only a few yellow-pigmented species)
Catalase +, Nonpigmented	
Motile	
β-hemolytic	*Listeria monocytogenes*
Nonhemolytic	*Arthrobacter, Kurthia*
Nonmotile	
Pink colonies	*Rhodococcus equi*
Nonpigmented colonies	*Actinomyces (catalase +), Arthrobacter, Brevibacterium, Corynebacterium, Dermabacter, Rothia, Turicella*
Catalase −	
H₂S in TSI slant	*Erysipelothrix rhusiopathiae*
Vancomycin-resistant	*Lactobacillus*
Branching rods in thioglycolate broth	*Actinomyces*
β-hemolytic, weak or narrow zone	*Arcanobacterium haemolyticum, Arcanobacterium pyogenes*
None of above characteristics	*Gardnerella, Microbacterium, Rothia*

*Species colonizing or infecting humans:
Catalase+: *A. naeslundii I* and *II, A. neuii* subsp. *anitratus* and *neuii, A. viscosus, A. radicidentis.*
Catalase−: *A. europaeus, A. funkei, A. georgiae, A. gerencseriae, A. graevenitzii, A. israelii, A. meyeri, A. odontolyticus, A. radingae, A. turicensis, A. urogenitalis.*
H₂S, production of hydrogen sulfide in triple sugar iron (TSI) agar.

Non–spore-forming gram-positive rods are preliminarily identified by a few key characteristics, including type of hemolysis, catalase production, and motility. In addition, colony morphology and Gram stain morphology are critical to the microbiologist's pathway of identification. The number of newly recognized and described genera and species of non–spore-forming bacilli, along with concomitant name changes, has made reliable identification harder to achieve without the addition of a greater number of biochemical tests or assistance from genetically based identification tools. Commercial panels that simultaneously test multiple biochemical reactions are now available to help identify diverse species of gram-positive bacilli, although they have met with variable success. Major pathogens that must be promptly recognized for optimal patient management include *L. monocytogenes, C. diphtheriae, Erysipelothrix rhusiopathiae, Actinomyces* spp., *Rhodococcus equi,* and *Corynebacterium jeikeium.* As can be seen from Table 15-10, many species of gram-positive rods can be encountered, some as normal flora, some as environmental contaminants, and occasionally, as opportunistic pathogens.

L. monocytogenes is vigorously catalase positive and should be recognized by its β-hemolytic colonies and its characteristic "tumbling" motility, as observed by hanging drop or "umbrella" motility at 25° C in semisolid motility medium. Other catalase-positive, motile, aerobic, gram-positive rods such as *Oerskovia* or *Leifsonia aquatica* (formerly *Corynebacterium aquaticum*) are not β-hemolytic and have yellow-pigmented colonies. Confirmation of *Listeria* can be achieved by additional biochemical reactions or by the use of certain commercially available biochemical panels, for which *Listeria* identification is usually highly reliable.

Except for *C. diphtheriae, Corynebacterium* species, including *C. jeikeium,* are commonly found on skin or mucosal surfaces. *C. diphtheriae* isolation and identification require previous notification of the laboratory because specific selective media and toxigenicity studies are needed for successful culturing and identification. The other corynebacteria and morphologically similar organisms that are catalase positive, nonmotile, and nonhemolytic are difficult for laboratories to identify to the species level. To date, at least 38 species of *Corynebacterium* have been determined to be of medical relevance.[46] As has been mentioned previously, some commercial panels are available for corynebacteria identification, although these are not in widespread use. Presumptive identification of *C. jeikeium* relies on colony and Gram stain morphology, although organisms such as *Corynebacterium urealyticum, Corynebacterium* Centers for Disease Control and Prevention (CDC)

group G2, and *Corynebacterium minutissimum* may appear similar. Antibiotic resistance profiles are used by many laboratories to confirm the identification of *C. jeikeium,* but *C. urealyticum* and CDC group G2 can also be resistant to multiple antibiotics.

R. equi, formerly *Corynebacterium equi,* can be a cause of serious, life-threatening pneumonia in patients with acquired immunodeficiency syndrome (AIDS). Like the corynebacteria, *R. equi* is nonmotile and catalase positive but can be distinguished by its mucoid, pink colony. Although it has been noted to be weakly acid fast, this characteristic should not be used as a screening test to identify this organism because acid-fastness is frequently very difficult to demonstrate. Other species of *Rhodococcus* may be variously pigmented and nonmucoid but have not been reported to cause fulminant pneumonia.

Clinically important catalase-negative aerobic gram-positive rods are generally nonmotile. Important pathogens include *E. rhusiopathiae, Actinomyces* spp., and occasionally, *Lactobacillus* spp. Both *E. rhusiopathiae* and *Lactobacillus* spp. have strains that may show in vitro vancomycin resistance. The production of H₂S in a triple sugar iron agar slant is a useful reaction that quickly provides presumptive evidence of *Erysipelothrix.* This organism should also be suspected if it is isolated from a skin lesion in a person with a history suggestive of fish handling or, on occasion, when isolated from a blood culture from a patient with subacute bacterial endocarditis. Confirmation of identification as *E. rhusiopathiae* requires additional biochemical reactions. Vancomycin-resistant lactobacilli should be differentiated from vancomycin-resistant *Leuconostoc* species, which may be coccobacillary and thus mistakenly thought to be a gram-positive rod like *Lactobacillus.*

The genus *Actinomyces* has expanded to include at least 21 genogroups, and it is likely that more will be added. They are found on the mucosal surfaces of humans and animals. Identification of the various *Actinomyces* species is not simple, although anaerobic identification panels are currently available that attempt to do species identification. *Actinomyces* is suspected by the observation of short, branching forms; frequently, these appear diphtheroidal on solid media but show more definitive branching when grown in thioglycollate broth. Although *Actinomyces israelii* and *Actinomyces naeslundii* are catalase negative, *Actinomyces viscosus, Actinomyces naeslundii* genomospecies II, and *Actinomyces neuii* are catalase positive. *A. israelii* usually requires anaerobic conditions for initial growth, whereas *A. naeslundii, A. viscosus,* and *Actinomyces odontolyticus* can initiate growth in an aerobic environment supplemented with CO₂. Although *A. israelii, A. naeslundii, A. odontolyticus,* and *A. viscosus* are better known species, other species are now more commonly encountered, including *Actinomyces turicensis* (genitourinary specimens), *Actinomyces radingae* (soft tissue abscesses of breast, chest, and back), and *Actinomyces europeus* (skin abscesses of back and genital areas).[47]

Gram-Negative Cocci

Aerobic gram-negative cocci belong to the genus *Neisseria* and do not produce coccobacillary forms. *Moraxella* and *Acinetobacter* are classified as gram-negative rods, although both genera are sometimes observed to appear as gram-negative cocci and thus need distinction from *Neisseria. Moraxella catarrhalis,* formerly *Neisseria catarrhalis* and *Branhamella catarrhalis,* has microscopic morphology similar to that of *Neisseria*; it occurs as diplococci with flattened adjacent edges and, upon division, forms packets of four cocci rather than chains of coccobacilli, as are formed by other *Moraxella* and *Acinetobacter* species. *M. catarrhalis* can be quickly identified, however, by either of two biochemical tests for which it is positive and *Neisseria* is negative, by DNAse production, or by butyrate esterase production. *Neisseria* spp. are oxidase positive, which readily distinguishes them from oxidase-negative *Acinetobacter* spp.

Traditional identification of *Neisseria* species relies on the pattern of acid production from four sugars—glucose, maltose, lactose, and sucrose—and on the ability of the organism to grow on nutrient agar and to grow at room temperature. *N. gonorrhoeae* produces acid from glucose only, while *N. meningitidis* produces acid from glucose and maltose only. The common nonpathogenic species either do not produce acid from any of the four sugars or may produce acid additionally from lactose, sucrose, or both. These features, along with colony color and morphology and ability to grow on Thayer-Martin selective agar, guide species identification. Various kits for the identification of *Neisseria* species are available; some rely on sugar patterns, but more recently developed tests use detection of specific enzymes. The chapters on *Neisseria* provides more detailed information.

Aerobic and Facultatively Anaerobic Gram-Negative Rods. Gram-negative rods are usually grouped into four major categories for identification purposes: (1) rapidly growing, glucose fermenting (facultatively anaerobic), (2) rapidly growing, nonfermentative, (3) fastidious or slow growing or both, and (4) strictly anaerobic gram-negative rods. Commercial companies have focused attention on accurate and timely identification of gram-negative rods because they constitute a large and important segment of clinically significant isolates. Although most of these identification products perform well and have been in use for many years, some are better than others, and some are better for certain groups of gram-negative rods but do poorly for others. To offer accurate identification, companies must regularly update their systems to incorporate name changes and to add new organisms. As a consequence of delays in updating, microbial identification panel names often lag behind accepted taxonomic changes.

The rapidly growing glucose fermenters, which are aerobic and facultatively anaerobic, include members of the Enterobacteriaceae and Vibrionaceae (including *Vibrio, Aeromonas,* and *Plesiomonas*). They are the most easily identified group; many different commercial panels do accurate identification within 4 to 6 hours or overnight. Vibrionaceae can be quickly distinguished from Enterobacteriaceae by their strong oxidase reaction. All of these organisms generally grow luxuriantly after overnight incubation and grow well on MacConkey agar. Rapid tests for indole production or methyl-umbelliferyl B-glucuronidase (MUG) are used by some laboratories for quick identification or confirmation of organisms such as *E. coli* or *Proteus mirabilis.* When screening stool cultures for enteric pathogens, most laboratories use a two-tube screen (triple sugar iron agar/urea or lysine-iron agar/urea) to select those isolates most suggestive of *Salmonella* or *Shigella* for further full biochemical evaluation.

Nonfermentative gram-negative rods are strictly aerobic and include many important pathogens such as *Pseudomonas, Burkholderia, Acinetobacter,* and *Stenotrophomonas,* as well as many that are opportunistic pathogens or environmental contaminants seen with regularity in clinical specimens. Tables 15-11 and 15-12 provide information on those nonfermentative species that produce yellow-pigmented colonies and those that do not. This initial pigment observation is a useful identification criterion, as are motility and the organism's ability to produce acid oxidatively from glucose. Most correct species identification, however, requires that multiple biochemical reactions be included in the analysis. The accuracy of different commercial panels in identifying these genera to the species level varies with both the panel and the specific organism. Organisms that have fairly distinctive biochemical properties are usually identified correctly, for example, *P. aeruginosa, Acinetobacter baumanii,* or *Stenotrophomonas maltophilia.* When the nonfermentative gram-negative rod is biochemically inert and has few characteristics useful for differentiation, identification panels may yield incorrect or ambiguous results, often necessitating extra tests for definitive identification (e.g., species of *Moraxella* or *Alcaligenes*). For some genera that contain multiple phenotypically similar species, such as *Burkholderia,* genetically based methods may be the only ones that afford reliably accurate species identification.

Fastidious gram-negative rods include a very wide range of organisms (Table 15-13). Early descriptions of some of the members of this group, primarily described because of their role in causing endocarditis, used the acronym HACEK, which refers to the first letter of each of the following species: *Haemophilus aphrophilus, Actinobacillus actinomycetemcomitans, Cardiobacterium hominis, Eikenella corrodens,* and *Kingella kingae.* For purposes of discussion here, the fastidious group includes these organisms, as well as many other gram-negative rods that either grow slowly or need enriched or special media for cultivation. This group comprises very significant pathogens, including *Haemophilus, Brucella, Francisella, Legionella, Bordetella,*

TABLE 15-11 Yellow-Pigmented* Nonfermentative Gram-Negative Rods: A Simplified Recognition Scheme

Oxidase Positive
  Acid from glucose and motile   **Burkholderia cepacia complex genomovar I**, *Brevundimonas vesicularis,*[†] *Agrobacterium* yellow group, CDC groups O1 and O2, **Sphingomonas paucimobilis/parapaucimobilis**

  Acid from glucose and nonmotile
    Indole-positive   *Chryseobacterium gleum, Chryseobacterium indologenes, Empedobacter brevis*
    Indole-negative   *Sphingobacterium,*[‡] CDC groups EF-4b,[§] EO3, EO4[‖]
  No acid from glucose   *Myroides odoratus/odoratimimus*

Oxidase Negative
  Acid from glucose   *Burkholderia gladioli,*[§] **Pseudomonas luteola, Pseudomonas oryzihabitans**
  No acid from glucose   *Massilia timonae*[**]

Organisms in bold print represent those more commonly found in clinical specimens.
*Yellow-pigmented colonies formed by insoluble pigment in >75% of isolates except those noted below.
[†]52% yellow-pigmented.
[‡]33-57% yellow-pigmented, depending on species.
[§]50% yellow-pigmented.
[‖]75% yellow-pigmented.
[¶]44% yellow-pigmented (some strains brown-pigmented).
[**]Only two described infections known.

Campylobacter, Capnocytophaga, Helicobacter, Pasteurella, and *Bartonella*. Extensive discussions of these pathogens are presented in separate chapters to follow. Identification of most of these organisms is often a challenge for the laboratory. Many cannot be identified with the use of simple, commercially available panels. For many of these organisms, the laboratory must be notified in advance to optimize isolation by including specific media, temperature, or growth conditions or extending incubation times. Organisms such as *Brucella* and *Francisella* are laboratory hazards once they start to grow, and they must be handled with caution. For a few of these fastidious species, simple tests are available to aid in identification. X factor (hemin) and V factor (nicotinamide adenine dinucleotide [NAD]) requirements or the ALA test (δ-aminolevulinic acid) is used to identify common respiratory species of *Haemophilus*. For a delicate, curved organism that grows well at 42° C from a stool culture, a positive hippurate hydrolysis reaction is regarded as sufficient for identification of the organism as *Campylobacter jejuni*, whereas a similarly curved gram-negative rod that is strongly urease positive and has been isolated from a gastric biopsy specimen is likely to be *H. pylori*. A faintly staining, slender, gram-negative rod that grows only on charcoal-yeast extract agar is presumptively identified as *Legionella*; this is usually confirmed by specific fluorescent antisera. *P. multocida* is one of the few organisms in the fastidious group that can be identified with the use of commercially available panels designed for fermentative gram-negative rods.

Anaerobic Bacteria

Strictly anaerobic bacteria are discussed extensively in the chapters on anaerobes in general, or in those that describe specific anaerobic groups.

TABLE 15-12   Nonfermentative Gram-Negative Rods with Nonpigmented Colonies: A Simplified Recognition Scheme for Clinically Encountered Genera or Species

Oxidase Negative	
Motile	*Burkholderia gladioli, Pandoraea,* **Stenotrophomonas maltophilia**
Nonmotile	**Acinetobacter,** *Bordetella holmesii, Bordetella parapertussis* CDC groups EO5, NO-1
Oxidase Positive	
Asaccharolytic,* motile	**Alcaligenes faecalis, Achromobacter,** *Bordetella avium,* **Bordetella bronchiseptica,** *Bordetella hinzii, Brevundimonas diminuta, Comamonas, Delftia acidovorans, Pandoraea,† Pseudomonas alcaligenes, Pseudomonas pseudoalcaligenes, Ralstonia gilardii, Ralstonia paucula*
Asaccharolytic, nonmotile	*Bergeyella zoohelcum,* **Moraxella,** *Myroides, Neisseria elongata, Neisseria weaveri, Oligella urethralis, Psychrobacter immobilis, Psychrobacter phenylpyruvicus, Weeksella virosa*
Saccharolytic,* motile	**Achromobacter,** *Brevundimonas vesicularis,* **Burkholderia,** *Ochrobactrum, Pandoraea,* **Pseudomonas,‡** *Ralstonia mannitolilytica,* **Ralstonia pickettii,** *Rhizobium radiobacter, Shewanella*
Saccharolytic, nonmotile	CDC groups EF-4b, EO2, *Chryseomonas meningosepticum, Psychrobacter immobilis*

Organisms in bold print represent those more commonly found in clinical specimens.

*Ability to produce acid by oxidative utilization of glucose.

†New genera comprise species formerly similar to *B. cepacia* and *R. pickettii*.

‡*P. aeruginosa* usually identified by production of pigments, pyocyanin, and fluorescein. Other common species include *P. fluorescens/putida* (produce only fluorescein) and *P. stutzeri*.

Identification by Means of Specific Antisera

In addition to biochemical methods of identification, laboratories use antisera for culture confirmation of certain organisms. Agglutination with the use of whole-organism suspensions or latex agglutination by means of antibody bound to latex beads is technically simple to perform and takes a few minutes to complete. Agglutination and latex agglutination tests are used on colony growth by some laboratories to identify *S. pneumoniae*, groups of β-hemolytic streptococci, serotypes of *H. influenzae*, serogroups of *N. meningitidis*, *E. coli* O157, and serogroups of *Salmonella* and *Shigella*. Detection of specific antigens by fluorescent antibody staining can also be used to identify colonies of *B. pertussis*, *S. pyogenes*, and the species and serotypes of *Legionella*, although lack of specificity of some antisera can lead to misidentification. The quellung reaction, which relies on the ability of specific antisera to interact with capsular polysaccharides of *S. pneumoniae*, can be used to confirm the identification and to determine the serotypes of these organisms, although this reaction is not routinely needed.

Identification by Means of Molecular Techniques

The first molecular identification techniques were probe-based tests that relied on detection of nucleic acid sequences that were specific for a particular genus or species. These probe assays (AccuProbe, Gen-Probe, San Diego, CA), when made available commercially, became the method of choice for rapid and accurate identification of mycobacterial species, particularly *M. tuberculosis* complex, but for other common mycobacterial species as well. Similar probe assays were developed for fungal pathogens and have provided a substantial improvement in terms of more timely and accurate identification of dimorphic fungal pathogens. Although a few probe assays were available for routine bacteria, use of probe technology as a clinical laboratory tool has been limited primarily to mycobacteria and fungi.

Sequence-based identification is another molecular technique that can be used to improve on both the speed and accuracy of identification of bacteria that are traditionally (i.e., phenotypically) difficult to identify, or those that grow either very poorly or very slowly. Analysis of organisms on the basis of nucleic acid sequencing of the 16S rRNA gene

TABLE 15-13   Fastidious, Aerobic, or Facultatively Anaerobic Gram-Negative Bacilli: Organisms That Show No Growth, Slow Growth, or Poor Growth on Blood Agar: A Simplified Recognition Scheme

Oxidase Positive	
Curved rods	*Arcobacter, Campylobacter, Helicobacter*
Straight rods	
Acid from glucose	
Straight rods or coccobacilli	*Actinobacillus hominis/ureae, Cardiobacterium, Haemophilus,* Kingella, Pasteurella, Suttonella, CDC Groups EF-4a, EF-4b*
Fusiform	*Capnocytophaga canimorsus/ cynodegmi*
No acid from glucose	*Afipia,† Bordetella pertussis,‡ Brucella, Eikenella, Legionella‡*
Oxidase Negative	
Acid from glucose	
Straight rods or coccobacilli	*Actinobacillus actinomycetemcomitans, Dysgonomonas, Haemophilus,* Streptobacillus*
Fusiform	*Capnocytophaga* (human species)
No acid from glucose	*Bartonella,‡ Francisella,§ Legionella‡*

*Most species of *Haemophilus* other than *H. aphrophilus/paraphrophilus* require chocolate agar and grow on horse but not on sheep blood agar.

†Requires prolonged incubation (>7 days); special cell culture methods enhance growth.

‡No growth on standard blood or chocolate agar, requires special enriched media for growth (e.g., buffered charcoal yeast extract [BCYE] agar).

§*F. tularensis* grows well on chocolate, BCYE, and Thayer-Martin agars; other media must be supplemented.

and DNA hybridization studies have been used by taxonomists to improve the classification of organisms so that it better reflects true phylogenetic relationships. Through the same type of analysis, identification of an unknown organism is obtained by comparing the organism's 16S rRNA gene sequence with those found in a large database of known organisms, and then determining the closest related organism. The ability of this sequence comparison to result in definitive identification is not absolute and will vary according to the specific genus or species being identified. In some instances, insufficient divergence among closely related species may make the sequence data alone insufficient for reliable identification.[37] In many instances, however, a leading choice is indicated, and if one is not clear-cut, the analysis is at least helpful in showing those with the closest relationships. Acceptance of sequence-based identification should also be validated by confirmation of the organism's conformance to known morphologic or other phenotypic characteristics of the proposed choice. Although sequencing of other genes could be used similarly for organism identification, the 16S rRNA gene sequence is the most widely used at present.

Beyond species identification, strain typing is another discipline in which molecular methodology has made significant inroads.[5,6] Phenotypic methods such as antibiograms and biochemical profiles had only limited usefulness owing to their lack of discriminatory power. Availability of accurate typing helps to control outbreaks more rapidly and can help in the identification of sources, carriers, and patterns of spread. The main genotypic methods that are currently in use include pulsed-field gel electrophoresis (PFGE), restriction fragment length polymorphism (RFLP) of chromosomal DNA, and PCR-based methods such as random amplification of polymorphic DNA (RAPD), although many other methods have been used successfully for specific organisms. PFGE is the accepted gold standard for many organisms. Multilocus sequence typing (MLST) is a recently introduced typing method that uses automated sequencing of alleles present at selected housekeeping genes that are responsible for metabolic functions.[5,48] MLST is relatively rapid to perform and provides unambiguous sequences that are electronically portable, which can be used to accurately compare isolates between different laboratories. Like the other typing methods, however, suitability of the method must be validated for each group of organisms. PCR- and sequence-based methods can be completed within 1 to 2 days; PFGE and RFLP analyses often take much longer. The different methods vary in reproducibility, ease of performance, turnaround time, robustness, and discriminatory power. Microbiology laboratories in research or university settings are fortunate to have molecular typing methods available in-house, whereas community hospitals must refer isolates to their county or state laboratories, which generally extends the time it takes to confirm an outbreak.

ANTIMICROBIAL SUSCEPTIBILITY TESTING

Susceptibility testing of a presumed pathogen is indicated when its response to antimicrobial agents is not predictable from its identification.[49-51] Unfortunately, with the continuing increase and dissemination of resistance mechanisms in bacteria, more and more species require at least some form of susceptibility testing. To ensure both clinical relevance and interlaboratory comparability of results, much effort has been devoted to the standardization of susceptibility testing. The basic problem is to demonstrate that in vitro growth inhibition of an infecting organism by a specific agent correlates with clinical response to that agent. The NCCLS has published several standards that pertain to various aspects of bacterial susceptibility testing; many of these standards are updated regularly.[49-57] Because these documents reflect consensus statements by a committee of experts, laboratories cannot readily deviate from NCCLS recommendations without excellent data to justify their procedures. The CLIA of 1988, as revised in the final rule, has also imposed stringent validation requirements on laboratories that perform procedures developed in-house, further encouraging the use of standardized procedures for which proficiency testing is available.[2,3] Unfortunately, as both the number of organisms requiring testing and the number of

available antimicrobial agents have increased, the NCCLS recommendations have become increasingly complex, with more and more organism- and drug-specific variables needing to be taken into account when susceptibility test results are obtained and reported. Each new edition of an NCCLS susceptibility testing document must be carefully reviewed to ensure that the laboratory has incorporated the latest changes into its testing methodology.

Nearly all the more common and nonfastidious organisms can be tested and the results reported with the use of NCCLS criteria. The NCCLS also provides recommendations regarding the selection of antimicrobial agents to be tested against specific organisms; those agents recommended for routine testing and those suggested for testing only under certain circumstances, such as the presence of a resistant strain in a particular institution, have been placed into separate groups. Agents solely or primarily useful for the treatment of urinary tract infection have also been placed in a separate group. For less common or more fastidious organisms, as well as for nonstandard organism/drug combinations, the NCCLS publications may not provide any specific guidance. This lack of guidance is partly a consequence of the NCCLS requirement that before interpretive breakpoints are provided for an organism–antimicrobial agent combination, adequate data should be available to substantiate clinical responsiveness at species-specific (or group-specific) minimal inhibitory concentrations (MICs) for that agent. Many organism/antibiotic combinations have inadequate clinical response data to help define sensitive and resistant MIC breakpoints. The consequent lack of interpretive criteria results in some vexing problems for both the laboratory and the clinician. For example, interpretive guidelines are not provided for organisms such as *Bacillus* (other than *B. anthracis), Corynebacterium,* and noncholera *Vibrio,* or for many fastidious or unusual species (e.g., *Eikenella, Capnocytophaga, Leuconostoc*). Many of these organisms may cause significant infections, and in the past, laboratories used more "generally applicable" breakpoints to help guide the clinician; these were usually based on known achievable serum levels and the clinical responses of other organisms with similar MICs. Currently, in following NCCLS recommendations, laboratories are more limited in what they can report because the guidelines specify both the organisms and the antimicrobial agents that can be reported. This lack of breakpoint criteria for a variety of organisms or organism/antimicrobial combinations becomes particularly problematic for organisms that are resistant to many different antibiotics, in which case the laboratory would like to test and report agents that may not be recommended by the NCCLS for that specific organism. For organisms not included in the NCCLS standards, "consultation with an infectious disease specialist is recommended for guidance in determining the need for susceptibility testing and in the interpretation of results."[53]

The results obtained by any form of in vitro antibiotic testing depend not only on the particular antibiotic and organism involved but also on a host of other performance variables as well, including the organism inoculum concentration, the medium used, and the time, atmosphere, and temperature of incubation. NCCLS documents provide detailed instructions for dealing with all the variables involved in susceptibility testing, including procedural modifications that may have to be made for specific organism–antimicrobial combinations. Also included are warnings regarding specific organism–antimicrobial agent combinations, the results of which should not be reported because in vitro data may be misleading.

Most bacterial species or groups of species have a susceptibility pattern characteristic for the species or group. Whenever an unusual susceptibility pattern for a particular species is obtained, it is worth checking to be sure that the susceptibility test was set up and interpreted correctly, that a pure culture was used, and that identification of the organism is correct.

Terminology

Susceptibility testing for most bacteria is performed either by a disk diffusion procedure or by a procedure (usually broth microdilution) that provides an MIC. A newer procedure (Etest, AB Biodisk, Solna,

Sweden) that uses a strip impregnated with a gradient of antimicrobial agent also provides an MIC. With the disk diffusion procedure, only a qualitative result (sensitive, intermediate, or resistant) is usually reported, whereas with MIC testing, both a quantitative result (the MIC) and a qualitative result (which "interprets" the MIC) may be reported. The MIC is the lowest concentration of a specific antimicrobial agent that prevents visible growth of the test organism.[50] MICs can also be determined by an agar dilution procedure in which dilutions of antimicrobial agents are incorporated into an agar-based medium rather than dissolved in broth. Similarly, the *minimal bactericidal concentration* (MBC) (also known as the minimal lethal concentration) is the lowest concentration of a specific antimicrobial agent that kills most (>99.9%) of the inoculum of test organism under defined conditions.[56] All of these minimal concentrations have units of weight or mass divided by volume—usually they are given in micrograms per milliliter. A *serum bactericidal titration* or *test,* also called a Schlichter test, is a measure of the extent to which a patient's body fluid (usually serum) can be diluted and still exert bactericidal activity against an infecting organism that is isolated from the patient. The result is reported as a titer or ratio and therefore has no units.[57] An *antimicrobial level* is the amount of a specific drug in a patient's body fluid; the result is generally expressed in micrograms per milliliter.

Traditional quantitative susceptibility testing has used twofold dilution steps for the antimicrobial agent because such a dilution sequence is easy to perform. Increasingly, however, commercially prepared microdilution trays are used that do not contain an entire sequence of dilutions, but only the most clinically relevant concentrations. This elimination of certain dilutions has consequences for the meaning of quantitative results. For example, if in a twofold dilution series of 2, 4, and 8 µg/mL, the 4-µg/mL dilution were to be omitted, an organism with an actual MIC between 2 and 4 µg/mL would be reported as having an MIC of 8 µg/mL, rather than the 4-µg/mL value that would be reported if the full twofold dilution series were used.

The following definitions of *susceptible, intermediate,* and *resistant* are taken from NCCLS documents.[49,50]

1. Susceptible. The "susceptible" category "implies that an infection due to the isolate may be appropriately treated with the dosage of antimicrobial agent recommended for that type of infection and infecting species, unless otherwise indicated."
2. Intermediate. The "intermediate" category "implies that an infection due to the isolate may be appropriately treated in body sites where the drugs are physiologically concentrated or when a high dosage of drug can be used; also indicates a 'buffer zone' that should prevent small, uncontrolled technical factors from causing major discrepancies in interpretations."
3. Resistant. "Resistant isolates are not inhibited by the usually achievable concentrations of the agent with normal dosage schedules and/or fall in the range where specific microbial resistance mechanisms are likely (e.g., β-lactamases), and clinical efficacy has not been reliable in treatment studies."

Specific Susceptibility Testing Procedures

Disk Diffusion Susceptibility Testing

Disk diffusion susceptibility testing,[49] still frequently referred to as the Kirby-Bauer procedure, should be used primarily for rapidly growing organisms. A disk that contains a certain amount of antibiotic is placed on an agar plate immediately after it has been inoculated with the test organism. After incubation for 16 to 18 hours, the diameter of the zone of inhibition around the disk is measured. Interpretation of the organism as sensitive, intermediate, or resistant to the antibiotic depends on the zone diameter criteria for the particular organism–antimicrobial combination. For example, for one of the Enterobacteriaceae, a zone diameter around an ampicillin disk of 17 mm or greater is considered susceptible, whereas for a *Staphylococcus* species, the zone diameter for ampicillin must be 29 mm or larger to be considered susceptible.

Zone diameter interpretive breakpoints are based on the inverse correlation of zone diameter with MIC, that is, the larger the zone diameter, the lower the MIC. The NCCLS lists the MIC correlates of its disk diffusion breakpoints in its tables. For example, for Enterobacteriaceae, the MIC equivalent to the zone diameter breakpoint for susceptibility to ampicillin is 8 µg/mL or less; for staphylococci, it is 0.25 µg/mL or less. However, with disk diffusion testing, it is standard practice to refrain from reporting an MIC; only an interpretive category should be reported.

Minimal Inhibitory Concentration Testing

MIC testing[50] is most often done by a broth microdilution technique that uses commercially available trays, which may also contain biochemical reactions used for organism identification. MIC testing may also be performed by broth macrodilution, by agar dilution, and by Etest.[58] All three dilution procedures involve the incorporation of known concentrations of antimicrobial agents into either broth or agar and subsequent checking for the presence or absence of organism growth after a suitable incubation period, generally 16 to 20 hours. Broth macrodilution testing is very labor intensive and is rarely performed in a diagnostic laboratory. Agar dilution testing is cost-effective if a large number of isolates are tested at the same time; with this procedure, many different organisms can be tested simultaneously on each plate. The Etest is a relatively new procedure that uses a strip impregnated with a gradient of antimicrobial agent; after inoculation of a plate with an organism, the strip is applied to the plate. After incubation, the plate is examined for growth; if the organism has been inhibited by the antimicrobial agent, an oval of growth inhibition is produced that is widest at the end of the strip with the highest drug concentration. The MIC of the drug for the organism is read off the strip at the point at which the oval of inhibition intersects the strip.

Testing for Bactericidal Activity

The NCCLS published an approved procedural guideline for the determination of bactericidal activity in 1999.[56] Determination of bactericidal activity is technically difficult and labor intensive; relatively few laboratories offer such testing on a routine, nonresearch basis. As the NCCLS document states, "Because of their specialized nature, complexity, and potential difficulty for interpretation, tests for bactericidal activity should be done in the context of consultation with the appropriate persons (such as the microbiology laboratory director) who are aware of the potential problems involved in such testing."

Serum Bactericidal Testing

The NCCLS published an approved guideline in 1999 that pertains to the serum bactericidal test.[57] With regard to this test, the relevant NCCLS document states, "Because of the complexity involved with the serum bactericidal test (including the particular method used, the proper collection of timed serum specimens, and the interpretation of results), and the lack of clinical data clearly documenting the usefulness of this test for most infections, it is recommended that consultation with the microbiology laboratory be obtained as a prerequisite for this test. . . .The clinical relevance of the serum bactericidal test remains controversial, and there are relatively few clinical situations in which the test is indicated." Foremost among potential problems with the serum bactericidal test is that the results may stimulate an attempt to achieve an arbitrary bactericidal titer through modification of a treatment regimen that is in fact already adequate.[59]

Synergy Testing

Because no standardized methodology for synergy testing exists, this procedure remains essentially a research tool. However, a standardized method (which is actually a surrogate test) is available for predicting synergism between aminoglycosides and cell wall–active agents against enterococci (see later under susceptibility testing problems with enterococci).

Important Susceptibility Testing Issues

Staphylococci

All species of staphylococci that are oxacillin (or methicillin) resistant should be considered resistant to all β-lactam antibiotics, including imipenem, regardless of the actual in vitro result.[52,53] For either MIC or disk testing of staphylococcal susceptibility to oxacillin and vancomycin, a full 24 hours of incubation at 35° C is required to maximize the likelihood of detection of resistance.[52,53] For oxacillin, the breakpoint for susceptibility is lower for coagulase-negative staphylococci than for *S. aureus*.[52,53] An agar screening test that uses Mueller-Hinton agar with 4% NaCl and 6 µg/mL of oxacillin is quite reliable for detecting oxacillin-resistant *S. aureus* after 24 hours of incubation.[53]

Streptococcus pneumoniae

If a disk diffusion procedure is used to screen isolates for susceptibility to penicillin and related agents, an oxacillin disk is used. However, no result for oxacillin itself should be reported. If the zone around the oxacillin disk is 20 mm or larger, the isolate should be reported as susceptible to penicillin. If the zone is 19 mm or smaller, MIC testing with penicillin, meropenem, and either cefotaxime or ceftriaxone should be done because isolates with such a zone size may prove to be susceptible, intermediate, or resistant to penicillin by MIC testing.[52] All CSF isolates of *S. pneumoniae* should be tested by an MIC method against cefotaxime or ceftriaxone, penicillin, and meropenem.[52]

Enterococci

Several issues pertain to susceptibility testing of enterococci:

1. Test results for the following agents should not be reported as susceptible because the agents have not been found to be clinically effective: Aminoglycosides (except for screening for high-level resistance), cephalosporins, clindamycin, and trimethoprim/sulfamethoxazole.[52,53]
2. Testing at high levels for gentamicin (500 µg/mL) and streptomycin (1000 or 2000 µg/mL, depending on methodology) susceptibility is useful for the purpose of predicting synergy with cell wall–active agents. For gentamicin, 24 hours of incubation is required; for streptomycin, 48 hours is required unless the isolate is already resistant at 24 hours. An isolate susceptible to either agent at these high levels should exhibit a synergistic response to that agent plus a cell wall–active antimicrobial such as ampicillin.[53]
3. Vancomycin resistance may be detected by means of a screening procedure that involves growth on brain-heart infusion agar that contains 6 µg/mL of vancomycin.[53] A full 24 hours of incubation is required. The MIC of organisms that grow on the screening medium or that are determined to be vancomycin resistant by a breakpoint method can be more precisely determined so that those with intermediate-level intrinsic *vanC*-mediated resistance can be distinguished from those with acquired, usually higher-level *vanA*- or *vanB*-mediated resistance.[53] Several other resistance genes, including *vanD*, *vanE*, and *vanG*, have been recognized; subtypes of most of these have also been described.[60] PCR can be used for the identification of most, if not all, of the resistance genes in enterococci. Also, one must be aware that automated identification systems may not be able to distinguish species with intermediate-level resistance such as *Enterococcus casseliflavus* and *Enterococcus gallinarum* from *E. faecium*.[61]

Anaerobes

Anaerobes require susceptibility testing procedures that are different from those for organisms that can be grown aerobically. The NCCLS has a separate standard, which has recently been extensively revised, that pertains to susceptibility testing of anaerobes.[51,54] Both an agar dilution and a broth microdilution procedure are described; however, the broth microdilution procedure has been standardized for use only for certain antimicrobial agents tested against members of the *Bacteroides fragilis* group. The NCCLS document and relevant chapters in this text can be consulted for a discussion of the circumstances under which anaerobic susceptibility testing may be warranted.

Extended-Spectrum β-Lactamase Detection

Extended-spectrum β-lactamase (ESBL)-producing strains of *E. coli*, *Klebsiella oxytoca*, and *Klebsiella pneumoniae* are of increasing concern and may be difficult to detect in the laboratory. The NCCLS recommends that isolates of these species be screened to determine if they have MICs of 4 µg/mL or greater for cefpodoxime, or 1 µg/mL or greater for ceftazidime, aztreonam, cefotaxime, or ceftriaxone.[53] Such MICs suggest possible ESBL production, and confirmatory testing should be done with both ceftazidime and cefotaxime (each drug should be tested both alone and in combination with clavulanic acid). Because ESBLs are inhibited by clavulanic acid, a sufficient decrease in MIC to either one of these two agents, when tested in combination with clavulanic acid, as compared with the MIC when tested without clavulanic acid, is considered to confirm ESBL production. (Disk testing can also be done in an analogous fashion.[52]) All confirmed ESBL producers should be reported as resistant to all penicillins, all cephalosporins, and aztreonam.[49,50] (The NCCLS documents contain glossaries that further define penicillins and cephalosporins; note that cephamycins such as cefoxitin are not considered by the NCCLS to be cephalosporins.)

Molecular Methods of Susceptibility Determination

The genetic basis for specific antimicrobial resistance in some organisms is now known, and it is possible for molecular methods to be used to reliably detect these resistance determinants.[60] A well-studied example concerns the *mecA* gene for oxacillin resistance in staphylococci. Some *S. aureus* strains that lack the *mecA* gene may be at least borderline oxacillin resistant on the basis of high levels of β-lactamase production.[60] Unfortunately, the absence of a gene or gene mutation known to confer resistance to an antimicrobial agent does not necessarily mean that an organism is susceptible to the agent, because other mechanisms of resistance might be present. Also, most molecular procedures for resistance determination are presently labor intensive, time consuming, and costly. Thus, because molecular methods are unable to determine susceptibility (as opposed to resistance) to specific agents, phenotypic procedures for susceptibility testing will continue to be required for the foreseeable future.

MYCOBACTERIA

Mycobacteria are aerobic, nonmotile, rod-shaped bacteria that are acid fast, that is, once stained with certain dyes, they resist decolorization with acid alcohol as a consequence of their cell wall structure.

Safety Issues

When direct smears are made, bleach (5% sodium hypochlorite) can be used to inactivate mycobacteria that may be present in patient specimens; such smears can be prepared without special containment facilities. Otherwise, processing of specimens, including digestion, decontamination, and planting, requires a BSL 2 facility and an appropriate biologic safety cabinet. Any procedure performed on a specimen that may contain *M. tuberculosis* complex that could result in aerosol production, as well as any manipulation of cultures of the organism, requires a BSL 3 facility. Such a facility includes a room with unidirectional airflow that preferably is entered through a series of two separate doors.[62]

Specimen Collection and Transport

Specimens for smear and culture for mycobacteria should be collected and transported in closed, leakproof, sterile containers. Containers contaminated with specimen on the outside are not acceptable because of the hazard posed to personnel. Gastric aspirates require pH neutralization soon after collection to ensure the viability of any mycobacteria that may be present; arrangements should be made with the laboratory in advance to ensure optimal specimen handling. Biopsies are preferable to swab specimens of tissue lesions for the isolation of mycobacteria. No special procedures are usually necessary for the collection and transport of sterile fluids, urine, and stool. However, organism concentrations in sterile fluids may be low, so a minimum of several milliliters (in the case of CSF, more than 3 mL if possible) should be obtained whenever mycobacterial infection is a serious consideration.[63] Blood may be collected for mycobacterial culture either in a blood collection tube that contains anticoagulant or in a lysis-centrifugation tube, or it may be inoculated directly into a special bottle for mycobacterial blood culture, depending on laboratory protocol. Twenty-four-hour collections of sputum and urine are unacceptable because of the likelihood of bacterial overgrowth. For sputum and urine, it is recommended that at least three first morning specimens be obtained, and that a minimum of 40 mL of midstream urine be processed for each culture.[63] Protocols for handling different specimen types vary significantly among laboratories, and it is important for physicians to be aware of the procedures used by each of the laboratories they use.

Direct Organism Detection

Mycobacteria may be detected directly in patient specimens through visualization of stained organisms or by detection of specific mycobacterial nucleic acids or other cellular constituents.

The Gram stain is insensitive for the detection of mycobacteria. If visible at all, mycobacteria may appear as finely beaded, gram-positive rods with only the beads visible (gram-positive) and the rest of the organism appearing gram-negative, or they may appear as negative images (rodlike clefts) in the specimen. Specific mycobacterial stains are based on the ability of mycobacteria to retain certain dyes after washing with an acid-alcohol decolorizer (hence, "acid fast"), unlike most other bacteria. The Ziehl-Neelsen and Kinyoun stains are both carbolfuchsin based and stain mycobacteria red. The Ziehl-Neelsen stain requires a heating step and has been largely replaced by the Kinyoun stain, which is a "cold" acid-fast stain. The auramine O and auramine-rhodamine stains use fluorescent compounds; although fluorescence microscopy is required for visualization of mycobacteria, these stains do not involve the use of an antibody but are based on the acid-fast properties of mycobacteria. Fluorescent stains are more sensitive for the detection of mycobacteria, particularly in direct specimens, because the organisms stain brightly and can be clearly distinguished from background material. In addition, because slides stained with a fluorescent dye can be examined reliably with an objective lens of lower magnification (25×) than with the oil immersion lens (100×) required for carbolfuchsin-stained smears, reading of slides can be done faster. Rapidly growing mycobacteria may be less avidly acid fast than are slow growers and may be more readily visualized with a modified acid-fast stain that uses a weaker decolorizing step than is used with a regular carbolfuchsin stain. Some species of mycobacteria differ from others in the length, width, or arrangement of individual cells. *Mycobacterium kansasii*, for example, tends to be long and broad, sometimes with a banded rather than a beaded appearance, whereas *Mycobacterium avium* complex may appear coccobacillary, especially on a smear from a liquid medium. Cells of *M. tuberculosis* often group together in "cords" that are composed of long strands of organisms with their long axes parallel. However, the microscopic appearance of individual cells and groups of cells should at best be considered only suggestive of a certain species or group of species.[63]

Amplification of mycobacterial nucleic acids can be used for the direct detection of mycobacteria in clinical material. Two commercially available procedures for the detection of organisms in the *M. tuberculosis* complex—the Gen-Probe MTD (AMPLIFIED Mycobacterium Tuberculosis Direct Test) and the Roche Amplicor—have been approved by the FDA for use with smear-positive respiratory specimens; the Gen-Probe procedure has also been approved for use with smear-negative respiratory specimens. An automated version of the Roche procedure is available. For smear-positive respiratory specimens, both procedures have a very high sensitivity; with such specimens, one comparative study found a sensitivity of 100% for the Gen-Probe procedure and 97% for the Roche procedure.[64] For smear-

negative respiratory specimens, the same study reported sensitivities of 87.5% for the Gen-Probe procedure and 66.7% for the Roche procedure.[64] A study of respiratory and nonrespiratory specimens analyzed by the Gen-Probe procedure found somewhat lower sensitivities for nonrespiratory as compared with respiratory specimens.[65] A study that used the automated Roche procedure found no significant differences in sensitivity and specificity for respiratory and nonrespiratory specimens.[66] Although direct detection of both mycobacterial antigens and tuberculostearic acid may have some usefulness for the diagnosis of tuberculosis, particularly tuberculous meningitis, such testing is not generally available.[67,68] Nucleic acid amplification may be more sensitive than tuberculostearic acid detection for the diagnosis of both pulmonary and meningeal tuberculosis.[69,70]

Specimen Processing and Planting

Specimens such as sputum, urine, and stool, which can be expected to contain considerable normal microbial flora, must be digested and decontaminated to prevent overgrowth of any mycobacteria present. These processing steps are inevitably somewhat toxic to mycobacteria, and a balance must be struck to minimize the loss of mycobacteria while simultaneously maximizing the elimination of as many other microorganisms as possible.[63] Concentration of the specimen occurs as part of the digestion and decontamination procedures, and smears of a specimen are prepared from such concentrates. The most commonly used digestion and decontamination procedure entails the use of a mixture of *N*-acetyl-L-cysteine and NaOH, although other procedures are occasionally used, such as the oxalic acid procedure for specimens heavily contaminated with *P. aeruginosa*.[63] Normally, sterile fluids such as CSF may be concentrated for smear preparation and planting, but they need not be subjected to digestion and decontamination. Biopsies obtained from normally sterile sites must be ground before planting but do not require digestion and decontamination. Blood processed by a lysis-centrifugation method can be planted onto solid media, from which quantitation of growth (organisms per milliliter) in the blood can be determined. Currently, several types of mycobacterial blood culture bottles that can be used with automated instruments are available for direct inoculation, but quantitation cannot be obtained with liquid culture media.[63,71]

It is recommended that a liquid in addition to a solid medium be used for planting specimens whenever practical; the liquid media may enhance both the sensitivity of culture and the rapidity of organism detection.[63,72] Most studies have shown improved mycobacterial isolation rates when both solid and liquid media are used. The benefit of using two different types of medium may derive from the preference of some mycobacterial isolates for one type of medium over another, or simply from the increased sensitivity obtained by the culturing of a larger volume of specimen. Use of a liquid medium often results in the isolation of *M. tuberculosis* within 2 weeks and isolation of other slowly growing mycobacteria in even less time.[63] Consequently, when one of these liquid media has been used, one cannot assume that an organism detected within a week of incubation is necessarily a rapid grower in the traditional sense. Solid media used for the initial isolation of mycobacteria are either egg based, such as Lowenstein-Jensen medium, or agar based, such as Middlebrook 7H11 medium. Antimicrobial agents may be added to solid media to help prevent overgrowth of contaminants; for example, Gruft is an egg-based medium that contains penicillin and nalidixic acid, whereas Mitchison's or selective 7H11 medium is an agar-based medium that contains polymyxin B, amphotericin B, carbenicillin, and trimethoprim. Many liquid-based systems use an instrument for automated detection of organism growth, but some nonautomated systems are also available. Detection is based on such features as liberation of radiolabeled carbon dioxide from a ^{14}C-labeled substrate (BACTEC 460 TB System, Becton Dickinson bioMérieux, Sparks, MD), nonradiolabeled carbon dioxide production (BacT/ALERT 3D, bioMérieux, Durham, NC), oxygen consumption with activation of a fluorescent compound (BACTEC 9000MB System and Mycobacteria Growth Indicator Tube [MGIT], Becton-Dickinson, Sparks, MD) or change in vial gas pressure as a result of organism metabolism (ESP

Culture System II, Trek Diagnostic Systems, Westlake, OH).[63] Liquid media inoculated with specimens that require digestion and decontamination are supplemented with an antimicrobial mixture as a further aid in suppressing bacterial overgrowth; an example is the addition of PANTA (polymyxin B, amphotericin B, nalidixic acid, trimethoprim, and azlocillin) to BACTEC medium.

Mycobacterial cultures are generally incubated at 36° C ± 1° C in an atmosphere of approximately 8% CO_2, the optimum conditions for isolation of *M. tuberculosis*. However, several species of pathogenic mycobacteria have different growth requirements or preferences that may have to be satisfied to ensure their isolation (Table 15-14).[63,73] To optimize conditions for possible mycobacterial pathogens, some decisions need to be made regarding the initial handling of each specimen. Given the preference of several skin and subcutaneous pathogens (including *Mycobacterium haemophilum, M. marinum, Mycobacterium ulcerans,* and rapid growers) to grow at 30° C, at least a portion of all skin biopsy specimens (and perhaps other specimen types obtained from cooler areas of the body such as the extremities) submitted for mycobacterial culture should be incubated at approximately 30° C.[63] It is also important that the clinician notify the laboratory if a pathogen with specific growth requirements, such as *M. haemophilum*, is suspected so that optimal culturing procedures can be used. *Mycobacterium avium* subsp. *paratuberculosis,* reported from some patients with Crohn's disease and the etiologic agent of Johne's disease in ruminants, cannot reliably be isolated in the routine diagnostic laboratory.[73]

Significance of Isolation of Mycobacteria from Clinical Specimens

Isolation of certain species of mycobacteria, such as *M. avium* complex or a rapidly growing mycobacterium, may represent colonization or specimen contamination rather than active disease, but the potential significance of repeated isolation of the same species from the same source requires careful evaluation.[74] Most isolates of *Mycobacterium gordonae,* a water organism, are regarded as contaminants; only rarely is it a proven pathogen.[75-79] Unfortunately, the specimen-processing steps required for mycobacterial culture make transfer of a mycobacterium from one specimen to another a rare but real possibility. Therefore, the significance even of the isolation of *M. tuberculosis* from a solitary smear-negative specimen, especially in the absence of consistent histopathology or a highly consistent clinical picture, requires careful consideration.[80] Laboratory cross-contamination, while fortunately rare, has been well documented and requires sustained vigilance for its detection and prevention.[81]

Mycobacterial Identification

Traditional Categories and Methods

A mycobacterial species is placed into one of several categories, depending on its growth rate and its pigment production in relation to light stimulation. Rapid growers take less than 7 days for growth after subculture to a solid medium from a dilute suspension; however, they generally also take less than 7 days to grow on solid or in liquid medium on initial isolation. Slowly growing mycobacteria are further divided into photochromogens, scotochromogens, and nonphotochromogens, depending on their ability to produce pigment and the relationship of pigment production to light stimulation. Photochromogens produce pigment after light stimulation, but not when grown continuously in the dark with no light exposure. Scotochromogens produce pigment when grown in the dark, as well as after light exposure. Nonphotochromogens do not produce pigment even after light stimulation. However, not all isolates of some species will fall into the same categories based on growth rate or pigment production. For example, most isolates of *M. avium* complex are nonphotochromogenic, but some are scotochromogenic; many isolates of *M. marinum* (a photochromogen) grow rapidly, and isolates of *Mycobacterium szulgai* are usually photochromogenic at 25° C but scotochromogenic at 36° C. These three categories (photochromogen, scotochromogen, and nonphotochromogen) correspond to the Runyoun groups I, II, and III, respectively, which, along with group IV (rapid growers), were initially established for the categorization of mycobacteria other than *M. tuberculosis*. The Runyoun numerical group designations are rarely used today. *M. tuberculosis* complex, although by definition not a member of any of the Runyoun groups, is in fact a nonphotochromogen. In addition to features of growth rate and pigment production, traditional identification of mycobacterial species is based on colony morphology and a variety of other phenotypic features.[63,82] *M. tuberculosis,* for example, in addition to the production of rough, buff colonies (which are considered nonpigmented), produces niacin, reduces nitrate, and hydrolyzes urea. By conventional biochemical methods, *M. avium* is essentially indistinguishable from *Mycobacterium intracellulare;* serologic techniques (not generally available) may help distinguish between the two species, but the distinction is best made by newer procedures such as cell wall– or nucleic acid–based analysis.

Rapid Methods

Three major categories of methods are available for the rapid identification of mycobacteria.

Nucleic Acid–Based Methods. Commercially available probes (AccuProbe [Gen-Probe, San Diego, CA]) are available for the identification of *M. avium* complex, *M. gordonae, M. kansasii,* and *M. tuberculosis* complex (See Table 15-11 for the species in each of the two complexes.) These chemiluminescent compound–labeled probes are DNA probes for rRNA; they can be used only with organisms grown in culture, not directly on patient specimens. The procedure can be performed within a matter of hours from the time of organism isolation.[82] The sensitivity of the procedure derives in part from the multiple copies of rRNA that exist in each bacterial cell, as opposed to a single copy of bacterial DNA. Laboratories not doing further testing of isolates of the *M. avium* complex and the *M. tuberculosis* complex should make it clear that their identifications have not gone beyond the level of the complex (e.g., they should report "*M. tuberculosis* complex," not "*M. tuberculosis*," unless additional appropriate testing such as niacin and nitrate reactions has been done). Other nucleic acid–based methods for identification of mycobacterial species include amplification of a species-specific portion of the genome and amplification of a portion of the genome common to all mycobacteria, followed by the use of species-specific probes, by RFLP analysis, or by sequencing of the amplified material.[82]

Analysis of Mycolic Acids. High-performance liquid chromatography (HPLC) allows rapid identification of many species of mycobac-

---

TABLE 15-14 Pathogenic Mycobacteria with Unusual Growth Requirements or Characteristics

Mycobacterium bovis
1. Growth said to be enhanced by 0.4% pyruvate, but there is no apparent need for supplementation with the use of newer media

Mycobacterium haemophilum
1. Requires ferric ion (provided as ferric ammonium citrate, hemin, or blood)
2. Requires approximately 30° C for initial growth

Mycobacterium genavense
1. Grows best in BACTEC media
2. May grow on Middlebrook 7H11 medium supplemented with mycobactin J, or on acidified Middlebrook medium supplemented with blood and charcoal

Mycobacterium marinum
1. May require approximately 30° C for initial growth

Mycobacterium paratuberculosis
1. May require many months to grow, even on special media
2. Cultivation is not feasible in the diagnostic laboratory
3. May be killed by routinely used digestion and decontamination procedures

Mycobacterium ulcerans
1. May require approximately 30° C for initial growth
2. Requires prolonged (up to 3 months) incubation for detection

Mycobacterium xenopi
1. Grows best at 42° C, but will grow, at least slowly, at 36° C

Rapidly-growing mycobacteria
1. Often grow best at approximately 30° C, but usually also grow well at 36° C

teria via analysis of cell wall mycolic acids.[82] Because of the equipment and expertise required, these chromatographic identification procedures are available primarily in larger, specialized laboratories.

NAP Test. The NAP test, based on the inhibition of growth of members of the *M. tuberculosis* complex by p-nitro-α-acetylamino-β-hydroxypropiophenone (NAP), can be used with the BACTEC system. It provides in approximately 5 days presumptive identification as *M. tuberculosis* complex or not *M. tuberculosis* complex. Caution must be used in interpreting test results in that occasional isolates of nontuberculous mycobacteria may have their growth delayed in the presence of NAP.[83]

Mycobacteria Isolated in the Clinical Laboratory

Table 15-15 lists most of the mycobacterial species that have been reported to date from clinical specimens and for which some data exist to support their pathogenicity; each species is placed in the category to which it is usually assigned.[63,84-88] Many of these species are rarely isolated, and some can be reliably identified at present only by the use of molecular methods. Unfortunately, some reports of unusual pathogens provide few, if any, data to substantiate identification of the species stated to be the infecting agent. Determination of the clinical significance of some of these species must await further resolution of their frequency of isolation, spectrum of illness, and therapeutic responsiveness. Within the group of rapid growers, certain organisms recently considered to be subspecies or biovariants are now regarded as separate species. With continuing use of molecular techniques, it can be anticipated that additional mycobacterial species will continue to be described for some time.

TABLE 15-15 Mycobacterial Species Isolated from Clinical Specimens*

Nonphotochromogens	Scotochromogens
M. avium complex	*M. bohemicum*[†]
M. avium	*M. doricum*[†]
M. intracellulare	*M. flavescens*
Other unnamed organisms	*M. gordonae*
M. branderi[†]	*M. heckeshornense*[†]
M. celatum[†]	*M. interjectum*[†]
M. conspicuum[†]	*M. kubicae*[†]
M. gastric	*M. lentiflavum*[†]
M. genavense[†]	*M. palustre*[†]
M. haemophilum	*M. scrofulaceum*
M. heidelbergense[†]	*M. szulgai*
M. lacus[†]	*M. tusciae*
M. malmoense	
M. paratuberculosis	**Rapid Growers**
M. shimoidei	*M. abscessus*
M. terrae complex	*M. alvei*
M. nonchromogenicum	*M. aurum*[†]
M. terrae	*M. chelonae*
M. triviale[‡]	*M. elephantis*[†]
M. triplex[†]	*M. fortuitum*
M. tuberculosis complex	*M. fortuitum, 3rd biovar*
M. africanum	*M. goodii*[†]
M. bovis	*M. hassiacum*[†]
M. canettii[†]	*M. immunogenum*[†]
M. microti[§]	*M. margeritense*[†]
M. tuberculosis	*M. mucogenicum*[†]
M. ulcerans	*M. neoaurum*
M. xenopi	*M. novocastrense*[†]
	M. peregrinum[†]
Photochromogens	*M. phlei*
M. asiaticum	*M. septicum*[†]
M. intermedium[†]	*M. smegmatis*
M. kansasii	*M. thermoresistible*
M. marinum	*M. vaccae*
M. simiae	*M. wolinskyi*[†]

*Includes most species of mycobacteria reported from human clinical specimens and thought to be possible pathogens; does not include *M. leprae*, which cannot be grown in vitro.
[†]Species newly described since 1990.
[‡]May never be a pathogen.[102]
[§]Primarily an animal pathogen and only very rarely implicated as a human pathogen.

Susceptibility Testing

In the United States, susceptibility testing of *M. tuberculosis* complex is done either by the proportion method using Middlebrook 7H10 agar or in a liquid medium.[55,89] It is currently recommended that all initial isolates of *M. tuberculosis* complex be tested, as well as isolates from patients who are still culture positive after 3 months of therapy or who are clinically failing to respond. The use of liquid medium is recommended for testing the four primary antituberculous drugs (ethambutol, isoniazid, pyrazinamide, and rifampin) because results are usually available within a week, as opposed to the 3 weeks required with solid medium. In the proportion method, an isolate is considered resistant to a specific concentration of antimicrobial if the number of colonies growing on the corresponding drug-containing quadrant of the plate is greater than 1% of the number of colonies on a drug-free quadrant. Testing that uses the liquid media has been adjusted to provide results that are in accordance with those obtained with the standardized procedure employing a solid medium. Testing of the "critical concentration" of each drug is considered most important.[89] These "critical" concentrations may differ somewhat between solid and liquid media for a given agent (e.g., the critical concentration for isoniazid in 7H10 agar is 0.2 µg/mL; in BACTEC 12B and ESP II liquid media, it is 0.1 µg/mL). The NCCLS has recently published an approved standard for susceptibility testing of *M. tuberculosis*, which also includes recommendations for the testing of most other pathogenic species of mycobacteria, as well as of aerobic actinomycetes.[55] The document includes discussions of the circumstances under which susceptibility testing of the various species may be most useful. Rapidly growing mycobacteria do not generally respond to agents used for the treatment of tuberculosis. The NCCLS document describes a modification of the broth microdilution procedure used for bacterial susceptibility testing for use with rapid growers, including a variety of species-specific procedural and interpretive guidelines.[55]

Epidemiology

Molecular typing can now be performed by a variety of methods to determine the relatedness of different isolates of *M. tuberculosis*.[82] The method still considered the most discriminatory is based on the insertion sequence IS*6110*, which is found in 0 to approximately 25 copies scattered in different locations in the chromosome in different strains.[82] The DNA fragments produced by a specific endonuclease (which cleaves at only one site in each insertion sequence) are separated by gel electrophoresis. A probe is then used to detect the fragments that contain the larger portion of the cleaved insertion sequence, and fragment patterns obtained from different isolates are compared to determine relatedness.[90] The procedure has been used for such purposes as investigating episodes of possible laboratory cross-contamination, tracing sources of infection in outbreak situations, determining whether a second episode of disease is due to a previously isolated strain or to a newly infecting strain, and determining whether an infection is caused by more than one strain of organism.[91] Other techniques can be used when the IS*6110*-based technique is not practicable, such as for isolates with too few copies of the insertion sequence. Among the molecular techniques used for evaluation of the strain relatedness of nontuberculous mycobacteria are PFGE and RAPD.[82]

Recommended Procedures and Target Times for Results for the Mycobacteriology Laboratory

To help control the resurgence of tuberculosis in the United States and to deal with the increase in isolation of drug-resistant *M. tuberculosis*, the recommendations summarized in Table 15-16 have been made regarding diagnostic mycobacteriology laboratory procedures.[55,72]

Latent Tuberculosis: Laboratory Diagnosis

The QuantiFERON-TB test (Cellestis Limited, Carnegie, Victoria, Australia) has been approved by the FDA for use in the diagnosis of latent *M. tuberculosis* infection. The test involves the quantitative measurement by an ELISA procedure of the interferon-γ released

TABLE 15-16   Turnaround Times for Diagnostic Mycobacteriology Laboratory Procedures for *Mycobacterium tuberculosis*[72,82]

Recommended Procedure	Turnaround Time for Recommended Procedure	Conventional Procedure and Turnaround Time
Fluorochrome stain	Within 24 hours of specimen receipt	Carbolfuchsin stain; within 24 hours of specimen receipt
Liquid medium for culture	Growth within approximately 2 weeks	Solid medium for culture; growth detected at approximately 3 to 6 weeks
Rapid method for identification	Within 24 hours (by probes or chromatography) or 5 days (NAP) of organism isolation	Phenotypic identification; requires 3 to 6 weeks after organism isolation and adequate organism growth
Susceptibility testing in a liquid medium	Results available approximately 1 week after organism isolation	Susceptibility testing on a solid medium; results available 3 weeks after adequate organism growth

from sensitized lymphocytes after overnight incubation with purified protein derivative from *M. tuberculosis*. Detailed guidelines on the use and interpretation of this test have been published recently by the CDC. Among the groups for which the CDC states that the test is contraindicated are those thought to have active tuberculosis, contacts of individuals with active tuberculosis, individuals younger than age 17, and others, such as those positive for HIV, who have a condition that increases their risk of progressing from latent to active tuberculosis.[92]

AEROBIC ACTINOMYCETES

Aerobic Actinomycetes are branching, gram-positive rods that grow best (or in many cases, only) under aerobic conditions. They are similar in certain respects to both corynebacteria and mycobacteria, which are often also included with the aerobic Actinomycetes.[93] The taxonomy of this group is under active revision, and considerable nomenclatural change is occurring. The morphologically similar anaerobic Actinomycetes (including the genus *Actinomyces*), which have a preference or requirement for anaerobic growth conditions, are included with gram-positive anaerobic bacteria. In addition to *Corynebacterium* and *Mycobacterium*, genera of aerobic Actinomycetes that contain species pathogenic for humans include *Actinomadura, Dermatophilus, Gordonia, Nocardia, Nocardiopsis, Rhodococcus, Streptomyces, Tropheryma,* and *Tsukamurella*.[93] *Tropheryma whipplei,* now generally considered the causative agent of Whipple's disease, is not cultivatable in the routine laboratory. Organisms in the genera *Gordonia, Nocardia, Rhodococcus,* and *Tsukamurella* are usually modified acid-fast positive; of these, only isolates of *Nocardia* regularly produce an aerial mycelium.[93] Although they are true bacteria and not molds, these organisms have traditionally been identified in the mycology section of the laboratory, perhaps because they resemble molds both in their relatively slow growth rate and in their tendency to form long, branched structures reminiscent of hyphae. Because these organisms are widespread in the environment, colonization and specimen contamination can occur. Single colonies of *Streptomyces,* especially from nonsterile sites and from nonmycetomatous lesions, are very likely to represent contamination. However, most aerobic actinomycetes are very uncommon as laboratory contaminants, and their isolation should not be too quickly dismissed as insignificant.

Specimen Collection and Transport

Collection and transport procedures suitable for bacterial and fungal cultures are also adequate for the aerobic actinomycetes, but refrigeration of specimens should be avoided because some *Nocardia* strains lose viability at low temperatures.[93] If infection with an organism in this group is strongly suspected, alerting the laboratory is advisable because special staining and planting procedures are useful for enhancing the likelihood that the organism will be detected. Because these organisms may cause deep-seated infections such as brain abscess, biopsy may be necessary for isolation. These organisms are not considered a safety hazard in the laboratory.

Direct Organism Detection

In some infections caused by these organisms, such as mycetoma, the organisms may grow in dense masses visible macroscopically as "grains" in purulent material. Detection of these "grains" may greatly facilitate isolation of the etiologic agent; hence, the laboratory should be notified in advance when such an infection is suspected. The only generally available means of direct detection of these organisms in patient specimens is staining. On Gram stain, many of these organisms appear as long, branching, somewhat beaded gram-positive rods. *Nocardia* tends to be especially thin and long and may appear to be composed mainly of tiny noncontiguous gram-positive beads. Organisms in other genera such as *Streptomyces* (and the anaerobic actinomycetes) tend to appear wider and more avidly gram positive, but a definite genus assignment of any organism other than *Dermatophilus* cannot be made with certainty on the basis of organism morphology alone. *Nocardia* may also be invisible on Gram stain or may appear only as negative images, and a modified acid-fast smear should always be requested if *Nocardia* infection is suspected. *Gordonia* and *Rhodococcus* spp. may be unbranched, much shorter than *Nocardia,* and overall more coryneform in appearance. *Dermatophilus congolensis,* the only species in the genus, produces branching filaments with divisions that occur both parallel and perpendicular to the long axis of the filament. In Gram-stained material, the organism may appear too darkly stained for adequate visualization of structural detail, and some other stain such as a Giemsa stain may be necessary.[93] The modified acid-fast stain for aerobic actinomycetes is similar to the Kinyoun stain for mycobacteria but differs particularly in that a weaker decolorizing solution, a shorter time period, or both are used for decolorization. The stain requires some expertise for performance and interpretation and should always be done with appropriate positive and negative controls. *Nocardia* spp. are weakly acid fast in that they retain carbolfuchsin only if a weak decolorization procedure is performed; they are not acid fast with the decolorizing procedure used for mycobacteria. In addition to being weakly acid fast, they tend to be only partially acid fast, particularly when they are stained from culture, which means that often only a small proportion of cells retain the carbolfuchsin dye.

Specimen Processing and Planting

No special specimen processing is required for isolation of the aerobic actinomycetes, which grow on many different types of media. However, they may not survive the specimen processing used to eliminate bacterial flora from specimens for mycobacterial culture. Because they may be present in low numbers and are relatively slowly growing, isolation of aerobic actinomycetes may be enhanced with the use of media that contain antimicrobial agents to suppress the normal flora. A medium that has been found to be particularly useful for the isolation of *Nocardia* is buffered charcoal-yeast extract agar with antibiotics.[93] Cultures for *Nocardia* should be held for up to 3 weeks.

Identification of Aerobic Actinomycetes

Colonies of *Nocardia* typically have a powdery, whitish surface because of the production of aerial mycelium and a tan to orange reverse surface. When stained from colonies, the organism often breaks up into coccobacillary fragments, with long, branching forms much less conspicuous than in direct patient material. Organisms stained from culture may be less acid fast than those in stains prepared from the original specimen.

The taxonomy of the genus *Nocardia* has become increasingly complex as new pathogenic species are recognized and formerly recognized species are subdivided into additional species. Species in the genus currently recognized as human pathogens include *N. abscessus, N. africana, N. asteroides, N. brasiliensis, N. brevicatena* (perhaps a complex of species), *N. farcinica, N. nova, N. otitidiscaviarum* (formerly called *N. caviae*), *N. paucivorans, N. pseudobrasiliensis, N. transvalensis* (a name applied to what may be four different species), and *N. veterana.*[91,94] Conventional identification procedures for *Nocardia* spp. as performed in most laboratories involve only a small number of phenotypic tests, and these are insufficient to distinguish accurately among the different species in the genus. Differences in the results of testing for susceptibility to certain antimicrobial agents may help in discriminating among some of these species, but such testing does not, for example, distinguish between *N. nova* and *N. veterana.*[93-95]

Colonies of *R. equi,* which is the principal pathogen in the genus *Rhodococcus,* most commonly are somewhat mucoid and acquire a pink color after 4 days of incubation; the organism has been isolated from a variety of sites, including the respiratory tract and blood.[93]

Molecular methods, such as amplification by PCR of a portion of the genome, followed by RFLP analysis or DNA sequencing of the 16S rRNA gene (and other genes), may prove to be the most rapid and reliable means of accurately identifying aerobic actinomycetes to the species level, but these techniques are not yet widely available.[95,96] Thus, for accurate identification of many of these organisms, referral to a specialized laboratory is necessary.

Susceptibility Testing

It is hoped that the use of the NCCLS-recommended procedure for susceptibility testing of aerobic actinomycetes will produce greater comparability of results from different laboratories, but experience with the procedure is needed to assure intralaboratory and interlaboratory reproducibility.[55] In the past, different investigators used different susceptibility testing procedures; caution must be used when one is attempting to compare published results obtained by differing methodologies. Sulfonamides have been the most widely used agents for the treatment of *Nocardia* infection; a recent report indicates that linezolid is also efficacious.[97] See Chapter 252 on *Nocardia* infections in this text for a discussion of treatment options.

Epidemiology

Because infection with aerobic actinomycetes generally occurs on a sporadic basis, epidemiologic investigations are only rarely needed. When epidemiologic analysis is needed, a variety of molecular techniques have been found useful.[93]

FUNGI

Like plants and animals, fungi are eukaryotic, a characteristic that distinguishes these three groups from bacteria. Fungi are now placed in their own separate kingdom. It is estimated that there may be several hundred thousand species of fungi, of which approximately 150 have been reported to be at least occasional human pathogens, with additional ones appearing in the literature regularly.[98] The genus *Pneumocystis,* formerly considered to be a parasite, is now thought to be a fungus, although the human pathogen *P. jirovecii* (until very recently known as *P. carinii* f. sp. [forma specialis, or special form] *hominis*) remains for all practical purposes uncultivatable in vitro.[99] Other fungal pathogens that have not yet been cultured in vitro include *Loboa loboi* and *Rhinosporidium seeberi.*[100] Organisms recovered from patients with hepatosplenic candidiasis, although often readily visible microscopically, are frequently uncultivatable in vitro.[101] The genus *Prototheca* is thought to be an achlorophyllous alga; organisms in this genus can be pathogenic and are usually included in discussions of fungi because they grow well on most fungal culture media.[100]

Terminology

The diagnostic mycology laboratory uses terminology that, although it has little taxonomic significance, is useful in terms of assessing both clinical relevance and identification possibilities.[98,100,102] *Yeasts* are organisms that grow as relatively smooth, creamy colonies, whereas *molds* produce fuzzy colonies because of the production of aerial hyphae. Some organisms may initially produce yeastlike colonies that become more moldlike with continued incubation. Microscopically, yeasts appear as round or oval cells that reproduce by budding. Many yeasts, such as most species of *Candida,* also produce hyphal structures. Hyphae are morphologically subdivided into pseudohyphae and true hyphae. *Pseudohyphae* resemble chains of sausages in that the hyphae tend to be constricted at the septa and each cell originates as a bud. The cell at the tip tends to be small and rounded, and a septum is often found at each branch point. In contrast, *true hyphae* tend to have straighter, more parallel walls without constrictions at the septa and usually without a septum at the branch point. True hyphae may be either *septate* or *aseptate.* True hyphae that are septate suggest organisms such as *Aspergillus, Fusarium,* and *Scedosporium.* True aseptate hyphae may be broad and have a ribbon-like appearance; their presence suggests one of the zygomycetes (aseptate molds) such as *Rhizomucor.* Brown pigment in hyphae suggests that the organism is a *dematiaceous* (black) mold; *hyaline* molds do not produce pigmented hyphae. These simplified distinctions are not absolute. Thus, some *Candida* species can form true hyphae, and the "aseptate" molds may have an occasional septum. *Dermatophytes* and *dimorphic* molds are usually considered separate categories of mold distinct from the other hyaline septate molds. The likelihood that an organism may be a dermatophyte is usually suggested by the specimen source (e.g., skin, hair, nails). Dimorphic molds have a nonmold form when they are growing in the patient but grow as a mold in the laboratory at 30° C. Table 15-17 summarizes some of the more significant and more commonly isolated genera and species according to the categories frequently used in the diagnostic laboratory. Of the clinically significant dimorphic molds, *Blastomyces dermatitidis, Histoplasma capsulatum, Paracoccidioides brasiliensis, Penicillium marneffei,* and *S. schenckii* grow as yeasts in the patient at 37° C and hence are thermally dimorphic. *Coccidioides* species most commonly grow in the patient as thick-walled spherules and require a special medium that is not widely available to be grown in this form in vitro; otherwise, these species grow as a mold both at 30° C and at 35° C, and hence are not thermally dimorphic. (Two species of *Coccidioides* are now recognized and are distinguished by molecular methods and by geographic location. *C. immitis* is found primarily in California, and the newly recognized species *C. posadasii* is found in the southwestern United States and in Central and South America, overlapping with *C. immitis* in southern California and parts of Mexico.[103])

Many molds have a morphologic form that results from sexual reproduction; these differ from the form that results from asexual reproduction. The form that results from sexual reproduction is known as the *teleomorph,* or perfect state; the form that results from asexual reproduction is known as the *anamorph,* or imperfect state. Traditionally, each form has been given a different scientific name; for example, the sexual form of *H. capsulatum* is named *Ajellomyces capsulatum,* and the sexual form of *Scedosporium apiospermum* is named *Pseudallescheria boydii.*

Safety Issues

Virtually all molds release their reproductive structures (conidia or spores) into the air, and for many fungal pathogens, the respiratory tract is the initial portal of entry. Thus, it is not surprising that certain organisms, particularly *Coccidioides* spp. and *H. capsulatum,* can be significant laboratory hazards. Containment facilities (BSL 2 for specimen handling, initial isolation, and identification; BSL 3 for further propagation of such agents) are needed to process specimens and to work with cultures of these organisms.[104] Because infectious spores are not present in patient specimens such as sputa or biopsy specimens, these specimens are not considered hazardous by the aerosol

TABLE 15-17 Laboratory Categorization of Selected Clinically Significant and/or Commonly Isolated Fungi

	Molds					Hyaline Aseptate
	Dematiaceous	Hyaline Septate				
Yeasts		Dermatophyte	Dimorphic	Other		Hyaline Aseptate
Candida	Alternaria	Epidermophyton	Blastomyces dermatitidis	Aspergillus		Cunninghamella
Cryptococcus	Bipolaris	Microsporum	Coccidioides species	Fusarium		Conidiobolus
Blastoschizomyces	Cladophialophora	Trichophyton	Histoplasma capsulatum	Paecilomyces		Mucor
Malassezia	Curvularia		Paracoccidioides brasiliensis	Penicillium		Rhizomucor
Saccharomyces	Exophiala		Penicillium marneffei	Scedosporium apiospermum*		Rhizopus
Rhodotorula	Wangiella		Sporothrix schenckii*	Scedosporium prolificans*		
Trichosporon						

*Often considered a dematiaceous mold.
Adapted from Koneman EW, Roberts GD. Practical Laboratory Mycology. 3rd ed. Baltimore: Williams & Wilkins; 1985.

route, but of course they would be infectious by accidental inoculation. In view of the fact that several of the dimorphic molds can be significant laboratory hazards when grown in mold phase, the clinician should alert laboratory personnel whenever a patient has a significant probability of a dimorphic mold infection. Such advance notification allows the laboratory to take additional precautions with the cultures of such patients' specimens.

Specimen Collection and Transport

The procedures used for the collection of specimens for bacterial culture will suffice for fungal culture. However, it is important to be sure that an adequate volume of specimen has been collected, as for example, in the cases of CSF (up to 5 mL or even 30 mL for chronic meningitis) and urine (up to 200 mL).[100] Twenty-four-hour collections of urine or sputa are not suitable for fungal culture because of bacterial overgrowth; first morning specimens are considered optimal. Aspirated material can be transported to the laboratory in an anaerobic transport vial; as long as the specimen is received and processed promptly by the laboratory, little loss of fungal viability appears to occur.[105] Blood culture performed by lysis-centrifugation is still considered to be the most sensitive procedure for the isolation of *H. capsulatum* from blood.[105] Commercially available broth and biphasic systems have been shown to be quite sensitive for the isolation of yeasts from blood[105] (Table 15-18). Certain specimen types are more useful than others for the detection of particular pathogens; these issues are dealt with in the chapters that pertain to specific organisms.

Direct Organism Detection

Fungi are detected in clinical specimens either by direct visualization of the organisms themselves or by detection of substances produced by or contained in the organism. Fungi may be visualized histopathologically or cytologically by a variety of special stains such as the methenamine silver, periodic acid–Schiff, and Papanicolaou stains. In the microbiology laboratory, fungi are usually visualized directly by a Gram stain, a potassium hydroxide (KOH) (wet) mount, or a calcofluor white stain.[106] With Gram stain, yeast cells and pseudohyphae of *Candida* species usually stain uniformly throughout as gram positive, whereas the cells of *C. neoformans* may be unevenly speckled with crystal violet and may be surrounded by an orange halo that is presumably capsular material. The true hyphae of organisms such as *Aspergillus* species are Gram negative, visible as unstained negative images, or Gram stain invisible. Although KOH wet mounts allow visualization of most fungi, organisms may actually be quite difficult to discern because they do not stand out prominently from the background; in addition, tissue components such as blood vessels can be mistaken for fungal elements, so considerable care and expertise are required for the reading of such preparations. In the calcofluor white stain, a fluorescent compound binds to certain cell wall polysaccharides found in all fungi; organisms stained by this dye can be readily visualized with the use of a fluorescence microscope.[106]

Among the procedures that can be used for visualization of *P. jirovecii* are calcofluor white, toluidine blue O, methenamine silver, Giemsa, and monoclonal antibody stains.[99] Calcofluor white, toluidine blue O, and methenamine silver stains stain only the cyst wall; a drawback of these stains is that they also stain yeast cells, which can be morphologically similar to *Pneumocystis* cysts. Giemsa stain allows visualization of intracystic structures and trophozoites, but the cyst wall appears only as a negative image. Monoclonal antibody stains allow the visualization of both cysts and trophozoites of *P. jirovecii*, but even with these stains, some expertise is required to recognize the various forms of the organism and to distinguish them from staining artifacts. The Giemsa stain is also useful for detecting *H. capsulatum* within macrophages.[106]

Antigen detection for *C. neoformans* and for *H. capsulatum* has been demonstrated to be of sufficient sensitivity to have considerable diagnostic usefulness.[107] The capsular polysaccharide antigen of

TABLE 15-18 Identification of Commonly Encountered Yeasts, Excluding Dimorphic Molds

Capsule +			
	Phenol oxidase*	+	Cryptococcus neoformans
		−	Cryptococcus sp., not neoformans
Capsule −			
	Germ tube/chlamydospore	+	Candida albicans (or C. dubliniensis)
		−	Pseudohyphae or hyphae seen
			Arthroconidia +, urea + Trichosporon spp.
			Arthroconidia +, urea − Blastoschizomyces spp. or Geotrichum spp.
			Arthroconidia − Candida spp.†
		−	Pseudohyphae or hyphae NOT seen
			Red or orange colonies Rhodotorula spp.
			White or cream colonies Candida glabrata or Malassezia spp. (lipid-requiring) or Saccharomyces sp. (ascospore +)

*Determined by either caffeic acid or birdseed agar test.
†*C. tropicalis, C. krusei, C. parapsilosis, C. lusitaniae,* and others.

C. neoformans may be detected by either latex agglutination or EIA techniques. These tests can be performed on both CSF and serum. Detection of cryptococcal antigen has been demonstrated to be a more sensitive technique for the diagnosis of cryptococcal meningitis than is examination of CSF for cryptococci by the India ink procedure. A test for detection of *Histoplasma* antigen in CSF, bronchoalveolar lavage fluid, serum, or urine for diagnosis of *H. capsulatum* infection is available from MiraVista Diagnostics in Indianapolis, Indiana.

The detection of galactomannan in blood has been found to be helpful for the diagnosis of invasive aspergillosis, and the FDA has recently approved the Platelia Aspergillus EIA (Bio-Rad, Redmond, Wash.) for the detection of galactomannan antigen in blood.[107,108] However, care is needed in interpreting the significance of these test results in that sensitivity and specificity are both less than 100% and have varied in different studies.

The development of molecular methods for the diagnosis of fungal infection is an area of active research.[107] An example is the use of real-time PCR for diagnosis of *Pneumocystis* pneumonia.[109] This sensitive assay may be useful for patients in whom respiratory specimens are negative for *Pneumocystis* by traditional stains, but in whom there is a high clinical suspicion of infection with *Pneumocystis*. The assay, which can detect *Pneumocystis* in oral washes or sputum, may also benefit patients who are too ill to undergo invasive procedures such as bronchoalveolar lavage.

Specimen Processing and Planting

No special processing of specimens is required for isolation of fungi from clinical specimens. Specimens from nonsterile sites are planted onto media that contain antibiotics such as chloramphenicol and gentamicin to inhibit bacterial growth; media used for the isolation of dermatophytes may also contain cycloheximide to inhibit yeasts. Media commonly used include inhibitory mold agar and brain-heart infusion agar. A source of fatty acids such as olive oil must be added to media to recover *Malassezia* spp.; clinicians should therefore notify the laboratory when the presence of this organism is suspected.[100] Fungal cultures are generally incubated at 30° C, and until recently, they were generally held for 4 weeks or even longer when the presence of a slowly growing mold such as *H. capsulatum* was suspected.[105] However, it has been shown that shorter periods of incubation suffice for the isolation of most fungal pathogens, depending on the type of specimen and the organisms being sought; these shorter incubation periods are likely to be used by a growing number of laboratories.[110,111] Thus, if a slowly growing mold such as *H. capsulatum* is suspected, it is useful for the clinician to notify the laboratory.

Significance of Isolation of Fungi from Clinical Specimens

It is often difficult to assess the significance of the isolation of fungi other than dimorphic molds from clinical specimens, particularly if they are isolated in small quantity from nonsterile sites such as the respiratory tract. It is usually impossible to attach clinical significance to the isolation of *Candida* from pulmonary material other than a lung biopsy because *Candida* can be part of the normal upper respiratory tract flora. Even *C. neoformans* may occasionally be a colonizer and not a pathogen in the respiratory tract.[100] Isolation of opportunistic pathogens such as *Aspergillus* from the respiratory tract of an immunocompromised patient presents a particularly difficult interpretive problem for which no unambiguous guidelines exist. In addition to the clinical and radiographic aspects of each situation, it may be useful to consider (1) whether the organism was seen directly in the specimen, (2) the quantity of organism that grew in culture, and (3) the particular genus or species recovered (e.g., *Aspergillus niger* is less likely to be a pathogen than is *Aspergillus fumigatus* or *Aspergillus flavus*[100]). *Penicillium* species other than *P. marneffei* are common laboratory contaminants; their isolation is almost never indicative of disease. However, because many different fungi are capable of causing at least occasional cases of infection, each situation needs to be assessed individually.

Identification of Fungi

Yeasts are identified by initially performing a simple test, such as a germ tube test, or a test based on the detection of preformed enzymes to identify *Candida albicans*, or a caffeic acid test for the presumptive identification of *C. neoformans*.[42] Figure 15-2 is a schematic diagram for identification of the various categories of yeast. With the use of a rapid and inexpensive test such as the germ tube for the presumptive identification of *C. albicans*, the most commonly isolated yeast in the diagnostic laboratory, the laboratory reduces the need for more time-consuming and expensive testing. It has recently been found, however, that another *Candida* species, *Candida dubliniensis*, is also germ tube positive. However, unlike most isolates of *C. albicans*, most isolates of *C. dubliniensis* will not grow at 45° C.[42] (The organism is geographically widespread and causes disease primarily in individuals infected with HIV, although HIV-negative patients may be infected. *C. dubliniensis* may develop resistance to azoles.[112]) Both manual kits and automated systems are available for the identification of clinically significant yeasts.[113] A cornmeal agar plate is inoculated along with any of these systems to confirm that the isolate's morphologic features are compatible with the identification. Identification of most molds is based largely on the morphologic features of the organism, but for certain organisms, other features such as the ability to grow at higher temperatures or the need for specific nutritional supplements are also used. For some fungi, assignment to a particular genus may be straightforward, whereas identification to the species level may require a mycologist with expertise in the particular group in question; examples include organisms that belong to the genera *Curvularia* and *Fusarium*. Chemiluminescent probes are available for the identification of isolates of *B. dermatitidis*, *Coccidioides* species, and *H. capsulatum*.[114] As with similar probes for mycobacterial identification, they are intended for use with isolates, not with direct patient specimens; the probe is a DNA probe for organism ribosomal RNA. These probes can be used with either the yeast or mold phase, thus allowing early identification of isolates and obviating the need for conversion of the mold to the yeast phase for *B. dermatitidis* and *H. capsulatum*. Use of these probes also eliminates the need for extensive manipulation of cultures of these hazardous organisms. Exoantigen testing for identification of most of the pathogenic dimorphic molds can also be done but requires an adequate amount of a mold-phase culture.[114]

Susceptibility Testing

The NCCLS has published standardized procedures for susceptibility testing of yeast and filamentous fungi.[115,116] For *Candida* species, interpretive guidelines are presently provided only for fluconazole, flucytosine, and itraconazole; for the azoles, these guidelines are based largely (fluconazole) or entirely (itraconazole) on results with mucosal infection. It is important to note that for the filamentous fungi, the NCCLS has not established any interpretive breakpoints; furthermore, the document that pertains to the susceptibility testing of these organisms specifically states the following: "The clinical relevance of testing this group of fungal pathogens remains uncertain."[116] Although it is not generally available in routine diagnostic laboratories, susceptibility testing of filamentous fungi can be performed by certain reference centers.

Epidemiology

A variety of molecular techniques have been applied to different fungal species for determination of strain relatedness.[113,117] Such studies are available only in larger laboratories or in reference centers.

Serology

The usefulness of serologic determinations for the diagnosis of infection has been investigated for many different fungi. Often, several different methodologies, such as complement fixation and immunodiffusion, have been developed for the same organism. Kits for detection of antibody to certain organisms are commercially available. Testing for the presence of antibody to assist in the diagnosis of invasive disease has been used for blastomycosis, coccidioidomycosis, histoplasmosis,

FIGURE 15-2. Schematic diagram for identification of commonly encountered yeasts, excluding dimorphic molds.

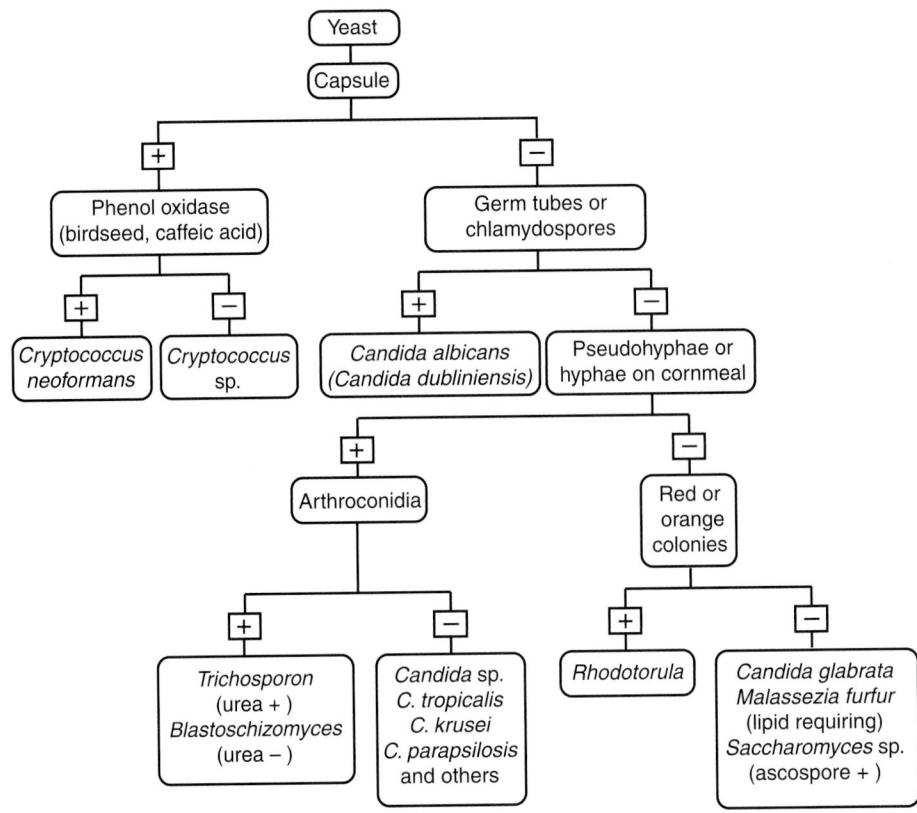

paracoccidioidomycosis, penicilliosis, and sporotrichosis[107,118]; at present, such testing may be particularly useful for the diagnosis of coccidioidomycosis and paracoccidioidomycosis.[107] Antibody testing for the diagnosis of invasive infection caused by other fungal pathogens generally has not been found to be useful.[107] However, testing for antibody in noninvasive disease has been found helpful for the diagnosis of allergic bronchopulmonary aspergillosis and aspergilloma.[117] For details regarding optimal diagnostic methodology for different agents and for problems relating to result interpretation, see relevant chapters in this text that pertain to specific etiologic agents.

VIRUSES

Virology Specimen Collection and Transport

Appropriate specimen collection and transport vary depending on the specimen site, the time of year, and the virus suspected. Many viruses enter through the upper respiratory tract, yet the disease caused by the virus may involve multiple or distant organs. In some cases, the optimal site for viral culture or detection may be different from the site at which the virus produces its major clinical impact. Infections with enteroviruses are a good example. Enteroviruses can cause a variety of infections such as aseptic meningitis, myocarditis, exanthems, and conjunctivitis, but the specimens of choice for diagnosis of these enterovirus infections are throat and nasopharyngeal aspirates. Specimen collection based on the suspicion of a specific virus should be done with caution because a request for a specific viral agent will probably eliminate testing to detect other viruses that may cause the same disease or syndrome. Unlike with many other groups of bacterial or fungal pathogens, the time of year is important to keep in mind when one is making a diagnosis of certain viral diseases. Influenza viruses, which circulate in the winter months, and arboviruses and enteroviruses, which circulate in the summer months, are unlikely to cause infection at other times of the year. Table 15-19 provides a guide

for selection of specimens for diagnosis of the more common viral syndromes or specific viral agents. One must remember that specimens should not be sent to the virology laboratory with the generalized request for "viral studies." Discussion of the patient's history, signs, and symptoms with the infectious diseases physician or the clinical microbiologist should help the caregiver decide on the most likely viral pathogens to suspect, which specimens to collect, and the appropriate laboratory test to order. This information should be included on the requisition that accompanies the specimens to the laboratory.

Timing is important when one is collecting specimens for the detection of viruses. Specimens should be collected as early as possible after the onset of symptoms. Enteroviruses are present in the respiratory tract shortly before and after the onset of symptoms, but within a few days, the virus can be detected only in stool specimens. Once viral shedding stops, serologic analysis may be the only way of diagnosing the viral pathogen. Acute and convalescent serum specimens collected 2 to 4 weeks apart are recommended. Swab and tissue specimens for viral culture should be placed in a viral transport medium that is buffered and contains protein (serum, albumin, or gelatin) and antibiotics. Because of the presence of antibiotics in viral transport media, separate specimens from the same site are needed if bacterial or fungal cultures are also being requested. Liquid specimens such as CSF, bronchoalveolar lavage fluid, or urine need not be sent in viral transport media. Isolation of virus from sputum, nasopharyngeal washes, or throat swabs can support the clinical diagnosis of a viral respiratory infection.[119] Isolation from bronchoscopic specimens or lung tissue is stronger evidence. Blood for viral diagnostic tests should be sent in a tube that contains an anticoagulant. Heparin, ethylenediaminetetraacetic acid (EDTA), and citrate are all acceptable for the detection of cytomegalovirus (CMV) by culture or antigenemia testing, but citrate should be used if other viruses are to be cultured. Heparin should not be used as an anticoagulant if PCR on blood is to be performed because it is a nonspecific ribonuclease inhibitor.[120] Citrate and EDTA are suitable anticoagulants for PCR

TABLE 15-19 Specimen Collection Guide for Viral Infections

Disease Category and Most Common Viral Agents	Season of Occurrence	Specimen Sources for Viral Detection	Serologic Diagnosis
Upper Respiratory Tract		Nasopharyngeal swab or wash, nasal wash, throat swab, stool (enterovirus), Stensen's duct (mumps virus)	
Rhinovirus	Y		No
Coronavirus	W, SP		No
Respiratory syncytial virus	W		Yes
Adenovirus	Y		Yes
Influenza virus	W		Yes
Parainfluenza virus	Y		No
Enterovirus	S, F		No
Mumps virus	SP		Yes
Lower Respiratory Tract		Endotracheal aspirate, bronchial wash, bronchoalveolar lavage, stool (enterovirus)	
Adenovirus	Y		Yes
Influenza virus	W		Yes
Parainfluenza virus	Y		No
Enterovirus	S, F		No
Cytomegalovirus	Y		Yes
Respiratory syncytial virus	W		Yes
Central Nervous System		Throat swab, cerebrospinal fluid, stool (enterovirus), urine (mumps virus), brain biopsy	
Meningitis			
Enterovirus	S, F		
Herpes simplex virus type 2	Y		Yes
Mumps virus	SP		Yes
Arboviruses	S, F		Yes
Cytomegalovirus	Y		Yes
Lymphocytic choriomeningitis virus	Y		Yes
Encephalitis		Throat swab, cerebrospinal fluid, stool (enterovirus), urine (mumps virus), brain biopsy	
Herpes simplex virus type 1	Y		Yes
Cytomegalovirus	Y		Yes
Mumps virus	SP		Yes
Arboviruses (includes West Nile)	S, F		Yes
Human polyomavirus (JC virus)	Y		Yes
Vesicular Lesions		Vesicle scraping, vesicle swab, throat swab (varicella-zoster, enterovirus), stool (enterovirus)	
Herpes simplex virus	Y		No
Enterovirus	S, F		No
Varicella-zoster virus	Y (varicella: W, SP)		No
Smallpox/monkeypox	Y		Yes
Exanthems		Throat swab, urine (measles, rubella), stool (enterovirus), amnionic fluid (parvovirus B19)	
Enterovirus	S, F		No
Parvovirus (B19)	Y		Yes
Measles Virus	Y		Yes
Rubella virus	Y		Yes
Human herpesvirus 6	Y		Yes
Ocular		Conjunctival swab or scraping, throat swab (adenovirus, enterovirus), stool (enterovirus), aqueous or vitreous humor (CMV), blood (CMV)	
Adenovirus	Y		No
Enterovirus	S, F		No
Herpes simplex virus	Y		No
Cytomegalovirus (CMV)	Y		No
Cardiac		Throat swab, stool, pericardial fluid, biopsy	
Enterovirus	S, F		Yes
Gastrointestinal Tract		Stool, throat swab (enterovirus)	
Rotavirus	W, SP		No
Adenovirus types 40, 41	Y		No
Norovirus (Norwalk-like virus)	S		No
Enterovirus	S		No
Genital		Vesicle scraping (HSV), endocervical swab, biopsy (HPV)	
Herpes simplex virus (HSV)	Y		No
Human papillomavirus (HPV)	Y		No
Congenital and Perinatal Disease		Throat, urine, skin lesions, cerebrospinal fluid, stool (enterovirus), biopsy, blood	
Cytomegalovirus (CMV)	Y		Yes
Herpes simplex virus	Y		Yes
Rubella virus	Y		Yes
Varicella-zoster virus	Y		Yes
Enterovirus	S, F		Yes
Posttransplantation Syndrome		Biopsy, blood (CMV), urine (CMV, adenovirus, BK virus)	
Adenovirus	Y		Yes
Human polyomavirus (BK virus)	Y		Yes
Cytomegalovirus (CMV)	Y		Yes
Herpes simplex virus (HSV)	Y		Yes
Human herpesvirus 6	Y		Yes
Epstein-Barr virus	Y		Yes

F, fall, S, summer, SP, spring, W, winter, Y, year round.

assay because they are less inhibitory and are easily removed during sample preparation. All specimens for virologic testing should be kept cold after collection and during transport to the laboratory and should be promptly transported to the laboratory. Delays in transport or processing may lead to loss of viral viability or possibly antigen or nucleic acid degradation. Specimens should not be frozen unless transport or processing is delayed by more than 5 days. Freezing at −70° C is preferable to freezing at −20° C.

Swabs can be used to collect a variety of specimens for viral detection such as from the throat, eye, skin, or rectum. Most fibers, including cotton, dacron, polyester, and rayon, are acceptable for the collection of specimens for viral studies. Calcium alginate has been demonstrated to inactivate HSV, may also act as an inhibitor of PCR, and should therefore not be used for viral culture or for viral PCR assays.[12] Swabs with metal or plastic shafts are preferable to those with wooden shafts because the latter may cause toxicity in cell cultures.[121]

Laboratory Methods for Diagnosis of Viral Infection

Respiratory Viruses

Although most viral respiratory infections are predominant during the colder months, viruses should be considered throughout the year in the differential workup of respiratory tract infections (see Table 15-19). Cell culture techniques allow detection of a wide range of viral pathogens and can allow detection of dual or mixed viral infections. Diagnostic virology laboratories must use more than one cell line for culture of respiratory viruses because influenza and parainfluenza viruses prefer to replicate in primary cell lines such as RhMK (primary rhesus monkey kidney) cells or heteroploid cell lines such as LLC-Mk2 (rhesus monkey kidney), whereas adenoviruses and respiratory syncytial virus (RSV) prefer to replicate in heteroploid cell lines such as A549 (human lung carcinoma) or Hep-2 (human epidermoid larynx carcinoma). Unfortunately, traditional cell culture techniques often do not provide a diagnosis until the patient is convalescing rather than during the acute stage of illness. Respiratory viruses may take up to 10 days to produce a cytopathic effect in cell culture. Moreover, influenza and parainfluenza viruses may produce little or no visible cytopathic effect and may be detected only after hemadsorption or hemagglutination with guinea pig red blood cells 3 to 7 days after inoculation of the cell culture monolayer. In contrast, some viruses such as RSV produce a distinctive cytopathic effect in 1 or 2 days in continuous cell lines such as HeLa or Hep-2 cells. Most diagnostic virology laboratories also use virus-specific fluorescent antibodies to identify viruses with an uncharacteristic or unrecognizable cytopathic effect in cell culture. Traditional viral cultures are held for 7 to 28 days, depending on the type of viral pathogen that is being cultured.

Shell vial spin amplification (SVA) cultures give a more rapid turnaround time than do traditional viral cultures for detection of the more common respiratory viruses. This system uses 1-dram vials that contain cell culture monolayers on 12-mm round coverslips immersed in tissue culture media. Multiple shell vials are required that contain different cell lines such as a primary cell line (RhMK) and a heteroploid cell line (A549 or Hep-2) for the system to detect influenza A and B; parainfluenza 1, 2, and 3; adenovirus; and RSV. Urine can be cultured for adenovirus in bone marrow transplant recipients with hemorrhagic cystitis. Specimens are added to the monolayer, centrifuged at low speed, and incubated. Instead of an examination for cytopathic effect, fluorescein-labeled monoclonal antibodies are used to detect viral antigens of replicating viruses. Shell vial cultures are incubated for up to 5 days, but most respiratory viruses can be detected in as little as 24 hours because visual cytopathic effect is not necessary for detection.[122] A pool of monoclonal antibodies is first used to detect the presence of a respiratory virus; individual monoclonal antibodies are then used to identify the specific virus. In an effort to reduce the number of shell vials (and therefore the cost) used in the SVA, investigators began using a combination of cells in a single vial. Mixtures of mink lung cells and A549 cells are available commercially and have been shown to perform as well as each cell line individually.[123]

A multiplex quantitative reverse transcription-PCR-enzyme hybridization assay for simultaneous detection of influenza virus types A and B, RSV types A and B, and parainfluenza virus types 1, 2, and 3 is available as a commercial kit (Hexaplex, Prodesse, Inc., Milwaukee, Wis.). Viral genomic RNA is first converted to cDNA, followed by PCR amplification by means of primer pairs to the seven viruses and amplicon detection with an enzyme hybridization assay with peroxidase-labeled DNA probes specific for each of the seven viruses. Sensitivities for the seven viruses have been reported to range from 91% to 100%, and specificities range from 97.4% to 100% compared with conventional viral culture and direct fluorescent antibody (DFA) testing.[124-126] The main drawbacks of this assay are that it is labor intensive, the assay takes 8 to 9 hours to complete and cannot be performed on a STAT basis, and it is considerably more expensive than viral culture and DFA panels.[125]

Rapid identification of RSV can be beneficial because it (1) permits timely cohorting of patients to prevent nosocomial spread of disease and (2) allows prompt initiation of ribavirin therapy if needed. Similarly, rapid identification of influenza A and B allows early administration of amantadine, rimantadine, zanamivir, or oseltamivir. In winter months when the incidence of respiratory infection is high and a corresponding increase in hospital admissions for viral respiratory infection is observed, traditional viral cultures and even SVA cultures are not rapid enough for expedient cohorting of patients. Detection of viral antigen provides for more rapid identification of RSV and influenza A and B; viral antigen tests include DFA assay and EIA. Results from these nonculture assays are often available within hours after receipt in the laboratory and may be particularly useful during the peak months of transmission. These assays have sensitivities of 6% to 80% and are highly specific (>95%).[126a] A note of caution regarding the use of rapid assays, however, is that most rapid assays target a single viral pathogen and, if used alone, an assay can make a specific diagnosis but will not allow the detection of other viruses. Dual or mixed viral infections have been reported to occur in 5% to 35% of patients.[127] The diagnostic virology laboratory should use rapid methods in conjunction with culture or other assays to facilitate the detection of a wider range of viruses in each specimen and to detect mixed viral infections.

Childhood Viral Infections

Many of the classic infections of childhood, especially the rash syndromes, are caused by viruses (Table 15-20). Laboratory diagnosis is usually not required for suspected cases of measles, mumps, or rubella unless complications of severe or atypical disease are present. Although virus culture is useful during the acute illness, serologic analysis can provide the diagnosis in retrospect and can also provide information on whether immunity is present. Serologic tests for childhood viral infections are most often performed with commercially available ELISA or immunofluorescence assays. Latex agglutination tests are available for detecting antibodies to VZV and rubella virus. Reference laboratories may offer complement fixation tests for measles, mumps, and VZV. Although VZV can be detected within cells collected from the base of newly formed vesicular lesions, such detection is done more frequently to diagnose zoster than chickenpox. The virus can be cultured by traditional cell culture or shell vial culture, or VZV-infected cells can be observed directly in specimens with the use of either the Tzanck test or specific fluorescent antibodies. VZV-specific fluorescent antibody stains are more sensitive than culture and more sensitive and specific than Tzanck smears.[128]

In addition to the childhood rash syndromes, erythema infectiosum, and papular-purpuric gloves-and-socks syndrome, parvovirus B19 can be a cause of polyarthropathy syndrome, hemolytic disease (primarily in patients with hemolytic anemia or who are immunocompromised), chronic bone marrow failure, and fetal hydrops.[128] Diagnosis of these manifestations of parvovirus B19 infection in immunocompetent patients can be made by using serologic assays for IgM. Nucleic acid hybridization assays performed on serum have been found to be most helpful for the diagnosis of chronic parvovirus B19

TABLE 15-20   Childhood Rash Syndromes

Disease Name(s)	Disease Number	Etiologic Agent(s)
Rubeola, measles	First disease	Measles virus
Scarlet fever	Second disease	*Streptococcus pyogenes*
Rubella German measles	Third disease	Rubella virus

Duke's disease
  Filatov-Duke's disease
  Pseudoscarlatina
	Fourth disease	Coxsackieviruses
		Echoviruses

Erythema infectiosum "Slapped cheek disease"	Fifth disease	Parvovirus B19

Roseola
  Exanthem subitum
  Roseola infantum
	Sixth disease	Human herpesvirus 6,7

Chickenpox Varicella	None	Varicella-zoster virus
Hand-foot-and-mouth syndrome	None	Coxsackieviruses Echoviruses
Papular-purpuric gloves-and-socks syndrome	None	Parvovirus B19

infection.[129] PCR detection on serum or other body fluids is performed by large reference laboratories and is useful for monitoring patient response to treatment with immunoglobulin, as well as for the diagnosis of congenital infection.

Enterovirus Infection

Enteroviruses are a common cause of mild febrile illness with minimal respiratory or gastrointestinal symptoms that may be accompanied by exanthems, enanthems, myopericarditis, or aseptic meningitis (see specific chapter). Most infections occur during the summer and early fall in temperate climates, but they are occasionally seen during the rest of the year. Enteroviruses are shed in the stool and oropharynx, often for prolonged periods, so isolation from these sites provides only circumstantial diagnostic evidence. Because of the large number of serotypes, serologic analysis is impractical for the diagnosis of polioviruses, group A coxsackieviruses, and echoviruses. A group-specific serologic test is available for group B coxsackieviruses. Until recently, laboratory diagnosis was usually made through the isolation of virus in cell culture. Echoviruses and group B coxsackieviruses usually grow well in primary human or monkey kidney cells and variably in a variety of cell culture strains and continuous cell lines. Group A coxsackieviruses generally grow poorly in cell culture and require inoculation in suckling mouse brain for isolation. Because enteroviruses may take 4 to 8 days to grow, enterovirus culture results are usually not available in time to affect patient management. Culture has a relatively low sensitivity, especially for diagnosis of central nervous system (CNS) infection (<75%).[130] Although no PCR kits for the detection of enteroviruses in clinical specimens are commercially available,

most reference laboratories offer "home-brew" PCR tests of sources such as throat swabs, rectal swab, stool, tissue, and CSF. PCR of CSF is the method of choice for the rapid diagnosis of enterovirus-caused aseptic meningitis. Sensitivity has been reported to range from 86% to 100%, and specificity has ranged from 92% to 100% when PCR of CSF has been compared with cell culture.[131]

Gastrointestinal Tract Infection

In addition to the viruses listed in Table 15-19, caliciviruses (including norovirus [Norwalk-like virus] and sapovirus [Sapporo-like virus]), astroviruses, and coronaviruses have been associated with diarrhea. Viral agents of diarrhea are not detectable by cell culture. Historically, viral gastrointestinal pathogens have been detected by electron microscopy during investigations of large outbreaks; this method is still useful today. Rotavirus infections account for approximately 50% of pediatric hospital admissions for diarrhea and dehydration in the cooler months of the year in the United States.[132] Each year, rotavirus epidemics follow a regional sequence from East to West. Outbreaks occur in November and December in the southwestern states and spread to the New England states in April and May.[133] Rapid detection of rotavirus aids not only in the diagnosis of gastroenteritis but also in the identification of infected individuals who may serve as sources of outbreaks in settings such as daycare centers and hospital wards. Commercial kits for the rapid detection of rotavirus antigen in stool specimens are now available and include ELISA, membrane EIA, and latex agglutination formats. Sensitivities range from 90% to 100% for ELISA and from 70% to 90% for latex tests.[132] Adenovirus serotypes 40 and 41 are second to rotaviruses as the most common cause of pediatric gastroenteritis, and a sensitive commercial EIA is available for their detection. Commercially available EIA kits for detection of astrovirus and norovirus in stool specimens are currently not approved by the FDA for use in the United States. Although PCR assays for adenovirus and reverse transcription PCR (RT-PCR) assays for RNA viruses such as norovirus and rotavirus have been described, PCR technology for the detection of gastrointestinal viruses has not yet made its way into diagnostic virology laboratories.

Arboviruses

Arboviruses (arthropod-borne viruses) not only are seasonal but also are regional in distribution as determined by the residences of the specific hematophagous arthropods that transmit the viruses to humans (Table 15-21). More than 500 arboviruses are recognized, and although approximately 150 can cause disease in humans, fewer than 50 are important human or veterinary pathogens worldwide.[134] Arbovirus infections are emerging or resurging throughout the world as a result of changes in public health policy, de-emphasis on prevention programs, demographic and societal changes, and genetic changes in pathogens.[135] For example, West Nile virus in the United States was first detected in 1999 during an epidemic of meningoencephalitis in

TABLE 15-21   Most Common Arboviruses in North America

Virus	Occurrence	Distribution	Vector	Clinical Disease
Eastern equine encephalitis*	Sporadic	Atlantic and Gulf Coasts, upper New York, Michigan, Canada	Mosquito (*Culiseta melanura*)	Encephalitis
Western equine encephalitis	Epidemic	Western USA and Canada	Mosquito (*Culex* sp.)	Encephalitis
St. Louis encephalitis	Epidemic	USA, Canada, Mexico	Mosquito (*Culex* sp.)	Encephalitis
Venezuelan encephalitis*	Sporadic	Florida, Texas, Mexico	Mosquito (*Culex* and *Aedes* sp.)	Encephalitis
LaCrosse encephalitis	Epidemic	North Central and Northeast USA	Mosquito (*Aedes triseriatus*)	Encephalitis
Dengue types 1–4†	Epidemic	Caribbean, Mexico	Mosquito (*Aedes* sp.)	Febrile illness and rash; hemorrhagic fever
Colorado tick fever	Frequent	Rocky Mountain states, Canada	Tick (*Dermacentor andersoni*)	Febrile illness and rash; hemorrhagic encephalitis
West Nile‡	Epidemic	USA—48 contiguous states, Canada	Mosquito (*Culex* sp.)	Febrile illness and weakness; meningoencephalitis

*Also prevalent in central and northern South America.
†Also prevalent in central and northern South America, Southeast Asia, Africa.
‡Also prevalent in Africa, Europe, Asia, Australia.

New York City, and its range has expanded rapidly throughout much of North America. Diagnosis of infection with an arbovirus can be difficult and delayed because symptoms may range from mild fever to encephalitis. The patient's travel history and exposure are important for laboratory diagnosis of arbovirus infection (see Table 15-21). The CDC and most state public health laboratories in the United States have a battery of monoclonal antibodies for arbovirus antigen detection in peripheral blood mononuclear cells or tissue sections that includes the viruses listed in Table 15-21, as well as Japanese encephalitis virus, yellow fever virus, Highlands J virus, and Murray Valley encephalitis, among others.[134] Serologic procedures are the primary methods used for laboratory diagnosis of arbovirus infection, including West Nile virus. For West Nile virus, the CDC recommends detection of IgM antibody in serum or CSF collected within 8 days of illness onset by means of the IgM-antibody–capture ELISA. Detection of IgM antibodies may allow the diagnosis of an arbovirus infection with a single specimen; however, paired acute and convalescent sera collected 2 to 4 weeks apart may be necessary. Virus culture and RT-PCR are of limited usefulness in the diagnosis of West Nile virus infection because virus is detectable in blood or CSF only during the first 4 days of illness.[136]

Herpesviruses

The herpesviruses are a diverse group of DNA viruses. CMV, HSV types 1 and 2, and VZV can be easily cultured from most sites by conventional cell culture or in the shell vial assay. In contrast, human herpesvirus 6 (HHV-6), HHV-7, HHV-8, and Epstein-Barr virus (EBV) cannot be cultivated in routine diagnostic virology laboratories. Currently, PCR is the method of choice for the detection of herpesviruses in CSF.[137,138] In the past, definitive diagnosis of CNS infection caused by herpesviruses relied on the use of brain biopsy. Because detection in CSF by PCR has been demonstrated to be as sensitive as stain of brain biopsy specimens, CSF PCR is now the recommended test for establishing this diagnosis.[137] Traditional laboratory methods for the detection of HSV, CMV, and VZV in CSF, such as cell culture, antigen detection, and CSF or serum antibody detection, are known to be insensitive and are no longer recommended.

In many hospital laboratories, HSV detection may be the only diagnostic virology service offered. Cell culture or the shell vial assay allows detection of HSV in as little as 1 or 2 days. Even more rapid is a detection system that uses a genetically engineered baby hamster kidney cell line in conjunction with an enzyme-linked virus-inducible system for the detection of HSV in 16 to 24 hours. The cells in this system contain a plasmid that encodes the *E. coli lacZ* gene (for the enzyme β-galactosidase), which has been engineered to be driven by the promoter of the HSV-1 ribonucleotide reductase gene.[139] The enzyme is synthesized only when cells are infected with HSV type 1 or 2. To detect infected cells, an enzyme substrate is added, the enzyme catalyzes the substrate, and a blue color is produced that can be detected by light microscopy. This rapid assay is reported to be as sensitive as traditional cell culture held for 5 to 7 days.[139] Diagnostic laboratories may also detect HSV antigen directly in clinical material with one of several commercially available ELISA, immunofluorescence, or immunoperoxidase kits, the sensitivities of which range from 73% to 94% compared with traditional cell culture.[132] The traditional Tzanck smear (scrapings from lesions stained with Giemsa or Wright stain) is still a useful presumptive method for rapid diagnosis of HSV skin or mucous membrane lesions, although it does not differentiate between HSV and VZV.

Detection of antibodies to CMV in serum from blood or organ donors and recipients is performed with ELISA or latex agglutination tests. The detection of IgM antibodies to CMV can be used to diagnose acute infection in neonates and pregnant women.[138] CMV antigen detection in tissue sections by immunofluorescence or immunoperoxidase is a valuable complement to and a more sensitive test than histopathologic diagnosis by means of hematoxylin and eosin staining.[138] Because CMV remains latent after an acute primary

infection and can cause recurrent disease in immunosuppressed patients, new methods are being developed to diagnose CMV disease and to monitor anti-CMV therapy in transplant recipients or AIDS patients.[140] Culture methods alone are not useful for the diagnosis of active CMV disease because shedding of CMV in urine or respiratory tract secretions may occur in immunosuppressed patients without development of CMV disease. However, isolation of CMV from the urine or saliva of neonates is still useful for the identification of congenital CMV infection.

Detection of either CMV antigen or CMV DNA in blood can reveal CMV when the viral load is low, which may be weeks before cultures become positive.[140] For the CMV antigenemia assay, monoclonal antibodies to the pp65 lower matrix protein antigen are used to detect the antigen in CMV-infected leukocytes. A fluorescent label allows infected cells to be detected and counted. Thus, the CMV antigenemia assay provides quantitative results that can be used either to determine the initiation of antiviral therapy or to monitor viral load during a course of treatment. Because different laboratories may examine different numbers of leukocytes, physicians must understand how the laboratory performs and reports the assay if interlaboratory comparisons are to be made. Quantitative or semiquantitative PCR assays are thought to be more useful than qualitative PCR assays for the detection of viremia and the diagnosis of disseminated CMV disease.[141] Semiquantitative PCR entails the use of serial dilutions of patient samples followed by PCR, whereas quantitative methods relate the PCR product to an internal control or to an external standard curve.[138] Commercial kits that rely on amplification of the signal rather than CMV DNA itself, such as the branched DNA assay from Chiron Corporation (Emeryville, Calif.), are also useful for the diagnosis of CMV disease in immunocompromised hosts. Qualitative PCR assays are adequate for the detection of CMV DNA in aqueous or vitreous humor for the diagnosis of retinitis, in biopsy specimens for demonstration of organ localization, and in other instances in which quantitation is not needed.[140]

Serologic methods are used for the diagnosis of primary EBV infection and for screening and monitoring of nasopharyngeal carcinoma, whereas molecular methods are used to diagnose EBV-associated lymphoma of the brain and EBV involvement in other organ lesions.[142] The most common test for the diagnosis of primary EBV infection—most frequently, infectious mononucleosis—is a heterophile antibody test. Heterophile antibodies are IgM antibodies that are reactive to antigens on heterologous erythrocytes. The antibodies are detected in a variety of assay formats, including detection of lysis of bovine erythrocytes in the presence of complement, agglutination reactions with horse or sheep erythrocytes or antigen-coated latex agglutination particles, and ELISA formats that use purified heterophile antigens.[142] A negative heterophile antibody test in the presence of a clinical mononucleosis syndrome should prompt the physician to consider tests for EBV-specific antibodies, CMV, or toxoplasmosis.[143] Specific antibodies used to diagnose EBV infection commonly include IgG and IgM to the viral capsid antigen, antibody to early antigen, and antibody to Epstein-Barr nuclear antigen. Assays to detect EBV-specific antibodies include indirect immunofluorescence, anticomplement immunofluorescence, and ELISA formats. Information concerning the interpretation of serologic tests for EBV can be found in the chapter on Epstein-Barr virus (Chapter 135). Reference laboratories offer EBV DNA detection in blood or CSF by PCR and EBV mRNA detection in tissue by in situ hybridization. Quantitation of EBV DNA in serum can be used to monitor patients at risk for EBV-associated lymphoproliferation.[144]

HHV-6, which is a cause of exanthem subitum (roseola infantum or sixth disease), has also been associated with an infectious mononucleosis–like syndrome in adults, interstitial pneumonitis, encephalitis, and bone marrow suppression.[145] HHV-6 is postulated to be an opportunistic pathogen in both bone marrow and solid organ transplant recipients.[146] Prompt recognition of HHV-6 disease in transplantation patients may prove to be important because this virus is susceptible to ganciclovir and foscarnet. The virus can be isolated in cell culture, but detection may take 5 to 21 days. Reference laboratories offer serologic testing for HHV-6

IgG and IgM by both ELISA and immunofluorescence methods. Detection of DNA by PCR is also available and should be performed on serum or plasma rather than leukocytes. Diagnostic methods that cannot distinguish between latent and active infection, such as serum IgG detection or PCR on leukocytes, may be inappropriate or even misleading for the diagnosis of HHV-6 disease.[147] Quantitative PCR, if available, may be more diagnostically useful than qualitative PCR, especially for monitoring response to antiviral therapy. HHV-6 has two major variants; the B variant is more frequent, except in patients with AIDS, who are more likely to have variant A.[145] Currently available laboratory tests do not distinguish between variants A and B. HHV-7 may be associated with some cases of exanthem subitum and may cause disease in transplant patients; HHV-8 has been associated with Kaposi's sarcoma, primary effusion lymphoma, and multicentric Castleman's disease.[145] Serologic assays for HHV-7 and serologic testing and PCR for HHV-8 are available from reference laboratories.

Hepatitis Viruses

The hepatitis viruses are a group of unrelated DNA and RNA viruses that cause liver disease as their major clinical manifestation. Laboratory diagnosis of these infections is usually made by serologic testing for a number of different antigenic markers associated with the viruses. Laboratories have tried to make hepatitis diagnosis easier by offering panel or profile testing that varies according to patient characteristics: exposure but asymptomatic, symptomatic with acute disease (<6 months), or symptomatic with chronic disease (>6 months) (Table 15-22). The most commonly used methods for serologic diagnosis are ELISA and immunofluorescence assays. The first generation of ELISA tests for hepatitis C lacked sensitivity and specificity, but second- and third-generation tests have shown greatly improved performance.[148] Similar to HIV testing, immunoblots performed with recombinant antigens (recombinant immunoblot [RIBAs]) are used to confirm positive sera detected by ELISA. Third-generation RIBA tests were approved by the FDA in 1999; these use synthetic c100 and c22 peptides with a significant reduction in the number of indeterminant RIBA results.[148] A rapid membrane ELISA test for the combined detection of hepatitis B virus surface antigen (HBsAg) and hepatitis B virus early antigen (HBeAg) has been produced, but it is currently unavailable in the United States. This test was recently reported to have a clinical sensitivity of 99.8% for HBsAg and 96.4% for HBeAg.[149] The rapid hepatitis B sAg/eAg test would be useful for identifying subjects who require vaccination (negative for both antigens) and patients who might benefit most from antiviral therapy (positive for both antigens). Molecular methods for the detection of hepatitis virus nucleic acids include DNA PCR and the branched DNA assay (bDNA) for hepatitis B virus and RT-PCR for hepatitis D and G viruses. Commercially available hepatitis C virus (HCV) RNA detection assay kits include qualitative assays that use RT-PCR and transcription-mediated amplification (TMA) and quantitative assays that use RT-PCR and the bDNA assay.[148] Hepatitis C genotyping by RT-PCR and RFLP analysis is also available from large reference laboratories. Details concerning the interpretation of results for hepatitis tests can be found in the chapters in which acute and chronic hepatitis are discussed and in individual chapters for each virus.

Human Retrovirus

Diagnostic testing for human immunodeficiency virus types 1 and 2 (HIV-1 and HIV-2) and for human T-cell lymphotropic virus types 1 and 2 (HTLV-1 and HTLV-2) requires various levels to meet different needs (e.g., population screening, home testing, detection in blood supplies, qualitative and quantitative assays for diagnosis or monitoring). Discussion of the types of available assays (serology, antigen detection, nucleic acid detection, virus isolation) and their suitability for specific needs can be found in the specific chapters devoted to these viruses.

Viral Agents of Bioterrorism

Variola (smallpox) virus and the diverse group of viruses that are capable of causing viral hemorrhagic fever syndrome (e.g., Ebola and Marburg viruses) are the viruses thought most likely to be used as agents of bioterrorism. Detailed information concerning these agents, the diseases they cause, differential diagnoses, specimen collection, and diagnostic testing options is found in other chapters of this book and at the CDC website (http://www.bt.cdc.gov). Smallpox must be differentiated from other illnesses that present with a rash, including VZV infection, acne, erythema multiforme, allergic dermatitis, drug rash, enterovirus infection, and complications of vaccination with vaccinia. If smallpox is suspected, the CDC recommends both an infectious disease and a dermatology consultation, with digital photographs sent to the CDC and specimens sent to the CDC or state public health laboratory. Most hospital laboratories offer the Tzanck smear or DFA to diagnose VZV or HSV infection, but these laboratories should not perform viral testing on specimens from patients thought to have smallpox (patients categorized as high risk according to the CDC criteria) or on environmental specimens. Specimens to rule out smallpox include lesion roofs and crusts, vesicular fluid, and biopsy and autopsy tissue. The CDC and state laboratories can perform PCR, electron microscopy, histopathology, or culture to detect the poxviruses and VZV. Diagnosis of viral hemorrhagic fever is made with the use of primarily clinical features. Specimens, which are accepted by the CDC only after previous consultation, include serum for serology, tissue for immunohistochemistry (formalin fixed or paraffin block), and tissue for PCR or virus isolation.

Miscellaneous Viruses

The human polyomaviruses BK virus and JC virus infect a large proportion of the general population and remain latent in the kidneys after primary infection.[150] Reactivation can occur when T-cell functions are deficient, for example, in recipients of bone marrow or organ transplant or patients with HIV infection. BK viruria has been implicated as a cause of hemorrhagic cystitis in bone marrow transplantation patients, whereas JC virus causes progressive multifocal leukoencephalopathy (PML), which is seen primarily in AIDS patients. Rapid detection of active BK virus may help in the medical management of these patients. Although BK virus can be detected by cytologic examination of exfoliated urinary epithelial cells, this method cannot differentiate BK and JC viruses, cytopathic effects caused by other viruses, or changes caused by malignancy.[150] Specific identification of BK virus in urine can be achieved by immunologic staining of exfoliated urinary cells, by ELISA, or by PCR. Serologic testing by hemagglutination inhibition or ELISA for the detection of IgM in serum or CSF may be useful for diagnosing active polyomavirus infection. Examination of CSF for JC virus DNA by PCR is the method of choice for the diagnosis of PML.[151] A negative PCR result does not rule out the diagnosis of PML, and for these patients, a brain biopsy specimen should be obtained for histopathologic or molecular diagnostic testing.[151]

TABLE 15-22 Examples of Test Panels of Serologic Markers Offered by Reference Laboratories for Diagnosis of Asymptomatic and Symptomatic Hepatitis Virus Infections

Hepatitis Exposure Panel (asymptomatic)	Acute Hepatitis Panel (symptomatic)	Chronic Hepatitis Panel (symptomatic)
Anti-HAV (IgG + IgM)	Anti-HAV (IgM)	HBsAg
Anti-HAV (IgM)*	HBsAg	Anti-HBc (IgG + IgM)
HBsAg	Anti-HBc (IgG + IgM)	Anti-HBc (IgM)*
Anti-HBc (IgG + IgM)	Anti-HBc (IgM)*	Anti-HBs
Anti-HBs	Anti-HCV	Anti-HCV
Anti-HCV		

*Assay for IgM is performed if the IgG + IgM assay is positive.

HAV, hepatitis A virus; HBsAg, hepatitis B surface antigen; HBc, hepatitis B core antigen; HCV, hepatitis C virus.

Although many human papillomavirus (HPV)-induced lesions are benign, certain HPV types have been strongly associated with cervical neoplasia. The assay offered by most laboratories is in situ hybridization performed on paraffin-embedded tissue, with results reported as positive or negative for groups of HPV type 6/11, 16/18, or 31/33/51. PCR may soon be the method of choice because it has greater sensitivity in that it is capable of detecting as few as 10 to 100 viral genome copies and it is faster and easier to perform than other methods.[152] More than 90% of cervical cancers detected by histologic examination of cervical biopsy specimens are positive for HPV DNA by PCR. HPV can be typed by PCR assays that incorporate specific DNA probes or by sequencing the PCR product and comparing the sequence with published HPV sequences.

Hantavirus infections are zoonoses transmitted to humans through contact with aerosolized rodent excreta that contain the virus or through infected rodent bites.[153] Hantaviruses are found worldwide, but hantavirus infections in the United States were not considered a major public health concern until an outbreak of severe pulmonary disease was reported by the New Mexico Department of Public Health in the Four Corners area of New Mexico, Arizona, Colorado, and Utah in 1993. The virus has been cultured by the CDC and by the U.S. Army Medical Research Institute of Infectious Disease and is the Sin Nombre virus of the genus Hantavirus in the family Bunyaviridae. Hantaviruses cause two clinical syndromes—hemorrhagic fever with renal syndrome and hantavirus pulmonary syndrome. Detection of IgG and IgM antibodies by ELISA is available at many state health laboratories or by referral from a state laboratory to the CDC; a Western blot assay is available at the University of New Mexico and the University of Alabama at Birmingham.[154] A hantavirus RIBA has been jointly developed by the University of New Mexico and the Chiron Corporation. This assay uses membrane-immobilized antigens in a dipstick-like format and requires minimal equipment and 5 hours to perform. The assay has performed well in preliminary studies and will enable field testing by state laboratories for better surveillance and detection of future outbreaks.[154]

Emerging Viral Pathogens

Many emerging viral pathogens have been identified in Southeast Asia, the western Pacific, and other parts of the world. Several are arboviruses such as Japanese encephalitis virus (Flaviviridae); and Barmah Forest virus, Ross River virus, and Chikungunya virus (all Togaviridae). Emerging zoonotic viruses include Hendra virus, Nipah virus, Menangle virus, and Tioman virus (all Paramyxoviridae); Australian bat lyssavirus (Rhabdoviridae); and Cercopithecine herpesvirus 1 (B-virus, Herpesviridae). Diagnosis of most emerging viral infectious diseases is done by serologic or molecular methods and is performed in research laboratories or national health laboratories such as the CDC; a BSL of 3 or 4 is required.

Two recently described respiratory viruses—human metapneumovirus (Paramyxoviridae) and the agent of severe acute respiratory syndrome (SARS, Coronaviridae)—are of global concern. Human metapneumovirus was first described in 2001 and has since been identified through serologic surveys as a common virus that is responsible for acute respiratory tract infection in all age-groups worldwide.[155,156] Symptoms of human metapneumovirus infection are similar to those associated with RSV infection. The virus can be propagated in primary monkey kidney, Vero, and A549 cells and therefore could be identified in most virology laboratories once proper reagents are available. The agent of SARS is a novel coronavirus (SARS-CoV) that was identified in 2003.[157] The initial appearance of human infection with SARS-CoV occurred as an outbreak of severe pneumonia in southern China in late 2002. The infection then spread to Hong Kong, Vietnam, and Canada during 2003, prompting the World Health Organization (WHO) to issue a global alert for this illness and to initiate worldwide surveillance.[158] Transmission to household members and health care workers and deaths associated with SARS-CoV infection were of immediate concern, as scientists worked quickly to identify the pathogen. From November of 2002 through the end of May of 2003, 8240 SARS cases had been reported to the WHO from 28 countries; 745 deaths resulted, for a case fatality proportion of 9.0%.[159] The complete genome sequence of SARS-CoV, which was completed by April of 2003, showed it to be a novel coronavirus.[158] By May of 2003, the CDC had reagents available for distribution to be used in antibody testing by EIA and immunofluorescence assay and also by RT-PCR testing (for serum, stool, and nasal secretions).[160] For more extensive information on SARS-CoV, consult the CDC and WHO websites.

Antiviral Susceptibility Testing

Antiviral drugs are available for the management of viral infections, including those caused by HIV-1, HSV types 1 and 2, CMV, VZV, influenza A and B virus, RSV, hepatitis B virus, and hepatitis C virus. The emergence of resistant viruses is inevitable in that antiviral agents are used frequently and widely.[161] Antiviral resistance is defined as a decrease in susceptibility to an antiviral agent established by in vitro testing and confirmed by genetic analysis of the viral genome and biochemical analysis of the altered enzymes.[162] Clinical failures may not always be due to the presence of a drug-resistant virus. Factors to consider in a patient with a poor clinical response to an antiviral agent include the patient's immunologic status and the pharmacokinetics of the drug in the individual patient (e.g., dose or route of administration).[162] The development of resistance is favored by long-term suppressive therapy, recurrent intermittent therapy, and the use of suboptimal doses of an antiviral agent.[161] Antiviral susceptibility testing is warranted for the following clinical situations: failure of HSV or VZV lesions to resolve or the appearance of new lesions during treatment with acyclovir, progression of CMV disease during ganciclovir therapy, continued shedding or transmission of influenza A virus during treatment or prophylaxis with amantadine or rimantadine, and increased HIV-1 RNA plasma levels or decreased CD4 cell counts in HIV-infected patients during antiretroviral therapy.[161]

Laboratory assays for antiviral susceptibility testing include phenotypic and genotypic assays. Phenotypic assays require growth of the virus in vitro; therefore, viruses for which in vitro culture systems are not available, such as hepatitis B virus, cannot be tested with these assays. Results from phenotypic assays may not be available within a time frame that is clinically relevant because they all require initial propagation of the virus to attain a standard inoculum concentration, followed by growth of the virus in the assay to obtain results. After up to a week of propagation to prepare inoculum, once the assay has been set up, results for HSV may be obtained in 48 hours. For CMV, results may take 8 to 14 days after several weeks of propagation. Results of phenotypic assays are reported as the drug concentration that causes a 50% inhibition (IC_{50}) or a 95% inhibition (IC_{95}) in growth of the virus.[161] Phenotypic assays are not standardized, so comparison of results from different laboratories is difficult. The most commonly used phenotypic antiviral susceptibility assay is the plaque reduction assay (PRA), which measures the ability of varying concentrations of an antiviral agent to inhibit the viral cytopathic effect as the end point. The NCCLS offers a proposed standard in an effort to standardize the PRA for HSV.[163] Other end points for phenotypic viral assays that have been developed in an effort to make phenotypic testing more rapid and sensitive include dye uptake by viable (noninfected) cells, DNA hybridization, ELISA, plaque autoradiography, and flow cytometry.[164]

Genotypic assays have been developed for the rapid detection of mutations that confer antiviral-drug resistance.[161] Results from these assays simply report the presence or absence of a mutation known to confer resistance to a specific antiviral agent. Most genotypic assays use PCR to amplify specific viral genes, followed by direct sequencing of the amplified products or hybridization to specific probes on membrane strips or gene chips to detect changes in the sequence known to be associated with resistance to antiviral agents. Genotypic assays for the detection of drug resistance in HSV and VZV reveal thymidine kinase mutations that confer resistance to acyclovir, famciclovir, penciclovir, and valacyclovir. Genotypic assays used for determining resistance to ganciclovir, foscarnet, and cidofovir in CMV detect mutations in the UL54, UL97, and DNA polymerase genes.[164]

Commercially available LineProbe assays (Innogenetics, Inc., Alpharetta, Ga.) are now available to detect resistance mutations in the HBV DNA polymerase gene and the 5′-untranslated region (5′ UTR) of the HCV genome.[165] Genotypic assays to detect resistance in HIV-1 strains identify mutations within the reverse transcriptase and protease genes and are commercially available as the LineProbe assay or as gene chip technology from Affymetrix in Santa Clara, California.

The major drawback of genotypic assays is that they can detect only resistance caused by known mutations. Both in-house and commercial assays must be continually updated as new mutations or resistance mechanisms are identified. If resistance to an antiviral agent can be caused by different gene mutations, multiple assays might be needed for optimal detection. Strains with new or different resistance genes would go undetected, so phenotypic assays will still be required to identify new mutations responsible for antiviral resistance.[163]

REFERENCES

1. Peterson LR, Hamilton JD, Baron EJ, et al. Role of clinical microbiology laboratories in the management and control of infectious diseases and the delivery of health care. Clin Infect Dis. 2001;32:605-611.
2. Health Care Financing Administration. Medicare, Medicaid and CLIA programs. Regulations implementing the Clinical Laboratory Improvement Amendments of 1988 (CLIA). Fed Register. 1992;57:7002-7186.
3. Medicare, Medicaid, and CLIA Programs. Laboratory requirements relating to quality systems and certain personnel qualifications. Fed Register. 2003;68:3639-3714.
4. Elder BL, Hansen SA, Kellogg JA, et al. Verification and Validation of Procedures in the Clinical Microbiology Laboratory. Cumitech 31. Washington, DC: American Society for Microbiology; 1997.
5. van Belkum A, Struelens M, de Visser A, et al. Role of genomic typing in taxonomy, evolutionary genetics, and microbial epidemiology. Clin Microbiol Rev. 2001; 14:547-560.
6. Gurtler V, Mayall BC. Genomic approaches to typing, taxonomy and evolution of bacterial isolates. Int J Syst Evol Microbiol. 2001;51:3-16.
7. Murray PR, ed-in-chief. Manual of Clinical Microbiology. 8th ed. Washington, DC: ASM Press; 2003.
8. Forbes BA, Sahm DF, Weissfeld AS. Bailey & Scott's Diagnostic Microbiology. 11th ed. St. Louis: Mosby; 2002.
9. Truant AL, ed. Manual of Commercial Methods in Clinical Microbiology. Washington, DC: ASM Press; 2002.
10. Bisno AL, Gerber MA, Gwaltney JM, et al. Practice guidelines for the diagnosis and management of group A streptococcal pharyngitis. Clin Infect Dis. 2002;35:113-125.
11. Snow V, Mottur-Pilson C, Cooper RJ, et al. Principles of appropriate antibiotic use for acute pharyngitis in adults. Ann Intern Med. 2001;134:506-508.
12. Cloud JL, Hymas W, Carroll KC. Impact of nasopharyngeal swab types on detection of Bordetella pertussis by PCR and culture. J Clin Microbiol. 2002;40:3838-3840.
13. Carroll KC. Laboratory diagnosis of lower respiratory tract infections: Controversy and conundrums. J Clin Microbiol. 2002;40:3115-3120.
14. Cantral DE, Tape TG, Reed EC, et al. Quantitative culture of bronchoalveolar lavage fluid for the diagnosis of bacterial pneumonia. Am J Med. 1993;95:601-607.
15. Kovacs JA, Ng V, Masur H, et al. Diagnosis of Pneumocystis carinii pneumonia: Improved detection in sputum using monoclonal antibodies. N Engl J Med. 1988;318:589-593.
16. Quinn TC. Diagnosis of atypical pneumonias: Legionella, Chlamydia, and Mycoplasma infections. Ann Intern Med. 1996;124:591-594.
17. Ieven M, Goossens H. Relevance of nucleic acid amplification techniques for diagnosis of respiratory tract infections in the clinical laboratory. Clin Microbiol Rev. 1997;10:242-256.
18. Benin AL, Benson RF, Besser RE. Trends in legionnaires disease, 1980-1998: Declining mortality and new patterns of diagnosis. Clin Infect Dis. 2002; 35:1039-1046.
19. Maki DG, Weise CE, Sarafin HW. A semiquantitative culture method for identifying intravenous-catheter related infection. N Engl J Med. 1977;296:1305-1309.
20. Wisplinghoff H, Seifert H, Wenzel RP, Edmond MB. Current trends in the epidemiology of nosocomial bloodstream infections in patients with hematological malignancies and solid neoplasms in hospitals in the United States. Clin Infect Dis. 2003; 36:1103-1110.
21. Richter SS, Beekmann SE, Croco JL, et al. Minimizing the workup of blood culture contaminants: Implementation and evaluation of a laboratory-based algorithm. J Clin Microbiol. 2002;40:2437-2444.
22. Morris AJ, Wilson ML, Mirrett S, Reller LB. Rationale for selective use of anaerobic blood cultures. J Clin Microbiol. 1993;31:2110-2113.
23. Goldstein EJC. Anaerobic bacteremia. Clin Infect Dis. 1996;23:1292-1301.
24. Collignon PJ, Soni N, Pearson IY, et al. Is semiquantitative culture of central vein catheter tips useful in the diagnosis of catheter-associated bacteremia? J Clin Microbiol. 1986;24:532-535.
25. Siegman-Igra Y, Anglim AM, Shapiro DE, et al. Diagnosis of vascular catheter-related bloodstream infection: A meta-analysis. J Clin Microbiol. 1997;35:928-936.
26. O'Grady NP, Alexander M, Dellinger EP, et al. Guidelines for the prevention of intravascular catheter-related infections. Clin Infect Dis. 2002;35:1281-1307.
27. Thomson RB, Bertram H. Laboratory diagnosis of central nervous system infections. Infect Dis Clin North Am. 2001;15:1047-1071.
28. Askari S, Cartwright CP. The changing epidemiology of bacterial meningitis: Implications for the clinical laboratory. Clin Microbiol Newsl. 1998;20:33-36.
29. Saravolatz LD, Manzor O, VanderVelde N, et al. Broad-range bacterial polymerase chain reaction for early detection of bacterial meningitis. Clin Infect Dis. 2003; 36:40-45.
30. Woods GS, Washington JA II. Comparison of methods for processing dialysate in suspected continuous ambulatory peritoneal-associated peritonitis. Diagn Microbiol Infect Dis. 1987;7:155-157.
31. Metz DC. Stool testing for Helicobacter pylori infection: Yet another noninvasive alternative. Am J Gastroenterol. 2000;95:546-548.
32. Hines J, Nachamkin I. Effective use of the clinical microbiology laboratory for diagnosing diarrheal diseases. Clin Infect Dis. 1996;23(Suppl 1):S97-S101.
33. Wilkins TD, Lyerly DM. Clostridium difficile testing: After 20 years, still challenging. J Clin Microbiol. 2003;41:531-534.
34. Morris AJ, Wilson ML, Reller LB. Application of rejection criteria for ovum and parasite examinations. J Clin Microbiol. 1992;30:3213-3216.
35. Amsel R, Totten PA, Spiegel CA, et al. Nonspecific vaginitis: Diagnostic criteria and microbial epidemiologic association. Am J Med. 1983;74:14-22.
36. Ismail TF, Smits H, Wasfy MO, et al. Evaluation of dipstick serologic tests for diagnosis of brucellosis and typhoid fever in Egypt. J Clin Microbiol. 2002;40:3509-3511.
37. Hayden R, Persing DH. Diagnostic molecular microbiology. Curr Clin Top Infect Dis. 2001;21:323-348.
38. Pfaller MA. Molecular approaches to diagnosing and managing infectious diseases: Practicality and costs. Emerg Inf Dis. 2001;7:312-318.
39. Ballagi-Pordány A, Belák S. The use of mimics as internal standards to avoid false negatives in diagnostic PCR. Mol Cell Probes. 1996;10:159-164.
40. NCCLS. Molecular Diagnostic Methods for Infectious Diseases: Approved Guideline. Document MM3-A. Wayne, Pa: NCCLS; 1999.
41. Krafft AE, Kulesh DA. Applying molecular biological techniques to detecting biological agents. Clin Lab Med. 2001;21:631-660.
42. NCCLS. Abbreviated Identification of Bacteria and Yeast: Approved Guideline. Document M35-A. Wayne, Pa: NCCLS; 2002.
43. Barros RR, Carvalho MDGS, Peralta JM, et al. Phenotypic and genotypic characterization of Pediococcus strains isolated from human clinical sources. J Clin Microbiol. 2001;39:1241-1246.
44. Facklam R. What happened to the streptococci: Overview of taxonomic and nomenclature changes. Clin Microbiol Rev. 2002;15:613-630.
45. Doern GV, Ferraro MJ, Brueggemann AB, Ruoff KL. Emergence of high rates of antimicrobial resistance among viridans group streptococci in the United States. Antimicrob Agents Chemother. 1996;40:891-894.
46. Funke G, Bernard KA. Coryneform gram positive rods. In: Murray PR, ed-in-chief. Manual of Clinical Microbiology. 8th ed. Washington, DC: ASM Press; 2003:472-501.
47. Clarridge JE, Zhang Q. Genotypic diversity of clinical Actinomyces species: Phenotype, source and disease correlation among genospecies. J Clin Microbiol. 2002;40:3442-3448.
48. Maiden MCJ, Bygraves JA, Feil E, et al. Multilocus sequence typing: A portable approach to the identification of clones within populations of pathogenic microorganisms. Proc Natl Acad Sci U S A. 1998;95:3140-3145.
49. NCCLS. Performance Standards for Antimicrobial Disk Susceptibility Tests. Approved Standard. 8th ed. NCCLS Document M2-A8. Wayne, Pa: NCCLS; 2003.
50. NCCLS. Methods for Dilution Antimicrobial Susceptibility Tests for Bacteria That Grow Aerobically. 6th ed. Approved Standard. NCCLS Document M7-A6. Wayne, Pa: NCCLS; 2003.
51. NCCLS. Methods for Antimicrobial Susceptibility Testing of Anaerobic Bacteria. 7th ed. Approved Standard. NCCLS Document M11-A5. Wayne, Pa: NCCLS; 2003.
52. NCCLS. Performance Standards for Antimicrobial Susceptibility Testing: 13th Informational Supplement. Disk Diffusion Supplemental Tables. NCCLS Document M100-S13 (M2). Wayne, Pa: NCCLS; 2003.
53. NCCLS Performance Standards for Antimicrobial Susceptibility Testing: 13th Informational Supplement. MIC Testing Supplemental Tables. NCCLS Document M100-S13 (M7). Wayne, Pa: NCCLS; 2003.
54. NCCLS Performance Standards for Antimicrobial Susceptibility Testing of Anaerobic Bacteria; Informational Supplement. NCCLS Document M100-S13 (M11). Wayne, Pa: NCCLS; 2003.
55. NCCLS. Susceptibility Testing of Mycobacteria, Nocardiae, and Other Aerobic Actinomycetes; Approved Standard. NCCLS Document M24-A. Wayne, Pa: NCCLS; 2003.
56. NCCLS. Methods for Determining Bactericidal Activity of Antimicrobial Agents; Approved Guideline. NCCLS Document M26-A. Wayne, Pa: NCCLS; 1999.
57. NCCLS. Methodology for the Serum Bactericidal Test; Approved Guideline. NCCLS Document M21-A. Wayne, Pa: NCCLS; 1999.
58. Jorgensen JH, Turnidge JD. Susceptibility test methods: Dilution and disk diffusion methods. In: Murray PR, ed-in-chief. Manual of Clinical Microbiology. 8th ed. Washington, DC: ASM Press; 2003:1108-1127.
59. Wolfson JS, Swartz MN. Serum bactericidal activity as a monitor of antibiotic therapy. N Engl J Med. 1985;312:968-975.
60. Rasheed JK, Tenover FC. Detection and characterization of antimicrobial resistance genes in bacteria. In: Murray PR, ed-in-chief. Manual of Clinical Microbiology. 8th ed. Washington, DC: ASM Press; 2003:1196-1212.

61. Hanson KL, Cartwright CP. Comparison of simple and rapid methods for identifying enterococci intrinsically resistant to vancomycin. J Clin Microbiol. 1999;37:815-817.

62. Richmond JY, McKinney RW, eds. Biosafety in Microbiological and Biomedical Laboratories. 4th ed. Washington, DC: U.S. Government Printing Office; 1999.

63. Pfyffer GE, Brown-Elliott BA, Wallace RJ Jr. *Mycobacterium*: General characteristics, isolation and staining procedures. In: Murray PR, ed-in-chief. Manual of Clinical Microbiology. 8th ed. Washington, DC: ASM Press; 2003:532-559.

64. Piersimoni C, Callegaro A, Nista D, et al. Comparative evaluation of two commercial amplification assays for direct detection of *Mycobacterium tuberculosis* complex in respiratory specimens. J Clin Microbiol. 1997;35:193-196.

65. O'Sullivan CE, Miller DR, Schneider PS, Roberts GD. Evaluation of Gen-Probe Amplified *Mycobacterium tuberculosis* Direct Test by using respiratory and nonrespiratory specimens in a tertiary care center laboratory. J Clin Microbiol. 2002; 40:1723-1727.

66. Reischl U, Lehn V, Wolf H, Naumann L. Clinical evaluation of the automated COBAS AMPLICOR MTB assay for testing respiratory and nonrespiratory specimens. J Clin Microbiol. 1998;36:2853-2860.

67. Daniel TM. Antibody and antigen detection for the immunodiagnosis of tuberculosis: Why not? What more is needed? Where do we stand today? J Infect Dis. 1988; 158:678-680.

68. Elias J, De Coning JP, Vorster SA, et al. The rapid and sensitive diagnosis of tuberculous meningitis by the detection of tuberculostearic acid in cerebrospinal fluid using gas chromatography-mass spectrometry with selective ion monitoring. Clin Biochem. 1989;22:463-467.

69. Savic B, Sjöbring U, Alugupalli S, et al. Evaluation of polymerase chain reaction, tuberculostearic acid analysis, and direct microscopy for the detection of *Mycobacterium tuberculosis* in sputum. J Infect Dis. 1992;166:1177-1180.

70. Pfyffer GE, Kissling P, Jahn EMI, et al. Diagnostic performance of Amplified *Mycobacterium tuberculosis* Direct Test with cerebrospinal fluid, other nonrespiratory, and respiratory specimens. J Clin Microbiol. 1996;34:834-841.

71. Crump JA, Tanner DC, Mirrett S, et al. Controlled comparison of BACTEC 13A, MYCO/F LYTIC, BacT/ALERT MB, and ISOLATOR 10 systems for detection of mycobacteremia. J Clin Microbiol. 2002;42:1987-1990.

72. Tenover FC, Crawford JT, Huebner RE, et al. The resurgence of tuberculosis: Is your laboratory ready? J Clin Microbiol. 1993;31:767-770.

73. Chamberlin W, Graham DY, Hulten K, et al. Review article: *Mycobacterium avium* subsp. *paratuberculosis* as one cause of Crohn's disease. Aliment Pharmacol Ther. 2001;15:337-346.

74. American Thoracic Society. Diagnosis and treatment of disease caused by nontuberculous mycobacteria. Am J Respir Crit Care Med. 1997;156(Suppl):S1-S25.

75. Weinberger M, Berg SL, Feuerstein IM, et al. Disseminated infection with *Mycobacterium gordonae*: Report of a case and critical review of the literature. Clin Infect Dis. 1992;14:1229-1239.

76. Bagarazzi ML, Watson B, Kim IK, et al. Pulmonary *Mycobacterium gordonae* infection in a two-year-old child: Case report. Clin Infect Dis. 1996;22:1124-1125.

77. Bonnet E, Massip P, Bauriaud R, et al. Disseminated *Mycobacterium gordonae* infection in a patient infected with human immunodeficiency virus. Clin Infect Dis. 1996;23:644-645.

78. Harro C, Braden GL, Morris AB, et al. Failure to cure *Mycobacterium gordonae* peritonitis associated with continuous ambulatory peritoneal dialysis. Clin Infect Dis. 1997;24:955-957.

79. Rusconi S, Gori A, Vago L, et al. Cutaneous infection caused by *Mycobacterium gordonae* in a human immunodeficiency virus-infected patient receiving antimycobacterial treatment. Clin Infect Dis. 1997;25:1490-1491.

80. CDC. Multiple misdiagnoses of tuberculosis resulting from laboratory error—Wisconsin, 1996. MMWR Morb Mortal Wkly Rep. 1997;46:797-801.

81. Jasmer RM, Roemer M, Hamilton J, et al. A prospective, multicenter study of laboratory cross-contamination of *Mycobacterium tuberculosis* cultures. Emerg Infect Dis. 2002;8:1260-1263.

82. Vincent V, Brown-Elliott BA, Jost KC Jr, Wallace RJ Jr. *Mycobacterium*: Phenotypic and genotypic identification. In: Murray PR, ed-in-chief. Manual of Clinical Microbiology. 8th ed. Washington, DC: ASM Press; 2003:560-584.

83. BACTEC NAP TB differentiation test kit. Sparks, Maryland: Becton Dickinson Microbiology Systems; 1998.

84. Esteban J, Fernández-Roblas R, Román A, et al. Catheter-related bacteremia due to *Mycobacterium aurum* in an immunocompromised host. Clin Infect Dis. 1998;26:496-497.

85. Fischer PR, Christenson JC, Pavia AT, et al. Postoperative *Mycobacterium flavescens* infection in a child. Infect Dis Clin Pract. 1997;6:263-265.

86. Hachem R, Raad I, Rolston KVI, et al. Cutaneous and pulmonary infections caused by *Mycobacterium vaccae*. Clin Infect Dis. 1996;23:173-175.

87. Brown-Elliott BA, Wallace RJ Jr. Clinical and taxonomic status of pathogenic nonpigmented or late pigmenting rapidly growing mycobacteria. Clin Microbiol Rev. 2002;15:716-746.

88. Tortoli E. Impact of genotypic studies on mycobacterial taxonomy: The new mycobacteria of the 1990s. Clin Microbiol Rev. 2003;16:319-354.

89. Inderlied CB, Pfyffer GE. Susceptibility test methods: Mycobacteria. In: Murray PR, ed-in-chief. Manual of Clinical Microbiology. 8th ed. Washington, DC: ASM Press; 2003:1149-1177.

90. van Embden JDA, Cave MD, Crawford JT, et al. Strain identification of *Mycobacterium tuberculosis* by DNA fingerprinting: Recommendations for a standardized methodology. J Clin Microbiol. 1993;31:406-409.

91. Behr MA, Small PM. Molecular fingerprinting of *Mycobacterium tuberculosis*: How can it help the clinician? Clin Infect Dis. 1997;25:806-810.

92. Mazurek GH, Villarino ME. Guidelines for using the QuantiFERON-TB test for diagnosing latent *Mycobacterium tuberculosis* infection. MMWR Morb Mortal Wkly Rep. 2003;52(RR-2):15-18.

93. Brown JM, McNeil MM. *Nocardia, Rhodococcus, Gordonia, Actinomadura, Streptomyces,* and other aerobic actinomycetes. In: Murray PR, ed-in-chief. Manual of Clinical Microbiology. 8th ed. Washington, DC: ASM Press; 2003:502-531.

94. Pottumarthy S, Limaye AP, Prentice JL, et al. *Nocardia veterana,* a new emerging pathogen. J Clin Microbiol. 2003;41:1705-1709.

95. Conville PS, Brown JM, Steigerwalt AG, et al. *Nocardia veterana* as a pathogen in North American patients. J Clin Microbiol. 2003;41:2560-2568.

96. Wilson RW, Steingrube VA, Brown BA, et al. Clinical application of PCR-restriction enzyme pattern analysis for rapid identification of aerobic actinomycete isolates. J Clin Microbiol. 1998;36:148-152.

97. Moylett EH, Pacheco SE, Brown-Elliott BA, et al. Clinical experience with linezolid for the treatment of *Nocardia* infection. Clin Infect Dis. 2003;36:313-318.

98. Fromtling RA, Rhodes JC, Dixon DM. Taxonomy, classification, and morphology of fungi. In: Murray PR, ed-in-chief. Manual of Clinical Microbiology, 8th ed. Washington, DC: ASM Press; 2003:1653-1658.

99. Cushion MT. *Pneumocystis.* In: Murray PR, ed-in-chief. Manual of Clinical Microbiology. 8th ed. Washington, DC: ASM Press; 2003:1712-1725.

100. Kwon-Chung KJ, Bennett JE. Medical Mycology. Philadelphia: Lea & Febiger; 1992.

101. Kontoyiannis DP, Luna MA, Samuels BI, Bodey GP. Hepatosplenic candidiasis. A manifestation of chronic disseminated candidiasis. Infect Dis Clin North Am. 2000; 14:721-739.

102. Larone DH. Medically Important Fungi: A Guide to Identification. 4th ed. Washington, DC: ASM Press; 2002.

103. Fisher MC, Koenig GL, White TJ, Taylor JW. Molecular and phenotypic description of *Coccidioides posadasii* sp. nov., previously recognized as the non-California population of *Coccidioides immitis*. Mycologia. 2002;94:73-84.

104. Voss A, Nulens E. Prevention and control of laboratory-acquired infections. In: Murray PR, ed-in-chief. Manual of Clinical Microbiology. 8th ed. Washington, DC: ASM Press; 2003:109-120.

105. Sutton DA. Specimen collection, transport, and processing: Mycology. In: Murray PR, ed-in-chief. Manual of Clinical Microbiology. 8th ed. Washington, DC: ASM Press; 2003:1659-1667.

106. Merz WG, Roberts GD. Algorithms for detection and identification of fungi. In: Murray PR, ed-in-chief. Manual of Clinical Microbiology. 8th ed. Washington, DC: ASM Press; 2003:1668-1685.

107. Yeo SF, Wong B. Current status of nonculture methods for diagnosis of invasive fungal infections. Clin Microbiol Rev. 2002;15:465-484.

108. Ascioglu S, Rex JH, dePauw B, et al. Defining opportunistic invasive fungal infections in immunocompromised patients with cancer and hematopoietic stem cell transplants: An international consensus. Clin Infect Dis. 2002;34:7-14.

109. Larsen HH, Masur H, Kovacs JA, et al. Development and evaluation of a quantitative touch-down, real-time PCR assay for diagnosing *Pneumocystis carinii* pneumonia. J Clin Microbiol. 2002;40:490-494.

110. Morris AJ, Byrne TC, Madden JF, et al. Duration of incubation of fungal cultures. J Clin Microbiol. 1996;34:1583-1585.

111. Labarca JA, Wagar EA, Grasmick AE, et al. Critical evaluation of 4-week incubation for fungal cultures: Is the fourth week useful? J Clin Microbiol. 1998;36:3683-3685.

112. Sebti A, Kiehn TA, Perlin D, et al. *Candida dubliniensis* at a cancer center. Clin Infect Dis. 2001;32:1034-1038.

113. Hazen KC, Howell SA. *Candida, Cryptococcus,* and other yeasts of medical importance. In: Murray PR, ed-in-chief. Manual of Clinical Microbiology. 8th ed. Washington, DC: ASM Press; 2003:1693-1711.

114. Walsh TJ, Larone DH, Schell WA, Mitchell TG. *Histoplasma, Blastomyces, Coccidioides,* and other dimorphic fungi causing systemic mycoses. In: Murray PR, ed-in-chief. Manual of Clinical Microbiology. 8th ed. Washington, DC: ASM Press; 2003:1781-1797.

115. NCCLS. Reference Method for Broth Dilution Antifungal Susceptibility Testing of Yeasts; Approved Standard—2nd ed. NCCLS Document M27-A2. Wayne, Pa: NCCLS; 2002.

116. NCCLS. Reference Method for Broth Dilution Antifungal Susceptibility Testing of Filamentous Fungi; Approved Standard. NCCLS Document M38-A. Wayne, Pa: NCCLS; 2002.

117. Sigler L, Verweij PE. *Aspergillus, Fusarium,* and other opportunistic moniliaceous fungi. In: Murray PR, ed-in-chief. Manual of Clinical Microbiology. 8th ed. Washington, DC: ASM Press; 2003:1726-1760.

118. Schell WA, Salkin IF, McGinnis MR. *Bipolaris, Exophiala, Scedosporium, Sporothrix,* and other dematiaceous fungi. In: Murray PR, ed-in-chief. Manual of Clinical Microbiology. 8th ed. Washington, DC: ASM Press; 2003:1820-1847.

119. Smith TF. Specimen requirements. In: Specter S, Lancz G, eds. Clinical Virology Manual. 2nd ed. New York: Elsevier; 1992:19-41.

120. Wang J-T, Wang T-H, Sheu J-C, et al. Effects of anticoagulants and storage of blood samples on efficacy of the polymerase chain reaction assay for hepatitis C virus. J Clin Microbiol. 1992;30:750-753.

121. Lennette DA. Collection and preparation of specimens for virological examination. In: Murray PR, Baron EJ, Pfaller MA, et al, eds. Manual of Clinical Microbiology. 6th ed. Washington, DC: ASM Press; 1995:868-875.

122. Engler HD, Preuss J. Laboratory diagnosis of respiratory virus infections in 24 hours by utilizing shell vial cultures. J Clin Microbiol. 1997;35:2165-2167.

123. Fong CKY, Lee M, Griffith BP. Evaluation of R-mix fresh cells in shell vials for detection of respiratory viruses. J Clin Microbiol. 2000;38:4660-4662.

124. Kehl S, Henrickson KJ, Hua W, Fan J. Evaluation of the Hexaplex assay for detection of respiratory viruses in children. J Clin Microbiol. 2001;39:1696-1701.

125. Hindiyeh M, Hillyard DR, Carroll KC. Evaluation of the Prodesse Hexaplex multiplex PCR assay for direct detection of seven respiratory viruses in clinical specimens. Am J Clin Pathol. 2001;116:218-224.

126. Liolios L, Jenney A, Spelman D, et al. Comparison of a multiplex reverse transcription-PCR-enzyme hybridization assay with conventional viral culture and immunofluorescence techniques for the detection of seven viral respiratory pathogens. J Clin Microbiol. 2001;39:2779-2783.

126a. Abramowitz M. Rapid diagnostic tests for influenza. Med Letter. 1999;41:121-122.

127. Waner JL. Mixed viral infections: Detection and management. Clin Microbiol Rev. 1994;7:143-151.

128. Mancini AJ. Exanthems in childhood: An update. Pediatr Ann. 1998;27:163-170.

129. Brown KE, Young NS. Parvovirus B19 in human disease. Ann Rev Med. 1997;48:59-67.

130. Sawyer MH. Enterovirus infections: Diagnosis and treatment. Curr Opin Pediatr. 2001;13:65-69.

131. Romero JR. Reverse-transcription polymerase chain reaction detection of the enteroviruses. Arch Pathol Lab Med. 1999;123:1161-1169.

132. Bruner TA, Fedorko DP. Opportunities for rapid viral diagnosis. Clin Microbiol Newsl. 1993;15:65-69.

133. LeBaron CW, Lew J, Glass RI, et al. Annual rotavirus epidemic patterns in North America. Results of a 5-year retrospective survey of 88 centers in Canada, Mexico, and the United States. JAMA. 1990;264:983-988.

134. Tsai T, Chandler LJ. Arboviruses. In: Murray PR, ed-in-chief. Manual of Clinical Microbiology. 8th ed. Washington, DC: ASM Press; 2003:1553-1569.

135. Gubler DJ. Resurgent vector-borne diseases as a global health problem. Emerg Infect Dis. 1998;4:442-450.

136. Campbell GL, Marfin AA, Lanciotti RS, Gubler DJ. West Nile virus. Lancet Infect Dis. 2002;2:519-529.

137. Lakeman FD, Whitley RJ, National Institute of Allergy and Infectious Diseases Collaborative Antiviral Study Group. Diagnosis of herpes simplex encephalitis: Application of polymerase chain reaction to cerebrospinal fluid from brain-biopsied patients and correlation with disease. J Infect Dis. 1995;171:857-863.

138. Ehrnst A. The clinical relevance of different laboratory tests in CMV diagnosis. Scand J Infect Dis Suppl. 1996;100:64-71.

139. Marcon MJ, Salamon D. Traditional and newer approaches to laboratory diagnosis of herpes simplex virus infections. Clin Microbiol Newsl. 1997;19:9-14.

140. Dal Monte P, Lazzarotto T, Ripalti A, Landini MP. Human cytomegalovirus infection: A complex diagnostic problem in which molecular biology has induced a rapid evolution. Intervirology. 1997;39:193-203.

141. Yan SS, Fedorko DP. Recent advances in laboratory diagnosis of human cytomegalovirus infection. Clin Applied Immunol Rev. 2002;2:155-167.

142. Linde A. Diagnosis of Epstein-Barr virus-related diseases. Scand J Infect Dis Suppl. 1996;100:83-88.

143. Wolfson WL. Immunology and serology. In: Jacobs DS, Kasten BL, DeMott WR, Wolfson WL, eds. Laboratory Test Handbook. 2nd ed. Baltimore: Williams & Wilkins; 1990:611.

144. Berger C, Day P, Meier G, et al. Dynamics of Epstein-Barr virus DNA levels in serum during EBV-associated disease. J Med Virol. 2001;64:505-512.

145. Levy JA. Three new human herpesviruses (HHV6, 7, and 8). Lancet. 1997;349:558-562.

146. Singh N, Carrigan DR. Human herpesvirus-6 in transplantation: An emerging pathogen. Ann Intern Med. 1996;124:1065-1071.

147. Lusso P. Human herpesvirus 6 (HHV-6). Antiviral Res. 1996;31:1-21.

148. Richter SS. Laboratory assays for diagnosis and management of hepatitis C virus infection. J Clin Microbiol. 2002;40:4407-4412.

149. Clement F, Dewint P, Leroux-Roels G. Evaluation of a new rapid test for the combined detection of hepatitis B virus surface antigen and hepatitis B virus e antigen. J Clin Microbiol. 2002;40:4603-4606.

150. Arthur RR. Polyomaviruses. In: Lennette EH, ed. Laboratory Diagnosis of Viral Infections. 2nd ed. New York: Marcel Dekker; 1992:613-625.

151. Fong IW, Britton CB, Luinstra KE, et al. Diagnostic value of detecting JC virus DNA in cerebrospinal fluid of patients with progressive multifocal leukoencephalopathy. J Clin Microbiol. 1995;33:484-486.

152. Wieland U, Pfister H. Molecular diagnosis of persistent human papillomavirus infections. Intervirology. 1996;39:145-157.

153. Schmaljohn C, Hjelle B. Hantaviruses: A global disease problem. Emerg Infect Dis. 1997;3:95-104.

154. Mertz GJ, Hjelle BL, Bryan RT. Hantavirus infection. Dis Mon. 1998;44:85-138.

155. Van Der Hoogen BG, DeJong JC, et al. A newly discovered pneumovirus isolated from young children with respiratory tract disease. Nature Med. 2001;7:719-724.

156. Falsey AR, Erdman D, Anderson LJ, et al. Human metapneumovirus infections in young and elderly adults. J Infect Dis. 2003;187:785-790.

157. Ksiazek TG, Erdman D, Goldsmith CS, et al. A novel coronavirus associated with severe acute respiratory syndrome. N Engl J Med. 2003;348:1953-1966.

158. Rota PA, Oberste MS, Monroe SS, et al. Characterization of a novel coronavirus associated with severe acute respiratory syndrome. Science. 2003;300:1394-1399.

159. CDC. Update: Severe acute respiratory syndrome—United States, 2003. MMWR Morb Mortal Wkly Rep. 2003;52:500-501.

160. CDC. Updated interim surveillance case definition for severe acute respiratory syndrome (SARS)—United States, April 29, 2003. MMWR Morb Mortal Wkly Rep. 2003;52:391-393.

161. Hodinka RL. What clinicians need to know about antiviral drugs and viral resistance. Infect Dis Clin North Am. 1997;11:945-967.

162. Swierkosz EM, Arens MG. Susceptibility test methods: Viruses. In: Murray PR, ed-in-chief. Manual of Clinical Microbiology. 8th ed. Washington, DC: ASM Press; 2003:1638-1649.

163. NCCLS. Antiviral Susceptibility Testing; Proposed Standard. NCCLS Document M33-P. Wayne, Pa: NCCLS; 2000.

164. Smith TF. Susceptibility testing. Viral pathogens. Infect Dis Clin North Am. 2001;15:1263-1294.

165. McSharry JJ. Antiviral drug susceptibility assays: Going with the flow. Antiviral Res. 1999;43:1-21.

CHAPTER **16**

Principles of Anti-infective Therapy

ROBERT C. MOELLERING, JR.
GEORGE M. ELIOPOULOS

Although the discovery of effective agents to prevent and treat infection caused by bacteria and other pathogenic microorganisms is one of the most important developments of modern medicine, the use of such agents is not limited to the present era. Substances with anti-infective potential have been applied medically for thousands of years. Indeed, more than 2500 years ago, the Chinese were aware of the therapeutic properties of moldy soybean curd applied to carbuncles, boils, and other infections,[1] and ancient Greek physicians, including Hippocrates, routinely used substances with antimicrobial activity, including wine, myrrh, and inorganic salts, in their treatment of wounds.[2] Until the discovery of the microbiologic basis of infections in the 19th century, however, the therapy for infections remained strictly empirical. Heavy metals such as arsenic and bismuth were found to be useful against a number of infections, including syphilis, in the early 1900s, but the modern era of chemotherapy did not really begin until the discovery and initial clinical use of the sulfonamides in 1936.[1] This was followed in the 1940s by the discovery of the therapeutic value of penicillin and streptomycin, and by 1950 the golden age of antimicrobial chemotherapy was well under way.

It is the relatively recent work in this area (since 1936) that forms the basis for this and each of the succeeding chapters on anti-infective therapy. The major emphasis in this chapter is on antibacterial agents, because more data are available on these drugs. However, many of the principles to be discussed can also be applied to the use of antifungal, antiviral, and, to some extent, antiparasitic drugs.

CHOICE OF THE PROPER ANTIMICROBIAL AGENT

In choosing the appropriate antimicrobial agent for therapy for a given infection, a number of factors must be considered. First, the identity of the infecting organism must be known, or at the very least it must be possible to arrive at a statistically reasonable guess as to its identity on the basis of clinical information. Second, the information about the antimicrobial susceptibility (or potential susceptibility) of the infecting organism must be as accurate as possible. Finally, a series of so-called host factors must be taken into consideration to arrive at the optimal choice of antimicrobial agent. Each of these items is considered in this section.

Identification of the Infecting Organism

Several methods for the rapid identification of pathogenic bacteria in clinical specimens are available. A Gram stain preparation is perhaps the simplest, least expensive, and most useful of all the rapid methods of identification of bacterial (and some fungal) pathogens. This technique can be used to identify the presence and morphologic features of microorganisms in body fluids that are normally sterile (cerebrospinal fluid, pleural fluid, synovial fluid, peritoneal fluid, urine). On occasion, Gram staining of a buffy coat preparation of blood reveals phagocytosed organisms in the polymorphonuclear leukocytes of patients with bacteremia or fungemia. Similar preparations of sputum are also helpful in revealing the nature of the infecting organism in patients with bacterial bronchitis or pneumonia.

A Gram stain of a stool specimen may produce useful information. The presence of polymorphonuclear leukocytes in the stool also provides a helpful clue to the cause of certain cases of diarrhea. Polymorphonuclear leukocytes are not found in normal stools. When present, they suggest the possibility of a bacterial gastroenteritis such as shigellosis, salmonellosis, or campylobacteriosis, or invasive *Escherichia coli* gastroenteritis. Polymorphonuclear leukocytes are not found in the stools of patients with viral gastroenteritis, food poisoning, cholera, and diarrhea due to noninvasive toxigenic *E. coli*.[3] *Campylobacter* may be identified in the stools of patients by its characteristic gull-wing appearance on smears of stool.[4]

Immunologic methods for antigen detection (such as enzyme-linked immunosorbent assay [ELISA] or latex agglutination) may also provide clues for the rapid identification of the infecting pathogens. New molecular techniques are also being applied to the detection and identification of antimicrobial agents. The polymerase chain reaction (PCR) has been used to identify RNA or DNA of viruses, bacteria, and other microorganisms in the blood of patients,[5,6] and this technique and others, including the use of DNA probes, have proved to be helpful in rapid identification of organisms that have been cultured in the laboratory.[7] Final and definitive identification of pathogenic organisms, therefore, usually requires cultural techniques. It is thus imperative that appropriate specimens be obtained for culture before beginning antimicrobial therapy. Once anti-infective therapy has been started, cultures often are rendered sterile, even though viable organisms remain in the host.

In many cases, it is impossible to determine the exact nature of the infecting organisms before the institution of antimicrobial therapy. In these cases, the use of bacteriologic statistics may be particularly helpful.[8,9] The term *bacteriologic statistics* refers to the application of knowledge of the organisms most likely to cause infection in a given clinical setting. For example, a person with normal host defense mechanisms who develops cellulitis of the arm after a minor abrasion most likely has an infection due to *Staphylococcus aureus* or group A streptococci, and antimicrobial therapy should be tailored accordingly, even though there is no material available for examination with Gram stain. Similarly, a young child with acute otitis media almost certainly has an infection due either to a virus or to one of four major bacterial pathogens: *Haemophilus influenzae, Streptococcus pneumoniae, Moraxella (Branhamella) catarrhalis*, or a group A streptococcus.

Determination of Antimicrobial Susceptibility of Infecting Organisms

Because different organisms vary in their susceptibility to antimicrobial agents, it is imperative that we have a way to determine the antimicrobial susceptibility of the actual (or presumed) infecting organism or organisms. If the pathogen is isolated from a culture, it can be subjected to direct susceptibility testing, as described in Chapter 15. A number of methods for determining antimicrobial susceptibility are available. The E test, for example, uses diffusion of a continuous concentration gradient of an antimicrobial agent from a plastic strip into an agar medium to yield quantitative measurements of antimicrobial susceptibility.[10]

Quantitative data are also provided by methods that incorporate serial dilutions of antimicrobials in agar-containing or broth culture media. The lowest concentration of the antimicrobial agent that prevents visible growth after an 18- to 24-hour incubation period is the minimal inhibitory concentration (MIC). The minimal bactericidal concentration (MBC), or minimal lethal concentration (MLC), may be determined in broth dilution tests by subculturing the containers that show no growth onto antibiotic-free agar-containing media. The lowest concentration of antimicrobial that totally suppresses growth on antibiotic-free media (or results in a 99.9% or greater decline in colony count) after overnight incubation is known as the MBC (or MLC). The aforementioned techniques are based on an 18- to 24-hour incubation period. A variety of rapid methods are available as well.[11] These are based on a determination of changes in bacterial growth rates caused by antimicrobial agents and can provide susceptibility information in 4 to 8 hours.

Susceptibility testing is particularly important for certain organisms such as *S. aureus* and the various facultative and aerobic gram-negative bacilli. The widespread clinical and agricultural use of antibiotics since the 1930s and 1940s has resulted in the emergence of many strains of bacteria that are resistant to one or more antimicrobial agents (see Chapter 17).[12,13] In most cases in which adequate studies have been done, it appears that the role of antimicrobial agents is to exert selective pressure that results in the emergence of resistant organisms. In some cases, the organisms are naturally resistant to the antibiotic used. Examples of the latter include gram-positive organisms such as staphylococci and streptococci, which are naturally resistant to nalidixic acid, aztreonam, and the polymyxins. Many gram-negative bacilli are naturally resistant to penicillin G, erythromycin, and clindamycin.

In other cases, the resistant bacterial strains have acquired genes encoded on transposons or plasmids that enable them to resist antimicrobial inhibition. These genes may provide the organisms with the ability to synthesize enzymes that modify or inactivate the antimicrobial agent, or they may result in changes in the bacterial cell's ability to accumulate the antimicrobial agent, or they may permit the cell to produce metabolic enzymes resistant to inhibition by the antimicrobial agent.[12] Examples of each of these mechanisms of resistance are well known. Most strains of *S. aureus* that are resistant to penicillin contain plasmids that enable them to produce an extracellular β-lactamase that hydrolyzes and inactivates penicillin G.[12] Many gram-negative bacilli that are resistant to aminoglycosides such as streptomycin, kanamycin, tobramycin, gentamicin, and amikacin contain genes on plasmids that code for the production of periplasmic enzymes that catalyze a modification of the aminoglycosides by phosphorylation, acetylation, or adenylation.[12] Efflux mechanisms (which may be plasmid or transposon mediated) in *S. aureus*, pneumococci, and gram-negative bacilli can cause resistance to tetracycline, the macrolides, and other agents.[14,15] *E. coli* resistant to trimethoprim has been found to contain R factors that enable it to synthesize a new dihydrofolate reductase (the enzyme specifically inhibited by trimethoprim) that is 10,000 times less susceptible to the in vitro effects of trimethoprim than is the host bacteria's own chromosomal enzyme.[12]

These developments provide the rationale for performing tests of antimicrobial susceptibility whenever there is reasonable doubt about the susceptibility of a given organism. In certain cases, routine susceptibility testing need not be done, but these cases make up an ever-diminishing list. All group A and other β-hemolytic streptococci remain susceptible to the penicillins and cephalosporins; virtually all anaerobes except *Bacteroides* species are susceptible to penicillin G. Thus, testing these organisms against these particular agents need not be carried out routinely at the present time. However, even a statement such as this is fraught with a certain amount of danger. The discoveries of penicillin-resistant meningococci, the emergence of fluoroquinolone-resistant gonococci in Asia, Africa, and the United States, the rapid spread of ampicillin-resistant (and even chloramphenicol-resistant) strains of *H. influenzae* in the United States and Europe, the proliferation of vancomycin-resistant enterococci and staphylococci, the recent identification of chloramphenicol-resistant meningococci in France and Southeast Asia, and the discovery of streptomycin-resistant *Yersinia pestis* in Madagascar make us realize that, in time, strains of virtually any organism may be found that are resistant to antimicrobial agents that previously had been effective against them.[16-19]

It is important to consider geographic differences in patterns of susceptibility of organisms when choosing antimicrobial agents. In many cases, there may be variations in susceptibility patterns between hospitals and the community or among hospitals themselves. The emergence of gram-negative bacilli that are resistant to gentamicin is a good example of this. Most aminoglycoside-resistant organisms are found in hospitals, whereas most isolates from nonhospitalized patients

remain susceptible to gentamicin.[12,20] Initially, cases of methicillin-resistant *S. aureus* (MRSA) were confined to hospitals, but that has changed, and community-acquired MRSA infections have been documented in a number of different countries.[21]

All of these facts must be considered when choosing initial therapy for various infections. Tables listing drugs of choice, such as those in the *Medical Letter on Drugs and Therapeutics,* must be updated frequently to keep up with changes in antimicrobial resistance patterns.[22,23]

Host Factors

It is clearly important to determine the identity and antimicrobial susceptibility of the organism or organisms causing a given infection. However, optimal therapy is impossible unless we also consider a number of host factors that may influence the efficacy and toxicity of antimicrobial agents.[24]

History of Previous Adverse Reactions to Antimicrobial Agents

Simply obtaining an adequate history of previous adverse reactions to drugs may prevent the inadvertent administration of an antimicrobial agent to which the patient is allergic. A failure to do so can have serious (and sometimes fatal) consequences (see Chapter 22).

Age

The age of the patient is a major factor in choosing an antimicrobial agent. Gastric acidity varies with age. The pH of gastric secretions is higher in young children and does not reach adult levels of acidity until approximately the age of 3 years. At the other end of the age spectrum, there is also a decline in gastric acidity: gastric achlorhydria is found in 5.3% of people 20 to 29 years of age, in 16% of those 40 to 49, and in 35.4% of those older than 60.[24] The absorption of a number of antimicrobials administered via the oral route depends on their acid stability and the pH of gastric secretions. Penicillin G is an excellent example of this phenomenon. The oral absorption of penicillin G is markedly reduced by gastric acid. However, in young children and in older achlorhydric patients, the absorption of the drug is markedly enhanced. As a result, various orally administered penicillins produce high serum levels in young children and in older patients who have achlorhydria. The absorption of other orally administered β-lactam antibiotics is probably also enhanced in achlorhydric patients; however, evidence is convincing only in the case of the penicillins.[25] Gastric acidity does not always have a negative influence on the absorption of antimicrobials. Drugs that are weak acids, such as ketoconazole, may be better absorbed at a low pH. Thus, absorption of ketoconazole is impaired by the administration of antacids, cimetidine, or even food.[26]

Renal function, likewise, varies with age. It is relatively diminished in premature and newborn children and reaches adult levels between 2 and 12 months of age.[24] Thus, the serum half-lives of drugs that are primarily excreted by the kidneys may be considerably increased in neonates. As a result, doses of antimicrobial agents such as penicillin G and its various semisynthetic derivatives, as well as the aminoglycosides, must be altered in neonates.

Aging results in the decline of a number of physiologic processes, including renal function.[25] Creatinine clearance may be significantly reduced in older patients even though they have normal blood urea nitrogen or serum creatinine concentrations. In view of this, high doses of the penicillins or cephalosporins or carbapenems such as imipenem must be given with caution to older adults to prevent the development of excessively high serum levels, which may produce severe neurotoxic reactions such as myoclonus, seizures, and coma.[24,25] Other adverse reactions to the penicillins, such as reversible neutropenia, may be dose related and may occur with increased frequency when high doses of such drugs are given to older patients with physiologic renal impairment.[25] This, however, has not been proven. Impaired renal excretion of the aminoglycoside antibiotics may result in elevated serum concentrations, which in turn may be associated with an increasing incidence of ototoxicity in older patients.[27]

In addition to the toxicity that may result from impaired renal excretion in neonates and older adult patients, other adverse effects of antimicrobial agents may also be age related.[25,28] Hepatic function in the neonate is underdeveloped by adult standards. This can result in difficulties if such patients are administered drugs that are normally excreted or inactivated by the liver. Chloramphenicol is inactivated by conjugation to the glucuronide form in the liver. However, in the neonate, hepatic levels of glucuronyl transferase are relatively insufficient. Thus, when neonates are given large doses of chloramphenicol, high serum levels of unconjugated chloramphenicol result. Such high concentrations of unconjugated chloramphenicol are toxic and can result in shock, cardiovascular collapse, and death (the so-called gray syndrome).[24,29] For this reason, chloramphenicol should be avoided if possible in the neonate. If it is necessary to use the drug, however, it may be administered safely if given in a dosage that has been reduced appropriately for the patient's age.[29,30]

The sulfonamides compete with bilirubin for binding sites on serum albumin. When given to neonates, they produce increased serum levels of unbound bilirubin that predispose the child to kernicterus.[29,30] Therefore, sulfonamides should not be administered to neonates. Hyperbilirubinemia per se may be associated with the administration of novobiocin to neonates,[29] because this drug inhibits hepatic glucuronyl transferase, which in turn diminishes the ability of the liver to conjugate and excrete bilirubin. Hence, novobiocin should be avoided in newborn infants.

The tetracyclines are avidly bound to developing bone and tooth structures. As they bind to developing teeth, they may cause a number of adverse effects ranging from purplish to brownish discoloration of the teeth to actual enamel hypoplasia.[24,29] The tetracyclines readily cross the placenta.[31] Thus, when administered during the latter half of pregnancy or from birth to the age of 6 months, they may cause these effects on the deciduous teeth of the infant. From the age of 6 months to 6 to 8 years, similar damage to the permanent teeth may occur. In view of this, tetracycline should be avoided, if possible, in young children.

The quinolone antimicrobials have been shown to cause cartilage damage and arthropathy in young animals. As a result, they are not currently recommended for use in prepubertal children.[32,33] More recent evidence, however, suggests that the risk of arthropathy is less than previously thought, opening the way for judicious use of fluoroquinolones in children.[34]

Adverse effects caused by a number of antimicrobial agents have been noted to occur with increased incidence in older adults.[25] In some cases (and perhaps in all if adequately studied), this relationship may be shown to be caused by specific disease states or by impairment of physiologic processes associated with aging, as noted earlier. However, in certain cases, no specific factors other than age can be identified. The hepatotoxicity associated with isoniazid administration is a good example of this. A small percentage of patients receiving isoniazid develop toxic hepatitis that may be fatal if not recognized in time.[35] Liver damage from isoniazid almost never occurs in patients younger than 20 years. In patients 20 to 34 years old, the incidence of isoniazid hepatotoxicity is 0.3%, and it rises steadily with age to reach 2.3% in patients 50 years of age or older.[36] Despite these data, many now feel that isoniazid prophylaxis has a positive risk-benefit ratio in older patients as long as liver function tests are monitored.[37,38]

Nephrotoxic reactions to certain antimicrobial agents likewise appear to be more frequent or to occur with lower doses of drugs among older adults. This has been demonstrated with cephaloridine[39] and colistin,[24,40] and it may be true for other nephrotoxic antimicrobials as well.

Finally, hypersensitivity reactions to antimicrobial agents also appear to be more common in older adults than in younger patients.[24] This seems to be because older patients are more likely to have been previously exposed, and thus sensitized, to these agents. In addition, prior exposure to drugs such as the aminoglycosides, which produce irreversible cochlear damage, can result in cumulative toxicity on repeat exposure.[25]

Genetic or Metabolic Abnormalities

The presence of genetic or metabolic abnormalities may also have a significant effect on the toxicity of a given antimicrobial agent. The rate at which isoniazid is conjugated and biologically inactivated by acetylation in the liver is determined genetically.[24] Rapid acetylators are found more commonly in Asian populations, whereas 45% to 65% of U.S. and northern European populations are slow acetylators. Several studies have suggested that polyneuritis is seen more frequently as a complication of isoniazid therapy in slow than in rapid acetylators.[24] It was once thought that hepatotoxicity due to isoniazid was related to the conversion of isoniazid to acetylhydrazine and other related hepatotoxic derivatives and was more common among rapid acetylators,[41] but this does not appear to be true.

A number of antimicrobial agents have been shown to be capable of provoking hemolysis in patients with glucose-6-phosphate dehydrogenase (G6PD) deficiency, including the sulfonamides, nitrofurantoin, furazolidone, diaminodiphenylsulfone, and chloramphenicol.[24] Sulfonamides may likewise cause hemolytic reactions in the presence of certain hemoglobinopathies, including hemoglobin Zurich and hemoglobin H.[24]

The presence of metabolic disorders such as diabetes mellitus may also pose problems in antimicrobial therapy. Certain agents such as the sulfonamides (especially the long-acting types) and chloramphenicol can potentiate the hypoglycemic activity of sulfonylurea hypoglycemic agents such as tolbutamide and chlorpropamide.[25] In the case of the sulfonamides, this action may be related to their being structurally similar to the sulfonylurea drugs. Chloramphenicol inhibits microsomal enzyme activity in the liver, and this impairs the metabolism of the sulfonylurea hypoglycemic agents. The dextrose load infused with intravenous antibiotics dissolved in dextrose-containing vehicles may be sufficient to produce hyperglycemia and glucosuria in diabetic patients. Another kind of "glucosuria" can occur in patients receiving antimicrobial agents. The cephalosporins, chloramphenicol, isoniazid, nalidixic acid, nitrofurantoin, penicillin, streptomycin, sulfanilamide, and the tetracyclines can all cause false-positive test results when urine sugar levels are determined by a method (e.g., the Benedict test or Clinitest) that measures reducing substances in the urine.[25] Tests that are specific for glucose (i.e., that use glucose oxidase) such as Dextrostix or Labstix are not affected by antimicrobial agents.[42]

The absorption of intramuscularly administered antibiotics may be impaired in diabetic patients. Diabetics with bacterial endocarditis who failed to respond to intramuscular penicillin have been described.[24] Administration of the same dose of penicillin by the intravenous route, however, resulted in bacterial eradication.[24] Because of the potential for impaired absorption of intramuscularly administered antimicrobial agents, it is probably prudent to initiate therapy by the intravenous route when using drugs such as the aminoglycosides to treat diabetic patients with gram-negative bacteremia (especially if accompanied by hypotension) or other serious infections.

The concomitant administration of chloramphenicol has been noted to delay the reticulocyte response to vitamin B_{12} or iron therapy in patients with pernicious anemia or iron deficiency anemia.[24] Patients with pernicious anemia and gastric achlorhydria may exhibit enhanced serum levels of antimicrobials such as penicillin G when chloramphenicol is given by the oral route.

Rifampin and other rifamycins may increase the hepatic metabolism and therefore decrease the effect of oral anticoagulants, oral contraceptives, barbiturates, and a number of other drugs including the protease inhibitors.[43]

Pregnancy

Patients who are pregnant and nursing mothers also pose certain problems in the selection of appropriate antimicrobial agents. All antimicrobial agents cross the placenta in varying degrees.[44,45] Thus, the use of such agents in pregnant women provides direct exposure of the fetus to adverse effects of the drug. Although there are few solid data on the teratogenic potential of most antimicrobial agents in humans, experience suggests that certain drugs such as the penicillins, the cephalosporins, the macrolides, and antituberculous drugs such as isoniazid, rifampicin, and ethambutol are unlikely to be teratogenic and are safe for pregnant women to use.[29,44-46] Metronidazole has been shown to be teratogenic in rodents and thus should be avoided in pregnancy.[47] The teratogenic potential of many other drugs in humans, including the fluoroquinolones, pyrazinamide, and trimethoprim, is unknown but is probably relatively low.

A number of antimicrobials have been shown to be deleterious in pregnancy, and the tetracyclines head the list. The possible adverse effects of these drugs on fetal dentition have already been noted. In addition, pregnant women receiving tetracycline are particularly vulnerable to certain toxic effects, including acute fatty necrosis of the liver, pancreatitis, and probably renal damage.[24] The liver damage may be severe and can result in death. When administered to patients with impaired renal function, these effects may be magnified, particularly if the agent is one of the tetracyclines that are primarily excreted by the kidneys. These adverse effects are dose related and may be more frequent after intravenous administration. Although it has been suggested that tetracyclines may be given to pregnant women by the oral route in doses of 1 g or less per 24 hours, it is probably safer to avoid these agents entirely in pregnancy.[24,29]

The aminoglycosides cross the placenta. Thus far, fetal toxicity has been reported only for streptomycin when used to treat tuberculosis in pregnant women. Even in that setting, the toxicity has been mild, detectable only by formal vestibular testing or by an audiogram.[48] Psychomotor retardation, myoclonus, and convulsions have been reported in a small uncontrolled series of children whose mothers received isoniazid for tuberculosis during pregnancy.[49] This observation has not been confirmed to date.

Another aspect of drug therapy in pregnancy has been examined. It has been found that serum levels after a given dose of ampicillin are lower in pregnant that in nonpregnant women.[50] This is related to more rapid clearance of the drug and to a greater volume of distribution (probably due to increased plasma volume) in pregnancy, Thus, higher doses of ampicillin are required to achieve therapeutic blood levels in pregnancy. It is likely that these observations also apply to other antimicrobial agents, but data on this are not available.

Virtually all antimicrobial agents appear in measurable concentrations in breast milk when administered in therapeutic doses to nursing women.[51] The amount of drug excreted into breast milk depends on its degree of ionization, its molecular weight, and its solubility in fat and water. Under usual circumstances, the concentrations of antibiotics found in breast milk are quite low. However, even these small amounts may cause significant adverse reactions in the nursing infant. Nalidixic acid and the sulfonamides in breast milk have been shown to cause hemolysis in infants with G6PD deficiency. Sulfonamides in breast milk may be dangerous to premature babies, because even small doses of ingested sulfonamides may produce increased levels of unbound bilirubin by displacing bilirubin from its albumin-binding sites. As noted previously, this predisposes the child to kernicterus.[51] The possibility that antimicrobial agents in breast milk can sensitize newborn children is a theoretical one and has not been convincingly demonstrated. Although tetracycline is excreted in breast milk, it is unlikely to produce damage to the nursing child's bones or teeth because the calcium in the milk forms an insoluble chelate with tetracyclines, and the chelate is not absorbable by the oral route.[51]

Renal and Hepatic Function

The ability of the patient to metabolize or excrete antimicrobial agents is one of the most important host factors to consider, especially when high serum or tissue concentrations of the administered drugs are potentially toxic. From a practical point of view, this means that one must assess the patient's renal and hepatic function carefully, because these organs serve as the major (and in most cases the *only*) routes of excretion and inactivation of antimicrobials. Renal excretion is the most important route of elimination of most antimicrobial agents.[52-57] Doses for drugs that require alteration in patients with impaired renal function can be found in the chapters dealing with the individual

agents and in Chapter 46. In general, agents that require no dosage change in impaired renal function are excreted effectively by extrarenal routes (usually the hepatobiliary system) in patients with renal failure. Their use in normal doses does not result in the appearance of toxic serum levels in this situation, although the urine levels of a number of these agents (e.g., doxycycline, moxifloxacin, and chloramphenicol) may be diminished significantly.

Toxic serum levels of certain agents may develop if they are used without dosage modification in patients with impaired renal function. Excessive serum levels of penicillin G or imipenem may be associated with neuromuscular hyperexcitability, myoclonus, seizures, or coma.[24] Excessive serum levels of semisynthetic penicillins (e.g., piperacillin) or of cephalothin may cause hemostatic defects in patients with impaired renal failure because of interference with platelet function.[58,59] Elevated serum levels of aminoglycosides or vancomycin may result in eighth nerve damage.[27,57] Neurotoxic reactions including respiratory arrest and death may occur in patients who have excessive serum levels of certain aminoglycosides or the polymyxins.[24,40] Bone marrow suppression may occur in patients with renal failure who receive inappropriately high doses of 5-fluorocytosine.[60] In all these situations, the possibility of toxic reactions can be lessened significantly or eliminated if the doses of the antimicrobial agents are appropriately reduced in the presence of renal insufficiency.

The tetracyclines (except doxycycline and possibly minocycline) are contraindicated in patients with impaired renal function because the elevated serum levels that result may produce a significant worsening of the uremic state because of their antianabolic effect. Moreover, they may cause enhanced hepatotoxicity in this situation.[24] The long-acting sulfonamides should be avoided in this situation because they are potentially nephrotoxic.

Certain antimicrobial agents, including erythromycin, azithromycin, dirithromycin, chloramphenicol, lincomycin, and clindamycin, should be used with caution in patients with impaired hepatic function.[61] These drugs are primarily excreted or detoxified in the liver. Bone marrow suppression due to chloramphenicol is much more likely to occur in patients with impaired hepatic function; because of this, it has been suggested that the dose of chloramphenicol be cut at least in half in patients with cirrhosis and other severe liver disease.[59,62] Because the serum half-life of clindamycin is increased in patients with severe liver disease, its dose should also be decreased in this situation. The tetracyclines may produce elevations in serum transaminase levels in patients recovering from viral hepatitis.[24] They should be avoided or used with extreme caution in patients with underlying liver disease. The serum half-lives of both rifampin and isoniazid are prolonged in patients with cirrhosis.[63] Other drugs that should be used with caution, or for which serum levels should be monitored in patients with severe liver disease, include metronidazole, ketoconazole, miconazole, fluconazole, itraconazole, nitrofurantoin, and pyrazinamide.[61] It has been suggested that β-lactam antibiotic–induced leukopenia occurs more frequently in patients with impaired hepatic function.[64] Hepatobiliary disease influences antimicrobic therapy in still another way. The biliary concentrations of many antimicrobial agents, including ampicillin and nafcillin, that are normally excreted in high concentration in the bile may be reduced significantly in patients with liver disease or biliary obstruction.[24]

Site of Infection

Of all the host factors to be considered in the choice of an antimicrobial agent, none is more important than the site of infection. The locus of the infectious process determines not only the choice of the agent but also its dose and the route by which it should be administered. For antimicrobial therapy to be effective, an adequate concentration of the drug must be delivered to the site of infection. In most cases, this means that the local concentration of the antimicrobial agent should at least equal the MIC of the infecting organism. Concentrations representing multiples of the MIC are generally believed more likely to be efficacious, but in many cases such local concentrations may be difficult or impossible to achieve. A failure to achieve local concentrations of antibiotics higher than the MIC of the infecting organism may not always be disastrous, however, because there is evidence that subinhibitory concentrations of drugs may produce antimicrobial effects that aid the host defenses against infections. It has been demonstrated clearly that subinhibitory concentrations of antibiotics can alter bacterial morphology,[65] adherence properties,[66] and opsonic requirements[67]; can enhance phagocytosis[68]; and can even aid intracellular killing of bacteria by polymorphonuclear leukocytes.[69] This may explain the clinical observation that, on occasion, doses of antimicrobials that produce seemingly inadequate serum levels may still result in clinical cure. In spite of such observations, most infectious disease clinicians feel that optimal therapy requires concentrations of antimicrobials that are above the MIC at the actual site of infection (see Chapter 18).

Serum concentrations of antimicrobial agents are relatively easy to determine and therefore are often used as a guide in the therapy. However, except in cases of bacteremia, antimicrobial efficacy is more likely determined by the tissue concentration than by the blood level, as noted earlier. Moreover, some agents such as spiramycin and certain macrolides such as azithromycin are effective in vivo despite an inability to achieve serum levels above the MIC of certain organisms.[70] This may be explained by their ability to achieve intracellular and tissue concentrations that far exceed those obtained in serum.[71,72] Binding to serum proteins may affect both the tissue distribution and the activity of antimicrobial agents in the blood.

Although much careful investigation has been done on protein binding, the precise clinical significance of this phenomenon remains to be determined. For example, it has been shown that only the unbound form of a given antimicrobial agent is active in vitro (and presumably also in vivo) against infecting organisms.[73] However, because protein binding is rapidly reversible,[74] the activity of even highly protein-bound agents may not be limited absolutely by protein binding. The penetration of antimicrobial agents into interstitial fluid and lymph is related to protein binding, because only the free form of the agent is able to pass through the capillary wall.[73] Penetration of antibiotics into fibrin clots (which may be analogous to the penetration of the drugs to reach the site of infection in patients with bacterial endocarditis) is likewise related to the amount of unbound antibiotic in the surrounding fluid.[75] Nevertheless, it is often difficult to correlate therapeutic outcome with in vitro susceptibility and protein binding unless several variables are carefully controlled.[76,77]

The reason for this is simply that it is the concentration of antibiotic at the site of infection that is the major determinant in the successful therapy. Such concentrations are often difficult to assess because they are the result of a complex interaction between local factors that may bind, inactivate, or enhance the activity of a given antimicrobial agent. The ability of an antibiotic to pass through membranes by nonionic diffusion is related to its lipid solubility. Thus, lipid-soluble agents such as chloramphenicol, rifampin, trimethoprim, and isoniazid are all more adept at penetrating membranes than are the more highly ionized compounds.[73] These agents rapidly cross the blood-brain barrier and produce better cerebrospinal fluid levels than do more highly ionized compounds such as the aminoglycosides. Except in neonates, none of the aminoglycosides produce effective cerebrospinal fluid levels when given parenterally. To be effective for the treatment of meningitis, they must be given via the intrathecal or intraventricular route in adults.[78] This is an excellent example of the importance of the site of infection in determining the most efficacious antimicrobial therapy.

For the treatment of bacterial meningitis in adults, there are two choices: (1) agents such as chloramphenicol or the third-generation cephalosporins (e.g., cefotaxime, ceftriaxone, or ceftazidime) or the fourth-generation agent cefepime, all of which cross the blood-brain barrier reasonably well, or (2) high parenteral doses of drugs such as penicillin G, ampicillin, or nafcillin, which penetrate into the cerebrospinal fluid only with difficulty. Agents such as the aminoglycosides and first-generation cephalosporins that produce inadequate cerebrospinal fluid levels even after high-dose parenteral therapy must be administered directly into the cerebrospinal fluid or must be avoided entirely.

The penetration of antimicrobial agents into the heart valve vegetations of bacterial endocarditis, into bones, and into devitalized tissue may be borderline or inadequate. Therefore, high-dose and prolonged parenteral therapy is usually required for the effective treatment of bacterial endocarditis and osteomyelitis. Biofilm produced by bacteria in these settings also serves to impair antimicrobial efficacy (see later). In some cases, we can take advantage of the physiologic handling of antimicrobials to achieve therapeutic success. Agents that are excreted by the liver and are concentrated in the bile, such as ampicillin and doxycycline, may be more effective in treating cholangitis than are agents such as the first-generation cephalosporins or aminoglycosides, which are not greatly concentrated in bile. The new fluoroquinolones may owe some of their effectiveness in the treatment of osteomyelitis to their ability to achieve superior concentrations in bone.[79] Likewise, these agents penetrate far more effectively into the prostate than the β-lactams or aminoglycosides, and this undoubtedly accounts for their superior therapeutic efficacy in prostatitis.[80,81]

Even the achievement of "therapeutic concentrations" of antimicrobial agents at the site of infection may not be sufficient for cure, because a number of local factors may influence the activity of antimicrobial agents. These, too, must be considered in designing an appropriate therapeutic regimen. Aminoglycosides and the polymyxins are bound to and inactivated by purulent material.[82] This is one of many reasons why surgical drainage is imperative when treating abscesses with agents such as these. Although penicillins may be more active in purulent material, clinical experience strongly suggests that appropriate drainage procedures greatly enhance the efficacy of these agents as well. Penicillin G is not inactivated by purulent material per se,[74] but the presence of β-lactamase–producing organisms such as *Bacteroides fragilis* in abscesses may result in local inactivation of penicillin G and other β-lactam antibiotics.[83]

Penicillins and tetracyclines are also bound by hemoglobin and thus may be less effective in the presence of significant hematoma formation.[73] In vitro, *Pseudomonas aeruginosa* is protected from the action of the aminoglycosides and polymyxins by high concentrations of calcium or magnesium in the culture medium.[84] The clinical significance of this observation, if any, remains to be determined. Local decreases in oxygen tension, such as occur in abscesses and intraperitoneal infections, may also have an effect on the activity of certain antimicrobial agents. The aminoglycosides, for example, are inactive against anaerobes and may also be less effective against facultative organisms under anaerobic conditions because oxygen is required for the transport of these agents into the bacterial cell.[85]

Local alterations in pH such as occur in abscesses and especially in the urine may have an important effect on the activity of a number of antimicrobial agents. Methenamine, nitrofurantoin, novobiocin, and chlortetracycline are more active at an acid pH, whereas alkalinization enhances the activity of erythromycin, azithromycin, dirithromycin, clarithromycin, lincomycin, clindamycin, and the aminoglycosides. Indeed, the aminoglycosides show a marked loss of activity at a low pH. These observations have occasionally been used to advantage in treating patients with urinary tract infections, a situation in which the local pH can be altered by the addition of acidifying or alkalinizing agents.[86,87]

The presence of foreign bodies also has a profound effect on the activity of antimicrobial agents. Thus, it is often necessary to remove the foreign material to cure an infection in the vicinity of a prosthetic heart valve or joint implant.[88] The mechanism by which foreign bodies potentiate infection is not clear, but they probably cause localized impairment of host defense mechanisms.[89] In addition, the foreign body often serves as a nidus on which organisms can adhere and produce extracellular substances such as glycocalyx or biofilm, which may interfere with phagocytosis.[90] Although it was originally thought that biofilm produces a barrier to penetration of antimicrobials, this is clearly not the case. The ineffectiveness of antibiotics against bacteria in biofilm is the result of an alteration in the metabolic state of these organisms that renders them relatively resistant to antibiotics.[90,91]

FIGURE 16-1. Antibacterial effects of antibiotic combinations. *Left:* Curve of A+B illustrates synergism (increased killing). *Center:* Curve of C+D illustrates antagonism (D is less effective when C is added). *Right:* Curve of E+F illustrates indifference, or additive effect (addition of E to F has no effect on F). *(From Moellering RC Jr. Use and abuse of antibiotic combinations. R I Med J. 1972;55:341.)*

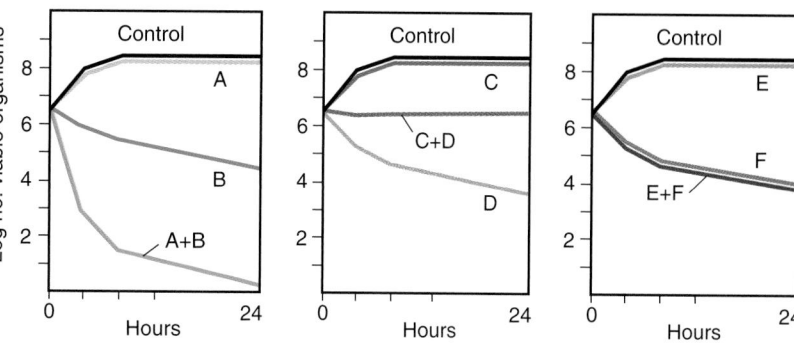

It has also been demonstrated that antimicrobial agents themselves may cause alterations in host defenses. Clinically achievable concentrations of many different agents have been shown to have adverse effects on leukocyte chemotaxis, lymphocyte transformation, monocyte transformation, delayed hypersensitivity, antibody production, phagocytosis, and the microbicidal action of polymorphonuclear leukocytes.[92-98] It is not clear, however, whether any of these effects (largely demonstrated by in vitro studies) are of clinical significance.[98] Nonetheless, the possibility that antimicrobial agents can cause immunosuppression exists, and this fact should discourage the indiscriminate use of antibiotics, especially in patients who are already immunosuppressed because of their underlying disease or because of their concomitant drug therapy.[96] Finally, antimicrobial agents such as the β-lactams that cause rapid lysis of bacteria may also release endotoxins or cell wall components that have potentially deleterious local or systemic effects, or both, in the host. The local inflammatory consequences of such activity have been clearly defined in experimental models of bacterial meningitis (and this forms the basis for the use of dexamethasone in bacterial meningitis),[99,100] but their significance in other settings such as gram-negative sepsis remains to be determined.[101]

ANTIMICROBIAL COMBINATIONS

Most infections in humans with normal host defenses can be treated with a single antimicrobial agent, but there are clear-cut (as well as borderline) indications for the use of combinations of (usually two) antimicrobials. Because combinations may provide more broad-spectrum coverage than single agents can, the physician is often tempted to use combinations of two or more antimicrobials for the sense of security they provide, even in situations in which they are not indicated. Such inappropriate use of antimicrobial combinations may have significantly deleterious effects. In this section, we examine indications for the use of combinations and the potential disadvantages of this approach to therapy. Although we consider briefly the use of combination therapy in neutropenic patients, this discussion does not attempt to deal with combination therapy in severely immunocompromised patients, such as those undergoing organ transplantation or those with severe immunodeficiency states (e.g., patients with human immunodeficiency virus infections). In these special circumstances, clinicians are often forced to use broad-spectrum combinations of antibacterial, antiviral, antifungal, and even, at times, antiparasitic agents.

In Vitro Results of Combination Therapy

When two antimicrobial agents are combined in vitro, they may have one of three types of activity against a given organism: (1) an additive effect (sometimes called an *indifferent effect*), (2) synergism, or (3) antagonism.[102] Two drugs are said to be additive when the activity of the drugs in combination is equal to the sum (or a partial sum) of their independent activities when studied separately. The combined effect of a synergistic pair of antimicrobials is greater than the sum of their independent activities when measured separately. If two drugs are antagonistic, the activity of the combination is less than the sum of their

independent effects when measured alone. These concepts are illustrated by the *time-kill curves* in Figure 16-1. The various methods used to determine the in vitro effects of antibiotic combinations are beyond the scope of this chapter but have been reviewed in detail.[103]

Indications for Clinical Use of Antimicrobial Combinations

Five reasons have been advanced to justify the use of antimicrobial combinations. The first three of these (preventing emergence of resistant organisms, polymicrobial infections, and initial therapy) are discussed in detail in other chapters (see Chapter 17) and given only brief mention here.

Prevention of the Emergence of Resistant Organisms

Preventing the emergence of resistant organisms would seem to be a major indication for the use of combination therapy; however, combination therapy has been documented as being clearly effective in preventing resistance only when resistance to the particular antimicrobials is the result of chromosomal mutations. The best example of the efficacy of combinations to prevent mutational resistance is in the treatment of tuberculosis (see Chapter 248). There is somewhat less epidemiologic evidence in support of this concept as it applies to the use of rifampin for the treatment of nonmycobacterial infections, but it nonetheless appears that one of the major benefits of using rifampin in combination with a second agent for treating staphylococcal infections, for example, is that the combination prevents the rapid emergence of resistance to rifampin, which is evident when this drug is used alone.[104,105] The effectiveness of combinations of rifampin and a fluoroquinolone for staphylococcal infections of prosthetic implants most likely results, at least in part, from the combination preventing the emergence of resistance to each drug, which is seen when either is used alone.[106] Combination therapy is also useful to prevent mutational resistance to macrolides and other antimicrobials in the treatment of infections due to *Helicobacter pylori*.[107]

Polymicrobial Infections

In most infections, even those caused by more than one organism, a single effective agent can be found. For example, cellulitis due to *S. aureus* and group A streptococci can be treated with a penicillinase-resistant penicillin alone. However, certain types of infections are caused by such a broad variety of organisms that more than one antimicrobial agent may be required to provide adequate coverage. Examples of such infections include intraperitoneal and pelvic infections caused by mixed aerobic and anaerobic organisms. However, many of the newer fluoroquinolones, carbapenems, and β-lactam–β-lactamase inhibitor combinations have such broad spectra of activity that they can be employed effectively as "monotherapy" for intra-abdominal and pelvic sepsis.[108,109]

Initial Therapy

In neutropenic patients or other patients with presumed infection in whom the nature of the infection is not clear, it may be reasonable to begin broad-spectrum coverage, usually with two agents such as an expanded-spectrum cephalosporin plus an aminoglycoside or fluoroquinolone while awaiting the results of cultures. In this setting, it is often possible to switch to a single drug after the results of cultures are available. The development of new drugs with broad spectra of activity makes it possible to use a single agent for most cases of initial therapy, but many clinicians still prefer combinations in this setting.[110]

Decreased Toxicity

Many of the drugs used in therapy for infections are potentially toxic (e.g., aminoglycosides). Therefore, a major goal of combination therapy has been to reduce the amount of drug required for treatment and, thus, to reduce dose-related toxicity. Unfortunately, data from clinical trials do not establish beyond doubt that combination therapy with different agents permits a reduction of the drug dose sufficient to reduce dose-related toxicity.

Synergism

The use of synergistic combinations of antimicrobial agents to treat infections due to resistant or relatively resistant organisms is most appealing. There are numerous examples of in vitro synergism, but thus far synergistic antimicrobial combinations have proved more effective than single agents in only a limited number of clinical settings.[111,112]

Perhaps the best known application of synergistic combinations of antimicrobial agents is in the treatment of enterococcal endocarditis. Treatment of this disease with penicillin alone results in an unacceptable relapse rate because enterococci are relatively resistant to penicillin.[113] Indeed, penicillin alone seems to act as a bacteriostatic and not a bactericidal agent.[114] The addition of an aminoglycoside such as streptomycin or gentamicin results in synergism both in vitro and in vivo and yields clinical cure rates comparable to those achieved for endocarditis caused by less resistant streptococci.[113,114] Penicillin enhances the uptake of aminoglycosides by enterococci, and the result of this interaction is the synergistic killing of the organisms.[115]

Some enterococci, however, have been found to be resistant to penicillin-streptomycin, penicillin-kanamycin, and penicillin-amikacin synergism because of high-level resistance (MIC >2000 µg/mL) to streptomycin, to kanamycin, or to both.[116] Strains may resist synergism if they are ribosomally resistant to streptomycin[117] or if they contain plasmid-mediated enzymes that inactivate streptomycin, kanamycin, gentamicin, or amikacin.[118] The prevalence of enterococci with high-level resistance to gentamicin appears to be increasing rapidly.[119-121] Moreover, the use of penicillin-gentamicin therapy in such patients may result in a failure to eradicate the infecting organisms.[122] Therefore, it is important to test for high-level resistance to streptomycin and gentamicin before embarking on a therapeutic regimen for enterococcal endocarditis or meningitis.

Penicillin-streptomycin combinations are also synergistic against viridans streptococci and have been used for the treatment of endocarditis caused by these organisms.[112] However, some viridans streptococci remain susceptible to penicillin, and penicillin alone has been used successfully for treatment of this kind of endocarditis.[123,124]

A similar type of synergism occurs when semisynthetic penicillinase-resistant penicillins, such as nafcillin, oxacillin, or vancomycin, are combined with gentamicin against S. aureus.[125] Thus far, the data have not documented that the use of combination therapy for S. aureus infections in humans has any advantage over therapy with a penicillin, cephalosporin, or vancomycin alone.[126]

Combinations of ticarcillin, mezlocillin, azlocillin, or piperacillin with gentamicin, tobramycin, or amikacin exhibit synergism against many strains of P. aeruginosa.[127,128] The mechanism of synergism in this setting is similar to that described for enterococci (i.e., enhanced uptake of the aminoglycoside in the presence of the antipseudomonal penicillin). Studies with experimental animals demonstrate the superiority of such combinations for the treatment of serious Pseudomonas infections.[129] Although the information available from limited human trials is also consistent with enhanced activity of these combinations for Pseudomonas infections, this form of therapy has not been subjected to definitive controlled study.[103] A large prospective (but uncontrolled) study of patients with Pseudomonas bacteremia documented

an increased survival in patients who received antimicrobial combinations compared with those who received single-drug therapy. Interestingly, the presence or absence of synergism seemed less important than administration of combination therapy (presumably to prevent emergence of resistance) in this population.[130]

Synergism occurs by a different mechanism when sulfonamides are combined with trimethoprim. In this case, the two agents are synergistic because they act to inhibit sequential steps in the microbial pathway of folic acid metabolism.[131] As a result, combinations of sulfonamides with trimethoprim are often useful for the treatment of infections caused by organisms that may be resistant to sulfonamides alone. A fixed combination of sulfamethoxazole and trimethoprim is available for clinical use and has been shown to be effective for the treatment and prevention of chronic urinary tract infections, even when they are caused by sulfonamide-resistant organisms.[132] The combination has also been shown to be useful for the treatment of typhoid fever and shigellosis caused by organisms resistant to ampicillin, chloramphenicol, or both; for the treatment of infections due to ampicillin-resistant H. influenzae; and for therapy for a wide variety of other infections as well.[103,133-135] Its usefulness, however, has now been eroded by the development of widespread resistance among enteric pathogens and even E. coli.[136]

Combinations of amphotericin B with a number of other agents, including 5-fluorocytosine, rifampin, and tetracycline, have been shown to result in enhanced in vitro antimicrobial activity against fungi.[137] The mechanism of synergism seems to involve damage to the fungal cell envelope by amphotericin B, with resultant enhanced intracellular penetration of 5-fluorocytosine and other agents.[137] Fluorocytosine and low-dose amphotericin B have been used successfully in treating candidiasis and cryptococcosis when the patient's isolate was susceptible to both drugs.[135,138] Combinations of triazoles, echinocandins, and amphotericin may also have enhanced activity against pathogenic yeast and even Aspergillus species.[139]

Synergism and Infections in Impaired Hosts. The clinical applications of antimicrobial combinations discussed thus far have all represented attempts to use a synergistic interaction for enhanced efficacy in the treatment of infections due to relatively resistant organisms. Another use of such therapy is to obtain enhanced antimicrobial activity in the treatment of infections due to susceptible organisms occurring in patients with abnormalities of host defense systems. Several groups have conducted randomized trials of various combinations of two agents chosen from among carbenicillin, ticarcillin, piperacillin, the cephalosporins, gentamicin, tobramycin, and amikacin for the treatment of severe infections in patients with impaired host defense mechanisms. Both Lau and colleagues[140] and Klastersky and associates[141] have demonstrated improved survival rates in patients treated with combinations that were synergistic against the infecting organisms compared with patients who received nonsynergistic combinations. These studies add strong support to the concept that synergistic combinations of antimicrobials may be an important determinant of success in the treatment of serious infections, especially when the infections are caused by gram-negative organisms in patients with impaired host defenses. However, there is no absolute proof that synergistic combinations are more effective in this setting than are single agents that have a sufficiently broad spectrum and that produce sufficiently high serum bactericidal titers against the infecting organisms.[142]

Disadvantages of Inappropriate Use of Antimicrobial Combinations

Although the clinical use of synergistic combinations of antimicrobial agents may have beneficial results, the inappropriate use of antimicrobial combinations may have important adverse effects, three of which are discussed here.

Antagonism

The medical literature contains a large number of reports of in vitro antagonism between antimicrobial agents.[111,112] In view of this, it is surprising that there are only a few well-documented clinical examples of antagonism. Perhaps the most impressive is the study of Lepper and Dowling, who demonstrated conclusively in 1951 that penicillin is more effective than the combination of penicillin and chlortetracycline for the treatment of pneumococcal meningitis.[143] The fatality among patients treated with penicillin alone was 21%, whereas that among patients treated with penicillin plus chlortetracycline was 79%. A study of childhood meningitis also demonstrated the superiority of single-drug therapy. Mathies and associates treated a group of children suffering from bacterial meningitis with either ampicillin alone or a combination of ampicillin, chloramphenicol, and streptomycidis.[144] The mortality among 140 children treated with ampicillin alone was 4.3%, whereas the mortality among 124 children receiving the antibiotic combination was 10.5%, a difference that reached statistical significance. There are several other reports of the influence of antagonism on the treatment of urinary tract infections and streptococcal pharyngitis, but none is particularly impressive.[111]

Considering the extensive clinical use of antimicrobial combinations and especially in view of the large number of reports of in vitro antagonism, it is surprising that there are so few reports of in vivo antagonism. This might be the result of a paucity of well-controlled studies in this area, or perhaps investigators have been reluctant to report adverse results. Another possible explanation is simply that clinically significant antagonism is not a common event. In most cases, in vitro antagonism results in the loss or partial loss of activity of the most active drug (e.g., the bactericidal activity of such an agent may be reduced to simple bacteriostasis), but the combination still retains some antimicrobial activity. As long as the patient receiving such therapy has normal host defense mechanisms, it is unlikely that adverse effects will be seen.

This has been the case in studies using an antagonistic combination of antibiotics (chloramphenicol plus gentamicin) to treat experimental infections caused by *Proteus mirabilis* in mice.[145] In healthy mice, in vivo antagonism could not be demonstrated, but after irradiation to render the animals neutropenic, gentamicin alone was more effective than gentamicin plus chloramphenicol. This combination has also been shown to be antagonistic in experimentally produced meningitis caused by *P. mirabilis* in rabbits.[146] Thus, it seems that clinically important antagonism is most likely to be manifested in patients with generalized impairment of host defense mechanisms (e.g., in leukemia patients and cancer patients who are neutropenic) or in patients with infections such as meningitis or endocarditis in whom localized host defenses may be inadequate.

The observation of in vivo antagonism in the treatment of bacterial meningitis raised some questions about recommendations for the use of ampicillin plus chloramphenicol in the initial treatment of childhood meningitis (see Chapter 80), because of the initial emergence of ampicillin-resistant strains of *H. influenzae*.[12] Combinations of penicillin plus chloramphenicol were shown to exhibit in vitro antagonism against pneumococci and other organisms.[112] However, this antagonism takes the form of lessened bactericidal activity of penicillin in the presence of chloramphenicol. Because chloramphenicol alone is quite active against the organisms likely to cause childhood meningitis (*H. influenzae, S. pneumoniae, Neisseria meningitidis*) and because there is no evidence that penicillin or ampicillin antagonizes the activity of chloramphenicol, it is not surprising that the use of ampicillin-chloramphenicol therapy for pediatric meningitis did not result in in vivo antagonism when used to treat these organisms.[112] Moreover, studies documenting the effectiveness of cephalosporins such as cefotaxime and ceftriaxone[147,148] for childhood meningitis make it unnecessary to continue to use combination therapy in this setting, as does the fact that use of the *H. influenzae* vaccine has virtually eliminated *H. influenzae* as a cause of childhood meningitis in Western countries.

Broad-spectrum β-lactams have been used in combination to obtain broad-spectrum coverage without exposing the patient to the possible toxicity of an agent such as chloramphenicol or an aminoglycoside.[149] In some cases, this seems reasonable. However, there is in vitro and in vivo evidence that some β-lactam–β-lactam combinations may be antagonistic against certain organisms such as *Enterobacter, Serratia,* or *Pseudomonas*. This antagonism seems to be the result of the induction or derepression of chromosomally mediated β-lactamases by one of the agents, leading to inactivation of the second.[150] The exact clinical significance of this phenomenon is not clear at present, but it must be kept in mind when considering the clinical use of such combinations. Again, the development of the newest broad-spectrum cephalosporins and β-lactam–β-lactamase inhibitor combinations and carbapenems now renders most earlier combinations obsolete.[110]

Most of the examples of in vitro antagonism are the result of interactions of the antimicrobial agents as they act at a subcellular level on a given microorganism. However, another type of antagonism may result from the direct interaction of drugs before they reach the microorganism. If chloramphenicol and erythromycin are inadvertently mixed together in the same parenteral infusion solution, they form insoluble precipitates and hence lose activity. The mixing of a penicillin such as piperacillin with an aminoglycoside results in the inactivation of the aminoglycoside.[151] Because the reaction occurs slowly, this is usually not a problem in vivo, provided the drugs are given by separate routes of administration. However, in uremic patients in whom the serum half-life of aminoglycosides is greatly prolonged, in vivo inactivation can occur.[152] The clinical significance of this observation, however, has not yet been elucidated.

Cost

With the possible exception of penicillin G, ampicillin, and certain of the macrolides, tetracyclines, and sulfonamides, antimicrobials are expensive drugs. Thus, the inappropriate use of antimicrobial combinations (when a single agent would be adequate) can add greatly to the cost of the patient's illness.

Adverse Effects

It has been estimated that approximately 5% of the patients receiving an antibiotic in the hospital experience some sort of adverse reaction that leads to excess length of stay, extra costs, and an almost twofold increased risk of death.[26,153,154] The possibility of such adverse reactions (including hypersensitivity reactions and direct toxic effects) is increased without any enhanced therapeutic benefit when one uses combinations of antimicrobial agents inappropriately. Moreover, when an adverse reaction occurs in a patient receiving more than one drug, it is often difficult to be certain of the agent that caused the reaction. This may mean that treatment with several or all drugs must be stopped. If combination drug therapy is to be used in such a patient, each drug must be tested carefully first to make certain that it was not the cause of the original adverse reaction. This is time consuming and expensive and may needlessly deprive the patient of the benefits of a useful agent.

DOSAGES AND EVALUATION OF EFFICACY

Route of Administration

Once the most appropriate drug has been determined for a given infection, a route of administration must be chosen that will maximize the benefits of therapy (see Chapter 18). In most cases, the choice is between oral and parenteral routes. In general, the oral route of administration is chosen for infections that are mild and can be treated on an outpatient basis. Not all antibiotics, however, can be administered in this way. Drugs such as vancomycin, the polymyxins, the aminoglycosides, and amphotericin B are absorbed so poorly from the gastrointestinal tract that they cannot be administered orally to treat systemic infections. When drugs are administered by the oral route, the physician must ascertain that the patient will take them as ordered. The absorption of certain agents such as penicillin G is markedly impaired if it is taken with meals, whereas the absorption of acid-stable penicillins such as penicillin V is not affected by food or gastric acidity. The concomitant administration of antacids or iron-containing preparations may severely impair the absorption of tetracycline, because this drug forms insoluble chelates in the presence of Mg^{2+}, Ca^{2+}, or Fe^{2+}. Antacids and histamine antagonists may also interfere with the absorption of the fluoroquinolones.[155] The oxazolidinones are well absorbed from the gastrointestinal tract (100% oral bioavailability) and produce equivalent serum concentrations whether given orally or parenterally.[156] More detailed information on the oral absorption of antimicrobial agents may be found in the chapters on the individual drugs.

The parenteral route of administration is used for agents that are inefficiently absorbed from the gastrointestinal tract and for the treatment of patients with serious infections that require higher serum concentrations of antimicrobial agents than can be reliably obtained by the oral route. The aminoglycosides and polymyxins may be given by intramuscular injection and are well tolerated when given this way. For most infections, adequate serum concentrations are achieved after intramuscular administration of these drugs.

In life-threatening infections, however, especially in the presence of shock (or in diabetic patients, as discussed earlier), intravenous administration is preferred. Intravenous administration allows large doses of drugs to be given with a minimum of discomfort to the patient when high serum concentrations are required for the effective treatment of disease processes such as meningitis, endocarditis, and osteomyelitis.

Dosing Regimen

Whether intravenously administered drugs should be given by continuous infusion or by intermittent bolus infusion was a matter of controversy in the past. The former method has the advantage of simplicity, and because pulses containing very high concentrations of drugs are avoided, it may result in less venous irritation and phlebitis. On the other hand, studies in animal models suggest that the concentration of drugs such as penicillins and cephalosporins in fibrin clots is related to the peak serum levels achieved, and greater concentrations of drugs seem to be achieved in the clots with intermittent bolus therapy.[157] These data may be applicable to therapy for infective endocarditis and other infections in which high tissue concentrations of antibiotics are required.

More recent evidence, based on modern pharmacodynamic studies, however, strongly suggests that the clinical effectiveness of β-lactams, macrolides, clindamycin, and linezolid is optimal when the concentration of these antimicrobial agents exceeds the MIC of the infecting organism for a prolonged period of time at the site of infection. This is expressed as "time above MIC."[158,159] These studies lend support to the concept of administering β-lactam antibiotics at shorter intervals or by continuous infusion for serious systemic infections.[160]

The aminoglycosides and fluoroquinolones, on the other hand, exhibit *concentration*-dependent killing.[158,159] In pharmacodynamic parlance, the two ratios of "peak/MIC" (peak serum concentrations over MIC) and "24-hr AUC/MIC" (24-hour area-under-serum-concentration curve over MIC) are major determinants of activity of these agents.[159,161] These ratios show that giving the fluoroquinolones and aminoglycosides by once-a-day administration is attractive from a pharmacodynamic point of view.[162] Thus, the high peak levels obtained after bolus dosing cause more rapid killing of the infecting pathogen. Peak/MIC ratios of 8 or more and 24-hr AUC/MIC ratios of greater than 100 are optimal for therapy of infections caused by gram-negative bacteria and to prevent emergence of resistance during therapy. It appears that AUC/MIC ratios of only 25 to 35 are sufficient for successful treatment of pneumococcal infections with fluoroquinolones or azithromycin.[158] Once-a-day dosing of aminoglycosides also leads to lower (or absent) trough levels, which may be advantageous in terms of potential toxicity.[162,163]

As discussed earlier, the intrathecal or intraventricular route of administration may be necessary for the treatment of meningeal infections with drugs such as the aminoglycosides, polymyxins, bacitracin, and possibly vancomycin, all of which cross the blood-brain barrier with considerable difficulty. The parenteral administration of antimicrobial agents results in adequate concentrations in pleural, peritoneal, pericardial, and synovial fluids.[164,165] Thus, direct instillation of antibiotics into these areas is not necessary.

Monitoring the Response of the Patient to Antimicrobial Therapy

Although several laboratory tests are available to assist in the monitoring of antimicrobial therapy, clinical assessment remains the most important method for determining the efficacy of treatment. It is not uncommon to see patients fail to respond in the face of laboratory studies that suggest adequate therapy is being given, and vice versa. The reasons are usually found among the many host factors that affect therapy.

Nonetheless, the measurement of serum concentrations of antimicrobial agents and the determination of serum bactericidal titers are of considerable use in some circumstances. The major value of the direct determination of serum concentrations of antimicrobial agents is to avoid toxicity from excessive levels of agents such as the aminoglycosides, especially in patients with impaired renal or hepatic function. These tests are also useful for determining inadequate serum levels that result from insufficient dosing or unusually rapid clearance.[166] Serum concentrations of vancomycin are frequently monitored to ensure safe and adequate dosing. However, following the standard nomograms for dosing in patients with various degrees of renal impairment makes it unnecessary to routinely monitor vancomycin serum levels.[166,167] Monitoring serum levels of other antibiotics is not generally necessary or helpful.

Another method used to monitor the effectiveness of antimicrobial therapy is the serum bactericidal titer (sometimes called the *serum antimicrobial dilution titer*). This test, originally described by Schlichter and MacLean as a guide for effective therapy for subacute bacterial endocarditis,[168] has been used to monitor therapy in patients with infective endocarditis, osteomyelitis, septic arthritis, empyema, and bacteremia.[141,169] Serial dilutions of the patient's serum are incubated with an inoculum of the infecting organism. After incubation, the highest dilution that inhibits or kills the organism is determined. Some investigators feel that a serum bactericidal titer of at least 1:8 can be correlated with a successful therapeutic outcome.[141,168,170,171] A multicenter study has suggested that peak and trough titers of at least 1:64 and 1:32, respectively, are good predictors of a successful therapeutic outcome in patients with infective endocarditis.[172] However, a lack of standardization and a lack of consistency in specifying the point (peak, trough, or midpoint serum levels) at which the test should be done have hindered attempts at more widespread application and evaluation of this test.[173-176]

REFERENCES

1. Weinstein L. General considerations. In: Goodman LS, Gilman A, eds. The Pharmacological Basis of Therapeutics. New York: Macmillan; 1970:1154.
2. Majno G. The Healing Hand: Man and Wound in the Ancient World. Cambridge: Harvard University Press; 1975:154, 215.
3. Harris JC, Dupont HL, Hornick RB. Fecal leukocytes in diarrheal illness. Ann Intern Med. 1972;76:697.
4. Ho D, Ault MJ, Ault MA, et al. *Campylobacter* enteritis: Early diagnosis with Gram's stain. Arch Intern Med. 1982;142:1858.
5. Zipeto D, Revello MG, Silini E, et al. Development and clinical significance of a diagnostic assay based on the polymerase chain reaction for detection of human cytomegalovirus DNA in blood samples from immunocompromised patients. J Clin Microbiol. 1992;30:527.
6. Peter J. The polymerase chain reaction: Amplifying our options. Rev Infect Dis. 1991;13:166.
7. Desmond EP. Molecular approaches to the identification of mycobacteria. Clin Microbiol Newslett. 1992;14:145.
8. Weinstein L. Common sense (clinical judgment) in the diagnosis and antibiotic therapy of etiologically undefined infections. Pediatr Clin North Am. 1968;15:141.
9. Moellering RC Jr. A rational approach to the choice of antimicrobial agents in bacterial infections. In: Seminar on Gram-Negative Infections. St Louis: Mosby; 1974:5.
10. Huang MB, Baker CN, Bannerjee S, Tenover FC. Accuracy of the E test for determining antimicrobial susceptibility of staphylococci, enterococci, *Campylobacter jejuni,* and gram-negative bacteria resistant to antimicrobial agents. J Clin Microbiol. 1992;30:3243.
11. Jorgensen JH. Antibacterial susceptibility tests: Automated or instrument-based methods. In: Balows A, Hausler WJ Jr, Herrmann KL, et al., eds. Manual of Clinical Microbiology. Washington, DC: American Society for Microbiology; 1991:1166.
12. Murray BE, Moellering RC Jr. Patterns and mechanisms of antibiotic resistance. Med Clin North Am. 1978;62:899.
13. Gold HS, Moellering RC Jr. Antimicrobial drug resistance. N Engl J Med. 1996; 335:1445.

14. Levy SB. Active efflux mechanisms for antimicrobial resistance. Antimicrob Agents Chemother. 1992;36:695.
15. Edelstein PH. Pneumococcal resistance to macrolides, lincosamides, ketolides and streptogramin B: Molecular mechanisms and resistance phenotypes. Clin Infect Dis. 2004;38(Suppl 4):S322.
16. Ruoff KL. Gram-positive vancomycin-resistant clinical isolates. Clin Microbiol Newslett. 1989;11:1.
17. Moellering RC Jr. Vancomycin-resistant enterococci. Clin Infect Dis. 1998;26:1196.
18. Galimand M, Guiyoule A, Gerbaud G, et al. Multidrug resistance in *Yersinia pestis* mediated by a transferable plasmid. N Engl J Med. 1997;337:677.
19. Tanaka M, Nakayama H, Haroaka M, et al. Antimicrobial resistance of *Neisseria gonorrhoeae* and high prevalence of ciprofloxacin-resistant isolates in Japan, 1993 to 1998. J Clin Microbiol. 2000;38:521.
20. Moellering RC Jr, Kunz LJ, Poitras JW, et al. Microbiologic basis for the rational use of antibiotics. South Med J. 1977;70(Suppl):8.
21. Salmenlinna S, Lyytikainen O, Vuopio-Varkila J. Community-acquired methicillin-resistant *Staphylococcus aureus*, Finland. Emerg Infect Dis. 2002;8:602.
22. Abramowicz M, ed. The choice of antibacterial drugs. Med Lett. 2001;43:69.
23. Gilbert DN, Moellering RC Jr, Sande MA. The Sanford Guide to Antimicrobial Therapy. Hyde Park, VT: Antimicrobial Therapy; 2003.
24. Weinstein L, Dalton AC. Host determinants of response to antimicrobial agents. N Engl J Med. 1968;279:467.
25. Moellering RC Jr. Factors influencing the clinical use of antimicrobial agents in elderly patients. Geriatrics. 1978;33:83.
26. Mannisto PT, Mantyla R, Nykanen S, et al. Impairing effect of food on ketoconazole absorption. Antimicrob Agents Chemother. 1982;21:730.
27. Jackson GG, Arcieri G. Ototoxicity of gentamicin in man: A survey and controlled analysis of clinical experience in the United States. J Infect Dis. 1969;119:432.
28. Calderwood S, Moellering RC Jr. Common adverse effects of antibacterial agents on major organ systems. Surg Clin North Am. 1980;60:65.
29. Moellering RC Jr. Antimicrobial agents in pregnancy and the postpartum period. Clin Obstet Gynecol. 1989;22:277.
30. McCracken GH Jr. Pharmacologic basis for antimicrobial therapy in newborn infants. Am J Dis Child. 1974;128:407.
31. Kline AH, Blattner RJ, Lunin M. Transplacental effect of tetracyclines on teeth. JAMA. 1964;118:178.
32. Hoyer D, Wolfson J. Adverse effects of quinolone antibiotics. In: Hooper D, Wolfson J, eds. Quinolone Antimicrobial Agents. Washington, DC: American Society for Microbiology; 1989:249-271.
33. Ball P. The quinolones: History and overview. In: Andriole VT, ed. The Quinolones. San Diego, Calif: Academic Press; 1998:2.
34. Khaliq Y, Zhanel GG. Fluoroquinolone-associated tendinopathy: A critical review of the literature. Clin Infect Dis. 2003;36:1404.
35. Garibaldi RA, Druish RE, Ferebee SH, et al. Isoniazid-associated hepatitis. Am Rev Respir Dis. 1972;106:357.
36. Rose DN, Schechter CB, Silver AL. The age threshold for isoniazid chemoprophylaxis. JAMA. 1986;256:2709.
37. Salpeter SR, Sanders GD, Salpeter EE, et al. Monitored isoniazid prophylaxis for low-risk tuberculin reactors older than 35 years of age: A risk-benefit and cost effectiveness analysis. Ann Intern Med. 1997;127:1051.
38. Nolan CM, Goldberg SV, Buskin SE. Hepatotoxicity associated with isoniazid preventative therapy. JAMA. 1999;281:1014.
39. Foord RD. Cephaloridine, cephalothin and the kidney. J Antimicrob Chemother. 1975;1(Suppl):119.
40. Koch-Weser J, Sidel VW, Federman EB, et al. Adverse effects of sodium colistimethate. Ann Intern Med. 1970;72:857.
41. Van Scoy RE. Antituberculous agents. Mayo Clin Proc. 1977;52:694.
42. Young DS, Thomas DW, Friedman RB, et al. Effects of drugs on clinical laboratory tests. Clin Chem. 1972;18:1041.
43. Anonymous. Updated guidelines for the use of rifabutin or rifampin for the treatment and prevention of tuberculosis among HIV-infected patients taking protease inhibitors or nonnucleoside reverse transcriptase inhibitors. MMWR Morb Mortal Wkly Rep. 2000;49:185.
44. Hamod KA, Khouzami VA. Antibiotics in pregnancy. In: Nietyl JR, ed. Drug Use in Pregnancy. Philadelphia: Lea & Febiger; 1982:31.
45. Meyer JM, Rodvold KA. Antimicrobials during pregnancy. Infect Med. 1995;12:420.
46. Blumberg HM, Hopewell PC, O'Brien JR. Treatment of tuberculosis. MMWR Morb Mortal Wkly Rep. 2003;52:1.
47. Anonymous. Is Flagyl dangerous? Med Lett. 1975;17:53-54.
48. Conway N, Birt BD. Streptomycin in pregnancy: Effect in foetal ear. Br Med J. 1965;2:260.
49. Monnet P, Kalb JC, Pujol M. Toxic influence of isoniazid on fetus. Lyon Med. 1967;218:431.
50. Philipson A. Pharmacokinetics of ampicillin during pregnancy. J Infect Dis. 1977;136:370.
51. Vorherr H. Drug excretion in breast milk. Postgrad Med. 1974;56:97.
52. Reeves DS. The effect of renal failure on the pharmacokinetics of antibiotics. J Antimicrob Chemother. 1988;21:5.
53. Jackson EA, McLeod DC. Pharmacokinetics and dosing of antimicrobial agents in renal impairment, part I. Am J Hosp Pharm. 1974;31:36.
54. Jackson EA, McLeod DC. Pharmacokinetics and dosing of antimicrobial agents in renal impairment, part II. Am J Hosp Pharm. 1974;31:137.

55. Moellering RC Jr, Eliopoulos GM. Principles of anti-infective therapy. In: Stein JH, ed. Internal Medicine. St. Louis: Mosby; 1998:1343.
56. Bennett WM, Aronoff GR, Morrison G, et al. Drug prescribing in renal failure: Dosing guidelines for adults. Am J Kidney Dis. 1983;3:155.
57. Cooper K, Bennett WM. Nephrotoxicity of common drugs used in clinical practice. Arch Intern Med. 1987;147:1213.
58. Natelson EA, Brown CH III, Bradshaw MW, et al. Influence of cephalosporin antibiotics on blood coagulation and platelet function. Antimicrob Agents Chemother. 1976;9:91.
59. Neu HC. Adverse effects of new cephalosporins. Ann Intern Med. 1983;98:415.
60. Kaufman CA, Frame PT. Bone marrow toxicity associated with 5-fluorocytosine therapy. Antimicrob Agents Chemother. 1977;11:244.
61. Davey PG. Pharmacokinetics in liver disease. J Antimicrob Chemother. 1988;21:1.
62. Suhrland LG, Weisberger AS. Chloramphenicol toxicity in liver and renal disease. Arch Intern Med. 1963;112:747.
63. Pessayre D, Allemand H, Benhamou J-P. Effets des maladies du foie et des voies biliaires sur le métabolisme des médicaments. Nouv Presse Med. 1977;35:3209.
64. Singh N, Yu VL, Mieles LA, et al. β-Lactam antibiotic-induced leukopenia in severe hepatic dysfunction: Risk factors and implications for dosing in patients with liver disease. Am J Med. 1993;94:251.
65. Lorian V, Atkinson B. Killing of oxacillin-exposed staphylococci in human polymorphonuclear leukocytes. Antimicrob Agents Chemother. 1980;18:807.
66. Ofek IE, Beachey H, Eisenstein BI, et al. Suppression of bacterial adherence by subminimal inhibitory concentration of β-lactam and aminoglycoside antibiotics. Rev Infect Dis. 1979;1:832.
67. Gemmell CG, Peterson PK, Schmeling DJ, et al. Potentiation of opsonization and phagocytosis of *Streptococcus pyogenes* following growth in the presence of clindamycin. J Clin Invest. 1981;67:1249.
68. Friedman HH, Warren GH. Enhanced susceptibility of penicillin-resistant staphylococci to phagocytosis after in vitro incubation with low dose of nafcillin. Proc Soc Exp Biol Med. 1974;146:707.
69. Elliott GR, Peterson PK, Verburg HA, et al. Influence of subinhibitory concentrations of penicillin, cephalothin, and clindamycin on *Staphylococcus aureus* growth in human phagocytic cells. Antimicrob Agents Chemother. 1982;22:781.
70. Moellering RC Jr. Revolutionary changes in the macrolide and azalide antibiotics. Am J Med. 1991;91:1s.
71. Smith CR. The spiramycin paradox. J Antimicrob Chemother. 1988;22(Suppl B):141.
72. Foulds G, Johnson RB. Selection of dose regimens of azithromycin. J Antimicrob Chemother. 1993;31(Suppl E):39.
73. Craig WA, Kunin CM. Significance of serum protein and tissue binding of antimicrobial agents. Annu Rev Med. 1976;27:287.
74. Peterson LR, Gerding DN. Interaction of cephalosporins with human and canine serum proteins. J Infect Dis. 1978;137:452.
75. Barza M, Samuelson T, Weinstein L. Penetration of antibiotics into fibrin loci in vivo. II. Comparison of nine antibiotics: Effect of dose and degree of protein binding. J Infect Dis. 1974;129:66.
76. Kunst MW, Mattie H. Cefazolin and cephradine. Relationship between antibacterial activity in vitro and in mice experimentally infected with *Escherichia coli*. J Infect Dis. 1978;137:391.
77. Merrikin DJ, Briant J, Rolinson GN. Effect of protein binding on antibiotic activity in vivo. J Antimicrob Chemother. 1983;11:233.
78. Kaiser AB, McGee ZA. Aminoglycoside therapy of gram-negative bacillary meningitis. N Engl J Med. 1975;293:1215.
79. Lew D, Waldvogel FW. Use of quinolones for treatment of osteomyelitis and septic arthritis. In: Hooper D, Wolfson J, eds. Quinolone Antimicrobial Agents. 2nd ed. Washington, DC: American Society for Microbiology; 1993:371-379.
80. Naber KG. The role of quinolones in the treatment of chronic bacterial prostatitis. In: Hooper D, Wolfson J, eds. Quinolone Antimicrobial Agents. 2nd ed. Washington, DC: American Society for Microbiology; 1993:285.
81. Nicolle L. Use of quinolones in urinary tract infection and prostatitis. In: Andriole VT, ed. The Quinolones. 2nd ed. San Diego, Calif: Academic Press; 1998:183.
82. Bryant RE, Howard D. Interaction of purulent material with antibiotics used to treat *Pseudomonas* infections. Antimicrob Agents Chemother. 1974;6:702.
83. O'Keefe JP, Tally FP, Barza M, et al. Inactivation of penicillin G during experimental infection with *Bacteroides fragilis*. J infect Dis. 1978;137:437.
84. Zimelis VM, Jackson GG. Activity of aminoglycoside antibiotics against *Pseudomonas aeruginosa:* Specificity and site of calcium, and magnesium antagonism. J Infect Dis. 1973;127:663.
85. Bryan LE, Van Den Elzen HM. Streptomycin accumulation in susceptible and resistant strains of *Escherichia coli* and *Pseudomonas aeruginosa*. Antimicrob Agents Chemother. 1976;9:928.
86. Zinner SH, Sabath LD, Casey JI, et al. Erythromycin and alkalinization of the urine in the treatment of urinary tract infection due to gram-negative bacilli. Lancet. 1971;1:1267.
87. Sabath LD, Gerstein DA, Leaf CD, et al. Increasing the usefulness of antibiotics: Treatment of infections caused by gram-negative bacilli. Clin Pharmacol Ther. 1970;11:161.
88. Karchmer AW, Dismukes WE, Buckley MJ, et al. Late prosthetic valve endocarditis. Am J Med. 1978;64:99.
89. Zimmerli W, Waldvogel FA, Vaudaux P, et al. Pathogenesis of foreign body infection: Description and characteristics of an animal model. J Infect Dis. 1982;146:487.
90. Dickinson GM, Bisno AL. Infections associated with indwelling medical devices. Antimicrob Agents Chemother. 1989;33:597.

91. Anderl JN, Zahller J, Roe F, et al. Role of nutrient limitation and stationary-phase existence in *Klebsiella pneumoniae* biofilm resistance to ampicillin and ciprofloxacin. Antimicrob Agents Chemother. 2003;47:1251.

92. Forsgren A, Schmeling D, Quie PG. Effect of tetracycline on the phagocytic function of human leukocytes. J Infect Dis. 1974;130:412.

93. Seklecki MM, Quintiliani R, Maderazo EG. Aminoglycoside antibiotics moderately impair granulocyte function. Antimicrob Agents Chemother. 1978;13:552.

94. Chaperon EA, Sanders WE Jr. Suppression of lymphocyte responses by cephalosporins. Infect Immun. 1978;19:378.

95. Mandell LA. Effects of antimicrobial and antineoplastic drugs on the phagocytic and microbicidal function of the polymorphonuclear leukocyte. Rev Infect Dis. 1982;4:683.

96. Hauser WE, Remington JS. Effect of antibiotics on the immune response. Am J Med. 1982;72:711.

97. Manzella JP, Clark JK. Effects of moxalactam and cefuroxime on mitogen-stimulated human mononuclear leukocytes. Antimicrob Agents Chemother. 1983;23:360.

98. Daschner FD. Antibiotics and host defense with special reference to phagocytosis by human polymorphonuclear leukocyte function in vivo. Antimicrob Agents Chemother. 1985;27:712.

99. Wispelwey B, Lesse AJ, Hansen EJ, et al. *Haemophilus influenzae* lipopolysaccharide-induced blood-brain barrier permeability during experimental meningitis in the rat. J Clin Invest. 1988;82:1339.

100. deGans J, van de Beek D. The European Dexamethasone in Adulthood Bacterial Meningitis Study Investigators. Dexamethasone in adults with bacterial meningitis. N Engl J Med. 2002;347:1549.

101. Evins ME, Pollack M. Effect of antibiotic class and concentration on the release of lipopolysaccharide from *Escherichia coli*. J Infect Dis. 1993;167:1336.

102. Jawetz E. Combined antibiotic action: Some definitions and correlations between laboratory and clinical results. Antimicrob Agents Chemother. 1967;7:203.

103. Eliopoulos GM, Moellering RC Jr. Antimicrobial combinations. In: Lorian V, ed. Antibiotics in Laboratory Medicine. 4th ed. Baltimore: Williams & Wilkins; 1996:330-396.

104. VanderAuwera P, Meunier-Carpentier F, Klastersky J. Clinical study of combination therapy with oxacillin and rifampin for staphylococcal infections. Rev Infect Dis. 1983;5(Suppl 3):515.

105. Karchmer AW, Archer GL, Dismukes WE. Rifampin treatment of prosthetic valve endocarditis due to *Staphylococcus epidermidis*. Rev Infect Dis. 1983;5(Suppl 3):543.

106. Zimmerli W, Widmer AF, Blatter M, et al. Role of rifampin for treatment of orthopedic implant-related staphylococcal infections: A randomized control trial. JAMA. 1998;279:1537.

107. Suerbaum S, Michetti P. Medical Progress: *Helicobacter pylori* infection. N Engl J Med. 2002;347:1175.

108. Solomkin JS, Dellinger EP, Christou NV, et al. Results of a multicenter trial comparing imipenem/cilastatin to tobramycin/clindamycin for intra-abdominal infections. Ann Surg. 1990;212:581.

109. Brismar B, Malmborg AS, Tunevall G, et al. Piperacillin-tazobactam versus imipenem-cilastatin for treatment of intra-abdominal infections. Antimicrob Agents Chemother. 1992;36:2766.

110. Moellering RC Jr. Antimicrobial combinations. Jpn J Clin Pharmacol Ther. 1993;24:293.

111. Moellering RC Jr. Use and abuse of antibiotic combinations. R I Med J. 1972;55:341.

112. Rahal JJ Jr. Antibiotic combinations: The clinical relevance of synergy and antagonism. Medicine (Baltimore). 1978;57:179.

113. Mandell GL, Kaye D, Levison ME, et al. Enterococcal endocarditis: An analysis of 38 patients observed at the New York Hospital-Cornell Medical Center. Arch Intern Med. 1970;125:258.

114. Moellering RC Jr, Wennersten C, Weinberg AN. Studies on antibiotic synergism against enterococci: I. Bacteriologic studies. J Lab Clin Med. 1971;77:821.

115. Moellering RC Jr, Weinberg AN. Studies on antibiotic synergism against enterococci: II. Effect of various antibiotics on the uptake of ^{14}C-labeled streptomycin by enterococci. J Clin Invest. 1971;50:2580.

116. Moellering RC Jr, Wennersten CBG, Medrek T, et al. Prevalence of high-level resistance to aminoglycosides in clinical isolates of enterococci. Antimicrob Agents Chemother. 1970;10:335.

117. Zimmermann RA, Moellering RC Jr, Weinberg AN. Mechanism of resistance to antibiotic synergism in enterococci. J Bacteriol. 1971;105:873.

118. Krogstad DJ, Korfhagen TR, Moellering RC Jr, et al. Aminoglycoside-inactivating enzymes: An explanation for resistance to penicillin-aminoglycoside synergism in enterococci. J Clin Invest. 1978;62:480.

119. Mederski-Samoraj BD, Murray BE. High-level resistance to gentamicin in clinical isolates of enterococci. J Infect Dis. 1983;147:751.

120. Moellering RC Jr. The enterococcus: High-level resistance to gentamicin and production of beta-lactamase. Clin Microbiol Newslett. 1988;10:129.

121. Moellering RC Jr. The enterococcus-a versatile pathogen. J Infect Chemother. 1997;3:1.

122. Fernandez-Guerrero ML, Barros C, Tudela JLR, et al. Aortic endocarditis caused by gentamicin-resistant *Enterococcus*. Eur J Clin Microbiol. 1988;7:525.

123. Wolfe JC, Johnson WD Jr. Penicillin-sensitive streptococcal endocarditis. Ann Intern Med. 1974;81:178.

124. Karchmer AW, Moellering RC Jr, Maki D, et al. Single antibiotic therapy of streptococcal endocarditis. JAMA. 1979;241:1801.

125. Watanakunakorn C, Glotzbecker C. Enhancement of the effects of antistaphylococcal antibiotics by aminoglycosides. Antimicrob Agents Chemother. 1974;6:802.

126. Korzeniowski O, Sande MA. The National Collaborative Endocarditis Study Group: Combination antimicrobial therapy for *Staphylococcus aureus* endocarditis in patients addicted to parenteral drugs and in nonaddicts. Ann Intern Med. 1982;97:496.

127. Smith CB, Dans PE, Wilfert JN, et al. Use of gentamicin in combination with other antibiotics. J Infect Dis. 1969;119:370.

128. Eliopoulos GM, Moellering RC Jr. Azlocillin, mezlocillin and piperacillin: New broad-spectrum penicillins. Ann Intern Med. 1982;97:755.

129. Andriole VT. Antibiotic synergy in experimental infection with *Pseudomonas:* II. The effect of carbenicillin, cephalothin or cephanone combined with tobramycin or gentamicin. J Infect Dis. 1974;129:124.

130. Hilf M, Yu VL, Sharp JA, et al. Antibiotic therapy for *Pseudomonas aeruginosa* bacteremia: Outcome correlations in a prospective study of 200 patients. Am J Med. 1989;87:540.

131. Then R. Synergism between trimethoprim and sulfonamides. Science. 1977; 197:1301.

132. Harding GKM, Ronald AR. A controlled study of antimicrobial prophylaxis of recurrent urinary tract infections in women. N Engl J Med. 1974;291:597.

133. Gilman RN, Terminel M, Levine MM, et al. Comparison of trimethoprim-sulfamethoxazole and amoxicillin in therapy of chloramphenicol-resistant and chloramphenicol-sensitive typhoid fever. J Infect Dis. 1975;132:630.

134. Chang MJ, Dunkle LM, Van Reken D, et al. Trimethoprim-sulfamethoxazole compared to ampicillin in the treatment of shigellosis. Pediatrics. 1977;59:726.

135. Quintiliani R, Levite RE, Nightingale CH. Potential role of trimethoprim-sulfamethoxazole in the treatment of serious hospital-acquired infections. Rev Infect Dis. 1987;9(Suppl 2):160.

136. Gupta K. Addressing antibiotic resistance. Am J Med. 2002;113(1A):29S.

137. Kwan CN, Medoff G, Kobayashi G, et al. Potentiation of the antifungal effects of antibiotics by amphotericin B. Antimicrob Agents Chemother. 1972;2:61.

138. Bennett J, Dismukes W, Duma R, et al. A comparison of amphotericin B alone with amphotericin B plus flucytosine in the treatment of cryptococcal meningitis. N Engl J Med. 1979;301:126.

139. Huang SS, Chan IT, Stone RM, et al. Successful treatment of angioinvasive aspergillosis during prolonged neutropenia with liposomal amphotericin, voriconazole, and caspofungin. Infect Dis Clin Practice. 2002;11:355.

140. Lau WK, Young LS, Block RE, et al. Comparative efficacy and toxicity of amikacin/carbenicillin versus gentamicin/carbenicillin in leukopenic patients. Am J Med. 1977;62:959.

141. Klastersky J, Hensgens C, Meunier-Carpentier F. Comparative effectiveness of combinations of amikacin with penicillin G and amikacin with carbenicillin in gram-negative septicemia: Double-blind clinical trial. J Infect Dis. 1976;134(Suppl):433.

142. Moellering RC Jr. Monotherapy with expanded-spectrum cephalosporins for empiric treatment of serious infections diseases. In: Hoepelman IM, Moellering RC Jr, eds. New Directions in Cephalosporin Therapy: The Expanded Spectrum Cephalosporins. Winchester, UK: Theracom; 1988:49.

143. Lepper MH, Dowling HF. Treatment of pneumococcic meningitis with penicillin compared with penicillin plus Aureomycin. Arch Intern Med. 1951;88:489.

144. Mathies AW Jr, Leedom JM, Ivier D, et al. Antibiotic antagonism in bacterial meningitis. Antimicrob Agents Chemother. 1967;7:218.

145. Sande MA, Overton JW. In vivo antagonism between gentamicin and chloramphenicol in neutropenic mice. J Infect Dis. 1973;128:247.

146. Strausbaugh LJ, Sande MA. Factors influencing the therapy of experimental *Proteus mirabilis* meningitis in rabbits. J Infect Dis. 1978;137:251.

147. Schaad UB, Suter S, Gianella-Borradori A, et al. A comparison of ceftriaxone and cefuroxime for the treatment of bacterial meningitis in children. N Engl J Med. 1990;322:141.

148. Del Rio MDL, Chrane D, Shelton S, et al. Ceftriaxone versus ampicillin and chloramphenicol for treatment of bacterial meningitis in children. Lancet. 1983;1:1241.

149. Moellering RC Jr. Rationale for the use of antibiotic combinations. Am J Med. 1983;75(2a):4.

150. Sanders CC. Novel resistance selected by the new expanded spectrum cephalosporins: A concern. J Infect Dis. 1983;147:585.

151. McLaughlin JE, Reeves DS. Clinical and laboratory evidence for inactivation of gentamicin by carbenicillin. Lancet. 1971;1:261.

152. Riff LJ, Jackson GG. Laboratory and clinical conditions for gentamicin inactivation by carbenicillin. Arch Intern Med. 1972;130:887.

153. Seidl LG, Thornton GF, Smith SW, et al. Studies on epidemiology of adverse drug reactions: III. Reactions in patients on general medical service. Bull Johns Hopkins Hosp. 1966;119:299.

154. Classen DC, Pestotnik SL, Evans RC, et al. Adverse drug events in hospitalized patients. JAMA. 1997;277:301.

155. Drusano GL. Pharmacokinetics of quinolone antimicrobial agents. In: Hooper D, Wolfson J, eds. Quinolone Antimicrobial Agents. Washington, DC: American Society for Microbiology; 1989:71-105.

156. Moellering RC Jr. Linezolid: The first oxazolidinone antimicrobial. Ann Intern Med. 2003;138:135.

157. Barza M, Brusch J, Bergeron M, et al. Penetration of antibiotics into fibrin loci in vivo: III. Intermittent versus continuous infusion and the effect of probenecid. J Infect Dis. 1974;129:73.

158. Craig WA. Pharmacokinetic/pharmacodynamic parameters: Rationale for antibacterial dosing of mice and men. Clin Infect Dis. 1998;26:1.

159. Craig WA. Does the dose matter? Clin Infect Dis. 2001;33(Suppl 3):S233.

160. Craig WA, Ebert SC. Continuous infusion of β-lactam antibiotics. Antimicrob Agents Chemother. 1992;36:2577.

161. Lacy MK, Nicolau DP, Nightingale CH, et al. The pharmacodynamics of the aminoglycosides. Clin Infect Dis. 1998;27:23.

162. Gilbert DN. Once-daily aminoglycoside therapy. Antimicrob Agents Chemother. 1991;35:399.

163. Beaucaire G. Does once-daily dosing prevent nephrotoxicity in all aminoglycosides equally? Clin Microbiol Infect. 2000;6:357.

164. Nelson JD. Antibiotic concentrations in septic joint effusions. N Engl J Med. 1971;284:349.

165. Gerding DN, Hall WH. The penetration of antibiotics into peritoneal fluid. Bull N Y Acad Med. 1975;51:1016.

166. Moellering RC Jr. Editorial: Monitoring serum vancomycin levels: Climbing the mountain because it is there? Clin Infect Dis. 1994;18:544.

167. Cantu TG, Yamanaka-Yuen NA, Lietman PS. Serum vancomycin concentrations: Reappraisal of their clinical value. Clin Infect Dis. 1994;18:533.

168. Schlichter JG, MacLean H. A method of determining the effective therapeutic level in the treatment of subacute bacterial endocarditis with penicillin. Am Heart J. 1947;34:209.

169. Reller LB, Stratton CW. Serum dilution test for bactericidal activity: II. Standardization and correlation with antimicrobial assays and susceptibility tests. J Infect Dis. 1977;136:196.

170. Carrizosa J, Kaye D. Antibiotic concentrations in serum, serum bactericidal activity, and results of therapy of streptococcal endocarditis in rabbits. Antimicrob Agents Chemother. 1977;12:479.

171. Levy J, Klastersky J. Serum bactericidal test: A review with emphasis on its role in the evaluation of antibiotic combination. In: Klastersky J, Staquet MJ, eds. Combination Antibiotic Therapy in the Compromised Host. New York: Raven Press; 1982:43.

172. Weinstein MP, Stratton CW, Ackley A, et al. Multicenter collaborative evaluation of a standardized serum bactericidal test as a prognostic indicator in infective endocarditis. Am J Med. 1985;78:262.

173. Pien FD, Vosti KL. Variation in performance of the serum bactericidal test. Antimicrob Agents Chemother. 1974;6:330.

174. Stratton CW, Reller LB. Serum dilution test for bactericidal activity. I. Selection of a physiologic diluent. J Infect Dis. 1977;136:187.

175. Mellors JW, Coleman DL, Andriole VT. Value of the serum bactericidal test in management of patients with bacterial endocarditis. Eur J Clin Microbiol. 1986;5:67.

176. Reller LB. The serum bactericidal test. Rev Infect Dis. 1986;8:803.

CHAPTER **17**

Molecular Mechanisms of Antibiotic Resistance in Bacteria

STEVEN M. OPAL

ANTONE A. MEDEIROS

MOLECULAR GENETICS OF ANTIBIOTIC RESISTANCE

Genetic variability is essential for microbial evolution to occur. The fitness of a microorganism depends on its capacity to adapt to changing environmental conditions.[1] Antimicrobial agents exert strong selective pressures on bacterial populations, favoring organisms that are capable of resisting them.[1,2] Genetic variability may occur by a variety of mechanisms. Point mutations may occur in a nucleotide base pair, which is referred to as *microevolutionary change*. These mutations may alter the target site of an antimicrobial agent, interfering with its activity. Point mutations at crucial locations on "old" β-lactamase genes (e.g., genes for TEM-1, SHV-1) are primarily responsible for the remarkable array of newly recognized extended-spectrum β-lactamases.[3,4]

A second level of genomic variability in bacteria is referred to as a *macroevolutionary change* and results in whole-scale rearrangements of large segments of DNA as a single event. These rearrangements may include inversions, duplications, insertions, deletions, or transposition of large sequences of DNA from one location of a bacterial chromosome or plasmid to another. These whole-scale rearrangements of large segments of the bacterial genome frequently are created by specialized genetic elements called *transposons* or *insertion sequences*, which have the capacity to move independently as a unit from the rest of the bacterial genome.[2]

A third level of genetic variability in bacteria is created by the acquisition of foreign DNA carried by plasmids, bacteriophages, naked sequences of DNA, or transposable genetic elements. Inheritance of foreign DNA from extrachromosomal elements further contributes to the organism's ability to cope with selection pressures imposed by antimicrobial agents.[5] These mechanisms endow bacteria with the seemingly unlimited capacity to develop resistance to any antimicrobial agent (Fig. 17-1). Examples of vancomycin-resistant *Staphylococcus aureus*,[6,7] multidrug-resistant *Yersinia pestis*,[8] and transferable quinolone resistance in enterobacteria[9] attest to the capacity of microorganisms to adapt to environmental stresses such as antibiotic exposure. When an antibiotic-resistance gene evolves, this resistance determinant may spread between bacteria by transformation, transduction, conjugation, or transposition. Favored clones of bacteria may proliferate in the flora of patients who receive antibiotics. Evidence exists that antibiotic-resistance genes were present in the pre–antibiotic therapy era.[3,10] Selection pressures placed on microbial populations by antibiotics favor the expansion of strains that have the capacity to resist the inhibitory effects of antibiotics. These resistant populations proliferate and spread antibiotic-resistance genes to other susceptible strains of bacteria. Some antibiotic-resistance genes may have derived from antibiotic-producing bacteria themselves.[3,4] Although some antibiotic-resistance genes place a metabolic "cost" on bacteria, many microorganisms evolved strategies to limit this cost by limiting expression, alternate gene products, or phase variation limiting expression. These strategies allow favorable but sometimes "costly" genes that mediate antibiotic resistance to persist in the absence of antibiotic selection pressure, yet rapidly express their resistance potential on exposure to antibiotics.[11]

Plasmids

Extrachromosomal elements were present in bacteria before the advent of antibiotics.[10] The introduction of antibiotics into clinical medicine in the 20th century created selection pressures, however, that favor the dissemination of resistance genes via mobile genetic elements. Plasmids are particularly well adapted to serve as agents of genetic evolution and resistance-gene dissemination.[12] Plasmids are extrachromosomal genetic elements that are made of circular double-stranded DNA molecules that range from less than 10 kilobase pairs to greater than 400 kilobase pairs and are extremely common in bacteria.[13] Although multiple copies of a specific plasmid, or multiple different plasmids, or both may be found in a single bacterial cell, closely related plasmids often cannot coexist in the same cell. This observation led to a classification scheme of plasmids based on incompatibility groups.[14]

Plasmids may determine a wide range of functions besides antibiotic resistance, including virulence and metabolic capacities. Plasmids are autonomous, self-replicating genetic elements that possess an origin for replication and genes that facilitate its stable maintenance in host bacteria. Conjugative plasmids require additional genes that can initiate self-transfer.[14]

The transfer of plasmid DNA between bacterial species is a complex process, and conjugative plasmids tend to be larger than nonconjugative ones. Some small plasmids may be able to use the conjugation apparatus of a coresident conjugative plasmid. Many plasmid-encoded functions enable bacterial strains to persist in the environment by resisting noxious agents, such as heavy metals. Mercury released from dental fillings may increase the number of antibiotic-resistant bacteria in the oral flora.[15] Compounds such as hexachlorophene are used as topical bacteriostatic agents, and plasmid-mediated resistance to these agents has increased significantly.[16]

Transposable Genetic Elements

Transposons can translocate from one area of the bacterial chromosome to another or between the chromosome and plasmid or bacteriophage DNA. Transposable genetic elements possess a specialized system of recombination that is independent of the generalized

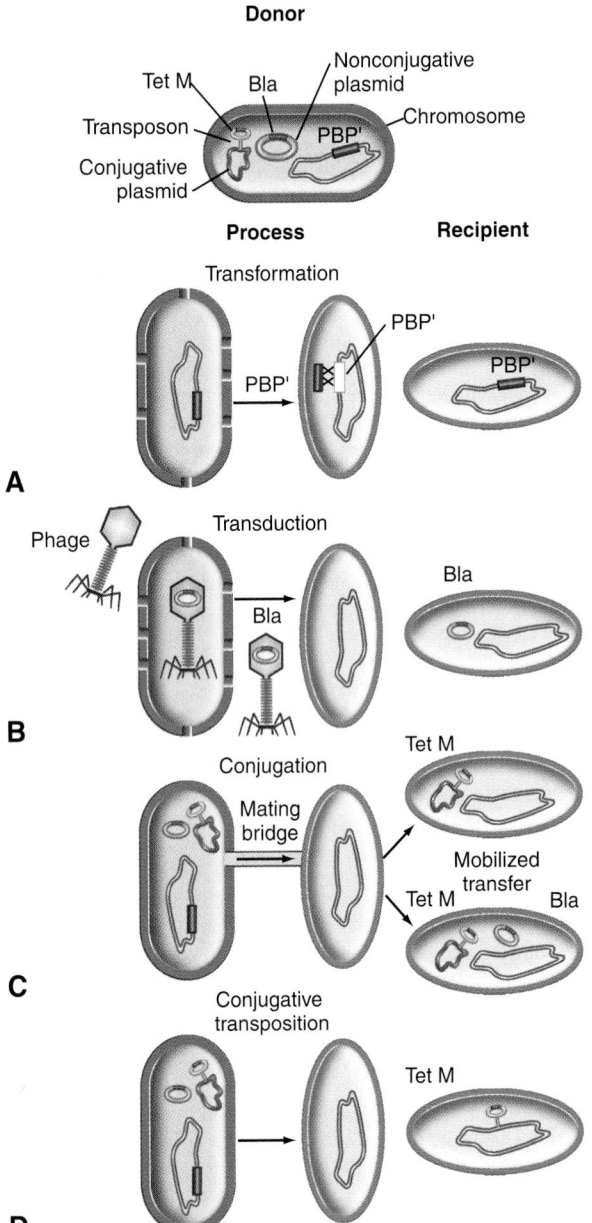

FIGURE 17-1. Examples of recombination events and molecular spread of antibiotic-resistance genes. The donor organism depicted here has three antibiotic-resistance genes: the first on the chromosome, designated as *PBP'*, a low-affinity penicillin-binding protein; the second (a β-lactamase gene labeled *Bla*) on a small nonconjugative plasmid; and the third (*Tet M*—a tetracycline resistance determinant) on a transposon residing on a large self-conjugative plasmid. **A,** Genetic exchange may occur by transformation (naked DNA transfer for dying bacteria to a competent recipient). This generally results in transfer of homologous genes located on the chromosome by recombination enzymes (*recA*). **B,** Transduction also may transfer antibiotic-resistance genes (usually from small plasmids) by imprecise packaging of nucleic acids by transducing bacteriophages. **C,** Conjugation is an efficient method of gene transfer requiring physical contact between donor and recipient. Self-transferable plasmids mediate direct contact by forming a mating bridge between cells. Smaller nonconjugative plasmids might be mobilized in this mating process and be transported into the recipient. **D,** Transposons are specialized sequences of DNA that possess their own recombination enzymes (transposases) allowing for transposition ("hopping") from one location to another independent of the recombination enzymes of the host (*recA*-independent). They may transpose to nonhomologous sequences of DNA and spread antibiotic-resistance genes to multiple plasmids or genomic locations throughout the host. Some transposons possess the ability to move directly from a donor to a recipient independent of other gene transfer events (conjugative transposons).

recombination system that classically permits recombination of largely homologous sequences of DNA by crossover events (the *recA* system of bacteria). The *recA*-independent recombination system ("transposase") of transposable elements usually occurs in a random fashion between nonhomologous sequences of DNA and results in whole-scale modifications of large sequences of DNA as a single event (Fig. 17-2).[2,5]

There are two types of transposable genetic elements, called *transposons* and *insertion sequences,* which have similar characteristics. Evidence from whole-genome sequencing projects indicates that bacterial chromosomes are replete with transposable elements.[17] These mobile sequences probably play an important physiologic role in genetic variation and evolution in prokaryotic organisms. Transposons differ from insertion sequences in that they mediate a recognizable phenotypic characteristic, such as an antibiotic-resistance marker. Either element can translocate as an independent unit. Both elements are flanked on either end by short identical sequences of DNA in reverse order (*inverted repeats*). These inverted-repeat DNA termini are

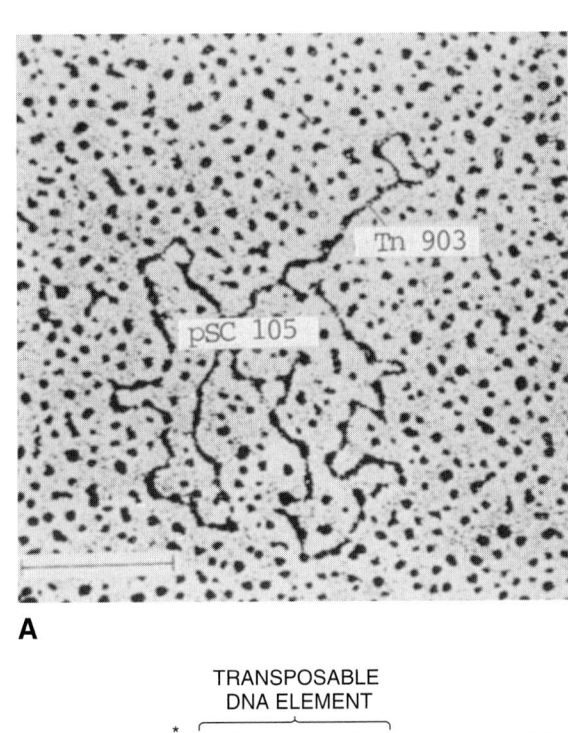

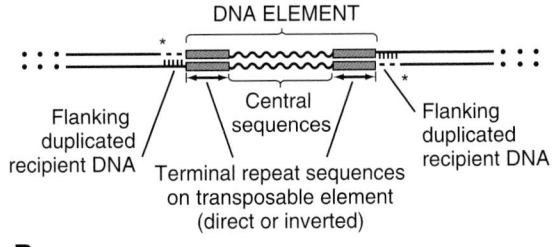

FIGURE 17-2. A, Characteristic appearance of a transposon by electron microscopy showing the stem-loop configuration. The kanamycin resistance transposon Tn903 is inserted into a small plasmid (pSC105). After denaturation, intrastrand annealing of the complementary 1000-bp, inverted repeat, terminal sequences of the transposon forms the stem structure. The kanamycin-resistance gene and the genes necessary for transposition are located in the central loop structure. **B,** Structure of a transposable element inserted into a recipient DNA sequence. The transposon (*rectangles* and *wavy lines*) consists of a central sequence containing the phenotypic marker gene(s) (antibiotic-resistance gene) and the "transposase" genes. The terminal-repeat sequences of the transposon flank the central sequences on both sides. Insertion of the transposon results in single-strand, staggered cuts in the recipient DNA (*asterisks*). Subsequent gap-filling DNA synthesis and ligation results in duplication of a short sequence of recipient DNA at either end of the transposon.

essential to the transposition process. Transposons and insertion sequences are incapable of autonomous self-replication and must exist on a replicon, such as the chromosome, bacteriophage, or plasmid, to be replicated and maintained in a bacterial population. Some transposons have the capability to move from one bacterium to another without being fixed within a plasmid or bacteriophage. These elements are referred to as *conjugative* transposons and have been found primarily in aerobic and anaerobic gram-positive organisms.[18]

Transposition usually results in the localized replication of the transposable element from the original donor sequence of DNA and the insertion of a copy of the transposable element into the recipient sequence of DNA (replicative transposition).[2,5] Transposition, similar to point mutation, is a continuous, ongoing process in bacterial populations. An example of this phenomenon is the spread of a tetracycline-resistance transposon among *Neisseria gonorrhoeae, Mycoplasma hominis,* and *Ureaplasma urealyticum.*[19,20] Transposons also are essential in the evolution of resistance plasmids that contain multiple antibiotic-resistance determinants.[16] High-level vancomycin resistance (vanA) in enterococci is mediated by a composite transposon that encodes a series of genes needed to express vancomycin resistance.[21] Single transposons may encode multiple antibiotic-resistance determinants within their inverted-repeat termini as well.[5]

Genetic exchange of antibiotic-resistance genes occurs between bacteria of widely disparate species and different genera.[22,23] Identical aminoglycoside-resistance genes occur in streptococci and *Campylobacter,*[23] and enterococci apparently have acquired aminoglycoside[24] and β-lactam[25] resistance from staphylococci. Given the highly variable environmental selection pressures created by antibiotics and the plasticity of bacterial genomes, the ongoing evolution of multiresistant species seems inevitable.[26-31]

DNA Integration Elements

The structural genes that mediate antibiotic resistance often are closely linked and may exist in tandem along the bacterial chromosome or plasmid. Genetic analysis of sequences of DNA adjacent to antibiotic-resistance genes has revealed that unique integration units often exist near promoter sites.[32]

These integration elements, called *integrons,*[33] function as recombinational "hot spots" for site-specific recombination events between largely nonhomologous sequences of DNA. Integrons facilitate the lateral transfer and integration of antibiotic-resistance genes from mobile gene cassettes. The integron provides its own unique integrase function[34] that facilitates *rec*A-independent recombination and a specialized attachment and integration site consisting of a variable length (57 to 141 base pairs [bp]) but often a 59-bp sequence of highly conserved DNA. This 59-bp element is preserved at the 3′ end of inserted antibiotic-resistance genes.[35,36]

Although these integration elements differ structurally and functionally from transposons,[37] they seem to be widespread in bacterial populations and play an important role in the dissemination of antibiotic-resistance genes.[38,39] Integrons do not transpose independently as a specific unit structure from one sequence of DNA to another. This capability of autonomous movement of large sequences of DNA is reserved primarily for transposons and insertion sequence elements. They may become flanked, however, by transposable elements and become integrated into an existing transposon. The principal role of integrons is to provide a convenient insertion site for antibiotic-resistance genes from foreign DNA sources.

There are five classes of integrons that encode antibiotic-resistance genes, with type I integrons being the most common in pathogenic microorganisms.[39] A schematic representation of a class I integron is shown in Figure 17-3. Integrons also serve as expression cassettes for antibiotic-resistance genes in that an efficient promoter site is provided in close proximity to the 5′ end of the newly inserted DNA sequence. The frequency of transcription of integrated cassettes of antibiotic-resistance genes depends on the proximity of the gene to the promoter at the 5′ upstream end of the integron. The level of expression of a resistance gene diminishes as the distance between the promoter and the specific antibiotic-resistance gene cassette increases.[34] Numerous clusters of different antibiotic-resistance genes have been identified that have evolved through specific insertions into common integrons.[35] Integrons have been found to possess five antibiotic-resistance genes in sequence from a single integron unit.[40]

MECHANISMS OF ANTIBIOTIC RESISTANCE

At least seven distinctive mechanisms of antibiotic resistance have been described in bacteria (Table 17-1).[37]

Enzymatic Inhibition

β-Lactamases

Resistance to β-lactam antibiotics is due mainly to the production of β-lactamases, enzymes that inactivate these antibiotics by splitting the amide bond of the β-lactam ring. Numerous β-lactamases exist, encoded either by chromosomal genes or by transferable genes located on plasmids or transposons.[3]

Four evolutionarily distinct classes of β-lactamases have been defined on the basis of amino acid and nucleotide sequence studies.[41] Class A β-lactamases have molecular weights around 29,000, possess a serine residue at their active site, and preferentially hydrolyze penicillins. An example is the TEM-1 β-lactamase, which is widely prevalent in gram-negative bacilli. Class B enzymes are metalloenzymes that have a zinc-binding thiol group required for β-lactamase activity. Class C includes the β-lactamase determined by the chromosomal *ampC* gene of *Escherichia coli* K-12, which shares extensive sequence homology with chromosomally mediated β-lactamases of *Shigella* and *Klebsiella* spp. These enzymes are large proteins (molecular weight about 39,000) with mainly cephalosporinase activity. They also have serine at their active site but share little homology with the class A β-lactamases.[42] The tertiary structures of class C β-lactamases show striking similarities to penicillin-binding proteins (PBPs), from which they may have evolved.[43-45] Class D β-lactamases are oxacillin-hydrolyzing enzymes.

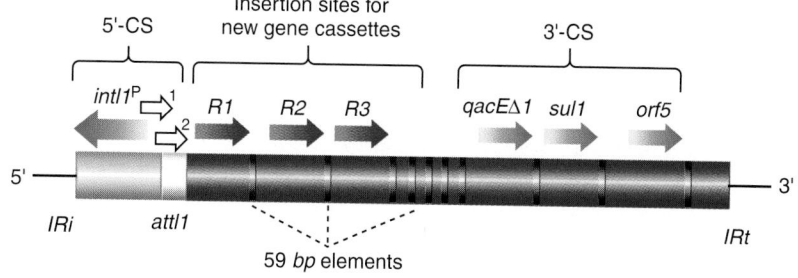

FIGURE 17-3. Organization of a hypothetical class I integron: The 5′ conserved sequence (5′-CS) contains a site-specific integrase (*intI1*); an attachment site (*attI1*), which functions as a receptor for new gene cassettes; and two potential promoter sites (P1 and P2). The promoter is the initiation site for the transcription of the multiple, potential, antibiotic gene cassettes (labeled *R1, R2, R3*) that are inserted downstream from the promoter. Repeated, variable-length, but usually 59-bp elements flank the central antibiotic-resistance gene cassettes. The conserved 3′ end of the integron (3′-CS) usually consists of a gene for resistance to quaternary ammonium compounds, a sulfonamide-resistance gene, and another open reading frame (*orf5*). The outer boundaries of the integron structure are flanked by a 25-bp inverted repeat sequence (noted as *IRi* and *IRt*).

TABLE 17-1 Major Mechanisms of Resistance by Antimicrobial Class

	β-lactams	Aminoglycosides	Chloramphenicol	Macrolides	Sulfonamides	Tetracyclines
Enzymatic inactivation	+++	+++	+++	+ (gram-negative)	−	+
Decreased permeability	+ (gram-negative)	+ (gram-negative)	+ (gram-negative)	++ (gram-negative)	−	+ (gram-negative)
Efflux	+	+	+	++	−	+++
Alteration of target site	++	++	−	+++	++	+ (H. pylori)
Protection of target site	−	−	−	−	−	++
Overproduction of target	−	−	−	−	++	−
Bypass of inhibited process	−	−	−	−	+	−

+++, most common mechanism; ++, common; + less common.

Gram-Positive Bacteria. Among gram-positive bacteria, staphylococci are the major pathogens that produce β-lactamase. Staphylococcal β-lactamases preferentially hydrolyze penicillins. Most are inducible and are excreted extracellularly.[3] The genes that determine staphylococcal β-lactamases usually are carried on small plasmids or transposons. Larger plasmids encoding β-lactamase and other resistances also exist and can transfer by conjugation, not only between strains of *S. aureus,* but also between *S. aureus* and *Staphylococcus epidermidis.*[46]

Enterococci produce a plasmid-determined β-lactamase that seems to be of staphylococcal origin.[47] Since the appearance of the first strain in Texas in 1981, β-lactamase–producing enterococci have been found throughout the United States and in South America.[48] The genes often coexist with genes that determine high-level resistance to gentamicin and may occur on transposons and on plasmids. These transposons are similar to staphylococcal β-lactamase transposons and may be derived from them.[49]

Gram-Negative Bacteria. Gram-negative bacteria produce a much greater variety of β-lactamases than do gram-positive bacteria. This diversity has led to several classification schemes. A classification by Bush and colleagues[41] groups β-lactamases according to substrate profiles and inhibition by clavulanic acid (Table 17-2). The relationships between these functional groups and the β-lactamase classes based on amino acid sequence are shown in Figure 17-4.

β-Lactamases encoded by plasmids are a special concern because the possibility of spread among different strains and different species of pathogens increases. Many types exist.[50,51] All are produced constitutively and can be grouped into seven broad classes, as follows:

1. Broad-spectrum enzymes that hydrolyze benzylpenicillin and cephaloridine at similar rates.
2. Oxacillinases that hydrolyze oxacillin and related penicillins rapidly.
3. Carbenicillinases that break down carbenicillin readily.

4. Extended-spectrum β-lactamases, mutant class A oxyimino-β-lactamases derived from the widely prevalent plasmid-determined TEM, SHV, or OXA β-lactamases.
5. Other class A oxyimino-β-lactamases not related to TEM, SHV, or OXA β-lactamases. Two subgroups in this class consist of six β-lactamases that have high sequence homology with the class A chromosomal β-lactamase of *Klebsiella oxytoca* and two novel β-lactamases, PER-1 and PER-2, that have little sequence similarity to any other known β-lactamases. The former tends to confer resistance to cefuroxime and aztreonam but not to ceftazidime, whereas the latter may confer resistance to ceftibuten, an unusual characteristic for class A β-lactamases.
6. Enzymes that break down cephamycins and oxyimino-β-lactams and are resistant to inhibition by clavulanate. The genes that encode these enzymes are similar in nucleotide sequence to chromosomal β-lactamase genes of *Enterobacter cloacae* (two enzymes) or *Citrobacter freundii* (four enzymes). Both types have caused outbreaks in hospitals in Greece and the United States. A group of five enzymes (FOX related) in this class have been isolated only from unique patient isolates so far and have no close nucleotide sequence similarity to any naturally occurring chromosomal β-lactamase outside the group.
7. Carbapenemases that confer resistance to imipenem or meropenem. Plasmid-mediated metalloenzymes have been identified in Japan. One (IMP-1) has spread in many hospitals around Tokyo. Two non–metallo-β-lactamases, not yet sequenced, that confer resistance to carbapenems have been found in isolates of *Acinetobacter* from Europe and Argentina. Properties of the plasmid-determined β-lactamases are summarized in Table 17-3.

Anaerobic Bacteria. β-Lactamases also contribute to the resistance of anaerobic bacteria to β-lactam antibiotics.[52,53] The β-lactamases of fusobacteria and clostridia are principally penicillinases.[54,55] The β-lactamases produced by *Bacteroides fragilis* are predominantly cephalosporinases, some of which have been found to hydrolyze

TABLE 17-2 The Bush-Jacoby-Medeiros Functional Classification Scheme for β-Lactamases

Group	Enzyme Type	Inhibition by Clavulanate	Molecular Class	No. of Enzymes	Examples*
1	Cephalosporinase	No	C	57	*Enterobacter cloacae* P99 (C), MIR-1 (P)
2a	Penicillinase	Yes	A	20	*Bacillus cereus* I, *Staphylococcus aureus* (B)
2b	Broad-spectrum	Yes	A	16	SHV-1 (B), TEM-1 (P)
2be	Extended-spectrum	Yes	A	81	*Klebsiella oxytoca* K1 (C), TEM-3 (P), SHV-2 (P)
2br†	Inhibitor-resistant	Diminished	A	13	TEM-30 (IRT-2) (P)
2c	Carbenicillinase	Yes	A	15	AER-1 (C), PSE-1 (P), CARB-3 (P)
2d	Cloxacillinase	Yes	D or A	21	*Streptomyces cacaoi* (C), OXA-1 (P)
2e	Cephalosporinase	Yes	A	19	*Proteus vulgaris* (C), FEC-1 (P)
2f†	Carbapenemase	Yes	A	3	IMI-1 (C), NMC-A (C), Sme-1 (C)
3	Carbapenemase	No	B	15	*Stenotrophomonas maltophilia* L1 (C), IMP-1 (P)
4	Penicillinase	No		7	*Burkholderia cepacia* (C), SAR-2 (P)

*B, both; C, chromosomal; P, plasmid.
†New groups.
From Bush K, Jacoby GA, Madeiros AA. A functional classification scheme for β-lactamases and its correlation with molecular structure. Antimicrob Agents Chemother. 1995;39:1211–1233.

Trimethoprim	Quinolones	Glycopeptides	Linosamides; Streptogramins	Rifampin	Polymyxim
–	–	–	–		–
+ (gram-negative)	+ (gram-negative)	++ (gram-negative)	+ (gram-negative)	–	+++ (gram-negative)
–	+	–		–	–
+++	+++	+++	+++	+++	–
–	+	–	–	–	–
++	–	+	–	–	–
+	–	–	–	–	–

cefoxitin and imipenem and may be transferable.[56-61] Most of the cephalosporinases are inhibited by clavulanate, sulbactam, or tazobactam. Some isolates of *Bacteroides* produce carbapenemases, metalloenzymes inhibited by ethylenediaminetetraacetic acid but not clavulanate, that confer resistance to imipenem.

Distribution in Clinical Isolates. The existence of β-lactamase genes on plasmids and transposons ensures that a β-lactamase originally confined to one group of bacteria sooner or later may appear in other groups. The widespread use of antibiotics fosters selection of the resistant organisms that rise in prevalence locally and spread worldwide. A prime example of this process occurred with the TEM-1 β-lactamase, which has spread from the Enterobacteriaceae to *Haemophilus influenzae*[62] and *N. gonorrhoeae*.[63] Clinical isolates may produce two or three plasmid-determined β-lactamases. In nearly all cases, TEM-1 is one of the β-lactamases produced. Many strains from South America and the Far East have had novel or multiple, or both, plasmid β-lactamases.[51] The OXA extended-spectrum β-lactamases and the plasmid-mediated metallocarbapenemase IMP-1 so far have proliferated only in certain regions of Turkey and Japan.

The success of the pharmaceutical industry in developing new β-lactams resistant to hydrolysis by β-lactamases led to the introduction into clinical use of the third-generation β-lactam antibiotics around 1978 in Europe and 1981 in the United States. These antibiotics were very resistant to hydrolysis by the known plasmid-determined β-lactamases. In 1983, in Germany, isolates of *Klebsiella pneumoniae* and other Enterobacteriaceae were discovered that produce a plasmid-determined β-lactamase that hydrolyzes cefotaxime and other newer cephalosporins. This new β-lactamase, called *SHV-2,* derived from a mutation in the well-known SHV-1 β-lactamase commonly found in *Klebsiella*. The mutation resulted in an enhanced affinity of the SHV-1 β-lactamase for cefotaxime.[64] Subsequently, ceftazidime-resistant strains of *K. pneumoniae* producing a novel plasmid-encoded ceftazidime-hydrolyzing β-lactamase, designated *CTX-1,* were isolated in several French hospitals.[65] Nucleotide sequencing studies showed that this enzyme differed from TEM-2 by only two amino acids. Since then, there has been a rapid increase in the number and variety of extended-spectrum β-lactamases.[66] The numbers of derivatives of the TEM and SHV β-lactamases proved to be unique by sequencing have reached greater than 60 for TEM and greater than 30 for SHV (see G. Jacoby and K. Bush, http://www.lahey.org/studies/webt.htm).[66,67] Several β-lactamases (SHV-2, SHV-4, SHV-5, TEM-6) occur in many countries, whereas others seem to occur more commonly in one or two countries. TEM-3 is prevalent in France, and TEM-10 and TEM-12 are prevalent in the United States and England.[66,68] The varied national patterns of antibiotic use in hospitals probably account for the differences in distribution of these enzymes. Several extended-spectrum β-lactamases derived from OXA enzymes have been found in *Pseudomonas aeruginosa* isolates from Turkey.[69,70] Most of the clinical isolates that produce extended-spectrum β-lactamases have come from hospitalized patients and frequently have caused nosocomial outbreaks, mostly due to *K. pneumoniae*. Surveys of hospital isolates of *K. pneumoniae* in England,[71] France,[72] and Portugal[73] show that 14% to 16% produce extended-spectrum β-lactamases. In France, the prevalence increased from less than 1% in 1985 to the current level by 1988. Extended-spectrum β-lactamases also are found in nearly all

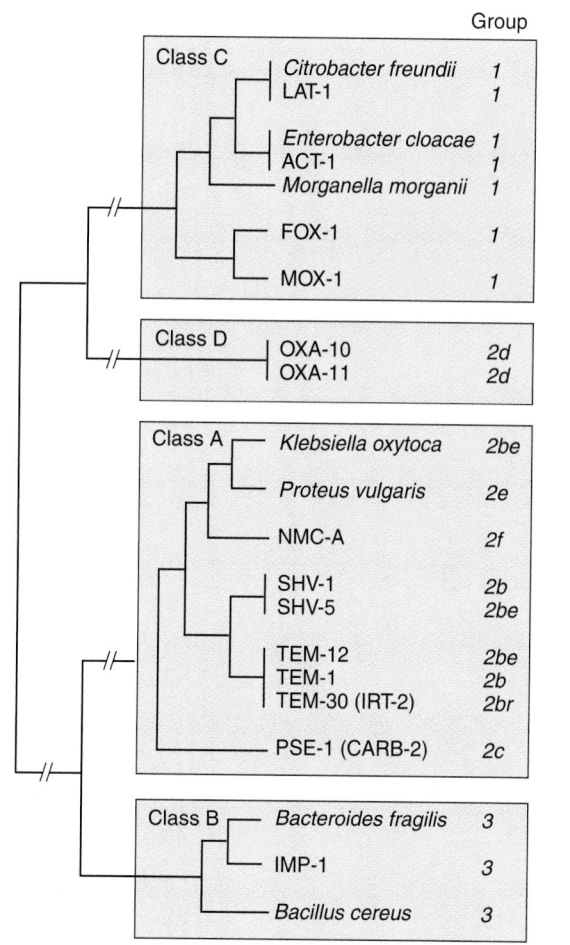

FIGURE 17-4. Correlation between amino acid sequences (Ambler classes) and functional properties of β-lactamases (Bush-Jacoby-Medeiros groups). *(Adapted from Philippon A, Dusart J, Doris B, Frère JM. The diversity, structure and regulation of β-lactamases. Cell Mol Life Sci. 1998;54:341-346.)*

other species of Enterobacteriaceae, but they occur infrequently. In a French survey, 2% to 3% of *Enterobacter* spp. and *K. oxytoca* but only 0.1% of *E. coli* produced extended-spectrum β-lactamases.[72] Surveys of strains isolated since 1988 in England and Portugal also document a low frequency in *E. coli*.[71,74] Reports of extended-spectrum β-lactamases in *Proteus mirabilis* have been relatively rare.[75-80] In *Proteus* spp., the spread of extended-spectrum β-lactamases may be limited by a low frequency of plasmid conjugation.[81]

Sporadic nosocomial outbreaks due to strains producing extended-spectrum β-lactamases seem to have led to an endemic problem in some hospitals. Sometimes patients from nursing homes and other long-term care institutions bring these strains into the hospital.[82,83] Selection pressure from widespread hospital use of a β-lactam apparently enhances

TABLE 17-3 Properties of Plasmid-Determined Beta-Lactamases

β-lactamase	pI	Prevalence	Host Bacteria	Specific Features
1. Broad Spectrum[51]				
HMS-1	5.2	Rare	Enterobacteriaceae	
TEM-1	5.4	Very common	Enterobacteriaceae *Pseudomonas aeruginosa* *Haemophilus influenzae* *Neisseria gonorrhoeae* *Vibrio cholerae*	Most common plasmid-determined β-lactamase in nearly all bacterial species
TLE-1	5.55	Rare	*Escherichia coli*	Closely related to TEM-1
TEM-2	5.6	Common	Enterobacteriaceae	Differs from TEM-1 by one amino acid, away from binding site
LCR-1	5.85 or 6.5	Rare	*P. aeruginosa*	Not inhibited by clavulanic acid
NPS-1	6.5	Rare	*P. aeruginosa*	Cefsulodin induces conformational change
TLE-2	6.5	Rare	*Klebsiella pneumoniae*	High affinity for cefsulodin and cefotetan
LXA-1	6.7	Uncommon	Enterobacteriaceae	Very low affinity for benzyl penicillin Confers low-level β-lactam resistance
OHIO-1	7.0	Uncommon	*Enterobacter cloacae* *Serratia marcescens*	Found only in isolates from Ohio Similar to SHV-1
SHV-1 (PIT-2)	7.6	Common	Enterobacteriaceae	Often encoded by chromosomal genes in *K. pneumoniae*
ROB-1	8.1	Uncommon	*H. influenzae* *Haemophilus pleuropneumoniae* *Pasteurella multocida*	Found in both human and animal isolates
2. Oxacillinase[51]				
OXA-9	6.9	Rare	*K. pneumoniae*	Encoded by *Tn 1331*
OXA-3	7.1	Uncommon	Enterobacteriaceae *P. aeruginosa*	
OXA-1	7.4	Common	Enterobacteriaceae *P. aeruginosa*	Second most common type in *E. coli*
OXA-4	7.45	Rare	Enterobacteriaceae	Closely related to OXA-1
OXA-8	7.6?	Rare	?	Encoded by p40Tn2
OXA-5	7.62	Rare	*P. aeruginosa*	
OXA-7	7.65	Rare	*E. coli*	
OXA-6	7.68	Rare	*P. aeruginosa*	
OXA-2	7.7	Common	Enterobacteriaceae *P. aeruginosa*	Second most common type in salmonellae
3. Carbenicillinase[51]				
CARB-4	4.3	Rare	*P. aeruginosa*	
SAR-1	4.9	Rare	*V. cholerae*	
PSE-4 (CARB-1)	5.3	Uncommon	*P. aeruginosa* Enterobacteriaceae	
BRO-1,2,3	Multiple bands (5.3-7.7)	Common	*Moraxella (Brahamella)*	Confers resistance to cefsulodin Confers resistance to ampicillin and cefaclor Found in *Moraxella catarrhalis*; may be on conjugative transposon
PSE-1 (CARB-2)	5.7	Common	*P. aeruginosa* Enterobacteriaceae	Most common type in *P. aeruginosa*
CARB-3	5.75	Rare	*P. aeruginosa*	
CARB-5	6.3	Rare	*Acinetobacter baumannii*	Susceptible to ticarcillin combined with clavulanate
PSE-3	6.9	Uncommon	*P. aeruginosa* Enterobacteriaceae	
Unnamed (N-29)	6.9 (6.93)	Rare	*Proteus mirabilis*	
4. Extended-Spectrum				
Class A β-lactamases related to TEM, SHV, or OXA—confer resistance to cefotaxime, ceftazidime or aztreonam[*]				
TEM-Derived TEM-3-TEM-29, TEM-42-TEM-43, TEM-46-TEM-67	5.2-6.5	Nosocomial outbreaks worldwide	*K. pneumoniae*; less common in other Enterobacteriaceae	One to four amino acid substitutions in TEM-1 or TEM-2 active site structure Confer resistance mainly to ceftazidime or aztreonam Susceptible to clavulanate
SHV-Derived SHV-2-SHV-12	7.0-8.2	Nosocomial outbreaks worldwide	*K. pneumoniae* Less common in other Enterobacteriaceae	One to three amino acid substitutions in SHV-1 active site; confer greater resistance to cefotaxime than TEM derivatives
Inhibitor-Resistant TEM-30-TEM-40, TEM-44–TEM-45	5.2-5.4	Nosocomial isolates from Europe	*E. coli*	One to two amino acid substitutions in TEM-1 or TEM-2 active site Resistant to inhibition by clavulanate but often more susceptible to cefazolin than TEM-1

[*]For full references, see Jacoby GA, Bush K. http://www.lahey.org/studies/webt.htm.

TABLE 17-3   Properties of Plasmid-Determined Beta-Lactamases—cont'd

β-lactamase	pI	Prevalence	Host Bacteria	Specific Features
OXA-Derived				
OXA-11, OXA-14-16	6.1-8.0	Nosocomial isolates from Turkey	*P. aeruginosa*	One or two amino acid substitutions in the OXA active site
5. Other Class A β-Lactamases Not Related to TEM, SHV, or OXA (confer resistance to cefuroxime)				
CTX-M-2[247]	5.5	Clinical isolates from Argentina	*Salmonella typhimurium, E. coli, V. cholerae*	Most common oxyimin-β-lactamase in *E. coli* in Argentina
Toho-1[248]	7.8	Clinical isolate from Japan	*E. coli*	
Toho-2[249]	?	Urinary isolate from Japan	*E. coli*	Inhibited by tazobactam more than clavulanate
MEN-1 (CTX-M-1)[247]	8.4	Clinical isolates from France and Germany	*E. coli*	
CTX-M-3[250]	8.4	Urinary isolates from hospital in Poland	*E. coli, Citrobacter freundii*	
CTX-M-4[251]	8.4	Six isolates from Russia	*S. typhimurium*	
PER-1[252]	5.4	Isolates from Turkey	*P. aeruginosa K. pneumoniae Acinetobacter*	Confer resistance to ceftibuten, PER-2 (86% homology)
PER-2[253]	5.4	Isolates from Argentina	*S. typhimurium* Other Enterobacteriaceae Not in *P. aeruginosa*	Hydrolyzes ceftibuten
6. Class C Cephamycinases (confer resistance to cefoxitin or cefotetan)				
Sequence Like E. cloacae *Chromosomal β-Lactamase*				
MIR-1[101]	8.4	Outbreak in Providence, RI	*K. pneumoniae*	
ACT-1[254]	9.0	Nosocomial isolates from New York City	*E. coli K. pneumoniae*	Confers resistance to imipenem in porin-deficient strain
Sequence Like C. freundii *Chromosomal β-Lactamase*				
BIL-1[255, 256]	8.8	Burn unit in Pakistan	*E. coli*	
CMY-2[257]	9.0	Urine isolates from Greece	*K. pneumoniae C. freundii*	
SAL-1[258]	9.0	Stool isolate from Nigeria	*Salmonella senftenberg*	
LAT-1[259]	9.4	Nosocomial isolates from Greece	*K. pneumoniae*	
LAT-2[260]	9.4, 9.1, 8.9	Nosocomial isolates from Greek hospitals	*K. pneumoniae E. coli, Enterobacter aerogenes*	
Sequence Like Morganella morganii *Chromosomal β-Lactamase*				
MOR-1[261]	?	Clinical isolate	*Salmonella enteritidis*	Encoded by integron-like structure
FOX-Related				
FOX-1[262]	6.8 or 7.2	Blood isolate from a Buenos Aires hospital	*K. pneumoniae*	No close nucleotide sequence similarity to any naturally occurring chromosomal β-lactamase
FOX-2[263]	6.7	Urinary isolate from Guatemala	*E. coli*	97% sequence identity with FOX-1
FOX-3[264]	7.25	Vaginal isolate from Italy	*Klebsiella oxytoca*	96% homology with FOX-1
CMY-1[265]	8.0	Wound isolate from Korea	*K. pneumoniae*	89% homology to MOX-1
MOX-1[266, 267]	8.9	Urinary isolate from Nagoya, Japan	*K. pneumoniae*	51% homology with *P. aeruginosa* PAO1, 69% with FOX-1
Unknown Source				
CEP-1[268]	8.0	Rare	*P. mirabilis*	
7. Carbapenemases Confers Resistance to Imipenem/Meropenem				
Metallo-enzymes (class B β-lactamases)				
IMP-1[104]	9.0	Isolates from hospitals in Japan	*P. aeruginosa S. marcescens Alcaligenes xylosoxidans Pseudomonas putida K. pneumoniae*	Hydrolyzes imipenem Resistant to clavulanate
			Bacteroides fragilis	Encoded on small self-transmissible plasmid Sequence identical to chromosomal CcrA (CfiA) β-lactamases in *Bacteroides* isolates from United States
Unnamed[269, 270]	?	Wound isolate from Japan		
ARI-1[106, 107]	6.65	Blood isolate from Scotland	*Acinetobacter baumanii*	Transferred to *Acinetobacter junii*
ARI-2[108]	~7.1	Outbreak in Buenos Aires, Argentina Also found in Europe and Southeast Asia	*Acinetobacter* spp	Inhibited by clavulanate

colonization of the digestive or respiratory tracts of other patients, and infection follows.[67,84] Outbreaks often have been associated with a prolonged hospital stay, surgery, or the presence of urinary or arterial catheters, especially in patients in intensive care units.[84]

Failure to control outbreaks has resulted in the appearance of new mutant-type, extended-spectrum β-lactamases in the same institution and sometimes in the same patient. In Clermont-Ferrand hospital, eight different extended-spectrum β-lactamases (TEM-3, TEM-5, TEM-8, TEM-12, TEM-24, TEM-16, SHV-4, and SHV-5) have appeared since the first surfaced in 1984.[85] Plasmid and strain dissemination have occurred. The finding of CAZ-7-producing *K. pneumoniae* and *E. coli* in the same patient led to the discovery that the CAZ-7 and amikacin genes were on a fragment that could translocate to different plasmids. Other extended-spectrum β-lactamase genes (i.e., genes for TEM-3 and TEM-12) are known to reside on transposons.[86-88] TEM-12 arose as the result of a single point mutation in a plasmid bearing the gene for TEM-1 that had been seen 12 years earlier in one hospital.[89] Apparently, single point mutations and recombinations between different β-lactamase genes are yielding new extended-spectrum β-lactamases in the "hot house" environments where these genes are endemic.[89,90]

Other genetic events also may be contributing to the resistance mediated by extended-spectrum β-lactamases. In many strains producing TEM-6 and other TEM variants, researchers have found IS1-like elements that insert into the promoter of the gene for TEM-6 and increase its strength, causing high-level production of these extended-spectrum β-lactamases.[91] Even the high-level production of the parent β-lactamase SHV-1 confers resistance to ceftazidime and aztreonam.[92]

Isolates of *E. coli* that produce a new class of TEM-derived, plasmid-borne β-lactamase have been found in France, Scotland, and Spain.[93-95] These so-called TRI or IRT β-lactamases confer resistance to β-lactamase inhibitors (clavulanate, sulbactam) but not to the oxyimino-β-lactams, such as cefotaxime, aztreonam, and ceftazidime.

β-Lactamases Determined by Chromosomal Genes. Virtually all gram-negative bacteria produce some chromosomally determined β-lactamase. The types of β-lactamases produced are often specific for species and sometimes for subspecies. β-Lactamase activity frequently is very low, particularly in ampicillin-susceptible isolates, but it may increase because of either induction or alteration in the number of β-lactamase genes on the chromosome.[96] Also, mutation of genes that regulate induction may lead to constitutive hyperproduction of inducible β-lactamases.[97] Selection of hyperproducer mutants caused the emergence of resistance to third-generation cephalosporins in 19% of patients receiving third-generation cephalosporins for *Enterobacter* bacteremia.[98] Most of the clinically relevant, chromosomally determined β-lactamases belonging to Bush group 1 preferentially hydrolyze cephalosporins and are resistant to inhibition by clavulanic acid. They inactivate many of the third-generation β-lactams that are resistant to hydrolysis by most of the plasmid-determined β-lactamases. The metallo-β-lactamases that hydrolyze carbapenems are a growing threat of great concern.[99]

Chromosomally determined β-lactamases nearly always differ in their biochemical properties from the plasmid-determined enzymes. The exception is a chromosomal β-lactamase found in many isolates of *K. pneumoniae* that is indistinguishable from the SHV-1 β-lactamase. It may be that the gene for SHV-1 β-lactamase evolved as a chromosomal gene in *Klebsiella* and later was incorporated into a plasmid.[100] No such ancestral chromosomal gene has been found for the much more common TEM-1 β-lactamase or for any of the other plasmid-determined β-lactamases.

Chromosomal genes have incorporated into plasmids, a long-feared threat. In Providence, Rhode Island, nosocomial isolates of *K. pneumoniae* and *E. coli* were found to produce the MIR-1 β-lactamase, a plasmid-determined *ampC*-type β-lactamase derived from *E. cloacae*.[101] Besides resistance to oxyimino-β-lactams, the strains also were highly resistant to the 7α-methoxy-β-lactams and the clavam and sulfone β-lactamase inhibitors. Nosocomial isolates of *E. coli* and *K. pneumoniae* producing ACT-1, an *E. cloacae*–like, plasmid-determined β-lactamase, caused an

outbreak in a New York hospital. In addition to resistance to cephamycins and oxyimino-cephalosporins, some porin-deficient isolates were resistant to imipenem as well.[94] Plasmid-borne genes determining *ampC*-type β-lactamases from *C. freundii* (CMY-2, BIL-1, SAL-1, LAT-1, and LAT-2), *Morganella morganii* (MOR-1), and *K. oxytoca* (MEN-1, CTX-M-2, CTX-M-3, CTX-M-4, TOHO-1, and TOHO-2) also have been found. The plasmids were in strains of *K. pneumoniae* and *E. coli* from France, Greece, and Pakistan, showing that the formidable threat posed by them is already worldwide. The discovery in Japan of a strain of *P. aeruginosa* producing a plasmid-mediated metallo-β-lactamase, IMP-1, that confers resistance to imipenem and all other β-lactams presents an even greater threat.[102] IMP-1 has spread to *Serratia* and other gram-negative bacilli, causing multifocal outbreaks in hospitals around Tokyo.[103-105] Reports of transferable carbapenemases (apparently non–metallo-β-lactamases) in *Acinetobacter* isolates from Scotland and Argentina are equally disturbing.[106-108]

Contribution of β-Lactamases to β-Lactam Antibiotic Resistance. The level of antibiotic resistance mediated by a particular β-lactamase in a population of bacteria is determined by several variables. The efficiency of the β-lactamase in hydrolyzing an antibiotic depends on its rate of hydrolysis and its affinity for the antibiotic. Other variables are the amount of β-lactamase produced by the bacterial cell, the susceptibility of the target protein (PBP) to the antibiotic, and the rate of diffusion of the antibiotic into the periplasm of the cell.

Within the bacterial cell, β-lactamases contribute to antibiotic resistance in several ways. The simplest model is that of penicillinase-producing staphylococci, in which the bacteria, on exposure to penicillin, begin to produce β-lactamase, which they excrete extracellularly. Two events then take place concurrently: (1) Penicillin lyses bacteria, and (2) β-lactamase hydrolyzes penicillin. If viable bacterial cells remain after the level of penicillin has declined to less than the minimal inhibitory concentration (MIC), regrowth of bacteria occurs.[40]

Another model is exemplified by gram-negative bacilli, which (1) produce a β-lactamase that remains trapped in the periplasmic space and (2) have no barrier to antibiotic penetration. An example is *H. influenzae* strains that produce the TEM-1 β-lactamase.[109] In this model and the first one discussed, a marked inoculum effect occurs in that the MIC for a large inoculum (10^6 organisms/mL) may be 1000-fold greater than that for a small inoculum (10^2 organisms/mL). The low level of resistance of single cells has made it possible for ampicillin to cure some infections caused by β-lactamase-producing strains of *H. influenzae* when the inoculum of infecting bacteria was low.

Another model is exemplified by ampicillin resistance of *E. coli* strains that produce the TEM-1 β-lactamase. These bacteria have a barrier to entry of β-lactam molecules (the outer membrane), and they produce a β-lactamase that remains localized to the periplasmic space. In this model, the kinetics are more complicated. The enzyme is situated strategically between the barrier to antibiotic penetration (outer membrane) and the antibiotic targets (penicillin-binding proteins on the cytoplasmic membrane). In this position, the enzyme can destroy antibiotic molecules sequentially as they make their way through the barrier, analogous to a sharpshooter with abundant ammunition who aims at targets passing through a single entry point. As a consequence, high levels of resistance occur with single bacterial cells, in contrast to the previous example.[40]

Variations on this model occur when the amount of β-lactamase produced increases with exposure to a β-lactam (induction), as occurs in *Enterobacter* and *Pseudomonas* spp. High levels of β-lactamase are produced only after a period of exposure to the inducing antibiotic, and resistance may be expressed late. When *Enterobacter* strains are exposed to two β-lactam antibiotics, one of which is a potent inducer (e.g., cefamandole), antagonism between the two antibiotics may result.[110]

Table 17-4 lists mechanisms of resistance to β-lactam antibiotics. Often these mechanisms work in concert and may accumulate in a single patient. An example is a 19-month-old child with aplastic anemia who over 3 months had nine blood isolates of *E. coli*, all derived from

TABLE 17-4 Mechanisms of Resistance to β-Lactam Antibiotics

I. Alter target site (PBP, penicillin-binding protein)
  A. Decrease affinity of PBP for β-lactam antibiotic
    1. Modify existing PBP
      a. Create mosaic PBP
        Insert nucleotides obtained from neighboring bacteria, e.g., penicillin-resistant *Streptococcus pneumoniae*
        Mutate structural gene of PBP(s), e.g., ampicillin-resistant β-lactamase–negative *Haemophilus influenzae*
    2. Import new PBP, e.g., mecA in methicillin-resistant *Staphylococcus aureus*
II. Destroy β-lactam antibiotic
  A. Increase production of β-lactamase
    1. Acquire more efficient promoter
      a. Mutate existing promoter
      b. Import new one
    2. Deregulate control of β-lactamase production
      a. Mutate regulator genes, e.g., *ampD* in "stably derepressed" *Enterobacter cloacae*
  B. Modify structure of resident β-lactamase
    1. Mutate its structural gene, e.g., extended-spectrum β-lactamases in *Klebsiella pneumoniae*
  C. Import new β-lactamase(s) with different spectrum of activity
III. Decrease concentration of β-lactam antibiotic inside cell
  A. Restrict its entry (loss of porins)
  B Pump it out (efflux mechanisms)

TABLE 17-5 Aminoglycoside-Modifying Enzymes

Enzymes	Usual Antibiotics Modified	Common Genera
Phosphorylation		
APH(2″)	K, T, G,	SA, SR
APH(3′)-I	K	E, PS, SA, SR
APH(3′)-III	K, ± A	E, PS, SA, SR
Acetylation		
AAC(2′)	G	PR
AAC(3)-I	±T, G	E, PS
AAC(3)-III,		
-IV, OR –V	K, T, G	E, PS
AAC(6′)	K, T, (A	E, PS, SA
Adenylation		
ANT(2″)	K, T, GE, PS	
ANT(4′)	K, T, A	SA

A, amikacin; AAC, aminoglycoside acetyltransferase; ANT, aminoglycoside nucleotidyltransferase; APH, aminoglycoside phosphotransferase; E, Enterobacteriaceae; G, gentamicin; K, karamycin; PR, *Providencia-Proteus*; PS, pseudomonids; SA, staphylococci; SR, streptococci; T, tobramycin.

a common ancestor, despite multiple courses of antibiotics including ceftazidime.[111] The first isolate produced a TEM-1 β-lactamase but was susceptible to ceftazidime (MIC 0.25 μg/mL). A subsequent isolate became resistant (MIC of ceftazidime 32 μg/mL) by acquiring a new plasmid-determined β-lactamase (SHV-1) linked to efficient promoter and turning off production of an outer membrane porin. An even higher level of resistance (MIC of ceftazidime ≥128 μg/mL) occurred when the SHV-1 β-lactamase mutated to form the extended-spectrum β-lactamase, SHV-8, which hydrolyzes ceftazidime much more rapidly. By turning off porin production to slow the rate of entry of ceftazidime into the periplasmic space and producing an extended-spectrum, ceftazidime-inactivating β-lactamase, the infecting *E. coli* used two mechanisms synergistically to achieve a high level of resistance to ceftazidime.

Aminoglycoside Resistance–Modifying Enzymes

Among aerobic bacteria, aminoglycoside resistance is most commonly due to modifying enzymes that are coded by genes on plasmids or the chromosome.[112] Several aminoglycoside-modifying enzymes have been shown to be carried on transposons.[18]

More than 30 aminoglycoside-modifying enzymes that have been identified are capable of three general reactions: *N*-acetylation, *O*-nucleotidylation, and *O*-phosphorylation. For each of these general reactions, there are several different enzymes that attack a specific amino or hydroxyl group. The nomenclature for these enzymes lists the molecular site where the modification occurs after the type of enzymatic activity. An aminoglycoside acetyltransferase (AAC) that acts at the 3′ site is designated *AAC (3′)* (Table 17-5).[45] There may be more than one enzyme that catalyzes the same reaction, however, and roman numerals may be necessary (e.g., AAC [3′]–IV).

Enzymatic aminoglycoside resistance is achieved by modification of the antibiotic in the process of transport across the cytoplasmic membrane.[112] Resistance to a particular aminoglycoside is a function of two different rates—that of drug uptake versus that of drug inactivation. An important factor in determining the level of resistance is the affinity of the modifying enzyme for the antibiotic. If an enzyme has a high affinity for the specific aminoglycoside, drug inactivation can occur at very low concentrations of the enzyme.

The differences in the worldwide distribution of aminoglycoside-modifying enzymes may be partially a function of antibiotic selection pressures and may have had profound implications on the choice of antibiotics used at specific medical centers. Aminoglycoside phospho-

transferase (APH) (3′) and APH (3″) are distributed widely among gram-positive and gram-negative species worldwide and have led to decreased use of kanamycin and streptomycin. The gene for aminoglycoside nucleotidyltransferase (ANT) (2″) has been associated with multiple nosocomial outbreaks in the 1990s across the United States. The gene for aminoglycoside acetyltransferase AAC (6′)–I has been found to be more prevalent in East Asia.[113] The AAC (3) group of enzymes have been responsible for outbreaks of antibiotic resistance in South America, western Europe, and the United States. Although each outbreak of aminoglycoside-resistant Enterobacteriaceae has its own pattern, the most typical manner of spread has been the appearance of a plasmid-carrying, aminoglycoside-resistant strain of *K. pneumoniae* usually carrying the ANT (2″) gene, with subsequent dissemination to other strains of the species and further spread later to other species and genera of Enterobacteriaceae.[114]

Major increases in plasmid-mediated aminoglycoside resistance have been noted among enterococci,[28,115,116] initially in the developing world[117] but increasingly in the United States and Europe.[118,119] The plasmids that carry the aminoglycoside-modifying genes in enterococcal outbreaks are heterogeneous.[120] Their clinical impact is exacerbated by the frequent cotransmission of β-lactamases, resulting in a loss of synergy when combination therapy is employed for serious enterococcal infections. *S. aureus* and *S. epidermidis* have become increasingly resistant to aminoglycosides because of the interspecies and intraspecies dissemination of plasmid-mediated, aminoglycoside-modifying enzymes.[121]

Chloramphenicol Acetyltransferase

Resistance to chloramphenicol in gram-positive and gram-negative organisms is mediated primarily by the inactivating enzyme *chloramphenicol acetyltransferase*. This is an intracellular enzyme that inactivates the drug by 3-*O*-acetylation[122] and is encoded by plasmid-borne or chromosomal genes. Despite homology at the active site of this enzyme, there is considerable diversity between chloramphenicol acetyltransferase enzymes isolated from gram-positive and gram-negative organisms.[123]

Macrolide, Lincosamide, Streptogramin, Inactivating Enzymes

Although resistance to erythromycin and other macrolides is frequently the result of alteration in the ribosomal target site or efflux pumps, several substrate-inactivating enzymes have been characterized.[124] Erythromycin esterases have been isolated from *E. coli* that hydrolyze the lactone ring of the antibiotic and result in its inactivation. This is a plasmid-mediated resistance determinant that is constitutively produced and results in high-level resistance to erythromycin (MIC >2000 μg/mL).[125] These resistance determinants may limit the utility of oral erythromycin in reducing the aerobic gram-negative flora of the intestinal tract before gastrointestinal surgical procedures. Other plasmid-mediated resistance genes generate specific inactivating enzymes in *Streptococcus hemolyticus* and *S. aureus* that adenylate[126] lincosamides or acetylate[127] or hydrolyze[128] streptogramins.

Tetracycline Inactivation

A tetracycline-inactivating enzyme called *tetX* has been described rarely in *Bacteroides* spp.[129] Most tetracycline resistance is mediated by other mechanisms, including efflux and ribosomal protection (see Table 17-6).

Decreased Permeability of Bacterial Membranes

Outer Membrane Permeability

It was recognized early in the history of antibiotic development that penicillin is effective against gram-positive bacteria but not against gram-negative bacteria.[130] This difference in susceptibility to penicillin is due in large part to the outer membrane, a lipid bilayer that acts as a barrier to the penetration of antibiotics into the cell.[131] Situated outside the peptidoglycan cell wall of gram-negative bacteria, this outer membrane is absent in gram-positive bacteria. The outer portion of this lipid bilayer is composed principally of lipopolysaccharide made up of tightly bound hydrocarbon molecules that impede the entry of hydrophobic antibiotics, such as nafcillin or erythromycin.[132,133] Agents that disrupt the integrity of the lipopolysaccharide layer, such as polymixin, or mutations that lead to the production of defective lipopolysaccharides result in increased permeability of hydrophobic antibiotics.[134]

The passage of hydrophilic antibiotics through this outer membrane is facilitated by the presence of porins, proteins that are arranged so as to form water-filled diffusion channels through which antibiotics may traverse.[135] Bacteria usually produce many porins; approximately 10^5 porin molecules are present in a single cell of *E. coli*. Bacteria are able to regulate the relative number of different porins in response to the osmolarity of the surrounding media. In hyperosmolar media, *E. coli* may repress production of the larger porins (OmpF), while continuing to express smaller ones (OmpC).[136]

The rate of diffusion of antibiotics through this outer membrane is a function not only of the numbers and properties of the porin channels, but also of the physicochemical characteristics of the antibiotic. Generally the larger the antibiotic molecule, the more negative the charges, and the greater the degree of hydrophobicity, the less likely it is to penetrate through the outer membrane.[131,137] Small hydrophilic molecules with a zwitterionic charge, such as imipenem, are highly permeable. Conversely, larger highly charged molecules, such as carbenicillin, are much less permeable.

Mutations resulting in the loss of specific porins can occur in clinical isolates and determine increased resistance to β-lactam antibiotics. A strain of *Salmonella typhimurium* obtained from a perirenal abscess became resistant to multiple cephalosporins during therapy with cephalexin.[138] The parent strain produced OmpF and OmpC proteins, but the mutant produced only OmpF. The mutant was resistant to β-lactam antibiotics only when tested in media of high osmolarity compared with that in the patient's tissues. Under these conditions, the production of the OmpF protein was repressed completely, leaving the microorganism devoid of either species of porin and impermeable to the cephalosporins. Resistance to aminoglycosides and carbapenems emerging during therapy also has been associated with a lack of production of outer membrane proteins.[139,140] In *P. aeruginosa*, resistance to imipenem seems to be due to an interplay between chromosomal β-lactamase activity and a loss of a specific entry channel, the D2 porin.[141]

Resistance to nalidixic acid and other quinolones has been associated with alterations of outer membrane proteins in *Serratia marcescens*[142] and *P. aeruginosa*. Single-step, high-level mutational resistance to nalidixic acid by aerobic gram-negative bacilli occurs with a 10^{-7} frequency, however, whereas only low-level resistance to the newer quinolones ($<10 \times$ MIC) usually is obtained with a single-

step selection of less than 10^{-9}.[143] Plasmid-mediated chloramphenicol resistance due to decreased permeability has been shown in *E. coli*.[144]

Inner Membrane Permeability

The rate of entry of aminoglycoside molecules into bacterial cells is a function of their binding to a usually nonsaturable anionic transporter, whereupon they retain their positive charge and subsequently are "pulled" across the cytoplasmic membrane by the internal negative charge of the cell.[145] This process requires energy and a threshold minimal level of internal negative charge of the cell that has to be present before significant transport occurs (*proton motive force*).[146] The level of the internal charge that is required may depend on the actual aminoglycoside concentration at a given time. The energy generation or the proton motive force that is required for substrate transport into the cell may be altered in mutants resistant to aminoglycosides.

These aminoglycoside-resistant isolates with altered proton motive force occur rarely but develop in the course of long-term aminoglycoside therapy.[147] These isolates usually have a "small colony" phenotype due to their reduced rate of growth. They may be unstable and revert to a sensitive phenotype in the absence of selective aminoglycoside pressure. The clinical significance of these isolates is not clear. They may retain some virulence[148] and rarely may cause fatal bacteremia.[149] Because oxidative metabolism is essential for aminoglycoside uptake action and cell growth and development, *Pseudomonas* mutants have been found that have been deficient in specific cytochromes.[145] Resistant mutants with defective electron transport systems have been described in *E. coli*, *S. aureus*, and *Salmonella* spp. Facultative organisms grown anaerobically are resistant to aminoglycosides because of a marked reduction of the uptake of the antibiotic.[112]

Promotion of Antibiotic Efflux

Tetracyclines

Active efflux of antimicrobial agents is recognized increasingly as a common mechanism of resistance in many clinically relevant pathogens. Some strains of *E. coli*, *Shigella*, and other enteric organisms express a membrane transporter system that leads to multidrug resistance by drug efflux.[150] Many of these are multicomponent, regulated, energy-dependent transporter systems that promote the active efflux of multiple classes of antibiotics. Specific efflux pumps also exist that promote the egress of single classes of antimicrobial agents.

The major mechanism of resistance to tetracycline found in enteric gram-negative organisms results from the decreased accumulation of tetracycline (Table 17-6). This reduced uptake is an energy-dependent process that is related to the generation of an inner membrane protein produced by the tetracycline-resistance determinant. The primary mechanism for the decreased accumulation of tetracycline is mainly through the active efflux of the antibiotic across the cell membrane.[151] Decreased uptake of tetracycline from the extracellular environment also accounts for decreased accumulation of tetracycline inside resistant cells. These resistance determinants may be found on the chromosome or plasmids and frequently are found on transposable genetic elements. Tetracycline-resistance genes are generally inducible by subinhibitory concentrations of tetracycline. There are more than 30 recognized tetracycline-resistance determinants, most of which mediate drug efflux.[152] They have been designated in the past by letters (e.g., tet A, tet B). Because there are now more determinants than letters in the English alphabet, new *tet* genes now are designated by numbers.

Macrolides and Streptogramins

In some strains of *S. pneumoniae*, *Staphylococcus pyogenes*, *S. aureus*, and *S. epidermidis*, an active efflux mechanism causes resistance to macrolides, streptogramins, and azalides.[153] This efflux mechanism is mediated by the *mef* (for *m*acrolide *ef*flux) genes in streptococci and

TABLE 17-6 Mechanisms of Tetracycline Resistance

Resistance Mechanism	Tet Determinant	Common Bacterial Species
Drug Efflux	Tet A-L, P*, V, Y, Z, otrB, tcr3, Tet 30	Enterobacteriaceae, Pseudomonas, Streptomyces, Staphylococcus, Streptococcus spp.
Ribosomal Protection	Tet M, O, P*, Q, S, T, W, otrA	Gram-positive and gram-negative anaerobes, Neisseria, Haemophilus, Enterococcus. Staphylococcus, Streptococcus spp.
Enzymatic Inactivation	Tet X	Bacteroides spp.
Unknown Mechanism	Tet U, otrC	Mycobacteria, Enterococcus spp.
Altered Ribosomal Target	—	Helicobacter pylori

*Tet P has two different genes mediating different mechanisms of resistance.

msr (for *m*acrolide *s*treptogramin *r*esistance) genes in staphylococci.[154] A similar efflux system, encoded by a gene called *mreA* (for *m*acrolide *r*esistance *e*fflux), has been described in group B streptococci.[155] This mechanism of resistance may be more prevalent in community-acquired infections than generally was appreciated.[156] Dissemination of these resistance genes among important bacterial pathogens is a considerable threat to the usefulness of macrolide antibiotics (see Table 17-7).

β-Lactams

Active efflux mechanisms also may contribute to the full expression of β-lactam resistance in *P. aeruginosa*. Multidrug efflux pumps in the inner and outer membrane of *P. aeruginosa* may act in concert with periplasmic β-lactamases and membrane permeability components to protect the bacterium from β-lactam agents.[157,158]

Fluoroquinolones

Active efflux of fluoroquinolones has been detected in enteric bacteria[159,160] and staphylococci.[156,161] This efflux may be related to a multiple antibiotic resistance transporter[156] (i.e., norA) or a specific quinolone efflux pump (i.e., EmrAB, AcrAB).

Altered Target Sites

Alteration of Ribosomal Target Sites

Macrolides, Lincosamides, Streptogramins. Resistance to a wide variety of antimicrobial agents, including tetracyclines, macrolides, lincosamides, streptogramins, and the aminoglycosides, may result from alteration of ribosomal binding sites. Failure of the antibiotic to bind to its target site or sites on the ribosome disrupts its ability to inhibit protein synthesis and cell growth. For macrolides, lincosamides, and streptogramin B, this is the principal mechanism of multiple-agent resistance among aerobic and anaerobic gram-positive organisms.[154] Resistance occurs as the result of at least eight classes of methylase enzymes (MLS$_B$-determinant) that dimethylate adenine residues on the 23-S ribosomal RNA of the 50-S subunit of the prokaryotic ribosome, disrupting the binding of MLS to the ribosome (Table 17-7). Different classes of this resistance determinant may be located on plasmids or on the bacterial chromosome.

MLS$_B$ resistance due to ribosomal methylation has been described in *S. aureus*, *Streptococcus sanguis*, *Bacteroides fragilis*, and *Clostridium perfringens*. MLS resistance may be constitutive or inducible by either older macrolides (e.g., erythromycin) or newer azalides. Inducible resistance in streptococci is generated by a variety of lincosamides and macrolides, resulting in cross-resistance to the MLS$_B$ antibiotics. In staphylococci, only 14 to 15 numbered macrolides induce MLS$_B$ methylation, and the organisms express resistance to macrolides only. Point mutations in ribosomal proteins L4 and L22 of the 50S subunit also have been described that render *S. pneumoniae* resistant to macrolides.[162]

Tetracyclines. Tetracycline resistance may be mediated by a variety of mechanisms (see Table 17-6). An unusual and previously unrecognized mechanism of tetracycline resistance by target resistance has been found in *Helicobacter pylori*.[163] This organism has been shown to possess a mutation in its 16S ribosomal RNA that limits tetracycline binding to its target site at the 30S subunit of the bacterial ribosome.

Aminoglycosides. Resistance to aminoglycosides also may be mediated at the ribosomal level. Mutations of the S12 protein of the 30S subunit have been shown to interfere with binding streptomycin to the ribosome. Ribosomal resistance to streptomycin may be a significant cause of streptomycin resistance among enterococcal isolates.[164] Ribosomal resistance to the 2-deoxystreptamine aminoglycosides (gentamicin, tobramycin, amikacin) seems to be uncommon and may require multiple mutations in that these aminoglycosides seem to bind to several sites on the 30S and 50S subunits of the prokaryotic ribosome.

TABLE 17-7 Resistance Mechanisms against the Macrolides, Lincosamides, and Streptogramins

Bacterial Species	Gene Designation	Phenotype	Resistance Mechanism	Resistance Pattern 14- or 15-Membered Ring	16-Membered Ring	Clindamycin	Streptogramin B
Streptococcus, Enterococcus spp.	erm(A,B)	MLS$_B$– inducible	Ribosomal methylation	(s) I or R	(s) I or R	(s) I or R	(s) I or R
	erm(A,B)	MLS$_B$– constitutive	Ribosomal methylation	R	R	R	R
	mef(A or E)	M	Efflux	I or R	S	S	S
	L4/L22 mut	M	Ribosomal mutation	R	R	S	S
	Inu (B)	L	inactivation	S	S	S-I	S
Staphylococcus spp.	erm(A,C)	MLS$_B$– inducible	Ribosomal methylation	R	(s)	(s)	(s)
	erm(A,C)	MLS$_B$– constitutive	Ribosomal methylation	R	R	R	R
	Msr(A or B)	MS$_B$	Efflux	R	S	S	R
	Vgb, vgbB	S$_B$	Inactivation	S	S	S	R
	Ere A or B	M	Inactivation	R	R	S	S
	Inu (A)	L	Inactivation	S	S	S-I	S

14- or 15-membered ring structures, erythromycin, clarithromycin, azithromycin; 16-membered ring structures, spiramycin; I, intermediate susceptibility; R, resistant; (s), appears susceptible in vitro but may select resistant clones in vivo; S, sensitive.

TABLE 17-8 Vancomycin Resistance in Enterococci and Staphylococci

	A	B	C	D	E	G
(MIC) Vanco (μg/mL)	64->500	4->500	2-32	64-128	16	12-16
Teico (μg/mL)	16->500	0.5-2	0.5-2	4-64	0.5	0.5
Expression	Inducible	Inducible	Constitutive, inducible	Constitutive	Inducible	ND
Genetic location	P, C	P, C	C	C	C	C
Target alteration	D-ala-D-lac	D-ala-D-lac	D-ala-D-Ser	D-ala-D-lac	D-ala-D-Ser	D-ala-D-Ser
Common species	Enterococcus faecalis, Enterococcus faecium, Staphylococcus aureus	E. faecalis, E. faecium	Enterococcus gallinarum (C-1) Enterococcus casseliflavus (C-2) Enterococcus flavescens (C-3)	E. faecium	E. faecalis	E. faecalis

C, chromosome; D-ala, D-alanine; D-lac, D-lactate; D-Ser, D-Serine; MIC, minimal inhibitory concentration; ND, not described; P, plasmid; Teico, teicoplanin; Vanco, vancomycin.

Ribosomal resistance often is associated with decreased intracellular accumulation of the drug.[165]

Alteration of Cell Wall Precursor Targets

Vancomycin and other glycopeptide antibiotics, such as teicoplanin, bind to D-alanine-D-alanine, which is present at the termini of peptidoglycan precursors. The large glycopeptide molecules prevent the incorporation of the precursors into the cell wall. Resistance of enterococci to vancomycin has been classified as A through G based on genotype, type of target site alterations, and levels of resistance to vancomycin and susceptibility or resistance to teicoplanin (Table 17-8).[166,167]

Strains of Enterococcus faecium and Enterococcus faecalis with high-level resistance to vancomycin and teicoplanin have class A resistance. Either vancomycin or teicoplanin can induce resistance in these strains. Class A resistance to glycopeptides transfers by conjugation from E. faecium to other gram-positive bacteria,[168] including E. faecalis,[169] S. pyogenes, S. sanguis, and Listeria monocytogenes. The vanA gene on the plasmid encodes an inducible protein that is related to the D-alanine-D-alanine ligases involved in cell wall synthesis in E. coli.[170] This protein synthesizes peptidoglycan precursors that have a depsipeptide terminus (D-alanine-D-lactate) instead of the usual D-alanine-D-alanine. The modified peptidoglycan binds glycopeptide antibiotics with reduced affinity, conferring resistance to vancomycin and teicoplanin.[171,172]

Strains of E. faecium and E. faecalis with class B resistance have levels of resistance to vancomycin that range from high (MIC 1024 μg/mL) to low (MIC 4 μg/mL) and are susceptible to teicoplanin. Vancomycin, but not teicoplanin, can induce resistance to vancomycin and teicoplanin in these strains. The genes determining the vanB phenotype are self-transferable by conjugation to other Enterococcus strains.[173,174]

All isolates of Enterococcus gallinarum, Enterococcus casseliflavus, and Enterococcus flavescens possess low-level resistance to vancomycin and are susceptible to teicoplanin (class C phenotype). The resistance is mediated by chromosomal genes known as Van C$_1$, Van C$_2$, or Van C$_3$.[175] The Van C gene complex gives rise to resistance to vancomycin by synthesis of an alternative dipeptide D-ala-D-Ser, in which a serine replaces the terminal alanine. Other variant genes known as Van E and Van G have been found in enterococcal species that also mediate various levels of glycopeptide resistance (see Table 17-8).

Since 1987, reports from the United States and Japan have documented outbreaks of vancomycin-resistant S. epidermidis,[176] S. haemolyticus,[177] and S. aureus.[178] The resistance patterns have been heterogeneous, and the underlying mechanisms still are being elucidated. Vancomycin-intermediate S. aureus expresses unusually thick peptidoglycan cell walls that are less completely cross-linked together.[179] The cell wall in some strains of vancomycin-intermediate S. aureus contains nonamidated glutamine precursors that provide an increased number of false binding sites to vancomycin.[180] The vancomycin molecules are absorbed to these excess binding sites, reducing vancomycin concentrations of the growth point of peptidoglycan synthesis along the inner surface of the cell wall. The specter of increasing outbreaks of vancomycin-resistant staphylococci has led the U.S. Centers for Disease Control and Prevention to develop vigorous interim guidelines to mitigate the spread of this serious nosocomial problem.[181]

Alteration of Target Enzymes

β-Lactams

β-Lactam antibiotics inhibit bacteria by binding covalently to PBPs in the cytoplasmic membrane. These target proteins catalyze the synthesis of the peptidoglycan that forms the cell wall of bacteria.[182] Alterations of PBPs can lead to β-lactam antibiotic resistance.[183]

In gram-positive bacteria, resistance to β-lactam antibiotics may be associated either with a decrease in the affinity of the PBP for the antibiotic[184] or with a change in the amount of PBP produced by the bacterium.[185] Multiple mechanisms seem to be present in some clinical isolates. Penicillin-resistant strains of S. pneumoniae isolated in South Africa have shown several changes in PBPs (i.e., decreased affinity of some PBPs, loss of others, and appearance of PBPs not present in the more susceptible cells).[186] The genes that encode these PBPs are mosaics, composed of segments from susceptible pneumococci and segments from resistant commensal streptococci.[187] In S. aureus[188-190] and E. faecium,[190,191] additional PBPs may be inducible (i.e., their production is stimulated by exposure of the microorganism to the β-lactam antibiotic). These inducible PBPs have a lower affinity for β-lactam antibiotics, making them less susceptible to inhibition by low concentrations of drug. Changes in the types of PBPs observed in susceptible and resistant strains also have been seen with the viridans streptococcal species Streptococcus mitis.[192]

Factors that regulate the induction of PBPs are poorly understood. The induction of a low-affinity PBP in methicillin-resistant S. aureus occurs to a larger extent when the microorganisms are grown at 32° C rather than at 37° C, conditions known to favor the expression of methicillin resistance.[193] There is evidence that the production of this inducible PBP is under the control of plasmid-borne genes that regulate staphylococcal penicillinase production. The structural gene (mecA) that determines the low-affinity PBP of methicillin-resistant S. aureus shares extensive sequence homology with a PBP of E. coli, and the genes that regulate the production of the low-affinity PBP have considerable sequence homology with the genes that regulate the production of staphylococcal penicillinase.[194] The production of this low-affinity PBP in methicillin-resistant S. aureus may be mediated by a fusion of gene segments from E. coli and S. aureus. Another gene (femA) also influences the expression of methicillin resistance by unknown mechanisms.[195]

The PBPs of β-lactamase-negative, penicillin-resistant strains of N. gonorrhoeae, Neisseria meningitidis, and H. influenzae have shown reduced penicillin-binding affinity.[196-199] Their PBPs seem to be encoded by hybrid genes containing segments of DNA scavenged from resistant strains of related species, similar to penicillin-resistant pneumococci.[200] Mutations leading to a loss of outer membrane proteins also may be associated with the acquisition of penicillin resistance in non–penicillinase-producing strains of *N. gonorrhoeae*, suggesting that altered permeability also may contribute to the resistance.[201] Permeability changes and decreased affinity of PBPs are mechanisms found jointly in clinical isolates of *P. aeruginosa*[202] and in non–β-lactamase-producing strains of *H. influenzae*.[203] Multiple mutations may be necessary to effect this type of resistance.

Quinolones

DNA gyrase (also called *bacterial topoisomerase II*) is necessary for the supercoiling of chromosomal DNA in bacteria to have efficient cell division.[204] Another related enzyme, topoisomerase IV, also is required for segregation of bacterial genomes into two daughter cells during cell division. These enzymes consist of two A subunits encoded by the *gyrA* gene and two B subunits encoded by the *gyrB* gene (or parC and parE for topoisomerase IV). Although spontaneous mutation in the *gyrA* locus is the most common cause of resistance to multiple fluoroquinolones in enteric bacteria, B-subunit alterations also may affect resistance to these drugs. Quinolone resistance may occur from decreased cell wall permeability, efflux, or enzyme protection mechanisms.[9]

DNA gyrase is the primary site of action in gram-negative bacteria, whereas topoisomerase IV is the principal target of quinolones in gram-positive bacteria. Mutations in a variety of chromosomal loci have been described that resulted in altered DNA gyrases resistant to nalidixic acid and the newer fluoroquinolones in Enterobacteriaceae and *P. aeruginosa*.[205,206] Many of these mutations involve the substitution of single amino acids at key enzymatic sites (located between amino acids 67 and 106 in the gyrase A subunit) that are involved in the generation of the DNA gyrase–bacterial DNA complex.[207,208] Clinical isolates of *C. freundii* in Japan have been found to be highly resistant to the newer quinolones via alterations in the DNA gyrase.[209] Alterations in the DNA gyrases of clinical isolates of other Enterobacteriaceae, particularly *E. coli*, have been described[210,211] and are thought to involve a mechanism that is similar to that found in quinolone-resistant *S. aureus* and other gram-positive species.

Sulfonamides

There are two common genes that mediate resistance to sulfa drugs in pathogenic bacteria: *sul1* and *sul2*. These genes give rise to altered forms of the target enzyme for sulfonamide, dihydropteroate synthase (DHPS).[212] This enzyme is essential for folic acid synthesis in susceptible bacteria. The altered DHPS enzymes mediated by the sulfonamide-resistance genes no longer bind to sulfa, yet continue to synthesize dihydropteroate from para-aminobenzoic acid substrate. The ubiquitous *sul1* gene is part of the class 1 integron family, giving rise to widespread resistance to sulfonamides.[38]

Trimethoprim

Trimethoprim is a potent inhibitor of bacterial dihydrofolate reductase (DHFR). Many altered DHFR enzymes with loss of inhibition by trimethoprim have been described from genes found primarily on resistance plasmids. These altered DHFR genes are widespread in gram-negative bacteria and are found in staphylococci (*dfrA* gene).[213,214]

Protection of Target Site

Tetracycline resistance also may occur by a mechanism that interferes with the ability of tetracycline to bind to the ribosome. The ubiquitous *tetM* resistance gene and related tetracycline-resistance determinants protect the ribosome from tetracycline action. The precise molecular site of action of this resistance mechanism is unclear at present. The *tetM* determinant is dispersed widely in gram-positive organisms in addition to *Mycoplasma*,[152] *Ureaplasma*,[20] *Campylobacter*,[152] and *Neisseria* spp.[19] The *tetM* gene generates protein with elongation factor–like activity that stabilizes ribosome transfer RNA interactions in the presence of tetracycline molecules.

The newly recognized plasmid-mediated, antibiotic-resistance gene mediating quinolone resistance seems to function as a target protection system.[9] The resistance mechanism seems to protect DNA gyrase from binding to quinolones, allowing the bacterium to resist quinolone inhibitory effects.

Overproduction of Target

Sulfonamides and Trimethoprim

Sulfonamides compete with para-aminobenzoic acid to bind the enzyme DHPS and halt the generation of pteridines and nucleic acids. Sulfonamide resistance may be mediated in some bacteria by the overproduction of the synthetic enzyme DHPS. The gene responsible for DHPS is *felP*, and strains of bacteria that produce excess DHPS can overwhelm sulfa inhibition.[212] Trimethoprim resistance may occur in a similar fashion, by making excess amounts of DHFR from the bacterial chromosomal gene *folA*.[213,214]

Bypass of Antibiotic Inhibition

Another mechanism for acquiring resistance to specific antibiotics is by the development of auxotrophs, which have growth factor requirements different from those of the wild strain. These mutants require substrates that normally are synthesized by the target enzymes, and if the substrates are present in the environment, the organisms are able to grow despite inhibition of the synthetic enzyme. For example, bacteria that lose the enzyme thymidylate synthetase are "thymine dependent" and cannot synthesize thymidylate in the usual way. They require exogenous supplies of thymidine to synthesize thymidylate via salvage pathways and are highly resistant to sulfa drugs and trimethoprim.[212,215]

CONTROL OF ANTIBIOTIC RESISTANCE

Although the emergence of antibiotic-resistant bacteria generally has been correlated with the rise and fall of specific antibiotic use in clinical practice, the chain of causality is not always clear-cut.[29,30,216,217] Bacterial strains contain complex aggregations of genes that may be linked together. The use of one antibiotic may select for the emergence of resistance to another. Mobile genetic elements and rapidly evolving integron cassettes with multiple antibiotic-resistance genes endow bacteria with a remarkable capacity to resist antibiotics.[218] Although the development of antibiotic resistance may be inevitable, the rate at which it develops may be diminished by the rational use of antibiotics.[29] Increasing evidence of multiple antibiotic-resistance mechanisms within the same bacterium against a single type of antibiotic[219] and cooperation between bacterial populations within biofilms[220,221] attest to the ingenuity of bacterial populations. Efflux pump activation and phenotypic alterations within biofilms promote antibiotic resistance on the surface of medical devices.[222-224]

The wider accessibility to computers and the ability to track antibiotic-resistance genes with molecular techniques have enhanced the ability to track the spread of antibiotic resistance. With the appropriate computerized surveillance, a hospital laboratory may be able to detect rapidly the emergence of a new type of resistance or the presence of a new microbial strain within a specific unit or patient population. Techniques such as restriction endonuclease digestion analyses of microbial genomes and genetic probes of antibiotic-resistance genes by polymerase chain reaction make it possible to confirm the presence of new genes in the environment. This information may be correlated with the phenotypic measures determined by the clinical microbiology surveillance system (Fig. 17-5).[225] Use of molecular techniques greatly augments surveillance data because large data sets may obscure subtle changes ("miniepidemics") that may be more amenable to the institution of stringent infection control measures.

The study of the genetics of antibiotic resistance, particularly the awareness of the great mobility of plasmids and transposons, leads one to the conclusion that ultimately each antibiotic used may alter its microenvironment inexorably, creating selective advantages for resistant organisms. Some bacterial strains have the ability to hypermutate in stressful environments, increasing the risk of acquisition of resistance mutations.[226,227] Because prokaryotic organisms all contribute to a common

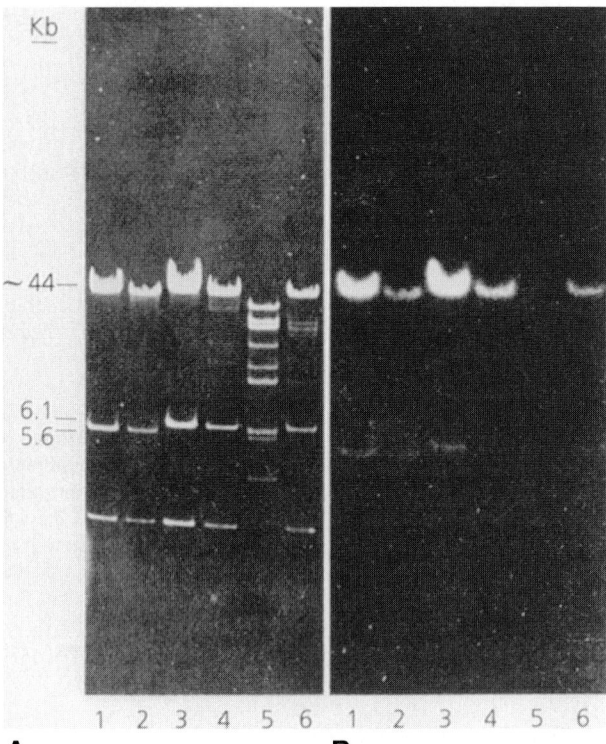

FIGURE 17-5. **A,** Agarose gel of *Eco*RI-digested plasmids derived from four isolates that contain a nosocomial trimethoprim-resistance plasmid (called *pBWH10*) from a Boston hospital (*lanes 1-4*). Another nosocomial plasmid from the same hospital that does not contain trimethoprim-resistance genes (*lane 5*) and one in which the trimethoprim-resistance and sensitive plasmids are present in the same isolate (*lane 6*) are shown. **B,** To show that the "fingerprints" from the trimethoprim-resistance plasmids in lanes 1 through 4 and 6 contain the same gene, DNA-DNA hybridization of the same six plasmids was performed using a type II dihydrofolate reductase probe. The probe and the restriction endonuclease analyses helped pinpoint the location and genetic homology of this trimethoprim-resistance gene.

"gene pool," favorable genes mediating antibiotic resistance may disseminate among bacterial populations. In less than a decade, newly used inexpensive drugs such as trimethoprim have gone from being highly effective in the treatment of dysentery in developing countries to becoming unusable in several of these areas.[228] Other examples of the emergence of multiresistant organisms have had clinical significance in the management of outpatient and nosocomial infections. The increased use of erythromycin for the management of streptococcal pharyngitis in Finland in the 1980s has been paralleled by a dramatic increase in the prevalence of multiresistant streptococci isolated from pharyngeal and blood cultures.[229] The clinical importance of this finding is that in β-lactam-intolerant or β-lactam-allergic patients, the range of effective antistreptococcal drugs is becoming increasingly limited. Even more worrisome is the specter of multiresistant enterococci as nosocomial pathogens,[230] as evidenced by their increasing resistance to β-lactams,[231] aminoglycosides,[232] vancomycin,[233] and other glycopeptides. Outbreaks of vancomycin-resistant *E. faecalis* and vancomycin/ampicillin–resistant *E. faecium* have occurred in London, New York, Philadelphia, and Providence, Rhode Island.[234-238]

Similar concerns exist regarding the management of staphylococcal infections, given the rapid spread of simultaneous β-lactam-resistant, aminoglycoside-resistant, and quinolone-resistant isolates.[239-241] Reports of vancomycin-resistant *S. aureus* in Japan and the United States suggest that common, invasive, microbial pathogens may become refractory to any chemotherapeutic agent in the future.[29]

Rational antibiotic usage policies suggest the curtailment of the unnecessary use of antibiotics in situations such as animal husbandry. The causal link between the use of antibiotics for animal growth promotion and their augmentation of the resistance in human pathogens has been disputed,[242] but more recent evidence is convincing that transfer of resistance genes occurs from the food humans consume.[242-244] New drug discoveries have allowed physicians to be one step ahead of the bacterial pathogens. Nonetheless, the rapid evolution of resistance has limited the duration of the effectiveness of specific agents against certain pathogens. The best hope for the future is the development of a greater understanding of how antimicrobial resistance spreads and the implementation of effective infection control strategies.[245] Newer antimicrobial agents have had a substantial impact in decreasing human morbidity and mortality rates over the past half century. It behooves us to expand our surveillance of antibiotic-resistance determinants and to exercise caution in dispensing antibiotics to maximize their continued efficacy.

REFERENCES

1. Rice W, Chippindale A. Sexual recombination and the power of natural selection. Science. 2001;294:555-559.
2. Kopecko D. Specialized genetic recombination systems in bacteria: Their involvement in gene expression and evolution. Prog Mol Subcell Biol. 1980;7:135-243.
3. Medeiros AA. Evolution and dissemination of β-lactamases accelerated by generations of β-lactam antibiotics. Clin Infect Dis. 1997;24:S19-S45.
4. Gold HS, Moellering RC Jr. Antimicrobial-drug resistance. N Engl J Med. 1996;335:1445-1453.
5. Lupski JR. Molecular mechanisms for transposition of drug-resistance genes and other movable genetic elements. Rev Infect Dis. 1987;9:357-368.
6. Hiramatsu K, Aritaka N, Hanaki H, et al. Dissemination in Japanese hospitals of strains of *Staphylococcus aureus* heterogeneously resistant to vancomycin (see comments). Lancet. 1997;350:1670-1673.
7. Chang S, Sievert DM, Hageman JE, et al. Infection with vancomycin-resistant *Staphylococcus aureus* containing the vanA resistance gene. N Engl J Med. 2003;348:1342-1347.
8. Galimand M, Guiyoule A, Gerbaud G, et al. Multidrug resistance in *Yersinia pestis* mediated by a transferable plasmid (see comments). N Engl J Med. 1997;337:677-680.
9. Tran JH, Jacoby GA. Mechanism of plasmid-mediated quinolone resistance. Proc Natl Acad Sci U S A. 2002;99:5638-5642.
10. Gardner P, Smith DH, Beer H, Moellering R. Recovery of resistance factors from a drug-free community. Lancet. 1969;2:774-776.
11. Massey RC, Buckling A, Peacock SJ. Phenotypic switching of antibiotic resistance circumvents permanent costs in *Staphylococcus aureus*. Curr Biol. 2001;11:1810-1814.
12. O'Brien TF, Pla MP, Mayer KH, et al. Intercontinental spread of a new antibiotic resistance gene on an epidemic plasmid. Science. 1985;230:87-88.
13. Timmis KN, Gonzalez-Carrero MI, Sekizaki T, Rojo F. Biological activities specified by antibiotic resistance plasmids. J Antimicrob Chemother. 1986;18(Suppl C):1-12.
14. Thompson R. R plasmid transfer. J Antimicrob Chemother. 1986;18(Suppl C):13-23.
15. Summers AO, Wireman J, Vimy MJ, et al. Mercury released from dental silver fillings provokes an increase in mercury-resistant and antibiotic-resistant bacteria in oral and intestinal floras of primates. Antimicrob Agents Chemother. 1993;37:825-834.
16. Foster TJ. Plasmid-determined resistance to antimicrobial drugs and toxic metal ions in bacteria. Microbiol Rev. 1983;47:361-409.
17. Blattner FR, Plunkett G 3rd, Bloch CA, et al. The complete genome sequence of *Escherichia coli* K-12 (comment). Science. 1997;277:1453-1474.
18. El Solh N, Allignet J, Bismuth R, et al. Conjugative transfer of staphylococcal antibiotic resistance markers in the absence of detectable plasmid DNA. Antimicrob Agents Chemother. 1986;30:161-169.
19. Morse SA, Johnson SR, Biddle JW, Roberts MC. High-level tetracycline resistance in *Neisseria gonorrhoeae* is result of acquisition of streptococcal tetM determinant. Antimicrob Agents Chemother. 1986;30:664-670.
20. Roberts MC, Kenny GE. Dissemination of the tetM tetracycline resistance determinant to *Ureaplasma urealyticum*. Antimicrob Agents Chemother. 1986;29:350-352.
21. Arthur M, Reynolds P, Courvalin P. Glycopeptide resistance in enterococci. Trends Microbiol. 1996;4:401-407.
22. Brisson-Noel A, Arthur M, Courvalin P. Evidence for natural gene transfer from gram-positive cocci to *Escherichia coli*. J Bacteriol. 1988;170:1739-1745.
23. Papadopoulou B, Courvalin P. Dispersal in *Campylobacter* spp. of aphA-3, a kanamycin resistance determinant from gram-positive cocci. Antimicrob Agents Chemother. 1988;32:945-948.
24. Courvalin P, Carlier C, Collatz E. Plasmid-mediated resistance to aminocyclitol antibiotics in group D streptococci. *J Bacteriol*. 1980;143:541-551.
25. Zscheck KK, Hull R, Murray BE. Restriction mapping and hybridization studies of a beta-lactamase-encoding fragment from *Streptococcus (Enterococcus) faecalis*. Antimicrob Agents Chemother. 1988;32:768-769.
26. Neu HC. The crisis in antibiotic resistance. Science. 1992;257:1064-1073.

27. Cohen ML. Epidemiology of drug resistance: Implications for a post-antimicrobial era (see comments). Science. 1992;257:1050-1055.

28. Salyers AA, Shoemaker NB, Stevens AM, et al. Conjugative transposons: an unusual and diverse set of integrated gene transfer elements. Microbiol Rev. 1985;49:679-690.

29. Levy SB. Antibiotic resistance: consequences of inaction. Clin Infect Dis. 2001;3:S124-129.

30. Summers AO. Generally overlooked fundamentals of bacterial genetics and ecology. Clin Infect Dis. 2002;3:S85-92.

31. Hawkey PM. The origins and molecular basis of antibiotic resistance. BMJ. 1998;317:657-660.

32. Recchia GD, Hall RM. Origins of the mobile gene cassettes found in integrons. Trends Microbiol. 1997;5:389-394.

33. Stokes HW, Hall RM. A novel family of potentially mobile DNA elements encoding site-specific gene-integration functions: Integrons. Mol Microbiol. 1989;3:1669-1683.

34. Collis CM, Hall RM. Expression of antibiotic resistance genes in the integrated cassettes of integrons. Antimicrob Agents Chemother. 1995;39:155-162.

35. Ouellette M, Bissonnette L, Roy PH. Precise insertion of antibiotic resistance determinants into Tn21-like transposons: Nucleotide sequence of the OXA-1 beta-lactamase gene. Proc Natl Acad Sci U S A. 1987;84:7378-7382.

36. Paulsen IT, Littlejohn TG, Radstrom P, et al. The 3′ conserved segment of integrons contains a gene associated with multidrug resistance to antiseptics and disinfectants. Antimicrob Agents Chemother. 1993;35:761-768.

37. Messier N, Roy PH. Integron integrases possess a unique additional domain necessary for activity. J Bacteriol. 2001;183:6699-6706.

38. Hall MAL, Block HEM, Donders RT, et al. Multidrug resistance among enterobacteriaceae is strongly associated with the presence of integrons and is independent of species or isolate origin. J Infect Dis. 2003;187:251-259.

39. Recchia GD, Hall RM. Gene cassettes: A new class of mobile element. Microbiology. 1995;141:3015-3027.

40. Naas T, Mikami Y, Imai T, Foirel L, Nordmann P. Characterization of In53, a class 1 plasmid- and composite transposon-located integron of Escherichia coli which carries an unusual array of gene cassettes. J Bacteriol. 2001;183:235-249.

41. Bush K, Jacoby GA, Medeiros AA. A functional classification scheme for β-lactamases and its correlation with molecular structure. Antimicrob Agents Chemother. 1995;39:1211-1233.

42. Sykes RB, Matthew M. The beta-lactamases of gram-negative bacteria and their role in resistance to beta-lactam antibiotics. J Antimicrob Chemother. 1976;2:115-157.

43. Joris B, Ghuysen J-M, Dive G, et al. The active-site-serine penicillin-recognizing enzymes as members of the Streptomyces R61 DD-peptidase family. Biochem J. 1988;250:313-324.

44. Herzberg O. Refined crystal structure of β-lactamase from Staphylococcus aureus PC1 at 2.0 Å resolution. J Mol Biol. 1991;217:701-719.

45. Kelly JA, Dideberg O, Charlier P, et al. On the origin of bacterial resistance to penicillin: Comparison of a beta-lactamase and a penicillin target. Science. 1986;231:1429-1431.

46. McDonnell RW, Sweeney HM, Cohen S. Conjugational transfer of gentamicin resistance plasmids intra- and interspecifically in Staphylococcus aureus and Staphylococcus epidermidis. Antimicrob Agents Chemother. 1983;23:151-160.

47. Zscheck KK, Murray BE. Genes involved in the regulation of beta-lactamase production in enterococci and staphylococci. Antimicrob Agents Chemother. 1993;37:1966-1970.

48. Murray BE. Beta-lactamase-producing enterococci. Antimicrob Agents Chemother. 1992;36:2355-2359.

49. Rice LB, Marshall SH. Evidence of incorporation of the chromosomal beta-lactamase gene of Enterococcus-faecalis-CH19 into a transposon derived from staphylococci. Antimicrob Agents Chemother. 1992;36:1843-1846.

50. Medeiros AA. Plasmid-determined beta-lactamases. In: Bryan LE, ed. Handbook of Experimental Pharmacology, v. 91. Berlin: Springer-Verlag; 1989:101-128.

51. Livermore DM. Beta-lactamases: quantity and resistance. Clin Microbiol Infect 1997;3(Suppl 4):10-19.

52. Nord CE. Mechanisms of beta-lactam resistance in anaerobic bacteria. Rev Infect Dis. 1986;8(Suppl 5):S543-S548.

53. Appelbaum PC. Patterns of resistance and resistance mechanisms in anaerobes. Clin Microbiol Newslett. 1992;14:49-53.

54. Appelbaum PC, Spangler SK, Pankuch GA, et al. Characterization of a beta-lactamase from Clostridium clostridioforme. J Antimicrob Chemother. 1994;33:33-40.

55. Tuner K, Lindqvist L, Nord CE. Purification and properties of a novel beta-lactamase from Fusobacterium nucleatum. Antimicrob Agents Chemother. 1985;27:943-947.

56. Cuchural GJ Jr, Tally FP, Storey JR, Malamy MH. Transfer of beta-lactamase-associated cefoxitin resistance in Bacteroides fragilis. Antimicrob Agents Chemother. 1986;29:918-920.

57. Cuchural GJ Jr, Malamy MH, Tally FP. Beta-lactamase-mediated imipenem resistance in Bacteroides fragilis. Antimicrob Agents Chemother. 1986;30:645-648.

58. Hedberg M, Edlund C, Lindqvist L, et al. Purification and characterization of an imipenem hydrolysing metallo-beta-lactamase from Bacteroides fragilis. J Antimicrob Chemother. 1992;29:105-113.

59. Yotsuji A, Minami S, Inoue M, Mitsuhashi S. Properties of novel beta-lactamase produced by Bacteroides fragilis. Antimicrob Agents Chemother. 1983;24:925-929.

60. Appelbaum PC, Philippon A, Jacobs MR, et al. Characterization of beta-lactamases from non-Bacteroides fragilis group Bacteroides spp. belonging to seven species and their role in beta-lactam resistance. Antimicrob Agents Chemother. 1990;34:2169-2176.

61. Jacobs MR, Spangler SK, Appelbaum PC. Beta-lactamase production and susceptibility to US and European anaerobic gram-negative bacilli to beta-lactams and other agents. Eur J Clin Microbiol Infect Dis. 1992;11:1081-1093.

62. Medeiros AA, O'Brien TF. Ampicillin-resistant Haemophilus influenzae type B possessing a TEM-type beta-lactamase but little permeability barrier to ampicillin. Lancet. 1975;1:716-719.

63. Elwell LP, Roberts M, Mayer LW, Falkow S. Plasmid-mediated beta-lactamase production in Neisseria gonorrhoeae. Antimicrob Agents Chemother. 1977;11:528-533.

64. Kliebe C, Nies BA, Meyer JF, et al. Evolution of plasmid-coded resistance to broad-spectrum cephalosporins. Antimicrob Agents Chemother. 1985;28:302-307.

65. Brun-Buisson C, Legrand P, Philippon A, et al. Transferable enzymatic resistance to third-generation cephalosporins during nosocomial outbreak of multiresistant Klebsiella pneumoniae. Lancet. 1987;2:302-306.

66. Jacoby GA, Medeiros AA. More extended-spectrum beta-lactamases. Antimicrob Agents Chemother. 1991;35:1697-1704.

67. Naumovski L, Quinn JP, Miyashiro D, et al. Outbreak of ceftazidime resistance due to a novel extended-spectrum beta-lactamase in isolates from cancer patients. Antimicrob Agents Chemother. 1992;36:1991-1996.

68. Sanders CC, Sanders WE. β-Lactam resistance in gram-negative bacteria-global trends and clinical impact. Clin Infect Dis. 1992;15:824-839.

69. Danel F, Hall LMC, Gur D, Livermore DM. OXA-15, an extended-spectrum variant of OXA-2 (-lactamase, isolated from a Pseudomonas aeruginosa strain. Antimicrob Agents Chemother. 1997;41:785-790.

70. Danel F, Hall LMC, Gur D, Livermore DM. OXA-14, another extended-spectrum variant of OXA-10 (PSE-2) β-lactamase from Pseudomonas aeruginosa. Antimicrob Agents Chemother. 1995;39:1881-1884.

71. Liu PY, Gur D, Hall LMC, Livermore DM. Survey of the prevalence of beta-lactamases amongst 1000 gram-negative bacilli isolated consecutively at the Royal London Hospital. J Antimicrob Chemother. 1992;30:429-447.

72. Sirot DL, Goldstein FW, Soussy CJ, et al. Resistance to cefotaxime and seven other beta-lactams in members of the family Enterobacteriaceae: A 3-year survey in France. Antimicrob Agents Chemother. 1992;36:1677-1681.

73. Ferreira HMN, Sousa JC, Peixe LM. Characterization of the beta-lactamases responsible for the resistance of hospital strains of Klebsiella pneumoniae to beta-lactam antibiotics [in Portuguese]. Rev Port Doencas Infecciosas 1992;15:207-209.

74. Sousa JC, Carneiro G, Peixe ML, et al. Characterization of beta-lactamases encoded by pathogenic strains of Escherichia coli from Portugal. J Antimicrob Chemother. 1991;27:437-440.

75. Watanabe Y, Yokota T, Higashi Y, et al. In vitro and in vivo transferrable beta-lactam resistance due to a new plasmid-mediated oxyiminocephalosporinase from a clinical isolate of Proteus mirabilis. Microbiol Immunol. 1991;35:87-97.

76. Espinasse F, Mariotte S, Labia R, Nicolas MH. Each epidemic cefotaxime (CTX) resistant strain of Proteus mirabilis is related to an extended spectrum beta-lactamase. Abstract 1272. In: Program Abstracts of the 32nd Interscience Conference on Antimicrobial Agents and Chemotherapy. Washington, DC: American Society for Microbiology; 1992:323.

77. Rossi MA, Gutkind G, Quinteros M, et al. A Proteus mirabilis with a novel extended spectrum beta-lactamase and 6 different aminoglycoside (AG) resistance genes. Abstract 939. In: Program and Abstracts of the 31st Interscience Conference on Antimicrobial Agents and Chemotherapy. Washington, DC: American Society for Microbiology; 1991:255.

78. Mariotte S, Nordmann P, Nicolas MH. Extended-spectrum beta-lactamase in Proteus mirabilis. J Antimicrob Chemother. 1994;33:925-935.

79. Bret L, Chanal-Claris C, Sirot D, et al. Chromosomally encoded AmpC-type β-lactamase in a clinical isolate of Proteus mirabilis. Antimicrob Agents Chemother. 1998;42:1110-1114.

80. Pitout JDD, Thomson KS, Hanson ND, et al. β-Lactamases responsible for resistance to expanded-spectrum cephalosporins in Klebsiella pneumoniae, Escherichia coli, and Proteus mirabilis isolates recovered in South Africa. Antimicrob Agents Chemother. 1998;42:1350-1354.

81. Mariotte S, Nordmann P, Nicolas MH. Spread of extended-spectrum beta-lactamases (ES Bla) in Proteus mirabilis (P.m.) may be limited by low frequency of plasmid conjugation. Abstract 940. In: Program and Abstracts of the 31st Interscience Conference on Antimicrobial Agents and Chemotherapy. Washington, DC: American Society for Microbiology; 1991:255.

82. Wiener J, Quinn J, Kowalczyk M, et al. Production of TEM-10 beta-lactamase in ceftazidime-resistant (CFZ-R) Enterobacteriaceae from multiple nursing homes (NHs). Abstract 641. In: Program Abstracts of the 32nd Interscience Conference on Antimicrobial Agents and Chemotherapy. Washington, DC: American Society for Microbiology; 1992:217.

83. Schiappa DA, Hayden MK, Matushek MG, et al. Ceftazidime-resistant Klebsiella pneumoniae and Escherichia coli bloodstream infection: A case-control and molecular epidemiologic investigation. J Infect Dis. 1996;174:529-536.

84. Lucet JC, Chevret S, Decre D, et al. Outbreak of multiply resistant Enterobacteriaceae in an intensive care unit: Epidemiology and risk factors for acquisition. Clin Infect Dis. 1996;22:430-436.

85. Sirot D, deChamps C, Chanal C, et al. Translocation of antibiotic resistance determinants including an extended-spectrum beta-lactamase between conjugative plasmids of Klebsiella pneumoniae and Escherichia coli. Antimicrob Agents Chemother. 1991;35:1576-1581.

86. Jiang H, Hopkins JD, Zieg J, et al. Origin and transposition of a gene encoding a TEM12 beta-lactamase on pBWH102 and pBWH501 in ceftazidime resistant (CAZ-R) isolates of Klebsiella pneumoniae at one U.S. medical center. Abstract 186. In: Program and Abstracts of the 30th Interscience Conference on Antimicrobial Agents and Chemotherapy. Washington, DC: American Society for Microbiology; 1990:117.

87. Heritage J, Hawkey PM, Todd N, Lewis IJ. Transposition of the gene encoding a TEM-12 extended-spectrum beta-lactamase. Antimicrob Agents Chemother. 1992;36:1981-1986.

88. Mabilat C, Lourencaovital J, Goussard S, Courvalin P. A new example of physical linkage between tn1 and tn21—the antibiotic multiple-resistance region of plasmid pCFF04 encoding extended-spectrum beta-lactamase TEM-3. Mol Gen Genet. 1992;235:113-121.

89. Jiang H, Zieg J, O'Brien TF. Observation of the acquisition of an amikacin resistance gene by an endemic nosocomial plasmid encoding a ceftazidime resistance gene. Abstract 442. In: Program Abstracts of the 32nd Interscience Conference on Antimicrobial Agents and Chemotherapy. Washington, DC: American Society for Microbiology; 1992:184.

90. Chanal C, Poupart MC, Sirot D, et al. Nucleotide sequences of CAZ-2, CAZ-6, and CAZ-7 beta-lactamase genes. Antimicrob Agents Chemother. 1992;36:1817-1820.

91. Goussard S, Sougakoff W, Mabilat C, et al. An IS1-like element is responsible for high-level synthesis of extended-spectrum beta-lactamase TEM-6 in Enterobacteriaceae. J Gen Microbiol. 1991;137:2681-2687.

92. Petit A, Ben Yaghlane-bouslama H, Sofer L, Labia R. Does high level production of SHV-type penicillinase confer resistance to ceftazidime in Enterobacteriaceae. FEMS Microbiol Lett. 1992;92:89-94.

93. Thomson CJ, Amyes SGB. TRC-1—emergence of a clavulanic acid-resistant TEM beta-lactamase in a clinical strain. FEMS Microbiol Lett. 1992;91:113-117.

94. Vedel G, Belaaouaj A, Gilly L, et al. Clinical isolates of Escherichia coli producing TRI beta-lactamases: Novel TEM-enzymes conferring resistance to beta-lactamase inhibitors. J Antimicrob Chemother. 1992;30:449-462.

95. Blazquez J, Baquero MR, Canton R, et al. Characterization of a new TEM-type beta-lactamase resistant to clavulanate, sulbactam, and tazobactam in a clinical isolate of Escherichia coli. Antimicrob Agents Chemother. 1993;37:2059-2063.

96. Sanders CC. Chromosomal cephalosporinases responsible for multiple resistance to newer beta-lactam antibiotics. Ann Rev Microbiol. 1987;41:573-593.

97. Korfmann G, Sanders CC, Moland ES. Altered phenotypes associated with ampD mutations in Enterobacter cloacae. Antimicrob Agents Chemother. 1991;35:358-364.

98. Chow JW, Fine MJ, Shlaes DM, et al. Enterobacter bacteremia—clinical features and emergence of antibiotic resistance during therapy. Ann Intern Med. 1991;115:585-590.

99. Livermore DM. Carbapenemases. J Antimicrob Chemother. 1992;29:609-612.

100. Nugent ME, Hedges RW. The nature of the genetic determinant for the SHV-1 beta-lactamase. Mol Gen Genet. 1979;175:239-243.

101. Papanicolaou GA, Medeiros AA, Jacoby GA. Novel plasmid-mediated beta-lactamase (MIR-1) conferring resistance to oxyimino- and alphamethoxy-beta-lactams in clinical isolates of Klebsiella pneumoniae. Antimicrob Agents Chemother. 1990;34:2200-2209.

102. Watanabe M, Iyobe S, Inoue M, Mitsuhashi S. Transferable imipenem resistance in Pseudomonas aeruginosa. Antimicrob Agents Chemother. 1991;35:147-151.

103. Ito H, Arakawa Y, Ohsuka S, et al. Plasmid-mediated dissemination of the metallo-β-lactamase gene bla_{IMP} among clinically isolated strains of Serratia marcescens. Antimicrob Agents Chemother. 1995;39:824-829.

104. Senda K, Arakawa Y, Ichiyama S, et al. PCR detection of metallo-β-lactamase gene (bla_{IMP}) in gram-negative rods resistant to broad-spectrum β-lactams. J Clin Microbiol. 1996;34:2909-2913.

105. Senda K, Arakawa Y, Nakashima K, et al. Multifocal outbreaks of metallo-β-lactamase-producing Pseudomonas aeruginosa resistant to broad-spectrum β-lactams, including carbapenems. Antimicrob Agents Chemother. 1996;40:349-353.

106. Scaife W, Young HK, Paton RH, Amyes SGB. Transferable imipenem-resistance in Acinetobacter species from a clinical source. J Antimicrob Chemother. 1995;36:585-586.

107. Paton R, Miles RS, Hood J, Amyes SGB. ARI 1: Beta-lactamase-mediated imipenem resistance in Acinetobacter baumannii. Int J Antimicrob Agents. 1993;2:81-88.

108. Brown S, Bantar C, Young HK, Amyes SGB. Limitation of Acinetobacter baumannii treatment by plasmid-mediated carbapenemase ARI-2. Lancet. 1998;351:186-187.

109. Moxon ER, Medeiros AA, O'Brien TF. Beta-lactamase effect on ampicillin treatment of Haemophilus influenzae B bacteremia and meningitis in infant rats. Antimicrob Agents Chemother. 1977;12:461-464.

110. Sanders CC, Sanders WE Jr, Goering RV. In vitro antagonism of beta-lactam antibiotics by cefoxitin. Antimicrob Agents Chemother. 1982;21:968-975.

111. Rasheed JK, Jay C, Metchock B, et al. Evolution of extended-spectrum beta-lactam resistance (SHV-8) in a strain of Escherichia coli during multiple episodes of bacteremia. Antimicrob Agents Chemother. 1997;41:647-653.

112. Bryan LE. Aminoglycoside resistance. In: Bryan LE, ed. Antimicrobial Drug Resistance. Orlando, FL: Academic Press; 1984:241-277.

113. Shimizu K, Kumada T, Hsieh WC, et al. Comparison of aminoglycoside resistance patterns in Japan, Formosa, and Korea, Chile, and the United States. Antimicrob Agents Chemother. 1985;28:282-288.

114. John JF Jr, Twitty JA. Plasmids as epidemiologic markers in nosocomial gram-negative bacilli: Experience at a university and review of the literature. Rev Infect Dis. 1986;8:693-704.

115. Horodniceanu T, Bougueleret L, El-Solh N, et al. High-level, plasmid-borne resistance to gentamicin in Streptococcus faecalis subsp. zymogenes. Antimicrob Agents Chemother. 1979;16:686-689.

116. Mederski-Samoraj BD, Murray BE. High-level resistance to gentamicin in clinical isolates of enterococci. J Infect Dis. 1983;147:751-757.

117. Murray BE, Tsao J, Panida J. Enterococci from Bangkok, Thailand, with high-level resistance to currently available aminoglycosides. Antimicrob Agents Chemother. 1983;23:799-802.

118. Zervos MJ, Kauffman CA, Therasse PM, et al. Nosocomial infection by gentamicin-resistant Streptococcus faecalis: An epidemiologic study. Ann Intern Med. 1987;106:687-691.

119. Hoffmann SA, Moellering RC Jr. The enterococcus: "Putting the bug in our ears." Ann Intern Med. 1987;106:757-761.

120. Patterson JE, Masecar BL, Kauffman CA, et al. Gentamicin resistance plasmids of enterococci from diverse geographic areas are heterogeneous. J Infect Dis. 1988;158:212-216.

121. Lyon BR, Skurray R. Antimicrobial resistance of Staphylococcus aureus: Genetic basis. Microbiol Rev. 1987;51:88-134.

122. Gaffney DF, Foster TJ, Shaw WV. Chloramphenicol acetyl transferases determined by R-plasmids from gram (−) bacteria. J Gen Microbiol. 1978;109:351-358.

123. Davies J. General mechanisms of antimicrobial resistance. Rev Infect Dis. 1979;1:23-29.

124. LeClercq R, Courvalin P. Resistance to macrolides, azalides, and streptogramins. In: Neu HC, Young LS, Zinner SH, eds. The New Macrolides, Azalides, and Streptogramins. New York: Marcel Dekker; 1993:33-40.

125. Andremont A, Gerbaud G, Courvalin P. Plasmid-mediated high-level resistance to erythromycin in Escherichia coli. Antimicrob Agents Chemother. 1986;29:515-518.

126. Brisson-Noel A, Delrieu P, Samain D, Courvalin P. Inactivation of lincosaminide antibiotics in Staphylococcus: Identification of lincosaminide O-nucleotidyltransferases and comparison of the corresponding resistance genes. J Biol Chem. 1988;263:15,880-15,887.

127. Le G'offic F, et al. Plasmid-mediated pristinamycin resistance: PH1A, a pristinamycin 1A hydrolase. Ann Microbiol. 1977;128:417-474.

128. Allignet J, Loncle V, Mazodier P, el Solh N. Nucleotide sequence of a staphylococcal plasmid gene, vgb, encoding a hydrolase inactivating the B components of virginiamycin-like antibiotics. Plasmid. 1988;20:271-275.

129. Speer BS, Bedzyk L, Salyers AA. Evidence that a novel tetracycline resistance gene found on two Bacteroides transposons encodes an NADP-oxidoreductase. J. Bacteriol. 1991;173:176-183.

130. Fleming A. On the antibacterial action of cultures of a penicillium, with special reference to their use in the isolation of B. influenzae. Br J Exp Pathol. 1929;10:226-236.

131. Nikaido H. Role of permeability barriers in resistance to beta-lactam antibiotics. Pharmacol Ther. 1985;27:197-231.

132. Labischinski H, Barnickel G, Bradaczek H, et al. High state of order of isolated bacterial lipopolysaccharide and its possible contribution to the permeation barrier property of the outer membrane. J Bacteriol. 1985;162:9-20.

133. Takeuchi Y, Nikaido H. Physical interaction between lipid A and phospholipids: A study with spin-labeled phospholipids. Rev Infect Dis. 1984;6:488-492.

134. Vaara M. Polymyxin B nonapeptide complexes with lipopolysaccharide (Letter). FEMS Microbiol Lett. 1983;18:117-121.

135. Nikaido H, Vaara M. Molecular basis of bacterial outer membrane permeability. Microbiol Rev. 1985;49:1-32.

136. Hasegawa Y, Yamada H, Mizushima S. Interactions of outer membrane proteins 0-8 and 0-9 with peptidoglycan sacculus of Escherichia coli K-12. J Biochem (Tokyo). 1976;80:1401-1409.

137. Yoshimura F, Nikaido H. Diffusion of beta-lactam antibiotics through the porin channels of Escherichia coli K-12. Antimicrob Agents Chemother. 1985;27:84-92.

138. Medeiros AA, O'Brien TF, Rosenberg EY, Nikaido H. Loss of OmpC porin in a strain of Salmonella typhimurium causes increased resistance to cephalosporins during therapy. J Infect Dis. 1987;156:751-757.

139. Goldstein FW, Gutmann L, Williamson R, et al. In vivo and in vitro emergence of simultaneous resistance to both beta-lactam and aminoglycoside antibiotics in a strain of Serratia marcescens. Ann Microbiol. 1983;134A:329-337.

140. Quinn JP, Dudek EJ, DiVincenzo CA, et al. Emergence of resistance to imipenem during therapy for Pseudomonas aeruginosa infections. J Infect Dis. 1986;154:289-293.

141. Livermore DM. Interplay of impermeability and chromosomal beta-lactamase activity in imipenem-resistant Pseudomonas aeruginosa. Antimicrob Agents Chemother. 1992;36:2046-2048.

142. Sanders CC, Sanders WE Jr, Goering RV, Werner V. Selection of multiple antibiotic resistance by quinolones, beta-lactams, and aminoglycosides with special reference to cross-resistance between unrelated drug classes. Antimicrob Agents Chemother. 1984;26:797-801.

143. Hooper DC, Wolfson JS, Ng EY, Swartz MN. Mechanisms of action of and resistance to ciprofloxacin. Am J Med. 1987;82:12-20.

144. Gaffney DF, Cundliffe E, Foster TJ. Chloramphenicol resistance that does not involve chloramphenicol acetyltransferase encoded by plasmids from gram-negative bacteria. J Gen Microbiol. 1981;125:113-121.

145. Bryan LE, Kwan S. Roles of ribosomal binding, membrane potential, and electron transport in bacterial uptake of streptomycin and gentamicin. Antimicrob Agents Chemother. 1983;23:835-845.

146. Mates SM, Eisenberg ES, Mandel LJ, et al. Membrane potential and gentamicin uptake in Staphylococcus aureus. Proc Natl Acad Sci U S A. 1982;79:6693-6697.

147. Rusthoven JJ, Davies TA, Lerner SA. Clinical isolation and characterization of aminoglycoside-resistant small colony variants of Enterobacter aerogenes. Am J Med. 1979;67:702-706.

148. Musher DM, Baughn RE, Merrell GL. Selection of small-colony variants of Enterobacteriaceae by in vitro exposure to aminoglycosides: Pathogenicity for experimental animals. J Infect Dis. 1979;140:209-214.

149. Funada H, Hattori KI, Kosakai N. Catalase-negative Escherichia coli isolated from blood. J Clin Microbiol. 1978;7:474-478.

150. Williams JB. Drug efflux as a mechanism of resistance. Br J Biomed Sci. 1996;53:290-293.

151. McMurry L, Petrucci RE Jr, Levy SB. Active efflux of tetracycline encoded by four genetically different tetracycline resistance determinants in *Escherichia coli*. Proc Natl Acad Sci U S A. 1980;77:3974-3977.

152. Levy SB, McMurry LM, Barbosa TM, et al. Nomenclature for new tetracycline resistance determinants. Antimicrob Agents Chemother. 1999;43:1523-1524.

153. Sutcliffe J, Tait-Kamradt A, Wandrack L. *Streptococcus pneumoniae* and *Streptococcus pyogenes* resistant to macrolide but sensitive to clindamycin: A common resistance pattern made by an efflux system. Antimicrob Agents Chemother. 1996;40:1817-1824.

154. Leclercq R. Mechanisms of resistance to macrolides and lincosamides: Nature of the resistance elements and their clinical implications. Clin Infect Dis. 2002;34:482-492.

155. Clancy J, Dib-Hajj F, Petitpas JW, Yuan W. Cloning and characterization of a novel macrolide efflux gene, *mreA*, from *Streptococcus agalactiae*. Antimicrob Agents Chemother. 1997;41:2719-2723.

156. Levy SB. Active efflux, a common mechanism for biocide and antibiotic resistance. J Appl Microbiol. 2002;92(Suppl1):65S-71S.

157. Srikumar R, Li XZ, Poole K. Inner membrane efflux components are responsible for β-lactam specificity of multidrug efflux pumps in *Pseudomonas aeruginosa*. J Bacteriol. 1997;179:7875-7881.

158. Masuda N, Sakagawa E, Ohya S, et al. Contribution of the Mex-X-MexY-oprM efflux system to intrinsic resistance in *Pseudomonas aeruginosa*. Antimicrob Agents Chemother. 2000;44:2242-2246.

159. Ghosh AS, Ahamed J, Chauhan KK, Kundu M. Involvement of an efflux system in high-level fluoroquinolone resistance of *Shigella dysenteriae*. Biochem Biophys Res Commun. 1998;242:54-56.

160. Cohen SP, Hooper DC, Wolfson JS, et al. Endogenous active efflux of norfloxacin in susceptible *Escherichia coli*. Antimicrob Agents Chemother. 1988;32:1187-1191.

161. Brown MH, Skurray RA. Staphylococcal multidrug efflux protein QacA. J Mol Microbiol Biotechnol. 2001;3:163-170.

162. Tait-Kamradt X, Davies T, Appelbaum PC, et al. Two new mechanisms of macrolide resistance in clinical strains of *Streptococcus pneumoniae* from Eastern Europe and North America. Antimicrob Agents Chemother. 2000;44:3395-3401.

163. Trieber GA, Taylor DE. Mutations in the 16S rRNA genes of *Helicobacter pylori* mediate resistance to tetracycline. J Bacteriol. 2002;184:2131-2140.

164. Eliopoulos GM, Farber BF, Murray BE, et al. Ribosomal resistance of clinical enterococcal to streptomycin isolates. Antimicrob Agents Chemother. 1984;25:398-399.

165. Ahmad MH, Rechenmacher A, Bock A. Interaction between aminoglycoside uptake and ribosomal resistance mutations. Antimicrob Agents Chemother. 1980;18:798-806.

166. Dutka-Malen S, LeClercq R, Coutant V, et al. Phenotypic and genotypic heterogeneity of glycopeptide resistance determinants in gram-positive bacteria. Antimicrob Agents Chemother. 1990;34:1875-1879.

167. McKessar SJ, Barry AM, Bell JM, et al. Genetic characterization of vanG, a novel vancomycin resistance locus for *Enterococcus faecalis*. Antimicrob Agents Chemother. 2000;44:3224-3228.

168. LeClercq R, Derlot E, Weber M, et al. Transferable vancomycin and teicoplanin resistance in *Enterococcus faecium*. Antimicrob Agents Chemother. 1989;33:10-15.

169. Shlaes DM, Bouvet A, Devine C, et al. Inducible, transferable resistance to vancomycin in *Enterococcus faecalis* A256. Antimicrob Agents Chemother. 1989;33:198-203.

170. Centers for Disease Control and Prevention. Vancomycin-resistant *Staphylococcus aureus*—Pennsylvania, 2002. MMWR Morb Mortal Wkly Rep. 2002;51:902.

171. Nicas TI, Cole CT, Preston DA, et al. Activity of glycopeptides against vancomycin-resistant gram-positive bacteria. Antimicrob Agents Chemother. 1989;33:1477-1481.

172. Bugg TD, Wright GD, Dutka-Malen S, et al. Molecular basis for vancomycin resistance in *Enterococcus faecium* BM4147: Biosynthesis of a depsipeptide peptidoglycan precursor by vancomycin resistance proteins VanH and VanA. Biochemistry. 1991;30:10,408-10,415.

173. LeClercq R, Dutka-Malen S, Brissonnoel A, et al. Resistance of enterococci to aminoglycosides and glycopeptides. Clin Infect Dis. 1992;15:495-501.

174. Quintiliani R, Evers S, Courvalin P. The *van*B gene confers various levels of self-transferable resistance to vancomycin in enterococci. J Infect Dis. 1993;167:1220-1223.

175. Fluit AC, Visser MR, Schmitz FJ. Molecular detection of antimicrobial resistance. Clin Microbiol Rev. 2001;14:836-871.

176. Schwalbe RS, Stapleton JT, Gilligan PH. Emergence of vancomycin resistance in coagulase-negative staphylococci. N Engl J Med. 1987;316:927-931.

177. Biavasco F, Vignaroli C, Lazzarini R, Varaldo PE. Glycopeptide susceptibility profiles of *Staphylococcus haemolyticus* blood stream isolates. Antimicrob Agents Chemother. 2000;44:3122-3126.

178. Centers for Disease Control and Prevention. Reduced susceptibility of *Staphylococcus aureus* to vancomycin—Japan, 1996. MMWR Morb Mortal Wkly Rep. 1997;46:624-635.

179. Geisel R, Schmitz FJ, Fluit AC, et al. Emergence, mechanism, and clinical implications of reduced glycopeptide susceptibility in *Staphylococcus aureus*. Eur J Clin Microbiol Infect Dis. 2001;20:685-697.

180. Cui L, Murakami H, Kuwahara-Arai K, et al. Contribution of a thickened cell wall and its glutamine nonamidated component to the vancomycin resistance expressed by *Staphylococcus aureus* M450. Antimicrob Agents Chemother. 2000;44:2276-2285.

181. Hospital Infection Control Practices Advisory Committee (HICPAC). Recommendations for preventing the spread of vancomycin resistance. Infect Control Hosp Epidemiol. 1995;16:105-113.

182. Waxman DJ, Strominger JL. Penicillin-binding proteins and the mechanism of action of beta-lactam antibiotics. Ann Rev Biochem. 1983;52:825-869.

183. Malouin F, Bryan LE. Modification of penicillin-binding proteins as mechanisms of beta-lactam resistance. Antimicrob Agents Chemother. 1986;30:1-5.

184. Williamson R. Resistance of *Clostridium perfringens* to beta-lactam antibiotics mediated by a decreased affinity of a single essential penicillin-binding protein. J Gen Microbiol. 1983;129:2339-2342.

185. Giles AF, Reynolds RE. *Bacillus megaterium* resistance to cloxacillin accompanied by a compensatory change in penicillin binding proteins. Nature. 1979;280:167-168.

186. Hakenbeck R, Tarpay M, Tomasz A. Multiple changes of penicillin-binding proteins in penicillin-resistant clinical isolates of *Streptococcus pneumoniae*. Antimicrob Agents Chemother. 1980;17:364-371.

187. Spratt BG, Dowson CG, Zhang Q-Y, et al. Mosaic genes, hybrid penicillin-binding proteins, and the origins of penicillin resistance in *Neisseria meningitidis* and *Streptococcus pneumoniae*. In: Pardee A, Campisi J, eds. Perspectives on Cellular Regulation: From Bacteria to Cancer. New York: Wiley-Liss; 1991:73-83.

188. Hartman BJ, Tomasz A. Low-affinity penicillin-binding protein associated with beta-lactam resistance in *Staphylococcus aureus*. J Bacteriol. 1984;158:513-516.

189. Ubukata K, Yamashita N, Konno M. Occurrence of a beta-lactam-inducible penicillin-binding protein in methicillin-resistant staphylococci. Antimicrob Agents Chemother. 1985;27:851-857.

190. Fontana R. Penicillin-binding proteins and the intrinsic resistance to beta-lactams in gram-positive cocci. J Antimicrob Chemother. 1985;16:412-416.

191. Fontana R, Grossato A, Rossi L, et al. Transition from resistance to hypersusceptibility to beta-lactam antibiotics associated with loss of a low-affinity penicillin-binding protein in a *Streptococcus faecium* mutant highly resistant to penicillin. Antimicrob Agents Chemother. 1985;28:678-683.

192. Farber BF, Eliopoulos GM, Ward JI, et al. Multiply resistant viridans streptococci: Susceptibility to beta-lactam antibiotics and comparison of penicillin-binding protein patterns. Antimicrob Agents Chemother. 1977;3(Suppl C):47-51.

193. Sabath LD. Chemical and physical factors influencing methicillin resistance of *Staphylococcus aureus* and *Staphylococcus epidermidis*. J Antimicrob Chemother. 1977;3(Suppl C):47-51.

194. Song MD, Wachi M, Doi M, et al. Evolution of an inducible penicillin-target protein in methicillin-resistant *Staphylococcus aureus* by gene fusion. FEBS Lett. 1987;221:167-171.

195. Berger-Bachi B, Barberis-Maino L, Strassle A, Kayser FH. FemA, a host-mediated factor essential for methicillin resistance in *Staphylococcus aureus*: Molecular cloning and characterization. Mol Gen Genet. 1989;219:263-269.

196. Dougherty TJ, Koller AE, Tomasz A. Penicillin-binding proteins of penicillin-susceptible and intrinsically resistant *Neisseria gonorrhoeae*. Antimicrob Agents Chemother. 1980;18:730-737.

197. Mendelman PM, Chaffin DO, Kalaitzoglou G. Penicillin-binding proteins and ampicillin resistance in *Haemophilus influenzae*. J Antimicrob Chemother. 1990;25:525-534.

198. Dougherty TJ. Genetic analysis and penicillin-binding protein alterations in *Neisseria gonorrhoeae* with chromosomally mediated resistance. Antimicrob Agents Chemother. 1986;30:649-652.

199. Mendelman PM, Campos J, Chaffin DO, et al. Relative penicillin G resistance in *Neisseria meningitidis* and reduced affinity of penicillin-binding protein 3. Antimicrob Agents Chemother. 1988;32:706-709.

200. Spratt BG, Zhang Q-Y, Jones DM, et al. Recruitment of a penicillin-binding protein gene from *Neisseria flavescens* during the emergence of penicillin resistance in *Neisseria meningitidis*. Proc Natl Acad Sci U S A. 1989;86:8988-8992.

201. Faruki H, Kohmescher RN, McKinney WP, Sparling PF. A community-based outbreak of infection with penicillin-resistant *Neisseria gonorrhoeae* not producing penicillinase (chromosomally mediated resistance). N Engl J Med. 1985;313:607-611.

202. Mirelman D, Nuchamowitz Y, Rubinstein E. Insensitivity of peptidoglycan biosynthetic reactions to beta-lactam antibiotics in a clinical isolate of *Pseudomonas aeruginosa*. Antimicrob Agents Chemother. 1981;19:687-695.

203. Parr TR Jr, Bryan LE. Mechanism of resistance of an ampicillin-resistant, beta-lactamase-negative clinical isolate of *Haemophilus influenzae* type b to beta-lactam antibiotics. Antimicrob Agents Chemother. 1984;25:747-753.

204. Wolfson JS, Hooper DC. The fluoroquinolones: Structures, mechanisms of action and resistance, and spectra of activity in vitro. Antimicrob Agents Chemother. 1985;28:581-586.

205. Hane MW, Wood TH. *Escherichia coli* K-12 mutants resistant to nalidixic acid: Genetic mapping and dominance studies. J Bacteriol. 1969;99:238-241.

206. Robillard NJ, Scarpa AL. Genetic and physiological characterization of ciprofloxacin resistance in *Pseudomonas aeruginosa* PAO. Antimicrob Agents Chemother. 1988;32:535-539.

207. Schmitz FJ, Higgins P, Meyer S, et al. Activity of quinolones against gram-positive cocci: mechanisms of drug action and bacterial resistance. Eur J Clin Microbiol Infect Dis. 2002;21:647-659.

208. Schmitz FJ, Jones ME, Hofmann B, et al. Characterization of grlA, grlB, gyrA and gyrB mutations in 116 unrelated isolates of *Staphylococcus aureus* in relation to minimal inhibitory concentrations of ciprofloxacin. Antimicrob Agents Chemother. 1998;42:1249-1252.

209. Aoyama H, Fujimaki K, Sato K, et al. Clinical isolate of *Citrobacter freundii* highly resistant to new quinolones. Antimicrob Agents Chemother. 1988;32:922-924.

210. Nakamura S, Nakamura M, Kojima T, Yoshida H. *gyrA* and *gyrB* mutations in quinolone-resistant strains of *Escherichia coli*. Antimicrob Agents Chemother. 1989;33:254-255.

211. Cullen ME, Wyke AW, Kuroda R, Fisher LM. Cloning and characterization of a DNA gyrase A gene from *Escherichia coli* that confers clinical resistance to 4-quinolones. Antimicrob Agents Chemother. 1989;33:886-894.

212. Enne VI, King A, Livermore DM, Hall LMC. Sulfonamide resistance in *Haemophilus influenzae* mediated by acquisition of sul2 or a short insertion in chromosomal folP. Antimicrob Agents Chemother. 2002;46:1934-1939.

213. Huovinen P. Trimethoprim resistance. Antimicrob Agents Chemother. 1987;31:1451-1456.

214. Steen R, Skold O. Plasmid-borne or chromosomally mediated resistance by Tn7 is the most common response to ubiquitous use of trimethoprim. Antimicrob Agents Chemother. 1985;27:933-937.

215. Maskell R, Okubadejo OA, Payne RH, Pead L. Human infections with thymine-requiring bacteria. J Med Microbiol. 1978;11:33-45.

216. Whitney CG, Farley MM, Hadler J, et al. Increasing prevalence of multidrug-resistant *Streptococcus pneumoniae* in the United States. N Engl J Med. 2000;343:1917-1924.

217. Hogan D, Kolter R. Why are bacteria refractory to antimicrobials? Curr Opin Microbiol. 2002;5:472-477.

218. Partridge SR, Brown HJ, Hall RM. Characterization and movement of the class I integron known as Tn2521 and Tn1405. Antimicrob Agents Chemother. 2002;46:1288-1294.

219. LeThomas I, Couetdio G, Clermont O, et al. In vivo selection of a target/efflux double mutant of *Pseudomonas aeruginosa* by ciprofloxacin therapy. J Antimicrob Chemother. 2001;48:553-555.

220. Mah TF, O'Tolle GA. Mechanisms of biofilm resistance to antimicrobial agents. Trends Micribiol. 2001;9:34-39.

221. Heal RD, Parsons AT. Novel intercullular communication in *Escherichia coli* that confers antibiotic resistance between physically separated populations. J Appl Microbiol. 2002;92:1116-1122.

222. DeKlevit T, Parkins M, Gillis R, et al. Multidrug efflux pumps: Expression patterns and contribution to antibiotic resistance in *Pseudomonas aeruginosa* biofilms. Antimicrob Agents Chemother. 2001;45:1761-1770.

223. Rand JD, Danby SG, Greenway DL, England R. Increased expression of the multidrug efflux genes acrAB occurs during slow growth of *Escherichia coli*. FEMS Microbiol Lett. 2002;207:91-95.

224. Drenkard E, Ausubel FM. *Pseudomonas* biofilm formation and antibiotic resistance are linked to phenotypic variation. Nature. 2002;416:740-743.

225. Mayer KH, Hopkins JD, Gilleece ES, et al. Computer-assisted correlations between antibiotypes of clinical isolates and the endonuclease restriction fragment of types of their plasmids. In: Mitsuhasi S, Rosival L, Krcmery V, eds. Transferrable Antibiotic Resistance: Plasmids and Gene Manipulation. Prague: Czechoslovak Press; 1984:163-169.

226. Rainey PB, Moxon ER. When being hyper keeps you fit. Science. 2000;288:1186-1187.

227. Tompkins JD, Nelson JL, Hazel JC, et al. Error-prone polymerase, DNA polymerase IV, is responsible for transient hypermutation during adaptive mutation in *Escherichia coli*. J Bacteriol. 2003;185:3469-3472.

228. Murray BE, Alvarado T, Kim KH, et al. Increasing resistance to trimethoprim-sulfamethoxazole among isolates of *Escherichia coli* in developing countries. J Infect Dis. 1985;152:1107-1113.

229. Seppala H, Nissinen A, Jarvinen H, et al. Resistance to erythromycin in group A streptococci (see comments). N Engl J Med. 1992;326:292-297.

230. Moellering RC Jr. Emergence of *Enterococcus* as a significant pathogen. Clin Infect Dis. 1992;14:1173-1176.

231. Grayson ML, Eliopoulos GM, Wennersten CB, et al. Increasing resistance to beta-lactam antibiotics among clinical isolates of *Enterococcus faecium*: A 22-year review at one institution. Antimicrob Agents Chemother. 1991;35:2180-2184.

232. Rhinehart E, Smith NE, Wennersten C, et al. Rapid dissemination of beta-lactamase-producing, aminoglycoside-resistant *Enterococcus faecalis* among patients and staff on an infant-toddler surgical ward (see comments). N Engl J Med. 1990;323:1814-1818.

233. Bugg TD, Dutka-Malen S, Arthur M, et al. Identification of vancomycin resistance protein VanA as a D-alanine:D-alanine ligase of altered substrate specificity. Biochemistry. 1991;30:2017-2021.

234. Rubin LG, Tucci V, Cercenado E, et al. Vancomycin-resistant *Enterococcus faecium* in hospitalized children. Infect Control Hosp Epidemiol. 1992;13:700-705.

235. Karanfil LV, Murphy M, Josephson A, et al. A cluster of vancomycin-resistant *Enterococcus faecium* in an intensive care unit (see comments). Infect Control Hosp Epidemiol. 1992;13:195-200.

236. Livornese LL, Dias S, Samel C, et al. Hospital-acquired infection with vancomycin-resistant *Enterococcus faecium* transmitted by electronic thermometers. Ann Intern Med. 1992;117:112-116.

237. Uttley AHC, Collins CH. Vancomycin-resistant enterococci. Lancet. 1988;1:57-58.

238. Boyce JM, Opal SM, Chow JW, et al. Outbreak of multidrug-resistant *Enterococcus faecium* with transferable vanB class vancomycin resistance. J Clin Microbiol. 1994;32:1148-1153.

239. Schaefler S. Methicillin-resistant strains of *Staphylococcus aureus* resistant to quinolones. J Clin Microbiol. 1989;27:335-336.

240. Shalit I, Berger SA, Gorea A, Frimerman H. Widespread quinolone resistance among methicillin-resistant *Staphylococcus aureus* isolates in a general hospital. Antimicrob Agents Chemother. 1989;33:593-594.

241. Banerjee SN, Emori TG, Culver DH, et al. Secular trends in nosocomial primary bloodstream infections in the United States, 1980-1989. National Nosocomial Infections Surveillance System. Am J Med. 1991;91:86S-89S.

242. White DG, Shao S, Sudler R, et al. The isolation of antibiotic-resistant *Salmonella* from retail ground meats. N Engl J Med. 2001;345:1147-1154.

243. Sørenson TL, Blom M, Monnet DL, et al. Transient intestinal carriage after ingestion of antibiotic-resistant *Enterococcus faecium* from chicken and pork. N Engl J Med. 2001;345:1161-1166.

244. McDonald LC, Rossiter S, Mackinson C, et al. Quinupristin-dalfopristin-resistant *Enterococcus faecium* on chicken and in human stool specimens. N Engl J Med. 2001;345:1155-1160.

245. McGowan JE Jr, Tenover FC. Control of antimicrobial resistance in the health care system. Infect Dis Clin North Am. 1997;11:297-311.

246. Philippon A, Dusart J, Joris B, Frère JM. The diversity, structure and regulation of β-lactamases. Cell Mol Life Sci. 1998;54:341-346.

247. Bauernfeind A, Stemplinger I, Jungwirth R, et al. Sequences of p-lactamase genes encoding CTX-M-1 (MEN-1) and CTX-M-2 and relationship of their amino acid sequences with those of other β-lactamases. Antimicrob Agents Chemother. 1996;40:509-513.

248. Ishii Y, Ohno A, Taguchi H, et al. Cloning and sequence of the gene encoding a cefotaxime-hydrolyzing class a β-lactamase isolated from *Escherichia coli*. Antimicrob Agents Chemother. 1995;39:2269-2275.

249. Ma L, Ishii Y, Ishiguro M, et al. Cloning and sequencing of the gene encoding Toho-2, a class A β-lactamase preferentially inhibited by tazobactam. Antimicrob Agents Chemother. 1998;42:1181-1186.

250. Gniadkowski M, Schneider I, Palucha A, et al. Cefotaxime-resistant Enterobacteriaceae isolates from a hospital in Warsaw, Poland: Identification of a new CTX-M-3 cefotaxime-hydrolyzing β-lactamase that is closely related to the CTX-M-1/MEN-1 enzyme. Antimicrob Agents Chemother. 1998;42:827-832.

251. Gazouli M, Tzelepi E, Sidorenko SV, Tzouvelekis LS. Sequence of the gene encoding a plasmid-mediated cefotaxime-hydrolyzing class A β-lactamase (CTX-M-4): Involvement of serine 237 in cephalosporin hydrolysis. Antimicrob Agents Chemother. 1998;42:1259-1262.

252. Nordmann P, Naas T. Sequence analysis of PER-1 extended-spectrum beta-lactamase from *Pseudomonas aeruginosa* and comparison with class A beta-lactamases. Antimicrob Agents Chemother. 1994;38:104-114.

253. Bauernfeind A, Stemplinger I, Jungwirth R, et al. Characterization of β-lactamase gene blaPER-2, which encodes an extended-spectrum class A β-lactamase. Antimicrob Agents Chemother. 1996;40:616-620.

254. Bradford PA, Urban C, Mariano N, et al. Imipenem resistance in *Klebsiella pneumoniae* is associated with the combination of ACT-1, a plasmid-mediated AmpC β-lactamase, and the loss of an outer membrane protein. Antimicrob Agents Chemother. 1997;41:563-569.

255. Payne DJ, Woodford N, Amyes SGB. Characterization of the plasmid mediated beta-lactamase BIL-1. J Antimicrob Chemother. 1992;30:119-127.

256. Fosberry AP, Payne DJ, Lawlor EJ, Hodgson JE. Cloning and sequence analysis of bla (BIL-1), a plasmid- mediated class C beta-lactamase gene in *Escherichia coli* BS. Antimicrob Agents Chemother. 1994;38:1182-1185.

257. Bauernfeind A, Stemplinger I, Jungwirth R, Giamarellou H. Characterization of the plasmidic β-lactamase CMY-2, which is responsible for cephamycin resistance. Antimicrob Agents Chemother. 1996;40:221-224.

258. Koeck JL, Arlet G, Philippon A, et al. Novel plasmid-mediated ampC-type β-lactamase (SAL-1) in a clinical isolate of *Salmonella senftenberg*. In: Program and Abstracts of the 36th Interscience Conference on Antimicrobial Agents and Chemotherapy. Washington, DC: American Society for Microbiology; 1996:39.

259. Tzouvelekis LS, Tzelepi E, Mentis AF. Nucleotide sequence of a plasmid-mediated cephalosporinase gene (blaLAT-1) found in *Klebsiella pneumoniae*. Antimicrob Agents Chemother. 1994;38:2207-2209.

260. Gazouli M, Tzouvelekis LS, Prinarakis E, et al. Transferable cefoxitin resistance in enterobacteria from Greek hospitals and characterization of a plasmid-mediated group 1 β-lactamase (LAT-2). Antimicrob Agents Chemother. 1998;42:1736-1740.

261. Verdet C, Arlet G, Barnaud G, et al. Novel integron carrying *ampC* and *ampR* genes on a plasmid from *Salmonella enteritidis*. Abstract C-125. In: Abstracts of the 37th Interscience Conference on Antimicrobial Agents and Chemotherapy. Washington, DC: American Society for Microbiology; 1997:68.

262. Gonzalez Leiza M, Perez-Diaz JC, Ayala J, et al. Gene sequence and biochemical characterization of FOX-1 from *Klebsiella pneumoniae*, a new AmpC-type plasmid-mediated beta-lactamase with two molecular variants. Antimicrob Agents Chemother. 1994;38:2150-2157.

263. Bauernfeind A, Wagner S, Jungwirth R, et al. A novel class C β-lactamase (FOX-2) in *Escherichia coli* conferring resistance to cephamycins. Antimicrob Agents Chemother. 1997;41:2041-2046.

264. Marchese A, Arlet G, Schito GC, et al. Characterization of FOX-3, an AmpC-type plasmid-mediated β-lactamase from an Italian isolate of *Klebsiella oxytoca*. Antimicrob Agents Chemother. 1998;42:464-467.

265. Bauernfeind A, Stemplinger I, Jungwirth R, et al. Comparative characterization of the cephamycinase blaCMY-1 gene and its relationship with other β-lactamase genes. Antimicrob Agents Chemother. 1996;40:1926-1930.

266. Horii T, Arakawa Y, Ohta M, et al. Plasmid-mediated ampC-type beta-lactamase isolated from *Klebsiella pneumoniae* confers resistance to broad-spectrum beta-lactams, including moxalactam. Antimicrob Agents Chemother. 1993;37:984-990.

267. Horii T, Arakawa Y, Ohta M, et al. Characterization of a plasmid-borne and constitutively expressed bla (MOX-1) gene encoding ampC-type beta-lactamase. Gene. 1994;139:93-98.

268. Bobrowski MM, Matthew M, Barth PT, et al. Plasmid-determined beta-lactamase indistinguishable from the chromosomal beta-lactamase of *Escherichia coli*. J Bacteriol. 1976;125:149-157.

269. Bandoh K, Watanabe K, Muto Y, et al. Conjugal transfer of imipenem resistance in *Bacteroides fragilis*. J Antibiot (Tokyo). 1992;45:542-547.

270. Rasmussen BA, Bush K. Carbapenem-hydrolyzing β-lactamases. Antimicrob Agents Chemother. 1997;41:223-232.

Pharmacokinetics and Pharmacodynamics of Anti-infective Agents

GUY W. AMSDEN

CHARLES H. BALLOW

JOSEPH S. BERTINO, JR.

ANGELA D. M. KASHUBA

***P**harmacology* is the knowledge base of a compound concerning its history, source, physical and chemical properties, compounding, biochemical and physiologic effects, mechanisms of action and resistance, absorption, distribution, metabolism, excretion, and therapeutic and other uses.[1] *Pharmacokinetics* encompasses all the ways that the body manipulates a drug, including absorption, distribution, metabolism, and excretion. *Pharmacodynamics* describes the biochemical and physiologic effects of the drug and its mechanism of action (Fig. 18-1). The terms defined in this chapter are summarized in Table 18-1.

PHARMACOKINETICS

Pharmacokinetic Modeling

Pharmacokinetic drug data may be analyzed by noncompartmental or compartmental methods. Noncompartmental analysis makes no assumption of the physiologic distribution or elimination of a drug. *Noncompartmental* analysis simply serves as a description of drug behavior in biologic fluids, most commonly serum or plasma. *Compartmental* analysis offers the potential to broaden the appreciation of the drug by providing more insight into physiologic distribution and potential elimination pathways. The latter may be linear, such as renal elimination, or nonlinear, such as hepatic elimination. Compartmental analysis can compensate best for errors in investigational procedures (i.e., sampling errors, missing values).

Compartmental analysis is more amenable to population analysis, in which prior information about the pharmacokinetic and pharmacodynamic behaviors of a drug in the target population is incorporated into the analysis.

Compartmental modeling requires exploration of several candidate models (e.g., one-compartment model, two-compartment model), which can be selected initially after visual inspection of the plots of drug concentration versus time. All models are defined by combinations of parameters depending on the route of administration, biologic fluids collected, chemical analyses performed, and other factors. The

TABLE 18-1   Quick Reference Pharmacologic Abbreviations and Their Definitions

Type of Term	Abbreviation	Definition
Pharmacokinetics		
Absorption	F	Bioavailability; absolute bioavailability
	Ka	Absorption rate constant
Distribution	V_d	Volume of distribution
	V_d/F	Apparent volume of distribution
	V_{ss}	Volume of distribution at steady-state
	V_{ss}/F	Apparent volume of distribution at steady-state
	CL_D	Distributional clearance
	CL_D/F	Apparent distributional clearance
Metabolism	Km	The drug concentration at which the rate that an enzyme system can metabolize a drug is half of Vm (Michaelis-Menten type metabolism [saturable metabolism])
	Vm	Maximal metabolic capacity (Michaelis-Menten type metabolism [saturable metabolism])
	CYP	Cytochrome P-450 enzyme systems
Elimination	CL_r	Renal clearance
	CL_{nr}	Nonrenal clearance
	CL_{nr}/F	Nonrenal oral clearance
	CL_T	Total clearance
	CL_T/F	Total oral clearance
	$T_{1/2}$	Half-life
Pharmacodynamics		
	MIC_{90}	Minimal inhibitory concentration for 90% of isolates
	EC_{50}	Effective concentration for 50% of all isolates
	MPC	Mutant prevention concentration
	MSW	Mutant selection window
	IC_{50}	Inhibitory concentration for 50% of isolates
	Cmax/MIC	Peak antimicrobial serum concentration-to-MIC ratio (concentration-dependent killers)
	AUC/MIC	24-hour area under the serum antimicrobial concentration versus time curve-to-MIC ratio
	AUIC	24-hour area under the inhibitory curve
	$T_{1/2}$	Half-life
	T>MIC	Time that serum antimicrobial concentrations are above the organism's MIC (time-dependent killers)
	SBT	Serum bactericidal titer (concentration)
	IQ	Inhibitory quotient = ratio of rough serum concentration to IC_{50}
	PAE	Postantibiotic effect

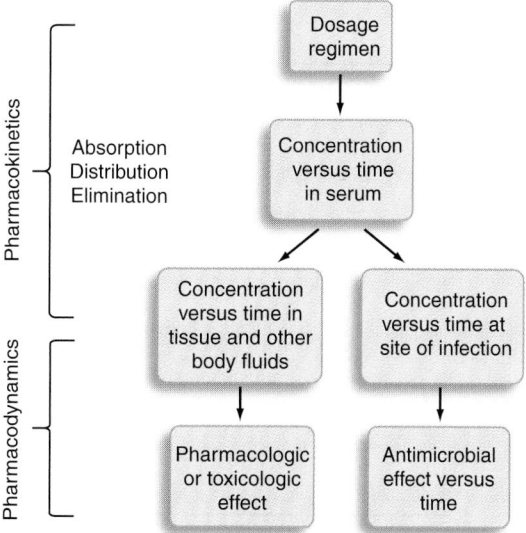

FIGURE 18-1. Overview of the interaction of pharmacokinetics and pharmacodynamics for anti-infective agents. *(From Craig WA. Pharmacokinetic/pharmacodynamic parameters: Rationale for antibacterial dosing of mice and men. Clin Infect Dis. 1998;26:1-12. Copyright © 1998 University of Chicago.)*

model that minimizes the statistical error in curve fitting ultimately is selected as the final model. The following sections describe commonly modeled parameters associated with the pharmacokinetics literature.

Absorption

Absorption of a drug into the systemic circulation occurs anywhere that it is administered except when it is administered directly into a physiologic fluid compartment (e.g., blood stream, cerebrospinal fluid). This definition includes intramuscular, subcutaneous, or topical administration and absorption from the gastrointestinal tract after oral, rectal, or tube administration. The amount of drug that reaches the systemic circulation is expressed as a percentage of the total amount that could have been absorbed. This percentage is defined as the drug's *bioavailability,* commonly described in the literature by the term *F.* It also may be reported as *absolute bioavailability,* a more accurate value that is determined by direct comparison of an intravenous form of the drug with the extravascularly administered form. By definition, most (but not all) intravenous forms of a drug are 100% bioavailable because all of the administered dose enters the blood stream. Many other pharmacokinetic values depend on bioavailability (e.g., clearance, volume of distribution) for drugs that need to be absorbed.

Absorption is a dynamic process. Depending on the form of administration, a drug's absorption and its bioavailability can vary. Although a paucity or lack of absorption channels or systems at the site of administration may decrease absorption, such a decrease also may be caused by the dose administered or the type of absorption channel or system. Many systems can be overwhelmed and go from absorbing everything passed on to them (*nonsaturable absorption*) to absorbing the compound only at a certain rate (*saturable* or *zero-order absorption*). In addition, concentration-dependent solubility may be interpreted as dose-dependent absorption. In any case, the rate at which the drug is absorbed is termed the *absorption rate constant* (Ka).

A factor commonly associated with a decrease in the bioavailability of a drug (i.e., the amount that gets into the systemic circulation) is the first-pass effect. Drugs that are absorbed from the small intestine can be affected by the first-pass effect of the liver because the circulation leading away from these sites (portal vein circulation) passes through the liver immediately. Drugs administered via other sites (e.g., rectally [variable], intramuscularly, intravenously) usually are not associated with a first-pass effect and can have higher bioavailability because they are not affected immediately by the liver's metabolic capacity. Additionally, drugs can be metabolized by drug-metabolizing enzymes in the gastrointestinal tract, reducing absorption of these compounds. Finally, transport proteins in the gastrointestinal tract can affect drug absorption. In general, inhibition of transport proteins increases gastrointestinal drug absorption (of specific transporter substrates), whereas induction reduces drug absorption. Other factors that can affect absorption and bioavailability are drug interactions with other compounds or food that may bind the drug and prevent it from being absorbed or a disease state that may affect adversely the site of absorption (i.e., diarrhea, parasites, ileus, ulcerative colitis).

Distribution

Distribution of a drug is described most commonly by the *volume of distribution* (V_d or V_d/F). The volume of distribution is not a real or physiologic value, but rather a value that relates drug concentration in the system to the amount of drug present in that system. Factors that alter the volume of distribution include lipid solubility, partition coefficient of the drug between different types of tissues, blood flow to tissues, pH, and binding to biologic material (e.g., plasma proteins, cellular components).[2]

Drugs with small distribution volumes have limited distribution, whereas drugs with large distribution volumes are distributed extensively throughout the body. A drug with a 5-L volume of distribution in an adult would be restricted to the circulatory system. If the volume of distribution is between 10 and 20 L, the drug distributes into extracellular compartments. If the volume of distribution is on the order of 25 to 30 L, intracellular distribution is implied. Distribution volumes

of approximately 40 L suggest distribution within whole-body fluid. In rare circumstances, distribution volumes may be measured in hundreds or even thousands of liters. These large volumes suggest either "deep" tissue deposition in peripheral compartments (e.g., fat) or extensive binding to biologic structures (e.g., tissue protein, organelles). When a steady state has been achieved after multiple doses of a medication, the *total volume of distribution* is referred to as the V_{ss}. This value represents the sum of the distribution volumes from each of the identified physiologic compartments.

After intravenous administration of a drug, the concentration rapidly reaches a peak before beginning to decline. Distribution and elimination are two factors that affect the extent of the peak concentration and the rate of decay. Usually distribution is completed sooner than elimination. This situation results in two phases in the concentration versus time plot (Fig. 18-2). The first phase, or α *phase*, is usually short and represents mixing of the drug throughout the circulatory system and distribution into rapidly equilibrating tissues. The second phase, or β *phase*, is usually a reflection of terminal elimination and is the phase from which the terminal half-life ($T_{1/2}$) is calculated. Occasionally, more than two phases may be observed; this usually indicates further distribution into slowly equilibrating tissues. An understanding of distribution and elimination is important when applying pharmacokinetics to therapeutic drug monitoring. An example is aminoglycosides. In the use of single daily dose therapy, nomograms and rules have been constructed to assist in dosing. These nomograms and rules were devised, however, using assumptions of distribution of the drugs based on smaller doses. With the use of larger doses of aminoglycosides, distribution time is increased, and many popular nomograms and rules for dosing these agents once a day are subsequently in error because the original assumptions do not apply to high doses.[3]

The rate at which a drug moves from the blood to tissues is described by the *distributional clearance* (CL_D or CL_D/F). Just as total body clearance describes the volume of blood from which a drug is eliminated per unit time, distributional clearance describes the volume of blood from which a drug is transferred into a tissue or compartment per unit of time. Distributional clearance is a bidirectional process reflecting the equilibrium in movement from blood to tissue and from tissue to blood. When the drug has moved into a tissue compartment, the local tissue concentration is a function of the amount of drug located in the tissue and the tissue volume of distribution, also known as the *volume of the peripheral compartment* (V_p). These volumes can be estimated only by mathematical modeling because it is unusual to be able to collect biologic specimens from peripheral compartments and assay the drug concentration.

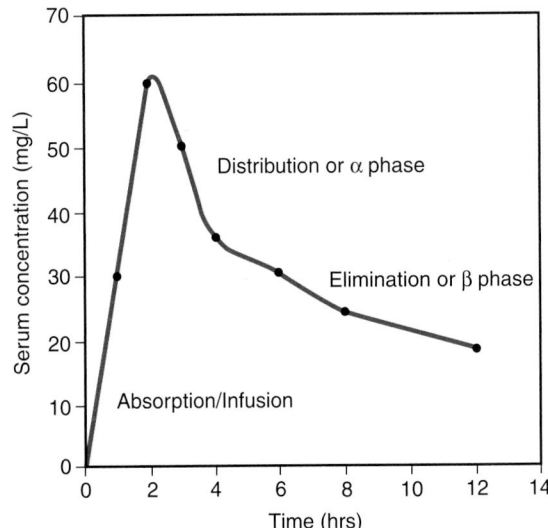

FIGURE 18-2. A graphic example of the serum concentration versus time profile of a typical two-phase or two-compartment drug during the absorptive-infusion, distributive, and elimination phases.

Many drugs bind to serum proteins, especially albumins or α_1-acid glycoprotein. Similar to other classes of drugs, antimicrobial agents range from highly to poorly protein bound. Theoretically, protein binding is an important consideration for antimicrobial agents because only unbound drug is available to exert antimicrobial activity.[4] Changes in the unbound fraction of drug may be caused by displacement from other drugs, changes in serum protein concentrations, or accumulation of endogenous substances, such as free fatty acids. Changes in the unbound fraction typically do not lead, however, to significant changes in free drug concentration due to various equilibrium processes. Although changes in protein binding may alter pharmacokinetic behavior of an antimicrobial agent, it is unlikely that substantial changes in pharmacodynamics would occur.[5]

Metabolism and Biotransformation

Drugs and other compounds are metabolized by a variety of reactions. Although traditionally drug metabolism was thought to occur in the liver, other organs also have the ability to metabolize drugs.

Because drug metabolism requires the presence of enzymes, the principles of Michaelis and Menten can be applied to drug metabolism. Michaelis and Menten showed approximately 90 years ago that enzyme systems have a finite capacity to metabolize substrate. Although all routes of drug metabolism are saturable, if the doses and concentrations at the site of metabolism do not exceed the maximal rate of metabolism, the metabolic system appears to follow linear pharmacokinetics. If the dose exceeds the amount that can be metabolized, drug accumulation can occur, leading to high serum concentrations and high tissue levels. These high levels can result in toxic side effects. If a daily dose is given that is lower than what the body can eliminate, low concentrations may be seen. These *dose-dependent kinetics* (also called *Michaelis-Menten, zero-order,* or *saturation kinetics*) mean that when saturation of the ability to metabolize the drug in a 24-hour period is reached, small dosage increases may produce large, disproportionate increases in serum concentrations. Conversely, if a daily dose is higher than what can be metabolized in 24 hours and results in high serum concentrations, small reductions in the dose may cause large reductions in the serum concentration.

Drug metabolism reactions are classified as either phase I or phase II reactions. *Phase I reactions* can inactivate, activate, or convert an active substrate into another active substrate with activity that is higher, lower, or equal to that of the parent compound. Generally, phase I reactions cause inactivation of substrate, with the resulting compound being more polar than the parent. Making the metabolite more polar facilitates its elimination from the body. Phase I reactions include dealkylation, hydroxylation, oxidation, and deamination.

Phase II reactions involve conjugation of the parent compound with larger molecules, which increases the polarity of the parent to ready it for excretion. Although phase II reactions generally lead to inactivation of the parent compound, occasionally conjugation increases the potency of the parent compound. When the conjugated compounds are secreted into the intestine, enzymatic cleavage may occur with release and reabsorption of the active parent compound, a phenomenon called *enterohepatic recirculation*. Conjugation reactions include glucuronidation, sulfation, and acetylation.

Cytochrome P-450 System

Phase I reactions generally are under the control of the *cytochrome P-450 (CYP) system*. CYP enzymes are heme-containing proteins that are localized in the endoplasmic reticulum of a variety of cell types, most abundantly in the liver. CYP enzymes are controlled by a superfamily of genes that are classified into families according to their amino acid sequences. Each family is divided further into subfamilies. The term *CYP3A4* designates a mammalian enzyme (CYP) family 3, subfamily A, gene 4. Fourteen families of CYPs have been found in mammals, including 26 subfamilies, of which 20 have been mapped in the human genome. Currently, data exist to describe 33 human CYP enzymes in 20 families.[6]

CYP enzymes are affected by many factors that stimulate or inhibit their ability to metabolize drugs. Genetic factors have been shown to result in a phenomenon called *polymorphism*. Simply put, polymorphism means that individuals vary in their genetically determined ability to metabolize CYP substrate. For some CYP enzymes, such as CYP2D6, distinct "poor" and "extensive" metabolic patterns exist in a population; in a white population, 4% to 6% are poor metabolizers, and the rest are extensive metabolizers. For other CYPs, such as CYP3A, polymorphism has been discovered; however, the significance of this continues to be elucidated. These phenomena have important implications for anti-infective agents, for which efficacy against infecting organisms and toxicity to the host are determined by the pharmacokinetics of the agent and its resultant pharmacodynamic effect.

Other factors that have been investigated for their effects on CYP enzymes include sex, disease state, age, and menstrual cycle. In general, differences related to sex and menstrual cycle (i.e., mid-follicular versus mid-luteal phase) have not been observed. Age and disease state effects are not clear, but it may be postulated that cytokines released during acute infection can cause inhibition of CYP activity. This may be the case with acute and chronic infections, such as human immunodeficiency virus (HIV).

Clinically, drug, food, disease, and herbal effects on the CYP system may translate into either inhibition or induction of metabolism. Induction of CYP results in increased production of the protein and a resultant increase in the ability to metabolize specific compounds. An example is the induction by rifampin of CYP3A with a subsequent increase in the metabolism of estrogens. Many inducers of CYP enzymes also induce phase II conjugation reactions. In addition, a phenomenon called *allosteric activation of drug-metabolizing enzymes* has been described. At present, it is unclear if classic inducers of drug-metabolizing enzymes also cause allosteric activation to increase the efficiency of these enzymes. The implication for increased substrate metabolism as it applies to anti-infective therapy is the development of resistance.

Inhibition of CYP activity occurs through reduction of enzyme production or competition for CYP substrate. Generally, persons with increased enzyme activity exhibit a greater inhibition of the CYP system with an inhibiting agent than do persons with less activity. Enzyme inhibition may result in increased pharmacodynamic effect, with the potential not only for greater efficacy, but also for greater toxicity. This inhibitory process may be used in the clinical setting advantageously. Ritonavir can be used to decrease the activity of CYP3A in the gut, allowing greater absorption of saquinavir (through a reduction in the first-pass effect) and reducing the overall cost of therapy. Clinically, a combination of ritonavir and lopinavir has been marketed to take advantage of this beneficial drug interaction.

Quantification of CYP activity has been performed through the use of genotyping and phenotyping. Genotyping identifies the alleles present in the DNA of an individual patient. From this allele identification, a prediction of genetically determined CYP activity can be made. Because genetically determined CYP activity also is affected by exogenous influences (e.g., drugs, environmental pollutants, cigarette smoke), however, phenotyping has shown more promise for determining individual CYP activity. A relatively innocuous agent is administered as a single dose to a subject, and urine, blood, or breath analysis ensues. These techniques, although still investigational, are beginning to be used in the clinical setting in an attempt to optimize drug dosing. Phenotyping of many drug-metabolizing enzymes can be performed simultaneously using a multidrug cocktail.[7]

To date, most drugs that are metabolized by phase I enzymes have been shown to be metabolized by five primary CYP enzymes. In decreasing order of potency for drug metabolism, they are CYP3A, CYP2D6, CYP2C, CYP1A2, and CYP2E1. Although a complete discussion of the CYP system is beyond the scope of this chapter, many of the newer anti-infectives, particularly antiretroviral agents, can induce or inhibit CYP enzymes, and in many cases they are substrates for CYP enzymes and are affected by changes in CYP activity. A thorough understanding of the CYP system is important to optimize efficacy and minimize toxicity of these agents.

As mentioned, the liver is not the only place in the body where metabolism occurs. Metabolism and detoxification of foreign substances can occur in many other systems.

Elimination

Elimination of a foreign substance from the body occurs via two main mechanisms of excretion. *Renal clearance* (CL_r) describes the rate at which the body eliminates a substance via the kidneys, through various methods, including glomerular filtration, tubular secretion, and passive diffusion. Different compounds are eliminated by one or more of these processes, and the degree to which a process is used may depend on the saturation of another process by the compound. Tubular secretion by the kidney is a saturable process, and dose-dependent pharmacokinetics can be shown for substances that undergo tubular secretion as their primary role of elimination. Elimination through a dialysis procedure (hemodialysis or peritoneal dialysis) also can be construed as a form of renal elimination because these processes are acting as an artificial kidney.

Nonrenal clearance (CL_{nr} or CL_{nr}/F) is a generic term that describes the sum of clearance pathways that do not involve the kidneys. These mechanisms may involve the biliary tree (e.g., ceftriaxone) or the intestine (e.g., azithromycin). Other, uncommon mechanisms can be used, such as elimination of alcohol through the skin and lungs (respiration) and ionization and inactivation of aminoglycosides by the sputum in cystic fibrosis patients with elimination through expectoration.

Renal and nonrenal clearance rates are combined to determine the rate at which a drug is eliminated from the body, known as *total body clearance* (CL_T, or CL_T/F for *total oral clearance*). Clearance also affects the *half-life*. The half-life of a compound is the amount of time required for the blood concentration of the compound to decrease by half. This time can be minutes or a day or more. Most pharmacologists consider that a *steady-state concentration* of a drug has been achieved when the patient has been taking the drug for a period equal to at least five to seven half-lives (e.g., 5 to 7 days for a drug with a half-life of 24 hours). Similarly, a drug is thought to have been eliminated almost completely when the time span of five to seven half-lives has passed since the final dose of the drug. Half-lives vary from patient to patient and often are reported as ranges. Changes in end-organ function or protein binding also can alter the half-life of a drug.

PHARMACODYNAMICS

Antimicrobial Activity

An antimicrobial agent may inhibit growth and replication (*static*) or cause bacterial cell death (*cidal*). Interference in the development of a bacterial cell wall or membrane (e.g., β-lactams, vancomycin) results in cell lysis and death from intolerably high internal osmotic pressure or destruction by autolytic enzymes. Antimicrobials that inhibit nucleic acid (e.g., quinolones) or protein synthesis (e.g., aminoglycosides, macrolides-azalides) also lead ultimately to cell death. In contrast, changes in bacterial physiology, such as inhibition of folic acid synthesis (e.g., sulfonamides), may cause only inhibition of bacterial growth.

Another factor that affects whether a drug is bacteriostatic or bactericidal is the antimicrobial concentration at the site of action. Antimicrobials may be bacteriostatic at low concentrations but bactericidal at high concentrations. These inhibitory and bactericidal concentrations have been used to quantitate the activity of an agent against an organism. Most commonly, the *minimal concentration that is inhibitory for 90% of all isolates* of a bacterial species (MIC_{90}) and the *inhibitory or effective concentration for 50% of all isolates* of a strain of virus (IC_{50} or EC_{50}) have been used. Although these parameters are helpful, they do not provide information on the time course of activity. In addition, they do not provide information on the potential for persistent anti-infective activity after the concentration at the site has decreased below the inhibitory level or on the interaction of the immune system with the drug.

A more recent concept in microbiologic testing is being discussed increasingly in the literature. The concept of the *mutant prevention concentration* and *mutant selection window* has been used to investigate the relationship of drug exposure to the development of resistance.[8] Mutant prevention concentration indicates the concentration that prevents bacterial mutation that leads to the development of resistance. Mutant prevention concentration appears to be different for different organisms and different drugs. Mutant selection window is the period of exposure that is below the mutant prevention concentration of the organism but above the MIC. It is thought that the time in the mutant selection window can determine the development of resistance for an organism to an antibiotic.[9,10] To date, much of this work has been performed with the concentration-dependent killing drugs in the fluoroquinolone class. Although interesting, these concepts have not been shown to date to apply to the clinical setting. Antimicrobial agents are given in combination for several reasons, including severe or life-threatening infections, empirical therapy when the pathogen is unknown, avoidance of resistance, and the desire for synergistic activity. Data on avoidance of resistance or the improved outcome in the use of antibiotic combinations are conflicting, however. *Synergism* is defined as activity of two antimicrobials given together that is greater than the sum of activity had the two agents been given separately. β-Lactams commonly are given in combination with aminoglycosides to take advantage of synergy against *Pseudomonas* or *Enterococcus* spp. Trimethoprim and sulfamethoxazole are combined to provide synergy through inhibition of sequential steps in folic acid synthesis.

Combinations of antimicrobial agents may not always be beneficial. *Antagonism* between agents occurs when one agent diminishes the activity of another. β-Lactams require a normally growing bacterium to inhibit cell wall synthesis. Concomitant administration with a bacteriostatic agent (e.g., a tetracycline) that inhibits cell growth prevents the β-lactam from exerting its bactericidal activity. In this case, the action of the β-lactam has been antagonized. Most antimicrobial combinations result in little or no change in activity of the two agents, an interaction termed *indifference*.

Methodology for the Study of Pharmacodynamic Effects of Anti-infective Agents

In Vitro Models

The traditional model used to study pharmacodynamic effects of anti-infective agents is the "hollow fiber model" system.[12] In this system, broth is used as a growth medium; bacteria are exposed to predetermined concentrations of antibiotics that are "eliminated" from the system in such a manner as to simulate pharmacokinetically determined excretion.[13] Although these models offer control over bacterial inoculum and drug exposure (in terms of concentration and time), they do not assess the effects of the immune system on organism killing or growth inhibition. They do assess, however, the relationship of free drug concentrations to effect, assisting in the development of relationships of protein-bound drug in humans.

Animal Models

Animals models have used a variety of species, often with the animals rendered neutropenic before infection. Craig and colleagues[14-16] showed that the presence of neutrophils may affect antibacterial activity with fluoroquinolones, penicillin, clindamycin, and doxycycline. Animal infectious disease models have been developed to mimic human infections. Animal models allow for frequent sampling of blood and tissue and allow a broad dosage range to be investigated along with a wide range of organism inocula, allowing investigators to study the effects of variation in a single parameter at a time. Problems with animal models include lack of standardization of inocula size (often large inocula are required to produce infection) and the faster rate of drug elimination in animals compared with humans, which leads to the use of unusual dosing regimens in an attempt to mimic human drug exposure.

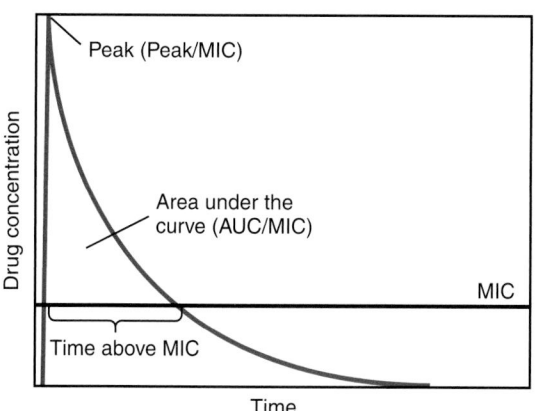

FIGURE 18-3. Common antibiotic pharmacokinetic and minimal inhibitory concentration (MIC) pharmacodynamic relationships.

Human Trials

To date, most human trials[17-28] reported have been retrospective analyses of prospectively collected data, with only one study, that of Preston and co-workers,[29] being performed prospectively. These trials have used three measures of assessment to relate antimicrobial pharmacokinetics to pharmacodynamics: (1) clinical outcome (cure/fail or improved); (2) eradication of bacteria from the site of infection or reduction in virus concentration (load) in blood, other sites, or both; and (3) improvement in surrogate markers of infection, such as temperature or leukocyte count. The disadvantage of these types of trials is the retrospective nature of their analyses; prospective trials using all three criteria are needed. Most retrospective trials that have been published have used one of three antimicrobial pharmacodynamic outcome parameters (defined and discussed later): Cmax/MIC, AUC/MIC, or T>MIC (Fig. 18-3). Few trials have focused on relationships of drug exposure to toxicity or on the development of resistance.

Concentration-Dependent Killing Agents

Concentration-dependent killing agents (e.g., fluoroquinolones, aminoglycosides, macrolides, azalides, ketolides, metronidazole) eliminate bacteria when their concentrations are well above the MIC of the organism. When the ratio of the concentration at the site of infection to the MIC is increased further, greater killing occurs. This concept is illustrated in Figure 18-4 for tobramycin and ciprofloxacin against *Pseudomonas aeruginosa*.[30] As the ratio of drug concentration to MIC increases from 0.25 to 64, bacterial killing continues to increase. In addition, these agents exhibit postantibiotic effect (PAE) (discussed later): Growth inhibition continues for a varying period after the concentration at the site of the bacteria has decreased below the MIC for the antimicrobial agent. In vivo the Cmax/MIC ratio—the maximal serum concentration of the drug (Cmax) divided by the MIC—is the clinical correlate used as the pharmacodynamic predictor for outcome for concentration-dependent killing agents. In clinical trials, the AUC/MIC ratio—the area under the 24-hour serum concentration versus time curve (AUC) divided by the MIC—also has been correlated with improved outcome.[17-29] This finding is not surprising because Cmax and AUC are covariates: When Cmax increases, AUC increases also. More recent data have suggested that for drugs such as fluoroquinolones, different goals for AUC/MIC ratios are required for gram-positive pathogens compared with gram-negative pathogens.[31-33] In general, free drug AUC/MIC ratios of 30 are desired for maximal kill of *Streptococcus pneumoniae*, whereas AUC/MIC ratios of greater than 100 are desired for gram-negative pathogens.

Time-Dependent (Concentration-Independent) Killing Agents

Time-dependent killing agents kill gram-negative bacteria only when the concentration at the site of the bacteria is higher than the MIC of the organism; this is shown for ticarcillin against *P. aeruginosa* in Figure 18-4. Generally, when the concentration at the bacterial site is more than four times higher than the MIC, the additional killing that occurs is modest.

Some authors have attempted to use the time during which the serum drug concentration is greater than the MIC (time above MIC [T >MIC]) as the dynamic parameter to predict efficacy for these anti-infectives.[10,25] One study in the neutropenic mouse model using *Klebsiella pneumoniae* lung infection and treatment with cefotaxime suggested a strong correlation of 0.94 in terms of reduction of bacterial colony counts versus T>MIC (Fig. 18-5).[34] An additional report of many animal studies with *S. pneumoniae* in which treatment was performed with penicillins or cephalosporins showed that when T>MIC was 20% or less of the dosing interval, mortality was 100%. In contrast, a mortality rate of 0% to 10% occurred when serum concentrations

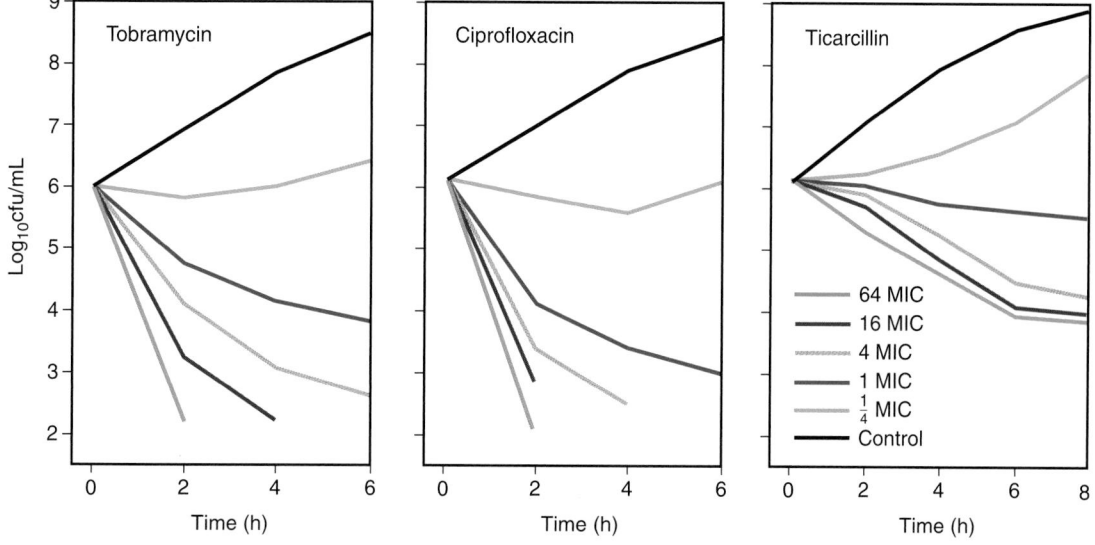

FIGURE 18-4. Time-kill curves for *Pseudomonas aeruginosa* ATCC 27853 with exposure to tobramycin, ciprofloxacin, and ticarcillin at concentrations from one fourth to 64 times the minimum inhibitory concentration (MIC). *(From Craig WA, Ebert SC. Killing and regrowth of bacteria in vitro: A review. Scand J Infect Dis. 1991;74:63-70.)*

were above the MIC for longer than 40% to 50% of the dosing interval.[10,35] Time-dependent killing agents include the penicillins, cephalosporins, aztreonam, vancomycin, carbapenems, macrolides, linezolid, and clindamycin.

Ratio of Maximal Serum Concentration to Minimal Inhibitory Concentration

The Cmax/MIC ratio has been used in animal studies and retrospective analyses of clinical trials to predict the outcome of antimicrobial therapy. This pharmacodynamic parameter applies to concentration-dependent killing agents, such as aminoglycosides and fluoroquinolones. In addition to the prediction of efficacy, the Cmax/MIC ratio has been used in vitro to predict the development of bacterial resistance.[13]

There have been five studies in humans using the Cmax/MIC ratio to predict outcome, four with aminoglycosides and one with levofloxacin. These trials used either clinical response (measured by improvement with therapy or by improvement of surrogate markers) or cure/fail as the outcome measure.

The trial by Keating and colleagues[17] examined neutropenic cancer patients. In this trial, patients were assigned randomly to receive continuous infusions of one of three aminoglycoside antibiotics plus carbenicillin. When the ratios of aminoglycoside concentration to MIC were examined, a relationship was noted for response rate. For mean ratios of 1 to 4, 4 to 10, and greater than 10, response rates were 57%, 67%, and 85%.

The study by Moore and colleagues[20] often is quoted as the basis for use of a Cmax/MIC ratio target of 10 or greater in the clinical setting. In this retrospective analysis of prospectively collected data, the investigators examined 236 patients with a variety of gram-negative infections treated with aminoglycoside antibiotics on an every-8-hour basis. They found that the odds ratio for improved clinical response increased as the Cmax/MIC ratio increased, with a mean ratio of 6.6 ± 3.9 in patients who responded and 4.6 ±3.6 in patients who did not respond. This trial had a majority of patients with urinary tract infections (approximately 60%), however. Because aminoglycosides are known to concentrate 5-fold to 100-fold in the urine, the relationship of Cmax to MIC in this study may be meaningless. It was impossible to separate patients with other disease states to determine the optimal Cmax/MIC ratio needed to elicit response. In addition, the authors did not consider concurrent antimicrobial therapy in their model, so it is difficult to assess the contribution of other antimicrobial agents to the response rate.

Deziel-Evans and associates[21] examined a variety of pharmacodynamic predictors in 45 adult patients treated with aminoglycosides. In this trial, a Cmax/MIC ratio greater than 4 was noted to improve clinical response.

A more recent study by Kashuba and co-workers[26] described the relationship between Cmax and MIC in 78 patients with documented gram-negative pneumonia. The authors examined cure or failure along with two surrogate markers of infection, temperature and leukocyte count. There was a high cure rate for well-documented gram-negative pneumonia (92%), and no pharmacodynamic variable could be correlated with cure/fail, probably because of the small number of failures. The researchers did examine the Cmax/MIC ratio, however, in relation to the time required for the patient to become afebrile (≤ 37.9° C) and the time to normalization of the leukocyte count. As shown by the probability graph in Figure 18-6, a strong relationship was noted between Cmax/MIC ratio and time to normalization of fever. A ratio of 10 or greater gave a 90% probability of normalization of temperature by day 7. Similar graphs can be constructed for earlier and later days into therapy. Generally, these probability graphs show that an increased Cmax/MIC ratio yields an earlier and greater chance of surrogate marker normalization; this does not take into account the probability of toxicity with higher Cmax/MIC ratios. One strength of this trial is that the authors statistically analyzed concurrent antibiotic therapy, which was not a significant variable for prediction of surrogate response or cure/fail.

To date, one study has addressed the use of the Cmax/MIC ratio with the quinolone levofloxacin. Preston and co-workers[29] prospectively examined 134 evaluable patients with bacterial infections of the respiratory tract, the urinary tract, or the skin who were treated with levofloxacin monotherapy. All 134 patients had serum concentrations obtained along with identified microorganisms with an MIC determined. In terms of clinical outcome, Cmax/MIC ratio and AUC/MIC ratio were found to be the most important predictors of outcome; the correlation of these two pharmacodynamic parameters was 0.942. The investigators did not find any failures in patients with urinary tract infections, illustrating that the Cmax/MIC ratio may not be a valid predictor in patients receiving drugs that concentrate in the urine. In terms of microbiologic response, the Cmax/MIC ratio was the most important predictor of bacterial eradication. In this study, 26% of infections were due to gram-positive organisms, however, and outcomes for gram-positive and gram-negative organisms were not separated. As shown by in vitro studies, breakpoints of pharmacodynamic indices for efficacy seem to be pathogen specific. AUC/MIC ratios that correlate to efficacy

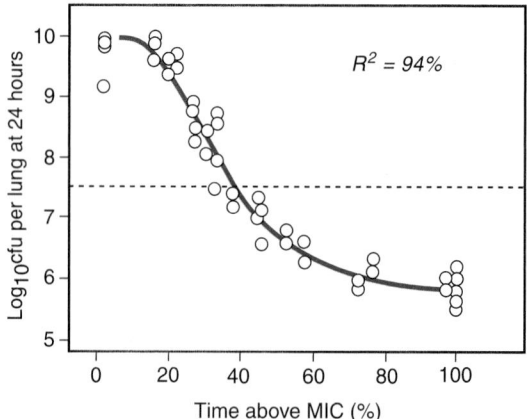

FIGURE 18-5. The relationship of time above the minimal inhibitory concentration (MIC) and the reduction in bacterial count in a neutropenic mouse model of *Klebsiella pneumoniae* for cefotaxime. *(From Craig WA. Interrelationship between pharmacokinetics and pharmacodynamics in determining dosage regimens for broad-spectrum cephalosporins. Diagn Microbiol Infect Dis. 1995;22:89-96.)*

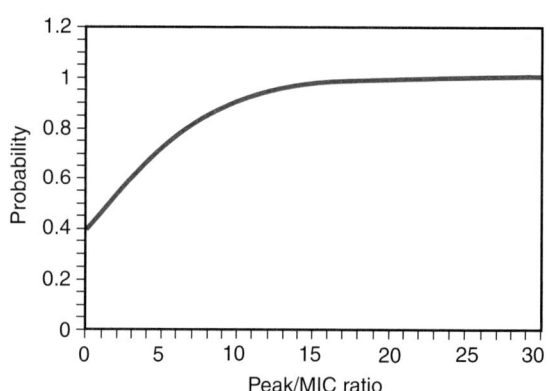

FIGURE 18-6. Probability graph for temperature normalization for peak antimicrobial serum concentration-to-minimal inhibitory concentration (Peak/MIC) ratio for aminoglycosides in 78 patients with culture-proven, nosocomial gram-negative pneumonia. *(Adapted from Kashuba ADM, Nafziger AN, Drusano GL, et al. Optimizing aminoglycoside therapy for nosocomial pneumonia caused by gram-negative bacteria. Antimicrob Agents Chemother. 1999;43:623-629.)*

are higher for gram-negative organisms compared with gram-positive organisms. As noted subsequently (AUC/MIC section), another study has correlated fluoroquinolone exposure as measured by AUC/MIC ratios to efficacy and bacterial eradication.

These retrospective analyses of prospective data illustrate the potential importance of the Cmax/MIC ratio for concentration-dependent killing agents. Because none of the four trials with aminoglycosides used single daily dosing of these agents, however, it is not possible to extrapolate these data to support this mode of administration.[36]

In terms of prevention of bacterial resistance, only in vitro data using the hollow fiber model exist relating the Cmax/MIC ratio to resistance. The study of Blaser and co-workers[13] examined the Cmax/MIC ratio for enoxacin and netilmicin against various gram-negative organisms. Regrowth of organisms occurred in all cultures when enoxacin or netilmicin attained ratios lower than 8. On redosing of these antibiotics after bacterial regrowth, no killing was seen because of the development of resistance. A similar study by Marchbanks and associates[37] using ciprofloxacin noted the development of resistant *P. aeruginosa* when the organism was exposed to a Cmax/MIC ratio of 6 compared with no resistance when the Cmax/MIC ratio was 12, even though both regimens showed adequate rates of bacterial killing. These in vitro data suggest that Cmax/MIC ratios may be influential in determining the development of bacterial resistance for aminoglycosides and quinolones. A disadvantage of these trials, however, is that they do not account for the role of the immune system in "cleaning up" small numbers of resistant bacteria before they can become pathogenic.

Although the Cmax/MIC ratios for aminoglycosides and quinolones may be useful, no data to date have examined drug toxicity with higher exposures. A prospective trial to evaluate efficacy and toxicity with pharmacodynamic dosage adjustments is needed.

Ratio of Area under the 24-Hour Serum Concentration Curve to Minimal Inhibitory Concentration

The AUC/MIC ratio is a measure of total exposure of bacteria to an antimicrobial agent. The AUC/MIC ratio encompasses peak concentration and prolonged exposure, which may be vital for drugs with a long half-life. Cmax/MIC and AUC/MIC ratios are difficult to separate in a scientifically designed clinical trial because when the Cmax/MIC ratio is high, the AUC/MIC ratio usually is high as well. Both would be found to be statistically predictive of outcome and indistinguishable in terms of which is of primary importance.

Several studies have defined the role of the AUC/MIC ratio as a predictor of bacterial or clinical success. Various pharmacodynamic predictors of outcome were evaluated in 74 acutely ill patients, mostly with nosocomial pneumonia, who were treated with ciprofloxacin. The AUC/MIC ratio, which represents the inverse serum inhibitory titer over time (SIT^{-1} • T), was identified as the factor most predictive of clinical and microbiologic success (Fig. 18-7). At an AUC/MIC ratio lower than 125 SIT^{-1} • hr (log^{10} = 2.1 = 125 SIT^{-1} • hr), the probabilities of clinical and microbiologic cure were 42% and 26%,

whereas at values greater than 125 SIT^{-1} • hr, the probabilities were 80% and 82%. At an AUC/MIC ratio lower than 125 SIT^{-1} • hr, between 125 and 250 SIT^{-1} • hr (log^{10} = 2.4 = 250 SIT^{-1} • hr), and higher than 250 SIT^{-1} • hr, the median time to eradication was more than 32 days, 6.6 days, and 1.9 days.[23] A similar analysis was performed for a small number of patients experiencing an acute exacerbation of chronic bronchitis treated with grepafloxacin.[28] At an AUC/MIC ratio less than 75 SIT^{-1} • hr, the probability of clinical cure was 71%, whereas with AUC/MIC ratios greater than 175 SIT^{-1} • hr, the probability of cure was 98%. Clear conclusions cannot be drawn from this study, however, because of the limited sample size.

A retrospective analysis by Ambrose and colleagues[38] in patients with community-acquired pneumonia due to *S. pneumoniae* noted microbiologic response in 64% with free drug AUC/MIC ratios less than 33.7 and 100% at ratios greater than 33.7. This finding is consistent with in vitro studies with *S. pneumoniae*. In addition, these researchers reported clinical cure of 70% when free drug AUC/MIC ratio was less than 40 and 92% when the AUC/MIC ratio was greater than 40. No patient-specific pharmacokinetic measures were obtained, however, and fluoroquinolone exposure was determined by using population-derived estimates of clearance.

At this time, it is clear that for different organisms, different free drug AUC/MIC ratios are desirable. Attempts to standardize exposure to one AUC/MIC ratio are erroneous.

The use of the AUC/MIC ratio for the prevention of bacterial resistance is limited to in vitro data. An in vitro study with gatifloxacin, grepafloxacin, levofloxacin, moxifloxacin, and trovafloxacin linked AUC/MIC ratios less than 31.7 with significant regrowth and resistance of ciprofloxacin-resistant *S. pneumoniae* strains.[39] An in vitro study by Fazili and associates[40] showed that an initial population of ciprofloxacin-sensitive *S. pneumoniae* became resistant to ciprofloxacin after 12 hours on ciprofloxacin treatment and after 48 hours on gatifloxacin treatment. Resistance was suppressed when gatifloxacin at an AUC/MIC ratio greater than 50 was used. Because different AUC/MIC ratios correlate with efficacy for gram-negative and gram-positive organisms, breakpoints for resistance with gram-negative organisms are generally higher compared with gram-positive organisms. In an in vitro study with garenoxacin, Tam and co-workers[41] showed that AUC/MIC ratios greater than 200 were needed to suppress resistance with *P. aeruginosa*, and ratios greater than 100 were needed with *K. pneumoniae*. AUC/MIC ratios less than 200 and less than 100 for *P. aeruginosa* and *K. pneumoniae* were selected for resistant subpopulations at 48 hours to garenoxacin and ciprofloxacin. In vitro studies with fluoroquinolones evaluating the emergence of resistance showed consistent results that suboptimal dosing of antibiotics may select resistant subpopulations to grow.

Clinical studies examining the emergence of resistance with AUC/MIC goals are limited. A retrospective study of 107 acutely ill patients with nosocomial lower respiratory tract infections examined resistance rates with the use of pharmacodynamics.[42] Bacterial isolates

FIGURE 18-7. Relationship between 24-hour area under the serum antimicrobial concentration versus time curve-to-minimal inhibitory concentration ratio (AUC/MIC) and clinical (**A**) or microbiologic (**B**) cure in 74 patients with nosocomial pneumonia. *(From Forrest A, Nix DE, Ballow CH, et al. Pharmacodynamics of intravenous ciprofloxacin in seriously ill patients. Antimicrob Agents Chemother. 1993;37:1073-1081.)*

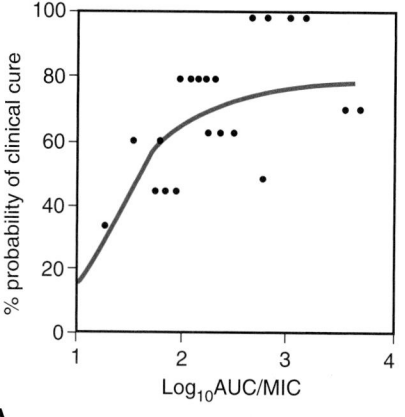

A

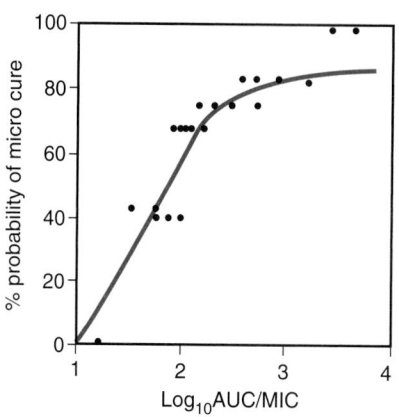

B

were separated into four groups: *Pseudomonas* spp., gram-negative organisms resistant to narrow-spectrum cephalosporins, gram-negative rods susceptible to cephalosporins, and a last group that contained the remainder of a diverse number of organisms. Five antimicrobial regimens were evaluated: ciprofloxacin, cefmenoxime, ceftazidime, ciprofloxacin plus piperacillin, and ceftazidime plus tobramycin. The likelihood of developing resistance was greater when ciprofloxacin was used to treat *P. aeruginosa* and at AUC/MIC ratios less than 100. The AUC/MIC ratio was applied to either monotherapy or combination therapy of antibiotics inappropriately, however. β-Lactams have been linked pharmacodynamically to T>MIC, and the use of a concentration-dependent pharmacodynamic index such as AUC/MIC may not be an accurate prediction of efficacy or resistance.

Time above Minimal Inhibitory Concentration

T>MIC is a pharmacodynamic parameter that measures how the time that serum drug concentrations stay higher than the MIC for the organism relates to outcomes. This definition usually refers to total drug concentration, although some authors have used free drug concentration in the definition. For intermittent bolus infusions, the parameters T>MIC, AUC/MIC ratio, and Cmax/MIC ratio are interrelated: As T>MIC increases, AUC/MIC and Cmax/MIC ratios do also. It may be difficult to separate the importance of these dynamic parameters, unless a study compares continuous versus intermittent infusions of antimicrobials.

Animal models have shown that T>MIC is an important pharmacodynamic predictor for penicillins, cephalosporins, carbapenems, monobactams, macrolides, and clindamycin.[10] Human studies are sparse, however, in defining this parameter as an important one. The study of Bodey and colleagues[18] examined the efficacy of intermittent versus continuous infusions of cefamandole plus intermittent infusions of carbenicillin in neutropenic patients. These investigators showed a slightly higher response rate in the continuous infusion group, but the difference was not significant. Analysis of a subset of patients with cefamandole-susceptible organisms revealed a significant benefit of continuous versus intermittent infusion, although the patient numbers were small.

Schentag and associates[19] also noted for cefmenoxime that T>dynamic response concentration (DRC) (analogous to T>MIC) correlated better than the AUC/DRC ratio (analogous to AUC/MIC ratio) for bacterial eradication from the lung. The results of the retrospective and prospective portions of the study were combined, however. In the retrospective study, no dose adjustments to cefmenoxime were made during treatment, whereas in the prospective study doses were adjusted to achieve time to eradication by day 4. Turnidge[43] reanalyzed the data to separate the results of the retrospective study and showed that T>MIC is the best predictor of outcome compared with the AUC/MIC ratio for this β-lactam. Because presently defined T>MIC is being extrapolated from neutropenic animal studies and limited clinical studies, establishing the optimal T>MIC for gram-positive and gram-negative organisms clinically requires further research.

A retrospective analysis by Craig and Andes[25] attempted to correlate the pharmacodynamics of antibiotics in the treatment of otitis media. Using retrospective data and free drug calculations, the authors examined T>MIC and bacteriologic cure for β-lactams, macrolides, and trimethoprim-sulfamethoxazole. They concluded that an 80% to 85% efficacy rate was achieved when the T>MIC was 40% to 50% of the dosing interval.

Data are available for staphylococcal infections and vancomycin in pediatric patients. Schaad and colleagues[44] noted that a peak *serum bactericidal titer* of 1:8 or greater was associated with cure in 16 of 20 patients. Louria and co-workers[45] noted cure of staphylococcal infections when the serum bactericidal titer was 1:8 or greater (six patients) and failure when the titer was less than 1:8 (three patients, although in one, cure was seen after dose escalation). Although animal and in vitro data suggest that for certain antibiotics T>MIC is an important pharmacodynamic predictor, few data in human studies exist to support this conclusion.

Postantibiotic Effect

During in vitro testing of antimicrobials, there may be a delay before microorganisms recover and reenter a log-growth period. This phenomenon is termed the *postantibiotic effect* (PAE). The exact duration of the PAE is species and drug dependent. Aminoglycosides and fluoroquinolones produce in vitro PAEs against gram-negative bacilli of approximately 2 to 6 hours. β-Lactam antibiotics (except for imipenem) produce little or no PAE against gram-negative organisms under identical experimental conditions but generally induce 2-hour PAEs against gram-positive organisms. Other factors that affect the in vitro PAE include combinations of antimicrobials, antimicrobial concentration, duration of antimicrobial exposure, and pH. Potential factors that also may affect the PAE include size of inoculum, type of growth medium, and bacterial growth phase.

Studies in animal models have verified that PAE is not an artifact of in vitro testing. Investigational animal models that have been studied include a neutropenic mouse thigh model, a rabbit meningitis model, a rat endocarditis model, and a guinea pig pneumonia model. These studies showed that an in vivo PAE exists against gram-negative organisms for aminoglycosides, fluoroquinolones, erythromycin, clindamycin, and tetracycline, but not for β-lactams. As in the in vitro studies, β-lactam agents do produce abbreviated PAEs against gram-positive organisms.

The mechanism of the PAE is unknown. Possible explanations include nonlethal bacterial damage induced by the antimicrobial agent and persistence of the antimicrobial at the site of action. When fresh organisms are injected into animals during the PAE period, however, there is rapid and immediate growth, suggesting that the PAE is not caused by persistence of the drug in tissue.

The presence or absence of a PAE has been used to alter antimicrobial dosing schedules. Theoretically, an agent with a long PAE can be dosed less frequently than an antimicrobial lacking a PAE. Alternatively, an agent with little or no PAE may be most effective if it is given as a continuous infusion so that the serum concentration always exceeds the MIC. Dosing strategies such as these are theoretical and require clinical investigation in human studies of sufficient size before implementation into clinical practice.

Antiretroviral Pharmacodynamics

Pharmacologic differences between patients is an important factor responsible for heterogeneity in the response to antiretroviral therapy. Although many antiretroviral agents are available, the number of treatment options is limited because these drugs generally are used in combinations of three or more. It has been shown that successive antiretroviral regimens do not perform as effectively or for as extensive a duration as the initial regimen. Optimizing success with the first regimen is crucial.

Many variables can confound the pure relationship between one antiretroviral drug and its pharmacodynamic response. Antagonism or synergy between antiretroviral agents, demonstrated in vitro cross-resistance, adherence patterns, and protein binding all can contribute to distort the true relationship between individual drugs and efficacy.[46] Despite these obstacles, numerous studies have shown correlations between antiretroviral drug exposure and outcome, as measured by changes in plasma HIV RNA concentrations or CD4+ T-lymphocyte changes.

Drug exposure is an important determinant of virologic outcome, particularly with protease inhibitors. Plasma clearance, peak plasma concentration (C_{max}), trough plasma concentration (C_{trough} or C_{min}), and AUC all have been proposed as determinants of virologic response, and all correlate with each other. Although no study has compared directly all three pharmacokinetic parameters as individual predictors of treatment efficacy, most attention has been focused on the role of trough plasma concentrations in determining virologic outcome.[47]

Large interindividual variability exists in the pharmacokinetics of protease inhibitors. Concentration-effect relationships have been shown, however, for indinavir,[48,49] saquinavir,[50-52] nelfinavir,[53] amprenavir,[54] and lopinavir.[55,56] Adverse effects have been linked to concentrations of indinavir[57] and amprenavir.[54] Pharmacokinetic-pharmacodynamic relationships also have been established for the nonnucleoside reverse transcriptase inhibitors nevirapine[58] (efficacy and toxicity), delavirdine,[59] and efavirenz.[60]

Defining concentration-effect relationships with nucleoside analogue reverse transcriptase inhibitors is more difficult because these drugs require intracellular phosphorylation to their active triphosphate moieties. Multiple intracellular rate-limited phosphorylation steps and potential cellular membrane efflux transporter activity[61,62] result in plasma parent drug concentrations that do not correlate well with intracellular drug concentrations.[63] Plasma concentration-effect relationships have been shown, however, in a few patients for zidovudine[64] and didanosine.[65] Concentration-toxicity relationships have been shown for zidovudine[66] and didanosine.[67] One investigation showed significant positive correlations between the rate of HIV-1 RNA decline and change in CD4+ T lymphocytes and intracellular concentrations of zidovudine and lamivudine triphosphate.[63]

Generally, most of these pharmacodynamic relationships are linear, with no obvious concentration target. It is not rational, however, to use the same drug exposure for patients with drug-sensitive virus as for patients with drug-resistant virus. It follows that relating drug concentrations to an individual patient's viral isolate might be a better option for optimizing antiretroviral exposure.

First described by Ellner and Neu,[68] the inhibitory quotient has been proposed as a predictor of clinical outcomes in HIV and integrates drug exposure and viral susceptibility measures. Drug exposure can be defined as AUC, C_{max} or C_{trough} (either as protein-unbound or as total drug concentration), and viral susceptibility can be expressed as the in vitro IC_{50}, IC_{90}, IC_{95}, or IC_{99}, with or without the presence of plasma proteins. The IC_{50} is used most commonly because it is associated with the least degree of error (due to the sigmoidal relationship between viral inhibition and drug concentration) and can be determined by a phenotypic assay or by the virtual phenotype.

The use of inhibitory quotients (IQ),[69] virtual inhibitory quotients (vIQ), or normalized inhibitory quotients (nIQ) currently is being evaluated[70] primarily for the protease inhibitors. IQ is defined as the ratio of the drug concentration at the end of the dosing interval (C_{trough}) to the in vitro concentration of drug resulting in 50% inhibition of virus: C_{trough}/IC_{50}. Although C_{trough} may not be the optimal measure of drug exposure, it is logistically simple to obtain in ambulatory patients. The virtual IQ is defined as the ratio of C_{trough} to the IC_{50} of wild-type virus multiplied by the virtual phenotype (a calculated fold-increase in concentration-response relationships determined from the individual patient viral genotype and matched phenotype in a large data base): C_{trough}/IC_{50} • virtual phenotype. The nIQ is the ratio of C_{trough} to the fold change of the virtual phenotype ($C_{trough}/fold$-change in IC_{50}), all divided by a fixed ratio of the mean antiretroviral C_{trough} in the population to the cutoff for resistance for the virtual phenotype (population $C_{trough}/fold$-change resistance cutoff).[71] This ratio was derived to eliminate protein binding confounding, but it may be effective only in choosing targets for wild-type virus.

The benefits of these ratios still are primarily theoretical. The IQ has been shown to predict virologic response with saquinavir.[72] The vIQ has been shown to be a significant predictor of virologic response in patients treated with indinavir/ritonavir[73] and amprenavir/lopinavir.[74] In one preliminary investigation, the nIQ for amprenavir correlated with change in plasma HIV RNA in patients receiving a multiple antiretroviral drug regimen.[75] Investigations into the clinical utility of the IQ, vIQ, and nIQ are ongoing.

Cautionary Note on Pharmacodynamic Indices

When studying an antibiotic and its pharmacodynamic properties when it is first introduced into development research or the market, it is common to note that multiple pharmacodynamic dosing indices may apply to the drug and that the one to follow is chosen as the one most statistically correlated.[29] Multiple indices may be correlated positively because MICs tend to be very low for susceptible isolates, and many of the pharmacokinetic parameters that are used in the index

equations are interrelated. Although the application of the chosen index may continue to validate the drug's use for a time, when MICs of previously susceptible organisms begin to rise, there will come a point at which the necessary index ratio breakpoint no longer is achieved. At this point, the index descriptions that have been discussed in this chapter would indicate that the drug would have to be abandoned because clinical and microbiologic outcomes no longer are optimal. What has not been discussed, however, is how to interpret the worth of these indices if the drug continues to work despite higher or even resistant MICs being encountered in which the pharmacodynamic index ratios are far from optimal. Whether the indices are wrong or just being applied to the wrong biologic matrix (all currently are based on antibiotic serum concentrations) is as yet unclear.

The best example of this quandary exists with community-acquired respiratory tract infections caused by *S. pneumoniae*. Pneumococcal isolates globally continue to show increasing incidences of resistance to all antibiotics that typically are used to treat pneumococcal infections, including penicillin (β-lactams in general), macrolides, and fluoroquinolones. Despite this show of resistance, the antibiotics all continue to prove successful clinically and continue to be recommended as first-line treatment options by a variety of treatment guideline groups throughout the world.[77-81] The answers to why this occurs most likely do lie within the indices described in this chapter. For β-lactams, whose extracellular, interstitial infection site concentrations would be in relative equilibrium with concurrent serum concentrations, the use of T>MIC for these drugs most likely is appropriate. Whether purposely or not, clinicians have continued to rely on this index and optimize it by using higher or more frequent doses of β-lactams for the treatment of pneumococcal infections, including resistant ones and ones in difficult-to-reach physiologic spaces.[82-84] The use of these higher doses keeps concentrations in the serum and in the interstitial space, where most of the pathogen load exists above the MIC of the pneumococcus for a greater portion of the dosing interval, optimizing their dynamics. For the fluoroquinolones and macrolides, the answer is less clear. Both classes of drugs have serum concentrations that are lower than either their interstitial fluid concentrations, especially those in an inflamed area, or the concentrations in the phagocytes that eventually clear the bacteria from the infection site. As a result, the use of serum concentrations in index ratio calculations most likely is flawed, as is evidenced by the following examples: (1) If the average Cmax achieved with steady-state intravenous levofloxacin is 8 mg/L[85] and the average levofloxacin pneumococcal MIC is 1 mg/L, and the desired ratio of the two for optimal activity is 12,[29] intravenous, let alone oral, levofloxacin should never be curative for pneumococcal infections because the ratio that is achieved is only 8. (2) If the average 24-hour AUC that is achieved with a 500-mg oral dose of azithromycin is 2 mg.h/L[86] and the average MICs of susceptible and resistant pneumococcal isolates are 0.25 mg/L and 32 mg/L and the desired ratio is greater than 30, azithromycin should never be curative not only for resistant pneumococcal isolates, but also for infections caused by susceptible isolates because the ratio that is achieved is only 8. Despite this index evidence to the contrary, both of these agents continue to work and be recommended on a regular basis at currently approved dosages. It may be postulated that although the index may be correct, the use of a different biologic matrix to determine the pharmacokinetic values for the index equations may be more appropriate. As an example, although the 24-hour serum AUC of azithromycin is only 2 mg.h/L, that inside of a neutrophil is approximately 1500 mg.h/L.[86] By applying this new value to the previous example, it may be possible to state that an MIC of 50 mg/L has the potential to be optimally treated. Whether this alteration of the equation to fit the distribution properties of the class of drugs and what the pathogen actually comes into contact with on its being cleared from the body turns out to be the appropriate manipulation of these index equations, or, whether a next generation of the pharmacodynamic model evolves that can actually use serum concentrations in all instances is something for further study.

REFERENCES

1. Benet LZ. General principles: Introduction. In: Hardman JG, Limbird LE, eds. Goodman and Gilman's the Pharmacological Basis of Therapeutics. 9th ed. New York: McGraw-Hill; 1996:1-3.

2. Benet LZ, Kroetz DL, Sheiner LB. Pharmacokinetics: The dynamics of drug absorption, distribution, and elimination. In: Hardman JG, Limbird LE, eds. Goodman and Gilman's the Pharmacological Basis of Therapeutics. 9th ed. New York: McGraw-Hill; 1996:3-28.

3. Wallace AW, Jones M, Bertino JS Jr. Evaluation of four once-daily aminoglycoside dosing nomograms. Pharmacotherapy. 2002;22:1077-1083.

4. Craig WA, Welling PG. Protein binding of antimicrobials: Clinical pharmacokinetic and therapeutic implications. Clin Pharmacokinet. 1977;2:252-268.

5. Sansom LN, Evans AM. What is the true significance of plasma protein binding displacement interactions? Drug Saf. 1995;12:227-233.

6. Rendic S, DiCarlo FJ. Human cytochrome-P450 enzymes: A status report summarizing their reactions, substrates, inducers and inhibitors. Drug Metab Rev. 1997;29:413-580.

7. Chainuvati S, Nafziger A, Leeder JS, et al. Combined phenotypic assessment of CYP1A2, CYP2C9, CYP2C19, CYP2D6, CYP3A, NAT2 and XO with the "Cooperstown 5+1 Cocktail." Clin Pharmacol Ther. 2002;71:P101.

8. Dong Y, Zhao X, Domagala J, et al. Effect of fluoroquinolone concentration on selection of resistant mutants. Antimicrob Agents Chemother. 1999;43:1756-1758.

9. Shao X, Drlica K. Restricting the selection of antibiotic-resistant mutants: A general strategy derived from fluoroquinolone studies. Clin Infect Dis. 2001;33(Suppl 3): S147-S156.

10. Craig WA. Pharmacokinetic/pharmacodynamic parameters: Rationale for antibacterial dosing of mice and men. Clin Infect Dis. 1998;26:1-12.

11. Thomas JK, Forrest A, Bhavnani SM, et al. Pharmacodynamic evaluation of factors associated with the development of bacterial resistance in acutely ill patients during therapy. Antimicrob Agents Chemother. 1998;42:521-527.

12. Blaser J, Stone BB, Zinner SH. Two compartment kinetic models with multiple artificial capillary units. J Antimicrob Chemother. 1985;15(Suppl. A):131-137.

13. Blaser J, Stone BB, Groner MC, et al. Comparative study with enoxacin and netilmicin in a pharmacodynamic model to determine importance of ratio of antibiotic peak concentration to MIC for bacterial activity and emergence of resistance. Antimicrob Agents Chemother. 1987;31:1055-1060.

14. Kiem S, Craig WA. Why do neutrophils markedly reduce the 24-hr AUC/MIC required for efficacy of fluoroquinolones against Streptococcus pneumoniae? (Abstract A-492). Program and Abstracts of the 42nd Interscience Conference on Antimicrobial Agents and Chemotherapy, September 2002.

15. Ambrose PG, Craig WA, Bhavnani SM, et al. Pharmacodynamic comparisons of different dosing regimens of penicillin G (PenG) against penicillin-susceptible and -resistant pneumococci (PSSP and PRSP) (Abstract A-1263). Program and Abstracts of the 42nd Interscience Conference on Antimicrobial Agents and Chemotherapy, September 2002.

16. Christianson JC, Craig WA, Kiem S, et al. Impact of neutrophils on pharmacodynamic activity of clindamycin (CLINDA) and doxycycline (DOXY) against Streptococcus pneumoniae (Abstract A-1267). Program and Abstracts of the 42nd Interscience Conference on Antimicrobial Agents and Chemotherapy, September 2002.

17. Keating MJ, Bodey GP, Valdivieso M, et al. A randomized comparative trial of three aminoglycosides: Comparison of continuous infusions of gentamicin, amikacin and sisomicin combined with carbenicillin in the treatment of infections in neutropenic patients with malignancies. Medicine (Baltimore). 1979;58:159-170.

18. Bodey GP, Ketchel SJ, Rodriguez V. A randomized study of carbenicillin plus cefamandole or tobramycin in the treatment of febrile episodes in cancer patients. Am J Med. 1979;67:608-611.

19. Schentag JJ, Smith IL, Swanson DJ, et al. Role for dual individualization with cefmenoxime. Am J Med. 1984;77(Suppl 6A):43-50.

20. Moore RD, Lietman PS, Smith CR. Clinical response to aminoglycoside therapy: Importance of the ratio of peak concentration to minimum inhibitory concentration. J Infect Dis. 1987;155:93-99.

21. Deziel-Evans JM, Murphy JE, Job ML. Correlation of pharmacokinetic indices with therapeutic outcome in patients receiving aminoglycosides. Clin Pharmacol. 1986;5:319-324.

22. Schentag JJ, Nix DE, Adelman MH. Mathematical examination of dual individualization principles (I): Relationships between AUC above MIC and area under the inhibitory curve for cefmenoxime, ciprofloxacin and tobramycin. Ann Pharmacother. 1991;25:1050-1057.

23. Forrest A, Nix DE, Ballow CH, et al. Pharmacodynamics of intravenous ciprofloxacin in seriously ill patients. Antimicrob Agents Chemother. 1993;37:1073-1081.

24. Goss TF, Forrest A, Nix DE, et al. Mathematical examination of dual individualization principles (II): The rate of bacterial eradication at the same area under the inhibitory curve is more rapid for ciprofloxacin than for cefmenoxime. Ann Pharmacother. 1994;28:863-868.

25. Craig WA, Andes D. Pharmacokinetics and pharmacodynamics of antibiotic in otitis media. Pediatr Infect Dis J. 1996;15:255-259.

26. Kashuba ADM, Nafziger AN, Drusano GL, et al. Optimizing aminoglycoside therapy for nosocomial pneumonia caused by gram-negative bacteria. Antimicrob Agents Chemother. 1999;43:623-629.

27. Hyatt JM, Luzier AB, Forrest A, et al. Modeling the response of pneumonia to antimicrobial therapy. Antimicrob Agents Chemother. 1997;41:1269-1274.

28. Forrest A, Chodosh S, Amantea MA, et al. Pharmacokinetics and pharmacodynamics of oral grepafloxacin in patients with acute bacterial exacerbations of chronic bronchitis. J Antimicrob Chemother. 1997;40(Suppl A):45-57.

29. Preston SL, Drusano GL, Berman AL, et al. Pharmacodynamics of levofloxacin: A new paradigm for early clinical trials. JAMA. 1998;279:125-129.

30. Craig WA, Ebert SC. Killing and regrowth of bacteria in vitro: A review. Scand J Infect Dis. 1991;74:63-70.

31. Lister PD, Sanders CC. Pharmacodynamics of levofloxacin and ciprofloxacin against Streptococcus pneumoniae. J Antimicrob Chemother. 1999;43:79-86.

32. Lister PD. Pharmacodynamics of gatifloxacin against Streptococcus pneumoniae in an in vitro pharmacokinetic model: Impact of area under the curve/MIC ratios on eradication. Antimicrob Agents Chemother. 2002;46:69-74.

33. Madaras-Kelly KJ, Ostergaard BE, Hovde LB, et al. Twenty-four-hour area under the concentration-time curve/MIC ratio as a generic predictor of fluoroquinolone antimicrobial effect by using three strains of Pseudomonas aeruginosa and an in vitro pharmacodynamic model. Antimicrob Agents Chemother. 1996;40:627-632.

34. Craig WA. Interrelationship between pharmacokinetics and pharmacodynamics in determining dosage regimens for broad-spectrum cephalosporins. Diagn Microbiol Infect Dis. 1995;22:89-96.

35. Craig WA. Antimicrobial resistance issues of the future. Diagn Microbiol Infect Dis. 1996;25:213-217.

36. Bertino JS Jr, Rotschafer JC. Single daily dosing of aminoglycosides: A concept whose time has not yet come. Clin Infect Dis. 1997;24:820-823.

37. Marchbanks CR, McKeil JR, Gilbert DH, et al. Dose ranging and fractionation of intravenous ciprofloxacin against Pseudomonas aeruginosa and Staphylococcus aureus in an in vitro model of infection. Antimicrob Agents Chemother. 1993;37:1756-1763.

38. Ambrose PG, Grasela DM, Grasela TH, et al. Pharmacodynamics of fluoroquinolones against Streptococcus pneumoniae in patients with community-acquired respiratory tract infections. Antimicrob Agents Chemother. 2001;45:2793-2797.

39. Coyle EA, Kaatz GW, Rybak MJ. Activities of newer fluoroquinolones against ciprofloxacin-resistant Streptococcus pneumoniae. Antimicrob Agents Chemother. 2001;45:1654-1659.

40. Fazili T, Louie A, Tam V, et al. Effect of inoculum on the pharmacodynamic breakpoint dosage that prevents selection of gatifloxacin resistance in ciprofloxacin-susceptible and -resistant Streptococcus pneumoniae (Abstract 445). Program and Abstracts of 41st Interscience Conference on Antimicrobial Agents and Chemotherapy, December 2001.

41. Tam VH, Louie A, Deziel MR, et al. Pharmacodynamics of BMS-284756 and ciprofloxacin against Pseudomonas aeruginosa and Klebsiella pneumoniae in hollow-fiber system (Abstract 443). Program and Abstracts of 41st Interscience Conference on Antimicrobial Agents and Chemotherapy, December 2001.

42. Thomas JK, Forrest A, Bhavnani S, et al. Pharmacodynamic evaluation of factors associated with the development of bacterial resistance in acutely ill patients during therapy. Antimicrob Agents Chemother. 1998;42:521-527.

43. Turnidge JD. The pharmacodynamics of beta-lactams. Clin Infect Dis. 1998;27:10-22.

44. Schaad UB, McCracken Jr GH, Nelson JD. Clinical pharmacology and efficacy of vancomycin in pediatric patients. J Pediatr. 1980;96:119-126.

45. Louria DB, Kaminski T, Buchman J. Vancomycin in severe staphylococcal infections. Arch Intern Med. 1961;107:225-240.

46. Patick AK, Boritzki TJ, Bloom LA. Activities of the human immunodeficiency virus type 1 (HIV-1) protease inhibitor nelfinavir mesylate in combination with reverse transcriptase and protease inhibitors against acute HIV-1 infection in vitro. Antimicrob Agents Chemother. 1997;41:2159-2164.

47. Deeks SG. Determinants of virological response to antiretroviral therapy: Implications for long-term strategies. Clin Infect Dis. 2000;30(Suppl 2):S177-S184.

48. Stein DS, Fish DG, Bilello JA, et al. A 24-week open-label phase I/II evaluation of the HIV protease inhibitor MK-639 (indinavir). AIDS. 1996;10:485-492.

49. Gatti G, Niganó A, Sala N, et al. Indinavir pharmacokinetics and pharmacodynamics in children with human immunodeficiency virus infection. Antimicrob Agents Chemother. 2000;44:752-755.

50. Vanhove GF, Gries JM, Verotta D, et al. Exposure-response relationships for saquinavir, zidovudine, and zalcitabine in combination therapy. Antimicrob Agents Chemother. 1997;41:2433-2438.

51. Gieschke R, Fotteler B, Buss N, et al. Relationships between exposure to saquinavir monotherapy and antiviral response in HIV-positive patients. Clin Pharmacokinet. 1999;37:75-86.

52. Schapiro JM, Winters MA, Stewart F, et al. The effect of high-dose saquinavir on viral load and CD4+ T-cell counts in HIV-infected patients. Ann Intern Med. 1996; 124:1039-1050.

53. Burger DM, Hugen PW, Aarnoutse RE, et al. Treatment failure of nelfinavir-containing triple therapy can largely be explained by low nelfinavir plasma concentrations. Ther Drug Monit. 2003;25:73-80.

54. Sadler BM, Gillotin C, Lou Y, et al. Pharmacokinetic and pharmacodynamic study of the human immunodeficiency virus protease inhibitor amprenavir after multiple oral dosing. Antimicrob Agents Chemother. 2001;45:30-37.

55. Hsu A, Isaacson J, Brun S, et al. Pharmacokinetic-pharmacodynamic analysis of lopinavir-ritonavir in combination with efavirenz and two nucleoside reverse transcriptase inhibitors in extensively pretreated human immunodeficiency virus-infected patients. Antimicrob Agents Chemother. 2003;47:350-359.

56. Moyle GJ, Back D. Principles and practice of HIV-protease inhibitor pharmacoenhancement. HIV Med. 2001;2:105-113.

57. Dieleman JP, Gyssens IC, van der Endeme, et al. Urological complaints in relation to indinavir plasma concentrations in HIV-infected patients. AIDS. 1999;13:473-478.

58. Havlir D, Cheeseman SH, McLaughlin M, et al. High-dose nevirapine: Safety, pharmacokinetics, and antiviral effect in patients with human immunodeficiency infection. J Infect Dis. 1995;171:537-545.

59. Para MF, Meehan P, Holden-Wiltse J, et al. ACTG 260: A randomized, phase I-II, dose-ranging trial of the anti-human immunodeficiency virus activity of delavirdine monotherapy. The AIDS Clinical Trials Group Protocol 260 Team. Antimicrob Agents Chemother. 1999;43:1373-1378.

60. Joshi AS, Barrett JS, Fiske WD, et al. Population pharmacokinetics of efavirenz in phase II studies and relationship with efficacy (Abstract 1201). Program and Abstracts of the 39th Interscience Conference on Antimicrobial Agents and Chemotherapy, September 1999.

61. Schuetz JD, Connelly MC, Sun D, et al. MRP4: A previously unidentified factor in resistance to nucleoside-based antiviral drugs. Nat Med. 1999;5:1048-1051.

62. Reid G, Wielinga P, Zelcer N, et al. Characterization of the transport of nucleoside analog drugs by the human multidrug resistance proteins MRP4 and MRP5. Mol Pharmacol. 2003;63:1094-1103.

63. Fletcher CV, Kawle SP, Kakuda TN, et al. Zidovudine triphosphate and lamivudine triphosphate concentration-response relationships in HIV-infected persons. AIDS. 2000;14:2137-2144.

64. Fletcher CV, Acosta EP, Henry K, et al. Concentration-controlled zidovudine therapy. Clin Pharmacol Ther. 1998;64:331-338.

65. Drusano GL, Yuen GJ, Lambert JS, et al. Relationship between dideoxyinosine exposure, CD4 counts, and p24 antigen levels in human immunodeficiency virus infection. Ann Intern Med. 1992;116:562-566.

66. Drusano GL, Balis FM, Gitterman SR, et al. Quantitative relationships between zidovudine exposure and efficacy and toxicity. Antimicrob Agents Chemother. 1994;38:1726-1731.

67. Beltangady M, Knupp CA, Gustafson N, et al. Relation between plasma concentrations of didanosine and markers of antiviral efficacy in adults with AIDS or AIDS-related complex. Clin Infect Dis. 1993;16(Suppl 1):S26-S31.

68. Ellner PD, Neu HC. The inhibitory quotient: A methods for interpreting minimum inhibitory concentration data. JAMA. 1981;246:1575-1578.

69. Back D, Gatti G, Fletcher C, et al. Therapeutic drug monitoring in HIV infection: Current status and future directions. AIDS. 2002;16(Suppl 1):S5-S37.

70. Back DJ, Khoo SH. The role of clinical pharmacology in optimizing antiretroviral therapy. Br J Clin Pharmacol. 2003;55:473-476.

71. Castagna AD, Hasson H, Boeri E, et al. The normalized inhibitory quotient (NIQ) of lopinavir is predictive of viral load response over 48 weeks in a cohort of highly experienced HIV-1-infected individuals (Abstract 128). Program and Abstracts of the 9th Conference on Retroviruses and Opportunistic Infections, 2002.

72. Fletcher CV, Cheng F, Fiscus CH, et al. The inhibitory quotient (IQ) for saquinavir (SQV) predicts virologic response to salvage therapy (Abstract 129). Program and Abstracts of 9th Conference on Retroviruses and Opportunistic Infections, 2002.

73. Shulman N, Zolopa A, Havlir D, et al. Virtual inhibitory quotient (IQ) for indinavir (SQV) predicts response to ritonavir boosting of indinavir-based therapy in human immunodeficiency virus-infected patients with ongoing viremia. Antimicrob Agents Chemother. 2002;46:3907-3916.

74. Phillips E, Tseng TA, Walker S, et al. The use of virtual inhibitory quotient (vIQ) in antiretroviral (ART)-experienced patients taking amprenavir/lopinavir combinations (Abstract 130). Program and Abstracts of 9th Conference on Retroviruses and Opportunistic Infections, 2002.

75. Piscitelli SC, Metcalf F, Hoetelmans MJ, et al. The normalized inhibitory quotient: A method for predicting response to amprenavir (Abstract 164). Program and Abstracts of the 8th European Conference on Clinical Aspects and Treatment of HIV, 2001.

76. Eagle H. Experimental approach to the problem of treatment failure with penicillin. Am J Med. 1952;11:389-399.

77. Niederman MS, Mandell LA, Anzueto A, et al. Guidelines for the management of adults with community-acquired pneumonia. Am J Respir Crit Care Med. 2001;163:1730-1754.

78. Bartlett JG, Dowell SF, Mandell LA, et al. Practice guidelines for the management of community-acquired pneumonia in adults: Guidelines from the Infectious Diseases Society of America. Clin Infect Dis. 2000;31:811-838.

79. Heffelfinger JD, Dowell SF, Jorgensen JH, et al. Management of community-acquired pneumonia in the era of pneumococcal resistance: a report from the Drug-Resistant Streptococcus pneumoniae Therapeutic Working Group. Arch Intern Med. 2000;160:1399-1408.

80. Macfarlane J, Boswell T, Douglas G, et al. BTS guidelines for the management of community acquired pneumonia in adults. Thorax. 2001;56(Suppl IV):iv1-iv64.

81. Memish ZA, Shibl AM, Ahmed QAA, The Saudi Arabian Community-Acquired Pneumonia Working Group: Guidelines for the management of community-acquired pneumonia in Saudi Arabia: A model for the Middle East region. Int J Antimicrob Agents. 2002;20(Suppl):S1-S12.

82. Pallares R, Linares J, Vadillo M, et al. Resistance to penicillin and cephalosporin and mortality from severe pneumococcal pneumonia in Barcelona, Spain. N Engl J Med. 1995;333:474-480.

83. Friedland IR. Comparison of the response to antimicrobial therapy of penicillin-resistant and penicillin-susceptible pneumococcal disease. Pediatr Infect Dis J. 1995;14:885-890.

84. Viladrich PF, Cabellos C, Pallares R, et al. High doses of cefotaxime in treatment of adult meningitis due to Streptococcus pneumoniae with decreased susceptibilities to broad-spectrum cephalosporins. Antimicrob Agents Chemother. 1996;40:218-220.

85. Amsden GW, Graci DM, Cabelus LJ, et al. A randomized, crossover design study of the pharmacology of extended-spectrum fluoroquinolones for pneumococcal infections. Chest. 1999;116:115-119.

86. Amsden GW, Nafziger AN, Foulds G. Pharmacokinetics in serum and leukocyte exposures of oral azithromycin, 1,500 milligrams, given over a 3- or 5-day period in healthy subjects. Antimicrob Agents Chemother. 1999;43:163-165.

Penicillins

HENRY F. CHAMBERS

Penicillin was discovered by Alexander Fleming in 1928.[1] The work of Florey, Chain, and associates made possible the commercial production of penicillin G. By the end of the 1940s, penicillin G was available for general use in the United States, initiating the modern antibiotic era.

CHEMISTRY

The basic structure of the majority of commercially available penicillins is a nucleus consisting of a thiazolidine ring, the β-lactam ring, and a side chain (Fig. 19-1). The core ring structures, particularly the β-lactam ring, are essential for antibacterial activity. The side chain determines in large part the antibacterial spectrum and pharmacologic properties of a particular penicillin.

The appearance of β-lactamase–producing organisms, particularly *Staphylococcus aureus*, prompted studies to develop compounds resistant to hydrolysis by β-lactamases and to find agents more active than penicillin G against gram-negative species. The isolation of the penicillin nucleus, 6-amino-penicillanic acid, from a precursor-depleted fermentation of *Penicillium chrysogenum* made possible the production and testing of numerous semisynthetic penicillins, including methicillin, active against β-lactamase–producing *S. aureus*; ampicillin, active against selected gram-negative bacilli; and carbenicillin, active against *Pseudomonas aeruginosa*. Since then, numerous agents with different pharmacologic and antimicrobial properties have been developed.

MECHANISM OF ACTION

The antibacterial activity of penicillin, like all β-lactam antibiotics, is due to its inhibition of bacterial cell wall synthesis.[2,3] However, the concept that penicillin kills bacteria simply by blocking cell wall synthesis is overly simplistic.[4-6] The precise mechanism by which penicillin kills bacterial cells is not known.

The cell wall of both gram-positive and gram-negative bacteria is a rigid structure of peptidoglycan that protects against osmotic rupture. The cell wall of gram-positive bacteria is a substantial layer 50 to 100 molecules in thickness, whereas in gram-negative bacteria it is only one or two molecules thick. An outer membrane lipopolysaccharide layer, not found in gram-positive bacteria, is present on top of the peptidoglycan in

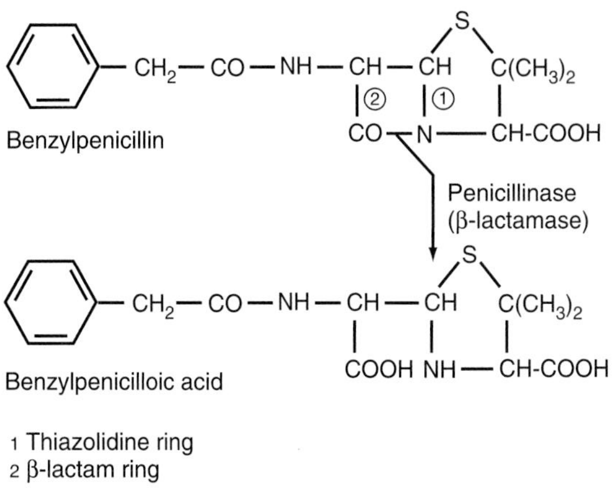

Benzylpenicillin

Penicillinase (β-lactamase)

Benzylpenicilloic acid

1 Thiazolidine ring
2 β-lactam ring

FIGURE 19-1. Structure of penicillin and site of β-lactamase attack.

gram-negative species. The cell wall of bacteria is assembled in a series of enzymatic steps involving at least 30 enzymes. The basic subunit of the peptidoglycan component is a disaccharide monomer of *N*-acetylglucosamine (NAG) and *N*-acetylmuramic (NAM) pentapeptide (Fig. 19-2). The cytoplasmic reactions that generate cell wall precursors and the disaccharide monomer subunit transport this subunit outside the cell, and the transglycosylase reaction that links the subunit to the peptidoglycan polymer is not sensitive to penicillin. Penicillin inhibits the final step in bacterial cell wall assembly, which is the formation of the cross-links that bridge peptidoglycan, giving it its structural integrity.

Peptidoglycan is composed of long polysaccharide chains of NAG and NAM pentapeptide. The pentapeptide consists of amino acid residues alternating between L- and D-stereoisomers and terminating in D-alanyl-D-alanine (see Fig. 19-2). A stem peptide of variable length and composition is attached to the third amino acid of this pentapeptide. Pentapeptides are then joined with stem peptides to form a cross-link between polysaccharide chains. This reaction is catalyzed by a transpeptidase that forms an amide bond between the terminal-free amine group of a stem peptide and the penultimate D-alanine of a pentapeptide, displacing the terminal D-alanine in the process. This transpeptidation reaction is sensitive to inhibition by penicillin. There are distinct transpeptidases that provide for anchoring of new peptidoglycan to old, that cross link special structures, and that direct formation of the cell wall septum. Although there are other penicillin-sensitive reactions, such as those catalyzed by carboxypeptidases, these reactions do not seem to be essential.

The penicillin-sensitive reactions are catalyzed by a family of closely related proteins, penicillin-binding proteins (PBPs).[7] Bacteria produce four types of PBPs, which structurally resemble and likely are derived from serine proteases. High-molecular-weight PBPs (i.e., >50 kD) and low-molecular-weight PBPs catalyze transpeptidation and carboxypeptidation reactions of cell wall assembly, respectively. Penicillin receptor PBPs transmit a transmembrane signal for induction of β-lactamases.[8,9] β-Lactamases are PBPs that catalyze hydrolysis of the β-lactam ring. Except for β-lactamases, which may be either secreted or membrane associated, PBPs are membrane bound. PBPs are inhibited by β-lactam antibiotics through covalent binding of the active site serine residue. Because the essential functions for survival of the cell generally reside with high-molecular-weight PBPs, it is binding to and inhibition of these PBPs that probably are responsible for the antibacterial activity of β-lactam antibiotics.

PBPs account for approximately 1% of membrane proteins. PBPs vary both in amounts present and in the physiologic functions they serve during cell wall assembly. They differ in their affinities for binding β-lactam antibiotics, which explains at least in part why the β-lactam antibiotics differ in their antibacterial properties and spectrum of activity. Spratt's[10] studies in *Escherichia coli* were the first to elucidate the different functions of PBPs. Inhibition of PBP 1b,

which has transpeptidase activity, or a substitute enzyme 1a, results in cell lysis.[11] PBP 1 is speculated to be important for cell elongation. Inhibition of PBP 2 results in formation of round cells that eventually lyse, suggesting that it has a role in an initial step in cell elongation and in determining the rod size and shape in *E. coli.*[12] Inhibition of PBP 3 produces long, filamentous cells, indicating that it is important for the ordered process of cross wall formation and cell division.[13] The functions performed by low-molecular-weight PBPs have not been well defined, but they probably play a role in the maintenance of cell shape.[14]

β-Lactam antibiotics produce their lethal effect on bacteria by inactivation of multiple PBPs simultaneously, but inhibition of cell wall synthesis by itself is not necessarily lethal. For example, nongrowing cells and cells that are osmotically protected survive in the presence of penicillin. Unopposed action of autolysins occurring when PBPs are inhibited by β-lactam antibiotics may contribute to the antibacterial effect in some organisms. Cell lysis, although it certainly is lethal and often accompanies cell wall inhibition, is also not required for cell death.[6] The lethal effect in both gram-positive and gram-negative organisms appears to be cell cycle–dependent,[4] with inhibition of PBPs leading to disruption of a crucial event probably at the time of cell division. This disturbed morphogenesis is hypothesized to initiate cell death.[5]

BACTERIAL RESISTANCE

Four mechanisms account for clinically significant bacterial resistance to penicillins, and other β-lactam antibiotics as well: (1) destruction of antibiotic by β-lactamase, (2) failure of antibiotic to penetrate the outer membrane of gram-negatives to reach PBP targets, (3) efflux of drug across the outer membrane of gram-negatives, and (4) low-affinity binding of antibiotic to target PBPs. β-Lactamase destruction of antibiotic is the most common. β-Lactamases covalently react with the β-lactam ring, rapidly hydrolyze it, and destroy activity of the drug.

β-Lactamases can be assigned to one of four classes, Ambler class A through D, based on amino acid sequence similarity and molecular structure[15,16] (Table 19-1). Class A, C, and D β-lactamases contain penicillin-binding motifs and are PBPs. They differ from other PBPs in that they typically are smaller in size, around 35 kD versus greater than 50 kD, and they are not cell wall synthetic enzymes. They react with penicillin through the same series of reactions as other PBPs. There is initial, reversible binding and formation of the Michaelis-Menton complex, followed by acylation of the active site serine and then followed by hydrolysis of the acyl intermediate in a deacylation reaction regenerating the active enzyme. Biochemically, the main distinction between cell wall synthetic PBPs and β-lactamases is the rate of deacylation: the deacylation rate of penicillin-bound cell wall synthetic PBP is relatively slow, amounting to irreversible inhibition of its activity, whereas the deacylation rate of β-lactamase usually is orders of magnitude faster,

FIGURE 19-2. Penicillin-binding protein (PBP) transpeptidation reaction that cross links bacterial cell wall. NAG, *N*-acetylglucosamine; NAM, *N*-acetylmuramic.

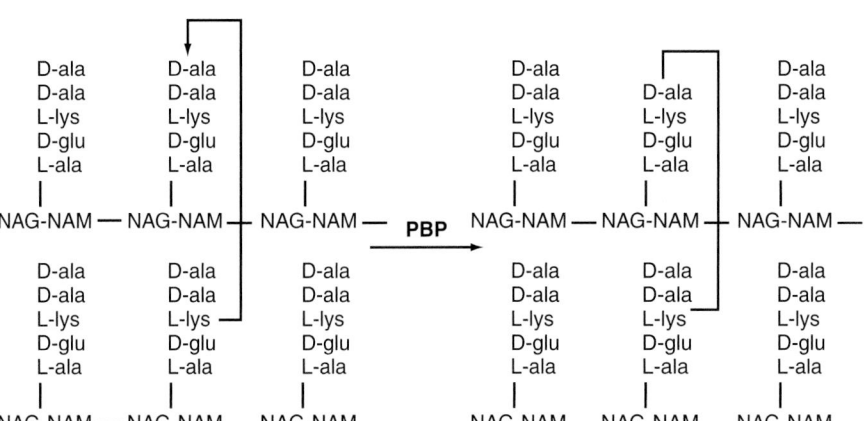

rapidly hydrolyzing and turning over β-lactam molecules. Class B enzymes, although they also hydrolyze the β-lactam ring, structurally are unrelated to PBPs. They are Zn^{2+}-dependent enzymes that use a different series of reactions to open the β-lactam ring.

The vast majority of the β-lactamases produced by clinical isolates are class A or class C. Class A enzymes are penicillinases, and some also have cephalosporinase activity. A few class A enzymes also have carbapenemase activity. They are inhibited by β-lactamase inhibitors such as clavulanic acid. Point mutations can render the enzyme inhibitor resistant or extend the spectrum of activity to include third-generation cephalosporins and monobactams (so-called extended spectrum β-lactamases [ESBLs]). Class C β-lactamase are cephalosporinases not inhibited by clavulanic acid. These β-lactamases frequently are encoded on the chromosome and inducible, although they may also be plasmid encoded and produced constitutively. Class B enzymes are the broadest-spectrum enzymes, are inhibited by chelating agents, and are able to hydrolyze all β-lactams except monobactams.

The outer membrane of gram-negative organisms is an important barrier to drug penetration and an important component of resistance.[17] β-Lactamases of gram-negative bacteria are located in the periplasmic space, which lies between the inner cytoplasmic membrane and outer lipopolysaccharide membrane, concentrating β-lactamases and strategically locating them to protect target PBPs from exposure to active β-lactam antibiotics. Small polar molecules (e.g., glucose, essential nutrients, β-lactam antibiotics) cross this barrier through protein channels called *porins*. Porins constrain entry of molecules into the cell according to size, structure, and charge. β-Lactam antibiotics that satisfy the entry requirements can traverse porin channels to the periplasmic space and bind to target PBPs. Absence or deletion of a critical porin, usually in the presence of a β-lactamase activity, can result in resistance.[18,19]

The third mechanism of resistance is efflux; the drug that enters the periplasmic space is pumped back across the outer membrane.[20-22] Efflux may operate independently of other mechanisms, but more often exclusion of antibiotic by porins, destruction of antibiotic by β-lactamases, or both also contribute to resistance by limiting periplasmic antibiotic concentration. Species differences in porins, pumps, β-lactamases, and target PBPs determine whether the organism is susceptible or resistant to a particular antibiotic. Mutations affecting protein structure or expression may cause a strain that was initially susceptible to a given β-lactam antibiotic to become resistant.

The fourth general type of resistance mechanism involves production of a PBP that has low affinity for binding of β-lactam antibiotic.[23] These may be the result of mutations in PBP genes that lower binding affinity, as in penicillin-resistant pneumococci or *Neisseria* spp., or due to the presence of an extra, low-affinity PBP, such as PBP 5 produced by *E. faecium* or PBP 2a produced by methicillin-resistant staphylococci.[24-28] Solution of the crystal structures of low-affinity PBPs have identified critical molecular features and interactions that are responsible for resistance.[29,30] In the case of PBP 2a, low-affinity binding of β-lactam antibiotic is mediated by structural changes that result in energetically unfavorable interactions between antibiotic and protein so that the active site serine is inactivated not at all or too slowly to effectively block cell wall synthesis and bacterial growth.

CLASSIFICATION

Penicillins can be conveniently divided into five classes on the basis of antibacterial activity with considerable overlap among the classes: (1) natural penicillins, penicillin G and penicillin; (2) penicillinase-resistant penicillins, methicillin, nafcillin, and isoxazolyl penicillins; (3) aminopenicillins, ampicillin and amoxicillin; (4) carboxypenicillins, carbenicillin and ticarcillin; and (5) acyl ureidopenicillins, azlocillin, mezlocillin, and piperacillin. The carboxypenicillins and ureidopenicillins are also referred to as antipseudomonal penicillins. Differences within a class are principally pharmacologic, although one compound in a class may be more active than another.

The susceptibility profiles of various species of microorganisms are given in Tables 19-2, 19-3, and 19-4. The natural penicillins are most active against non–β-lactamase–producing gram-positive bacteria, anaerobes, and selected gram-negative cocci, such as *Neisseria*. Gram-positive bacteria inhibited by natural penicillins tend to be more susceptible to these penicillins than to semisynthetic penicillins.[31,32] Penicillin V (used orally) can be substituted for penicillin G, except against gram-negative species because it is less active than penicillin G against *Neisseria* and *Haemophilus*. Semisynthetic penicillinase-resistant penicillins are the drugs of choice only for penicillin-resistant *Staphylococcus aureus* and *Staphylococcus epidermidis*, although they also are active against streptococci but not against enterococci. Aminopenicillins possess the same spectrum as penicillin G, plus they are active against gram-negative cocci and Enterobacteriaceae that do not produce β-lactamase.[33] Carboxypenicillins and ureidopenicillins have activity against gram-negative aerobic rods, such as *P. aeruginosa*,

TABLE 19-1   Classification of β-Lactamases

Ambler Molecular Class	Major Subtypes*	Preferred Substrates	Inhibitor†	Main Genetic Localization
A	Gram-positive β-lactamase 2a	Penicillins	Clavulanate	Chromosomal or plasmid, inducible
	Gram-negative β-lactamase (e.g., TEM-1 and SHV-1) 2b	Penicillins, some cephalosporins	Clavulanate	Plasmid or chromosomal
	Extended spectrum β-lactamase 2be	Penicillins, narrow-spectrum and third-generation cephalosporins, monobactams	Clavulanate	Plasmid
	Inhibitor-resistant TEM β-lactamase 2br	Penicillins	Clavulanate ±	Plasmid
	Carbenicillin-hydrolyzing β-lactamase 2c	Penicillins, carbenicillin	Clavulanate ±	Plasmid
	Cephalosporin hydrolyzing β-lactamase 2e	Cephalosporins	Clavulanate	Chromosome, inducible
	Carbapenem hydrolyzing β-lactamase 2f	Penicillins, cephalosporins, carbapenems	Clavulanate	Chromosomal
B	Metallo-β-lactamase 3	All β-lactams except monobactam	EDTA, divalent cation chelators	Chromosomal
C	AmpC-type cephalosporinase 1	Cephalosporins, penicillins	Cloxacillin, monobactams	Chromosomal (inducible); constitutive, plasmid-encoded enzymes increasingly reported
D	Cloxacillin-hydrolyzing β-lactamase 2d	Penicillins, cloxacillin	Clavulanate ±	Plasmid

*Bush-Jacoby-Medeiros group is indicated in parentheses.
†Tazobactam and sulbactam have activities similar to those of clavulanate.

TABLE 19-2 Usual Minimal Inhibitory Concentrations (MICs) for Penicillins against Cocci

Organism	Penicillin G	Penicillin V	Ampicillin, Amoxicillin	Methicillin	Oxacillin, Cloxacillin, Dicloxacillin	Nafcillin	Ticarcillin	Azlocillin, Mezlocillin, Piperacillin
				Mean MIC (μg/mL)				
Streptococcus pneumoniae	0.01*	0.02*	0.02*	0.1*	0.04	0.02	0.4	0.02
Streptococcus pyogenes	0.005	0.01	0.02	0.2	0.04	0.02	0.2	0.02
Streptococcus agalactiae	0.005	0.01	0.02	0.2	0.06	0.02	0.2	0.15
Viridans streptococci	0.01	0.01	0.05	0.1	0.1	0.06	0.2	0.12
Enterococcus faecalis	3.0	6.0	1.5†	>25	>25	>25	50	1.5
Peptostreptococcus	0.2	0.5	0.2	2.0	0.6	0.5	0.4	0.8
Staphylococcus aureus								
Penicillinase negative	0.02	0.02	0.05	1.0	0.3	0.25	1.2	0.8
Penicillinase positive	>25	>25	>25	2.0	0.4	0.25	25	25
Staphylococcus epidermidis	0.02‡	0.02‡	0.05‡	0.8‡	0.2‡	0.2‡	0.8‡	1.6‡
Neisseria gonorrhoeae§	0.01‡	0.1	0.3‡	12.0	12.0	12.0	0.3‡	0.05‡
Neisseria meningitidis	0.05	0.25	0.05	6.0	6.0	6.0	0.1	0.05

*Rare isolates resistant to penicillin have been found with MIC >5 μg/mL.
†Amoxicillin has a mean MIC of 0.4.
‡Many isolates resistant.
§MIC can range from 0.005 to 100.

TABLE 19-3 Activity of Penicillins against Selected Bacilli and Anaerobic Organisms

Organism	Penicillin G	Ampicillin, Amoxicillin	Oxacillin*	Ticarcillin†	Azlocillin, Mezlocillin, Piperacillin†
		Mean Minimal Inhibitory Concentration (μg/mL)			
Clostridium perfringens	0.5	0.05	>0.5	0.5	0.05
Corynebacterium diphtheriae	0.1	0.02	>0.1	0.1	1.0
Listeria monocytogenes	0.5	0.5	>4.0	4	0.5
Haemophilus influenzae‡	0.8	0.5	>25	0.5	0.1
Prevotella melaninogenica	0.5	0.5	>25	0.5	0.2
Fusobacterium nucleatum	0.5	0.1	>100	0.5	0.5
Bacteroides fragilis	32	32	>500	64	32

*Oxacillin is used as representative of isoxazolyl penicillins.
†Minor differences do occur.
‡β-Lactamase–producing strains occur and are resistant to the penicillins

which are resistant to ampicillin. Carboxypenicillins are less active than the ureidopenicillins against streptococci and *Haemophilus* spp. Ureidopenicillins generally are more active against gram-negative bacteria other than *Pseudomonas*. Many anaerobic gram-positive species are susceptible to the penicillins. Gram-negative anaerobic bacteria are susceptible to most penicillins (with the exception of isolates of *Bacteroides fragilis*, other *Bacteroides* spp., and some *Prevotella* spp., which produce chromosomal class A β-lactamase) and are inhibited by high levels of penicillin G or the semisynthetic anti-*Pseudomonas* agents—azlocillin, carbenicillin, mezlocillin, piperacillin, and ticarcillin.[34,35] Strains of *Fusobacterium varium* often are resistant to all penicillins.

TABLE 19-4 Activity of Penicillins against Enterobacteriaceae and *Pseudomonas*

Organism	Penicillin G	Ampicillin, Amoxicillin	Oxacillin*	Ticarcillin	Azlocillin,† Mezlocillin, Piperacillin
		Mean Minimal Inhibitory Concentration (μg/mL)			
Escherichia coli‡	100	3	>1000	6	8
Proteus mirabilis	50	3	>1000	1.5	1
Klebsiella spp.	>400	200	>1000	>400	16
Enterobacter spp.	>500	>500	>1000	50	16
Citrobacter diversus	>500	>100	>1000	12	8
Citrobacter freundii	>500	50	>1000	12	32
Serratia	>500	>500	>1000	100	32
Salmonella‡	10	1.5	>1000	3	4
Shigella‡	20	1.5	>1000	3	8
Proteus vulgaris	>500	>500	>1000	12	16
Providencia	>500	>500	>1000	12	8
Morganella	>500	200	>1000	25	8
Pseudomonas, other	>500	>500	>500	100	>100
Acinetobacter	>500	250	>1000	25	32
Pseudomonas aeruginosa	>500	>500	>1000	50	16*

*Used as representative anti-staphylococcal penicillin.
†Some isolates, particularly *Klebsiella*, are resistant to azlocillin but susceptible to mezlocillin and piperacillin.
‡Amoxicillin is twofold more active against *Salmonella* and twofold less active against *Shigella*. Strains containing the TEM plasmid β-lactamase are resistant.

TABLE 19-5   Pharmacokinetic Properties of Penicillins

Antibiotic	Oral Adsorption (%)	Food Decreases Adsorption	Protein Binding (%)	Amount of Dose Metabolized (%)	Serum Level* Total Drug (µg/mL)	Serum Level* Free Drug (µg/mL)	Serum T½ (hr)† Normal (Ccr >90 mL/min)	Serum T½ (hr)† With Renal Failure (Ccr <10 mL/min)	Liver Impairment Increases T½	Na⁺ Content‡ (mEq/g)
Penicillin G	20	Yes	55	20	2	0.9	0.5	10	+	2.7
Penicillin V	60	No	80	55	4	0.8	1	4		
Methicillin	Nil		35	10			0.5	4		3.1
Oxacillin	30	Yes	93	45	6	0.4	0.5	1		
Cloxacillin	50	Yes	94	20	10	0.6	0.5	1	++	
Dicloxacillin	50	Yes	97	10	15	0.45	0.5	1.5	++	
Nafcillin	Erratic	Yes	87				0.5	1.5	+++	
Ampicillin	40	Yes	17	10	3.5	2.9	1	8	++	3.4
Amoxicillin	75	No	17	10	7.5	6.2	1	8	+	
Indanyl carbenicillin	30	No	50		15	7.5	1.1	15	++	
Ticarcillin	Nil		50	15			1.2	15	++, 18-20 h	4.7
Mezlocillin	Nil		50				1.1	4	++	1.8
Piperacillin	Nil		50				1.3	4	++	1.8
Azlocillin	Nil		20				0.8	4	++	2.2

*After 500-mg dose taken fasting.
†Values have been rounded off to approximate values.
‡Na⁺ content based on intravenous preparations.
C$_{cr}$, Creatinine clearance; T½, serum half-life.

PHARMACOLOGIC PROPERTIES

Penicillins differ markedly in their oral absorption (Table 19-5). Acid-labile compounds, penicillin G, methicillin, and antipseudomonal penicillins are poorly absorbed. Acid-stable compounds can have major differences in oral absorption. Semisynthetic penicillins, except nafcillin, are well absorbed. Ampicillin is only partially absorbed, 30% to 60%, and food decreases absorption, whereas amoxicillin is almost totally absorbed. Although carbenicillin is not absorbed, the ester form, indanyl carbenicillin, is adequately absorbed to provide urinary concentration to treat urinary tract infections.

Orally absorbed penicillins yield peak concentrations 1 to 2 hours after ingestion. Peak serum levels are delayed after ingestion with food and peak levels also are lower, except for amoxicillin. Procaine penicillin G and benzathine penicillin, repository forms of penicillin G, are absorbed more slowly from intramuscular sites than are the crystalline salts. Procaine or lidocaine can also be used as a diluent for intramuscular injection of antipseudomonal penicillins, but the half-life of these drugs is not prolonged by these agents.

Penicillins are bound to serum proteins in varying degrees, ranging from 17% for the aminopenicillins to 97% for dicloxacillin (see Table 19-5). The major protein to which they bind is albumin.[31] Only unbound drug exerts antibacterial activity. However, protein binding is a reversible process, and it is possible for bound penicillin to be released and then to kill bacteria in tissue or in the blood stream. The major mechanism by which most of these drugs are removed from the body is by excretion as intact molecules via the kidney. Penicillins are metabolized to a minor degree.[36] Even minor differences in metabolism can result in clinically significant differences in half-life in the presence of renal failure. Biliary excretion of penicillins does occur, but it probably is important only for nafcillin and the antipseudomonal penicillins.

Penicillins are rapidly excreted into urine by renal tubular cells, and hence they have a short half-life, ranging from less than 30 minutes for penicillin to 70 minutes for carbenicillin. The ability of the renal tubular cells to excrete penicillin varies with the agents, but up to 4 g of penicillin G per hour can be excreted. This excretion can be blocked by probenecid, an inhibitor of organic acid secretion by tubular cells, which prolongs the serum half-life of all the penicillins. Probenecid also competes for binding sites on albumin; hence, there is more free drug in the presence of probenecid. Renal excretion of all penicillins in newborns is markedly less than in older children, because tubular function is not fully developed at birth. Hence, the dosage programs for penicillins must be modified when these drugs are given to newborns or low-birth-weight infants.

Reduction in renal function must be taken into account in the administration of certain penicillins (e.g., ticarcillin). For creatinine clearance above 10-20 mL/min, only minor adjustments in the dosage of other penicillins are required. In the presence of anuria, reduction is necessary in total daily dose of the natural penicillins, of many of the penicillinase-resistant penicillins, and of the aminopenicillins (Table 19-6).

Peritoneal dialysis removes variable amounts of the penicillins. In general, after peritoneal dialysis only the dosage regimens of ticarcillin need to be adjusted. After hemodialysis, which yields a creatinine clearance of approximately 10 to 15 mL/min, and during continuous venovenous hemofiltration, with a 25 mL/min creatinine clearance, the dose of penicillin G, ampicillin, amoxicillin, ticarcillin, azlocillin, mezlocillin, and piperacillin must be adjusted, but the dose of nafcillin or the isoxazolyl penicillins need not be adjusted.

TABLE 19-6   Antibiotic Dosage Change in Renal Disease and after Dialysis

Agent	Dosage Change in Renal Failure* Creatinine Clearance (30-50 mL/min)	Dosage Change in Renal Failure* Creatinine Clearance (<10-20 mL/min)	Dosage Change After Hemodialysis
Penicillin G	NC	1.6 × 10⁶ units/6 h	Yes (1.6 × 10⁶ units)
Penicillin V	NC	250 mg/6 h	Yes (250 mg)
Methicillin	NC	2 g/8 h	Slight (2 g)
Oxacillin	NC	NC	Slight (as in uremia)
Cloxacillin	NC	NC	Slight (as in uremia)
Dicloxacillin	NC	NC	Slight (as in uremia)
Nafcillin	NC	NC	Slight (as in uremia)
Ampicillin	NC	0.5-1 g/8 h	Yes (500 mg)
Amoxicillin	NC	500 mg/12 h	Yes (250 mg)
Ticarcillin†	2 g/4h	2 g/12 h	Yes (2 g)
Indanyl carbenicillin†	NC	Avoid	
Azlocillin	NC	3 g/8-12 h	Yes (2 g)
Mezlocillin	NC	3 g/8-12 h	Yes (2 g)
Piperacillin	NC	3 g/8-12 h	Yes (2 g)

*Refers to maximum dose used.
†Only carbenicillin and ticarcillin need adjustment of dosage after peritoneal dialysis.
NC, no change.

Penicillins are well distributed to most tissues, including lung, liver, kidney, muscle, bone, and placenta. The levels of penicillins in abscesses, middle ear, and pleural, peritoneal, and synovial fluids are sufficient in the presence of inflammation to inhibit most susceptible bacteria. Most penicillins are relatively insoluble in lipid and penetrate cells relatively poorly. Distribution of all the penicillins to eye, brain, cerebrospinal fluid, or prostate is nil in the absence of inflammation.[37] Inflammation alters normal barriers, permitting entry of penicillins; most achieve concentrations in cerebrospinal fluid that range between 1% and 5% of serum concentrations, except for ampicillin, for which the range is 5% to 10%. Penicillins with low rates of protein binding reach levels in fetal serum equivalent to levels in maternal serum 30 to 60 minutes after injection. In contrast, the highly protein-bound semisynthetic penicillins achieve low concentrations in both amniotic fluid and fetal serum.[38]

Urinary concentrations of all penicillins are high, even in the presence of moderately reduced renal function, but in people with rates of creatinine clearance below 10 mL/min, the urinary levels may not exceed those in the blood. Cortical and medullary concentrations of penicillins exceed serum levels.

Most penicillins are actively secreted into the bile, yielding biliary concentrations well in excess of those in serum. The biliary levels of penicillin G and ampicillin are at least 10 times those in the serum, and the levels of nafcillin and mezlocillin in bile are as high as 100 times the simultaneous serum level. In the presence of common duct obstruction, the levels of all penicillins in bile are markedly reduced. Because the biliary transport system is a saturable one, with drug doses producing very high serum levels, the biliary levels are not significantly increased over those measured at lower serum levels.

UNTOWARD REACTIONS

The major adverse effects of the penicillins are hypersensitivity reactions, which range in severity from rash to immediate anaphylaxis[39] (Table 19-7) (see Chapter 22). Penicillins are capable of acting as haptens to combine with proteins contaminating the solution or with human protein after the penicillin has been administered to humans. Penicilloyl and penicillanic acid derivatives are the major determinants of penicillin allergy. The penicilloyl determinant, which is produced through opening of the β-lactam ring, thereby allowing amide linkage to body proteins (Fig. 19-3), is the most important antigenic component. Penicillanic acid and derivatives of penicillanic acid are produced when reconstituted penicillins break down in solution owing to acidity or temperature elevation. Minor determinants of allergy are benzyl penicillin itself and sodium benzyl penicilloate, which can act either as sensitizing agents or on their own elicit an allergic reaction. Both major and minor determinants may be involved in anaphylactic reactions, as well as in urticarial reactions. These reactions are mediated by immunoglobulin E (IgE) antibody. Minor determinants are the major cause of anaphylactic reactions. A person who has been sensitized by the hapten-carrier complex can have a reaction to penicillin alone or to penicillin that has formed dimers or polymers in solution. Anaphylactic reactions to penicillins are uncommon, occurring in only 0.2% of 10,000 courses of treatment, with a fatality rate of 0.001% of 100,000 courses.[40]

Serum sickness does occur with penicillins, but it is very uncommon. It probably is due to IgG antibodies against the benzyl penicilloyl hapten. The illness is characterized by fever, urticaria, joint pains, and angioneurotic edema. Exfoliative dermatitis and Stevens-Johnson syndrome are rare forms of allergic reactions to penicillins. The morbilliform eruptions that develop after penicillin therapy probably are due to IgM antibody to the benzyl penicilloyl hapten and to the minor determinants. In many patients, these rashes disappear, even if the penicillin is continued, owing to the production of IgG-blocking antibody. There is a risk, however, that the rash could progress to generalized desquamation. If an allergic reaction does occur, epinephrine given intramuscularly or intravenously usually aborts the reaction. Antihistamines and corticosteroids have not been shown to be of benefit.

TABLE 19-7 Adverse Reactions to Penicillins*		
Type of Reaction	**Frequency (%)**	**Occurs Most Frequently With***
Allergic		
IgE antibody	0.004-0.4	Penicillin G
Anaphylaxis		
Early urticaria (<72 h)		
Cytotoxic antibody	Rare	Penicillin G
Hemolytic anemia		
Antigen-antibody complex disease	Rare	Penicillin G
Serum sickness		
Delayed hypersensitivity	4-8	Ampicillin
Contact dermatitis		
Idiopathic	4-8	Ampicillin
Skin rash		
Fever		
Late-onset urticaria		
Gastrointestinal	2-5	
Diarrhea	2-5	Ampicillin
Enterocolitis	<1	Ampicillin
Hematologic		
Hemolytic anemia	Rare	Penicillin G
Neutropenia	1-4	Penicillin G, nafcillin, oxacillin, piperacillin
Platelet dysfunction	3	Carbenicillin, ticarcillin
Hepatic		
Elevated serum aspartate transaminase level	1-4	Oxacillin, nafcillin, carbenicillin
Electrolyte disturbance		
Sodium overload	Variable	Ticarcillin
Hypokalemia	Variable	Ticarcillin
Hyperkalemia—acute	Rare	Penicillin G
Neurologic		
Seizures	Rare	Penicillin G
Bizarre sensations		Procaine penicillin
Renal		
Interstitial nephritis	1-2	Methicillin
Hemorrhagic cystitis	Rare	Methicillin

*All the reactions can occur with any of the penicillins.

Another allergic reaction to penicillins is that of allergic vasculitis with the development of cutaneous and visceral lesions similar to that found with periarteritis nodosa. This reaction is extremely rare.

Hematologic toxicity is rare, although neutropenia has been encountered with the use of all types of penicillins, particularly when large doses are used. The mechanism of the neutropenia is unknown, and white blood cell counts return to normal rapidly if the offending agent is discontinued. Sometimes a lower dose of drug can be used without production of neutropenia. Coombs-positive hemolytic anemia occurs rarely.[41] All penicillins at high concentrations, particularly carbenicillin and ticarcillin, bind to the adenosine diphosphate receptor site in platelets, preventing normal platelet aggregation. Clinically significant bleeding occurs relatively infrequently.[34,42]

Renal toxicity from penicillins is variable, ranging from allergic angiitis to interstitial nephritis.[43] Interstitial nephritis, most common with methicillin, is seen with all penicillins. The clinical syndrome is one of fever, macular rash, eosinophilia, proteinuria, eosinophiluria, and hematuria. Initially the reaction is one of nonoliguric renal failure with a decrease in creatinine clearance and a rise in serum urea nitrogen and serum creatinine concentrations. This reaction can progress to anuria and renal failure. Biopsy specimens of the kidney show an interstitial infiltrate of mononuclear and eosinophilic cells with tubular damage but no glomerular lesions. Discontinuation of the penicillin results in the return of renal function to normal in most cases.

Administration of massive doses of any penicillin, but most often carbenicillin and ticarcillin, may result in hypokalemia owing to the large dose of nonreabsorbable anion presented to the distal renal tubules, which alters H^+ excretion and secondarily results in K^+ loss.

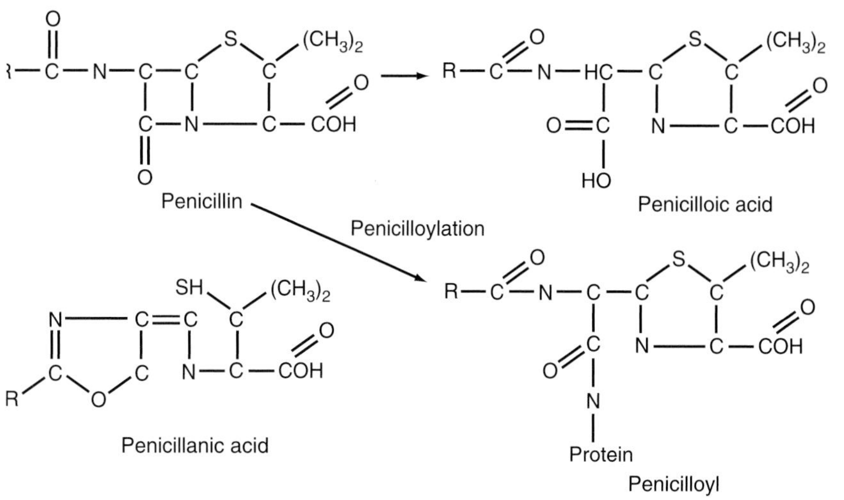

FIGURE 19-3. Mechanisms for formation of antigens from penicillins.

Central nervous system toxicity in the form of myoclonic seizures can follow the administration of massive doses of penicillin G or ampicillin. If there is reduced renal function, the drugs accumulate, and this form of toxicity becomes more likely.[44] Direct instillation of small doses of methicillin, oxacillin, or nafcillin into the ventricles at the time of surgery for placement of atrioventricular shunts has not resulted in seizures. Direct application of penicillin to the cortex provokes seizure activity.

Gastrointestinal disturbances may follow the use of any of the oral forms but are most pronounced with ampicillin. Antibiotic-associated colitis due to *Clostridium difficile* has followed the use of each of the penicillins (see Chapter 92). All penicillins used at high doses for prolonged periods abolish normal bacterial flora, with resulting colonization with resistant gram-negative bacilli or with fungi such as *Candida*. Abnormalities in liver function test results such as elevation of the alkaline phosphatase and aminotransferase (transaminase) levels have been reported, most often after the use of oxacillin and carbenicillin. The pathogenesis of the hepatic reaction is unknown. Major hepatic injury is very uncommon, and liver enzymes return to normal values within a few days of stopping therapy.

CLINICAL USE

Some uses of penicillins are given in Table 19-8. Penicillin G remains the primary agent for treatment of infections due to *Streptococcus pyogenes*, penicillin-susceptible strains of *Streptococcus pneumoniae*, and enterococci. Intravenous penicillin G remains the treatment of choice for pneumococcal and meningococcal meningitis, streptococcal and enterococcal endocarditis (in the latter case in combination with gentamicin), and neurosyphilis. None of the newer penicillins or agents in other classes has been shown to be more effective. Penicillin-susceptible strains of *S. pneumoniae* are inhibited at concentrations less than 0.1 μg of penicillin G/mL. Other penicillins also are highly active, although minimal inhibitory concentrations (MICs) usually exceed that of penicillin G.[45] This hierarchy of activity of the penicillins is maintained against penicillin-resistant strains of *S. pneumoniae*, albeit at higher MICs. Penicillin, ampicillin, and amoxicillin are the most active compounds, with MICs rarely exceeding 4 μg/mL, versus MICs of 128 μg/mL or greater for ticarcillin against highly penicillin-resistant strains. Except in pneumococcal meningitis, for which clinical failures with penicillin are well documented, infections caused by penicillin-resistant pneumococci appear to respond to penicillin G, provided a sufficiently high dose is used.[46,47] For serious pneumococcal infections caused by penicillin-resistant strains with MICs greater than 1 μg/mL, particularly in immuno-compromised patients, vancomycin or another non–β-lactam may be preferred over a penicillin or other β-lactam antibiotic.[48]

Penicillin should be used to treat pneumococcal meningitis only if the isolate is fully penicillin susceptible.[49]

Nearly all *Neisseria meningitidis* strains are susceptible to penicillin G. *Neisseria gonorrhoeae* strains vary in susceptibility to penicillin G; resistance can be due to β-lactamase production or to altered PBPs. Penicillin G is the drug of choice for syphilis at all stages. Puerperal infections due to anaerobic streptococci or group B streptococci *(Streptococcus agalactiae)*, as well as genital clostridial infections, are treated with penicillin G. Infections produced by anaerobic mouth flora including gram-positive and gram-negative cocci and actinomycetes can be treated with penicillin G, although penicillin-resistant strains of *Prevotella melaninogenica* that produce a β-lactamase are being encountered.

The penicillinase-resistant penicillins are indicated solely for the treatment of infections caused by methicillin-susceptible strains of staphylococci for which they are the agents of choice. They also cover viridans streptococci, *S. pyogenes* and other hemolytic streptococci, penicillin-susceptible strains of *S. pneumoniae*, anaerobic gram-positive cocci, and anaerobic gram-positive bacilli, but penicillin is slightly more active against these organisms and is the preferred drug. These compounds are inactive against *Listeria monocytogenes*, *Enterococcus* spp., and methicillin-resistant strains of staphylococci. The basis of methicillin resistance in staphylococci is the production of PBP 2a, which has low affinity for binding methicillin. They lack gram-negative activity.

Aminopenicillins are indicated for treatment of upper respiratory tract infections, lower respiratory tract infections, bacterial gastroenteritis (ampicillin only), bacterial endocarditis, meningitis, and urinary tract infections caused by susceptible (i.e., non–β-lactamase–producing) organisms. Amoxicillin, because of its excellent bioavailability, is the preferred agent for oral administration in most situations; it is well tolerated even in high doses up to 2 g (50 to 90 mg/kg/day in children) administered two or three times a day.[50,51] Amoxicillin is also recommended as one component of a triple-drug combination regimen for treatment of ulcers and gastric infections caused by *Helicobacter pylori*.[52]

The antipseudomonal and extended-spectrum penicillins are indicated for the treatment of infections caused by resistant gram-negative bacilli, especially *P. aeruginosa*. They should be used in combination with another antipseudomonal agent, typically an aminoglycoside, for non–urinary tract pseudomonal infections, at least for the first few days. The ureidopenicillins, piperacillin in particular, are active against many strains of *Klebsiella* spp., *Enterobacter* spp., *Serratia marcescens*, and *Providentia*, and can be used to treat infections caused by the organisms. Carbenicillin and ticarcillin are less active against enterococci than ureidopenicillins and ampicillin and should not be used to treat documented infections caused by these organisms. Carbenicillin and ticarcillin have fallen into disuse, and even piperacillin, which is still widely used, is often given as a combination with tazobactam (see Chapter 21) because of

TABLE 19-8 Antimicrobial Spectrum of Penicillin*

Infecting Organism	Penicillin of Choice	Alternative Acceptable Penicillin	Frequency of Resistance to Penicillins (%)
Gram-positive cocci			
Streptococcus pneumoniae	G	V	20-25
Streptococcus pyogenes (A)	G	V	None
Streptococcus agalactiae (B)	G	Ampicillin	None
Viridans streptococci	G		10-20
Streptococcus bovis (D)	G		Rare
Enterococcus faecalis	Ampicillin	Mezlocillin	10-20
Staphylococcus aureus (non–penicillinase producing)	G	Penicillinase resistant	Rare†
Staphylococcus aureus (penicillinase producing)	Penicillinase resistant		25%‡
Staphylococcus aureus (methicillin resistant)	None	None	100
Staphylococcus epidermidis	Penicillinase resistant		80‡
Staphylococcus epidermidis (methicillin resistant)	None	None	100
Gram-negative cocci			
Neisseria meningitidis	G	Ampicillin	Very rare
Neisseria gonorrhoeae	G	Ampicillin	1-40
Gram-positive bacilli			
Bacillus anthracis	G		None
Corynebacterium diphtheriae	G		None
Listeria monocytogenes	Ampicillin	G	None
Anaerobic species			
Peptostreptococcus	G	Ampicillin	None
Actinomyces israelii	G	V	None
Prevotella melaninogenica	G	C, T	10
Fusobacterium spp.	G	Ampicillin	1-10
Bacteroides fragilis	M, P A		75
Clostridium spp.	G	Ampicillin	<1
Gram-negative bacilli			
Haemophilus spp.	Ampicillin		5-30
Escherichia coli	Ampicillin		30
Proteus mirabilis	Ampicillin		<5
Salmonella typhi	Ampicillin		20
Salmonella, other spp.	Ampicillin		20
Klebsiella spp.	None		95
Enterobacter spp.	M, P, T		70
Citrobacter freundii	M, P, T		80
Proteus, indole-positive spp.	M, P, T		20
Serratia spp.	M, P, T		90
Pseudomonas aeruginosa	A, P, T		20-30
Pseudomonas, other spp.	None		95
Acinetobacter spp.	T	A, G, P	50
Providencia spp.	M, P, T		20-30
Stenotrophomonas maltophilia	None		95
Other organisms infrequently encountered			
Erysipelothrix spp.	G	Ampicillin	None
Pasteurella multocida	G	Ampicillin*	Rare, <1
Streptobacillus moniliformis	G		None
Spirillum minus	G		None
Treponema pallidum	G		None

*In each case, it is assumed that a route of administration would be used that would achieve levels in serum and tissue to eradicate the organism. If there is no entry in the alternative column, it means that an antibiotic in another class would be a more appropriate choice. Amoxicillin can be used in place of ampicillin in all situations except with *Shigella* infections.

†Most non–penicillinase-producing strains are methicillin-susceptible.

‡Approximate frequency of methicillin-resistant strains among penicillinase-producing strains.

A, azlocillin; M, mezlocillin; P, piperacillin; T, ticarcillin.

the prevalence of β-lactamase–producing strains. However, the activity of piperacillin against many of the gram-negative species, such as *P. aeruginosa*, *Enterobacter*, *Citrobacter*, *Serratia*, and *Providentia*, is usually not improved by tazobactam because these organisms typically produce a class C β-lactamase, which is not inhibited by β-lactamase inhibitors, and piperacillin can be used without tazobactam for infections caused by these organisms.

PROPHYLACTIC USE

Penicillins have been used in a number of situations for prevention of infection. The oral administration of 200,000 units of penicillin G or penicillin V every 12 hours has resulted in a significant reduction in recurrences of rheumatic fever. Because of the problems with compliance with oral therapy, intramuscular injections of 1.2 or 2.4 million units of benzathine penicillin given once each month have also been used with excellent results. Outbreaks of streptococcal infection due to *S. pyogenes* have been aborted by the use of oral penicillin G or V (200,000 units) given twice a day for 5 days, by single injections of procaine penicillin daily, or by administration of benzathine penicillin.

Ampicillin or amoxicillin has been administered orally to asplenic children or to children with agammaglobulinemia to prevent infections caused by *Haemophilus influenzae* and *S. pneumoniae*. It is recommended as a single 2-g oral dose for prophylaxis of bacterial endocarditis.[53] Penicillin prophylaxis has not been of benefit in the prevention of meningococcal infection, bacterial infection after viral respiratory infection, or pneumonia after coma, shock, or congestive heart failure.

TABLE 19-9 Dosage of Penicillins

| Compound | Dosage* | | |
	Oral	Intramuscular	Intravenous
Penicillin G			25,000-500,000 units/kg/day, 6 divided doses
Procaine		300,000-600,000 units q12h	
Benzathine		1.2-2.4 million units q5-20d	
Penicillin V	Infant: 50 mg/kg/day, 3 divided doses		
		Adult: 125-500 mg/kg qid	
Ampicillin	25-50 mg/kg/day, 4 divided doses	100-200 mg/kg/day, 4 divided doses	100-300 mg/kg/day, 6 divided doses
Amoxicillin	25-50 mg/kg/day, 2-3 divided doses		
Oxacillin		100 mg/kg/day, 4 divided doses	100-300 mg/kg/day, 6 divided doses
Nafcillin			
Cloxacillin	25-100 mg/kg/day, 4 divided doses		
Dicloxacillin	12-25 mg/kg/day, 4 divided doses		
Ticarcillin		50-100 mg/kg/day, 4 divided doses	50-300 mg/kg/day, 6 divided doses
Indanyl carbenicillin	50-65 mg/kg/day, 4 divided doses		
Azlocillin		50-100 mg/kg/day, 4 divided doses	200-300 mg/kg/day, 4 divided doses
Mezlocillin		50-100 mg/kg/day, 4 divided doses	200-300 mg/kg/day, 4 divided doses
Piperacillin		50-100 mg/kg/day, 4 divided doses	200-300 mg/kg/day, 4 divided doses

*For mg/kg/day the number of doses shown indicates the number of doses into which the total daily dose should be divided.

PROPERTIES OF INDIVIDUAL PENICILLINS

Dosage guidelines for the penicillins are given in Tables 19-9 and 19-10.

Natural Penicillins

Penicillin G

Penicillin G, or benzyl penicillin G (Fig. 19-4), is available as salts for oral and parenteral administration and as repository salts for intramuscular injection. Because penicillin G is unstable in acid, penicillin V (or amoxicillin) should be used for oral administration.

Crystalline penicillin G in aqueous solution has been used intramuscularly, subcutaneously, intravenously, and intrathecally. Given intramuscularly as an aqueous solution, penicillin G is very rapidly cleared from the body, and it may be preferable to use a repository form. It is available as sterile dry powder in ampules or vials containing 200,000 to 20 million units per vial. Each million units of penicillin G contain 1.7 mEq of sodium or potassium.

Repository penicillins provide tissue depots from which the drug is absorbed over hours in the case of procaine penicillin or over days in the case of benzathine penicillin. Repository penicillins are only for intramuscular use and cannot be used intravenously or subcutaneously or to irrigate wounds. Procaine penicillin is a mixture of equal molar parts of procaine and penicillin; thus, 300,000 units contain 120 mg of procaine. The use of this suspension delays the peak of activity but provides serum and tissue levels for at least 12 hours. Doubling the dose of procaine penicillin given at a single injection site does not double the serum level. To increase the peak level, it is necessary to use two body sites, as is done in the treatment of gonorrhea—for example, with 2.4 million units of procaine penicillin given in each buttock.

Benzathine penicillin is a repository form of penicillin that combines 1 mol of penicillin and 2 mol of an ammonium base. It provides detectable serum levels for 15 to 30 days, depending on the size of the dose. Concentrations of penicillin G in the cerebrospinal fluid after use of benzathine penicillin may be inadequate to treat neurosyphilis.

Penicillin V

Phenoxymethyl penicillin (see Fig. 19-4) is available only for oral use as a sodium or a potassium salt in suspension or tablets in doses of 125, 250, and 500 mg. The usual dosage for children is 25 to 50 mg/kg/day and for adults, 1 to 4 g/day in three or four divided doses. The potassium salt produces higher blood levels than the other salts. Serum levels are from two to five times those obtained with oral penicillin G. Blood levels after 500 mg administered to an adult are equivalent to the levels achieved with 600,000 units of procaine penicillin administered intramuscularly. Penicillin V can be substituted for penicillin G in most situations in which it is reasonable to treat an infection by the oral route. However, penicillin V is less active than penicillin G against *Haemophilus, Neisseria,* and enteric organisms.

Penicillinase-Resistant Penicillins

The antibacterial spectra of all penicillinase-resistant penicillins are identical (Fig. 19-5). They are active against methicillin-susceptible strains of staphylococci; penicillin-susceptible strains of streptococci, including *S. pneumoniae*; and most anaerobic gram-positive cocci. None are active against methicillin-resistant staphylococci, high-level penicillin-resistant streptococci, enterococci, *Listeria monocytogenes,* aerobic gram-negative cocci or bacilli, or anaerobic gram-negative bacteria.

Methicillin

Methicillin (2,6-dimethoxyphenylpenicillin) was the first of several penicillins developed that are resistant to hydrolysis by staphylococcal β-lactamase. Methicillin is the least active of the penicillinase-resistant

TABLE 19-10 Dosage of Antibiotics in Newborn Infants

| Agent | Infants <1 Week Old | | Infants 1 Week to 1 Month Old | |
	Dosage (per kg/day)	Interval between Doses (hr)	Dosage (per kg/day)	Interval between Doses (hr)
Penicillin G	50,000-100,000 units	12	100,000 units	8
Ampicillin	100 mg	12	200 mg	6
Oxacillin	100 mg	12	200 mg	6
Nafcillin	100 mg	12	200 mg	6
Ticarcillin	150 mg	8	300 mg	6
Mezlocillin	75 mg	12	300 mg	6
Azlocillin	75-100 mg	12	300 mg	6

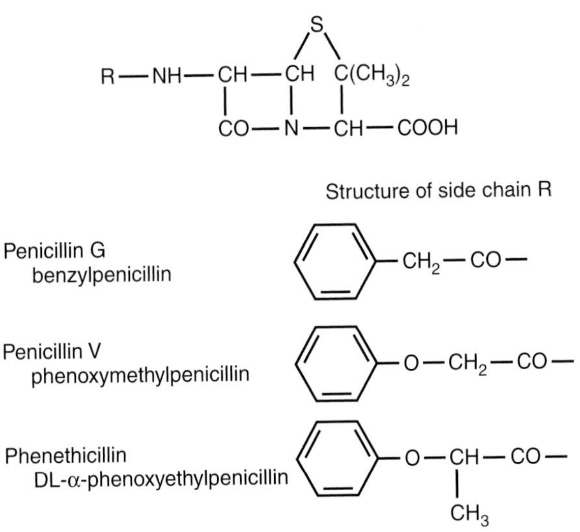

FIGURE 19-4. The structures of penicillin G and penicillin V.

penicillins by weight; it is acid-labile and therefore can be administered only parenterally. It is more likely to cause interstitial nephritis than are the other penicillinase-resistant penicillins. For these reasons, methicillin is no longer used clinically.

Nafcillin

Nafcillin (2-ethoxy-1-naphthylpenicillin) has more intrinsic activity than methicillin against susceptible organisms. It is highly protein bound. Oral absorption of nafcillin is erratic[54] and levels after intramuscular injection are low; therefore, the only practical route of administration is intravenous. The antibiotic is primarily excreted by the liver and to a lesser extent by the kidney. Serum levels are elevated and the half-life is prolonged by probenecid. The usual dosage of nafcillin is 6 to 12 g/day, depending on the severity of the infection, and 100 to 200 mg/kg/day for children.

Isoxazolyl Penicillins

Isoxazolyl penicillins, oxacillin, cloxacillin, and dicloxacillin, are absorbed after oral administration, but absorption is adversely affected by food. Although dicloxacillin yields the highest total drug serum concentrations, because of differences in protein binding free-drug concentrations are nearly identical for all three compounds (see Table 19-5). After intravenous infusion of 1 g over 15 minutes, serum levels are 25 μg/mL 1 hour later and less than 1 μg/mL at 6 hours. The isoxazolyl penicillins undergo some metabolism but are excreted primarily by the kidney, with slight biliary excretion. Oxacillin undergoes more rapid degradation in the body than does cloxacillin or dicloxacillin.

Oxacillin is available as a sodium salt for oral use in 250- and 500-mg capsules and as a powder for suspension at 250 mg/5 mL. It should be taken 1 to 2 hours before meals. The daily dosage for adults is 1 to 4 g taken in four parts. The dosage for children is 50 to 100 mg/kg/day taken in four parts. Oxacillin sodium for injection may be given intramuscularly or intravenously. The adult dosage is 2 to 12 g/day, and for children, 100 to 300 mg/kg/day given every 4 to 6 hours. Oxacillin may be associated with a higher incidence of hepatotoxicity and rash than nafcillin or other antistaphylococcal agents.[55]

Cloxacillin sodium is available in the United States only as an oral solution (125 mg/5 mL) or capsules of 250 and 500 mg. The dosage for children is 50 to 100 mg/kg/day given as four equal doses, and the dosage for adults is 1 to 4 g/day given as four equal doses.

Dicloxacillin sodium is available as a suspension (62.5 mg/5 mL) and as capsules of 125 and 250 mg. The dosage for children less than 40 kg is 25 mg/kg/day given as four doses. For adults, a dosage of 250 mg to 1 g every 6 hours can be given, depending on the severity of the infection.

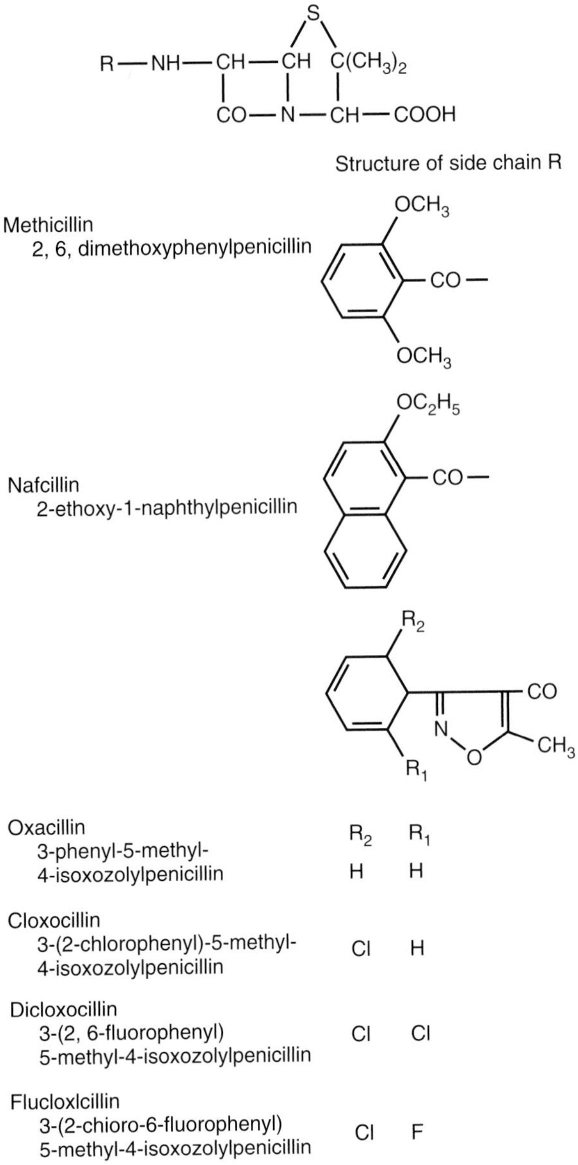

FIGURE 19-5. Antistaphylococcal penicillins.

Aminopenicillins

The antibacterial activities of all aminopenicillins (Fig. 19-6) are similar. They are not stable to β-lactamases. For practical purposes, the activity of aminopenicillins is virtually identical to that of penicillin G against penicillin-susceptible organisms, except that aminopenicillins are slightly more active against enterococci. Non–β-lactamase–producing strains of *H. influenzae* and *Haemophilus parainfluenzae* are susceptible. Strains of *E. coli*, *Shigella sonnei*, and *Salmonella* spp., including many strains of *Salmonella typhi*, once uniformly susceptible to aminopenicillins, often are resistant due to β-lactamase production. *Klebsiella* spp., *Serratia*, *Acinetobacter*, indole-positive *Proteus*, *Pseudomonas* spp., and strains of *Bacteroides fragilis* are resistant to aminopenicillins.

Ampicillin

Ampicillin is moderately well absorbed after oral administration, but peak levels are delayed and lowered if it is ingested with food. Peak blood levels of 3 μg/mL occur 1 to 2 hours after ingestion of 0.5 g; levels peak later in diabetic patients with neurologic disease and in patients with renal failure. After intramuscular injection of 0.5 g, peak

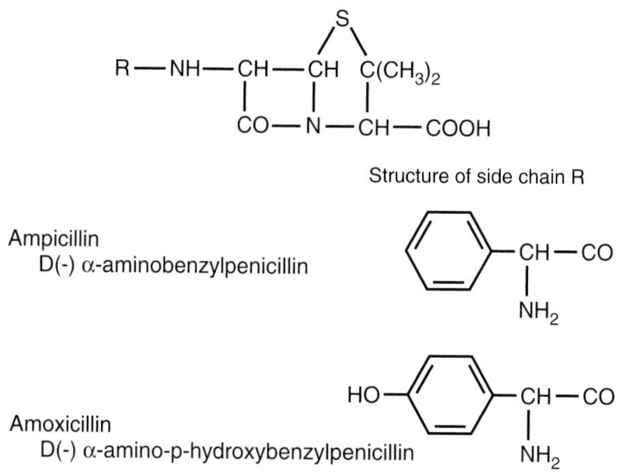

R—NH—CH—CH C(CH₃)₂ ... structure

Structure of side chain R

Ampicillin
D(-) α-aminobenzylpenicillin

—CH—CO
|
NH₂

Amoxicillin
D(-) α-amino-p-hydroxybenzylpenicillin

HO—⟨⟩—CH—CO
|
NH₂

FIGURE 19-6. Aminopenicillins.

levels of 10 μg are achieved at 1 hour. The elimination half-life is approximately 80 minutes. Probenecid increases the magnitude of peak levels and the area-under-the-concentration curve. Ampicillin is well distributed to body compartments and achieves therapeutic concentrations in cerebrospinal fluid and in pleural, joint, and peritoneal fluids in the presence of inflammation after parenteral administration. The drug undergoes enterohepatic circulation and significant levels appear in bile and stool. Urinary levels are high even in the presence of markedly reduced renal function. Peritoneal dialysis is ineffective in removing the drug, but hemodialysis removes approximately 40% in a 6-hour period. The half-life of ampicillin is about 3 hours during continuous venovenous hemofiltration.

Ampicillin is available for oral use as the sodium salt as 250-mg or 500-mg capsules and oral suspensions of 125 or 250 mg/5 mL. The sodium salt can be used for either intramuscular or intravenous administration. For most indications, oral ampicillin has been abandoned in favor of oral amoxicillin because of the greater bioavailability of the latter. Ampicillin is effective for upper and lower respiratory tract infections caused by S. pneumoniae, β-hemolytic streptococci, and non–β-lactamase–producing strains of H. influenzae. It is effective in the treatment of meningitis caused by group B streptococci, Listeria monocytogenes, N. meningitidis, and penicillin-susceptible strains of S. pneumoniae. Although formerly useful in treating urinary tract infections caused by E. coli and gastroenteritis caused by Salmonella enterica or Shigella spp., due to the high prevalence of β-lactamase–producing strains, ampicillin should not be used until susceptibility has been documented.

Dosage varies with the age of the patient, the status of renal function, and the severity of the disease. For children above 1 month of age, the oral dosage is 50 to 100 mg/kg/day in four doses; the intramuscular or intravenous dosage is 100 to 300 mg/kg/day in four or six doses. For adults, the oral dosage is 2 to 4 g/day given in divided doses every 6 hours. For severe infection, the parenteral dosage is 6 to 12 g/day given in divided doses every 4 hours. See Chapter 21 for a discussion of ampicillin-sulbactam.

Amoxicillin

Amoxicillin differs from ampicillin only in the presence of a hydroxyl group in the *para* position of the benzene side chain. Its in vitro activity is identical to that of ampicillin. It is significantly better absorbed when given by mouth compared with ampicillin, and for this reason it is preferred for most indications. Peak blood levels are from 2 to 2.5 times those achieved with a similar dose of ampicillin, and food does not decrease absorption. Oral amoxicillin produces blood levels similar to those produced by intramuscularly administered sodium ampicillin or ampicillin trihydrate. The elimination half-life averages 80 minutes in adults with normal renal function. Urinary excretion of

amoxicillin is greater than that of ampicillin, and tissue distribution is similar to that of ampicillin. Parenteral amoxicillin, which is available in Europe but not the United States, is pharmacologically identical to parenterally administered ampicillin.

Clinical studies with amoxicillin have been extensive; it has been used in the treatment of otitis media, bronchitis, pneumonia, typhoid, gonorrhea, and urinary tract infections. Among the oral penicillins and cephalosporins, amoxicillin can achieve concentrations that exceed MICs effective for nonmeningeal infections caused by penicillin-resistant strains of S. pneumoniae.[56,57] In vitro, clavulanate may enhance the activity of amoxicillin against penicillin-resistant strains of pneumococci.[58] Amoxicillin is not useful for the treatment of shigellosis.

Side effects of amoxicillin are similar to those seen with ampicillin, although diarrhea may be less common than with ampicillin. The usual dosage for children is 20 to 40 mg/kg/day, and as high as 90 mg/kg/day given in two or three divided doses every 8 hours; for adults, the dosage is 0.5 to 1 g every 8 to 12 hours,[57,59] although it has been used in doses up to 1 g every 4 hours. See Chapter 21 for a discussion of amoxicillin-clavulanate.

Carboxypenicillins

Carbenicillin

Carbenicillin was the first penicillin with activity against P. aeruginosa, Enterobacter, Morganella, and Proteus-Providencia spp. because it is relatively stable against hydrolysis by the β-lactamases of these species (Fig. 19-7). Because of the large doses required, the greater potential for toxicity, and the availability of more potent alternatives, it should no longer be used.

Indanyl carbenicillin is an α-carboxy ester of carbenicillin. It is a prodrug with no intrinsic activity of its own, but it is highly acid-stable and relatively well absorbed from the gastrointestinal tract. The ester is immediately hydrolyzed to free carbenicillin, and only trace amounts of ester are found in serum or urine. Ingestion with food may actually enhance absorption. Peak serum levels after 1 g taken orally are 10 μg at 1 to 2 hours. Urine levels are 300 to 1000 μg/mL, with 30% of a dose recovered in the first 6 hours. The compound does not provide adequate serum or tissue levels for efficacy in systemic infections, and it is useful only for the treatment of urinary tract infections. In the presence of decreased renal function, urine levels are lower and may be inadequate to treat Pseudomonas infections. Side effects are those of all the penicillins, but gastrointestinal irritation has been a problem in some people. The usual dosage is 1 g every 6 hours for adults. Quinolones have largely replaced this agent for the treatment of urinary tract infections and prostatitis.

Ticarcillin

The antibacterial spectrum for ticarcillin is similar to that for carbenicillin, except that it is from two to four times more active against P. aeruginosa. It is less active than aminopenicillins against penicillin-resistant streptococci and relatively inactive against enterococci. The pharmacokinetics and side effect profiles of ticarcillin and carbenicillin are also similar. Ticarcillin is not absorbed by mouth but can be given by intramuscular or intravenous administration. After an intramuscular dose of 1 g, peak serum levels of 20 μg/mL are reached in 1 hour. Serum levels of 150 to 200 μg/mL are maintained when it is given at dosages of 100 mg/kg over 1 to 2 hours. Ticarcillin is excreted by renal tubules. Probenecid delays renal excretion and increases serum concentrations. Tissue distribution is similar to that of ampicillin, but cerebrospinal fluid concentrations are not adequate for treatment of meningitis. Its half-life is approximately 70 minutes, and it accumulates in the presence of renal failure. Greater accumulation occurs if there is combined hepatic and renal dysfunction. Hemodialysis and continuous venovenous hemofiltration reduce plasma concentrations. Side effects are similar to those seen with penicillins and in addition can interfere with platelet function because it binds to the adenosine diphosphate (ADP) receptor site on platelets

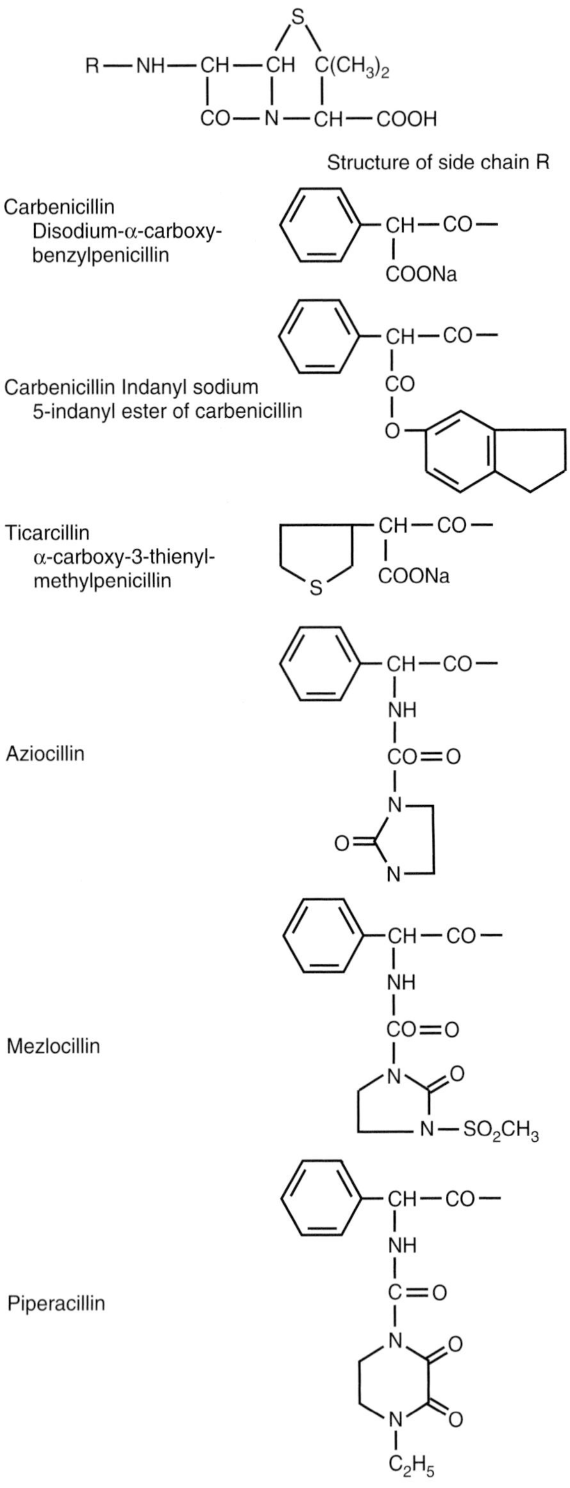

FIGURE 19-7. Penicillins active against gram-negative bacteria.

and prevents normal contraction. Bleeding may occur in the presence of high serum levels and in the presence of renal failure.

Ticarcillin can be used at dosages of 200 to 300 mg/kg/day. Ticarcillin is indicated for treatment of infections caused by *P. aeruginosa*. Like ampicillin, it is susceptible to hydrolysis by class A β-lactamases; therefore, it is rarely used alone and most often is administered as a fixed combination of ticarcillin-clavulanate (see Chapter 21).

Ureidopenicillins

Azlocillin

Azlocillin is an acyl ureidopenicillin that is 8 to 16 times more active than carbenicillin against *P. aeruginosa* and is less active against indole-positive *Proteus* spp. It has the same activity as ampicillin against streptococcal species.[60] It is destroyed by β-lactamases of both gram-positive and gram-negative bacteria. It is not orally absorbed and must be given via the intravenous route to provide adequate serum levels to treat *Pseudomonas* infection. The half-life is approximately 50 minutes, and administration of 4 g yields peak levels of 285 μg/mL.

Azlocillin shows nonlinear pharmacokinetics; peak serum concentrations and the area-under-the-drug curve are not proportional. A 4-g dose produces serum levels that are higher than four 1-g doses. The drug thus could be administered in larger doses at intervals of 6 hours. Azlocillin does not accumulate in renal failure to the same degree as do carbenicillin and ticarcillin, because its half-life rises only to approximately 4 hours with creatinine clearances below 10 mL/min. Azlocillin enters the cerebrospinal fluid in the presence of meningeal inflammation, producing levels that are 10% of the serum level. Azlocillin has less affinity for the ADP receptor site and is commonly associated with platelet dysfunction. Azlocillin is used primarily to treat *Pseudomonas* infections.[33]

Mezlocillin

Mezlocillin is an acyl ureidopenicillin similar in antibacterial spectrum to ticarcillin except that it is more active in vitro against *E. faecalis, Klebsiella* spp., and *H. influenzae*. Like azlocillin and piperacillin, mezlocillin shows dose-related nonlinear kinetics: peak serum levels, half-life, and area-under-the-time curve are greater with larger doses. Administration of 4 g produces peak levels of 300 μg/mL.[61] Its half-life increases only to 4 hours in patients with advanced renal failure. Mezlocillin is the least likely of the broad-spectrum penicillins to alter bleeding times. Clinical studies in the United States and Europe have shown that it is an effective agent for treatment of respiratory, urinary, gynecologic, and surgical infections. Usual dosages have been 12 to 18 g/day for adults.

Piperacillin

Piperacillin is an acyl ureidopenicillin derivative that is similar to ampicillin in activity against gram-positive species. It has excellent activity against streptococcal species and against *Neisseria* and *Haemophilus* and many members of the family Enterobacteriaceae. It also has excellent activity against anaerobic species of both cocci and bacilli. It inhibits 60% to 90% of *P. aeruginosa* strains at concentrations less than 16 μg/mL. Like ampicillin, it is hydrolyzed by class A β-lactamases. Although it is hydrolyzed by class C β-lactamases produced by *P. aeruginosa* and *Enterobacter* spp., it is not an inducer, which accounts for its activity against the majority of strains of these and related species. Emergence of resistance to piperacillin is often due to selection of mutants that constitutively express high levels of ampC β-lactamase.[18] Piperacillin acts synergistically against *Pseudomonas* and against some of the Enterobacteriaceae species when it is combined with aminoglycosides[62,63]; the antibacterial activity is mostly additive when combination with a fluoroquinolone.[64]

The human pharmacology of piperacillin is similar to that of azlocillin and mezlocillin.[34] Administration of 4 g via the intravenous route produces peak serum drug levels above 350 μg/mL. Piperacillin shows kinetics that are dose dependent. It accumulates in renal failure to a lesser degree than does carbenicillin, and its half-life is only 4 to 6 hours at creatinine clearances less than 10 mL/min. It is removed through hemodialysis and should be dosed after dialysis. The half-life with continuos venovenous hemofiltration is approximately 5 hours, and 4 g administered twice daily is recommended.[65]

Piperacillin has shown adverse reactions similar to those for the other penicillins noted earlier. After prolonged administration at high doses, neutropenia has been reported. Alteration of bleeding time and hypokalemia occur infrequently. Clinical studies have shown that it is a useful agent in the treatment of a variety of infections.[33,34] It is administered to adults in daily doses of 12 to 18 g. As with ticarcillin, piperacillin is usually administered empirically as piperacillin-tazobactam (see Chapter 21) to retain activity of the drug against class A β-lactamase–producing strains. Tazobactam generally does not improve the activity of piperacillin against *Ps. aeruginosa* or other class C β-lactamase–producing strains.

REFERENCES

1. Fleming A. On the antibacterial action of cultures of a penicillium, with special reference to their use in the isolation of *B. influenzae*. Br J Exp Pathol. 1929;10:226.
2. Tipper DJ. Mode of action of beta-lactam antibiotics. Rev Infect Dis. 1979;1:39-54.
3. Tipper DJ. Mode of action of beta-lactam antibiotics. Pharmacol Ther. 1985;27:1-35.
4. Maidhof H, et al. Onset of penicillin-induced bacteriolysis in staphylococci is cell cycle dependent. J Bacteriol. 1989;171:2252-2257.
5. Giesbrecht P, et al. Staphylococcal cell wall: Morphogenesis and fatal variations in the presence of penicillin. Microbiol Mol Biol Rev. 1998;62:1371-1414.
6. Moreillon P, et al. Two bactericidal targets for penicillin in pneumococci: Autolysis-dependent and autolysis-independent killing mechanisms. Antimicrob Agents Chemother, 1990;34:33-39.
7. Ghuysen JM. Molecular structures of penicillin-binding proteins and beta-lactamases. Trends Microbiol. 1994;2:372-380.
8. Hardt K, et al. The penicillin sensory transducer, BlaR, involved in the inducibility of beta-lactamase synthesis in Bacillus licheniformis is embedded in the plasma membrane via a four-alpha-helix bundle. Mol Microbiol. 1997;23:935-944.
9. Zhang HZ, et al. A proteolytic transmembrane signaling pathway and resistance to beta- lactams in staphylococci. Science. 2001;291:1962-1965.
10. Spratt BG. Distinct penicillin binding proteins involved in the division, elongation, and shape of Escherichia coli K12. Proc Natl Acad Sci U S A. 1975;72:2999-3003.
11. Terrak M, et al. The catalytic, glycosyl transferase and acyl transferase modules of the cell wall peptidoglycan-polymerizing penicillin-binding protein 1b of Escherichia coli. Mol Microbiol. 1999;34:350-364.
12. Den Blaauwen T, et al. Penicillin-binding protein PBP2 of Escherichia coli localizes preferentially in the lateral wall and at mid-cell in comparison with the old cell pole. Mol Microbiol. 2003;47:539-547.
13. Mercer KL, Weiss DS. The Escherichia coli cell division protein FtsW is required to recruit its cognate transpeptidase, FtsI (PBP3), to the division site. J Bacteriol. 2002;184:904-912.
14. Nelson DE, Young KD. Contributions of PBP 5 and DD-carboxypeptidase penicillin binding proteins to maintenance of cell shape in Escherichia coli. J Bacteriol. 2001;183:3055-3064.
15. Bush K, Jacoby GA, Medeiros AA. A functional classification scheme for beta-lactamases and its correlation with molecular structure. Antimicrob Agents Chemother. 1995;39:1211-1233.
16. Bush K. New beta-lactamases in gram-negative bacteria: Diversity and impact on the selection of antimicrobial therapy. Clin Infect Dis. 2001;32:1085-1089.
17. Nikaido H. Prevention of drug access to bacterial targets: Permeability barriers and active efflux. Science. 1994;264:382-388.
18. Bonfiglio G, et al. In vitro activity of piperacillin/tazobactam against 615 Pseudomonas aeruginosa strains isolated in intensive care units. Chemotherapy. 1998;44:305-312.
19. Crowley B, Benedi VJ, Domenech-Sanchez A. Expression of SHV-2 beta-lactamase and of reduced amounts of OmpK36 porin in Klebsiella pneumoniae results in increased resistance to cephalosporins and carbapenems. Antimicrob Agents Chemother. 2002;46:3679-3682.
20. Bonfiglio G, et al. Mechanisms of beta-lactam resistance amongst Pseudomonas aeruginosa isolated in an Italian survey. J Antimicrob Chemother. 1998;42:697-702.
21. Zgurskaya HI, Nikaido H. Multidrug resistance mechanisms: Drug efflux across two membranes. Mol Microbiol. 2000;37:219-225.
22. Mazzariol A, Cornaglia G, Nikaido H. Contributions of the AmpC beta-lactamase and the AcrAB multidrug efflux system in intrinsic resistance of Escherichia coli K-12 to beta-lactams. Antimicrob Agents Chemother. 2000;44:1387-1390.
23. Spratt BG. Resistance to antibiotics mediated by target alterations. Science. 1994;264:388-393.
24. Ameyama S, et al. Mosaic-like structure of penicillin-binding protein 2 gene (penA) in clinical isolates of Neisseria gonorrhoeae with reduced susceptibility to cefixime. Antimicrob Agents Chemother. 2002;46:3744-3749.
25. Sibold C, et al. Mosaic pbpX genes of major clones of penicillin-resistant Streptococcus pneumoniae have evolved from pbpX genes of a penicillin-sensitive Streptococcus oralis. Mol Microbiol. 1994;12:1013-1023.
26. Hartman BJ, Tomasz A. Low-affinity penicillin-binding protein associated with beta-lactam resistance in Staphylococcus aureus. J Bacteriol. 1984;158:513-516.
27. Rybkine T, et al. Penicillin-binding protein 5 sequence alterations in clinical isolates of Enterococcus faecium with different levels of beta-lactam resistance. J Infect Dis. 1998;178:159-163.
28. Sifaoui F, et al. Role of penicillin-binding protein 5 in expression of ampicillin resistance and peptidoglycan structure in Enterococcus faecium. Antimicrob Agents Chemother. 2001;45:2594-2597.
29. Sauvage E, et al. The 2.4-A crystal structure of the penicillin-resistant penicillin-binding protein PBP5fm from Enterococcus faecium in complex with benzylpenicillin. Cell Mol Life Sci. 2002;59:1223-1232.
30. Lim D, Strynadka NC. Structural basis for the beta lactam resistance of PBP2a from methicillin-resistant Staphylococcus aureus. Nat Struct Biol. 2002;9:870-876.
31. Rolinson GN, Sutherland R. Semisynthetic penicillins. Adv Pharmacol Chemother. 1973;11:151-220.
32. Marcy SM, Klein JO. The isoxazolyl penicillins: Oxacillin, cloxacillin, and dicloxacillin. Med Clin North Am. 1970;54:1127-1143.
33. Wright AJ. The penicillins. Mayo Clin Proc. 1999;74:290-307.
34. Tan JS, File TM Jr. Antipseudomonal penicillins. Med Clin North Am. 1995;79:679-693.
35. Hedberg M, Nord CE. Beta-lactam resistance in anaerobic bacteria: A review. J Chemother. 1996;8:3-16.
36. Cole M, Kenig MD, Hewitt VA. Metabolism of penicillins to penicilloic acids and 6-aminopenicillanic acid in man and its significance in assessing penicillin absorption. Antimicrob Agents Chemother. 1973;3:463-468.
37. Fishman RA. Blood-brain and CSF barriers to penicillin and related organic acids. Arch Neurol. 1966;15:113-124.
38. Depp R, et al. Transplacental passage of methicillin and dicloxacillin into the fetus and amniotic fluid. Am J Obstet Gynecol. 1970;107:1054-1057.
39. Levine BB, et al. Penicillin allergy and the heterogenous immune responses of man to benzylpenicillin. J Clin Invest. 1966;45:1895-1906.
40. Idsoe O, et al. Nature and extent of penicillin side-reactions, with particular reference to fatalities from anaphylactic shock. Bull World Health Organ. 1968;38:159-188.
41. Kerr RO, et al. Two mechanisms of erythrocyte destruction in penicillin-induced hemolytic anemia. N Engl J Med. 1972;287:1322-1325.
42. Fass RJ, et al. Platelet-mediated bleeding caused by broad-spectrum penicillins. J Infect Dis. 1987;155:1242-1248.
43. Appel GB, Neu HC. The nephrotoxicity of antimicrobial agents (first of three parts). N Engl J Med. 1977;296:663-670.
44. Barrons RW, Murray KM, Richey RM. Populations at risk for penicillin-induced seizures. Ann Pharmacother. 1992;26:26-29.
45. Schreiber JR, Jacobs MR. Antibiotic-resistant pneumococci. Pediatr Clin North Am. 1995;42:519-537.
46. Garau J. Treatment of drug-resistant pneumococcal pneumonia. Lancet Infect Dis. 2002;2:404-415.
47. Cunha BA. Clinical relevance of penicillin-resistant Streptococcus pneumoniae. Semin Respir Infect. 2002;17:204-214.
48. Bartlett JG, et al. Community-acquired pneumonia in adults: Guidelines for management. The Infectious Diseases Society of America. Clin Infect Dis. 1998;26:811-838.
49. Quagliarello VJ, Scheld WM. Treatment of bacterial meningitis. N Engl J Med. 1997;336:708-716.
50. Oliveira CH, et al. Comparative bioavailability of 4 amoxicillin formulations in healthy human volunteers after a single dose administration. Int J Clin Pharmacol Ther. 2001;39:167-172.
51. Schrag SJ, et al. Effect of short-course, high-dose amoxicillin therapy on resistant pneumococcal carriage: A randomized trial. JAMA. 2001;286:49-56.
52. Peterson WL, et al. Helicobacter pylori-related disease: Guidelines for testing and treatment. Arch Intern Med. 2000;160:1285-1291.
53. Dajani AS, et al. Prevention of bacterial endocarditis. Recommendations by the American Heart Association. JAMA. 1997;277:1794-1801.
54. Neu HC. Antistaphylococcal penicillins. Med Clin North Am. 1982;66:51-60.
55. Maraqa NF, et al. Higher occurrence of hepatotoxicity and rash in patients treated with oxacillin, compared with those treated with nafcillin and other commonly used antimicrobials. Clin Infect Dis. 2002;34:50-54.
56. Blumer JL. Pharmacokinetics and pharmacodynamics of new and old antimicrobial agents for acute otitis media. Pediatr Infect Dis J. 1998;17:1070-5; discussion 1099-1100.
57. Fonseca W, et al. Comparing pharmacokinetics of amoxicillin given twice or three times per day to children older than 3 months with pneumonia. Antimicrob Agents Chemother. 2003;47:997-1001.
58. Martin M, et al. Effect of clavulanic acid and/or polymorphonuclear neutrophils on amoxicillin bactericidal activity against Streptococcus pneumoniae. Eur J Clin Microbiol Infect Dis. 1997;16:512-516.
59. Calver AD, et al. Dosing of amoxicillin/clavulanate given every 12 hours is as effective as dosing every 8 hours for treatment of lower respiratory tract infection. Lower Respiratory Tract Infection Collaborative Study Group. Clin Infect Dis. 1997;24:570-574.
60. Fu KP, Neu HC. Azlocillin and mezlocillin: New ureido penicillins. Antimicrob Agents Chemother. 1978;13:930-938.
61. Meyers BR, et al. Pharmacokinetic properties of mezlocillin in ambulatory elderly subjects. J Clin Pharmacol. 1987;27:678-681.
62. Hoogkamp-Korstanje JA, Westerdaal NA. Activity and synergy of ureido penicillins and aminoglycosides against Pseudomonas aeruginosa. Infection. 1982;10(suppl 3):S257-S261.
63. Baltch AL, et al. Synergy with cefsulodin or piperacillin and three aminoglycosides or aztreonam against aminoglycoside resistant strains of Pseudomonas aeruginosa. J Antimicrob Chemother. 1991;27:801-808.
64. Burgess DS, Nathisuwan S. Cefepime, piperacillin/tazobactam, gentamicin, ciprofloxacin, and levofloxacin alone and in combination against Pseudomonas aeruginosa. Diagn Microbiol Infect Dis. 2002;44:35-41.
65. Capellier G, et al. Removal of piperacillin in critically ill patients undergoing continuous venovenous hemofiltration. Crit Care Med. 1998;26:88-91.

CHAPTER **20**

Cephalosporins

DAVID R. ANDES

WILLIAM A. CRAIG

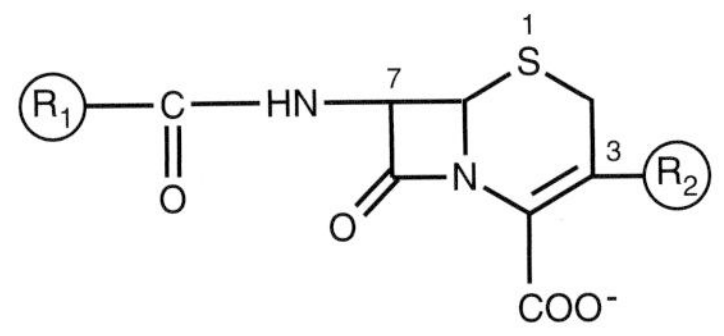

FIGURE 20-1. Basic cephalosporin nucleus.

Although the discovery of the cephalosporin antibiotic class was reported in 1945, it took nearly two decades for this class to achieve clinical utility. Giuseppe Brotzu is widely credited for discovery of the broad-spectrum inhibitory effects of sewage outflow in Sardinia, Italy.[1] Professor Brotzu subsequently isolated the mold *Cephalosporin acremonium* (now *Acremonium chrysogenum*) and demonstrated antimicrobial activity of culture filtrates against both gram-positive and gram-negative bacteria. He also demonstrated the in vivo activity of these culture filtrates in both animal infection models and several patients. The filtrate was used both locally by injection into skin abscesses and systemically for the therapy of brucella and typhoid fever.

A decade after the initial discovery, the cephalosporin substances were isolated and identified as fermentation products of the mold.[2] Investigators at Oxford, including Florey and Abraham, systematically studied the physical, chemical, and structural characteristics of cephalosporins as they had those of the penicillin class a decade earlier. Three substances, cephalosporins P, N, and C, were identified. Each of the products possessed antimicrobial activity. However, only cephalosporin C demonstrated activity against both gram-negative and -positive bacteria. In addition, it had advantageous stability in the presence of acid and penicillinases.[2] Cephalosporin C became the foundation of subsequent drug development.

The first cephalosporin, cephalothin, was introduced for clinical use in 1964. There are more than 20 cephalosporin antibiotics in use today. The cephalosporin class is among the most widely prescribed antimicrobial classes because of its broad spectrum of activity, low toxicity, ease of administration, and favorable pharmacokinetic profile.

CHEMISTRY

Most of the available cephalosporins are semisynthetic derivatives of cephalosporin C. The basic structure of the cephem nucleus includes a β-lactam ring fused to a six-member sulfur-containing dihydrothiazine ring (Fig. 20-1). The cephem nucleus is chemically distinct from the penicillin nucleus, which in contrast contains a five-member thiazolidine ring. Basic structure numbering of the cephalosporin ring system begins within the dihydrothiazine ring at the sulfur moiety. The starting material utilized as the nucleus for current cephalosporin development is 7-aminocephalosporanic acid (7-ACA). Attempts to alter the physiochemical and biologic properties of the cephalosporins by chemical side chain modifications were based upon similar success with structural changes at the 6-aminopenicillanic acid side chain of penicillin.[3] Chemical modifications of the basic cephem structure by substitution of constituents at positions 1, 3, and 7 have led to the various cephalosporin compounds in use today.[4,5] Alterations in positions C7 and C3 are also commonly referred to as R1 and R2, respectively. In general, changes at R1 affect the microbial spectrum of activity. These modifications often affect the stability of the compound to enzymatic destruction by β-lactamases or the affinity of the compound for the drug target. Modification at R2 often alters the pharmacology of the compound. Changes in the R2 constituent may influence the ability of the compound to reach certain infection sites such as the central nervous system or may simply prolong the elimination half-life of the drug.

The predominant changes at R1 (position 7) include the addition of an acyl side chain and the substitution of the hydrogen with a methoxy group.[5] This R1 methoxy substitution led to the development of the cephamycin group of compounds, such as cefoxitin, cefmetazole, and cefotetan. This alteration enhanced resistance to β-lactamase pro-

duced by gram-negative anaerobic and aerobic bacteria.[5,6] These compounds, however, have lower affinity for the penicillin-binding protein (PBP) target in gram-positive bacteria.[7] The cephamycin group is structurally related to the cephalosporins but originated as a metabolite from *Streptomyces lactamdurans*.[6] The basic building block of the cephamycin group is cephamycin C. Hydrolysis of cephamycin C, however, produces the 7-ACA nucleus.

Many modifications of the acyl side chain have been undertaken. The first compounds resulting from addition of a thienyl ring or a tetrazole structure at R1 included the first-generation cephalosporins,

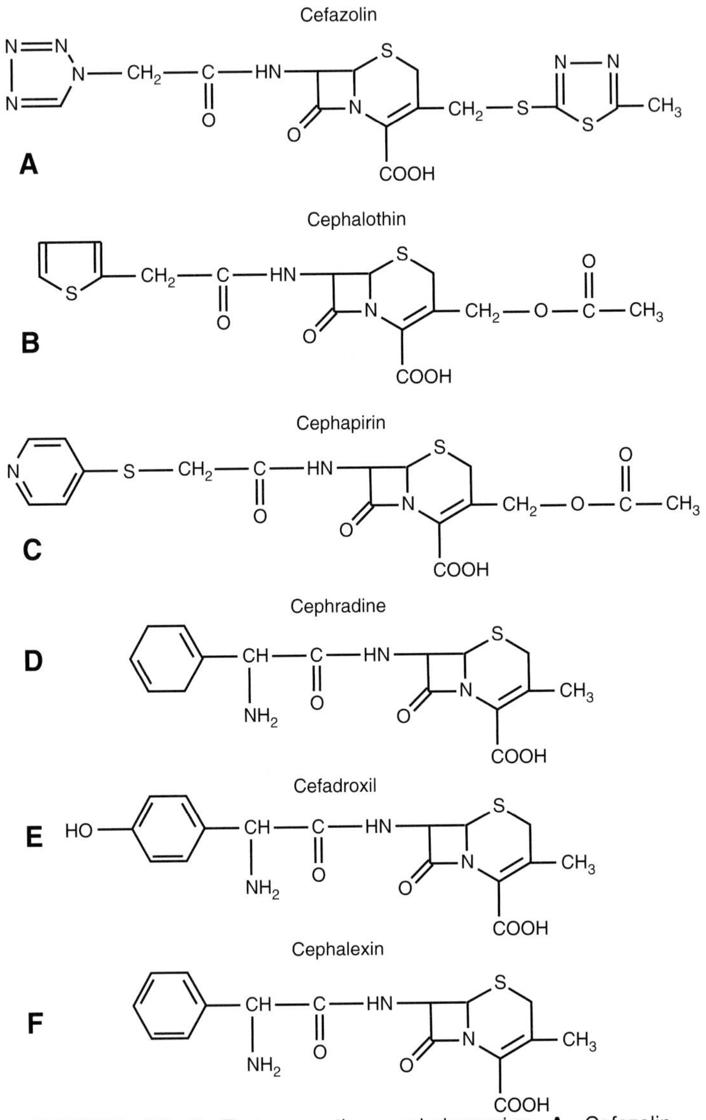

FIGURE 20-2. First-generation cephalosporins. **A,** Cefazolin. **B,** Cephalothin. **C,** Cephapirin. **D,** Cephradine. **E,** Cefadroxil. **F,** Cephalexin.

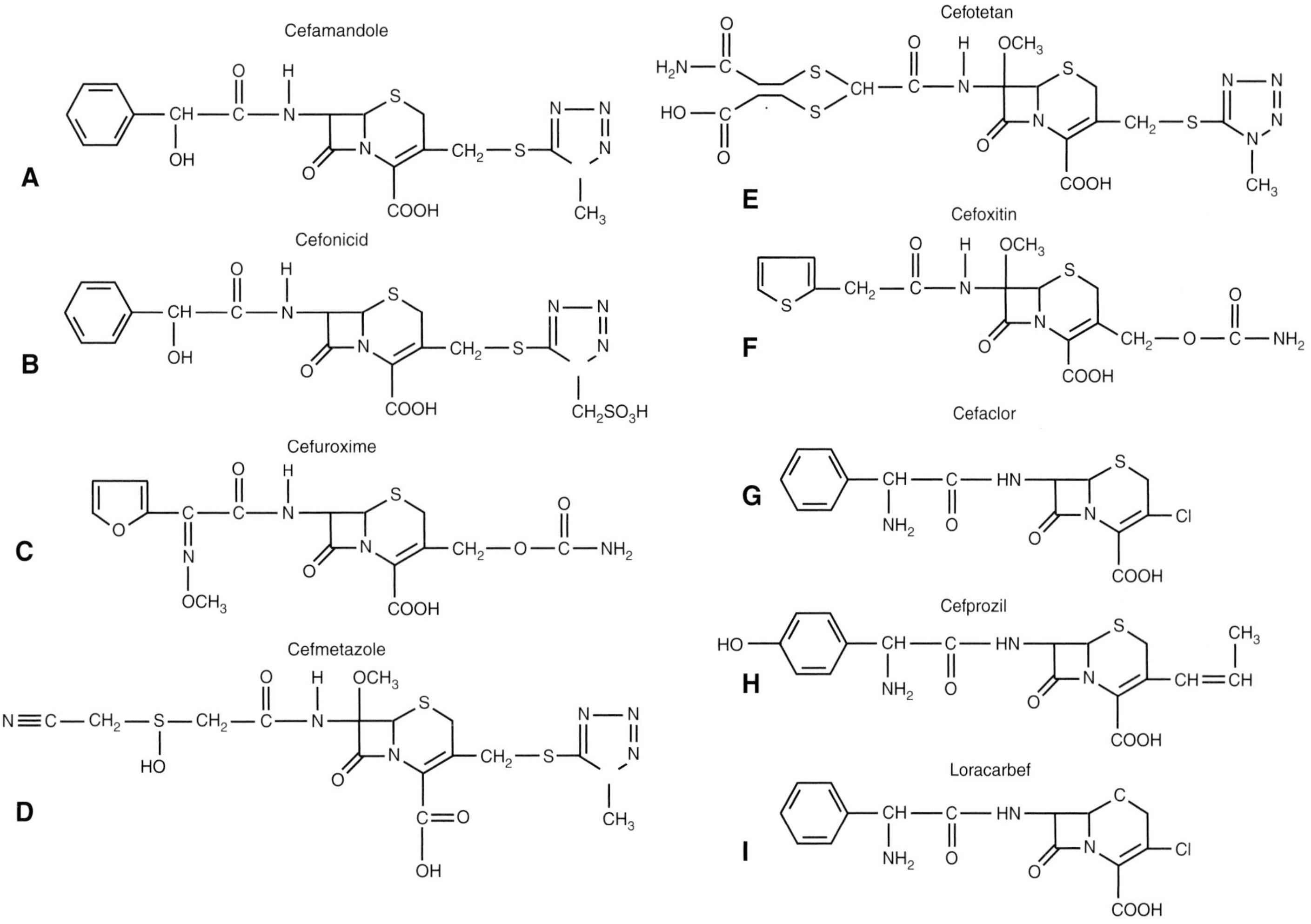

FIGURE 20-3. Second-generation cephalosporins. **A,** Cefamandole. **B,** Cefonicid. **C,** Cefuroxime. **D,** Cefmetazole. **E,** Cefotetan. **F,** Cefoxitin. **G,** Cefaclor. **H,** Cefprozil. **I,** Loracarbef.

cephalothin, cephaloridine, and cefazolin (Fig. 20-2). The simple substitution of an aminobenzyl group in the 7 position is important for oral absorption of the cephalosporins.[5] Cephalexin, cephradine, cefaclor, cefprozil, and loracarbef all have this structure or a closely related one (Fig. 20-3). Absorption of later generation cephalosporins is enhanced by the production of ester formulations. Axetil, proxetil, or pivoxyl esters of cefuroxime, ceftamet, cefpodoxime, and cefditoren are currently available.

The majority of the chemical modifications in cephalosporin development, which have resulted in changes in microbiologic spectrum, are due to alterations at the α-carbon of the acyl side chain.[5] These changes have ranged from the relatively simple addition of a hydroxyl group to the addition of large synthetic moieties. Each of the acyl side chain alterations has led to enhanced gram-negative potency because of improved β-lactamase stability. The addition of a hydroxyl group at the α-carbon led to the second-generation cephalosporin cefamandole. The second-generation cephalosporin cefuroxime resulted from the addition of a methoxyimino group in the α position along with a furyl ring at the β-acyl side chain. Addition of a 2-aminothiazol group to the 7-β-acyl side chain and a methoxyimino group to the α-carbon led to many of the third- and fourth-generation cephalosporins (Figs. 20-4 and 20-5).[8,9] Cefotaxime, ceftizoxime, ceftriaxone, cefepime, cefpirome, and cefpodoxime all have a similar structure at the 7 position. Ceftazidime differs from these drugs by replacing the methoxyimino group with a dimethylacetic acid moiety attached to the imino group.[8] This alteration enhances activity against *Pseudomonas aeruginosa* but

reduces activity against staphylococci. Two other modifications that have resulted in compounds with increased activity against *P. aeruginosa* are an ureido-2,3-dioxopiperazine group and a carboxyl group on the α-carbon with cefoperazone and moxalactam, respectively.[5] These changes are similar to those with piperacillin and carbenicillin.

Numerous modifications at R2 or the 3 position have also played a significant role in the development of the current cephalosporins. An acetoxy side chain is present in cephalothin, cephapirin, and cefotaxime.[5] Cephalosporins with this structure can be metabolized in both the serum and liver to a less active desacetyl derivative. Such drugs also tend to have a short half-life. A chloride substitution at R2 enhanced the gram-negative spectrum of activity and led to the development of cefaclor, an early second-generation cephalosporin. The unique pharmacology of ceftriaxone results from an R2 modification. Substitution of a heterocyclic thiomethyl group at the 3 position increases its biliary secretion and remarkably prolongs the elimination half-life of the compound because of protein binding.[5,10] The addition of positively charged quaternary ammonium moieties in the 3 position contributed to the development of the fourth-generation cephalosporins cefepime and cefpirome.[9] The chemical modification produces a zwitterion, which enhances the ability of the compound to penetrate the outer membrane of gram-negative organisms. Not all modifications have led to desired effects. The placement of a thiomethyl tetrazole ring (MTT) at the R2 position not only enhanced antibacterial activity but also resulted in two important adverse effects that have limited use of these compounds.[11,12] Cefamandole, cefotetan, and

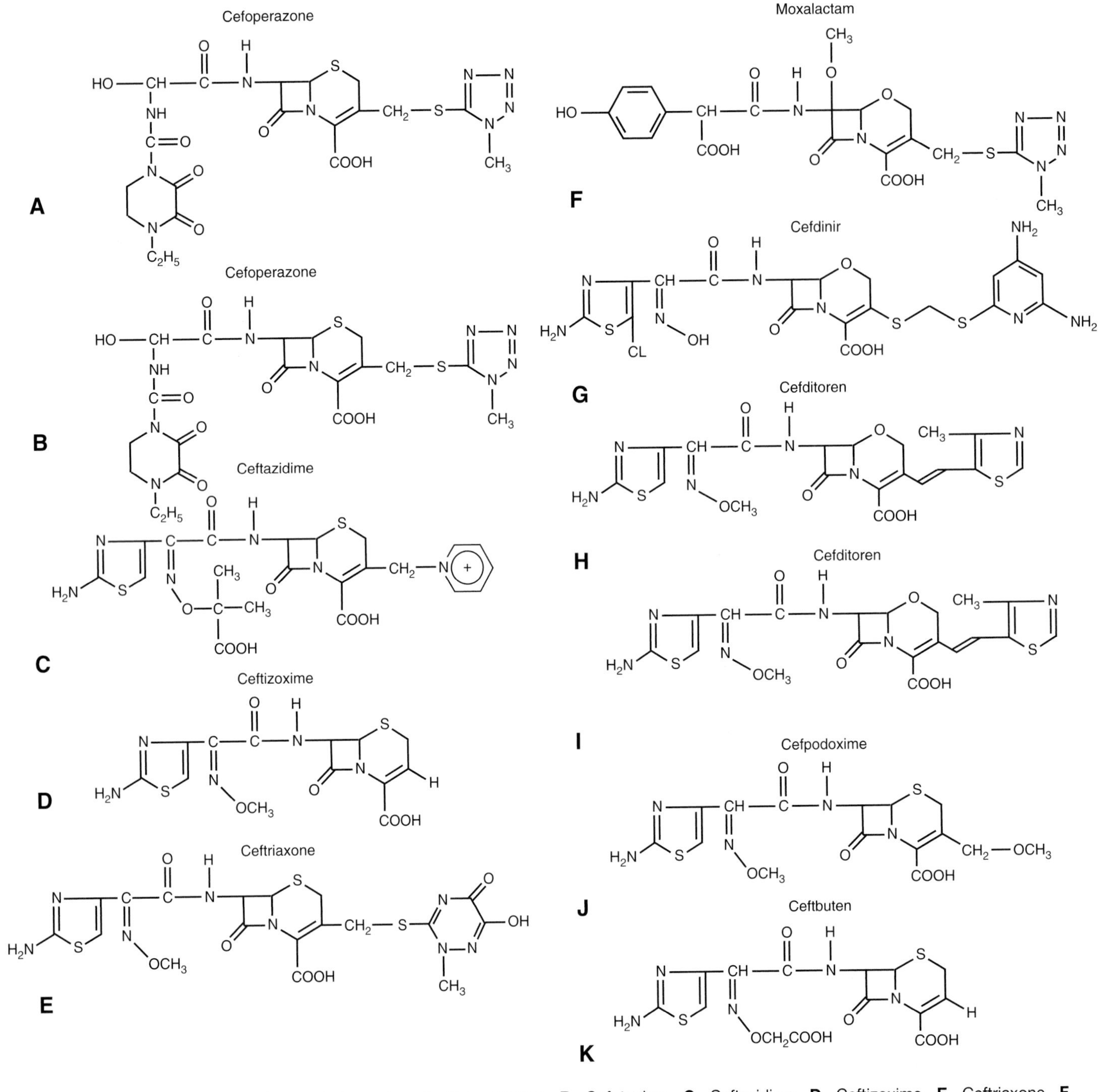

FIGURE 20-4. Third-generation cephalosporins. **A**, Cefoperazone. **B**, Cefotaxime. **C**, Ceftazidime. **D**, Ceftizoxime. **E**, Ceftriaxone. **F**, Moxalactam. **G**, Cefdinir. **H**, Cefditoren. **I**, Cefixime. **J**, Cefpodoxime. **K**, Ceftibuten.

cefoperazone contain this MTT side chain, which is responsible for coagulation abnormalities related to antagonism of vitamin K action. This side chain is also responsible for the disulfiram-like properties of these compounds.

More recently, cephalosporins with enhanced activity against methicillin-resistant *Staphylococcus aureus* (MRSA) have been developed. A variety of structural alterations at the 3 and 7 positions have increased stability to β-lactamase inactivation and increased binding to the altered PBP 2a'.[13-15] Because some of these compounds require more lipophilicity at the 3 position for activity, prodrugs have been required to enhance aqueous solubility.[16]

CLASSIFICATION

There are several microbiologic and pharmacologic differences that could serve as a basis for classification in the cephalosporin drug class. The most widely accepted classification includes four divisions or generations based loosely on the microbial spectrum of activity (Table 20-1). The first-generation cephalosporins exhibit activity focused primarily on gram-positive bacteria. The second-generation drugs have enhanced activity against gram-negative bacilli but maintain varying degrees of activity against gram-positive cocci. The cephamycin group is included in the second-generation classification as well. The

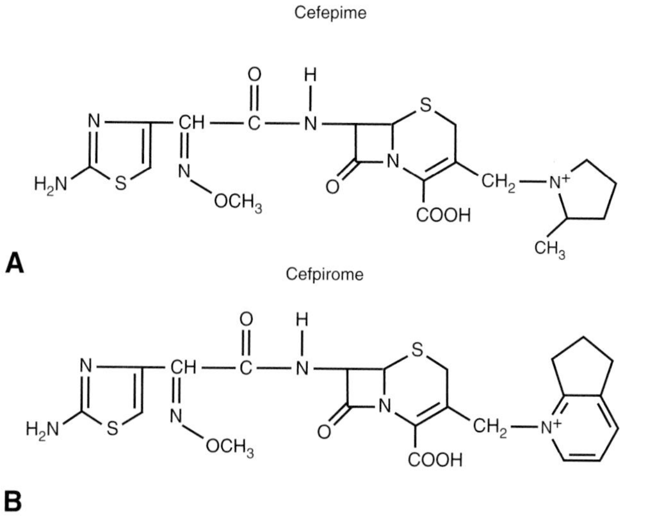

Cefepime

A

Cefpirome

B

FIGURE 20-5. Fourth-generation cephalosporins. **A,** Cefepime. **B,** Cefpirome.

cephamycins are noted for their additional activity against gram-negative anaerobic bacteria, such as *Bacteroides* spp. The third-generation group has markedly increased potency against gram-negative bacilli. However, for some compounds in the third-generation class, activity against gram-positive cocci is reduced. Among the third-generation group, a few compounds, such as ceftazidime, are considered separately for activity against *P. aeruginosa*. The fourth generation has the widest spectrum of activity of the groups. These drugs, such as cefepime and cefpirome, have activity against most gram-negative bacilli including *P. aeruginosa* and maintain their potency against gram-positive cocci. The third- and fourth-generation drugs combined are also called the extended-spectrum cephalosporins. When the MRSA-active cephalosporins are approved for clinical use, a fifth group or generation will need to be created.

MECHANISM OF ACTION

The mechanism of antibacterial activity of cephalosporins is similar to that of other β-lactam drugs. Bacterial growth is inhibited by interfering with the synthesis of the cell wall. The primary target of these compounds within the cell wall is the peptidoglycan cross-linkage structure.[17] Peptidoglycans are polysaccharide chains consisting of alternating *N*-acetylglucosamine and *N*-acetylmuramic acid residues. The polysaccharide chains are cross-linked at the pentapeptide side chain of the *N*-acetylmuramic acid residues to form a netlike structure. These structures are inserted into the cytoplasmic membrane from the

cytoplasm by the action of a group of enzymes that includes transpeptidases, carboxypeptidases, and endopeptidases. The lactam ring provides for penicillins and cephalosporins a conformation similar to the terminal D-alanine-D-alanine of the pentapeptide.[18] These antibiotics bind covalently to these enzymes, in particular the transpeptidases, resulting in the loss of enzyme activity.[19] The enzyme drug targets are referred to as PBPs.[19,20]

The location of the PBPs relative to the extracellular space differs between gram-positive and gram-negative bacteria. The peptidoglycan of gram-positive bacteria is located on the outer surface of the cell. A complex lipopolysaccharide structure is located on the outermost surface of gram-negative bacteria. Cephalosporins must first penetrate or diffuse across the lipopolysaccharide membrane to reach the PBPs of gram-negative bacteria. The PBP targets within bacteria vary by type and amount. These targets are numbered by convention on the basis of molecular weight. Letters differentiate proteins of similar molecular weight. Gram-positive and gram-negative cocci typically have 3 to 5 PBPs; gram-negative bacilli usually contain 7 to 10 PBPs. The cephalosporin drugs can vary in affinity for each of these drug targets. At low concentrations, cephalosporins preferentially bind to PBP 3 in gram-negative bacilli, resulting in filament formation with septa.[21] The events following the covalent binding of cephalosporins to the PBP targets that lead to cell lysis and death are not entirely understood.

In general, cephalosporins are considered bactericidal drugs. The rate of killing of bacteria by cephalosporins exhibits minimal dependence on the concentration of the antibiotic.[22] Maximal bacterial killing is observed at concentrations four times the minimal inhibitory concentration (MIC). Cephalosporins produce persistent suppression of bacterial growth (i.e., the postantibiotic effect) of several hours' duration with gram-positive bacteria but induce very short or no postantibiotic effects with gram-negative bacilli.[23,24] The duration of time that the drug concentrations exceed the MIC is the major determinant of the antibacterial activity of the cephalosporins.[24,25]

SPECTRUM OF ACTIVITY

The cephalosporins are active against a wide variety of aerobic and anaerobic bacteria (Tables 20-2 and 20-3).[26-55] Most drugs are active against streptococci and staphylococci. Some of the differences in potency among the agents are magnified by their activity against penicillin-resistant pneumococci. Cefditoren, ceftriaxone, cefotaxime, cefepime, and cefpirome have the greatest potency against those organisms. The cephamycins, ceftazidime, cefixime, and ceftibuten have the poorest activity against methicillin-susceptible staphylococci. Although methicillin-resistant staphylococci are resistant to all the current cephalosporins, the new MRSA cephalosporins exhibit MICs of about 1 to 4 g/mL with such strains.[56,57] Enterococci have also consistently been resistant to the cephalosporins with most MICs greater

TABLE 20-1	**Classification of Parenteral and Oral Cephalosporins**				
Cephalosporins	*First Generation*	*Second Generation*	*Cephamycins*	*Third Generation*	*Fourth Generation*
Parenteral	Cefazolin (Ancef, Kefzol)	Cefamandole (Mandol)	Cefmetazole (Zefazone)	Cefoperazone (Cefobid)	Cefepime (Maxipime)
	Cephalothin (Keflin, Seffin)	Cefonicid (Monocid)	Cefotetan (Cefotan)	Cefotaxime (Claforan)	Cefpirome
	Cephapirin (Cefadyl)	Cefuroxime (Kefurox, Zinacef)	Cefoxitin (Mefoxin)	Ceftazidime (Fortaz)	
	Cephradine (Velosef)			Ceftizoxime (Cefizox)	
				Ceftriaxone (Rocephin)	
				Moxalactam	
Oral	Cefadroxil (Duricef, Ultracef)	Cefaclor (Ceclor)		Cefdinir (Omnicef)	
	Cephalexin (Keflex, Biocef, Keftab)	Cefprozil (Cefzil)		Cefditoren (Spectracef)	
	Cephradine (Velosef)	Cefuroxime-axetil (Ceftin)		Cefixime (Suprax)	
		Loracarbef (Lorabid)		Cefpodoxime (Vantin)	
				Ceftibuten (Cedax)	

TABLE 20-2 In Vitro Activity of Cephalosporins against Selected Gram-Positive Cocci, *Haemophilus influenzae*, *Moraxella catarrhalis*, and *Neisseria* Species

	Streptococcus pneumoniae (PSSP)	Streptococcus pneumoniae (PRSP)	Streptococcus pyogenes	Streptococcus agalactiae	Viridans Streptococci Group	Staphylococcus aureus (MSSA)	Staphylococcus epidermidis	Haemophilus influenzae	Moraxella catarrhalis	Neisseria meningitidis	Neisseria gonorrhoeae
First Generation											
Cefazolin	0.5/4	32/>32	0.12/0.12	0.12/0.12	0.12/0.12	0.5/2	0.5/>32	4/16	2/4	—	16/32
Cephalothin	0.12/0.25	8/16	0.05/0.10	0.12/0.5	0.25/0.50	0.12/0.5	0.5/32	4/8	4/8	0.25/0.5	8/32
Cefadroxil (O)	2/4	>32	0.12/0.25	0.25/2	—	2/8	4/>32	16/>32	2/4	—	8/64
Cephalexin (O)	1/2	>32	0.25/2	0.5/4	—	2/4	1/>32	8/16	2/8	2/2	4/16
Cephradine (O)	2/4	>32	0.25/2	0.5/2	—	1/4	4/>32	4/16	2/4	—	8/16
Second Generation											
Cefamandole	0.12/0.5	8/>32	0.12/0.12	0.12/0.5	0.12/4	1/1	0.5/>32	2/8	1/4	0.12/0.12	0.25/4
Cefonicid	0.5/1	4/>32	0.12/0.12	0.12/2	0.12/8	1/2	2/>32	0.5/1	1/4	0.12/2	0.06/0.5
Cefuroxime	0.12/0.25	4/>32	0.12/0.12	0.12/0.12	0.12/0.5	1/2	0.5/>32	1/2	0.5/2	0.12/2	0.015/0.25
Cefaclor (O)	0.5/1	16/>32	0.06/0.5	0.5/2	—	1/8	1/>32	2/32	0.5/2	0.06/0.25	0.25/16
Cefprozil (O)	0.12/0.5	8/>32	0.03/0.12	0.06/0.25	—	0.5/2	0.25/32	2/16	1/8	—	0.12/4
Loracarbef (O)	0.5/2	>32	0.5/2	0.5/2	—	1/4	4/>32	1/4	0.5/4	0.12/0.25	0.5/4
Cephamycins											
Cefmetazole	2/16	>32	0.5/0.5	2/2	2/4	4/16	8/>32	1/4	0.12/0.5	0.12/0.12	0.25/4
Cefotetan	8/16	>32	2/4	4/8	2/8	8/16	32/>32	1/2	0.12/2	0.12/0.25	0.25/2
Cefoxitin	2/4	32/>32	1/2	2/2	4/16	4/8	2/>32	1/4	0.25/0.5	0.12/0.25	0.25/4
Third Generation											
Cefoperazone	0.06/0.12	4/16	0.12/0.12	0.12/0.25	0.5/1	2/4	2/>32	0.015/0.25	0.12/2	0.12/0.5	0.03/0.06
Cefotaxime	0.015/0.06	0.5/2	0.015/0.015	0.03/0.25	0.06/0.25	2/2	4/>32	0.008/0.015	0.5/1	0.004/0.008	0.004/0.008
Ceftazidime	0.25/1	16/>32	0.12/0.25	0.25/0.5	1/2	8/32	8/>32	0.06/0.12	0.03/0.5	0.015/0.06	0.03/0.06
Ceftizoxime	0.25/1	16/32	0.015/0.015	0.12/0.12	0.25/2	4/8	4/>32	0.015/0.03	0.03/0.5	0.008/0.03	0.008/0.015
Ceftriaxone	0.03/0.06	0.5/2	0.015/0.03	0.03/0.06	0.06/0.25	2/4	8/>32	0.008/0.015	0.25/0.5	0.008/0.015	0.002/0.004
Moxalactam	1/1	2/8	1/2	—	—	8/16	16/>32	0.03/0.12	0.03/0.12	0.008/0.06	0.015/0.06
Cefdinir (O)	0.06/0.12	2/8	0.015/0.03	0.03/0.06	—	0.25/0.5	0.25/>32	0.12/0.5	0.06/0.25	0.06/0.25	0.008/0.06
Cefditoren (O)	0.015/0.03	0.5/2	0.008/0.015	0.06/1	—	0.25/1	0.25/>32	0.008/0.015	0.25/1	<0.06/0.06	0.004/0.06
Cefixime (O)	0.25/1	32/>32	0.06/0.25	0.12/0.25	—	16/>32	16/>32	0.015/0.12	0.03/0.5	<0.06/0.06	0.015/0.06
Cefpodoxime (O)	0.015/0.06	2/>32	0.06/0.12	0.03/0.12	—	2/4	2/32	0.015/0.12	1/2	<0.06/0.06	0.06/0.06
Ceftibuten (O)	4/8	>32	0.5/2	4/16	—	16/>32	16/32	0.06/0.12	2/4	0.06/0.25	0.015/0.5
Fourth Generation											
Cefepime	0.06/0.12	0.5/2	0.015/0.12	0.05/0.05	0.016/0.03	2/4	2/>32	0.06/0.12	1/4	0.03/0.06	0.03/0.06
Cefpirome	0.03/0.12	0.5/2	0.008/0.06	.06/.06	0.06/0.25	1/2	1/>32	0.06/0.12	0.5/2	0.06/0.06	0.015/0.12

MSSA, methicillin-susceptible *S. aureus*; (O), oral; PRSP, penicillin-resistant *S. pneumoniae*; PSSP, penicillin-susceptible *S. pneumoniae*.

TABLE 20-3 In Vitro Activity of Cephalosporins against Selected Aerobic and Anaerobic Gram-Negative Bacilli

Cephalosporins	Escherichia coli	Klebsiella pneumoniae	Proteus mirabilis	Enterobacter aerogenes	Enterobacter cloacae	Citrobacter freundii	Serratia sp.	Pseudomonas aeruginosa	Morganella sp.	Bacteroides fragilis	Salmonella sp.	Shigella sp.
First Generation												
Cefazolin	2/16	2/>16	4/16	>32	>32	>32	>32	>32	>32	>32	2/4	2/8
Cephalothin	4/8	1/16	8/16	>32	>32	>32	>32	>32	>32	>32	2/4	4/8
Cefadroxil (O)	4/>16	8/>16	16/>32	>32	>32	>32	>32	>32	>32	>32	8/>16	4/16
Cephalexin (O)	8/>16	8/32	16/>32	>32	>32	>32	>32	>32	>32	>32	4/16	8/>16
Cephradine (O)	4/>16	4/>16	16/>32	>32	>32	>32	>32	>32	>32	>32	4/>16	8/>16
Second Generation												
Cefamandole	1/2	1/8	1/2	4/>32	2/>32	2/>32	16/>32	>32	4/>32	32/>32	0.5/4	0.5/2
Cefonicid	2/8	2/8	1/2	4/>32	8/>32	8/>32	>32	>32	16/>32	32/>32	2/8	2/8
Cefuroxime	2/8	2/16	2/4	8/>32	8/>32	8/>32	>32	>32	32/>32	8/>32	4/8	2/4
Cefaclor (O)	2/>16	2/32	2/4	>32	>32	>32	>32	>32	>32	>32	2/8	4/16
Cefprozil (O)	2/8	1/>32	2/2	>32	>32	16/>32	16/>32	>32	16/>32	>32	2/8	4/16
Loracarbef (O)	1/>16	0.5/8	0.5/2	16/>32	16/>32	4/>32	>32	>32	32/>32	>32	0.5/8	0.25/8
Cephamycins												
Cefmetazole	0.5/1	1/2	2/4	>32	>32	>32	16/>32	>32	4/8	8/>32	0.5/2	1/2
Cefotetan	0.12/0.5	0.12/0.5	0.12/0.5	32/>32	8/>32	0.5/>32	1/8	>32	2/4	8/>32	0.12/0.12	0.12/0.5
Cefoxitin	2/8	2/8	2/4	>32	>32	>32	16/>32	>32	8/16	8/32	2/4	2/4
Third Generation												
Cefoperazone	0.12/8	0.25/8	0.5/1	0.25/8	0.25/8	0.5/32	2/8	4/>32	1/8	32/>32	0.5/4	0.25/1
Cefotaxime	0.06/0.25	0.06/0.25	0.06/0.25	0.12/16	0.25/32	0.25/>32	0.25/2	16/>32	0.25/4	8/>32	0.06/0.12	0.06/0.25
Ceftazidime	0.06/0.25	0.25/1	0.06/0.5	0.25/32	0.25/32	0.5/>32	0.25/2	2/16	0.12/0.5	>32	0.12/0.5	0.06/0.25
Ceftizoxime	0.03/0.12	0.03/0.12	0.008/0.015	0.06/16	0.06/16	0.25/>32	0.12/0.5	32/>32	0.25/2	16/>32	0.015/0.25	0.008/0.25
Ceftriaxone	0.06/0.12	0.06/0.25	0.008/0.03	0.25/16	0.25/>32	0.12/>32	0.25/4	32/>32	0.008/0.25	8/>32	0.06/0.25	0.03/0.12
Moxalactam	0.12/0.25	0.12/0.25	0.25/0.5	0.25/16	0.5/8	0.25/8	0.25/4	32/>32	0.25/0.5	2/32	0.12/0.25	0.12/0.25
Cefdinir (O)	0.25/0.5	0.06/0.25	0.06/0.12	0.5/>32	0.5/>32	0.25/>32	4/32	16/>32	4/16	16/>32	0.25/0.5	0.25/0.5
Cefditoren (O)	0.12/0.25	0.25/1	0.12/1	0.5/>32	1/>32	1/>32	2/32	>32	-	4/>32	0.06/0.25	0.25/0.5
Cefixime (O)	0.12/0.25	0.03/0.12	0.008/0.03	0.5/>32	0.12/>32	2/>32	2/>32	>32	2/32	16/>32	0.06/0.25	0.12/0.25
Cefpodoxime (O)	0.25/1	0.5/2	0.06/0.12	2/>32	4/>32	2/>32	1/8	>32	2/>32	16/>32	0.5/1	0.12/0.25
Ceftibuten (O)	0.12/0.25	0.06/0.25	0.015/0.03	1/32	2/>32	1/>32	0.5/8	>32	0.25/8	16/>32	0.06/0.25	0.06/0.25
Fourth Generation												
Cefepime	0.03/0.06	0.03/0.25	0.06/0.12	0.06/0.5	0.06/2	0.06/2	0.12/0.5	2/16	0.03/0.12	>32	0.06/0.12	0.03/0.06
Cefpirome	0.06/0.12	0.06/0.25	0.06/0.12	0.06/0.5	0.12/4	0.03/2	0.25/2	2/16	0.03/0.12	32/>32	0.06/0.25	0.06/0.12

(O), oral.

than 32 μg/mL. However, the new MRSA-active cephalosporins have much lower MICs for ampicillin-susceptible strains. These have ranged from 0.12 to 4 g/mL for most of these drugs.[56,57]

The first-generation cephalosporins are not very active against *Haemophilus influenzae* and *Moraxella catarrhalis*. In comparison, the second-generation drugs are about fourfold more potent against these respiratory pathogens. The third-generation cephalosporins have the lowest MICs for *H. influenzae* and *M. catarrhalis*, which are 10 to 100 times lower than those of the second-generation drugs. The first-generation cephalosporins are also not as active against *Neisseria* species as the second-, third-, and fourth-generation drugs.

Although all of the cephalosporins are considered active against *Escherichia coli*, *Klebsiella pneumoniae*, and *Proteus mirabilis*, the potency of the third- and fourth-generations drugs is 10- to 100-fold greater than that of the first- and second-generation cephalosporins. The increased potency of the later generation drugs extends to strains of *Enterobacter*, *Serratia*, *Citrobacter*, and *Morganella* species, which are usually resistant to the first- and second-generation drugs. Several cephalosporins, such as ceftazidime, cefoperazone, ceftizoxime, cefepime, and cefpirome, are active against most strains of *P. aeruginosa*. The third- and fourth-generation cephalosporins also exhibit enhanced potency against strains of *Salmonella* and *Shigella*.

Many cephalosporins are active against penicillin-susceptible gram-positive anaerobes, such as peptostreptococci.[58,59] Against *Bacteroides fragilis*, drugs such as the cephamycins, cefotaxime, ceftriaxone, and ceftizoxime have the best activity. Many of the drugs are active against spirochetes including the agents of Lyme disease and syphilis.[60,61] As a group, the cephalosporins have very poor activity against *Chlamydia*, *Mycoplasma*, and *Listeria* species.[62-64]

MECHANISMS OF RESISTANCE

Four general mechanisms can result in resistance to cephalosporin antibiotics: (1) antibiotic destruction by hydrolyzing β-lactamase enzymes, (2) reduced penetration of the antibiotic through the lipopolysaccharide membrane to the PBP target, (3) enhanced efflux of the drug from the periplasmic space, and (4) alteration in the PBP target resulting in reduced binding affinity. Most often resistance in a bacterial population is due to a single mechanism; however, an increasing percentage of organisms are exhibiting multiple mechanisms.[65]

Production of β-lactamase enzymes that hydrolyze the β-lactam ring is a predominant resistance mechanism for many gram-negative bacteria. With staphylococci, most cephalosporins, with the exception of cephaloridine, are poorly hydrolyzed by staphylococcal penicillinases. Resistance to cephalosporins in these organisms is due almost entirely to reduced binding affinity of the PBPs. Although all gram-negative bacilli produce β-lactamase enzymes, the type and amount of enzyme vary among organisms. These enzymes are located in the periplasmic space between the outer lipopolysaccharide membrane and the inner cell membrane. Drugs that are able to penetrate the outer membrane can be degraded before reaching the PBP target. The net antimicrobial activity of cephalosporins against gram-negative bacilli is dependent upon the rate of penetration across the outer membrane and the stability of the drug to the various hydrolyzing β-lactamases. The penetration of drugs across the outer membrane is through water-filled channels formed by various membrane proteins, termed porins. Movement through porin channels is dependent upon the size, shape, charge, and hydrophilic properties of the compound. The concentration of a drug with a slow rate of penetration is low relative to the amount of β-lactamase within the periplasmic space. The relatively high β-lactamase concentration can enhance antibiotic inactivation. For a drug that can penetrate rapidly, the converse is true. For example, the zwitterion of cefepime enhances movement across the membrane, resulting in high concentrations in the periplasmic space and a relative net resistance to drug hydrolysis.[66]

The number of unique β-lactamases is markedly increasing. These proteases may be genetically encoded chromosomally or extrachromosomally. Stable derepression of a chromosomal mutation is the most common genotypic scenario. This is observed predominantly in *Enterobacter* species, *Serratia* species, *Citrobacter freundii*, and *P. aeruginosa*.[67] The Bush type 1 AmpC cephalosporinase is capable of inactivating almost all current cephalosporins including the cephamycins. Emergence of this type of resistance is frequent when infections resulting from these organisms are treated only with broad-spectrum cephalosporins.[67-69] Extrachromosomal propagation is most often through plasmids but can occur through transposons. Some of these newer enzymes represent variants of the common plasmid-encoded TEM-1, TEM-2, and SHV-1 β-lactamases. These enzymes have been observed most commonly in *K. pneumoniae* and *E. coli* and are referred to as extended-spectrum β-lactamases (ESBLs) because they are capable of inactivating many third- and fourth-generation cephalosporins.[70,71] These enzymes are the result of amino acid substitutions related to point mutations in the common β-lactamase genes (i.e., TEM- and SHV-). SHV ESBLs are the most common ESBLs found in *K. pneumoniae*.[72] Other newer plasmid β-lactamases include variants of the chromosomal AmpC β-lactamase.[73] These enzymes have also been observed primarily in *K. pneumoniae* and *E. coli*.

The different β-lactamase enzymes can vary significantly in their affinity for drugs within the cephalosporin class. For example, cefepime and cefpirome are less susceptible than other cephalosporins to inactivation by Bush type 1 AmpC cephalosporinases.[74,75] Cephalothin, cefamandole, and cefoperazone are most susceptible to inactivation by the common plasmid-encoded TEM-1, TEM-2, and SHV-1 β-lactamases.[67,68] The cephamycins are not susceptible to inactivation by ESBLs. Ceftazidime and cefpodoxime generally exhibit high sensitivity to inactivation by ESBLs.[70,76] On the other hand, cefepime, cefpirome, and even cefotaxime and ceftriaxone may exhibit only modest inactivation and still be considered susceptible by standard susceptibility testing. Tests using ceftazidime, cefpodoxime, and cefotaxime or ceftriaxone, or both, to identify strains of *K. pneumoniae* and *E. coli* producing ESBLs have been devised for clinical laboratories by the National Committee for Clinical Laboratory Standards.[77] Their recommendation is that all such strains should be called resistant to cephalosporins other than the cephamycins even if they are susceptible on standard susceptibility tests.[77] A large prospective observational study of patients with *Klebsiella* bacteremia observed a significantly poorer outcome in patients treated with third- and fourth-generation cephalosporins than with carbapenems.[78] The poorer outcome was observed primarily in strains with MICs greater than 2 μg/mL. Thus, strains with ESBLs that have low MICs are still probably treatable with cephalosporins. Identification of ESBLs in the clinical laboratory is also complicated by new emerging ESBLs called the CTX-M enzymes, which hydrolyze ceftazidime much less than other third- and fourth-generation cephalosporins and exhibit susceptibility to ceftazidime in standard susceptibility testing.[72,79,80]

It is unlikely that deletion or mutation of porin proteins causes primary resistance to cephalosporins. However, such changes can alter the relationship between the concentrations of drug and β-lactamase in the periplasmic space resulting in much more hydrolysis of the cephalosporin. For example, strains of *K. pneumoniae* containing ESBLs have been shown to be resistant to cephamycins because of the lack of an outer-membrane porin protein.[81] Porin-deficient strains are especially high in *Enterobacter aerogenes*.[82]

The endogenous AcrAB multidrug efflux system in *E. coli* affects the potency of penicillins but has little effect on the activity of cephalosporins.[83] However, the MexAB-OprM efflux pump in *P. aeruginosa* has been associated with resistance to both third- and fourth-generation drugs.[84,85] The difference between these organisms in the impact of somewhat similar pumps is probably due to a markedly higher outer-membrane permeability in *E. coli* than in *P. aeruginosa*.[86]

Changes in the PBP target are responsible for reduced cephalosporin affinity and subsequent drug resistance for

Streptococcus pneumoniae, methicillin-resistant *S. aureus*, *H. influenzae*, and some *Neisseria gonorrhoeae* strains. Changes in the PBP target may result from amino acid substitutions or insertions. Nearly 40 amino acid substitutions in PBP 2b have been described in the pneumococcus.[87,88] Resistance in *S. pneumoniae* and several other pathogens has also resulted from insertion of resistance sequences from other related species. For example, the reduced affinity PBP in *S. aureus* responsible for methicillin resistance is thought to represent a fusion product of an *E. coli* PBP region and the regulatory region of the staphylococcal β-lactamase sequence.[89]

PHARMACOLOGIC PROPERTIES

The pharmacologic properties of selected cephalosporins are listed in Table 20-4.[90-115] Cephalosporins are polar, water-soluble compounds. Within each of the first-, second-, and third-generation classifications there are both oral and parenteral formulations. The only fourth-generation compounds in clinical use are available for parenteral use only. The parenteral formulations are available for both intravenous and intramuscular administration. All of the parenteral formulations with the exception of cephradine are stable in solution at room temperature for 24 hours or longer.[116,117] Drug stability at room temperature facilitates use of these compounds for home intravenous therapy including continuous infusions. Many of the parenteral compounds can also be administered by the intraperitoneal route for therapy of peritoneal infections associated with continuous ambulatory peritoneal dialysis.[118] Formulations of the oral cephalosporins are available as tablets or capsules and as suspensions.

In contrast to many other β-lactams, oral preparations of the cephalosporins are stable in the acid milieu of the upper gastrointestinal tract. Cephalosporins can be actively absorbed if their structure mediates transport by the di- and tripeptide transport systems in the brush border membrane in the small intestine.[119] Cephalexin, cephradine, cefadroxil, cefaclor, cefprozil, and loracarbef have an aminobenzyl group or a similar group in the 7 position and have high oral bioavailability (80% to 95%). Ceftibuten, cefixime, and cefdinir have

TABLE 20-4 Pharmacokinetics of Cephalosporins

Cephalosporin	Adult Dose	Peak Serum Concentration (µg/mL)	Half-life (hr)	Serum Protein Binding (%)	Route of Excretion	Cerebrospinal Fluid Concentration Range (µg/mL)	Cerebrospinal Fluid Penetration (%)	Stability at Room Temperature (hr) or Oral Bioavailability (%)
First Generation								
Cefazolin	0.5-1 g q8h	193 (1 g)	1.9	74-86	R (65-100%)	<0.7	0-4	24
Cephalothin	0.5-2 g q4-6h	64 (1 g)	0.5-1.0	50-80	R (50-70%)	0.16-0.31	1	24
Cephapirin	0.5-2 g q4-6h	70 (1 g)	0.6	50-60	R (60-85%)	NA	NA	24
Cephradine	0.5-1 g q6h	50 (1 g)	0.7	8-17	R (75-100%)	NA	NA	2-10
Second Generation								
Cefamandole	0.5-2 g q6h	88 (1 g)	0.7-1.3	50-78	R (80%)	0.35-7.4	0-8.6	24
Cefonicid	0.5-1 g q24h	221 (1 g)	4.4	98	R (95%)	NA	NA	24
Cefuroxime	0.75-1.5 g q8h	39 (1 g)	1.2-1.8	33-50	R (70-100%)	0.35-22.5	11.6-13.7	24
Cephamycins								
Cefmetazole	2 g q8h	143 (2 g)	1.3-1.8	68	R (75-85%)	NA	NA	24
Cefotetan	1-2 g q12h	158 (2 g)	3.5	76-90	R (80%)	1.1-4.8	0.8-3.6	24
Cefoxitin	1-2 g q6h	110 (1 g)	0.8-1	41-79	R (90%)	1.2-22	0.8-35	24
Third Generation								
Cefoperazone	1-3 g q8-12h	153 (1 g)	1.6-2.1	90	H (80%) R (20%)	<0.8-119	2.5-5.9	12
Cefotaxime	1-2 g q12h	102 (1 g)	1-1.2	35-40	R (50-80%)	1-83	4-55	24
Ceftazidime	1-2 g q8-12h	107 (1 g)	1-2	17	R (80-90%)	1.4-30	14-45	24
Ceftizoxime	1-2 g q6-12h	113 (1 g)	1.4-1.7	31	R (70-100%)	<0.5-29	3-22.6	24
Ceftriaxone	1-2 g q12-24h	145 (1 g)	6.4	85-95	R (50%) H (40%)	2-20	1.5-7	72
Moxalactam	1-2 g q8h	70 (1 g)	2.2	50	R (67-88%)	0.8-39	12-69	24
Fourth Generation								
Cefepime	1-2 g q12h	79 (1 g)	2	16-19	R (85%)	5.7	11.8	24
Cefpirome	1-2 g q12h	80 (1 g)	2	10	R (90%)	0.8-4.2	5-67%	24
Oral—First Generation								
Cefadroxil	0.5-1 g q12h	15 (0.5 g)	1.3-1.6	20	R (90%)	NA	NA	80%
Cephalexin	0.5-1 g q6h	5.8 (250 mg)	0.5-1.2	6-15	R (80-100%)	NA	NA	90%
Cephradine	0.5-1g q6h	15 (0.5 g)	1-2	10-20	R (80-90%)	NA	NA	95%
Oral—Second Generation								
Cefaclor	250-500 mg q8h	6 (250 mg)	0.5-1	25-50	R (50-80%)	NA	NA	50-90% FE
	375 mg q12h	19.2 (400 mg)						
Cefprozil	500 mg q12h	9.3 (500 mg)	1.3	35-45	R (61%)	NA	NA	95%
Cefuroxime (axetil)	250-500 mg q12h	4.6 (250 mg)	1.2	33-50	R (66-100%)	NA	NA	52-68% FE
Loracarbef	200-400 mg q12h	8 (200 mg)	1.0	25	R (87%)	NA	NA	90%
Oral—Third Generation								
Cefdinir	300 mg q12h	2.9	1.5-1.7	60-73	R (18%)	NA	NA	25%
Cefditoren (pivoxil)	200-400 mg q12h	2.5 (200 mg)	0.8-1.6	88	R (16-22%)	NA	NA	17% FE
Cefixime	200-400 mg q12-24h	2.8 (200 mg)-4.5 (400 mg)	3-4	65-70	R (50%) H (5%)	NA	NA	40-50%
Cefpodoxime (proxetil)	200 mg q12h	2.2 (200 mg)	2.2-2.7	18-40	R (29-33%)	NA	NA	50-80% FE
Ceftibuten	400 mg q24h	15 (400 mg)	2.4	65-77	R (57%)	NA	NA	75-90%

FE, food enhances; H, hepatic; NA, not applicable; R, renal.

other groups in the 7 position and exhibit more variable bioavailability after oral dosing. Absorption by the di- and tripeptide transport systems appears to be both pH and calcium dependent.[119] Drugs that have low oral bioavailability can be esterified to enhance absorption. The ester prodrug is hydrolyzed after absorption in the intestinal epithelial cells. The esters commonly used include axetil, proxetil, and pivoxil formulations.[120] Ester prodrug formulations exist for cefuroxime, cefditoren, and cefpodoxime. Absorption of the ester is still not complete. In fact, the percent oral bioavailability of ester formulations is lower than that of most nonesterified compounds. Absorption of the ester formulations is enhanced by concomitant food intake.[120] Food within the stomach delays gastric emptying and prolongs contact with the mucosal surface.

Distribution of cephalosporins within the body is governed by the lipid solubility of the drug and the extent of protein binding. β-Lactams bind almost exclusively to albumin. The extent of protein binding can vary from less than 10% to as much as 98%.[108] Because only unbound drug can pass through capillary pores into interstitial fluid or across cell membranes into intracellular fluid, avidly bound compounds tend to exhibit high serum concentrations and low tissue concentrations. In general, the cephalosporins are largely confined to the extracellular compartment. Drug concentrations in subcutaneous blisters, a model for extracellular drug penetration, are similar to those found in serum.[108,121] Techniques measuring extracellular drug concentrations in human tissues, such as microdialysis, have demonstrated that concentrations of unbound drug in interstitial fluid are also similar to those in serum.[122] The cephalosporins have relatively poor intracellular concentrations. Tissue homogenates, which mix intracellular and extracellular fluid, always provide concentrations that are lower than serum because of dilution by the larger intracellular volume.[121] This group of compounds does not achieve intracellular concentrations adequate for therapy for most intracellular pathogens such as *Legionella* spp.[123]

In the absence of infection, drug concentrations in the cerebrospinal fluid (CSF) and the vitreous humor are low. None of the oral cephalosporins achieve therapeutic concentrations in the CSF. Penetration of most parenteral drugs from the first- and second-generation groups is similarly poor. Parenteral cefuroxime is one exception, and this drug also has the lowest MICs for common meningeal pathogens among the first- and second-generation cephalosporins.[109] The parenteral third- and fourth-generation drugs, such as ceftriaxone, cefotaxime, ceftazidime, and cefepime, achieve concentrations that would allow therapy for central nervous system infections.[110-115,124] The presence of an active transport system that transports many cephalosporins from the CSF back to serum contributes to the low drug levels in the CSF with many of the earlier generation drugs. The transport protein involved in this system is similar to the protein involved in renal secretion of β-lactam antibiotics.[124] Ceftriaxone, cefotaxime, ceftazidime, and cefepime exhibit minimal renal tubular secretion and are poor substrates for the choroid plexus pump, contributing to higher CSF concentrations. Probenecid is a competitive substrate for this pump and can produce higher concentrations with drugs that are effluxed by

TABLE 20-5 Dosing Adjustment of Cephalosporins in Patients with Renal Insufficiency

Cephalosporin	Usual Adult Dosing Regimen	Dosing Regimen with Renal Insufficiency			Dosing Regimen with Dialysis	
		GFR < 10 mL/min	GFR 10-50 mL/min	GFR 50-90 mL/min	Hemodialysis	CAPD
First Generation						
Cefazolin	1 g q8h	0.5-1 g q24h	0.5-1 g q12h	NC	0.5-1 g after	0.5 g q12h
Cephalothin	1 g q4-6h	0.5 g q8h	0.5 g q6h	NC	0.5 g after	1 g q12h
Cephapirin	1 g q4-6h	0.5 g q8h	0.5 g q6h	NC	0.5 g after	1 g q12h
Cephradine	1 g q4-6h	0.5 g q8h	0.5 g q6h	NC	0.5 g after	1 g q12h
Second Generation						
Cefamandole	1 g q6h	1 g q12h	1 g q8h	NC	0.5 g after	1 g q12h
Cefonicid	1 g q24h	0.125 g q24h	0.5 g q24h	NC	None	0.125 g q24h
Cefuroxime	1.5 g q8h	0.75 g q24h	0.75 g q8-12h	NC	0.75 g after	0.75 g q24h
Cephamycins						
Cefmetazole	2 g q8-12h	1 g q24h	2 g q24h	NC	1 g after	1 g q24h
Cefotetan	2 g q12h	1 g q24h	2 g q24h	NC	1 g after	1 g q24h
Cefoxitin	2 g q6h	1 q q12h	2 g q12h	2 g q8h	1 g after	1 g q12h
Third Generation						
Cefoperazone	1 g q8h	NC	NC	NC	None	NC
Cefotaxime	2 g q8h	2 g q24h	2 g q12h	NC	1 g after	1 g q24h
Ceftazidime	2 g q8h	0.5 g q24h	2 g q24h	2 g q12h	1 g after	0.5 g q24h
Ceftizoxime	1 g q8h	0.5 g q24h	1 g q24h	NC	1 g after	0.5 g q24h
Ceftriaxone	1 g q24h	NC	NC	NC	None	NC
Moxalactam	1 g q8h	0.2 g q24h	0.35 g q24h	0.5 g q8h	1 g after	0.25 g q24h
Fourth Generation						
Cefepime	2 g q12h	0.5-1 g q24h	1 g q24h	NC	1 g after	0.5-1 g q24h
Oral—First Generation						
Cefadroxil	500 mg q12h	500 mg q24h	500 mg q24h	NC	500 mg after	500 mg q24h
Cephalexin	500 mg q6h	250 mg q12h	500 mg q12h	NC	500 mg after	500 mg q12h
Cephradine	500 mg q6h	250 mg q12h	250 mg q6h	NC	500 mg after	500 mg q12h
Oral—Second Generation						
Cefaclor	500 mg q8h	500 mg q12h	NC	NC	500 mg after	500 mg q12h
Cefprozil	500 mg q12h	250 mg q24h	500 mg q24h	NC	500 mg after	250 mg q24h
Cefuroxime (axetil)	500 mg q8h	500 mg q24h	500 mg q12h	NC	500 mg after	500 mg q24h
Loracarbef	400 mg q12h	200 mg q24h	200 mg q12h	NC	400 mg after	400 mg q24h
Oral—Third Generation						
Cefdinir	300 mg q12h	300 mg q24h	NC	NC	300 mg after	300 mg q24h
Cefditoren	400 mg q12h	200 mg q24h	200 mg q12h	NC	None	200 mg q24h
Cefixime	400 mg q12h	200 mg q24h	300 mg q24h	NC	300 mg after	200 mg q24h
Cefpodoxime	200 mg q12h	200 mg q24h	NC	NC	200 mg after	200 mg q24h
Ceftibuten	400 mg q24h	100 mg q24h	200 mg q24h	NC	300 mg after	100 mg q24h

CAPD, continuous ambulatory peritoneal dialysis; GFR, glomerular filtration rate; NC, no change.

this transport system.[125] Infection results in higher CSF levels because inflammation can enhance penetration as well as interfere with efflux by active transport.

Few drugs from the cephalosporin class are extensively metabolized. The three exceptions are cefotaxime, cephalothin, and cephapirin, which undergo deacetylation of the acetoxymethyl side chain in the liver.[113,126] The metabolic desacetyl products still possess modest microbiologic activity. The elimination half-life of desacetyl-cefotaxime is significantly longer than that of the parent compound, allowing less frequent administration of this otherwise short-half-life drug.[113] The remaining drugs in the cephalosporin class are excreted from the body unchanged.

Most cephalosporins are eliminated by the kidney with half-lives of 1 to 2 hours. The major mechanism for renal excretion of many compounds is tubular secretion. This active transport process is largely unaffected by protein binding.[108] Probenecid inhibits this organic acid transport system and can prolong the half-life of these compounds. For several compounds, glomerular filtration is more important and protein binding can significantly prolong their elimination half-life.[127] For some drugs the elimination half-life is 3 to 8 hours, allowing 12- and 24-hour dosing intervals. A few compounds with high protein binding and high molecular weights, such as ceftriaxone and cefoperazone, are eliminated to a large extent by the biliary route.[128] From 50% to 70% of active parent compound may be recovered in the bile and eventually the feces.

The maximal daily doses of agents eliminated primarily by the kidney need to be reduced in renal impairment. Most often this adjustment includes both a reduction in dose level and lengthening of the dosing interval. Recommended dose adjustments for various degrees of renal impairment and for patients receiving dialysis are listed in Table 20-5.[129,130] For drugs eliminated by the biliary system, such as ceftriaxone and cefoperazone, dose adjustments are unnecessary unless concomitant severe hepatic insufficiency and renal insufficiency are present.[129] The majority of cephalosporins eliminated by the renal route are eliminated by hemodialysis. From 20% to 50% of the parent compound is removed after a usual dialysis session. It is recommended that the drug be given again after hemodialysis. On the other hand, few cephalosporins are removed to any significant extent (less than 10%) by peritoneal dialysis. Additional dosing is not recommended after a peritoneal dialysis session. Continuous venous hemofiltration (CVH) is being used more frequently in critically ill patients. Compounds eliminated by the kidneys and hemodialysis are removed with CVH. Most often the efficiency of drug removal is thought to be similar to a creatinine clearance of 10 to 30 mL/min, and appropriate dosing modification is recommended.[131]

ADVERSE REACTIONS AND TOXICITIES

The safety profile of the cephalosporins as a class is generally favorable. The incidence of specific adverse reactions for these compounds is relatively similar among drugs within the class with few exceptions (Table 20-6). Hypersensitivity reactions are the most common adverse effect associated with cephalosporin therapy, as with other β-lactam drugs.[132,133] The frequency of hypersensitivity reactions to cephalosporins is less than that to penicillins. Various cutaneous rashes, often associated with eosinophilia and occasionally fever, occur in 1% to 7% of patients receiving these drugs.[134] More severe hypersensitivity reactions such as serum sickness, anaphylaxis, or angioedema occur infrequently. These immunoglobulin E (IgE)–mediated reactions are estimated to occur in less than 1 in 100,000 patients.[135,136] However, there have been reports of a strong association between serum sickness in children and use of cefaclor.[137,138] The specific cephalosporin product responsible for eliciting the various skin reactions has not been clearly delineated. Although it is thought that these reactions are hapten mediated, as with related penicillin reactions, the specific haptens are not known. Cross-reactivity among drugs from the cephalosporin class and other β-lactams has been extensively investigated, yet controversy remains regarding the reported rates of cross-reactivity. Reports from early studies suggested a much higher frequency of reactions than more recent reports. Most current estimates suggest a cross-reaction frequency of 5% or less.[139]

Because of the large number of potential haptens thought to be potentially involved, a reliable skin test has not yet been developed. Use of the penicillin skin test to predict cephalosporin reactions is unreliable. For example, in a study of nearly 100 individuals with a history of reaction to the penicillin determinants used in skin testing, only a single patient who received a cephalosporin had a reaction.[140] The practical clinical decision to use a cephalosporin in a patient with a prior history of reaction to either a penicillin or other cephalosporin should be guided by the severity of the prior reaction. Use of cephalosporins in patients with prior nonsevere, non–IgE-mediated reactions to other β-lactams is considered safe.[132,133] Although the risk of a similar reaction is increased, the reactions are rarely severe. However, in the setting of a prior IgE-mediated reaction with another β-lactam compound, use of a cephalosporin would be discouraged.

Immunologically mediated reactions to cephalosporins may also be manifest as hematologic or renal toxicities. Eosinophilia is the most commonly reported laboratory abnormality.[141] Cytopenias associated with cephalosporin use are rare.[142] Cytotoxic reactions from immunoglobulin antibodies can rarely result in either neutropenia, thrombocytopenia, or anemia.[142] Although Coombs laboratory tests have been reported to be positive in a significant percentage of patients receiving many of the cephalosporins, these patients most often do not have hemolytic anemia.[143] This is a false-positive reaction related to cross-reactivity that occurs in up to 3% of patients. A similar cytotoxic reaction can result in renal damage because of interstitial nephritis.[144] The frequency of this reaction appears to be less than with drugs from the penicillin class.

Nonimmunologic hematologic and renal toxicities have been reported with a similarly low frequency. Bleeding abnormalities have been reported with increased frequency related to two mechanisms. Impaired adenosine diphosphate–induced platelet aggregation has been reported with moxalactam.[145] This abnormality is not observed

TABLE 20-6 Potential Adverse Effects of Cephalosporins

Type	Specific	Frequency
Hypersensitivity	Rash	1-3%
	Urticaria	<1%
	Serum sickness	<1%
	Anaphylaxis	0.01%
Gastrointestinal		
	Diarrhea	1-19%
	Nausea, vomiting	1-6%
	Transient transaminase elevation	1-7%
	Biliary sludge	20-46%*
Hematologic		
	Eosinophilia	1-10%
	Neutropenia	<1%
	Thrombocytopenia	<1-3%
	Hypoprothrombinemia	<1%
	Impaired platelet aggregation	<1%
	Hemolytic anemia	<1%
Renal		
	Interstitial nephritis	<1%
Central nervous system		
	Seizures	<1%
False positive laboratory		
	Coombs positive	3%
	Glucosuria	Rare
	Serum creatinine	Rare
Other		
	Drug fever	Rare
	Disulfiram-like reaction†	Rare
	Superinfection	Rare
	Phlebitis	Rare

*Ceftriaxone.
†Cephalosporins with thiomethyl tetrazole ring (MTT) side chain.

with other cephalosporins. Another coagulopathy is specifically associated with the MTT side chain present on cefamandole, cefotetan, cefoperazone, and moxalactam.[11] The MTT side chain can dissociate from the parent cephalosporin and act as a competitive inhibitor of the vitamin K–dependent carboxylase responsible for converting clotting factors II, VII, IX, and X to active forms.[146] In addition, the side chain (like warfarin) may inhibit vitamin K 2,3-epoxide reductase, which converts vitamin K to its active form.[147] These reactions can lead to prolongation of the prothrombin time and clinically significant bleeding. Patients with poor nutritional status, advanced age, and recent surgery on the gastrointestinal tract are at increased risk for clinically significant bleeding.[148-151] In addition, patients with renal failure may be at increased risk for bleeding because of the accumulation of the side chain.[152] Vitamin K administration rapidly reverses the abnormality in 24 to 36 hours. The MTT side chain can also produce a disulfiram-like reaction with ethanol ingestion that may persist for several days after antibiotic administration.[12,153] The disulfiram reaction is manifest with flushing, tachycardia, headache, sweating, nausea, vomiting, hypotension, confusion, or blurred vision. The reaction is due to a block in alcohol metabolism at the acetaldehyde step resulting in the accumulation of acetaldehyde and subsequent symptoms.

A variety of adverse reactions in the gastrointestinal tract have been reported with variable frequency. Diarrhea is the most commonly reported side effect, with rates ranging from 1% to 20%.[134,154] Upper gastrointestinal symptoms occur much less frequently. Mild and transient hepatic toxicity has been reported with most compounds from the class, manifest as two- to fourfold elevations in transaminase levels in up to 7% of patients.[155] Obstructive biliary toxicity has also been reported with ceftriaxone.[156,157] The high biliary ceftriaxone concentrations have resulted in crystallization of a ceftriaxone-calcium salt and the clinical syndrome of biliary pseudolithiasis. This biliary abnormality has been reported most commonly in children receiving high ceftriaxone doses and in patients with preexisting biliary abnormalities.[158] The syndrome is reversible and in most reports has cleared in 10 to 60 days after discontinuing the drug.

Adverse reactions in the nervous system are uncommon and are similar to those reported with other β-lactams. Seizures have been reported in patients with renal insufficiency receiving high doses of these drugs.[159] Decreased protein binding and inhibition of the choroid plexus pump occur with uremia and may contribute to enhanced toxicity in patients with renal impairment. Local phlebitis reactions related to intravenous administration of the parenteral compounds have been reported with variable frequency ranging from 1% to 5%.[160] On the other hand, pain associated with intramuscular administration is common with all of the parenteral compounds.[161] The local discomfort can be reduced by use of 1% lidocaine in diluent. With the exception of once-daily intramuscular ceftriaxone, most parenteral cephalosporins are administered by the intravenous route.

The cephalosporins have not been studied extensively in pregnancy. All drugs in the cephalosporin group are placed in pregnancy class B.[162,163] All of the compounds are secreted to a small degree into breast milk, but as a class they are considered safe for use in this situation.[162]

In addition to the false-positive Coombs test, laboratory abnormalities in urine glucose and serum creatinine have been reported with certain cephalosporins. A false-positive glucosuria test performed by the copper reduction technique (Clinitest) has been reported with cefaclor, cefadroxil, cefamandole, cefonicid, cefotaxime, cefoxitin, and ceftazidime.[164] Similarly, a false increase in serum creatinine has been reported in patients receiving cefoxitin and cephalothin in laboratories utilizing the Jaffe technique.[165]

Because the cephalosporins have broad-spectrum activity, superinfection or overgrowth of *Candida* in the gastrointestinal and vaginal tracts can occur.[166,167] Similarly, overgrowth of *Clostridium difficile* in the gastrointestinal tract with diarrhea and less commonly colitis has been associated with cephalosporin use.[168] However, the incidence of these superinfections is similar to rates reported with drugs from other antibiotic classes.

CLINICAL USE OF SPECIFIC DRUGS

The usual dosing regimens for adults and children for the various cephalosporins by generation are listed in Table 20-7. The daily doses to use for serious infections are also listed.

First-Generation Cephalosporins

The first-generation cephalosporins have been extensively used as alternatives to penicillin for staphylococcal and nonenterococcal streptococcal infections. Most commonly, these include skin and soft tissue infections. Among the parenteral first-generation cephalosporins, *cephalothin* and *cephapirin* are no longer available in the United States. Both drugs were metabolized and rapidly eliminated by renal excretion and required frequent dosing. *Cefazolin* is not metabolized and is eliminated more by glomerular filtration than by tubular excretion.[127] Its moderate protein binding slows the glomerular filtration of the drug, resulting in a half-life of 1.5 to 2 hours, which allows 8- and 12-hourly dosing. With co-administration of probenecid, cefazolin has been effective in skin and soft tissue infections with once-daily dosing.[169] Cefazolin is still recommended in penicillin-allergic patients for more serious staphylococcal infections, such as endocarditis, even though the drug is more readily hydrolyzed by staphylococcal β-lactamase than other first-generation cephalosporins.[170-172] Cefazolin is recommended as the prophylactic antibiotic of choice for foreign-body implantation and many clean and clean contaminated surgical procedures in which there is a high risk of infection.[173,174] These include cardiac and vascular surgery, insertion of orthopedic devices, head and neck surgery that crosses the oropharyngeal mucosal barrier, vaginal and abdominal hysterectomy, high-risk cesarean sections, and high-risk gastroduodenal and biliary tract procedures. Because of its poor activity against *Bacteroides* species, cefazolin alone is not recommended for intraabdominal procedures that involve the intestine.

The oral first-generation cephalosporins, *cephalexin*, *cephradine*, and *cefadroxil*, have very high oral bioavailability. Cefadroxil has a slightly longer half-life than cephalexin and cephradine, which allows twice-daily dosing instead of the usual four times a day.[91] These drugs provide appropriate outpatient therapy for many skin and soft tissue infections. However, these drugs are not effective for animal bites and scratches involving *Pasteurella multocida*.[175] The drugs are quite active against *Streptococcus pyogenes* and provide effective therapy in streptococcal pharyngitis.[176,177] They have poor activity against penicillin-resistant pneumococci, *H. influenzae*, and *M. catarrhalis*, and are not recommended for sinusitis, otitis media, and lower respiratory tract infections. The drugs are effective in uncomplicated urinary tract infections. However, they are less effective than trimethoprim-sulfamethoxazole and fluoroquinolones.[178,179]

Second-Generation Cephalosporins

This group includes the cephamycins as well as true cephalosporins. The two groups of drugs have different spectra of antimicrobial activity and clinical uses. The true cephalosporins have increased activity against *H. influenzae*, *M. catarrhalis*, and *Neisseria* species and comparable activity against staphylococci and nonenterococcal streptococci. On the other hand, the cephamycins have inferior activity against staphylococci but enhanced antibacterial activity against certain Enterobacteriaceae. The cephamycins are especially noted for their activity against anaerobic bacteria, especially *B. fragilis*. They also demonstrate good in vitro activity against ESBL-producing strains of *E. coli* and *K. pneumoniae*. However, their reliability in treating infections caused by ESBL-producing strains has not been proved.

Because of their activity against *S. pneumoniae*, *H. influenzae*, and *M. catarrhalis*, the true second-generation cephalosporins have been used extensively for treatment of various respiratory tract infections in hospitalized patients.[180-182] *Cefuroxime* has become the preferred agent, compared with *cefamandole* and *cefonicid*, because of its lower serum protein binding and improved central nervous system penetration. Cefuroxime can be used to treat meningitis caused by penicillin-susceptible pneumococci, *H. influenzae*, and *Neisseria meningitidis*.[183]

TABLE 20-7 Dosing Regimens of Cephalosporins in Adults and Children

| Cephalosporin | Adults | | Children |
	Usual Dose	Severe Disease	Usual Dose
First Generation			
Cefazolin	0.5-1 g q8-12h	2 g q6-8h	12.5-33 mg/kg q6-8h
Cephalothin	0.5-1 g q6h	2 g q4-6h	20-25 mg/kg q6h
Cephapirin	0.5-1 g q6h	2 g q4-6h	10-20 mg/kg q6h
Cephradine	0.5-1 g q6h	2 g q4-6h	12.5-25 mg/kg q6h
Second Generation			
Cefamandole	1 g q6h	2 g q4h	12.5-25 mg/kg q4-6h
Cefonicid	1 g q24h	2 g q24h	50 mg/kg q24h
Cefuroxime	0.75-1.5 g q8h	1.5 g q8h	12.5-60 mg/kg q6-8h
Cephamycins			
Cefmetazole	1-2 g q8h	2 g q6h	Not recommended
Cefotetan	1-2 g q12h	2-3 g q12h	Not recommended
Cefoxitin	1-2 g q6h	2 g q4-6h	20-25 mg/kg q4-6h
Third Generation			
Cefoperazone	1-2 g q12h	2-4 g q8h	Not recommended
Cefotaxime	1 g q8-12h	2 g q4-8h	25-30 mg/kg q4-6h
Ceftazidime	1 g q8-12h	2 g q8h	30-50 mg/kg q8h
Ceftizoxime	1 g q8-12h	2 g q8-12h	50 mg/kg q6-8h
Ceftriaxone	1 g q24h	2 g q12-24h	50-100 mg/kg q24h
Moxalactam	1 g q8h	2 g q8h	Not recommended
Fourth Generation			
Cefepime	1 g q12h	2 g q8-12h	50 mg/kg q8h
Cefpirome	1 g q12h	2 g q12h	Not recommended
Oral—First Generation			
Cephalexin	250-500 mg qid	1 g qid	6.25-25 mg/kg qid
Cephradine	250-500 mg qid	500 mg qid	6.25-25 mg/kg qid
Cefadroxil	500 mg bid	1 g bid	15 mg/kg bid
Oral—Second Generation			
Cefaclor	250 mg tid or 375 mg bid	500 gm tid	8.3-16.7 mg/kg tid
Cefprozil	250-500 mg bid	500 mg bid	7.5-15 mg/kg bid
Cefuroxime (axetil)	250-500 mg bid	500 mg bid	10-15 mg/kg bid
Loracarbef	200 mg bid	400 mg bid	7.5-15 mg/kg bid
Oral—Third Generation			
Cefdinir	300 mg bid or 600 mg qd	300 mg bid or 600 mg qd	7 mg/kg bid or 14 mg/kg qd
Cefditoren	200-400 mg bid	400 mg bid	Not recommended
Cefixime	200 mg bid or 400 mg qd	400 mg bid	4 mg/kg bid or 8 mg/kg qd
Cefpodoxime	200-400 mg bid	400 mg bid	5 mg/kg bid
Ceftibuten	400 mg qd	400 mg qd	9 mg/kg qd

However, it has been largely replaced by third-generation cephalosporins that result in faster eradication of bacteria from the CSF.[184] Cefuroxime has been one of the recommended agents for empirical therapy of community-acquired pneumonia in hospitalized patients.[185,186] Although cefuroxime has good activity against penicillin-susceptible and penicillin-intermediate strains of *S. pneumoniae*, its activity against most penicillin-resistant strains is suboptimal. In an observational study of 844 patients with pneumococcal bacteremia, mostly related to pneumonia, resistance to cefuroxime was associated with significantly greater mortality.[187] The latest recommendations on community-required pneumonia no longer include cefuroxime as a recommended agent for initial empirical therapy.[188] Cefuroxime, cefamandole, and cefonicid provide effective therapy for other serious infections caused by susceptible pathogens, including skin and soft tissue infections, epiglottitis, complicated sinusitis, and gynecologic infections.[181,182,189] Cefamandole is more susceptible to β-lactamase inactivation by β-lactamase–positive strains of *H. influenzae*.[181] Cefonicid, which has slow elimination because of its very high protein binding of 98%, can be administered once daily. However, failures have occurred in more serious infections, primarily *S. aureus* bacteremia.[182] None of these cephalosporins should be considered for empirical therapy of nosocomial pneumonia or other nosocomial infections because of their poor activity against most strains of *Enterobacter, Citrobacter, Serratia, Morganella,* and *P. aeruginosa*.

The oral second-generation cephalosporins, including *cefuroxime axetil, cefprozil, cefaclor,* and *loracarbef,* are effective for treatment of a variety of mild to moderate community-acquired infections. Double-tap studies in acute otitis media and acute maxillary sinusitis have demonstrated that bacterial eradication is related to the drug's ability to produce serum concentrations that exceed the MIC of the infecting pathogen for 40% to 50% of the dosing interval.[190-193] In this regard, cefuroxime axetil and cefprozil are the best agents for *S. pneumoniae* and are effective against penicillin-susceptible isolates and most penicillin-intermediate strains. Cefaclor and loracarbef are primarily active only against penicillin-susceptible strains. None of the oral second-generation cephalosporins provide optimal therapy for penicillin-resistant pneumococci. For *H. influenzae* and *M. catarrhalis,* cefuroxime axetil would be a more optimal choice than cefprozil, cefaclor, and loracarbef. Clinical and bacteriologic outcomes have demonstrated that 5- to 10-day courses of therapy with the second-generation cephalosporins are equivalent to or more effective than 10 days of therapy with penicillin V for the treatment of group A, β-hemolytic streptococcal pharyngitis.[194-196] Cefuroxime axetil is also a recommended alternative to doxycycline and penicillin for treatment of early Lyme disease.[197]

The cephamycins, *cefoxitin, cefotetan,* and *cefmetazole,* have provided effective therapy for a variety of infections involving aerobic gram-negative and anaerobic organisms, especially *B. fragilis*. These infections include intra-abdominal, pelvic, and gynecologic infections; infected decubitus ulcers; diabetic foot infections; and mixed aerobic-anaerobic soft tissue infections.[198-201] Cefoxitin and cefotetan are the agents primarily used. Cefotetan has a half-life of 3 to 4 hours because of its high protein binding and can be administered twice daily rather than every 8 hours with cefmetazole and every 6 hours with cefoxitin. Cefmetazole and cefotetan both contain the MTT side chain, which increases their potential for hypoprothrombinemia and disulfiram reactions. In terms of antimicrobial activity, cefotetan is more active than cefoxitin and cefmetazole against gram-negative bacilli but is less active against non–*B. fragilis* members of the *B. fragilis* group.[202,203] The significance of these differences is not clear. Of more importance, as many as 15% of *B. fragilis* strains can be resistant to the various cephamycins, and drugs with better anaerobic activity should be used for empirical therapy of serious *Bacteroides* infections.[202] All of the cephamycins are active against *N. gonorrhoeae,* including penicillin-resistant strains. However, recommended therapy for infections with this organism is with ceftriaxone, which is effective as a single dose.[203] Cefoxitin and cefotetan, in combination with doxycycline, provide effective therapy for pelvic inflammatory disease.[204,205] For antimicrobial prophylaxis during surgery, cefoxitin and cefotetan are recommended over cefazolin only for colorectal procedures and appendectomies.[173,174] For elective colorectal surgery, cefoxitin or cefotetan is still commonly administered even when an oral bowel preparation with erythromycin and neomycin is used.

Third-Generation Cephalosporins

The third-generation cephalosporins are major drugs for the treatment of many important infections because of their high antibacterial potency, wide spectrum of activity, low potential for toxicity, and favorable pharmacokinetics, such as enhanced drug concentrations in the CSF. They have been especially useful in infections resulting from gram-negative bacilli that are resistant to other β-lactam antibiotics. However, their superior activity against the Enterobacteriaceae is being challenged by the increasing frequency of organisms with β-lactamase–mediated resistance. New AmpC β-lactamases and ESBLs, which inactivate third-generation cephalosporins, may represent a distinct threat to the continued utility of these agents.

Cefotaxime, ceftriaxone, ceftizoxime, and *ceftazidime* are the major parenteral third-generation cephalosporins in clinical use for the treatment of nosocomial infections caused by susceptible gram-negative bacilli. Cefotaxime and ceftriaxone are also two of the most potent cephalosporins against penicillin-resistant pneumococci. Because of its high protein binding, ceftriaxone has the longest half-life and is usually administered once daily. Ceftizoxime and ceftazidime are given two or three times daily, and effective dosing of cefotaxime, which has the shortest half-life, has varied from every 4 hours to twice daily. Ceftazidime is usually reserved for infections that are likely to involve *P. aeruginosa. Cefoperazone* is another third-generation cephalosporin with modest activity against strains of *P. aeruginosa.*[206] The availability of the drug in the United States has declined. It differs from the other third-generation cephalosporins in that the majority of the drug is eliminated by biliary secretion. *Moxalactam* is an oxacephem that has a methoxy group at position 7 similar to that in the cephamycins. The drug has activity against gram-negative bacilli similar to that of other third-generation cephalosporins.[207] Both cefoperazone and moxalactam have the MTT group at position 3. Moxalactam also has an acyl carboxyl group that produces a defect in platelet aggregation. Significant bleeding complications have been observed with its use, especially when administered three times a day.[208] The drug is not available for use in the United States.

Monotherapy with cefotaxime, ceftriaxone, and ceftizoxime has provided effective treatment for a variety of nosocomial infections caused by susceptible gram-negative bacilli, including complicated skin and soft tissue infections, pneumonia, complicated urinary tract infections, and intra-abdominal infections, such as peritonitis.[209-214] However, cephalosporin monotherapy for infections caused primarily by *Enterobacter, Citrobacter*, and *Serratia* species can be complicated

by the emergence of stably derepressed resistant mutants.[215,216] Combination antimicrobial therapy may be beneficial in reducing this emergence of resistance resulting from increased chromosomal β-lactamase production.[216] Organisms containing ESBLs have also been observed to fail therapy with cephalosporins even when the organism tested susceptible in laboratory tests.[78] The carbapenems are the recommended drugs for these ESBL-producing strains.

Cefotaxime, ceftriaxone, and, to a lesser degree, ceftizoxime have provided effective therapy for meningitis caused by a variety of different bacteria.[217-221] They are the drugs of choice for meningitis caused by *H. influenzae* and various Enterobacteriaceae.[222] Cefotaxime and ceftriaxone also provide effective therapy for meningitis caused by *N. meningitidis* and by pneumococci that have MICs of 0.5 g/mL or less. Organisms with higher MICs have failed monotherapy with these cephalosporins. As a result, empirical therapy with cefotaxime or ceftriaxone is combined with vancomycin (with or without rifampin) until the laboratory determines the susceptibility of the pneumococcal isolate.[222] If the organism is susceptible to cefotaxime or ceftriaxone, the vancomycin (and rifampin) can be discontinued. Treatment of meningitis requires maximal doses of these cephalosporins, such as 2 g every 12 hours in adults and 50 mg/kg twice daily or 100 mg/kg once daily in children for ceftriaxone and 2 g every 4 to 6 hours in adults and 100 to 150 mg/kg every 4 to 6 hours in children for cefotaxime.

Cefotaxime and ceftriaxone continue to be active against most bacteria producing community-acquired pneumonia. In a large observational study of pneumococcal bacteremia, resistance to cefotaxime and ceftriaxone was not associated with higher mortality.[187] Cefotaxime and ceftriaxone were also effective in treating patients with nonmeningeal pneumococcal infections, mostly pneumonia, caused by strains with MICs as high as 2 μg/mL.[223] The National Committee for Clinical Laboratory Standards has created higher susceptibility and resistance breakpoints for pneumococci causing nonmeningeal infections than for *S. pneumoniae* causing meningitis.[224,225] As a result of these changes, cefotaxime and ceftriaxone are active against most penicillin-resistant pneumococci and are recommended, in combination with a macrolide, for empirical therapy for community-acquired pneumonia requiring hospitalization.[185,186,188] Single intramuscular doses of ceftriaxone are also highly effective in eradicating *H. influenzae* and penicillin-susceptible strains of *S. pneumoniae* from middle ear fluid.[226] However, three daily doses of ceftriaxone were required in one study to eradicate penicillin-resistant pneumococci.[227]

The oral third-generation cephalosporins, which include *cefdinir, cefditoren pivoxyl, cefixime, cefpodoxime proxetil,* and *ceftibuten,* are approved for oral therapy of mild to moderate respiratory infections, such as otitis media, sinusitis, and acute exacerbations of chronic bronchitis. These drugs have potent activity against *H. influenzae,* but their activity against pneumococci is more variable.[228-231] Cefdinir, cefditoren, and cefpodoxime have activity similar to that of cefuroxime and cefprozil and are active against penicillin-susceptible and most penicillin-intermediate strains of *S. pneumoniae.* Cefixime is active only against penicillin-susceptible strains, and ceftibuten is even marginal with penicillin-susceptible pneumococci. Short courses of most of these drugs have also provided equivalent rates of eradication in group A, β-hemolytic streptococcal pharyngitis.[232-235] Their increased potency over other oral cephalosporins for *E. coli, K. pneumonia,* and *Enterobacter, Citrobacter,* and *Serratia* species enhances their utility for treatment of complicated urinary tract infections.[236]

Ceftazidime is the third-generation cephalosporin used for serious infections in which *P. aeruginosa* is documented or highly likely. It is one of the recommended drugs, either alone or in combination with an aminoglycoside, for initial empirical management of febrile neutropenic patients.[237] However, ESBLs and AmpC β-lactamases have reduced the utility of ceftazidime for monotherapy. Continuous infusion of ceftazidime has been used to increase trough concentrations. However, trials of intermittent versus continuous administration have not demonstrated any significant difference in efficacy.[238,239] Ceftazidime has been effective for the treatment of acute exacerbations of chronic pulmonary infections in patients with cystic fibrosis.[240] The drug penetrates into CSF and is the treatment of choice for meningitis caused by *P. aeruginosa*.[241]

Third-generation cephalosporins have also become established therapy for a variety of specific infections. Ceftriaxone is highly active against *N. gonorrhoeae*, including penicillin- and quinolone-resistant strains. It is the drug of choice for all forms of gonococcal infection and is used in combination with doxycycline for pelvic inflammatory disease, proctitis, and proctocolitis.[204,242] A single oral dose of cefixime is also highly effective for uncomplicated gonococcal infections of the cervix, urethra, and rectum.[243,244] Single-dose intramuscular ceftriaxone is recommended therapy for chancroid.[204] Ceftriaxone and cefotaxime are recommended therapy for treatment of early Lyme disease in patients with neurologic involvement or third-degree atrioventricular heart block.[245] These drugs are also recommended for patients with both arthritis and objective evidence of neurologic disease and those with late neurologic disease affecting the central or peripheral nervous system. Although several small studies have suggested that ceftriaxone is effective therapy for syphilis in penicillin-allergic patients, tetracyclines are the currently recommended alternative therapy.[246,247] Ceftriaxone is a recommended alternative therapy for typhoid fever and for severe infections with *Shigella* species and nontyphi species of *Salmonella*.[248,249] Third-generation cephalosporins have provided effective therapy for focal salmonella infections, brain abscess caused by gram-negative bacilli, and endocarditis caused by fastidious gram-negative coccobacilli.[250,251] Single doses of ceftriaxone are highly effective in eradicating nasopharyngeal carriage of *N. meningitidis*.[252,253] The long half-life of ceftriaxone, which allows once-daily dosing, has enhanced its use in the outpatient setting for both streptococcal and staphylococcal infections. Ceftriaxone has been effective for the outpatient treatment of staphylococcal and streptococcal skin and soft tissue infections including osteomyelitis.[254,255] The drug is also effective as monotherapy for the outpatient treatment of nonenterococcal streptococcal endocarditis.[256]

Fourth-Generation Cephalosporins

The fourth-generation cephalosporins have the widest spectrum of all the cephalosporins. They have enhanced activity against certain gram-negative bacilli, such as *Enterobacter*, *Citrobacter*, and *Serratia* species. These drugs are zwitterions, which cross the outer membrane of gram-negative bacilli more rapidly than other cephalosporins.[257] They are also less susceptible to inactivation by AmpC β-lactamases.[258] Thus, about 75% to 80% of the Enterobacteriaceae resistant to ceftazidime are susceptible to the fourth-generation drugs. They are active against *P. aeruginosa* and, unlike ceftazidime, maintain good potency against gram-positive cocci. Only two agents have been developed so far. *Cefepime* has a slightly longer half-life than ceftazidime and is usually administered twice daily, although 8-hour dosing is recommended for documented *P. aeruginosa* infections. *Cefpirome*, which is not available in the United States, has a pharmacokinetic profile very similar to that of cefepime. Both of these agents maintain excellent activity against methicillin-susceptible *S. aureus*, *S. pneumoniae* (including most penicillin-resistant strains), and other streptococci.[259,260]

The role of fourth-generation cephalosporins, in relation to the third-generation drugs, has not yet been determined. At some hospitals, the fourth-generation agents have largely replaced the third-generation cephalosporins for treatment of serious gram-negative bacillary infections. They have proved to be effective in a variety of serious gram-negative infections such as bacteremia, pneumonia, skin and soft tissue infections, and complicated urinary tract infections.[258,261,262] With continuous infusion of cefepime, optimal efficacy was observed when serum concentrations were at least fourfold above the MIC.[263] Comparative trials with ceftazidime or other agents have generally demonstrated equivalent efficacy.[264-268] Still, cefepime has demonstrated efficacy against organisms with reduced susceptibility or resistance to ceftazidime.[269] Cefepime is recommended as monotherapy or in combination with an aminoglycoside for initial empirical therapy in febrile neutropenic patients.[237,270] Cefepime appears to require the addition of vancomycin less frequently than with ceftazidime. The drug is one of the recommended agents for the empirical treatment of severe community-acquired pneumonia when *P. aeruginosa* is suspected.[188] The drug's activity against pneumococci is similar to that of ceftriaxone. Cefepime has demonstrated results comparable to those with ceftriaxone in patients with community-acquired pneumonia requiring hospitalization.[271,272] The drug penetrates well into CSF and produces outcomes similar to those with cefotaxime in acute bacterial meningitis.[273,274] Although emergence of resistance during therapy may be less of a problem with the fourth-generation cephalosporins, it does occur. Many of the new ESBLs, especially the new CTX-M enzymes, can inactivate these fourth-generation drugs.

REFERENCES

1. Bo G. Giuseppe Brotzu and the discovery of cephalosporins. Clin Microbiol Infect. 2000;6(Suppl 3):6-9.
2. Sykes RB. From moulds to drugs. Clin Microbiol Infect. 2000;6(Suppl 3)10-12.
3. Rolinson GN. The influence of 6-aminoenicillanic acid on antibiotic development. J Antimicrob Chemother. 1988;22:5-14.
4. Neu HC. Structure-activity relations of new β-lactam compounds and in vitro activity against common bacteria. Rev Infect Dis. 1983;5(Suppl 2):S319-S336.
5. Neu HC. β-Lactam antibiotics: Structural relationships affecting in vitro activity and pharmacologic properties. Rev Infect Dis. 1986;8(Suppl 3):S237-S259.
6. Onishi HR, Daoust DR, Zimmerman SB, et al. Cefoxitin, a semisynthetic cephamycin antibiotic: Resistance to β-lactamase inactivation. Antimicrob Agents Chemother. 1974;5:38-48.
7. Stapley EO, Birnbaum J. Chemistry and microbiological properties of the cephamycins. In: Salton MRJ, Shockman GD, eds. Beta-Lactam Antibiotics. New York: Academic Press; 1981:327-351.
8. Dunn GL. Ceftizoxime and other third generation cephalosporins: Structure-activity relationships. J Antimicrob Chemother. 1982;10(Suppl C):l-10.
9. Naito T, Aburki S, Kamachi H, et al. Synthesis and structure activity relationship of a new series of cephalosporins, BMY-28142 and related compounds. J Antibiot. 1986;39:1092-1107.
10. Turnidge JD, Craig WA. Beta-lactam pharmacology in liver disease. J Antimicrob Chemother. 1983;11:499-501.
11. Bechtold H, Andrassy K, Jahnchen E, et al. Evidence for impaired hepatic vitamin K metabolism in patients treated with N-methyl-thiotetrazole cephalosporins. Thomb Haemost. 1984;51:358-361.
12. Buening MK, Wold JS, Israel KS, et al. Disulfiram-like reactions to β-lactams. JAMA. 1981;245:2027.
13. Hanaki H, Akagi H, Nomura S, et al. Structure-activity relationships of cephalosporin derivatives against methicillin-resistant *Staphylococcus aureus* and *Enterococcus faecalis*. J Antibiot. 1996;49:402-404.
14. Hecker SJ, Cho IS, Glinka TW, et al. Discovery of MC-02,331, a new cephalosporin exhibiting potent activity against methicillin resistant *Staphylococcus aureus*. J Antibiot. 1998;51:722-734.
15. Yoshizawa H, Itani H, Ishikura K, et al. S-3578, a new broad spectrum parenteral cephalosporin exhibiting potent activity against both methicillin-resistant *Staphylococcus aureus* (MRSA) and *Pseudomonas aeruginosa*: Synthesis and structure-activity relationships. J Antibiot. 2002;55:975-992.
16. Hecker SJ, Calkins T, Price ME, et al. Prodrugs of cephalosporin RWJ-333441 (MC-04,546) with improved aqueous solubility. Antimicrob Agents Chemother. 2003;47:2043-2046.
17. Wise EM Jr, Park JT. Penicillin: Its basic site of action as an inhibitor of a peptide cross-linking reaction in cell wall mucopeptide synthesis. Proc Natl Acad Sci USA. 1965;54:75-81.
18. Virudachalam R, Rao VS. Theoretical studies on beta-lactam antibiotics. I. Conformational similarity of penicillin and cephalosporins to X-D-alanyl-D-alanine and correlation of their structure with activity. Int J Peptide Protein Res. 1977;10:51-59.
19. Waxman DJ, Strominger JL. Penicillin binding proteins and the mechanism of action of beta-lactam antibiotics. Annu Rev Biochem. 1983;52:825-869.
20. Spratt BG. Distinct penicillin-binding protein involved in the division, elongation and shape of *Escherichia coli* K12. Proc Natl Acad Sci USA. 1975;72:2999-3003.
21. Spratt BG. Properties of the penicillin-binding proteins of *Escherichia coli* K12. Eur J Biochem. 1977;72:341-352.
22. Vogelman B, Craig WA. Kinetics of antimicrobial activity. J Pediatr. 1986;108: 835-840.
23. Bundtzen RW, Gerber AU, Cohn D, Craig WA. Post-antibiotic suppression of bacterial growth. Rev Infect Dis. 1981;3:28-37.
24. Craig WA. Interrelationship between pharmacokinetics and pharmacodynamics in determining dosage regimens for broad-spectrum cephalosporins. Diagn Microbiol Infect Dis. 1995;22:89-96.
25. Craig WA. Pharmacokinetic/pharmacodynamic parameters: Rationale for antibacterial dosing of mice and men. Clin Infect Dis. 1998;26:1-12.
26. Bergeron MG, Bausch JL, Barza M, et al. Bactericidal activity and pharmacology of cefazolin. Antimicrob Agents Chemother. 1973;4:396-401.
27. Sabath LD, Wilcox C, Garner C, et al. In vitro activity of cefazolin against recent clinical bacterial isolates. J Infect Dis. 1973;128(Suppl):S320-S326.

28. Bill NJ, Washington JA. Comparison of in vitro activity of cephalexin, cephradine and cefaclor. Antimicrob Agents Chemother. 1977;11:470-474.

29. Sanders CC. In vitro studies with cefaclor, a new oral cephalosporin. Antimicrob Agents Chemother. 1977;12:490-497.

30. Hartstein AI, Patrick KE, Jones SR, et al. Comparison of pharmacologic antimicrobial properties of cephadroxil and cephalexin. Antimicrob Agents Chemother. 1977;12:93-97.

31. Birnbaum J. Stapley EO, Miller AK, et al. Cefoxitin, a semi-synthetic cephamycin: A microbiologic overview. J Antimicrob Chemother. 1978;4:15-32.

32. Eickhoff TC, Ehret JM. In vitro comparison of cefoxitin, cefamandole, cephalexin, and cephalothin. Antimicrob Agents Chemother. 1976;9:994-999.

33. Greenwood D, Pearson N, Eley A, et al. Comparative in-vitro activities of cefotaxime and ceftizoxime (FK 749): New cephalosporins with exceptional potency. Antimicrob Agents Chemother. 1980;17:397-401.

34. Acuna G, Johnston J, Young LS, et al. In-vitro studies with ceftazidime against aerobic gram-negative bacilli and Bacteroides fragilis group. J Antimicrob Chemother. 1981;8(Suppl B):83-89.

35. Cleeland R, Squires E. Antimicrobial activity of ceftriaxone, a review. Am J Med. 1984;77:3-11.

36. Ayers LW, Jones RN, Barry AL, et al. Cefotetan, a new cephamycin: Comparison of in vitro antimicrobial activity with other cephems, beta-lactamase stability, and preliminary recommendations for disk diffusion testing. Antimicrob Agents Chemother. 1982;22:859-877.

37. Jones RN. Review of the in-vitro spectrum and characteristics of cefmetazole (CS-1170). J Antimicrob Chemother. 1989;12(Suppl D):1-12.

38. Goldstein EJC, Citron DM. Annual incidence, epidemiology and comparative in vitro susceptibilities to cefoxitin, cefotetan, cefmetazole and ceftizoxime of recent community-acquired isolates of the Bacteroides fragilis group. J Antimicrob Chemother. 26:2361-2366.

39. Barry AL, Jones RN. Cefixime: Spectrum of antibacterial activity against 16016 clinical isolates. Pediatr Infect Dis J. 1987;6:954-957.

40. King A, Boothman C, Phillips I. Comparative in vitro activity of cefpirome and cefepime, two new cephalosporins. Eur J Clin Microbiol Infect Dis. 1990;9:677-685.

41. Arguedas AG, Arrieta AC, Sutman HR, et al. In-vitro activity of cefprozil (BMY 28100) and loracarbef (LY 163892) against pathogens obtained from middle ear fluid. J Antimicrob Chemother. 1991;27:311-318.

42. Bragman SGL, Casewell MW. The in-vitro activity of ceftibuten against 475 clinical isolates of gram-negative bacilli, compared with cefuroxime and cefadroxil. J Antimicrob Chemother. 1990;25:221-226.

43. Jones RN, Barry AL, Collaborative Antimicrobial Susceptibility Testing Group. Ceftibuten (7432-S, SCH 39720): Comparative antimicrobial activity against 4735 clinical isolates, beta-lactamase stability and broth microdilution quality control guidelines. Eur J Clin Microbiol Infect Dis. 1988;7:802-807.

44. Debbia EA, Pesce A, Chiesa M, et al. Microbiological profile of ceftibuten, a new oral cephalosporin. Drugs Exp Clin Res. 1992;18:129-139.

45. Briggs BN, Jones RN, Erwin ME, et al. In vitro activity evaluations of cefdinir (FK482, Cl-983, and PD134393): A novel orally administered cephalosporin. Diagn Microbiol Infect Dis. 1991;14:425-434.

46. Jones RN, Biedenbach DJ, Croco MAT, et al. In vitro evaluation of a novel orally administered cephalosporin (cefditoren) tested against 1249 recent clinical isolates of Haemophilus influenzae, Moraxella catarrhalis, and Streptococcus pneumoniae. Diagn Microbiol Infect Dis. 1998;31:573-578.

47. Clark CE, Naomi K, Dewasse BE, et al. Activity of cefditoren against respiratory pathogens. Int J Antimicrob Agents. 2002;50:33-41.

48. Jones RN, Pfaller MA, Doern GV, et al. Antimicrobial activity and spectrum investigation of eight broad-spectrum beta-lactam drugs: A 1997 surveillance trial in 102 medical centers in the United States. Cefepime Study Group. Diagn Microbiol Infect Dis. 1998;30:215-228.

49. Karlowsky JA, Jones MY, Hayfield DC, et al. Ceftriaxone activity against gram-positive and gram-negative pathogens isolated in US clinical microbiology laboratories from 1996 to 2000: Results from The Surveillance Network (TSN) Database-USA. Int J Antimicrob Agents. 2002;19:413-426.

50. Jones RN, Kirby IT, Beach ML, et al. Geographic variations in activity of broad-spectrum beta-lactams against Pseudomonas aeruginosa: Summary of the worldwide SENTRY Antimicrobial Surveillance Program (1997-2000). Diagn Microbiol Infect Dis. 2002;43:239-243.

51. Spangler SK, Jacobs MR, Pankuch GA, et al. Susceptibility of 170 penicillin-susceptible and penicillin-resistant pneumococci to six oral cephalosporins, four quinolones, desacetyl cefotaxime, Ro 23-9424 and RP 67829. J Antimicrob Chemother. 1993;31:273-280.

52. Thornsberry C, Ogilvie P, Kahn J, et al. Surveillance of antimicrobial resistance in Streptococcus pneumoniae, Haemophilus influenzae, and Moraxella catarrhalis in the United States in 1996-97 respiratory season. Diagn Microbial Infect Dis. 1997;29:249-257.

53. Doern GV, Jones RN, Pfaller MA, Kugler K. Haemophilus influenzae and Moraxella catarrhalis from patients with community-acquired respiratory tract infections: Antimicrobial susceptibility patterns from the SENTRY antimicrobial Surveillance Program (United States and Canada, 1997). Antimicrob Agents Chemother. 1999;43:385-389.

54. Hoban D, Waites K, Felmingham D. Antimicrobial susceptibility of community-acquired respiratory tract pathogens in North America in 1999-2000: Findings of the PROTEKT surveillance study. Diagn Microbiol Infect Dis. 2003;45:251-259.

55. Karlowsky JA, Critchley IA, Blosser-Middleton RS, et al. Antimicrobial surveillance of Haemophilus influenzae in the United States during 2000-2001 leads to detection of clonal dissemination of a beta-lactamase–negative and ampicillin-resistant strain. J Clin Microbiol. 2002;40:1063-1066.

56. Glinka T, Huie K, Cho A, et al. Relationships between structure, antibacterial activity, serum stability, pharmacokinetics and efficacy in 3-(heteroarylthio)cephems. Discovery of RWJ-333441 (MC-04,546). Bioorg Med Chem 2003;11:591-600.

57. Fung-Tomc JC, Clark J, Minassian B, et al. In vitro and in vivo activities of a novel cephalosporin, BMS-247243, against methicillin-resistant and -susceptible staphylococci. Antimicrob Agents Chemother. 2002;46:971-976.

58. Chow AW, Finegold SM. In-vitro activity of ceftizoxime against anaerobic bacteria and comparison with other cephalosporins. J Antimicrob Chemother. 1982;10 (Suppl C):45-50.

59. Murray RP, Jones RN, Allen SD, et al. Multilaboratory evaluation of the in vitro activity of 13 β-lactam antibiotics against 1474 clinical isolates of aerobic and anaerobic bacteria. Diagn Microbiol Infect Dis. 1993;16:191-203.

60. Ferrari M, Galla F, Pagnes P. In vitro antitreponemic activity of twelve cephalosporins. Chemotherapy. 1965;10:305-311.

61. Hunfeld KP, Rodel R, Wichelhaus TA. In vitro activity of eight oral cephalosporins against Borrelia burgdorferi. Int J Antimicrob Agents. 2003;21:313-318.

62. Segreti J, Kapell KS, Trenholme GM. In vitro activity of beta-lactam drugs and sulbactam against Chlamydia trachomatis. Diagn Microbiol Infect Dis. 1992;15:371-373.

63. Cormican MG, Jones RN. Antimicrobial activity of cefotaxime tested against infrequently isolated pathogenic species (unusual pathogens). Diagn Microbiol Infect Dis. 1995;22:43-48.

64. Stewart SM, Burnet ME, Young JE. In vitro sensitivity of strains of mycoplasmas from human sources to antibiotics and to sodium aurothiomalate and tylosin tartrate. J Med Microbiol. 1969;2:287-292.

65. Livermore DM. Mechanisms of resistance to cephalosporin antibiotics. Drugs. 1987;34(Suppl 2):64-88.

66. Sanders CC. Cefepime. Clin Infect Dis. 1993;17:369-379.

67. Sanders CC. β-Lactamases of gram-negative bacteria: New challenges for new drugs. Clin Infect Dis. 1992;14:1089-1099.

68. Sanders WE Jr, Sanders CC. Inducible β-lactamases: Clinical and epidemiologic implications for use of newer cephalosporins. Rev Infect Dis. 1988;10:830-838.

69. Medeiros AA. Evolution and dissemination of β-lactamases accelerated by generations of β-lactam antibiotics. Clin Infect Dis. 1997;24(Suppl 1):Sl9-S45.

70. Jacoby GA, Han P. Detection of extended-spectrum beta-lactamases in clinical isolates of Klebsiella pneumoniae and Escherichia coli. J Clin Microbiol. 1996;34: 908-911.

71. Babini GS, Livermore DM. Antimicrobial resistance amongst Klebsiella spp. collected from intensive care units in Southern and Western Europe in 1997-1998. J Antimicrob Chemother. 2000;45:183-189.

72. Paterson DL, Hujer KM, Hujer AM, et al, International Klebsiella Study Group. Extended-spectrum beta-lactamases in Klebsiella pneumoniae bloodstream isolates from seven countries: Dominance and widespread prevalence of SHV- and CTX-M-type beta-lactamases. Antimicrob Agents Chemother. 2003;47:3554-3560.

73. Jacoby GA, Medeiros AA. More extended-spectrum β-lactamases. Antimicrob Agents Chemother. 1991;35:1697-1704.

74. Pfaller MA, Jones RN. Antimicrobial susceptibility of inducible AmpC beta-lactamase–producing Enterobacteriaceae from the meropenem yearly susceptibility test information collection (MYSTIC) programme, Europe 1997-2000. Int J Antimicrob Agents. 2002;19:383-388.

75. Biedenbach DJ, Johnson DM, Jones RN. In vitro evaluation of cefepime and other broad-based beta-lactams in eight medical centers in Thailand. The Thailand Antimicrobial Resistance Group. Diagn Microbiol Infect Dis. 1999;35:325-331.

76. Emery CL, Weymouth LA. Detection and clinical significance of extended-spectrum beta-lactamases in a tertiary-care medical center. J Clin Microbiol. 1997;35:2061-2067.

77. National Committee for Clinical Laboratory Standards. MIC testing supplemental tables. Document M100-S13 (M7). National Committee for Clinical Laboratory Standards, Wayne, Pa, January 2003.

78. Paterson DL, Ko WC, Gottberg A, et al. Outcome of cephalosporin treatment for serious infections due to apparently susceptible organisms producing extended-spectrum beta-lactamases: Implications for the clinical microbiology laboratory. J Clin Microbiol. 2001;39:2206-2212.

79. Poirel L, Naas T, le Thomas I, et al. CTX-M-type extended-spectrum β-lactamase that hydrolyzes ceftazidime through a single amino acid substitution in the omega loop. Antimicrob Agents Chemother. 2001;45:3355-3361.

80. Chanawong A, M'Zali FH, Heritage J, et al. Three cefotaximases, CTX-M-9, CTX-M-13, and CTX-M-14, among Enterobacteriaceae in the People's Republic of China. Antimicrob Agents Chemother. 2002;46:630-637.

81. Martinez-Martinez L, Hernandez-Alles S, Alberti S, et al. In vivo selection of porin-deficient mutants of Klebsiella pneumoniae with increased resistance to cefoxitin and expanded-spectrum cephalosporins. Antimicrob Agents Chemother. 1996;40:342-348.

82. Charrel RN, Pages JM, De Micco P, Mallea M. Prevalence of outer membrane porin alteration in beta-lactam-antibiotic–resistant Enterobacter aerogenes. Antimicrob Agents Chemother. 1996;40:2854-2858.

83. Mazzariol A, Cornaglia G, Nikaido H. Contributions of the AmpC β-lactamase and the AcrAB multidrug efflux system in intrinsic resistance of Escherichia coli K-12 to β-lactams. Antimicrob Agents Chemother. 2000;44:1387-1390.

84. Li XZ, Nikaido H, Poole K. Role of MexA-MexB-OprM in antibiotic efflux in Pseudomonas aeruginosa. Antimicrob Agents Chemother. 1995;39:1948-1953.

85. Srikumar R, Li XZ, Poole K. The inner membrane efflux components are responsible for the β-lactam specificity of multidrug efflux pumps in Pseudomonas aeruginosa. J Bacteriol. 1997;179:7875-7881.

86. Nikaido H. Multidrug efflux pumps of gram-negative bacteria. J Bacteriol. 1996;178:5853-5859.

87. Nagai K, Davies TA, Jacobs MR, Appelbaum PC. Effects of amino acid alterations in penicillin-binding proteins (PBPs) 1a, 2b, and 2x on PBP affinities of penicillin, ampicillin, amoxicillin, cefditoren, cefuroxime, cefprozil, and cefaclor in 18 clinical isolates of penicillin-susceptible, -intermediate, and -resistant pneumococci. Antimicrob Agents Chemother. 2002;46:1273-1280.

88. du Plessis M, Smith AM, Klugman KP. Analysis of penicillin-binding protein 1b and 2a genes from *Streptococcus pneumoniae*. Microb Drug Resist. 2000;6:127-131.

89. Hartman BJ, Tomasz A. Low affinity penicillin binding proteins associated with β-lactam resistance in *Staphylococcus aureus*. J Bacteriol. 1984;158:513-516.

90. Barza M, Melethil S, Berger S, et al. Comparative pharmacokinetics of cefamandole, cephapirin, and cephalothin in healthy subjects and effect of repeated dosing. Antimicrob Agents Chemother. 1976;10:421-425.

91. Pfeffer M, Jackson A, Ximenes J, et al. Comparative human oral clinical pharmacology of cefadroxil, cephalexin, and cephradine. Antimicrob Agents Chemother. 1977;11:331-338.

92. Korzeniowski OM, Scheld WM, Sande MA. Comparative pharmacology of cefaclor and cephalexin. Antimicrob Agents Chemother. 1977;12:157-162.

93. Patel IH, Chen S, Parsonnet M, et al. Pharmacokinetics of ceftriaxone in humans. Antimicrob Agents Chemother. 1981;20:634-640.

94. Brogard JM, Conte E. Pharmacokinetics of the new cephalosporins. Antibiot Chemother. 1982;31:145-210.

95. Cutler RE, Blair AD, Burgess ED. Pharmacokinetics of ceftizoxime. J Antimicrob Chemother. 1982;10(Suppl C):91-97.

96. Barriere SL, Flaherty JR. Third generation cephalosporins: A critical evaluation. Clin Pharm. 1984;3:351-373.

97. Browning MJ, Holt HA, White LO, et al. Pharmacokinetics of cefotetan in patients with end-stage renal failure on maintenance dialysis. J Antimicrob Chemother. 1986;18:103-106.

98. Faulkner RD, Bohaychuk W, Haynes JD, et al. The pharmacokinetics of cefixime in the fasted and fed state. Eur J Clin Pharmacol. 1988;34:525-528.

99. Barbhaiya RH, Shukla UA, Gleason CR, et al. Comparison of the effects of food on the pharmacokinetics of cefprozil and cefaclor. Antimicrob Agents Chemother. 1990;34:1210-1213.

100. Wise R. The pharmacokinetics of the oral cephalosporins—A review. J Antimicrob Chemother. 1990;26(Suppl E):13-20.

101. Barr WH, Lin CC, Radwanski E, et al. The pharmacokinetics of ceftibuten in humans. Diagn Microbiol Infect Dis. 1991;14:93-100.

102. Barbhaiya RH, Forgue ST, Gleason CR: Pharmacokinetics of cefepime after single and multiple intravenous administrations in healthy subjects. Antimicrob Agents Chemother. 1992;36:552-557.

103. DeSante KA, Zeckel ML. Pharmacokinetic profile of loracarbef. Am J Med. 1992;92 (Suppl 6A):16S-25S.

104. Craig WA. The pharmacokinetics of cefpirome—Rationale for a twelve-hour dosing regimen. Scand J Infect Dis Suppl. 1993;91:33-40.

105. Nix DE, Symonds WT, Hyatt JM, et al. Comparative pharmacokinetics of oral ceftibuten, cefixime, cefaclor, and cefuroxime axetil in healthy volunteers. Pharmacotherapy. 1997;17:121-125.

106. Li JT, Hou F, Lu H, et al. Phase I clinical trial of cefditoren pivoxil (ME 1207): Pharmacokinetics in healthy volunteers. Drugs Under Exp Clin Res. 1997;23: 145-150.

107. Guay DR. Cefdinir: An advanced-generation, broad-spectrum oral cephalosporin. Clin Ther. 2002;24:473-489.

108. Craig WA, Suh B. Protein binding and the antimicrobial effects. Methods for the determination of protein binding. In: Lorian V, ed. Antibiotics in Laboratory Medicine. Baltimore: Williams & Wilkins; 1991:367-402.

109. Friedrich H, Haensel-Friedrich G, Langmaak H, et al. Investigations of cefuroxime levels in the cerebrospinal fluid of patients with and without meningitis. Chemotherapy. 1980;26:91-97.

110. Cable D, Edralin G, Overturf GD. Human cerebrospinal fluid pharmacokinetics and treatment of bacterial meningitis with ceftizoxime. J Antimicrob Chemother. 1982;10 (Suppl C):121-127.

111. Chandrasekar PH, Rolston KV, Smith BR, et al. Diffusion of ceftriaxone into the cerebrospinal fluid of adults. J Antimicrob Chemother. 1984;14:427-430.

112. Cherubin CE, Eng RHK, Norrby R, et al. Penetration of newer cephalosporins into cerebrospinal fluid. Rev Infect Dis. 1989;11:526-548.

113. Chin NX. Neu HC. Cefotaxime and desacetyl cefotaxime: An example of advantageous antimicrobial metabolism. Diagn Microbial Infect Dis. 1984;2(3 Suppl):21S-31S.

114. Fong IW, Tomkins KB. Penetration of ceftazidime into the cerebrospinal fluid of patients with and without evidence of meningeal inflammation. Antimicrob Agents Chemother. 1984;26:115-116.

115. Wolff M, Chavanet P, Kazmierczak A, et al. Diffusion of cefpirome into the cerebrospinal fluid of patients with purulent meningitis. J Antimicrob Chemother. 1992;29 (Suppl. A):59-62.

116. Andes D, Craig WA. Pharmacokinetics and pharmacodynamics of outpatient intravenous antimicrobial therapy. Infect Dis Clinics North Am. 1998;12:849-859.

117. Strehl E, Kees F. Pharmacological properties of parenteral cephalosporins: Rationale for ambulatory use. Drugs. 2000;59(Suppl 3):9-18.

118. Johnson CA, Zimmerman SW, Rogge M. The pharmacokinetics of antibiotics used to treat peritoneal dialysis–associated peritonitis. Am J Kidney Dis. 1984;4:3-17.

119. Groneberg DA, Doring F, Eynott PR, et al. Intestinal peptide transport: Ex vivo uptake studies and localization of peptide carrier PEPT1. Am J Physiol. 2001;281:697-704.

120. Saab AN, Dittert LW, Hussain AA. Isomerization of cephalosporin esters: Implications for the prodrug ester approach to enhancing the oral bioavailabilities of cephalosporins. J Pharm Sci. 1988;77:906-907.

121. Redington J, Ebert SC, Craig WA. Role of antimicrobial pharmacokinetics and pharmacodynamics in surgical prophylaxis. Rev Infect Dis. 1991;13(Suppl 10):S790-S799.

122. Joukhadar C, Derendorf H, Muller M. Microdialysis. A novel tool for clinical studies of anti-infective agents. Eur J Clin Pharmacol. 2001;57:211-219.

123. Higa F, Kusano N, Tateyama M, et al. Simplified quantitative assay system for measuring activities of drugs against intracellular *Legionella pneumophila*. J Clin Microbiol. 1998;36:1392-1398.

124. Andes D, Craig WA. Pharmacokinetics and pharmacodynamics of antibiotics in meningitis. Infect Dis Clin North Am. 1999;13:595-617.

125. Dacey RG, Sande MA. Effect of probenecid on cerebrospinal fluid concentrations of penicillin and cephalosporin derivatives. Antimicrob Agents Chemother. 1974;6:437-441.

126. Jones RN. A review of cephalosporin metabolism: A lesson to be learned for future chemotherapy. Diagn Microbiol Infect Dis. 1989;12:25-31.

127. Craig WA. Pharmacokinetics of antibiotics with special emphasis on cephalosporins. Clin Microbiol Infect. 2000;6(Suppl 3):46-49.

128. Craig WA, Vogelman B. Changing patterns of hospital infections: Implications for therapy. Changing concepts and new applications of antibiotic pharmacokinetics. Am J Med. 1984;77(Suppl 1B):24-28.

129. Aronoff GR, Bennett WM, Berns JS, et al. Drug Prescribing in Renal Failure: Dosing Guidelines for Adults. 4th ed. Philadelphia: American College of Physicians–American Society of Internal Medicine; 1999.

130. Livornese LL Jr, Slavin D, Benz RL, et al. Use of antibacterial agents in renal failure. Infect Dis Clin North Am. 2000;14:371-390.

131. Bressolle F, Kinowski JM, de la Coussaye JE, et al. Clinical pharmacokinetics during continuous haemofiltration. Clin Pharmacokinet. 1994;26:457-471.

132. Baumgart KW, Baldo BA. Cephalosporin allergy. N Engl J Med. 2002;346:380-381.

133. Macy E. Cephalosporin allergy. N Engl J Med. 2002;346:380-381.

134. Norrby SR. Side effects of cephalosporins. Drugs. 1987;34(Suppl 2):105-120.

135. Romano A, Mayorga C, Torres MJ, et al. Immediate allergic reactions to cephalosporins: Cross-reactivity and selective responses. J Allergy Clin Immunol. 2000;106:1177-1183.

136. Saxon A, Beall GN, Rohr AS, et al. Immediate hypersensitivity reactions to beta-lactam antibiotics. Ann Intern Med. 1987;107:204-215.

137. Hama R, Mori K. High incidence of anaphylactic reactions to cefaclor. Lancet. 1988;1:1331.

138. Hebert AA, Sigman ES, Levy ML. Serum sickness–like reactions from cefaclor in children. J Am Acad Dermatol. 1991;25:805-808.

139. Novalbos A, Sastre J, Cuesta J, et al. Lack of allergic cross-reactivity to cephalosporins among patients allergic to penicillins. Clin Exp Allergy. 2001;31: 438-443.

140. Nugent JS, Quinn JM, McGrath CM, et al. Determination of the incidence of sensitization after penicillin skin testing. Ann Allergy Asthma Immunol. 2003;90:398-403.

141. Smith CR. Considerations regarding clinical safety and tolerability of antibiotics in serious and nosocomial infections. Clin Ther. 1981;4(Suppl A):133-145.

142. Bang N, Kammer RB. Hematological complications associated with beta-lactam antibiotics. Rev Infect Dis. 1983;5(Suppl 2):S380-S393.

143. Molthan L, Reidenberg MM, Eichman MF. Positive direct Coombs tests due to cephalothin. N Engl J Med. 1967;277:123-125.

144. Barza M. Nephrotoxicity of cephalosporins: An overview. J Infect Dis. 1978;137 (Suppl):S60-S73.

145. Ingalls CS, Freimer EH. Detection of antibiotic-induced platelet dysfunction in whole blood using flow cytometry. J Antimicrob Chemother. 1992;29:313-321.

146. Barza M, Furie B, Brown AK, et al. Defects in vitamin K–dependent carboxylation associated with moxalactam treatment. J Infect Dis. 1986;153:1166-1169.

147. Shearer MJ, Bechtold H, Andrassy K, et al. Mechanism of cephalosporin-induced hypoprothrombinemia: Relation to cephalosporin side chain, vitamin K metabolism, and vitamin K status. J Clin Pharmacol. 1988;28:88-95.

148. Conly JM, Ramotar K, Chubb H, et al. Hypoprothrombinemia in febrile, neutropenic patients with cancer: Association with antimicrobial suppression of intestinal microflora. J Infect Dis. 1984;150:202-212.

149. Fainstein V, Bodey GP, McCredie KB, et al. Coagulation abnormalities induced by beta-lactam antibiotics in cancer patients. J Infect Dis. 1983;148:745-750.

150. Nichols RL, Wikler MA, McDevitt JT, et al. Coagulopathy associated with extended-spectrum cephalosporins in patients with serious infections. Antimicrob Agents Chemother. 1987;31:281-285.

151. McCloskey RV. Spontaneous reports of bleeding: Comparison of *N*-methylthiotetrazole side chain (MTT) and non-MTT cephalosporins. J Infect Dis. 1988;158:1405.

152. Aronoff GR, Wolen RL, Obermeyer BD, Black HR. Pharmacokinetics and protein binding of cefamandole and its 1-methyl-1 H-tetrazole-5-thiol side chain in subjects with normal and impaired renal function. J Infect Dis. 1986;153:1069-1074.

153. Foster RS, Raehl CL, Wilson HD. Disulfiram-like reactions associated wish a parenteral cephalosporin. Am J Hosp Pharm. 1980;37:858-859.

154. Platt R, Dreis MW, Kennedy DL, et al. Serum sickness–like reactions to amoxicillin, cefaclor, cephalexin, and trimethoprim-sulfamethoxazole. J Infect Dis. 1988;158:474-477.

155. Thiim M, Freidman LS. Hepatotoxicity of antibiotics and antifungals. Clin Liver Dis. 2003;7:381-399.

156. Heim-Duthoy KL, Caperton EM, Pollock R, et al. Apparent biliary pseudolithiasis during ceftriaxone therapy. Antimicrob Agents Chemother. 1990;34:1146-1149.

157. Park HZ, Lee SP, Schy A, et al. Ceftriaxone-associated gallbladder sludge. Gastroenterology. 1991;100:1665-1670.

158. Schaad UB, Wedgwood-Krucko J, Tschaeppeler H. Reversible ceftriaxone-associated biliary pseudo-lithiasis in children. Lancet. 1988;2:1411-1413.

159. Martinez-Rodriguez JE, Barriga FJ, Santamaria J, et al. Nonconvulsive status epilepticus associated with cephalosporins in patients with renal failure. Am J Med. 2001;111:115-119.

160. Inagaki J, Bodey GP. Phlebitis associated with cephalosporins: Cephapirin versus cephalothin. Curr Ther Res Clin Exp. 1973;15:37-43.

161. Thompson JW, Jacobs RF. Adverse effects of newer cephalosporins. An update. Drug Saf. 1993;9:132-142.

162. Briggs GG, Freeman RK, Yaffee SJ. Drugs in Pregnancy and Lactation: A Reference Guide to Fetal and Neonatal Risk. 2nd ed. Baltimore: Williams & Wilkins; 1986.

163. Berkowitz RL, Coustan DR, Mochizuki TK. Handbook for Prescribing Medications During Pregnancy. Boston: Little, Brown; 1981.

164. McManus MC, Barriere SL. Interaction between newer cephalosporins and Clinitest, Diastix, and Tes-Tape. Am J Hosp Pharm. 1983;40:1544-1545.

165. Letellier G, Desjarlais F. Analytical interference of drugs in clinical chemistry: II—The interference of three cephalosporins with the determination of serum creatinine concentration by the Jaffe reaction. Clin Biochem. 1985;18:352-356.

166. Thomakos N, Maraki S, Liakakos T, et al. Effect of cefamandole, cefuroxime and cefoxitin on yeast fecal flora of surgical patients. Chemotherapy. 1998;44:324-327.

167. MacDonald TM, Beardon PH, McGilchrist MM, et al. The risks of symptomatic vaginal candidiasis after oral antibiotic therapy. J Med. 1993;86:419-424.

168. Bartlett JG, Willey SH, Chang TW, et al. Cephalosporin-associated pseudomembranous colitis due to *Clostridium difficile*. JAMA. 1979;242:2683-2685.

169. Grayson ML, McDonald M, Gibson K, et al. Once-daily intravenous cefazolin plus oral probenecid is equivalent to once-daily intravenous ceftriaxone plus oral placebo for the treatment of moderate-to-severe cellulitis in adults. Clin Infect Dis. 2002;34:1440-1448.

170. Regamey C, Lobke RD, Engelking ER, et al. Inactivation of cefazolin, cephaloridine, and cephalothin by methicillin-sensitive and methicillin-resistant strains of *Staphylococcus aureus*. J Infect Dis. 1975;131:291-294.

171. Fong IW, Engelking ER, Kirby WMM. Relative inactivation by *Staphylococcus aureus* of eight cephalosporin antibiotics. Antimicrob Agents Chemother. 1976;9:939-944.

172. Quinn EL, Pohlod D, Madhavan T, et al. Clinical experience with cefazolin and other cephalosporins in bacterial endocarditis. J Infect Dis. 1983;128(Suppl):S386-S391.

173. Antimicrobial prophylaxis in surgery. Med Lett Drugs Ther. 1999;41:75-79.

174. Woods RK, Dellinger EP. Current guidelines for antibiotic prophylaxis of surgical wounds. Am Fam Physician. 1998;57:2731-2740.

175. Weber DJ, Wofson JS, Swartz MN, et al. *Pasteurella multocida* infections: Report of 3 cases and review of the literature. Medicine (Baltimore). 1984;63:133-154.

176. Milatovic D. Evaluation of cefadroxil, penicillin and erythromycin in the treatment of streptococcal tonsillopharyngitis. Pediatr Infect Dis J. 1991;10(Suppl 10):S61-S63.

177. Disney FA, Dillon H, Blumer JL, et al. Cephalexin and penicillin in the treatment of group A ß-hemolytic streptococcal throat infections. Am J Dis Child. 1992;146:1324-1327.

178. Warren JW, Abrutyn E, Hebel JR, et al. Guidelines for antimicrobial treatment of uncomplicated acute bacterial cystitis and acute pyelonephritis in women. Clin Infect Dis. 1999;29:745-758.

179. Norby SR. Short-term treatment of uncomplicated lower urinary tract infections in women. Rev Infect Dis. 1990;12:458-467.

180. Mehtar S, Parr JH, Morgan DJR. A comparison of cefuroxime and cotrimoxazole in severe respiratory tract infections. J Antimicrob Chemother. 1982;9:479-484.

181. Delgado DG, Crau CJ, Cobbs CG, et al. Clinical and laboratory evaluation of cefamandole in therapy of *Haemophilus* sp. bronchopulmonary infections. Antimicrob Agents Chemother. 1979;15:807-812.

182. Jacob LS, Layne P. Cefonicid: An overview of clinical studies in the United States. Rev Infect Dis. 1984;6(Suppl 4):S791-S802.

183. Marks WA, Stutman HR, Marks ML, et al. Cefuroxime versus ampicillin plus chloramphenicol childhood bacterial meningitis: A multicenter randomized controlled trial. J Pediatr. 1986;109:123-130.

184. Schaad UB, Suter S, Gianella-Borradori A, et al. A comparison of ceftriaxone and cefuroxime for the treatment of bacterial meningitis in children. N Engl J Med. 1990;322:141-147.

185. Bartlett JG, Dowell SF, Mandell LA, et al. Practice guidelines for the management of community-acquired pneumonia in adults. Clin Infect Dis. 2000;31:347-382.

186. Niederman MS, Mandell LA, Anzueto A, et al. Guidelines for the management of community-acquired pneumonia. Am J Respir Crit Care Med. 2001;123:S1-S32.

187. Vu VL, Chiou CCC, Feldman C, et al. An international prospective study of pneumococcal bacteremia: Correlation with in vitro resistance, antibiotics administered, and clinical outcome. Clin Infect Dis. 2003;37:230-237.

188. Mandell LA, Bartlett JG, Dowell SF, et al. Update of practice guidelines for the management of community-acquired pneumonia in immunocompetent adults. Clin Infect Dis. 2003;37:1405-1433.

189. Gibbs RS, Huff RW. Cefamandole therapy of endomyometritis following cesarean section. Am J Obstet Gynecol. 1980;136:32-37.

190. Klein JO. Microbiologic efficacy of antibacterial drugs for acute otitis media. Pediatr Infect Dis J. 1993;12:973-975.

191. Craig WA, Andes D. Pharmacokinetics and pharmacodynamics of antibiotics in otitis media. Pediatr Infect Dis J. 1966;15:255-259.

192. Craig WA. Basic pharmacodynamics of antibacterials with clinical applications to the use of β-lactams, glycopeptides, and linezolid. Infect Dis Clin North Am. 2003;17:479-501.

193. Dagan R, Klugman KP, Craig WA, Baquero F. Evidence to support the rationale that bacterial eradication in respiratory tract infection is an important aim of antimicrobial therapy. J Antimicrob Chemother. 2001;47:129-140.

194. Bisno AL, Gerber MA, Gwaltney JM Jr, et al. Practice guidelines for the diagnosis and management of group A streptococcal pharyngitis. Clin Infect Dis. 2002;35:113-125.

195. McCarty JM, Renteria A. Treatment of pharyngitis and tonsillitis with cefprozil: Review of three multicenter trials. Clin Infect Dis. 1992;14(Suppl 2):S224-S230.

196. McCarty J. Loracarbef versus penicillin VK in the treatment of streptococcal pharyngitis and tonsillitis in an adult population. Am J Med. 1992;92(Suppl 6A):74S-79S.

197. Nadelman RB, Luger SW, Frank E, et al. Comparison of cefuroxime axetil and doxycycline in the treatment of early Lyme disease. Ann Intern Med. 1992;117:273-280.

198. Poindexter AN, Sweet R, Ritter M. Cefotetan in the treatment of obstetric and gynecologic infections. Am J Obstet Gynecol. 1986;154:946-950.

199. Wilson SE, Boswick JA, Duma RJ, et al. Cephalosporin therapy in intraabdominal infections: A multicenter randomized, comparative study of cefotetan, moxalactam and cefoxitin. Am J Surg. 1988;155(Suppl 5A):61-66.

200. Sweet R, Gall SA, Gobbs RS, et al. Multicenter clinical trial comparing cefotetan with moxalactam or cefoxitin as therapy for obstetric gynecologic infections. Am J Surg. 1988;155(Suppl 5A):S56-S60.

201. Griffith DL, Novak E, Greenwald CA, et al. Clinical experience with cefmetazole sodium in the United States: An overview. J Antimicrob Chemother. 1989;23 (Suppl D):S21-S33.

202. Appelman MD, Haseltine PNR, Cherubin CE. Epidemiology, antimicrobial susceptibility, pathogenicity, and significance of *Bacteroides fragilis* group organisms isolated at Los Angeles County–University of Southern California Medical Center. Rev Infect Dis. 1991;13:12-18.

203. Morel C, Vergnaud M, Lengeard MM, et al. Cefotetan: Comparative study in vitro against 266 gram-negative clinical isolates. J Antimicrob Chemother. 1983;11(Suppl A):31-36.

204. Sexually transmitted diseases treatment guidelines 2002. Centers for Disease Control and Prevention. MMWR Recomm Rep. 2002;51(RR-6):1-78.

205. Peterson HB, Galaid EI, Zenilman JM. Pelvic inflammatory disease: Review of treatment options. Rev Infect Dis. 1990;12(Suppl 6):S656-S664.

206. Jones RN, Barry AL. Cefoperazone: A review of its antimicrobial spectrum, beta-lactamase stability, enzyme inhibition, and other in vitro characteristics. Rev Infect Dis. 1983;5(Suppl):S108-S126.

207. Kurtz TO, Winston DJ, Hindler JA, et al. Comparative in vitro activity of moxalactam, cefotaxime, cefoperazone, piperacillin, and aminoglycosides against gram-negative bacilli. Antimicrob Agents Chemother. 1980;18:645-648.

208. Weitekamp MR, Aber RC. Prolonged bleeding times and bleeding diathesis associated with moxalactam administration. JAMA. 1983;249:69-71.

209. Counts GW, Hill CD, Hooton TM, et al. Ceftizoxime treatment of pneumonia, cellulitis and other infections in 120 hospitalized patients. J Antimicrob Chemother. 1982;10(Suppl C):201-207.

210. Trenholme GM, Schmitt BA, Nelson JA, et al. Comparative study of three different dosing regimens of cefotaxime for gram-negative bacteremia. Diagn Microbiol Infect Dis. 1989;12:107-112.

211. Young JPW, Husson JM, Bruch K, et al. The evaluation of efficacy and safety of cefotaxime: A review of 2500 cases. J Antimicrob Chemother. 1980;6(Suppl A):293-300.

212. Daikos GK, Kosmidis J, Giamarellou H, et al. Evaluation of cefotaxime in a hospital with high antibiotic resistance rates. J Antimicrob Chemother. 1980;6(Suppl A):255-261.

213. Scully BE, Neu HC. The use of ceftizoxime in the treatment of critically ill patients infected with multiply resistant bacteria. J Antimicrob Chemother. 1982;10(Suppl C):141-150.

214. Eron LJ, Park CH, Goldenberg RI, et al. Ceftriaxone therapy of serious bacterial infections. J Antimicrob Chemother. 1983;12:65-78.

215. Chow JW, Fine MJ, Shlaes DM, et al. *Enterobacter* bacteremia: Clinical features and emergence of antibiotic resistance during therapy. Ann Intern Med. 1991;115:585-590.

216. Thomas JK, Forrest A, Bhavnani SM, et al. Pharmacodynamic evaluation of factors associated with the development of bacterial resistance in acutely ill patients during therapy. Antimicrob Agents Chemother. 1998;42:521-527.

217. Congeni BL, Bradley J, Hammerschlag MR. Safety and efficacy of once daily ceftriaxone for the treatment of bacterial meningitis. Pediatr Infect Dis. 1986;5:293-297.

218. Overturf GD, Cable DC, Forthal DN, et al. Treatment of bacterial meningitis with ceftizoxime. Antimicrob Agents Chemother. 1984;25:258-262.

219. Jacobs RJ, Wells TO, Steele RW, et al. A prospective randomized comparison of cefotaxime vs. ampicillin and chloramphenicol for bacterial meningitis in children. Pediatr Infect Dis. 1986;4:362-368.

220. Mullaney DT, John IF. Cefotaxime therapy: Evaluation of its effects on bacterial meningitis, CSF drug levels, and bactericidal activity. Arch Intern Med. 1983;143:1705-1708.

221. del Rio M, McCracken GH Jr, Nelson JD, et al. Pharmacokinetics and cerebrospinal fluid bactericidal activity of ceftriaxone in the treatment of pediatric patients with bacterial meningitis. Antimicrob Agents Chemother. 1982;22:622-627.

222. Quagliarello VJ, Scheld WM. Treatment of bacterial meningitis. N Engl J Med. 1997;336:708-716.

223. Pallares R, Capdevila Q, Linares J, et al. The effect of cephalosporin resistance on mortality in adult patients with nonmeningeal systemic pneumococcal infections. Am J Med. 2002;113:120-126.

224. Jones RN, Mutnick AH, Vamam DJ. Impact of modified nonmeningeal *Streptococcus pneumoniae* interpretive criteria (NCCLS M100-S12) on the susceptibility patterns of five parenteral cephalosporins: Report from the SENTRY antimicrobial surveillance program (1997 to 2001). J Clin Microbiol. 2002;40:4332-4333.

225. Sahm DF, Thornsberry C, Mayfield DC, et al. In vitro activities of broad-spectrum cephalosporins against nonmeningeal isolates of *Streptococcus pneumoniae*: MIC interpretation using NCCLS M100-S12 recommendations. J Clin Microbiol. 2002;40:669-674.

226. Leibovitz E, Piglansky L, Raiz S, et al. Efficacy of a three-day intramuscular ceftriaxone regimen in nonresponsive acute otitis media. Pediatr Infect Dis J. 1998;17:1126-1131.
227. Leibovitz E, Piglansky L, Raiz S, et al. Bacteriologic and clinical efficacy of one day vs. three day intramuscular ceftriaxone for treatment of nonresponsive acute otitis media in children. Pediatr Infect Dis J. 2000;19:1040-1050.
228. Blumer JL, McLinn SE, Deabate CA, et al. Multinational multicenter controlled trial comparing ceftibuten with cefaclor for the treatment of acute otitis media. Pediatr Infect Dis J. 1995;14:S115-S120.
229. Harrison CJ, Chartrand SA, Pichichero ME. Microbiologic and clinical aspects of a trial of once daily cefixime compared with twice daily cefaclor for treatment of acute otitis media in infants and children. Pediatr Infect Dis J. 1993;12:62-69.
230. Mandel EM, Casselbrant ML, Kurs-Lasky M, et al. Efficacy of ceftibuten compared with amoxicillin for otitis media with effusion in infants and children. Pediatr Infect Dis J. 1996;15:409-414.
231. Piippo T, Stefansson S, Pitkajarvi T, et al. Double-blind comparison of cefixime and cefaclor in the treatment of acute otitis media in children. Scand J Infect Dis. 1991;23:459-465.
232. Block SL, Hedrick JA, Tyler RD. Comparative study of the effectiveness of cefixime and penicillin V for the treatment of streptococcal pharyngitis in children and adolescents. Pediatr Infect Dis J. 1992;11:919-925.
233. Peyramond D, Tigaud S, Bremard-Oury C, et al. Multicenter comparative trial of cefixime and phenoxymethylpenicillin for group A beta-hemolytic streptococcal tonsillitis. Curr Ther Res. 1994;55:14-21.
234. Pichichero ME, Gooch WM III. Comparison of cefdinir and penicillin V in the treatment of pediatric streptococcal tonsillopharyngitis. Pediatr Infect Dis J. 2000;19:8171-8173.
235. Pichichero ME, McLinn SE, Gooch WM III, et al. Ceftibuten vs penicillin V in group A beta-hemolytic streptococcal pharyngitis. Pediatr Infect Dis J. 1995;14(Suppl 7):S102-S107.
236. Banfi A, Gavriele G, Hill-Juarez JM, et al, Ceftibuten Urinary Tract Infection International Study Group. Multinational comparative trial of ceftibuten and trimethoprim-sulfamethoxazole in the treatment of children with complicated or recurrent urinary tract infections. Pediatr Infect Dis. 1993;12(Suppl):S84-S91.
237. Hughes WT, Armstrong D, Bodey GP, et al. 2002 guidelines for the use of antimicrobial agents in neutropenic patients with cancer. Clin Infect Dis. 2002;34:730-751.
238. Nicolau D, McNabb J, Lacey M. Continuous versus intermittent administration of ceftazidime in intensive care unit patients with nosocomial pneumonia. Int J Antimicrob Agents. 2001;17:497-504.
239. Egerer G, Goldschmidt H, Salwender H, et al. Efficacy of continuous infusion of ceftazidime for patients with neutropenic fever after high-dose chemotherapy and peripheral blood stem cell transplantation. Int J Antimicrob Agents. 2000;15:119-123.
240. Blumer JL, Stern RC, Klinger JD. Ceftazidime therapy in patients with cystic fibrosis and multiply-drug-resistant pseudomonas. Am J Med. 1985;79(Suppl 2A):37-46.
241. Fong IW, Tompkins KB. Review of *Pseudomonas aeruginosa* meningitis with special emphasis on treatment with ceftazidime. Rev Infect Dis. 1985;7:604-612.
242. Arredondo JL, Diaz V, Gaitan H, et al. Oral clindamycin and ciprofloxacin versus intramuscular ceftriaxone and oral doxycycline in the treatment of mild-to-moderate pelvic inflammatory disease in outpatients. Clin Infect Dis. 1997;24:170-178.
243. Handsfield HH, McCormack WM, Hook EW, et al. A comparison of single-dose cefixime with ceftriaxone as treatment for uncomplicated gonorrhea. N Engl J Med. 1991;325:1337-1341.
244. Asbach HW. Single dose oral administration of cefixime 400mg in the treatment of acute uncomplicated cystitis and gonorrhoea. Drugs. 1991;42(Suppl 4):10-13.
245. Wormser GP, Nadelman RP, Dattwyler RJ, et al. Practice guidelines for the treatment of Lyme disease. Clin Infect Dis. 2000;31:S1-S14.
246. Augenbraun M, Workowski K. Ceftriaxone therapy for syphilis: Report from the emerging infections network. Clin Infect Dis. 1999;29:1337-1338.
247. Marra CM, Boutin P, McArthur JC, et al. A pilot study evaluating ceftriaxone and penicillin G as treatment agents for neurosyphilis in human immunodeficiency virus–infected individuals. Clin Infect Dis. 2000;30:540-544.
248. Guerrant RL, van Gilder T, Steiner TS, et al. Practice guidelines for the management of infectious diarrhea. Clin Infect Dis. 2001;32:331-351.
249. Ti TY, Monteiro EH, Lam S, et al. Ceftriaxone therapy in bacteremic typhoid fever. Antimicrob Agents Chemother. 1985;28:540-543.
250. Finch RG. Third-generation cephalosporins in the treatment of rare infections. Am J Med. 1990;88(Suppl 4A):25S-31S.
251. Wilson WR, Karchmer AW, Dajani AS, et al. Antibiotic treatment of adults with infective endocarditis due to streptococci, enterococci, staphylococci, and HACEK microorganisms. JAMA. 1995;274:1706-1713.
252. Simmons G, Jones N, Calder L. Equivalence of ceftriaxone and rifampicin in eliminating nasopharyngeal carriage of serogroup B *Neisseria meningitidis*. J Antimicrob Chemother. 2000;45:909-911.
253. Martin MJ, Hutchinson NA, Eltringham IJ, et al. Secondary prevention of meningococcal disease. Ceftriaxone or ciprofloxacin should be considered as first line prophylaxis. BMJ. 1996;312:1536-1537.
254. Bradsher RW, Snow RM. Ceftriaxone treatment of skin and soft tissue infections in a once daily regimen. Am J Med. 1984;77(Suppl C):63-67.
255. Tice AD, Hoaglund PA, Shoultz DA. Outcomes of osteomyelitis among patients treated with outpatient parenteral antimicrobial therapy. Am J Med. 2003;114:723-728.
256. Sexton DJ, Tenenbaum MJ, Wilson WR, et al, Endocarditis Treatment Consortium Group. Ceftriaxone once daily for four weeks compared with ceftriaxone plus gentamicin once daily for two weeks for treatment of endocarditis due to penicillin-susceptible streptococci. Clin Infect Dis. 1998;27:1470-1474.
257. Bryskier A. New concepts in the field of cephalosporins: C-3′ quaternary ammonium cephem (group IV). Clin Microbiol Infect. 1997;3(Suppl 1):S1-S6.
258. Garau J, Wilson W, Wood M, Carlet J. Fourth generation cephalosporins: A review of in vitro activity, pharmacokinetics, pharmacodynamics, and clinical utility. Clin Microbiol Infect. 1997;3(Suppl 1):S87-S101.
259. Neu HC, Chin NX, Labthavilul P. The in vitro activity and beta lactamase stability of cefpirome (HR 810), a pyridine cephalosporin agent active against staphylococci Enterobacteriaceae, and *Pseudomonas aeruginosa*. Infection. 1985;13:146-155.
260. King A, Boothman C, Phillips I. Comparative in vitro activity of cefpirome and cefepime, two new cephalosporins. Eur J Clin Microbiol Infect Dis. 1990;9:677-685.
261. Jauregui L, Matzke D, Scott M, et al. Cefepime as treatment for osteomyelitis and other severe bacterial infections. J Antimicrob Chemother. 1993;32(Suppl B):141-149.
262. Arguedas AG, Stutman HR, Zaleska M, et al. Cefepime: Pharmacokinetics and clinical response in patients with cystic fibrosis. Am J Dis Child. 1992;146:797-802.
263. Tam VH, McKinnon PS, Akins RL, et al. Pharmacodynamics of cefepime in patients with gram-negative infection. J Antimicrob Chemother. 2002;50:425-428.
264. Hoepelman AI, Kieft H, Aoun M, et al. International comparative study of cefepime and ceftazidime in the treatment of serious bacterial infections. J Antimicrob Chemother. 1993;32(Suppl B):175-186.
265. Chandrasekar PH, Arnow PM. Cefepime versus ceftazidime as empiric therapy for fever in neutropenic patients with cancer. Ann Pharmacother. 2000;34:989-995.
266. Cordonnier C, Herbrecht R, Pico JL, et al. Cefepime/amikacin versus ceftazidime/amikacin as empirical therapy for febrile episodes in neutropenic patients: A comparative study. Clin Infect Dis. 1997;24:41-51.
267. Kieft H, Hoepelman AIM, Arska MR, et al. Cefepime compared with ceftazidime as initial therapy for serious bacterial infections and sepsis syndrome. Antimicrob Agents Chemother. 1994;38:415-421.
268. Cordonnier C, Herbrecht R. Pico JL, et al. Cefepime/amikacin versus ceftazidime/amikacin as empirical therapy for febrile episodes in neutropenic patients: A comparative study. Clin Infect Dis. 1997;24:41-51.
269. Sanders WE Jr, Tenney JH, Kessler RE. Efficacy of cefepime in the treatment of infections due to multiply resistant *Enterobacter* species. Clin Infect Dis. 1996;23:454-461.
270. Biron P, Fuhrmann C, Cure H, et al. Cefepime versus imipenem-cilastatin as empirical monotherapy in 400 febrile patients with short duration neutropenia. J Antimicrob Chemother. 1998;32:511-518.
271. Barckow D, Schwigon CD. Cefepime versus cefotaxime in the treatment of lower respiratory tract infections. J Antimicrob Chemother. 1993;32(Suppl B):187-193.
272. Zervos M, Nelson M, Cefepime Study Group. Cefepime versus ceftriaxone for empiric treatment of hospitalized patients with community-acquired pneumonia. Antimicrob Agents Chemother. 1998;42:729-733.
273. Saez-Llorens X, Castano E, Garcia R, et al. Prospective randomized comparison of cefepime and cefotaxime for treatment of bacterial meningitis in infants and children. Antimicrob Agents Chemother. 1995;39:937-940.
274. Saez-Llorens X, O'Ryan M. Cefepime in the empiric treatment of meningitis in children. Pediatr Infect Dis J. 2001;20:356-361.

CHAPTER **21**

Other β-Lactam Antibiotics

HENRY F. CHAMBERS

CARBAPENEMS

Three carbapenems—imipenem, meropenem, and ertapenem—are approved for clinical use in the United States. A fourth, panipenem, which is not discussed here, is approved in Japan, China, and South Korea. Carbapenems have the broadest antibacterial spectrum of the β-lactam class largely because they are so β-lactamase stable. They are derivatives of thienamycin, a compound produced by *Streptomyces cattleya*.

Chemistry

The carbapenem core nucleus is differentiated from penicillins by a methylene replacement for sulfur and a double bond in the five-membered α-ring structure (Fig. 21-1). Penicillins and cephalosporins also contain an acylamino side chain attached to the β-ring in a *cis* configuration, whereas carbapenems have a hydroxyethyl side chain in a *trans* configuration at position C-6. This *trans* conformation is responsible for the excellent β-lactamase stability of this group of com-

FIGURE 21-1. Core structure and substituents for carbapenem antibiotics.

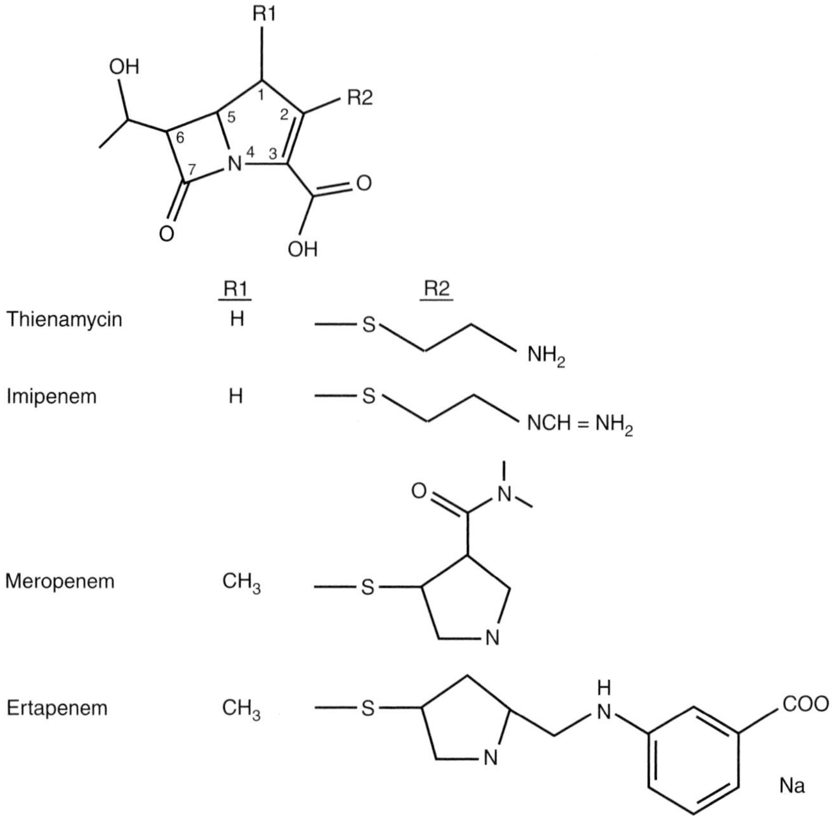

pounds. Thienamycin is too chemically unstable to be clinically useful. Imipenem, the *N*-formimidoyl derivative of thienamycin, is chemically much more stable but is substrate for mammalian renal dehydropeptidase I (DHP-I) and must be coadministered with a DHP-I inhibitor. Meropenem and ertapenem are β-1-methyl, 2-thio pyrrolidinyl derivatives of thienamycin. The β-1-methyl substituent confers stability to DHP-I; these compounds, in contrast to imipenem, do not require coadministration of a DHP-I inhibitor to prevent hydrolysis.

Mechanism of Action

Carbapenems bind with high affinity to most high-molecular-weight, penicillin-binding proteins (PBPs) of gram-positive and gram-negative bacteria. Carbapenems, particularly imipenem, traverse the outer membrane barrier of gram-negative bacteria through a specific outer membrane protein, OprD, rather than OmpC or OmpF, which are used by cephalosporins or penicillins.[1,2] Their unique outer membrane permeability feature and excellent β-lactamase stability compared with other β-lactams largely accounts for the broad antibacterial spectrum of carbapenems and relative lack of cross-resistance between carbapenems and the other members of the β-lactam antibiotic class. They are not hydrolyzed, or only very slowly hydrolyzed, by the most common penicillinases and cephalosporinases (Ambler class A and C enzymes), including those produced by *Staphylococcus aureus, Escherichia coli, Enterobacter cloacae, Citrobacter freundii, Proteus rettgeri, Serratia marcescens, Proteus vulgaris, Klebsiella oxytoca, Pseudomonas aeruginosa,* and *Bacteroides fragilis.* Carbapenems are hydrolyzed by Ambler class B enzymes, which are zinc-dependent metalloenzymes found in *Stenotrophomonas maltophilia,* some *Bacillus* spp. (e.g., *B. cereus* and *B. anthracis*), and other species. A few class A enzymes with carbapenemase activity have been described.[2-5]

Resistance

Resistance is due to one of four mechanisms: (1) production of a low-affinity PBP target; (2) diminished permeability, often due to absence of OprD (in gram-negative bacteria, usually in conjunction with pro-

duction of a β-lactamase); (3) efflux of drug across the outer membrane in gram-negative bacteria; and (4) production of a β-lactamase that hydrolyzes carbapenems (and other β-lactams). Resistance in gram-negative bacteria is usually an interplay involving impaired drug entry, efflux, and a β-lactamase (which need not be particularly efficient if drug entry is slow enough), which together produce a concentration of drug in the periplasmic space that is too low to inactivate target PBPs.

Downregulated production or absence of OprD by selection for mutation is responsible for emergence of resistance to imipenem in *P. aeruginosa, Enterobacter* spp., and other gram-negative bacteria, usually in conjunction with β-lactamase expression.[6,7] Resistance to imipenem reduces the activity of other carbapenems as well, although minimal inhibitory concentrations (MICs) still may fall within the susceptible range, suggesting that some carbapenems (e.g., meropenem) do not rely exclusively on OprD for entry into the cell.[8]

Meropenem is a substrate for the multidrug efflux system, MexA-MexB-OprM, present in *P. aeruginosa.*[7,9] MexB is a cytoplasmic membrane efflux pump protein linked via MexA to the outer membrane protein, OprM, through which meropenem, penicillins, cephalosporins, and fluoroquinolones can be effluxed from the cell. Overexpression of this efflux system raises the MIC of meropenem and other substrate antibiotics, but not imipenem. In the presence of a β-lactamase or reduced permeability from downregulation of a critical outer membrane protein, frank resistance to meropenem can occur. A similar efflux mechanism for imipenem has been identified in *Enterobacter aerogenes.*[10]

Production of a low-affinity PBP or PBPs mediates β-lactam class resistance, including carbapenem resistance, of high-level, penicillin-resistant pneumococci and viridans group streptococci, methicillin-resistant staphylococci, and ampicillin-resistant (non–β-lactamase producing) enterococci, particularly *Enterococcus faecium.*

Antibacterial Activity

Carbapenems are similar in their antibacterial spectra.[11-16] Imipenem is slightly more active against gram-positive bacteria than meropenem

TABLE 21-1   Comparative Activity of Imipenem and Meropenem against Aerobic and Anaerobic Bacteria

Organism	MIC₉₀ (μg/mL)	
	Imipenim	Meropenem
Staphylococcus aureus*†	0.03	0.3
Coagulase-negative staphylococci*†	0.1	1
Streptococcus pyogenes	0.03	0.1
Streptococcus agalactiae	0.03	0.1
Streptococcus pneumoniae	0.02	0.03
Enterococcus faecalis	2	8
Haemophilus influenzae	2	0.1
Neisseria gonorrhoeae	0.1	0.03
Neisseria meningitidis	0.1	0.01
Listeria monocytogenes	0.3	0.3
Klebsiella pneumoniae*	0.3	0.1
Enterobacter cloacae*	1	0.1
Enterobacter aerogenes*	1	0.1
Escherichia coli*	0.1	0.03
Klebsiella oxytoca*	1	0.03
Aeromonas hydrophila*	8	0.3
Citrobacter freundii	1	0.1
Citrobacter diversus*	0.5	0.02
Serratia marcescens*	4	0.1
Proteus mirabilis	4	0.1
Morganella morganii*	4	0.2
Proteus vulgaris*	4	0.1
Acinetobacter anitratus	0.5	1
Pseudomonas aeruginosa*	4	2
Stenotrophomonas maltophilia	>50	>50
Burkholderia cepacia	16	32
Bacteroides fragilis	2	1
Prevotella melaninogenicus	0.1	0.1
Clostridium difficile	4	2
Clostridium perfringens	0.1	0.02
Anaerobic gram-positive cocci	0.5	0.3
Campylobacter jejuni	0.03	0.02

*Both β-lactamase- and non-β-lactamase–containing strains.
†Methicillin-susceptible strains; methicillin-resistant strains are also resistant to imipenem and meropenem.

and ertapenem; meropenem and ertapenem are slightly more active against gram-negative aerobic species. All have excellent in vitro activity against aerobic hemolytic streptococci with MIC values of 0.2 μg/mL or less (Table 21-1); penicillin-susceptible *Streptococcus pneumoniae*, with MICs less than 0.1 μg/mL; and methicillin-susceptible strains of *S. aureus* and *Staphylococcus epidermidis*, which are inhibited by less than 0.5 μg/mL. Methicillin-resistant staphylococci are resistant to currently available carbapenems. *Listeria* and *Bacillus* spp., including *B. anthracis*, are inhibited by less than 1 μg/mL. Penicillin-intermediate (penicillin MICs 0.1 to 1 μg/mL) and resistant strains of *S. pneumoniae* (penicillin MIC ≥ 2 μg/mL) are inhibited by less than or equal to 0.5 μg/mL and 0.5 to 4 μg/mL. Penicillin-susceptible strains of *Enterococcus faecalis* are susceptible to imipenem, with MICs less than or equal to 2 μg/mL, but resistant to meropenem and ertapenem. Similar to penicillin, imipenem is bacteriostatic, not bactericidal, against susceptible enterococci. Strains of *E. faecium* are resistant to all carbapenems. *Corynebacterium* spp. are inhibited at concentrations less than 1 μg/mL.

Neisseria gonorrhoeae and *Neisseria meningitidis* are highly susceptible with MICs typically less than 0.1 μg/mL. MICs of *Haemophilus influenzae* and other *Haemophilus* spp. are less than or equal to 0.1 μg/mL for ertapenem and meropenem and less than or equal to 2 μg/mL for imipenem. Most of the Enterobacteriaceae are inhibited by imipenem at concentrations less than or equal to 1 μg/mL; some *Morganella* and *Proteus* strains have MIC values of 2 to 4 μg/mL. Corresponding MICs of meropenem and ertapenem are less than or equal to 0.1 μg/mL. *Citrobacter, Enterobacter,* and *Providencia* spp. are inhibited at ertapenem or meropenem concentrations of less than 0.5 μg/mL compared with imipenem concentrations of 2 to 4 μg/mL. Meropenem is the most active carbapenem against *P. aeruginosa,* including strains resistant to antipseudomonal penicillins and cephalosporins, with MICs less than or equal to 2 μg/mL; imipenem

is slightly less active with MICs of 4 to 8 μg/mL. Ertapenem is not active against *P. aeruginosa. Acinetobacter* organisms are inhibited by less than or equal to 2 μg/mL of imipenem or meropenem, but resistant to ertapenem with MICs greater than 8 μg/mL. *S. maltophilia* and *Burkholderia cepacia* are intrinsically resistant to all carbapenems. Carbapenems as a class are highly active against most anaerobic species, including anaerobic gram-positive cocci, *B. fragilis,* non-fragilis species of *Bacteroides, Clostridium* spp. (with the exception of *C. difficile,* which generally are resistant), *Fusobacterium* spp., *Prevotella* spp., *Eubacterium* spp., *Porphyromonas* spp., and others with MICs less than or equal to 1 μg/mL.[17-21]

Nocardia spp. are inhibited by meropenem or imipenem. Although few isolates have been tested, *Actinomyces* seem generally susceptible to carbapenems. Carbapenems have variable activity against *Mycobacterium* spp.

Pharmacology

Imipenem, meropenem, and ertapenem are absorbed poorly after oral ingestion and must be administered parenterally. All are cleared renally. Imipenem is formulated for coadministration with an equivalent amount of the DHP-I inhibitor, cilastatin. Cilastatin has no antibacterial activity, and it does not affect activity of imipenem. It prolongs the half-life of imipenem, maintains therapeutic urinary concentrations, and prevents the nephrotoxic effects of imipenem and its metabolites. Meropenem and ertapenem are stable to DHP-I and require no inhibitor.

Imipenem and meropenem are pharmacologically similar. A 30-minute infusion of 500 mg of either agent produces mean peak serum concentrations of approximately 30 μg/mL.[22,23] A 1-g dose of ertapenem administered intravenously produces peak serum concentrations of approximately 150 μg/mL; the same dose given intramuscularly results in peak serum concentrations at 2 hours of approximately 70 μg/mL.[24-26] The plasma half-life is 1 hour for imipenem and for meropenem and 4 hours for ertapenem in healthy people. The relatively long half-life of ertapenem permits once-daily dosing, whereas imipenem typically is administered every 6 hours, and meropenem is given every 8 hours. Carbapenems require dosage adjustment in patients with reduced renal function but not in patients with impaired liver function. Carbapenems are removed by continuous venovenous hemofiltration, hemodialysis, and very minimally by peritoneal dialysis.

The carbapenems are well distributed to various body compartments and penetrate well into most tissues. They all penetrate inflamed meninges, producing cerebrospinal fluid (CSF) concentrations of 1 to 5 $\mu g/mL$.[27,28]

Adverse Reactions

Carbapenems generally have been well tolerated. β-Lactam class allergic reactions are the most common adverse events, including rash, urticaria, immediate hypersensitivity, and cross-reactions with penicillins. There seems to be no particular propensity for these antibiotics to cause major adverse effects, such as diarrhea, pseudomembranous colitis, coagulation abnormalities, nephrotoxicity, or hepatotoxicity, which occur with frequencies similar to comparators. Imipenem produces nausea if infused too rapidly, and it can cause seizures, an infrequent side effect that occurs most often in patients receiving high doses with underlying central nervous system pathology and in patients with decreased renal function in whom dose adjustment has not been made.[29,30] The toxicity profiles of meropenem and ertapenem are similar to that of imipenem except that they seem less likely to cause seizures.

Clinical Use

Carbapenems, because of their broad antibacterial spectrum covering gram-positive, gram-negative, and anaerobic bacteria, are useful for treatment of a wide variety of infections, including bacteremia, bone and soft tissue infections, obstetric and gynecologic infections, complicated urinary tract infections, intra-abdominal sepsis, and pneumonia.[29,31] Imipenem and meropenem are most appropriate as treatment of infections caused by cephalosporin-resistant Enterobacteriaceae, particularly *S. marcescens*, *Providencia* spp., *C. freundii*, and *Enterobacter* spp.; as empirical therapy in the treatment of serious infections in patients previously treated with multiple antibiotics, because of the high likelihood of encountering organisms resistant to more conventional β-lactams; as a single agent in the treatment of febrile, neutropenic patients[32,33]; and as treatment of polymicrobial infections in which otherwise multiple-drug regimens of higher cost and potentially more adverse side effects would be necessary. Meropenem and imipenem are therapeutically equivalent and interchangeable[34] in most situations, of which bacterial meningitis is an important exception. Meropenem is approved by the U.S. Food and Drug Administration for treatment of bacterial meningitis in children 3 months old and older[35] and is efficacious in adults.[36] Ertapenem and imipenem are not approved by the Food and Drug Administration for meningitis, and imipenem probably should be avoided because of its propensity to cause seizures. Imipenem and meropenem are appropriate for use in the treatment of nosocomial infections because they also are active against *P. aeruginosa* and *Acinetobacter* spp. As with other antibiotics, single-drug therapy for serious *P. aeruginosa* infections has been accompanied by emergence of resistance to meropenem. Although it is uncertain whether emergence of resistance may be prevented and outcome improved, combination therapy should be used whenever possible to treat serious infections caused by *P. aeruginosa*. The recommended adult dose of imipenem for patients with creatinine clearance greater than 50 mL/min is 250 to 500 mg intravenously every 6 to 8 hours. The pediatric dose is 15 to 25 mg/kg every 6 to 8 hours. The recommended adult dose of meropenem for patients with creatinine clearance greater than 50 mL/min is 500 to 1000 mg intravenously every 8 hours, although doses of 6 g/day seem to be safe.[36] The pediatric dose is 20 to 40 mg/kg, with the higher dose indicated for treatment of meningitis, every 8 hours. Dosage adjustment is required for either drug for creatinine clearance of less than 50 mL/min.

Ertapenem differs from imipenem and meropenem in two important respects: It has a long half-life so that it can be given as a once-daily dose, and it has relatively poor activity against *P. aeruginosa* and *Acinetobacter*. Ertapenem is indicated for the treatment of intra-abdominal infections, obstetric and gynecologic infections, community-acquired pneumonia, complicated skin and skin structure infections, and urinary tract infections.[2,37-39] Similar to imipenem and meropenem, ertapenem has excellent antianaerobic activity and so is especially useful in a single daily dosage regimen for polymicrobial infections. Ertapenem also is active against cephalosporin-resistant Enterobacteriaceae, particularly *S. marcescens*, *Providencia* spp., *C. freundii*, and *Enterobacter* spp. and can be used for infections caused by these organisms. Although it penetrates into CSF, ertapenem is not approved for treatment of bacterial meningitis. The recommended adult dose of ertapenem or patients with creatinine clearance greater than 30 mL/min is 1000 mg intravenously or intramuscularly once a day and 500 mg once daily for patients with creatinine clearance less than 30 mL/min or on dialysis. No pediatric dose or indications have been established.

MONOBACTAMS

Many bacteria, particularly *Gluconobacter* and *Acinetobacter*, produce monocyclic β-lactam antibiotics with antibacterial activity.[40] Monobactams are active only against gram-negative aerobic bacteria.[41] Aztreonam is the only monobactam currently on the market.

Aztreonam is a monocyclic β-lactam (Fig. 21-2) that is a modified form of a compound produced by *Chromobacterium violaceum*. It has no useful antibacterial activity against gram-positive or anaerobic bacteria because it does not bind to PBPs in these species. Aztreonam readily passes through the outer membrane of gram-negative species, and it binds primarily to PBP 3 in Enterobacteriaceae, *P. aeruginosa*, and other gram-negative aerobic organisms producing nonviable, long filamentous structures. It is resistant to hydrolysis by most plasmid and chromosomal β-lactamases and class B enzymes, although it is inactivated by many class C β-lactamases that also inactivate third-generation cephalosporins.

Antibacterial Activity

Aztreonam inhibits most Enterobacteriaceae at concentrations less than 0.5 $\mu g/mL$ (Table 21-2); some *P. aeruginosa*, *E. cloacae*, and *C. freundii* strains are resistant. Most *P. aeruginosa* organisms are inhibited by less than 16 $\mu g/mL$. Most *B. cepacia* and *S. maltophilia* are resistant, as are many *Acinetobacter* spp.; *Haemophilus* and *Neisseria*, including β-lactamase-producing isolates, are inhibited by less than 0.2 $\mu g/mL$. *Yersinia* and *Aeromonas* are inhibited by less than 0.5 $\mu g/mL$. Enterobacteriaceae and *P. aeruginosa* can be resistant owing to a failure to penetrate the outer membrane or destruction by β-lactamases.

Pharmacokinetics

Aztreonam is not absorbed from the gastrointestinal tract. It is absorbed rapidly and completely after intramuscular administration, with peak serum concentrations attained within 1 hour.[42] A 500-mg

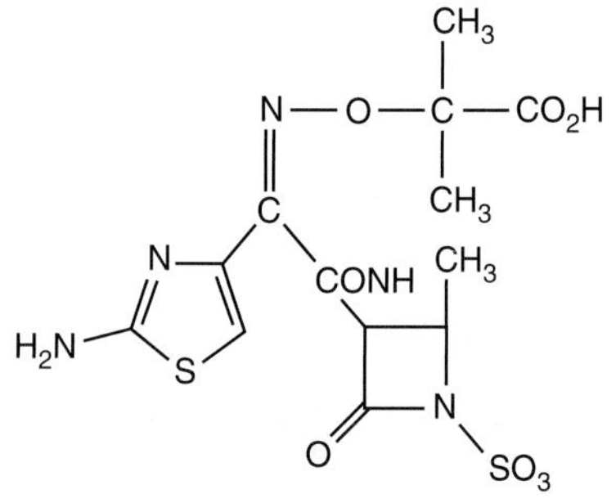

FIGURE 21-2. Aztreonam.

intramuscular dose of aztreonam produces serum concentrations of 21 to 27 μg/mL at 1 hour and 4 to 6 μg/mL at 6 hours. After intravenous infusion of a single dose of 0.5 g of aztreonam in healthy adults over 30 minutes, serum concentrations immediately after completion of the infusion average 55 to 65 μg/mL; serum concentrations 1 hour after an intramuscular dose are the same as after an intravenous dose.

Aztreonam achieves therapeutic levels in tissues and fluids throughout the body.[42] CSF concentrations in the presence of inflamed meninges after a 2-g dose are approximately 3 to 7 μg/mL, and higher concentrations can be achieved after multiple doses.[43,44]

Aztreonam is excreted by glomerular filtration and tubular secretion. In adults with normal renal and hepatic function, the elimination half-life is approximately 2 hours. In neonates 7 days old and weighing less than 2.5 kg, the half-life of aztreonam ranges from 5.5 to 9.9 hours. In adults with renal impairment, the half-life of aztreonam increased to 8 hours at creatinine clearances of 10 mL/min. The half-life of aztreonam is prolonged only slightly in patients with hepatic impairment. Aztreonam is removed by continuous venovenous hemofiltration, hemodialysis, and, to a lesser extent, peritoneal dialysis.

Adverse Reactions

No major adverse reactions to aztreonam have been reported. Skin rashes can occur. Aztreonam can be used safely in patients with rashes or immediate hypersensitivity reactions to penicillins or other β-lactams because cross-reactivity does not occur. Hematologic, gastrointestinal, nephrotoxic, or neurotoxic reactions have not been noted.

Clinical Use

Aztreonam has been used in children and in adults for the treatment of a variety of infections, such as cystitis, pyelonephritis, lower respiratory tract infections including pneumonia and bronchitis, septicemia, skin and skin structure infections, infections of postoperative wounds or ulcers and burns, intra-abdominal infection including peritonitis, and gynecologic infections including endometritis and pelvic cellulitis caused by gram-negative aerobic bacteria.[45,46] The usual dose is 1 to 2 g every 6 to 8 hours intravenously or intramuscularly, with a daily dose for serious infection of 6 g. The pediatric dose is 30 mg/kg every 6 to 8 hours.

Because aztreonam has a spectrum of activity limited to aerobic gram-negative bacteria, the drug should not be used alone for empirical therapy in seriously ill patients if there is any possibility that the infection may be caused by gram-positive aerobic bacteria or if a mixed aerobic-anaerobic bacterial infection is suspected. An anti-infective agent effective against the suspected organism or organisms should be used concomitantly. Aztreonam has been used safely and effectively in conjunction with clindamycin, erythromycin, metronidazole, penicillins, and vancomycin.

β-LACTAMASE INHIBITORS

β-Lactamase inhibitors are clavulanic acid and penicillanic acid sulfone derivatives. These compounds, which have weak antibacterial activity, are potent inhibitors of many plasmid-encoded and some chromosomal β-lactamases. These compounds can restore antibacterial activity of amoxicillin, ampicillin, piperacillin, mezlocillin, and cefoperazone, all of which can be destroyed by β-lactamases commonly produced by gram-positive and gram-negative bacteria (Table 21-3). Although competitive inhibition is seen, β-lactamase inhibitors primarily act as a suicide substrate that forms a stable intermediate, rendering the enzyme inactive.

Three β-lactamase inhibitors are in clinical use: clavulanic acid, sulbactam, and tazobactam. Each inhibitor is available only as a fixed-combination preparation that includes an active β-lactam antibiotic as the companion agent. There are minor differences in potency, activity, and pharmacology among the β-lactamase inhibitors, but clinically they can be considered therapeutically equivalent except for some *Klebsiella* spp., in which clavulanate inhibits isolates resistant to sulbactam and tazobactam. The antibacterial activity of the inhibitor-antibiotic combination is determined by the spectrum of the companion β-lactam antibiotic. The three parenteral combinations—ampicillin-sulbactam, ticarcillin-clavulanate, and piperacillin-tazobactam—although differing in bacterial spectrum and pharmacology, have similar indications, including treatment of pneumonia, complicated skin and skin tissue infections, and intra-abdominal infections.

β-Lactamase inhibitors are effective only against Ambler class A β-lactamases, that is, penicillinases, which often are plasmid-encoded,

TABLE 21-2 In Vitro Activity of Aztreonam

Organism	MIC_{90} (μg/mL)
Escherichia coli	0.25
Klebsiella pneumoniae	1
Klebsiella oxytoca	1
Enterobacter cloacae	16
Enterobacter aerogenes	8
Enterobacter agglomerans	1
Citrobacter freundii	8
Citrobacter diversus	0.25
Serratia marcescens	4
Proteus mirabilis	0.01
Proteus vulgaris	0.12
Proteus rettgeri	0.12
Morganella morganii	0.25
Providencia	0.025
Salmonella enteritidis	0.25
Shigella spp.	0.12
Arizona hinshawi	0.12
Aeromonas hydrophila	0.12
Aeromonas shigelloides	0.12
Yersinia enterocolitica	2
Pasteurella multocida	0.12
Salmonella typhi	0.12
Haemophilus influenzae	0.12
Neisseria gonorrhoeae	0.25
Neisseria meningitidis	0.025
Pseudomonas aeruginosa	16
Stenotrophomonas maltophilia	>128
Pseudomonas spp., other (*P. diminuta, P. stutzeri, P. fluorescens*)	>128
Burkholderia cepacia	>128
Streptococcus pyogenes	16
Streptococcus pneumoniae	16
Enterococcus spp.	>128
Clostridium spp.	>128
Bacteroides spp.	>128

MIC_{90}, minimal inhibitory concentration for 90% of isolates.
Data from Edwards JR, Turner PJ, Wannop C, et al. In vitro antibacterial activity of SM-7338, a carbapenem antibiotic with stability to dehydropeptidase I. Antimicrob Agents Chemother. 1989;33:215-222; and Sentochnik DE, Eliopoulos GM, Ferraro MJ, et al. Comparative in vitro activity of SM7338, a new carbapenem antimicrobial agent. Antimicrob Agents Chemother. 1989;33:1232-1236.

TABLE 21-3 Activity of Amoxicillin-Clavulanate against Amoxicillin-Resistant Organisms

Organism	Amoxicillin	Augmentin*
Staphylococcus aureus	256	1
Staphylococcus epidermidis	256	2
S. aureus (MRSA)	256	16
Haemophilus influenzae	64	0.5
Branhamella catarrhalis	16	0.25
Neisseria gonorrhoeae	128	1
Escherichia coli	>256	8
Klebsiella pneumoniae	128	4
Proteus mirabilis	>256	4
Proteus vulgaris	>256	2
Bacteroides fragilis	32	0.5
Enterobacter, Citrobacter, Serratia spp. and *Pseudomonas aeruginosa*	>128	>128

*Contains amoxicillin and clavulanate in a 2:1 ratio.
MRSA, methicillin-resistant *S. aureus*.

produced by *S. aureus, H. influenzae, Branhamella catarrhalis, Bacteroides* spp. (the β-lactamases are chromosomal in the latter two species), and Enterobacteriaceae, which produce the closely related TEM and SHV β-lactamases. Chromosomal β-lactamases, which typically are Ambler class C β-lactamases (i.e., amp C cephalosporinases) of *Serratia* spp., *C. freundii, Enterobacter* spp., *P. aeruginosa,* and some Enterobacteriaceae, are not inhibited by β-lactamase inhibitors. They do inhibit extended-spectrum β-lactamases, however, reflecting the fact that these enzymes are mutants of class A β-lactamases. β-Lactamase inhibitors do not inhibit class B metallo-β-lactamases, which are structurally unrelated to the other β-lactamase classes.

Clavulanate

The β-lactamase inhibitor clavulanate (Fig. 21-3) was found in cultures of *Streptomyces clavuligerus*. The compound had only weak antibacterial activity, but when combined with penicillin G, inhibition of a *Klebsiella* isolate normally resistant to penicillin was noted. Clavulanate subsequently was found to inhibit certain types of β-lactamases from many clinically important gram-positive and gram-negative organisms. It is a weak inducer of chromosomal β-lactamases.[47] Clavulanate in combination with amoxicillin is available for oral administration. It also is available as a parenteral preparation in many countries, but not in the United States. Clavulanate in combination with ticarcillin is available for intravenous administration in the United States.

Pharmacology

Clavulanate is moderately well absorbed from the gastrointestinal tract. Peak serum concentration of 4 μg/mL in children and adults occurs 40 to 120 minutes after ingestion of 125 mg.[48] Combining clavulanate with amoxicillin does not alter significantly the pharmacologic parameters of either drug. The absorption of clavulanate is unaffected by the simultaneous administration of food, milk, or aluminum hydroxide–containing antacids. After intravenous infusion of clavulanate combined with either amoxicillin or ticarcillin, the drug is distributed rapidly, producing peak serum concentrations of approximately 8 μg/mL after a 100-mg intravenous dose. The serum half-life of clavulanate is about 1 hour and slightly less than that of amoxicillin. No accumulation of clavulanate occurs until creatinine clearance is less than 10 mL/min.[48] Dose adjustment is made on the basis of the desired dose for amoxicillin or ticarcillin. Clavulanate is degraded in vivo, with metabolites being excreted via lung, feces, and urine; only 20% to 60% appears unchanged in urine 6 hours after an oral dose. Urinary levels after a 125-mg dose of clavulanate are greater than 40 μg/mL for 4 to 6 hours after dosing.

Clavulanate produces therapeutic levels in bile, middle ear fluid, and tonsil tissue. Clavulanate crosses the placenta and may be found in the cord blood of newborns and in the amniotic fluid, but no clavulanate can be detected in breast milk. Clavulanate does not penetrate noninflamed meninges. In patients with meningitis, CSF levels of clavulanate have been in the range of 0.25 μg/mL.[49] Clavulanate concentrations of less than 1 μg/mL are achieved in sputum after the oral administration of amoxicillin-clavulanate, but pleural fluid levels are 46% to 91% of peak serum levels. There is rapid penetration of clavulanate into peritoneal fluid, with mean peritoneal fluid levels of clavulanate equaling 66% of serum levels.

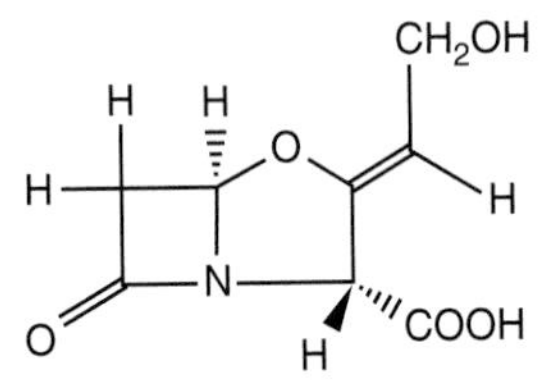

Adverse Reactions

No new or major adverse reactions to the use of clavulanate combined with either amoxicillin or ticarcillin have been reported. The incidence of skin reactions has been similar to that seen when penicillin is used alone. Diarrhea has occurred after the use of 250 mg of clavulanate given three times daily, and some nausea has occurred with this dosage program. Accordingly the oral dose of clavulanate is recommended not to exceed 125 mg two or three times a day. Parenterally administered clavulanate combinations have not caused undue diarrhea.

Amoxicillin-Clavulanate

Amoxicillin-clavulanate (Augmentin) has been used in many different clinical settings. The combination has proved useful as therapy for treatment of acute otitis media in children that is caused by β-lactamase-producing *H. influenzae* and *B. catarrhalis*.[50,51] It also has been used to treat sinusitis or pneumonia caused by susceptible β-lactamase-producing or non–β-lactamase-producing bacteria. It is particularly useful to treat polymicrobial infections in which β-lactamase-producing organisms may be present, including bite wounds of human or animal origin and diabetic foot infections.[52,53] Skin structure infections caused by streptococci and staphylococci have responded to amoxicillin-clavulanate with results comparable to those achieved with oral antistaphylococcal agents and oral cephalosporins.

The agent is formulated as tablets containing 250, 500, or 875 mg of amoxicillin combined with 125 mg of clavulanate. The usual dose is 250 mg of amoxicillin every 8 hours to 875 mg every 12 hours by mouth. In children, the dose is 20 to 45 mg/kg/day in two or three divided doses; a variety of oral suspensions and chewable tablets are available. The twice-daily formulation (875 mg of amoxicillin and 125 mg of clavulanate by tablet for adults; 400 mg and 57 mg in suspension for children) is as effective as the thrice-daily formulation.[54,55]

Ticarcillin-Clavulanate

Ticarcillin-clavulanate (Timentin) has been used for treatment of community-acquired and hospital-acquired pneumonia, particularly in cases involving aspiration of oral secretions and aerobic gram-negative bacilli, intra-abdominal infections, gynecologic infections, skin and skin structure infections, and osteomyelitis.[56] The usual dose is 3.1 g administered every 4 to 6 hours.

Sulbactam

Sulbactam (Fig. 21-4) is a 6-desaminopenicillin sulfone. Sulbactam is a broader spectrum β-lactamase inhibitor than clavulanic acid, but less potent. It does not induce chromosomal β-lactamases. Sulbactam is available in the United States only in combination with ampicillin (Unasyn), in a ratio of 0.5 g of sulbactam to 1 g of ampicillin as a parenteral formulation for intravenous administration.

FIGURE 21-3. Clavulanate.

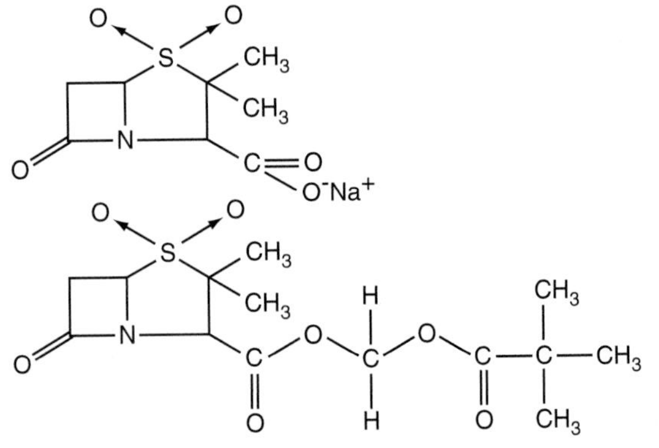

FIGURE 21-4. Sulbactam *(top)* and sulbactam oral ester *(bottom)*.

Pharmacology

Sulbactam has pharmacokinetics in humans similar to those of ampicillin.[57] The average peak serum level after intravenous infusion of 1 g is 68 μg/mL. The serum half-life is 1 hour. Sulbactam is excreted by the kidney and has a urinary recovery rate of 70% to 80% of a dose. Biliary excretion is minimal, and metabolism is less than 25%. Renal excretion is blocked by probenecid. The half-life is not altered significantly until the creatinine clearance decreases to less than 30 mL/min. The half-life is 9.2 hours at clearances of 5 to 15 mL/min and 20 hours in anuria. Dosage adjustment is required for creatinine clearance less than 50 mL/min and is based on the ampicillin component. Concentrations of sulbactam in interstitial fluid and peritoneal secretions are comparable to levels in serum. Penetration of sulbactam into inflamed meninges is low, with levels of 0.1 to 10 μg/mL found in the CSF after an infusion of 1 g.

Adverse Reactions

Clinical studies of the combination of sulbactam plus ampicillin have revealed no major hematologic, renal, hepatic, or central nervous system reactions. Diarrhea has not been a major problem after intravenous use. Skin reactions are similar to those found for ampicillin, and there is occasional elevation of transaminase levels.

Clinical Use

Ampicillin-sulbactam and amoxicillin-clavulanate have the same spectrum of antibacterial activity. Ampicillin-sulbactam has been used in the treatment of mixed bacterial infections, such as intra-abdominal infections, obstetric and gynecologic infections, and soft tissue and bone infections.[58]

Tazobactam

Tazobactam is a penicillanic acid sulfone β-lactamase inhibitor with a structure similar to that of sulbactam (Fig. 21-5). Its spectrum of β-lactamase inhibition is similar to that of sulbactam, but its potency is more like that of clavulanic acid. It is not an inducer of chromosomal β-lactamases.[59] It is available for parenteral administration only in combination with piperacillin (Zosyn) in an 8:1 ratio of piperacillin to tazobactam by weight.

Pharmacology

Mean peak serum concentration after a 30-minute intravenous infusion of 375 mg of tazobactam in combination with piperacillin is 25 μg/mL in healthy subjects. Tazobactam is cleared primarily renally, and dosage should be adjusted for creatinine clearances of less than 40 mL/min. Combining tazobactam with piperacillin reduces clearance of tazobactam, but the clearance of piperacillin is not affected. Clearances of piperacillin and tazobactam are similar in subjects with normal renal function. Peak serum concentrations are approximately 50% higher in patients with end-stage renal disease.[60] The half-life of tazobactam is 1 hour in subjects with normal renal function, increasing to 3.6 hours (compared with 2 hours for piperacillin) in subjects with a creatinine clearance of less than 20 mL/min. The half-life of tazobactam is approximately 7 hours in patients with end-stage renal disease. These differences in pharmacokinetics of piperacillin and tazobactam do not require adjustment of the dose of tazobactam independent of piperacillin; the dose is adjusted based on the pharmacokinetics of piperacillin.

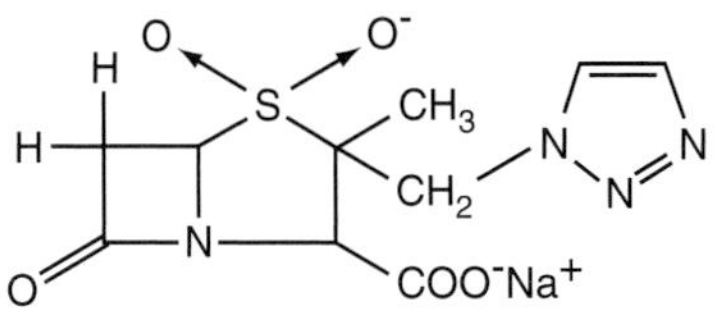

Tissue levels of tazobactam reflect a percent penetration that is similar to that of piperacillin for each tissue type.[61] Tazobactam penetrates inflamed meninges. CSF concentrations of piperacillin and tazobactam were 16% and 32% of simultaneous serum concentrations in a rabbit meningitis model.[62]

Adverse Reactions

Limited clinical data do not indicate any new or unusual toxicity unique to tazobactam.

Clinical Use

Piperacillin-tazobactam has the broadest spectrum of the three parenteral β-lactamase inhibitor combinations. Published clinical studies have been conducted mainly in adults; experience with this combination for treatment of serious infections in children indicates that it is safe and effective.[63] In general, the antibacterial spectrum of piperacillin-tazobactam is similar in vitro to that of ticarcillin-clavulanate. Piperacillin-tazobactam is slightly more active than ticarcillin-clavulanate for some strains (including enterococci), presumably because of the greater intrinsic activity of piperacillin.[64] In clinical trials, the efficacy of piperacillin-tazobactam has been equivalent, and occasionally superior, to similarly broad-spectrum comparator drugs (e.g., ticarcillin-clavulanate, carbapenems, third-generation cephalosporins) for treatment of pneumonia, skin and soft tissue infections, intra-abdominal infections, polymicrobial infections, and febrile neutropenia in combination with an aminoglycoside.[65,66] As with other antibiotics, piperacillin-tazobactam should be used in combination with another agent (e.g., an aminoglycoside) for treatment of pneumonia caused by *P. aeruginosa*. The usual adult dose is 12 g of piperacillin/1.5 g of tazobactam administered at a dose of 3.375 g (3 g piperacillin, 0.375 g of tazobactam) every 6 hours or 4.5 g every 8 hours for creatinine clearance greater than 40 mL/min.

REFERENCES

1. Trias J, Nikaido H. Outer membrane protein D2 catalyzes facilitated diffusion of carbapenems and penems through the outer membrane of *Pseudomonas aeruginosa*. Antimicrob Agents Chemother. 1990;34:52-57.
2. Bonfiglio G, Russo G, Nicoletti G. Recent developments in carbapenems. Expert Opin Invest Drugs. 2002;11:529-544.
3. Bush K. New beta-lactamases in gram-negative bacteria: Diversity and impact on the selection of antimicrobial therapy. Clin Infect Dis. 2001;32:1085-1089.
4. Yigit H, et al. Novel carbapenem-hydrolyzing beta-lactamase, KPC-1, from a carbapenem-resistant strain of *Klebsiella pneumoniae*. Antimicrob Agents Chemother. 2001;45:1151-1161.
5. Yigit H, et al. Carbapenem resistance in a clinical isolate of *Enterobacter aerogenes* is associated with decreased expression of OmpF and OmpC porin analogs. Antimicrob Agents Chemother. 2002;46:3817-3822.
6. Ballestero S, et al. Carbapenem resistance in *Pseudomonas aeruginosa* from cystic fibrosis patients. J Antimicrob Chemother. 1996;38:39-45.
7. Kohler T, et al. Carbapenem activities against *Pseudomonas aeruginosa*: Respective contributions of OprD and efflux systems. Antimicrob Agents Chemother. 1999;43:424-427.
8. Sumita Y, Fukasawa M. Meropenem resistance in *Pseudomonas aeruginosa*. Chemotherapy. 1996;42:47-56.
9. Li XZ, Zhang L, Poole K. Interplay between the MexA-MexB-OprM multidrug efflux system and the outer membrane barrier in the multiple antibiotic resistance of *Pseudomonas aeruginosa*. J Antimicrob Chemother. 2000;45:433-436.
10. Bornet C, et al. Imipenem and expression of multidrug efflux pump in *Enterobacter aerogenes*. Biochem Biophys Res Commun. 2003;301:985-990.
11. Sentochnik DE, et al. Comparative in vitro activity of SM7338, a new carbapenem antimicrobial agent. Antimicrob Agents Chemother. 1989;33:1232-1236.
12. Edwards JR, et al. In vitro antibacterial activity of SM-7338, a carbapenem antibiotic with stability to dehydropeptidase I. Antimicrob Agents Chemother. 1989;33:215-222.
13. Jones RN. Review of the in vitro spectrum of activity of imipenem. Am J Med. 1985;78:22-32.
14. Iaconis JP, et al. Comparison of antibacterial activities of meropenem and six other antimicrobials against *Pseudomonas aeruginosa* isolates from North American studies and clinical trials. Clin Infect Dis. 1997;24(Suppl 2):S191-196.
15. Fuchs PC, Barry AL, Brown SD. In vitro activities of ertapenem (MK-0826) against clinical bacterial isolates from 11 North American medical centers. Antimicrob Agents Chemother. 2001;45:1915-1918.
16. Livermore DM, et al. In vitro activities of ertapenem (MK-0826) against recent clinical bacteria collected in Europe and Australia. Antimicrob Agents Chemother. 2001;45:1860-1867.

FIGURE 21-5. Tazobactam.

17. Goldstein EJ, et al. Comparative susceptibility of the *Bacteroides fragilis* group species and other anaerobic bacteria to meropenem, imipenem, piperacillin, cefoxitin, ampicillin/sulbactam, clindamycin and metronidazole. J Antimicrob Chemother. 1993;31:363-372.

18. Goldstein EJ, et al. Comparative in vitro activities of ertapenem (MK-0826) against 1,001 anaerobes isolated from human intra-abdominal infections. Antimicrob Agents Chemother. 2000;44:2389-2394.

19. Goldstein EJ, et al. Comparative in vitro activity of ertapenem and 11 other antimicrobial agents against aerobic and anaerobic pathogens isolated from skin and soft tissue animal and human bite wound infections. J Antimicrob Chemother. 2001;48:641-651.

20. Goldstein EJ, et al. Comparative in vitro activities of ertapenem (MK-0826) against 469 less frequently identified anaerobes isolated from human infections. Antimicrob Agents Chemother. 2002;46:1136-1140.

21. Hoellman DB, et al. In vitro antianaerobic activity of ertapenem (MK-0826) compared to seven other compounds. Antimicrob Agents Chemother. 2002;46:220-224.

22. Drusano GL, Standiford HC. Pharmacokinetic profile of imipenem/cilastatin in normal volunteers. Am J Med. 1985;78:47-53.

23. Leroy A, et al. Pharmacokinetics of meropenem (ICI 194,660) and its metabolite (ICI 213,689) in healthy subjects and in patients with renal impairment. Antimicrob Agents Chemother. 1992;36:2794-2798.

24. Majumdar AK, et al. Pharmacokinetics of ertapenem in healthy young volunteers. Antimicrob Agents Chemother. 2002;46:3506-3511.

25. Odenholt I. Ertapenem: A new carbapenem. Expert Opin Invest Drugs. 2001; 10:1157-1166.

26. Musson DG, et al. Pharmacokinetics of intramuscularly administered ertapenem. Antimicrob Agents Chemother. 2003;47:1732-1735.

27. Mouton JW, et al. Comparative pharmacokinetics of the carbapenems: clinical implications. Clin Pharmacokinet. 2000;39:185-201.

28. Cottagnoud P, et al. Activities of ertapenem, a new long-acting carbapenem, against penicillin-sensitive or -resistant pneumococci in experimental meningitis. Antimicrob Agents Chemother. 2003;47:1943-1947.

29. Balfour JA, Bryson HM, Brogden RN. Imipenem/cilastatin: An update of its antibacterial activity, pharmacokinetics and therapeutic efficacy in the treatment of serious infections. Drugs. 1996;51:99-136.

30. Koppel BS, et al. Seizures in the critically ill: The role of imipenem. Epilepsia. 2001;42:1590-1593.

31. Wiseman LR, et al. Meropenem: A review of its antibacterial activity, pharmacokinetic properties and clinical efficacy. Drugs 1995;50:73-101.

32. Vandercam B, et al. Meropenem versus ceftazidime as empirical monotherapy for febrile neutropenic cancer patients. Ann Hematol. 2000;79:152-157.

33. Deaney NB, Tate H. A meta-analysis of clinical studies of imipenem-cilastatin for empirically treating febrile neutropenic patients. J Antimicrob Chemother. 1996; 37:975-986.

34. Colardyn F, Faulkner KL. Intravenous meropenem versus imipenem/cilastatin in the treatment of serious bacterial infections in hospitalized patients. Meropenem Serious Infection Study Group. J Antimicrob Chemother. 1996;38:523-537.

35. Klugman KP, Dagan R. Randomized comparison of meropenem with cefotaxime for treatment of bacterial meningitis. Meropenem Meningitis Study Group. Antimicrob Agents Chemother. 1995;39:1140-1146.

36. Schmutzhard E, et al. A randomised comparison of meropenem with cefotaxime or ceftriaxone for the treatment of bacterial meningitis in adults. Meropenem Meningitis Study Group. J Antimicrob Chemother. 1995;36(Suppl A):85-97.

37. Gesser RM, et al. Efficacy of ertapenem in the treatment of serious infections caused by Enterobacteriaceae: Analysis of pooled clinical trial data. J Antimicrob Chemother. 2003;51:1253-1260.

38. Solomkin JS, et al. Ertapenem versus piperacillin/tazobactam in the treatment of complicated intraabdominal infections: Results of a double-blind, randomized comparative phase III trial. Ann Surg. 2003;237:235-245.

39. Graham DR, et al. Ertapenem once daily versus piperacillin-tazobactam 4 times per day for treatment of complicated skin and skin-structure infections in adults: Results of a prospective, randomized, double-blind multicenter study. Clin Infect Dis. 2002; 34:1460-1468.

40. Wells JS, et al. Distribution of beta-lactam and beta-lactone producing bacteria in nature. J Antibiot (Tokyo). 1982;35:814-821.

41. Barry AL, et al. Aztreonam: Antibacterial activity, beta-lactamase stability, and interpretive standards and quality control guidelines for disk-diffusion susceptibility tests. Rev Infect Dis. 1985;7(Suppl 4):S594-604.

42. Swabb EA. Review of the clinical pharmacology of the monobactam antibiotic aztreonam. Am J Med. 1985;78:11-18.

43. Greenman RL, et al. Penetration of aztreonam into human cerebrospinal fluid in the presence of meningeal inflammation. J Antimicrob Chemother. 1985;15:637-640.

44. Modai J, et al. Penetration of aztreonam into cerebrospinal fluid of patients with bacterial meningitis. Antimicrob Agents Chemother. 1986;29:281-283.

45. Brogden RN, Heel RC. Aztreonam: A review of its antibacterial activity, pharmacokinetic properties and therapeutic use. Drugs. 1986;31:96-130.

46. Bosso JA, Black PG. The use of aztreonam in pediatric patients: A review. Pharmacotherapy. 1991;11:20-25.

47. Lister PD, Gardner VM, Sanders CC. Clavulanate induces expression of the *Pseudomonas aeruginosa* AmpC cephalosporinase at physiologically relevant concentrations and antagonizes the antibacterial activity of ticarcillin. Antimicrob Agents Chemother. 1999;43:882-889.

48. Munch R, et al. Human pharmacokinetics and CSF penetration of clavulanic acid. J Antimicrob Chemother. 1981;8:29-37.

49. Bakken JS, et al. Penetration of amoxicillin and potassium clavulanate into the cerebrospinal fluid of patients with inflamed meninges. Antimicrob Agents Chemother. 1986;30:481-484.

50. Marchant CD, et al. A randomized controlled trial of amoxicillin plus clavulanate compared with cefaclor for treatment of acute otitis media. J Pediatr. 1986;109: 891-896.

51. Dagan R, et al. Bacteriologic and clinical efficacy of high dose amoxicillin/clavulanate in children with acute otitis media. Pediatr Infect Dis J. 2001;20:829-837.

52. Brakenbury PH, Muwanga C. A comparative double blind study of amoxycillin/clavulanate vs placebo in the prevention of infection after animal bites. Arch Emerg Med. 1989;6:251-256.

53. Abrahamian FM. Dog bites: Bacteriology, management, and prevention. Curr Infect Dis Rep. 2000;2:446-453.

54. Hoberman A, et al. Equivalent efficacy and reduced occurrence of diarrhea from a new formulation of amoxicillin/clavulanate potassium (Augmentin) for treatment of acute otitis media in children. Pediatr Infect Dis J. 1997;16:463-470.

55. Calver AD, et al. Dosing of amoxicillin/clavulanate given every 12 hours is as effective as dosing every 8 hours for treatment of lower respiratory tract infection. Lower Respiratory Tract Infection Collaborative Study Group. Clin Infect Dis. 1997;24: 570-574.

56. Hart SM, Bailey EM. A practical look at the clinical usefulness of the beta-lactam/beta-lactamase inhibitor combinations. Ann Pharmacother. 1996;30: 1130-1140.

57. Foulds G. Pharmacokinetics of sulbactam/ampicillin in humans: A review. Rev Infect Dis. 1986;8(Suppl 5):S503-511.

58. Campoli-Richards DM, Brogden RN. Sulbactam/ampicillin: A review of its antibacterial activity, pharmacokinetic properties, and therapeutic use. Drugs. 1987; 33: 577-609.

59. Akova M, Yang Y, Livermore DM. Interactions of tazobactam and clavulanate with inducibly- and constitutively-expressed class I beta-lactamases. J Antimicrob Chemother. 1990;25:199-208.

60. Johnson CA, et al. Single-dose pharmacokinetics of piperacillin and tazobactam in patients with renal disease. Clin Pharmacol Ther. 1992;51:32-41.

61. Sorgel F, Kinzig M. The chemistry, pharmacokinetics and tissue distribution of piperacillin/tazobactam. J Antimicrob Chemother. 1993;31(Suppl A):39-60.

62. Kern W, et al. Evaluation of piperacillin-tazobactam in experimental meningitis caused by a beta-lactamase-producing strain of K1-positive *Escherichia coli*. Antimicrob Agents Chemother. 1990;34:697-701.

63. Maltezou HC, et al. Piperacillin/tazobactam versus cefotaxime plus metronidazole for treatment of children with intra-abdominal infections requiring surgery. Eur J Clin Microbiol Infect Dis. 2001;20:643-646.

64. Kuck NA, et al. Comparative in vitro and in vivo activities of piperacillin combined with the beta-lactamase inhibitors tazobactam, clavulanic acid, and sulbactam. Antimicrob Agents Chemother. 1989;33:1964-1969.

65. Perry CM, Markham A. Piperacillin/tazobactam: An updated review of its use in the treatment of bacterial infections. Drugs. 1999;57:805-843.

66. Schoonover LL, et al. Piperacillin/tazobactam: A new beta-lactam/beta-lactamase inhibitor combination. Ann Pharmacother. 1995;29:501-514.

CHAPTER **22**

β-Lactam Allergy

MICHAEL E. WEISS

N. FRANKLIN ADKINSON, Jr.

CLASSIFICATION OF β-LACTAM REACTIONS

Since the introduction of penicillin by Fleming in the mid-1940s, the number of β-lactam antibiotics has grown dramatically. Other than allergy, these drugs have remarkably low toxicity when used in correct doses. In fact, the principal toxicity of β-lactam antibiotics is allergic reactions. The first case of anaphylaxis related to penicillin was reported in 1946,[1] and the first reported death from an allergic reaction was in 1949.[2] Allergic reactions occur in 7 to 40 of every 1000 penicillin treatment courses.[3,4] Studies have indicated that as many as half of all allergic drug reactions occurring in hospitalized patients are attributable to β-lactam antibiotics.[5] A wide range of allergic reactions have been caused by β-lactam antibiotics. It is possible to classify these reactions by the Gell and Coombs immunopathologic classification system[6]; by Levine's classification system,[7] which is based on

TABLE 22-1 Classification of Immunopathologic Reactions According to the Scheme of Gell and Coombs

Types of Reaction	Description	Antibody	Cells	Other	Clinical Reactions
I	Anaphylactic (reagenic), immediate hypersensitivity	IgE	Basophils, mast cells	—	Anaphylaxis, urticaria
II	Cytotoxic or cytolytic	IgG, IgM	Any cell with isoantigen	C', RES	Hemolytic anemia, cytopenias, nephritis
III	Immune complex disease	Soluble immune complexes (Ag-Ab)	None directly	C'	Serum sickness, drug fever
IV	"Delayed" or cell-mediated hypersensitivity	None known	Sensitized T lymphocytes	—	Contact dermatitis
Other	Idiopathic		?	?	Maculopapular eruptions
			?	?	Eosinophilia
			?	?	Stevens-Johnson syndrome
			?	?	Exfoliative dermatitis

Ag-Ab, antigen-antibody; C', complement; Ig, immunoglobulin; RES, reticuloendothelial system; ? immunopathologic mechanism is in doubt.
Modified from Weiss ME, Adkinson NF Jr. Immediate hypersensitivity reactions to penicillin and related antibiotics. Clin Allergy 1988;18:515-540.

time of onset of the reaction; or on the basis of the predominant clinical manifestation.

Gell and Coombs Classification

Gell and Coombs distinguished four types of immunopathologic reactions, all of which have been seen with β-lactam antibiotics (Table 22-1).

Type I—Immediate Hypersensitivity. These reactions result from the interaction of β-lactam antigens with preformed β-lactam–specific immunoglobulin E (IgE) antibodies that are bound to tissue mast cells or circulating basophils through high-affinity IgE receptors. Cross-linking of two or more IgE receptors by β-lactam antigens leads to the release of both preformed mediators (histamine, proteases, and chemotactic factors) and newly formed mediators (prostaglandins, leukotrienes, and platelet-activating factor), which are generated by the metabolism of arachidonic acid (Fig. 22-1; see Fig. 22-4).[8] Release of these mediators can lead to urticaria, laryngeal edema, and bronchospasm with or without cardiovascular collapse. Anaphylactic reactions occur in 4 to 15 of every 100,000 penicillin treatment courses.[4-9] Fatality caused by β-lactam anaphylaxis has been reported to occur once in every 32,000 to 100,000 treatment courses.[4,9]

The use of β-adrenergic antagonists may increase the risk of death if anaphylaxis occurs because treatment of the anaphylactic reaction is made more difficult.[10] IgE type I acute allergic reactions cause the greatest clinical concern because of the risk of life-threatening anaphylaxis.

Type II—Cytotoxic Antibodies. These reactions result when β-lactam–specific cytotoxic antibodies, usually IgG or IgM, become attached to circulating blood cells or renal interstitial cells that have β-lactam antigens bound to their cell surface. This antigen-antibody interaction activates the complement system, resulting in cell lysis. Type II reactions may also be complement independent. IgG or IgM antibody may bind to β-lactam antigens on cell membranes, resulting in neutrophil or macrophage attachment and activation through IgG or IgM Fc receptors. This opsonization can result in injury to the antigen-laden cell. Examples include hemolytic anemia, leukopenia, thrombocytopenia, and drug-induced nephritis. Long-term, high-dose β-lactam treatment is usually required for this form of allergic reaction to occur.

Type III—Immune Complexes (Arthus Reaction). β-Lactam–specific IgG or IgM antibodies may form circulating complexes with β-lactam antigens. These circulating complexes can fix

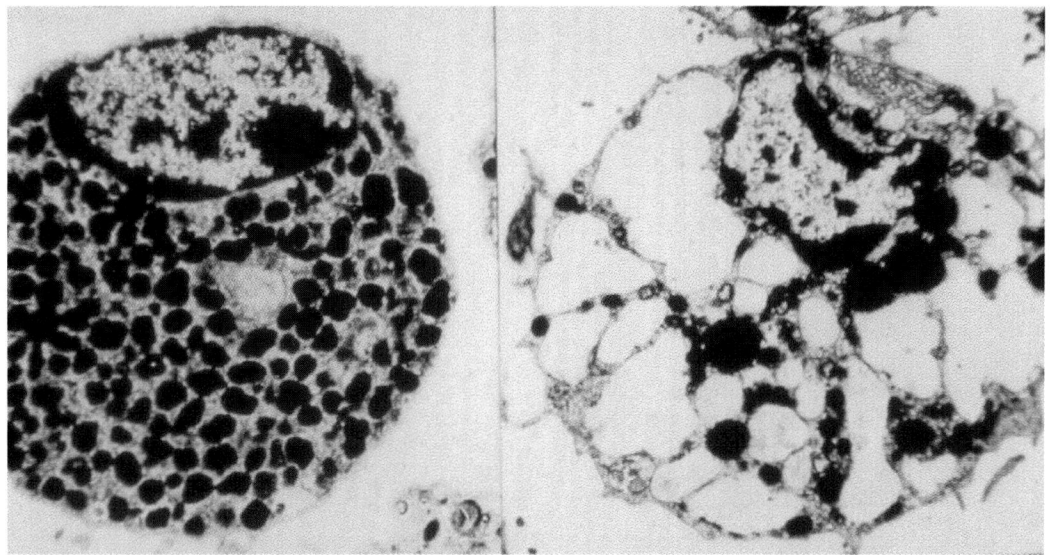

FIGURE 22-1. Electron micrograph of resting mast cell *(left)* and degranulated mast cell *(right)* after drug introduced in vitro to mast cell laden with drug-specific immunoglobulin E antibodies.

complement and then lodge in tissue sites, causing serum sickness–like reactions and possibly drug fever. In children, serum sickness is 15 times more likely to occur after administration of cefaclor than after amoxicillin.[11] These reactions typically occur 7 to 14 days after initiation of the β-lactam therapy. The syndrome can occur even after the termination of therapy. Preliminary data, obtained with sera from a small number of patients, suggest that cefaclor serum sickness may be predicted using a microsome metabolite lymphotoxic assay.[12]

Type IV—Cell-Mediated Hypersensitivity. These reactions are not mediated by an antibody but rather by T lymphocytes. A T lymphocyte recognizes the β-lactam antigen through an antigen-specific T-cell receptor. This recognition triggers the T cell to release cytokines that orchestrate an immune response by recruiting and stimulating proliferation of other lymphocytes and mononuclear cells, ultimately causing tissue inflammation and injury. Contact dermatitis is a clinical manifestation of a type IV reaction. The high rate of penicillin-related contact dermatitis (5% to 10%) in the 1940s led to the discontinuation of its use as a topical antibiotic.

Idiopathic Reactions

Some reactions to β-lactam antibiotics have an obscure pathogenesis and are not included in the Gell and Coombs classification system. These reactions include pruritus, maculopapular (morbilliform) exanthems, erythema multiforme, erythema nodosum, photosensitivity reactions, fixed drug reactions, and exfoliative dermatitis. The common maculopapular rash appears late in the treatment course in 2% to 3% of penicillin treatments. Rashes induced by ampicillin (and amoxicillin) occur with much greater frequency: 5.2% to 9.5% of treatment courses in uncomplicated cases.[5,13,14] When ampicillin or amoxicillin is given during infections with Epstein-Barr virus or cytomegalovirus or to patients with acute lymphocytic leukemia, a much higher incidence of rash (69% to 100%) occurs.[15]

Other reactions caused by unknown mechanisms include the Stevens-Johnson syndrome, involving rash (usually erythema multiforme) plus involvement of two or more mucous membranes, and Lyell's syndrome, also known as toxic epidermal necrolysis. Patients who have had Stevens-Johnson or Lyell's syndrome associated with β-lactam antibiotics should not receive β-lactam drugs in the future. Attempts to desensitize patients to the β-lactam antibiotics that caused these syndromes are also not recommended. Pseudoanaphylactic reactions have been observed after intramuscular or inadvertent intravenous injection of procaine penicillin. These reactions are probably caused by a combination of toxic and embolic phenomena resulting from procaine.[16]

Levine's Classification

Levine[7] classified reactions to penicillin according to their time of onset (Table 22-2). Immediate reactions occur within the first hour after β-lactam administration, and they are almost all IgE mediated (anaphylaxis and urticaria). Accelerated reactions occur 1 to 72 hours after initial treatment with β-lactams; they most commonly involve urticaria. Late reactions occur more than 72 hours after onset of therapy. Anaphylaxis does not occur later in the course of continuous β-lactam therapy; maculopapular reactions are most common, but type II, III, and IV reactions also occur during this time frame. Allergic reactions may also be classified according to their predominant clinical manifestations, as listed in Table 22-3.

IMMUNOCHEMISTRY OF β-LACTAM ANTIBIOTICS

Penicillins consist of a β-lactam ring, on which antimicrobial activity depends, and a five-membered thiazolidine ring (Fig. 22-2). Because penicillin is a low-molecular-weight compound (356 Da), it must first combine covalently with tissue macromolecules (presumably proteins) to produce multivalent hapten-protein complexes, which are required for both the induction of an immune response and the later elicitation of an allergic reaction (Figs. 22-3 and 22-4).[17] The most common form of haptenization by penicillin is in the penicilloyl configuration. Because the penicilloyl determinant is the most abundant derivative of penicillin in vivo, it has been labeled the *major determinant*. Although the formation of the penicilloyl group has been shown to occur spontaneously under physiologic conditions, evidence suggests that penicillin haptenization may be facilitated by serum molecules.[18,19] This reaction occurs with the prototype benzylpenicillin and

TABLE 22-2 Classification of Allergic Reactions to β-Lactam Antibiotics Based on Their Time of Onset

Reaction Type	Onset (hr)	Clinical Reactions
Immediate	0-1	Anaphylaxis
		Hypotension
		Laryngeal edema
		Urticaria, angioedema
		Wheezing
Accelerated	1-72	Urticaria, angioedema
		Laryngeal, edema
		Wheezing
Late	>72	Morbilliform rash
		Interstitial nephritis
		Hemolytic anemia
		Neutropenia
		Thrombocytopenia
		Serum sickness
		Drug fever
		Stevens-Johnson syndrome
		Exfoliative dermatitis

Adapted from Levine BB. Immunologic mechanisms of penicillin allergy: A haptenic model system for the study of allergic diseases of man. N Engl J Med. 1966;275:1115-1125.

TABLE 22-3 Classification of Reactions to β-Lactam Antibiotics According to Their Predominant Clinical Manifestations

Reaction	Manifestation
Anaphylaxis	Laryngeal edema
	Hypotension
	Bronchospasm
Cutaneous reactions	Urticaria, angioedema
	Vasculitis
	Stevens-Johnson syndrome
	Exfoliative dermatitis
	Contact sensitivity
	Fixed drug eruption
	Toxic epidermal necrolysis
	Pruritus
	Maculopapular (morbilliform) rash
	Erythema multiforme
	Erythema nodosum
	Photosensitivity reactions
Destruction of formed elements of blood	Hemolytic anemia
	Neutropenia
	Thrombocytopenia
Renal reactions	Interstitial nephritis
	Glomerulonephritis
	Nephrotic syndrome
Serum sickness	—
Drug fever	—
Systemic vasculitis	—
Lymphadenopathy	—

FIGURE 22-2. Structures of four classes of β-lactam antibiotics in use in the United States.

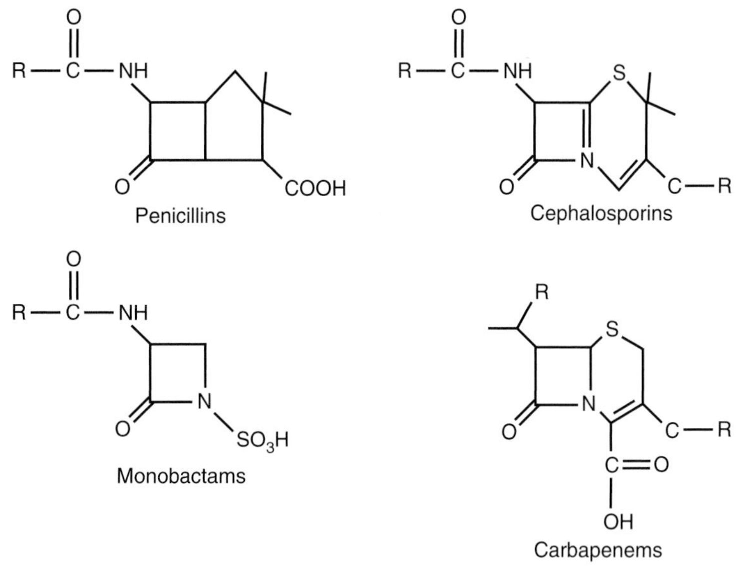

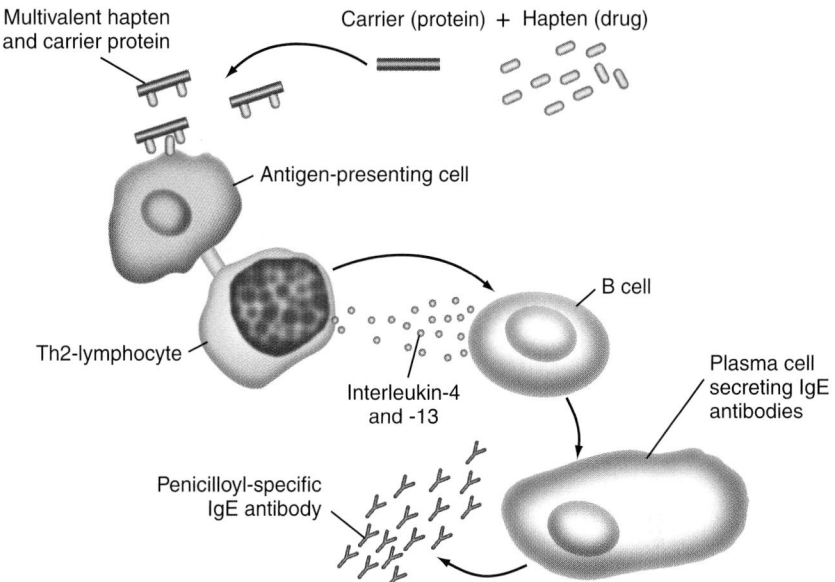

Penicillins

Cephalosporins

Monobactams

Carbapenems

FIGURE 22-3. Illustration of drug hapten combining with carrier molecule to induce immunoglobulin E (IgE) antibody production against drug (sensitization). An antigen-presenting cell stimulates a type 2 helper T cell (Th2) lymphocyte to drive a B lymphocyte to switch from IgG to IgE antibody production under the influence of interleukin-4 (IL-4) and IL-13.

Multivalent hapten and carrier protein

Carrier (protein) + Hapten (drug)

Antigen-presenting cell

B cell

Th2-lymphocyte

Interleukin-4 and -13

Plasma cell secreting IgE antibodies

Penicilloyl-specific IgE antibody

FIGURE 22-4. On subsequent exposure, the drug combines with drug-specific immunoglobulin E (IgE) bound to the mast cell through high-affinity IgE receptors. This causes mast cell degranulation of potent proinflammatory mediators leading to an allergic reaction.

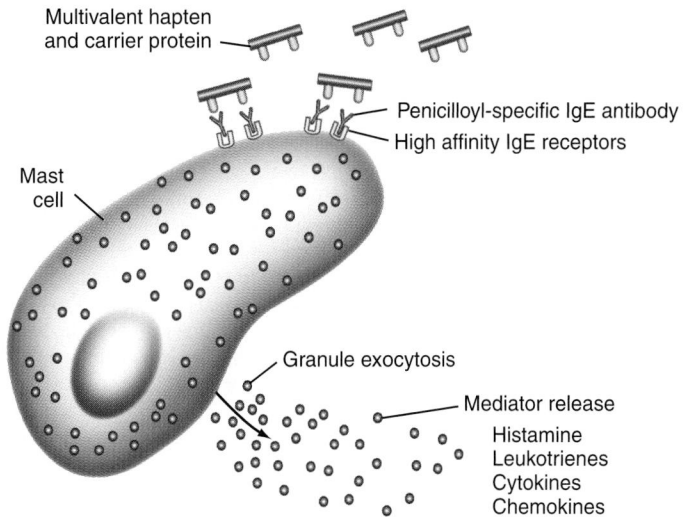

Multivalent hapten and carrier protein

Penicilloyl-specific IgE antibody

High affinity IgE receptors

Mast cell

Granule exocytosis

Mediator release
Histamine
Leukotrienes
Cytokines
Chemokines

virtually all semisynthetic penicillins. Penicillin can also be degraded by other metabolic pathways to form additional antigenic determinants.[20] These derivatives are formed in small quantities and stimulate a variable immune response; hence, they have been termed the *minor determinants*. Known precursors of minor determinants of penicillin include benzylpenicillin, its alkaline hydrolysis product (benzylpenicilloate), and an acid hydrolysis product (benzylpenilloate), collectively called the *minor determinant mixture* (MDM).

Therefore, for penicillin and other β-lactam antibiotics, IgE antibodies can be produced against a number of haptenic determinants (i.e., major and minor determinants). Anaphylactic reactions to penicillin are usually mediated by IgE antibodies directed against minor determinants, although some anaphylactic reactions have occurred in patients with only penicilloyl-specific IgE antibodies.[7,20,21] Accelerated and late urticarial reactions are usually mediated by penicilloyl-specific IgE antibodies (major determinant).[7]

RISK FACTORS FOR β-LACTAM REACTIONS

Immune responses to β-lactam antibiotics occur in only a small percentage of exposed patients, and clinical expression of β-lactam allergy occurs in only a fraction of the patients demonstrating an immune response. The generation of a sustained immune response to a β-lactam antibiotic is probably controlled in part by the genetic makeup of the individual.[22] The half-life of β-lactam IgE antibodies has been shown to range from as short as 10 days to an indeterminately long interval (more than 1000 days).[23] A person whose β-lactam–specific IgE antibody response persists is at greater cumulative risk for allergic reactions to β-lactam antibiotics than one whose IgE antibody quickly disappears.

Parenteral administration of β-lactam antibiotics produces more allergic reactions than oral administration.[24] However, this may be more related to dose than to route of administration. When higher oral doses are given, as in the treatment of gonorrhea, the incidence of allergic reactions is no different from that seen with intramuscular procaine penicillin at a comparable dose.[25]

A history of atopy (allergic rhinitis, asthma, atopic dermatitis) does not seem to be an independent risk factor for the development of β-lactam allergy,[23,26] although atopic individuals, especially those with asthma, seem to be predisposed to severe and fatal reactions should anaphylaxis occur.[9]

Persons with a history of penicillin reactions have a fourfold to sixfold increased risk of subsequent reactions to β-lactam antibiotics compared with those without previous reaction histories.[26] The risk is particularly pronounced if the previous reaction was anaphylaxis or urticaria.[23] However, because most serious and fatal allergic reactions to β-lactam antibiotics occur in persons who have never had an allergic reaction, a negative history of β-lactam allergy should not lead to a false sense of security. Sensitization in these patients probably resulted from their last therapeutic course of penicillin. A randomized, controlled trial of routine penicillin skin testing in history-negative patients was shown not to be cost-effective, and therefore skin testing at this time is recommended only for patients with a prior history of β-lactam allergy.[27]

In general, the likelihood of sustaining IgE-specific β-lactam antibodies declines with time since the previous reaction. Sullivan and collaborators[28] reported that skin tests done within the first 1 or 2 months after an acute allergic reaction were positive 80% to 90% of the time. Thereafter, there was a time-dependent decline in the rate of positive skin tests, to less than 20% by 10 years.[28] Patients who have had serum sickness–like reactions to β-lactam antibiotics often persist with an intense antibody response and may remain at high risk for allergic reactions for many years.

Despite sparse evidence, it is generally thought that penicillin reactions occur less frequently in children and in elderly persons than in nonelderly adults.[26,29] Although the frequency of anaphylactic reactions may be less in elderly persons, fatal outcomes are more commonly owing to compromised cardiopulmonary reserve.

DIAGNOSING β-LACTAM ALLERGY

An important question facing clinicians is how to assess a patient with a history of β-lactam reaction who has a current clinical need for β-lactam antibiotics. Approximately 5% to 20% of patients give a history of reactions to β-lactam antibiotics. By current medical standards, all of these subjects would be denied therapy with β-lactam antibiotics for the rest of their lives unless further evaluation were undertaken. The most useful single piece of information in assessing an individual's risk for a type I, IgE-mediated reaction (anaphylaxis and urticaria) is the skin test response to major and minor penicillin determinants.

The major (penicilloyl) determinant of penicillin can be assessed by skin testing with penicilloyl polylysine (PPL). This commercially available skin test reagent (Pre-Pen, Hollister-Stein, Spokane, WA) contains multiple penicilloyl molecules synthetically coupled to a weakly immunogenic polylysine carrier. Minor determinants of penicillin are not commercially available in the United States at present, although that may change in the future. In the meantime, benzylpenicillin alone (10,000 U/mL) can be substituted as a less efficient minor determinant reagent in patients without a history of anaphylactic sensitivity.

Skin testing should proceed first with an epicutaneous (prick-puncture) test for safety. If there is no induration (or systemic symptoms) after 15 minutes, intradermal injections are placed, raising 3- to 4-mm blebs in duplicate on the forearm. Testing should be done with PPL, MDM, a positive control (histamine), and a negative diluent control. The diameter of induration at 15 to 20 minutes is read; if it is greater than 5 mm, the test is considered positive.[30] Antihistamines, tricyclic antidepressants, and adrenergic drugs, all of which may inhibit skin test results, should be discontinued at least 48 hours before skin testing. Antihistamines with long half-lives need to be discontinued for appropriate intervals.

When properly performed with due consideration for preliminary epicutaneous tests and appropriate dilutions, skin testing with penicillin reagents can almost always be accomplished safely. Systemic reactions occur in about 1% of those tested[31,32]; these are usually mild but can be serious. Therefore, skin tests should be done in the presence of a physician and with immediate access to medications needed to treat anaphylaxis.

In numerous studies in which both PPL and minor determinant skin tests were performed, only 7% to 35% of patients who gave histories of penicillin allergy were skin test positive to either reagent,[33,34] although one study found a positive skin test rate of 63%.[28] In general, with increasing time since the allergic reaction, the prevalence of positive skin tests to penicillin determinants decreases, although some patients have penicillin antibodies indefinitely.[28,35] In patients who give a history of penicillin allergy, skin tests confirm that 65% to 93% can safely be given a β-lactam antibiotic. With a negative history of penicillin allergy, the rate of positive skin tests is about 2%.[27,32]

Extensive worldwide experience involving more than 20,000 patients has shown that persons with a history of penicillin reaction can be re-treated safely with penicillin or related antibiotics if intradermal skin tests with PPL and a suitable MDM are negative.[32,36] When therapeutic doses of penicillin are given to patients with a history of penicillin allergy but negative skin tests to PPL and MDM, IgE-mediated reactions occur in 2% to 15%, depending on the clinical history; such reactions are almost always mild and self-limited. Penicillin anaphylaxis has not been reported in skin test–negative patients in the United States. When penicillin is given after negative skin tests, about 1% to 3% of patients have urticarial or other mild cutaneous reactions.[33] If the major determinant penicillin is used alone as a skin test reagent, approximately 10% to 25% of all potential positive reactions are missed.[28] If benzylpenicillin G, diluted to a concentration of 10,000 U/mL (10^{-2} mol/L), is used as the sole minor determinant, about 5% to 10% of skin test–positive patients are missed.[28] Mendelson and associates[37] studied more than 200 children who had a history of penicillin allergy but were skin test negative to penicillin reagents. After negative skin tests, a 10-day course of oral penicillin was given, and repeated skin testing 1 month later showed that less than 1% of the children became skin test positive to penicillin reagents. Solensky and colleagues[38] studied 46 individuals with history of penicillin allergy who, when skin tests were negative, were given multiple courses of penicillin to see if resensitization occurred. They found that after three consecutive 10-day courses of oral penicillin, skin tests continued to be negative in 100% of patients. This finding suggests that penicillin skin tests can be done electively and that negative skin tests still have a useful negative predictive value at a later date.

In contrast, Parker and colleagues[39] found that 3 (20%) of 15 patients with a history of penicillin allergy who were skin test negative became resensitized (skin tests to penicillin turned positive) after they were treated with high-dose intravenous penicillin in the hospital. Therefore, it may be prudent to retest patients with clear, impressive histories of penicillin allergy who were skin test negative and subsequently treated with intravenous high-dose penicillin.

A limited number of skin test–positive patients have been treated with therapeutic doses of penicillin. The risk of an acute immediate or accelerated allergic reaction ranges from about 10% in history-negative subjects to 50% to 70% in history-positive subjects.[33] Therefore, if skin tests are positive, an equally effective, non–cross-reacting antibiotic should be substituted if possible. Patients with a history of exfoliative dermatitis, Stevens-Johnson syndrome, or Lyell's syndrome, reactions that constitute absolute contraindications for penicillin administration, should not be evaluated by skin testing. Skin tests have no predictive value in non–IgE-mediated reactions such as drug fever, serum sickness, cytopenias, interstitial nephritis, contact dermatitis, or maculopapular exanthems. Penicillin skin tests are indeterminate (usually erythema without wheal or discordant duplicates) in about 0.6% to 3% of patients with histories of penicillin allergy.[32,36] The meaning of such results is unclear.

Type II reactions, such as hemolytic anemias, cytopenias, and interstitial nephritis, usually follow high-dose, long-term β-lactam therapy. Anecdotal experience suggests that short courses of β-lactam therapy in moderate doses can be tolerated by most, if not all, patients with such histories. Penicillin skin testing is important to rule out concomitant type I sensitivity but would not be predictive of type II or type III reactions. If skin tests are negative in these patients and β-lactam antibiotics are strongly indicated, gradual dose escalation under careful medical observation can be prudently attempted. If cytopenia, hemolytic anemia, hematuria, or proteinuria develops, therapy should be promptly stopped and high-dose glucocorticoids administered. However, most subjects can be re-treated without recurrence, especially if the history of reaction is remote.

Solid-phase immunoassays such as the radioallergosorbent test (RAST) have been developed to detect serum IgE antibodies directed against the penicilloyl determinant. At present, there is no in vitro RAST for minor determinant antibodies.[30] Because it is more time consuming, more expensive, and less sensitive than skin testing for detection of the major determinant IgE antibodies and presently unavailable for minor determinant antibody detection, the RAST and other in vitro analogues have limited clinical utility at this time.

SEMISYNTHETIC PENICILLINS WITH SPECIAL REFERENCE TO AMPICILLIN OR AMOXICILLIN

Semisynthetic penicillins have the same nuclear structure as benzylpenicillin with different side chains. Because allergic reactions are thought to be caused by neoantigens formed by interaction of the β-lactam nucleus with native proteins, it has generally been considered unnecessary to perform skin tests with specific derivatives of semisynthetic penicillins. Hapten inhibition theory predicts that antibodies directed against the unmodified side chain will not cause allergic reactions because of overwhelming hapten inhibition from unconjugated univalent drug.[40,41] Earlier studies showed that skin testing with derivatives of semisynthetic penicillins in addition to benzylpenicillin derivatives was not needed.[42] Blanca and colleagues,[43,44] in Spain, questioned this dogma and suggested that skin testing with major and minor

determinants of benzylpenicillin may not identify all patients with ampicillin- or amoxicillin-specific allergy. Silviu-Dan and co-workers[45] subsequently reported that skin testing with derivatives of ampicillin or amoxicillin detected nine patients who were otherwise skin test negative to benzylpenicillin reagents. These nine represented almost half of all skin test–positive persons tested. This study did not provide any information about benzylpenicillin skin test–negative and ampicillin or amoxicillin skin test–positive persons challenged with a β-lactam.

Macy and associates[46] studied 215 patients who had a history of penicillin allergy but negative skin tests to benzylpenicillin reagents. These subjects were given a one-time 250-mg oral challenge dose of amoxicillin. Only 5% had mild reactions, and only 0.9% had possible IgE-mediated reactions. Mendelson and colleagues (personal communication) studied 443 patients with a history of penicillin allergy who were skin test negative to PPL and to an MDM of benzylpenicillin. The 443 patients tolerated a 10-day penicillin challenge, but when they were given amoxicillin for 10 days, 18.7% had cutaneous reactions. Therefore, amoxicillin or ampicillin seems to have a greater propensity for causing cutaneous allergic reactions. It has been postulated that the diamino acyl side chain contained in ampicillin and amoxicillin more readily allows the formation of linear polymers of varying lengths, which may explain the higher cutaneous reaction rate seen with ampicillin and amoxicillin.[47] Except for isolated reports from Spain (Blanca and colleagues,[44] Martin and colleagues[48]), there have been no reports of any patient with negative skin tests to PPL and an MDM of benzylpenicillin, subsequently treated with amoxicillin or ampicillin, who had anything more than a cutaneous reaction. Studies in the 1960s showed that patients with late-occurring maculopapular rashes from ampicillin or amoxicillin could safely be re-treated with these antibiotics without any increased risk for acute allergic reactions. In such patients, skin testing with PPL and MDM may be useful to rule out concomitant type I, IgE-mediated sensitivity. Studies by Romano and co-workers[49] and by Terrados and associates[50] presented evidence that the maculopapular exanthems seen in some amoxicillin reactions may be related to delayed-type hypersensitivity reactions involving T cells. Diagnostic tests that are presently being evaluated include delayed intradermal skin tests using native amoxicillin, measuring induration at 48 hours, and possibly a patch test using native amoxicillin.

β-LACTAM DESENSITIZATION

Effective, non–cross-reacting alternative antibiotics are usually available for patients with positive skin tests to penicillin. If alternative drugs fail, induce unacceptable side effects, or are clearly less effective, the administration of a β-lactam antibiotic using a desensitization protocol may be justified. Infections in which this may be considered include endocarditis caused by enterococci, brain abscess, bacterial meningitis, serious infections caused by *Staphylococcus* or *Pseudomonas* organisms, *Listeria* infections, neurosyphilis, or syphilis during pregnancy. Use of a desensitization protocol for penicillin skin test–positive patients markedly reduces the risk of anaphylaxis.

β-Lactam desensitization of patients with prior anaphylactic reactions should be performed only in an intensive care setting. All β-adrenergic antagonists, including ophthalmologic drops, should be discontinued. Asthmatic patients should be under optimal control. An intravenous line should be established, and baseline electrocardiography and spirometry should be performed. Continuous electrocardiographic monitoring should be instituted.

Protocols have been developed for β-lactam desensitization using both the oral and the parenteral route (Tables 22-4 and 22-5).[51] If an oral preparation is available and the patient has a functional gastrointestinal tract, the oral route may be preferable for desensitization. Results of oral desensitization have shown that approximately one third of patients have a transient allergic reaction during desensitization, and two thirds have a reaction during penicillin treatment after desensitization. These reactions are usually mild and self-limited in nature, but they can be serious.[24]

TABLE 22-4 Protocol for Oral Densensitization of β-Lactam Antibiotic-Allergic Patients

Step	β-Lactam Drug (mg/mL)	Amount* (mL)	Dose*† (mg)	Cumulative Dose (mg)
1	0.5	0.1	0.05	0.05
2	0.5	0.2	0.10	0.15
3	0.5	0.4	0.20	0.35
4	0.5	0.8	0.40	0.75
5	0.5	1.6	0.80	1.55
6	0.5	3.2	1.60	3.15
7	0.5	6.4	3.20	6.35
8	5.0	1.2	6.00	12.35
9	5.0	2.4	12.00	24.35
10	5.0	4.8	24.00	48.35
11	50.0	1.0	50.00	98.35
12	50.0	2.0	100.00	198.35
13	50.0	4.0	200.00	398.35
14	50.0	8.0	400.00	798.35

15: Observe patient for 30 min; then administer 1 g of same agent intravenously.

*Drug suspension diluted in 30 mL of water for ingestion.
†Internal between doses: 15 min.
From Sullivan TJ. Drug allergy. In: Middleton E, Reed C, Ellis E, et al, eds. Allergy: Principles and Practice, 4th ed. St. Louis: CV Mosby; 1993: 1523-1534.

During desensitization, any dose that causes mild systemic reactions (e.g., pruritus, fleeting urticaria, rhinitis, mild wheezing) should be repeated until the patient tolerates the dose without systemic symptoms or signs. More serious reactions (e.g., hypotension, laryngeal edema, asthma) require appropriate treatment, and if desensitization is continued the dose should be decreased by at least 10-fold and withheld until the patient is stable.[52]

After desensitization, the patient's treatment with penicillin must not lapse or the risk of an allergic reaction increases. If the patient requires a β-lactam antibiotic in the future and still remains skin test positive to penicillin reagents, desensitization is required again. Patients have been maintained with long-term, low-dose oral penicillin therapy (usually two or three times daily) to sustain a chronic state of desensitization.[53]

TABLE 22-5 Protocol for Parenteral Desensitization of β-Lactam Antibiotic-Allergic Patients

Step	β-Lactam Drug (mg/mL)	Amount* (mL)	Dose*† (mg)	Cumulative Dose (mg)
1	0.1	0.1	0.01	0.01
2	0.1	0.2	0.02	0.03
3	0.1	0.4	0.04	0.07
4	0.1	0.8	0.08	0.15
5	1.0	0.16	0.16	0.31
6	1.0	0.32	0.32	0.63
7	1.0	0.64	0.64	1.27
8	10	0.12	1.20	2.47
9	10	0.24	2.40	4.87
10	10	0.48	4.80	10
11	100	0.10	10	20
12	100	0.20	20	40
13	100	0.40	40	80
14	100	0.80	80	160
15	1000	0.16	160	320
16	1000	0.32	320	640
17	1000	0.65	640	1280

18: Observe patient for 30 min; then administer 1 g of same agent intravenously.

*Dose administered subcutaneously (or intramuscularly or intravenously).
†Internal between doses: 15 min.
From Sullivan TJ. Drug allergy. In: Middleton E, Reed C, Ellis E, et al., eds. Allergy: Principles and Practice. 4th ed. St. Louis: CV Mosby; 1993: 1523-1534.

CROSS-REACTIVITY AMONG β-LACTAM ANTIBIOTICS

Cephalosporins

Like penicillins, cephalosporins have a β-lactam ring, but the five-membered thiazolidine ring is replaced by a six-membered dihydrothiazine ring (see Fig. 22-2). Shortly after cephalosporins came into clinical use, allergic reactions were reported in penicillin-allergic patients and the question of cross-reactivity between cephalosporins and penicillins was raised.[54] To date, the degree of cross-reactivity between penicillins and cephalosporins remains a matter of considerable uncertainty. Complicating matters, the early cephalosporins were contaminated with trace amounts of penicillin, potentially leading to overestimates of the degree of cross-reactivity. Nevertheless, studies in both animals and humans clearly demonstrated cross-reactivity between penicillins and first-generation cephalosporins when immunoassays and bioassays were used to evaluate IgE, IgM, and IgG antibodies.[55-57] In general, the degree of clinical cross-reactivity is much lower than the in vitro cross-reactivity between penicillins and cephalosporins. Small numbers of penicillin skin test–positive patients have been treated with cephalosporin antibiotics without allergic reactions.[58,59] Novalbos and colleagues[60] treated 41 patients with well-characterized penicillin allergy (including positive skin tests to penicillin) with three cephalosporins that do not share the same side chain to penicillin (cefazolin, cefuroxime, and ceftriaxone), and none of the 41 patients challenged had adverse reactions to the three cephalosporins. Too few cephalosporin skin test–positive individuals have been challenged with cephalosporins to allow estimation of the predictive value of a positive skin test. Because major determinant analogues of cephalosporins are not currently available as skin test reagents, the utility of skin testing for cephalosporin allergy is limited.

Cephalosporin antibiotics are widely prescribed for common infections and are also administered as first-line prophylaxis for many types of surgical procedures. When a patient with a history of penicillin allergy requires a cephalosporin antibiotic, three options are presently available:

1. *Use a non–β-lactam antimicrobial agent that has no cross-reactivity with penicillin.* Many patients need prophylactic antimicrobial coverage preoperatively, and the antibiotic of choice is often cefazolin. Vancomycin is often substituted preoperatively in patients with a history of penicillin allergy, yet resistance to antibiotics, in particular vancomycin resistance, is an important problem worldwide. Emergence of antimicrobial-resistant organisms demands that the selection of antibiotics such as vancomycin be made only after careful evaluation.

2. *Use a cephalosporin antibiotic without penicillin skin testing.* In this strategy, the risk of anaphylaxis from a reaction to cephalosporin is not considered high enough to warrant either the selection of a non–β-lactam antibiotic or further evaluation.[61] The appeal of this approach is that serious reactions to cephalosporins are rare. However, review of the literature suggests that patients with a history of penicillin allergy who are treated with various cephalosporins have an approximately fourfold higher reaction rate than patients without a history of penicillin allergy receiving cephalosporins.

3. *Do penicillin skin testing, and in patients with a negative skin test to penicillin administer cephalosporin and in patients with positive skin tests to penicillin choose a non–β-lactam antimicrobial agent or desensitize to β-lactam antibiotics if needed.* Li and colleagues[62,63] showed that skin testing preoperatively in an orthopedic unit with penicillin in patients who had a history of penicillin allergy reduced the rate of vancomycin administration preoperatively from 30% to 3%. Therefore, when penicillin skin testing was done before surgery, 97% of the patients were able to receive cefazolin preoperatively, decreasing vancomycin use and its associated health care costs and risk for antimicrobial resistance.

The incidence of clinically relevant cross-reactivity between the penicillins and cephalosporins is probably small, but rare cases of life-threatening anaphylactic reactions have occurred. The risk of administering a first-generation cephalosporin to a penicillin skin test–positive patient is lower than that of administering a penicillin antibiotic, but it is not negligible. Antibodies to the second- and third-generation cephalosporins are often directed against the side chains rather than the ring structures, and therefore cross-reactivity with penicillins is less than with first-generation cephalosporins.[51] Patients with positive skin test results to any penicillin reagent probably should not receive cephalosporin antibiotics unless alternative drugs are clearly less desirable. If cephalosporin drugs are to be used, they should be administered with caution and with adequate precautions.

Carbapenems

These are a third class of β-lactam antibiotics of which imipenem is the prototype (see Fig. 22-2). Studies have shown that approximately 50% of penicillin skin test–positive patients have positive skin reactions to analogous imipenem determinants,[64] suggesting appreciable cross-reactivity and indicating that these β-lactam antibiotics are relatively contraindicated in patients with positive penicillin skin tests.

Monobactams

The monobactams are a class of β-lactam antibiotics that contain a monocyclic ring structure rather than the bicyclic structure of the penicillins, cephalosporins, and carbapenems (see Fig. 22-2). The prototype monobactam licensed in the United States is aztreonam. In preclinical studies, negligible cross-reactivity in rabbits and in human subjects between aztreonam and penicillins or cephalosporins was found.[65] When subjects with positive penicillin skin tests were skin tested with analogous aztreonam reagents, appreciable cross-reactivity was not found.[66] In a subsequent trial, 20 patients with a positive penicillin skin test were treated with therapeutic doses of aztreonam, and none had IgE-mediated reactions.[67] Taken together, these data suggest weak cross-reactivity between aztreonam and other β-lactam antibiotics and indicate that aztreonam may be safely administered to most, if not all, penicillin-allergic subjects. "There have been a small number of patients with allergic reactions to aztreonam. In these cases, the antibody response is directed against the side chain and not the beta lactam ring. Because the side chain on aztreonam is the same as that of ceftazidime, it would be prudent not to administer ceftazidime to individuals with allergic reactions to aztreonam and vice versa."[68,69]

UNANSWERED QUESTIONS

Important clinical questions remain for future research in β-lactam allergy. These include (1) the further elucidation of when side chain–specific allergies may be the cause of β-lactam reactions, (2) the possible identification of genetic factors that predispose to β-lactam allergy, (3) the validation of testing procedures to evaluate clinical cross-reactivity between cephalosporin and penicillin antibiotics, and (4) the potential relation of penicillin allergy to other medication reactions involving structurally unrelated drugs.

REFERENCES

1. Gorevic PD. Drug-induced autoimmune disease. In: Kaplan A, ed. Allergy. New York: Churchill Livingstone; 1985:480.
2. Schwartz HJ, Sher TH. Anaphylaxis to penicillin in a frozen dinner. Ann Allergy. 1984;52:342-343.
3. Parker CW. Drug therapy (first of three parts). N Engl J Med. 1975;292:511-514.
4. International Rheumatic Fever Study Group. Allergic reactions to long-term benzathine penicillin prophylaxis for rheumatic fever. Lancet. 1993;337:1308-1310.
5. Arndt KA, Jick H. Rates of cutaneous reactions to drugs: A report from the Boston Collaborative Drug Surveillance Program. JAMA. 1976;235:918-922.
6. Gell PGH, Coombs RRA. Classification of allergic reactions responsible for clinical hypersensitivity and disease. In: Gell PGH, Coombs RRA, Hachmann PJ, eds. Clinical Aspects of Immunology. Oxford: Blackwell Scientific Publications; 1975:761-781.
7. Levine BB. Immunologic mechanisms of penicillin allergy: A haptenic model system for the study of allergic diseases of man. N Engl J Med. 1966;275:1115-1125.
8. Ishizaka T. Mechanisms of IgE-mediated hypersensitivity. In: Middleton E Jr, Reed CE, Ellis EF, et al., eds. Allergy: Principles and Practice. St. Louis: CV Mosby; 1988:71-93.
9. Idsoe O, Guthe T, Willcox RR, et al. Nature and extent of penicillin side-reactions, with particular reference to fatalities from anaphylactic shock. Bull World Health Organ 1968;38:159-188.
10. Jacobs RL, Geoffrey WR Jr, Fournier DC, et al. Potentiated anaphylaxis in patients with drug-induced beta-adrenergic blockade. J Allergy Clin Immunol. 1981;68:125-127.
11. Heckbert SR, Stryker WS, Coltin KL, et al. Serum sickness in children after antibiotic exposure: Estimates of occurrence and morbidity in a health maintenance organization population. Am J Epidemiol. 1990;132:336-342.
12. Wheeler JG, Childress SH, Kearns GL. Cefaclor serum sickness: In vitro identification using microsome cytotoxicity and flow cytometry (Abstract). J Allergy Clin Immunol. 1993;91:363.
13. Levine B. Skin rashes with penicillin therapy: Current management. N Engl J Med. 1972;286:42-43.
14. Shapiro S, Siskin V, Slone D, et al. Drug rash with ampicillin and other penicillins. Lancet. 1969;2:969-972.
15. Kerns DL, Shira JE, Go S, et al. Ampicillin rash in children: Relationship to penicillin allergy and infectious mononucleosis. Am J Dis Child. 1973;125:187-190.
16. Galpin JE, Chow AW, Yoshikawa TT, et al. "Pseudoanaphylactic" reactions from inadvertent infusion of procaine penicillin G. Ann Intern Med. 1974;81:358-359.
17. Eisen HN. Hypersensitivity to simple chemicals. In: Lawrence HS, ed. Cellular and Humoral Aspects of the Hypersensitive States. New York: PB Hoeber; 1959:111-116.
18. DiPiro JT, Hamilton RG, Adkinson NF Jr. Facilitation of penicilloation of proteins by serum cofactors (Abstract). J Allergy Clin Immunol. 1990;85:192.
19. Sullivan TJ. Facilitated haptenation of human proteins by penicillin (Abstract). J Allergy Clin Immunol. 1989;83:255.
20. Levine BB, Redmond AP. Minor haptenic determinant-specific reagins of penicillin hypersensitivity in man. Int Arch Allergy. 1969;35:445-455.
21. Levine BB, Redmond AP, Fellner MJ, et al. Penicillin allergy and the heterogeneous immune responses of man to benzylpenicillin. J Clin Invest. 1966;45:1895-1906.
22. Levine BB. Effect of combinations of inbred strain, antigen, and antigen dose on immune responsiveness and reagin production in the mouse: A potential mouse model for immune aspects of human atopic allergy. Int Arch Allergy Appl Immunol. 1970;39:156-171.
23. Adkinson NF Jr. Risk factors for drug allergy. J Allergy Clin Immunol. 1984;74:567-572.
24. Sullivan TJ, Yecies LD, Shatz GS, et al. Desensitization of patients allergic to penicillin using orally administered beta-lactam antibiotics. J Allergy Clin Immunol. 1982;69:275-282.
25. Adkinson NF Jr, Wheeler B. Risk factors for IgE-dependent reactions to penicillin. In: Kerr JW, Ganderton MA, eds. XI International Congress of Allergology and Clinical Immunology. London: Macmillan; 1983:55-59.
26. Sogn DD. Prevention of allergic reactions to penicillin. J Allergy Clin Immunol. 1987;78:1051-1052.
27. Gadde J, Space M, Wheeler B, Adkinson NF Jr. Clinical experience with penicillin skin testing in a large inner-city STD clinic. JAMA. 1993;270:2456-2463.
28. Sullivan TJ, Wedner HJ, Shatz GS, et al. Skin testing to detect penicillin allergy. J Allergy Clin Immunol. 1981;68:171-180.
29. Sogn DD. Penicillin allergy. J Allergy Clin Immunol. 1984;74:589-593.
30. Adkinson NF Jr. Tests for immunological drug reactions. In: Rose NF, Friedman H, eds. Manual of Clinical Immunology. Washington, DC: American Society for Microbiology; 1986:692-697.
31. Sullivan TJ. Penicillin allergy. In: Lichtenstein LM, Fauci A, eds. Current Therapy in Allergy. St. Louis: CV Mosby; 1985:57-61.
32. Gadde J, Spence M, Wheeler B, et al. Clinical experience with penicillin skin testing in a large inner city STD clinic. JAMA. 1993;270:2456-2463.
33. Weiss ME, Adkinson NF Jr. Immediate hypersensitivity reactions to penicillin and related antibiotics. Clin Allergy. 1988;18:515-540.
34. Pichichero M, Pichichero D. Diagnosis of penicillin, amoxicillin and cephalosporin allergy: Reliability of examination assessed by skin testing and oral challenge. J Pediatr. 1998;132:137-143.
35. Chandra RK, Joglekar SA, Tomas E. Penicillin allergy: Anti-penicillin IgE antibodies and immediate hypersensitivity skin reactions employing major and minor determinants of penicillin. Arch Dis Child. 1980;55:857-860.
36. Sogn DD, Casale TB, Condemi JJ, et al. Results of the NIAID collaborative clinical trial to test the predictive value of skin testing with major and minor penicillin derivatives in hospitalized adults. Arch Intern Med. 1992;152:1025-1032.
37. Mendelson LML, Ressler C, Rosen JP, et al. Routine elective penicillin allergy skin testing in children and adolescents: Study of sensitization. J Allergy Clin Immunol. 1984;73:76-81.
38. Solensky R, Earl HS, Gruchalla RS. Lack of penicillin resensitization in patients with a history of penicillin allergy after receiving repeated penicillin courses. Arch Intern Med 2002;162:822-826.
39. Parker P, Parrinello, JT, Condemi J, et al. Penicillin resensitization among hospitalized patients. J Allergy Clin Immunol. 1991;88:213-217.
40. De Weck AL, Schneider CH. Specific inhibition of allergic reactions to penicillin in man by a monovalent hapten: II. Clinical studies. Int Arch Allergy Immunol. 1972;42:798-815.
41. De Weck AL, Schneider CH. Specific inhibition of allergic reactions to penicillin in man by a monovalent hapten. Int Arch Allergy Immunol. 1972;42:782-797.
42. Warrington RJ, Simons FER, Ho HW, et al. Diagnosis of penicillin allergy by skin testing: The Manitoba experience. Can Med Assoc J. 1978;11:787-791.
43. Blanca M, Vega JM, Garcia J, et al. Allergy to penicillin with good tolerance to other penicillins: Study of the incidence in subjects allergic to beta-lactams. Clin Exp Allergy. 1990;20:475-481.
44. Blanca M, Perez E, Garcia J, et al. Anaphylaxis to amoxicillin but good tolerance for benzylpenicillin. Allergy. 1988;43:508-510.

45. Silviu-Dan F, McPhillips S, Warrington R. The frequency of skin test reactions to side-chain penicillin determinants. J Allergy Clin Immunol. 1993;91:694-701.

46. Macy E, Richter P, Falkoff R, et al. Clinical aspects of allergic disease: Skin testing with penicilloate and penilloate prepared by an improved method. Amoxicillin oral challenge in patients with negative skin test responses to penicillin reagents. J Allergy Clin Immunol. 1997;100:586-591.

47. Adkinson NF Jr. Side-chain specific beta-lactam allergy. Clin Exp Allergy. 1990; 20:445-447.

48. Martin J, Igea J, Fraj J, et al. Allergy to amoxicillin in patients who tolerated benzylpenicillin, aztreonam, and ceftazidime. Clin Infect Dis. 1992;14:592-593.

49. Romano A, Quaratino D, DiFonso M, et al. A diagnostic protocol for evaluating non-immediate reactions to aminopenicillins. J Allergy Clin Immunol. 1999;103: 1186-1190.

50. Terrados S, Blanca M, Garcia J, et al. Nonimmediate reactions to betalactams: Prevalence and role of the different penicillins. Allergy. 1995;50:563-567.

51. Sullivan TJ. Drug allergy. In: Middleton E, Reed C, Ellis E, et al., eds. Allergy: Principles and Practice. 4th ed. St. Louis: CV Mosby; 1993:1523-1534.

52. Adkinson NF Jr. Penicillin allergy. In: Lichtenstein LM, Fauci A, eds. Current Therapy in Allergy, Immunology and Rheumatology. Ontario: BS Decker; 1983: 57-62.

53. Naclerio R, Mizrahi EA, Adkinson NF Jr. Immunologic observations during desensitization and maintenance of clinical tolerance to penicillin. J Allergy Clin Immunol. 1983;71:294-301.

54. Grieco MH. Cross-allergenicity of the penicillins and the cephalosporins. Arch Intern Med. 1967;119:141-146.

55. Petz L. Immunologic cross-reactivity between penicillins and cephalosporins: A review. J Infect Dis. 1978;137:S74-S79.

56. Shibata K, Atsumi T, Itorivchi Y, et al. Immunological cross-reactivities of cephalothin and its related compounds with benzylpenicillin (penicillin G). Nature. 1966;212:419-420.

57. Abraham GN, Petz LD, Fudenberg HH. Immunohaematological cross-allergenicity between penicillin and cephalothin in humans. Clin Exp Immunol. 1968;3:343-357.

58. Solley GO, Gleich GJ, Van Dellen RG. Penicillin allergy: Clinical experience with a battery of skin-test reagents. J Allergy Clin Immunol. 1982;69:238-244.

59. Saxon A, Beall GN, Rohr AS, et al. Immediate hypersensitivity reactions to beta-lactam antibiotics. Ann Intern Med. 1987;107:204-215.

60. Novalbos A, Sastre J, Cuesta J, et al. Lack of allergic cross-reactivity to cephalosporins among patients allergic to penicillins. Clin Exp Allergy 2000;31: 438-443.

61. Goodman EJ, Morgan MJ, Johnson PA, et al. Cephalosporins can be given to penicillin-allergic patients who do not exhibit an anaphylactic response. J Clin Anesth 2001;13:561-564.

62. Li JTC, Markus PJ, Osmon DR, et al. Reduction of vancomycin use in orthopedic patients with a history of antibiotic allergy. Mayo Clin Proc 2000;75:902-906.

63. Kelkar PS, Li JTC. Cephalosporin allergy. N Engl J Med. 2001;345:804-809.

64. Saxon A, Beall GW, Rohr AS, Adelman DS. Immediate hypersensitivity reactions to beta-lactam antibiotics. Ann Intern Med. 1987;107:204-215.

65. Adkinson NF Jr, Swabb EA, Sugerman AA. Immunology of the monobactam aztreonam. Antimicrob Agents Chemother. 1984;25:93-97.

66. Saxon A, Hassner A, Swabb EA, et al. Lack of cross-reactivity between aztreonam, a monobactam antibiotic, and penicillin in penicillin-allergic subjects. J Infect Dis. 1984;149:16-22.

67. Adkinson NF Jr, Wheeler B, Swabb EA. Clinical tolerance of the monobactam aztreonam in penicillin allergic subjects (Abstract WS-26-4). Presented at the 14th International Congress of Chemotherapy, Kyoto, Japan, June 23-28, 1985.

68. Pimiento P, Martinez G, Mena M, et al. Aztreonam and ceftazidime: Evidence of in vivo cross-allergenicity. Allergy. 1998;50:524-525.

69. de la Fuente Prieto R, Armentia Medina A, Sanchez Palla P, et al. Urticaria caused by sensitization to aztreonam. Allergy. 1993;48:634-636.

CHAPTER **23**

Fusidic Acid

LIONEL A. MANDELL

STRUCTURE

Fusidic acid, a member of the fusidane class, is derived from the fungus *Fusidium coccineum* and is related chemically to the antibiotics helvolic acid and cephalosporin P_1.[1] Despite its steroid-like structure, fusidic acid does not have steroid activity. The sodium salt of fusidic acid (Fucidin) was developed by Leo Laboratories in Denmark and first was introduced into clinical practice in 1962.

MECHANISM OF ACTION

Fusidic acid is usually bacteriostatic but at higher concentrations may be bactericidal. It exerts its antibacterial effect by inhibiting protein synthesis, but the exact mechanisms by which this inhibition occurs have not been elucidated fully.

Bacterial protein synthesis depends on the translocation of petidyl-transfer RNA from the ribosomal acceptor site to the peptidyl site. This translocation requires protein elongation factor G and hydrolysis of guanosine triphosphate (GTP). At least part of fusidic acid's action reflects its ability to stabilize ribosome-elongation factor—GTP plus inorganic phosphate complexes—inhibiting GTP hydrolysis and blocking elongation of the nascent polypeptide chain.[2]

Resistance to fusidic acid may occur through a variety of mechanisms. Strains of *Staphylococcus aureus* may exhibit chromosome-mediated or plasmid-mediated resistance. Fusidic acid resistance in *S. aureus* results from point mutations within the chromosomal *fus* A gene, which encodes for elongation factor G.[3] Chromosomal mutations occur at a frequency of 1 in 10^{-6} to 10^{-7},[4,5] and result in alteration at the target site (i.e., elongation factor G). In the presence of fusidic acid and rifampin, however, mutants are not recoverable.[6] Plasmid-mediated resistance may be due to reduced permeability to the antibiotic.[7]

ANTIMICROBIAL ACTIVITY

Fusidic acid has a unique spectrum of antimicrobial activity, and susceptible organisms include select aerobes and anaerobes. Although there are no official National Committee for Clinical Laboratory Standards guidelines for in vitro susceptibility testing, a study determined the minimal inhibitory concentrations (MICs) and zone diameters for fusidic acid using standard National Committee for Clinical Laboratory Standards methods.[8] The proposed break points for fusidic acid against staphylococci are listed in Table 23-1.

Fusidic acid is most active against *S. aureus* and *Staphylococcus epidermidis,* including strains that are methicillin resistant. These organisms are generally sensitive to fusidic acid because there is no cross-resistance between this agent and β-lactam antimicrobials. MICs for methicillin-resistant *S. aureus* range from 0.03 to 0.8 mg/L, but in one study of bacteremic isolates, the MIC_{90} was 0.2 mg/L.[9] Only a short in vitro postantibiotic effect of 1 to 2 hours has been shown. Fusidic acid is considerably less active against *Staphylococcus saprophyticus* strains and streptococci. *Corynebacterium* spp. are generally sensitive, as are *Neisseria gonorrhoeae* and *Meningococcus* spp. Aerobic gram-negative bacilli seem to be resistant.[4]

With the exception of *Fusobacterium necrophorum,* anaerobic organisms are generally quite sensitive to fusidic acid. Gram-positive anaerobes generally are very susceptible, with MIC_{90} values ranging from 0.25 to 1 mg/L.[5] MIC_{90} values for *Clostridium difficile* are higher at 2 mg/L. Gram-negative anaerobes are a little more variable in their susceptibility. The *Bacteroides* spp. *B. distasonis, B. ovatus, B. thetaiotaomicron,* and *B. fragilis* exhibit MIC_{90} values ranging from 2 to 16 mg/L, whereas for *B. ureolyticus* and *B. vulgatus,* MIC_{90} values range from only 0.25 to 1 mg/L. MICs are increased markedly in the presence of serum, and antimicrobial activity is reduced in alkaline media.

Reports of the effects of antimicrobial combinations containing fusidic acid have been inconsistent. One study of drug combinations involving fusidic acid with either vancomycin or rifampin against isolates of methicillin-resistant, coagulase-positive and coagulase-

TABLE 23-1 Proposed Break Points for Fusidic Acid against Staphylococci

	Minimal Inhibitory Concentration (mg/L)	*Zone Diameter (mm)*
Susceptible	≤0.25	≥22
Intermediate	0.5-1	>17-<22
Resistant	≥2	≤17

negative staphylococci suggested a synergistic effect.[10,11] In vitro antagonism between fusidic acid and fluoroquinolones (levofloxacin, ciprofloxacin, ofloxacin, moxifloxacin) was shown using clinical isolates of *S. aureus* and coagulase-negative staphylococci.[12]

Some data suggest that fusidic acid may be active in vitro against mycobacteria, including *Mycobacterium leprae*.[13,14] MIC_{90} values of 16 mg/L and 30 mg/L have been reported for *Mycobacterium tuberculosis* and *Mycobacterium bovis*.

PHARMACOLOGY

Fusidic acid may be used parenterally as an intravenous formulation, or it may be given orally or applied topically. Various formulations, dosages, and frequencies of administration are listed in Table 23-2. The sodium salt intravenous formulation may be administered over 2 to 4 hours.

The drug is virtually completely absorbed after oral administration, achieving levels of 71 mg/L with repeated thrice-daily dosing. With repeated intravenous infusions, peak plasma concentrations of 123 mg/L have been recorded. The drug is highly protein bound (95% to 97%), exhibits nonlinear kinetics, and has a half-life of approximately 14 hours. Although the standard frequency of administration has been three times a day, because of the drug's long half-life, it has been suggested that dosing could be changed to a twice-daily schedule.[5,15] This has been my practice for the past several years, and it seems to reduce gastrointestinal intolerance without altering efficacy.

Fusidic acid is distributed widely to such tissues as synovial fluid, bone, subcutaneous fat, kidney, bronchial secretions, cardiac tissue, and aqueous humor.[16] This drug also crosses the placenta.

Fusidic acid is metabolized by the liver and is eliminated primarily by biliary excretion of various conjugative and cytochrome P-450 (CYP450) oxidative metabolites. Approximately 2% of fusidic acid can be recovered unchanged in the stool, but very little is recovered in urine. Dosage modification is not necessary for patients with renal failure or for patients on hemodialysis. Little is known about the use of fusidic acid in patients with hepatic impairment, and the drug probably is best avoided in such circumstances.

Fusidic acid also has in vitro and in vivo immunosuppressive functions. This drug has been found to have activity similar to that of cyclosporine. In animal models and in preliminary human trials, it has been shown either to protect against the development of insulin-dependent diabetes mellitus or to have an ameliorating effect on the disease.[17-19]

ADVERSE REACTIONS

Adverse reactions depend on the route of administration of fusidic acid. With the intravenous formulation, thrombophlebitis and reversible jaundice have been noted. Reversible jaundice also is seen with the oral preparation, but to a lesser extent (6% versus 17%).[20]

Because fusidic acid is avidly bound to albumin, it competes with bilirubin for binding sites. It should be used with caution, if at all, in newborns, particularly if they are icteric, acidotic, or premature.[20] Oral use generally is well tolerated but has been associated with mild gastrointestinal upset. The ophthalmic preparations occasionally may cause mild-to-moderate local symptoms, such as itching or stinging. A drug-induced, reversible immune-mediated thrombocytopenia has been described in which a fusidic acid–dependent, platelet-reactive antibody binds platelets but only in the presence of the drug.[21]

DRUG INTERACTIONS

Drug interactions may exist in a variety of forms and can result in significant problems for patients. Effects on the hepatic CYP450 enzyme system have implications for the many drugs that interact at the CYP450 level. Fusidic acid was found to have a time-dependent activating effect on this system when used for 28 days but not when used for 14 days.[22] The clinical significance of this finding has yet to be determined.

Protease inhibitors generally are known to have inhibitory effects on the CYP450 system. Elevated levels of ritonavir, saquinavir, and fusidic acid, possibly resulting from mutual inhibition of metabolism, were found in a 32-year-old patient with acquired immunodeficiency syndrome.[23] Rhabdomyolysis has been reported in patients taking atorvastatin or simvastatin and fusidic acid.[24,25]

CLINICAL USE

Fusidic acid has been used in systemic (intravenous, oral) and topical (ophthalmic, skin preparations) formulations primarily for the treatment of staphylococcal infections. It is not available in the United States, although it may be obtained through compassionate release. The foci of infection, with and without associated bacteremia, have included acute and chronic osteomyelitis, septic arthritis, endocarditis, soft tissue infections including burns, and lower respiratory tract infections in patients with cystic fibrosis.[26-29]

Endocarditis has been treated with some success using fusidic acid in combination with a second drug. Fusidic acid has been given with a penicillinase-resistant semisynthetic penicillin, such as flucloxacillin, for staphylococcal endocarditis and with erythromycin for endocarditis caused by *Corynebacterium* spp.[30,31]

Application of fusidic acid cream to the nostrils of patients with lepromatous leprosy reduced the morphologic index of the nose-blow smear. Nine lepromatous leprosy patients showed clinical improvement when treated with fusidic acid for 12 weeks.[32,33]

Given the increased incidence of methicillin-resistant *S. aureus* and *S. epidermidis* infections, fusidic acid may offer advantages over currently available agents. Topical use has been limited to external eye infections and superficial skin infections, including erythrasma caused by *Corynebacterium minutissimum*.

TABLE 23-2 Dosage and Administration of Fusidic Acid

Route of Administration	Formulation	Dosage	Frequency of Administration
IV	Fusidate sodium	>50 kg BW, 500 mg*	tid
		<50 kg BW, 7 mg/kg	tid
PO (film-coated tablets)	Fusidate sodium	500 mg	tid
PO (suspension)	Hemihydrate	0-1 yr, 0.3 mg/kg BW	tid
		1-5 yr, 5 mL	tid
		6-12 yr, 10 mL	tid
		Adults, 15 mL	tid
Topical			
Cream (2%)	Fusidic acid		bid
Ointment (2%)	Fusidate sodium		bid
Gel (2%)	Fusidate sodium		bid
Ophthalmic			
Viscous eye drops (1%)	Fusidic acid		bid

*500 mg of fusidate sodium = 480 mg of fusidic acid.
BW, body weight.

Initial concerns about the emergence of resistant strains during therapy led to the practice of combining fusidic acid with a second drug. Resistance may be more likely to occur in the setting of chronic infections if the drug is used alone.[4,34] Experience over the past few decades has shown, however, that when the drug is used alone for the treatment of acute infections, resistance is seen in only 0 to 2% of patients, whereas resistance occurs in less than 1% of patients treated with combination therapy.

REFERENCES

1. Godtfredsen W, Roholt K, Tybring L. Fusidin: A new orally active antibiotic. Lancet. 1962;1:928-931.
2. Von Daehne W, Godtfredsen WO, Rasmussen PR. Structure-activity relationships in fusidic acid-type antibiotics. Adv Appl Microbiol. 1979;25:95-146.
3. Besier S, Ludwig A, Brade V, Wichelhaus T. Molecular analysis of fusidic acid resistance in Staphylococcus aureus. Mol Microbiol. 2003;47:463-469.
4. Verbist L. The antimicrobial activity of fusidic acid. J Antimicrob Chemother. 1990;25(Suppl B):1-5.
5. Steinkraus GE, McCarthy LR. In vitro activity of sodium fusidate against anaerobic bacteria. Antimicrob Agents Chemother. 1979;16:120-122.
6. O'Neill A, Cove J, Chopra I. Mutation frequencies for resistance to fusidic acid and rifampin in Staphylococcus aureus. J Antimicrob Chemother. 2001;47:647-650.
7. Shanson DC. Clinical relevance of resistance to fusidic acid in Staphylococcus aureus. J Antimicrob Chemother. 1990;25(Suppl B):15-21.
8. Coutant C, Olden D, Bell J, Turnidge J. Disk diffusion interpretive criteria for fusidic acid susceptibility testing of staphylococci by the National Committee for Clinical Laboratory Standards method. Diagn Mocrobiol Infect Dis. 1996;25:9-13.
9. Van der Auwera P, Godard C, Denis C, et al. In vitro activities of new antimicrobial agents against multiresistant Staphylococcus aureus isolated from septicemic patients during a Belgian national survey from 1983 to 1985. Antimicrob Agents Chemother. 1990;34:2260-2262.
10. Foldes M, Munro R, Sorrell TC, et al. In-vitro effects of vancomycin, rifampicin and fusidic acid, alone and in combination, against methicillin-resistant Staphylococcus aureus. J Antimicrob Chemother. 1983;11:21-26.
11. Farber BF, Yee YC, Karchmer AW. Interaction between rifampin and fusidic acid against methicillin-resistant coagulase-positive and negative staphylococci. Antimicrob Agents Chemother. 1986;30:174-175.
12. Ertek M, Yazgi H, Erol S, Altoparlak U. Demonstration of in vitro antagonism between fusidic acid and quinolones. J Int Med Res. 2002;30:525-528.
13. Fuurstd K, Askgaard D, Faber V. Susceptibility of strains of the mycobacterium tuberculosis complex to fusidic acid. APMIS. 1992;100:663-667.
14. Franzblau S, Biswas A, Harris E. Fusidic acid is highly active against extracellular and intracellular Mycobacterium leprae. Antimicrob Agents Chemother. 1992;36:92-94.
15. Carr WD, Wall AR, Georgala-Zervogiani S, et al. Fusidic acid tablets in patients with skin and soft tissue infection: A dose finding study. Eur J Clin Res. 1994;5:87-95.
16. Reeves DS. The pharmacokinetics of fusidic acid. J Antimicrob Chemother. 1987;20:467-476.
17. Nicoletti F, Meroni PL, Bendtzen K. Fusidic acid and insulin-dependent diabetes mellitus. Autoimmunology. 1996;24:187-197.
18. Nicoletti F, Zaconne P, Di Marco R, et al. Effects of sodium fusidate in animal models of insulin dependent diabetes mellitus and septic shock. Immunology. 1995;85:645-650.
19. Nicoletti F, Marco R, Morrone S, et al. Reduction of spontaneous autoimmune diabetes in diabetes-prone BB rats with the novel immunosuppressant fusidic acid: Effect on T-cell proliferation and production of interferon-γ. Immunology. 1994;81:317-321.
20. Brodersen R. Fusidic acid binding to serum albumin and interaction with binding of bilirubin. Acta Paediatr Scand. 1985;74:874-880.
21. El-Kassar N, Kalfon F, Fromont P, et al. Fusidic acid induced acute immunologic thrombocytopenia. Br J Haematol. 1996;93:427-431.
22. Reimann G, Barthel B, Rockstroh J, et al. Effect of fusidic acid on the hepatic cytochrome P450 enzyme system. Int J Clin Pharmacol Ther. 1999;37:562-566.
23. Khaliq Y, Gallicano K, Leger R, et al. A drug interaction between fusidic acid and a combination of ritonavir and saquinavir. Br J Clin Pharmacol. 2000;50:83-84.
24. Dromer C, Vedrenne C, Billey T, et al. Rhabdomyolysis due to simvastatin: Apropos of a case with review of the literature. Rev Rhum Mal Osteoartic. 1992;59:281-283.
25. Wenisch C, Krause R, Fladerer P, et al. Acute rhabdomyolysis after atorvastatin and fusidic acid therapy (Letter). Am J Med. 2000;109:78.
26. Gransden WR, Eykyn SJ, Phillips I. Staphylococcus aureus bacteremia: 400 episdes in St. Thomas's Hospital. BMJ. 1984;288:300-303.
27. O'Brien T, McManus F, MacAuley PH, Ennis JT. Acute haematogenous osteomyelitis. J Bone Joint Surg Br. 1982;64:450-453.
28. Eykyn SJ. Staphylococcal bacteremia and endocarditis and fusidic acid. J Antimicrob Chemother. 1990;25(Suppl B):33-38.
29. Wright GLT, Harper J. Fusidic acid and lincomycin therapy in staphylococcal infections in cystic fibrosis. Lancet. 1970;1:9-14.
30. Moy RJD, George RH, de Giovanni JV, Silove ED. Improving survival in bacterial endocarditis. Arch Dis Child. 1986;61:394-399.
31. Jackson G, Saunders K. Prosthetic valve diphtheroid endocarditis treated with sodium fusidate and erythromycin. Br Heart J. 1973;35:931-936.
32. Mahajan PM, Jadhav VH, Jogaikar DG, Mehta JM. Intranasal administration of fusidic acid cream in leprosy. Indian J Lepr. 2000;72:451-455.
33. Franzblau S, Chan G, Garcia-Ignacio B, et al. Clinical trial of fusidic acid for lepromatous leprosy. Antimicrob Agents Chemother. 1994;38:1651-1654.
34. Faber M, Rosdahl VT. Susceptibility to fusidic acid among Danish Staphylococcus aureus strains and fusidic consumption. J Antimicrob Chemother. 1990;25 (Suppl B):7-14.

Aminoglycosides

DAVID N. GILBERT

Aminoglycoside antibiotics have been an important part of the antibacterial drug arsenal since the 1940s. They demonstrate concentration-dependent bactericidal activity against susceptible organisms. Several members of the aminoglycoside family have predictable in vitro activity against *Pseudomonas aeruginosa* and the vast majority of other aerobic gram-negative bacilli. Some aminoglycosides have useful activity against mycobacteria; one (paromomycin) has been used to treat selected colonic protozoan pathogens, and a related antibiotic, spectinomycin, has been used to treat infections with *Neisseria gonorrhoeae*. The aminoglycoside antimicrobial activity may be additive to or synergistic with that of penicillins or cephalosporins against infection by aerobic gram-negative bacilli or aerobic gram-positive cocci. The prevalence of aminoglycoside resistance has remained low and emergence of bacterial resistance during therapy rare.

The aminoglycoside family shares the potential for nephrotoxicity, ototoxicity, and, rarely, neuromuscular blockade. The risk of toxicity may be decreasing as mechanisms are understood, new dosage strategies introduced, concomitant risk factors avoided, and shorter drug courses used. Allergic reactions are rare. With patent expirations, the cost of many aminoglycosides is low. Although new β-lactams and fluoroquinolones share the same antibacterial spectrum, the efficacy of the aminoglycosides and resistance problems with the newer drugs presage a continued need.

NAMES AND SOURCES

In the 1940s, soil actinomycetes (bacteria) were systematically screened for the elaboration of antimicrobial substances. Streptomycin was the first aminoglycoside found (Table 24-1).[1] Streptomycin was produced by a *Streptomyces* species, and subsequent drugs were derived from either *Streptomyces* spp. or *Micromonospora* spp. The suffix indicates the source; that is, aminoglycosides with names ending in *-mycin* derive directly or indirectly from *Streptomyces*, whereas aminoglycosides with names ending in *-micin* derive directly or indirectly from *Micromonospora*.

Neomycin, kanamycin, and gentamicin are fermentation products with two or three chemical constituents. Amikacin, netilmicin, dibekacin, and isepamicin are semisynthetic derivatives of the natural product. Nine aminoglycosides (including spectinomycin) are commercially available in the United States. Sisomicin, dibekacin, and isepamicin are approved for human use in Japan, Europe, and elsewhere.

STRUCTURE

All aminoglycosides have an essential six-membered ring with amino group substituents, hence the name *aminocyclitol*.[1] The descriptor *aminoglycoside* results from the glycosidic bonds between the aminocyclitol and two or more amino-containing or non–amino-containing sugars. Spectinomycin differs in that there is an aminocyclitol ring but there are no amino sugars and no glycosidic bonds.

The central aminocyclitol for streptomycin is streptidine, whereas for all other current aminoglycosides it is 2-deoxystreptamine (Fig. 24-1).

TABLE 24-1 The Family of Aminoglycosides in Clinical Use*

Names				
Generic	Proprietary	Source	Year Reported	Chemistry
Streptomycin	None	*Streptomyces griseus*	1944	Unique central aminocyclitol ring
Neomycin	Mycifradin, Neobiotic	*Streptomyces fradiae*	1949	Roughly equal proportions of neomycin B and C
Kanamycin	Kantrex	*Streptomyces kanamyceticus*	1957	Mixture of 95% kanamycin A and 5% kanamycin B
Paromomycin	Humatin	*Streptomyces fradiae*	1959	Part of "neomycin" family
Gentamicin	Garamycin	*Micromonospora purpurea* and *Micromonospora echinospora*	1963	Roughly equal proportions of gentamicin C$_1$, C$_{1a}$, C$_2$
Tobramycin	Nebcin	*Streptomyces tenebrarius*	1967	Natural 3'-deoxy derivative of kanamycin B
Amikacin†	Amikin	*Streptomyces kanamyceticus*	1972	Semisynthetic derivative of kanamycin A Netilmicin†
Netilmicin†	Netromycin	*Micromonospora inyoensis*	1975	*N*-Ethyl derivative of sisomicin
Spectinomycin	Trobicin	*Streptomyces spectabilis*	1961	Chemically distinct but closely related to aminoglycosides
Sisomicin‡	Siseptin	*Micromonospora inyoensis*	1970	Dehydro analogue of gentamicin C$_{1a}$
Dibekacin†,‡		*Streptomyces kanamyceticus*	1971	Dideoxy derivative of kanamycin B
Isepamicin†,‡		*Micromonospora purpurea*	1978	I-*N*-*S*-α-Hydroxy B amino propionyl derivative of gentamicin B

*The drugs are listed by the year in which they were described with comments on their chemistry.[1]
†Semisynthetic aminoglycosides.
‡Approved for human use in countries other than the United States.

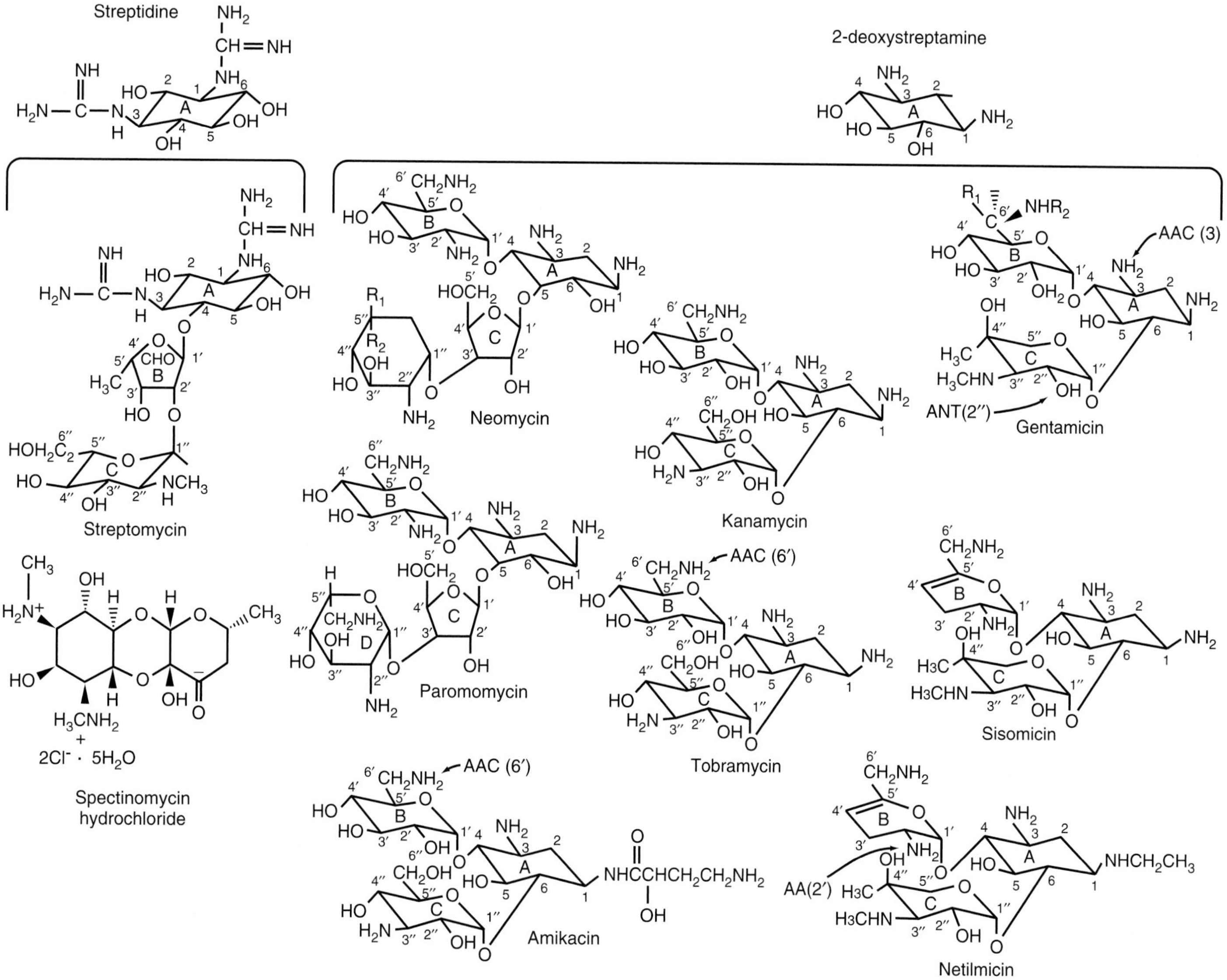

FIGURE 24-1. Chemical structure of the aminoglycosides and spectinomycin. Neomycin contains approximately equal amounts of neomycin B (R$_1$ = H; R$_2$ = CH$_2$NH$_2$) and neomycin C (R$_1$ = CH$_2$NH$_2$; R$_2$ = H). Kanamycin is principally kanamycin A, as shown. Gentamicin is gentamicin C complex with roughly equal amounts of C$_1$ (R$_1$ = R$_2$ = CH$_3$), C$_{1a}$ (R$_1$ = R$_2$ = H), and C$_2$ (R$_1$ = CH$_3$; R$_2$ = H). The sites of action of four inactivating enzymes are shown: three acetyltransferases (AAC [3], AAC [2'], and AAC [6']) and one adenyltransferase (ANT [2'']).

TABLE 24-2 Chemical Families of Aminoglycoside Antibiotics

Family	Member
Streptomycin	Streptomycin
Kanamycin	Kanamycin A
	Kanamycin B
	Amikacin
	Tobramycin
	Dibekacin
Gentamicin	Gentamicin C_1, C_{1a}, C_2
	Sisomicin
	Netilmicin
	Isepamicin
Neomycin	Neomycin
	Paromomycin
Spectinomycin*	

*An aminocyclitol, no glycosidic bonds.

The standard numbering convention is illustrated in Figure 24-1. Note the counterclockwise numbering of the aminocyclitol ring and the clockwise numbering of linked sugar molecules. Figure 24-1 also illustrates the structural basis of the aminoglycoside subgroups. Neomycin and paromomycin are derived from *Streptomyces* spp. and link to cyclic sugars at positions 4 and 5 of 2-deoxystreptamine. Both drugs contain a distinctive pentose linkage as well as linkage to two hexose sugars. Note that of the commonly used aminoglycosides, neomycin contains the largest number, six, of free amino groups.

Kanamycin, tobramycin, amikacin, and dibekacin constitute the kanamycin family (Table 24-2). All derive from *Streptomyces* spp. and link to cyclic sugars at positions 4 and 6 of 2-deoxystreptamine. Tobramycin is 3'-deoxykanamycin B. Amikacin is kanamycin A with the semisynthetic addition of 2-hydroxy-4-aminobutyric acid to the amino group at position 1 of the aminocyclitol.

Gentamicin is a mixture of three closely related constituents, C_1, C_{1a}, and C_2, elaborated by *Micromonospora* spp. with glycosidic linkages at positions 4 and 6. Sisomicin is the dihydro analogue of gentamicin C_{1a}; netilmicin is derived from sisomicin by the addition of an ethyl group to the amino group at position 1 of the aminocyclitol.

Structure and Antimicrobial Activity

Aminoglycoside antibiotics bind with high avidity to a region of highly conserved nucleotides in the messenger RNA (mRNA) decoding region of the 30S subunit of prokaryotic ribosomes. The critical translation of the mRNA codon and the anticodon of the aminoacyl-transfer RNA occurs at the A (acceptance) site.[2,3] The A site is in the 16S reverse transfer RNA portion of the 30S ribosomal subunit.

Nuclear magnetic resonance (NMR) spectroscopy studies demonstrate changes consistent with aminoglycoside binding to an asymmetric interval loop (U1406-A1408, A1492-U1495) within the A site (Fig. 24-2).[4] The binding induces a conformational change in two adenine residues (A1492 and A1493) that results in interference with mRNA translation and translocation.

Aminoglycoside antibiotics preferentially bind to prokaryotic ribosomes.[4] In prokaryotes, the 1408 position is an adenosine. In eukaryotic cytosolic ribosomes, the adenosine is replaced by a guanosine with a concomitant reduction in binding of aminoglycosides. An A1408G mutation in *Escherichia coli* results in a high level of resistance to selected aminoglycosides. It is speculated that the difference in binding is due to access to the target. The double adenosine nucleotides in prokaryotic ribosomes create an internal bulge and a larger groove that allows access to the ribosomal binding site.[5] Aminoglycoside interaction with eukaryotic ribosomes may prove useful in therapy for selected genetic diseases (see later).

Avidity of binding varies with the aminoglycoside. One variable is the number of amino groups and their state of protonation.[6]

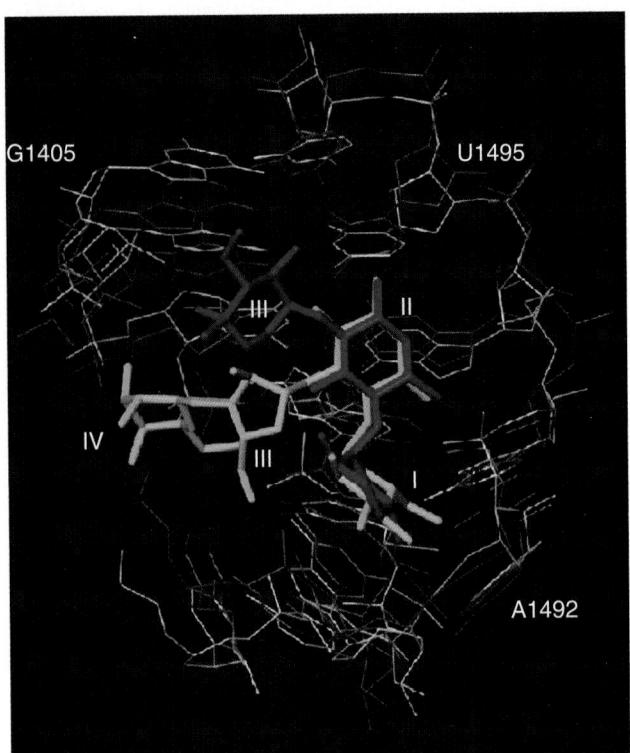

FIGURE 24-2. Three-dimensional structures of the aminoglycoside antibiotics paromomycin (yellow) and gentamicin C_{1a} (red) bound to *Escherichia coli* 16S ribosomal RNA (light and dark tans, respectively). Rings I and II of the two drugs, which are required for antibiotic activity, bind in the same mode in both complexes; the additional rings (III and IV in paromomycin and III in gentamicin C_{1a}), which are less important for drug activity, make diverse contacts with the RNA. *(Courtesy of Joseph D. Puglisi, Director, Stanford Magnetic Resonance Laboratory, Stanford University School of Medicine.)*

OTHER AMINOGLYCOSIDE BIOLOGIC ACTIVITIES

The aminoglycosides have a variety of other biologic activities that are the subject of ongoing study. Some genetic diseases arise, in part, from point mutations that result in premature stop codons in important coding sequences. Examples include the transmembrane conductance regulator protein of cystic fibrosis (CF), Duchenne's muscular dystrophy, the Hurler syndrome, and nephrogenic diabetes insipidus. In vitro and in vivo studies and even one preliminary clinical trial in CF indicate that aminoglycosides can suppress premature stop codons and restore physiologically active amounts of functional protein (see "Cystic Fibrosis").[7-12] The mechanism of the suppression of the stop codons is under study.

Aminoglycosides bind to, and modulate the function of, a wide variety of other RNA or RNA-related molecules. Examples include the hairpin ribozyme, the hammerhead ribozyme, the ribonuclease P ribonucleoprotein, and the Rev response element transcribed activator region from human immunodeficiency virus that contains the binding site for the Rev protein.[13,14] The latter studies employ aminoglycosides as probes to allow better understanding of physiology. The new knowledge of structure-activity relationships will improve our understanding of the antibacterial and toxic potential of the aminoglycosides.

CHEMICAL CHARACTERISTICS

Aminoglycosides are highly soluble in water and insoluble in organic solvents.[15] The latter property correlates with the limited ability of aminoglycosides to cross lipid-containing cellular membranes.

Aminoglycosides have a molecular size in the range of 445 to 600 daltons.[15] The molecular structure is unchanged by freezing, heating to 100° C for up to 4 hours, or changes in solution pH ranging from 3.0 to 12 over several hours.[16-18] Using NMR spectroscopy, the pK_a values of the individual amino groups can be determined.[6] The overall pK_a for gentamicin is about pH 8.4.[15] Hence, at pH 7.4, the aminoglycosides have a very high positive charge and are cationic.

The overall positive charge contributes to both antimicrobial activity and toxicity. Antibacterial activity is enhanced in media with an alkaline pH and reduced in media with an acidic pH.[18] The positively charged aminoglycosides bind to the negatively charged RNA backbone, cell wall lipopolysaccharide (LPS), cell membrane phospholipids, and other anionic molecules.[19]

Of interest, cationic aminoglycosides interact chemically with β-lactam antibiotics.[20-22] The reaction results in a nucleophilic opening of the β-lactam ring with acylation of an amino group of the aminoglycoside and mutual loss of antibacterial activity. In vitro, gentamicin and tobramycin are inactivated with greater ease than netilmicin, amikacin, or isepamicin. Perhaps because their dosage is in grams rather than milligrams, the antipseudomonal penicillins (e.g., carbenicillin, ticarcillin, piperacillin, mezlocillin, and azlocillin) are the β-lactams most susceptible to the reaction. As the reaction requires several hours in vitro, the clinical import is limited. Nonetheless, penicillins and aminoglycosides should not be mixed in the same solution before infusion. Serum specimens for drug level determination from patients receiving both drugs should be assayed immediately or frozen. If patients with renal failure are administered a concomitant aminoglycoside and an antipseudomonal penicillin, there is a 10% to 20% reduction in the serum aminoglycoside concentration compared with the levels observed when each drug is administered alone.[23] The interaction is molecular to molecular, and, because of the 40-fold difference in dosage, there is no discernible decrement in the serum concentration of the penicillin.

ENZYMATIC INACTIVATION

Aminoglycosides are subject to modification and loss of antimicrobial activity by enzymes derived from both gram-positive and gram-negative bacterial pathogens.[1] The three recognized classes of enzyme effects are (1) ATP-dependent phosphorylation of a hydroxyl group by a phosphotransferase, (2) ATP-dependent adenylation of a hydroxyl group by a nucleotidyltransferase, and (3) acetyl coenzyme A–dependent acetylation of an amino group by an acetyltransferase. Examples of sites of enzyme activity are shown in Figure 24-1. Enzyme modification results in loss of antibacterial activity.

MECHANISM OF ANTIMICROBIAL ACTIVITY

Binding of aminoglycosides to prokaryotic ribosomes is a prerequisite for the drugs' antimicrobic activity. However, the exact mechanism or mechanisms of cidal activity remain unknown.[1] The binding to ribosomes is reversible, which usually results in a bacteriostatic rather than a bactericidal effect.[1] Ribosomal binding results in a measurable decrease in protein synthesis as a result of misreading of mRNA. Chloramphenicol and other drugs that inhibit protein synthesis are bacteriostatic and not bactericidal, which suggests additional unidentified mechanisms of bactericidal activity.

There is initial electrostatic binding of aminoglycosides to the cell surface followed by two energy-dependent uptake phases and binding to ribosomes.[24-26] The initial binding is rapid and not energy dependent.[27,28] In gram-negative bacteria, the cationic aminoglycosides bind to negatively charged residues in the LPS, polar heads of phospholipids, and anionic outer-membrane proteins.[25,29] The aminoglycosides displace competitively cell wall Mg^{2+} and Ca^{2+} bridges that normally link adjacent LPS molecules.[30-31] The result is a rearrangement of LPS with subsequent bleeding of the outer membrane, formation of transient holes in the cell wall, and disruption of the cell wall's normal permeability function.[32]

ENERGY-DEPENDENT PHASE

Subsequent transport across the bacterial cytoplasmic membrane is energy dependent and divided into phases: an initial slow energy-dependent phase (EDP-I) and a subsequent rapid energy-dependent phase, EDP-II.[24-26,33-35] EDP-I transports drug into the cytosol. EDP-I is inhibited by divalent cations, elevated osmolarity, low pH, and anaerobic conditions. EDP-II is rapid and represents binding to the ribosomes.

The source of energy is an electrochemical gradient of protons generated by proton extrusion during respiration or by the hydrolysis of ATP.[24] The electrochemical gradient is calculated from the additive effects of the electrical potential difference across the membrane plus the proton concentration across the membrane.

The onset of bacterial killing is coincident with the transition from EDP-I to EDP-II.[25,26] Most bacterial cells manifest lethal injury after only 25% of the maximum EDP-II uptake.[34] The higher the external concentration of aminoglycoside, the quicker the intracellular drug level reaches levels necessary to trigger EDP-II uptake, which in turn forecasts death of the organism.[36]

The mechanisms of the intracellular accumulation of high concentrations of drug and of cell death are unclear. It is suggested that the high intracellular concentrations of drug result from aminoglycoside closure of voltage-gated channels with subsequent trapping of drug.[37] There are many consequences of the accumulation of large concentrations of aminoglycoside inside bacterial cells: binding to ribosomes with mistranslation of mRNA yielding abnormal proteins, loss of cell membrane integrity with efflux of intracellular ions, and inhibition of DNA replication. One theory suggests that misfolded nonfunctional proteins disrupt normal function of the cell membrane.[1] In short, aminoglycosides require aerobic energy to enter the cell and bind to ribosomes. Subsequent cell death may result from some combination of trapping of high concentrations of drug, RNA mistranslation with aberrant protein production, and cell membrane dysfunction.

AMINOGLYCOSIDE RESISTANCE

Intrinsic Resistance

As with other antimicrobials, resistance to aminoglycosides may be intrinsic or acquired.[1]

Intrinsic resistance may be nonenzymatic or enzymatic. For aminoglycosides to enter a bacterial cell, there must be an active electron transport chain sufficient to generate an electrical potential difference across the membrane. Thus, anaerobic bacteria are intrinsically resistant to aminoglycosides.

Mutations at the 16S ribosomal RNA (rRNA) can result in resistance. The best known example is resistance of *Mycobacterium tuberculosis* to streptomycin as a result of point mutations in ribosomal protein S12 and in the 16S rRNA. Resistance of *Mycobacterium abscessus* and *Mycobacterium chelonae* to amikacin is the result of a 16S rRNA point mutation.

Enzymatic intrinsic resistance is exemplified by the methylating enzymes that modify the 16S rRNA. To date, these enzymes have been described in aminoglycoside-producing organisms in nature but have not been identified in aminoglycoside-resistant clinical isolates.

Acquired Resistance: Reduced Entry or Efflux or Both

Acquired resistance to aminoglycosides results from some combination of decreased drug uptake, efflux pump activity, or enzymatic modification of the drug.[38-42]

Current data suggest that previously reported low-level aminoglycoside resistance attributed to impaired cell wall permeability may be the result of drug efflux mechanisms. Several groups have identified multidrug, including aminoglycoside, efflux pumps in *P. aeruginosa*. The pumps are named Mex XY or AmrAB.[38] The Mex XY pump is necessary for the inhibitory effect of divalent cations on the antibacterial activity of aminoglycosides versus *P. aeruginosa*.[39]

Activation of the Mex XY efflux pump also appears to explain adaptive resistance. Adaptive resistance is defined as a transient resistance to aminoglycosides that follows the rapid, early concentration-dependent killing of susceptible bacteria.[28,40] The refractory state lasts beyond the postantibiotic effective period into the time of regrowth. This phenomenon is termed *adaptive resistance* rather than *emergence of unstable mutants*. Adaptive resistance has been documented in vitro in animal modes and in patients with CF.[41,43] The effect lasts only a few hours. The implications for treatment are discussed later under "Once-Daily Therapy."

Exposure of susceptible bacteria to aminoglycosides can select for two types of drug-resistant subpopulations. One subpopulation results from activation of the Mex XY efflux pump and the phenomenon of adaptive resistance. The second subpopulation results from small colony variants with deficient energy-dependent uptake of aminoglycosides that may result in clinical treatment failure.[44,45]

Acquired Resistance: Enzymatic Modification

Three covalent modifications of aminoglycosides are recognized.[1,46] The amino groups can be modified by N-acetyltransferases (AAC) that use acetyl-coenzyme A as the donor. The hydroxyl groups can be modified by either O-nucleotidyltransferases (ANT) or O-phosphotransferases (APH). The latter use ATP as the donor. The enzymatically modified drugs bind poorly to ribosomes and result in high levels of resistance. In addition, the aminoglycoside may bind directly to a modifying enzyme in lieu of the ribosomal target.[47]

Specific enzymes are categorized by a nomenclature published in 1993.[1,48] Each enzyme is described by its class (AAC, ANT, or APH), a number in parentheses describing the location of modification of the drug, and a Roman numeral indicating a unique aminoglycoside resistance profile. Distinct genes resulting in identical resistance phenotypes are indicated by a lowercase letter after the Roman numeral. For example, aac (6')-Ia describes an acetylating enzyme that modifies aminoglycosides at the 6' position (see Fig. 24-1); the resistance profile would be the same as that of aac (6')-Ib but the enzyme protein is unique. A summary of modifying enzymes and their profile, source, and phenotype is available elsewhere.[1] Modifying enzyme genes are spread by plasmids or transposons, or both. Some are chromosomal. However, the plasmid-transposon genes can result in the rapid spread of drug-resistant phenotypes both within and between bacterial species. The resistance genes in gram-negative pathogens are diverse. In gram-positive pathogens, resistance is limited to a unique bifunctional enzyme, aac (6')-aph (2''), aph (3')-IIIa, and ant (6). In gram-negative organisms, a complex pattern of aac (6')-I genes combined with aac (3) and ant (2'') and others is observed.

Aminoglycoside Resistance in Enterococci

All enterococci have intrinsic resistance to aminoglycosides with minimal inhibitory concentrations (MICs) ranging from 4 to 256 μg/mL.[49] The resistance is attributed to the facultative anaerobic metabolism of enterococci that in turn reduces the transmembrane potential and hence limits drug intake. Concomitant exposure of enterococci to a cell wall–active drug, such as ampicillin or vancomycin, facilitates access of aminoglycosides to their ribosomal target site and classical synergistic bactericidal activity.

Acquisition of genes that encode aminoglycoside-modifying enzymes leads to high-level aminoglycoside resistance with loss of synergistic activity with penicillins or vancomycin.[50] At least nine genes have been described that mediate resistance to aminoglycoside synergism in enterococci.[50] The most important is the bifunctional gene aac (6')-Ie-aph (2'')-Ia, which encodes the bifunctional enzyme Aac (6')-Ie-Aph (2'')-Ia. Presence of the enzyme results in high-level resistance of gram-positive cocci to all aminoglycosides except streptomycin. A similar gene has been described in amikacin-resistant gram-negative bacterial clinical isolates from Europe.[51]

Resistance to streptomycin can result from acquisition of one of two nucleotidyltransferase genes, ant (3'')-Ia or ant (6')-Ia, or from a single-step ribosomal target mutation. Further, it is common for clini-

cal enterococcal isolates to have three or more resistance genes. A combination of resistance genes can result in a failure of synergism with all aminoglycosides available in the United States. Arbekacin, a derivative of dibekacin available only in Japan, shows somewhat promising results in the presence of a variety of modifying enzymes.[50]

The current threshold for detection of high-level resistance to gentamicin in vitro is an MIC of 500 μg/mL or more and to streptomycin is an MIC of 2000 μg/mL or more. The latter levels of resistance were chosen as surrogate markers for predicting synergism on the basis of the presence or absence of the aac (6')-Ie-aph (2'')-Ia bifunctional gene. Different MIC criteria are needed as surrogate markers for the presence of one or more of the other eight known resistance genes (enzymes).

Clinical Epidemiology of Aminoglycoside Resistance

In vitro resistance of clinical isolates of aerobic gram-negative bacilli to aminoglycosides varies with the specific drug, the target organism, the nature of the population of patients and their underlying disease or diseases, and local or regional patterns of physicians' use of specific aminoglycosides. A surveillance network of up to 270 clinical microbiology laboratories analyzed in vitro susceptibility data of selected Enterobacteriaceae and two nonfermentative gram-negative bacilli from 1998 to 2001. Portions of the data relevant to aminoglycoside susceptibility are summarized in Table 24-3.[52,53] The original data are subdivided into isolates from patients in intensive care units and patients not in intensive care units; the data in Table 24-3 are only for patients not in intensive care units.

Amikacin susceptibility exceeded that of gentamicin against all 10 species of Enterobacteriaceae tested and against *Acinetobacter baumannii* and *P. aeruginosa*. Tobramycin was not tested. Gentamicin susceptibility among the Enterobacteriaceae varied by less than 2% from 1998 to 2001; small stepwise decreases in susceptibility were most evident for *Enterobacter cloacae*.

The nonfermentative organisms are less susceptible than the Enterobacteriaceae to aminoglycosides. Again, a substantively higher percentage of isolates of *A. baumannii* and *P. aeruginosa* were sensitive to amikacin as compared with gentamicin.

A 1997 surveillance study included the in vitro susceptibility of blood-stream isolates of gram-negative bacilli from Canada, Latin America, and the United States.[54] Nearly 4300 isolates were roughly equally divided among the three geographic regions. The percentages of susceptibility and the somewhat greater percent susceptibility of amikacin were similar between isolates from the United States and Canada and similar to the surveillance data in Table 24-3. However, isolates from Latin America were substantively more resistant. The following are percent susceptible data for amikacin (the most active aminoglycoside) for Latin American isolates: *E. coli* 97%, *Klebsiella* species 76%, *Enterobacter* species 82%, *P. aeruginosa* 84%, and *Acinetobacter* species 40%.

The reasons for different patterns of resistance are complex and go beyond local or regional usage patterns. In the first 20 years of aminoglycoside use, gentamicin was the most frequently prescribed amino-

TABLE 24-3 In Vitro Susceptibility of Enterobacteriaceae, *Pseudomonas aeruginosa*, and *Acinetobacter baumannii* to Amikacin and Gentamicin from 1981 to 2001[52,53]

Organism	% Susceptible (No. of Isolates)	
	Amikacin	Gentamicin
Escherichia coli	99.6 (82,309)	95.8 (158,512)
Klebsiella pneumoniae	98.7 (32,107)	94.7 (55,921)
Enterobacter cloacae	99 (14,082)	91.2 (23,383)
All Enterobacteriaceae*	99 (170,745)	94.3 (309,183)
Acinetobacter baumannii	78.8 (3698)	45.7 (5321)
Pseudomonas aeruginosa	92 (44,186)	78.2 (60,910)

*Does not include isolates from intensive care unit patients.

glycoside in the United States and the most frequent mechanism of resistance was enzymatic alteration by ANT (2'')-I. ANT (2'')-I adenylates gentamicin but not amikacin.[55] During the same time in Japan, amikacin was used more often than gentamicin. In Japan, production of AAC (6')-I was found in 50% of the resistant isolates. AAC (6') acetylates amikacin and not gentamicin.[55]

Two different groups, employing more than 20 gene probes for aminoglycoside resistance enzymes, have documented the increasing complexity of mechanisms of resistance.[55-57] For example, in 148 aminoglycoside-nonsusceptible aerobic gram-negative bacillus blood isolates, 179 resistance mechanisms were found including 150 genes encoding aminoglycoside-modifying enzymes and 29 genes encoding permeability mechanisms.[57] In nine isolates, it was not possible to identify a genetic mechanism for the observed phenotypic resistance.

In distinction to β-lactams with activity against aerobic gram-negative bacilli, resistance rarely emerges during the course of aminoglycoside therapy. In a study of *Enterobacter* bacteremia in 129 adults, emergence of antimicrobial resistance during 4 to 18 days of therapy occurred in 6 of 31 patients administered a third-generation cephalosporin (19%) and in 1 of 89 patients administered an aminoglycoside (1%) ($P = .001$).[58] Concomitant administration of an aminoglycoside did not decrease the emergence of resistance to the third-generation cephalosporin. This and other studies document the emergence of cephalosporin-resistant aerobic gram-negative bacilli during therapy; in contrast, the evolution of aminoglycoside resistance appears to require either long periods of exposure or a very large inocula of organisms, as found in patients with burns or CF.

IN VITRO ANTIMICROBIAL ACTIVITY

Clinical Microbiology

The in vitro spectrum of activity of the aminoglycosides is compared with that of selected β-lactams and fluoroquinolones in Table 24-4.[59] The aminoglycosides demonstrate concentration-dependent bactericidal activity against a broad spectrum of aerobic and facultative gram-negative bacilli. Susceptible organisms in the spectrum of activity range from members of the family Enterobacteriaceae to *Pseudomonas* spp. to *Haemophilus* spp. Methicillin-susceptible but not methicillin-resistant *Staphylococcus aureus* strains are inhibited. Streptomycin has the greatest activity in vitro against *M. tuberculosis*, whereas amikacin is more active against *Mycobacterium avium-intracellulare* and other atypical mycobacteria. Streptomycin is the drug of choice for *Yersinia pestis* infection, and success with both streptomycin and gentamicin has been reported for *Francisella tularensis* infections. Compared with the other 2-deoxystreptamine aminoglycosides, the spectrum of kanamycin is limited by the absence of predictable activity against *P. aeruginosa* and the development of resistant Enterobacteriaceae. Equally important are the other bacteria against which the aminoglycosides have no predictable in vitro activity, such as *Streptococcus pneumoniae*, *Stenotrophomonas maltophilia*, *Burkholderia (Pseudomonas) cepacia*, *Bacteroides* spp., *Clostridium* spp., and other anaerobic organisms. Resistance to aminoglycosides is one characteristic used to identify *S. maltophilia* and *B. cepacia* in clinical specimens. There is no clinically significant activity against rickettsiae, fungi, or viruses.

Although the spectrum of activity of streptomycin and kanamycin is limited, the activity spectra of gentamicin, tobramycin, amikacin, and netilmicin are virtually identical. Table 24-4 defines *sensitive* as an in vitro MIC or minimal bactericidal concentration (MBC) that is within the range of blood concentrations achieved clinically with traditional twice- or three-times-daily dosing. Table 24-4 does not indicate relative degrees of in vitro potency. The MIC or MBC of gentamicin against *Serratia* spp. is consistently twofold lower than that of the other aminoglycosides, and the MIC or MBC of tobramycin versus *P. aeruginosa* is also consistently twofold lower than that of the other aminoglycosides. Although tobramycin is more active in animal models of pneumonia, to date no clinical efficacy data have been presented that parallel these in vitro differences.

Aminoglycosides have in vitro activity against *Haemophilus* spp. and *Legionella* spp. but are not used clinically for infections with these organisms. Legionellae are intracellular pathogens, and the intracellular antimicrobic activity of the aminoglycosides is hampered by their concentration in the acidic lysosomal compartment.[60] Nonetheless, aminoglycosides are used successfully in the treatment of other intracellular infections such as brucellosis, chronic forms of bartonellosis, tuberculosis, tularemia, and yersiniosis.[59-61]

Only spectinomycin has been used clinically for infections with *N. gonorrhoeae*.[59] Aminoglycosides in combination with other drugs have been used successfully to treat infections with staphylococci, streptococci, enterococci, *Listeria*, and mycobacteria.

Not shown in Table 24-4 is the activity of the aminoglycoside paromomycin against intestinal parasites. Paromomycin is too toxic for parenteral administration. Because the drug is not absorbed from the intestinal tract, it can be used safely as an alternative therapy for infection by *Entamoeba histolytica*.[59]

As Table 24-4 indicates, many extended-spectrum penicillins (with and without a β-lactamase inhibitor), the monobactam aztreonam, the carbapenems, extended-spectrum cephalosporins, and the fluoroquinolones share with aminoglycosides the virtue of in vitro activity against a wide spectrum of fermentative and some nonfermentative aerobic gram-negative bacilli. Some differences are apparent when other facets of in vitro antimicrobial sensitivity testing are considered.

Aminoglycosides are little influenced by the size of the test inoculum of bacteria; the MIC for 90% of test strains (MIC_{90}) is unchanged whether the initial inoculum is 10^5 or 10^7 bacteria per milliliter.[18] In contrast, an increase in test inoculum often results in a substantive increase in the MIC_{90} of extended-spectrum penicillins or cephalosporins. Depending on the method used, the percentage of aminoglycoside that is protein bound ranges between 0 and 30 and is considered inconsequential.[62] The higher the cation content of the test medium, the higher the MIC-MBC results versus *P. aeruginosa* and, to a lesser degree, other gram-negative bacilli. Early in the evaluation of gentamicin it was recognized that the Ca^{2+}, Mg^{2+}, and to a lesser extent sodium concentrations of standard agar culture media varied widely from lot to lot.[63] Broth medium has very low concentrations of Ca^{2+} and Mg^{2+}. Subsequently, broth culture media have been standardized as Mueller-Hinton broth supplemented with physiologic concentrations of calcium (50 mg/L) and magnesium (25 mg/L).[64] Because netilmicin activity against *P. aeruginosa* is more influenced by the medium cation concentration than the activity of other aminoglycosides, some authors recommend separate media with lower cation supplementation for netilmicin MIC testing.[65] No similar standards have been set for the cation content of test agar.[66] Some laboratories incorporate *p*-nitrophenylglycerol into agar susceptibility test media to prevent swarming of *Proteus* organisms. *p*-Nitrophenylglycerol is reported to increase the MIC of aminoglycosides against strains of *P. aeruginosa*.[67] An alkaline medium yields an erroneously low MIC, whereas an acid medium yields an erroneously high MIC.[18]

Urine is known to inhibit the activity of aminoglycosides against urinary tract pathogens. Inhibition is believed to result from the low pH and high osmolality caused by the high salt and glucose concentrations. In addition, present data support the hypothesis that betaines, normally found in urine, permit the expression of increased aminoglycoside resistance.[68] To date, betaine concentrations have not been standardized in test media.

The other drugs listed in Table 24-4 were selected because their spectrum includes activity against aerobic gram-negative bacilli. Note the absence of activity of ampicillin-sulbactam, ceftriaxone, kanamycin, and trimethoprim-sulfamethoxazole against *P. aeruginosa*.

Time Course of In Vitro Antimicrobial Activity

"Time-kill" curves are not practical for routine susceptibility testing but do illustrate three facets of aminoglycoside antibacterial activity: concentration-dependent killing, the presence of a postantibiotic effect (PAE), and synergism with other drugs.[69]

TABLE 24-4 Comparison of the "Usual" In Vitro Spectrum of Activity of Aminoglycosides with Other Classes of Antimicrobial Agents against Selected Microorganisms

Organism	Aminoglycosides							ESP	
	Streptomycin	Kanamycin	Gentamicin	Tobramycin	Amikacin	Netilmicin	Spectinomycin	Ticarcillin	Piperacillin
Gram-Negative									
Escherichia coli		+	+	+	+	+	0	+	+
Proteus mirabilis	+	+	+	+	+	+	0	+	+
Klebsiella sp.	+	+	+	+	+	+	0	0	+
Enterobacter sp.	0	+	+	+	+	+	0	±	+
Morganella sp.	+	+	+	+	+	+	0	+	+
Citrobacter sp.		+	+	+	+	+	0	+	+
Serratia sp.	+	+	+	+	+	+	0	+	0
Salmonella sp.								+	+
Providencia sp.		+	+	+	+	+	0	+	+
Aeromonas sp.		+	+	+	+	+	0		+
Acinetobacter sp.			0	±	0			0	0
Pseudomonas aeruginosa	0	+	+	+	+	+	0	+	+
Burkholderia cepacia	0	0	0	0	0	0	0	0	
Stenotrophomonas maltophilia	0	0	0	0	0	0	0		0
Neisseria gonorrhoeae	0	0	0	0	0	0	+	+	+
Haemophilus influenzae	+	+	+	+	+	+	0	0	±
Yersinia pestis	+		+						
Francisella tularensis	+	+	+						
Gram-Positive									
Streptococcus pneumoniae	0	0	0	0	0	0	0	+	+
Staphylococcus aureus (MSSA)	+	+	+	+	+	+	0	0	0
Staphylococcus aureus (MRSA)	0	0	0	0	0	0	0	0	0
Miscellaneous									
Mycobacterium tuberculosis	+	0	0	0	+	0	0	0	0
Mycobacterium avium-intracellulare	0	0	0	0	+	0	0		0
Bacteroides fragilis	0	0	0	0	0	0	0	0	0

+ , Sensitive (relative degrees of sensitivity are not indicated); ±, variable; 0, resistant; blank, data not available; Amp/Sulb, ampicillin-sulbactam; ESC, representative extended-spectrum cephalosporins; ESP, representative extended-spectrum penicillins; FQ, fluoroquinolones; MRSA, methicillin-resistant S. *aureus;* MSSA, methicillin-sensitive S. *aureus;* Piper/Tazo, piperacillin-tazobactam; Ticar/Clav, ticarcillin-clavulanate; TMP/SMX, trimethoprim-sulfamethoxazole.

Adapted from Gilbert DN, Moellering RC, Sande MA. Sanford Guide to Antimicrobial Therapy. 34th ed. Hyde Park, Vt: Antimicrobial Therapy, Inc; 2004.

Aminoglycosides are rapidly bactericidal, and their rate of bacterial killing increases as the antibiotic concentration is increased regardless of the inoculum.[70] Standard in vitro test systems have a static drug concentration. In vitro kinetic models allow fluctuations in drug concentration that mimic in vivo pharmacokinetics. For netilmicin and amikacin in the latter model, exposure of test bacteria to the 24-hour aminoglycoside dose as a single bolus with the associated high peak drug concentration resulted in faster killing and a larger magnitude of bactericidal activity than exposure to the same total dose administered in smaller increments at regular intervals.[71] In years past, high concentrations of aminoglycosides were avoided because of concern about toxicity. Now, transient high concentrations are considered a virtue and serve as a part of the rationale for once-daily dosing of aminoglycosides. Of interest, β-lactams do not exhibit concentration-dependent killing; bactericidal activity depends on maintaining drug concentrations at or above the target organism's MIC.[72,73]

Postantibiotic Effect

The PAE is persistent suppression of bacterial growth after short antimicrobial exposure.[74] PAE can be measured in vitro or in animal models of infection. In vitro, the aminoglycosides consistently demonstrate a PAE that varies from 1 to 3 hours in broth and serum for *P. aeruginosa* and from 0.9 to 2.0 hours for other Enterobacteriaceae.[75] An aminoglycoside PAE can be demonstrated after incubation with *S. aureus* but not after contact with *S. pneumoniae*.[73,74] The higher the aminoglycoside concentration, the longer the PAE. The smaller the inoculum and the higher the oxygen tension, the longer the PAE.[74-76] The lower the pH of the test medium, the shorter the PAE.[74] For the aerobic or facultative gram-negative rods tested, the combination of a β-lactam and an aminoglycoside resulted in a PAE of the aminoglycoside.[74] An exception is imipenem; imipenem plus tobramycin or gentamicin enhanced the PAE of the aminoglycoside alone.[77] Rifampin was associated with synergistic enhancement of the PAE induced in *P. aeruginosa* by tobramycin.[75]

An aminoglycoside-induced PAE is the second part of the rationale for once-daily dosing of aminoglycosides. The last part is an attenuated risk of toxicity, as discussed later. In contrast, β-lactam antibiotics, other than the carbapenems, have not demonstrated a PAE against aerobic and facultative gram-negative bacilli.[72-76]

In vitro, the tobramycin-induced PAE against *E. coli* correlated with inhibition of protein synthesis but not DNA or RNA synthesis.[78]

Antimicrobial Synergy

The synergy between an aminoglycoside and a cell wall–active antimicrobial (e.g., penicillin, cephalosporin, monobactam, carbapenem, glycopeptide) is a desirable interaction.[69-79] The effect of the drugs in combination is greater than the anticipated results based on the effect of each individual drug. In short, the effect is more than additive.

Several laboratory procedures are used to study drug combinations for evidence of synergism. Although cumbersome and labor intensive, only the time-kill curve (or killing curve) method detects and quantifies bactericidal activity. The following comments and the data summarized in Table 24-5 are based on results from time-kill curves.[69] A great many additional studies describe synergism by using "checkerboard" or other techniques that indicate bacteriostatic activity as an end point and are hence excluded from the table.

ESP			Monobactam	ESC		Carbapenems		FQ		
Amp/Sulb	Ticar/Clav	Piper/Tazo	Aztreonam	Ceftriaxone	Ceftazidime	Imipenem	Meropenem	Levofloxacin	Ciprofloxacin	TMP/SMX
+	+	+	+	+	+	+	+	+	+	+
+	+	+	+	+	+	+	+	+	+	+
+	+	+	+	+	+	+	+	+	+	+
+	+	+	+	+	+	+	+	+	+	+
+	+	+	+	+	+	+	+	+	+	+
+	+	+	+	+	+	+	+	+	+	+
+	+	+	+	+	+	+	+	+	+	
+	+	+	+	+	+	+	+	+	+	
	+	+	+		+	+	+	+	+	
±	+	+	0	+	+	+	+	+	+	0
0	+	+	+	0	+	+	+	+	+	0
0		+	0	+	+	+	+	0	0	+
0		+	0	0	0	0	0	0	0	+
+	+	+	+	+	+	+	+	+	+	
+	+	+	+	+	+	+	+	+	+	
+	+	+	0	+	+	+	+	+	±	+
+	+	+	0	+	0	+	+	+	+	+
0	0	0	0	0	0	0	0	0	0	0
0	0	0	0	0	0	0	0	0	0	0
0	0	0	0	0	0	+	0	+	0	0
+	+	+	0	0	0	+	+	0	0	0

The mechanism of aminoglycoside synergistic activity may not be the same for all target organisms. Study of the enterococcus indicates that intracellular accumulation of labeled streptomycin is significantly enhanced in the presence of penicillin or other cell wall–active drugs (e.g., bacitracin, vancomycin).[69] Similar enhanced aminoglycoside uptake in the presence of a cell wall–active drug has been demonstrated with viridans streptococci, *S. aureus*, and *P. aeruginosa*.[69]

The enterococci have been studied extensively since the original description of penicillin-streptomycin synergy in 1947.[80] Subsequently, the concept was extended to viridans streptococci and group B streptococci. Note that no combination of aminoglycoside and cell wall–active drug is indicated as effective for methicillin-resistant *S. aureus*. Some laboratories have reported synergy between cephalothin and kanamycin and between high concentrations of either oxacillin or cephalothin and gentamicin.[69] Unfortunately, the latter regimens have not proved useful clinically.

Many time-kill curve studies have documented synergism against *P. aeruginosa* and Enterobacteriaceae.[69,79] Because of the rapid bactericidal activity of high aminoglycoside concentrations, low to moderate aminoglycoside concentrations are used to detect synergistic activity. The clinical inference might be that lower doses of aminoglycoside could be effectively combined with the cell wall–active drug; from the opposite perspective, higher doses are desirable to maximize the concentration-dependent bactericidal activity of aminoglycosides.

Of equal import, the bactericidal activity of aminoglycosides can be antagonized by bacteriostatic agents such as chloramphenicol and tetracycline.[69] The mechanism is unclear. Postulates include inhibition of the energy-dependent uptake of aminoglycosides and interference with movement of the ribosome along mRNA.

ANTIBACTERIAL EFFICACY IN ANIMAL MODELS OF INFECTION

Historical Perspective

An idealistic goal is an animal model that mimics human infection so that the efficacy of aminoglycoside therapy, alone or in combination, can be maximized while simultaneously minimizing the risk of toxicity.[81] In a critical review of the literature published through 1980, the use of aminoglycosides alone was not found very effective in animal models of pyelonephritis, osteomyelitis, endocarditis, peritonitis, and meningitis.[82] Aminoglycosides were more effective in experimental models of pneumonia.[82] In retrospect, the studies reviewed did not consider the influence of dosing regimens, the pretreatment interval, and combination therapy with drugs that have different targets of activity.

Aminoglycosides Alone

Several infection models have been used to study the influence of aminoglycoside pharmacokinetics on drug efficacy.[72,74] In the infected mouse thigh model, successful outcome of treatment of aerobic gram-negative rod infection correlated with the presence of granulocytes and with the peak serum aminoglycoside concentration.[72,74,75]

The growth of *P. aeruginosa* in thigh muscle increases rapidly in neutropenic mice as opposed to a plateau number of organisms in non-neutropenic animals.[83] Gentamicin therapy results in a rapid and continuing response in normal mice, whereas neutropenic mice display an

TABLE 24-5 Selected Examples of In Vitro Synergism of an Aminoglycoside Combined with a Cell Wall–Active Antimicrobial*

Organism	Aminoglycoside(s)	Cell Wall–Active Drug(s)
Enterococci	Streptomycin, kanamycin, gentamicin, tobramycin, netilmicin, sisomicin, amikacin	Penicillin, ampicillin, nafcillin, vancomycin
Viridans streptococci	Streptomycin	Penicillin
Streptococcus pyogenes	Gentamicin	Penicillin, ampicillin
Staphylococcus aureus, MSSA	Kanamycin, gentamicin, tobramycin, netilmicin, sisomicin	Nafcillin, oxacillin, cephalothin, vancomycin
Staphylococcus aureus, MRSA		Teicoplanin (+ rifampin)
Staphylococcus epidermidis, MSSE	Gentamicin, tobramycin	Vancomycin (+ rifampin)
Staphylococcus epidermidis, MRSE		
Entero-bacteriaceae	Gentamicin, tobramycin, amikacin	Piperacillin, cephalothin, cefoxitin, cefotaxime
Pseudomonas aeruginosa	Gentamicin, tobramycin, amikacin, netilmicin, sisomicin	Antipseudomonal penicillins,† aztreonam, ceftazidime, imipenem
Listeria monocytogenes	Streptomycin, gentamicin	Penicillin, ampicillin, imipenem
Corynebacteria JK	Gentamicin, tobramycin	Vancomycin, teicoplanin

*Inclusion required killing curve data demonstrating bactericidal activity.

†Includes ticarcillin, mezlocillin, azlocillin, piperacillin.

MRSA, methicillin resistant *S. aureus*; MRSE, methicillin resistant *S. epidermidis*; MSSA, methicillin sensitive *S. aureus*; MSSE, methicillin sensitive *S. epidermidis*.

Modified from Eliopoulos GM, Moellering RC. Antimicrobial combinations. In: Lorian V, ed. Antibiotics in Laboratory Medicine. 4th ed. Baltimore: Williams & Wilkins; 1996:330-383.

initial response followed by, despite continued gentamicin therapy, regrowth with organisms resistant to gentamicin. Overgrowth of these small colonies of resistant mutants is prevented by concomitant administration of an active antipseudomonal penicillin (e.g., ticarcillin).

In the neutropenic thigh model, the therapeutic efficacy of aminoglycosides correlated with the peak serum concentration and the area under the concentration curve over time.[84] Because the half-life of aminoglycosides in small animals is short (less than 1 hour), it is possible to separate the influence of the peak serum concentration from the area under the curve.[72] The short drug half-life also predicts a long interval of sub-MIC serum levels, implying an in vivo PAE.

The in vivo PAE of aminoglycosides has been studied in at least five animal models.[74,85,86] In a study of the neutropenic mouse thigh infected with 15 clinical isolates of Enterobacteriaceae, the in vivo PAE after gentamicin therapy varied from 1.4 to 6.9 hours. In the same model infected with *P. aeruginosa*, increasing the dose of tobramycin fivefold increased the PAE from 2.2 to 7.3 hours.[85] The in vivo PAE is prolonged further in non-neutropenic animals. In experimental thigh infections with *Klebsiella pneumoniae* treated with an aminoglycoside, the PAE ranged from 2.6 hours in granulocytopenic animals to 12.8 hours in non-neutropenic mice.[79] The PAE is more prolonged in renally impaired neutropenic animals than in neutropenic mice with normal renal function.[86] Guinea pigs with *P. aeruginosa* pneumonia were treated with once-daily tobramycin.[87] Although drug levels were not directly measured, on the basis of assumed serum levels and quantitation of lung bacteria, the PAE is estimated as 12 or more hours. Animal models are influenced by other factors as well. In a model of *K. pneumoniae* empyema in rabbits, gentamicin alone effected a

cure rate of 60%.[88] The cure rate increased to 100% in a shorter time when animals were maintained in a hyperbaric oxygen chamber.[88] The time between experimental infection and treatment had a major influence. In both normal and granulocytopenic mice, a pretreatment interval of 6 or more hours abolished the bactericidal activity of gentamicin against *P. aeruginosa* in the thigh.[89]

In short, current animal data on the efficacy of aminoglycosides alone support the administration of large, appropriately spaced doses rather than frequent small doses. In neutropenic animals, concomitant administration of an active β-lactam antibiotic was necessary to avoid selection of resistant mutants.

Combination Therapy

The organisms in which in vitro synergy can be demonstrated between an aminoglycoside and a cell wall–active antimicrobial are summarized in Table 24-5.[69] Many of the same combinations have been evaluated in animal models of endocarditis, meningitis, pneumonia, peritonitis-bacteremia, pyelonephritis, osteomyelitis, myositis (mouse thigh), subcutaneous infection with and without a foreign body, and more.[69,82,90-93] The results can be reviewed by the organ or tissue infected[75] (e.g., endocarditis) or by the etiologic organism.[90] The latter approach is summarized in Table 24-6. In general, when the etiologic organism is susceptible to both the aminoglycoside and the companion drug, antibacterial activity is enhanced. Note the lack of synergy of amikacin plus pefloxacin (a fluorinated quinolone) in a mouse peritonitis model. Although active against different targets, both classes of drugs have an intracellular target; virtually all studies showing effectiveness of combined therapy used a cell wall–active drug (β-lactam or glycopeptide) with the aminoglycoside.

Import of the Dosing Regimen

For drug-organism combinations without a PAE, evidence is increasing in support of β-lactam dosage regimens that maintain serum levels above the MIC for the infecting organism for the entire dosage interval.[72,73,94] In contrast, the optimal dosing regimen for aminoglycosides depends on the specific microbial target. For experimental enterococcal endocarditis, results are mixed.[95] Some studies reported greater efficacy with multiple daily doses, whereas others were unable to demonstrate a difference in efficacy between a once-daily and a three-times-a-day aminoglycoside in combination with a penicillin. For penicillin-susceptible streptococcal endocarditis, combinations of penicillin and tobramycin were reported to be equally effective regardless of the total daily dose or dosing regimen.[95] The bactericidal activity of penicillin alone is a likely explanation.

For experimental infections with aerobic gram-negative bacilli, a single daily dose of aminoglycoside was reported to be as efficacious as the same total dose divided into multiple administrations.[96,97] The results are consistent with the known concentration-dependent killing and the long in vivo PAE of aminoglycosides. In neutropenic animals, the PAE of aminoglycosides is much shorter. In contrast, an effective blood level of a β-lactam must be continuously present to ensure efficacy.[73,94] Of interest, in the neutropenic murine thigh model, the in vivo PAE was prolonged in animals given combination therapy for infections with *S. aureus*, *E. coli*, *K. pneumoniae*, and *P. aeruginosa* provided that both the aminoglycoside and the companion drug demonstrated a PAE when used alone.[98]

Prevention of Emergence of Drug Resistance

An aminoglycoside as part of combination therapy may prevent or delay the emergence of bacteria resistant to either the aminoglycoside or the companion drug. In a series of studies, aminoglycosides were shown to reduce but not fully prevent the emergence of quinolone-resistant strains of Enterobacteriaceae or *P. aeruginosa* in a murine model of peritonitis.[99-101]

The concomitant use of an active β-lactam appears to prevent the emergence of gentamicin-resistant subpopulations in neutropenic animals.[83] Another example is the treatment of *P. aeruginosa* soft tissue infection in the neutropenic mouse with carbenicillin or gentamicin

TABLE 24-6 Use of Aminoglycosides as Part of a Combination Therapy against Selected Bacteria in Animal Models of Infection

Organism	Infection (Animal)	Aminoglycoside*	Drug(s) Combined with Aminoglycoside	Results
Enterococcus faecalis	Endocarditis (rat, rabbit)			
Penicillin susceptible		S, G	Penicillin/ampicillin	Combination synergistic
Penicillin resistant		S, G	Vancomycin	Combination synergistic
HLR streptomycin, kanamycin		G	Penicillin/ampicillin	Combination synergistic
HLR gentamicin		S	Penicillin/ampicillin	
Enterococcus faecium				
Penicillin susceptible		G	Penicillin	Combination synergistic
Penicillin resistant		G	Penicillin or vancomycin	Penicillin combination failed; vancomycin effective
Vancomycin resistant, high level		G	Teicoplanin	Combination more effective
Viridans streptococci	Endocarditis (rabbit)	S	Penicillin	Combination synergistic
Staphylococcus aureus	Endocarditis (rabbit)			
MSSA		G	Nafcillin	Combination synergistic
MRSA		None	Vancomycin (+ rifampin)	Combination effective
Staphylococcus epidermidis	Endocarditis (rabbit)			
MRSE		G	Vancomycin (+ rifampin)	Triple combination more effective
MGRSE		N,A	Amoxicillin/clavulanic acid	Triple combination more effective
Enterobacteriaceae	Peritonitis (mouse)			
Variety of organisms		G,T	Ticarcillin, carbenicillin	Enhanced activity of combination
Escherichia coli	Endocarditis (rabbit)	G	Ceftriaxone + sulbactam	Combination effective
Klebsiella pneumoniae	Peritonitis (rat)	A	Imipenem	Enhanced survival with combination
Pseudomonas aeruginosa				
Serratia marcescens				
Klebsiella pneumoniae	Pneumonia (neutropenic mice)	G	Ceftazidime	Modest enhanced efficacy
Pseudomonas aeruginosa	Peritonitis (rat, mouse; neutropenic and non-neutropenic)	G,T	Ticarcillin, carbenicillin	Enhanced activity of combination
	Peritonitis (mouse)	A	Pefloxacin	No benefit of combination
	SQ chamber (rabbit)	A	Azlocillin	Combination more effective
	Infected thigh (neutropenic mice)	N	Azlocillin	Combination more effective
	Osteomyelitis (rabbit)	Sis	Carbenicillin	Combination synergistic
	Pneumonia (guinea pig)	T	Ceftazidime	Enhanced activity of combination
Listeria monocytogenes	Meningitis (rabbit)	G	Ampicillin	Enhanced activity of combination

*A, amikacin; G, gentamicin; N, netilmicin; S, streptomycin; Sis, sisomicin; T, tobramycin.

HLR, high-level resistance; MGRSE, methicillin/gentamicin-resistant *S. epidermidis*; MRSA, methicillin-resistant *S. aureus*; MRSE, methicillin-resistant *S. epidermidis*; MSSA, methicillin-susceptible *S. aureus*.

Data from references 69, 82, 90-93.

plus carbenicillin.[102] In vivo synergism was believed to result from suppression by carbenicillin of the emergence of gentamicin-resistant subpopulations.

EXPERIMENTAL INTRA-ABDOMINAL PERITONITIS OR ABSCESS

Experimental models of intraperitoneal infection differ in that the bacterial inoculum is purposely a polymicrobial mixture of the aerobic and anaerobic flora of the colon. Human or rat pooled colonic content was placed intraperitoneally, and shortly thereafter therapy was initiated.[103] In untreated animals, a two-stage disease developed. In the first few days, 37% of the rats died of acute peritonitis and associated bacteremia; intra-abdominal abscesses developed in all the survivors.[104] The early stage is primarily due to aerobic or facultative gram-negative bacilli; the late stage requires both aerobic and anaerobic gram-negative bacilli. The former includes Enterobacteriaceae and *P. aeruginosa*, whereas the latter is usually due to *Bacteroides fragilis*, especially heavily encapsulated strains.[105]

Treatment of infected animals with gentamicin markedly reduced mortality but had virtually no influence on the incidence of abscess formation.[103-105] Treatment with clindamycin or metronidazole reduced the incidence of abscess formation but had no effect on peritonitis-bacteremia or lethality.[106] Combination therapy reduced both acute mortality and late abscess formation.

The role of enterococci in intra-abdominal infections has been controversial. In the rat model, intraperitoneal implantation of only enterococci and *B. fragilis* resulted in abscess formation.[107] The clinical implications are discussed later.

The efficacy of the aminoglycosides has been surprising. Their activity is significantly reduced at low pH, at low oxygen tension, and in the presence of drug-binding purulent debris.[18,19,108] The latter conditions characterize the murine intra-abdominal infection model, and yet beneficial aminoglycoside activity is demonstrable. The treatment of clinical peritonitis is discussed subsequently.

PHARMACOLOGY

Administration

Aminoglycosides are administered intravenously over a 15- to 30-minute period. If large single daily doses are prescribed, it is reasonable to extend the infusion to 30 to 60 minutes to diminish the theoretical risk of a rapid rise in serum concentration that might precipitate neuromuscular blockade. Aminoglycoside administered intramuscularly is absorbed completely, with maximal serum levels achieved between 30 and 90 minutes.[109] Absorption may be delayed in patients with hypotension and impaired tissue perfusion.

Aminoglycosides are minimally absorbed from the gastrointestinal tract.[110] Nonetheless, instances of deafness have resulted from administration of oral neomycin to patients with hepatic encephalopathy and impaired renal function.[111] Also, increased absorption in the presence of concomitant inflammatory bowel disease is of theoretical concern. In contrast, patients with acquired immunodeficiency syndrome and severe cryptosporidiosis have ingested large amounts of paromomycin over protracted periods without evidence of toxicity. Other exposures may lead to systemic toxicity. Topical application of aminoglycoside on inflamed skin leads to no or minimal absorption. However, patients with extensive burns or other severe dermal injury may absorb drug and be at risk for toxicity.[112] Aminoglycosides can be instilled into either the pleural space or the peritoneal cavity. Absorption is rapid, with resultant serum concentrations proportionate to the concentration of drug instilled. The use of aminoglycosides in abdominal irrigation solutions is not recommended because rapid absorption with subsequent neuromuscular blockade has been reported.[113] In contrast, aminoglycosides have been administered as a bladder irrigant, as an aerosol, and by direct instillation into the lumbar sac or lateral ventricles without evidence of detectable concentrations in the blood.[114-116]

Distribution

As anticipated for drugs with a low level of protein binding (approximately 10%) and a high level of solubility in water, the aminoglycosides are distributed freely in the vascular space and relatively freely in the interstitial spaces of most tissues.[93] The mean aminoglycoside concentration of interstitial fluids approximates the mean plasma concentration as achieved at steady state after repetitive dosing. Interstitial peak concentrations are lower, oscillations between peak and trough levels are less frequent, and the rate of elimination is slower.[117] In the absence of disease or infection, or both, the volume of distribution is 0.2 to 0.3 L/kg.[118] The volume of distribution increases in edematous states including ascites, in patients with burns, in patients with optic fibrosis, and in some severe infections. The volume of distribution decreases in obese individuals.[118] Because of their size, polycationic charge, and lipid insolubility, aminoglycosides cross biologic membranes poorly, with the exception of renal tubular cells and perhaps inner ear cells that appear to have an inherent transport mechanism. The cells of the renal proximal convoluted tubule can concentrate aminoglycosides to levels that exceed those of plasma or interstitial fluid.[119]

Parenteral aminoglycoside administration results in low concentrations of active drug in bronchial secretions.[116] Much higher concentrations can be achieved by administration through aerosol.[120] For success, it is necessary to use an aerosol generator that produces droplets 1 to 3 μm in diameter.

Aminoglycosides traverse the blood–cerebrospinal fluid and blood-brain barriers poorly.[121] Penetration is somewhat better in newborns. Lumbar sac administration yields high local cerebrospinal fluid levels but poor intraventricular levels, whereas intraventricular administration results in high concentrations in both ventricular and spinal fluid.[122,123] Hence, the intraventricular route is recommended for meningitis caused by aerobic gram-negative bacilli in adults in the rare cases in which this therapy is necessary. In the newborn, intraventricular aminoglycoside is no more effective and perhaps more toxic than the drug given intravenously.[124]

Urine concentrations of aminoglycosides exceed peak plasma levels 25- to 100-fold within 1 hour of drug administration.[125,126] Because of renal tubular cell absorption and subsequent release, urine concentrations remain above therapeutic levels for several days after a single dose. After termination of a multiple-dose regimen, urine levels remain above therapeutic levels for days, with a terminal half-life of 48 to 200 hours.[126-128]

Aminoglycosides enter synovial fluid easily, with subsequent levels only slightly less than simultaneous serum concentrations.[129] The biliary tract is poorly penetrated by aminoglycosides, with bile drug levels only 30% of concomitant serum concentrations.[130] The peak concentrations are twice as high with once-daily dosing.[131] Aminoglycoside penetration into the tissues of the eye has been studied intensively.[132] Mean vitreous levels are only about 40% of serum levels over a 12-hour period.[133] In humans, subconjunctival injections yield high aqueous humor levels,[134] but neither systemic nor subconjunctival administration in single doses produces reliable levels in the vitreous humor of humans.[135] Direct intravitreal injection is recommended for the treatment of endophthalmitis.[132]

Metabolism

No evidence of in vivo metabolism of the aminoglycosides has been reported.

Excretion

Of a parenteral dose of aminoglycosides, 99% is excreted unchanged by the kidney. Less than 1% is eliminated in the feces and 1% in saliva.[136] Aminoglycosides undergo glomerular filtration. In animals, approximately 5% binds to the brush border of renal proximal tubular cells and is reabsorbed.[119,137-139] Tubular cell handling of the drug is discussed under "Toxicity." Reabsorbed drug is returned to the tubular lumen and excreted. With normal renal function in adults, more than 90% of an administered dose is recovered in urine unchanged during the first 24 hours.[136,140] The remainder is slowly recycled to the tubular lumen, with a tissue half-life of 30 to 700 hours.[140,141] Drug can be detected in urine for 20 days or longer after discontinuation of therapy.

Pharmacokinetics

All the aminoglycosides have similar pharmacokinetics. The pharmacokinetics occur in three interrelated phases.[142] The first (α or distributive) phase is the result of drug distribution from the vascular to the extravascular space. This phase occurs with a half-life of 15 to 30 minutes.[142] It is suggested that "peak" aminoglycoside serum levels be checked 30 minutes after the end of an intravenous infusion. Because the drug is often infused over a 15- to 30-minute period, it is convenient to request that the serum sample be collected 1 hour after the start of the drug administration.

The second (or β) phase of elimination results from excretion of drug from plasma and the extravascular space. The second phase is determined by the glomerular filtration rate and is hence of greatest import in clinical dosage regimens. In adults and infants older than 6 months with normal renal function, the half-lives of all the aminoglycosides are similar and range from 1.5 to 3.5 hours.[143] The half-life in infants younger than 1 week or in low-birth-weight premature infants can be 8 to 11 hours. The half-life in neonates who weigh more than 2 kg is roughly 5 hours.[144] The half-life is shortened in febrile illnesses and progressively prolonged with any process that decreases renal function. Prolongation of the half-life in elderly people is the result of age-related decrements in renal function.[145]

The third (or γ) phase consists of prolonged and slow elimination of drug that has accumulated in the kidney. The third phase is not considered in dosage calculations. Clinical dosing procedures are presented in later sections.

TOXICITY

With the exception of the aminocyclitol spectinomycin, aminoglycoside antibiotics share the potential for causing injury to the renal proximal convoluted tubules, damage to the cochlea or vestibular apparatus or both, and neuromuscular blockade (Table 24-7). The inherent toxicity and relative toxic potential of the aminoglycosides correlate with their positive electrical charge at physiologic pH.[15]

Also important are untoward effects that are encountered rarely. Hypersensitivity reactions are uncommon, and the aminoglycosides do not provoke inflammation. Hence, phlebitis at intravenous infusion sites is rare; intramuscular injection sites do not become painful; instillation into the pleural space, abdominal cavity, and cerebrospinal fluid causes no irritation; and incorporation of an aminoglycoside into

TABLE 24-7 Estimated Frequency of Serious Clinical Adverse Reactions after Administration of Aminoglycoside Antibiotics*

Adverse Reaction	Estimated Frequency, %
Nephrotoxicity	0-50[211-218]
Ototoxicity	
Cochlear	0-62[234-236]
Vestibular	0-19[234,257,258]
Neuromuscular blockade	Exceedingly rare[113,270]

*See text for explanation of large range.

methyl methacrylate prosthetic joint cement is well tolerated over protracted periods. The aminoglycosides are not hepatotoxic, do not induce photosensitivity, and have no identified adverse influence on hematopoiesis or the coagulation cascade.

Nephrotoxicity

Experimental Nephrotoxicity

Pathogenesis. The precise mechanism or mechanisms of aminoglycoside-induced injury to renal proximal tubular cells remain incompletely understood. Nonetheless, largely on the basis of animal studies, a reasonable postulate is possible (Fig. 24-3). Not shown are as yet unidentified genetic factors. There are major differences in susceptibility to nephrotoxicity between animal species and between inbred strains of a specific animal.[146]

The data support uptake of aminoglycosides by the process of endocytosis.[147] The drugs bind to phospholipids in the apical plasma membrane. However, the phospholipid binding does not explain the localized uptake. Subsequently, the endocytotic receptor megalin was identified.[148]

Megalin and the attached receptor cubilin are very important in the endocytotic uptake of proteins in the renal proximal tubule.[148] A large number of ligands, including aminoglycosides, bind specifically to megalin. The affinity for binding to megalin is higher than that for binding to phospholipids. Further, in megalin receptor knockout mice, there was no renal uptake of aminoglycosides.[149.]

It was proposed that the cationic aminoglycoside binds to the anionic megalin in clathrin-coated pits.[147,150] The aminoglycosides are then transferred to endosomes while the megalin is returned to the apical plasma membrane.

A portion of drug-containing endosomes fuse with lysosomes. The aminoglycosides inhibit lysosomal phospholipases, resulting in lysosomal whorl-like membrane changes that, because of their morphologic appearance, have been termed myeloid bodies.[147] The term cytosegresome is used to describe the same structures. At least a portion of the altered lysosomes (myeloid bodies) are excreted in the urine.

In addition, some of the aminoglycoside-containing endosomes move rapidly to the Golgi apparatus.[151] The time frame correlates with the observed rapid decrease in cellular protein synthesis after aminoglycoside exposure.[152-155]

The aminoglycoside-megalin interaction may ultimately explain a variety of other facets of toxicity. Megalin is involved in many facets of calcium metabolism, such as reabsorption of vitamin D binding protein and calcium.[148-150] Calcium metabolism influences aminoglycoside nephrotoxicity.[156-161] Little is known about the possible role of megalin in ototoxicity. The presence of megalin in the cells of the rat cochlear duct has been reported.[162]

In cells that internalize aminoglycosides, it takes time for cellular necrosis to occur. During this time, a variety of abnormalities are demonstrable.[147] Cellular respiration by mitochondria is disturbed.[156] The tubular cells leak apical brush border enzymes into the urine.[163] Membrane transporter molecules fail to function properly.[164,165] There is decreased reabsorption of calcium and perhaps magnesium from the glomerular filtrate.[157,166] The apoptotic pathway is activated with subsequent necrosis of the cells of the proximal tubules.[167]

FIGURE 24-3. A proposed pathway of the renal handling of aminoglycosides by the kidney.

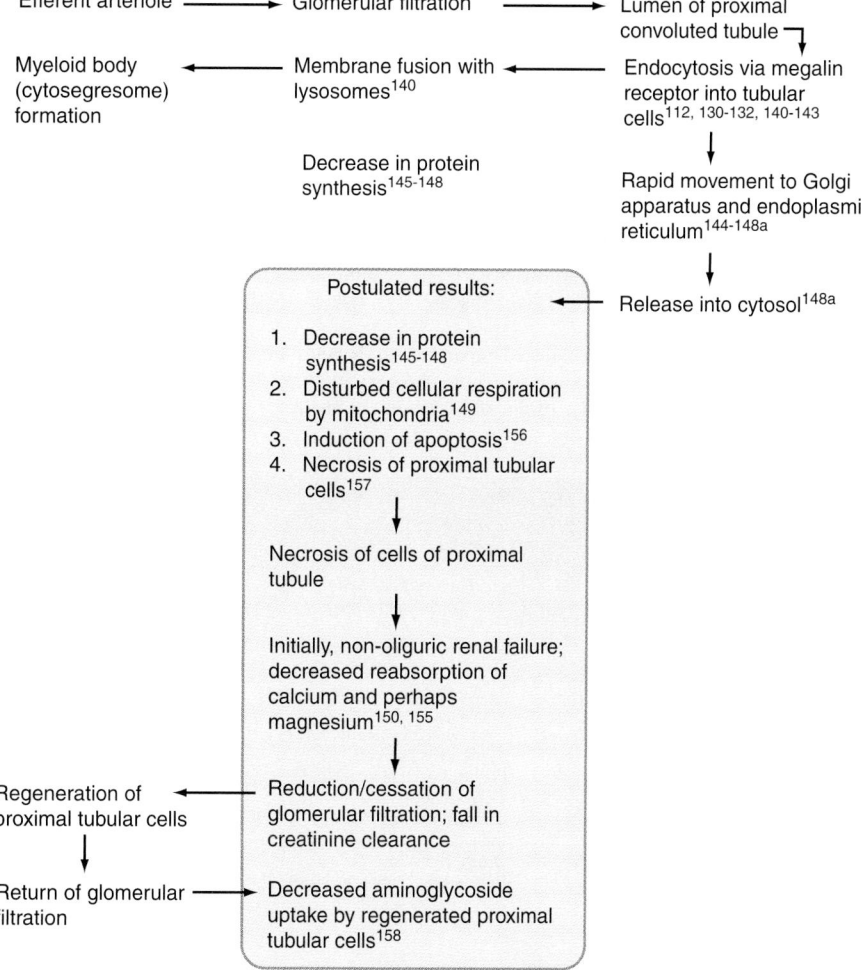

Initially, the animals, as do human patients, manifest nonoliguric renal failure.[168] After several days, there is a fall in glomerular filtration. The cells of the proximal tubule can regenerate with return of glomerular filtration. Of interest, the regeneration occurs even if there is continued administration of the aminoglycoside.[169] In animals, the regenerated tubular cells have a reduced capacity to take up aminoglycosides.

Variables. Animal models, particularly rat models, have been studied to delineate variables that may have clinical import or to elucidate the pathophysiology. Selected examples are summarized in Table 24-8. A hierarchy of nephrotoxic potential exists among the aminoglycosides.[170,171] Neomycin is the most toxic aminoglycoside, and parenteral administration is precluded. Streptomycin is the least nephrotoxic, perhaps because the drug does not accumulate in the renal cortex. The influence of dosage regimens has been tested in multiple types of animals administered a variety of aminoglycosides. For a given total daily dose of a specific drug, the magnitude of toxicity is greatest when the dose is divided into multiple small increments and least when given as a single daily dose.[171,172] Older animals either are more susceptible to injury or have a reduced capacity for cellular regeneration.[174] The enhanced susceptibility of male rats is of interest inasmuch as retrospective analysis of clinical studies suggests an increased susceptibility of human females.[175-177] Depletion of vascular volume, sodium, or both and systemic acidosis worsen renal injury, but volume or salt loading does not prevent or lessen renal injury.[178,179] The influence of an induced alkalosis is unclear; some studies suggest blunting of renal injury, whereas another demonstrated marked kidney calcification.[178,180,181] Potassium depletion worsens and potassium loading attenuates renal injury.[182,183] The mechanism may be related to changes in Na^+,K^+-adenosine triphosphatase activity.[183] A similar mechanism is suggested for the reduced renal injury observed after thyroid administration.[184] Loop diuretics may amplify toxicity through volume depletion, hypokalemia, or acceleration of drug uptake by renal cells.[185]

Dietary calcium loading ameliorates gentamicin-induced acute renal failure and the associated decline in mitochondrial function.[158-160] The mechanism of protection remains unclear.[161]

The influence of experimental liver disease on aminoglycoside nephrotoxicity is also unclear. One report described amplification of drug-induced renal injury by experimental extrahepatic cholestasis.[186] A second study found no influence of experimental cirrhosis on the severity of aminoglycoside nephrotoxicity.[187] The accumulated clinical data indicate that concomitant liver disease is a risk factor for nephrotoxicity.[188]

Animals with streptozotocin-induced experimental diabetes are reported to have attenuated aminoglycoside nephrotoxicity.[189,190] The mechanism and clinical relevance of this observation are unclear.

Various drugs influence the severity of experimental aminoglycoside nephrotoxicity. Vancomycin and the related drug teicoplanin amplify experimental aminoglycoside nephrotoxicity.[191,192] Neither drug alone exhibits a toxic potential. Of interest, vancomycin interacts with the kidney at sites other than the proximal tubular cell.[193] Extended-spectrum penicillins lower the risk of kidney injury.[194] Some data suggest that the protection is the result of the high sodium content of the penicillin salts.[195]

Polymers of aspartic acid dramatically reduce renal tubular injury despite the accumulation of very high renal concentrations of aminoglycoside.[199-209] It is postulated that the anionic polyaspartic acid complexes the cationic aminoglycoside in cytoplasmic vacuoles and thereby precludes movement of aminoglycoside to an intracellular site or sites of toxicity.[208] Despite the dramatic results in animal models, at present little interest has been shown in clinical evaluation of these drugs.

Although differences were noted between species, animal experiments with an aminoglycoside plus cephalothin, cefazolin, or cefamandole indicate either no effect or an attenuation of nephrotoxicity compared with those using an aminoglycoside plus placebo.[210] These results contrast with those of clinical studies suggesting amplification of toxicity with some cephalosporins.

Clinical Nephrotoxicity

The reported incidence of nephrotoxicity varies from 0% to 50%, with most reports in the 5% to 25% range (see Table 24-8).[211-218] The variability results from differences in the definition of nephrotoxicity, the frequency of and the particular tests used to measure renal function, and the clinical setting in which the drugs are administered. The incidence in a small group of healthy young volunteers who received a single daily infusion of tobramycin for 11 days was zero; the incidence in infected older patients with multisystem disease and exposure to other potential nephrotoxins ranged as high as 35% to 50%.[210,211] In prospective randomized studies with definitions of nephrotoxicity that reflect a substantive decrement in the glomerular filtration rate in seriously ill patients, the reported incidence of nephrotoxicity varied between 5% and 10% of patients' courses.[213-218]

In studies of the etiology of acute renal failure, medication-induced renal injury is reported as a major cause. In an analysis of more than 2000 hospitalized patients, almost 100 experienced renal insufficiency, and seven episodes were attributed to aminoglycoside therapy.[219]

In general, the aminoglycoside-induced decrement in the glomerular filtration rate is small. Most patients have a nonoliguric fall in creatinine clearance; progression to dialysis-dependent oliguric-anuric renal failure is rare. As in animal models, the tubular injury is reversible, and in a few patients, recovery of renal function has been documented despite continued administration of the aminoglycoside.[220]

Reported clinical risk factors for aminoglycoside nephrotoxicity are summarized in Table 24-9.[176,177,211,212,221] The factors listed can be grouped as related to the patient, to the aminoglycoside, and to the influence of the selected concomitant drug. Many of the factors identified in clinical trials concur with data from animal models of nephrotoxicity. Female gender was identified as a risk factor in one study but not confirmed in others.[176,211,217,218] In a retrospective analysis, male gender was a risk factor.[216] Reported clinical studies with cephalosporins do not include an aminoglycoside-only group of patients, and hence it is not possible to ascertain whether the cephalosporins had no influence on or increased or decreased the risk of nephrotoxicity. Based on the urinary excretion of tubular cell brush border enzymes, ceftazidime increased the enzymuria seen with gentamicin alone in human volunteers.[219]

The correlation of increased risk of toxicity with age, preexisting renal disease, or both may be misleading. It is unclear whether a risk exists when the dosing regimen is adjusted for a preexisting decrease in the glomerular filtration rate.

Hypotensive patients, especially those with septic shock or sepsis syndrome, have an increased incidence of renal insufficiency. The role of aminoglycosides is unclear in that infection-induced low perfusion pressures, consumptive coagulopathy, cytokine-mediated endothelial

---

TABLE 24-8 Variables Reported to Increase or Decrease the Severity of Experimental Aminoglycoside Nephrotoxicity

Factors That Increase Severity of Injury	Factors That Reduce Severity of Injury
More toxic aminoglycoside	Less toxic aminoglycoside[170,171]
Frequent dosing[172]	Once-daily dosing[172,173]
Old male Fischer rats[174]	Young female Sprague-Dawley rats[175]
Infected, volume sodium-depleted, acidotic rats[178,179]	Uninfected euvolemic, role of alkalosis unclear[178-181]
Hypokalemia[182,183]	Potassium supplements[182,183]
Magnesium depletion	Thyroid hormone[184]
Experimental liver disease[186-188]	Calcium loading[158-161]
Drugs	Induced diabetes mellitus[179,180]
Vancomycin, teicoplanin[191-193]	Drugs
Methoxyflurane[196]	Extended-spectrum penicillins*[194,195]
Cyclosporine[197,198]	Polyaspartic acid[200-209]
Cis-platinum[199]	? Cephalothin[210]

*For example, ticarcillin, piperacillin.

damage, and other factors may be etiologic in the fall in the glomerular filtration rate.

Liver disease was identified as a risk factor in the retrospective analysis of two large clinical trials and was then validated in two additional prospective trials.[188] Further support derives from a retrospective review of aminoglycoside treatment in patients with biliary obstruction, cholangitis, or both.[221]

The significance of recent aminoglycoside therapy is hard to define. In animals, the pattern of injury is cyclic. Administration of more aminoglycoside during the renal saturation phase may increase risk, whereas risk may be decreased if more drug is given when the tubular cells are in a regenerative phase.

Clinical trial data support the concept of a need for several days of therapy to cause nephrotoxicity of clinical consequence. In contrast, accidental massive overdosage of 1 day or less has not resulted in acute tubular necrosis.[222,223]

In the rat model of nephrotoxicity, tobramycin was found to be less nephrotoxic than gentamicin.[171] This hypothesis was tested in a randomized prospective clinical trial. The results indicated a lower incidence of nephrotoxicity in tobramycin recipients, but controversy surrounds the study methods and data interpretation.[214] The results of subsequent trials were mixed. Amikacin and gentamicin were found to be equivalent with respect to the risk of nephrotoxicity.[213] One study reported a lower incidence of renal injury in netilmicin recipients than in patients administered tobramycin.[217]

On the basis of 26 published clinical trials and 8 meta-analyses of those trials, a single daily dose of aminoglycoside appears to be a safe and efficacious treatment method.[221] Single daily dosing does not prevent drug toxicity but may reduce the risk. This subject is amplified later.

The influence of concomitant drugs is difficult to interpret in patients with serious or complex disease states who are receiving multiple pharmaceuticals. Nonetheless, the majority of studies suggest an increased risk of a fall in the glomerular filtration rate when the drugs listed in Table 24-9 are administered concomitantly with aminoglycosides.[176,177,211,212,216] The data are not always conclusive in that many studies suffer from the absence of a matched population of patients given only an aminoglycoside. Three prospective studies, one of which was double blind, found the combination of cephalothin plus aminoglycoside more nephrotoxic than a penicillin derivative plus an

aminoglycoside.[224-226] Subsequent multiple logistic regression risk factor analysis identified a variety of cephalosporins as risk factors. These results are consistent with ceftazidime enhancement of gentamicin enzymuria in healthy volunteers.[219] Two studies evaluated concomitant vancomycin administration; one analysis included a control group that received only an aminoglycoside.[227,228] Both studies indicated that vancomycin was a risk factor. In children, vancomycin was not found to be a risk factor.[229]

In febrile neutropenic patients administered gentamicin or tobramycin plus carbenicillin or ticarcillin, the reported incidence of nephrotoxicity is 2% to 6% compared with 10% to 15% or higher when the aminoglycoside is combined with other β-lactam antibiotics.[224,225] Of interest, a risk factor analysis found an increased risk with concomitant piperacillin but not carbenicillin or ticarcillin.[195] The authors speculated that the lower sodium content of piperacillin may explain the difference.[195]

The identification of some concomitant drugs as risk factors intuitively made sense because a drug may have its own inherent potential kidney toxicity (e.g., amphotericin B), some drugs may act indirectly by altering intravascular volume or electrolyte concentrations (e.g., furosemide), some are of theoretical concern because of their own inherent toxicity potential (e.g., foscarnet, intravenous radiocontrast agents), and some statistically identified risk factors defy explanation at present (e.g., clindamycin). Finally, it should be noted that two drugs that amplify aminoglycoside experimental nephrotoxicity, cyclosporine and cisplatin, do not appear to increase the risk of clinical nephrotoxicity in their clinical application.[197-199,230,231]

If deterioration in renal function occurs, it is advisable to discontinue aminoglycoside therapy. Spontaneous recovery occurs within a few days in the absence of other nephrotoxins, hypotension, renal cortical necrosis of another etiology, or other clinical factors. Progression to anuric renal failure is uncommon. In patients in whom it is inadvisable to discontinue therapy (e.g., those with *P. aeruginosa* endocarditis), the aminoglycoside dosage is adjusted and therapy continued. Recovery of renal function concomitant with continued aminoglycoside therapy has been reported.[220]

Serum Levels and Nephrotoxicity

Note that serum levels are not included as a risk factor, although they are frequently identified as such.[176,177,216] In experimental animals and presumably in patients, the higher the dose of aminoglycoside, the higher the serum levels, the greater the area under the time-concentration curve, and the greater the risk of toxicity. Measurement of peak serum concentrations is indicated to ensure that enough drug was given for antibacterial efficacy and to avoid a large overdosage. Trough levels are measured to ensure adequacy of renal clearance of drug. A high trough concentration is a reflection of impaired renal clearance of drug and indicates a need to adjust the dosage regimen as discussed later.

Ototoxicity

Aminoglycoside antibiotics can cause cochlear and vestibular damage in both experimental animals and humans. Streptomycin-induced hearing loss and dizziness were included in the first clinical report of the drug's efficacy.[233] Ototoxicity is of particular concern because it is usually irreversible and can appear after the end of treatment and repeated exposure engenders cumulative risk.[234] Because the target sites of injury are small and buried in bone, studies dealing with pathophysiology are fewer in number than those addressing nephrotoxicity. A given patient may suffer just cochlear damage or just vestibular damage, or, rarely, both organs are injured. Of interest, it is unusual to have both ototoxicity and nephrotoxicity in the same patient; in addition, it is unusual to have both cochlear and vestibular toxicity in the same patient.

Cochlear Toxicity

Incidence. Few recipients of aminoglycoside therapy complain of hearing loss, and yet the reported incidence is as high as 62% when

TABLE 24-9 Risk Factors for Clinical Aminoglycoside Nephrotoxicity

Factors That Increase Risk of Toxicity	Factors That Decrease Risk of Toxicity
Patient-related factors	Patient-related factors
Older patients	Younger patients
Preexisting renal disease	Normal renal function
Female gender[175]	
Male gender[216]	
Volume depletion, hypotension	Normotensive
Hepatic dysfunction	No hepatic dysfunction
Aminoglycoside factors	Aminoglycoside factors
Recent aminoglycoside therapy	No recent aminoglycoside therapy
Larger doses	Smaller doses
Treatment of 3 or more days	Treatment less than 3 days
Drug choice (e.g., gentamicin)[214]	Drug choice (e.g., tobramycin)[214]
Frequent dosing interval[97,221]	Once-daily dosing[97,221]
Concomitant drugs	Concomitant drugs
Vancomycin[a][227-229]	Extended-spectrum penicillins[224,225]
Amphotericin B	
Furosemide	
Clindamycin	
Piperacillin	
Cephalosporins[219,224-226]	
Methoxyflurane[232]	
Foscarnet	
Intravenous radiocontrast agents	

Data from references 176, 177, 212, 216, and references included in the table.

asymptomatic high-frequency audiograms are performed repeatedly.[235] An overall incidence has been reported as 3% to 14%.[236]

Normal sound perception extends to frequencies of 20 kHz. The outer hair cells in the basal turn of the cochlea are most susceptible to aminoglycoside damage; the basal turn is the site of detection of high-frequency sound.[234] Perception of human speech requires sound detection in the 0.3- to 3-kHz range. Even in the speech frequency range, a loss of hearing threshold of 25 to 30 dB is necessary before the patient is aware of the deficit. Hence, considerable cochlear damage can occur without the patient's recognition. Furthermore, detection is difficult in ill patients with impaired cognition. Finally, many audiometers do not test frequencies above 8 kHz.

Another problem in ascertaining incidence is the absence of a universally accepted definition for drug-induced ototoxicity. A commonly used definition is an increase in auditory threshold of 15 dB or greater at any of two or more frequencies.[234]

Controlled data on cochlear toxicity are sparse. In healthy adult male volunteers administered kanamycin sulfate, cochlear toxicity developed in 17%.[237] In contrast, ototoxicity was reported in 7.4% of infected patients treated with cefotaxime.[212] Also as a comparison, hearing deficits developed in 15 of 27 patients admitted to the hospital without exposure to antimicrobials or other known ototoxins.[238] In a series of prospective clinical studies that examined the efficacy and toxicity of gentamicin, tobramycin, and amikacin in combination with β-lactam antibiotics, 22% of the aminoglycoside recipients had documented audiometric toxicity; all but one patient had hearing loss at 4 or 8 kHz.[239] Frequencies over 8 kHz were not tested. In a different study of 53 subjects administered gentamicin, tobramycin, or amikacin for at least 4 days who were tested at frequencies up to 20 kHz, 33 of the 53 patients suffered either a 20-dB or greater loss at one frequency, a 10-dB or greater loss at two consecutive frequencies, or loss of response at three consecutive frequencies.[235] Of the ears with damage, 62% demonstrated hearing loss initially at or above 9 kHz.[235] Loss was unilateral in 55% and bilateral in 45% of patients. Treatment ranged from 4 to 32 days, and hearing loss was initially detected after a mean of 9 days of therapy.

Pathophysiology. The site of aminoglycoside toxicity is initially the outer hair cells of the organ of Corti.[234,240] The specifics of the interaction are unclear. In experimental animals, aminoglycosides can be detected in inner ear fluid, but the concentration never exceeds serum levels.[240,241] Inner ear tissues are saturated with gentamicin roughly 3 hours after administration, but cochlear damage, as measured by brain stem evoked potentials, requires 3 weeks of daily injections.[240,241]

As in renal proximal tubular cells, lysosomal changes (myeloid bodies) are visible within the hair cells of treated animals. Attempts to study intracellular trafficking are consistent with endocytotic uptake and lysosomal accumulation.[242,243] The glycoprotein megalin is the endocytotic receptor for aminoglycosides in renal proximal tubular cells.[149] Megalin is present in the inner ear, but it is unclear whether it binds aminoglycosides.[148,150]

Mechanism.[244] The precise mechanism of cochlear toxicity has eluded detection. Nonetheless, clues abound, some of which have implication for treatment or prevention, or both.

The aminoglycosides bind strongly to the negatively charged polyphosphoinositides. The degree of binding correlates with the rank order ototoxic potential of the drugs.[244]

There is evidence that cochlear injury results from drug-induced formation of free radicals.[244] Gentamicin can initiate free radical formation by the chelation of iron. In animals, depletion of the antioxidant glutathione in inner ear tissues enhances aminoglycoside toxicity. Gentamicin-induced cochlear toxicity is enhanced by iron supplementation and attenuated by iron chelation and antioxidant therapy. There is, at present, no suitable safe and efficacious antioxidant drug for use in clinical trials. Of interest, salicylate protected guinea pigs against gentamicin-induced hearing loss. Salicylate activity includes free radical scavenging and metal chelation.

A series of studies postulate aminoglycoside-induced overstimulation of the cochlear hair cells at the junction of the cells and the fibers of the eighth cranial nerve. It is hypothesized that aminoglycosides overstimulate N-methyl-D-aspartate receptors, resulting in an overload of cellular calcium and cell death.[245] However, the pathology in other disease processes implicated in excitotoxicity does not match that induced by aminoglycosides.[244]

As in renal tubular cells, there is evidence for aminoglycoside-induced apoptotic cell death in cells of both the organ of Corti and the vestibular apparatus. Apoptosis can be attenuated by neurotropins, growth factors, or inhibitors of the apoptotic cascade.[246] The clinical implications remain theoretical.

Hair cell loss has been considered irreversible. However, animal studies in nonmammals and mammals document potential regeneration.[247-249]

Inherited Risk. The greatest risk may be genetic predisposition.[250] Numerous families are reported wherein deafness developed in multiple members after receiving an aminoglycoside. Likewise, macaque monkeys are resistant to dihydrostreptomycin toxicity and patas monkeys are highly sensitive to cochlear toxicity.

Multiple family pedigrees have been studied. In three Chinese families, a specific mutation was identified in the 12S mitochondrial rRNA. The mitochondrial locus is consistent with a matrilineal pattern of inheritance. The abnormality is an A-to-G substitution at nucleotide position 1555. The same A-to-G substitution has been reported in Japanese families, Mongolian families, and an Israeli-Arab kindred. Forty-one ethnically diverse U.S. patients were studied after aminoglycoside-induced deafness developed; seven (17%) of the patients had the nucleotide 1555 A-to-G mutation. Of clinical import, four of the seven had a family history of aminoglycoside-induced ototoxicity. Overall, 17% to 33% of patients with cochlear toxicity carry the mutation. In addition, a second mitochondrial 12S rRNA mutation has been identified: ΔT961Cn.[251] Commercial testing for the presence of the A1555G mutation is available: www.athenadiagnostics.com. To date, no genetic predisposition to aminoglycoside vestibular or renal toxicity has been identified.

In vitro constructs of normal and mutant 12S rRNA have been reported.[252] The mutant rRNA bound aminoglycosides, whereas the normal construct did not. Of interest, the binding was tighter for the clinically more toxic drugs (paromomycin, neomycin) than for gentamicin and tobramycin.[252]

Other Risk Factors. Risk factors have been assessed in animal models of cochlear injury. Many of the results parallel those observed in the rat model of nephrotoxicity. To wit, toxicity is related to the dose and duration of aminoglycoside therapy.[234] A hierarchy of toxic potential has been established, with neomycin being the most toxic, followed in descending order by gentamicin, tobramycin, amikacin, and netilmicin. Drug structure makes a difference. Streptomycin's potential to cause neurosensory hearing loss is well known. Changing an aldehyde group of streptomycin to an alcohol yields dihydrostreptomycin. Dihydrostreptomycin has little cochlear toxicity but causes damage to the vestibular apparatus.

Concomitant "loop" diuretics, vancomycin, and loud ambient noise increase the risk of toxicity.[234,253-255] Once-daily dosing decreases the risk compared with the same total daily dose administered at frequent intervals or by continuous infusion.[256]

Risk factor analysis of human trials is difficult to assess in that patients were not studied for high-frequency hearing loss and baseline data cannot be obtained with confidence in ill, febrile patients. Nonetheless, retrospective stepwise discriminant analysis of data for 135 patients enrolled in prospective double-blind clinical trials of aminoglycoside therapy identified treatment duration, associated bacteremia, hypovolemia, degree of temperature elevation, and liver dysfunction as risk factors.[257] One group used multivariate analysis and identified only age as a risk factor.[258] With the currently available data, it is difficult to ascertain measurable differences in the risk of cochlear toxicity between gentamicin, tobramycin, amikacin, and netilmicin.[236-259] In one study, netilmicin was found to be less cochleotoxic than tobramycin.[217] The development of renal impairment for whatever reason and failure to lower the aminoglycoside daily dose or to discontinue aminoglycoside therapy result in higher serum levels, greater perilymph drug concentrations, and an increased risk of toxicity.[260]

Clinical Features. Cochlear toxicity may be unilateral or bilateral.[244,260] Injury may occur days to weeks after termination of drug administration. Cochlear injury may be independent of vestibular injury and nephrotoxicity. The cumulative dose and duration of therapy are more important than serum concentrations.

The risk of either cochlear or vestibular toxicity is greater in patients with renal impairment.[260] The use of neomycin, regardless of the route of administration (e.g., oral, intraperitoneal, topical on open wounds, or bladder irrigation), is particularly hazardous.[260]

High-frequency hearing loss can occur with no symptoms. Conversational hearing loss can occur without warning. Some patients complain of tinnitus or a sensation of "fullness in the ears," which may represent early injury.

Vestibular Toxicity

The target of drug toxicity is the type I hair cell of the summit of the ampullary cristae.[261] The true incidence of vestibular toxicity in ill patients is virtually impossible to determine. Because vestibular injury can be compensated by visual and proprioceptive cues, patients can suffer considerable injury before the appearance of symptoms or clinical findings. Suspicion is raised at the bedside by complaints of nausea, vomiting, and true vertigo.[262] Visual blurring with head movement (i.e., oscillopsia) may occur. Symptoms are exacerbated in the dark, when the eyes are closed, with moving or uneven surfaces, or in other situations that block compensatory pathways. Nystagmus may be evident. Systematic surveillance of patients with electronystagmography is seldom performed; in one clinical study using electronystagmographic surveillance, abnormalities were found in 4% to 6% of patients receiving gentamicin or amikacin.[217,218] There are no data that compare, in a controlled fashion, the toxic potential of the commonly prescribed aminoglycosides.

Vestibular injury can be unilateral or bilateral and mild or severe.[262] Functional recovery, even with bilateral damage, is reported to occur in up to 53% of patients 10 days to 9 months after cessation of drug exposure.[262-265] In addition to visual and proprioceptive compensation, recovery may be due to hair cell regeneration as demonstrated in animal models.[266,267] The relevance of the latter to humans is unclear.

Vestibular hair cells are purposely damaged by gentamicin as treatment of Meniere's disease that fails to respond to conservative measures.[268] Injection into the middle ear allows gentamicin to pass through the round window membrane, penetrate the labyrinth, and destroy hair cells. A single injection is reported to effect good control of vertigo in 75% of patients with minimal sensorineural hearing loss.[269]

Prevention

When aminoglycoside therapy is indicated, the risk of ototoxicity can be minimized by as short a duration of therapy as is clinically appropriate and by periodic assessments of renal function to avoid rising serum concentrations. If high-frequency audiometric testing is available, the patient's mental state allows valid responses to auditory stimuli, and a treatment duration of more than 4 days is likely, it seems reasonable to monitor serially the ability of the patient to hear high-frequency sound.

Neuromuscular Blockade

Neuromuscular blockade after aminoglycoside administration is a rare but serious and potentially lethal adverse effect. Neuromuscular blockade has been described in patients administered neomycin, streptomycin, kanamycin, tobramycin, gentamicin, amikacin, or netilmicin.[113,270] In general, blockade has occurred in clinical situations in which a disease state or a concomitant drug interferes with neuromuscular transmission.[270] A rapid rise in serum drug concentrations is also a risk factor.

Clinical manifestations of blockade may include weakness of respiratory musculature, flaccid paralysis, and dilated pupils. Deep tendon reflexes may be absent, hypoactive, or present. Drug exposure may have been a result of intraperitoneal, intravenous, intramuscular, intrapleural, oral, topical, or retroperitoneal administration.[113,270] Both in vitro and in vivo, the greater the positive charge, the greater the propensity to cause blockade; hence, neomycin is the most potent of the aminoglycosides.[271]

The risk of blockade is amplified in patients also administered D-tubocurarine, succinylcholine, or similar agents.[270] Hypomagnesemia, hypocalcemia, and perhaps calcium channel blockers amplify the risk.[272] Patients with infant botulism are at risk.[273] Reports are conflicting regarding the risk in patients with myasthenia gravis.[274,275]

Blockade results from inhibition of the presynaptic release of acetylcholine and blockage of postsynaptic receptor sites of acetylcholine. Aminoglycosides can prevent internalization of calcium into the presynaptic region of the axon.[276] Calcium internalization must occur before acetylcholine release. The drugs also blunt the response of postsynaptic receptors to acetylcholine. Neomycin is more apt to inhibit presynaptic release, whereas streptomycin and netilmicin are the most active drugs at the postsynaptic site.[277,278] The neuromuscular blockade is rapidly reversed by the intravenous administration of calcium gluconate.[279] The response to neostigmine has been variable.

Blockade is preventable by intravenously infusing aminoglycoside over a period of 20 to 30 minutes or more, especially in patients administered large doses once per day. No clear indication is recognized for instillation of high concentrations of aminoglycoside into the peritoneal cavity or pleural space.

CLINICAL INDICATIONS

The clinical indications for aminoglycosides are divided into empirical, specific, and prophylactic categories. Empirical and specific uses are respectively summarized in Tables 24-10 and 24-11.

Empirical Therapy

The aminoglycosides (gentamicin, tobramycin, amikacin) are effective in the empirical treatment of infections suspected to be due to or due to aerobic gram-negative bacilli, including *P. aeruginosa*. Aminoglycosides have in vitro activity against *S. aureus*, but resistant small colony variants appear within 24 hours unless a concomitant antistaphylococcal β-lactam or vancomycin is administered. Activity against *Enterococcus* spp. requires a concomitant active penicillin or vancomycin. It is emphasized that aminoglycosides have no practical activity against pneumococci or anaerobic organisms. For reasons of anticipated spectrum of activity or to achieve an additive or synergistic effect, aminoglycosides are often combined with a β-lactam antibiotic, vancomycin, or a drug active against anaerobic bacteria. Except for selected mycobacterial infections, there is no reason to combine an aminoglycoside with a fluoroquinolone.

Other classes of antimicrobials, alone or in combination, may be equally efficacious in the empirical treatment of the infections listed in Table 24-10. Examples include the antipseudomonal penicillins (e.g., piperacillin), a penicillin combined with a β-lactamase inhibitor (e.g., ampicillin-sulbactam, ticarcillin–clavulanic acid, piperacillin-tazobactam), the extended-spectrum cephalosporins (e.g., ceftriaxone, ceftazidime), a carbapenem (e.g., imipenem-cilastatin, meropenem), or the fluorinated quinolones (e.g., ciprofloxacin, trovafloxacin).

The efficacy of empirical aminoglycoside therapy is documented in published symposia describing the results of clinical trials that served as the basis for licensure as well as in subsequent trials that compared one aminoglycoside with another or with a β-lactam.[213,214,217,293-297] In febrile neutropenic patients, a high failure rate was experienced after monotherapy with an aminoglycoside, and hence the aminoglycosides are administered in combination with a β-lactam antibiotic active against aerobic gram-negative bacilli.[283] To avoid the toxic potential of the aminoglycosides, a fluoroquinolone active against aerobic gram-negative bacilli,

TABLE 24-10 Examples of Empirical Indications for Aminoglycosides

Type of Infection	Examples; Other Pertinent Chapters	Initial Use in Combination with Other Antimicrobials
Bacteremia, possible	Fever without obvious source; Chapter 48	Yes
Burn wound	Burn wound infection; Chapter 315	Yes
Endocarditis, infective[281,282]	Streptococcal, enterococcal, staphylococcal; Chapter 74	Yes
Intra-abdominal infections[283,298]	Appendicitis, diverticulitis, cholecystitis, peritonitis; Chapter 67	Yes
Meningitis[59]	Post-trauma, postoperative; Chapter 80	Yes
Neutropenia and fever[284]	Postchemotherapy; Chapter 306	Yes
Ocular[132,135]	Endophthalmitis; Chapter 108	Yes
Osteomyelitis, septic arthritis[59,280,285]	Postoperative or post-trauma; Chapters 90, 91	Yes
Otitis[59,280]	Malignant, external otitis in a diabetic patient; Chapter 53	Yes
Pneumonia[59,280,286]	Nosocomial pneumonia; Chapter 299	Yes
Pyelonephritis[59,280]	Patients with chronic Foley catheter; Chapter 65	Yes
Sexually transmitted disease[287]	Pelvic inflammatory disease; Chapter 104	Yes
Skin, subcutaneous tissue	Infected diabetic foot; Chapter 86	Yes

Data from references 59, 69, 259, 280, and references included in the table.

such as ciprofloxacin or levofloxacin, may be substituted for the aminoglycoside in combination with a β-lactam. Current guidelines suggest, if possible, avoidance of aminoglycosides and, instead, empirical monotherapy with imipenem-cilastatin or ceftazidime.[283]

Current guidelines on the empirical therapy of community-acquired intra-abdominal infection of moderate or high severity do not recommend the combination of an aminoglycoside with metronidazole.[283,298] This judgment is based on both the toxic potential of the aminoglycosides and the availability of equally efficacious regimens. An aminoglycoside with metronidazole is considered a first-choice option in patients with severe health care–associated intra-abdominal infection.[283] The other first-choice option is a carbapenem, such as imipenem-cilastatin or meropenem. Hence, the aminoglycoside regimen is helpful in patients unable to receive a carbapenem. The weight of evidence suggests that the virulence of *Enterococcus* is insufficient to warrant inclusion of an aminoglycoside in empirical therapy.[283,298] An exception may be patients with underlying valvular heart disease.

TABLE 24-11 The Specific Indications for Aminoglycosides and Spectinomycin

Selected Pathogens	Aminoglycoside	Drugs Used in Combination
Aerobic Gram-Negative Bacillus		
Klebsiella spp.[288,289]	A, G, N, T	APP, ESC
Enterobacter aerogenes	A, G, N, T	APP, ESC
Serratia marcescens	G	APP, ESC
Pseudomonas aeruginosa	T	APP, APC
Francisella tularensis[290]	St, G	No
Brucella abortus[291]	G or St	Doxycycline
Yersinia pestis[292]	St, G	No
Vibrio vulnificus[293]	A, G, N, T	Esc
Aerobic Gram-Positive Coccus		
Viridans streptococci	G	Penicillin G
Enterococcus faecalis	G	Penicillin G
Staphylococcus aureus	G	Nafcillin
Staphylococcus epidermidis	G	Vancomycin (+ rifampin)
Neisseria gonorrhoeae	Sp	No
Mycobacterium avium-intracellulare	A	Multiple
Mycobacterium tuberculosis	St	Multiple
Entamoeba histolytica	P	No
Cryptosporidium parvum	P	No

A, amikacin; APC, antipseudomonal cephalosporin; APP, antipseudomonal penicillin; ESC, extended-spectrum cephalosporin; G, gentamicin; N, netilmicin; P, paromomycin; Sp, spectinomycin; St, streptomycin; T, tobramycin.

Data from references 59, 280, and references included in the table.

Specific Therapy

After 1 or 2 days, when the patient is stabilized, the disease process is better understood, and the results of cultures performed on admission are available, it may be possible to increase the specificity of the patient's antimicrobial therapy (see Table 24-11). If *P. aeruginosa* is isolated, an aminoglycoside is often continued with an antipseudomonal penicillin (e.g., piperacillin) or an antipseudomonal cephalosporin (e.g., ceftazidime). If active, a fluoroquinolone could substitute for the aminoglycoside. Occasionally, rifampin may be added to enhance antipseudomonal therapy.[299] Enterobacteriaceae producing extended-spectrum β-lactamases have emerged. *E. coli* and *Klebsiella* species are most often involved. They often carry plasmids that also mediate resistance to aminoglycosides.[289] In a non-neutropenic patient with a urinary tract infection of mild severity, monotherapy with an aminoglycoside may suffice. Because of greater activity in vitro and in animal models, tobramycin is the preferred aminoglycoside for *P. aeruginosa* infection. Because gentamicin displays greater in vitro activity against *Serratia* spp., gentamicin is preferred when *Serratia* is the pathogen. For other aerobic gram-negative bacilli, amikacin, gentamicin, netilmicin, and tobramycin appear to be of equivalent efficacy.

Streptomycin and gentamicin have proved efficacious in the treatment of plague and tularemia, as has gentamicin plus doxycycline in the treatment of brucellosis.[291,292,300] Other aminoglycosides may be effective, but no experience with their use has been reported.

The aminoglycosides are most often used in combination therapy as indicated in Table 24-11. With an increasing armamentarium of drugs of different classes that have predictable activity against aerobic gram-negative bacilli, it is now possible and often advisable to discontinue aminoglycoside therapy after 2 or 3 days. Such a strategy takes advantage of the efficacy of aminoglycosides and, because of the short duration of therapy, minimizes the risk of aminoglycoside toxicity. Initiating empirical therapy with one of the nonaminoglycoside drugs is another treatment strategy. The emergence of resistant Enterobacteriaceae during the first few days of therapy with extended-spectrum cephalosporins is a concern.[301,302] It is theorized that this problem is inoculum dependent and hence less likely to occur after a few days of aminoglycoside or combined therapy including an aminoglycoside.

Prophylaxis

Genitourinary and gastrointestinal surgical procedures place the patient at risk for enterococcal bacteremia. If the patient has underlying valvular heart disease, antimicrobial prophylaxis with the combination of ampicillin and gentamicin is recommended. Vancomycin is substituted for ampicillin in penicillin-allergic patients.

The risk of infection after elective colectomy is reduced by mechanical cleansing of the bowel plus oral administration of neomycin and erythromycin. One gram of each is given three times during the 18 to 24 hours before surgery.

DOSING OF AMINOGLYCOSIDES

The aminoglycosides are licensed for multiple administrations per day to patients with normal renal function, that is, twice a day for streptomycin and amikacin and three times a day for gentamicin, tobramycin, netilmicin, and amikacin. As an alternative, aminoglycosides can be administered once a day. Both methods are described here as they apply to adults. Dosing in the pediatric population and in other selected circumstances is reviewed separately.

Multiple Daily Dosing

Loading Dose

The treatment regimen is divided into an initial (loading) dose and maintenance doses (Table 24-12). The purpose of the initial dose is to achieve rapidly a "therapeutic" peak plasma concentration. The targeted range of peak levels represents a compromise between the efficacy that correlates with higher concentrations and the desirability of excreting potentially toxic drug before the next dose. The indicated trough levels reflect the intent to maintain trough concentrations at or above the MIC for the majority of susceptible aerobic gram-negative bacilli for the entire dosage interval.

Calculation of the loading dose is based on ideal body weight in kilograms as derived from the following formulas:

Females: 45 kg + 2.3 kg per inch of height over 5 feet
Males: 50 kg + 2.3 kg per inch of height over 5 feet

The loading dose is independent of renal function. The peak serum level obtained is dependent on the volume of distribution. Because the volume of distribution is less in adipose tissue than in lean body mass, the initial dose is adjusted in patients with an actual body weight that is more than 30% above ideal weight. The ideal body weight is added to 40% of the excess weight and the total used as a basis for calculating the loading dose: ideal body weight + 0.4 (total body weight − ideal body weight).[118] Adjustment for excess adiposity is particularly important in the "morbidly" obese.[303]

Volume of distribution is increased in patients with severe burns, ascites, other edematous states, and, at least in theory, any disease process that results in a capillary "leak" syndrome. The volume of distribution of aminoglycosides is reported as 0.2 to 0.3 L/kg.[304] Conversely, dehydration or muscle wasting decreases the apparent volume of distribution. The latter conditions vary widely from patient to patient and hour to hour in critically ill patients.[305] Hence, it is recommended that after either the initial dose or the first maintenance dose a "peak" serum drug level be obtained.

A rough estimate of the predicted serum level (micrograms per milliliter) can be calculated from the following formula:

$$\frac{[\text{Dose (mg/kg)}] \times (\text{kg body weight})}{[\text{Volume of distribution (L/kg)}] \times (\text{kg body weight})}$$

The definition of the time of a target peak drug level varies from author to author.[306,307] For the clinician, a precise definition is not necessary. For patients treated intravenously, the loading dose is infused over a 15- to 30-minute period. Ideally, peak serum levels are obtained 30 minutes after the end of the infusion. Such careful timing is often not feasible or practical, and it is acceptable and easier to time the serum collection for 1 hour from the start of the 15- to 30-minute infusion. After intramuscular administration, serum is collected 1 hour later. The ranges of desired peak and trough concentrations are summarized in Table 24-12.

Maintenance Dose

Calculation of the maintenance dosage regimen requires an estimation of renal function inasmuch as aminoglycoside excretion correlates directly with glomerular filtration. Glomerular filtration falls normally with aging and as a result of some disease states. The glomerular filtration rate is reflected by the endogenous creatinine clearance. The endogenous creatinine clearance (C_{cr}) is estimated from the equation of Cockcroft and Gault.[308]

$$C_{cr} = \frac{(140 - \text{age})(\text{weight in kg})}{(\text{Serum creatinine}) \times 72}$$

To adjust for females, the calculated creatinine clearance is multiplied by 0.85.

Disease states that result in significant loss of muscle mass are associated with low serum creatinine values. In such patients, the estimated creatinine clearance formula may seriously overestimate the glomerular clearance of aminoglycosides. Thus, it is suggested that the minimum serum creatinine concentration used in the formula just presented be 0.8 μg/mL.[309] Not as widely used is an alternative method of estimating the glomerular filtration rate based on the serum creatinine, age, sex, race, blood urea nitrogen, and serum albumin.[310]

Normal Renal Function. Suggested loading doses, maintenance doses, and desirable serum concentrations in patients with an estimated creatinine clearance above 90 mL/minute are summarized in Table 24-12.[59,304,306,307] It is desirable to measure peak and trough serum aminoglycoside levels after the first or second maintenance dose and adjust the maintenance dosage accordingly. Subsequently, serum creatinine should be measured every 3 to 5 days. If the creatinine level is stable, it is not necessary to repeat serum aminoglycoside measurements. If renal function changes, the dosage is recalculated, and serum levels are repeated after initiation of the new regimen.

Peak serum aminoglycoside levels are obtained to ensure that enough drug was administered for therapeutic efficacy. Data from infected animals and analysis of clinical trial data support the correlation between high peak levels and antibacterial efficacy.[87,97,311,312]

Among other risk factors, the larger the total daily dose and the longer the duration of therapy, the greater the risk of renal toxicity and ototoxicity.[176,212,216] Trough levels are a measure of renal function, as is the serum creatinine concentration, and do not predict nephrotoxicity per se. If the dosage calculation is in error and the dosage administered

---

TABLE 24-12 Suggested Loading Doses, Maintenance Doses, and Desirable Serum Concentrations of Aminoglycosides Administered Multiple Times per Day to Adult Patients with an Estimated Creatinine Clearance above 90 mL/min

| Drug* | Loading Dose | Daily Maintenance Dose | | Desired Serum Concentrations (μg/mL) | |
		Total mg/kg	Divided as mg/kg	Peak	Trough
Gentamicin	2	5.1	1.7 q8h	4-10	1-2
Tobramycin	2	5.1	1.7 q8h	4-10	1-2
Netilmicin	2	6	2 q8h	4-10	1-2
Amikacin	7.5	15	7.5 q12h	15-30	5-10
Streptomycin†	7.5	15	7.5 q12h	15-30	5-10

*All drugs, including streptomycin, can be given intramuscularly or intravenously.
†Maximum daily dose, 2.0 g.0 g can be administered 1.0 g IM (or IV) daily for tuberculosis.
Data from references 304-306.

exceeds renal excretory capacity, the overdosage is reflected by a high trough concentration.

Impaired Renal Function. The two general methods of dosage adjustment are either continuation of the same dose and extending the dosage interval or reduction of the dose and continuing the every-8-hour dosage interval for gentamicin-tobramycin and every-12-hour dosage interval for amikacin. Extension of the dosage interval is favored in that higher peak levels are achieved with enhanced bactericidal activity. Suggested intervals are summarized by the degree of renal impairment in Table 24-13.

Alternatively, after a loading dose, the maintenance dose can be decreased while maintaining the standard dosage interval at every 8 to 12 hours.[313,314] The maintenance dose is calculated as follows:

$$(\text{Estimated } C_{Cr}) \times$$

$$\frac{(\text{mg/kg maintenance dose used for } C_{Cr} \text{ over 80 mL/minute})}{(100)}$$

Recall that serum creatinine concentrations below 0.8 mg/dL may overestimate renal clearance of gentamicin.[309]

Dosing of Dialysis Patients. Patients with end-stage renal disease are usually assisted by either hemodialysis or continuous ambulatory peritoneal dialysis. Critically ill patients may require continuous arteriovenous hemofiltration. All three procedures enhance the clearance of aminoglycosides. The suggested amount of supplementation is summarized in Table 24-13. The data in Table 24-13 do not refer to the use of aminoglycosides in the treatment of peritonitis complicating continuous ambulatory peritoneal dialysis; the latter is discussed later.

The supplements suggested for patients undergoing hemodialysis are based on the assumption that roughly two thirds of circulating aminoglycoside is removed per hemodialysis. However, aminoglycoside clearance can vary widely depending on the characteristics of the dialysis membrane, duration of dialysis, patient's blood pressure during dialysis, and other variables. Hence, it is suggested, especially in critically ill patients, that a peak serum aminoglycoside concentration be determined after the postdialysis dose of aminoglycoside.

Continuous arteriovenous hemofiltration (CAVH) is used in the management of critically ill patients with acute renal failure.[315] Depending on variables related to both the patient and the filter, continuous hemofiltration results in the equivalent of a creatinine clearance of 10 to 50 mL/min.[304] The filtered fluid is continuously replaced by administration of parenteral fluid. For patients undergoing continuous ambulatory peritoneal dialysis (CAPD) who have a systemic infection and are receiving an IV dose of aminoglycoside every 2 to 3 days, it is necessary to give small daily IV supplements to replace the drug lost in the dialysate (see footnote, Table 24-13). For patients on hemodialysis, a full dose is given every 48 to 72 hrs and, on the day of

hemodialysis, an additional one-half of the full dose is given, after dialysis, to replace drug that was removed by the dialysis. Because of individual variability, serum levels should be measured. Suggested doses for gentamicin, tobramycin, and amikacin are summarized in Table 24-13.

Individualized Dosing

It remains unclear whether every patient administered an aminoglycoside requires an individual pharmacokinetic evaluation.[316] Individualized dosing is essential in the critically ill patient with altered volume of distribution of drug and changing unstable renal function. At the other extreme is the otherwise healthy patient with normal renal function and no significant comorbid conditions who is expected to receive 3 or fewer days of therapy. The latter patient may not require any serum levels. Many patients are in between these extremes; they are initially unstable and require close attention to serum levels but, when stable, may require only periodic creatinine determinations. It has been difficult to prove that individualized dosing results in greater efficacy or reduced toxicity, or both, when compared with the normogram approach.[317] In practice, serious and critically ill patients have peak or trough serum levels, or both, determined frequently until they are stable.

Once-Daily Administration

Premise

The concept of once-daily aminoglycoside therapy evolved from three separate but related observations.[97-312] First, experimental nephrotoxicity and ototoxicity were less severe in animals administered a daily dose of drug as a single injection as opposed to the same daily dosage administered in two or three divided doses. Animals given a single daily dose accumulated less drug in the renal cortex. The same result was observed in patients who agreed to receive an aminoglycoside before elective nephrectomy. Patients given standard doses every 8 hours had lower renal tissue concentrations of tobramycin, netilmicin, and amikacin than recipients given an equivalent amount of drug by continuous intravenous infusion.[318,319] Second, the aminoglycosides demonstrate a PAE against aerobic gram-negative bacilli both in vitro and in vivo.[76,85,86] The duration of the PAE is greater the higher the peak aminoglycoside concentration. In animals, the duration of the PAE is much longer in intact animals than in animals rendered neutropenic. Finally, once-daily dosing obviates concern about the adaptive resistance phenomenon. During the period of undetectable aminoglycoside at the end of the once-daily dosage interval, the adaptive resistance phenomenon disappeared in vitro, in an animal model of endocarditis, and in the sputum of patients with CF.[320-322] Hence, the serum level of aminoglycoside can fall below the MIC for the pathogenic bacteria without loss of efficacy. Third, antibacterial efficacy of

TABLE 24-13 Multiple Daily Dosing Method: Adjustment of Dosage of Aminoglycoside Antibiotics in Patients with Variable Degrees of Impaired Renal Function by the Method of Prolongation of the Dosage Interval Combined with Dosage Reduction*

Drug	Dose for Normal Renal Function (mg/kg)	Dose Adjustment for Renal Failure (% Decrease in Normal Dose and Increased Dose Interval by Estimated Creatinine Clearance [CrCl], ml/min)			Hemodialysis Patients	CAPD Patients (mg lost/L of dialysate/day)†
		>50-90	10-50	<10		
Gentamicin & Tobraymcin	1.7 mg/kg q8h	60-90% q8-12h	30-70% q12h Use this dose for CAVH‡	20-30% q24-48h	Dose for CrCl <10 & give extra ½ of dose after dialysis	3-4ᵃ
Amikacin	7.5 mg/kg q12h	60-90% q12h	30-70% q12-18h Use this dose for CAVH‡	20-30% q24-48h	Dose for CrCl <10 & give extra ½ dose after dialysis	15-20ᵇ

*Dose recommendations are guidelines. In critically ill patients, serum aminoglycoside levels should be monitored.
†CAPD = Continuous ambulatory peritoneal dialysis. Replace intravenously drug lost in dialysate.
ᵃFor gentamicin and tobramycin: (3-4 mg per liter of dialysate) × (8 L of dialysate/day) = 24-32 mg lost per day. Replace by IV administration.
ᵇFor Amikacin: (15-20 mg per liter of dialysate) × (8 L of dialysate/day) = 120-160 mg lost per day. Replace by IV administration.
‡CAVH = Continuous arteriovenous hemofiltration.

the aminoglycosides is enhanced with high peak drug concentrations.[70,76,312] Thus, once-a-day dosing offers the potential of both reducing the risk of ototoxicity and nephrotoxicity and not sacrificing antibacterial efficacy.

Once-daily therapy proved safe and efficacious in infected animal models. Nephrotoxicity was delayed in onset and less severe in rats with subcutaneous abscesses given once-daily doses than in rats given multiple daily doses.[323] In guinea pigs with pneumonia secondary to *P. aeruginosa*, once-daily dosing was as efficacious as multiple daily doses.[87] In neutropenic animals, once-daily aminoglycoside therapy was less efficacious unless the drug was combined with a β-lactam active against *P. aeruginosa*.[87]

Two small groups of healthy volunteers received a single dose of aminoglycoside. No evidence of nephrotoxicity or ototoxicity was detected.[324,325]

Clinical Trials

There are more than 55 published clinical trials, including 31 prospective randomized trials deemed suitable for 8 published meta-analyses.[326-367] The controlled trials plus experience with large numbers of patients not part of controlled trials include treatment of all the commonly encountered infections and virtually all populations of patients: neonates,[368-370] children,[337,339,354,364,371,372] elderly people,[342,355] febrile neutropenic patients,[328,343,350,355,366] critically ill patients,[329,337,355] and patients with variable levels of renal insufficiency.[335,355,373,366] The overview of the large, published, extensively analyzed experience in patients indicates that once-daily aminoglycoside administration[367]:

1. Is as efficacious as the traditional multiple-dose method (see later for exceptions).
2. May lower but not eliminate the risk of drug-induced nephrotoxicity and ototoxicity.
3. Is simpler, less time consuming, and more cost-effective than multiple-dose regimens.
4. Probably should not be used in patients with enterococcal endocarditis.[312]
5. Needs further study in selected populations of patients, for example, in pregnancy, CF (see later), meningitis caused by aerobic gram-negative bacilli, and osteomyelitis.[373]

6. Does not worsen neuromuscular function even in critically ill ventilated patients. Nonetheless, rapid intravenous infusion should be avoided.[374]

Once-Daily-Dose Regimens

At present, no consensus has been reached regarding the details of a once-daily dosing regimen. The two methods used most often are summarized in Tables 24-14, 24-15, and 24-16 and are discussed in the following sections.

Total Daily Dose—Normal Renal Function. Normal renal function is defined as an estimated creatinine clearance of 80 mL/minute. This calculation may be invalid in patients with reduced muscle mass reflected by a serum creatinine level of 0.5 mg/dL.

One approach uses the sum of the Food and Drug Administration–approved multiple-dose regimens; for example, gentamicin or tobramycin is approved for up to 1.7 mg/kg per dose for three doses per day for a total daily dose of 5.1 mg/kg/day (see Table 24-14).[355,375] For netilmicin the total would be 6.0 mg/kg/day and for amikacin, 15 mg/kg/day (see Table 24-15).[375] The advantage of this method is confidence that the serum level will fall below 1 μg/mL between 12 and 18 hours after the dose and hence lower the risk of nephrotoxicity. The disadvantage is the potential failure to achieve the targeted peak serum concentration (for gentamicin-tobramycin) of 16 to 24 μg/mL because of an increased volume of drug distribution as encountered in patients with edematous states (e.g., congestive heart failure, ascites) or "leaky" capillaries as a result of bacteremia. In one clinical study that included a high percentage of critically ill patients, the peak serum gentamicin concentration after the first dose of 5.1 mg/kg was below 16 μg/mL in 48% of the patients.[355] Hence, in critically ill patients, it is reasonable to give an initial dose of 7.0 mg/kg.

A second method increases the daily dose of gentamicin or tobramycin to 7 mg/kg/day to increase the average peak serum concentration and hence further facilitate concentration-dependent bactericidal activity (see Table 24-16).[365,366] The higher dose has a clear advantage in patients with an increased volume of drug distribution, and neuromuscular blockade has not been reported. No controlled studies have compared 5 versus 7 mg/kg/day of gentamicin or tobramycin, but clinical experience with the 7 mg/kg/day dosage is substantial.[365,366] With the exception of patients with CF, the clinical use

---

TABLE 24-14 Suggested Once-Daily Dosage Regimens of Gentamicin and Tobramycin in Patients with Estimated Creatinine Clearance between 20 and 100 mg/min and Every-Other-Day Regimens for Creatinine Clearance below 20 mL/min*

Estimated CrCl† (mL/min)	Dosage Interval (hr)	Dose (mg/kg)	T₁/₂ (hr)	Estimated Serum Level (μg/mL) at			
				1 hr	*12 hr*	*18 hr*	*24 hr*
100	24	5 (7)‡	2.5	20 (28)	1.0 (1.4)	<1	<1
90	24	5 (7)	3.1	20 (28)	2.0 (2.3)	<1	<1
80	24	5 (7)	3.4	20 (28)	2.5 (2.9)	<1	<1
70	24	4 (5.5)	3.9	16	2.0	<1	<1
60	24	4 (5.5)	4.5	16	3.0	1.5	<1
50	24	3.5 (5.0)	5.3	14	3.5	1.0	<1
40	24	2.5 (3.5)	6.5	10	3.0	1.5	<1
30	24	2.5 (3.5)	8.4	10	4.0	2.5	1.5
				1 hr	*24 hr*	*36 hr*	*48 hr*
20	48	4.0 (5.5)	11.9	16	4.0	2.0	1.0
10	48	3.0 (4.0)	20.4	12	5.0	3.0	2.0
0§ (hemodialysis)	48	2.0 (4.0)	69.3	8	7.0	6.0	5.0

*Predicted peak and trough serum levels are shown. Peak levels are calculated as follows:

$$\frac{\text{mg/kg administered} \times \text{kg body weight}}{V_D \text{ (L/kg)} \times \text{kg body weight}}$$

Trough levels are calculated from peak concentration and published half-life (T₁/₂) in hours at varying levels of renal function (V_D, volume of distribution).
†The estimated creatinine clearance assumes a minimum serum creatinine of 0.8 mg/dL.
‡Initial 7 mg/kg dose recommended for patients with anticipated increased volume of drug distribution; see the text.
§Example values are for patient receiving hemodialysis every other day. The actual peak depends on the efficiency of dialysis. The dose is given after dialysis.
Data from Gilbert DN, Lee BL, Dworkin RJ, et al. A randomized comparison of the safety and efficacy of once-daily gentamicin or thrice-daily gentamicin in combination with ticarcillin-clavulanate. Am J Med. 1998;105:182-191; and Gilbert DN, Bennett WM. Use of antimicrobial agents in renal failure. Infect Dis Clin North Am. 1989;3:517-531.

TABLE 24-15 Suggested Once-Daily Dosage Regimens of Netilmicin, Amikacin, Kanamycin, and Streptomycin in Patients with Estimated Creatinine Clearance between 20 and 90 mL/min and Every-Other-Day Regimen for Creatinine Clearance below 20 mg/min[*]

Estimated CrCl[†] (mL/min)	Dosage Interval (hr)	Dose (mg/kg)	$T_{1/2}$ (hr)	Estimated Serum Level (μg/mL) at			
				1 hr	12 hr	18 hr	24 hr
Netilmicin							
90	24	6.5	3.1	26	2	<1	<1
70	24	5.0	3.9	20	2.5	1.0	<1
50	24	4.0	5.3	16	4	1	<1
30	24	2.0	8.4	8	3	2	1
				1 hr	*24 hr*	*36 hr*	*48 hr*
20	48	3.0	11.9	13	3.0	1.5	0.75
10	48	2.5	20.4	10	4.0	3	2
0[‡] (hemodialysis)	48	2.0	69.3	8	7.0	6	5
Amikacin, kanamycin, streptomycin				*1 hr*	*12 hr*	*18 hr*	*24 hr*
90	24	15	3.1	60	6.0	<1	<1
70	24	12	3.9	48	9.0	2.5	<1
50	24	7.5	5.3	30	7.0	3.5	1.0
30	24	4.0	8.4	20	7.5	5.0	3.0
				1 hr	*24 hr*	*36 hr*	*48 hr*
20	48	7.5	11.9	30	7.5	3.3	1.6
10	48	4.0	20.4	16	12	5.0	3.0
0[‡] (hemodialysis)	48	3.0	69.3	20	16	15	12

[*]Predicted peak and trough serum levels are shown. Peak levels are calculated as follows:

$$\frac{\text{mg/kg administered} \times \text{kg body weight}}{V_D \text{ (L/kg)} \times \text{kg body weight}}$$

Trough levels are calculated from peak concentration and published half-life ($T_{1/2}$) in hours at varying levels of renal function (V_D, volume of distribution).
[†]The estimated creatinine clearance assumes a minimum serum creatinine of 0.8 mg/dL.
[‡]Example values are for a patient receiving hemodialysis every other day. The actual peak depends on the efficiency of dialysis. The dose is given after dialysis.
Data from Gilbert DN, Bennett WM. Use of antimicrobial agents in renal failure. Infect Dis Clin North Am. 1989;3:517-531.

of single doses of amikacin or netilmicin exceeding the licensed total daily dose has not been reported. Neonates and patients with CF have altered aminoglycoside kinetics and are discussed separately. As for multiple daily dosing, the dose calculation is based on ideal body weight with an adjustment for obesity if needed (see earlier).

For emphasis, for critically ill patients, it is recommended that the initial dose of gentamicin or tobramycin be 7 mg/kg, with confirmation of a peak serum level between 16 and 24 μg/mL. Assuming clinical improvement and continued normal renal function, the dose could be decreased to 5.1 mg/kg/day during the first few days of therapy.

Total Daily Dose—Abnormal Renal Function. Dosing in patients with reduced renal function and, hence, decreased drug clearance is unsettled. One method gradually lowers the daily dose in proportion to the fall in creatinine clearance (see Tables 24-14 and 24-15). The dosage interval is maintained at 24 hours for patients with an estimated creatinine clearance between 30 and 80 mL/minute with prolongation to every 48 hours when the creatinine clearance falls below 30 mL/minute. Note that for creatinine clearances of 40 mL/minute or less, the theoretical advantage of once-daily dosing is gone; that is, the peak serum level is 10 μg/mL and drug is detectable in serum throughout the 24-hour dosing interval. This dose reduction method has the advantage of convenient timing of doses and maintaining some time period of no detectable drug in serum for patients with mild to moderate renal impairment.

The second method prolongs the dosage interval without altering the total daily dosage (see Table 24-16).[365,366] The published tables are based on a gentamicin-tobramycin daily dosage of 7 mg/kg. The advantage is achievement of high peak serum levels regardless of the degree of impairment in renal function. One disadvantage is implementation of an every-36-hour dosage interval in patients with an estimated creatinine clearance between 40 and 60 mL/minute. Perhaps more substantive is the longer duration of high aminoglycoside levels and the theoretical concern that the risk of nephrotoxicity and ototoxicity may be increased.

Summary of Once-Daily Dosing Regimens

Subject to data from controlled trials, I prefer a total daily dosage that achieves targeted peak serum concentrations for a given level of renal function. For patients with an expanded volume of distribution, the first few daily doses should be larger, as indicated in Table 24-14. For prolonged treatment in patients with normal renal function, for example, osteomyelitis, 5 mg/kg/day for gentamicin-tobramycin, 6 mg/kg/day for netilmicin, and 15 mg/kg/day for amikacin should be efficacious.

In summary, when renal function is impaired, the total daily dose may be reduced or the dosage interval prolonged. On practical and theoretical grounds, the former method is preferred pending new data.

Serum Level Monitoring with Once-Daily Regimens

It is necessary to obtain serum levels early in a course of therapy. Peak serum levels are obtained to ensure efficacy; trough serum levels are

TABLE 24-16 Alternative Once-Daily Aminoglycoside Dosage Regimen in Adults Based on Constant Dose and Interval Prolongation

Estimated CrCl (mL/min)	Administer 7 mg/kg at time interval (hr) as indicated
≥60	Every 24 hr
40-60	Every 36 hr
20-40	Every 48 hr
	After initial dose, follow blood levels.
<20	Redose when level <1 μg/mL

Data from Nicolau DP, Freeman CD, Bellineau PP, et al. Experience with a once-daily aminoglycoside program administered to 2184 adult patients. Antimicrob Agents Chemother. 1995;39:650-655; and Freeman CD, Nicolau DP, Belliveau PP, et al. Once-daily dosing of aminoglycosides: Review and recommendations for clinical practice. J Antimicrob Chemother. 1997;39:677-686.

obtained to reduce the risk of toxicity. In critically ill patients, a peak level should be obtained after the first dose. The serum is collected 60 minutes after the start of a 30- to 45-minute infusion. Alternatively, serum can be obtained later after infusion and a formula used to back-calculate an idealized peak serum concentration. The distribution time is prolonged with doses of 7 mg/kg and hence peak samples should be obtained no sooner than 30 minutes after the end of the infusion to avoid overestimation of the peak concentration.[375]

The timing of determining trough serum levels has not been standardized. I have found 18 hours after dosing to be convenient; the goal in patients with creatinine clearance values of 70 mL/minute is a trough level of less than 1 μg/mL (undetectable) (see Table 24-14). If the estimated creatinine clearance is between 40 and 60 mL/minute, a reasonable target is a serum level of less than 1 μg/mL 23 to 24 hours after the dose.

Another approach, based on a fixed daily dosage of 7 mg/kg, uses serum drawn between 6 and 14 hours after a dose. The serum level is applied to a nomogram to determine the recommended fixed-dose dosage interval.[365,366]

In patients with stable renal function who require more than 3 days of therapy, additional serum levels are not needed. Instead, it is recommended that serum creatinine levels be measured once or twice per week. A change in creatinine concentration leads to a change in dosage and the need to revalidate serum levels.

Special Circumstances

Children

The pharmacokinetics of aminoglycosides in newborns and infants differ from the pharmacokinetics in adults in at least two ways.[144,376] The renal clearance of aminoglycosides is reduced in newborns with a resultant prolongation of the half-life and need for a reduction in the aminoglycoside dosage.[376] The half-life is even further prolonged in low-birth-weight infants. By 7 days in newborns with normal birth weight, the serum half-life is approaching adult values.

Furthermore, the volume of distribution of aminoglycosides is larger, as a percentage of body weight, in newborns than in adults. This larger volume of distribution compensates, but only in a modest way, for the reduction in renal clearance. Because of the unpredictable pharmacokinetics, particularly in low-birth-weight newborns, it is necessary to obtain peak and trough serum levels.

Multiple-daily-dose regimens for the three most commonly used aminoglycosides are presented in Table 24-17. Note that neither kanamycin nor streptomycin is listed in Table 24-17, the former because of the frequency of resistance among Enterobacteriaceae and the latter because of the risk of ototoxicity. Nonetheless, streptomycin therapy may prove necessary in patients with multidrug-resistant tuberculosis.

There are fewer studies with once-daily dosing in neonates and children. Studies to date include a total of roughly 700 patients.[377] Safety and efficacy appear similar to those with traditional multiple dosing regimens. Most studies have compared traditional dosage with a once-daily dose that is a multiple of the three-times-a-day dosage, for example, 5.1 mg/kg once daily versus 1.7 mg/kg every 8 hours.

One author has proposed a once-daily dosing regimen for neonates and children given gentamicin or tobramycin based on days of life and body weight.[378]

Cystic Fibrosis

Aminoglycosides are of import to patients with CF for two reasons. First, the mechanism of disease in 5% to 10% of CF patients is mutations that stop the process of translating the mRNA of the CF transmembrane conductance regulator (CFTR) protein.[7-9,379] The prevalence of the stop mutation is as high as 85% in CF patients of Ashkenazi Jewish descent. In vitro aminoglycosides allow translation to proceed past the stop codon.[380] Further, gentamicin nose drops given to CF patients with stop mutations resulted in functional CFTR channels.[381] This treatment approach requires further study.

Of immediate clinical import, patients with advanced CF suffer airway colonization with *P. aeruginosa*. As the disease progresses, there is an increase in the frequency of episodes of *P. aeruginosa* tracheobronchitis and pneumonia necessitating treatment with the combination of an antipseudomonal β-lactam antibiotic and an aminoglycoside.[382,383] Reviews of treatment with critical analysis of data are published periodically by CF foundations and the Cochrane Database.[384-386]

The standard therapy for acute exacerbations of chronic endobronchial *P. aeruginosa* consists of intravenous administration of an active β-lactam and an aminoglycoside, chest physiotherapy, and nutrition.[382,383] Combination therapy is reported to decrease the density of *P. aeruginosa* more than monotherapy. The use of an aminoglycoside combination, compared with an active β-lactam alone, prolonged the time between readmissions.[383] Frequent assessments of culture and sensitivity results are necessary to ensure both absence of resistance of *P. aeruginosa* and absence of an aminoglycoside-resistant pathogen, for example, *Burkholderia (Pseudomonas) cepacia.*

Of the aminoglycosides commercially available in the United States, tobramycin is usually one-tube dilution more active than gentamicin or amikacin.

Parenteral Therapy. CF patients demonstrate altered aminoglycoside pharmacokinetics manifest as an increase in glomerular clearance, with a resultant shortened serum half-life, plus an increased volume of distribution.[387,388] The mechanism is unclear. Nevertheless, the altered kinetics result in a need for much larger doses of drug to achieve therapeutic serum levels.

The initial adult and pediatric dosage of tobramycin and gentamicin is 3.3 mg/kg intravenously every 8 hours, assuming normal renal function.[384-387] The adult dosage of amikacin is 45 mg/kg every 12 hours. Targeted peak and trough serum levels are the same in children and adults.

Once-Daily Therapy. The rationale for once-daily aminoglycoside therapy was summarized earlier. The Cochrane Database of Systemic Reviews analyzed 10 studies that compared once-daily with multiple daily doses of aminoglycoside in CF patients.[389] In a total of 175 patients, there was no difference in either measurement of efficacy or the incidence of nephrotoxicity and ototoxicity. The reported studies vary in doses used, clinical end points, and duration of therapy. Caution is necessary because of the small numbers of patients reported.

Toxicity. It is not possible to ascertain the frequency of nephrotoxicity as the data come from trials comparing dosage regimens and anecdotal case reports. The consensus is that the frequency of nephrotoxicity in CF patients is less than that in non-CF patients.[390]

The prevalence of hearing loss after aminoglycosides in young (10 to 18 years old) and adult (18 to 37 years old) CF patients is 17%, which is roughly the same as that in non-CF patients. However, the risk per course of treatment is 2% in CF patients compared with 7.5% in patients without CF.[391] If this is true, it is unclear how CF protects against aminoglycoside cochlear toxicity.

Aerosol Therapy. Aerosol therapy has many advantages: the prospect of higher concentrations of drug in sputum, less systemic exposure to drug, self-administration by the patient at home, and

TABLE 24-17 Multiple Daily Dosing Regimens of Aminoglycosides Based on Postconceptual Age

Aminoglycoside (IV, IM)	Dosage (mg/kg) and Time Interval of Administration Based on Gestational Age plus Weeks of Life			
	≤26	27-34	28-42	≥43
Amikacin	7.5 q24h	7.5 q18h	10 q12h	10 q8h
Gentamicin	2.5 q24h	2.5 q18h	2.5 q12h	2.5 q8h
Tobramycin	2.5 q24h	2.5 q18h	2.5 q12h	2.5 q8h

Data from Hickey SM, McCracken GH Jr. Antibacterial therapeutic agents. In: Feigin RD, Cherry JD, eds. Textbook of Pediatric Infectious Diseases, 4th ed. Philadelphia: WB Saunders; 1998:2614-2649.

improvement in lung function coincident with a reduced burden of *P. aeruginosa*. When compared with placebo, 600 mg of tobramycin in saline delivered by nebulizer three times per day improved pulmonary function and reduced the sputum density of *P. aeruginosa* over a 28-day study period.[392] The dosage recommended by the Food and Drug Administration for both adults and children 6 years of age and older is 300 mg by one of two approved nebulizers twice a day for 28 days.[393] After 28 days, inhaled tobramycin therapy ceases for 28 days and then the cycle repeats. The Cochrane Database analyzed 10 placebo-controlled trials of nebulized antipseudomonal antibiotics that included 758 patients.[394] Despite variations in study design, the patients receiving treatment had a 12% increase in forced expiratory volume in 1 second (95% confidence interval 8.1 to 15.6) and a reduced odds ratio of 0.69 (95% confidence interval 0.5 to 0.96) needing hospitalization. Over time, there was more aminoglycoside-resistant *P. aeruginosa* in the treatment group.

Ten minutes after inhalation, sputum tobramycin concentrations are variable but range up to several thousand micrograms per milliliter. Within 2 hours after the dose, sputum concentrations fall to approximately 14% of the levels found 10 minutes after inhalation.[393]

Absorption into serum is low. The average serum drug concentration 1 hour after inhalation was 1.0 μg/mL with a range of 0.2 to 3.0 μg/mL.[395] Ototoxicity has not been reported, but transient tinnitus occurred in a few individuals during clinical trials. Nephrotoxicity has not been observed. Inhaled therapy is expensive: roughly, more than $2000 for the drug per 28-day cycle plus the expense of the nebulizer.

Infective Endocarditis

A detailed analysis of use of aminoglycosides in the treatment of bacterial endocarditis has been published.[396] The use of aminoglycosides in combination with a β-lactam or vancomycin is of benefit for patients with streptococcal or enterococcal endocarditis. The standard dosage to achieve a synergistic effect is 1 mg/kg intravenously every 8 hours with no benefit from larger doses. For viridans streptococcal endocarditis, thrice-daily and once-daily regimens appear of equal efficacy in animal model studies and in reported clinical trials.

The use of a once-daily regimen in patients with enterococcal endocarditis is more problematic. The animal model data are mixed; there are reports of greater reductions in bacteria within vegetations with thrice-daily regimens compared with once-daily regimens. Other animal model studies could demonstrate no difference. There are no controlled clinical trials. At present, it is suggested that once-daily therapy not be employed for the treatment of enterococcal endocarditis.

Peritonitis during Continuous Ambulatory Peritoneal Dialysis

Aminoglycosides are often used in peritoneal dialysis fluid to treat peritoneal dialysis–associated peritonitis resulting from aminoglycoside-susceptible organisms.[397] This method of drug administration is not recommended for patients with systemic infection. The aminoglycoside is added to the peritoneal dialysis fluid. It may be added in a "therapeutic" concentration to each bag of dialysis fluid, or the aminoglycoside may be added in a higher concentration to only one of the usual four daily exchanges of peritoneal dialysis fluid (Table 24-18). The once-a-day regimen is analogous to once-daily parenteral aminoglycoside therapy.

Spectinomycin and Gonorrhea

Spectinomycin is used exclusively to treat gonococcal infections.[287] It is not effective in the treatment of infections with *Treponema pallidum* or *Chlamydia trachomatis*. The drug does not achieve therapeutic concentrations in saliva and hence does not eliminate pharyngeal gonococci. The drug is neither nephrotoxic nor ototoxic. Spectinomycin is effective in the treatment of uncomplicated urethral, cervical, or disseminated gonorrhea. It is an alternative therapy in patients allergic to penicillin or in patients infected with penicillinase-producing strains of gonococci. For infection of the cervix or urethra, the dose is 2 g given as a single intramuscular injection. For gonococcemia, the suggested dose is 2 g intramuscularly every 12 hours for 3 days. No intravenous form of the drug is available.

TABLE 24-18   Dosage of Aminoglycosides Added to Dialysis Bags to Treat CAPD Peritonitis

Drug	*Intermittent Method:* Dose Added to One Bag/Day (mg/kg)	*Continuous Method:* mg Drug/L of All Bags (mg/L)	
		Loading Dose	*Maintenance Dose*
Amikacin	2	25	12
Gentamicin, netilmicin, tobramycin	0.6	8	4

CAPD, continuous ambulatory peritoneal dialysis.

REFERENCES

1. Wright GD, Berghuis AM, Mobashery S. Aminoglycoside antibiotics. Structures, functions, and resistance. In: Rosen BP, Mobashery S, eds. Resolving the Antibiotic Paradox: Progress in Understanding Drug Resistance and Development of New Antibiotics. New York: Plenum; 1998:27-69.
2. Walter F, Vicens Q, Westhof E. Aminoglycoside-RNA interactions. Curr Opin Chem Biol. 1999;3:694-704.
3. Lynch SR, Recht MI, Puglisi JD. Biochemical and nuclear magnetic resonance studies of aminoglycoside-RNA complexes. Methods Enzymol. 2000;317:240-261.
4. Lynch SR, Puglisi JD. Structural origins of aminoglycoside specificity for prokaryotic ribosomes. J Mol Biol. 2001;306:1037-1058.
5. Ryers DH, Rando RR. Aminoglycoside binding to human and bacterial A-site rRNA decoding region constructs. Bioorg Med Chem. 2001;9:2601-2608.
6. Kaul M, Barbieri CM, Kerrigan JE, et al. Coupling of drug protonation to the specific binding of aminoglycosides to the A site of 16S rRNA: Elucidation of the number of drug amino groups involved and their identities. J Mol Biol. 2003;326:1373-1387.
7. Bedwell DM, Kaerijak A, Benos DJ, et al. Suppression of a CFTR premature stop mutation in a bronchial epithelial cell line. Nat Med. 1997;3:1280-1284.
8. Clancy JP, Bebok Z, Ruiz F, et al. Evidence that systemic gentamicin suppresses premature stop mutations in patients with cystic fibrosis. Am J Respir Crit Care Med. 2001;163:1683-1692.
9. Du M, Jones JR, Lanier J, et al. Aminoglycoside suppression of a premature stop mutation in a Cftr-1-mouse carrying a human CFTR-G542A transgene. J Mol Med. 2002;380:595-604.
10. Howard MT, Shirts BH, Petros LM, et al. Sequence specificity of aminoglycoside-induced stop codon readthrough: Potential implication for treatment of Duchenne muscular dystrophy. Ann Neurol. 2000;48:164-169.
11. Keeling KM, Brooks DA, Hopwood JJ, et al. Gentamicin-mediated suppression of Hurler syndrome stop mutations restores a low level of α-2-iduronidase activity and restores lysosomal glycosaminoglycan accumulation. Hum Mol Genet. 2001;10:291-299.
12. Schulz A, Sangkuhl K, Lennert T, et al. Aminoglycoside pretreatment partially restores the function of truncated V2 vasopressin receptors found in patients with nephrogenic diabetes insipidus. J Clin Endocrinol Metab. 2002;87:5247-5257.
13. Schroeder R, Waldsich C, Wank H. Modulation of RNA function by aminoglycoside antibiotics. EMBO J. 2000;19:1-9.
14. Cho J, Rando RR. Specificity in the binding of aminoglycosides to HIV-RRE RNA. Biochemistry. 1999;38:8548-8554.
15. Berdy J, Aszalos A, Bostian M, et al. CRC Handbook of Antibiotic Compounds, v. 1. Carbohydrate Antibiotics. Boca Raton, Fla: CRC Press; 1980.
16. Weinstein MJ, Wagman GH, Oden EM, et al. Biological activity of the antibiotic components of the gentamicin complex. J Bacteriol. 1967;94:789-790.
17. Gilbert DN, Kohlhepp SJ. New sodium hydroxide digestion method for measurement of renal tobramycin concentrations. Antimicrob Agents Chemother. 1986;30:361-365.
18. Moellering RC Jr. In vitro antibacterial activity of the aminoglycoside antibiotics. Rev Infect Dis. 1983;5(Suppl):S212-S232.
19. Rocque WJ, Fesik SW, Haug A, et al. Polycation binding to isolated lipopolysaccharide from antibiotic-hypersusceptible mutant strains of *Escherichia coli*. Antimicrob Agents Chemother. 1988;32:308-313.
20. McLaughlin JE, Reeves DS. Clinical and laboratory evidence for inactivation of gentamicin by carbenicillin. Lancet. 1971;1:261-264.
21. Pickering LK, Rutherford I. Effect of concentration and time upon inactivation of tobramycin, gentamicin, netilmicin, mezlocillin, and piperacillin. J Pharmacol Exp Ther. 1981;217:345-349.

22. Walterspiel JN, Feldman S, Van R, et al. Comparative inactivation of isepamicin, amikacin, and gentamicin by nine beta-lactams and two beta-lactamase inhibitors, cilastatin and heparin. Antimicrob Agents Chemother. 1991;35:1875-1878.

23. Halstenson CE, Wong MU, Herman CS, et al. Effect of concomitant administration of piperacillin on the dispositions of isepamicin and gentamicin in patients with end-stage renal disease. Antimicrob Agents Chemother. 1992;36:1832-1836.

24. Bryan LE, Kawan S. Roles of ribosomal binding, membrane potential, and electron transport in bacterial uptake of streptomycin and gentamicin. Antimicrob Agents Chemother. 1983;23:835-845.

25. Taber HW, Muller JP, Arrow AS. Bacterial uptake of aminoglycoside antibiotics. Microbiol Rev. 1987;51:439-457.

26. Hancock RE, Bellido F. Antibiotic uptake: Unusual results for unusual molecules. J Antimicrob Chemother. 1992;29:235-239.

27. Hurwitz C, Rosano CL, Landau JV. Kinetics of loss of viability of Escherichia coli exposed to streptomycin. J Bacteriol. 1962;83:1210-1216.

28. Jackson GE, Lolans VT, Daikos GL. The inductive role of ionic binding in the bactericidal and postexposure effects of aminoglycoside antibiotics with implications for dosing. J Infect Dis. 1990;162:408-413.

29. Laurent G, Kishore BK, Tulkens PM. Aminoglycoside-induced renal phospholipidosis and nephrotoxicity. Biochem Pharmacol. 1990;40:2383-2392.

30. Hancock REW. Alterations in outer membrane permeability. Annu Rev Microbiol. 1984;38:237-264.

31. Peterson AA, Hancock REW, McGroarty EJ. Binding of polycationic antibiotics and polyamines to lipopolysaccharides of Pseudomonas aeruginosa. J Bacteriol. 1985;164:1256-1261.

32. Martin NL, Beveridge TJ. Gentamicin interaction with Pseudomonas aeruginosa. Antimicrob Agents Chemother. 1986;29:1079-1087.

33. Hancock REW. Aminoglycoside uptake and mode of action with special reference to streptomycin and gentamicin. I. Antagonists and mutants. J Antimicrob Chemother. 1981;8:249-276.

34. Hancock REW. Aminoglycoside uptake and mode of action with special reference to streptomycin and gentamicin. II. Effects of aminoglycosides on cells. J Antimicrob Chemother. 1981;8:429-445.

35. Bryan LE. Mechanisms of action of aminoglycoside antibiotics. In: Root RK, Sande MA, eds. Contemporary Issues in Infectious Diseases, v. 1. New Dimensions in Antimicrobial Therapy. New York: Churchill Livingstone; 1984:17-36.

36. Nicas TI, Hancock REW. Outer membrane protein H1 of Pseudomonas aeruginosa: Involvement in adaptive and mutational resistance to ethylenediamine tetraacetate, polymyxin B, and gentamicin. J Bacteriol. 1980;143:872-878.

37. Lavitan IM, Fraimow HS, Carrasco N, et al. Tobramycin uptake in Escherichia coli in membrane vesicles. Antimicrob Agents Chemother. 1995;39:467-475.

38. Hocquet D, Vogue C, El Garch F, et al. MexXY-OprM efflux pump is necessary for adaptive resistance of Pseudomonas aeruginosa to aminoglycosides. Antimicrob Agents Chemother. 2003;47:1371-375.

39. Mao W, Warren MS, Lee A, et al. MexXY-OprM efflux pump is required for antagonism of aminoglycosides by divalent cation in Pseudomonas aeruginosa. Antimicrob Agents Chemother. 2001;45:2001-2007.

40. Daikos GL, Jackson GG, Lolans VT, et al. Adaptive resistance to aminoglycoside antibiotics from first-exposure down-regulation. J Infect Dis. 1990;162:414-420.

41. Xiong Y-Q, Caillon J, Kergueris MF, et al. Adaptive resistance of Pseudomonas aeruginosa induced by aminoglycosides and killing kinetics in a rabbit endocarditis model. Antimicrob Agents Chemother. 1997;41:823-826.

42. Bush K, Miller GH. Bacterial enzymatic resistance: β-Lactamases and aminoglycoside-modifying enzymes. Curr Opin Microbiol. 1998;1:509-515.

43. Barclay ML, Begg EJ, Chambers ST, et al. Adaptive resistance to tobramycin in Pseudomonas aeruginosa lung infection in cystic fibrosis. J Antimicrob Chemother. 1996;37:1155-1164.

44. Gilleland LB, Gilleland HE, Gibson JA, et al. Adaptive resistance to aminoglycoside antibiotics in Pseudomonas aeruginosa. J Med Microbiol. 1984;29:41-50.

45. Häubler SB, Tümmler B, Weibbrodt M, et al. Small colony variants of Pseudomonas aeruginosa in cystic fibrosis. Clin Infect Dis. 1999;29:621-625.

46. Mingeot-Leclerqe M-P, Glupczynski Y, Tulkins P. Aminoglycosides: Activity and resistance. Antimicrob Agents Chemother. 1999;43:727-737.

47. Fong DH, Berghuis AM. Substrate promiscuity of an aminoglycoside antibiotic resistance enzyme via target mimicry. EMBO J. 2002;21:2323-2331.

48. Shaw KJ, Rather PN, Hare RS. Molecular genetics of aminoglycoside resistance genes and familial relationships of the aminoglycoside-modifying enzymes. Microbiol Rev. 1993;57:138-163.

49. Moellering RC. The enterococcus: A classic example of the impact of antimicrobial resistance on therapeutic options. J Antimicrob Chemother. 1991;28:1-12.

50. Chow JW. Aminoglycoside resistance in enterococci. Clin Infect Dis. 2000;31:586-589.

51. Vakulenko SB, Donabedian SM, Voskresensky AM, et al. Multiplex PCR for detection of aminoglycoside resistance genes in enterococci. Antimicrob Agents Chemother. 2003;47:1423-1426.

52. Karlowsky JA, Jones ME, Thornsberry CT, et al. Trends in antimicrobial susceptibilities among Enterobacteriaceae isolated from hospitalized patients in the United States from 1998 to 2001. Antimicrob Agents Chemother. 2003;47:1672-1680.

53. Karlowsky JA, Draghi DC, Jones ME, et al. Surveillance for antimicrobial susceptibility among clinical isolates of Pseudomonas aeruginosa and Acinetobacter baumannii from hospitalized patients in the United States, 1998 to 2001. Antimicrob Agents Chemother. 2003;47:1681-1688.

54. Diekema DJ, Pfaller MA, Jones RN, et al. Survey of bloodstream infections due to gram-negative bacilli: Frequency of occurrence and antimicrobial susceptibility of isolates collected in the United States, Canada, and Latin America for the SENTRY Antimicrobial Surveillance program, 1997. Clin Infect Dis. 1999;29:595-607.

55. Miller GH, Sabatelli FJ, Hare RS, et al. The most frequent aminoglycoside resistance mechanisms—Changes with time and geographic area: a reflection of aminoglycoside usage patterns? Aminoglycoside Resistance Study Groups. Clin Infect Dis. 1997;24(Suppl 1):S46-S62.

56. Chow JW, Kak V, You I, et al. The changing nature of aminoglycoside resistance mechanisms and prevalence of newly recognized resistance mechanisms in Turkey. Clin Microbiol Infect. 2001;7:470-478.

57. Vanhoof R, Nyseen HJ, Bossuyt EV, et al. Aminoglycoside resistance in gram-negative blood isolates from various hospitals in Belgium and the Grand Duchy of Luxembourg. J Antimicrob Chemother. 1999;44:483-488.

58. Chow JW, Fine MJ, Shlaes DM, et al. Enterobacter bacteremia: Clinical features and emergence of antibiotic resistance during therapy. Ann Intern Med. 1991;115:585-590.

59. Gilbert DN, Moellering RC, Sande MA. Sanford Guide to Antimicrobial Therapy. 33rd ed. Hyde Park, Vt: Antimicrobial Therapy; 2003.

60. Maurin M, Raoult D. Use of aminoglycosides in treatment of infections due to intracellular bacteria. Antimicrob Agents Chemother. 2001;45:2977-2986.

61. Rolain J-M, Maurin M, Raoult D. Bactericidal effect of antibiotics on Bartonella and Brucella spp: Clinical implications. J Antimicrob Chemother. 2000;46:811-814.

62. Craig WA, Suh B. Protein binding and the antimicrobial effects: Methods for the determination of protein binding. In: Lorian V, ed. Antibiotics in Medicine. 3rd ed. Baltimore: Williams & Wilkins; 1991:367-402.

63. Gilbert DN, Kutscher E, Ireland P, et al. Effect of the concentrations of magnesium and calcium on the in vitro susceptibility of Pseudomonas aeruginosa to gentamicin. J Infect Dis. 1971;124:537-544.

64. Reller LB, Schoenknecht FD, Kenny MA, et al. Antibiotic susceptibility testing of Pseudomonas aeruginosa: Selection of a control strain and criteria for magnesium and calcium content in media. J Infect Dis. 1979;130:454-463.

65. Barry AL, Miller GH, Thornsberry C, et al. Influence of cation supplements on activity of netilmicin against Pseudomonas aeruginosa in vitro and in vivo. Antimicrob Agents Chemother. 1987;31:1514-1518.

66. Barry AL, Acar JF, Goldstein FW. Disk susceptibility testing. In: Lorian V, ed. Antibiotics in Laboratory Medicine. 4th ed. Baltimore: Williams & Wilkins; 1996:1-51.

67. Ward PB, Palladino S, Looker JC, et al. P-nitrophenylglycerol in susceptibility testing media alters the MICs of antimicrobials for Pseudomonas aeruginosa. J Antimicrob Chemother. 1993;31:489-496.

68. Peddie BA, Chambers ST. Effects of betaines and urine on the antibacterial activity of aminoglycosides. J Antimicrob Chemother. 1993;31:481-488.

69. Eliopoulos GM, Moellering RC. Antimicrobial combinations. In: Lorian V, ed. Antibiotics in Laboratory Medicine. 4th ed. Baltimore: Williams & Wilkins; 1996:330-383.

70. Vogelman B, Craig WA. Kinetics of antimicrobial activity. J Pediatr. 1986;108:835-840.

71. Dudley MN, Zinner SH. Single daily dosing of amikacin in an in vitro model. J Antimicrob Chemother. 1991;27(Suppl C):15-19.

72. Drusano GL. Role of pharmacokinetics in the outcome of infections. Antimicrob Agents Chemother. 1988;32:289-297.

73. Craig WA, Ebert SC. Continuous infusion of beta-lactams. Antimicrob Agents Chemother. 1992;36:2577-2583.

74. Craig WA, Gudmundsson S. Postantibiotic effect. In: Lorain V, ed. Antibiotics in the Laboratory. 4th ed. Baltimore: Williams & Wilkins; 1996:296-329.

75. Fantin B, Ebert S, Leggett J, et al. Factors influencing the duration of in vivo postantibiotic effect for aminoglycosides against gram-negative bacilli. J Antimicrob Chemother. 1990;27:829-386.

76. Craig WA, Ebert SC. Killing and regrowth of bacteria in vitro: A review. Scand J Infect Dis Suppl. 1991;74:63-70.

77. Hessen MT, Pitsakis PG, Levison ME. Absence of a postantibiotic effect in experimental Pseudomonas endocarditis treated with imipenem, with or without gentamicin. J Infect Dis. 1988;158:542-548.

78. Barmada S, Kohlhepp S, Leggett J, et al. Correlation of tobramycin-induced inhibition of protein synthesis with postantibiotic effect in Escherichia coli. Antimicrob Agents Chemother. 1993;27:2678-2683.

79. Holm SE. Interaction between β-lactam and other antibiotics. Rev Infect Dis. 1986;8(Suppl 3):S305-S314.

80. Hunter TH. Use of streptomycin in the treatment of bacterial endocarditis. Am J Med. 1947;2:436-442.

81. Zak O, O'Reilly T. Animal models in the evaluation of antimicrobial agents. Antimicrob Agents Chemother. 1991;35:1527-1531.

82. Andriole VT. Aminoglycoside antibiotics: Antibacterial efficacy in animal models of infection. J Infect Dis. 1983;5(Suppl 2):S233-S249.

83. Vastola AP, Brandel J, Craig WA. Selection of aminoglycoside-resistant variants of Pseudomonas aeruginosa in an in vivo model. J Infect Dis. 1982;146:691-697.

84. Gerber AU, Feller-Segessenmann C. In vivo assessment of in vitro killing patterns of Pseudomonas aeruginosa. J Antimicrob Chemother. 1985;15:201-206.

85. Vogelman B, Gudmundsson S, Turnidge J, et al. In vivo postantibiotic effect in a thigh infection in neutropenic mice. J Infect Dis. 1988;157:287-298.

86. Craig WA. Post-antibiotic effects in experimental infection models: Relationship to in vitro phenomena and to treatment of infections in man. J Antimicrob Chemother. 1993;31(Suppl D):S149-S158.

87. Kapusnik JE, Hackbarth CJ, Chambers HF, et al. Single, large daily dosing vs intermittent dosing of tobramycin for treating experimental *Pseudomonas aeruginosa* pneumonia. J Infect Dis. 1988;158:7-12.

88. Sohet I, Yellin A, Meyerovitch J, et al. Pharmacokinetics and therapeutic efficacy of gentamicin in an experimental pleural empyema rabbit model. Antimicrob Agents Chemother. 1987;31:982-985.

89. Gerber AU, Grestes U, Segesseman C, et al. The impact of the pre-treatment interval on antimicrobial efficacy in a biological model. J Antimicrob Chemother. 1993;31(Suppl D):S29-S39.

90. Fantin B, Carbon C. In vivo antibiotic synergism. Contribution of animal models. Antimicrob Agents Chemother. 1992;36:907-912.

91. Chavanet P, Colin F, Muggeo E, et al. The in vivo activity of co-amoxiclav with netilmicin against experimental methicillin and gentamicin resistant *Staphylococcus epidermidis* infection in rabbits. J Antimicrob Chemother. 1993;31:129-138.

92. Trautman M, Bruckner O, Marre R, et al. Comparative efficacy of ciprofloxacin, ceftazidime and gentamicin, given alone or in combination, in a model of experimental septicemia due to *Klebsiella pneumoniae* in neutropenic mice. Infection. 1988;16:49-53.

93. Chadwick EK, Shulman ST, Yogev R. Correlation of antibiotic synergy in vitro and in vivo: Use of an animal model of neutropenic gram-negative sepsis. J Infect Dis. 1986;154:670-675.

94. Craig WA. Pharmacokinetic/pharmacodynamic parameters: Rationale for antibacterial dosing of mice and men. Clin Infect Dis. 1998;26:1-10.

95. Graham JC, Gould FK. Role of aminoglycosides in the treatment of bacterial endocarditis. J Antimicrob Chemother. 2002;49:437-444.

96. Fantin B, Pangon B, Potel G, et al. Ceftriaxone-netilmicin combination in single-daily-dose treatment of experimental *Escherichia coli* endocarditis. Antimicrob Agents Chemother. 1989;33:767-770.

97. Gilbert DN. Once daily aminoglycoside therapy. Antimicrob Agents Chemother. 1991;35:339-405.

98. Gudmundsson S, Einarsson S, Erlendstotter H, et al. The postantibiotic effect of antimicrobial combinations in a neutropenic murine thigh infection model. J Antimicrob Chemother. 1993;31(Suppl D):S177-S191.

99. Michea Hamzehpour M, Auckenthaler R, Regamey P, et al. Resistance occurring after fluoroquinolone therapy of experimental *Pseudomonas aeruginosa* peritonitis. Antimicrob Agents Chemother. 1987;31:1803-1808.

100. Michea-Hamzehpour M, Pechere JC, Marchou B, et al. Combination therapy: A way to limit emergence of resistance? Am J Med. 1986;80(Suppl 6B):S138-S142.

101. Pechere JC, Marchou B, Michea-Hamzehpour M, et al. Emergence of resistance after therapy with antibiotics used alone or combined in a murine model. J Antimicrob Chemother. 1986;17(Suppl A):S11-S18.

102. Gerber AU, VaStola AP, Brandel J, et al. Selection of aminoglycoside-resistant variants of *Pseudomonas aeruginosa* in an in vivo model. J Infect Dis. 1982;146:691-697.

103. Weinstein WM, Onderdonk AB, Bartlett JG, et al. Antimicrobial therapy of experimental intra-abdominal sepsis. J Infect Dis. 1975;132:282-286.

104. Weinstein WM, Onderdonk AB, Bartlett JG, et al. Experimental intra-abdominal abscesses in rats: Development of an experimental model. Infect Immun. 1974; 10:1250-1255.

105. Onderdonk AB, Kasper DL, Cisneros RL, et al. The capsular polysaccharide of *Bacteroides fragilis* as a virulence factor: Comparison of the pathogenic potential of encapsulated and unencapsulated strains. J Infect Dis. 1977;136:82-89.

106. Nichols RL, Smith JW. Wound and intra-abdominal infections: Microbiological considerations and approaches to treatment. Clin Infect Dis. 1993;16(Suppl 4): S266-S277.

107. Onderdonk AB, Bartlett JG, Louie T, et al. Microbial synergy in experimental intra-abdominal abscess. Infect Immun. 1976;13:22-26.

108. Vandaux P, Waldvogel FA. Gentamicin inactivation in purulent exudates: Role of cell lysis. J Infect Dis. 1980;142:586-593.

109. Barza M, Lauermann M. Why monitor serum levels of gentamicin? Clin Pharmacokinet. 1978;3:202-215.

110. Kunin CM, Chalmers TC, Leevy CM, et al. Absorption of orally administered neomycin and kanamycin. N Engl J Med. 1960;262:380-385.

111. Breen KJ, Bryant RE, Levinson JD, et al. Neomycin absorption in man. Ann Intern Med. 1972;76:211-218.

112. Bamford MFM, Jones LF. Deafness and biochemical imbalance after burns treatment with topical antibiotics in young children. Arch Dis Child. 1978;53:326-329.

113. Pittinger CB, Adamson R. Antibiotic blockade of neuromuscular function. Annu Rev Pharmacol. 1972;12:169-184.

114. Chamberlain G, Needham P. The absorption of antibiotics from the bladder. J Urol. 1976;116:172-173.

115. Lifschitz MI, Denning CR. Safety of kanamycin aerosol. Clin Pharmacol Ther. 1971;12:91-95.

116. Odio W, VanLeier E, Klastersky J. Concentrations of gentamicin in bronchial secretions after intramuscular and endotracheal administration. J Clin Pharmacol. 1975; 15:518-524.

117. Van Etta LL, Kravitz GR, Russ TE, et al. Effect of method of administration on extravascular penetration of four antibiotics. Antimicrob Agents Chemother. 1982;21:873-880.

118. Schwartz SN, Pazin GJ, Lyon JA, et al. A controlled investigation of the pharmacokinetics of gentamicin and tobramycin in obese subjects. J Infect Dis. 1978;138: 499-505.

119. Kunar MJ, Mak LL, Lietman PS. Localization of ³H-gentamicin in the proximal renal tubule of the mouse. Antimicrob Agents Chemother. 1979;15:131-133.

120. Ramsey BW, Dorkin HL, Eisenberg JD, et al. Efficacy of aerosolized tobramycin in patients with cystic fibrosis. N Engl J Med. 1993;328:1740-1746.

121. Rahal JJ Jr, Hyams PJ, Simberkoff MS, et al. Combined intrathecal and intramuscular gentamicin for gram-negative meningitis. N Engl J Med. 1974;290:1394-1398.

122. Kaiser AB, McGee ZA. Aminoglycoside therapy of gram-negative bacillary meningitis. N Engl J Med. 1975;293:1215-1220.

123. Wirt TC, McGee ZA, Oldfield EH, et al. Intraventricular administration of amikacin for complicated gram-negative meningitis and ventriculitis. J Neurosurg. 1979;50: 95-99.

124. Cracken GH Jr, Mize S, Threlkeld N. Intraventricular gentamicin therapy in gram-negative bacillary meningitis of infancy. Lancet. 1980;1:787-791.

125. Wood MJ, Farrell W. Comparison of urinary excretion of tobramycin and gentamicin in adults. J Infect Dis. 1976;134(Suppl):S133-S136.

126. Kahlmeter G, Kamme G. Prolonged excretion of gentamicin in a patient with unimpaired renal function. Lancet. 1975;1:286.

127. Kahlmeter G. Netilmicin: Clinical pharmacokinetics and aspects of dosage schedules. An overview. Scand J Infect Dis. 1980;23:74-81.

128. Laskin OL, Longstreth JA, Smith CR, et al. Netilmicin and gentamicin multidose kinetics in normal subjects. Clin Pharmacol Ther. 1983;34:644-650.

129. Dee TH, Kozin F. Gentamicin and tobramycin penetration into synovial fluid. Antimicrob Agents Chemother. 1977;12:548-549.

130. Pitt HA, Roberts RB, Johnson WD Jr. Gentamicin levels in the human biliary tract. J Infect Dis. 1973;127:299-302.

131. Reckziegel R, Maguilnik I, Goldami LZ. Gentamicin concentration in bile after once-daily versus thrice-daily dosing of 4 mg/kg/day. J Antimicrob Chemother. 2001;48:327-329.

132. Baum J. Infections of the eye. Clin Infect Dis. 1995;21:479-488.

133. Barza M, Kane A, Baum J. Comparison of the effects of continuous and intermittent systemic administration on the penetration of gentamicin into infected rabbit eyes. J Infect Dis. 1983;147:144-148.

134. Gorden TB, Cunningham RD. Tobramycin levels in aqueous humor after subconjunctival injection in humans. Am J Ophthalmol. 1982;93:107-110.

135. Rubenstein E, Goldfarb J, Keren G, et al. The penetration of gentamicin into the vitreous humor in man. Invest Ophthalmol Vis Sci. 1983;24:637-639.

136. Wilson TW, Mahon WA, Inaba T, et al. Elimination of tritiated gentamicin in normal human subjects and in patients with severely impaired renal function. Clin Pharmacol Ther. 1973;14:815-822.

137. Collier VU, Lietman PS, Mitch WE. Evidence for luminal uptake of gentamicin in perfused rat kidney. J Pharmacol Exp Ther. 1979;210:247-251.

138. Silberblatt FJ, Kuehn C. Autoradiography of gentamicin uptake by the rat proximal tubular cell. Kidney Int. 1979;15:335-345.

139. Beauchamp D, Gourde P, Bergeron MG. Subcellular distribution of gentamicin in proximal tubular cells, determined by immunogold labeling. Antimicrob Agents Chemother. 1991;35:2173-2179.

140. Fabre J, Rudhardt M, Blanchard P, et al. Persistence of sisomicin and gentamicin in renal cortex and medulla compared with other organs and serum of rats. Kidney Int. 1976;10:444-449.

141. Schentag JJ, Jusko WJ. Renal clearance and tissue accumulation of gentamicin. Clin Pharmacol Ther. 1977;22:364-370.

142. Laskin OL, Longstreth JA, Smith CR, et al. Netilmicin and gentamicin multidose kinetics in normal subjects. Clin Pharmacol Ther. 1983;34:644-650.

143. Barza M, Brown RB, Shen D, et al. Predictability of blood levels of gentamicin in man. J Infect Dis. 1975;132:165-174.

144. McCracken GH, Freij BJ. Clinical pharmacology of antimicrobial agents. In: Remington JS, Klein JO, eds. Infectious Diseases of the Fetus and Newborn Infant. 3rd ed. Philadelphia: WB Saunders; 1990:1020-1076.

145. Welling PG, Baumueller A, Lau CC, et al. Netilmicin pharmacokinetics after single intravenous doses to elderly male patients. Antimicrob Agents Chemother. 1977;12:328-334.

146. Reinhard MK, Hottendorf GH, Powell FD. Differences in the sensitivity of Fischer and Sprague-Dawley rats to aminoglycoside nephrotoxicity. Toxicol Pathol. 1991;19:66-71.

147. Mingeot-Leclercq M-P, Tulkens PM. Aminoglycosides: nephrotoxicity. Antimicrob Agents Chemother. 1999;43:1005-1012.

148. Verroust PJ, Birn H, Nielsen R, et al. The tandem endocytic receptors megalin and cubilin are important proteins in renal pathology. Kid Int. 2002;62:745-756.

148a. Sandoval RM, Molitoris BA. Gentamicin traffics retrograde through the secretory pathway and is released in the cytosol via the endoplasmic reticulum. Am J Physiol Renal Physiol. 2004;286:F617-F624.

149. Schmitz C, Hilpert J, Jacobsen C, et al. Megalin deficiency offers protection from renal aminoglycoside accumulation. J Biol Chem. 2002;277:618-622.

150. Verroust PJ, Christensen EI. Megalin and cubilin—The story of two multipurpose receptors unfolds. Nephrol Dial Transplant. 2002;17:1867-1871.

151. Sandoval RM, Dunn KW, Molitoris BA. Gentamicin traffics rapidly and directly to the Golgi complex in LLC-PK1 cells. Am J Physiol. 2000;279:F884-F890.

152. Bennett WM, Mela-Riker L, Houghton DC, et al. Microsomal protein synthesis inhibition: An early manifestation of gentamicin nephrotoxicity. Am J Physiol. 1988;255:F265-F269.

153. Gilbert DN, Bennett WM. Progress in the elucidation of aminoglycoside nephrotoxicity. Contemp Issues Infect Dis. 1984;1:121-152.

154. Buss WC, Piatt MK. Gentamicin administered in vivo reduces protein synthesis in microsomes subsequently isolated from rat kidney but not from rat brain. J Antimicrob Chemother. 1985;15:715-721.

155. Loveless MO, Kohlhepp SJ, Gilbert DN. The influence of aminoglycoside antibiotics on the in vitro function of rat liver ribosomes. J Lab Clin Med. 1984;103:94-303.

156. Sastrasink M, Weinberg JM, Humes HD. The effect of gentamicin on calcium uptake by renal mitochondria. Life Sci. 1982;30:2309-2315.

157. Elliott C, Newman N, Madon A. Gentamicin effects on urinary electrolyte excretion in healthy subjects. Clin Pharmacol Ther. 2000;67:16-21.

158. Bennett WM, Elliott WC, Houghton DC, et al. Reduction of experimental gentamicin nephrotoxicity in rats by dietary calcium loading. Antimicrob Agents Chemother. 1982;22:508-512.

159. Quarum ML, Houghton DC, Gilbert DN, et al. Increasing dietary calcium moderates experimental gentamicin nephrotoxicity. J Lab Clin Med. 1984;103:104-114.

160. Humes HD, Sastrasink M, Weinberg JM. Calcium is a competitive inhibitor of gentamicin renal membrane binding interactions and dietary calcium supplementation protects against gentamicin nephrotoxicity. J Clin Invest. 1984;73:134-147.

161. Ernst S. Model of gentamicin induced nephrotoxicity and its amelioration by calcium and thyroxine. Med Hypoth. 1989;30:195-202.

162. Mizuta K, Saito A, Watanabe T, et al. Ultrastructural localization of megalin in the rat cochlear duct. Hear Res. 1999;129:83-91.

163. Scherbeich JE, Mondorf WA. Nephrotoxic potential of antiinfective drugs as assessed by tissue-specific proteinuria of renal antigens. Int J Clin Pharm Ther. 1998;36: 152-158.

164. Lipsky JJ, Lietman PS. Neomycin inhibition of adenosine triphosphate: Evidence for a neomycin phospholipid interaction. Antimicrob Agents Chemother. 1980;18: 532-535.

165. Sorribas V, Halaikel N, Puttaparthi K, et al. Gentamicin causes endocytosis of Na/Pi cotransporter protein (NaPi-2). Kidney Int. 2001;59:1024-1036.

166. von Vigier RO, Truttman AC, Zindler-Schmocker K, et al. Aminoglycosides and renal magnesium homeostasis in humans. Nephrol Dial Transplant. 2000;15:822-826.

167. Mohammed EM, Laurent G, Mingeot-Leclercq M-P, et al. Apoptosis in renal proximal tubules of rats treated with low does of aminoglycosides. Antimicrob Agents Chemother. 2000;44:665-675.

168. Appel GB. Aminoglycoside nephrotoxicity. Am J Med. 1990;88(Suppl C):S16-S20.

169. Gilbert DN, Houghton DC, Bennett WM, et al. Reversibility of gentamicin nephrotoxicity in rats: Recovery during continuous drug administration. Proc Soc Exp Biol Med. 1979;160:99-103.

170. Luft FC, Bennett WM, Gilbert DN. Experimental aminoglycoside nephrotoxicity: Accomplishments and future potential. Rev Infect Dis. 1983;5(Suppl 2):S268-S293.

171. Gilbert DN, Plamp C, Starr P, et al. Comparative nephrotoxicity of gentamicin and tobramycin in rats. Antimicrob Agents Chemother. 1979;13:34-40.

172. Bennett WM, Plamp CE, Gilbert DN, et al. The influence of dosage regimen on experimental gentamicin nephrotoxicity: Dissociation of peak serum levels from renal failure. J Infect Dis. 1979;140:576-580.

173. Powell SH, Thompson WL, Luthe MA, et al. Once daily vs continuous aminoglycoside dosing: Efficacy and toxicity in animal and clinical studies of gentamicin, netilmicin, and tobramycin. J Infect Dis. 1983;147:918-923.

174. Beauchamp D, Gourde P, Thereault G, et al. Age-dependent gentamicin experimental nephrotoxicity. J Pharmacol Exp Ther. 1992;260:444-449.

175. Bennett WM, Parker RA, Elliott WB, et al. Sex: A determinant of susceptibility to gentamicin nephrotoxicity in the rat. J Infect Dis. 1982;145:370-373.

176. Moore RD, Smith CR, Lipsky JJ et al. Risk factors for nephrotoxicity in patients treated with aminoglycosides. Ann Intern Med. 1984;100:352-357.

177. Sawyers CL, Moore RD, Lerner SA, et al. A model for predicting nephrotoxicity in patients treated with aminoglycosides. J Infect Dis. 1985;153:1062-1068.

178. Elliott WB, Parker RA, Houghton DC, et al. Effect of sodium bicarbonate and ammonium chloride ingestion in experimental gentamicin nephrotoxicity in rats. Res Commun Pathol Pharmacol. 1980;28:483-496.

179. Bennett WM, Hartnett MN, Gilbert D, et al. Effect of sodium intake on gentamicin nephrotoxicity in the rat. Proc Soc Exp Biol Med. 1976;151:736-738.

180. Peterson LN, Borzecki JS. Inhibition of tobramycin reabsorption in nephron segments by metabolic alkalosis. Kidney Int. 1990;37:1492-1499.

181. Chiu PJS, Miller GH, Long JF, et al. Renal uptake and nephrotoxicity of gentamicin during urinary alkalinization in rats. Clin Exp Pharmacol Physiol. 1979;6:317-326.

182. Thompson JR, Simonsen R, Spindler MA, et al. Protective effect of KCl loading in gentamicin nephrotoxicity. Am J Kidney Dis. 1990;15:583-591.

183. Rodriquez HJ, Hogan WC, Hellman RN, et al. Mechanism of activation of renal Na$^+$-K$^+$-ATPase in the rat: Effects of potassium loading. Am J Physiol. 1980;238: F315-F323.

184. Cronin RE, Newman JA. Protective effect of thyroxine but not parathyroidectomy on gentamicin nephrotoxicity. Am J Physiol. 1985;248:F332-F339.

185. Adelman RD, Spangler WL, Beasom F, et al. Furosemide enhancement of experimental gentamicin nephrotoxicity: Comparison of functional and morphological changes with activities of urinary enzymes. J Infect Dis. 1979;140:342-342.

186. Vakil N, Abu-Alfa A, Mujais SK. Gentamicin nephrotoxicity in extrahepatic cholestasis: Modulation by dietary calcium. Hepatology. 1989;9:519-524.

187. Camps J, Sola X, Rimola A, et al. Comparative study of aminoglycoside nephrotoxicity in normal rats and rats with experimental cirrhosis. Hepatology. 1988;8: 837-844.

188. Lietman PS. Liver disease, aminoglycoside antibiotics, and renal dysfunction. Hepatology. 1988;4:966-968.

189. Teixeira RB, Kelley J, Alpert H, et al. Complete protection from gentamicin-induced acute renal failure in the diabetes mellitus rat. Kidney Int. 1982;21:600-612.

190. Elliott WB, Houghton DC, Gilbert DN, et al. Experimental gentamicin nephrotoxicity: Effect of streptozotocin-induced diabetes. J Pharmacol Exp Ther. 1985;233: 264-270.

191. Wood CA, Kohlhepp SJ, Kohnen PW, et al. Vancomycin enhancement of experimental tobramycin nephrotoxicity. Antimicrob Agents Chemother. 1985;30:20-24.

192. Kohlhepp SJ, Gilbert DN, Kohnen PW, et al. Teicoplanin enhancement of experimental tobramycin nephrotoxicity (Abstract). Proceedings of the 31st Interscience Conference on Antimicrobial Agents Chemotherapy. Washington, DC: American Society for Microbiology; 1991.

193. Golper TA, Noonan HM, Elzinga L, et al. Vancomycin pharmacokinetics, renal handling and non-renal clearance in normal human subjects. Clin Pharmacol Ther. 1988;43:565-570.

194. English J, Gilbert DN, Kohlhepp SJ, et al. Attenuation of experimental tobramycin nephrotoxicity by ticarcillin. Antimicrob Agents Chemother. 1985;276:897-902.

195. Sabra R, Branch RA. Role of sodium in protection by extended spectrum penicillins against tobramycin-induced nephrotoxicity. Antimicrob Agents Chemother. 1990;340:1020-1025.

196. Barr GA, Mazze RI, Cousins MJ, et al. An animal model for combined methoxyflurane and gentamicin nephrotoxicity. Br J Anaesth. 1973;45:306-331.

197. Whiting PH, Simpson JG. The enhancement of cyclosporin-A induced nephrotoxicity by gentamicin. Biochem Pharmacol. 1983;32:2025-2028.

198. Ryffel B, Muller AM, Mihatsch MJ. Experimental cyclosporine nephrotoxicity: Risk of concomitant chemotherapy. Clin Nephrol. 1988;25(Suppl 1):S121-S125.

199. Jongejan HTM, Provoost AP, Molenaar JC. Potentiated nephrotoxicity of cisplatin when combined with amikacin comparing young and adult rats. Pediatr Nephrol. 1989;31:290-5.

200. Williams PD, Hottdenford GH. Inhibition of renal membrane binding and nephrotoxicity of gentamicin by polyasparagine and polyaspartic acid in the rat. Res Commun Chem Pathol Pharmacol. 1985;47:317-320.

201. Gilbert DN, Wood CA, Kohlhepp SJ, et al. Polyaspartic acid prevents experimental aminoglycoside nephrotoxicity. J Infect Dis. 1989;159:945-953.

202. Swan SK, Kohlhepp SJ, Kohnen PW, et al. Long-term protection of polyaspartic acid in experimental gentamicin nephrotoxicity. Antimicrob Agents Chemother. 1991;35:2591-2595.

203. Gilbert DN, Kohlhepp SJ, Swan SK, et al. Pharmacologic limits of polyaspartic acid's protective effect on experimental gentamicin nephrotoxicity. Antimicrob Agents Chemother. 1993;37:347-348.

204. Swan SK, Gilbert DN, Kohlhepp SJ, et al. Duration of the protective effect of polyaspartic acid on experimental gentamicin nephrotoxicity. Antimicrob Agents Chemother. 1992;36:2556-2558.

205. Ramsammy LS, Josepovitz C, Lane BP, et al. Polyaspartic acid protects against gentamicin nephrotoxicity in the rat. J Pharmacol Exp Ther. 1989;250:149-153.

206. Beauchamp D, Laurent G, Maldague P, et al. Protection against gentamicin-induced early renal alterations (phospholipidosis and increased DNA synthesis) by coadministration of poly-L-aspartic acid. J Pharmacol Exp Ther. 1990;255:858-866.

207. Kishore BK, Ibrahim S, Lambrict P, et al. Comparative assessment of poly-L-aspartic and poly-L-glutamic acids as protectants against gentamicin-induced renal lysosomal phospholipidosis, phospholipiduria and cell proliferation in rats. J Pharmacol Exp Ther. 1992;262:424-432.

208. Kohlhepp SJ, McGregor D, Gilbert DN. Determinants of the in vitro interaction of polyaspartic acid and aminoglycoside antibiotics. J Pharmacol Exp Ther. 1992;263:1464-1470.

209. Ramsammy L, Josepovitz C, Lane B, et al. Polyaspartic acid inhibits gentamicin-induced perturbations of phospholipid metabolism. Am J Physiol. 1990; 58: C1141-C1149.

210. Luft FC. Cephalosporin and aminoglycoside interactions: Clinical and toxicologic implications. In: Whelton A, Neu HC, eds. The Aminoglycosides. New York: Marcel Dekker; 1982:387-399.

211. Kahlmeter G, Dahlager JI. Aminoglycoside toxicity—A review of clinical studies published between 1975 and 1982. J Antimicrob Chemother. 1984;13(Suppl A): S9-S22.

212. Lietman PS, Smith CR. Aminoglycoside nephrotoxicity in humans. Rev Infect Dis. 1983;5(Suppl 2):S284-S292.

213. Smith CR, Baughman KL, Edwards CQ, et al. Controlled comparison of amikacin and gentamicin. N Engl J Med. 1977;296:349-353.

214. Smith CR, Lipsky JJ, Laskin OL, et al. Double-blind comparison of the nephrotoxicity and auditory toxicity of gentamicin and tobramycin. N Engl J Med. 1980;302:1106-1109.

215. Smith CR, Ambinder R, Lipsky JJ, et al. Cefotaxime compared with nafcillin plus tobramycin for serious bacterial infections. Ann Intern Med. 1984;101:469-477.

216. Bertino JS, Booker LA, Franck PA, et al. Incidence of and significant risk factors for aminoglycoside-associated nephrotoxicity in patients dosed by using individualized pharmacokinetic monitoring. J Infect Dis. 1993;167:173-179.

217. Lerner AM, Cone LA, Jansen W, et al. Randomized, controlled trial of the comparative efficacy, auditory toxicity and nephrotoxicity of tobramycin and netilmicin. Lancet. 1983;1:1123-1126.

218. Lerner SA, Schmitt BA, Seligsohn R, et al. Comparative study of ototoxicity and nephrotoxicity in patients randomly assigned treatment with amikacin and gentamicin. Am J Med. 1986;80(Suppl 5B):S98-S104.

219. Hou SH, Bushinsky DA, Wish JB, et al. Hospital-acquired renal insufficiency: A prospective study. Am J Med. 1983;74:243-248.

220. Trollfors B. Gentamicin-associated changes in renal function reversible during continued treatment. J Antimicrob Chemother. 1983;12:285-287.

221. Gilbert DN. Meta-analyses are no longer required for determining the efficacy of single daily dosing of aminoglycosides. Clin Infect Dis. 1997;24:816-819.

222. Green FJ, Lavelle KJ, Aronoff GR, et al. Management of amikacin overdose. Am J Kidney Dis. 1981;1:110-112.

223. Ho PW, Pien FD, Kominami N. Massive amikacin "overdose." Ann Intern Med. 1979;91:227-228.

224. The EORTC International Antimicrobial Therapy Project Group. Three antibiotic regimens in the treatment of infection in febrile granulocytopenic patients with cancer. J Infect Dis. 1978;137:14-29.

225. Klastersky J, Hensgens C, Debusscher I. Empiric therapy for cancer patients: Comparative study of ticarcillin-tobramycin, ticarcillin-cephalothin, and cephalothin-tobramycin. Antimicrob Agents Chemother. 1975;7:640-645.

226. Wade JC, Smith CR, Petty BG, et al. Cephalothin plus an aminoglycoside is more nephrotoxic than methicillin plus an aminoglycoside. Lancet. 1978;3:604-606.

227. Farber BF, Moellering RC. Retrospective study of the toxicity of preparations of vancomycin from 1974-1981. Antimicrob Agents Chemother. 1983;23:138-141.

228. Rybak MJ, Albrecht LM, Boike SC, et al. Nephrotoxicity of vancomycin alone and with an aminoglycoside. J Antimicrob Chemother. 1990;25:679-687.

229. Nahata MC. Lack of nephrotoxicity in pediatric patients receiving vancomycin and aminoglycoside therapy. Chemotherapy. 1987;33:302-304.

230. Cooper B, Creger RJ, Soegiarso W, et al. Renal dysfunction during high-dose cisplatin therapy and autologous hematopoietic stem cell transplantation: Effect of aminoglycoside therapy. Am J Med. 1993;94:497-504.

231. Leach CT, Kuhls TL, Brill JE, et al. Use of aminoglycosides during cyclosporine A immunosuppression after liver transplantation in children. Pediatr Infect Dis J. 1989;8:354-357.

232. Mazze RI, Cousins MJ. Combined nephrotoxicity of gentamicin and methoxyflurane in man. Br J Anaesth. 1973;45:394-398.

233. Hinshaw HC, Feldman WH. Streptomycin in treatment of clinical tuberculosis: A preliminary report. Proc Staff Meet Mayo Clin. 1945;20:313-318.

234. Brummett RE, Fox KE. Aminoglycoside induced hearing loss in humans. Antimicrob Agents Chemother. 1989;33:797-800.

235. Fausti SA, Henry JA, Schaffer HI, et al. High-frequency audiometric monitoring for early detection of aminoglycoside ototoxicity. J Infect Dis. 1992;165:1026-1032.

236. Govaerts PJ, Claes PH, DeHeyring PHV, et al. Aminoglycoside-induced ototoxicity. Toxicol Lett. 1990;52:227-251.

237. Sataloff J, Wagner S, Menduke H. Kanamycin ototoxicity in healthy men. Arch Otolaryngol. 1964;80:413-417.

238. Davey PG, Jabeen F, Harpur ES, et al. The use of pure-tone audiometry in the assessment of gentamicin auditory toxicity. Br J Audiol. 1982;16:151-154.

239. Moore RD, Smith CR, Lietman PS. Risk factors for the development of auditory toxicity in patients receiving aminoglycosides. J Infect Dis. 1984;149:23-30.

240. Hutchin T, Cortopassi G. Proposed molecular and cellular mechanism of aminoglycoside ototoxicity. Antimicrob Agents Chemother. 1994;38:2517-2520.

241. Tran Ba Huy P, Bernard P, Schacht J. Kinetics of gentamicin uptake and release in the rat. Comparison of inner ear tissues and fluids with other organs. J Clin Invest. 1986;77:1492-1500.

242. de Groot JCMJ, Meeuwsen F, Ruizendaal WE, et al. Ultrastructural localization of gentamicin in the cochlear. Hear Res. 1990;50:35-42.

243. Hashino E, Shero M, Salvi RJ. Lysosomal targeting and accumulation of aminoglycoside antibiotics in sensory hair cells. Brain Res. 1997;777:75-85.

244. Forge A, Schacht J. Aminoglycoside antibiotics. Audiol Neurootol. 2000;5:3-22.

245. Duan M, Agerman K, Ernfors P, et al. Complementary roles of neurotrophin 3 and a N-methyl-D-aspartate antagonist in the protection of noise and aminoglycoside-induced ototoxicity. Proc Natl Acad Sci U S A. 2000; 97:2597-2602.

246. Takumida M, Anniko M, Shimizu A, et al. Neuroprotection of vestibular sensory cells from gentamicin ototoxicity obtained using nitric oxide synthase inhibitors, reactive oxygen species scavengers, brain-derived neurotrophic factors and calpain inhibitors. Acta Otolaryngol. 2003;123:8-13.

247. Hashino E, Tanaka Y, Salvi RJ, et al. Hair cell regeneration in the adult budgerigar after kanamycin ototoxicity. Hear Res. 1992;59:46-58.

248. Lombarte A, Yan HY, Popper AN, et al. Damage and regeneration of hair cell ciliary bundles in a fish ear following treatment with gentamicin. Hear Res. 1993;64:166-174.

249. Forge A, Li L, Corwin JT, et al. Ultrastructural evidence for hair cell regeneration in the mammalian inner ear. Science. 1993;259:1616-1621.

250. Fischel-Ghodsian N. Genetic factors in aminoglycoside toxicity. Ann NY Acad Sci. 1999;884:99-109.

251. Tang H-Y, Hucheson E, Neill S, et al. Genetic susceptibility to aminoglycoside ototoxicity: How many are at risk? Genet Med. 2002;4:336-345.

252. Hamasaki K, Rando RR. Specific binding of aminoglycoside to a human rRNA construct based on a DNA polymorphism which causes aminoglycoside-induced deafness. Biochemistry. 1997;36:12323-12328.

253. Brummett RE, Fox KE. Vancomycin- and erythromycin-induced hearing loss in humans. Antimicrob Agents Chemother. 1989;33:791-796.

254. Tan C-T, Hsu C-J, Lee S-Y, et al. Potentiation of noise-induced hearing loss by amikacin in guinea pigs. Hear Res. 2001;161:72-80.

255. Brummett RE, Fox KE, Kempton JB. Quantitative relationships of the interaction between sound and kanamycin. Arch Otolaryngol Head Neck Surg. 1992;118:498-500.

256. Tran Ba Huy PT, Deffrennes D. Aminoglycoside ototoxicity: Influence of dosage regimen on drug uptake and correlation between membrane binding and some clinical features. Acta Otolaryngol. 1988;105:511-515.

257. Moore RD, Smith CR, Lietman PS. Risk factors for the development of auditory toxicity in patients receiving aminoglycosides. J Infect Dis. 1984;149:23-30.

258. Gatell JM, Ferran F, Araujo V, et al. Univariate and multivariate analyses of risk factors predisposing to auditory toxicity in patients receiving aminoglycosides. Antimicrob Agents Chemother. 1987;31:1383-1387.

259. Buring JE, Evans DA, Mayrent SL, et al. Randomized trials of aminoglycoside antibiotics: Quantitative overview. Rev Infect Dis. 1988;10:951-957.

260. Manian FA, Stone WJ, Alford R. Adverse antibiotic effects associated with renal insufficiency. Rev Infect Dis. 1990;12:236-249.

261. Amiko M, Bagger-Sjoback D, Wersall J, et al. Gentamicin binding to the isolated crista ampullaris of the guinea pig. Res Commun Chem Pathol Pharmacol. 1982;37:333-342.

262. Minor LB. Gentamicin-induced bilateral vestibular hypofunction. JAMA. 1998;279:541-544.

263. Black FO, Gianna-Poulin C, Pesznecker SC. Recovery from vestibular ototoxicity. Otol Neurol. 2001;22:662-671.

264. Fee WE. Aminoglycoside ototoxicity in the human. Laryngoscope. 1980;90(Suppl 24):1-9.

265. Walsh RM, Bath AP, Bance ML. Reversible tobramycin-induced bilateral high-frequency vestibular toxicity. ORL J Otorhinolaryngol Relat Spec. 2000;62:156-159.

266. Forge A, Li L, Corwin JT, Nevill G. Ultrastructural evidence for hair-cell regeneration in the mammalian inner ear. Science. 1993;259:1616-1619.

267. Rubel EW, Dew LA, Roberson DW: Mammalian vestibular hair-cell regeneration. Science. 1995;267:701-703.

268. Harner SG, Driscoll CL, Facer GW, et al. Long-term followup of transtympanic gentamicin for Meniere's syndrome. Otol Neurol. 2001;22:210-214.

269. Perez N. Martin E, Garcia-Tapia R. Intratympanic gentamicin for intractable Meniere's disease. Laryngoscope. 2003;113:456-464.

270. Snavely SR, Hodges GR. The neurotoxicity of antibacterial agents. Ann Intern Med. 1984;101:92-104.

271. Talbot PA. Potentiation of aminoglycoside-induced neuromuscular blockade by protons in vitro and in vivo. J Pharmacol Exp Ther. 1987;241:686-694.

272. Del-Pozo E, Baezem JM. Effects of calcium channel blockers on neuromuscular blockade induced by aminoglycoside antibiotics. Eur J Pharmacol. 1986;128:49-54.

273. Gay CT, Marks WA, Riley HD Jr, et al. Infantile botulism. South Med J. 1988;81:457-460.

274. Sanders DB, Kim YI, Howard JR Jr, et al. Intercostal muscle biopsy studies in myasthenia gravis: Clinical correlations and the direct effects of drugs and myasthenic serum. Ann NY Acad Sci. 1981;377:544-566.

275. Hokkanen E. The aggravating effect of some antibiotics on the neuromuscular blockade in myasthenia gravis. Acta Neurol Scand. 1964;40:346-352.

276. Wright JM, Collier B. The effects of neomycin upon transmitter release and action. J Pharmacol Exp Ther. 1977;200:576-587.

277. Lee C, DeSilva AJ. Acute and subchronic neuromuscular blocking characteristics of streptomycin: A comparison with neomycin. Br J Anaesth. 1979;51:431-434.

278. Caputy AJ, Kim YI, Sanders DB. The neuromuscular blocking effects of therapeutic concentrations of various antibiotics on normal rat skeletal muscle: A quantitative comparison. J Pharmacol Exp Ther. 1981;217:369-378.

279. Singh YN, Harvey AL, Marshall IG. Antibiotic-induced paralysis of the mouse phrenic nerve-hemidiaphragm preparation, and reversibility by calcium and by neostigmine. Anesthesiology. 1978;48:418-424.

280. Choice of antibacterials. Med Lett. 2001;43:69-78.

281. Wilson WR, Karchmer AW, Dajani AS, et al. Antibiotic treatment of adults with infective endocarditis due to streptococci, enterococci, staphylococci and HACEK microorganisms. JAMA. 1995;274:1706-1173.

282. Mylonakes E, Calderwood SB. Infective endocarditis in adults. N Engl J Med. 2001;345:1318-1330.

283. Solomkin JS, Mazuski JE, Baron EJ et al. Guidelines for the selection of anti-infective agents for complicated intra-abdominal infections. Clin Infect Dis. 2003;37:997-1005.

284. Hughes WT, Armstrong D, Bodey GP, et al. 2002 guidelines for the use of antimicrobial agents in neutropenic patients with cancer. Clin Infect Dis. 2002;34:730-751.

285. Lew DP, Waldvogel FA. Osteomyelitis. N Engl J Med. 1997;336:999-1007.

286. Craig WA, Andes D. Aminoglycosides are useful for severe respiratory tract infections. Semin Respir Infect. 1997;12:271-277.

287. Guidelines for treatment of sexually transmitted diseases. MMWR Morb Mortal Wkly Rep. 2002;51(Suppl RR-6):1-80.

288. Korvick JA, Bryan CS, Farber B, et al. Prospective observational study of Klebsiella bacteremia in 230 patients: Outcome for antibiotic combinations versus monotherapy. Antimicrob Agents Chemother. 1992;36:2639-2644.

289. Rupp ME, Fey PD. Extended-spectrum beta-lactamase (ESBL)-producing Enterobacteriaceae: Considerations for diagnosis, prevention and drug treatment. Drugs. 2003;63:353-365.

290. Dennis DT, Inglesby TV, Henderson DA, et al. Tularemia as a biological weapon: Medical and public health management. JAMA. 2001;285:2763-2773.

291. Corbel MJ. Brucellosis: An overview. Emerg Infect Dis. 1997;3:213-221.

292. Inglesby TV, Dennis DT, Henderson DA, et al. Plague as a biological weapon. JAMA. 2000;283:2281-2290.

293. Chuang YC, Yuan CY, Liu CY, et al. Vibrio vulnificus infection in Taiwan: Report of 28 cases and review of clinical manifestations and treatment. Clin Infect Dis. 1992;15:271-276.

294. Jackson GG, Finland M, eds. International Symposium on Gentamicin. J Infect Dis. 1969;119:341-540.

295. Finland M, Hewitt WL, eds. Second International Symposium on Gentamicin. J Infect Dis. 1971;124:S1-S300.

296. Finland M, Neu HC, eds. Tobramycin. J Infect Dis. 1976;134(Suppl):S1-S234.

297. Hewitt WL, Young LS. Symposium perspective. Am J Med. 1977;62:863-867.

298. Ho JL, Barza M. Role of aminoglycoside antibiotics in the treatment of intra-abdominal infection. Antimicrob Agents Chemother. 1987;31:485-491.

299. Korvick JA, Peacock JE, Muder RR, et al. Addition of rifampin to combination antibiotic therapy for Pseudomonas aeruginosa bacteremia: Prospective trial using the Zelen protocol. Antimicrob Agents Chemother. 1992;36:620-625.

300. Young EJ. An overview of brucellosis. Clin Infect Dis. 1995;21:283-290.

301. Bouza E, Cercenado E. *Klebsiella* and *Enterobacter* antibiotic resistance and treatment implications. Semin Respir Infect. 2002;17:215-230.
302. Jones RN. Important and emerging beta-lactamase–mediated resistances in hospital-based pathogens: The Amp C enzymes. Diagn Microbiol Infect Dis. 1998;31:461-466.
303. Voytovich RM, Massaro MJ, Titus DL, et al. An aminoglycoside dosing regimen in a morbidly obese patient (Letter). DICP. 1990;24:100-102.
304. Aronoff GR, ed. Drug Prescribing in Renal Failure. 4th ed. Philadelphia: American College of Physicians; 1999.
305. Hickling KG, Begg EJ, Perry RE, et al. Serum aminoglycoside clearance is predicted as poorly by renal aminoglycoside clearance as by creatinine clearance in critically ill patients. Crit Care Med. 1991;19:1041-1047.
306. McCormack JP, Jewesson PJ. A critical reevaluation of the "therapeutic range" of aminoglycoside. Clin Infect Dis. 1992;14:320-329.
307. Edwards C, Bent AJ, Venables CW, et al. Sampling time for serum gentamicin levels. J Antimicrob Chemother. 1992;29:575-578.
308. Cockcroft DW, Gault MH. Prediction of creatinine clearance from serum creatinine. Nephron. 1976;16:31-41.
309. Reichley RM, Ritchie DJ, Bailey TC. Analysis of various creatinine clearance formulas in predicting gentamicin elimination in patients with low serum creatinine. Pharmacotherapy. 1995;15:625-630.
310. Levey AS, Bosch JP, Lewis JB, et al. A more accurate method to estimate glomerular filtration rate from serum creatinine: New prediction equation. Ann Intern Med. 1999;130:461-470.
311. Moore RD, Lietman PS, Smith CR. Clinical response to aminoglycoside therapy: Importance of the ratio of peak concentration to minimal inhibitory concentrations. J Infect Dis. 1987;155:93-99.
312. Craig WA. Pharmacokinetic/pharmacodynamic parameters: Rationale for antibacterial dosing of mice and men. Clin Infect Dis. 1998;26:1-10.
313. Sarubbi FA, Hull H. Amikacin serum concentrations: Prediction of levels and dosage guidelines. Ann Intern Med. 1978;89:612-618.
314. Vreede D. Infections by gram-negative bacilli. In: Humoral Defense of the Host and Antimicrobial Therapy. Utrecht: Drukkerij Elinkwijg BV; 1988:143-165.
315. Reetze-Bonorden P, Bohler J, Keller E. Drug dosage in patients during continuous renal replacement therapy. Clin Pharmacokinet. 1993;24:362-379.
316. Wallace AW, Jones M, Bertino JS. Evaluation of four once-daily aminoglycoside dosing nomograms. Pharmacotherapy. 2002;22:1077-1083.
317. Streetman DS, Nafziger AN, Destache CJ, et al. Individualized pharmacokinetic monitoring results in less aminoglycoside-associated nephrotoxicity and fewer associated costs. Pharmacotherapy. 2001;21:443-451.
318. Verpooten GA, Giuliano RA, Verbist L, et al. Once-daily dosing decreases renal accumulation of gentamicin and netilmicin. Clin Pharmacol Ther. 1989;45:22-27.
319. De Broe ME, Verbist L, Verpooten GA. Influence of dosage schedule on renal cortical accumulation of amikacin and tobramycin in man. J Antimicrob Chemother. 1991;27(Suppl C):S41-S47.
320. Karlowsky J, Zhanel GG, Davidson RJ, et al. Postantibiotic effect in *Pseudomonas aeruginosa* following single and multiple aminoglycoside exposures in vitro. J Antimicrob Chemother. 1994;33:937-947.
321. Xiong Y, Caillon J, Kergueris MF, et al. Adaptive resistance of *Pseudomonas aeruginosa* induced by aminoglycosides and killing kinetics in a rabbit endocarditis model. Antimicrob Agents Chemother. 1997;41:823-826.
322. Barclay ML, Begg EJ, Chambers ST, et al. Adaptive resistance to tobramycin in *Pseudomonas aeruginosa* lung infection in cystic fibrosis. J Antimicrob Chemother. 1996;37:1155-1164.
323. Wood CA, Norton DR, Kohlhepp SJ, et al. The influence of tobramycin dosage regimen on nephrotoxicity, ototoxicity and antibacterial efficacy in a rat model of subcutaneous abscess. J Infect Dis. 1988;158:13-22.
324. Pierre C, Blanchet F, Seta N, et al. Tolerance of once daily dosing of netilmicin and teicoplanin alone or in combination in healthy volunteers. Clin Pharmacol Ther. 1988;44:458-466.
325. Proctor L, Petty B, Lietman P, et al. Study of potential vestibulotoxic effects of one daily versus thrice daily administrations of tobramycin. Laryngoscope. 1987;97:1443-1449.
326. Klastersky J, Prevost JM, Meunier-Carpentier F, et al. Comparative trials of single dose vs twice daily sisomicin in bacteriuric patients. J Clin Pharmacol. 1997;17:520-528.
327. Nordstrom L, Ringberg H, Cronberg S, et al. Does administration of an aminoglycoside in single daily dose affect its efficacy and toxicity? J Antimicrob Chemother. 1990;25:159-173.
328. Hansen M, Achen F, Carstensen C, et al. Once- versus thrice-daily dosing of netilmicin in febrile immunocompromised patients: A randomized, controlled study of efficacy and safety. J Drug Dev. 1988;1(Suppl 3):S119-S124.
329. Muijsken MA, Vreede RW, Van Dijk WC, et al. A randomized clinical study of efficacy and safety of once daily versus conventional dosing of netilmicin in patients with severe infections. J Drug Dev. 1988;1(Suppl 3):S145-S146.
330. Tulkens PM, Clerckx-Braun F, Donnez J, et al. Safety and efficacy of aminoglycosides once-a-day: Experimental data and randomized, controlled evaluation in patients suffering from pelvic inflammatory disease. J Drug Dev. 1988;1(Suppl 3):S71-S83.
331. Hollender LF, Bahnini J, DeManzini N, et al. A multicentric study of netilmicin once daily versus thrice daily in patients with appendicitis and other intra-abdominal infections. J Antimicrob Chemother. 1989;23:773-783.

332. Mauracher EH, Lau WY, Kartowisastro H, et al. Comparison of once-daily and thrice-daily netilmicin regimens in serious system infections: A multicenter study in six Asian countries. Clin Ther. 1989;11:604-613.
333. Strum AW. Netilmicin in the treatment of gram-negative bacteremia: Single daily versus multiple daily dosage. J Infect Dis. 1989;159:931-937.
334. DeVries PJ, Verkooyen RP, Leguit P, et al. Prospective randomized study of once-daily versus thrice-daily netilmicin regimens in patients with intra-abdominal infections. Eur J Clin Microbiol Infect Dis. 1990;9:161-168.
335. Ter Braak EW, deVried PJ, Bouter KP, et al. Once-daily dosing regimen for aminoglycoside plus β-lactam combination therapy of serious bacterial infections: Comparative trial with netilmicin plus ceftriaxone. Am J Med. 1990;89:58-66.
336. Giamarellou H, Yiallouros K, Petrikkos G, et al. Comparative kinetics and efficacy of amikacin administered once or twice daily in the treatment of systemic gram-negative infections. J Antimicrob Chemother. 1991;27(Suppl C):S73-S79.
337. Marik PE, Lipman J, Kobilski S, et al. A prospective randomized study comparing once- versus twice-daily amikacin dosing in critically ill adult and pediatric patients. J Antimicrob Chemother. 1991;28:753-764.
338. Van de Auwera P, Meunier J, Ibrahim S, et al. Pharmacodynamic and toxicity of netilmicin (5 mg/kg/day) given once daily or in three divided doses to cancer patients with urinary tract infections. Antimicrob Agents Chemother. 1991;35:640-647.
339. Vigano A, Prinicipi N, Brivio L, et al. Comparison of 5 mg of netilmicin per kilogram of body weight once daily versus 2 mg per kilogram thrice daily for treatment of gram-negative pyelonephritis in children. Antimicrob Agents Chemother. 1992;36:1499-1503.
340. Gonzalez P, Aguado JM, Martin MA, et al. Once-daily aminoglycoside dosing (Letter). Lancet. 1993;341:895.
341. Maller R, Ahrne H, Holmen C, et al. Once- versus twice-daily amikacin regimen. Efficacy and safety in systemic gram-negative infections. J Antimicrob Chemother. 1993;31:939-948.
342. Vanhaeverbeek M, Siska G, Douchamps J, et al. Comparison of the efficacy and safety of amikacin once or twice-a-day in the treatment of severe gram-negative infections in the elderly. Int J Clin Pharmacol Ther Toxicol. 1993;31:153-156.
343. Gibson J, Johnson L, Snowson L, et al. Single daily ceftriaxone and tobramycin in the empirical management of febrile neutropenic patients: A randomized trial. Int J Hematol. 1993;58:63-72.
344. Mendes da Costa P, Kaufman L. Amikacin once daily plus metronidazole versus amikacin twice daily plus metronidazole in colorectal surgery. Hepato-gastroenterology. 1992;39:350-354.
345. Fan ST, Lau WY, Teoh-Chan CH, et al. Once daily administration of netilmicin compared with thrice daily, both in combination with metronidazole, in gangrenous and perforated appendicitis. J Antimicrob Chemother. 1988;22:69-74.
346. Prins JM, Buller HP, Kuijper EJ, et al. Once versus thrice daily gentamicin in patients with serious infection. Lancet. 1993;341:335-339.
347. Raz R, Adawi M, Romano S. Intravenous administration of gentamicin once daily versus thrice daily in adults. Eur J Clin Microb Infect Dis. 1995;14:88-91.
348. Rozdzinsk E, Kern WV, Reichle A, et al. Once-daily versus thrice-daily dosing of netilmicin in combination with beta-lactam antibiotics as empirical therapy for febrile neutropenic patients. J Antimicrob Chemother. 1993;31:585-598.
349. Ibrahim S, Derde MP, Kaufman L, et al. Safety, pharmacokinetics and efficacy of once-a-day netilmicin and amikacin versus their conventional schedules in patients suffering from pelvic inflammatory disease. Ren Fail. 1990;12:199-203.
350. International Antimicrobial Therapy Cooperative Group of the European Organization for Research and Treatment of Cancer. Efficacy and toxicity of single daily doses of amikacin and ceftriaxone versus multiple daily doses of amikacin and ceftazidime for infection in patients with cancer and granulocytopenia. Ann Intern Med. 1993;199:584-593.
351. Maller R, Isaksson B, Nilsson L, et al. A study of amikacin given once versus twice daily in serious infections. J Antimicrob Chemother. 1998;22:75-79.
352. Blaser J, Simmen HP, Thrunheer U, et al. Nephrotoxicity, high frequency ototoxicity, efficacy and serum kinetics of once versus thrice daily dosing of netilmicin in patients with serious infections. J Antimicrob Chemother. 1995;36:803-814.
353. Koo J, Tight R, Rajkumar V, et al. Comparison of once-daily versus pharmacokinetic dosing of aminoglycosides in elderly patients. Am J Med. 1996;101:177-183.
354. Elhanan K, Siplovich L, Ra R. Gentamicin once-daily versus thrice-daily in children. J Antimicrob Chemother. 1995;35:327-332.
355. Gilbert DN, Lee BL, Dworkin RJ, et al. A randomized comparison of the safety and efficacy of once-daily gentamicin or thrice-daily gentamicin in combination with ticarcillin-clavulanate. Am J Med. 1998;105:182-191.
356. Bailey TC, Little JR, Littenberg B, et al. A meta-analysis of extended interval dosing versus multiple daily dosing of aminoglycosides. Clin Infect Dis. 1997;24:786-795.
357. Ali MZ, Goetz B. Meta-analysis of the relative efficacy and toxicity of once-daily versus multiple daily dosing of aminoglycosides. Clin Infect Dis. 1997;24:796-809.
358. Hatala R, Dinh TT, Cook DJ. Once-daily aminoglycoside dosing for immunocompromised adults: A systematic review. Clin Infect Dis. 1997;24:810-815.
359. Barza M, Ioannidis JPA, Cappelleri JC, et al. Single or multiple daily doses of aminoglycosides: A meta-analysis. BMJ. 1996;312:338-345.
360. Munckhof WJ, Grayson JL, Turnide JD. A meta-analysis of studies on the safety and efficacy of aminoglycosides given either once daily or as divided doses. J Antimicrob Chemother. 1996;37:645-663.
361. Hatala R, Dinh T, Cook DJ. Once-daily aminoglycoside dosing in immunocompetent adults: A meta-analysis. Ann Intern Med. 1996;124:717-725.
362. Galloe AM, Gaudal N, Christensen HR, et al. Aminoglycosides: Single or multiple daily dosing: A meta-analysis on efficacy and safety. Eur J Clin Pharmacol. 1995;48:39-43.

363. Ferriols-Lisart R, Alos-Alminana M. Effectiveness and safety of once-daily amino-glycosides: A meta-analysis. Am J Health Syst Pharm. 1996;53:1141-1150.

364. Vigano A, Principi N, Brivio L, et al. Comparison of 5 mg of netilmicin per kilo-gram of body weight once daily versus 2 mg per kilogram thrice for treatment of gram negative pyelonephritis in children. Antimicrob Agents Chemother. 1992;36:1499-1503.

365. Nicolau DP, Freeman CD, Bellineau PP, et al. Experience with a once-daily amino-glycoside program administered to 2184 adult patients. Antimicrob Agents Chemother. 1995;39:650-655.

366. Freeman CD, Nicolau DP, Belliveau PP, et al. Once-daily dosing of aminoglycosides: Review and recommendations for clinical practice. J Antimicrob Chemother. 1997;39:677-686.

367. Gilbert DN. Editorial response: Meta-analyses are no longer required for determining the efficacy of single daily dosing of aminoglycosides. Clin Infect Dis. 1997;24:816-819.

368. Thureen PJ, Reiter RD, Gresores A, et al. Once- versus twice-daily gentamicin dos-ing in neonates ≤ 34 weeks gestation: Cost-effectiveness analysis. Pediatrics 1999;103:594-598.

369. Rastogi A, Agarwal G, Pyati S, et al. Comparison of two gentamicin dosing sched-ules in very low birth weight infants. Pediatr Infect Dis. 2002;21:234-240.

370. Chattopadhyay B. Newborns and gentamicin—How much and how often? J Antimicrob Chemother. 2002;49:13-16.

371. Carapetis JR, Jaquiery AL, Buttery JP, et al. Randomized, controlled trial comparing once daily and three times daily gentamicin in children with urinary tract infections. Pediatr Infect Dis J. 2001;20:240-246.

372. Chong C-Y, Tan AS-L, Ng W, et al. Treatment of urinary tract infection with gen-tamicin once or three times daily. Acta Pediatr. 2003;92:291-296.

373. Akmed H, Paris MM, Trujillo M, et al. Once daily gentamicin therapy for experi-mental *Escherichia coli* meningitis. Antimicrob Agents Chemother. 1997;41:49-53.

374. Wong J, Brown G. Does once-daily dosing of aminoglycosides affect neuromuscular function? J Clin Pharm Ther. 1996;21:407-411.

375. Gilbert DN, Bennett WM. Use of antimicrobial agents in renal failure. Infect Dis Clin North Am. 1989;3:517-31.

376. Hickey SM, McCracken GH Jr. Antibacterial therapeutic agents. In: Feigin RD, Cherry JD, eds. Textbook of Pediatric Infectious Diseases. 4th ed., Philadelphia: WB Saunders; 1998:2614-2649.

377. Knoderer CA, Everett JA, Buss WF. Clinical issues surrounding once daily amino-glycoside dosing in children. Pharmacotherapy. 2003;23:44-56.

378. Avent ML, Kinney JS, Istre GR, et al. Gentamicin and tobramycin in neonates: Comparison of a new extended dosing interval regimen with a traditional multiple daily dosing regimen. Am J Perinatol. 2002;19:413-419.

379. Davis PB, Drumm M, Konstan MW. Cystic fibrosis. Am J Respir Crit Care Med. 1996;154:1229-56.

380. Howard M, Frizzell RA, Bedwell DM. Aminoglycoside antibiotics restore CFTR function by overcoming premature stop mutations. Nat Med. 1996;2:467-469.

381. Wilschanski M, Famini C, Blau H, et al. A pilot study of the effect of gentamicin on nasal potential difference measurements in cystic fibrosis patients carrying stop mu-tations. Am J Respir Crit Care Med. 2000;161:860-65.

382. Denton M, Wilcox MH. Antimicrobial treatment of pulmonary colonization and in-fection by *Pseudomonas aeruginosa* in cystic fibrosis patients. J Antimicrob Chemother. 1997;40:468-474.

383. Smith AL, Doershuk C, Goldman D, et al. Comparison of a β-lactam alone versus β-lactam and an aminoglycoside for pulmonary exacerbation in cystic fibrosis. J Pediatr. 1999;413-421.

384. Antibiotic Treatment for Cystic Fibrosis. Kent, England: Cystic Fibrosis Trust; September 2002.

385. Cochrane Database of Systematic Reviews. The Cochrane Collaboration; 2003. http://www.cochrane.org

386. Döreng G, Conway SP, Heijerman HGM, et al. Antibiotic therapy against *Pseudomonas aeruginosa* in cystic fibrosis: A European consensus. Eur Respir J. 2000;16:749-767.

387. Zebner R, Quinn JP. Antimicrobials in cystic fibrosis: Emergence of resistance and implications for treatment. Semin Respir Infect. 1992;7:210-7.

388. deGroot R, Smith AL. Antibiotic pharmacokinetics in cystic fibrosis: Differences and clinical significance. Clin Pharmacokinet. 1987;13:228-253.

389. Tan K, Bunn H. Once daily versus multiple daily dosing with intravenous aminogly-cosides for cystic fibrosis. Cochrane Database Syst Rev. 2000;(4):CD002009.

390. Tan KH, Mulheran M, Knox AJ, Smyth AR. Aminoglycoside prescribing and sur-veillance in cystic fibrosis. Am J Respir Crit Care Med. 2003;167:819-823.

391. Mulheran M, Degg C, Morgan DW, et al. The occurrence and risk of cochleotoxicity in cystic fibrosis patients receiving repeated high dose aminoglycoside therapy. Antimicrob Agents Chemother. 2001;45:2502-2509.

392. Ramsey BW, Dorkin HL, Eisenberg JD, et al. Efficacy of aerosolized tobramycin in patients with cystic fibrosis. N Engl J Med. 1993;328:1740-1746.

393. Package insert prescribing information for Tobramycin Solution for Inhalation. Pathogenesis Corporation, January 1998.

394. Ryan G, Mukhopadhyay S, Singh M. Nebulized anti-pseudomonal antibiotics for cys-tic fibrosis. Cochrane Database Syst Rev. 2003;(3):CD001021.

395. Touw DJ, Jacobs FAH, Brimicombe RW, et al. Pharmacokinetics of aerosolized to-bramycin in adult patients with cystic fibrosis. Antimicrob Agents Chemother. 1997;41:184-187.

396. Graham JC, Gould FK. Role of aminoglycosides in the treatment of bacterial endo-carditis. J Antimicrob Chemother. 2002;49:437-444.

397. Keane WF, Everett ED, Golper TA, et al. Peritoneal dialysis related peritonitis treat-ment recommendations. 2000 update. Perit Dial Int. 2000;20:396-411.

Tetracyclines and Chloramphenicol

BURT MEYERS
MIRELLA SALVATORE

TETRACYCLINES

Tetracyclines are a class of broad-spectrum bacteriostatic antibiotics active against gram-positive and gram-negative bacteria as well as against intracellular organisms such as chlamydiae, mycoplasma, rick-ettsiae, and protozoan parasites. These characteristics, together with the low cost and the paucity of major side effects—except in children and pregnant women—have made the tetracyclines a widely used class of antibiotics. Moreover, the discovery that tetracyclines can be used as growth promoters has resulted in their use in animal feeds.[1] Since the 1970s, the identification of an increasing number of tetracycline-resistant pathogens has limited their usefulness in clinical practice. However, a new generation that retains the broad spectrum of activity and is also active against resistant bacteria is being developed.

History and Classification of Tetracyclines

The first tetracyclines were discovered in the 1950s by screening or-ganisms obtained from the soil for their antimicrobial properties. Benjamin M. Duggar found that an organism (*Streptomyces aureofa-ciens*) produced an antimicrobial product that he named Aureomycin (chlortetracycline). Oxytetracycline was derived in 1950, and tetracy-cline was produced by the catalytic dehalogenation of chlortetracy-cline in 1953. Tetracycline, chlortetracycline, and oxytetracycline are short-lasting compounds, and demeclocycline and methacycline are intermediate acting. In the late 1960s, a second generation of long-acting compounds, doxycycline (in 1966) and minocycline (in 1967), were semisynthetically derived. Finally, during the early 1990s, to overcome the problem of growing resistance to earlier compounds, a third generation of tetracyclines, the glycylcyclines, was developed. Glycylcyclines are minocycline derivatives with a specific modifica-tion in position 9 that have the antibacterial effects of tetracyclines even in resistant strains.[2,3] The clinical candidate of the class is tigecy-cline (GAR-936), the long-acting 9-*t*-butylglycylamido derivative of minocycline that is currently undergoing clinical trials.[4,5]

Tetracycline molecules are composed of a hydronaphthacene nu-cleus containing four fused rings, to which a variety of functional groups are attached. The simplest tetracycline with antibacterial activ-ity is 6-deoxy-6-demethyltetracycline. The generic names of the ana-logues are determined by the substitutions on the basic structure of tetracycline (Fig. 25-1). Table 25-1 lists the tetracyclines currently available in the United States and their dosages. Tetracycline HCl and doxycycline have emerged as the most useful clinically. Chlortetracycline (Aureomycin) is no longer available except for top-ical use, and methacycline (Rondomycin) has been withdrawn from the market.

Mechanism of Action

Tetracyclines inhibit bacterial protein synthesis by binding the 30S ri-bosomal subunit. The binding to the ribosome is reversible, explaining the bacteriostatic nature of these compounds. This binding blocks the association of the aminoacyl-transfer RNA to the acceptor site on the messenger RNA–ribosome complex,[6] thus preventing the addition of new amino acids into the growing peptide chain. Tetracyclines enter the outer membrane of gram-negative bacteria by passive diffusion

This chapter is based, in part, on the chapter prepared by Dr. H. C. Standiford for the 5th edition.

FIGURE 25-1. Structures of the tetracyclines. *(From Chopra I. New developments in tetracycline antibiotics: Glycylcyclines and tetracyclines efflux pump inhibitors. Drug Resist Updat. 2002;5:119-125).*

Name
(date of discovery)

7-chlortetracycline
(1948)

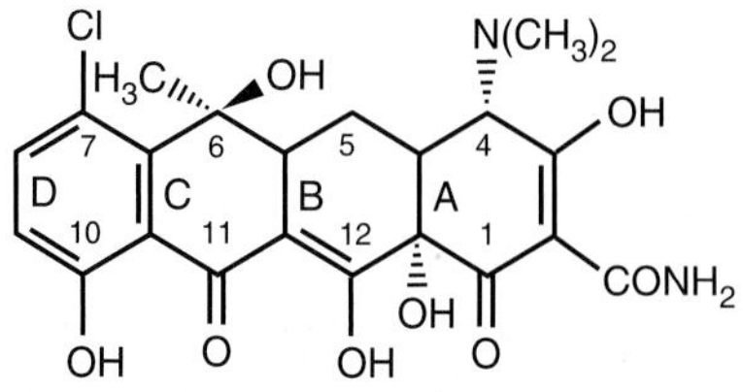

Tetracycline
(1953)

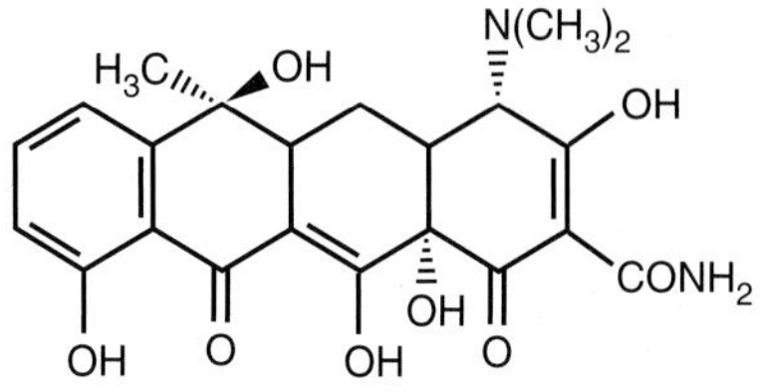

7-dimethylamino 6-demethyl-
6-deoxy-tetracycline
(minocycline)
(1973)

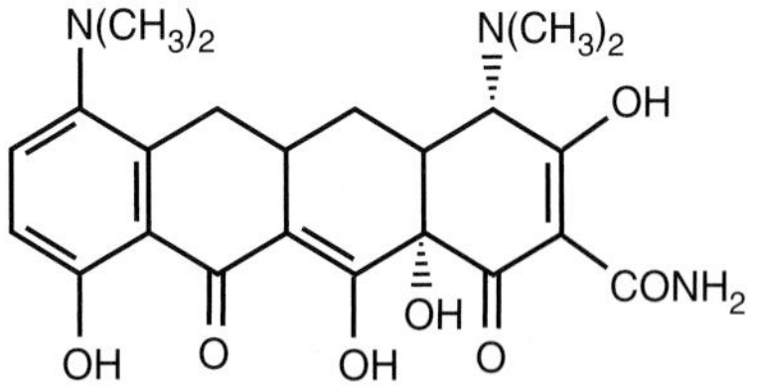

9-(*N,N*-dimethylglycylamido)-
6-demethyl-6-
deoxytetracycline
(1993)

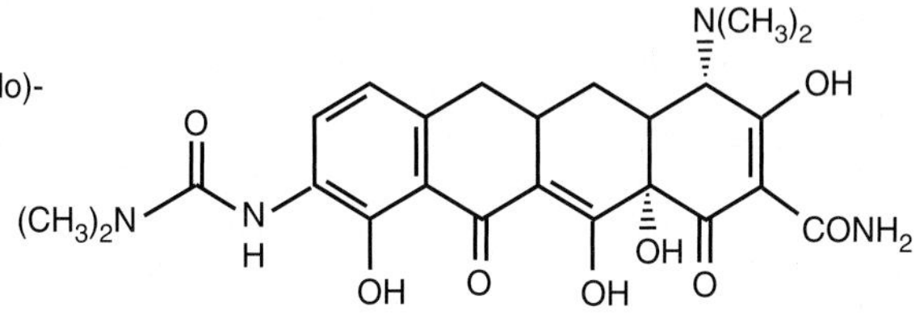

9-(*N,N*-dimethylglycylamido)-
minocycline
(1993)

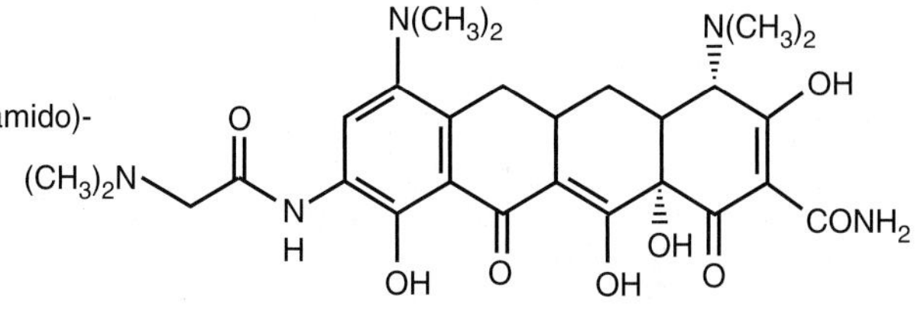

9-(*t*-butylglycylamido)-
minocycline (GAR-936)
(1993)

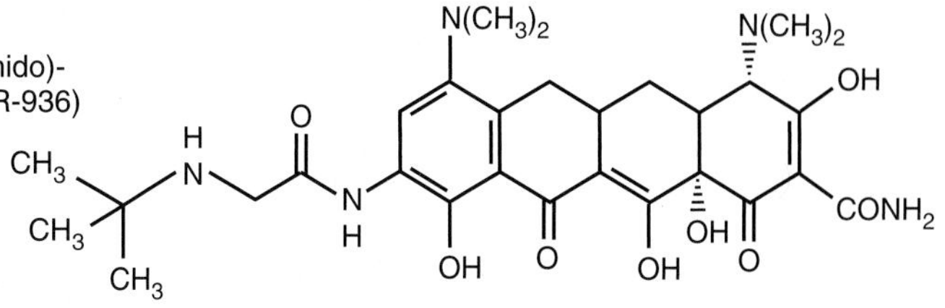

through porin channels OmpF and OmpC, probably as positively charged molecules associated with magnesium. Once in the periplasmic space, the complex dissociates and tetracyclines enter the inner membrane by diffusion (tetracyclines are lipophilic). Similarly, the lipophilic form enters the cytoplasmic space of gram-positive bacteria driven by a process dependent on the ΔpH.[7]

The tetracyclines have a high affinity for bacterial ribosomal subunit 30S. The interaction with the 80S ribosomal subunit of eukaryotes is very weak, explaining the absence of accumulation and toxic effects in eukaryotes.[8] Tetracyclines also inhibit mitochondrial protein synthesis by binding the 70S ribosome subunits in mitochondria, which has been cited to help explain the efficacy of tetracyclines in eukary-

otic parasites. However, the antiprotozoan activity is retained also in other organisms that do not have mitochondria. The mechanism of this activity is still unknown.

Spectrum of Activity In Vitro

The antimicrobial spectra of all the tetracyclines are almost identical, but some differences in the degree of activity against different organisms do exist among the analogues. However, it is recommended (for cost reasons) that the clinical microbiology laboratory use tetracycline to evaluate susceptibility for all the analogues.[9] Minimal inhibitory concentrations of tetracycline, minocycline, and tigecycline for selected bacteria are given in Table 25-2.

TABLE 25-1 Tetracycline Formulations Currently Available in the United States

Generic Name	Major Brand Name (Company)	Oral Preparations	Usual Adult Oral Dosage	Notes
Short-Acting				
Oxytetracycline	Terramycin (Pfizer)	Capsules: 125, 250 mg Syrup: 125 mg/5 mL	500 mg q6h	No longer widely used
Tetracycline HCl	—	Capsules: 250, 500 mg Syrup: 125 mg/5 mL	500 mg q6h	—
Intermediate-Acting				
Demeclocycline HCl	Declomycin (Wyeth)	Tablets: 150, 300 mg	300 mg q12h	Used for SIADH
Long-Acting				
Doxycycline	Vibramycin (Pfizer)	Capsules (hyclate): 50, 100 mg Tablets: 50, 100 mg Syrup (calcium): 50 mg/5 mL Syrup (monohydrate): 25 mg/5 mL	200 mg (or 100 mg q12h) for first day, then 100 mg q24h	—
Minocycline	Minocin (Wyeth)	Capsules and tablets: 50, 100 mg Suspension: 50 mg/5 mL	200 mg, then 100 mg q12h	—
Long-Acting, Third-Generation				
Tigecycline	(Wyeth)	NA	NA	Investigational

SIADH, syndrome of inappropriate antidiuretic hormone.

Although many aerobic and facultative anaerobic organisms are within the spectrum of the first and second generation of tetracyclines, more effective agents are available for the treatment of infections caused by most of these bacteria. However, the data available on tigecycline, the last generation of tetracyclines, look quite promising.[5,10-19] Pneumococci and *Haemophilus influenzae* can be inhibited by concentrations of tetracyclines achieved in the serum, and this provides a rationale for their use in sinusitis and acute exacerbations of chronic bronchitis.[20] Pneumococci resistant to penicillin are generally more resistant to tetracyclines; doxycycline is the more active congener available on the market.[16,17,21] Gonococci and meningococci are extremely susceptible; unfortunately, gonococci resistant to penicillin G also tend to be resistant to tetracycline.[18,22-24] In most cases, *Escherichia coli* acquired outside the hospital setting can be inhibited by concentrations achieved in the urine, if not the serum. Tetracycline, therefore, is a useful agent for the treatment of acute, uncomplicated urinary tract infections and the acute urethral syndrome. *Pseudomonas pseudomallei* is generally sensitive, and this has therapeutic importance, as does the high degree of susceptibility of *Brucella* species.[25] *Vibrio cholerae, Vibrio vulnificus,* and other vibrios are generally susceptible; tetracyclines are important therapeutic agents for diseases caused by this group of organisms.[26] Although *Campylobacter* species are generally susceptible, a high percentage of resistant isolates has been noted in some countries.[27] Therefore, it is not the drug of choice for infections caused by these bacteria. *Shigella* organisms have become increasingly resistant.[28] *Mycobacterium marinum* is susceptible and appears to respond clinically.[19]

The tetracyclines have activity against many anaerobic organisms (Table 25-3).[15,29] Their activity against *Actinomyces* is relevant clinically.[17] Doxycycline is more active against *Bacteroides fragilis* than tetracycline is, but other classes are preferred for infections caused by this organism. The activity of the tetracyclines against anaerobic bacteria, however, may be partially responsible for the effectiveness of the neomycin-tetracycline combination and doxycycline alone as alternative oral presurgical bowel preparations.[30,31] Many pathogenic spirochetes are susceptible, including *Borrelia burgdorferi,* the agent of Lyme disease.[32] Other organisms generally inhibited by this group of antibiotics include rickettsiae, chlamydiae, mycoplasmas, and, to a limited degree, protozoans (*Plasmodium* spp. and *Entamoeba histolytica*).[33]

Tigecycline has potent in vitro activity against a wide variety of clinical isolates (see Tables 25-2 and 25-3), including organisms resistant to older tetracyclines, vancomycin-resistant *Enterococcus* (VRE), methicillin-resistant *Staphylococcus aureus* (MRSA), and resistant pneumococci, but with the exception of *Proteus mirabilis* and indole-positive *Proteus* species. The efficacy in vivo correlates to the activity in vitro, and tigecycline is effective against lethal infections caused by *E. coli, Klebsiella pneumoniae, S. aureus, Streptococcus pneumoniae,* and *Enterococcus faecium* in mice.

Mechanisms of Resistance

The widespread use of tetracycline, both for human therapy in and animal feeds to promote growth, has been followed in recent years by an increased number of resistant strains.[1] This resistance is mediated by the acquisition of genes on mobile elements. Thirty-three different genes of tetracycline resistance have been identified, 29 of them belonging to the tetracycline *(tet)* family and three belonging to the oxytetracycline resistance gene family *(otr).* In some rare cases, resistance is caused by point mutations in ribosomal RNA (e.g., in propionibacteria) or by the activity of innate bacterial efflux proteins that confer resistance to multiple antibiotics including tetracyclines.[7] Moreover, low levels of resistance can also result from mutations or from a decrease in the porin content of the outer membrane, with consequent decreased tetracycline uptake.[7]

The tetracycline resistance genes code for proteins that confer resistance by two main mechanisms: efflux pump or ribosomal protection, or sometimes both. In addition, resistance to tetracyclines may be mediated by enzymatic inactivation; this mechanism is known only for the product of the resistance gene *tet*(X). The *tet*(X) gene, found only in *Bacteroides,* codes for a protein that in the presence of NADPH and O_2 modifies tetracyclines.[34] The mechanisms of resistance for the products of the genes *tet*(U) and *otr*(C) have not been determined. The distribution of *tet* resistance genes among gram-negative bacteria, along with their mechanism of resistance, can be found in Table 25-4.

Efflux pumps are membrane-associated proteins that export tetracyclines from the cell, reducing the intracellular concentrations and therefore making them ineffective. Most of them confer resistance to the earlier tetracyclines but not to the second-generation doxycycline and minocycline. These proteins can be found in both gram-positive and gram-negative bacteria (Tables 25-5 and 25-6). Six different classes of efflux proteins have been described on the basis of their amino acid sequence identity.[35] Group 1 is found in gram-negative species, except for Tet C. These proteins have similarities with other efflux proteins involved in multidrug, chloramphenicol, and quinolone resistance. Group 2 includes Tet K and Tet L and is mainly found in gram-positive bacteria. (Information on efflux proteins can be found in refs. 7 and 35.)

TABLE 25-2 Minimal Inhibitory Concentrations (MICs) of Tetracyclines for Common Bacteria and Nontuberculous Mycobacteria

Organism (No. of Isolates Tested)	Antibiotic	MIC (µg/mL) Range	MIC (µg/mL) 50%	MIC (µg/mL) 90%
Staphylococcus aureus (methicillin sensitive) (639)	Tetracycline	0.25-128	128	128
	Minocycline	0.03-0.12	0.12	0.12
	Tigecycline	≤0.06-0.5	0.25	0.25
S. aureus (methicillin resistant) (504)	Tetracycline	0.25-128	128	128
	Minocycline	0.03-16	4	8
	Tigecycline	≤0.06-1	0.25	0.5
Enterococcus faecalis (vancomycin resistant) (45)	Tetracycline	0.25-128	32	64
	Minocycline	≤0.06-32	2	8
	Tigecycline	0.03-0.25	0.12	0.12
Enterococcus faecium (vancomycin resistant) (81)	Tetracycline	0.25-128	16	128
	Minocycline	≤0.06-16	0.12	8
	Tigecycline	0.015-0.25	0.06	0.125
Streptococcus pneumoniae (penicillin resistant) (303)	Tetracycline	<0.016-0.125	0.06	0.125
	Minocycline	<0.25-128	32	64
	Tigecycline	<0.016-0.125	0.06	0.125
S. pneumoniae (penicillin susceptible) (201)	Tetracycline	<0.016-64	0.25	32
	Minocycline	<0.06-16	0.06	8
	Tigecycline	<0.016-0.125	0.03	0.125
Haemophilus influenzae (319)	Tetracycline	0.25-4	0.5	1
	Minocycline	0.25-4	0.5	1
	Tigecycline	0.25-4	1	2
Escherichia coli (243)	Tetracycline	0.5->128	>128	>128
	Minocycline	0.25-128	8	16
	Tigecycline	0.06-2	0.25	0.5
Enterobacter cloacae (149)	Tetracycline	2->128	16	>128
	Minocycline	2->128	4	128
	Tigecycline	0.25-32	2	4
Klebsiella pneumoniae (279)	Tetracycline	1->128	4	>128
	Minocycline	0.25-128	8	16
	Tigecycline	0.5-16	0.5	2
Shigella (26)	Tetracycline	1->32	>32	>32
	Minocycline	0.16-0.25	2	4
	Tigecycline	0.12-1	0.25	0.5
Pseudomonas aeruginosa (195)	Tetracycline	1-128	16	62
	Minocycline	2-128	128	128
	Tigecycline	4-32	16	32
Mycobacterium fortuitum (10)	Tetracycline	16-64	16	32
	Minocycline	2->64	32	32
	Tigecycline	≤0.06-0.12	≤0.06	≤0.12
Mycobacterium abscessus (18)	Tetracycline	32->128	128	>128
	Minocycline	0.25->64	>64	>64
	Tigecycline	<0.06-1	≤0.12	0.25
Mycobacterium chelonae (22)	Tetracycline	16-128	32	>128
	Minocycline	2->64	16	>64
	Tigecycline	≤0.06-0.12	≤0.06	≤0.12

Data adapted from references 5, 10-14, 16-18, 29.

The ribosomal protection proteins (RPPs) are cytoplasmic proteins that protect the ribosome from the action of both first- and second-generation tetracyclines, thereby conferring a wider spectrum of resistance than the efflux proteins. RPPs release tetracyclines from their target site by a GDP-dependent mechanism.[7,8] The binding to the ribosome determines a conformational modification that prevents tetracycline binding without interfering with protein synthesis. RPPs are found mainly in gram-positive bacteria and in some nonenteric gram-negative bacteria and anaerobes (see Tables 25-5 and 25-6).

A large majority of bacterial strains isolated from hospital-acquired infections carry one, and in some cases two, tetracycline resistance genes. To restore the therapeutic utility of tetracyclines against resistant strains, another generation of tetracyclines, the glycylcycline derivatives, has been developed. These drugs and tigecycline are active against bacterial strains carrying both efflux pump and ribosomal protection proteins.[36,37] Glycylcyclines have higher binding affinities for the ribosome than earlier agents, overcoming the ribosomal protection mechanism of resistance.[38] Tet efflux mechanisms, however, may not recognize the glycylcycline or may not be able to export the new analogue across the membrane.[39] At present, resistance has not been seen to tigecycline, but resistant strains may emerge with clinical use of the drug. Recently, an increased frequency of mutations, up to 1000-fold higher than normal, in bacterial strains such as *E. coli, Pseudomonas aeruginosa, Neisseria meningitidis,* and *Helicobacter pylori* has been found. In some cases, these hypermutators account for up to 20% of clinical isolates.[39] These strains constitute a new concern and may be responsible for increasing antibiotic resistance.

Future attempts to prevent resistance include the development of efflux pump inhibitors, but this is complicated by the existence of different classes of efflux proteins and the simultaneous presence of efflux and ribosomal resistance systems.

Interestingly, no tetracycline resistance has yet been described in protozoa. A possible explanation may be the relatively limited use of tetracyclines as antiprotozoan agents. Also, for the obligate intracellular pathogens *Chlamydia* and *Rickettsia,* no resistant strains have been described in humans. However, tetracycline-resistant strains of *Chlamydia suis* have been described in pigs that were given low doses of tetracyclines in their feed.

TABLE 25-3 In Vitro Activity of Tetracyclines against Selected Anaerobic and Atypical Isolates

Organism (No. of Isolates Tested)	Antibiotic	MIC (μg/mL)		
		Range	50%	90%
Bacteroides spp. (425)	Minocycline	≤0.06-8	8	8
	Tigecycline	0.015-32	1	4
Clostridium perfringens (30)	Tetracycline	0.032-32	0.064	8
	Minocycline	≤0.06	0.016	0.125
	Tigecycline	0.032-2	0.032	0.25
Clostridium difficile (50)	Tetracycline	0.064-8	0.064	0.125
	Minocycline	0.008-4	0.032	0.032
	Tigecycline	0.016-0.032	0.032	0.032
Chlamydophila pneumoniae (10)				
	Doxycycline	<0.06-2	0.25	0.25
	Tigecycline	0.12-0.25	0.12	0.12
Fusobacterium spp. (16)	Tetracycline	0.015-1	0.25	0.25
	Doxycycline	0.015-0.125	0.06	0.125
	Minocycline	0.015-0.125	0.06	0.06
	Tigecycline	0.015-0.06	0.03	0.06
Mycoplasma pneumoniae (30)	Tetracycline	0.5-2	0.5	1
	Minocycline	0.25-1	0.5	1
	Tigecycline	0.06-0.25	0.12	0.25
Prevotella spp. (19)	Tetracycline	0.125-16	0.25	16
	Minocycline	0.03-8	0.06	8
	Doxycycline	0.06-8	0.125	8
	Tigecycline	0.06-0.25	0.125	0.25

Data adapted from references 5, 10, 13-15, 29.

Pharmacology

Absorption of Tetracyclines

Absorption occurs primarily in the proximal small bowel and produces peak serum concentrations 1 to 3 hours after administration. Some of the pharmacokinetic properties of the tetracyclines are compared in Table 25-7.[40-45] Thrombophlebitis is a frequent complication of the intravenous preparations. Intramuscular preparations are available for the short-acting compounds but are not recommended because of the severe pain produced on injection even when mixed with local anesthetics.

The high levels obtained orally with tetracycline compared with other short-acting agents are primarily the result of better absorption from the gastrointestinal tract. The long-acting analogues doxycycline and minocycline are highly bioavailable (taken with or without food);

TABLE 25-4 Mechanisms of Resistance to Tetracyclines for Characterized *tet* and *otr* Genes

Mechanism	Genes
Efflux	tet(A), tet(B), tet(C), tet(D), tet(E), tet(G), tet(H), tet(I), tet(J), tet(Z), tet(30),* tet(31)*
	tet(K), tet(L)
	otr(B), tcr3
	tetP(A)
	tet(V)
	tet(Y)
Ribosomal protection	tet(M), tet(O), tet(S), tet(W)
	tet(Q), tet(T)
	otr(A), tetP(B),† tet
Enzymatic	tet(X)
Unknown‡	tet(U), otr(C)

*The first numbered genes.
†The *tet*P(B) gene is not found alone, and *tet*P(A) and *tet*P(B) are counted as one gene.
‡The *tet*(U) gene has been sequenced but does not appear to be related to either efflux or ribosomal protection proteins; *otr*(C) has not been sequenced.
From Chopra I, Roberts M. Tetracycline antibiotics: Mode of action, applications, molecular biology, and epidemiology of bacterial resistance. Microbiol Mol Biol Rev. 2001;65:232-260, with permission. Genes are grouped according to McMurry LM, Levy SB. Tetracycline resistance in gram-positive bacteria, In: Fischetti VA, Novick RP, Ferretti JJ, et al, eds. Gram-Positive Pathogens. Washington, DC: American Society for Microbiology; 2000:660-677.

in contrast, tetracycline bioavailability can be decreased up to 50% if taken with food. The absorption of all the tetracyclines can be reduced by the concomitant administration of multivalent cations (e.g., calcium, iron, and magnesium), which chelate the tetracyclines and prevent or decrease their absorption. Some data suggest that the absorption of doxycycline may be unaffected by administration of cations.[45]

The tetracyclines can be differentiated into three groups on the basis of their half-lives. Doxycycline has the longest half-life, allowing therapeutic levels to be maintained with a single daily dose, although twice-daily regimens are frequently recommended. The 8-hour half-life of tetracycline suggests that its dosage interval could be 8 hours when it is used to treat minor infections.[44] Half-lives of most of these compounds are determined mainly by the rate of excretion by the kidneys. Chlortetracycline is an exception: it has a short half-life despite a slow rate of clearance as a result of its marked instability in vitro as well as in vivo.[44]

Pharmacokinetic studies after intravenous administration in mice demonstrated a dose-dependent maximum serum concentration of tigecycline between 0.42 μg/mL (for a dose of 3 μg/kg) and 11.1 μg/mL (for a dose of 48 μg/kg) and a serum protein binding of 59%. These data and data from healthy human volunteers support the possibility of daily therapeutic administration in humans of 300 mg intravenously.[46,47]

Adequate therapeutic concentrations of all the tetracyclines, with the possible exception of chlortetracycline and minocycline, are achieved in the urine for the treatment of urinary tract infections caused by sensitive organisms. The degree of protein binding of the analogues varies with the method used for the determination, but it tends to be greater for the intermediate- and long-acting compounds. This may be one of the factors that determine their slow rate of renal excretion. The apparent volume of distribution for most of the tetracyclines is greater than that of extracellular body water, indicating sequestration in tissues, presumably the liver.[44] Minocycline and doxycycline have the smallest volume of distribution, another factor that tends to enhance their serum levels.

Tissue Distribution

The tetracyclines can be found in small amounts in many tissues and fluids, including the lung, liver, kidney, brain, sputum, and mucosal fluid (see Table 25-7). For tetracycline, levels in the cerebral spinal fluid are approximately 10% to 26% of the serum levels,[48,49] whereas concentrations in synovial fluid and the maxillary sinus mucosa approach serum levels.[50,51] All the tetracyclines are concen-

TABLE 25-5 **Distribution of *tet* Resistance Genes among Gram-Negative Bacteria**

Efflux Pump				Ribosomal Protection* and/or Efflux Pump			
One Gene		Two or More Genes		One Gene		Two or More Genes	
Genus	Gene	Genus	Genes	Genus	Gene	Genus	Genes
Actinobacillus	*tet*(B)	*Edwardsiella*	*tet*(A), *tet*(D)	*Eikenella*	*tet*(M)	*Butyrivibrio*†	*tet*(O), *tet*(W)
Erwinia	*tet*(B)	*Providencia*	*tet*(B), *tet*(E), *tet*(I)	*Kingella*	*tet*(M)	*Mitsuokella*†	*tet*(Q), *tet*(W)
Moraxella	*tet*(B)	*Plesiomonas*	*tet*(A), *tet*(B), *tet*(D)	*Neisseria*	*tet*(M)	*Selenomonas*†	*tet*(Q), *tet*(W)
Pantoea	*tet*(B)	*Enterobacter*	*tet*(B), *tet*(C), *tet*(D)	*Campylobacter*	*tet*(O)	*Porphyromonas*†	*tet*(Q), *tet*(W)
Treponema‡	*tet*(B)	*Mannheimia*	*tet*(B), *tet*(G), *tet*(H)	*Capnocytophaga*†	*tet*(Q)	*Bacteroides*†	*tet*(M), *tet*(Q), *tet*(X)
Yersinia	*tet*(D)	*Proteus*	*tet*(A), *tet*(B), *tet*(C), *tet*(J)				
				Prevotella†	*tet*(Q)	*Fusobacterium*†	*tet*(L), *tet*(M), *tet*(W)
Alcaligenes	*tet*(E)	*Pseudomonas*	*tet*(A), *tet*(C), *tet*(E), *tet*(G)			*Haemophilus*	*tet*(B), *tet*(K), *tet*(M)
Eubacterium†	*tet*(K)	*Serratia*	*tet*(A), *tet*(B), *tet*(C), *tet*(E)			*Veillonella*†	*tet*(L), *tet*(M), *tet*(Q)
Agrobacterium	*tet*(30)§	*Citrobacter*	*tet*(A), *tet*(B), *tet*(C), *tet*(D)			*Pasteurella*	*tet*(B), *tet*(D), *tet*(H), *tet*(G), *tet*(M)
		Klebsiella	*tet*(A), *tet*(B), *tet*(C), *tet*(D)				
		Shigella	*tet*(A), *tet*(B), *tet*(C), *tet*(D)				
		Salmonella	*tet*(A), *tet*(B), *tet*(C), *tet*(D), *tet*(G)				
		Aeromonas	*tet*(A), *tet*(B), *tet*(D), *tet*(E), *tet*				
		Vibrio	*tet*(A), *tet*(B), *tet*(C), *tet*(D), *tet*(E), *tet*(G)				
		Escherichia	*tet*(A), *tet*(B), *tet*(C), *tet*(D), *tet*(E), *tet*(I), *tet*(Y)				

*Ribosomal protection genes have not yet been found in enteric genera, and when these genes are cloned into *E. coli,* the level of resistance conferred is relatively low.

†Anaerobic species.

‡*T. denticola* is anaerobic, but not all species in the genus are anaerobes.

§Beginning with this gene, designations are numerals.

From Chopra I, Roberts M. Tetracycline antibiotics: Mode of actions, applications, molecular biology and epidemiology of bacterial resistance. Microbiol Mol Biol Rev. 2001;65:232-260, with permission.

trated in unobstructed bile and produce levels in this fluid 5 to 20 times those obtained in the serum. It has been suggested that lipid solubility is a primary determinant for the diffusion in many tissues. Minocycline is about five times more lipophilic at a physiologic pH than tetracycline, and it is followed by doxycycline. This may explain why minocycline reaches sufficient concentrations in saliva and tears to eradicate the meningococcal carrier state, whereas the other tetracyclines do not.[52]

Crossing the Placenta and Excretion in Breast Milk

The tetracyclines cross the placenta and achieve concentrations in umbilical cord plasma and amniotic fluid of 60% and 20% of the levels in the maternal circulation, respectively. They accumulate in fetal bone and teeth and therefore should not be given during pregnancy. They are excreted in breast milk; however, they form an insoluble complex with calcium, and their concentrations in the infant's serum are below detectability.

TABLE 25-6 **Distribution of Tetracycline Resistance Genes among Gram-Positive (and Other) Bacteria**

One Determinant		Two Determinants		Three or More Determinants	
Genus	Gene	Genus	Genes	Genus	Genes
Abiotrophia	*tet*(M)	*Actinomyces*	*tet*(L), *tet*(M)	*Eubacterium*	*tet*(K), *tet*(M), *tet*(Q)
Bacterionema	*tet*(M)	*Aerococcus*	*tet*(M), *tet*(O)	*Bacillus*	*tet*(K), *tet*(L), *tet*(M)
Gemella	*tet*(M)	*Bifidobacterium*	*tet*(M), *tet*(W)	*Listeria*	*tet*(K), *tet*(L), *tet*(M), *tet*(S)
Mycoplasma	*tet*(M)	*Gardnerella*	*tet*(M), *tet*(Q)	*Staphylococcus*	*tet*(K), *tet*(L), *tet*(M), *tet*(O)
Ureaplasma	*tet*(M)	*Lactobacillus*	*tet*(O), *tet*(Q)	*Clostridium*	*tet*(K), *tet*(L), *tet*(M), *tet*(P), *tet*(Q)
Nocardia	*tet*(K)	*Mobiluncus*	*tet*(O), *tet*(Q)	*Peptostreptococcus*	*tet*(K), *tet*(L), *tet*(M), *tet*(O), *tet*(Q)
		Corynebacterium	*tet*(M), *tet*(Z)	*Enterococcus*	*tet*(K), *tet*(L), *tet*(M), *tet*(O), *tet*(S), *tet*(U)
				Streptococcus	*tet*(K), *tet*(L), *tet*(M), *tet*(O), *tet*(Q), *tet*(T)
				Mycobacterium	*tet*(K), *tet*(L), *tet*(V), *otr*(A), *otr*(B)
				Streptomyces	*tet*(K), *tet*(L), *otr*(A), *otr*(B), *otr*(C), *tcr*3,* *tet**

*The *tet* and *tcr* genes have not been given number designations.

From Chopra I, Roberts M. Tetracycline antibiotics: Mode of actions, applications, molecular biology and epidemiology of bacterial resistance. Microbiol Mol Biol Rev. 2001;65:232-260, with permission.

TABLE 25-7 Pharmacologic Properties of Tetracyclines

	Tetracycline	Doxycycline	Minocycline
Serum drug concentrations	500 mg PO q6h: 4-5 µg/mL 250 mg PO q6h: 2-2.5 µg/mL	200 mg PO q24h: 4.4 µg/mL	200 mg PO in 1 dose followed by 100 mg PO bid: 2.3-3.5 µg/mL
Cmax	PO: 4 µg/mL after a 500-mg dose IV: 8 µg/mL	PO: 3 µg/mL after a 200-mg dose for nonfasting adults 5.0-5.4 µg/mL for fasting adults IV: 5-10 µg/mL after a 200-mg dose	PO: 2.1 to 5.1 (2 × 100 mg) PO: 0.74 (capsule) IV: 2.52-6.63 (200 mg)
Time to peak	Oral: 1.5-4 hr	Oral: 1.5-4 hr	Oral: 1.5-4 hr
Protein binding	20%-67%	80%-93%	76%
Bioavailability	60%-80% when taken on an empty stomach Food may reduce absorption by 50%.	90%-100% absorbed in fasting adults. Food or milk may reduce absorption by 20%, but effect not clinically significant.	90%-100% absorbed in fasting adults. Food or milk may reduce absorption by 20%, but effect not clinically significant.
Tissue distribution	**Excellent** Periodontal tissue **Good** Pleural fluid Ascitic fluid Synovial fluid Maxillary sinuses **Moderate** Sputum **Poor** Tears Saliva CNS (one tenth of serum concentration)	Doxycycline is more lipophilic than tetracycline and penetrates into most body tissues. **Excellent** Sinuses **Good** Peritoneal fluid, 75% Gingival fluid Bronchial secretions Tears Saliva Lung tissue **Moderate** Prostatic tissue 60% CNS Aqueous humor **Poor** Pleural fluid 25% Bone Skin Sputum	Minocycline is more lipophilic than doxycycline and penetrates body tissue better than all other tetracyclines. **Excellent** Prostate Uterus Ovaries Fallopian tubes Skin Sinuses Gingival fluid **Good/moderate** Aqueous humor Thyroid Lung Liver Intestinal tract Gallbladder/bile Tears Saliva Sputum (60% of serum levels) **Poor** CNS (noninflamed meninges; better than all other tetracyclines)
Volume of distribution	108 L	50 L	60 L
Metabolism	Liver: minimal	Liver: approximately 50% metabolized	Liver: principally metabolized to six inactive metabolites
Elimination	Kidney: 60% unchanged Bile: up to 10-25 times the concentration found in serum	Kidney: 20%-30% Feces: 70%-80% Bile: 14 µg/mL	Kidney: 10%-13% Feces: 19% Bile: 76 µg/mL
Elimination t$_{1/2}$	6-12 hr	15-24 hr	11-22 hr
Pregnancy category	Pregnancy category D* Crosses the placenta May cause inhibition of bone growth	Pregnancy category D* Crosses the placenta May cause inhibition of bone growth	Pregnancy category D* Crosses the placenta May cause inhibition of bone growth
Breastfeeding	Penetrates well into breast milk	Penetrates well into breast milk	Penetrates well into breast milk

*Positive evidence of human fetal risk but maternal benefits may outweigh fetal risk in serious or life-threatening situations.
Data from references 42-44, 48-51, 73.

Routes of Elimination

Routes of elimination differ for the drugs of this class. Tetracycline is eliminated in the urine via glomerular filtration. Minocycline is metabolized by the liver to inactive metabolites, and only 10% to 13% is excreted by the kidney, and a very small quantity appears in the feces; however, there is no drug accumulation in hepatic diseases. Doxycycline is eliminated mainly in the feces (70% to 80%) and the remainder is eliminated in the urine by glomerular filtration.

Renal and Hepatic Insufficiency

Except for doxycycline, the tetracyclines should not be used in patients with renal failure. Doxycycline's pharmacokinetics, half-life, and therapeutic levels do not vary with alterations in renal function.[53] The tetracyclines are slowly removed by hemodialysis but not effectively by peritoneal dialysis. Administration of tetracycline in patients with altered renal function can result in accumulation of the active drug and hepatotoxicity. Hepatic disease is not known to cause elevated serum levels of the tetracyclines. However, they should be used very cautiously in such situations, because they have been noted to cause hepatic toxicity. For dosages in patients with decreased renal function, see Table 25-8.

Toxicity

Side effects to tetracyclines are listed in Table 25-9.

Allergy, Photosensitivity, and Pigmentation Changes

Hypersensitivity reactions, including anaphylaxis, urticaria, periorbital edema, fixed drug eruptions, and morbilliform rashes, occur with tetracyclines but are not common.[54] A patient who is allergic to one analogue should be considered to be allergic to all. A number of recent reports describe a systemic lupus erythematosus–like syndrome seen in association with minocycline. These patients have antinuclear antibody. Symptoms disappear in most patients when the antibiotic is discontinued and recur with rechallenge.[55-57] Photosensitivity reactions (a red rash on areas exposed to sunlight, frequently associated with onycholysis) are most common in patients receiving demeclocycline but occur with all analogues.[58] They appear to be a toxic rather than an allergic reaction. Prolonged administration of minocycline has been noted rarely to cause nail, skin, and scleral pigmentation, which is usually reversible, as well as an asymptomatic black pigmentation of the thyroid.[59,60] A blue or blue-black discoloration of the gums has also been reported; this appears to be secondary to bone pigmen-

TABLE 25-8 Dosages of Tetracyclines for Patients with Decreased Renal Function

Drug	CrCl > 50 mL/min	CrCl 10-50 mL/min	CrCl < 10 mL/min	HD	PD	CVVH CAVH
Tetracycline	250-500 mg IV q8-12h	250-500 mg q12 to q24h	Not recommended In patients with ESRD, tetracyclines result in liver toxicity.	Not recommended	Not recommended	Not recommended
Demeclocycline	150-300 mg q12 to q24h	Avoid	Avoid	Avoid	Avoid	Avoid
Doxycycline	100 mg IV/PO q12h	No adjustment	No adjustment	No adjustment	No adjustment	No adjustment
Minocycline	200 mg IV once, then 100 mg q12h	No adjustment	No adjustment	No adjustment	No adjustment	No adjustment

CAVH, continuous arteriovenous hemofiltration; CrCl, creatinine clearance; CVVH, continuous venous-venous hemofiltration; ESRD, end-stage renal disease; HD, hemodialysis; PD, peritoneal dialysis.

tation, which is visible through the oral mucosal tissues. This pigmentation is permanent.[61,62]

Teeth and Bones

A gray-brown to yellow discoloration of the teeth has been noted in children taking tetracyclines.[63] This side effect is permanent and may be associated with hypoplasia of the enamel[64] and depression of skeletal growth in premature infants.[65] The darkening effect of tetracyclines on permanent teeth appears to be related to the total dose of the antibiotic administered. In a retrospective study, cosmetically noticeable but mild darkening of the permanent teeth occurred in 3 of 14 children receiving five courses of tetracycline, whereas 4 of 6 children receiving eight courses had moderate darkening of the enamel. Primary teeth generally show more darkening than do the larger, thicker, and more opaque permanent teeth. Since there is some variability in staining with similar tetracycline exposure, it is prudent not to administer these agents to pregnant women and to children up to the age of 8 years, the period when tooth enamel is being formed. For this reason, the U.S. Food and Drug Administration has withdrawn from the market the concentrated liquid dosage forms (drops) specifically intended for pediatric

TABLE 25-9 Common Side Effects of Tetracyclines

	Tetracycline	Doxycycline	Minocycline
Hematologic toxicity	Mild leukopenia (rare) Thrombocytopenia Vascular purpura (associated with thrombocytopenia) Hemolytic anemia Eosinophilia	Eosinophilia	Eosinophilia
Neurotoxicity	Dizziness, tinnitus Visual disturbances Neuromuscular blockade at high concentrations Bulging fontanels in infants Pseudotumor cerebri	Bulging fontanels in infants Pseudotumor cerebri	Bulging fontanels in infants Pseudotumor cerebri Headache, dizziness Vertigo-vestibular dysfunction Memory disturbances Neuromuscular blockade
Gastrointestinal	Anorexia, nausea, vomiting Diarrhea Glossitis, esophagitis, esophageal ulceration Acute pancreatitis Enterocolitis Tongue discoloration	GI side effects less common. Anorexia, nausea, vomiting Diarrhea Glossitis, esophagitis, esophageal ulceration	GI side effects most common. Anorexia, nausea, vomiting (40%-50%) Diarrhea Glossitis Tongue discoloration
Superinfection	Antibiotic-associated colitis Monilia	Antibiotic-associated colitis (less frequent) Monilia	Antibiotic-associated colitis Monilia
Kidney	Azotemia Increased serum creatinine Fanconi-like syndrome (outdated tetracycline)	Lower risk of nephrotoxicity	Lower risk of nephrotoxicity Interstitial nephritis
Liver	Hepatitis Fatty liver	Hepatitis (rare)	Hepatitis (rare)
Skeletal	Gray/yellow discoloration of teeth	Gray/yellow discoloration of teeth (less risk compared to other tetracyclines)	Gray/yellow discoloration of teeth
Skin	Photosensitivity	Photosensitivity	Photosensitivity Gray pigmentation of skin (sites of inflammation—i.e., scars), nails, sclerae, and conjunctiva
Endocrine	Antianabolic	Antianabolic	Antianabolic
Hypersensitivity	Uncommon Urticaria, asthma exacerbation, facial edema, contact dermatitis Jarisch-Herxheimer reaction	Uncommon Urticaria, asthma exacerbation, facial edema, contact dermatitis Jarisch-Herxheimer reaction	Uncommon Urticaria, asthma exacerbation, facial edema, contact dermatitis Jarisch-Herxheimer reaction SLE-like syndrome

SLE, systemic lupus erythematosus.

use. However, a single course of tetracycline therapy is administered to young children for specifically defined indications when the alternative regimen might produce more severe toxicity. Doxycycline binds less with calcium than do other tetracyclines and may cause dental changes less frequently in children.[66]

Gastrointestinal Symptoms

The tetracyclines are irritative substances and frequently produce gastrointestinal symptoms after oral administration. Esophageal ulcerations that are manifested as retrosternal pain exacerbated by swallowing have been clearly documented after tetracycline and doxycycline administration. In most cases, the patients were taking the capsules with little or no fluid just before going to bed. The complication may also occur in patients with esophageal obstruction or motility disorders.[67,68] Nausea, vomiting, and epigastric distress are dose related and limit the dose of most of the analogues. The administration of food with doxycycline, minocycline, or oxytetracycline may ameliorate some of these symptoms, but food seriously decreases the absorption of the other tetracyclines. Diarrhea, most often associated with analogues that are poorly absorbed, appears to be related to alterations in the enteric flora. Doxycycline produces less of an effect on bowel flora than does tetracycline. The diarrhea usually subsides when treatment with the antibiotic is stopped, but prolonged symptoms due to pseudomembranous colitis have been reported. Tetracycline also has been noted, rarely, to cause pancreatitis with or without overt liver disease.[69]

Liver

The hepatotoxicity of the tetracyclines, first described in patients receiving intravenous chlortetracycline but now described with other analogues, appears pathologically as a fine-droplet fatty metamorphosis and results in a high mortality.[70] The administration of less than 2 g/day intravenously is not associated with liver dysfunction or injury except in pregnant women, who are particularly at risk,[71] and in patients with an excessive serum level due to renal failure.[72] This toxicity is rarely reported with doxycycline.[73]

Renal Function

The tetracyclines aggravate preexisting renal failure by inhibiting protein synthesis, which increases the azotemia from amino acid metabolism.[74] Nephrogenic diabetes insipidus is produced by demeclocycline, a side effect that has been used therapeutically to reverse chronic inappropriate antidiuretic hormone secretion[75]; renal failure has complicated its use for this purpose in patients with cirrhosis.[76] Outdated tetracycline has produced a reversible Fanconi-like syndrome with renal tubular acidosis, but tetracycline formulations producing this syndrome have been modified. It is unlikely that this complication will recur.

Nervous and Sensory Systems

Vertigo is a side effect unique to minocycline. Symptoms of lightheadedness, loss of balance, dizziness, and tinnitus usually begin on the second or third day of therapy and have been noted more frequently in women (70%) than in men (28%). The symptoms are reversible within several days after discontinuation of therapy, but this side effect has seriously limited the use of minocycline. Benign intracranial hypertension (pseudotumor cerebri) has been described in infants and adults with many of the analogues[77,78] and has often been associated with the medium- or long-term use of minocycline for acne vulgaris.[79,80] Intracranial hypertension due to the tetracycline antibiotics (including doxycycline) occurs in both sexes, at almost any age, and without concomitant obesity. Recently, acute onset of severe intracranial hypertension with visual loss has been reported to be associated with doxycycline used for malaria prophylaxis.[81] In a recent study, 25% of the 57 patients with minocycline-induced intracranial hypertension had notable visual field loss.[82] Therefore, patients who

TABLE 25-10 Significant Food-Drug and Drug-Drug Interactions with Tetracyclines			
Interacting Agent	Effect	Comments	References
Food	**Tetracycline** Food may reduce absorption by 50%.	Bioavailability is 60%-80% when taken on an empty stomach.	42, 196
	Doxycycline May be reduced by up to 20% when taken with food or milk.	Food effect is not clinically significant.	
	Minocycline May be reduced by up to 20% when taken with food or milk.	Food effect is not clinically significant.	
Divalent or trivalent cations: aluminum, calcium, magnesium, iron, zinc Kaolin and pectin Bismuth subsalicylate	Significant reduction of all tetracyclines	Should not be administered concurrently with foods or drugs containing divalent or trivalent cations—i.e., antacids, sucralfate, didanosine, multivitamins. Separate administration of tetracycline from divalent or trivalent cations by 2 hours.	196, 198, 199
Sodium bicarbonate	May decrease absorption of tetracycline	—	200
Cimetidine	Decreased tetracycline absorption	Effect not clinically significant	201
Carbamazepine, phenytoin, barbiturates	Decreased half-life of doxycycline	Increases the hepatic metabolism	202, 203
Chronic ethanol ingestion	Decreased half-life of doxycycline but not tetracycline	Possible mechanism: induction of hepatic microsomal enzymes	204
Methoxyflurane or fluorinated anesthetic agents	Nephrotoxicity when administered with tetracyclines	—	205, 206
Diuretics	Increased blood urea nitrogen (BUN)	Volume depletion may increase the nephrotoxic effects of tetracycline by unknown mechanisms.	207
Oral anticoagulants	Increased risk of bleeding	Tetracyclines may impair utilization of prothrombin; may decrease vitamin K production by intestinal bacteria.	—
Oral contraceptives	Reduced levels when administered with tetracyclines	Women should use an additional (mechanical) form of birth control. Possible mechanism: reduction in bacterial hydrolysis of conjugated estrogen in the intestine	208
Anti-infectives	May reduce antimicrobial activity of aminoglycosides and penicillins	Rare reports of in vitro antagonism. Some clinicians recommend that the drugs not be used concomitantly.	83

complain of headache after using tetracycline should be examined carefully, with special attention to their visual acuity and with formal testing of the visual fields and funduscopy to look for papilledema.

Superinfection

Colonization by tetracycline-resistant organisms is a frequent occurrence during tetracycline therapy and is generally of little clinical significance. Rarely, a fulminating diarrhea resulting from pseudomembranous colitis caused by *Clostridium difficile* or from staphylococcal enteritis may occur after oral or parenteral therapy. More often and less serious, oral or vaginal moniliasis complicates treatment, and this complication may require specific therapy (see Table 25-9).

Significant Food and Drug Interactions

Significant interactions between tetracyclines and other drugs or food are summarized in Table 25-10.

Combination with Penicillins

The antagonistic effect that is seen when a primarily inhibitory anti-infective agent is combined with a bactericidal agent appears to account for the poor outcome observed in the treatment of pneumococcal meningitis when penicillin and chlortetracycline were used together.[83] In that case, the association was less effective than penicillin alone. Whether this can be generalized to other indications is not known.

Indications

The tetracyclines are the drugs of choice or an effective alternative therapy for a wide variety of bacterial, chlamydial, mycoplasmal, and rickettsial infections (Table 25-11).[7,8,40,84-97] Tetracycline and doxycycline can be used interchangeably for most of these indications. However, compliance may be better with doxycycline since it can be taken twice daily without regard to meals, and cost is no longer an im-

portant factor. Doxycycline is also preferred by most when intravenous administration is required. Although the tetracyclines have no primary role in the treatment of viral or fungal diseases, earlier studies showed some increased activity of amphotericin B against *Aspergillus* spp. in vitro when combined with minoglycine.[98]

In recent years, the increasing number of resistant strains has significantly reduced the use of tetracyclines and in some cases they are no longer drugs of choice.[7]

For the management of community-acquired pneumonia (CAP), the practice guidelines of the Infectious Diseases Society of America (2000)[84] and of the Canadian Infectious Diseases Society and the Canadian Thoracic Society (2000)[85] consider doxycycline to be one of the equivalent alternative regimens for outpatients who lack modifying factors. However, it is still controversial whether doxycycline should be used as first line of treatment. The tetracyclines are active in vitro against the atypical organisms, including *Mycoplasma pneumoniae, Chlamydophila pneumoniae,* and *Legionella,*[86] and against *S. pneumoniae* and *H. influenzae.* The latter two organisms have been quite susceptible to these agents in the past,[87] but 15% to 59% of pneumococci are now resistant, with up to 40% of strains showing high-level resistance.[88,89] The recent focus on agents of bioterrorism has increased the role of tetracyclines as therapeutic and as prophylactic agents in anthrax, plague, and tularemia.[90]

The new role of tetracycline as part of a triple therapy for management of gastritis and peptic ulcer disease associated with *Helicobacter pylori* may increase as more clarithromycin- and metronidazole-resistant *H. pylori* isolates are encountered. Moreover, the activity of tetracyclines against malaria has unexpectedly become important for prophylaxis after the rapid increase of mefloquine-resistant *Plasmodium falciparum* strains.[33] Mefloquine is the most effective and most recommended antimalarial agent, but its side effects have begun to limit its acceptance. Doxycycline is being used increasingly in areas where

---

TABLE 25-11   Therapeutic Indications for Tetracyclines

Major Indications
Anaplasma (formerly *Ehrlichia*) *phagocytophila* infection
Anthrax inhalation, cutaneous postexposure
Bacillary angiomatosis in HIV patients (*Bartonella henselae* and *Bartonella quintana*)
Balantidium coli infection (infectious colitis)
Bartonellosis: Oroya fever and *Verruga peruana* (*Bartonella bacilliformis*)
Brucellosis (plus rifampin, streptomycin, or gentamicin)
Cat-scratch fever (*B. henselae*)
Cervicitis due to *Chlamydia trachomatis*
Cholera
Community-acquired pneumonia
Ehrlichia chaffeensis infection
Peptic ulcer (with other agents) (*Helicobacter pylori*)
Granuloma inguinale (*Calymmatobacterium granulomatis*)
Inclusion conjunctivitis (*C. trachomatis*)
Lyme disease (*Borrelia burgdorferi*)
Lymphogranuloma venereum (*C. trachomatis*)
Mycobacterial infections caused by *Mycobacterium marinum* and some isolates of *Mycobacterium fortuitum* and *Mycobacterium chelonae*
Nongonococcal urethritis
Pneumonia caused by *Chlamydophila pneumoniae*
Pelvic inflammatory disease
Periodontitis
Psittacosis and ornithosis (*Chlamydia psittaci*)
Q fever (*Coxiella burnetii*)
Relapsing fever, both louse- and tick-borne
Rickettsial infections (spotted fever group and rickettsialpox)
Scrub typhus (*Orientia tsutsugamushi*)
Trachoma (*C. trachomatis*)
Trench fever (*B. quintana*)
Urethral infections caused by *C. trachomatis* or *Ureaplasma urealyticum*
Vibrio vulnificus infection

Second-Line Treatment
Acinetobacter baumannii infections (sensitive strains)
Acne
Actinomyces israelii when penicillin is contraindicated
Acute intestinal amebiasis (as adjunct therapy)
Campylobacter fetus infections
Clostridium infections when penicillin is contraindicated
Eikenella corrodens infection
Leptospirosis if penicillin contraindicated
Mycobacterium leprae (only minocycline is active)
Nocardia (minocycline)
Pasteurella multocida
Burkholderia mallei (glanders) infections (only in combination with other drugs)
Burkholderia pseudomallei (melioidosis) (only in combination with other drugs)
Rat-bite fever (*Spirillum minus, Streptobacillus moniliformis*)
Syphilis, primary and secondary: (patients with penicillin allergy) (*Treponema pallidum*)
U. urealyticum infection
Vincent's angina
Yaws caused by *Treponema pertenue* when penicillin is contraindicated
Whipple disease (*Tropheryma whipplei*)

Prophylaxis
Anthrax (*Bacillus anthracis*) prophylaxis
Colonic surgery prophylaxis
Lyme disease, post–tick bite prophylaxis
Malaria prophylaxis
Plague (*Yersinia pestis*) prophylaxis
Traveler's diarrhea prophylaxis
Tularemia (*Francisella tularensis*) prophylaxis
Treatment of asymptomatic carriers of *Neisseria meningitidis* to eliminate meningococci from the nasopharynx: minocycline

Parasites
Entamoeba histolytica
Giardia lamblia

HIV, human immunodeficiency virus.

there is resistance to, or in patients who have side effects to, mefloquine. Tetracyclines have been used to treat other parasitic diseases in humans (see Table 25-11) and were effective for the treatment of filarial nematode infections, suggesting that tetracycline may be beneficial for treatment of humans infected with filarial nematodes.[7,8,91]

Use in Noninfectious Conditions

Recent studies have identified the effectiveness of tetracycline in a variety of noninfectious conditions. A number of its nonantibacterial effects, including its anti-inflammatory properties, immunosuppression, inhibition of lipase and collagenase activity, enhancement of gingival fibroblast cell attachment, and wound healing, make tetracycline a good agent for treating diseases such as acne, rosacea, and periodontal diseases. Its ability to reduce inflammation explains the subtherapeutic doses of tetracyclines that are effective in acne treatment. Minocycline may be used for early (within the first year of disease) rheumatoid arthritis and tetracycline is administered intrapleurally for the control of malignant pleural effusions.[100-102]

CHLORAMPHENICOL

Soon after chloramphenicol was released in the United States in 1949, reports linked this highly effective agent with aplastic anemia, and it quickly fell into disuse. Increased awareness of the pathogenicity of anaerobic organisms and the development of ampicillin-resistant *H. influenzae* accounted for a brief resurgence, but the availability of other agents has markedly reduced the need for this antibiotic. Since it is readily available (often over the counter) and inexpensive, it is still used as first-line therapy for enteric fever and other infections in many parts of the developing world. In the United States and other developed nations, chloramphenicol remains a useful antibiotic, but only as alternative therapy in seriously ill patients and for patients infected with organisms that are highly resistant to antibiotics, and possibly as an alternative therapy for anthrax or plague during a bioterrorism event.

Structure and Preparations

Chloramphenicol was discovered by screening organisms for their antimicrobial activity. Isolated independently by Burkholder from a mulched field near Caracas, Venezuela,[103] and by workers at the University of Illinois from compost,[104] the organism producing the active compound was named *Streptomyces venezuelae*. The structure of chloramphenicol is shown in Figure 25-2. It was the first antibiotic whose chemical synthesis was economically and technically practical for large-scale production. In many countries, chloramphenicol is available in 250-mg capsules, as a suspension (150 mg/5 mL), and as a parenteral formulation (1-g powder). It is also available as Chloromycetin ophthalmic ointment (1%), Chloromycetin ophthalmic (25-mg powder to prepare ophthalmic solution), and Chloromycetin otic (drops). In the United States, the oral Chloromycetin Kapseals (250 mg) and Chloromycetin Palmitate are no longer manufactured (since 1991). No oral products are currently available in the United States.

Thiamphenicol, not available in the United States, is an analogue in which the *p*-nitro group on the benzene ring is replaced by a methyl-

sulfonyl group. Its spectrum of activity is similar to that of chloramphenicol, but it has not been reported to cause aplastic anemia.

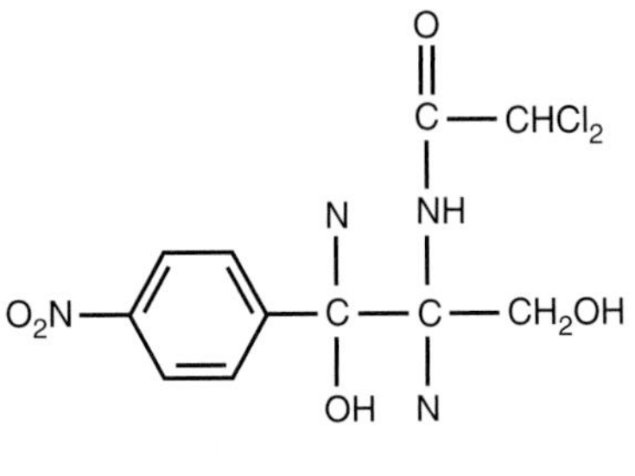

Mechanism of Action

Chloramphenicol appears to enter the cell by an energy-dependent process.[105] Once within the cell, it inhibits protein synthesis by reversibly binding to the larger 50S subunit of the 70S ribosome at a locus that prevents the attachment of the amino acid–containing end of the aminoacyl-transfer RNA to its binding region. Without this attachment, the association of the amino acid substrate with peptidyltransferase does not occur, and peptide bond formation is prevented. This block in protein synthesis produces a static effect against most sensitive microorganisms. However, chloramphenicol is bactericidal against some meningeal pathogens, such as *H. influenzae, S. pneumoniae,* and *Neisseria meningitidis,* but not against group B streptococci or enteric gram-negative bacilli at concentrations that can be achieved therapeutically.[106-108] Although mammalian cells contain primarily 80S ribosomes that are unaffected by chloramphenicol, the mitochondria do contain 70S particles. The effect of chloramphenicol on these has been suggested as a cause for the dose-related bone marrow suppression of the compound but not for the idiosyncratic aplastic anemia.

In Vitro Activity

Chloramphenicol is extremely active against a variety of organisms, including bacteria, spirochetes, rickettsiae, chlamydiae, and mycoplasmas. The percentages of strains of bacteria inhibited at various concentrations of this antibiotic are listed in Table 25-12. Most gram-positive and gram-negative aerobic bacteria are inhibited by concentrations easily achieved in the serum of patients, but more active or less toxic therapeutic agents are available for most of these pathogens. Salmonellae including *Salmonella typhi* are generally susceptible. However, since 1989, chloramphenicol-resistant strains have rapidly spread in India, Korea, Vietnam, Peru, Mexico, and Thailand.[109] The resistance gene was carried on a plasmid and associated with resistance to ampicillin, chloramphenicol, and trimethoprim/sulfamethoxazole. In 1990-91, 78.4% of the *S. typhi* isolates collected in India were multidrug-resistant (MDR).[110] Although MDR strains of *S. typhi* are still common in many part of Asia, recent reports found the reemergence of chloramphenicol-sensitive strains in India (91.8% of isolates were sensitive in 1998)[111] and Egypt (95% of isolates were sensitive).[112] In the United States, resistant strains occasionally occur,[113] but imported strains may be highly resistant.

In the 1990s, the spread of an MDR clonal strain of *Salmonella typhimurium* was extremely worrisome.[114] Its resistance phenotype was linked to the phage type 104 (DT 104), which has a chromosomal gene cluster that codes resistance to ampicillin, chloramphenicol, streptomycin, sulfonamides, and tetracycline.[115] Recent data suggest that the emergence of this MDR strain in humans and animals may have been the result of the dissemination of a strain already present in the United States rather than the introduction of a new strain.[116]

The three most common organisms that cause meningitis in childhood (*H. influenzae, S. pneumoniae,* and *N. meningitidis*) are susceptible to chloramphenicol,[117,118] although resistant strains of each species have been reported. The overall rate of *H. influenzae* resistance among clinical strains in the United States is approximately 0.6%.[119] Also, in Canada, more than 99.2% of isolates are sensitive to chloramphenicol, regardless of the presence of β-lactamase.[120] Indeed, strains of *H. influenzae* that cause clinical infections and are resistant to both chloramphenicol and ampicillin have been isolated in several parts of the world.[121-123] These resistant isolates are rare in the United States and Canada but rather frequent in Spain.[124-126] Recent data on respiratory isolates of *S. aureus* and *S. pneumoniae* report that 81.6% and 91% of the isolates, respectively, are sensitive to chloramphenicol.[127] Chloramphenicol is one of the most effective antibiotics against anaerobic bacteria, including the *B. fragilis* group. A recent survey showed that all *Bacteroides* strains tested between 1997 and 2000 were sensitive to chloramphenicol,[128] but other agents have be-

FIGURE 25-2. Chemical structure of chloramphenicol.

come more clinically important for treating infections caused by these bacteria.[129-131] Bacteria develop resistance to chloramphenicol by several mechanisms: reduced permeability or uptake, ribosomal mutation, and production of an enzyme, acetyltransferase, that acetylates the antibiotic to an inactive diacetyl derivative.[132,133] Such resistance may be associated with resistance to other drugs such as the tetracyclines.

The third mechanism, production of acetyltransferase, has been shown to be R-factor mediated and responsible for widespread epidemics of chloramphenicol-resistant typhoid fever and *Shigella* dysentery in Central and South America, Vietnam, India, and other countries.[134-136] It has been suggested that unrestricted over-the-counter sales of chloramphenicol in these countries may have provided antibiotic pressure for the development of resistant strains.[136] In the United States, chloramphenicol resistance in *Salmonella* has been traced to the use of chloramphenicol on dairy farms.

Pharmacology

Serum levels of chloramphenicol achieved by different routes of administration are shown in Figure 25-3. In the encapsulated form, chloramphenicol is well absorbed from the gastrointestinal tract and produces peak serum levels of 12 μg/mL of active antibiotic after a 1-g dose.[137] Chloramphenicol palmitate ester oral preparation is available in some countries; it is inactive and must be hydrolyzed in the upper intestinal tract to produce active chloramphenicol. The biovailability of chloramphenicol palmitate in the current formulation is the same as that in the capsules.[138] The intravenous preparation of the drug is the soluble but inactive chloramphenicol succinate ester that is rapidly hydrolized within the body to become biologically active chloramphenicol. This preparation produces active chloramphenicol levels in the serum that are 70% of those obtained after oral administration because of incomplete hydrolysis.[137]

Intramuscular injection is well tolerated and in most studies produces peak serum levels and areas under the serum-level curve similar to those of intravenous administration.[140,141] In adults with enteric fever, however, peak concentrations of only one half to two thirds of those obtained by the intravenous route were obtained, and this was associated with a delayed therapeutic response and increased relapse rate of typhoid fever.[142] Lower chloramphenicol serum levels were also found in children treated with intravenous chloramphenicol for enteric fever compared with other diseases.[139] Since 30% of the unhydrolyzed inactive succinate ester is found in the urine regardless of which parenteral route is used, the lower serum levels produced by in-

TABLE 25-12 Activity of Chloramphenicol against Selected Bacteria*

Bacterium	No. of Strains	Cumulative Inhibition (%) at Indicated Concentration (μg/mL)				
		0.4	0.8	1.6	3.2	6.4
Aerobic Bacteria						
Gram Positive						
Staphylococcus aureus	291	0	0	0	5	55
S. aureus (methicillin resistant)	22	0	0	0	0	20
Streptococcus pyogenes	303	0	0	20	92	99
Streptococci, group B	146	0	0	0	85	99
Viridans streptococci	193	0	0	0	60	90
Enterococci	382	0	0	0	0	0
Streptococcus pneumoniae	78	—	—	—	50	100
Gram Negative						
Haemophilus influenzae	17	—	—	50	100	—
Neisseria meningitidis	7	—	50	—	100	—
Neisseria gonorrhoeae	106	5	52	97	100	—
Escherichia coli	71	0	0	5	30	75
Klebsiella pneumoniae	35	0	0	6	70	75
Enterobacter	10	0	0	0	10	20
Serratia marcescens	111	0	0	0	5	—
Proteus mirabilis	209	0	0	0	20	60
Proteus (indole positive)	32	0	0	0	10	40
Salmonella typhi	81	0	0	0	50	95
Salmonella paratyphi A	31	—	—	—	28	97
Shigella spp.	44	—	20	30	75	90
Vibrio cholerae	64	—	—	—	—	84
Brucella spp.	25	0	0	28	92	100
Pseudomonas aeruginosa	11	0	0	0	0	0
Pseudomonas pseudomallei	10	0	0	0	0	50
Bordetella pertussis	31	20	45	85	97	99
Anaerobic Bacteria						
Gram Positive						
Peptococcus spp.	145	8	25	67	97	98
Peptostreptococcus spp.	72	11	37	63	96	100
Propionibacterium acnes	16	12	31	94	100	—
Eubacterium lentum	14	14	14	28	71	100
Clostridium perfringens	34	0	0	15	100	—
Other Clostridium species	17	12	12	53	88	100
Gram Negative						
Veillonella spp.	13	23	46	85	100	—
Bacteroides fragilis	195	0	1	2	23	98
Prevotella melaninogenica	29	14	31	93	96	100
Fusobacterium spp.	18	39	44	56	89	100

*The National Committee for Laboratory Standards recommends that 8 μg/mL or less be considered susceptible, 16 μg/mL intermediate, and 32 μg/mL or greater be considered resistant. For *Haemophilus*, ≥2 μg/mL is sensitive, 4 μg/mL intermediate, and ≥8 μg/mL resistant. For testing *S. pneumoniae,* the breakpoints are ≤4, 8, and ≥16 μg/mL.[9]

Data from references 113, 117, 118, 120, 122-126, 129-131, 209-221.

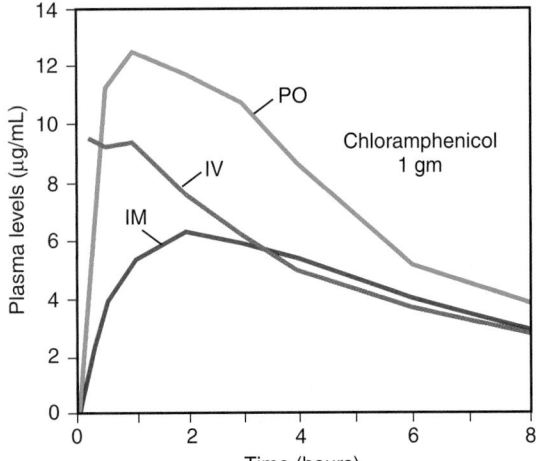

FIGURE 25-3. Plasma levels of chloramphenicol vary with time and the route of administration.

tramuscular injection appear to be due to delayed absorption of the ester from the site of injection rather than to decreased hydrolysis.[137,142] The intramuscular route should be used cautiously.

Chloramphenicol is metabolized primarily by the liver (about 90%), where it is conjugated with glucuronic acid, forming monoglucoronide that is water soluble but inactive. This compound is excreted in the bile into the small intestine, hydrolyzed by bacterial enzymes to aglycone, reabsorbed, and conjugated with glucuronic acid again. This enterohepatic circulation eventually results in about 80 to 90% of the monoglucoronide being excreted in this inactive form by the kidney. Only about 5 to 10% of the administered dose is recovered in the urine as biologically active chloramphenicol. Nevertheless, in the absence of renal disease, concentrations of 150 to 200 μg/mL of active drug are achieved, which is sufficient to treat urinary tract infections if necessary. Urinary concentrations are markedly diminished, however, in patients with renal failure, and more active chloramphenicol is available for conversion to the active form.

The use of chloramphenicol in children has led to a better understanding of its pharmacokinetics. It is clear that there is a wide variation in the metabolism and excretion in that age group. Dosage requirements may vary threefold in children of the same age, with even greater variation noted in newborn and young infants. Because newborns metabolize the antibiotic at a slow rate, the initial dose for those younger than 1 week should be 25 mg/kg every 24 hours and for infants from 1 to 4 weeks old, 25 mg/kg every 12 hours instead of the usual 50 mg/kg/day divided into 6-hour dosing intervals for older children and adults. However, the wide variation makes monitoring serum levels imperative.[145,146]

Chloramphenicol has a half-life in adults of 4.1 hours after single intravenous injections, is not highly bound to protein (25 to 50%), and has an apparent volume of distribution of 100 liters.[137,147] The high degree of lipid solubility and low protein binding and small molecular size allow chloramphenicol to diffuse well into many tissues and body fluids. Levels in the cerebrospinal fluid even without inflamed meninges are generally 30 to 50% of serum concentrations, much higher than those of most other antibiotics. Therapeutic levels are obtained in pleural, ascitic, and synovial fluids.[149] Chloramphenicol also penetrates well in all parts of the eye. The antibiotic crosses the placenta to the fetal circulation but produces negligible amounts in the amniotic fluid. Only small amounts of active chloramphenicol are recovered in the bile (0.14% of a 1-g dose).[103]

Renal and Hepatic Insufficiency

The half-life of biologically active chloramphenicol in patients with renal disease differs only slightly from that in healthy subjects, whereas the concentrations of its metabolites increase markedly. However, the dose should not be modified if therapeutic levels of the active drug are to be maintained. Fortunately, the metabolites do not appear to be as toxic as the active compound. Neither peritoneal dialysis nor hemodialysis alters serum levels sufficiently to require dose alterations.[147,150] Chloramphenicol is only slightly dialyzable and does not require supplemental dosing during hemo- or peritoneal dialysis, or during continuous arteriovenous (CAVH) or venous-venous (CVVH) hemofiltration.

Patients with hepatic failure, as evidenced by jaundice or ascites, conjugate chloramphenicol at a slower rate. Serum levels of active chloramphenicol increase to levels capable of bone marrow suppression.[151] The regimen suggested for adults with hepatic insufficiency is an initial 1-g loading dose followed by 500 mg every 6 hours. The course of therapy should be limited when possible to 10 to 14 days, and levels should be monitored.

Assay

Because of the narrow therapeutic-to-toxic ratio, it is important to monitor serum levels of this antibiotic, particularly in newborn and premature infants, in patients with hepatic disease, and in patients taking interacting drugs. A number of very effective assays can be used, including bioassays, radioenzymatic assays, competitive enzyme-linked immunoassays, and high-performance chromatography.[152] Peak serum levels should be maintained between 15 and 25 μg/mL, and trough levels between 5 and 15 μg/mL, in patients with meningitis. Levels should be maintained between 10 and 20 μg/mL in patients with other infections. Concentrations of greater than 40 μg/mL result in toxicity.

Toxicity

Hematologic

The most important toxic effects of chloramphenicol occur in the bone marrow. The effects can be divided into two types. The more common is a reversible bone marrow depression that is a direct pharmacologic effect of the antibiotic and results from inhibition of mitochondrial protein synthesis. It is manifested by reticulocytopenia, anemia, leukopenia, thrombocytopenia, or any combination thereof. Serum iron levels increase in association with a reduced uptake of radioactive iron by the red blood cells, indicating diminished hemoglobin synthesis. The bone marrow reveals vacuolization of the erythroid and myeloid precursors, but these changes are not specific for chloramphenicol. This type of toxicity is extremely common, occurs during the course of therapy, and is dose related.[153] It is more likely to occur in patients receiving 4 g/day or more, or in patients in whom serum levels are above 25 μg/mL, a level that may occur in patients with severe liver disease who are receiving usual doses. It is reversible when treatment with the antibiotic is discontinued.[154]

The second type of hematologic toxicity is a rare but generally fatal "idiosyncratic" response that is most frequently manifested as aplastic anemia.[155] Indeed, at one time chloramphenicol toxicity was the most common cause of this syndrome. According to the best epidemiologic studies in the United States, aplastic anemia occurs once in 24,500 to 40,800 patients who receive the antibiotic, a risk about 13 times greater than that for aplastic anemia in the general population.[156] The aplastic anemia most commonly occurs weeks to months after the completion of therapy and is not necessarily dose related. It appears that this toxic effect is caused by a mechanism different from the direct bone marrow suppression previously described. Although the pathogenesis of this idiosyncratic response is not known, observations and theories have suggested that the toxicity is very complex, involving interactions of the host and toxic intermediates of the antibiotic. This type of toxicity has occurred in identical twins, which suggests a genetic predisposition.[157] Morley and co-workers have observed that mice given chloramphenicol after treatment with busulfan had a progressive decrease in the number of pluripotential stem cells, whereas control mice did not, suggesting that the aplastic anemia might result in patients with unrecognized preexisting residual marrow damage either genetic or acquired.[157a] In 1967, Holt observed that the aplastic anemia occurred only after oral administration of the antibiotic.[157b] He postulated that the fatal reaction may be caused by the absorption of toxic products produced by enzymatic degradation of chloramphenicol, perhaps as a result of specific types of bacteria colonizing the gut of affected people. Supporting this hypothesis, Jimenez and colleagues have shown that one of chloramphenicol's metabolites, dehydrochloramphenicol, is 10- to 20-fold more cytotoxic than chloramphenicol yet is only one third as effective in inhibiting protein synthesis,[158] which suggests that this metabolite and perhaps others may play a significant role in this toxicity. These toxic metabolites may undergo further metabolic transformation in the bone marrow with on-site production of toxic intermediates.[159] Although the number of cases reported is greater after oral therapy, some cases of aplastic anemia from parenteral chloramphenicol, even after the administration of eye drops, have also been reported.[160,161] These latter cases have prompted considerable debate but are very rare; estimates of serious hematologic toxicity appear to be no more than 3 in 442,543 patients and most likely many fewer.[162,163] In a review of 426 cases of aplastic anemia, none of the patients used chloramphenicol eye drops.[164]

Although most cases of aplastic anemia from chloramphenicol become apparent after the completion of therapy, it should be emphasized that 22% of the cases occur concurrently with antibiotic administration.[99,155,161] Whether some of these episodes can be prevented by checking the blood counts of patients is not known. Until the pathogenesis of the toxicity is clearly understood, it is recommended that a complete blood count be obtained twice a week from all patients receiving chloramphenicol. If the white blood cell count decreases below 2500/mm^3, it is desirable to discontinue antibiotic treatment if the clinical condition allows. It should be recognized, however, that low numbers of white blood cells may occur in illnesses for which chloramphenicol is used, such as typhoid fever.

Also of concern are reports of childhood leukemia after the use of chloramphenicol. Although these cases are generally preceded by aplastic anemia, a population-based case-control interview study of 309 childhood leukemia cases and 618 age- and sex-matched controls showed a significant dose-response relationship between chloramphenicol and the risk for both acute lymphocytic and nonlymphocytic leukemia, particularly after treatment for more than 10 days in children without prior aplastic anemia. Until this is more clearly defined, it seems prudent to change therapy as quickly as possible to equally effective and less toxic antibiotics.[165]

Chloramphenicol may also produce a hemolytic anemia in patients with the Mediterranean form of glucose-6-phosphate dehydrogenase deficiency. This apparently does not occur with the milder type A glucose-6-phosphate dehydrogenase deficiency, which is the more common form in blacks.

Gray Baby Syndrome

The gray baby syndrome of neonates is characterized by abdominal distention, vomiting, flaccidity, cyanosis, circulatory collapse, and death. This side effect results from the neonate's diminished ability to conjugate chloramphenicol and to excrete the active form in the urine.[166] If chloramphenicol is necessary in premature infants and neonates, the dose should be reduced to 25 mg/kg/day and the antibiotic levels should be monitored. This syndrome has also been recognized in toddlers and after accidental overdoses in adults.[167] It is generally associated with serum concentrations of chloramphenicol of greater than 50 μg/mL and may occur with unexplained metabolic acidosis.[168] Large-volume exchange transfusions and charcoal hemoperfusion have been used to accelerate drug removal. This syndrome is caused in part by impaired myocardial contractility related to direct interference of myocardial tissue respiration and oxidative phosphorylation.[169-171]

Optic Neuritis

Optic neuritis resulting in decreased visual acuity has been described in patients receiving prolonged chloramphenicol therapy.[172] The symptoms are generally reversible, but loss of vision has occurred. Other neurologic sequelae such as peripheral neuritis, headache, depression, ophthalmoplegia, and mental confusion have also been described.

Other Reactions

Hypersensitivity reactions (including rashes and drug fevers) and anaphylaxis are rare. Herxheimer-like responses during therapy for syphilis, brucellosis, and typhoid fever have been observed. Symptoms involving the gastrointestinal tract, including nausea, vomiting and diarrhea, glossitis, and stomatitis, occur but have not been a major problem. Prolonged oral administration of chloramphenicol may induce bleeding, either by bone marrow depression or by reducing the intestinal flora with consequent inhibition of vitamin K synthesis. Chloramphenicol has been associated with acute attacks of porphyria and is considered unsafe in porphyric patients. Chloramphenicol may also interfere with the development of immunity and it should not be given during active immunization.

Significant Drug Interactions

Significant interactions between chloramphenicol and other drugs are listed in Table 25-13. Chloramphenicol prolongs the half-life of tolbutamide, chlorpropamide, phenytoin, cyclophosphamide, and warfarin (Coumadin), apparently by inhibiting hepatic microsomal enzymes.[173-176] Severe toxicity and death have occurred. Phenytoin, rifampin, and phenobarbital have been observed to decrease the serum concentration and increase the total body clearance of chloramphenicol, perhaps by inducing hepatic microsomal enzymes. Serum concentrations should

TABLE 25-13	Important Drug-Drug Interactions with Chloramphenicol	
Object Drug	*Effect*	*Reference*
Phenobarbital	Reduced serum concentration of chloramphenicol by 30%-40%	
	Increased serum concentration of phenobarbital by up to 50%	222, 223
Phenytoin	Can increase or decrease chloramphenicol serum concentration	223, 224
(and fosphenytoin)	Chloramphenicol can inhibit the metabolism of phenytoin, resulting in increased serum concentration of phenytoin	
Cyclosporine	Increased concentration of cyclosporine due to inhibition of metabolism by chloramphenicol	
	Increased risk of renal dysfunction, cholestasis, paresthesias	225, 226
Cimetidine	Possible additive or synergistic bone marrow suppressant effects with concomitant administration	
	Two case reports of fatal aplastic anemia	227, 228
Cyclophosphamide	Reduced effectiveness of cyclophosphamide due to decreased metabolism to active cyclophosphamide metabolite by chloramphenicol	173
Rifampin/rifabutin	Decreased serum concentrations of chloramphenicol due to induction of chloramphenicol metabolism	177
Tacrolimus	Increased blood concentrations of tacrolimus due to decreased metabolism of chloramphenicol	229

be monitored when these drugs are administered concurrently.[177] When administering this agent, the physician should be on the alert for toxicity from other agents that are metabolized by the liver and should monitor serum levels when these drugs are administered concurrently. Chloramphenicol may delay the response of anemias to iron, folic acid, and vitamin B_{12}.[174] Chloramphenicol is primarily a bacteriostatic agent, and in vitro antagonizes the bactericidal activity of the penicillins, cephalosporins, and aminoglycoside antibiotics. This has doubtful clinical significance in most instances. However, care should be exercised in the use of such combinations for infections that require bactericidal activity for efficacy, such as for infections in the granulocytopenic host or in the treatment of endocarditis.[175] In the treatment of meningitis, the bacteriostatic activity of chloramphenicol against group B streptococci and its in vitro antagonism with ampicillin against this organism are of concern and should be considered in selecting therapy when this organism is likely to be a pathogen.[174]

Indications

With the possible exception of typhoid fever in areas where cost and availability make it the primary therapy, chloramphenicol is no longer the drug of choice for any specific infection. Chloramphenicol-resistant typhoid fever associated with the high-molecular-weight, self-transferable, IncHI plasmid has been a major problem is Asia and South America for many years.[109] However, chloramphenicol, amoxicillin, and trimethoprim-sulfamethoxazole remain appropriate for the treatment of typhoid fever in areas of the world where the bacterium is still fully susceptible to these drugs and where the fluoroquinolones are not available or affordable. Moreover, reemergence of chloramphenicol-sensitive strains after decreased usage of this drug has been reported.[111,112]

Third-generation cephalosporins have superseded chloramphenicol for the treatment of bacterial meningitis in infants and children, although chloramphenicol is still used for this indication in penicillin-allergic patients.[177] In a recent study in Papua New Guinea, children who had meningitis and were treated with cephalosporins had a better outcome than those treated with chloramphenicol, because the latter acquired infections with chloramphenicol-resistant *Haemophilus influenzae*.[178]

Chloramphenicol resistance in *H. influenzae* is also found in a global distribution.[121,179] A study found that 6.7% of patients in Salvador, Brazil, developed meningitis due to strains resistant to ampicillin and chloramphenicol, antibiotics used routinely for the empirical treatment of bacterial meningitis in Brazil.[180] A review of the literature related to *Salmonella* meningitis, a leading cause of gram-negative bacterial meningitis in the developing world, showed that chloramphenicol and conventional antibiotics had a cure rate of 41.2%, a relapse rate of 11.8%, and an associated mortality of 44.7%, whereas fluoroquinolones and third-generation cephalosporins had cure rates of 88.9% and 84.6%, respectively, with no associated mortality.[180a] Moreover, meningococci that are resistant to chloramphenicol have been described in Vietnam and France.[181,182] Occasionally, chloramphenicol is useful when the differential diagnosis includes both meningococcemia and Rocky Mountain spotted fever, diseases that may be difficult to distinguish on clinical characteristics. Of note is the occasional use of chloramphenicol for the treatment of infections caused by multiply resistant organisms.[183-185] However, the treatment of penicillin-resistant pneumococcal meningitis with chloramphenicol was shown to have poor clinical outcome.[186,187]

In a recent study[188] chloramphenicol was comparable to gentamicin and benzylpenicillin as first-line treatment of severe pneumonia in children in Papua New Guinea.

Chloramphenicol was found to be effective against vancomycin-resistant *Enterococcus faecium*,[189-191] and a retrospective analysis of the outcomes of six patients with bacteremia due to vancomycin-resistant *E. faecium* concluded that chloramphenicol was effective and should be considered as a treatment option.[192] However, it has to be considered a second-line drug compared to the newer drugs available.

Chloramphenicol is active against plague, anthrax, and tularemia. Because these agents may be used as biologic threats or weapons, the Working Group on Civilian Biodefense suggested that chloramphenicol may be an effective alternative treatment in such a setting.[193-195]

Acknowledgment

The authors want to thank Umberto Conte, Pharm.D., for his helpful suggestions and contribution to the pharmacology sections of this chapter.

REFERENCES

1. Rapoport MI, Calia FM. The use of antibiotics in animal feeds. JAMA. 1974;229:1212.
2. Testa RT, Petersen PJ, Jakobus NL, et al. In vivo and in vivo antibacterial activity of the glycylcyclines, a new class of semisynthetic tetracyclines. Antimicrob Agents Chemother. 1993;37:2270-2277.
3. Sum PE, Lee VJ, Testa RT, et al. Glycylcyclines: 1. A new generation of potent antibacterial agents through modification of 9 aminotetracyclines. J Med Chem. 1994;37:184-188.
4. Sum PE, Petersen P. Synthesis and structure-activity relationship leading to the discovery of GAR-936. Bioorg Med Chem Lett. 1999;9:1459-1462.
5. Petersen PJ, Jakobus NV, Weiss WJ, et al. In vitro and in vivo antibacterial activities of a novel glycylcycline, the 9-t-butylglycylamido derivative of minocycline (GAR-936). Antimicrobial Agents Chemother. 1999;43:738-744.
6. Craven GR, Gavin R, Fanning T. The transfer RNA binding site of the 30S ribosome and the site of tetracycline inhibition. Symp Quant Biol. 1969;34:129.
7. Chopra I, Roberts M. Tetracycline antibiotics: Mode of action, applications, molecular biology, and epidemiology of bacterial resistance. Microbiol Mol Biol Rev. 2001;65:232-260.
8. Roberts MC. Tetracycline therapy: Update. Clin Infect Dis. 2003;36:462-467.
9. National Committee for Clinical Laboratory Standards. Sixth Informational Supplement: Performance Standards for Antimicrobial Susceptibility Testing: Approved Standard. NCCLS publications M2-AS, M2-A3, and MH-A3. Villanova, Pa: NCCLS; 1995.
10. Betriu C, Rodriguez-Avial I, Sanchez BA, et al. In vitro activities of tigecycline (GAR-936) against recently isolated clinical bacteria in Spain. Antimicrob Agents Chemother. 2002;46:892-895.
11. Biedenbach DJ, Beach ML, Jones RN. In vitro antimicrobial activity of GAR-936 tested against antibiotic-resistant gram-positive blood stream infection isolates and strains producing extended-spectrum beta-lactamases. Diagn Microbiol Infect Dis. 2001;40:173-177.
12. Boucher HW, Wennersten CB, Eliopoulos GM. In vitro activities of the glycylcycline GAR-936 against gram-positive bacteria. Antimicrob Agents Chemother. 2000;44:2225-2229.
13. Gales AC, Jones RN. Antimicrobial activity and spectrum of the new glycylcycline, GAR-936 tested against 1,203 recent clinical bacterial isolates. Diagn Microbiol Infect Dis. 2000;36:19-36.
14. Milatovic D, Schmitz FJ, Verhoef J, Fluit AC. Activities of the glycylcycline tigecycline (GAR-936) against 1,924 recent European clinical bacterial isolates. Antimicrob Agents Chemother. 2003;47:400-404.
15. Goldstein EJ, Citron DM, Merriam CV, et al. Comparative in vitro activities of GAR-936 against aerobic and anaerobic animal and human bite wound pathogens. Antimicrob Agents Chemother. 2000;44:2747-2751.
16. Hoellman DB, Pankuch GA, Jacobs MR, Appelbaum PC. Antipneumococcal activities of GAR-936 (a new glycylcycline) compared to those of nine other agents against penicillin-susceptible and -resistant pneumococci. Antimicrob Agents Chemother. 2000;44:1085-1088.
17. Patel R, Rouse MS, Piper KE, Steckelberg JM. In vitro activity of GAR-936 against vancomycin-resistant enterococci, methicillin-resistant *Staphylococcus aureus* and penicillin-resistant *Streptococcus pneumoniae*. Diagn Microbiol Infect Dis. 2000;38:177-179.
18. Deshpande LM, Gales AC, Jones RN. GAR-936 (9-t-butylglycylamido-minocycline) susceptibility test development for streptococci, *Haemophilus influenzae* and *Neisseria gonorrhoeae*: Preliminary guidelines and interpretive criteria. Int J Antimicrob Agents. 2001;18:29-35.
19. Wallace RJ Jr, Brown-Elliott BA, Crist CJ, et al. Comparison of the in vitro activity of the glycylcycline tigecycline (formerly GAR-936) with those of tetracycline, minocycline, and doxycycline against isolates of nontuberculous mycobacteria. Antimicrob Agents Chemother. 2002;46:3164-3167.
20. Poulsen RK, Knudsen JC, Petersen MB. In vitro activity of 6 macrolides, clindamycin, and tetracycline on *Streptococcus pneumoniae* with different penicillin susceptibilities. APMIS. 1996;104:227-233.
21. Shea KW, Cunha BA. Doxycycline activity against penicillin-resistant *Streptococcus pneumoniae*. Chest. 1995;108:1775-1776.
22. Centers for Disease Control. Antibiotic-resistant strains of *Neisseria gonorrhoeae*. MMWR Morb Mortal Wkly Rep. 1987;36(Suppl 55):1-18.
23. Kobayashi I, Kanayama A, Saika T, et al. Tendency toward increase in the frequency of isolation of beta-lactamase-nonproducing *Neisseria gonorrhoeae* exhibiting penicillin resistance, and recent emergence of multidrug-resistant isolates in Japan. J Infect Chemother. 2003;9:126-130.

24. Arreaza L, Salcedo C, Alcala B, et al. Antibiotic resistance of *Neisseria gonorrhoeae* in Spain: Trends over the last two decades. J Antimicrob Chemother. 2003;51: 153-156.

25. Farrell ID, Hinchliffe PM, Robertson L. Susceptibility of *Brucella* spp. to tetracycline and its analogues. J Clin Pathol. 1976;29:1097.

26. Morris JG Jr, Black RE. Cholera and other vibrioses in the United States. N Engl J Med. 1985;312:343-350.

27. Michel J, Rogol M, Dickman D. Susceptibility of clinical isolates of *Campylobacter jejuni* to sixteen antimicrobial agents. Antimicrob Agents Chemother. 1983;23:796.

28. Gordon RC, Thompson TR, Carlson W, et al. Antimicrobial resistance of shigellae isolated in Michigan. JAMA. 1975;231:1159.

29. Edlund C, North CE. In-vitro susceptibility of anaerobic bacteria to GAR-936, a new glycylcycline. Clin Microbiol Infect. 2000;6:159-163.

30. Washington JA, Dearing WH, Judd ES, et al. Effect of preoperative antibiotic regimen on development of infection after intestinal surgery: Prospective, randomized, double-blind study. Ann Surg. 1974;180:567.

31. Hojer H, Wetterfors J. Systemic prophylaxis with doxycycline in surgery of the colon and rectum. Ann Surg. 1978;187:362.

32. Levin JM, Nelson JA, Segreti J, et al. In vitro susceptibility of *Borrelia burgdorferi* to 11 antimicrobial agents. Antimicrob Agents Chemother. 1993;37:1444-1446.

33. Pang LW, Limsomwong N, Boudreau EF, et al. Doxycycline prophylaxis for falciparum malaria. Lancet. 1987;1:1161-1164.

34. Speer BS, Bedzyk L, Salyers AA. Evidence that a novel tetracycline resistance gene found on two *Bacteroides* transposons encodes an NADP-requiring oxidoreductase. J Bacteriol. 1991;173:176-183.

35. McMurry LM, Levy SB. Tetracycline resistance in gram-positive bacteria, In: Fischetti VA, Novick RP, Ferretti JJ, et al, eds. Gram-Positive Pathogens. Washington, DC: American Society for Microbiology; 2000:660-677.

36. Petersen PJ, Jakobus NV, Weiss WJ, et al. In vitro and in vivo antibacterial activities of a novel glycylcycline, the 9-t-butylglycylamido derivative of minocycline (GAR-936). Antimicrobial Agents Chemother. 1999;43:738-744.

37. Petersen PJ, Weiss WJ, Labthavikul P, Bradford PA. The post-antibiotic effects and time kill kinetics of the glycylcyclines, GAR-936 (TGB-MINO) and PAM-MINO. Presented in the abstracts of the 38th Interscience Conference on Antimicrobial Agents and Chemotherapy, 1998.

38. Bergeron J, Ammirati M, Danley D, et al. Glycylcyclines bind to the high affinity tetracycline ribosomal binding site and evade Tet(M)- and Tet(O)-mediated ribosomal protection. Antimicrobial Agent Chemother. 1996;40:2226-2228.

39. Chopra I. New developments in tetracyclines antibiotics: Glycylcyclines and tetracyclines efflux pump inhibitors. Drug Resist Updat. 2002;5:119-125.

40. Kucers A, Crowe S, Grayson ML, Hoy J. The use of antibiotics in a clinical review of antibacterial, antifungal and antiviral drugs. 1997:719-761.

41. American Hospital Formulary Service (AHFS). Drug information: Tetracyclines. 2002:432-452.

42. Welling PG, Koch PA, Lau CC, Craig WA. Bioavailability of tetracycline and doxycycline in fasted and nonfasted subjects. Antimicrob Agents Chemother. 1977;11:462-469.

43. Fabre J, Pitton JS, Junz JP, et al. Distribution and excretion of doxycycline in man. Chemotherapia. 1966;11:73.

44. Kunin CM, Dornbush AC, Finland M. Distribution and excretion of four tetracycline analogues in normal young men. J Clin Invest. 1959;38:1950.

45. Saivin S, Houin G. Clinical pharmacokinetics of doxycycline and minocycline. Clin Pharmacokinet. 1988;15:355-366.

46. van Ogtrop ML, Andes D, Stamstad TJ, et al. In vivo pharmacodynamic activities of two glycylcyclines (GAR-936 and WAY 152,288) against various gram-positive and gram-negative bacteria. Antimicrobial Agents Chemother. 2000;44:943-949.

47. Muralidhan G, Getsy J, Mayer P, et al. Pharmacokinetics, safety and tolerability of GAR-936, a novel glycylcycline antibiotics, in healthy subjects. Abstract of the 39th conference on Antimicrobial Agents and Chemotherapy (ICAAC), Sept. 26-29. Washington, DC: American Society for Microbiology; 1999:303.

48. Wood WS, Kipnis GP. The concentrations of tetracycline, chlortetracycline and oxytetracycline in the cerebrospinal fluid after intravenous administration. In: Welch H, Marti-Ibanez F, eds. Antibiotics Annual, 1953-1954. New York: Medical Encyclopedia; 1953:98-101.

49. Yim CW, Flynn NM, Fitzgerald FT. Penetration of oral doxycycline into the cerebrospinal fluid of patients with latent or neurosyphilis. Antimicrob Agents Chemother. 1985;28:347.

50. Parker RH, Schmid F. Antimicrobial activity of synovial fluid during therapy of septic arthritis. Arthritis Rheum. 1971;14:96.

51. Lundberg C, Malmburg A, Ivemark BI. Antibiotic concentrations in relation to structural changes in maxillary sinus mucosa following intramuscular or peroral treatment. Scand J Infect Dis. 1974;6:187.

52. Hoeprich PD, Warshauer DM. Entry of four tetracyclines into saliva and tears. Antimicrob Agents Chemother. 1974;5:330.

53. Whelton A. Tetracyclines in renal insufficiency: Resolution of a therapeutic dilemma. Bull N Y Acad Med. 1978;54:223.

54. Tilles S, Slatore C. Hypersensitivity reactions to non-beta-lactam antibiotics. Clin Rev Allergy Immunol. 2003;3:221-228.

55. Byrne PAC, Williams BD, Pritchard MH. Minocycline-related lupus. Br J Rheumatol. 1994;33:674-676.

56. Gough A, Chapman S, Wagstaff K, et al. Minocycline induced autoimmune hepatitis and systemic lupus erythematosus-like syndrome. BMJ. 1996;312:169-172.

57. Singer SJ, Piazza-Hepp TD, Girardi LS, Moledina NR. Lupus-like reaction associated with minocycline. JAMA. 1997;277:295-296.

58. Frost P, Weinstein GD, Gomez EC. Phototoxic potential of minocycline and doxycycline. Arch Dermatol. 1972;105:681.

59. Angeloni VL, Salasche SJ, Ortiz R. Nail, skin and scleral pigmentation induced by minocycline. Cutis. 1987;40:229-233.

60. Atwood HD, Dennet X. A black thyroid and minocycline treatment. Br Med J. 1976;2:1109.

61. Siller GM, Tod MA, Savage NW. Minocycline-induced oral pigmentation. J Am Acad Dermatol. 1994;30:350-354.

62. Odell EW, Hodgson RP, Haskell R. Oral presentation of minocycline-induced black bone disease. Oral Surg Oral Med Oral Pathol Oral Radiol Endod. 1995;79:459-461.

63. Brearley LJ, Storey E. Tetracycline-induced tooth changes: Part 2. Prevalence, localization and nature of staining in extracted deciduous teeth. Med J Aust. 1968;2:714.

64. Witkop CJ, Wolf RO. Hypoplasia and intrinsic staining of enamel following tetracycline therapy. JAMA. 1963;185:1008.

65. Cohan S, Bevelander G, Tiamsic T. Growth inhibition of prematures receiving tetracycline. Am J Dis Child. 1963;105:453.

66. Forti G, Benincori C. Doxycycline and the teeth. Lancet. 1969;1:782.

67. Schneider R. Doxycycline esophageal ulcers. Am J Dig Dis. 1977;22:805.

68. Winckler K. Tetracycline ulcers of the oesophagus: Endoscopy, histology, and roentgenology in two cases, and review of the literature. Endoscopy. 1981;13:225.

69. Elmore MF, Rogge JD. Tetracycline-induced pancreatitis. Gastroenterology. 1981;81:1134.

70. Lepper MH, Wolfe CK, Zimmerman HJ, et al. Effect of large doses of Aureomycin on human liver. Arch Intern Med. 1951;88:271.

71. Whalley PJ, Adams RH, Combes B. Tetracycline toxicity in pregnancy: Liver and pancreatic dysfunction. JAMA. 1964;189:357.

72. Damjanov I, Arnold R, Faour M. Tetracycline toxicity in a non-pregnant woman. JAMA. 1968;204:934.

73. Vial T, Biour M, Descotes J, Trepo C. Antibiotic-associated hepatitis: Update from 1990. Ann Pharmacother. 1997;31:304-320.

74. Shils ME. Renal disease and the metabolic effects of tetracycline. Ann Intern Med. 1963;58:389.

75. Forrest JN, Cox M, Hong C, et al. Superiority of demeclocycline over lithium in the treatment of chronic syndrome of inappropriate secretion of antidiuretic hormone. N Engl J Med. 1978;298:173.

76. Carrilho F, Bosch J, Arroyo V, et al. Renal failure associated with demeclocycline in cirrhosis. Ann Intern Med. 1977;87:195.

77. Koch-Weser J, Gilmore EB. Benign intracranial hypertension in an adult after tetracycline therapy. JAMA. 1967;200:345-347.

78. Walters BN, Gubbay SS. Tetracycline and benign intracranial hypertension: Report of five cases. Br Med J (Clin Res Ed). 1981;282:19-20.

79. Lander CM. Minocycline-induced BIH. Clin Exp Neurol. 1989;26:161-167.

80. Nagarajan L, Lam GC. Tetracycline-induced benign intracranial hypertension. J Paediatr Child Health. 2000;36:82-83.

81. Lochhead J, Elston JS. Lesson of the week: Doxycycline induced intracranial hypertension. BMJ. 2003;326:641-642.

82. Corbett JJ, Savino PJ, Thompson HS, et al. Visual loss in pseudotumor cerebri: Follow-up of 57 patients from five to 41 years and a profile of 14 patients with permanent severe visual loss. Arch Neurol. 1982;39:461-474.

83. Lepper MH, Dowling HF. Treatment of pneumococcal meningitis with penicillin compared with penicillin plus Aureomycin. Arch Intern Med. 1951;88:489.

84. Bartlett JG, Dowell SF, Mandell LA, et al. Practice guidelines for the management of community-acquired pneumonia in adults. Infectious Diseases Society of America. Clin Infect Dis. 2000;31:347-382.

85. Mandell LA, Marrie TJ, Grossman RF, et al. Canadian guidelines for the initial management of community-acquired pneumonia: An evidence-based update by the Canadian Infectious Diseases Society and the Canadian Thoracic Society. The Canadian Community-Acquired Pneumonia Working Group. Clin Infect Dis. 2000;31:383-421.

86. File TM Jr, Segreti J, Dunbar L, et al. A multicenter, randomized study comparing the efficacy and safety of intravenous and/or oral levofloxacin versus ceftriaxone and/or cefuroxime axetil in treatment of adults with community-acquired pneumonia. Antimicrob Agents Chemother. 1997;41:1965-1972.

87. Shea KW, Cunha BA, Ueno Y, et al. Doxycycline activity against *Streptococcus pneumoniae*. Chest. 1995;108:1775-1776.

88. Doern GV, Pfaller MA, Kugler K, et al. Prevalence of antimicrobial resistance among respiratory tract isolates of *Streptococcus pneumoniae* in North America: 1997 results from the SENTRY antimicrobial surveillance program. Clin Infect Dis. 1998;27:764-770.

89. Lederman ER, Gleeson TD, Driscoll T, Wallace MR. Doxycycline sensitivity of *S. pneumoniae* isolates. Clin Infect Dis. 2003;36:1091.

90. Inglesby TV, O'Toole T, Henderson DA, et al. Consensus Statement: Anthrax as a biological weapon, 2002—Updated recommendations for management. JAMA. 2002;287:2236-2252.

91. Smith HL, Rajan TV. Tetracycline inhibits development of the infective-stage larvae of filarial nematodes in vitro. Exp Parasitol. 2000;95:265-270.

92. White NJ. Melioidosis. Lancet. 2003;361:1715-1722.

93. Koehler JE, Tappero JW. Bacillary angiomatosis and bacillary peliosis in patients infected with human immunodeficiency virus. Clin Infect Dis. 1993;17:612-624.

94. Dutta D, Bhattacharya SK, Bhattacharya MK, et al. Efficacy of norfloxacin and doxy-cycline for treatment of vibrio cholerae 0139 infection. J Antimicrob Chemother. 1996;37:575-581.
95. Anonymous. The choice of antibacterial drugs. Med Lett Drugs Ther. 1996;38:25-34.
96. Ljungberg B, Christensson B, Grubb R. Failure of doxycycline treatment in aquar-ium-associated Mycobacterium marinum infections. Scand J Infect Dis. 1987;19:539-543.
97. Cannon WR. Whipple's disease, genomics, and drug therapy. Lancet. 2003;361:1916.
98. Hughes CE, Harris C, Peterson LR, Gerding DN. Enhancement of the in vitro activ-ity of amphotericin B against Aspergillus spp. by tetracycline analogs. Antimicrob Agents Chemother. 1984;26:837-840.
99. Farber BF, Brody JP. Rapid development of aplastic anemia after intravenous chlo-ramphenicol and cimetidine therapy. South Med J. 1981;74:1257-1258.
100. O'Dell JR, Haure CE, Palmer W, et al. Treatment of early rheumatoid arthritis with minocycline or placebo: Results of a randomized, double-blind, placebo-controlled trial. Arthritis Rheum. 1997;40:794-796.
101. Pillemer SR, Fowler SE, Tilley BC, et al. Meaningful improvement criteria sets in a rheumatoid arthritis clinical trial. Minocycline in Rheumatoid Arthritis trial group. Arthritis Rheum. 1997;40:419-425.
102. Walker-Renard PB, Vaughan LM, Sahn SA. Chemical pleurodesis for malignant pleural effusions. Ann Intern Med. 1994;120:56-64.
103. Ehrlich J, Bartz QR, Smith RM, et al. Chloromycetin, a new antibiotic from a soil actinomycete. Science. 1947;106:417.
104. Carter HE, Gottliebb D, Anderson HW. Comments and communications. Science. 107;113:947.
105. Abdel-Sayed S. Transport of chloramphenicol into sensitive strains of Escherichia coli and Pseudomonas aeruginosa. J Antimicrob Chemother. 1987;19:7-20.
106. Turk DC. A comparison of chloramphenicol and ampicillin as bactericidal agents for Haemophilus influenzae type B. J Med Microbiol. 1977;10:127.
107. Rahal JJ, Simberkoff MS. Bactericidal and bacteriostatic action of chloramphenicol against meningeal pathogens. Antimicrob Agents Chemother. 1979;16:13.
108. Weeks JL, Mason EO Jr, Baker CJ. Antagonism of ampicillin and chloramphenicol for meningeal isolates of group B streptococci. Antimicrob Agents Chemother. 1981;20:281.
109. Parry CM, Hien TT, Dougan G, et al. Medical progress: Typhoid fever. N Engl J Med. 2002;347:1770-1782.
110. Rao PS, Rajasekhar V, Varghese GK, Shivananda PG. Emergence of multidrug-resis-tant Salmonella typhi in rural southern India. Am J Trop Med Hyg. 1993;48:108-111.
111. Sood S, Kapil A, Das B, et al. Re-emergence of chloramphenicol-sensitive Salmonella typhi. Lancet. 1999;353:1241-1242.
112. Wasfy MO, Frenck R, Ismail TF, et al. Trends of multiple-drug resistance among Salmonella serotype Typhi isolates during a 14-year period in Egypt. Clin Infect Dis. 2002;35:1265-1268.
113. Cherubin CE, Neu HC, Rahal JJ, et al. Emergence of resistance to chloramphenicol in Salmonella. J Infect Dis. 1977;135:807.
114. Glynn MK, Bopp C, Dewitt W, et al. Emergence of multidrug-resistant Salmonella enterica serotype typhimurium DT104 infections in the United States. N Engl J Med. 1998;338:1333-1338.
115. Sandvang D, Aarestrup FM, Jensen LB. Characterisation of integrons and antibiotic resistance genes in Danish multiresistant Salmonella enterica typhimurium DT104. FEMS Microbiol Lett. 1998;160:37-41.
116. Ribot EM, Wierzba RK, Angulo FJ, Barrett TJ. Salmonella enterica serotype Typhimurium DT104 isolated from humans, United States, 1985, 1990, and 1995. Emerg Infect Dis. 2002;8:387-391.
117. Long SS, Phillips SE. Chloramphenicol-resistant Haemophilus influenzae. J Pediatr. 1976;90:1030.
118. Doern GV, Jorgensen JH, Thornsberry C, et al. Prevalence of antimicrobial resistance among clinical isolates of Haemophilus influenzae: A collaborative study. Diagn Microbiol Infect Dis. 1986;4:95-107.
119. Hoban DJ, Doern GV, Fluit AC, et al. Worldwide prevalence of antimicrobial resis-tance in Streptococcus pneumoniae, Haemophilus influenzae, and Moraxella ca-tarrhalis in the SENTRY Antimicrobial Surveillance Program, 1997-1999. Clin Infect Dis. 2001;32(Suppl 2):S81-93.
120. MacMahon P, Sills J, Hall E, et al. Haemophilus influenzae type B resistant to both chloramphenicol and ampicillin in Britain. BMJ. 1982;24:1229.
121. Johnson AW, Mookkolu OA, Onile BA. Chloramphenicol-resistant Haemophilus in-fluenzae meningitis in young urban Nigerian children. Acta Paediatr. 1992;81:941-943.
122. Bergeron MC, Claveau S, Simard P. Limited in vitro activity of cefamandole against 100 beta-lactamase and non-beta-lactamase-producing Haemophilus influenzae strains: Comparison of moxalactam, chloramphenicol and ampicillin. Antimicrob Agents Chemother. 1981;19:101.
123. Kenny JF, Isburg CD, Michaels RH. Meningitis due to Haemophilus influenzae type b resistant to both ampicillin and chloramphenicol. Pediatrics. 1980;66:14.
124. Campos J, Garcia-Tornel S, San Feliu I. Susceptibility studies of multiply resistant Haemophilus influenzae isolated from pediatric patients and contacts. Antimicrob Agents Chemother. 1984;25:706.
125. Williams JD, Mossdeen F. Antibiotic resistance in Haemophilus influenzae. Epidemiology, mechanisms, and therapeutic possibilities. Rev Infect Dis. 1986;8(Suppl 5):555-561.
126. Kabani A, Joffe A, Jadavji T. Haemophilus influenzae type B resistant to ampicillin and chloramphenicol. Pediatr Infect Dis J. 1991;9:681.
127. Hoban DJ, Biedenbach DJ, Mutnick AH, Jones RN. Pathogen of occurrence and sus-ceptibility patterns associated with pneumonia in hospitalized patients in North America: results of the SENTRY Antimicrobial Surveillance Study (2000). Diagn Microbiol Infect Dis. 2003;45:279-285.
128. Snydman DR, Jacobus NV, McDermott LA, et al. National survey on the susceptibil-ity of Bacteroides Fragilis Group: report and analysis of trends for 1997-2000. Clin Infect Dis. 2002;35(Suppl 1):S126-134.
129. Cuchural GJ Jr, Talley FP, Jacobus NV, et al. Susceptibility of the Bacteroides frag-ilis group in the United States: Analysis by site of isolation. Antimicrob Agents Chemother. 1988;32:717-722.
130. Finegold SM, Wexler HM. Therapeutic implications of bacteriologic findings in mixed aerobic-anaerobic infections. Antimicrob Agents Chemother. 1988;32:611-616.
131. Snydman DR, McDermott L, Cuchural G Jr, et al. Analysis of trends in antimicrobial resistance patterns among clinical isolates of Bacteroides fragilis group species from 1990 to 1994. Clin Infect Dis. 1996;23(Suppl 1):S54-S65.
132. Okamoto S, Mizuno D. Mechanism of chloramphenicol and tetracycline resistance in Escherichia coli. J Gen Microbiol. 1964;35:125.
133. Okamoto S, Suzuki Y. Chloramphenicol-, dihydrostreptomycin-, and kanamycin-in-activating enzymes from multiple drug-resistant Escherichia coli carrying episome "R." Nature. 1965;208:1301.
134. Gangarosa EJ, Bennett JV, Wyatt C, et al. An epidemic-associated episome? J Infect Dis. 1972;126:215.
135. Butler T, Linh NN, Arnold K, et al. Chloramphenicol-resistant typhoid fever in Vietnam associated with R-factor. Lancet. 1973;2:983.
136. Halder KK, Dalal BS, Ghose E, Samyal S. Chloramphenicol resistant Salmonella ty-phi: The cause of recent outbreak of enteric fever in Calcutta. Indian J Pathol Microbiol. 1992;35:11-17.
137. Glazko AJ, Dill WA, Kinkel AW, et al. Absorption and excretion of parenteral doses of chloramphenicol sodium succinate in comparison with peroral doses of chloram-phenicol (Abstract). Clin Pharmacol Ther. 1977;21:104.
138. Pickering LK, Hoecker JL, Kramer WG, et al. Clinical pharmacology of two chlo-ramphenicol preparations in children: Sodium succinate (IV) and palmitate (oral) es-ters. J Pediatr. 1980;96:757.
139. Bhutta ZA, Niazi SK, Suria A. Chloramphenicol clearance in typhoid fever: Implications for therapy. Indian J Pediatr. 1992;59:213-219.
140. Shann F, Linnenmann V, MacKenzie A, et al. Absorption of chloramphenicol sodium succinate after intramuscular administration in children. N Engl J Med. 1985;313:410-414.
141. DuPont HL, Hornick RB, Weiss CF, et al. Evaluation of chloramphenicol acid succi-nate therapy of induced typhoid fever and Rocky Mountain spotted fever. N Engl J Med. 1970;282:53.
142. Acharya GP, Davis TME, Ho M, et al. Factors affecting the pharmacokinetics of par-enteral chloramphenicol in enteric fever. J Antimicrob Chemother. 1997;40:91-98.
143. Holt DE, Hurley R, Harvey D. A reappraisal of chloramphenicol metabolism: Detection and quantification of metabolites in the sera of children. J Antimicrob Chemother. 1995;35:115-127.
144. Lindberg AA, Nilsson LH, Bucht H, et al. Concentration of chloramphenicol in the urine and blood in relation to renal function. Br Med J. 1966;2:724.
145. Kauffman RE, Miceti JN, Strebel L, et al. Pharmacokinetics of chloramphenicol and chloramphenicol succinate in infants and children. J Pediatr. 1981;98:315.
146. Kauffman RE, Thirumoorthi MC, Buckley JA, et al. Relative bioavailability of intra-venous chloramphenicol succinate and oral chloramphenicol palmitate in infants and children. J Pediatr. 1981;99:363.
147. Kunin CM. A guide to use of antibiotics in patients with renal disease. Ann Intern Med. 1967;67:151.
148. Kramer PW, Griffith RS, Campbell RL, et al. Antibiotic penetration of the brain: A comparative study. J Neurosurg. 1969;31:295.
149. Rapp GF, Griffith RS, Hebble WM. The permeability of traumatically inflamed syn-ovial membrane to commonly used antibiotics. J Bone Joint Surg Am. 1966;48:1534.
150. Kunin CM, Glazko AJ, Finland M. Persistence of antibiotics in blood of patients with acute renal failure: II. Chloramphenicol and its metabolic products in the blood of pa-tients with severe renal disease or hepatic cirrhosis. J Clin Invest. 1959;38:1498.
151. Suhrland LG, Weisberger AS. Chloramphenicol toxicity in liver and renal disease. Arch Intern Med. 1963;112:161.
152. Hammett-Stabler CA, Johns T. Laboratory guidelines for monitoring of antimicrobial drugs. National Academy of Clinical Biochemistry. Clin Chem. 1998;44:1129-1140.
153. Yunis AA. Chloramphenicol-induced bone marrow suppression. Semin Hematol. 1973;10:225.
154. Scott JL, Finegold SM, Belkin GA, et al. A controlled double-blind study of the hematologic toxicity of chloramphenicol. N Engl J Med. 1965;272:1137.
155. Best WR. Chloramphenicol-associated blood dyscrasias: A review of cases submitted to the American Medical Association Registry. JAMA. 1967;201:181.
156. Wallerstein RO, Condit PK, Kasper CK, et al. Statewide study of chloramphenicol therapy and fatal aplastic anemia. JAMA. 1969;208:2045.
157. Nagao T, Mauer AM. Concordance for drug-induced aplastic anemia in identical twins. N Engl J Med. 1969;281:7.
157a. Morley A, Trailor K, Remes J. Residual marrow damage: Possible explanation for idiosyncrasy to chloramphenicol. Br J Haematol. 1976;32:525.
157b. Holt R. The bacterial degradation of chloramphenicol. Lancet 1967;1:1259.
158. Jimenez JJ, Arimura GK, Abou-Khalil WH, et al. Chloramphenicol-induced bone marrow injury: Possible role of bacterial metabolites of chloramphenicol. Blood. 1987;70:1180-1185.

159. Jimenez JJ, Jimenez JG, Daghistani D, Yunis AA. Interaction of chloramphenicol and metabolites with colony stimulating factors: Possible role in chloramphenicol-induced bone marrow injury. Am J Med Sci. 1990;300:350-353.

160. Plaut ME, Best WR. Aplastic anemia after parenteral chloramphenicol: Warning renewal (Letter). N Engl J Med. 1982;306:1486.

161. Daum RS, Cohen DL, Smith AL. Fatal aplastic anemia following apparent "dose-related" chloramphenicol toxicity. J Pediatr. 1979;94:403.

162. Lancaster T, Stewart AM, Jick H. Risk of serious hematological toxicity with use of chloramphenicol eye drops in a British general practice database. BMJ. 1998;316:667.

163. Doona M, Walsh JB. Use of chloramphenicol as topical eye medication: Time to cry halt (Editorial) (see comments)? BMJ. 1995;310:1217-1218.

164. Wiholm BE, Kelly JP, Kaufman D, et al. Relation of aplastic anaemia to use of chloramphenicol eye drops in two international case-control studies. BMJ. 1998;316:666.

165. Shu XO, Linet MS, Gao RN, et al. Chloramphenicol use and childhood leukaemia in Shanghai. Lancet. 1987;2:934-937.

166. Burns LE, Hodgman JE, Cass AB. Fatal circulatory collapse in premature infants receiving chloramphenicol. N Engl J Med. 1959;261:1318.

167. Thompson WL, Anderson SE, Lipsky JJ, et al. Overdoses of chloramphenicol. JAMA. 1975;234:149.

168. Evans LS, Kleiman MB. Acidosis as a presenting feature of chloramphenicol toxicity. J Pediatr. 1986;108:475-477.

169. Suarez CR, Ow EP. Chloramphenicol toxicity associated with severe cardiac dysfunction. Pediatr Cardiol. 1992;13:48-51.

170. Stevens DC, Kleinman MB, Lietman PS, et al. Exchange transfusion in acute chloramphenicol toxicity. J Pediatr. 1981;99:651.

171. Freundlick M, Cynamon H, Tamer A, et al. Management of chloramphenicol intoxication in infancy by charcoal hemoperfusion. J Pediatr. 1983;103:485.

172. Anonymous. Chloramphenicol blindness (Editorial). Br Med J. 1965;1:1511.

173. Faber OK, Mouridsen HT, Skovsted L, et al. The effect of chloramphenicol and sulphaphenazole on the biotransformation of cyclophosphamide in man. Br J Clin Pharmacol. 1975;2:281.

174. Christensen LK, Skovsted L. Inhibition of drug metabolism by chloramphenicol. Lancet. 1969;2:1397.

175. Petitpierre B, Fabre J. Chlorpropamide and chloramphenicol. Lancet. 1970;1:789.

176. Rose JQ, Choi HK, Schentag JJ. Intoxication caused by interaction of chloramphenicol and phenytoin. JAMA. 1977;237:2630.

177. Prober CG. Effect of rifampin on chloramphenicol levels. N Engl J Med. 1985;312:788-789.

178. Duke T, Michael A, Mokela D, et al. Chloramphenicol or ceftriaxone, or both, as treatment for meningitis in developing countries? Arch Dis Child. 2003;88:536-539.

179. Fujita K, Shang DH, Sakata H, et al. Antibiotic susceptibility of type b Haemophilus influenzae and Streptococcus pneumoniae, and antibiotic concentration in cerebrospinal fluid. Acta Paediatr Jpn. 1990;32:132-138.

180. Reis JN, Lima JB, Ribeiro GS, et al. Antimicrobial resistance in Haemophilus influenzae isolated during population-based surveillance for meningitis in Salvador, Brazil. Antimicrob Agents Chemother. 2002;46:3641-3643.

180a. Owusu-Ofori A, Scheld WM. Treatment of Salmonella meningitis. Two case reports and a review of the literature. Int J Infect Dis. 2003;7:53-60.

181. Galimand M, Gerband G, Guibourdenche M, et al. High level chloramphenicol resistance in Neisseria meningitidis. N Engl J Med. 1998;339:868-874.

182. Klugman KP, Madhi SA. Emergence of drug resistance: Impact on bacterial meningitis. Infect Dis Clin North Am. 1999;13:637-646.

183. Klass PE, Klein JO. Therapy of bacterial sepsis, meningitis and otitis media in infants and children: 1992 poll of directors of programs in pediatric infectious diseases. Pediatr Infect Dis J. 1992;11:702-705.

184. Messick CR, Pendland SL. In vitro activity of chloramphenicol alone and in combination with vancomycin, ampicillin, or RP 59500 (quinupristin/dalfopristin) against vancomycin-resistant enterococci. Diagn Microbiol Infect Dis. 1997;29:203-205.

185. Mundlein E, von Baum H, Geiss HK, et al. Life-threatening infection with multiresistant Staphylococcus epidermidis in a patient with end-stage renal disease: Cure with chloramphenicol and quinupristin/dalfopristin (RP 59500). Infection. 1997;25:252-254.

186. Friedland IR, Klugman KP: Failure of chloramphenicol therapy in penicillin-resistant pneumococcal meningitis. Lancet. 1992;339:405-408.

187. Bradley JS, Scheld WM. The challenge of penicillin-resistant Streptococcus pneumoniae meningitis: Current antibiotic therapy in the 1990s. Clin Infect Dis. 1997;24(Suppl 2):S213-S221.

188. Duke T, Poka H, Dale F, et al. Chloramphenicol versus benzylpenicillin and gentamicin for the treatment of severe pneumonia in children in Papua New Guinea: A randomised trial. Lancet. 2002;359:474-480.

189. Norris AH, Reilly JP, Edelstein PH, et al. Chloramphenicol for the treatment of vancomycin-resistant enterococcal infections. Clin Infect Dis. 1995;20:1137-1144.

190. Papanicolaou GA, Meyers BR, Meyers J, et al. Nosocomial infections with vancomycin-resistant Enterococcus faecium in liver transplant recipients: Risk factors for acquisition and mortality. Clin Infect Dis. 1996;23:760-766.

191. Mato SP, Robinson S, Bégué AE. Vancomycin-resistant Enterococcus faecium meningitis successfully treated with chloramphenicol. Pediatr Infect Dis J. 1999;18:483-484.

192. Ricaurte JC, Boucher HW, Turett GS, et al. Chloramphenicol treatment for vancomycin-resistant Enterococcus faecium bacteremia. Clin Microbiol Infect. 2001;7:17-21.

193. Dennis DT, Inglesby TV, Henderson DA, et al. Tularemia as a biological weapon: Medical and public health management. JAMA. 2001;285:2763-2773.

194. Inglesby TV, Dennis DT, Henderson DA, et al. Plague as a biological weapon: Medical and public health management. JAMA. 2000;283:2281-2290.

195. Inglesby TV, O'Toole T, Henderson DA, et al. Consensus Statement: Anthrax as a biological weapon, 2002; updated recommendations for management. JAMA. 2002;287:2236-2252.

196. Leyden JJ. Absorption of minocycline hydrochloride and tetracycline hydrochloride: Effect of food, milk, and iron. J Am Acad Dermatol. 1985;12:308-312.

197. MacArthur CG, Johnson AJ, Allen ES, et al. The absorption and sputum penetration of doxycycline. J Antimicrob Chemother. 1978;4:509-514.

198. Neuvonen PJ, Gothoni G, Hackman R, et al. Interference of iron with the absorption of tetracycline in man. Br Med J. 1970;4:532.

199. Gugler R, Allgayer H. Effects of antacids on the clinical pharmacokinetics of drugs: An update. Clin Pharmacokinet. 1990;18:210-219.

200. Bar WH, Adir J, Garrettson L. Decrease of tetracycline in man by sodium bicarbonate. Clin Pharmacol Ther. 1971;12:779.

201. Fisher P, House F, Inns P, et al. Effect of cimetidine on the absorption of orally administered tetracycline. Br J Clin Pharmacol. 1980;9:153.

202. Neuvonen PJ, Penttila O. Interaction between doxycycline and barbiturates. Br Med J. 1974;1:535.

203. Penttila O, Neuvonen PJ, Lehtovaara R. Interaction between doxycycline and some antiepileptic drugs. Br Med J. 1974;2:470.

204. Neuvonen PJ, Penttila O, Roos M. Effect of long-term alcohol consumption on the half-life of tetracycline and doxycycline in man. Int J Clin Pharmacol. 1976;14:303.

205. Kuzucu EY. Methoxyflurane, tetracycline and renal failure. JAMA. 1970;211:1162.

206. Semel JD. Renal failure and multiple organ toxicity associated with tetracycline operative prophylaxis. Infect Surg. 1988;June:405-408.

207. Boston Collaborative Drug Surveillance Program. Tetracycline and drug-attributed rises in blood urea nitrogen. JAMA. 1972;220:377.

208. Bacon JF, Chenfield GM. Pregnancy attributable to interaction between tetracycline and oral contraceptives. BMJ. 1980;280:293.

209. Steigbigel NH, Reed CR, Finland M. Susceptibility of common pathogenic bacteria to seven tetracycline antibiotics in vitro. Am J Med Sci. 1968;255:179.

210. Finland M. Changing patters of susceptibility of common bacterial pathogens to antimicrobial agents. Ann Intern Med. 1972;76:1009.

211. Sabath LD, Stumpf LL, Wallace SJ, et al. Susceptibility of Diplococcus pneumoniae, Haemophilus influenzae, and Neisseria meningitidis to 23 antibiotics. Antimicrob Agents Chemother. 1970;10:53-56.

212. Poulsen RK, Knudsen JC, Petersen MB. In vitro activity of 6 macrolides, clindamycin, and tetracycline on Streptococcus pneumoniae with different penicillin susceptibilities. APMIS. 1996;104:227-233.

213. Chow AW, Patten V, Dominick B. Susceptibility of Campylobacter fetus to twenty-two antimicrobial agents. Antimicrob Agents Chemother. 1978;13:416.

214. Woodward TE, Wisseman CL. Chloromycetin (chloramphenicol). New York: Medical Encyclopedia; 1958.

215. McGowan JE, Garner C, Wilcox C, et al. Antibiotic susceptibility of gram negative bacilli isolated from blood cultures: Results of tests with 35 agents and strains from 169 patients at Boston City Hospital during 1972. Am J Med. 1974;57:225.

216. Yow EM, Spink WW. Experimental studies on the action of streptomycin, Aureomycin and Chloromycetin on Brucella. J Clin Invest. 1949;28:871.

217. Robertson RP, Wahab MFA, Raasch FO. Evaluation of chloramphenicol and ampicillin in Salmonella enteric fever. N Engl J Med. 1968;278:171.

218. Rubinstein E, Shainberg B. In vitro activity of cinoxacin, ampicillin, and chloramphenicol against Shigella and non-typhoid Salmonella. Antimicrob Agents Chemother. 1977;11:173.

219. Wells EB, Chang SM, Jackson GG, et al. Antibiotic spectrum of Hemophilus pertussis. J Pediatr. 1950;36:752.

220. Mathies AW Jr. Penicillins in the treatment of bacterial meningitis. J R Coll Physicians Lond. 1972;6:139.

221. Martin WJ, Gardner M, Washington JA II. In vitro antimicrobial susceptibility of anaerobic bacteria isolated from clinical specimens. Antimicrob Agents Chemother. 1972;1:148.

222. Bloxham RA, Durbin GM, Johnson T, Winterborn MH. Chloramphenicol and phenobarbitone: A drug interaction. Arch Dis Child. 1979;54:76-77.

223. Krasinski K, Kusmiesz H, Nelson JD. Pharmacologic interactions among chloramphenicol, phenytoin and phenobarbital. Pediatr Infect Dis. 1982;1:232-235.

224. Powell DA, Nahata MC, Durrell DC, et al. Interactions among chloramphenicol, phenytoin and phenobarbital in a pediatric patient. J Pediatr. 1981;98:1001.

225. Steinfort CL, McConachy KA. Cyclosporin-chloramphenicol drug interaction in a heart-lung transplant recipient. Med J Aust. 1994;161:455.

226. Bui LL, Huang DD. Possible interaction between cyclosporine and chloramphenicol. Ann Pharmacother. 1999;33:252.

227. Farber BF, Brody JP. Rapid development of aplastic anemia after intravenous chloramphenicol and cimetidine therapy. South Med J. 1981;74:1257-1258.

228. West BC, DeVault GA Jr, Clement JC, Williams DM. Aplastic anemia associated with parenteral chloramphenicol: Review of 10 cases, including the second case of possible increased risk with cimetidine. Rev Infect Dis. 1988;10:1048-1051.

229. Schulman SL, Shaw LM, Jabs K, et al. Interaction between tacrolimus and chloramphenicol in a renal transplant recipient. Transplantation. 1998;65:1397-1398.

CHAPTER 26

Rifamycins

DAVID P. CALFEE

The rifamycin class of antimicrobial agents was discovered in 1957 when a group of substances with antimicrobial activity was isolated from *Streptomyces mediterranei* (now *Nocardia mediterranei*).[1] The name of this group of substances, collectively referred to as the rifamycin complex, was derived from a French movie, *Rififi*, popular at that time.[2] Introduced in 1963, rifamycin SV, a derivative of rifamycin B, was the first compound in this class to be used clinically. Further chemical modifications of rifamycin SV were made to improve its oral bioavailability and to achieve more prolonged and potent antibacterial activity. Rifampicin, or rifampin, was developed and first was introduced into clinical practice in Italy in 1968. Rifampin first was approved for use in the United States in 1971 for treatment of pulmonary tuberculosis and meningococcal carriage. Additional semisynthetic rifamycins, with variations in pharmacokinetic properties and some differences in antimicrobial activity compared with rifampin, subsequently have been introduced. These agents include rifabutin (a spiro-piperidyl rifamycin also called *ansamycin*), rifapentine (a cyclo-pentyl–substituted rifamycin of the piperazinyl hydrazone class), and rifaximin, which is available in Europe. Other rifamycin derivatives (e.g., rifalazil) currently are undergoing clinical evaluation. The rifamycins are broad-spectrum antibacterial agents, with the greatest activity being against mycobacteria and gram-positive organisms (Table 26-1). All of the rifamycins have an ansa structure, which is an aromatic nucleus spanned by an aliphatic bridge. The chemical structures of rifampin, rifabutin, and rifapentine are shown in Figure 26-1.

MECHANISM OF ACTION

The rifamycin derivatives exert their antimicrobial activity by inhibiting the β-subunit of DNA-dependent RNA polymerase, which is highly conserved among prokaryotic organisms. Crystal structure analysis of the rifampin–RNA polymerase complex has shown that rifampin binds deep within the main DNA/RNA channel of the polymerase, where it sterically blocks the elongating RNA transcript when it reaches a length of two or three nucleotides, leading to abortive transcription.[3] Mammalian RNA polymerase is not inhibited at clinically achievable concentrations.

MECHANISMS OF RESISTANCE

Acquired resistance to the rifamycins is the result of one of several single-step mutations within the *rpoB* gene that encodes the β-subunit of the RNA polymerase. The frequency with which rifampin resistance–conferring mutations occurs is approximately 10^{-8}. Most *rpoB* mutations that lead to rifampin resistance are missense mutations, which lead to amino acid substitutions within the rifampin-binding pocket of the RNA polymerase.[3,4] The resistance phenotype (i.e., the minimal inhibitory concentration [MIC] and the degree of cross-resistance among the various rifamycin derivatives) that results from an individual mutation depends on the mutation position and the type of substitution that occurs.[5,6] In approximately 96% of rifampin-resistant isolates of *Mycobacterium tuberculosis,* mutations can be identified within a small region of the gene,[7-9] allowing for the development of molecular tests that provide rapid detection of rifampin resistance in *M. tuberculosis.*[10]

Not all resistance to the rifamycins is the result of a mutation in the *rpoB* gene. Some organisms, such as the *Mycobacterium avium* complex (MAC), show reduced permeability to the rifamycins. This reduced permeability results in variable degrees of resistance despite susceptibility of the RNA polymerase to the inhibitory effects of the rifamycins in vitro.[11,12]

PHARMACOLOGIC PROPERTIES

The pharmacokinetic properties of the individual rifamycins vary considerably from one compound to another. These differences have been reviewed in detail elsewhere.[13] Rifampin is absorbed rapidly and reaches peak serum concentrations of 8 to 20 µg/mL within 1 to 2 hours of a standard 600-mg oral dose.[14] The pharmacokinetics of rifampin are optimized with single daily dosing. A 300-mg oral dose of rifabutin reaches a peak serum concentration of 0.25 to 0.6 µg/mL within 2 to 4 hours of ingestion,[15] whereas 600 mg of rifapentine results in a peak serum concentration of 8 to 30 µg/mL 4 to 6 hours after ingestion.[16,17] The effect of food on drug absorption varies considerably among the individual agents in this class. When rifampin is administered with food, the maximal serum concentration (Cmax) and the area under the concentration time curve (AUC) to 8 hours may each be decreased by more than 20% in 37% of individuals,[18] although the AUC_{0-8} has been found to be reduced by only 6%.[19] Administration of rifabutin after a high-fat meal results in a slowing of the rate of absorption with no change in the overall extent of absorption.[20] Rifapentine bioavailability is increased by approximately 50% when administered with food.[21] Antacids seem to have no substantial effect on the absorption of rifampin and rifabutin,[19,22] although individual cases of impaired absorption of rifabutin when administered with the buffered formulation of didanosine have been reported.[23] The proportion of drug that is protein bound in serum is 71%, 80%, and 97.7% for rifabutin, rifampin, and rifapentine.[14,21,24]

TABLE 26-1   Antibacterial Activity of Rifampin

Species	MIC Range (µg/mL)	MIC_{50} (µg/mL)	MIC_{90} (µg/mL)
Staphylococcus aureus	0.008-0.015	0.015	0.015
Staphylococcus epidermidis	0.004-0.015	0.015	0.015
Group A streptococci	0.03-0.12	0.12	0.12
Group B streptococci	0.25-1	1	1
Streptococcus pneumoniae	0.06-32	0.12	0.12
Viridans group streptococci	0.03-8	0.06	0.12
Enterococcus faecalis	1-8	2	8
Haemophilus influenzae	0.5-64	1	1
Neisseria gonorrhoeae	0.06-2	0.25	0.5
Neisseria meningitidis	0.015-1	0.03	0.5
Listeria monocytogenes	≤0.12-0.25	≤0.12	0.25
Mycobacterium fortuitum	16->64	>64	>64
Mycobacterium chelonei	>64	>64	>64
Escherichia coli	8-16	8	16
Klebsiella pneumoniae	16-32	32	32
Enterobacter agglomerans	8-64	32	64
Enterobacter cloacae	16-64	64	64
Enterobacter aerogenes	16-64	32	64
Citrobacter freundii	32	32	32
Citrobacter diversus	32	32	32
Proteus mirabilis	4-8	4	8
Proteus vulgaris	8-32	16	32
Morganella morganii	8-32	16	32
Providencia rettgeri	8-64	16	32
Providencia stuartii	4-16	8	16
Serratia marcescens	32-64	64	64
Acinetobacter spp.	4-16	8	8
Pseudomonas aeruginosa	32->64	32	64
Pseudomonas spp.	4->64	8	32
Legionella spp.		≤0.25*	

*Geometric mean MIC.

MIC, minimal inhibitory concentration; MIC_{50}, minimal inhibitory concentration for 50% of isolates; MIC_{90}, minimal inhibitory concentration for 90% of isolates.

Adapted from Thornsberry C, Hill BC, Swenson JM, McDougal LK. Rifampin: Spectrum of antibacterial activity. Rev Infect Dis. 1983;5(Suppl 3):S412-S417.

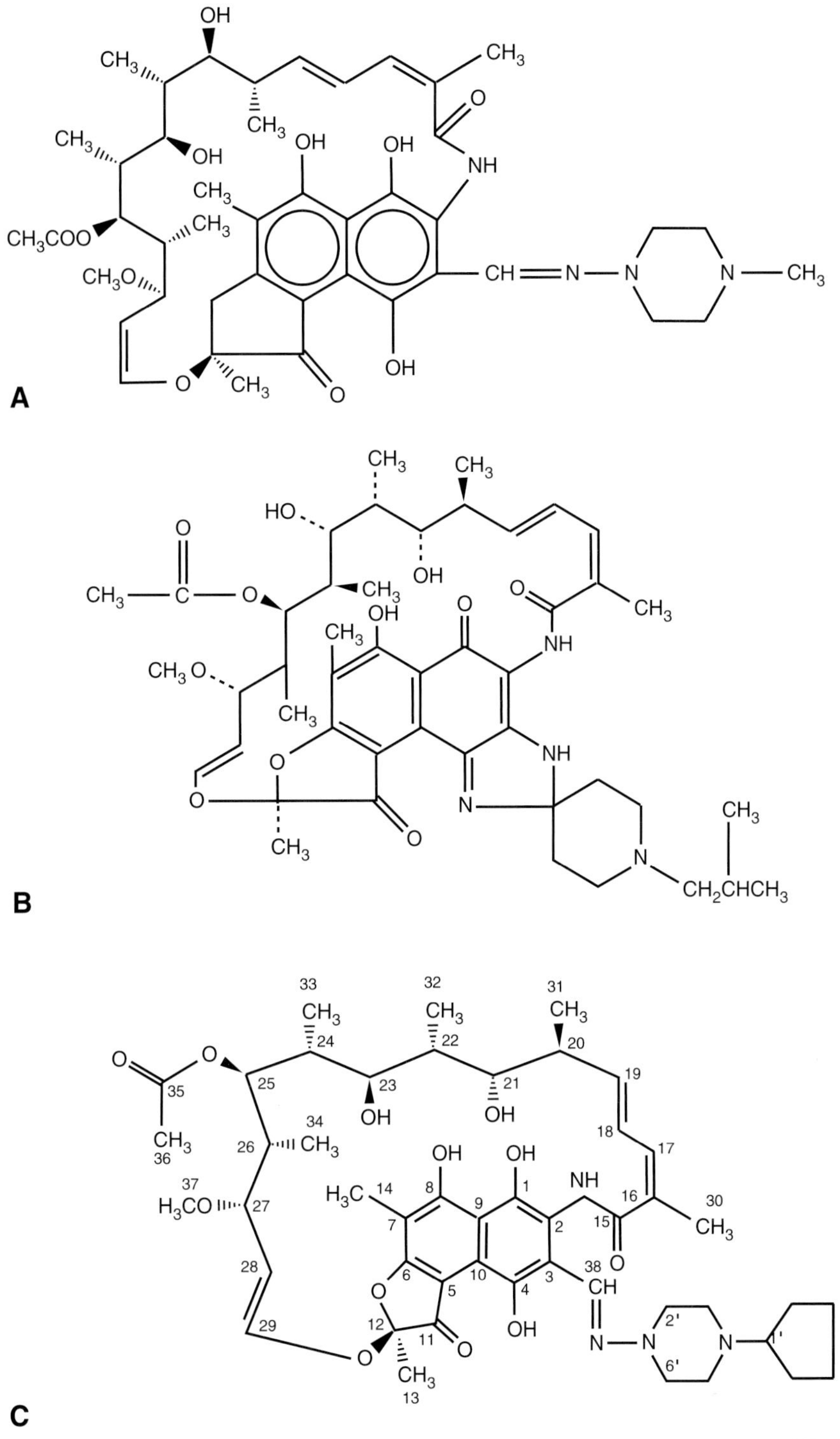

FIGURE 26-1. Chemical structures of rifampin **(A)**, rifabutin **(B)**, and rifapentine**(C)**.

The rifamycins are metabolized through hepatic and intestinal processes. Rifampin and rifabutin undergo metabolism by the hepatic and intestinal microsomal system, notably the cyotchrome P-450 3A4 oxidase, and exhibit a substantial hepatic first-pass effect with excretion into the bile. This system is saturable, however, and when the transport maximum is surpassed, higher doses of drug lead to greater than proportional increases in serum concentrations. Rifapentine is metabolized primarily by esterases with additional metabolism occur-

ring through nonenzymatic hydrolysis. Most rifapentine and its metabolites are excreted in the feces.[25]

The rifamycins are potent, but not equivalent, inducers of hepatic microsomal enzymes; rifampin is a more potent inducer than rifapentine, which is a much more potent inducer than rifabutin.[26-28] The 3A isoenzyme of the cytochrome P-450 (CYP3A) oxidase system is affected most notably.[29] Hepatic microsomal enzyme activity has been shown to return to baseline values within 2 weeks of the discontinuation of rifapentine.[27,28] Rifampin and rifabutin induce their own metabolism, a process that seems to be complete by the end of 1 week of daily administration.[24,29] Rifapentine, which primarily undergoes nonoxidative metabolism, does not induce its own metabolism.[27]

Dose adjustment of rifampin is not necessary in the setting of renal insufficiency or hemodialysis. A dose reduction of 50% is recommended when administering rifabutin to individuals with a creatinine clearance less than 30 mL/min.[30] A pharmacokinetic study of rifabutin administered using this reduced dose (i.e., 150 mg/day) in a patient with end-stage renal disease determined that such dose reductions may not be necessary and that rifabutin is not removed substantially by hemodialysis.[31]

The lipophilic properties of these drugs allow them to cross cell membranes readily. The lipophilic properties of these compounds allows them to achieve extensive distribution into tissues and body fluids, including urine, tears, saliva, sweat, and aqueous humor, resulting in an orange-red discoloration of these body fluids. Drug concentrations in many tissues exceed plasma concentrations within several hours of administration. Indirect evidence suggests that rifampin penetrates into tuberculous pulmonary cavities[32] and reaches therapeutic concentrations in bacterial abscess cavities.[33] Bone concentrations ranging from 0 to 8.2 μg/g of bone have been detected after administration of therapeutic doses of rifampin to animals and humans.[34-36] Higher rifampin concentrations are achieved in diseased bone than in normal bone and in cancellous bone than in cortical bone. In inflamed meninges, rifampin reaches concentrations in cerebrospinal fluid that are approximately 20% of serum levels.[37] Penetration into the cerebrospinal fluid is reduced in the absence of meningeal inflammation.

DRUG INTERACTIONS

As previously mentioned, the rifamycins, particularly rifampin, are potent inducers of the cytochrome P-450 microsomal enzyme system. Administration of the rifamycins can increase the metabolism of other drugs that are metabolized by this pathway, leading to subtherapeutic levels of these drugs. These drug interactions have been described in detail elsewhere.[38] Table 26-2 lists some drugs that can be affected by co-administration of rifampin and other rifamycins. Close clinical monitoring, therapeutic drug monitoring, and selection of an alternative agent may be required.

Rifabutin is a substrate and an inducer of the cytochrome P-450 3A isoenzyme. Concomitant administration of one or more drugs that inhibit this enzyme (e.g., fluconazole, clarithromycin, ritonavir, and other human immunodeficiency virus [HIV] protease inhibitors) can result in substantial increases in rifabutin exposure,[39,40] which can result in an increased risk of drug toxicity (Table 26-3).

Because of the frequent indication for use of the rifamycins in patients with HIV infection and acquired immunodeficiency syndrome (AIDS) (e.g., for treatment or prevention of mycobacterial diseases), one particularly concerning group of drug interactions is that which occurs between these agents and many antiretroviral medications, particularly protease inhibitors and non-nucleoside reverse transcriptase inhibitors. These interactions are complex because of various degrees of induction or inhibition of CYP3A by these antiretroviral drugs. In addition, some of these agents also are substrates of CYP3A allowing for bidirectional interactions. The pharmacokinetic interactions between these agents have been described in detail elsewhere.[41] Guidelines for the use of rifampin and rifabutin in patients taking protease inhibitors or non-nucleoside reverse transcriptase inhibitors are available.[42]

ADVERSE REACTIONS

The rifamycins are associated with many adverse reactions. The frequency with which rifampin is discontinued owing to adverse effects is relatively low (1.9%), however, and most of these treatment discontinuations are unnecessary.[43] Although as a group the rifamycins have

TABLE 26-2 Drugs for Which Serum Concentrations Can Be Reduced Substantially by Rifampin-Mediated Induction of Hepatic and Intestinal Microsomal Enzymes

Type of Drug	Specific Drug
Anticoagulants	Warfarin
Anticonvulsants	Phenytoin
Antimicrobial agents	Chloramphenicol
	Clarithromycin
	Dapsone
	Doxycycline
	Fluconazole
	Itraconazole
	Ketoconazole
	Non-nucleoside reverse transcriptase inhibitors
	Protease inhibitors
Cardiovascular agents	β-Blockers
	Digoxin
	Diltiazem
	Disopyramide
	Losartan
	Nifedipine
	Quinidine
	Tocainide
	Verapamil
Immunosuppressive agents	Cyclosporine
	Tacrolimus
Neuropsychiatric agents and opioids	Diazepam
	Haloperidol
	Methadone
	Midazolam and triazolam
	Nortriptyline
	Phenytoin
Endocrine-related agents	Glucocorticoids
	Oral contraceptives
	Sulfonylureas
Miscellaneous	Theophylline

Adapted from Finch CK, Chrisman CR, Baciewicz AM, Self TH. Rifampin and rifabutin drug interactions: An update. Arch Intern Med. 2002;162:985-992.

a similar side-effect profile, the cross-toxicity of the various rifamycins has not been established clearly. Case reports have documented tolerance of rifabutin by patients who have had various reactions to rifampin, including anaphylaxis, influenza-like syndrome, thrombocytopenia, and gastrointestinal symptoms,[44,45] but administration of rifabutin in this situation should be undertaken with caution and under close observation.

The adverse reactions attributable to the rifamycins have been separated into two groups: reactions that can arise during daily therapy (e.g., cutaneous reactions, gastrointestinal symptoms, hepatic injury, and mild hematologic abnormalities) and reactions that mainly occur with highly intermittent administration (less frequently than twice per week) or on reintroduction of rifampin after a long drug-free period (e.g., influenza-like syndrome, hemolytic anemia, acute renal failure, and shock).[46] Although this classification is not absolute, it can be use-

TABLE 26-3 Drugs That Can Increase Substantially Serum Concentrations of Rifabutin

Type of Drug	Specific Drug
Antifungal agents	Fluconazole
	Ketoconazole
HIV non-nucleoside reverse transcriptase inhibitors	Delavirdine
HIV protease inhibitors	Amprenavir
	Indinavir
	Nelfinavir
	Ritonavir
Macrolide antibiotics	Clarithromycin

HIV, human immunodeficiency virus.

ful in understanding the pathophysiology underlying particular reactions. The adverse events associated with intermittent administration often are due to the development of rifampin-dependent antibodies that result in complement-mediated cell damage.

Anaphylaxis

Anaphylactic reactions to the rifamycins have been reported. In some cases, an immediate-type hypersensitivity reaction has been documented by the presence of antirifampin IgE antibodies or an urticarial response to skin testing or both.[44] Similar testing in other cases has been negative. Oral desensitization therapy has allowed some individuals with hypersensitivity reactions to rifampin to complete therapy.[47]

Gastrointestinal

Gastrointestinal symptoms, such as abdominal pain or cramping, nausea, vomiting, and diarrhea, are relatively common among individuals treated with rifamycins and are among the most commonly reported side effects resulting in treatment discontinuation or dose adjustment.[43,48] Rare cases of *Clostridium difficile* pseudomembranous colitis have been reported in association with rifampin.

Hepatic

Mild, transient elevations in serum bilirubin often are noted within hours of oral administration of rifampin. This elevation is thought to be the result of inhibition of bilirubin excretion rather than true hepatic toxicity and to be of no clinical significance.[49] Elevations of serum hepatic transaminase levels also can occur during therapy with rifampin and other rifamycins. The incidence of this complication is relatively low but has varied among different patient populations, with the highest rates reported among individuals with chronic liver disease or predisposing conditions, such as alcohol abuse or co-administration of other potentially hepatotoxic medications. A meta-analysis reported the incidence of hepatitis among adults receiving rifampin without isoniazid to be 1.1% (range 0.6% to 2.7%).[50] Spontaneous resolution of these abnormalities despite ongoing administration of the drug is common.[51,52]

More severe hepatitis requiring discontinuation of rifamycin therapy also can occur. Many cases of severe liver injury, including several deaths, have been reported in association with administration of rifampin and pyrazinamide for the treatment of latent tuberculosis infection.[53-58] No underlying liver disease has been present in most subjects in whom hepatotoxicity has developed. The incidence of this complication is not known with certainty, but several investigators have reported rates of hepatotoxicity ranging from 1.2% to 13% among recipients of this combination regimen.[56-61] The unexpectedly high rate of hepatotoxicity associated with this combination regimen has resulted in updated recommendations regarding the use and monitoring of this regimen for the treatment of latent tuberculosis infection.[54]

Hematologic

Thrombocytopenia, leukopenia, and granulocytopenia are relatively common during rifamycin therapy but in most cases these changes are mild and are not clinically significant. These abnormalities resolve on discontinuation of the drug, and dose adjustment usually is not required. The more severe hematologic complications of rifamycin therapy (e.g., hemolytic anemia and profound thrombocytopenia) are thought to be the result of rifampin-dependent antibodies that result in complement-mediated cell damage due to interaction with the I antigen expressed on the surface of erythrocytes and platelets.[62-65] Similar to other antibody-mediated adverse effects of the rifamycins, these complications usually occur during highly intermittent therapy or on reintroduction of the drug after a prolonged drug-free period. The onset of hemolysis typically is within hours of drug administration and often is accompanied by fever, joint and muscle pain, malaise, and headache. Acute renal failure also may occur. Continued administration of the drug can be fatal.[62] In antibody-mediated thrombocytopenia, the platelet count typically begins to decrease within hours of rifampin administration and usually returns to normal over 1 to 2 days, although clinically sig-

nificant bleeding complications can occur.[66] Rechallenge with rifampin is not recommended in patients who previously have developed hemolytic anemia or significant thrombocytopenia.

Renal

Acute renal failure associated with administration of rifampin most commonly has been described in highly intermittent dosing regimens or on reinstitution of rifampin after a drug-free interval.[65,67,68] In these cases, patients often report acute onset of fever, chills, myalgias, nausea, or vomiting within hours of reintroduction of rifampin. Laboratory abnormalities, in addition to those produced by acute renal failure, can include anemia with or without evidence of intravascular hemolysis, leukocytosis, thrombocytopenia, and elevations in serum levels of hepatic transaminases. Most cases of acute renal failure in this setting have been attributed to acute tubular necrosis[68] or acute interstitial nephritis.[67] Rifampin-dependent antibodies have been detected in the serum of most patients in whom testing was performed. Renal damage is thought to be due to the interaction between rifampin-dependent antibodies and the I antigen expressed on renal tubular epithelium with subsequent complement-mediated cell damage.[68] The prognosis of this type of rifampin-associated renal failure is excellent, and nearly all reported patients have had full recovery of renal function within several weeks.[67,69] Administration of rifampin to a patient with a history of rifampin-associated renal failure is not recommended.

Acute renal failure also can occur during continuous dosing, but this is much less common, and the pathophysiology seems to be different. In these cases, tests for rifampin-dependent antibodies typically have been negative, and various causes of acute renal failure (e.g., acute interstitial nephritis or rapidly progressive glomerulonephritis) have been reported.

Uveitis

Uveitis has been reported as a complication of rifabutin-containing regimens for the prophylaxis or treatment of MAC infection. Most episodes have been reported among patients receiving rifabutin in combination with clarithromycin or fluconazole, drugs that are known to cause substantial increases in serum rifabutin levels.[39,70] The reported incidence of uveitis has varied substantially among reports, which may reflect differences in drug dosage or concurrently administered medications among the populations studied. In two large trials of rifabutin monotherapy (300 mg/day) for the prevention of MAC disease in patients with AIDS, there were no reported cases of uveitis.[71] Among subjects treated with 600 mg of rifabutin in combination with clarithromycin and ethambutol for the treatment of MAC bacteremia, the 6-month overall risk of uveitis was 43%.[72] After reducing the dose of rifabutin to 300 mg/day (the currently recommended dose), the 6-month risk of uveitis decreased to 13%, with a relative risk of 0.13 compared with subjects receiving rifabutin at the higher dose.

Uveitis typically presents with the acute onset of unilateral or bilateral eye pain and redness and decreased visual acuity. The anterior chamber is the usual site of involvement, and hypopyon sometimes is present. The onset of uveitis usually is 1 to 4 months after initiation of therapy, but cases have been reported 14 months after the introduction of rifabutin.[72-74] The mechanism by which rifampin-associated uveitis develops is not completely understood. It is presumed that this condition represents either an augmented inflammatory response to bacterial cell wall components or direct drug toxicity.[74] With timely diagnosis and therapy, which typically includes discontinuation of rifabutin and topical corticosteroids and cycloplegics, the prognosis of rifabutin-associated uveitis is excellent. Reintroduction of rifabutin after an episode of uveitis generally is thought to be safe,[75,76] but recurrence has been reported.[73]

Cutaneous

Cutaneous reactions, such as maculopapular rashes or hypersensitivity reactions (e.g., urticaria or diffuse erythema), can result from administration of the rifamycins. Skin rash was found to be one of the most common reasons for discontinuation of rifampin, often unnecessarily, among individuals treated for tuberculosis in New York City.[43] Most skin reactions resolve spontaneously and do not require permanent discontinuation of the medication. Treatment with antihistamines or desensitization therapy has allowed continuation of rifamycin therapy in some patients with cutaneous hypersensitivity reactions.[77]

Lupus-like Syndrome

A drug-induced lupus syndrome has been reported during daily therapy with standard doses of rifampin and rifabutin. Many of these patients also were receiving medications that inhibit the cytochrome P-450 enzyme responsible for the metabolism of rifampin and rifabutin,[51,78,79] suggesting that this syndrome may be the result of excessively high rifamycin levels. The lupus syndrome is characterized by arthralgias, arthritis, edema, and malaise. Symptoms typically resolve after discontinuation of the rifamycin, although symptomatic therapy initially may be necessary. Antinuclear antibodies are present during the acute illness and decline over time after discontinuation of the rifamycin.[79]

Influenza-like Syndrome

Influenza-like syndrome, which occurs predominantly during intermittent rifampin therapy or with the administration of high doses of rifampin (>1200 mg/day), is thought to be due to a rifampin-dependent, antibody-mediated process.[64] The onset of symptoms typically is within 1 to 2 hours of ingestion of rifampin. These symptoms, which include fever, rigors, headache, arthralgias, and myalgias, may last 8 hours.[64,65] Changing to daily administration usually prevents subsequent reactions and may allow continuation of therapy. Anaphylactic reactions have been reported, however, in a few patients rechallenged in this manner.[44]

Immunosuppression

In vitro and animal studies have shown that rifampin can lead to inhibition of delayed-type hypersensitivity reactions and lymphocyte stimulation.[80] Studies of the immune-modulating effects of rifampin in humans have produced inconsistent results, but there is no strong evidence that clinically significant immunosuppressive effects occur in humans receiving standard doses of rifampin.[64]

Other

Rifampin causes an orange-red discoloration of tears, sweat, urine, and other body fluids. Permanent staining of clothing and contact lenses can occur.

THERAPEUTIC USES

Tuberculosis

Rifampin is highly active against *M. tuberculosis* with an MIC_{90} value of less than or equal to 0.25 μg/mL.[81-83] The minimal bactericidal concentration (MBC) of rifampin for *M. tuberculosis* has been reported to range from 0.12 to 1 μg/mL.[82,84] The bactericidal activity of rifampin has allowed for the development of highly effective, short-course (6- to 9-month) multidrug regimens for the treatment of active tuberculosis due to drug-susceptible *M. tuberculosis*. Although isoniazid is responsible for most sterilizing activity during the first 2 to 4 days of combination therapy, rifampin has been shown to provide the bulk of bactericidal activity after the first few days of treatment, likely as a result of its better ability to act against more slowly growing organisms.[85] Because of the crucial bactericidal activity that rifampin provides in short-course treatment regimens, infections caused by rifampin-resistant strains of *M. tuberculosis* require a longer duration of treatment and are associated with higher rates of treatment failure than infections caused by drug-susceptible strains.[86,87]

The MIC_{90} of rifabutin for *M. tuberculosis* is lower than that of rifampin, but the Cmax/MIC ratio is similar for these two drugs. In vitro studies have shown that rifabutin has activity against intracellular *M. tuberculosis* and shows a prolonged postantibiotic effect.[82] Strains of *M. tuberculosis* that are susceptible to rifampin also are susceptible to

rifabutin; however, cross-resistance between rifampin and rifabutin is not complete. The likelihood of cross-resistance to rifabutin seems to be associated with the location of the *rpoB* mutation and to be correlated with the level of rifampin resistance.[6,81,88] Although susceptible to rifabutin by MIC testing, the rifabutin MIC/MBC ratio for rifampin-resistant strains may be greater than that of rifampin-susceptible strains, and the concentration of rifabutin necessary for bactericidal activity may not be clinically achievable.[89]

Clinical studies comparing rifabutin with rifampin in the treatment of newly diagnosed, drug-susceptible pulmonary tuberculosis in HIV-seronegative individuals found similar clinical and microbiologic efficacy with rifabutin-based and rifampin-based multidrug regimens.[90,91] Bacteriologic cure rates at the last valid observation ranged from 89% to 90% for rifampin and 92% to 95% for rifabutin. Rifabutin also has been found to be as effective as rifampin in the treatment of HIV-associated tuberculosis.[92]

In vitro tests have shown that rifapentine has greater inhibitory activity and either equivalent or greater bactericidal activity than rifampin against clinical isolates of *M. tuberculosis*.[83,93] The greatest difference in activity between rifampin and rifapentine seems to be against intracellular bacteria, for which the MICs and MBCs of rifapentine are twofold to eightfold lower than those of rifampin. This difference most likely is due to higher intracellular concentration of rifapentine within monocytes, exceeding that of rifampin by fourfold to fivefold.[94] Rifampin-resistant strains of *M. tuberculosis* typically show resistance to rifapentine as well.

The long half-life and extensive intracellular accumulation of rifapentine have resulted in evaluation of this drug in once-weekly treatment regimens for tuberculosis. In an animal model, weekly administration of rifapentine had significant bactericidal activity, although less than that observed with daily administration of rifampin.[95] The first human study of rifapentine in the continuation phase of treatment of pulmonary tuberculosis compared the combination of rifapentine and isoniazid administered either once every week or 2 out of every 3 weeks with a standard regimen of rifampin plus isoniazid administered three times per week.[96] After 5 years of follow-up, the rates of treatment failure or relapse were 10.8% and 11.7% in the two rifapentine-containing groups and 4.2% in the rifampin group ($P = .92$ and $P = .009$). More than half of the subjects randomized to the rifapentine groups received a formulation of the drug that subsequently was found to have poor bioavailability. In the subgroup of subjects who received rifapentine at a dose that had been adjusted to achieve desired concentrations, the risk of relapse or failure still was 3.39 compared with the control group (0.06).

A second study compared 600 mg of rifapentine plus 900 mg of isoniazid once per week with 600 mg of rifampin plus 900 mg of isoniazid twice per week in HIV-seronegative individuals.[97] The rates of treatment failure or relapse in the two groups were 9.2% and 5.6% (relative risk 1.64, $P = .04$). Risk factors independently associated with treatment failure or relapse included having positive sputum cultures at 2 months, having cavitary pulmonary lesions on chest radiography, having bilateral pulmonary involvement, being underweight, and being a non-Hispanic white person. When individuals with cavitary disease were excluded from the analysis, the failure or relapse rates in the two groups were 2.9% and 2.5% ($P = .81$). In patients with HIV-related tuberculosis, treatment with once-weekly doses of rifapentine plus isoniazid during the continuation phase of therapy compared with twice-weekly doses of rifampin and isoniazid was associated with relapse with rifamycin-monoresistant tuberculosis.[98] Based on the available data, more recent guidelines for the treatment of tuberculosis recommend limiting the use of rifapentine to the continuation phase of treatment of HIV-seronegative adults with noncavitary, drug-susceptible pulmonary tuberculosis who have negative sputum smears at the end of 8 weeks of induction therapy and in whom a once-weekly regimen is desired.[99] The recommended dose of rifapentine is 10 mg/kg, with a maximum dose of 600 mg, administered orally once per week.

Nontuberculous Mycobacterial Infections

Mycobacterium leprae

Rifampin is active against *Mycobacterium leprae* and is more rapidly bactericidal than dapsone and other antileprosy drugs.[100-102] Using the mouse footpad method, the MIC and MBC of rifampin for *M. leprae* have been estimated to be 0.2 to 0.3 μg/mL and 1 to 2 μg/mL.[100,102] In vivo studies have confirmed the antilepromatous activity of rifampin. Clinical and microbiologic responses with the combination of rifampin and dapsone have been more rapid than the responses seen with dapsone monotherapy.[101,103] Because of its rapid bactericidal activity and proven clinical efficacy in treating human leprosy, rifampin is included in the multidrug therapy regimens currently recommended by the World Health Organization for the treatment of leprosy.[104] As in other mycobacterial infections, development of rifampin resistance by *M. leprae* has been reported in association with rifampin monotherapy, and rifampin should not be administered as a single agent for the treatment of leprosy.

Mycobacterium avium Complex

The bactericidal activity of the rifamycins is significantly lower against MAC than it is against *M. tuberculosis*.[84] This is thought to be the result of differences in permeability rather than differences in the RNA polymerase.[11] Rifabutin, which is more lipophilic than rifampin, has greater in vitro inhibitory effects than rifampin against MAC.[81,105] Agar dilution MIC_{90} values of 1 μg/mL and 4 μg/mL were determined for rifabutin and rifampin using 20 clinical isolates of *Mycobacterium intracellulare*.[106] Strains that are highly resistant to rifampin (i.e., resistant at a rifampin concentration of 10 μg/mL) are more likely to be resistant to rifabutin than strains resistant only to 1 μg/mL of rifampin.[81] Despite relatively low MICs, the concentrations of rifabutin necessary for bactericidal activity are quite high (MBC/MIC ratios of 8:256) and often exceed clinically achievable serum concentrations of rifabutin.[84,107]

Clinical trials have evaluated the efficacy of rifampin alone and in combination with other antimycobacterial drugs for the prevention of MAC disease in patients with AIDS. Administration of 300 mg of rifabutin per day significantly reduced the risk of MAC bacteremia compared with placebo (relative risk 0.43 to 0.47) in randomized trials of patients with AIDS and CD4 counts equal to or greater than 200.[71,108] Among the subjects of these trials in whom MAC bacteremia developed while receiving rifabutin prophylaxis, no rifabutin-resistant strains were detected. At least one case of rifampin-resistant *M. tuberculosis* has been reported, however, in a patient receiving rifabutin prophylaxis for MAC disease.[108] In a randomized, double-blind, placebo-controlled comparison of clarithromycin (500 mg twice daily), rifabutin (450 mg daily), or both for the prevention of MAC disease in patients with AIDS, rifabutin monotherapy was significantly less effective than clarithromycin or combination therapy.[109] Combination therapy was no more effective than clarithromycin monotherapy but was associated with more adverse effects.

Rifabutin also has been evaluated for its use in the treatment of MAC disease. AIDS patients with MAC bacteremia who were treated with rifabutin (600 mg daily) were significantly more likely to have negative blood cultures or an equal to or greater than 0.5 log reduction in the number of colony-forming units of MAC per milliliter of blood after 14 days of treatment than patients treated with placebo (70% versus 8%, $P = .002$).[110] In a randomized trial of ethambutol plus clofazimine with or without rifabutin, clinical responses were similar between the two groups, but the group treated with rifabutin had a greater bacteriologic response to therapy (odds ratio 1.99 to 2.58).[111] A similar study compared isoniazid, ethambutol, and clofazimine with or without rifabutin in the treatment of MAC or *Mycobacterium xenopi* bacteremia in patients with AIDS.[112] No differences were observed in rates of clinical improvement or mortality. The median time to culture conversion was shorter (43 days versus 69 days) and rates of culture conversion at 12 weeks were higher (45% versus 38%) in subjects treated with rifabutin, but these differences did not reach statistical

significance. Finally, a randomized, placebo-controlled study compared clarithromycin (500 mg twice daily) plus ethambutol (1200 mg daily) with and without rifabutin (300 mg daily) for the treatment of MAC bacteremia in patients with AIDS.[113] Microbiologic and clinical responses and survival were similar between the two groups. Clarithromycin-resistant MAC was isolated from only 1 (2%) of 44 rifabutin recipients, however, compared with 6 (14%) of 42 placebo recipients ($P = .055$), suggesting that although rifabutin did not improve outcomes, it may have prevented development of clarithromycin resistance during therapy. The role of rifampin in the treatment of MAC pulmonary disease in HIV-seronegative patients has not been evaluated in controlled clinical studies.

Other Nontuberculous Mycobacteria

The rifamycins show in vitro activity against several other nontuberculous mycobacteria, including *M. kansasii*, *M. marinum*, *M. xenopi*, *M. terrae* complex, and *M. gordonae*.[81] Rapidly growing mycobacteria, such as *M. fortuitum* and *M. chelonae*, are naturally resistant to the rifamycins.[81,114,115]

Staphylococcal Infections

The rifamycins are highly active against staphylococci, showing significant inhibitory and bactericidal activity. Rifampin is significantly more effective than other antistaphylococcal antibiotics in killing intracellular *Staphylococcus aureus* at clinically achievable drug concentrations.[116-119] This effectiveness is thought to be due to the lipid solubility of rifampin, which allows it to cross membranes readily and reach high concentrations within the cell.

In vivo, the use of rifampin as a single agent for the treatment of *S. aureus* infections has been limited by a high rate of development of rifampin resistance during therapy. When administered alone, resistance to rifampin can develop within the first 24 to 48 hours of exposure. Concurrent administration of other antistaphylococcal antibiotics has been shown to reduce the development of rifampin resistance in vitro and in vivo. Even with this approach, however, rifampin resistance can develop during therapy. In clinical practice, development of rifampin resistance during combination therapy seems to be more likely to occur in the setting of high bacterial burdens and low local antibiotic concentrations, such as in endocarditis and large abscesses.[120-122]

In vitro studies of the effect of rifampin on the inhibitory and bactericidal activity of other antistaphylococcal antibiotics have not provided consistent results. The observed interactions have ranged from synergy to indifference to antagonism. These interactions seem to depend on many factors, including the ratio of the concentrations of rifampin and other drugs, size of the inoculum, sampling time, testing method and definitions of synergy, and growth phase of the organism. The results of in vitro synergy testing do not predict in vivo responses to combination antimicrobial regimens. In clinical trials, higher rates of bacteriologic cure have been observed among subjects with various staphylococcal infections receiving rifampin in addition to an antistaphylococcal penicillin, but this has not always been associated with improvements in clinical outcomes.[123,124] There are no conclusive data to support the use of rifampin in the routine management of staphylococcal skin and soft tissue infections.

Staphylococcus aureus Endocarditis

The definitive role of rifampin in the treatment of *S. aureus* endocarditis is unclear. In a rabbit model of penicillin-susceptible *S. aureus* endocarditis, the combination of penicillin plus rifampin administered for 6 to 10 days was less effective in sterilizing vegetations than penicillin alone, although treatment with rifampin alone or penicillin plus rifampin led to more rapid sterilization of renal tissue than did treatment with penicillin, vancomycin, cefazolin, clindamycin, or penicillin plus gentamicin.[125] Using a similar model, rifampin had a variable effect on the bacterial killing activity of cloxacillin, as determined by quantitative cultures of cardiac valve vegetations after 3 days of treatment, that was dependent on the concentrations of each antibiotic.[126] Peak serum bactericidal titers often were predictive of the in vivo findings. At concentrations of rifampin that typically are achieved in humans, the effect was primarily indifferent. In vitro tests of synergy have failed to predict the antagonistic effect of rifampin on the bactericidal activity of cephalosporins that has been observed in animal models of *S. aureus* endocarditis.[127] An antagonistic effect also has been shown in animals when rifampin-fluoroquinolone combinations were administered on a short-term basis (4 to 6 days).[128,129] The combination of quinupristin-dalfopristin plus rifampin was found to have a synergistic effect in the rabbit model of quinupristin-susceptible *S. aureus* endocarditis.[130]

Animal models of methicillin-resistant *S. aureus* (MRSA) endocarditis also have yielded conflicting results. In one study, the combination of vancomycin and rifampin was found to be significantly more effective than either drug alone in reducing cardiac valve bacterial titers and sterilizing valve vegetations, although the combination regimen was similar to vancomycin alone in preventing death and sterilizing renal abscesses.[131] Other studies have found, however, that the addition of rifampin to vancomycin provides no benefit regarding survival, resolution of bacteremia, or sterilization of heart valve vegetations.[132,133]

Only limited human data are available to support the use of rifampin in *S. aureus* endocarditis. In humans, the addition of rifampin to vancomycin has been reported to improve the response to therapy in cases of endocarditis due to vancomycin-tolerant *S. aureus*.[134,135] This observed clinical response to combination therapy may not have been due to true synergy between the two drugs, but rather to the bactericidal activity of rifampin with vancomycin acting to prevent the emergence of rifampin-resistant mutants.[134] In a randomized study of MRSA endocarditis, the addition of rifampin provided no significant advantage over vancomycin alone in terms of duration of bacteremia or fever or cure after 28 days of treatment.[136] A small noncomparative study suggested that ciprofloxacin plus rifampin may provide a viable option for an orally administered treatment regimen for right-sided *S. aureus* endocarditis, providing cure rates of 76% to 100%.[137] These findings subsequently were supported by the results of a small randomized study that compared enteral ciprofloxacin plus rifampin with intravenous vancomycin.[138] After 28 days of therapy, cure rates of 95% and 88% were observed for the ciprofloxacin-rifampin and vancomycin groups. The incidence of drug toxicity, including hepatotoxicity, was significantly lower in the ciprofloxacin-rifampin group. The emergence of resistance to ciprofloxacin and rifampin has been reported during unsupervised treatment with this combination regimen.[139]

Staphylococcus epidermidis Endocarditis

Rifampin has been shown to be more effective than vancomycin or gentamicin in sterilizing cardiac valve vegetations caused by *S. epidermidis*, but the use of rifampin as a single agent results in emergence of rifampin-resistant mutants.[140] In one study, many combination regimens (including vancomycin-rifampin, gentamicin-rifampin, and vancomycin-gentamicin-rifampin) were found to have similar efficacy, however, in reducing bacterial densities in cardiac valve vegetations compared with vancomycin alone.[141] Several other studies have suggested the superiority of treatment with a glycopeptide plus rifampin for 3 to 10 days compared with a glycopeptide alone in experimental *S. epidermidis* endocarditis.[142-144] In a study in which infected rabbits were treated for only 48 hours, the combination of rifampin-gentamicin-vancomycin was superior to rifampin-vancomycin and vancomycin alone with valve sterilization rates of 71%, 29%, and 0%.[145] The combination of ciprofloxacin plus rifampin also has been shown in animal models to be superior to therapy with vancomycin alone.[146]

Retrospective human data suggest that the combination of rifampin (900 to 1200 mg/day) plus vancomycin with or without an aminoglycoside may be better than vancomycin alone in the treatment of *S. epidermidis* prosthetic valve endocarditis.[147,148] These combination regimens have shown higher serum bactericidal titers than titers measured during vancomycin monotherapy. Cure rates also have been higher, but because of small sample sizes, the differences were not statistically significant. The emergence of rifampin resistance has been observed during combination therapy in this setting.

Staphylococcal Osteomyelitis and Orthopedic Implant Infections

Animal models of *S. aureus* osteomyelitis have suggested that infected bone may be sterilized more frequently during treatment with rifampin-containing combination antimicrobial regimens than by treatment with a β-lactam antibiotic or vancomycin alone, although rifampin-resistant staphylococci have been isolated from the bone of animals treated with combination regimens in which bone sterilization did not occur.[35,149] Human data supporting the use of rifampin in uncomplicated staphylococcal osteomyelitis are limited. In a small study of chronic methicillin-susceptible *S. aureus* osteomyelitis, human subjects were assigned randomly to receive treatment with intravenous nafcillin with or without rifampin (600 to 1200 mg/day) for 42 days.[150] The rate of a favorable clinical response was higher among subjects treated with nafcillin plus rifampin than subjects treated with nafcillin alone (80% versus 50%, P = .2) In a small, uncontrolled trial of oral combination therapy for chronic staphylococcal osteomyelitis, treatment with rifampin plus a second antibiotic (determined by the susceptibility profile of the infecting strain) for 6 months resulted in cure of only 6 (43%) of 14 subjects.[151] True bacteriologic failure was documented in only one case, however. The remaining seven subjects had clinical failure with no evidence of persistent staphylococcal infection. This failure was thought to be the result of polymicrobial infections that had not been treated adequately by an antistaphylococcal antibiotic regimen.

Rifampin possesses several characteristics that suggest a potential role for this agent in the treatment of foreign body–associated infections, such as orthopedic implant–related infections, including intracellular bactericidal activity; the ability to penetrate biofilms produced by bacteria that frequently cause foreign body infections (e.g., *S. epidermidis*); and bactericidal activity against nongrowing organisms.[152-154] Animal studies have found that combinations of rifampin with vancomycin, teicoplanin, or a fluoroquinolone are more effective than any of these agents alone or any of these agents in combination with an aminoglycoside for the treatment of device-related infections.[155] More recently, combinations of rifampin and vancomycin or quinupristin-dalfopristin were found to be similar in efficacy, and both combinations were significantly more effective than monotherapy with either agent in an animal model of *S. aureus* prosthetic joint infection.[156]

Cure rates of 82% have been observed in association with the administration of rifampin with either a β-lactam antibiotic or ciprofloxacin to patients with staphylococcal or streptococcal orthopedic device infections from whom the infected device could not be removed.[157] In another study, the combination of rifampin (900 mg/day) plus ofloxacin (600 mg/day) was evaluated in patients with staphylococcal infections of an orthopedic implant.[158] After a minimum of 6 months of post-treatment follow-up, successful outcomes were seen in 81%, 69%, and 69% of patients with prosthetic hip, prosthetic knee, and bone plate infections. Device removal in a one- or two-stage procedure had been performed in 45%, 60%, and 50%. A similar study reported overall success rates of 55% and 50% after treatment with rifampin plus fusidic acid and rifampin plus ofloxacin.[159] Finally, the combination of oral ciprofloxacin plus rifampin (450 mg twice daily) for 3 to 6 months was compared with ciprofloxacin plus placebo in a randomized trial of the treatment of culture-proven, staphylococcal infections of stable orthopedic implants.[160] All subjects underwent an initial débridement procedure, then received a 2-week course of flucloxacillin or vancomycin plus rifampin or placebo before beginning the oral treatment regimen. The reported cure rates were 100% in the ciprofloxacin-rifampin group and 58% in the ciprofloxacin-placebo group after a minimum of 15 months of follow-up (P = .02). Ciprofloxacin resistance developed in four subjects in the ciprofloxacin-placebo group, suggesting that one role of rifampin in the combination regimen was in the prevention of emergence of ciprofloxacin resistance. Because the subjects of this trial had symptoms and signs of infection for a median of only 4 to 5 days, the efficacy of ciprofloxacin plus rifampin in the treatment of more chronic infections of orthopedic device–related infections remains to be determined.

Eradication of *Staphylococcus aureus* Colonization

Short courses of rifampin with or without intranasal bacitracin have been shown to reduce nasal carriage of methicillin-susceptible *S. aureus* among individuals with renal failure requiring long-term hemodialysis or peritoneal dialysis. Recurrent colonization has been common, however, after a single 5-day course of therapy.[161] Administration of rifampin for 5 days every 3 months has been shown to reduce the incidence of peritonitis and catheter loss secondary to *S. aureus*[162] and to reduce the frequency of dialysis catheter–related infections[163]; however, the emergence of rifampin-resistant *S. aureus* may limit the long-term utility of this prophylactic regimen.

The efficacy of rifampin in eliminating colonization with MRSA also has been evaluated. Rifampin alone has been unsuccessful in eradicating MRSA carriage.[164] Combinations of rifampin with other antistaphylococcal antibiotics (e.g., minocycline or trimethoprim-sulfamethoxazole) with or without topical antimicrobial therapy have been more successful. The combination of rifampin (600 mg/day) plus minocycline administered for 2 weeks in addition to intranasal application of mupirocin for 5 days resulted in clearance of MRSA colonization in 10 of 11 patients in a spinal cord injury unit as determined by nasal cultures obtained 4 days after the end of treatment.[165] Five of these 10 subjects were reevaluated 3 to 4 months later, and all remained culture negative. A randomized study of rifampin (600 mg twice daily for 5 days), minocycline (100 mg twice daily for 5 days), rifampin plus minocycline, or no treatment in MRSA-colonized residents of a long-term care facility found that the combination of rifampin plus minocycline was more effective in eliminating MRSA carriage than was minocycline alone.[166] A retrospective review of the combination of oral trimethoprim-sulfamethoxazole and rifampin with or without intranasal bacitracin reported that 40 of 47 subjects were culture negative during the first 4 days after the completion of treatment.[167] Subsequent relapse was documented in nine of these patients. Similar rates of relapse had been reported previously.[168] A cohort study of MRSA-colonized hospital patients found an initial eradication rate of 64% after completion of a 5-day course of oral trimethoprim-sulfamethoxazole and rifampin.[169] Among patients in whom colonization initially was eradicated, the probability of remaining MRSA culture negative after 32 days was 65%.

Prevention of Foreign Body Infections

Rifampin also has been evaluated for its potential use in the prevention of foreign body–related infections, particularly infections resulting from temporary central vascular catheters. Catheters coated with minocycline-rifampin have been shown to have activity against gram-positive bacteria, gram-negative bacteria, and *Candida albicans* that persist for at least 2 weeks.[170-172] In vitro studies have shown that the combination of minocycline plus rifampin prevents colonization with slime-producing strains of *S. epidermidis* and *S. aureus*.[170] Randomized clinical trials have determined that central venous catheters treated with rifampin-minocycline significantly reduce the frequency of catheter colonization and catheter-related blood stream infection compared with untreated catheters[172,173] and catheters impregnated with chlorhexidine and silver sulfadiazine on the external surface.[174] Serum concentrations of rifampin and minocycline have been undetectable in patients during the period of catheterization,[172] and so far no rifampin or minocycline resistance has been detected among staphylococci isolated from the coated catheters after removal. In vitro studies indicate that there is some risk that bacteria may develop resistance to the antibiotics used to coat such catheters,[175] but the clinical implications of this finding have not been determined.

Randomized clinical trials also have shown the efficacy of minocycline-rifampin–coated urinary bladder and external ventricular drain catheters in reducing the risk of device-associated, gram-positive bacteriuria and cerebrospinal fluid infections.[176,177] In vitro and animal models have suggested a role for rifampin-minocycline coating to prevent infections related to prosthetic heart valves[178] and subcutaneously placed silicone implants.[179,180] Rifampin also is being evaluated alone and in combination with antimicrobial agents other than minocycline for use in preventing foreign body infections.

Streptococcal and Enterococcal Infections

Studies using the time-kill curve method have shown synergistic bactericidal activity against some clinical isolates of nutritionally deficient streptococci with the combination of vancomycin plus rifampin.[181] There was no evidence of antagonism, and synergistic activity was observed against some strains. Although enhanced bactericidal activity might increase the rate of successful treatment of endocarditis caused by nutritionally deficient streptococci, there are no clinical data to confirm these in vitro observations.

Rifampin often is incompletely bactericidal against enterococci.[182] In vitro testing has not revealed consistent evidence of synergy for the combinations of ampicillin or vancomycin plus rifampin against enterococci.[182-184] Some studies have suggested an antagonistic interaction.[185,186] In an animal model of enterococcal pyelonephritis, there was no significant outcome difference between ampicillin and ampicillin plus rifampin.[183] Human data are lacking. Currently, there is no clear role for the use of rifampin in the treatment of enterococcal infections.

Meningitis Chemoprophylaxis

Neisseria meningitidis

Studies performed in military recruits, college students, and close contacts of individuals with invasive meningococcal disease have shown the efficacy of rifampin in eradicating oropharyngeal colonization with *Neisseria meningitidis*.[52,187-194] Eradication rates ranging from 75% to 98% have been reported using a variety of rifampin dosing regimens. Current recommendations from the Centers for Disease Control and Prevention's Advisory Committee for Immunization Practices for chemoprophylaxis of contacts of sporadic cases of meningococcal disease include twice-daily administration of rifampin for 2 days.[195] The recommended dose is 600 mg twice daily for adults, 10 mg/kg twice daily for children 1 month of age or older, and 5 mg/kg for children less than 1 month of age. One concern regarding the use of rifampin for eradication of the meningococcal carrier state is the development of rifampin-resistant strains in 63% of post-treatment meningococcal isolates.[52,189,190] The clinical significance of this finding is uncertain, but it does suggest that long-term use of rifampin to prevent meningococcal carriage or disease in high-risk groups, such as military recruits, should be avoided. Alternative agents with demonstrated efficacy in eradication of meningococcal carriage include ciprofloxacin, ceftriaxone, and minocycline.

Haemophilus influenzae

Before routine immunization against *Haemophilus influenzae* type B, nasopharyngeal colonization with this organism could be detected in 49% of daycare contacts of children with invasive disease[196] with a secondary attack rate of approximately 2% in children younger than 5 years old.[197] To reduce the risk of secondary cases of *H. influenzae* type B infection, various antimicrobials have been administered to eradicate nasopharyngeal colonization among contacts of an index case. Administration of rifampin at 20 mg/kg/day for 4 days has eradicated nasopharyngeal carriage in 87.5% to 100% of colonized contacts[196,198-202] with only one small study reporting an eradication rate less than 95%.[196] Eradication rates have been substantially lower when shorter courses of rifampin were administered. Emergence of rifampin resistance during eradication therapy has been documented.[203]

Although routine immunization with *H. influenzae* type B conjugate vaccine has reduced dramatically the incidence of invasive disease and the number of at-risk children, chemoprophylaxis still is indicated in certain situations. All household contacts of a primary case of invasive *H. influenzae* disease should receive prophylaxis if there are any infants younger than 12 months in the household or if there are any children 1 to 3 years old in the household who are inadequately vaccinated.[204] Similar recommendations have been made for daycare attendees and staff contacts of cases of invasive disease. The recommended dose is 20 mg/kg (maximal dose 600 mg) in a single daily dose for 4 days. In infants younger than 1 month old, a daily dose of 10 mg/kg is recommended.

Rhodococcus equi Infections

Rhodococcus equi is an opportunistic, intracellular pathogen of immunocompromised hosts, particularly individuals with AIDS. Rifampin inhibits the growth of *R. equi* at concentrations less than 1 µg/mL[205] but may fail to provide bactericidal activity.[206] In vitro, synergy has been shown when rifampin is combined with erythromycin and minocycline.[206] Indifferent interactions have been observed between rifampin and other agents. For the treatment of *R. equi* infections in humans, rifampin has been used in combination with several antibiotics, including vancomycin, erythromycin, and a fluoroquinolone.

Pseudomonas aeruginosa and Burkholderia cepacia Infections

The minimal concentration of rifampin required to inhibit the growth of *Pseudomonas aeruginosa* in vitro frequently exceeds clinically achievable serum concentrations.[115,207] This "natural" resistance is thought to be the result of a membrane barrier to the rifamycins.[208] Some in vitro and animal studies have reported increased antibacterial activity of the combination of an antipseudomonal penicillin or cephalosporin plus an aminoglycoside after the addition of rifampin.[209-212] Small case series have described clinical improvement after the addition of rifampin to traditional antipseudomonal combination therapies,[213] but clinical data to support the use of these triple-drug combinations are limited. A randomized trial of an antipseudomonal β-lactam and an aminoglycoside with or without rifampin (600 mg every 8 hours for 72 hours, then every 12 hours for the next 7 days) for the treatment of *P. aeruginosa* bacteremia reported a higher frequency of bacteriologic cure and a lower rate of breakthrough bacteremia in the rifampin group.[214] Survival was similar between the two groups, however.

In vitro tests of synergy have identified synergistic interactions between rifampin and a carbapenem, a carbapenem plus ciprofloxacin, a carbapenem plus ticarcillin, and a carbapenem plus tobramycin against some clinical isolates of *Burkholderia cepacia*.[215,216] Clinical data are lacking.

Chlamydia and Chlamydophila Infections

Rifampin is highly active against *Chlamydia* and *Chlamydophila* spp., but resistance emerges during exposure to rifampin alone.[217-219] Some in vitro studies have suggested that the combination of rifampin with azithromycin provides synergistic activity against *Chlamydia trachomatis*[217] and *Chlamydophila pneumoniae*[220] and that the combination prevents the emergence of rifampin resistance.[217,219] Clinical data to support the use of rifampin for the treatment of chlamydial infections in humans are lacking.

Legionellosis

Rifampin is highly active against *Legionella* spp.[115] Synergy between rifampin and erythromycin has been shown in vitro,[221] and retrospective human data suggest better outcomes with the use of this combination compared with erythromycin alone.[222] More recent treatment guidelines recommend single-drug therapy with a newer macrolide or azalide (i.e., azithromycin), a fluoroquinolone, or doxycycline.[223] In vitro and in vivo data suggest that these agents are more effective than erythromycin and that use of these agents in combination with rifampin provides no additional benefit compared with monotherapy.[222,224,225]

Helicobacter pylori Infection

Rifampin and rifabutin have been shown to possess activity against *Helicobacter pylori* in vitro.[226,227] In open trials, administration of rifabutin plus amoxicillin and a proton-pump inhibitor for 1 week eradicated *H. pylori* from 72% to 86% of individuals who previously had failed standard eradication therapy.[228,229] Subsequent randomized trials confirmed the efficacy of this combination as a second-line treatment option for *H. pylori* infection, with reported eradication rates of 91%.[230,231]

Mediterranean Spotted Fever

Many of the *Rickettsia* spp. that cause human disease are susceptible to clinically achievable concentrations of rifampin.[232,233] The rifampin MIC for *Rickettsia conorii,* the agent of Mediterranean spotted fever, is 0.06 to 1 µg/mL. Although doxycycline remains the drug of choice for infections caused by most of these organisms, alternative treatment regimens sometimes are needed. A randomized trial performed in Spain compared doxycycline (two 200-mg doses 12 hours apart) with rifampin (10 mg/kg twice daily for 5 days) in patients with Mediterranean spotted fever.[234] Although all subjects were afebrile by day 7, subjects treated with rifampin had a significantly longer duration of fever, suggesting that the antibacterial action of rifampin was slower than that of doxycycline.

Q Fever

In vitro, rifampin seems to be highly effective in eliminating *Coxiella burnetii,* the agent of Q fever, from chronically infected cells at a concentration of 1 µg/mL.[235] The activity of rifampin may be only bacteriostatic, however.[236] Rifampin has been used clinically in combination with doxycycline for the treatment of Q fever, although other treatment regimens now are used more commonly.

Ehrlichiosis

At therapeutic concentrations, rifampin and rifabutin possess bactericidal activity against Ehrlichiae.[237] At an extracellular concentration of 0.125 µg/mL, rifampin reduces the number of *Ehrlichia chaffeensis* organisms in infected cells within 72 hours of treatment.[238] These in vitro findings suggest that the rifamycins may be one alternative treatment option when doxycycline, the drug of choice, cannot be used. Successful treatment of human ehrlichiosis with rifampin has been reported.[239]

Brucellosis

The intracellular killing activity of the rifamycins has made these agents of particular interest in treating infectious processes, such as those caused by *Brucella* spp., which are characterized by intracellular pathogens. Rifampin has been shown to be active against *Brucella* in vitro, and clinically achievable concentrations typically provide bactericidal activity.[240,241] The in vitro activity of rifapentine is similar to that of rifampin.[241] Studies evaluating the efficacy of a 6-week course of doxycycline plus rifampin in the treatment of human brucellosis have reported therapeutic success rates ranging from 76% to 97%.[242-249] Although this regimen, compared with standard treatment with doxycycline plus streptomycin, has the advantage of oral administration, many prospective trials and a meta-analysis of six randomized studies found higher rates of initial treatment failure or relapse with the rifampin-containing regimen.[242,246,249-251] At least one study suggested that the presence of spondylitis may increase the risk of treatment failure in patients receiving doxycycline-rifampin.[245] Two relatively small studies found that combination therapy with a fluoroquinolone plus rifampin has efficacy similar to that of doxycycline-rifampin in the treatment of human brucellosis.[247,252]

Clostridium difficile Infections

Rifampin is active against most strains of *C. difficile*.[253,254] In vitro testing has indicated an additive or partially synergistic antibacterial effect with the combinations of rifampin and vancomycin or metronidazole.[253] The combination of rifampin-bacitracin synergistically inhibited most tested strains of *C. difficile*. The combination of oral vancomycin-rifampin has been used to treat a few patients with relapsing *C. difficile*–associated diarrhea.[255]

Fungal Infections

Although rifampin alone does not possess significant antifungal activity at clinically achievable concentrations, in vitro studies have shown potentiation of the activity of several antifungal drugs, such as amphotericin B, ketoconazole, and 5-fluorocytosine, against many fungal pathogens (e.g., *Aspergillus* spp., *Candida* spp., *Cryptococcus neoformans, Coccidioides immitis,* and *Histoplasma capsulatum*) by the addition of rifampin.[256-262] In murine models of aspergillosis, histoplasmosis, and blastomycosis that used relatively low doses of amphotericin B (0.5 mg/kg), the combination of amphotericin B-rifampin was more effective than either drug given alone.[263,264] Animal models of candidiasis and coccidioidomycosis showed no therapeutic benefit, however, of the addition of rifampin to standard antifungal regimens.[259,260,265] Combination therapy may have been less effective than treatment with amphotericin B alone. There are no human data to support the addition of rifampin to standard regimens for treatment of fungal infections.

Cryptosporidium parvum Infection

Prospective, observational clinical data suggest that rifabutin is protective against cryptosporidiosis in patients with AIDS.[266] Patients receiving rifabutin for the treatment or prophylaxis of MAC disease were significantly less likely to develop cryptosporidiosis than patients not receiving rifabutin (relative hazard 0.15). This finding is supported by in vitro studies showing that the parasite-reducing activity of the combination of rifabutin-nitazoxanide was greater than that of nitazoxanide alone.[267] Clinical studies assessing the efficacy of rifabutin in the treatment of cryptosporidiosis have not been performed.

Pruritus of Cholestasis

The ability of rifampin to relieve the pruritus associated with chronic cholestasis has been shown in many open trials and randomized, crossover studies.[268-274] Other studies have not found rifampin to be effective for the relief of pruritus associated with these conditions.[275] The antipruritic effect typically is seen within days of initiation of therapy,[268] and its effect can persist for at least 8 months.[270,271] The exact mechanism by which this effect occurs is unknown, but it has been hypothesized that this may be the result of inhibition of hepatic bile acid uptake or of detoxification of hepatic bile acids owing to induction of mixed-function oxidases.[268] In one series, 7.3% of rifampin recipients developed significant hepatitis.[276] Because of this and other potential side effects, rifampin is considered a second-line agent for the treatment of pruritus of chronic cholestasis.

OTHER RIFAMYCINS

Rifaximin

Rifaximin is a poorly absorbed rifamycin derivative that currently is available in Europe. Oral administration of 400 mg every 12 hours for 3 days produces fecal concentrations of 4000 to 8000 μg/g.[277,278] Systemic exposure to the drug does not seem to be increased by the presence of even moderate-to-severe ulcerative colitis. The spectrum of activity of rifaximin is similar to that of rifampin, with its greatest activity being against many gram-positive bacteria.[279] Although the minimal concentration of rifaximin required to inhibit the growth of many of the bacterial causes of traveler's diarrhea is relatively high, the lack of absorption of the drug allows it to reach concentrations in the feces that are often 50 to 500 times higher than the MICs of these organisms.[277,278,280,281] Other gastrointestinal pathogens against which rifaximin has in vitro activity include *H. pylori*[282,283] and *C. difficile*.[284]

The poor absorption of this drug and the ability to achieve high concentrations in the gastrointestinal tract has led to its development for use in the treatment of hepatic encephalopathy, gastrointestinal infections, and inflammatory bowel disease. In human studies, rifaximin produced significantly greater reductions in H_2 production and symptoms compared with chlortetracycline in subjects with small intestinal overgrowth.[285] Rifaximin also has been shown to reduce colonic ammonia production significantly in patients with cirrhosis[286] and to be at least as effective as neomycin in reducing blood ammonia levels in patients with hepatic encephalopathy.[287,288] Studies performed in children and adults with infectious diarrhea have shown that the efficacy of rifaximin is similar to that of paromomycin and ciprofloxacin for the treatment of these conditions.[278,289] In patients with moderate-to-severe ulcerative colitis refractory to corticosteroids, there was no overall difference in the frequency of a positive response to therapy between the rifaximin and placebo groups, but subjects randomized to the rifaximin group had significantly greater reductions in stool frequency, rectal bleeding, and sigmoidoscopic score.[290]

Rifalazil (KRM-1648)

Rifalazil, a benzoxazinorifamycin, is a highly lipophilic rifamycin derivative with extensive tissue distribution and a long elimination half-life.[291] In contrast to rifampin and rifabutin, rifalazil is not an inducer of the cytochrome P-450 microsomal enzyme system.[292] Rifalazil has in vitro antimycobacterial inhibitory activity similar to or greater than that of other rifamycins and in vivo intracellular killing activity greater than that of rifampin for many mycobacterial species, including some rifampin-resistant strains of *M. tuberculosis*.[6,7,88,293-296] The greater intracellular activity of rifalazil is thought to be the result of its greater intracellular accumulation, which is 50-fold to 100-fold higher than that of rifampin.[296] Animal models have shown the efficacy of rifalazil in the treatment of *M. tuberculosis* and MAC infection.[295,297-299] Human experience with rifalazil for the treatment of mycobacterial infections is limited. In vitro and animal studies also have shown that rifalazil is as active or more active than rifampin against gram-positive pathogens such as *S. aureus, S. epidermidis,* and streptococci.[300] Some strains of rifampin-resistant *S. aureus* remain susceptible to rifalazil.[301] Although it has minimal activity against most gram-negative organisms, rifalazil exhibits substantial activity against *H. pylori*.[283] Activity against *Chlamydia* spp. also has been shown.[302]

REFERENCES

1. Sensi P. Rifampicin. In: Bindra J, Lednicer D, eds. Chronicles of Drug Discovery. New York: Wiley; 1982:201-221.
2. Sensi P. History of the development of rifampin. Rev Infect Dis. 1983;5:S402-S406.
3. Campbell EA, Korzheva N, Mustaev A, et al. Structural mechanism for rifampicin inhibition of bacterial RNA polymerase. Cell. 2001;104:901-912.
4. Williams D, Waguespack C, Eisenach K, et al. Characterization of rifampin resistance in pathogenic mycobacteria. Antimicrob Agents Chemother. 1994;38:2380-2386.
5. Bodmer T, Zurcher G, Imboden P, Telenti A. Mutation position and type of substitution in the B-subunit of the RNA polymerase influence in-vitro activity of rifamycins in rifampicin-resistant *Mycobacterium tuberculosis*. J Antimicrob Chemother. 1995;35:345-348.
6. Yang B, Koga H, Ohno H, et al. Relationship between antimycobacterial activities of rifampicin, rifabutin and KRM-1648 and *rpoB* mutations of *Mycobacterium tuberculosis*. J Antimicrob Chemother. 1998;42:621-628.
7. Moghazeh SL, Pan X, Arain T, et al. Comparative antimycobacterial activities of rifampin, rifapentine, and KRM-1648 against a collection of rifampin-resistant *Mycobacterium tuberculosis* isolates with known *rpoB* mutations. Antimicrob Agents Chemother. 1996;40:2655-2657.
8. Heep M, Rieger U, Beck D, Lehn N. Mutations in the beginning of the *rpoB* gene can induce resistance to rifamycins in both *Helicobacter pylori* and *Mycobacterium tuberculosis*. Antimicrob Agents Chemother. 2000;44:1075-1077.
9. Heep M, Brandstatter B, Rieger U, et al. Frequency of *rpoB* mutations inside and outside the cluster I region in rifampin-resistant clinical *Mycobacterium tuberculosis* isolates. J Clin Microbiol. 2001;39:107-110.
10. Van Der Zanden A, Te Keppele-Vije E, Vijaya Bhanu N, et al. Use of DNA extracts from Ziehl-Neelsen-stained slides for molecular detection of rifampin resistance and spoligotyping of *Mycobacterium tuberculosis*. J Clin Microbiol. 2003;41:1101-1108.
11. Hui J, Gordon N, Kajioka R. Permeability barrier to rifampin in mycobacteria. Antimicrob Agents Chemother. 1977;11:773-779.
12. Fujii K, Saito H, Tomioka H, et al. Mechanism of action of antimycobacterial activity of the new benzoxazinorifamycin KRM-1648. Antimicrob Agents Chemother. 1995;39:1489-1492.
13. Burman WJ, Gallicano K, Peloquin C. Comparative pharmacokinetics and pharmacodynamics of the rifamycin antibacterials. Clin Pharmacokinet. 2001;40:327-341.

14. Acocella G. Pharmacokinetics and metabolism of rifampin in humans. Rev Infect Dis. 1983;5:S428-S432.

15. Skinner MH, Blaschke TF. Clinical pharmacokinetics of rifabutin. Clin Pharmacokinet. 1995;28:115-125.

16. Conte JE Jr, Golden JA, McQuitty M, et al. Single-dose intrapulmonary pharmacokinetics of rifapentine in normal subjects. Antimicrob Agents Chemother. 2000;44:985-990.

17. Keung A, Eller MG, McKenzie KA, Weir SJ. Single and multiple dose pharmacokinetics of rifapentine in man: Part II. Int J Tuberc Lung Dis. 1999;3:437-444.

18. Zent C, Smith P. Study of the effect of concomitant food on the bioavailability of rifampicin, isoniazid and pyrazinamide. Tuber Lung Dis. 1995;76:109-113.

19. Peloquin C, Namdar R, Singleton M, Nix D. Pharmacokinetics of rifampin under fasting conditions, with food, and with antacids. Chest. 1999;115:12-18.

20. Narang PK, Lewis RC, Bianchine JR. Rifabutin absorption in humans: Relative bioavailability and food effect. Clin Pharmacol Ther. 1992;52:335-341.

21. Jarvis B, Lamb HM. Rifapentine. Drugs. 1998;56:607-616.

22. Sahai J, Narang PK, Hawley-Foss N, et al. A phase I evaluation of concomitant rifabutin and didanosine in symptomatic HIV-infected patients. J Acquir Immune Defic Syndr Hum Retrovirol. 1995;9:274-279.

23. Marzolini C, Chave JP, Telenti A, et al. Impaired absorption of rifabutin by concomitant administration of didanosine. AIDS. 2001;15:2203-2204.

24. Skinner MH, Hsieh M, Torseth J, et al. Pharmacokinetics of rifabutin. Antimicrob Agents Chemother. 1989;33:1237-1241.

25. Reith K, Keung A, Toren P, et al. Disposition and metabolism of ^{14}C-rifapentine in healthy volunteers. Drug Metab Dispos. 1998;26:732-738.

26. Perucca E, Grimaldi R, Frigo GM, et al. Comparative effects of rifabutin and rifampicin on hepatic microsomal enzyme activity in normal subjects. Eur J Clin Pharmacol. 1988;34:595-599.

27. Keung A, Reith K, Eller M, et al. Enzyme induction observed in healthy volunteers after repeated administration of rifapentine and its lack of effect on steady-state rifapentine pharmacokinetics: Part I. Int J Tuberc Lung Dis. 1999;3:426-436.

28. Vital Durand D, Hampden C, Boobis AR, et al. Induction of mixed function oxidase activity in man by rifapentine (MDL 473), a long-acting rifamycin derivative. Br J Clin Pharmacol. 1986;21:1-7.

29. Strolin BM, Dostert P. Induction and autoinduction properties of rifamycin derivatives: A review of animal and human studies. Environ Health Perspect. 1994;102:101-105.

30. Package insert. Kalamazoo, MI: Pharmacia & Upjohn Company; 2002.

31. Bassilios N, Launay-Vacher V, Hamani AA, et al. Pharmacokinetics and dosage adjustment of rifabutin in a haemodialysis patient. Nephrol Dial Transplant. 2002;17:531-532.

32. Tsukamura M. Permeability of tuberculous cavities to antituberculosis drugs. Tubercle. 1972;53:47-52.

33. Suter F, Maserati R, Concia E, et al. Rifampicin in collections of pus—a kinetic study in human abscesses. J Antimicrob Chemother. 1984;13:43-47.

34. Roth B. Penetration of parenterally administered rifampicin into bone tissue. Chemotherapy. 1984;30:358-365.

35. Norden C. Experimental osteomyelitis: IV. Therapeutic trials with rifampin alone and in combination with gentamicin, sisomicin, and cephalothin. J Infect Dis. 1975;132:493-499.

36. Cluzel RA, Lopitaux R, Sirot J, Rampon S. Rifampicin in the treatment of osteoarticular infections due to staphylococci. J Antimicrob Chemother. 1984;13:23-29.

37. D'Oliveira JJG. Cerebrospinal fluid concentrations of rifampin in meningeal tuberculosis. Am Rev Respir Dis. 1972;106:432-437.

38. Finch CK, Chrisman CR, Baciewicz AM, Self TH. Rifampin and rifabutin drug interactions: An update. Arch Intern Med. 2002;162:985-992.

39. Trapnell CB, Narang PK, Li R, Lavelle JP. Increased plasma rifabutin levels with concomitant fluconazole therapy in HIV-infected patients. Ann Intern Med. 1996;124:573-576.

40. Jordan MK, Polis MA, Kelly G, et al. Effects of fluconazole and clarithromycin on rifabutin and 25-O-desacetylrifabutin pharmacokinetics. Antimicrob Agents Chemother. 2000;44:2170-2172.

41. Burman WJ, Gallicano K, Peloquin C. Therapeutic implications of drug interactions in the treatment of human immunodeficiency virus-related tuberculosis. Clin Infect Dis. 1999;28:419-429.

42. Centers for Disease Control and Prevention. Updated guidelines for the use of rifabutin or rifampin for the treatment and prevention of tuberculosis among HIV-infected patients taking protease inhibitors or nonnucleoside reverse transcriptase inhibitors. MMWR Morb Mortal Wkly Rep. 2000;49:185-189.

43. Cook SV, Fujiwara PI, Frieden TR. Rates and risk factors for discontinuation of rifampicin. Int J Tuberc Lung Dis. 2000;4:118-122.

44. Martinez E, Collazos J, Mayo J. Hypersensitivity reactions to rifampin: Pathogenetic mechanisms, clinical manifestations, management strategies, and review of the anaphylactic-like reactions. Medicine. 1999;78:361-369.

45. Tattevin P, Revest M, Dupont M, et al. A regimen containing rifabutin for the treatment of tuberculosis in patients intolerant to rifampin. Clin Infect Dis. 2003;36:127-128.

46. Girling DJ. Adverse reactions to rifampicin in antituberculosis regimens. J Antimicrob Chemother. 1977;3:115-132.

47. Holland CL, Malasky C, Ogunkoya A, Bielory L. Rapid oral desensitization to isoniazid and rifampin. Chest. 1990;98:1518-1519.

48. Hong Kong Chest Service/British Medical Research Council. Acceptability, compliance, and adverse reactions when isoniazid, rifampin, and pyrazinamide are given as a combined formulation or separately during three-times-weekly antituberculosis chemotherapy. Am Rev Respir Dis. 1989;140:1618-1622.

49. Cohn H. Clinical studies with a new rifamycin derivative. J Clin Pharmacol. 1969;9:118-125.

50. Steele MA, Burk RF, DesPrez RM. Toxic hepatitis with isoniazid and rifampin: A meta-analysis. Chest 1991;99:465-471.

51. Griffith D, Brown B, Girard W, Wallace R. Adverse events associated with high-dose rifabutin in macrolide-containing regimens for the treatment of *Mycobacterium avium* complex lung disease. Clin Infect Dis. 1995;21:594-598.

52. Weidmer CE, Dunkel TB, Pettyjohn FS, et al. Effectiveness of rifampin in eradicating the meningococcal carrier state in a relatively closed population: Emergence of resistant strains. J Infect Dis. 1971;124:172-178.

53. Fatal and severe hepatitis associated with rifampin and pyrazinamide for the treatment of latent tuberculosis infection—New York and Georgia, 2000. MMWR Morb Mortal Wkly Rep 2000;50:289-291.

54. Update: Fatal and severe liver injuries associated with rifampin and pyrazinamide for latent tuberculosis infection, and revisions in American Thoracic Society/CDC recommendations—United States, 2001. MMWR Morb Mortal Wkly Rep. 2001;50:733-735.

55. Medinger A. Death associated with rifampin and pyrazinamide 2-month treatment of latent *Mycobacterium tuberculosis*. Chest. 2002;121:1710-1712.

56. Jasmer RM, Saukkonen JJ, Blumberg HM, et al. Short-course rifampin and pyrazinamide compared with isoniazid for latent tuberculosis infection: A multicenter clinical trial. Ann Intern Med. 2002;137:640-647.

57. McNeill L, Allen M, Estrada C, Cook P. Pyrazinamide and rifampin vs isoniazid for the treatment of latent tuberculosis: Improved completion rates but more hepatotoxicity. Chest. 2003;123:102-106.

58. Stout J, Engemann J, Cheng A, et al. Safety of 2 months of rifampin and pyrazinamide for treatment of latent tuberculosis. Am J Respir Crit Care Med. 2003;167:824-827.

59. Bock NN, Rogers T, Tapia JR, et al. Acceptability of short-course rifampin and pyrazinamide treatment of latent tuberculosis infection among jail inmates. Chest. 2001;119:833-837.

60. Chaisson RE, Armstrong J, Stafford J, et al. Safety and tolerability of intermittent rifampin/pyrazinamide for the treatment of latent tuberculosis infection in prisoners. JAMA. 2002;288:165-166.

61. Jasmer R, Daley C. Rifampin and pyrazinamide for treatment of latent tuberculosis infection: Is it safe? Am J Respir Crit Care Med. 2003;167:809-810.

62. Ahrens N, Genth R, Salama A. Belated diagnosis in three patients with rifampicin-induced immune haemolytic anaemia. Br J Haematol. 2002;117:441-443.

63. Pereira A, Sanz C, Cervantes F, Castillo R. Immune hemolytic anemia and renal failure associated with rifampicin-dependent antibodies with anti-I specificity. Ann Hematol. 1991;63:56-58.

64. Grosset J, Leventis S. Adverse effects of rifampin. Rev Infect Dis. 1983;5:S440-S446.

65. Poole G, Stradling P, Worlledge S. Potentially serious side effects of high-dose twice-weekly rifampicin. BMJ. 1971;3:343-347.

66. Blajchman MA, Lowry RC, Pettit JE, Stradling P. Rifampicin-induced immune thrombocytopenia. BMJ. 1970;3:24-26.

67. Muthukumar T, Jayakumar M, Fernando EM, Muthusethupathi MA. Acute renal failure due to rifampicin: A study of 25 patients. Am J Kidney Dis. 2002;40:690-696.

68. De Vriese AS, Robbrecht DL, Vanholder RC, et al. Rifampicin-associated acute renal failure: Pathophysiologic, immunologic, and clinical features. Am J Kidney Dis. 1998;31:108-115.

69. Covic A, Goldsmith DJ, Segall L, et al. Rifampicin-induced acute renal failure: A series of 60 patients. Nephrol Dial Transplant. 1998;13:924-929.

70. Hafner R, Bethel J, Power M, et al. Tolerance and pharmacokinetic interactions of rifabutin and clarithromycin in human immunodeficiency virus-infected volunteers. Antimicrob Agents Chemother. 1998;42:631-639.

71. Nightingale S, Cameron D, Gordin F, et al. Two controlled trials of rifabutin prophylaxis against *Mycobacterium avium* complex infection in AIDS. N Engl J Med. 1993;329:828-833.

72. Shafran SD, Singer J, Zarowny DP, et al. Determinants of rifabutin-associated uveitis in patients treated with rifabutin, clarithromycin, and ethambutol for *Mycobacterium avium* complex bacteremia: A multivariate analysis. Canadian HIV Trials Network Protocol 010 Study Group. J Infect Dis. 1998;177:252-255.

73. Havlir D, Torriani F, Dube M. Uveitis associated with rifabutin prophylaxis. Ann Intern Med. 1994;121:510-512.

74. Saran B, Maguire A, Nichols C, et al. Hypopyon uveitis in patients with acquired immunodeficiency syndrome treated for systemic *Mycobacterium avium* complex infection with rifabutin. Arch Ophthalmol. 1994;112:1159-1165.

75. Nichols CW. *Mycobacterium avium* complex infection, rifabutin, and uveitis—is there a connection? Clin Infect Dis. 1996;22:S43-S47.

76. Centers for Disease Control and Prevention. Uveitis associated with rifabutin therapy. MMWR Morb Mortal Wkly Rep. 1994;43:658.

77. Matz J, Borish L, Routes J, Rosenwasser L. Oral desensitization to rifampin and ethambutol in mycobacterial disease. Am J Respir Crit Care Med. 1994;149:815-817.

78. Siegal FP, Eilbott D, Burger H, et al. Dose-limiting toxicity of rifabutin in AIDS-related complex: Syndrome of arthralgia/arthritis. AIDS. 1990;4:433-441.

79. Berning SE, Iseman MD. Rifamycin-induced lupus syndrome. Lancet. 1997;349:1521-1522.

80. Grassi GG, Pozzi E. Effect of rifampicin on delayed-hypersensitivity reactions. J Infect Dis. 1972;126:542-544.

81. Heifets L, Iseman M. Determination of in vitro susceptibility of mycobacteria to ansamycin. Am Rev Respir Dis. 1985;132:710-711.

82. Luna-Herrera J, Reddy MV, Gangadharam PR. In-vitro and intracellular activity of rifabutin on drug-susceptible and multiple drug-resistant (MDR) tubercle bacilli. J Antimicrob Chemother. 1995;36:355-363.

83. Bemer-Melchior P, Bryskier A, Drugeon HB. Comparison of the in vitro activities of rifapentine and rifampicin against *Mycobacterium tuberculosis* complex. J Antimicrob Chemother. 2000;46:571-576.
84. Heifets L, Lindhold-Levy P, Flory M. Bactericidal activity in vitro of various rifamycins against *Mycobacterium avium* and *Mycobacterium tuberculosis*. Am Rev Respir Dis. 1990;141:626-630.
85. Mitchison DA. Role of individual drugs in the chemotherapy of tuberculosis. Int J Tuberc Lung Dis. 2000;4:796-806.
86. Mitchison DA, Nunn AJ. Influence of initial drug resistance on the response to short-course chemotherapy of pulmonary tuberculosis. Am Rev Respir Dis. 1986;133:423-430.
87. Goble M, Iseman MD, Madsen LA, et al. Treatment of 171 patients with pulmonary tuberculosis resistant to isoniazid and rifampin. N Engl J Med. 1993;328:527-532.
88. Williams D, Spring L, Miller L, et al. Contribution of *rpoB* mutations to development of rifamycin cross-resistance in *Mycobacterium tuberculosis*. Antimicrob Agents Chemother. 1998;42:1853-1857.
89. Heifets L, Lindhold-Levy P, Iseman M. Rifabutine: minimal inhibitory and bactericidal concentrations for *Mycobacterium tuberculosis*. Am Rev Respir Dis. 1988;137:719-721.
90. Gonzalez-Montaner LJ, Natal S, Yongchaiyud P, Olliaro P. Rifabutin for the treatment of newly-diagnosed pulmonary tuberculosis: A multinational, randomized, comparative study versus rifampicin. Tuber Lung Dis. 1994;75:341-347.
91. McGregor MM, Olliaro P, Wolmarans L, et al. Efficacy and safety of rifabutin in the treatment of patients with newly diagnosed pulmonary tuberculosis. Am J Respir Crit Care Med. 1996;154:1462-1467.
92. Schwander S, Rusch-Gerdes S, Mateega A, et al. A pilot study of antituberculosis combinations comparing rifabutin with rifampicin in the treatment of HIV-1 associated tuberculosis: A single-blind randomized evaluation in Ugandan patients with HIV-1 infection and pulmonary tuberculosis. Tuber Lung Dis. 1995;76:210-218.
93. Rastogi N, Goh KS, Berchel M, Bryskier A. Activity of rifapentine and its metabolite 25-O-desacetylrifapentine compared with rifampicin and rifabutin against *Mycobacterium tuberculosis, Mycobacterium africanum, Mycobacterium bovis* and *M. bovis* BCG. J Antimicrob Chemother. 2000;46:565-570.
94. Mor N, Simon B, Mezo N, Heifets L. Comparison of activities of rifapentine and rifampin against *Mycobacterium tuberculosis* residing in human macrophages. Antimicrob Agents Chemother. 1995;39:2073-2077.
95. Grosset J, Lounis N, Truffot-Pernot C, et al. Once-weekly rifapentine-containing regimens for treatment of tuberculosis in mice. Am J Respir Crit Care Med. 1998;157:1436-1440.
96. Tam CM, Chan SL, Kam KM, et al. Rifapentine and isoniazid in the continuation phase of a 6-month regimen: Final report at 5 years: prognostic value of various measures. Int J Tuberc Lung Dis. 2002;6:3-10.
97. Benator D, Bhattacharya M, Bozeman L, et al. Rifapentine and isoniazid once a week versus rifampicin and isoniazid twice a week for treatment of drug-susceptible pulmonary tuberculosis in HIV-negative patients: A randomised clinical trial. Lancet. 2002;360:528-534.
98. Vernon A, Burman W, Benator D, et al. Acquired rifamycin monoresistance in patients with HIV-related tuberculosis treated with once-weekly rifapentine and isoniazid. Tuberculosis Trials Consortium. Lancet. 1999;353:1843-1847.
99. Blumberg HM, Burman WJ, Chaisson RE, et al. American Thoracic Society/Centers for Disease Control and Prevention/Infectious Diseases Society of America: Treatment of tuberculosis. Am J Respir Crit Care Med. 2003;167:603-662.
100. Holmes I, Hilson G. The effect of rifampicin and dapsone on experimental *Mycobacterium leprae* infections: Minimum inhibitory concentrations and bactericidal action. J Med Microbiol. 1972;5:251-261.
101. Waters M, Rees R, Pearson J, et al. Rifampicin for lepromatous leprosy: Nine years' experience. BMJ. 1978;1:133-136.
102. Franzblau SG. In vitro activities of aminoglycosides, lincosamides, and rifamycins against *Mycobacterium leprae*. Antimicrob Agents Chemother. 1991;35:1232-1234.
103. Dietrich M, Gaus W, Kern P, Meyers WM. An international randomized study with long-term follow-up of single versus combination chemotherapy of multibacillary leprosy. Antimicrob Agents Chemother. 1994;38:2249-2257.
104. WHO Expert Committee on Leprosy. World Health Organ Tech Rep Ser. 1998;874: 1-43.
105. Woodley C, Kilburn J. In vitro susceptibility of *Mycobacterium avium* complex and *Mycobacterium tuberculosis* strains to a spiro-piperidyl rifamycin. Am Rev Respir Dis. 1982;126:586-587.
106. Cynamon M. Comparative in vitro activities of MDL 473, rifampin, and ansamycin against *Mycobacterium intracellulare*. Antimicrob Agents Chemother. 1985;28:440-441.
107. Yajko DM, Nassos PS, Hadley WK. Therapeutic implications of inhibition versus killing of *Mycobacterium avium* complex by antimicrobial agents. Antimicrob Agents Chemother. 1987;31:117-120.
108. Maslo C, Bure-Rossier A, Girard PM, et al. Clinical and bacteriologic impact of rifabutin prophylaxis for *Mycobacterium avium* complex infection in patients with human immunodeficiency virus infection. Clin Infect Dis. 1997;24:344-349.
109. Benson CA, Williams PL, Cohn DL, et al. Clarithromycin or rifabutin alone or in combination for primary prophylaxis of *Mycobacterium avium* complex disease in patients with AIDS: A randomized, double-blind, placebo-controlled trial. The AIDS Clinical Trials Group 196/Terry Beirn Community Programs for Clinical Research on AIDS 009 Protocol Team. J Infect Dis. 2000;181:1289-1297.
110. Dautzenberg B, Castellani P, Pellegrin JL, et al. Early bactericidal activity of rifabutin versus that of placebo in treatment of disseminated *Mycobacterium avium* complex bacteremia in AIDS patients. Antimicrob Agents Chemother. 1996;40:1722-1725.
111. Sullam P, Gordin F, Wynne B, and the Rifabutin Treatment Group. Efficacy of rifabutin in the treatment of disseminated infection due to *Mycobacterium avium* complex. Clin Infect Dis. 1994;19:84-86.
112. Dautzenberg B, Olliaro P, Ruf B, et al. Rifabutin versus placebo in combination with three drugs in the treatment of nontuberculous mycobacterial infection in patients with AIDS. Clin Infect Dis. 1996;22:705-708.
113. Gordin FM, Sullam PM, Shafran SD, et al. A randomized, placebo-controlled study of rifabutin added to a regimen of clarithromycin and ethambutol for treatment of disseminated infection with *Mycobacterium avium* complex. Clin Infect Dis. 1999;28:1080-1085.
114. Woodley CL, Kilburn JO, David HL, Silcox VA. Susceptibility of mycobacteria to rifampin. Antimicrob Agents Chemother. 1972;2:245-249.
115. Thornsberry C, Hill BC, Swenson JM, McDougal LK. Rifampin: Spectrum of antibacterial activity. Rev Infect Dis. 1983;5:S412-S417.
116. Mandell GL, Vest TK. Killing of intraleukocytic *Staphylococcus aureus* by rifampin: In-vitro and in-vivo studies. J Infect Dis. 1972;125:486-490.
117. Hand W, King-Thompson N. Contrasts between phagocyte antibiotic uptake and subsequent intracellular bactericidal activity. Antimicrob Agents Chemother. 1986;29:135-140.
118. Bamberger DM, Herndon BL, Dew M, et al. Efficacies of ofloxacin, rifampin, and clindamycin in treatment of *Staphylococcus aureus* abscesses and correlation with results of an in vitro assay of intracellular bacterial killing. Antimicrob Agents Chemother. 1997;41:1178-1181.
119. Nielsen SL, Black FT. Extracellular and intracellular killing in neutrophil granulocytes of *Staphylococcus aureus* with rifampicin in combination with dicloxacillin or fusidic acid. J Antimicrob Chemother. 1999;43:407-410.
120. Simon GL, Smith RH, Sande MA. Emergence of rifampin-resistant strains of *Staphylococcus aureus* during combination therapy with vancomycin and rifampin: A report of two cases. Rev Infect Dis. 1983;5:S507-S508.
121. Eng RH, Smith SM, Buccini FJ, Cherubin CE. Differences in ability of cell-wall antibiotics to suppress emergence of rifampicin resistance in *Staphylococcus aureus*. J Antimicrob Chemother. 1985;15:201-207.
122. Acar JF, Goldstein FW, Duval J. Use of rifampin for the treatment of serious staphylococcal and gram-negative bacillary infections. Rev Infect Dis. 1983;5:S502-S506.
123. Van der Auwera P, Thys J, Meunier-Carpentier F, Klastersky J. The combination of oxacillin with rifampicin in staphylococcal infections: A review of laboratory and clinical studies of the Institut Jules Bordet. J Antimicrob Chemother. 1984;13:31-42.
124. Van der Auwera P, Klastersky J, Thys JP, et al. Double-blind, placebo-controlled study of oxacillin combined with rifampin in the treatment of staphylococcal infections. Antimicrob Agents Chemother. 1985;28:467-472.
125. Sande MA, Johnson ML. Antimicrobial therapy of experimental endocarditis caused by *Staphylococcus aureus*. J Infect Dis. 1975;131:367-375.
126. Zak O, Scheld W, Sande M. Rifampin in experimental endocarditis due to *Staphylococcus aureus* in rabbits. Rev Infect Dis. 1983;5:S481-S490.
127. Brandt CM, Rouse MS, Tallan BM, et al. Failure of time-kill synergy studies using subinhibitory antimicrobial concentrations to predict in vivo antagonism of cephalosporin-rifampin combinations against *Staphylococcus aureus*. Antimicrob Agents Chemother. 1994;38:2191-2193.
128. Kaatz GW, Seo SM, Barriere SL, et al. Ciprofloxacin and rifampin, alone and in combination, for therapy of experimental *Staphylococcus aureus* endocarditis. Antimicrob Agents Chemother. 1989;33:1184-1187.
129. Chambers HF, Xiang Q, Liu QX, et al. Efficacy of levofloxacin for experimental aortic-valve endocarditis in rabbits infected with viridans group streptococcus or *Staphylococcus aureus*. Antimicrob Agents Chemother. 1999;43:2742-2746.
130. Zarrouk V, Bozdogan B, Leclercq R, et al. Activities of the combination of quinupristin-dalfopristin with rifampin in vitro and in experimental endocarditis due to *Staphylococcus aureus* strains with various phenotypes of resistance to macrolide-lincosamide-streptogramin antibiotics. Antimicrob Agents Chemother. 2001;45:1244-1248.
131. Bayer AS, Lam K. Efficacy of vancomycin plus rifampin in experimental aortic-valve endocarditis due to methicillin-resistant *Staphylococcus aureus*: In vitro-in vivo correlations. J Infect Dis. 1985;151:157-165.
132. Perdikaris G, Giamarellou H, Pefanis A, et al. Vancomycin or vancomycin plus netilmicin for methicillin- and gentamicin-resistant *Staphylococcus aureus* aortic valve experimental endocarditis. Antimicrob Agents Chemother. 1995;39:2289-2294.
133. Hessen MT, Pitsakis PG, Kaye D. Oral temafloxacin versus vancomycin for therapy of experimental endocarditis caused by methicillin-resistant *Staphylococcus aureus*. Antimicrob Agents Chemother. 1990;34:1143-1145.
134. Faville RJ Jr, Zaske DE, Kaplan EL, et al. *Staphylococcus aureus* endocarditis: Combined therapy with vancomycin and rifampin. JAMA. 1978;240:1963-1965.
135. Massanari R, Donta S. The efficacy of rifampin as adjunctive therapy in selected cases of staphylococcal endocarditis. Chest. 1978;73:371-375.
136. Levine DP, Fromm BS, Reddy BR. Slow response to vancomycin or vancomycin plus rifampin in methicillin-resistant *Staphylococcus aureus* endocarditis. Ann Intern Med. 1991;115:674-680.
137. Dworkin RJ, Lee BL, Sande MA, Chambers HF. Treatment of right-sided *Staphylococcus aureus* endocarditis in intravenous drug users with ciprofloxacin and rifampicin. Lancet 1989;2:1071-1073.
138. Heldman AW, Hartert TV, Ray SC, et al. Oral antibiotic treatment of right-sided staphylococcal endocarditis in injection drug users: Prospective randomized comparison with parenteral therapy. Am J Med. 1996;101:68-76.
139. Tebas P, Martinez RR, Roman F, et al. Early resistance to rifampin and ciprofloxacin in the treatment of right-sided *Staphylococcus aureus* endocarditis. J Infect Dis. 1991;163:204-205.
140. Vazquez G, Archer G. Antibiotic therapy of experimental *Staphylococcus epidermidis* endocarditis. Antimicrob Agents Chemother. 1980;17:280-285.
141. Lowy F, Wexler M, Steigbigel N. Therapy of methicillin-resistant *Staphylococcus epidermidis* experimental endocarditis. J Lab Clin Med. 1982;100:94-104.

142. Galetto DW, Boscia JA, Kobasa WD, Kaye D. Teicoplanin compared with vancomycin for treatment of experimental endocarditis due to methicillin-resistant *Staphylococcus epidermidis*. J Infect Dis. 1986;154:69-75.

143. Tuazon CU, Washburn D. Teicoplanin and rifampicin singly and in combination in the treatment of experimental *Staphylococcus epidermidis* endocarditis in the rabbit model. J Antimicrob Chemother. 1987;20:233-237.

144. Brandt CM, Rouse MS, Tallan BM, et al. Effective treatment of cephalosporin-rifampin combinations against cryptic methicillin-resistant beta-lactamase-producing coagulase-negative staphylococcal experimental endocarditis. Antimicrob Agents Chemother. 1995;39:1815-1819.

145. Kobasa W, Kaye K, Shapiro T, Kaye D. Therapy for experimental endocarditis due to *Staphylococcus epidermidis*. Rev Infect Dis. 1983;5:S533-S537.

146. Rouse MS, Wilcox RM, Henry NK, et al. Ciprofloxacin therapy of experimental endocarditis caused by methicillin-resistant *Staphylococcus epidermidis*. Antimicrob Agents Chemother. 1990;34:273-276.

147. Karchmer AW, Archer GL, Dismukes WE. Rifampin treatment of prosthetic valve endocarditis due to *Staphylococcus epidermidis*. Rev Infect Dis. 1983;5:S543-S548.

148. Karchmer AW, Archer GL, Dismukes WE. *Staphylococcus epidermidis* causing prosthetic valve endocarditis: Microbiologic and clinical observations as guides to therapy. Ann Intern Med. 1983;98:447-455.

149. Norden C. Experimental chronic staphylococcal osteomyelitis in rabbits: Treatment with rifampin alone and in combination with other antimicrobial agents. Rev Infect Dis. 1983;5:S491-S494.

150. Norden CW, Bryant R, Palmer D, et al. Chronic osteomyelitis caused by *Staphylococcus aureus*: Controlled clinical trial of nafcillin therapy and nafcillin-rifampin therapy. South Med J. 1986;79:947-951.

151. Norden CW, Fierer J, Bryant RE. Chronic staphylococcal osteomyelitis: Treatment with regimens containing rifampin. Rev Infect Dis. 1983;5:S495-S501.

152. Widmer A, Frei R, Rajacic A, Zimmerli W. Correlation between in vivo and in vitro efficacy of antimicrobial agents against foreign body infections. J Infect Dis. 1990;162:96-102.

153. Dunne WM Jr, Mason EO Jr, Kaplan SL. Diffusion of rifampin and vancomycin through a *Staphylococcus epidermidis* biofilm. Antimicrob Agents Chemother. 1993;37:2522-2526.

154. Zheng Z, Stewart PS. Penetration of rifampin through *Staphylococcus epidermidis* biofilms. Antimicrob Agents Chemother. 2002;46:900-903.

155. Blaser J, Vergères P, Widmer A, Zimmerli W. In vivo verification of in vitro model of antibiotic treatment of device-related infection. Antimicrob Agents Chemother. 1995;39:1134-1139.

156. Saleh-Mghir A, Ameur N, Muller-Serieys C, et al. Combination of quinupristin-dalfopristin (Synercid) and rifampin is highly synergistic in experimental *Staphylococcus aureus* joint prosthesis infection. Antimicrob Agents Chemother. 2002;46:1122-1124.

157. Widmer AF, Gaechter A, Ochsner PE, Zimmerli W. Antimicrobial treatment of orthopedic implant-related infections with rifampin combinations. Clin Infect Dis. 1992;14:1251-1253.

158. Drancourt M, Stein A, Argenson JN, et al. Oral rifampin plus ofloxacin for treatment of *Staphylococcus*-infected orthopedic implants. Antimicrob Agents Chemother. 1993;37:1214-1218.

159. Drancourt M, Stein A, Argenson JN, et al. Oral treatment of *Staphylococcus* spp. infected orthopaedic implants with fusidic acid or ofloxacin in combination with rifampicin. J Antimicrob Chemother. 1997;39:235-240.

160. Zimmerli W, Widmer AF, Blatter M, et al. Role of rifampin for treatment of orthopedic implant-related staphylococcal infections: A randomized controlled trial. Foreign-Body Infection (FBI) Study Group. JAMA. 1998;279:1537-1541.

161. Yu VL, Goetz A, Wagener M, et al. *Staphylococcus aureus* nasal carriage and infection in patients on hemodialysis: Efficacy of antibiotic prophylaxis. N Engl J Med. 1986;315:91-96.

162. Bernardini J, Piraino B, Holley J, et al. A randomized trial of *Staphylococcus aureus* prophylaxis in peritoneal dialysis patients: Mupirocin calcium ointment 2% applied to the exit site versus cyclic oral rifampin. Am J Kidney Dis. 1996;27:695-700.

163. Zimmerman SW, Ahrens E, Johnson CA, et al. Randomized controlled trial of prophylactic rifampin for peritoneal dialysis-related infections. Am J Kidney Dis. 1991;18:225-231.

164. Canawati H, Tuddenham W, Sapico F, Montgomerie J. Failure of rifampin to eradicate methicillin-resistant *Staphylococcus aureus* colonization. Clin Ther. 1982;4:526-531.

165. Darouiche R, Wright C, Hamill R, et al. Eradication of colonization by methicillin-resistant *Staphylococcus aureus* by using oral minocycline-rifampin and topical mupirocin. Antimicrob Agents Chemother. 1991;35:1612-1615.

166. Muder RR, Boldin M, Brennen C, et al. A controlled trial of rifampicin, minocycline, and rifampicin plus minocycline for eradication of methicillin-resistant *Staphylococcus aureus* in long-term care patients. J Antimicrob Chemother. 1994;34:189-190.

167. Roccaforte J, Bittner M, Stumpf C, Preheim L. Attempts to eradicate methicillin-resistant *Staphylococcus aureus* colonization with the use of trimethoprim-sulfamethoxazole, rifampin, and bacitracin. Am J Infect Control. 1988;16:141-146.

168. Ellison RT III, Judson FN, Peterson LC, et al. Oral rifampin and trimethoprim/sulfamethoxazole therapy in asymptomatic carriers of methicillin-resistant *Staphylococcus aureus* infections. West J Med. 1984;140:735-740.

169. Asensio A, Guerrero A, Quereda C, et al. Colonization and infection with methicillin-resistant *Staphylococcus aureus*: Associated factors and eradication. Infect Control Hosp Epidemiol. 1996;17:20-28.

170. Raad I, Darouiche R, Hachem R, et al. Antibiotics and prevention of microbial colonization of catheters. Antimicrob Agents Chemother. 1995;39:2397-2400.

171. Raad I, Darouiche R, Hachem R, et al. The broad-spectrum activity and efficacy of catheters coated with minocycline and rifampin. J Infect Dis. 1996;173:418-424.

172. Raad II, Darouiche RO, Hachem R, et al. Antimicrobial durability and rare ultrastructural colonization of indwelling central catheters coated with minocycline and rifampin. Crit Care Med. 1998;26:219-224.

173. Raad I, Darouiche R, Dupuis J, et al. Central venous catheters coated with minocycline and rifampin for the prevention of catheter-related colonization and bloodstream infections: A randomized, double-blind trial. Ann Intern Med. 1997;127:267-274.

174. Darouiche RO, Raad II, Heard SO, et al: A comparison of two antimicrobial-impregnated central venous catheters. N Engl J Med. 1999;340:1-8.

175. Tambe SM, Sampath L, Modak SM. In vitro evaluation of the risk of developing bacterial resistance to antiseptics and antibiotics used in medical devices. J Antimicrob Chemother. 2001;47:589-598.

176. Darouiche RO, Smith JA Jr, Hanna H, et al. Efficacy of antimicrobial-impregnated bladder catheters in reducing catheter-associated bacteriuria: A prospective, randomized, multicenter clinical trial. Urology. 1999;54:976-981.

177. Zabramski J, Whiting D, Darouiche R, et al. Efficacy of antimicrobial-impregnated external ventricular drain catheters: A prospective, randomized, controlled trial. J Neurosurg. 2003;98:725-730.

178. Darouiche RO, Meade R, Mansouri M, Raad II. In vivo efficacy of antimicrobial-coated fabric from prosthetic heart valve sewing rings. J Heart Valve Dis. 1998;7:639-646.

179. Darouiche RO, Mansouri MD, Raad II. Efficacy of antimicrobial-impregnated silicone sections from penile implants in preventing device colonization in an animal model. Urology. 2002;59:303-307.

180. Darouiche RO, Meade R, Mansouri MD, Netscher DT. In vivo efficacy of antimicrobe-impregnated saline-filled silicone implants. Plast Reconstr Surg. 2002;109:1352-1357.

181. Stein DS, Libertin CR. Time kill curve analysis of vancomycin and rifampin alone and in combination against nine strains of nutritionally deficient streptococci. Diagn Microbiol Infect Dis. 1988;10:139-144.

182. Moellering RC Jr, Wennersten C. Therapeutic potential of rifampin in enterococcal infections. Rev Infect Dis. 1983;5:S528-S532.

183. Oill P, Kalmanson G, Guze L. Rifampin, ampicillin, streptomycin, and their combinations in the treatment of enterococcal pyelonephritis in rats. Antimicrob Agents Chemother. 1981;20:491-492.

184. Tuazon CU, Miller H. Comparative in vitro activities of teichomycin and vancomycin alone and in combination with rifampin and aminoglycosides against staphylococci and enterococci. Antimicrob Agents Chemother. 1984;25:411-412.

185. Iannini PB, Ehret J, Eickhoff TC. Effects of ampicillin-amikacin and ampicillin-rifampin on enterococci. Antimicrob Agents Chemother. 1976;9:448-451.

186. Watanakunakorn C, Tisone JC. Effects of a vancomycin-rifampin combination on enterococci. Antimicrob Agents Chemother. 1982;22:915-916.

187. Deal WB, Sanders E. Efficacy of rifampin in treatment of meningococcal carriers. N Engl J Med. 1969;281:641-645.

188. Devine LF, Johnson DP, Hagerman CR, et al. Rifampin: Levels in serum and saliva and effect on the meningococcal carrier state. JAMA. 1970;214:1055-1059.

189. Guttler R, Counts G, Avent C, Beaty H. Effect of rifampin and minocycline on meningococcal carrier rates. J Infect Dis. 1971;124:199-205.

190. Beam WE Jr, Newberg NR, Devine LF, et al. The effect of rifampin on the nasopharyngeal carriage of *Neisseria meningitidis* in a military population. J Infect Dis. 1971;124:39-46.

191. Munford R, Sussuarana de Vasconcelos Z, Phillips C, et al. Eradication of carriage of *Neisseria meningitidis* in families: A study in Brazil. J Infect Dis. 1974;129:644-649.

192. Schwartz B, Al Tobaiqi A, Al Ruwais A, et al. Comparative efficacy of ceftriaxone and rifampin in eradicating pharyngeal carriage of group A *Neisseria meningitidis*. Lancet. 1988;1:1239-1242.

193. Cuevas LE, Kazembe P, Mughogho GK, et al. Eradication of nasopharyngeal carriage of *Neisseria meningitidis* in children and adults in rural Africa: A comparison of ciprofloxacin and rifampicin. J Infect Dis. 1995;171:728-731.

194. Simmons G, Jones N, Calder L. Equivalence of ceftriaxone and rifampicin in eliminating nasopharyngeal carriage of serogroup B *Neisseria meningitidis*. J Antimicrob Chemother. 2000;45:909-911.

195. Control and prevention of meningococcal disease: Recommendations of the Advisory Committee on Immunization Practices (ACIP). MMWR Morb Mortal Wkly Rep. 1997;46:1-10.

196. Granoff D, Gilsdorf J, Gessert C, Basden M. *Haemophilus influenzae* type b disease in a day care center: Eradication of carrier state by rifampin. Pediatrics. 1979;63:397-401.

197. Daum RS, Glode MP, Goldmann DA, et al. Rifampin chemoprophylaxis for household contacts of patients with invasive infections due to *Haemophilus influenzae* type b. J Pediatr. 1981;98:485-491.

198. Horner D, McCracken G, Ginsburg C, Zweighaft T. A comparison of three antibiotic regimens for eradication of *Haemophilus influenzae* type b from the pharynx of infants and children. Pediatrics. 1980;66:136-138.

199. Gessert C, Granoff D, Gilsdorf J. Comparison of rifampin and ampicillin in day care center contacts of *Haemophilus influenzae* type b disease. Pediatrics. 1980;66:1-4.

200. Shapiro E, Wald E. Efficacy of rifampin in eliminating pharyngeal carriage of *Haemophilus influenzae* type b. Pediatrics. 1980;66:5-8.

201. Cox F, Trincher R, Rissing JP, et al. Rifampin prophylaxis for contacts of *Haemophilus influenzae* type b disease. JAMA. 1981;245:1043-1045.

202. Murphy TV, Chrane DF, McCracken GH Jr, Nelson JD. Rifampin prophylaxis v placebo for household contacts of children with *Hemophilus influenzae* type b disease. Am J Dis Child. 1983;137:627-632.

203. Murphy TV, McCracken GH Jr, Zweighaft TC, Hansen EJ. Emergence of rifampin-resistant *Haemophilus influenzae* after prophylaxis. J Pediatr. 1981;99:406-409.

204. *Haemophilus influenzae* type B. 7. Atlanta: Centers for Disease Control and Prevention, U.S. Department of Health and Human Services, 2003.

205. Arlotti M, Zoboli G, Moscatelli GL, et al. *Rhodococcus equi* infection in HIV-positive subjects: A retrospective analysis of 24 cases. Scand J Infect Dis. 1996;28:463-467.

206. Nordmann P, Ronco E. In-vitro antimicrobial susceptibility of *Rhodococcus equi*. J Antimicrob Chemother. 1992;29:383-393.

207. Finland M, Garner C, Wilcox C, Sabath LD. Susceptibility of "enterobacteria" to penicillins, cephalosporins, lincomycins, erythromycin, and rifampin. J Infect Dis. 1976;134:S75-S96.

208. Yee YC, Kisslinger B, Yu VL, Jin DJ. A mechanism of rifamycin inhibition and resistance in *Pseudomonas aeruginosa*. J Antimicrob Chemother. 1996;38:133-137.

209. Zuravleff JJ, Yu VL, Yee RB. Ticarcillin-tobramycin-rifampin: In vitro synergy of the triplet combination against *Pseudomonas aeruginosa*. J Lab Clin Med. 1983;101:896-902.

210. Chin NX, Neu HC. Synergy of imipenem—a novel carbapenem, and rifampin and ciprofloxacin against *Pseudomonas aeruginosa*, *Serratia marcescens* and *Enterobacter* species. Chemotherapy. 1987;33:183-188.

211. Traub WH, Spohr M, Bauer D. *Pseudomonas aeruginosa*: In vitro susceptibility to antimicrobial drugs, single and combined, with and without defibrinated human blood. Chemotherapy. 1988;34:284-297.

212. Ghani M, Soothill JS. Ceftazidime, gentamicin, and rifampicin, in combination, kill biofilms of mucoid *Pseudomonas aeruginosa*. Can J Microbiol. 1997;43:999-1004.

213. Yu VL, Zuravleff JJ, Peacock JE, et al. Addition of rifampin to carboxypenicillin-aminoglycoside combination for the treatment of *Pseudomonas aeruginosa* infection: Clinical experience with four patients. Antimicrob Agents Chemother. 1984;26:575-577.

214. Korvick JA, Peacock JE Jr, Muder RR, et al. Addition of rifampin to combination antibiotic therapy for *Pseudomonas aeruginosa* bacteremia: Prospective trial using the Zelen protocol. Antimicrob Agents Chemother. 1992;36:620-625.

215. Kumar A, Wofford-McQueen R, Gordon RC. In vitro activity of multiple antimicrobial combinations against *Pseudomonas cepacia* isolates. Chemotherapy. 1989;35:246-253.

216. Kumar A, Wofford-McQueen R, Gordon RC. Ciprofloxacin, imipenem and rifampicin: In-vitro synergy of two and three drug combinations against *Pseudomonas cepacia*. J Antimicrob Chemother. 1989;23:831-835.

217. Dreses-Werringloer U, Padubrin I, Zeidler H, Kohler L. Effects of azithromycin and rifampin on *Chlamydia trachomatis* infection in vitro. Antimicrob Agents Chemother. 2001;45:3001-3008.

218. Treharne J, Yearsley P, Ballard R. In vitro studies of *Chlamydia trachomatis* susceptibility and resistance to rifampin and rifabutin. Antimicrob Agents Chemother. 1989;33:1393-1394.

219. Jones RB, Ridgway GL, Boulding S, Hunley KL. In vitro activity of rifamycins alone and in combination with other antibiotics against *Chlamydia trachomatis*. Rev Infect Dis. 1983;5:S556-S561.

220. Freidank H, Losch P, Vogele H, Wiedmann-Al-Ahmad M. In vitro susceptibilities of *Chlamydia pneumoniae* isolates from German patients and synergistic activity of antibiotic combinations. Antimicrob Agents Chemother. 1999;43:1808-1810.

221. Baltch A, Smith R, Ritz W. Inhibitory and bactericidal activities of levofloxacin, ofloxacin, erythromycin, and rifampin used singly and in combination against *Legionella pneumophila*. Antimicrob Agents Chemother. 1995;39:1661-1666.

222. Dournon E, Mayaud C, Wolff M, et al. Comparison of the activity of three antibiotic regimens in severe Legionnaires' disease. J Antimicrob Chemother. 1990;26 (Suppl):39.

223. Bartlett J, Dowell S, Mandell L, et al. Practice guidelines for the management of community-acquired pneumonia in adults. Clin Infect Dis. 2000;31:347-382.

224. Reda C, Quaresima T, Castellani Pastoris M. In-vitro activity of six intracellular antibiotics against *Legionella pneumophila* strains of human and environmental origin. J Antimicrob Chemother. 1994;33:757-764.

225. Saito A, Koga H, Shigeno H, et al. The antimicrobial activity of ciprofloxacin against *Legionella* species and the treatment of experimental *Legionella* pneumonia in guinea pigs. J Antimicrob Chemother. 1986;18:251-260.

226. Kunin CM. Antimicrobial activity of rifabutin. Clin Infect Dis. 1996;22:S3-S14.

227. Heep M, Beck D, Bayerdörffer E, Lehn N. Rifampin and rifabutin resistance mechanisms in *Helicobacter pylori*. Antimicrob Agents Chemother. 1999;43:1497-1499.

228. Perri F, Festa V. Treatment of antibiotic-resistant *Helicobacter pylori* infection. N Engl J Med. 1998;339:53.

229. Bock H, Koop H, Lehn N, Heep M. Rifabutin-based triple therapy after failure of *Helicobacter pylori* eradication treatment: Preliminary experience. J Clin Gastroenterol. 2000;31:222-225.

230. Perri F, Festa V, Clemente R, et al. Randomized study of two "rescue" therapies for *Helicobacter pylori*-infected patients after failure of standard triple therapies. Am J Gastroenterol. 2001;96:58-62.

231. Wong W, Gu Q, Lam S, et al. Randomized controlled study of rabeprazole, levofloxacin and rifabutin triple therapy vs. quadruple therapy as second-line treatment for *Helicobacter pylori* infection. Aliment Pharmacol Ther. 2003;17:553-560.

232. Rolain JM, Maurin M, Vestris G, Raoult D. In vitro susceptibilities of 27 rickettsiae to 13 antimicrobials. Antimicrob Agents Chemother. 1998;42:1537-1541.

233. Raoult D, Roussellier P, Vestris G, Tamalet J. In vitro antibiotic susceptibility of *Rickettsia rickettsii* and *Rickettsia conorii*: Plaque assay and microplaque colorimetric assay. J Infect Dis. 1987;155:1059-1062.

234. Bella F, Espejo E, Uriz S, et al. Randomized trial of 5-day rifampin versus 1-day doxycycline therapy for Mediterranean spotted fever. J Infect Dis. 1991;164:433-434.

235. Yeaman MR, Mitscher LA, Baca OG. In vitro susceptibility of *Coxiella burnetii* to antibiotics, including several quinolones. Antimicrob Agents Chemother. 1987;31:1079-1084.

236. Raoult D, Drancourt M, Vestris G. Bactericidal effect of doxycycline associated with lysosomotropic agents on *Coxiella burnetii* in P388D1 cells. Antimicrob Agents Chemother. 1990;34:1512-1514.

237. Klein MB, Nelson CM, Goodman JL. Antibiotic susceptibility of the newly cultivated agent of human granulocytic ehrlichiosis: Promising activity of quinolones and rifamycins. Antimicrob Agents Chemother. 1997;41:76-79.

238. Brouqui P, Raoult D. In vitro antibiotic susceptibility of the newly recognized agent of ehrlichiosis in humans, *Ehrlichia chaffeensis*. Antimicrob Agents Chemother. 1992;36:2799-2803.

239. Buitrago M, Ijdo J, Rinaudo P, et al. Human granulocytic ehrlichiosis during pregnancy treated successfully with rifampin. Clin Infect Dis. 1998;27:213-215.

240. Corbel MJ. Determination of the in vitro sensitivity of *Brucella* strains to rifampicin. Br Vet J. 1976;132:266-275.

241. Garcia-Rodriguez JA, Munoz Bellido JL, Fresnadillo MJ, Trujillano I. In vitro activities of new macrolides and rifapentine against *Brucella* spp. Antimicrob Agents Chemother. 1993;37:911-913.

242. Colmenero Castillo JD, Hernandez MS, Reguera Iglesias JM, et al. Comparative trial of doxycycline plus streptomycin versus doxycycline plus rifampin for the therapy of human brucellosis. Chemotherapy. 1989;35:146-152.

243. Acocella G, Bertrand A, Beytout J, et al. Comparison of three different regimens in the treatment of acute brucellosis: A multicenter multinational study. J Antimicrob Chemother. 1989;23:433-439.

244. Lubani MM, Dudin KI, Sharda DC, et al. A multicenter therapeutic study of 1100 children with brucellosis. Pediatr Infect Dis J. 1989;8:75-78.

245. Ariza J, Gudiol F, Pallares R, et al. Treatment of human brucellosis with doxycycline plus rifampin or doxycycline plus streptomycin: A randomized, double-blind study. Ann Intern Med. 1992;117:25-30.

246. Montejo JM, Alberola I, Glez-Zarate P, et al. Open, randomized therapeutic trial of six antimicrobial regimens in the treatment of human brucellosis. Clin Infect Dis. 1993;16:671-676.

247. Akova M, Uzun O, Akalin HE, et al. Quinolones in treatment of human brucellosis: Comparative trial of ofloxacin-rifampin versus doxycycline-rifampin. Antimicrob Agents Chemother. 1993;37:1831-1834.

248. Colmenero JD, Fernández-Gallardo LC, Agúndez JA, et al. Possible implications of doxycycline-rifampin interaction for treatment of brucellosis. Antimicrob Agents Chemother. 1994;38:2798-2802.

249. Solera J, Rodríguez-Zapata M, Geijo P, et al. Doxycycline-rifampin versus doxycycline-streptomycin in treatment of human brucellosis due to *Brucella melitensis*. Antimicrob Agents Chemother. 1995;39:2061-2067.

250. Solera J, Medrano F, Rodriguez M, et al. A comparative therapeutic and multicenter trial of rifampicin and doxycycline versus streptomycin and doxycycline in human brucellosis. Med Clin. 1991;96:649-653.

251. Solera J, Martinez-Alfaro E, Saez L. Meta-analysis of the efficacy of the combination of rifampicin and doxycycline in the treatment of human brucellosis. Med Clin. 1994;102:731-738.

252. Agalar C, Usubutun S, Turkyilmaz R. Ciprofloxacin and rifampicin versus doxycycline and rifampicin in the treatment of brucellosis. Eur J Clin Microbiol. 1999;18:535-538.

253. Bacon AE, McGrath S, Fekety R, Holloway WJ. In vitro synergy studies with *Clostridium difficile*. Antimicrob Agents Chemother. 1991;35:582-583.

254. Barbut F, Decre D, Burghoffer B, et al. Antimicrobial susceptibilities and serogroups of clinical strains of *Clostridium difficile* isolated in France in 1991 and 1997. Antimicrob Agents Chemother. 1999;43:2607-2611.

255. Buggy BP, Fekety R, Silva J Jr. Therapy of relapsing *Clostridium difficile*-associated diarrhea and colitis with the combination of vancomycin and rifampin. J Clin Gastroenterol. 1987;9:155-159.

256. Kitahara M, Seth V, Medoff G, Kobayashi G. Activity of amphotericin B, 5-fluorocytosine, and rifampin against six clinical isolates of *Aspergillus*. Antimicrob Agents Chemother. 1976;9:915-919.

257. Hughes CE, Harris C, Moody JA, et al. In vitro activities of amphotericin B in combination with four antifungal agents and rifampin against *Aspergillus* spp. Antimicrob Agents Chemother. 1984;25:560-562.

258. Beggs WH, Sarosi GA, Walker MI. Synergistic action of amphotericin B and rifampin against *Candida* species. J Infect Dis. 1976;133:206-209.

259. Graybill J, Ahrens J. Interaction of rifampin with other antifungal agents in experimental murine candidiasis. Rev Infect Dis. 1983;5:S620-S625.

260. Huppert M, Pappagianis D, Sun SH, et al. Effect of amphotericin B and rifampin against *Coccidioides immitis* in vitro and in vivo. Antimicrob Agents Chemother. 1976;9:406-413.

261. Fujita NK, Edwards JE Jr. Combined in vitro effect of amphotericin B and rifampin on *Cryptococcus neoformans*. Antimicrob Agents Chemother. 1981;19:196-198.

262. Kobayashi GS, Medoff G, Schlessinger D, et al. Amphotericin B potentiation of rifampicin as an antifungal agent against the yeast phase of *Histoplasma capsulatum*. Science. 1972;177:709-710.

263. Kitahara M, Kobayashi G, Medoff G. Enhanced efficacy of amphotericin B and rifampin combined in treatment of murine histoplasmosis and blastomycosis. J Infect Dis. 1976;133:663-668.

264. Arroyo J, Medoff G, Kobayashi G. Therapy of murine aspergillosis with amphotericin B in combination with rifampin or 5-fluorocytosine. Antimicrob Agents Chemother. 1977;11:21-25.

265. Ernst JD, Rusnak M, Sande MA. Combination antifungal chemotherapy for experimental disseminated candidiasis: Lack of correlation between in vitro and in vivo observations with amphotericin B and rifampin. Rev Infect Dis. 1983;5:S626-S630.

266. Holmberg S, Moorman A, Von Bargen J, et al. Possible effectiveness of clarithromycin and rifabutin for cryptosporidiosis chemoprophylaxis in HIV disease. JAMA. 1998;279:384-386.

267. Giacometti A, Cirioni O, Barchiesi F, et al. Activity of nitazoxanide alone and in combination with azithromycin and rifabutin against *Cryptosporidium parvum* in cell culture. J Antimicrob Chemother. 2000;45:453-456.

268. Ghent CN, Carruthers SG. Treatment of pruritus in primary biliary cirrhosis with rifampin: Results of a double-blind, crossover, randomized trial. Gastroenterology. 1988;94:488-493.

269. Cynamon HA, Andres JM, Iafrate RP. Rifampin relieves pruritus in children with cholestatic liver disease. Gastroenterology. 1990;98:1013-1016.

270. Podesta A, Lopez P, Terg R, et al. Treatment of pruritus of primary biliary cirrhosis with rifampin. Dig Dis Sci. 1991;36:216-220.

271. Bachs L, Pares A, Elena M, et al. Effects of long-term rifampicin administration in primary biliary cirrhosis. Gastroenterology. 1992;102:2077-2080.

272. Gregorio GV, Ball CS, Mowat AP, Mieli-Vergani G. Effect of rifampicin in the treatment of pruritus in hepatic cholestasis. Arch Dis Child. 1993;69:141-143.

273. Price TJ, Patterson WK, Olver IN. Rifampicin as treatment for pruritus in malignant cholestasis. Support Care Cancer. 1998;6:533-535.

274. Yerushalmi B, Sokol RJ, Narkewicz MR, et al. Use of rifampin for severe pruritus in children with chronic cholestasis. J Pediatr Gastroenterol Nutr. 1999;29:442-447.

275. Woolf GM, Reynolds TB. Failure of rifampin to relieve pruritus in chronic liver disease. J Clin Gastroenterol. 1990;12:174-177.

276. Prince MI, Burt AD, Jones DE. Hepatitis and liver dysfunction with rifampicin therapy for pruritus in primary biliary cirrhosis. Gut. 2002;50:436-439.

277. Jiang ZD, Ke S, Palazzini E, et al. In vitro activity and fecal concentration of rifaximin after oral administration. Antimicrob Agents Chemother. 2000;44:2205-2206.

278. DuPont HL, Jiang ZD, Ericsson CD, et al. Rifaximin versus ciprofloxacin for the treatment of traveler's diarrhea: A randomized, double-blind clinical trial. Clin Infect Dis. 2001;33:1807-1815.

279. Hoover WW, Gerlach EH, Hoban DJ, et al. Antimicrobial activity and spectrum of rifaximin, a new topical rifamycin derivative. Diagn Microbiol Infect Dis. 1993;16:111-118.

280. Sierra JM, Navia MM, Vargas M, et al. In vitro activity of rifaximin against bacterial enteropathogens causing diarrhoea in children under 5 years of age in Ifakara, Tanzania. J Antimicrob Chemother. 2001;47:904-905.

281. Sierra JM, Ruiz J, Navia MM, et al. In vitro activity of rifaximin against enteropathogens producing traveler's diarrhea. Antimicrob Agents Chemother. 2001;45:643-644.

282. Holton J, Vaira D, Menegatti M, Barbara L. The susceptibility of *Helicobacter pylori* to the rifamycin, rifaximin. J Antimicrob Chemother. 1995;35:545-549.

283. Akada J, Shirai M, Fujii K, et al. In vitro anti-*Helicobacter pylori* activities of new rifamycin derivatives, KRM-1648 and KRM-1657. Antimicrob Agents Chemother. 1999;43:1072-1076.

284. Marchese A, Salerno A, Pesce A, et al. In vitro activity of rifaximin, metronidazole and vancomycin against *Clostridium difficile* and the rate of selection of spontaneously resistant mutants against representative anaerobic and aerobic bacteria, including ammonia-producing species. Chemotherapy. 2000;46:253-266.

285. Di Stefano M, Malservisi S, Veneto G, et al. Rifaximin versus chlortetracycline in the short-term treatment of small intestinal bacterial overgrowth. Aliment Pharmacol Ther. 2000;14:551-556.

286. Testa R, Eftimiadi C, Sukkar GS, et al. A non-absorbable rifamycin for treatment of hepatic encephalopathy. Drugs Exp Clin Res. 1985;11:387-392.

287. Pedretti G, Calzetti C, Missale G, Fiaccadori F. Rifaximin versus neomycin on hyperammoniemia in chronic portal systemic encephalopathy of cirrhotics: A double-blind, randomized trial. Ital J Gastroenterol. 1991;23:175-178.

288. Miglio F, Valpiani D, Rossellini SR, Ferrieri A. Rifaximin, a non-absorbable rifamycin, for the treatment of hepatic encephalopathy: A double-blind, randomised trial. Curr Med Res Opin. 1997;13:593-601.

289. Frisari L, Viggiano V, Pelagalli M. An open, controlled study of two non-absorbable antibiotics for the oral treatment of paediatric infectious diarrhoea. Curr Med Res Opin. 1997;14:39-45.

290. Gionchetti P, Rizzello F, Ferrieri A, et al. Rifaximin in patients with moderate or severe ulcerative colitis refractory to steroid-treatment: A double-blind, placebo-controlled trial. Dig Dis Sci. 1999;44:1220-1221.

291. Hosoe K, Mae T, Konishi E, et al. Pharmacokinetics of KRM-1648, a new benzoxazinorifamycin, in rats and dogs. Antimicrob Agents Chemother. 1996;40:2749-2755.

292. Mae T, Hosoe K, Yamamoto T, et al. Effect of a new rifamycin derivative, rifalazil, on liver microsomal enzyme induction in rat and dog. Xenobiotica. 1998;28:759-766.

293. Saito H, Tomioka H, Sato K, et al. In vitro antimycobacterial activities of newly synthesized benzoxazinorifamycins. Antimicrob Agents Chemother. 1991;35:542-547.

294. Tomioka H, Saito H, Fujii K, Sato K, Hidaka T. In vitro antimicrobial activity of benzoxazinorifamycin, KRM-1648, against *Mycobacterium avium* complex, determined by the radiometric method. Antimicrob Agents Chemother. 1993;37:67-70.

295. Hirata T, Saito H, Tomioka H, et al. In vitro and in vivo activities of the benzoxazinorifamycin KRM-1648 against *Mycobacterium tuberculosis*. Antimicrob Agents Chemother. 1995;39:2295-2303.

296. Mor N, Simon B, Heifets L. Bacteriostatic and bactericidal activities of benzoxazinorifamycin KRM-1648 against *Mycobacterium tuberculosis* and *Mycobacterium avium* in human macrophages. Antimicrob Agents Chemother. 1996;40:1482-1485.

297. Tomioka H, Saito H, Sato K, et al. Chemotherapeutic efficacy of a newly synthesized benzoxazinorifamycin, KRM-1648, against *Mycobacterium avium* complex infection induced in mice. Antimicrob Agents Chemother. 1992;36:387-393.

298. Klemens S, Grossi M, Cynamon M. Activity of KRM-1648, a new benzoxazinorifamycin, against *Mycobacterium tuberculosis* in a murine model. Antimicrob Agents Chemother. 1994;38:2245-2248.

299. Klemens S, Cynamon M. Activity of KRM-1648 in combination with isoniazid against *Mycobacterium tuberculosis* in a murine model. Antimicrob Agents Chemother. 1996;40:298-301.

300. Fujii K, Tsuji A, Miyazaki S, Yamaguchi K, Goto S. In vitro and in vivo antibacterial activities of KRM-1648 and KRM-1657, new rifamycin derivatives. Antimicrob Agents Chemother. 1994;38:1118-1122.

301. Wichelhaus T, Schafer V, Brade V, Boddinghaus B. Differential effect of *rpoB* mutations on antibacterial activities of rifampicin and KRM-1648 against *Staphylococcus aureus*. J Antimicrob Chemother. 2001;47:153-156.

302. Roblin P, Reznik T, Kutlin A, Hammerschlag M. In vitro activities of rifamycin derivatives ABI-1648 (Rifalazil, KRM-1648), ABI-1657, and ABI-1131 against *Chlamydia trachomatis* and recent clinical isolates of *Chlamydia pneumoniae*. Antimicrob Agents Chemother. 2003;47:1135-1136.

CHAPTER **27**

Metronidazole*

MIRELLA SALVATORE
BURT MEYERS

OVERVIEW

Metronidazole is a nitroimidazole drug with the chemical formula 1-(2-hydroxyethyl)-2-methyl-5-nitroimidazole. It was introduced for the first time in 1959 for the treatment of *Trichomonas vaginalis* infections but was then found to be bactericidal for most anaerobic and facultative anaerobic bacteria and protozoa. Because it is an extremely active and well-tolerated drug that penetrates well into tissues including the central nervous system, it is used for treatment of many anaerobic bacterial infections, *Helicobacter pylori* infections, amebiasis, giardiasis, trichomoniasis, Crohn's disease, as well as a prophylactic antibiotic prior to surgical interventions.

MECHANISM OF ACTION

Metronidazole can be considered a prodrug that needs to be activated in susceptible organisms. It has a low molecular weight (171 kd), enters the cells by diffusion, and exerts its cytotoxic effects by production of free radicals. The bactericidal effect is rapid and the killing rate is proportional to the concentration of the drug[1,2] both in susceptible anaerobic bacteria, in *Entamoeba histolytica* and *T. vaginalis*.[3,4]

Metronidazole enters the cell membrane by passive diffusion (the details of this process are still not known) and is activated by reduction of its nitro group that accepts electrons donated by electron transport proteins, such as flavoproteins in mammal cells and ferredoxins in bacteria. In the case of obligate anaerobes, in which the environment has a very low negative redox potential, this process occurs as a single reduction step and involves the transfer of just an electron. This reaction is catalyzed by a nitroreductase, such as the pyruvate:ferredoxin oxidoreductase that is the anaerobic bacterial homologue of pyruvate dehydrogenase. This enzyme normally generates adenosine triphosphate (ATP) via oxidative decarboxylation of pyruvate capturing electrons that would usually be transferred to ferredoxin(s). Reduction of metronidazole is thought to create a concentration gradient that determines the increased

---

*This chapter is based, in part, on the chapter prepared by Dr. Sydney M. Finegold for the fifth edition.

uptake of the drug, and promotes formation of metronidazole radicals.[5,6,7] These highly reactive reduced intermediate compounds are unstable and before decaying into inactive end products[8] interact with nucleic acids, causing breakage and destabilization,[9,10] and with proteins and eventually cause the death of the bacterium. Metronidazole is also active against facultative anaerobes such as *H. pylori* and *Gardnerella vaginalis,* but the mechanism of action appears to be different. In anaerobic microorganisms with low redox potential, metronidazole is reduced to its active metabolite by a one-electron transfer step. In *H. pylori* metronidazole metabolites formed by a one-electron transfer are readily reoxidized in the microaerophilic environment. This process is called "futile cycling" and is accompanied by the formation of toxic oxygen radicals that are neutralized by an active scavenger system. It has been shown that in *H. pylori* metronidazole is activated by an oxygen-insensitive NAPDH nitroreductase encoded by the rdxA gene. This activation occurs by a two-electron transfer step and produces a toxic metabolite that cannot be retransformed into the parental compound in presence of oxygen, thus preventing futile cycling and enabling the action of metronidazole in a microaerophilic environment.[11]

Parasites such as *Giardia* or *Entamoeba* have no mitochondria, and their metabolism is glycolytic with the final step being executed by the pyruvate:ferredoxin oxidoreductase; this enzyme is also responsible for the activation of metronidazole. Purified pyruvate:ferredoxin oxidoreductase and ferredoxin from *Giardia* are able to activate metronidazole in vitro.[12-14] The protozoan parasite *T. vaginalis* also lacks mitochondria. Its energy requirements are provided by the glycolysis of glucose followed by further conversion of the pyruvate and maleate in an organelle called hydrogenosome. This organelle contains electron transport components linked to the pyruvate:ferredoxin oxidoreductase that is probably responsible for the activation of metronidazole.[14]

SPECTRUM OF ACTIVITY

Metronidazole is active against a variety of anaerobic bacteria as well as microaerophilic bacteria and protozoa (Table 27-1). Sensitivity to metronidazole may be difficult to assess because sensitivity testing for anaerobes is not performed routinely. In a multicenter 3-year analysis of 1108 anaerobic isolates,[15] metronidazole was active for all clinically important species. Large-scale studies did not show metronidazole resistance in bacteria of the *Bacteroides fragilis* group or *B. fragilis* itself.[16-19] However, resistant *Bacteroides* isolates have been described.[20-26] Gram-negative anaerobes such as *Prevotella* and *Fusobacterium* are usually sensitive, but resistant *Prevotella* strains have been described.[27] Approximately 70% to 75% of *Actinomyces* species and *Propionibacterium propionica,* are resistant to metronidazole.[28,29] *Propionibacterium acnes* is highly resistant.[30,31] Susceptibility of *Mobiluncus* is variable; *Mobiluncus curtisii* is usually resistant to metronidazole, while *Mobiluncus mulieris* are often sensitive.[32,33] A recent study showed that the majority of the periodontal pathogens—whether β-lactamase producers or not—are inhibited by metronidazole at a concentration of less than or equal to 8 mg/L except for the *Actinomyces* species.[34] *Capnocytophaga* species are usually sensitive with 7% to 10% of the isolates reported resistant. The facultative anaerobes *Actinobacillus actinomycetemcomitans* and *Eikenella corrodens* are typically resistant.[35,36] *G. vaginalis,* also a facultative anaerobe, is variably sensitive to metronidazole; however, the hydroxymetabolite of metronidazole is two to eight times more active against both *Gardnerella* and *A. actinomycetemcomitans* than the parental compound.[37] *H. pylori,* a microaerophilic organism, is usually sensitive to metronidazole; however, resistant strains (minimal inhibitory concentration [MIC] greater than 8 μg/mL) are becoming an increasing problem.[38] *Clostridium* species are usually sensitive but *Clostridium ramosum* may require higher concentrations for inhibition.[39,40] *Treponema pallidum,* oral spirochetes, *Campylobacter fetus, T. vaginalis, Giardia lamblia,* and *E. histolytica* are also sensitive to metronidazole.[41]

MECHANISMS OF RESISTANCE TO METRONIDAZOLE

Resistance to metronidazole develops rarely, and a combination of several mechanisms may be required for emergence of high-level resistance.[42] A large study did not show any significant change in the overall activity and spectrum of metronidazole during a 4-year period, with the overall resistance rate of the tested species varying only between 1.8% and 2.5% according to the testing method used.[15] In general, failure to test metronidazole susceptibility under strict anaerobic conditions may lead to reports of false resistance. Although both plasmid-mediated and chromosomally mediated resistance have been described,

TABLE 27-1 Antianaerobic Organism Activity of Metronidazole Tested (Agar Dilution and Etest) against 1108 Clinical Isolates from Five or More Medical Centers in the United States in 1994, 1996, and 1997

Organisms (Number Tested by Year)	Metronidazole MIC$_{50}$/MIC$_{90}$ (μg/mL)			Percent Susceptible		
	1994	1996	1997	1994	1996	1997
Clinically Indicated Species						
Bacteroides fragilis group						
B. fragilis (104/120/101)	1/2	0.5/1	0.75/2-3*	98.5	100	98.5
B. distasonis (24/19/19)	1-0.75-2-3	0.5-1/2	1/4-6	97.9	100	100
B. ovatus (26/19/19)	1-1.5/2-3	0.5-1/1.5-2	1.5-2/6-8	98.1	100	100
B. theataiotaomicron (45/17/18)	1-1.5/2-3	0.5/2	1/2	97.8	100	100
B. vulgatus (38/16/17)	0.5-1/1.5-2	0.38-1/0.75-1	0.5/2-4	100	100	100
Fusobacterium spp. (31/18/15)	0.25-0.125/0.5-1	0.047-0.25/2-4	0.012-0.25/1-2	100	97.2	93.3
Eubacterium spp. (15/12/14)	0.25-0.5/≥32	0.125-0.25/1->32	0.19-0.25/0.25-0.5	86.7	100/66.7†	92.6
Clostridium spp. (113/20/16)	0.38-0.5/2	0.5-1/2	0.75-1/2-3	100	95	100
Anaerobic gram-positive cocci‡ (60/18/21)	0.25-0.5/2	0.125-0.25/16->32	0.25-1/ >32†	96.7	88.8	80.9
Additional Species/Genera						
B. fragilis group, other§ (39/12/5)	0.75-1/2	0.38-1/1-1.5	0.38-0.5/NT‖	97.4	100	100
Prevotella spp.¶ (41/20/17)	1-2/4-8	0.5-1/8-16	0.75-1/4-12	100/90.2	90/85	100/82.4

*If a range is shown it indicates that different values for the Etest and the reference test were obtained (reference/Etest).
†If two percentages are listed, a difference in spectrum was detected (agar dilution/Etest spectrum).
‡Includes species peptostreptococci and those previously designated as peptoccocci. Includes one or more of the following *Bacteroides* spp.: *B. uniformis* (one strain), *B. caccae* (one strain), *B. eggerthii* (one strain), *B. pyogenes* (one strain).
§*B. stercoralis* (one strain).
‖NT = MIC$_{90}$ not tabulated because of fewer than 10 strains.
¶Includes *Prevotella* spp. *P. bivia, P. disiens, P. baccae, P. buccalis, P. ovalis, P. denticola,* and *P. intermedia.*

the transfer to metronidazole-sensitive *Bacteroides* species does not yet appear to be a problem.[43] It has been suggested that resistance is conferred by different degrees of reduction in pyruvate:ferredoxin oxidoreductase activity with decreased uptake and altered activation of metronidazole. Resistant bacteria compensate for reduced action of pyruvate:ferredoxin oxidoreductase by increasing pyruvate dehydrogenase activity.[44] The recent report of *Bacteroides* strains with multiple antibiotic resistances is, however, of concern.[26] This resistance has been attributed to novel transferable genes (*nimA* to *nimD*).[45,46] The same nim genes are responsible for resistance to metronidazole in bacteria of the *B. fragilis* group and in other anaerobes.[47,48]

Resistance of *H. pylori* to metronidazole is also an increasing problem. The acquisition of resistance is associated with mutational inactivation of the *rdxA* gene, which encodes an oxygen-insensitive NADPH nitroreductase. Inactivation of *frxA* (NADPH flavin oxidoreductase), *fdxB* (ferredoxin-like protein) and possibly other reductase-encoding genes may also contribute to the resistant phenotype.[11,49] Many cases of metronidazole-resistant *T. vaginalis* isolates have been reported in the literature[50-52] and clinical resistance of *Giardia* to metronidazole can be as prevalent as 20% of isolates. Metronidazole resistance in *Trichomonas* and *Giardia* is multifactorial. Resistant isolates probably have reduced activation of metronidazole, as suggested by the downregulation and decreased activity of the enzyme pyruvate:ferredoxin oxidoreductase and/or a reduced transcription of the ferredoxin gene with decreased intracellular levels of ferredoxin, as reported in resistant *Trichomonas*[53] and *Giardia*.[13,54] In addition, pyruvate is preferentially metabolized to lactate in the cytosol via lactate dehydrogenase, instead of being metabolized within hydrogenosomes.[5,55] In addition, a second oxidase that does not donate electrons to ferredoxins and does not activate metronidazole (2 oxoacid oxidoreductase) would substitute the decreased activity of pyruvate:ferredoxin oxidoreductase.[53] Other mechanisms including transport changes and gene rearrangements also

appear to be involved in the development of resistance in *Giardia*.[14] In case of amebae resistant to metronidazole, an increase in iron containing superoxide dismutase without a significant decrease of the pyruvate:ferredoxin oxidoreductase has been described.[14]

PHARMACOLOGY

Pharmacokinetics

Pharmacokinetic data regarding metronidazole are summarized in Table 27-2. When given orally, metronidazole is absorbed rapidly and almost completely.[56] Blood levels are proportional to the administered dose. Absorption of metronidazole is not affected by the ingestion of food, but peak levels may be markedly delayed. The standard intravenous dosage regimen that has been used in the United States consists of a loading dose of 15 mg/kg of body weight followed by 7.5 mg/kg every 6 hours. This results in peak and trough steady-state plasma levels averaging 25 and 18 µg/mL, respectively. The half-life is 8 hours. Metronidazole mostly circulates as a free drug (80%). The apparent volume of distribution is equivalent to about 80% of body weight and it reaches all tissues and fluids. Therapeutic levels are achieved in amniotic fluid, polymorphonuclear leukocytes, the unobstructed biliary tract, pancreas, alveolar bone, cerebrospinal fluid (CSF) and brain abscess contents, cord blood, pleural empyema fluid, peritoneal fluid, hepatic abscesses, middle ear discharge, middle ear mucosa, breast milk, pelvic tissues (concentrations attained in the myometrium and fallopian tubes are nearly the same as concomitant serum levels), colonic mucosa, saliva, seminal fluid, and vaginal secretions. Levels achieved in the aqueous humor are between one third and one half those attained in the serum.[57] In patients without meningeal inflammation, CSF levels approximate 45% of corresponding serum concentrations.[58] Those with meningitis experience similar CSF and serum concentrations. Metronidazole exhibits excellent penetration

---

TABLE 27-2   Pharmacologic Properties of Metronidazole

Time to peak concentration	Intravenous: end of infusion Oral: 1-2 hr Rectal: 3 hr Topical: 8-12 hr	
Peak plasma concentrations	IV: 25 µg/mL peak and 18 µg/mL steady state PO: 6, 12, 21.4, and 40 µg/mL Rectal: 18.5 µg/mL Topical: 27.6 ng/mL	After a loading dose of 15 mg/kg IV plus 7.5 mg/Kg µg/mL q6h After single oral doses of 250, 500, 750, and 2000 mg, respectively Suppositories of 500 mg Topical application of 1% cream
Total protein binding	Less than 20%	
Sites of distribution	Appendix tissue: high Bile: high Bronchial secretions: approximates serum concentrations Cerebrospinal fluid approximates serum concentrations Saliva approximates serum concentrations Abscesses: high Peritoneal fluid: high	
Volume of distribution	0.25-0.85 L/kg	
Elimination half-life	8 hr	
Bioavailability	Oral: >98% Rectal: 59%-94% Topical: minimal Topical 25% gel applied to inflamed periodontal pockets Vaginal: 2%-56% of oral dose	
Metabolism	Liver: severe hepatic disease reduces the metabolism with accumulation of metabolites	
Major metabolites	1-2-hydroxyethyl-2-hydroxy-methyl-5-nitroimidazole (hydroxymetabolite), biologic activity, 30%-65% of the activity 2-methyl-5-nitroimidazole-1-acetic acid (acetic acid metabolite), inactive	
Excretion	Renal: 60%-80%. Approximately 6% to 18% as unchanged drug Hydroxymetabolite is entirely excreted in the urine feces, 6%-15%	Renal failure results in accumulation of metabolites
Pregnancy	Category B	Avoid administration during first trimester
Lactation	Not recommended	Concentrations in breast milk approach those in serum following therapeutic doses

TABLE 27-3 Metronidazole Dose Adjustments in Patients with Decreased Renal Function

Normal renal function	7.5 mg IV q6-8h
CrCl <50	Usual dose
ClCr <10 mL/min	50% usual dose q12h
Hemodialysis	Usual dose + 50% of normal dose supplement after hemodialysis
Peritoneal dialysis	50% usual dose q12h
CVVH, CAVH	Usual dose
Liver—mild	Usual dose
— end stage	50% usual dose q12h

CAVH, continuous arteriovenous hemofiltration; CVVH, continuous venous-venous hemofiltration.

into brain abscesses, where concentrations approximate that of the serum.[59] The drug penetrates well in the gallbladder and the biliary systems when the cystic duct is patent; however, little or no metronidazole is recovered from gallbladder bile among patients who had a stone blocking the cystic duct.[60]

The oxidation of the aliphatic side chains of metronidazole in humans is the principal metabolic pathway. The metabolism is dose dependent. Metronidazole is metabolized by the human liver through the cytochrome P-450 (CYP) family of enzymes to five major products including a hydroxymetabolite, which has 30% to 65% of the activity of the parent compound.[61] In addition, there is an acid metabolite, acetylmetronidazole, metronidazole glucuronide, and the glucuronide conjugate of hydroxymetronidazole. A sulfate conjugate may also be found on occasion. Metronidazole and particularly its metabolites are eliminated primarily in the urine (60% to 80% of the dose), unchanged in 6% to 18%. From 6% to 15% are excreted in the feces.

The elimination half-life of metronidazole in patients with no renal function is the same as in healthy people. However, the hydroxymetabolite may accumulate in patients with absent renal function, and although dosage adjustment is usually not considered necessary in the absence of hepatic disease, consideration might be given to dosage adjustment in patients initially receiving large doses.[62] The clearance of metronidazole is increased during hemodialysis, and metronidazole half-life is shortened to only 2 to 3 hours.[62,63] The pharmacokinetics of metronidazole and its metabolites are not appreciably affected by chronic ambulatory peritoneal dialysis, with peritoneal dialysis accounting for only 8.9% of total body clearance.[64] In patients with hepatic failure[65,66] the half-life of the drug may be extended to 18 to 20 hours. It is recommended that doses should be reduced by at least 50% in this patient population.[65] Suggested dose adjustments in patients with decreased renal or hepatic function are summarized in Table 27-3.

Elimination of metronidazole is significantly decreased among premature neonates, with clearance and half-life correlating with gestational age. Careful dosage adjustments are thus recommended for this patient population.

Topical Preparations

After vaginal administration of vaginal suppositories and vaginal gel metronidazole is absorbed to varying degrees, depending upon formulation, but peak serum levels have generally been low. The commercial 0.75% intravaginal gel produced peak serum concentrations of 0.2 to 0.3 mg/L and vaginal suppository peak serum concentrations of 1.1 to 1.9 mg/L, significantly less than the peak concentration of 8 to 13 mg/L after a single 500 mg oral dose.[66] Absorption after rectal administration is quite good, although peak serum levels occur approximately 3 hours after insertion.

After the application of gel to skin lesions (such as acne rosacea) systemic absorption is negligible.[66] Metronidazole is rapidly transferred across the placenta; peak serum levels in the fetus are equivalent to maternal levels after intravenous administration to pregnant women.[67]

Administration and Dosage

Table 27-4 gives dosage recommendations for the major indications for metronidazole therapy. The intravenous route is recommended ini-

TABLE 27-4 Major Indications for Metronidazole: Administration and Dosage

Indication	Route of Administration	Dosage
Susceptible anaerobic infections	IV	Loading dose of 15 mg/kg, then 7.5 mg/kg q6h 500 mg q 6/8h max 4 g/day
	PO	1-2 g/d in 2-4 doses q6-12h
Clostridium difficile colitis	PO	250 mg qid or 500 mg tid for 10-14 d
Helicobacter pylori eradication	PO	250 mg with meals at bedtime for 14 d in combination with another antibiotic and a proton pump inhibitor or H₂ blocker
Bacterial vaginosis	PO	500 mg bid for 7 d
	Intravaginally	1 applicator (3.75 g of metronidazole) intravaginal gel bid or at bedtime only × 5 d
Trichomonas vaginitis	PO	250-500 mg tid for 7 d 2 g in single dose *or*
Amebiasis (intestinal or extraintestinal)	IV or PO	500-750 mg tid for 10 d followed by paromomycin 500 mg PO tid × 7 d
Giardiasis	PO	250 mg bid or tid for 5-7 d refractory cases: 750 PO and quinacrine 100 mg PO, both tid for 14 d
Acne rosacea	Topical	Apply a thin film twice daily; results should be noticed within 3 wk, improvement for 9 wk
Prophylactic use Perioperative for contaminated or potentially contaminated surgery	IV	15 mg/kg over 30-60 min 1 hr before surgery and (if necessary) 7.5 mg/kg at 6 and 12 hr after the initial dose
Sexual assault victim	PO	2 g in single dose (in conjunction with 125 mg IM of ceftriaxone and 1 g PO azytromycine in a single dose or 100 mg of doxycycline bid for 7 d)

tially for seriously ill patients. Because oral therapy gives blood levels comparable to those achieved by the intravenous route, one may switch when conditions warrant.

As noted, the standard regimen in the United States for intravenous administration has been a loading dose of 15 mg/kg of body weight followed by a maintenance schedule of 7.5 mg/kg every 6 hours. Clearly, the half-life of the drug could warrant administration at longer intervals such as every 8 or even every 12 hours. The manufacturer recommends that intravenous infusions be administered over a period of 1 hour. However, a number of foreign investigators have administered the drug in as little as 20 minutes without any apparent adverse effects. The maximal daily dose recommended is 4 g. The duration of therapy varies according to the organisms/syndromes being treated.

Adverse Reactions and Precautions

In general, metronidazole is well tolerated. There is an interesting report of an accidental 10-fold overdose on three occasions in a preterm neonate that resulted in a peak serum level of 140 mg/L and a level of 40 mg/L 33.75 hours later but with no clinical signs of toxicity.[68] The most serious adverse effects are those involving *the central nervous system*. These are rare unless prolonged therapy or large doses, or both, are used. Two cases of acute onset of ataxia, dysarthria, and lesions of the cerebellar dentate nucleus associated with use of metronidazole have been described. These symptoms started approximately 1 month after the initiation of metronidazole for treatment of cerebral/epidural abscess and were reversible with the interruption of the drug.[69] Peripheral neuropathy has been described in an individual who received repeated short courses of the drug. The peripheral neuropathy is generally reversible but may take a considerable period of time to resolve. Metronidazole should be used with caution in people with a history of seizures or other central nervous system disorders. Other adverse reactions include headache, dizziness, syncope, vertigo, impaired sleep, confusion, excitation, or depression. There is also one report of metronidazole-induced psychosis of 2 weeks' duration. If abnormal neurologic symptoms are observed, treatment with the drug must be discontinued immediately.

The most common side effects involve the *gastrointestinal tract* and include nausea, epigastric distress, anorexia, and, less commonly vomiting, diarrhea or constipation, pancreatitis,[70] and hepatitis.

An unpleasant metallic taste is often experienced by those taking metronidazole systemically. There may also be furring of the tongue, glossitis, stomatitis, dry mouth with candidal overgrowth. Although the drug is active against *Clostridium difficile,* cases of *C. difficile* colitis have rarely been reported among patients receiving metronidazole.[71] However, the drug has proved effective for this condition and is comparable to vancomycin in effectiveness. Allergic reactions have also been described and include urticaria, maculopapular rash, pustular eruption, flushing, bronchospasm, and serum sickness.[72] No significant irritant or sensitization reactions have been reported with topical formulations.

Genitourinary reactions commonly include transient darkening of the urine to a deep red-brown. Dysuria, cystitis, incontinence, and decreased libido have also been reported less commonly.

Other side effects include fever, reversible neutropenia,[73] and occasionally overgrowth of *Candida* in the oral cavity or vagina. Thrombophlebitis has been reported with intravenous infusion but is seldom seen now with proper buffering of the preparation. There is one report of an immediate rhinoconjunctivitis.

Mutagenic Properties

There has been concern about mutagenicity in the Ames *Salmonella* mutant system and carcinogenicity of metronidazole. Reduction of the nitro group of the compound is necessary for both antibacterial and mutagenic activity. Mutagenic activity has been detected in the urine of patients receiving 750 mg/day of metronidazole. When a mutant *Salmonella* strain that did not possess nitroreductase was used in the mutagenic testing system, metronidazole could not be demonstrated to be a mutagen. Thus, not the drug itself but rather one or more reduction products of it is mutagenic. Some protozoa, bacteria (including facultative anaerobes), and fungi possess nitroreductase activity. Eukaryotic tissues have very little nitroreductase activity. It has been suggested that during metronidazole therapy some reduction products of the drug might escape from the bacterial cells and serve as mutagens to the host's mammalian tissue. However, these active derivatives are very short lived and either promptly bind to macromolecules within the bacterial cell or are promptly reduced to compounds that are not mutagenic or carcinogenic. The drug has been studied specifically for mutagenic potential in eukaryotic test systems (human lymphocytes in vitro and lymphocytes of patients receiving metronidazole therapy) as well as in animal models with conflicting results.

Long-term follow-up of a cohort of 771 women who received low doses of metronidazole therapy for the treatment of vaginal trichomoniasis did not show an increased incidence of malignancy.[74] An anecdotal observation raises the possibility of carcinogenicity in three patients with Crohn's disease who had received prolonged therapy with metronidazole. A larger study with 5222 pairs of randomly selected patients who used metronidazole on an outpatient basis matched for age, gender, and year of enrollment to nonusers, and followed for an average of 12.6 years, also failed to show an association between metronidazole use and cancer.[75] However, some authors observed that the cancer incidence diverged between the two groups after 15 years of follow-up and that the relative risk also increased with time, without reaching a significant value for any period. Therefore, the authors question if with a longer follow-up this difference would have possibly achieved a statistical significance.[76] Although metronidazole ap-

pears to be safe, the long-term effects of high-dose prolonged therapy are not completely known.

Metronidazole crosses the placental barrier, and concerns have been raised about possible teratogenic effects in light of the evidence for mutagenicity in bacterial systems. Studies in pregnant women who had received metronidazole during pregnancy for the treatment of vaginal trichomoniasis have not shown an increased incidence of stillbirths, small-for-gestational-age infants, premature infants, or teratogenicity.[77] A meta-analysis failed to find any relationship between metronidazole exposure during the first trimester of pregnancy and birth defects.[78] A retrospective study of a cohort of 328,846 children younger than 5 years who had been exposed to metronidazole in utero[79] did not find an increased incidence of cancer at any site in children. However, there was a 2.5-fold increase in the relative risk of neuroblastoma; nevertheless, it was not statistically significant. The authors suggested that the relationship between metronidazole treatment and neuroblastoma needed further investigation. (For a review on metronidazole and carcinogenesis see Bendesky and colleagues.[76])

The use of metronidazole during pregnancy should be reserved for situations in which it is clearly needed. Metronidazole during the first trimester should be avoided. Because metronidazole is excreted into breast milk, nursing should be discontinued during and for 2 days after therapy with metronidazole.

DRUG INTERACTIONS AND INTERFERENCE WITH LABORATORY TESTS

Major food-metronidazole and drug-metronidazole interactions are listed in Table 27-5.

Metronidazole also interferes with certain chemical analyses for the serum enzyme glutamic oxaloacetic transaminase, which results in falsely low values.

EFFECT ON NORMAL FECAL FLORA

Early studies showed that in people with a healthy gastrointestinal tract who are not receiving other drugs, metronidazole has very little effect on the fecal flora. This is thought to be due to the drug being rapidly reduced by the bowel flora under the usual anaerobic conditions in the colon. Why this reduction would not have an impact on the organisms carrying out the reduction, as it does in the course of treating infections, is not at all clear. In patients on high-dosage regimens, in patients with diarrhea, and in patients receiving certain other antimicrobial agents concurrently, there may be a significant impact of metronidazole on the fecal flora. For example, when oral neomycin or kanamycin (active primarily against nonanaerobes) is given with metronidazole, there is a significant negative impact on both the anaerobic and aerobic flora. Thus, it has been feasible to use metronidazole for therapy in certain conditions such as ileal bypass enteropathy and for preoperative "bowel preparation" along with an oral aminoglycoside.[80]

METRONIDAZOLE AND VANCOMYCIN-RESISTANT ENTEROCOCCUS

Vancomycin-resistant enterococcus (VRE), first described in the early 1980s, is now an important pathogen. Studies have tried to correlate the use of different antibiotic agents with the emergence of nosocomial VRE. The previous use of metronidazole—as well vancomycin, cephalosporins, and quinolones—is associated with an increased incidence of VRE infections.[81-83] In a recent matched case-control study, it was found that use of parenteral metronidazole as well as of third-generation cephalosporins were highly significant and independent risk factors for VRE.[84] The suppression of gastrointestinal anaerobic flora is the presumed mechanism for the association between metronidazole and VRE. In a study comparing the risk factors for VRE bacteremia versus bacteremia with vancomycin-sensitive enterococcus found that VRE-infected patients were less likely to have undergone recent surgery or have polymicrobial bacteremia and instead had a sig-

TABLE 27-5 Significant Food-Drug and Drug-Drug Interactions with Metronidazole

Alcohol	Disulfiram-like reaction: flushing, tachycardia, palpitations, nausea, and vomiting	
	Acute psychosis or confusional state	
Alcohol or disulfiram	Sudden death	
Cimetidine	May increase metronidazole levels	
Aluminum- or magnesium-containing antacids	Reduces plasma concentrations of metronidazole	15%-20% decreased bioavailability of metronidazole
Cisapride	Inhibits metabolism of cisapride	
Cyclosporine, tacrolimus	Increases cyA and tacrolimus serum concentrations	
Lithium	Increases lithium levels	Renal retention
Phenytoin	Increases phenytoin concentrations	Inhibits aromatic oxidase reactions in the liver with decreased clearance of phenytoin
Phenytoin, rifampin, prednisone	Reduces plasma concentrations of metronidazole	Enhanced hepatic clearance of metronidazole
Warfarin	Increases warfarin levels	Same
		Monitor closely anticoagulant effect by prothrombin time

From Alexander I. "Alcohol-Antabuse" syndrome in patients receiving metronidazole during gynaecological treatment. Br J Clin Pract. 1985;39:292-293; Heath MJ, Pachar JV, Perez MA, Toseland PA. An exceptional case of lethal disulfiram-alcohol reaction. Forensic Sci Int. 1992;56:45-50; Zylber-Katz E, Rubinger D, Berlatzky Y. Cyclosporine interactions with metronidazole and cimetidine [letter]. Drug Intell Clin Pharm. 1988;22:504-505; Herzig K, Johnson DW. Marked elevation of blood cyclosporin and tacrolimus levels due to concurrent metronidazole therapy [letter]. Nephrol Dial Transplant. 1999;14:521-523; Teicher MH, Altesman RI, Cole JO, Schatzberg AF. Possible nephrotoxic interaction of lithium and metronidazole [letter]. JAMA. 1987;257:3365-3366; Lassen E. Effects of acute and short-time antibiotic treatment on renal lithium elimination and serum lithium levels in the rat. Acta Pharmacol et Toxicol. 1985;56:273-277; Blyden GT, Scavone JM, Greenblatt DJ. Metronidazole impairs clearance of phenytoin but not of alprazolam or lorazepam. J Clin Pharmacol. 1988;28:240-245; Eradiri O, Jamali F, Thomson AB. Interaction of metronidazole with phenobarbital, cimetidine, prednisone, and sulfasalazine in Crohn's disease. Biopharm Drug Dispos. 1988;9:219-927; Mead PB, Gibson M, Schentag JJ, Ziemniak JA. Possible alteration of metronidazole metabolism by phenobarbital. N Engl J Med. 1982;306:1490; O'Reilly RA. The stereoselective interaction of warfarin and metronidazole in man. N Engl J Med. 1976;295:354-357.

nificantly higher incidence of prior exposure to metronidazole. These data support the animal studies suggesting that metronidazole potentiates enterococcal overgrowth in the gastrointestinal tract and translocation into the blood stream.[85]

Clinical Uses

Parasitic Infections

Metronidazole has been used successfully for therapy for *T. vaginitis* since the 1960s with a cure rate of approximately 95%.[86] A topical preparation is available. However, there are increased numbers of cases of metronidazole-resistant trichomoniasis. Many of these patients will respond to increased doses or multiple courses of administration. Tinidazole (not available in the United States) is more active in vitro against resistant strains.[87]

Metronidazole treatment of pregnant women with asymptomatic trichomoniasis failed to prevent preterm delivery.[88]

Metronidazole is also an effective agent for therapy of amebic liver abscess and has been used with generally good results in intestinal amebiasis. Symptoms usually resolve within 2 to 3 days and the therapy is continued for 14 days. Metronidazole is effective against luminal cysts in only about half of cases; therefore, to eradicate the parasite, it must be followed by a course of paromomycin or another luminal antiamebic agent.[89] The drug is also effective against giardiasis, being at least as active as quinacrine for this purpose. In immunocompromised patients with refractory giardiasis, a combination of the two drugs succeeded in eradicating the parasite in five out of six cases.[90] Metronidazole has been used effectively in treating *Dientamoeba fragilis* infections in children. Metronidazole may be beneficial in the management of dracunculiasis, providing symptomatic relief. It is also thought to weaken the anchorage of the worms within subcutaneous tissue, thus allowing them to be removed more quickly. Some workers have felt that metronidazole has been effective in *Balantidium coli* infection but this indication is not well established. Metronidazole has been used in the treatment of cutaneous leishmaniasis, although it appears to be less effective than other available agents.

Anaerobic Infections

The excellent distribution of metronidazole throughout the body, including the central nervous system, and the impressive bactericidal activity of this compound, even against organisms that are not actively multiplying, make it an excellent choice for a number of serious infections, including brain abscess and other central nervous system infections involving anaerobes and endocarditis due to anaerobic bacteria.[91]

Metronidazole has been useful against other types of anaerobic infections, including bacteremia, infections of bones and joints, soft tissue infections, oral and dental infections, and head and neck and tetanus.[92] Metronidazole is, however, not effective in the treatment of actinomycosis and infections with *Propionebacterium acnes*. Metronidazole alone is not optimal therapy for anaerobic lung abscess, probably because of the presence of aerobic gram-positive cocci that are not susceptible to metronidazole.

Metronidazole has also provided good results in therapy for bacterial vaginosis, a condition in which various anaerobes or *G. vaginalis*, or both, may be important.[93] However, a short course of metronidazole was found to be ineffective in reducing the risk of preterm delivery in women with bacterial vaginosis.[94] Metronidazole is effective in the management of pseudomembranous colitis due to *C. difficile*.[95] Limited studies have shown that in patients with active colitis, fecal levels of metronidazole may be attained by using either the oral or parenteral route of administration.[96,97] The parenteral route may be especially useful in patients who have *C. difficile*–induced toxic megacolon and are unable to take oral medications.

H. pylori is clearly linked to peptic ulcer disease; metronidazole, in combination with various other agents such as tetracycline or other antibiotics, histamine (H_2) receptor antagonists, or proton pump inhibitors, appears to be effective therapy and markedly decreases the incidence of relapse. Moreover, such therapy has led to regression of gastric lymphoma of mucosa-associated lymphoid tissue.

Other Therapeutic Uses

Metronidazole is activated in hypoxic cells of animals and it has been used experimentally in very high doses as a hypoxic cell sensitizer in radiotherapy of human tumors.[98] Activated metronidazole is thought to interact directly with deoxyribonucleic acid (DNA), and the resultant complex can no longer function as an effective primer for DNA and ribonucleic acid (RNA) polymerases; however, it has not yet been properly proved.

Metronidazole was found to be useful in a number of types of bowel bacterial overgrowth syndromes such as for complications of jejunoileal bypass for obesity and dysfunction of the continent ileostomy,[99] and for pouchitis after pouch construction for ulcerative colitis. Early studies suggested a role for metronidazole in the prevention of intrahepatic cholestasis associated with total parenteral nutrition.[100] This seems to be supported by a recent experimental study in rabbits showing that ursodeoxycholic acid therapy during total parenteral nutrition reduces bilirubin levels and improves the markers of cholestasis, and that this effect is more marked when combined with metronidazole.[101]

It appears that metronidazole has had a beneficial effect in Crohn's disease, lessening diarrhea (in patients with colonic involvement) and promoting healing of perianal lesions and erythema nodosum.[102,103] Prolonged use of the drug, however, may result in a significant incidence of metronidazole-induced peripheral neuropathy,[104] and concerns have been raised about possible carcinogenic effects of the drug.

Recent studies showed that metronidazole administration improves clinical symptoms of children with inherited metabolic defects that results in excess methylmalonic[105,106] and propionic[107] acid in blood or urine. Metronidazole reduced the excretion of fecal propionate and urinary methylmalonate, suggesting that propionic acid derived from fecal bacterial metabolism contributes substantially to methylmalonate production. Therefore, the beneficial effect of metronidazole is due to the antimicrobial effect on gut anaerobes that are involved in propionate production.[108] Metronidazole is beneficial in the treatment of acne rosacea whether used orally or topically.[109,110] According to some investigators[111] but not others,[112,113] treatment with metronidazole is effective in cyclosporin-induced gingival hyperplasia.

Metronidazole administration has also been used in perioral dermatitis, childhood granulomatous periorificial dermatitis, acute necrotizing gingivitis, decubitus ulcers, and malodorous infected malignant processes. Some earlier reports[114] noted decreased serum cholesterol and triglyceride levels in patients receiving metronidazole for other indications. The activity of metronidazole as a lipid-lowering agent is also supported by a recent open-label crossover trial that shows decreased cholesterol (total and low-density lipoprotein [LDL]) and triglyceride levels accompanied by increased high-density lipoprotein [HDL] cholesterol in 30 patients treated with oral metronidazole (250 mg every 8 hours) for 14 days.[115]

Prophylactic Use

Several groups have carried out prospective controlled studies of metronidazole, alone or in combination with other agents, for prophylaxis of infections in patients undergoing elective colonic surgery, gynecologic surgery, emergency appendectomy, or esophageal surgery. Oral metronidazole is an effective prophylactic agent in both simple and complicated appendicitis.[116] Metronidazole is effective alone and in combination for colorectal surgery prophylaxis, and this is an approved indication for the drug in the United States. It has also been suggested that metronidazole in combination with gentamicin could be used in developing countries before emergency cesarean section because of its low cost.[117]

A multicenter observational study in Germany[80] of 2513 patients who received infection prophylaxis prior to elective colonic resection found that postoperative infection rates were higher when metronidazole was not added to the antibiotic prophylaxis.

REFERENCES

1. Stratton CW, Weeks LS, Aldridge KE. Comparison of the bactericidal activity of clindamycin and metronidazole against cefoxitin-susceptible and cefoxitin-resistant isolates of the *Bacteroides fragilis* group. Diagn Microbiol Infect Dis. 1991;14:377-382.
2. Stratton CW, Weeks LS, Aldridge KE. Inhibitory and bactericidal activity of selected beta-lactam agents alone and in combination with beta-lactamase inhibitors compared with that of cefoxitin and metronidazole against cefoxitin-susceptible and cefoxitin-resistant isolates of the *Bacteroides fragilis* group. Diagn Microbiol Infect Dis. 1992;15:321-330.
3. Ravdin JI, Skilogiannis J. In vitro susceptibilities of *Entamoeba histolytica* to azithromycin, CP-63,956, erythromycin, and metronidazole. Antimicrob Agents Chemother. 1989;33:960-962.
4. Nix DE, Tyrrell R, Muller M. Pharmacodynamics of metronidazole determined by a time-kill assay for *Trichomonas vaginalis*. Antimicrob Agents Chemother. 1995;39:1848-1852.
5. Edwards DI. Nitroimidazole drugs—Action and resistance mechanisms. I. Mechanisms of action. J Antimicrob Chemother. 1993;31:9-20.
6. Edwards DI. Reduction of nitroimidazoles in vitro and DNA damage. Biochem Pharmacol. 1986;35:53-58.

7. Muller M. Reductive activation of nitroimidazoles in anaerobic microorganisms. Biochem Pharmacol. 1986;35:37-41.
8. Goldman P, Koch RL, Yeung TC. Comparing the reduction of nitroimidazoles in bacteria and mammalian tissues and relating it to biological activity. Biochem Pharmacol. 1986;35:43-51.
9. Tocher JH, Edwards DI. The interaction of reduced metronidazole with DNA bases and nucleosides. Int J Radiat Oncol Biol Phys. 1992;22:661-663.
10. Tocher JH, Edwards DI. Evidence for the direct interaction of reduced metronidazole derivatives with DNA bases. Biochem Pharmacol. 1994;48:1089-1094.
11. Van Der Wouden E-J, Thijs JC, Kusters JG, et al. Mechanism and clinical significance of metronidazole resistance in *Helicobacter pylori*. Scand J Gastroenterol. 2001;36:10-14.
12. Upcroft P. Drug resistance in *Giardia*: Clinical versus laboratory isolates. Drug Resist Updates. 1998;1:166-168.
13. Townson SM, Upcroft JA, Upcroft P. Characterisation and purification of pyruvate:ferredoxin oxidoreductase from *Giardia duodenalis*. Mol Biochem Parasitol. 1996;79:183-193.
14. Upcroft P, Upcroft JA. Drug targets and mechanisms of resistance in the anaerobic protozoa. Clin Microbiol Rev. 2001;14:150-164.
15. Erwin ME, Fix AM, Jones RN. Three independent yearly analyses on the spectrum and potency of metronidazole: A multicenter study of 1,108 contemporary anaerobic clinical isolates. Diagn Microbiol Infect Dis. 2001;39:129-132.
16. Snydman DR, Jacobus NV, McDermott LA, et al. National survey on the susceptibility of *Bacteroides fragilis* group: Report and analysis of trends for 1997-2000. CID. 2002;35:S126-S134.
17. Aldridge KE, Ashcraft D, O'Brien M, Sanders CV. Bacteremia due to *Bacteroides fragilis* group: Distribution of species, beta-lactamase production, and antimicrobial susceptibility patterns. Antimicrob Agents Chemother. 2003;47:148-153.
18. Aldridge KE, Ashcraft D, Cambre K, et al. Multicenter survey of the changing in vitro antimicrobial susceptibilities of clinical isolates of *Bacteroides fragilis* group, *Prevotella, Fusobacterium, Porphyromonas,* and *Peptostreptococcus* species. Antimicrob Agents Chemother. 2001;45:1238-1243.
19. Aldridge KE. Ertapenem (MK-0826), a new carbapenem: Comparative in vitro activity against clinically significant anaerobes. Diagn Microbiol Infect Dis. 2002;44:181-186.
20. Elsaghier AA, Brazier JS, James EA. Bacteraemia due to *Bacteroides fragilis* with reduced susceptibility to metronidazole. J Antimicrob Chemother. 2003;6:1436-1437.
21. Brazier JS, Stubbs SL, Duerden BI. Metronidazole resistance among clinical isolates belonging to the *Bacteroides fragilis* group: Time to be concerned? J Antimicrob Chemother. 1999;44:580-581.
22. O'Donoghue MA, Potter J, Allen KD. Metronidazole-resistant *Bacteroides fragilis* infection. J Infect. 1992;25:211-214.
23. Hickey MM, Davies UM, Dave J, et al. Metronidazole resistant *Bacteroides fragilis* infection of a prosthetic hip joint. J Infect. 1990;20:129-133.
24. Brogan O, Garnett PA, Brow R. *Bacteroides fragilis* resistant to metronidazole, clindamycin and cefoxitin. J Antimicrob Chemother. 1989;23:660-662.
25. Lamothe F, Fijalkowski C, Malouin F, et al. *B. fragilis* resistant to both metronidazole and imipenem. J Antimicrob Chemother. 1986;18:642-643.
26. Turner P, Edward SR, Weston V, et al. Simultaneous resistance to metronidazole, co-amoxiclav, and imipenem in clinical isolate of *Bacteroides fragilis*. Lancet. 1995;345:1275-1277.
27. Sandoe JA, Struthers JK, Brazier JS. Subdural empyema caused by *Prevotella loescheii* with reduced susceptibility to metronidazole. J Antimicrob Chemother. 2001;47:366-367.
28. Pankuch GA, Jacobs MR, Appelbaum PC. Susceptibilities of 428 gram-positive and -negative anaerobic bacteria to Bay y3118 compared with their susceptibilities to ciprofloxacin, clindamycin, metronidazole, piperacillin, piperacillin-tazobactam, and cefoxitin. Antimicrob Agents Chemother. 1993;37:1649-1654.
29. Sheikh W, Pitkin DH, Nadler H. Antibacterial activity of meropenem and selected comparative agents against anaerobic bacteria at seven North American centers. CID. 1993;16:S361-S366.
30. Smith MA, Alperstein P, France K, et al. Susceptibility testing of *Propionibacterium acnes* comparing agar dilution with E test. J Clin Microbiol. 1996;34:1024-1026.
31. Dali P, Giugliano ER, Vellozzi EM, Smith MA. Susceptibilities of *Propionibacterium acnes* ophthalmic isolates to moxifloxacin. Antimicrob Agents Chemother. 2001;45:2969-2970.
32. Jones BM, Geary I, Lee ME, Duerden BI. Comparison of the in vitro activities of fenticonazole, other imidazoles, metronidazole, and tetracycline against organisms associated with bacterial vaginosis and skin infections. Antimicrob Agents Chemother. 1989;33:970-972.
33. Spiegel CA. Susceptibility of *Mobiluncus* species to 23 antimicrobial agents and 15 other compounds. Antimicrob Agents Chemother. 1987;31:249-252.
34. Milazzo I, Blandino G, Caccamo F, et al. Speciale A faropenem, a new oral penem: Antibacterial activity against selected anaerobic and fastidious periodontal isolates. J Antimicrob Chemother. 2003;51:721-725.
35. Muller HP, Holderrieth S, Burkhardt U, Hoffler U. In vitro antimicrobial susceptibility of oral strains of *Actinobacillus actinomycetemcomitans* to seven antibiotics. J Clin Periodontol. 2002;29:736-742.
36. Sheng WS, Hsueh PR, Hung CC, et al. Clinical features of patients with invasive *Eikenella corrodens* infections and microbiological characteristics of the causative isolates. Eur J Clin Microbiol Infect Dis. 2001;20:231-236.
37. Bannatyne RM, Jackowski J, Cheung R, Biers K. Susceptibility of *Gardnerella vaginalis* to metronidazole, its bioactive metabolites, and tinidazole. Am J Clin Pathol. 1987;87:640-641.

38. Sobel JD, Nagappan V, Nyirjesy P. Metronidazole-resistant vaginal trichomoniasis—An emerging problem. Lancet. 1999;341:292-293.

39. Alexander CJ, Citron DM, Brazier JS, Goldstein EJ. Identification and antimicrobial resistance patterns of clinical isolates of *Clostridium clostridioforme, Clostridium innocuum,* and *Clostridium ramosum* compared with those of clinical isolates of *Clostridium perfringens.* J Clin Microbiol. 1995;33:3209-3215.

40. Brazier JS, Levett PN, Stannard AJ, et al. Antibiotic susceptibility of clinical isolates of clostridia. J Antimicrob Chemother. 1985;15:181-185.

41. Kucers A, Crowe S, Grayson ML, Hoy J. The use of antibiotics in a clinical review of antibacterial, antifungal and antiviral drugs. 1997 pp 936-958.

42. Rasmussen BA, Bush K, Tally FP. Antimicrobial resistance in *Bacteroides.* CID. 1993;16:S390-S400.

43. Reysset G, Haggoud A, Sebald M. Genetics of resistance of *Bacteroides* species to 5-nitroimidazole. CID. 1993;16:S401-S403.

44. Narikawa S, Suzuki T, Yamamoto M, Nakamura M. Lactate dehydrogenase activity as a cause of metronidazole resistance in *Bacteroides fragilis* NCTC 11295. J Antimicrob Chemother. 1991;28:47-53.

45. Reysset G. Genetics of 5-nitroimidazole resistance in *Bacteroides* species. Anaerobe 1996;2:59-69.

46. Carlier JP, Sellier N, Rager M-N, Reysset G. Metabolism of a 5-nitroimidazole in susceptible and resistant isogenic strains of *Bacteroides fragilis.* Antimicrob Agents Chemother. 1997;41:1495-1499.

47. Lubbe MM, Stanley K, Chalkley LJ. Prevalence of *nim* genes in anaerobic/facultative anaerobic bacteria isolated in South Africa. FEMS Microbiol Lett. 1999;172:79-83.

48. Fang H, Edlund C, Hedberg M, Nord CE. New findings in beta-lactam and metronidazole resistant *Bacteroides fragilis* group. Int J Antimicrob Agents. 2002;19:361-370.

49. Jenks PJ, Edwards DI. Metronidazole resistance in *Helicobacter pylori.* Int J Antimicrob Agents. 2002;19:1-7.

50. Krajden S, Lossick JG, Wilk E, et al. Persistent *Trichomonas vaginalis* infection due to a metronidazole-resistant strain. Can Med Assoc J. 1986;134:1373-1374.

51. Muller M, Meingassner JG, Miller WA, Ledger WJ. Three metronidazole-resistant strains of *Trichomonas vaginalis* from the United States. Am J Obstet Gynecol. 1980;138:808-812.

52. Dombrowski MP, Sokol RJ, Bronsteen RA. Intravenous therapy of metronidazole-resistant *Trichomonas vaginalis.* Obstet Gynecol. 1987;69:524-525.

53. Brown DM, Upcroft JA, Dodd HN, et al. Alternative 2-ketoacid oxidoreductase activities in *Trichomonas vaginalis.* Mol Biochem Parasitol. 1999;98:203-214.

54. Liu S, Brown D, O'Donoghue P et al. Ferredoxin involvement in metronidazole resistance of *Giardia duodenalis.* Mol Biochem Parasitol. 2000;108:137-140.

55. Quon, DV, d'Oliveira, CE, Johnson, PJ. Reduced transcription of the ferredoxin gene in metronidazole-resistant *Trichomonas vaginalis.* Proc Natl Acad Sci U S A. 1992;89:4402-4406.

56. Lau, AH, Lam, NP, Piscitelli SC, et al. Clinical pharmacokinetics of metronidazole and other nitroimidazole anti-infectives. Clin Pharmacokinet. 1992;23:328-364.

57. Mattila J, Nerdrum K, Rouhiainen H, et al. Penetration of metronidazole and tinidazole into the aqueous humor in man. Chemotherapy. 1983;29:188-191.

58. Jokipii AM, Myllyla VV, Hokkanen E, Jokipii L. Penetration of the blood brain barrier by metronidazole and tinidazole. J Antimicrob Chemother. 1977;3:239-245.

59. Warner JF, Perkins RL, Cordero L. Metronidazole therapy of anaerobic bacteremia, meningitis, and brain abscess. Arch Intern Med. 1979;139:167-169.

60. Nielsen ML, Justesen T. Excretion of metronidazole in human bile. Investigations of hepatic bile, common duct bile, and gallbladder bile. Scand J Gastroenterol. 1977;12:1003-1008.

61. Jensen JC, Gugler R. Single- and multiple-dose metronidazole kinetics. Clin Pharmacol Ther. 1983;34:481-487.

62. Kreeft JH, Ogilvie RI, Dufresne LR. Metronidazole kinetics in dialysis patients. Surgery 1983;93:149-153.

63. Lau AH, Chang CW, Sabatini S. Hemodialysis clearance of metronidazole and its metabolites. Antimicrob Agents Chemother. 1986;29:235-238.

64. Guay DR, Meatherall RC, Baxter H, et al. Pharmacokinetics of metronidazole in patients undergoing continuous ambulatory peritoneal dialysis. Antimicrob Agents Chemother. 1984;25:306-310.

65. Lau AH, Evans R, Chang CW, Seligsohn R. Pharmacokinetics of metronidazole in patients with alcoholic liver disease. Antimicrob Agents Chemother. 1987;31:1662-1664.

66. Lamp KC, Freeman CD, Klutman NE, Lacy MK. Pharmacokinetics and pharmacodynamics of the nitroimidazole antimicrobials. Clin Pharmacokinet. 1999;36:353-373.

67. Visser AA, Hundt HKL. The pharmacokinetics of a single intravenous dose of metronidazole in pregnant patients. J Antimicrob Chemother. 1984;13:279-283.

68. Lentelink MB, de Vries TW, van Dijk KN. Accidental metronidazole overdose in a preterm newborn. Clin Pharmacokinet. 1997;32:496-497.

69. Woodruff BK, Eelco FM, Wijdicks MD, et al. Reversible metronidazole-induced lesions of the cerebellar dentate nuclei. N Engl J Med. 2002;346:68-69.

70. Celifarco A, Warschauer C, Burakoff R. Metronidazole-induced pancreatitis. Am J Gastroenterol. 1989;84:958-960.

71. Saginur R, Hawley CR, Bartlett JG. Colitis associated with metronidazole therapy. J Infect Dis. 1980;141:772-774.

72. Knowles S, Choudhury T, Shear NH. Metronidazole hypersensitivity. Ann Pharmacother. 1994;28:325-326.

73. Smith JA. Neutropenia associated with metronidazole therapy. CMAJ. 1980;123:202.

74. Beard CM, Noller KL, O'Fallon WM, et al. Cancer after exposure to metronidazole. Mayo Clin Proc. 1988;63:147-153.

75. Falagas ME, Walker AM, Jick H, et al. Late incidence of cancer after metronidazole use: A matched metronidazole user/nonuser study. Clin Infect Dis. 1998;26:384-388.

76. Bendesky A, Menéndez D, Ostrosky-Wegman P. Is metronidazole carcinogenic? Mutat Res/Reviews in Mutation Research. 2002;511:133-144.

77. Robbie MO, Sweet RL. Metronidazole use in obstetrics and gynecology: A review. Am J Obstet Gynecol. 1983;145:865-881.

78. Caro-Paton T, Carvajal A, Martin de Diego I, et al. Is metronidazole teratogenic? A meta-analysis. Br J Clin Pharmacol. 1997;44:179-182.

79. Thapa PB, Whitlock JA, Brockman Worrell KG, et al. Prenatal exposure to metronidazole and risk of childhood cancer: A retrospective cohort study of children younger than 5 years. Cancer. 1998;83:1461-1468.

80. Mittelkotter U. Antimicrobial prophylaxis for abdominal surgery: Is there a need for metronidazole? J Chemother. 2001;13:27-34.

81. Morris JG Jr, Shay DK, Hebden JN, et al. Enterococci resistant to multiple antimicrobial agents, including vancomycin. Establishment of endemicity in a university medical center. Ann Intern Med. 1995;123:250-259.

82. Tornieporth NG, Roberts RB, John J, et al. Risk factors associated with vancomycin-resistant *Enterococcus faecium* infection or colonization in 145 matched case patients and control patients. CID. 1996;23:767-772.

83. Bonten MJ, Hayden MK, Nathan C, et al. Epidemiology of colonization of patients and environment with vancomycin-resistant enterococci. Lancet. 1996;348:1615-1619.

84. Carmeli Y, Eliopoulos GM, Samore MH. Antecedent treatment with different antibiotic agents as a risk factor for vancomycin-resistant *Enterococcus.* Emerg Infect Dis. 2002;8:802-807.

85. Lucas GM, Lechtzin N, Puryear DW, et al. Vancomycin-resistant and vancomycin-susceptible enterococcal bacteremia: Comparison of clinical features and outcomes. CID. 1998;26:1127-1133.

86. Centers for Disease Control and Prevention. Sexually transmitted diseases treatment guidelines. MMWR Morb Mortal Wkly Rep 1993;42(RR-14):70-72.

87. Crowell AL, Sanders-Lewis KA, Secor WE. In vitro metronidazole and tinidazole activities against metronidazole-resistant strains of *Trichomonas vaginalis.* Antimicrob Agents Chemother. 2003;4:1407-1409.

88. Klebanoff MA, Carey V, Hauth JC, et al. Failure of metronidazole to prevent preterm delivery among pregnant women with asymptomatic *Trichomonas vaginalis* infection. N Engl J Med. 2001;345:487-493.

89. Goessling W, Chung RT. Amebic liver abscess. Curr Treat Options Gastroenterol. 2002;5:443-449.

90. Nash TE, Ohl CA, Thomas E, et al. Treatment of patients with refractory giardiasis. Clin Infect Dis. 2001;33:22-28.

91. Bisharat N, Goldstein L, Raz R, Elias M. Gram-negative anaerobic endocarditis: Two case reports and review of the literature. Eur J Clin Microbiol Infect Dis. 2001;20(9):651-654.

92. Ahmadsyah I, Salim A. Treatment of tetanus: An open study to compare the efficacy of procaine penicillin and metronidazole. BMJ. 1985;291:648-650.

93. Biswas NJ. Bacterial vaginosis. Clin Obstet Gynecol. 1993;36:166-176.

94. Carey JC, Klebanoff M, Hauth JC, et al. Metronidazole to prevent perterm delivery in pregnant women with asymptomatic bacterial vaginosis. N Engl J Med. 2000;24:534-540.

95. Vasa CV, Glatt AE. Effectiveness and appropriateness of empiric metronidazole for *Clostridium difficile*–associated diarrhea. Am J Gastroenterol. 2003;98:354-358.

96. Kleinfeld DI, Sharpe RJ, Donta ST. Parenteral therapy for antibiotic-associated pseudomembranous colitis. J Infect Dis. 1988;157:389.

97. Bolton RP, Culshaw MA. Faecal metronidazole concentrations during oral and intravenous therapy for antibiotic associated colitis due to *Clostridium difficile.* Gut. 1986;27:1169-1172.

98. Skoropad VY, Berdov BA, Zagrebin VM. Preoperative radiotherapy in combination with metronidazole for resectable gastric cancer: Long-term results of a phase 2 study. Eur J Surg Oncol. 2003;29:166-170.

99. Kelly DG, Phillips SF, Kelly KA, et al. Dysfunction of the continent ileostomy: Clinical features and bacteriology. Gut. 1983;24:193-201.

100. Capron J-P, Herve M-A, Gineston J-L, et al. Metronidazole in prevention of cholestasis associated with total parenteral nutrition. Lancet. 1983;1:446-447.

101. Gunsar C, Melek M, Karaca I, et al. The biochemical and histopathological effects of ursodeoxycholic acid and metronidazole on total parenteral nutrition–associated hepatic dysfunction: An experimental study. Hepatogastroenterology. 2002;49:497-500.

102. Rutgeerts P, Hiele M, Geboes K, et al. Controlled trial of metronidazole treatment for prevention of Crohn's recurrence after ileal resection. Gastroenterology. 1995;108:1617-1621.

103. Prantera C, et al. An antibiotic regimen for the treatment of active Crohn's disease: A randomized, controlled clinical trial of metronidazole plus ciprofloxacin. Am J Gastroenterol. 1996;91:328-332.

104. Duffy LF, Daum F, Fisher SE, et al. Peripheral neuropathy in Crohn's disease patients treated with metronidazole. Gastroenterology. 1985;88:681-684.

105. Koletzko B, Bachmann C, Wendel U. Antibiotic therapy for improvement of metabolic control in methylmalonic aciduria. J Pediatr. 1990;117:99-101.

106. Thompson GN, Chalmers RA, Walter JH, et al. The use of metronidazole in management of methylmalonic and propionic acidaemias. Eur J Pediatr. 1990;149:792-796.

107. Mellon AF, Deshpande SA, Mathers JC, Bartlett K. Effect of oral antibiotics on intestinal production of propionic acid. Arch Dis Child. 2000;82:169-172.

108. Bain MD, Jones M, Borriello SP, et al. Contribution of gut bacterial metabolism to human metabolic disease. Lancet. 1988;3:1078-1079.

109. McClellan KJ, Noble S. Topical metronidazole: A review of its use in rosacea. Am J Clin Dermatol. 2000;1:191-199.

110. Dahl MV, Jarratt M, Kaplan D. Once-daily topical metronidazole cream formulations in the treatment of the papules and pustules of rosacea. J Am Acad Dermatol. 2001;45:723-730.

111. Wong W, et al. Resolution of cyclosporin-induced gingival hypertrophy with metronidazole. Lancet. 1994;343:986.

112. Aufricht C, Hogan EL, Ettenger RB. Oral metronidazole does not improve cyclosporine A-induced gingival hyperplasia. Pediatr Nephrol. 1997;11:552-555.

113. Mesa FL, Osuna A, Aneiros J, et al. Antibiotic treatment of incipient drug-induced gingival overgrowth in adult renal transplant patients. J Periodontal Res. 2003;38:141-146.

114. Davis JL, Schultz TA, Mosley CA. Metronidazole lowers serum lipids. Ann Intern Med. 1983;99:43-44.

115. Shamkhani K, Azarpira M, Akbar MH. An open label crossover trial of effects of metronidazole on hyperlipidaemia. Int J Cardiol. 2003;90:141-145.

116. Banani SA, Talei A. Can oral metronidazole substitute parenteral drug therapy in acute appendicitis? A new policy in the management of simple or complicated appendicitis with localized peritonitis: A randomized controlled clinical trial. Am Surg. 1999;65:411-416.

117. Kayihura V, Osman NB, Bugalho A, Bergstrom S. Choice of antibiotics for infection prophylaxis in emergency cesarean sections in low-income countries: A cost-benefit study in Mozambique. Acta Obstet Gynecol Scand. 2003;82:636-641.

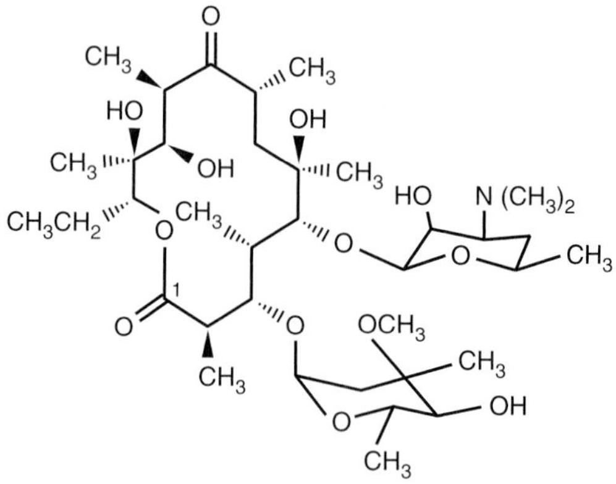

FIGURE 28-1. Erythromycin base.

CHAPTER **28**

Macrolides, Clindamycin, and Ketolides

SUMATHI SIVAPALASINGAM

NEAL H. STEIGBIGEL

The macrolide antibiotics (erythromycin, azithromycin, clarithromycin, and others) and the lincosamide antibiotics (lincomycin and clindamycin) are chemically unrelated but possess many similar biologic properties in terms of mechanisms of action and resistance, antimicrobial activity, and clinical pharmacology. Erythromycin, the macrolide in longest use, has several primary indications in therapy and is sometimes useful as an alternative to penicillin G and other antibiotics. It is one of the safest antibiotics in clinical use, although it may be associated with some important drug interactions. Azithromycin and clarithromycin have some advantages over erythromycin related to their antimicrobial activity, their pharmacokinetics, their fewer gastrointestinal side effects, and their effectiveness in certain infections. Some of the macrolides possess interesting anti-inflammatory activities. Some preliminary clinical studies of macrolides in patients with coronary artery disease have shown beneficial results, which must be confirmed. That effect, if established, may be related to anti-inflammatory activity or activity against *Chlamydophila pneumoniae*, the latter of which has been associated with coronary artery disease. The ketolides are a new class of antibiotics derived from erythromycin that are important because of their increased activity against many bacterial strains that are resistant to macrolides. Telithromycin is the first member of that class to be used. Clindamycin has been restricted in use by its potential gastrointestinal toxicity, but it remains particularly important in the treatment of certain anaerobic infections. Lincomycin is now mainly of historic interest.

ERYTHROMYCIN

Derivation, Chemistry, and Preparations

Erythromycin was derived in 1952 from a strain of *Saccharopolyspora erythraea* (originally named *Streptomyces erythreus*) obtained from soil from the Philippines. It consists of a mixture of antibiotics in which erythromycin A is the active component. The structure (Fig. 28-1) of erythromycin A consists of a 14-member macrocyclic lactone ring—therefore the class name *macrolide*—attached to two sugar moieties, desosamine and L-cladinose. Erythromycin base is poorly soluble in water, has a pK of 8.8, is rapidly inactivated by gastric acid, and is often inconsistently absorbed after oral administration.

Pharmaceutical preparations for oral use have been made with an aim to diminish destruction by gastric acid and to promote better absorption. Six preparations for oral use are available: enteric-coated tablets, enteric-coated pellets in capsules for delayed release, and "film"-coated tablets of the base; the stearate salt (formed in association with the amino group on desosamine), available as film-coated tablets; the ethylsuccinate ester (formed with the hydroxyl group on desosamine), available in tablet, chewable, and liquid forms; and the lauryl sulfate salt of the propionyl ester (the estolate), available in tablet, capsule, or liquid form. There are two water-soluble salts of erythromycin prepared for intravenous use, erythromycin gluceptate and erythromycin lactobionate. The drug is not given intramuscularly because of pain on injection. Erythromycin base is also available in 1.5% and 2% topical solutions, gels, and creams for treatment of acne vulgaris, and in an ophthalmic ointment for treatment of bacterial conjunctivitis and prevention of neonatal gonococcal and chlamydial conjunctivitis.

Mechanisms of Action

Erythromycin inhibits RNA-dependent protein synthesis at the step of chain elongation in susceptible prokaryotic organisms. X-ray crystallography studies indicate that several functional groups on erythromycin A bind to sequences on domain V of the 23S rRNA that is a component of the 50S subunit of the bacterial ribosome.[1,2] That binding site is near the peptidyltransferase center, and peptide chain elongation is thereby prevented by blocking of the polypeptide exit tunnel.[1,2,2a] As a result, peptidyl-tRNA is dissociated from the ribosome.[1,2] Data provided by macrolide-resistant mutants indicate that there are also important interactions between macrolides and specific ribosomal proteins or bases of the 50S subunit near the peptidyltransferase center.[2a,3]

Studies in *Escherichia coli* and *S. aureus* have demonstrated that erythromycin also inhibits the formation of the 50S ribosomal subunit.[1,2a,4] In some bacteria, erythromycin interferes with the ribosomal binding of other macrolides, lincomycin, and chloramphenicol, suggesting common or overlapping binding sites for these antibiotics.

Antimicrobial Activity

The antimicrobial activity of erythromycin is broad in spectrum, being exhibited against gram-positive and gram-negative bacteria, including actinomycetes and mycobacteria, as well as against treponemes, mycoplasmas, *Chlamydia,* and rickettsiae. Depending on drug concentration, bacterial species, phase of growth, and density of the inoculum, erythromycin may be primarily bacteriostatic or bactericidal. Bacterial killing is favored by higher antibiotic concentrations, lower bacterial density, and rapid growth.[5] The activity of erythromycin, which is a weak base, increases markedly with increasing pH over the range 5.5 to 8.5 for both gram-positive and gram-negative bacteria,[6,7] possibly reflecting increased entry into the bacterial cell of the un-ionized drug that is more plentiful at the higher pH.

The in vitro susceptibilities of potential pathogens to erythromycin are listed in Table 28-1.[3,8-32] Erythromycin shows high activity against the majority of pneumococci and group A streptococci isolated in the United States; however, resistant clinical isolates have been increasingly encountered worldwide, especially in *Streptococcus pneumoniae* and particularly, in the latter species, if the strain shows resistance to penicillin.[8,33-36] In the United States (1999-2000), the prevalence of erythromycin resistance ranged from 17.1% to 36.1%.[33] In another study of strains from the United States, approximately 37% of strains of intermediate resistance to penicillin (minimal inhibitory concentration [MIC], 0.12 to 1.0 μg/mL) and 69% of strains showing high-level resistance to penicillin (MIC, >2.0 μg/mL) were resistant to erythromycin.[37] The prevalence of clinical isolates of *S. pneumoniae* in Taiwan not susceptible to erythromycin ranged from 67% to 100%.[35] *S. pneumoniae* strains demonstrate complete cross-resistance among the macrolides,[38,39] but cross-resistance extending from the macrolides to clindamycin is variable, depending on whether the resistance mechanism is of the MLS$_B$ or M phenotype (see later discussion).[39,40] The M phenotype is the predominant one for *S. pneumoniae* in the United States, accounting for 83% of isolates[34]; it is usually associated with low levels of erythromycin resistance (MIC, 1 to 32 μg/mL) and usually does not extend to clindamycin.[41] The MLS$_B$ phenotype is the predominant one in most of Europe[42,43] and Asia[44] for *S. pneumoniae,* and it is associated with a high level of erythromycin resistance (MIC, 128 to >1024 μg/mL)[41] and generally with clindamycin resistance.

Since the first description of group A streptococcus resistance to erythromycin in 1955[45] in the United Kingdom, a rapid increase in macrolide resistance occurred in the 1980s and continued in the 1990s.[36,46] Worldwide, erythromycin resistance in *Streptococcus pyogenes* is demonstrated in approximately 14% of isolates,[47] although prevalence of resistance varied regionally: 39% in Italy in 1998,[48] 24% in Spain in 1998,[49] and 9.6% in France in 1999.[50] A longitudinal study in one elementary school in Pittsburgh in 2001 documented an outbreak of erythromycin-resistant group A streptococcus infections due to a single clone; laboratory surveillance in the surrounding community revealed that 38% of the 100 isolates tested were also resistant to erythromycin.[36] In Finland, where there had been a great increase in the use of erythromycin in the 1980s through 1991, resistance to that antibiotic was found in up to 44% of clinical isolates of group A streptococci from some communities in 1990.[51] However, nationwide policies in Finland reduced the use of macrolides for respiratory and skin infections in outpatients after 1991, and erythromycin resistance among clinical isolates steadily dropped, from 16.5% in 1992 to 8.6% in 1996.[52] As with *S. pneumoniae,* there is cross-resistance among the macrolides in *S. pyogenes;* however, resistance does not extend to clindamycin if resistance is due to the M phenotype.[46,49] The M-phenotype is more prevalent in the Americas than in the Asia-Pacific or Europe, where the MLS$_B$ phenotype is predominant.[47] Spain, where the M-phenotype predominates, is an exception.[53]

The emergence of resistance to erythromycin encountered in clinical isolates of these organisms from patient populations treated with this antibiotic is consistent with in vitro studies of pneumococci and streptococci subcultured sequentially in the presence of erythromycin, which demonstrate the selection of erythromycin resistance and often cross-resistance to other macrolides. Similar in vitro results are ob-

TABLE 28-1 In Vitro Susceptibilities* to Erythromycin, Azithromycin, Clarithromycin, and Telithromycin

Organism	Erythromycin		Azithromycin		Clarithromycin		Telithromycin	
	MIC$_{50}$	MIC$_{90}$	MIC$_{50}$	MIC$_{90}$	MIC$_{50}$	MIC$_{90}$	MIC$_{50}$	MIC$_{90}$
Streptococcus pneumoniae								
Penicillin-susceptible (MIC ≤ 0.06 μg/mL)	0.03	1.0	0.125	1.0	0.016	0.25	0.016	0.03
Penicillin-intermediate (MIC = 0.12-1.0 μg/mL)	0.03	>64.0	0.125	>64.0	0.03	>64.0	0.016	0.06
Penicillin-resistant (MIC ≥ 2.0 μg/mL)	1.0	>64.0	1.0	>64.0	0.5	>64.0	0.03	0.25
Streptococcus pyogenes	0.06	0.06	0.12	0.25	0.03	0.06	0.015	0.015
Streptococcus agalactiae	≤0.06	8	0.06	0.12	0.03	0.06	0.015	0.06
Viridans streptococci	0.12	>128	2.0	8.0	0.5	8	0.06	0.12
Enterococcus spp.								
Vancomycin-sensitive	1	2	>8	>8	0.5	1	0.03	0.06
Vancomycin-resistant	>128	>128	>8	>8	>128	>128	8	32
Staphylococcus aureus								
Methicillin-sensitive	0.25	>128	—	—	0.06	>128	0.06	0.25
Methicillin-resistant	>128	>128	>128	>128	>128	>128	0.25	0.5
Staphylococcus epidermidis	32	>128	16	>128	16	>128	0.06	>128
Corynebacterium diphtheriae	0.015	0.026	0.044	0.058	0.006	0.008	0.004	0.008
Listeria monocytogenes	0.125	0.25	1	1	0.06	0.125	0.03-0.125	0.03-0.25
Moraxella catarrhalis	≤0.25	≤0.25	≤0.06	≤0.06	≤0.25	≤0.25	0.06	0.12
Haemophilus influenzae	4	8	1	2	8	16	1	2
Bordetella pertussis	0.03	0.06	0.03	0.06	0.06	0.06	0.015	0.03
Neisseria gonorrhoeae	0.5	2	0.12	0.25	0.25	1	0.06	0.12
Neisseria meningitidis	1	1	0.5	1	0.12	0.5	0.015	0.12
Campylobacter jejuni	0.5-2	1-4	0.25	0.12-0.5	0.5-2	1-8	—	—
Helicobacter pylori	0.12	0.25	0.25	0.5	0.008	0.015	—	0.5
Mycoplasma pneumoniae	≤0.015	≤0.015	≤0.015	≤0.015	≤0.015	≤0.015	≤0.015	≤0.015
Chlamydia trachomatis	—	≤0.25[†]	—	≤0.25[†]	—	≤0.015[†]	—	—
Chlamydophila pneumoniae	0.125	0.25	0.125	0.25	NA	0.03	0.06	0.25
Legionella pneumophila	0.125	0.5	0.12	0.5	0.032	0.046	0.032	0.125
Bacteroides fragilis	32	>32	>32	>32	4	8	16	32
Peptococcus, Peptostreptococcus	2	16	1	>64	1	4	0.03	0.03
Clostridium perfringens	2	2	4	4	0.125	0.125	0.25	0.25
Propionibacterium spp.	≤0.06	0.5	0.125	2	≤0.06	≤0.06	≤0.06	≤0.06
Mycobacterium avium complex	—	≥64	8[‡]	—	2[‡]	—	>128	>128

*MIC$_{50}$ (MIC$_{90}$), minimal inhibitory concentration for 50% (90%) of isolates (μg/mL); values are ranges reported in referenced publications.[3,8-32]
[†]Reported as MIC$_{100}$.
[‡]Reported as median MIC.

tained with staphylococci.[54] Resistance to erythromycin by *Staphylococcus aureus* may be selected by its use in hospitals.[55] Most methicillin-resistant strains and many methicillin-sensitive clinical isolates are now resistant to this agent.[56-58] In addition, there is a potential for the emergence, during treatment in an individual patient, of erythromycin resistance by *S. aureus*.[59,60] These strains may demonstrate the emergence of one-step high-level resistance to erythromycin alone, or they may show cross-resistance to other macrolides and to lincomycin and clindamycin. In addition, staphylococci isolated from patients treated with erythromycin may exhibit a phenomenon called *dissociated resistance* by Garrod.[61] Only a small proportion of the population of such staphylococcal isolates exhibit resistance when grown in large concentrations of erythromycin; however, in the presence of lower concentrations of erythromycin, almost the entire population demonstrates resistance to erythromycin, to other macrolides, and often to the lincosamide antibiotics.

The viridans group of streptococci has traditionally been considered generally susceptible to erythromycin. Recent studies have shown that macrolide resistance may be increasing in some areas, with the percentage of resistant isolates from blood being 32% and 53% in Taiwan and 42% in Canada.[62,63] The majority of strains of *Listeria monocytogenes*, and *Corynebacterium diphtheriae* show appreciable susceptibility to erythromycin.[16,64] Many strains of *Clostridium perfringens* may be only moderately sensitive.[27] Appreciable in vitro activity has been demonstrated against *Actinomyces israelii*[65] and against *Nocardia asteroides* when combined with ampicillin.[66] Both clarithromycin and azithromycin are more active than erythromycin against mycobacteria.[67]

With gram-negative bacteria, erythromycin displays excellent activity against *B. pertussis*,[68] moderate activity against *Neisseria meningitidis*[69] and *Neisseria gonorrhoeae*,[21] and fair to poor activity against *Haemophilus influenzae*.[21] Resistance to erythromycin in isolates of *Bordetella pertussis* was first reported in the United States in Arizona in 1994, but this continues to be rare.[70] Strains of *N. gonorrhoeae* that are resistant to erythromycin, with MICs up to 32 μg/mL, are occasionally encountered,[71] and such strains have also been isolated from patients with prior exposure to azithromycin.[72] However, National Committee on Clinical Laboratory Standards (NCCLS) criteria for resistance and susceptibility to erythromycin have not been established for *N. gonorrhoeae* and a single-drug, single-dose therapy with erythromycin is not advised.[73] Failure rates in treatment of *N. gonorrhoeae* with erythromycin have correlated with reduced in vitro susceptibility; with an MIC of 0.25 μg/mL, the failure rate was 12.5%, and at a MIC of 2 μg/mL it was 80%.[71] In 2000, only 1% of *Campylobacter jejuni* isolates tested in the United States were resistant (MIC, >8) to erythromycin.[74] Breakpoint interpretive criteria for macrolide activity against anaerobic bacteria has not been established, but erythromycin generally has moderate activity against some species of gram-negative anaerobes, such as *Prevotella* and *Porphyromonas*, but *Bacteroides fragilis* strains are usually resistant.[75] The Enterobacteriaceae are usually resistant, except as the pH rises to 8.5.[7]

The extensive spectrum of activity of erythromycin is also demonstrated by its clinically useful activity against such diverse organisms as *Legionella pneumophila*,[26] *Mycoplasma pneumoniae*,[26] *Ureaplasma urealyticum*,[76] some strains of *Rickettsia*, *Chlamydia trachomatis*,[23] and *Chlamydophila pneumoniae*.[77] Erythromycin is about 30 times more potent against *M. pneumoniae* than is levofloxacin[26] and 50 times more potent than tetracycline.[78] Erythromycin-resistant variants of *M. pneumoniae* have been isolated in the laboratory and from a patient.[79] Extracellular and intracellular *L. pneumophila* strains show substantial susceptibility to erythromycin.[26,80]

Mechanisms of Resistance

Decreased Microbial Entry or Export of Drug

Enterobacteriaceae exhibit decreased permeability of the outer cell envelope to macrolides; cell-free systems and protoplasts of these organisms are susceptible to the drug.[81-83] This intrinsic resistance is also exhibited by *Pseudomonas* spp. and *Acinetobacter* spp. In addi-

tion, chromosomally encoded efflux pumps of several families can provide macrolide and in some cases, lincosamide and streptogramin resistance.[3] These pumps are energized by the proton motive force or by ATP hydrolysis. For example, plasmid-mediated erythromycin resistance in *Staphylococcus epidermidis* and *S. aureus* caused by active efflux of the drug is encoded by the *msr*(A) gene and is carried out by an adenosine triphosphatase–binding protein working together with additional transmembrane domains to complete the transporter functions.[81,84] A different efflux system for erythromycin and other 14- and 15-member macrolides (but not 16-member macrolides, lincosamides, or analogues of streptogramin B), called the M phenotype, has been elucidated in erythromycin-resistant strains of *S. pyogenes*, *S. pneumoniae*, and group C streptococci. That efflux system is encoded by the *mef*(A) gene, a transposable element, and consists of transmembrane domains across the cytoplasmic membrane that are driven by the proton motive force.[1] The M phenotype resistance is expressed by *S. pneumoniae* at moderate levels with erythromycin MICs of 1 to 64 μg/mL.

Target Site Alterations

Mutations in genes for 50S ribosomal proteins or bases of critical domains of the 23S rRNA receptor site confer resistance to erythromycin and sometimes to other macrolides, lincomycin, and clindamycin; in some but not all strains, this is associated with a decreased binding affinity for erythromycin.[1,2a,3,85,86] This type of resistance may be of a high level and has been demonstrated in some strains of *S. pneumoniae*, *H. pylori*, *M. avium*, *B. subtilis*, *S. pyogenes*, *Campylobacter* spp., *Mycoplasma pneumoniae*, *E. coli*, and *S. aureus*.

Alteration in the 23S ribosomal RNA of the 50S ribosomal subunit by methylation of adenine, at a defined position[1,2a,87,88] is associated with resistance to erythromycin and most other macrolides (M), lincosamides (L, lincomycin, and clindamycin), and streptogramin type B (S$_B$). This pattern of resistance, referred to as the MLS$_B$ phenotype, is mediated by the *erm* (erythromycin ribosome methylation) gene (*erm*[A], *erm*[B], *erm*[C]) on plasmids or transposons on chromosomes. The resistance results from decreased binding of the antibiotics to their overlapping targets on the ribosome, which is probably altered in conformation by methylation. It can be exhibited by strains of *S. aureus*, streptococci (including *S. pneumoniae*), *Enterococcus* spp., *C. diphtheriae*, *Campylobacter* spp., *B. fragilis*, *C. perfringens*, *Listeria* spp., *M. pneumoniae*, and *Legionella* spp. This phenomenon may be constitutive or inducible by subinhibitory concentrations of erythromycin that bring about induction of the methylating enzyme. The inducible mechanism seems to explain the phenomenon of dissociated resistance, described earlier under Antimicrobial Activity.

Drug Inactivation

Enzymatic inactivation of erythromycin and some other 14-, 15-, and 16-member ring macrolides by phosphotransferases has been described in strains of *S. aureus*, *E. coli*, and *Nocardia* spp. and is encoded by genes designated *mph*(A), *mph*(B), and *mph*(C).[3] Esterase genes (*ere*[A] and *ere*[B]) on plasmids encode for the hydrolysis of the macrocyclic lactone of erythromycin and have been found in strains of *E. coli*, *Klebsiella* spp., *Citrobacter* spp., *Proteus* spp., *Enterobacter* spp., and rare strains of *S. aureus*.[3]

Polymerase chain reaction methods have been developed that allow for relatively rapid detection of the different mechanisms of macrolide resistance among clinical isolates (genotypic testing).[89] A given bacterial strain may possess more than one type of macrolide resistance mechanism, resulting in complex resistant phenotypes.

Other Activities of Erythromycin

Erythromycin and other 14-member ring macrolides have a gastrointestinal motility–stimulating effect.[90] In this regard, erythromycin acts as a motilin receptor agonist in the gut and gallbladder.[91] These prokinetic effects are being studied for their potential in the treatment of diabetic gastroparesis,[92] postvagotomy gastroparesis,[93] gastroparesis in critically ill patients receiving mechanical ventilation,[94] and intestinal dysmotility in young infants.[95] Other 14-member ring macrolides, such as clarithromycin, have similar promotility effects, but the latter requires more than double the dose of erythromycin.[96] Development of new macrolide agents with enhanced activity on gastrointestinal motility but lacking antimicrobial properties, so-called motilide agents, is currently underway.[97]

There has been appreciable interest in the anti-inflammatory activities of erythromycin and other macrolides. These include interference with oxidant production by neutrophils (in which the cladinose moiety of erythromycin was found to be the key structure[98]), acceleration of neutrophil apoptosis, suppression of the release of proinflammatory cytokines, and promotion of the release of nitric oxide from endothelial cells.[98,99] At the molecular level, macrolides appear to modulate inflammation at the transcriptional level by inhibiting two transcription factors, nuclear factor kappa B (NF-κB) and activation protein-1 (AP-1),[100,101] both of which are important regulators of, among others, expression of interleukin-8, a chemokine that acts as a major recruiter of neutrophils in chronic airway disease.[102] The anti-inflammatory protective effects of erythromycin appear to be a slow process as demonstrated by the requirement of at least a 28-day pretreatment with erythromycin to suppress an inflammatory response in zymosan-induced peritonitis in rats.[103] The 14-member ring macrolides have been effective in animal models in preventing the acute exacerbation of interstitial pneumonia and acute lung injury, such as after the use of bleomycin.[104]

In vitro studies have demonstrated that erythromycin and other macrolides at subinhibitory concentrations reduce the adherence of various pathogenic bacterial species to host cells; however, the clinical significance of these observations is unknown.[105]

Clinical Pharmacology

The peak serum levels obtained after single doses of various erythromycin preparations are given in Table 28-2.[106-108] Erythromycin base is subject to destruction by gastric acid, and preparations of the base have been made with an acid-resistant coating to delay dissolution of the drug until it reaches the small bowel. The esters and ester salts of erythromycin are more acid stable, form a stable suspension in water, and are tasteless. These characteristics are used in the liquid suspension for children. Erythromycin base (absorbed intact), stearate (absorbed as the base), and ethylsuccinate (absorbed both as the intact ester and as the free base after hydrolysis in the intestine) are usually absorbed more completely in the fasting state, although one study demonstrated increased absorption of a stearate preparation when it was taken with a meal.[108] After absorption, about 45% of the ethylsuccinate preparation is present in the serum as the inactive ester and about 55% as the active base.

Average serum levels achieved under fasting conditions with these preparations are similar; however, results with the base may be erratic.

Erythromycin base has become available in a capsule containing enteric-coated granules; this preparation is promoted as giving more uniform absorption,[109,110] but some enteric-coated tablets may provide similar blood levels.[111] The absorption of the estolate is not affected by food, and the resulting peak serum level consists of both free base (20% to 30%, active form) and estolate (70% to 80%, much less active); the level of base achieved is similar to that achieved by the other oral preparations taken in comparable doses in the fasting state. The clinical significance of the much less active esterified form of the drug that is present in serum in appreciable concentration is controversial. It would seem that in treatment of infections of only moderate severity by organisms highly sensitive to erythromycin, differences in therapeutic results using the various oral preparations would be insignificant. Limited clinical comparisons confirm that suspicion.[112] However, in the treatment of group A streptococcal pharyngitis in children, substantially higher rates of bacteriologic eradication and lower rates of gastrointestinal side effects have been reported with the estolate preparation in comparison with the ethylsuccinate formulation.[113] Intravenous preparations of erythromycin achieve appreciably higher serum levels and should be used to treat serious infections requiring erythromycin.

Erythromycin is distributed through total body water.[114] Values given for protein binding vary from 40% to 90%; however, the significance of such binding is speculative. The drug persists in tissues longer than in the blood. The ratios of tissue or body fluid concentrations to simultaneous serum concentrations (usually at peak) are as follows: aqueous humor, 0.3; ascites, 0.4; bile, 28; middle ear exudate in otitis media, 0.3 to 0.7; pleural fluid, 0.7; prostatic fluid, 0.4; cerebrospinal fluid without meningitis, 0 to 0.02, and with meningitis, 0.05 to 0.1; infected maxillary paranasal sinus, 0.4 to 0.8; tonsil, 0.3. Concentrations achieved in the middle ear in otitis media are adequate to treat pneumococcal and group A streptococcal infections involving sensitive strains of these species but are not adequate to consistently eradicate *H. influenzae*.[115,116] High concentrations of erythromycin are achieved in alveolar macrophages[117] and polymorphonuclear leukocytes[118] compared with those in extracellular fluid.

There are very limited data on concentrations of erythromycin achieved in the cerebrospinal fluid of patients with meningitis that suggest that large parenteral doses may be effective against meningeal infection by highly susceptible organisms such as *S. pneumoniae*.[119] Limited data from patients with septic arthritis suggest poor penetration of synovial fluid. Erythromycin is transferred across the placenta; fetal serum concentrations are about 2% of those in maternal serum, but higher concentrations accumulate in fetal tissue and amniotic fluid.[120] The drug is excreted in breast milk.

Up to 4.5% of an oral dose and 15% of a parenteral dose of erythromycin are recoverable in the urine. Urine concentrations after oral doses are often high but quite variable. Erythromycin is concentrated by the liver and excreted into the bile in high concentrations; however, only

TABLE 28-2 Serum Levels of Erythromycin in Adults			Peak Serum Levels	
Preparation	*Dose (mg)*	*Route*	*Hours after Dose*	*Concentration (μg/mL)*
Base	250	Oral	4	0.3-1.0*
	500			0.3-1.9
Stearate	250 (fasting)	Oral	3	0.2-1.3
	500 (fasting)		3	0.4-1.8
	500 (after food)		3	0.1-0.4†
Ethylsuccinate	500	Oral	0.5-2.5	1.5‡ (0.6§)
Estolate	250	Oral	2-4	1.4-1.7
	500		3.5-4	4.2‡ (1.1§)
Lactobionate	200	Intravenous	Immediately	3-4
	500		1	9.9
Gluceptate	250	Intravenous	Immediately	3.5-10.7
	1000		1	9.9

*Somewhat higher levels reported with some enteric-coated preparation after repeated doses.[63,64]
†One study demonstrated higher levels (to 2.8 μg/mL) with dose taken during a meal.[62]
‡Total drug (inactive ester and free base).
§Free base.

about 1.5% of the dose of the base and 0.2% of the ester can be recovered from bile in the first 8 hours, and some of this is reabsorbed from the intestine.[121] The higher serum levels achieved by the estolate have been attributed to both better absorption and lower biliary excretion. After an oral dose, large concentrations of the antibiotic are found in feces, probably representing ingested drug that was never absorbed as well as some that was excreted in bile. A large proportion of absorbed drug cannot be accounted for by urinary or biliary excretion or by tissue binding and may be inactivated in the liver by demethylation.[122]

The normal serum half-life of erythromycin is 1.4 hours, and appreciable serum levels are maintained for 6 hours. In anuric patients, the half-life is prolonged to about 5 hours, but dosage reduction in patients with renal failure is generally not necessary.[123] Erythromycin is not removed by peritoneal dialysis or hemodialysis.

Adverse Reactions

Erythromycin is one of the safest antibiotics in clinical use. Untoward reactions caused by the drug itself, except for pseudomembranous colitis and ventricular arrhythmias (with intravenous use), are not life-threatening and, with the exception of the irritative reactions, they are rare.

Irritative reactions include dose-related abdominal cramps, nausea, vomiting, diarrhea, and gas; these reactions occur more commonly in children and young adults than in older persons and may be associated with either intravenous or oral administration. They result from the motility-stimulating effects of erythromycin discussed previously. Enteric coating of erythromycin base in the form of pellets in a capsule (e.g., ERYC) does not reduce the common dose-related gastrointestinal side effects of oral erythromycin.[124] Thrombophlebitis with intravenous use can be decreased by appropriate dilution of the dose in at least 250 mL of solution and by avoidance of rapid infusions. Infusion should take place over 45 to 60 minutes.

Allergic reactions include skin rash, fever, and eosinophilia.

Cholestatic hepatitis occurs rarely,[125] almost always with the estolate preparation and chiefly in adults.[126] The syndrome typically begins after 20 days of therapy, but more rapidly in those previously treated, and consists of nausea, vomiting, and abdominal pain followed by jaundice, fever, and abnormal liver function tests consistent with cholestatic hepatitis. These findings are sometimes accompanied by rash, leukocytosis, and eosinophilia. The abnormalities usually clear within days to a few weeks after the drug is stopped but may return rapidly on rechallenge. The syndrome appears to represent a hypersensitivity reaction to the specific structure of the estolate compound.[127] However, hepatocyte toxicity induced by the drug or its metabolites, and allergy to altered hepatocyte components, may be contributory.[128] Milder forms of the syndrome occur with the estolate and may be more common in pregnant women.[129] It must be distinguished from false-positive serum glutamic-oxaloacetic transaminase (AST) elevations that occur in patients taking the estolate.[130] The latter may be found when AST is determined by colorimetric procedures rather than by an enzymatic method and seems to result from an interfering substance present in the blood in association with estolate administration. Reversible hepatotoxicity, including jaundice, has occurred with the stearate salt and with the ethylsuccinate ester of erythromycin.[131]

Transient hearing loss has been reported rarely in association with the use of large intravenous doses of erythromycin lactobionate or large doses of oral erythromycin.[132,133] This may occur more commonly in older adults with renal insufficiency.[134,135] The ototoxicity depends on the serum concentration of the drug.[136]

Polymorphic ventricular tachycardia with QT prolongation (torsades de pointes) has been reported rarely in association with treatment with intravenous erythromycin.[137,138] The drug has been shown to effect repolarization in the isolated heart and to block electrical current in guinea pig ventricular myocytes in a way consistent with the observed arrhythmia.[139] The possibility for interaction with potential-lengthening drugs (classes Ia and III antiarrhythmics) and for increased risk in the presence of electrolyte abnormality or prolonged QT interval should be kept in mind.

Superinfection, especially of the gastrointestinal tract or vagina, with *Candida* species or gram-negative bacilli may occur, as with other antibiotics.

Pseudomembranous colitis caused by overgrowth of toxin-producing *Clostridium difficile* occurs rarely with the use of erythromycin.[140]

Infantile hypertrophic pyloric stenosis has been epidemiologically linked to very early exposure to erythromycin in children. It has been hypothesized that erythromycin interacts with motilin receptors, inducing strong gastric and pyloric contractions leading to pyloric hypertrophy.[141,142] There is no substantive evidence of a risk associated with prenatal exposure.[143]

Drug Interactions

Incompatibility during administration between intravenous preparations of erythromycin and other drugs has been reported; the latter include vitamin B complex and vitamin C, cephalothin, tetracycline, chloramphenicol, colistin, heparin, metraminol, and diphenylhydantoin.

Erythromycin may produce interactions with other drugs by interfering with their hepatic metabolism through the cytochrome P-450 enzyme (CYP3A subclass) system.[144,145] This may occur because erythromycin metabolites are capable of forming inactive complexes with cytochrome P-450 enzymes.[145,146] The resulting raised level of drug may result in serious toxicity (Table 28-3).[147] For example, elevations of terfenadine or astemizole serum concentrations have led to serious ventricular arrhythmias, and the same phenomenon with midazolam has led to unconsciousness.

Erythromycin can increase the bioavailability of digoxin, possibly by interfering with its inactivation by gut flora.[144] Erythromycin may inhibit the assay organism used in some determinations of serum folic acid. Sequential use of erythromycin and clindamycin should be avoided when possible because of the potential for the development of cross-resistance or dissociated resistance.

Uses of Erythromycin

Erythromycin has a few indications for use as the drug of choice and some important applications as an alternative drug to penicillin G and other antibiotics (Table 28-4).[3,73,148-159] When given to adults by the oral route, preparations other than the estolate are generally preferable be-

TABLE 28-3 Potentially Clinically Significant Drug Interactions Produced by Macrolides[*]

Drug	Interactions
Erythromycin	Alfentanil, astemizole, buspirone, bromocriptine, carbamazepine, cilostazol, cisapride, clomipramine plus rispiridone, clozapine, colchicine, cyclosporine, digoxin, disopyramide, dofetilide, ergot alkaloids, felodipine, lidocaine, loratadine, lovastatin, methylprednisolone, midazolam, pimozide, phenytoin, quinidine, repaglinide, rifabutin, ropivacaine, saquinavir, sertraline, sildenafil, simvastatin, tacrolimus, terfenadine, theophylline, triazolam, valproate, verapamil, warfarin
Clarithromycin	Carbamazepine, cisapride, cyclosporine, digoxin, disopyramide, disulfiram, dofetilide, ergot alkaloids, lidocaine, loratadine, lovastatin, midazolam, pimozide, repaglinide, rifampin, rifabutin, ritonavir, saquinavir, simvastatin, sildenafil, tacrolimus, terfenadine, theophylline, verapamil, warfarin, zidovudine
Azithromycin	Cyclosporine (one case)

[*]Interactions generally lead to increased levels of the listed drugs caused by interaction of the macrolide with CYP-450 hepatic metabolism. Exceptions are digoxin, in which the raised levels are caused by interference with digoxin inactivation by gut flora, and zidovudine, in which serum concentrations may be decreased by unknown mechanisms. Rifampin and rifabutin may lower the levels of clarithromycin, and clarithromycin may raise the levels of rifampin and rifabutin. Ritonavir may raise clarithromycin levels. Clarithromycin may produce modest reduction of zidovudine levels.

Modified from Kim RB and the Editors of the Medical Letter. The Medical Letter Handbook of Adverse Drug Interactions. New Rochelle, NY: The Medical Letter on Drugs and Therapeutics, 2003.

TABLE 28-4 Major Indications for Use of Macrolides

Infections in Which Macrolides Are the Drugs of Choice	Macrolide	Adult Dosages*
Bartonella henselae (cat-scratch bacillus)	Azithromycin	500 mg PO on day 1, then 250 mg PO on days 2-5
	Erythromycin	1 g q 6h IV for 7-14 days
Bartonella henselae or B. quintana (bacillary angiomatosis)	Erythromycin	0.5 g qid PO for 12 weeks
	Azithromycin	500 mg qd PO for 4-6 weeks (Patients with endocarditis should receive treatment for 4-6 mo)
Bordetella pertussis	Erythromycin	40 to 50 mg/kg/day (maximum, 2 g/day) in four doses for 14 days
	Azithromycin	10 mg/kg/day qd for 5 days
	Clarithromycin	10 mg/kg/day bid for 7 days
Campylobacter jejuni†	Erythromycin	250 mg qid PO for 5-7 days
	Azithromycin	500 mg PO on day 1, then 250 mg PO on days 2-5
Chlamydophila pneumoniae	Azithromycin	500 mg qd PO/IV for 1-2 days, then 500 mg PO qd to complete 7-10 days‡
(TWAR strain)	Clarithromycin	250-500 mg bid PO for 7-10 days
	Erythromycin	0.5 g tid-qid PO for 7-10 days
Chlamydia trachomatis (inclusion conjunctivitis)§	Erythromycin	Erythromycin base or ethylsuccinate 50 mg/kg/day PO divided into four doses daily for 14 days
Chlamydia trachomatis (pneumonia)§	Erythromycin	Erythromycin base or ethylsuccinate 50 mg/kg/day PO divided into four doses daily for 14 days
Chlamydia trachomatis (trachoma)	Azithromycin	1 g PO, single dose
Chlamydia trachomatis (urethritis or cervicitis)	Azithromycin	1 g PO, single dose
Diphtheria‖	Infection: erythromycin	125-500 mg qid PO for 14 days
	Carrier: erythromycin	250 mg qid PO for 7-10 days
Helicobacter pylori	Clarithromycin (+ amoxicillin +omeprazole)	500 mg bid PO for 7-10 days
Haemophilus ducreyi (chancroid)	Azithromycin	1 g, single dose
Legionella spp. pneumonia	Azithromycin ± rifampin (or a fluoroquinolone ± rifampin)	500 mg qd IV or PO for 5-10 days
Mycobacterium avium complex (MAC) disseminated disease	Clarithromycin (+ ethambutol ± rifabutin)	500 mg PO bid for indefinite duration¶
	Azithromycin (+ ethambutol ± rifabutin)	500 mg qd PO for indefinite duration¶
Mycobacterium avium complex prophylaxis	Azithromycin	1200 mg once weekly
	Clarithromycin	500 mg bid
Mycobacterium avium complex pulmonary infiltrative disease	Clarithromycin (+ ethambutol ± rifabutin)	500 mg bid PO for 1 year after sputum cultures are negative
	Azithromycin (+ ethambutol ± rifabutin)	500 mg qd PO for 1 year after sputum cultures are negative
Mycobacterium fortuitum/chelonae complex	Clarithromycin (+ amikacin)	500 mg bid PO for 4-6 mo
Mycoplasma pneumoniae	Azithromycin	500 mg PO qd for 5-10 days
	Clarithromycin	250 mg PO bid for 14 days
	Erythromycin	0.5 g tid-qid PO for 14-21 days
Nongonococcal urethritis in men (C. trachomatis or Ureaplasma urealyticum)	Azithromycin	1 g PO, single dose
	Erythromycin	0.5 g qid PO for 7 days

Infections in Which Macrolides Are an Important Alternative Drug	Macrolides and Adult Dosages*	Drug of Choice
Groups A, C, G streptococcal infection	Erythromycin 250-500 mg qid PO** Azithromycin 500 mg PO on day 1, then 250 mg PO on days 2-5 Clarithromycin 250 mg bid PO††	Penicillin G or V
Streptococcus pneumoniae infection	Erythromycin 250-500 mg qid PO†† Azithromycin 500 mg qid†† Clarithromycin 250-500 mg bid††	Penicillin G, ceftriaxone, or cefotaxime
Moraxella catarrhalis	Azithromycin 500 mg PO on day 1, then 250 mg PO on days 2-5 Erythromycin 250-500 mg qid PO Clarithromycin 250-500 mg bid	Cefuroxime; a fluoroquinolone
Haemophilus influenzae (upper respiratory infection and bronchitis)	Azithromycin 500 mg PO on day 1, then 250 mg PO on days 2-5 Clarithromycin 250-500 mg bid PO	Trimethoprim-sulfamethoxazole
Salmonella typhi	Azithromycin 500 mg qd PO for 5-7 days	Fluoroquinolone or ceftriaxone
Shigella	Azithromycin 500 mg on day 1, then 250 mg on days 2-5	Fluoroquinolone
Prevention of infection after colorectal surgery	1 g PO each of neomycin and erythromycin base at 1, 2, and 11 PM on the day before 8 AM surgery (combined with vigorous purgation over the 2nd day before surgery)	Cefoxitin or cefotetan
Rheumatic fever prophylaxis	Erythromycin 250 mg bid PO	Penicillin G
Anthrax	Erythromycin 500 mg qid PO for 10 days‡‡	Ciprofloxacin, doxycycline, penicillin G, amoxicillin
Lymphogranuloma venereum	Erythromycin 500 mg qid PO for 21 days	A tetracycline
Acne vulgaris	Erythromycin 250 mg qid PO or topical preparation	A tetracycline PO and a number of topical drugs
Borrelia burgdorferi (Lyme disease)	Erythromycin 250 mg qid PO for 14-21 days	Doxycycline
Babesia microti	Azithromycin 500 mg on day 1 and 250 mg on days 2-7 + atovaquone 750 mg q 12 hr	Clindamycin and quinine

*Intravenous therapy should be used in serious illness or when oral therapy is not possible or reliable.
†In some areas, such as in Thailand, macrolide- and fluoroquinolone-resistant strains have become common.
‡Mild to moderate severity: azithromycin 500 mg PO on day 1, then 250 mg PO on days 2-5.
§Diseases of infants.
‖Antitoxin is essential primary therapy for disease.
¶May be discontinued after >1 year with MAC treatment, when CD4 cell count is greater than 100 cells/mm³ for 3-6 mo on highly active antiretroviral therapy (HAART), and patient is asymptomatic.
**Treatment should be continued for 10 days for group A.
††Resistance to macrolides is increasing and is particularly frequent in penicillin-resistant strains.
‡‡Therapy may need to be continued for prolonged periods until vaccination is completed in those infected by the pulmonary route.

cause they have less risk of cholestatic hepatitis. Absorption, particularly with the enteric-coated base, stearate, or ethylsuccinate preparations taken in the fasting state or before meals, is usually adequate. The estolate preparation should be particularly avoided during pregnancy, when hepatotoxicity may be more common.[129] When higher serum levels are needed in more severe infections requiring erythromycin therapy, the drug should be given intravenously.

Although erythromycin continues to be useful in the treatment of community-acquired respiratory infections, its usefulness has become more limited in areas in which the incidence of penicillin-resistant pneumococci has become substantial. Such strains are often resistant to erythromycin, as discussed.[160-162] Treatment of *M. pneumoniae* infection with erythromycin, as with tetracycline, shortens the clinical course of the infection, even if started late in the course of illness; radiologic clearing of pulmonary lesions occurs earlier with erythromycin.[163,164]

Clinical experience and studies in vitro and in guinea pigs suggest that erythromycin is very effective in treating pneumonia caused by *L. pneumophila* or *L. micdadei*[165]; however, the newer macrolides, azithromycin and clarithromycin, are at least as active as erythromycin in vitro, clinically efficacious, and more easily tolerated when given orally.[166] The U.S. Food and Drug Administration (FDA) has approved azithromycin and levofloxacin for the treatment of legionellosis and they are now considered preferable to erythromycin, especially when given orally.[153,167]

Early treatment of pertussis with erythromycin is associated with clinical improvement, a rapid clearance of *B. pertussis* from the nasopharynx, and a reduction in secondary transmission in households. Erythromycin is also recommended for postexposure prophylaxis of pertussis.[168,169] Treatment of infants with erythromycin for pneumonia or conjunctivitis caused by *C. trachomatis* is approximately 80% effective, although a second course of antimicrobial therapy may be required.[170] Because of reports of an association between oral erythromycin and infantile hypertrophic pyloric stenosis (IHPS), monitoring for signs and symptoms of IHPS should be implemented in treated infants who are less than 6 weeks of age.[142]

Erythromycin treatment of patients with gastroenteritis caused by *C. jejuni* hastens the eradication of the organism from the feces but does not appear to alter the clinical course of uncomplicated infection when therapy begins 4 days or more after the onset of symptoms.[171] However, earlier treatment of young children with acute dysentery associated with *C. jejuni* has been shown to shorten the course of diarrhea and fecal excretion of the organism.[172] Nevertheless, in an institutional setting in Thailand, where *C. jejuni* strains were frequently resistant to erythromycin in vitro, early treatment of infants with diarrhea caused by this organism was not beneficial.[173] Erythromycin base given orally together with neomycin on the day before colorectal surgery and combined with vigorous purgation is about as effective as parenteral cephalosporin administration just before surgery in decreasing the incidence of septic complications.[174] No advantage has been demonstrated for the use of a combination of oral and intravenous antibiotics.[175] In the presence of bowel obstruction or when there is need for emergency surgery, the parenteral antibiotic regimen should be used.[176] Erythromycin remains the drug of choice in treating bacillary angiomatosis in immunocompromised patients.[177]

A comparative study involving a small number of children with cholera, who were all treated with rehydration solutions, showed that erythromycin or trimethoprim-sulfamethoxazole was effective and superior to treatment without an antimicrobial agent.[178] Erythromycin may be used as an alternative antibiotic in the treatment of anthrax and in infections by *Moraxella catarrhalis* and *Eikenella corrodens*. Erythromycin is not consistently effective in treatment of infections caused by *H. influenzae*.[115,116] In view of the availability of more effective alternative drugs, erythromycin should not be used alone in the treatment of deep-seated staphylococcal infections because of the potential for the emergence of resistant strains during therapy.[54,60,179] The results of treating syphilis with erythromycin during pregnancy must be considered uncertain at best; fetal syphilis may not be eradicated,[180] and this treatment is no longer recommended when pregnant women

with syphilis have a history of penicillin allergy.[170] Erythromycin may occasionally be useful in treating urinary tract infections caused by gram-negative bacilli that might otherwise require the use of more toxic agents.[181] Urine pH must generally be raised to 8.0 or above to achieve effective activity at urinary concentrations against the gram-negative bacilli.

Diffuse panbronchiolitis, a chronic inflammatory disease of the airways, particularly encountered in Japan, is associated with an increase in survival of patients treated with erythromycin at a low dose (400 to 600 mg/day) and for a prolonged course.[182] The beneficial effect is generally attributed to the anti-inflammatory activity of the macrolide.

AZITHROMYCIN AND CLARITHROMYCIN

Azithromycin and clarithromycin were developed to improve the qualities of erythromycin. They have better oral absorption, longer half-life, fewer gastrointestinal side effects, and a greater antimicrobial spectrum of activity than erythromycin.

Derivation, Chemistry, and Preparations

Azithromycin is derived from erythromycin, differing in having a methyl-substituted nitrogen in its 15-member lactone ring (Fig. 28-2). It is therefore an azalide antibiotic. Clarithromycin, having a 14-member ring structure, is produced by modifying position C6 of the lactone ring of erythromycin to possess a methoxy group (Fig. 28-3). These changes increase the stability of these compounds in gastric acid, improving absorption by the oral route.[183]

Azithromycin is available in capsules for oral use as azithromycin dihydrate equivalent to 250 mg of azithromycin, in film-coated tablets of 250 mg and 600 mg, as a powder for oral suspension, and in vials of 500 mg for intravenous infusion. Clarithromycin is provided in 250- or 500-mg film-coated tablets and as granules for oral suspension.

Mechanisms of Action and Resistance

Limited studies suggest that azithromycin, clarithromycin, and erythromycin bind to the same receptor on the bacterial 50S ribosomal subunit and inhibit RNA-dependent protein synthesis by the same mechanism.[2,184] Azithromycin has greater activity than the 14-member macrolides erythromycin and clarithromycin against gram-negative bacteria (especially for *M. catarrhalis* and *H. influenzae*) and therefore appears to better penetrate the outer envelope of those organisms.[185] Like other macrolides, azithromycin and clarithromycin are generally considered to be bacteriostatic agents; however, bactericidal activity is easily demonstrated in vitro against such species as *S. pyogenes*, *S. pneumoniae*, and *H. influenzae*.[184,185] In vitro activity of the newer macrolides increases with rising pH, as with erythromycin.

Mechanisms of resistance to azithromycin or clarithromycin are the same as or similar to those for erythromycin.[1,2a,3] There is complete cross-resistance between erythromycin, azithromycin, and clarithromycin for gram-positive organisms showing resistance to erythromycin by the MLS$_B$ phenotype, because the methylation mechanism already described operates for all of the 14- and 15-member macrolides.[87] Cross-resistance among the 14- and 15-member macrolides is also characteristic of the M phenotype and is the result of an efflux system for the drugs. Clarithromycin-resistant strains of *Helicobacter pylori* with point mutations in the 23S rRNA genes that presumably result in diminished binding of the drug to the ribosomal target have been isolated from patients with peptic ulcer disease treated with that antibiotic.[186] Further studies with such strains suggest that horizontal transfer of the mutated gene can occur.[187] Similar point mutations in the 23S rRNA gene associated with macrolide resistance in *Mycobacterium avium* complex have been selected in patients undergoing clarithromycin or azithromycin monotherapy for disseminated infections.[188]

Antimicrobial Activity

Clarithromycin is highly active against gram-positive bacteria, being twofold to fourfold more active than erythromycin against most streptococci, including *S. pneumoniae* and *S. pyogenes,* and methicillin-sensitive *S. aureus*.[33,183,184] However, azithromycin is about twofold to fourfold less active than erythromycin against those organisms.[183,184] Streptococci and staphylococci that are resistant to erythromycin are resistant to clarithromycin and azithromycin.[38,39,184,189] The emergence of macrolide resistance in clinical isolates of *S. pneumoniae* and *S. pyogenes* was discussed in the section on erythromycin. Most methicillin-resistant staphylococci are resistant to the newer macrolides.[56,57] The activity of clarithromycin against many gram-negative bacteria is similar to that of erythromycin,[3,184] although it is slightly more active against *M. catarrhalis.* An active metabolite of clarithromycin, 14-hydroxyclarithromycin, has slightly greater activity than the parent compound against *S. aureus, S. pneumoniae, H. influenzae,* and *M. catarrhalis* and is additive in vitro to the activity of clarithromycin.[3,189] Azithromycin is more active than erythromycin or clarithromycin against gram-negative bacteria, especially against *H. influenzae* and *M. catarrhalis.*[183,190] The greater activity of azithromycin against the Enterobacteriaceae is of questionable clinical significance. However, it is of interest that prolonged incubation of *Pseudomonas aeruginosa* strains with macrolides at clinically achievable concentrations is associated with decreased viability and diminished protein synthesis.[191] Azithromycin is the most potent in that regard.

Azithromycin and clarithromycin have equal or slightly better in vitro activities than erythromycin against *L. pneumophila.*[26,80] In guinea pigs infected with *L. pneumophila,* azithromycin was found to be a more effective treatment than clarithromycin or erythromycin.[192] All three of those macrolides have good activity against *M. pneumoniae* and *Chlamydophila pneumoniae.*[26,76,189] Both of the newer macrolides have significantly greater activity than erythromycin against *C. trachomatis* and *U. urealyticum,*[23,76] and somewhat greater activity against *B. burgdorferi.*[184,185] The small in vitro differences in potency among these macrolides may not have any clinical significance with regard to efficacy.[193]

The macrolides show little activity against *Mycobacterium tuberculosis.*[194] In contrast, clarithromycin shows substantial activity against *Mycobacterium leprae* and is superior in this respect to erythromycin and azithromycin.[184,189]

Clarithromycin and azithromycin have appreciable activities against *M. avium* complex. Clarithromycin is about fourfold more active than azithromycin against this organism in vitro[31] and is somewhat more active in slowing its replication in infected human macrophages.[195] However, macrolide-resistant populations of *M. avium* emerge frequently after treatment of experimentally infected beige mice with clarithromycin or azithromycin.[196] Both of these macrolides also have significant and approximately equal activity against *Toxoplasma gondii* in tissue culture systems.[197]

The interesting and potentially useful anti-inflammatory actions of the macrolides (aside from their antimicrobial activity) were discussed under Erythromycin, earlier.

Clinical Pharmacology

Clarithromycin is well absorbed after oral administration, with or without food, and is approximately 50% bioavailable.[184] Mean peak serum concentrations in the steady state with oral doses of 250 and 500 mg every 12 hours are 1 and 2 to 3 µg/mL, respectively. The elimination half-lives for those two regimens are 3 to 4 and 5 to 7 hours, respectively. Clarithromycin is appreciably metabolized in the liver by oxidation and hydrolysis to a number of compounds, accounting for a recovery of 78%. The major metabolite, 14-hydroxyclarithromycin, has antibacterial activity and accounts for 20% of the metabolites.[184] With the 250-mg oral dose given every 12 hours, about 20% of the drug is excreted into the urine unchanged and 10% to 15% as the hydroxy metabolite. With the 500-mg dose given at the same interval, about 30% is excreted into the urine unchanged and 10% to 15% as the major metabolite. At higher doses, there is some nonlinearity of half-life, apparently because of saturation of metabolic mechanisms with a higher proportion of unchanged drug eliminated in the urine.[184] About 65% to 70% of the drug is bound to protein in the serum. With renal insufficiency involving creatinine clearances of less than 30 mL/min, there is a marked increase in half-life of clarithromycin.[189] Dose adjustment is suggested in patients with severe renal failure, including recommendations for a 500-mg loading dose followed by 250 mg once or twice daily depending on the type of infection being treated.[189] In the face of severe hepatic disease, there is an increase in the renal clearance of clarithromycin associated with a decrease in metabolic clearance, to the extent that no dosage adjustment is recommended at present.[189]

Clarithromycin is widely distributed and penetrates well into various tissues, generally exceeding peak maximum serum levels by severalfold.[189] Concentrations of clarithromycin and its 14-hydroxy metabolite in middle ear fluids of children with acute otitis media exceeded the plasma concentrations by approximately ninefold and fourfold, respectively, 12 hours after the sixth dose when the drug was given every 12 hours.[198] Concentrations generally exceed the MIC of most strains of middle ear pathogens, except for highly penicillin-resistant *S. pneumoniae.* Limited data indicate minimal penetration of clarithromycin and its 14-hydroxy metabolite into cerebrospinal fluid in patients without meningitis.[199] The levels achieved were below the MIC for the usual pathogens associated with bacterial meningitis and were 1% to 2% of the corresponding plasma levels. Clarithromycin, like the other macrolides, penetrates well into phagocytic cells.[200]

The oral bioavailability of azithromycin after a single 500-mg dose is 37%.[201] Food decreases the absorption by 50%; therefore, the dose should be taken at least 1 hour before or 2 hours after a meal.[202] The drug should not be taken simultaneously with magnesium- or aluminum-containing antacids, which decrease the rate of absorption and therefore the peak serum concentration but do not change the extent of absorption (i.e., the area under the curve).[203] The maximum serum concentration achieved after a single 500-mg

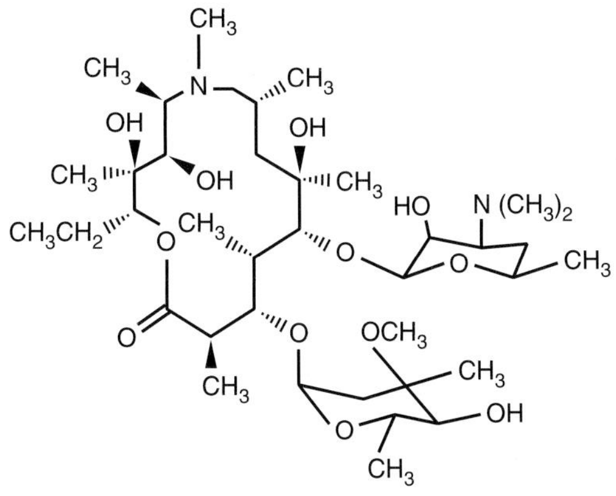

FIGURE 28-2. Azithromycin base.

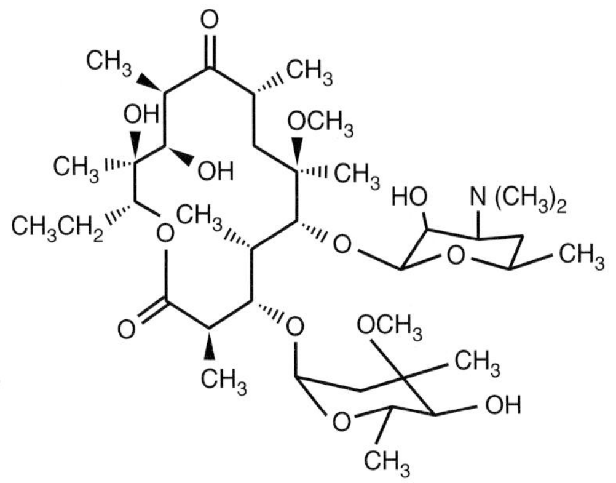

FIGURE 28-3. Clarithromycin base.

oral dose was 0.41 μg/mL; after a 500-mg loading dose on day 1 followed by 250 mg daily for 4 additional days, it was 0.24 μg/mL; after 500 mg twice on day 1 followed by 500 mg daily for 5 additional days, it was 0.62 μg/mL.[184] Protein binding of azithromycin in serum varies between 7% and 50% depending on the drug concentration.[184] Azithromycin is widely distributed in tissues, and for most the drug concentration exceeds that in serum by 10- to 100-fold,[201] particularly in sputum and lung. Very high concentrations were found in alveolar macrophages and neutrophils.[204] The extensive tissue uptake of azithromycin has been attributed to cell uptake of this basic compound into relatively acidic lysosomes because of ionic trapping.[204] Very low concentrations were noted in cerebrospinal fluid in patients without meningitis and in the aqueous humor of the uninflamed eye.[205] However, appreciable concentrations of azithromycin have been detected in the brains of patients undergoing resections of brain tumors after they received 500 mg orally.[205] The average half-life in many tissues is between 2 and 4 days,[201] so that it is estimated that significant antibacterial activity against many pathogens persists in tissue for at least 5 days after a 5-day course of treatment.[201] The average terminal half-life is 68 hours, consistent with a slow release of drug from tissues followed by elimination from the vascular compartment. About 6% of an oral dose appears as unchanged drug in the urine within 1 week of administration, and another small proportion is metabolized to inactive compounds, particularly by demethylation.[201] Most of the drug that is absorbed remains unmetabolized and is probably eliminated in feces by way of biliary excretion and possibly transintestinal elimination.[201] Biliary concentrations of azithromycin are higher than in the serum, and most of the drug in the bile is unchanged.[201] There are no data available on dose adjustments required with severe renal or hepatic failure.

Adverse Reactions

Adverse reactions to clarithromycin and azithromycin at the usual doses have been rare.[183,184,202] The most common complaints are gastrointestinal (diarrhea, nausea, abdominal pain), and discontinuance of therapy is rarely required. This is in contrast to the relatively common abdominal complaints encountered with erythromycin, which not infrequently leads to cessation of therapy.[183,184] Abnormalities in liver function are occasionally encountered in patients treated with these drugs, and reversible cholestatic hepatitis has been reported with azithromycin.[206] With the high doses of these drugs used in the treatment of *M. avium* complex, tinnitus, dizziness, and reversible hearing loss have been reported.[207,208] Rarely, severe allergic reactions have occurred with the use of azithromycin. One case of ventricular tachycardia that was probably caused by clarithromycin has been reported.[209] The risk of macrolide-associated torsade de pointes (a polymorphic ventricular tachycardia) has been associated with increasing age, female sex, and concomitant drug use, especially with cisapride.[210] Acute psychosis or "mania" has been noted in a few patients receiving clarithromycin.[137,138] High doses of clarithromycin in animals have been associated with teratogenic effects.

Drug Interactions

Clarithromycin has been reported to be associated with increased concentrations of several drugs that undergo hepatic metabolism by the CYP3A system (see Table 28-3).[147] As with erythromycin, these interactions can lead to serious toxicity. It is not yet clear whether the clarithromycin interactions can occur with all the drugs that interact with erythromycin, but a conservative clinical approach would be to consider that potential. These interactions with the hepatic metabolism of other drugs have not been documented with azithromycin, which does not appear to induce or bind and inactivate the CYP-450 enzymes, probably because of its different azalide structure.[145,146] Clarithromycin may decrease the serum concentration of zidovudine by unknown mechanisms when the two drugs are taken at the same time.[211] However, in another study, with a somewhat different design, there was no significant alteration of zidovudine bioavailability in volunteers with acquired immunodeficiency syndrome (AIDS) who took the two drugs 2 hours apart.[212]

Clarithromycin, like erythromycin, may occasionally lead to digoxin toxicity, possibly by diminishing the bacterial metabolism of digoxin in the gut.[213]

Uses of Clarithromycin and Azithromycin

Clarithromycin and azithromycin have several indications for use as the drug of choice and some important applications as an alternative drug (see Table 28-4).[3,73,148-159] Clarithromycin and azithromycin were as effective as other commonly used antimicrobial agents when employed in randomized multicenter trials for the treatment of pharyngitis, sinusitis, community-acquired pneumonia (including *M. pneumoniae* and *C. pneumoniae* pneumonia), and skin infections.[162,183,184,214] Clarithromycin or azithromycin have been considered alternatives to penicillin in treating group A β-hemolytic streptococcal pharyngitis, especially in patients with penicillin allergies.[215] Treatment with a 10- to 14-day course of either clarithromycin (250 mg twice daily) or penicillin VK (250 mg every 6 hours) is equally effective.[184,216] Azithromycin administered for 5 days (500 mg on day 1 followed by 250 mg daily for 4 days) is effective in eradicating group A streptococci from the pharynx,[217] although shorter courses of 3-day treatment with azithromycin were associated with lower levels of bacteriologic eradication when compared to a 10-day course of penicillin V.[218] Clinical studies have demonstrated equal or superior tolerability and clinical and bacterial efficacy of azithromycin (12 mg/kg, once daily for 5 days) compared with a 10-day therapy with penicillin V in the treatment of pediatric streptococcal pharyngitis.[219] However, the effectiveness of short-course azithromycin in preventing acute rheumatic fever is unknown.[220] Moreover, with the rising prevalence of macrolide resistance by group A streptococci, the effectiveness of these agents in treating such infections when the susceptibility of the organism is unknown should be questioned.

Azithromycin administered for 5 days or clarithromycin for 7 to 10 days for the treatment of acute otitis media in children has been effective.[221,222] Side effects, mostly gastrointestinal, were more common with clarithromycin in those studies, but similar to azithromycin in one study that directly compared the two macrolides.[222] As with other antimicrobial agents, bacterial meningitis may develop during oral therapy with macrolides for otitis media in children, particularly when the susceptibility of the pathogen is not optimal and spinal fluid penetration of the drug is limited.[223] The dosage of clarithromycin recommended for adults for those conditions is 250 mg orally twice daily for 7 to 14 days, except with sinusitis or bronchitis caused by *H. influenzae,* in which case 500 mg twice daily is suggested. The recommended azithromycin dosage for the same conditions in adults is 500 mg orally on day 1 and 250 mg on days 2 through 5 for a 5-day course of therapy. The 5-day course is used because of the prolonged persistence of good concentrations of azithromycin in tissues.[184] In children, the recommended total dose of azithromycin administered over 5 days is 30 mg/kg (10 mg/kg on day 1 and 5 mg/kg on days 2 to 5) to treat acute otitis media. At present, the consideration to use these newer agents rather than erythromycin for those aforementioned conditions must balance the potential advantages of a low incidence of side effects and infrequent dosing with the disadvantages of no increased effectiveness and a higher cost. Azithromycin can be given effectively for a shorter duration than clarithromycin and may be associated with fewer gastrointestinal disturbances, especially in children. However, with the substantial and rising prevalence of macrolide-resistant *S. pneumoniae* strains, poor response to treatment of acute otitis media can be expected in some patients treated with a macrolide alone.

Guidelines available for the treatment of adult outpatients with community-acquired pneumonia include the use of a macrolide as a first-line agent.[224-226] Erythromycin administered orally is poorly tolerated because of gastrointestinal side effects; therefore, the more expensive macrolides, azithromycin and clarithromycin, are often used instead. All three macrolides have good activity against most pathogens that commonly cause community-acquired pneumonia, many strains of

S. pneumoniae, and almost all strains of *M. pneumonia, C. pneumoniae, Legionella* species, and *Moraxella catarrhalis* (see Table 28-1).[33] However, the rising prevalence, already discussed, of macrolide resistance by strains of *S. pneumoniae,* especially those that are penicillin resistant, requires caution in the use of any of the macrolides as a sole agent when that organism may be causing pneumonia. That concern would be greatest for older adults or persons with underlying medical conditions. Macrolides, with their ability to concentrate intracellularly, are effective against intracellular pathogens, including *C. pneumoniae, Legionella* species, and *C. burnetii* (the agent of Q fever).[227] Treatment with macrolides of lower respiratory tract infection with *M. pneumoniae* and *C. pneumoniae* in children shortens the clinical course of infection.[228] In the treatment of patients with nonpneumococcal pneumonia, erythromycin and azithromycin were equally effective (76% and 79%, respectively) in achieving clinical and radiologic resolution.[193] The longer half-life of azithromycin allows a shorter duration of therapy, and in one retrospective study, a 3-day course of azithromycin (daily dose, 500 mg) was as effective as a 5-day course (500 mg in a single dose the first day, followed by 250 mg daily for 4 days) in the treatment of atypical pneumonia.[229]

The generally recommended empirical therapy for community-acquired pneumonia requiring hospitalization includes the combination of a macrolide and a β-lactam; this recommendation is based on observational studies that indicated that treatment with this combination as the initial regimen was associated with briefer hospital stays and a lower mortality rate than treatment with a cephalosporin alone.[230,231] In addition, two retrospective studies found that in cases of bacteremic pneumococcal pneumonia, dual antimicrobial therapy, including a macrolide, reduced mortality.[232,233] A study by Martinez and colleagues suggests that a benefit of lower mortality is achieved with combination therapy, including a macrolide, in community-acquired pneumonia associated with *S. pneumoniae,* including penicillin-susceptible strains, although sample size was small and the study was retrospective in design.[234] The possible benefit of adding a macrolide to a β-lactam agent in the treatment of bacteremic pneumococcal pneumonia may result from several factors,[234a] including antimicrobial synergism, macrolide-induced attenuation of cytokine production,[100] diminished adherence of pneumococci to respiratory epithelial cells,[42] and the coexistence of atypical pathogens. However, in vitro studies have not shown antimicrobial synergism,[235] and one study demonstrated in vitro and in vivo (in a mouse peritonitis model) antagonism between penicillin and erythromycin against *S. pneumoniae,* possibly caused by the inhibitory activity of erythromycin on the growth rate of the bacteria, attenuating the bacterial activity of penicillin.[236]

Although macrolides are becoming less reliable in the treatment of pneumococcal pneumonia, clarithromycin and azithromycin show increasing promise in the treatment of *Legionella* pneumonia.[153,167] Azithromycin showed superior results in an animal model of that infection,[192] and its lower likelihood of drug interactions compared with the other macrolides gives it a potential advantage, especially in the treatment of immunodeficient patients, who often are receiving multiple medications, and including those undergoing hepatic metabolism by the CYP-450 system. The suggested dosage of azithromycin for this condition for adults is 500 mg orally or intravenously for 5 to 10 days.[153]

Bordetella pertussis is susceptible in vitro to azithromycin and clarithromycin,[19] but limited studies are available on their clinical effectiveness.[237] In a study involving a small number of children with pertussis in Japan, a 5-day course of azithromycin and a 7-day course of clarithromycin were as effective in eradicating *B. pertussis* from cultures 1 week after treatment as in historical control subjects who had been treated with erythromycin for 2 weeks.[150] Until more data from clinical studies evaluating clarithromycin and azithromycin are available, the American Academy of Pediatrics recommends erythromycin as the antimicrobial agent of choice for treatment of and prophylaxis against pertussis, and clarithromycin (15 to 20 mg/kg/day orally in two divided doses, with a maximum of 1g/day, for 10 to 14 days) and azithromycin (10 to 12 mg/kg/day orally in one dose, with a maximum of 500 mg/day, for 5 to 7 days) as alternatives for patients who cannot tolerate erythromycin.[238]

Clarithromycin (500 mg orally twice daily) or azithromycin (500 mg orally once daily) in addition to ethambutol with or without rifabutin are now considered the drugs of choice in the treatment of disseminated *M. avium* complex infections in patients with AIDS.[176] Relatively few mutations are associated with macrolide resistance in mycobacteria, and all are in genes encoding the peptidyltransferase region of the 23S rRNA.[239] Therefore, the use of the macrolides alone is often associated with clinical relapse and the emergence of macrolide-resistant organisms.[240] In AIDS patients with CD4+ T-lymphocyte counts lower than 100 cells/mm^3, prophylaxis of disseminated *M. avium* complex infection with clarithromycin (500 mg orally once or twice daily) or azithromycin (1200 mg orally once weekly) is effective.[241,242] Clarithromycin prophylaxis of this condition has been demonstrated to increase survival.[241] Discontinuation of a macrolide-based prophylaxis for *M. avium* complex infection may be possible in patients who have been given prophylaxis for at least 1 year and whose CD4+ counts have increased to greater than 100 cells/μL on highly active antiretroviral therapy.[243] In patients who develop disseminated infection despite prophylaxis, macrolide-resistant isolates are frequently found.[241]

A single oral dose of azithromycin (20 mg/kg, up to 1 g) is highly effective in treating trachoma and has become the treatment of choice.[176,244] A single oral 1-g dose of azithromycin has been as effective as a 1-week course of doxycycline in the treatment of *C. trachomatis* urethritis and cervicitis[154] and acute nongonococcal urethritis (caused by *C. trachomatis* or *Ureaplasma urealyticum*) in men.[245] Azithromycin (1-g single oral dose) is as effective as ceftriaxone (250-mg intramuscular dose) in treating chancroid.[246]

The majority of patients with peptic ulcer disease can now be cured with short courses of antimicrobial agents combined with an acid-reducing agent, often a proton pump inhibitor or ranitidine bismuth citrate.[247] Clarithromycin (500 mg orally daily) with either metronidazole, amoxicillin, or tetracycline given for 7 days, together with the aforementioned acid-reducing agents, is very effective.[247] Failure is often associated with primary resistance by *H. pylori* strains to one of these antimicrobials (relatively common to metronidazole and rare to clarithromycin in several studies) or with the emergence of secondary resistance, which occurs more frequently if only one antimicrobial agent is used or if two are used in the presence of primary resistance to one of them.[248,249]

Azithromycin is an effective alternative to ciprofloxacin in the treatment of *Campylobacter* enteritis, but in some areas azithromycin-resistant strains are common.[151,250] Azithromycin treatment for 5 days was found to be as effective as ciprofloxacin in the treatment of shigellosis in a randomized controlled trial and can be considered a good alternative therapy for that condition, especially for children and pregnant women.[156,176]

Clarithromycin has been used effectively in a variety of mycobacterial infections other than tuberculosis and infections caused by *M. avium* complex. It can serve as the central drug or as an alternative in treating infections caused by *Mycobacterium chelonae,*[251] *M. fortuitum, M. genavense,* and *M. kansasii.*[176] In deep-seated infections and in immunocompromised patients with these infections, it is suggested that therapy be carried out with more than one active agent to decrease the chance for the emergence of resistant strains.[252] Clarithromycin has had a limited trial suggesting its effectiveness in treating leprosy and can serve as an alternative drug for that disease.[176,253]

Several studies suggest that clarithromycin (500 mg twice daily for 21 days) or azithromycin (for 7 to 10 days) is effective in treating most cases of early Lyme disease.[254,255] One of those studies demonstrated that azithromycin (500 mg daily for 7 days) was less effective than amoxicillin (500 mg three times daily for 20 days).[255] In some situations, such as allergy to β-lactam antibiotics in pregnant women or allergy to both β-lactam and tetracycline antibiotics, azithromycin may be an effective alternative treatment for Lyme disease. In addition, azithromycin (when given with atovaquone) is as effective as clindamycin and quinine for the treatment of *Babesia microti* infections, a frequent coinfecting agent with *B. burgdorferi.*[159] Although clindamycin and quinine remains the preferred regimen in severe cases of babesiosis, atovaquone and azithromycin is an effective treatment regimen for non–life-threatening babesiosis in immunocompetent adult patients.[159]

Azithromycin has been shown to have antimalarial activity similar to that of doxycycline in animal models.[256] Two human volunteer studies suggested that azithromycin has potential in the prevention of chloroquine-resistant *Plasmodium falciparum* infection.[256,257] Two field trials on the use of azithromycin as a single agent for malaria prophylaxis demonstrated only moderate efficacy (70% to 90%) for *P. falciparum* compared with high efficacy for *Plasmodium vivax.*[258,259] Azithromycin in combination with other antimalarial agents, such as chloroquine or quinine, produces synergistic interactions in vitro.[260]

In an uncontrolled study, nine patients with AIDS and chronic cryptosporidiosis were treated with azithromycin at a variety of doses for 30 to 360 days (mean, 129 days) and in seven there was a "complete" clinical response, with a major decrease (five patients) or eradication (two patients) of parasites in the stool.[261] However, in another limited study of azithromycin, given for shorter periods for the same condition, results were poor.[262] In one study, the use of clarithromycin for prophylaxis for *Mycobacterium avium* complex was highly protective against development of cryptosporidiosis in immune-suppressed HIV-infected persons, whereas no protective effect was seen in the 54 patients reporting taking azithromycin.[263] With the availability in some communities of highly active antiretroviral therapy for AIDS, the relative role of a drug with activity against cryptosporidia in improving diarrheal disease in these patients needs to be interpreted with data from appropriate control groups.

There has been great interest in the potential role of chronic infections (especially those caused by *C. pneumoniae*) in potentiating atherosclerosis and vascular thromboses, including coronary artery disease. In this regard, azithromycin has been investigated because of its activity against *C. pneumoniae* and its ability to accumulate in high concentrations in atherosclerotic plaques.[264] One study in a small number of men who had survived myocardial infarction demonstrated a significant decrease in subsequent adverse cardiovascular events in those who had substantial titers of antibody to *C. pneumoniae* and were given azithromycin (500 mg daily for 3 or 6 days), compared with a similar group of men who were not treated with azithromycin.[265] However, clinical trials have not shown a benefit of macrolide use in preventing recurrent events in patients with acute coronary syndromes.[266,267] Assuming a real effect of the macrolide on such cardiac events, it is uncertain whether the result is related to its antimicrobial activity, its anti-inflammatory activity on atheromata or thrombogenesis (discussed earlier under Erythromycin, Antimicrobial Activity), both of these activities, or other unknown effects. A large randomized, placebo-controlled trial of stable patients with previous myocardial infarction and IgG antibodies to *C. pneumoniae* treated with azithromycin for 12 weeks and followed for a median of 14 months did not demonstrate a significant reduction of clinical sequelae of coronary heart disease.[267a]

KETOLIDES

Ketolides are a new class of semisynthetic agents derived from erythromycin A that have increased acid stability, that have increased antibacterial potency against many bacteria resistant to macrolides, and that are unable to induce the MLS_B methylase type of resistance. Telithromycin (HMR 3647, or Ketek), which has been approved for clinical use in the United States and is already in use in Europe (since 2001) and some Latin American countries, is the first member of this new class.

Derivation, Chemistry, and Preparations

Ketolides are derived from erythromycin A, differing in having a replacement of the L-cladinose moiety that is present at position 3 in other 14-member macrolides with a ketone group. This is the only chemical modification necessary to classify a ketolide. The name ketolide is derived from *keto* (3-keto group) and *olide* (lactone).[268] Telithromycin (Fig. 28-4) has additional modifications, including a 11,12-cyclic carbamate linkage in place of two hydroxyl groups of erythromycin A. The latter ring also has a butyl imidazolyl pyridinyl side chain. In addition, a methoxy group replaces a hydroxyl group at position 6 of the lactone ring of telithromycin.

The alterations in structure of telithromycin are related to its improved antimicrobial properties. The replacement of L-cladinose with a 3-keto function prevents induction of MLS_B resistance.[1,268,269] In conjunction with the 3-keto group, the addition of a methoxy group at position C6 of erythromycin A prevents internal hemiketalization, thereby making ketolides more acid stable.[268,270] Substitution of the C_{11}-C_{12} hydroxyl groups of the erythronolide A ring by a carbamate residue results in enhanced antibacterial activity when compared with erythromycin A, and increases stability in an acid medium.[268] The butyl imidazolyl pyridinyl side chain of the cyclic carbamate is responsible for tighter binding to ribosomes and thereby greater potency as well as diminished susceptibility to bacterial efflux systems.[268,270,271]

Once marketed in the United States, telithromycin will be available in 400-mg film-coated tablets. An adult intravenous and a pediatric formulation of telithromycin are in development.

Mechanisms of Action and Resistance

Ketolides, specifically telithromycin, have a mechanism of action essentially similar to that of erythromycin A and other macrolides—that is, to inhibit bacterial protein synthesis by interacting closely to the peptidyl transferase site of the 50S ribosomal subunit,[1,2] and to interfere with the formation of the 50S ribosomal subunit.[4] The difference between the mechanisms of action of telithromycin and macrolides is in the nature of their interaction with the ribosome: telithromycin has a higher binding affinity and mechanisms that may sometimes overcome the methylation of binding sites on the peptidyl transferase loop.

The 23S rRNA molecule in the 50S ribosomal subunit contains six distinct structural domains, with domains II and V being the most important sites for interaction with macrolides and ketolides. Although the major site of interaction of traditional macrolides is domain V, at nucleotides A2058 and A2059,[271] ketolides are also able to interact with domain II of 23S rRNA, at nucleotide A752.[271] This additional interaction is mainly due to the heteroaromatic ring side chain of the C_{11}-C_{12} cyclic carbamate. The dual interaction between telithromycin and domains V and II allows a higher overall binding affinity for telithromycin than for traditional macrolides. That property allows telithromycin to have greater potency and often greater and significant activity compared to traditional macrolides against bacterial strains exhibiting the M type (drug efflux) and MLS_B (ribosomal methylase) types of resistance.

In addition to inhibiting protein synthesis by directly interfering with elongation of polypeptide chains, telithromycin is able to inhibit the formation of the 50S ribosomal subunit, and at high enough concentrations, unlike macrolides, it is also able to inhibit the formation of the 30S ribosomal subunit.[272]

Resistance to telithromycin is as yet uncommon. Telithromycin is a poor inducer or poor substrate for bacterial strains expressing efflux mechanisms of resistance. The telithromycin MICs for such strains are sometimes higher than for strains without efflux pumps but generally remain in the therapeutic range.[268] Ketolides are also poor inducers of the MLS_B methylase genes, and telithromycin retains good activity against strains of *S. pneumoniae, S. pyogenes,* and *S. aureus* with inducibly expressed MLS_B resistance, but strains of *S. aureus* harboring a constitutive *erm* gene are resistant.[268,273] Among *S. pyogenes* isolates harboring a constitutive *erm*B gene, and therefore resistant to erythromycin A, telithromycin MIC values ranged from 4 to 64 µg/mL.[274] In contrast, telithromycin remains potent against *S. pneumoniae* isolates with the constitutive *erm* gene.[274] Structural differences in the ribosomes of bacteria may explain this difference in activity of telithromycin against strains harboring a constitutive *erm*

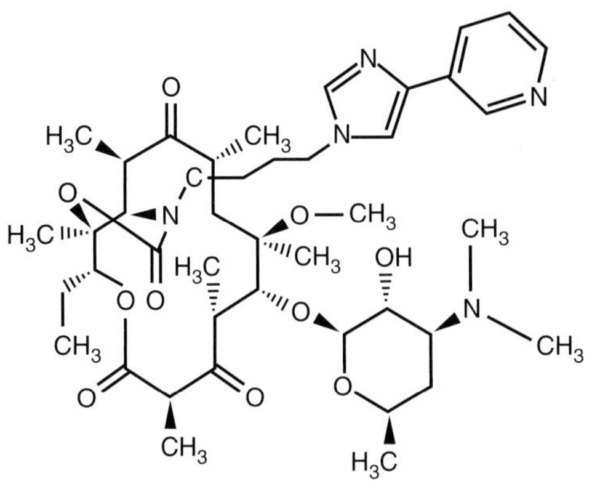

FIGURE 28-4. Telithromycin.

gene.[274] Rare bacterial strains have shown increased MICs to telithromycin caused by mutations in the bases of 23S rRNA of the 50S ribosomal subunit or in ribosomal proteins; most have been laboratory isolates,[268] but these may predict future clinical isolates that will be ketolide resistant. *Nocardia* species are capable of inactivating telithromycin by glycosylating or phosphorylating the hydroxyl group on the desosamine sugar.[268]

Antimicrobial Activity

Compared to macrolides, the ketolides have improved in vitro activity against a majority of gram-positive aerobic bacteria.[275] Ketolides show greater activity than clarithromycin and azithromycin against erythromycin-susceptible strains of *S. pneumoniae*.[276] Against erythromycin-resistant strains of *S. pneumoniae*, ketolides have higher MIC values (compared to erythromycin-susceptible strains) but retain good activity.[274] Ketolides are highly active against erythromycin-resistant strains of *S. pyogenes* when resistance is of the M or inducible MLS$_B$ phenotype, but their activity is reduced when resistance is of the constitutive MLS$_B$ phenotype.[277] Ketolides show excellent activity against *S. aureus* isolates that are erythromycin susceptible or with inducible erythromycin resistance (including most strains of methicillin-resistant *S. aureus*); however, the ketolide shows little activity against *S. aureus* isolates with constitutive erythromycin resistance.[13,278] Ketolides are more potent than macrolides against erythromycin-susceptible and erythromycin-resistant *Enterococcus faecalis* isolates but exhibit poor activity against *Enterococcus faecium* strains.[278]

Enterobacteriaceae are intrinsically resistant to macrolide antibiotics, and the same is true for ketolides.[268] However, the activity of ketolides against *H. influenzae* is similar to that of azithromycin.[279] In addition, ketolides demonstrate consistent activity against *M. catarrhalis*[280] and *B. pertussis*.[19] Telithromycin has shown good in vitro activity against *Propionibacterium* and peptostreptococcal species but poor activity against *B. fragilis* and *Fusobacterium* species.[268]

Ketolides are similar to, or slightly more active than, the macrolides against *C. pneumoniae, L. pneumophila,* and *M. pneumoniae*.[22,24,281]

Ketolides have poor in vitro activity against *M. tuberculosis* and are less potent than clarithromycin against *M. avium*.[282]

Clinical Pharmacology

Telithromycin is well absorbed after oral administration with or without food, and it is approximately 60% bioavailable in both young and older persons.[11] The maximum concentration (Cmax) after 7 days of once-daily dosing with 800 mg telithromycin is approximately 2.27 mg/L,[283] well above MICs of common respiratory pathogens. Telithromycin concentrates well in both extracellular tissue and intracellular compartments, such as in alveolar macrophages and polymorphonuclear granulocytes.[14] Approximately 70% of telithromycin is metabolized, mainly by the cytochrome CYP 450 3A4 enzyme system

in the liver.[14] The elimination half-life is approximately 9.5 hours.[283] No dosage adjustment is necessary in patients with mild to moderate renal impairment, although in the presence of severe renal impairment, the dose should be reduced by 50%.[11]

Adverse Reactions

Clinical trials suggest that telithromycin has a safety profile similar to that of clarithromycin and azithromycin, with complaints involving mainly the gastrointestinal tract (diarrhea, nausea, vomiting).[283,284] Abnormalities in liver function are occasionally encountered in patients treated with telithromycin, but they resolve with discontinuation of the drug.[284]

More serious adverse reactions observed in clinical trials are less common (0.4%); they include allergic reactions, liver injury, pseudomembranous colitis, erythema multiforme, blurred vision, and severe gastroenteritis and vomiting.[284] Telithromycin showed no significantly increased risk of QT prolongation when used at therapeutic dosages.[284]

Several reports, beginning in early 2003, of exacerbation of myasthenia gravis in patients treated with telithromycin, including one death, led to a drug warning to European physicians calling for extreme caution in the use of telithromycin in patients with that condition. Patients with myasthenia gravis experienced worsening dyspnea and muscle weakness within hours of first taking telithromycin.[285] The cause of this serious side effect is unknown, but the effect may be similar to the problems with ciliary body function that can lead to difficulties in visual accommodation, causing blurred vision in apparently healthy young persons.

Drug Interactions

Ketolide use is associated with increased concentrations of several drugs that undergo hepatic metabolism by the CYP 450 3A4 system.[284] As with some macrolides, these interactions can lead to serious toxicity. For example, telithromycin slows the metabolism of simvastatin, leading to increased concentrations. Although rhabdomyolysis has not been specifically observed with the concomitant use of telithromycin and simvastatin, the combination is to be avoided.[284] Because co-administration of cisapride with telithromycin can lead to increased serum cisapride concentrations and prolongation of the QT interval, this combination is also contraindicated.[284] The full range of drug interactions is likely to become more evident upon introduction of telithromycin into clinical practice. At present, it should be assumed that drug interactions involving telithromycin will be similar to those that have been observed with erythromycin and clarithromycin (see Table 28-3).

Potential Uses for Telithromycin

In community-acquired pneumonia, telithromycin administered orally (800 mg daily for 7 to 10 days) has comparable efficacy (clinical cure rate, 93% to 94%) to amoxicillin (1 g three times a day for 10 days), clarithromycin (500 mg twice a day for 10 days), and trovafloxacin (200 mg once daily for 10 days).[284] Telithromycin was also efficacious in treating community-acquired pneumonia in older adults, and in treating severe disease, including pneumococcal bacteremia.[284] When analyzed by pathogens, telithromycin was highly efficacious in patients with community-acquired pneumonia caused by penicillin- or macrolide-resistant *S. pneumoniae* and atypical pathogens such as *C. pneumoniae, Legionella,* and *M. pneumoniae*.[284] Telithromycin administered orally (800 mg daily for 5 days) was efficacious in treating acute exacerbations of chronic bronchitis, and this was comparable to a 10-day regimen of cefuroxime axetil (500 mg twice daily), and to amoxicillin/clavulanic acid (500/125 mg three times daily).[284] A 5-day course of telithromycin was as effective as a 10-day course in treating adults with acute maxillary sinusitis, and it was comparable in efficacy to a 10-day regimen of amoxicillin/clavulanic acid (500/125 mg three times daily) in patients with acute sinusitis.[284] In adults and adolescents with group A β-hemolytic streptococci pharyngitis or tonsillitis, a 5-day regimen of telithromycin was as effective as a 10-day regimen of clarithromycin 250 mg twice daily.[284]

The FDA has approved telithromycin at an 800-mg oral dose daily for the treatment of community-acquired pneumonia, acute bacterial exacerbation of chronic bronchitis, acute sinusitis, and group A β-hemolytic *Streptococcus* tonsillitis or pharyngitis in adults.[284] With the increase in the prevalence of erythromycin-resistant strains of common bacterial respiratory pathogens, such as *S. pneumoniae* and group A streptococci, ketolides are likely to become important alternative antibacterial drugs for these circumstances. The convenience of the once-daily dosage regimen of telithromycin and its activity against many penicillin- and macrolide-resistant respiratory pathogens will make it a potentially useful alternative for treatment of community-acquired respiratory tract infections. However, factors that may limit its use include emerging knowledge of potentially serious adverse events involving muscle function, high drug cost, the potential for drug interactions involving the hepatic microsomal system, and the potential emergence of resistant organisms as a result of ribosomal mutations or constitutive ribosomal methylation mechanisms.

DIRITHROMYCIN

Dirithromycin, a semisynthetic 14-member macrolide antibiotic, is a prodrug that is rapidly converted to erythromycylamine by nonenzymatic hydrolysis after intestinal absorption. The latter differs from erythromycin in having an amino group instead of a carbonyl group at the C9 position of the lactone ring. Dirithromycin became available for pharmaceutical use in the United States in 1995 and is provided in 250-mg enteric-coated tablets. Its mechanism of action is the same as that of the other macrolides. The antimicrobial activity of dirithromycin against gram-positive bacteria is about the same or half that of erythromycylamine, which is usually fourfold to eightfold less active than erythromycin against *S. pneumoniae, H. influenzae,* and *M. catarrhalis.*[286,287] Strains of *H. influenzae* are often resistant to achievable serum concentrations of dirithromycin. Dirithromycin is less active than erythromycin against *L. pneumophila, M. pneumoniae,* and *C. pneumoniae.*[286,288,289] There is complete cross-resistance between erythromycin and dirithromycin.

Erythromycylamine, the active product of hydrolysis of the prodrug after absorption, reaches peak serum concentrations in 4 to 5 hours, achieving levels lower than those of other macrolides (<1 µg/mL).[286] About 10% of an oral dose is bioavailable. The drug is widely distributed and achieves much higher levels in tissue than in serum. There are no data on cerebrospinal fluid penetration. Erythromycylamine, and a smaller amount of dirithromycin, are eliminated in the bile and feces, with a half-life of 30 to 44 hours. About 2% of the orally administered dose is recovered in the urine. There is little or no hepatic metabolism, and slow elimination allows once-daily dosing, with 500 mg suggested in adults.

In a limited number of studies, dirithromycin was similar to erythromycin in clinical and bacteriologic effectiveness in the treatment of community-acquired pneumonia caused by *S. pneumoniae, H. influenzae, L. pneumophila, M. pneumoniae,* or *C. pneumoniae.*[287,290] The drug was also effective in treating acute bacterial exacerbations of bronchitis, streptococcal pharyngitis, and skin and soft tissue infections.

The adverse effects of dirithromycin have mainly been limited to gastrointestinal symptoms, especially abdominal pain and nausea, probably similar in incidence to the effects associated with erythromycin. Dirithromycin does not inhibit the CYP-450 hepatic enzyme system and has not been implicated in the drug interactions typical of erythromycin in relation to that system.[291] Its limited in vitro antimicrobial activity and the clinical studies of effectiveness preclude a recommendation for its widespread use.

OTHER MACROLIDES

Troleandomycin, an ester of the 14-member ring macrolide oleandomycin, is still marketed, although it has no advantages over erythromycin and may occasionally cause cholestatic hepatitis. It is a potent inhibitor of the cytochrome P-450 enzyme system.[146] Roxithromycin is a 14-member ring macrolide that, like dirithromycin, has a modification at the C9 position. It is an investigational drug in the United States, with in vitro antibacterial activity somewhat less than or similar to that of erythromycin but with a longer half-life.[183,286] In a double-blind, randomized, placebo-controlled trial in patients with unstable angina or non–Q-wave myocardial infarction, those who received roxithromycin (150 mg orally twice daily for 3 to 30 days) had significantly decreased rates of severe recurrent ischemia, acute myocardial infarction, or death from cardiac ischemia when assessed at day 31.[292] The authors attributed the results to an antichlamydial or an anti-inflammatory effect of the macrolide on atheromata.

LINCOMYCIN AND CLINDAMYCIN

Derivation, Chemistry, and Preparations

Lincomycin was isolated in 1962 from an organism, *Streptomyces lincolnensis,* obtained from soil near Lincoln, Nebraska. Many of its biologic properties are similar to those of erythromycin, but it is chemically unrelated, consisting of an amino acid linked to an amino sugar (Fig. 28-5). Chemical modification provided clindamycin (7-chloro-7-deoxy-lincomycin) (see Fig. 28-5) with increased antibacterial potency and absorption after oral administration.[293] Because there are no therapeutic advantages for lincomycin over clindamycin, the discussion here concentrates on the latter, although both are still marketed as pharmaceuticals. Both are weak bases that are readily water soluble when provided as salts.

Lincomycin (Lincocin) is available as the hydrochloride salt in 250- and 500-mg capsules and syrup for oral administration and in solution (300 mg/mL) for parenteral use. Clindamycin (Cleocin) is prepared as the hydrochloride salt of the base in 75-, 150-, and 300-mg capsules and of the palmitate ester for pediatric suspension. It is supplied as the phosphate ester for intramuscular or intravenous use (150 mg/mL). It is also available in a topical solution, gel, and lotion for the treatment of acne vulgaris, and in a concentration of 2% in a vaginal cream for the treatment of bacterial vaginosis.

Mechanism of Action

The lincosamide antibiotics have, in susceptible organisms, the same or overlapping 50S ribosomal binding sites as those for the macrolides and chloramphenicol, and they may compete with these drugs for binding.[1] Protein synthesis is inhibited primarily in early chain elongation by interference with the transpeptidation reaction,[1] possibly by blocking of the P (peptidyl donor) site. Like the macrolides, the lincosamide antibiotics may also stimulate the dissociation of peptidyl-tRNA from ribosomes.

Antimicrobial Activity and Mechanisms of Resistance

In vitro susceptibilities to clindamycin are given in Table 28-5.[27,47,49,56,62,293-295] Clindamycin is more potent than lincomycin but similar in degree of activity to erythromycin against staphylococci, pneumococci, *S. pyogenes,* and streptococci of the viridans group. However, although erythromycin demonstrates at least moderate activity against *Enterococcus, H. influenzae,* and *N. meningitidis,* clindamycin is generally inactive against these organisms at clinically achievable concentrations. In contrast, clindamycin shows significantly greater activity than erythromycin against most clinically significant anaerobic bacteria, particularly *B. fragilis*[75] and some erythromycin-resistant strains of *S. aureus.*[296] Clindamycin has been one of the most active antibiotics available against *B. fragilis,* but documented increases in resistance have been reported.[297] A recent survey of the susceptibility of *B. fragilis* group isolates collected in the United States from 1997 to 2000 revealed clindamycin resistance in 23% of strains.[297] Resistance to clindamycin by that group of organisms is significantly more likely when the infection is acquired in hospital or when the patient has received prior antimicrobial therapy.[298] Clindamycin resistance to anaerobes can show substantial variation among hospitals as well as across geographic regions.[299] Resistance to clindamycin by anaerobes also includes 10% to 20% of clostridial species other than *C. perfringens,*[300] 8% of peptostreptococci, 9% of *Fusobacterium* species, and

11% of *Prevotella* strains.[295] All the Enterobacteriaceae are resistant to clindamycin.

Clindamycin provides high activity against pneumococci and group A streptococci; however, clinical isolates showing resistance to clindamycin and erythromycin have been increasingly reported from different areas, as already discussed under Erythromycin. However, in the United States, most macrolide-resistant *S. pneumoniae* and *S. pyogenes* strains are of the M phenotype, which does not show cross-resistance to clindamycin.[39] One study of isolates of *S. pneumoniae* from middle ears and nasal sinuses of infected children in Houston showed that more than 90% of strains that had in vitro susceptibilities to penicillin classified as intermediate or highly resistant were sensitive to clindamycin.[301] In a more recent study, 70% of erythromycin-resistant *S. pneumoniae* isolates collected from 1994 through 1999 were sensitive to clindamycin (MIC, <1 μg/mL).[40] In a study involving group A streptococcal clinical strains from Italy, 5% of 303 isolates from 1993 and approximately 17% of 799 isolates from 1995 were resistant to clindamycin.[302]

The antibacterial activity of clindamycin against *S. pyogenes* displays several characteristics that have the potential to be clinically advantageous and are less prominently demonstrated or absent in the penicillin family. Subinhibitory concentrations of clindamycin diminish encapsulation of group A streptococci,[303] production of M protein,[304] pyrogenic exotoxin A, and promitogenic activity[305] in broth cultures of *S. pyogenes*. In a mouse model of *S. pyogenes* myositis, clindamycin administration was more effective than penicillin in limiting bacterial growth and bringing about survival.[306,307]

Clindamycin continues to have substantial activity against methicillin-sensitive *S. aureus*, with only 1% to 5% of strains collected in 1997 from the United States, Canada, and Latin America showing resistance; however, against methicillin-resistant isolates from the same study, 57% to 85% of isolates were resistant.[56] Cross-resistance of *S. aureus* between lincomycin and clindamycin is complete. The MICs of clindamycin and erythromycin in vitro are generally similar for *S. aureus* strains that are sensitive to both agents; however, resistance can be selected in vitro by serial subculture in the presence of subinhibitory concentrations of either drug, and it occurs slowly for clindamycin and more rapidly for erythromycin.[293,308] In contrast, strains that are sensitive to clindamycin and resistant to erythromycin can be rapidly selected for clindamycin resistance by serial subculture on clindamycin. Consistent with these in vitro observations, the emergence of clindamycin-resistant *S. aureus* has been noted in clindamycin-treated patients, in particular when the organisms had demonstrated erythromycin resistance at the onset of treatment (i.e., the dissociated resistance of Garrod [inducible MLS$_B$]).[293,308] The bacterial strains possessing the dissociated resistance mechanism can often be detected in the laboratory with the D test—a double-disk diffusion test in which the zone of inhibition around the clindamycin disk is blunted on the side facing the erythromycin disk.[308a]

The antibacterial activity of lincomycin and clindamycin has been shown, in limited in vitro studies, to be bactericidal for *S. pneumoniae*, *S. pyogenes*, and *S. aureus*. Its killing activity is similar to that of erythromycin and therefore probably varies with the concentration, bacterial species, and inoculum. It is more slowly bactericidal for *S. aureus* than are the penicillins,[310] and it is inconsistently bactericidal for *B. fragilis*.[311]

Clindamycin has substantial in vitro activity against *T. gondii* in infected human fibroblasts.[312] Clindamycin and its three major metabolites are inhibitory against *P. falciparum*.[313]

There are several mechanisms of resistance to the lincosamide antibiotics. First, alteration in particular 50S ribosomal proteins of the receptor site confers resistance to erythromycin and often to the lincosamides[1]; this mechanism was previously discussed for erythromycin. Second, alteration in the 23S ribosomal RNA of the 50S ribosomal subunit by methylation of adenine[1,88] has also been discussed. It is usually plasmid mediated and provides the MLS$_B$ type of resistance, which includes that exhibited by some strains of *S. aureus* and *B. fragilis* to clindamycin. Third, resistance is conferred through inactivation of lincomycin and clindamycin by a few isolates of staphylococci (including *S. aureus*) that possess a plasmid-mediated 3-lincomycin 4-clindamycin 0-nucleotidyltransferase that catalyzes the nucleotidylation of the hydroxyl group in position 4 of clindamycin.[81,314] This adenylation of the lincosamides is associated with high-level resistance to lincomycin, but clindamycin resistance may not be detected by routine methods. The adenylation of clindamycin is associated with impaired bactericidal activity and decreased activity at high inoculum levels. The nucleotide sequences of the plasmid-mediated genes *linA* and *linA'*, which encode for the inactivating enzymes, have been determined.[314] Finally, Enterobacteriaceae, *Pseudomonas* spp., and *Acinetobacter* spp. are intrinsically resistant to clindamycin, apparently because of poor permeability of the cellular outer envelope to the drug.[81]

Clinical Pharmacology

Peak serum levels achieved after oral administration of clindamycin occur earlier and are at least twice as high as those of lincomycin. Absorption of clindamycin is about 90% and is slightly delayed, but not decreased, by ingestion of food, whereas that of lincomycin is markedly decreased.[293] Mean peak serum concentrations of clindamycin in adults after single oral doses of 150 and 300 mg occur at 1 hour and are 2.5 and 3.6 μg/mL, respectively; at 6 hours, they are 0.7 and 1.1 μg/mL, respectively. The esters clindamycin palmitate in suspension for oral use and clindamycin phosphate for parenteral use are absorbed as the inactive ester and are rapidly hydrolyzed in the blood to the active base. After intramuscular administration, which causes little pain, mean peak serum levels are reached in 3 hours and are about 6 μg/mL after a 300-mg dose and 9 μg/mL after a 600-mg

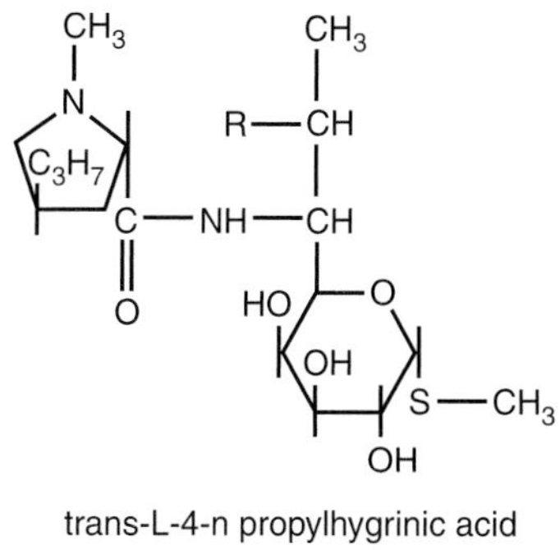

trans-L-4-n propylhygrinic acid

FIGURE 28-5. The lincosamide antibiotics. Lincomycin, R = OH; clindamycin, R = Cl.

TABLE 28-5 In Vitro Susceptibilities to Clindamycin

Organism	Minimal Inhibitory Concentration (μg/mL)	
	Range	*MIC$_{50}$*
Streptococcus pneumoniae	≤0.25-≥128	≤0.25
Streptococcus pyogenes	≤0.06->64	≤0.06
Viridans streptococci	≤0.06->256	≤0.06-0.12
Enterococcus	0.12->8	>8
Staphylococcus aureus	≤0.06->8	0.25
Staphylococcus epidermidis	<0.12->8	0.12
Clostridium perfringens	≤0.06->4	1
Neisseria gonorrhoeae	0.01-6.3	3.1
Haemophilus influenzae	0.4-50	12.5
Bacteroides fragilis group	0.25-16	1
Bacteroides melaninogenicus	≤0.1-1	<0.1
Fusobacterium spp.	≤0.008->16	0.015
Peptococcus spp.	≤0.1->100	≤0.5
Peptostreptococcus spp.	≤0.06->32	0.125
Mycoplasma pneumoniae	1.6-3.1	3.1

MIC$_{50}$, μg/mL; minimal inhibitory concentration for 50% of isolates.

dose; at 12 hours, they are 0.7 and 0.9 μg/mL, respectively.[315] In adult healthy volunteers, immediately after 20- to 45-minute intravenous infusions of 600, 900, or 1200 mg of clindamycin phosphate, serum levels of base are 10, 11, and 14 μg/mL, respectively. Higher levels after intravenous infusion have been reported in infected patients under treatment.[316] Dose regimens of intravenous clindamycin using 900 mg every 8 hours or 600 mg every 6 hours are considered acceptable.[317]

Limited studies have demonstrated good penetration of most tissues by the lincosamides, except for clinically insignificant entry of clindamycin into the cerebrospinal fluid, even with meningitis.[318] The concentration in bone compared with serum is particularly high.[319] Clindamycin administered to pregnant women readily passes the placental barrier and enters fetal blood and tissues.[120] Clindamycin is actively transported into polymorphonuclear leukocytes and macrophages[320] and is present in relatively high concentrations, compared with peak serum levels, in experimental abscesses.[321]

The normal half-life of clindamycin is 2.4 hours. Most of the absorbed drug is metabolized, probably by the liver, to products with variable antibacterial activity, including N-demethyl-clindamycin (more active than the parent compound) and clindamycin sulfoxide (less active), which have been detected in bile and urine but not in serum.[315] High bioactivity is found in bile, mostly as the N-demethyl metabolite; this represents a minor route of excretion and accounts for the activity assayed in feces after parenteral administration.[315,322] Clindamycin activity in feces persists for at least 5 days after 48 hours of parenteral administration and is associated with a major reduction in the population of sensitive bacteria in the colon that lasts for up to 14 days.[323] Clindamycin concentration in bile is markedly diminished or absent when the common bile duct is obstructed.[324] High clindamycin bioactivity, also mostly in the N-demethyl form, is found in the urine and persists for up to 4 days after a single dose, suggesting slow release from tissues.[316] Accurate data on the proportion of absorbed clindamycin that is excreted in the urine are not available because of the variable activity of the metabolites and their unknown proportions in urine.

The half-life of clindamycin is increased from 2.4 to about 6 hours in patients with severe renal failure, and peak blood levels after parenteral administration are about twice those in healthy people.[325] If modified at all, parenteral doses should be halved in such patients. Some prolongation of clindamycin activity in serum is noted in patients with severe liver disease.[326] Appreciable dose modification should be made when a patient exhibits concomitant severe renal and hepatic disease. Neither hemodialysis nor peritoneal dialysis removes significant amounts of clindamycin.

Adverse Reactions

Allergic reactions include a variety of rashes, fever, and rare cases of erythema multiforme and anaphylaxis. Diarrhea occurs in up to 20% of patients and is more common with oral administration. However, the major toxicity of lincomycin and clindamycin that now appreciably limits their use is the occurrence of pseudomembranous colitis caused by a toxin secreted by *C. difficile* that overgrows in the presence of these antibiotics.[327] This has been reported to occur in 0.01% to 10% of clindamycin-treated patients.[328] The syndrome may occur in association with administration of other antibiotics but does so less frequently; it is not related to the dose and may occur after oral or parenteral therapy. It has been reported after the use of clindamycin vaginal cream in a patient being treated for bacterial vaginosis.[329] The variable incidence of colitis in different reports has been ascribed to different diagnostic methods and the variable epidemiology of *C. difficile*.[328] Studies suggest that variabilities in the presence of humoral immunity (antitoxin) among individual patients account for some of the differences in susceptibility or recurrence of this infection.[330] It may begin during or as long as several weeks after a course of lincomycin or clindamycin therapy and is characterized by diarrhea, sometimes bloody, with fever and cramps and the appearance of yellow-white plaques on the colonic mucosa, seen by proctoscopy. The toxins of *C. difficile* can be detected in the stool of most patients with antibiotic-associated pseudomembranous colitis by using tissue cul-

ture cells and assaying for cytotoxicity, or enzyme-linked immunosorbent assays (ELISAs) for the toxins.[331] The cytotoxic effect can be prevented by neutralization of the toxin in the stool extract with *Clostridium sordellii* antitoxin. The syndrome can be protracted and may end fatally. Prompt cessation of the antibiotic is essential. Use of antiperistaltic drugs should be avoided because they may worsen the condition. Vancomycin given by mouth and oral metronidazole are effective in treatment.[327] Metronidazole is preferred to limit the selective pressure that potentiates the emergence of vancomycin-resistant enterococci in the environment. Relapse after treatment may occur when the immune reaction has been inadequate.

Minor reversible elevation of transaminase levels, unassociated with other evidence of liver abnormality, has commonly been observed in patients receiving clindamycin, especially by the parenteral route. Some of these may have been false-positive reactions associated with colorimetric rather than specific enzymatic measurements.[293] However, rare cases of frank hepatotoxicity, including jaundice associated with hepatocellular damage, have been observed.[332]

Isolated cases of reversible neutropenia, thrombocytopenia, and agranulocytosis associated with lincomycin or clindamycin therapy have been reported; their relation to the administration of the antibiotic was uncertain.

Hypotension and electrocardiographic changes have occasionally been reported, and cardiopulmonary arrest rarely, when large intravenous doses of lincomycin were given rapidly. These effects have not been reported with clindamycin.

Local irritative reactions are rare with these drugs. Intramuscular or intravenous administration is generally well tolerated.

Drug Interactions

Clindamycin may block neuromuscular transmission and may enhance the action of other blocking agents.[147] Clindamycin may decrease the effect of cyclosporine.[147] Clindamycin phosphate in solution is physically incompatible with ampicillin, diphenylhydantoin, barbiturates, aminophylline, calcium gluconate, and magnesium sulfate.

Uses of Clindamycin

The higher activity and absorption properties of clindamycin compared with lincomycin, along with no greater potential for toxicity, favor the former in all indications for use of these antibiotics. The lincosamides have been used in a variety of infections, often with good effect; however, appreciation of the potential for serious or even fatal toxicity with pseudomembranous colitis and the availability of safer alternative antibiotics should now generally limit the use of clindamycin to a few indications.[176]

The most important use of clindamycin is in the treatment of infections that are outside of the central nervous system and are likely to involve *B. fragilis* or other penicillin-resistant anaerobic bacteria. These particularly involve polymicrobial intra-abdominal or gynecologic pelvic infections. Clindamycin is likely to be beneficial where there is spillage of fecal flora associated with tissue damage, as in cases involving bowel damage or perforation. In these situations, studies of experimental animal models and patients with infection suggest that clindamycin decreases the likelihood of abscess formation involving fecal organisms, especially *B. fragilis*.[333] In these conditions, clindamycin is administered together with an aminoglycoside, a third-generation cephalosporin, or aztreonam because additional activity is required against Enterobacteriaceae. The beneficial effect of clindamycin in preventing or ameliorating morbidity from fecal abscess formation or other infections appears to be superior to that of penicillin, cephalothin, or aminoglycosides.[334] However, in comparative trials of therapy for intra-abdominal or pelvic sepsis, clindamycin, cefoxitin, metronidazole, imipenem, meropenem, ticarcillin-clavulanic acid, and chloramphenicol have shown similar effectiveness.[335-337] Although increasing resistance by the *B. fragilis* group to clindamycin has been reported,[297] there has not been good documentation correlating that with clinical failure of treatment,[338] probably because of the complex nature of those infections, which are usually polymicrobial and often are treated with broad-spectrum regimens combined with mechanical drainage.

Clindamycin may offer some advantage over penicillin G in the treatment of anaerobic bronchopulmonary infections,[339] and, in addition, it may serve as an alternative in patients who are allergic to penicillin. In a prospective, randomized study of 39 patients with community-acquired putrid lung abscess, clindamycin was more effective than penicillin in the time until eradication of fever and fetid sputum and in the "overall response" to treatment.[340] The study involved small numbers of patients and had some flaws in the analysis;[341] however, the superiority of clindamycin for some patients was demonstrated and may relate to observations that 15% to 25% of anaerobic pulmonary infections involve β-lactamase–producing strains of *B. fragilis, B. melaninogenicus, Prevotella ruminicola,* and *Bacteroides ureolyticus,* which are resistant to penicillin.[341] Another similar study also demonstrated a higher failure rate with penicillin than with clindamycin and attributed it to penicillin-resistant anaerobes.[342] That study was problematic in that penicillin oral therapy was used to complete the course of treatment of some patients in the penicillin group. Nevertheless, clindamycin may be preferable for treatment of this condition, particularly in seriously ill patients and in those who have responded poorly to penicillin.

Clindamycin is useful as an alternative to penicillin in treatment of *C. perfringens* infections. Clindamycin was more effective than penicillin in reducing mortality in a mouse model of *C. perfringens* gas gangrene and in vitro in suppressing the alpha toxin activity produced by that organism.[343,344]

Clindamycin may sometimes be useful as an alternative to penicillin in the treatment of staphylococcal infections. However, its more limited bactericidal rate for staphylococci than that of the penicillins, and particularly the real potential for the emergence of clindamycin-resistant strains in treated patients, are disadvantages. The latter problem, noted especially but not only with erythromycin-resistant strains, appreciably limits its effectiveness as therapy for deep-seated staphylococcal infections, particularly endocarditis.[309] Vancomycin or a cephalosporin is usually a better alternative to the penicillins for the latter. Although high concentrations of clindamycin are achieved in bone, an advantage of clindamycin for the treatment of osteomyelitis has not been established.[319]

The topical clindamycin/benzoyl peroxide gel is more effective in the treatment of acne vulgaris than topical clindamycin alone.[345] However, pseudomembranous colitis associated with the use of topical clindamycin has been reported.[346] In the treatment of bacterial vaginosis, clindamycin vaginal cream (2%) appears to be similar in efficacy and in the incidence of side effects to oral metronidazole (both used for 7 days).[347] The case report of *C. difficile* colitis associated with clindamycin vaginal cream has already been noted.[329] Bacterial vaginosis is a risk factor for preterm delivery, and studies have shown that while intravaginal clindamycin treatment in pregnancy eradicates bacterial vaginosis, it fails to reduce the risk of preterm delivery, possibly because of lack of endometrial activity of intravaginal drugs.[348] Several studies have evaluated the use of oral clindamycin during pregnancy in reducing the risk of preterm delivery. Two studies did not show benefit from treatment.[349,350] In contrast, a more recent study demonstrated that treatment with oral clindamycin (300 mg twice daily for 5 days) of asymptomatic women with abnormal vaginal flora and bacterial vaginosis early in the second trimester significantly reduced the rate of late miscarriage and preterm birth.[351] In the latter study, patients were treated earlier in pregnancy and with oral clindamycin for a longer course than in previous studies.

Clindamycin is effective in treating experimental animals and when combined with pyrimethamine in treating patients with toxoplasmosis of the central nervous system.[352] A randomized, controlled study found pyrimethamine-clindamycin therapy for that condition in AIDS patients to be less effective in preventing relapses than a pyrimethamine-sulfadiazine regimen.[353]

Clindamycin in combination with primaquine is an effective and well-tolerated regimen for the treatment of mild and moderately severe *Pneumocystis jirovecii* pneumonia in patients with AIDS. In a comparative trial, this combination showed an efficacy similar to that of trimethoprim with sulfamethoxazole or trimethoprim with dapsone.[354]

Clindamycin in combination with quinine is effective in the treatment of falciparum malaria.[176] That regimen used for 4 days was found to be superior to quinine used alone for 7 days in a randomized trial in Gabonese children with severe disease.[355] The same combination has also been reported to be useful in the treatment of babesiosis.[176,356]

The coexistence of β-lactamase-producing *S. aureus* or *Bacteroides* species, and group A streptococci may be associated with the failure of penicillin to eradicate the latter, resulting in recurrent tonsillitis. Limited evidence suggests that recurrence rates may be lowered when clindamycin is used.[357] In a more recent study, patients with group A streptococcal pharyngitis in whom the organisms with the same T protein type persisted (in some with symptoms and signs as well) after 10 days of treatment with phenoxymethyl penicillin were randomly allocated to retreatment for 10 days with phenoxymethyl penicillin or clindamycin.[358] Group A streptococci were not recovered from any of the patients receiving clindamycin, but the same T type was cultured from 64% of those retreated with the penicillin. However, widespread use of clindamycin for this common problem is likely to lead to a substantial number of cases of pseudomembranous colitis, as well as selection for clindamycin-resistant strains of group A streptococci.

Although penicillin has been the traditional drug of choice for the treatment of group A streptococcal infections, clindamycin must be considered as potentially more effective in serious soft tissue infections, based on data, already discussed, from the treatment of experimental infections in mice and the effectiveness of that agent compared with penicillin in decreasing the in vitro production of several of the virulence factors of the pathogen. However, there are as yet no data from clinical trials to substantiate such an advantage for clindamycin, and, because some strains of *S. pyogenes* may be resistant to clindamycin, that drug should be used in combination with penicillin for the empirical treatment of life-threatening group A streptococcal infections, until sensitivity data are available.[359] Limited in vitro data suggest that the addition of penicillin to clindamycin does not antagonize the bactericidal effects of the latter.[360]

The dosage of clindamycin for adults depends on the site and severity of infection and the condition of the patient. Oral doses are usually 150 to 450 mg every 6 hours, and parenteral doses, given every 6 to 12 hours, usually total 600 to 2700 mg/day, occasionally higher.

REFERENCES

1. Leclercq R, Courvalin P. Resistance to macrolides and related antibiotics in *Streptococcus pneumoniae.* Antimicrob Agents Chemother. 2002;46:2727-34.
2. Allen N. Effects of macrolide antibiotics on ribosome function. In: Schonfeld W, Kirst HA, eds. Macrolide Antibiotics. Boston: Birkhauser Verlag; 2002:261-280.
2a. Edelstein PH. Pneumococcal resistance to macrolides, linasamides, ketolides and streptomycin B agents: Molecular mechanisms and resistance phenotypes. Clin Infect Dis. 2004;38(Suppl 4):S322-S327.
3. Sutcliffe J, Leclercq R. Mechanisms of resistance to macrolides, lincosamides, and ketolides. In: Schonfeld W, Kirst HA, eds. Macrolide Antibiotics. Boston: Birkhauser Verlag; 2002:281-317.
4. Chittum HS, Champney WS. Erythromycin inhibits the assembly of the large ribosomal subunit in growing *Escherichia coli* cells. Curr Microbiol. 1995;30:273-279.
5. Haight T, Finland M. Observations on mode of action of erythromycin. Proc Soc Exp Biol Med. 1952;81:188-193.
6. Haight T, Finland M. The antibacterial action of erythromycin. Proc Soc Exp Biol Med. 1952;81:175-183.
7. Sabath L, Gerstein DA, Loder PB, et al. Excretion of erythromycin and its enhanced activity in urine against gram-negative bacilli with alkalinization. J Lab Clin Med. 1968;72:916-923.
8. Pankuch GA, Visalli MA, Jacobs MR, Appelbaum PC. Susceptibilities of penicillin- and erythromycin-susceptible and -resistant pneumococci to HMR 3647 (RU 66647), a new ketolide, compared with susceptibilities to 17 other agents. Antimicrob Agents Chemother. 1998;42:624-30.
9. Canton R, Loza E, Morosini MI, Baquero F. Antimicrobial resistance amongst isolates of *Streptococcus pyogenes* and *Staphylococcus aureus* in the PROTEKT antimicrobial surveillance programme during 1999-2000. J Antimicrob Chemother. 2002;50(Suppl S1):9-24.
10. Aracil B, Minambres M, Oteo J, et al. Susceptibility of strains of *Streptococcus agalactiae* to macrolides and lincosamides, phenotype patterns and resistance genes. Clin Microbiol Infect. 2002;8:745-748.
11. Zhanel GG, Walters M, Noreddin A, et al. The ketolides: A critical review. Drugs. 2002;62:1771-1804.

12. Alcaide F, Benitez MA, Carratala J, et al. In vitro activities of the new ketolide HMR 3647 (telithromycin) in comparison with those of eight other antibiotics against viridans group Streptococci isolated from blood of neutropenic patients with cancer. Antimicrob Agents Chemother. 2001;45:624-626.

13. Hamilton-Miller JM, Shah S. Comparative in-vitro activity of ketolide HMR 3647 and four macrolides against gram-positive cocci of known erythromycin susceptibility status. J Antimicrob Chemother. 1998;41:649-653.

14. Shain CS, Amsden GW. Telithromycin: The first of the ketolides. Ann Pharmacother. 2002;36:452-464.

15. Boswell FJ, Andrews JM, Ashby JP, et al. The in-vitro activity of HMR 3647, a new ketolide antimicrobial agent. J Antimicrob Chemother. 1998;42:703-709.

16. Engler KH, Warner M, George RC. In vitro activity of ketolides HMR 3004 and HMR 3647 and seven other antimicrobial agents against Corynebacterium diphtheriae. J Antimicrob Chemother. 2001;47:27-31.

17. Martinez-Martinez L, Pascual A, Suarez AI, Perea EJ. In vitro activities of ketolide HMR 3647, macrolides, and clindamycin against coryneform bacteria. Antimicrob Agents Chemother. 1998;42:3290-3292.

18. Hoban DJ. Prevalence and characterization of macrolide resistance in clinical isolates of Streptococcus pneumoniae and Streptococcus pyogenes from North America. J Chemother. 2002;14(Suppl 3):25-30.

19. Hoppe JE, Bryskier A. In vitro susceptibilities of Bordetella pertussis and Bordetella parapertussis to two ketolides (HMR 3004 and HMR 3647), four macrolides (azithromycin, clarithromycin, erythromycin A, and roxithromycin), and two ansamycins (rifampin and rifapentine). Antimicrob Agents Chemother. 1998;42:965-966.

20. Vanhoof R, Gordts B, Dierickx R, et al. Bacteriostatic and bactericidal activities of 24 antimicrobial agents against Campylobacter fetus subsp. jejuni. Antimicrob Agents Chemother. 1980;18:118-121.

21. Nilius AM, Bui MH, Almer L, et al. Comparative in vitro activity of ABT-773, a novel antibacterial ketolide. Antimicrob Agents Chemother. 2001;45:2163-2168.

22. Bebear CM, Renaudin H, Bryskier A, Bebear C. Comparative activities of telithromycin (HMR 3647), levofloxacin, and other antimicrobial agents against human mycoplasmas. Antimicrob Agents Chemother. 2000;44:1980-1982.

23. Samra Z, Rosenberg S, Soffer Y, Dan M. In vitro susceptibility of recent clinical isolates of Chlamydia trachomatis to macrolides and tetracyclines. Diagn Microbiol Infect Dis. 2001;39:177-179.

24. Roblin PM, Hammerschlag MR. In vitro activity of a new ketolide antibiotic, HMR 3647, against Chlamydia pneumoniae. Antimicrob Agents Chemother. 1998;42:1515-1516.

25. Edelstein PH, Edelstein MA. In vitro activity of the ketolide HMR 3647 (RU 6647) for Legionella spp., its pharmacokinetics in guinea pigs, and use of the drug to treat guinea pigs with Legionella pneumophila pneumonia. Antimicrob Agents Chemother. 1999;43:90-95.

26. Critchley IA, Jones ME, Heinze PD, et al. In vitro activity of levofloxacin against contemporary clinical isolates of Legionella pneumophila, Mycoplasma pneumoniae and Chlamydia pneumoniae from North America and Europe. Clin Microbiol Infect. 2002;8:214-221.

27. Citron DM, Appleman MD. Comparative in vitro activities of ABT-773 against 362 clinical isolates of anaerobic bacteria. Antimicrob Agents Chemother. 2001;45:345-348.

28. Ednie LM, Jacobs MR, Appelbaum PC. Comparative antianaerobic activities of the ketolides HMR 3647 (RU 66647) and HMR 3004 (RU 64004). Antimicrob Agents Chemother. 1997;41:2019-2022.

29. Bermudez LE, Inderlied CB, Kolonoski P, et al. Telithromycin is active against Mycobacterium avium in mice despite lacking significant activity in standard in vitro and macrophage assays and is associated with low frequency of resistance during treatment. Antimicrob Agents Chemother. 2001;45:2210-2214.

30. Alvarez-Elcoro S, Enzler MJ. The macrolides: Erythromycin, clarithromycin, and azithromycin. Mayo Clin Proc. 1999;74:613-634.

31. Steele-Moore L, Stark K, Holloway WJ. In vitro activities of clarithromycin and azithromycin against clinical isolates of Mycobacterium avium-M. intracellulare. Antimicrob Agents Chemother. 1999;43:1530.

32. Saez-Nieto JA, Vazquez JA. In vitro activities of ketolides HMR 3647 [correction of HRM 3647] and HMR 3004 [correction of HRM 3004], levofloxacin, and other quinolones and macrolides against Neisseria spp. and Moraxella catarrhalis. Antimicrob Agents Chemother. 1999;43:983-984.

33. Thornsberry C, Sahm DF, Kelly LJ, et al. Regional trends in antimicrobial resistance among clinical isolates of Streptococcus pneumoniae, Haemophilus influenzae, and Moraxella catarrhalis in the United States: Results from the TRUST Surveillance Program, 1999-2000. Clin Infect Dis. 2002;34(Suppl 1):S4-S16.

34. Hyde TB, Gay K, Stephens DS, et al. Macrolide resistance among invasive Streptococcus pneumoniae isolates. JAMA. 2001;286:1857-1862.

35. Hsueh PR, Liu CY, Luh KT. Current status of antimicrobial resistance in Taiwan. Emerg Infect Dis. 2002;8:132-137.

36. Martin JM, Green M, Barbadora KA, Wald ER. Erythromycin-resistant group A streptococci in schoolchildren in Pittsburgh. N Engl J Med. 2002;346:1200-1206.

37. Thornsberry C, Ogilvie PT, Holley HP Jr, Sahm DF. Survey of susceptibilities of Streptococcus pneumoniae, Haemophilus influenzae, and Moraxella catarrhalis isolates to 26 antimicrobial agents: A prospective U.S. study. Antimicrob Agents Chemother. 1999;43:2612-2623.

38. Ednie LM, Visalli MA, Jacobs MR, Appelbaum PC. Comparative activities of clarithromycin, erythromycin, and azithromycin against penicillin-susceptible and penicillin-resistant pneumococci. Antimicrob Agents Chemother. 1996;40:1950-1952.

39. Sutcliffe J, Tait-Kamradt A, Wondrack L. Streptococcus pneumoniae and Streptococcus pyogenes resistant to macrolides but sensitive to clindamycin: A common resistance pattern mediated by an efflux system. Antimicrob Agents Chemother. 1996;40:1817-1824.

40. Gay K, Baughman W, Miller Y, et al. The emergence of Streptococcus pneumoniae resistant to macrolide antimicrobial agents: A 6-year population-based assessment. J Infect Dis. 2000;182:1417-1424.

41. Corso A, Severina EP, Petruk VF, et al. Molecular characterization of penicillin-resistant Streptococcus pneumoniae isolates causing respiratory disease in the United States. Microb Drug Resist. 1998;4:325-337.

42. Lagrou K, Peetermans WE, Verhaegen J, et al. Macrolide resistance in Belgian Streptococcus pneumoniae. J Antimicrob Chemother. 2000;45:119-21.

43. Marchese A, Tonoli E, Debbia EA, Schito GC. Macrolide resistance mechanisms and expression of phenotypes among Streptococcus pneumoniae circulating in Italy. J Antimicrob Chemother. 1999;44:461-464.

44. Wang M, Zhang Y, Zhu D, Wang F. Prevalence and phenotypes of erythromycin-resistant Streptococcus pneumoniae in Shanghai, China. Diagn Microbiol Infect Dis. 2001;39:187-189.

45. Lowbury E, Jurst L. The sensitivity of staphylococci and other wound bacteria to erythromycin, oleandomycin and spiramycin. J Clin Pathol. 1959;12:163-164.

46. Hsueh PR, Teng LJ, Lee LN, et al. Increased prevalence of erythromycin resistance in streptococci: Substantial upsurge in erythromycin-resistant M phenotype in Streptococcus pyogenes (1979-1998) but not in Streptococcus pneumoniae (1985-1999) in Taiwan. Microb Drug Resist. 2002;8:27-33.

47. Gordon KA, Beach ML, Biedenbach DJ, et al. Antimicrobial susceptibility patterns of beta-hemolytic and viridans group streptococci: Report from the SENTRY Antimicrobial Surveillance Program (1997-2000). Diagn Microbiol Infect Dis. 2002;43:157-162.

48. Avanzini C, Bosio K, Volpe G, et al. Streptococcus pyogenes collected in Torino (northwest Italy) between 1983 and 1998: Survey of macrolide resistance and trend of genotype by RAPD. Microb Drug Resist. 2000;6:289-295.

49. Alos JI, Aracil B, Oteo J, et al. High prevalence of erythromycin-resistant, clindamycin/miocamycin-susceptible (M phenotype) Streptococcus pyogenes: Results of a Spanish multicentre study in 1998. Spanish Group for the Study of Infection in the Primary Health Care Setting. J Antimicrob Chemother. 2000;45:605-609.

50. Weber P, Filipecki J, Bingen E, et al. Genetic and phenotypic characterization of macrolide resistance in group A streptococci isolated from adults with pharyngo-tonsillitis in France. J Antimicrob Chemother. 2001;48:291-294.

51. Seppala H, Nissinen A, Jarvinen H, et al. Resistance to erythromycin in group A streptococci. N Engl J Med. 1992;326:292-297.

52. Seppala H, Klaukka T, Vuopio-Varkila J, et al. The effect of changes in the consumption of macrolide antibiotics on erythromycin resistance in group A streptococci in Finland. Finnish Study Group for Antimicrobial Resistance. N Engl J Med. 1997;337:441-446.

53. Baquero F, Garcia-Rodriguez JA, de Lomas JG, Aguilar L. Antimicrobial resistance of 914 beta-hemolytic streptococci isolated from pharyngeal swabs in Spain: Results of a 1-year (1996-1997) multicenter surveillance study. The Spanish Surveillance Group for Respiratory Pathogens. Antimicrob Agents Chemother. 1999;43:178-180.

54. Haight T, Finland M. Resistance of bacteria to erythromycin. Proc Soc Exp Biol Med. 1952;81:183-188.

55. Westh H, Rosdahl VT, Friis H. Erythromycin resistance in Danish Staphylococcus aureus hospital strains with emphasis on erythromycin consumption. APMIS. 1989;97:1121-4.

56. Pfaller MA, Jones RN, Doern GV, et al. Survey of blood stream infections attributable to gram-positive cocci: Frequency of occurrence and antimicrobial susceptibility of isolates collected in 1997 in the United States, Canada, and Latin America from the SENTRY Antimicrobial Surveillance Program. SENTRY Participants Group. Diagn Microbiol Infect Dis. 1999;33:283-297.

57. Schmitz FJ, Verhoef J, Fluit AC. Prevalence of resistance to MLS antibiotics in 20 European university hospitals participating in the European SENTRY surveillance programme. Sentry Participants Group. J Antimicrob Chemother. 1999;43:783-792.

58. Almer LS, Shortridge VD, Nilius AM, et al. Antimicrobial susceptibility and molecular characterization of community-acquired methicillin-resistant Staphylococcus aureus. Diagn Microbiol Infect Dis. 2002;43:225-232.

59. Lepper M, Dowling HF, Jackson GG, et al. Effect of antibiotic usage in the hospital on the incidence of antibiotic-resistant strains among personnel carrying staphylococci. J Lab Clin Med. 1953;42:832.

60. Haight TH FM. Laboratory and clinical studies on erythromycin. N Engl J Med. 1952;247:227-232.

61. Garrod L. The erythromycin group of antibiotics. Br Med J. 1957;2:57-63.

62. Wu JJ, Lin KY, Hsueh PR, et al. High incidence of erythromycin-resistant streptococci in Taiwan. Antimicrob Agents Chemother. 1997;41:844-846.

63. Gershon AS, de Azavedo JC, McGeer A, et al. Activities of new fluoroquinolones, ketolides, and other antimicrobials against blood culture isolates of viridans group streptococci from across Canada, 2000. Antimicrob Agents Chemother. 2002;46:1553-1556.

64. Hof H, Nichterlein T, Kretschmar M. Management of listeriosis. Clin Microbiol Rev. 1997;10:345-357.

65. Goldstein EJ, Citron DM, Merriam CV, et al. Activities of telithromycin (HMR 3647, RU 66647) compared to those of erythromycin, azithromycin, clarithromycin, roxithromycin, and other antimicrobial agents against unusual anaerobes. Antimicrob Agents Chemother. 1999;43:2801-2805.

66. Finland M, Bach MC, Garner C, Gold O. Synergistic action of ampicillin and erythromycin against Nocardia asteroides: Effect of time of incubation. Antimicrob Agents Chemother. 1974;5:344-353.

67. Rapp RP, McCraney SA, Goodman NL, Shaddick DJ. New macrolide antibiotics: Usefulness in infections caused by mycobacteria other than Mycobacterium tuberculosis. Ann Pharmacother. 1994;28:1255-1263.

68. Korgenski EK, Daly JA. Surveillance and detection of erythromycin resistance in Bordetella pertussis isolates recovered from a pediatric population in the Intermountain West region of the United States. J Clin Microbiol. 1997;35:2989-2991.

69. Angyo IA, Okpeh ES. Changing patterns of antibiotic sensitivity and resistance during an outbreak of meningococcal infection in Jos, Nigeria. J Trop Pediatr. 1998;44:263-265.

70. Lewis K, Saubolle MA, Tenover FC, et al. Pertussis caused by an erythromycin-resistant strain of Bordetella pertussis. Pediatr Infect Dis J. 1995;14:388-391.

71. Ehret JM, Nims LJ, Judson FN. A clinical isolate of Neisseria gonorrhoeae with in vitro resistance to erythromycin and decreased susceptibility to azithromycin. Sex Transm Dis. 1996;23:270-272.

72. Young H, Moyes A, McMillan A. Azithromycin and erythromycin resistant Neisseria gonorrhoeae following treatment with azithromycin. Int J STD AIDS 1997;8:299-302.

73. Centers for Disease Control and Prevention. Sexually Transmitted Disease Surveillance 2001 Supplement: Gonococcal Isolate Surveillance Project (GISP) Annual Report, 2001. Atlanta, Georgia: U.S. Department of Health and Human Services, 2002.

74. Centers for Disease Control and Prevention. National antimicrobial resistance monitoring system: Enteric bacteria 2000 annual report. NARMS. Atlanta: Centers for Disease Control and Prevention, 2000.

75. Ednie LM, Spangler SK, Jacobs MR, Appelbaum PC. Antianaerobic activity of the ketolide RU 64004 compared to activities of four macrolides, five beta-lactams, clindamycin, and metronidazole. Antimicrob Agents Chemother. 1997;41:1037-1041.

76. Kenny GE, Cartwright FD. Susceptibilities of Mycoplasma hominis, M. pneumoniae, and Ureaplasma urealyticum to GAR-936, dalfopristin, dirithromycin, evernimicin, gatifloxacin, linezolid, moxifloxacin, quinupristin-dalfopristin, and telithromycin compared to their susceptibilities to reference macrolides, tetracyclines, and quinolones. Antimicrob Agents Chemother. 2001;45:2604-2608.

77. Roblin PM, Reznik T, Kutlin A, Hammerschlag MR. In vitro activities of gemifloxacin (SB 265805, LB20304) against recent clinical isolates of Chlamydia pneumoniae. Antimicrob Agents Chemother. 1999;43:2806-7.

78. Jao RL. Susceptibility of Mycoplasma pneumoniae to 21 antibiotics in vitro. Am J Med Sci. 1967;253:639-650.

79. Nittu Y, Hasegawa S, Kubota H. In vitro development of resistance to erythromycin, other macrolide antibiotics, and lincomycin in Mycoplasma pneumoniae. Antimicrob Agents Chemother. 1974;5:513-519.

80. Segreti J, Meyer P, Kapell K. In vitro activity of macrolides against intracellular Legionella pneumophila. Diagn Microbiol Infect Dis. 1996;25:123-126.

81. Leclercq R, Courvalin P. Intrinsic and unusual resistance to macrolide, lincosamide, and streptogramin antibiotics in bacteria. Antimicrob Agents Chemother. 1991;35:1273-1276.

82. Mao JC, Putterman M. Accumulation in gram-positive and gram-negative bacteria as a mechanism of resistance to erythromycin. J Bacteriol. 1968;95:1111-1117.

83. Taubeneck U. Susceptibility of Proteus mirabilis and its stable L-forms to erythromycin and other macrolides. Nature. 1962;196:195-196.

84. Ross JI, Eady EA, Cove JH, Baumberg S. Minimal functional system required for expression of erythromycin resistance by msrA in Staphylococcus aureus RN4220. Gene. 1996;183:143-148.

85. Prunier AL, Malbruny B, Laurans M, et al. High rate of macrolide resistance in Staphylococcus aureus strains from patients with cystic fibrosis reveals high proportions of hypermutable strains. J Infect Dis. 2003;187:1709-1716.

86. Farrell DJ, Douthwaite S, Morrissey I, et al. Macrolide resistance by ribosomal mutation in clinical isolates of Streptococcus pneumoniae from the PROTEKT 1999-2000 Study. Antimicrob Agents Chemother. 2003;47:1777-1783.

87. Leclercq R, Courvalin P. Bacterial resistance to macrolide, lincosamide, and streptogramin antibiotics by target modification. Antimicrob Agents Chemother. 1991;35:1267-1272.

88. Weisblum B. Erythromycin resistance by ribosome modification. Antimicrob Agents Chemother. 1995;39:577-585.

89. Sutcliffe J, Grebe T, Tait-Kamradt A, Wondrack L. Detection of erythromycin-resistant determinants by PCR. Antimicrob Agents Chemother. 1996;40:2562-2566.

90. Itoh Z, Suzuki T, Nakaya M, et al. Structure-activity relation among macrolide antibiotics in initiation of interdigestive migrating contractions in the canine gastrointestinal tract. Am J Physiol. 1985;248:G320-325.

91. Catnach SM, Fairclough PD. Erythromycin and the gut. Gut. 1992;33:397-401.

92. Annese V, Lombardi G, Frusciante V, et al. Cisapride and erythromycin prokinetic effects in gastroparesis due to type 1 (insulin-dependent) diabetes mellitus. Aliment Pharmacol Ther. 1997;11:599-603.

93. Kendall BJ, Chakravarti A, Kendall E, et al. The effect of intravenous erythromycin on solid meal gastric emptying in patients with chronic symptomatic post-vagotomy-antrectomy gastroparesis. Aliment Pharmacol Ther. 1997;11:381-385.

94. Dive A, Miesse C, Galanti L, et al. Effect of erythromycin on gastric motility in mechanically ventilated critically ill patients: A double-blind, randomized, placebo-controlled study. Crit Care Med. 1995;23:1356-1362.

95. Nogami K, Nishikubo T, Minowa H, et al. Intravenous low-dose erythromycin administration for infants with feeding intolerance. Pediatr Int. 2001;43:605-610.

96. Bortolotti M, Annese V, Mari C, et al. Dose-related stimulatory effect of clarithromycin on interdigestive gastroduodenal motility. Digestion. 2000;62:31-37.

97. Netzer P, Schmitt B, Inauen W. Effects of ABT-229, a motilin agonist, on acid reflux, oesophageal motility and gastric emptying in patients with gastro-oesophageal reflux disease. Aliment Pharmacol Ther. 2002;16:1481-1490.

98. Abdelghaffar H, Vazifeh D, Labro MT. Erythromycin A-derived macrolides modify the functional activities of human neutrophils by altering the phospholipase D-phosphatidate phosphohydrolase transduction pathway: L-cladinose is involved both in alterations of neutrophil functions and modulation of this transductional pathway. J Immunol. 1997;159:3995-4005.

99. Ianaro A, Ialenti A, Maffia P, et al. Anti-inflammatory activity of macrolide antibiotics. J Pharmacol Exp Ther. 2000;292:156-163.

100. Aoki Y, Kao PN. Erythromycin inhibits transcriptional activation of NF-kappaB, but not NFAT, through calcineurin-independent signaling in T cells. Antimicrob Agents Chemother. 1999;43:2678-2684.

101. Desaki M, Takizawa H, Ohtoshi T, et al. Erythromycin suppresses nuclear factor-kappaB and activator protein-1 activation in human bronchial epithelial cells. Biochem Biophys Res Commun. 2000;267:124-128.

102. Yamamoto T, Kajikawa O, Martin TR, et al. The role of leukocyte emigration and IL-8 on the development of lipopolysaccharide-induced lung injury in rabbits. J Immunol. 1998;161:5704-5709.

103. Mikasa K, Kita E, Sawaki M, et al. The anti-inflammatory effect of erythromycin in zymosan-induced peritonitis of mice. J Antimicrob Chemother. 1992;30:339-348.

104. Li Y, Azuma A, Takahashi S, et al. Fourteen-membered ring macrolides inhibit vascular cell adhesion molecule 1 messenger RNA induction and leukocyte migration: Role in preventing lung injury and fibrosis in bleomycin-challenged mice. Chest 2002;122:2137-2145.

105. Shryock TR, Mortensen JE, Baumholtz M. The effects of macrolides on the expression of bacterial virulence mechanisms. J Antimicrob Chemother. 1998;41:505-512.

106. Kucers A. Chloramphenicol, erythromycin, vancomycin, tetracyclines. Lancet. 1982;2:425-429.

107. Bechtol L, Stephens VC, Pugh CT, et al. Erythromycin esters: Comparative in vivo hydrolysis and bioavailability. Curr Ther Res. 1976;20:610-622.

108. Malmborg AS. Effect of food on absorption of erythromycin: A study of two derivatives, the stearate and the base. J Antimicrob Chemother. 1979;5:591-599.

109. McDonald PJ, Mather LE, Story MJ. Studies on absorption of a newly developed enteric-coated erythromycin base. J Clin Pharmacol. 1977;17:601-606.

110. Yakatan GJ, Rasmussen CE, Feis PJ, Wallen S. Bioinequivalence of erythromycin ethylsuccinate and enteric-coated erythromycin pellets following multiple oral doses. J Clin Pharmacol. 1985;25:36-42.

111. DiSanto AR, Chodos DJ. Influence of study design in assessing food effects on absorption of erythromycin base and erythromycin stearate. Antimicrob Agents Chemother. 1981;20:190-196.

112. Janicki RS, Garnham JC, Worland MC, et al. Comparison of erythromycin ethyl succinate, stearate and estolate treatments of group A streptococcal infections of the upper respiratory tract. Clin Pediatr (Phila). 1975;14:1098-1107.

113. Ginsburg CM, McCracken GH Jr, Crow SD, et al. Erythromycin therapy for group A streptococcal pharyngitis: Results of a comparative study of the estolate and ethyl-succinate formulations. Am J Dis Child. 1984;138:536-539.

114. Osono T, Umezawa H. Pharmacokinetics of macrolides, lincosamides and streptogramins. J Antimicrob Chemother. 1985;16(Suppl A):151-166.

115. Bass JW, Steele RW, Wiebe RA, Dierdorff EP. Erythromycin concentrations in middle ear exudates. Pediatrics. 1971;48:417-422.

116. Howard JE, Nelson JD, Clahsen J, Jackson LH. Otitis media of infancy and early childhood: A double-blind study of four treatment regimens. Am J Dis Child. 1976;130:965-970.

117. Hand WL, Corwin RW, Steinberg TH, Grossman GD. Uptake of antibiotics by human alveolar macrophages. Am Rev Respir Dis. 1984;129:933-937.

118. Miller MF, Martin JR, Johnson P, et al. Erythromycin uptake and accumulation by human polymorphonuclear leukocytes and efficacy of erythromycin in killing ingested Legionella pneumophila. J Infect Dis. 1984;149:714-718.

119. Romansky M, Nasou JP, Davis DS, et al. The treatment of 171 patients with erythromycin, including 132 with bacterial pneumonia. Antibiot Annu. 1955-1956;3:48-62.

120. Philipson A, Sabath LD, Charles D. Transplacental passage of erythromycin and clindamycin. N Engl J Med. 1973;288:1219-1221.

121. Hammond J, Griffith RS. Factors affecting the absorption and biliary excretion of erythromycin and two of its derivatives in humans. Clin Pharmacol Ther. 1961;2:308-312.

122. Mao J-H, Tardrew PL. Demethylation of erythromycin by rabbit tissues in vitro. Biochem Pharmacol. 1965;14:1049-1058.

123. Kunin CM. A guide to use of antibiotics in patients with renal disease: A table of recommended doses and factors governing serum levels. Ann Intern Med. 1967;67:151-158.

124. Ellsworth AJ, Christensen DB, Volpone-McMahon MT. Prospective comparison of patient tolerance to enteric-coated vs nonenteric-coated erythromycin. J Fam Pract. 1990;31:265-270.

125. Inman WH, Rawson NS. Erythromycin estolate and jaundice. Br Med J (Clin Res Ed). 1983;286:1954-1955.

126. Braun P. Hepatotoxicity of erythromycin. J Infect Dis. 1969;119:300-306.

127. Tolman KG, Sannella JJ, Freston JW. Chemical structure of erythromycin and hepatotoxicity. Ann Intern Med. 1974;81:58-60.

128. Pessayre D, Larrey D, Funck-Brentano C, Benhamou JP. Drug interactions and hepatitis produced by some macrolide antibiotics. J Antimicrob Chemother. 1985;16(Suppl A):181-194.

129. McCormack WM, George H, Donner A, et al. Hepatotoxicity of erythromycin estolate during pregnancy. Antimicrob Agents Chemother. 1977;12:630-635.

130. Sabath LD, Gerstein DA, Finland M. Serum glutamic oxalacetic transaminase: False elevations during administration of erythromycin. N Engl J Med. 1968;279:1137-1139.

131. Carson JL, Strom BL, Duff A, et al. Acute liver disease associated with erythromycins, sulfonamides, and tetracyclines. Ann Intern Med. 1993;119:576-583.

132. Karmody CS, Weinstein L. Reversible sensorineural hearing loss with intravenous erythromycin lactobionate. Ann Otol Rhinol Laryngol. 1977;86:9-11.

133. Eckman MR, Johnson T, Riess R. Partial deafness after erythromycin (Letter). N Engl J Med. 1975;292:649.

134. Taylor R, Schofield IS, Ramos JM, et al. Ototoxicity of erythromycin in peritoneal dialysis patients. Lancet. 1981;2:935-936.

135. Haydon RC, Thelin JW, Davis WE. Erythromycin ototoxicity: Analysis and conclusions based on 22 case reports. Otolaryngol Head Neck Surg. 1984;92:678-684.

136. Swanson DJ, Sung RJ, Fine MJ, et al. Erythromycin ototoxicity: Prospective assessment with serum concentrations and audiograms in a study of patients with pneumonia. Am J Med. 1992;92:61-68.

137. Katapadi K, Kostandy G, Katapadi M, et al. A review of erythromycin-induced malignant tachyarrhythmia—torsade de pointes: A case report. Angiology. 1997;48:821-826.

138. Schoenenberger RA, Haefeli WE, Weiss P, Ritz RF. Association of intravenous erythromycin and potentially fatal ventricular tachycardia with Q-T prolongation (torsades de pointes). BMJ. 1990;300:1375-1376.

139. Daleau P, Lessard E, Groleau MF, Turgeon J. Erythromycin blocks the rapid component of the delayed rectifier potassium current and lengthens repolarization of guinea pig ventricular myocytes. Circulation. 1995;91:3010-3016.

140. Gantz NM, Zawacki JK, Dickerson WJ, Bartlett JG. Pseudomembranous colitis associated with erythromycin. Ann Intern Med. 1979;91:866-867.

141. SanFilippo J. Infantile hypertrophic pyloric stenosis related to ingestion of erythromycin estolate: A report of five cases. J Pediatr Surg. 1976;11:177-180.

142. Cooper WO, Griffin MR, Arbogast P, et al. Very early exposure to erythromycin and infantile hypertrophic pyloric stenosis. Arch Pediatr Adolesc Med. 2002;156:647-650.

143. Cooper WO, Ray WA, Griffin MR. Prenatal prescription of macrolide antibiotics and infantile hypertrophic pyloric stenosis. Obstet Gynecol. 2002;100:101-106.

144. Ludden TM. Pharmacokinetic interactions of the macrolide antibiotics. Clin Pharmacokinet. 1985;10:63-79.

145. Amsden GW. Macrolides versus azalides: A drug interaction update. Ann Pharmacother. 1995;29:906-917.

146. Periti P, Mazzei T, Mini E, Novelli A. Pharmacokinetic drug interactions of macrolides. Clin Pharmacokinet. 1992;23:106-131.

147. Kim R. The Medical Letter Handbook of Adverse Drug Interactions. New Rochelle, NY: The Medical Letter on Drugs and Therapeutics; 2003.

148. Bass JW, Freitas BC, Freitas AD, et al. Prospective randomized double blind placebo-controlled evaluation of azithromycin for treatment of cat-scratch disease. Pediatr Infect Dis J. 1998;17:447-452.

149. Ohl ME, Spach DH. *Bartonella quintana* and urban trench fever. Clin Infect Dis. 2000;31:131-135.

150. Aoyama T, Sunakawa K, Iwata S, et al. Efficacy of short-term treatment of pertussis with clarithromycin and azithromycin. J Pediatr. 1996;129:761-764.

151. Kuschner RA, Trofa AF, Thomas RJ, et al. Use of azithromycin for the treatment of *Campylobacter enteritis* in travelers to Thailand, an area where ciprofloxacin resistance is prevalent. Clin Infect Dis. 1995;21:536-541.

152. Bailey RL, Arullendran P, Whittle HC, Mabey DC. Randomised controlled trial of single-dose azithromycin in treatment of trachoma. Lancet. 1993;342:453-456.

153. Stout JE, Yu VL. Legionellosis. N Engl J Med. 1997;337:682-687.

154. Martin DH, Mroczkowski TF, Dalu ZA, et al. A controlled trial of a single dose of azithromycin for the treatment of chlamydial urethritis and cervicitis. The Azithromycin for Chlamydial Infections Study Group. N Engl J Med. 1992;327:921-925.

155. Girgis NI, Butler T, Frenck RW, et al. Azithromycin versus ciprofloxacin for treatment of uncomplicated typhoid fever in a randomized trial in Egypt that included patients with multidrug resistance. Antimicrob Agents Chemother. 1999;43:1441-1444.

156. Khan WA, Seas C, Dhar U, et al. Treatment of shigellosis: V. Comparison of azithromycin and ciprofloxacin. A double-blind, randomized, controlled trial. Ann Intern Med. 1997;126:697-703.

157. Mabey D, Peeling RW. Lymphogranuloma venereum. Sex Transm Infect. 2002;78:90-92.

158. Steere AC. Lyme disease. N Engl J Med. 2001;345:115-125.

159. Krause PJ, Lepore T, Sikand VK, et al. Atovaquone and azithromycin for the treatment of babesiosis. N Engl J Med. 2000;343:1454-1458.

160. Thornsberry C, Ogilvie P, Kahn J, Mauriz Y. Surveillance of antimicrobial resistance in *Streptococcus pneumoniae*, *Haemophilus influenzae*, and *Moraxella catarrhalis* in the United States in 1996-1997 respiratory season. The Laboratory Investigator Group. Diagn Microbiol Infect Dis. 1997;29:249-257.

161. Hofmann J, Cetron MS, Farley MM, et al. The prevalence of drug-resistant *Streptococcus pneumoniae* in Atlanta. N Engl J Med. 1995;333:481-486.

162. Bartlett JG, Breiman RF, Mandell LA, File TM Jr. Community-acquired pneumonia in adults: Guidelines for management. The Infectious Diseases Society of America. Clin Infect Dis. 1998;26:811-838.

163. Rasch J, Mogabgab WJ. Therapeutic effect of erythromycin on *Mycoplasma pneumoniae* pneumonia. Antimicrob Agents Chemother. 1965;5:399.

164. Shames JM, George RB, Holliday WB, et al. Comparison of antibiotics in the treatment of mycoplasmal pneumonia. Arch Intern Med. 1970;125:680-684.

165. Edelstein PH, Meyer RD. Susceptibility of *Legionella pneumophila* to twenty antimicrobial agents. Antimicrob Agents Chemother. 1980;18:403-408.

166. Kuzman I, Soldo I, Schonwald S, Culig J. Azithromycin for treatment of community acquired pneumonia caused by *Legionella pneumophila*: A retrospective study. Scand J Infect Dis. 1995;27:503-505.

167. Fields BS, Benson RF, Besser RE. *Legionella* and Legionnaires' disease: 25 years of investigation. Clin Microbiol Rev. 2002;15:506-526.

168. Sprauer MA, Cochi SL, Zell ER, et al. Prevention of secondary transmission of pertussis in households with early use of erythromycin. Am J Dis Child. 1992;146:177-181.

169. Centers for Disease Control and Prevention. Guidelines for the control of pertussis outbreaks. Atlanta, Ga: Centers for Disease Control and Prevention; 2000.

170. Centers for Disease Control and Prevention. Sexually transmitted diseases treatment guidelines. MMWR Morbid Mortal Wkly Rep. 2002;51(RR-6):1-77.

171. Anders BJ, Lauer BA, Paisley JW, Reller LB. Double-blind placebo controlled trial of erythromycin for treatment of *Campylobacter enteritis*. Lancet. 1982;1:131-132.

172. Salazar-Lindo E, Sack RB, Chea-Woo E, et al. Early treatment with erythromycin of *Campylobacter jejuni*-associated dysentery in children. J Pediatr. 1986;109:355-360.

173. Taylor DN, Blaser MJ, Echeverria P, et al. Erythromycin-resistant *Campylobacter* infections in Thailand. Antimicrob Agents Chemother. 1987;31:438-442.

174. Clarke JS, Condon RE, Bartlett JG, et al. Preoperative oral antibiotics reduce septic complications of colon operations: Results of prospective, randomized, double-blind clinical study. Ann Surg. 1977;186:251-259.

175. Stellato TA, Danziger LH, Gordon N, et al. Antibiotics in elective colon surgery. A randomized trial of oral, systemic, and oral/systemic antibiotics for prophylaxis. Am Surg. 1990;56:251-254.

176. Handbook of Antimicrobial Therapy. The Medical Letter on Drugs and Therapeutics. New Rochelle, NY: Medical Letter; 2002.

177. Gasquet S, Maurin M, Brouqui P, et al. Bacillary angiomatosis in immunocompromised patients. AIDS. 1998;12:1793-1803.

178. Kabir I, Khan WA, Haider R, et al. Erythromycin and trimethoprim-sulphamethoxazole in the treatment of cholera in children. J Diarrhoeal Dis Res. 1996;14:243-247.

179. Prunier AL, Malbruny B, Tande D, et al. Clinical isolates of *Staphylococcus aureus* with ribosomal mutations conferring resistance to macrolides. Antimicrob Agents Chemother. 2002;46:3054-3056.

180. Fenton LJ, Light IJ. Congenital syphilis after maternal treatment with erythromycin. Obstet Gynecol. 1976;47:492-494.

181. Zinner SH, Sabath LD, Casey JI, Finland M. Erythromycin and alkalinisation of urine in the treatment of urinary-tract infections due to gram-negative bacilli. Lancet. 1971;1:1267-1268.

182. Kudoh S, Azuma A, Yamamoto M, et al. Improvement of survival in patients with diffuse panbronchiolitis treated with low-dose erythromycin. Am J Respir Crit Care Med. 1998;157:1829-1832.

183. Bahal N, Nahata MC. The new macrolide antibiotics: Azithromycin, clarithromycin, dirithromycin, and roxithromycin. Ann Pharmacother. 1992;26:46-55.

184. Piscitelli S, Danziger LH, Rodvold KA. Clarithromycin and azithromycin: New macrolide antibiotics. Clin Pharm. 1992;11:137-152.

185. Neu HC. Clinical microbiology of azithromycin. Am J Med. 1991;91:12S-18S.

186. Versalovic J, Shortridge D, Kibler K, et al. Mutations in 23S rRNA are associated with clarithromycin resistance in *Helicobacter pylori*. Antimicrob Agents Chemother. 1996;40:477-480.

187. Taylor DE, Ge Z, Purych D, et al. Cloning and sequence analysis of two copies of a 23S rRNA gene from *Helicobacter pylori* and association of clarithromycin resistance with 23S rRNA mutations. Antimicrob Agents Chemother. 1997;41:2621-2628.

188. Nash KA, Inderlied CB. Genetic basis of macrolide resistance in *Mycobacterium avium* isolated from patients with disseminated disease. Antimicrob Agents Chemother. 1995;39:2625-2630.

189. Hardy DJ, Guay DR, Jones RN. Clarithromycin, a unique macrolide: A pharmacokinetic, microbiological, and clinical overview. Diagn Microbiol Infect Dis. 1992;15:39-53.

190. Credito KL, Lin G, Pankuch GA, et al. Susceptibilities of *Haemophilus influenzae* and *Moraxella catarrhalis* to ABT-773 compared to their susceptibilities to 11 other agents. Antimicrob Agents Chemother. 2001;45:67-72.

191. Tateda K, Ishii Y, Matsumoto T, et al. Potential of macrolide antibiotics to inhibit protein synthesis of *Pseudomonas aeruginosa*: Suppression of virulence factors and stress response. J Infect Chemother. 2000;6:1-7.

192. Fitzgeorge RB, Lever S, Baskerville A. A comparison of the efficacy of azithromycin and clarithromycin in oral therapy of experimental airborne Legionnaires' disease. J Antimicrob Chemother. 1993;31(Suppl E):171-176.

193. Bohte R, van't Wout JW, Lobatto S, et al. Efficacy and safety of azithromycin versus benzylpenicillin or erythromycin in community-acquired pneumonia. Eur J Clin Microbiol Infect Dis. 1995;14:182-187.

194. Yew WW, Piddock LJ, Li MS, et al. In-vitro activity of quinolones and macrolides against mycobacteria. J Antimicrob Chemother. 1994;34:343-351.

195. Perronne C, Gikas A, Truffot-Pernot C, et al. Activities of sparfloxacin, azithromycin, temafloxacin, and rifapentine compared with that of clarithromycin against multiplication of *Mycobacterium avium* complex within human macrophages. Antimicrob Agents Chemother. 1991;35:1356-1359.

196. Bermudez LE, Petrofsky M, Kolonoski P, Young LS. Emergence of *Mycobacterium avium* populations resistant to macrolides during experimental chemotherapy. Antimicrob Agents Chemother. 1998;42:180-183.

197. Derouin F, Chastang C. Activity in vitro against *Toxoplasma gondii* of azithromycin and clarithromycin alone and with pyrimethamine. J Antimicrob Chemother. 1990;25:708-711.

198. Gan VN, McCarty JM, Chu SY, Carr R. Penetration of clarithromycin into middle ear fluid of children with acute otitis media. Pediatr Infect Dis J. 1997;16:39-43.

199. Sanche S, Williams K, Stein K. Cerebrospinal fluid penetration of clarithromycin and 14-hydroxyclarithromycin (Abstract 728). Thirty-third Interscience Conference on Antimicrobial Agents and Chemotherapy, New Orleans, La, October, 1993.

200. Anderson R, Joone G, van Rensburg CE. An in-vitro evaluation of the cellular uptake and intraphagocytic bioactivity of clarithromycin (A-56268, TE-031), a new macrolide antimicrobial agent. J Antimicrob Chemother. 1988;22:923-933.

201. Schentag JJ, Ballow CH. Tissue-directed pharmacokinetics. Am J Med. 1991;91:5S-11S.

202. Hopkins S. Clinical toleration and safety of azithromycin. Am J Med. 1991;91:40S-45S.

203. Foulds G, Hilligoss DM, Henry EB, Gerber N. The effects of an antacid or cimetidine on the serum concentrations of azithromycin. J Clin Pharmacol. 1991;31:164-167.

204. Ballow CH, Amsden GW. Azithromycin: The first azalide antibiotic. Ann Pharmacother. 1992;26:1253-1261.

205. Jaruratanasirikul S, Hortiwakul R, Tantisarasart T, et al. Distribution of azithromycin into brain tissue, cerebrospinal fluid, and aqueous humor of the eye. Antimicrob Agents Chemother. 1996;40:825-826.

206. Chandrupatla S, Demetris AJ, Rabinovitz M. Azithromycin-induced intrahepatic cholestasis. Dig Dis Sci 2002;47:2186-2188.
207. Wallace RJ Jr, Brown BA, Griffith DE. Drug intolerance to high-dose clarithromycin among elderly patients. Diagn Microbiol Infect Dis. 1993;16:215-221.
208. Kolkman W, Groeneveld JH, Baur HJ, Verschuur HP. Ototoxicity induced by clarithromycin. Ned Tijdschr Geneeskd. 2002;146:1743-1745.
209. Kundu S, Williams SR, Nordt SP, Clark RF. Clarithromycin-induced ventricular tachycardia. Ann Emerg Med. 1997;30:542-544.
210. Shaffer D, Singer S, Korvick J, Honig P. Concomitant risk factors in reports of torsades de pointes associated with macrolide use: Review of the United States Food and Drug Administration Adverse Event Reporting System. Clin Infect Dis. 2002;35:197-200.
211. Polis MA, Piscitelli SC, Vogel S, et al. Clarithromycin lowers plasma zidovudine levels in persons with human immunodeficiency virus infection. Antimicrob Agents Chemother. 1997;41:1709-1714.
212. Vance E, Watson-Bitar M, Gustavson L, Kazanjian P. Pharmacokinetics of clarithromycin and zidovudine in patients with AIDS. Antimicrob Agents Chemother. 1995;39:1355-1360.
213. Nawarskas JJ, McCarthy DM, Spinler SA. Digoxin toxicity secondary to clarithromycin therapy. Ann Pharmacother. 1997;31:864-866.
214. Hammerschlag MR, Roblin PM, Bebear CM. Activity of telithromycin, a new ketolide antibacterial, against atypical and intracellular respiratory tract pathogens. J Antimicrob Chemother. 2001;48(Suppl T1):25-31.
215. Bisno AL, Gerber MA, Gwaltney JM Jr, et al. Practice guidelines for the diagnosis and management of group A streptococcal pharyngitis. Infectious Diseases Society of America. Clin Infect Dis. 2002;35:113-125.
216. Still JG, Hubbard WC, Poole JM, et al. Comparison of clarithromycin and penicillin VK suspensions in the treatment of children with streptococcal pharyngitis and review of currently available alternative antibiotic therapies. Pediatr Infect Dis J. 1993;12:S134-141.
217. Hooton TM. A comparison of azithromycin and penicillin V for the treatment of streptococcal pharyngitis. Am J Med. 1991;91:23S-26S.
218. Schaad UB, Kellerhals P, Altwegg M. Azithromycin versus penicillin V for treatment of acute group A streptococcal pharyngitis. Pediatr Infect Dis J. 2002;21:304-308.
219. Hamill J. Multicentre evaluation of azithromycin and penicillin V in the treatment of acute streptococcal pharyngitis and tonsillitis in children. J Antimicrob Chemother. 1993;31(Suppl E):89-94.
220. Ghirga G, Palazzi C, Ghirga P, et al. Inefficacy of a 3-day course of azithromycin in preventing acute rheumatic fever after group A streptococcal infection (scarlet fever) in an 8-year-old child. J Pediatr. 1999;134:123-124.
221. Aronovitz G. A multicenter, open label trial of azithromycin vs. amoxicillin/clavulanate for the management of acute otitis media in children. Pediatr Infect Dis J. 1996;15:S15-19.
222. Arguedas A, Loaiza C, Rodriguez F, et al. Comparative trial of 3 days of azithromycin versus 10 days of clarithromycin in the treatment of children with acute otitis media with effusion. J Chemother. 1997;9:44-50.
223. Bochud PY, Calandra T, Moreillon P, et al. Breakthrough *Streptococcus pneumoniae* meningitis during clarithromycin therapy for acute otitis media. Eur J Clin Microbiol Infect Dis. 2001;20:136-137.
224. Mandell LA, Marrie TJ, Grossman RF, et al. Canadian guidelines for the initial management of community-acquired pneumonia: An evidence-based update by the Canadian Infectious Diseases Society and the Canadian Thoracic Society. The Canadian Community-Acquired Pneumonia Working Group. Clin Infect Dis. 2000;31:383-421.
225. Bartlett JG, Dowell SF, Mandell LA, et al. Practice guidelines for the management of community-acquired pneumonia in adults. Infectious Diseases Society of America. Clin Infect Dis. 2000;31:347-382.
226. Niederman MS, Mandell LA, Anzueto A, et al. Guidelines for the management of adults with community-acquired pneumonia: Diagnosis, assessment of severity, antimicrobial therapy, and prevention. Am J Respir Crit Care Med. 2001;163:1730-1754.
227. Gikas A, Kofteridis DP, Manios A, et al. Newer macrolides as empiric treatment for acute Q fever infection. Antimicrob Agents Chemother. 2001;45:3644-3646.
228. Principi N, Esposito S, Blasi F, Allegra L. Role of *Mycoplasma pneumoniae* and *Chlamydia pneumoniae* in children with community-acquired lower respiratory tract infections. Clin Infect Dis. 2001;32:1281-1289.
229. Socan M. Treatment of atypical pneumonia with azithromycin: Comparison of a 5-day and a 3-day course. J Chemother. 1998;10:64-68.
230. Gleason PP, Meehan TP, Fine JM, et al. Associations between initial antimicrobial therapy and medical outcomes for hospitalized elderly patients with pneumonia. Arch Intern Med. 1999;159:2562-2572.
231. Houck PM, MacLehose RF, Niederman MS, Lowery JK. Empiric antibiotic therapy and mortality among Medicare pneumonia inpatients in 10 western states: 1993, 1995, and 1997. Chest. 2001;119:1420-1426.
232. Mufson MA, Stanek RJ. Bacteremic pneumococcal pneumonia in one American city: A 20-year longitudinal study, 1978-1997. Am J Med. 1999;107:34S-43S.
233. Waterer GW, Somes GW, Wunderink RG. Monotherapy may be suboptimal for severe bacteremic pneumococcal pneumonia. Arch Intern Med. 2001;161:1837-1842.
234. Martinez JA, Horcajada JP, Almela M, et al. Addition of a macrolide to a beta-lactam-based empirical antibiotic regimen is associated with lower in-hospital mortality for patients with bacteremic pneumococcal pneumonia. Clin Infect Dis. 2003;36:389-395.
234a. Martinez FJ. Monotherapy versus dual therapy for community-acquired pneumonia in hospitalized patients. Clin Infect Dis. 2004;38(Suppl 4):5328-5340.
235. Lin E, Stanek RJ, Mufson MA. Lack of synergy of erythromycin combined with penicillin or cefotaxime against *Streptococcus pneumoniae* in vitro. Antimicrob Agents Chemother. 2003;47:1151-1153.
236. Johansen HK, Jensen TG, Dessau RB, et al. Antagonism between penicillin and erythromycin against *Streptococcus pneumoniae* in vitro and in vivo. J Antimicrob Chemother. 2000;46:973-980.
237. Hoppe JE, Haug A. Treatment and prevention of pertussis by antimicrobial agents (Part II). Infection. 1988;16:148-152.
238. American Academy of Pediatrics. Pertussis. Red Book: Report of the Committee on Infectious Diseases. In: Pickering LK, ed. Elk Grove Village, Ill: American Academy of Pediatrics; 2000.
239. Meier A, Heifets L, Wallace RJ Jr, et al. Molecular mechanisms of clarithromycin resistance in *Mycobacterium avium:* Observation of multiple 23S rRNA mutations in a clonal population. J Infect Dis. 1996;174:354-360.
240. Chaisson RE, Benson CA, Dube MP, et al. Clarithromycin therapy for bacteremic *Mycobacterium avium* complex disease: A randomized, double-blind, dose-ranging study in patients with AIDS. AIDS Clinical Trials Group Protocol 157 Study Team. Ann Intern Med. 1994;121:905-911.
241. Pierce M, Crampton S, Henry D, et al. A randomized trial of clarithromycin as prophylaxis against disseminated *Mycobacterium avium* complex infection in patients with advanced acquired immunodeficiency syndrome. N Engl J Med. 1996;335:384-391.
242. Havlir DV, Dube MP, Sattler FR, et al. Prophylaxis against disseminated *Mycobacterium avium* complex with weekly azithromycin, daily rifabutin, or both. California Collaborative Treatment Group. N Engl J Med. 1996;335:392-398.
243. Aberg JA, Williams PL, Liu T, et al. A study of discontinuing maintenance therapy in human immunodeficiency virus-infected subjects with disseminated *Mycobacterium avium* complex: AIDS Clinical Trial Group 393 Study Team. J Infect Dis. 2003;187:1046-1052.
244. Tabbara KF, Abu-el-Asrar A, al-Omar O, et al. Single-dose azithromycin in the treatment of trachoma: A randomized, controlled study. Ophthalmology. 1996;103:842-846.
245. Stamm WE, Hicks CB, Martin DH, et al. Azithromycin for empirical treatment of the nongonococcal urethritis syndrome in men: A randomized double-blind study. JAMA. 1995;274:545-549.
246. Martin DH, Sargent SJ, Wendel GD Jr, et al. Comparison of azithromycin and ceftriaxone for the treatment of chancroid. Clin Infect Dis. 1995;21:409-414.
247. Ulmer H, Beckerling A, Gatz G. Recent use of proton pump inhibitor-based therapies for the eradication of *H. pylori:* A broad data review. Helicobacter. 2003;8:95-104.
248. Tompkins DS, Perkin J, Smith C. Failed treatment of *Helicobacter pylori* infection associated with resistance to clarithromycin. Helicobacter. 1997;2:185-187.
249. Buckley MJ, Xia HX, Hyde DM, et al. Metronidazole resistance reduces efficacy of triple therapy and leads to secondary clarithromycin resistance. Dig Dis Sci. 1997;42:2111-2115.
250. Hoge CW, Gambel JM, Srijan A, et al. Trends in antibiotic resistance among diarrheal pathogens isolated in Thailand over 15 years. Clin Infect Dis. 1998;26:341-345.
251. Wallace RJ Jr, Tanner D, Brennan PJ, Brown BA. Clinical trial of clarithromycin for cutaneous (disseminated) infection due to *Mycobacterium chelonae*. Ann Intern Med. 1993;119:482-486.
252. Vemulapalli RK, Cantey JR, Steed LL, et al. Emergence of resistance to clarithromycin during treatment of disseminated cutaneous *Mycobacterium chelonae* infection: Case report and literature review. J Infect. 2001;43:163-168.
253. Ji B, Jamet P, Perani EG, et al. Powerful bactericidal activities of clarithromycin and minocycline against *Mycobacterium leprae* in lepromatous leprosy. J Infect Dis. 1993;168:188-190.
254. Dattwyler RJ, Grunwaldt E, Luft BJ. Clarithromycin in treatment of early Lyme disease: A pilot study. Antimicrob Agents Chemother. 1996;40:468-469.
255. Luft BJ, Dattwyler RJ, Johnson RC, et al. Azithromycin compared with amoxicillin in the treatment of erythema migrans: A double-blind, randomized, controlled trial. Ann Intern Med. 1996;124:785-791.
256. Andersen SL, Ager AL, McGreevy P, et al. Efficacy of azithromycin as a causal prophylactic agent against murine malaria. Antimicrob Agents Chemother. 1994;38:1862-1863.
257. Anderson SL, Berman J, Kuschner R, et al. Prophylaxis of *Plasmodium falciparum* malaria with azithromycin administered to volunteers. Ann Intern Med. 1995;123:771-773.
258. Andersen SL, Oloo AJ, Gordon DM, et al. Successful double-blinded, randomized, placebo-controlled field trial of azithromycin and doxycycline as prophylaxis for malaria in western Kenya. Clin Infect Dis. 1998;26:146-150.
259. Taylor WR, Richie TL, Fryauff DJ, et al. Malaria prophylaxis using azithromycin: A double-blind, placebo-controlled trial in Irian Jaya, Indonesia. Clin Infect Dis. 1999;28:74-81.
260. Ohrt C, Willingmyre GD, Lee P, et al. Assessment of azithromycin in combination with other antimalarial drugs against Plasmodium falciparum in vitro. Antimicrob Agents Chemother. 2002;46:2518-2524.
261. Dionisio D, Orsi A, Sterrantino G, et al. Chronic cryptosporidiosis in patients with AIDS: Stable remission and possible eradication after long-term, low dose azithromycin. J Clin Pathol. 1998;51:138-142.
262. Blanshard C, Shanson DC, Gazzard BG. Pilot studies of azithromycin, letrazuril and paromomycin in the treatment of cryptosporidiosis. Int J STD AIDS. 1997;8:124-129.
263. Holmberg SD, Moorman AC, Von Bargen JC, et al. Possible effectiveness of clarithromycin and rifabutin for cryptosporidiosis chemoprophylaxis in HIV disease. HIV Outpatient Study (HOPS) Investigators. JAMA. 1998;279:384-386.
264. Schneider CA, Diedrichs H, Riedel KD, et al. In vivo uptake of azithromycin in human coronary plaques. Am J Cardiol. 2000;86:789-791, A9.

265. Gupta S, Leatham EW, Carrington D, et al. Elevated *Chlamydia pneumoniae* antibodies, cardiovascular events, and azithromycin in male survivors of myocardial infarction. Circulation. 1997;96:404-407.

266. Cercek B, Shah PK, Noc M, et al. Effect of short-term treatment with azithromycin on recurrent ischaemic events in patients with acute coronary syndrome in the Azithromycin in Acute Coronary Syndrome (AZACS) trial: A randomised controlled trial. Lancet. 2003;361:809-813.

267. Muhlestein JB, Anderson JL, Carlquist JF, et al. Randomized secondary prevention trial of azithromycin in patients with coronary artery disease: Primary clinical results of the ACADEMIC study. Circulation. 2000;102:1755-1760.

267a. O'Connor CM, Dunne MW, Pfeffer MA, et al. Azithromycin for the secondary prevention of coronary heart disease events. The WIZARD Study: A randomized controlled trial. JAMA 2003;290:1459-1466.

268. Bryskier A, Denis A. Ketolides: Novel antibacterial agents designed to overcome resistance to erythromycin A within gram positive cocci. In: Schonfeld W, Kirst HA, eds. Macrolide Antibiotics. Boston: Birkauser Verlag; 2002:97-140.

269. Bonnefoy A, Girard AM, Agouridas C, Chantot JF. Ketolides lack inducibility properties of MLS(B) resistance phenotype. J Antimicrob Chemother. 1997;40:85-90.

270. Douthwaite S. Structure-activity relationships of ketolides vs. macrolides. Clin Microbiol Infect. 2001;7:11-17.

271. Hansen LH, Mauvais P, Douthwaite S. The macrolide-ketolide antibiotic binding site is formed by structures in domains II and V of 23S ribosomal RNA. Mol Microbiol. 1999;31:623-631.

272. Champney WS, Tober CL. Structure-activity relationships for six ketolide antibiotics. Curr Microbiol. 2001;42:203-210.

273. Malathum K, Coque TM, Singh KV, Murray BE. In vitro activities of two ketolides, HMR 3647 and HMR 3004, against gram-positive bacteria. Antimicrob Agents Chemother. 1999;43:930-936.

274. Jalava J, Kataja J, Seppala H, Huovinen P. In vitro activities of the novel ketolide telithromycin (HMR 3647) against erythromycin-resistant *Streptococcus* species. Antimicrob Agents Chemother. 2001;45:789-793.

275. Schulin T, Wennersten CB, Moellering RC Jr, Eliopoulos GM. In-vitro activity of the new ketolide antibiotic HMR 3647 against gram-positive bacteria. J Antimicrob Chemother. 1998;42:297-301.

276. Wootton M, Bowker KE, Janowska A, et al. In-vitro activity of HMR 3647 against *Streptococcus pneumoniae, Haemophilus influenzae, Moraxella catarrhalis* and beta-haemolytic streptococci. J Antimicrob Chemother. 1999;44:445-453.

277. Giovanetti E, Montanari MP, Marchetti F, Varaldo PE. In vitro activity of ketolides telithromycin and HMR 3004 against Italian isolates of *Streptococcus pyogenes* and *Streptococcus pneumoniae* with different erythromycin susceptibility. J Antimicrob Chemother. 2000;46:905-908.

278. Okamoto H, Miyazaki S, Tateda K, et al. Comparative in vitro activity of telithromycin (HMR 3647), three macrolides, amoxicillin, cefdinir and levofloxacin against gram-positive clinical isolates in Japan. J Antimicrob Chemother. 2000;46:797-802.

279. Barry AL, Fuchs PC, Brown SD. In vitro activities of the ketolide HMR 3647 against recent gram-positive clinical isolates and *Haemophilus influenzae*. Antimicrob Agents Chemother. 1998;42:2138-2140.

280. Hoban DJ, Zhanel GG, Karlowsky JA. In vitro activity of the novel ketolide HMR 3647 and comparative oral antibiotics against Canadian respiratory tract isolates of *Streptococcus pneumoniae, Haemophilus influenzae*, and *Moraxella catarrhalis*. Diagn Microbiol Infect Dis. 1999;35:37-44.

281. Schulin T, Wennersten CB, Ferraro MJ, et al. Susceptibilities of *Legionella* spp. to newer antimicrobials in vitro. Antimicrob Agents Chemother. 1998;42:1520-1523.

282. Rastogi N, Goh KS, Berchel M, Bryskier A. In vitro activities of the ketolides telithromycin (HMR 3647) and HMR 3004 compared to those of clarithromycin against slowly growing mycobacteria at pHs 6.8 and 7.4. Antimicrob Agents Chemother. 2000;44:2848-2852.

283. Namour F, Wessels DH, Pascual MH, et al. Pharmacokinetics of the new ketolide telithromycin (HMR 3647) administered in ascending single and multiple doses. Antimicrob Agents Chemother. 2001;45:170-175.

284. Pharma A. Ketek (telithromycin) briefing document for the FDA anti-infective drug products advisory committee [executive summary]. Bridgewater, NJ: Aventis Pharma; 2001. Available at http://www.fda.gov/ohrms/dockets/ac/03/briefing/3919B1_01_Aventis-KETEK.pdf.

285. Anonymous. Aventis urges extreme caution with Ketek in patients with myasthenia gravis. Clin Infect Dis. 2003;36:i

286. Bryskier A, Butzler JP. Macrolides. In: Finch RG, Greenwood D, Ragnar Norrby S, Whitley RJ, eds. Antibiotic and Chemotherapy. Edinburgh: Churchill Livingstone; 2003:310-325.

287. Visalli MA, Jacobs MR, Appelbaum PC. Susceptibility of penicillin-susceptible and -resistant pneumococci to dirithromycin compared with susceptibilities to erythromycin, azithromycin, clarithromycin, roxithromycin, and clindamycin. Antimicrob Agents Chemother. 1997;41:1867-1870.

288. Stout JE, Arnold B, Yu VL. Activity of azithromycin, clarithromycin, roxithromycin, dirithromycin, quinupristin/dalfopristin and erythromycin against Legionella species by intracellular susceptibility testing in HL-60 cells. J Antimicrob Chemother. 1998;41:289-291.

289. Roblin PM, Kutlin A, Sokolovskaya N, Hammerschlag MR. In-vitro activity of dirithromycin against *Chlamydia pneumoniae*. J Antimicrob Chemother. 1997;39:647-649.

290. Jacobson K. Clinical efficacy of dirithromycin in pneumonia. J Antimicrob Chemother. 1993;31(Suppl C):121-129.

291. Watkins VS, Polk RE, Stotka JL. Drug interactions of macrolides: Emphasis on dirithromycin. Ann Pharmacother. 1997;31:349-356.

292. Gurfinkel E, Bozovich G, Daroca A, et al. Randomised trial of roxithromycin in non-Q-wave coronary syndromes: ROXIS Pilot Study. ROXIS Study Group. Lancet. 1997;350:404-407.

293. McGehee R, Smith CB, Wilcox C, et al. Comparative studies of antibacterial activity in vitro and absorption and excretion of lincomycin and clindamycin. Am J Med Sci. 1968;256:279-292.

294. Low DE, de Azavedo J, Weiss K, et al. Antimicrobial resistance among clinical isolates of *Streptococcus pneumoniae* in Canada during 2000. Antimicrob Agents Chemother. 2002;46:1295-1301.

295. Aldridge KE, Ashcraft D, Cambre K, et al. Multicenter survey of the changing in vitro antimicrobial susceptibilities of clinical isolates of *Bacteroides fragilis* group, *Prevotella, Fusobacterium, Porphyromonas*, and *Peptostreptococcus* species. Antimicrob Agents Chemother. 2001;45:1238-1243.

296. Frank AL, Marcinak JF, Mangat PD, et al. Clindamycin treatment of methicillin-resistant *Staphylococcus aureus* infections in children. Pediatr Infect Dis J. 2002;21:530-534.

297. Snydman DR, Jacobus NV, McDermott LA, et al. National survey on the susceptibility of *Bacteroides fragilis* group: Report and analysis of trends for 1997-2000. Clin Infect Dis. 2002;35:S126-134.

298. Dalmau D, Cayouette M, Lamothe F, et al. Clindamycin resistance in the *Bacteroides fragilis* group: Association with hospital-acquired infections. Clin Infect Dis. 1997;24:874-877.

299. Rasmussen BA, Bush K, Tally FP. Antimicrobial resistance in anaerobes. Clin Infect Dis. 1997;24(Suppl 1):S110-120.

300. Sutter VL. In vitro susceptibility of anaerobes: Comparison of clindamycin and other antimicrobial agents. J Infect Dis. 1977;135(Suppl):S7-12.

301. Nelson CT, Mason EO Jr, Kaplan SL. Activity of oral antibiotics in middle ear and sinus infections caused by penicillin-resistant *Streptococcus pneumoniae*: Implications for treatment. Pediatr Infect Dis J. 1994;13:585-589.

302. Cornaglia G, Ligozzi M, Mazzaroil A, et al. Rapid increase of resistance to erythromycin and clindamycin in *Streptococcus pyogenes* in Italy, 1993-1995. The Italian Surveillance Group for Antimicrobial Resistance. Emerg Infect Dis. 1996;2:339-342.

303. Brook I, Gober AE, Leyva F. In vitro and in vivo effects of penicillin and clindamycin on expression of group A beta-hemolytic streptococcal capsule. Antimicrob Agents Chemother. 1995;39:1565-1568.

304. Gemmell CG, Peterson PK, Schmeling D, et al. Potentiation of opsonization and phagocytosis of *Streptococcus pyogenes* following growth in the presence of clindamycin. J Clin Invest. 1981;67:1249-1256.

305. Sriskandan S, McKee A, Hall L, Cohen J. Comparative effects of clindamycin and ampicillin on superantigenic activity of *Streptococcus pyogenes*. J Antimicrob Chemother. 1997;40:275-277.

306. Stevens DL, Gibbons AE, Bergstrom R, Winn V. The Eagle effect revisited: Efficacy of clindamycin, erythromycin, and penicillin in the treatment of streptococcal myositis. J Infect Dis. 1988;158:23-28.

307. Stevens DL, Yan S, Bryant AE. Penicillin-binding protein expression at different growth stages determines penicillin efficacy in vitro and in vivo: An explanation for the inoculum effect. J Infect Dis. 1993;167:1401-1405.

308. Duncan IB. Development of lincomycin resistance by staphylococci. Antimicrobial Agents Chemother. 1967;7:723-729.

308a. Siberry GK, Tekle T, Carroll K, et al. Failure of clindamycin treatment of methicillin-resistant *Staphylococcus aureus* expressing inducible clindamycin resistance in vitro. Clin Infect Dis. 2003;37:1257-1260.

309. Watanakunakorn C. Clindamycin therapy of *Staphylococcus aureus* endocarditis: Clinical relapse and development of resistance to clindamycin, lincomycin and erythromycin. Am J Med. 1976;60:419-425.

310. Sande MA, Johnson ML. Antimicrobial therapy of experimental endocarditis caused by *Staphylococcus aureus*. J Infect Dis. 1975;131:367-375.

311. Nastro LJ, Finegold SM. Bactericidal activity of five antimicrobial agents against *Bacteroides fragilis*. J Infect Dis. 1972;126:104-107.

312. Pfefferkorn ER, Nothnagel RF, Borotz SE. Parasiticidal effect of clindamycin on *Toxoplasma gondii* grown in cultured cells and selection of a drug-resistant mutant. Antimicrob Agents Chemother. 1992;36:1091-1096.

313. Seaberg LS, Parquette AR, Gluzman IY, et al. Clindamycin activity against chloroquine-resistant *Plasmodium falciparum*. J Infect Dis. 1984;150:904-911.

314. Leclercq R, Brisson-Noel A, Duval J, Courvalin P. Phenotypic expression and genetic heterogeneity of lincosamide inactivation in *Staphylococcus* spp. Antimicrob Agents Chemother. 1987;31:1887-1891.

315. DeHaan RM, Metzler CM, Schellenberg D, Vandenbosch WD. Pharmacokinetic studies of clindamycin phosphate. J Clin Pharmacol. 1973;13:190-209.

316. Fass RJ, Saslaw S. Clindamycin: Clinical and laboratory evaluation of parenteral therapy. Am J Med Sci. 1972;263:368-382.

317. Townsend RJ, Baker RP. Pharmacokinetic comparison of three clindamycin phosphate dosing schedules. Drug Intell Clin Pharm. 1987;21:279-281.

318. Panzer JD, Brown DC, Epstein WL, et al. Clindamycin levels in various body tissues and fluids. J Clin Pharmacol New Drugs. 1972;12:259-262.

319. Nicholas P, Meyers BR, Levy RN, Hirschman SZ. Concentration of clindamycin in human bone. Antimicrob Agents Chemother. 1975;8:220-221.

320. Prokesch RC, Hand WL. Antibiotic entry into human polymorphonuclear leukocytes. Antimicrob Agents Chemother. 1982;21:373-380.

321. Joiner KA, Lowe BR, Dzink JL, Bartlett JG. Antibiotic levels in infected and sterile subcutaneous abscesses in mice. J Infect Dis. 1981;143:487-494.

322. McCall CE, Steigbigel NH, Finland M. Lincomycin: Activity in vitro and absorption and excretion in normal young men. Am J Med Sci. 1967;254:144-155.

323. Kager L, Liljeqvist L, Malmborg AS, Nord CE. Effect of clindamycin prophylaxis on the colonic microflora in patients undergoing colorectal surgery. Antimicrob Agents Chemother. 1981;20:736-740.

324. Brown RB, Martyak SN, Barza M, et al. Penetration of clindamycin phosphate into the abnormal human biliary tract. Ann Intern Med. 1976;84:168-170.

325. Joshi AM, Stein RM. Altered serum clearance of intravenously administered clindamycin phosphate in patients with uremia. J Clin Pharmacol. 1974;14:140-144.

326. Williams DN, Crossley K, Hoffman C, Sabath LD. Parenteral clindamycin phosphate: Pharmacology with normal and abnormal liver function and effect on nasal staphylococci. Antimicrob Agents Chemother. 1975;7:153-158.

327. Bartlett JG. *Clostridium difficile*-associated enteric disease. Curr Infect Dis Rep. 2002;4:477-483.

328. Tedesco FJ. Clindamycin and colitis: A review. J Infect Dis. 1977;135 (Suppl):S95-98.

329. Meadowcroft AM, Diaz PR, Latham GS. *Clostridium difficile* toxin-induced colitis after use of clindamycin phosphate vaginal cream. Ann Pharmacother. 1998;32:309-311.

330. Salcedo J, Keates S, Pothoulakis C, et al. Intravenous immunoglobulin therapy for severe *Clostridium difficile* colitis. Gut. 1997;41:366-370.

331. Moyenuddin M, Williamson JC, Ohl CA. *Clostridium difficile*-associated diarrhea: Current strategies for diagnosis and therapy. Curr Gastroenterol Rep. 2002;4:279-286.

332. Elmore M, Rissing JP, Rink L, Brooks GF. Clindamycin-associated hepatotoxicity. Am J Med. 1974;57:627-630.

333. Weinstein WM, Onderdonk AB, Bartlett JG, et al. Antimicrobial therapy of experimental intraabdominal sepsis. J Infect Dis. 1975;132:282-286.

334. diZerega G, Yonekura L, Roy S, et al. A comparison of clindamycin-gentamicin and penicillin-gentamicin in the treatment of post-cesarean section endomyometritis. Am J Obstet Gynecol. 1979;134:238-42.

335. Solomkin JS, Dellinger EP, Christou NV, Busuttil RW. Results of a multicenter trial comparing imipenem/cilastatin to tobramycin/clindamycin for intra-abdominal infections. Ann Surg. 1990;212:581-591.

336. Sirinek KR, Levine BA. A randomized trial of ticarcillin and clavulanate versus gentamicin and clindamycin in patients with complicated appendicitis. Surg Gynecol Obstet. 1991;172:30-35.

337. Condon RE, Walker AP, Sirinek KR, et al. Meropenem versus tobramycin plus clindamycin for treatment of intraabdominal infections: Results of a prospective, randomized, double-blind clinical trial. Clin Infect Dis. 1995;21:544-550.

338. Bartlett JG. Intra-abdominal sepsis. Med Clin North Am. 1995;79:599-617.

339. Bartlett JG, Gorbach SL. Treatment of aspiration pneumonia and primary lung abscess: Penicillin G vs clindamycin. JAMA. 1975;234:935-937.

340. Levison ME, Mangura CT, Lorber B, et al. Clindamycin compared with penicillin for the treatment of anaerobic lung abscess. Ann Intern Med. 1983;98:466-471.

341. Bartlett JG, Gorbach SL. Penicillin or clindamycin for primary lung abscess? Ann Intern Med. 1983;98:546-548.

342. Gudiol F, Manresa F, Pallares R, et al. Clindamycin vs penicillin for anaerobic lung infections. High rate of penicillin failures associated with penicillin-resistant *Bacteroides melaninogenicus*. Arch Intern Med. 1990;150:2525-2529.

343. Stevens DL, Maier KA, Mitten JE. Effect of antibiotics on toxin production and viability of *Clostridium perfringens*. Antimicrob Agents Chemother. 1987;31:213-218.

344. Stevens DL, Maier KA, Laine BM, Mitten JE. Comparison of clindamycin, rifampin, tetracycline, metronidazole, and penicillin for efficacy in prevention of experimental gas gangrene due to *Clostridium perfringens*. J Infect Dis. 1987;155:220-228.

345. Leyden JJ, Berger RS, Dunlap FE, et al. Comparison of the efficacy and safety of a combination topical gel formulation of benzoyl peroxide and clindamycin with benzoyl peroxide, clindamycin and vehicle gel in the treatments of acne vulgaris. Am J Clin Dermatol. 2001;2:33-39.

346. Parry MF, Rha CK. Pseudomembranous colitis caused by topical clindamycin phosphate. Arch Dermatol. 1986;122:583-584.

347. Schmitt C, Sobel JD, Meriwether C. Bacterial vaginosis: Treatment with clindamycin cream versus oral metronidazole. Obstet Gynecol. 1992;79:1020-1023.

348. Kurkinen-Raty M, Vuopala S, Koskela M, et al. A randomised controlled trial of vaginal clindamycin for early pregnancy bacterial vaginosis. BJOG. 2000;107:1427-1432.

349. McDonald HM, O'Loughlin JA, Vigneswaran R, et al. Impact of metronidazole therapy on preterm birth in women with bacterial vaginosis flora *(Gardnerella vaginalis)*: A randomised, placebo controlled trial. Br J Obstet Gynaecol. 1997;104:1391-1397.

350. Carey JC, Klebanoff MA, Hauth JC, et al. Metronidazole to prevent preterm delivery in pregnant women with asymptomatic bacterial vaginosis. National Institute of Child Health and Human Development Network of Maternal-Fetal Medicine Units. N Engl J Med. 2000;342:534-540.

351. Ugwumadu A, Manyonda I, Reid F, Hay P. Effect of early oral clindamycin on late miscarriage and preterm delivery in asymptomatic women with abnormal vaginal flora and bacterial vaginosis: A randomised controlled trial. Lancet. 2003;361:983-988.

352. Dannemann B, McCutchan JA, Israelski D, et al. Treatment of toxoplasmic encephalitis in patients with AIDS: A randomized trial comparing pyrimethamine plus clindamycin to pyrimethamine plus sulfadiazine. The California Collaborative Treatment Group. Ann Intern Med. 1992;116:33-43.

353. Katlama C, De Wit S, O'Doherty E, et al. Pyrimethamine-clindamycin vs. pyrimethamine-sulfadiazine as acute and long-term therapy for toxoplasmic encephalitis in patients with AIDS. Clin Infect Dis. 1996;22:268-275.

354. Safrin S, Finkelstein DM, Feinberg J, et al. Comparison of three regimens for treatment of mild to moderate *Pneumocystis carinii* pneumonia in patients with AIDS: A double-blind, randomized, trial of oral trimethoprim-sulfamethoxazole, dapsone-trimethoprim, and clindamycin-primaquine. ACTG 108 Study Group. Ann Intern Med. 1996;124:792-802.

355. Kremsner PG, Radloff P, Metzger W, et al. Quinine plus clindamycin improves chemotherapy of severe malaria in children. Antimicrob Agents Chemother. 1995;39:1603-1605.

356. Wittner M, Rowin KS, Tanowitz HB, et al. Successful chemotherapy of transfusion babesiosis. Ann Intern Med. 1982;96:601-604.

357. Brook I, Hirokawa R. Treatment of patients with a history of recurrent tonsillitis due to group A beta-hemolytic streptococci: A prospective randomized study comparing penicillin, erythromycin, and clindamycin. Clin Pediatr (Phila). 1985;24:331-336.

358. Orrling A, Stjernquist-Desatnik A, Schalen C, Kamme C. Clindamycin in persisting streptococcal pharyngotonsillitis after penicillin treatment. Scand J Infect Dis. 1994;26:535-541.

359. American Academy of Pediatrics, Committee on Infectious Diseases. Severe invasive group A streptococcal infections: A subject review. Pediatrics. 1998;101:136-140.

360. Stevens DL, Madaras-Kelly KJ, Richards DM. In vitro antimicrobial effects of various combinations of penicillin and clindamycin against four strains of *Streptococcus pyogenes*. Antimicrob Agents Chemother. 1998;42:1266-1268.

CHAPTER **29**

Glycopeptides (Vancomycin and Teicoplanin), Streptogramins (Quinupristin-Dalfopristin), and Lipopeptides (Daptomycin)

BARBARA E. MURRAY

ESTEBAN C. NANNINI

GLYCOPEPTIDES

Vancomycin

Vancomycin, the first glycopeptide antibiotic developed for clinical use, was isolated from *Amycolatopsis orientalis* (known first as *Streptomyces orientalis*, and later as *Nocardia orientalis*) found in a soil sample from Borneo in the mid 1950s.[1] In 1958, vancomycin was introduced into clinical practice as an agent active against penicillin-resistant *Staphylococcus aureus*.[2] However, a few years later, the use of vancomycin was relegated to patients allergic to β-lactam antibiotics because of the availability of new penicillinase-resistant β-lactams, methicillin and cephalothin, and the high rate of toxicity observed with the initial vancomycin formulation. Indeed, early lots of vancomycin (compound 05865) were called "Mississippi mud," owing to the color provided by their large quantity of impurities; later manufacturing procedures markedly improved purification. Since the early 1980s, a steady rise in vancomycin use has occurred (e.g., in the United States, from 2000 kg/year in 1984 to 11,200 kg/year in 1996[3]), which has likely contributed to the increase in organisms with decreased glycopeptide susceptibility.

Structure and Mechanism of Action

Vancomycin is a complex tricyclic glycopeptide that consists of a seven-membered peptide chain forming the tricyclic structure, and an attached disaccharide composed of vancosamine and glucose.[4] The molecular weight is 1485.73, much higher than that of other antimicrobials.[4]

The primary effect of glycopeptides is inhibition of bacterial cell wall synthesis, although inhibition of RNA synthesis and the cytoplasmic membrane in *S. aureus* isolates has also been described.[5] The target of glycopeptides is murein monomers, which are peptidoglycan precursors composed of two amino sugars, *N*-acetylmuramic acid and *N*-acetylglucosamine, with a D-alanyl-D-alanine terminating pentapeptide. After crossing the cell membrane, monomers are normally added to the growing peptidoglycan chain in a process known as transglycosylation. The large glycopeptide molecules bind to the D-alanyl-D-alanine terminus of the pentapeptide after these precursors cross the cell membrane, forming a stable complex.[6] This complex cannot be accessed by the enzyme glycosyltransferase, leading to inhibition of incorporation of the murein monomers into the growing peptidoglycan chain and thus to interruption of cell wall synthesis.

Antimicrobial Activity

Vancomycin has broad activity against gram-positive microorganisms. Staphylococci (including *S. aureus, Staphylococcus epidermidis, Staphylococcus saprophyticus, Staphylococcus haemolyticus, Staphylococcus hominis, Staphylococcus warneri,* and other coagulase-negative staphylococci) are susceptible to vancomycin with minimal inhibitory concentrations (MIC) less than or equal to 4 μg/mL and minimal bactericidal concentrations (MBC) within twofold the MIC.[7] Glycopeptides remain active against most *Enterococcus faecalis* and a variable percent of *Enterococcus faecium,* but are not bactericidal even against susceptible isolates, with MBCs more than 32 times the MICs[8]; however, as with other cell-wall agents, the addition of an aminoglycoside (if the strain is not highly aminoglycoside resistant) increases the bactericidal activity.[9] All strains of *Streptococcus pneumoniae* and *Streptococcus pyogenes* are susceptible to vancomycin, as are virtually all *Streptococcus agalactiae,* group C and group G streptococci, *Streptococcus bovis, Streptococcus mutans* and viridans streptococci,[10-12] although rare isolates of streptococci (*S. bovis* group) have acquired *vanB* genes typical of VanB type enterococci. Vancomycin also shows good in vitro activity against *Granulicatella adiacens* and *Abiotrophia defectiva* (formerly members of the nutritionally variant streptococci).[13]

Listeria monocytogenes is susceptible to vancomycin, although strains with high MBCs have been reported.[14] Vancomycin also displays good in vitro activity against *Bacillus anthracis* isolates,[15] *Bacillus cereus,* and other *Bacillus* spp.,[16] with MICs less than or equal to 2 μg/mL. Against *Corynebacterium* spp., including *Corynebacterium jeikeium,* vancomycin has good activity and is the drug of choice for serious infections caused by these organisms until susceptibilities are known.[17] *Rhodococcus equi* is also susceptible to vancomycin.[17] The typical susceptibility to vancomycin of *Lactobacillus acidophilus* helps differentiate this organism from other *Lactobacillus* spp.,[18] which are intrinsically vancomycin resistant.

Among the gram-positive anaerobes, *Peptostreptococcus* species, *Actinomyces* spp., and *Propionibacterium* spp. are usually susceptible to vancomycin,[19] as are most *Clostridium* spp., including *Clostridium difficile,*[20] except some strains of *Clostridium ramosum* and *Clostridium innocuum.*[10]

Vancomycin displays no in vitro activity against gram-negative organisms, except for some nongonococcal *Neisseria* spp.[21] A few reports of its successful use in combination with rifampin (and/or ciprofloxacin) against *Chrysobacterium* (formerly, *Flavobacterium*) *meningosepticum* have been described,[22,23] although this gram-negative bacillus shows high MICs of vancomycin by broth microdilution method[24]; vancomycin should not be administered as monotherapy for infections caused by this organism.

Mechanisms of Resistance

Development of resistance to vancomycin by mutations was predicted to be a rare occurrence in the clinical setting because the MIC of vancomycin against staphylococcal isolates increased only modestly after serial passages in the presence of the drug, compared with 100,000-fold when penicillin was used.[25] Although higher MICs and MBCs of vancomycin are noted when using high inocula (10[7] colony forming units [CFU]/mL) of *S. epidermidis* isolates,[26] it was not until the mid 1980s that the first clinical isolates of (methicillin-resistant) *S. epidermidis* with reduced susceptibility to glycopeptides were described.[27] Several years later vancomycin-resistant enterococci (VRE) (MIC ≥32 μg/mL) isolates were reported in Europe and, subsequently, the rest of the world. In 1997, the first clinical isolate of *S. aureus* with diminished susceptibility to vancomycin was described from Japan.[28,29] This strain displayed a vancomycin MIC of 8 μg/mL, which is in the range of intermediate susceptibility (8 to 16 μg/mL) per the National Committee for Clinical Laboratory Studies (NCCLS) breakpoints,[30] and thus was

referred to in this country as vancomycin-intermediate *S. aureus* (VISA) or glycopeptide-intermediate *S. aureus* (GISA). However, based on the breakpoints of the British Society for Antimicrobial Chemotherapy (BSAC), which classifies a vancomycin MIC of 8 μg/mL as resistant,[31] this strain has also been called vancomycin-resistant *S. aureus* (see Table 29-1 for staphylococcal susceptibility breakpoints recommended by NCCLS and BSAC).[28] This initial report was followed by others from various countries.[32] In 2002, two clinical isolates of vancomycin-resistant *S. aureus* (MIC ≥ 32 μg/mL) were described, both containing the enterococcal *vanA* genes.[33,34]

Enterococci. Among enterococci, six types of glycopeptide resistance have been described (VanA, VanB, VanC, VanD, VanE, and VanG), that are named based on their specific ligase genes (e.g., *vanA, vanB,* etc.). A related gene cluster, *vanF,* has been found in *Paenibacillus* (formerly *Bacillus*) *popilliae* strains (a biopesticide used in the United States to suppress Japanese beetle populations).[35] The common end point of these phenotypes is the formation of a peptidoglycan precursor with decreased affinity for glycopeptides, resulting in decreased inhibition of peptidoglycan synthesis. Peptidoglycan precursors ending in the depsipeptide D-alanyl-D-lactate are produced in VanA, VanB, and VanD strains, whereas VanC and VanE isolates produce precursors terminating in D-alanyl-D-serine, instead of the normally occurring D-alanyl-D-alanine.

Glycopeptide resistance in enterococci is classified as either intrinsic (as a species characteristic) or acquired. The former is a characteristic of the motile species *Enterococcus gallinarum* and *Enterococcus casseliflavus/flavescens,* members of which all carry the naturally occurring *vanC-1,* and *vanC-2/vanC-3* genes, respectively.[36] These enterococci show variable MICs of vancomycin, with many falling in the susceptible range, and clinical failures have been reported following vancomycin use.[37] In general, the isolation of these species does not require strict infection control isolation procedures, unless they are highly resistant, suggesting the added presence of potentially transferable *vanA* or *vanB* genes.[38]

Acquired glycopeptide resistance is found most often in *E. faecium,* followed by *E. faecalis,* and is much less common in other enterococcal species. VanA and VanB account for the vast majority of glycopeptide resistance. VanA isolates show high MICs of vancomycin and teicoplanin, whereas VanB strains often have lower MICs of vancomycin and, typically, are susceptible to teicoplanin.

Expression of the *vanA* gene cluster is regulated by a membrane-associated sensor kinase (VanS) that senses glycopeptides in the medium and activates the cytoplasmic response regulator (VanR), which triggers transcription of the resistance as well as the regulatory genes. Similarly, the *vanB* gene cluster has VanS$_B$ and VanR$_B$[39]; the VanB sensor kinase (VanS$_B$) does not appear to recognize teicoplanin, which explains the typical susceptibility of VanB VRE.[40]

The epidemiology, spread, and impact of VRE strains in Europe and the United States have notable differences. In the European Union, the glycopeptide avoparcin was frequently fed to animals as a growth enhancer, apparently selecting for the VRE commonly found in the intestinal flora of animals.[41] The contamination of food from animals, such as poultry products,[41] presumably led to the VRE colonization seen in healthy volunteers from European countries.[42] However, the prevalence of VRE in hospitalized patients of most European countries has not reached the epidemic magnitude found in the United States,[43] where glycopeptides have never been approved for animal feed use and VRE carriage has been largely undetected (except the endogenously resistant species *E. gallinarum* and *E. casseliflavus*) outside the health care setting.[44] The widespread use of vancomycin in the hospital setting is likely one of the culprits for the rapid selection and proliferation of VRE within this environment. The proportion of VRE among enterococcal isolates from nosocomial infections has continued to rise during recent years, as reported by the Centers for Disease Control and Prevention (CDC).[45]

Another phenomenon described in *E. faecalis* and *E. faecium* is the existence of strains that can only sustain growth in the presence of vancomycin, so-called vancomycin-dependent enterococci (VDE), or when supplemented with the dipeptide D-alanyl-

D-alanine.[46] VDE strains have an inactive D-alanine:D-alanine ligase (and thus do not produce D-alanine-D-alanine) but, under vancomycin-inducing conditions, are able to synthesize cell-wall utilizing D-alanine:D-lactate ligase produced from their *vanA* or *vanB* gene cluster. When vancomycin is not present, these precursors are not produced and the organism cannot survive. Discontinuation of vancomycin may not suffice to cure VDE infections because these strains can revert to vancomycin-independent growth.[47]

Staphylococcus aureus. The exact mechanism and genetic basis underlying the decreased susceptibility to vancomycin of VISA isolates is a subject of active investigation, but none of these strains carry the vancomycin-resistant genes found in enterococci.[48] *S. aureus* derivatives with four- to eightfold increases in the MICs of vancomycin and significant thickening of the cell wall can be generated in the laboratory by serial passage in the presence of vancomycin.[49] Clinical VISA isolates also have a thicker cell wall when grown in glycopeptides and an increased amount of D-alanyl-D-alanine residues, which may be the result of increased synthesis of cell wall precursors[48] or decreased cell wall turnover[50]; these extra residues appear to trap glycopeptides, keeping them from reaching their actual target sites near the cytoplasmic membrane.[51] A positive correlation has been found between cell wall thickness and the MICs of vancomycin and teicoplanin.[52]

Because VISA isolates are not detected in vitro by the disk diffusion methodology, MIC determinations by agar or broth dilution and/or by E-test® strips are recommended for confirmation of vancomycin susceptibility.[53,54] It is also recommended to contact the CDC for any *S. aureus* isolates with an MIC of vancomycin greater than or equal to 4 μg/mL.[55] Several VISA isolates have been recovered from patients failing therapy with vancomycin,[56] and, as expected, poor response to vancomycin has been documented in the experimental endocarditis model using these strains.[57]

Another form of decreased susceptibility to vancomycin in *S. aureus* is a phenomenon called heteroresistance. Heteroresistance means that only a subpopulation of bacterial cells (sometimes as few as 1 in 100,000 bacteria) can grow on vancomycin-containing agar; when recultured, greater than or equal to 8 μg/mL is required for inhibition.[56] These heteroresistant strains are considered precursors of VISA isolates.[51] Conventional susceptibility tests cannot identify heteroresistant cells, and population analysis (determination of the number of surviving cells at increasing antibiotic concentrations) is needed. The spread of heteroresistant strains has been confirmed in Japanese hospitals,[58] but the extent of the dissemination of these strains in the United States still appears to be minimal.[59] A few cases of vancomycin failures in patients infected with heteroresistant strains have been reported[60,61] and in the endocarditis model response to vancomycin is significantly affected when heteroresistant *S. aureus* derivative strains are used.[61] However, the overall clinical significance and impact of heteroresistant strains are still unknown, and screening for their detection is not recommended.[62] Typically VISA isolates also display decreased susceptibility to teicoplanin (MIC ≥8 μg/mL).[51] In addition, *S. aureus* strains with decreased susceptibility to teicoplanin, although remaining susceptible to vancomycin, were reported before the emergence of VISA isolates.[63]

As of 2002, two truly vancomycin-resistant *S. aureus* (VRSA) clinical isolates were described.[33,34] The MICs of vancomycin were 1024 μg/mL and 32 to 64 μg/mL for the first and second isolate, respectively.[33,64] These isolates were epidemiologically unrelated to each other, and in both the enterococcal *vanA* gene was amplified; in one patient, a *vanA* containing *E. faecalis* strain was also isolated, the presumed source of the *vanA* gene cluster.[33,34] Infection control measures appear to have controlled the spread of these isolates.[64]

Coagulase-Negative Staphylococci. In vitro studies in the 1980s found higher MICs of teicoplanin, sometimes within the resistance range, against methicillin-resistant *S. haemolyticus*.[65] Overall, MICs of teicoplanin against coagulase-negative staphylococci show a wide range, occasionally higher than the NCCLS resistance breakpoint

(MIC ≥32 μg/mL).[66,67] MICs of vancomycin are generally less variable and within the susceptible range,[68] although resistant *S. haemolyticus* and *S. epidermidis* strains have been reported.[69,70]

Streptococcus pneumoniae. Historically, *S. pneumoniae* isolates have been susceptible to the bactericidal activity of vancomycin; however, the relatively recent description of vancomycin tolerance in *S. pneumoniae* raises some concern. Such strains appear to have a defect in the control process for triggering autolysis, which may be secondary to the loss of function of part of a sensor-regulatory system,[71] although other mechanisms have been proposed.[72] Three percent of 116 clinical pneumococcal isolates were tolerant to vancomycin in a time-kill assay,[73] whereas another study, using similar methods, did not find vancomycin-tolerance among 120 clinical isolates.[74] The clinical implications of this phenomenon are difficult to assess; an apparent vancomycin (with cefotaxime) therapeutic failure for pneumococcal meningitis caused by a vancomycin-tolerant strain has been reported.[75]

Other Gram-Positive Bacteria. Although less often associated with human disease, the genera *Leuconostoc* and *Pediococcus*, and certain *Lactobacillus* spp. (*Lactobacillus rhamnosus*, *Lactobacillus casei*, and *Lactobacillus plantarum*) are intrinsically resistant to glycopeptides.[76] The mechanism of resistance apparently involves production of peptidoglycan precursors that terminate in D-alanyl-D-lactate.[77] The D-alanine:D-lactate ligase of these organisms, however, is not closely related to the VanA or VanB ligase found in VRE strains.[78] Another gram-positive organism, *Erysipelothrix rhusiopathiae,* is also typically vancomycin resistant.[79] The gram-positive and glycopeptide-producing organisms *Amycolatopsis orientalis* and *Streptomyces toyocaensis* have been proposed as the remote ancestor of some of the vancomycin-resistant genes found in VRE because of the homology found in the proteins from these organisms and those from VRE.[80]

Clinical Pharmacodynamics and Pharmacokinetics

A considerable number of studies have found that the bactericidal activity of vancomycin is concentration independent once a concentration of four or five times the MIC for the organism is reached, and that the pharmacodynamic parameters that best express its activity are the time that the vancomycin concentration is greater than the MIC and the 24-hour area under the concentration-time curve (AUC)/MIC ratio.[81] The in vitro postantibiotic effect of vancomycin against staphylococci and enterococci has been described mostly as of short duration.[81] The activity of vancomycin is affected, at least to some degree, by the presence of biofilm,[82] which is often seen in the setting of medical device–related infection, likely due to metabolic differences.

Vancomycin is given intravenously for the treatment of systemic infections caused by susceptible organisms. In certain circumstances, vancomycin can be administered through oral, intraperitoneal, intrathecal or intraventricular, and intraocular routes, but intramuscular injection is not used because it causes severe local pain. Oral administration of vancomycin results in high levels within the gut lumen, but not usually in measurable serum concentrations[83]; occasionally, in the presence of diffuse colonic inflammation and renal insufficiency, detectable levels of vancomycin are obtained in serum.[84]

Distribution. Vancomycin concentrations achieved in serum in normal volunteers 2 hours after an intravenous dose of 0.5 g and 1 g are about 10 μg/mL and 25 μg/mL, respectively.[2,25] These levels decrease to 2 μg/mL by 6 to 8 hours after 0.5 g and by 12 hours after 1 g.[25] Vancomycin pharmacokinetics are best described by a two-[2,85] or three-compartment model.[86] After intravenous dosing of vancomycin, the drug shows a short distribution phase of about 7 minutes and then an intermediate phase of serum decline (half-life of 30 to 90 minutes). This is followed by a highly variable elimination phase of 3 to 11 hours (averaging 6 hours) in subjects with normal renal function[87-89]; in this phase, the vancomycin concentration is inversely affected by the creatinine clearance. The volume of distribution of vancomycin at steady state ranges from 390 to 970 mL/kg in studies including adults, children, and infants[90] and the percent protein binding in serum varies between 30% and 55%[88,91] with no differences noted in patients with various degrees of renal impairment.[91]

Penetration of vancomycin into the cerebrospinal fluid (CSF) is minimal in the absence of meningeal inflammation.[2,89,92] In adults with ventriculitis, CSF penetration ranges from 5% to 10% after intravenous administration,[93] whereas in children with meningitis, the vancomycin concentration in CSF has ranged from 14% to 28% (mean, 21%) of that in serum after a vancomycin dose of 60 mg/kg/day in conjunction with dexamethasone[94]; this concentration is considered adequate and predictable.[94] Dexamethasone, through reduction of meningeal inflammation, decreases vancomycin CSF penetration, which was associated with delayed CSF sterilization in experimental meningitis,[95,96] although with higher doses, therapeutic CSF levels were achieved.[96] Low vancomycin CSF levels have been associated with clinical failures in adults with pneumococcal meningitis.[97]

Animal studies have documented high concentrations of vancomycin in kidney, liver, and spleen of rats[98] but data on concentrations in human organs are limited. A relatively good concentration was found in kidney, liver, aorta, lung, heart tissue, and in abscess fluid in a patient after several vancomycin doses.[99] Concentrations in heart valve, subcutaneous tissue, and muscle were found to be 52%, 29%, and 27% of the concomitant serum level, respectively, 6 hours after a single vancomycin dose.[100] Penetration of vancomycin into vegetations has been demonstrated in experimental endocarditis models.[101] Vancomycin concentrations are generally adequate to treat susceptible organisms in fluids from the pericardial, ascitic, pleural, and synovial spaces,[2,89,92] but are relatively low in lung tissue.[102] Although vancomycin appears to penetrate into bile,[2] it is not concentrated there.[92] Vancomycin, like many other antimicrobials, penetrates very poorly into the aqueous humor of the eye.[103]

Human studies evaluating the concentration of vancomycin reached in infected and uninfected bone have reported highly variable results.[104] A mean concentration of vancomycin in the sternum of 10.4 μg/g 60 minutes after administration of 15 mg/kg has been documented in subjects undergoing cardiac surgery.[105] Nonetheless, it has been difficult to find a correlation between antibiotic bone concentrations and clinical outcome.[106]

Transplacental passage of vancomycin during the second trimester of pregnancy has been documented,[107] and the concentration of vancomycin in breast milk 4 hours after intravenous infusion was 12.7 μg/mL,[108] which could lead to a potential infant oral dose of 1.9 mg/kg/day.[109]

Excretion. Vancomycin is primarily excreted unchanged via the kidneys by glomerular filtration, with no direct evidence of tubular secretion or resorption.[89] A linear correlation between creatinine clearance and vancomycin levels was recognized early on in patients with varying degrees of renal dysfunction.[85,92,110] Some investigators report a lower rate of vancomycin clearance in patients with hepatic dysfunction.[111] However, nonrenal clearance does not appear to account for more than 5% of the total drug clearance, and, therefore, dosage adjustment in patients with hepatic dysfunction alone is unlikely to be necessary.[90]

Administration. For intravenous administration, vancomycin is generally diluted in 100 to 250 mL of 5% dextrose or 0.9% saline solution with a concentration of less than or equal to 5 mg/mL and infused at a rate not exceeding 15 mg/minute (i.e., 0.5 g and 1 g in 30 and 60 minutes, respectively) to minimize the occurrence of infusion-related toxicities.[88] Antihistamines may be used to reduce the incidence of "red man" or "red-neck" syndrome, which, when seen, is usually associated with rapid infusion of a high vancomycin dose.[112] The usual recommended intravenous dose in adults with normal renal function is 30 mg/kg daily divided into two or four doses (typically, 500 mg every 6 hours or 1 g every 12 hours); continuous infusion at a dose of 30 mg/kg/day after a loading dose of 15 mg/kg also has been used.[113] Morbidly obese patients should receive vancomycin based on their actual total body weight instead of their ideal weight, and, in order to avoid very high peak values, a frequent dosing schedule should be considered[114]; serum level measurements may be worthwhile.[115] Significantly higher vancomycin clearance has been shown in burn patients, suggesting also the need for higher and more frequent doses in

this group of patients.[116] Even though a significant decrease of serum vancomycin levels during cardiopulmonary bypass has been documented,[117] concentrations are maintained within the therapeutic range after a 15 mg/kg dose of this drug administered intravenously 1 hour before skin incision.[117] No dosage adjustment appears to be necessary during pregnancy,[108] although a higher dose (1250 mg every 8 hours) was needed in a pregnant woman with endocarditis.[118] The dose of intravenous vancomycin for children with non–central nervous system (CNS) infections should be 10 mg/kg every 6 hours and, for infections involving the CNS and other serious infections, 15 mg/kg every 6 hours.[119,120] Newborns and young infants appear to have a lower vancomycin clearance rate; for newborns of less than a week of age, the recommended dose is 15 mg/kg every 12 hours, and for those between 1 week and 30 days of age, 15 mg/kg every 8 hours.[119]

Vancomycin is also an alternative choice for prophylaxis of endocarditis and the recommended intravenous dose is 1 g and 20 mg/kg in adults and children, respectively.[121] The infusion should be completed within 30 minutes of the beginning of the procedure.[121]

Vancomycin for oral administration is formulated in capsules and oral solution and can be given by mouth or, as needed in case of ileus or toxic megacolon, by nasogastric tube and even via rectal tube (intracolonic administration) or ileostomy.[122] The recommended oral dose for pseudomembranous colitis in adults has ranged from 125 mg to 500 mg every 6 hours, depending on the severity of the colitis.[123] In children, the usual dose is 40 mg/kg/day (not exceeding 2 g per day) divided in three or four doses. For the intracolonic administration, 500 mg of vancomycin dissolved in 1 to 2 L of 0.9% saline solution has been infused as a retention enema several times (two to six) a day.[122]

After intraperitoneal administration of vancomycin in patients on continuous ambulatory peritoneal dialysis (CAPD), therapeutic levels in serum can be obtained[124] and the concentrations of vancomycin in serum and in the dialysate can be therapeutic (7 ± 1.2 μg/mL and 3.6 ± 1.1 μg/mL for serum and dialysate, respectively) up to 7 days after the intraperitoneal administration of 30 mg/kg (in 2 L of dialysate, with 6 hours' retention/settling).[125] The peak serum concentration with this dose given intraperitoneally occurred at about 6 hours after the dose and the serum half-life was 105 ± 36 hours.[125] Others have suggested the use of continuous treatment, with vancomycin (1.5 mg/kg) added in each dialysate exchange.[125] Conversely, the peritoneal dialysate concentration of vancomycin after intravenous administration does not reliably provide adequate levels to treat peritonitis caused by susceptible organisms.[89,124]

Because of concern that CSF levels of vancomycin may be inadequate to treat ventriculitis, even with active infection, intrathecal or intraventricular administration of vancomycin has been advocated, particularly when vancomycin is used as monotherapy.[2,89] The recommended initial dose for the treatment of ventriculitis or shunt-related infections is 5 to 10 mg/day in infants and 10 to 20 mg/day in children and adults[126,127]; however, further adjustments based on CSF levels should be made because of variable and unpredictable kinetics.[127] The recommended optimal vancomycin trough concentration in CSF ranges from 5 μg/mL to 10 to 20 μg/mL,[127,128] which is greater than the MBC of most vancomycin-susceptible pathogens. A peak CSF concentration that is four- to eightfold higher than the MBC for the infecting organism was adequate for bacterial clearance in an experimental model, if the concentration was maintained at more than the MBC for the majority of the time interval.[96] For administration of vancomycin into the CSF, the drug should be diluted up to 2 mL in 0.9% saline solution to a concentration of 2.5 to 25 mg/mL.[127]

The use of intravenous vancomycin in patients with postoperative endophthalmitis results in subtherapeutic concentrations in the vitreous.[129] However, after intraocular administration of 1 mg of vancomycin, vitreous concentrations are in the therapeutic range for at least 3 days.[129]

Dosing in Renal Insufficiency. Because vancomycin is not removed by hemodialysis[130] and the serum half-life of vancomycin in anephric patients is 7.5 days,[85] the recommended dose of vancomycin in these patients has been 15 mg/kg every 7 to 10 days.[89,131] However, if high-flux membranes are used, a significant reduction of vancomycin serum levels might occur.[132] In this setting, Barth and colleagues suggested a loading dose of 20 mg/kg followed by supplementation with 500 mg after each dialysis; this schedule led to a mean trough concentration of 15.9 μg/mL.[132] CAPD also can decrease the elimination half-life of vancomycin,[124,133] leading to a need for a modest increase in the intravenous dose.

There are several nomograms and formulas to determine the dosing schedule in patients with decreased creatinine clearance. The total daily dose of vancomycin (in mg) needed to achieve a mean steady-state serum level of 15 μg/mL was established by Moellering and associates,[134] using a graph derived from the following formula:

$$\text{Dose (mg/day)} = 15.4 \times \text{creatinine clearance (mL/min)}$$

These authors also recommended not using the nomogram for anephric patients; instead, a dose of 1.9 mg/kg/day should be given after a loading dose of 15 mg/kg.[134]

Another approach is to lengthen the interval between doses, which may result in a more convenient regimen than the daily dosing schedule.[110] A fixed loading dose (25 mg/kg) followed by a maintenance dose (19 mg/kg) administered intravenously at a calculated interval should result in an approximate serum peak value of 30 μg/mL and a trough of 7.5 μg/mL. The interval is calculated from the following formula[110]:

$$\text{Interval} = \text{normal interval (86 mL/min} \div [0.689 \times \text{creatinine clearance mL/min} + 3.66])$$

For example, for a creatinine clearance of 60 mL/min, the interval would be 12 hours times 1.9, which results in 22.9 hours, meaning that after a loading dose of 25 mg/kg, the patient should receive a dose of 19 mg/kg every approximately 23 hours.

Clearance of vancomycin in patients with acute renal failure undergoing continuous venovenous hemofiltration (CVVH) or continuous venovenous hemodialysis (CVVHD) is significantly increased.[135,136] This clearance depends on operational factors such as the ultrafiltration flow rate and the type of hemofilter.[135] The recommended doses have ranged from 0.5 g to 1.5 g every 24 hours for CVVH and from 0.8 g to 1.75 g every 24 hours for CVVHD.[135] Measurements of vancomycin levels may be required due to patient-related factors and changes in the operational characteristics of CVVH or CVVHD.[136]

Adverse Reactions

One of the first reports of the clinical use of vancomycin included six cases with severe ototoxicity.[137,138] Most of these patients were receiving 1 to 2 g of vancomycin per day despite renal insufficiency[137] and, when vancomycin levels were measured, values between 80 and 100 μg/mL were observed.[138] These findings led to recommendations for a serum target level less than 40 to 50 μg/mL.[139] However, after more than 40 years of clinical use of vancomycin and with purified material, relatively few cases of confirmed vancomycin-related ototoxicity have been reported; this has led to the conclusion that vancomycin-related ototoxicity is a rare reaction.[90,140,141] Animal studies have also failed to show evidence of vancomycin-induced hearing damage[142] and, although augmentation of the ototoxic effects of aminoglycosides by the co-administration with vancomycin has been reported,[143] this has been difficult to prove in humans.[144] When ototoxicity develops, it generally appears to be reversible after drug discontinuation.[140] Vertigo and tinnitus are also rarely reported during vancomycin therapy[141,145] and may precede hearing loss.

Nephrotoxicity associated with vancomycin has been reported since the beginning of its clinical use, and thought to be related, at least in part, to impurities in the early preparations.[90] Initial studies also noted renal toxicity in animals when high doses of vancomycin were administered.[146] However, and despite its old reputation as a nephrotoxic agent, vancomycin use alone has been associated with a low rate of renal dysfunction in clinical studies that avoided the inclusion of confounding factors. Most prospectively designed studies report an incidence of renal function impairment between zero and

7%.[147,148] However, confirming previously reported synergistic nephrotoxic effects between vancomycin and aminoglycosides in animal studies,[146] the nephrotoxicity rate increases to 14% to more than 20% when vancomycin is co-administered with an aminoglycoside.[147,148] A case of acute interstitial nephritis associated with vancomycin use has also been reported.[149]

Infusion-related reactions are the most common side effects seen with vancomycin. A rapid onset of an erythematous rash and/or pruritus affecting the head, face, neck, and upper trunk, with or without associated angioedema and hypotension (anaphylactoid reaction), commonly known as "red-neck" or "red man syndrome," has been reported during the infusion of vancomycin with variable frequency, ranging from 3.4% to 11.2%.[90,150] More severe hypotension[151] and even cardiac arrest[152] have also been reported during vancomycin infusion. The mechanism for these effects is probably related to histamine release from basophils and mast cells.[112,153] These reactions usually subside soon after stopping the infusion without other measures. The incidence of these side effects can be reduced by decreasing the infusion rate or the concentration,[153] and by using antihistamines (H_1 receptor antagonists).[112] Local reactions, such as phlebitis, have been reported in 3% to 14% of patients receiving vancomycin.[139,148,154]

Neutropenia is also observed with vancomycin with a frequency of about 1% to 2%,[139,148] although this rate increases with long-term vancomycin therapy; one study showed a rate of 13% in patients treated with vancomycin for a mean of 6.2 months.[145] Neutropenia usually resolves after discontinuation of the drug,[131,139] and it is recommended to monitor leukocyte count in patients receiving vancomycin for more than 2 weeks.[90] Thrombocytopenia associated with vancomycin use is very rarely reported,[131] and probably secondary to immune-mediated platelet destruction.[155]

Presumptive vancomycin-induced maculopapular or erythematous skin rash and drug-related fever were noted in 3% and 2% of patients receiving vancomycin, respectively.[139] Reports of more severe reactions, such as erythema multiforme, toxic epidermal necrolysis, and Stevens-Johnson syndrome have also been reported.[156,157] Despite the clinical efficacy of oral vancomycin for treating *C. difficile*–related diarrhea, cases of *C. difficile* colitis attributed to the use of intravenous vancomycin have been reported.[158]

Even though an episode of reversible decreased consciousness[159] and two cases of CSF eosinophilia[160] have been reported after intraventricular administration of vancomycin, this route is regarded as generally safe.[161] Intraperitoneal administration of vancomycin is rarely associated with chemical peritonitis.[162]

Scarce published data exist on the use of vancomycin during pregnancy and it is classified as pregnancy category C. Infants born to mothers that received a course of vancomycin during the second or third trimester of pregnancy had no nephrotoxicity or sensorineural hearing loss.[108] However, because no reports exist on vancomycin use during the first trimester, it is unknown if this drug produces fetal harm. This drug should be used only when clearly needed considering the maternal benefit and the possible fetal risk. Vancomycin is excreted in human milk,[108] resulting in potential exposure of infants to this agent.

Drug Interactions

Precipitation has been noted with a highly concentrated solution of vancomycin mixed with ceftazidime,[163] and the use of different syringes for the intraocular administration of these two antibiotics for the treatment of endophthalmitis has been recommended.[164] Vancomycin has also been reported to be incompatible in intravenous solutions with other compounds, such as chloramphenicol, methicillin, corticosteroids, aminophylline, barbiturates, thiazides, diphenylhydantoin, sodium bicarbonate, and sulfisoxazole.[131] Precipitation with decreased activity of vancomycin was reported when infused together with heparin,[165] although others were unable to detect an effect of heparin on vancomycin stability or activity.[166] Even though co-administration of vancomycin and anesthetic agents was thought to produce a higher incidence of anaphylactoid reactions and hypotension, a blinded study could not validate this interaction.[167] Anion-exchange resins such as cholestyramine can bind to vancomycin, decreasing the activity of vancomycin in the gut lumen when orally administered.[168]

Drug Dosage Monitoring

Even though some studies have documented a higher rate of nephrotoxicity in subjects with vancomycin trough levels greater than 10 µg/mL or 15 µg/mL,[147,169] the close relationship between glomerular function and vancomycin levels makes it very difficult to discern which event occurred first.[140] The correlation between vancomycin levels and clinical outcome is even more difficult to establish. One study reported that patients with gram-positive bacteremia became afebrile sooner if vancomycin peak and trough levels were greater than 20 µg/mL and 10 µg/mL, respectively,[170] although no effect on mortality or outcome was noted. Another study found that vancomycin levels did not predict outcome in cancer patients with gram-positive bacteremia.[169]

Some investigators previously proposed that measurement of vancomycin levels in serum should be used to optimize therapy[87]; however, a number of investigators[86,140,171,172] have firmly taken a position against the routine measurement of vancomycin serum levels. This opinion is based on the relative lack of studies showing a correlation between serum levels and clinical outcome or toxicity.[86,154] Most researchers do agree, however, that in special circumstances, it is prudent to measure vancomycin concentrations. These situations include, for the most part, patients concomitantly receiving another nephrotoxic agent, especially aminoglycosides; patients receiving high-dose vancomycin; patients with rapidly changing renal function; and subjects undergoing hemodialysis, especially if high-flux membranes are used, including patients on CVVH or CVVHD. Other situations include the measurement of CSF levels in patients receiving vancomycin for CNS infection, whether by intrathecal, intraventricular,[127] or intravenous routes; vancomycin administration in neonates, in which measurement of trough and not peak levels has been suggested[173]; and in extremely ill patients or in the face of possible therapeutic failure, to ensure adequate drug presence.[174] A peak serum concentration of 30 to 40 µg/mL, a trough of 5 to 10 µg/mL, and an average steady state of 15 µg/mL have been proposed as optimal targets when vancomycin levels are measured.[87,134] Others have used a targeted trough of 10 to 15 µg/mL with intermittent dosing and a targeted plateau concentration of 20 to 25 µg/mL with continuous infusion for critically ill patients with severe infections.[113] If serum vancomycin levels are to be measured, it should be noted that trough concentrations less than 15 µg/ml have been highly correlated with peak levels no more than 40 µg/mL in adults with normal renal function.[175]

The detection of vancomycin degradation products, which accumulate in renal failure, can result in an overestimate of the (active) vancomycin concentration if levels are measured by fluorescence polarization immunoassay (FPIA) using polyclonal antibodies.[176] Enzyme multiplied immunoassay technique (EMIT) and modified FPIA,[176,177] both utilizing monoclonal antibodies, are the suggested methods of choice in this setting.

Clinical Uses

Endocarditis. Vancomycin is generally the drug of choice for bacteremia, endocarditis, and other serious infections caused by methicillin-resistant staphylococci. In subjects with a history of significant allergic reactions to β-lactams, vancomycin is frequently used for the therapy for endocarditis caused by gram-positive bacteria.[178] If vancomycin is to be administered for the treatment of staphylococcal endocarditis, a course of 4 to 6 weeks is recommended.[178] Treatment failures have been reported with this glycopeptide in the treatment of staphylococcal endocarditis,[179,180] and its effectiveness has been questioned based on the high rate of unsatisfactory response among intravenous drug users with S. aureus endocarditis,[181] the slow response (median duration of bacteremia, 7 days) in patients with methicillin-resistant S. aureus (MRSA) endocarditis,[182] and the higher failure rate in a 14-day course therapy for right-sided methicillin-susceptible

S. aureus (MSSA) endocarditis when vancomycin or teicoplanin were compared with cloxacillin (both co-administered with gentamicin).[183] These studies suggest that vancomycin is not as effective as penicillinase-stable penicillins for the treatment of MSSA endocarditis. For this reason, vancomycin should not be used purely for its dosing convenience,[178] and in patients with MSSA endocarditis with a suspicious history of immediate hypersensitivity reaction to β-lactam antibiotics, skin testing for penicillin allergy should be performed.[184]

The addition of gentamicin (1 mg/kg intramuscularly or intravenously every 8 hours) to vancomycin is regarded as an optional regimen for the treatment of MRSA native valve endocarditis,[178] based on in vitro data enhancement between vancomycin and aminoglycosides (gentamicin and tobramycin) against some S. aureus isolates[185] and on a reduced duration of bacteremia obtained with the addition of gentamicin to nafcillin in patients with MSSA endocarditis.[186] However, due to synergism between vancomycin and aminoglycosides in terms of nephrotoxicity[187] and the lack of clinical studies showing the benefits of this combination, the addition of gentamicin should be restricted to the initial 3 to 5 days of therapy and probably not be given if the S. aureus isolate is resistant to the aminoglycoside.[178] The addition of rifampin to vancomycin in the treatment of native valve endocarditis caused by S. aureus was successful in a few reports[180] and in an animal model,[188] but was not better than vancomycin alone in a randomized clinical trial (rifampin administered at a dose of 600 mg every 24 hours).[182]

A 4-week course of vancomycin has been recommended for β-lactam–allergic patients with native valve endocarditis caused by viridans streptococci, G. adiacens and A. defectiva (both formerly classified within the group of nutritionally variant streptococci), and S. bovis.[178] The addition of gentamicin does not seem to be necessary, except for Granulicatella spp. or Abiotrophia spp.[178]

For the treatment of enterococcal endocarditis, vancomycin may be considered if the infecting strain is highly ampicillin resistant (typically an E. faecium isolate) or the patient is allergic to β-lactam antibiotics (preferably confirmed by skin test); in these instances, vancomycin should be combined with gentamicin or streptomycin in order to achieve bactericidal activity (if the organism does not display high-level resistance to the aminoglycoside).[189,190]

For prosthetic valve endocarditis due to methicillin-resistant staphylococci, vancomycin in combination with rifampin (300 mg orally every 8 hours) for 6 weeks, together with gentamicin (1 mg/kg intramuscularly or intravenously every 8 hours) for the first 2 weeks (if the strain is susceptible) is a recommended regimen.[178] This combination was particularly effective against S. epidermidis.[191] The same antibiotic combination has been recommended for MRSA prosthetic valve endocarditis despite lack of proven clinical benefit[178] because of the poor prognosis associated with this condition; also for the latter reason, surgical treatment should be undertaken whenever possible.

Vancomycin also plays an important role in the treatment of endocarditis caused by diphtheroids, including C. jeikeium, which typically affects patients with prosthetic valves.[192,193] The addition of rifampin has been suggested,[194] although without much clinical evidence. Vancomycin has also been effective in a few reported cases of penicillin- and cephalosporin-resistant S. pneumoniae endocarditis[195] and in the experimental model of endocarditis caused by this organism.[196] Vancomycin in combination with gentamicin can be used for the treatment of L. monocytogenes bacteremia and endocarditis,[197] although ampicillin (with or without gentamicin) is preferred.[197]

Meningitis/Ventriculitis. Vancomycin in combination with cefotaxime or ceftriaxone is the treatment of choice for empirical therapy of patients with suspected or proven pneumococcal meningitis until susceptibility data are available, in areas where infections caused by penicillin-resistant S. pneumoniae have been documented.[198,199] If pneumococcal meningitis is confirmed and the isolate shows an MIC of ceftriaxone/cefotaxime of greater than or equal to 1 µg/mL (considered nonsusceptible for meningeal isolates by the NCCLS), the administration of vancomycin and ceftriaxone or cefotaxime should continue.[199] In children, rifampin might be added to this regimen if the S. pneumoniae isolate shows an MIC of ceftriaxone/cefotaxime of greater than or equal to 4 μg/mL.[198] In adults, the addition of rifampin to the regimen appears justified in cases caused by ceftriaxone nonsusceptible *S. pneumoniae* strains when dexamethasone is also administered, although the clinical benefit of this approach has not been evaluated. Vancomycin as the only antimicrobial agent with concomitant administration of dexamethasone has been associated with a high failure rate[97] in adults with pneumococcal meningitis; in children, the higher vancomycin dose usually given appears to overcome the negative effect of dexamethasone on the vancomycin CSF concentration.[94,96]

Vancomycin has a major role in the treatment of infections related to CSF shunts, the most common cause being *S. epidermidis.* Intravenous with or without intraventricular antibiotic administration, together with shunt hardware removal followed by external drainage and placement of a new shunt after confirmed CSF sterility, appears to be the most appropriate treatment modality.[200] Intravenous administration of vancomycin has been successful,[93] although others favor additional intraventricular dosing as well.[93,126,128] Determination of vancomycin levels in the CSF is recommended to ensure adequate concentrations. The addition of rifampin to the regimen should be contemplated for susceptible organisms when bacterial eradication is not achieved with vancomycin alone.

Osteomyelitis. Vancomycin is the agent of choice for methicillin-resistant staphylococci and it is an alternative for methicillin-susceptible strains in patients with intolerance or with allergic reactions to β-lactam agents. Intravenous vancomycin plus radical bone débridement was associated with successful outcome in 8 of 10 post-traumatic MRSA osteomyelitis cases, with a follow-up of 2 to 3.5 years.[201] Animal models, however, have shown poor results using vancomycin for the treatment of experimental MRSA osteomyelitis,[202,203] in which the co-administration of rifampin has been consistently associated with improved response.[202,203] The addition of rifampin to 2 weeks of flucloxacillin or vancomycin followed by long-term therapy with rifampin plus a fluoroquinolone was superior to therapy without rifampin in a randomized clinical trial of orthopedic implant-related staphylococcal infections of short duration.[204] It should be noted, however, that development of resistance to rifampin can occur promptly, even if co-administered with vancomycin.[205] Four to 6 weeks is the recommended length of therapy in adults with osteomyelitis and complete surgical débridement is critical for a successful outcome.

Pseudomembranous Colitis. Oral vancomycin was used historically for the treatment of pseudomembranous colitis caused by *C. difficile* and pseudomembranous enterocolitis caused by *S. aureus*, now a rare disease. Oral metronidazole and oral vancomycin, administered for 7 to 10 days, have similar failure and relapse rates in the treatment of *C. difficile* colitis.[206] Because of the cost of vancomycin and concern about selection of vancomycin-resistant enterococci, this drug should be used for the treatment of *C. difficile* colitis only when there is no clinical response or intolerance to metronidazole, or when the infected woman is pregnant.[207] Because of the poor concentration in stools after intravenous administration, vancomycin should not be used solely via this route.[207] In cases of severe disease and/or in the presence of ileus or toxic megacolon, increasing the dose of vancomycin from 125 mg to 500 mg every 6 hours[123,207] or intracolonic administration of this glycopeptide antibiotic[122,207] is probably an effective measure.

Febrile Neutropenia. The use of vancomycin in febrile neutropenic patients has been a controversial issue for a number of years. No differences in morbidity and mortality have been detected with the use of vancomycin as part of the initial regimen, even if a gram-positive organism was initially isolated.[208] The inclusion of vancomycin for patients with febrile neutropenia is recommended in only specific clinical situations, as reviewed by Hughes and associates.[209]

Prophylaxis. Vancomycin is recommended for prophylaxis of endocarditis when genitourinary or gastrointestinal (excluding esophageal) procedures are performed in subjects with cardiac conditions considered as risks for endocarditis and who are allergic to ampicillin.[121] Patients at high risk should also receive gentamicin.[121] Vancomycin is also recommended as a prophylactic agent for β-lactam–allergic patients undergoing cardiovascular surgery or or-

thopedic procedures with hardware placement and for surgical procedures requiring prophylaxis in centers with a high prevalence of MRSA,[210,211] although the clinical benefit from the latter has not been confirmed in a recent study.[212] Due to the relatively high infection rate observed in some series of CSF shunt placement, preoperative intraventricular administration of this agent (10 mg diluted in 1 mL) with gentamicin has been suggested, although this approach has not been evaluated in a clinical trial.[213]

Oral vancomycin has been used by some for prevention of endogenous gram-positive infections in cancer patients undergoing chemotherapy[214] and systemically in bone marrow transplant patients.[215] However, such use of vancomycin, as well as its use for routine prophylaxis in hemodialysis and CAPD patients or prior to insertion of central venous catheters, is discouraged due to the risk of selecting resistant organisms.[131]

Other Uses. Vancomycin is active against the majority of the agents that cause post-traumatic and postoperative endophthalmitis and is the recommended agent for gram-positive coverage in the empirical intraocular treatment of this disease. Animal models of endophthalmitis have also demonstrated the usefulness of vancomycin in this setting.[216] Bacterial peritonitis, the most frequent complication seen in patients undergoing CAPD, usually involves coagulase-negative staphylococci or *S. aureus*, among other gram-positive organisms, and in this setting, therapy with weekly doses of intravenous vancomycin has been associated with a high relapse rate[217] (see "Clinical Pharmacodynamics and Pharmacokinetics" earlier). Intraperitoneal administration of vancomycin, in either an intermittent (weekly) or continuous (in each dialysate exchange) dosing schedule has proven to be efficacious in this setting.[218] Vancomycin has been considered the drug of choice for MRSA pneumonia; however, in a randomized double-blind trial of patients with nosocomial pneumonia, a trend toward poorer response was observed in the vancomycin group compared with the linezolid group.[219] Moreover, in an observational study, vancomycin was associated with lower efficacy than cloxacillin in patients with MSSA bacteremic pneumonia.[220] Empirical treatment of catheter-related infections should include a glycopeptide antibiotic because methicillin-resistant coagulase-negative staphylococci, *S. aureus,* or other gram-positive organisms are frequently found, and clinical trials have shown the effectiveness of vancomycin in this setting.[221] Vancomycin was also shown to be effective when it was part of antibiotic-lock therapy in nonrandomized trials of uncomplicated catheter-related infections, avoiding the need for catheter removal[222] and in combination with heparin, has been relatively successful as prevention of central venous catheter-related infections in cancer patients.[223]

Teicoplanin

Teicoplanin (formerly known as teichomycin A$_2$) was obtained through fermentation of an actinomycete strain isolated from a soil sample in India in 1978, thereafter named *Actinoplanes teichomyceticus.*[224] This compound is currently commercially available in many countries in Europe, Asia, and North and South America but not in the United States. Teicoplanin is actually a mixture of different but related glycopeptide analogues with a basic structure characterized by a linear heptapeptide, the distinct carbohydrates D-mannose and D-glycosamine, and an acyl residue that carries various fatty acids, which define the members of the teicoplanin complex.[224,225] Teicoplanin has a molecular weight estimated as 1900 daltons.

Antimicrobial Activity and Resistance

Teicoplanin inhibits cell wall synthesis by a mechanism similar to that described for vancomycin, although some differences, mostly quantitative, exist. For instance, MICs of teicoplanin against coagulase-negative staphylococci tend to be more variable, especially for *S. haemolyticus* isolates, with some MICs above the susceptible breakpoint (Table 29-1).[67,226,227] On the other hand, the MICs of teicoplanin for *Enterococcus* spp., *S. pneumoniae*, *S. bovis*, viridans streptococci, and other streptococci are usually a few dilutions lower than those of vancomycin.[226-229] Despite low MICs against susceptible enterococci,[230] this drug appears to require the addition of an aminoglycoside for optimal

TABLE 29-1　MIC Susceptibility Breakpoints and Interpretation for Vancomycin, Teicoplanin, and Quinupristin-Dalfopristin against Staphylococci Based on the National Committee for Clinical Laboratory Standards (NCCLS) and the British Society for Antimicrobial Chemotherapy (BSAC) Recommendations

	NCCLS			BSAC		
	Susceptible	Intermediate	Resistant	Susceptible	Intermediate	Resistant
Vancomycin	≤4	8-16	≥32	≤4	—	≥8
Teicoplanin	≤8	16	≥32	≤4	—	≥8
Quinupristin-dalfopristin	≤1	2	≥4	≤2	—	≥4

bactericidal activity.[27] Activity similar to that reported with vancomycin has been described for teicoplanin against *L. monocytogenes*, *Corynebacterium* spp. (including *C. jeikeium*), and gram-positive anaerobes such as *Clostridium* spp. (including *C. difficile*), *Peptostreptococcus* spp., *Actinomyces* spp., and *Propionibacterium* spp.[226,229]

Strains of *S. aureus* susceptible to vancomycin but displaying high MICs of teicoplanin were reported before the description of VISA isolates,[231] and high MICs of teicoplanin are subsequently found in VISA isolates as well.[51] VanA-type VRE strains are resistant to teicoplanin, whereas VanB, VanE, and VanG strains typically show low MICs of teicoplanin. This agent, however, should be used very cautiously (if at all) to treat infections caused by such VRE strains, due to the risk for development of resistance while on therapy.[232]

Clinical Pharmacokinetics

The favorable pharmacokinetic properties of teicoplanin allow its administration by intravenous bolus or by the intramuscular route. As with vancomycin, however, this agent is not significantly absorbed when administered orally. In healthy volunteers, the mean peak concentrations of teicoplanin in serum are 53.5 μg/mL and 7.1 μg/mL (at 2 hours) after 3 mg/kg administered via intravenous and intramuscular routes, respectively, and 111.8 μg/mL after an intravenous dose of 6 mg/kg.[228] Trough levels are 4 μg/mL after the 6 mg/kg intravenous dose and 2 μg/mL after both intramuscular and intravenous administration of 3 mg/kg.[228] The steady-state trough teicoplanin mean concentrations were 14 μg/mL and 23 μg/mL following intravenous administration of 6 mg/kg and 12 mg/kg, respectively.[233] The distribution of teicoplanin is best described by a three-compartment kinetic model[234] and its volume of distribution at steady state ranges from 800 to 1600 mL/kg.[235] Teicoplanin is approximately 90% bound to serum proteins (albumin) and highly bound in tissues,[235] which may explain its low clearance and long half-life, which has ranged from 83 to 168 hours.[235]

Animal studies have reported better bone concentrations with teicoplanin than with vancomycin after equivalent intravenous infusion.[236] Clinical studies including patients undergoing joint replacement have confirmed its good penetration into bone.[237] Penetration into heart, pericardium, mediastinal tissue, lung, and synovial, pleural, peritoneal, and pericardial fluid is also considered adequate.[238,239] In experimental endocarditis, teicoplanin appears to be concentrated only at the periphery of the vegetation.[240] After intravenous infusion, significant concentrations of teicoplanin are generally not achieved in vitreous samples[241] or in the CSF, even in the presence of meningitis.[242]

Teicoplanin is almost entirely eliminated by renal mechanisms,[227,243] and even though this agent used to be regarded as a nondialyzable drug,[243] hemodialysis using high-flux membranes and CVVHD (depending on the ultrafiltration rate) removes significant quantities.[244] Teicoplanin levels seem not to be significantly modified in subjects undergoing cardiopulmonary bypass surgery.[245]

The oral dose of teicoplanin for the treatment of *C. difficile* pseudomembranous colitis ranges from 100 mg to 400 mg twice daily for 10 days.[206] The parenteral teicoplanin dose depends on the patient's age and renal function, the suspected or known microorganism, and the infected site. A loading regimen of 6 mg/kg every 12 hours for three doses is recommended, regardless of the renal function, in order to reach steady state sooner.[235] Then, in adults with normal renal func-

tion, 6 mg/kg every 24 hours is the usual maintenance dose. A higher dose (12 mg/kg every 12 hours for three times and then every 24 hours) is recommended for more difficult infections, such as endocarditis caused by *S. aureus* (especially when aminoglycosides are not co-administered), septic arthritis, and in burn patients.[235] The recommended dose for neonates is 16 mg/kg initially, followed by 8 mg/kg daily, and for children more than 2 months old, 10 mg/kg every 12 hours for three doses, and then every 24 hours.[235] In subjects with creatinine clearance between 40 and 60 mL/minute and in those with more severe renal failure or in hemodialysis with conventional membranes, the chosen dose (6 or 12 mg/kg) should be administered every 48 hours and 72 hours, respectively.[235] The maintenance daily dose can be calculated by multiplying the regular dose (i.e., 400 mg) by the ratio between the patient's creatinine clearance and the normal creatinine clearance.[243] Another way is to lengthen the interval between the doses, which, in days, results from dividing the normal creatinine clearance by the patient's clearance.[243] In patients undergoing CVVHD, 800 mg on day 1, 400 mg on days 2 and day 3, followed by 400 mg every 48 or 72 hours is the suggested dosing scheme, though measurement of serum levels is suggested.[244]

Peritoneal administration of teicoplanin results in serum concentrations similar to those achieved by intravenous concentration[243]; however, after intravenous administration, penetration of teicoplanin into the peritoneal dialysate does not achieve local therapeutic levels.[246] Teicoplanin has been administered in doses of 20 mg/L in each bag for the first week, in alternate bags during the second week, and only in the overnight dwell bag in the third week.[247] Another more practical and apparently effective approach is to dose 20 mg/L in each exchange (four times daily) for 10 days or for 5 days after clearing bacteria from the dialysate.[248]

Monitoring of teicoplanin serum levels is not generally needed with doses less than 12 mg/kg/day. Intravenous drug abusers with endocarditis have a higher clearance rate of teicoplanin, suggesting a need for serum level measurements in this population.[249] Other clinical scenarios in which measurement of teicoplanin serum levels might be appropriate include the following: patients not responding to treatment, patients with severe burns, and patients with rapidly changing renal function or on CVVHD.

Adverse Events

Teicoplanin is generally regarded as a safe drug.[250,251] Higher rates of all adverse events and nephrotoxicity are reported in individuals receiving vancomycin (21.9% and 10.7%, respectively) than those receiving teicoplanin (13.9% and 4.8%, respectively).[250] Teicoplanin is nephrotoxic in animals, although at much higher doses than those used in humans.[235] This antibiotic also appears to have less nephrotoxic synergism with aminoglycosides than vancomycin.[252] The most common side effects associated with teicoplanin are maculopapular or erythematous rash and drug-related fever, described in approximately 7% and 6% of patients, respectively,[253] which are more frequent in patients receiving doses of more than 12 mg/kg/day.[254] Cases of allergic cross reactions between vancomycin and teicoplanin have been reported, but vancomycin-allergic patients also have been successfully treated with teicoplanin.[253] The anaphylactoid reaction typically described with vancomycin intravenous administration (known as "red man," or "redneck" syndrome) is extremely uncommon with the infusion of teicoplanin. Ototoxicity related to teicoplanin is also rare.[251] Thrombocytopenia can occur at a similar rate to that found with vancomycin use, and also appears to be more frequent at higher doses (more than 12 mg/kg/day).[253] Other hematologic effects, such as neutropenia and eosinophilia, are infrequently reported.[253]

Clinical Uses

Several trials have explored the efficacy of teicoplanin in the treatment of severe staphylococcal infections. A failure rate of more than 50% was found in initial studies using low-doses of teicoplanin (3 mg/kg/day), including in patients with bacteremia, endocarditis, and osteomyelitis.[255,256] Even at higher doses (6 mg/kg/day and 10 mg/kg/day), teicoplanin was associated with a significantly poorer response compared with vancomycin in patients with endocarditis or intravascular infection caused by *S. aureus*.[257,258] Of note, in one of these studies, teicoplanin trough levels less than 20 µg/mL were correlated with treatment failure.[258] Teicoplanin, however, performed as well as vancomycin in the treatment of staphylococcal bacteremia related to catheter infection or from other sources.[257] Higher doses of teicoplanin, sometimes more than 12 mg/kg/day, appear to be needed in patients with staphylococcal arthritis.[254,258] Long-term (minimum of 4 months) intramuscular administration of teicoplanin (400 mg/day) was reported to cure 70 out of 76 MRSA episodes of chronic osteomyelitis.[259]

Two reports have shown that teicoplanin might be an efficacious alternative in the treatment of native valve endocarditis caused by viridans streptococci and enterococci, in doses of 6 mg/kg/day and 600 mg/day.[260,261] Interesting, against enterococci, several patients were cured receiving teicoplanin monotherapy.[260] In an experimental model of enterococcal endocarditis, teicoplanin showed to be as effective as ampicillin[262] and more effective than vancomycin.[263] In this model the addition of an aminoglycoside to teicoplanin resulted in enhanced activity.[262]

Teicoplanin has been shown to be effective in the treatment of susceptible organisms causing skin and soft tissue infections[264] (the 6 mg/kg/day dose more so than the 3 mg/kg/day dose[258]), lower respiratory tract infections,[227,252] and urinary tract infections.[260] Teicoplanin is also an option for the treatment of catheter-related infections[221] and was equivalent to vancomycin in a study of neutropenic patients with persistent fever.[265] Oral teicoplanin results in response and relapse rates similar to those observed with metronidazole and vancomycin in patients with *C. difficile* colitis.[206] Intraperitoneal administration of teicoplanin has been successfully used for the treatment of CAPD-related peritonitis.[218,247,248] Small series of cases of CSF shunt-related infections treated with intraventricular teicoplanin have been reported, using doses of 10 to 20 mg every 24 to 48 hours.[266,267]

Teicoplanin (400 mg intravenous dose at the time of anesthesia induction) is as effective as first-generation cephalosporins in the prevention of hip or knee implant-related infections.[268] However, it seems to be not as successful as other agents (flucloxacillin plus tobramycin in one study and cefazolin in another) as a prophylactic agent in patients undergoing cardiac[269] and prosthetic vascular surgeries.[270] The intravenous administration of teicoplanin reduces the rate of streptococcal bacteremia in patients undergoing dental extraction[271] and, in some European countries, teicoplanin is recommended as an option for prophylaxis of infective endocarditis in patients allergic to penicillin.[272]

STREPTOGRAMINS

Quinupristin-Dalfopristin

The group of antibiotics named *streptogramins* is composed of different compounds, including mikamycin, virginiamycin, pristinamycin, and, more recently, quinupristin-dalfopristin.[273] Three of these antibiotics (virginiamycin, pristinamycin, and quinupristin-dalfopristin) have been used in animal feeds or as a therapeutic agent in human or veterinary medicine. Each of these streptogramin antibiotics contains two macrocyclic lactone peptolide components referred to as streptogramin A and streptogramin B. The former are polyunsaturated cyclic peptolides and the latter, cyclic hexadepsipeptide.[273,274] Virginiamycin, a secreted product from *Streptomyces virginiae*, includes virginiamycin M (a strep-

togramin A) and virginiamycin S (a streptogramin B) and has been utilized mainly in animals as a growth promoter. Pristinamycin, a naturally occurring mixture produced by *Streptomyces pristinaespiralis*, also contains a streptogramin A (pristinamycin II_A) and a streptogramin B (pristinamycin I_A) component, and has been used orally in some European countries, mainly France, for the treatment of skin and soft tissue infections caused by streptococci and staphylococci.[275] Quinupristin-dalfopristin (Synercid, formerly RP 59500) is a water-soluble combination in a 30:70 ratio suitable for intravenous administration. Quinupristin, a derivative of pristinamycin I_A, is the streptogramin B constituent and dalfopristin, a derivative of pristinamycin II_B, is the streptogramin A component. The molecular weights for quinupristin and dalfopristin are 1022.24 and 690.85, respectively.[276]

Mechanism of Action

Streptogramins exert their action within the 50S ribosomal subunit of the 70S unit in the second phase, or elongation stage, of protein synthesis. Type A streptogramins (i.e., dalfopristin) appear to bind to the free arms of the peptidyl transferase in the 50S ribosomal subunit, blocking the addition of new amino acids from the aminoacyl-tRNA molecule to the growing peptide chain,[277] inhibiting therefore the earliest process of elongation. Quinupristin (a streptogramin B compound), like macrolides, works at a later phase of protein synthesis, preventing further peptide elongation and causing release of incomplete peptide chains.[277] In the absence of specific resistance mechanisms, the affinity of quinupristin for the 50S ribosomal subunit is considerably enhanced by a conformational change produced within it by the binding of dalfopristin, explaining the synergistic antimicrobial activity observed between the two streptogramin components.[274] The irreversibility of the complex formed results in bactericidal activity against most susceptible organisms. The blockage of different steps of the protein synthesis pathway may also help explain this synergistic activity.[277]

Antimicrobial Activity

Quinupristin-dalfopristin is active against most gram-positive (with the notable exception of *E. faecalis*) and some gram-negative organisms. Each compound separately displays bacteriostatic activity, and the bactericidal activity that can be observed with the combination may be diminished if resistance to one or both components is present.[278] Against *E. faecium* isolates, quinupristin-dalfopristin generally displays MICs of less than or equal to 1 µg/mL, including against vancomycin- and erythromycin-resistant isolates,[230,279, 280] and is primarily bacteriostatic, although a slow bactericidal effect has been reported for some strains under specific conditions.[281,282] The MIC_{90}s of this agent against *E. faecalis* strains are typically greater than or equal to 16 µg/mL[279-283] and this species is considered inherently resistant to quinupristin-dalfopristin,[284] although some exceptions exist. The in vitro activity of quinupristin-dalfopristin against other enterococcal species is variable, with approximately 50% of isolates displaying an MIC below the NCCLS susceptibility breakpoint.[285]

The MIC_{90}s of quinupristin-dalfopristin against *S. aureus* and *S. epidermidis* are less than or equal to 2 µg/mL, regardless of the methicillin, vancomycin, erythromycin, or clindamycin resistance pattern (see Table 29-1 for susceptibility breakpoints).[280,283,286,287] Ninety percent of *S. pyogenes*, *S. agalactiae*, group C and group G streptococci, *S. pneumoniae*, and viridans streptococci are inhibited by less than or equal to 1 µg/mL of quinupristin-dalfopristin.[280, 283,286,288] *Corynebacterium* spp., including *C. jeikeium*[289] and *L. monocytogenes*[290] are also susceptible, as are *Bacillus* spp.,[291] *Leuconostoc* spp., *Lactobacillus* spp., *Pediococcus* spp., and *Erysipelothrix rhusiopathiae*.[292] Against gram-positive anaerobes, MICs of quinupristin-dalfopristin of less than or equal to 1 µg/mL for *Peptostreptococcus* spp., *Propionebacterium* spp., and *Actinomyces* spp. are usually observed.[289,293] Most strains of clostridial species are inhibited by less than or equal to 2 µg/mL,[293,294] although high MICs against *C. difficile* strains have been reported.[289]

The MIC_{90}s of quinupristin-dalfopristin against *Haemophilus influenzae*, *Moraxella catarrhalis*, *Neisseria gonorrhoeae*, and *Neisseria meningitidis* are 4 µg/mL, 1 µg/mL, 1 µg/mL, and 0.5 µg/mL, respectively.[286,290] Against the intracellular pathogens *Legionella* spp., *Mycoplasma* spp., and *Ureaplasma urealyticum*, MICs are between 0.05 μg/mL and 2 μg/mL.[295] Despite moderate in vitro activity of quinupristin-dalfopristin against some anaerobes, fastidious gram-negatives, and intracellular pathogens, breakpoints for susceptibilities have not been defined and in vivo studies have not been performed. Quinupristin-dalfopristin displays no activity against Enterobacteriaceae, *Pseudomonas aeruginosa*, and *Acinetobacter* spp.[286]

Resistance

Because quinupristin and dalfopristin are chemically distinct compounds and their specific target sites within the 50S ribosomal subunit are different, the mechanisms leading to resistance to these components are specific for each one. The three general types of resistance to these compounds are through a conformational change in the target site decreasing the binding affinity of the drug (quinupristin), by enzymatic inactivation (quinupristin and dalfopristin) and, through active transport of the compounds out of the cell (quinupristin and dalfopristin).

The species *E. faecalis* is naturally resistant to quinupristin-dalfopristin due to the presence of an apparently intrinsic gene, named *lsa*, which encodes a homologue of ATP binding cassette transporter-related proteins and likely causes resistance to lincosamides and streptogramins A via efflux.[284] Reflecting the lack of activity of quinupristin-dalfopristin against *E. faecalis*, superinfection with this enterococcal species has been reported in patients receiving this agent.[296] *E. faecium* clinical isolates with a quinupristin-dalfopristin MIC greater than or equal to 4 μg/mL are infrequently reported and the majority remain susceptible to ampicillin and/or glycopeptides.[297] Higher rates of resistance are found among *E. faecium* strains isolated from animals in some European countries and the United States, probably related to the use of virginiamycin in animal feeds.[298] *Staphylococcus* spp. and *S. pyogenes* strains with high MICs of quinupristin-dalfopristin have been rare,[288,299] although a recent study from Taiwan reported that 8% of the *S. pyogenes* strains isolated in 2001 were nonsusceptible (MICs ≥2 μg/mL).[300]

The most common mechanism of resistance to streptogramin B in gram-positive cocci is through modification of the ribosomal target site, known as MLS$_B$ (conferring resistance to *m*acrolides, *l*incosamides, and *s*treptogramins *B*); this phenotype is encoded by various *erm* (erythromycin ribosome methylation) genes. Dalfopristin is not affected by MLS$_B$ resistance. The *erm* genes encode methylases that add one or two methyl groups (methylation) to a specific adenine residue (A2058) in the 23S ribosomal RNA within the 50S ribosomal subunit,[301] which results in reduced binding affinity of MLS$_B$ antibiotics for their specific target.[301] The *erm* genes are often located on conjugative or nonconjugative transposons and can reside on the chromosome or on plasmids. These genes can be constitutively expressed or inducible and are found in many species including staphylococci, streptococci, enterococci, *Clostridium* spp., and *Bacillus* spp., among others.[302] In staphylococci, the presence of 14-membered (such as erythromycin and clarithromycin) and 15-membered ring macrolides (azithromycin), after binding to ribosomes, causes a conformational change in the mRNA upstream of the specific *erm* gene (e.g., *erm*[C]), which then unblocks Erm translation and results in synthesis of the Erm methylase at an increased efficiency.[303] The genes conferring MLS$_B$ resistance typically found in staphylococci are *erm*(A), *erm*(B), *erm*(C), and *erm*(Y).[301] Staphylococcal strains with inducible MLS$_B$ (iMLS$_B$) resistance are resistant to inducer macrolides (e.g., erythromycin) and susceptible to noninducer macrolides, such as the 16-membered ring macrolides, josamycin and spiramycin, lincosamides (clindamycin), and streptogramins B (quinupristin).[278,304] However, deletions, duplications, and multiple or single point mutations in the *erm* regulatory region can lead to constitutive expression, that is, constant synthesis of the Erm methylase, which results in resistance to all the MLS$_B$ antibiotics, including clindamycin and quinupristin.[303] Constitutive mutants can be selected from iMLS$_B$ strains in vitro at a frequency of 10^{-7} to 10^{-8} by non-MLS$_B$ inducer agents[278] and clinical failures using clindamycin have been reported during treatment of

such staphylococcal strains.[305] Among nosocomial MRSA isolates, expression of constitutively MLS$_B$ (cMLS$_B$) resistance is much more common than iMLS$_B$-type which, on the other hand, is more frequent in MSSA isolates[306] and also among recent isolates from community-onset MRSA infections. Despite causing resistance to quinupristin, the presence of the cMLS$_B$ phenotype alone has no effect on the MICs of quinupristin-dalfopristin against staphylococci, but decreases the bactericidal activity, as observed by minimal bactericidal concentration and time-kill experiments.[278,304] Moreover, in the experimental model of endocarditis, quinupristin-dalfopristin shows decreased efficacy when the *S. aureus* strain expresses cMLS$_B$; increased MICs of quinupristin[304] and of clindamycin[307] appear to be a useful tool for screening for the decreased bactericidal activity of quinupristin-dalfopristin.

In enterococci, MLS$_B$ resistance is most frequently related to the presence of *erm*(B) and is often iMLS$_B$-type.[308] However, unlike with staphylococci, all the MLS$_B$ antibiotics can act as inducers of the MLS$_B$ resistance system[302]; thus resistance is expected to all MLS$_B$ antibiotics whether MLS$_B$ resistance is inducible or constitutively expressed. In the experimental endocarditis model, quinupristin-dalfopristin is less efficacious when the infecting *E. faecium* strain has the iMLS$_B$-resistance phenotype (versus an MLS$_B$-lacking strain), although different degrees of diffusion of the two streptogramins into the vegetation may partially explain these results.[309] The bactericidal activity of quinupristin-dalfopristin against *S. pneumoniae*, *S. pyogenes*, *S. agalactiae*, and viridans streptococci appears not to be affected by the presence of MLS$_B$ resistance.[310]

Hydrolysis of streptogramin B compounds is another mechanism of resistance to this agent. The *vgb*(A) gene responsible for inactivation has been identified, rarely, in *E. faecium*[311] and in *S. epidermidis* strains.[306] Efflux systems coding for ATP-binding transporters such as *msr*(A) can pump macrolides and streptogramin B compounds out of the cell and are found in some staphylococci species.[306] Streptogramin A compounds can be inactivated by acetyltransferases—encoded by the genes *vat*(A), *vat*(B), and *vat*(C) in staphylococci,[306] and *vat*(D) and *vat*(E) in *E. faecium*[312]—and are subjected to the action of efflux pumps encoded by the *vga*(A) and *vga*(B) genes in staphylococci.[301] High MICs of quinupristin-dalfopristin generally require the presence of more than one gene conferring resistance to the individual components.[306,313] Organisms with decreased susceptibility, *E. faecium* more so than *S. aureus* isolates, have been recovered from subjects failing therapy,[297,314,315] most likely due to mutation(s).

Clinical Pharmacodynamics and Pharmacokinetics

Quinupristin-dalfopristin displays a postantibiotic effect against many gram-positive organisms[316] with a mean of 2.8 hours for pneumococci and 4.7 hours for staphylococci, although it is shorter for isolates with cMLS$_B$ expression.[317] For *E. faecium* isolates, the postantibiotic effect averages 2.6 and 8.5 hours for vancomycin-resistant and vancomycin-susceptible strains, respectively.[317] In an experimental model of staphylococcal endocarditis, the area under the concentration-time curve (AUC)/MBC ratio was the pharmacodynamic parameter that best predicted response to quinupristin-dalfopristin.[304]

Distribution and Elimination

The mean peak concentration of quinupristin-dalfopristin was 0.95 μg/mL, 4.96 μg/mL, and 29.4 μg/mL after the infusion of doses of 1.4 mg/kg, 7 mg/kg, and 29.4 mg/kg, respectively.[318] The terminal half-lives of quinupristin and dalfopristin are relatively short, ranging from 0.93 to 0.96 hour and from 0.39 to 0.91 hour, respectively.[319] Quinupristin-dalfopristin has a wide volume of distribution (540 to 1800 mL/kg), is excreted mainly in the feces and only partially in the urine, does not reach therapeutic levels in CSF, and appears not to cross the placenta.[319] Excretion into breast milk was detected in lactating rats, although no data exist in women.[276] Approximately 90% of the drug is plasma protein bound.[281] Both streptogramins are metabolized in the liver, resulting in metabolites with antimicrobial activity. Studies in monkeys found high levels of drug in bile, gallbladder, liver, and kidney tissues after infusion of radiolabeled quinupristin-dalfopristin.[319] Quinupristin and dalfopristin diffuse differently into infected vegetations; quinupristin is homogeneously distributed, whereas dalfopristin concentrates only in the periphery,[320] which may hinder clinical efficacy because both drugs are required to obtain synergism and bactericidal activity.[309]

Administration and Dosing

The recommended intravenous dosing for quinupristin-dalfopristin is 7.5 mg/kg every 8 hours for the treatment of vancomycin-resistant *E. faecium* and 7.5 mg/kg every 12 hours for complicated skin and skin structure infections, respectively. The same doses have been safely used in pediatric patients.[321] Reconstituted drug should be diluted in 5% dextrose (not in saline) to a concentration of about 2 mg/mL and then infused over 60 minutes.[322] If significant venous irritation is noted, the solution can be further diluted or the drug administered through a central line,[322] the preferred route.

A mild increase in the concentration of quinupristin-dalfopristin is observed in patients with low creatinine clearance, which does not appear to require dosage adjustment in patients with renal failure whether or not they are receiving hemodialysis.[323,324] The lack of data in subjects undergoing CVVH precludes making dosing recommendations in this setting. Despite an apparent increase of serum levels in patients with liver insufficiency, dosage adjustment is not recommended in this population until further studies are performed.[322] Quinupristin-dalfopristin penetrates poorly into the peritoneal fluid of patients undergoing CAPD.[325]

Adverse Events and Drug Interactions

More than 30% of the patients experience irritation at the venous site when quinupristin-dalfopristin is administered through peripheral veins.[296,314] Arthralgias (9.1%) and myalgias (6.6%), sometimes severe and typically with normal creatine phosphokinase (CPK) levels, are the side effects that most commonly lead to drug discontinuation; these can be severe but usually resolve after cessation of therapy.[296,326] Risk factors associated with the development of these symptoms are chronic liver disease, elevated bilirubin at baseline, being a liver transplant recipient, and concomitant use of cyclosporine or mycophenolate.[327] Other less common adverse events associated with quinupristin-dalfopristin are nausea, vomiting, diarrhea, skin rash, pruritus, headache, and asthenia,[296,322] whereas laboratory abnormalities are mostly increased liver enzymes and total and conjugated bilirubin, which appear to be secondary to competition for excretion between bilirubin and this agent.[296,322] These laboratory abnormalities are rarely severe enough to cause discontinuation of this drug.[296,322] Quinupristin-dalfopristin has not been associated with significant teratogenic abnormalities in animal studies, but there are no data on the use of this antibiotic in pregnant women or in nursing woman, for whom this drug should be used only in situations in which there are no other therapeutic alternatives.[322]

Quinupristin-dalfopristin produces significant inhibition of the cytochrome P-450 3A4 isoenzyme system, resulting in increased levels of drugs that are metabolized through it; a few examples include diazepam, verapamil, "statins," most of the HIV-1 protease inhibitors, as well as nevirapine and delavirdine, vinca alkaloids, cyclosporine, tacrolimus, methylprednisolone, quinidine, lidocaine, and disopyramide.[322] Drugs that are metabolized through the cytochrome P-450 3A4 isoenzyme system that can produce prolongation of the QTc interval should not be co-administered with quinupristin-dalfopristin.[322]

Clinical Uses

Quinupristin-dalfopristin is currently approved in the United States for the treatment of vancomycin-resistant *E. faecium* infections and skin and skin structure infections caused by MSSA or *S. pyogenes*. In open-label trials, this drug showed a response rate between 75% to 86% in subjects with urinary tract infections, catheter-related bacteremia, and bone and joint infections caused by vancomycin-resistant *E. faecium*

isolates.[297,314] Slightly lower response rates were attained for individuals with skin and skin structure infections, intra-abdominal infections, and bacteremia of unknown origin; only about 25% of patients with endocarditis had a successful outcome.[297,314] In another study including mostly liver transplant recipients with vancomycin-resistant *E. faecium* infections at diverse sites, an initial favorable response was seen in approximately 80% of patients, although 4 out of 23 patients later experienced bacteriologic and clinical relapse.[328] Some patients with shunt-related meningitis caused by vancomycin-resistant *E. faecium* have been successfully treated with the addition of intraventricular quinupristin-dalfopristin[329,330]; in one, lethargy developed after the third 5 mg/day dose, which resolved upon discontinuation of the drug.[329] Based on pharmacokinetics of quinupristin-dalfopristin in the CSF, 1 to 2 mg/day appears to be the appropriate intraventricular dose.[330] Intravenous plus intraperitoneal quinupristin-dalfopristin (25 mg/L in alternate dialysate bags) has been effective in a few cases of vancomycin-resistant *E. faecium* CAPD-related peritonitis.[331]

In other open-label clinical trials, quinupristin-dalfopristin was evaluated for the treatment of patients with MRSA infections (bone and joint infections accounted for almost half of them) that were intolerant or were not responding to other therapies.[326] Clinical success rates of more than 70% were observed for skin and skin structure infections, bone and joint infections, and respiratory infections, and 54% for endocarditis cases (although neither of two bacteriologic evaluable patients responded favorably).[326] A randomized trial including patients with nosocomially acquired pneumonia (aztreonam was given for gram-negative coverage), in which *S. aureus* was the most common isolated organism, reported a clinical success rate of 56% for quinupristin-dalfopristin and 58% for vancomycin,[315] suggesting that quinupristin-dalfopristin can be efficacious for the treatment of staphylococcal nosocomial pneumonia.

LIPOPEPTIDES

Daptomycin

Daptomycin (formerly LY146032, now Cidecin), a fermentation product of *Streptomyces roseosporus*, is a cyclic 13-member amino acid lipopeptide antibiotic with a lipophilic tail that was discovered in the early 1980s.[332] In 1991, despite showing some efficacy in clinical trials, skeletal muscle toxicity was observed with twice-daily doses in phase II trials, which led to discontinuation of clinical studies. Subsequently, the rights to daptomycin were obtained by another company that, because of escalating multidrug-resistant gram-positive organisms, pursued clinical development using a different dosing regimen, resulting in FDA approval in late 2003 for complicated skin and soft tissue infections.

Mechanism of Action, Antimicrobial Activity, and Resistance

The exact mechanism for the antimicrobial activity of daptomycin is not fully known, although it is different from that of other antibiotics. This agent binds to the cell membrane of gram-positive organisms in a calcium-dependent process, and, without entering the bacterial cytoplasm, disrupts the bacterial cell membrane potential.[333,334] Daptomycin-resistant mutants have an increased voltage difference across the cytoplasmic membrane compared with a susceptible parental strain, supporting the hypothesis of the membrane as the primary target.[335]

The spectrum of antimicrobial activity of daptomycin closely overlaps that of glycopeptides, except that daptomycin maintains its activity against relevant organisms with decreased susceptibility to glycopeptides. The in vitro activity of this drug is dependent on the presence of calcium cations in the medium, which led to the 2003 NCCLS guidelines recommending the addition of calcium to the standard cation-adjusted Mueller-Hinton broth (CAMHB) for microdilution susceptibility testing with daptomycin in order to achieve 50 μg/mL of calcium.[336] The inclusion of extra calcium is associated with two- to fourfold lower MICs.[337] FDA-approval breakpoints for daptomycin using calcium-supplemented CAMHB are less than or equal to 1 μg/mL (susceptible) for staphylococci and streptococci and ≤4 μg/mL for

E. faecalis (susceptible).[338] MIC$_{90}$s of daptomycin are less than or equal to 0.5 μg/mL for MRSA and MSSA, coagulase-negative staphylococci, *S. agalactiae*, *S. pyogenes*, group C, group G, and group F β-hemolytic streptococci, *S. pneumoniae* (including penicillin-resistant isolates), *Bacillus* spp., and *Corynebacterium* spp. strains.[230,337,339] Slightly higher MICs are observed for viridans streptococci (MIC$_{90}$, 1 to 2 μg/mL).[337,339] Against enterococci, MIC$_{90}$s of daptomycin are usually of 2 μg/mL and 4 μg/mL for *E. faecalis* and *E. faecium*, respectively, regardless of the vancomycin susceptibility pattern.[230,337,339] The MIC$_{90}$s for other enterococcal species and *Lactobacillus* spp. are usually 4 μg/mL.[230,337,339] Daptomycin has activity against gram-positive anaerobes, such as *Peptostreptococcus* spp. (MIC$_{90}$, ≤1 μg/mL), *Clostridium perfringens* (MIC$_{90}$, 0.5 μg/mL), and *C. difficile* (MIC$_{90}$, 1 μg/mL), whereas some other clostridial species require higher concentrations for inhibition.[340] Importantly, daptomycin shows rapid, concentration-dependent bactericidal activity against staphylcococci, pneumococci,[341] and *E. faecalis* and *E. faecium*,[342,343] including MRSA, vancomycin-intermediate *S. aureus*, and vancomycin-resistant enterococci isolates.[343,344]

Development of resistance to daptomycin was rare in clinical trials as well as in vitro.[332,335] Although some strains with decreased susceptibility have been obtained after serial passage, these displayed growth defects and were attenuated in an animal model.[335]

Clinical Pharmacodynamics, Pharmacokinetics, and Uses

The pharmacodynamic parameter that appears to predict in vivo outcome of daptomycin therapy is the AUC/MIC ratio,[345] which, together with a prolonged postantibiotic effect observed against several gram-positive bacteria,[342] support once-daily dosing of this drug. The mean daptomycin peak serum concentrations are 54.6, 86.4, and 116.3 μg/mL after a single intravenous dose (infused over 30 minutes) of 4, 6, and 8 mg/kg, respectively.[346] Daptomycin exhibits a long terminal half-life (from 7.4 to 9.6 hours) and small volume of distribution (92 to 104 mL/kg), suggesting distribution mainly into plasma and interstitial fluid.[346] Daptomycin has significant affinity for plasma proteins (91.7% protein bound)[346] but low affinity for tissue proteins,[332] and is eliminated primarily through renal excretion, largely as unchanged drug.[332] Increases in the terminal half-life and AUC are observed in subjects with a creatinine clearance of less than 30 mL/minute, including patients on hemodialysis and on peritoneal dialysis.[347] Daptomycin undergoes little hepatic metabolism implying a low risk for drug-drug interactions.[332]

Doses of 3 mg/kg every 12 hours were well tolerated in early clinical trials[332]; however, when 4 mg/kg every 12 hours was assessed, two out of five participants developed myalgias and weakness associated with elevation in the serum levels of CPK, which returned to normal a few days after stopping the drug. Subsequent animal studies showed that this toxicity is more related to the frequency than to the total daily dose of the drug.[348] More recently, asymptomatic, mild elevations of CPK (MM isoenzyme) were observed in 2 out of 18 subjects receiving doses up to 8 mg/kg of daptomycin once a day.[346] During clinical trials, other adverse events, comparable to conventional therapy, were observed, including phlebitis, rash, headache, nausea, constipation, and diarrhea.[332]

Phase III trials for the treatment of complicated skin and soft tissue infections at doses of 2 mg/kg and 4 mg/kg every 24 hours showed efficacy comparable to that of conventional therapy,[349] leading to recent U.S. Food and Drug Administration (FDA) approval of the latter dose for these infections; a 2 mg/kg/day dosing schedule was less efficacious than the comparator arm in the treatment of deep-seated infections.[332] Based on these results and efficacy in endocarditis models caused by *S. aureus* and enterococci,[350,351] studies of daptomycin for the treatment of endocarditis have been initiated at 6 mg/kg/day.

REFERENCES

1. Griffith RS. Introduction to vancomycin. Rev Infect Dis. 1981;3(Suppl):S200-204.
2. Geraci JE, Heilman FR, Nichols DR, et al. Some laboratory and clinical experiences with a new antibiotic, vancomycin. Proc Staff Meet Mayo Clin. 1956;31:564-582.
3. Kirst HA, Thompson DG, Nicas TI. Historical yearly usage of vancomycin. Antimicrob Agents Chemother. 1998;42:1303-1304.
4. Pfeiffer RR. Structural features of vancomycin. Rev Infect Dis. 1981;3(Suppl): S205-209.
5. Jordan DC, Inniss WE. Selective inhibition of ribonucleic acid synthesis in *Staphylococcus aureus* by vancomycin. Nature. 1959;184:1894-1895.
6. Perkins HR, Nieto M. The chemical basis for the action of the vancomycin group of antibiotics. Ann N Y Acad Sci. 1974;235:348-363.
7. Watanakunakorn C. Mode of action and in-vitro activity of vancomycin. J Antimicrob Chemother. 1984;14(Suppl D):7-18.
8. Krogstad DJ, Pargwette AR. Defective killing of enterococci: A common property of antimicrobial agents acting on the cell wall. Antimicrob Agents Chemother. 1980;17:965-968.
9. Moellering RC, Weinberg AN. Studies on antibiotic syngerism against enterococci. II. Effect of various antibiotics on the uptake of 14 C-labeled streptomycin by enterococci. J Clin Invest. 1971;50:2580-2584.
10. Watanakunakorn C. The antibacterial action of vancomycin. Rev Infect Dis. 1981;3(Suppl):S210-215.
11. Pankuch GA, Jacobs MR, Appelbaum PC. Bactericidal activity of daptomycin against *Streptococcus pneumoniae* compared with eight other antimicrobials. J Antimicrob Chemother. 2003;51:443-446.
12. Gordon KA, Beach ML, Biedenbach DJ, et al. Antimicrobial susceptibility patterns of beta-hemolytic and viridans group streptococci: Report from the SENTRY Antimicrobial Surveillance Program (1997-2000). Diagn Microbiol Infect Dis. 2002;43:157-162.
13. Tuohy MJ, Procop GW, Washington JA. Antimicrobial susceptibility of *Abiotrophia adiacens* and *Abiotrophia defectiva*. Diagn Microbiol Infect Dis. 2000;38:189-191.
14. Tuazon CU, Shamsuddin D, Miller H. Antibiotic susceptibility and synergy of clinical isolates of *Listeria monocytogenes*. Antimicrob Agents Chemother. 1982;21:525-527.
15. Mohammed MJ, Marston CK, Popovic T, et al. Antimicrobial susceptibility testing of *Bacillus anthracis*: Comparison of results obtained by using the National Committee for Clinical Laboratory Standards broth microdilution reference and Etest agar gradient diffusion methods. J Clin Microbiol. 2002;40:1902-1907.
16. Weber DJ, Saviteer SM, Rutala WA, et al. In vitro susceptibility of *Bacillus* spp. to selected antimicrobial agents. Antimicrob Agents Chemother. 1988;32:642-645.
17. Soriano F, Zapardiel J, Nieto E. Antimicrobial susceptibilities of *Corynebacterium* species and other non-spore-forming gram-positive bacilli to 18 antimicrobial agents. Antimicrob Agents Chemother. 1995;39:208-214.
18. Hamilton-Miller JM, Shah S. Vancomycin susceptibility as an aid to the identification of lactobacilli. Lett Appl Microbiol. 1998;26:153-154.
19. Goldstein EJ, Citron DM, Merriam CV, et al. In vitro activities of daptomycin, vancomycin, quinupristin-dalfopristin, linezolid, and five other antimicrobials against 307 gram-positive anaerobic and 31 *Corynebacterium* clinical isolates. Antimicrob Agents Chemother. 2003;47:337-341.
20. Brazier JS, Levett PN, Stannard AJ, et al. Antibiotic susceptibility of clinical isolates of clostridia. J Antimicrob Chemother. 1985;15:181-185.
21. Geraci JE, Wilson WR. Vancomycin therapy for infective endocarditis. Rev Infect Dis. 1981;3(Suppl):S250-258.
22. Tizer KB, Cervia JS, Dunn AM, et al. Successful combination vancomycin and rifampin therapy in a newborn with community-acquired *Corynebacterium meningosepticum* neonatal meningitis. Pediatr Infect Dis J. 1995;14:916-917.
23. Di Pentima MC, Mason EO, Jr., Kaplan SL. In vitro antibiotic synergy against *Flavobacterium meningosepticum*: Implications for therapeutic options. Clin Infect Dis. 1998;26:1169-1176.
24. Fraser SL, Jorgensen JH. Reappraisal of the antimicrobial susceptibilities of *Chryseobacterium* and *Flavobacterium* species and methods for reliable susceptibility testing. Antimicrob Agents Chemother. 1997;41:2738-2741.
25. Griffith RS. Vancomycin use—An historical review. J Antimicrob Chemother. 1984;14(Suppl D):1-5.
26. Siebert WT, Moreland N, Williams TW, Jr. Synergy of vancomycin plus cefazolin or cephalothin against methicillin-resistance *Staphylococcus epidermidis*. J Infect Dis. 1979;139:452-457.
27. Tuazon CU, Miller H. Comparative in vitro activities of teichomycin and vancomycin alone and in combination with rifampin and aminoglycosides against staphylococci and enterococci. Antimicrob Agents Chemother. 1984;25:411-412.
28. Hiramatsu K, Hanaki H, Ino T, et al. Methicillin-resistant *Staphylococcus aureus* clinical strain with reduced vancomycin susceptibility. J Antimicrob Chemother. 1997;40:135-136.
29. CDC. Reduced susceptibility of *Staphylococcus aureus* to vancomycin—Japan, 1996. MMWR Morb Mortal Wkly Rep. 1997;46:624-626.
30. Standards NCCLS. MIC testing—Supplemental tables. NCCLS document M100-S13 (M7). National Committee for Clinical Laboratory Standards, Wayne, Pa. 2003.
31. MacGowan AP, Wise R. Establishing MIC breakpoints and the interpretation of in vitro susceptibility tests. J Antimicrob Chemother. 2001;48(Suppl 1):17-28.
32. Smith TL, Pearson ML, Wilcox KR, et al. Emergence of vancomycin resistance in *Staphylococcus aureus*. Glycopeptide-Intermediate *Staphylococcus aureus* Working Group. N Engl J Med. 1999;340:493-501.

33. CDC. Vancomycin–resistant *Staphylococcus aureus*—Pennsylvania, 2002. MMWR Morb Mortal Wkly Rep. 2002;51:902.

34. CDC. *Staphylococcus aureus* resistant to vancomycin—United States, 2002. MMWR Morb Mortal Wkly Rep. 2002;51:565-567.

35. Rippere K, Patel R, Uhl JR, et al. DNA sequence resembling *vanA* and *vanB* in the vancomycin-resistant biopesticide *Bacillus popilliae*. J Infect Dis. 1998;178:584-588.

36. Navarro F, Courvalin P. Analysis of genes encoding D-alanine-D-alanine ligase-related enzymes in *Enterococcus casseliflavus* and *Enterococcus flavescens*. Antimicrob Agents Chemother. 1994;38:1788-1793.

37. Reid KC, Cockerill IF, Patel R. Clinical and epidemiological features of *Enterococcus casseliflavus/flavescens* and *Enterococcus gallinarum* bacteremia: A report of 20 cases. Clin Infect Dis. 2001;32:1540-1546.

38. Dutka-Malen S, Blaimont B, Wauters G, et al. Emergence of high-level resistance to glycopeptides in *Enterococcus gallinarum* and *Enterococcus casseliflavus*. Antimicrob Agents Chemother. 1994;38:1675-1677.

39. Arthur M, Quintiliani R, Jr. Regulation of VanA- and VanB-type glycopeptide resistance in enterococci. Antimicrob Agents Chemother. 2001;45:375-381.

40. Evers S, Courvalin P. Regulation of VanB-type vancomycin resistance gene expression by the VanS(B)-VanR (B) two-component regulatory system in *Enterococcus faecalis* V583. J Bacteriol. 1996;178:1302-1309.

41. Bates J, Jordens JZ, Griffiths DT. Farm animals as a putative reservoir for vancomycin-resistant enterococcal infection in man. J Antimicrob Chemother. 1994; 34:507-514.

42. Van der Auwera P, Pensart N, Korten V, et al. Influence of oral glycopeptides on the fecal flora of human volunteers: Selection of highly glycopeptide-resistant enterococci. J Infect Dis. 1996;173:1129-1136.

43. Schouten MA, Hoogkamp-Korstanje JA, Meis JF, et al. Prevalence of vancomycin-resistant enterococci in Europe. Eur J Clin Microbiol Infect Dis. 2000;19:816-822.

44. Coque TM, Tomayko JF, Ricke SC, et al. Vancomycin-resistant enterococci from nosocomial, community, and animal sources in the United States. Antimicrob Agents Chemother. 1996;40:2605-2609.

45. NNIS. National Nosocomial Infections Surveillance (NNIS) System Report, Data Summary from January 1992-June 2001, issued August 2001. Am J Infect Control. 2001;29:404-421.

46. Fraimow HS, Jungkind DL, Lander DW, et al. Urinary tract infection with an *Enterococcus faecalis* isolate that requires vancomycin for growth. Ann Intern Med. 1994;121:22-26.

47. Van Bambeke F, Chauvel M, Reynolds PE, et al. Vancomycin-dependent *Enterococcus faecalis* clinical isolates and revertant mutants. Antimicrob Agents Chemother. 1999;43:41-47.

48. Hanaki H, Kuwahara-Arai K, Boyle-Vavra S, et al. Activated cell-wall synthesis is associated with vancomycin resistance in methicillin-resistant *Staphylococcus aureus* clinical strains Mu3 and Mu50. J Antimicrob Chemother. 1998;42:199-209.

49. Daum RS, Gupta S, Sabbagh R, et al. Characterization of *Staphylococcus aureus* isolates with decreased susceptibility to vancomycin and teicoplanin: Isolation and purification of a constitutively produced protein associated with decreased susceptibility. J Infect Dis. 1992;166:1066-1072.

50. Sieradzki K, Tomasz A. Inhibition of cell wall turnover and autolysis by vancomycin in a highly vancomycin-resistant mutant of *Staphylococcus aureus*. J Bacteriol. 1997;179:2557-2566.

51. Hiramatsu K. Vancomycin-resistant *Staphylococcus aureus*: A new model of antibiotic resistance. Lancet Infect Dis. 2001;1:147-155.

52. Cui L, Ma X, Sato K, et al. Cell wall thickening is a common feature of vancomycin resistance in *Staphylococcus aureus*. J Clin Microbiol. 2003;41:5-14.

53. CDC. Laboratory capacity to detect antimicrobial resistance, 1998. MMWR Morb Mortal Wkly Rep. 2000;48:1167-1171.

54. Tenover FC, Lancaster MV, Hill BC, et al. Characterization of staphylococci with reduced susceptibilities to vancomycin and other glycopeptides. J Clin Microbiol. 1998;36:1020-1027.

55. CDC. Interim guidelines for prevention and control of staphylococcal infection associated with reduced susceptibility to vancomycin. MMWR Morb Mortal Wkly Rep. 1997;46:626-628, 635.

56. Tenover FC, Biddle JW, Lancaster MV. Increasing resistance to vancomycin and other glycopeptides in *Staphylococcus aureus*. Emerg Infect Dis. 2001;7:327-332.

57. Patron RL, Climo MW, Goldstein BP, et al. Lysostaphin treatment of experimental aortic valve endocarditis caused by a *Staphylococcus aureus* isolate with reduced susceptibility to vancomycin. Antimicrob Agents Chemother. 1999;43:1754-1755.

58. Hiramatsu K, Aritaka N, Hanaki H, et al. Dissemination in Japanese hospitals of strains of *Staphylococcus aureus* heterogeneously resistant to vancomycin. Lancet. 1997;350:1670-1673.

59. Hubert SK, Mohammed JM, Fridkin SK, et al. Glycopeptide-intermediate *Staphylococcus aureus*: Evaluation of a novel screening method and results of a survey of selected U.S. hospitals. J Clin Microbiol. 1999;37:3590-3593.

60. Wong SS, Ng TK, Yam WC, et al. Bacteremia due to *Staphylococcus aureus* with reduced susceptibility to vancomycin. Diagn Microbiol Infect Dis. 2000;36:261-268.

61. Moore MR, Perdreau-Remington F, Chambers HF. Vancomycin treatment failure associated with heterogeneous vancomycin-intermediate *Staphylococcus aureus* in a patient with endocarditis and in the rabbit model of endocarditis. Antimicrob Agents Chemother. 2003;47:1262-1266.

62. Tenover FC. Implications of vancomycin-resistant *Staphylococcus aureus*. J Hosp Infect. 1999;43(Suppl):S3-7.

63. Brunet F, Vedel G, Dreyfus F, et al. Failure of teicoplanin therapy in two neutropenic patients with staphylococcal septicemia who recovered after administration of vancomycin. Eur J Clin Microbiol Infect Dis. 1990;9:145-147.

64. Chang S, Sievert DM, Hageman JC, et al. Infection with vancomycin-resistant *Staphylococcus aureus* containing the *vanA* resistance gene. N Engl J Med. 2003; 348:1342-1347.

65. Del Bene VE, John JF, Jr., Twitty JA, et al. Anti-staphylococcal activity of teicoplanin, vancomycin, and other antimicrobial agents: The significance of methicillin resistance. J Infect Dis. 1986;154:349-352.

66. Arioli V, Pallanza R. Teicoplanin-resistant coagulase-negative staphylococci. Lancet. 1987;1:39.

67. Biavasco F, Vignaroli C, Lazzarini R, et al. Glycopeptide susceptibility profiles of *Staphylococcus haemolyticus* bloodstream isolates. Antimicrob Agents Chemother. 2000;44:3122-3126.

68. Biavasco F, Vignaroli C, Varaldo PE. Glycopeptide resistance in coagulase-negative staphylococci. Eur J Clin Microbiol Infect Dis. 2000;19:403-417.

69. Veach LA, Pfaller MA, Barrett M, et al. Vancomycin resistance in *Staphylococcus haemolyticus* causing colonization and bloodstream infection. J Clin Microbiol. 1990;28:2064-2068.

70. Sanyal D, Johnson AP, George RC, et al. In-vitro characteristics of glycopeptide resistant strains of *Staphylococcus epidermidis* isolated from patients on CAPD. J Antimicrob Chemother. 1993;32:267-278.

71. Novak R, Henriques B, Charpentier E, et al. Emergence of vancomycin tolerance in *Streptococcus pneumoniae*. Nature. 1999;399:590-593.

72. Robertson GT, Zhao J, Desai BV, et al. Vancomycin tolerance induced by erythromycin but not by loss of *vncRS*, *vex3*, or *pep27* function in *Streptococcus pneumoniae*. J Bacteriol. 2002;184:6987-7000.

73. Henriques Normark B, Novak R, Ortqvist A, et al. Clinical isolates of *Streptococcus pneumoniae* that exhibit tolerance of vancomycin. Clin Infect Dis. 2001;32:552-558.

74. Anton N, Blazquez R, Gomez-Garces JL, et al. Study of vancomycin tolerance in 120 strains of *Streptococcus pneumoniae* isolated in 1999 in Madrid, Spain. J Antimicrob Chemother. 2001;47:902-903.

75. McCullers JA, English BK, Novak R. Isolation and characterization of vancomycin-tolerant *Streptococcus pneumoniae* from the cerebrospinal fluid of a patient who developed recrudescent meningitis. J Infect Dis. 2000;181:369-373.

76. Swenson JM, Facklam RR, Thornsberry C. Antimicrobial susceptibility of vancomycin-resistant *Leuconostoc*, *Pediococcus*, and *Lactobacillus* species. Antimicrob Agents Chemother. 1990;34:543-549.

77. Billot-Klein D, Gutmann L, Sable S, et al. Modification of peptidoglycan precursors is a common feature of the low-level vancomycin-resistant VANB-type *Enterococcus* D366 and of the naturally glycopeptide-resistant species *Lactobacillus casei*, *Pediococcus pentosaceus*, *Leuconostoc mesenteroides*, and *Enterococcus gallinarum*. J Bacteriol. 1994;176:2398-2405.

78. Elisha BG, Courvalin P. Analysis of genes encoding D-alanine:D-alanine ligase-related enzymes in *Leuconostoc mesenteroides* and *Lactobacillus* spp. Gene. 1995;152:79-83.

79. Venditti M, Gelfusa V, Tarasi A, et al. Antimicrobial susceptibilities of *Erysipelothrix rhusiopathiae*. Antimicrob Agents Chemother. 1990;34:2038-2040.

80. Marshall CG, Lessard IA, Park I, et al. Glycopeptide antibiotic resistance genes in glycopeptide-producing organisms. Antimicrob Agents Chemother. 1998;42:2215-2220.

81. Lowdin E, Odenholt I, Cars O. In vitro studies of pharmacodynamic properties of vancomycin against *Staphylococcus aureus* and *Staphylococcus epidermidis*. Antimicrob Agents Chemother. 1998;42:2739-2744.

82. Souli M, Giamarellou H. Effects of slime produced by clinical isolates of coagulase-negative staphylococci on activities of various antimicrobial agents. Antimicrob Agents Chemother. 1998;42:939-941.

83. Bryan CS, White WL. Safety of oral vancomycin in functionally anephric patients. Antimicrob Agents Chemother. 1978;14:634-635.

84. Spitzer PG, Eliopoulos GM. Systemic absorption of enteral vancomycin in a patient with pseudomembranous colitis. Ann Intern Med. 1984;100:533-534.

85. Cunha BA, Quintiliani R, Deglin JM, et al. Pharmacokinetics of vancomycin in anuria. Rev Infect Dis. 1981;3(Suppl):S269-272.

86. Freeman CD, Quintiliani R, Nightingale CH. Vancomycin therapeutic drug monitoring: Is it necessary? Ann Pharmacother. 1993;27:594-598.

87. Rotschafer JC, Crossley K, Zaske DE, et al. Pharmacokinetics of vancomycin: Observations in 28 patients and dosage recommendations. Antimicrob Agents Chemother. 1982;22:391-394.

88. Krogstad DJ, Moellering RC, Greenblatt DJ. Single-dose kinetics of intravenous vancomycin. J Clin Pharmacol. 1980; 20:197-201.

89. Moellering RC. Pharmacokinetics of vancomycin. J Antimicrob Chemother. 1984;14(Suppl D):43-52.

90. Matzke GR, Zhanel GG, Guay DR. Clinical pharmacokinetics of vancomycin. Clin Pharmacokinet. 1986;11:257-282.

91. Rodvold KA, Blum RA, Fischer JH, et al. Vancomycin pharmacokinetics in patients with various degrees of renal function. Antimicrob Agents Chemother. 1988;32:848-852.

92. Moellering RC, Krogstad DJ, Greenblatt DJ. Pharmacokinetics of vancomycin in normal subjects and in patients with reduced renal function. Rev Infect Dis. 1981; 3(Suppl):S230-235.

93. Pfausler B, Spiss H, Beer R, et al. Treatment of staphylococcal ventriculitis associated with external cerebrospinal fluid drains: A prospective randomized trial of intravenous compared with intraventricular vancomycin therapy. J Neurosurg. 2003;98:1040-1044.

94. Klugman KP, Friedland IR, Bradley JS. Bactericidal activity against cephalosporin-resistant *Streptococcus pneumoniae* in cerebrospinal fluid of children with acute bacterial meningitis. Antimicrob Agents Chemother. 1995;39:1988-1992.

95. Cabellos C, Martinez-Lacasa J, Martos A, et al. Influence of dexamethasone on efficacy of ceftriaxone and vancomycin therapy in experimental pneumococcal meningitis. Antimicrob Agents Chemother. 1995;39:2158-2160.

96. Ahmed A, Jafri H, Lutsar I, et al. Pharmacodynamics of vancomycin for the treatment of experimental penicillin- and cephalosporin-resistant pneumococcal meningitis. Antimicrob Agents Chemother. 1999;43:876-881.

97. Viladrich PF, Gudiol F, Linares J, et al. Evaluation of vancomycin for therapy of adult pneumococcal meningitis. Antimicrob Agents Chemother. 1991;35:2467-2472.

98. Engineer MS, Ho DH, Bodey GP, Sr. Comparison of vancomycin disposition in rats with normal and abnormal renal functions. Antimicrob Agents Chemother. 1981;20:718-722.

99. Torres JR, Sanders CV, Lewis AC. Vancomycin concentration in human tissues—preliminary report. J Antimicrob Chemother. 1979;5:475-477.

100. Daschner FD, Frank U, Kummel A, et al. Pharmacokinetics of vancomycin in serum and tissue of patients undergoing open-heart surgery. J Antimicrob Chemother. 1987;19:359-362.

101. Nicolau DP, Freeman CD, Nightingale CH, et al. Minocycline versus vancomycin for treatment of experimental endocarditis caused by oxacillin-resistant *Staphylococcus aureus*. Antimicrob Agents Chemother. 1994;38:1515-1518.

102. Cruciani M, Gatti G, Lazzarini L, et al. Penetration of vancomycin into human lung tissue. J Antimicrob Chemother. 1996;38:865-869.

103. Bouvet A, Cremieux AC, Contrepois A, et al. Comparison of penicillin and vancomycin, individually and in combination with gentamicin and amikacin, in the treatment of experimental endocarditis induced by nutritionally variant streptococci. Antimicrob Agents Chemother. 1985;28:607-611.

104. Graziani AL, Lawson LA, Gibson GA, et al. Vancomycin concentrations in infected and noninfected human bone. Antimicrob Agents Chemother. 1988;32:1320-1322.

105. Kitzes-Cohen R, Farin D, Piva G, et al. Pharmacokinetics of vancomycin administered as prophylaxis before cardiac surgery. Ther Drug Monit. 2000;22:661-667.

106. Mader JT, Shirtliff ME, Bergquist SC, et al. Antimicrobial treatment of chronic osteomyelitis. Clin Orthop. 1999:47-65.

107. Bourget P, Fernandez H, Delouis C, et al. Transplacental passage of vancomycin during the second trimester of pregnancy. Obstet Gynecol. 1991;78:908-911.

108. Reyes MP, Ostrea EM, Jr., Cabinian AE, et al. Vancomycin during pregnancy: Does it cause hearing loss or nephrotoxicity in the infant? Am J Obstet Gynecol. 1989;161:977-981.

109. Chin KG, Mactal-Haaf C, McPherson CE. Use of anti-infective agents during lactation: Part 1—Beta-lactam antibiotics, vancomycin, quinupristin-dalfopristin, and linezolid. J Hum Lact. 2000;16:351-358.

110. Matzke GR, McGory RW, Halstenson CE, et al. Pharmacokinetics of vancomycin in patients with various degrees of renal function. Antimicrob Agents Chemother. 1984;25:433-437.

111. Brown N, Ho DH, Fong KL, et al. Effects of hepatic function on vancomycin clinical pharmacology. Antimicrob Agents Chemother. 1983;23:603-609.

112. Wallace MR, Mascola JR, Oldfield EC, 3rd. Red man syndrome: Incidence, etiology, and prophylaxis. J Infect Dis. 1991;164:1180-1185.

113. Wysocki M, Delatour F, Faurisson F, et al. Continuous versus intermittent infusion of vancomycin in severe staphylococcal infections: Prospective multicenter randomized study. Antimicrob Agents Chemother. 2001;45:2460-2467.

114. Blouin RA, Bauer LA, Miller DD, et al. Vancomycin pharmacokinetics in normal and morbidly obese subjects. Antimicrob Agents Chemother. 1982;21:575-580.

115. Penzak SR, Gubbins PO, Rodvold KA, et al. Therapeutic drug monitoring of vancomycin in a morbidly obese patient. Ther Drug Monit. 1998;20:261-265.

116. Rybak MJ, Albrecht LM, Berman JR, et al. Vancomycin pharmacokinetics in burn patients and intravenous drug abusers. Antimicrob Agents Chemother. 1990;34:792-795.

117. Miglioli PA, Merlo F, Grabocka E, et al. Effects of cardiopulmonary bypass on vancomycin plasma concentration decay. Pharmacol Res. 1998;38:275-278.

118. Salzman C, Weingold AB, Simon GL. Increased dose requirements of vancomycin in a pregnant patient with endocarditis. J Infect Dis. 1987;156:409.

119. Kaplan EL. Vancomycin in infants and children: A review of pharmacology and indications for therapy and prophylaxis. J Antimicrob Chemother. 1984;14(Suppl D):59-66.

120. Glover ML, Cole E, Wolfsdorf J. Vancomycin dosage requirements among pediatric intensive care unit patients with normal renal function. J Crit Care. 2000;15:1-4.

121. Dajani AS, Taubert KA, Wilson W, et al. Prevention of bacterial endocarditis: Recommendations by the American Heart Association. Clin Infect Dis. 1997;25:1448-1458.

122. Apisarnthanarak A, Razavi B, Mundy LM. Adjunctive intracolonic vancomycin for severe *Clostridium difficile* colitis: Case series and review of the literature. Clin Infect Dis. 2002;35:690-696.

123. Fekety R, Silva J, Kauffman C, et al. Treatment of antibiotic-associated *Clostridium difficile* colitis with oral vancomycin: Comparison of two dosage regimens. Am J Med. 1989;86:15-19.

124. Bunke CM, Aronoff GR, Brier ME, et al. Vancomycin kinetics during continuous ambulatory peritoneal dialysis. Clin Pharmacol Ther. 1983;34:631-637.

125. Morse GD, Farolino DF, Apicella MA, et al. Comparative study of intraperitoneal and intravenous vancomycin pharmacokinetics during continuous ambulatory peritoneal dialysis. Antimicrob Agents Chemother. 1987;31:173-177.

126. Pfausler B, Haring HP, Kampfl A, et al. Cerebrospinal fluid (CSF) pharmacokinetics of intraventricular vancomycin in patients with staphylococcal ventriculitis associated with external CSF drainage. Clin Infect Dis. 1997;25:733-735.

127. Luer MS, Hatton J. Vancomycin administration into the cerebrospinal fluid: A review. Ann Pharmacother. 1993;27:912-921.

128. Bayston R. Epidemiology, diagnosis, treatment, and prevention of cerebrospinal fluid shunt infections. Neurosurg Clin N Am. 2001;12:703-708, viii.

129. Ferencz JR, Assia EI, Diamantstein L, et al. Vancomycin concentration in the vitreous after intravenous and intravitreal administration for postoperative endophthalmitis. Arch Ophthalmol. 1999;117:1023-1027.

130. Lindholm DD, Murray JS. Persistence of vancomycin in the blood during renal failure and its treatment by hemodialysis. N Engl J Med. 1966;274:1047-1051.

131. Cunha BA. Vancomycin. Med Clin North Am. 1995;79:817-831.

132. Barth RH, DeVincenzo N. Use of vancomycin in high-flux hemodialysis: Experience with 130 courses of therapy. Kidney Int. 1996;50:929-936.

133. Blevins RD, Halstenson CE, Salem NG, et al. Pharmacokinetics of vancomycin in patients undergoing continuous ambulatory peritoneal dialysis. Antimicrob Agents Chemother. 1984;25:603-606.

134. Moellering RC, Krogstad DJ, Greenblatt DJ. Vancomycin therapy in patients with impaired renal function: A nomogram for dosage. Ann Intern Med. 1981;94:343-346.

135. Joy MS, Matzke GR, Frye RF, et al. Determinants of vancomycin clearance by continuous venovenous hemofiltration and continuous venovenous hemodialysis. Am J Kidney Dis. 1998;31:1019-1027.

136. Boereboom FT, Ververs FF, Blankestijn PJ, et al. Vancomycin clearance during continuous venovenous haemofiltration in critically ill patients. Intensive Care Med. 1999;25:1100-1104.

137. Dutton AA, Elmes PC. Vancomycin: Report on treatment of patients with severe staphylococcal infections. Br Med J. 1959;1:1144-1149.

138. Geraci JE, Heilman FR, Nichols DR, et al. Antibiotic therapy of bacterial endocarditis. VII. Vancomycin for acute micrococcal endocarditis. Proc Staff Meet Mayo Clin. 1958;33:172-181.

139. Farber BF, Moellering RC. Retrospective study of the toxicity of preparations of vancomycin from 1974 to 1981. Antimicrob Agents Chemother. 1983;23:138-141.

140. Cantu TG, Yamanaka-Yuen NA, Lietman PS. Serum vancomycin concentrations: Reappraisal of their clinical value. Clin Infect Dis. 1994;18:533-543.

141. Mellor JA, Kingdom J, Cafferkey M, et al. Vancomycin toxicity: A prospective study. J Antimicrob Chemother. 1985;15:773-780.

142. Tange RA, Kieviet HL, von Marle J, et al. An experimental study of vancomycin-induced cochlear damage. Arch Otorhinolaryngol. 1989;246:67-70.

143. Brummett RE, Fox KE, Jacobs F, et al. Augmented gentamicin ototoxicity induced by vancomycin in guinea pigs. Arch Otolaryngol Head Neck Surg. 1990;116:61-64.

144. Brummett RE. Ototoxicity of vancomycin and analogues. Otolaryngol Clin North Am. 1993;26:821-828.

145. Bernard E, Perbost I, Carles M, et al. Efficacy and safety of vancomycin constant-rate infusion in the treatment of chronic gram-positive bone and joint infections. Clin Microbiol Infect. 1997;3:440-446.

146. Wold JS, Turnipseed SA. Toxicology of vancomycin in laboratory animals. Rev Infect Dis. 1981;3(Suppl):S224-229.

147. Rybak MJ, Albrecht LM, Boike SC, et al. Nephrotoxicity of vancomycin, alone and with an aminoglycoside. J Antimicrob Chemother. 1990;25:679-687.

148. Downs NJ, Neihart RE, Dolezal JM, et al. Mild nephrotoxicity associated with vancomycin use. Arch Intern Med. 1989;149:1777-1781.

149. Wai AO, Lo AM, Abdo A, et al. Vancomycin-induced acute interstitial nephritis. Ann Pharmacother. 1998;32:1160-1164.

150. O'Sullivan TL, Ruffing MJ, Lamp KC, et al. Prospective evaluation of red man syndrome in patients receiving vancomycin. J Infect Dis. 1993;168:773-776.

151. Southorn PA, Plevak DJ, Wright AJ, et al. Adverse effects of vancomycin administered in the perioperative period. Mayo Clin Proc. 1986;61:721-724.

152. Dajee H, Laks H, Miller J, et al. Profound hypotension from rapid vancomycin administration during cardiac operation. J Thorac Cardiovasc Surg. 1984;87:145-146.

153. Polk RE, Healy DP, Schwartz LB, et al. Vancomycin and the red-man syndrome: Pharmacodynamics of histamine release. J Infect Dis. 1988;157:502-507.

154. Elting LS, Rubenstein EB, Kurtin D, et al. Mississippi mud in the 1990s: Risks and outcomes of vancomycin-associated toxicity in general oncology practice. Cancer. 1998;83:2597-2607.

155. Govindarajan R, Baxter D, Wilson C, et al. Vancomycin-induced thrombocytopenia. Am J Hematol. 1999;62:122-123.

156. Marik PE, Ferris N. Delayed hypersensitivity reaction to vancomycin. Pharmacotherapy. 1997;17:1341-1344.

157. Laurencin CT, Horan RF, Senatus PB, et al. Stevens-Johnson-type reaction with vancomycin treatment. Ann Pharmacother. 1992;26:1520-1521.

158. Miller SN, Ringler RP. Vancomycin-induced pseudomembranous colitis. J Clin Gastroenterol. 1987;9:114-115.

159. Golledge CL, McKenzie T. Monitoring vancomycin concentrations in CSF after intraventricular administration. J Antimicrob Chemother. 1988;21:262-263.

160. Grabb PA, Albright AL. Intraventricular vancomycin-induced cerebrospinal fluid eosinophilia: Report of two patients. Neurosurgery. 1992;30:630-634; discussion 634-635.

161. Lutsar I, McCracken GH, Jr., Friedland IR. Antibiotic pharmacodynamics in cerebrospinal fluid. Clin Infect Dis. 1998;27:1117-1127, quiz 1128-1129.

162. Freiman JP, Graham DJ, Reed TG, et al. Chemical peritonitis following the intraperitoneal administration of vancomycin. Perit Dial Int. 1992;12:57-60.

163. Wazny LD, Blake PG. Incompatibility of vancomycin and ceftazidime for intraperitoneal use. Perit Dial Int. 2002;22:93-94.

164. Fiscella RG. Physical incompatibility of vancomycin and ceftazidime for intravitreal injection. Arch Ophthalmol. 1993;111:730.

165. Barg NL, Supena RB, Fekety R. Persistent staphylococcal bacteremia in an intravenous drug abuser. Antimicrob Agents Chemother. 1986;29:209-211.

166. Vaughan LM, Poon CY. Stability of ceftazidime and vancomycin alone and in combination in heparinized and nonheparinized peritoneal dialysis solution. Ann Pharmacother. 1994;28:572-576.

167. von Kaenel WE, Bloomfield EL, Amaranath L, et al. Vancomycin does not enhance hypotension under anesthesia. Anesth Analg. 1993;76:809-811.

168. Taylor NS, Bartlett JG. Binding of *Clostridium difficile* cytotoxin and vancomycin by anion-exchange resins. J Infect Dis. 1980;141:92-97.

169. Kralovicova K, Spanik S, Halko J, et al. Do vancomycin serum levels predict failures of vancomycin therapy or nephrotoxicity in cancer patients? J Chemother. 1997;9:420-426.

170. Zimmermann AE, Katona BG, Plaisance KI. Association of vancomycin serum concentrations with outcomes in patients with gram-positive bacteremia. Pharmacotherapy. 1995;15:85-91.

171. Moellering RC. Monitoring serum vancomycin levels: Climbing the mountain because it is there? Clin Infect Dis. 1994;18:544-546.

172. Saunders NJ. Vancomycin administration and monitoring reappraisal. J Antimicrob Chemother. 1995;36:279-282.

173. de Hoog M, Schoemaker RC, Mouton JW, et al. Vancomycin population pharmacokinetics in neonates. Clin Pharmacol Ther. 2000;67:360-367.

174. Begg EJ, Barclay ML, Kirkpatrick CM. The therapeutic monitoring of antimicrobial agents. Br J Clin Pharmacol. 2001;52(Suppl 1):35S-43S.

175. Saunders NJ. Why monitor peak vancomycin concentrations? Lancet. 1994;344:1748-1750.

176. Follin SL, Mueller BA, Scott MK, et al. Falsely elevated serum vancomycin concentrations in hemodialysis patients. Am J Kidney Dis. 1996;27:67-74.

177. Kingery JR, Sowinski KM, Kraus MA, et al. Vancomycin assay performance in patients with end-stage renal disease receiving hemodialysis. Pharmacotherapy. 2000;20:653-656.

178. Wilson WR, Karchmer AW, Dajani AS, et al. Antibiotic treatment of adults with infective endocarditis due to streptococci, enterococci, staphylococci, and HACEK microorganisms. American Heart Association. JAMA. 1995;274:1706-1713.

179. Gopal V, Bisno AL, Silverblatt FJ. Failure of vancomycin treatment in *Staphylococcus aureus* endocarditis. In vivo and in vitro observations. JAMA. 1976;236:1604-1606.

180. Faville RJ, Jr., Zaske DE, Kaplan EL, et al. *Staphylococcus aureus* endocarditis. Combined therapy with vancomycin and rifampin. JAMA. 1978;240:1963-1965.

181. Small PM, Chambers HF. Vancomycin for *Staphylococcus aureus* endocarditis in intravenous drug users. Antimicrob Agents Chemother. 1990;34:1227-1231.

182. Levine DP, Fromm BS, Reddy BR. Slow response to vancomycin or vancomycin plus rifampin in methicillin-resistant *Staphylococcus aureus* endocarditis. Ann Intern Med. 1991;115:674-680.

183. Fortun J, Navas E, Martinez-Beltran J, et al. Short-course therapy for right-side endocarditis due to *Staphylococcus aureus* in drug abusers: Cloxacillin versus glycopeptides in combination with gentamicin. Clin Infect Dis. 2001;33:120-125.

184. Dodek P, Phillips P. Questionable history of immediate-type hypersensitivity to penicillin in staphylococcal endocarditis: Treatment based on skin-test results versus empirical alternative treatment—A decision analysis. Clin Infect Dis. 1999;29:1251-1256.

185. Watanakunakorn C, Tisone JC. Synergism between vancomycin and gentamicin or tobramycin for methicillin-susceptible and methicillin-resistant *Staphylococcus aureus* strains. Antimicrob Agents Chemother. 1982;22:903-905.

186. Korzeniowski O, Sande MA. Combination antimicrobial therapy for *Staphylococcus aureus* endocarditis in patients addicted to parenteral drugs and in nonaddicts: A prospective study. Ann Intern Med. 1982;97:496-503.

187. Goetz MB, Sayers J. Nephrotoxicity of vancomycin and aminoglycoside therapy separately and in combination. J Antimicrob Chemother. 1993;32:325-334.

188. Bayer AS, Lam K. Efficacy of vancomycin plus rifampin in experimental aortic-valve endocarditis due to methicillin-resistant *Staphylococcus aureus*: In vitro-in vivo correlations. J Infect Dis. 1985;151:157-165.

189. Watanakunakorn C, Bakie C. Synergism of vancomycin-gentamicin and vancomycin-streptomycin against enterococci. Antimicrob Agents Chemother. 1973;4:120-124.

190. Murray BE. The life and times of the *Enterococcus*. Clin Microbiol Rev. 1990;3:46-65.

191. Karchmer AW, Archer GL, Dismukes WE. *Staphylococcus epidermidis* causing prosthetic valve endocarditis: Microbiologic and clinical observations as guides to therapy. Ann Intern Med. 1983;98:447-455.

192. Murray BE, Karchmer AW, Moellering RC. Diphtheroid prosthetic valve endocarditis. A study of clinical features and infecting organisms. Am J Med. 1980;69:838-848.

193. Vanbosterhaut B, Surmont I, Vandeven J, et al. *Corynebacterium jeikeium* (group JK diphtheroids) endocarditis. A report of five cases. Diagn Microbiol Infect Dis. 1989;12:265-268.

194. Sande MA, Scheld WM. Combination antibiotic therapy of bacterial endocarditis. Ann Intern Med. 1980;92:390-395.

195. Siegel M, Timpone J. Penicillin-resistant *Streptococcus pneumoniae* endocarditis: A case report and review. Clin Infect Dis. 2001;32:972-974.

196. Lopez Fornas F, Martinez Garcia F, Perez Salmeron J, et al. Comparative study of treatment with penicillin, ceftriaxone, trovafloxacin, quinupristin-dalfopristin and vancomycin in experimental endocarditis due to penicillin- and ceftriaxone-resistant *Streptococcus pneumoniae*. J Antimicrob Chemother. 2001;47:623-629.

197. Temple ME, Nahata MC. Treatment of listeriosis. Ann Pharmacother. 2000;34:656-661.

198. Kaplan SL. Management of pneumococcal meningitis. Pediatr Infect Dis J. 2002;21:589-591; discussion 613-584.

199. Saez-Llorens X, McCracken GH, Jr. Antimicrobial and anti-inflammatory treatment of bacterial meningitis. Infect Dis Clin North Am. 1999;13:619-636, vii.

200. Schreffler RT, Schreffler AJ, Wittler RR. Treatment of cerebrospinal fluid shunt infections: A decision analysis. Pediatr Infect Dis J. 2002;21:632-636.

201. Fitzpatrick DJ, Cafferkey MT, Toner M, et al. Osteomyelitis with methicillin-resistant *Staphylococcus aureus*. J Hosp Infect. 1986;8:24-30.

202. Norden CW, Shaffer M. Treatment of experimental chronic osteomyelitis due to *Staphylococcus aureus* with vancomycin and rifampin. J Infect Dis. 1983;147:352-357.

203. Dworkin R, Modin G, Kunz S, et al. Comparative efficacies of ciprofloxacin, pefloxacin, and vancomycin in combination with rifampin in a rat model of methicillin-resistant *Staphylococcus aureus* chronic osteomyelitis. Antimicrob Agents Chemother. 1990;34:1014-1016.

204. Zimmerli W, Widmer AF, Blatter M, et al. Role of rifampin for treatment of orthopedic implant-related staphylococcal infections: A randomized controlled trial. Foreign-Body Infection (FBI) Study Group. JAMA. 1998;279:1537-1541.

205. Eng RH, Smith SM, Tillem M, et al. Rifampin resistance. Development during the therapy of methicillin-resistant *Staphylococcus aureus* infection. Arch Intern Med. 1985;145:146-148.

206. Wenisch C, Parschalk B, Hasenhundl M, et al. Comparison of vancomycin, teicoplanin, metronidazole, and fusidic acid for the treatment of *Clostridium difficile*-associated diarrhea. Clin Infect Dis. 1996;22:813-818.

207. Bartlett JG. Clinical practice. Antibiotic-associated diarrhea. N Engl J Med. 2002;346:334-339.

208. Anonymous. Vancomycin added to empirical combination antibiotic therapy for fever in granulocytopenic cancer patients. European Organization for Research and Treatment of Cancer (EORTC) International Antimicrobial Therapy Cooperative Group and the National Cancer Institute of Canada-Clinical Trials Group. J Infect Dis. 1991;163:951-958.

209. Hughes WT, Armstrong D, Bodey GP, et al. 2002 guidelines for the use of antimicrobial agents in neutropenic patients with cancer. Clin Infect Dis. 2002;34:730-751.

210. Maki DG, Bohn MJ, Stolz SM, et al. Comparative study of cefazolin, cefamandole, and vancomycin for surgical prophylaxis in cardiac and vascular operations. A double-blind randomized trial. J Thorac Cardiovasc Surg. 1992;104:1423-1434.

211. Dellinger EP, Gross PA, Barrett TL, et al. Quality standard for antimicrobial prophylaxis in surgical procedures. Infectious Diseases Society of America. Clin Infect Dis. 1994;18:422-427.

212. Finkelstein R, Rabino G, Mashiah T, et al. Vancomycin versus cefazolin prophylaxis for cardiac surgery in the setting of a high prevalence of methicillin-resistant staphylococcal infections. J Thorac Cardiovasc Surg. 2002;123:326-332.

213. Antimicrobial prophylaxis in neurosurgery and after head injury. Infection in Neurosurgery Working Party of the British Society for Antimicrobial Chemotherapy. Lancet. 1994;344:1547-1551.

214. Bodey GP. Antibiotic prophylaxis in cancer patients: Regimens of oral, nonabsorbable antibiotics for prevention of infection during induction of remission. Rev Infect Dis. 1981;3(Suppl):S259-268.

215. Attal M, Schlaifer D, Rubie H, et al. Prevention of gram-positive infections after bone marrow transplantation by systemic vancomycin: A prospective, randomized trial. J Clin Oncol. 1991;9:865-870.

216. Aguilar HE, Meredith TA, Drews C, et al. Comparative treatment of experimental *Staphylococcus aureus* endophthalmitis. Am J Ophthalmol. 1996;121:310-317.

217. Mulhern JG, Braden GL, O'Shea MH, et al. Trough serum vancomycin levels predict the relapse of gram-positive peritonitis in peritoneal dialysis patients. Am J Kidney Dis. 1995;25:611-615.

218. Schaefer F, Klaus G, Muller-Wiefel DE, et al. Intermittent versus continuous intraperitoneal glycopeptide/ceftazidime treatment in children with peritoneal dialysis-associated peritonitis. The Mid-European Pediatric Peritoneal Dialysis Study Group (MEPPS). J Am Soc Nephrol. 1999;10:136-145.

219. Wunderink RG, Cammarata SK, Oliphant TH, et al. Continuation of a randomized, double-blind, multicenter study of linezolid versus vancomycin in the treatment of patients with nosocomial pneumonia. Clin Ther. 2003;25:980-992.

220. Gonzalez C, Rubio M, Romero-Vivas J, et al. Bacteremic pneumonia due to *Staphylococcus aureus*: A comparison of disease caused by methicillin-resistant and methicillin-susceptible organisms. Clin Infect Dis. 1999;29:1171-1177.

221. Rolston KV, Nguyen H, Amos G, et al. A randomized double-blind trial of vancomycin versus teicoplanin for the treatment of gram-positive bacteremia in patients with cancer. J Infect Dis. 1994;169:350-355.

222. Carratala J. The antibiotic-lock technique for therapy of "highly needed" infected catheters. Clin Microbiol Infect. 2002;8:282-289.

223. Carratala J, Niubo J, Fernandez-Sevilla A, et al. Randomized, double-blind trial of an antibiotic-lock technique for prevention of gram-positive central venous catheter-related infection in neutropenic patients with cancer. Antimicrob Agents Chemother. 1999;43:2200-2204.

224. Bardone MR, Paternoster M, Coronelli C. Teichomycins, new antibiotics from *Actinoplanes teichomyceticus* nov. sp. II. Extraction and chemical characterization. J Antibiot (Tokyo). 1978;31:170-177.

225. Parenti F. Structure and mechanism of action of teicoplanin. J Hosp Infect. 1986;7(Suppl A):79-83.

226. Greenwood D. Microbiological properties of teicoplanin. J Antimicrob Chemother. 1988;21(Suppl A):1-13.

227. Brogden RN, Peters DH. Teicoplanin. A reappraisal of its antimicrobial activity, pharmacokinetic properties and therapeutic efficacy. Drugs. 1994;47:823-854.

228. Verbist L, Tjandramaga B, Hendrickx B, et al. In vitro activity and human pharmacokinetics of teicoplanin. Antimicrob Agents Chemother. 1984;26:881-886.

229. Shea KW, Cunha BA. Teicoplanin. Med Clin North Am. 1995;79:833-844.

230. Critchley IA, Draghi DC, Sahm DF, et al. Activity of daptomycin against susceptible and multidrug-resistant gram-positive pathogens collected in the SECURE study (Europe) during 2000-2001. J Antimicrob Chemother. 2003;51:639-649.

231. Kaatz GW, Seo SM, Dorman NJ, et al. Emergence of teicoplanin resistance during therapy of Staphylococcus aureus endocarditis. J Infect Dis. 1990;162:103-108.

232. Hayden MK, Trenholme GM, Schultz JE, et al. In vivo development of teicoplanin resistance in a VanB Enterococcus faecium isolate. J Infect Dis. 1993;167:1224-1227.

233. Thompson GA, Smithers JA, Kenny MT, et al. Pharmacokinetics of teicoplanin upon multiple dose intravenous administration to normal healthy male volunteers. Biopharm Drug Dispos. 1992;13:213-220.

234. Danese A, Bernareggi A, Rosina R, et al. Model choice for teicoplanin kinetics in man. Eur J Drug Metab Pharmacokinet. 1991;Spec No 3:250-255.

235. Wilson AP. Clinical pharmacokinetics of teicoplanin. Clin Pharmacokin. 2000;39:167-183.

236. Drago L, De Vecchi E, Fassina MC, et al. Serum and bone concentrations of teicoplanin and vancomycin: Study in an animal model. Drugs Exp Clin Res. 1998;24:185-190.

237. Lazzarini L, Novelli A, Marzano N, et al. Regional and systemic prophylaxis with teicoplanin in total knee arthroplasty: A tissue penetration study. J Arthroplasty. 2003;18:342-346.

238. Martin C, Bourget P, Alaya M, et al. Teicoplanin in cardiac surgery: Intraoperative pharmacokinetics and concentrations in cardiac and mediastinal tissues. Antimicrob. Agents Chemother. 1997;41:1150-1155.

239. Miglioli PA, Merlo F, Fabbri A, et al. Teicoplanin concentrations in serum, pericardium, pericardial fluid and thoracic wall fat in patients undergoing cardiopulmonary bypass surgery. J Antimicrob Chemother. 1997;39:229-233.

240. Cremieux AC, Maziere B, Vallois JM, et al. Evaluation of antibiotic diffusion into cardiac vegetations by quantitative autoradiography. J Infect Dis. 1989;159:938-944.

241. Briggs MC, McDonald P, Bourke R, et al. Intravitreal penetration of teicoplanin. Eye. 1998;12(Pt 2):252-255.

242. Stahl JP, Croize J, Wolff M, et al. Poor penetration of teicoplanin into cerebrospinal fluid in patients with bacterial meningitis. J Antimicrob Chemother. 1987;20:141-142.

243. Bonati M, Traina GL, Rosina R. Pharmacokinetics of a single intravenous dose of teicoplanin in subjects with various degrees of renal impairment. J Antimicrob Chemother. 1988;21(Suppl A):29-37.

244. Wolter K, Claus M, Wagner K, et al. Teicoplanin pharmacokinetics and dosage recommendations in chronic hemodialysis patients and in patients undergoing continuous veno-venous hemodialysis. Clin Nephrol. 1994;42:389-397.

245. Mini E, Mazzei T, Reali EF, et al. Pharmacokinetics of teicoplanin during cardiopulmonary bypass surgery. Int J Clin Pharmacol Res. 1989;9:287-292.

246. Stamatiadis D, Papaioannou MG, Giamarellos-Bourboulis EJ, et al. Pharmacokinetics of teicoplanin in patients undergoing continuous ambulatory peritoneal dialysis. Perit Dial Int. 2003;23:127-131.

247. Neville LO, Baillod RA, Brumfitt W, et al. Efficacy and safety of teicoplanin in gram-positive peritonitis in patients on peritoneal dialysis. J Antimicrob Chemother. 1988;21(Suppl A):123-131.

248. Finch RC, Holliday AP, Innes A, et al. Pharmacokinetic behavior of intraperitoneal teicoplanin during treatment of peritonitis complicating continuous ambulatory peritoneal dialysis. Antimicrob Agents Chemother. 1996;40:1971-1972.

249. Rybak MJ, Lerner SA, Levine DP, et al. Teicoplanin pharmacokinetics in intravenous drug abusers being treated for bacterial endocarditis. Antimicrob Agents Chemother. 1991;35:696-700.

250. Wood MJ. The comparative efficacy and safety of teicoplanin and vancomycin. J Antimicrob Chemother. 1996;37:209-222.

251. Davey PG, Williams AH. A review of the safety profile of teicoplanin. J Antimicrob Chemother. 1991;27(Suppl B):69-73.

252. Lewis P, Garaud JJ, Parenti F. A multicentre open clinical trial of teicoplanin in infections caused by gram-positive bacteria. J Antimicrob Chemother. 1988;21(Suppl A):61-67.

253. Wilson AP. Comparative safety of teicoplanin and vancomycin. Int J Antimicrob Agents. 1998;10:143-152.

254. Greenberg RN. Treatment of bone, joint, and vascular-access-associated gram-positive bacterial infections with teicoplanin. Antimicrob Agents Chemother. 1990;34:2392-2397.

255. Calain P, Krause KH, Vaudaux P, et al. Early termination of a prospective, randomized trial comparing teicoplanin and flucloxacillin for treating severe staphylococcal infections. J Infect Dis. 1987;155:187-191.

256. Galanakis N, Giamarellou H, Vlachogiannis N, et al. Poor efficacy of teicoplanin in treatment of deep-seated staphylococcal infections. Eur J Clin Microbiol Infect Dis. 1988;7:130-134.

257. Gilbert DN, Wood CA, Kimbrough RC. Failure of treatment with teicoplanin at 6 milligrams/kilogram/day in patients with Staphylococcus aureus intravascular infection. The Infectious Diseases Consortium of Oregon. Antimicrob Agents Chemother. 1991;35:79-87.

258. Wilson AP, Gruneberg RN, Neu HC. A critical review of the dosage of teicoplanin in Europe and the USA. Int J Antimicrob Agents. 1994;4(Suppl 1):S1-30.

259. Testore GP, Uccella I, Sarrecchia C, et al. Long-term intramuscular teicoplanin treatment of chronic osteomyelitis due to oxacillin-resistant Staphylococcus aureus in outpatients. J Chemother. 2000;12:412-415.

260. Schmit JL. Efficacy of teicoplanin for enterococcal infections: 63 cases and review. Clin Infect Dis. 1992;15:302-306.

261. Presterl E, Graninger W, Georgopoulos A. The efficacy of teicoplanin in the treatment of endocarditis caused by gram-positive bacteria. J Antimicrob Chemother. 1993;31:755-766.

262. Sullam PM, Tauber MG, Hackbarth CJ, et al. Therapeutic efficacy of teicoplanin in experimental enterococcal endocarditis. Antimicrob Agents Chemother. 1985;27:135-136.

263. Eliopoulos GM, Thauvin-Eliopoulos C, Moellering RC, Jr. Contribution of animal models in the search for effective therapy for endocarditis due to enterococci with high-level resistance to gentamicin. Clin Infect Dis. 1992;15:58-62.

264. Turpin PJ, Taylor GP, Logan MN, et al. Teicoplanin in the treatment of skin and soft tissue infections. J Antimicrob Chemother. 1988;21(Suppl A):117-122.

265. Chow AW, Jewesson PJ, Kureishi A, et al. Teicoplanin versus vancomycin in the empirical treatment of febrile neutropenic patients. Eur J Haematol Suppl. 1993;54:18-24.

266. Cruciani M, Navarra A, Di Perri G, et al. Evaluation of intraventricular teicoplanin for the treatment of neurosurgical shunt infections. Clin Infect Dis. 1992;15:285-289.

267. Fernandez Guerrero ML, de Gorgolas M, Fernandez Roblas R, et al. Treatment of cerebrospinal fluid shunt infections with teicoplanin. Eur J Clin Microbiol Infect Dis. 1994;13:1056-1058.

268. Periti P, Stringa G, Mini E. Comparative multicenter trial of teicoplanin versus cefazolin for antimicrobial prophylaxis in prosthetic joint implant surgery. Italian Study Group for Antimicrobial Prophylaxis in Orthopedic Surgery. Eur J Clin Microbiol Infect Dis. 1999;18:113-119.

269. Wilson AP, Treasure T, Gruneberg RN, et al. Antibiotic prophylaxis in cardiac surgery: A prospective comparison of two dosage regimens of teicoplanin with a combination of flucloxacillin and tobramycin. J Antimicrob Chemother. 1988; 21:213-223.

270. Marroni M, Cao P, Fiorio M, et al. Prospective, randomized, double-blind trial comparing teicoplanin and cefazolin as antibiotic prophylaxis in prosthetic vascular surgery. Eur J Clin Microbiol Infect Dis. 1999;18:175-178.

271. Shanson DC, Shehata A, Tadayon M, et al. Comparison of intravenous teicoplanin with intramuscular amoxycillin for the prophylaxis of streptococcal bacteraemia in dental patients. J Antimicrob Chemother. 1987;20:85-93.

272. Leport C, Horstkotte D, Burckhardt D. Antibiotic prophylaxis for infective endocarditis from an international group of experts towards a European consensus. Group of Experts of the International Society for Chemotherapy. Eur Heart J. 1995;16 (Suppl B):126-131.

273. Cocito C. Antibiotics of the virginiamycin family, inhibitors which contain synergistic components. Microbiol Rev. 1979;43:145-192.

274. Aumercier M, Bouhallab S, Capmau ML, et al. RP 59500: A proposed mechanism for its bactericidal activity. J Antimicrob Chemother. 1992;30(Suppl A):9-14.

275. Dancer SJ, Robb A, Crawford A, et al. Oral streptogramins in the management of patients with methicillin-resistant Staphylococcus aureus (MRSA) infections. J Antimicrob Chemother. 2003;51:731-735.

276. Synercid, package insert. Monarch Pharmaceuticals Inc.: Bristol, Tenn, 2002.

277. Vannuffel P, Cocito C. Mechanism of action of streptogramins and macrolides. Drugs. 1996;51(Suppl 1):20-30.

278. Leclercq R, Nantas L, Soussy CJ, et al. Activity of RP 59500, a new parenteral semisynthetic streptogramin, against staphylococci with various mechanisms of resistance to macrolide-lincosamide-streptogramin antibiotics. J Antimicrob Chemother. 1992;30(Suppl A):67-75.

279. Eliopoulos GM, Wennersten CB, Gold HS, et al. Characterization of vancomycin-resistant Enterococcus faecium isolates from the United States and their susceptibility in vitro to dalfopristin-quinupristin. Antimicrob Agents Chemother. 1998;42:1088-1092.

280. Bouanchaud DH. In-vitro and in-vivo antibacterial activity of quinupristin/dalfopristin. J Antimicrob Chemother. 1997;39(Suppl A):15-21.

281. Hill RL, Smith CT, Seyed-Akhavani M, et al. Bactericidal and inhibitory activity of quinupristin/dalfopristin against vancomycin- and gentamicin-resistant Enterococcus faecium. J Antimicrob Chemother. 1997;39(Suppl A):23-28.

282. Williams JD, Maskell JP, Whiley AC, et al. Comparative in-vitro activity of quinupristin/dalfopristin against Enterococcus spp. J Antimicrob Chemother. 1997;39 (Suppl A):41-46.

283. Finch RG. Antibacterial activity of quinupristin/dalfopristin. Rationale for clinical use. Drugs. 1996;51(Suppl 1):31-37.

284. Singh KV, Weinstock GM, Murray BE. An Enterococcus faecalis ABC homologue (Lsa) is required for the resistance of this species to clindamycin and quinupristin-dalfopristin. Antimicrob Agents Chemother. 2002;46:1845-1850.

285. Critchley IA, Blosser-Middleton RS, Jones ME, et al. Baseline study to determine in vitro activities of daptomycin against gram-positive pathogens isolated in the United States in 2000-2001. Antimicrob Agents Chemother. 2003;47:1689-1693.

286. Verbist L, Verhaegen J. Comparative in-vitro activity of RP 59500. J Antimicrob Chemother. 1992;30(Suppl A):39-44.

287. Rybak MJ, Hershberger E, Moldovan T, et al. In vitro activities of daptomycin, vancomycin, linezolid, and quinupristin-dalfopristin against staphylococci and enterococci, including vancomycin-intermediate and -resistant strains. Antimicrob Agents Chemother. 2000;44:1062-1066.

288. Gordon KA, Beach ML, Biedenbach DJ, et al. Antimicrobial susceptibility patterns of [beta]-hemolytic and viridans group streptococci: Report from the SENTRY Antimicrobial Surveillance Program (1997-2000). Diagnostic Microbiology and Infectious Disease. 2002;43:157-162.

289. Goldstein EJ, Citron DM, Merriam CV, et al. In vitro activities of daptomycin, vancomycin, quinupristin-dalfopristin, linezolid, and five other antimicrobials against 307 gram-positive anaerobic and 31 *Corynebacterium* clinical isolates. Antimicrob Agents Chemother. 2003; 47:337-341.

290. Neu HC, Chin NX, Gu JW. The in-vitro activity of new streptogramins, RP 59500, RP 57669 and RP 54476, alone and in combination. J Antimicrob Chemother. 1992;30(Suppl A):83-94.

291. Brumfitt W, Hamilton-Miller JM, Shah S. In-vitro activity of RP 59500, a new semi-synthetic streptogramin antibiotic, against gram-positive bacteria. J Antimicrob Chemother. 1992;30(Suppl A):29-37.

292. Collins LA, Malanoski GJ, Eliopoulos GM, et al. In vitro activity of RP59500, an injectable streptogramin antibiotic, against vancomycin-resistant gram-positive organisms. Antimicrob Agents Chemother. 1993;37:598-601.

293. Ednie LM, Rattan A, Jacobs MR, et al. Antianaerobe activity of RBX 7644 (Ranbezolid), a new oxazolidinone, compared with those of eight other agents. Antimicrob Agents Chemother. 2003;47:1143-1147.

294. Appelbaum PC, Spangler SK, Jacobs MR. Susceptibility of 539 gram-positive and gram-negative anaerobes to new agents, including RP59500, biapenem, trospectomycin and piperacillin/tazobactam. J Antimicrob Chemother. 1993;32:223-231.

295. Bebear C, Bouanchaud DH. A review of the in-vitro activity of quinupristin/dalfopristin against intracellular pathogens and mycoplasmas. J Antimicrob Chemother. 1997;39(Suppl A):59-62.

296. Moellering RC, Linden PK, Reinhardt J, et al. The efficacy and safety of quinupristin/dalfopristin for the treatment of infections caused by vancomycin-resistant *Enterococcus faecium*. Synercid emergency-use study group. J Antimicrob Chemother. 1999;44:251-261.

297. Low DE, Keller N, Barth A, et al. Clinical prevalence, antimicrobial susceptibility, and geographic resistance patterns of enterococci: Results from the SENTRY Antimicrobial Surveillance Program, 1997-1999. Clin Infect Dis. 2001;32(Suppl 2):S133-145.

298. McDonald LC, Rossiter S, Mackinson C, et al. Quinupristin-dalfopristin-resistant *Enterococcus faecium* on chicken and in human stool specimens. N Engl J Med. 2001;345:1155-1160.

299. Diekema DJ, Pfaller MA, Schmitz FJ, et al. Survey of infections due to *Staphylococcus* species: Frequency of occurrence and antimicrobial susceptibility of isolates collected in the United States, Canada, Latin America, Europe, and the Western Pacific region for the SENTRY Antimicrobial Surveillance Program, 1997-1999. Clin Infect Dis. 2001;32(Suppl 2):S114-132.

300. Hsueh P-R, Teng L-J, Lee C-M, et al. Telithromycin and quinupristin-dalfopristin resistance in clinical isolates of *Streptococcus pyogenes*: SMART Program 2001 Data. Antimicrob. Agents Chemother. 2003; 47:2152-2157.

301. Roberts MC, Sutcliffe J, Courvalin P, et al. Nomenclature for macrolide and macrolide-lincosamide-streptogramin B resistance determinants. Antimicrob Agents Chemother. 1999;43:2823-2830.

302. Leclercq R, Courvalin P. Bacterial resistance to macrolide, lincosamide, and streptogramin antibiotics by target modification. Antimicrob Agents Chemother. 1991;35:1267-1272.

303. Weisblum B. Insights into erythromycin action from studies of its activity as inducer of resistance. Antimicrob Agents Chemother. 1995;39:797-805.

304. Fantin B, Leclercq R, Merle Y, et al. Critical influence of resistance to streptogramin B-type antibiotics on activity of RP 59500 (quinupristin-dalfopristin) in experimental endocarditis due to *Staphylococcus aureus*. Antimicrob Agents Chemother. 1995;39:400-405.

305. Drinkovic D, Fuller ER, Shore KP, et al. Clindamycin treatment of *Staphylococcus aureus* expressing inducible clindamycin resistance. J Antimicrob Chemother. 2001;48:315-316.

306. Lina G, Quaglia A, Reverdy ME, et al. Distribution of genes encoding resistance to macrolides, lincosamides, and streptogramins among staphylococci. Antimicrob Agents Chemother. 1999;43:1062-1066.

307. Fuchs PC, Barry AL, Brown SD. Bactericidal activity of quinupristin-dalfopristin against *Staphylococcus aureus*: Clindamycin susceptibility as a surrogate indicator. Antimicrob. Agents Chemother. 2000;44:2880-2882.

308. Rosato A, Vicarini H, Leclercq R. Inducible or constitutive expression of resistance in clinical isolates of streptococci and enterococci cross-resistant to erythromycin and lincomycin. J Antimicrob Chemother. 1999;43:559-562.

309. Fantin B, Leclercq R, Garry L, et al. Influence of inducible cross-resistance to macrolides, lincosamides, and streptogramin B-type antibiotics in *Enterococcus faecium* on activity of quinupristin-dalfopristin in vitro and in rabbits with experimental endocarditis. Antimicrob Agents Chemother. 1997;41:931-935.

310. Betriu C, Redondo M, Palau ML, et al. Comparative in vitro activities of linezolid, quinupristin-dalfopristin, moxifloxacin, and trovafloxacin against erythromycin-susceptible and -resistant streptococci. Antimicrob. Agents Chemother. 2000;44:1838-1841.

311. Jensen LB, Hammerum AM, Aerestrup FM, et al. Occurrence of *satA* and *vgb* genes in streptogramin-resistant *Enterococcus faecium* isolates of animal and human origins in the Netherlands. Antimicrob Agents Chemother. 1998;42:3330-3331.

312. Soltani M, Beighton D, Philpott-Howard J, et al. Mechanisms of resistance to quinupristin-dalfopristin among isolates of *Enterococcus faecium* from animals, raw meat, and hospital patients in Western Europe. Antimicrob Agents Chemother. 2000;44:433-436.

313. Bozdogan B, Leclercq R. Effects of genes encoding resistance to streptogramins A and B on the activity of quinupristin-dalfopristin against *Enterococcus faecium*. Antimicrob Agents Chemother. 1999;43:2720-2725.

314. Linden PK, Moellering RC, Jr., Wood CA, et al. Treatment of vancomycin-resistant *Enterococcus faecium* infections with quinupristin/dalfopristin. Clin Infect Dis. 2001;33:1816-1823.

315. Fagon J, Patrick H, Haas DW, et al. Treatment of gram-positive nosocomial pneumonia. Prospective randomized comparison of quinupristin/dalfopristin versus vancomycin. Nosocomial Pneumonia Group. Am J Respir Crit Care Med. 2000;161:753-762.

316. Ling TK, Fung KS, Cheng AF. In vitro activity and post-antibiotic effect of quinupristin/dalfopristin (Synercid). Chemotherapy. 2001;47:243-249.

317. Pankuch GA, Jacobs MR, Appelbaum PC. Postantibiotic effect and postantibiotic sub-MIC effect of quinupristin-dalfopristin against gram-positive and -negative organisms. Antimicrob Agents Chemother. 1998;42:3028-3031.

318. Etienne SD, Montay G, Le Liboux A, et al. A phase I, double-blind, placebo-controlled study of the tolerance and pharmacokinetic behaviour of RP 59500. J Antimicrob Chemother. 1992;30(Suppl A):123-131.

319. Bergeron M, Montay G. The pharmacokinetics of quinupristin/dalfopristin in laboratory animals and in humans. J Antimicrob Chemother. 1997;39(Suppl A):129-138.

320. Fantin B, Leclercq R, Ottaviani M, et al. In vivo activities and penetration of the two components of the streptogramin RP 59500 in cardiac vegetations of experimental endocarditis. Antimicrob Agents Chemother. 1994;38:432-437.

321. Loeffler AM, Drew RH, Perfect JR, et al. Safety and efficacy of quinupristin/dalfopristin for treatment of invasive gram-positive infections in pediatric patients. Pediatr Infect Dis J. 2002;21:950-956.

322. Rubinstein E, Prokocimer P, Talbot GH. Safety and tolerability of quinupristin/dalfopristin: Administration guidelines. J Antimicrob Chemother. 1999;44:37-46.

323. Chevalier P, Rey J, Pasquier O, et al. Pharmacokinetics of quinupristin/ dalfopristin in patients with severe chronic renal insufficiency. Clin Pharmacokinet. 2000;39:77-84.

324. Schwenger V, Mundlein E, Dagrosa EE, et al. Treatment of life-threatening multiresistant staphylococcal and enterococcal infections in patients with end-stage renal failure with quinupristin/dalfopristin: Preliminary report. Infection. 2002;30:257-261.

325. Johnson CA, Taylor CA, 3rd, Zimmerman SW, et al. Pharmacokinetics of quinupristin-dalfopristin in continuous ambulatory peritoneal dialysis patients. Antimicrob Agents Chemother. 1999;43:152-156.

326. Drew RH, Perfect JR, Srinath L, et al. Treatment of methicillin-resistant *Staphylococcus aureus* infections with quinupristin-dalfopristin in patients intolerant of or failing prior therapy. For the Synercid Emergency-Use Study Group. J Antimicrob Chemother. 2000;46:775-784.

327. Carver PL, Whang E, VandenBussche HL, et al. Risk factors for arthralgias or myalgias associated with quinupristin-dalfopristin therapy. Pharmacotherapy. 2003;23:159-164.

328. Winston DJ, Emmanouilides C, Kroeber A, et al. Quinupristin/dalfopristin therapy for infections due to vancomycin-resistant *Enterococcus faecium*. Clin Infect Dis. 2000;30:790-797.

329. Kanchanapoom T, Koirala J, Goodrich J, et al. Treatment of central nervous system infection by vancomycin-resistant *Enterococcus faecium*. Diagn Microbiol Infect Dis. 2003;45:213-215.

330. Garey KW, Tesoro E, Muggia V, et al. Cerebrospinal fluid concentrations of quinupristin-dalfopristin in a patient with vancomycin-resistant *Enterococcus faecium* [correction of *faecalis*] ventriculitis. Pharmacotherapy. 2001;21:748-750.

331. Lynn WA, Clutterbuck E, Want S, et al. Treatment of CAPD-peritonitis due to glycopeptide-resistant *Enterococcus faecium* with quinupristin/dalfopristin. Lancet. 1994;344:1025-1026.

332. Tally FP, Zeckel M, Wasilewski MM, et al. Daptomycin: A novel agent for gram-positive infections. Exp Opin Investig Drugs. 1999;8:1223-1238.

333. Allen NE, Alborn WE, Jr., Hobbs JN, Jr. Inhibition of membrane potential-dependent amino acid transport by daptomycin. Antimicrob Agents Chemother. 1991;35:2639-2642.

334. Alborn WE, Jr, Allen NE, Preston DA. Daptomycin disrupts membrane potential in growing *Staphylococcus aureus*. Antimicrob Agents Chemother. 1991;35:2282-2287.

335. Silverman JA, Oliver N, Andrew T, et al. Resistance studies with daptomycin. Antimicrob Agents Chemother. 2001;45:1799-1802.

336. National Committee for Clinical Laboratories Standards (NCCLS). MIC testing-Supplemental tables. NCCLS document M100-S13 (M7). National Committee for Clinical Laboratory Standards, Wayne, Pa., 2003.

337. Barry AL, Fuchs PC, Brown SD. In vitro activities of daptomycin against 2,789 clinical isolates from 11 North American medical centers. Antimicrob Agents Chemother. 2001;45:1919-1922.

338. Jones RN, Barry AL. Antimicrobial activity and spectrum of LY146032, a lipopeptide antibiotic, including susceptibility testing recommendations. Antimicrob Agents Chemother. 1987;31:625-629.

339. Critchley IA, Blosser-Middleton RS, Jones ME, et al. Baseline study to determine in vitro activities of daptomycin against gram-positive pathogens isolated in the United States in 2000-2001. Antimicrob Agents Chemother. 2003;47:1689-1693.

340. Goldstein EJ, Citron DM, Merriam CV, et al. In vitro activities of daptomycin, vancomycin, quinupristin-dalfopristin, linezolid, and five other antimicrobials against 307 gram-positive anaerobic and 31 *Corynebacterium* clinical isolates. Antimicrob Agents Chemother. 2003;47:337-341.

341. Pankuch GA, Jacobs MR, Appelbaum PC. Bactericidal activity of daptomycin against *Streptococcus pneumoniae* compared with eight other antimicrobials. J Antimicrob Chemother. 2003;51:443-446.

342. Hanberger H, Nilsson LE, Maller R, et al. Pharmacodynamics of daptomycin and vancomycin on *Enterococcus faecalis* and *Staphylococcus aureus* demonstrated by studies of initial killing and postantibiotic effect and influence of Ca^{2+} and albumin on these drugs. Antimicrob Agents Chemother. 1991;35:1710-1716.

343. Akins RL, Rybak MJ. Bactericidal activities of two daptomycin regimens against clinical strains of glycopeptide intermediate-resistant *Staphylococcus aureus*, vancomycin-resistant *Enterococcus faecium*, and methicillin-resistant *Staphylococcus aureus* isolates in an in vitro pharmacodynamic model with simulated endocardial vegetations. Antimicrob Agents Chemother. 2001;45:454-459.

344. Rybak MJ, Hershberger E, Moldovan T, et al. In vitro activities of daptomycin, vancomycin, linezolid, and quinupristin-dalfopristin against staphylococci and enterococci, including vancomycin- intermediate and -resistant strains. Antimicrob Agents Chemother. 2000;44:1062-1066.

345. Louie A, Kaw P, Liu W, et al. Pharmacodynamics of daptomycin in a murine thigh model of *Staphylococcus aureus* infection. Antimicrob. Agents Chemother. 2001;45:845-851.

346. Dvorchik BH, Brazier D, DeBruin MF, et al. Daptomycin pharmacokinetics and safety following administration of escalating doses once daily to healthy subjects. Antimicrob Agents Chemother. 2003;47:1318-1323.

347. Dvorchik BH, Sica D, Gehr T. Pharmacokinetics and safety of single-dose daptomycin in subjects with graded renal insufficiency and end-stage renal disease. 42nd Interscience Conference on Antimicrobial Agents and Chemotherapy (ICAAC); American Society for Microbiology, Washington, D.C. Abstract A-1387, p. 18. ASM Press.

348. Oleson FB, Jr., Berman CL, Kirkpatrick JB, et al. Once-daily dosing in dogs optimizes daptomycin safety. Antimicrob Agents Chemother. 2000;44:2948-2953.

349. Arbeit RD, DeBruin MF. Daptomycin, a novel lipopeptide antibiotic, in the treatment of complicated skin and soft tissue infections: Combined results of two phase III studies (99-01 and 98-01). In: 41st Interscience Conference on Antimicrobial Agents and Chemotherapy (ICAAC); American Society for Microbiology, Washington, D.C. Abstract UL-19. ASM Press.

350. Sakoulas G, Eliopoulos GM, Alder J, et al. Efficacy of daptomycin in experimental endocarditis due to methicillin-resistant *Staphylococcus aureus*. Antimicrob Agents Chemother. 2003;47:1714-1718.

351. Eliopoulos GM, Thauvin-Eliopoulos C, Moellering RC, Jr. Contribution of animal models in the search for effective therapy for endocarditis due to enterococci with high-level resistance to gentamicin. Clin Infect Dis. 1992;15:58-62.

Polymyxins (Polymyxin B and Colistin)

KEITH S. KAYE

DONALD KAYE

The polymyxins are old drugs, discovered in 1947. They were used parenterally from 1962 until anti-*Pseudomonas* aminoglycosides (such as gentamicin) came into common use after the middle to late 1960s.

The polymyxins fell into disuse by 1980 because of their nephrotoxicity and subsequently have been reserved mainly for topical and oral use.[1-5] However, the increasing emergence of *Pseudomonas aeruginosa* and other gram-negative bacilli resistant to all other antimicrobial agents has resulted in the occasional need for use of an injectable polymyxin. The two parenteral polymyxins that have been used are polymyxin B and polymyxin E (colistin, usually formulated as colistimethate sodium). Colistimethate sodium is less active in vitro than polymyxin B and colistin and is less nephrotoxic than polymyxin B.[6] In past years, these agents were used to treat patients with bacteremia, pneumonia, and other systemic infections.[5] More recently, series of patients treated with colistimethate sodium have been reported in the literature much more frequently than series of patients treated with polymyxin B.

STRUCTURE AND SOURCE

The polymyxins are cyclic cationic polypeptide detergents with molecular weights greater than or equal to 1000. Polymyxin B is derived from products of strains of *Bacillus polymyxa*, and colistin (polymyxin E) is derived from products of *Bacillus colistinus*. The sulfomethylated formulation of colistin (colistimethate sodium) must be hydrolyzed to be active as an antibiotic. Hydrolysis occurs at body temperature and in in vitro testing systems.[5]

MECHANISM OF ACTION

The polymyxins are surface-active amphipathic agents containing both lipophilic and lipophobic groups. They penetrate into cell membranes, interact with phospholipids in the membranes, and quickly disrupt the membranes. They are rapidly bactericidal in a concentration-dependent manner and have a post-antibiotic effect.[6] They also bind to the lipid A portion of endotoxin or lipopolysaccharide and, in animal studies, block many of the biologic effects of endotoxin.[7] Resistance of gram-negative bacteria is most likely related to decreased permeability across the outer membrane.

ANTIMICROBIAL ACTIVITY

The polymyxins are active against a broad array of gram-negative aerobic bacilli with the notable exception of *Proteus* species, most of which are highly resistant. They also have poor activity against *Providencia*, *Burkholderia*, and *Serratia*.[4,8] Most gram-negative bacilli are inhibited by 1 µg/mL; *P. aeruginosa* strains are more resistant, but the majority of strains are inhibited by 2 µg/mL. Gram-positive organisms and most anaerobes are resistant. The antibacterial activity of the polymyxins is decreased by the presence of divalent cations such as calcium and magnesium. The polymyxins have retained activity against many multidrug-resistant (MDR) gram-negative bacilli such as MDR *P. aeruginosa* and *Acinetobacter baumannii*. There is complete cross-resistance between the polymyxins.

PREPARATIONS

Polymyxin B is available for topical use (see Chapter 35). There is also a parenteral preparation that can be given intramuscularly and intravenously.

Colistin has been available as colistin sulfate for use topically and orally and as colistimethate sodium for intramuscular and intravenous use.

PHARMACOLOGY

None of the polymyxins are absorbed when given orally. After intramuscular injection of 2 to 4 mg/kg polymyxin B, peak serum levels of 1 to 8 µg/mL are achieved. There are few or no reliable data on serum levels after intravenous administration of polymyxin B. When colistimethate, 2.5 mg/kg, is given intramuscularly to adults, a peak serum level of 5 to 7 µg/mL is achieved. When colistimethate is given intravenously, the peak is about 20 µg/mL at 10 minutes. The excretion of both polymyxin B and colistin is primarily by glomerular filtration. There is a 12- to 24-hour lag period after the initial dose of polymyxin B (but not colistimethate) before significant amounts appear in the urine. With subsequent doses, urine levels of both polymyxin B and colistimethate exceed 15 µg/mL for at least 6 hours after injection. The half-life of polymyxin B in serum is about 4.5 to 6 hours and that of colistimethate is about 3 hours[9]; half-lives are much longer in patients with renal insufficiency. Accumulation of both drugs occurs with repeated dosing. Distribution to the cerebrospinal fluid, biliary tract, pleural fluid, and joint fluid is poor. The polymyxins are poorly dialyzed.

TOXICITY

Hypersensitivity is unusual. There is dose-related nephrotoxicity, which is usually reversible after discontinuing the drug. There is also dose-related reversible neurotoxicity manifested by neuromuscular blockade, which can result in muscle weakness and even apnea. Neuromuscular blockade is most likely to occur with drug overdosage and in patients with renal insufficiency or those who are receiving curariform drugs. With respiratory paralysis, support of respiratory function is required until the effects of the polymyxin wear off. Aminoglycosides may potentiate the neurotoxic effects.

Paresthesias around the lips, tongue, and extremities; peripheral neuropathy; and other neurotoxic side effects are not uncommon.[9]

CLINICAL USE

Polymyxin B is very painful when given intramuscularly, and this route of administration should be avoided; if necessary, the usual intramuscular dose is 2.5 to 3 mg/kg/day in divided doses every 4 to 6 hours. The intravenous dose is 1.5 to 2.5 mg/kg/day by continuous intravenous infusion or in divided doses every 12 hours over a period of 60 to 90 minutes. For treatment of gram-negative bacillary meningitis, polymyxin B has been given intrathecally in doses of 5 to 10 mg/day for the initial 3 days of therapy and then every other day.

The recommended dosage of colistimethate in patients with normal renal function is 2.5 to 5 mg/kg (depending on the severity of infection) each day intramuscularly or intravenously in two to four divided doses. The dose should be based on ideal body weight and should not exceed 300 mg/day. Doses must be decreased in patients with impaired renal function to avoid drug accumulation and toxicity. When given intravenously, colistimethate is administered over 3 to 5 minutes. Administration of doses as high as 8 mg/kg/day has been reported.[10]

Colistin sulfate has been used for intestinal decontamination. The oral preparation is not available in the United States.

Inhalation therapy with aerosolized colistimethate has been used with varying results to treat colonization or infection of the bronchial system in patients with cystic fibrosis, especially with MDR *P. aeruginosa*.[11,12] Systemic blood levels are not achieved with inhalation therapy.

Colistimethate has been used parenterally to treat systemic infections caused by MDR gram-negative bacilli, mainly ventilator-associated pneumonia.[2,5] In contrast to the past experience, more recent reports mention little in the way of nephrotoxicity or neurotoxicity.[2,5,10,13] However, more experience is necessary before colistimethate can be considered a relatively nontoxic systemic agent. Modern reports of use of polymyxin B have been sparse.[14]

In the 1960s, one of us found that polymyxin B and colistimethate were relatively ineffective in the treatment of *P. aeruginosa* bacteremia in neutropenic patients. These agents were also more toxic and less effective in the treatment of gram-negative bacillary infection than aminoglycosides such as gentamicin. Parenteral polymyxin B and colistimethate should be reserved for use when no other less toxic or potentially more effective drug is available.

REFERENCES

1. Wolinsky E, Hines JD. Neurotoxic and nephrotoxic effects of colistin in patients with renal disease. N Engl J Med. 1962;266:759-762.
2. Garnacho-Montero J, Ortiz-Leyba C, Jimenez-Jimenez FJ, et al. Treatment of multidrug-resistant *Acinetobacter baumannii* ventilator-associated pneumonia (VAP) with intravenous colistin: A comparison with imipenem-susceptible VAP. Clin Infect Dis. 2003;36:1111-1118.
3. Koch-Weser J, Sidel VW, Federman EB, et al. Adverse effects of sodium colistimethate. Manifestations and specific reaction rates during 317 courses of therapy. Ann Intern Med. 1970;72:857-868.
4. Gales AC, Reis AO, Jones RN. Contemporary assessment of antimicrobial susceptibility testing methods for polymyxin B and colistin: Review of available interpretative criteria and quality control guidelines. J Clin Microbiol. 2001;39:183-190.
5. Levin AS, Barone AA, Penco J, et al. Intravenous colistin as therapy for nosocomial infections caused by multidrug-resistant *Pseudomonas aeruginosa* and *Acinetobacter baumannii*. Clin Infect Dis. 1999;28:1008-1011.
6. Li J, Turnidge J, Milne R, et al. In vitro pharmacodynamic properties of colistin and colistin methanesulfonate against *Pseudomonas aeruginosa* isolates from patients with cystic fibrosis. Antimicrob Agents Chemother. 2001;45:781-785.
7. From AH, Fong JS, Good RA. Polymyxin B sulfate modification of bacterial endotoxin: Effects on the development of endotoxin shock in dogs. Infect Immun. 1979;23:660-664.
8. Catchpole CR, Andrews JM, Brenwald N, et al. A reassessment of the in-vitro activity of colistin sulphomethate sodium. J Antimicrob Chemother. 1997;39:255-260.
9. Reed MD, Stern RC, O'Riordan MA, et al. The pharmacokinetics of colistin in patients with cystic fibrosis. J Clin Pharmacol. 2001;41:645-654.
10. Beringer P. The clinical use of colistin in patients with cystic fibrosis. Curr Opin Pulm Med. 2001;7:434-440.
11. Hodson ME, Gallagher CG, Govan JR. A randomised clinical trial of nebulised tobramycin or colistin in cystic fibrosis. Eur Respir J. 2002;20:658-664.
12. Hamer DH. Treatment of nosocomial pneumonia and tracheobronchitis caused by multidrug-resistant *Pseudomonas aeruginosa* with aerosolized colistin. Am J Respir Crit Care Med. 2000;162:328-330.
13. Conway SP, Pond MN, Watson A, et al. Intravenous colistin sulphomethate in acute respiratory exacerbations in adult patients with cystic fibrosis. Thorax. 1997;52:987-993.
14. Ouderkirk JP, Nord JA, Turett GS, et al. Polymyxin B nephrotoxicity and efficacy against nosocomial infections caused by multiresistant gram-negative bacteria. Antimicrob Agents Chemother. 2003;47:2659-2662.

CHAPTER **31**

Oxazolidinones

GERALD R. DONOWITZ

The oxazolidinones are a class of antibiotics prepared completely by organic synthesis. In 1978, a patent was issued to E. I. DuPont de Nemours and Company for a series of 5-(halomethyl)-3-aryl-2-oxazolidinones that had antimicrobial activity against plant pathogens. Further manipulation of the molecule led to the development of two agents that displayed activity against human pathogens.[1] These two agents, DuP 105 and DuP 721, were orally absorbed and displayed activity against a variety of streptococcal and staphylococcal species

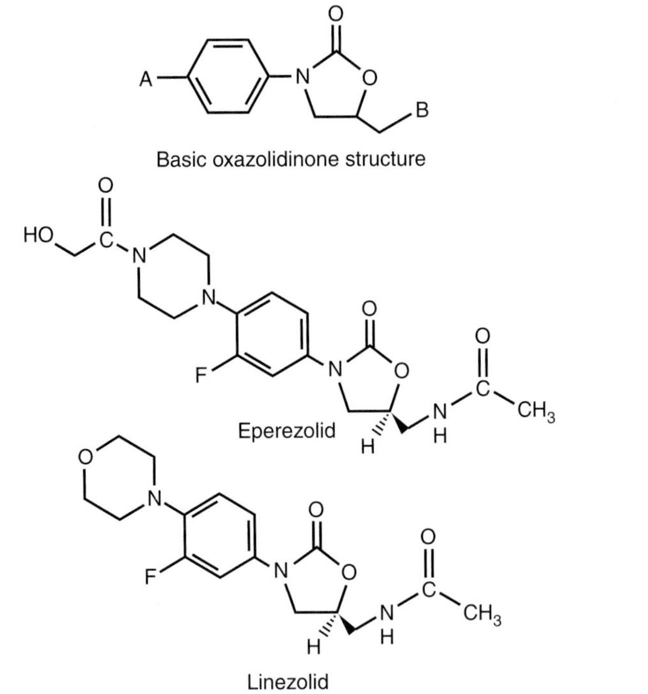

FIGURE 31-1. Top, The basic molecular structure of the oxazolidinones. Bottom, The molecular structure of linezolid.

comparable to that of vancomycin and β-lactam agents. Further manipulation of these compounds led to the development of eperezolid (PNU-100592) and linezolid (PNU-100766). A number of oxazolidinones are being investigated; however, at present only linezolid (Zyvox) is available for clinical use.

CHEMICAL STRUCTURE

The basic molecular structure of the oxazolidinones is shown in the top part of Figure 31-1. Initial chemical manipulation included the incorporation of a piperazine moiety into the basic structure at site A. Antibacterial activity was increased by the addition of a hydroxyacetyl group to the heterocyclic nitrogen at site B.[2] Further antibacterial activity was derived by fluorine substitution at the phenyl 3 position. Only the enantiomers with a 5S acetamidomethyl configuration have antibacterial activity. The molecular structure of linezolid is shown in Figure 31-1, bottom. The unique chemical structure of the compound makes cross-resistance with more commonly used compounds such as β-lactams and vancomycin, as well as subsequently developed agents such as streptogramins, unlikely.

MECHANISM OF ACTION

The oxazolidinones are inhibitors of protein synthesis and are bacteriostatic against most bacteria. The mechanism of activity is thought to be unique, involving inhibition of the earliest steps of bacterial protein synthesis.[3-5] These agents bind to the 50S ribosome at its interface with the 30S unit, thereby preventing the formation of the 70S initiation complex. Some data have shown that production of the 50S subunit may also be inhibited in some bacteria.[6] Binding is competitively inhibited by chloramphenicol and lincomycin, which suggests either shared or overlapping binding sites. It has been shown that oxazolidinones do not inhibit the formation of initiator transfer RNA (*N*-formylmethionyl-tRNA). It has been postulated that the ribosomal peptidyltransferase center is the major site of action of the drug.[7]

TABLE 31-1 In Vitro Susceptibility to Linezolid of Common Aerobic Gram-Positive Organisms

Organism	MIC_{90}* ($\mu g/mL$)	Susceptible % of Strains
Staphylococcus aureus		
Methicillin-susceptible	2-4	100[†]
Methicillin-resistant	1-4	100
Coagulase-Negative Staphylococci		
Oxacillin-susceptible	0.5-4	100
Oxacillin-resistant	0.5-4	100
β-Hemolytic Streptococci		
Streptococcus pyogenes	2	100
Streptococcus agalactiae	2	100
Other species	1-4	100
α-Hemolytic Streptococci		
Streptococcus pneumoniae	2	100
Penicillin-susceptible	1	100
Penicillin-resistant	1	100
Other species	1-2	100
Enterococcus faecium		
Vancomycin-susceptible	1-4	96.5
Vancomycin-resistant	2-4	95.6-77
Enterococcus faecalis		
Vancomycin-susceptible	2-4	96.5
Vancomycin-resistant	2-4	95.6

*Minimal concentration at which 90% of strains are inhibited.
[†]A resistant strain has been reported.

ANTIMICROBIAL ACTIVITY

Linezolid has consistent activity against the majority of clinically important gram-positive organisms including *Staphylococcus aureus* (methicillin-susceptible and -resistant strains), coagulase-negative staphylococci, *Enterococcus faecium* and *Enterococcus faecalis* (vancomycin-susceptible and -resistant strains), and streptococci (including penicillin-resistant strains of *Streptococcus pneumoniae*) (Table 31-1).[3,8-15] The distribution of linezolid's minimal inhibitory concentrations for most of these organisms is unimodal with ranges of 1 to 4 $\mu g/mL$ noted for staphylococci, 1 to 2 $\mu g/mL$ for enterococci, and 0.5 to 1 $\mu g/mL$ for streptococci. Although linezolid is usually bacteriostatic, it has been shown to be bactericidal against strains of *S. pneumoniae* and *Streptococcus pyogenes*.[13]

Other gram-positive organisms appear to be susceptible to linezolid, although fewer strains have been evaluated. These include *Corynebacterium* spp., *Listeria monocytogenes*, *Bacillus* spp., *Micrococcus* spp., *Erysipelothrix rhusiopathiae*, *Leuconostoc* spp., *Rhodococcus equi*, and *Pediococcus* spp.[8,12,15]

Linezolid has demonstrated activity against *Neisseria* spp., inconsistent activity against *Haemophilus influenzae*,[8,16] and virtually no activity against other gram-negative organisms. Linezolid resistance in organisms such as *Escherichia coli* appears to be related to an efflux pump mechanism that effectively removes the drug from within the bacteria.[17] Limited information has been generated concerning linezolid's activity against anaerobes. Linezolid has activity against *Bacteroides fragilis*, *Clostridium* spp. including *Clostridium difficile*, *Fusobacterium*, and anaerobic cocci.[8,12,18,19]

Mycoplasma pneumoniae and *Ureaplasma urealyticum* are usually resistant to linezolid, and *Mycoplasma hominis* is susceptible.[20] Linezolid has activity against a wide number of strains of *Nocardia* with minimal inhibitory concentrations at which 90% of strains are inhibited of 2 to 4 $\mu g/mL$.[21] Virtually all strains tested have proved susceptible. Finally, linezolid has demonstrated activity against *Mycobacterium tuberculosis*, *Mycobacterium marinum*, and strains of rapidly growing *Mycobacterium*.[22-24]

PHARMACOLOGY

Absorption after ingestion is rapid, with peak serum levels occurring after 1 to 2 hours. Bioavailability approaches 100%. With oral doses of 375 and 625 mg twice daily, steady-state peak values of 12 to 18 $\mu g/mL$, respectively, have been observed.[25,26] Intravenous dosing at 500 and 625 mg twice daily maintains serum levels above 4 $\mu g/mL$ throughout the dosing interval.[25] At the present oral dose regimen of 400 and 600 mg twice daily, peak serum levels of 11.0 and 21.2 $\mu g/mL$, respectively, are observed. Intravenous dosing of 600 mg twice daily yields peak concentrations of 15.1 $\mu g/mL$.[27] The elimination half-life of linezolid is approximately 5.5 hours.

Linezolid is metabolized by oxidation and does not appear to interact with the cytochrome P-450 enzyme.[27] Urinary excretion accounts for approximately 85% of drug elimination, with 30% to 40% of drug excreted unchanged. Fecal excretion accounts for most of the remaining drug.[28] No dose adjustment has yet been suggested for patients with renal or hepatic insufficiency. Linezolid and its metabolites are removed by dialysis, and although data are not conclusive, it is suggested that linezolid be administered after hemodialysis.

Protein binding for linezolid is 31%.[27] Penetration of linezolid into various body sites has been documented in small numbers of patients. Trough cerebrospinal fluid concentrations of linezolid in patients after neurosurgery and a patient with meningitis ranged from 1.46 to 7.0 $\mu g/mL$[29,30] with cerebrospinal fluid/plasma ratios greater than 1.[29] Peak cerebrospinal fluid levels in patients with meningitis of 3.12 to 12.5 $\mu g/mL$ have been documented.[30,31] Levels of drug adequate to treat most relevant pathogens have been documented in pulmonary epithelial lining fluid, alveolar cells, pancreatic secretions, and bone.[32] Although concentrations of linezolid within neutrophils have been observed, intracellular killing of bacteria has not been demonstrated.[33]

The approved dose of linezolid for adults and adolescents is 600 mg intravenously or orally every 12 hours for serious infections, with a dose of 400 mg every 12 hours for uncomplicated skin and soft tissue infections. An animal model of methicillin-resistant *S. aureus* (MRSA) endocarditis suggested that continuous infusion may lead to bactericidal rather than bacteriostatic activity.[34]

Most studies have not documented significant synergy of linezolid and other antimicrobials. However, when used with gentamicin, linezolid demonstrated bactericidal rather than bacteriostatic activity against streptococci. This finding was not observed with staphylococci.[35]

CLINICAL USE

Linezolid has been approved by the Food and Drug Administration since April 2000 for use in a variety of clinical situations involving gram-positive organisms that may or may not be resistant to more commonly used agents (Table 31-2).[27] Supporting data for these indications have involved only limited numbers of highly statistically powered, well-controlled, double-blind studies, although single case reports and small case series have been more numerous.

In general, linezolid appears to be useful for infections involving MRSA, methicillin-susceptible *S. aureus* (MSSA), vancomycin-

TABLE 31-2 Linezolid: U.S. Food and Drug Administration–Approved Indications for Clinical Use (2003)

Infections with vancomycin-resistant *Enterococcus faecium*
  Including those with associated bacteremia
Nosocomial pneumonia caused by:
  Staphylococcus aureus (methicillin-susceptible and -resistant strains)
  Streptococcus pneumoniae (penicillin-susceptible strains)
Uncomplicated skin and skin structure infections caused by:
  Staphylococcus aureus (methicillin-susceptible strains only)
  Streptococcus pyogenes
Complicated skin and skin structure infections (without osteomyelitis) caused by:
  Staphylococcus aureus (methicillin-susceptible and -resistant strains)
  Streptococcus pyogenes
  Streptococcus agalactiae
Community-acquired pneumonia caused by:
  Streptococcus pneumoniae (penicillin-susceptible strains)
  Staphylococcus aureus (methicillin-susceptible strains)

resistant enterococci (VRE), *S. pneumoniae*, and other streptococcal species. Therapy of infections caused by specific organisms includes the following.

Staphylococcus aureus and Other Staphylococcal Species

Linezolid has been shown to be as effective as intravenous oxacillin changed to oral dicloxacillin in patients with complicated skin and soft tissue infections including susceptible strains of staphylococci and streptococci.[36] Reviews of phase II and III trials of linezolid for skin and soft tissue infections have shown overall response rates of 85% or higher.[37] In infections with MRSA, linezolid was shown to be comparable to vancomycin for therapy of skin and soft tissue infections, pneumonia, and urinary tract infections with or without bacteremia.[38] Similarly, in a randomized, double-blind study, linezolid in combination with azithromycin proved comparable to vancomycin plus azithromycin for therapy of nosocomial pneumonia in which *S. aureus* (both methicillin-susceptible and -resistant strains) and *S. pneumoniae* were the most commonly isolated gram-positive pathogens.[39]

In a relatively large series involving compassionate use in patients with staphylococcal infections, in which standard drug failure or intolerance was documented, linezolid produced an 83.9% clinical cure rate. Infections involved bone and joint, skin and soft tissue, blood stream, and lower respiratory tract.[40,41]

Case reports and small series have shown linezolid to be effective in treating MRSA and methicillin-resistant coagulase-negative staphylococci in pulmonary infections, bone and joint infections, infections of a renal allograft, parotitis, ventriculitis, meningitis, epidural abscesses, bacteremias, and a variety of localized infections.[42] There are inadequate data to recommend linezolid for infection with coagulase-negative staphylococci.

Linezolid failure has been noted in two cases of endocarditis caused by MRSA.[43] Interestingly, animal models have suggested that serum levels of linezolid higher than are possible with present dosing regimens are required for successful therapy.[44] A linezolid failure in a patient with an MRSA-infected vascular graft was associated with low blood levels of the drug despite the standard drug schedule suggested for severe infection.[45]

Because linezolid can be given orally, the possibility of shorter hospital stays and less overall costs of therapy with linezolid versus more commonly used agents such as vancomycin has been suggested.[46]

Vancomycin-Resistant Enterococci

Case reports and small series document the efficacy of linezolid in the therapy of vancomycin-resistant enterococcal infections. Successful therapy of VRE bacteremias,[47-49] endocarditis,[49,50] intra-abdominal infections, and osteomyelitis[51] has been reported. A series of case reports and reviews of the literature have documented the successful therapy of a small number of central nervous system infections caused by vancomycin-resistant *E. faecium* including postoperative meningitis and ventriculitis.[30,31,52,53]

Streptococcus pneumoniae

The efficacy of linezolid against *S. pneumoniae* has been demonstrated in open-label trials involving community-acquired pneumonia in hospitalized adults and children[54] and in a controlled multicenter study.[54] Only small numbers of penicillin-intermediate or -resistant strains were identified, with linezolid clearing 76% of these strains compared with 100% for the control regimen.[54]

Although linezolid has been approved for therapy for susceptible strains of pneumococcus in community-acquired pneumonia, it has been noted that because linezolid has minimal activity against *H. influenzae* and inconsistent activity against *M. pneumoniae* and *Chlamydophila pneumoniae*, it should not be considered as first-line empirical therapy.[55] There are few data concerning the efficacy of linezolid therapy of central nervous system infection involving pneumococcal disease. A single case of a postsurgical cerebral abscess caused by *S. pneumoniae* was reported to be treated successfully with linezolid.[56]

Miscellaneous Infections

Case reports have suggested that linezolid, alone or in combination with other agents, may be used successfully in treating nontuberculous mycobacterial infections and *Nocardia* infections.[57-59] Infections with *Nocardia* have included disseminated disease and brain abscess.

RESISTANCE TO LINEZOLID

Despite the relatively recent introduction of linezolid into clinical use, resistance among strains of VRE and MRSA has already been reported.[60-66] Resistance was first noted among strains of VRE with both VAN A and VAN B genotypes.[60] Subsequently, a single strain of MRSA resistant to linezolid was described.[61,63] In general, linezolid resistance has been associated with prior exposure to the drug and with long duration of therapy.[62] However, resistance without prior exposure to linezolid has been described.[66] Mutation in the 23S RNA domain V region appears to be the major cause of linezolid resistance in both VRE and MRSA.[63,64] The impact of resistance on the overall clinical utility of linezolid remains to be determined.

UNTOWARD REACTIONS

General Toxicities

In general, linezolid is relatively well tolerated with gastrointestinal symptoms of diarrhea, nausea, and vomiting predominating in the larger clinical trials.[38-41] Headache and hypertension have also been observed. In a review of phase II and III studies, insomnia, constipation, rash, and dizziness were all noted in at least 2% of patients.[27] Other important untoward reactions include the following.

Hematologic Toxicities

Myelosuppression, which is reversible, has been clearly documented and related to linezolid use.[67,68] Thrombocytopenia, pure red blood cell aplasia, and pancytopenia have all been described. Therapy duration greater than 2 weeks appears to be associated with this effect, with thrombocytopenia being more likely to occur than anemia and neutropenia being the least likely hematologic toxicity.[67] Anemia appears to be due to suppression of normal erythropoiesis, similar to the marrow effect of chloramphenicol. Thrombocytopenia appears to be due to an immune-mediated mechanism.[69] Although up to 47% of patients receiving 10 days or more of linezolid therapy developed thrombocytopenia, similar toxicity has been observed with shorter durations of therapy.[68] Serial monitoring of hematologic parameters, especially platelet count, has been suggested.

Monoamine Oxidase Inhibition

Linezolid is a monoamine oxidase inhibitor and has been associated with the development of the serotonin syndrome (fever, agitation, mental status changes, tremors) in patients taking concurrent selective serotonin receptor inhibitors.[70] Small increases in systolic blood pressure have been documented in patients receiving tyramine concurrently with linezolid.[71] The change has not been significant enough to warrant restriction of tyramine-containing foods when linezolid is used. Similarly, a mild blood pressure increase has been noted in patients taking pseudoephedrine and phenylpropanolamine hydrochloride, leading to the recommendation that dosing of these and similar compounds be titered when patients receive linezolid.

Miscellaneous Toxicity

In small numbers of cases, peripheral and optic neuropathy and lactic acidosis have been associated with prolonged durations of linezolid therapy.[72,73]

Other Oxazolidinones

Linezolid is the only member of the oxazolidinones currently marketed. Other agents of the same class are being evaluated. Eperezolid, which was developed at the same time as linezolid, has not gone beyond phase I study. Other agents, such as AZD2563, VRC3808, and

PNU100766, have in vitro activities similar to those of linezolid but are not yet entered into clinical trials.[8,12,35]

REFERENCES

1. Slee AM, Wuonola MA, McRipley RJ, et al. Oxazolidinones, a new class of synthetic antibacterial agents: In vitro and in vivo activities of DuP105 and DuP721. Antimicrob Agents Chemother. 1987;31:1791-1797.
2. Brickner SJ, Hutchinson DK, Barbachyn MR, et al. Synthesis and antibacterial activity of U-100592 and U-100766, two oxazolidinone antibacterial agents for the potential treatment of multidrug-resistant gram-positive bacterial infections. J Med Chem. 1996;39:673-679.
3. Dresser LD, Rybek MJ. The pharmacologic and bacteriologic properties of oxazolidinones, a new class of synthetic antimicrobials. Pharmacotherapy. 1998;18:456-462.
4. Lin AH, Murray RW, Vidmar TJ, Marotti KR. The oxazolidinone eperezolid binds to the 50S ribosomal subunit and competes with binding of chloramphenicol and lincomycin. Antimicrob Agents Chemother. 1997;41:2127-2131.
5. Swaney SM, Aoki H, Ganoza MC, Shinabanger DC. The oxazolidinone linezolid inhibits initiation of protein synthesis in bacteria. Antimicrob Agents Chemother. 1998;42:3251-3255.
6. Champney WS, Miller M. Linezolid is a specific inhibitor of 50S ribosomal subunit formation in Staphylococcus aureus cells. Curr Microbiol. 2002;44:350-356.
7. Colca JR, McDonald WG, Waldon DJ, et al. Crosslinking in the living cell locates the site of action of oxazolidinone antibiotics. J Biol Chem. 2003;278:21972-21979.
8. Zurenko GE, Yagi BH, Schaadt RD, et al. In vitro activities of U-100592 and U-100766, novel oxazolidinone antibacterial agents. Antimicrob Agents Chemother. 1996;40:839-845.
9. Jorgensen JH, McElmeel ML, Trippy CW. In vitro activities of the oxazolidinone antibiotics U-100592 and U-100766 against Staphylococcus aureus and coagulase-negative Staphylococcus species. Antimicrob Agents Chemother. 1997;41:465-467.
10. Rybak MJ, Cappelletty DM, Moldovan T, et al. Comparative in vitro activities and post-antibiotic effects of the oxazolidinone compounds eperezolid (PNU-100592) and linezolid (PNU-100766) versus vancomycin against Staphylococcus aureus and Enterococcus faecium. Antimicrob Agents Chemother. 1998;42:721-724.
11. Jones RN, Johnson DM, Erwin ME. In vitro antimicrobial activities and spectra of U-100592 and U-0100766, two novel fluorinated oxazolidinones. Antimicrob Agents Chemother. 1996;40:720-726.
12. Diekema D, Jones R. Oxazolidinone antibiotics. Lancet. 2001;358:1975-1982.
13. Bain KT, Wittbrodt ET. Linezolid for the treatment of resistant gram-positive cocci. Ann Pharmacother. 2001;35:566-575.
14. Ballow DH, Jones RN, Biedenbach DJ, et al. A multicenter evaluation of linezolid antimicrobial activity in North America. Diagn Microbiol Infect Dis. 2002;43:75-83.
15. Mutnick AH, Biedenbach DJ, Turnidge JD, Jones RN. Spectrum and potency evaluation of a new oxazolidinone, linezolid: Report from the SENTRY antimicrobial surveillance program, 1998-2000. Diagn Microbiol Infect Dis. 2002;43:65-73.
16. Biedenbach DJ, Jones RN. In vitro activity of linezolid (U-100766) against Haemophilus influenzae measured by three different susceptibility testing methods. Diagn Microbiol Infect Dis. 2001;39:49-53.
17. Hamel JC, Stapert D, Moerman JK, Ford CW. Linezolid, critical characteristics. Infection. 2000;28:60-64.
18. Pelaez T, Alonso R, Perez C, et al. In vitro activity of linezolid against Clostridium difficile. Antimicrob Agents Chemother. 2002;46:1617-1618.
19. Goldstein EJ, Citron DM, Merriam CV. Linezolid activity compared to those of selected macrolides and other agents against aerobic and anaerobic pathogens isolated from soft tissue bite infections in humans. Antimicrob Agents Chemother. 1999;43:1469-1474.
20. Kenny GE, Cartwright FD. Susceptibilities of Mycoplasma hominis, M. pneumoniae, and Ureaplasma urealyticum to GAR-936, dalfopristin, dirithromycin, evernimicin, gatifloxacin, linezolid, moxifloxacin, quinupristin-dalfopristin, and telithromycin compared to their susceptibilities to reference macrolides, tetracyclines, and quinolones. Antimicrob Agents Chemother. 2001;45:2604-2608.
21. Brown-Elliott BA, Ward SC, Crist CJ, et al. In vitro activities of linezolid against multiple Nocardia species. Antimicrob Agents Chemother. 2001;45:1295-1297.
22. Ashtekar DR, Costa-Periera R, Shrinivasan T, et al. Oxazolidinones, a new class of synthetic antituberculosis agent: In vitro and in vivo activities of DuP-721 against Mycobacterium tuberculosis. Diagn Microbiol Infect Dis. 1991;14:465-471.
23. Wallace RJ, Brown-Elliott BA, Ward SC, et al. Activities of linezolid against rapidly growing mycobacteria. Antimicrob Agents Chemother. 2001;45:764-767.
24. Brown-Elliott BA, Crist DJ, Mann LB, et al. In vitro activity of linezolid against slowly growing nontuberculous mycobacteria. Antimicrob Agents Chemother. 2003;47:1736-1738.
25. Stalker DJ, Wajszczuk CP, Batts DH. Linezolid safety, tolerance, pharmacokinetics following oral dosing twice daily for 14.5 days. Abstract A-115. Presented at the Thirty-seventh Interscience Conference on Antimicrob Agents Chemother, Toronto, September 28 to October 1, 1997.
26. Schaadt RD, Batts DH, Daley-Yates PT, et al. Serum inhibitory titers and serum bactericidal titers for human subjects receiving multiple doses of the antibacterial oxazolidinones eperezolid and linezolid. Diagn Microbiol Infect Dis. 1997;28:201-204.
27. Pharmacia and Upjohn. Zyvox. Physicians' Desk Reference. 57th ed. Montvale, New Jersey: Thompson PDR;2003:2801.
28. Slatter JG, Stalker DJ, Feenstra KL, et al. Pharmacokinetics, metabolism, and excretion of linezolid following an oral dose of [¹⁴C]linezolid to healthy human subjects. Drug Metab Dispos. 2001;29:1136-1145.
29. Villani P, Regazzi MG, Marubbi F, et al. Cerebrospinal fluid linezolid concentrations in postneurosurgical central nervous system infections. Antimicrob Agents Chemother. 2002;46:936-937.
30. Zeana C, Kubin CJ, Della-Latta P, Hammer SM. Vancomycin-resistant Enterococcus faecium meningitis successfully managed with linezolid: Case report and review of the literature. Clin Infect Dis. 2001;33:477-482.
31. Shaikh ZH, Peloquin CA, Ericsson CD. Successful treatment of vancomycin-resistant Enterococcus faecium meningitis with linezolid: Case report and literature review. Scand J Infect Dis. 2001;33:375-379.
32. Lovering AM, Zhang J, Bannister GC, et al. Penetration of linezolid into bone, fat, muscle and haematoma of patients undergoing routine hip replacement. J Antimicrob Chemother. 2002;50:73-77.
33. Pascual A, Ballesta S, Garcia I, Perea EJ. Uptake and intracellular activity of linezolid in human phagocytes and nonphagocytic cells. Antimicrob Agents Chemother. 2002;46:4013-4015.
34. Jacqueline C, Batard E, Perez L, et al. In vivo efficacy of continuous infusion verus intermittent dosing of linezolid compared to vancomycin in a methicillin-resistant Staphylococcus aureus rabbit endocarditis model. Antimicrob Agents Chemother. 2002;46:3706-3711.
35. Jones RN, Anderegg TR, Deshpande LM. AZD2563, a new oxazolidinone: Bactericidal activity and synergy studies combined with gentamicin or vancomycin against staphylococci and streptococcal strains. Diagn Microbiol Infect Dis. 2002;43:87-90.
36. Stevens DL, Smith LG, Bruss JB, et al. Randomized comparison of linezolid (PNU-100766) versus oxacillin-dicloxacillin for treatment of complicated skin and soft tissue infections. Antimicrob Agents Chemother. 2000;44:3408-3413.
37. Hau T. Efficacy and safety of linezolid in the treatment of skin and soft tissue infections. Eur J Clin Microbiol Infect Dis. 2002;21:491-498.
38. Stevens DL, Herr D, Lampiris H, et al. Linezolid versus vancomycin for the treatment of methicillin-resistant Staphylococcus aureus infections. Clin Infect Dis. 2002;34:1481-1490.
39. Rubinstein E, Cammarata SK, Oliphant TH, et al. Linezolid (PNU-100766) versus vancomycin in the treatment of hospitalized patients with nosocomial pneumonia: A randomized, double-blind, multicenter study. Clin Infect Dis. 2001;32:402-412.
40. Moise PA, Forrest A, Birmingham MC, Schentag JJ. The efficacy and safety of linezolid as treatment for Staphylococcus aureus infections in compassionate use patients who are intolerant of, or who have failed to respond to, vancomycin. J Antimicrob Chemother. 2002;50:1017-1026.
41. Birmingham MC, Rayner CR, Meagher AK, et al. Linezolid for the treatment of multidrug-resistant, gram-positive infections: Experience from a compassionate-use program. Clin Infect Dis. 2003;36:159-168.
42. Gill CJ, Murphy MA, Hamer DH. Treatment of Staphylococcus epidermidis ventriculo-peritoneal shunt infection with linezolid. J Infect. 2002;45:129-132.
43. Ruiz ME, Guerrero IC, Tuazon CU. Endocarditis caused by methicillin-resistant Staphylococcus aureus: Treatment failure with linezolid. Clin Infect Dis. 2002;35:1018-1020.
44. Dailey CF, Dileto-Fang CL, Buchanan LV, et al. Efficacy of linezolid in treatment of experimental endocarditis caused by methicillin-resistant Staphylococcus aureus. Antimicrob Agents Chemother. 2001;45:2304-2308.
45. Sperber S, Levine JF, Gross PA. Persistent MRSA bacteremia in a patient with low linezolid levels. Clin Infect Dis. 2003;36:675-676.
46. Siegel RE. Linezolid to decrease length of stay in the hospital for patients with methicillin-resistant Staphylococcus aureus infection. Clin Infect Dis. 2003;36:124-125.
47. Soto-Hernandez JL. Successful treatment of vertebral osteomyelitis with linezolid in a patient receiving hemodialysis and with persistent methicillin-resistant Staphylococcus aureus and vancomycin-resistant Enterococcus bacteremias. Clin Infect Dis. 2000;31:208-209.
48. McNeil SA, Clark NM, Chandrasekar PH, Kauffman CA. Successful treatment of vancomycin-resistant Enterococcus faecium bacteremia with linezolid after failure of treatment with Synercid (quinupristin/dalfopristin). Clin Infect Dis. 2000;30:403-404.
49. Babcock HM, Ritchie DJ, Christiansen E, et al. Successful treatment of vancomycin-resistant Enterococcus endocarditis with oral linezolid. Clin Infect Dis. 2001;32:1373-1375.
50. Rao N, White GJ. Successful treatment of Enterococcus faecalis prosthetic valve endocarditis with linezolid. Clin Infect Dis. 2002;35:902-904.
51. Till M, Wixson RL, Pertel PE. Linezolid treatment for osteomyelitis due to vancomycin-resistant Enterococcus faecium. Clin Infect Dis. 2002;34:1412-1414.
52. Steinmetz MP, Vogelbaum MA, De Georgia MA, et al. Successful treatment of vancomycin-resistant enterococcus meningitis with linezolid: Case report and review of the literature. Crit Care Med. 2001;29:2383-2385.
53. Graham PK, Ampofo K, Saiman L. Linezolid treatment of vancomycin-resistant Enterococcus faecium ventriculitis. Pediatr Infect Dis J. 2002;21:798-800.
54. San Pedro GS, Cammarata SK, Oliphant TH, et al. Linezolid versus ceftriaxone/cefpodoxime in patients hospitalized for the treatment of Streptococcus pneumoniae pneumonia. Scand J Infect Dis. 2002;34:720-728.
55. Moellering RC Jr. Linezolid: The first oxazolidinone antimicrobial. Ann Intern Med. 2003;138:135-142.
56. Viale P, Pagani L, Cristini F, et al. Linezolid for the treatment of central nervous system infections in neurosurgical patients. Scand J Infect Dis. 2002;34:456-459.
57. Brown-Elliott BA, Wallace RJ, Blinkhorn R, et al. Successful treatment of disseminated Mycobacterium chelonae infection with linezolid. Clin Infect Dis. 2001;33:1433-1434.
58. Nannini EC, Keating M, Binstock P, et al. Successful treatment of refractory disseminated Mycobacterium avium complex infection with the addition of linezolid and mefloquine. J Infect. 2002;44:201-203.
59. Moylett EH, Pacheco SE, Brown-Elliot BA, et al. Clinical experience with linezolid for the treatment of Nocardia infection. Clin Infect Dis. 2003;36:313-318.

60. Jones RN, Della-Latta P, Lee LV, Biedenbach DJ. Linezolid-resistant *Enterococcus faecium* isolated from a patient without prior exposure to an oxazolidinone: Report from the SENTRY antimicrobial surveillance program. Diagn Microbiol Infect Dis. 2002;42:137-139.

61. Tsiodras S, Gold HS, Sakoulas G, et al. Linezolid resistance in a clinical isolate of *Staphylococcus aureus*. Lancet. 2001;358:207-208.

62. Gonzales RD, Schreckenberger PC, Graham MB, et al. Infections due to vancomycin-resistant *Enterococcus faecium* resistant to linezolid. Lancet. 2001;357:1179.

63. Pillai SK, Sakoulas G, Wennersten C, et al. Linezolid resistance in *Staphylococcus aureus*: Characterization and stability of resistant phenotype. J Infect Dis. 2002;186:1603-1607.

64. Prystowsky J, Siddiqui F, Chosay J, et al. Resistance to linezolid: Characterization of mutations in rRNA and comparison of their occurrences in vancomycin-resistant enterococci. Antimicrob Agents Chemother. 2001;45:2154-2156.

65. Boo TW, Hone R, Sheehan G, Walsh M. Isolation of linezolid-resistant *Enterococcus faecalis*. J Hosp Infect. 2003;53:312-313.

66. Rahim S, Pillai SK, Gold HS, et al. Linezolid-resistant, vancomycin-resistant *Enterococcus faecium* infection in patients without prior exposure to linezolid. Clin Infect Dis. 2003;36:E146-E148.

67. Gerson SL, Kaplan SL, Bruss JB, et al. Hematologic effects of linezolid: Summary of clinical experience. Antimicrob Agents Chemother. 2002;46:2723-2726.

68. Orrick JJ, Johns T, Janelle J, Ramphal R. Thrombocytopenia secondary to linezolid administration: What is the risk? Clin Infect Dis. 2002;35:348-349.

69. Bernstein WB, Trotta RF, Rector JT, et al. Mechanisms for linezolid-induced anemia and thrombocytopenia. Ann Pharmacother. 2003;37:517-520.

70. Wigen CL, Goetz MB. Serotonin syndrome and linezolid. Clin Infect Dis. 2002;4:1651-1652.

71. Antal EJ, Hendershot PE, Batts DH, et al. Linezolid, a novel oxazolidinone antibiotic: Assessment of monoamine oxidase inhibition using pressor response to oral tyramine. J Clin Pharmacol. 2001;41:552-562.

72. Corallo CE, Paull AE. Linezolid-induced neuropathy. Med J Aust. 2002;177:332.

73. Apodaca AA, Rakita RM. Linezolid-induced lactic acidosis. N Engl J Med. 2003;348:86-87.

CHAPTER **32**

Sulfonamides and Trimethoprim

STEPHEN H. ZINNER
KENNETH H. MAYER

The modern era of antimicrobial chemotherapy began in 1932 with the first reports by Domagk of the protective activity of sulfachrysoidine (Prontosil) against murine streptococcal infections. This drug was developed initially by the German dye industry and had been available commercially since the early 20th century. Sulfachrysoidine exerted its antibacterial activity through the release in vivo of para-aminobenzenesulfonamide (sulfanilamide). This was the first antibacterial agent used in the United States, in July 1935, in an unsuccessful attempt to treat a 10-year-old girl late in the course of meningitis and sepsis caused by *Haemophilus influenzae*.[1] During the late 1930s, the basic sulfanilamide compound was modified to remove unpleasant side effects and expand its spectrum of activity. More recent modifications resulted in compounds of specific usefulness—for example, in urinary infections (compounds that are highly soluble) or within the gastrointestinal tract (nonabsorbable sulfonamides).

Trimethoprim is a 2,4-diamino-pyrimidine and, as such, inhibits the enzyme dihydrofolate reductase, resulting in interference in folic acid and subsequent pyrimidine synthesis in the bacterial cell. Trimethoprim is one of several such compounds synthesized and studied by Hitchings and co-workers in the 1950s and 1960s. The use of trimethoprim as a potentiator of sulfonamide activity was introduced by Bushby and Hitchings[2] in 1968. In the subsequent decade, the combination of trimethoprim-sulfamethoxazole (TMP-SMX) was introduced clinically and gained a place in chemotherapy for many infectious diseases. These agents, available in a fixed drug combination, show true antibacterial synergism against a wide variety of organisms.

SULFONAMIDES

Structure

The clinically useful sulfonamides are derived from sulfanilamide, which is similar in structure to para-aminobenzoic acid (PABA), a factor required by bacteria for folic acid synthesis (Fig. 32-1). A free amino group at the 4-carbon position is associated with enhanced activity. Increased activity due to increased PABA inhibition is associated with substitutions at the sulfonyl radical (SO_2), which is attached to the 1-carbon, as seen with sulfadiazine, sulfisoxazole, and sulfamethoxazole, all of which are more active than the parent compound, sulfanilamide. The nature of these substitutions determines other pharmacologic properties of the drug, such as absorption, solubility, and gastrointestinal tolerance. Substitutions at the 4-amino group result in decreased absorption from the gastrointestinal tract (e.g., phthalylsulfathiazole).

Derivation and Nomenclature

Since the introduction of sulfonamides into clinical medicine, dozens of compounds have been used. Relatively few survive today, however. The various compounds can be classified as (1) short-acting or medium-acting sulfonamides, (2) long-acting sulfonamides, (3) sulfonamides limited to the gastrointestinal tract, and (4) topical sulfonamides. Many branded sulfonamide preparations have been discontinued or replaced by generic products.

Short-Acting or Medium-Acting Sulfonamides

Sulfisoxazole (*United States Pharmacopeia* [USP]; sulphafurazole [*British Pharmacopeia*]; 3,4-dimethyl-5-sulfanilamidoisoxazole; Pediazole in combination with erythromycin) is a highly soluble drug especially useful in urinary tract infections. Sulfamethoxazole USP

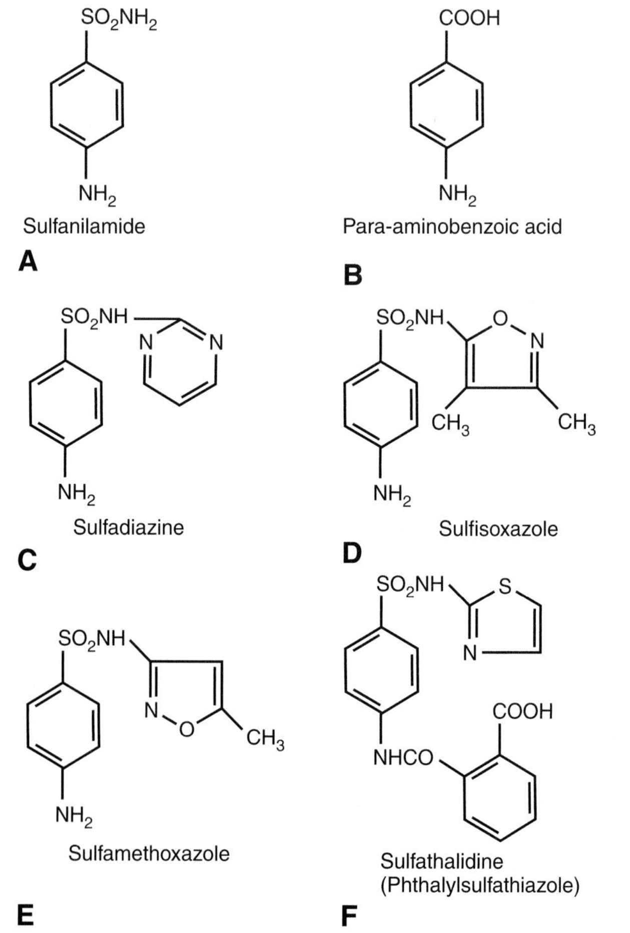

FIGURE 32-1. A-F, Structural formulas of selected sulfonamides.

(5-methyl-3-sulfanilamidoisoxazole) is less soluble than sulfisoxazole and yields higher blood levels. It is the sulfonamide most frequently combined with trimethoprim. Sulfadiazine USP (2-sulfanilamidopyridine) is highly active, attains high blood and cerebrospinal fluid levels, and is associated with low protein binding and lower solubility than the previously mentioned drugs. Sulfamethizole USP (2-sulfanilamide-5-methyl-1:3:4-thiazole) is used for urinary tract infections. Sulfadimidine and sulfacarbamide are available in the United Kingdom.

Short-acting sulfonamides also are available in several combinations. Sulfisoxazole and sulfamethoxazole have been combined with phenazopyridine, a urinary analgesic. Phenazopyridine also is present with sulfamethizole and oxytetracycline in Urobiotic.

Long-Acting Sulfonamides

Sulfamethoxypyridazine (3-sulfanilamido-5-methoxy-pyridazine) and sulfameter (4-amino-*N*-[5-methoxy-2-pyrimidinyl] benzene-sulfonamide) are no longer available for single-daily-dose therapy because they were associated with hypersensitivity reactions such as Stevens-Johnson syndrome. Neither sulfadimethoxine (Madribon) nor any other long-acting sulfonamides other than sulfadoxine currently are available in the United States.

Sulfadoxine, originally known as *sulformethoxine* (*N'*-[5,6-dimethoxy-4-pyrimidyl]sulfanilamide) is a very long-acting sulfonamide that, combined with pyrimethamine, formerly was available in the United States as Fansidar. Sulfadoxine has a half-life of 100 to 230 hours and reaches a peak serum level of 51 to 76 μg/mL 2.5 to 6 hours after an oral dose of 500 mg. The combination is active in the treatment and prophylaxis of malaria caused by chloroquine-resistant *Plasmodium falciparum*.[3] Because of the unknown teratogenic potential of pyrimethamine, this combination should not be recommended for prophylaxis of pregnant women, and its use has been associated with Stevens-Johnson syndrome. Also, some strains of *P. falciparum* from Southeast Asia and South America are resistant.

Sulfonamides Limited to the Gastrointestinal Tract

Sulfaguanidine (*N'*-amidinosulfanilamide), sulfasuxidine (2-[para-succinylsulfanilamido]-thiazole, succinylsulfathiazole), and sulfathalidine (2[para-phthalyl-sulfanilamido]-thiazole) are relatively poorly absorbed from the gastrointestinal tract. They have been used in the past to suppress the susceptible bowel flora before surgery. Salicylazosulfapyridine (sulfasalazine, Azulfidine) is a sulfonamide derivative used to treat ulcerative colitis. This drug is absorbed in its parent form as sulfapyridine, and significant blood levels of this compound are measurable.

Topical Sulfonamides

Mafenide acetate (para-aminomethylbenzene sulfonamide, Sulfamylon cream) is available for use in the topical treatment of burns. Its use has been limited, however, by metabolic acidosis caused by carbonic anhydrase inhibition. Silver sulfadiazine (Silvadene cream) has fewer side effects and is used extensively for burns.[4] In this formulation, the sulfonamide acts primarily as a vehicle for release of silver ions that exert an antibacterial effect. Outbreaks of silver-resistant infections in burn units ultimately may limit its usefulness.[5] Various combinations of other sulfonamides are available as vaginal creams or suppositories (e.g., AVC cream and suppositories). A variety of ophthalmic ointments and solutions of sulfacetamide sodium USP (a highly soluble sulfonamide) are available for use in the treatment of conjunctivitis caused by susceptible bacteria and as adjunctive therapy for trachoma (e.g., Blephamide).

Mechanisms of Action

Although a wide variety of chemical modifications of the sulfonamides have been synthesized, all basically share the same mechanism of action. The sulfonamides are bacteriostatic in that they inhibit bacterial growth by interfering with microbial folic acid synthesis. More specifically, sulfonamides inhibit competitively the incorporation of PABA into tetrahydropteroic acid,[6] and they may be incorporated into dihydropteroate.[7] Sulfonamides may have a higher affinity for the microbial enzyme tetrahydropteroic acid synthetase than the natural substrate PABA. Richmond[8] suggested that sulfonamides may act on bacterial repressor genes or by feedback inhibition to decrease formation of new enzyme. The ultimate result of decreased folic acid synthesis is a decrease in bacterial nucleotides, with subsequent inhibition of bacterial growth.

Antimicrobial Activity In Vitro

Sulfonamides exhibit in vitro inhibitory activity against a broad spectrum of gram-positive and gram-negative bacteria and *Actinomyces, Chlamydia, Plasmodium,* and *Toxoplasma* spp. (Table 32-1). The in vitro antimicrobial sensitivity of sulfonamides is influenced strongly by the size of the inoculum and the composition of the test medium. High concentrations of PABA and thymidine inhibit sulfonamide activity.

Antimicrobial Resistance

Resistance to sulfonamides is widespread and increasingly common in community-acquired and nosocomial strains of bacteria, including streptococci, staphylococci, Enterobacteriaceae, *Neisseria* spp., and *Pseudomonas* spp.[9] Cross-resistance among different sulfonamides is common.

Organisms may develop resistance or partial resistance by mutation, resulting in either microbial overproduction of PABA[10] or structural change in dihydropteroate synthetase that produces an enzyme with lowered affinity for sulfonamide.[11] PABA overproduction has been implicated in resistant strains of *Neisseria gonorrhoeae* and *Staphylococcus aureus*[10]; altered dihydropteroate synthetase has been found in strains of *Escherichia coli*.[12] Resistance also may be mediated by plasmids that code for the production of drug-resistant enzymes, such as dihydropteroate synthetase,[13] or decrease bacterial cell permeability to sulfonamides.[14] Plasmid transfer can occur in the gastrointestinal tract and in vitro and has been seen especially with multiple species of Enterobacteriaceae.[15]

Transformational exchanges of dihydropteroate synthetase among *Neisseria* spp. raise the specter of wider dissemination of sulfonamide resistance by chromosomal and plasmid genes.[16] Sulfonamide resistance genes also have been found in a common *Pseudomonas aeruginosa* integron, which may be facilitating the spread of resistance

TABLE 32-1 In Vitro Activity of Sulfonamides against Representative Organisms

Organism	Range of MIC[a] (μg/mL)
Gram-Positive Organisms	
Staphylococcus aureus	2-512
Streptococcus pneumoniae	4-128
Streptococcus pyogenes	0.5-16
Enterococcus faecalis	32-512
Corynebacterium diphtheriae	25-75
Listeria monocytogenes	3-75
Bacillus anthracis	12-100
Gram-Negative Organisms	
Escherichia coli	0.5-512
Klebsiella spp.	4-512
Proteus mirabilis	2-512
Serratia marcescens	25->1000
Salmonella spp.	16-128
Shigella spp.	≤65-≥4096
Haemophilus influenzae	2-320
Neisseria gonorrhoeae	0.25-≥64
Neisseria meningitidis	2-128
Pseudomonas aeruginosa	>100-200
Other Organisms	
Chlamydia trachomatis	0.1
Nocardia asteroides	2-16

[a]Range is expressed for a variety of sulfonamide compounds. The acquisition of plasmids may increase MICs. Local susceptibilities are likely to vary, and MICs may be higher.
MIC, minimal inhibitory concentration.
Data from references 24-29.

among aerobic gram-negative bacilli.[17] More than one resistance mechanism may be operating simultaneously.[18]

Plasmid-mediated sulfonamide resistance has increased greatly in more recent years, often in conjunction with trimethoprim resistance. In the 1980s, more than one fourth of the uropathogens and one half of the clinical *Shigella* isolates studied in Sweden,[19] England, and the United States[20] were sulfonamide resistant. *Salmonella* resistance to sulfonamides also has increased, often in conjunction with resistance to other antibiotic classes. A report from Barcelona showed 80% to 100% sulfonamide resistance in *Salmonella* and 53% to 90% in *Shigella*.[21] The increase in sulfonamide-resistant *Haemophilus ducreyi* in Asia and Africa has been associated with a plasmid related to plasmids found in Enterobacteriaceae.[22] Bacterial resistance to sulfonamides has increased among human immunodeficiency virus (HIV)–infected patients during the era of increased use of TMP-SMX prophylaxis.[23]

Pharmacology

Routes of Administration

Sulfonamides usually are administered orally, although sulfadiazine and sulfisoxazole are available for use as intravenous or subcutaneous preparations. These latter forms are used rarely, if at all. Sulfacetamide is available as ophthalmic preparations; silver sulfadiazine and mafenide acetate are applied topically in burn patients and are associated with significant absorption of sulfonamide percutaneously. Vaginal preparations are available for topical application.

Absorption

Most of the short-acting and medium-acting sulfonamides are absorbed rapidly and almost completely in the un-ionized state from the small intestine and stomach. Compounds with N-1 substitutions are absorbed poorly, as are more acidic compounds (e.g., phthalylsulfathiazole; see Fig. 32-1F). Long-acting sulfonamides also are absorbed rapidly but have a much slower excretion rate. Topical sulfonamides are absorbed and may be detectable in blood.

Distribution

The sulfonamides generally are well distributed throughout the body, entering the cerebrospinal fluid and synovial, pleural, and peritoneal fluids with concentrations approaching 80% of serum levels. Blood and tissue levels are related to the degree of protein binding (Table 32-2) and lipid solubility. Sulfonamides administered in pregnancy readily cross the placenta and are present in the fetal blood and amniotic fluid.[31]

Excretion

Acetylation and glucuronidation occur in the liver, and free and metabolized drug appears in the urine. Glomerular filtration is probably a route of excretion, although partial reabsorption and active tubular secretion also are involved, especially at low creatinine clearance rates. Urinary excretion is more rapid for sulfonamides with low pK_a values (e.g., sulfamethizole, sulfisoxazole), and alkalinization of the urine in-

creases excretion by this route. Plasma half-lives vary widely; they are related inversely to lipid solubility and directly to pK_a values but are not related clearly to the degree of protein binding.[30] Small amounts of sulfonamides are found in bile, human milk, prostatic secretions, saliva, and tears.

Protein Binding and Blood or Tissue Levels

Sulfonamides are bound variably and not irreversibly to plasma albumin, and the bound drug is inactive (see Table 32-2). Levels obtainable in cerebrospinal fluid and other body fluids are related inversely to the degree of protein binding. The amount of free drug in plasma is related directly to pK_a.[30]

Use in Renal Insufficiency

Sulfonamides can be used in renal failure, but therapeutic serum levels persist longer because of reduced excretion, and the dosage must be reduced and the interval between doses extended in proportion to the degree of renal impairment. Protein binding of sulfonamides is decreased in severe renal insufficiency.[32] The N-4 acetylated metabolite of sulfonamides can accumulate in patients with renal failure, especially during prolonged therapy. This derivative loses its antibacterial effect but still may have toxic properties. Plasma levels of sulfonamide should be measured every 3 days, and peak concentrations of sulfamethoxazole should be less than 120 µg/mL.

Toxicity and Adverse Reactions

Sulfonamides can cause nausea, vomiting, diarrhea, rash, fever, headache, depression, jaundice, hepatic necrosis, drug-induced lupus,[33] and a serum sickness–like syndrome. Earlier, less soluble compounds (sulfadiazine, sulfathiazole) used in excessively high doses were associated with crystalluria and tubular deposits of sulfonamide crystals. These complications could be minimized by maintenance of high urine flow and alkalinization of the urine. This complication usually is not seen with modern, soluble sulfonamides. Tubular necrosis, interstitial nephritis, and necrotizing angiitis may be associated rarely with sulfonamide sensitivity. Acute pancreatitis has been attributed to sulfonamide.[34]

More serious adverse reactions caused by sulfonamides may include acute hemolytic anemia sometimes related to a deficiency in erythrocyte glucose-6-phosphate dehydrogenase, aplastic anemia, agranulocytosis, thrombocytopenia, and leukopenia. In one study, glucose-6-phosphate dehydrogenase–deficient patients who received TMP-SMX did not have hemolytic reactions during therapy.[35]

Sulfonamides should not be administered during the last month of pregnancy because they compete for bilirubin-binding sites on plasma albumin and may increase fetal blood levels of unconjugated bilirubin, increasing the risk of kernicterus. Also, because of the immature fetal acetyltransferase system, blood levels of free sulfonamide may be increased, further adversely affecting the risk of kernicterus.[30]

Finally, significant hypersensitivity reactions can occur with sulfonamides administered via any route. The most important of these reactions are erythema nodosum, erythema multiforme (including Stevens-Johnson syndrome), drug eruption, vasculitis similar to periarteritis nodosa, and anaphylaxis. One report suggested that cutaneous reactions, including toxic epidermal necrolysis, may be related to an inherited constitutional defect in detoxification of metabolites.[36] Long-acting sulfonamides have been associated with fatal hypersensitivity reactions, especially in children, and this severely limits their use. Locally applied sulfonamides (e.g., to skin) may be associated with any of these adverse reactions.

Many HIV-infected patients who have adverse reactions to sulfa drugs can be desensitized by gradual dose escalation or may tolerate rechallenges without severe adverse reactions.[37] Patients who are not desensitized successfully to sulfa drugs have tolerated changing their regimen to dapsone with or without pyrimethamine.[38,38a] The acute onset of hypotension and fever rarely has been associated with TMP-SMX therapy in HIV infection.[39]

TABLE 32-2 Blood Levels, Cerebrospinal Fluid Levels, Plasma Half-life, and Protein Binding of Some Sulfonamides

Drug	Peak Blood Level* (µg/mL)	Level in CSF (%)	Plasma Half-life (hr)	Protein Binding (%)
Sulfadiazine	30-60	40-80	17	45
Sulfisoxazole	40-50	30-50	5-6	92
Sulfamethoxazole	80-100	25-30	11	70
Sulfadoxine	50-75	20-30	100-230	80-98

*Approximate free sulfonamide level after a 2-g oral dose.
CSF, cerebrospinal fluid.
Data from references 24 and 30.

Drug Interactions

Sulfonamides may displace from albumin-binding sites drugs such as warfarin, increasing the effective activity of the displaced drug. Anticoagulant dosage should be reduced during sulfonamide therapy. Sulfonamides also displace methotrexate from its bound protein, increasing methotrexate toxicity. An increased hypoglycemic effect of chlorpropamide and tolbutamide may occur during sulfonamide therapy, possibly because of the same mechanism or structural similarities. Sulfonamides may potentiate the action of some thiazide diuretics, phenytoin, and uricosuric agents. Conversely, sulfonamides themselves can be displaced from binding sites by indomethacin, phenylbutazone, salicylates, probenecid, and sulfinpyrazone, resulting in increased sulfonamide activity.

The activity of sulfonamides may be decreased by procaine and other local anesthetics derived from PABA. Methenamine compounds should not be used with sulfonamides because of the formation of insoluble urinary precipitates. Intravenous solutions of sulfonamides are physically incompatible with chloramphenicol, aminoglycosides, lincomycin, methicillin, tetracyclines, vancomycin, norepinephrine, insulin, procaine, Ringer's lactate solution, and others. Sulfonamides may decrease protein-bound iodine and ^{131}I uptake and may produce false-positive Benedict tests for urine glucose and false-positive sulfosalicylic acid tests for urine proteins.[40,41]

Major Clinical Use

Sulfonamides are used primarily in the treatment of acute urinary tract infections, but increasing resistance has diminished their effectiveness. Most first episodes of infection in the unobstructed urinary tract are caused by *E. coli,* which usually were sensitive to sulfonamides. Sulfisoxazole is administered orally in a usual dosage of 1 g four times daily. Because the infecting organism of any urinary tract infection no longer may be sensitive to sulfonamides, the choice of therapy should be based on appropriate sensitivity tests (see Chapter 66).

Sulfonamides also are effective in the treatment of infections caused by *Nocardia asteroides.* Therapy must include 4 to 6 g or more daily after a loading dose of 4 g and should be continued for 4 to 6 months or longer if necessary (see Chapter 252). A report showed increasing sulfonamide resistance in strains of *N. asteroides* isolated from the soil in Kuwait.[42] Sulfonamides may be useful in combination with other antimycobacterial drugs for the management of infections caused by rifampin-resistant *Mycobacterium kansasii.*[43]

Sulfonamides were effective for prophylaxis against recurrent attacks of rheumatic fever associated with group A β-hemolytic streptococcal infections, but they are not effective as therapy for established streptococcal pharyngitis or in the eradication of these organisms from the upper respiratory tract.[44] Streptococcal TMP-SMX resistance is increasing.[45] Sulfonamide prophylaxis of close contacts of patients with meningitis caused by *Neisseria meningitidis* is effective if the infecting organism is known to be sulfonamide sensitive; the adult dose for sulfadiazine is 1 g every 12 hours for 2 days. Rifampin or ciprofloxacin is preferred, however.

Sulfonamides have been used to treat toxoplasmosis in patients with or without acquired immunodeficiency syndrome (AIDS) and chloroquine-sensitive or chloroquine-resistant *P. falciparum* malaria (with pyrimethamine). The optimal treatment for toxoplasmic encephalitis is the combination of pyrimethamine plus sulfadiazine or, for patients intolerant to sulfonamides, pyrimethamine plus clindamycin. In most studies, both regimens seem equally efficacious.[38a] The pyrimethamine/sulfadiazine regimen begins with a 4- to 8-week induction course of pyrimethamine (100 to 200 mg once daily for 1 day followed by 50 to 75 mg once daily) plus sulfadiazine (1 to 2 g four times daily). Leucovorin (5 to 50 mg once daily) is administered to prevent pyrimethamine-associated folinic acid deficiency. More recent findings indicate that sulfadiazine may be given twice daily (2 g) even during induction therapy.[45a] Sulfonamide desensitization has been effective for patients with cerebral toxoplasmosis and allergies to sulfonamides.[46] For people with advanced HIV disease (CD4 counts < 100 cells/mm^3) and without access to antiretrovirals, primary toxo-

plasmosis prophylaxis may be instituted using a fixed dose of pyrimethamine, 25 mg, combined with sulfadoxine, 500 mg, plus folinic acid, 15 mg. Of 74 patients in one study who had antitoxoplasma IgG antibodies, one patient, who did not adhere to the regimen, developed toxoplasmic encephalitis after 24 months.[47]

Melioidosis, dermatitis herpetiformis, lymphogranuloma venereum, and chancroid have responded to sulfonamides. Nongonococcal urethritis due to *Chlamydophila,* but not that due to *Ureaplasma urealyticum,* responded to sulfonamide therapy (see Chapter 102). Sulfasalazine is used in the treatment of inflammatory bowel diseases.[48] Currently, sulfonamides are used most frequently in combination with trimethoprim (see later discussion).

TRIMETHOPRIM

Structure and Derivation

Trimethoprim is a 2,4-diamino-5-(3′,4′,5′-trimethoxybenzyl) pyrimidine (Fig. 32-2). This drug was synthesized by Bushby and Hitchings[2] as a dihydrofolate reductase inhibitor thought to potentiate the activity of sulfonamides by sequential inhibition of folic acid synthesis. In the United States, trimethoprim now is available as a single agent and in combination with sulfamethoxazole (co-trimoxazole) (see later discussion). Trimethoprim has antibacterial activity of its own.

Mechanism of Action

Trimethoprim owes its activity to powerful inhibition of bacterial dihydrofolate reductase, which is the enzyme step after the step in folic acid synthesis blocked by sulfonamides. Trimethoprim is 50,000 to 100,000 times more active against bacterial dihydrofolate reductase than against the human enzyme. Trimethoprim interferes with the conversion of dihydrofolate to tetrahydrofolate, the precursor of folinic acid and ultimately of purine and DNA synthesis (Fig. 32-3). The sequential blockage of the same biosynthetic pathway by sulfonamides and trimethoprim results in a high degree of synergistic activity against a wide spectrum of microorganisms. Humans do not synthesize folic acid but require it in their diet, and human purine synthesis is not affected significantly by the enzyme inhibition of trimethoprim.[49]

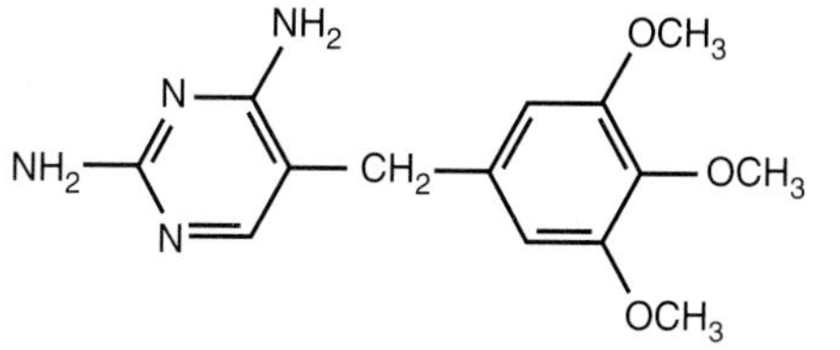

(2,4-diamino-5-(3′,4′,5′ - trimethoxybenzyl) pyrimidine)

FIGURE 32-2. Chemical structure of trimethoprim.

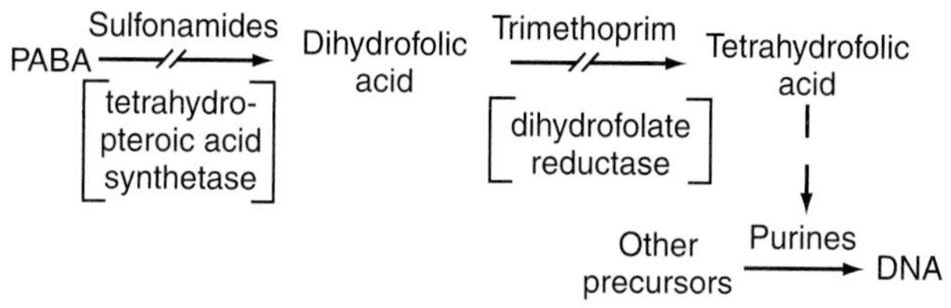

FIGURE 32-3. Action of sulfonamides and trimethoprim on the metabolic pathway of bacterial folic acid synthesis.

Antimicrobial Activity

Trimethoprim is active in vitro against many gram-positive cocci and most gram-negative rods except for *P. aeruginosa* and *Bacteroides* spp. (Table 32-3). *Treponema pallidum, Mycobacterium tuberculosis, Mycoplasma* spp., and most anaerobes are resistant. Thymidine inhibits the in vitro activity of trimethoprim, but the addition of thymidine phosphorylase or 5% lysed horse blood to Mueller-Hinton medium or other sensitivity media removes this inhibition. The minimal inhibitory concentration (MIC) varies considerably with the medium used.[55] Trimethoprim alone has good in vitro activity against *H. influenzae* (most strains have MICs ≤ 0.25 μg/mL, but higher MICs now are reported[29]) and *Streptococcus pyogenes* (MICs ≤ 2 μg/mL).[45]

Potentiation of the action of trimethoprim is seen in combination with sulfamethoxazole (see Table 32-3). Antibacterial synergism has been shown in vitro for trimethoprim and polymyxins[56] and for trimethoprim and aminoglycosides against some gram-negative bacilli.[57] The combination of trimethoprim and sulfamethoxazole (TMP-SMX, co-trimoxazole) is active in vitro against many isolates of *S. aureus*,[58] *S. pyogenes* (MIC for 90% of isolates [MIC_{90}] = 0.5 μg/mL), *Streptococcus pneumoniae* (MIC_{90} = 1 μg/mL),[45] *Moraxella catarrhalis, E. coli, Proteus mirabilis, Burkholderia cepacia, Burkholderia pseudomallei, Yersinia enterocolitica* (but 28% resistance reported in Spain[21]), *N. gonorrhoeae* (resistance rates >20% reported[59]), and *Stenotrophomonas maltophilia*. TMP-SMX-resistant strains of *S. maltophilia* may occur in severely ill patients and carry serious morbidity.[60] Studies of children in areas of high incidence of penicillin-resistant pneumococci showed TMP-SMX resistance in 40% of isolates.[61] Similar resistance rates for TMP-SMX were found in an area of Mexico with low rates of penicillin resistance.[62] Of pneumococci carried in the nasopharynx of children treated for malaria with a sulfonamide or TMP-SMX, 50% were resistant to TMP-SMX.[63]

A study suggests that the E test might not be reliable for the determination of TMP-SMX-resistant pneumococci.[64] Increased resistance of *Salmonella* and *Shigella* spp. has been reported; rates approach 50% to 90% in some areas.[21] A report from Taiwan showed 85% TMP-SMX resistance in penicillin-susceptible *S. pneumoniae* and 100% resistance in non–penicillin-susceptible pneumococci.[65]

Variable bactericidal effects have been noted when enterococci are tested against TMP-SMX,[66] but TMP-SMX is not clinically useful. The susceptibility of Enterobacteriaceae may vary greatly among locations and within the same location from year to year, owing to the spread of trimethoprim-resistant plasmids and transposons. Almost all strains of *P. aeruginosa* are resistant in vitro to TMP-SMX.[58]

Trimethoprim combined with sulfamethoxazole or dapsone has been effective in the treatment of *Pneumocystis carinii* pneumonia in immunocompromised patients (see later discussion). *Listeria monocytogenes*,[67] *Moraxella catarrhalis*,[68] and atypical mycobacteria[69] have been shown to be susceptible to TMP-SMX.

The optimal ratio for in vitro synergism of TMP-SMX in combination is 1:20, but this ratio does not always obtain in vivo. The synergism seen depends on the sensitivity of the organism to each drug.

Resistance to Trimethoprim

Bacteria may develop trimethoprim resistance by several mechanisms, which can be chromosomal or plasmid mediated. Clinical resistance has increased. A decrease in the ratio of strains resistant to sulfamethoxazole and trimethoprim compared with strains resistant only to trimethoprim may reflect an increase in independent trimethoprim resistance, and this might be a useful monitoring parameter in hospitals.[70] Concomitant resistance to sulfonamides has increased greatly in eastern Asia.

Trimethoprim resistance may be caused by changes in cell permeability, loss of bacterial drug-binding capacity, and overproduction of or alterations in dihydrofolate reductase. Clinically the most important mechanism is plasmid-mediated dihydrofolate reductases that are resistant to trimethoprim.[71] Distinctive dihydrofolate reductases have been described in Enterobacteriaceae, *P. aeruginosa*, *H. influenzae*, and *S. aureus*.[72,73] They frequently are plasmid mediated[58,71-73] and may be disseminated by highly mobile transposons (e.g., Tn7) with wide host-species ranges.[74] Outbreaks caused by trimethoprim-resistant conjugative plasmids have been noted in western and eastern Europe,[71,72,74] eastern Asia, South America, and the United States.[75] Many of the outbreaks occurred in immunocompromised hosts, associated with resistance to multiple other antibiotic groups. Two groups of mutations in dihydrofolate reductase genes of *S. pneumoniae* were reported from South Africa. These changes were highly conserved and might have resulted from recombination by transformation.[76]

Local increases in trimethoprim resistance, particularly among Enterobacteriaceae, have been especially marked in developing countries,[77] with 20% of nosocomial clinical isolates resistant to trimethoprim. Also, fecal isolates from outpatient settings and daycare centers are increasingly resistant to trimethoprim.[78] With more than one third of the *E. coli* and *Salmonella* isolates resistant to trimethoprim in several South American and Asian nations, the use of this low-cost agent for the treatment of urinary tract infections and serious enteric infections is imperiled. Whether the clinical use of trimethoprim alone in some countries has resulted in increasing resistance to TMP-SMX is unclear. Concomitant trimethoprim and sulfonamide resistance may limit the utility of TMP-SMX against methicillin-resistant *S. aureus* and *Staphylococcus epidermidis*.[79] In association with the increased use of TMP-SMX in HIV-infected patients, increasing TMP-SMX resistance has been seen in *S. aureus* and many Enterobacteriaceae.[23] Multiple drug resistance is common now in *E. coli* isolated from the urinary tract, and 93% of *E. coli* may be resistant to TMP-SMX.[80]

Permeability changes may occur in the bacterial cell and result in resistance to trimethoprim and sulfonamides. Thymine-requiring auxotrophs also may account for clinically significant resistance to both drugs. These mutants lack thymidylate synthetase and probably are less virulent than are sensitive strains.[81] The clinical utility of trimethoprim,

TABLE 32-3 In Vitro Activity of Trimethoprim against Representative Organisms

Organism	MIC Alone* (μg/mL)	MIC with Sulfamethoxazole (μg/mL, 1:20)†
Gram-Positive Organisms		
Staphylococcus aureus	0.03-128	0.125-512
Staphylococcus epidermidis	0.125-4	0.25-8
Streptococcus pneumoniae	0.5-2	1-32
Streptococcus pyogenes	0.5-1	0.03->32
Enterococcus faecalis	0.06-128	0.015->32
Corynebacterium diphtheriae	0.15-0.5	0.05-0.15
Listeria monocytogenes	0.05-1.5	0.015-0.15
Clostridium perfringens	2-50	—
Gram-Negative Organisms		
Escherichia coli	0.01-≥128	0.06-512
Klebsiella spp.	0.15-≥128	0.25-512
Proteus mirabilis	0.15-≥128	0.05-512
Serratia marcescens	0.125-128	0.4-512
Salmonella spp.	0.05-0.5	0.05-16
Shigella spp.	0.125-≥128	1-128
Citrobacter freundii	0.125-128	0.06-512
Vibrio cholerae	0.2	—
Haemophilus influenzae	0.06-32	0.004-64
Neisseria gonorrhoeae	0.2-128	0.15-128
Neisseria meningitidis	3.1-50	0.01-1.6
Pseudomonas aeruginosa	50-1000	3.1-100
Burkholderia cepacia	1-2	<0.06-8
Stenotrophomonas maltophilia	1->32	0.25->64
Bacteroides fragilis	≥4.0	—
Other Organisms		
Nocardia asteroides	3-100	1.5
Chlamydia trachomatis	20	—

*MIC varies with the method, inoculum size, and medium used. Acquisition of resistant plasmids may increase MICs. Local susceptibilities may vary. Resistance has increased significantly since the 1990s.
†Minimal bactericidal concentration may be much higher.[66]
MIC, minimal inhibitory concentration.
Data from references 24-27, 45, and 50-54.

sulfonamides, and TMP-SMX has declined significantly due to resistance.[82] *E. coli* resistance varies from 10% to 70% and is higher in elderly patients and in the developing world. Almost all *Shigella* spp. are resistant, and *Salmonella* spp., *Campylobacter* spp., *S. pneumoniae, M. catarrhalis,* and *S. pyogenes* all are increasing in resistance. *P. carinii* also may develop sulfonamide and trimethoprim resistance mutations in the course of therapy of immunocompromised HIV-infected patients, resulting in treatment failure.[83]

Pharmacology

Routes of Administration

Trimethoprim is available as 100-mg tablets for oral use. Trimethoprim is absorbed readily and almost completely from the gastrointestinal tract. Peak serum levels appear 1 to 4 hours after ingestion of 100 mg and approach 1 μg/mL. The coadministration of sulfamethoxazole does not affect the rate of absorption or serum levels of trimethoprim.

Trimethoprim also is available in fixed combination with sulfamethoxazole in a ratio of 1:5 for oral use (trimethoprim, 80 mg; sulfamethoxazole, 400 mg [Bactrim, Septra]). Double-strength and quarter-strength pediatric tablets are available, as is an oral suspension containing 40 mg of trimethoprim and 200 mg of sulfamethoxazole per 5 mL. Intravenous trimethoprim (16 mg/mL) plus sulfamethoxazole (80 mg/mL) is available. When administered intravenously, 10 mL or 160 mg of trimethoprim (with 800 mg of sulfamethoxazole) produces a peak serum trimethoprim concentration of 3.4 μg/mL in 1 hour. After repeated doses, the peak trimethoprim concentration may approach 9 μg/mL.[84] Similar peak levels may be reached with oral therapy, but at 2 to 4 hours after administration.[85,86]

Distribution

Trimethoprim is distributed widely in tissues and may appear in kidney, lung, and sputum in higher concentrations than in plasma and in bile, saliva, human breast milk, and seminal fluid.[87] Trimethoprim also is found in prostatic fluid at two to three times the serum concentration, but lower levels may be present in patients with chronic prostatitis.[88] Cerebrospinal fluid concentrations are about 40% of serum levels.

Metabolism and Excretion

Approximately 60% to 80% of an administered dose of trimethoprim is excreted in the urine via tubular secretion within 24 hours. The remainder of the drug is excreted by the kidney in one of four oxide or hydroxyl derivatives. The urinary metabolites are bacteriologically inactive.[84] Trimethoprim also is excreted in the bile. The serum half-life ranges from 9 to 11 hours in healthy subjects and is prolonged in patients with renal insufficiency. In contrast to sulfamethoxazole, the excretion rate of trimethoprim is increased with acidification of the urine, and serum protein binding (65% to 70%) does not decrease significantly with increasing degrees of uremia.[32] Urine concentrations in healthy subjects (60 to 1000 μg/mL) are usually greater than the MIC of most urinary pathogens.[32] TMP-SMX can be given in the usual doses to patients with creatinine clearances of 30 mL/min or greater. One half of the usual daily dose can be given to patients with creatinine clearances of 15 to 30 mL/min, but TMP-SMX is not recommended for use in patients with creatinine clearances less than 15 mL/min.[32,89,90] Trimethoprim and nonacetylated sulfamethoxazole are removed by hemodialysis.[32] Patients needing long-term peritoneal dialysis can receive the equivalent of one double-strength TMP-SMX tablet every 48 hours.

Toxicity and Side Effects

The toxic and undesired effects of TMP-SMX include all the effects discussed previously for sulfonamides. Nausea, vomiting, diarrhea, anorexia, and hypersensitivity reactions are the most common.[91] Rash and other adverse reactions, including hypouricemia (after high-dose therapy)[92] and Sweet's syndrome (acute febrile neutrophilic dermatosis),[93] have been noted frequently in patients with

AIDS.[94] In one report, 40% of HIV-infected children had adverse reactions, including erythema multiforme, neutropenia, and Stevens-Johnson syndrome.[95] Patients have been desensitized successfully with the use of oral regimens.[96,97] Also, in patients with AIDS, transient diffuse pulmonary infiltrates and hypotension have been described after reexposure to TMP-SMX.[98] Other dermatologic manifestations, including fixed drug eruptions, toxic epidermal necrolysis, and nail loss, have been reported.[99-101]

In addition, impaired folate usage may be seen in humans with prolonged administration. This impaired usage usually manifests as a megaloblastic marrow, with hypersegmented polymorphonuclear leukocytes. Also, leukopenia, thrombocytopenia, and granulocytopenia may be seen. One study suggested that this occurs in one case per 18,000 prescriptions and that elderly patients are at greater risk.[102] The administration of folinic acid usually prevents or treats effectively the antifolate effects of trimethoprim, and trimethoprim's antibacterial efficacy is not impaired except possibly against enterococci.

Pseudomembranous colitis has been described with TMP-SMX but is uncommon.[103] Renal dysfunction may occur in patients with preexisting renal disease, but this is reversible with dose reduction. Hyperkalemia also has been noted, especially after high doses and in patients with renal insufficiency,[102,104,105] and TMP-SMX may cause an increase in measured serum creatinine.[106] Hyperkalemia may occur at standard doses as well.[107-109] Interstitial nephritis attributable to TMP-SMX has been described in transplant recipients.[110] Drug-induced hepatitis has been reported,[111] and prolonged cholestasis with pruritus may occur rarely.[112] Fulminant hepatic failure and pancreatitis have been reported.[113] TMP-SMX-induced meningitis has been described,[114,115] and meningoencephalitis confirmed by magnetic resonance imaging has been reported.[116] Although other central nervous system effects are seen primarily in HIV-infected patients, a case report described TMP-SMX-associated tremor in an immunocompetent patient that reversed when the drug was discontinued.[117] Renal tubular acidosis has been reported in children undergoing treatment for acute lymphocytic leukemia.[118] Drug-induced hypoglycemia may occur,[119,120] and rhabdomyolysis has been described in an HIV-infected patient.[121] Anterior uveitis and retinal hemorrhage have been described with trimethoprim alone and with TMP-SMX[122] as have reversible myopia and angle-closure glaucoma.[123]

Drug Interactions

Active levels of phenytoin may be increased markedly by TMP-SMX.[124] Also, concomitant administration of TMP-SMX and methotrexate results in decreased renal clearance of free methotrexate.[125] Severe pancytopenia may result.[125] Reversible inhibition of tubular creatinine excretion may be caused by trimethoprim in the presence of cyclosporine.[126] Digoxin levels may be increased,[127] and sulfonylureas may be potentiated with resulting hypoglycemia.[128] Serum rifampin levels may increase during concomitant therapy with TMP-SMX.[129] Through its inhibition of cytochrome P-450, fluconazole may decrease hypersensitivity reactions to TMP-SMX caused by hydroxylamine or other metabolites.[130] Although TMP-SMX may inhibit metabolism of some antiretroviral drugs, including lamivudine, saquinavir, and delavirdine,[131] the effect is minimal and does not require adjustment of antiretroviral drug dosage.

Trimethoprim Plus Other Antimicrobial Agents

Other sulfonamides, such as sulfamoxole, sulfadiazine, sulfadimidine, and sulfametrole, have been combined with trimethoprim, but clinical experience is limited.[132] Combinations of trimethoprim with other agents, such as rifampin,[133] polymyxin,[56] amikacin,[134,135] and metronidazole,[136] have been suggested or used. Extensive clinical experience with these combinations is lacking. Reports suggest that trimethoprim-dapsone is more efficacious for the treatment of *P. carinii* pneumonia than is dapsone alone.[137] A randomized, controlled trial of HIV-infected patients with mild-to-moderate *P. carinii* pneumonia found that trimethoprim-dapsone was comparable to TMP-SMX in terms of overall activity and tolerability.[138] Because it is the cheapest and most carefully studied regimen, TMP-SMX continues to be first-line therapy for HIV-associated *P. carinii* pneumonia.

Clinical Use

The increasing worldwide rates of TMP-SMX resistance have limited seriously the clinical usefulness of co-trimoxazole and its components.

Urinary Tract Infections

TMP-SMX is useful in the treatment of recurrent or chronic urinary tract infections caused by sensitive organisms. Many Enterobacteriaceae are sensitive to the combined action of TMP-SMX. The combination also is effective in acute pyelonephritis and cystitis (see Chapter 66), although either antibiotic alone could be appropriate for susceptible isolates. More recent reports caution, however, against their routine use if rates of resistance approach 10% to 20%.[139,140] Because trimethoprim accumulates in prostatic secretions, TMP-SMX often is effective in bacterial prostatitis[88] and in orchitis and epididymitis caused by susceptible bacteria.

The usual adult dosage for the treatment of acute prostate or urinary infection is 2 tablets every 12 hours or 1 double-strength tablet every 12 hours. The pediatric dose for urinary tract infection is 150 to 185 mg/m^2 for trimethoprim and 750 to 925 mg/m^2 for sulfamethoxazole daily in two divided doses. Single-dose therapy with 1 or 2 double-strength tablets may be effective in some women with uncomplicated lower urinary tract infection,[141] but a trial suggested that 7 days of TMP-SMX was better than single-dose ofloxacin and was equivalent to 3-day treatment with the quinolone.[142] In patients with chronic tissue-invasive urinary tract infections, longer term therapy of 6 weeks may be required.

TMP-SMX has been shown to be useful in the long-term suppressive therapy of adults and children with chronic or recurrent urinary infections, and extremely low doses (½ to 1 tablet at bedtime or every other night) are effective.[143] This approach has been effective in preventing recurrent urinary tract infections in children with vesicoureteral reflux.[144] Postcoital prophylactic TMP-SMX effectively reduces recurrent urinary tract infections related to intercourse.[145] Trimethoprim is thought to achieve effective concentrations in the vaginal secretions, and it is believed by some authors that it exerts its protective effect on reducing the number of recurrent infections in this manner despite the fact that TMP-SMX-resistant organisms may be present in the vaginal and stool flora.[146] Trimethoprim alone is effective therapy for uncomplicated and recurrent urinary infections in women. Usual doses are 100 to 200 mg twice daily, and nightly doses of 100 mg may be effective suppressive therapy.[147] Increasing rates of trimethoprim and TMP-SMX resistance should militate against widespread use of these drugs, unless bacterial susceptibility is known.

Respiratory Tract Infections

TMP-SMX is effective in the treatment of acute bronchitis and pneumonitis caused by sensitive organisms, although it is not the treatment of choice for any single organism. TMP-SMX may be as effective as tetracyclines in the reduction of acute exacerbations in patients with chronic bronchitis,[148] but full doses should be used. Although not usually considered for use in seriously ill patients with pneumonia, intravenously administered TMP-SMX may be effective in patients with infections caused by susceptible gram-negative bacteria.[149]

TMP-SMX was as effective as ampicillin for the treatment of otitis media in an early study,[150] and it was effective in otitis externa[151] and sinusitis even with a 3-day course.[152] A more recent report strongly suggested, however, that TMP-SMX no longer should be considered appropriate as a first-line choice for acute otitis media, especially when resistant respiratory tract pathogens predominate.[153] Ampicillin-resistant strains of *H. influenzae* and *M. catarrhalis* may or may not be susceptible. TMP-SMX plus prednisone produced short-term but not long-term resolution of this condition.[154]

Gastrointestinal Infections

Although antibiotics per se prolong the carrier state in acute gastroenteritis caused by *Salmonella* spp., TMP-SMX was effective in eliminating chronic *Salmonella* carriage, including carriage of *Salmonella typhi*, especially in patients older than 2 years of age. Typhoid fever also was treated successfully with this combination, although the development of resistant strains has been reported increasingly.[77] TMP-SMX was effective in shigellosis,[155] especially that caused by ampicillin-resistant strains; however, susceptibility testing is necessary given reports of plasmid-mediated outbreaks of resistant organisms and the almost universal resistance now.[156] TMP-SMX also was effective in treating diarrhea caused by enteropathogenic *E. coli* and in the treatment and prophylaxis of traveler's diarrhea with or without loperamide[157] if the prevalence of resistant strains in the area to be visited was low. The combination may be a useful adjunct to fluids in the treatment of cholera[158]; however, plasmid-mediated trimethoprim resistance has been reported in eastern Asia.[159] Huovinen[82] suggested that with the exception of this possible second-line or third-line use in cholera, TMP-SMX no longer is indicated for *Salmonella*, *Shigella*, *Campylobacter*, or enterotoxigenic *E. coli* infections.

Sexually Transmitted Diseases

TMP-SMX had been effective in the treatment of uncomplicated gonorrhea when used in several dosage regimens (e.g., 2 tablets orally twice daily for 5 days, 4 tablets for 2 days, and a single dose of 8 tablets).[160] For pharyngeal gonorrhea, especially that caused by penicillinase-producing *N. gonorrhoeae*, 9 tablets per day for 5 days had been recommended previously, but these regimens no longer are included in the Centers for Disease Control and Prevention guidelines for treatment of sexually transmitted diseases. TMP-SMX is ineffective for syphilis. As a result of increased resistance, TMP-SMX no longer is indicated in the treatment of gonorrhea, chancroid, or *Chlamydia trachomatis* infections.

Other Infections

TMP-SMX was useful against brucellosis (long-term therapy for 6 weeks),[161] but resistance is increasing. Sulfonamides and TMP-SMX are useful in nocardiosis,[162,163] including *Nocardia* keratitis.[164] Successful responses to combination therapy have been described for melioidosis[165] and *B. cepacia* bacteremia.[166] Trimethoprim and sulfonamides have been used successfully in Whipple's disease,[167] *S. maltophilia* infection,[168] and Wegener's granulomatosis alone or as adjunctive therapy, but clinical responses vary with disease stage.[169-171] TMP-SMX can be used to treat infections caused by *Mycobacterium chelonae*, *Mycobacterium fortuitum*, and *Cyclospora cayetanensis*.

Intravenous TMP-SMX has been useful in treating gram-negative rod bacteremia and staphylococcal bacteremia and endocarditis, although other agents may be preferred.[136,172] Reports have described nosocomial *S. aureus* infections with TMP-SMX-resistant strains.[173] TMP-SMX plus extended-spectrum β-lactams, aminoglycosides, or both provides effective broad-spectrum antimicrobial coverage in the management of febrile neutropenic patients.[174] Meningitis due to susceptible organisms may be treated successfully,[175] but other agents usually are preferred. The combination is effective in meningitis caused by *L. monocytogenes*.[67] Lyme disease has been treated successfully by the combination of TMP-SMX and roxithromycin.[176] One daily dose of TMP-SMX given 5 days/wk may prevent spontaneous bacterial peritonitis in patients with cirrhosis.[177] *M. kansasii*, *Mycobacterium marinum*, and *Mycobacterium scrofulaceum* are inhibited in vitro by TMP-SMX, and several clinical successes have been reported, often in combination with other agents.[43,69,178-180] TMP-SMX is used in combination with isoniazid and rifampin to treat leprosy.[181]

TMP-SMX has been used in the treatment of susceptible *P. falciparum* infections, although this combination is not active against multiple-drug–resistant strains. HIV-infected patients with *Isospora belli* enteritis have had clinical responses after receiving TMP-SMX[182]; however, relapse after treatment is common, necessitating long-term suppressive therapy. TMP-SMX has been shown to decrease the duration of oocyst excretion in children with *C. cayetanensis* infection[183] and is more effective than ciprofloxacin in HIV-infected adults with cyclosporiasis or isosporiasis.[184] TMP-SMX has no activity against other related coccidial parasites, such as *Cryptosporidium parvum.*

TMP-SMX is active against *Toxoplasma gondii* in vitro and has been used clinically,[185] but is not superior to first-line therapy with pyrimethamine-sulfadiazine. TMP-SMX prophylaxis in HIV-infected patients protects against toxoplasmosis and may reduce the incidence of bacterial infections.[186] A more recent abstract reported a study that suggested oral TMP-SMX with topical permethrin might be more effective against refractory head lice infestation than either drug alone.[187] Two cases of *Acanthamoeba* meningitis were treated successfully with combination therapy that included TMP-SMX.[188]

Pneumocystis carinii Infections

TMP-SMX has been highly efficacious in the treatment of *P. carinii* pneumonia in immunocompromised patients with and without AIDS and is considered first-line therapy for both indications. TMP-SMX therapy for HIV-infected patients with *P. carinii* pneumonia had been associated with a better safety and toxicity profile than trimetrexate[189] and a higher survival rate than atovaquone (see also Chapter 268).[38a,190,191] Patients with AIDS frequently respond to therapy but have a higher incidence of adverse reactions, particularly neutropenia and rash. TMP-SMX may be administered orally (2 double-strength tablets every 8 hours) or intravenously (5 mg/kg of TMP plus 25 mg/kg of SMX every 8 hours) for 3 weeks. Patients were more likely to manifest a hypersensitivity reaction while receiving TMP-SMX if they were less immunocompromised (i.e., had higher CD4+ T-lymphocyte counts) and were treated for longer than 2 weeks, suggesting a role for intact cell-mediated immunity in the pathogenesis of these reactions.[192] The toxicities of a 3-week course of parenteral TMP-SMX for *P. carinii* pneumonia may be decreased if serum trimethoprim levels are monitored and maintained between 5 and 8 μg/mL.[193] Trimethoprim also has been used successfully with dapsone for treatment of mild-to-moderate *P. carinii* pneumonia.[137,194] The development of TMP-SMX resistance mutations has been associated with *P. carinii* treatment failures.[83] The clinical significance of *P. carinii* mutations has been debated,[195,196] so there is no indication at this time to monitor prospectively *P. carinii* resistance mutations.

TMP-SMX has been used successfully for primary and secondary chemoprophylaxis of *P. carinii* pneumonia[197] and generally is selected as the first-line agent, but long-term use may be limited by toxicities, such as rash or leukopenia.[39] All HIV-infected patients with CD4+ counts less than or equal to 200 cells/mm³, thrush, or prior *P. carinii* pneumonia should be started on TMP-SMX unless sulfa-allergic. A prospective study showed that a double-strength tablet taken every other day had comparable efficacy to daily TMP-SMX with fewer side effects.[198] AIDS patients receiving *P. carinii* prophylaxis with TMP-SMX had fewer serious bacterial infections than patients who received aerosolized pentamidine,[199,200] and TMP-SMX is comparable in tolerability and efficacy to second-line regimens and is much cheaper. Based on more recent studies, current guidelines suggest discontinuing primary prophylaxis for patients who have sustained CD4+ counts greater than 200 cells/mm³ for at least 3 months after the initiation of highly active antiretroviral therapy.[201,202]

In randomized studies, TMP-SMX, 160 mg of trimethoprim and 800 mg of sulfamethoxazole, given daily was more effective than monthly aerosolized pentamidine for prophylaxis after an initial episode of *P. carinii* pneumonia,[203] and half of this daily dose was more efficacious in patients with less than 200 CD4+ cells/mm³ and no prior *P. carinii* pneumonia.[204] *P. carinii* pneumonia prophylaxis in conjunction with antiretroviral therapy has been associated with markedly enhanced survival in patients with AIDS.[205,206]

P. carinii pneumonia prophylaxis with TMP-SMX confers cross-protection against toxoplasmosis.[207,208] TMP-SMX is the recommended prophylactic agent for toxoplasmosis for all patients with CD4+ counts less than 100 cells/mm³ and a previous episode of toxoplasmic encephalitis.

Prophylactic Therapy in Immunocompromised Patients

Several studies have presented evidence of a striking reduction in gram-negative rod bacteremia in neutropenic patients treated prophylactically with TMP-SMX ($\geq$ 2 tablets twice daily until stools are free of Enterobacteriaceae) compared with untreated control neutropenic patients.[209] Other studies have not shown universal benefit in preventing bacteremia in neutropenic patients with acute myelocytic leukemia.[210] Oral prophylaxis with TMP-SMX decreased the incidence of serious bacterial infections in patients with multiple myeloma.[211] TMP-SMX plus colistin compared favorably with ciprofloxacin except for gram-negative rod bacteremia in a prophylactic trial,[212] but in another study it was less effective than penicillin G in preventing viridans group streptococcal bacteremia.[213] TMP-SMX may prolong recovery from induction chemotherapy–induced neutropenia, as has been reported in some, but not all, studies,[214] and it may be associated with *Clostridium difficile*–related diarrhea[215] or with the emergence of resistant organisms.[216] More recent publications caution against the routine use of TMP-SMX prophylaxis in these patients.[217] In another report, 68% of bacteremic isolates of viridans streptococci were resistant to TMP-SMX.[218] Effective prophylactic use of TMP-SMX in chronic granulomatous disease has been reported.[219]

Trimethoprim Use in Pregnancy

The teratogenicity of trimethoprim in humans is not defined clearly, but this drug is not recommended for use in pregnancy. A report showed an increased risk of neural tube defects, oral clefts, and cardiovascular defects in infants whose mothers received difolate reductase inhibitors including trimethoprim early in pregnancy.[220] Trimethoprim is well tolerated, however, in pediatric patients.[221]

REFERENCES

1. Carithers HA. The first use of an antibiotic in America. Am J Dis Child. 1974;128:207-211.
2. Bushby SRM, Hitchings GH. Trimethoprim, a sulphonamide potentiator. Br J Pharmacol Chemother. 1968;33:72-90.
3. Pearson RD, Hewlett EL. Use of pyrimethamine-sulfadoxine (Fansidar) in prophylaxis against chloroquine-resistant *Plasmodium falciparum* and *Pneumocystis carinii.* Ann Intern Med. 1987;106:714-718.
4. Ballin JC. Evaluation of a new topical agent for burn therapy: Silver sulfadiazine (Silvadene). JAMA. 1974;230:1184-1185.
5. Mayer KH, Hopkins JD, Gilleece ES, et al. Molecular evolution, species distribution, and clinical consequences of an endemic aminoglycoside resistance plasmid. Antimicrob Agents Chemother. 1986;29:628-633.
6. Woods DD. Relation of p-aminobenzoic acid to mechanism of action of sulphanilamide. Br J Exp Pathol. 1940;21:74-90.
7. Brown GH. The biosynthesis of pteridines. Adv Enzymol. 1971;35:35-77.
8. Richmond MH. Structural analogy and chemical reactivity in the action of antibacterial compounds. In: Biochemical Studies of Antimicrobial Drugs. Proceedings of the Sixteenth Symposium of the Society of General Microbiology. London: Cambridge University Press; 1966:301.
9. Mennish ML, Salam MA, Hossain MA, et al. Antimicrobial resistance of *Shigella* isolates in Bangladesh, 1983-1990: Increasing frequency of strains multiply resistant to ampicillin, trimethoprim-sulfamethoxazole, and nalidixic acid. Clin Infect Dis. 1992;14:1055-1060.
10. Landy M, Larkun NW, Oswald EJ, et al. Increased synthesis of p-aminobenzoic acid associated with the development of resistance in *Staphylococcus aureus.* Science. 1943;97:265-267.
11. Wolf B, Hotchkiss RD. Genetically modified folic acid synthesising enzymes in *Pneumococcus.* Biochemistry. 1940;2:145-150.
12. Swedberg G, Castenssos S, Sköld O. Characterization of mutationally altered dihydropteroate synthase and its ability to form a sulfonamide-containing dihydrofolate analog. J Bacteriol. 1979;137:129-136.
13. Sköld O. R-factor mediated resistance to sulfonamides by a plasmid-borne, drug-resistant dihydropteroate synthase. Antimicrob Agents Chemother. 1976;9:49-54.
14. Kabins SA, Panse MV, Cohen S. Role of R-factor and bacterial host in sulfonamide resistance mediated by R-factor in *Escherichia coli.* J Infect Dis. 1971;123:158-168.
15. Watanabe T. Infective heredity of multiple drug resistance in bacteria. Bacteriol Rev. 1963;27:87-115.
16. Radstrom P, Fermer C, Kristiansen BE, et al. Transformational exchanges in the dihydropteroate synthase gene of *Neisseria meningitidis:* A novel mechanism for acquisition of sulfonamide resistance. J Bacteriol. 1992;174:6386-6393.
17. Bissonnette L, Roy PH. Characterization of InO of *Pseudomonas aeruginosa* plasmid pVS1, an ancestor of integrons of multiresistance plasmids and transposons of gram-negative bacteria. J Bacteriol. 1992;174:1248-1257.

18. Then RL. Mechanisms of resistance to trimethoprim, the sulfonamides and trimethoprim-sulfamethoxazole. Rev Infect Dis. 1982;4:261-269.

19. Hansson HB, Walder M, Juhlin I. Susceptibility of shigellae to mecillinam, nalidixic acid, trimethoprim, and five other antimicrobial agents. Antimicrob Agents Chemother. 1981;19:271-274.

20. Gordon RC, Thompson TR, Carlson W, et al. Antimicrobial resistance of shigellae isolated in Michigan. JAMA. 1975;231:1159-1164.

21. Prats G, Mirelis B, Llovett T, et al. Antibiotic resistance trends in enteropathogenic bacteria isolated in 1985-1987 and 1995-1998. Antimicrob Agents Chemother. 2000;44:1140-1145.

22. Albritton WL, Brunton JL, Slaney L, Maclean I. Plasmid-mediated sulfonamide resistance in Haemophilus ducreyi. Antimicrob Agents Chemother. 1982;21:159-166.

23. Martin J, Rose DA, Hadley WK, et al. Emergence of trimethoprim-sulfamethoxazole resistance in the AIDS era. J Infect Dis. 1999;180:1809-1819.

24. Garrod LP, Lambert HP, O'Grady F. Antibiotic and Chemotherapy. 4th ed. Edinburgh: Churchill Livingstone; 1973.

25. Bushby SRM. Trimethoprim-sulfamethoxazole: In vitro microbiologic aspects. J Infect Dis. 1973;128:S442-S462.

26. Bach MC, Finland M, Gold W, et al. Susceptibility of recently isolated pathogenic bacteria to trimethoprim and sulfamethoxazole separately and combined. J Infect Dis. 1973;128:S508-S533.

27. Wiedemann B, Grimm H. Susceptibility to antibiotics: Species incidence and trends. In: Lorian V, ed. Antibiotics in Laboratory Medicine. 4th ed. Baltimore: Williams & Wilkins; 1996:900-1168.

28. Trallero EP, Garcia Arenzana JM, Ayestaran I, Munoz Baroja I. Comparative activity in vitro of 16 antimicrobial agents against penicillin-susceptible menigococci and meningococci with diminshed susceptibility to penicillin. Amtimicrob Agents Chemother. 1989;33:1622-1623.

29. Zhanel GG, Karlowsky JA, Low DE, Hoban DJ, The Canadian Respiratory Infection Study Group. Antibiotic resistance in respiratory tract isolates of Haemophilus influenzae and Moraxella catarrhalis collected from across Canada in 1997-1998. J Antimicrob Chemother. 2000;45:655-662.

30. Anand N. Sulfonamides and sulfones. In: Corcoran JW, Hahn FE, eds. Antibiotics III: Mechanism of Action of Antimicrobial and Antitumor Agents. Berlin: Springer-Verlag; 1975:668.

31. Sparr RA, Pritchard JA. Maternal and newborn distribution and excretion of sulfamethoxypyridazine (Kynex). Obstet Gynecol. 1958;12:131-134.

32. Craig WA, Kunin CM. Trimethoprim-sulfamethoxazole: Pharmacodynamic effects of urinary pH and impaired renal function. Ann Intern Med. 1973;78:491-497.

33. Price EJ, Venables PJ. Drug-induced lupus. Drug Saf. 1995;12:283-290.

34. Bartels RH, van der Spek JA, Oosten HR. Acute pancreatitis due to sulfamethoxazole-trimethoprim. South Med J. 1992;85:1006-1007.

35. Markowitz N, Saravolatz LD. Use of trimethoprim-sulfamethoxazole in a glucose-6-phosphate dehydrogenase-deficient population. Rev Infect Dis. 1987;9:S218-S225.

36. Wolkenstein P, Charue D, Laurent P, et al. Metabolic predisposition to cutaneous adverse drug reactions: Role in toxic epidermal necrolysis caused by sulfonamides and anticonvulsants. Arch Dermatol. 1995;131:544-551.

37. Leoung GS, Stanford JF, Giordano MF, et al. Trimethoprim-sulfamethoxazole (TMP-SMX) dose escalation versus direct rechallenge for Pneumocystis carinii pneumonia prophylaxis in human immunodeficiency virus-infected patients with a previous adverse reaction to TMP-SMX. J Infect Dis. 2001;184:992-997.

38. Para MF, Finkelstein D, Becker S, et al. Reduced toxicity with gradual initiation of trimethoprim-sulfamethoxazole as primary prophylaxis for Pneumocystis carinii pneumonia. ACTG 268. J Acquir Immune Defic Syndr. 2000;24:337-343.

38a. HHS panel. 2001 USPHS/IDSA guidelines for the prevention of opportunistic infections in persons infected with human immunodeficiency virus. November 28, 2001. Available at: http://www.hivaids.org/guidelines/other/OIs/OIGNov27.pdf.

39. Kelly JW, Dooley DP, Lattuada CP, et al. A severe, unusual reaction to trimethoprim-sulfamethoxazole in patients infected with human immunodeficiency virus. Clin Infect Dis. 1992;14:1034-1039.

40. Dunea G, Freedman P. Proteinuria. JAMA. 1968;203:973-984.

41. Stockley IH. Drug Interactions. 2nd ed. Oxford: Blackwell Scientific Publications; 1991.

42. Khan Z, Al-Sayer H, Chugh TD, et al. Antimicrobial susceptibility profile of soil isolates of Nocardia asteroides from Kuwait. Clin Microbiol Infect. 2000;6:94-98.

43. Ahn CH, Wallace RJ Jr, Steel LC, et al. Sulfonamide-containing regimens for disease caused by rifampin-resistant Mycobacterium kansasii. Am Rev Respir Dis. 1987;135:10-16.

44. Gerber MA. Antibiotic resistance: Relationship to persistence of group A streptococci in the upper respiratory tract. Pediatrics. 1996;97:971-975.

45. Eliopoulos GM, Wennersten CB. In vitro activity of trimethoprim alone compared with trimethoprim-sulfamethoxazole and other antimicrobials against bacterial species associated with upper respiratory tract infections. Diag Microbiol Infect Dis. 1997;29:33-38.

45a. Jordan MK, Barstein AH, Alfaro D, et al. Twice-daily sulfadiazine is bioequivalent to four times per day administration in HIV-infected patients. Presented at the Forty-first Interscience Conference on Antimicrobial Agents and Chemotherapy, Chicago, Ill, 2001.

46. Tenant-Flowers M, Boyle MJ, Carey D, et al. Sulfadiazine desensitization in patients with AIDS and cerebral toxoplasmosis. AIDS. 1991;5:311-315.

47. Schurmann D, Bergmann F, Albrecht H, et al. Effectiveness of twice-weekly pyrimethamine-sulfadoxine as primary prophylaxis of Pneumocystis carinii pneumonia and toxoplasmic encephalitis in patients with advanced HIV infection. Eur J Clin Microbiol Infect Dis. 2002;21:353-361.

48. Peppercorn MA. Sulfasalazine: Pharmacology, clinical use, toxicity, and related new drug development. Ann Intern Med. 1984;3:377-384.

49. Hitchings GT. The biochemical basis for the antimicrobial activity of septrin. In: Bernstein LS, Salter AJ, eds. Trimethoprim/Sulphamethoxazole in Bacterial Infections. Edinburgh: Churchill Livingstone; 1973:7-16.

50. Phillips I, Warren C. Activity of sulfamethoxazole and trimethoprim against Bacteroides fragilis. Antimicrob Agents Chemother. 1976;9:736-740.

51. Trehane JD, Day J, Yeo CK, et al. Susceptibility of chlamydiae to chemotherapeutic agents. In: Hobsen D, Holmes KK, eds. Nongonococcal Urethritis and Related Infections. Washington, DC: American Society for Microbiology; 1977:214-222.

52. Lu DC-T, Chang S-C, Chen Y-C, et al. In vitro activities of antimicrobial agents, alone and in combinations, against Burkholderia cepacia isolated from blood. Diagn Microbiol Infect Dis. 1997;28:187-191.

53. Spangler SK, Visalli MA, Jacobs MR, Appelbaum PC. Susceptibilities of non-Pseudomonas aeruginosa gram-negative nonfermentative rods to ciprofloxacin, ofloxacin, levofloxacin, D-ofloxacin, sparfloxacin, ceftazidime, piperacillin, piperacillin-tazobactam, trimethoprim-sulfamethoxazole, and imipenem. Antimicrob Agents Chemother.1996;40:772-775.

54. Kaplan EL, Johnson DR, Del Rosario MC, Horn DL. Susceptibility of group A beta-hemolytic streptococci to thirteen antibiotics: Examination of 301 strains isolated in the United States between 1994 and 1997. Pediatr Infect Dis J. 1999;18:1069-1072.

55. Dornbusch K, Moore WB. The effects of different media on the response of bacteria to sulphonamides and trimethoprim using the disc-diffusion method and regression line analysis. In: Bernstein LS, Salter AJ, eds. Trimethoprim/Sulphamethoxazole in Bacterial Infections. Edinburgh: Churchill Livingstone; 1973:39-51.

56. Simmons NA. Colistin, sulphamethoxazole and trimethoprim in synergy against gram-negative bacilli. J Clin Pathol. 1970;23:757-764.

57. Parsley TL, Provonchee RB, Glicksman C, et al. Synergistic activity of trimethoprim and amikacin against gram-negative bacilli. Antimicrob Agents Chemother. 1977;12:349-354.

58. Bushby SRM. Sensitivity patterns and use of a combined disc of trimethoprim-sulphamethoxazole. In: Bernstein LS, Salter AJ, eds. Trimethoprim/Sulphamethoxazole in Bacterial Infections. Edinburgh: Churchill Livingstone; 1973:31-38.

59. Van Dyck E, Karita E, Abdellati S, et al. Antimicrobial susceptibilities of Neisseria gonorrhoeae in Kigali, Rwanda, and trends of resistance between 1986 and 2000. Sex Transm Dis. 2000;28:539-545.

60. Tsiodras S, Pieete D, Carmeli Y, et al. Clinical implications of Stenotrophomonas maltophilia resistant to trimethoprim-sulfamethoxazole: A study of 69 patients at 2 university hospitals. Scand J Infect Dis. 2000;32:651-656.

61. Mainous AG 3rd, Evans ME, Hueston WJ, et al. Patterns of antibiotic-resistant Streptococcus pneumoniae in children in a day-care setting. J Fam Pract. 1998;46:142-146.

62. Miranda Novales MG, Solorzano Santos F, Guiscaafre Gallardo H, et al. Streptococcus pneumoniae: Low frequency of penicillin resistance and high resistance to trimethoprim-sulfamethoxazole in nasopharyngeal isolates from children in a rural area in Mexico. Arch Med Res. 1997;28:559-563.

63. Feikin DR, Dowell SF, Nwanyanwu OC, et al. Increased carriage of trimethoprim/sulfamethoxazole-resistant Streptococcus pneumoniae in Malawian children after treatment for malaria with sulfadoxine/pyrimethamine. J Infect Dis. 2000;181:1501-1515.

64. Lovgren M, Dell'acqua L, Palcio R, et al. Determination of trimethoprim-sulfamethoxazole resistance in Streptococcus pneumoniae by using the E test with Mueller-Hinton agar supplemented with sheep or horse blood may be unreliable. J Clin Microbiol. 1999;37:215-217.

65. Hsueh P, Teng L, Lee L, et al. Extremely high incidence of macrolide and trimethoprim-sulfamethoxazole resistance among clinical isolates of Streptococcus pneumoniae in Taiwan. J Clin Microbiol. 1999;37:897-901.

66. Najjar A, Murray BE. Failure to demonstrate a consistent in vitro bactericidal effect of trimethoprim-sulfamethoxazole against enterococci. Antimicrob Agents Chemother. 1987;31:808-810.

67. Armstrong RW, Slater B. Listeria monocytogenes meningitis treated with trimethoprim-sulfamethoxazole. Pediatr Infect Dis J. 1986;5:712-713.

68. Doern GV, Brueggemann AB, Pierce AG, et al. Prevalence of antimicrobial resistance among 723 outpatient clinical isolates of Moraxella catarrhalis in the United States in 1994 and 1995: Results of a 30-center national surveillance study. Antimicrob Agents Chemother. 1996;40:2884-2886.

69. Wallace RJ Jr, Swanson JM, Silcox VA, et al. Treatment of nonpulmonary infections due to Mycobacterium fortuitum and Mycobacterium chelonei based on in vitro susceptibility. J Infect Dis. 1985;152:500-514.

70. O'Brien TF, Acar JF, Altmann G, et al. Laboratory surveillance of synergy between and resistance to trimethoprim and sulfonamides. Rev Infect Dis. 1982;4:351-357.

71. Houvinen P. Trimethoprim resistance. Antimicrob Agents Chemother. 1987;31:1451-1456.

72. Goldstein FW, Labigne-Roussel A, Gerbaud G, et al. Transferable plasmid-mediated antibiotic resistance in Acinetobacter. Plasmid. 1983;10:138-147.

73. Jorgensen JH. Update on mechanisms and prevalence of antimicrobial resistance in Haemophilus influenzae. Clin Infect Dis. 1992;14:1119-1123.

74. Steen R, Sköld O. Plasmid-borne or chromosomally mediated resistance by Tn7 is the most common response to ubiquitous use of trimethoprim. Antimicrob Agents Chemother. 1985;27:933-937.

75. Mayer KH, Fling ME, Hopkins JD, et al. Trimethoprim resistance in multiple genera of Enterobacteriaceae at a U.S. hospital: Spread of the type II dihydrofolate reductase gene by a single plasmid. J Infect Dis. 1985;5:783-789.

76. Adrian PV, Klugman KP. Mutations in the dihydrofolate reductase gene of trimethoprim-resistant isolates of Streptococcus pneumoniae. Antimicrob Agents Chemother. 1997;41:2406-2413.

77. Murray BE, Alvardo T, Kim K-H, et al. Increasing resistance to trimethoprim-sulfamethoxazole among isolates of *Escherichia coli* in developing countries. J Infect Dis. 1985;152:1107-1113.

78. Reves RR, Fong M, Pickering LK, et al. Risk factors for fecal colonization with trimethoprim-resistant and multiresistant *Escherichia coli* among children in day-care centers in Houston, Texas. Antimicrob Agents Chemother. 1990;34:1429-1434.

79. Then RL, Kohl I, Burdeska A. Frequency and transferability of trimethoprim sulfonamide resistance in methicillin-resistant *Staphylococcus aureus* and *Staphylococcus epidermidis*. J Chemother. 1992;4:67-71.

80. Sahm DF, Thornsberry C, Mayfield DC, et al. Multidrug-resistant urinary tract isolates of *Escherichia coli*: Prevalence and patient demographics in the United States in 2000. Antimicrob Agents Chemother. 2001;45:1402-1406.

81. Smith HW, Tucker JF. The virulence of trimethoprim resistant thymine-requiring strains of Salmonella. J Hyg (Lond). 1976;76:97-108.

82. Huovinen P. Resistance to trimethoprim-sulfamethoxazole. Clin Infect Dis. 2001;32:1608-1614.

83. Kazanjian P, Armstrong W, Hossler PA, et al. *Pneumocystis carinii* mutations are associated with duration of sulfa prophylaxis and with sulfa treatment failure in AIDS patients. J Infect Dis. 2000;182:551-557.

84. Grose WE, Bodey GP, Loo TL. Clinical pharmacology of intravenously administered trimethoprim-sulfamethoxazole. Antimicrob Agents Chemother. 1979;15:447-451.

85. Bach MC, Gold O, Finland M. Absorption and urinary excretion of trimethoprim, sulfamethoxazole, and trimethoprim-sulfamethoxazole: Results with single doses in normal young adults and preliminary observations during therapy with trimethoprim-sulfamethoxazole. J Infect Dis. 1973;128:S584-S598.

86. Kaplan SA, Weinfeld RE, Abruzzo CW, et al. Pharmacokinetic profile of trimethoprim-sulfamethoxazole in man. J Infect Dis. 1973;128:S547-S555.

87. Pater RB, Welling PG. Clinical pharmacokinetics of co-trimoxazole (trimethoprim/sulfamethoxazole). Clin Pharmacokinet. 1980;5:405-423.

88. Meares EM Jr. Prostatitis: Review of pharmacokinetics and therapy. Rev Infect Dis. 1982;4:475-483.

89. Welling PG, Craig WA, Amidon GL, et al. Pharmacokinetics of trimethoprim and sulfamethoxazole in normal subjects and in patients with renal failure. J Infect Dis. 1974;128(Suppl):556-566.

90. Salter AJ. Trimethoprim-sulfamethoxazole: An assessment of more than 12 years of use. Rev Infect Dis. 1982;4:196-236.

91. Jick H. Adverse reactions to trimethoprim-sulfamethoxazole in hospitalized patients. Rev Infect Dis. 1982;4:426-428.

92. Chertow GM, Seifter JL, Christiansen CL, O'Donnell WJ. Trimethoprim-sulfamethoxazole and hypouricemia. Clin Nephrol. 1996;46:193-198.

93. Walker DC, Cohen PR. Trimethoprim-sulfamethoxazole-associated acute febrile neutrophilic dermatosis: Case report and review of drug-induced Sweet's syndrome. J Am Acad Dermatol. 1996;34:918-923.

94. van der Ven AJ, Koopmans PP, Vree TB, et al. Adverse reaction to cotrimoxazole in HIV infection. Lancet. 1991;338:431-433.

95. Reider MJ, King SM, Read S. Adverse reactions to trimethoprim-sulfamethoxazole among children with human immunodeficiency virus infection. Pediatr Infect Dis J. 1997;16:1028-1031.

96. Kalanadhabhatta V, Muppidi D, Sahni H, et al. Successful oral desensitization to trimethoprim-sulfamethoxazole in acquired immune deficiency syndrome. Ann Allergy Asthma Immunol. 1996;77:394-400.

97. Gluckstein D, Ruskin J. Rapid oral desensitization to trimethoprim-sulfamethoxazole (TMP-SMX): Use in prophylaxis for *Pneumocystis carinii* pneumonia in patients with AIDS who were previously intolerant to TMP-SMX. Clin Infect Dis. 1995;20:849-853.

98. Kelly JW, Dooley DP, Lattuada CP, et al. A severe, unusual reaction to trimethoprim-sulfamethoxazole in patients infected with human immunodeficiency virus. Clin Infect Dis. 1992;14:1034-1039.

99. Ozkaya-Bayazit E, Bayazit H, Ozarmagan G. Topical provocation in 27 cases of cotrimoxazole-induced fixed drug eruption. Contact Dermatitis. 1999;41:185-189.

100. Lipozencic J, Milavec-Puretic V, Kotrulja L, et al. Toxic epidermal necrolysis due to cotrimoxazole. J Eur Acad Dermatol Venereol. 2002;16:182-183.

101. Canning DA. A suspected case of trimethoprim-sulfamethoxazole-induced loss of fingernails and toenails. J Urol. 2000;163:1386-1387.

102. Keisu M, Wiholm BE, Palmblad J. Trimethoprim-sulphamethoxazole-associated blood dyscrasias: Ten years experience of the Swedish spontaneous reporting system. J Intern Med. 1990;228:353-356.

103. Cameron A, Thomas M. Pseudomembranous colitis and co-trimoxazole. BMJ. 1977;1:1321.

104. Alappan R, Perazella MA, Buller GK. Hyperkalemia in hospitalized patients treated with trimethoprim-sulfamethoxazole. Ann Intern Med. 1996;124:316-320.

105. Perazella MA, Mahnensmith RL. Trimethoprim-sulfamethoxazole: Hyperkalemia is an important complication regardless of dose. Clin Nephrol. 1996;46:187-192.

106. Trollfors B, Wahl M, Alestig K. Co-trimoxazole, creatinine and renal function. J Infect. 1980;2:221-226.

107. Koc M, Bihorac A, Oener CI, et al. Severe hyperkalemia in two renal transplant recipients treated with standard dose of trimethoprim-sulfamethoxazole. Am J Kidney Dis. 2000;36:E18.

108. Marinella MA. Trimethoprim-induced hyperkalemia: An analysis of reported cases. Gerontology. 1999;45:209-212.

109. Alappan R, Buller GK, Perazella MA. Trimethoprim-sulfamethoxazole therapy in outpatients: Is hyperkalemia a significant problem? Am J Nephrol. 1999;19:389-394.

110. Josephson MA, Chiu MY, Woodle ES, et al. Drug-induced acute interstitial nephritis in renal allografts: Histopathologic features and clinical course in six patients. Am J Kidney Dis. 199;34:540-548.

111. Vial T, Biour M, Descotes J, Trepo C. Antibiotic-associated hepatitis: Update from 1990. Ann Pharmacother. 1997;31:204-220.

112. Kowdley KV, Keefe EB, Fawaz KA. Prolonged cholestasis due to trimethoprim-sulfamethoxazole. Gastroenterology. 1992;102:2148-2150.

113. Brett AS, Shaw SV. Simultaneous pancreatitis and hepatitis associated with trimethoprim-sulfamethoxazole. Am J Gastroenterol. 1999;94:267-268.

114. Derhes SJ. Trimethoprim-induced aseptic meningitis. JAMA. 1984;252:2865-2867.

115. Capra C, Monza GM, Meazza G, Ramella G. Trimethoprim-sulfamethoxazole-induced aseptic meningitis: Case report and literature review. Intensive Care Med. 2000;26:212-214.

116. Blumenfeld H, Cha JH, Cudkowicz ME. Trimethoprim and sulfonamide-associated meningoencephalitis with MRI correlates. Neurology. 1996;36:556-558.

117. Patterson GR, Couchenour RL. Trimethoprim-sulfamethoxazole-induced tremor in an immunocompetent patient. Pharmacotherapy. 1999;9:1456-1458.

118. Murphy JL. Renal tubular acidosis in children treated with trimethoprim-sulfamethoxazole during therapy for acute lymphoid leukemia. Pediatrics. 1992;89:1072-1074.

119. Lee AJ, Maddix DS. Trimethoprim/sulfamethoxazole-induced hypoglycemia in a patient with acute renal failure. Ann Pharmacother. 1997;31:727-732.

120. Mathews WA, Manint JE, Kleiss J. Trimethoprim-sulfamethoxazole-induced hypoglycemia as a cause of altered mental status in an elderly patient. J Am Board Fam Pract. 2000;13:211-214.

121. Singer SJ, Racoosin JA, Viraraghavan R. Rhabdomyolysis in human immunodeficiency virus-positive patients taking trimethoprim-sulfamethoxazole. Clin Infect Dis. 1998;26:233-234.

122. Kristinsson JK, Hannesson OB, Sveinsson O. Bilateral anterior uveitis and retinal haemorrhages after administration of trimethoprim. Acta Ophthalmol Scand. 1997;75:314-315.

123. Postel EA, Assalian A, Epstein DL. Drug-induced transient myopia and angle-closure glaucoma associated with supraciliary choroidal effusion. Am J Ophthalmol. 1996;122:110-112.

124. Hansen JM, Kampmann JP, Siersback-Nielsen K, et al. The effect of different sulfonamides on phenytoin metabolism in man. Acta Med Scand. 1979;624(Suppl):106-110.

125. Ferrazzini G, Klein J, Sulh H, et al. Interaction between trimethoprim-sulfamethoxazole and methotrexate in children with leukemia. J Pediatr. 1990;117:823-826.

126. Maki DG, Fox BC, Kuntz J, et al. A prospective, randomized, double-blind study of trimethoprim-sulfamethoxazole for prophylaxis of infection in renal transplantation: Side effects of trimethoprim-sulfamethoxazole, interaction with cyclosporine. J Lab Clin Med. 1991;119:11-24.

127. Brumfitt W, Hamilton-Miller J. Limitations of and indications for the use of co-trimoxazole. J Chemother. 1994;6:3-11.

128. Chan JCN, Cockram CS, Critchley AJH. Drug-induced disorders of glucose metabolism: Mechanisms and management. Drug Saf. 1996;15:135-151.

129. Bhatia RS, Uppal R, Malhi R, et al. Drug interaction between rifampicin and cotrimoxazole in patients with tuberculosis. Hum Exp Toxicol. 1991;10:419-421.

130. Gill HJ, Maggs JL, Madden S, et al. The effect of fluconazole and ketoconazole on the metabolism of sulphamethoxazole. Br J Clin Pharmacol. 1996;42:347-353.

131. Taburet AM, Singlas E. Drug interactions with antiviral drugs. Clin Pharmacokinet. 1996;30:385-401.

132. Bernstein LS. Combination of trimethoprim with sulfonamides other than sulfamethoxazole. Rev Infect Dis. 1982;4:411-418.

133. Alvarez S, DeMaria A Jr, Kulkarni R, et al. Interactions of rifampin and trimethoprim in vitro. Rev Infect Dis. 1982;4:390-401.

134. Zinner SH, Lagast H, Kasry A, et al. Synergism of trimethoprim combined with aminoglycosides in vitro and in serum of volunteers. Eur J Clin Microbiol. 1982;1:144-148.

135. Engervall P, Gunther G, Ljungman P, et al. Trimethoprim-sulfamethoxazole plus amikacin versus ceftazidime monotherapy as empirical treatment in patients with neutropenia and fever. Scand J Infect Dis. 1996;28:297-303.

136. Salter AJ. Trimethoprim-sulfamethoxazole in treatment of severe infections. Rev Infect Dis. 1982;4:338-350.

137. Glatt A, Chirgwin K. *Pneumocystis carinii* pneumonia in human immunodeficiency virus-infected patients. Arch Intern Med. 1990;50:271-279.

138. Safrin S, Finkelstein DM, Feinberg J, et al. Comparison of three regimens for treatment of mild to moderate *Pneumocystis carinii* pneumonia in patients with AIDS: A double-blind, randomized, trial of oral trimethoprim-sulfamethoxazole, dapsone-trimethoprim, and clindamycin-primaquine. Ann Intern Med. 1996;124:792-802.

139. Gupta K, Hooton TM, Stamm WE. Increasing antimicrobial resistance and the management of uncomplicated community acquired urinary tract infections. Ann Intern Med. 2001;135:41-50.

140. Raz R, Chazan B, Kennes Y, et al. Empiric use of trimethoprim-sulfamethoxazole (TMP-SMX) in the treatment of women with uncomplicated urinary tract infections in a geographical area with a high prevalence of TMP-SMX resistant uropathogens. Clin Infect Dis. 2000;34:1165-1169.

141. Tolkoff-Rubin NE, Weber D, Fang LST, et al. Single dose therapy with trimethoprim-sulfamethoxazole for urinary infection in women. Rev Infect Dis. 1982;4:444-448.

142. Hooton TM, Johnson C, Winter C, et al. Single-dose and three-day regimens of ofloxacin versus trimethoprim-sulfamethoxazole for acute cystitis in women. Antimicrob Agents Chemother. 1991;35:1479-1483.

143. Harding GKM, Ronald AR, Nicolle LE, et al. Long-term antimicrobial prophylaxis for recurrent urinary tract infection in women. Rev Infect Dis. 1982;4:438-443.

144. Hori C, Hiraoka M, Tsukahara H, et al. Intermittent trimethoprim-sulfamethoxazole in children with vesicoureteral reflux. Pediatr Nephrol. 1997;11:328-330.

145. Stapleton A, Latham RH, Johnson C, et al. Postcoital antimicrobial prophylaxis for recurrent urinary tract infection: A randomized, double-blind, placebo-controlled trial. JAMA. 1990;264:703-706.

146. Brumfitt W, Pursell R. Double-blind trial to compare ampicillin, cephalexin, co-trimoxazole and trimethoprim in treatment of urinary infection. BMJ. 1972;2:673-674.

147. Stamm WE, Counts GW, Wagner KR, et al. Antimicrobial prophylaxis of recurrent urinary tract infections. Ann Intern Med. 1980;92:770-775.

148. Pandy GJ. Trimethoprim/sulphamethoxazole and doxycycline in acute exacerbations of chronic bronchitis in general practice: A comparative study. Med J Aust. 1979;1:264-266.

149. Schmidt U, Sen P, Kapila R, et al. Clinical evaluation of intravenous trimethoprim sulfamethoxazole for serious infections. Rev Infect Dis. 1982;4:332-337.

150. Shurin PA, Pelton SI, Donner A, et al. Trimethoprim-sulfamethoxazole compared with ampicillin in the treatment of acute otitis media. J Pediatr. 1980;96:1081-1087.

151. Yelland MJ. The efficacy of oral cotrimoxazole in the treatment of otitis externa in general practice. Med J Aust. 1993;158:697-699.

152. Williams JW Jr, Holleman DR Jr, Samsa GP, et al. Randomized controlled trial of 3 vs 10 days of trimethoprim/sulfamethoxazole for acute maxillary sinusitis. JAMA. 1995;273:1015-1021.

153. Leiberman A, Leibovitz E, Piglansky L, et al. Bacteriologic and clinical efficacy of trimethoprim-sulfamethoxazole for treatment of acute otitis media. Pediatr Infect Dis J. 2001;20:260-264.

154. Daly K, Giebink GS, Batalden PB, et al. Resolution of otitis media with effusion with the use of a stepped treatment regimen of trimethoprim-sulfamethoxazole and prednisone. Pediatr Infect Dis J. 1991;10:500-506.

155. Nelson JD, Kusmiesz H, Shelton S. Oral or intravenous trimethoprim-sulfamethoxazole therapy for shigellosis. Rev Infect Dis. 1982;4:546-550.

156. Reploge MC, Fleming DW, Cieslak PR. Emergence of antimicrobial-resistant shigellosis in Oregon. Clin Infect Dis. 2000;30:515-519.

157. Ericsson CD, Nicholls-Vasquez I, DuPont HL, et al. Optimal dosing of trimethoprim-sulfamethoxazole when used with loperamide to treat traveler's diarrhea. Antimicrob Agents Chemother. 1992;36:2821-2824.

158. Kabir I, Khan WA, Haider R, et al. Erythromycin and trimethoprim-sulphamethoxazole in the treatment of cholera in children. J Diarrhoeal Dis Res. 1996;14:243-247.

159. Threlfall EJ, Rowe B, Huq I. Plasmid-encoded multiple antibiotic resistance in Vibrio cholerae El Tor from Bangladesh (Letter). Lancet. 1980;1:1247-1248.

160. Svindland HB. Treatment of gonorrhoea with sulphamethoxazole-trimethoprim: Lack of effect on concomitant syphilis. Br J Vener Dis. 1973;49:50-53.

161. Shehabi A, Shakir K, el-Khateeb M, et al. Diagnosis and treatment of 106 cases of human brucellosis. J Infect. 1990;20:5-10.

162. Wallace RJ, Septimus EJ, Williams JH, et al. Use of trimethoprim-sulfamethoxazole for the treatment of infections due to Nocardia. Rev Infect Dis. 1982;4:315-325.

163. Roberts SA, Franklin JC, Mijch A, Spelman D. Nocardia infection in heart-lung transplant recipients at Alfred Hospital, Melbourne, Australia. Clin Infect Dis. 2000;31:968-972.

164. Lee LH, Zaidman GW, Van Horn K. Topical bactrim versus trimethoprim and sulfonamide against nocardia keratitis. Cornea. 2001;20:179-182.

165. Macher AM. Chronic melioidosis. Proc R Soc Med. 1970;63:239-249.

166. Neu HC, Garvey GJ, Bleach MP. Successful treatment of Pseudomonas cepacia endocarditis in a heroin addict with trimethoprim-sulfamethoxazole. J Infect Dis. 1973;128(Suppl):768-770.

167. Durand DV, Lecomte C, Cathebras P, et al. Whipple disease: Clinical review of 52 cases. Medicine (Baltimore). 1997;76:170-184.

168. Munoz JL, Garcia MI, Munoz S, et al. Activity of trimethoprim/sulfamethoxazole plus polymyxin B against multiresistant Stenotrophomonas maltophilia. Eur J Clin Microbiol Infect Dis. 1996;15:879-882.

169. Stegeman CA, Cohen Tervaert JW, de John PE, et al. Trimethoprim-sulfamethoxazole (co-trimoxazole) for the prevention of relapses of Wegener's granulomatosis: Dutch co-trimoxazole Wegener study group. N Engl J Med. 1996;335:16-20.

170. Reinhold-Keller E, De Groot K, Rudert H, et al. Response to trimethoprim/sulfamethoxazole in Wegener's granulomatosis depends on the phase of disease. QJM. 1996;89:15-23.

171. Ohtake T, Kobayashi S, Honjoy Y, et al. Generalized Wegner's granulomatosis responding to sulfamethoxazole-trimethoprim monotherapy. Intern Med. 2001;40:666-670.

172. Quintiliani R, Levitz RE, Nightingale CH. Potential role of trimethoprim-sulfamethoxazole in the treatment of serious hospital-acquired infections. Rev Infect Dis. 1987;9:S160-S165.

173. Alonso R, Padilla B, Sanchez-Carrillo C, et al. Outbreak among HIV-infected patients of Staphylococcus aureus resistant to cotrimoxazole and methicillin. Infect Control Epidemiol. 1997;18:617-621.

174. Engervall PA, Stiernstedt GT, Gunther GC, et al. Trimethoprim-sulfamethoxazole plus amikacin as first-line therapy and imipenem/cilastatin as second empirical therapy in febrile neutropenic patients with hematological disorders. J Chemother. 1992;4:99-106.

175. Levitz RE, Quintiliani R. Trimethoprim-sulfamethoxazole for bacterial meningitis. Ann Intern Med. 1984;100:881-890.

176. Gasser R, Reisinger E, Sedij B, et al. Oral treatment of late Lyme borreliosis with a combination of roxithromycin and co-trimoxazole: A pilot study on 18 patients. Acta Med Aust. 1996;23:99-101.

177. Singh N, Gayowski AT, Yu VL, et al. Trimethoprim-sulfamethoxazole for the prevention of spontaneous bacterial peritonitis in cirrhosis: A randomized trial. Ann Intern Med. 1995;122:595-598.

178. Guay DRP. Nontuberculous mycobacterial infections. Ann Pharmacol. 1996;30:819-830.

179. Jacobson K, Garcia R, Libshitz H, et al. Clinical and radiological features of pulmonary disease caused by rapidly growing mycobacteria in cancer patients. Eur J Clin Microbiol Infect Dis. 1998;7:615-621.

180. Woods GL, Bergmann JS, Witebsky FG, et al. Multisite reproducibility of Etest for susceptibility testing of Mycobacterium abscessus, Mycobacterium chelonae, and Mycobacterium fortuitum. J Clin Microbiol. 2000;38:656-661.

181. Freerksen E, Alvarenga AE, Legguizamo O, et al. A new short-term combination therapy of leprosy. Chemotherapy. 1991;37:353-363.

182. Gellin BG, Soave R. Coccidian infections in AIDS: Toxoplasmosis, cryptosporidiosis, and isosporiasis. Med Clin North Am. 1992;76:205-234.

183. Madico G, McDonald J, Gilman RH, et al. Epidemiology and treatment of Cyclospora cayetanensis infection in Peruvian children. Clin Infect Dis. 1997;24:977-981.

184. Verdier RI, Fitzgerald DW, Johnson WD Jr, Pape JW. Trimethoprim-sulfamethoxazole compared with ciprofloxacin for treatment and prophylaxis of Isospora belli and Cyclospora cayetanesis infection in HIV-infected patients: A randomized, controlled trial. Ann Intern Med. 2000;132:885-888.

185. Canessa A, DelBono V, De Leo P, et al. Cotrimoxazole therapy of Toxoplasma gondii encephalitis in AIDS patients. Eur J Clin Microbiol Infect Dis. 1992;11:125-130.

186. Dworkin MS, Williamson J, Jones JL, Kaplan JE. Prophylaxis with trimethoprim-sulfamethoxazole for human immunodeficiency virus-infected patients: Impact on risk for infectious disease. Clin Infect Dis. 2001;33:393-398.

187. Hipolito RB, Mallorca FG, Zuniga-Macaraig ZO, et al. Head lice infestation: Single drug versus combination therapy with one percent permethrin and trimethoprim/sulfamethoxazole. Pediatrics. 2001;107:e30.

188. Singhal T, Bajpai A, Kalra V, et al. Successful treatment of Acanthamoeba meningitis with combination of oral antimicrobials. Pediatr Infect Dis J. 2001;20:623-627.

189. Sattler F, Frame P, Davis R, et al. Trimetrexate with leucovorin versus trimethoprim-sulfamethoxazole for moderate to severe episodes of Pneumocystis carinii pneumonia in patients with AIDS: A prospective, controlled multicenter investigation of the ACTG 029/031. J Infect Dis. 1994;170:165-172.

190. Hughes W, Leoung G, Kramer F, et al. Comparison of atovaquone (566C80) and trimethoprim-sulfamethoxazole to treat Pneumocystis carinii pneumonia in patients with AIDS. N Engl J Med. 1993;328:1521-1527.

191. Kovacs JA, Masur H. Prophylaxis for Pneumocystis carinii pneumonia in patients infected with human immunodeficiency virus. Clin Infect Dis. 1992;14:1005-1009.

192. Carr A, Swanson C, Penny R, et al. Clinical and laboratory markers of hypersensitivity to trimethoprim-sulfamethoxazole in patients with Pneumocystis carinii pneumonia and AIDS. J Infect Dis. 1993;167:180-185.

193. Sattler FR, Cowan R, Nielsen DM. Trimethoprim/sulfamethoxazole compared with pentamidine for treatment of Pneumocystis carinii pneumonia in acquired immunodeficiency syndrome: Prospective, noncrossover study. Ann Intern Med. 1988;109:280-287.

194. Safrin S, Finkelstein DM, Feinberg J, et al. Comparison of three regimens for treatment of mild to moderate Pneumocystis carinii pneumonia in patients with AIDS: A double-blind, randomized trial of oral trimethoprim-sulfamethoxazole, dapsone-trimethoprim, and clindamycin-primaquine. Ann Intern Med. 1996;124:792-802.

195. Helweg-Larsen J, Benfield TL, Eugen-Olsen J, et al. Effects of mutations in Pneumocystis carinii dihydropteroate synthase gene on outcome of AIDS-associated P. carinii pneumonia. Lancet. 1999;354:1347-1351.

196. Navin TR, Beard CB, Huang L, et al. Effect of mutations in Pneumocystis carinii dihydropteroate synthase gene on outcome of P carinii pneumonia in patients with HIV-1: A prospective study. Lancet. 2001;358:545-549.

197. Anonymous. Recommendations for prophylaxis against Pneumocystis carinii pneumonia for adults and adolescents infected with human immunodeficiency virus. MMWR Morb Mortal Wkly Rep. 1992;41:1-11.

198. El-Sadr W, Luskin-Hawk R, Yurik TM, et al. A randomized trial of daily and thrice weekly trimethoprim-sulfamethoxazole for the prevention of Pneumocystis carinii pneumonia in human immunodeficiency-infected persons. Clin Infect Dis. 1999;29:775-783.

199. Tabet SR, Krone MR, Hooton TM, et al. Bacterial infections in adult patients hospitalized with AIDS: Case-control study of prophylactic efficacy of trimethoprim-sulfamethoxazole versus aerosolized pentamidine. Int J STD AIDS. 1997;8:563-569.

200. Edge MD, Rimland D. Community-acquired bacteremia in HIV-positive patients: Protective benefit of co-trimoxazole. AIDS. 1996;10:1635-1639.

201. Koletar SL, Heald AE, Finkelstein D, et al. A prospective study of discontinuing primary and secondary Pneumocystis carinii pneumonia prophylaxis after CD4 cell count increase to >200 cells/mm^3. AIDS. 2001;15:1509-1515.

202. Ledergerber B, Mocroft A, Reiss P, et al. Discontinuation of secondary prophylaxis against Pneumocystis carinii pneumonia in patients with HIV infection who have a response to antiretroviral therapy: Eight European study groups. N Engl J Med. 2001;344:168-174.

203. Hardy WD, Feinberg J, Finkelstein DM, et al. A controlled trial of trimethoprim-sulfamethoxazole or aerosolized pentamidine for secondary prophylaxis of Pneumocystis carinii pneumonia in patients with the acquired immunodeficiency syndrome. AIDS Clinical Trials Group Protocol 021. N Engl J Med. 1992;327:1842-1848.

204. Schneider MM, Hoepelman IM, Eeftininck Schattenkerk JK, et al. A controlled trial of aerosolized pentamidine or trimethoprim-sulfamethoxazole as primary prophylaxis against Pneumocystis carinii pneumonia in patients with human immunodeficiency virus infection. The Dutch AIDS Treatment Group. N Engl J Med. 1992;327:1836-1841.

205. Chaisson RE, Keruly J, Richman DD, et al. *Pneumocystis* prophylaxis and survival in patients with advanced human immunodeficiency virus infection treated with zidovudine. The Zidovudine Epidemiology Group. Arch Intern Med. 1992;152: 2009-2013.

206. Goldie SJ, Kaplan JE, Losina E, et al. Prophylaxis for human immunodeficiency virus-related *Pneumocystis carinii* pneumonia: Using simulation modeling to inform clinical guidelines. Arch Intern Med. 2002;162:921-928.

207. Carr A, Tindall B, Brew BJ, et al. Low-dose trimethoprim-sulfamethoxazole prophylaxis for toxoplasmic encephalitis. Ann Intern Med. 1992;117:106-111.

208. Ruskin J, LaRiviere M. Low-dose co-trimoxazole for prevention of *Pneumocystis carinii* pneumonia in human immunodeficiency virus disease. Lancet. 1991;337: 468-471.

209. Gualtieri RJ, Donowitz GR, Kaiser DC, et al. Double-blind randomized study of prophylactic trimethoprim/sulfamethoxazole in granulocytopenic patients with hematologic malignancies. Am J Med. 1983;74:934-940.

210. EORTC International Antimicrobial Therapy Project Group. Trimethoprim-sulfamethoxazole in the prevention of infection in neutropenic patients. J Infect Dis. 1984;150:372-379.

211. Oken MM, Pomeroy C, Weisdorf D, et al. Prophylactic antibiotics for the prevention of early infection in multiple myeloma. Am J Med. 1996;100:624-628.

212. Donnelly JP, Maschmeyer G, Daenen S. Selective oral antimicrobial prophylaxis for the prevention of infection in acute leukaemia: Ciprofloxacin versus co-trimoxazole plus colistin. The EORTC-Gnotobiotic Project Group. Eur J Cancer. 1992;28A: 873-878.

213. Guiot HF, van der Meer JW, van den Broek PJ, et al. Prevention of viridans-group streptococcal septicemia in oncohematologic patients: A controlled comparative study on the effect of penicillin G and cotrimoxazole. Ann Hematol. 1992;64: 260-265.

214. Wade JC, de Jongh CA, Newman KA, et al. Selective antimicrobial modulations as prophylaxis against infection during granulocytopenia: Trimethoprim-sulfamethoxazole vs. nalidixic acid. J Infect Dis. 1983;147:624-634.

215. Lew MA, Kehoe K, Ritz J, et al. Ciprofloxacin versus trimethoprim/sulfamethoxazole for prophylaxis of bacterial infections in bone marrow transplant recipients: A randomized, controlled trial. J Clin Oncol. 1995;13:239-250.

216. Ward TT, Thomas RG, Fye CL, et al. Trimethoprim-sulfamethoxazole prophylaxis in granulocytopenic patients with acute leukemia: Evaluation of serum antibiotic levels in a randomized, double-blind, placebo-controlled Department of Veterans Affairs Cooperative Study. Clin Infect Dis. 1993;17:323-332.

217. Tunkel AR, Sepkowitz KA. Infections caused by viridans streptococci in patients with neutropenia. Clin Infect Dis. 2002;34:1524-1529.

218. Wisplinghoff H, Reinert RR, Cornely O, Seifert H. Molecular relationships and antimicrobial susceptibility of viridans group streptococci isolated from blood of neutropenic cancer patients. J Clin Microbiol. 1999;37:1876-1880.

219. Margolis DM, Melnick DA, Alling DW, Gallin JI. Trimethoprim-sulfamethoxazole prophylaxis in the management of chronic granulomatous disease. J Infect Dis. 1990;162:723-726.

220. Hernandez-Diaz S, Werler MM, Walker AM, Mitchell AA. Folic acid antagonists during pregnancy and the risk of birth defects. N Engl J Med. 2000;343:1608-1614.

221. Overturf GD. Use of trimethoprim-sulfamethoxazole in pediatric infections: Relative merits of intravenous administration. Rev Infect Dis. 1987;9:S168-S173.

CHAPTER **33**

Quinolones

DAVID C. HOOPER

The first member of the quinolone class of antimicrobial agents, nalidixic acid, is a 1,8-naphthyridine structure that was identified by Lesher and associates in 1962 among the byproducts of chloroquine synthesis. Oxolinic acid and cinoxacin were developed in the 1970s, but it was the identification in the 1980s of the fluorine- and piperazinyl-substituted derivatives with substantially greater potency and expanded spectrum that began a resurgence in development and a rapid and steady expansion of this class of compounds. A broad spectrum of activity, good oral absorption, and generally good overall tolerability has resulted in extensive clinical use of the newer fluoroquinolones. Several quinolones, however, including temafloxacin, sparfloxacin, grepafloxacin, and trovafloxacin, were removed from clinical use after approval because of toxicities, which were uncommon but severe. In this chapter, the focus will be on those quinolones currently in clinical use.

CHEMICAL STRUCTURES

All quinolone derivatives currently in clinical use have a dual ring structure with a nitrogen at position 1, a carbonyl group at position 4, and a carboxyl group attached to the carbon at the 3 position of the first ring (Fig. 33-1). Several different dual ring structures (cinnoline [nitrogens at positions 1 and 2], pyridopyrimidine rings [nitrogens at positions 1, 6, and 8], and 2-pyridone rings [a dual ring structure with the nitrogen located at the junction of the two rings]) have been developed, but quinolones, which themselves have a carbon at position 8 in the second ring, and naphthyridines, which contain a nitrogen at position 8, have been most widely successful. Both quinolones and naphthyridines, however, are commonly referred to as quinolones.

Nalidixic acid is a 1,8-naphthyridine with 1-ethyl and 7-methyl substituents (see Fig. 33-1). Oxolinic acid (quinolone ring) (see Fig. 33-1) and cinoxacin (cinnoline ring; not shown in Fig. 33-1) also have 1-ethyl substituents, as well as a dioxolo ring bridging positions 6 and 7. Potency is greatly improved by the addition of a fluorine at position 6, and potency against gram-negative bacteria is further enhanced by the addition of a piperazinyl (norfloxacin, enoxacin, ciprofloxacin), methyl-piperazinyl (pefloxacin, ofloxacin, lomefloxacin, fleroxacin, temafloxacin, levofloxacin, grepafloxacin, gatifloxacin), or dimethyl-piperazinyl (sparfloxacin) substituent at position 7.[1] Methyl substituents on the piperazine ring generally result in improved oral bioavailability. These structural features are common to most of the newer quinolone derivatives now in clinical use. Pyrrolidinyl (tosufloxacin, clinafloxacin, gemifloxacin) or dual ring substituents (trovafloxacin, moxifloxacin, sitafloxacin) at position 7 enhance activity against gram-positive bacteria. A number of newer compounds (sparfloxacin, gatifloxacin, moxifloxacin, gemifloxacin) use the 1-cyclopropyl group, which to date represents the substituent at position 1 with the greatest enhancement in potency, particularly against gram-negative bacteria, and which was originally identified for ciprofloxacin. The 1-difluorophenyl group found in temafloxacin, tosufloxacin, and trovafloxacin adds potency against gram-positive bacteria. An additional ring structure bridging positions 1 and 8 is found in ofloxacin and levofloxacin; the additional ring of ofloxacin contains an asymmetric carbon, resulting in stereoisomeric forms. Thus, ofloxacin is a racemic mixture of the two stereoisomers, one of which is responsible for most of the potency against bacteria and purified DNA gyrase. Levofloxacin is the more potent of the ofloxacin stereoisomers and thus predictably has twice the potency of ofloxacin in vitro. At position 5, replacement of the hydrogen by an amino group (sparfloxacin) or a methyl group (grepafloxacin) results in some enhancement of activity against gram-positive bacteria. At position 8, addition of a halide (chlorine [clinafloxacin], fluorine [sparfloxacin and sitafloxacin]) or a methoxy group (gatifloxacin, moxifloxacin) enhances activity against anaerobic bacteria. Halides at position 8 increase the risk of phototoxicity, but methoxy groups at this position reduce risks of phototoxicity, even relative to compounds with a hydrogen at position 8.

Coming full circle in structural modifications, newer "desfluoro" quinolones (garenoxacin) have been recently identified with excellent potency—similar to that of their fluorinated counterparts but with possible reductions in joint toxicities.[2,3] More extensive discussion of the relationships between structure and activity of the quinolone class is beyond the scope of this chapter. The reader is referred to recent reviews of this subject.[4]

MECHANISM OF ACTION

The quinolones rapidly inhibit bacterial DNA synthesis, an event that is followed by rapid bacterial cell death. The molecular events that underlie these actions are understood in part, but key details remain to be defined.[5]

Quinolones inhibit the enzymatic activities of two members of the topoisomerase class of enzymes, DNA gyrase and topoisomerase IV, and promote the cleavage of DNA in these enzyme–DNA

FIGURE 33-1. Structures of selected quinolones in clinical use or under development. *Circle* indicates the asymmetric carbon resulting in the stereoisomers that make up the racemic mixture in ofloxacin. Levofloxacin is the more active of the two stereoisomers of ofloxacin.

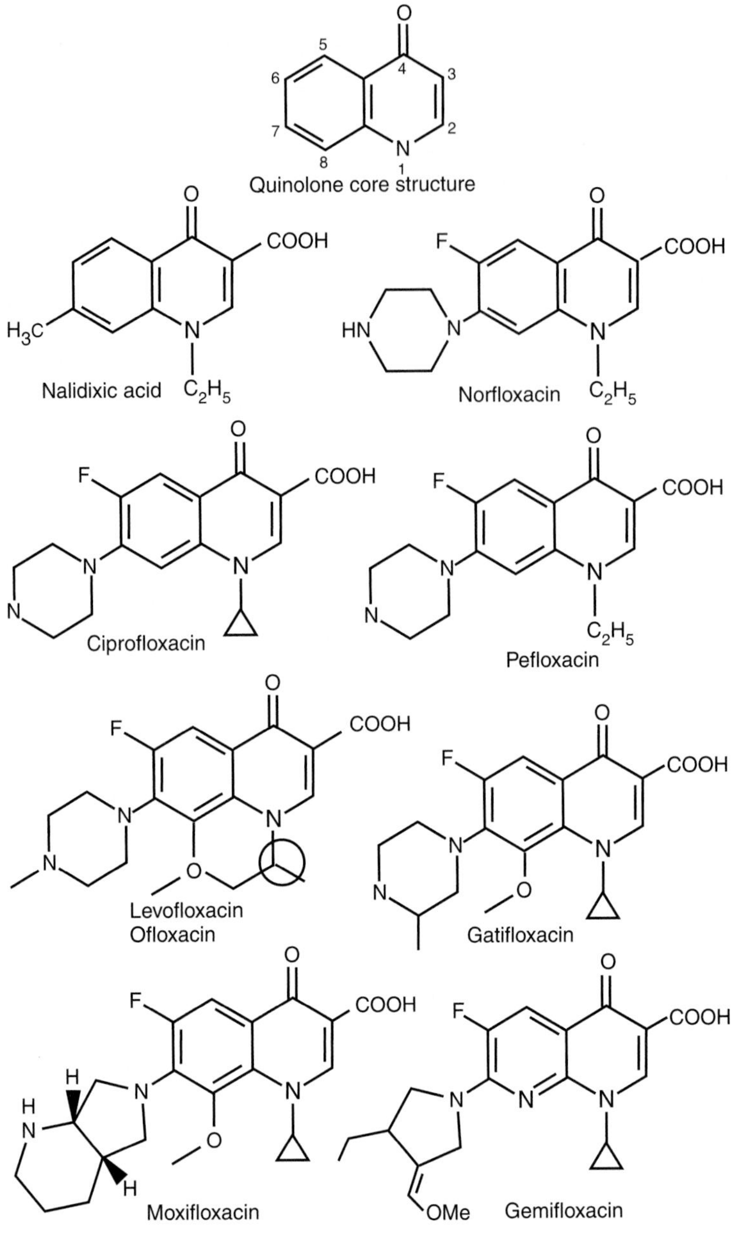

complexes. DNA gyrase, which was first recognized as a target of quinolones, is an essential bacterial enzyme composed of two A and two B subunits, products of *gyrA* and *gyrB* genes, respectively.[6,7] DNA gyrase uniquely catalyzes the introduction of negative superhelical twists into closed covalently circular chromosomal and plasmid DNA within the bacterial cell. The superhelical state of intracellular DNA is regulated by the actions of DNA gyrase and topoisomerase I, which removes DNA superhelical twists but is not inhibited by quinolones. DNA superhelicity affects the initiation of DNA replication and transcription of many genes. DNA gyrase is also responsible for removing positive superhelical twists that accumulate ahead of the DNA replication fork. These activities result from the enzyme's coordinated breaking of both strands of duplex DNA, passage of another segment of DNA through the break, and resealing of the break, a mechanism that defines type 2 topoisomerases.

Quinolones also inhibit the activities of topoisomerase IV, another type 2 topoisomerase that is composed of two subunits encoded by the *parC* and *parE* genes. Topoisomerase IV and DNA gyrase are structurally related; *parC* is homologous to *gyrA,* and *parE* is homologous to *gyrB*.[8] Topoisomerase IV functions to resolve (decatenate) interlinked (catenated) daughter DNA molecules that are the products of completion of a round of DNA replication to allow their segregation into daughter cells. Thus, DNA gyrase and topoisomerase IV have distinct essential roles in bacterial DNA replication.[9] Although gyrase can mediate the functions of topoisomerase IV (albeit as a less efficient decatenase), topoisomerase IV lacks the ability to introduce negative supercoils into DNA, a function that is unique to DNA gyrase.

Quinolones appear to function by trapping or stabilizing the enzyme–DNA complexes after strand breakage and before resealing of DNA. This trapped complex appears to function as a cellular poison, possibly by generating a DNA break that the cell is able to repair only poorly.[5] Quinolones have been shown to bind specifically to the complex of DNA gyrase and DNA rather than to DNA gyrase alone.[10] The importance of the interaction of quinolones with the gyrase–DNA complex for the antibacterial activities of the quinolones in *Escherichia coli* is indicated by the identification of bacterial single *gyrA* or *gyrB* mutants that are resistant to quinolones and produce gyrase–DNA complexes with reduced quinolone binding (see "Mechanisms of Acquired Bacterial Resistance," later).[11] In contrast to this interaction in *E. coli,* which is also similar to that in other gram-negative bacteria studied, the interactions of quinolones with topoisomerase IV in *Staphylococcus aureus* and *Streptococcus pneumoniae* have been shown to determine antibacterial activity by the identification of *parC* (*grlA* in *S. aureus*) and *parE* (*grlB* in *S. aureus*), single mutants that have reduced quinolone activity.[12] On the basis of studies of mutants of this type, a general pattern has emerged. For most gram-negative bacteria, DNA gyrase is the primary quinolone target, and for many gram-positive bacteria, topoisomerase IV is the primary target with gyrase being the secondary target. There are exceptions, however, that depend on the quinolone studied.[13] These patterns appear to result from the relative sensitivities of these two topoisomerases to a given quinolone, with the more sensitive of the two enzymes defining the primary target of a particular quinolone.[14] Some quinolones under development appear to have similar potencies against both DNA gyrase and topoisomerase IV in some bacterial species.[15,16]

Quinolone inhibition of bacterial DNA replication may be dissociated from bacterial killing under some conditions, suggesting that events in addition to the initial interaction of quinolones with the topoisomerase–DNA complex may be required for cell killing. In particular, inhibitors of RNA and protein synthesis reduce the bactericidal activity of some quinolones but do not affect their ability to inhibit bacterial DNA synthesis.[17] Thus, inhibition of bacterial DNA synthesis per se is not sufficient to account for bacterial killing, and newly synthesized gene products may also be necessary. This effect may account for the observations that at high concentrations of quinolones, which also secondarily inhibit protein synthesis, cell killing is reduced.[5]

The nature of the gene products (in addition to DNA gyrase and topoisomerase IV) that contribute to killing, however, has yet to be defined. The gene products in the RecA-SOS DNA repair and recombination system, the expression of which is known to be induced by the damage to bacterial DNA caused by quinolones, appear to function at least in part to repair quinolone-induced DNA damage, because *rec* mutants with defective function are hypersusceptible to killing by quinolones.[18] Certain *hip* mutants exhibit a *hi*gher fraction of *p*ersisters, or surviving cells, after treatment with bactericidal antimicrobial agents without exhibiting major differences in the concentrations of drug that inhibit bacterial growth. Those *hipA* mutants selected for reduced killing by ampicillin have alterations in the cell wall and are also killed less well by quinolones, and *hipQ* mutants selected for reduced killing by quinolones also exhibit selective reduced killing by β-lactams.[19,20] The function of the *hipA* and *hipQ* gene products are not known, but the overlap in reduced killing by both β-lactams and quinolones suggests that after the interaction of these classes of drugs with their different targets, there may be common overlapping pathways that are necessary for bacterial lethality.

Differences among quinolones in the magnitude of bacterial killing in the presence of rifampin (an inhibitor of RNA synthesis), phosphate-buffered saline, and anaerobiasis have led to the suggestion that some quinolones may have more than one mechanism of killing,[21] but the molecular events underlying these phenomena are not yet understood, except that killing is dependent on drug interaction with DNA gyrase and topoisomerase IV.[5]

Eukaryotic cells also contain topoisomerases, and eukaryotic topoisomerase II, which is a homodimeric enzyme, has limited primary amino acid sequence homology with DNA gyrase and topoisomerase IV.[22,23] Current antibacterial quinolones have only minimal activity against mammalian topoisomerase II,[24] but other quinolone structures (containing a 7-hydroxyphenyl substituent or an isothiazolo ring bridging positions 2 and 3) have been shown to have substantially enhanced potency against the mammalian enzyme.[23]

MECHANISMS OF ACQUIRED BACTERIAL RESISTANCE

Bacteria acquire resistance to quinolones by spontaneously occurring mutations in chromosomal genes that either alter the target enzymes (DNA gyrase and topoisomerase IV) or alter drug permeation across the bacterial cell membranes.[25] As yet, no specific quinolone-degrading or quinolone-inactivating enzymes have been identified, but certain fungi *(Gloeophyllum striatum)* have been shown to degrade quinolones by metabolic pathways.[26] Recently, plasmid-mediated quinolone resistance has been identified in clinical isolates of *Klebsiella pneumoniae* and *E. coli,* and the product of the plasmid-encoded gene *qnr* has been shown to protect DNA gyrase and topoisomerase IV from quinolone action.[27,28]

Resistant chromosomal mutants may be selected in the laboratory by plating bacteria on drug-containing agar. The frequency of occurrence of spontaneous mutants differs with the selecting drug concentration and the drug. For gram-negative bacteria selected with the newer fluoroquinolones, frequencies range, in general, from 10^{-6} or higher at twofold above the minimum inhibitory concentration (MIC) to undetectable ($<10^{-10}$) at 16- to 32-fold above the MIC. With a similar selection using nalidixic acid, mutants are detected more frequently when selected at a similar factor above the MIC, because single mutations can cause a higher level of increase in resistance (>30-fold) relative to ciprofloxacin (eightfold) and other fluoroquinolones. This difference results in part because the magnitude of the increase in resistance conferred by a single target mutation is modified by the interaction of drug with the second target enzyme. For example, for nalidixic acid, which has little activity against topoisomerase IV, a common mutation in the *gyrA* subunit of DNA gyrase causes a 30-fold increase in MIC. In contrast, for ciprofloxacin, which has activity against topoisomerase IV (albeit less than its activity against gyrase), the same *gyrA* mutation causes only an eightfold increase in MIC, despite the fact that both drugs exhibit similar loss of activity against purified DNA gyrase reconstituted with the resistant *gyrA* subunit.[29] Thus, quinolone interaction with a second target enzyme puts a ceiling on the magnitude of the increase in resistance due to mutation in the first enzyme target. For some quinolones that have similar potency against both target enzymes, frequencies of selection of first-step mutants may be particularly low because single target mutations produce little or no increment in resistance. Thus, for such quinolones, mutations in both targets are needed to produce substantial increments in MIC. Serial passage of bacteria on increasing concentrations of quinolones selects mutants with high levels of resistance resulting from the additive effects of several mutations involving both enzyme targets.[30]

Alterations in the A subunit of DNA gyrase that cause quinolone resistance have now been defined in a substantial number of clinical and laboratory isolates of *E. coli.* These alterations are clustered between amino acids 67 and 106 in the amino terminus of the A protein near the active site of the enzyme (tyrosine-122).[25] In particular, changes in serine-83 (to leucine or tryptophan) are most common and cause the largest increment in resistance as well as reduced binding of drug to the gyrase-DNA complex in vitro. Leucine-83 causes a 128-fold increase in resistance to nalidixic acid but lesser increases in resistance to the newer fluoroquinolones (16- to 32-fold), thus likely accounting for the greater ease of selection of resistant mutants with nalidixic acid. Similar changes in the A subunit have been associated with resistance in many species of gram-negative bacteria. Single amino acid changes in the midportion of the gyrase B protein have also been found to cause lower levels of resistance to nalidixic acid and fluoroquinolones.[25,31]

Resistance mutations in the *parC* gene of topoisomerase IV in *S. aureus* and *S. pneumoniae* have been most commonly found at position 80 in which a wild-type serine (homologous to serine-83 of DNA gyrase) is replaced by phenylalanine or tyrosine.[12,32] These mutations cause eightfold increases in resistance to several fluoroquinolones. Resistance mutations have also been found less commonly in the *parE* gene, often in positions similar to those of resistance mutations in *gyrB*.[25]

Stepwise increasing resistance occurs by sequential mutations in the *gyrA* (or *gyrB*) and *parC* (or *parE*) genes, with the first target mutation occurring in a gene for the more sensitive target enzyme. The level of susceptibility of the first-step mutant is then usually determined by the intrinsic level of sensitivity of the secondary target enzyme. A second mutation in a gene for the secondary target then further increases resistance to a level that is determined by the already mutant primary enzyme target. This finding implies that the drug concentration above which two mutations will be required for resistance will decrease to the extent that the similarity of sensitivities of DNA gyrase and topoisomerase IV to a given quinolone approach the same value. In the most highly resistant clinical strains of both gram-positive and gram-negative bacteria, one or more mutations in each of *gyrA* and *parC* have been commonly found. Some species, including *Mycobacterium tuberculosis*, *Helicobacter pylori*, and *Treponema pallidum* appear to lack genes for topoisomerase IV.[25] Thus, gyrase or another enzyme may carry out the functions of topoisomerase IV in these organisms, and target resistance may occur more readily in the absence of a second drug target to limit the effects of resistance mutations in gyrase.

The routes of quinolone permeation across bacterial cell membranes are not fully defined, but the hydrophilic congeners appear to diffuse across the gram-negative bacterial outer membrane through porin channels. In *E. coli* and *Pseudomonas aeruginosa*, resistance mutations in genes that affect expression of outer membrane proteins have been described.[33,34] In both cases, resistance cannot be explained by reduced diffusion alone, and reduced drug accumulation in some mutants is energy dependent, being abolished by agents that collapse proton-motive force. In *E. coli*, resistance of Mar mutants, which exhibit reduced porin channels, is dependent on the AcrAB efflux pump, which is linked to the TolC outer membrane protein.[35,36] Overexpression of AcrAB has also been associated with quinolone resistance in clinical isolates.[37] In *P. aeruginosa*, resistance has been shown to be caused by increased expression of one of several sets of three genes that appear to encode an efflux pump in the inner membrane, a periplasm-spanning membrane fusion protein, and a linked outer membrane protein (e.g., MexAB-OprM [composed of MexA, a membrane fusion protein; MexB, inner membrane efflux pumps; and OprM, an outer membrane protein]),[25,33,38] and such increased expression of one or more pump complexes is found commonly, along with *gyrA* mutations, in quinolone-resistant clinical isolates of *P. aeruginosa*.[39] Regulation of expression appears to be complex, and overexpression has in some cases been shown to be due to mutations in specific regulators. Resistance in many mutants of this type is pleiotropic, with additional low levels of resistance to tetracycline, chloramphenicol, and some β-lactams, because of the broad substrate profiles of most such pumps—hence the term *multidrug resistance* (MDR) is often applied to these efflux pumps.[33]

MDR efflux pumps of this type appear to be present in most, if not all, bacteria, and in many cases, multiple pumps, which may vary in their relative levels of expression under different conditions of growth or antibiotic exposure and selection, are present in a given species. For example, in *P. aeruginosa*, the MexAB-OprM pump complex is normally expressed, but selection with different quinolones can result in mutants that overexpress the MexCD-OprJ or MexEF-OprN pump complexes, presumably reflecting the particular ability of the overexpressed pump to remove the selecting quinolone from the cell.[40]

Physiologic overexpression of pumps (without regulatory mutations) occurring during infection but not during laboratory growth conditions could also affect outcomes of therapy in a way not necessarily predicted by in vitro methods for susceptibility testing. Compounds that can inhibit all of the known MDR pumps of *P. aeruginosa* have been identified, with the idea of combining such compounds with quinolones or other antimicrobial agents to improve activity in wild-type bacteria and to reduce resistance due to pump overexpression, a concept analogous to the combination of β-lactams with β-lactamase inhibitors.[41] As yet, no such MDR pump inhibitor–containing combinations are available for clinical use.

In gram-positive bacteria, which lack an outer membrane, overexpression of endogenous efflux pumps has also been shown to cause low-level quinolone resistance. The *S. aureus norA* gene encodes a native membrane protein that pumps hydrophilic quinolones driven by the proton gradient across the cell membrane,[42] and overexpression of NorA due to mutation in its promoter region or in other regulators causes resistance to norfloxacin, ciprofloxacin, and levofloxacin, in order of decreasing magnitude of the effect on MICs.[43] Some quinolones such as sparfloxacin and moxifloxacin are not affected by NorA overexpression. Recent data, however, suggest that other, less well studied pumps can cause resistance to these quinolones as well.[44] In *S. pneumoniae*, PmrA, a pump with a structure similar to NorA, can also contribute to reduced quinolone susceptibility.[45] Reserpine, an inhibitor of several efflux pumps in gram-positive bacteria, improves MICs of some quinolones in clinical isolates of *S. pneumoniae* and viridans streptococci.[46] It is likely that further study of potential MDR pumps in *S. aureus*, *S. pneumoniae*, and other gram-positive bacteria, aided by the increasing number of species with completely sequenced genomes, will identify additional quinolone resistance mechanisms resulting from overexpression of other as yet undefined MDR efflux pumps.

Plasmid-mediated quinolone resistance, long thought not to occur, was first identified and verified in multidrug-resistant, clinical isolates of *K. pneumoniae* from Alabama.[47] Used as donors, these isolates transferred plasmids by conjugation to a recipient laboratory *E. coli* with selection for resistance to β-lactams. Unexpectedly, the recipients acquired low-level resistance to quinolones as well. The plasmid-encoded gene responsible for quinolone resistance, *qnr*, was located on class I integrons flanked by other resistance genes, which can transfer multidrug resistance en bloc with the plasmid.[27] The *qnr* gene encodes a protein of the pentapeptide repeat family that is able to protect purified DNA gyrase and topoisomerase IV from quinolone action. How this protection occurs at the molecular level has not yet been defined. Plasmid-mediated quinolone resistance associated with *qnr* has recently been found in quinolone-resistant *E. coli* isolates from China and in resistant isolates of *K. pneumoniae* from other parts of the United States.[28] Although resistance mediated by *qnr* alone is usually low level, *qnr* plasmids, which are broad in their host range, are usually found in strains of *E. coli* and *K. pneumoniae* with additional chromosomal mutations, and the presence of *qnr* has been shown to increase the frequency of selection of chromosomal quinolone resistance mutations, presumably by reducing the quinolone therapeutic index.

ANTIMICROBIAL ACTIVITY

Current quinolones are most active against aerobic gram-negative bacilli, particularly members of the family *Enterobacteriaceae* and species of *Haemophilus*, and against gram-negative cocci such as *Neisseria* species and *Moraxella (Branhamella) catarrhalis* (Table 33-1).[48-50] Relative to nalidixic acid, the fluoroquinolones also have additional activity against gram-negative bacilli such as *P. aeruginosa* (see Table 33-1) and against staphylococci (Table 33-2). Ciprofloxacin remains the most potent marketed fluoroquinolone against gram-negative bacteria, and it and levofloxacin are the only available quinolones with sufficient potency for use against susceptible strains of *P. aeruginosa*. Resistance may emerge easily, however, when these quinolones are used alone for treatment of serious pseudomonal infections. For norfloxacin, ciprofloxacin, and ofloxacin, activity against streptococci and many anaerobes is limited (Table 33-3, and see Table 33-2). Agents released subsequently in the United States (levofloxacin, gatifloxacin, moxifloxacin, and

TABLE 33-1 Activity of Selected Quinolones against Selected Gram-Negative, Mycoplasmal, and Chlamydial Pathogens In Vitro

Organism	Nalidixic Acid	Norfloxacin	Pefloxacin	Ciprofloxacin	Ofloxacin	Levofloxacin	Gatifloxacin	Moxifloxacin	Gemifloxacin
				Representative MIC_{90} (μg/mL) (range)					
Acinetobacter spp.	(32-256)	(8-64)	(1-8)	0.25-2 (0.25->128)	0.25->8	0.05-32	0.03-8	>0.25-16	4-32 (0.008-32)
Aeromonas spp.	0.5	0.03	0.03	0.008-≤0.06	0.03-≤0.06	≤0.015-0.03	0.03	0.03	0.03
Burkholderia cepacia	16	8 (8-50)	—	(2->256)	4-25	4-256	12.5-256	4-256	64
Campylobacter jejuni	8	(0.25-2)	0.5	0.12-64	0.25-32	0.12-32	0.25-4	0.06-0.13	—
Chlamydia trachomatis	—	≥16	—	0.5-2	1-2	0.25-0.5	0.06	0.06	—
Chlamydophila pneumoniae	—	—	—	2	1	0.5-1	0.12	0.06-1	0.25
Citrobacter spp.	8	0.5 (<0.25-50)	0.4-1	0.06-0.25	0.25-1	0.13-0.5	0.25-2	0.25-2	2 (0.004-16)
Enterobacter aerogenes	8	0.5 (0.2-2)	0.25	0.5 (0.03->16)	0.25 (0.1-1)	0.5 (0.06-16)	1 (1-16)	2 (0.25->16)	0.25 (0.008-2)
Enterobacter cloacae	8	0.5 (<0.25-2)	0.5	0.25 (0.025-2)	1 (0.12-1)	0.5 (0.05-2)	0.5 (0.06-1)	1 (0.06-2)	0.25-1 (0.008-16)
Escherichia coli	4	0.12 (0.01-0.5)	0.12-0.25	0.25 (0.015->128)	0.25 (0.06-0.25)	0.5 (0.025-32)	0.25 (0.016-8)	0.25 (0.008-32)	0.016-0.03 (0.004-32)
Haemophilus influenzae	1	0.06	0.06	≤0.015-0.06	0.05-0.12	0.015-≤0.5	0.013-0.03	0.03-0.06	≤0.004-0.03
Klebsiella pneumoniae	8-16	0.5 (0.2-2)	2 (0.5-2)	0.5 (0.05-0.5)	2 (0.25-2)	0.5 (0.05-1)	1 (0.1-1)	1 (0.13-1)	0.25 (0.008-32)
Legionella spp.	1	(0.2-2)	—	0.016-0.06	0.03-0.12	0.016-0.03	0.03	0.06	0.003-0.008
Moraxella catarrhalis	2	0.4	0.25	≤0.015-0.12	0.06-0.12	≤0.03-≤0.5	≤0.03-0.05	≤0.015-0.12	≤0.004-0.015
Morganella morganii	8	0.12 (<0.06-25)	(0.25-4)	0.06 (0.015-1)	0.25 (0.12-0.25)	0.12 (0.06-1)	0.5 (0.25-2)	0.5 (0.13-4)	0.12 (0.016-8)
Mycoplasma hominis	>256	8-16	4	0.5-4	0.5-8	0.5-2	0.12	0.06-0.12	—
Mycoplasma pneumoniae	—	12	4	1-5	1	0.5-2.5	0.13-0.5	0.12-0.3	0.25
Neisseria gonorrhoeae	1	0.06	0.06	0.001-2	0.03-2	≤0.008-0.016	0.004-0.025	0.015-1	0.002
Neisseria meningitidis	0.5	0.03	0.03	0.004-0.008	0.03	≤0.008	≤0.008	≤0.008-0.016	
Proteus mirabilis	8	0.1 (0.12-0.5)	0.25	0.12 (0.025-4)	0.25 (0.12-0.5)	0.12 (0.05-4)	0.25 (0.2-4)	0.5 (0.25-16)	0.12-0.5 (0.03-8)
Proteus vulgaris	8	0.1 (0.12-0.5)	0.25	0.06 (0.03-0.12)	0.5 (0.12-0.5)	0.12 (0.06-0.25)	0.39 (0.25-0.5)	1 (0.5-1)	0.12 (0.03-0.12)
Providencia rettgeri	16	2 (0.25-3.1)	0.5	0.5 (0.025-4)	2-4	1 (0.1-4)	0.5	1 (0.5-2)	—
Providencia stuartii	32	2 (<0.25-2)	4	4-8 (0.12->16)	>8 (1->16)	4 (0.25->16)	0.5	1 (0.5-2)	0.25-16 (0.015-1)
Pseudomonas aeruginosa	16	2 (2-16)	2	0.5-128	4->128	2-128	>4-32	8->128	4-8 (0.03-256)
Salmonella spp.	2-4	≤0.06 (≤0.06-0.25)	0.12	0.01-0.25	0.12-0.5	0.03-0.25	0.06-0.25	0.12-0.25	0.015-0.12
Serratia marcescens	≥100	1 (0.025-50)	1 (1-8)	2 (0.5-12.5)	4 (1-25)	2 (0.25-8)	4 (2-12.5)	4 (0.5-8)	1-2 (0.008-4)
Shigella spp.	8	≤0.06-0.12	0.25	0.008-≤0.06	0.06-0.12	0.016-0.03	0.016-0.03	0.03-0.06	≤0.015-0.25
Stenotrophomonas maltophilia	16	2 (2-25)	4	>2-32	8-64	2-32	2-32	1-128	4 (0.016-16)
Yersinia enterocolitica	2	≤0.12	0.25	0.016-0.06	0.12-0.25	0.03-0.06	0.06	0.06-0.12	0.015-0.03

MIC_{90}, minimal concentration that inhibits 90% of strains.

Data from Eliopoulos CT, Eliopoulos GM. Activity in vitro of the quinolones. In: Hooper DC, Rubinstein E, eds. Quinolone Antimicrobial Agents. 3rd ed. Washington, DC: ASM Press; 2003:91-111; and Eliopoulos GM, Eliopoulos CT. Activity in vitro of the quinolones. In: Hooper DC, Wolfson JS, eds. Quinolone Antimicrobial Agents. 2nd ed. Washington, DC: American Society for Microbiology; 1993:161-193.

TABLE 33-2 Activity of Selected Quinolones against Selected Gram-Positive Bacteria In Vitro

Organism	Nalidixic acid	Norfloxacin	Pefloxacin	Ciprofloxacin	Ofloxacin	Levofloxacin	Gatifloxacin	Moxifloxacin	Gemifloxacin
Staphylococcus aureus, methicillin susceptible	100	2 (1-4)	0.5 (0.1-2)	0.5 (0.03-2)	0.5 (0.25-1)	0.25 (0.25-0.5)	0.12 (0.10-0.25)	0.12 (0.06-0.25)	0.06 (0.03-0.06)
Staphylococcus aureus, methicillin resistant	—	—	—	≥32 (25-128)	32 (62.5-50)	16 (8->32)	16 (4->32)	4 (2-16)	8 (1-8)
Coagulase-negative staphylococci, methicillin susceptible	100	2 (0.4->4)	1 (0.5-4)	2 (0.25-16	0.5	1 (0.5-2)	(0.25-4)	0.13 (0.12-1)	0.3 (0.015-0.03)
Coagulase-negative staphylococci, methicillin resistant	—	—	—	>16 (0.39-64)	32 (>8-32)	(0.39-16)	(0.25-8)	4 (0.13-8)	2 (0.25-2)
Streptococcus pneumoniae	>128	16 (4-16)	12 (8-16)	2 (1-8)	2 (1-8)	1 (1-2)	0.5 (0.25-1)	0.25 (0.06-0.5)	0.06 (0.03-0.06)
Streptococcus pyogenes	>100	4 (2-16)	8 (8-16)	2 (0.5-3.1)	2 (1-4)	1 (0.5-2)	0.5 (0.39-0.5)	0.25 (0.12-0.25)	0.06 (0.015-0.06)
Streptococcus agalactiae	>128	16 (4-16)	32	2 (0.5-2)	4 (1-4)	1	0.5	0.5 (0.12-0.5)	0.12 (0.03-0.25)
Streptococcus spp.	>64	16 (4-32)	>12.5	4 (1-8)	4 (2-8)	2 (1-2)	0.5 (0.5-1)	0.25 (0.25-2)	0.12
Enterococcus faecalis	>64	8 (4-32)	4-8	(1-128)	(2-32)	(2-50)	(1.4)	(0.5-16)	2 (2-4)
Enterococcus faecium	>64	≥12.5	—	(2->128)	(4-100)	(2-64)	(3->32)	(4-≥32)	8
Listeria monocytogenes	>64	8 (4-16)	6-8	1 (0.5-4)	4 (2-4)	1 (1-2)	0.5	0.5	0.25 (0.12-0.25)
Corynebacterium spp.	—	4 (4->128)	8 (8->128)	1 (0.05-128)	1 (0.5-64)	(2->16)	>4	2	(0.5-16)
Bacillus spp.	—	1	—	0.25 (0.06-1)	0.5	0.25 (0.06-2)	0.25	—	—
Nocardia spp.	>128	64	64	(1.4->25)	(2.6->25)	—	—	8	—

MIC90, minimal concentration that inhibits 90% of strains.
Data from Eliopoulos CT, Eliopoulos GM. Activity in vitro of the quinolones. In: Hooper DC, Rubinstein E, eds. Quinolone Antimicrobial Agents. 3rd ed. Washington, DC: ASM Press; 2003:91-111; and Eliopoulos GM, Eliopoulos CT. Activity in vitro of the quinolones. In: Hooper DC, Wolfson JS, eds. Quinolone Antimicrobial Agents. 2nd ed. Washington, DC: American Society for Microbiology; 1993:161-193.

gemifloxacin), however, have greater potency against these organisms, with gemifloxacin being especially potent against *S. pneumoniae.* For the fluoroquinolones that are used for treatment of infections outside the urinary tract, the MICs listed in Table 33-1 should be interpreted in relationship to peak drug concentrations in serum that range from 1.1 to 6.4 μg/mL (with usual dosing) and in relationship to drug concentrations in urine that are many-fold higher for many quinolones except those that are largely excreted by nonrenal mechanisms (see "Pharmacology," later). For highly suscepti-

ble organisms, MICs may be 10- to 30-fold below achievable serum concentrations.

Fluoroquinolones also have activity against mycobacteria (see Table 33-3).[48,51] Ciprofloxacin, ofloxacin, levofloxacin, gatifloxacin, and moxifloxacin are active against *M. tuberculosis, Mycobacterium fortuitum, Mycobacterium kansasii,* and some strains of *Mycobacterium chelonae* but have only fair or poor activity against *Mycobacterium avium-intracellulare.* Ofloxacin and pefloxacin have activity against *Mycobacterium leprae* in animal models.

TABLE 33-3 Activity of Selected Quinolones against Selected Anaerobic Bacteria and Mycobacteria In Vitro

Organism	Nalidixic acid	Norfloxacin	Pefloxacin	Ciprofloxacin	Ofloxacin	Levofloxacin	Gatifloxacin	Moxifloxacin	Gemifloxacin
Bacteroides fragilis	512	>128	16	4-64	2-12.5	2->16	0.25-8	0.5-8	0.5-4
Bacteroides spp.	512	128	—	16->64	2-32	4-16	2-8	8	—
Fusobacterium spp.	256	16	32	2-4	2-16	0.39	—	2	0.5
Clostridium spp.	256	2	1	1-16	1-8	(0.12-4)	—	—	—
Clostridium perfringens	64	8	8	0.5-1.56	0.5-8	0.39	0.39-1	1	0.12
Clostridium difficile	>128	128	64	6.25-12.5	12.5-16	6.25-128	1.56-2	2-16	2
Anaerobic gram-positive cocci	256-512	16-64	16	2-6.25	2-8	0.39-0.78	2	1-2	0.125-0.5
Mycobacterium tuberculosis	—	8	8	1	0.8-1.3	0.5-1	0.12-0.5	0.125	8
Mycobacterium avium complex	—	≥16	>64	16	10-100	(1-8)	—	—	—
Mycobacterium chelonae	—	>16	>64	8	>20	(1-4)	—	—	—
Mycobacterium fortuitum	—	2	2	0.3	1-3.2	0.25	—	—	—
Mycobacterium kansasii	—	8	4	8	1-3.2	0.25	—	—	—

MIC90, minimal concentration that inhibits 90% of strains.
Data from Eliopoulos CT, Eliopoulos GM. Activity in vitro of the quinolones. In: Hooper DC, Rubinstein E, eds. Quinolone Antimicrobial Agents. 3rd ed. Washington, DC: ASM Press; 2003:91-111; and Eliopoulos GM, Eliopoulos CT. Activity in vitro of the quinolones. In: Hooper DC, Wolfson JS, eds. Quinolone Antimicrobial Agents. 2nd ed. Washington, DC: American Society for Microbiology; 1993:161-193.

Other bacteria are also inhibited by quinolones in vitro (see Table 33-1). Ciprofloxacin, ofloxacin, levofloxacin, gatifloxacin, moxifloxacin, and gemifloxacin all have activity against the agents of atypical pneumonias, including *Legionella pneumophila, Mycoplasma pneumoniae,* and *Chlamydophila pneumoniae,* and against genital pathogens such as *Chlamydia trachomatis, Ureaplasma urealyticum,* and *Mycoplasma hominis. Treponema pallidum* is resistant to ofloxacin in animal models, and no other quinolone has been shown to have activity against this spirochete. Gatifloxacin and moxifloxacin among available quinolones and sitafloxacin among quinolones under development all have increased potency against anaerobes. Trovafloxacin also had antianaerobic activity.

Activity in vitro is reduced in the presence of urine but generally not in the presence of serum. Activity is also reduced at pH values below 7 and in the presence of magnesium concentrations at 8 to 16 mM. Both of these factors often contribute to the reduced quinolone activity observed in the presence of urine. Low pH and elevated concentrations of magnesium are associated with reduced drug accumulation in *E. coli.*[49]

Minimal bactericidal concentrations of quinolones are usually within two- to fourfold of the MIC, and the magnitude of bacterial killing increases with further increases in drug concentration, reaching a maximum at about 30-fold above the MIC. Above this maximal killing concentration, paradoxical reductions in killing are observed and are associated with additional inhibition of protein synthesis by high concentrations of quinolones.[5,52]

The postantibiotic effect (PAE) reflects the period of time required for bacteria surviving a brief exposure to an antimicrobial agent to resume growth. Although the PAE may be relevant in estimating the proper interval for drug dosing, its clinical importance, which may be greatest in patients with compromised host defenses, has not been proven. For quinolones, the duration of the PAE has been in the range of 1 to 2 hours and tends to increase with increasing drug concentration and length of exposure to the drug.

Combinations of quinolones with other antimicrobial agents have been extensively studied, and interactions with β-lactams and aminoglycosides as measured by fractional inhibitory or bactericidal concentrations or time-kill curve studies have generally been found to be indifferent or additive.[48] Synergistic interactions were found in a minority of strains, although for *P. aeruginosa* in some studies, synergy with ciprofloxacin in combination with imipenem or azlocillin was seen in a substantial minority (30% to 50%) of strains. Antagonistic interactions of quinolones with other antimicrobial agents have been rare. Rifampin reduced the bactericidal activity of ciprofloxacin and pefloxacin against *S. aureus* in some studies.[53]

PHARMACOLOGY

Absorption

The quinolones are well absorbed from the upper gastrointestinal tract, with bioavailability exceeding 50% for all compounds and approaching 100% for several (Table 33-4).[54,55] Peak concentrations in serum are usually attained within 1 to 3 hours of administering a dose. Neither food nor achlorhydria substantially affects the extent of quinolone absorption, but food may delay the time to reach peak drug concentrations in serum.[56,57] Enteral feedings given orally, however, may reduce absorption.[58] Absorption is good when ciprofloxacin is given by nasogastric or jejunostomy tube[59] but may be decreased by concurrent enteral feedings given through these tubes.[58]

Peak fluoroquinolone concentrations in serum after a 200- to 500-mg dose range from 1.4 to 1.5 μg/mL for gemifloxacin and norfloxacin to 5.7 μg/mL for levofloxacin (see Table 33-4). A 1-g dose of nalidixic acid produces concentrations of 20 to 50 μg/mL of serum. Drug binding to serum proteins is generally low, 20% to 50%; binding of gemifloxacin to serum proteins is somewhat higher, 55% to 70%.

Distribution in Tissues

The volumes of distribution of quinolones are high and in most cases exceed the volume of total body water (see Table 33-4), indicating accumulation in some tissues. Concentrations in prostate tissue, stool, bile, lung, and neutrophils and macrophages usually exceed serum concentrations (Table 33-5). Concentrations in urine and kidney tissue are high for quinolones with a major renal route of elimination (particularly so for gatifloxacin and levofloxacin and substantially less for moxifloxacin, which has a major route of nonrenal elimination). Concentrations of quinolones in saliva, prostatic fluid, bone, and cerebrospinal fluid (CSF) are usually lower than drug concentrations in serum. Active transport systems appear to be involved in reducing concentrations of levofloxacin, grepafloxacin, and sparfloxacin in CSF.[60]

Penetration into ascitic fluid in patients with liver failure has been found for pefloxacin (72% of serum concentration) and ofloxacin (120%).[61] Penetration into human breast milk has also been documented for ciprofloxacin, ofloxacin, and pefloxacin.[62]

Elimination

The terminal half-lives of elimination from serum range from 3 hours for norfloxacin and ciprofloxacin to 11 hours for pefloxacin, allowing twice- or once-daily dosing (Table 33-6, and see Table 33-4). The principal routes of elimination differ among quinolones. Ofloxacin, levofloxacin, and gatifloxacin are eliminated predominantly by the kidneys, whereas nalidixic acid, pefloxacin, and moxifloxacin are eliminated predominantly by nonrenal pathways. Most other quinolones have mixed excretion by both renal and nonrenal routes.

Renal clearances of norfloxacin, ciprofloxacin, ofloxacin, and levofloxacin exceed glomerular filtration rates (GFR), indicating net tubular secretion. In support of tubular secretion, renal clearances of norfloxacin and ciprofloxacin are reduced by probenecid, but drug accumulation does not occur. In contrast, the renal clearance of pefloxacin is below or equal to the GFR, suggesting net tubular reabsorption.[63]

TABLE 33-4 Pharmacokinetics of Selected Quinolones

Pharmacokinetic parameter	Norfloxacin	Pefloxacin	Ciprofloxacin	Ofloxacin	Levofloxacin	Gatifloxacin	Moxifloxacin	Gemifloxacin
Dose (mg) PO	400	400	500	400	500	400	400	320
C_{max} (μg/mL) PO	1.5	3.2	2.4	4.6	5.7	3.4	4.3	1.4
Dose (mg) IV	—	400	400	400	500	400	400	—
C_{max} (μg/mL) IV	—	5.8	3.4-6.7	5.5	5.7	4.5	4.5	—
Serum protein binding (%)	—	—	30	—	24-52	20	39-52	55-73
Half-life (h)	3.3	11	4	4-5	6-8	6.5	9.5	7
Oral bioavailability (%)	(50)	>95	70	>95	99	96	86-100	71
V_D (liters)	—	112	231	102	102	110	122	280
Cl_r (mL/min)	234	20	358	195	116	153	30	193
Renal excretion (% of dose)	27	—	40	73	77	77	20	36

Cl_r, renal clearance; C_{max}, peak plasma concentration; V_D, volume of distribution.

TABLE 33-5 Body Tissues, Fluids, and Cells in Which Quinolone Concentrations Exceed Quinolone Concentrations in Serum

Site	Fold Increment
Prostate tissue	0.9-2.3
Feces	100-1000
Bile	2-20
Lung tissue	1.6-6
Macrophages and neutrophils	2->100

Hepatic metabolism accounts for the majority of the elimination of pefloxacin and nalidixic acid. In these cases, however, active metabolites contribute to antibacterial effects. The desmethylpiperazinyl derivative of pefloxacin is norfloxacin, and hydroxynalidixic acid is more active than its parent compound. These metabolites and inactive glucuronide conjugated to the 3-carboxyl group are excreted in the urine. Conversion of norfloxacin and ciprofloxacin to less active metabolites accounts for 10% to 20% of elimination. There is minimal hepatic biotransformation (<10%) of ofloxacin and levofloxacin. Hepatic metabolism and biliary excretion are the principal routes of elimination of moxifloxacin (>60% of dose; 38% sulfoconjugation and 14% glucuronide conjugation). In addition to glucuronide conjugates and desmethylpiperazinyl derivatives, other metabolites of quinolones that have been identified have predominantly had alterations of the piperazine ring, including N-oxide, N-sulfo, N-formyl, and desethylene derivatives.[54,63]

Transintestinal secretion has been identified after intravenous administration of ciprofloxacin and accounts for about 10% to 15% of drug excretion.[63] This effect may be mediated by P-glycoprotein and other intestinal transporters.[54]

Dosage Adjustments in Renal and Hepatic Insufficiency

As expected from differences in the routes of excretion, increases in drug half-life in the presence of severe renal insufficiency are greatest for ofloxacin and levofloxacin (four- to fivefold) and least for pefloxacin, grepafloxacin, trovafloxacin, and moxifloxacin (no change), with other quinolones exhibiting intermediate effects (about twofold) (see Table 33-6). To prevent excessive drug accumulation, dosage reduction (increasing the dose interval from 12 to 24 hours or halving the daily dose for those quinolones normally given once daily) is indicated at creatinine clearances below 50 mL/min for ofloxacin and levofloxacin, below 40 mL/min for gatifloxacin and gemifloxacin, and below 30 mL/min for norfloxacin and ciprofloxacin. No dosage reduction is indicated for nalidixic acid, pefloxacin, and moxifloxacin. Clearance by hemodialysis is low (<14% of plasma clearance) for norfloxacin, ciprofloxacin, ofloxacin, and levofloxacin and is somewhat greater (28%) for pefloxacin. Similarly, peritoneal dialysis contributes little to the clearance of ciprofloxacin and ofloxacin.[64] Continuous venovenous hemofiltration (CVVH) in patients with severe renal failure consti-

tutes 16% to 70% clearance of levofloxacin and 6% to 37% clearance of ciprofloxacin.[65,66] In patients on CVVH, levofloxacin is administered at 250 mg/day and ciprofloxacin at 400 mg/day.

Fewer data are available on the effects of hepatic insufficiency on quinolone half-lives. For pefloxacin but not norfloxacin, ciprofloxacin, or ofloxacin, threefold increases in half-life were seen in some patients with cirrhosis, but there was substantial variation.[67] Changes in renal function that accompany severe liver disease may, however, affect ciprofloxacin and ofloxacin elimination to a lesser extent. Specific parameters of liver function that predict effects on pefloxacin clearance have not yet been defined, but in patients with severe liver disease, reduction of pefloxacin dose (possibly a twofold increase in dose interval) with monitoring of drug levels in serum may be indicated. No dosage adjustment is recommended for gatifloxacin, moxifloxacin, or gemifloxacin in patients with Childs classes A and B cirrhosis.

Interactions with Other Drugs

When co-administered by mouth with aluminum-, magnesium-, or, to a lesser extent, calcium-containing antacids, quinolones have markedly reduced oral bioavailability, presumably because of the formation of cation–quinolone complexes that are poorly absorbed.[68,69] Sucralfate, which contains large amounts of aluminum ions, also reduces absorption of quinolones. Although staggering of doses of antacids and quinolones may reduce this interaction, there is sufficient variability to suggest that this maneuver may not be fully reliable in an individual patient. Generally H_2-receptor antagonists and proton pump inhibitors do not have important effects on absorption of quinolones. Concurrent administration of quinolones with $FeSO_4$, multivitamin-mineral regimens containing zinc, and the buffered formulation of dideoxyinosine have also been reported to reduce quinolone absorption.[70] Nutritional supplements given by nasogastric tube may reduce the absorption of quinolones given concurrently by the same route, most likely because these supplements also contain multivalent cations such as iron and zinc. Concomitant administration of morphine decreases maximum serum concentrations of oral ciprofloxacin by 35% to 50%.

For intravenous formulations of ciprofloxacin and pefloxacin, precipitates have been reported when these quinolones were infused through the same intravenous tubing with aminophylline, amoxicillin with and without clavulanate, or flucloxacillin. Separate infusions are indicated.

Quinolones vary in the extent to which they impair the elimination of the methylxanthines theophylline and caffeine. The effects appear to result from inhibition by some quinolones of hepatic cytochrome P450 isozyme 1A2 (CYP1A2),[71] which is involved in theophylline and caffeine metabolism. Enoxacin and clinafloxacin exhibit the greatest effect and may produce two- to threefold increases in theophylline concentrations in serum, associated with a 40% to 65% reduction in total theophylline clearance without alterations in renal clearance of theophylline. Similar effects of a lesser magnitude are seen with grepafloxacin (30% increase in maximum serum concentrations of theophylline), ciprofloxacin (30% reduction in clearance and 20% to

TABLE 33-6 Dosages of Quinolones in Patients with Normal and Reduced Renal Function

Quinolone	Normal Renal Function		Renal Failure		Removal by Dialysis?
	Oral	Intravenous	GFR 10-50 mL/min	GFR<10 mL/min	
Norfloxacin	400 mg q12h	—	1 × dose q24h	1 × dose q24h	No (H, P)
Pefloxacin	400 mg q12h	400 mg q12h	No change	No change	No (H)
Ciprofloxacin	250-750 mg q12h	200-400 mg q12h	1 × dose q18h	1 × dose q24h	No (H, P)
Ofloxacin	200-400 mg q12h	200-400 mg q12h	1 × dose q24h	½ dose q24h	No (H, P)
Levofloxacin	250-750 mg q24h	250-750 mg q24h	½ dose q24h	½ dose q48h	No (H, P)
Gatifloxacin	400 mg q24h	400 mg q24h	½ dose q24h	½ dose q24h	No (H, P)
Moxifloxacin	400 mg q24h	400 mg q24h	No change	No change	No information
Gemifloxacin	320 mg q24h	—	½ dose q24h	½ dose q24h	20%-30% (H)

GFR, glomerular filtration rate; H, hemodialysis; P, peritoneal dialysis.

90% increases in serum concentrations of theophylline), and pefloxacin (30% reduction in clearance), but norfloxacin, ofloxacin, levofloxacin, gatifloxacin, moxifloxacin, and gemifloxacin had little or no effect (2% to 11% increases in serum concentrations of the-ophylline).[69,72,73] In patients receiving ciprofloxacin in combination with theophylline, serum levels of theophylline should be monitored and reductions in the dose of theophylline considered. No such ad-justments should be needed in patients receiving theophylline concur-rently with other fluoroquinolones.

Clozapine and methadone are also metabolized by CYP1A2. Low doses of ciprofloxacin have increased serum levels of clozapine, and one patient has been reported to develop symptoms of methadone over-dose while taking ciprofloxacin.[74] Thus, the effects of ciprofloxacin on clozapine and methadone (and possibly other drugs affected by CYP1A2, such as haloperidol, mexiletine, cimetidine, paroxetine) should be monitored the same way the methylxanthines are.

Another hepatic P450 enzyme, CYP3A4, is affected by many classes of antimicrobials, which can be inhibitors, inducers, or sub-strates of this metabolism enzyme. Such antimicrobials include macrolides, streptogramins, rifampin, azoles, and a variety of anti-retroviral agents, but not quinolones. Thus, the occasional case reports of apparent interactions of quinolones with other drugs inter-acting with CYP3A4 are difficult to assess for their importance or predictive value. Such case reports include those associating ciprofloxacin with increased cyclosporine levels and nephrotoxicity or increased levels of diazepam.[69]

In direct studies of interactions between warfarin and quinolones, in general no effects on coagulation tests were seen, and in those cases in which a drug interaction was seen (enoxacin, ciprofloxacin, and clinafloxacin), there was an increase in the relatively inactive R enantiomer of warfarin, which is metabolized by CYP2C9, and no effect on the active S enantiomer or prothrombin times.[75] Case reports of patients who developed bleeding while on warfarin and ciprofloxacin have appeared, however, suggesting that in uncommon, special settings quinolone promotion of an anticoagulant effect of warfarin may occur, possibly confounded by other concomitant ther-apies or promoted by the underlying disease conditions or genetic predispositions, which would not be reflected in data collected in con-trolled clinical studies. As a precaution, prothrombin times should be rechecked in patients on warfarin after initiation of quinolones or other antimicrobial agents.

Disturbances of glucose metabolism have been rarely reported with quinolones, but there have been recent case reports of elevated gly-buride levels and hypoglycemia in a diabetic patient given ciprofloxacin and in several patients receiving gatifloxacin and hypo-glycemic agents.[76] These effects were unexpected and not fully ex-plained. Glyburide may be metabolized by CYP2C9, which is not known to be affected by quinolones, and when this was directly tudied there was no detectable effect of gatifloxacin on glyburide me-tabolism or glucose tolerance in diabetic volunteers. Furthermore, hypoglycemia has been reported in patients receiving gatifloxacin and clinafloxacin without concomitant hypoglycemic agents, and hyper-glycemia has also been reported in patients receiving gatifloxacin. Thus, effects in addition to potential drug interactions are likely to contribute to the occurrences.

Nonsteroidal anti-inflammatory drugs (NSAIDs) may affect the central nervous system stimulant effects of some quinolones. Seizures were reported in a group of Japanese patients receiving enoxacin and the NSAID fenbufen. Potentiation of seizures by combinations of quinolones and NSAIDs has also been reported in animals. Assays of the displacement of the inhibitory neurotransmitter γ-aminobutyric acid (GABA) or a related molecule from GABA receptors in rat brain tissue have demonstrated displacement of GABA by quinolones and enhancement of this displacement by fenbufen and by the-ophylline.[77,78] Clinical experience does not suggest, however, that con-current use of quinolones (other than enoxacin) with other NSAIDs will result in central nervous system toxicities, but patients receiving

both classes of drugs should be cautioned about and monitored for these potential adverse effects.

Although probenecid reduces the renal clearance of norfloxacin and fleroxacin, no quinolone accumulation occurred. The effect of probenecid might be predicted to be greater with quinolones such as ofloxacin and lomefloxacin, for which renal clearance includes tubu-lar secretion and is the predominant mode of clearance, but data are lacking.

CLINICAL USES

Earlier quinolones such as nalidixic acid, oxolinic acid, and cinoxacin were used almost exclusively for treatment of urinary tract infections, although nalidixic acid was also used for treatment of shigellosis. With the development of the more potent fluoroquinolones, an increasingly broad array of infections are treated with members of the fluoro-quinolone class.

Urinary Tract Infections

Although the low pH and magnesium concentrations present in urine may reduce quinolone activity, the concentrations of many quinolones in urine are usually sufficient to provide substantial therapeutic ratios of urinary drug concentration to the MIC of most urinary pathogens. Lower urinary concentrations are expected with sparfloxacin, grepafloxacin, and trovafloxacin because of their predominantly non-renal clearance.

For uncomplicated urinary tract infections, usually in sympto-matic young women with cystitis caused by highly susceptible or-ganisms such as E. coli, most quinolones are likely to be highly ef-fective when given for brief courses of 3 to 10 days,[79,80] and norfloxacin, ciprofloxacin, and ofloxacin have been found to be comparable to trimethoprim-sulfamethoxazole.[67,80] Usually, the low-est dose in the dosage range (see Table 33-6) is sufficient for treat-ment of these infections. Three-day regimens of norfloxacin, ciprofloxacin, ofloxacin, and gatifloxacin result in cure rates of 81% to 96%.[80] An extended-release formulation of ciprofloxacin (500 mg PO once a day) was comparable to conventional ciprofloxacin (250 mg PO twice a day) when both were given for 3 days.[81] Limited data on single-dose therapies with ciprofloxacin, ofloxacin, and nor-floxacin indicate eradication in 75% to 96% of patients.[82,83] Single-dose norfloxacin (800 mg) was equivalent to a 3-day regimen for E. coli infections,[84] but for Staphylococcus saprophyticus infections, a 7-day regimen is preferred because of failures with shorter courses.[85,86] Women with uncomplicated acute pyelonephritis given norfloxacin, ciprofloxacin, or ofloxacin for 7 to 10 days have bacteriologic cure rates comparable to or better than those with trimethoprim-sulfamethoxazole, and levofloxacin and ciprofloxacin are compa-rable to each other with 95% eradication rates.[87] Guidelines of the Infectious Diseases Society of America (IDSA) recommend a fluo-roquinolone as first-line treatment for this condition because of in-creasing of resistance to trimethoprim-sulfamethoxazole among uropathogenic E. coli strains that has been associated with clinical failures.[88] For prophylaxis of recurrent infections in women, nor-floxacin (200 mg at bedtime) was highly effective and superior to ni-trofurantoin,[89] and low doses of ofloxacin (100 mg), norfloxacin (200 mg), and ciprofloxacin (125 mg) given after coitus have also been effective as prophylaxis.[90] Once-weekly pefloxacin has also been shown to be effective.[91] Other agents, such a nitrofurantoin or trimethoprim-sulfamethoxazole, are preferred for this indication, however, because of expense and the risks of potential pregnancy.

Cystitis occurring in older women is more often complicated by comorbid conditions and is more likely to be caused by pathogens in addition to E. coli that are less susceptible to antimicrobial agents.[92] For such infections, ofloxacin and ciprofloxacin given for 7 days have high eradication rates.[93]

Complicated urinary tract infections occurring in men and in pa-tients with catheters or structural or functional abnormalities of the urinary tract are often caused by more resistant pathogens and have a higher frequency of relapse and reinfection. Bacteriologic cure rates for ciprofloxacin were superior to those for trimethoprim-sulfamethoxazole and aminoglycosides shortly after completion of a 7- to 10-day course, but the low fractions of patients who continued to have sterile urine were similar by 4 to 6 weeks after therapy.[67,94] Sparfloxacin (200 mg loading dose followed by 100 mg/day) and ciprofloxacin (500 mg twice daily) given for 10 to 14 days were equivalent in clinical response, but eradication of bacteriuria was lower for sparfloxacin, possibly reflecting its lower concentrations in urine.[95] High cure rates were seen with both ofloxacin and levofloxacin.[96,97] In collected noncomparative trials, infections caused by *P. aeruginosa* were eradicated in 70% of patients given ciprofloxacin and in 83% given norfloxacin. Development of bacterial resistance has been associated with therapeutic failure in about 2% of patients overall, but resistance rates (10% to 20%) are often higher for *P. aeruginosa* infections and resistance can be selected with fluoroquinolone therapy.[98] Ciprofloxacin is the preferred fluoroquinolone for treatment of *P. aeruginosa* infections and when chosen, dosages of at least 500 mg PO twice a day should be used. In patients with bladder dysfunction due to spinal cord injury who used intermittent suprapubic taps or self-catheterization for bladder emptying, ciprofloxacin (100 mg at bedtime) reduced episodes of infection about 10-fold relative to placebo.[99] Whereas infections in the placebo group represented a mixture of enteric and nonenteric bacteria and enterococci, breakthrough infections in the ciprofloxacin group were largely nonenteric bacteria, particularly *P. aeruginosa*, which were often resistant.

Fluoroquinolones are now commonly used as prophylaxis in urologic surgery, and single-dose ciprofloxacin (500 mg) has been shown to be effective in reducing urinary tract infection rates after transurethral prostate resection and transrectal prostate biopsies.[100-102] Prophylaxis of urinary tract infection in renal transplant recipients is routinely done because of high risk for infection. Although ciprofloxacin is effective,[103] trimethoprim-sulfamethoxazole is often used as prophylaxis against opportunistic pathogens in this patient group.

Prostatitis

Fluoroquinolones concentrate in prostatic tissue, with lower levels in prostatic fluid. In one small comparative study of men with predominantly *E. coli* infections, norfloxacin given for 4 to 6 weeks was superior (92% eradication) to trimethoprim-sulfamethoxazole (67% eradication) at the 1-month follow-up.[104] In open studies, similar courses of norfloxacin, ciprofloxacin, and ofloxacin have produced eradication rates of 60% to 86% at follow-up ranging from 1 to 13 months.[105] With 2-week courses of therapy and infections caused by less susceptible organisms such as *P. aeruginosa* and enterococci, failures appear to be more frequent.[67,106]

Sexually Transmitted Diseases

Quinolones have activity in vitro against the major sexually transmitted pathogens *N. gonorrhoeae, C. trachomatis,* and *Haemophilus ducreyi,* but they appear to lack activity against *T. pallidum.*[107]

Uncomplicated gonococcal urethritis and cervicitis are effectively eradicated by single doses of quinolones (norfloxacin, 800 mg; ciprofloxacin, 250 mg; ofloxacin, 400 mg; trovafloxacin 100 mg, and gatifloxacin 400 mg).[108-111] Rectal infections appear to have virtually complete cures with all of these quinolones, and pharyngeal infections have similarly high rates of cure by ciprofloxacin, ofloxacin, and gatifloxacin.[109,111,112] Single doses of ciprofloxacin (500 mg), ofloxacin (400 mg), or levofloxacin (250 mg) are considered as alternative regimens for treatment of gonorrhea at genital and nongenital sites in guidelines from the Centers for Disease Control and Prevention (CDC).[113] Small numbers of patients with gonococcal salpingitis have been cured with 10- to 14-day courses of sequential intravenous and oral ciprofloxacin or oral ofloxacin,[114,115] and intravenous regimens of ciprofloxacin (400 mg every 12 hours), ofloxacin (400 mg every 12 hours), and levofloxacin (250 mg every 24 hours) may be used for disseminated infection, with a switch to oral therapy after improvement

to complete a 1-week course.[113] Gonococci resistant to quinolones have emerged in large numbers in the Far East[116] and have now begun to appear in Europe and parts of the United States,[117-119] with the result that in some areas quinolones can no longer be used as empiric therapy for gonorrhea.

Single doses of quinolones are ineffective for genital chlamydial infections.[67] Seven-day courses of therapy with norfloxacin and ciprofloxacin have failed, but 7-day courses of ofloxacin and levofloxacin were comparable to a similar course of doxycycline for treatment of chlamydial infections,[120-123] and ofloxacin (300 mg twice a day for 7 days) or levofloxacin (500 mg/day for 7 days) are recommended alternative regimens for chlamydial infections and nongonococcal urethritis.[113] There are only limited data on the use of ofloxacin for treatment of patients with chlamydial salpingitis.[115]

In patients with chancroid, *H. ducreyi* was eradicated from genital ulcers by ciprofloxacin, 500 mg twice a day for 3 days, in 100% of patients, a result comparable to that with trimethoprim-sulfamethoxazole.[124] A single dose of 500 mg or 250 mg for 5 days resulted in cure in 88% of patients.[125] The 3-day ciprofloxacin regimen is an option for treatment of chancroid in the CDC guidelines.[113]

For treatment of pelvic inflammatory disease (PID), a syndrome with mixed microbiology including gonococci, chlamydia, enteric bacteria, and anaerobes, clinical response rates for ofloxacin (400 mg twice a day for 10 days) and cefoxitin (2 g IM once) plus doxycycline (100 mg twice a day for 10 days) were similar, and ofloxacin was highly effective in eradicating gonococci and chlamydia.[126] Ciprofloxacin (250 mg twice a day) plus clindamycin (300 mg three times a day) given for 14 days was also comparable to ceftriaxone plus doxycycline with high clinical cure rates.[127] The CDC now recommends ofloxacin (400 mg twice a day) or levofloxacin (500 mg/day) with or without metronidazole (500 mg twice a day) given for 14 days as a preferred oral regimen for treatment of PID.[113] These two quinolones are also part of recommended alternative IV regimens. Two cases of gonococcal septic arthritis have responded to ciprofloxacin. For bacterial vaginosis, ofloxacin was less effective than metronidazole.[128] There are no data on treatment of syphilis with quinolones in humans, but in experimentally infected rabbits ofloxacin lacked efficacy.

Gastrointestinal and Abdominal Infections

All bacterial pathogens known to cause gastroenteritis are generally susceptible to quinolones in vitro. Although fecal material may decrease the activity of quinolones, drug concentrations in feces are exceedingly high. The penetration of quinolones into macrophages (see Table 33-5) may also be important for their effectiveness in systemic *Salmonella* infections.

Bacterial gastroenteritis is often a self-limited disease, but in a number of circumstances quinolones have been shown to shorten the duration of diarrhea and to eradicate pathogens from stools.[129] In traveler's diarrhea, which is often caused by enterotoxigenic *E. coli* and *Shigella* species, norfloxacin, 400 mg twice a day for 3 days, and ciprofloxacin, 500 mg twice a day for 5 days, begun shortly after the onset of diarrhea, have shortened the duration of loose stools by 1 to 3 days relative to placebo and have been comparable to trimethoprim-sulfamethoxazole.[130,131] Because of resistance to trimethoprim-sulfamethoxazole among *E. coli* strains in many parts of the developing world, quinolones are often the preferred therapeutic agents in travelers.[132] Single-dose therapies, including ciprofloxacin (500 mg or 1 g)[133,134] and ofloxacin (400 mg),[135] are also effective with or without loperamide for this indication. When given as prophylaxis to travelers, quinolones have produced protection rates that ranged from 68% to 92% compared with placebo controls, although routine use of quinolones or other antimicrobials is not recommended for prevention of diarrhea in travelers.[129,136,137] Contingency treatment at the onset of diarrhea is preferred for travelers, and with this approach norfloxacin (400 mg twice a day for 3 days)[138] and ciprofloxacin (500 mg single dose)[134] were shown to shorten diarrhea by 1 to 3 days relative to placebo.

In patients with shigellosis, for whom antimicrobials are generally indicated, 5-day courses of norfloxacin, ciprofloxacin, and ofloxacin have been highly effective and generally at least as effective as comparator agents, including ampicillin, trimethoprim-sulfamethoxazole, azithromycin, and ceftriaxone.[129,139] Addition of loperamide to ciprofloxacin may further shorten the duration of diarrhea.[140] Even a single dose of ciprofloxacin, 750 mg, may be effective in shigellosis, except in those cases caused by *Shigella dysenteriae* type 1, the most virulent of *Shigella* types.[141]

In patients with nontyphoidal *Salmonella* gastroenteritis, symptoms were shortened with ciprofloxacin or norfloxacin in some[142,143] but not all studies.[144] Eradication of stool carriage of *Salmonella* is generally transient,[143,145] but carriage is not necessarily prolonged relative to no treatment.[146] Treatment of *Salmonella* gastroenteritis is generally not indicated, except in immunocompromised individuals and older adults because of the risk of invasive disease. In immunocompromised hosts, systemic, nontyphoidal *Salmonella* infections have been successfully treated with ciprofloxacin, but there have been no comparative trials and some relapses have occurred in patients with acquired immunodeficiency syndrome (AIDS).[147]

For *Campylobacter jejuni* gastroenteritis, studies of treatment with quinolones have had variable results. Ciprofloxacin (500 mg twice a day for 5 days)[148] and norfloxacin (400 mg twice a day for 5 days)[143] were superior to placebo. Clinical and microbiologic failures have been associated with development of resistant *C. jejuni* in some[133,149] but not all studies using ciprofloxacin.[146] Quinolone resistance in *C. jejuni* is now highly prevalent in Europe and Latin America and is increasing in the United States.[150]

For treatment of patients with cholera, norfloxacin (400 mg twice a day for 3 days) has been shown to be superior to trimethoprim-sulfamethoxazole, a single dose of doxycycline, and placebo in shortening diarrhea,[151,152] and 3 days of ciprofloxacin (250 mg/day) and a standard tetracycline regimen (500 mg four times a day) were comparable.[153] A single dose of ciprofloxacin (1 g) or two 500-mg doses of ciprofloxacin has been effective and superior to doxycycline in shortening diarrhea and eradicating *Vibrio cholerae* from stool.[154,155] In patients with diarrhea caused by *Yersinia enterocolitica, Plesiomonas shigelloides,* and *Aeromonas* species, quinolones have eradicated the organisms from stool but have not yet been clearly shown to shorten clinical illness.[129]

In noncomparative studies of patients with enteric fever caused predominantly by *Salmonella enterica* serovar Typhi or serovar Paratyphi, ciprofloxacin cured 92% of patients, and ofloxacin cured 96% of patients, with resolution of fever within 5 days.[156,157] Three- to 5-day courses of ofloxacin (200 mg twice a day; 10 mg/kg/day in pediatric patients) have been highly effective and in adults shown to be superior to ceftriaxone given for 3 days for patients with enteric fever.[111,112] Ciprofloxacin was also shown to be superior to ceftriaxone.[158] Because of their effectiveness in short-course regimens and the common occurrence of resistance to other antimicrobials in *S. enterica* isolates in some areas of the developing world, ciprofloxacin and ofloxacin are now considered the agents of choice for treatment of patients with enteric fever. Although fluoroquinolone resistance in *S. enterica* isolates is rare, resistance to nalidixic acid is common in parts of the developing world, and such isolates have reduced susceptibility to fluoroquinolones. Clinical failures and delayed defervescence after short courses of ofloxacin are more frequent in patients with nalidixic acid–resistant strains than in those with nalidixic acid–susceptible strains.[159] Chronic fecal carriage of *S. enterica* serovar Typhi has been eradicated in 83% to 93% of small numbers of patients, including a few with gallstones, given norfloxacin, ciprofloxacin, or ofloxacin for 4 weeks.[160,161]

Although active against *Helicobacter pylori* in vitro, quinolones have failed to eradicate this organism from gastric mucosa, and failures have been associated with acquisition of quinolone resistance.[67] Data are quite limited on the use of quinolones for treatment of biliary tract infections. In a single small study, 83% of patients with cholecystitis and cholangitis, most associated with *E. coli* bacteremia, responded to intravenous and then oral ciprofloxacin.[162] In patients with biliary stents, late blockage has been thought to be due in part to bacterial adherence to the stent with biofilm formation. In small studies, ciprofloxacin (250 mg PO twice a day) and ofloxacin (200 mg twice a day) were not shown to delay stent blockage.[163]

For patients with complicated intra-abdominal infections due to disruption of the integrity of the gastrointestinal tract, a mixture of anaerobes and facultative gram-negative aerobes, with or without enterococci, are usually involved. In a randomized, double-blind trial, ciprofloxacin (400 mg IV every 12 hours, or 500 mg PO every 12 hours) plus metronidazole (500 mg IV or PO every 6 hours) was compared to imipenem (500 mg every 6 hours) for patients with complicated infections largely due to disease of the colon, small bowel, and appendix.[164] Ciprofloxacin and metronidazole were given either entirely IV or with a switch to PO after initial response. Clinical outcomes were highly similar in all three arms of the study. There was, however, regardless of treatment, a significantly higher rate of treatment failure if enterococci were isolated from the site of infection (28%) than if they were not (14%), suggesting that additional agents active against enterococci should be considered if culture results dictate. Ciprofloxacin plus metronidazole also appeared superior to piperacillin-tazobactam in another double-blind trial, although analysis of treatment failures was incomplete,[165,166] and a smaller study found no differences when ciprofloxacin plus metronidazole was compared to ceftriaxone plus metronidazole.[167]

Trovafloxacin, which has activity against gram-negative bacilli similar to that of ciprofloxacin and additional activity against anaerobic bacteria, was studied as a single agent (alatrofloxacin [the prodrug of trovafloxacin] 300 mg/day IV followed by trovafloxacin 200 mg/day PO) in comparison to imipenem (1 g IV every 8 hours) followed by amoxicillin-clavulanate (500 mg PO three times a day), both regimens given for up to 14 days.[168] Clinical cure or improvement occurred in 83% and 84% of patients in the two arms, high rates of response that would be expected because of the low Acute Physiology and Chronic Health Evaluation (APACHE) II scores (means, 6.4 and 7.0 versus 8 to 10 in the two other comparative trials) of the patients studied. Although gatifloxacin and moxifloxacin have activity against anaerobic bacteria in vitro that is similar to or slightly less than that of trovafloxacin,[48] no clinical data are yet available on their use for treatment of patients with intra-abdominal infections.

The use of quinolones in peritonitis has been evaluated most in patients undergoing chronic ambulatory peritoneal dialysis (CAPD) and in patients with cirrhosis. Oral ofloxacin, 300 mg/day, and ciprofloxacin, 500 mg/day, have cured episodes of peritonitis in CAPD patients, but failures in infections caused by the common coagulase-negative staphylococci have occurred. Higher concentrations of ciprofloxacin have been achieved by adding drug (20 to 50 μg/mL) to the dialysate, with outcomes similar to those with standard regimens of intraperitoneal vancomycin plus gentamicin.[169] A combination of intraperitoneal ciprofloxacin (50 mg/L) and rifampin (50 mg/L) produced a 65% cure rate, which was superior to that with intraperitoneal cephradine.[170] When intraperitoneal vancomycin was used, oral levofloxacin was inferior to an intraperitoneal aminoglycoside in patients with gram-negative CAPD infections, a limitation that appeared to be related to the prevalence of levofloxacin resistance in these organisms.[171] Spontaneous bacterial peritonitis in cirrhotic patients responds similarly to IV (200 mg twice a day) or oral (500 mg twice a day) ciprofloxacin (cure in 77%),[172] but there have been no comparisons to other regimens, such as third-generation cephalosporins, which are often used. In patients with cirrhosis at high risk for recurrent spontaneous bacterial peritonitis, norfloxacin 400 mg/day given as prophylaxis reduced recurrences by threefold.[173] Ciprofloxacin 750 mg given once weekly has also been effective.[174] Prolonged use of norfloxacin was, however, later associated with increasing occurrence of quinolone-resistant bacteria,[175] and patients who have been on this prophylaxis and develop peritonitis should be treated with agents other than a fluoroquinolone, because the risk of quinolone resistance is high in this group.[176]

Thus, the risks of selecting resistant enteric bacteria must be considered before embarking on prolonged use in prophylaxis.

Respiratory Tract Infections

A range of respiratory tract pathogens are susceptible to a number of quinolones in vitro. *Haemophilus influenzae, Moraxella catarrhalis,* and enteric gram-negative bacilli are highly susceptible. Ciprofloxacin and ofloxacin also have activity against the agents of atypical pneumonias, *Mycoplasma pneumoniae, Chlamydophila pneumoniae,* and *Legionella pneumophila,* and against *S. aureus* and *M. tuberculosis.* High intracellular concentrations of quinolones is quite likely advantageous for intracellular pathogens, such as *L. pneumophila* and *M. tuberculosis.* Least susceptible among common pathogens is *Streptococcus pneumoniae,* but levofloxacin, sparfloxacin, grepafloxacin, trovafloxacin, gatifloxacin, moxifloxacin, and gemifloxacin have improved activity.

Patients with acute bacterial exacerbations of chronic bronchitis have been treated with many different quinolones, which have generally been effective in eradicating *H. influenzae* from sputum.[177] In studies with ciprofloxacin, eradication rates for *S. pneumoniae* and *P. aeruginosa* were lower, and some failures have been associated with the development of bacterial resistance. In comparative trials, clinical responses have usually been similar to or better than those with ampicillin, amoxicillin, and cefaclor. In a randomized community-based study, ciprofloxacin (500 mg PO twice a day) resulted in similar clinical outcomes compared to usual treatment (agents chosen at the discretion of investigator and dominated by macrolides, cefuroxime, and amoxicillin with or without clavulanate), but it was somewhat more expensive, except in those patients with the greatest frequency of recurrent episodes for whom ciprofloxacin was more cost-effective.[178] Microbiologic eradication rates were not determined.

For available quinolones with enhanced pneumococcal activity, in randomized comparative trials, clinical and microbiologic outcomes were similar for levofloxacin (500 mg/day) compared with cefuroxime axetil,[179-181] gatifloxacin (400 mg/day) compared with cefuroxime axetil,[182,183] moxifloxacin (400 mg/day) compared with clarithromycin[184,185] or azithromycin,[186] and gemifloxacin (320 mg/day) compared with clarithromycin[187] or trovafloxacin.[188] Five- or 7-day courses seemed to be sufficient, with clinical response rates of 85% to 95%, and 5- and 10-day courses of moxifloxacin were comparable to each other (94% responses).[185] Moxifloxacin and gemifloxacin were superior to clarithromycin in eradicating *H. influenzae* from sputum, most likely because of the lesser activity of clarithromycin against this organism.[184,187]

In a study of more severely ill, hospitalized patients with acute exacerbation of chronic bronchitis, gemifloxacin (320 mg/day PO for 5 days) had better clinical responses in the intent-to-treat analysis and a shorter time to hospital discharge relative to ceftriaxone (1 g IV daily for ≤3 days) followed by cefuroxime axetil (500 mg PO twice a day for ≤7 days).[189] Time to next recurrent exacerbation was lengthened after treatment with ciprofloxacin as compared with clarithromycin[190] but was comparable to that after treatment with cefuroxime axetil,[191] and average infection-free intervals were not different in both comparisons. The proportion of patients without a recurrence after treatment of an exacerbation with gemifloxacin was significantly lower than that after treatment with clarithromycin (71% versus 58% at 26 weeks).[187]

In patients with community-acquired pneumonias, ciprofloxacin and ofloxacin have consistently eradicated *H. influenzae* and *M. catarrhalis.*[50] Cures of pneumococcal pneumonias, including a few cases with bacteremia, have been reported with intravenous and then oral ciprofloxacin[192] and ofloxacin[193,194] and with oral ofloxacin alone,[195] but some failures with both drugs have occurred, and pneumococcal bacteremia has developed during ciprofloxacin therapy of pneumonia.[67] For available quinolones with enhanced activity against pneumococci, similar or better clinical and microbiologic efficacies have been found for levofloxacin (500 mg IV or PO daily) versus ceftriaxone with or without erythromycin followed by cefuroxime axetil,[196] ceftriaxone alone,[197] or amoxicillin-clavulanate.[198] Comparable outcomes with generally high cure rates have also been seen in comparisons of gatifloxacin (400 mg IV or PO daily) versus ceftriaxone (with or without erythromycin) followed by clarithromycin,[199,200] levofloxacin,[201] or clarithromycin[202]; moxifloxacin (400 mg/day PO) versus clarithromycin[203] or amoxicillin[204]; and gemifloxacin (320 mg/day PO) versus ceftriaxone followed by cefuroxime axetil.[205] In addition to the initial study with levofloxacin,[196] a few studies, one with moxifloxacin[206] and another with gemifloxacin,[207] have also demonstrated superiority relative to the comparator agents. In hospitalized patients requiring initial parenteral therapy, moxifloxacin (400 mg IV or PO daily) was superior to amoxicillin-clavulanate (IV or PO) with or without clarithromycin, with more rapid defervescence, higher rates of clinical success (93% versus 85%), and higher rates of bacteriologic eradication of sputum (94% versus 82%).[206] Gemifloxacin (320 mg/day PO) produced modestly better clinical success in comparison to trovafloxacin (200 mg/day PO) in an intent-to-treat analysis (88% versus 81%), but responses were similar in the per-protocol analysis (96% versus 94%).[207]

Clinical responses in the subgroups of patients (usually numbering 10 to 20 patients, except for a study of 136 patients treated with gatifloxacin[208]) with pneumococci isolated from sputum from various trials were usually similar to the overall response rates (levofloxacin [81% to 100%],[196,201] gatifloxacin [95% to 100%],[199,201,208] moxifloxacin [100%],[203,206] and gemifloxacin [90% to 100%]).[205,207] Most studies have included patients with mild to moderate pneumonia, but those with gatifloxacin,[199,201] levofloxacin,[201] and gemifloxacin[205] included patients with severe pneumonia by clinical criteria similar to those used for stratification of risk for death,[209] with 96%, 91%, and 87% clinical cures, respectively. Outcomes in patients with pneumococcal bacteremia and pneumonia, a more severe test of drug efficacy, were excellent with levofloxacin (9 of 9 cured),[196] moxifloxacin (11 of 11 cured),[206] and gemifloxacin (12 of 12 cured).[205] Clinical failures associated with prior or acquired quinolone resistance in pneumococci have been reported with levofloxacin therapy but have not yet been associated with the less extensive use of gatifloxacin, moxifloxacin, or gemifloxacin.[210]

Among atypical pneumonias, smaller numbers of patients with pneumonias caused by *Legionella,*[211,212] *Mycoplasma,*[50] and *C. pneumoniae*[213] have also responded to ciprofloxacin and ofloxacin, but some apparent failures were seen in patients with *M. pneumoniae* and *C. pneumoniae* infection treated with ofloxacin.[194] Clinical responses to levofloxacin,[196] gatifloxacin, moxifloxacin,[206,214] and gemifloxacin[205,207] in usually small numbers (except for the larger number in the trial of gemifloxacin)[207] of patients with *C. pneumoniae, M. pneumoniae,* and *Legionella pneumophila* infection usually diagnosed serologically have generally been high. In some cases, particularly with *M. pneumoniae* infections, which may improve without treatment, assessment of responses is difficult because study designs often do not compare the rapidity of symptomatic improvement. Respiratory quinolones appear to be at least as good if not superior to macrolides for treatment of *L. pneumophila.*[215]

Hospital-acquired pneumonias, which are commonly caused by gram-negative bacilli, have responded to intravenous ciprofloxacin[67,216] and ofloxacin,[193] and responses to ciprofloxacin correlated with the level of susceptibility of the infecting organism, with better bacteriologic responses in infections caused by *Haemophilus* species and members of the *Enterobacteriaceae* than in infections caused by the less susceptible *P. aeruginosa.* Comparative trials of imipenem versus ciprofloxacin[217] or levofloxacin[218] for treatment of patients with nosocomial pneumonia have been published. For hospitalized patients with severe pneumonia, ciprofloxacin in high dose (400 mg IV every 8 hours) was compared to imipenem (1000 mg IV every 8 hours) in a multicenter, randomized, double-blind trial.[217] Most of the patients (78%) had nosocomial pneumonia and most (79%) were mechanically ventilated. Clinical and microbiologic response rates were somewhat higher in the ciprofloxacin (69% and 69%) than the imipenem (56% and 59%) group, and bacterial eradication rates were highest for members of the Enterobacteriaceae. Substantially poorer responses in both treatment groups were seen in patients with *P. aeruginosa* infection, and for both *P. aeruginosa* and *S. aureus,* persistence in sputum was substantial (60% to 67%, and 35% of patients, respectively) and was associated with development of resistance. For these reasons, combination therapy and use of maximal approved doses of ciprofloxacin, 750 mg PO or 400 mg IV every 12 hours to every 8 hours, may be preferred when quinolones are used in patients with *P. aeruginosa* infection.

In a multicenter, randomized, open-label trial, high-dose levofloxacin (750 mg IV or PO) produced clinical responses similar to those with imipenem (500 mg to 1 g, every 6 to 8 hours) followed by ciprofloxacin (750 mg PO every 12 hours) when both regimens were given for 7 to 15 days (66% [135/204] versus 69% [143/206] intent-to-treat analysis; 59% [70/118] versus 62% [70/112] clinically evaluable at 3 to 15 days after treatment), including a severely ill subset of patients with APACHE II scores greater than 20 (mean APACHE II scores were 15.0 and 14.8, respectively, in the two treatment groups).[218] Patients also received adjunctive therapy if they had documented infection with methicillin-resistant *S. aureus* (MRSA) (vancomycin for both arms) or *P. aeruginosa* (ceftazidime for levofloxacin arm and amikacin for imipenem arm). Microbiologic eradication rates were also similar overall. In patients with *P. aeruginosa* infection, however, there was a trend toward better clinical and microbiologic responses in the levofloxacin arm, suggesting that levofloxacin plus ceftazidime might be somewhat better than imipenem plus amikacin for these infections. No data were included about emergence of bacterial resistance.

Mild to moderate respiratory exacerbations in patients with cystic fibrosis and *P. aeruginosa* in the sputum respond clinically to oral ciprofloxacin, 750 mg twice a day, and ofloxacin, 400 mg twice a day, similar to the response to conventional parenteral therapies that use an antipseudomonal β-lactam and tobramycin.[67] In patients with more severe exacerbations, however, conventional parenteral combination therapy may be superior. Rarely is *P. aeruginosa* eliminated from sputum by any regimen in patients with cystic fibrosis. Rotating the use of different regimens may reduce the selective pressure for persistence of resistant bacteria that may emerge with either type of regimen.

Acute purulent sinusitis acquired in the community is often caused by a similar group of pathogens that causes acute bacterial exacerbations of chronic bronchitis, and it may be seen as a complication of viral upper respiratory infections. Anaerobic bacteria are usually present in only a small percentage of patients and are more likely if sinusitis is chronic or associated with dental infections. Establishing drainage of the infected sinus cavity by use of nasal decongestants is an important adjunctive therapy in addition to antimicrobial agents. A number of trials compared quinolones with other therapies in patients with acute purulent sinusitis, including ciprofloxacin (500 mg PO twice a day) versus cefuroxime axetil,[219] levofloxacin (500 mg/day PO) versus amoxicillin-clavulanate[220] or clarithromycin,[221] gatifloxacin (400 mg/day PO) versus clarithromycin,[222] and moxifloxacin (400 mg PO daily) versus cefuroxime axetil.[223,224] In all of these studies, the clinical responses are comparable between the quinolone and its comparator, with generally high response rates (87% to 96%). In these or other studies in which microbiologic samples were obtained by sinus puncture or nasal endoscopy prior to therapy, *H. influenzae* and *S. pneumoniae* were the predominant pathogens, and clinical responses in the subset of patients from whom *S. pneumoniae* was isolated were high, 100% for levofloxacin,[225] 97% for gatifloxacin,[226] and 97% for moxifloxacin.[224] Thus, these quinolones may be an alternative to but offer no advantage over nonquinolone therapies for treatment of acute community-acquired sinusitis.

Invasive otitis externa in diabetic patients is usually caused by *P. aeruginosa* and may respond to oral ciprofloxacin, 750 mg twice a day given for 6 weeks.[227,228] No studies comparing quinolones with conventional parenteral therapies have been reported.

Bone and Joint Infections

The prolonged antimicrobial therapy usually employed for bone and joint infections is facilitated by effective oral agents, and quinolones may fill this role in some cases.[229] For treatment of chronic os-

teomyelitis, there have been noncomparative trials using ciprofloxacin, ofloxacin, pefloxacin, or levofloxacin, in which treatment was usually for 6 or more weeks and follow-up was for at least 6 months after completion of therapy.[50,67,230,231] Clinical cures after oral ciprofloxacin, 750 mg twice a day, were 75% overall in infections in which gram-negative bacilli predominated, and similar rates of cure were reported in the smaller subgroups of patients with *P. aeruginosa* and methicillin-susceptible *S. aureus* (MSSA) infections. Failures were associated with incomplete débridement, the presence of foreign bodies, and the development of resistance in *P. aeruginosa, S. aureus,* and *Serratia marcescens.* Levofloxacin (500 mg/day) was effective in 9 of 15 patients (60%), with largely polymicrobial (*S. aureus* in seven and *P. aeruginosa* in three; all but three had other organisms as well) infections; in four cases, failures were thought to have resulted from inadequate débridement.[230] Three months of treatment with ciprofloxacin produced a cure rate of 60% in one study of osteomyelitis in the feet of diabetic patients[232]; ofloxacin produced a similar response rate.[233] Calcaneal osteochondritis caused by nail puncture wounds of the foot is often due to *P. aeruginosa.* Local débridement in combination with ciprofloxacin (400 mg IV every 12 hours, then 750 mg PO twice a day) given for 14 days appears to be highly effective for this condition, with cures in all 18 patients with *P. aeruginosa* infection and the two with *S. aureus* infection.[234]

In four small comparative trials, ciprofloxacin (750 mg twice a day) and ofloxacin (400 mg twice a day) have generally produced apparent rates of cure similar to those of conventional parenteral therapies using β-lactams with or without an aminoglycoside,[67,235] but the power of these studies to detect differences between the regimens has been small. For ofloxacin, cures of MSSA infections were 80% (10 of 12), but cures of *P. aeruginosa* infections were only 25% (1 of 4).[235]

For septic arthritis of prosthetic joints, standard therapy involves staged prosthesis removal and débridement, prolonged antibiotic treatment, and prosthesis reimplantation. Infections of prosthetic joints due to *S. aureus* and coagulase-negative staphylococci have been treated with ofloxacin (200 mg PO three times a day) plus rifampin (900 mg/day) for 6 to 9 months using the standard approach as well as débridement, with retention of the prosthesis in patients for whom removal was not possible.[236] With prolonged follow-up after completion of therapy, response rates were high in patients after the standard approach (81% to 93%) and unexpectedly high in the patients with retained prostheses (54% to 70%). Similar results have been reported for ciprofloxacin plus rifampin that also document the importance of rifampin in the antimicrobial regimen, as failure rates were high when ciprofloxacin was used alone.[237] Ceftazidime (1.5 g every 12 hours) given for 6 weeks plus ciprofloxacin (500 mg PO every 8 hours) given for 6 months also appeared to cure *P. aeruginosa*–infected orthopedic implants without prosthesis removal.[238]

There are few other data on the treatment of septic arthritis with quinolones, and most of those studies are with ciprofloxacin or ofloxacin.[50] Infections caused by *N. gonorrhoeae* and *E. coli* have responded to oral therapy. Failures have been seen in infections of prosthetic joints and infections caused by *S. aureus* and *P. aeruginosa.*

Skin and Soft Tissue Infections

Although the most common causes of cellulitis and pyoderma are streptococci and *S. aureus,* in patients with diabetes and peripheral vascular disease, decubitus ulcers, and some surgical wound infections, soft tissues may become infected with a mixture of bacteria that includes, in addition to streptococci and staphylococci, aerobic gram-negative bacteria and anaerobes. Quinolones have been evaluated as treatment for skin and soft tissue infections in some of these subgroups of patients.[239,240]

For uncomplicated skin infections, comparable clinical response rates (usually 90% or higher in both arms) have been reported for ofloxacin (400 mg PO twice a day) versus cephalexin,[241] levofloxacin (500 mg/day PO) versus ciprofloxacin (500 mg PO twice a day),[242] gatifloxacin (400 mg/day PO) versus levofloxacin,[243] and moxifloxacin (400 mg/day PO) versus cephalexin.[244] *S. aureus* and *Streptococcus pyogenes* were the dominant pathogens in these studies, but MRSA strains, which are commonly resistant to quinolones, were infrequently reported. Levofloxacin was significantly better than ciprofloxacin in eradicating *S. aureus* in one study.[242] In these and noncomparative studies,[50] failures have been seen with infections caused by *P. aeruginosa* (11%), streptococci (6%), and *S. aureus* (5%) and have been associated with the development of resistant organisms, which for *P. aeruginosa* may be more frequent in diabetic patients.[239]

For complicated skin infections, comparisons of oral ciprofloxacin, 750 mg twice a day,[245,246] and ofloxacin, 400 mg twice a day,[247] with intravenous cefotaxime or ceftazidime given for 9 to 12 days to patients with mixed infections in which gram-negative bacilli predominated, showed similar rates of clinical and bacteriologic efficacy, in the range of 79% to 98% clinical cure. *S. aureus* and *P. aeruginosa* were the most common pathogens in these studies, with few MRSA strains identified. In diabetic foot infections without osteomyelitis, the overall rate for complete healing using ciprofloxacin alone was 50%.[232] The polymicrobial nature of these infections that may include anaerobes may be a limiting factor. Trovafloxacin (200 mg/day PO), which had activity against many anaerobes, when given for 14 days produced clinical responses in 93% of patients.[248] Use of additional antimicrobial agents with activity against anaerobes should be considered in these patients. No data are yet available on the use of gatifloxacin or moxifloxacin, both of which have some antianaerobic activity but lack activity against *P. aeruginosa*, for treatment of diabetic foot infections.

The role of quinolones in the treatment of cutaneous and other forms of anthrax received considerable attention as a result of bioterrorism cases of anthrax in the United States in 2001. Activity in vitro is excellent for a number of fluoroquinolones, and ciprofloxacin (500 mg PO twice a day) is the recommended regimen for cutaneous disease and prophylaxis after exposure to anthrax spores.[249] Inhalational anthrax is treated with IV ciprofloxacin in combination with other agents. Ongoing animal studies of other quinolones may also support their efficacy.

For patients with uncomplicated cellulitis or pyoderma in whom staphylococci and streptococci are the most likely pathogens, conventional therapies with penicillin, semisynthetic penicillins, and cephalosporins, either oral or parenteral, remain the therapies of choice. For infections with MRSA, for which the quinolones were initially hoped to be valuable oral therapies, rapid emergence of quinolone resistance has become a particular problem, and resistance is now highly prevalent in many medical centers.[250]

Other Uses

There are limited data on the use of quinolones for treatment of mycobacterial infections. In patients with multidrug-resistant pulmonary tuberculosis, ofloxacin, 300 or 800 mg/day, has been used in combination with other second-line agents, with sputum conversions and apparent clinical cures,[251] but in cases in which ofloxacin was the only active drug, there was failure of sputum conversion and development of ofloxacin resistance.[251,252] Ciprofloxacin (750 mg/day PO) has been compared to rifampin when used together with three other agents—isoniazid, pyrazinamide, and streptomycin—for short-course (6-month) therapy. Somewhat poorer responses were seen in the ciprofloxacin-containing regimen than in the rifampin-containing regimen (3 of 18 [17%] versus 1 of 17 [6%] bacteriologic relapses).[253] Ciprofloxacin (750 mg/day) combined with rifampin and isoniazid was also associated with a slower rate of conversion of sputum to negative and a higher rate of relapse than a regimen of isoniazid, rifampin, pyrazinamide, and ethambutol, a difference that was particularly apparent in the group of patients with HIV infection.[254] Thus, ciprofloxacin appears to be less effective than first-line antituberculous agents, but its activity and that of ofloxacin may be valuable when second-line agents are needed because of resistance to first-line agents.

For nontuberculous mycobacteria, ciprofloxacin, 750 mg twice a day or 500 mg three times a day, has been used in three-drug (with clarithromycin plus amikacin)[255] and four-drug (with rifampin, ethambutol, and clofazimine)[256] regimens in patients with AIDS and *M. avium-intracellulare* complex bacteremia. Improvement in symptoms occurred with both regimens, but clearance of bacteremia appeared better with the clarithromycin-containing three-drug regimen.[257] In cutaneous *Mycobacterium fortuitum* infections, ciprofloxacin used alone was followed by relapse and the development of drug resistance,[67] but ofloxacin has been used successfully in some sternotomy infections caused by *M. fortuitum*.[258] Preliminary studies have also documented bactericidal activity in vivo and clinical improvement in patients with lepromatous leprosy given ofloxacin, 400 mg/day, and pefloxacin, 800 mg/day.[259]

For patients with bacteremias, intravenous ciprofloxacin and ofloxacin have been effective in cases caused by enteric gram-negative bacilli, although responses have been poor for *P. aeruginosa* bacteremias when these drugs were used in relatively low doses (200 mg twice a day).[260,261] In neutropenic patients with fever, ciprofloxacin in combination with aminoglycosides produced defervescence and cure of documented infections comparably to standard β-lactam–aminoglycoside combinations,[262] but ciprofloxacin monotherapy was less effective than such combinations[263] and should not be used. Although lower doses were used in earlier studies, more recent studies have used regimens of ciprofloxacin 400 mg IV every 8 hours (in one case, followed by 750 mg PO twice a day) either alone[264] or in combination with piperacillin.[265] Ciprofloxacin alone was comparable to ceftazidime plus amikacin, and ciprofloxacin plus piperacillin was comparable to tobramycin plus piperacillin in resolution of fever, but changes in therapy were necessary in over half of patients in both arms of both studies. Use of quinolones in this setting should be with caution and should be considered principally as an alternative regimen when there are reasons for not choosing standard regimens with combinations of β-lactams and aminoglycosides.

Recently, there has been increased interest in defining low-risk groups of neutropenic patients who might be safe candidates for oral antimicrobial therapy for fever, because of the potential for increased convenience and reduced costs. Quinolones have been components of such oral regimens.[266,267] These trials evaluated a combination of oral ciprofloxacin and amoxicillin-clavulanate compared to intravenous ceftazidime in one trial[267] and to intravenous ceftriaxone plus amikacin in the other[266] in patients with fever and neutropenia from cancer chemotherapy who were able to take oral medications and were considered to be at low risk based on the absence of other diseases and documented infection and a projected duration of neutropenia of less than 10 days. Successes of treatment in patients given the oral and parenteral regimens were similar in both studies, although the oral regimen was associated unexpectedly with a higher incidence of adverse effects (16% versus 1%), largely nausea and vomiting.[267] Renal failure reported in an earlier trial of ciprofloxacin plus clindamycin for treatment of a similar group of patients was not seen in these trials.[268] Whether oral therapy can also be safely translated into outpatient therapy for rigorously defined low-risk patients remains to be determined. Early trials using ofloxacin,[269,270] or in pediatric patients, ciprofloxacin (in comparison to ceftazidime),[271] suggest that it may be possible to manage low-risk patients safely outside the hospital. These studies were too small, however, to detect clinically important differences in preventable bad outcomes in the outpatients.

Oral ciprofloxacin (500 mg twice a day), ofloxacin (300 mg twice a day), and norfloxacin (400 mg twice a day) given as prophylaxis in neutropenic patients have consistently reduced the occurrence of gram-negative bacteremia and in some cases prolonged the time to first fever, but breakthrough gram-positive bacteremias have occurred, particularly streptococcal bacteremias in bone marrow transplant recipients.[272,273] Ciprofloxacin and ofloxacin appear superior to norfloxacin,[274,275] with lower rates of gram-negative and, in the case of ofloxacin, streptococcal bacteremias. Addition of penicillin to norfloxacin reduced breakthrough streptococcal bacteremias,[276] and addition of rifampin to ofloxacin reduced staphylococcal bacteremias.[275] Breakthrough bacteremias with quinolone-resistant viridans streptococci have also been reported when levofloxacin alone was used as prophylaxis in recipients of autologous stem-cell transplants.[277]

Quinolones should not be used for treatment of fever in neutropenic patients who have received a quinolone as prophylaxis because of the risk of quinolone resistance, which has occurred in hematology units in which prophylaxis was used.[278]

There is limited experience in using quinolones for treatment of endocarditis.[279] One study has reported good responses in intravenous drug abusers with right-sided MSSA endocarditis who complied with the full course of ciprofloxacin, 300 mg IV twice a day for 1 week, then 750 mg PO twice a day for 3 weeks, plus rifampin, 300 mg PO twice a day for 4 weeks.[280] An additional study compared 28 days of inpatient therapy with ciprofloxacin (750 mg PO twice a day) plus rifampin (300 mg PO twice a day) versus IV oxacillin or vancomycin plus gentamicin (given for the first 5 days) for similar patients, with similar response rates for the two regimens when patients were evaluated at 6 to 7 days after completion of therapy.[281] Drug resistance, however, has occurred in this setting, and there have been failures in patients with left-sided *S. aureus* endocarditis. There have been a number of single case reports of patients with gram-negative bacillary endocarditis whose infections have been suppressed with oral quinolones, but there have been failures. Q fever endocarditis, which responds poorly to conventional antimicrobial therapy, has been successfully cured with prolonged courses of ciprofloxacin (12 weeks)[282] or ofloxacin plus doxycycline (4 years).[283] Doxycycline combined with hydroxychloroquine was, however, superior to ofloxacin plus doxycycline.[283] Use of quinolones for endocarditis should currently be limited to circumstances in which established therapies are not possible.

Quinolones vary in their penetration across the blood-brain barrier into CSF.[284] In the presence of meningeal inflammation, concentrations in CSF have reached as high as 39%, 90%, and 60% of serum concentrations for ciprofloxacin, ofloxacin, and pefloxacin, respectively. Trovafloxacin achieves CSF concentrations that are 25% of those in serum in the absence of meningeal inflammation. In two small studies of patients with predominantly gram-negative bacillary meningitis, pefloxacin, 800 mg IV every 12 hours, cured 12 of 16 neurosurgical patients, many of whom had failed to respond to β-lactam therapies,[285] and ciprofloxacin, 200 mg IV every 12 hours, cured 18 of 20 similar patients.[286] Ten of 12 neonates with gram-negative bacillary meningitis (and in some cases mixed infections) were also reported to have been cured with IV ciprofloxacin (10 to 60 mg/kg/day).[287] Treatment of *P. aeruginosa* meningitis with ciprofloxacin may require very high doses in some patients (800 mg every 8 hours).[288] Trovafloxacin was shown to have high cure rates and comparability to ceftriaxone (90% and 89%, respectively) in African children with epidemic meningococcal meningitis.[289] Use of these quinolones for treatment of meningitis should be considered only in those circumstances in which standard therapies are not possible or have failed. Trovafloxacin has been removed from clinical use because of toxicities, and other quinolones, although very active in vitro, have not been adequately studied for treatment of meningococcal meningitis. Ciprofloxacin has been used successfully in the treatment of brain abscess caused by *Salmonella enterica* serovar Enteritidis in a small number of case reports.[284] For eradication of nasopharyngeal carriage of *N. meningitidis,* which is indicated in the setting of close contact with patients who have meningococcal meningitis, ciprofloxacin (750 mg) or ofloxacin (400 mg) given as a single dose has been highly effective,[290,291] and ciprofloxacin had efficacy similar to those of rifampin (600 mg twice a day for 2 days) and ceftriaxone (2 g IM).[292]

Quinolones have been used for treatment of a variety of other infections in small numbers of patients. A few patients with tularemia have responded to ciprofloxacin or levofloxacin,[293,294] and several patients with cat-scratch disease improved more rapidly after ciprofloxacin treatment than might be expected without treatment.[295] Patients with Mediterranean spotted fever caused by *Rickettsia conorii* and Q fever caused by *Coxiella burnetii* may respond to ciprofloxacin or ofloxacin, but doxycycline remains the preferred therapy.[283,296,297] Attempts to treat patients with brucellosis with quinolones have been complicated by a high frequency of relapses,[298] but a combination of ofloxacin (400 mg/day) and rifampin (600 mg/day) for 6 weeks

resulted in a low relapse rate and was comparable to doxycycline plus rifampin.[299] Patients with falciparum malaria have had inconsistent responses to quinolones.[300,301]

PROBLEMS WITH QUINOLONE RESISTANCE DURING CLINICAL USE

Development of bacterial resistance among pathogens during clinical use of quinolones is predicted to occur more often in settings in which there are large numbers of bacteria at the site of infection and the therapeutic index at this site is below 8,[302] because spontaneous chromosomal resistance mutations causing resistance increments of four- to eightfold for fluoroquinolones may occur at frequencies of 10^{-8} to 10^{-10}.[25] Therapeutic indices below 8 are more likely in infections caused by less susceptible pathogens such as *P. aeruginosa* and *S. aureus* and at sites of infection at which drug delivery or host eradication mechanisms may be compromised and in patients who receive inadequate drug doses. The plasmid-mediated, low-level resistance mechanism found recently in clinical isolates of *K. pneumoniae* and *E. coli*[28] may act to facilitate selection of additional chromosomal mutations by lowering the therapeutic index.[303] Epidemiologic factors also affect the extent to which resistant pathogens can spread and thereby amplify the prevalence of resistance.[304]

General surveys of resistance patterns occurring over time have found resistance to increase after the introduction of fluoroquinolones and to occur most often with *Pseudomonas* species and staphylococci and in soft tissue infections and infections associated with foreign bodies.[305-307] In many medical centers, ciprofloxacin resistance has increased markedly (to over 90%) among MRSA but not MSSA strains.[308,309] Resistance appears to have been selected in patients colonized with MRSA and given ciprofloxacin for other infections.[308] Clonal dissemination may also contribute to spread of resistance during outbreaks. A similar difference between methicillin-resistant and methicillin-susceptible strains has been seen for ciprofloxacin resistance in coagulase-negative staphylococci, and in this setting cross-selection by exposure to other antibiotics in addition to direct quinolone selection appears to augment ciprofloxacin resistance in MRSA strains, which are usually also multidrug resistant.[310,311]

More surprising has been the emergence of substantial quinolone resistance in initially more highly susceptible species of bacteria, particularly *N. gonorrhoeae, C. jejuni,* and *E. coli.* Fluoroquinolone resistance in *N. gonorrhoeae* has also become substantial in some countries in the Far East,[312] and outbreaks of strains with reduced susceptibility have been also been reported. In some areas of the United States, these were sufficient to lead to modification of the recommendation for inclusion of quinolones for empiric therapy.[119] In one outbreak, reduced susceptibility was associated with reduced rates of positive Gram stains of urethral discharge, thereby probably resulting in decreased detection and enhanced spread.[117]

Resistance emerged in *C. jejuni* in human and poultry populations in parallel after quinolone use in both groups in Europe.[313] In the United States, travel to Spain or Latin America was a risk factor for acquiring resistant *C. jejuni,* and the occurrence of domestically acquired cases in patients without prior treatment with a fluoroquinolone also increased. Strain typing has shown an overlap in resistant *C. jejuni* strains from humans and poultry, and contamination of food products with resistant *C. jejuni* has been demonstrated,[150,314] suggesting contaminated poultry products as the source of some resistant infections in humans. Resistance acquired by an initially susceptible isolate of *C. jejuni* during treatment of *Campylobacter* gastroenteritis with a quinolone has also been reported.[149]

Quinolone-resistant strains of *E. coli* have emerged in Spain and the Far East. Risk factors in Spanish patients with resistant urinary isolates have included use of quinolones, complicated infections, and use of urinary catheters.[315] Clinically important resistance in *E. coli* has also developed in some hematology-oncology units in Spain and Germany in which quinolones were used as prophylaxis during periods of neutropenia,[316,317] as well as in non-neutropenic patients in

Spain.[318] In these units, breakthrough bacteremias with quinolone-resistant *E. coli* have become problems. These bacteremias, as well as colonization of the fecal flora with quinolone-resistant *E. coli,*[319] have been associated with quinolone use as prophylaxis and were caused by distinct strains rather than representing clonal spread within the units. Additionally, some patients not receiving quinolones were found to be colonized with quinolone-resistant *E. coli,*[319] and a survey suggested that 25% of the population in Spain may have fecal colonization with such strains.[320] These findings, in conjunction with earlier findings of high rates of colonization of poultry with resistant *E. coli* in Spain,[321] raise the possibility that contamination of the food supply with resistant *E. coli* could be a contributing factor in these areas.[322]

With increasing use of quinolones for treatment of patients with respiratory tract infections, there are concerns about the emergence of quinolone resistance in *S. pneumoniae*. In Canada, ciprofloxacin resistance in isolates of *S. pneumoniae* was 0%, 1.7%, and 1.4% in 1993, 1997-98,[323] and 2000,[324] respectively, with the increase between 1993 and 1997-98 preceded by increasing use of quinolones, largely ciprofloxacin. Rates of resistance as high as 15.2% in Northern Ireland, 12.1% in Hong Kong, and 5.3% in Spain[311] have also been reported. Resistant isolates were generally reported in adults but not children, who would be less likely to have received a quinolone. Resistant isolates in Hong Kong were clonal, indicating spread from person to person, but those in Canada and Spain were polyclonal. Worrisome was the observation that among the Spanish isolates, 30% of the strains belonged to one of two international, epidemic, multidrug resistance clones, France[9V]-3 and Spain[23F]-1, raising concerns of possible future spread. In the United States, fluoroquinolone resistance in *S. pneumoniae* has generally remained below 1%.[325] There has, however, been a rise in strains that contain single *parC* resistance mutations (from 0.4% in 1992-96 to 4.5% in 1999-2000) in one survey[326] but not another.[327] These strains, which may be the progenitors of fully resistant strains with dual mutations in *parC* and *gyrA,* would be classified as susceptible and thus are difficult to detect with routine testing.[328] Because children are a major reservoir of pneumococci, concerns have been raised that future, extensive use of quinolones in children could increase the rate of development of resistance to quinolones in *S. pneumoniae.*[329]

Resistance to quinolones should be monitored, and strategies for minimizing its occurrence, including focused quinolone use, should be employed to avoid compromising the future utility of the class. The inverse relationship between quinolone concentration and the frequency of selection of resistant mutants in vitro and in vivo[330,331] also argues that underdosing of quinolones should be avoided to minimize opportunities for selection of resistant bacteria.

ADVERSE EFFECTS

The tolerability of the fluoroquinolones is best assessed in double-blind randomized trials in which the effects of patient populations, methods of ascertainment, and possible bias can be controlled. In some cases, however, such trials may not have the power to detect adverse effects occurring at low frequency or in more diverse patient populations, as evidenced in the United States by unexpected toxicity profiles (see later) and unexpectedly high rates of adverse drug effect reporting for temafloxacin and trovafloxacin shortly after their release for clinical use.[332] In an analysis of 56 such trials in which fluoroquinolones were compared with placebo or other antimicrobial agents, most studies found similar adverse effect profiles.[333] In six studies, there were significantly fewer adverse events with fluoroquinolones relative to the comparison agent (ciprofloxacin versus trimethoprim-sulfamethoxazole and ampicillin; norfloxacin versus trimethoprim-sulfamethoxazole and cefadroxil; ofloxacin versus erythromycin). On the other hand, adverse events were more frequent with the fluoroquinolone in seven studies (ciprofloxacin versus doxycycline; norfloxacin versus placebo; temafloxacin versus cefadroxil; fleroxacin versus amoxicillin and placebo). In a number of instances, increasing doses and durations of therapy were associated with higher rates of adverse effects.

The most frequent category of adverse effects involves the gastrointestinal tract, occurring in 3% to 17% of patients reported in clinical trials. In most patients, anorexia, nausea, vomiting, and abdominal discomfort, when they occur, are mild. Diarrhea is less frequent, and antibiotic-associated colitis has been rare, possibly because most current quinolones have little or no effect on the anaerobic bowel flora.[332]

The next most frequent category of adverse effects involves the central nervous system, occurring in 0.9% to 11% of patients.[334] Symptoms of mild headache and dizziness have predominated, followed by insomnia and alterations in mood. Distinctively, dizziness was reported by the manufacturer in up to 11% of patients receiving trovafloxacin at 200 PO mg/day. Hallucinations, delirium, and seizures are rare. Seizures may have resulted in some but not all cases from theophylline accumulation or from the ability of theophylline and NSAIDs to augment the ability of quinolones to displace GABA from its receptors.[335]

Allergic and skin reactions have occurred in 0.4% to 2.8% of patients in clinical trials overall. Unspecified rashes have been the most frequent of these. With gemifloxacin, rashes developed in 2.8% of patients in clinical trials, but in young women receiving gemifloxacin for 7 days or longer, a self-limited, maculopapular rash without evidence of vasculitis occurred in 14%. Whether the occurrence of this unusual rash predicts the occurrence of allergic reactions with later exposure to other quinolones is not certain. Phototoxicity reactions are uncommon with most quinolones but can occur in some patients after exposure to ultraviolet A (UVA; 320 to 400 nm) light and were more frequent with lomefloxacin, pefloxacin, fleroxacin, sparfloxacin, and clinafloxacin.[336,337] All of these agents except pefloxacin have a halide substituent at the 8 position, which is known to increase phototoxicity. Drug fever, urticaria, angioedema, vasculitis, serum sickness–like syndromes, and anaphylactoid reactions have been uncommon. Acute interstitial nephritis, most likely allergic in origin, also occurs infrequently and has been associated with eosinophiluria but generally not crystalluria. Infiltrates of lymphocytes and eosinophils have been found in the renal interstitium on renal biopsies.[332]

Arthropathy with cartilage erosions and noninflammatory effusions occurs in the weight-bearing joints of juvenile animals given quinolones.[338] Experience with use of quinolones in children has increased, particularly in children with cystic fibrosis given ciprofloxacin.[339] These children and others receiving nalidixic acid, norfloxacin, and ciprofloxacin have only uncommonly had joint symptoms, which have been reversible.[339,340] Studies to identify subclinical cartilage damage by nuclear magnetic resonance imaging of joints of treated children have also been negative.[341] In cystic fibrosis patients given pefloxacin, however, arthralgia and joint swelling developed in 14%.[342] Because of concerns about cartilage toxicity in children, quinolones have not been recommended for routine pediatric use, but there is an evolving view based on absence of human arthropathy seen over the past decade of fluoroquinolone use, that in some children, particularly those with cystic fibrosis, the benefit of quinolones outweighs what appears to be a small, short-term risk of joint toxicity, and expanded use of quinolones in pediatrics is under consideration.[339,343] Tendinitis with tendon rupture has been reported uncommonly in adults given norfloxacin, ofloxacin, ciprofloxacin, and pefloxacin.[344,345] The risks are highest in older patients and those on corticosteroids.

To varying extents, quinolones can block the potassium channels and thereby delay repolarization in cardiac tissue, an effect that underlies their ability to prolong the QT interval on the electrocardiogram. Prolongation of QT interval can predispose to ventricular arrhythmias such as torsades de pointes.[346] QT interval prolongation of a magnitude similar to that seen with erythromycin has been reported for patients receiving sparfloxacin, and there have been rare (3 of 750,000) cases of ventricular arrhythmias associated with its use.[346] Grepafloxacin also prolongs the QT interval and was withdrawn from clinical use after the occurrence of unexpected cardiac events. Although QT prolongation of a lesser magnitude was also found with gatifloxacin and moxifloxacin, arrhythmias have not been noted to be a problem with the use of these quinolones. Additive effects on QT prolongation may occur when quinolones are given together with other agents that prolong the QT interval. Thus, quinolones should be avoided or used with caution in patients also receiving class III (block potassium channel; e.g., amiodarone, sotalol) or class IA (block potassium and sodium channels; e.g., quinidine, procainamide) antiarrhythmics, or other agents that prolong the QT interval. Risk is also potentially increased in the presence of cardiomyopathy, bradycardia, hypokalemia, and hypomagnesemia.

Leukopenia and eosinophilia generally occur in less than 1% of patients, and mild elevations in serum transaminases occur in less than 1% to 3% of patients receiving quinolones; these abnormalities are rarely of sufficient severity to require cessation of therapy. An exception occurred with trovafloxacin, which was associated with elevated transaminases in about 10% of patients receiving a 4-week course for prostatitis. After release of trovafloxacin for clinical use, rare reports of idiosyncratic, symptomatic hepatitis (reporting incidence of 1 in 17,000) were identified in postmarketing surveillance, some of which were associated with eosinophilic infiltrates and sufficiently severe to cause hepatic failure requiring liver transplantation.[332,347] Although occurring more often in patients receiving more than 14 days of therapy, severe hepatotoxicity occurred in one case after a single dose.[332] These events led to the restriction of trovafloxacin use and later to its withdrawal from clinical use.

Earlier, in a similar set of circumstances, temafloxacin was also found through postmarketing surveillance shortly after its release to be associated with rare cases of hemolytic anemia, thrombocytopenia, and renal failure at a reporting incidence of 1 in 5000. These occurrences led the manufacturer to remove temafloxacin from the market.[348] The mechanisms of these rare but severe toxic effects of trovafloxacin and temafloxacin are not known.

Although there have been occasional reports of hypoglycemia associated with the use of ciprofloxacin, levofloxacin, and moxifloxacin, cases of severe hypoglycemia associated with the use of gatifloxacin in diabetic patients receiving oral hypoglycemics have recently appeared.[76] Modest reductions of glucose and increases in insulin were also reported in one study of gatifloxacin in diabetic patients not on hypoglycemics.[349] Interestingly, hyperglycemia has also been reported in older nondiabetic patients receiving gatifloxacin. Various quinolones have been shown to stimulate release of insulin from rat pancreatic islet cells. Although the frequency of these effects appears to be low overall, the relative risk with use of various quinolones remains to be determined.

Safety in pregnancy[332] has not been established for any of the quinolones, but studies of babies born to women exposed to norfloxacin or ciprofloxacin during the first trimester identified no increase in teratogenic risks.[350,351] In one prospective case-control study comparing 200 women exposed to fluoroquinolones and 200 women exposed to known nonembryotoxic antibiotics, there were no differences in birth defects, spontaneous abortions, prematurity, or fetal distress, but there was a higher rate of therapeutic abortions, suggesting that concerns about teratogenic risks may exceed the actual risks.[351] Because quinolones can be excreted in breast milk, they should be avoided for nursing mothers.

REFERENCES

1. Domagala JM. Structure-activity and structure-side-effect relationships for the quinolone antibacterials. J Antimicrob Chemother. 1994;33:685-706.
2. Rolston KVI, Frisbee-Hume S, LeBlanc BM, et al. Antimicrobial activity of a novel des-fluoro (6) quinolone, garenoxacin (BMS-284756), compared to other quinolones, against clinical isolates from cancer patients. Diagn Microbiol Infect Dis. 2002;44:187-194.
3. Kappel EM, Shakibaei M, Bello A, Stahlmann R. Effects of the des-F(6)-quinolone garenoxacin (BMS-284756), in comparison to those of ciprofloxacin and ofloxacin, on joint cartilage in immature rats. Antimicrob Agents Chemother. 2002;46:3320-3322.
4. Domagala JM, Hagen SE. Structure-activity relationships of the quinolone antibacterials in the new millennium: Some things change and some do not. In: Hooper DC, Rubinstein E, eds. Quinolone Antimicrobial Agents. 3rd ed. Washington, DC: ASM Press; 2003:3-18.
5. Drlica K, Hooper DC. Mechanisms of quinolone action. In: Hooper DC, Rubinstein E, eds. Quinolone Antimicrobial Agents. 3rd ed. Washington, DC: ASM Press; 2003:19-40.
6. Wang JC. DNA topoisomerases. Annu Rev Biochem. 1996;65:635-692.
7. Drlica K, Zhao XL. DNA gyrase, topoisomerase IV, and the 4-quinolones. Microbiol Rev. 1997;61:377-392.
8. Kato J, Nishimura Y, Imamura R, et al. New topoisomerase essential for chromosome segregation in E. coli. Cell. 1990;63:393-404.
9. Ullsperger C, Cozzarelli NR. Contrasting enzymatic activities of topoisomerase IV and DNA gyrase from Escherichia coli. J Biol Chem. 1996;271:31549-31555.
10. Shen LL, Kohlbrenner WE, Weigl D, Baranowski J. Mechanism of quinolone inhibition of DNA gyrase. Appearance of unique norfloxacin binding sites in enzyme-DNA complexes. J Biol Chem. 1989;264:2973-2978.
11. Willmott CJ, Maxwell A. A single point mutation in the DNA gyrase A protein greatly reduces binding of fluoroquinolones to the gyrase-DNA complex. Antimicrob Agents Chemother. 1993;37:126-127.
12. Ng EY, Trucksis M, Hooper DC. Quinolone resistance mutations in topoisomerase IV: Relationship of the flqA locus and genetic evidence that topoisomerase IV is the primary target and DNA gyrase the secondary target of fluoroquinolones in Staphylococcus aureus. Antimicrob Agents Chemother. 1996;40:1881-1888.
13. Pan XS, Fisher LM. Targeting of DNA gyrase in Streptococcus pneumoniae by sparfloxacin: Selective targeting of gyrase or topoisomerase IV by quinolones. Antimicrob Agents Chemother. 1997;41:471-474.
14. Blanche F, Cameron B, Bernard FX, et al. Differential behaviors of Staphylococcus aureus and Escherichia coli type II DNA topoisomerases. Antimicrob Agents Chemother. 1996;40:2714-2720.
15. Pan XS, Fisher LM. DNA gyrase and topoisomerase IV are dual targets of clinafloxacin action in Streptococcus pneumoniae. Antimicrob Agents Chemother. 1998;42:2810-2816.
16. Ince D, Zhang X, Silver LC, Hooper DC. Dual targeting of DNA gyrase and topoisomerase IV: Target interactions of garenoxacin (BMS-284756, T3811ME), a new desfluoroquinolone. Antimicrob Agents Chemother. 2002;46:3370-3380.
17. Dietz WH, Cook TM, Goss WA. Mechanism of action of nalidixic acid on Escherichia coli: III. Conditions required for lethality. J Bacteriol. 1966;91:768-773.
18. McDaniel LS, Rogers LH, Hill WE. Survival of recombination-deficient mutants of Escherichia coli during incubation with nalidixic acid. J Bacteriol. 1978;134:1195-1198.
19. Moyed HS, Bertrand KP. hipA, a newly recognized gene of Escherichia coli K-12 that affects frequency of persistence after inhibition of murein synthesis. J Bacteriol. 1983;155:768-775.
20. Wolfson JS, Hooper DC, McHugh GL, et al. Mutants of Escherichia coli K-12 exhibiting reduced killing by both quinolone and beta-lactam antimicrobial agents. Antimicrob Agents Chemother. 1990;34:1938-1943.
21. Lewin CS, Morrissey I, Smith JT. The mode of action of quinolones: The paradox in activity of low and high concentrations and activity in the anaerobic environment. Eur J Clin Microbiol Infect Dis. 1991;10:240-248.
22. Lynn R, Giaever G, Swanberg SL, Wang JC. Tandem regions of yeast DNA topoisomerase II share homology with different subunits of bacterial gyrase. Science. 1986;233:647-649.
23. Gootz TD, Osheroff N. Quinolones and eukaryotic topoisomerases. In: Hooper DC, Rubinstein E, eds. Quinolone Antimicrobial Agents. 3rd ed. Washington, DC: ASM Press; 2003:69-89.
24. Hussy P, Maass G, Tummler B, et al. Effect of 4-quinolones and novobiocin on calf thymus DNA polymerase alpha primase complex, topoisomerases I and II, and growth of mammalian lymphoblasts. Antimicrob Agents Chemother. 1986;29:1073-1078.
25. Hooper DC. Mechanisms of quinolone resistance. In: Hooper DC, Rubinstein E, eds. Quinolone Antimicrobial Agents. 3rd ed. Washington, DC: ASM Press; 2003:41-67.
26. Wetzstein HG, Schmeer N, Karl W. Degradation of the fluoroquinolone enrofloxacin by the brown rot fungus Gloeophyllum striatum: Identification of metabolites. Appl Environ Microbiol. 1997;63:4272-4281.
27. Tran JH, Jacoby GA. Mechanism of plasmid-mediated quinolone resistance. Proc Natl Acad Sci U S A. 2002;99:5638-5642.
28. Wang M, Tran JH, Jacoby GA, et al. Plasmid-mediated quinolone resistance in clinical isolates of Escherichia coli from Shanghai, China. Antimicrob Agents Chemother. 2003;47:2242-2248.
29. Ince D, Zhang X, Silver LC, Hooper DC. Topoisomerase targeting with and resistance to gemifloxacin in Staphylococcus aureus. Antimicrob Agents Chemother. 2003;47:274-282.
30. Hooper DC, Wolfson JS, Souza KS, et al. Genetic and biochemical characterization of norfloxacin resistance in Escherichia coli. Antimicrob Agents Chemother. 1986;29:639-644.
31. Yoshida H, Bogaki M, Nakamura M, et al. Quinolone resistance-determining region in the DNA gyrase gyrB gene of Escherichia coli. Antimicrob Agents Chemother. 1991;35:1647-1650.
32. Pan XS, Ambler J, Mehtar S, Fisher LM. Involvement of topoisomerase IV and DNA gyrase as ciprofloxacin targets in Streptococcus pneumoniae. Antimicrob Agents Chemother. 1996;40:2321-2326.
33. Poole K. Efflux-mediated resistance to fluoroquinolones in gram-negative bacteria. Antimicrob Agents Chemother. 2000;44:2233-2241.
34. Poole K. Efflux-mediated resistance to fluoroquinolones in gram-positive bacteria and the mycobacteria. Antimicrob Agents Chemother. 2000;44:2595-2599.
35. Okusu H, Ma D, Nikaido H. AcrAB efflux pump plays a major role in the antibiotic resistance phenotype of Escherichia coli multiple-antibiotic-resistance (Mar) mutants. J Bacteriol. 1996;178:306-308.

36. Murakami S, Nakashima R, Yamashita E, Yamaguchi A. Crystal structure of bacterial multidrug efflux transporter AcrB. Nature. 2002;419:587-593.

37. Wang H, Dzink-Fox JL, Chen MJ, Levy SB. Genetic characterization of highly fluoroquinolone-resistant clinical *Escherichia coli* strains from China: Role of *acrR* mutations. Antimicrob Agents Chemother. 2001;45:1515-1521.

38. Poole K, Tetro K, Zhao QX, et al. Expression of the multidrug resistance operon *mexA-mexB-oprM* in *Pseudomonas aeruginosa*: *mexR* encodes a regulator of operon expression. Antimicrob Agents Chemother. 1996;40:2021-2028.

39. Jalal S, Wretlind B. Mechanisms of quinolone resistance in clinical strains of *Pseudomonas aeruginosa*. Microb Drug Resist. 1998;4:257-261.

40. Köhler T, Michea-Hamzehpour M, Plesiat P, et al. Differential selection of multidrug efflux systems by quinolones in *Pseudomonas aeruginosa*. Antimicrob Agents Chemother. 1997;41:2540-2543.

41. Lomovskaya O, Warren MS, Lee A, et al. Identification and characterization of inhibitors of multidrug resistance efflux pumps in *Pseudomonas aeruginosa*: Novel agents for combination therapy. Antimicrob Agents Chemother. 2001;45:105-116.

42. Yoshida H, Bogaki M, Nakamura S, et al. Nucleotide sequence and characterization of the *Staphylococcus aureus norA* gene, which confers resistance to quinolones. J Bacteriol. 1990;172:6942-6949.

43. Ng EY, Trucksis M, Hooper DC. Quinolone resistance mediated by *norA*: Physiologic characterization and relationship to *flqB*, a quinolone resistance locus on the *Staphylococcus aureus* chromosome. Antimicrob Agents Chemother. 1994;38:1345-1355.

44. Truong-Bolduc QC, Zhang X, Hooper DC. Characterization of NorR protein, a multifunctional regulator of *norA* expression in *Staphylococcus aureus*. J Bacteriol. 2003;185:3127-3138.

45. Brenwald NP, Gill MJ, Wise R. Cloning of a novel efflux pump gene associated with fluoroquinolone resistance in *Streptococcus pneumoniae* (Abstract). 38th Interscience Conference on Antimicrobial Agents and Chemotherapy, 1998:LB-4.

46. Brenwald NP, Gill MJ, Wise R. The effect of reserpine, an inhibitor of multidrug efflux pumps, on the in-vitro susceptibilities of fluoroquinolone-resistant strains of *Streptococcus pneumoniae* to norfloxacin. J Antimicrob Chemother. 1997;40:458-460.

47. Martínez-Martínez L, Pascual A, Jacoby GA. Quinolone resistance from a transferable plasmid. Lancet. 1998;351:797-799.

48. Eliopoulos CT, Eliopoulos GM. Activity in vitro of the quinolones. In: Hooper DC, Rubinstein E, eds. Quinolone Antimicrobial Agents. 3rd ed. Washington, DC: ASM Press; 2003:91-111.

49. Eliopoulos GM, Eliopoulos CT. Activity in vitro of the quinolones. In: Hooper DC, Wolfson JS, eds. Quinolone Antimicrobial Agents. 2nd ed. Washington, DC: American Society for Microbiology; 1993:161-193.

50. Wolfson JS, Hooper DC. Fluoroquinolone antimicrobial agents. Clin Microbiol Rev. 1989;2:378-424.

51. Jacobs MR. Activity of quinolones against mycobacteria. Drugs. 1999;58:19-22.

52. Howard BM, Pinney RJ, Smith JT. 4-Quinolone bactericidal mechanisms. Arzneimittel-Forschung. 1993;43:1125-1129.

53. Hackbarth CJ, Chambers HF, Sande MA. Serum bactericidal activity of rifampin in combination with other antimicrobial agents against *Staphylococcus aureus*. Antimicrob Agents Chemother. 1986;29:611-613.

54. Dudley MN. Pharmacokinetics of fluoroquinolones. In: Hooper DC, Rubinstein E, eds. Quinolone Antimicrobial Agents. 3rd ed. Washington, DC: ASM Press; 2003:115-132.

55. Lode H, Hoffken G, Boeckk M, et al. Quinolone pharmacokinetics and metabolism. J Antimicrob Chemother. 1990;26(Suppl B):41-49.

56. Sorgel F, Kinzig M. Pharmacokinetics of gyrase inhibitors: Part 1. Basic chemistry and gastrointestinal disposition. Am J Med. 1993;94:44S-55S.

57. Staib AH, Beermann D, Harder S, et al. Absorption differences of ciprofloxacin along the human gastrointestinal tract determined using a remote-control drug delivery device (HF-capsule). Am J Med. 1989;87:66S-69S.

58. Healy DP, Brodbeck MC, Clendening CE. Ciprofloxacin absorption is impaired in patients given enteral feedings orally and via gastrostomy and jejunostomy tubes. Antimicrob Agents Chemother. 1996;40:6-10.

59. Yuk JH, Nightingale CH, Sweeney KR, et al. Relative bioavailability in healthy volunteers of ciprofloxacin administered through a nasogastric tube with and without enteral feeding. Antimicrob Agents Chemother. 1989;33:1118-1120.

60. Tamai I, Yamashita J, Kido Y, et al. Limited distribution of new quinolone antibacterial agents into brain caused by multiple efflux transporters at the blood-brain barrier. J Pharmacol Exp Ther. 2000;295:146-152.

61. Montay G, Gaillot J. Pharmacokinetics of fluoroquinolones in hepatic failure. J Antimicrob Chemother. 1990;26(Suppl B):61-67.

62. Giamarellou H, Kolokythas E, Petrikkos G, et al. Pharmacokinetics of three newer quinolones in pregnant and lactating women. Am J Med. 1989;87:49S-51S.

63. Sorgel F, Kinzig M. Pharmacokinetics of gyrase inhibitors: Part 2. Renal and hepatic elimination pathways and drug interactions. Am J Med. 1993;94:56S-69S.

64. Fillastre JP, Leroy A, Moulin B, et al. Pharmacokinetics of quinolones in renal insufficiency. J Antimicrob Chemother. 1990;26(Suppl B):51-60.

65. Malone RS, Fish DN, Abraham E, Teitelbaum I. Pharmacokinetics of levofloxacin and ciprofloxacin during continuous renal replacement therapy in critically ill patients. Antimicrob Agents Chemother. 2001;45:2949-2954.

66. Traunmuller F, Thalhammer-Scherrer R, Locker G, et al. Single-dose pharmacokinetics of levofloxacin during continuous veno-venous haemofiltration in critically ill patients. J Antimicrob Chemother. 2001;47:229-231.

67. Hooper DC, Wolfson JS. Fluoroquinolone antimicrobial agents. N Engl J Med. 1991;324:384-394.

68. Radandt JM, Marchbanks CR, Dudley MN. Interactions of fluoroquinolones with other drugs: Mechanisms, variability, clinical significance, and management. Clin Infect Dis. 1992;14:272-284.

69. Qaqish R, Polk RE. Drug-drug interactions. In: Hooper DC, Rubinstein E, eds. Quinolone Antimicrobial Agents. 3rd ed. Washington, DC: ASM Press; 2003:133-146.

70. Polk RE, Healy DP, Sahai J, et al. Effect of ferrous sulfate and multivitamins with zinc on absorption of ciprofloxacin in normal volunteers. Antimicrob Agents Chemother. 1989;33:1841-1844.

71. Fuhr U, Strobl G, Manaut F, et al. Quinolone antibacterial agents: Relationship between structure and in vitro inhibition of the human cytochrome P450 isoform CYP1A2. Mol Pharmacol. 1993;43:191-199.

72. Schwartz J, Jauregui L, Lettieri J, Bachmann K. Impact of ciprofloxacin on theophylline clearance and steady-state concentrations in serum. Antimicrob Agents Chemother. 1988;32:75-77.

73. Robson RA. The effects of quinolones on xanthine pharmacokinetics. Am J Med. 1992;92:22S-25S.

74. Raaska K, Neuvonen PJ. Ciprofloxacin increases serum clozapine and *N*-desmethylclozapine: A study in patients with schizophrenia. Eur J Clin Pharmacol. 2000;56:585-589.

75. Israel DS, Stotka J, Rock W, et al. Effect of ciprofloxacin on the pharmacokinetics and pharmacodynamics of warfarin. Clin Infect Dis. 1996;22:251-256.

76. Anonymous. Hypoglycemia and hyperglycemia with fluoroquinolones. Med Lett Drugs Ther. 2003;45:64.

77. Hori S, Shimada J, Saito A, et al. Comparison of the inhibitory effect of new quinolones on 46gamma-aminobutyric acid receptor binding in the presence of anti-inflammatory drugs. Rev Infect Dis. 1989;11:S1397-S1398.

78. Norrby SR. Central nervous system toxicity. In: Hooper DC, Rubinstein E, eds. Quinolone Antimicrobial Agents. 3rd ed. Washington, DC: ASM Press; 2003:461-465.

79. Wolfson JS, Hooper DC. Treatment of genitourinary tract infections with fluoroquinolones: Activity in vitro, pharmacokinetics, and clinical efficacy in urinary tract infections and prostatitis. Antimicrob Agents Chemother. 1989;33:1655-1661.

80. Gupta K, Naber K, Stamm W. Treatment of urinary tract infections. In: Hooper DC, Rubinstein E, eds. Quinolone Antimicrobial Agents. 3rd ed. Washington, DC: ASM Press; 2003:159-170.

81. Henry DC Jr, Bettis RB, Riffer E, et al. Comparison of once-daily extended-release ciprofloxacin and conventional twice-daily ciprofloxacin for the treatment of uncomplicated urinary tract infection in women. Clin Ther. 2002;24:2088-2104.

82. Raz R, Rottensterich E, Hefter H, et al. Single-dose ciprofloxacin in the treatment of uncomplicated urinary tract infection in women. Eur J Clin Microbiol Infect Dis. 1989;8:1040-1042.

83. Pfau A, Sacks TG. Single dose quinolone treatment in acute uncomplicated urinary tract infection in women. J Urol. 1993;149:532-534.

84. Saginur R, Nicolle LE. Single-dose compared with 3-day norfloxacin treatment of uncomplicated urinary tract infection in women. Canadian Infectious Diseases Society Clinical Trials Study Group. Arch Intern Med. 1992;152:1233-1237.

85. The Urinary Tract Infection Study Group. Coordinated multicenter study of norfloxacin versus trimethoprim-sulfamethoxazole of symptomatic urinary tract infections. J Infect Dis. 1987;155:170-177.

86. Raz R, Rottensterich E, Leshem Y, Tabenkin H. Double-blind study comparing 3-day regimens of cefixime and ofloxacin in treatment of uncomplicated urinary tract infections in women. Antimicrob Agents Chemother. 1994;38:1176-1177.

87. Richard GA, Klimberg IN, Fowler CL, et al. Levofloxacin versus ciprofloxacin versus lomefloxacin in acute pyelonephritis. Urology. 1998;52:51-55.

88. Warren JW, Abrutyn E, Hebel JR, et al. Guidelines for antimicrobial treatment of uncomplicated acute bacterial cystitis and acute pyelonephritis in women. Infectious Diseases Society of America (IDSA). Clin Infect Dis. 1999;29:745-758.

89. Raz R, Boger S. Long-term prophylaxis with norfloxacin versus nitrofurantoin in women with recurrent urinary tract infection. Antimicrob Agents Chemother. 1991;35:1241-1242.

90. Pfau A, Sacks TG. Effective postcoital quinolone prophylaxis of recurrent urinary tract infections in women. J Urol. 1994;152:136-138.

91. Krcméry S, Hromec J, Tvrdikova M, et al. Newer quinolones in the long term prophylaxis of recurrent urinary tract infections (UTI). Drugs. 1999;58:99-102.

92. Gupta K, Sahm DF, Mayfield D, Stamm WE. Antimicrobial resistance among uropathogens that cause community-acquired urinary tract infections in women: A nationwide analysis. Clin Infect Dis. 2001;33:89-94.

93. Raz R, Naber KG, Raizenberg C, et al. Ciprofloxacin 250 mg twice daily versus ofloxacin 200 mg twice daily in the treatment of complicated urinary tract infections in women. Eur J Clin Microbiol Infect Dis. 2000;19:327-331.

94. Fang GD, Brennen C, Wagener M, et al. Use of ciprofloxacin versus use of aminoglycosides for therapy of complicated urinary tract infection: prospective, randomized clinical and pharmacokinetic study. Antimicrob Agents Chemother. 1991;35:1849-1855.

95. Naber KG, Di Silverio F, Geddes A, Guibert J. Comparative efficacy of sparfloxacin versus ciprofloxacin in the treatment of complicated urinary tract infection. J Antimicrob Chemother. 1996;37:135-144.

96. Peng MY. Randomized, double-blind, comparative study of levofloxacin and ofloxacin in the treatment of complicated urinary tract infections. J Microbiol Immunol Infect. 1999;32:33-39.

97. Pisani E, Bartoletti R, Trinchieri A, Rizzo M. Lomefloxacin versus ciprofloxacin in the treatment of complicated urinary tract infections: A multicenter study. J Chemother. 1996;8:210-213.

98. Nakano M, Yasuda M, Yokoi S, et al. In vivo selection of *Pseudomonas aeruginosa* with decreased susceptibilities to fluoroquinolones during fluoroquinolone treatment of urinary tract infection. Urology. 2001;58:125-128.

99. Biering-Sørensen F, Høiby N, Nordenbo A, et al. Ciprofloxacin as prophylaxis for urinary tract infection: Prospective, randomized, cross-over, placebo controlled study in patients with spinal cord lesion. J Urol. 1994;151:105-108.

100. Christiano AP, Hollowell CMP, Kim H, et al. Double-blind randomized comparison of single-dose ciprofloxacin versus intravenous cefazolin in patients undergoing outpatient endourologic surgery. Urology. 2000;55:182-185.

101. Klimberg IW, Malek GH, Cox CE, et al. Single-dose oral ciprofloxacin compared with cefotaxime and placebo for prophylaxis during transurethral surgery. J Antimicrob Chemother. 1999;43:77-84.

102. Isen K, Kupeli B, Sinik Z, et al. Antibiotic prophylaxis for transrectal biopsy of the prostate: A prospective randomized study of the prophylactic use of single dose oral fluoroquinolone versus trimethoprim-sulfamethoxazole. Int Urol Nephrol. 1999;31:491-495.

103. Moyses Neto M, Costa RS, Reis MA, et al. Use of ciprofloxacin as a prophylactic agent in urinary tract infections in renal transplant recipients. Clin Transplantation. 1997;11:446-452.

104. Sabbaj J, Hoagland VL, Cook T. Norfloxacin versus co-trimoxazole in the treatment of recurring urinary tract infections in men. Scand J Infecti Dis Suppl. 1986;48:48-53.

105. Naber KG, Weidner W. Chronic prostatitis: An infectious disease? J Antimicrob Chemother. 2000;46:157-161.

106. Schaeffer AJ, Darras FS. The efficacy of norfloxacin in the treatment of chronic bacterial prostatitis refractory to trimethoprim-sulfamethoxazole and/or carbenicillin. J Urol. 1990;144:690-693.

107. Peeling RW, Ronald AR. Use of quinolones for treatment of sexually transmitted diseases. In: Hooper DC, Rubinstein E, eds. Quinolone Antimicrobial Agents. 3rd ed. Washington, DC: ASM Press; 2003:171-192.

108. Hooper DC, Wolfson JS. Treatment of genitourinary tract infections with fluoroquinolones: Clinical efficacy in genital infections and adverse effects. Antimicrob Agents Chemother. 1989;33:1662-1667.

109. Thorpe EM, Schwebke JR, Hook EW, et al. Comparison of single-dose cefuroxime axetil with ciprofloxacin in treatment of uncomplicated gonorrhea caused by penicillinase-producing and non-penicillinase-producing *Neisseria gonorrhoeae* strains. Antimicrob Agents Chemother. 1996;40:2775-2780.

110. Jones RB, Schwebke J, Thorpe EM Jr, et al. Randomized trial of trovafloxacin and ofloxacin for single-dose therapy of gonorrhea. Am J Med. 1998;104:28-32.

111. Stoner BP, Douglas JM, Martin DH, et al. Single dose gatifloxacin compared with ofloxacin for the treatment of uncomplicated gonorrhea. Sex Transm Dis. 2000;28:136-42.

112. Lutz FB Jr. Single-dose efficacy of ofloxacin in uncomplicated gonorrhea. Am J Med. 1989;87:69S-74S.

113. Centers for Disease Control and Prevention. Guidelines for treatment of sexually transmitted diseases. Morb Mortal Wkly Rep. 2002;51:1-78.

114. Crombleholme WR, Schachter J, Ohm-Smith M, et al. Efficacy of single-agent therapy for the treatment of acute pelvic inflammatory disease with ciprofloxacin. Am J Med. 1989;87:142S-147S.

115. Wendel GDJ, Cox SM, Bawdon RE, et al. A randomized trial of ofloxacin versus cefoxitin and doxycycline in the outpatient treatment of acute salpingitis. Am J Obstet Gynecol. 1991;164:1390-1396.

116. Knapp JS, Fox KK, Trees DL, Whittington WL. Fluoroquinolone resistance in *Neisseria gonorrhoeae*. Emerg Infect Dis. 1997;3:33-39.

117. Gordon SM, Carlyn CJ, Doyle LJ, et al. The emergence of *Neisseria gonorrhoeae* with decreased susceptibility to ciprofloxacin in Cleveland, Ohio: Epidemiology and risk factors. Ann Intern Med. 1996;125:465-470.

118. Centers for Disease Control and Prevention. Fluoroquinolone-resistance in *Neisseria gonorrhoeae* in Hawaii, 1999, and decreased susceptibility to azithromycin in *N. gonorrhoeae*, Missouri 1999. Morb Mortal Wkly Rep. 2000;49:833-837.

119. Centers for Disease Control and Prevention. Increases in fluoroquinolone-resistant *Neisseria gonorrhoeae*—Hawaii and California, 2001. Morb Mortal Wkly Rep. 2002;51:1041-1044.

120. Bosleyo JW, Hicks CB, Greenup R, et al. A prospective randomized trial of ofloxacin vs. doxycycline in the treatment of uncomplicated male urethritis. Sex Transm Dis. 1988;15:186-191.

121. Hooton TM, Batteiger BE, Judson FN, et al. Ofloxacin versus doxycycline for treatment of cervical infection with *Chlamydia trachomatis*. Antimicrob Agents Chemother. 1992;36:1144-1146.

122. Kitchen VS, Donegan C, Ward H, et al. Comparison of ofloxacin with doxycycline in the treatment of non-gonococcal urethritis and cervical chlamydial infection. J Antimicrob Chemother. 1990;26(Suppl D):99-105.

123. Mikamo H, Sato Y, Hayasaki Y, et al. Adequate levofloxacin treatment schedules for uterine cervicitis caused by *Chlamydia trachomatis*. Chemotherapy. 2000;46:150-152.

124. Naamara W, Plummer FA, Greenblatt RM, et al. Treatment of chancroid with ciprofloxacin: A prospective, randomized clinical trial. Am J Med. 1987;82:317-320.

125. Behets FM, Liomba G, Lule G, et al. Sexually transmitted diseases and human immunodeficiency virus control in Malawi: A field study of genital ulcers. J Infect Dis. 1995;171:451-455.

126. Martens MG, Gordon S, Yarborough DR, et al. Multicenter randomized trial of ofloxacin versus cefoxitin and doxycycline in outpatient treatment of pelvic inflammatory disease. South Med J. 1993;86:604-610.

127. Arredondo JL, Diaz V, Gaitan H, et al. Oral clindamycin and ciprofloxacin versus intramuscular ceftriaxone and oral doxycycline in the treatment of mild-to-moderate pelvic inflammatory disease in outpatients. Clin Infect Dis. 1997;24:170-178.

128. Covino JM, Black JR, Cummings M, et al. Comparative evaluation of ofloxacin and metronidazole in the treatment of bacterial vaginosis. Sex Transm Dis. 1993;20: 262-264.

129. Bennish ML. Treatment and prophylaxis of gastroenteritis. In: Hooper DC, Rubinstein E, eds. Quinolone Antimicrobial Agents. 3rd ed. Washington, DC: ASM Press; 2003:193-216.

130. Wiström J, Jertborn M, Hedstrom SA, et al. Short-term self-treatment of travellers' diarrhoea with norfloxacin: A placebo-controlled study. J Antimicrob Chemother. 1989;23:905-913.

131. Ericsson CD, Johnson PC, DuPont HL, et al. Ciprofloxacin or trimethoprim-sulfamethoxazole as initial therapy for travelers' diarrhea: A placebo-controlled, randomized trial. Ann Intern Med. 1987;106:216-220.

132. Gomi H, Jiang ZD, Adachi JA, et al. In vitro antimicrobial susceptibility testing of bacterial enteropathogens causing traveler's diarrhea in four geographic regions. Antimicrob Agents Chemother. 2001;45:212-216.

133. Petruccelli BP, Murphy GS, Sanchez JL, et al. Treatment of travelers' diarrhea with ciprofloxacin and loperamide. J Infect Dis. 1992;165:557-560.

134. Salam I, Katelaris P, Leigh-Smith S, Farthing MJG. Randomised trial of single-dose ciprofloxacin for travellers' diarrhoea. Lancet. 1994;344:1537-1539.

135. Ericsson CD, DuPont HL, Mathewson JJ. Single dose ofloxacin plus loperamide compared with single dose or three days of ofloxacin in the treatment of traveler's diarrhea. J Travel Med. 1997;4:3-7.

136. DuPont HL, Ericsson CD. Prevention and treatment of traveler's diarrhea. N Engl J Med. 1993;328:1821-1827.

137. Heck JE, Staneck JL, Cohen MB, et al. Prevention of travelers' diarrhea: Ciprofloxacin versus trimethoprim/sulfamethoxazole in adult volunteers working in Latin America and the Caribbean. J Travel Med. 1994;1:136-142.

138. Mattila L, Peltola H, Siitonen A, et al. Short-term treatment of traveler's diarrhea with norfloxacin: A double-blind, placebo-controlled study during two seasons. Clin Infect Dis. 1993;17:779-782.

139. Khan WA, Seas C, Dhar U, et al. Treatment of shigellosis: V. Comparison of azithromycin and ciprofloxacin. A double-blind, randomized, controlled trial. Ann Intern Med. 1997;126:697-703.

140. Murphy GS, Bodhidatta L, Echeverria P, et al. Ciprofloxacin and loperamide in the treatment of bacillary dysentery. Ann Intern Med. 1993;118:582-586.

141. Bennish ML, Salam MA, Khan WA, Khan AM. Treatment of shigellosis: III. Comparison of one- or two-dose ciprofloxacin with standard 5-day therapy. A randomized, blinded trial. Ann Intern Med. 1992;117:727-734.

142. Pichler HE, Diridl G, Wolf D. Ciprofloxacin in the treatment of acute bacterial diarrhea: A double blind study. Eur J Clin Microbiol. 1986;5:241-243.

143. Wiström J, Jertborn M, Ekwall E, et al. Empiric treatment of acute diarrheal disease with norfloxacin. A randomized, placebo-controlled study. Swedish Study Group. Ann Intern Med. 1992;117:202-208.

144. Sanchez C, Garcia-Restoy E, Garau J, et al. Ciprofloxacin and trimethoprim-sulfamethoxazole versus placebo in acute uncomplicated *Salmonella* gastroenteritis: A double-blind trial. J Infect Dis. 1993;168:1304-1307.

145. Neill MA, Opal SM, Heelan J, et al. Failure of ciprofloxacin to eradicate convalescent fecal excretion after acute salmonellosis: Experience during an outbreak in health care workers. Ann Intern Med. 1991;114:195-199.

146. Dryden MS, Gabb RJ, Wright SK. Empirical treatment of severe acute community-acquired gastroenteritis with ciprofloxacin. Clin Infect Dis. 1996;22:1019-1025.

147. Hung CC, Hsieh SM, Hsiao CF, et al. Risk of recurrent non-typhoidal *Salmonella* bacteraemia after early discontinuation of ciprofloxacin as secondary prophylaxis in AIDS patients in the era of highly active antiretroviral therapy. AIDS. 2001;15:645-647.

148. Pichler HE, Diridl G, Stickler K, Wolf D. Clinical efficacy of ciprofloxacin compared with placebo in bacterial diarrhea. Am J Med. 1987;82:329-332.

149. Goodman LJ, Trenholme GM, Kaplan RL, et al. Empiric antimicrobial therapy of domestically acquired acute diarrhea in urban adults. Arch Intern Med. 1990;150:541-546.

150. Smith KE, Besser JM, Hedberg CW, et al. Quinolone-resistant *Campylobacter jejuni* infections in Minnesota, 1992-1998. N Engl J Med. 1999;340:1525-1532.

151. Bhattacharya SK, Bhattacharya MK, Dutta P, et al. Double-blind, randomized, controlled clinical trial of norfloxacin for cholera. Antimicrob Agents Chemother. 1990;34:939-940.

152. Dutta D, Bhattacharya SK, Bhattacharya MK, et al. Efficacy of norfloxacin and doxycycline for treatment of *Vibrio cholerae* O139 infection. J Antimicrob Chemother. 1996;37:575-581.

153. Gotuzzo E, Seas C, Echeverria P, et al. Ciprofloxacin for the treatment of cholera: A randomized, double-blind, controlled clinical trial of a single daily dose in Peruvian adults. Clin Infect Dis. 1995;20:1485-1490.

154. Khan WA, Bennish ML, Seas C, et al. Randomised controlled comparison of single-dose ciprofloxacin and doxycycline for cholera caused by *Vibrio cholerae* 01 or 0139. Lancet. 1996;348:296-300.

155. Usubutun S, Agalar C, Diri C, Turkyilmaz R. Single dose ciprofloxacin in cholera. Eur J Emerg Med. 1997;4:145-149.

156. Wang F, Gu XJ, Zhang MF, Tai TY. Treatment of typhoid fever with ofloxacin. J Antimicrob Chemother. 1989;23:785-788.

157. Uwaydah AK, Al Soub H, Matar I. Randomized prospective study comparing two dosage regimens of ciprofloxacin for the treatment of typhoid fever. J Antimicrob Chemother. 1992;30:707-711.

158. Wallace MR, Yousif AA, Hahroos GA, et al. Ciprofloxacin versus ceftriaxone in the treatment of multiresistant typhoid. Eur J Clin Microbiol Infect Dis. 1993;12:907-910.

159. Wain J, Hoa NT, Chinh NT, et al. Quinolone-resistant *Salmonella typhi* in Viet Nam: Molecular basis of resistance and clinical response to treatment. Clin Infect Dis. 1997;25:1404-1410.

160. Gotuzzo E, Guerra JG, Benavente L, et al. Use of norfloxacin to treat chronic typhoid carriers. J Infect Dis. 1988;157:1221-1225.

161. Ferreccio C, Morris JGJ, Valdivieso C, et al. Efficacy of ciprofloxacin in the treatment of chronic typhoid carriers. J Infect Dis. 1988;157:1235-1239.

162. Chrysanthopoulos CJ, Skoutelis AT, Starakis JC, et al. Use of ciprofloxacin in biliary sepsis. Infection. 1988;16:249-250.

163. Sung JJ, Sollano JD, Lai CW, et al. Long-term ciprofloxacin treatment for the prevention of biliary stent blockage: A prospective randomized study. Am J Gastroenterol. 1999;94:3197-3201.

164. Solomkin JS, Reinhart HH, Dellinger EP, et al. Results of a randomized trial comparing sequential intravenous oral treatment with ciprofloxacin plus metronidazole to imipenem cilastatin for intra-abdominal infections. Ann Surg. 1996;223:303-315.

165. Solomkin JS. Treatment of intra-abdominal infections. In: Hooper DC, Rubinstein E, eds. Quinolone Antimicrobial Agents. 3rd ed. Washington, DC: ASM Press; 2003:217-225.

166. Cohn SM, Lipsett PA, Buchman TG, et al. Comparison of intravenous/oral ciprofloxacin plus metronidazole versus piperacillin/tazobactam in the treatment of complicated intraabdominal infections. Ann Surg. 2000;232:254-262.

167. Starakis I, Karravias D, Asimakopoulos C, et al. Results of a prospective, randomized, double blind comparison of the efficacy and the safety of sequential ciprofloxacin (intravenous/oral)+metronidazole (intravenous/oral) with ceftriaxone (intravenous)+metronidazole (intravenous/oral) for the treatment of intra-abdominal infections. Int J Antimicrob Agents. 2003;21:49-57.

168. Donahue PE, Smith DL, Yellin AE, et al. Trovafloxacin in the treatment of intra-abdominal infections: Results of a double blind, multicenter comparison with imipenem/cilastatin. Am J Surg. 1998;176:53S-61S.

169. Friedland JS, Iveson TJ, Fraise AP, et al. A comparison between intraperitoneal ciprofloxacin and intraperitoneal vancomycin and gentamicin in the treatment of peritonitis associated with continuous ambulatory peritoneal dialysis (CAPD). J Antimicrob Chemother. 1990;26:77-81.

170. de Fijter CW, ter Wee PM, Oe LP, Verbrugh HA. Intraperitoneal ciprofloxacin and rifampicin versus cephradine as initial treatment of (C)APD-related peritonitis: A prospective randomized multicenter comparison (CIPPER trial). Perit Dial Int. 2001;21:480-486.

171. Cheng IK, Fang GX, Chau PY, et al. A randomized prospective comparison of oral levofloxacin plus intraperitoneal (IP) vancomycin and IP netromycin plus IP vancomycin as primary treatment of peritonitis complicating CAPD. Perit Dial Int. 1998;18:371-375.

172. Terg R, Cobas S, Fassio E, et al. Oral ciprofloxacin after a short course of intravenous ciprofloxacin in the treatment of spontaneous bacterial peritonitis: Results of a multicenter, randomized study. J Hepatol. 2000;33:564-569.

173. Gines P, Rimola A, Planas R, et al. Norfloxacin prevents spontaneous bacterial peritonitis recurrence in cirrhosis: Results of a double-blind, placebo-controlled trial. Hepatology. 1990;12:716-724.

174. Rolachon A, Cordier L, Bacq Y, et al. Ciprofloxacin and long-term prevention of spontaneous bacterial peritonitis: Results of a prospective controlled trial. Hepatology. 1995;22:1171-1174.

175. Dupeyron C, Mangeney N, Sedrati L, et al. Rapid emergence of quinolone resistance in cirrhotic patients treated with norfloxacin to prevent spontaneous bacterial peritonitis. Antimicrob Agents Chemother. 1994;38:340-344.

176. Cereto F, Molina I, Gonzalez A, et al. Role of immunosuppression in the development of quinolone-resistant *Escherichia coli* spontaneous bacterial peritonitis and in the mortality of *E. coli* spontaneous bacterial peritonitis. Aliment Pharmacol Ther. 2003;17:695-701.

177. Ball P, Mandell L. Treatment of community-acquired respiratory tract infections. In: Hooper DC, Rubinstein E, eds. Quinolone Antimicrobial Agents. 3rd ed. Washington, DC: ASM Press; 2003:227-243.

178. Grossman R, Mukherjee J, Vaughan D, et al. A 1-year community-based health economic study of ciprofloxacin vs usual antibiotic treatment in acute exacerbations of chronic bronchitis—The Canadian Ciprofloxacin Health Economic Study Group. Chest. 1998;113:131-141.

179. DeAbate CA, Russell M, McElvaine P, et al. Safety and efficacy of oral levofloxacin versus cefuroxime axetil in acute bacterial exacerbation of chronic bronchitis. Respir Care. 1997;42:206-213.

180. Shah PM, Maesen FP, Dolmann A, et al. Levofloxacin versus cefuroxime axetil in the treatment of acute exacerbation of chronic bronchitis: Results of a randomized, double-blind study. J Antimicrob Chemother. 1999;43:529-539.

181. Davies BI, Maesen FPV. Clinical effectiveness of levofloxacin in patients with acute purulent exacerbations of chronic bronchitis: The relationship with in vitro activity. J Antimicrob Chemother. 1999;43:83-90.

182. Ramirez A, Molina J, Dolmann A, et al. Gatifloxacin treatment in patients with acute exacerbations of chronic bronchitis: Clinical trail results. J Resp Dis. 1999;20:S30-S39.

183. DeAbate CA, McIvor RA, McElvaine P, et al. Gatifloxacin vs cefuroxime axetil in patients with acute exacerbations of chronic bronchitis. J Resp Dis. 1999;20:S23-S29.

184. Wilson R, Kubin R, Ballin I, et al. Five day moxifloxacin therapy compared with 7 day clarithromycin therapy for the treatment of acute exacerbations of chronic bronchitis. J Antimicrob Chemother. 1999;44:501-513.

185. Chodosh S, DeAbate CA, Haverstock D, et al. Short-course moxifloxacin therapy for treatment of acute bacterial exacerbations of chronic bronchitis. The Bronchitis Study Group. Respir Med. 2000;94:18-27.

186. DeAbate CA, Mathew CP, Warner JH, et al. The safety and efficacy of short course (5-day) moxifloxacin vs. azithromycin in the treatment of patients with acute exacerbation of chronic bronchitis. Respir Med. 2000;94:1029-1037.

187. Wilson R, Schentag JJ, Ball P, Mandell L. A comparison of gemifloxacin and clarithromycin in acute exacerbations of chronic bronchitis and long-term clinical outcomes. Clin Ther. 2002;24:639-652.

188. Ball P, Wilson R, Mandell L, et al. Efficacy of gemifloxacin in acute exacerbations of chronic bronchitis: A randomised, double-blind comparison with trovafloxacin. J Chemother. 2001;13:288-298.

189. Wilson R, Langan C, Ball P, et al. Oral gemifloxacin once daily for 5 days compared with sequential therapy with i.v. ceftriaxone/oral cefuroxime (maximum of 10 days) in the treatment of hospitalized patients with acute exacerbations of chronic bronchitis. Respir Med. 2003;97:242-249.

190. Chodosh S, Schreurs A, Siami G, et al. Efficacy of oral ciprofloxacin vs. clarithromycin for treatment of acute bacterial exacerbations of chronic bronchitis. Clin Infect Dis. 1998;27:730-738.

191. Chodosh S, McCarty J, Farkas S, et al. Randomized, double-blind study of ciprofloxacin and cefuroxime axetil for treatment of acute bacterial exacerbations of chronic bronchitis. Clin Infect Dis. 1998;27:722-729.

192. Chrysanthopoulos CJ, Starakis JC, Skoutelis AT, et al. Sequential intravenous/oral therapy with ciprofloxacin in severe infection. Am J Med. 1989;87:225S-227S.

193. Gentry LO, Rodriguez-Gomez G, Kohler RB, et al. Parenteral followed by oral ofloxacin for nosocomial pneumonia and community-acquired pneumonia requiring hospitalization. Am Rev Resp Dis. 1992;145:31-35.

194. Plouffe JF, Herbert MT, File TM Jr, et al. Ofloxacin versus standard therapy in treatment of community-acquired pneumonia requiring hospitalization. Antimicrob Agents Chemother. 1996;40:1175-1179.

195. Sanders WE Jr, Morris JF, Alessi P, et al. Oral ofloxacin for the treatment of acute bacterial pneumonia: Use of a nontraditional protocol to compare experimental therapy with "usual care" in a multicenter clinical trial. Am J Med. 1991;91:261-266.

196. File TM Jr, Segreti J, Dunbar L, et al. A multicenter, randomized study comparing the efficacy and safety of intravenous and/or oral levofloxacin versus ceftriaxone and/or cefuroxime axetil in treatment of adults with community-acquired pneumonia. Antimicrob Agents Chemother. 1997;41:1965-1972.

197. Norrby SR, Petermann W, Willcox PA, et al. A comparative study of levofloxacin and ceftriaxone in the treatment of hospitalized patients with pneumonia. Scand J Infect Dis. 1998;30:397-404.

198. Carbon C, Ariza H, Rabie WJ, et al. Comparative study of levofloxacin and amoxicillin-clavulanic acid in adults with mild-to-moderate community-acquired pneumonia. Clin Microbiol Infect. 1999;5:724-732.

199. Fogarty C, Dowell ME, Ellison WT, et al. A prospective, randomized, double-blind study treating community-acquired pneumonia in hospitalized patients: Gatifloxacin vs ceftriaxone/clarithromycin. J Resp Dis. 1999;20:S60-S69.

200. Correa JC, Badaro R, Bumroongkit C, et al. Randomized, open-label, parallel-group, multicenter study of the efficacy and tolerability of IV gatifloxacin with the option for oral stepdown gatifloxacin versus IV ceftriaxone (with or without erythromycin or clarithromycin) with the option for oral stepdown clarithromycin for treatment of patients with mild to moderate community-acquired pneumonia requiring hospitalization. Clin Ther. 2003;25:1453-1468.

201. Sullivan JG, McElroy AD, Honsinger RW, et al. A double-blind, randomized study of safety and efficacy treating community-acquired pneumonia with once-daily gatifloxacin vs once-daily levofloxacin. J Resp Dis. 1999;20:S49-S59.

202. Ramirez JA, Nguyen T-H, Tellier G, et al. A prospective, randomized, double-blind, comparative study treating community-acquired pneumonia with once-daily gatifloxacin vs twice-daily clarithromycin. J Resp Dis. 1999;20:S40-S48.

203. Fogarty C, Grossman C, Williams J, et al. Efficacy and safety of moxifloxacin vs clarithromycin for community-acquired pneumonia. Infect Med. 1999;16:748-763.

204. Petitpretz P, Arvis P, Marel M, et al. Oral moxifloxacin vs high-dosage amoxicillin in the treatment of mild- to-moderate, community-acquired, suspected pneumococcal pneumonia in adults. Chest. 2001;119:185-195.

205. Lode H, File TM Jr, Mandell L, et al. Oral gemifloxacin versus sequential therapy with intravenous ceftriaxone/oral cefuroxime with or without a macrolide in the treatment of patients hospitalized with community-acquired pneumonia: A randomized, open-label, multicenter study of clinical efficacy and tolerability. Clin Ther. 2002;24:1915-1936.

206. Finch R, Schürmann D, Collins O, et al. Randomized controlled trial of sequential intravenous (i.v.) and oral moxifloxacin compared with sequential i.v. and oral co-amoxiclav with or without clarithromycin in patients with community-acquired pneumonia requiring initial parenteral treatment. Antimicrob Agents Chemother. 2002;46:1746-1754.

207. File TM Jr, Schlemmer B, Garau J, et al. Efficacy and safety of gemifloxacin in the treatment of community-acquired pneumonia: A randomized, double-blind comparison with trovafloxacin. J Antimicrob Chemother. 2001;48:67-74.

208. Jones RN, Andes DR, Mandell LA, et al. Gatifloxacin used for therapy of outpatient community-acquired pneumonia caused by *Streptococcus pneumoniae*. Diagn Microbiol Infect Dis. 2002;44:93-100.

209. Fine MJ, Auble TE, Yealy DM, et al. A prediction rule to identify low-risk patients with community-acquired pneumonia. N Engl J Med. 1997;336:243-250.

210. Davidson R, Cavalcanti R, Brunton JL, et al. Resistance to levofloxacin and failure of treatment of pneumococcal pneumonia. N Engl J Med. 2002;346:747-750.

211. Mouton Y, Leroy O, Beuscart C, et al. Efficacy of intravenous ofloxacin: A French multicentre trial in 185 patients. J Antimicrob Chemother. 1990;26 Suppl D:115-121.

212. Unertl KE, Lenhart FP, Forst H, et al. Ciprofloxacin in the treatment of legionellosis in critically ill patients including those cases unresponsive to erythromycin. Am J Med. 1989;87:128S-131S.

213. Lipsky BA, Tack KJ, Kuo CC, et al. Ofloxacin treatment of *Chlamydia pneumoniae* (strain TWAR) lower respiratory tract infections. Am J Med. 1990;89:722-724.

214. Fogarty C, Grossman C, Williams J, et al. Efficacy and safety of moxifloxacin vs clarithromycin for community-acquired pneumonia. Infect Med. 1999;16:748-763.

215. Edelstein PH. Antimicrobial chemotherapy for Legionnaire's disease: Time for a change. Ann Intern Med. 1998;129:328-330.

216. Peloquin CA, Cumbo TJ, Nix DE, et al. Evaluation of intravenous ciprofloxacin in patients with nosocomial lower respiratory tract infections: Impact of plasma concentrations, organism, minimum inhibitory concentration, and clinical condition on bacterial eradication. Arch Intern Med. 1989;149:2269-2273.

217. Fink MP, Snydman DR, Niederman MS, et al. Treatment of severe pneumonia in hospitalized patients: Results of a multicenter, randomized, double-blind trial comparing intravenous ciprofloxacin with imipenem-cilastatin. Antimicrob Agents Chemother. 1994;38:547-557.

218. West M, Boulanger BR, Fogarty C, et al. Levofloxacin compared with imipenem/cilastatin followed by ciprofloxacin in adult patients with nosocomial pneumonia: A multicenter, prospective, randomized, open-label study. Clin Ther. 2003;25:485-506.

219. Johnson PA, Rodriguez HP, Wazen JJ, et al. Ciprofloxacin versus cefuroxime axetil in the treatment of acute bacterial sinusitis. Sinusitis Infection Study Group. J Otolaryngol. 1999;28:3-12.

220. Adelglass J, DeAbate CA, McElvaine P, et al. Comparison of the effectiveness of levofloxacin and amoxicillin-clavulanate for the treatment of acute sinusitis in adults. Otolaryngol Head Neck Surg. 1999;120:320-327.

221. Adelglass J, Jones TM, Ruoff G, et al. A multicenter, investigator-blinded, randomized comparison of oral levofloxacin and oral clarithromycin in the treatment of acute bacterial sinusitis. Pharmacother. 1998;18:1255-1263.

222. Fogarty C, McAdoo M, Paster RZ, et al. Gatifloxacin vs clarithromycin in the management of acute sinusitis. J Resp Dis. 1999;20:S17-S22.

223. Burke T, Villanueva C, Mariano H Jr, et al. Comparison of moxifloxacin and cefuroxime axetil in the treatment of acute maxillary sinusitis. Sinusitis Infection Study Group. Clin Ther. 1999;21:1664-1677.

224. Siegert R, Gehanno P, Nikolaidis P, et al. A comparison of the safety and efficacy of moxifloxacin (BAY 12-8039) and cefuroxime axetil in the treatment of acute bacterial sinusitis in adults. The Sinusitis Study Group. Respir Med. 2000;94:337-344.

225. Sydnor TA, Kopp EJ, Anthony KE, et al. Open-label assessment of levofloxacin for the treatment of acute bacterial sinusitis in adults. Ann Allergy Asthma Immunol. 1998;80:357-362.

226. Sisniega JAL, Jones RW, Kaminszczik G, et al. An open-label, multicenter, noncomparative study treating acute, uncomplicated sinusitis with gatifloxacin. J Resp Dis. 1999;20:S11-S16.

227. Grandis JR, Yu VL. Treatment of infections of the ears, nose, and throat and nasal carriage. In: Hooper DC, Rubinstein E, eds. Quinolone Antimicrobial Agents. 3rd ed. Washington, DC: ASM Press; 2003:245-250.

228. Levenson MJ, Parisier SC, Dolitsky J, Bindra G. Ciprofloxacin: Drug of choice in the treatment of malignant external otitis (MEO). Laryngoscope. 1991;101:821-824.

229. Gentry LO. Oral antimicrobial therapy for osteomyelitis. Ann Intern Med. 1991;114:986-987.

230. Greenberg RN, Newman MT, Shariaty S, Pectol RW. Ciprofloxacin, lomefloxacin, or levofloxacin as treatment for chronic osteomyelitis. Antimicrob Agents Chemother. 2000;44:164-166.

231. Bernard L, Waldvogel F, Lew D. Treatment of osteomyelitis and septic arthritis. In: Hooper DC, Rubinstein E, eds. Quinolone Antimicrobial Agents. 3rd ed. Washington, DC: ASM Press; 2003:251-258.

232. Peterson LR, Lissack LM, Canter K, et al. Therapy of lower extremity infections with ciprofloxacin in patients with diabetes mellitus, peripheral vascular disease, or both. Am J Med. 1989;86:801-808.

233. Lipsky BA, Baker PD, Landon GC, Fernau R. Antibiotic therapy for diabetic foot infections: Comparison of two parenteral-to-oral regimens. Clin Infect Dis. 1997;24:643-648.

234. Raz R, Miron D. Oral ciprofloxacin for treatment of infection following nail puncture wounds of the foot. Clin Infect Dis. 1995;21:194-195.

235. Gentry LO, Rodriguez-Gomez G. Ofloxacin versus parenteral therapy for chronic osteomyelitis. Antimicrob Agents Chemother. 1991;35:538-541.

236. Drancourt M, Stein A, Argenson JN, et al. Oral rifampin plus ofloxacin for treatment of Staphylococcus-infected orthopedic implants. Antimicrob Agents Chemother. 1993;37:1214-1218.

237. Zimmerli W, Widmer AF, Blatter M, et al. Role of rifampin for treatment of orthopedic implant-related staphylococcal infections: A randomized controlled trial. Foreign-Body Infection (FBI) Study Group. JAMA. 1998;279:1537-1541.

238. Brouqui P, Rousseau MC, Stein A, et al. Treatment of Pseudomonas aeruginosa-infected orthopedic prostheses with ceftazidime-ciprofloxacin antibiotic combination. Antimicrob Agents Chemother. 1995;39:2423-2425.

239. Gentry LO. Review of quinolones in the treatment of infections of the skin and skin structure. J Antimicrob Chemother. 1991;28(Suppl C):97-110.

240. Karchmer AW. Treatment of skin and soft tissue infections. In: Hooper DC, Rubinstein E, eds. Quinolone Antimicrobial Agents. 3rd ed. Washington, DC: ASM Press; 2003:311-321.

241. Powers RD, Schwartz R, Snow RM, Yarbrough DR III. Ofloxacin versus cephalexin in the treatment of skin, skin structure, and soft-tissue infections in adults. Clin Ther. 1991;13:727-736.

242. Nichols RL, Smith JW, Gentry LO, et al. Multicenter, randomized study comparing levofloxacin and ciprofloxacin for uncomplicated skin and skin structure infections. South Med J. 1997;90:1193-1200.

243. Tarshis GA, Miskin BM, Jones TM, et al. Once-daily oral gatifloxacin versus oral levofloxacin in treatment of uncomplicated skin and soft tissue infections: Double-blind, multicenter, randomized study. Antimicrob Agents Chemother. 2001;45:2358-2362.

244. Parish LC, Routh HB, Miskin B, et al. Moxifloxacin versus cephalexin in the treatment of uncomplicated skin infections. Int J Clin Pract. 2000;54:497-503.

245. Gentry LO, Ramirez-Ronda CH, Rodriguez-Noriega E, et al. Oral ciprofloxacin vs parenteral cefotaxime in the treatment of difficult skin and skin structure infections: A multicenter trial. Arch Intern Med. 1989;149:2579-2583.

246. Fass RL, Plouffe JF, Russell JA. Intravenous/oral ciprofloxacin versus ceftazidime in the treatment of serious infections. Am J Med. 1989;18:153-157.

247. Gentry LO, Rodriguez-Gomez G, Zeluff BJ, et al. A comparative evaluation of oral ofloxacin versus intravenous cefotaxime therapy for serious skin and skin structure infections. Am J Med. 1989;87:57S-60S.

248. Daniel R, The Trovafloxacin Study Group. Trovafloxacin once daily vs. flucloxacillin four times daily in the treatment of uncomplicated skin and skin-structure infections. Drugs. 1999;58:293-294.

249. Bartlett JG, Inglesby TV, Borio L. Management of anthrax. Clin Infect Dis. 2002;35:851-858.

250. Trucksis M, Hooper DC, Wolfson JS. Emerging resistance to fluoroquinolones in staphylococci: An alert. Ann Intern Med. 1991;114:424-426.

251. Yew WW, Kwan SY, Ma WK, et al. In-vitro activity of ofloxacin against Mycobacterium tuberculosis and its clinical efficacy in multiply resistant pulmonary tuberculosis. J Antimicrob Chemother. 1990;26:227-236.

252. Tsukamura M, Nakamura E, Yoshii S, Amano H. Therapeutic effect of a new antibacterial substance ofloxacin (DL8280) on pulmonary tuberculosis. Am Rev Resp Dis. 1985;131:352-356.

253. Mohanty KC, Dhamgaye TM. Controlled trial of ciprofloxacin in short-term chemotherapy for pulmonary tuberculosis. Chest. 1993;104:1194-1198.

254. Kennedy N, Berger L, Curram J, et al. Randomized controlled trial of a drug regimen that includes ciprofloxacin for the treatment of pulmonary tuberculosis. Clin Infect Dis. 1996;22:827-833.

255. de Lalla F, Maserati R, Scarpellini P, et al. Clarithromycin-ciprofloxacin-amikacin for therapy of Mycobacterium avium-Mycobacterium intracellulare bacteremia in patients with AIDS. Antimicrob Agents Chemother. 1992;36:1567-1569.

256. Kemper CA, Meng TC, Nussbaum J, et al. Treatment of Mycobacterium avium complex bacteremia in AIDS with a four-drug oral regimen: Rifampin, ethambutol, clofazimine, and ciprofloxacin. The California Collaborative Treatment Group. Ann Intern Med. 1992;116:466-472.

257. Shafran SD, Singer J, Zarowny DP, et al. A comparison of two regimens for the treatment of Mycobacterium avium complex bacteremia in AIDS: Rifabutin, ethambutol, and clarithromycin versus rifampin, ethambutol, clofazimine, and ciprofloxacin. N Engl J Med. 1996;335:377-383.

258. Yew WW, Kwan SY, Ma WK, et al. Ofloxacin therapy of Mycobacterium fortuitum infection: Further experience. J Antimicrob Chemother. 1990;25:880-881.

259. Grosset JH, Ji BH, Guelpa-Lauras CC, et al. Clinical trial of pefloxacin and ofloxacin in the treatment of lepromatous leprosy. Int J Lepr Other Mycobact Dis. 1990;58:281-295.

260. Bouza E, Diaz-Lopez MD, Bernaldo de Quiros JC, Rodriguez-Creixems M. Ciprofloxacin in patients with bacteremic infections. The Spanish Group for the Study of Ciprofloxacin. Am J Med. 1989;87:228S-231S.

261. Regamey C, Steinbach-Lebbin C. Severe infections treated with intravenous ofloxacin: A prospective clinical multicentre Swiss study. J Antimicrob Chemother. 1990;26(Suppl D):107-114.

262. Chan CC, Oppenheim BA, Anderson H, et al. Randomized trial comparing ciprofloxacin plus netilmicin versus piperacillin plus netilmicin for empiric treatment of fever in neutropenic patients. Antimicrob Agents Chemother. 1989;33:87-91.

263. Meunier F, Zinner SH, Gaya H, et al. Prospective randomized evaluation of ciprofloxacin versus piperacillin plus amikacin for empiric antibiotic therapy of febrile granulocytopenic cancer patients with lymphomas and solid tumors. The European Organization for Research on Treatment of Cancer International Antimicrobial Therapy Cooperative Group. Antimicrob Agents Chemother. 1991;35:873-878.

264. Giamarellou H, Bassaris HP, Petrikkos G, et al. Monotherapy with intravenous followed by oral high-dose ciprofloxacin versus combination therapy with ceftazidime plus amikacin as initial empiric therapy for granulocytopenic patients with fever. Antimicrob Agents Chemother. 2000;44:3264-3271.

265. Peacock JE, Herrington DA, Wade JC, et al. Ciprofloxacin plus piperacillin compared with tobramycin plus piperacillin as empirical therapy in febrile neutropenic patients: A randomized, double-blind trial. Ann Intern Med. 2002;137:77-87.

266. Kern WV, Cometta A, de Bock R, et al. Oral versus intravenous empirical antimicrobial therapy for fever in patients with granulocytopenia who are receiving cancer chemotherapy. N Engl J Med. 1999;341:312-318.

267. Freifeld A, Marchigiani D, Walsh T, et al. A double-blind comparison of empirical oral and intravenous antibiotic therapy for low-risk febrile patients with neutropenia during cancer chemotherapy. N Engl J Med. 1999;341:305-311.

268. Rubenstein EB, Rolston K, Benjamin RS, et al. Outpatient treatment of febrile episodes in low-risk neutropenic patients with cancer. Cancer. 1993;71:3640-3646.

269. Malik IA, Khan WA, Karim M, et al. Feasibility of outpatient management of fever in cancer patients with low-risk neutropenia: Results of a prospective randomized trial. Am J Med. 1995;98:224-231.

270. Hidalgo M, Hornedo J, Lumbreras C, et al. Outpatient therapy with oral ofloxacin for patients with low risk neutropenia and fever: A prospective, randomized clinical trial. Cancer. 1999;85:213-219.

271. Mullen CA, Petropoulos D, Roberts WM, et al. Outpatient treatment of fever and neutropenia for low risk pediatric cancer patients. Cancer. 1999;86:126-134.

272. Winston DJ. Use of quinolone antimicrobial agents in immunocompromised patients. In: Hooper DC, Wolfson JS, eds. Quinolone Antimicrobial Agents. 2nd ed. Washington, DC: American Society for Microbiology; 1993:435-471.

273. Jansen J, Cromer M, Akard L, et al. Infection prevention in severely myelosuppressed patients: A comparison between ciprofloxacin and a regimen of selective antibiotic modulation of the intestinal flora. Am J Med. 1994;96:335-341.

274. Anonymous. Prevention of bacterial infection in neutropenic patients with hematologic malignancies: A randomized, multicenter trial comparing norfloxacin with ciprofloxacin. The GIMEMA Infection Program. Gruppo Italiano Malattie Ematologiche Maligne dell'Adulto. Ann Intern Med. 1991;115:7-12.

275. Bow EJ, Mandell LA, Louie TJ, et al. Quinolone-based antibacterial chemoprophylaxis in neutropenic patients: Effect of augmented gram-positive activity on infectious morbidity. Ann Intern Med. 1996;125:183-190.

276. Broun ER, Wheat JL, Kneebone PH, et al. Randomized trial of the addition of gram-positive prophylaxis to standard antimicrobial prophylaxis for patients undergoing autologous bone marrow transplantation. Antimicrob Agents Chemother. 1994;38:576-579.

277. Razonable RR, Litzow MR, Khaliq Y, et al. Bacteremia due to viridans group streptococci with diminished susceptibility to levofloxacin among neutropenic patients receiving levofloxacin prophylaxis. Clin Infect Dis. 2002;34:1469-1474.

278. Kern WV. Epidemiology of fluoroquinolone-resistant Escherichia coli among neutropenic patients. Clin Infect Dis. 1998;27:235-237.

279. Le TP, Yeaman MR, Bayer AS. Treatment of experimental and human bacterial endocarditis with quinolone antimicrobial agents. In: Hooper DC, Rubinstein E, eds. Quinolone Antimicrobial Agents. 3rd ed. Washington, DC: ASM Press; 2003:259-273.

280. Dworkin RJ, Lee BL, Sande MA, Chambers HF. Treatment of right-sided Staphylococcus aureus endocarditis in intravenous drug abusers with ciprofloxacin and rifampin. Lancet. 1989;2:1071-1072.

281. Heldman AW, Hartert TV, Ray SC, et al. Oral antibiotic treatment of right-sided staphylococcal endocarditis in injection drug users: Prospective randomized comparison with parenteral therapy. Am J Med. 1996;101:68-76.

282. Yebra M, Ortigosa J, Albarran F, Crespo MG. Ciprofloxacin in a case of Q fever endocarditis. N Engl J Med. 1990;323:614.

283. Raoult D, Houpikian P, Dupont HT, et al. Treatment of Q fever endocarditis: Comparison of 2 regimens containing doxycycline and ofloxacin or hydroxychloroquine. Arch Intern Med. 1999;159:167-173.

284. Tunkel AR, Scheld WM. Treatment of bacterial meningitis and other central nervous system infections. In: Hooper DC, Rubinstein E, eds. Quinolone Antimicrobial Agents. 3rd ed. Washington, DC: ASM Press; 2003:275-289.

285. Segev S, Rosen N, Joseph G, et al. Pefloxacin efficacy in gram-negative bacillary meningitis. J Antimicrob Chemother. 1990;26(Suppl B):187-192.

286. Schonwald S, Beus I, Lisic M, et al. Ciprofloxacin in the treatment of gram-negative bacillary meningitis. Am J Med. 1989;87:248S-249S.

287. Krcméry V Jr, Filka J, Uher J, et al. Ciprofloxacin in treatment of nosocomial meningitis in neonates and in infants: Report of 12 cases and review. Diagn Microbiol Infect Dis. 1999;35:75-80.

288. Wong-Beringer A, Beringer P, Lovett MA. Successful treatment of multidrug-resistant Pseudomonas aeruginosa meningitis with high-dose ciprofloxacin. Clin Infect Dis. 1997;25:936-937.

289. Hopkins S, Williams D, Dunne M, et al. A randomized, controlled trial of oral or IV trovafloxacin vs. ceftriaxone in the treatment of epidemic meningococcal meningitis. Proceedings and Abstracts of the 36th Interscience Conference on Antimicrobial Agents and Chemotherapy. 1996. Washington, DC: American Society for Microbiology.

290. Dworzack DL, Sanders CC, Horowitz EA, et al. Evaluation of single-dose ciprofloxacin in the eradication of Neisseria meningitidis from nasopharyngeal carriers. Antimicrob Agents Chemother. 1988;32:1740-1741.

291. Gilja OH, Halstensen A, Digranes A, et al. Use of single-dose ofloxacin to eradicate tonsillopharyngeal carriage of Neisseria meningitidis. Antimicrob Agents Chemother. 1993;37:2024-2026.

292. Cuevas LE, Kazembe P, Mughogho GK, et al. Eradication of nasopharyngeal carriage of Neisseria meningitidis in children and adults in rural Africa: A comparison of ciprofloxacin and rifampicin. J Infect Dis. 1995;171:728-731.

293. Limaye AP, Hooper CJ. Treatment of tularemia with fluoroquinolones: Two cases and review. Clin Infect Dis. 1999;29:922-924.

294. Chocarro A, Gonzalez A, García I. Treatment of tularemia with ciprofloxacin. Clin Infect Dis. 2000;31:623.

295. Holley HP Jr. Successful treatment of cat-scratch disease with ciprofloxacin. JAMA. 1991;265:1563-1565.

296. Raoult D, Drancourt M. Antimicrobial therapy of rickettsial diseases. Antimicrob Agents Chemother. 1991;35:2457-2462.

297. Rolain JM, Raoult D. Treatment of intracellular infections. In: Hooper DC, Rubinstein E, eds. Quinolone Antimicrobial Agents. 3rd ed. Washington, DC: ASM Press; 2003:323-335.

298. Lang R, Rubinstein E. Quinolones for the treatment of brucellosis. J Antimicrob Chemother. 1992;29:357-360.

399. Akova M, Uzun O, Akalin HE, et al. Quinolones in treatment of human brucellosis: Comparative trial of ofloxacin-rifampin versus doxycycline-rifampin. Antimicrob Agents Chemother. 1993;37:1831-1834.

300. McClean KL, Hitchman D, Shafran SD. Norfloxacin is inferior to chloroquine for falciparum malaria in northwestern Zambia: A comparative clinical trial. J Infect Dis. 1992;165:904-907.

301. Watt G, Shanks GD, Edstein MD, et al. Ciprofloxacin treatment of drug-resistant falciparum malaria. J Infect Dis. 1991;164:602-604.

302. Blaser J, Stone BB, Groner MC, Zinner SH. Comparative study with enoxacin and netilmicin in a pharmacodynamic model to determine importance of ratio of antibiotic peak concentration to MIC for bactericidal activity and emergence of resistance. Antimicrob Agents Chemother. 1987;31:1054-1060.

303. Martínez-Martínez L, Pascual A, García I, et al. Interaction of plasmid and host quinolone resistance. J Antimicrob Chemother. 2003;51:1037-1039.

304. Low DE. Quinolone resistance and its clinical relevance. In: Hooper DC, Rubinstein E, eds. Quinolone Antimicrobial Agents. 3rd ed. Washington, DC: ASM Press; 2003:355-386.

305. Parry MF, Panzer KB, Yukna ME. Quinolone resistance: Susceptibility data from a 300-bed community hospital. Am J Med. 1989;87:12S-16S.

306. Kresken M, Wiedemann B. Development of resistance to nalidixic acid and the fluoroquinolones after the introduction of norfloxacin and ofloxacin. Antimicrob Agents Chemother. 1988;32:1285-1288.

307. Coronado VG, Edwards JR, Culver DH, Gaynes RP. Ciprofloxacin resistance among nosocomial Pseudomonas aeruginosa and Staphylococcus aureus in the United States. Infect Control Hosp Epidemiol. 1995;16:71-75.

308. Blumberg HM, Rimland D, Carroll DJ, et al. Rapid development of ciprofloxacin resistance in methicillin-susceptible and -resistant Staphylococcus aureus. J Infect Dis. 1991;163:1279-1285.

309. Schmitz FJ, Jones ME, Hofmann B, et al. Characterization of grlA, grlB, gyrA, and gyrB mutations in 116 unrelated isolates of Staphylococcus aureus and effects of mutations on ciprofloxacin MIC. Antimicrob Agents Chemother. 1998;42:1249-1252.

310. Pegues DA, Colby C, Hibberd PL, et al. The epidemiology of resistance to ofloxacin and oxacillin among clinical coagulase-negative staphylococcal isolates: Analysis of risk factors and strain types. Clin Infect Dis. 1998;26:72-79.

311. Hooper DC. Fluoroquinolone resistance among gram-positive cocci. Lancet Infect Dis. 2002;2:530-538.

312. Tanaka M, Matsumoto T, Kobayashi I, et al. Emergence of in vitro resistance to fluoroquinolones in Neisseria gonorrhoeae isolated in Japan. Antimicrob Agents Chemother. 1995;39:2367-2370.

313. Endtz HP, Ruijs GJ, van Klingeren B, et al. Quinolone resistance in Campylobacter isolated from man and poultry following the introduction of fluoroquinolones in veterinary medicine. J Antimicrob Chemother. 1991;27:199-208.

314. Endtz HP, Mouton RP, van der Reyden T, et al. Fluoroquinolone resistance in Campylobacter spp. isolated from human stools and poultry products. Lancet. 1990;335:787.

315. Ena J, Amador C, Martinez C, Ortiz de la Tabla V. Risk factors for acquisition of urinary tract infections caused by ciprofloxacin resistant Escherichia coli. J Urol. 1995;153:117-120.

316. Carratala J, Fernandez-Sevilla A, Tubau F, et al. Emergence of quinolone-resistant Escherichia coli bacteremia in neutropenic patients with cancer who have received prophylactic norfloxacin. Clin Infect Dis. 1995;20:557-560.

317. Oethinger M, Conrad S, Kaifel K, et al. Molecular epidemiology of fluoroquinolone-resistant Escherichia coli bloodstream isolates from patients admitted to European cancer centers. Antimicrob Agents Chemother. 1996;40:387-392.

318. Pena C, Albareda JM, Pallares R, et al. Relationship between quinolone use and emergence of ciprofloxacin-resistant Escherichia coli in bloodstream infections. Antimicrob Agents Chemother. 1995;39:520-524.

319. Carratala J, Fernandez-Sevilla A, Tubau F, et al. Emergence of fluoroquinolone-resistant Escherichia coli in fecal flora of cancer patients receiving norfloxacin prophylaxis. Antimicrob Agents Chemother. 1996;40:503-505.

320. Garau J, Xercavins M, Rodríguez-Carballeira M, et al. Emergence and dissemination of quinolone-resistant Escherichia coli in the community. Antimicrob Agents Chemother. 1999;43:2736-2741.

321. Blanco JE, Blanco M, Mora A, Blanco J. Prevalence of bacterial resistance to quinolones and other antimicrobials among avian Escherichia coli strains isolated from septicemic and healthy chickens in Spain. J Clin Microbiol. 1997;35:2184-2185.

322. Hooper DC. New uses for new and old quinolones and the challenge of resistance. Clin Infect Dis. 2000;30:243-254.

323. Chen DK, McGeer A, de Azavedo JC, et al. Decreased susceptibility of Streptococcus pneumoniae to fluoroquinolones in Canada. N Engl J Med. 1999;341:233-239.

324. Low DE, De Azavedo J, Weiss K, et al. Antimicrobial resistance among clinical isolates of Streptococcus pneumoniae in Canada during 2000. Antimicrob Agents Chemother. 2002;46:1295-1301.

325. Sahm DF, Peterson DE, Critchley IA, Thornsberry C. Analysis of ciprofloxacin activity against Streptococcus pneumoniae after 10 years of use in the United States. Antimicrob Agents Chemother. 2000;44:2521-2524.

326. Davies TA, Evangelista A, Pfleger S, et al. Prevalence of single mutations in topoisomerase type II genes among levofloxacin-susceptible clinical strains of Streptococcus pneumoniae isolated in the United States in 1992 to 1996 and 1999 to 2000. Antimicrob Agents Chemother. 2002;46:119-124.

327. Brueggemann A, Coffman SL, Rhomberg P, et al. Fluoroquinolone resistance in Streptococcus pneumoniae in United States since 1994-1995. Antimicrob Agents Chemother. 2002;46:680-688.

328. Richardson DC, Bast D, McGeer A, Low DE. Evaluation of susceptibility testing to detect fluoroquinolone resistance mechanisms in Streptococcus pneumoniae. Antimicrob Agents Chemother. 2001;45:1911-1914.

329. Mandell LA, Peterson LR, Wise R, et al. The battle against emerging antibiotic resistance: Should fluoroquinolones be used to treat children? Clin Infect Dis. 2002;35:721-727.

330. Thomas JK, Forrest A, Bhavnani SM, et al. Pharmacodynamic evaluation of factors associated with the development of bacterial resistance in acutely ill patients during therapy. Antimicrob Agents Chemother. 1998;42:521-527.

331. Drusano GL, Johnson DE, Rosen M, Standiford HC. Pharmacodynamics of a fluoroquinolone antimicrobial agent in a neutropenic rat model of Pseudomonas sepsis. Antimicrob Agents Chemother. 1993;37:483-490.

332. Lode H, Rubinstein E. Adverse effects. In: Hooper DC, Rubinstein E, eds. Quinolone Antimicrobial Agents. 3rd ed. Washington, DC: ASM Press; 2003:407-419.

333. Hooper DC, Wolfson JS. Adverse effects. In: Hooper DC, Wolfson JS, eds. Quinolone Antimicrobial Agents. 2nd ed. Washington, DC: American Society for Microbiology; 1993:489-512.

334. Norrby SR. Central nervous system toxicity. In: Hooper DC, Rubinstein E, eds. Quinolone Antimicrobial Agents. 3rd ed. Washington, DC: ASM Press; 2003:461-465.

335. Halliwell RF, Davey PG, Lambert JJ. Antagonism of GABA_A receptors by 4-quinolones. J Antimicrob Chemother. 1993;31:457-462.

336. Ferguson J. Fluoroquinolone photosensitization: A review of clinical and laboratory studies. Photochem Photobiol. 1995;62:954-958.

337. Ferguson J. Phototoxicity due to fluoroquinolones. In: Hooper DC, Rubinstein E, eds. Quinolone Antimicrobial Agents. 3rd ed. Washington, DC: ASM Press; 2003:451-460.

338. Stahlmann R. Effects on connective tissue structures. In: Hooper DC, Rubinstein E, eds. Quinolone Antimicrobial Agents. 3rd ed. Washington, DC: ASM Press; 2003:441-449.

339. Burkhardt JE, Walterspiel JN, Schaad UB. Quinolone arthropathy in animals versus children. Clin Infect Dis. 1997;25:1196-1204.

340. Adam D. Use of quinolones in pediatric patients. Rev Infect Dis. 1989;11 (Suppl 5):S1113-S1116.

341. Schaad UB, Wedgwood J. Lack of quinolone-induced arthropathy in children. J Antimicrob Chemother. 1992;30:414-416.

342. Pertuiset E, Lenoir G, Jehanne M, et al. [Joint tolerance of pefloxacin and ofloxacin in children and adolescents with cystic fibrosis.] Rev Rhum Mal Osteoartic. 1989;56:735-740.

343. Schaad UB, abdus Salam M, Aujard Y, et al. Use of fluoroquinolones in pediatrics: Consensus report of an International Society of Chemotherapy commission. Pediatr Infect Dis J. 1995;14:1-9.

344. Zabraniecki L, Negrier I, Vergne P, et al. Fluoroquinolone induced tendinopathy: Report of 6 cases. J Rheumatol. 1996;23:516-520.

345. Van der Linden PD, Sturkenboom MCJM, Herings RMC, et al. Increased risk of Achilles tendon rupture with quinolone antibacterial use, especially in elderly patients taking oral corticosteroids. Arch Intern Med. 2003;163:1801-1807.

346. Yap YG, Camm AJ. QT prolongation with quinolone antimicrobial agents. In: Hooper DC, Rubinstein E, eds. Quinolone Antimicrobial Agents. 3rd ed. Washington, DC: ASM Press; 2003:421-440.

347. Ball P, Mandell L, Niki Y, Tillotson G. Comparative tolerability of the newer fluoroquinolone antibacterials. Drug Saf. 1999;21:407-421.

348. Blum MD, Graham DJ, McCloskey CA. Temafloxacin syndrome: Review of 95 cases. Clin Infect Dis. 1994;18:946-950.

349. Gajjar DA, LaCreta FP, Kollia GD, et al. Effect of multiple-dose gatifloxacin or ciprofloxacin on glucose homeostasis and insulin production in patients with noninsulin-dependent diabetes mellitus maintained with diet and exercise. Pharmacotherapy. 2000;20:76S-86S.

350. Berkovitch M, Pastuszak A, Gazarian M, et al. Safety of the new quinolones in pregnancy. Obstet Gynecol. 1994;84:535-538.

351. Loebstein R, Addis A, Ho E, et al. Pregnancy outcome following gestational exposure to fluoroquinolones: A multicenter prospective controlled study. Antimicrob Agents Chemother. 1998;42:1336-1339.

CHAPTER **34**

Urinary Tract Agents: Nitrofurantoin and Methenamine

DAVID C. HOOPER

Two antimicrobial agents in clinical use are employed exclusively for treatment or prophylaxis of urinary tract infections because of their pharmacologic and chemical properties. At tolerated doses, nitrofurantoin achieves adequate concentrations only in kidney tissues and urine. Methenamine, which lacks antimicrobial activity itself, becomes active only after chemical degradation in acidic bladder urine to generate its active breakdown product, formaldehyde.

NITROFURANTOIN

Chemical Structure

Nitrofurantoin (N-[5-nitro-2-furfurylidene]-1-aminohydantoin) is a weak acid (pK_a, 7.2) (Fig. 34-1) and a member of a group of synthetic nitrofuran compounds that also includes furazolidone, which is avail-

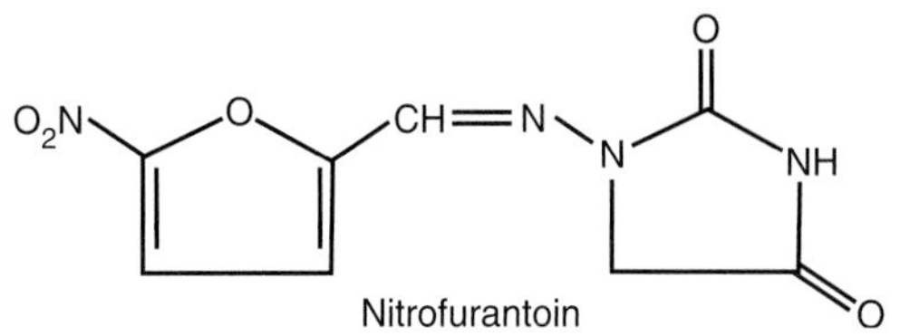

FIGURE 34-1. Structure of nitrofurantoin.

able in Europe but not in the United States, and nitrofurazone, which has been impregnated into some urinary catheters.[1] Three oral formulations of nitrofurantoin were developed. A microcrystalline form was introduced in 1953, and macrocrystalline forms were introduced in 1967. Mixtures of macrocrystalline and microcrystalline forms (Macrobid [25 mg macrocrystals plus 75 mg monohydrate form], Procter & Gamble; generic capsules [Mylan]) and macrocrystals alone (Macrodantin, Procter & Gamble) are currently available.

Mechanisms of Drug Action and Bacterial Resistance

The mechanism of action of nitrofurantoin is poorly understood, but activity in many cases appears to require enzymatic reduction within the bacterial cell.[2] The reduced derivatives appear to be capable of binding to ribosomal proteins. Nitrofurans have been shown to inhibit the synthesis of inducible enzymes by blocking translation,[3] and also to inhibit bacterial respiration and pyruvate metabolism. Antibacterial activity has also been shown under conditions in which nitroreductase activity was inhibited, suggesting that nitrofurantoin may act in part without reduction to active metabolites.[4] The nitrofurans, like the quinolones, appear to damage bacterial DNA,[5] and they induce bacterial DNA repair systems.[6] Mutants with defective DNA repair functions are hypersusceptible.[7] Nitrofurantoin may antagonize the bacterial activity of quinolones against Proteus and Enterobacter.[8] The principal drug action that determines the bactericidal activity of nitrofurantoin, however, remains to be defined.

Resistant strains of Escherichia coli with chromosomal or plasmid-mediated resistance have been associated with inhibition of nitrofuran reductase enzyme activity, thereby decreasing the production of the active derivative(s).[9-11] In clinical use, however, the emergence of nitrofurantoin-resistant variants from initially susceptible pathogens has been rare despite many years of clinical use of this agent.[12,13]

Spectrum of Activity

Susceptibility breakpoints are based on urinary concentrations of nitrofurantoin and have been correlated with eradication of bacteriuria in patients with urinary tract infections.[14,15] Bacterial strains with a minimal inhibitory concentration (MIC) of 32 μg/mL or less are considered clinically susceptible. For strains having an MIC of 64 μg/mL, clinical responses may be more variable.[16] MIC values of greater than 500 μg/mL are uniformly correlated with clinical failure.[14] On the basis of these criteria, more than 90% of clinical strains of E. coli, and Citrobacter species are susceptible. Group B streptococci are also usually susceptible. Recent surveys have found a persisting low prevalence of resistance to nitrofurantoin (1.9% to 7.7%) among urinary E. coli isolates,[17] including those resistant to trimethoprim-sulfamethoxazole or ciprofloxacin.[18] Group B streptococci are usually susceptible, as are Staphylococcus saprophyticus, Enterococcus faecalis, and Enterococcus faecium. Many vancomycin-resistant strains of enterococci (VRE) are also susceptible.[19]

In contrast, only a minority of strains of Enterobacter species (20% to 50%) and Klebsiella species (45%) are susceptible, and members of the genera Proteus, Providencia, Morganella, Serratia, Acinetobacter, and Pseudomonas are almost always resistant.[15,16] Among uropathogens causing catheter-associated urinary tract infections, overall resistance to nitrofurantoin is around 28% and has been stable over time.[1,20]

Other organisms that are uncommonly associated with urinary tract infections but that may be susceptible to nitrofurantoin in vitro include *Salmonella* species, *Shigella* species, *Staphylococcus aureus,* coagulase-negative staphylococci, *Streptococcus pneumoniae, Streptococcus pyogenes, Corynebacterium* species, and *Bacteroides* species.[21-23]

Pharmacology

Absorption. The completeness of absorption of orally administered nitrofurantoin as determined from drug recovery in the urine is about 40% to 50%, and absorption is enhanced when the drug is taken with food.[24,25] Absorption occurs principally and rapidly in the small intestine. Two formulations of nitrofurantoin differ in the rate of drug absorption. The slower rate of dissolution and absorption of the macrocrystalline form relative to the microcrystalline form was associated with a lower occurrence of gastrointestinal adverse effects, a minimal reduction in overall absorption (36% versus 43%), and no change in efficacy (see later). Although parenteral preparations of nitrofurantoin have been evaluated, they are not generally available for clinical use.

Distribution. Serum concentrations of nitrofurantoin are low or undetectable (≤ 1 µg/mL) with standard oral doses of 100 mg four times daily. After administration of intravenous nitrofurantoin, serum half-life has been estimated to be 30 minutes or less. In animals given intravenous nitrofurantoin, a high volume of distribution (0.7 L/kg) suggested drug distribution into extracellular and intracellular compartments, but enzymatic degradation of nitrofurantoin in situ is thought to contribute to low drug levels in most tissues.[24,26] Therapeutic concentrations are not detected in prostatic secretions,[27] and only low concentrations have been detected in human breast milk.[28] Nitrofurantoin concentrations in bile may be equal to or greater than those in serum.[24] Drug concentrations in urine are substantial (50 to 250 µg/mL) and exceed the MIC for susceptible organisms.[29]

Excretion. Nitrofurantoin is eliminated predominantly in the urine. Renal elimination involves glomerular filtration, tubular secretion, and tubular reabsorption.[24] Tubular handling is by the weak acid transport system. Reabsorption is decreased in the presence of alkaline urine, because at alkaline pH the equilibrium of nonionized and ionized drug is shifted toward the ionized form, which diffuses back across the renal tubular epithelium less well than the nonionized form. Urine alkalinization does not enhance antibacterial activity in the urine, however, because nitrofurantoin may be less active at alkaline pH.[12] In patients with renal failure, nitrofurantoin excretion is decreased in proportion to decreases in creatinine clearance, and urinary drug concentrations become subtherapeutic.[30] In severe renal failure, there may also be modest increases in serum concentrations of nitrofurantoin (≤ 6 µg/mL).[30] Thus, nitrofurantoin should not be used in patients with renal insufficiency (creatinine clearance of <40 mL/min).

With normal renal function, metabolism and biliary excretion are minor pathways of nitrofurantoin elimination that are less well understood.[12] No dosage adjustment is required in patients with liver disease without alterations in renal function.

Dosing. For therapy of established urinary tract infections, nitrofurantoin is given orally at 50 to 100 mg four times daily. For use as prophylaxis for recurrent urinary tract infections, it is usually given at 50 to 100 mg once daily.

Clinical Uses

Nitrofurantoin is indicated only for the treatment and prophylaxis of urinary tract infections.

Acute Uncomplicated Cystitis

In earlier noncomparative studies, bacteriologic and clinical responses in patients with acute uncomplicated cystitis ranged from 61% to 100%,[12] although in a number of these studies, follow-up periods were brief. Infections caused by *E. coli* generally responded well, and infections caused by *Proteus* species and *Pseudomonas aeruginosa* responded poorly if at all. When given for 7 days to young women, ni-

trofurantoin and trimethoprim (200 mg PO once daily) produced similar rates of eradication of infections caused by *E. coli* (66 of 78 [84%] versus 72 of 77 [93%]) and *S. saprophyticus* (7/8 [87%] versus 10/12 [83%]), but the smaller numbers of infections caused by *Klebsiella* species and *Proteus* species responded better to trimethoprim.[31] With 3-day courses of therapy for acute cystitis in young women, nitrofurantoin (100 mg four times daily) produced cure rates at the 6-week follow-up evaluation similar to the rates for cefadroxil and amoxicillin (61%) but lower than that of trimethoprim-sulfamethoxazole (82%).[32] Persistence of bacteriuria was also lower for trimethoprim-sulfamethoxazole (noted in 3% of patients) than for nitrofurantoin (in 16%). In both studies, suppression of potential pathogens in the periurethral, vaginal, and rectal flora occurred significantly more often with trimethoprim than with nitrofurantoin, a finding that may have contributed to the higher success rate noted in the trimethoprim-sulfamethoxazole group. A 7-day course of nitrofurantoin is thus preferred over a 3-day course. In contrast, 3 days of trimethoprim-sulfamethoxazole or a fluoroquinolone is usually sufficient for treatment of uncomplicated cystitis.[33] A modified-release formulation of nitrofurantoin that can be given twice daily was comparable to trimethoprim-sulfamethoxazole for treatment of women with uncomplicated cystitis in a general practice population.[34]

A more recent randomized, double-blind trial of uncomplicated urinary tract infections in women (largely caused by *E. coli*) found clinical responses and initial rates of bacterial eradication with nitrofurantoin (100 mg twice daily for 7 days), ciprofloxacin (100 mg twice daily for 3 days), and trimethoprim-sulfamethoxazole (160 to 800 mg twice daily for 7 days) to be similar.[35] However, eradication at the 4- to 6-week follow-up was greater with ciprofloxacin (91%, versus 79% for trimethoprim-sulfamethoxazole and 82% for nitrofurantoin).

Nitrofurantoin has also been used for the treatment of lower urinary tract infections in pregnant women[36] and children.[22] In young girls with cystitis, responses to nitrofurantoin given for 3 days were similar to responses to a 7-day course.[37] Because 15% to 20% of urinary isolates causing acute uncomplicated cystitis may be resistant to nitrofurantoin, and because responses to this agent in infections caused by susceptible pathogens may be less satisfactory and require longer courses of therapy than treatment with trimethoprim-sulfamethoxazole or fluoroquinolones,[36] nitrofurantoin should be considered an alternative rather than a first-line therapeutic agent for this clinical syndrome.[33]

Acute Uncomplicated Pyelonephritis and Complicated Urinary Tract Infections

Patients with acute pyelonephritis respond inconsistently to nitrofurantoin, and bacteremias have occurred during nitrofurantoin treatment, presumably because serum concentrations are inadequate.[12] Thus, nitrofurantoin should not be used for treatment of patients with pyelonephritis. In addition, complicated urinary tract infections, which are defined as those associated with structural or functional abnormalities of the urinary tract, are often associated with pyelonephritis and are often caused by pathogens resistant to nitrofurantoin. In general, nitrofurantoin is not indicated for treatment of these infections, and it is specifically contraindicated in cases that are complicated by resistant pathogens, pyelonephritis, renal failure, or prostatic infection. An earlier study of older men with recurring bacteriuria showed that nitrofurantoin given for long-term suppressive therapy reduced recurrences of bacteriuria by about 40% relative to placebo,[38] but drugs that penetrate the prostate (trimethoprim or fluoroquinolones) are more likely to eradicate bacteriuria in these patients.

Because nitrofurantoin is active against many strains of VRE and because there are few other agents available for treatment of VRE lower urinary tract infections, nitrofurantoin could be considered in patients with these infections. Published clinical data suggest efficacy but are quite limited.[19] Removal of urinary catheters is an important adjunct for management of these infections and may be sufficient for eradication without antimicrobial therapy in some patients.

Prophylaxis of Recurrent Urinary Tract Infections

In young women with two or more episodes of symptomatic bacteriuria within 12 months, once-daily nitrofurantoin (100 mg) was highly effective and comparable to trimethoprim-sulfamethoxazole (40 to 200 mg) in preventing recurrent urinary tract infections without emergence of resistant organisms.[39] Infections recurred at the same rate when prophylaxis was stopped after 6 months. In two trials in a more heterogeneous population of women with a history of four or more symptomatic urinary tract infections in the preceding 12 months, nitrofurantoin (50 to 100 mg at bedtime) was comparable to cefaclor (250 mg at bedtime)[40] or norfloxacin (200 mg at bedtime)[41] in increasing the interval between symptomatic episodes (fivefold to sevenfold). In both trials, nitrofurantoin was somewhat less well tolerated than the comparison agent.

For women in whom recurrence of infection is associated with sexual intercourse, a single dose of nitrofurantoin (100 mg) taken shortly after intercourse has also been highly effective in preventing symptomatic infection.[42] Postcoital prophylaxis was also effective in pregnant women with a history of recurrent urinary tract infections before pregnancy.[43]

In postmenopausal women with recurrent urinary tract infections, nitrofurantoin (100 mg every day) was more effective than an estriol-containing vaginal pessary in preventing symptomatic and asymptomatic bacteriuria.[44] Nitrofurantoin has reduced the rates of bacteriuria in patients undergoing intermittent catheterization in some[45] but not all[46] studies. In one study of children with neurogenic bladders receiving intermittent catheterization, nitrofurantoin was effective in preventing only *E. coli* infections, and with usage the occurrence of resistant uropathogens increased.[47] Antimicrobial prophylaxis is not of value in patients with long-term indwelling catheters.[36]

Adverse Effects

Gastrointestinal and Skin Reactions

The overall tolerability of nitrofurantoin is determined by gastrointestinal adverse effects, the rates of which are dose related and differ for the two formulations.[29] In a randomized, double-blind comparison, the microcrystalline formulation (100 mg four times daily) was associated with adverse effects (predominantly nausea and vomiting) in 39% of patients, compared with 17% of patients receiving the macrocrystalline formulation in the same dose.[48] With long-term prophylaxis, a higher rate of side effects and cessation of therapy has been reported with the microcrystalline than with the macrocrystalline formulation.[49] Slower dissolution of the macrocrystalline formulation is thought to be responsible for its lower frequency of gastrointestinal side effects. In a double-blind study, ciprofloxacin (100 mg twice daily for 3 days) had significantly fewer episodes of nausea than nitrofurantoin (100 mg twice daily for 7 days) (3% versus 11%), but nitrofurantoin was less likely to cause rash than trimethoprim-sulfamethoxazole (160 to 800 mg twice daily for 7 days) (4% versus 0.4%).[35]

Rashes, presumably of an allergic nature, have been reported in about 1% of hospitalized patients receiving nitrofurantoin.[22] Other, less common but more serious, toxic effects of nitrofurantoin have received considerable attention.[22,29]

Pulmonary Reactions

Pulmonary reactions have been classified into acute, subacute, and chronic forms[22] and in the United States appear to occur at a frequency of one or fewer cases per 100,000 courses of treatment.[29] The chronic form of pulmonary reactions appears to be less common than the acute form, at least in part because fewer patients receive the extended courses of therapy that precede the chronic form.

The acute reaction appears to be a reversible hypersensitivity phenomenon and may occur within hours to weeks of drug exposure, with a shorter time to onset of symptoms after drug reexposure.[50,51] The clinical presentation is characterized by the rapid onset of fever, cough, dyspnea, and myalgia. These symptoms are usually accompanied by peripheral blood eosinophilia (in 83% of cases) and lower-lobe infiltrates (in 94%) with (in 20%) or without pleural effusions on chest radiographs. Alveolar exudates, interstitial inflammation, and vasculitis have been found on lung biopsy. In addition, rash, pruritus, chest discomfort, and sputum production may also be present. Improvement is generally rapid after discontinuation of the drug, and acute reactions do not generally progress to the chronic form.

It is not clear whether the subacute and chronic forms of nitrofurantoin pulmonary reactions are distinct from each other except that the former has an onset after 1 month of drug therapy and the latter after 6 or more months.[51] These reactions are thought to result from toxic effects on the lung, possibly related to oxidant injury of the type that has been demonstrated in rat lung explants treated with nitrofurantoin.[52] In both the subacute and chronic forms, clinical features include the gradual onset of progressive nonproductive cough and dyspnea and interstitial infiltrates on chest radiographs. Fever is variably present. Eosinophilia is uncommon, but abnormalities on liver function testing may be seen in up to 40% of patients, and positive results on assays for antinuclear antibodies have been reported.[50] Regression often occurs with discontinuation of nitrofurantoin, but in the more chronic cases, irreversible pulmonary fibrosis and fatal reactions have occurred. A pattern consistent with bronchiolitis obliterans and organizing pneumonia has also been reported.[53] A widespread reticular pattern can be seen on high-resolution chest tomography, but this finding does not necessarily indicate irreversible lung disease.[54] A beneficial effect of corticosteroid therapy has not been convincingly demonstrated in patients with the chronic form of nitrofurantoin pulmonary reactions.

Hepatic Reactions

Hepatic reactions appear to occur with a frequency similar to that of the chronic form of pulmonary reactions.[55] In some cases, findings have included both hepatitis and pulmonary infiltrates.[56] Acute hepatitis with or without cholestasis associated with short-term use of nitrofurantoin is generally self-limited and reversible.[57] Prolonged use of nitrofurantoin, however, has been associated with chronic active hepatitis, cirrhosis, and death.[56] In such cases, hyperglobulinemia and antinuclear antibodies were commonly present, but eosinophilia was an inconsistent finding.

Hematologic Reactions

Hemolytic anemia has occurred rarely in patients receiving nitrofurantoin and most often, but not always, in those with deficiency of glucose-6-phosphate dehydrogenase (G6PD).[28,58] Decreases in cellular NADPH in such patients result in diminished cellular levels of reduced glutathione. Nitrofurantoin may inhibit glutathione reductase, further compromising the ability of the cell to generate reduced glutathione,[59] and it may also generate the release of superoxide from oxyhemoglobin in the presence of oxygen,[60] thereby further contributing to oxidant stresses.[22] Patients with deficiencies in enolase and glutathione peroxidases have developed nitrofurantoin-induced hemolysis as well. Folic acid–responsive megaloblastic anemia has also been reported.[61] Eosinophilia is seen as a feature of the acute pulmonary reactions and some hepatic reactions, but leukopenia and aplastic anemia have been only rarely reported.

Peripheral Neuropathy

A peripheral sensorimotor neuropathy of unclear mechanism has been reported uncommonly, less often than pulmonary reactions have been. Neuropathy has been seen in patients receiving nitrofurantoin for prolonged periods as well as in patients with renal failure.[29,55] The onset of neuropathy is often insidious, with the occurrence of paresthesias and dysesthesias in a stocking-and-glove distribution. Distal weakness and centripetal spread may also occur.[62] Histopathologic findings have included demyelination and axonal degeneration.[63] The reversibility of the deficits after cessation of drug therapy may be slow and variable.

Uses in Pediatrics and in Pregnancy

Toxic effects of nitrofurantoin appear to be similar in children and adults,[64] but the drug is not recommended for use in neonates. It may be used for treatment of urinary tract infections in pregnancy when clearly indicated but should not be used at term.[8,36] Nitrofurantoin crosses the placenta, but very low concentrations are reached in amniotic fluid.[65] Although it is mutagenic in some bacterial tests in vitro,[66] results of tests for teratogenicity and carcinogenicity in animals have been negative.[8,29] Review of adverse events in a total of 165 pregnant patients who received nitrofurantoin therapy in each of the three trimesters of pregnancy found no increased incidence of fetal loss or fetal abnormality over that in the population in general.[67,68] Other studies have also found no evidence for nitrofurantoin teratogenicity.[61,69] Healthy infants with G6PD deficiency have been born to mothers treated with nitrofurantoin during pregnancy.[29]

METHENAMINE

Chemical Structure

Methenamine (hexamethylenetetramine) (Fig. 34-2) is available as a salt of mandelic acid (α-hydroxybenzene-acetic acid) (Mandelamine, Warner Chilcott; Uroquid-Acid No. 2, Beach) or hippuric acid (benzoylamino-acetic acid) (Hipprex, Aventis) or without these acids (Urised, Polymedic; Prosed DS, Star; Urimax, Integrity).

Mechanism of Action and Antimicrobial Activity

Methenamine itself has little antibacterial activity, but at acid pH, each moleculare of methenamine that is hydrolyzed generates four molecules of ammonia and six molecules of formaldehyde, as shown in the following equation[25,70]:

$$(N_4[CH_2])_6 + 6H_2O + 4H^+ \longleftrightarrow 4NH_4^+ + 6HCHO$$

Increased concentrations of H+ and diffusional loss of NH_3 drive the reaction to the right. Formaldehyde, the active product, is a nonspecific denaturant of proteins and nucleic acids and has broad-spectrum antimicrobial activity. Free formaldehyde concentrations greater than 25 μg/mL may be bactericidal. Microbial resistance to formaldehyde has not been described.[70] Antimicrobial activity in urine is correlated with urinary concentrations of formaldehyde.[71] Although formaldehyde has activity against *Proteus* species, an alkaline urine may be generated by the urease activity of these organisms, preventing conversion of methenamine to formaldehyde. Inhibitors of urease may prevent this effect in laboratory simulations of *Proteus* growing in urine.[72] Hippuric and mandelic acids themselves have only limited antibacterial activity at concentrations achieved with usual doses of their respective methenamine salts.[73]

Pharmacology

Absorption and Distribution. Methenamine itself is rapidly absorbed after oral administration, and 82% to 88% is recovered in the urine of normal volunteers in the 24 hours after a 1-g dose,[74] indicating excellent bioavailability. Methenamine may be partially degraded in the presence of gastric acid before absorption.[75] This degradation is avoided with enteric-coated formulations, but absorption is slower. The volume of distribution (0.56 L/kg) suggests a relatively broad distribution in tissues. Methenamine crosses the placenta, and concentrations in breast milk are similar to those in plasma.[76]

Excretion. The half-life of elimination of methenamine from serum is 3 to 4 hours with normal renal function. Renal clearance is 95% of total clearance from serum, indicating a predominant renal route of excretion.[74] Hippuric and mandelic acids are also excreted renally by both glomerular filtration and tubular secretion.[25,77] The extent to which methenamine and hippuric and mandelic acids accumulate in patients with renal failure is not known.

Factors Affecting Formaldehyde Concentrations in Urine. The concentration of formaldehyde in bladder urine determines antimicrobial activity and is a function of (1) methenamine concentrations in urine, (2) the rate of hydrolysis of methenamine to formaldehyde, and (3) the rate of urine loss from the bladder by voiding or drainage. At constant rates of renal clearance, methenamine concentrations in urine decrease with increasing urine volumes, but with repetitive dosing, concentrations of greater than 150 μg/mL are usually maintained.[74] Conversion of methenamine to formaldehyde occurs as a first-order reaction, with higher rates of conversion in the presence of higher concentrations of methenamine.[78] The relative rate constant for conversion increases with decreasing urine pH and is 13-fold higher at pH 5.2 than at pH 6.5[78]; no hydrolysis occurs above pH 6.8. At methenamine concentrations of 1000 μg/mL, the time needed to generate formaldehyde concentrations in excess of 25 μg/mL is more than 6 hours at pH 6.5, 3 hours at pH 5.85, and 1.5 to 2 hours at pH 5.6.[79] At such concentrations of formaldehyde, bacterial exposure for at least 2 hours appears to be necessary for antibacterial activity. Thus, increases in the frequency of voiding or bladder drainage will reduce antibacterial effects by removing formaldehyde and by reducing the time of exposure of bladder bacteria to formaldehyde.[80] For these reasons, methenamine is ineffective in the presence of indwelling bladder catheters and may be ineffective when intermittent catheterization is performed frequently. Similarly, the brief time in which methenamine resides in the renal tissues and the upper urinary tract obviates efficacy in pyelonephritis.

Acidification of the Urine during Methenamine Treatment. Maintaining urinary pH below 6 is necessary for generating antibacterial activity from methenamine, and in many patients, urine pH is sufficiently low without additional measures. The amounts of hippuric and mandelic acids given with usual doses of methenamine hippurate and methenamine mandelate, however, do not contribute importantly to urine acidification.[75] Ascorbic acid has been given to aid urine acidification, but doses as high as 12 g/day may be required.[25] The value of acetohydroxamic acid, an inhibitor of urease, as an adjunctive agent in patients with an alkaline urine associated with *Proteus* infections is suggested by in vitro data,[72] but it is unclear in vivo.

Dosing. With equimolar mixtures of methenamine and their respective acids, 1 g of methenamine mandelate contains 480 mg methenamine, and 1 g of methenamine hippurate contains 440 mg of methenamine. For adults and children older than 12 years, methenamine mandelate and methenamine hippurate are usually given in a dose of 1 g PO twice daily, but up to 4 g/day (1 g four times daily) may be given. For children between 6 and 12 years, the dose is 500 mg to 1 g twice daily. An oral suspension (methenamine mandelate, 500 mg/5 mL and 250 mg/5 mL) is available for younger children; for children younger than 6 years, the usual dose is 250 mg per 30 pounds body weight PO four times daily.

Clinical Uses

The efficacy of methenamine for treatment of established cystitis has not been adequately documented in comparative clinical trials, and methenamine is not effective for treatment of pyelonephritis. Methenamine thus should not be used for treatment of established urinary tract infections.

Methenamine has been shown, however, to be effective for suppression or prophylaxis of recurrent lower urinary tract infections. In a double-blind, placebo-controlled, crossover trial in young, otherwise healthy women with recurrent cystitis, 1 g of methenamine hippurate twice daily reduced recurrent symptomatic infections by 73%.[81] A similar significant reduction (56%) was seen in another comparative

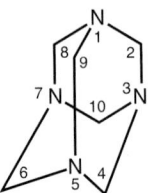

Methenamine

FIGURE 34-2. Structure of methenamine.

study of a similar population of young women and girls given methenamine mandelate (500 mg four times daily) and ascorbic acid (2 g daily).[82] Trimethoprim-sulfamethoxazole (40 to 200 mg at bedtime), however, was significantly better than methenamine in reducing the frequency of recurrent infections in this study,[82] as was trimethoprim alone in another study.[83] Trimethoprim-sulfamethoxazole was more effective than methenamine in reducing periurethral colonization with gram-negative bacilli, a potential reservoir of recurring pathogens.[82] Although less well tolerated, nitrofurantoin was also more effective than methenamine hippurate in preventing symptomatic infections in another trial.[84]

Methenamine has also prevented episodes of recurring bacteriuria in children[85,86] and has suppressed chronic bacteriuria in men.[38] It has not been shown, however, that methenamine is superior to other agents such as trimethoprim-sulfamethoxazole for these uses.

Attempts to prevent recurring infections in patients with indwelling bladder catheters by use of methenamine have not been successful,[87] as might be expected because sufficient concentrations of formaldehyde cannot be generated under these conditions. The results of prophylaxis in patients undergoing intermittent catheterization have been variable.[87,88] In a double-blind, randomized, placebo-controlled trial in patients with neurogenic bladders undergoing bladder retraining, urinary acidification was augmented with ammonium chloride in the methenamine group (both agents given as 1 g every 6 hours), and catheterization (usually every 6 hours), voiding, and drinking schedules were specifically controlled. Over the 21 days of the study, bacteriuria occurred at a significantly lower rate in the methenamine group—53% (9 of 17 patients)—than in the placebo group—86% (19 of 22 patients).[88] For patients undergoing intermittent catheterization for longer periods, however, antimicrobial regimens may only delay episodes of bacteriuria. The effectiveness of methenamine-containing regimens is probably inversely related to the frequency of catheterization and voiding.

Adverse Effects

Methenamine is generally well tolerated,[25,82] and in double-blind studies,[88] side effects have been few, mild, and reversible, and the incidence of such effects is comparable to that reported with placebo. In nonblinded studies, most commonly encountered have been gastrointestinal side effects (nausea, vomiting) and rashes or pruritus.[25] Symptoms of bladder irritation have been reported in patients with sterile urine receiving methenamine suppression.[38] With high doses of methenamine, increased gastrointestinal intolerance and hemorrhagic cystitis[89] may occur, possibly related to increased local concentrations of formaldehyde.

Methenamine salts may predispose to the development of urate crystals in the urine of patients with gout and may cause precipitation of sulfonamides in the urine of patients concurrently receiving these drugs.

Because conversion of methenamine to formaldehyde also releases ammonia, methenamine should be avoided in patients with hepatic insufficiency. The safety of methenamine itself in patients with renal failure is unclear; because of the potential risk of increased systemic acidosis, acidifying agents should be avoided in such patients.[90] Limited data suggest that methenamine may be given safely in the second and third trimesters of pregnancy.[91]

REFERENCES

1. Guay DR. An update on the role of nitrofurans in the management of urinary tract infections. Drugs. 2001;61:353-364.
2. McCalla DR, Reuvers A, Kaiser C. Mode of action of nitrofurazone. J Bacteriol. 1970;104:1126-1134.
3. Herrlich P, Schweiger M. Nitrofurans, a group of synthetic antibiotics, with new mode of action: discrimination of specific messenger RNA classes. Proc Natl Acad Sci U S A. 1976;73:3386-3390.
4. McOsker CC, Fitzpatrick PM. Nitrofurantoin: Mechanism of action and implications for resistance development in common uropathogens. J Antimicrob Chemother. 1994;33:23-30.
5. Tu Y, McCalla DR. Effect of activated nitrofurans on DNA. Biochim Biophys Acta. 1975;402:142-149.
6. Rahman MS, Pal AK. Induction of SOS like responses by nitrofurantoin in Vibrio cholerae El Tor cells. Arch Microbiol. 1993;159:98-100.
7. Jenkins ST, Bennett PM. Effect of mutations in deoxyribonucleic acid repair pathways on the sensitivity of Escherichia coli K-12 strains to nitrofurantoin. J Bacteriol. 1976;125:1214-1216.
8. Shah S, Greenwood D. Interactions between antibacterial agents of the quinolone group and nitrofurantoin. J Antimicrob Chemother. 1988;21:41-48.
9. McCalla DR, Kaiser C, Green MHL. Genetics of nitrofurazone resistance in Escherichia coli. J Bacteriol. 1978;133:10-16.
10. Breeze AS, Obaseiki-Ebor EE. Nitrofuran reductase activity in nitrofurantoin-resistant strains of Escherichia coli K-12: Some with chromosomally determined resistance and others carrying R-plasmids. J Antimicrob Chemother. 1983;12:543-547.
11. Breeze AS, Obaseiki-Ebor EE. Transferable nitrofuran resistance conferred by R-plasmids in clinical isolates of Escherichia coli. J Antimicrob Chemother. 1983;12:459-467.
12. Richards WA, Riss E, Kass EH, et al. Nitrofurantoin: Clinical and laboratory studies in urinary tract infections. Arch Intern Med. 1955;96:437-450.
13. Gupta K, Scholes U, Stamm WE. Increasing prevalence of antimicrobial resistance among uropathogens causing acute uncomplicated cystitis in women. JAMA. 1999;281:736-738.
14. Winn WR, Silton J, Finegold SM. In vitro sensitivity to nitrofurantoin compared with clinical bacteriological response. Antimicrob Agents Chemother. 1964;10:582-590.
15. Turck M, Ronald AR, Petersdorf RG. Susceptibility of Enterobacteriaceae to nitrofurantoin correlated with eradication of bacteriuria. Antimicrob Agents Chemother. 1966;6:446-452.
16. Barry AL. Nitrofurantoin susceptibility test criteria. J Antimicrob Chemother. 1990;25:711-713.
17. Karlowsky JA, Thornsberry C, Jones ME, Sahm DF. Susceptibility of antimicrobial-resistant urinary Escherichia coli isolates to fluoroquinolones and nitrofurantoin. Clin Infect Dis. 2003;36:183-187.
18. Sahm DF, Thornsberry C, Mayfield DC, et al. Multidrug-resistant urinary tract isolates of Escherichia coli prevalence and patient demographics in the United States in 2000. Antimicrob Agents Chemother. 2001;45:1402-1406.
19. Zhanel GG, Hoban DJ, Karlowsky JA. Nitrofurantoin is active against vancomycin-resistant enterococci. Antimicrob Agents Chemother. 2001;45:324-326.
20. Wazait HD, Patel HR, Veer V, et al. Catheter-associated urinary tract infections: prevalence of uropathogens and pattern of antimicrobial resistance in a UK hospital (1996-2001). BJU Int. 2003;91:806-809.
21. Schroeder SA, Terry PM, Bennett JV. Antibiotic resistance and transfer factor in Salmonella, United States 1967. JAMA. 1968;205:903-906.
22. Gleckman R, Alvarez S, Joubert DW. Drug therapy reviews: Nitrofurantoin. Am J Hosp Pharm. 1979;36:342-351.
23. Brumfitt W, Reynolds AV, Hamilton-Miller JM. Activity of nitrofurantoin and nifuratel against anaerobic gram-negative bacilli (Letter). Lancet. 1975;1:460.
24. Conklin JD. The pharmacokinetics of nitrofurantoin and its related bioavailability. Antibiot Chemother. 1978;25:233-252.
25. Gleckman R, Alvarez S, Joubert DW, et al. Drug therapy review: Methenamine mandelate and methenamine hippurate. Am J Hosp Pharm. 1979;36:1509-1512.
26. Schmidt FH. Inactivation of nitrofuran derivatives by mammalian tissue. Klinische Wochenschrift. 1966;44:653-654.
27. Dunn BL, Stamey TA. Antibacterial concentrations in prostatic fluid, 1-nitrofurantoin. J Urol. 1967;97:505-507.
28. Varsano I, Fischl J, Shochet SB. The excretion of orally ingested nitrofurantoin in human milk. J Pediatr. 1973;82:886-887.
29. D'Arcy PF. Nitrofurantoin. Drug Intell Clin Pharm. 1985;19:540-547.
30. Sachs J, Geer J, Noell P, et al. Effect of renal function on urinary recovery of orally administered nitrofurantoin. N Engl J Med. 1968;278:1032-1035.
31. Iravani A, Richard GA, Baer H. Trimethoprim once daily vs. nitrofurantoin in treatment of acute urinary tract infections in young women, with special reference to periurethral, vaginal, and fecal flora. Rev Infect Dis. 1982;4:378-387.
32. Hooton TM, Winter C, Tiu F, Stamm WE. Randomized comparative trial and cost analysis of 3-day antimicrobial regimens for treatment of acute cystitis in women. JAMA. 1995;273:41-45.
33. Warren JW, Abrutyn E, Hebel JR, et al. Guidelines for antimicrobial treatment of uncomplicated acute bacterial cystitis and acute pyelonephritis in women. Infectious Diseases Society of America (IDSA). Clin Infect Dis. 1999;29:745-758.
34. Spencer RC, Moseley DJ, Greensmith MJ. Nitrofurantoin modified release versus trimethoprim or co-trimoxazole in the treatment of uncomplicated urinary tract infection in general practice. J Antimicrob Chemother. 1994;33:121-129.
35. Iravani A, Klimberg I, Briefer C, et al. A trial comparing low-dose, short-course ciprofloxacin and standard 7 day therapy with co-trimoxazole or nitrofurantoin in the treatment of uncomplicated urinary tract infection. J Antimicrob Chemother. 1999;43:67-75.
36. Stamm WE, Hooton TM. Management of urinary tract infections in adults. N Engl J Med. 1993;329:1328-1334.
37. Lohr JA, Hayden GF, Kesler RW, et al. Three-day therapy of lower urinary tract infections with nitrofurantoin macrocrystals: a randomized clinical trial. J Pediatr. 1981;99:980-983.
38. Freeman RB, Smith WM, Richardson JA, et al. Long-term therapy for chronic bacteriuria in men. U.S. Public Health Service Cooperative Study. Ann Intern Med. 1975;83:133-147.

39. Stamm WE, Counts GW, Wagner KF, et al. Antimicrobial prophylaxis of recurrent urinary tract infections: A double-blind, placebo-controlled trial. Ann Intern Med. 1980;92:770-775.

40. Brumfitt W, Hamilton-Miller JM. A comparative trial of low dose cefaclor and macrocrystalline nitrofurantoin in the prevention of recurrent urinary tract infection. Infection. 1995;23:98-102.

41. Brumfitt W, Hamilton-Miller JM, Smith GW, Al-Wali W. Comparative trial of norfloxacin and macrocrystalline nitrofurantoin (Macrodantin) in prophylaxis of recurrent urinary tract infections in women. Q J Med. 1991;81:811-820.

42. Vosti KL. Recurrent urinary tract infections: Prevention by prophylactic antibiotics after sexual intercourse. JAMA. 1975;231:934-940.

43. Pfau A, Sacks TG. Effective prophylaxis for recurrent urinary tract infections during pregnancy. Clin Infect Dis. 1992;14:810-814.

44. Raz R, Colodner R, Rohana Y, et al. Effectiveness of estriol-containing vaginal pessaries and nitrofurantoin macrocrystal therapy in the prevention of recurrent urinary tract infection in postmenopausal women. Clin Infect Dis. 2003;36:1362-1368.

45. Anderson RU. Prophylaxis of bacteriuria during intermittent catheterization of acute neurogenic bladder. J Urol. 1980;123:364-366.

46. Kuhlemeier KV, Stover SL, Lloyd LK. Prophylactic antibacterial therapy for preventing urinary tract infections in spinal cord injury patients. J Urol. 1985;134:514-517.

47. Schlager TA, Anderson S, Trudell J, Hendley JO. Nitrofurantoin prophylaxis for bacteriuria and urinary tract infection in children with neurogenic bladder on intermittent catheterization. J Pediatr. 1998;132:704-708.

48. Kalowski S, Radford N, Kincaid-Smith P. Crystalline and macrocrystalline nitrofurantoin in the treatment of urinary-tract infection. N Engl J Med. 1974;290:385-387.

49. Brumfitt W, Hamilton-Miller JM. Efficacy and safety profile of long-term nitrofurantoin in urinary infections: 18 years' experience. J Antimicrob Chemother. 1998;42:363-371.

50. Holmberg L, Boman G. Pulmonary reactions to nitrofurantoin: 447 cases reported to the Swedish Adverse Drug Reaction Committee 1966-1976. Eur J Resp Dis. 1981;62:180-189.

51. Sovijärvi ARA, Lemola M, Stenius B, et al. Nitrofurantoin-induced acute, subacute and chronic pulmonary reactions. Scand J Resp Dis. 1977;58:41-50.

52. Martin WJ. Nitrofurantoin: Evidence for the oxidant injury of lung parenchymal cells. Am Rev Resp Dis. 1983;127:482-486.

53. Cameron RJ, Kolbe J, Wilsher ML, Lambie N. Bronchiolitis obliterans organising pneumonia associated with the use of nitrofurantoin. Thorax. 2000;55:249-251.

54. Sheehan RE, Wells AU, Milne DG, Hansell DM. Nitrofurantoin-induced lung disease: Two cases demonstrating resolution of apparently irreversible CT abnormalities. J Comput Assist Tomogr. 2000;24:259-261.

55. Holmberg L, Boman G. Adverse reactions to nitrofurantoin: Analysis of 921 reports. Am J Med. 1980;69:733-738.

56. Sharp JR, Ishak KG, Zimmerman HJ. Chronic active hepatitis and severe hepatic necrosis associated with nitrofurantoin. Ann Intern Med. 1980;92:14-19.

57. Goldstein LI, Ishak KG, Burns W. Hepatic injury associated with nitrofurantoin therapy. Am J Digest Dis. 1974;19:987-998.

58. Gait JE. Hemolytic reactions to nitrofurantoin in patients with glucose-6-phosphate dehydrogenase deficiency: Theory and practice. DICP. 1990;24:1210-1213.

59. Buzard JA, Kopko F, Paul MF. Inhibition of glutathione reductase by nitrofurantoin. J Lab Clin Med. 1960;56:885-890.

60. Dershwitz M, Novak RF. Studies of the mechanism of nitrofurantoin-mediated red cell toxicity. J Pharmacol Exp Ther. 1982;222:430-434.

61. Shah RR, Wade G. Reappraisal of the risk/benefit of nitrofurantoin: Review of toxicity and efficacy. Adverse Drug React Acute Poisoning Rev. 1989;8:183-201.

62. Toole J, Parrish M. Nitrofurantoin polyneuropathy. Neurology. 1973;23:554-559.

63. Yiannikas C, Pollard JD, McLeod JG. Nitrofurantoin neuropathy. Aust N Z J Med. 1981;11:400-405.

64. Corragio MJ, Gross TP, Roscelli JD. Nitrofurantoin toxicity in children. Pediatr Infect Dis J. 1989;8:163-166.

65. Perry JE, LeBlanc AL. Transfer of nitrofurantoin across the human placenta. Tex Rep Biol Med. 1967;25:265-269.

66. Wang CY, Benson RC Jr, Bryan GT. Mutagenicity for *Salmonella typhimurium* of urine obtained from human receiving nitrofurantoin. J Natl Cancer Inst. 1977;58:871-873.

67. Hailey FJ, Fort H, Williams JC, et al. Foetal safety of nitrofurantoin macrocrystals therapy during pregnancy: a retrospective analysis. J Int Med Res. 1983;11:364-369.

68. Kass EH. Pyelonephritis and bacteriuria: A major problem in preventive medicine. Ann Intern Med. 1962;56:46-53.

69. Czeizel AE, Rockenbauer M, Sorensen HT, Olsen J. Nitrofurantoin and congenital abnormalities. Eur J Obstet Gynecol Reprod Biol. 2001;95:119-126.

70. Duca CJ, Scudi JV. Some antibacterial properties of Mandelamine (methenamine mandelate). Proc Soc Exp Biol Med. 1947;66:123-126.

71. Gandelman AL. Methenamine mandelate: Antimicrobial activity in urine and correlation with formaldehyde levels. J Urol. 1967;97:533-536.

72. Musher DM, Griffith DP, Templeton BG. Further observations on the potentiation of the antibacterial effect of methenamine by acetohydroxamic acid. J Infect Dis. 1976;133:564-567.

73. Hamilton-Miller JM, Brumfitt W. Methenamine and its salts as urinary tract antiseptics: Variables affecting the antibacterial activity of formaldehyde, mandelic acid, and hippuric acid in vitro. Invest Urol. 1977;14:287-291.

74. Klinge E, Männistö P, Mäntylä R, et al. Pharmacokinetics of methenamine in healthy volunteers. J Antimicrob Chemother. 1982;9:209-216.

75. Mayrer AR, Andriole VT. Urinary tract antiseptics. Med Clin N Am. 1982;66:199-208.

76. Allgén L-G, Holmberg G, Persson B, et al. Biological fate of methenamine in man. Absorption, renal excretion and passage into umbilical cord blood, amniotic fluid and breast milk. Acta Obstet Gynecol Scand. 1979;58:287-293.

77. Knoefel PK, Huang KC. Biochemorphology of renal tubular transport: Hippuric acid and related substances. J Pharmacol Exp Ther. 1959;126:296-303.

78. Strom JG, Jun HW. Effect of urine pH and ascorbic acid on the rate of conversion of methenamine to formaldehyde. Biopharmaceut Drug Dispos. 1993;14:61-69.

79. Musher DM, Griffith DP. Generation of formaldehyde from methenamine: Effect of pH and concentration, and antibacterial effect. Antimicrob Agents Chemother. 1974;6:708-711.

80. Musher DM, Griffith DP, Richie Y. The generation of formaldehyde from methenamine. Effect of urinary flow and residual volume. Invest Urol. 1976;13:380-382.

81. Cronberg S, Welin C-O, Henriksson L, et al. Prevention of recurrent acute cystitis by methenamine hippurate: Double blind controlled crossover long term study. BMJ. 1987;294:1507-1508.

82. Harding GKM, Ronald AR. A controlled study of antimicrobial prophylaxis of recurrent urinary tract infection in women. N Engl J Med. 1974;291:597-601.

83. Kasanen A, Junnila SYT, Kaarsalo E, et al. Secondary prevention of recurrent urinary tract infections: Comparison of the effect of placebo, methenamine hippurate, nitrofurantoin and trimethoprim alone. Scand J Infect Dis. 1982;14:293-296.

84. Brumfitt W, Cooper J, Hamilton-Miller JM. Prevention of recurrent urinary tract infections in women: A comparative trial between nitrofurantoin and methenamine hippurate. J Urol. 1981;126:71-74.

85. Holland NH, West CD. Prevention of recurrent urinary tract infections in girls. J Dis Child. 1963;105:560-567.

86. Elo J, Sarna S, Ahava K, et al. Methenamine hippurate in urinary tract infections in children: prophylaxis, treatment and side effects. J Antimicrob Chemother. 1978;4:355-365.

87. Vainrub B, Musher DM. Lack of effect of methenamine in suppression of, or prophylaxis against, chronic urinary tract infection. Antimicrob Agents Chemother. 1977;12:625-629.

88. Kevorkian CG, Merritt JL, Ilstrup DM. Methenamine mandelate with acidification: An effective urinary antiseptic in patients with neurogenic bladder. Mayo Clin Proc. 1984;59:523-529.

89. Ross RR, Conway GF. Hemorrhagic cystitis following accidental overdose of methenamine mandelate. Am J Dis Child. 1970;119:86-87.

90. Kasanen A, Mustakallio EK, Koskinen EH. Methenamine hippurate in the treatment of urinary tract infections. Ann Clin Res. 1974;6:279-284.

91. Furness MB, McDonald PJ, Beasley NV. Urinary antiseptics in asymptomatic bacteriuria of pregnancy. N Z Med J. 1974;81:417-419.

CHAPTER **35**

Topical Antibacterials

JUDITH A. O'DONNELL

ALLAN R. TUNKEL

Topical antibacterial therapy has an important but often undervalued role to play in the prevention and management of specific infections. Topical antibacterial agents can be subdivided into two types: topical antimicrobials and topical antiseptics. The topical *antimicrobial* agents usually have a primary target site and mechanism of action. They include bacitracin, neomycin, mupirocin, clindamycin, erythromycin, and metronidazole, and they may be administered concomitantly with other antimicrobial agents that have an oral or intravenous route of delivery. Topical antimicrobials have been used to prevent wound infections, in the treatment of superficial skin and soft tissue infections, and to eradicate carriage of undesirable bacteria such as *Staphylococcus aureus*. More recently, these agents have been utilized to prevent postoperative infections and catheter-related infections in certain patient populations. The topical *antiseptics* (such as chlorhexidine gluconate, povidone-iodine, alcohol, and triclosan) have multiple target sites of action against bacteria and are sometimes referred to as biocides.[1] For the purposes of this chapter, the term *topical antibacterials* will refer to both types of agents.

Topical antibacterial therapy has several potential advantages over oral or parenteral administration of antibacterial agents in specific clin-

TABLE 35-1 Advantages of Topical Antibacterial Therapy
Ease of administration
Lower potential for adverse reactions
Lower risk of noncompliance
Delivery of high drug concentrations to site of infection
Decreased risk of bacterial resistance or antimicrobial cross-resistance
Cost savings (depending on agent used)

ical settings (Table 35-1).[2] After the application of small amounts directly to an infection or wound, very high local drug concentrations are achieved, levels that would be toxic if they had to be reached by systemic administration. When administered topically, these agents first enter the skin (the first target organ), and then a variable quantity is distributed throughout the body and is finally eliminated. Concentrations of a topical antibacterial decline from the skin surface to the subcutis (after systemic administration, the opposite occurs).[3] Therefore, topical administration is favored if the pathologic process is in the epidermis or papillary dermis, as the highest doses are delivered directly to the site of infection. For infection in the lower dermis or subcutis, one needs to determine whether topical antibacterial administration yields the necessary drug concentrations to effectively eradicate the infection. Topical preparations formulated to contain combinations of topical antibacterial agents may offer the benefits of synergism and may delay the selection of resistant microorganisms. In this chapter, we review the general uses of topical antibacterial agents in the therapy and prevention of infections. Topical agents are also effective in treating eye (Chapters 106 and 107) and ear (Chapter 54) infections.

GENERAL USES OF TOPICAL ANTIBACTERIALS

Disinfecting the Skin

Skin disinfection is a critical component of effective patient care, whether it is disinfection of the patient's skin to provide a sterile environment for procedures, or disinfection of the health care worker's skin to prevent transmission of pathogenic bacteria through contact with patients. Some topical antibacterial agents, in particular the topical antiseptics noted earlier, are very effective at decreasing the number of bacteria on the skin. The ideal antiseptic agent should have the following properties: a broad antimicrobial spectrum; rapid bactericidal activity; persistent activity on the skin; an absence of irritating, allergic, or toxic reactions; an absence of systemic absorption; activity in the presence of body fluids (e.g., blood); and cosmetic acceptance.[2] Unfortunately, no single compound meets all these criteria. Depending on the specific clinical situation, however, only certain properties may be required. For example, for repeated hand washings (e.g., by medical personnel), lack of irritation and persistence of activity are essential properties. In contrast, for preparation of operative sites, rapid bactericidal activity is needed.

Several topical antiseptic agents have been used as skin disinfectants. Hexachlorophene, despite its remarkable persistence on the skin when used regularly, has lost favor as a skin disinfecting agent. It is not very effective against gram-negative organisms and absorption, with resultant toxicity (especially in newborns), has been a concern. The iodophors, in particular povidone-iodine, are widely used as skin antiseptics. Povidone-iodine is an organic complex of polyvinylpyrrolidone and tri-iodine ions (the antimicrobial component) that slowly liberate iodine on reduction. Iodophors have a broad antimicrobial spectrum, but antibacterial activity does not persist for prolonged periods on the skin, in wounds, or on mucous membranes, and iodophors may be inactivated by body fluids. Their microbicidal effects are the result of cell wall penetration, oxidation, and substitution of microbial contents with free iodine. Povidone-iodine has been widely used for many years in preoperative skin preparation, preparation of skin for blood culture phlebotomy and certain catheter placements, hand scrubbing, and the treatment and prevention of skin infections.[2] Recently, recommendations have been made to switch from povidone-iodine to chlorhexidine compounds for skin preparation for intravascular catheter placement and for obtaining blood cultures (see later).[4]

Povidone-iodine in a 5% cream preparation has recently been studied for its in vitro activity against various strains of *S. aureus,* including methicillin-resistant strains (MRSA) and mupirocin-resistant strains. It has also been evaluated for its bioavailability in human nasal secretions. One study demonstrated rapid bactericidal activity against all *S. aureus* strains tested, and good bioavailability within the human nares.[5] The cream formulation may have a future role in the prevention of infection and eradication of nasal colonization by *S. aureus.*

Alcohols are rapidly bactericidal, but older preparations have been criticized for their transient antiseptic action, local irritation, and excessive drying, especially when associated with repeated use or when applied to damaged skin. Recently, however, several new waterless, alcohol-based hand hygiene products have been brought to market in the United States. These products contain 90% alcohol as the active antiseptic ingredient, but they also contain emollients to make them nondrying and nonirritating to skin[6]; they also differ from older preparations in that their antiseptic action is more prolonged. Because these products are waterless, they can be made widely available in and around patient care areas without the need for a sink or paper towels, which encourages more widespread use. The most recent guidelines on hand hygiene recommend that these products be used preferentially over soap and water as the first line of defense for cleaning nonsoiled hands prior to and after patient encounters.[7]

Chlorhexidine, a cationic biguanide that achieves its antiseptic activity by causing disruption of microbial cell membranes and precipitation of cell contents, is the most ideal agent for skin cleaning and surgical scrubs. Its valuable properties include persistent activity on the skin when used regularly, rapid bactericidal activity, a broad antibacterial spectrum, little evidence of irritancy or allergy, activity in the presence of body fluids, and minimal absorption. Chlorhexidine-containing products have been more widely available in the United States since 2000 when the U.S. Food and Drug Administration (FDA) approved a 2% tincture of a chlorhexidine preparation for use as a skin antiseptic. In a study comparing 2% chlorhexidine, povidone-iodine, and 70% alcohol for sterile skin preparation of central venous and arterial catheter sites, the 2% chlorhexidine lowered rates of subsequent blood-stream infections significantly more than the other preparations.[8] It is important to note that preparations containing smaller amounts of chlorhexidine might not be as effective as the 2% chlorhexidine products. Chlorhexidine-containing preparations are not currently recommended for use in children 2 months of age or younger. Partly on the basis of these results, recent guidelines on the prevention of vascular catheter–related infections recommend chlorhexidine gluconate for preparation of skin prior to catheter insertion.[4] In addition, chlorhexidine is recommended for skin preparation prior to phlebotomy for blood cultures.

Triclosan (2,4,4′-trichloro-2′-hydroxydiphenyl ether) is a synthetic bisphenol antimicrobial agent active against a broad range of gram-positive and gram-negative bacteria. It has been used extensively for many years in dental hygiene products and soaps. More recently, its physiochemical properties have facilitated the incorporation of triclosan into plastic kitchenware products, toys, and tea towels.[9,10] Triclosan is considered a biocide with multiple target sites of antibacterial action. Although theoretical concerns have been raised that its chronic use and its presence in certain products may lead to resistance to it and to other antimicrobials, this has yet to be proven.[9] In the most recent guidelines regarding hand hygiene, triclosan-containing products are considered as acceptable, active antiseptic agents.

Prophylaxis of Infection in Clean Wounds

When a wound leads to disruption of epidermal integrity (e.g., secondary to abrasions, cuts, or bites), the application of a topical antibacterial agent to prevent infection from developing can be considered. However, no antibacterial formulation has ever been proven to be efficacious in the prophylaxis of clean wounds, because so few clean wounds become infected. Studies of topical preparations (e.g., neomycin, alone or in combination with bacitracin or polymyxin, or both) have shown efficacy in the prevention of infection in some circumstances, although these studies have been criticized because of the absence of control groups.[11] Controlled studies are unlikely to be performed, however, because the number of patients required to be studied would be extremely large.

To avoid the difficulties in performing a large, randomized controlled trial, a human skin infection model was developed to test the efficacy of topical antibiotic formulations in the prophylaxis of minor skin infections.[11] After the induction of abrasion-type wounds in human volunteers, the wounds were inoculated with either 10^5 organisms of *S. aureus* or 10^7 organisms of *Streptococcus pyogenes* and covered with an impermeable dressing for 6 hours. Both neomycin and bacitracin were highly effective in preventing infection with both *S. aureus* and *S. pyogenes* compared with the bland ointment vehicle. The treated wounds did not develop pus and reepithelialized within 3 to 5 days. Other investigators have also found that use of either topical neomycin-bacitracin-polymyxin ointment or bacitracin alone enhanced epidermal healing of wounds[12] and significantly reduced streptococcal skin colonization and subsequent infection of small skin traumas in children.[13] In one placebo-controlled trial, the efficacy of a novel topical antimicrobial gel containing cetrimide, bacitracin, and polymyxin B was studied with regard to the prevention of infections in minor wounds.[14] The preparation showed therapeutic action and reduced the incidence of clinical infection from 12.5% to 1.6%.

Despite these studies, the efficacy of topical antibacterials in the prevention of infections in clean wounds and wound healing remains questionable. The use of topical antibacterials in superficial wounds for a few days, until the integrity of the epidermis is reestablished, has been recommended, because the longer the epidermal barrier remains defective, the more likely it is that infection will occur. An important principle is that the agent do no harm and not be irritating, toxic, sensitizing, or lead to the development of organisms resistant to therapeutically important antimicrobial agents.

The use of topical antibacterials in nonhealing, noninfected chronic wounds such as pressure ulcers has been recommended by the U.S. Agency for Health Care Policy and Research.[15] The goal of such therapy is to decrease the bacterial burden in such wounds, and possibly to promote healing. However, there is no substantial evidence in the published medical literature that this goal has been achieved.[16] Moreover, chronic use of topical antibacterials is likely to promote bacterial resistance and should thus be avoided. None of the currently marketed topical antibacterials has been labeled for use specifically in the setting of chronic nonhealing wounds.[16] Thus, the use of topical antibacterials for chronic nonhealing wounds should not be promoted.

Prophylaxis of Recurrent Skin and Soft Tissue Infections

Some patients with recurrent furuncles, carbuncles, and other skin and soft tissue infections caused by *S. aureus* may have persistent nasal carriage of this organism. It has been suggested that eradication of *S. aureus* from the nares could reduce the recurrence of these infections. In one study, 34 such patients were treated with a 5-day course of intranasal mupirocin; 17 patients were then randomized to successive monthly therapy for 1 year, and the other 17 received placebo.[17] The investigators found a significant reduction in the number of recurrent skin infections among those patients treated with monthly maintenance mupirocin; one patient became colonized with an isolate that had low-level mupirocin resistance. The small size of the study precluded the authors from making definitive recommendations for the management of recurrent furunculosis and folliculitis in staphylococcal carriers. However, the results provide some support for the common clinical practice of maintenance mupirocin in patients with persistent *S. aureus* nasal colonization. Well-controlled clinical trials are needed to clarify this issue.

Prophylaxis of Infection in Operative Wounds

There is good evidence from both controlled and uncontrolled trials that topical antibacterials are efficacious in the prevention of postoperative wound infections, and a significant decrease in wound infec-

tions has been reported in treated patients.[3] In one study involving more than 6000 cases over a 4-year period, a declining rate of infection was documented with the increased use of a neomycin-bacitracin-polymyxin spray during operations. When the neomycin-bacitracin-polymyxin spray was compared with no prophylaxis in 851 surgical wounds, a significant decrease in wound infection was noted in the treatment group. Other investigators have noted similar results in prospective, randomized clinical trials, indicating the importance of preoperative topical neomycin-bacitracin-polymyxin spray in the prophylaxis of operative wound infections.

Several recent studies have been performed in a variety of surgical patients to evaluate the effectiveness of intranasal mupirocin, applied preoperatively, on the subsequent rate of postoperative surgical site infections. The largest double-blind, randomized, placebo-controlled trial enrolled 4030 patients undergoing general, cardiothoracic, neurosurgical, and gynecologic surgical procedures.[18] Patients received either intranasal mupirocin or placebo twice daily for up to 5 days prior to their surgical procedure; 83% received three or more doses prior to surgery. Of the 3864 patients included in the intent-to-treat analysis, 2.3% of mupirocin-treated patients developed a surgical site infection, compared with 2.4% of the placebo recipients. In a secondary analysis of 891 patients who were noted to have *S. aureus* nasal carriage prior to surgery, those patients treated with mupirocin had a subsequent surgical site infection rate of 4% as compared with their placebo-treated counterparts who had a 7.7% rate of subsequent infection. This difference, however, did not achieve statistical significance. It has been suggested that the lack of a statistically significant outcome in this study resulted, in part, from the fact that the sample size calculation had an 85% power to detect a relative reduction of 50% in the rate of *S. aureus* surgical site infections.[19] Moreover, because fewer patients than anticipated remained in the study and there were less than the expected number of *S. aureus* surgical site infections in the placebo group, there may have been as much as a 25% likelihood that study results would be negative even if the mupirocin were effective.

Several additional studies have assessed the effectiveness of preoperative intranasal mupirocin therapy in a variety of surgical patients. In two open trials performed in patients undergoing open heart surgery, patients were treated with preoperative intranasal mupirocin and compared with historical controls.[20,21] The patients in the treatment group had a statistically significant decrease in subsequent postoperative sternal wound infections. In another large open trial in which 1044 orthopedic surgery patients in The Netherlands were treated with preoperative intranasal mupirocin and compared with 1260 historical controls, the mupirocin-treated patients had a statistically significant decrease in postoperative wound infections.[22]

In a randomized, double-blind, placebo-controlled trial in orthopedic surgery patients in whom prosthetic material would be used, intranasal mupirocin or placebo ointment was applied 1 day before and on the day of surgery; there were 315 patients in the treatment arm with an *S. aureus* carriage rate of 30% and 299 patients in the placebo arm with an *S. aureus* nasal carriage rate of 29%.[23] There were a total of 13 infections with *S. aureus*, five in the mupirocin group and eight in the placebo group. Of the five patients in the mupirocin group, two had documented nasal carriage of *S. aureus*, and only one had a postoperative infection with the endogenous *S. aureus* strain. This compared with the eight patients in the placebo group, five of whom had documented *S. aureus* nasal carriage, and all of whom had a postoperative infection with the endogenous strain. Endogenous infections were five times less likely to occur in the mupirocin-treated patients, but this difference did not achieve statistical significance. Additionally, there was no difference in overall numbers of postoperative infections in either group and no difference in length of hospital stay. A potential limitation of this study was that it was underpowered to identify a lesser treatment effect than the planned 75% reduction in infection.[24] Moreover, patients received an average of only two doses of mupirocin prior to surgery, which may not have been adequate to prevent the development of subsequent staphylococcal infections.

Although numerous studies support the notion that nasal colonization with *S. aureus* is an important risk factor for the development of postoperative infections and that its eradication can prevent such sequelae, the effectiveness of preoperative intranasal mupirocin remains unclear. Although all of the open trials demonstrate the effectiveness of *S. aureus* eradication, the use of historical controls is a limitation in interpretation of study results. The two randomized, double-blind, placebo-controlled trials failed to show a statistically significant decrease in postoperative surgical site infection rates, but they may have been underpowered to demonstrate a true clinical effect. Based on cost-effectiveness analyses, it appears that it may be cost effective to utilize preoperative intranasal mupirocin in patients undergoing cardiothoracic surgery.[19,25] However, more studies are needed to determine the best regimen and the potential impact, if any, of resistance or change in flora on development of subsequent infections.

Prophylaxis of Vascular Catheter–Related Infections

Many authorities have recommended the use of topical antibacterial agents for prophylaxis against bacterial colonization of central and peripheral intravascular catheter sites, although the efficacy of this practice in the prevention of catheter-associated bacteremia remains unclear. In one prospective evaluation of 827 random catheter insertions employing three regimens of catheter care (neomycin-bacitracin-polymyxin at insertion and every 48 hours, versus iodophor ointment at insertion and every 48 hours, versus no ointment), no differences in catheter-acquired sepsis (two patients in each group) or local inflammation (38.9% versus 41.9% versus 41.7%, respectively) were noted.[26] The only differences were in semiquantitative cultures of catheter tips, with 6 positive cultures in the neomycin-bacitracin-polymyxin group, 10 in the iodophor group, and 18 in the no-treatment group. In contrast, a randomized controlled trial of povidone-iodine in the prevention of infection in subclavian vein hemodialysis catheters found that povidone-iodine was associated with a significant decrease in the incidence of septicemia (5% versus 18%; $p < .02$).[27]

Another study comparing skin preparation with either 2% chlorhexidine, 70% alcohol, or 10% povidone-iodine found that chlorhexidine was superior to the other two disinfectants in the reduction of both local infection and catheter-related bacteremias.[8] Another study evaluated a novel antiseptic solution (composed of 0.25% chlorhexidine gluconate, 0.025% benzalkonium chloride, and 4% benzyl alcohol) and found it was more effective than 10% povidone-iodine for insertion site care of short-term central venous and arterial catheters[28]; this effect appeared to be related to a more efficacious prevention of gram-positive bacterial infections. Further studies are needed, however, to determine the optimal regimen for the prophylaxis of catheter-related infections.

Prophylaxis of Dialysis Catheter Infections

Catheter-associated infections in patients undergoing either hemodialysis or peritoneal dialysis are one of the most common reasons for hospitalization and catheter removal in this patient population. In patients who undergo peritoneal dialysis, a few strategies have demonstrated efficacy in the prophylaxis against exit site and tunnel infections. In the absence of prophylaxis, the average rates of *S. aureus* exit site infections range from 0.34 to 0.41 per patient per year.[29] Patients with *S. aureus* nasal colonization have exit site infection rates that are significantly higher (>0.5 infections per year).[30] Moreover, the rates of peritonitis in patients with one or more positive nares cultures for *S. aureus* have been shown to be significantly higher than in patients never colonized (0.24 per year versus 0.08 per year).[30] With the use of some prophylaxis regimen, rates of infection can be reduced to less than half of these numbers.[31]

The application of povidone-iodine at the exit site of the peritoneal dialysis catheter was shown to be effective in reducing subsequent infection rates in some published studies.[32] However, other studies using this strategy have failed to demonstrate effectiveness.[31] Intranasal mupirocin twice daily for 5 days for the treatment of *S. aureus* nasal carriage was shown to be an effective strategy in decreasing *S. aureus*

catheter infections in those patients who are proven nasal carriers.[33-35] Therapy must be repeated monthly or, if routine cultures are performed, whenever cultures return positive for *S. aureus*. In a prospective open trial of intranasal mupirocin, peritoneal dialysis patients were treated with mupirocin when nares cultures were positive for *S. aureus*.[34] Compared with historical controls, exit site infections were significantly decreased from 0.22 per patient-year among controls to 0.09 per patient-year in the mupirocin-treated patients. Topical intranasal mupirocin also resulted in a significant decrease in subsequent rates of *S. aureus* peritonitis in this study, although the rates of peritonitis caused by gram-negative organisms increased over the study period. The only randomized, double-blind, placebo-controlled trial of monthly intranasal mupirocin was performed by the Mupirocin Study Group in nine centers throughout Europe.[36] Peritoneal dialysis patients with positive nares cultures for *S. aureus* were randomized to receive twice-daily intranasal mupirocin or placebo for 5 days every 4 weeks, and followed for 18 months. Although the rate of *S. aureus* exit site infections was significantly lower in the mupirocin group in this study, the total rate of exit site infections, tunnel infections, and peritonitis was not significantly different between treated and placebo recipients. Of note, in a cost-effectiveness analysis, it was not cost effective to use prophylactic topical intranasal mupirocin in chronic peritoneal dialysis patients.[37]

Another prophylactic strategy is application of topical mupirocin to the exit site as part of routine daily care of the peritoneal dialysis catheter. In a prospective, randomized study comparing oral rifampicin with topical mupirocin applied daily to the exit site, rates of infection were compared with historical controls.[38] The rates of *S. aureus* exit site infections, tunnel infections, peritonitis, and catheter loss caused by *S. aureus* infections were not statistically different between the two treatment groups, but they were significantly lower than rates in the historical control groups. In another prospective, historically controlled study in which a group of peritoneal dialysis patients were treated with topical mupirocin at the exit site three times weekly,[39] there was a significant reduction in *S. aureus* exit site infections (21 versus 3 episodes) and *S. aureus* peritonitis (35 versus 11 episodes); patients were not screened for *S. aureus* carrier status, however. Several smaller studies (none of which were randomized, placebo-controlled, or blinded) also employed topical mupirocin to the exit site either daily or three times weekly, and their results were similar with respect to decreased rates of peritoneal dialysis catheter–related infections.[31,40,41] However, no cost-effectiveness analyses have been performed for the use of topical mupirocin in this patient population.

As a result of the findings in these studies, and despite the fact that there has not been a definitive, well-designed, large, multicenter, randomized, placebo-controlled trial to date, topical mupirocin has been advocated and prescribed at many centers in Europe and North America as part of the routine peritoneal dialysis catheter management. This practice has led to concerns about long-term use of mupirocin and the emergence of resistance, as well as to concerns about changing the predominant pathogen in peritoneal dialysis catheter–associated infections from staphylococci to gram-negative bacteria.[31] One study revealed the emergence of colonization with *S. aureus* strains exhibiting high-level resistance to mupirocin in patients who had been using mupirocin as part of their routine catheter care for 4 years.[42] Although topical mupirocin is generally very well tolerated, has an extremely low side effect profile, and has been safely used in patients for prolonged periods of time, there have been a few case reports of spontaneous rupture of polyurethane peritoneal dialysis catheters, possibly linked to this topical agent (see later).[43]

In contrast to the peritoneal dialysis patients, there are few studies that assess potential prophylactic strategies in patients with hemodialysis catheters. Prophylactic strategies that have been evaluated in the hemodialysis catheter population include intranasal mupirocin, topical mupirocin applied to catheter exit site, and povidone-iodine application to the exit site.[31] There is only one double-blind, randomized, placebo-controlled study published that examined the prophylaxis of catheter infection in hemodialysis patients.[44] This study assessed intranasal mupirocin given three times daily for 2 weeks after catheter insertion, followed by three times weekly as a maintenance regimen, versus placebo.[44] All patients were positive for *S. aureus* nasal carriage prior to enrollment and were followed for 9 months. The authors observed a significant decrease in nasal colonization in the mupirocin-treated group, as well as a significant decrease in the rate of *S. aureus* infections. However, rates of *S. aureus* bacteremia did not differ between the treated group and the placebo recipients.

A subsequent prospective open trial study, performed by the same group, utilized intranasal mupirocin in hemodialysis patients three times weekly for 6 months followed by once weekly for 6 months.[45] Study patients were compared with historical controls and were found to have a statistically significant decrease in *S. aureus* bacteremias over the study period. Another prospective open trial assessing intranasal mupirocin applied once weekly in hemodialysis patients showed significantly decreased rates of *S. aureus* bacteremia in the mupirocin-treated study patients when compared with historical controls.[46] A single cost-effectiveness analysis of intranasal mupirocin in hemodialysis patients suggested that such a strategy was cost effective.[47]

A single prospective, randomized, open trial study evaluated the use of povidone-iodine at the exit site of the hemodialysis catheter along with a sterile dressing, compared with a sterile dressing alone[48]; at the onset of this study, 22% of patients in the treatment group and 32% of patients in the placebo group were positive for *S. aureus* nasal carriage. There was a statistically significant decrease in subsequent rates of bacteremias, exit site infections, and positive catheter-tip cultures in the group receiving povidone-iodine ointment to the catheter site along with the sterile dressing. Additional studies using povidone-iodine ointment as part of the catheter site care are clearly warranted. On the basis of the results of this single small study, however, no specific recommendations can be made regarding this prophylactic strategy.

A single randomized, controlled, open-label trial of topical exit site mupirocin application in patients with tunneled, cuffed hemodialysis catheters was recently published.[49] A total of 50 hemodialysis patients were randomized to topical mupirocin applied to the catheter exit site three times weekly, or no treatment. The rates of *S. aureus* nasal carriage in the two groups were similar. Compared with controls, the mupirocin-treated patients had significantly fewer catheter-related bacteremias (7% versus 35%) and had a longer time interval to first bacteremia. Median catheter survival was also significantly longer in the treated group. More research needs to be performed on this prophylactic strategy before it can be widely recommended, however, especially in view of concerns about emergence of resistant strains.

Prophylaxis of Infection in Burn Wounds

Prevention of infection in the burned patient is extremely difficult because burn wound sites are favorable for bacterial overgrowth, the epidermal barrier is often defective for extended periods, and the patients are in the hospital where multiple antibiotic–resistant organisms are found.[2] Frequent débridement and the establishment of an epidermis, or a surrogate such as a skin graft or skin substitute, are essential for the prevention of infection. As a result of the pathogenesis and pathophysiology of the burn wound, the delivery of systemic antimicrobial therapy to the deepest, most severely ischemic areas of the wound cannot be relied on because gradient diffusion from the wound periphery is the sole means of access.[50]

The use of topical antibacterial agents for burned patients is well established. Before the development of effective topical burn wound chemotherapy, burn wound sepsis was diagnosed as the principal cause of death in 60% of burn patients who died[51]; the use of mafenide acetate has reduced to 28% the incidence of burn wound sepsis as a cause of death. After administration, high antimicrobial concentrations are found on the wound surface where the risk of bacterial contamination is the greatest. In patients with deep, extensive wounds, dense bacterial colonization, particularly by gram-positive cocci, often occurs within 24 hours; aerobic gram-negative bacilli typically appear within 3 to 7 days. If this initial bacterial colonization is not treated, deeper spread and ultimate systemic invasion of pathogenic bacteria

can occur. Therefore, topical antibacterial therapy should be initiated as soon as possible to delay or prevent these processes.

There is evidence that effective topical antibacterial therapy delays colonization of the burn wound for a variable period (measured in days, not weeks); maintains the wound bacterial density at lower levels than can otherwise be achieved and for appreciable intervals (measured in weeks); and tends to result in a relatively homogeneous and less diverse wound flora than would otherwise be expected.[50] The specific antimicrobial agent chosen for topical therapy should have a broad in vitro spectrum of activity against gram-positive cocci (staphylococci, streptococci, and enterococci) and the aerobic gram-negative flora (including *Pseudomonas aeruginosa*). Ideally, the agent should penetrate the eschar, but as it may be absorbed, it must have low toxicity[52]; the agent must also remain active in the presence of serum and necrotic debris. Furthermore, with increasing use of cultured skin grafts in the therapeutic approach to the burned patient, topical antibacterials may be required to prevent microbial colonization and destruction of grafts containing cultured skin cells. Successful use of topical agents prevents the bacterial conversion of superficial burns to deeper injury, results in spontaneous healing of wounds that initially appeared clinically to be full thickness, and decreases the frequency of episodes of systemic sepsis.[20] Specific topical agents for use in burned patients are discussed in Chapter 317.

Treatment of Pyodermas

The major pyoderma in which topical antibacterials have been utilized is impetigo. Impetigo is a superficial infection of the skin caused by group A streptococci (see Chapter 195) or *S. aureus,* or both. Bullous impetigo is usually caused by *S. aureus.* One of the goals of antimicrobial therapy in impetigo is to prevent the spread of infection to uninvolved skin.[2] Early uncontrolled and controlled trials of topical antibacterial therapy in patients with impetigo suggested the efficacy of topical antibacterials, although other studies found that systemic antimicrobial therapy was more efficacious.[53] Despite this controversy, it appears that systemic antimicrobial therapy is somewhat superior to topical therapy in the management of streptococcal pyoderma, with swifter healing and fewer failures. However, topical therapy may be used early in infection, when the number of lesions is small and when there is a reasonable chance that these agents will be scrupulously and skillfully applied.[53] Exclusions to the use of topical antibacterials in pyodermas include the following: bullous impetigo (because the pathogenesis of this exfoliative infection may lead to continuing infection, rapid spread, or recurrence, or all of these, unless *S. aureus* is promptly eradicated); extensive pyoderma, regardless of the clinical form or bacterial cause; and children with poststreptococcal pyodermal nephritis and their infected contacts.[54] However, systemic antimicrobial therapy for streptococcal pyoderma does not guarantee the prevention of poststreptococcal glomerulonephritis,[53] although prompt eradication of nephritogenic streptococci may lessen the risk of spread to others, with the subsequent prevention of secondary cases. A newer topical antibacterial, mupirocin, has been shown to be as efficacious as systemic antibiotics in the therapy of limited impetigo (see later).

Topical antibacterial agents may have some efficacy in the therapy of secondary pyodermas, although the available studies generally did not include control groups.[53] Despite organism eradication, the underlying process persisted. Therefore, cure, in the sense of complete healing, was not achieved. Because topical antibacterials can lower the bacterial colony counts in acute dermatitis, the use of these agents in combination with topical glucocorticoids is a logical treatment regimen.[2] There is no role for topical antibacterials in the treatment of erysipelas, cellulitis, or furuncles.

Treatment of Erythrasma and Rosacea

Erythrasma is a cutaneous eruption caused by the bacterium *Corynebacterium minutissimum.* The rash of erythrasma is commonly found in intertriginous areas including axillae, inframammary areas, interspaces of toes, and intergluteal and crural folds. Once the diagnosis is confirmed, systemic antibacterial therapy with erythromycin is usually prescribed as first line therapy.[55] However, there is an important role for topical antibacterial therapy in the management of this dermatologic infection. Most experts recommend the addition of a topical agent to systemic therapy in patients with intertriginous area involvement, and the exclusive use of topical therapy in those patients intolerant of the recommended active systemic therapies.[55] Topical 2% clindamycin has been shown to be effective in the treatment of erythrasma and, when it is in an alcohol-based formulation, has the additional advantage of a drying effect.[56] The fusidic acid preparation, sodium fusidate ointment, has also been shown to be effective as a topical therapy for erythrasma, although it is not available in the United States.[55] Topically administered erythromycin, tetracycline, and chloramphenicol have all been evaluated and found not to be effective in the treatment of erythrasma.[55]

Rosacea is a dermatologic condition with several disease phases that include flushing, followed by erythrosis, papulopustular rosacea, and finally phimosis. The etiology of rosacea remains somewhat controversial and is considered to be multifactorial, depending on the phase of disease. *Helicobacter pylori* has been implicated as a potential causative factor by some authorities, and the *Demodex* mite has been implicated as a significant contributing factor of papulopustular rosacea.[57] There are no clear data that rosacea has a bacterial etiology, although the disease clearly responds to both systemic and topical treatment with antibacterial agents. Topical metronidazole, either in a 1% cream or a 0.75% gel, is the topical therapy that has been most widely evaluated in the treatment of papulopustular rosacea and the preceding erythrosis. Numerous randomized controlled trials have been published that confirm the tolerability and superior efficacy of topical metronidazole.[58,59] As topical metronidazole has no anti-inflammatory effects, its mechanism of action with respect to cure of rosacea remains unknown. Azelaic acid in a 20% cream formulation is an acceptable topical alternative.[57]

Treatment of Acne Vulgaris

Topical antibacterials are helpful for inflammatory acne.[60,61] The proliferation of *Propionibacterium acnes* is considered critical for the development of inflammatory lesions. The blocked follicles become an ideal anaerobic culture medium filled with nutrients in the form of lipid substrates; *P. acnes* metabolize the lipid, producing free fatty acids, and this may be the triggering mechanism that leads to retention hyperkeratosis and microcomedone formation. Benzoyl peroxide exerts its effects by bacteriostatic activity on the proliferation of *P. acnes*. Oxygen is liberated when the drug is decomposed by cysteine in the skin, and bacterial proteins are thus oxidized. After 2 weeks of daily application, a 10% benzoyl peroxide preparation reduces concentrations of free fatty acids by about 50%, and *P. acnes* by about 98%, comparable to the levels obtained after 4 weeks of treatment with other antibiotics.

Topical antibiotics are also used almost universally by dermatologists for the treatment of acne vulgaris.[60,61] These agents also exert their beneficial effects by decreasing the population of *P. acnes* in the follicle, although not as effectively or rapidly as benzoyl peroxide, and they also inhibit the production of proinflammatory mediators by organisms that are not killed.[60] Preparations containing clindamycin and erythromycin are most commonly used[60,61]; topical tetracyclines have also been utilized but are less effective than either clindamycin or erythromycin. Topical azelaic acid, a dicarboxylic acid derivative that is bacteriostatic for *P. acnes*, has been shown to reduce colony counts of *P. acnes* by about the same degree as clindamycin. However, the most effective topical antibacterial regimens against *P. acnes* are the combination formulations that include benzoyl peroxide and either erythromycin or clindamycin. A randomized 10-week trial comparing the efficacy of benzoyl peroxide (5%)–erythromycin (3%) gel with that of erythromycin (4%)–zinc (1.2%) solution in 72 acne vulgaris patients revealed that both inflammatory lesions and comedones showed a significantly greater percentage reduction from baseline in those patients receiving the benzoyl peroxide–erythromycin combination[62]; both physician and patient efficacy evaluations were also more favorable

for this regimen. Additional studies have also demonstrated the efficacy of the combination formulation of benzoyl peroxide with erythromycin, and this regimen had been considered the most effective in the treatment of acne.

Recently, the combination formulation of 1% clindamycin and 5% benzoyl peroxide gel has been marketed and evaluated for its effectiveness in the treatment of acne vulgaris.[63] Several clinical trials have demonstrated that twice-daily application of this product for 10 to 16 weeks was more effective in reducing the number of inflammatory lesions than 5% benzoyl peroxide, 1% clindamycin, or vehicle in patients with mild to moderately severe acne.[64,65] In another multicenter blinded trial, clindamycin–benzoyl peroxide gel was directly compared with benzoyl peroxide alone and the benzoyl peroxide–erythromycin combination formulation.[66] The clindamycin–benzoyl peroxide was significantly more effective in reducing the mean number of inflammatory lesions than benzoyl peroxide alone, and it was similar in efficacy to benzoyl peroxide–erythromycin. Both patient and physician assessments at the end of the study indicated that global improvement was significantly greater with clindamycin–benzoyl peroxide as compared with benzoyl peroxide alone, and similar to that identified with benzoyl peroxide–erythromycin. Thus, the clindamycin–benzoyl peroxide and erythromycin–benzoyl peroxide formulations are equally efficacious and can both be considered first-line topical therapies in the treatment of acne vulgaris.

Strains of *P. acnes* have emerged that are less sensitive to the antimicrobial agents used to treat acne. Several studies have been performed to assess the clinical significance of this antimicrobial resistance and to monitor the acquisition of resistant strains during therapy[67]; in these trials, topical antibacterials were used alone or in combination with either zinc or benzoyl peroxide. Generally, these studies have demonstrated a marked reduction in the colony counts of *P. acnes*, although there was emergence of antimicrobial-resistant strains. Combinations of benzoyl peroxide and erythromycin have a greater in vivo activity against *P. acnes* than erythromycin alone and bring about clinical improvement in acne patients who have high numbers of erythromycin-resistant strains.[68] It has been suggested clindamycin–benzoyl peroxide be considered an alternative therapy in those patients with erythromycin-resistant strains of *P. acnes*.[63] However, there have been no studies to evaluate this, nor have there been studies to evaluate the frequency of clindamycin resistance in *P. acnes*. These areas require further investigation.

Elimination of *Staphylococcus aureus* Nasal Carriage

Approximately 20% to 40% of healthy persons carry *S. aureus* in their anterior nares. In hospitalized patients, serious infection caused by *S. aureus* may occur from autoinoculation onto susceptible sites or transfer of organisms from another patient or staff member who is a carrier. Attempts to control these outbreaks have included methods to eradicate nasal carriage of offending staphylococci by means of systemic or topical antimicrobial agents; recolonization is frequent, however, and the development of resistance has been reported. Numerous topical antibacterial agents have been utilized in the nasal eradication of *S. aureus*, with varied degrees of success.

Mupirocin can eliminate nasal carriage of *S. aureus*. In four blinded, placebo-controlled trials conducted in health care workers with *S. aureus* nasal carriage, virtually all persons treated with mupirocin were initially cleared of the carrier state, compared with a 0% to 18% rate of clearance after treatment with placebo[69-72]; in one of the studies, a corresponding effect on the eradication of hand carriage at 72 hours of therapy was also found.[70] However, relapse after therapy occurred in 19% to 59% of persons after 4 to 12 weeks of evaluation. Relapses could have resulted from reinoculation of the nares with staphylococci from an untreated site (e.g., skin, perineum, rectum) or by reinfection with new staphylococcal strains after the completion of therapy.

Mupirocin has been evaluated in acute carrier outbreaks of epidemic MRSA colonization.[73-75] Mupirocin was effective in clearing MRSA from nearly all patients and staff, although these studies were uncontrolled and it is difficult to know whether the development of negative cultures in these patients can be attributed to therapy with mupirocin or to a transient carrier state. Recently, mupirocin has been evaluated in the control of MRSA in facilities for rehabilitation and long-term care.[76,77] Mupirocin was effective in the elimination of chronic nasal MRSA colonization, although in one study transient recolonization occurred in about 44% of patients.[77] In another study of 65 patients colonized with MRSA at a Veterans Affairs long-term care facility, mupirocin (applied to the nares for the first 7 months and to the nares and wounds for the second 5 months) rapidly eliminated MRSA at treated sites in most patients by the end of the first week.[78] Despite weekly maintenance mupirocin therapy, 40% of patients had recurrences of MRSA colonization. In contrast, a 5-day treatment course of mupirocin of all infants, colonized and noncolonized, their parents, and the personnel working with the colonized infants in a neonatal intensive care unit, failed to eradicate the organism.[79]

SPECIFIC TOPICAL ANTIBACTERIALS

Numerous topical antibacterial agents are available for clinical use in various concentrations, vehicles, and mixtures (Table 35-2). The following sections discuss the more common topical antibacterials in general use. Antimicrobial agents such as clindamycin, erythromycin, tetracycline, and gentamicin, although used as topical agents, are covered in other chapters of this book.

Bacitracin

Mechanism of Action. Bacitracin is a polypeptide antibiotic produced by *Bacillus subtilis*. There are three bacitracin subgroups: A, B, and C. Subgroup A is the major constituent of commercial preparations.[80] Bacitracin contains a thiazoline ring and peptide side chains. After administration, it forms a complex with C_{55}-isoprenyl pyrophosphate, a component of the bacterial cell wall. This molecule acts as a carrier involved in the transfer of polysaccharides, peptidoglycans, and lipopolysaccharides to the growing cell wall. Thus, formation of the bacterial cell wall is stunted.

In Vitro Spectrum of Activity. The activity of bacitracin is primarily against gram-positive organisms: staphylococci, streptococci, corynebacteria, and clostridia.[80] Development of resistance to bacitracin is rare, although it has been reported in *S. aureus*.

Clinical Uses. Topical bacitracin has been used for many years, although its efficacy in controlled clinical trials has never been shown. In impetigo, bacitracin ointment was shown to be 80% effective in clearing pathogenic organisms,[54] although slow or delayed healing

was noted in one third of those patients cured. Bacitracin was least effective for bullous impetigo, in which four of six patients continued to develop new lesions, requiring systemic erythromycin therapy. Furthermore, in a recent trial comparing topical bacitracin to topical mupirocin or oral cephalexin for the treatment of impetigo, the treatment failed in most patients (six of nine) treated with bacitracin.[81] Bacitracin has also been evaluated in the eradication of nasal carriage of *S. aureus*, although its efficacy has never been shown.[82] For topical use, bacitracin is often formulated with neomycin or polymyxin B, or both (see Table 35-2).

Adverse Effects. Toxicity with bacitracin is minimal. Minor skin irritation may occur. Cases of anaphylaxis have been reported after the topical administration of bacitracin to open lesions[80]; these patients had multiple previous exposures to the drug. Additionally, there have been rare reports of anaphylaxis after the use of bacitracin as an irrigating solution in the intraoperative setting, and when used topically in conjunction with nasal packing after a rhinoplasty.[83,84] Ready access to the systemic circulation appears to be a prerequisite for the development of anaphylaxis from this externally applied agent. Rarely, an allergic contact dermatitis has been reported. As bacitracin and polymyxin B are both derived from *Bacillus* species, cross-reactivity between the two agents may occur.

Neomycin

Mechanism of Action. Neomycin is an aminoglycoside antibiotic isolated from cultures of *Streptomyces fradiae*.[80] The mechanism of action involves inhibition of protein synthesis by binding to the 30S subunit of the bacterial ribosome, leading to misreading of the genetic code; neomycin may also inhibit the bacterial DNA polymerase.

In Vitro Spectrum of Activity. Neomycin has in vitro activity against many gram-positive and gram-negative bacteria, including *Escherichia coli, Haemophilus influenzae, Proteus* species, *S. aureus*, and *Serratia* species. *Pseudomonas aeruginosa* is generally resistant.[85] There is minimal in vitro activity against streptococci, although at the high concentrations achieved on the skin, *S. pyogenes* organisms are probably killed by topical neomycin preparations.[2] Resistance to neomycin has been reported in both gram-positive and gram-negative bacteria[53,80] and can be plasmid mediated; resistance to other aminoglycosides such as kanamycin and gentamicin may be on the same plasmid.

Clinical Uses. Neomycin is widely used in combination with other antibiotics, antifungals, and corticosteroids because of its availability, relatively low cost, and perceived efficacy.[11,53] There are few well-controlled clinical trials documenting the efficacy and safety of

TABLE 35-2 Selected Topical Antibacterial Agents in Clinical Use			
Topical Antibacterial (Trade Name)	*Concentration*	*Frequency*	*Indication*
Azelaic acid (Azelex)	20% cream	Twice daily	Acne vulgaris
Benzoyl peroxide	2.5%-10%	Once to twice daily	Acne vulgaris
Clindamycin (Cleocin,* Clindagel)	1%, 2%	Twice daily	Acne vulgaris; bacterial vaginosis
Clindamycin–benzoyl peroxide (BenzaClin)	1%-5%	Twice daily	Acne vulgaris
Erythromycin (Emgel)	2%	Twice daily	Acne vulgaris
Erythromycin–benzoyl peroxide (Benzamycin)	3%-5%	Twice daily	Acne vulgaris
Fusidic acid (Fucidin)†	2%	Three times daily	Skin infections; eradication of nasopharyngeal carriage of *Staphylococcus aureus*
Mafenide (Sulfamylon)	—	Twice daily	Burns
Metronidazole (MetroGel, MetroCream, MetroLotion, Noritate)‡	.075%	Once to twice daily	Inflammatory pustules, papules, and rosacea; bacterial vaginosis
Mupirocin (Bactroban)	2% ointment	Three times daily	Skin infections; elimination of nasopharyngeal carriage of *S. aureus*
Polymyxin B–bacitracin–neomycin (Neosporin)§	5000 units/g–400 units/g–3.5 mg/g	One to three times daily	Prevention of infection in minor cuts, scrapes, burns
Polymyxin B–neomycin–hydrocortisone (Cortisporin)	10,000 units/g–3.5 mg/g–0.5%	Two to four times daily	Corticosteroid-responsive dermatoses with secondary infection
Silver sulfadiazine (SSD; Silvadene)	1%	Once to twice daily	Burns

*The 2% formulation is recommended for bacterial vaginosis.
†Not licensed in the United States.
‡Supplied in a 1% cream and given once daily for inflammatory lesions and erythema of rosacea.
§Maximal strength formulation contains 10,000 units/g polymyxin B, 500 units/g bacitracin, and 3.5 mg/g neomycin.

topical neomycin.[54] Neomycin has been shown to enhance reepithelialization in wound healing.[12] However, in view of its well-documented contact sensitivity, possible systemic toxicity, and cross-reactivity with other antibiotics, and because of the emergence of resistance, it is difficult to recommend the use of topical neomycin in the treatment of superficial skin infections.[80]

Adverse Reactions. Neomycin is not absorbed through intact skin, although application to denuded or damaged epithelium can lead to sensitization and systemic toxicity.[85] After systemic absorption, neomycin is excreted by the kidney. Patients with decreased renal function may develop ototoxicity that is irreversible and may progress after discontinuation of the drug. Allergic contact sensitivity is widely reported, with a prevalence of 1% to 6% and an incidence of 3% to 6%.[85,86] The incidence of hypersensitivity, as assessed by patch testing, in 390 patients with suspected contact dermatitis to topical medications, was approximately 36%.[87] Sensitivity is most likely to occur with chronic use on inflamed skin. Sensitivity to neomycin was reported in 49% of patients with a history of allergy to any topical agent.[80] Neomycin may also cause mast cell degranulation and histamine release.

Polymyxin B

Mechanism of Action. Polymyxin B is isolated from the aerobic gram-positive rod Bacillus *polymyxa,* a soil organism (see Chapter 30). The polymyxins are cationic branched cyclic decapeptides that destroy bacterial membranes with a surface detergent-like mechanism by interacting with membrane phospholipids and increasing cellular permeability.

In Vitro Spectrum of Activity. The spectrum of activity of polymyxin B is almost exclusively limited to gram-negative organisms. The agent is bactericidal against many aerobic gram-negative organisms including *P. aeruginosa,* but it is not active against *Proteus* species, and it is poorly active against *Providencia, Burkholderia,* and *Serratia* species. There is no in vitro activity against gram-positive organisms. Although *Pseudomonas* is usually sensitive, the in vitro activity of polymyxin B against *Pseudomonas* is promptly neutralized by divalent cations at concentrations in body fluids. Organisms resistant to polymyxin B have cell walls that prevent access of the drug to the bacterial cell membrane. There is no cross-resistance with other antimicrobial agents, and resistance rarely develops during therapy.

Clinical Uses. Polymyxin B is used primarily in the prevention and treatment of minor skin infections. It is most often added to neomycin and bacitracin (see earlier) to broaden coverage against gram-negative organisms.

Adverse Effects. Because polymyxin B binds to cell membranes with very high affinity, there is little systemic absorption and there are few reactions even when applied to open wounds. Contact sensitization has been reported.

Mupirocin

Structure and Mechanism of Action. Mupirocin has a chemical structure unlike that of any other antimicrobial agent (Fig. 35-1).[88,89] It contains a short fatty acid side chain (9-hydroxy-nonanoic acid) linked to monic acid by an ester linkage. Mupirocin is formulated in a bland water-miscible ointment base consisting of polyethylene glycol 400 and polyethylene glycol 3350. Mupirocin used to be called pseudomonic acid because its major metabolite is derived from submerged fermentation by *Pseudomonas fluorescens.* Pseudomonic acid A represents 90% to 95% of the pseudomonic acid family and is responsible for most of the antibacterial activity; three other minor metabolites of similar chemical structure and antimicrobial spectrum have been denoted as pseudomonic acids B, C, and D.[88] Mupirocin inhibits bacterial RNA and protein synthesis by binding to bacterial isoleucyl–transfer RNA (tRNA) synthetase, which catalyzes the formation of isoleucyl-tRNA from isoleucine and tRNA.[88,89] This prevents the incorporation of isoleucine into protein chains of the bacterial cell wall, leading to the arrest of protein synthesis. Because of this unique mechanism of action, mupirocin does not cross react with other antimicrobial agents.

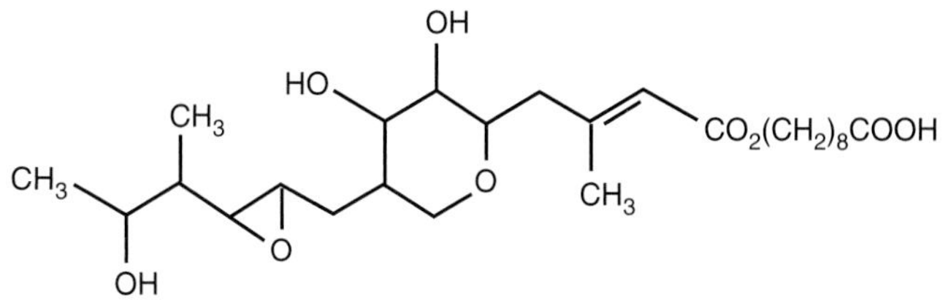

FIGURE 35-1. Structure of mupirocin.

In Vitro Spectrum of Activity. The antibacterial spectrum of mupirocin is shown in Table 35-3.[88] Mupirocin is bacteriostatic at low concentrations near the minimal inhibitory concentration (MIC) for *S. aureus,* but it is bactericidal at concentrations achieved by topical administration (20,000 μg/mL with the 2% formulation) after 24 to 36 hours of exposure.[88] It is highly active in vitro against MRSA, staphylococcal strains resistant to other antibacterials (e.g., penicillin, streptomycin, neomycin, erythromycin, fusidic acid, lincomycin, chloramphenicol, and tetracycline), and streptococci that are associated

TABLE 35-3 Antibacterial Activity of Mupirocin against Selected Bacteria

Organism and Strain	MIC (μg/mL)
Gram-Positive Cocci	
Streptococcus pyogenes 421	0.12
Streptococcus pneumoniae 1959	0.12
Staphylococcus aureus ATCC 25923	0.25
Staphylococcus epidermidis 54815	0.5
Streptococcus agalactiae 9579	0.5
Streptococcus sanguis	1
Peptostreptococcus anaerobius 3395	32
Enterococcus faecium 98-D	32
Enterococcus faecalis I	64
Peptococcus prevotii 372.5	>128
Micrococcus luteus ATCC 9341	>128
Gram-Positive Bacilli	
Bacillus subtilis ATCC 6633	0.12
Erysipelothrix rhusiopathiae	8
Listeria monocytogenes NCTC 5348	8
Clostridium difficile 12328	32
Clostridium sporogenes 532	32
Bacillus anthracis NCTC 8234	64
Corynebacterium hofmannii M8	64
Corynebacterium xerosis 9755	>128
Corynebacterium jekeium	>128
Propionibacterium acnes 10162	>128
Gram-Negative Cocci	
Neisseria gonorrhoeae WHO V	0.05
Neisseria meningitidis 1990	0.05
Moraxella catarrhalis 1502	0.2
Gram-Negative Bacilli	
Bordetella pertussis 2420	0.02
Haemophilus influenzae Q1	0.12
Pasteurella multocida 1633	0.25
Proteus vulgaris X	64
Enterobacter cloacae 10005	64
Enterobacter aerogenes T660	128
Citrobacter freundii W18	128
Escherichia coli NCTC 10418	128
Klebsiella pneumoniae A	128
Proteus mirabilis 889	128
Serratia marcescens US9	1600
Morganella morganii F	6400
Pseudomonas aeruginosa R3	6400
Bacteroides fragilis BC4	>6400

ATCC, American Type Culture Collection; MIC, Minimal inhibitory concentration; NCTC, National Collection of Type Cultures.
Data from Pappa KA. The clinical development of mupirocin. J Am Acad Dermatol. 1990;22:873-879; Leyden JJ. Mupirocin: A new topical antibiotic. Semin Dermatol. 1987;6:48-54; and Sutherland R, Boon RJ, Griffin KE, et al. Antibacterial activity of mupirocin (pseudomonic acid), a new antibiotic for topical use. Antimicrob Agents Chemother. 1985;27:495-498.

with primary and secondary skin infections.[88] The exception to the antistreptococcal activity of mupirocin is the enterococcus. Mupirocin is inactive in vitro against *P. aeruginosa,* anaerobes, fungi, and the Enterobacteriaceae. An important feature of mupirocin's antibacterial spectrum is its weaker in vitro activity against the normal skin flora (e.g., *Micrococcus, Corynebacterium,* and *Propionibacterium*), which are part of the skin's natural defense against infection. The in vitro antibacterial activity of mupirocin is greatest at an acidic pH, which is advantageous because of the low pH of the skin; in one study, mupirocin was fourfold to eightfold more active in vitro at pH 6 than at pH 7.

Long-term therapy with mupirocin can lead to the development of resistant staphylococci,[88,90] an effect that is irreversible. Staphylococcal isolates with low- or intermediate-level resistance have MICs in the range of 8 to 256 μg/mL, whereas isolates with MICs at or above 512 μg/mL demonstrate high-level resistance. This resistance can be induced in *S. aureus* by subculturing the organisms onto media containing increasing concentrations of the drug. Naturally occurring clones of staphylococci with low-level resistance to mupirocin have been described, although their clinical significance is unclear because the concentration of mupirocin in ointment exceeds 20,000 μg/mL. High-level mupirocin resistance, associated with clinical treatment failure, has emerged in both MRSA and *Staphylococcus epidermidis.*[91] In one study, resistance emerged in three patients treated with mupirocin for months and, in addition, from patients never treated with mupirocin, suggesting the possibility of cross-infection. In another study of 144 patients with epidermolysis bullosa, many of whom received continuous application of mupirocin for as long as 4 consecutive years, five isolates of *S. aureus* were resistant to mupirocin[88]; four of the five patients with resistant isolates had a less favorable response to mupirocin and required systemic antistaphylococcal therapy. Most mupirocin-resistant staphylococcal isolates have been found in patients with chronic skin infections, many of whom had been treated with prolonged courses of mupirocin.[89] It has recently been reported from France that a 5-day course of intranasal mupirocin for decolonization of a patient with a glycopeptide-intermediate *S. aureus* (GISA) failed to eradicate this isolate, even though the strain was susceptible in vitro to mupirocin.[92] The patient went on to develop a nosocomial pneumonia with the GISA strain and, on repeat testing, the strain had developed resistance to mupirocin. The use of mupirocin against GISA requires additional study.

Several mechanisms have been advanced to explain mupirocin resistance in staphylococci. Low-level resistance is most likely mediated by altered access to binding sites on isoleucyl-tRNA synthetase, whereas high-level resistance appears to be mediated by a transferable plasmid on the *mupA* gene that codes for a modified isoleucyl-tRNA synthetase.[89] It has been suggested that high-level resistance may have evolved by the conjugate transfer of plasmids from enterococci,[93] which are inherently resistant to mupirocin; conjugate transfer of high-level mupirocin resistance has also been observed among coagulase-negative staphylococci.[94] A recent study has demonstrated that two different isoleucyl-tRNA synthetase enzymes are present in highly mupirocin-resistant *S. aureus* isolates (MIC≥512 μg/mL), whereas only a chromosomally encoded isoleucyl-tRNA synthetase was detected in strains expressing intermediate levels of resistance (MIC between 8 and 256 μg/mL). Commercially available E-tests to detect mupirocin resistance in *S. aureus* are available and are quite accurate in differentiating low-level from high-level resistance patterns.[95] E-tests compare favorably with the more traditional disk diffusion method and MIC determination in the detection of resistance.[96]

Pharmacokinetics. After systemic administration, mupirocin is immediately metabolized to monic acid, which is bacteriologically inactive and rapidly eliminated (plasma half-life of <30 minutes). Mupirocin is not appreciably absorbed after topical administration to intact skin. In one study, a mean of 0.24% of applied radiolabeled ointment was absorbed through intact skin after 24 hours of occlusion.[97] Greater penetration of mupirocin is expected in damaged or diseased skin. Any drug that is absorbed, however, is converted to monic acid, formed by deesterification of mupirocin at the ester linkage between the side chain and the nucleus, and rapidly eliminated in the urine.[80] Skin can also metabolize mupirocin to its inactive metabolite, but at a rate below 3%. Therefore, because only small amounts of mupirocin penetrate skin and equally small amounts are degraded, most of the drug is available to act at the skin level. Because mupirocin is highly protein bound (approximately 95%), its activity decreases in the presence of serum.[88]

Clinical Uses. Mupirocin is used primarily in skin infections such as impetigo and folliculitis, which are usually caused by *S. aureus* and *S. pyogenes,* to decolonize the nares in outbreak settings, and as prophylaxis against a variety of catheter-related and surgical site infections. In trials of mupirocin alone in the therapy of impetigo (772 evaluable patients),[98-100] clinical cure rates ranged from 81% to 100% and bacterial elimination rates from 67% to 100%. Several trials have shown mupirocin to be more effective in the treatment of impetigo than its polyethylene glycol vehicle, which also has antibacterial activity. Clinical cure and bacterial elimination rates have ranged from 85% to 100% and from 80% to 95%, respectively, for mupirocin, versus from 12% to 84% and from 12% to 63%, respectively, for the vehicle.[98-101] As impetigo is a self-limiting condition, bacteriologic results are a more appropriate assessment of efficacy because elimination of pathogens can be used to ascertain infection resolution. Of eight comparative trials of mupirocin versus several other topical antibacterials (neomycin, fusidic acid, chlortetracycline, polymyxin B–bacitracin–neomycin),[98,102,103] six found mupirocin to be the more effective agent. Multiple studies have also compared topical mupirocin to systemic antibiotics (erythromycin, cloxacillin, dicloxacillin, flucloxacillin, ampicillin, cephalexin) in the therapy of impetigo, and topical mupirocin was found to be as, or more, effective than the oral agent.[81,98] In many of these studies, however, the entry criteria excluded patients who, in the judgment of the investigator, had too many lesions to allow reliable compliance with topical therapy.[104] No studies have shown that topical therapy is as effective as systemic antimicrobial therapy for the treatment of widespread, extensive lesions.

Mupirocin is effective for the treatment of secondarily infected eczema, burns, lacerations, and leg ulcers. In a study in which 33 centers contributed a total of 1030 cases,[105] mupirocin ointment produced significantly better bacteriologic and clinical responses than its vehicle in the treatment of secondary skin infections. Of 851 evaluable patients with 1131 pathogens, mupirocin eliminated 87% (505/583) of pathogens, versus only 53% (288/548) for the vehicle. In a double-blind, vehicle-controlled study, mupirocin successfully eradicated 85% of *S. aureus* in 33 patients, compared with a 6% eradication rate in the vehicle-treated group[106]; for all pathogens, the success rate of mupirocin versus the vehicle was 69% versus 14%, respectively. Comparative trials have also demonstrated the efficacy of mupirocin compared with other topical antibacterials and systemic antimicrobial agents in the treatment of secondary skin infections.

The use of mupirocin to eliminate nasal carriage of *S. aureus* in a variety of settings including outbreaks, preoperative patients, and chronic dialysis patients was discussed earlier. The development of mupirocin resistance in MRSA has become a problem since widespread use of nasal mupirocin. In one study at a Veterans Affairs long-term care facility where patients were treated with nasal mupirocin for 1 year, mupirocin-resistant MRSA organisms were identified in 11% of patients.[78] In another study, resistance among MRSA isolates after the use of nasal mupirocin increased from 2.7% to 65% between 1990 and 1993.[107] A resistance rate of 63% was also observed in a study of MRSA strains in Rio de Janeiro, where there was extensive use of topical mupirocin.[108] In contrast, in another study of blanket use of intranasal mupirocin for outbreak control and long-term prophylaxis of endemic MRSA colonization in an open ward, no mupirocin resistance was observed.[109] Although there are conflicting results from clinical trials, prolonged use of nasal mupirocin should be discouraged; instead, it should be used primarily in outbreak situations and not in facilities with endemic MRSA colonization.[89]

Adverse Effects. Mupirocin is not associated with substantial toxicity in humans because of its very low affinity for mammalian isoleucyl-tRNA synthetase. The propylene glycol base may irritate mucous membranes and eroded skin. There is minimal potential for inducing allergic contact dermatitis; only two cases have been reported.[110] The drug is not phototoxic. Local effects such as itching, stinging, or rash have been reported when mupirocin is used on broken skin or mucous membranes. As has been mentioned, chronic exposure to topical mupirocin has been rarely associated with polyurethane peritoneal dialysis catheter rupture, which may be caused by the vehicle portion of the preparation interacting with the polyurethane in the catheter.[43] No photosensitivity reactions have occurred. In experimental rat and rabbit models, mupirocin has been shown to be without teratogenic effects, embryotoxicity, or effects on fertility and reproduction in doses up to 160 mg/kg/day.[105] Prolonged use may lead to overgrowth of nonsusceptible organisms such as fungi.

Fusidic Acid

Mechanism of Action. Fusidic acid is isolated from culture media of the fungus Fusidium *coccineum*.[80] Chemically, it is a carboxylic acid belonging to the group of tetracycline triterpenes. Fusidic acid is lipophilic. It penetrates intact epidermis at approximately the same rate as glucocorticoids and penetrates both intact and damaged skin. Fusidic acid inhibits bacterial protein synthesis primarily by interfering with elongation factor G (translocase) (see Chapter 23).[111]

In Vitro Spectrum of Activity. Fusidic acid has a narrow antibacterial spectrum, mainly against gram-positive bacteria. It has exceptionally high in vitro activity against *S. aureus* (MIC range, 0.04 to 0.16 µg/mL). There is also in vitro activity against corynebacteria and clostridia. Streptococci are 100 times less sensitive (MIC range, 4.2 to 16 µg/mL) to fusidic acid when compared with staphylococci, but at concentrations given topically it is efficacious against both organisms. Reports from Europe have documented staphylococcal resistance to fusidic acid, although general levels of resistance have remained low (about 1% to 2%).[112] In one report of 8176 *S. aureus* strains isolated from cases of bacteremia between 1963 and 1987 in Denmark, 1% or less of strains were resistant to fusidic acid (MIC ≥ 2 µg/mL).[113] After topical use of fusidic acid, a rate of staphylococcal resistance of 43% has been reported, although other authors have not observed the emergence of resistance.[114] In vitro evidence suggests that resistance to *S. aureus* is less likely to occur after exposure to high concentrations of fusidic acid, reflecting the situation with topical use.

Clinical Uses. Fusidic acid has the remarkable ability to penetrate both intact and damaged skin, making it useful for treating deep infections such as paronychia and boils.[80] It also penetrates crust and cellular debris as seen in impetigo and pyoderma. In comparative trials of fusidic acid for the therapy of primary and secondary skin infections, fusidic acid has been found to be equivalent or inferior to mupirocin.[98] In one study, the combination of topical fusidic acid and oral cotrimoxazole was found to be as efficacious as topical mupirocin in the eradication of nasal carriage of MRSA.[114] The drug is not available in the United States but has been used in Europe and Canada.

Adverse Effects. Because the structure of fusidic acid differs markedly from that of other antibiotics, it is unlikely to produce cross-sensitivity. There are a few reports of contact sensitivity. Although the ring structure of fusidic acid is remarkably similar to that of the glucocorticoids, there is no evidence of suppressive activity on the pituitary axis.

REFERENCES

1. Russell AD. Plasmids and bacterial resistance to biocides. J Appl Microbiol. 1997;83:155-165.
2. Feingold DS. Antibacterial agents. In: Fitzpatrick TB, Eisen AZ, Wolff K, et al, eds. Dermatology in General Medicine. 3rd ed. New York: McGraw-Hill; 1987;2550-2552.
3. Kaye ET, Kaye KM. Topical antibacterial agents. Infect Dis Clin North Am. 1995;9:547-559.
4. Centers for Disease Control and Prevention. Guidelines for the prevention of intravascular catheter-related infections. MMWR Morb Morbid Wkly Rep. 2002;51(RR10):1-29.
5. Hill RLR, Casewell MW. The in-vitro activity of povidone-iodine cream against *Staphylococcus aureus* and its bioavailability in nasal secretions. J Hosp Infect. 2000;45:198-205.
6. Pittet D, Hugonnet S, Harbath S, et al. Effectiveness of a hospital-wide program to improve compliance with hand hygiene. Lancet. 2000;356:1307-1312.
7. Centers for Disease Control and Prevention. Guideline for hand hygiene in health-care settings. MMWR Morb Morbid Wkly Rep. 2002;52(RR16):1-44.
8. Maki DG, Ringer M, Alvarado CJ. Prospective randomised trial of povidone-iodine, alcohol, and chlorhexidine for prevention of infection associated with central venous and arterial catheters. Lancet. 1991;338:339-343.
9. Suller MTE, Russell AD. Triclosan and antibiotic resistance in *Staphylococcus aureus*. J Antimicrob Chemother. 2000;46:11-18.
10. Bamber AI, Neal TJ. An assessment of triclosan susceptibility in methicillin-resistant and methicillin-sensitive *Staphylococcus aureus*. J Hosp Infect. 1999;41:1079.
11. Leyden JJ, Sulzberger MB. Topical antibiotics and minor skin trauma. Am Fam Physician. 1981;23:121-125.
12. Eaglstein WH, Mertz P, Alvarez OM. Effect of topically applied agents on healing wounds. Clin Dermatol. 1984;2:112-115.
13. Maddox JS, Ware JC, Dillon HC Jr. The natural history of streptococcal skin infection: Prevention with topical antibiotics. J Am Acad Dermatol. 1985;13:207-212.
14. Langford JH, Artemi P, Benrimoj SI. Topical antimicrobial prophylaxis in minor wounds. Ann Pharmacother. 1997;31:559-563.
15. Eaglstein WH, Falanga V. Chronic wounds. Surg Clin North Am. 1997;77:689-700.
16. Filius PM, Gyssens IC. Impact of increasing antimicrobial resistance on wound management. Am J Clin Dermatol. 2002;3:1-7.
17. Raz R, Miron D, Colodner R, et al. A 1-year trial of nasal mupirocin in the prevention of recurrent staphylococcal nasal colonization and skin infection. Arch Intern Med. 1996;156:1109-1112.
18. Perl TM, Cullen JJ, Wenzel RP, et al. Intranasal mupirocin to prevent postoperative *Staphylococcus aureus* infections. N Engl J Med. 2002;346:1871-1877.
19. Farr BM. Mupirocin to prevent *S. aureus* infections (Editorial). N Engl J Med. 2002;346:1905-1906.
20. Cimochowski GE, Harostock MD, Brown R, et al. Intranasal mupirocin reduces sternal wound infection after open heart surgery in diabetics and nondiabetics. Ann Thorac Surg. 2001;71:1572-1579.
21. Kluytmans JA, Mouton JW, Vandenbergh MF, et al. Reduction in surgical site infections in cardiothoracic surgery by elimination of nasal carriage of *Staphylococcus aureus*. Infect Control Hosp Epidemiol. 1996;17:780-785.
22. Gernaat-van der Sluis AJ, Hoogenboom-Verdegaal AM, Edixhoven PJ, Spies-van Rooijen NH. Prophylactic mupirocin could reduce orthopedic wound infections. Acta Orthop Scand. 1998;69:412-414.
23. Kalmeijer MD, Coertjens H, van Niewland-Bollen PM, et al. Surgical site infections in orthopedic surgery: the effect of mupirocin nasal ointment in a double-blind, randomized, placebo-controlled study. Clin Infect Dis. 2002;35:353-358.
24. Laupland KB, Conly JM. Treatment of *Staphylococcus aureus* colonization and prophylaxis for infection with topical intranasal mupirocin: An evidence-based review. Clin Infect Dis. 2003;37:933-938.
25. vanden Bergh MF, Kluytmans JA, van Hout BA, et al. Cost-effectiveness of perioperative mupirocin nasal ointment in cardiothoracic surgery. Infect Control Hosp Epidemiol. 1996;17:786-792.
26. Maki DG, Band JD. A comparative study of polyantibiotic and iodophor ointments in prevention of vascular catheter-related infection. Am J Med. 1981;70:739-744.
27. Levin A, Mason AJ, Jindal KK, et al. Prevention of hemodialysis subclavian vein catheter infections by topical povidone-iodine. Kidney Int. 1991;40:934-938.
28. Mimoz O, Pieroni L, Lawrence C, et al. Prospective, randomized trial of two antiseptic solutions for prevention of central venous or arterial catheter colonization and infection in intensive care unit patients. Crit Care Med. 1996;24:1818-1823.
29. Gokal R. Peritoneal dialysis: Prevention and control of infection. Drugs Aging. 2000;17:269-282.
30. Piraino B, Perlmutter JA, Holley JL, Bernardini J. *Staphylococcus aureus* peritonitis is associated with *Staphylococcus aureus* nasal carriage in peritoneal dialysis patients. Perit Dial Int. 1992;13:5332-5334.
31. Herwaldt LA. Reduction of *Staphylococcus aureus* nasal carriage and infection in dialysis patients. J Hosp Infect. 1998;40:513-523.
32. Wilson AP, Lewis C, O'Sullivan A, et al. The use of povidone-iodine in exit site care for patients undergoing CAPD. J Hosp Infect. 1997;35:287-293.
33. Bending M, Mellotte G, Hashmi C, et al. Nasal mupirocin prevents *S. aureus* exit site infection during peritoneal dialysis. J Am Soc Nephrol. 1996;7:2403-2408.
34. Perez-Fontan M, Garcia-Falcon T, Rodrigues-Carmona A, et al. Treatment of *Staphylococcus aureus* nasal carriage in continuous ambulatory peritoneal dialysis (CAPD) with mupirocin: Long term results. Am J Kid Dis. 1993;22:700-712.
35. Thodis E, Passadakis P, Vargemezis V, Oreopoulos DG. Prevention of catheter-related infections in patients on CAPD. Int J Artif Organs. 2001;24:671-682.
36. Mupirocin Study Group. Nasal mupirocin prevents *Staphylococcus aureus* exit-site infections during peritoneal dialysis. J Am Soc Nephrol. 1996;7:2403-2408.
37. Davey P, Craig AM, Hau C, Malek M. Cost-effectiveness of prophylactic nasal mupirocin in patients undergoing peritoneal dialysis based on a randomized, placebo-controlled trial. J Antimicrob Chemother. 1999;43:105-112.
38. Bernardini J, Piraino B, Holley J, et al. A randomized trial of *Staphylococcus aureus* prophylaxis in peritoneal dialysis patients: Mupirocin calcium ointment 2% applied to the exit site versus cyclic oral rifampin. Am J Kidney Dis. 1996;27:695-700.
39. Thodis E, Passadakis P, Panagoutsos S, et al. The effectiveness of mupirocin preventing *Staphylococcus aureus* in catheter-related infections in peritoneal dialysis. Adv Perit Dial. 2000;16:257-261.
40. Thodis E, Bhaskaran S, Passadakis P, et al. Decrease in *Staphylococcus aureus* exit-site infections and peritonitis in CAPD patients by local application of mupirocin ointment at the catheter exit site. Perit Dial Int. 1998;18:261-270.

41. Casey M, Taylor J, Clinard P, et al. Application of mupirocin cream at the catheter exit site reduces exit-site infections and peritonitis in peritoneal dialysis patients. Perit Dial Int. 2000;20:566-574.

42. Annigeri R, Conly J, Vas SI, et al. Emergence of mupirocin-resistant Staphylococcus aureus in chronic peritoneal dialysis patients using mupirocin prophylaxis to prevent exit-site infection. Perit Dial Int. 2001;21:554-559.

43. Riu S, Ruiz C, Martinez-Vea C, et al. Spontaneous rupture of polyurethane peritoneal catheter: A possible deleterious effect of mupirocin ointment. Nephrol Dial Transplant. 1998;13:1870-1871.

44. Boelaert JR, de Smedt RA, de Bacre YA, et al. The influence of calcium mupirocin nasal ointment on the incidence of Staphylococcus aureus infections in haemodialysis patients. Nephrol Dial Transplant. 1989;4:278-281.

45. Boelaert JR, van Landuyt HW, Godard CA, et al. Nasal mupirocin ointment decreases the incidence of Staphylococcus aureus bacteremias in haemodialysis patients. Nephrol Dial Transplant. 1993;8:235-239.

46. Kluytmans JAJW, Manders MJ, van Bommel E, Verbrugh H. Elimination of nasal carriage of Staphylococcus aureus in hemodialysis patients. Infect Control Hosp Epidemiol. 1996;17:793-797.

47. Bloom BS, Fendrick AM, Chernew ME, Patel P. Clinical and economic effects of mupirocin calcium in preventing Staphylococcus aureus infection in hemodialysis patients: A decision analysis. Am J Kidney Dis. 1996;27:687-694.

48. Fong IW. Prevention of haemodialysis and peritoneal dialysis catheter-related infection by topical povidone-iodine. Postgrad Med J. 1993;69:515-517.

49. Johnson DW, MacGinley R, Kay TD, et al. A randomized trial of topical exit site mupirocin application in patients with tunneled, cuffed, haemodialysis catheters. Nephrol Dial Transplant. 2002;17:1802-1807.

50. Monafo WW, Freedman B. Topical therapy for burns. Surg Clin North Am. 1987;67:133-145.

51. Pruitt BA Jr, McManus AT, Kim SH, Goodwin CW. Burn wound infections: Current status. World J Surg. 1998;22:135-145.

52. Andreassi L, Flori L. Pharmacologic treatment of burns. Clin Dermatol. 1992;9:453-458.

53. Leyden JJ, Kligman AM. Rationale for topical antibiotics. Cutis. 1978;22:515-528.

54. Dillon HC Jr. Topical and systemic therapy for pyodermas. Int J Dermatol. 1980;19:443-451.

55. Holdiness MR. Management of cutaneous erythrasma. Drugs. 2002;62:1131-1141.

56. Cochran RJ, Rosen D, Landers T. Topical treatment for erythrasma. Int J Dermatol. 1981;20:562-564.

57. Rebora A. The management of rosacea. Am J Clin Dermatol. 2002;3:489-496.

58. Breneman D, Stewart D, Hevia O, et al. A double blind multicenter clinical trial comparing efficacy of once daily metronidazole 1% cream to vehicle in patients with rosacea. Cutis. 1998;61:44-47.

59. Jorizzo J, Lebwohl M, Tobey R. The efficacy of metronidazole 1% cream once daily compared with metronidazole cream 1% twice daily and their vehicles in rosacea: A double-blind clinical trial. J Am Acad Dermatol. 1998;395:502-504.

60. Leyden JJ. Therapy for acne vulgaris. N Engl J Med. 1997;336:1156-1162.

61. Weiss JS. Current options for the topical treatment of acne vulgaris. Pediatr Dermatol. 1997;14:480-488.

62. Chu A, Huber FJ, Plott RT. The comparative efficacy of benzoyl peroxide 5%/erythromycin 3% gel and erythromycin 4%/zinc 1.2% solution in the treatment of acne vulgaris. Br J Dermatol. 1997;136:235-238.

63. Warner GT, Plosker GL. Clindamycin/benzoyl peroxide gel. Am J Clin Dermatol. 2002;3:349-360.

64. Lookingbill DT, Chalker DK, Lindholm JS, et al. Treatment of acne with a combination clindamycin/benzoyl peroxide gel compared with clindamycin gel, benzoyl peroxide gel and vehicle gel: Combined results of two double-blind investigations. J Am Acad Dermatol. 1997;4:590-595.

65. Tschen EH, Katz HI, Jones TM, et al. A combination benzoyl peroxide and clindamycin topical gel compared with benzoyl peroxide, clindamycin phosphate, and vehicle in the treatment of acnes vulgaris. Cutis. 2001;67:165-169.

66. Leyden JJ, Hickman JG, Jarratt MT, et al. The efficacy and safety of a combination benzoyl peroxide/clindamycin topical gel compared with benzoyl peroxide alone and a benzoyl peroxide/erythromycin combination product. J Cutan Med Surg. 2001;5:37-42.

67. Thiboutot DM. Acne: An overview of clinical research findings. Dermatol Clin. 1997;15:97-109.

68. Eady EA, Bojar RA, Jones CE, et al. The effects of acne treatment with a combination of benzoyl peroxide and erythromycin on skin carriage of erythromycin-resistant propionibacteria. Br J Dermatol. 1996;134:107-113.

69. Casewell MW, Hill RLR. Elimination of nasal carriage of Staphylococcus aureus with mupirocin ("pseudomonic acid"): A controlled study. J Antimicrob Chemother. 1986;17:365-372.

70. Reagan DR, Doebbeling BN, Pfaller MA, et al. Elimination of coincident Staphylococcus aureus nasal and hand carriage with intranasal application of mupirocin calcium ointment. Ann Intern Med. 1991;114:101-106.

71. Scully BE, Briones F, Gu JW, et al. Mupirocin treatment of nasal staphylococcal colonization. Arch Intern Med. 1992;152:353-356.

72. Fernandez C, Gaspar C, Torrellas A, et al. A double-blind, placebo-controlled clinical trial to evaluate the safety and efficacy of mupirocin calcium ointment for eliminating nasal carriage of Staphylococcus aureus among hospital personnel. J Antimicrob Chemother. 1995;35:399-408.

73. Hill RLR, Duckworth GJ, Casewell MW. Elimination of nasal carriage of methicillin-resistant Staphylococcus aureus with mupirocin during a hospital outbreak. J Antimicrob Chemother. 1988;22:377-384.

74. Vandenbroucke-Grauls CM, Frenay HME, van Klingeren B, et al. Control of epidemic methicillin-resistant Staphylococcus aureus in a Dutch university hospital. Eur J Clin Microbiol Infect Dis. 1991;10:6-11.

75. Barrett SP. The value of nasal mupirocin in containing an outbreak of methicillin-resistant Staphylococcus aureus in an orthopedic ward. J Hosp Infect. 1990;15:137-142.

76. Dariouche R, Wright C, Hamill R, et al. Eradication of colonization by methicillin-resistant Staphylococcus aureus by using oral minocycline-rifampin and topical mupirocin. Antimicrob Agents Chemother. 1991;35:1612-1615.

77. Cederna JE, Terpenning MS, Ensberg M, et al. Staphylococcus aureus nasal colonization in a nursing home: Eradication with mupirocin. Infect Control Hosp Epidemiol. 1990;11:13-16.

78. Kauffman CA, Terpenning MS, He X, et al. Attempts to eradicate methicillin-resistant Staphylococcus aureus from a long-term-care facility with use of mupirocin ointment. Am J Med. 1993;94:371-378.

79. Back NA, Linnemann CC Jr, Staneck JL, et al. Control of methicillin-resistant Staphylococcus aureus in a neonatal intensive-care unit: Use of intensive microbiologic surveillance and mupirocin. Infect Control Hosp Epidemiol. 1996;17:227-231.

80. Winkelman W, Gratton D. Topical antibacterials. Clin Dermatol. 1989;7:156-162.

81. Bass JW, Chan DS, Creamer KM, et al. Comparison of oral cephalexin, topical mupirocin and topical bacitracin for treatment of impetigo. Pediatr Infect Dis J. 1997;16:708-710.

82. Yu VL, Goetz A, Wagener M, et al. Staphylococcus aureus nasal carriage and infection in patients on hemodialysis: Efficacy of antibiotic prophylaxis. N Engl J Med. 1986;315:91-96.

83. Blas M, Briesacher KS, Lobato E. Bacitracin irrigation: A cause of anaphylaxis in the operating room. Anesth Analg. 2000;91:1027-1028.

84. Gall R, Blakley B, Warrington R, Bell DD. Intraoperative anaphylactic shock from bacitracin nasal packing after septorhinoplasty. Anesthesiology. 1999;91:1545.

85. MacDonald RH, Beck M. Neomycin: A review with particular reference to dermatological usage. Clin Exp Dermatol. 1983;8:249-258.

86. Gette MT, Marks JG Jr, Maloney ME. Frequency of postoperative allergic contact dermatitis to topical antibiotics. Arch Dermatol. 1992;128:365-367.

87. Bajaj AK, Gupta SC. Contact hypersensitivity to topical antibacterial agents. Int J Dermatol. 1986;25:103-105.

88. Pappa KA. The clinical development of mupirocin. J Am Acad Dermatol. 1990;22:873-879.

89. Bradley SF. Effectiveness of mupirocin in the control of methicillin-resistant Staphylococcus aureus. Infect Med. 1993;10:23-31.

90. Eltringham I. Mupirocin resistance and methicillin-resistant Staphylococcus aureus (MRSA). J Hosp Infect. 1997;35:1-8.

91. Smith GE, Kennedy CTC. Staphylococcus aureus resistant to mupirocin. J Antimicrob Chemother. 1988;21:141-142.

92. Decousser JW, Pina P, Ghnassia JC, et al. First report of clinical and microbiologic failure in the eradication of glycopeptide-intermediate methicillin-resistant Staphylococcus aureus carriage by mupirocin. Eur J Clin Microbiol Infect Dis. 2003;22:318-319.

93. Cookson BD. Mupirocin resistance in staphylococci. J Antimicrob Chemother. 1990;25:497-503.

94. Udo EE, Jacob LE, Mokadas EM. Conjugate transfer of high-level mupirocin resistance from Staphylococcus haemolyticus to other staphylococci. Antimicrob Agents Chemother. 1997;41:693-695.

95. Mondino PJJ, Netto dos Santos KR, do Carmo de Freire Bastos M, Giambiagi-deMarral M. Improvement of mupirocin E-test for susceptibility testing of Staphylococcus aureus. J Med Microbiol. 2003;52:385-387.

96. Reshpane LM, Fix AM, Pfaller MA, et al. Emerging elevated mupirocin resistance rates among staphylococcal isolates in the SENTRY antimicrobial surveillance program (2000): Correlations of results from disk diffusion, E-test and reference dilution methods. Diagn Microbiol Infect Dis. 2002;42:283-290.

97. Ward A, Campoli-Richards DM. Mupirocin: A review of its antibacterial activity, pharmacokinetic properties and therapeutic use. Drugs. 1986;32:425-444.

98. Booth JH, Benrimoj SI. Mupirocin in the treatment of impetigo. Int J Dermatol. 1992;31:1-9.

99. Bork K, Brauers J, Kresken M. Efficacy and safety of 2% mupirocin ointment in the treatment of primary and secondary skin infections: An open multicentre trial. Br J Clin Pract. 1989;43:284-288.

100. De la Brassinne M, De Bersaques J, Vossaert K, et al. Efficacy of mupirocin 2% ointment in skin infection: Belgian prospective open multicentre study. Dermatologica. 1988;177:397-400.

101. Eells LD, Mertz PM, Piovanetti Y, et al. Topical antibiotic treatment of impetigo with mupirocin. Arch Dermatol. 1986;122:1273-1276.

102. Wilkinson RD, Carey WD. Topical mupirocin versus topical neosporin in the treatment of cutaneous infections. Int J Dermatol. 1988;27:514-515.

103. Gilbert M. Topical 2% mupirocin versus 2% fusidic acid ointment in the treatment of primary and secondary skin infections. J Am Acad Dermatol. 1989;20:1083-1087.

104. Leyden JJ. Review of mupirocin ointment in the treatment of impetigo. Clin Pediatr. 1992;31:549-553.

105. Leyden JJ. Mupirocin: A new topical antibiotic. Semin Dermatol. 1987;6:48-54.

106. Breneman DL. Use of mupirocin ointment in the treatment of secondarily infected dermatoses. J Am Acad Dermatol. 1990;22:886-892.

107. Miller MA, Dascal A, Portnoy J, et al. Development of mupirocin resistance among methicillin-resistant Staphylococcus aureus after widespread use of nasal mupirocin ointment. Infect Control Hosp Epidemiol. 1996;17:811-813.

108. Dos Santos KRN, de Souza L, Filho PPG. Emergence of high-level mupirocin resistance in methicillin-resistant Staphylococcus aureus isolated from Brazilian university hospitals. Infect Control Hosp Epidemiol. 1996;17:813-816.

109. Mayall B, Martin R, Keenan AM, et al. Blanket use of intranasal mupirocin for outbreak control and long-term prophylaxis of endemic methicillin-resistant *Staphylococcus aureus* in an open ward. J Hosp Infect. 1996;32:257-266.
110. Zappi E, Brancaccio RR. Allergic contact dermatitis from mupirocin ointment. J Am Acad Dermatol. 1997;36:266.
111. Verbist L. The antimicrobial activity of fusidic acid. J Antimicrob Chemother. 1990;25:1-5.
112. Shanson DC. Clinical relevance of resistance to fusidic acid in *Staphylococcus aureus*. J Antimicrob Chemother. 1990;25:15-21.
113. Faber M, Rosdahl VT. Susceptibility to fusidic acid among Danish *Staphylococcus aureus* strains and fusidic acid consumption. J Antimicrob Chemother. 1990;25:7-14.
114. Parras F, del Carmen Guerrero M, Bouza E, et al. Comparative study of mupirocin and oral co-trimoxazole plus topical fusidic acid in eradication of nasal carriage of methicillin-resistant *Staphylococcus aureus*. Antimicrob Agents Chemother. 1995;39:175-179.

CHAPTER **36**

Antimycobacterial Agents

RICHARD J. WALLACE, JR.

DAVID E. GRIFFITH

Drugs for mycobacterial infections are discussed in three groups: those primarily for the treatment of infections caused by *Mycobacterium tuberculosis*, drugs for nontuberculous (*atypical*) mycobacterial infections, and agents principally for the treatment of leprosy.

Approaches to antituberculous chemotherapy have been affected by the spread of multidrug-resistant *M. tuberculosis* (MDR-TB), defined as resistance to at least isoniazid (INH) and rifampin,[1-4] and by the special impact on *M. tuberculosis* of those infected with the human immunodeficiency virus (HIV).[5,6]

MDR-TB strains having various combinations of resistance to INH, rifampin, streptomycin, or ethambutol have necessitated the use of drugs that were considered second-line agents as well as drugs that must be administered by injection.[2] The list of agents active against MDR-TB is quite limited, emphasizing both the need for universal supervised therapy[7] and the need for new antituberculous agents.[8]

MDR-TB infections are of increased concern in persons immunologically disabled by HIV with or without acquired immunodeficiency syndrome (AIDS) because the host contribution to controlling the infection is severely diminished. HIV-infected individuals have a number of other special problems. They are especially susceptible to adverse drug reactions.[9] The susceptibility of protease inhibitors to hepatic metabolism induced by rifampin has introduced the continued need for treatment regimens that exclude rifampin.[10] In addition, malabsorption of antituberculous drugs can occur in AIDS patients.[11]

The early years of HIV disease saw a dramatic increase in the prevalence and severity of *Mycobacterium avium* and other nontuberculous mycobacterial infections, especially in their disseminated forms. Fortunately, the combination of the macrolide-azalide group with ethambutol was active against *M. avium* and other mycobacteria, even in patients with markedly impaired cell-mediated immune defenses. In the past 5 years, with great advancement in antiretroviral therapy, the incidence of disseminated mycobacterial disease in advanced HIV has markedly declined. The effects of HIV and AIDS on leprosy and its chemotherapy do not appear to be as great as expected.

Traditionally, antimicrobials for tuberculosis have been classified as *first-line* drugs, having superior efficacy with acceptable toxicity, and *second-line* drugs, having either less efficacy, greater toxicity, or both. Several excellent reviews of antimycobacterial agents and therapy are available,[12-18] including guidelines for therapy of MDR-TB.[17,18]

Antituberculous drugs differ in their mechanism of bactericidal action and in their delivery to tuberculous lesions.[12] Three of the first-line agents—INH, rifampin, and ethambutol—are active against the large populations of tubercle bacilli in cavities. Streptomycin (now considered a second-line agent), other aminoglycosides, and capreomycin penetrate cells poorly and are inactive at acidic pH. Pyrazinamide (PZA) (the fourth first-line agent), inactive at the neutral or slightly alkaline pH that may occur extracellularly, is active only in acidic environments. Slowly replicating organisms in necrotic foci are killed by rifampin and somewhat less readily by INH.

First-line antituberculous agents, except ethambutol, are bactericidal. The bactericidal activities of both INH and rifampin against tubercle bacilli in cavitary, intracellular, or necrotic foci provide the basis for the efficacy of short-course INH-rifampin regimens. A combination of three bactericidal agents active against intracellular organisms—INH, rifampin, and PZA—is fundamental for the standard 6-month regimen currently recommended for drug-susceptible disease in the United States. A residual population consisting of virtually non-replicating dormant tubercle bacilli within necrotic foci is especially difficult to eradicate, perhaps explaining the minimum of approximately 4 months of therapy needed even in persons with competent immune defenses.

FIRST-LINE ANTITUBERCULOUS DRUGS

Isoniazid

Derivation and Structure. Isoniazid, isonicotinic acid hydrazide (INH), a synthetic agent, was introduced in 1952.

Mechanism of Action. INH is bactericidal against actively growing *M. tuberculosis* and bacteriostatic against nonreplicating organisms. It acts by inhibition of synthetic pathways of mycolic acid, an important constituent of mycobacterial cell walls. It also probably inhibits the catalase-peroxidase (*katG*) enzyme.

Antimicrobial Activity and Resistance. Against *M. tuberculosis*, 0.025 to 0.05 μg/mL of INH is inhibitory, and higher concentrations are bactericidal against replicating organisms. When INH is administered alone, resistance tends to emerge. Initially susceptible isolates become resistant in more than 70% of cases treated with INH monotherapy for 3 months. Resistance results from selection under antimicrobic pressure of resistant mutants of *M. tuberculosis* that number 1 in 10^6 among untreated bacillary populations. Large populations such as the 10^9 to 10^{10} bacilli in pulmonary cavities are especially likely to contain significant numbers of inherently resistant tubercle bacilli. Low-level INH resistance is most commonly associated with point mutations or short deletions within the catalase-peroxidase gene (*katG*), which still produces some enzymatic activity, whereas high-level resistance is associated with major deletions within the gene with loss of all enzymatic activity.[19,20] Resistance in the regulatory region of a second gene involved in mycolic acid synthesis (*inhA*) also confers INH resistance.[19,20] The prevalence of INH resistance among new cases of tuberculosis in1997 was 8% among more than 12,000 isolates in the United States,[4] with higher rates encountered in selected populations including immigrants from Southeast Asia and Central America, where resistance is more common.[1-4,21]

Pharmacology. INH is well absorbed orally or intramuscularly and is distributed throughout the body. Cerebrospinal fluid (CSF) levels are generally about 20% of plasma concentrations but may approach plasma levels in the presence of meningeal inflammation. Coadministration with vitamin C appears to inactivate INH suspensions markedly.[22]

Metabolism of INH occurs initially by liver *N*-acetyltransferase. Diminished acetylation capacity is inherited as an autosomal recessive trait that varies from a 5% prevalence rate in Canadian Eskimos to 83% in Egyptians. Ten percent to 15% of Asians are "slow" acetylators, as are 58% of American whites. Six hours after a 4 mg/kg oral dose, slow acetylators exhibit plasma INH levels of more than 0.8 μg/mL and rapid acetylators levels of less than 0.2 μg/mL.[13] The striking bimodal distribution of plasma half-lives of INH depending on acetylator status generally does not affect the outcome with daily therapy because plasma levels are maintained well above inhibitory concentrations. Metabolically altered INH is principally excreted in urine along with lesser amounts of unaltered drug. Dosage modification in renal insufficiency is not usually necessary. The benefit of dosage adjustment with significant hepatic disease is not established. Table 36-1 summarizes dosage modifications for INH and other antituberculous drugs in hepatic or renal failure.

Adverse Reactions

Hepatitis. INH has infrequent major toxicities, most notably hepatitis. Approximately 10% to 20% of INH recipients have asymptomatic minor elevations in serum aspartate aminotransferase levels that usually resolve even with continued therapy.[23] A meta-analysis of six studies estimated the rate of clinical (symptomatic) hepatitis in patients given INH alone to be approximately 0.6%.[24] Data indicate that the incidence of clinical hepatitis is even lower. Hepatitis occurred in only 0.1% to 0.15% of 11,141 persons receiving INH alone as treatment for latent tuberculosis infection (LTBI) in an urban tuberculosis control program.[25] Early estimates of the incidence of severe or major INH hepatotoxicity were provided from the results of a large multicenter trial sponsored by the National Institutes of Health. Fatal hepatitis occurred in 8 of nearly 14,000 patients receiving INH.[26] All but one of the deaths occurred in one study center, and patients did not receive routine monitoring for toxicity during the trial.[26] More recent studies, however, suggest that the rate of fatal INH-related hepatitis is substantially lower.[25,27,28] The likely explanation is the adoption in the early 1980s of uniform clinical toxicity monitoring for patients receiving INH for treatment of LTBI.[28]

Hepatotoxicity can occur at any time but is most likely 4 to 8 weeks after treatment is begun. INH hepatotoxicity is clearly correlated with age, presumably because of a diminished capacity for repair of INH-induced hepatocellular damage in elderly persons. Undernutrition may also play a role in the expression of INH hepatotoxicity.[29] Hepatotoxicity is increased in alcoholic patients with preexisting liver damage,[26] in pregnant women,[30] in combination with acetaminophen,[31] and in patients receiving other antituberculosis agents such as rifampin.[28] Histologically, hepatocellular damage can progress to submassive necrosis. Although endemic viral hepatitis has been considered a possible factor contributing to INH hepatotoxicity,[32,33] INH has been safely administered to some with acute hepatitis[34] and for LTBI to persons chronically infected with hepatitis B.[35,36] Educating patients about the recognition of symptoms of INH-induced liver disease is key in preventing its progression.

As noted, routine clinical monitoring of patients receiving INH is now considered mandatory.[28] Routine monitoring of serum hepatic enzyme concentrations is not routinely indicated for all patients at the start of treatment for LTBI. Baseline testing is recommended for patients whose initial evaluation suggests a liver disorder, patients infected with HIV, pregnant women and those in the immediate postpartum period (i.e., within 3 months of delivery), persons with a history of liver disease (e.g., hepatitis B or C, alcoholic hepatitis, or cirrhosis), persons who use alcohol regularly, and others who are at risk for chronic liver disease.[28] Baseline testing is no long routinely indicated in persons older than 35 years.[28] Laboratory monitoring during treatment of LTBI is indicated for patients whose baseline liver function tests are abnormal and for other persons at risk for hepatic disease.[28,37] INH-related death has been associated with continued administration of INH despite onset of symptoms of hepatitis; therefore, patients should be advised to discontinue INH therapy at the onset of symptoms consistent with incipient hepatitis, such as nausea, loss of appetite, and dull midabdominal pain. Generally, hepatotoxicity subsides after INH discontinuation. Cautious readministration of INH after resolution of hepatitis has been reported to be well tolerated and safe,[38] although consideration should be given in these patients to alternative therapies for LTBI. Recognition of the frequency and severity[39] of INH hepatotoxicity has not curtailed therapeutic usage but has led to a revision of indications for treatment of LTBI with special caution indicated in those, especially black and Hispanic women, older than 35 years.[28,40]

Neurotoxicity. Peripheral neuropathy has been described in 17% of recipients of INH at 6 mg/kg/day but is less frequent when adults receive the standard dose of 300 mg/day. Poor nutrition or underlying alcoholism, diabetes mellitus, or uremia predisposes to neuropathy, which is more frequent in slow acetylators who have higher plasma levels of unaltered drug. Increased pyridoxine excretion is promoted by INH. Pyridoxine, 10 to 50 mg daily, can ameliorate the neuropathy without interfering with the antimycobacterial effect.

INH-induced central nervous system (CNS) toxicity can produce aberrations ranging from memory loss to psychosis or seizures. Particular caution is indicated when administering INH to those with a seizure disorder. Optic neuropathy has been reported. Toxic CNS reactions are not necessarily related to pyridoxine deficiency but have responded to its administration.[13]

Hypersensitivity Reactions. Fever, which may be sustained or "spiking," skin eruptions, or hematologic abnormalities can occur. INH recipients can develop positive antinuclear antibody reactions and rarely manifest a lupus-like syndrome that is reversible on discontinuation of the INH.

Miscellaneous Adverse Reactions. INH-associated arthritic disorders have included Dupuytren's contracture and shoulder-hand syndrome. Pellagra can occur in malnourished INH recipients.[13,41] Pyridoxine deficiency–related anemia can occur in children or adults.[42]

Overdose. Accidental ingestion of INH by children or ingestion during a suicide attempt may result in metabolic acidosis, hyperglycemia, seizures, and coma. High-dose pyridoxine usually reverses these toxicities.

Significant Drug Interactions. Phenytoin (Dilantin) toxicity is potentiated by INH. Mental changes, nystagmus, and ataxia can result, especially in slow acetylators whose high INH levels inhibit phenytoin metabolism. Theophylline toxicity has been reported with coadministration of INH. Combined INH and rifampin therapy predisposes to elevation of plasma hepatic enzymes. Plasma INH concentrations are increased by *para*-aminosalicylic acid (PAS) through interference with acetylation.

Usage. INH is indicated for all clinical forms of tuberculosis. It is used alone for therapy of LTBI for selected purified protein derivative skin test reactors at high risk for developing active tuberculosis disease.[28] The latest Centers for Disease Control and Prevention/American Thoracic Society (CDC/ATS) guidelines state that INH is considered safe in pregnancy, but the risk of hepatitis may be increased immediately before or after delivery. Supplementation with pyridoxine is recommended if INH is administered during pregnancy.[18] It is approved for treating active tuberculosis in pregnant patients but should be given with caution and then only for selected high-risk patients with LTBI (such as HIV seropositive patients).

Availability and Dosage. INH is available generically (tablets, syrup, injectable solutions) and under brand names—INH tablets or

TABLE 36-1 Need for Dosage Modification for Antituberculous Drugs in Hepatic or Renal Failure

Antimicrobial Drug	*Modify in Hepatic Failure*	*Modify in Renal Failure*
Isoniazid	???	Minor
Pyrazinamide	Yes	Yes
Ethambutol	No	Yes
Rifampin	?Yes	No
Rifabutin	?Yes	No
Amikacin	No	Yes
Capreomycin	No	Yes
Kanamycin	No	Yes
Streptomycin	No	Yes
Quinolones	No	Yes
para-Aminosalicylic acid	No	Yes
Ethionamide	Yes	No
Cycloserine	No	Yes

Nydrazid injectable solution. Dosage forms include 100- and 300-mg tablets; syrup containing 10 mg/mL; 100 mg/mL solution for parenteral injection; and combination capsules combining 150 mg of INH with 300 mg of rifampin (Rifamate) or tablets of 50 mg with 120 mg of rifampin and 300 mg of PZA (Rifater). The usual adult dosage is 5 mg/kg/day (preferably 300 mg once daily). A higher dosage (10 mg/kg/day) has been recommended for special situations such as meningitis and for infants and children.

With the move toward the use of directly observed therapy for all patients, twice-weekly high-dose INH (15 mg/kg orally) is combined with rifampin (600 mg orally) and PZA (50 mg/kg, not to exceed 3 g) after an initial period of daily drug therapy for drug-susceptible isolates. For areas with a greater than 5% risk of drug-resistant tuberculosis, these drugs are combined with streptomycin (15 mg/kg up to 1.0 g intramuscularly) or ethambutol (50 mg/kg orally) twice weekly until susceptibilities are available. A reliable urine test is available to confirm INH ingestion.[43]

Although the preferred parenteral route is intramuscular injection, INH for injection can be administered safely intravenously.[44]

Rifampin

Derivation and Structure. Rifampin (termed *rifampicin* in the United Kingdom) is a semisynthetic derivative of a complex macrocyclic antibiotic, rifamycin B, produced by *Streptomyces mediterranei*. It was introduced for clinical trials in tuberculosis in 1967.

Mechanism of Action. Rifampin inhibits DNA-dependent RNA polymerase; human RNA polymerase is insensitive.

Antimicrobial Activity and Resistance. Rifampin is bactericidal against actively replicating *M. tuberculosis* to a degree comparable to that of INH with minimal inhibitory concentrations (MICs) of 0.005 to 0.2 μg/mL. It is also active against intracellular, slowly replicating bacilli and somewhat active against nearly dormant organisms in necrotic foci. Unlike other two-drug combinations, rifampin plus INH sterilizes tissues in experimental murine tuberculosis. Rifampin's efficacy is indicated in susceptible pulmonary tuberculosis by sputum conversion 2 weeks earlier with rifampin-containing regimens than with regimens without the drug. Resistance emerges rapidly if the drug is given as monotherapy. Primary resistance among isolates of *M. tuberculosis* is currently 3% in the United States but more than 10% in Southeast Asia and some Central American countries. Approximately 95% of resistance to rifampin results from a point mutation or deletion within an 81-bp region of the gene encoding the (β-subunit of RNA polymerase (*rpoB*).[20,45] The prevalence of rifampin resistance among new cases of tuberculosis in 1997 was 1.7% in the United States.[4] Isolated resistance to rifampin in the United States is strongly associated with HIV infection.[46] Resistance to rifampin is associated in all instances with cross-resistance to rifapentine and in most instances with rifabutin, especially in the presence of high-level resistance. Rifampin resistance coupled with resistance to INH and other antituberculous agents now characterizes many MDR-TB isolates.[2]

Pharmacology. Rifampin is well absorbed orally, yielding peak plasma concentrations of 7 to 8 μg/mL after a dose of 600 mg. It is widely distributed throughout the body. CSF concentrations range from undetectable to 0.5 μg/mL in healthy persons and reach 50% of plasma concentrations with meningeal inflammation. Rifampin's high lipid solubility enhances phagosomal penetration. Rifampin is deacetylated to an active form that undergoes biliary excretion and enterohepatic recirculation. Because of autoinduction of rifampin metabolism (cytochrome P-450 coupled),[47] biliary excretion increases with continued therapy. Induction of rifampin's metabolism with consequent reduction in its half-life and plasma concentrations becomes maximal after approximately six doses.[48] Excretion is primarily into the gastrointestinal tract, with lesser amounts in the urine. The plasma concentration and urinary excretion increase in hepatic failure. Probenecid blocks hepatic uptake, causing decreased biliary excretion. Liver failure requires a moderate dosage reduction, but the full dosage can be given in renal insufficiency. Rifampin is removed by hemodialysis or peritoneal dialysis.[49]

Adverse Reactions. Minor adverse reactions are rather frequent with rifampin, but in only 6 of 372 patients taking the drug for 20 weeks was cessation of therapy necessary because of adverse effects.[50]

Hepatitis. Rifampin's major adverse effect is hepatitis, which reportedly caused 16 deaths in 500,000 recipients.[13] Minimal abnormalities in liver function tests are common in those taking rifampin and usually resolve, possibly because of autoinduction of its metabolism even with continuation of the drug. Characteristically, elevations of bilirubin and alkaline phosphatase levels result, whereas elevation of hepatocellular enzyme concentrations can be caused by rifampin, INH, or both. Alcoholic patients with preexisting liver damage appear to be especially susceptible to rifampin-induced liver reactions.

Effects on Immune Parameters. Rifampin has widespread effects on humoral and cell-mediated immunity, but they appear to be of no clinical significance.

Hypersensitivity Reactions. Flushing, fever, pruritus without rash, urticaria, cutaneous vasculitis, eosinophilia, thrombocytopenia, hemolysis, or renal failure related to interstitial nephritis can occur because of rifampin. A systemic flulike syndrome, at times associated with thrombocytopenia, has been described almost exclusively with intermittent, high-dose therapy. Regimens of 600 mg of rifampin twice weekly have infrequently produced the flulike syndrome.

Miscellaneous Adverse Reactions. Widespread distribution of rifampin is reflected in an orange color appearing in urine, feces, saliva, sputum, pleural effusions, tears, soft contact lenses, sweat, semen, and CSF. With overdosage, a "red man syndrome" of skin discoloration has been described. Gastrointestinal upset is frequent but is usually ameliorated by a temporary reduction in dosage.

Significant Drug Interactions. By induction of microsomal cytochrome P-450–mediated enzymatic activities, rifampin causes increased hepatic metabolism of many substances. Rifampin interaction with more than 100 drugs has been described.[51-53] A partial compilation of this expanding list of compounds is given in Table 36-2. The induction period with rifampin may last for weeks after the drug is discontinued. The introduction of the protease inhibitors for the treatment of HIV infection has complicated the treatment of tuberculosis in this setting. Because rifampin induces metabolism of the protease inhibitors and non-nucleoside reverse transcriptase inhibitors, rifampin should not be coadministered with these agents.[10,54] As new antiretroviral agents and more pharmacokinetic data become available, treatment recommendations are likely to be modified. Up-to-date information can be obtained from the CDC website, http://www.cdc.gov/nchstp/tb/. Updated information on antiretroviral drugs and drug interactions, compiled by Medscape, can be found at http://www.medscape.com/updates/quickguide. In general, the coadministration of antituberculosis drugs and

TABLE 36-2 Commonly Used Compounds Having Rifampin-Induced Reduction in Plasma Concentrations

Antimicrobials	Hormonal Agents
Clarithromycin	Estrogens
Fluconazole	Oral contraceptives
Itraconazole	Prednisone-glucocorticoids
Ketoconazole	**Miscellaneous**
Indinavir	Barbiturates
Nelfinavir	Cyclosporine
Ritonavir	Diazepam
Saquinavir	Haloperidol
Cardiovascular Agents	Methadone
Digitoxin	Nortriptyline
Digoxin	Phenytoin
Diltiazem	Sulfonylurea
Metoprolol	Theophylline
Propranolol	
Quinidine	
Tocainide	
Verapamil	
Warfarin	

antiretroviral drugs should be initiated and guided by clinicians experienced in the treatment of these patients and familiar with the potential drug-drug interactions.

Competition for excretion with contrast agents used for biliary tract imaging may cause failure to visualize the gallbladder. Probenecid interferes with renal excretion, whereas PAS may interfere with gastrointestinal absorption.

Usage. Rifampin is indicated for treatment of all forms of pulmonary and extrapulmonary tuberculosis. It is recommended for treatment of LTBI when INH cannot be used.[28] Rifampin in combination with PZA was shown to be effective in HIV-positive patients for prophylaxis when given for only 2 months[55] and was subsequently included in recommendations as an option for treatment of LTBI.[28] For reasons that have yet to be elucidated, the combination of rifampin and PZA for treatment of LTBI has been associated with an unanticipated high rate (almost 6%) of severe or fatal hepatotoxicity, especially in HIV-seronegative patients.[56-58] As a consequence, rifampin-PZA is no longer recommended as an alternative for treatment of LTBI. If used, this regimen should be limited to carefully selected patients with close clinical and biochemical monitoring and supervision by experienced clinicians. Rifampin is a category C drug but is approved for use in pregnant patients with active tuberculosis. It should be used in pregnancy (as with INH) only for high-risk patients with LTBI, and then only if INH is not appropriate.

Availability and Dosage. Rifampin is supplied in the United States as Rifadin, available in 150- or 300-mg capsules and in combination 300-mg capsules with 150 mg of INH (Rifamate) or in 120-mg tablets with 50 mg of INH and 300 mg of PZA (Rifater). Rifampin for intravenous infusion (600 mg per vial, Rifadin) should not be used intramuscularly. The usual oral dosage is 600 mg once daily for adults and 10 to 20 mg/kg/day for children (not to exceed 600 mg/day). Twice-weekly 900- or 1200-mg dosage regimens have largely been abandoned because of toxic reactions. A 600-mg twice-weekly schedule generally has been well tolerated. Rifampin from opened capsules can be suspended (usually 10 mg/mL) in simple or flavored sugar syrups that should not include ascorbic acid, which can inactivate rifampin.[21] Suspensions can be refrigerated for up to 2 weeks.

Pyrazinamide

Derivation and Structure. PZA is a synthetic pyrazine analogue of nicotinamide.

Mechanism of Action. The mechanism of action of PZA remains unknown.

Antimicrobial Activity and Resistance. PZA is bactericidal for tubercle bacilli at 12.5 μg/mL. Its optimal activity appears to be against semidormant organisms in an acid pH environment such as that existing intracellularly in phagolysosomes. Despite good activity at acid pH in vitro and inhibitory concentrations within monocytes,[59] PZA exhibits low activity alone in pretreated macrophages.[60] Resistance rapidly evolves if PZA is used alone. Primary resistance is seen in less than 1% of isolates, but nearly 50% of INH-rifampin–resistant MDR-TB isolates are PZA resistant.[2] Most isolates resistant to PZA have mutations in the gene encoding pyrazinamidase (*pncA*) (Table 36-3).[61,62] This mutation results in loss of activity of pyrazinamidase, an enzyme that converts PZA to the active form of pyrazinoic acid.

Pharmacology. Well absorbed orally, PZA is widely distributed throughout the body, attaining concentrations above that needed to inhibit tubercle bacilli. Peak plasma concentrations are approximately 50 μg/mL, with a half-life of 12 hours, making once-daily or less frequent dosing practical. PZA crosses inflamed meninges and has been recommended in combination regimens for tuberculous meningitis.[63] It is metabolized by the liver, and metabolic products, including principally pyrazinoic acid, are excreted mainly by the kidneys, requiring dosage modification in renal failure. PZA is dialyzable, and supplemental dosage may be advisable after dialysis sessions.[49]

Adverse Reactions. The most common side effects are nausea and vomiting. Hepatotoxicity occurred in nearly 15% of PZA recipients in early trials that employed dosages of 40 to 50 mg/kg/day for prolonged periods. Current regimens of 20 to 25 mg/kg/day are much safer.[64] Patients with preexisting liver disease should have symptoms and hepatic function tests monitored closely. Other adverse reactions (1% of patients or less) include interstitial nephritis,[65] rhabdomyolysis with myoglobinuric renal failure,[66] nonincapacitating polymyalgia, photosensitivity, and rash. Asymptomatic urate retention occurs in 50% of PZA recipients.[64]

Significant Drug Interactions. As noted earlier, the combination of rifampin and PZA for treatment of LTBI is associated with a high rate of severe or fatal hepatotoxicity.[56-58] There are no other significant drug interactions with PZA.

Usage. PZA is included as an essential component of multidrug 6-month short-course chemotherapy.[12,17,64] Without PZA for the first 2 months, relapse rates are unacceptable.[65] Efficacy with its administration as infrequently as once weekly makes PZA suitable for directly observed therapy regimens. PZA is a class C drug and should be used with caution in pregnancy. Although PZA is recommended for routine use in pregnant women by the World Health Organization, the drug has not been recommended for general use in pregnant women in the United States by the CDC because of insufficient data to determine safety.[18] The practical consequence of this policy is that pregnant women in the United States with active tuberculosis require 9 months of therapy because PZA is not included in the first 2 months of therapy.

Availability and Dosage. PZA is available in 500-mg tablets or as 300-mg tablets in combination with INH (50 mg) and rifampin (120 mg) (Rifater). Dosage is 20 to 25 mg/kg/day (often 1.5 to 2.0 g) orally once or in two divided doses. PZA has been well tolerated in a twice-weekly dosage of 50 mg/kg (not to exceed 3 g/day) for short-course regimens. It has even been administered safely once weekly in a dose of 90 mg/kg.

Ethambutol

Derivation and Structure. Ethambutol (ethylenediiminobutanol) was discovered in 1961 among synthetic compounds screened for antituberculous activity.

TABLE 36-3 Mechanism of Action and Recognized Mutational Resistance in Commonly Used Antituberculous Agents

Drug	Mechanism of Action	Site of Mutational Resistance (gene)
Isoniazid	Inhibits mycolic acid synthesis Catalase/peroxidase enzyme	*inhA* (regulatory region) (mycolic acid gene) *katG* (catalase/peroxidase gene)
Rifampin	Inhibits RNA polymerization	β-subunit *rpoB* (RNA polymerase gene)
Pyrazinamide	Unknown	*pncA* (pyrazinamidase gene)
Ethambutol	Inhibits cell wall synthesis (blocks arabinosyl transferase)	*embB* (gene for arabinosyl transferase enzyme)
Streptomycin	Inhibits protein synthesis	*rpsL* (gene for ribosomal S12 protein); 16S ribosomal RNA gene
Amikacin	Inhibits protein synthesis	16S ribosomal RNA gene (? amikacin binding site)
Capreomycin	Inhibits cell wall synthesis	Unknown
Quinolones	Inhibits DNA structure	*gyrA* (gyrase A gene)

Mechanism of Action. Ethambutol inhibits arabinosyl transferase enzymes that are involved in arabinogalactan and lipoarabinomannan biosynthesis within the cell wall.[67]

Antimicrobial Activity and Resistance. Ethambutol is bacteriostatic in vitro or within macrophages[59] at concentrations of 1 μg/mL against susceptible strains of *M. tuberculosis*. Primary ethambutol resistance in the United States is only 2%.[4] Ethambutol's principal role has been as a "companion" drug to curtail resistance. However, resistance rates as high as 80% for ethambutol in INH-rifampin–resistant isolates from New York City apparently indicate limited utility against MDR-TB.[2] Ethambutol resistance is related to point mutations in the arabinosyl transferase enzyme EmbB, which is coded for by the *embB* gene.[68]

Pharmacology. Ethambutol administered orally is 75% to 80% absorbed, yielding peak plasma concentrations of 5 μg/mL after a dose of 25 mg/kg. It is distributed throughout the body, including the CSF. Although little ethambutol crosses normal meninges, levels 10% to 50% of those in plasma occur in CSF with meningeal inflammation. After conversion of approximately 25% of absorbed ethambutol to inactive metabolites, 80% of the parent together with metabolites is excreted in urine. Consequently, it becomes necessary to modify the dosage in significant renal failure.

Adverse Reactions

Optic Neuritis and Visual Loss. The major toxicity of ethambutol is neuropathy. Peripheral neuropathy is infrequent; retrobulbar optic neuritis is more common. Characteristically, patients complain of bilateral blurry vision and are found to have impairment of visual acuity and red-green color vision. Common in association with high-dose (50 mg/kg/day) therapy with prolonged administration and more common with 25 mg/kg/day than with 15 mg/kg/day dosing, retrobulbar neuritis is usually slowly reversible. Visual loss has rarely occurred in elderly persons receiving as little as 15 mg/kg/day.[69] The administration of ethambutol at 25 mg/kg three times weekly appears to be associated with a reduced risk of visual toxicity in this population of patients compared with daily dosing at 15 mg/kg.[70] This is important because baseline visual acuity is often impaired in elderly persons and associated with other diseases such as cataracts that are frequently associated with blurred vision. Recipients of ethambutol should be instructed to report symptoms of blurry vision promptly and to discontinue the drug until confirmatory visual testing can be done. Visual acuity and red-green color perception testing is recommended at baseline, whenever a change in visual symptoms occurs, and every 4 to 6 weeks in those taking 25 mg/kg/day. Monthly testing in patients receiving 15 mg/kg can be useful in establishing the range of visual abnormalities in those already visually impaired.

Miscellaneous Adverse Reactions. Gastrointestinal intolerance is infrequent. Hyperuricemia occurs because of decreased renal uric acid excretion. Hypersensitivity reactions are rare and include dermatitis, arthralgias, and fever.

Significant Drug Interactions. There are no significant drug interactions with ethambutol.

Usage. Ethambutol is commonly included as the fourth drug along with INH, rifampin, and PZA in patients with tuberculosis at high risk for drug resistance. It is also routinely used in treatment regimens for patients with isolates resistant to INH or rifampin, or both. Ethambutol has no detectable effects on the fetus but has no pregnancy classification.

Availability and Dosage. Ethambutol is available as ethambutol hydrochloride (Myambutol) supplied in 100- or 400-mg tablets. The usual dosage is 15 to 25 mg/kg/day initially, followed after 60 days by 15 mg/kg/day as a single daily dose.

Streptomycin

Derivation, Structure, and Pharmacology. Streptomycin, an aminoglycoside antibiotic introduced in the 1940s, was the first drug to reduce tuberculosis mortality. Its structure, mechanism of action, and pharmacology are covered in other chapters. Briefly, intramuscular injection of 1 g yields peak plasma concentrations of 25 to 45 μg/mL. It is virtually excluded from the CNS.

Antimicrobial Activity and Resistance. Streptomycin is bactericidal against *M. tuberculosis* in vitro but is inactive against intracellular tubercle bacilli. Concentrations of 4 to 10 μg/mL of plasma are inhibitory. The rapid emergence of resistance to streptomycin was quickly recognized as a consequence of single-drug therapy. Approximately 1 in 10[6] tubercle bacilli is spontaneously resistant to streptomycin. Primary resistance to streptomycin is seen most often in populations of patients with a high incidence of INH resistance. In MDR-TB outbreaks, approximately 80% of INH-rifampin–resistant isolates are also streptomycin resistant.[2] Streptomycin resistance is related to mutational changes involving ribosomal binding protein or the ribosomal binding site.[20,71,72] Isolates resistant to streptomycin are not cross-resistant to amikacin, kanamycin, or capreomycin.

Adverse Reactions. Streptomycin toxicity is like that of other aminoglycoside antibiotics but with less renal and auditory toxicity and greater vestibular toxicity than more commonly used aminoglycosides. Patients receiving streptomycin should be instructed to be aware of tinnitus, decreased hearing, and problems with balance, and they should be instructed to notify their caregiver immediately if such reactions occur.

Significant Drug Interactions. There are no significant drug interactions with streptomycin.

Usage. Streptomycin is indicated as the fourth drug along with INH, rifampin, and PZA in patients at significant risk for drug resistance. It is also used for multidrug therapy of drug-resistant tuberculosis. Dosages greater than 1 g/day should be avoided. Reduction of dosage or frequency of administration, or both, is indicated in patients older than 50 years, those with low body weight, and those in whom renal function is impaired. Special care must be taken when streptomycin is used in combination with other nephrotoxic or ototoxic drugs such as capreomycin or amikacin. It is a category D drug in pregnancy because of fetal ototoxicity.

Availability and Dosage. Streptomycin sulfate for intramuscular injection is provided in 1-g single-injection vials. The recommended dosage in adults with normal renal function is 0.5 to 1 g daily for the first several months and then 1 g twice weekly. For persons 60 years of age or older the dose should be 10 mg/kg/day up to 750 mg. Children receive 20 to 40 mg/kg/day in divided doses every 12 hours (maximum 1.0 g/day). Although not approved for such use, the drug can be safely given intravenously when needed. Streptomycin is currently available in the United States, but its supply has been interrupted in the past.

Alternatives to Rifampin

Rifabutin

Derivation, Pharmacology. Several spiropiperidyl rifamycins have activity against mycobacteria, including *M. tuberculosis*, *Mycobacterium avium-intracellulare* complex, and *Mycobacterium kansasii*.[73-77] Rifabutin (Mycobutin), a derivative of rifamycin-S, is more active in vitro and more effective on a weight basis in experimental murine tuberculosis than rifampin.[76] The mechanism of action is inhibition of RNA polymerase, as it is with rifampin. It has a long plasma half-life (45 hours) in humans and marked tissue tropism, producing tissue concentrations 5- to 10-fold greater than in serum. Peak serum concentrations of rifampin (5 to 10 μg/mL) are 5- to 10-fold higher than those of rifabutin (0.5 μg/mL).[78]

Adverse Reactions. A polymyalgia syndrome, a yellowish-tan discoloration of the skin (*pseudojaundice*), and anterior uveitis have occurred in patients taking rifabutin, usually at doses exceeding 300 mg daily.[79,80] Almost all persons with these side effects have also been receiving clarithromycin, fluconazole, or ritonavir. Symptoms of uveitis include ocular pain and blurred vision. Neutropenia occurs infrequently when rifabutin is used to treat tuberculosis but has been reported in one third of patients receiving therapy for pulmonary *M. avium* complex disease.[81] The incidence of rash, hepatitis, and gastrointestinal distress appears comparable to that with rifampin. It can also produce an orange-red discoloration of urine, saliva, tears, and contact lenses similar to that of rifampin.

Significant Drug Interactions. Rifabutin induces the hepatic cytochrome P-450 system but only about 50% of that seen with rifampin. This induction produces lowered serum levels of numerous drugs normally metabolized in the liver, including the protease inhibitors. Concurrent administration of ritonavir and saquinavir with rifabutin is not recommended for this reason.[82] Rifabutin is also metabolized by the same system, and enzyme inhibitors such as the protease inhibitors, fluconazole, and clarithromycin increase plasma rifabutin concentrations.[78,82]

Usage. Rifabutin appears as effective as rifampin in the treatment of drug-susceptible tuberculosis,[83,84] but experience with it is limited. In patients receiving protease inhibitors for HIV infection, rifabutin at 150-300 mg is recommended in place of rifampin at 600 mg because it has less effect on the metabolism of the protease inhibitors.[10] Rifabutin's potential for treatment of MDR-TB is under investigation.[85,86] Approximately 25% of rifampin-resistant tuberculosis strains are inhibited by low concentrations of rifabutin.

Rifapentine

Derivation, Pharmacology. With the microbiologic success of rifabutin but problems with low serum levels and complex adverse reactions, investigators searched for other rifamycin compounds. The two most promising agents are rifapentine[87-89] and KRM-1648.[90] In the study leading to licensure in 1998, rifapentine, 600 mg twice weekly, was compared with rifampin, 450 to 600 mg, when both were given with daily INH, PZA, and ethambutol for 2 months, followed by rifapentine, 600 mg, plus INH once weekly or rifampin, 450 to 600 mg, plus INH twice weekly. Results at 6 months follow-up were comparable, although the relapse rate with rifapentine was slightly higher (10% versus 5%).[89] When it is given with a fatty meal, peak blood levels after the administration of 600 mg of rifapentine are 15 μg/mL of native drug and 6 μg/mL of 25-desacetyl rifapentine, the active metabolite. The half-life of both compounds is 13 hours.

Adverse Drug Reactions. The adverse effects of rifapentine are similar to those associated with rifampin.

Significant Drug Interactions.

Rifapentine appears to be a more potent inducer of the cytochrome P-450 system than rifabutin but less than rifampin. It, therefore, may increase metabolism of coadministered drugs that are metabolized by these enzymes.

Usage. Rifapentine has been approved for once-weekly use with INH in the continuation phase of therapy for HIV-negative patients without cavitation on chest radiography and negative acid-fast bacilli smears at 2 months.[18] The drug should be avoided in HIV-positive patients because of interaction with protease inhibitors and the unexplained development of rifamycin monoresistance in some patients.[91]

Availability and Dosage. Rifapentine is available in 150-mg tablets. The recommended dosage for adults in the continuation phase of therapy for tuberculosis is 10 mg/kg or a maximum 600 mg/week. The drug is not approved for use in children or pregnant women. The pharmacokinetics of rifapentine have not been evaluated in patients with renal impairment. Only about 17% of an administered dose is excreted by the kidneys. The clinical significance of impaired renal function in the disposition of rifapentine is unknown. Similarly, the clinical significance of impaired hepatic function in the disposition of rifapentine and its 25-desacetyl metabolite is not known.

Other Rifamycins

KRM-1648 is available as Priftin in 150-mg tablets. KRM-1648 is not yet approved by the U.S. Food and Drug Administration.

SECOND-LINE ANTITUBERCULOUS DRUGS

Quinolones

Mechanism of Action. Emerging outbreaks of MDR-TB[1-3] have stimulated the investigation of fluorinated quinolones for their activity against mycobacteria.[92-98] Some are bactericidal against *M. tuberculosis*, presumably by inhibition of its DNA gyrase at concentrations within achievable serum levels.[93]

Antimicrobial Activity and Resistance. Ciprofloxacin and ofloxacin inhibit more than 90% of strains of drug-susceptible tubercle bacilli at concentrations of 0.5 and 1.0 μg/mL, respectively.[94-96] Fluoroquinolones, particularly sparfloxacin,[97] have produced additive effects with other antituberculous drugs in vitro and in animals. Clinical trials of ofloxacin in combination with INH and rifampin indicate activity comparable to that of ethambutol.[98] Ofloxacin used alone in a dose of 300 mg/day in patients with MDR-TB has produced decreases in sputum colony counts, with sputum conversion in 26%.[99] In nonconverters, ofloxacin resistance emerged. Usage as a single agent in animal models or in human trials with inactive drugs has led to the rapid emergence of resistance. Resistance appears to result from mutations in the genes responsible for DNA configuration (DNA gyrase).[20,100]

Of the fluoroquinolones, levofloxacin, moxifloxacin, and gatifloxacin have the most activity against *M. tuberculosis*.[101] Cross-resistance has been demonstrated among ciprofloxacin, ofloxacin, and levofloxacin. Whether some strains retain susceptibility to the newer 8-methoxyquinolones gatifloxacin and moxifloxacin awaits additional studies.

Usage. Quinolones are now routinely incorporated into treatment regimens for MDR-TB along with other agents. The usual dosage is levofloxacin 500 to 1000 mg/day and ciprofloxacin 750 mg or ofloxacin 400 mg, both given twice daily. The use of fluoroquinolones in children and adolescents has not been approved, but most experts agree that the drugs should be considered for children with multidrug-resistant tuberculosis. This class of drugs should be avoided in pregnancy. Fluoroquinolones are cleared primarily by the kidney and dosage adjustment is recommended if creatinine clearance is less than 50 mL/minute. They are not cleared by hemodialysis, and supplemental doses after dialysis are not necessary. Drug levels are not affected by hepatic disease.

Adverse Reactions. The adverse effects of levofloxacin (these apply to most of the quinolones) include nausea and bloating, dizziness, insomnia, tremulousness, headache, rash, pruritus, and photosensitivity. There are limited data on the safety and tolerability of long-term moxifloxacin and gatifloxacin at 400 mg/day. One issue of long-term safety for the newer quinolones is their cardiac effect on the QT interval, resulting in a ventricular tachycardia known as torsades de pointes. The concern varies among the newer quinolones and is more of an issue with the newer quinolones.

Significant Drug Reactions. Because antacids and other medications containing divalent cations markedly decrease absorption of fluoroquinolones, it is important that fluoroquinolone not be administered within 2 hours of such medication.

Linezolid

Linezolid is an oxazolidinone introduced for its activity against drug-resistant gram-positive bacteria. It has been shown to inhibit all strains of *M. tuberculosis* at concentrations less than 1 μg/mL in vitro, but no animal or human studies of the treatment of tuberculosis are yet available. However, it has exciting potential for therapy of tuberculosis, especially MDR-TB. It is marketed as Zyvox and is available as 600-mg tablets and infusions. The usual daily dose for bacterial infections has been 600 mg twice daily, while 600 mg once or twice daily has been used for tuberculosis. The oral form is almost 100% bioavailable. Mutational resistance has not been described but is likely to occur as the drug inhibits the ribosome and *M. tuberculosis* has only one copy of this gene. The high cost of the drug and bone marrow toxicity associated with long-term administration are likely to prohibit any routine use of the drug.

Capreomycin, Amikacin, and Kanamycin

Capreomycin, amikacin, and kanamycin are considered as a group because all are administered by intramuscular or intravenous injection, have similar pharmacokinetics and toxicities, and are excreted by the renal route. These drugs have been used principally as alternative agents for MDR-TB. All have additive ototoxicity and nephrotoxicity and in that regard should be given cautiously, as with streptomycin or other aminoglycosides.

Capreomycin

Antimicrobial Activity and Resistance. Capreomycin, a polypeptide antibiotic obtained from *Streptomyces capreolus,* is active against *M. tuberculosis,* including most MDR-TB strains,[2] at concentrations of 1 to 50 μg/mL (usually 10 μg/mL). Average peak plasma concentrations of 30 μg/mL are achievable. There is no cross-resistance between streptomycin and capreomycin,[102] but some isolates resistant to kanamycin or amikacin are cross-resistant to capreomycin. The site of mutational change resulting in capreomycin resistance is unknown.

Adverse Reactions. Capreomycin can cause hearing loss, tinnitus, and decreased renal function but is considered less toxic than amikacin and especially kanamycin.

Significant Drug Interactions. There are no significant drug interactions with capreomycin.

Usage. Capreomycin has emerged as the first-line injectable agent in regimens for the treatment of drug-resistant tuberculosis, especially when there is streptomycin resistance.

Availability and Dosage. Capreomycin sulfate is supplied as Capastat. The dosage is the same as with streptomycin, with a range of 500 mg to 1 g deep intramuscularly five times weekly for 2 to 4 months in those younger than 50 years and having normal renal function. The dose is thereafter reduced to 1 g two to three times weekly. It is a category C pregnancy drug.

Amikacin

Antimicrobial Activity and Resistance. In vitro and in animals, amikacin is among the most active aminoglycosides against *M. tuberculosis.* There is limited experience with amikacin in human tuberculosis. Because of its expense and greater toxicity, it is generally considered the third-line agent after streptomycin and capreomycin for the treatment of MDR-TB. It has generally replaced kanamycin in the United States. Resistance to amikacin and kanamycin results from an A-to-G change at base pair 1408 of the 16S ribosomal RNA gene.[103]

Adverse Reactions. Common side effects include tinnitus, hearing loss, and nonoliguric renal failure. Hypersensitivity events are rare.

Usage. Amikacin is an alternative injectable agent for the treatment of resistant *M. tuberculosis* infections. The customary dose is 7 to 10 mg/kg (not to exceed 1 g) five times weekly. Because most pathology laboratories can determine blood levels of amikacin but not kanamycin, streptomycin, or capreomycin, amikacin is especially suited when parenteral therapy is required in patients with renal failure or in elderly patients with preexisting hearing loss. It is a category D drug in pregnancy.

Kanamycin

Kanamycin is an aminoglycoside that has activity against most strains of streptomycin-resistant tubercle bacilli. Except for its lower cost, kanamycin offers no advantage over amikacin in combination therapy and has substantial ototoxicity. In addition, serum levels are not readily available.

Availability and Dosage. Kanamycin sulfate is available as Kantrex, 0.5 g/2 mL, 1 g/3 mL, or 75 mg/2 mL (pediatric formulation) for intramuscular injection. The usual dose is 10 mg/kg, generally limited to 500 mg/day in adults because of ototoxicity.

Para-Aminosalicylic Acid

Derivation, Structure, and Pharmacology. As a calcium or sodium salt, this synthetic compound inhibits the growth of tubercle bacilli by impairment of folate synthesis. PAS is incompletely absorbed orally. A 4-g dose yields plasma concentrations of 70 to 80 μg/mL. Eighty-five percent of absorbed PAS is excreted in urine as various metabolic products.

Adverse Reactions. Chief among PAS side effects is gastrointestinal intolerance, which is often severe and results in poor compliance. PAS can cause reversible drug-induced lupus-like reactivity and, when given as the sodium salt, sodium overload. It can produce lymphoid hyperplasia, and recipients can develop mononucleosis-like syndromes with fever, rash, hepatosplenomegaly, occasionally toxic hepatitis, and adenopathy. Hypersensitivity to PAS is frequent.

Usage. PAS has retained a limited role in multidrug therapy in developing countries because of its low cost. However, it is becoming less favored because of poor compliance and primary resistance. Its use in the United States is limited to the treatment of MDR-TB.

Availability and Dosage. In the United States, PAS is available from the CDC (website: www.cdc.gov). Dosage forms include 500-mg tablets and 4-g resin packets. The usual dosage is 10 to 12 g/day in three or four divided doses for adults (6 to 8 g/day of the sodium-potassium–free ascorbate) and, in children, 200 to 300 mg/kg/day in divided doses.

Cycloserine

Derivation, Mechanism of Action. By virtue of inhibiting cell wall synthesis, cycloserine has antimicrobial activity against a broad range of prokaryotic organisms including mycobacteria. From 5 to 20 μg/mL inhibits susceptible *M. tuberculosis* in vitro.

Pharmacology. Cycloserine is readily absorbed orally, producing peak plasma concentrations of 20 to 50 μg/mL. It is widely distributed among tissues, and there is no blood-brain barrier to cycloserine.[13] Little of the drug is metabolized, and approximately two thirds is excreted unchanged by the kidneys.

Adverse Reactions. Cycloserine can cause peripheral neuropathy or CNS dysfunction, including confusion, irritability, somnolence, headache, nervousness, vertigo, dysarthria, and seizures. Behavioral alterations include severe depression with suicidal ideation. Cycloserine is contraindicated in patients with a history of seizures or those with severe underlying depression. Because the CNS toxicity appears to be dose related and only a few specialized laboratories can determine serum drug levels, the drug is generally avoided, even by experienced TB clinicians.

Usage. Cycloserine is one of several alternatives for re-treatment regimens or for treatment of primary drug-resistant *M. tuberculosis.* It does not appear to have great activity against MDR-TB strains.[2] It is classified as a category C drug in pregnancy.

Availability and Dosage. Cycloserine is provided in the United States as Seromycin in 250-mg pulvules. The usual dosage is 500 to 1000 mg/day in two divided doses, with 500 mg/day commonly used.

Ethionamide

Derivation, Mechanism of Action, and Resistance. Ethionamide, a derivative of isonicotinic acid, was first synthesized in 1956. It is tuberculostatic at 0.6 to 2.5 μg/mL against susceptible strains, presumably by inhibition of oxygen-dependent mycolic acid synthesis.[104] The mechanism of ethionamide resistance is unknown, but some isolates are resistant to both INH and ethionamide and harbor mutations in the region of the *inhA* gene, which is involved in mycolic acid biosynthesis.[20]

Pharmacology. Ethionamide is absorbed well orally, yielding peak plasma concentrations of 20 μg/mL. It is widely distributed and penetrates both normal and inflamed meninges to yield CSF concentrations equivalent to those in plasma. It is metabolized by the liver, with metabolites renally excreted. Ethionamide interferes with INH acetylation.

Adverse Reactions. Gastrointestinal distress with nausea and vomiting frequently leads to poor compliance and drug discontinuance. Various neurologic disorders have been caused by ethionamide, including peripheral neuropathy and psychiatric disturbances. Neurologic side effects have been reported to be alleviated by pyridoxine or nicotinamide. Reversible hepatotoxicity occurs in approximately 5% of ethionamide recipients. A hypersensitivity-type rash and poor diabetic control are infrequent complications.

Usage. Ethionamide is among the agents that can be chosen for the treatment of resistant tuberculosis. It appears to be active against most MDR-TB isolates.[2] Its usage is limited by a high frequency of severe gastrointestinal intolerance.

Availability and Dosage. Ethionamide is available in the United States as Trecator-SC in 250-mg coated tablets. The initial dosage is 250 mg twice daily (or as a single dose at bedtime), which is increased by 250 mg daily until 1 g/day in divided doses is reached. Usually, 500 to 750 mg is the maximal tolerated dose.

β-Lactams

All mycobacteria produce β-lactamase. Several β-lactamase–resistant β-lactam antibiotics or combinations of a β-lactam with β-lactamase inhibitors such as clavulanic acid are active in vitro against *M. tuberculosis*[105,106] and various nontuberculous mycobacteria.[107] Unfortunately, activity of β-lactam agents against intracellular mycobacteria is generally poor.[59,108,109] In concentrations as high as 50 μg/mL in a macrophage model, ceforanide, active in vitro, was unable to inhibit tubercle bacilli.[59]

Amithiozone

Amithiozone (thiacetazone), a thiosemicarbazole, is active against many strains of *M. tuberculosis*.[13,14] Because of its low cost, amithiozone has been employed as a first-line drug, particularly in East Africa.[14] However, because of severe toxicity in HIV-infected recipients there, clinical usage no longer appears appropriate.[6,9]

MAJOR DRUGS FOR THE TREATMENT OF NONTUBERCULOUS MYCOBACTERIAL INFECTIONS

Nontuberculous (atypical or environmental) mycobacteria vary greatly in susceptibility to antimicrobics. Some, such as *M. kansasii*, are susceptible to agents used principally for the treatment of tuberculosis; others, such as *Mycobacterium fortuitum* and *Mycobacterium chelonae*, respond to antibiotics used more commonly for pyogenic bacterial infections[110]; and still others, especially *M. avium-intracellulare*, are broadly resistant. Susceptibility testing of the nontuberculous mycobacteria has been greatly facilitated by the publication of national guidelines for testing by the National Committee for Clinical Laboratory Standards (NCCLS).[111] Hence, chemotherapy for nontuberculous mycobacterial infections based on susceptibility results is now feasible for many species. An important exception is that susceptibility testing has no clinically predictive value in infections with *M. avium-intracellulare* except for the newer macrolide clarithromycin.[54]

Macrolides

Antimicrobial Activity and Resistance. Pretreatment strains of *M. kansasii*, *Mycobacterium scrofulaceum*, *Mycobacterium marinum*, *Mycobacterium haemophilum*, *Mycobacterium malmoense*, *M. avium-intracellulare*, *M. chelonae*, and *Mycobacterium abscessus* are susceptible to achievable therapeutic concentrations of the newer macrolides, clarithromycin and azithromycin. This susceptibility has resulted in a dramatic change in therapy for nontuberculous mycobacteria, with a macrolide now part of the treatment regimen for most species. Clarithromycin inhibits almost all species with the exception of 20% of *M. fortuitum* and *Mycobacterium simiae* at 4 μg/mL or less.[112,113] Initial therapeutic results have indicated that these agents are clinically efficacious as well, including efficacy against both pulmonary and disseminated *M. avium-intracellulare* infections.[114-118] Both macrolides have proved efficacious for the prevention of disseminated *M. avium* infection in patients with AIDS.[119,120] These agents should not be used as monotherapy because of the rapid emergence of resistance, which results from a point mutation at adenine 2058 or 2059 on the 23S ribosomal RNA, the presumed macrolide-binding site, and produces cross-resistance to all macrolides.[121,122]

Pharmacology. Clarithromycin is metabolized in the liver, and significant concentrations of the 14-OH metabolite are detectable in the serum.[123] Clarithromycin is also excreted in part by the kidneys, and a reduction in dosage is required in elderly patients, patients with low body weights, and those with reduced renal function.

Adverse Reactions. The most common side effects are nausea, vomiting, and diarrhea, which are generally dose related.[124] A toxic hepatitis occurs with daily doses above 1.0 g and is associated with elevated levels of alkaline phosphatase and γ-glutamyl transferase.[124] Temporary hearing loss may also occur with high-dose azithromycin.[125]

Significant Drug Interactions. Clarithromycin is metabolized by the cytochrome P-450 enzyme system, and serum levels are dramatically reduced by enzyme inducers such as rifampin.[123] Clarithromycin is an inhibitor of the P-450 enzyme system, and its use results in increased serum levels and potential increased toxicities of multiple drugs metabolized by these enzymes, including rifabutin,[79,80] carbamazepine, cisapride, astemizole, terfenadine, and theophylline. Clarithromycin inhibits the metabolism of protease inhibitors as well.[82] In contrast, azithromycin is not metabolized by the cytochrome P-450 system and has no significant drug interactions.

Dosage. The usual therapeutic doses are 500 mg twice daily for clarithromycin and 250 mg once daily for azithromycin. For *M. avium* complex lung disease, the usual clarithromycin dose is 500 mg in the morning and evening and for azithromycin 500 mg given three times weekly. For disseminated *M. avium* prophylaxis, the dosage of azithromycin is 1200 mg once a week.[120]

Rifampin

Antimicrobial Activity. Rifampin is employed for the treatment of many nontuberculous mycobacterial infections. In vitro, all untreated strains of *M. kansasii*, *M. marinum*, *M. haemophilum*, and *Mycobacterium xenopi* are inhibited by 0.25 to 1.0 μg/mL.[54,126,127] Other species are much less susceptible. Only one half of *M. avium-intracellulare* strains are inhibited in vitro by 4 to 16 μg/mL of rifampin. Synergy between rifampin and other agents has been demonstrable for a number of species in vitro. Its role as a single agent is discouraged because resistance occurs.[128]

Pharmacology, Adverse Events, and Significant Drug Interactions. See the earlier discussion in the section on tuberculosis.

Usage. The excellent response of *M. kansasii* infections to rifampin-containing regimens has made rifampin a recommended component of most treatment regimens.[54] For patients with HIV infection receiving protease inhibitors, rifabutin (150 mg/day) or clarithromycin (500 mg twice daily) is recommended over rifampin[54] because of its lesser effect on the cytochrome P-450 system.

Rifabutin

Antimicrobial Activity. Rifabutin is inhibitory against 90% of strains of *M. avium-intracellulare* at a concentration of 2 μg/mL.[76,77] It is concentrated several fold in tissue and, like rifampin, has gastrointestinal toxicity as its most common adverse effect. Rifabutin at a dose of 300 mg/day has been shown to reduce by 50% the incidence and rate of dissemination of *M. avium-intracellulare* infections in AIDS patients with CD4 counts less than 200,[128] although it is probably not as effective as the newer macrolides.

Pharmacology, Adverse Events, and Significant Drug Interactions. See the earlier discussion in the section on tuberculosis.

Usage. Rifabutin is used in place of rifampin in patients with HIV receiving protease inhibitors, although it is not recommended with saquinavir or retonavir.[82] Rifabutin is frequently used in the multidrug regimen for treatment of *M. avium-intracellulare* lung disease, especially in patients who may not have responded to a regimen containing rifampin.[54] However, for disseminated disease in patients with AIDS, a placebo-controlled study showed that through 16 weeks of follow-up, a dose of 300 mg daily did not increase the culture conversion rate over that with clarithromycin and ethambutol alone.[129]

Aminoglycosides

Aminoglycoside antibiotics have been used extensively for the treatment of nontuberculous mycobacterial infections. Among *M. kansasii* strains, 86% demonstrated streptomycin susceptibility, as did 93% of *M. scrofulaceum* strains. Forty-four percent of strains of *M. avium-intracellulare* have been streptomycin susceptible. *M. fortuitum* complex isolates are resistant.

Amikacin is the most active aminoglycoside against the nontuberculous mycobacteria.[54,130-132] However, marked variability exists between mycobacterial species in susceptibility to amikacin. Virtually all strains of *M. marinum, M. kansasii,* and *M. fortuitum* are susceptible to 4 μg/mL or less,[126,131,132] whereas isolates of *M. chelonae, M. abscessus,* and *M. avium-intracellulare* are more resistant but are usually inhibited by 8 to 32 μg/mL of amikacin.[131,132] Tobramycin is the most active aminoglycoside and is the recommended aminoglycoside for treatment of *M. chelonae.*[131,132] Other aminoglycosides are less active and are generally not clinically useful.

Mutational resistance to amikacin during therapy is rare, probably because of relatively high toxicity, which limits therapy. Resistance has been described with *M. abscessus* and results from the same 16S ribosomal RNA mutation described with *M. tuberculosis.*[103,133]

Ethambutol

Ethambutol has good in vivo activity against *M. avium* complex and is included as part of treatment regimens for these organisms.[54] It also has activity against most other slowly growing nontuberculous mycobacteria, including *M. kansasii, M. marinum,* and *M. xenopi.* Species of rapidly growing mycobacteria are all highly resistant with the exception of the *Mycobacterium smegmatis* group.

LESS FREQUENTLY USED MISCELLANEOUS ANTIMICROBIALS FOR TREATMENT OF NONTUBERCULOUS MYCOBACTERIA

Isoniazid

Drugs such as INH used principally for treatment of *M. tuberculosis* were evaluated relatively early for their activity against nontuberculous mycobacteria. INH inhibits nearly 90% of strains of *M. kansasii* at concentrations of 1 to 5 μg/mL, in contrast to only 10% to 30% of *M. avium-intracellulare* strains. At present, INH is included routinely in therapy for *M. kansasii* in the United States,[54] *M. xenopi,* and *Mycobacterium szulgai.* It has generally been replaced by more active agents in therapy for other species, including *M. avium-intracellulare.*

Tetracyclines

Approximately 50% of isolates of the rapidly growing species *M. fortuitum* and 20% of *M. chelonae* are tetracycline susceptible.[132] Minocycline and doxycycline are two- to fourfold more active than tetracycline[131] and have been effective in therapy when the isolates were susceptible in vitro.[109] Minocycline and doxycycline are also active against *M. marinum*[126,134,135] and have been used successfully in *M. marinum* infections.[54,134]

Sulfonamides

Sulfamethoxazole is active against *M. fortuitum* but not against *M. chelonae* or *M. abscessus.*[131,132] Localized infections have been cured with sulfamethoxazole alone or in combination with trimethoprim.[109] *M. marinum* infections have responded to therapy with trimethoprim-sulfamethoxazole,[54] but strains are susceptible in vitro only against a low inoculum.[135]

Both *M. marinum* and *M. kansasii* exhibit similar drug susceptibilities. Sulfamethoxazole is also active against isolates of *M. kansasii.* It has been curative in combination regimens used for the treatment of rifampin-resistant *M. kansasii* infections.[127]

Limited experience indicates some in vitro activity and clinical efficacy of sulfonamides against *Mycobacterium terrae* complex, *M. haemophilum, M. simiae,* and *M. avium-intracellulare.*[54]

Quinolones

The newer fluorinated quinolones (ciprofloxacin, ofloxacin, sparfloxacin) have in vitro activity against a number of nontuberculous mycobacteria at achievable serum levels.[93,94,96,132,136] *M. fortuitum* strains are the most susceptible, with ciprofloxacin MICs of 0.25 μg/mL or less and good responses clinically.[136] Studies have shown levofloxacin to have activity comparable to that of ciprofloxacin, and the newer quinolone gatifloxacin has two- to fourfold lower MICs than these older agents.[137] A number of species are inhibited by intermediate concentrations of ciprofloxacin (1 to 4 μg/mL). These include *M. chelonae* (25%), *M. malmoense, M. marinum, M. xenopi, M. kansasii, M. haemophilum,* and some strains of *M. avium-intracellulare.* Again, the newer quinolones gatifloxacin and moxifloxacin are more active than ciprofloxacin.[137] The clinical efficacy of the quinolones for these species has yet to be established. Resistance to ciprofloxacin after monotherapy has been described[137] and presumably involves the same DNA gyrase mutations observed with quinolone resistance with *M. tuberculosis.*[100]

Linezolid

Studies have shown that many nontuberculous mycobacteria are inhibited by 8 μg/mL (susceptible MICs) of linezolid, including *M. fortuitum, M. kansasii, M. marinum,* and *M. haemophilum.* Isolates of *M. chelonae* are all susceptible or have intermediate susceptibility to linezolid, and it is the best oral drug available for this species after the macrolides. Isolates of *M. avium* complex and *M. simiae* are usually resistant.[138]

β-Lactams

All mycobacteria produce β-lactamase, although it can be difficult to detect in *M. avium* complex. β-Lactams or combinations of β-lactam–β-lactamase inhibitor have been shown to be active or useful clinically, but only for the *M. fortuitum* complex. Cefoxitin, cefmetazole, and imipenem-cilastatin are active in vitro against approximately 80% of *M. fortuitum* strains and most isolates of *M. abscessus* at clinically achievable plasma concentrations.[107]

Clofazimine

Discussed more fully later under "Drugs for Treatment of Leprosy (Hansen's Disease)," clofazimine (Lamprene) has in vitro activity against *M. chelonae, M. abscessus,* and *M. avium-intracellulare.* Most strains are inhibited by 1.6 to 2.0 μg/mL.[75,139] Clinical experience with clofazimine in therapy against *M. avium* in AIDS has been disappointing.[75]

Susceptibility Tests

Standardized methods for susceptibility testing of the nontuberculous mycobacteria were approved for the first time in 2003 by the NCCLS.[111] In vitro susceptibility of nontuberculous mycobacterial drugs is no guarantee of therapeutic efficacy. Previously cited failures of clofazimine in *M. avium-intracellulare* infections indicate limitations in extrapolating in vitro data to clinical experience. As a rule, favorable therapeutic results are likely when drugs are used to which nontuberculous mycobacteria are susceptible in vitro, and poor outcomes can be anticipated when there is in vitro resistance. Least predictable are outcomes of *M. avium-intracellulare* infections, for which routine susceptibility testing is *not* recommended except for clarithromycin (or azithromycin).[54,111]

DRUGS FOR TREATMENT OF LEPROSY (HANSEN'S DISEASE)

Background

The special parasite-host relationship of *Mycobacterium leprae* (Hansen's bacillus), characterized by persistence of the organism in tissue for years, has mandated prolonged chemotherapy to prevent relapse. For years, chemotherapy for leprosy consisted mainly of dapsone alone, which produced gratifying clinical results and was affordable. However, because of self-supervised monotherapy, resistance of leprosy bacilli, both secondary and now primary, became a problem worldwide.[140] Currently, multidrug therapy is the rule for both multibacillary and paucibacillary disease and has markedly increased cure rates and decreased the incidence of drug resistance. The principal agents used in therapeutic multidrug regimens are dapsone, rifampin, and clofazimine.

Dapsone

Derivation and Structure. Dapsone (diaminophenyl sulfone), a synthetic compound, was demonstrated to be effective in rat leprosy in 1941 and soon thereafter was used successfully in human trials.

Mechanism of Action. Sulfones inhibit bacterial dihydropteroate synthase, as do sulfonamides, and presumably inhibit *M. leprae* by the same mechanism.

Antimicrobial Activity. From mouse footpad inoculation, as little as 0.003 μg/ml of dapsone is estimated to inhibit multiplication of *M. leprae*. Dapsone has been described as "weakly bactericidal" for susceptible leprosy bacilli. In humans, it has been estimated that 99.9% of bacillary populations are killed after 3 to 4 months of dapsone therapy.[141] In patients with lepromatous (multibacillary) leprosy receiving monotherapy, secondary dapsone resistance often emerges 5 to 24 *years* after commencing therapy.[142] Before the usage of current standard multidrug regimens, secondary resistance occurred in approximately 20% of cases.

Pharmacology. Dapsone is well absorbed orally. It is distributed throughout body fluids, and tissue concentrations are approximately 2 μg/mL. The plasma half-life of dapsone is 21 to 44 hours, with some drug retention for up to 3 weeks. Dapsone becomes acetylated, with 70% to 80% excreted as metabolites in urine. The dosage should be reduced accordingly in renal failure.

Adverse Reactions. An oxidant drug, dapsone produces dose-dependent hemolysis, which is not of clinical consequence in patients without a hematologic disorder taking dapsone at 50 to 100 mg daily. Hemolysis is greatly enhanced in patients with glucose-6-phosphate dehydrogenase deficiency, especially in its severe forms. Gastrointestinal intolerance occurs with resulting anorexia, nausea, or vomiting. Hematuria, fever, pruritus, skin rashes, and granulocytopenia can occur.

Dapsone is now being used in AIDS as prophylaxis and for treatment of *Pneumocystis jirovecii* pneumonia. These patients usually have preexisting anemia, making dapsone-induced hemolysis less well tolerated. Conversion of up to 20% of erythrocyte hemoglobin to methemoglobin can occur with dapsone doses of 100 mg daily. Although methemoglobinemia is usually asymptomatic, it may become of clinical consequence if the patient experiences hypoxemia from lung disease. Rash is common in this population of patients. In one study using dapsone, 100 mg daily, for prophylaxis, 33 of 47 patients discontinued the drug.[143]

In patients with leprosy, reactions with dapsone may be difficult to extricate from the reactions associated with the disease itself.[144] A sulfone syndrome occurring 5 to 6 weeks after the initiation of therapy can be characterized by fever, jaundice, dermatitis, and lymphadenopathy—a presentation not unlike that of infectious mononucleosis.[145] During initial dapsone therapy, erythema nodosum leprosum reactions commonly become manifest in those with multibacillary disease.

Usage. Dapsone and rifampin are the principal therapeutic agents for the treatment of both multibacillary and paucibacillary *M. leprae* infections. Usage in prophylaxis or treatment of *Pneumocystis jirovecii* pneumonia is discussed in Chapter 266. Dapsone is also useful in dermatitis herpetiformis, a subject beyond the scope of this chapter.

Availability and Dosage. Dapsone is available generically in tablets of 25 or 100 mg. The adult daily dosage is 100 mg, and for children it is 1 to 1.5 mg/kg/day. It is administered daily for 6 months in paucibacillary disease and for a minimum of 2 years in multibacillary disease.

Rifampin

Mechanism of Action and Resistance. The mechanism of action of rifampin is presumed to be inhibition of *M. leprae* DNA-dependent RNA polymerase, which produces a relatively rapid bactericidal effect. Its inhibitory concentration for human strains of *M. leprae* tested in mice is 0.3 μg/mL. Acquired rifampin resistance is caused by mutational changes in RNA polymerase.[146]

Usage. Clinical usage of rifampin has confirmed that it is more bactericidal by several orders of magnitude than all other antileprosy drugs alone or in combination. It is considered the only rapidly bactericidal drug against *M. leprae*. In a skin biopsy assay, a single 1500-mg dose of rifampin was determined to reduce the viability of leprosy bacilli to undetectable levels by 3 to 5 days.[147] Despite such a dramatic impact on numbers of tissue *M. leprae*, rifampin must be employed with one or more companion drugs to prevent the development of resistance.[141] The high cost of rifampin has discouraged daily usage in economically disadvantaged regions. However, once-monthly therapy with 600 to 1200 mg of rifampin in combination drug regimens has produced satisfactory clinical responses with a minimum of adverse reactions.[148] Current recommendations are that rifampin be administered in a single monthly supervised dose of 600 mg. This dosage is continued for 6 months in paucibacillary disease and for a minimum of 2 years in multibacillary disease. In the United States, rifampin is given as a 600-mg daily dose in both of the settings described. Reversal and erythema nodosum leprosum reactions with rifampin have been comparable to or less severe than those with sulfones alone. Daily rifampin treatment may reduce both the serum levels and subsequently the beneficial effects of corticosteroids for reactions by inducing hepatic microsomal enzymes.

Clofazimine (Lamprene)

Derivation and Structure. Clofazimine is a phenazine dye.

Mechanism of Action and Antimicrobial Activity. Clofazimine's precise mechanism of action is unknown. Highly lipophilic and bound to mycobacterial DNA, clofazimine is weakly bactericidal against *M. leprae*. Its action may be related to iron chelation with resulting production of nascent oxygen radicals intracellularly.[149] The inhibitory concentration of clofazimine in mouse tissue is between 0.1 and 1 mg/kg. A delay of some 50 days ensues before tissue antimicrobic activity can be demonstrated in humans.

Pharmacology. Clofazimine pharmacokinetics are complex. Absorption is quite variable, with 9% to 74% of an administered dose appearing in feces. Oral administration results in plasma concentrations of 0.4 to 3 μg/mL with a half-life of approximately 70 days. Clofazimine is widely distributed throughout reticuloendothelial tissues, especially liver, spleen, lung, adrenals, adipose tissue, and skin lesions. Red-orange phagocytized crystals of clofazimine are observed microscopically in macrophages. It is largely unmetabolized and subsequently slowly excreted with less than 1% in urine. Biliary excretion appears to be the major route of excretion. Excretion also occurs in breast milk. Dosage of 100 mg/day has been calculated to result eventually in a total accumulation of at least 10 g in human tissue.

Adverse Reactions. Gastrointestinal intolerance (anorexia, diarrhea, abdominal pain) is the most common therapy-limiting side effect and is generally dose related. Dry mouth and skin may occur. Skin pigmentation is quite common, resulting from drug accumulation and producing red-brown to nearly black discoloration, especially in dark-skinned persons.

Usage. Clofazimine's current role is principally in combination with rifampin and dapsone for multibacillary disease. It is also used in combination for sulfone-resistant infections and for individuals who are sulfone intolerant, usually because of severe sulfone-associated erythema nodosum leprosum or reversal reactions. Such reactions occur much less often with clofazimine than with dapsone,[150] possibly because of the anti-inflammatory properties of clofazimine.

Availability and Dosage. Clofazimine is supplied in 50- and 100-mg capsules. For multibacillary disease, it is administered in a dosage of 50 mg/day for a minimum of 2 years in combination with rifampin and dapsone. A dapsone alternative dosage has usually been 100 to 300 mg/day.

Additional or Second-Line Drugs

Thiacetazone (Amithiozone)

Thiacetazone's efficacy is greater in tuberculoid (paucibacillary) than in lepromatous (multibacillary) disease. It can be administered when sulfones are not tolerated. Considerable cross-resistance occurs with sulfones. Thiacetazone is unavailable in the United States.

Ethionamide and Prothionamide

Ethionamide (Trecator-SC) is described in "Second-Line Antituberculous Drugs." It and its congener prothionamide (not available in the United States) possess similar pharmacokinetics and dosing and provide alternatives to clofazimine in multidrug regimens for multibacillary disease in those who are unable to tolerate clofazimine or refuse it because of skin pigmentation. Ethionamide and prothionamide are apparently weakly bactericidal against *M. leprae*. Ethionamide is provided in 250-mg tablets. The usual dosage is 250 mg daily. Both agents are expensive and cause considerable gastrointestinal intolerance and occasional hepatitis.

Other Substituted Rifamycins

Rifabutin (Mycobutin) and rifapentine (Priftin) are substituted rifamycins active against *M. leprae*. Both are approved by the Food and Drug Administration in the United States. In mice, these compounds are even more active than rifampin,[151] which raises interest in their use, especially in intermittent regimens.

Other Sulfones

Acedapsone. Acedapsone (4,4'-diacetyldiaminodiphenyl sulfone) is a long-acting intramuscular repository derivative of dapsone. The parent compound possesses little activity against *M. leprae* but is metabolized into active dapsone. Its half-life is 46 days, and that of the derived dapsone is 43 days.[152] A 300-mg intramuscular dose maintains dapsone levels in volunteers above the inhibitory concentration for *M. leprae* for approximately 100 days. Microbiologic and clinical responses are somewhat slower than those for daily dapsone. Long-term studies with acedapsone administered by injection five times yearly have yielded encouraging results. Acedapsone shows promise especially in regions where, or in patients in whom, long-term oral therapy is not practical.

Sulfoxone. Less well absorbed and more expensive than dapsone, sulfoxone, a disubstituted sulfone, may be better tolerated gastrointestinally. It is formulated in 165-mg enteric-coated tablets, with a usual daily dosage of 300 mg.[13]

Newer Agents. Several other agents have shown promising activity against *M. leprae* in mouse footpad models and early clinical trials. Among these are minocycline (Minocin),[153] clarithromycin (Biaxin),[153] and fluorinated quinolones—pefloxacin, ofloxacin (Floxin),[154,155] and especially sparfloxacin.[155] Their roles in replacing drugs in existing multidrug regimens remain to be determined, although none of these agents appear to be as bactericidal against *M. leprae* as rifampin. Current efforts with these newer agents are also focusing on short-course therapy[156] rather than the current standard 2-year regimens.

Chemotherapy-Associated Reactions in Leprosy

Febrile reactions in leprosy can be ameliorated with acetylsalicylic acid (aspirin) in conventional dosage. Immunologic reactions are common during chemotherapy. "Reversal" reactions associated with swelling and edema in preexisting skin lesions or peripheral neuropathy in more severe reactions usually occur in the first year of therapy. Corticosteroids such as prednisone at 40 to 80 mg/day initially with subsequent tapering of dosage have been reasonably efficacious for reversal reactions.

For patients with erythema nodosum leprosum reactions, thalidomide in an initial dosage of 400 mg daily may be the treatment of choice. Its beneficial effect for these reactions appears to be mediated by the inhibition of tumor necrosis factor-α.[157] It should be tapered over the first week, with a maintenance dose of 50 to 100 mg/day. Thalidomide is commercially available for the treatment of leprosy, but its usage is tightly regulated. Because of its marked teratogenicity, thalidomide should never be administered to women of childbearing *potential*. In patients with erythema nodosum leprosum for whom thalidomide is unacceptable, high-dose prednisone offers an alternative. Patients who manifest puzzling or severe reactions are best managed by specialists such as those at the National Hansen's Disease Program in Baton Rouge, Louisiana (1-800-642-2477 or www.bphc.hrsa.gov/nhdp).[144]

REFERENCES

1. Frieden TR, Sterling T, Pablos-Méndez A, et al. The emergence of drug-resistant tuberculosis in New York City. N Engl J Med. 1993;328:521-526.
2. Goble M, Iseman MD, Madsen LA, et al. Treatment of 171 patients with pulmonary tuberculosis resistant to isoniazid and rifampin. N Engl J Med. 1993;328:527-532.
3. Centers for Disease Control and Prevention. Outbreak of multidrug-resistant tuberculosis at a hospital-New York City, 1991. MMWR Morb Mortal Wkly Rep. 1993;42:427-434.
4. Espinal MA, Laszlo A, Simonsen L, et al. Global trends in resistance to antituberculosis drugs. N Engl J Med. 2001;344:1294-1303.
5. Laraque F, Riley LW. Tuberculosis in HIV-infected patients. AIDS Reader. 1992;September-October:171-180.
6. Eriki PP, Okera A, Aisu T, et al. The influence of human immunodeficiency virus infection on tuberculosis in Kampala, Uganda. Am Rev Respir Dis. 1991;143:185-187.
7. Iseman MD, Cohn DL, Sbarbaro JA. Directly observed treatment of tuberculosis. N Engl J Med. 1993;328:576-578.
8. Sensi P. Approaches to the development of new antituberculosis drugs. Rev Infect Dis. 1989;11(Suppl 2):S467-S470.
9. Pozniak AL, MacLeod GA, Mahari M, et al. The influence of HIV status on single and multiple drug reactions to antituberculous therapy in Africa. AIDS. 1992;6:809-814.
10. Centers for Disease Control and Prevention. Impact of HIV protease inhibitors on the treatment of HIV-infected tuberculosis patients with rifampin. MMWR Morb Mortal Wkly Rep. 1996;45:921-925.
11. Gordon SM, Horsburgh CR, Peloquin CA, et al. Low serum levels of oral antimycobacterial agents in patients with disseminated *Mycobacterium avium* complex disease. J Infect Dis. 1993;168:1559-1562.
12. Bass JB Jr, Farer LS, Hopewell PC, et al. Treatment of tuberculosis and tuberculosis infection in adults and children. American Thoracic Society Statement. Am J Respir Crit Care Med. 1994;149:1359-1374.
13. Mandell GL, Sande MA. Drugs used in the chemotherapy of tuberculosis and leprosy. In: Gilman AS, Rall TW, Nies AS, et al, eds. The Pharmacological Basis of Therapeutics. 8th ed. New York: Pergamon; 1990:1146-1164.
14. Kucers A, Bennett NM. Drugs mainly for tuberculosis. Part III. In: The Use of Antibiotics. 4th ed. Philadelphia: JB Lippincott; 1987:1351-1437.
15. Davidson PT, Hahn QL. Drug treatment of tuberculosis-1992. Drugs. 1992;43:651-673.
16. Starke JR. Current chemotherapy for tuberculosis in children. Infect Dis Clin North Am. 1992;6:215-238.
17. Centers for Disease Control and Prevention. Initial therapy for tuberculosis in the era of multidrug resistance. Recommendations of the Advisory Council for the Elimination of Tuberculosis. MMWR Morb Mortal Wkly Rep. 1993;42:1-8.
18. American Thoracic Society/Centers for Disease Control and Prevention/Infectious Diseases Society of America: Treatment of tuberculosis. Am J Respir Crit Care Med. 2003;167:602-662.
19. Musser JM, Kapur V, Williams DL, et al. Characterization of the catalase-peroxidase gene *(katG)* and *inhA* locus in isoniazid-resistant and -susceptible strains of *Mycobacterium tuberculosis* by automated DNA sequencing: Restricted array of mutations associated with drug resistance. J Infect Dis. 1996;173:196-202.
20. Musser JM. Antimicrobial agent resistance in mycobacteria: Molecular genetic insights. Clin Microbiol Rev. 1995;8:496-514.
21. Ormerod LP, Harrison JM, Wright PA. Drug resistance trends in *Mycobacterium tuberculosis*: Blackburn 1985-89. Tubercle. 1990;71:283-285.
22. Seifart HI, Parkin DP, Donald PR. Stability of isoniazid, rifampin and pyrazinamide in suspensions used for the treatment of tuberculosis in children. Pediatr Infect Dis J. 1991;10:827-831.
23. Mitchell JR, Zimmerman HJ, Ishak KG, et al. Isoniazid liver injury: Clinical spectrum, pathology and probably pathogenesis. Ann Intern Med. 1976;84:181-192.
24. Steele MA, Burk RF, DesPrez RM. Toxic hepatitis with isoniazid and rifampin. Chest. 1991;99:465-471.
25. Nolan CM, Goldberg SV, Buskin SE. Hepatotoxicity associated with isoniazid preventive therapy. JAMA. 1999;281:1014-1018.
26. Kopanoff DE, Snider DE, Caras GJ. Isoniazid-related hepatitis. Am Rev Respir Dis. 1978;117:991-1001.
27. Salpeter S. Fatal isoniazid-induced hepatitis: Its risk during chemoprophylaxis. West J Med. 1993;159:560-564.
28. American Thoracic Society/Centers for Disease Control and Prevention. Targeted tuberculin testing and treatment of latent tuberculosis infection. Am J Respir Crit Care Med. 2000;161:S221-S247.
29. Krishnaswamy K, Prasad CE, Murthy KJ. Hepatic dysfunction in undernourished patients receiving isoniazid and rifampicin. Trop Geogr Med. 1991;43:156-160.

30. Franks AL, Binkin NJ, Snider DE Jr, et al. Isoniazid hepatitis among pregnant and postpartum Hispanic patients. Public Health Rep. 1989;104:151-155.
31. Murphy R, Swartz R, Watkins PB. Severe acetaminophen toxicity in a patient receiving isoniazid. Ann Intern Med. 1990;113:799-800.
32. Wu JC, Lee SD, Yeh PF, et al. Isoniazid-rifampin-induced hepatitis in hepatitis B carriers. Gastroenterology. 1990;98:502-504.
33. Kumar A, Misra PK, Mehotra R, et al. Hepatotoxicity of rifampin and isoniazid. Is it all drug-induced hepatitis? Am Rev Respir Dis. 1991;143:1350-1352.
34. Deshpande DV, Nachne D, Koyande D, et al. Anti-tubercular treatment in patients with hepatitis. J Assoc Physicians India. 1991;143:1350-1352.
35. McGlynn KA, Lustbader ED, Sharrar RE, et al. Isoniazid prophylaxis in hepatitis B carriers. Am Rev Respir Dis. 1986;134:666-668.
36. Gangadharam PRJ. Isoniazid, rifampin, and hepatotoxicity. Am Rev Respir Dis. 1986;133:963-965.
37. Woo J, Chan HS. Therapeutic problems in the management of elderly patients with tuberculosis. Adverse Drug React Toxicol Rev. 1992;11:13-18.
38. Ansari MM, Beg MH, Haleem S. Hepatitis in patients with surgical complications of pulmonary tuberculosis. Indian J Chest Dis Allied Sci. 1991;33:133-138.
39. Centers for Disease Control and Prevention. Severe isoniazid-associated hepatitis–New York, 1991-1993. MMWR Morb Mortal Wkly Rep. 1993;42:545-547.
40. Jordan TJ, Lewit EM, Reichman LB. Isoniazid preventive therapy for tuberculosis. Decision analysis considering ethnicity and gender. Am Rev Respir Dis. 1991;144:1357-1360.
41. Ishii N, Nishibara Y. Pellagra encephalopathy among tuberculous patients: Its relation to isoniazid therapy. J Neurol Neurosurg Psychiatry. 1985;48:628-634.
42. Pellock JM, Howell J, Kendig EL Jr, et al. Pyridoxine deficiency in children treated with isoniazid. Chest. 1985;87:658-661.
43. Schraufnagel DE, Stoner R, Whiting E, et al. Testing for isoniazid. An evaluation of the Arkansas method. Chest. 1990;98:314-316.
44. Koestner JA, Jones LK, Polk WH, et al. Prolonged use of intravenous isoniazid and rifampin. Drug Intell Clin Pharm. 1989;23:48-50.
45. Telenti A, Imboden P, Marchesi F, et al. Detection of rifampicin-resistance mutations in *Mycobacterium tuberculosis*. Lancet. 1993;341:647-650.
46. Centers for Disease Control and Prevention. Acquired rifamycin resistance in persons with advanced HIV disease being treated for active tuberculosis with intermittent rifamycin-based regimens. MMWR Morb Mortal Wkly Rep. 2002;51:214-215.
47. Venkatesan K. Pharmacokinetic drug interactions with rifampin. Clin Pharmacokinet. 1992;22:47-65.
48. Immanuel C, Jayasankar K, Narayana AS, et al. Induction of rifampicin metabolism during treatment of tuberculous patients with daily and fully intermittent regimens containing the drug. Indian J Chest Dis Allied Sci. 1989;31:251-257.
49. Woo J, Leung A, Chan K, et al. Pyrazinamide and rifampicin regimens for patients on maintenance dialysis. Int J Artif Organs. 1988;11:181-185.
50. Newman R, Doster BE, Murray FJ, et al. Rifampin in initial treatment of pulmonary tuberculosis. A US Public Health Service tuberculosis therapy trial. Am Rev Respir Dis. 1974;109:216-232.
51. Mehta M, ed. Physicians' Desk Reference Guide to Drug Interactions, Side Effects, Indications. Montvale, NJ: Medical Economics Data; 1992:797-799.
52. Strayhorn VA, Baciewicz AM, Self TH. Update on rifampin drug interactions. III. Arch Intern Med. 1997;157:2453-2458.
53. Borcherding SM, Baciewicz AM, Self TH. Update on rifampin drug interactions. II. Arch Intern Med. 1992;152:711-716.
54. Wallace RJ Jr, Glassroth J, Griffith DE, et al. American Thoracic Society Statement: Diagnosis and treatment of disease caused by nontuberculous mycobacteria. Am Rev Respir Crit Care Med. 1997;156:S1-S25.
55. Gordin F, et al. Prevention and treatment of opportunistic infections (Abstract LB5). Presented at the 5th Retrovirus Conference, Washington, DC, 1998.
56. Jasmer RM, Saukkonen JJ, Blumberg HM, et al. Short course rifampin and pyrazinamide compared with isoniazid for latent tuberculosis infection: A multicenter clinical trial. Ann Intern Med. 2002;137:640-647.
57. Stout JE, Engemann JJ, Cheng AC, et al. Safety of 2 months of rifampin and pyrazinamide for treatment of latent tuberculosis. Am J Respir Crit Care Med. 2003;167:824-827.
58. Jasmer RM, Daley CL. Rifampin and pyrazinamide for treatment of latent tuberculosis infection. Is it safe? Am J Respir Crit Care Med. 2003;167:809-810.
59. Crowle AJ. Studies of antituberculosis chemotherapy with an in vitro model of human tuberculosis. Semin Respir Infect. 1986;1:262-264.
60. Rastogi N, Potar M, David HL. Pyrazinamide is not effective against intracellularly growing *Mycobacterium tuberculosis*. Antimicrob Agents Chemother. 1988;31:287.
61. Scorpio A, Lindholm-Levy P, Heifets L, et al. Characterization of *pncA* mutations in pyrazinamide-resistant *Mycobacterium tuberculosis*. Antimicrob Agents Chemother. 1997;41:540-543.
62. Sreevatsan S, Pan X, Zhang Y, et al. Mutations associated with pyrazinamide resistance in *pncA* of *Mycobacterium tuberculosis* complex organisms. Antimicrob Agents Chemother. 1997;41:636-640.
63. Donald PR, Seifart H. Cerebrospinal fluid pyrazinamide concentrations in children with tuberculous meningitis. Pediatr Infect Dis J. 1988;7:469-471.
64. Zierski M, Bek E. Side effects of drug regimens used in short-course chemotherapy for pulmonary tuberculosis. A controlled clinical study. Tubercle. 1980;61:41-49.
65. Ssanwijarja S, Kauffmann RH, te Velde J, et al. Tubulointerstitial nephritis associated with pyrazinamide. Neth J Med. 1989;34:40-46.
66. Namba S, Igari T, Nishiyama K, et al. A case of pyrazinamide-associated myoglobinuric renal failure. Jpn J Med. 1991;30:468-472.
67. Belanger AE, Besra GS, Ford ME, et al. The *embAB* genes of *Mycobacterium avium* encode an arabinosyl transferase involved in cell wall arabinan biosynthesis that is the target for the antimycobacterial drug ethambutol. Proc Natl Acad Sci U S A. 1996;93:11919-11924.
68. Alcaide F, Pfyffer GE, Telenti A. Role of *embB* in natural and acquired resistance to ethambutol in mycobacteria. Antimicrob Agents Chemother. 1997;41:2270-2273.
69. Chatterjee VK, Buchanan OR, Friedman AI, et al. Ocular toxicity following ethambutol in standard dosage. Br J Dis Chest. 1986;80:288-291.
70. Griffith DE, Brown-Elliott BA, McLarty J, et al. Ethambutol (EMB) ocular toxicity during therapy for *Mycobacterium avium* complex (MAC) lung disease. Am J Respir Crit Care Med. 2001;A763.
71. Meier A, Sander P, Schaper K-J, et al. Correlation of molecular resistance mechanisms and phenotypic resistance levels in streptomycin-resistant *Mycobacterium tuberculosis*. Antimicrob Agents Chemother. 1996;40:2452-2454.
72. Honoré N, Cole ST. Streptomycin resistance in mycobacteria. Antimicrob Agents Chemother. 1994;38:238-242.
73. Dautzenberg B, Castellani P, Pellegrin J-L, et al. Early bactericidal activity of rifabutin versus that of placebo in treatment of disseminated *Mycobacterium avium* complex bacteremia in AIDS patients. Antimicrob Agents Chemother. 1996;40:1722-1725.
74. Heifets LB, Iseman MD, Lindholm-Levy PJ, et al. Determination of ansamycin MICs for *Mycobacterium avium* complex in liquid medium by radiometric and conventional methods. Antimicrob Agents Chemother. 1985;28:570-575.
75. Masur H, Tuazon C, Gill V, et al. Effect of combined clofazimine and ansamycin therapy on *Mycobacterium avium-Mycobacterium intracellulare* bacteremia in patients with AIDS. J Infect Dis. 1987;155:127-129.
76. O'Brien RJ, Lyle MA, Snider DE Jr. Rifabutin (ansamycin LM 427): A new rifamycin-S derivative for the treatment of mycobacterial diseases. Rev Infect Dis. 1987;9:519-530.
77. Woodley CL, Kilburn JO. In vitro susceptibility of *Mycobacterium avium* complex and *Mycobacterium tuberculosis* strains to a spiro-piperidyl rifamycin. Am Rev Respir Dis. 1992;126:586-587.
78. Blaschke TF, Skinner MH. The clinical pharmacokinetics of rifabutin. Clin Infect Dis. 1996;22(Suppl 1):S15-S22.
79. Shafran SD, Deschenes J, Phillips P, et al. Uveitis and pseudojaundice during a regimen of clarithromycin, rifabutin, and ethambutol. N Engl J Med. 1994;330:438-439.
80. Frank MO, Graham MB, Wispelway B. Rifabutin and uveitis. N Engl J Med. 1994;330:868.
81. Griffith DE, Brown BA, Girard WM, et al. Adverse events associated with high-dose rifabutin in macrolide-containing regimens for the treatment of *Mycobacterium avium* complex lung disease. Clin Infect Dis. 1995;21:594-598.
82. Flexner C. HIV-protease inhibitors. N Engl J Med. 1998;338:1281-1291.
83. Grassi C, Peona V. Use of rifabutin in the treatment of pulmonary tuberculosis. Clin Infect Dis. 1996;22(Suppl 1):S50-S54.
84. Chan SL, Yew WW, Ma WK, et al. The early bactericidal activity of rifabutin measured by sputum viable counts in Hong Kong patients with pulmonary tuberculosis. Tubercle Lung Dis. 1992;73:33-38.
85. Hong Kong Chest Service/British Medical Research Council. A controlled study of rifabutin and an uncontrolled study of ofloxacin in the re-treatment of patients with pulmonary tuberculosis resistant to isoniazid, streptomycin and rifampicin. Tubercle Lung Dis. 1992;73:59-67.
86. Pretet S, Lebaeaut A, Parrot R, et al, and the Group for the Study and Treatment of Resistant Mycobacterial Infections. Combined chemotherapy including rifampicin for rifampicin and isoniazid resistant pulmonary tuberculosis. Eur Respir J. 1992;5:680-684.
87. Grosset J, Lounis N, Truffot-Pernot C, et al. Once-weekly rifapentine-containing regimens for treatment of tuberculosis in mice. Am J Respir Crit Care Med. 1998;157:1436-1440.
88. Tam CM, Chan SL, Lam CW, et al. Rifapentine and isoniazid in the continuation phase of treating pulmonary tuberculosis. Am J Respir Crit Care Med. 1998;157:1726-1733.
89. Rifapentine-A long acting rifamycin for tuberculosis. Med Lett Drugs Ther. 1999;41:21-22.
90. Klemens SP, Cynamon MH. Activity of KRM-1648 in combination with isoniazid against *Mycobacterium tuberculosis* in murine model. Antimicrob Agents Chemother. 1996;40:298-301.
91. Vernon A, Khan A, Bozeman L, et al. Update on US Public Health Service (USPHS) Study 22: A trial of once weekly isoniazid (NIH) and rifapentine (RPT) in the continuation phase of TB treatment. The USPHS Rifapentine Trial Group. Am J Respir Crit Care. 1998;157(S):A467.
92. Yew WW, Kwan SY, Ma WK, et al. In-vitro activity of ofloxacin against *Mycobacterium tuberculosis* and its clinical efficacy in multiply resistant pulmonary tuberculosis. J Antimicrob Chemother. 1990;26:227-236.
93. Leysen DC, Haemers A, Pattyn SR. Mycobacteria and the new quinolones. Antimicrob Agents Chemother. 1989;33:1-5.
94. Gay JD, DeYoung DR, Roberts GD. In vitro activities of norfloxacin and ciprofloxacin against *Mycobacterium tuberculosis*, *M. avium* complex, *M. chelonei*, *M. fortuitum*, and *M. kansasii*. Antimicrob Agents Chemother. 1984;26:94-96.
95. Chen CH, Shih JF, Lindholm-Levy PJ, et al. Minimal inhibitory concentrations of rifabutin, ciprofloxacin, and ofloxacin against *Mycobacterium tuberculosis* isolated before treatment of patients in Taiwan. Am Rev Respir Dis. 1989;140:987-989.
96. Caekenberghe DV. Comparative in vitro activities of ten fluoroquinolones and fusidic acid against *Mycobacterium* spp. J Antimicrob Chemother. 1990;26:381-386.

97. LaLande V, Truffot-Pernot C, Paccaly-Moulin A, et al. Powerful bactericidal activity of sparfloxacin (AT-4140) against *Mycobacterium tuberculosis* in mice. Antimicrob Agents Chemother. 1993;37:407-413.

98. Kohno S, Koga H, Kaku M, et al. Prospective comparative study of ofloxacin or ethambutol for the treatment of pulmonary tuberculosis. Chest. 1992;102:1815-1818.

99. Tsukamura M, Nakamura E, Yoshii S, et al. Therapeutic effect of new antibacterial substance ofloxacin (DL 8280) on pulmonary tuberculosis. Am Rev Respir Dis. 1985;131:352-356.

100. Takiff HE, Salazar L, Guerrero C, et al. Cloning and nucleotide sequence of *Mycobacterium tuberculosis* gyrA and gyrB genes and detection of quinolone resistance mutations. Antimicrob Agents Chemother. 1994;38:773-780.

101. Ginsburg AS, Grosset JH, Bishai WR. Fluoroquinolones, tuberculosis, and resistance. Lancet (Infect Dis). 2003;3:432-442 (http://infection.thelancet.com).

102. McClatchy JK, Kanes W, Davidson PT, et al. Cross-resistance in *M. tuberculosis* to kanamycin, capreomycin, and viomycin. Tubercle. 1977;58:29-34.

103. Alangaden GJ, Kreiswirth BN, Aouad A, et al. Mechanism of resistance to amikacin and kanamycin in *Mycobacterium tuberculosis*. Antimicrob Agents Chemother. 1998;42:1295-1297.

104. Quemard A, Laneelle G, Lacave C. Mycolic acid synthesis: A target for ethionamide in mycobacteria? Antimicrob Agents Chemother. 1992;36:1316-1321.

105. Cynamon MH, Palmer GS. In vitro activity of amoxicillin in combination with clavulanic acid against *Mycobacterium tuberculosis*. Antimicrob Agents Chemother. 1983;24:429-431.

106. Chambers HF, Kocagöz T, Sipit T, et al. Activity of amoxicillin/clavulanate in patients with tuberculosis. Clin Infect Dis. 1998;26:874-877.

107. Wallace RJ Jr, Brown BA, Onyi GO. Susceptibilities of *Mycobacterium fortuitum* biovar *fortuitum* and the two subgroups of *Mycobacterium chelonae* to imipenem, cefmetazole, cefoxitin, and amoxicillin-clavulanic acid. Antimicrob Agents Chemother. 1991;35:773-775.

108. Nozawa RT, Kato H, Yokota T, et al. Susceptibility of intra- and extracellular *Mycobacterium avium-intracellulare* to cephem antibiotics. Antimicrob Agents Chemother. 1985;27:132-134.

109. Kernodle DS. β-Lactam drugs and tuberculosis. Clin Infect Dis. 1998;26:878-879.

110. Wallace RJ Jr, Swenson JM, Silcox VA, et al. Treatment of nonpulmonary infections due to *Mycobacterium fortuitum* and *Mycobacterium chelonei* on the basis of in vitro susceptibilities. J Infect Dis. 1985;152:500-514.

111. National Committee for Clinical Laboratory Standards. Susceptibility testing of mycobacteria, nocardia and other aerobic actinomycetes. Tentative Standard. 2nd ed. NCCLS document M24-T2. Wayne, PA: NCCLS; 2000.

112. Brown BA, Wallace RJ Jr, Onyi GO. Activities of clarithromycin against eight slowly growing species of nontuberculous mycobacteria, determined by using a broth microdilution MIC system. Antimicrob Agents Chemother. 1992;36:1987-1990.

113. Brown BA, Wallace RJ Jr, Onyi GO, et al. Activities of four macrolides, including clarithromycin, against *Mycobacterium fortuitum*, *Mycobacterium chelonae*, and *Mycobacterium chelonae*-like organisms. Antimicrob Agents Chemother. 1992;36:1987-1990.

114. Laing RBS, Wynn RF, Leen CLS. New antimicrobials against *Mycobacterium marinum* infection. Br J Dermatol. 1994;131:914.

115. Wallace RJ Jr, Tanner D, Brennan PJ, et al. Clinical trial of clarithromycin for cutaneous (disseminated) infection due to *Mycobacterium chelonae*. Ann Intern Med. 1993;119:482-486.

116. Saubolle MA, Kiehn TE, White MH, et al. *M. haemophilum*: Microbiology and expanding clinical and geographic spectra of disease in humans. Clin Microbiol Rev. 1996;9:435-447.

117. Dautzenberg B, Truffot C, Legris S, et al. Activity of clarithromycin against *Mycobacterium avium* infection in patients with the acquired immune deficiency syndrome. A controlled clinical trial. Am Rev Respir Dis. 1991;144:564-569.

118. Young LS, Wiviott L, Wu M, et al. Azithromycin for treatment of *Mycobacterium avium-intracellulare* complex infection in patients with AIDS. Lancet. 1991;338:1107-1109.

119. Pierce M, Crampton S, Henry D, et al. A randomized trial of clarithromycin as prophylaxis against disseminated *Mycobacterium avium* complex infection in patients with advanced acquired immunodeficiency syndrome. N Engl J Med. 1996;335:384-391.

120. Oldfield EC III, Fessel J, Dunne MW, et al. Once weekly azithromycin therapy for prevention of *Mycobacterium avium* complex infection in patients with AIDS: A randomized, double-blind, placebo-controlled multicenter trial. Clin Infect Dis. 1998;26:611-619.

121. Meier A, Kirschner P, Springer B, et al. Identification of mutations in 23S rRNA gene of clarithromycin-resistant *Mycobacterium intracellulare*. Antimicrob Agents Chemother. 1994;38:381-384.

122. Wallace RJ Jr, Meier A, Brown BA, et al. Genetic basis for clarithromycin resistance among isolates of *Mycobacterium chelonae* and *Mycobacterium abscessus*. Antimicrob Agents Chemother. 1996;40:1676-1681.

123. Wallace RJ Jr, Brown BA, Griffith DE, et al. Reduced serum levels of clarithromycin in patients treated with multidrug regimens including rifampin or rifabutin for *Mycobacterium avium-M. intracellulare* infection. J Infect Dis. 1995;171:747-750.

124. Brown BA, Wallace RJ Jr, Griffith DE, et al. Clarithromycin-induced hepatotoxicity. Clin Infect Dis. 1995;20:1073-1074.

125. Brown BA, Griffith DE, Girard W, et al. Relationship of adverse events to serum drug levels in patients receiving high-dose azithromycin for mycobacterial lung disease. Clin Infect Dis. 1997;24:958-964.

126. Sanders WJ, Wolinsky E. In vitro susceptibility of *Mycobacterium marinum* to eight antimicrobial agents. Antimicrob Agents Chemother. 1980;18:529-531.

127. Wallace RJ Jr, Dunbar D, Brown BA, et al. Rifampin-resistant *Mycobacterium kansasii*. Clin Infect Dis. 1994;18:736-743.

128. Nightingale SD, Cameron DW, Gordin FM, et al. Two controlled trials of rifabutin prophylaxis against *Mycobacterium avium* complex infection in AIDS. N Engl J Med. 1993;329:828-833.

129. Gordin FM, Sullam PM, Shafran SD, et al. Disseminated infections with *Mycobacterium avium* complex. Clin Infect Dis. 1999;28:1080-1085.

130. Nozawa RT, Kato H, Yokota T. Intra- and extracellular susceptibility of *Mycobacterium avium-intracellulare* complex to aminoglycoside antibiotics. Antimicrob Agents Chemother. 1984;26:841-844.

131. Swenson JM, Thornsberry C, Silcox VA. Rapidly growing mycobacteria: Testing of susceptibility to 34 antimicrobial agents by broth microdilution. Antimicrob Agents Chemother. 1982;22:186-192.

132. Swenson JM, Wallace RJ Jr, Silcox VA, et al. Antimicrobial susceptibility of five subgroups of *Mycobacterium fortuitum* and *Mycobacterium chelonae*. Antimicrob Agents Chemother. 1985;28:807-811.

133. Prammananan T, Sander P, Brown BA, et al. A single 16S ribosomal RNA substitution is responsible for resistance to amikacin and other 2-deoxystreptamine aminoglycosides in *Mycobacterium abscessus* and *Mycobacterium chelonae*. J Infect Dis. 1998;177:1573-1581.

134. Donta ST, Smith PW, Levitz RE, et al. Therapy of *Mycobacterium marinum* infections. Use of tetracyclines vs rifampin. Arch Intern Med. 1986;146:902-904.

135. Stone MS, Wallace RJ Jr, Swenson JM, et al. Agar disk elution method for susceptibility testing of *Mycobacterium marinum* and *Mycobacterium fortuitum* complex to sulfonamides and antibiotics. Antimicrob Agents Chemother. 1983;24:486-493.

136. Wallace RJ Jr, Bledsole G, Sumter G, et al. Activities of ciprofloxacin and ofloxacin against rapidly growing mycobacteria with demonstration of acquired resistance following single-drug therapy. Antimicrob Agents Chemother. 1990;34:65-70.

137. Brown-Elliott BA, Wallace RJ Jr, Crist CJ, et al. Comparison of in vitro activities of gatifloxacin and ciprofloxacin against four taxa of *Mycobacterium avium* complex. Antimicrob Agents Chemother. 2002;46:3283-3285.

138. Brown-Elliott BA, Crist CJ, Man LB, et al. In vitro activity of linezolid against slowly growing nontuberculous mycobacteria. Antimicrob Agents Chemother. 2003;47:1736-1738.

139. Gangadharam PRJ, Candler ER. Activity of some antileprosy compounds against *Mycobacterium intracellulare* in vitro. Am Rev Respir Dis. 1977;115:705-708.

140. Centers for Disease Control and Prevention. Increase in prevalence of leprosy caused by dapsone-resistant *Mycobacterium leprae*. MMWR Morb Mortal Wkly Rep. 1982;30:637-638.

141. Hastings RC, Franzblau SG. Chemotherapy of leprosy. Annu Rev Pharmacol Toxicol. 1988;28:231-245.

142. Pearson JMH, Rees RJW, Waters MFR. Sulphone resistance in leprosy. A review of one hundred proven clinical cases. Lancet. 1975;2:69-72.

143. Blum RA, Miller LA, Gaggini LC, Cohn DL. Comparative trial of dapsone versus trimethoprim/sulfamethoxazole for primary prophylaxis of *Pneumocystis carinii* pneumonia. J Acquir Immune Defic Syndr. 1992;5:341-347.

144. Case records of the Massachusetts General Hospital. Weekly clinicopathological exercises. Case 49-1985. Erythema nodosum leprosum reaction in patient with lepromatous leprosy. N Engl J Med. 1985;313:1464-1472.

145. Adverse reactions to dapsone (Editorial). Lancet. 1981;2:184-185.

146. Honore N, Cole ST. Molecular basis of rifampin resistance in *Mycobacterium leprae*. Antimicrob Agents Chemother. 1993;37:414-418.

147. Shepard CC, Levy L, Fasal P. Further experience with the rapid bactericidal effect of rifampin on *Mycobacterium leprae*. Am J Trop Med Hyg. 1974;23:1120-1124.

148. Yawalkar SJ, Languillon J, Hajra SK, et al. Once-monthly rifampicin plus dapsone in initial treatment of lepromatous leprosy. Lancet. 1982;1:1199-1202.

149. Niwa Y, Sakance T, Miyachi Y, et al. Oxygen metabolism in phagocytes of leprotic patients: Enhanced endogenous superoxide dismutase activity and hydroxyl radical generation by clofazimine. J Clin Microbiol. 1984;20:837-842.

150. Spaced clofazimine therapy of lepromatous leprosy. Am J Trop Med Hyg. 1976;25:437-440.

151. Pattyn SR. Rifabutin and rifapentine compared with rifampin against *Mycobacterium leprae* in mice. Antimicrob Agents Chemother. 1987;31:134.

152. Peters JH, Murray JF, Gordon GR, et al. Acedapsone treatment of leprosy patients: Response versus drug disposition. Am J Trop Med Hyg. 1977;26:127-136.

153. Ji B, Jamet P, Perani EG, et al. Powerful bactericidal activities of clarithromycin and minocycline against *Mycobacterium leprae* in lepromatous leprosy. J Infect Dis. 1993;168:188-190.

154. Ji B, Perani EG, Petinom C, et al. Clinical trial of ofloxacin alone and in combination with dapsone plus clofazimine for treatment of lepromatous leprosy. Antimicrob Agents Chemother. 1994;38:662-667.

155. Gelber RH, Iranmanesh A, Murray L, et al. Activities of various quinolone antibiotics against *Mycobacterium leprae* in infected mice. Antimicrob Agents Chemother. 1992;36:2522-2527.

156. Ji B, Jamet P, Sow S, et al. High relapse rate among lepromatous leprosy patients treated with rifampin plus ofloxacin daily for 4 weeks. Antimicrob Agents Chemother. 1997;41:1953-1956.

157. Sampaio EP, Kaplan G, Miranda A. The influence of thalidomide on the clinical and immunologic manifestation of erythema nodosum leprosum. J Infect Dis. 1993;168:404-414.

CHAPTER 37

Systemic Antifungal Agents

JOHN H. REX

DAVID A. STEVENS

Systemic antifungal agents and their use to treat invasive mycoses are discussed in this chapter. Many of these agents also can be used to treat the mucocutaneous forms of candidiasis; these usages are discussed in detail in Chapter 255 and are mentioned only in passing here. Likewise, the therapy of the various forms of tinea and onychomycosis with topical agents and systemic agents is discussed in Chapter 265. Although *Pneumocystis jirovecii* (formerly, *Pneumocystis carinii*) now is classified among the fungi, the drugs used to treat it principally are used to treat parasitic infections. Those drugs and their uses are discussed in Chapters 41 and 268.

AMPHOTERICIN B–BASED PREPARATIONS

Mechanism of Action

Amphotericin B is available in a formulation with deoxycholate and in three lipid-associated formulations. For all preparations, the active component is amphotericin B produced by *Streptomyces nodosus.* Amphotericin B is a lipophilic molecule (Fig. 37-1) that exerts its antifungal effect by insertion into the fungal cytoplasmic membrane, probably orienting as head-to-tail oligomers perpendicular to the plane of the membrane.[1] The drug exists as aggregates in the cytoplasmic membrane and is bound closely to sterols, such as ergosterol. Amphotericin B causes membrane permeability to increase (Fig. 37-2). At lower drug concentrations, potassium channel activity is increased.[2] At higher concentrations, pores are formed in the membrane. Loss of intracellular potassium and other molecules impairs fungal viability. The onset of action is rapid and unrelated to the growth rate, consistent with the concept that the drug acts at preformed sites, and no metabolic processing is required before a target is exposed. Amphotericin B also has effects on oxidation that may enhance antifungal activity.

Spectrum of Activity and Mechanisms of Resistance

Amphotericin B is active against most fungi, and its spectrum of activity is not influenced by the choice of formulation. Where resistance occurs, it generally is attributed to reductions in ergosterol biosynthesis and synthesis of alternative sterols that lessen the ability of amphotericin B to interact with the fungal membrane.[3-5] Primary resistance is common for *Aspergillus terreus, Scedosporium apiospermum, Scedosporium prolificans,* and *Trichosporon* spp.[6] Among the *Candida* spp., primary resistance is noted at meaningful frequencies most often for *Candida lusitaniae.* Development of resistance in isolates of normally susceptible species is uncommon but has been described for essentially all common pathogens. Although these isolates may exhibit altered growth and reduced pathogenicity,[7] invasive and lethal infections are well described. Identification of amphotericin B–resistant isolates by standardized susceptibility testing methods is difficult, and optimal methods are as yet undefined.[6] In studies of amphotericin B deoxycholate as therapy for candidiasis, the principal pharmacodynamic driver of in vivo response has been ratio of the peak achieved serum concentration to the minimal inhibitory concentration (MIC).[8]

Available Formulations

There are four commercially available amphotericin B formulations. Amphotericin B deoxycholate (Fungizone) was licensed in 1959 in the United States.[9] More recently, three lipid-associated formulations have been marketed: amphotericin B colloidal dispersion (Amphotec,

Amphocil), amphotericin B lipid complex (Abelcet), and liposomal amphotericin B (AmBisome).[10] In attempts to produce less expensive lipid-associated formulations, some authors have advocated mixing amphotericin B deoxycholate with a parenteral fat emulsion at an amphotericin B deoxycholate concentration of 1 to 2 mg/mL. Although less nephrotoxicity in adults has been observed with this preparation at a dose of 1 mg/kg/day than with infusions of amphotericin B deoxycholate in 5% dextrose,[11] no advantage was found in children.[12] Also, serum amphotericin B concentrations were lower with the fat emulsion, raising the possibility that amphotericin B simply was aggregating in the fat emulsion, but the cloudiness could not be perceived in the milky-looking lipid. Use of these preparations should be reserved for investigational settings.

Amphotericin B Deoxycholate

Formulation. Amphotericin B deoxycholate is insoluble in water at physiologic pH. The drug is marketed for intravenous use as a powder containing 50 mg of amphotericin B, 41 mg of sodium deoxycholate, and 25.2 mg of sodium phosphate buffer. Although a clear yellow solution forms when the powder is hydrated, the colloidal nature of amphotericin B deoxycholate is easy to show. If a filter with a 0.22-μ pore diameter is placed in the infusion line, considerable drug is removed by the filter. The addition of electrolyte aggregates the colloids so that the solution becomes cloudy when saline or sodium bicarbonate is added to an amphotericin B deoxycholate solution. Amphotericin B deoxycholate currently is produced by many different generic manufacturers, and significant differences in amphotericin A contamination and the ability of the product to induce interleukin-1β production have been reported and may be part of the cause of the intersubject variation in toxicities observed with this compound.[13]

Pharmacology. Concentrations of amphotericin B in biologic fluids usually have been measured by bioassay,[14] but high-pressure liquid chromatography,[15] immunoassay,[16] and radiometric respirometry[17] have been described. Despite the proliferation of methods, routine determination of amphotericin B serum, urine, or cerebrospinal fluid concentrations has no definite clinical value. Nonetheless, amphotericin B assays have revealed some remarkable pharmacologic properties of amphotericin B deoxycholate. When colloidal amphotericin B is admixed in serum, deoxycholate separates from amphotericin B, and more than 95% of the latter binds to serum proteins, principally to β-lipoprotein. Presumably the drug is bound to the cholesterol carried on this protein. Most of the drug leaves the circulation promptly, perhaps bound to cholesterol-containing cytoplasmic membranes. Amphotericin B is stored in the liver and other organs; the drug seems to reenter the circulation slowly. Most of the drug is degraded in situ, with only a small percentage being excreted in urine or bile. Blood levels are uninfluenced by hepatic or renal failure. Hemodialysis does not alter blood levels except in an occasional patient with lipemic plasma, who may be losing drug by adherence to the dialysis membrane. Concentrations of amphotericin B in fluid from inflamed areas, such as pleura, peritoneum, joint, vitreous humor, and aqueous humor, are roughly two thirds of the trough serum level. Cord blood from one infant contained an amphotericin B concentration of 0.37 μg/mL, half the simultaneous maternal trough blood level. Amphotericin B penetrates poorly into either normal or inflamed meninges, saliva, bronchial secretions, brain, pancreas, muscle, bone, vitreous humor, or normal amniotic fluid. Urine concentrations are similar to serum concentrations. Peak serum concentrations with conventional intravenous doses are roughly 0.5 to 2 μg/mL and rapidly decrease initially to approach slowly a plateau of roughly 0.2 to 0.5 μg/mL.[14] The initial half-life is about 24 hours; the β-phase half-life is roughly 15 days. Serum concentrations can be detected for at least 7 weeks after the end of therapy, presumably reflecting release from cell membranes. The drug also has complex immunomodulatory properties, potentially of clinical significance but presently undefined.

Nephrotoxicity. Amphotericin B deoxycholate causes a dose-dependent decrease in the glomerular filtration rate. The direct vasoconstrictive effect of amphotericin B on afferent renal arterioles

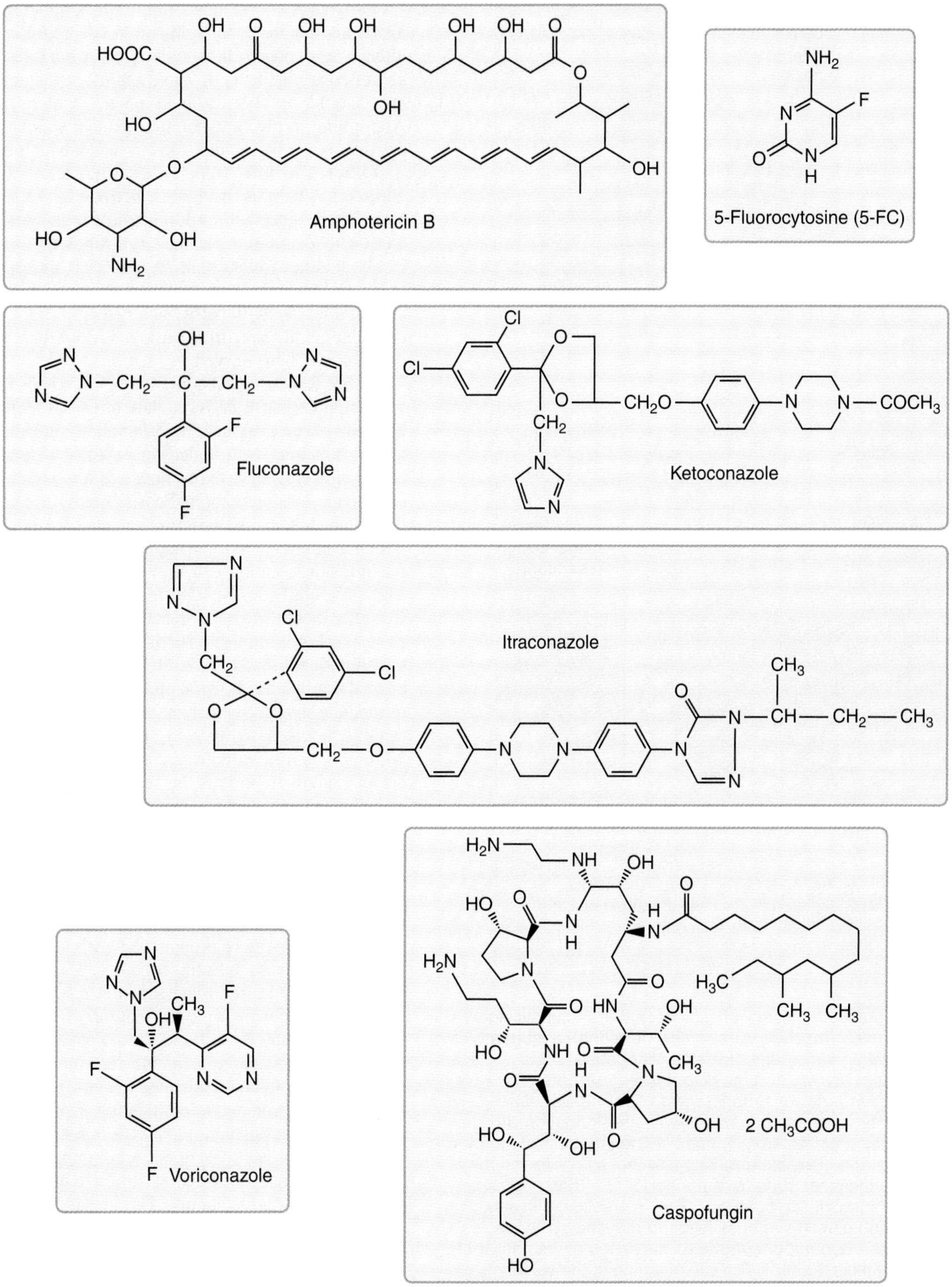

FIGURE 37-1. Structures of the systemic antifungal agents.

results in reduced glomerular and renal tubular blood flow.[18] Other primary or secondary effects on the kidney include potassium, magnesium, and bicarbonate wasting and decreased erythropoietin production. Permanent loss of renal function is related to the total dose, not the level of temporary azotemia, and is due to destruction of renal tubular cells, disruption of tubular basement membrane, and loss of functioning nephron units. Saline loading, such as infusion of 1 L of saline before amphotericin B deoxycholate, has been associated with reduced nephrotoxicity in some, but not all, studies.[19] Potassium wasting often requires supplemental oral or intravenous

potassium. Renal tubular acidosis from bicarbonate wasting rarely requires base replacement, but other drugs and diseases that promote acidosis may act synergistically.

Azotemia caused by amphotericin B is often worse in patients taking other nephrotoxic drugs, such as cyclosporine or aminoglycosides. Hypotension, intravascular volume depletion, renal transplantation, and other preexisting renal disease all magnify the management problems associated with amphotericin B–induced azotemia. These toxicities are lessened by use of the lipid-associated formulations of amphotericin B (see later).

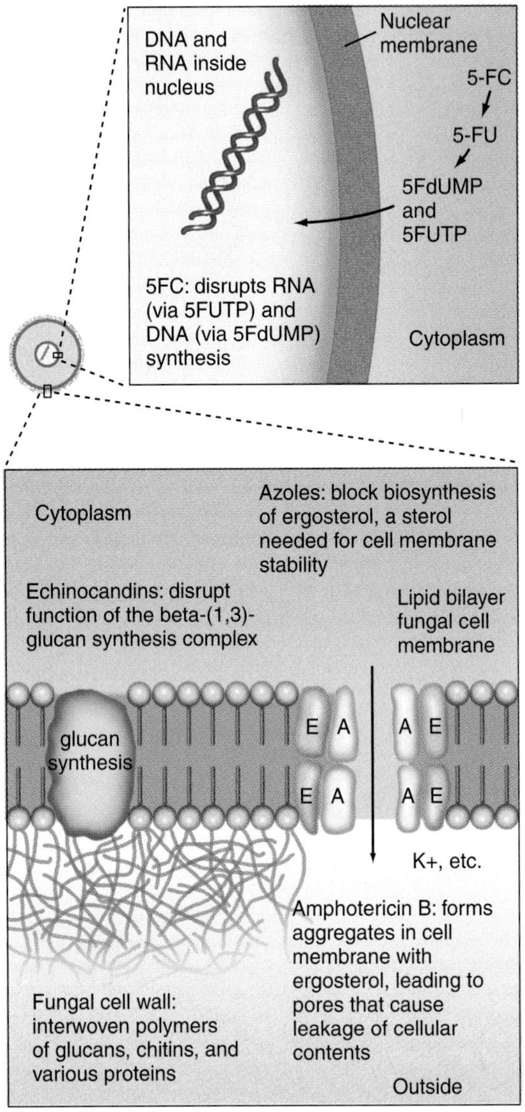

FIGURE 37-2. Mechanisms of action of the antifungal agents. Shown are the major mechanism and site of action for currently licensed antifungal agents. Many of the precise details of the physical interactions are not known, and the diagram is at best an approximation. The interaction between amphotericin B (A) and ergosterol (E) in the fungal cell membrane is consistent with the formation of pores with a diameter of approximately 0.8 nm.[152] The structure of the pore is not known, but the available data suggest that amphotericin molecules would line the inner surface of the pore.[153,154] These pores permit leakage of intracellular contents. The interaction between the echinocandins and glucan synthase leads to reduced synthesis of β-(1,3)-glucan, a crucial component of the interwoven glucan polymers that form the fungal cell wall.[137] The site of action of the echinocandin and molecular mechanism of the inhibition are unknown, however. The azole antifungal agents act within the cell to inhibit 14-α-demethylase and to reduce synthesis of ergosterol,[155] a sterol that is crucial to cell membrane function. Flucytosine is converted into 5-fluorouridine triphosphate (5FUTP), is incorporated into fungal RNA, and becomes an inhibitor of fungal protein synthesis or converted into 5-fluorodeoxyuridine monophosphate (5FdUMP), an inhibitor of thymidylate synthetase and of DNA synthesis.[156] These compounds presumably are created in the cytoplasm with subsequent diffusion into the nucleus. 5-FC, 5-fluorocytosine; 5-FU, 5-fluorouracil.

Early in a course of therapy with amphotericin B deoxycholate, azotemia may increase rapidly, often decreases a little, then stabilizes after several days. Adults with no other renal disease have an average serum creatinine level of 2 to 3 mg/dL at therapeutic doses, and therapy should not be withheld unless azotemia exceeds this level. Attempting to give amphotericin B deoxycholate to an adult without causing azotemia usually leads to inadequate therapy.

Other Chronic Toxicity. Nausea, anorexia, and vomiting are common. Phlebitis occurs if peripheral vein catheters are used. Normocytic normochromic anemia occurs gradually and is associated with decreased plasma erythropoietin levels. The hematocrit rarely declines to less than 20% to 25%, unless other causes of anemia are present. Rarely, thrombocytopenia, modest leukopenia, arrhythmias, coagulopathy, hemorrhagic enteritis, tinnitus, vertigo, encephalopathy, seizures, hemolysis, and dysesthesia of the soles of the feet may be observed.

Acute Reactions. About 30 to 45 minutes after beginning the first few amphotericin B deoxycholate infusions, chills, fever, and tachypnea may occur, peak in 15 to 30 minutes, and slowly abate over 2 to 4 hours. A patient with underlying cardiac or pulmonary disease may have hypoxemia. These reactions are less common in young children or patients receiving adrenal corticosteroids. Subsequent infusions of the same dose cause progressively milder reactions. Premedication with acetaminophen or the addition of hydrocortisone, 25 to 50 mg, to the infusion solution can diminish the reactions. Meperidine given early in a chill shortens the rigors but may induce nausea or emesis. Concern about this kind of reaction in an unstable patient had led some physicians to use a test dose of 1 mg given over 15 minutes to assess the subsequent reaction over 1 hour before deciding whether the next dose should be a full therapeutic dose of at least 0.5 mg/kg or an intermediate dose. Whether or not a test dose is given, patients with rapidly progressive mycoses should receive a full therapeutic dose within 24 hours, without any delay entailed by test or intermediate doses. Equally important, this reaction should not be mistaken for anaphylaxis or otherwise considered a contraindication to further amphotericin B deoxycholate. True allergic reactions are extremely rare.

Administration. Amphotericin B deoxycholate is infused in 5% dextrose over a 2- to 4-hour infusion interval. Infusions 1 hour in duration seem generally to be safe for persons who have tolerated slower infusions and may be advantageous for outpatient therapy.[20,21] Early in therapy, fever is more pronounced with infusion intervals of only 45 minutes than infusion lasting 4 hours.[22] Rapid infusion in patients with severely compromised renal function may lead to acute, marked hyperkalemia and ventricular fibrillation.

When therapy is well under way, patients receiving a stable daily dose may be changed to a double dose on alternate days to reduce the frequency of infusion-associated toxicity, particularly anorexia, and as a convenience for outpatient therapy. Doses greater than 1.5 mg/kg generally are not given on this schedule because the toxicity of these infusions is not well described. A common misconception is that amphotericin B may be switched to alternate-day administration at the same dose as daily therapy. This dosage results in reduced trough serum concentrations and may lead to serious underdosing. Based on limited data, continuous infusion of amphotericin B with doses up to 2 mg/kg/24 hours has been described as another approach to reduce toxicity,[23] but this approach is not consistent with the observation that the principal pharmacodynamic driver of efficacy for amphotericin B is peak drug concentration.[24]

Dosage. Daily amphotericin B deoxycholate doses of 0.3 mg/kg often suffice for esophageal candidiasis. A dose of 0.5 mg/kg is appropriate for blastomycosis, disseminated histoplasmosis, and extracutaneous sporotrichosis. Patients with cryptococcal meningitis generally are given doses of 0.6 to 0.8 mg/kg; patients with coccidioidomycosis may require doses of 1 mg/kg. Patients with mucormycosis or invasive aspergillosis are given daily doses of 1 to 1.5 mg/kg until improvement is clearly present. Doses of 0.5 to 1 mg/kg often are used in neutropenic patients receiving empirical amphotericin B (see Chapter 308).[25] Local instillation of amphotericin B into cerebrospinal fluid, joints, or pleura rarely is indicated. One exception is coccidioidal meningitis, which is treated with intrathecal amphotericin B because it may produce superior results, particularly in the long-term, although with far greater toxicity than seen with systemic azole therapy. Intraocular administration for fungal endophthalmitis occasionally is used; doses of 10 μg seem to avoid retinal toxicity. Corneal baths with 1 mg/mL in sterile water are useful for fungal keratitis but are irritating. Bladder irrigation with 50 μg/mL in sterile water is useful for patients with *Candida* cystitis and a Foley catheter, particularly as preparation for genitourinary surgery. Equivalent results may be obtained with oral fluconazole.

Lipid-Associated Formulations of Amphotericin B

The three lipid-associated formulations of amphotericin B are licensed in the United States for a variety of indications and at a range of doses. When using these agents, it is crucial to be aware of the ease with which their names can be confused. Only one of the products (AmBisome) is a liposomal formulation. The other two, amphotericin B lipid complex (Abelcet) and amphotericin B colloidal dispersion (tradenames of both Amphotec and Amphocil), are aggregates of lipid and amphotericin B rather than liposomes. The problem is that the phrase *liposomal amphotericin B* often is used mistakenly as a label for the entire class of compounds. This chapter uses the phrase *lipid-associated formulation of amphotericin B* as a general label for the class. Because the tolerance to one product does not always translate into tolerance for another, it is important that the physician use an unambiguous name when prescribing these compounds.

Amphotericin B lipid complex is licensed in the United States for treatment of invasive fungal infections in patients who are refractory to or intolerant of conventional amphotericin B therapy (5 mg/kg/day). Liposomal amphotericin B is licensed for empirical therapy for presumed fungal infection in febrile, neutropenic patients (3 mg/kg/day); treatment of cryptococcal meningitis in human immunodeficiency virus (HIV)–infected patients (6 mg/kg/day); treatment of patients with *Aspergillus* spp., *Candida* spp., or *Cryptococcus* spp. infections refractory to amphotericin B deoxycholate or of patients with these infections in whom renal impairment or unacceptable toxicity precludes the use of amphotericin B deoxycholate (3 to 5 mg/kg/day); and treatment of visceral leishmaniasis (3 to 4 mg/kg/day). Amphotericin B colloidal dispersion is licensed for treatment of invasive aspergillosis in patients in whom renal impairment or unacceptable toxicity precludes the use of amphotericin B deoxycholate in effective doses or in whom prior amphotericin B deoxycholate therapy has failed (3 to 4 mg/kg/day). All formulations must be infused in 5% dextrose with no electrolytes added. Infusion bottles need not be protected from light.

Pharmacology and Toxicity. The three lipid-associated formulations of amphotericin B have different pharmacokinetic patterns.[9,10] When compared on the basis of equal mg/kg dosages, the lipid-associated formulations of amphotericin B produce tissue amphotericin B concentrations that range from 90% lower to 500% higher than the concentrations seen for amphotericin B deoxycholate,[9] with the most consistent relative reduction seen in the kidney (80% to 90% reduction). Because the lipid-associated formulations of amphotericin B typically are given at mg/kg doses that are sixfold to 12-fold higher than the doses used for amphotericin B deoxycholate, the relevance of these comparisons is uncertain, although it is generally clear that all three lipid-associated formulations of amphotericin B require higher doses in experimental animals to achieve the same therapeutic effect as amphotericin B deoxycholate.

These higher but equipotent doses of the lipid-associated formulations of amphotericin B are notably better tolerated than amphotericin B deoxycholate, with reductions in the frequency and the severity of acute infusion-related reactions and chronic nephrotoxicity. An exception to this rule is amphotericin B colloidal dispersion, which generally shows acute infusion-related reactions similar to those for amphotericin B deoxycholate.

Amphotericin B Colloidal Dispersion. Amphotericin B colloidal dispersion, which contains cholesterol sulfate in equimolar amounts to amphotericin B, forms disklike colloidal particles about 122 ± 48 nm in diameter. Similar to amphotericin B deoxycholate, it forms a clear yellow solution when hydrated. A randomized, prospective, double-blind comparison of amphotericin B deoxycholate, 0.8 mg/kg/day, and amphotericin B colloidal dispersion, 4 mg/kg/day, was done in neutropenic patients whose fever had not abated after 72 hours of antibacterial therapy.[26] Efficacy was the same in the 98 patients receiving amphotericin B colloidal dispersion as in the 95 patients receiving amphotericin B deoxycholate, with 53% and 58% becoming afebrile after 48 hours and 14% compared with 15% having a suspected or documented mycosis emerge during amphotericin B therapy. Acute febrile reactions were significantly more common with amphotericin B colloidal dispersion than with amphotericin B deoxycholate, with hypoxia developing in 15% and 3%. The percentage of patients having amphotericin B therapy discontinued because of some toxicity was the same in the two arms (14% and 15%), with the amphotericin B deoxycholate discontinuations being due much more often to azotemia. In a randomized, double-blind study of amphotericin B colloidal dispersion (6 mg/kg/day) versus amphotericin B deoxycholate (1 to 1.5 mg/kg/day) as therapy for invasive aspergillosis,[27] response rates for the two therapies were similar (52% versus 51%) with reduced rates of nephrotoxicity noted with amphotericin B colloidal dispersion (25% versus 49%). Infusion-related chills and fever were more common, however, with amphotericin B colloidal dispersion than with amphotericin B deoxycholate. The recommended dose for adults and children is 3 to 4 mg/kg once daily infused as 0.6 mg/mL at a rate of 1 mg/kg/hr. The infusion can be speeded to a duration of 2 hours for patients who tolerate the drug well. Premedication with acetaminophen has not been studied prospectively but should be considered.

Amphotericin B Lipid Complex. Amphotericin B lipid complex is a complex of almost equimolar concentrations of amphotericin B and lipid, the latter being a 7:3 mixture of dimyristoylphosphatidylcholine and dimyristoylphosphatidylglycerol. The drug is shipped as a cloudy suspension with particles 1.6 to 11 μm in diameter. Particle shape is ribbon-like rather than globular. The manufacturer provides a device for the pharmacy to filter out aggregates larger than 5 μm before dispensing in 5% dextrose solution. The only efficacy data are from the manufacturer's open-label, noncomparative studies of 556 adult and pediatric patients[28] and of 111 pediatric patients.[29] All patients in these studies either had failed prior amphotericin B deoxycholate therapy or were intolerant of amphotericin B deoxycholate therapy. Of the enrolled patients, only 345 were considered to have a documented mycosis and had sufficient data to evaluate the drug's therapeutic effect. If all the mycoses are considered together, a complete response to amphotericin B lipid complex was judged to have occurred in 28% and a partial response in 32%, for an overall response rate of 60%.

Liposomal Amphotericin B. Liposomal amphotericin B is a unilamellar liposome about 55 to 75 nm in diameter that contains roughly one molecule of amphotericin B per nine molecules of lipid. The latter is a mixture of hydrogenated soy lecithin-cholesterol-distearoylphosphatidylglycerol in a 10:5:4 ratio. In contrast to the other lipid-associated amphotericins, serum concentrations are not lower than concentrations obtained with the same dose of amphotericin B deoxycholate. A randomized three-way comparison of liposomal amphotericin B, 3 mg/kg/day; liposomal amphotericin B, 6 mg/kg/day; and amphotericin B deoxycholate, 0.7 mg/kg/day, for cryptococcal meningitis enrolled 267 HIV-infected subjects and reported global response rates of 66%, 75%, and 66%.[30] A randomized comparison of liposomal amphotericin B at 3 mg/kg/day versus amphotericin B deoxycholate at 0.7 mg/kg/day for histoplasmosis in HIV-infected subjects reported superior efficacy for liposomal amphotericin B (89% response versus 59% response; *P* = .01).[31] Open-label efficacy data in patients with invasive mycoses (mostly candidiasis and aspergillosis) not responding to or intolerant of amphotericin B deoxycholate also have been reported.[32-35] Of the patients in these studies with defined mycoses and evaluable outcomes, 118 of 161 (73%) were judged to have a complete or partial response to therapy. The European Organization for Research and Treatment of Cancer conducted a prospective randomized comparison of liposomal amphotericin B, 1 mg/kg and 4 mg/kg, in 120 patients with proven and probable aspergillosis.[36] Of the 87 evaluable patients, responses were the same in the 41 receiving 1 mg/kg as the 46 receiving 4 mg/kg, although the group receiving the higher dosage contained the greater proportion of subjects with proven (rather than probable) aspergillosis.

Three prospective randomized studies comprising adults and children have compared liposomal amphotericin B with amphotericin B deoxycholate in neutropenic patients with fever not responsive to 96 hours of antibacterial antibiotics. The U.S. study compared 343 patients receiving 1.5 to 6 mg/kg of liposomal amphotericin B daily and 344 adults receiving 0.3 to 1.2 mg/kg of amphotericin B deoxycholate daily.[37] Although some patients received subtherapeutic doses of amphotericin B deoxycholate, the two regimens had identical efficacy. A subset analysis of possible and proven mycoses emerging during therapy suggested an advantage for liposomal amphotericin B. A report of two combined studies in Europe that compared amphotericin B deoxycholate, 1 mg/kg, with liposomal amphotericin B, 3 mg/kg, also found equal efficacy in neutropenic patients failing 96 hours of antibacterial therapy.[38] No difference was noted in mycoses emerging during empirical therapy.

The above-mentioned studies generally suggest that liposomal amphotericin B causes less nephrotoxicity and less severe hypokalemia than amphotericin B deoxycholate, a result supported by a direct comparison of these two formulations.[39] Infusion as 1 to 2 mg/mL over 2 hours is recommended. Infusion intervals can be shortened to 60 minutes for patients in whom the treatment is well tolerated. A triad of infusion-related reactions—symptoms from the categories of (1) chest pain, dyspnea, and hypoxia; (2) severe pain in the abdomen, flank, or leg; and (3) flushing and urticaria—has been reported to occur, most often within the first 5 minutes of infusion and apparently unrelated to infusion speed.[40] These reactions are managed effectively by diphenhydramine administration and brief interruption of the liposomal amphotericin B infusion. Liposomal amphotericin B is the only lipid-associated amphotericin B formulation that does not contraindicate the use of an in-line filter, although pore size should be at least 1 μm.

Comparison of Amphotericin B Deoxycholate and Lipid-Associated Formulations of Amphotericin B

Randomized clinical trials comparing amphotericin B deoxycholate as therapy for a defined mycosis are limited to the demonstrations for liposomal amphotericin B of similar efficacy for cryptococcal meningitis[30] and greater efficacy for histoplasmosis.[31] Randomized comparisons with amphotericin B deoxycholate as therapy in the persistently neutropenic and febrile cancer patient provide consistent demonstrations of a generally better tolerability profile but few data on differential antifungal effect other than a subset analysis showing a reduced rate of breakthrough infections in one study.[37] Consistent with these results, the aggregate open-label data efficacy rates for the lipid-associated formulations of amphotericin B are similar to the rates for amphotericin B deoxycholate.[9] Although the lipid-associated formulations of amphotericin B are notably more costly than amphotericin B deoxycholate (10-fold to 60-fold more), the purchase cost of the compound must be balanced against the morbidity and financial costs of monitoring, treating, and managing amphotericin B deoxycholate–related nephrotoxicity. Importantly, this toxicity may be well tolerated in an outpatient with few other comorbidities, whereas amphotericin B deoxycholate–related nephrotoxicity (50% increase in baseline creatinine to a minimum of 2 mg/dL) was associated with a 6.6-fold increased odds of death and an absolute increase in mortality from 16% to 54%.[41]

FLUCYTOSINE

Formulation and Pharmacology

Flucytosine, or 5-fluorocytosine (Ancobon), is the fluorine analogue of a normal body constituent, cytosine (see Fig. 37-1). Flucytosine is moderately soluble in water, stable in dry storage, and marketed as 250- and 500-mg capsules. Absorption from the gastrointestinal tract

is rapid and complete, and approximately 90% is excreted unchanged in the urine. Protein binding is barely measurable.[42] Cerebrospinal fluid concentrations approximate 74% of simultaneous serum concentrations. Limited data suggest that flucytosine also penetrates well into aqueous humor, joints, bronchial secretions, peritoneal fluid, brain, bile, and bone. The drug is cleared readily by hemodialysis[42] and peritoneal dialysis.

The half-life of the drug in the serum of patients with normal renal function is 3 to 5 hours and higher in newborns. Abnormal hepatic function has no influence, but decreased renal function prolongs the half-life.

Mechanisms of Action and Resistance

Isolates of *Candida* spp. other than *C. krusei* are usually susceptible to flucytosine,[43] as are most current isolates of *Cryptococcus neoformans*.[44] Flucytosine is often active against isolates of *Aspergillus* spp. and against the melanin-pigmented molds that cause chromoblastomycosis. The mechanism of flucytosine's antifungal action seems to be by deamination to 5-fluorouracil, then conversion through several steps to 5-fluorodeoxyuridylic acid monophosphate, a noncompetitive inhibitor of thymidylate synthetase, which interferes with DNA synthesis, or through its conversion to 5-fluouridine triphosphate, which causes aberrant transcription RNA (see Fig. 37-2).[3] In studies of therapy of candidiasis, the principal pharmacodynamic driver of response was the proportion of the time the blood level exceeded the MIC.[8] Resistance may be due to loss of the cytosine permease that permits flucytosine to cross the fungal cell membrane or loss of the any of the enzymes that lead to its conversion into the forms that interfere with DNA or RNA synthesis. Induction of resistance during monotherapy is sufficiently frequent and rapid that flucytosine essentially always is used as part of combination therapy.

Administration and Dosage

Flucytosine usually is administered by mouth at 100 to 150 mg/kg/day in four divided doses. Patients with a serum creatinine level of 1.7 mg/dL or greater usually require dose reduction. As an approximation, the total daily dose should be reduced to 75 mg/kg with a creatinine clearance of 26 to 50 mL/min and to 37 mg/kg when the creatinine clearance is 13 to 25 mL/min.[45] Ideally the blood level should be measured in azotemic patients 2 hours after the last dose and immediately before the next dose. These values should range between 20 and 100 μg/mL. Patients requiring hemodialysis may be given a single postdialysis dose of 37.5 mg/kg. Further doses are adjusted by blood level. Reliable biologic,[46] enzymatic,[47] and physical[48] methods are available to assay flucytosine, even in the presence of amphotericin B.

Flucytosine given alone to patients with normal renal, hematologic, and gastrointestinal function is associated with infrequent adverse effects, including rash, diarrhea, and, in about 5%, hepatic dysfunction. In the presence of azotemia, such as that caused by concomitant amphotericin B, leukopenia, thrombocytopenia, and enterocolitis may appear and can be fatal. These complications seem to be far more frequent among patients whose flucytosine blood levels attain, and especially if they exceed, 100 to 125 μg/mL.[45] Patients receiving flucytosine whose renal function is changing should have serum flucytosine concentrations determined twice per week and the leukocyte count, platelet count, alkaline phosphatase, and aminotransferase levels at a similar frequency. Patients in whom loose stools or dull abdominal pain suddenly develops or who have laboratory evidence consistent with flucytosine toxicity should have flucytosine blood levels determined and consideration given to withholding therapy with the drug until the situation is clarified. Patients with bone marrow and gastrointestinal toxicity from flucytosine often tolerate the drug at reduced dosage. Patients with rash or hepatotoxicity have not been rechallenged. Uncommonly, vomiting, bowel perforation, confusion, hallucinations, headache, sedation, and euphoria have been reported. Flucytosine is teratogenic for rats and is contraindicated in pregnancy.

Conversion of flucytosine to 5-fluorouracil within the human body occurs in sufficient degree to be a possible explanation for toxicity to bone marrow and the gastrointestinal tract.[49] It is likely that the drug is secreted into the gut, where flucytosine becomes deaminated by intestinal bacteria and is reabsorbed as 5-fluorouracil.[50]

Flucytosine has a beneficial effect in patients with cryptococcosis,[51] candidiasis, and chromoblastomycosis. It is not the drug of choice for any infection because (1) its clinical efficacy in the first two mycoses is inferior to that of amphotericin B, (2) primary drug resistance is common in *Candida* infection, and (3) secondary drug resistance is common in cryptococcosis and chromoblastomycosis.

Flucytosine and amphotericin B are at least additive in their effects in vitro and in mice experimentally infected with doubly sensitive isolates of *Candida* spp. and *Cryptococcus* spp. Results with *Aspergillus* infection are contradictory.[52-54] In animals, the combination has never been better than an optimal dose of amphotericin B alone. Flucytosine permitted a lower dose of amphotericin B to be used to gain the same therapeutic effect, and amphotericin B prevented the emergence of secondary drug resistance. The same advantages have been confirmed in two large multicenter studies of cryptococcal meningitis.[55] Experience with candidiasis is limited.[56]

Flucytosine is more difficult to manage in patients with diminished bone marrow reserve. Leukopenia and diarrhea are difficult to manage in patients with acquired immunodeficiency syndrome (AIDS), as is leukopenia and thrombocytopenia in patients after bone marrow transplantation or in patients with leukemia or other hematologic malignancies. Oral flucytosine may not be ingested reliably by patients who are confused or vomiting. Intravenous flucytosine no longer is available in the United States but is used at the same dose as the capsule formulation. The incidence of diarrhea or leukopenia is not lower with intravenous administration.

Flucytosine resistance has occurred, albeit uncommonly, during combination therapy. Use of the combination in these patients incurs the risk of toxicity without evidence that flucytosine adds to the therapeutic effect. Whenever flucytosine is used to treat a patient who has received that drug before, the isolate should be tested for susceptibility.[6] In most laboratories, an MIC of 20 μg/mL or less is considered susceptible.

AZOLE ANTIFUNGAL AGENTS

Mechanism of Action

The imidazole ring (see Fig. 37-1) confers antifungal activity on a variety of synthetic organic compounds. In contrast to the 5-nitroimidazoles, such as metronidazole, activity against bacteria and protozoa, although measurable, has not been clinically significant. Most of the imidazoles reaching clinical trials have had similar in vitro activity against a broad range of superficial and deep pathogens.[57] Methods for in vitro susceptibility testing are increasingly available as standardized tools. Standardization has facilitated the establishment of clinically predictive interpretive breakpoints for susceptibility testing results.[6]

N-substitution of imidazoles has created a family of drugs called *triazoles* that have the same mechanism of action as imidazoles, a similar or broader spectrum of activity, and less effect on human sterol synthesis. Imidazoles and triazoles inhibit C-14α demethylation of lanosterol in fungi by binding to one of the cytochrome P-450 enzymes, which leads to the accumulation of C-14α methylsterols and reduced concentrations of ergosterol, a sterol essential for a normal fungal cytoplasmic membrane (see Fig. 37-2). Inhibition of cytochrome P-450 also decreases the synthesis of testosterone and glucocorticoids in mammals. In studies of candidiasis, the principal pharmacodynamic driver for response to the triazole antifungal agents has been the ratio of total drug exposure (area under the curve) to the MIC.[8] By studying cytochrome P-450 inhibition in vitro, new drugs can be selected that have better antifungal specificity. Some azoles, in addition to blocking ergosterol synthesis, have an immediate effect of damaging the fungal cytoplasmic membrane.

Newer triazoles have properties that make them preferable to ketoconazole—not only less hormonal inhibition, but also fewer drug interactions (parenteral and oral formulations), a broader spectrum, better distribution into body fluids, less gastrointestinal distress, and less hepatotoxicity. The ideal triazole has not arrived because none has all these properties yet, and resistance to azoles in previously susceptible species is emerging. Resistance mechanisms include increased drug efflux and altered or increased C-14α demethylase.[3-5] Development of fluconazole resistance has been documented in *Candida albicans,* and increased resistance has been seen in *Candida glabrata. C. krusei, C. glabrata, Candida norvegensis,* and *Candida inconspicua* are intrinsically more resistant to azoles.[58] Increased isolation of *C. glabrata* and *C. krusei* has been observed in patients receiving long-term azoles. Isolates resistant to fluconazole are variably cross-resistant to itraconazole and ketoconazole.[4]

Ketoconazole

Formulations and Pharmacology

The synthetic agent ketoconazole (Nizoral) differs from its closely related congener miconazole in its solubility at pH less than 3. Solubility in acidic aqueous solutions is conferred in large part by the basic piperazine ring. Ketoconazole is available as scored 200-mg tablets. Ketoconazole is metabolized in the liver and excreted as inactive drug in bile and, to a small extent, in urine.[57] Little biologically active drug appears in urine. Serum protein binding is greater than 90%. The drug is not removed significantly by hemodialysis or peritoneal dialysis. Decreased renal or hepatic function does not alter plasma drug levels. Based on studies of oral ingestion by volunteers, the initial half-life is approximately 2 hours, with a β-phase half-life of about 9 hours starting 8 to 12 hours after ingestion.

Oral absorption of ketoconazole differs among individuals. Serious gastrointestinal disease, such as the graft-versus-host reaction,[59] may lead to low blood levels. H₂ receptor blocking agents or other inhibitors of gastric acid secretion, such as omeprazole, should not be given to patients taking ketoconazole because blood levels of the latter drug are reduced drastically. Citrus fruit juices or cola beverages administered with ketoconazole improve absorption in hypochlorhydric patients. Antacids can be given to patients taking ketoconazole but should follow ketoconazole by 1 to 2 hours. Rifampin causes a substantial lowering of ketoconazole blood levels, probably by accelerating metabolism. Isoniazid possibly has the same effect. Occasional patients have had elevated phenytoin or oral anticoagulant levels while taking ketoconazole. Cyclosporine blood levels should be monitored during ketoconazole therapy because these levels usually increase and cause nephrotoxicity. Penetration into cerebrospinal fluid is poor, even in the presence of inflammation. Low concentrations are found in vaginal secretions, saliva, and breast milk, but penetration into inflamed joints is better.

Uses

When used as two tablets daily (400 mg), the drug is effective in chronic mucocutaneous candidiasis, coccidioidomycosis, histoplasmosis, paracoccidioidomycosis, and blastomycosis in nonimmunosuppressed hosts.[60] Therapy is continued for 6 to 12 months or longer, when the response is slow, to prevent relapse. Improvement may require weeks to months to be evident. Although the dose can be advanced to 600 or 800 mg daily in patients not responding to therapy, more evidence of increased toxicity than increased efficacy has been observed.[61,62] If mycosis involves the meninges, ketoconazole requires doses greater than 400 mg/day and produces limited efficacy.

Ketoconazole has limited value in nonmeningeal cryptococcosis and is of no value in meningeal cryptococcosis. Some patients with chromoblastomycosis and cutaneous sporotrichosis respond, but itraconazole is preferable. Ketoconazole has been used in Old World leishmaniasis and was useful in *Leishmania major* but not in *Leishmania tropica* or *Leishmania aethiopica* infections (see Chapter 273). Studies on New World leishmaniasis are not encouraging.

Aspergillosis does not respond to ketoconazole. Additionally, based on experience with mice, concern exists that subsequent use of amphotericin B may be antagonized.[63] The agents of mucormycosis all have been resistant to imidazoles and triazoles in vitro, discouraging clinical use for that indication.

Adverse Effects

The most frequent toxic effects of ketoconazole are anorexia, nausea, and vomiting. These reactions occurred in 17% of 71 patients taking 400 mg/day and in 29% of patients taking 800 mg/day.[60] Gastrointestinal distress is most common when the drug is first begun and can be controlled partially by taking the tablets with food. Dividing doses greater than 400 mg/day has not been recommended because hormonal suppression is prolonged. Ketoconazole causes a dose-dependent depression in serum testosterone-stimulated and adrenocorticotropic hormone–stimulated cortisol response.[64,65] Although this effect is reversible after 24 hours at 400 mg once daily, doses of 800 to 1200 mg/day cause a profound enough effect to have prompted trials in the treatment of Cushing's syndrome and prostatic cancer. Hypertension has been seen in a few of these high-dose patients in association with increased mineralocorticoid precursors. Gynecomastia, oligospermia, and menstrual irregularities also may be seen during prolonged therapy. Allergic rash and pruritus have been noted in 4% to 10% of patients.[60,66]

Perhaps the gravest complication of ketoconazole therapy is hepatitis.[67] This complication is quite rare; it is estimated to occur in 1 in 15,000 exposed individuals. Asymptomatic slight elevation of transaminase levels occurs in 5% to 15% and is generally transient. This event is distinguished from the potentially lethal hepatitis by the presence of symptoms and the progressive course. Ketoconazole-associated hepatitis begins as anorexia, malaise, nausea, and vomiting. Abnormalities of either or both serum transaminase and alkaline phosphatase become increasingly profound and soon are accompanied by jaundice. Of cases, 80% occur within the first 3 months, but onset can occur at any time. Progression can be swift. Patients should be instructed to discontinue ketoconazole therapy if they experience the aforementioned symptoms and to call their physician. If hepatotoxicity is suspected, serum transaminase and alkaline phosphatase levels should be measured within 1 to 2 days of discontinuing therapy. Rechallenge should be done with great caution. Some authorities have recommended that liver function be measured periodically.[67] This procedure does not protect a patient who has a rapid onset of hepatitis in the interval between tests but does require that all patients with abnormalities be contacted to inquire about symptoms and to arrange for repeat testing.

Itraconazole

Formulations and Pharmacology

Itraconazole (Sporanox) is marketed as a 100-mg capsule, as an oral suspension of 100 mg/10 mL in cyclodextrin, an oligosaccharide ring, and a solution in cyclodextrin for intravenous administration. The ring entraps the hydrophobic, water-insoluble drug. The drug is made soluble and is released at the lipid membrane of the enterocyte after oral administration or directly into tissues after intravenous administration. The solution makes possible delivery of the drug through a nasogastric tube in intubated patients and makes dosing of infants and small children more convenient. Oral absorption of the capsule is enhanced significantly by food, although absorption of the solution is best on an empty stomach.[68] Bioavailability of the capsule is 55% when ingested after breakfast, and the area under the time-concentration curve is increased 30% if the capsules are taken with food or if the solution is used. Bioavailability increases a further 25% to 30% with the solution in a fasting state.[69-72] Coadministration of a cola beverage with itraconazole capsules almost doubled the area under the plasma concentration-time curve.[73] Peak levels with either preparation are achieved 4 to 6 hours after a dose. Steady state is achieved only after 13 to 15 days, at which time the β-elimination half-life is about 19 to 22 hours. Absorption of the capsules in patients with AIDS is about half that in normal volunteers.[74] Absorption of the capsule is depressed markedly in bone marrow transplant recipients, probably because of

hypochlorhydria, mucositis, and graft-versus-host intestinal changes, but the depressed absorption can be alleviated by using the solution.[68]

The intravenous solution of itraconazole is given at 200 mg every 12 hours for four doses (2 days) and then at 200 mg/day. This regimen produces blood levels comparable to those achieved with 200 mg twice daily of the capsules or oral solution. Because the cyclodextrin component is cleared by renal excretion, use of this formulation is not recommended in patients with a creatinine clearance less than 30 mL/min.

For deep mycoses, an initial itraconazole dose of 200 mg three times per day is recommended for the first 3 days to achieve high serum and tissue levels quickly. Hydroxyitraconazole, a metabolite of itraconazole, appears in blood in amounts roughly twice that of the parent drug and has antifungal activity and pharmacokinetics similar to those of the parent compound.[75]

Bioassays of itraconazole give much higher concentrations than high-pressure liquid chromatography does, the difference depending on the susceptibility of the bioassay organism to hydroxyitraconazole. Tissue, pus, and bronchial secretion concentrations of itraconazole are generally higher than plasma concentrations, but cerebrospinal fluid concentrations are usually unmeasurable, even in patients with meningitis. Ocular levels are low. Saliva concentrations persist for 8 hours after the solution and provide a possible benefit in treating oral disease or eradicating oral colonization. The drug is metabolized in the liver and excreted in feces as metabolites. Of the cyclodextrin liquid administered, 50% to 64% is secreted intact in feces, with most of the remainder broken down by gut bacteria amylases; less than 0.5% is absorbed. No significant amount of bioactive itraconazole appears in urine. Plasma concentrations do not increase in patients with renal insufficiency or decrease with hemodialysis. The half-life is prolonged in patients with cirrhosis. About 99% of serum itraconazole is bound to plasma proteins.

Adverse Effects

The most common adverse effect is dose-related nausea and abdominal discomfort, but symptoms rarely necessitate stopping therapy.[76] Dividing the dose into twice-daily administration improves tolerance and absorption. Hypokalemia and edema may occur at 400 mg/day or higher doses. Allergic rash is seen occasionally. Therapy is contraindicated during pregnancy and in nursing mothers. Itraconazole is infrequently hepatotoxic and does not suppress adrenal or testicular function at the dosages recommended. Flavoring in the solution ameliorates the unpleasant taste of cyclodextrin. Diarrhea, nausea, and other gastrointestinal complaints are more frequent with the solution. This increased toxicity is probably due to the osmotic effect or bile salt complexing by unmetabolized cyclodextrin.

Interactions

Blood levels are reduced by about half in patients taking drugs that decrease gastric acidity, such as H_2 blockers and drugs blocking the gastric proton pump.[77] Simultaneous ingestion of itraconazole capsules with antacids and, most likely, with buffered didanosine decreases absorption. Rifampin, rifabutin, isoniazid, phenytoin, carbamazepine, phenobarbital, and cisapride decrease itraconazole blood levels. Itraconazole decreases rifampin blood levels and increases blood levels of the antihistamines terfenadine[78] and astemizole, potentially causing polymorphic ventricular tachycardia (torsades de pointes). It also increases levels of cisapride, warfarin, benzodiazepines, hepatic hydroxymethylglutaryl coenzyme A reductase cholesterol-lowering agents,[79] dihydropyridine calcium channel blockers,[80] digoxin, quinidine, cyclosporine, tacrolimus, methylprednisolone, HIV protease inhibitors (ritonavir, indinavir), and vinca alkaloids (vincristine, vinblastine).[81]

Uses

Itraconazole is useful for treatment of invasive aspergillosis,[82] allergic bronchopulmonary aspergillosis,[83] blastomycosis,[84] histoplasmosis,[84] meningeal[85] and nonmeningeal[86] coccidioidomycosis, paracoccidioidomycosis, sporotrichosis,[87,88] phaeohyphomycosis, ringworm including onychomycosis,[89] and tinea versicolor. Itraconazole also is useful for the prevention of relapse in AIDS patients with disseminated histoplasmosis.[90] Itraconazole may be useful for prophylaxis against fungal infections during neutropenia[91-93] and possibly reduced the rate of invasive aspergillosis in one study.[91] A comparison of itraconazole with amphotericin B as therapy of persistent fever in 384 neutropenic patients (56% of whom had acute myelogenous leukemia and 38% of whom had received marrow transplantation) found that itraconazole was similarly effective and less toxic.[94] The solution shows promise for the treatment of oral and esophageal candidiasis when used at 100 to 200 mg daily.[95,96] *L. major* infections respond poorly.[97]

Fluconazole

Formulations and Pharmacology

Fluconazole (Diflucan) is currently available in 50-, 100-, 150-, and 200-mg tablets; a powder for oral suspension; and an intravenous formulation of either 200 or 400 mg, both as 2 mg/mL. Fluconazole is well absorbed from the gastrointestinal tract.[98] After ingestion of fluconazole, more than 80% of the drug can be found in the circulation. Of the oral dose, 60% to 75% appears unchanged in the urine, and 8% to 10% appears unchanged in the feces. Oral absorption is not decreased in patients with AIDS or patients taking H_2 blocking agents.[99] Only 11% of serum fluconazole is protein-bound.

Concentrations of fluconazole in cerebrospinal fluid are approximately 70% of simultaneous blood levels, whether or not the meninges are inflamed and the drug penetrates into the brain. Penetration into saliva, sputum, urine, and other body fluids also has been excellent.[97] Local instillation into the cerebrospinal fluid, bladder, or another site is unnecessary because of excellent penetration of the drug into body compartments.

The half-life in patients with normal renal function is 27 to 34 hours and increases to 59 hours and 98 hours in groups with creatinine clearances of 35 mL/min and 14 mL/min. According to the manufacturer, the normal dose should be reduced to 50% when the creatinine clearance is reduced to 50 mL/min and to 25% when creatinine clearance is less than 20 mL/min. A loading dose of twice the daily dose is recommended. Patients receiving hemodialysis should have one daily dose after each session. A dose of 6 mg/kg every 3 days has been advocated for premature infants in the first week of life, with dosing every 2 days during the second week of life.[100]

Drug Interactions

Fluconazole can cause significant increases in the blood level of phenytoin, glipizide, glyburide, tolbutamide, warfarin, rifabutin,[101] or cyclosporine. This interaction is most obvious in adults given 400 mg daily or in azotemic patients given lower doses. Rifampin lowers fluconazole blood levels by about one fourth.[102]

Side Effects

Adverse effects are uncommon.[103] Even with long-term therapy, including doses greater than 400 mg/day, headache, hair loss, and anorexia were the most common symptoms, each occurring in 3% of patients, whereas 10% had increases in aspartate aminotransferase levels. Alopecia is reversible, even in some instances when the drug is continued at lower doses.[104] Neurotoxicity has been described after heroic doses of 2000 mg daily. Rarely, anaphylaxis after the first dose or Stevens-Johnson syndrome has been observed.

Indications

Candidiasis. Fluconazole, 50 to 100 mg once daily, is one of the most effective agents for the treatment of oropharyngeal candidiasis. Daily doses of 100 mg are effective for esophageal candidiasis.[105] A single dose of 150 mg is approximately as effective as topical treatment of vulvovaginal candidiasis. Patients with candidemia who are not neutropenic or otherwise seriously immunosuppressed respond as well to intravenous fluconazole therapy as to amphotericin B, provided that they do not have fluconazole-resistant *Candida* spp.[106] A study comparing fluconazole with a combination of fluconazole plus amphotericin as initial therapy of candidemia suggested that the combination might produce more rapid clearance of the bloodstream, but this result was confounded by differences in severity of illness between the two study groups.[107] Although the subject of some debate,[108] changing potentially infected central intravenous catheters in candidemic patients is believed by most authorities to be an important part of therapy.[105] In a few patients with *Candida* endocarditis, long-term fluconazole therapy has been used to prevent relapse after amphotericin B therapy.[105] For immunosuppressed patients and rapidly progressing or severely ill patients with deep candidiasis, amphotericin B or caspofungin is preferable.

Cryptococcal Meningitis. Fluconazole has been used for the initial treatment of AIDS patients with cryptococcal meningitis who are neurologically intact and judged to have a good prognosis.[109] Many authorities recommend amphotericin B or amphotericin B plus flucytosine for at least the first 2 weeks. Therapy can be changed to fluconazole, 400 mg daily for 2 months, if the patient has remained clinically stable. The propensity of AIDS patients to relapse has led to lifelong maintenance therapy with fluconazole, 200 mg daily.[110] Itraconazole capsules, 200 mg daily, are inferior to fluconazole, 200 mg daily, for maintenance therapy.[111] So far, relapse because of fluconazole resistance has been rare. Fluconazole is effective for the eradication of genitourinary foci. For initial treatment, fluconazole at doses of 800 mg[112] or given with flucytosine[113] has been advocated, but insufficient data exist to recommend these regimens (see Chapter 261). For patients without AIDS, fluconazole is useful for patients who have completed a course of amphotericin B and seem to have a high risk of relapse. At present, there are few firm data to guide selection of either dose or duration of fluconazole therapy for non-AIDS patients with cryptococcosis.

Other Mycoses. Fluconazole is useful for coccidioidal meningitis and for disseminated nonmeningeal coccidioidomycosis,[104,114] but a direct comparison with itraconazole found a trend favoring itraconazole that was driven by superior efficacy of itraconazole for skeletal infections.[86] The two drugs were similarly efficacious for soft tissue and pulmonary infection. Cutaneous sporotrichosis,[104,115] ringworm, histoplasmosis,[116] and blastomycosis may respond, but the results are inferior to the results with itraconazole. Fluconazole is not indicated for aspergillosis, mucormycosis, or scedosporiosis (pseudallescheriasis).

Prophylaxis in Neutropenic Patients. In a multicenter trial, administration of fluconazole, 400 mg daily, decreased the incidence of death from deep mycoses in bone marrow transplant recipients, most of whom had received allogeneic transplants, from 10 per 177 placebo recipients to 1 per 179 fluconazole recipients.[117] All the protection afforded seemed to be in deep candidiasis, not aspergillosis. This result was confirmed in a similar study of bone marrow transplant recipients.[118] Fluconazole resulted in decreased use of empirical amphotericin B in one study[118] but not the other.[117] Reduction in deep mycoses has not been shown convincingly in other groups, such as patients with acute leukemia.[119,120] In a long-term follow-up on one of the aforementioned studies, bone marrow transplant recipients who received at least 75 days of fluconazole prophylaxis also had improved survival.[121] Use for prophylaxis may result in shifts in the treated patients to less susceptible species.[122,123]

Prophylaxis in Patients with Acquired Immunodeficiency Syndrome. Fluconazole, 200 or 400 mg once per week, has reduced the incidence of oral and vulvovaginal candidiasis in patients with advanced HIV infection, but this regimen has not been shown to prevent histoplasmosis, cryptococcosis, or esophageal candidiasis in this population.[124,125] Prophylaxis with 200 mg daily reduces the incidence of oropharyngeal and esophageal candidiasis and cryptococcosis in patients with a CD4+ count less than 200/mm³. Cost, lack of effect on survival, and the possibility of azole resistance has led the U.S. Public Health Service Infectious Disease Society of America's advisory committee to recommend against fluconazole prophylaxis in AIDS patients. Fluconazole is an alternative to itraconazole for maintenance therapy in AIDS patients with prior disseminated histoplasmosis.[126]

Voriconazole

Formulations and Pharmacology

Voriconazole (Vfend) is marketed as a 50-mg tablet, a 200-mg tablet, and a solution in sulfobutyl ether β-cyclodextrin for intravenous administration. The oral bioavailability of voriconazole is approximately 96%, and plasma protein binding is approximately 58%.[127,128] Detailed tissue distribution data are not available, but voriconazole's volume of distribution (4.6 L/kg) greatly exceeds that of water, suggesting extensive distribution into tissues. Voriconazole is cleared by hepatic metabolism with less than 2% of the dose excreted unchanged in the urine. Hepatic clearance is via the cytochrome P-450 system. Voriconazole exhibits significantly nonlinear pharmacokinetics due to saturation of the clearance pathways at higher doses. The principal enzyme involved in clearance is CYP2C19. This enzyme has significant genetic polymorphisms that permit any given individual to be a homozygous extensive metabolizer, a homozygous poor metabolizer, or a heterozygous intermediate metabolizer. A heterozygous metabolizer has, on average, a twofold higher total voriconazole exposure relative to a homozygous extensive metabolizer. A homozygous poor metabolizer has a fourfold higher drug exposure on average. Fifteen percent to 20% of Asians but only 3% to 5% of whites and blacks are homozygous poor metabolizers. Despite these differences in metabolism, the achieved plasma levels overlap across the three possible groups, and dose adjustment based on genotype or racial group is not recommended.

Standard loading dosing regimens followed by maintenance doses that are 50% of normal are recommended for individuals with mild-to-moderate hepatic cirrhosis (Child-Pugh class A and B). No data are available, however, on rates of clearance in individuals with severe hepatic cirrhosis (Child-Pugh class C). Dosage adjustments are not required for renal dysfunction, and voriconazole is not cleared significantly by hemodialysis. In children age 2 to 12 years old, a dose of 4 mg/kg every 12 hours was found to produce systemic exposures comparable to those produced by a dose of 3 mg/kg every 12 hours in adults.

Drug Interactions

Voriconazole has many drug interactions. Rifampin, carbamazepine, and long-acting barbiturates induce the hepatic enzymes responsible for the clearance of voriconazole and may reduce voriconazole levels to essentially zero. Rifabutin and voriconazole alter the clearance of each other, and coadministration is contraindicated in the United States but permitted in Europe with a dose adjustment. Voriconazole inhibits the activity of CYP2C19, CYP2C9, and CYP3A4. As a consequence, sirolimus levels are increased dramatically, and coadministration is not recommended. Reduction in clearance of terfenadine, astemizole, cisapride, pimozide, and quinidine is predicted to be sufficient to place the patient at risk for Q-T$_c$ interval prolongation. Reduction in the clearance of ergot alkaloids could lead to ergotism. Cyclosporine, tacrolimus, warfarin, oral coumarins, lipid-lowering statin agents, benzodiazepines, calcium channel blockers, sulfonylureas, and vinca alkaloids may be coadministered with voriconazole, but the dosage of these drugs may need to be reduced, and suitable clinical or laboratory monitoring or deliberate dose reduction is suggested. Phenytoin increases the clearance of voriconazole, whereas voriconazole decreases the clearance of phenytoin. A higher dose of voriconazole and a lower dose of phenytoin may be required during coadministration. Voriconazole significantly reduces the rate of clearance of omeprazole, and the dose of omeprazole should be reduced 50% during coadministration if the dosage of omeprazole is 40 mg or more. Other interactions are possible, and any drug that is a known CYP3A4 substrate, CYP3A4 inhibitor, CYP2C19 inhibitor, or general cytochrome P-450 inducer should be considered possibly to have an interaction with voriconazole.

Side Effects

Voriconazole generally is well tolerated and has a side-effect profile that is similar to other triazoles. The most frequently reported adverse event is a visual disturbance that seems to be unique to voriconazole. In the clinical studies reported to date, approximately 30% of patients reported altered or enhanced light perception beginning approximately 30 minutes after a dose and lasting for approximately 30 minutes. The visual alteration is described as blurred vision, color vision change, or photophobia. The effect is mild, only rarely resulted in discontinuation of therapy, and was uniformly reversible. Despite extensive studies, the mechanism for this side effect is unknown. Although the effect is usually transient, patients should be advised to avoid activities that require keen visual acuity while experiencing visual changes. Hallucinations and confusion also have been reported.

Indications

Aspergillosis. Voriconazole was licensed for treatment of invasive aspergillosis on the basis of a randomized, unblinded comparative trial in which patients with invasive aspergillosis were randomized to receive initial therapy with either voriconazole (two intravenous doses of 6 mg/kg on day 1, two intravenous doses of 4 mg/kg daily for at least the next 7 days, then 200 mg by mouth twice daily) or amphotericin B deoxycholate (1 to 1.5 mg/kg/day).[129] After initial randomization, patients could be switched to other licensed therapies as dictated by clinical events. After 12 weeks, 53% of the patients randomized to voriconazole but only 32% of patients randomized to amphotericin B deoxycholate had a successful outcome. In addition, the survival rate of the voriconazole group was 71% versus only 58% for patients randomized to amphotericin B deoxycholate. These results show the efficacy of voriconazole for aspergillosis and its superiority over amphotericin B deoxycholate and are supported as well by data from open-label studies of therapy of aspergillosis with voriconazole.[130]

Other Mycoses. Voriconazole also is licensed for treatment of invasive fusariosis and scedosporiosis based on data submitted to the U.S. Food and Drug Administration showing a 43% (9 of 21 patients) and 63% (15 of 24 patients) response rate for these two diseases. Although not licensed for esophageal candidiasis, voriconazole (200 mg twice daily by mouth) was at least as effective as fluconazole (200 mg once daily) in a randomized, blinded trial but was associated more often with adverse events.[131] Promising open-label data in invasive candidiasis[132] and in refractory candidiasis[133] have been reported. A comparative trial of voriconazole as therapy for invasive candidiasis currently is under way.

Fever and Neutropenia. Voriconazole was compared with liposomal amphotericin B as empirical antifungal therapy for persistent fever in neutropenic cancer patients in a large open-label, randomized study.[134] The results were mixed, but the most conservative analyses found voriconazole to be possibly inferior to liposomal amphotericin B. The U.S. Food and Drug Administration did not approve voriconazole for this indication.[135]

Investigational Triazoles

Posaconazole and ravuconazole are two additional triazoles currently in the later stages of development.[136] Posaconazole seems to possess a broad spectrum of activity against molds. Less information currently is available about ravuconazole.

ECHINOCANDIN ANTIFUNGAL AGENTS

General Features

The echinocandin antifungal agents act by inhibiting the synthesis of 1,3-β-D glucan. Along with 1,6-β-D glucan, chitin (a polymer of N-acetyl glucosamine), and cell wall proteins, 1,3-β-D glucan is one of the fibrillar and interwoven macromolecules that form the fungal cell wall.[137] 1,3-β-D Glucans are the predominant component of the cell wall of the ascomycetous fungi, provide much of the rigidity of the wall, and are synthesized by a transmembrane glucan synthase complex. Although the precise mechanism of action is unknown, the echinocandins inhibit the functioning of this complex (see Fig. 37-2). Disruption of 1,3-β-D glucan synthesis leads to reduced wall integrity, abnormal cell morphology, and finally cell rupture and death. In studies to date of echinocandins as therapy for candidiasis, the principal pharmacodynamic driver of in vivo response has been the ratio of the peak achieved concentration to the MIC.[8]

At present, there is one licensed echinocandin (caspofungin). Two others are at advanced stages of clinical development (micafungin and anidulafungin). All are cyclic lipopeptides (see Fig. 37-1) that must be given intravenously.

The spectra of activity of these agents are similar.[138] All are broadly active and generally fungicidal against the isolates of all *Candida* spp., including isolates resistant to other agents. All have reduced activity against isolates of *Candida parapsilosis* and *Candida guilliermondii*, but this lesser activity does not seem to be clinically relevant in studies on caspofungin reported to date. All are active against *Aspergillus* spp., but activity is limited to growing and dividing hyphal elements; resting forms are not killed.[139] These agents are not active against *C. neoformans,* and their activity against other fungi is variable, with complete resistance noted in many cases. These agents presently are limited to therapy of candidiasis and aspergillosis. Because susceptibility varies little across isolates and reliably predictive methods are unknown, susceptibility testing of clinical isolates is not routine.

Caspofungin

Formulations and Pharmacology

Caspofungin (Cancidas) is marketed in 50-mg and 70-mg dose units as a powder to be reconstituted in water or saline for intravenous infusion.[140] In a murine study, caspofungin tissue levels were higher than serum levels in liver and kidney; lower in the heart, brain, and thigh; and similar in lung and spleen.[141] Caspofungin is 97% bound to serum albumin. The clearance of caspofungin is through a combination of spontaneous chemical degradation, hydrolysis, and *N*-acetylation. Dose adjustments are not required for renal function because caspofungin is neither excreted by the kidney nor cleared by hemodialysis. The clearance of caspofungin is modestly reduced in subjects with moderate hepatic insufficiency (Child-Pugh score of 7 to 9), and a reduction from the usual daily dose of 50 mg/day to 35 mg/day is recommended. No data are available in individuals with more advanced hepatic insufficiency. Limited data are available for dosing in children. A study of two pediatric liver transplant recipients found that doses of 1 mg/kg/day seemed appropriate,[142] but a study of nine patients suggested that 50 mg/m² would provide a systemic exposure similar to that produced in adults with 50 mg/day.[143] No data have been reported to guide usage in neonates.

Drug Interactions

Caspofungin is not an inhibitor or inducer of the hepatic cytochrome metabolism enzymes and has few meaningful drug interactions. Cyclosporine coadministration increases caspofungin exposure and has been associated with increased hepatic transaminase levels in volunteers. As a consequence, concomitant usage of caspofungin and cyclosporine is not recommended unless the potential benefit outweighs the potential risk to the patient. Caspofungin coadministration reduces tacrolimus exposure by approximately 20%, and dosage adjustments may be required. Rifampin reduces caspofungin blood levels by approximately 30%, and the daily dosage of caspofungin should be increased from 50 mg to 70 mg if these drugs are coadministered. Likewise, limited data with other inducers of drug clearance (efavirenz, nevirapine, phenytoin, dexamethasone, and carbamazepine) suggest that reduced caspofungin levels are possible and that an increase in the daily dose to 70 mg should be considered.

Side Effects

Adverse reactions with caspofungin overall have been infrequent and minor. Symptoms possibly related to histamine release have been reported. Caspofungin does not seem to be significantly hepatotoxic or nephrotoxic.

Indications

Candidiasis. In the United States, caspofungin is indicated for the treatment of invasive candidiasis and of esophageal candidiasis.[144] This licensure was based primarily on a randomized, double-blind, placebo-controlled comparison of caspofungin (70-mg loading dose followed by 50 mg daily) versus amphotericin B deoxycholate (0.6 to 1 mg/kg/day) as therapy for invasive candidiasis in adults, with 80% of the subjects enrolled for candidemia.[145] Both study arms permitted a switch to oral fluconazole after 10 days of intravenous therapy. The success rates were not statistically different but showed a trend favoring caspofungin (73% success) over amphotericin B (62%), with far fewer adverse events noted in the caspofungin-treated group. Responses for the two study regimens were similar for each of the *Candida* spp. causing meaningful numbers of infections (*C. albicans, C. parapsilosis, Candida tropicalis,* and *C. glabrata*). The results are entirely consistent with the efficacy and safety data shown in three related studies of caspofungin as therapy of esophageal candidiasis,[146-148] including disease due to fluconazole-resistant isolates.[149]

Aspergillosis. Caspofungin also is licensed in the United States as therapy for invasive aspergillosis in patients who are refractory to or intolerant of other therapies. The dosage is the same as for candidiasis. This indication is based on a series of open-label cases of proven invasive aspergillosis.[140,150] An overall success rate of approximately 40% was reported in a series of patients in whom neutropenia, malignancy, and concomitant immunosuppressive therapy were common.

Investigational Echinocandins

Based on data presented to date, anidulafungin and micafungin are similar in most aspects to caspofungin. In contrast to caspofungin, neither has been reported to have a clinically meaningful drug interaction with cyclosporine.

OTHER AGENTS

Drugs still being evaluated in preclinical studies include sordarins, which inhibit protein synthesis by their effect on fungal elongation factor 2; nikkomycins, which inhibit chitin synthesis; and various peptides with unknown mechanisms of action.[136] Immunomodulators hold promise, but insufficient clinical data exist to determine where and how these drugs might be used.[151]

REFERENCES

1. Balakrishnan AR, Easwaran KR. CD and NMR studies on the aggregation of amphotericin B in solution. Biochim Biophys Acta. 1993;1148:269-277.
2. Hsu SF, Burnette RR. The effect of amphotericin B on the K-channel activity of MDCK cells. Biochim Biophys Acta. 1993;1152:189-191.
3. Vanden Bossche H, Marichal P, Odds FC. Molecular mechanisms of drug resistance in fungi. Trends Microbiol. 1994;2:393-400.
4. White TC. Mechanisms of resistance to antifungal agents. In: Murray PR, Baron EJ, Jorgensen JH, et al, eds. Manual of Clinical Microbiology. Washington, DC: ASM Press; 2003:1869-1879.
5. Loeffler J, Stevens DA. Antifungal drug resistance. Clin Infect Dis. 2003;36:S31-S41.
6. Rex JH, Pfaller MA. Has antifungal susceptibility testing come of age? Clin Infect Dis. 2002;35:982-989.
7. Merz WG. *Candida lusitaniae*: Frequency of recovery, colonization, infection, and amphotericin B resistance. J Clin Microbiol. 1984;20:1194-1195.
8. Andes D. In vivo pharmacodynamics of antifungal drugs in treatment of candidiasis. Antimicrob Agents Chemother. 2003;47:1179-1186.
9. Ostrosky-Zeichner L, Marr KA, Rex JH, Cohen SH. Amphotericin B: Time for a new gold standard. Clin Infect Dis. 2003;37:415-425.
10. Wong-Beringer A, Jacobs RA, Guglielmo BJ. Lipid formulations of amphotericin B: Clinical efficacy and toxicities. Clin Infect Dis. 1998;27:603-618.
11. Chavanet PY, Garry I, Charlier N, et al. Trial of glucose versus fat emulsion in preparation of amphotericin for use in HIV infected patients with candidiasis. BMJ. 1992;305:921-925.
12. Nath CE, Shaw PJ, Gunning R, et al. Amphotericin B in children with malignant disease: A comparison of the toxicities and pharmacokinetics of amphotericin B administered in dextrose versus lipid emulsion. Antimicrob Agents Chemother. 1999;43:1417-1423.
13. Cleary JD, Rogers PD, Chapman SW. Variability in polyene content and cellular toxicity among deoxycholate amphotericin B formulations. Pharmacotherapy. 2003;23:572-578.

14. Bindschadler DD, Bennett JE, Abernathy RS. A pharmacologic guide to the clinical use of amphotericin B. Br J Infect Dis. 1969;120:427-436.

15. Mayhew JW, Fiore C, Murray T, Barza M. An internally-standardized assay for amphotericin B in tissues and plasma. J Chromatogr. 1983;274:271-279.

16. Cleary JD, Chapman SW, Hardin TC, et al. Amphotericin B enzyme-linked immunoassay for clinical use: Comparison with bioassay and HPLC. Ann Pharmacother. 1997;31:39-44.

17. Merz WG, Fay D, Thumar B, Dixon D. Susceptibility testing of filamentous fungi to amphotericin B by a rapid radiometric method. J Clin Microbiol. 1984;19:54-56.

18. Sawaya BP, Weihprecht H, Campbell WR, et al. Direct vasoconstriction as a possible cause for amphotericin B-induced nephrotoxicity in rats. J Clin Invest. 1991;87:2097-2107.

19. Anderson CM. Sodium chloride treatment of amphotericin B nephrotoxicity: Standard of care? West J Med. 1995;162:313-317.

20. Cruz JM, Peacock JE Jr, Loomer L, et al. Rapid intravenous infusion of amphotericin B: A pilot study. Am J Med. 1992;93:123-130.

21. Drutz DJ. Rapid infusion of amphotericin B: Is it safe, effective, and wise? Am J Med. 1992;93:119-121.

22. Ellis ME, Al-Hokail AA, Clink HM, et al. Double-blind randomized study of the effect of infusion rates on toxicity of amphotericin B. Antimicrob Agents Chemother. 1992;36:172-179.

23. Imhof A, Walter RB, Schaffner A. Continuous infusion of escalated doses of amphotericin B deoxycholate: An open-label observational study. Clin Infect Dis. 2003;36:943-951.

24. Andes D, Stamsted T, Conklin R. Pharmacodynamics of amphotericin B in a neutropenic-mouse disseminated-candidiasis model. Antimicrob Agents Chemother. 2001;45:922-926.

25. Pizzo PA. Management of fever in patients with cancer and treatment-induced neutropenia. N Engl J Med. 1993;328:1323-1332.

26. White MH, Bowden RA, Sandler ES, et al. Randomized, double-blind clinical trial of amphotericin B colloidal dispersion vs. amphotericin B in the empirical treatment of fever and neutropenia. Clin Infect Dis. 1998;27:296-302.

27. Bowden R, Chandrasekar P, White MH, et al. A double-blind, randomized, controlled trial of amphotericin B colloidal dispersion versus amphotericin B for treatment of invasive aspergillosis in immunocompromised patients. Clin Infect Dis. 2002;35:359-366.

28. Walsh TJ, Hiemenz JW, Seibel NL, et al. Amphotericin B lipid complex for invasive fungal infections: Analysis of safety and efficacy in 556 cases. Clin Infect Dis. 1998;26:1383-1396.

29. Walsh TJ, Seibel NL, Arndt C, et al. Amphotericin B lipid complex in pediatric patients with invasive fungal infections. Pediatr Infect Dis J. 1999;18:702-708.

30. Hamill RJ, Sobel J, El-Sadr W, et al. Randomized double-blind trial of AmBisome (liposomal amphotericin B) and amphotericin B in acute cryptococcal meningitis in AIDS patients (Abstract No. 1161). Presented at Thirty-ninth Interscience Conference on Antimicrobial Agents and Chemotherapy, San Francisco, Calif, 1999.

31. Johnson PC, Wheat LJ, Cloud GA, et al. Safety and efficacy of liposomal amphotericin B compared with conventional amphotericin B for induction therapy of histoplasmosis in patients with AIDS. Ann Intern Med. 2002;137:105-109.

32. Ng TT, Denning DW. Liposomal amphotericin B (AmBisome) therapy in invasive fungal infections: Evaluation of United Kingdom compassionate use data. Arch Intern Med. 1995;155:1093-1098.

33. Mills W, Chopra R, Linch DC, Goldstone AH. Liposomal amphotericin B in the treatment of fungal infections in neutropenic patients: A single-center experience of 133 episodes in 116 patients. Br J Haematol. 1994;86:754-760.

34. Tollemar J, Ringden O, the Ambisome Users Group. Early pharmacokinetic and clinical results from a noncomparative multicentre trial of amphotericin B encapsulated in a small unilamellar liposome (AmBisome). Drug Invest. 1992;4:232-238.

35. Ringden O, Meunier F, Tollemar J, et al. Efficacy of amphotericin B encapsulated in liposomes (AmBisome) in the treatment of invasive fungal infections in immunocompromised patients. J Antimicrob Chemother. 1991;28(Suppl B):73-82.

36. Ellis M, Spence D, de Pauw B, et al. An EORTC international multicenter randomized trial (EORTC number 19923) comparing two dosages of liposomal amphotericin B for treatment of invasive aspergillosis. Clin Infect Dis. 1998;27:1406-1412.

37. Walsh TJ, Finberg RW, Arndt C, et al. Liposomal amphotericin B for empirical therapy in patients with persistent fever and neutropenia. N Engl J Med. 1999;340:764-771.

38. Prentice HG, Hann IM, Herbrecht R, et al. A randomized comparison of liposomal versus conventional amphotericin B for the treatment of pyrexia of unknown origin in neutropenic patients. Br J Haematol. 1997;98:711-718.

39. Wingard JR, White MH, Anaissie E, et al. A randomized, double-blind comparative trial evaluating the safety of liposomal amphotericin B versus amphotericin B lipid complex in the empirical treatment of febrile neutropenia. Clin Infect Dis. 2000;31:1155-1163.

40. Roden MM, Nelson LD, Knudsen TA, et al. Triad of acute infusion-related reactions associated with liposomal amphotericin B: Analysis of clinical and epidemiological characteristics. Clin Infect Dis. 2003;36:1213-1220.

41. Bates DW, Su L, Yu DT, et al. Mortality and costs of acute renal failure associated with amphotericin B therapy. Clin Infect Dis. 2001;32:686-693.

42. Block ER, Bennett JE, Livoti LG, et al. Flucytosine and amphotericin B: Hemodialysis effects on the plasma concentration and clearance: Studies in man. Ann Intern Med. 1974;80:613-617.

43. Pfaller MA, Messer SA, Boyken L, et al. In vitro activities of 5-fluorocytosine against 8,803 clinical isolates of Candida spp.: Global assessment of primary resistance using National Committee for Clinical Laboratory Standards susceptibility testing methods. Antimicrob Agents Chemother. 2002;46:3518-3521.

44. Brandt ME, Pfaller MA, Hajjeh RA, et al. Trends in antifungal drug susceptibility of Cryptococcus neoformans isolates in the United States: 1992 to 1994 and 1996 to 1998. Antimicrob Agents Chemother. 2001;45:3065-3069.

45. Stamm AM, Diasio RB, Dismukes WE, et al. Toxicity of amphotericin B plus flucytosine in 194 patients with cryptococcal meningitis. Am J Med. 1987;83:236-242.

46. Kaspar RL, Drutz DJ. Rapid, simple bioassay for 5-fluorocytosine in the presence of amphotericin B. Antimicrob Agents Chemother. 1975;7:462-465.

47. Huang CM, Kroll MH, Ruddel M, et al. An enzymatic method for 5-fluorocytosine. Clin Chem. 1988;34:59-62.

48. Harding SA, Johnson GF, Solomon HM. Gas-chromatographic determination of 5-fluorocytosine in human serum. Clin Chem. 1976;22:772-776.

49. Diasio RB, Lakings DE, Bennett JE. Evidence for conversion of 5-fluorocytosine to 5-fluorouracil in humans: Possible factor in 5-fluorocytosine clinical toxicity. Antimicrob Agents Chemother. 1978;14:903-908.

50. Harris BE, Manning BW, Federle TW, Diasio RB. Conversion of 5-fluorocytosine to 5-fluorouracil by human intestinal microflora. Antimicrob Agents Chemother. 1986;29:44-48.

51. Hospenthal DR, Bennett JE. Flucytosine monotherapy for cryptococcosis. Clin Infect Dis. 1998;27:260-264.

52. Kitahara M, Seth VK, Medoff G, Kobayashi GS. Activity of amphotericin B, 5-fluorocytosine, and rifampin against six clinical isolates of Aspergillus. Antimicrob Agents Chemother. 1976;9:915-919.

53. Polak A, Scholer HJ, Wall M. Combination therapy of experimental candidiasis, cryptococcosis and aspergillosis in mice. Chemotherapy. 1982;28:461-479.

54. Denning DW, Hanson LH, Perlman AM, Stevens DA. In vitro susceptibility and synergy studies of Aspergillus species to conventional and new agents. Diagn Microbiol Infect Dis. 1992;15:21-34.

55. Dismukes WE, Cloud G, Gallis HA, et al, National Institute of Allergy and Infectious Diseases Mycoses Study Group. Treatment of cryptococcal meningitis with combination amphotericin B and flucytosine for four as compared with six weeks. N Engl J Med. 1987;317:334-341.

56. Smego RA Jr, Perfect JR, Durack DT. Combined therapy with amphotericin B and 5-fluorocytosine for Candida meningitis. Rev Infect Dis. 1984;6:791-801.

57. Heel RC, Brogden RN, Carmine A, et al. Ketoconazole: a review of its therapeutic efficacy in superficial and systemic fungal infections. Drugs. 1982;23:1-36.

58. Rex JH, Rinaldi MG, Pfaller MA. Resistance of Candida species to fluconazole. Antimicrob Agents Chemother. 1995;39:1-8.

59. Vu Van H, Piens MA, Archimbaud E, et al. Serum levels of ketoconazole in bone marrow transplanted patients. Nouv Rev Fr Hematol. 1983;25:241-244.

60. National Institute of Allergy and Infectious Diseases Mycoses Study Group. Treatment of blastomycosis and histoplasmosis with ketoconazole: Results of a prospective, randomized clinical trial. Ann Intern Med. 1985;103:861-872.

61. Galgiani JN, Stevens DA, Graybill JR, et al. Ketoconazole therapy of progressive coccidioidomycosis: Comparison of 400- and 800-mg doses and observations at higher doses. Am J Med. 1988;84:603-610.

62. Sugar AM, Alsip SG, Galgiani JN, et al. Pharmacology and toxicity of high-dose ketoconazole. Antimicrob Agents Chemother. 1987;31:1874-1878.

63. Schaffner A, Frick PG. The effect of ketoconazole on amphotericin B in a model of disseminated aspergillosis. J Infect Dis. 1985;151:902-910.

64. Pont A, Graybill JR, Craven PC, et al. High-dose ketoconazole therapy and adrenal and testicular function in humans. Arch Intern Med. 1984;144:2150-2153.

65. Stevens DA. Ketoconazole metamorphosis: An antimicrobial becomes an endocrine drug. Arch Intern Med. 1985;145:813-815.

66. Dismukes WE, Stamm AM, Graybill JR, et al. Treatment of systemic mycoses with ketoconazole: Emphasis on toxicity and clinical response in 52 patients. National Institute of Allergy and Infectious Diseases Collaborative Antifungal Study. Ann Intern Med. 1983;98:13-20.

67. Lewis JH, Zimmerman HJ, Benton GD, Ishak KG. Hepatic injury associated with ketoconazole therapy: Analysis of 33 cases. Gastroenterology. 1984;86:503-513.

68. Stevens DA. Itraconazole in cyclodextrin solution. Pharmacotherapy. 1999;19:603-611.

69. Barone JA, Moskovitz BL, Guarnieri J, et al. Enhanced bioavailability of itraconazole in hydroxypropyl-beta-cyclodextrin solution versus capsules in healthy volunteers. Antimicrob Agents Chemother. 1998;42:1862-1865.

70. de Repentigny L, Ratelle J, Leclerc JM, et al. Repeated-dose pharmacokinetics of an oral solution of itraconazole in infants and children. Antimicrob Agents Chemother. 1998;42:404-408.

71. Saag M. Itraconazole oral solution: Pharmacokinetics and absorption. AIDS Patient Care STDS. 1997;11:S16-S17.

72. Reynes J, Bazin C, Ajana F, et al. Pharmacokinetics of itraconazole (oral solution) in two groups of human immunodeficiency virus-infected adults with oral candidiasis. Antimicrob Agents Chemother. 1997;41:2554-2558.

73. Jaruratanasirikul S, Kleepkaew A. Influence of an acidic beverage (Coca-Cola) on the absorption of itraconazole. Eur J Clin Pharmacol. 1997;52:235-237.

74. Smith D, van de Velde V, Woestenborghs R, Gazzard BG. The pharmacokinetics of oral itraconazole in AIDS patients. J Pharm Pharmacol. 1992;44:618-619.

75. Hostetler JS, Heykants J, Clemons KV, et al. Discrepancies in bioassay and chromatography determinations explained by metabolism of itraconazole to hydroxyitraconazole: Studies of interpatient variations in concentrations. Antimicrob Agents Chemother. 1993;37:2224-2227.

76. Tucker RM, Haq Y, Denning DW, Stevens DA. Adverse events associated with itraconazole in 189 patients on chronic therapy. J Antimicrob Chemother. 1990;26:561-566.

77. Lim SG, Sawyerr AM, Hudson M, et al. Short report: The absorption of fluconazole and itraconazole under conditions of low intragastric acidity. Aliment Pharmacol Ther. 1993;7:317-321.

78. Crane JK, Shih H-T. Syncope and cardiac arrhythmia due to an interaction between intraconazole and terfenadine. Am J Med. 1993;95:445-446.

79. Neuvonen PJ, Jalava KM. Itraconazole drastically increases plasma concentrations of lovastatin and lovastatin acid. Clin Pharmacol Ther. 1996;60:54-61.

80. Jalava KM, Olkkola KT, Neuvonen PJ. Itraconazole greatly increases plasma concentrations and effects of felodipine. Clin Pharmacol Ther. 1997;61:410-415.

81. Buggia I, Zecca M, Alessandrino EP, et al. Itraconazole can increase systemic exposure to busulfan in patients given bone marrow transplantation. GITMO (Gruppo Italiano Trapianto di Midollo Osseo). Anticancer Res. 1996;16:2083-2088.

82. Stevens DA, Lee JY. Analysis of compassionate use itraconazole therapy for invasive aspergillosis by the NIAID Mycoses Study Group criteria. Arch Intern Med. 1997;157:1857-1862.

83. Stevens DA, Schwartz HJ, Lee JY, et al. A randomized trial of itraconazole in allergic bronchopulmonary aspergillosis. N Engl J Med. 2000;342:756-762.

84. Mangino JE, Pappas PG. Itraconazole for the treatment of histoplasmosis and blastomycosis. Int J Antimicrob Agents. 1995;5:219-225.

85. Tucker RM, Denning DW, Dupont B, Stevens DA. Itraconazole therapy for chronic coccidioidal meningitis. Ann Intern Med. 1990;112:108-112.

86. Galgiani JN, Cloud GA, Catanzaro A, et al, NIAID—Mycoses Study Group. A comparison of oral fluconazole or itraconazole for progressive, nonmeningeal coccidioidomycosis. Ann Intern Med. 2000;133:676-686.

87. Badley AD, Van Scoy RE. Long-term follow-up of multifocal osteoarticular sporotrichosis treated with itraconazole. Clin Infect Dis. 1996;23:394-395.

88. Sharkey-Mathis PK, Kauffman CA, Graybill JR, et al, other members of the NIAID Mycoses Study Group. Treatment of sporotrichosis with itraconazole. Am J Med. 1993;95:279-285.

89. Van Hecke E, Van Cutsem J. Double-blind comparison of itraconazole with griseofulvin in the treatment of tinea pedis and tinea manuum. Mycoses. 1988;31:641-649.

90. Hecht FM, Wheat J, Korzun AH, et al. Itraconazole maintenance treatment for histoplasmosis in AIDS: A prospective, multicenter trial. J Acq Immune Defic Syndr Hum Retrovirol. 1997;16:100-107.

91. Morgenstern GR, Prentice AG, Prentice HG, et al, U.K. Multicentre Antifungal Prophylaxis Study Group. A randomised controlled trial of itraconazole versus fluconazole for the prevention of fungal infections in patients with haematological malignancies. Br J Haematol. 1999;105:901-911.

92. Nucci M, Biasoli I, Akiti T, et al. A double-blind, randomized, placebo-controlled trial of itraconazole capsules as antifungal prophylaxis for neutropenic patients. Clin Infect Dis. 2000;30:300-305.

93. Menichetti F, Del Favero A, Martino P, et al. Itraconazole oral solution as prophylaxis for fungal infections in neutropenic patients with hematologic malignancies: A randomized, placebo-controlled, double-blind, multicenter trial. Clin Infect Dis. 1999;28:250-255.

94. Boogaerts M, Winston DJ, Bow EJ, et al. Intravenous and oral itraconazole versus intravenous amphotericin B deoxycholate as empirical antifungal therapy for persistent fever in neutropenic patients with cancer who are receiving broad-spectrum antibacterial therapy—a randomized, controlled trial. Ann Intern Med. 2001;135:412-422.

95. Wilcox CM, Darouiche RO, Laine L, et al. A randomized, double-blind comparison of itraconazole oral solution and fluconazole tables in the treatment of esophageal candidiasis. J Infect Dis. 1997;176:227-232.

96. Graybill JR, Vazquez J, Darouiche RO, et al. Randomized trial of itraconazole oral solution for oropharyngeal candidiasis in HIV/AIDS patients. Am J Med. 1998;104:33-39.

97. Momeni AZ, Jalayer T, Emamjomeh M, et al. Treatment of cutaneous leishmaniasis with itraconazole: Randomized double-blind study. Arch Dermatol. 1996;132:784-786.

98. Zervos M, Meunier F. Fluconazole (Diflucan): A review. Int J Antimicrob Agents. 1993;3:147-170.

99. DeMuria D, Forrest A, Rich J, et al. Pharmacokinetics and bioavailability of fluconazole in patients with AIDS. Antimicrob Agents Chemother. 1993;37:2187-2192.

100. Saxen H, Hoppu K, Pohjavuori M. Pharmacokinetics of fluconazole in very low birth weight infants during the first two weeks of life. Clin Pharmacol Ther. 1993;54:269-277.

101. Trapnell CB, Narang PK, Li R, Lavelle JP. Increased plasma rifabutin levels with concomitant fluconazole therapy in HIV-infected patients. Ann Intern Med. 1996;124:573-576.

102. Baciewicz AM, Baciewicz FA. Ketoconazole and fluconazole drug interactions. Arch Intern Med. 1993;153:1970-1976.

103. Stevens DA, Diaz M, Negroni R, et al, Fluconazole Pan-American Study Group. Safety evaluation of chronic fluconazole therapy. Chemotherapy. 1997;43:371-377.

104. Diaz M, Negroni R, Montero-Gei F, et al. A Pan-American 5-year study of fluconazole therapy for deep mycoses in the immunocompetent host. Pan-American Study Group. Clin Infect Dis. 1992;14(Suppl 1):S68-S76.

105. Rex JH, Walsh TJ, Sobel JD, et al. Practice guidelines for the treatment of candidiasis. Clin Infect Dis. 2000;30:662-678.

106. Rex JH, Bennett JE, Sugar AM, et al, the Candidemia Study Group, the NIAID Mycoses Study Group. A randomized trial comparing fluconazole with amphotericin B for the treatment of candidemia in patients without neutropenia. N Engl J Med. 1994;331:1325-1330.

107. Rex JH, Pappas PG, Karchmer AW, et al. A randomized and blinded multicenter trial of high-dose fluconazole plus placebo versus fluconazole plus amphotericin B as therapy for candidemia and its consequences in nonneutropenic subjects. Clin Infect Dis. 2003;36:1221-1228.

108. Nucci M, Anaissie E. Should vascular catheters be removed from all patients with candidemia? An evidence-based review. Clin Infect Dis. 2002;34:591-599.

109. Saag MS, Powderly WG, Cloud GA, et al. Comparison of amphotericin B with fluconazole in the treatment of acute AIDS-associated cryptococcal meningitis. N Engl J Med. 1992;326:83-89.

110. Van der Horst CM, Saag MS, Cloud GA, et al, National Institute of Allergy and Infectious Diseases Mycoses Study Group, AIDS Clinical Trials Group. Treatment of cryptococcal meningitis associated with the acquired immunodeficiency syndrome. N Engl J Med. 1997;337:15-21.

111. Powderly WG, Saag MS, Cloud GA, et al. A controlled trial of fluconazole or amphotericin B to prevent relapse of cryptococcal meningitis in patients with the acquired immunodeficiency syndrome. N Engl J Med. 1992;326:793-798.

112. Haubrich RH, Haghighat D, Bozzette SA, et al, the California Collaborative Treatment Group. High-dose fluconazole for treatment of cryptococcal disease in patients with human immunodeficiency virus infection. J Infect Dis. 1994;170:238-242.

113. Larsen RA, Bozzette SA, Jones BE, et al. Fluconazole combined with flucytosine for treatment of cryptococcal meningitis in patients with AIDS. Clin Infect Dis. 1994;19:741-745.

114. Catanzaro A, Galgiani JN, Levine BE, et al, the NIAID Mycoses Study Group. Fluconazole in the treatment of chronic pulmonary and nonmeningeal disseminated coccidioidomycosis. Am J Med. 1995;98:249-256.

115. Castro LGM, Belda W, Cucé LC, et al. Successful treatment of sporotrichosis with oral fluconazole: A report of three cases. Br J Dermatol. 1993;128:352-356.

116. McKinsey DS, Kauffman CA, Pappas PG, et al, National Institutes of Allergy and Infectious Diseases Mycoses Study Group. Fluconazole therapy for histoplasmosis. Clin Infect Dis. 1996;23:996-1001.

117. Goodman JL, Winston DJ, Greenfield RA, et al. A controlled trial of fluconazole to prevent fungal infections in patients undergoing bone marrow transplantation. N Engl J Med. 1992;326:845-851.

118. Slavin MA, Osborne B, Adams R, et al. Efficacy and safety of fluconazole prophylaxis for fungal infections after bone marrow transplantation: A prospective, randomized, double-blind study. J Infect Dis. 1995;171:1545-1552.

119. Menichetti F, Del Favero A, Martino P, et al. Preventing fungal infection in neutropenic patients with acute leukemia: Fluconazole compared with oral amphotericin B. The GIMEMA Infection Program. Ann Intern Med. 1994;120:913-918.

120. Winston DJ, Chandrasekar PH, Lazarus HM, et al. Fluconazole prophylaxis of fungal infections in patients with acute leukemia: Results of a randomized placebo-controlled, double-blind, multicenter trial. Ann Intern Med. 1993;118:495-503.

121. Marr KA, Seidel K, Slavin MA, et al. Prolonged fluconazole prophylaxis is associated with persistent protection against candidiasis-related death in allogeneic marrow transplant recipients: Long-term follow-up of a randomized, placebo-controlled trial. Blood 2000;96:2055-2061.

122. Wingard JR, Merz WG, Rinaldi MG, et al. Increase in *Candida krusei* infection among patients with bone marrow transplantation and neutropenia treated prophylactically with fluconazole. N Engl J Med. 1991;325:1274-1277.

123. Wingard JR, Merz WG, Rinaldi MG, et al. Association of *Torulopsis glabrata* infections with fluconazole prophylaxis in neutropenic bone marrow transplant patients. Antimicrob Agents Chemother. 1993;37:1847-1849.

124. Havlir DV, Dube MP, McCutchan JA, et al. Prophylaxis with weekly versus daily fluconazole for fungal infections in patients with AIDS. Clin Infect Dis. 1998;27:1369-1375.

125. Schuman P, Capps L, Peng G, et al. Weekly fluconazole for the prevention of mucosal candidiasis in women with HIV infection: A randomized, double-blind, placebo-controlled trial. Terry Beirn Community Programs for Clinical Research on AIDS. Ann Intern Med. 1997;126:689-696.

126. Norris S, Wheat J, McKinsey D, et al. Prevention of relapse of histoplasmosis with fluconazole in patients with acquired immunodeficiency syndrome. Am J Med. 1994;96:504-508.

127. Anonymous. VFEND Tables (voriconazole). VFEND I.V. (voriconazole for injection). Product Information. New York: Pfizer; 2002.

128. Muijsers RBR, Goa KL, Scott LJ. Voriconazole in the treatment of invasive aspergillosis. Drugs. 2002;62:2655-2665.

129. Herbrecht R, Denning DW, Patterson TF, et al. Voriconazole versus amphotericin B for primary therapy of invasive aspergillosis. N Engl J Med. 2002;347:408-415.

130. Denning DW, Ribaud P, Milpied N, et al. Efficacy and safety of voriconazole in the treatment of acute invasive aspergillosis. Clin Infect Dis. 2002;34:563-571.

131. Ally R, Schurmann D, Kreisel W, et al. A randomized, double-blind, double-dummy, multicenter trial of voriconazole and fluconazole in the treatment of esophageal candidiasis in immunocompromised patients. Clin Infect Dis. 2001;33:1447-1454.

132. Ostrosky-Zeichner L, Oude Lashof AML, Boucher HW, et al. Voriconazole salvage treatment of invasive candidiasis: Experience from open-label compassionate use protocols (Abstract No. 352). Presented at Fortieth Annual Meeting of the Infectious Diseases Society of America, Chicago, Ill, 2002.

133. Perfect JR, Marr KA, Walsh TJ, et al. Voriconazole treatment for less-common, emerging, or refractory fungal infections. Clin Infect Dis. 2003;36:1122-1131.

134. Walsh TJ, Pappas P, Winston DJ, et al. Voriconazole compared with liposomal amphotericin B for empirical antifungal therapy in patients with neutropenia and persistent fever. N Engl J Med. 2002;346:225-234.

135. Powers JH, Dixon CA, Goldberger MJ. Voriconazole versus liposomal amphotericin B in patients with neutropenia and persistent fever. N Engl J Med. 2002;346:289-290.

136. Arikan S, Rex JH. New agents for the treatment of systemic fungal infections-current status. Expert Opin Emerging Drugs. 2002;7:3-32.

137. Kurtz MB, Rex JH. Glucan synthase inhibitors as antifungal agents. Adv Protein Chem. 2001;56:463-475.

138. Denning DW. Echinocandins: A new class of antifungal. J Antimicrob Chemother. 2002;49:889-891.
139. Bowman JC, Hicks PS, Kurtz MB, et al. The antifungal echinocandin caspofungin acetate kills growing cells of *Aspergillus fumigatus* in vitro. Antimicrob Agents Chemother. 2002;46:3001-3012.
140. Anonymous. Cancidas (caspofungin acetate) for injection. Whitehouse Station, NJ: Merck & Co; 2003.
141. Hajdu R, Thompson R, Sundelof JG, et al. Preliminary animal pharmacokinetics of the parenteral antifungal agent MK-0991 (L-743,872). Antimicrob Agents Chemother. 1997;41:2339-2344.
142. Neely M, Blumer J. Pharmacokinetic characteristics of caspofungin in two pediatric liver transplant patients. Curr Ther Res. 2003;64:127-136.
143. Walsh TJ, Adamson PC, Seibel NL, et al. Pharmacokinetics of caspofungin in pediatric patients (Abstract No. M-896). Presented at Forty-second Interscience Conference on Antimicrobial Agents and Chemotherapy, San Diego, Calif, 2002.
144. Deresinski SC, Stevens DA. Caspofungin. Clin Infect Dis. 2003;36:1445-1457.
145. Mora-Duarte J, Betts R, Rotstein R, et al, Caspofungin Invasive Candidiasis Study Group. Comparison of caspofungin and amphotericin B for invasive candidiasis. N Engl J Med. 2002;347:2020-2029.
146. Villanueva A, Gotuzzo E, Arathoon E, et al. A randomized double-blind study of caspofungin versus fluconazole for the treatment of esophageal candidiasis. Am J Med. 2002;113:294-299.
147. Villanueva A, Arathoon EG, Gotuzzo E, et al. A randomized double-blind study of caspofungin versus amphotericin for the treatment of candidal esophagitis. Clin Infect Dis. 2001;33:1529-1535.
148. Arathoon EG, Gotuzzo E, Noriega LM, et al. Randomized, double-blind, multicenter study of caspofungin versus amphotericin B for treatment of oropharyngeal and esophageal candidiasis. Antimicrob Agents Chemother. 2002;46:451-457.
149. Kartsonis N, DiNubile MJ, Bartizal K, et al. Efficacy of caspofungin in the treatment of esophageal candidiasis resistant to fluconazole. J Acq Immune Defic Syndr Hum Retrovirol. 2002;31:183-187.
150. Hiemenz J, Raad I, Boogaerts M, et al. Efficacy of caspofungin as salvage therapy in invasive aspergillosis compared to standard therapy in historical cohort (Abstract No. 22). Presented at Focus on Fungal Infections 11, Washington, DC, 2001.
151. Stevens DA. Combination immunotherapy and antifungal chemotherapy. Clin Infect Dis. 1998;26:1266-1269.
152. Hamilton-Miller JM. Fungal sterols and the mode of action of the polyene antibiotics. Adv Appl Microbiol. 1974;17:109-134.
153. Gale EF. Perspectives in chemotherapy. BMJ. 1973;4:33-38.
154. Pratt WB. Chemotherapy of Infection. New York: Oxford University Press; 1977:462.
155. Vanden Bossche H, Warnock DW, Dupont B, et al. Mechanisms and clinical impact of antifungal drug resistance. J Med Vet Mycol. 1994;32(Suppl 1):189-202.
156. Francis P, Walsh TJ. Evolving role of flucytosine in immunocompromised patients—new insights into safety, pharmacokinetics, and antifungal therapy. Clin Infect Dis. 1992;15:1003-1018.

CHAPTER **38**

Antiviral Drugs (Other Than Antiretrovirals)

FREDERICK G. HAYDEN

GENERAL PRINCIPLES

Antiviral drugs with proven therapeutic (Table 38-1) and prophylactic effectiveness are available for a number of common and some life-threatening viral infections. In part as a response to human immunodeficiency virus (HIV) infection, transplantation-related viral infections, and recently emerging viral threats including poxviruses, severe acute respiratory syndrome (SARS) coronavirus, and potential bioweapon agents, the search for new antiviral agents and therapeutic approaches for managing viral diseases continues to intensify. More than four dozen antiviral agents are approved for use in the United States, and a number of others are in advanced clinical development. This chapter reviews antiviral agents used for infections caused by viruses other than HIV. Antiretroviral drugs are reviewed in Chapter 124. Please see earlier editions of this chapter for references published before 1990.

Mechanisms of Action

Chemotherapeutic agents for viral infections can be categorized into three broad groups: agents that directly inactivate intact viruses (virucides), those that inhibit viral replication at the cellular level (antivirals), and those that augment or modify the host response to infection (immunomodulators). Virucidal agents may cause direct inactivation in a single step, examples including detergents, organic solvents such as ether or chloroform, and ultraviolet light, or in multiple steps, as with photodynamic inactivation. However, such interventions have not proved clinically useful in the treatment of mucocutaneous herpes simplex virus (HSV) infections. Treatments that destroy both host tissues and virus simultaneously, such as cryotherapy, laser, or podophyllin treatment of warts, are useful only in discrete mucocutaneous infections. One potential use of virucidal agents may be in preventing transmission of certain viral infections.

Antivirals. Because viral replication depends primarily on host cell metabolic functions, useful antiviral agents must inhibit virus-specific events, such as attachment to the cell, uncoating of the viral genome, or assembly of progeny virions, or preferentially inhibit virus-directed (as contrasted to host cell–directed) macromolecular synthesis. Consequently, antiviral agents typically have a restricted spectrum of activity. Although many compounds exist that exhibit antiviral activity in vitro, most affect some host cell function and are associated with low therapeutic ratios or unacceptable toxicity in humans. Most current antivirals target viral nucleic acid synthesis. In addition, because these agents inhibit ongoing replication at the host cell level, replication may resume when the drug is removed. Similarly, current antiviral agents are not effective in the elimination of nonreplicating or latent viruses.

Few susceptibility assays for viruses are standardized, and results depend on various factors including the assay system, cell line, viral inoculum, and laboratory. Several commercial laboratories offer phenotypic susceptibility testing of selected herpesviruses.

Host Immune Responses. Intact host immunologic responses remain essential for recovery from virus infections. Immunosuppression resulting from organ transplantation, cancer chemotherapy, or HIV infection has been associated with high rates of recrudescent or chronic viral infections. Antiviral prophylaxis and preemptive therapy have become standard practice in immunocompromised patients such as bone marrow and solid-organ transplant recipients.[1] Responses to antiviral treatment may be delayed, and the risk of selecting drug-resistant viruses is higher in such patients. In addition, some antiviral agents may blunt host immune responses by direct immunosuppressive effects[2] or by altering humoral and cellular immune responses indirectly through reductions in viral antigen exposure. Factors other than inhibition of viral replication alone are important in treating certain viral diseases, such as orofacial HSV infections or rhinovirus colds in normal hosts and cytomegalovirus (CMV) pneumonia in bone marrow transplant recipients; in these diseases, it has been possible to demonstrate antiviral effects without clinical benefit.

Immunomodulating agents used to treat viral infections include those that replace deficient host immune responses (e.g., exogenous antibody in chronic echovirus infection, cytotoxic T lymphocytes in CMV infection of marrow transplant recipients) and those that enhance endogenous ones. Chemical agents that appear to augment cell-mediated immune responses have been used with variable success and remain largely investigational. One topical immune response modifier, imiquimod, is useful in treating anogenital papillomavirus infections.[3]

Drug Resistance

Drug-resistant viruses have been recognized increasingly during clinical use of various antiviral agents.[2] Indeed, the laboratory selection of a drug-resistant strain of virus implies that the drug has a specific antiviral mechanism. The development of resistance results from mutations within the viral genome, and the presence of selective drug pressure leads to the emergence of a resistant virus population. Resistant subpopulations often exist naturally in clinical isolates, but spontaneous mutations may also arise during drug exposure. Single

TABLE 38-1 Antiviral Agents of Established Therapeutic Effectiveness

Viral Infection	Drug	Route	Usual Adult Dosage
Cytomegalovirus (CMV)			
Retinitis	Ganciclovir	IV	5 mg/kg/12 hr in 1-hr infusion for 14-21 days*
	Valganciclovir	PO	900 mg bid for 21 days*
	Cidofovir	IV	5 mg/kg once wkly × 2, then every other wk
	Fomivirsen	Intravitreal	330 μg every 2 wk × 2, then every 4 wk
	Foscarnet	IV	60 mg/kg/8 hr in 1-2–hr infusion for 14-21 days†
Hepatitis Viruses			
Chronic hepatitis C	Peg-interferon-α-2a *or*	SC	180 μg wkly for 48 wk
(genotypes 1 and 4)	Peg-interferon-α-2b	SC	1.5 μg/kg wkly for 48 wk
	plus ribavirin‡	PO	1000-1200 mg/day depending on weight
Chronic hepatitis B	Interferon-α-2b	SC/IM	5 MU/day or 10 MU 3 times wkly for 16 wk
	Lamivudine§	PO	100 mg/day
	Adefovir	PO	10 mg/day
Herpes Simplex Virus (HSV)			
Genital herpes	Acyclovir	PO‖	400 mg tid or 200 mg 5 times/day for 7-10 days
First episode	Famciclovir	PO	250 mg tid for 7-10 days
	Valacyclovir	PO	1 g bid for 7-10 days
Recurrent	Acyclovir	PO	800 mg tid for 2 days or 400 mg tid or 200 mg 5 times/day or 800 mg bid for 5 days
	Famciclovir	PO	125 mg bid for 5 days
	Valacyclovir	PO	500 mg bid for 3 days or 1 g/day for 5 days
Suppression¶	Acyclovir	PO	400 mg bid or 200 mg tid
	Famciclovir	PO	250 mg bid
	Valacyclovir	PO	500 mg/day or 1 g/day (≥10 episodes/yr) or 250 mg bid
Encephalitis	Acyclovir**	IV	10-15 mg/kg/8 hr in 1-hr infusions for 14-21 days
Mucocutaneous disease in	Acyclovir†	IV	5 mg/kg/8 hr for 7-14 days‡‡
immunocompromised hosts		PO	400 mg 5 times/day for 7-14 days
	Valacyclovir§§	PO	500 mg or 1 g bid for 7-10 days
	Penciclovir§§	IV	5 mg/kg/8-12 hr for 7 days
	Famciclovir	PO	500 mg bid for 7-10 days
Orolabial herpes	Penciclovir 1%	Topical	Apply cream every 2 hr while awake for 4 days
	Acyclovir 5%	Topical	Apply cream 5 times/day for 4 days
	Docosanol 10%	Topical	Apply cream 5 times/day until healing
	Valacyclovir	PO	2 g repeated once at 12 hr for 1 day
	Acyclovir§§	PO	400 mg tid/day for 5 days
Neonatal	Acyclovir§§,‖‖	IV	10-20 mg/kg/8 hr for 14-21 days
Keratoconjunctivitis	Trifluridine¶¶	Topical	1 drop of 1% solution topically, q2h up to 9 drops/day
	Vidarabine	Topical	½-inch ribbon of 3% ointment 5 times daily
Influenza Viruses			
Influenza A and B viruses	Oseltamivir	PO	75 mg bid for 5 days***
	Zanamivir	Inhalation	10 mg bid by inhaler for 5 days†††
Influenza A virus	Amantadine	PO	100 mg bid for 5 days for treatment‡‡‡
	Rimantadine	PO	100 mg bid for 5 days for treatment§§§
Papillomavirus			
Condyloma acuminatum	Imiquimod 5%	Topical	Apply cream 3 times wkly to maximum 16 wk; wash off at 6-10 hr after each application
	Interferon-α-2b‖‖‖	Intralesional	1 MU/0.1 mL injected in up to 5 warts 3 times/wk for 3 wk
Respiratory Syncytial Virus	Ribavirin	Aerosol	Aerosol treatment 18 hr/day for 3 to 7 days¶¶¶
Varicella-Zoster Virus			
Varicella in normal children	Acyclovir	PO	20 mg/kg (up to 800 mg) qid for 5 days
Varicella in immunocompromised hosts	Acyclovir	IV	10 mg/kg/8 hr or 500 mg/m²/8 hr for 7-10 days****
Herpes zoster in immunocompromised hosts	Acyclovir	IV	10 mg/kg/8 hr in 1-h infusion for 7-10 days****
Herpes zoster in normal hosts	Acyclovir	PO	800 mg 5 times daily for 7-10 days
	Valacyclovir	PO	1 g tid for 7 days
	Famciclovir	PO	500 mg tid for 7 days

NOTE: Please consult text and manufacturer's product prescribing information for dosage adjustments in renal or hepatic insufficiency and in other circumstances.

*In patients with AIDS or who are otherwise highly immunocompromised, chronic suppression with valganciclovir 900 mg/day is recommended after acute treatment. Intravenous ganciclovir 5 mg/kg given 7 day/wk or 6 mg/kg given 5 day/wk or oral ganciclovir 1 g tid are alternatives for suppression. These dosages are also approved for prevention of CMV disease in transplant recipients. An intraocular insert is also available.

†Chronic suppression with daily infusion of 90 to 120 mg/kg over 2 hr is recommended after initial treatment in patients with AIDS.

‡Combination therapy is approved for patients with compensated liver disease for initial treatment and for those who have relapsed after interferon therapy. For genotypes 2 and 3, 24 weeks of pegIFN-α2a therapy and ribavirin dose of 800 mg appear adequate.351a Ribavirin is not currently approved for this indication in children; dosage should be adjusted according to weight in children.86 Monotherapy with pegylated interferon is a less effective alternative for ribavirin-intolerant persons.

§Dosage in children ≥2 years of age is 3 mg/kg/day to a maximum of 100 mg/day.

‖For severe initial genital herpes and in patients unable to tolerate oral medicines, IV acyclovir 5 mg/kg/8 hr for 5 to 7 days is recommended before a switch to an oral agent.

¶Famciclovir 500 mg bid and valacyclovir 500 mg bid are effective in reducing recurrences in HIV-infected persons.

**Both higher dosages and 21 days of intravenous therapy are recommended by some authorities. The possible value of additional oral valacyclovir treatment afterwards is under study.

††In acyclovir-resistant HSV or VZV infections, IV foscarnet 40 mg/kg/8 hr appears beneficial. Duration of therapy depends on the clinical response. For limited cutaneous infections in immunocompromised patients, 5% acyclovir ointment can be applied to lesions every 3 hr, up to 6 times daily for 7 days (about ½-inch ribbon per 4 square inches), using a finger cot or glove.

‡‡Higher dosages (30 mg/kg/day) are recommended in progressive or visceral infections. Suggested pediatric dosage in children <12 years is 10 mg/kg/8 hr for 7 days per manufacturer.

§§Not approved by FDA for this indication (January 2004). IV penciclovir is not available in USA.

‖‖The high dosage (20 mg/kg/8 hr) is recommended by experts,86 and appears superior in disseminated and CNS disease in neonates.

¶¶An ophthalmic ointment of 3% acyclovir is available in some countries. Idoxuridine 0.1% solution, q1h while awake and q2h at night, or 0.5% ointment 5 times/day is a less effective alternative. Treatment of HSV ocular infections should be supervised by an ophthalmologist.

***Pediatric dosages are weight adjusted: 30 mg bid for <15 kg, 45 mg bid for 16-23 kg, 60 mg bid for 24-40 kg, and 75 mg bid for >40 kg. Prophylactic dosage is given once daily (one half of total daily treatment dosage). Not FDA approved currently for prophylaxis in children <13 yr or treatment in children <1 yr.

†††FDA approved at same dosage for treatment to age 7 yr. Prophylactic dosage is 10 mg inhaled once daily. Not FDA approved for prophylaxis.

‡‡‡The maximum recommended dosage for older adults (aged ≥65 yr) is 100 mg/day. The recommended pediatric dosage is 5 mg/kg/day up to a maximum of 150 mg/day in divided doses. For prophylaxis, the same daily dosage should be given for period at risk.

§§§Pediatric dosage is 5 mg/kg up to a maximum of 150 mg/day in divided doses. Not approved by FDA for treatment in children <13 yr. For prophylaxis, the same daily dosage should be given for period at risk.

‖‖‖Other interferons are also approved for this indication.

¶¶¶Reservoir concentration of 20 mg/mL. Requirements: special aerosol-generating device (available from manufacturer) and expert respiratory therapy monitoring for administration. Higher reservoir concentration (60 mg/mL) given for 2 hr tid is an alternative.

****Pediatric dosage of 500 mg/m²/8 hr for 7-10 day for children ≥1 year, although some experts recommend the 10-mg/kg/8-hr dosage for these children.86

AIDS, acquired immunodeficiency syndrome; FDA, U.S. Food and Drug Administration; HIV, human immunodeficiency virus; IM, intramuscular; IV, intravenous; PO, oral; SC, subcutaneous.

nucleotide mutations leading to critical amino acid substitutions in a target protein are often sufficient to cause antiviral resistance.

The possibility of drug resistance is usually recognized because of a lack of clinical and virologic response to treatment. However, clinical failures of antiviral therapy may involve drug-sensitive viruses in immunocompromised hosts who are unable to mount effective host responses. Factors favoring the emergence of resistant variants include high viral replicative load, as in infections with prolonged and rapid viral turnover; high intrinsic viral mutation rate, which is generally greater in RNA than in DNA viruses; degree of selective drug pressure, which is higher with prolonged or repeated courses of drug therapy; and an antiviral target that can mutate without adversely affecting viral fitness. Consequently, most drug-resistant viruses (including HSV, varicella-zoster virus [VZV], CMV, and HIV-1) are recovered from immunocompromised patients, although resistant influenza A virus and hepatitis B virus (HBV) occur in immunocompetent persons.

The consequences of the emergence of resistance may include a reduction or alteration (e.g., different clinical syndromes) in viral pathogenicity, although such viruses are able to cause severe disease in immunocompromised hosts. Whether resistant variants are at some biologic disadvantage with respect to transmissibility, ability to establish chronic or latent infection, or persistence in the absence of selective drug pressure depends on the particular virus and drug.

Drug Administration

Clinical efficacy depends on achieving effective antiviral concentrations at the site of infection, usually adequate intracellular concentrations of an agent or its active metabolites. Many antivirals, particularly nucleoside analogues, are inactive until they are metabolized within the cell to phosphorylated derivatives, which compete with natural nucleosides for viral and sometimes host cell enzymes. The state of activation or stage of differentiation of the cell can affect the intracellular pools of the phosphorylated antiviral and its competing natural substrate and thereby affect inhibitory activity and toxicity.[4]

Human pharmacokinetic studies that define absorption, stability in body fluids, tissue and cellular distribution, and metabolic fate of antiviral drugs are important in selecting proper dosage. Because predictive relationships between the drug concentrations that are active in vitro, those that are achieved in blood or other body fluids, and clinical response have not been established for most antiviral agents, pharmacodynamic studies that examine correlations of in vivo antiviral activity, dosage, and drug kinetics are particularly useful. Although animal models are useful in the testing of antiviral agents, they may differ from the corresponding human infection in regard to pathogenesis, drug susceptibility of the virus, and drug pharmacology or toxicity.

Topical application of an antiviral agent to the cornea, skin, mucus membranes, or respiratory tract is intended to provide high concentrations at the site of infection and to avoid the possible toxicity of systemic administration. However, topically applied drugs must be able to penetrate such barriers as stratified epithelium or local secretions to reach the site of active viral replication. Several topically applied agents are available for treating orolabial herpes and inhalation of antivirals has proven useful in several respiratory viral infections (see Table 38-1).

Combinations of antiviral agents with different mechanisms of action are used as a means of increasing antiviral activity, reducing drug dosage and the associated risk for toxicity, and preventing or modifying the development of drug resistance. Individual drugs may act preferentially on different cell types or in different tissues to enhance antiviral effects. Viral isolates from treated patients may be genetically heterogeneous with respect to mixtures of sensitive and resistant viruses or viruses with different resistance mutations, so that combinations may be able to provide broader activity than single agents. Combination antiviral therapy is the standard of care in HIV and hepatitis C virus (HCV) infections and is likely to become increasingly used in other viral infections. In addition, interactions with other drugs commonly used in immunocompromised hosts (chemotherapeutic or immunosuppressive agents) may sometimes increase the risk for toxi-

cities and possibly alter antiviral effects (e.g., mycophenolate potentiates the antiherpes activities of acyclovir, penciclovir, and ganciclovir by depletion of competing guanosine nucleotides).[5]

ACYCLOVIR AND VALACYCLOVIR

Spectrum

Acyclovir (9-[(2-hydroxyethoxy)methyl]-9H-guanine) (acycloguanosine, Zovirax) is a deoxyguanosine analogue that has an acyclic side chain lacking the 3′-hydroxyl group, instead of the cyclic base of natural nucleosides (Fig. 38-1A). Valacyclovir (Valtrex) is the L-valyl ester prodrug of acyclovir. Acyclovir's clinically useful antiviral spectrum is limited to herpesviruses. It is approximately 10 times more potent against HSV-1 and HSV-2 than against VZV, and it is even less active against CMV (Table 38-2).[6,7] Acyclovir inhibits the replication of Epstein-Barr virus (EBV) in productively infected cells but does not affect latent or persistent infection. Acyclovir has shown antiviral activity in experimental HSV infection when administered topically, parenterally, or orally and in simian varicella when given systemically.[6] Enhanced antiherpesvirus activity occurs when acyclovir is given in combination with interferons and other antiviral agents in vitro and in animal models.[6]

Growth of uninfected mammalian cells is generally unaffected by high acyclovir concentrations. Acyclovir (20 μg/mL) does not reproducibly alter cell-mediated immune responses of human peripheral blood leukocytes or affect human granulocyte progenitor cell growth in vitro.[8]

Mechanism of Action

Acyclovir is the prototype of a group of antiviral agents that are activated by viral thymidine kinase (TK) to become inhibitors of viral DNA polymerase and block viral DNA synthesis.[6,7,9] Acyclovir uptake and intracellular phosphorylation to the monophosphate derivative are facilitated by HSV TK. Cellular enzymes convert the monophosphate to acyclovir triphosphate, which is present in 40- to 100-fold higher concentrations in HSV-infected than in uninfected cells. Acyclovir triphosphate competitively inhibits viral DNA polymerase, and to a much smaller extent cellular DNA polymerases, with respect to deoxyguanosine triphosphate. Acyclovir triphosphate is also incorporated into viral DNA, where it acts as a chain terminator because of the lack of the 3′-hydroxyl group. Formation of a complex between the terminated DNA template containing acyclovir and the enzyme may lead to irreversible inactivation of the DNA polymerase. The DNA polymerases of various herpesviruses differ in their degree of inhibition by acyclovir triphosphate; the polymerases of EBV and CMV appear to be especially sensitive.

Resistance

Acyclovir-resistant HSV, often defined by an in vitro inhibitory concentration greater than 2 to 3 μg/mL, can be readily selected by passage in the presence of acyclovir and also is present in native virus populations, with an approximate frequency of 1 in 10^{-3} to 10^{-4} infectious virions.[9-11] Three basic resistance mechanisms have been identified: absent or low production of viral TK, altered TK substrate specificity (e.g., phosphorylation of thymidine but not of acyclovir), and altered viral DNA polymerase. Changes in these viral enzymes relate to point mutations or base insertions or deletions in the corresponding genes.[12,13] The most common mechanism found in clinical HSV isolates is absent or deficient TK activity.[9,14] Less commonly, resistant isolates have altered TK activity, and DNA polymerase mutants are rare in clinical strains. Heterogeneous mixtures are not uncommonly found. TK-negative variants are cross-resistant to other agents activated by viral TK (e.g., penciclovir, ganciclovir), but TK-altered and DNA polymerase mutants variably retain susceptibility.[9]

The prevalence of acyclovir-resistant HSV isolates in immunocompetent hosts is about 0.1% to 0.7% but increases to approximately 4% to 14% in immunocompromised patients.[9,12,15] During several decades of use, no increase in the prevalence of acyclovir-resistant

FIGURE 38-1. Chemical structures of acyclovir (**A**), penciclovir (**B**), ganciclovir (**C**), and the nucleoside deoxyguanosine (**D**).

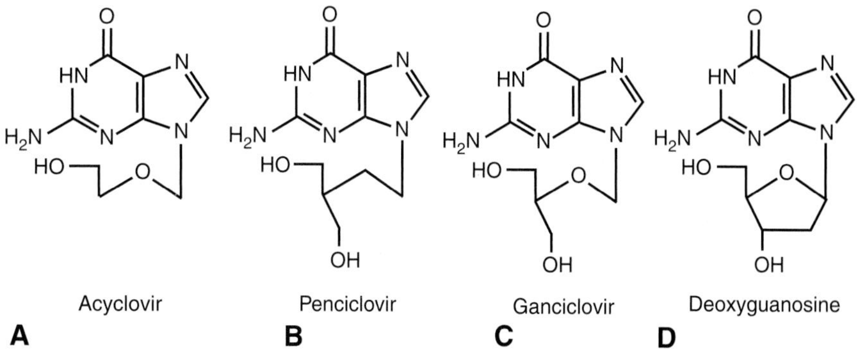

	Acyclovir	Penciclovir	Ganciclovir	Deoxyguanosine
	A	**B**	**C**	**D**

variants has occurred in immunocompetent persons.[9] Resistant HSV-2 has been found in 0.2% of HIV-negative and 5.3% of HIV-positive persons with genital herpes[16] and has been recovered from 11% to 17% of those with the acquired immunodeficiency syndrome (AIDS) or transplantation patients receiving acyclovir treatment for 2 weeks or longer.[17] Most isolates recovered during oral suppressive therapy of genital HSV remain susceptible. After chronic acyclovir suppression of genital HSV, the frequency of resistant HSV is comparable to that before treatment or in unexposed patients.[18] In contrast, progressive HSV disease associated with recovery of acyclovir-resistant virus and poor response to acyclovir therapy is well recognized in immunocompromised patients. Painful ulcerating perirectal lesions, often indolent and necrotizing, caused by HSV-2 represent the most common pattern in patients with AIDS, and orofacial disease due to HSV-1 is most common in transplant recipients. The risk factors for resistance emergence include degree of immunosuppression, size of lesions, repeated or prolonged use of acyclovir for treatment rather than prophylaxis, and, possibly, the use of topical acyclovir in genital herpes.[16]

TK-negative HSVs are less neurovirulent than wild-type strains and unable to reactivate from latency in animal models, although they may cause extensive mucocutaneous disease in immunocompromised hosts.[9,11] TK-deficient, TK-altered, or DNA polymerase mutants have variable decreases in pathogenicity. Acyclovir-resistant HSV recurrent genital or ocular infections have been found rarely in immunocompetent hosts.[9] One possible person-to-person spread of resistant HSV has been reported. Recurrences after cessation of acyclovir are usually caused by sensitive virus.[9] However, in patients with AIDS, persistent shedding of resistant HSV at the site of initial infection and recurrences with acyclovir-resistant variants have been found in the absence of selective drug pressure.[19] Visceral disease is uncommon, but pneumonitis, meningoencephalitis, esophagitis, hepatitis, retinal necrosis, and disseminated infection have occurred with resistant variants, including instances in neonates.[9,17,20]

Depending on the degree of immunosuppression, resistant HSV infections may undergo spontaneous healing during or after cessation of acyclovir therapy. In patients with progressive disease, intravenous foscarnet therapy is effective, but vidarabine is not.[19] Intravenous cidofovir also appears effective. High-dose, continuous infusion of acyclovir,[21]

topical trifluridine, topical interferon (IFN)-α2 alone or in combination with topical trifluridine,[22] topical foscarnet,[23] topical cidofovir gel, and topical imiquimod[24] have been used with variable success.[25]

Acyclovir resistance in VZV isolates, associated with 20- to 40-fold increases in inhibitory concentrations, is usually related to mutations in VZV TK with inability to phosphorylate acyclovir, or, less often, to mutations in viral DNA polymerase. Although rare, resistant isolates, including the Oka VZV vaccine strain,[26] have been recovered from highly immunocompromised children and adults with chronic (months) disseminated, hyperkeratotic or verrucous papular lesions that failed to heal with intravenous acyclovir.[27,28] Invasive disease with resistant variants occurs. Chronic suppressive therapy with subtherapeutic dosages of acyclovir appears to be a risk factor. Intravenous foscarnet or cidofovir may be effective for acyclovir-resistant VZV infections.[29]

Pharmacokinetics

The bioavailability of oral acyclovir is low (15% to 21%) and decreases with increasing dosages.[6] Peak plasma concentrations average 0.4 to 0.8 μg/mL after 200-mg oral doses and increase to about 1.6 μg/mL with 800-mg doses. Bioavailability is lower in transplant recipients, in whom doses of 400 mg provide peak levels of 0.7 to 0.9 μg/mL. A liquid suspension has somewhat lower oral bioavailability; peak plasma concentrations average 1.0 μg/mL in children receiving dosages of 600 mg/m². In neonates and infants younger than 2 years, oral bioavailability averages 12%, acyclovir kinetics are affected by prematurity and age less than 1 month, and weight-adjusted dosing is essential.[30] Peak and trough plasma concentrations average 9.8 and 0.7 μg/mL, respectively, after intravenous administration of 5 mg/kg every 8 hours, and 20.7 and 2.3 μg/mL, respectively, after 10 mg/kg every 8 hours. Peak concentrations average 10.3 and 20.7 μg/mL after intravenous dosages of 250 mg/m² and 500 mg/m², respectively, in children.

After oral administration, valacyclovir is readily absorbed, most likely via human peptide transporter 1 (hPEPT1), and rapidly converted to acyclovir during first-pass enzymatic hydrolysis in the liver and intestine by an enzyme designated valacyclovir hydrolase.[31] The relative bioavailability of acyclovir is three to five times greater after ingestion of valacyclovir, and the absolute bioavailability averages 54% to 70%.[32] Estimated bioavailability is 48% in hospitalized immunocompromised children 5 years old or older.[33] Peak plasma levels of valacyclovir are 0.4 μg/mL or less after 1000-mg doses. Peak plasma acyclovir levels average 5.0 and 8.5 μg/mL after doses of 1000 and 2000 mg, respectively, in adults and are estimated to be 7 to 8 μg/mL after doses of 30 mg/kg valacyclovir in children.[33] Total acyclovir exposure is similar to that seen with intravenous acyclovir, although peak plasma concentrations are twofold to fourfold lower.[34] In older adults, peak plasma concentrations increase 15% to 20% and overall acyclovir exposure increases 30% to 50%,[31] probably because of reduced renal clearance in this population.

Acyclovir is distributed widely in body fluids. Plasma protein binding is less than 20%. Concentrations over time in noninflamed cerebrospinal fluid (CSF) average 20% of those in serum.[35] Salivary con-

TABLE 38-2 Representative In Vitro Inhibitory Concentrations of Acyclic Nucleosides and Nucleotides for Clinical Isolates of Herpesviruses in Human Cells

Virus	Inhibitory Concentration (μg/mL)			
	Acyclovir	*Penciclovir*	*Ganciclovir*	*Cidofovir*
Herpes simplex virus 1	0.02-1.9	0.2-1.8	0.05-0.6	0.4-3
Herpes simplex virus 2	0.3-2.9	0.3-2.4	0.05-0.6	0.4-3
Varicella-zoster virus	0.8-5.2	0.9-5.1	0.2-2.8	0.25
Cytomegalovirus	2-57	52	0.2-2.8	0.2-0.9
Epstein-Barr virus	1.6	—	1.5	<0.03

Data from references 11, 13, 150, 152, 155, 192, 194, 262, 287, and 288.

centrations average 13% of plasma levels, but concentrations in vaginal secretions range from 15% to 170% of those in plasma. Zoster vesicular fluid levels are similar to those in plasma. Aqueous humor levels average 37% of concurrent plasma values. Acyclovir is concentrated in breast milk at approximately threefold higher levels than in maternal serum. Plasma levels in newborns are similar to maternal ones, and amniotic fluid and placental concentrations are several-fold higher.[36] Percutaneous absorption of acyclovir after topical administration appears to be low.

The mean plasma elimination half-life ($T_{1/2 elim}$) of acyclovir is about 2.5 to 3 hours (range, 1.5 to 6.3 hours) in adults with normal renal function; it is slightly longer (3.8 hours) in neonates and increases to 19.5 hours in anuric patients.[36,37] Renal excretion of unmetabolized acyclovir by glomerular filtration and tubular secretion accounts for 60% to 91% of an administered dose, whereas less than 15% is excreted as 9-carboxymethoxymethylguanine or minor metabolites.[38] Dosage reduction is indicated in patients with a creatinine clearance (CrCl) of less than 50 mL/min (Table 38-3). Hemodialysis removes 33% to 60% of acyclovir during a 6-hour session, whereas peritoneal dialysis removes very little.[39] Dosing is recommended after hemodialysis but supplementation is not needed during continuous ambulatory peritoneal dialysis. Bioavailability is about 61% after intraperitoneal dosing.[40]

Dosage adjustments for valacyclovir in patients with impaired renal function are presented in Table 38-4.

Interactions

Severe somnolence and lethargy may occur with combinations of zidovudine and acyclovir.[41] Concomitant use of cyclosporine and probably of other nephrotoxic agents enhances the risk for nephrotoxicity. Probenecid and cimetidine slow valacyclovir metabolism, decrease renal acyclovir clearance, and increase overall acyclovir exposure by 48% and 27%, respectively.[42] By competing for the organic acid secretory pathway, acyclovir may decrease the renal clearance of other drugs eliminated by active renal secretion, such as methotrexate. Thiazide diuretics or the hPEPT1 substrate cephalexin do not substantially alter valacyclovir pharmacokinetics.[31]

Toxicity

Topical acyclovir may cause transient burning when it is applied to genital lesions. The polyethylene glycol base of topical acyclovir may cause mucosal irritation and is not approved for intravaginal use. Acyclovir cream uncommonly causes allergic contact dermatitis.[6]

Intravenous acyclovir is generally well tolerated,[6] although inflammation, phlebitis, and, rarely, vesicular eruption can occur at the injection site after extravasation of the alkaline solution (pH 9 to 11). Uncommon side effects include rash, diaphoresis, hematuria, hypotension, headache, and nausea. Approximately 1% to 4% of patients receiving intravenous acyclovir have manifested neurotoxicity, characterized by lethargy, confusion, obtundation, tremor, myoclonus, hallucinations, delirium, seizures, extrapyramidal signs, autonomic instability, and/or coma.[43] Diffuse electroencephalographic abnormalities and increased CSF concentrations of myelin basic protein may occur. Symptoms of neurotoxicity usually develop within 1 to 3 days after starting treatment. Most of these patients have acute renal dysfunction or preexisting renal disease, and neurotoxicity occurs in association with high serum acyclovir concentrations (>25 µg/mL). Neurotoxicity occurs after oral acyclovir and more often after valacyclovir. Neurologic side effects usually resolve within several days after drug concentrations decrease. Hemodialysis may be useful in severe cases.

Reversible renal dysfunction has been observed in approximately 5% of patients, and a higher proportion of children, treated with intravenous acyclovir.[6] Acyclovir can cause a crystalline nephropathy and, rarely, interstitial nephritis.[44] Acyclovir solubility decreases to 2.5 mg/mL at 37° C, and crystalluria has been described in adult and pediatric patients. Obstructive nephropathy may be manifested by nausea, emesis, flank pain, and increasing azotemia. Bolus infusion, dehydration, preexisting renal insufficiency, high doses, and high acyclovir plasma levels are risk factors. Nephrotoxicity usually resolves with drug cessation and volume expansion.

Oral acyclovir has been associated infrequently with nausea, diarrhea, rash, and headache, and uncommonly with renal insufficiency or neurotoxicity. Immediate hypersensitivity reactions to acyclovir are rare but may be managed with oral desensitization.[45] Long-term acyclovir suppression for frequently recurring genital or mucocutaneous infections appears well tolerated for up to 10 years of use,[46,47] and no adverse effects on sperm production or peripheral blood lymphocyte cytogenetics have been detected.[48] However, oral acyclovir can cause neutropenia in infants.[49] High-dose valacyclovir (8 g/day) is associated with gastrointestinal intolerance, azotemia, and possibly thrombotic microangiopathy in patients with AIDS[50] and with confusion and hallucinations in transplant patients.[51] Tolerance at lower doses is comparable to that of acyclovir.

Acyclovir has shown mutagenic activity in some in vitro assays at high concentrations, but no significant immunosuppressive activity, carcinogenicity, or teratogenicity has been noted in animal studies. High doses decrease spermatogenesis and cause testicular atrophy in animals. Acyclovir is classified in pregnancy category B and is present in breast milk. No excess frequency of congenital abnormalities has been recognized in infants born to women exposed to acyclovir during pregnancy, although whether exposure may increase the risk for spontaneous abortion is unresolved.[46,52]

Clinical Studies

Acyclovir is the agent of choice for management of many types of HSV and VZV infections because of its efficacy, safety, and ease of administration (see Table 38-1).[6,7] Valacyclovir is comparably effective in most of the conditions in which oral acyclovir is used and offers more convenient dosing regimens at higher cost.

Herpes Simplex Virus. Acyclovir by various routes is effective in initial genital HSV infections.[53] Topical acyclovir is less effective than oral or intravenous administration, and its use is discouraged. Intravenous acyclovir markedly reduces viral shedding, time to healing, and duration of symptoms in patients hospitalized with severe primary genital HSV infections. In outpatients, oral acyclovir (200 mg five times daily for 10 days) is associated with significant reductions in virus shedding, symptoms, and time to healing. Higher doses of oral acyclovir do not increase efficacy,[53] and valacyclovir (1 g twice daily for 10 days) is comparable to acyclovir in efficacy and tolerability for treating first-episode genital herpes.[54] None of these regimens has

TABLE 38-3 Acyclovir Dosage Adjustments Suggested for Patients with Impaired Renal Function

Creatinine Clearance (mL/min/ 1.73 m²)	Intravenous		Oral*	
	Standard Dose (%)	Dosing Interval (hr)	Dose (mg)	Dosing Interval (hr)
>50	100	8	800	4
25-50	100	12	800	4
10-25	100	24	800	8
0-10†	50	24	800	12‡

*Oral acyclovir dosage adjustments are needed for severe renal insufficiency. Recommendations are based on high-dose oral regimen (4000 mg/day). For the low-dose (1000 mg/day) oral regimen, the suggested dosage is 200 mg q12h when creatinine clearance is less than 10 mL/min/1.73 m².

†An alternative in patients with end-stage renal disease is administration of 14% of standard dosage q8h after loading with 37% of the standard dosage. In hemodialysis, use 60% to 100% of the standard dosage after the hemodialysis run only.

‡In dialysis-dependent patients, a further dosage reduction to 200 mg/12 hr and 400 mg after dialysis is recommended to avoid toxic levels. A dosage of 800 mg PO q24h has been suggested for those on continuous ambulatory peritoneal dialysis.[546]

Adapted from Blum MR, Liao SH, de Miranda P. Overview of acyclovir pharmacokinetic disposition in adults and children. Am J Med. 1982;73:186-192; Laskin OL, Longstreth JA, Whelton A, et al. Effect of renal failure on the pharmacokinetics of acyclovir. Am J Med. 1982;73: 197-201.

been associated with consistent reductions in the risk for recurrent genital lesions. Acyclovir therapy decreases the humoral and cellular immune response to HSV after first-episode genital herpes. Higher oral dosages (400 mg five times daily for 10 days) provide similar benefit in first-episode HSV proctitis.

In recurrent genital HSV infections, patient-initiated oral acyclovir (200 mg five times daily for 5 days) during the prodrome or at the first sign of lesions is associated with reductions of 1.5 to 2 days in the duration of shedding and time to healing. A 2-day regimen of high-dose acyclovir (800 mg three times daily) is also associated with 2-day reductions in duration of lesions and symptoms.[55] Valacyclovir (500 mg twice daily for 5 days) is comparable to acyclovir and superior to placebo in the treatment of recurrent genital herpes.[56,57] A 3-day course of valacyclovir is as effective as a 5-day one.[58] Topical acyclovir offers no significant clinical benefit in this condition. In patients with frequently recurring genital herpes, long-term oral acyclovir (400 to 1000 mg/day in divided doses) reduces the frequency of clinical recurrences by about 90%, protects 65% to 85% of patients from recurrence, and reduces the frequency of subclinical viral shedding and viral DNA detectability.[47,59] Dosages of 400 mg twice daily are effective for longer than 5 years. Once-daily or weekend-only use of acyclovir is inadequate, whereas once-daily valacyclovir (500 mg, or 1000 mg if frequent recurrences) appears to be effective and well tolerated.[60] Valacyclovir suppression (500 mg daily) reduces the risk of transmitting HSV-2 infection to serosusceptible partners by approximately 50% in mismatched couples.[61] Asymptomatic shedding may occur during suppression, and transmission to sexual partners has occurred. After cessation of acyclovir, patients generally return to their previous pattern of recurrent infection. Oral acyclovir suppression during late pregnancy reduces virus shedding, recurrences, and possibly cesarean delivery rates for HSV after a first episode occurring during pregnancy and in women with recurrent genital herpes.[62,63]

Long-term suppression may be useful in other patients with disabling recurrences of herpes whitlow or HSV-related erythema multiforme. In patients with recurrent herpes labialis or ocular HSV disease, prolonged oral acyclovir (400 mg twice daily) or valacyclovir (500 mg once daily) reduces the number of recurrences by about one half.[64-66] In patients with a history of sun-induced recurrences, short-term prophylaxis (400 to 800 mg twice daily) inconsistently reduces the risk for recurrence.[67] Short-term prophylaxis during outbreaks in daycare centers may be effective in preventing primary infections in children,[68] but the efficacy of postexposure prophylaxis remains to be established.

In recurrent orolabial HSV infections in immunocompetent persons, topical acyclovir ointment is not beneficial. Topical 5% acyclovir cream is available in many countries outside of the United States, and patient-initiated treatment reduces the duration of an episode by about 0.5 day.[69] High-dose, patient-initiated oral valacyclovir (2 g twice in 1 day) reduces the duration of orolabial herpes episodes and healing time by about 1 day.[70] Oral acyclovir (200 to 400 mg five times daily for 5 days) provides modest clinical benefit in orolabial HSV but appears to be efficacious in recurrent whitlow.[71] Acyclovir (15 mg/kg five times daily to a maximum of 200 mg/dose for 7 days) is beneficial for treating primary HSV gingivostomatitis in children,[72] and chronic suppression reduces cutaneous recurrences after neonatal infection. Acyclovir combined with prednisone appears superior to prednisone alone for the treatment of Bell's palsy.[73]

Acyclovir in various regimens and valacyclovir have been used successfully for both prevention and treatment of mucocutaneous HSV infections in immunosuppressed patients.[1,7] Intravenous acyclovir (250 mg/m^2 every 8 to 12 hours, or 125 mg/m^2 every 6 hours), begun before transplantation and continuing for several weeks, is highly effective in reducing the incidence of HSV disease in seropositive bone marrow transplant recipients.[2] For patients who can tolerate oral medications, oral acyclovir (400 mg five times daily or 600 mg every 6 hours) or valacyclovir (500 mg twice daily) is effective in marrow transplant recipients, and long-term oral acyclovir (400 mg three times daily for 6 months) also reduces the risk for VZV infection.[75] Low doses of oral acyclovir (200 mg every 6 to 8 hours) appear to be effective in renal transplant recipients. Valacyclovir (500 mg twice daily) is effective for suppression of recurrent genital herpes in HIV-infected persons.[76]

In immunocompromised patients with established mucocutaneous HSV infection, intravenous acyclovir (250 mg/m^2 every 8 hours for 7 days) shortens healing time, duration of pain, and virus shedding,[1,77] although recurrences are common after cessation of therapy. Oral acyclovir (800 mg five times daily) is also effective.[78] Intravenous acyclovir may be beneficial in cases of viscerally disseminating HSV in pregnant women and transplant recipients.[79,80]

In HSV encephalitis, acyclovir reduces mortality to 19% to 28%, compared with 50% to 54% with vidarabine.[7] In neonates, in immunosuppressed patients, and, uncommonly, in apparently healthy persons, early relapse of encephalitis may follow initial acyclovir therapy; higher doses and longer courses of intravenous treatment are warranted in central nervous system (CNS) infections (see Table 38-1), and chronic oral suppression studies are in progress. High-dose intravenous acyclovir (60 mg/kg/day for 21 days) appears more effective than the dosage approved by the U.S. Food and Drug Administration (FDA) for neonatal CNS and disseminated HSV disease.[81] Acyclovir also appears to be effective in the acute retinal necrosis syndrome.[82]

Varicella-Zoster Virus Infections. High-dose oral acyclovir is effective treatment for herpes zoster in older adults, for zoster ophthalmicus, and, if begun within 24 hours after rash onset, for varicella in children,[83] adolescents,[84] and adults.[85] In children, acyclovir's effects include reductions of about 1 day in fever and of 15% to 30% in the severity of other illness measures, so routine use for uncomplicated varicella in otherwise healthy children younger than 13 years is not recommended.[86] In adults with varicella, oral acyclovir (800 mg five times daily for 7 days), initiated within 24 hours after the onset of rash, reduces fever and the time to total crusting of lesion by approximately 2 days; it does not affect the course of illness if begun later.[85] Postcontact prophylaxis with oral acyclovir (40 mg/kg daily in divided doses), beginning 9 to 11 days after exposure, may reduce the risk for varicella in household contacts.[87]

In immunocompetent older adults with herpes zoster, intravenous acyclovir reduces virus shedding, time to healing of skin lesions, and duration of acute pain. Oral acyclovir (800 mg five times daily for 7 to 10 days) also reduces acute pain and healing time in older adults, if treatment can be initiated within 72 hours after rash onset, and particularly within 1 or 2 days. A reduction in ocular complications, particularly keratitis and anterior uveitis, occurs with oral acyclovir or valacyclovir (1 g three times daily for 7 days) treatment of zoster ophthalmicus.[88] However, no consistent effect on the incidence or severity of postherpetic neuralgia has been found. Compared with acy-

TABLE 38-4 Dosage Adjustments of Valacyclovir in Patients with Impaired Renal Function

Creatinine Clearance (mL/min/1.73 m^2)	Herpes Zoster		Recurrent Genital HSV		Recurrent Orolabial Herpes	
	Dose	*Interval*	*Dose*	*Interval*	*Dosage*	*Interval*
>50	1 g	8 hr	500 mg	12 hr	2 g × 2	12 hr
30-49	1 g	12 hr	500 mg	12 hr	1 g × 2	12 hr
10-29	1 g	24 hr	500 mg	24 hr	500 mg × 2	12 hr
<10	500 mg	24 hr	500 mg	24 hr	500 mg	Once

Based on manufacturer's recommendations. Reductions are also indicated for other dosage regimens (e.g., for genital herpes suppression and initial treatment).

clovir, oral valacyclovir (1 g three times daily for 7 days) speeds resolution of zoster-associated pain and decreases the frequency of persistent pain.[34]

Intravenous acyclovir is effective for varicella and herpes zoster in immunocompromised patients. It also appears to be effective in varicella pneumonia or encephalitis in previously healthy adults.[89] In immunocompromised patients with herpes zoster, intravenous acyclovir (500 mg/m^2 every 8 hours for 7 days) reduces the risk for cutaneous dissemination and visceral complications. In immunosuppressed children with varicella, intravenous acyclovir reduces the risk for visceral complications and time to full crusting. Early relapse of infection may occur after cessation of therapy, and treatment may be ineffective in visceral disease. Early treatment with oral acyclovir (800 mg five times daily for 7 days) may be effective in immunocompromised children.[90]

Cytomegalovirus. Acyclovir is therapeutically ineffective in established CMV infections. High-dose intravenous acyclovir (500 mg/m^2 every 8 hours), beginning 5 days before allogeneic bone marrow transplantation and continuing for 30 days afterward, is associated with a delayed risk for CMV infection and, when followed by oral acyclovir (800 mg four times daily for 6 months), improved overall survival.[91,92] In seropositive allogeneic bone marrow or stem cell transplant recipients, valacyclovir (2 g four times a day after initial intravenous acyclovir) was more effective than high-dose oral acyclovir (800 mg four times a day)[93] and comparable to intravenous ganciclovir[93a] in preventing CMV reactivation.

High-dose oral acyclovir also reduces the risk for CMV disease in renal and liver transplant recipients but appears to be less effective than ganciclovir.[1,94,95] It has not proved effective in liver transplant recipients receiving OKT3 therapy or in lung transplant recipients. High-dose valacyclovir prophylaxis (2 g four times a day for 90 days) reduces the risk for CMV disease and of graft rejection in renal transplant recipients, including CMV seronegative recipients of seropositive grafts,[51] and appears effective in preventing CMV reactivation after heart transplantation.[96]

Other Viruses. Valacyclovir is recommended in managing herpes virus B (Cercopithecine herpesvirus 1) exposures and high-dose intravenous acyclovir (12.5 to 15 mg/kg/8 hr) or ganciclovir for treating non-CNS herpes virus B infections; intravenous ganciclovir is advised for CNS infection.[74] High-dose acyclovir has been reported to provide a modest survival benefit in advanced HIV infection, although this remains controversial.[97] High-dose valacyclovir, but not acyclovir, reduces CMV disease risk in advanced HIV infection but is less well tolerated and is associated with higher mortality.[50]

In infectious mononucleosis, acyclovir is associated with transient suppression of salivary EBV excretion but no important effects on illness parameters.[98] High-dose acyclovir is not effective in patients with the chronic fatigue syndrome. Some cases of severe EBV infection or EBV-related polyclonal lymphoproliferation may respond to acyclovir, and long-term acyclovir or related antivirals possibly reduce the risk for AIDS-related lymphoma.[99] EBV-related oral hairy leukoplakia usually regresses with oral acyclovir or valacyclovir treatment.[100]

Neither intravenous nor oral acyclovir enhances the response to IFN in patients with chronic hepatitis B. Long-term acyclovir does not reduce neurologic deterioration in multiple sclerosis.[101]

ADEFOVIR

Spectrum

Adefovir dipivoxil (9-[2-(phosphonomethoxy)ethyl]adenine; bis-POM, PMEA; Hepsera) is a diester prodrug of adefovir, an acyclic phosphonate nucleotide analogue of adenosine monophosphate (Fig. 38-2A). It is active in vitro against a range of DNA and RNA viruses, including hepatitis B, HIV, pox, and herpesviruses.[102,103] In cell culture, inhibitory concentrations for HBV range from 0.2 to 1.2 μM, whereas those inhibiting growth of uninfected cells are generally greater than 100 μM. Adefovir retains activity against lamivudine-resistant HBV strains and shows dose-dependent inhibition of hepadnavirus replication in animal models.[102] Combinations of adefovir with lamivudine or penciclovir show enhanced antihepadnavirus activity in vitro.[104]

Mechanism of Action

After intracellular transport, adefovir is converted by cellular enzymes to the diphosphate, which acts as a competitive inhibitor of viral DNA polymerases and reverse transcriptases with respect to deoxyadenosine triphosphate (dATP) and also serves as a chain terminator of DNA synthesis.[104,105] Its selectivity relates higher affinity for HBV DNA polymerase than for host cell polymerases. The prodrug is taken up intracellularly much more readily than the parent. The intracellular T$_{1/2}$ of the diphosphate is prolonged, ranging from 5 to 18 hours in different cells, which makes once-daily dosing feasible.[105]

Resistance

Adefovir resistance in HBV has been difficult to develop in the laboratory. No resistant variants have been detected during 48 to 60 weeks use in chronically infected patients.[106,107] After 144 weeks of dosing, 3.9% of patients show a novel HBV DNA polymerase mutation (N236T or A181V) that confers reduced susceptibility.[102] The consequences of resistance emergence remain to be determined, and lamivudine is inhibitory for such variants.

Pharmacology

Adefovir has low oral bioavailability (<12%).[105,108] In contrast, oral adefovir dipivoxil is rapidly absorbed and hydrolyzed to the parent compound by esterases in the intestine and/or blood, with liberation of pivalic acid. The bioavailability of adefovir ranges from approximately 30% to 60%, and after 10-mg doses of adefovir dipivoxil, peak serum concentrations average 0.02 μg/mL. No intact prodrug is detectable in the blood. Ingestion with food does not affect bioavailability. Adefovir has low protein binding (<5%) and has a volume of distribution approximating body water (approximately 0.4 L/kg).

Adefovir is eliminated unchanged by renal excretion through a combination of glomerular filtration and tubular secretion. After intravenous dosing, more than 98% is recovered in urine within 24 hours.[108] After oral administration of adefovir dipivoxil, about 30% to 45% of the dose is recovered within 24 hours, and the serum T$_{1/2elim}$ is approximately 5 to 7.5 hours. HIV-infected children have higher clearance than adults.

The peak plasma levels increase and clearance decreases with decreasing renal function, so that dosage reductions are indicated (Table

FIGURE 38-2. Chemical structures of adefovir (**A**) and lamivudine (**B**).

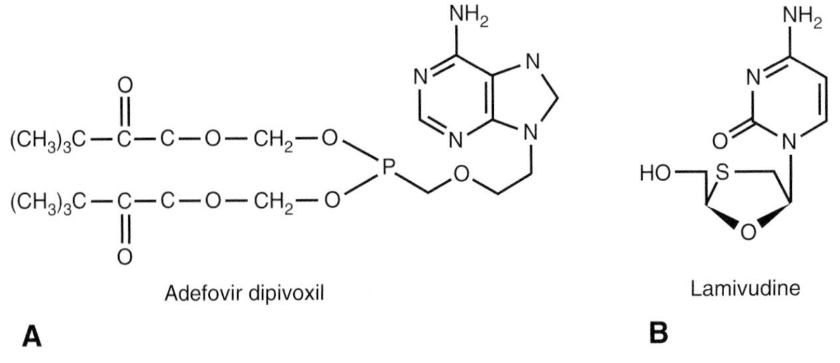

Adefovir dipivoxil

Lamivudine

A

B

38-5). Adefovir is removed by hemodialysis (approximately 35% of the dose during a 4-hour session), but the effects of peritoneal dialysis are unknown. The pharmacokinetics of adefovir in severe hepatic insufficiency are unreported.

Interactions

No clinically important drug interactions have been recognized to date, although drugs that reduce renal function or compete for active tubular secretion could decrease adefovir clearance. Ibuprofen increases adefovir exposure somewhat, but no interactions with lamivudine, acetaminophen, or trimethoprim-sulfa have been found. An increased risk for lactic acidosis and steatosis may exist when used in conjunction with nucleoside analogues or other antiretrovirals.

Toxicity

Nephrotoxicity at higher doses was the primary adverse event leading to discontinuation of HIV clinical studies in 1999. Adefovir is efficiently transported into tubular epithelium by a probenecid-sensitive human organic anion transporter (hOAT1), and inhibitory effects of the diphosphate on renal adenyl cyclase may contribute to nephrotoxicity. In HIV trials utilizing dosages of 60 mg daily, a Fanconi-like disorder with elevations of serum creatinine, decreases in serum phosphorus and bicarbonate, glycosuria, and proteinuria developed gradually after 20 weeks of dosing. It was generally mild-moderate in severity, and usually reversible after a median duration of 4 months. Older age and preexisting renal insufficiency appeared to be risk factors.

In studies of chronic hepatitis B, a lower dose (10 mg daily) has been associated with few adverse events (headache, abdominal discomfort, diarrhea, asthenia) and minimal renal toxicity compared with a higher one (30 mg).[106,109] Adverse events lead to premature discontinuation in about 2% of patients. At 96 weeks of dosing, the estimated risks of a rise in serum creatinine of 0.3 or greater and of a rise of 0.5 mg/dL or greater are 10% and 2%, respectively, but the risk is substantially higher in those with preexisting renal insufficiency. During therapy, marked increases in aminotransferase levels (>10 times the upper limit of normal) occur less often in adefovir recipients (10%) than placebo. Acute, sometimes severe exacerbations of hepatitis can occur in patients who stop adefovir or other anti-HBV therapies. Close monitoring is necessary and resumption of therapy may be required.

Pivalic acid, a product of adefovir dipivoxil metabolism, can esterify free carnitine and cause reduced free carnitine levels. Although L-carnitine was administered in some HIV studies, supplementation is generally not recommended at the dosages used in chronic hepatitis B.

In preclinical studies, adefovir is genotoxic and high doses cause renal tubular nephropathy, hepatotoxicity, and toxicity to lymphoid tissues in animals. Carcinogenicity studies in rodents are negative. Adefovir dipivoxil is not associated with reproductive toxicity, although high intravenous doses of adefovir cause maternal toxicity and embryotoxicity with fetal malformations in rats. It is classified as pregnancy category C.

Clinical Studies

Adefovir dipivoxil is approved for treatment of chronic hepatitis B and causes dose-dependent inhibition of HBV replication within 1 week of starting administration. In patients with chronic hepatitis B and positive for the e antigen (HB$_e$Ag), adefovir (10 mg daily for 48 weeks) results

in improved hepatic histology in 53%, reduced serum HBV DNA levels (>3.5 log$_{10}$ copies/mL), normal aminotransferase levels in 48%, and a 12% rate of HB$_e$Ag seroconversion.[109] Continued therapy is associated with sustained viral suppression and increasing frequencies of normalization of aminotransferase and HB$_e$Ag loss and seroconversion.[102,109] Similarly, in patients with HB$_e$Ag-negative chronic hepatitis B (pre-core mutants), adefovir dipivoxil (10 mg daily for 48 weeks) is associated with significant reductions in HBV DNA (nearly 4 log$_{10}$), normalization of transaminase levels in 72%, and histologic improvement in 64%.[106] Regression of cirrhosis may occur in some patients.[102]

In patients with lamivudine-resistant HBV infections, adefovir dipivoxil monotherapy results in sustained reductions in serum HBV DNA levels comparable to reductions seen with the combination of adefovir and lamivudine, whereas lamivudine monotherapy is ineffective.[109a] In patients with dual HIV and lamivudine-resistant HBV infections, adefovir dipivoxil (10 mg daily) causes sustained decreases in HBV DNA levels.[110] Adefovir dipivoxil has also been used successfully in patients with lamivudine-resistant HBV infections both before and after liver transplantation,[111] in whom approximately 4 log$_{10}$ reductions in HBV DNA levels, improved biochemical markers, and stable or improved histology have been observed.

The optimal duration of treatment in different populations, possible long-term effects on HBV complications, and combined use with other anti-HBV agents are under study.

AMANTADINE AND RIMANTADINE

Spectrum

Amantadine (1-adamantanamine hydrochloride; Symmetrel) and rimantadine (alpha-methyl-1-adamantane methylamine hydrochloride; Flumadine) are symmetric tricyclic amines (Fig. 38-3A and B) that specifically inhibit the replication of influenza A viruses at low concentrations (<1.0 µg/mL). By plaque assay, inhibitory concentrations of the drugs range from 0.1 to 0.4 µ/mL or less for human influenza A viruses. Rimantadine is 4 to 10 times more active than amantadine in some assay systems. Both are inhibitory for virus containing the M protein from the 1918 pandemic strain.[112]

Higher concentrations (10 to 50 µg/mL) have in vitro inhibitory activity against other enveloped viruses, including parainfluenza, influenza B, rubella, and dengue, but these concentrations are not achievable clinically and can be cytotoxic and immunosuppressive in vitro.[113] Rimantadine has pH-dependent trypanocidal activity at concentrations of approximately 1 µg/mL.[114] Amantadine may transiently inhibit HCV replication in humans.[115]

These agents have both prophylactic and therapeutic activity in experimental influenza A virus infection of animals after oral or parenteral dosing. Combinations of M2 inhibitors and neuraminidase inhibitors, ribavirin, interferons, or protease inhibitors show enhanced antiviral and therapeutic effects in vitro and/or in animal models of influenza.[116,117]

TABLE 38-5 Dosage Adjustments of Adefovir Dipivoxil in Renal Impairment

Creatinine Clearance (mL/min)	Oral Dose	Interval
≥50	10 mg	q24h
20-49	10 mg	q48h
10-19	10 mg	q72h
Hemodialysis	10 mg	q7day after dialysis

Dosage is based on manufacturer's recommendations.

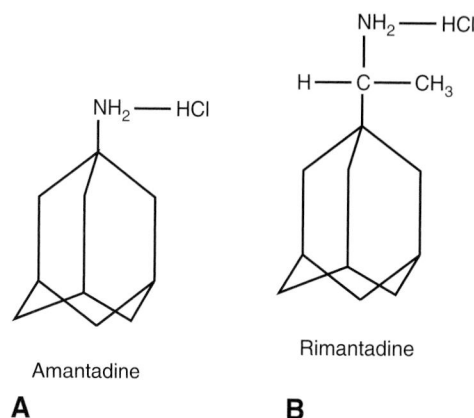

FIGURE 38-3. Chemical structures of amantadine hydrochloride (**A**) and rimantadine hydrochloride (**B**).

Mechanism of Action

Amantadine and rimantadine share two concentration-dependent mechanisms of anti-influenza action. Low concentrations inhibit the ion channel function of the M2 protein of influenza A viruses, which affects two different stages in virus replication.[118-120] The primary effect involves inhibition of viral uncoating or disassembly of the virion during endocytosis. For subtype H5 and H7 viruses, a late effect on hemagglutinin (HA) maturation and viral assembly is presumably mediated through altered pH regulation of the trans-Golgi network. Amantadine and rimantadine block proton permeation and prevent M2-mediated changes in pH. This action probably accounts for both inhibition of the acid-mediated dissociation of the matrix protein from the ribonucleoprotein complex within endosomes early in replication and potentiation of acidic pH–induced alterations in the hemagglutinin during its transport late in infection.

Amantadine and rimantadine are also concentrated in the lysosomal fraction of mammalian cells. Drug-mediated increases in lysosomal pH may inhibit virus-induced membrane fusion events and account for the broader antiviral spectrum at higher concentrations. In contrast, the selective anti-influenza A virus effects are quickly lost after removal of the drug from the surrounding medium, which suggests that drug must be present in extracellular fluid early in the replicative cycle.

Amantadine inhibits the ion channel activity of expressed HCV p7 protein at low concentrations,[121] an effect that might account for its reported anti-HCV effects in vivo. Neither agent inhibits HCV enzyme functions or internal ribosome entry in biochemical assays.[122]

Resistance

Contemporary epidemic strains have been M2 inhibitor sensitive, but resistant virus is readily selected by virus passage in the presence of drug. Resistance with more than 100-fold increases in inhibitory concentrations has been associated with single amino acid substitutions at critical sites (positions 26, 27, 30, 31, 34) in the transmembrane region of the M2 protein.[118] Amantadine and rimantadine share cross-resistance with each other and with other M2 inhibitors. In avian models, resistant viruses are virulent, genetically stable, and able to compete with wild-type virus, so that transmission of drug-resistant virus may occur after cessation of drug use.

A small fraction of untreated patients (<1%) have infection with resistant virus.[123] Approximately 30% of drug-treated ambulatory children and adults and up to 80% of hospitalized children or immunocompromised patients shed resistant virus.[124-126] Immunocompetent persons shedding resistant virus resolve their illness promptly,[127] whereas prolonged shedding and illness may occur in immunocompromised hosts.[125] Transmission of M2 inhibitor–resistant virus, associated with failure of drug prophylaxis, occurs in household contacts of treated index cases and in nursing home residents.[128] Resistant variants can cause typical influenza illness. It is prudent to avoid contact between treated patients and susceptible high-risk contacts and to avoid use of both treatment (specifically of young children) and postexposure prophylaxis in the same household.

Ribavirin and the neuraminidase inhibitors zanamivir and oseltamivir carboxylate are active in vitro against M2 inhibitor–resistant strains.

Pharmacokinetics

Amantadine. Amantadine is well absorbed after oral administration of capsule, tablet, or syrup forms.[113] Steady-state peak plasma concentrations average 0.5 to 0.8 µg/mL with a 100-mg twice daily regimen in healthy young adults. Older adults require only one half of the weight-adjusted dosage needed for young adults to achieve equivalent trough plasma levels of 0.3 µg/mL. Plasma protein binding of amantadine is about 67%, and amantadine's volume of distribution is large (4 to 5 L/kg). Nasal secretion and salivary levels of amantadine approximate those found in the serum. CSF levels are 52% to 96% of those in plasma, and amantadine is excreted in breast milk.

Amantadine is eliminated largely unchanged in the urine by glomerular filtration and probably tubular secretion. The plasma $T_{1/2elim}$ is about 12 to 18 hours, ranges widely, and correlates with creatinine clearance. Because of age-related declines in renal function, $T_{1/2elim}$ increases up to twofold in older adults and even more in patients with impaired renal function. Dosage reductions are required in renal insufficiency (Table 38-6). Amantadine is inefficiently cleared in patients receiving hemodialysis or continuous ambulatory peritoneal dialysis (CAPD), and additional doses are not required. Monitoring of plasma concentrations in such patients is desirable but impractical.

Rimantadine. Rimantadine is well but slowly absorbed, with the time to peak plasma concentration averaging 2 to 6 hours. Absorption does not appear to be decreased by food. With multiple doses of 100 mg twice daily, the steady-state peak and trough plasma concentrations in healthy adults are approximately 0.4 to 0.5 and 0.2 to 0.4 µg/mL, respectively. In infants receiving dosages of 3 mg/kg each day, peak serum levels range from 0.1 to 0.6 µg/mL. No important age-related changes in pharmacokinetics have been found in healthy older adults or in children. However, steady-state plasma concentrations in older nursing home residents receiving 100 mg twice daily average more than twofold higher (mean, 1.2 µg/mL) than those observed in healthy adults, which indicates the need for lower dosages in these patients. Plasma protein binding is about 40%. Rimantadine has a very large volume of distribution (about 12 L/kg), and concentrations in nasal mucus average 50% higher than those in plasma.

In contrast to amantadine, rimantadine undergoes extensive metabolism by hydroxylation, conjugation, and glucuronidation before renal excretion.[113] The plasma $T_{1/2elim}$ of rimantadine averages 24 to 36 hours. No clinically important differences in pharmacokinetics are found in patients with chronic liver disease without significant hepatocellular dysfunction. In hemodialysis patients with severe renal failure, the clearance of rimantadine is decreased by 40% and the $T_{1/2elim}$ is about 55% longer. Reducing dosages by one half (e.g., to 100 mg/day) is recommended for marked hepatic or renal insufficiency (CrCl <10 mL/min). Hemodialysis removes only a small amount of rimantadine, so supplemental doses are not required.

Interactions

The risks of CNS adverse effects with amantadine and possibly with rimantadine are increased by concomitant ingestion of antihistamines,

TABLE 38-6 Amantadine Dosage Regimens for Prophylaxis and Alterations in Renal Failure

Condition	Suggested Dosage
No Renal Insufficiency	
Children, 1-9 yr	5 mg/kg/day in 2 divided doses, up to 150 mg/day
Ages 10-64 yr	100 mg twice daily
Ages ≥65 yr	100 mg once daily*
Creatinine Clearance (mL/min/1.73 m²)†	
≥80	100 mg (1.4 mg/kg) twice daily
79-35	100 mg once daily
34-25	100 mg q2d
24-15	100 mg q3d
<15	100 mg q7d
Older Adults and Creatinine Clearance (mL/min/1.73 m²)‡	
≥80	100 mg daily
60-79	100 mg and 50 mg on alternate days
40-59	100 mg q2d
30-39	100 mg twice wkly
20-29	50 mg twice wkly
10-19	100 mg and 50 mg on alternate wk

*Use weight-adjusted dosing for smaller patients (<50 kg). Dosages of 1.4 mg/kg/day have been suggested.[113]

†Based on adult dosage of 200 mg/day. Proportionate reductions should be made for older adults receiving lower dosages and for children.

‡This dosing schedule for older adults with renal insufficiency is taken from the Canadian guidelines and has been found to be reasonably well tolerated.[133]

Adapted from Wu MJ, Ing TS, Soung LS, et al. Amantadine hydrochloride pharmacokinetics in patients with impaired renal function. Clin Nephrol. 1982;17:19-23.

antidepressants, anticholinergic drugs, and other drugs affecting CNS function. Concurrent use of trimethoprim-sulfamethoxazole or of triamterene-hydrochlorothiazide has been associated with CNS toxicity resulting from decreased renal clearance of amantadine. Cimetidine is associated with 15% to 20% increases, and aspirin or acetaminophen with 10% decreases in plasma rimantadine concentrations, but such changes are unlikely to be of significance.

Toxicity

The most common side effects related to amantadine ingestion are minor, dose-related gastrointestinal and CNS complaints. These include nervousness, lightheadedness, difficulty concentrating, confusion, insomnia, and loss of appetite or nausea.[129] Complaints typically develop within the first week of administration, often resolve despite continued ingestion, and are reversible on drug discontinuation. CNS side effects occur in approximately 5% to 33% of amantadine recipients at dosages of 200 mg/day but are significantly less frequent with rimantadine. When used for influenza prophylaxis in ambulatory adults, dosages of 200 mg/day are associated with excess withdrawals in 6% to 11% of recipients because of drug side effects. Dosages of 100 mg/day are better tolerated and may be protective against influenzal illness. Amantadine dosage reductions are required in older adults (100 mg/day), but 20% to 40% of nursing home residents experience significant adverse effects on this lower dosage despite some adjustment for renal insufficiency.[130-132] Consequently, further dosage reductions based on CrCl are warranted in this population.[133]

In the setting of renal insufficiency or high dosages, serious neurotoxic reactions, including delirium, hostility, hallucinations, tremor, myoclonus, seizures, or coma; cardiac arrhythmias; and death can occur in association with elevated amantadine plasma concentrations (1.0 to 5.0 μg/mL).[134] Neurotoxic reactions may be transiently reversed by physostigmine administration, and lidocaine has been used to treat ventricular arrhythmias. Long-term amantadine ingestion has been associated with livedo reticularis, peripheral edema, orthostatic hypotension, and, rarely, congestive heart failure, vision loss, or urinary retention. Patients with preexisting seizure disorders have an increased frequency of major motor seizures during amantadine use, and dosage reductions are advised. Psychiatric side effects in patients with Parkinson's disease and psychotic exacerbations in patients with schizophrenia may occur with addition of amantadine. Rash and leukopenia have been described rarely.

Rimantadine administration is associated with dose-related side effects similar to those observed with amantadine, although the risk for CNS side effects is lower with rimantadine at dosages of 200 or 300 mg/day in ambulatory adults.[113] During prophylaxis, excess withdrawal rates are usually less than 5%. In older nursing home residents, 200 mg/day dosages are associated with higher side effect rates, whereas 100 mg/day dosages appear to be better tolerated.[130,135] Rimantadine may uncommonly cause exacerbations of seizures in those not receiving anticonvulsants and was associated with an unexplained excess mortality in one nursing home study.[135]

The clinical observations of dry mouth, pupillary dilation, toxic psychosis, and urinary retention in acute amantadine overdose suggest that anticholinergic activity is present in humans. Amantadine demonstrates activity on the adrenergic nervous system by affecting accumulation, release, and reuptake of catecholamines in the CNS and in the peripheral nervous system. Malignant ventricular arrhythmia after amantadine overdose has been described in humans.

Both amantadine and rimantadine lack mutagenicity in vitro; carcinogenicity studies have not been reported for either. Amantadine is teratogenic and embryotoxic in rats, and rimantadine may cause teratogenic effects in rabbits, as well as maternal toxicity and embryotoxicity at high dosages in rodents. Both drugs are classified in pregnancy category C. Birth defects have been reported after amantadine exposure during pregnancy,[136] and the safety of either drug has not been established in pregnancy. Because of excretion in breast milk, use is not recommended in nursing mothers.

Clinical Studies

Influenza A. The clinical usefulness of amantadine and rimantadine is limited currently to the prevention and treatment of influenza A virus infections.[113,129,137] Both drugs, at a dosage of 200 mg/day in adults, are about 70% to 90% protective against clinical illness caused by various influenza A subtypes, including pandemic strains.[138] Prophylaxis is effective in preventing nosocomial influenza and possibly in curtailing nosocomial outbreaks. Protection appears to be additive to that provided by vaccine.[139] Rimantadine administration to school-aged children (5 mg/kg/day) decreases the risk for influenza A illness in recipients and possibly in their family contacts. However, postexposure prophylaxis with these drugs provides inconsistent protection to family contacts, in part depending on whether ill index children are treated.[124] Dosages of 100 mg/day appear to be protective against influenza A illness and are well tolerated in adults.[140]

Amantadine and rimantadine are also effective therapies in uncomplicated influenza A illness,[113,127] but it remains uncertain whether treatment reduces the risk for complications in high-risk patients or is useful in patients with established pulmonary complications. Early treatment in ambulatory adults (200 mg/day for 5 days) reduces the duration of fever and systemic complaints by 1 to 2 days, decreases virus shedding, and shortens time to resumption of usual activities.[127] In illness caused by H3N2-subtype influenza viruses, certain abnormalities of peripheral airways function, but not of airway hyperreactivity, resolve more quickly in amantadine-treated patients. Therapeutic benefits occur in older influenza patients treated with rimantadine. Amantadine or rimantadine treatment in adults with leukemia or stem cell transplant may reduce the risk for pneumonia.[141] In children, rimantadine treatment is associated with lower symptom burden, fever, and viral titers during the first 2 days of treatment, compared with acetaminophen administration, but rimantadine-treated children have more prolonged shedding of virus. Treatment generally does not appear to affect immune responses to infection but may blunt secretory antibody levels.[142]

Intermittent aerosol administration of amantadine or rimantadine appears to be therapeutically useful in uncomplicated influenza. An injectable formulation of either drug is not available in the United States.

Other Viruses. Amantadine has been used in multiple trials for treatment of chronic hepatitis C with inconsistent evidence for increases in sustained viral response (SVR). In treatment-naïve patients, the addition of amantadine (200 mg daily in single or divided doses) to interferon[143,144] or to IFN plus ribavirin[145] may modestly increase biochemical responses and the likelihood of SVR. In retreatment of IFN nonresponders, the combination of IFN plus amantadine is not effective,[146] but the addition of amantadine to the combination of IFN plus ribavirin may be associated with SVR in 10% to 25%.[147] Amantadine plus combined pegylated interferon (pegIFN) and ribavirin may increase SVR modestly in treatment-experienced patients compared with pegIFN plus ribavirin.[148] Reports of possible activity in bornavirus infections and associated neuropsychiatric symptoms require confirmation.

CIDOFOVIR

Spectrum

Cidofovir (S)-1-[3-hydroxy-2-(phosphomethoxy) propyl] cytosine dihydrate); (HPMPC, Vistide) is an acyclic phosphonate nucleotide analogue of deoxycytidine monophosphate (Fig. 38-4A) with inhibitory activity against human herpesviruses, including CMV, EBV, human herpesvirus-6 (HHV-6), and HHV-8, and other DNA viruses, including papillomaviruses, polyomaviruses, poxviruses, and adenoviruses.[102,149-151] In vitro inhibitory concentrations range from less than 0.2 to 0.7 μg/mL for CMV,[152] 0.4 to 33 μg/mL for HSV,[153] and 0.02 to 17 μg/mL for adenoviruses.[154] Because phosphorylation does not depend on virus-specified enzymes, cidofovir is inhibitory for acyclovir-resistant, TK-deficient, or TK-altered HSV strains and ganciclovir-resistant CMV strains with UL97 mutations, although not for those with UL54 mutations. TK mutants of HSV show up to 20-fold enhanced susceptibility to cidofovir compared with wild-type HSV,

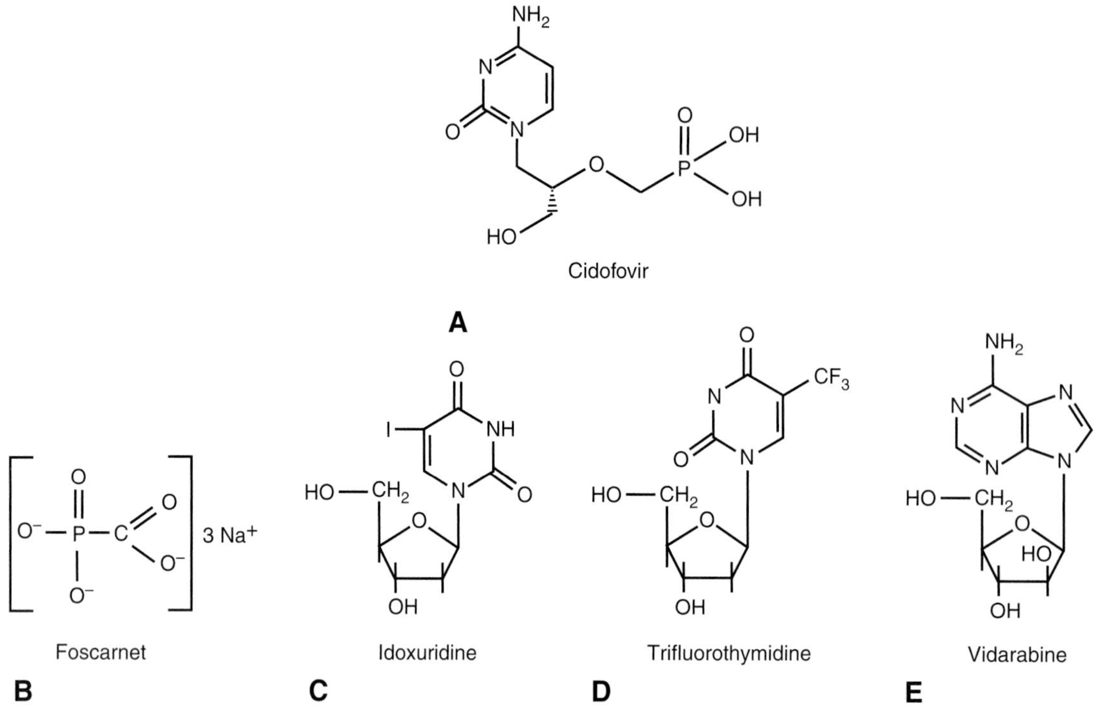

FIGURE 38-4. Chemical structures of other antiherpesvirus antiviral agents: cidofovir (**A**), foscarnet (**B**), idoxuridine (**C**), trifluorothymidine (**D**), and vidarabine (**E**).

because mutant viruses induce smaller elevations in competing deoxycytidine triphosphate (dCTP) pools in infected cells.[155] In vitro, cidofovir shows synergistic inhibition of CMV in combination with ganciclovir or foscarnet.[150] The prolonged intracellular half-life of the diphosphate is associated with persistent antiviral activity and enables infrequent dosing regimens. Cidofovir is active in animal models of herpesvirus, papillomavirus, and, given systemically or by aerosol, poxvirus infections.[156-158] Topical cidofovir is active against ocular adenovirus infection in rabbits but is associated with local irritation.[159]

Mechanism of Action

Cidofovir inhibits viral DNA synthesis. Cidofovir is metabolized intracellularly to its active diphosphate form by cellular enzymes, and the levels of phosphorylated metabolites are similar in infected and uninfected cells. The diphosphate acts both as a competitive inhibitor with respect to dCTP and as an alternative substrate for viral DNA polymerase. Incorporation of cidofovir slows chain elongation and abrogates it if two consecutive cidofovir molecules are introduced. The diphosphate has a prolonged intracellular half-life, averaging 17 to 65 hours depending on the cell type, and it competitively inhibits CMV and HSV DNA polymerase at concentrations 8- to 600-fold lower than those inhibitory for human DNA polymerases.[149,160] An adduct with prolonged intracellular half-life (>2 days) may serve as a reservoir of drug.

Alkoxyalkyl ester prodrugs of cidofovir have enhanced cellular uptake, are more potent poxvirus inhibitors than the parent, are well absorbed orally, and are not renally concentrated.[103] Two ether lipid esters, hexadecyloxypropyl-cidofovir (HDP-CDV) and octadecyloxyethyl-cidofovir (ODE-CDV), administered orally are highly active in experimental poxvirus and CMV infections in animals.[161]

Resistance

Resistance to cidofovir selected by in vitro passage of CMV, poxviruses, and adenovirus relates to point mutations in viral DNA polymerase. Highly ganciclovir-resistant clinical isolates of CMV that possess UL54 mutations show cross-resistance to cidofovir in vitro with 8- to 16-fold reductions in inhibitory concentrations.[162] Foscarnet-resistant CMV and HSV isolates may retain susceptibility to cidofovir, but multidrug-resistant CMV variants with DNA poly-

merase mutations occur.[163] The development of resistance to cidofovir as a result of cidofovir therapy appears to be uncommon and low level (less than eightfold change in susceptibility).[152,164] In patients with CMV retinitis, reduced cidofovir susceptibility has been detected in about 5% before treatment and in 29% by 3 months of therapy.[165] Poxviruses selected for resistance to cidofovir in vitro (8- to 27-fold reduced susceptibility) appear less virulent than wild-type viruses but are resistant to cidofovir in vivo.[166]

Pharmacokinetics

Oral bioavailability is low (<5%).[105] After intravenous infusion, plasma levels are proportional to dose and decline in a biphasic pattern, with a terminal $T_{1/2}$ that averages about 2.6 hours.[167] The maximum plasma concentration averages 19.6 µg/mL after a 5 mg/kg dose in conjunction with probenecid.[105] Plasma protein binding is low (<7%), and the volume of distribution approximates total body water (0.5 L/kg). CSF penetration is low.[105] Cidofovir is cleared by the kidney via glomerular filtration and active tubular secretion. More than 90% of the dose is recovered unchanged in the urine, and no significant metabolism has been recognized in humans. High-dose probenecid (2 g 3 hours before and 1 g 2 and 8 hours after each infusion) reduces renal clearance (by blocking tubular secretion of cidofovir) and increases blood levels. Clearance correlates with CrCl, and the $T_{1/2elim}$ increases to 32.5 hours in patients receiving CAPD.[105] About 50% of a dose is removed by hemodialysis or CAPD. After application of cidofovir gel, systemic absorption is low (peak plasma concentrations, <0.5 µg/mL) and is related to lesion size.[153]

Interactions

Probenecid but not cidofovir alters zidovudine pharmacokinetics, and zidovudine dosages should be reduced on administration days. Probenecid may interact with a variety of drugs (e.g., β-lactams, nonsteroidal anti-inflammatory drugs [NSAIDs], lorazepam, furosemide, methotrexate, theophylline, rifampin) and necessitate reductions in their dosage.[105] Concomitant therapy with other nephrotoxic agents is contraindicated during cidofovir therapy, and an interval of at least 7 days is recommended after aminoglycoside, intravenous pentamidine, amphotericin B, foscarnet, NSAID, or contrast dye exposure.

Toxicity

Dose-related nephrotoxicity is the principal side effect of intravenous cidofovir.[150] It is characterized by proximal tubular dysfunction including proteinuria, azotemia, glycosuria, metabolic acidosis, and, uncommonly, Fanconi's syndrome. Nephrotoxicity appears as a result of a cidofovir-avid renal organic anion transport protein that causes drug accumulation in the renal cortex. Concomitant oral probenecid and vigorous saline prehydration reduce, whereas prior foscarnet therapy and concurrent use of other nephrotoxic agents increase, the risk for renal toxicity. On maintenance dosing (5 mg/kg every other week), approximately 12% to 39% of patients develop proteinuria and 15% to 24% have elevated serum creatinine. Severe nephrotoxicity requiring dialysis sometimes occurs. Initiation of cidofovir is relatively contraindicated in those with CrCl <55 mL/min or with significant proteinuria (2+). Dosage reductions (3 mg/kg) are indicated for minor rises in serum creatinine (0.3 to 0.4 mg/dL), and cessation of administration for greater creatinine rises or development of proteinuria of 3+ or higher.

Neutropenia develops in approximately 24%, and regular monitoring of neutrophil counts is necessary. Fever, nausea, emesis, diarrhea, headache, rash, asthenia, iritis, uveitis, and ocular hypotony may occur during combined therapy with cidofovir and probenecid.[150,168] Maintenance is withdrawn in approximately 25% to 35% of patients with AIDS because of intolerance.

Mucosal application is associated with dose-related application site reactions (burning, pain, pruritus) in up to one third of patients, and occasionally with ulceration, but no evidence of systemic toxicity has been reported.[153] Intravitreal cidofovir may cause iritis, vitreitis, reduced intraocular pressure, and visual loss.[168a] Conjunctival application causes local irritation; persistent epiphora related to lacrimal canalicular blockade has developed in some patients.

Preclinical studies indicate that cidofovir has mutagenic, gonadotoxic, embryotoxic, and teratogenic effects. Because cidofovir causes carcinomas in rats, this agent is considered a potential human carcinogen. Safety during pregnancy is uncertain, and it is classified in pregnancy category C.

Clinical Studies

Intravenous cidofovir is approved for the treatment of CMV retinitis in patients with AIDS. Intravenous cidofovir (5 mg/kg once a week for 2 weeks, followed by every-other-week dosing) significantly increases the time to progression of CMV retinitis in previously untreated patients and in those failing or intolerant of ganciclovir and foscarnet therapy.[150,169,170] Maintenance dosages of 5 mg/kg every other week are more effective but less well tolerated than 3 mg/kg dosages.[171] Clearance of viruria but not viremia has been demonstrated.[172] Intravenous cidofovir appears comparable to a combined regimen of oral ganciclovir plus implant in preventing retinitis progression and mortality.[173] When used as preemptive therapy for post-transplant CMV infection or treatment of established disease, including CMV pneumonia, cidofovir has been associated with responses in 50% or more of allogeneic stem cell recipients.[174,175]

Intravenous cidofovir has been used to treat acyclovir- or foscarnet-resistant mucocutaneous HSV infection.[102,176,177] Early treatment is often effective in controlling invasive adenoviral infections of transplant recipients,[178,178a] although altered dosage schedules (e.g., 1 mg/kg thrice weekly) may be needed to reduce nephrotoxicity.[179] Low dosages (0.25 to 1.0 mg/kg every 2 to 3 weeks, without probenecid) have been used in treating refractory BK virus–associated nephropathy in renal transplant patients.[180] The addition of intravenous cidofovir to highly active antiretroviral therapy (HAART) has inconsistent effects on neurologic outcomes and survival in HIV-associated progressive multifocal leukoencephalopathy.[181,182] Cidofovir did not reduce human herpesvirus (HHV)-8 viral load in peripheral blood mononuclear cells or prevent progression in Kaposi's sarcoma in one small trial.[183]

Topical cidofovir gel formulated in polyethylene glycol reduces pain, virus shedding, and lesion healing time in HIV-infected patients with acyclovir-resistant mucocutaneous HSV infections.[153] Intralesional cidofovir induces remissions in respiratory papillomatosis,[184,185] and topical cidofovir has been used for the treatment of recurrent genital herpes, anogenital warts, refractory condyloma in HIV-infected persons, and the orf poxvirus lesion.[102,186] Topical and intravenous preparations have been used in recalcitrant molluscum contagiosum in immunosuppressed patients.[102] Intravitreal cidofovir injection may be effective for treatment of CMV retinitis[168a] but is contraindicated because of toxicity. A 1% ophthalmic solution reduced the risk for corneal opacities in adenoviral keratoconjunctivitis but was associated with severe, dose-dependent local toxicity.[187]

DOCOSANOL

Docosanol (n-docosanol or behenyl alcohol, Abreva) is a saturated 22-carbon aliphatic alcohol that is inhibitory for a broad range of lipid-enveloped viruses, including HSV-1 and -2, at millimolar concentrations in vitro.[188] Docosanol is not directly virucidal and its principal anti-HSV mechanism of action in vitro apparently relates to interference with viral fusion to host cell membranes early in replication, although other inhibitory effects may be possible.[188] A nonantiviral mechanism of action resulting from anti-inflammatory effects has been described. However, in a guinea pig model of cutaneous HSV, topical docosanol does not show antiviral or therapeutic benefits and is less active than topical penciclovir and acyclovir.[189] No resistance emergence has been described to date.

Docosanol 10% cream is available over the counter for treatment of recurrent herpes labialis in immunocompetent persons. Early treatment (five applications daily until healing, up to maximum of 10 days) shortens the time to complete healing by about 0.7 day and time to resolution of symptoms by 0.5 day.[190] Application site reactions occur in about 2% and its use is generally well tolerated. Whether combined treatment with docosanol and topical nucleosides might provide greater therapeutic effects remains to be determined.

FAMCICLOVIR AND PENCICLOVIR

Spectrum

Penciclovir (9-[4-hydroxy-3-hydroxymethylbut-1-yl] guanine, Denavir) is an acyclic guanosine analogue (see Fig. 38-1B) similar to acyclovir in its spectrum of activity and potency against herpesviruses (see Table 38-2).[191,192] Famciclovir (Famvir) is a prodrug, the diacetyl ester of 6-deoxy penciclovir, and lacks intrinsic antiviral activity. Because of its dependence on viral TK for initial phosphorylation, penciclovir is inactive against TK-deficient strains of HSV or VZV but may be active against some TK-altered or polymerase mutants that are resistant to acyclovir, and against some foscarnet-resistant HSV isolates.[193,194] Penciclovir is also inhibitory for HBV and shows enhanced inhibition in combination with lamivudine or adefovir in vitro.[104,195] Topical, parenteral, and oral penciclovir and oral famciclovir are active in experimental HSV infections.[196]

Mechanism of Action

Penciclovir is an inhibitor of viral DNA synthesis. In infected cells, penciclovir is preferentially phosphorylated to its active form, penciclovir triphosphate, which serves as a competitive inhibitor of viral DNA polymerase.[197] Unlike acyclovir, it is not an obligate chain terminator. Although penciclovir triphosphate is approximately 100-fold less potent in inhibiting viral DNA polymerase than acyclovir triphosphate, it is present in much higher concentrations and for more prolonged periods in infected cells. The prolonged intracellular $T_{1/2}$ of penciclovir-triphosphate, which ranges from 7 to 20 hours, is associated with a sustained antiviral effect in cell culture and in animal models.[198] This effect may allow for infrequent dosing during clinical use. Although not preferentially phosphorylated in HBV-infected cells, penciclovir triphosphate is also a potent inhibitor of HBV DNA polymerase–reverse transcriptase.[199]

Resistance

Penciclovir-resistant variants of HSV selected by in vitro passage have mutations in viral TK or DNA polymerase. Acyclovir-resistant, TK-negative mutants are resistant to penciclovir, but some variants with altered TK substrate specificity or with DNA polymerase mutations are susceptible.[9,200] Resistant HSV is detected in about 0.3% of patients with orolabial herpes, and emergence during clinical use has been very low in immunocompetent hosts.[10,201,202] As seen with acyclovir, higher rates have been observed in immunocompromised patients.[9] Resistance of HBV to penciclovir is associated with point mutations in viral DNA polymerase, particularly L528M.[203] Lamivudine resistance is associated with this mutation and predicts poor virologic response to famciclovir.[204]

Pharmacokinetics

Famciclovir is a prodrug that is well absorbed orally and is rapidly converted to penciclovir by deacetylation and oxidation of the purine. This occurs during and after absorption through the intestinal wall and in the liver.[191] Although penciclovir itself is poorly absorbed, its bioavailability averages 77% after oral administration of famciclovir.[205] Little or no famciclovir is detectable in blood or urine. Penciclovir is less than 20% bound to plasma proteins. The volume of distribution is approximately double that of body water. After single 250- and 500-mg doses of oral famciclovir, the peak plasma concentration of penciclovir averages 1.6 to 1.9 and 2.7 to 4.0 μg/mL, respectively.[205] Food reduces peak plasma concentrations but does not significantly alter overall bioavailability. After intravenous infusion of penciclovir (10 mg/kg), peak plasma levels average 12 μg/mL.[206]

The plasma $T_{1/2elim}$ of penciclovir averages 2 to 3 hours, and approximately 70% is recovered unchanged in the urine.[206] About 5% is excreted as the 6-deoxy precursor. Its rapid renal clearance suggests elimination by both filtration and active tubular secretion. Nonrenal clearance accounts for about 30% of the dose, primarily by fecal excretion of penciclovir and its 6-deoxy precursor. The plasma elimination rate is reduced approximately fourfold and penciclovir exposure is increased 10-fold in those with severe renal failure (CrCl <30 mL/min).[207] Dosage reductions are indicated in moderate or advanced renal failure (Table 38-7). In patients with compensated liver disease, peak plasma levels are reduced by approximately 40%, but overall penciclovir exposure is unchanged and dosage adjustments are not necessary.[207] Older adults have approximately 40% higher penciclovir exposure because of lower renal clearance.

Interactions

No clinically important drug interactions have been identified to date. Famciclovir does not interact pharmacokinetically with cimetidine, theophylline, allopurinol, digoxin, or zidovudine to a clinically significant extent.[208]

Toxicity

Oral famciclovir is well tolerated but may be associated with headache, nausea, fatigue, and diarrhea.[209] The frequencies of such complaints are generally comparable to those seen with placebo or acyclovir. Urticaria, rash, and, predominantly in older adults, hallucinations or confusional states have been reported. Neutropenia and elevated transaminase values occur in less than 5% of patients. The safety and efficacy of famciclovir are not established in children younger than 18 years.

Famciclovir reduces spermatogenesis and fertility in rodents and dogs, but long-term administration (1 year) does not affect spermatogenesis in men.[210] No teratogenic effects have been observed in animals, but safety during pregnancy has not been established (pregnancy category B). Very high penciclovir concentrations are mutagenic, and long-term administration of high-dose famciclovir is associated with mammary tumors in female rats but not in mice. The clinical significance of these observations is uncertain. Penciclovir is excreted in the breast milk of animals.

Topical penciclovir, which is formulated in 40% propylene glycol and a cetomacrogol base, is associated with application site reactions at low rates (approximately 1%), comparable to the vehicle.

Clinical Studies

Topical penciclovir and oral famciclovir are approved for clinical use in the United States, and intravenous penciclovir has been approved in some countries. In immunocompetent persons with recurrent orolabial HSV, patient-initiated topical 1% penciclovir cream (applied every 2 hours while awake for 4 days) shortens healing time and symptoms by nearly 1 day.[211] Oral famciclovir (250 mg three times daily for 5 to 10 days) is as effective as acyclovir in treating first-episode genital herpes.[212] In patients with recurrent genital HSV, patient-initiated famciclovir treatment (125 mg twice daily for 5 days) reduces healing time and symptoms by approximately 1 day and is comparable to acyclovir treatment.[213,214] Suppressive therapy (250 mg twice daily) for up to 1 year is effective in persons with frequent recurrences, but single daily doses are not as effective.[201,215] Famciclovir suppression (500 mg twice daily) reduces clinical HSV recurrences and asymptomatic viral shedding in HIV-infected persons.[202] Famciclovir (500 mg twice daily for 7 days) is comparable to acyclovir (400 mg five times daily) in the treatment of mucocutaneous HSV infections in HIV-infected patients.[216] Intravenous penciclovir (5 mg/kg every 8 or 12 hours for 7 days) is comparable to intravenous acyclovir in efficacy and tolerance for treatment of HSV infections in non–HIV-infected, immunocompromised hosts.[217]

In immunocompetent adults with herpes zoster of 3 days' duration or less, famciclovir (500 mg three times daily for 7 days) is at least as effective as acyclovir (800 mg five times daily) and superior to placebo in reducing both acute manifestations and the duration of postherpetic neuralgia, particularly in patients older than 50 years.[218,219] Famciclovir and valacyclovir provide comparable therapeutic effects in treating zoster in immunocompetent adults aged 50 years or older.[220] Famciclovir is comparable to high-dose oral acyclovir in the treatment of ophthalmic herpes zoster in immunocompetent adults[221] and, given for 10 days, in the treatment of nonophthalmic, localized zoster in immunocompromised patients.[222]

Famciclovir is associated with dose-related reductions in HBV DNA and transaminase levels in patients with chronic hepatitis B[223] but is less effective than lamivudine, with less than 10% of patients experiencing a greater than 100-fold drop in HBV DNA levels after 12 weeks.[224] Famciclovir also induces HBV resistance and is usually not effective in treating lamivudine-resistant infections.[204] It is not effective in chronic delta hepatitis[225] but has been used to treat recurrent HBV infection after liver transplantation, with reductions in HBV DNA levels for longer than 18 months in some patients.[226]

FOMIVIRSEN

Fomivirsen (ISIS 2922, Vitravene) is a 21-nucleotide phosphorothioate oligonucleotide that inhibits human CMV replication through an antisense mechanism.[227] Fomivirsen is complementary to a sequence in the messenger RNA (mRNA) transcripts of the major immediate-early region 2 of CMV, which encodes proteins responsible for regulation of viral gene expression. Other mechanisms of antiviral

TABLE 38-7 Dosage Adjustment of Famciclovir for Renal Insufficiency

Standard Dosage*	Creatinine Clearance (mL/min)†	Adjusted Dosage
500 mg q8h or q12h	40-59	500 mg q12h
	20-39	500 mg q24h
	<20	250 mg q24h
250 mg q12h	≥40	250 mg q12h
	20-39	125 mg q12h
	<20	125 mg q24h
125 mg q12h	≥40	125 mg q12h
	20-39	125 mg q24h
	<20	125 mg q24h

*Dosage is based on manufacturers' recommendations.
†For hemodialysis patients, give the adjusted dosage for creatinine clearance <20 mL/min after dialysis.

action may include nonantisense, sequence-dependent inhibition of virus replication, and sequence-independent inhibition of virus absorption to the cell.[228] With persistent in vitro passage, it has been possible to isolate CMV clones with 10-fold less susceptibility to inhibition of replication.[229] Fomivirsen, because of its novel mechanism of antiviral action, retains activity against CMV strains that are resistant to ganciclovir, foscarnet, or cidofovir.

Fomivirsen is administered by intravitreal injection. In human eyes, concentrations at 1 hour after injection of 165 or 330 μg doses average 5.5 and 11.6 μmol/L, respectively.[230] Clearance is first order with a $T_{1/2}$ of approximately 55 hours. The major route of elimination from the eye is metabolism by exonucleases, and systemic exposure is not detectable. Like other phosphorothioate oligonucleotides, fomivirsen binds readily to proteins.

Fomivirsen is indicated for the intravitreal treatment of CMV retinitis in HIV-infected patients who are intolerant of, have not responded to, or have contraindications to other treatments.[227] Intravitreous injection is associated with delays in time to progression in those with peripheral retinitis (dosages of 165 μg weekly for 3 weeks, followed by every 2 weeks).[231] In those with retinitis that reactivated or was persistent despite alternative agents, a comparison of two regimens (330 μg weekly for 3 weeks followed by every 2 weeks versus 330 μg on days 1 and 15 followed by every 4 weeks) found that the less intense regimen was better tolerated, more convenient, and apparently effective.[232] Dose-dependent inflammation, including iritis, uveitis, and vitritis, is the commonest adverse ocular effect but usually responds to topical corticosteroids. Increased intraocular pressure is common and needs close monitoring. Retinal pigment epitheliopathy and detachments have been described. Fomivirsen is not recommended for use in patients who have received cidofovir within 2 to 4 weeks because of the increased risk for ocular inflammation.

FOSCARNET

Spectrum

Foscarnet (trisodium phosphonoformate, Foscavir) is an inorganic pyrophosphate analogue (see Fig. 38-4B) that is inhibitory for herpesviruses and HIV.[233] In vitro inhibitory concentrations vary widely among clinical isolates but are generally 100 to 300 μmol/L for CMV and 80 to 200 μmol/L for HSV, VZV, EBV, and HHV-8.[234] Foscarnet is inhibitory for most ganciclovir-resistant CMV and acyclovir-resistant HSV and VZV strains. Combinations of foscarnet and ganciclovir or acyclovir synergistically inhibit CMV infection in vitro.[235] Foscarnet also acts synergistically with zidovudine in inhibiting HIV replication.

Concentrations of 500 to 1000 μmol/L reversibly inhibit the proliferation and/or cellular DNA synthesis of uninfected cells. Foscarnet is active in animal models of herpesvirus and hepadnavirus infection.[233]

Mechanism of Action

Unlike nucleosides, foscarnet does not undergo significant intracellular metabolism and directly inhibits herpesvirus DNA polymerase or HIV reverse transcriptase. Foscarnet reversibly blocks the pyrophosphate binding site of the viral polymerase in a noncompetitive manner with respect to deoxynucleotide triphosphates (dNTPs) and inhibits cleavage of pyrophosphate from dNTPs.[233,236] Concentrations that inhibit cell-free viral polymerases are many times lower than those required for inhibition of viral replication in cell culture,[233] and cellular uptake is slow. Foscarnet's selectivity relates to its 100-fold greater inhibitory effects against herpesvirus DNA polymerases or HIV reverse transcriptase, compared with cellular DNA polymerase-α.[236]

Resistance

Resistance to foscarnet is caused by point mutations in DNA polymerase of HSV and CMV or in reverse transcriptase of HIV, which confer threefold to over 10-fold increases in inhibitory concentrations in clinical isolates.[12,237,238] Foscarnet-selected CMV mutations generally do not cause cross-resistance to ganciclovir or cidofovir, but simultaneous resistance to all three drugs has occurred.[237] Foscarnet-

resistant CMV variants, defined by 50% inhibitory concentrations (IC_{50}) greater than 400 μmol/L in plaque reduction or greater than 600 μmol/L in DNA hybridization assays, develop in 37% of foscarnet recipients by 12 months of therapy and are associated with progressive retinitis.[239] Foscarnet-resistant HSV mucocutaneous and CNS infections have developed on therapy, including dually acyclovir- and foscarnet-resistant variants.[240,241] Some foscarnet-resistant CMV infections respond to ganciclovir or cidofovir, and resistant HSV strains usually remain susceptible to cidofovir. Foscarnet resistance in HIV can phenotypically reverse zidovudine resistance.[242]

Pharmacokinetics

Oral bioavailability is low, averaging 7% to 9%. After an infusion of 60 mg/kg every 8 hours, peak and trough plasma concentrations range broadly but average approximately 450 to 575 and 80 to 150 μmol/L, respectively. Peak concentrations range from 490 to 2600 μmol/L after dosages of 90 mg/kg/day. Plasma protein binding is about 15%, and the volume of distribution is moderate (0.4 to 0.7 L/kg). CSF concentrations vary widely but average 66% of plasma values at steady state.[243] Vitreous concentrations average 1.4 times higher than concurrent plasma ones.[244]

Foscarnet is eliminated renally, and more than 80% of the dose is excreted unchanged by glomerular filtration and tubular secretion. Plasma clearance is highly correlated with creatinine clearance, so that dosage adjustments are indicated for small decreases in renal function (Table 38-8). Initial plasma $T_{1/2elim}$ averages 2 to 3 hours in those with normal renal function but increases to greater than 100 hours in those with CrCl of less than 25 mL/min.[245] Plasma elimination is complex, with a prolonged terminal $T_{1/2elim}$ averaging 88 hours, which is attributed to bone deposition that is estimated to account for 15% to 20% of a dose. A hemodialysis run removes about 38% of a dose[245]; dosing after dialysis is recommended. Peritoneal dialysis clears foscarnet to a limited extent.[246]

Interactions

Administration of foscarnet with amphotericin B or other nephrotoxic agents (e.g., aminoglycosides, intravenous pentamidine, intravenous acyclovir, cyclosporine) may cause enhanced renal toxicity[233] and, with calcineurin inhibitors, neurotoxicity. Probenecid does not affect renal excretion. The risk for symptomatic hypocalcemia is increased by concomitant intravenous pentamidine. Ganciclovir does not alter foscarnet pharmacokinetics. Foscarnet and zidovudine do not affect each other's clearance, but the risk for anemia is higher with the combination.

Toxicity

Foscarnet has a narrow therapeutic index. Nephrotoxicity with azotemia, proteinuria, and sometimes acute tubular necrosis is the major dose-limiting side effect.[233,247] Approximately one third of patients develop significant renal impairment (serum creatinine 2.0 mg/dL or greater). Increases in serum creatinine usually occur during the 2nd week of therapy and are reversible within 2 to 4 weeks after cessation in most patients. High dosages, rapid or continuous infusion, dehydration, and concurrent use of nephrotoxic drugs are risk factors. Extra saline hydration before and during infusion appears to reduce the risk for nephrotoxicity.[247,248] Crystalluria, crystalline glomerulopathy, renal tubular acidosis, nephrogenic diabetes insipidus, and interstitial nephritis have also been described.

Foscarnet is a potent chelator of divalent cations, and metabolic abnormalities are common, including hypocalcemia (15% to 35%), hypomagnesemia (15% to 44%), hypokalemia (10% to 16%), and hypercalcemia, hypophosphatemia, and hyperphosphatemia.[249] Decreased serum ionized calcium may cause paresthesias, arrhythmias, tetany, seizures, and other CNS disturbances.[250] Intravenous magnesium sulfate does not prevent ionized hypocalcemia. Intravenous foscarnet should be administered at a fixed rate (maximum, 1 mg/kg/min) by infusion pump, to minimize the possibility of acute metabolic abnormalities. Close monitoring with electrolyte supplementation and foscarnet dosage adjustments are often required during induction therapy.

CNS side effects include headache in about one fourth of patients, seizures in up to 10%, tremor, irritability, and hallucinosis. Other re-

TABLE 38-8   Foscarnet Dosage Reduction in Renal Insufficiency

| Creatinine Clearance (mL/min/kg) | Induction Dosages | | Maintenance Dosages | |
	60 mg/kg/8 hr	90 mg/kg/12 hr	90 mg/kg/day	120 mg/kg/day
>1.4	60 q8h	90 q12h	90 q24h	120 q24h
>1.0-1.4	45 q8h	70 q12h	70 q24h	90 q24h
>0.8-1.0	50 q12h	50 q12h	50 q24h	65 q24h
>0.6-0.8	40 q12h	80 q24h	80 q48h	105 q48h
>0.5-0.6	60 q24h	60 q24h	60 q48h	80 q48h
≥0.4-0.5	50 q24h	50 q24h	50 q48h	65 q48h
<0.4	Not recommended	Not recommended	Not recommended	Not recommended

Dosages expressed in mg/kg. Recommendations taken from Aweeka FT, Jacobson MA, Martin-Munley S, et al. Effect of renal disease and hemodialysis on foscarnet pharmacokinetics and dosing recommendations. J Acquir Immune Defic Syndr Hum Retrovirol. 1999;20:350-357.

ported side effects are fever, generalized rash, diarrhea in 30%, nausea or emesis in up to one half, abnormal liver function tests, anxiety, fatigue, and painful genital ulcerations.[249] These ulcerations may be caused by high urinary foscarnet concentrations and usually resolve within weeks after therapy is stopped. Although anemia may develop in 20% to 50% of patients with AIDS, granulocytopenia is uncommon. Heart block and electrocardiographic changes occur in 5% or less of patients. Oral foscarnet causes dose-related gastrointestinal disturbances.

Preclinical studies indicate that high concentrations are mutagenic and that foscarnet causes fetal skeletal anomalies in rodents and rabbits. It may cause tooth and skeletal developmental abnormalities in growing animals. Safety in pregnancy (pregnancy category C) or in childhood is uncertain. Foscarnet is excreted in the breast milk of animals.

Clinical Studies

Intravenous foscarnet is approved for treatment of CMV retinitis in patients with AIDS and of acyclovir-resistant mucocutaneous HSV infections. With the usual foscarnet regimen (60 mg/kg every 8 hours for 14 to 21 days, followed by chronic maintenance at 90 to 120 mg/kg/day), about 90% of patients with retinitis experience clinical stabilization, and a smaller portion of patients cease CMV excretion.[233,251,252] An induction regimen of 100 mg/kg twice daily also is effective but is associated with a higher risk for penile ulceration. Maintenance dosages of 120 mg/kg/day appear to be more effective in prolonging survival and controlling retinitis.[253] Comparing it with ganciclovir, one study found that foscarnet provides comparable control of CMV retinitis in patients with AIDS but improved survival, although patients had to be switched from foscarnet more than three times as often because of side effects.[254] In patients with persistently active or relapsed retinitis, combined foscarnet (90 mg/kg/day) and ganciclovir (5 mg/kg/day) delay progression significantly longer than higher dosages of either single agent.[255] Intravitreal foscarnet has been used.

Foscarnet is useful in treating ganciclovir-resistant CMV retinitis and other CMV syndromes,[251] including gastrointestinal and pulmonary infections in patients with AIDS,[256] but not CMV pneumonia in bone marrow transplant recipients. In CMV-infected allogeneic stem cell transplant recipients, preemptive foscarnet therapy (60 mg/kg every 12 hours for 2 weeks, followed by 90 mg/kg/day for 5 days per week) is as effective as intravenous ganciclovir in clinical and antiviral effects and associated with less neutropenia.[248] Combinations of foscarnet and ganciclovir have been used to treat allogeneic transplant recipients with high CMV loads[257] and solid-organ transplant recipients with ganciclovir resistance.[258]

In acyclovir-resistant mucocutaneous HSV infections, lower dosages (40 mg/kg every 8 hours) are associated with complete healing in about 75% of patients.[19] Other dosage regimens (e.g., 90 mg/kg every 12 hours) appear to be effective. Foscarnet is also effective in acyclovir-resistant VZV infections in patients with AIDS.[29] Foscarnet has been used to treat severe primary HHV-8 infection after transplantation and may reduce the risk for Kaposi's sarcoma in HIV-infected persons with CMV disease.[259,260] In patients with AIDS, foscarnet administration significantly reduces p24

antigen and HIV RNA levels without clear increases in CD4 counts.[261] In recurrent orolabial or genital herpes infections of immunocompetent hosts, topically applied foscarnet is not associated with reproducible clinical benefits.

GANCICLOVIR AND VALGANCICLOVIR

Spectrum

Ganciclovir (9-[1,3-dihydroxy-2-propoxymethyl] guanine, Cytovene) is a deoxyguanosine analogue that differs from acyclovir in that it has an additional hydroxymethyl group on the acyclic side chain (see Fig. 38-1C). Valganciclovir (Valcyte) is the L-valyl ester of ganciclovir and is rapidly converted to ganciclovir after oral administration. Ganciclovir has inhibitory activity against herpesviruses (see Table 38-2), but its unique characteristic is potent inhibition of CMV replication.[262] Inhibitory concentrations are 10- to more than 50-fold lower than acyclovir for human CMV strains. Combinations of ganciclovir and foscarnet synergistically inhibit CMV replication in vitro.[235] Ganciclovir is about twofold more active than acyclovir for herpes B virus (Cercopithecine herpesvirus 1), with an inhibitory concentration of 9 μg/mL.[74] Ganciclovir inhibits some adenoviruses in vitro, and inhibition of HBV occurs in vivo.[263] Systemic ganciclovir is effective at relatively low dosages in animal models of CMV and HSV infections.

Although high concentrations are needed to inhibit the growth of uninfected cells, inhibitory concentrations for human bone marrow progenitor cells are similar to those that are inhibitory for CMV replication. Inhibition of human lymphocyte proliferative responses to mitogen and antigen occurs at concentrations of 1 to 10 μg/mL, so immune responses requiring active DNA synthesis may be depressed at therapeutic ganciclovir concentrations.[8] Cells transfected by viral TK are readily killed on exposure to ganciclovir, and this antitumor strategy is being explored.

Mechanism of Action

Ganciclovir inhibits viral DNA synthesis.[262,264] Intracellular ganciclovir is phosphorylated to the monophosphate derivative by a virus-induced enzyme, the viral TK during HSV infection, and by a viral protein kinase homologue encoded by the UL97 gene during CMV infection.[265,266] Ganciclovir diphosphate and triphosphate are formed through the action of cellular enzymes. At least 10-fold higher concentrations of ganciclovir triphosphate are present in CMV-infected than in uninfected cells. Intracellular ganciclovir triphosphate concentrations are also more than 10-fold higher than those of acyclovir triphosphate in CMV-infected cells, and the intracellular $T_{1/2}$ of ganciclovir triphosphate is prolonged (16.5 to more than 24 hours). These differences may account in part for ganciclovir's greater anti-CMV activity and explain how single daily doses are effective in suppressing human CMV infections.

Ganciclovir triphosphate is a competitive inhibitor of deoxyguanosine triphosphate (dGTP) incorporation into DNA and preferentially inhibits viral more than host cellular DNA polymerases. Incorporation of ganciclovir triphosphate into viral DNA causes a slowing and subsequent cessation of viral DNA chain elongation.[12] Unlike acyclovir, ganciclovir is not an obligate chain terminator, and continued viral

TABLE 38-9 Ganciclovir Dosage Adjustments in Renal Insufficiency

Creatinine Clearance* (mL/min)	IV Ganciclovir Induction Dose (mg/kg)	Dosing Interval (hr)	IV Ganciclovir Maintenance Dose (mg/kg)	Dosing Interval (hr)	Ganciclovir Capsule Dose
≥70	5.0	12	5.0	24	1000 mg tid
50-69	2.5	12	2.5	24	1500 mg qd or 500 mg tid
25-49	2.5	24	1.25	24	1000 mg qd or 500 mg bid
10-24	1.25	24	0.625	24	500 mg qd
<10	1.25	3 times/wk after hemodialysis	0.625	3 times /wk after hemodialysis	500 mg 3 times per wk, after hemodialysis

Dosing suggestions are based on manufacturer's recommendations.

DNA synthesis results in intranuclear accumulation of short, noninfectious viral DNA fragments.[267] Ganciclovir is incorporated into both host cell and viral DNA.

Resistance

Resistance in CMV isolates, often defined by inhibitory concentrations greater than 1.5 to 3 μg/mL in vitro, has been related to two mechanisms: (1) reduced intracellular ganciclovir phosphorylation caused by point mutations or deletions in the phosphotransferase encoded by the UL97 gene and (2) point mutations in viral DNA polymerase (UL54).[12,268,269] Most resistant clinical isolates with 4- to 20-fold increases in inhibitory concentrations have single or sometimes multiple UL97 mutations and usually remain susceptible to foscarnet and cidofovir.[162] Highly resistant CMV strains (inhibitory concentrations greater than 10 μg/mL) typically harbor both UL97 and UL54 mutations and are cross-resistant to cidofovir but usually susceptible to foscarnet.[162,163,270]

Ganciclovir resistance is rare in ganciclovir-naïve patients but has been recognized clinically by progressive disease and persistent CMV viremia on therapy.[251] Risk factors include prolonged ganciclovir exposure, primary infection, and higher immunosuppression including use of antilymphocyte globulin. In patients with AIDS receiving ganciclovir for retinitis, resistant CMV is detectable in about 7% by 3 months and in 28% by 9 months.[271] During the HAART era, a 15% frequency of UL97 mutations has been found by 18 months in valganciclovir recipients.[272] Emergence of resistance, sometimes within several weeks, also occurs with ganciclovir use in stem cell and solid-organ transplant recipients.[273] Ganciclovir-resistant CMV disease developed in 7% of mismatched solid-organ transplant recipients receiving ganciclovir prophylaxis.[274] Mismatched lung transplant recipients are at particular risk for resistance emergence.[275] The transmissibility of ganciclovir-resistant CMV strains is undefined, but patients with such strains may have invasive disease, including retinitis, enteritis, polyradiculopathy, or pneumonia.[12,276] Foscarnet or cidofovir therapy may benefit patients with ganciclovir-resistant CMV infections.[251]

Ganciclovir is more than 40 times less active against acyclovir-resistant, TK-deficient HSV strains than against wild-type strains.

Pharmacokinetics

The oral bioavailability of ganciclovir is about 5% under fasting conditions. Food increases bioavailability to 6% to 9%, so dosing with meals is recommended.[277,278] Peak and trough plasma levels average about 0.9 to 1.2 and 0.2 to 0.5 μg/mL, respectively, on an oral regimen of 1000 mg every 8 hours. Valganciclovir is a monovalyl ester prodrug that is well absorbed, most likely by intestinal peptide transporter 1, and rapidly hydrolyzed to the parent by intestinal and hepatic esterases. After administration of oral valganciclovir (900 mg) with food, ganciclovir bioavailability is approximately 60%, prodrug blood levels are low (1% to 2% of ganciclovir), ganciclovir peak plasma concentrations average 5.9 to 6.7 μg/mL, and overall ganciclovir exposure is comparable to intravenous dosing of ganciclovir at 5 mg/kg.[279] Valganciclovir has essentially supplanted oral ganciclovir.

After intravenous administration of 5 mg/kg doses, peak and trough plasma concentrations average 8 to 11 and 0.6 to 1.2 μg/mL, respectively.[262,280] Subcutaneous and intramuscular administration are too irritating for clinical use. Plasma protein binding is only 1% to 2%. After intravenous dosing, aqueous, vitreous, and subretinal fluid levels are similar to those in serum.[244,281] CSF levels are 24% to 70%, and brain tissue levels are 38% of those in plasma.[280] The plasma $T_{1/2elim}$ averages 2 to 4 hours in patients with normal renal function but increases almost linearly as creatinine clearance declines, increasing to 28 to 40 hours in those with severe renal insufficiency. Most ganciclovir is eliminated unmetabolized by renal excretion (>90% of dose) by both glomerular filtration and tubular secretion. Dosage reductions of ganciclovir (Table 38-9) and valganciclovir (Table 38-10) are necessary in patients with creatinine clearance of less than 80 mL/min. A single hemodialysis session reduces the plasma levels of ganciclovir by approximately 50% to 60%, and dosing after dialysis is recommended.[282]

The intravitreal ganciclovir implant is designed to release the drug at a rate of approximately 1 μg/hour over a period of 5 to 8 months.[283]

Interactions

Concurrent oral ganciclovir doubles the overall exposure to didanosine, increases zidovudine exposure by a much smaller extent, and may increase the risk for didanosine concentration–related toxicities.[284] Ganciclovir exposure is reduced about 20% when it is ingested 2 hours after but not simultaneously with didanosine. Ganciclovir antagonizes the anti-HIV activity of didanosine and zidovudine in vitro,[285] and zidovudine antagonizes the anti-CMV effects of ganciclovir,[286,287] but the clinical significance of these observations is unknown.

Zidovudine and probably other cytotoxic agents increase the risk for ganciclovir-induced myelosuppression, as do nephrotoxic or other agents (probenecid, trimethoprim-sulfa) that impair ganciclovir excretion. In animals, zidovudine (but not amphotericin B, ketoconazole, dapsone, or trimethoprim-sulfa) antagonizes the anti-CMV effects of ganciclovir.[286,288] Renal dysfunction may occur in patients given concurrent ganciclovir and either amphotericin B or cyclosporine, and ganciclovir may increase cyclosporine levels.

Toxicity

Myelosuppression is the principal dose-limiting toxicity of ganciclovir and its prodrug. The most common adverse events are neutropenia in 24% to 40% and thrombocytopenia in 15% to 20% of patients with AIDS receiving intravenous ganciclovir or oral valganciclovir.[262] The

TABLE 38-10 Dosage* Adjustments for Valganciclovir in Renal Insufficiency

Creatinine Clearance (mL/min)	Induction Dose	Maintenance Dose
≥60	900 mg bid	900 mg qd
40-59	450 mg bid	450 mg qd
25-39	450 mg qd	450 mg q2d
10-24	450 mg q2d	450 mg 2 × /wk
<10†	Not recommended	Not recommended
Hemodialysis†	Not recommended	Not recommended

*Dosage suggestions are based on manufacturer's recommendations.
†Dose less than 450-mg tablet is needed. Use intravenous ganciclovir.

risk for these toxicities is lower in transplant recipients. Neutropenia occurs in approximately one fourth of those receiving oral ganciclovir. Neutropenia is most commonly observed during the second week of treatment and is reversible in most patients within 1 week after drug cessation. Recombinant granulocyte-macrophage colony-stimulating factor may be useful in treating ganciclovir-induced neutropenia.[289]

CNS side effects, ranging in severity from headache to behavioral changes with confusion or psychosis, to convulsions and coma, have been described in 5% to 15% of patients. Up to one third of patients receiving intravenous ganciclovir interrupt or prematurely stop therapy because of bone marrow or CNS toxicity, and catheter-related complications are common. Approximately 25% of valganciclovir recipients discontinue maintenance therapy within 10 months for toxicity or other reasons.[290] Increased rates of azotemia occur in transplant recipients receiving intravenous ganciclovir prophylaxis.[291] Oral valganciclovir and ganciclovir are associated with diarrhea and possibly with mild nephrotoxicity.[292]

Anemia, rash, fever, liver function test abnormalities, nausea or vomiting, and eosinophilia have also been reported. Phlebitis at the infusion site may be caused by the alkaline pH of the solution. In the event of massive overdosage, hemodialysis and hydration may be effective in reducing plasma ganciclovir levels. Placement of the intravitreal insert may be associated with visual changes, hemorrhage, infection, and retinal detachment.

Ganciclovir is mutagenic, carcinogenic, and immunosuppressive, and it causes irreversible reproductive toxicity in animals and possibly humans.[262] Teratogenicity, embryotoxicity, testicular atrophy, and bone marrow hypocellularity have been observed in animals at ganciclovir exposures comparable to those in humans. Ganciclovir may be teratogenic in humans (classified in pregnancy category C), and mothers should avoid breast-feeding while receiving ganciclovir or valganciclovir.

Clinical Studies

Ganciclovir is currently approved for treatment and chronic suppression of CMV retinitis in immunocompromised patients and prevention of CMV disease in transplant recipients. Valganciclovir is approved for management of CMV retinitis. Because of their toxicities, administration is usually limited to patients at risk for or having life-threatening or sight-threatening CMV infections. With initial or induction intravenous dosages of 2.5 mg/kg every 8 hours or 5 mg/kg every 12 hours for 10 to 21 days, about 85% of CMV retinitis patients improve or stabilize their disease, and funduscopic improvement is usually evident by 10 to 14 days.[262,293] Ganciclovir is comparable to foscarnet in initial control of retinitis.[254] Oral valganciclovir (900 mg twice daily for 3 weeks) is as effective as intravenous ganciclovir for initial treatment of non–sight-threatening disease.[279] Almost all patients with AIDS who respond to initial treatment relapse within weeks without suppressive therapy.[293] High dosages of intravenous ganciclovir (30 to 35 mg/kg/week), but not low dosages (10 to 20 mg/kg/week), and oral valganciclovir (900 mg daily)[279] are effective for chronic suppression. Oral ganciclovir suppression (1 g three times daily) appears to be comparably effective to intravenous dosing.[294] Retinal detachments are common during long-term follow-up. Combined ganciclovir and foscarnet is superior to monotherapy and may be effective when single-agent therapy fails.[255] Intraocular sustained-release ganciclovir implants[283,295] and repeated intravitreal injections are effective in controlling retinitis but do not prevent CMV disease in the other eye or in other sites.

Clinical improvement and virologic responses are also seen in CMV pneumonia and gastrointestinal infections in patients with AIDS and in solid-organ transplant recipients.[264,293] CNS syndromes respond less predictably and may progress despite therapy.[296] In biopsy-proven CMV colitis in patients with AIDS, ganciclovir (5 mg/kg every 12 hours for 14 days) is associated with significant antiviral effects, stabilization of weight loss, and lower incidence of extracolonic CMV disease but no differences in symptoms compared with placebo.[297] In bone marrow transplant recipients, virologic responses (but no reduction in mortality) occur in patients with CMV pneumonia treated with

ganciclovir alone or in combination with corticosteroids. In contrast, ganciclovir combined with intravenous immunoglobulin or CMV immunoglobulin reduces the mortality rate among bone marrow transplant recipients with CMV pneumonia, from 80% to 90% to 30% to 50%. Prolonged ganciclovir treatment may reduce the risk for hearing loss in symptomatic infants with congenital CMV disease.[298]

Intravenous ganciclovir prophylaxis appears to be effective and reasonably well tolerated in preventing CMV disease in bone marrow[299,300] and solid-organ transplant recipients.[1,24,291] Preemptive ganciclovir treatment (5 mg/kg every 12 hours for 7 to 14 days, followed by 5 mg/kg/day until days 100 to 120 after transplantation) when CMV is isolated from bronchoalveolar lavage fluid[299] or from other body sites[300] is highly effective in preventing CMV pneumonia and appears to reduce mortality in bone marrow transplant recipients. In seropositive bone marrow transplant recipients, initiation of ganciclovir at the time of engraftment also markedly reduces CMV shedding and disease rates but does not improve survival, in part because of neutropenia-related infections.[301,302]

Short-term ganciclovir administration after transplantation reduces the risk for CMV disease in seropositive allograft recipients undergoing heart, lung, or liver transplantation.[1,291,303] More prolonged administration (to day 100) provides sustained protection, but late-onset CMV disease may occur after cessation. Longer term prophylaxis is under study. Preemptive intravenous ganciclovir during antilymphocyte antibody treatment for up to 2 weeks reduces the risk for disease.[304] Ganciclovir is also effective in preventing HSV infection[302] and results in clearance of EBV from oropharyngeal secretions, although a rapid rebound in excretion occurs after cessation of therapy.[305]

Oral ganciclovir (1 g three times daily to day 98) prophylaxis markedly reduces the risk for invasive CMV disease in liver transplant recipients, including the high-risk group comprising seronegative recipients of seropositive donors.[292] Ganciclovir (1 g three times daily for 12 weeks) is also effective in renal transplant recipients.[306] Compared with oral ganciclovir (1 g three times daily), valganciclovir (900 mg once daily) to day 100 is associated with a lower rate of CMV viremia on prophylaxis and comparable rates of CMV viremia and disease at 6 months in high-risk mismatched solid-organ transplant recipients.[307] The optimal duration of prophylaxis remains to be established, and studies of lower doses are in progress. Preemptive therapy with oral ganciclovir (1 g three times daily for 8 weeks) when CMV DNA is detectable protects against CMV disease in liver transplant recipients.[308] Oral ganciclovir (1 g every 8 hours) prophylaxis appears to decrease incidence of disease in HIV-infected patients with CD4 T-cell counts lower than 100 cells/mm³,[309] although not when administered with didanosine.[310]

Intravenous ganciclovir (5 mg/kg every 12 hours) is recommended for initial treatment of herpes B virus infections, particularly those with central nervous system involvement.[74] Intravenous ganciclovir reduces biochemical abnormalities and hepatitis B virus DNA levels by 90% in post-transplantation HBV infection.[263] Topical 0.15% ganciclovir ophthalmic gel is comparable to acyclovir ointment in treating HSV keratitis.[311]

IDOXURIDINE

Idoxuridine (5-iodo-2′-deoxyuridine, IDU; Herplex) is an iodinated thymidine analogue (see Fig. 38-4C) that inhibits replication of various DNA viruses in vitro, particularly herpesviruses and poxviruses.[312] Plaque production by most clinical isolates of HSV type 1 is inhibited by concentrations of 2 to 10 μg/mL. Idoxuridine's antiviral mechanism of action is not completely defined, but the phosphorylated derivatives interfere with various enzyme systems. The triphosphate inhibits viral DNA synthesis and is incorporated into both viral and cellular DNA. Resistance to idoxuridine readily develops under laboratory conditions[313] and occurs in viral isolates recovered from idoxuridine-treated patients with HSV keratitis.

In humans, extremely low plasma concentrations of idoxuridine (0.1 to 0.4 ppm) are detected in about one half of patients treated topically with 40% idoxuridine in the penetration-enhancing agent dimethylsulfoxide (DMSO). Idoxuridine is teratogenic, mutagenic, tumor-promoting, and immunosuppressive in preclinical testing. DMSO is teratogenic and can cause adverse ocular effects in laboratory animals.

In the United States, idoxuridine is approved only for topical treatment of HSV keratitis, whereas idoxuridine in DMSO is available in Europe for treatment of herpes labialis, genitalis, and zoster. In ocular HSV infections, topical idoxuridine is more effective in epithelial infections, especially initial episodes, than in stromal infections.[314] Adverse reactions include pain, pruritus, inflammation, or edema involving the eye or lids and, rarely, allergic reactions.

Topical idoxuridine alone is ineffective in mucocutaneous herpesvirus infections. Frequent topical application of 5% to 40% idoxuridine dissolved in DMSO appears to hasten healing and shorten pain duration in localized herpes zoster. Topical 30% idoxuridine in DMSO may shorten the duration of viral shedding in recurrent or primary genital HSV infections, but it does not reduce the duration of symptoms or healing time. Topical 15% idoxuridine in DMSO reduces the duration of pain and healing time in recurrent herpes labialis.[315] Mild local burning and aftertaste are common after topical application of DMSO, and headache, dizziness, sedation, nausea, and localized and generalized dermatitis have also been reported.

IMIQUIMOD

Imiquimod (Aldara) is an imidazoquinoline compound that is a topical immune response modifier lacking direct antiviral effects. Imiquimod exposure causes activation of immune cells (monocytes, macrophages, natural killer cells) to produce antiviral cytokines, particularly IFN-α and tumor necrosis factor (TNF)-α as well as interleukin (IL)-12, IL-10, IL-1, IL-6, and IL-8.[316,317] Imiquimod indirectly enhances acquired immune responses through activation of antigen-presenting dendritic cells including Langerhans' cells and helper T-cell 1 (Th1) lymphocytes. IFN-γ production from T cells stimulates cytotoxic T lymphocytes important in clearance of virally infected cells. Clinical responses in anogenital warts are associated with decreases in HPV DNA copies and RNA transcripts in treated skin.[318] Resiquimod is a structurally related compound associated with greater stimulation of cytokines and with activating dendritic cells.

Topical imiquimod 5% cream is approved for patient-applied treatment of anogenital warts and has been used in other mucocutaneous infections and dermatologic conditions.[316] In immunocompetent patients, imiquimod (three overnight applications [for approximately 8 hours] weekly for up to 16 weeks) leads to complete wart clearance in 37% to 52%.[316,319] Clearance rates are higher in women than men and substantially lower (<15%) in HIV-infected persons.[320,321] The time to clearance averages 8 to 10 weeks. Recurrences are less common (14% to 19%) than after ablative therapies, and retreatment is frequently successful.[316] Imiquimod may be useful as an adjunct to laser or surgical ablative therapies.[316]

Imiquimod has been used in other types of HPV-related conditions and for warts at nongenital sites.[317] It appears beneficial in refractory cutaneous leishmaniasis in combination with other drugs[322] and, depending on the level of immunocompetence, in molluscum contagiosum.[316,317] Imiquimod has been used in AIDS-associated chronic, acyclovir-unresponsive genital herpes, but no beneficial effects on lesions or recurrences are seen in immunocompetent adults with genital herpes.[323] Because of encouraging preliminary findings, topical resiquimod is under study for treatment of recurrent genital herpes in an effort to reduce recurrences.[324]

Patients need to wash the affected area upon awakening to remove residual drug. About two thirds of those treated experience local erythema. Application site reactions with erythema, irritation, pruritus, burning, tenderness, and scabbing (and less often with erosion or ulceration at the wart site and other exposed areas) are generally mild to moderate in intensity. These usually resolve within 2 weeks of cessation of the drug. The frequency of local reactions relates to frequency of application, and use in genital herpes may delay healing.[323] Severe local reactions including pain, erythema, or scarring are very uncommon.[320] No systemic toxicity has been recognized, but safety during pregnancy has not been established (pregnancy category B). Preclinical studies indicate that imiquimod is not genotoxic or teratogenic.

INTERFERONS

Classification

Since their discovery in 1957 as mediators of the phenomenon of viral interference (i.e., inhibition of growth of one virus by another), IFNs have become recognized as potent cytokines that are associated with complex antiviral, immunomodulating, and antiproliferative actions.[325,326] IFNs are proteins that are synthesized by eukaryotic cells in response to various inducers and that in turn cause biochemical changes leading to a nonselective antiviral state in exposed cells of the same species. Formerly designated on the basis of the cell types from which they were derived, three major classes of human IFNs are currently in clinical use (Table 38-11). Each type is immunologically distinct and has different producer cells, inducers, and biologic effects, as well as unique physicochemical characteristics.[326,327]

IFN-α and IFN-β are produced by almost all cells in response to viral infection and a variety of other stimuli, including double-stranded RNA, bacteria, protozoa, mycoplasmas, polyanions, several low-molecular-weight organic compounds, and certain cytokines and growth factors such as IL-1, IL-2, and TNF. IFN-γ production is restricted to T lymphocytes and natural killer cells responding to antigenic stimuli, mitogens, and certain cytokines such as IL-2. The principal antiviral interferons, IFN-α and IFN-β, are approximately 30% homologous at the amino acid level. Human IFN-αs are actually a family of multiple species that share a high degree of amino acid sequence homology (> 70%) but have differing in vitro antiviral and biologic effects on human cells.[328] Compared with IFN-α/β, IFN-γ has less antiviral activity but more potent immunoregulatory effects, particularly with respect to macrophage activation, expression of class II major histocompatibility complex (MHC) antigens, and mediation of local inflammatory responses. Most IFNs in clinical use are produced by recombinant DNA techniques (see Table 38-11).

Mechanisms of Action

A wide range of animal viruses are sensitive to the antiviral actions of IFNs, although many DNA viruses are relatively insensitive and considerable differences in potency exist among viruses and assay systems. IFN activity is usually measured in terms of antiviral effects in cell culture. Typically, one unit of IFN activity is the amount present in a sample dilution that causes a 50% reduction in virus replication or expression in certain cell lines; this is generally expressed as international units (IU) relative to National Institutes of Health or World Health Organization reference standards.

IFNs are not directly antiviral but cause elaboration of effector proteins in exposed cells, which contribute to a state of viral resistance.[325,329,330] The initial step involves IFN binding to specific cell surface receptors, which are shared between IFN-α and IFN-β but are different for IFN-γ. IFN receptors are linked to the JAK-STAT signaling pathways, which, through a multistep process, activate transcription factors that bind selectively to and upregulate approximately 100 IFN-regulated genes.[331,332] The distinct pattern of STAT proteins activated by different IFNs is one mechanism for eliciting different cellular responses. For IFN-α/β, a three-protein complex known as IFN-stimulated gene factor 3 (ISGF-3) localizes to the nucleus and binds to a cis-acting DNA element (designated IRSE) that activates transcription of the target genes.[325] A family of IFN regulatory factors (IRFs) exists, and other pathways may contribute to regulation of the IFN response. Of note, microarray analysis shows that a number of genes are upregulated by IFN-β but not by IFN-α or IFN-γ in vitro.[331] The onset of IFN-induced antiviral action is rapid, and IFN exposure leads to production of more than two dozen cellular proteins. For many viruses, the primary antiviral effect of IFN in vitro is mediated by inhibition of viral protein synthesis. Depending on the virus and cell

TABLE 38-11   Nomenclature and Classification of Human Interferons (IFNs)

Characteristic	Class* α	β	γ
Other designations	Type I, leukocyte	Type I, fibroblast	Type II, immune
No. species	>12	1	1
No. amino acids	165-172	166	143
Apparent molecular weight (kDa)[†]	16-27.6	20-23	15.5-25
Disulphide bonds	2	1	0
Glycosylation	Variable[‡]	Yes	Yes
Acid stability (pH 2)	Stable[§]	Stable	Labile
Chromosome coding for receptor	21	21	6
Commercial formulations	rIFN-α-2b (Intron A)		
	IFN-α-2a (Roferon A)		
	Le-IFN-αn3 (Alferon N)		
	Ly-IFN-αn1 (Wellferon)[∣]		
	rIFNalfacon-1 (Infergen)		
	PEG-IFN-α-2a (Pegasys)		
	PEG-IFN-α-2b (Peg-Intron)	rIFN-β-1b (Betaseron)	rIFN-γ-1b (Actimmune)
		rIFN-β-1a (Avonex, Rebif)	rIFN-γ (Immuneron)

*One IFN-ω subtype is included in type I IFNs.

[†]Range of molecular weights relates to post-translation modifications, including formation of dimers, glycosylation, and protein binding. Molecular weight of nonglycosylated recombinant IFN-α is approximately 19.5 kDa.

[‡]Generally not glycosylated, but several minor species are.

[§]Acid-labile IFN-α species occur in certain pathologic states, including human immunodeficiency virus infection, systemic lupus erythematosus, rheumatoid arthritis, and pemphigus.

[∣]No longer available in United States.

Adapted from Zoon KC. Human interferons: Structure and function. In: Anonymous. Interferon 9. London: Academic Press; 1987:1-12, and Greenberg SB. Human interferon in viral diseases. Infect Dis Clin North Am. 1987;1:383-423.

type, the antiviral actions of IFN may also include inhibition of viral penetration or uncoating, synthesis or methylation of mRNA, or viral assembly and release.

Among the better characterized IFN-induced proteins are unique 2′-5′-oligoadenylate (2-5[A]) synthetases and the protein kinase PKR, either of which can inhibit protein synthesis in the presence of double-stranded RNA (dsRNA).[325] The 2-5(A) synthetase produces adenylate oligomers that activate a latent cellular endoribonuclease (RNase L) to cleave both cellular and viral single-stranded RNAs, leading to inhibition of protein synthesis. Activated PKR selectively phosphorylates and inactivates eukaryotic initiation factor (eIF)-2 to impede translation. Activated PKR also phosphorylates the transcription factor inhibitor IκB and mediates dsRNA-induced activation of nuclear factor (NF)-κB, which in turn is required for IFN-β synthesis. IFN may also block mRNA capping by inhibiting transmethylation reactions. IFN also induces human guanylate binding protein-1 that mediates antiviral activity for several RNA viruses, the soluble form of the low-density lipoprotein receptor inhibitory for rhabdovirus assembly,[333] the MxA protein (a guanosine triphosphatase with activity against orthomyxoviruses and certain RNA viruses),[334] and the RNA-specific adenosine deaminase ADR1 that modifies RNA transcripts after transcription.[325] IFN also inhibits HCV internal ribosome entry site-dependent RNA translation in vitro.[335] Induction of nitric oxide synthase appears to mediate a substantial antiviral effect of IFN-γ.[336] Increased levels of 2-5(A) activity and MxA protein or mRNA in peripheral leukocytes are also used as a marker for IFN exposure or endogenous release.[334]

Except possibly for the Mx proteins and influenza viruses and for 2-5(A) synthetase/RNase-L and picornaviruses, no consistent correlations exist between induction of a particular protein and resistance to a specific virus across a range of cell types.[330] A particular virus may be inhibited at several steps, and the principal inhibitory effect differs among virus families. Many viruses are able to counter IFN effects by blocking signaling and production or activity of selected IFN-inducible proteins.[325,330] For example, the NS5A protein of HCV represses the function of the IFN-induced PKR,[337] and another HCV protein E2 competitively inhibits PKR kinase activity. The NS1 gene of influenza is an IFN antagonist that binds dsRNA to inhibit IFN production and dsRNA-activated pathways. IFN exposure may also reduce the expression of certain cellular genes, including selected oncogenes and those involved in collagen synthesis.

The viral and immune IFN systems are functionally nonredundant,[325] and complex interactions exist between IFNs and between IFNs and other parts of the immune system.[327,338] IFNs upregulate MHC class I expression and promote cytotoxic T-cell responses; regulate the expression of cytokines (IL-12, IL-15, IFN-γ) and chemokines that affect T-cell responses; alter expression of Toll receptors; enhance natural killer (NK) cell cytotoxicity; and promote the differentiation of dendritic cells and Th1 lymphocytes.[329,338] IFN-α is produced by macrophages and also can modify macrophage functions, increasing phagocytosis and cytolytic activity. Consequently, IFNs may ameliorate viral infections by exerting direct antiviral effects and by modifying the immune response to infection. For example, IFN-induced expression of MHC antigens may contribute to the antiviral actions of IFN by enhancing antigen presentation and the lytic effects of cytotoxic T lymphocytes. Both IFN-α/β and IFN-γ lead to increased expression of class I MHC molecules, but only IFN-γ efficiently induces class II MHC molecules.[325] Several viruses, including CMV and VZV, antagonize IFN-γ–induced MHC expression. In addition, both proapoptotic and antiapoptotic genes are induced by IFNs,[331] and IFN-α and IFN-β are important mediators of apoptosis, including induction of p53.[325,339]

IFN titers generally appear at the sites of viral replication just after peak titers of virus and before humoral antibody responses. IFNs may mediate some of the systemic symptoms associated with viral infections and contribute to immunologically mediated tissue damage in certain viral diseases. High IFN titers are usually followed by a reduction of virus titers, although persistently elevated IFN titers have been recognized in certain chronic and acute viral infections (e.g., hemorrhagic fevers). Unusual acid-labile IFN-α has been observed in patients with certain autoimmune disorders and AIDS, in which its presence appears to predict disease progression.

Pharmacokinetics

The prolonged biologic effects of IFN are not easily related to serum concentrations or other conventional pharmacokinetic parameters. After intramuscular or subcutaneous injection of IFN-α, absorption exceeds 80%.[340,341] Plasma levels are dose related, peaking at 4 to 10 hours and returning to baseline by 18 to 36 hours. Levels of 2-5(A) synthetase in peripheral blood mononuclear cells, which have been used as an index of biologic responsiveness to IFN, show increases beginning at 6 hours and lasting through 4 days after a single dose. An antiviral state in these cells is detectable at 1 hour, peaks at 24 hours, and slowly decreases to baseline by 6 days after injection. Intramuscular or subcutaneous injections of IFN-β result in negligible plasma levels, although increases in 2-5(A) synthetase may occur. Oral administration does not result in detectable serum IFN levels or increases in 2-5(A) synthetase activity in peripheral blood mononuclear cells.[342]

After systemic administration, low levels of IFN are detected in respiratory secretions, CSF, eye, and brain. After intravenous dosing, CSF levels average less than 1% of serum concentrations.[343] IFN-α is relatively stable in most body fluids, whereas IFN-β and IFN-γ appear to lose activity readily. However, it is unknown whether measurable IFN levels at a particular site accurately reflect its antiviral or other biologic activities. Both IFN-α and IFN-β are cleared rapidly in a complex fashion. Leukocyte and recombinant IFN-α species have a plasma $T_{1/2elim}$ of approximately 3 to 8 hours. The clearance of IFN includes inactivation by various body fluids, cellular uptake, and metabolism by body organs, primarily the kidney, although negligible biologically active IFN is excreted in the urine. Clearance of IFN-α2 is reduced by 64% to 79% in hemodialysis patients.[344]

The attachment of polyethylene glycol (PEG) to IFN slows absorption, decreases clearance, increases $T_{1/2elim}$, and results in higher and more sustained serum concentrations, so that once-weekly dosing is effective. Two pegylated IFN-αs are approved currently: pegIFN-α2a has a 40-kDa branched PEG moiety attached by a stable amide bond to lysine residues within the IFN protein, and pegIFN-α2b has a 12-kDa linear moiety attached to histidine residues. PegIFN-α2a is more stable and dispensed in solution, whereas pegIFN-α2b requires reconstitution prior to use. PegIFN-α2a is cleared primarily by the liver, whereas about 30% of pegIFN-α2b is cleared renally.[344] For pegIFN-α2a (multiple 180-μg doses), a peak serum concentration of 26 ng/mL occurs at about 45 hours after the dosing, and $T_{1/2elim}$ is about 80 to 90 hours. Steady-state serum levels are attained 5 to 8 weeks after initiation of weekly dosing.[148] Moderate renal impairment and presence of cirrhosis do not affect pharmacokinetics, although clearance is reduced by 25% to 45% in those with renal failure on hemodialysis.[148] For pegIFN-α2b, dose-related maximum plasma concentrations (1.4 ng/mL with multiple doses of 1.5 μg/kg) occur at 15 to 44 hours after dosing and decline with a $T_{1/2elim}$ of approximately 30 to 40 hours, or about 10-fold longer than for IFN-α2b.[344] Some accumulation occurs with repetitive dosing. Dosage reductions in both pegylated IFNs are indicated in end-stage renal disease.

Interactions

IFN and its inducers reduce the metabolism of various drugs by the hepatic cytochrome P-450–dependent mixed-function oxidase system and specifically decrease CYP1A2-mediated clearance of theophylline. IFNs may increase the neurotoxic, hematotoxic, or cardiotoxic effects of other drugs, including increased risk for anemia with ribavirin.

Toxicity

Both purified natural and recombinant IFNs are associated with dose-related immediate and late-onset toxicities.[345] Adverse effects are generally mild and reversible at dosages of less than 5 million IU (MU) per day.[341] Intramuscular and subcutaneous injection of IFN doses of 1 to 2 MU or more are usually associated with an acute influenza-like syndrome including fever, chills, headache, malaise, myalgia, arthralgia, and nausea, vomiting, and diarrhea, especially during the first week of therapy. Symptoms begin several hours after administration and are most prominent between 8 to 24 hours after dosing. Despite more prolonged blood levels, the duration of influenza-like symptoms after pegIFN is similar to that after conventional IFNs.[344] Tolerance develops in most patients within several weeks. Febrile responses can be moderated by pretreatment with various antipyretics. Up to one half of patients receiving intralesional therapy for genital warts experience the influenza-like illness. Intralesional IFN also causes discomfort at the injection site and leukopenia. Local reactions consisting of tender-

ness and erythema also occur after subcutaneous injection, and intranasal IFN causes local irritation.

Major toxicities that limit dosage and duration of therapy are bone marrow suppression with granulocytopenia and thrombocytopenia; neuropsychiatric disturbance manifested by depression, anxiety, somnolence, confusion, behavioral disturbance, electroencephalographic changes, and, rarely, seizures; reversible neurasthenia with profound fatigue and anorexia, weight loss, and myalgia; thyroid dysfunction and autoimmune thyroiditis; and cardiotoxicity with hypotension, arrhythmias, and reversible cardiomyopathy. Psychiatric disturbance and depression are more common in patients with preexisting disorders but can also occur in otherwise healthy persons. Elevations in hepatic enzymes and triglycerides and retinopathy are common.[346] IFN may lead to the development of or exacerbate various immunologically mediated disorders, including sarcoidosis, systemic lupus erythematosus, psoriasis, vitiligo, lichen planus, and eczematoid skin lesions. Rare pulmonary manifestations include interstitial pneumonia, bronchiolitis obliterans organizing pneumonia, asthma, and pleural effusion.[347] Alopecia, proteinuria, renal insufficiency, interstitial nephritis, autoantibody formation, bacterial infections, and hepatotoxicity occur.[348] Acute allergic reactions are rare. Patients with autoimmune chronic hepatitis, who may have false-positive enzyme immunoassay tests for anti-HCV antibodies, can worsen if treated with IFN.[349]

The adverse effects of pegylated IFNs are similar to those with conventional IFNs, although dose-related neutropenia and thrombocytopenia and injection site reactions are more common. About one half of pegIFN-treated patients with chronic hepatitis C develop fatigue and systemic symptoms after injections, 20% to 30% experience depression or other psychiatric reactions, and approximately 10% to 16% discontinue treatment because of adverse events, most commonly psychiatric disorders.[350,351] PegIFN-α2a may be associated with lesser frequency of depression.[351]

The development of serum neutralizing antibodies to exogenous IFNs varies with the IFN type, dosage, and route of administration but may be more common with IFN-α-2a.[352] Neutralizing antibodies may be associated infrequently with loss of clinical responsiveness.[341] Pegylation may reduce the immunogenicity of IFNs, and anti-PEG antibody appears to be very uncommon.

IFN may impair fertility and alter hormone levels in females. IFN is an abortifacient in monkeys at high dosages and has been used in small numbers of pregnant women, so that safety during pregnancy is not established.[353] It is classified as pregnancy category C.

Clinical Studies

Clinical use of IFNs has been limited by their relative lack of potency, their side effects, and the availability of competing antiviral agents. Depending on the IFN type, recombinant and natural IFN-α (see Table 38-11) are approved in the United States for treatment of condyloma acuminatum, chronic hepatitis C, chronic hepatitis B, Kaposi's sarcoma in HIV-infected patients, and other malignancies. IFN-β is approved for management of multiple sclerosis, and recombinant IFN-γ for treatment of chronic granulomatous disease.

Hepatitis B Virus. Chronic HBV infections are associated with deficient IFN production and often with decreased responsiveness to IFN. HBV polymerase is able to inhibit cellular responses to IFN-α and IFN-γ in vitro.[354] For patients with chronic hepatitis B, parenteral administration of various IFNs is associated with loss of HBV DNA, loss of HBeAg and development of anti-HBeAg antibody, and biochemical and histologic improvement in about 25% to 40% of patients.[341,355] Lasting responses require moderately high IFN dosages and prolonged administration (about 5 MU/day or 5 to 10 MU three times a week for 4 to 6 months). PegIFN-α2a (90 or 180 μg thrice weekly) may be superior to conventional IFN-α2a, although higher dosages (270 μg) are associated with more side effects and no greater response rates than the lower dosage.[356] Further studies of pegylated IFNs are in progress.

Responses with seroconversion to anti-HBeAg are usually associated with transaminase elevations and often a hepatitis-like illness during the 2nd or 3rd month of therapy, presumably related to immune clearance of infected hepatocytes. An increased risk for clinical deterioration exists in patients with poor or decreasing hepatic synthetic function, and lower dosages have been suggested for such patients. Factors associated with reduced response rates include high plasma HBV DNA levels (>200 pg/mL), long-standing infection, male sex, low transaminase levels, inactive histology, immunosuppressive therapy, and HIV infection.

Remissions in chronic hepatitis B induced by IFN are sustained in more than 80% of patients and are frequently followed by later loss of hepatitis B surface antigen (HBsAg) and improved long-term clinical outcomes.[357-360] Patients with pre-core mutants of HBV may have higher relapse rates.[361] IFN-γ is less effective than IFN-α/β, and combinations do not appear to enhance antiviral effects.[362,363] Some nonresponders to IFN-α may respond to a course of IFN-β.[364] Combinations of IFNs and lamivudine have not been shown to provide consistently greater antiviral effects or clinical benefits than monotherapy.[365,366]

IFN may improve HBV-associated nephrotic syndrome and glomerulonephritis in some patients.[367] Antiviral effects and improvements occur in about one half of patients with chronic hepatitis D,[368] but relapse is common unless HBsAg disappears. IFN does not appear to be beneficial in acute HBV or hepatitis D virus infections.

Hepatitis C Virus. In acute hepatitis C infection, high-dose INF monotherapy (IFN-α2b 5 MU daily for 4 weeks, then thrice weekly for 20 weeks) markedly reduces the risk for chronicity.[369] Lower-dose regimens appear less effective.[370] In chronic HCV infection, the combination of a pegylated IFN and oral ribavirin provides the highest SVR rates and has become the current standard of therapy for most patients.[371] Although IFN-α monotherapy (3 MU three times a week for 6 to 12 months) is associated with serum aminotransferase normalization[372,373] and loss of detectable serum HCV RNA in about 40% to 60% of patients,[374] more than 50% of responding patients relapse 1 to 2 months after treatment is stopped, and less than 20% have an SVR predictive of long-term biochemical and histologic improvement.[375-378]

Combined IFN and oral ribavirin (1000 to 1200 mg daily in divided doses) increases the likelihood of SVR to 35% to 45% and is superior to IFN monotherapy in both initial treatment and retreatment after IFN failure or relapse, especially in those with high HCV RNA levels or genotype 1 infections.[379,380] Combined IFN and ribavirin treatment benefits HCV-related systemic vasculitis, cryoglobulinemia, and glomerulonephritis.[381,382] Combined IFN and ribavirin, but not IFN alone, may reduce the risk for recurrent HCV infection after liver transplantation, but treatment results in an SVR in only 21% and is not well tolerated.[383]

Pegylated IFNs are more effective than standard ones in treating chronic hepatitis C. Monotherapy with pegIFN provides SVR rates of 30% to 39%, including stable cirrhotic patients,[375,376] and is a treatment option in patients unable to take ribavirin. No obvious difference in efficacy is apparent between the two available pegylated IFNs. Combined therapy with pegIFN-α2a (180 μg once weekly for 48 weeks) and ribavirin (1000 or 1200 mg daily in divided doses) gives an overall SVR rate of 56%, compared with 44% for IFN/ribavirin, and is more effective in genotype 1 infections (46% versus 36%) in previously untreated patients.[351] Similarly, combined pegIFN-α2b (1.5 μg/kg once weekly for 48 weeks) and ribavirin (800 mg daily) gives an overall SVR of 54%, compared with 47% for IFN/ribavirin.[350] Higher, weight-adjusted doses of ribavirin are more effective, particularly in genotype 1 infections. A shorter duration of therapy (24 weeks) and lower ribavirin dose (800 mg daily) are effective in genotype 2 and 3 infections (84% SVR), but prolonged therapy is needed for genotypes 1 and 4.[351a] Failure to achieve an early viral response (nondetectable HCV RNA or reduction of ≥2 log$_{10}$ at 12 weeks) is highly predictive of lack of SVR after further therapy.[384] Treatment is associated with reductions in steatosis and fibrosis progression, and histologic improvement may occur in patients who do not achieve SVRs. In patients with compensated cirrhosis, treatment may reverse cir-

rhotic changes and possibly reduce the risk for hepatocellular carcinoma.[385-387] Retreatment for 48 weeks may clear infection in those relapsing after an initial course.[148] However, only 15% to 20% of nonresponders to combined IFN/ribavirin achieve SVR with pegIFN/ribavirin therapy.[371] Long-term dosing studies with pegIFN maintenance therapy are in progress.

Age (<40 years), genotype other than 1, body weight (<75 kg), disease duration (<5 years), absence of cirrhosis, serum levels of HCV RNA (<2 × 10^6 copies/mL), and ribavirin dosage (>10.6 mg/kg) are predictors of response to IFNs.[350,351] Differences in genotype and, for genotype 1, mutations within an IFN sensitivity–determining region of the NS5A gene affect virologic responses.[388,389] HIV coinfected persons also appear to respond better to combined pegIFN/ribavirin therapy and can achieve SVRs.[148,371] Concurrent hepatitis G virus infection does not influence response and itself may resolve with IFN in a minority of patients.[390] Safety and efficacy remain to be established in uncompensated liver disease (see Chapters 112 and 150).

Herpesviruses. Although IFN is associated with antiviral effects, no consistent reductions in symptoms or lesion duration have been observed with topical or systemic IFN treatment of genital herpes.[391] Topical IFN appears to have some activity in combination with trifluridine in drug-resistant mucocutaneous HSV infections. In superficial HSV keratitis, combined administration of topical IFN-α with trifluridine or acyclovir appears to be more effective than single-agent therapy.

In localized herpes zoster in cancer patients, early treatment with high-dose IFN-α (about 36 MU/day for 5 to 7 days) reduces the risk for cutaneous or visceral dissemination, but systemic reactions are frequent, and more effective antivirals are available. IFN is not effective in preventing CMV infection in bone marrow recipients or in treating CMV pneumonia.

Human Immunodeficiency Virus. HIV-infected patients frequently have detectable IFN levels, and plasma inhibitors of IFN activity are often present during AIDS. High doses of IFN-α induce 10% to 40% response rates in patients with Kaposi's sarcoma without benefitting concurrent herpesvirus infections or immune functions.[392] IFN treatment is associated with dose-related antiretroviral effects, particularly in early-stage infection, but also with adverse effects.[393] IFN appears to benefit HIV-related thrombocytopenia[394] and eosinophilic folliculitis.

Papillomavirus. Both intralesional and systemic administrations of IFN produce some regression of anogenital warts,[395] although more cost-effective and better tolerated modalities are available.[319] Intralesional injection of various natural and recombinant IFNs is associated with complete clearance of injected warts in 42% to 62% of patients within 12 to 20 weeks.[396] Responders have relatively low relapse rates (approximately 20% to 30%). Responsiveness is poor in HIV-infected patients and those with chronic lesions. Intralesional IFN does not reliably increase the response to other local therapies.[396] Mild to moderate systemic side effects (8% to 10% dropout rate), pain and irritation at injection site, and leukopenia (up to 30%) are common with intralesional IFN. Topical IFN gel provides inconsistent effects and does not appear to substantially reduce the recurrence rate after ablative therapies.[319]

Systemic IFN may provide adjunctive benefit in recurrent juvenile laryngeal papillomatosis. The majority of children have some initial decrease in lesions, but recurrence rates are high after cessation of therapy, and the long-term response to parenteral IFN-α is variable.[397] Laryngeal disease in older patients appears to be more responsive.

Respiratory Viruses. Except for adenovirus, IFNs have broad-spectrum antiviral activity against respiratory viruses in vitro, including SARS coronavirus.[398] In experimentally induced infections in humans, intranasal administration of leukocyte or recombinant IFN-α is protective against rhinovirus, coronavirus 229E, respiratory syncytial virus (RSV), and, to a lesser extent, influenza virus infections.[399] However, under natural conditions, prophylactic intranasal IFN-α is protective only against rhinovirus colds, and chronic use is limited by the occurrence of nasal side effects. Intranasal IFN-α is ineffective in treating rhinovirus colds. IFN-α β, and γ inhibit SARS coronavirus replication in vitro,[398] and systemic alfa IFNs have been used to treat SARS coronavirus illness.[400,401]

LAMIVUDINE

Lamivudine (3TC, Epivir) is an L-configuration deoxycytidine analogue with a β-oxathiolane ring that is inhibitory for HIV and HBV (see Fig. 38-2B). Its use as an HIV reverse transcriptase inhibitor is discussed in more detail in Chapter 124 (Antiretroviral Therapy). The triphosphate moiety is also a potent inhibitor of the DNA polymerase–reverse transcriptase of HBV, and oral lamivudine is active in animal models of hepadnavirus infection. Lamivudine shows enhanced antiviral activity in combination with adefovir or penciclovir against hepadnaviruses.[104]

Resistance

Point mutations in the YMDD motif of HBV DNA polymerase (M550I/V, others) result in more than 40- to 10⁴-fold reduced in vitro susceptibility.[402-404] Lamivudine resistance confers cross-resistance to related agents such as emtricitabine and clevudine and is often associated with an additional non-YMDD mutation at codon L526M that confers cross-resistance to famciclovir.[203,405] Lamivudine-resistant HBV retains susceptibility to adefovir and entecavir.[107,405,406]

The frequency of lamivudine-resistant variants increases progressively with continued drug administration, and cumulative frequencies of 14% to 32%, 38%, 53%, and 67% have been found after 1, 2, 3, and 4 years of treatment in chronic hepatitis B, respectively.[107,407] The majority of lamivudine-resistant variants possess L526M/M550V mutations, followed by M550I and L526M/M550I.[406] The risk is higher in post-transplant infections, and HIV/HBV-coinfected patients have 50% and 90% frequencies of resistance at 2 and 4 years of lamivudine therapy, respectively.[408,409]

Viruses bearing YMDD mutations are less replication competent in vitro than wild-type HBV and may be associated with lower HBV DNA levels on therapy.[407] However, lamivudine resistance is associated with rise in HBV DNA levels, decreased likelihood of HBeAg loss or seroconversion, and sometimes biochemical and histologic deterioration, as well as graft failure in transplant recipients.[403,410,411] Emergence of resistant variants may be associated with hepatitis exacerbations in up to 67% of patients[411a] and with rapid deterioration, progressive fibrosis, and graft loss in patients with recurrent HBV after liver transplantation.

Toxicity

At the dosages used for chronic hepatitis B, lamivudine has been well tolerated, including by children, with adverse event and laboratory abnormalities being similar to those of placebo.[412] Rises in aminotransferase after therapy occur more often in lamivudine recipients, and substantial post-treatment aminotransferase elevations (>500 IU/mL) occur in about 15% of patients after cessation.[407]

Clinical Studies

In adults with chronic hepatitis B, lamivudine is associated with dose-related, reversible decreases in serum HBV DNA levels.[413] Dosages of 100 mg/day for 1 year suppress HBV DNA levels by 95% to 99%, normalize aminotransferase levels in 41% or more of patients, and reduce hepatic inflammation in 52% to 56%.[407,411] Seroconversion with detectable antibody to HBeAg occurs in only 15% to 17% of adults after 1 year. In children aged 2 to 17 years, lamivudine (3 mg/kg daily for 1 year) is associated with HBeAg loss in 26%, normalization of aminotransferase levels in 55%, and undetectable HBsAg with anti-HBe in 22%.[412] In those without emergence of YMDD variants, prolonged therapy is associated with sustained suppression of HBV DNA, normalization of aminotransferases, continued histologic improvement, and an increased proportion of patients experiencing a virologic response (loss of HBeAg and undetectable HBV DNA).[410] Combined use of IFN (10 MU three times weekly for 16 weeks) and lamivudine may be associated with higher HBeAg seroconversion rates than either

monotherapy, although not biochemical or histologic improvement,[365] and further studies are needed. In HIV-coinfected persons, higher lamivudine dosages are associated with reductions of HBV replication, reversal of hepatic decompensation, and, in a minority, anti-HBeAg seroconversion.[408] Administration before and after liver transplantation appears useful in preventing or suppressing recurrent HBV infection.[414] The use of lamivudine in chronic HBV infection is discussed in more detail in Chapter 112 (Chronic Viral Hepatitis) and Chapter 142 (Hepatitis B Virus and Hepatitis Delta Virus).

OSELTAMIVIR

Spectrum

Oseltamivir phosphate (Tamiflu) is the ethyl ester prodrug of oseltamivir carboxylate, a sialic acid analogue (Fig. 38-5A) that is a potent, specific inhibitor of the neuraminidases of influenza A and B viruses.[415,416] Oseltamivir carboxylate competitively and reversibly interacts with the active enzyme site to inhibit neuraminidase activity at low nanomolar concentrations.[417] Inhibitory concentrations for neuraminidase inhibitors in cell culture range broadly (1000-fold or more), depend on the assay method, and may not correlate with in vivo activity.[418,419] Oseltamivir carboxylate is active against viruses containing all nine influenza A neuraminidase subtypes recognized in nature, including recent pathogenic avian viruses (H5N1, H7N7, H9N2), reassortant virus containing neuraminidase from the 1918 pandemic strain, and M2 inhibitor-resistant strains.[112,116] The carboxylate is not cytotoxic and inhibits neuraminidases from mammalian sources or other pathogens only at 10⁶-fold higher concentrations. Oral oseltamivir is active in murine and ferret models of influenza.[416,418] Neuraminidase inhibitors and M2 inhibitors show enhanced antiviral activity in vitro and in animal models of influenza A virus infection.[116]

Mechanism of Action

Influenza neuraminidase cleaves terminal sialic acid residues on glycoconjugates and destroys the receptors recognized by viral hemagglutinin on cells, on newly released virions, and on respiratory tract mucins. This action is essential for release of virus from infected cells and for spread within the respiratory tract.[420] Inhibition of neuraminidase action causes newly formed virions to adhere to the cell surface and to form viral aggregates. Inhibitors limit spread of virus within the respiratory tract and may also prevent virus penetration of respiratory secretions to initiate replication.

Resistance

Resistant variants selected by in vitro passage with oseltamivir carboxylate or zanamivir have point mutations in the viral hemagglutinin and/or neuraminidase genes.[419,421] Hemagglutinin variants generally have mutations in or near the receptor binding site that make them less dependent on neuraminidase action for release from cells in vitro and that confer cross-resistance among neuraminidase inhibitors. Most of these variants retain full susceptibility in vivo.[419] Neuraminidase variants contain single amino acid substitutions in the framework or catalytic residues of the active enzyme site that alter drug binding and cause approximately 30- to over 1000-fold reduced susceptibility in enzyme inhibition assays.[417] Influenza A variants selected by oseltamivir carboxylate are subtype specific, most commonly Arg292Lys in N2 and His274Try in N1, and some remain susceptible to zanamivir. The altered neuraminidases have reduced activity or stability in vitro, and these variants usually show decreased infectivity and transmissibility in animals.[421,422]

Oseltamivir therapy has been associated with recovery of viruses with reduced susceptibility in about 1% of immunocompetent adult and 5.5% of pediatric recipients.[423,424] Generally, emergence of resistant variants has not been associated with clinical worsening, although prolonged recovery of resistant variants, sometimes in combination with M2 inhibitor resistance, has been uncommonly found in highly immunocompromised hosts.[425] Transmission of oseltamivir resistance has not been documented to date.

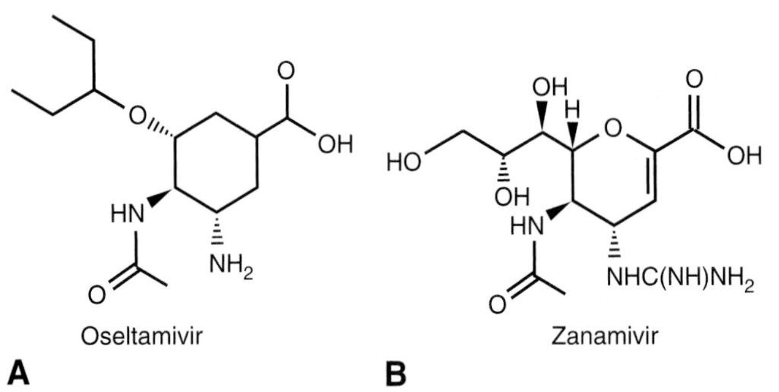

FIGURE 38-5. Chemical structures of oseltamivir carboxylate (**A**) and zanamivir (**B**).

Pharmacokinetics

Oral oseltamivir is rapidly absorbed and metabolized by esterases in the gastrointestinal tract, liver, and blood to the active carboxylate. The estimated bioavailability of the carboxylate is approximately 80%,[426] and its time to maximum plasma concentrations averages 2 to 4 hours. Only low blood levels of the prodrug are detectable. Ingestion with food delays absorption slightly but does not decrease overall bioavailability. Peak and trough plasma concentrations average 0.35 and 0.14 μg/mL, respectively, after 75-mg doses.[427] In children 1 to 12 years old given dosages of 2 mg/kg, systemic exposure to the carboxylate increased gradually as a function of age and at 5 to 8 years of age was similar to that in adults given 75 mg.[427] Overall drug exposure is about 25% greater in healthy older adults compared with healthy young adults, most likely because of differences in renal elimination. Uncomplicated influenza illness does not appear to alter the pharmacokinetics of oseltamivir.

Plasma protein binding of the prodrug (42%) and the carboxylate (<3%) is low.[426] The volume of distribution is moderate (23 to 26 L). In animals, lower respiratory tract levels are similar to or exceed those in blood,[428] and in humans the carboxylate is detectable in middle ear and maxillary sinus fluid at concentrations similar to those in plasma.[429] No carboxylate was detected in CSF in one child.[430] After oral oseltamivir, the plasma $T_{1/2elim}$ of the carboxylate averages 6 to 10 hours in healthy adults. Both the prodrug and carboxylate are excreted primarily unchanged through the kidney; the carboxylate is eliminated by glomerular filtration and tubular secretion via a probenecid-sensitive anionic transporter. Clearance varies linearly with CrCl, such that $T_{1/2elim}$ increases to 22 hours in those with CrCl less than 30 mL/min and dosage reductions are needed.[426] Oseltamivir is removed by hemodialysis.

Interactions

Probenecid reduces renal clearance of oseltamivir by about 50%. No other clinically important drug interactions have been recognized to date. Specific studies have found no interactions with antacids, acetaminophen, aspirin, or known inhibitors of selected renal tubular secretion pathways, amoxicillin, or cimetidine.

Toxicity

Oseltamivir is generally well tolerated, and no serious end-organ toxicity has been recognized.[418,431] Oral administration is associated with nausea, epigastric distress, or emesis in about 10% to 15% of treated patients. Gastrointestinal complaints are usually mild-moderate in intensity, resolve despite continued dosing, and are ameliorated by administration with food. Discontinuation rates of 1% to 2% were observed in controlled treatment studies. The mechanism is uncertain, but the risk appears to be lower in older adults. Long-term prophylaxis has not been associated with an increased risk for adverse events,[418] although headache may occur in older recipients. Erythematous skin

rashes and rare instances of severe eruptions or Stevens-Johnson syndrome, hepatic inflammation, anaphylaxis, CNS adverse events (loss of consciousness, hallucinosis, extrapyramidal signs), and thrombocytopenia have been reported but are of uncertain relationship to oseltamivir.

Preclinical studies have found no evidence of mutagenic, teratogenic, or oncogenic effects. High-dose oseltamivir causes renal tubular mineralization in mice and maternal toxicity in rabbits. It is classified as pregnancy category C.

Clinical Studies

Oral oseltamivir is highly protective against experimental human influenza, and early treatment is associated with reductions in viral titers, symptoms, nasal cytokines, and middle ear pressure abnormalities.[418] Early oseltamivir treatment of acute influenza in otherwise healthy adults and children aged 1 to 12 years reduces the time to illness alleviation by 1 to 1.5 days, fever duration, and viral titers in the upper respiratory tract.[423,432-434] Early treatment reduces time to functional recovery by 3 days or more.[435] Treatment of children also reduces the risk for otitis media and decreases overall antibiotic use.[423] In healthy and high-risk adults, early treatment decreases the risk for lower respiratory tract complications leading to antibiotics and to hospitalization.[436,437] It is unknown whether treatment reduces the risk for transmission.

Prophylactic administration of once-daily oral oseltamivir (75 mg) is highly effective in reducing the risk for developing febrile illness during influenza season in unimmunized adults (efficacy, 84%)[438] and immunized nursing home residents (efficacy, 92%).[439] Prevention of influenza reduces secondary complications in institutionalized older adults.[439] Once-daily oseltamivir for 7 to 10 days is also effective for postexposure prophylaxis in household contacts, including children, and when ill index cases receive concurrent treatment.[440,441] Oseltamivir chemoprophylaxis has been used to control institutional outbreaks of influenza A continuing despite M2 inhibitor use and of influenza B.[437]

RIBAVIRIN

Spectrum

Ribavirin (1-β-D-ribofuranosyl-1,2,4-thiazole-3-carboxamide; Virazole, Rebetol, Copegus) is a guanosine analogue (Fig. 38-6A) in which both the base and the D-ribose sugar are necessary for antiviral activity. Ribavirin inhibits the in vitro replication of a wide range of RNA and DNA viruses, including myxoviruses, paramyxoviruses, arenaviruses, flaviviruses, bunyaviruses, coronaviruses, togaviruses, reoviruses, herpesviruses, adenoviruses, poxviruses, and retroviruses. By plaque assay, inhibitory concentrations range from 3 to 10 μg/mL for influenza, parainfluenza, and RSV. High concentrations inhibit group C adenoviruses[442] and pathogenic flaviviruses,[442a] including West Nile virus in neural cells. Ribavirin does not inhibit SARS coronavirus in vitro.[443]

Low concentrations of ribavirin (1 to 10 μg/mL) reversibly inhibit macromolecular synthesis and the proliferation of rapidly dividing cells.[8] Ribavirin decreases nucleic acid and protein synthesis, inhibits IFN-γ release, and increases apoptosis in human peripheral blood mononuclear cells in vitro,[8,444] but it does not adversely affect polymorphonuclear leukocyte functions.[445] Ribavirin has been postulated to enhance cell-mediated immune responses by increasing type 1 and suppressing type 2 cytokine responses in T cells,[445] as well as to decrease proinflammatory cytokine elaboration and inflammatory cell numbers. Inhibition of mast cell secretory responses occurs in vitro.

Aerosol administration is more effective than parenteral dosing in animal models of influenza and RSV infection. Parenteral ribavirin has antiviral and therapeutic activity in animal models of Lassa virus, other arenaviruses, and bunyavirus infections. Combinations of ribavirin with immunoglobulin in RSV infection and with M2 or neuraminidase inhibitors in influenza A or with neuraminidase inhibitors in influenza B infections show enhanced antiviral activity.[117]

Mechanism of Action

The antiviral mechanisms of action of ribavirin are complex and most likely vary for different viruses. Ribavirin causes alterations of cellular nucleotide pools, inhibits viral RNA synthesis, and may cause lethal mutagenesis of certain RNA virus genomes.[445-447] Intracellular phosphorylation to the mono-, di-, and triphosphate derivatives is mediated by host cell enzymes. In both uninfected and RSV-infected cells, the predominant derivative (>80%) is the triphosphate, which is rapidly lost, with an intracellular $T_{1/2}$ of less than 2 hours.

Ribavirin monophosphate competitively inhibits inosine monophosphate dehydrogenase and interferes with the synthesis of GTP and therefore with nucleic acid synthesis. Decreased concentrations of competing GTP very likely potentiate ribavirin's other antiviral effects. Ribavirin triphosphate inhibits influenza virus RNA polymerase activity and the GTP-dependent 5'-capping of viral mRNA. The monophosphate is incorporated inefficiently into viral RNA genomes, and this may lead to lethal mutagenesis and contribute to antiviral activity.[446] HCV RNA polymerase incorporates ribavirin monophosphate into viral RNA, which causes mutations and inhibits viral RNA synthesis.[448] Ribavirin diphosphates and triphosphates also inhibit HIV reverse transcriptase activity.[449]

Ribavirin has immunosuppressive effects in experimental animals and shows therapeutic activity against transplantable virus-induced tumors and certain autoimmune diseases. Ribavirin increases type 1 cytokine–mediated immune responses in vivo, an effect that may contribute to its therapeutic activities,[445] and appears to augment type 1 cytokine responses ex vivo in peripheral blood mononuclear cells from patients with chronic hepatitis C.[447]

Resistance

Antiviral resistance to ribavirin has been documented only in Sindbis virus and hepatitis C virus to date. One HCV RNA polymerase variant (F415Y) selected in genotype 1a–infected, ribavirin-treated patients has been associated with ribavirin resistance in vitro.[450] No ribavirin-resistant RSVs have been detected during aerosol therapy of children.

Pharmacokinetics

Oral ribavirin is well absorbed but bioavailability averages 45% to 65% in adults because of first-pass metabolism.[451-454] Administration with food increases absorption and peak plasma concentrations by 70%.[451] After single oral doses of 600, 1200, or 2400 mg, peak plasma concentrations occur at 1 to 2 hours and average 1.3, 2.5, and 3.2 μg/mL, respectively. Plasma concentrations average approximately 24 μg/mL and 17 μg/mL after intravenous doses of 1000 and 500 mg, respectively, in patients with Lassa fever. During long-term administration, overall exposure and $T_{1/2elim}$ increase substantially.[451] Steady-state plasma levels of about 1.0 to 4.0 μg/mL with weight-adjusted dosing in chronic hepatitis C occur by about 4 weeks, and higher concentrations at 4 weeks correlate with both decline in hemoglobin and likelihood of SVR.[455] Plasma protein binding is negligible, and ribavirin has a large volume of distribution (>2000 L). At steady state, CSF levels are about 70% of those in plasma.[453]

The disposition of ribavirin is complex, involving both renal elimination and metabolism. After rapid initial distribution, there is a prolonged terminal $T_{1/2elim}$ of 37 to 79 hours.[451-453] Ribavirin triphosphate concentrates in erythrocytes with an erythrocyte-to-plasma ratio of 40:1 or greater, and erythrocyte levels gradually decrease, with an apparent $T_{1/2}$ of 40 days. Renal excretion accounts for approximately 30% to 60% of ribavirin's overall clearance, but hepatic metabolism is contributory. About 5% to 10% is recovered unchanged in the urine, and a much greater fraction is excreted as triazole carboxamide and carboxylic acid metabolites.[451] Plasma clearance is reduced threefold in those with advanced renal impairment (CrCl ≤30 mL/min). Dosage adjustments are needed for renal insufficiency, and ribavirin should be used with caution in those with CrCl less than 50 mL/min. Hemodialysis and hemofiltration remove small amounts of drug. Higher initial blood levels occur in severe hepatic dysfunction.[454]

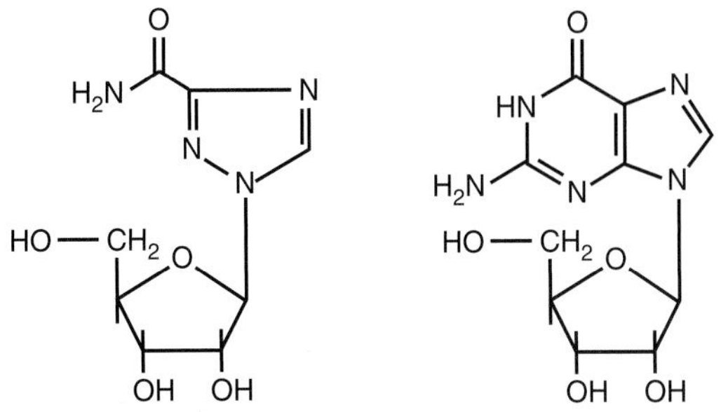

FIGURE 38-6. Chemical structures of ribavirin (**A**) and the nucleoside guanosine (**B**).

With aerosol administration, systemic absorption is low (<1% of deposited dose). Peak plasma levels range from 0.5 to 2.2 μg/mL after 8 hours exposure, and from 0.8 to 3.3 μg/mL after 20 hours in pediatric patients. Respiratory secretion levels often exceed 1000 μg/mL and persist with a half-life of 1.4 to 2.5 hours. A special aerosol generator (SPAG-2, ICN Pharmaceuticals) is needed to produce particles of proper aerodynamic size to reach the lower respiratory tract. The delivered dose is twice as high in infants (1.8 mg/kg/hour) than in adults, and various other factors influence dosage.

Toxicity

Systemic ribavirin causes dose-related anemia because of extravascular hemolysis and, at higher dosages, suppression of bone marrow release of erythroid elements.[456] Reversible increases of serum bilirubin (in up to one quarter of recipients), serum iron, and uric acid concentrations occur during short-term oral administration. Chronic oral ribavirin at dosages greater than 800 mg daily causes hemoglobin falls of 2 to 4 g/dL in most recipients, usually within 4 weeks. When used in combination with IFN, hemoglobin levels below 11 g/dL develop in 25% to 30% of patients.[457] Renal impairment increases the risk for hemolysis. Severe anemia requires dosage reduction or cessation, although erythropoietin has been used effectively.[457] Other reported side effects include pruritus, myalgia, rash, nausea, depression, nervousness, and cough or respiratory symptoms.[458] High-dose intravenous ribavirin is associated with headache, hypomagnesemia, and hypocalcemia.[459] Bolus intravenous dosing may cause rigors, and infusion over 10 to 15 minutes is advised.

Aerosolized ribavirin may cause conjunctival irritation, rash, bronchospasm, reversible deterioration in pulmonary function, and, rarely, acute water intoxication. No adverse hematologic effects have been associated with aerosolized ribavirin. The drug may precipitate on contact lenses, so that they should not be worn during aerosol exposure. Ribavirin exposure may occur in health care workers working in the environment of aerosol-treated infants.[460,461] Health care worker exposure is higher during delivery by oxygen hood than by ventilator or vacuum-exhausted hood systems.[460] Use of aerosol containment and scavenging systems, turning off the aerosol generator before providing routine care, and use of personal protective equipment have been recommended.[461]

When ribavirin is used in conjunction with mechanical ventilation, in-line filters, modified circuitry, and frequent monitoring are required to prevent plugging of ventilator valves and tubing with precipitates of ribavirin. The possible effects of such modifications on drug delivery to the lower respiratory tract are undefined.

In preclinical studies, ribavirin is mutagenic, gonadotoxic, and teratogenic.[456] Low oral dosages have been teratogenic or embryotoxic in multiple species. Its use is relatively contraindicated during pregnancy, and pregnant women should not directly care for patients receiving ribavirin aerosol. Ribavirin is categorized as pregnancy category X, and effective means of contraception for both men and women are recommended for at least 6 months after discontinuation of treatment or exposure.

Interactions

Antacids slightly decrease the bioavailability of ribavirin. Ribavirin antagonizes the anti-HIV-1 effects of zidovudine but enhances the activity of purine dideoxynucleosides. Ribavirin use in persons who are coinfected with HIV and HCV and on antiretroviral drugs, particularly combined with didanosine, appears to increase the risk for mitochondrial toxicity and lactic acidosis. Ribavirin may inhibit the effect of warfarin.

Clinical Studies

Ribavirin aerosol is approved in the United States for treatment of RSV bronchiolitis and pneumonia in hospitalized children, and oral ribavirin for treatment of chronic hepatitis C in combination with various IFNs.

Hepatitis C Virus. In adults with chronic hepatitis C, long-term oral ribavirin therapy (600 mg twice daily) reversibly reduces serum transaminase elevations, hepatic inflammation, and fatigue, without significantly affecting serum HCV RNA concentrations.[458,462] The mechanism of this benefit is uncertain but may relate to its immunomodulatory properties. The combination of oral ribavirin and conventional or pegylated IFNs significantly increases the frequency of sustained biochemical and virologic responses compared with IFN monotherapy.[379,463] Increases in sustained responses also occur in those nonresponsive to, or relapsing after, previous IFN monotherapy.[148,380,463] (See "Interferons," earlier, and Chapter 150.)

Respiratory Syncytial Virus. Aerosolized ribavirin (18-hour exposure daily for 3 to 6 days) variably shortens the duration of virus shedding and may improve certain clinical measures in infants hospitalized with RSV illness.[464] However, no consistent reductions in need for ventilatory support or duration of hospitalization have been documented. In infants receiving mechanical ventilation for RSV-related respiratory failure, no significant reductions in duration of ventilatory support, hospitalization, or mortality have been found.[464,465] Intermittent, high-dose therapy (2-hour exposures three times daily for 5 days) is well tolerated and may be as effective as prolonged exposure.[466]

Use of aerosolized ribavirin is limited by concerns regarding its efficacy, ease of administration, risk of occupational exposure, and cost. The American Academy of Pediatrics states that aerosol treatment for RSV infection "generally is not recommended" and that decisions about its administration should be based on clinical circumstances and physician experience.[86] Decreased RSV-specific serum neutralizing antibody titers, as well as diminished nasopharyngeal secretion RSV-specific IgE and IgA responses, may occur in ribavirin-treated children. No long-term adverse or beneficial effects of ribavirin therapy have been documented in children.[467]

Combinations of aerosolized ribavirin and intravenous immunoglobulin or palivizumab appear to be beneficial in treating RSV pneumonia in bone marrow transplant recipients,[468,469] whereas intravenous ribavirin alone is ineffective.[470] Aerosolized ribavirin may prevent progression from upper to lower respiratory tract illness in such patients, as might high oral dosages.[471]

Respiratory Viruses. Intravenous and aerosolized ribavirin have been used to treat severe influenza virus infections.[472] Aerosolized ribavirin inconsistently reduces viral titers and illness measures in adults with uncomplicated influenza A or B and has modest efficacy in children hospitalized with influenza.[473] Oral doses of 1.0 g/day have no activity in uncomplicated influenza, whereas a high-dose oral regimen may provide clinical benefit. Intravenous or aerosolized ribavirin, or both, have also been used in immunosuppressed patients with severe parainfluenza (PIV), measles, vaccinia, or adenovirus infections with inconsistent clinical benefits.[472,475-478] Intravenous ribavirin has been used in treating adenovirus-associated hemorrhagic cystitis, pneumonia, and invasive infections in immunocompromised patients, but it does

not appear particularly effective in severe disease.[477] Aerosolized ribavirin has been used in treating PIV infections in solid-organ transplant recipients but appears ineffective in PIV pneumonia in stem cell transplant recipients.[475] Intravenous dosing may benefit some patients failing aerosolized ribavirin. Ribavirin has been used extensively in treating SARS coronavirus infections without proven antiviral effects in vitro[443] or in patients[479] and has been associated with frequent adverse effects.[459]

Other Viruses. In patients with Lassa fever who are at high risk for death because of elevated serum aspartate aminotransferase levels or high-titer viremia, intravenous or oral ribavirin significantly reduces mortality, especially when therapy is initiated during the first 6 days of illness. High-dosage intravenous ribavirin (33 mg/kg load, 16 mg/kg every 6 hours for 4 days, 8 mg/kg every 8 hours for 3 days) reduces mortality and the risk for oliguria or hemorrhage in hemorrhagic fever with renal syndrome.[480] Intravenous ribavirin has been associated with benefit in other arenavirus hemorrhagic fevers.[481,482] High-dosage oral ribavirin appears to reduce mortality in treating Crimean-Congo hemorrhagic fever[483,484] and has been used for prophylaxis in contacts of those patients and in Lassa fever. An open-label trial suggested that it may possibly reduce mortality in Nipah virus encephalitis (see Chapter 158).[474] Intravenous ribavirin has been used in LaCrosse virus encephalitis,[485] but it appears ineffective in treatment of hantavirus cardiopulmonary syndrome.[486] In HIV-infected patients, chronic oral ribavirin at tolerable dosages has no consistent benefits on CD4 T-lymphocyte counts or HIV RNA levels.[487]

TRIFLURIDINE

Trifluridine (trifluorothymidine, 5-trifluoromethyl-2′-deoxyuridine; Viroptic) is a fluorinated pyrimidine nucleoside (see Fig. 38-4D) that has in vitro inhibitory activity against HSV types 1 and 2, CMV, vaccinia, and, to lesser extent, certain adenoviruses. Concentrations of 0.2 to 10 μg/mL inhibit replication of herpesviruses, including acyclovir-resistant HSV strains.[22]

Its antiviral mechanism of action involves inhibition of viral DNA synthesis. Trifluridine monophosphate irreversibly inhibits thymidylate synthetase, and the triphosphate competitively inhibits DNA polymerases with respect to thymidine triphosphate. Trifluridine is incorporated into viral and, to a lesser extent, cellular DNA, and it inhibits cellular DNA synthesis at relatively low concentrations. It also exhibits mutagenic, teratogenic, and antineoplastic activities in experimental systems. Trifluridine-resistant HSV with altered TK substrate specificity can be selected on laboratory passage.[313] The clinical significance of this observation is uncertain.

Trifluridine's clinical use is limited to topical therapy for HSV infections, and it is approved in the United States for treatment of primary keratoconjunctivitis and recurrent epithelial keratitis due to HSV types 1 and 2 (see Table 38-1).[314] Topical trifluridine is more active than idoxuridine in HSV ocular infections, but trials comparing its efficacy with that of topical vidarabine or acyclovir have generally found no important differences.[488] Topical trifluridine is effective in some patients who have not responded clinically to idoxuridine or vidarabine. Adverse reactions include discomfort on instillation, palpebral edema, and, uncommonly, hypersensitivity reactions, irritation, and superficial punctate or epithelial keratopathy.

Topical trifluridine also appears to benefit some patients with acyclovir-resistant HSV cutaneous infections.[489] Combinations of trifluridine and IFN-α synergistically inhibit HSV replication in vitro and have been used to treat both ocular and drug-resistant mucocutaneous HSV infections.[22]

VIDARABINE

Vidarabine (9-β-D-ribofuranosyladenine; ara-A, adenine arabinoside; Vira-A) is an analogue of adenosine (see Fig. 38-4E), which has in vitro antiviral activity against herpesviruses, poxviruses, rhabdoviruses, and some RNA tumor viruses. Plaque formation by most HSV and VZV strains is completely inhibited by 3.0 μg/mL or less of vidarabine, and it is inhibitory for idoxuridine- and acyclovir-resistant strains.

Vidarabine is phosphorylated by cellular enzymes to the triphosphate, which competitively inhibits the activity of viral and, to a lesser extent, cellular DNA polymerases. Vidarabine triphosphate is incorporated into both cellular and viral DNA. Vidarabine triphosphate inhibits other host cell enzyme systems, including ribonucleoside reductase, RNA polyadenylation, and S-adenosylhomocysteine hydrolase. Resistant variants resulting from mutations in viral DNA polymerase can be selected under laboratory conditions, but drug resistance is not a recognized clinical problem.

Little systemic absorption occurs after ophthalmic application. Absorbed vidarabine is rapidly converted to its hypoxanthine metabolite (araHx) which has 30- to 50-fold less antiviral activity. Excretion of vidarabine and araHx occurs by the kidneys.

Vidarabine has been shown to be mutagenic, teratogenic, and oncogenic in preclinical testing. Hypersensitivity reactions, including pruritus, erythema, ocular pain, and foreign body sensation may occur after ocular application. Other reported effects include photophobia, keratitis after exposure to ultraviolet light, and increased lacrimation.

Intravenous vidarabine has activity in certain life-threatening herpesvirus infections, including herpes simplex encephalitis, neonatal HSV, varicella in immunocompromised persons, and chronic EBV,[490] but not smallpox. It was discontinued in the United States in 1992. An ophthalmic ointment of vidarabine is superior to idoxuridine in HSV keratoconjunctivitis (see Table 38-1),[314] and is effective in patients who cannot receive idoxuridine because of allergy, toxicity, or drug resistance.

ZANAMIVIR

Spectrum

Zanamivir (4-guanidino-2,4-dideoxy-N-acetylneuraminic acid, Relenza) is a sialic acid analogue (see Fig. 38-5B) that is a potent and specific inhibitor of the neuraminidases of influenza A and B viruses.[491] It inhibits influenza neuraminidase activity at nanomolar concentrations but has a much broader range of inhibitory concentrations in cell culture.[492,493] Compared to oseltamivir carboxylate, zanamivir is more active against influenza B but less active against influenza A/N2 neuraminidases of clinical isolates,[494] although the clinical importance of such differences is uncertain. Zanamivir is inhibitory for certain influenza A neuraminidase variants that are resistant to oseltamivir carboxylate.[417] It is not cytotoxic and inhibits neuraminidases from mammalian sources or other pathogens only at 10^6-fold higher concentrations. Millimolar concentrations inhibit parainfluenza virus 3 in cell culture, most likely by blocking attachment.[495] Topical zanamivir is active in murine and ferret models of influenza.[492]

Resistance

The mechanisms of antiviral action and resistance are essentially the same as those for oseltamivir. Hemagglutinin variants resistant in cell culture generally remain susceptible in vivo.[419] Zanamivir-selected neuraminidase variants have active site substitutions that diminish drug binding (Glu119Gly, Ala, or Asp) or alter one of the catalytic residues (Arg152Lys, Arg292Lys). The altered neuraminidases have reduced activity or stability, and the mutated viruses have decreased infectivity in animals.[496] Resistance emergence has not been documented with zanamivir in immunocompetent hosts to date.[492] One variant, cross-resistant to oseltamivir carboxylate and possessing both hemagglutinin and neuraminidase substitutions (Arg152Lys) has been recovered from an immunocompromised child with prolonged virus excretion despite receiving nebulized zanamivir.[496]

Pharmacokinetics

The oral bioavailability of zanamivir is low (<5%), and the approved formulation is a dry powder containing a lactose carrier and delivered by oral inhalation with a proprietary Diskhaler device. After inhalation of the dry powder, approximately 15% is deposited in the lower respiratory tract and the remainder in the oropharynx.[492] In uninfected persons, median zanamivir levels in induced sputum are 1.34, 0.30, and 0.05 μg/mL at 6, 12, and 24 hours after dosing, respectively, and the pulmonary $T_{1/2}$ is estimated to be 2.8 hours.[497] Approximately 4% to 17% of a dose is absorbed systemically, and peak plasma levels are low, averaging 0.04 to 0.05 μg/mL.[492] After intravenous dosing, the plasma $T_{1/2elim}$ of zanamivir averages 1.6 hours, and about 90% is eliminated unchanged in the urine.[492] Because of the low bioavailability, dosage adjustments are not indicated in renal insufficiency.

The proprietary inhaler device for delivering zanamivir is breath-activated and requires a cooperative, trained patient. The use of the Diskhaler device is not reliable in young children, very infirm or elderly persons, or those cognitively impaired. Although the inhaler has been used effectively in most older adults,[498] over one half of hospitalized older adults could not correctly use the device after instruction.[499]

Interactions

No clinically significant drug interactions have been recognized for inhaled zanamivir.

Toxicity

Inhaled zanamivir is generally well tolerated, and the frequencies of complaints are not significantly different from those in placebo recipients among adults and children aged 5 years or older.[492,500,501] Most reported symptoms appear to be the result of the underlying illness. Similarly, in high-risk patients receiving zanamivir or placebo, no differences in adverse reactions have been seen in controlled trials.[502,503] In patients with mild-moderate asthma or chronic obstructive pulmonary disease (COPD), inhaled zanamivir is associated with fewer bronchitis episodes, similar measurements of forced expired volume in 1 second (FEV_1), and more rapid improvement in peak expiratory flow rate (PEFR) than with inhaled placebo.[504] However, postmarketing reports indicate a potential risk for acute bronchospasm, respiratory arrest, or worsening of COPD accompanied by pulmonary edema, after zanamivir inhalation, particularly in persons with underlying airway disease.[505] Apparent declines in respiratory function have also been rarely reported in those without recognized airway disease. Consequently, use in patients with underlying airway disease is not generally recommended in the United States, although treatment in at-risk patients is used in other countries.[506] If used in patients with obstructive airway disease, zanamivir should be administered cautiously under close observation and with availability of fast-acting bronchodilators.

Preclinical studies of zanamivir found no evidence of mutagenic, teratogenic, or oncogenic effects. It is classified as a pregnancy category C agent.

Clinical Studies

Intranasal and intravenous zanamivir are highly protective against experimental human influenza, and early treatment is associated with reductions in viral titers, symptoms, and middle ear pressure abnormalities.[433,492,507] Early inhaled zanamivir (10 mg twice daily for 5 days) treatment of uncomplicated influenza in previously healthy adults and children aged 5 to 12 years shortens the times to illness resolution and return to usual activities by 1 to 3 days.[501,508,509] Treatment benefits appear to be greater in those with severe symptoms at entry, in those older than 50 years, and in higher-risk patients.[510] Inhaled zanamivir treatment in adults is associated with a 40% reduction in lower respiratory tract events leading to antibiotic use and a 28% overall reduction in antibiotic prescriptions.[511] In high-risk patients with primarily mild-moderate asthma or other chronic cardiopulmonary conditions, zanamivir treatment reduces illness duration and the incidence of complications leading to antibiotic use.[504,512] It has been used to treat immunocompromised hosts with influenza A and B infections.[513]

Prophylactic administration of once-daily inhaled zanamivir (10 mg) is protective against febrile influenza illness during influenza season (84% efficacy)[514] or when used for postexposure prophylaxis in households with or without treatment of the ill index case (82% efficacy).[515,516] One study found that 2 weeks of inhaled zanamivir was superior to oral rimantadine in preventing influenza A infection in nursing home residents, in part because of a high frequency of rimantadine resistance,[517] and inhaled zanamivir has been used to curtail transmission of amantadine-resistant influenza A in nursing homes.[498] However, inhaled zanamivir is not approved for chemoprophylaxis in the United States or most countries.

AGENTS OF INVESTIGATIVE INTEREST

Progress continues to be made in determining the optimal dosing regimens for many of the available antiviral agents. However, a large number of viral infections exist for which no effective antiviral treatment is available, either because of lack of an agent with sufficient potency and selectivity or because active viral replication is not central to the pathogenesis of disease manifestations. Many agents have toxicity, poor oral bioavailability, and/or high cost. Although several antivirals can suppress reactivations of infection, none can eradicate viral latency. Gene inhibition therapy (e.g., antisense oligonucleotides, ribozymes) may eventually be able to accomplish this goal.

A novel antiviral strategy increasingly used in laboratory studies is RNA interference, a process of gene silencing in which introduced double-stranded RNA (dsRNA) leads to sequence-specific degradation of mRNA. Naturally occurring RNA interference is modulated by a dsRNA-specific endonuclease, termed Dicer-RDE-1, that cleaves longer dsRNA into fragments 21 to 25 bases in length. These short or small interfering RNAs (siRNAs) are incorporated into a host protein–enzyme complex that degrades the targeted mRNA or inhibits its translation. Intracellular introduction of synthetic 21- to 23-nucleotide siRNA duplexes into cells can inhibit expression of a variety of target genes, including essential viral ones, and does not induce interferon responses.[518] Inhibition of viral replication has been shown in transfected cell cultures for a range of viruses, including HCV, influenza, SARS CoV RSV, and picornaviruses.[518,519] Of note, intravenous administration of siRNA can reduce gene expression in vivo,[520] but in vivo application of this approach is limited by the technical challenges of achieving intracellular delivery of sufficient siRNA. Expression of small-hairpin RNAs is also effective in inducing gene suppression in vivo.[521] The clinical potential of RNA interference remains to be determined.

Current investigation remains focused heavily on antiretroviral agents, but there are a substantial number of candidate agents of clinical interest, particularly for hepatitis B infections.[408] In addition to agents with improved pharmacokinetic properties, greater potency, or improved toxicity profiles, the use of drug combinations will continue to receive greater emphasis. The areas in which advances are likely to provide more effective treatments include the identification of new viral targets (e.g., virus-specific enzymes, regulatory proteins); new drug delivery techniques to improve pharmacokinetic properties (e.g., oral prodrugs) or to target delivery to particular tissues; the use of agents to modulate the effects of immunopathologic responses or host inflammatory mediators; and the use of immunomodulators or specific immunotherapies (e.g., monoclonal antibodies, therapeutic vaccines). Several representative agents of recent investigative interest are outlined in the following paragraphs.

Brivudin

Brivudin ([E]-5-[2-bromovinyl]-2'-deoxyuridine) is a halogenated thymidine nucleoside analogue that is licensed for treatment of herpes zoster in several European Union countries but not the United States (Fig. 38-7A).[522] Brivudin potently and selectively inhibits replication of VZV and to a lesser extent HSV-1 in vitro. In vitro inhibitory concentrations of brivudin average 0.0033 μM for clinical VZV isolates and are over 100-fold lower than those for acyclovir and penciclovir.[523] When used for early treatment of nonophthalmic herpes zoster in immunocompetent adults, oral brivudin (125 mg once daily for 7 days) is generally comparable to acyclovir (800 mg 5 times daily) in effects on acute pain and

healing of lesions, although it may accelerate cessation of new lesion formation to a slightly greater extent.[522] In adults 50 years old and older, brivudin treatment appears to reduce modestly the frequency, although not the duration, of postherpetic neuralgia, compared with acyclovir.[524] Treatment-related adverse effects are similar to those of acyclovir, with low frequencies of gastrointestinal upset, headache, and dizziness.[524] The main metabolite of brivudin is bromovinyluracil, which interferes with the catabolism of fluorinated pyrimidines such as 5-fluorouracil, with the result that potentially serious drug interactions can occur.

Clevudine

Clevudine (L-FMAU) is a fluorinated L-arabinofuranosyl nucleoside analogue that is inhibitory for hepadnaviruses and EBV. Clevudine is about 10-fold more potent than lamivudine against HBV in cell culture, although it is not inhibitory for most lamivudine-resistant variants.[406] Once-daily oral administration reduces woodchuck hepatitis virus replication, including hepatocyte covalently closed circular (ccc) DNA levels.[525]

In patients with chronic HBV infection, clevudine (10 to 200 mg once daily for 4 weeks) reduces HBV DNA levels by 2.5 to 3.0 $\log_{10}$ copies/mL and is associated with sustained biochemical and antiviral effects at 6 months after dosing.[526] Tolerance has been good to date, and further studies are in progress.

Emtricitabine

Emtricitabine ([−]FTC) is a 5'-fluorinated derivative of lamivudine recently approved for treatment of HIV infection (see Fig. 38-7B). Emtricitabine's potency and selectivity for HBV are comparable to lamivudine in cell culture, and it is not inhibitory for lamivudine-resistant HBV variants.[406] Emtricitabine is phosphorylated by cellular enzymes to the triphosphate that inhibits HBV DNA polymerase. Once-daily emtricitabine reduces viremia in chronically infected woodchucks with effects similar to those of lamivudine. In humans, emtricitabine is rapidly absorbed and has a plasma $T_{1/2elim}$ of about 6 to 9 hours.[527] Once-daily dosing (25 to 300 mg for 8 weeks) is associated with nearly dose proportional steady-state plasma concentrations (peak 1.7 μg/mL with 100-mg doses) and rapid antiviral effects with approximate 3 $\log_{10}$ reductions in HBV DNA levels.[527] Resistance mutations develop in 19% of patients within 2 years of treatment.[408] Further studies are in progress. See Chapter 124 for use in HIV infection.

Entecavir

Entecavir is a cyclopentyl 2'-deoxyguanosine nucleoside analogue that potently and selectively inhibits hepadnaviruses (see Fig. 38-7C). It is inhibitory for HBV replication at nanomolar concentrations and is from 30- to greater than 1000-fold more active than lamivudine in cell culture, depending on the assay.[402,406,528] Entecavir is also inhibitory for lamivudine-resistant HBV variants possessing M550I or M550V/L526M mutations, although at 20- to 30-fold or higher concentrations.[402,406] After intracellular phosphorylation by cellular enzymes, the triphosphate inhibits several viral DNA polymerase functions, including priming, reverse transcription, and synthesis of positive-strand DNA. The triphosphate accumulates intracellularly at approximately 10- to 30-fold higher concentrations relative to extracellular entecavir levels and persists with a $T_{1/2}$ of about 15 hours. Oral entecavir is active in several animal models of hepadnavirus infection; prolonged administration for 3 years in hepatitis virus–infected woodchucks results in sustained viral suppression without resistance emergence, in reductions in hepatocyte ccc DNA levels, and in partial protection against hepatocellular carcinoma.[529]

In humans, administration of 0.5-mg doses results in steady-state plasma concentrations of approximately 2.4 nM. Short-term administration (0.05 to 1.0 mg daily for 4 weeks) is associated with approximately 2 to 3 $\log_{10}$ suppression of serum HBV DNA levels and at higher doses (0.5 and 1.0 mg) delay in return of levels to baseline.[530] Entecavir (0.1 or 0.5 mg once daily for 24 weeks) reduces HBV DNA levels by over 4 $\log_{10}$ copies/mL, or about 10-fold more than lamivudine.[531] Sustained inhibition of lamivudine-resistant HBV infections

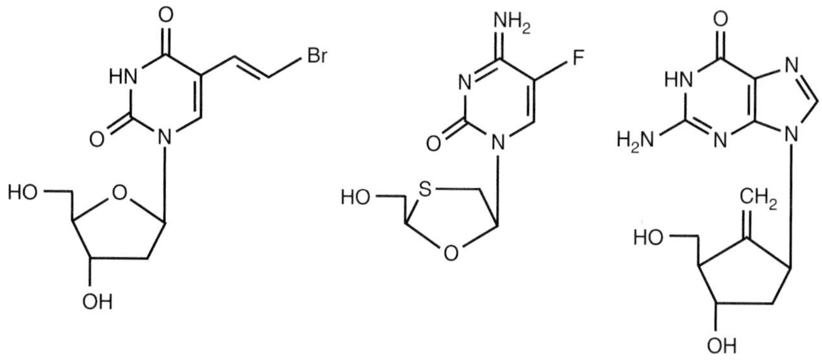

FIGURE 38-7. Chemical structures of the investigational agents brivudin (**A**), emtricitabine (**B**), and entecavir (**C**).

Brivudin

A

Emtricitabine

B

Entecavir

C

occurs at dosages of 0.5 or 1.0 mg given daily for 48 weeks.[528] Entecavir is active in those with liver transplant reinfection.[528] Possible adverse effects include headache, dizziness, lethargy, gastrointestinal upset (abdominal discomfort, nausea, and diarrhea), and photosensitivity. Long-term studies are in progress.

Levovirin and Viramidine

Several ribavirin analogues have been developed in efforts to reduce hematologic toxicity while retaining or enhancing other effects of the drug in treatment of chronic hepatitis C.[447] Viramidine, the carboxamidine analogue of ribavirin, is a prodrug that is converted by host deaminases to ribavirin, principally in the liver of experimental animals. Hepatic targeting may reduce systemic exposure and increase actions at the site of HCV replication. Levovirin, the L-enantiomer of ribavirin, does not undergo intracellular phosphorylation and avoids the anemia induced by ribavirin while apparently retaining ribavirin's immunomodulatory, although not its antiviral, properties. Clinical studies with such agents are in progress.

Maribavir

Maribavir is a L-ribofuranosyl benzimidazole (5,6-dichloro-2-isopropylamino-1-(β-L-ribofuranosyl)-1H-benzimadazole) that is inhibitory for CMV and EBV, but not other human herpesviruses, in vitro (Fig. 38-8A).[532] It inhibits replication of clinical isolates of CMV at concentrations of less than 1 μM to approximately 15 μM in cell culture, including most variants resistant to ganciclovir, cidofovir, and/or foscarnet.[532,533] Maribavir has a novel mechanism of anti-CMV action that does not require intracellular phosphorylation and that resistance selection studies map both to the UL97 protein kinase and to the UL27 protein.[534,535] Maribavir appears to inhibit viral DNA synthesis and to block nuclear egress of virions. Inhibition of UL97 function reduces the phosphorylation of several viral proteins, including UL44, which is essential for CMV DNA replication.[535]

Oral maribavir is rapidly absorbed and shows dose-proportional kinetics.[533] A high-fat meal decreases absorption by 30%.[536] Maribavir is highly bound to plasma proteins (>97%). The plasma $T_{1/2elim}$ is about 3 to 6 hours, and 30% to 40% of the dose is cleared in the urine as an N-alkylated metabolite and less than 2% as the parent.[536] In HIV-infected adults, maribavir (330 to 2400 mg daily in divided doses for 28 days) is associated with approximately 3 $\log_{10}$ or greater reductions in semen CMV titers.[533] Dose-related taste disturbance and diarrhea occur, and other possible adverse effects include rash, pruritus, headache, nausea, and fever. Studies for CMV prophylaxis in transplant recipients are expected.

Pleconaril

Pleconaril (3-[3,5-dimethyl-4([3-(3-methyl-5-isoxazoyl)propyl]oxy) phenyl]-5-[trifluoromethyl]-1,2,4-oxadiazole) is an orally active antipicornavirus agent (see Fig. 38-8B). Pleconaril inhibits picornavirus replication by binding to a specific hydrophobic pocket within the viral capsid and preventing viral attachment and/or uncoating of the genome. In cell culture, pleconaril inhibits replication of almost all commonly isolated enterovirus serotypes[537] and approximately 90% of rhinovirus clinical isolates.[538] Pleconaril is active in murine and human models of coxsackievirus infection.[537,539]

In adults, oral bioavailability is about 70% in the fed state, and peak plasma concentrations average 2.2 μg/mL after doses of 400 mg.[540] Pleconaril undergoes hepatic metabolism, and less than 1% is excreted unchanged in the urine. The initial plasma $T_{1/2elim}$ averages 2 to 3 hours, but there is a prolonged terminal $T_{1/2elim}$ of approximately 180 hours.[540] Single oral doses of 5 mg/kg in children provide maximal plasma concentrations of 1.3 μg/mL and approximately 40% lower overall drug exposure because of a larger volume of distribution and more rapid clearance. Neonates appear to require higher dosages in part because of lower bioavailability.[541]

Pleconaril has been generally well tolerated, and the most common adverse events have been headache, nausea, diarrhea, and abdominal discomfort. However, pleconaril induces cytochrome P450 3A isoenzymes and consequently has the potential for multiple drug interactions, including with oral contraceptives.[542] In children or adults with enteroviral meningitis, pleconaril has inconsistent effects on headache and illness duration.[540] Pleconaril (400 mg three times a day for 5 days) reduces the duration of uncomplicated rhinovirus colds by about 1 day[542] but was not approved by the FDA for this indication. Pleconaril treatment (15 mg/kg/day [children] and 600 to 1200 mg/day [adults] in divided doses for 7 to 10 days) appears to be beneficial in some patients

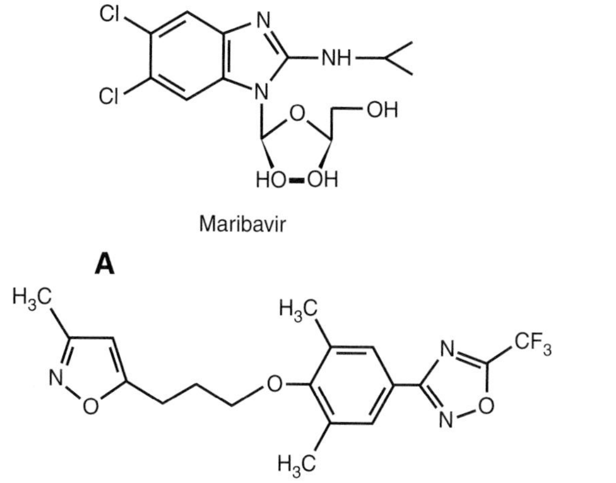

Maribavir

A

Pleconaril

B

FIGURE 38-8. Chemical structures of the investigational agents maribavir (**A**) and pleconaril (**B**).

with severe or life-threatening enteroviral syndromes, including chronic enteroviral meningoencephalitis in agammaglobulinemic patients and possibly neonatal enteroviral sepsis.[540,543] Intranasal pleconaril is under study.

Telbivudine

Telbivudine or L-deoxythymidine (LdT), is a potent inhibitor of HBV replication. A 1-year dose-ranging study found that oral doses of 400 mg and 600 mg per day, alone or in combination with lamivudine, were well tolerated and associated with $\geq 6.0 \log_{10}$ copies/mL reductions in HBV DNA, compared to a $4.7 \log_{10}$ reduction for standard lamivudine therapy.[545] Combining telbivudine and lamivudine did not enhance antiviral or biochemical effects. Phase III trials of telbivudine are underway.

Tenofovir

Tenofovir is an acyclic nucleotide analogue reverse transcriptase inhibitor with activity against HIV and HBV replication, including lamivudine-resistant variants.[102] The orally administered prodrug, tenofovir disoproxil fumarate, is widely used in treatment of HIV (see Chapter 124) and appears generally well tolerated. Tenofovir treatment (245 or 300 mg daily) of patients coinfected with HIV and HBV, including those with documented lamivudine resistance mutations, results in approximately $4 \log_{10}$ reductions in serum HBV DNA levels by 24 weeks and biochemical improvement.[408,409,544] Treatment to 52 weeks shows sustained anti-HBV effects, and some patients experience anti-HBe seroconversion.[409] HBV resistance emergence is not observed during short-term administration. The effects of prolonged therapy remain to be determined, but tenofovir appears to be an especially promising treatment for coinfected patients in the context of HAART therapy. Monotherapy in coinfected persons is discouraged because of the potential for selecting HIV resistance.[408]

REFERENCES

1. Avery R, Blumberg E, Burroughs M, et al. American Society of Transplantation Infectious Disease Community Practice Infectious Disease Guidelines. Am J Trans. In press.
2. Richman DD, ed. Antiviral Drug Resistance. Chichester, UK: Wiley; 1996.
3. Beutner KR, Ferenczy A. Therapeutic approaches to genital warts. Am J Med. 1997;102:28-37.
4. Sommadossi JP. Nucleoside analogs: Similarities and differences. Clin Infect Dis. 1993;16(Suppl 1):S7-15.
5. Neyts J, Andrei G, De Clercq E. The novel immunosuppressive agent mycophenolate mofetil markedly potentiates the antiherpesvirus activities of acyclovir, ganciclovir, and penciclovir in vitro and in vivo. Antimicrob Agents Chemother. 1998;42:216-222.
6. Wagstaff AJ, Faulds D, Goa KL. Aciclovir: A reappraisal of its antiviral activity, pharmacokinetic properties and therapeutic efficacy. Drugs. 1994;47:153-205.
7. Whitley RJ, Gnann JJ. Acyclovir: A decade later. N Engl J Med. 1992;327:782-789.
8. Heagy W, Crumpacker C, Lopez PA, Finberg RW. Inhibition of immune functions by antiviral drugs. J Clin Invest. 1991;87:1916-1924.
9. Bacon TH, Levin MJ, Leary JJ, et al. Herpes simplex virus resistance to acyclovir and penciclovir after two decades of antiviral therapy. Clin Microbiol Rev. 2003;16:114-128.
10. Shin YK, Weinberg A, Spruance S, et al. Susceptibility of herpes simplex virus isolates to nucleoside analogues and the proportion of nucleoside-resistant variants after repeated topical application of penciclovir to recurrent herpes labialis. J Infect Dis. 2003;187:1241-1245.
11. Chatis PA, Crumpacker CS. Resistance of herpesviruses to antiviral drugs. Antimicrob Agents Chemother. 1992;36:1589-1595.
12. Gilbert C, Bestman-Smith J, Boivin G. Resistance of herpesviruses to antiviral drugs: Clinical impacts and molecular mechanisms. Drug Resist Updat. 2002;5:88-114.
13. Gaudreau A, Hill E, Balfour HH, et al. Phenotypic and genotypic characterization of acyclovir-resistant herpes simplex viruses from immunocompromised patients. J Infect Dis. 1998;178:297-303.
14. Hill EL, Hunter GA, Ellis MN. In vitro and in vivo characterization of herpes simplex virus clinical isolates recovered from patients infected with human immunodeficiency virus. Antimicrob Agents Chemother. 1991;35:2322-2328.
15. Christophers J, Clayton J, Craske J, et al. Survey of resistance of herpes simplex virus to acyclovir in northwest England. Antimicrob Agents Chemother. 1998;42:868-872.
16. Reyes M, Shaik NS, Graber JM, et al. Acyclovir-resistant genital herpes among persons attending sexually transmitted disease and human immunodeficiency virus clinics. Arch Intern Med. 2003;163:76-80.
17. Englund JA, Zimmerman ME, Swierkosz EM, et al. Herpes simplex virus resistant to acyclovir: A study in a tertiary care center. Ann Intern Med. 1990;112:416-422.
18. Fife KH, Crumpacker CS, Mertz GJ, et al. Recurrence and resistance patterns of herpes simplex virus following cessation of > or = 6 years of chronic suppression with acyclovir. Acyclovir Study Group. J Infect Dis. 1994;169:1338-1341.
19. Safrin S, Crumpacker C, Chatis P, et al. A controlled trial comparing foscarnet with vidarabine for acyclovir-resistant mucocutaneous herpes simplex in the acquired immunodeficiency syndrome. The AIDS Clinical Trials Group. N Engl J Med. 1991;325:551-555.
20. Ljungman P, Ellis MN, Hackman RC, et al. Acyclovir-resistant herpes simplex virus causing pneumonia after marrow transplantation. J Infect Dis. 1990;162:244-248.
21. Engel JP, Englund JA, Fletcher CV, Hill EL. Treatment of resistant herpes simplex virus with continuous-infusion acyclovir. JAMA. 1990;263:1662-1664.
22. Birch CJ, Tyssen DP, Tachedjian G, et al. Clinical effects and in vitro studies of trifluorothymidine combined with interferon-alpha for treatment of drug-resistant and -sensitive herpes simplex virus infections. J Infect Dis. 1992;166:108-112.
23. Javaly K, Wohlfeiler M, Kalayjian R, et al. Treatment of mucocutaneous herpes simplex virus infections unresponsive to acyclovir with topical foscarnet cream in AIDS patients: A phase I/II study. J Acquir Immune Defic Syndr. 1999;21:301-306.
24. Gilbert J, Drehs MM, Weinberg JM. Topical imiquimod for acyclovir-unresponsive herpes simplex virus 2 infection. Arch Dermatol. 2001;137(8):1015-1017.
25. Chilukuri S, Rosen T. Management of acyclovir-resistant herpes simplex virus. Dermatol Clin. 2003;21:311-320.
26. Levin MJ, Dahl KM, Weinberg A, et al. Development of resistance to acyclovir during chronic infection with the Oka vaccine strain of varicella-zoster virus, in an immunosuppressed child [comment]. J Infect Dis. 2003;188(7):954-959.
27. Saint-Leger E, Caumes E, Breton G, et al. Clinical and virologic characterization of acyclovir-resistant varicella-zoster viruses isolated from 11 patients with acquired immunodeficiency syndrome. Clin Infect Dis. 2001;33:2061-2067.
28. Jacobson MA, Berger TG, Fikrig S, et al. Acyclovir-resistant varicella zoster virus infection after chronic oral acyclovir therapy in patients with the acquired immunodeficiency syndrome (AIDS). Ann Intern Med. 1990;112:187-191.
29. Safrin S, Berger TG, Gilson I, et al. Foscarnet therapy in five patients with AIDS and acyclovir-resistant varicella-zoster virus infection. Ann Intern Med. 1991;115:19-21.
30. Tod M, Lokiec F, Bidault R, et al. Pharmacokinetics of oral acyclovir in neonates and in infants: A population analysis. Antimicrob Agents Chemother. 2001;45:150-157.
31. Wang LH, Schultz M, Weller S, et al. Pharmacokinetics and safety of multiple-dose valaciclovir in geriatric volunteers with and without concomitant diuretic therapy. Antimicrob Agents Chemother. 1996;40:80-85.
32. Soul-Lawton J, Seaber E, On N, et al. Absolute bioavailability and metabolic disposition of valaciclovir, the L-valyl ester of acyclovir, following oral administration to humans. Antimicrob Agents Chemother. 1995;39:2759-2764.
33. Nadal D, Leverger G, Sokal EM, et al. An investigation of the steady-state pharmacokinetics of oral valacyclovir in immunocompromised children. J Infect Dis. 2002;186(Suppl 1):S123-S130.
34. Beutner KR, Friedman DJ, Forszpaniak C, et al. Valaciclovir compared with acyclovir for improved therapy for herpes zoster in immunocompetent adults. Antimicrob Agents Chemother. 1995;39:1546-1553.
35. Lycke J, Malmestrom C, Stahle L. Acyclovir levels in serum and cerebrospinal fluid after oral administration of valaciclovir. Antimicrob Agents Chemother. 2003;47:2438-2441.
36. Frenkel LM, Brown ZA, Bryson YJ, et al. Pharmacokinetics of acyclovir in the term human pregnancy and neonate. Am J Obstet Gynecol. 1991;164:569-576.
37. Hintz M, Connor JD, Spector SA, et al. Neonatal acyclovir pharmacokinetics in patients with herpes virus infections. Am J Med. 1982;73:210-214.
38. de Miranda P, Good SS, Krasny HC, et al. Metabolic fate of radioactive acyclovir in humans. Am J Med. 1982;73:215-220.
39. Stathoulopoulou F, Dhillon S, Thodis H, et al. Evaluation of valaciclovir dosage reduction in continuous ambulatory peritoneal dialysis patients. Nephron. 2002;91:164-166.
40. Burgess ED, Gill MJ. Intraperitoneal administration of acyclovir in patients receiving continuous ambulatory peritoneal dialysis. J Clin Pharmacol. 1990;30:997-1000.
41. Cooper DA, Pehrson PO, Pedersen C, et al. The efficacy and safety of zidovudine alone or as cotherapy with acyclovir for the treatment of patients with AIDS and AIDS-related complex: A double-blind randomized trial. European-Australian Collaborative Group. AIDS. 1993;7:197-207.
42. De Bony F, Tod M, Bidault R, et al. Multiple interactions of cimetidine and probenecid with valaciclovir and its metabolite acyclovir. Antimicrob Agents Chemother. 2002;46:458-463.
43. Haefeli WE, Schoenenberger RA, Weiss P, Ritz RF. Acyclovir-induced neurotoxicity: Concentration-side effect relationship in acyclovir overdose. Am J Med. 1993;94:212-215.
44. Rashed A, Azadeh B, Abu RH. Acyclovir-induced acute tubulo-interstitial nephritis. Nephron. 1990;56:436-438.
45. Henry RE, Wegmann JA, Hartle JE, Christopher GW. Successful oral acyclovir desensitization. Ann Allergy. 1993;70:386-388.
46. Tyring SK, Baker D, Snowden W. Valacyclovir for herpes simplex virus infection: Long-term safety and sustained efficacy after 20 years' experience with acyclovir. J Infect Dis. 2002;186(Suppl 1):S40-S46.
47. Goldberg LH, Kaufman R, Kurtz TO, et al. Long-term suppression of recurrent genital herpes with acyclovir: A 5-year benchmark. Acyclovir Study Group. Arch Dermatol. 1993;129:582-587.
48. Clive D, Corey L, Reichman RC, et al. A double-blind, placebo-controlled cytogenetic study of oral acyclovir in patients with recurrent genital herpes. J Infect Dis. 1991;164:753-757.
49. Kimberlin D, Powell D, Gruber W, et al. Administration of oral acyclovir suppressive therapy after neonatal herpes simplex virus disease limited to the skin, eyes and mouth: Results of a phase I/II trial. Pediatr Infect Dis J. 1996;15:247-254.

50. Feinberg JE, Hurwitz S, Cooper D, et al. A randomized, double-blind trial of valaciclovir prophylaxis for cytomegalovirus disease in patients with advanced human immunodeficiency virus infection. AIDS Clinical Trials Group Protocol 204/Glaxo Wellcome 123-014 International CMV Prophylaxis Study Group. J Infect Dis. 1998;177:48-56.

51. Lowance D, Neumayer H, Legendre CM, et al. Valacyclovir for the prevention of cytomegalovirus disease after renal transplantation. N Engl J Med. 1999;340:1462-1470.

52. Ratanajamit C, Vinther S, Jepsen P, et al. Adverse pregnancy outcome in women exposed to acyclovir during pregnancy: A population-based observational study. Scand J Infect Dis. 2003;35:255-259.

53. Wald A, Benedetti J, Davis G, et al. A randomized, double-blind, comparative trial comparing high- and standard-dose oral acyclovir for first-episode genital herpes infections. Antimicrob Agents Chemother. 1994;38:174-176.

54. Fife KH, Barbarash RA, Rudolph T, et al. Valaciclovir versus acyclovir in the treatment of first-episode genital herpes infection: Results of an international, multicenter, double-blind, randomized clinical trial. The Valaciclovir International Herpes Simplex Virus Study Group. Sex Transm Dis. 1997;24:481-486.

55. Wald A, Carrell D, Remington M, et al. Two-day regimen of acyclovir for treatment of recurrent genital herpes simplex virus type 2 infection. Clin Infect Dis. 2001;34:944-948.

56. Bodsworth NJ, Crooks RJ, Borelli S, et al. Valaciclovir versus aciclovir in patient initiated treatment of recurrent genital herpes: A randomised, double blind clinical trial. International Valaciclovir HSV Study Group. Genitourin Med. 1997;73:110-116.

57. Spruance SL, Tyring SK, Degregorio B, et al. A large-scale, placebo-controlled, dose-ranging trial of peroral valaciclovir for episodic treatment of recurrent herpes genitalis. Valaciclovir HSV Study Group. Arch Intern Med. 1996;156:1729-1735.

58. Leone PA, Trottier S, Miller JM. Valacyclovir for episodic treatment of genital herpes: A shorter 3-day treatment course compared with 5-day treatment. Clin Infect Dis. 2001;34:958-962.

59. Wald A, Corey L, Cone R, et al. Frequent genital herpes simplex virus 2 shedding in immunocompetent women: Effect of acyclovir treatment. J Clin Invest. 1997;99:1092-1097.

60. Reitano M, Tyring S, Lang W, et al. Valaciclovir for the suppression of recurrent genital herpes simplex virus infection: A large-scale dose range-finding study. J Infect Dis. 1998;178:603-610.

61. Corey L, Wald A, Patel R, et al. Once daily valacyclovir to reduce the risk of transmission of genital herpes. N Engl J Med. 2004;350:11-20.

62. Sheffield JS, Hollier LM, Hill JB, et al. Acyclovir prophylaxis to prevent herpes simplex virus recurrence at delivery: A systematic review. Obstet Gynecol. 2003;102(6):1396-1403.

63. Scott LL, Sanchez PJ, Jackson GL, et al. Acyclovir suppression to prevent cesarean delivery after first-episode genital herpes. Obstet Gynecol. 1996;87:69-73.

64. Baker D, Eisen D. Valacyclovir for prevention of recurrent herpes labialis: 2 double-blind, placebo-controlled studies. Cutis. 2003;71:239-242.

65. Rooney JF, Straus SE, Mannix ML, et al. Oral acyclovir to suppress frequently recurrent herpes labialis: A double-blind, placebo-controlled trial. Ann Intern Med. 1993;118:268-272.

66. The Herpetic Eye Disease Study Group. Acyclovir for the prevention of recurrent herpes simplex virus eye disease. N Engl J Med. 1998;339:300-306.

67. Raborn GW, Martel AY, Grace MG, McGaw WT. Oral acyclovir in prevention of herpes labialis: A randomized, double-blind, multi-centered clinical trial. Oral Surg Oral Med Oral Pathol Oral Radiol Endod. 1998;85:55-59.

68. Kuzushima K, Kudo T, Kimura H, et al. Prophylactic oral acyclovir in outbreaks of primary herpes simplex virus type 1 infection in a closed community. Pediatrics. 1992;89:379-383.

69. Spruance SL, Nett R, Marbury T, et al. Acyclovir cream for treatment of herpes simplex labialis: Results of two randomized, double-blind, vehicle-controlled, multicenter clinical trials. Antimicrob Agents Chemother. 2002;46:2238-2243.

70. Spruance SL, Jones TM, Blatter MM, et al. High-dose, short-duration, early valacyclovir therapy for episodic treatment of cold sores: Results of two randomized, placebo-controlled, multicenter studies. Antimicrob Agents Chemother. 2003;47:1072-1080.

71. Gill MJ, Bryant HE. Oral acyclovir therapy of recurrent herpes simplex virus type 2 infection of the hand. Antimicrob Agents Chemother. 1991;35:382-383.

72. Amir J, Harel L, Smetana Z, Varsano I. Treatment of herpes simplex gingivostomatitis with aciclovir in children: A randomised double blind placebo controlled study. BMJ. 1997;314:1800-1803.

73. Adour KK, Ruboyianes JM, Von DG, et al. Bell's palsy treatment with acyclovir and prednisone compared with prednisone alone: A double-blind, randomized, controlled trial. Ann Otol Rhinol Laryngol. 1996;105:371-378.

74. Cohen JI, Davenport DS, Stewart JA, et al. Recommendations for prevention of and therapy for exposure to B virus (Cercopithecine herpesvirus 1). Clin Infect Dis. 2002;35:1191-1203.

75. Eisen D, Essell J, Broun ER, et al. Clinical utility of oral valacyclovir compared with oral acyclovir for the prevention of herpes simplex virus mucositis following autologous bone marrow transplantation or stem cell rescue therapy. Bone Marrow Transplant. 2003;31:51-55.

76. DeJesus E, Wald A, Warren T, et al. Valacyclovir for the suppression of recurrent genital herpes in human immunodeficiency virus-infected subjects. J Infect Dis. 2001;188:1009-1016.

77. Wade JC, Newton B, McLaren C, et al. Intravenous acyclovir to treat mucocutaneous herpes simplex virus infection after marrow transplantation: A double-blind trial. Ann Intern Med. 1982;96:265-269.

78. Shepp DH, Newton BA, Dandliker PS, et al. Oral acyclovir therapy for mucocutaneous herpes simplex virus infections in immunocompromised marrow transplant recipients. Ann Intern Med. 1985;102:783-785.

79. Klein NA, Mabie WC, Shaver DC, et al. Herpes simplex virus hepatitis in pregnancy: Two patients successfully treated with acyclovir. Gastroenterology. 1991;100:239-244.

80. Kusne S, Schwartz M, Breinig MK, et al. Herpes simplex virus hepatitis after solid organ transplantation in adults. J Infect Dis. 1991;163:1001-1007.

81. Kimberlin DW, Lin CY, Jacobs RF, et al. Safety and efficacy of high-dose intravenous acyclovir in the management of neonatal herpes simplex virus infections. Pediatrics. 2001;108:230-238.

82. Palay DA, Sternberg PJ, Davis J, et al. Decrease in the risk of bilateral acute retinal necrosis by acyclovir therapy. Am J Ophthalmol. 1991;112:250-255.

83. Dunkle LM, Arvin AM, Whitley RJ, et al. A controlled trial of acyclovir for chickenpox in normal children. N Engl J Med. 1991;325:1539-1544.

84. Balfour HJ, Rotbart HA, Feldman S, et al. Acyclovir treatment of varicella in otherwise healthy adolescents. The Collaborative Acyclovir Varicella Study Group. J Pediatr. 1992;120:627-633.

85. Wallace MR, Bowler WA, Murray NB, et al. Treatment of adult varicella with oral acyclovir: A randomized, placebo-controlled trial. Ann Intern Med. 1992;117:358-363.

86. Committee on Infectious Diseases, American Academy of Pediatrics. Red Book: 2003 Report of the Committee on Infectious Diseases. 26th ed. Elk Grove Village, Ill.: American Academy of Pediatrics, 2003.

87. Lin TY, Huang YC, Ning HC, Hsueh C. Oral acyclovir prophylaxis of varicella after intimate contact. Pediatr Infect Dis J. 1997;16:1162-1165.

88. Colin J, Prisant O, Cochener B, et al. Comparison of the efficacy and safety of valaciclovir and acyclovir for the treatment of herpes zoster ophthalmicus. Ophthalmology. 2000;107:1507-1511.

89. Mohsen AH, McKendrick M. Varicella pneumonia in adults (Review). Eur Respir J. 2003;21:886-891.

90. Meszner Z, Nyerges G, Bell AR. Oral acyclovir to prevent dissemination of varicella in immunocompromised children. J Infect. 1993;26:9-15.

91. Prentice HG, Gluckman E, Powles RL, et al. Long-term survival in allogeneic bone marrow transplant recipients following acyclovir prophylaxis for CMV infection. The European Acyclovir for CMV Prophylaxis Study Group. Bone Marrow Transplant. 1997;19:129-133.

92. Prentice HG, Gluckman E, Powles RL, et al. Impact of long-term acyclovir on cytomegalovirus infection and survival after allogeneic bone marrow transplantation. European Acyclovir for CMV Prophylaxis Study Group. Lancet. 1994;343:749-753.

93. Ljungman P, de La Camara R, Milpied N, et al. Randomized study of valacyclovir as prophylaxis against cytomegalovirus reactivation in recipients of allogeneic bone marrow transplants. Blood. 2003;99:3050-3056.

93a. Winston DJ, Yeager AM, Chandrasekar PH, et al. Randomized comparison of oral valacyclovir and intravenous ganciclovir for prevention of cytomegalovirus disease after allogeneic bone marrow transplantation. Clin Infect Dis. 2003;36(6):749-758.

94. Winston DJ, Busuttil RW. Randomized controlled trial of oral ganciclovir versus oral acyclovir after induction with intravenous ganciclovir for long-term prophylaxis of cytomegalovirus disease in cytomegalovirus-seropositive liver transplant recipients. Transplantation. 2003;75:229-233.

95. Fiddian P, Sabin CA, Griffiths PD. Valacyclovir provides optimum acyclovir exposure for prevention of cytomegalovirus and related outcomes after organ transplantation. J Infect Dis. 2002;186(Suppl 1):S110-S115.

96. Egan JJ, Carroll KB, Yonan N, et al. Valacyclovir prevention of cytomegalovirus reactivation after heart transplantation: A randomized trial. J Heart Lung Transplant. 2002;21:460-466.

97. Ioannidis JP, Collier AC, Cooper D, et al. Clinical efficacy of high-dose acyclovir in patients with human immunodeficiency virus infection: A meta-analysis of randomized individual patient data. J Infect Dis. 1998;178:349-359.

98. Tynell E, Aurelius E, Brandell A, et al. Acyclovir and prednisolone treatment of acute infectious mononucleosis: A multicenter, double-blind, placebo-controlled study. J Infect Dis. 1996;174:324-331.

99. Fong IW, Ho J, Toy C, et al. Value of long-term administration of acyclovir and similar agents for protecting against AIDS-related lymphoma: Case-control and historical cohort studies (Comment). Clin Infect Dis. 2000;30:757-761.

100. Walling DM, Flaitz CM, Nichols CM. Epstein-Barr virus replication in oral hairy leukoplakia: Response, persistence, and resistance to treatment with valacyclovir. J Infect Dis. 2003;188:883-890.

101. Lycke J, Svennerholm B, Hjelmquist E, et al. Acyclovir treatment of relapsing-remitting multiple sclerosis: A randomized, placebo-controlled, double-blind study. J Neurol. 1996;243:214-224.

102. De Clercq E. Clinical potential of the acyclic nucleoside phosphonates cidofovir, adefovir, and tenofovir in treatment of DNA virus and retrovirus infections. Clin Microbiol Rev. 2003;16:569-596.

103. Kern ER. In vitro activity of potential anti-poxvirus agents. Antiviral Res. 2003;57:35-40.

104. Colledge D, Civitico G, Locarnini S, Shaw T. In vitro antihepadnaviral activities of combinations of penciclovir, lamivudine, and adefovir. Antimicrob Agents Chemother. 2000;44:551-560.

105. Cundy KC. Clinical pharmacokinetics of the antiviral nucleotide analogues cidofovir and adefovir. Clin Pharmacokinet. 1999;36:127-143.

106. Hadziyannis SJ, Tassopoulos NC, Heathcote EJ, et al. Adefovir dipivoxil for the treatment of hepatitis B e antigen-negative chronic hepatitis B. N Engl J Med. 2003;348:800-807.

107. Yang H, Westland CE, Delaney WE, et al. Resistance surveillance in chronic hepatitis B patients treated with adefovir dipivoxil for up to 60 weeks. Hepatology. 2002;36:464-473.

108. Cundy KC, Barditch-Crovo P, Walker RE, et al. Clinical pharmacokinetics of adefovir in human immunodeficiency virus type 1-infected patients. Antimicrob Agents Chemother. 1995;39:2401-2405.

109. Marcellin P, Chang TT, Lim SG, et al. Adefovir dipivoxil for the treatment of hepatitis B e antigen-positive chronic hepatitis B. N Engl J Med. 2003;348:808-816.

109a. Peters MG, Hann H, Martin P, et al. Adefovir dipivoxil alone or in combination with lamivudine in patients with lamivudine-resistant chronic hepatis B [see comment]. Gastroenterology. 2004;126(1):91-101.

110. Benhamou Y, Bochet M, Thibault V, Calvez V, Fievet MH, Vig P et al. Safety and efficacy of adefovir dipivoxil in patients co-infected with HIV-1 and lamivudine-resistant hepatitis B virus: An open-label pilot study. Lancet. 2001;358:718-723.

111. Walsh KM, Woodall T, Lamy P, et al. Successful treatment with adefovir dipivoxil in a patient with fibrosing cholestatic hepatitis and lamivudine resistant hepatitis B virus. Gut. 2001;49:436-440.

112. Tumpey TM, Garcia-Sastre A, Mikulasova A, et al. Existing antivirals are effective against influenza viruses with genes from the 1918 pandemic virus. Proc Natl Acad Sci U S A. 2002;99:13849-13854.

113. Hayden FG, Aoki FY. Amantadine, rimantadine, and related agents. In: Yu VL, Merigan TC, White NJ, Barriere S, eds. Antimicrobial Therapy and Vaccines. Baltimore: Williams & Wilkins; 1999:1344-1365.

114. Kelly JM, Miles MA, Skinner AC. The anti-influenza virus drug rimantadine has trypanocidal activity. Antimicrob Agents Chemother. 1999;43:985-987.

115. Chan J, O'Riordan K, Wiley TE. Amantadine's viral kinetics in chronic hepatitis C infection. Dig Dis Sci. 2002;47:438-442.

116. Leneva IA, Roberts N, Govorkova EA, et al. The neuraminidase inhibitor GS4104 (oseltamivir phosphate) is efficacious against A/Hong Kong/156/97 (H5N1) and A/Hong Kong/1074/99 (H9N2) influenza viruses. Antiviral Res. 2000;48:101-115.

117. Madren LK, Shipman C Jr, Hayden FG. In vitro inhibitory effects of combinations of anti-influenza agents. Antivir Chem Chemother. 1995;6:109-113.

118. Takeda M, Pekosz A, Shuck K, et al. Influenza A virus M2 ion channel activity is essential for efficient replication in tissue culture. J Virol. 2002;76(3):1391-1399.

119. Hay AJ. Amantadine and rimantadine: Mechanisms. In: Richman DD, ed. Antiviral Drug Resistance. Chichester, UK: Wiley; 1996:43-58.

120. Pinto LH, Holsinger LJ, Lamb RA. Influenza virus M2 protein has ion channel activity. Cell. 1992;69:517-528.

121. Griffin SD, Beales LP, Clarke DS, et al. The p7 protein of hepatitis C virus forms an ion channel that is blocked by the antiviral drug, amantadine. FEBS Lett. 2003;535:34-38.

122. Jubin R, Murray MG, Howe AY, et al. Amantadine and rimantadine have no direct inhibitory effects against hepatitis C viral protease, helicase, ATPase, polymerase, and internal ribosomal entry site-mediated translation. J Infect Dis. 2000;181:331-334.

123. Ziegler T, Hemphill ML, Ziegler ML, et al. Low incidence of rimantadine resistance in field isolates of influenza A viruses. J Infect Dis. 1999;180:935-939.

124. Hayden FG. Amantadine and rimantadine: Clinical aspects. In: Richman DD, ed. Antiviral Drug Resistance. Chichester, UK: Wiley; 1996:59-77.

125. Englund JA, Champlin RE, Wyde PR, et al. Common emergence of amantadine and rimantadine resistant influenza A viruses in symptomatic immunocompromised adults. Clin Infect Dis. 1998;26:1418-1424.

126. Shiraishi K, Mitamura K, Sakai-Tagawa Y, et al. High frequency of resistant viruses harboring different mutations in amantadine-treated children with influenza. J Infect Dis. 2003;188:57-61.

127. Hayden FG, Sperber SJ, Belshe RB, et al. Recovery of drug-resistant influenza A virus during therapeutic use of rimantadine. Antimicrob Agents Chemother. 1991;35:1741-1747.

128. Mast EE, Harmon MW, Gravenstein S, et al. Emergence and possible transmission of amantadine-resistant viruses during nursing home outbreaks of influenza A (H3N2). Am J Epidemiol. 1991;134:988-997.

129. Douglas RGJ. Prophylaxis and treatment of influenza. N Engl J Med. 1990;322:443-450.

130. Keyser LA, Karl M, Nafziger AN, Bertino JS Jr. Comparison of central nervous system adverse effects of amantadine and rimantadine used as sequential prophylaxis of influenza A in elderly nursing home patients. Arch Intern Med. 2000;160:1485-1488.

131. Degelau J, Somani SK, Cooper SL, Irvine PW. Occurrence of adverse effects and high amantadine concentrations with influenza prophylaxis in the nursing home. J Am Geriatr Soc. 1990;38:428.

132. Stange KC, Little DW, Blatnik B. Adverse reactions to amantadine prophylaxis of influenza in a retirement home. J Am Geriatr Soc. 1991;39:700-705.

133. Kolbe F, Sitar DS, Papaioannou A, Campbell G. An amantadine hydrochloride dosing program adjusted for renal function during an influenza outbreak in elderly institutionalized patients. Can J Clin Pharmacol. 2003;10:119-122.

134. Pimentel L, Hughes B. Amantadine toxicity presenting with complex ventricular ectopy and hallucinations. Pediatr Emerg Care. 1991;7:89-92.

135. Monto AS, Ohmit SE, Hornbuckle K, Pearce CL. Safety and efficacy of long-term use of rimantadine for prophylaxis of type A influenza in nursing homes. Antimicrob Agents Chemother. 1995;39(10):2224-2228.

136. Pandit PB, Chitayat D, Jefferies AL, et al. Tibial hemimelia and tetralogy of Fallot associated with first trimester exposure to amantadine. Reprod Toxicol. 1994;8:89-92.

137. Wintermeyer SM, Nahata MC. Rimantadine: A clinical perspective. Ann Pharmacother. 1995;29:299-310.

138. Hayden FG. Perspectives on antiviral use during pandemic influenza. Philos Trans R Soc Lond B Biol Sci. 2001;356:1877-1884.

139. Libow LS, Neufeld RR, Olson E, et al. Sequential outbreak of influenza A and B in a nursing home: Efficacy of vaccine and amantadine. J Am Geriatr Soc. 1996;44:1153-1157.

140. Brady MT, Sears SD, Pacini DL, et al. Safety and prophylactic efficacy of low-dose rimantadine in adults during an influenza A epidemic. Antimicrob Agents Chemother. 1990;34:1633-1636.

141. La Rosa AM, Malik S, Englund JA, et al. Influenza A in hospitalized adults with leukemia and hematopoietic stem call transplant (HSCT) recipients: Risk factors for progression to pneumonia. Abstract 418. Presented at the 39th Annual Meeting of the Infectious Diseases Society of America, San Francisco, Calif, October 25-28, 2001.

142. Clover RD, Waner JL, Becker L, Davis A. Effect of rimantadine on the immune response to influenza A infections. J Med Virol. 1991;34:68-73.

143. Zeuzem S, Teuber G, Naumann U, et al. Randomized, double-blind, placebo-controlled trial of interferon alfa2a with and without amantadine as initial treatment for chronic hepatitis C. Hepatology. 2000;32:835-841.

144. Helbling B, Stamenic I, Viani F, et al. Interferon and amantadine in naive chronic hepatitis C: A double-blind, randomized, placebo-controlled trial. Hepatology. 2002;35:447-454.

145. Berg T, Kronenberger B, Hinrichsen H, et al. Triple therapy with amantadine in treatment-naive patients with chronic hepatitis C: A placebo-controlled trial. Hepatology. 2003;37:1359-1367.

146. Younossi ZM, Mullen KD, Zakko W, et al. A randomized, double-blind controlled trial of interferon alpha-2b and ribavirin vs. interferon alpha-2b and amantadine for treatment of chronic hepatitis C non-responder to interferon monotherapy. J Hepatol. 2001;34:128-133.

147. Adinolfi LE, Utili R, Tonziello A, Ruggiero G. Effects of alpha interferon induction plus ribavirin with or without amantadine in the treatment of interferon non-responsive chronic hepatitis C: A randomised trial. Gut. 2003;52:701-705.

148. Keating GM, Curran MP. Peginterferon-alpha-2a (40kD) plus ribavirin: A review of its use in the management of chronic hepatitis C. Drugs. 2003;63:701-730.

149. Hitchcock MJ, Jaffe HS, Martin JC, Stagg RJ. Cidofovir, a new agent with potent anti-herpesvirus activity. Antivir Chem Chemother. 1996;7:115-127.

150. Safrin S, Cherrington JM, Jaffe HS. Clinical uses of cidofovir. Rev Med Virol. 1997;7:145-156.

151. Andrei G, Snoeck R, Vandeputte M, de Clercq CE. Activities of various compounds against murine and primate polyomaviruses. Antimicrob Agents Chemother. 1997;41:587-593.

152. Cherrington JM, Miner R, Hitchcock MJ, et al. Susceptibility of human cytomegalovirus to cidofovir is unchanged after limited in vivo exposure to various regimens of drug. J Infect Dis. 1996;173:987-992.

153. Lalezari J, Schacker T, Feinberg J, et al. A randomized, double-blind, placebo-controlled trial of cidofovir gel for the treatment of acyclovir-unresponsive mucocutaneous herpes simplex virus infection in patients with AIDS. J Infect Dis. 1997;176:892-898.

154. Gordon YJ, Romanowski E, Araullo-Cruz T, et al. Inhibitory effect of (S)-HPMPC, (S)-HPMPA, and 2'-nor-cyclic GMP on clinical ocular adenoviral isolates is serotype-dependent in vitro. Antiviral Res. 1991;16:11-16.

155. Mendel DB, Barkhimer DB, Chen MS. Biochemical basis for increased susceptibility to cidofovir of herpes simplex viruses with altered or deficient thymidine kinase activity. Antimicrob Agents Chemother. 1995;39:2120-2122.

156. Bray M, Martinez M, Smee DF, et al. Cidofovir protects mice against lethal aerosol or intranasal cowpox virus challenge. J Infect Dis. 2000;181:10-18.

157. Smee DF, Bailey KW, Wong MH, Sidwell RW. Effects of cidofovir on the pathogenesis of a lethal vaccinia virus respiratory infection in mice. Antiviral Res. 2001;52(1):55-62.

158. Soike KF, Huang JL, Zhang JY, et al. Evaluation of infrequent dosing regimens with (S)-1-(3-hydroxy-2-[phosphonylmethoxy]propyl)-cytosine (S-HPMPC) on simian varicella infection in monkeys. Antiviral Res. 1991;16:17-28.

159. de Oliveira CB, Stevenson D, LaBree L, et al. Evaluation of cidofovir (HPMPC, GS-504) against adenovirus type 5 infection in vitro and in a New Zealand rabbit ocular model. Antiviral Res. 1996;31:165-172.

160. Ho HT, Woods KL, Bronson JJ, et al. Intracellular metabolism of the antiherpes agent (S)-1-(3-hydroxy-2-[phosphonylmethoxy]propyl)cytosine. Molec Pharmacol. 1992;41:197-202.

161. Quenelle DC, Collins DJ, Wan WB, et al. Oral treatment of cowpox and vaccinia virus infections in mice with ether lipid esters of cidofovir. Antimicrob Agents Chemother. 2004;48:404-412.

162. Erice A. Resistance of human cytomegalovirus to antiviral drugs. Clin Microbiol Rev. 1999;12:286-297.

163. Tatarowicz WA, Lurain NS, Thompson KD. A ganciclovir-resistant clinical isolate of human cytomegalovirus exhibiting cross-resistance to other DNA polymerase inhibitors. J Infect Dis. 1992;166:904-907.

164. Cherrington JM, Fuller MD, Lamy PD, et al. In vitro antiviral susceptibilities of isolates from cytomegalovirus retinitis patients receiving first- or second-line cidofovir therapy: Relationship to clinical outcome. J Infect Dis. 1998;178:1821-1825.

165. Jabs DA, Enger C, Forman M, Dunn JP. Incidence of foscarnet resistance and cidofovir resistance in patients treated for cytomegalovirus retinitis. The Cytomegalovirus Retinitis and Viral Resistance Study Group. Antimicrob Agents Chemother. 1998;42:2240-2244.

166. Smee DF, Sidwell RW, Kefauver D, et al. Characterization of wild-type and cidofovir-resistant strains of camelpox, cowpox, monkeypox, and vaccinia viruses. Antimicrob Agents Chemother. 2002;46:1329-1335.

167. Cundy KC, Petty BG, Flaherty J, et al. Clinical pharmacokinetics of cidofovir in human immunodeficiency virus-infected patients. Antimicrob Agents Chemother. 1995;39:1247-1252.

168. Neau D, Renaud-Rougier MB, Viallard JF, et al. Intravenous cidofovir-induced iritis. Clin Infect Dis. 1999;28:157-158.

168a. Kirsch LS, Arevalo JF, Chavez dE, et al. Intravitreal cidofovir (HPMPC) treatment of cytomegalovirus retinitis in patients with acquired immune deficiency syndrome [published erratum appears in Ophthalmology. 1995;102:702]. Ophthalmology. 1995;102:533-542.
169. Lalezari JP, Stagg RJ, Kuppermann BD, et al. Intravenous cidofovir for peripheral cytomegalovirus retinitis in patients with AIDS: A randomized, controlled trial. Ann Intern Med. 1997;126:257-263.
170. Lalezari J, Holland GN, Kramer F, et al. Randomized, controlled study of the safety and efficacy of intravenous cidofovir for the treatment of relapsing cytomegalovirus retinitis in patients with AIDS. J Acquir Immune Defic Syndr Hum Retrovirol. 1998;17:339-344
171. Anonymous. Parenteral cidofovir for cytomegalovirus retinitis in patients with AIDS: The HPMPC peripheral cytomegalovirus retinitis trial. A randomized, controlled trial. Studies of Ocular Complications of AIDS Research Group in Collaboration with the AIDS Clinical Trials Group. Ann Intern Med. 1997;126:264-274.
172. Polis MA, Spooner KM, Baird BF, et al. Anticytomegaloviral activity and safety of cidofovir in patients with human immunodeficiency virus infection and cytomegalovirus viruria. Antimicrob Agents Chemother. 1995;39:882-886.
173. The Studies of Ocular Complications of AIDS Research Group. The ganciclovir implant plus oral ganciclovir versus parenteral cidofovir for the treatment of cytomegalovirus retinitis in patients with acquired immunodeficiency syndrome: The Ganciclovir Cidofovir Cytomegalovirus Retinitis Trial. Am J Ophthalmol. 2001;131:457-467.
174. Chakrabarti S, Collingham KE, Osman H, et al. Cidofovir as primary pre-emptive therapy for post-transplant cytomegalovirus infections. Bone Marrow Transplant. 2001;28:879-881.
175. Ljungman P, Deliliers GL, Platzbecker U, et al. Cidofovir for cytomegalovirus infection and disease in allogeneic stem cell transplant recipients. The Infectious Diseases Working Party of the European Group for Blood and Marrow Transplantation. Blood. 2001;97:388-392.
176. Bryant P, Sasadeusz J, Carapetis J, et al. Successful treatment of foscarnet-resistant herpes simplex stomatitis with intravenous cidofovir in a child. Pediatr Infect Dis J. 2001;20:1083-1086.
177. Lalezari JP, Drew WL, Glutzer E, et al. Treatment with intravenous (S)-1-[3-hydroxy-2-(phosphonylmethoxy)propyl]-cytosine of acyclovir-resistant mucocutaneous infection with herpes simplex virus in a patient with AIDS. J Infect Dis. 1994;170:570-572.
178. Leruez-Ville M, Minard V, Lacaille F, et al. Real-time blood plasma polymerase chain reaction for management of disseminated adenovirus infection. Clin Infect Dis. 2004;38:45-52.
178a. Ljungman P, Ribaud P, Eyrich M, et al. Cidofovir for adenovirus infections after allogeneic hematopoietic stem cell transplantation: A survey by the Infectious Diseases Working Party of the European Group for Blood and Marrow Transplantation. Bone Marrow Transplant. 2003;31(6):481-486.
179. Hoffman JA, Shah AJ, Ross LA, Kapoor N. Adenoviral infections and a prospective trial of cidofovir in pediatric hematopoietic stem cell transplantation. Biol Blood Marrow Transplant. 2001;7:388-394.
180. Vats A, Shapiro R, Singh R, et al. Quantitative viral load monitoring and cidofovir therapy for the management of BK virus-associated nephropathy in children and adults. Transplantation. 2003;75:105-112.
181. De Luca A, Giancola ML, Ammassari A, et al. Potent anti-retroviral therapy with or without cidofovir for AIDS-associated progressive multifocal leukoencephalopathy: Extended follow-up of an observational study. J Neurovirol. 2001;7:364-368.
182. Marra CM, Rajicic N, Barker DE, et al. A pilot study of cidofovir for progressive multifocal leukoencephalopathy in AIDS. AIDS. 2002;16:1791-1797.
183. Little RF, Merced-Galindez F, Staskus K, et al. A pilot study of cidofovir in patients with kaposi sarcoma. J Infect Dis. 2001;187:149-153.
184. Pransky SM, Brewster DF, Magit AE, Kearns DB. Clinical update on 10 children treated with intralesional cidofovir injections for severe recurrent respiratory papillomatosis. Arch Otolaryngol Head Neck Surg. 2000;126:1239-1243.
185. Bielamowicz S, Villagomez V, Stager SV, Wilson WR. Intralesional cidofovir therapy for laryngeal papilloma in an adult cohort. Laryngoscope. 2002;112:696-699.
186. Snoeck R, Bossens M, Parent D, et al. Phase II double-blind, placebo-controlled study of the safety and efficacy of cidofovir topical gel for the treatment of patients with human papillomavirus infection. Clin Infect Dis. 2001;33:597-602.
187. Hillenkamp J, Reinhard T, Ross RS, et al. The effects of cidofovir 1% with and without cyclosporin a 1% as a topical treatment of acute adenoviral keratoconjunctivitis: A controlled clinical pilot study. Ophthalmology. 2002;109:845-850.
188. Pope LE, Marcelletti JF, Katz LR, et al. The anti-herpes simplex virus activity of n-docosanol includes inhibition of the viral entry process. Antiviral Res. 1998;40:85-94.
189. McKeough MB, Spruance SL. Comparison of new topical treatments for herpes labialis: Efficacy of penciclovir cream, acyclovir cream, and n-docosanol cream against experimental cutaneous herpes simplex virus type 1 infection. Arch Dermatol. 2001;137:1153-1158.
190. Sacks SL, Thisted RA, Jones TM, et al. Clinical efficacy of topical docosanol 10% cream for herpes simplex labialis: A multicenter, randomized, placebo-controlled trial. J Am Acad Dermat. 2001;45:222-230.
191. Vere Hodge RA. Antiviral portraits series, No. 3. Famciclovir and penciclovir: The mode of action of famciclovir including its conversion to penciclovir. Antivir Chem Chemother. 1993;4:67-84.
192. Weinberg A, Bate BJ, Masters HB, et al. In vitro activities of penciclovir and acyclovir against herpes simplex virus types 1 and 2. Antimicrob Agents Chemother. 1992;36:2037-2038.
193. Talarico CL, Phelps WC, Biron KK. Analysis of the thymidine kinase genes from acyclovir-resistant mutants of varicella-zoster virus isolated from patients with AIDS. J Virol. 1993;67:1024-1033.
194. Boyd MR, Kern ER, Safrin S. Penciclovir: A review of its spectrum of activity, selectivity and cross-resistance pattern. Antivir Chem Chemother. 1993;4(Suppl 1):3-11.
195. Korba BE, Boyd MR. Penciclovir is a selective inhibitor of hepatitis B virus replication in cultured human hepatoblastoma cells. Antimicrob Agents Chemother. 1996;40:1282-1284.
196. Thackray AM, Field HJ. Famciclovir and valaciclovir differ in the prevention of herpes simplex virus type 1 latency in mice: A quantitative study. Antimicrob Agents Chemother. 1998;42:1555-1562.
197. Earnshaw DL, Bacon TH, Darlison SJ, et al. Mode of antiviral action of penciclovir in MRC-5 cells infected with herpes simplex virus type 1 (HSV-1), HSV-2, and varicella-zoster virus. Antimicrob Agents Chemother. 1992;36:2747-2757.
198. Goldthorpe SE, Boyd MR, Field HJ. Effects of penciclovir and famciclovir in a murine model of encephalitis induced by intranasal inoculation of herpes simplex virus type 1. Antivir Chem Chemother. 1992;3:37-47.
199. Shaw T, Mok SS, Locarnini SA. Inhibition of hepatitis B virus DNA polymerase by enantiomers of penciclovir triphosphate and metabolic basis for selective inhibition of HBV replication by penciclovir. Hepatology. 1996;24:996-1002.
200. Pelosi E, Mulamba GB, Coen DM. Penciclovir and pathogenesis phenotypes of drug-resistant Herpes simplex virus mutants. Antiviral Res. 1998;37:17-28.
201. Mertz GJ, Loveless MO, Levin MJ, et al. Oral famciclovir for suppression of recurrent genital herpes simplex virus infection in women: A multicenter, double-blind, placebo-controlled trial. Collaborative Famciclovir Genital Herpes Research Group. Arch Intern Med. 1997;157:343-349.
202. Schacker T, Hui-lin H, Koelle DM, et al. Famciclovir for the suppression of symptomatic and asymptomatic herpes simplex virus reactivation in HIV-infected persons. Ann Intern Med. 1998;128:21-28.
203. Seigneres B, Pichoud C, Ahmed SS, et al. Evolution of hepatitis B virus polymerase gene sequence during famciclovir therapy for chronic hepatitis B. J Infect Dis. 2000;181:1221-1233.
204. Mutimer D, Pillay D, Cook P, et al. Selection of multiresistant hepatitis B virus during sequential nucleoside-analogue therapy. J Infect Dis. 2000;181:713-716.
205. Perry CM, Wagstaff AJ. Famciclovir: A review of its pharmacological properties and therapeutic efficacy in herpesvirus infections. Drugs. 1995;50:396-415.
206. Fowles SE, Pierce DM, Prince WT, Staniforth D. The tolerance to and pharmacokinetics of penciclovir (BRL 39,123A), a novel antiherpes agent, administered by intravenous infusion to healthy subjects. Eur J Clin Pharmacol. 1992;43:513-516.
207. Boike SC, Pue M, Audet PR, et al. Pharmacokinetics of famciclovir in subjects with chronic hepatic disease. J Clin Pharmacol. 1994;34:1199-1207.
208. Daniels S, Schentag JJ. Drug interaction studies and safety of famciclovir in healthy volunteers: A review. Antivir Chem Chemother. 1993;4(Suppl 1):57-64.
209. Saltzman R, Jurewicz R, Boon R. Safety of famciclovir in patients with herpes zoster and genital herpes. Antimicrob Agents Chemother. 1994;38:2454-2457.
210. Sacks SL, Sasadeusz JJ, Shafran SD. Effect of long-term famciclovir treatment on sperm parameters in patients with recurent genital herpes. Abstract 22022. Presented at the 8th International Congress on Infectious Diseases, Boston, 1998.
211. Raborn GW, Martel AY, Lassonde M, et al. Effective treatment of herpes simplex labialis with penciclovir cream: Combined results of two trials. J Am Dent Assoc. 2002;133:303-309.
212. Loveless M, Sacks SL, Harris RJ. Famciclovir in the management of first-episode genital herpes. Infect Dis Clin Pract. 1997;6(Suppl 1):S12-S16.
213. Chosidow O, Drouault Y, Leconte-Veyriac F, et al. Famciclovir vs. aciclovir in immunocompetent patients with recurrent genital herpes infections: A parallel-groups, randomized, double-blind clinical trial. Br J Dermatol. 2001;144:818-824.
214. Sacks SL, Aoki FY, Diaz-Mitoma F, et al. Patient-initiated, twice-daily oral famciclovir for early recurrent genital herpes: A randomized, double-blind multicenter trial. Canadian Famciclovir Study Group [see comments]. JAMA. 1996;276:44-49.
215. Diaz-Mitoma F, Sibbald RG, Shafran SD, et al. Oral famciclovir for the suppression of recurrent genital herpes: A randomized controlled trial. Collaborative Famciclovir Genital Herpes Research Group [see comments]. JAMA. 1998;280:887-892.
216. Romanowski B, Aoki FY, Martel AY, et al. Efficacy and safety of famciclovir for treating mucocutaneous herpes simplex infection in HIV-infected individuals. Collaborative Famciclovir HIV Study Group. AIDS. 2000;14:1211-1217.
217. Lazarus HM, Belanger R, Candoni A, et al. Intravenous penciclovir for treatment of herpes simplex infections in immunocompromised patients: Results of a multicenter, acyclovir-controlled trial. The Penciclovir Immunocompromised Study Group. Antimicrob Agents Chemother. 1999;43:1192-1197.
218. Tyring S, Barbarash RA, Nahlik JE, et al. Famciclovir for the treatment of acute herpes zoster: Effects on acute disease and postherpetic neuralgia—A randomized, double-blind, placebo-controlled trial. Collaborative Famciclovir Herpes Zoster Study Group [see comments]. Ann Intern Med. 1995;123:89-96.
219. Degreef H, Famciclovir Herpes Zoster Clinical Study Group. Famciclovir, a new oral antiherpes drug: Results of the first controlled clinical study demonstrating its efficacy and safety in the treatment of uncomplicated herpes zoster in immunocompetent patients. Int J Antimicrob Agents. 1994;4:241-246.
220. Tyring SK, Beutner K, Tucker BA, et al. Antiviral therapy for herpes zoster. Arch Fam Med. 2000;9:863-869.
221. Tyring S, Engst R, Corriveau C, et al. Famciclovir for ophthalmic zoster: A randomised aciclovir controlled study. Br J Ophthalmol. 2001;85:576-581.
222. Tyring S, Belanger R, Bezwoda W, et al. A randomized, double-blind trial of famciclovir versus acyclovir for the treatment of localized dermatomal herpes zoster in immunocompromised patients. Cancer Invest. 2001;13-22.
223. Trepo C, Jezek P, Atkinson GF, et al. Famciclovir in chronic hepatitis B: Results of a dose-finding study. Hepatology. 2000;32:1011-1018.
224. Lai CL, Yuen MF, Hui CK, et al. Comparison of the efficacy of lamivudine and famciclovir in Asian patients with chronic hepatitis B: Results of 24 weeks of therapy. J Med Virol. 2002;67:334-338.

225. Yurdaydin C, Bozkaya H, Gurel S, et al. Famciclovir treatment of chronic delta hepatitis. J Hepatol. 2002;37:266-271.

226. Manns MP, Neuhaus P, Atkinson GF, et al. Famciclovir treatment of hepatitis B infection following liver transplantation: A long-term, multi-centre study. Transplant Infect Dis. 2001;3:16-23.

227. Perry CM, Balfour JAB. Formivirsen. Drugs. 1999;57:375-380.

228. Anderson KP, Fox MC, Brown-Driver V, et al. Inhibition of human cytomegalovirus immediate-early gene expression by an antisense oligonucleotide complementary to immediate-early RNA. Antimicrob Agents Chemother. 1996;40:2004-2011.

229. Mulamba GB, Hu A, Azad RF, et al. Human cytomegalovirus mutant with sequence-dependent resistance to the phosphorothioate oligonucleotide fomivirsen (ISIS 2922). Antimicrob Agents Chemother. 1998;42:971-973.

230. Geary RS, Henry SP, Grillone LR. Fomivirsen: Clinical pharmacology and potential drug interactions. Clin Pharmacokinet. 2002;41:255-260.

231. Vitravene Study Group. A randomized controlled clinical trial of intravitreous fomivirsen for treatment of newly diagnosed peripheral cytomegalovirus retinitis in patients with AIDS. Am J Ophthalmol. 2002;133:467-474.

232. Vitravene Study Group. Randomized dose-comparison studies of intravitreous fomivirsen for treatment of cytomegalovirus retinitis that has reactivated or is persistently active despite other therapies in patients with AIDS. Am J Ophthalmol. 2002;133:475-483.

233. Wagstaff AJ, Bryson HM. Foscarnet: A reappraisal of its antiviral activity, pharmacokinetic properties and therapeutic use in immunocompromised patients with viral infections. Drugs. 1994;48:199-226.

234. Kedes DH, Ganem D. Sensitivity of Kaposi's sarcoma-associated herpesvirus replication to antiviral drugs: Implications for potential therapy. J Clin Invest. 1997;99:2082-2086.

235. Manion DJ, Vibhagool A, Chou TC, et al. Susceptibility of human cytomegalovirus to two-drug combinations in vitro. Antivir Ther. 1996;1:237-245.

236. Crumpacker CS. Mechanism of action of foscarnet against viral polymerases. Am J Med. 1992;92:3S-7S.

237. Baldanti F, Gerna G. Human cytomegalovirus resistance to antiviral drugs: Diagnosis, monitoring and clinical impact. J Antimicrob Chemother. 2003;52:324-330.

238. Baldanti F, Underwood MR, Stanat SC, et al. Single amino acid changes in the DNA polymerase confer foscarnet resistance and slow-growth phenotype, while mutations in the UL97-encoded phosphotransferase confer ganciclovir resistance in three double-resistant human cytomegalovirus strains recovered from patients with AIDS. J Virol. 1996;70:1390-1395.

239. Weinberg A, Jabs DA, Chou S, Martin BK, Lurain NS, Forman MS et al. Mutations conferring foscarnet resistance in a cohort of patients with acquired immunodeficiency syndrome and cytomegalovirus retinitis. J Infect Dis. 2001;187:777-784.

240. Saijo M, Yasuda Y, Yabe H, Kato S, Suzutani T, De C et al. Bone marrow transplantation in a child with Wiskott-Aldrich syndrome latently infected with acyclovir-resistant (ACV(r)) herpes simplex virus type 1: Emergence of foscarnet-resistant virus originating from the ACV(r) virus. J Med Virol. 2002;68:99-104.

241. Read RC, Vilar FJ, Smith TL. AIDS-related herpes simplex virus encephalitis during maintenance foscarnet therapy. Clin Infect Dis. 1998;26:513-514.

242. Tachedjian G, Mellors J, Bazmi H, Birch C, Mills J. Zidovudine resistance is suppressed by mutations conferring resistance of human immunodeficiency virus type 1 to foscarnet. J Virol. 1996;70:7171-7181.

243. Hengge UR, Brockmeyer NH, Malessa R, et al. Foscarnet penetrates the blood-brain barrier: Rationale for therapy of cytomegalovirus encephalitis. Antimicrob Agents Chemother. 1993;37:1010-1014.

244. Arevalo JF, Gonzalez C, Capparelli EV, et al. Intravitreous and plasma concentrations of ganciclovir and foscarnet after intravenous therapy in patients with AIDS and cytomegalovirus retinitis. J Infect Dis. 1995;172:951-956.

245. Aweeka FT, Jacobson MA, Martin-Munley S, et al. Effect of renal disease and hemodialysis on foscarnet pharmacokinetics and dosing recommendations. J Acquir Immune Defic Syndr Hum Retrovirol. 1999;20:350-357.

246. Alexander AC, Akers A, Matzke GR, et al. Disposition of foscarnet during peritoneal dialysis. Ann Pharmacother. 1996;30(10):1106-1109.

247. Deray G, Martinez F, Katlama C, et al. Foscarnet nephrotoxicity: Mechanism, incidence and prevention. Am J Nephrol. 1989;9:316-321.

248. Reusser P, Einsele H, Lee J, et al. Randomized multicenter trial of foscarnet versus ganciclovir for preemptive therapy of cytomegalovirus infection after allogeneic stem cell transplantation. Blood. 2002;99:1159-1164.

249. Jayaweera DT. Minimising the dosage-limiting toxicities of foscarnet induction therapy. Drug Saf. 1997;16:258-266.

250. Jacobson MA, Gambertoglio JG, Aweeka FT, et al. Foscarnet-induced hypocalcemia and effects of foscarnet on calcium metabolism. J Clin Endocrinol Metab. 1991;72:1130-1135.

251. Jacobson MA, Drew WL, Feinberg J, et al. Foscarnet therapy for ganciclovir-resistant cytomegalovirus retinitis in patients with AIDS. J Infect Dis. 1991;163:1348-1351.

252. Palestine AG, Polis MA, De Smet MD, et al. A randomized, controlled trial of foscarnet in the treatment of cytomegalovirus retinitis in patients with AIDS [see comments]. Ann Intern Med. 1991;115:665-673.

253. Jacobson MA, Causey D, Polsky B, et al. A dose-ranging study of daily maintenance intravenous foscarnet therapy for cytomegalovirus retinitis in AIDS. J Infect Dis. 1993;168:444-448.

254. Anonymous. Mortality in patients with the acquired immunodeficiency syndrome treated with either foscarnet or ganciclovir for cytomegalovirus retinitis. Studies of Ocular Complications of AIDS Research Group, in collaboration with the AIDS Clinical Trials Group [published erratum appears in N Engl J Med. 1992;326:1172]. N Engl J Med. 1992;326:213-220.

255. Anonymous. Combination foscarnet and ganciclovir therapy vs monotherapy for the treatment of relapsed cytomegalovirus retinitis in patients with AIDS. The Cytomegalovirus Retreatment Trial. The Studies of Ocular Complications of AIDS Research Group in Collaboration with the AIDS Clinical Trials Group. Arch Ophthalmol. 1996;114:23-33.

256. Youle M, Chanas A, Gazzard B. Treatment of acquired immune deficiency syndrome (AIDS)-related pneumonitis with foscarnet: A double-blind placebo controlled study. J Infect. 1990;20:41-50.

257. Bacigalupo A, Bregante S, Tedone E, et al. Combined foscarnet -ganciclovir treatment for cytomegalovirus infections after allogeneic hemopoietic stem cell transplantation (HSCT). Bone Marrow Transplant. 1996;18(Suppl 2):110-114.

258. Mylonakis E, Kallas WM, Fishman JA. Combination antiviral therapy for ganciclovir-resistant cytomegalovirus infection in solid-organ transplant recipients. Clin Infect Dis. 2002;34:1337-1341.

259. Glesby MJ, Hoover DR, Weng S, Graham NM, Phair JP, Detels R et al. Use of anti-herpes drugs and the risk of Kaposi's sarcoma: Data from the Multicenter AIDS Cohort Study. J Infect Dis. 1996;173:1477-1480.

260. Jones JL, Hanson DL, Chu SY, et al. AIDS-associated Kaposi's sarcoma. Science. 1995;267:1078-1079.

261. Bergdahl S, Jacobsson B, Moberg L, Sonnerborg A. Pronounced anti-HIV-1 activity of foscarnet in patients without cytomegalovirus infection. J Acquir Immune Defic Syndr Hum Retrovirol. 1998;18:51-53.

262. Faulds D, Heel RC. Ganciclovir: A review of its antiviral activity, pharmacokinetic properties and therapeutic efficacy in cytomegalovirus infections. Drugs. 1990;39:597-638.

263. Gish RG, Lau JY, Brooks L, et al. Ganciclovir treatment of hepatitis B virus infection in liver transplant recipients. Hepatology. 1996;23:1-7.

264. Crumpacker CS. Ganciclovir. N Engl J Med. 1996;335:721-729.

265. Sullivan V, Talarico CL, Stanat SC, et al. A protein kinase homologue controls phosphorylation of ganciclovir in human cytomegalovirus-infected cells [published errata appear in Nature. 1992;359:85 and 1993;366:756]. Nature. 1992;358:162-164.

266. Littler E, Stuart AD, Chee MS. Human cytomegalovirus UL97 open reading frame encodes a protein that phosphorylates the antiviral nucleoside analogue ganciclovir. Nature. 1992;358:160-162.

267. Hamzeh FM, Lietman PS. Intranuclear accumulation of subgenomic noninfectious human cytomegalovirus DNA in infected cells in the presence of ganciclovir. Antimicrob Agents Chemother. 1991;35:1818-1823.

268. Erice A. Resistance of human cytomegalovirus to antiviral drugs. Clin Microbiol Rev. 1999;12(2):286-297.

269. Chou S, Guentzel S, Michels KR, et al. Frequency of UL97 phosphotransferase mutations related to ganciclovir resistance in clinical cytomegalovirus isolates. J Infect Dis. 1995;172:239-242.

270. Smith IL, Cherrington JM, Jiles RE, et al. High-level resistance of cytomegalovirus to ganciclovir is associated with alterations in both the UL97 and DNA polymerase genes. J Infect Dis. 1997;176:69-77.

271. Jabs DA, Enger C, Dunn JP, Forman M. Cytomegalovirus retinitis and viral resistance: Ganciclovir resistance. CMV Retinitis and Viral Resistance Study Group. J Infect Dis. 1998;177:770-773.

272. Boivin G, Gilbert C, Gaudreau A, et al. Rate of emergence of cytomegalovirus (CMV) mutations in leukocytes of patients with acquired immunodeficiency syndrome who are receiving valganciclovir as induction and maintenance therapy for CMV retinitis. J Infect Dis. 2001;184:1598-1602.

273. Wolf DG, Yaniv I, Honigman A, et al. Early emergence of ganciclovir-resistant human cytomegalovirus strains in children with primary combined immunodeficiency. J Infect Dis. 1998;178:535-538.

274. Limaye AP, Corey L, Koelle DM, et al. Emergence of ganciclovir-resistant cytomegalovirus disease among recipients of solid-organ transplants. Lancet. 2000;356:645-649.

275. Limaye AP, Raghu G, Koelle DM, et al. High incidence of ganciclovir-resistant cytomegalovirus infection among lung transplant recipients receiving preemptive therapy. J Infect Dis. 2001;185:20-27.

276. Tokumoto JI, Hollander H. Cytomegalovirus polyradiculopathy caused by a ganciclovir-resistant strain [see comments]. Clin Infect Dis. 1993;17:854-856.

277. Lavelle J, Follansbee S, Trapnell CB, et al. Effect of food on the relative bioavailability of oral ganciclovir. J Clin Pharmacol. 1996;36:238-241.

278. Anderson RD, Griffy KG, Jung D, et al. Ganciclovir absolute bioavailability and steady-state pharmacokinetics after oral administration of two 3000-mg/d dosing regimens in human immunodeficiency virus- and cytomegalovirus-seropositive patients. Clin Therapeut. 1995;17:425-432.

279. Martin DF, Sierra-Madero J, Walmsley S, et al. A controlled trial of valganciclovir as induction therapy for cytomegalovirus retinitis. N Engl J Med. 2002;346:1119-1126.

280. Fletcher C, Sawchuk R, Chinnock B, et al. Human pharmacokinetics of the antiviral drug DHPG. Clin Pharmacol Therapeut. 1986;40:281-286.

281. Kuppermann BD, Quiceno JI, Flores-Aguilar M, et al. Intravitreal ganciclovir concentration after intravenous administration in AIDS patients with cytomegalovirus retinitis: Implications for therapy. J Infect Dis. 1993;168:1506-1509.

282. Swan SK, Munar MY, Wigger MA, Bennett WM. Pharmacokinetics of ganciclovir in a patient undergoing hemodialysis. Am J Kidney Dis. 1991;17:69-72.

283. Marx JL, Kapusta MA, Patel SS, et al. Use of the ganciclovir implant in the treatment of recurrent cytomegalovirus retinitis. Arch Ophthalmol. 1996;114:815-820.

284. Cimoch PJ, Lavelle J, Pollard R, et al. Pharmacokinetics of oral ganciclovir alone and in combination with zidovudine, didanosine, and probenecid in HIV-infected subjects. J Acquir Immune Defic Syndr Hum Retrovirol. 1998;17:227-234.

285. Medina DJ, Hsiung GD, Mellors JW. Ganciclovir antagonizes the anti-human immunodeficiency virus type 1 activity of zidovudine and didanosine in vitro. Antimicrob Agents Chemother. 1992;36:1127-1130.

286. Feng JS, Crouch JY, Tian PY. Zidovudine antagonizes the antiviral effects of ganciclovir against cytomegalovirus infection in cultured cells and in guinea pigs. Antivir Chem Chemother. 1993;4:19-25.

287. Freitas VR, Fraser-Smith EB, Chiu S, et al. Efficacy of ganciclovir in combination with zidovudine against cytomegalovirus in vitro and in vivo. Antiviral Res. 1993;21:301-315.

288. Freitas VR, Fraser-Smith EB, Matthews TR. Efficacy of ganciclovir in combination with other antimicrobial agents against cytomegalovirus in vitro and in vivo. Antiviral Res. 1993;20:1-12.

289. Hardy WD. Combined ganciclovir and recombinant human granulocyte-macrophage colony-stimulating factor in the treatment of cytomegalovirus retinitis in AIDS patients. J Acquir Immune Defic Syndr. 1991;4(Suppl 1):S22-S28.

290. Lalezari J, Lindley J, Walmsley S, et al. A safety study of oral valganciclovir maintenance treatment of cytomegalovirus retinitis. J Acquir Immune Defic Syndr. 2001;30:392-400.

291. Merigan TC, Renlund DG, Keay S, et al. A controlled trial of ganciclovir to prevent cytomegalovirus disease after heart transplantation. N Engl J Med. 1992;326:1182-1186.

292. Gane E, Saliba F, Valdecasas GJC, et al. Randomized trial of efficacy and safety of oral ganciclovir in the prevention of cytomegalovirus disease in liver-transplant recipients. Lancet. 1997;350:1729-1733.

293. Drew WL. Cytomegalovirus infection in patients with AIDS. Clin Infect Dis. 1992;14:608-615.

294. Drew WL, Ives D, Lalezari JP, et al. Oral ganciclovir as maintenance treatment for cytomegalovirus retinitis in patients with AIDS. Syntex Cooperative Oral Ganciclovir Study Group. N Engl J Med. 1995;333:615-620.

295. Musch DC, Martin DF, Gordon JF, et al. Treatment of cytomegalovirus retinitis with a sustained-release ganciclovir implant. The Ganciclovir Implant Study Group. N Engl J Med. 1997;337:83-90.

296. Berman SM, Kim RC. The development of cytomegalovirus encephalitis in AIDS patients receiving ganciclovir. Am J Med. 1994;96:415-419.

297. Dieterich DT, Kotler DP, Busch DF, et al. Ganciclovir treatment of cytomegalovirus colitis in AIDS: A randomized, double-blind, placebo-controlled multicenter study. J Infect Dis. 1993;167:278-282.

298. Michaels MG, Greenberg DP, Sabo DL, Wald ER. Treatment of children with congenital cytomegalovirus infection with ganciclovir. Pediatr Infect Dis J. 2003;22:504-509.

299. Schmidt GM, Horak DA, Niland JC, et al. A randomized, controlled trial of prophylactic ganciclovir for cytomegalovirus pulmonary infection in recipients of allogeneic bone marrow transplants;The City of Hope-Stanford-Syntex CMV Study Group [see comments]. N Engl J Med. 1991;324:1005-1011.

300. Goodrich JM, Mori M, Gleaves CA, et al. Early treatment with ganciclovir to prevent cytomegalovirus disease after allogeneic bone marrow transplantation. N Engl J Med. 1991;325:1601-1607.

301. Winston DJ, Ho WG, Bartoni K, et al. Ganciclovir prophylaxis of cytomegalovirus infection and disease in allogeneic bone marrow transplant recipients: Results of a placebo-controlled, double-blind trial. Ann Intern Med. 1993;118:179-184.

302. Goodrich JM, Bowden RA, Fisher L, et al. Ganciclovir prophylaxis to prevent cytomegalovirus disease after allogeneic marrow transplant. Ann Intern Med. 1993;118:173-178.

303. Duncan SR, Paradis IL, Dauber JH, et al. Ganciclovir prophylaxis for cytomegalovirus infections in pulmonary allograft recipients. Am Rev Respir Dis. 1992;146:1213-1215.

304. Hibberd PL, Tolkoff-Rubin NE, Conti D, et al. Preemptive ganciclovir therapy to prevent cytomegalovirus disease in cytomegalovirus antibody-positive renal transplant recipients: A randomized controlled trial. Ann Intern Med. 1995;123:18-26.

305. Preiksaitis JK, Diaz-Mitoma F, Mirzayans F, et al. Quantitative oropharyngeal Epstein-Barr virus shedding in renal and cardiac transplant recipients: Relationship to immunosuppressive therapy, serologic responses, and the risk of posttransplant lymphoproliferative disorder. J Infect Dis. 1992;166:986-994.

306. Brennan DC, Garlock KA, Singer GG, et al. Prophylactic oral ganciclovir compared with deferred therapy for control of cytomegalovirus in renal transplant recipients. Transplantation. 1997;64:1843-1846.

307. Paya CV. A randomized, double-blind, double-dummy, active-comparator controlled multi-center sudy of the efficacy and safety of valganciclovir vs oral ganciclovir for prevention of CMV disease in 372 high-risk (D+/R-) heart, liver and kidney recipients: Poster presented on behalf of the Valganciclovir Solid Organ Transplant Study Group. Abstract LB-4. Presented at the 42nd ICAAC Late-Breaker Program/Abstracts and Exhibits Addendum, September 27-30, San Diego, Calif, 2002:9.

308. Paya CV, Wilson JA, Espy MJ, et al. Preemptive use of oral ganciclovir to prevent cytomegalovirus infection in liver transplant patients: A randomized, placebo-controlled trial. J Infect Dis. 2001;185:854-860.

309. Spector SA, McKinley GF, Lalezari JP, et al. Oral ganciclovir for the prevention of cytomegalovirus disease in persons with AIDS. Roche Cooperative Oral Ganciclovir Study Group. N Engl J Med. 1996;334:1491-1497.

310. Brosgart CL, Louis TA, Hillman DW, et al. A randomized, placebo-controlled trial of the safety and efficacy of oral ganciclovir for prophylaxis of cytomegalovirus disease in HIV-infected individuals. Terry Beirn Community Programs for Clinical Research on AIDS. AIDS. 1998;12:269-277.

311. Hoh HB, Hurley C, Claoue C, et al. Randomised trial of ganciclovir and acyclovir in the treatment of herpes simplex dendritic keratitis: A multicentre study. Br J Ophthalmol. 1996;80:140-143.

312. Prusoff WH. Idoxuridine or how it all began. In: DeClercq E, ed. Clinical Use of Antiviral Drugs. Boston: Martinus Nijhoff; 1988:15-24.

313. Fardeau C, Langlois M, Mathys B, et al. Emergence of cross-resistant herpes simplex virus following topical drug therapy in rabbit keratitis. Curr Eye Res. 1991;10(Suppl):151-158.

314. Pavan-Langston D. Major ocular viral infections. In: Galasso GJ, Whitley RJ, Merigan TC, eds. Antiviral Agents and Viral Diseases of Man. New York: Raven Press; 1990:183-233.

315. Spruance SL, Stewart JC, Freeman DJ, et al. Early application of topical 15% idoxuridine in dimethyl sulfoxide shortens the course of herpes simplex labialis: A multicenter placebo-controlled trial. J Infect Dis. 1990;161:191-197.

316. Garland SM. Imiquimod. Curr Opin Infect Dis. 2003;16:85-89.

317. Skinner RBJ. Imiquimod. Dermatol Clin. 2003;21:291-300.

318. Tyring SK, Arany I, Stanley MA, et al. A randomized, controlled, molecular study of condylomata acuminata clearance during treatment with imiquimod. J Infect Dis. 1998;178:551-555.

319. Wiley DJ, Douglas J, Beutner K, et al. External genital warts: Diagnosis, treatment, and prevention. Clin Infect Dis. 2002;35(Suppl 2):S210-S224.

320. Gilson RJ, Shupack JL, Friedman-Kien AE, et al. A randomized, controlled, safety study using imiquimod for the topical treatment of anogenital warts in HIV-infected patients. Imiquimod Study Group. AIDS. 1999;13:2397-2404.

321. Sauder DN, Skinner RB, Fox TL, Owens ML. Topical imiquimod 5% cream as an effective treatment for external genital and perianal warts in different patient populations. Sex Transm Dis. 2003;30:124-128.

322. Arevalo I, Ward B, Miller R, et al. Successful treatment of drug-resistant cutaneous leishmaniasis in humans by use of imiquimod, an immunomodulator. Clin Infect Dis. 2001;33:1847-1851.

323. Schacker TW, Conant M, Thoming C, et al. Imiquimod 5-percent cream does not alter the natural history of recurrent herpes genitalis: A phase II, randomized, double-blind, placebo-controlled study. Antimicrob Agents Chemother. 2002;46:3243-3248.

324. Spruance SL, Tyring SK, Smith MH, Meng TC. Application of a topical immune response modifier, resiquimod gel, to modify the recurrence rate of recurrent genital herpes: A pilot study. J Infect Dis. 2001;184:196-200.

325. Samuel CE. Antiviral actions of interferons. Clin Microbiol Rev. 2001;14:778-809.

326. Baron S, Coppenhaver DH, Doanzani F. Introduction to the interferon system. In: Baron S, ed. Interferon: Principles and Medical Applications. Galveston, Tex: UTMN; 1992:1-15.

327. Dianzani F, Antonelli G. Mechanisms of action of the interferons: Biological basis. In: Stuart-Harris R, Penny R, eds. Clinical Applications of the Interferons. London: Chapman & Hall; 1997:20-31.

328. Finter NB. Why are there so many subtypes of alpha-interferons? J Interferon Res. 1991;(Special Issue):185-194.

329. Brierley MM, Fish EN. Review: IFN-alpha/beta receptor interactions to biologic outcomes—Understanding the circuitry. J Interferon Cytokine Res. 2002;22:835-845.

330. Sen GC, Ransohoff RM. Interferon-induced antiviral actions and their regulation. Adv Virus Res. 1993;42:57-102.

331. Der SD, Zhou A, Williams BR, Silverman RH. Identification of genes differentially regulated by interferon alpha, beta, or gamma using oligonucleotide arrays. Proc Natl Acad Sci U S A. 1998;95:15623-15628.

332. Pfeffer LM, Mullersman JE, Pfeffer SR, et al. STAT3 as an adapter to couple phosphatidylinositol 3-kinase to the IFNAR1 chain of the type I interferon receptor. Science. 1997;276:1418-1420.

333. Fischer DG, Tal N, Novick D, et al. An antiviral soluble form of the LDL receptor induced by interferon. Science. 1993;262:250-253.

334. Roers A, Hochkeppel HK, Horisberger MA, et al. MxA gene expression after live virus vaccination: A sensitive marker for endogenous type I interferon. J Infect Dis. 1994;169:807-813.

335. Kato J, Kato N, Moriyama M, et al. Interferons specifically suppress the translation from the internal ribosome entry site of hepatitis C virus through a double-stranded RNA-activated protein kinase-independent pathway. J Infect Dis. 2002;186:155-163.

336. Karupiah G, Xie QW, Buller RM, et al. Inhibition of viral replication by interferon-gamma-induced nitric oxide synthase. Science. 1993;261:1445-1448.

337. Gale MJ, Korth MJ, Tang NM, et al. Evidence that hepatitis C virus resistance to interferon is mediated through repression of the PKR protein kinase by the nonstructural 5A protein. Virology. 1997;230:217-227.

338. Biron CA. Interferons alpha and beta as immune regulators: A new look. Immunity. 2001;14:661-664.

339. Takaoka A, Hayakawa S, Yanai H, et al. Integration of interferon-alpha/beta signalling to p53 responses in tumour suppression and antiviral defence. Nature. 2003;424:516-523.

340. Wills RJ. Clinical pharmacokinetics of interferons. Clin Pharmacokinet. 1990;19:390-399.

341. Haria M, Benfield P. Interferon-alpha-2a: A review of its pharmacological properties and therapeutic use in the management of viral hepatitis. Drugs. 1995;50:873-896.

342. Witt PL, Goldstein D, Storer BE, et al. Absence of biological effects of orally administered interferon-beta ser. J Interferon Res. 1992;12:411-413.

343. Smith RA, Norris F, Palmer D, et al. Distribution of alpha interferon in serum and cerebrospinal fluid after systemic administration. Clin Pharmacol Therapeut. 1985;37:85-88.

344. Glue P, Fang JW, Rouzier-Panis R, et al. Pegylated interferon-alpha2b: Pharmacokinetics, pharmacodynamics, safety, and preliminary efficacy data. Hepatitis C Intervention Therapy Group. Clin Pharmacol Therapeut. 2000;68:556-567.

345. Quesada JR. Toxicity and side effects of interferons. In: Baron S, ed. Interferon: Principles and Medical Applications. Galveston, Tex.: University of Texas Medical Branch; 1992:426-432.

346. Kawano T, Shigehira M, Uto H, et al. Retinal complications during interferon therapy for chronic hepatitis C. Am J Gastroenterol. 1996;91:309-313.

347. Kumar KS, Russo MW, Borczuk AC, et al. Significant pulmonary toxicity associated with interferon and ribavirin therapy for hepatitis C. Am J Gastroenterol. 2002;97:2432-2440.

348. Bayraktar Y, Bayraktar M, Gurakar A, et al. A comparison of the prevalence of autoantibodies in individuals with chronic hepatitis C and those with autoimmune hepatitis: The role of interferon in the development of autoimmune diseases. Hepatogastroenterology. 1997;44:417-425.

349. Papo T, Marcellin P, Bernuau J, et al. Autoimmune chronic hepatitis exacerbated by alpha-interferon. Ann Intern Med. 1992;116:51-53.

350. Manns MP, McHutchison JG, Gordon SC, et al. Peginterferon alfa-2b plus ribavirin compared with interferon alfa-2b plus ribavirin for initial treatment of chronic hepatitis C: A randomised trial. Lancet. 2001;358:958-965.

351. Fried MW, Shiffman ML, Reddy KR, et al. Peginterferon alfa-2a plus ribavirin for chronic hepatitis C virus infection. N Engl J Med. 2002;347:975-982.

351a. Hadziyannis SJ, Sette JH, Morgan TR, et al. Peginterferon-alpha2a and ribavirin combination therapy in chronic hepatitis C: A randomized study of treatment duration and ribavirin dose [see comment]. Ann Intern Med. 2004;140(5):346-355.

352. Antonelli G, Currenti M, Turriziani O, Dianzani F. Neutralizing antibodies to interferon-alpha: Relative frequency in patients treated with different interferon preparations. J Infect Dis. 1991;163:882-885.

353. Ozaslan E, Yilmaz R, Simsek H, Tatar G. Interferon therapy for acute hepatitis C during pregnancy. Ann Pharmacother. 2002;36:1715-1718.

354. Foster GR, Ackrill AM, Goldin RD, et al. Expression of the terminal protein region of hepatitis B virus inhibits cellular responses to interferons alpha and gamma and double-stranded RNA [published erratum appears in Proc Natl Acad Sci U S A. 1995;92:3632]. Proc Natl Acad Sci U S A. 1991;88:2888-2892.

355. Hoofnagle JH, Di Bisceglie AM. Drug therapy: The treatment of chronic viral hepatitis. N Engl J Med. 1997;336:347-356.

356. Cooksley WG, Piratvisuth T, Lee SD, et al. Peginterferon alpha-2a (40 kDa): An advance in the treatment of hepatitis B e antigen-positive chronic hepatitis B. J Viral Hepat. 2003;10:298-305.

357. Korenman J, Baker B, Waggoner J, et al. Long-term remission of chronic hepatitis B after alpha-interferon therapy. Ann Intern Med. 1991;114:629-634.

358. Perrillo RP, Schiff ER, Davis GL, et al. A randomized, controlled trial of interferon alfa-2b alone and after prednisone withdrawal for the treatment of chronic hepatitis B. The Hepatitis Interventional Therapy Group [see comments]. N Engl J Med. 1990;323:295-301.

359. Niederau C, Heintges T, Lange S, et al. Long-term follow-up of HBeAg-positive patients treated with interferon alfa for chronic hepatitis B. N Engl J Med. 1996;334:1422-1427.

360. Lau DT, Everhart J, Kleiner DE, et al. Long-term follow-up of patients with chronic hepatitis B treated with interferon alfa. Gastroenterology. 1997;113:1660-1667.

361. Fattovich G, McIntyre G, Thursz M, et al. Hepatitis B virus precore/core variation and interferon therapy. Hepatology. 1995;22:1355-1362.

362. Di Bisceglie AM, Rustgi VK, Kassianides C, et al. Therapy of chronic hepatitis B with recombinant human alpha and gamma interferon. Hepatology. 1990;11:266-270.

363. Kakumu S, Ishikawa T, Mizokami M, et al. Treatment with human gamma interferon of chronic hepatitis B: Comparative study with alpha interferon. J Med Virol. 1991;35:32-37.

364. Ruiz-Moreno M, Fernandez P, Leal A, et al. Pilot interferon-beta trial in children with chronic hepatitis B who had previously not responded to interferon-alpha therapy. Pediatrics. 1997;99:222-225.

365. Schalm SW, Heathcote J, Cianciara J, et al. Lamivudine and alpha interferon combination treatment of patients with chronic hepatitis B infection: A randomised trial [see comments]. Gut. 2000;46:562-568.

366. Sangfelt P, Uhnoo I, Hollander A, et al. Lamivudine and famciclovir combination therapy with or without addition of interferon-alpha-2b for HBeAg-positive chronic hepatitis B: A pilot study. Scand J Infect Dis. 2002;34:505-511.

367. Lai KN, Li PK, Lui SF, et al. Membranous nephropathy related to hepatitis B virus in adults. N Engl J Med. 1991;324:1457-1463.

368. Farci P, Mandas A, Coiana A, et al. Treatment of chronic hepatitis D with interferon alfa-2a. N Engl J Med. 1994;330:88-94.

369. Jaeckel E, Cornberg M, Wedemeyer H, et al. Treatment of acute hepatitis C with interferon alfa-2b. N Engl J Med. 2001;345:1452-1457.

370. Alberti A, Boccato S, Vario A, Benvegnu L. Therapy of acute hepatitis C. Hepatology. 2002;36(Suppl 1):S195-S200.

371. Seeff LB, Hoofnagle JH. National Institutes of Health Consensus Development Conference Statement: Management of hepatitis C: 2002. Hepatology. 2002;36(Suppl 1):S1-S2.

372. Di Bisceglie AM, Martin P, Kassianides C, et al. Recombinant interferon alfa therapy for chronic hepatitis C: A randomized, double-blind, placebo-controlled trial. N Engl J Med. 1989;321:1506-1510.

373. Davis GL, Balart LA, Schiff ER, et al. Treatment of chronic hepatitis C with recombinant interferon alfa: A multicenter randomized, controlled trial. Hepatitis Interventional Therapy Group. N Engl J Med. 1989;321:1501-1506.

374. Shindo M, Di Bisceglie AM, Cheung L, et al. Decrease in serum hepatitis C viral RNA during alpha-interferon therapy for chronic hepatitis C. Ann Intern Med. 1991;115:700-704.

375. Zeuzem S, Feinman V, Rasenack J, et al. Peginterferon alfa-2a in patients with chronic hepatitis C. N Engl J Med. 2000;343:1666-1672.

376. Heathcote J, Shiffman ML, Cooksley GE, et al. Peginterferon alfa-2a in patients with chronic hepatitis C and cirrhosis. N Engl J Med. 2000;343:1673-1680.

377. Marcellin P, Boyer N, Gervais A, et al. Long-term histologic improvement and loss of detectable intrahepatic HCV RNA in patients with chronic hepatitis C and sustained response to interferon-alpha therapy. Ann Intern Med. 1997;127:875-881.

378. Poynard T, Bedossa P, Chevallier M, et al. A comparison of three interferon alfa-2b regimens for the long-term treatment of chronic non-A, non-B hepatitis: Multicenter Study Group [see comments] [published erratum appears in N Engl J Med. 1996;334:1143]. N Engl J Med. 1995;332:1457-1462.

379. McHutchison JG, Gordon SC, Schiff ER, et al. Interferon alfa-2b alone or in combination with ribavirin as initial treatment for chronic hepatitis C: Hepatitis Interventional Therapy Group. N Engl J Med. 1998;339:1485-1492.

380. Davis GL, Esteban-Mur R, Rustgi V, et al. Interferon alfa-2b alone or in combination with ribavirin for the treatment of relapse of chronic hepatitis C: International Hepatitis Interventional Therapy Group [see comments]. N Engl J Med. 1998;339:1493-1499.

381. Cacoub P, Lidove O, Maisonobe T, et al. Interferon-alpha and ribavirin treatment in patients with hepatitis C virus-related systemic vasculitis. Arthrit Rheum. 2002;46:3317-3326.

382. Misiani R, Bellavita P, Fenili D, et al. Interferon alfa-2a therapy in cryoglobulinemia associated with hepatitis C virus. N Engl J Med. 1994;330:751-756.

383. Samuel D, Bizollon T, Feray C, et al. Interferon-alpha 2b plus ribavirin in patients with chronic hepatitis C after liver transplantation: A randomized study. Gastroenterology. 2003;124:642-650.

384. Davis GL, Wong JB, McHutchison JG, et al. Early virologic response to treatment with peginterferon alfa-2b plus ribavirin in patients with chronic hepatitis C. Hepatology. 2003;38:645-652.

385. Poynard T, McHutchison J, Manns M, et al. Impact of pegylated interferon alfa-2b and ribavirin on liver fibrosis in patients with chronic hepatitis C. Gastroenterology. 2002;122:1303-1313.

386. Nishiguchi S, Kuroki T, Nakatani S, et al. Randomised trial of effects of interferon-alpha on incidence of hepatocellular carcinoma in chronic active hepatitis C with cirrhosis. Lancet. 1995;346:1051-1055.

387. International Interferon-α Hepatocellular Carcinoma Study Group. Effect of interferon-alpha on progression of cirrhosis to hepatocellular carcinoma: A retrospective cohort study. Lancet. 1998;351:1535-1539.

388. Schiappa DA, Mittal C, Brown JA, Mika BP. Relationship of hepatitis C genotype 1 NS5A sequence mutations to early phase viral kinetics and interferon effectiveness. J Infect Dis. 2001;185:868-877.

389. Enomoto N, Sakuma I, Asahina Y, Kurosaki M, Murakami T, Yamamoto C et al. Mutations in the nonstructural protein 5A gene and response to interferon in patients with chronic hepatitis C virus 1b infection. N Engl J Med. 1996;334:77-81.

390. Martinot M, Marcellin P, Boyer N, et al. Influence of hepatitis G virus infection on the severity of liver disease and response to interferon-alpha in patients with chronic hepatitis C. Ann Intern Med. 1997;126:874-881.

391. Lebwohl M, Sacks S, Conant M, et al. Recombinant alpha-2 interferon gel treatment of recurrent herpes genitalis. Antiviral Res. 1992;17:235-243.

392. Krown SE. The role of interferon in the therapy of epidemic Kaposi's sarcoma. Semin Oncol. 1987;14(Suppl 3):27-33.

393. Berglund O, Engman K, Ehrnst A, et al. Combined treatment of symptomatic human immunodeficiency virus type 1 infection with native interferon-alpha and zidovudine. J Infect Dis. 1991;163:710-715.

394. Marroni M, Gresele P, Landonio G, et al. Interferon-alpha is effective in the treatment of HIV-1-related, severe, zidovudine-resistant thrombocytopenia: A prospective, placebo-controlled, double-blind trial. Ann Intern Med. 1994;121:423-429.

395. Frazer IH, McMillan AJ. Papillomatosis and condylomata acuminata. In: Stuart-Harris R, Penny R, eds. Clinical Applications of the Interferons. London: Chapman & Hall; 1997:79-90.

396. Beutner KR, Wiley DJ, Douglas JM, et al. Genital warts and their treatment. Clin Infect Dis. 1999;28(Suppl 1):S37-S56.

397. Leventhal BG, Kashima HK, Mounts P, et al. Long-term response of recurrent respiratory papillomatosis to treatment with lymphoblastoid interferon alfa-N1. Papilloma Study Group. N Engl J Med. 1991;325:613-617.

398. Cinatl J, Morgenstern B, Bauer G, et al. Treatment of SARS with human interferons. Lancet. 2003;362:293-294.

399. Higgins PG, Barrow GI, Tyrrell DA, et al. The efficacy of intranasal interferon alpha-2a in respiratory syncytial virus infection in volunteers. Antiviral Res. 1990;14:3-10.

400. Loutfy MR, Blatt LM, Siminovitch KA, et al. Interferon alfacon-1 plus corticosteroids in severe acute respiratory syndrome: A preliminary study. JAMA. 2003;290:3222-3228.

401. Zhao Z, Zhang F, Xu M, et al. Description and clinical treatment of an early outbreak of severe acute respiratory syndrome (SARS) in Guangzhou, PR China. J Med Microbiol. 2003;52:715-720.

402. Levine S, Hernandez D, Yamanaka G, et al. Efficacies of entecavir against lamivudine-resistant hepatitis B virus replication and recombinant polymerases in vitro. Antimicrob Agents Chemother. 2002;46:2525-2532.

403. Bartholomew MM, Jansen RW, Jeffers LJ, et al. Hepatitis-B-virus resistance to lamivudine given for recurrent infection after orthotopic liver transplantation. Lancet. 1997;349:20-22.

404. Allen MI, Deslauriers M, Andrews CW, et al. Identification and characterization of mutations in hepatitis B virus resistant to lamivudine. Lamivudine Clinical Investigation Group. Hepatology. 1998;27:1670-1677.

405. Ono-Nita SK, Kato N, Shiratori Y, et al. Susceptibility of lamivudine-resistant hepatitis B virus to other reverse transcriptase inhibitors. J Clin Invest. 1999;103:1635-1640.

406. Ono SK, Kato N, Shiratori Y, et al. The polymerase L528M mutation cooperates with nucleotide binding-site mutations, increasing hepatitis B virus replication and drug resistance. J Clin Invest. 2001;107:449-455.

407. Dienstag JL, Schiff ER, Wright TL, et al. Lamivudine as initial treatment for chronic hepatitis B in the United States. N Engl J Med. 1999;341:1256-1263.

408. Nunez M, Puoti M, Camino N, Soriano V. Treatment of chronic hepatitis B in the human immunodeficiency virus-infected patient: Present and future. Clin Infect Dis. 2003;37:1678-1685.

409. Nelson M, Portsmouth S, Stebbing J, et al. An open-label study of tenofovir in HIV-1 and Hepatitis B virus co-infected individuals. AIDS. 2003;17:F7-F10.

410. Dienstag JL, Goldin RD, Heathcote EJ, et al. Histological outcome during long-term lamivudine therapy. Gastroenterology. 2003;124:105-117.

411. Lai CL, Chien RN, Leung N, et al. A one-year trial of lamivudine for chronic hepatitis B. N Engl J Med. 1998;339:61-68.

411a. Liaw YF, Chien RN, Yeh CT. No benefit to continue lamivudine therapy after emergence of YMDD mutations. Antiviral Ther. 2004;9:257-262.

412. Jonas MM, Kelly DA, Mizerski J, et al. Clinical trial of lamivudine in children with chronic hepatitis B. N Engl J Med. 2002;346:1706-1713.

413. Lai CL, Ching CK, Tung AK, et al. Lamivudine is effective in suppressing hepatitis B virus DNA in Chinese hepatitis B surface antigen carriers: A placebo-controlled trial. Hepatology. 1997;25:241-244.

414. Grellier L, Mutimer D, Ahmed M, et al. Lamivudine prophylaxis against reinfection in liver transplantation for hepatitis B cirrhosis [published erratum appears in Lancet. 1997;349:364]. Lancet. 1996;348:1212-1215.

415. Kim CU, Lew W, Williams MA, et al. Influenza neuraminidase inhibitors possessing a novel hydrophobic interaction in the enzyme active site: Design, synthesis, and structural analysis of carbocyclic sialic acid analogues with potent anti-influenza activity. J Am Chem Soc. 1997;119:681-690.

416. Mendel DB, Tai CY, Escarpe PA, et al. Oral administration of a prodrug of the influenza virus neuraminidase inhibitor GS4071 protects mice and ferrets against influenza infection. Antimicrob Agents Chemother. 1998;42:640-646.

417. Wetherall NT, Trivedi T, Zeller J, et al. Evaluation of neuraminidase enzyme assays using different substrates to measure susceptibility of influenza virus clinical isolates to neuraminidase inhibitors: Report of the neuraminidase inhibitor susceptibility network. J Clin Microbiol. 2003;41:742-750.

418. McClellan K, Perry CM. Oseltamivir: A review of its use in influenza. Drugs. 2001;61:263-283.

419. Tisdale M. Monitoring of viral susceptibility: New challenges with the development of influenza NA inhibitors. Rev Med Virol. 2000;10:45-55.

420. Colman PM. Influenza virus neuraminidase: Structure, antibodies, and inhibitors. Protein Sci. 1994;3:1687-1696.

421. Zambon M, Hayden FG. Position statement: Global neuraminidase inhibitor susceptibility network. Antiviral Res. 2001;49:147-156.

422. Carr J, Ives J, Kelly L, et al. Influenza virus carrying neuraminidase with reduced sensitivity to oseltamivir carboxylate has altered properties in vitro and is compromised for infectivity and replicative ability in vivo. Antiviral Res. 2002;54:79-88.

423. Whitley RJ, Hayden FG, Reisinger K, et al. Oral oseltamivir treatment of influenza in children. Pediatr Infect Dis J. 2001;20(2):127-133.

424. Jackson HC, Roberts N, Wang Z, Belshe R. Management of influenza: Use of new antivirals and resistance in perspective. Clin Drug Invest. 2000;20:447-454.

425. Weinstock DM, Gubareva LV, Zuccotti G. Prolonged shedding of multidrug-resistant influenza A virus in an immunocompromised patient. N Engl J Med. 2003;348:867-868.

426. He G, Massarella J, Ward P. Clinical pharmacokinetics of the prodrug oseltamivir and its active metabolite Ro 64-0802. Clin Pharmacokinet. 1999;37:471-484.

427. Oo C, Barrett J, Hill G, et al. Pharmacokinetics and dosage recommendations for an oseltamivir oral suspension for the treatment of influenza in children. Paediatr Drugs. 2001;3:229-236.

428. Eisenberg G, Bidgood A, Lynch G, et al. Penetration of GS4071, a novel influenza neuraminidase inhibitor, into rat bronchoalveolar lining fluid following oral administration of the prodrug GS4104. Antimicrob Agents Chemother. 1997;41:1949-1952.

429. Kurowski M, Barrett J, Waalberg E, Wiltshire H. Oral oseltamivir rapidly delivers active drug levels to middle ear and sinuses in humans. Abstract 509. Presented at the 40th Interscience Conference on Antimicrobial Agents and Chemotherapy, Toronto, September 17-20, 2000:19.

430. Straumanis JP, Tapia M, King J. Influenza B infection associated with encephalitis: Treatment with oseltamivir. Pediatr Infect Dis J. 2003;21:173-175.

431. Enger C, Nordstrom BL, Thakrar B, et al. Health outcomes among patients receiving oseltamivir. Pharmacoepidemiol Drug Saf. 2003;12:1-11.

432. Treanor JJ, Hayden FG, Vrooman PS, et al. Efficacy and safety of the oral neuraminidase inhibitor oseltamivir in treating acute influenza. JAMA. 2000;283:1016-1024.

433. Cooper NJ, Sutton AJ, Abrams KR, et al. Effectiveness of neuraminidase inhibitors in treatment and prevention of influenza A and B: Systematic review and meta-analyses of randomised controlled trials. BMJ. 2003;326:1235-1239.

434. Boivin G, Coulombe Z, Wat C. Quantification of the influenza virus load by real-time polymerase chain reaction in nasopharyngeal swabs of patients treated with oseltamivir. J Infect Dis. 2003;188:578-580.

435. Aoki FY, Macleod MD, Paggiaro P, et al. Early administration of oral oseltamivir increases the benefits of influenza treatment. J Antimicrob Chemother. 2003;51:123-129.

436. Kaiser L, Wat C, Mills T, et al. Impact of oseltamivir treatment on influenza-related lower respiratory tract complications and hospitalizations. Arch Intern Med. 2003;163:1667-1672.

437. Bowles SK, Lee W, Simor AE, et al. Use of oseltamivir during influenza outbreaks in Ontario nursing homes, 1999-2000. J Am Geriatr Soc. 2002;50:608-616.

438. Hayden FG, Atmar RL, Schilling M, et al. Use of the selective oral neuraminidase inhibitor oseltamivir to prevent influenza. N Engl J Med. 1999;341:1336-1343.

439. Peters PH, Gravenstein S, Norwood P, et al. Long-term use of oseltamivir for the prophylaxis of influenza in a vaccinated frail older population. J Am Geriatr Soc. 2001;49:1-7.

440. Welliver R, Monto AS, Carewicz O, et al. Effectiveness of oseltamivir in preventing influenza in household contacts: A randomized controlled trial [see comments]. JAMA. 2001;285:748-754.

441. Hayden FG, Belshe R, Villanueva C, et al. Management of influenza in households: A prospective, randomized comparison of oseltamivir treatment with or without postexposure prophylaxis. J Infect Dis. 2004;189:440-449.

442. Morfin F, Dupuis-Girod S, Carrington D, et al. Adenovirus susceptibility to antiviral drugs is genogroup-dependent (poster V-282). 43rd Interscience Conference on Antimicrobial Agents and Chemotherapy, Chicago, Ill., September 14-17, 2003:9-14.

442a. Crance JM, Scaramozzino N, Jouan A, Garin D. Interferon, ribavirin, 6-azauridine and glycyrrhizin: Antiviral compounds active against pathogenic flaviviruses. Antiviral Res. 2003;58:73-79.

443. Cinatl J, Morgenstern B, Bauer G, et al. Glycyrrhizin, an active component of liquorice roots, and replication of SARS-associated coronavirus. Lancet. 2003;361:2045-2046.

444. Meier V, Burger E, Mihm S, et al. Ribavirin inhibits DNA, RNA, and protein synthesis in PHA-stimulated human peripheral blood mononuclear cells: Possible explanation for therapeutic efficacy in patients with chronic HCV infection. J Med Virol. 2003;69:50-58.

445. Tam RC, Lau JYN, Hong Z. Mechanisms of action of ribavirin in antiviral therapies. Antivir Chem Chemother. 2002;12:261-272.

446. Graci JD, Cameron CE. Quasispecies, error catastrophe, and the antiviral activity of ribavirin. Virology. 2002;298:175-180.

447. Hong Z, Cameron CE. Pleiotropic mechanisms of ribavirin antiviral activities. Prog Drug Res. 2002;59:41-69.

448. Vo NV, Young KC, Lai MM. Mutagenic and inhibitory effects of ribavirin on hepatitis C virus RNA polymerase. Biochemistry. 2003;42:10462-10471.

449. Fernandez-Larsson R, Patterson JL. Ribavirin is an inhibitor of human immunodeficiency virus reverse transcriptase. Molec Pharmacol. 1990;38:766-770.

450. Young KC, Lindsay KL, Lee KJ, et al. Identification of a ribavirin-resistant NS5B mutation of hepatitis C virus during ribavirin monotherapy. Hepatology. 2003;38:869-878.

451. Glue P. The clinical pharmacology of ribavirin. Semin Liver Dis. 1999;19(Suppl 1):17-24.

452. Preston SL, Drusano GL, Glue P, et al. Pharmacokinetics and absolute bioavailability of ribavirin in healthy volunteers as determined by stable-isotope methodology. Antimicrob Agents Chemother. 1999;43:2451-2456.

453. Laskin OL, Longstreth JA, Hart CC, et al. Ribavirin disposition in high-risk patients for acquired immunodeficiency syndrome. Clin Pharmacol Therapeut. 1987;41:546-555.

454. Glue P, Schenker S, Gupta S, et al. The single dose pharmacokinetics of ribavirin in subjects with chronic liver disease. J Clin Pharmacol. 2000;49:417-421.

455. Jen JF, Glue P, Gupta S, et al. Population pharmacokinetic and pharmacodynamic analysis of ribavirin in patients with chronic hepatitis C. Ther Drug Monit. 2000;22:555-565.

456. ICN Pharmaceuticals ICMC. Investigational Drug Brochure, Intravenous Ribavirin IND 9,076, February, 2001.

457. Dieterich DT, Spivak JL. Hematologic disorders associated with hepatitis C virus infection and their management. Clin Infect Dis. 2003;37:533-541.

458. Di Bisceglie AM, Conjeevaram HS, Fried MW, et al. Ribavirin as therapy for chronic hepatitis C: A randomized, double-blind, placebo-controlled trial. Ann Intern Med. 1995;123:897-903.

459. Knowles SR, Phillips EJ, Dresser L, Matukas L. Common adverse events associated with the use of ribavirin for severe acute respiratory syndrome in Canada. Clin Infect Dis. 2003;37:1139-1142.

460. Bradley JS, Connor JD, Compogiannis LS, Eiger LL. Exposure of health care workers to ribavirin during therapy for respiratory syncytial virus infections. Antimicrob Agents Chemother. 1990;34:668-670.

461. Shults RA, Baron S, Decker J, et al. Health care worker exposure to aerosolized ribavirin: Biological and air monitoring. J Occup Environ Med. 1996;38:257-263.

462. Bodenheimer HJ, Lindsay KL, Davis GL, et al. Tolerance and efficacy of oral ribavirin treatment of chronic hepatitis C: A multicenter trial. Hepatology. 1997;26:473-477.

463. Medina J, Garcia-Buey L, Moreno-Monteagudo JA, et al. Combined antiviral options for the treatment of chronic hepatitis C. Antiviral Res. 2003;60:135-143.

464. Randolph AG, Wang EE. Ribavirin for respiratory syncytial virus lower respiratory tract infection: A systematic overview. Arch Pediatr Adolesc Med. 1996;150:942-947.

465. Guerguerian AM, Gauthier M, Lebel MH, et al. Ribavirin in ventilated respiratory syncytial virus bronchiolitis: A randomized, placebo-controlled trial. Am J Respir Crit Care Med. 1999;160:829-834.

466. Englund JA, Piedra PA, Jefferson LS, et al. High-dose, short-duration ribavirin aerosol therapy in children with suspected respiratory syncytial virus infection. J Pediatr. 1990;117:313-320.

467. Long CE, Voter KZ, Barker WH, Hall CB. Long term follow-up of children hospitalized with respiratory syncytial virus lower respiratory tract infection and randomly treated with ribavirin or placebo. Pediatr Infect Dis J. 1997;16:1023-1028.

468. Small TN, Casson A, Malak SF, et al. Respiratory syncytial virus infection following hematopoietic stem cell transplantation. Bone Marrow Transplant. 2002;29:321-327.

469. Boeckh M, Berrey MM, Bowden RA, et al. Phase 1 evaluation of the respiratory syncytial virus-specific monoclonal antibody palivizumab in recipients of hematopoietic stem cell transplants. J Infect Dis. 2001;184:350-354.

470. Lewinsohn DM, Bowden RA, Mattson D, Crawford SW. Phase I study of intravenous ribavirin treatment of respiratory syncytial virus pneumonia after marrow transplantation. Antimicrob Agents Chemother. 1996;40:2555-2557.

471. Chakrabarti S, Collingham KE, Holder K, et al. Pre-emptive oral ribavirin therapy of paramyxovirus infections after haematopoietic stem cell transplantation: A pilot study. Bone Marrow Transplant. 2001;28:759-763.

472. Hayden FG, Sable CA, Connor JD, Lane J. Intravenous ribavirin by constant infusion for serious influenza and parainfluenzavirus infection. Antiviral Ther. 1996;1:51-56.

473. Rodriguez WJ, Hall CB, Welliver R, et al. Efficacy and safety of aerosolized ribavirin in young children hospitalized with influenza: A double-blind, multicenter, placebo-controlled trial. J Pediatr. 1994;125:129-135.

474. Chong HT, Kamarulzaman A, Tan CT, et al. Treatment of acute Nipah encephalitis with ribavirin. Ann Neurol. 2001;49:810-813.

475. Nichols WG, Corey L, Gooley T, et al. Parainfluenza virus infections after hematopoietic stem cell transplantation: Risk factors, response to antiviral therapy, and effect on transplant outcome. Blood. 2001;98:573-578.

476. Kaplan LJ, Daum RS, Smaron M, McCarthy CA. Severe measles in immunocompromised patients. JAMA. 1992;267:1237-1241.

477. Gavin PJ, Katz BZ. Intravenous ribavirin treatment for severe adenovirus disease in immunocompromised children. Pediatrics. 2002;110:E9.

478. Kesson AM, Ferguson JK, Rawlinson WD, Cunningham AL. Progressive vaccinia treated with ribavirin and vaccinia immune globulin. Clin Infect Dis. 1997;25:911-914.

479. Mazzulli T, Farcas GA, Poutanen SM, et al. Severe acute respiratory syndrome–associated coronavirus in lung tissue. Emerg Infect Dis (Online). Jan 1, 2004. Available at http://www.cdc.gov/ncidod/EID/vol10no1/03-0404.htm.

480. Huggins JW, Hsiang CM, Cosgriff TM, et al. Prospective, double-blind, concurrent, placebo-controlled clinical trial of intravenous ribavirin therapy of hemorrhagic fever with renal syndrome. J Infect Dis. 1991;164:1119-1127.

481. Borio L, Inglesby T, Peters CJ, et al. Hemorrhagic fever viruses as biological weapons: Medical and public health management. JAMA. 2002;287:2391-2405.

482. Kilgore PE, Ksiazek TG, Rollin PE, et al. Treatment of Bolivian hemorrhagic fever with intravenous ribavirin. Clin Infect Dis. 1997;24:718-722.

483. Mardani M, Jahromi MK, Naieni KH, Zeinali M. The efficacy of oral ribavirin in the treatment of crimean-congo hemorrhagic fever in Iran. Clin Infect Dis. 2003;36:1613-1618.

484. Fisher-Hoch SP, Khan JA, Rehman S, et al. Crimean Congo-haemorrhagic fever treated with oral ribavirin. Lancet. 1995;346:472-475.

485. McJunkin JE, Khan R, de los Reyes EC, et al. Treatment of severe La Crosse encephalitis with intravenous ribavirin following diagnosis by brain biopsy. Pediatrics. 1997;99:261-267.

486. Chapman LE, Mertz GJ, Peters CJ, et al. Intravenous ribavirin for Hantavirus pulmonary syndrome: Safety and tolerance during 1 year of open-label experience. Ribavirin Study Group. Antivir Ther. 1999;4:211-219.

487. Japour AJ, Lertora JJ, Meehan PM, et al. A phase-I study of the safety, pharmacokinetics, and antiviral activity of combination didanosine and ribavirin in patients with HIV-1 disease. AIDS Clinical Trials Group 231 Protocol Team. J Acquir Immune Defic Syndr Hum Retrovirol. 1996;13:235-246.

488. Wilhelmus KR. Interventions for herpes simplex virus epithelial keratitis. Cochrane Database Syst Rev. 2003;3:CD002898.

489. Kessler HA, Hurwitz S, Farthing C, et al. Pilot study of topical trifluridine for the treatment of acyclovir-resistant mucocutaneous herpes simplex disease in patients with AIDS (ACTG 172). AIDS Clinical Trials Group. J Acquir Immune Defic Syndr Hum Retrovirol. 1996;12:147-152.

490. Kimura H, Morita M, Tsuge I, et al. Vidarabine therapy for severe chronic active Epstein-Barr virus infection. J Pediatr Hematol Oncol. 2001;23:294-299.

491. von Itzstein M, Wu WY, Kok GB, et al. Rational design of potent sialidase-based inhibitors of influenza virus replication. Nature. 1993;363:418-423.

492. Cheer SM, Wagstaff AJ. Zanamivir: An update of its use in influenza. Drugs. 2002;62:71-106.

493. Woods JM, Bethell RC, Coates JA, et al. 4-Guanidino-2,4-dideoxy-2,3-dehydro-N-acetylneuraminic acid is a highly effective inhibitor both of the sialidase (neuraminidase) and of growth of a wide range of influenza A and B viruses in vitro. Antimicrob Agents Chemother. 1993;37:1473-1479.

494. McKimm-Breschkin J, Trivedi T, Hampson A, et al. Neuraminidase sequence analysis and susceptibilities of influenza virus clinical isolates to zanamivir and oseltamivir. Antimicrob Agents Chemother. 2003;47:2264-2272.

495. Murrell M, Porotto M, Weber T, et al. Mutations in human parainfluenza virus type 3 hemagglutinin-neuraminidase causing increased receptor binding activity and resistance to the transition state sialic acid analog 4-GU-DANA (Zanamivir). J Virol. 2003;77:309-317.

496. Gubareva LV, Matrosovich MN, Brenner MK, et al. Evidence for zanamivir resistance in an immunocompromised child infected with influenza B virus. J Infect Dis. 1998;178:1257-1262.

497. Peng AW, Milleri S, Stein DS. Direct measurement of the anti-influenza agent zanamivir in the respiratory tract following inhalation. Antimicrob Agents Chemother. 2000;44:1974-1976.

498. Lee C, Loeb M, Phillips A, et al. Zanamivir use during transmission of amantadine-resistant influenza A in a nursing home. Infect Control Hosp Epidemiol. 2000;21:700-704.

499. Diggory P, Fernandez C, Humphrey A, et al. Comparison of elderly people's technique in using two dry powder inhalers to deliver zanamivir: Randomised controlled trial. BMJ. 2001;322:1-4.

500. Freund B, Gravenstein S, Elliott M, Miller I. Zanamivir: A review of clinical safety. Drug Saf. 1999;21:267-281.

501. Hedrick JA, Barzilai A, Behre U, et al. Zanamivir for treatment of symptomatic influenza A and B infection in children five to twelve years of age: A randomized controlled trial. Pediatr Infect Dis J. 2000;19:410-417.

502. Gravenstein S, Johnston SL, Loeschel E. Zanamivir: A review of clinical safety in individuals at high risk of developing influenza-related complications. Drug Saf. 2001;24:1113-1125.

503. Gravenstein S, Johnston SL, Loeschel E, Webster A. Zanamivir: A review of clinical safety in individuals at high risk of developing influenza-related complications. Drug Saf. 2001;24:1113-1125.

504. Murphy K, Eivindson A, Pauksens K, et al. Efficacy and safety of inhaled zanamivir for the treatment of influenza in patients with asthma or chronic obstructive pulmonary disease. Clin Drug Invest. 2000;20:337-349.

505. FDA Public Health Advisory. Safe and appropriate use of influenza drugs. January 12, 2000. Available at www.fda.gov/cder/drug/advisory/influenza.htm.

506. Fleming D. Zanamivir in the treatment of influenza. Expert Opin Pharmacother. 2003;4:799-805.

507. Walker JB, Hussey EK, Treanor JJ, et al. Effects of the neuraminidase inhibitor zanamivir on otologic manifestations of experimental human influenza. J Infect Dis. 1997;176:1417-1422.

508. Hayden FG, Osterhaus ADME, Treanor JJ, et al. Efficacy and safety of the neuraminidase inhibitor zanamivir in the treatment of influenza virus infections. N Engl J Med. 1997;337:874-879.

509. MIST (Management of Influenza in the Southern Hemisphere Trialists) Study Group. Randomized trial of efficacy and safety of inhaled zanamivir in treatment of influenza A and B virus infections. Lancet. 1998;352:1877-1881.

510. Monto AS, Webster A, Keene O. Randomized, placebo-controlled studies of inhaled zanamivir in the treatment of influenza A and B: Pooled efficacy analysis. J Antimicrob Chemother. 1999;44:23-29.

511. Kaiser L, Keene ON, Hammond J, et al. Impact of zanamivir on antibiotics use for respiratory events following acute influenza in adolescents and adults. Arch Intern Med. 2000;160:3234-3240.

512. Lalezari JP, Elliott M, Keene O. Zanamivir for the treatment of influenza A and B infection in high-risk patients (abstract). Arch Intern Med. 2001;161:212-217.

513. Johny AA, Clark A, Price N, et al. The use of zanamivir to treat influenza A and B infection after allogeneic stem cell transplantation. Bone Marrow Transplant. 2002;29:113-115.

514. Monto AS, Robinson DP, Herlocher L, et al. Zanamivir in the prevention of influenza among healthy adults. JAMA. 1999;282:31-36.

515. Hayden FG, Gubareva LV, Monto AS, et al. Inhaled zanamivir for preventing influenza in families. N Engl J Med. 2000;343:1282-1289.

516. Monto AS, Pichichero ME, Blanckenberg SJ, et al. Zanamivir prophylaxis: An effective strategy for the prevention of influenza types A and B within households. J Infect Dis. 2002;186:1582-1588.

517. Gravenstein S, Drinka P, Osterweil D, et al. A multicenter prospective double-blind ramdomized controlled trial comparing the relative safety and efficacy of zanamivir to rimantadine for nursing home influenza outbreak control. Abstract 1155. Presented at the 40th Interscience Conference on Antimicrobial Agents and Chemotherapy, Toronto, September 17-20, 2000:270.

518. Gitlin L, Karelsky S, Andino R. Short interfering RNA confers intracellular antiviral immunity in human cells. Nature. 2002;418:430-434.

519. Ge Q, McManus MT, Nguyen T, et al. RNA interference of influenza virus production by directly targeting mRNA for degradation and indirectly inhibiting all viral RNA transcription. Proc Natl Acad Sci U S A. 2003;100:2718-2723.

520. Song E, Lee SK, Wang J, et al. RNA interference targeting Fas protects mice from fulminant hepatitis. Nat Med. 2003;9:347-351.

521. McCaffrey AP, Meuse L, Pham TT, et al. RNA interference in adult mice. Nature. 2002;418:38-39.

522. Wassilew SW, Wutzler P. Oral brivudin in comparison with acyclovir for improved therapy of herpes zoster in immunocompetent patients: Results of a randomized, double-blind, multicentered study. Antiviral Res. 2003;59:49-56.

523. Andrei G, Snoeck R, Reymen D, et al. Comparative activity of selected antiviral compounds against clinical isolates of varicella-zoster virus. Eur J Clin Microbiol Infect Dis. 1995;14:318-328.

524. Wassilew SW, Wutzler P. Oral brivudin in comparison with acyclovir for herpes zoster: A survey study on postherpetic neuralgia. Antiviral Res. 2003;59:57-60.

525. Peek SF, Cote PJ, Jacob JR, et al. Antiviral activity of clevudine (L-FMAU, [1-(2-fluoro-5-methyl-beta, L-arabinofuranosyl) uracil]) against woodchuck hepatitis virus replication and gene expression in chronically infected woodchucks (Marmota monax). Hepatology. 2001;33:254-266.

526. Marcellin P, Sacks S, Lau GK, et al. A dose-escalating trial evaluating the safety and antiviral activity of clevudine in patients with chronic HBV infection. Dig Dis Week. Presented May 20, 2003.

527. Gish RG, Leung NW, Wright TL, et al. Dose range study of pharmacokinetics, safety, and preliminary antiviral activity of emtricitabine in adults with hepatitis B virus infection. Antimicrob Agents Chemother. 2002;46:1734-1740.

528. Honkoop P, de Man RA. Entecavir: A potent new antiviral drug for hepatitis B. Expert Opin Investig Drugs. 2003;12:683-688.

529. Colonno RJ, Genovesi EV, Medina I, et al. Long-term entecavir treatment results in sustained antiviral efficacy and prolonged life span in the woodchuck model of chronic hepatitis infection. J Infect Dis. 2001;184:1236-1245.

530. de Man RA, Wolters L, Nevens F, et al. Safety and efficacy of oral entecavir given for 28 days in subjects with chronic hepatitis B. Hepatology 2001;34:578-582.

531. Lai CL, Rosmawati M, Lao J, et al. Entecavir is superior to lamivudine in reducing hepatitis B virus DNA in patients with chronic hepatitis B infection. Gastroenterology. 2002;123:1831-1838.

532. Williams SL, Hartline CB, Kushner NL, et al. In vitro activities of benzimidazole D- and L-ribonucleosides against herpesviruses. Antimicrob Agents Chemother. 2003;47:2186-2192.

533. Lalezari JP, Aberg JA, Wang LH, et al. Phase I dose escalation trial evaluating the pharmacokinetics, anti-human cytomegalovirus (HCMV) activity, and safety of 1263W94 in human immunodeficiency virus-infected men with asymptomatic HCMV shedding. Antimicrob Agents Chemother. 2002;46:2969-2976.

534. Komazin G, Ptak RG, Emmer BT, et al. Resistance of human cytomegalovirus to the benzimidazole L-ribonucleoside maribavir maps to UL27. J Virol. 2003;77:11499-11506.

535. Krosky PM, Baek MC, Jahng WJ, et al. The human cytomegalovirus UL44 protein is a substrate for the UL97 protein kinase. J Virol. 2003;77:7720-7727.

536. Wang LH, Peck RW, Yin Y, et al. Phase I safety and pharmacokinetic trials of 1263W94, a novel oral anti-human cytomegalovirus agent, in healthy and human immunodeficiency virus-infected subjects. Antimicrob Agents Chemother. 2003;47:1334-1342.

537. Pevear DC, Tull TM, Seipel ME, Groarke JM. Activity of pleconaril against enteroviruses. Antimicrob Agents Chemother. 1999;43:2109-2115.

538. Kaiser L, Crump CE, Hayden FG. In vitro activity of pleconaril and AG7088 against selected serotypes and clinical isolates of human rhinoviruses. Antiviral Res. 2000;47:215-220.

539. Schiff GM, Sherwood JR. Clinical activity of pleconaril in an experimentally induced coxackievirus A21 respiratory infection. J Infect Dis. 2000;181:20-26.

540. Florea NR, Maglio D, Nicolau DP. Pleconaril, a novel antipicornaviral agent. Pharmacotherapy. 2003;23:339-348.

541. Kearns GL, Bradley JS, Jacobs RF, et al. Single dose pharmacokinetics of pleconaril in neonates. Pediatric Pharmacology Research Unit Network. Pediatr Infect Dis J. 2000;19:833-839.

542. Hayden FG, Herrington DT, Coats TL, et al. Efficacy and safety of oral pleconaril for treatment of picornavirus colds in adults: Results of two double-blind, randomized, placebo-controlled trials. Clin Infect Dis. 2003;36:1523-1532.

543. Rotbart HA, Webster AD. Treatment of potentially life-threatening enterovirus infections with pleconaril. Clin Infect Dis. 2001;32:228-235.

544. Benhamou Y, Tubiana R, Thibault V. Tenofovir disoproxil fumarate in patients with HIV and lamivudine-resistant hepatitis B virus. N Engl J Med. 2003;348:177-178.

545. Lai CL, Leung NWY, Teo EK, et al. Results of a one-year international phase IIB comparative trial of telbivudine, lamivudine, and the combination, in patients with chronic hepatitis B (Abstract). Hepatology. 2003;262A.

546. Stathoulopoulou F, Almond MK, Dhillon S, Raftery MJ. Clinical pharmacokinetics of oral acyclovir in patients on continuous ambulatory peritoneal dialysis. Nephron. 1996;74:337-341.

Immunomodulators[*]

W. CONRAD LILES

Antimicrobial agents and vaccines represent the traditional strategies employed for treatment and prevention of infectious diseases. Although both approaches have yielded considerable therapeutic success, many infectious disorders remain difficult clinical problems. Treatment success may be compromised by defects of the immune system resulting from an underlying disease or treatment thereof. In such circumstances, enhancement of the host immune response may

be therapeutically beneficial. In contrast, in diseases such as sepsis, in which an overactive host immune response mediates inflammatory tissue damage, downregulation of the host immune response may be potentially beneficial.

An immunomodulator (also known as a biologic response modifier or biologic therapeutic) is a biologic or nonbiologic agent that affects host response via direct or indirect effects on one or more components of the immunoregulatory network. This network is a complex and intricate system, involving both the innate and acquired immune systems, as well as a wide variety of cell types and cytokines. With increasing knowledge of the system and its regulation, novel, rational, and therapeutic approaches to modulate its activity are emerging. Potential therapeutic agents include antibodies, cytokines, and synthetic agents targeted to selectively modulate immune function in a manner beneficial to the host during infection and inflammation. However, it is important to note that many of these agents are expensive, and cost-effective use is a critical issue in their application to clinical medicine.

Immunomodulators can be divided into six main groups: (1) naturally occurring cytokines, many of which are produced by recombinant deoxyribonucleic acid (DNA) technology, including the colony-stimulating factors (CSFs), interferons (IFNs), interleukins (ILs), chemokines, and thymic hormones; (2) monoclonal antibodies and receptor antagonists that block proinflammatory cytokines; (3) immunoglobulins, used either as replacement therapy in immunoglobulin-deficient individuals or as true immunomodulators to upregulate or downregulate the immune response; (4) glucocorticosteroids; (5) synthetic compounds with immunomodulatory activity, such as pentoxifylline imiquimod, and thalidomide; and (6) anti-coagulant proteins with associated anti-inflammatory properties, such as recombinant activated protein C (APC), which represents the first agent to be approved by the U.S. Food and Drug Administration (FDA) specifically for the treatment of severe sepsis. Agents that have been investigated for sepsis therapy in randomized clinical trials, such as antibodies to endotoxin (bacterial lipopolysaccharide [LPS]) and strategies to block the effects of proinflammatory cytokines, are discussed briefly in this chapter. The topic of sepsis therapeutics is discussed more comprehensively in Chapter 67.

This chapter focuses on agents that have been used in an effort to manipulate the immune system for the treatment or prevention of infection in humans. Many potentially useful immunomodulators have been investigated in vitro or in experiments involving animal models of infection. However, because of the complexity of the host immune response, in vitro data often do not correlate with in vivo results. Furthermore, animal models, although useful for preliminary studies, have inherent limitations compromising their applicability to human disease states. Therefore, this chapter is limited to immunomodulatory agents that have been investigated in clinical trials in humans. Table 39-1 lists cytokine immunomodulators that have been approved by the FDA for the prevention or treatment of infectious diseases. The field of immunomodulatory therapy continues to evolve. As our understanding of the molecular pathogenesis of inflammation, immunity, and infection continues to develop, one can expect emergence of novel immunomodulatory therapeutics and refinement of current immunomodulatory approaches in the future.

COLONY-STIMULATING FACTORS

CSFs are a group of naturally occurring glycoprotein cytokines that regulate the production, differentiation, survival, and activation of hematopoietic cells. Erythropoietin stimulates red blood cell production and is widely employed clinically for the treatment of anemia. Thrombopoietin plays a key regulatory role in the growth and differentiation of megakaryocytes. IL-5 stimulates the growth and survival of eosinophils and basophils. Stem cell factor (SCF; former designations: *Steel* factor, *c-kit* ligand) and IL-3 (former designations: multi-colony-stimulating factor, hematopoietic cell growth factor) serve as stimuli for multiple hematopoietic cell lineages. Granulocyte colony-

[*]This chapter is based in part on the chapter for the fifth edition by Michael O. Frank and Gerald L. Mandell.

TABLE 39-1   U.S. FDA-Approved Uses of Cytokines to Prevent or Treat Infection

Cytokine	Indications
Granulocyte colony-stimulating factor (G-CSF; filgrastim)	Following myelosuppressive chemotherapy associated with a clinically significant incidence of febrile neutropenia
	Following induction or consolidation chemotherapy for AML
	Myeloid reconstitution after HSCT
	Severe chronic neutropenia
Pegylated G-CSF	Following myelosuppressive chemotherapy for nonmyeloid malignancies associated with a clinically significant incidence of febrile neutropenia
Granulocyte-macrophage colony-stimulating factor (GM-CSF; sargramostim)	Following induction chemotherapy for AML in patients older than 55 years of age
	Following transplantation of autologous PBSC
	Myeloid reconstitution after autologous or allogeneic HSCT
	HSCT failure or engraftment delay
Interferon-α (IFN-α)	Treatment of chronic HBV infection
	Treatment of chronic HBC infection
	Treatment of condyloma acuminatum
	Treatment of HIV-related Kaposi's sarcoma
Pegylated IFN-α	Treatment of chronic HCV infection
Interferon-γ (IFN-γ)	Chronic granulomatous disease

AML, acute myelogenous leukemia; *FDA*, Food and Drug Administration; *HBV*, hepatitis B virus; *HCV*, hepatitis C virus; *HSCT*, hematopoietic stem cell transplantation; *PBSC*, peripheral blood stem cell.

stimulating factor (G-CSF), granulocyte-macrophage colony-stimulating factor (GM-CSF), and macrophage colony-stimulating factor (M-CSF) serve as growth factors for specific cell types in the myeloid series. These cytokines have attracted considerable interest for their potential role in immunomodulation.

Granulocyte Colony-Stimulating Factor

G-CSF is a glycoprotein that predominantly affects neutrophils (polymorphonuclear leukocytes [PMNs]) and neutrophilic precursors.[1] Nagata and colleagues isolated cDNA, encoding a 177-amino acid sequence from a squamous cell line.[2] Because of alternative mRNA splicing sites, Souza and associates isolated a different cDNA for G-CSF, encoding a 174-amino acid polypeptide from a bladder carcinoma cell line.[3] Endogenous G-CSF is produced predominantly by monocytes/macrophages, fibroblasts, and endothelial cells.[1] G-CSF serves as a potent stimulus to both increase and accelerate neutrophil production. Its essential role in normal regulation of neutrophil development has been clearly demonstrated in studies conducted with G-CSF "knock-out" mice. Mice rendered G-CSF deficient by targeted disruption of the G-CSF gene in embryonic stem cells develop chronic neutropenia with a 50% reduction in the number of bone marrow granulocyte precursor cells. G-CSF–deficient mice also have increased susceptibility to experimental *Listeria monocytogenes* infection and fail to develop sepsis-related neutrophilia.[4] In addition to its critical role in the regulation of granulopoiesis, G-CSF modulates the functional activity of developing and mature neutrophils. In vitro, G-CSF has been reported to upregulate multiple physiologic activities of neutrophils, including the inducible oxidative (respiratory) burst, phagocytosis, and chemotaxis. Furthermore, G-CSF prolongs neutrophil survival via delay of spontaneous apoptosis. Many of the modulatory effects observed in vitro have been confirmed when G-CSF has been administered in vivo to human subjects and neutrophil function subsequently measured ex vivo.[3]

G-CSF is available for clinical use in recombinant form as filgrastim in the United States and as lenograstim outside the United States. Lenograstim is a glycoprotein produced in Chinese hamster ovary cells, whereas filgrastim is produced in *Escherichia coli* and is thus nonglycosylated. A pegylated form of filgrastim, pegfilgrastim (with a greatly prolonged half-life compared with conventional filgrastim, has been recently released for clinical use in the United States. Clinical trials have reported similar therapeutic and adverse effects for both filgrastim and lenograstim.[1,3,5] G-CSF initially causes a transient decrease in the peripheral blood neutrophil count, which is followed by a sustained dose-dependent increase in neutrophil count over the subsequent 5- to 6-day period. The neutrophil count stabilizes or decreases slightly if G-CSF is continued for a 2-week course, then returns to baseline over a 4- to 7-day period when G-CSF is discontinued. The increase in neutrophil count results primarily in an increase in the rate of production with a shortened maturation time. At G-CSF doses greater than 10 μg/kg/day, slight increases in monocyte and lymphocyte counts occur, and relatively modest declines in platelet counts have been observed at doses greater than 30 μg/kg/day for 2 weeks.[5]

Because of its potent ability to increase neutrophil counts and thereby improve clinical outcome, treatment with G-CSF has emerged as an important therapeutic approach for a variety of neutropenic conditions. Clinical benefits observed include decreases in incidence and sequelae of bacterial and opportunistic fungal infections, hospitalizations, and days of antibiotics. The clinical benefits observed have led to widespread consensus that prolonged G-CSF therapy represents the standard of care for relatively rare primary (congenital) neutropenic disorders, such as severe congenital neutropenia, cyclic neutropenia (cyclic hematopoiesis), and symptomatic idiopathic neutropenia.[6] In cases of severe congenital neutropenia that prove refractory to standard G-CSF treatment, combination therapy with glucocorticosteroids and G-CSF may be beneficial.[7]

The first FDA-approved use of G-CSF was for the treatment of neutropenia after cancer chemotherapy, in which the risk of infection is related to both the degree and duration of neutropenia. Opportunistic bacterial and fungal infections continue to be a major cause of morbidity and mortality in patients with cancer who receive myelosuppressive therapy. Currently, G-CSF is widely used clinically to prevent febrile neutropenia and/or to shorten the duration of neutropenia associated with cancer chemotherapy, radiotherapy, or myelosuppressive drugs. On the basis of randomized clinical trials of patients with chemotherapy-induced neutropenia, G-CSF has been approved for acceleration of myeloid recovery in patients following administration of standard-dose and dose-intensive chemotherapy for solid tumors and hematologic malignancies.[8] When used prophylactically for individuals undergoing chemotherapy in clinical trials, G-CSF has significantly reduced the resulting period of neutropenia and decreased the incidence of febrile neutropenia in high-risk patients.[8] No clinical evidence indicates that G-CSF increases the relapse rate when used in patients undergoing treatment for leukemia. However, because of its high cost and relatively modest effects on overall survival, the routine use of G-CSF after chemotherapy remains controversial. The American Society of Clinical Oncology has published recommendations regarding the use of G-CSF after cancer chemotherapy. The expert panel recommended that G-CSF be reserved for use in patients receiving chemotherapy regimens associated with a 40% or greater risk of febrile neutropenia, or in patients with additional risk factors including previous episodes of febrile neutropenia.[8]

G-CSF is also used after allogeneic and autologous hematopoietic stem cell transplantation (HSCT), where it has been shown to shorten the duration of neutropenia post-transplantation and decrease days of parenteral antibiotic therapy without adverse effects on graft-versus-host disease (GVHD), relapse, or graft failure.[9,10] One economic analysis reported a 3% reduction in overall costs when G-CSF was used after autologous bone marrow transplantation.[11]

G-CSF is often used with antibiotics for treatment (as opposed to prevention) of febrile neutropenia. Despite several randomized trials designed to address this issue, the proper role of G-CSF in the treatment of febrile neutropenia remains controversial.[12] Rather than being a homogeneous group, patients with febrile neutropenia vary in terms of clinical prognosis. Prospectively validated risk factors for complications and poor clinical outcome include serious independent comorbid conditions, uncontrolled malignant disease, and prior hospitalization. Subset analysis in one clinical trial suggested that G-CSF yielded the greatest benefit in patients with an absolute neutrophil count (ANC) less than 100 cells/μL and/or documented infection.[12] In another prospective, multicenter, randomized clinical trial involving 210 patients with solid tumors and high-risk febrile neutropenia, G-CSF treatment, when added to empiric broad-spectrum antibiotic therapy, was associated with shortened duration of neutropenia, decreased number of days of antibiotics and hospitalization, and reduced overall costs of hospitalization.[13]

Neutropenia is a relatively common complication of human immunodeficiency virus (HIV) infection, occurring in 35% to 75% of patients with acquired immunodeficiency syndrome (AIDS), especially in individuals receiving zidovudine or ganciclovir.[14,15] The etiology of HIV-related neutropenia is multifactorial and includes depressed production of myeloid growth factors, bone marrow infiltration and infection, myelosuppressive drug regimens, autoimmune mechanisms, and accelerated spontaneous neutrophil apoptosis.[14,15] Neutropenia has been shown to be a significant risk factor for bacterial infection in HIV-infected individuals.[14,15] Furthermore, numerous physiologic deficits are present in neutrophils of HIV-infected individuals, including microbicidal activity.[14] G-CSF has been shown to partially ameliorate both HIV-related neutropenia and functional neutrophil impairment. In clinical trials its use has been associated with a reduced incidence of bacterial infections and a decrease in the number of attributable days of hospitalization and antibiotic use.[14-16] G-CSF treatment does not appear to affect HIV viral loads. It can be effectively employed to support the use of other myelosuppressive medications in HIV-infected patients.[16] One report documents successful treatment of HIV-related refractory aphthous ulcers with G-CSF.[17]

G-CSF has also received interest as a potential therapeutic immunomodulator in a number of non-neutropenic disease states. A double-blind, controlled, multicenter trial involving 756 patients was performed to examine the clinical efficacy of G-CSF (300 μg/day for up to 10 days) as adjunctive therapy for treatment of community-acquired pneumonia. Administration of G-CSF was well tolerated and safe in this patient population. It increased the peripheral blood neutrophil count threefold but failed to significantly affect the clinical course, mortality, or length of hospitalization. However, radiographic infiltrates resolved more rapidly in the group of patients that received G-CSF. Interestingly, the development of acute respiratory distress syndrome was significantly decreased in the G-CSF-treated group ($P = 0.017$). The beneficial effects of G-CSF appeared to be more pronounced in the subgroup of 261 patients with multilobar pneumonia, in which 17.1% of the placebo group developed organ dysfunction or empyema compared with 5.8% of the G-CSF-treated group.[18] These observations prompted subsequent trials of G-CSF therapy for multilobar pneumonia and pneumonia with sepsis syndrome. In 480 patients with multilobar community-acquired pneumonia, G-CSF failed to improve overall clinical outcome, although there was a trend toward reduced mortality in the subpopulation of patients with pneumococcal pneumonia that received G-CSF.[19] Likewise, G-CSF did not appear to be efficacious in reducing either mortality or complications when used in two clinical trials to treat septic patients with pneumonia.[20,21]

In a randomized, double-blind, placebo-controlled trial performed at a single center, 40 type 1 diabetes patients with severe foot infections were randomized to receive G-CSF ($n = 20$) or placebo ($n = 20$) for 7 days. More rapid healing was reported in the group receiving G-CSF in addition to standard antibiotics and débridement.[22] In a study of 37 patients following liver transplantation, G-CSF-treated patients reportedly experienced decreased episodes of sepsis, sepsis-related mortality, and acute rejection compared with historical controls.[23] A randomized, placebo-controlled, double-blind multicenter phase II study was performed to determine whether G-CSF reduced the frequency of nosocomial infections in patients with either acute traumatic brain injury or cerebral hemorrhage. Although G-CSF was found to be safe in this patient population and appeared to reduce the risk of primary bacteremia, no beneficial effects were observed on mortality, length of hospitalization, or other nosocomial infections.[24] Similar results were reported when G-CSF was studied as a strategy to reduce postoperative infections in patients undergoing esophagectomy for esophageal carcinoma.[25] There are also case reports of the combined use of G-CSF and antifungal therapy for treatment of life-threatening opportunistic fungal infections in both neutropenic and nonneutropenic patients.[26]

During the past decade, considerable interest has emerged regarding the use of G-CSF to mobilize CD34+ hematopoietic stem cells from bone marrow to peripheral blood (peripheral blood stem cells [PBSC]) for use in lieu of bone marrow cells in HSCT protocols.[4] The ability of G-CSF to significantly elevate blood neutrophil counts in normal individuals has also rekindled interest in granulocyte (neutrophil) transfusion therapy for treatment of serious opportunistic bacterial and fungal infections in individuals with neutropenia or inherited disorders of neutrophil dysfunction, such as chronic granulomatous disease (CGD) and leukocyte adhesion deficiency (LAD).[27] Planning is under way for a multicenter, randomized phase III clinical trial to test the clinical efficacy of granulocyte transfusion therapy in neutropenic cancer patients and following HSCT.

In summary, G-CSF has been approved by the FDA for treatment of patients with cancer receiving myelosuppressive chemotherapy, after induction chemotherapy for acute myelogenous leukemia (AML), for acceleration of myeloid reconstitution after HSCT, for mobilization and collection of PBSC for transplantation, and for individuals with severe chronic neutropenia. Preliminary clinical studies have suggested potential utility of G-CSF as a therapeutic agent to reduce sequelae of infections in not only neutropenic but also non-neutropenic patient populations. However, positive results from pilot studies have generally not been confirmed in larger randomized controlled clinical trials in disease states such as pneumonia and sepsis.

Dosage

The recommended dosage of G-CSF for high-risk patients after cytotoxic cancer chemotherapy is 5 μg/kg/day subcutaneously or intravenously, starting 24 hours after the last chemotherapy dose. Subsequent dosing should be adjusted depending on the neutrophil response. After HSCT, the recommended dosage is 10 μg/kg/day subcutaneously or intravenously until the ANC is greater than 1000 cells/μL for 3 consecutive days, then a reduction in dose to 5 μg/kg/day until discontinuation at the time when the ANC is stable. For cyclic or idiopathic neutropenia, an initial dose of 5 μg/kg/day is recommended, with adjustment per the individual ANC response. Effective treatment of severe congenital neutropenia often requires higher doses, and thus therapy is usually initiated at a dose of 6 to 10 μg/kg/day. In HIV-infected patients with neutropenia, lower doses are often sufficient, and therapy can be started at 1 μg/kg/day subcutaneously, with increases up to 10 μg/kg/day as needed. Dosing should be adjusted on an individual basis to maintain an ANC greater than 1000 cells/μL. Often, 1 μg/kg or less administered two or three times per week is sufficient to maintain a satisfactory therapeutic response. Pegfilgrastim is approved by the FDA for prophylaxis of neutropenia in patients receiving myelosuppressive chemotherapy for nonmyeloid malignancies. The recommended dosage is 6 mg subcutaneously, administered once for each chemotherapy cycle. Pegfilgrastim should not be given during the 24-day period prior to initiation of chemotherapy and for 24 hours after completion of chemotherapy.

Adverse Effects

G-CSF is usually well tolerated. The most common adverse effect is mild to moderate bone and/or musculoskeletal pain, which occurs in 20% to 30% of individuals.[1] Aside from musculoskeletal pain, there are relatively few adverse effects, even after years of administration for severe chronic neutropenia.[6] Other reported adverse effects include mild local erythema at injection sites, headache, anemia, splenomegaly, mild to moderate thrombocytopenia, and asymptomatic elevations of lactate dehydrogenase, alkaline phosphatase, and leukocyte alkaline phosphatase.[1] Rare adverse events include cutaneous neutrophilic vasculitis (Sweet's syndrome), G-CSF–induced lung toxicity after cancer chemotherapy, and splenic rupture in apparently otherwise healthy individuals after G-CSF–based regimens for harvest of PBSC.[28] Individuals with severe congenital neutropenia are at increased risk for development of myelodysplastic syndrome and progression to AML. No evidence exists indicating that G-CSF therapy is a cause of malignant transformation in severe congenital neutropenia.[29] Administration of G-CSF to individuals with sickle cell disease is contraindicated because of the risk of precipitating an occlusive sickle cell crisis.

Granulocyte-Macrophage Colony-Stimulating Factor

GM-CSF is a 127-amino acid glycoprotein available in recombinant form produced in yeast as sargramostim. Other forms of recombinant human GM-CSF include molgramostim produced in *E. coli* and regramostim produced in mammalian cells. The principal cellular sources of endogenous GM-CSF are T lymphocytes, monocytes/macrophages, fibroblasts, and endothelial cells.[1] GM-CSF raises peripheral blood counts of neutrophils, monocytes, and eosinophils and stimulates a variety of functional activities in these target cells.[1] Unlike G-CSF, it does not appear to play an essential in normal neutrophil development. Mice lacking GM-CSF as a result of targeted genetic disruption develop alveolar proteinosis, but steady-state hematopoiesis is not impaired.[30]

The predominant clinical use of GM-CSF has been to accelerate myeloid recovery in oncology patients following myelosuppressive treatment regimens.[1] GM-CSF was first shown to be beneficial in patients undergoing autologous bone marrow transplantation (BMT) for lymphoma, in which it accelerated neutrophil recovery, decreased antibiotic use, and shortened hospitalization when given for 3 weeks following the procedure. However, there was no change in rate of infection, incidence of fever, or overall survival.[31] Similar results were reported for GM-CSF in autologous BMT for nonlymphoid malignancies, autologous BMT, and PBSC transplantation.[1,32] The benefit of GM-CSF in allogeneic BMT is less clear, although the theoretical concern that GM-CSF might exacerbate GVHD does not appear to be justified. Although GM-CSF is approved by the FDA for administration to enhance myeloid recovery following induction chemotherapy for AML, variable results on its impact on incidence of infections in this clinical setting have been reported.[33,34] Like G-CSF, GM-CSF has been studied for acceleration of myeloid recovery after chemotherapy for solid tumors.[1] However, despite reports of decreased duration of neutropenia, number of infections, and length of hospitalizations, GM-CSF has not received FDA approval for this indication.[35] GM-CSF was evaluated as an adjunct to antibiotic therapy for the treatment of febrile neutropenia in a prospective randomized trial of 107 cancer patients. Although the response rate was reportedly significantly improved by GM-CSF treatment, the difference was not statistically significant in an intention-to-treat analysis.[36] In a small, uncontrolled travel trial, neutropenic patients with documented opportunistic fungal infections received GM-CSF plus amphotericin B. Of the eight evaluable patients, a favorable clinical response was reported for six, including four individuals who experienced complete resolution of infection. The same study also reported positive clinical responses in patients with bacterial infections that received GM-CSF.[37] Another uncontrolled, retrospective study of patients who received GM-CSF following cancer chemotherapy also suggested a potential antifungal effect.[38]

GM-CSF is effective in raising peripheral blood levels of granulocytes and monocytes in HIV-infected individuals, and administration has been reported to correct HIV-associated functional neutrophil defects.[14,15,39] Its use in patients with AIDS has been controversial because of early data suggesting that HIV replication in monocytes might be increased. This effect appears to be counterbalanced by concomitant use of antiretroviral therapy.[40] Variable results have been reported when GM-CSF has been studied as an immunomodulatory agent for treatment of HIV-related disseminated *Mycobacterium avium-intracellulare* complex (MAC) infection.[41] Use of GM-CSF has also been reported as beneficial in the treatment of small numbers of patients with AIDS-related cryptococcal meningitis and antimicrobial-refractory oropharyngeal candidiasis.[42,43]

In summary, GM-CSF is FDA approved for the following indications: (1) following induction chemotherapy for AML; (2) following transplantation of autologous PBSC; (3) mobilization and collection of PBSC for transplantation; (4) myeloid reconstitution after autologous or allogeneic HSCT; and (5) HSCT failure or engraftment delay. For reasons of relative efficacy and toxicity, its use has largely been supplanted by G-CSF in clinical practice. A number of clinical studies have suggested a potential therapeutic role for GM-CSF in addition to these approved indications. Most of these studies, however, have involved relatively small numbers of patients.

Dosage

The manufacturer's current dosing recommendation for use in bone marrow transplantation is 250 μg/m^2/day, administered intravenously, over 2 to 4 hours starting 2 to 4 hours after bone marrow infusion and continuing until the absolute neutrophil count is greater than 1500 cells/μL for 3 consecutive days. The same dosing is recommended after PBSC transplantation, administered either intravenously over 24 hours or subcutaneously, starting immediately after PBSC infusion. For treatment following induction chemotherapy for AML, GM-CSF therapy is started 4 days after completion of chemotherapy.

Adverse Effects

Compared with G-CSF, GM-CSF–associated toxicity is more frequent and severe, possibly due to stimulation of proinflammatory responses in monocytes/macrophages. The most frequent adverse effect is fever, which occurs in more than 20% of patients. Flulike symptoms of myalgias and malaise commonly accompany fever.[1] First-dose reactions, consisting of dyspnea, hypoxemia, hypotension, tachycardia, flushing, musculoskeletal pain, nausea, and vomiting, have been reported in 5% of patients receiving GM-CSF.[44] Adverse effects are more common when GM-CSF is administered intravenously and with doses greater than 3 μg/kg. High doses (20 μg/kg/day) of GM-CSF have been reported to cause a generalized capillary leak syndrome. Reactivation of autoimmune diseases, such as idiopathic thrombocytopenic purpura and rheumatoid arthritis, has also been reported.[1]

Macrophage Colony-Stimulating Factor

M-CSF is a glycoprotein that was first cloned and produced in recombinant form in 1985. It is produced endogenously by monocytes/macrophages, fibroblasts, and endothelial cells. M-CSF acts specifically on cells of the monocyte/macrophage lineage to stimulate their production and enhance their functional activity.[45] In contrast to G-CSF and GM-CSF, clinical experience with M-CSF has been limited primarily to its role as a potential adjuvant for the treatment of opportunistic fungal infections complicating prolonged neutropenia. In a phase I trial, 24 patients with invasive fungal infection after bone marrow transplantation received M-CSF, in doses ranging from 100 to 2000 μg/m^2/day intravenously, in addition to standard treatment with conventional antifungal agents. The only significant toxicity reported was transient dose-related thrombocytopenia. No M-CSF–mediated effects were noted on GVHD or neutrophil, monocyte, or lymphocyte counts. Fungal disease reportedly resolved in 6 of 12 evaluable patients.[46] The authors treated an additional 22 patients and pooled the two sets of data for long-term follow-up and comparison with historical controls. Overall survival was significantly improved in the M-CSF–treated patients compared with historical controls (27% versus 5%); however, subgroup analysis revealed that survival was improved only in the subgroup of patients with Karnofsky scores greater than 20 and *Candida* infections. No difference in survival was apparent in patients with invasive aspergillosis or Karnofsky scores less than 20.[47] No prospective, randomized, controlled clinical trials of M-CSF for adjunctive therapy of infections have been published.

INTERFERONS

IFNs are a class of cytokines, distinguished by their intrinsic antiviral properties, that are produced by cells in response to a variety of stimuli, including viruses, certain intracellular pathogens, and bacterial toxins. IFNs play complex, pivotal roles in the host immune response, often augmenting the effects of other cytokines. There are three main classes of IFNs: IFN-α and IFN-β are produced by many cell types but primarily by leukocytes and fibroblasts, respectively; IFN-γ is produced by T lymphocytes. Whereas IFN-α and IFN-β are primarily antiviral interferons, IFN-γ functions to activate macrophages and stimulate innate immunity. Interferon beta-1b is FDA approved for treatment of relapsing-remitting multiple sclerosis and is not discussed further in this chapter.

Interferon-α

The antiviral activity of IFN-α is discussed in Chapter 4. IFN-α actually refers to a class of molecules, of which there are more than 25 members. Currently, IFN-α is available for clinical use in the United States as recombinant interferon-alfa-2a and interferon-alfa-2, which differ by a single amino acid, natural interferon-alfa-n3, which is a mixture of subtypes of IFN-α purified from human leukocytes, and interferon-alfacon-1, a bioengineered form of IFN-α based on a "consensus" amino acid sequence of the most common forms of naturally occurring IFN-α. Pegylated forms of interferon-alfa-2a and interferon-alfa-2b are now available with extended biologic half-lives. IFN-α is approved by the FDA for use in chronic hepatitis B virus (HBV) and hepatitis C (HCV) infections, condyloma acuminatum, common warts (papillomavirus), and Kaposi's sarcoma (although Roche removed the Kaposi's indication in November 2003). It has been investigated for use in a variety of other infections, including viral upper respiratory tract infections.

Combination therapy with systemic IFN-α and ribavirin is currently the standard of care for treatment patients with symptomatic chronic HCV infection (see Chapters 112 and 150).[48,49] Treatment is recommended for individuals who are positive for HCV ribonucleic acid (RNA) in peripheral blood, have persistent elevations in serum alanine aminotransferase (ALT), and have findings of fibrosis and at least moderate inflammation on liver biopsy. Therapeutic efficacy varies depending on the HCV genotype causing infection. Unfortunately HCV genotype 1 is the most common in the United States (>90% of cases) and the least responsive to therapy.[48,49] Recent clinical trials have demonstrated the superior efficacy of pegylated IFN-α plus ribavirin over standard IFN-α plus ribavirin or pegylated IFN-α alone.[50,51] For treatment of chronic HCV infection caused by genotype 1, a 48-week course of therapy is recommended with either pegylated interferon-alfa-2a (180 μg subcutaneously each week) or pegylated interferon-alfa-2b (1.5 μg/kg subcutaneously each week), combined with oral ribavirin with the dose adjusted for patient weight (<75 kg: 400 mg every morning and 600 mg every evening; >75 kg: 600 mg twice daily). For treatment of chronic HCV infection caused by genotype 2 or 3 (nongenotype 1), a 24-week course of therapy with either pegylated IFN-α or standard IFN-α (3×10^6 U subcutaneously three times per week), both combined with ribavirin, is an acceptable alternative to the 48-week regimen above. With combination IFN-α/ribavirin treatment, a sustained viral response is achieved in 42% to 51% of patients infected with genotype 1 after 48-week therapy and in 76% to 82% of patients infected with genotypes 2 and 3 after 24-week therapy.[48-51] No data exist regarding treatment with IFN-α with or without ribavirin for postexposure prophylaxis of HCV infection. Recent evidence suggests that combination therapy with IFN-α (either standard or pegylated formulations) and ribavirin may be effective for acute HCV infection, but generalized use for this purpose is currently controversial.[52,53]

IFN-α is also an effective therapeutic option for treatment of chronic HBV infection (see Chapters 112 and 142).[54] Recommended regimens include conventional IFN-α at doses of 5×10^6 U subcutaneously daily or 10×10^6 U subcutaneously three times per week for a total duration of 16 weeks. In general, treatment of chronic HBV in-

fection should be considered for individuals with compensated liver disease who have persistent elevation of serum levels of hepatic aminotransferases, detectable levels of circulating HBsAg, HBeAg and HBV DNA in serum for at least 6 months, and evidence of hepatitis on liver biopsy. Predictors of response to therapy include high pretreatment serum levels of ALT, low serum levels of HBV DNA, and infection in adulthood. Predictors of nonresponse to therapy include normal serum ALT levels, high serum HBV DNA levels, absence of serum HBeAg, childhood infection, and immunosuppression.[54] In individuals with HBeAg-positive chronic HBV infection, a meta-analysis of randomized, controlled clinical trials demonstrated a significantly higher response rate with IFN-α compared with placebo. IFN-α treatment was associated with 21% and 6% increases in clearance of HBeAg and HBsAg, respectively.[55] Long-term follow-up studies have shown that durable response was achieved in 76% to 94% of responders and was associated with more favorable clinical outcomes, in terms of reductions in liver-related complications (e.g., cirrhosis, hepatoma) and survival.[56,57] The use of steroid priming in an effort to increase response rate has not been shown to be beneficial.[58] Recent evidence from a European trial suggests that sustained response rates might be improved by extending the duration of IFN-α from 16 weeks to 32 weeks.[59] Clinical studies are under way, investigating the use of pegylated IFN-α and combination IFN-α/lamivudine (3TC) therapy for treatment of chronic HBV infection.[60] In individuals with HBeAg-negative chronic HBV infection, the therapeutic response to IFN-α is decreased and the relapse rate is high.[61] IFN-α treatment of chronic HBV infection is contraindicated for individuals with decompensated cirrhosis.

IFN-α is an effective therapy for condyloma acuminatum (genital warts) caused by papillomavirus (see Chapter 140). Injection of intralesional interferon-alfa-2b, 1 to 5×10^6 U (1×10^6 U in each wart, up to five warts at a time) three times per week for 3 consecutive weeks, was effective in 60% to 70% of patients with recurrences after use of other therapeutic agents or methods.[62] Systemic IFN-α may also be an effective adjunctive modality for recurrent respiratory papillomatosis.[63] IFN-α has also been investigated as a potential therapeutic agent for the common cold (rhinovirus infection; see Chapters 50 and 171). When used as a nasal spray for prophylaxis, IFN-α has been shown to decrease upper respiratory tract infections caused by rhinovirus but not those caused by coronaviruses, influenza viruses, or parainfluenza viruses.[64,65] However, when used alone, IFN-α nasal spray causes inflammatory rhinitis. IFN-α has therapeutic potential as an adjunctive immunomodulatory agent when combined with antiviral agents. A combination of topical trifluorothymidine and IFN-α was reported to be effective in three HIV-infected individuals with severe cutaneous herpes simplex virus infection refractory to treatment with acyclovir or foscarnet.[66] Combined use of IFN-α with foscarnet was reportedly successful in treating a single case of severe acyclovir-resistant perianal herpes simplex virus infection in an individual with advanced HIV disease.[67] Interferon-alfa-2b was also combined with systemic IL-2 therapy in a small phase I study in an effort to increase CD4+ lymphocyte counts in individuals with advanced HIV infection. Although transient increases in CD4+ lymphocyte counts were observed, 8 of 17 patients enrolled in the study were unable to complete the 21-day course of therapy (IFN-α: $5-15 \times 10^6$ U/day; IL-2: $3-12 \times 10^6$ U/day) because of treatment-related toxicity, including pancreatitis, cytopenia, mental status changes, elevated serum levels of hepatic aminotransferases, and flulike symptoms.[68]

IFN-α has also been investigated as a potential therapeutic adjunctive immunomodulator for treatment of pulmonary tuberculosis. In a small study involving 20 individuals (10 received antimycobacterial chemotherapy alone; 10 received antimycobacterial therapy plus aerosolized IFN-α: 3×10^6 U three times weekly for 8 weeks), treatment with IFN-α was associated with earlier resolution of clinical signs of infection, radiographic abnormalities, sputum smears, and cellularity in bronchoalveolar lavage fluid samples.[69] Another report described the use of subcutaneous IFN-α (3×10^6 U three times weekly for 12 weeks) for treatment of multidrug-resistant pulmonary tuberculosis. Of the five patients treated, two reportedly cleared infection, one experienced sputum smear conversion but remained culture positive, and two had no change in status of infection.[70]

The major adverse effects of systemic IFN-α therapy are dose related and consist of flulike symptoms, including fever, headache, myalgias, arthralgias, nausea, and anorexia. These symptoms are usually alleviated by pretreatment with acetaminophen or nonsteroidal anti-inflammatory agents and generally decrease in severity over a period of several weeks, especially at doses of less than 10×10^6 U/day. At higher doses, bone marrow suppression (reported frequency: 3% to 69%, depending on dose), neuropsychiatric effects (reported frequency: 20%, with depression, paresthesias, or change in mental status most common), and elevated serum hepatic aminotransferase levels (reported frequency: 10% to 80%) are observed. Intralesional IFN-γ can cause local discomfort, inflammation, and mild systemic effects, especially when multiple injections are given concurrently.

Interferon-γ

Recombinant human IFN-γ is available as interferon-gamma-1b (Actimmune). IFN-γ is produced endogenously by three major types of lymphocytes: CD4+ cells, CD8+ cells, and natural killer (NK) cells.[1,71] The major target cells of IFN-γ are monocytes, macrophages, and neutrophils, but its effects extend beyond the conventional cells of the immune system to nonprofessional host defense cells, such as endothelial cells, fibroblasts, hepatocytes, astrocytes, and microglia cells.[1,71] IFN-γ plays a critical regulatory role in macrophage-mediated killing of important intracellular pathogens, including *Mycobacterium, Leishmania, Rickettsia, Legionella,* and *Chlamydia* species.[1,71] Granuloma formation in response to intracellular pathogens has been shown to be an IFN-γ–dependent process.[71] Mice with targeted disruption of either the IFN-γ or IFN-γ receptor genes have increased susceptibility to intracellular pathogens, such as viruses, *Mycobacterium tuberculosis,* bacillus Calmette-Guérin, and *Listeria monocytogenes.*[72,73] Recent evidence indicates that individuals who are functionally IFN-γ deficient are highly susceptible to infections caused by atypical mycobacteria and *Salmonella* spp.[74,75]

IFN-γ is FDA approved for the prophylactic treatment of individuals with chronic granulomatous disease (CGD). Based on the in vitro observation that, using CGD cells, IFN-γ can stimulate human monocyte bactericidal activity, 128 patients with CGD were enrolled in a study in which half of the individuals received IFN-γ (50 μg/m²) subcutaneously three times a week. The IFN-γ–treated group developed significantly fewer infections (both total and serious) and required fewer days of hospitalization. No change in phagocyte-mediated superoxide production was observed in the IFN-γ–treated group, suggesting that IFN-γ enhanced nonoxidative mechanisms of host defense. Toxicity was relatively mild, requiring withdrawal of only 4 patients from the study protocol. The therapeutic benefit of IFN-γ was independent of age, use of prophylactic antibiotics, or genotype of CGD.[76,77]

IFN-γ may also have therapeutic potential as an immunomodulatory agent for management of other specific immunodeficiency syndromes. Hyperimmunoglobulin E syndrome (hyper-IgE syndrome; Job's syndrome) is a distinct primary (congenital) immunodeficiency syndrome characterized by recurrent skin and pulmonary abscesses, pneumonia, eczema, eosinophilia, and elevated serum IgE levels. *Staphylococcus aureus* is the major pathogen responsible for infectious complications in individuals with hyper-IgE syndrome. Although the molecular basis of hyper-IgE syndrome remains unclear, several investigators have reported impairment of in vitro chemotactic responses in neutrophils from affected individuals.[78] Furthermore, lymphocytes of patients with hyper-IgE syndrome have been reported to have a depressed response to interleukin-12 (IL-12), resulting in decreased IFN-α production in response to bacterial antigens.[79] Based on these observations, a small, uncontrolled trial was performed, which suggested possible improvement in the clinical course of hyper-IgE patients when treated with systemic IFN-γ therapy.[80]

During the past two decades, systemic IFN-γ has been administered as adjunctive therapy to a number of patients with chronic infections caused by intracellular pathogens, including cutaneous and visceral leishmaniasis, disseminated atypical mycobacterial infection, and lepromatous leprosy (Hansen's disease).[1,71,81] Administration of IFN-γ at a dose of 100 to 400 μg/m²/day intramuscularly for 10 to 40 days with pentavalent antimony to patients with visceral leishmaniasis was reported to significantly improve the response rate compared with historical groups treated with pentavalent antimony alone.[82] However, no prospective, randomized, controlled trial has been reported. Adjunctive IFN-γ has also been reported to be effective for treatment of cutaneous leishmaniasis when combined with meglumine antimonate therapy.[83]

When given to patients with lepromatous leprosy, IFN-γ has been shown to increase macrophage responses to *Mycobacterium leprae* and enhance clearance of mycobacteria from skin.[84] Systemic IFN-γ therapy has also been reported to decrease mycobacterial organism burden in disseminated MAC infection in HIV-infected individuals, especially when given concomitantly with antimicrobial therapy.[85] When administered at a dose of 50 μg/m² subcutaneously three times per week, systemic IFN-γ therapy, combined with conventional antimicrobial therapy, also led to substantial clinical improvement in seven HIV-negative patients with antimicrobial-refractory disseminated MAC or *Mycobacterium kansasii* infection.[86]

Because IFN-γ activates alveolar macrophages, which play an important role in the host immune response against *M. tuberculosis,* aerosolized IFN-γ therapy has been used for treatment of a limited number of patients with multidrug-resistant pulmonary tuberculosis. In an open-label pilot study, five individuals with sputum smear–positive disease received aerosolized IFN-γ via inhalation three times per week for 2 months. Sputum smears for acid-fast bacilli converted from positive to negative in all five patients within 1 month. Treatment for 2 months resulted in a reduction in the size of cavitary lesions in each patient. However, sputum smears reverted to positive in four of the patients within 1 month of discontinuation of IFN-γ therapy.[87] A limited number of patients with antimicrobial refractory pulmonary infection with atypical (nontuberculous) mycobacteria have also been treated with adjunctive aerosolized IFN-γ with reported success.[88]

IFN-γ has also been investigated for potential utility as a prophylactic immunomodulator agent to decrease risk of infection in high-risk patient populations. Several large multicenter studies, however, failed to demonstrate that administration of systemic IFN-γ could effectively protect burn or trauma patients from infectious morbidity or mortality.[89,90]

Adverse effects of systemic IFN-γ administration include fever, myalgias, and headache, which occur in 15% to 50% of treated individuals. Although IFN-γ–associated flulike symptoms are typically mild, decrease over time, and can usually be managed with prophylactic antipyretics, these adverse effects are largely avoided when IFN-γ is administered via inhalation for treatment of pulmonary infections.[1,71] Although reversible neutropenia can occur, clinically significant hematologic abnormalities are infrequent, even when patients receive IFN-γ therapy for years.[1,71] Although systemic treatment with IFN-γ has been reported to produce beneficial effects in patients with rheumatoid arthritis and systemic sclerosis, it has been reported to exacerbate multiple sclerosis.[71] Therefore, caution should be exercised when using systemic IFN-γ therapy in patients with noninfectious inflammatory diseases.

OTHER CYTOKINES

Interleukin-1

Clinical interest in IL-1 has focused primarily on strategies to block its proinflammatory activity in rheumatologic diseases, such as rheumatoid arthritis and inflammatory bowel disease, and to dampen its activity in sepsis (see below and Chapter 67).

Interleukin-2

IL-2 plays an important role in the proliferation, differentiation, and activation of lymphocytes, including T cells, B cells, and NK cells.[15] Recombinant human IL-2 was approved by the FDA in 1992 for treatment of metastatic renal cell carcinoma and melanoma and is available under the generic name of aldesleukin. IL-2 has also attracted attention as an investigational immunomodulatory agent for treatment of several infectious diseases. In patients with lepromatous leprosy receiving antimycobacterial agents, low-dose subcutaneous IL-2 (10 μg every 12 hours for 18 days) caused marked erythema at the sites of injection with a subsequent decrease in cutaneous mycobacteria compared with treatment with antimycobacterial agents alone.[91] In another small trial, subcutaneous IL-2 (12.5 μg twice daily for 30 days) was administered to patients with treatment-refractory multidrug-resistant pulmonary tuberculosis. Short-term treatment resulted in increased NK and T-cell numbers and activation, rapid sputum smear conversion to negative, and overall improvement in the appearance of chest radiographs. These effects persisted for at least 4 months after discontinuation of IL-2 therapy.[92] Subsequent studies of short-term IL-2 therapy have reported an overall positive clinical response (decrease in mycobacterial burden in sputum) in approximately 60% of treated patients, but durable cures have yet to be reported.[93]

IL-2 therapy has also been investigated as a treatment modality to enhance CD4+ cell activity and to eliminate latently infected CD4+ reservoirs in HIV-infected individuals.[15,94] Initially IL-2 was administered as a continuous intravenous infusion, which resulted in significant toxicity (fever, myalgias, arthralgias, fatigue, and/or capillary leak syndrome).[95] In an effort to decrease toxicity and optimize therapeutic benefit, alternative formulations and routes of administration of IL-2 in HIV-infected individuals have been examined in a number of subsequent studies. Overall, administration of intermittent subcutaneous IL-2 or intravenous pegylated IL-2 appears to be less effective in increasing CD4+ cell counts than continuous intravenous infusion of nonmodified IL-2. Moreover, the magnitude of the IL-2–induced increase in CD4+ cell counts appears to be decreased in individuals receiving highly active antiretroviral therapy (HAART) compared with non-HAART recipients.[96] More recent trials have been designed to determine the effects of IL-2 therapy, via induction of HIV expression, to eliminate latent reservoirs of infection in CD4+ cells from patients receiving HAART. Although intermittent IL-2 therapy resulted in virtual elimination of replication-competent HIV in resting CD4+ cells or lymph node specimens in some patients, rapid rebound in viral replication was observed following discontinuation of HAART.[97] Currently, IL-2 therapy of HIV-infected patients remains promising but investigational. Based on published experience, administration of intermittent, subcutaneous IL-2 therapy in the ambulatory setting appears to be relatively safe and effective in increasing CD4+ cell counts in HAART recipients to a greater extent than caused by HAART alone. The most promising results have been observed in patients with elevated CD4+ cell counts (>250 cells/μL) and undetectable viremia. Because of the potential for IL-2 to induce transient elevations in HIV viremia, IL-2 therapy should probably be considered only for HIV-infected individuals receiving HAART with undetectable viral loads.[15]

Interleukin-10

Endogenous IL-10 is produced primarily by T cells and acts to suppress functional activity of macrophages. A clinical trial examining administration of multiple subcutaneous doses of recombinant human IL-10 to HIV-infected subjects over a 4-week period failed to demonstrate a beneficial effect on plasma viral load or CD4+ cell counts.[98]

Interleukin-12

IL-12 plays an essential role in the interaction and integration of innate immunity and acquired immunity. Endogenous IL-12 is produced primarily by macrophages, dendritic cells, and B lymphocytes and regulates activation and cytotoxicity of T cells and NK cells.[99] Although initial studies suggested a critical role for IL-12 in defense against infection by a variety of intracellular pathogens, recent evidence indicates that the role of IL-12 in host defense is largely redundant.[100] Nonetheless, considerable interest has been directed toward its potential role in cancer therapeutics and as tumor vaccine adjuvant.[99] IL-12 therapy has also been studied for possible treatment benefit in several infectious diseases. Despite early promising results, immunomodulatory therapy with recombinant human IL-12 for treatment of chronic HBV and HCV infections has not proven to be efficacious and may be associated with serious toxicity, including fulminant liver failure.[101,102] Phase I trials of IL-12 therapy in HIV-infected subjects have not shown positive treatment effects.[103] However, favorable case reports do suggest that use of adjuvant recombinant IL-12 may be beneficial in selected cases of antimicrobial-refractory mycobacterial disease in humans.[104]

IMMUNOGLOBULINS

Commercially available preparations of immunoglobulin (immune globulin) are derived from pooled human blood. Formulations are available for both intravenous use and traditional intramuscular use. Intravenous immune globulin (IGIV) has been used for the treatment of primary and secondary antibody deficiencies for more than 25 years.[105,106] Currently, there are several FDA-licensed "nonspecific," pooled IgG products available in the United States (Table 39-2). A number of other hyperimmune IgG preparations are available for passive immunization against specific infectious diseases. Pooled IGIV products vary in terms of the protocol used to isolate IgG and the additives used for stabilization. However, for most clinical situations they are generally believed to be therapeutically equivalent.[105,106] All are prepared from plasma obtained from at least 1000 donors per lot and contain more than 90% intact IgG with normal ratios of IgG subclasses. In the past, several preparations used in Europe and a single commercial product in the United States were documented to have transmitted non-A, non-B hepatitis or HCV infection.[107] Subsequent to the episodes of IGIV-transmitted infections during 1994 in the United States, viral inactivation procedures have been required in the production of all IGIV products. Moreover, input plasma is now screened by minipool nucleic acid testing (NAT) for HBV, HCV, and HIV to exclude lots contaminated with viral blood-borne pathogens.[108,109]

One of the oldest uses of immunoglobulin therapy is to provide specific antibodies that are lacking in the recipient. Intramuscular IgG has traditionally been used to prevent hepatitis A in travelers, as well as measles in selected patients. Intramuscular hyperimmune (high specific titer) IgG preparations are available for passive prophylaxis and treatment of a number of infectious diseases in selected patients, including hepatitis B, varicella, rabies, and tetanus.[105] IGIV therapy represents the cornerstone of treatment strategies for a number of primary immunodeficiency disorders, including X-linked agammaglobulinemia, severe combined immunodeficiency, hyper-IgM syndrome, Wiskott-Aldrich syndrome, and common variable immunodeficiency (CVID).[106] In a recent study of CVID patients, IGIV therapy was shown to substantially reduce the incidence of pneumonia, a common infectious complication in affected individuals.[110]

Despite normal or even elevated immunoglobulin levels, infants and young children with HIV infection often have depressed antibody infections and an associated increased incidence of bacterial and viral infections. Infants and children with AIDS have been shown to benefit

TABLE 39-2 Licensed Polyclonal, Human Plasma-Derived Intravenous Immune Globulin Products Available in the United States

Product	
Gamimune-N	Polygam S/D
Gammagard S/D	Sandoglobulin
Gammar-P-IV	Venoglobulin
Iveegam	
Panglobulin	

from IGIV therapy in combination with antiretroviral therapy if they have hypogammaglobulinemia (IgG <250 mg/dL) or have experienced two or more serious bacterial infections in the previous year.[105,111] A hyperimmune IGIV product has also been prepared, but it is unclear whether its administration to pregnant HIV-infected women reduced mother-infant HIV transmission compared with treatment with zidovudine alone.[112] In adults, although a randomized open-label trial failed to demonstrate significant clinical benefit in HIV-infected individuals, IGIV is effective for treatment of HIV-related parvovirus B19–associated pure red cell aplasia ("aplastic crisis").[113,114]

Following bone marrow transplantation, IGIV appears not only to provide antibodies for host defense but also play an immunomodulatory role. In a randomized controlled trial of bone marrow transplantation patients, IGIV (500 mg/kg) administered weekly until day 90 then monthly until day 360 post-transplantation decreased the incidence of acute GVHD, cytomegalovirus (CMV) pneumonia, and overall infection. However, no difference in overall mortality or relapse rate was observed.[115] IGIV has also been reported to be effective in preventing infection in chronic lymphocytic leukemia, although the cost effectiveness of its routine use for this indication is controversial.[116]

CMV hyperimmune globulin (CMVIG) was licensed in 1991. Both standard IGIV and CMVIG have been shown to reduce the incidence of CMV disease in patients at risk after both bone marrow transplantation and solid organ transplantation.[117,118] Although expensive and not completely effective in preventing CMV infections, several studies have shown that CMVIG infusions moderately reduce serious CMV disease associated with renal and liver transplantation and improve survival of infected patents.[119,120] Prophylaxis or treatment of CMV disease with the combination of ganciclovir and either CMVIG or standard IGIV appears to only slightly improve clinical outcome compared with treatment with ganciclovir alone.[121,122]

Clinical trials examining the use of IGIV to prevent infections in high-risk postsurgical, trauma, and burn patients have yielded equivocal results.[123,124] In adults, clinical trials evaluating IGIV-based treatment and prophylaxis strategies for bacterial sepsis have also yielded inconsistent results. A recent systematic review concluded that current evidence is inconclusive regarding clinical benefit of adjunctive IGIV therapy for the treatment of sepsis and septic shock, despite the promising results of several small trials.[125] Likewise, clinical trials have failed to demonstrate clear clinical benefit of IGIV therapy for prevention of infections in preterm or low-birth-weight infants.[126,127]

Exotoxins such as streptococcal pyrogenic exotoxin A and toxic shock syndrome toxin-1 play central roles as superantigens in the pathogenesis of the streptococcal and staphylococcal toxic shock syndromes, respectively. In vitro studies demonstrating the ability of pooled immunoglobulin to rapidly neutralize these exotoxins suggest a potential role for IGIV therapy in the management of bacterial toxic shock syndromes (see Chapters 3, 192, and 195).[128] However, conclusive clinical data defining a definitive role for IGIV therapy in either streptococcal or staphylococcal toxic shock syndrome are currently lacking. A recent European randomized, double-blind, placebo-controlled trial investigating IGIV therapy in streptococcal toxic shock syndrome was prematurely terminated because of poor patient enrollment and failed to demonstrate a statistically significant benefit of IGIV therapy.[129] Similarly, conflicting results have been reported when IGIV has been used to treat patients with toxic epidermal necrolysis or Stevens-Johnson syndrome.[130] Despite early optimistic reports, follow-up studies of IGIV therapy for treatment of chronic fatigue syndrome have been inconclusive.[131] In contrast, a regimen of IGIV plus aspirin is now considered the standard of care for treatment of Kawasaki's syndrome (see Chapter 288).[132]

Palivizumab is the first FDA-approved "humanized" mouse monoclonal antibody and has replaced the previous formulation of high-titered human polyclonal respiratory syncytial virus (RSV) IGIV for prevention of RSV pulmonary infections in high-risk patients, especially infants and young children. Rather than reducing RSV infection rates, monthly intramuscular administration of palivizumab (15 mg/kg) results in a significant decrease in RSV infection severity,

manifested as a reduction in hospitalization rate and duration of hospitalization in treated high-risk infants.[133,134] Currently, palivizumab is recommended for RSV prophylaxis for infants and children younger than 2 years old with chronic lung disease who have required medical therapy for chronic lung disease within 6 months of the next anticipated RSV season.[105] Clinical trials are being conducted to determine whether palivizumab may benefit other immunocompromised patient populations, including adult cancer and transplantation patients, who are also at high risk for serious RSV infections.[105]

IGIV is being used increasingly for a variety of infectious and noninfectious disorders, including acute inflammatory disorders, hematologic disorders, autoimmune diseases, and neuroimmunologic disorders. An expert panel has published consensus guidelines for the use of therapeutic IGIV.[135] The recommended dosage of IGIV for prophylactic treatment in primary immunodeficiency syndromes is 100 to 400 mg/kg/month, depending on the preparation used. The dosage can be adjusted according to the resulting clinical response and/or serum level of IgG achieved. For bone marrow transplantation, the recommended dosage is 500 mg/kg given on days 7 and 2 before transplantation and then weekly to day 90 following transplantation. Higher doses of IGIV are often used for acute treatment of autoimmune disease. Adverse effects of IGIV occur in less than 10% of patients and are usually related to the rate of administration. Headache is the most common adverse effect. Other relatively common side effects include myalgias, arthralgias, fatigue, and malaise. Transient acute renal insufficiency can occur. Because of the risk of anaphylaxis due to the possible presence of anti-IgA antibodies, IGIV is contraindicated in individuals with selective IgA deficiency. Rarely, administration of IGIV is associated with hypotension, fever, diaphoresis, and chest tightness, especially when the recommended rate of infusion is exceeded and in primary immunodeficiency patients who have not received previous IGIV infusion or who have not received an infusion within the preceding 8 weeks. Aseptic meningitis has been reported primarily in patients receiving high doses of IGIV for treatment of autoimmune disease.

GLUCOCORTICOSTEROIDS

Glucocorticosteroids have prominent anti-inflammatory effects on a variety of cells involved in the inflammatory response and are potent inhibitors of the host immune response. When used for management of infectious diseases, glucocorticosteroids are often employed to contain an overactive immune response that is contributing to the pathology of an infection. Examples of infectious diseases in which glucocorticosteroid therapy has proven to be beneficial to overall clinical outcome when combined with effective antimicrobial therapy include pneumonia due to *Pneumocystis jirovecii* (formerly *P. carinii*; PCP) in HIV-infected individuals and tuberculosis. In HIV-infected individuals with PCP and moderate-severe hypoxia (arterial Po_2 <70 mm Hg), clinical studies have conclusively demonstrated that initiation of glucocorticosteroid therapy within 72 hours of initiation of antibiotics significantly increases arterial oxygenation and decreases the incidence of respiratory failure and mortality (see Chapters 118, 125, and 268).[136,137] The recommended regimen for adjunctive treatment of PCP is oral prednisone, 40 mg twice daily for 5 days, then 40 mg once daily for 5 days, then 20 mg once daily for 11 days. Intravenous methylprednisolone can be substituted for oral prednisone if an individual is unable to take oral medications.

Complications of tuberculosis are often included as indications for adjunctive glucocorticosteroid therapy. Moreover, patients with tuberculosis occasionally experience unusual paradoxical reactions during the course of appropriate antimycobacterial therapy, often resulting in transient worsening of existing lesions or development of new lesions.[138] Tuberculous meningitis is typically a basilar meningitis associated with considerable inflammation and a consequent risk for hydrocephalus. An open-label prospective study was performed in Egypt investigating adjunctive steroid use in patients with tuberculous meningitis treated with intramuscular isoniazid, ethambutol, and streptomycin. Adjunctive dexamethsone therapy decreased overall morbidity and mortality.[139] One recommended regimen for patients with tuberculous meningitis complicated by increased intracranial pressure, focal neurologic deficits, or altered mental status is prednisone at a dose of 60 mg daily for 1 to 2 weeks, followed by tapered dosing over the subsequent 4 to 6 weeks.[140] No data are currently available on the use of adjunctive glucocorticosteroid therapy in HIV-infected individuals with tuberculous meningitis.[141] Relatively small clinical trials suggest that adjunctive glucocorticosteroid therapy may reduce morbidity and mortality in tuberculous pericarditis (see Chapters 77 and 248) and tuberculous peritonitis, in both HIV-negative and HIV-positive individuals.[142,143] Similar evidence suggests a potential role for adjunctive steroid therapy in the management of inflammatory complications of pulmonary tuberculosis, including tuberculous pleurisy and pleural effusion (see Chapters 62 and 248).[144,145]

Glucocorticosteroids were the first immunomodulatory agents studied in patients with sepsis. Although randomized clinical trials have clearly shown that a short course of high-dose glucocorticosteroid therapy is ineffective, and potentially deleterious, in patients with severe sepsis, recent evidence suggests that low-dose steroid therapy may be beneficial in patients with catecholamine-dependent septic shock and relative adrenal insufficiency. In a placebo-controlled, randomized double-blind trial performed in 19 intensive care units in France involving 300 adult patients with septic shock, a 7-day course of low-dose hydrocortisone (50 mg intravenously every 6 hours) and fludrocortisone (50 µg orally once daily) significantly reduced the risk of death in patients with relative adrenal insufficiency, defined as less than a 9-µg/mL increase in serum cortisol in response to a cosyntropin-stimulation test. Specifically, steroid treatment decreased 28-day mortality in patients with documented adrenal insufficiency by 10% and decreased the requirement for vasopressor therapy.[146] An exception to the general proscription against high-dose steroid therapy for treatment of septic shock may be typhoid fever, in which mortality was reduced approximately 50% by high-dose dexamethasone treatment (3 mg/kg followed by 1 mg/kg every 6 hours for eight doses) of seriously ill patients in a randomized, double-blind, placebo-controlled trial conducted in Indonesia.[147]

Short courses of high-dose glucocorticosteroid therapy have also been shown to be ineffective, and possibly harmful, in clinical trials to prevent development of acute respiratory distress syndrome (ARDS) in patients with severe sepsis or in patients with established ARDS.[148,149] However, case reports and one relatively small, randomized, placebo-controlled trial suggest a beneficial effect of prolonged glucocorticosteroid therapy in late ARDS.[150] The beneficial effect is presumed to result from inhibition of a fibroproliferative response in the late stages of ARDS.[148] To further investigate the potential therapeutic role of steroid therapy in late ARDS, a National Institutes of Health (NIH)–sponsored multicenter trial is being conducted under the auspices of the National Heart, Lung, and Blood Institute (NHLBI) ARDS clinical trials network, examining treatment with intravenous methylprednisolone (2 mg/kg bolus followed by 2 mg/kg/day in divided doses) for patients with nonresolving ARDS at days 7 through 28 following ARDS onset.[148]

In 1988, a pivotal study was reported in which adjunctive dexamethasone treatment of infants and children with bacterial meningitis significantly decreased sensorineural hearing loss in those subjects with meningitis caused by Haemophilus influenzae.[151] The benefits of adjunctive steroid therapy in pediatric meningitis caused by other pathogens and in adults with bacterial meningitis have been less straightforward (see Chapter 80). Subsequent clinical trials of adjunctive dexamethasone for bacterial meningitis in children and adults have produced conflicting results.[152] In 2002, a prospective, randomized, double-blind multicenter trial of adjunctive dexamethasone for treatment of adults with bacterial meningitis was reported. The results showed that early treatment with dexamethasone (10 mg administered 15-20 minutes before or with the first dose of antibiotics, followed by 10 mg every 6 hours for 4 days) reduced mortality, improved overall clinical outcome, and did not increase gastrointestinal bleeding in adults with acute

bacterial meningitis. The benefits of steroid therapy were most pronounced in patients with pneumococcal meningitis.[153] Based on available evidence, it is now recommended that adjunctive dexamethasone be given, with or immediately following the first dose of antimicrobials, to most adults with suspected pneumococcal meningitis. If the causative pathogen is found not to be Streptococcus pneumoniae, then discontinuation of dexamethasone therapy is advised.[154] It should also be noted that glucocorticosteroid therapy remains the treatment of choice for eosinophilic meningitis caused by infections with helminths, principally Angiostrongylus cantonensis and Gnathostoma spinigerum.[155] In contrast, glucocorticosteroid therapy has been shown to worsen clinical outcome and is contraindicated for treatment of cerebral malaria.[156]

Soon after initiation of HAART for treatment of HIV infection, some patients experience paradoxical clinical deterioration due to restoration of proinflammatory immune responses against preexisting infectious and noninfectious antigens. This phenomenon is generally referred to as the "immune reconstitution syndrome."[157] Case reports suggest that systemic glucocorticosteroid therapy can be helpful in suppressing the inflammatory manifestations of the immune reconstitution syndrome.[158] Although the potential deleterious effects of immunosuppressive glucocorticosteroid therapy during ongoing HIV infection is a concern, a recent study reported no significant adverse outcomes caused by short-term therapy in advanced HIV infection.[158]

ANTI-INFLAMMATORY THERAPEUTIC APPROACHES FOR THE TREATMENT OF SEPSIS

Over the past two decades, more than 30 double-blind, placebo-controlled, multicenter, phase II or III trials have been performed to investigate experimental therapeutic agents for the treatment of sepsis and septic shock.[158,159] Approaches that have ultimately failed to demonstrate convincing evidence of clinical efficacy include endotoxin neutralization agents,[161,162] anti-TNF strategies,[163,164] recombinant IL-1 receptor antagonist,[165] platelet activating factor (PAF) antagonists,[166] bradykinin antagonist (deltibant),[167] antithrombin III,[168] and recombinant tissue factor pathway inhibitor (tifacogin).[169] Recombinant human APC (drotrecogin alfa [activated]) is the first immunomodulatory agent that has proved effective for the treatment of severe sepsis, including septic shock. In the landmark PROWESS trial, administration of APC to patients with sepsis resulted in a statistically significant 6.1% absolute decrease in 28-day mortality (i.e., 19.4% reduction in relative risk of death).[170] The efficacy of APC in treatment of sepsis has been attributed to its combined anti-inflammatory and anticoagulant activities.[171] However, critics have questioned its generalized use for the treatment of sepsis based on concerns regarding safety, cost-effectiveness, and long-term outcomes in treated patients.[172-174] It should also be noted that recombinant bactericidal/permeability-increasing protein has shown promise as a clinically useful immunomodulatory agent in a study of children with meningococcal sepsis.[175] The pathophysiology and management of sepsis are discussed in more detail in Chapter 67.

OTHER IMMUNOMODULATORY AGENTS

Imiquimod is a heterocyclic amine that stimulates production of IFN-α and other cytokines. It is available as a 5% cream (Aldara) and approved for topical treatment of external genital and perianal condyloma acuminatum. Multicenter, double-blind, vehicle-controlled trials have demonstrated topical imiquimod effectively clears warts in both immunocompetent and HIV-infected individuals.[177] As with other treatments for warts, recurrences are relatively common. Localized erythema, erosion, and/or flaking occurs in up to 60% of patients, but only 1% of patients discontinue use of imiquimod cream because of adverse effects. Imiquimod cream should be applied to warts three times per week, allowed to remain for 6 to 10 hours before washing off, for a maximum of 16 weeks. Case reports suggest that imiquimod cream may be effective for treatment of refractory warts at other anatomic sites and molluscum contagiosum.[177]

Pentoxifylline and a related compound, lisofylline, are methylxanthine derivatives that have been shown to inhibit production of TNF by monocytes in vitro and to inhibit the effects of TNF and other proinflammatory cytokines on neutrophil activation. Although pentoxifylline demonstrated efficacy in a murine model of malaria, it has been shown to be ineffective in the treatment of severe falciparum malaria.[178] Despite early promising reports, intravenous pentoxifylline failed to prevent transplant-related morbidity (i.e., mucositis, hepatic failure, or renal failure) or mortality in allogeneic bone marrow transplant recipients.[179] In a randomized, double-blind trial comparing pentoxifylline versus placebo in 140 patients with cadaveric kidney grafts receiving cyclosporine and prednisone, pentoxifylline was shown to decrease allograft rejection, possibly as a result of downregulation of TNF production.[180] Pentoxifylline has been evaluated for the treatment of sepsis. In a prospective, controlled trial involving 51 adult patients with severe sepsis, intravenous pentoxifylline improved cardiopulmonary dysfunction but did not change mortality.[181] In premature infants with sepsis, a randomized, double-blind, placebo-controlled trial reported that pentoxifylline significantly reduced both mortality and proinflammatory cytokine production.[182] Pentoxifylline has also been evaluated as a potential immunomodulator in patients with HIV infection and in the treatment of erythema nodosum leprosum.[183,184] Treatment with lisofylline was reported to reduce the incidence of infections and improve 100-day survival in a multicenter, randomized, placebo-controlled trial of 60 patients receiving related-donor bone marrow transplantation.[185] However, lisofylline failed to decrease mortality when used for early treatment of acute lung injury and ARDS in a prospective, randomized, double-blind, placebo-controlled multicenter study of 235 patients.[186]

Thalidomide functions as an immunomodulator via selective inhibition of TNF-α production by monocytes/macrophages.[187] It is well established as an effective treatment for erythema nodosum leprosum, an inflammatory process that can occur in patients being treated for lepromatous leprosy.[187] Thalidomide has also been shown to be effective in the treatment of HIV-associated wasting syndrome, as well as HIV-associated aphthous ulcers and idiopathic esophageal ulcers.[188-190] Thalidomide has also shown promise as an antiangiogenic factor for the treatment of HIV-related Kaposi's sarcoma.[191] The most common adverse effects of short-term thalidomide therapy are sedation (24%-79% of patients) and rash. Other adverse effects include constipation and dry mouth. Peripheral neuropathy is a relatively common adverse effect associated with long-term use of thalidomide. The severe teratogenicity of thalidomide is well known. Both male and female patients must use barrier contraceptive methods. In the United States, thalidomide is available only through pharmacists participating in System for Thalidomide Education and Prescribing Safety (STEPS).

Thymosin-α$_1$ is a 28-amino acid protein member of a group of peptides produced by the thymus, which exerts effects on the neuroendocrine and immune systems. It has been sequenced and synthesized and found to induce expression of the cytokines IL-1, IL-2, IFN-α, and IFN-γ. Thymosin-α$_1$ has been investigated predominantly for immunomodulatory treatment of chronic HBV infection and chronic HCV infection. Despite early observations suggesting treatment efficacy, subsequent clinical studies have failed to validate thymosin-α$_1$ as effective monotherapy for chronic HBV infection.[192] Preliminary studies suggest possible utility as an adjunct immunomodulator in the treatment of HBV when combined with either interferon-alfa-2b or famciclovir.[193,194] Limited success has been reported in preliminary trials investigating combination therapy with thymosin-α$_1$ plus INF-α for the treatment of chronic HCV infection.[195] Although the combination of thymosin-α$_1$ and pegylated IL-2 was well tolerated in a small study of 12 patients with HIV infection, thymosin-α$_1$ did not increase the CD4+ count beyond that produced by pegylated IL-2 alone.[196]

PGG-glucan (poly-[1-6]-βD-glucopyranosyl-[1-3]-β-D-glucopyranose; Betafectin) is an immunomodulatory agent derived from yeast cell walls, which promotes phagocytosis and intracellular killing of bacteria by phagocytes and has been shown to improve wound healing and improve mortality from experimental peritonitis in animal models. In a multicenter, prospective, randomized, double-blind, placebo-controlled phase III trial of 1249 high-risk surgical patients undergoing colorectal or noncolorectal surgery, perioperative administration of PGG-glucan reduced serious postoperative infections or death by 39% in patients undergoing noncolorectal surgery.[197]

INFECTION RISK ASSOCIATED WITH ANTICYTOKINE THERAPY

Cytokines play critical roles in the regulation of host defense against infection. Thus it is not surprising that infectious risk may be increased in individuals receiving anticytokine therapy. Increasing numbers of patients are being treated with anti-TNF therapy (e.g., infliximab and etanercept) for rheumatoid arthritis, Crohn's disease, and other chronic inflammatory diseases. Anti-TNF treatment appears to increase the risk for development of serious infections, especially tuberculosis. Active tuberculosis should be treated appropriately before initiation of an anti-TNF agent, and treatment of latent tuberculosis should be strongly considered for individuals with a positive tuberculin skin test who are receiving anti-TNF therapy.[198]

REFERENCES

1. Hubel K, Dale DC, Liles WC. Therapeutic use of cytokines to modulate phagocyte function for the treatment of infectious diseases: Current status of granulocyte colony-stimulating factor, granulocyte-macrophage colony-stimulating factor, macrophage colony-stimulating factor, and interferon-γ. J Infect Dis. 2002;185:1490-1501.
2. Nagata S, Tsuchiya M, Asano S, et al. Molecular cloning and expression of cDNA for human granulocyte colony-stimulating factor. Nature. 1986;319:415-418.
3. Souza LM, Boone TC, Grabilove J, et al. Recombinant human granulocyte colony-stimulating factor: Effects on normal and leukemic myeloid cells. Science. 1986;232:61-65.
4. Lieschke GJ, Grail D, Hodgson G, et al. Mice lacking granulocyte colony-stimulating factor have chronic neutropenia, granulocyte and macrophage progenitor cell deficiency, and impaired neutrophil mobilization. Blood. 1994;84:1737-1746.
5. Welte K, Gabrilove J, Bronchud MH, et al. Filgrastim (r-metHuG-CSF): The first 10 years. Blood 1996;88:1907-1929.
6. Dale DC, Cottle TE, Flier CJ, et al. Severe chronic neutropenia: Treatment and follow-up of patients in the Severe Chronic Neutropenia International Registry. Am J Hematol. 2003;72:82-93.
7. Dror Y, Ward AC, Touw IP, Freedman EJ. Combined corticosteroid/granulocyte colony-stimulating factor (G-CSF) therapy in the treatment of severe congenital neutropenia unresponsive to G-CSF: Activated glucocorticoid receptors synergize with G-CSF signals. Exp Hematol. 2000;28:1381-1389.
8. American Society of Clinical Oncology. Update of recommendations for the use of hematopoietic colony-stimulating factors: Evidence-based, clinical practice guidelines. J Clin Oncol. 1996;14:1957-1960.
9. Masaoka T, Takaku F, Kato S, et al. Recombinant human granulocyte colony-stimulating factor in allogeneic bone marrow transplantation. Exp Hematol. 1989;17:1047-1050.
10. Sheridan WP, Morstyn G, Wolf M, et al. Granulocyte colony-stimulating factor and neutrophil recovery after high-dose chemotherapy and autologous bone marrow transplantation. Lancet. 1989;2:891-895.
11. Souetre E, Qing W, Penelaud PF. Economic analysis of the use of recombinant human granulocyte colony-stimulating factor in autologous bone marrow transplantation. Eur J Cancer. 1996;32A:1162-1165.
12. Maher DW, Lieschke GJ, Green M, et al. Filgrastim in patients with chemotherapy-induced febrile neutropenia: A double-blind, placebo-controlled trial. Ann Intern Med. 1994;121:492-501.
13. Garcia-Carbonero R, Mayordomo JI, Tornamira MV, et al. Granulocyte colony-stimulating factor in the treatment of high-risk febrile neutropenia: A multicenter randomized trial. J Natl Cancer Inst. 2001;93:31-38.
14. Kuritzkes DR. Neutropenia, neutrophil dysfunction, and bacterial infection in patients with human immunodeficiency virus disease: The role of granulocyte colony-stimulating factor. Clin Infect Dis. 2000;30:256-260.
15. Armstrong WS, Kazanjian P. Use of cytokines in human immunodeficiency virus-infected patients: Colony-stimulating factors, erythropoietin, and interleukin-2. Clin Infect Dis. 2001;32:766-773.
16. Hermans P, Rozenbaum W, Moreno J, et al. Filgrastim to treat neutropenia and support myelosuppressive medication dosing in HIV infection. AIDS. 1996;10:1627-1633.
17. Manders SM, Kostman JR, Mendez L, et al. Thalidomide-resistant HIV-associated aphthae successfully treated with granulocyte colony-stimulating factor. J Am Acad Dermatol. 1995;33:380-382.
18. Nelson S, Belknap SM, Carlson RW, et al. A randomized controlled trial of filgrastim as an adjunct to antibiotics for treatment of hospitalized patients with community-acquired pneumonia. CAP study group. J Infect Dis. 1998;178:1075-1080.
19. Nelson S, Heyder AM, Stone J, et al. A randomized controlled trial of filgrastim for the treatment of hospitalized patients with multilobar pneumonia. J Infect Dis. 2000;182:970-973.
20. Wunderink R, Leeper K, Schein R, et al. Filgrastim in patients with pneumonia and severe sepsis or septic shock. Chest. 2001;119:523-529.

21. Root RK, Lodato RF, Patrick W, et al. Multicenter, double-blind, placebo-controlled study of filgrastim in patients hospitalized with pneumonia and severe sepsis. Crit Care Med. 2003;31:367-373.
22. Gough A, Claperton M, Rolando N, et al. Randomized placebo-controlled trial of granulocyte colony-stimulating factor in diabetic foot infection. Lancet. 1997;182:970-973.
23. Foster PF, Mital D, Sankary HN, et al. The use of granulocyte colony-stimulating factor after liver transplantation. Transplantation. 1995;59:1557-1563.
24. Heard SO, Fink MP, Gamelli RL, et al. Effect of prophylactic administration of recombinant human granulocyte colony-stimulating factor (filgrastim) on the frequency of nosocomial infections in patients with acute traumatic brain injury or cerebral hemorrhage. Crit Care Med. 1998;26:748-754.
25. Schafer H, Hubel K, Bohlen H, et al. Perioperative treatment with granulocyte colony-stimulating factor (G-CSF) in patients with esophageal cancer stimulates granulocyte function and reduces infectious complications after esophagectomy. Ann Hematol. 2000;79:143-151.
26. Gaviria JM, Grohskopf LA, Barnes R, Root RK. Successful treatment of rhinocerebral zygomycosis: A combined strategy approach. Clin Infect Dis. 1999;28:160-161.
27. Hubel K, Dale DC, Engert A, Liles WC. Current status of granulocyte (neutrophil) transfusion therapy for infectious diseases. J Infect Dis. 2001;183:321-328.
28. Hilbe W, Nussbaumer W, Bonatti H, et al. Unusual adverse events following peripheral blood stem cell (PBSC) mobilisation using granulocyte colony stimulating factor (G-CSF) in healthy donors. Bone Marrow Transplant. 2000;26:811-813.
29. Freedman MH, Bonilla MA, Fier C, et al. Myelodysplasia syndrome and acute myeloid leukemia in patients with congenital neutropenia receiving G-CSF therapy. Blood. 2000;96:429-436.
30. Dranoff G, Crawford AD, Sadelain M, et al. Involvement of granulocyte-macrophage colony-stimulating factor in pulmonary hemostasis. Science. 1994;264:713-716.
31. Nemunaitis J, Rabinowe SN, Singer JW, et al. Recombinant granulocyte-macrophage colony-stimulating factor after autologous bone marrow transplant for lymphoid cancer. N Engl J Med. 1991;324:1173-1178.
32. Nemunaitis J, Rosenfeld C, Ash R, et al. Phase III randomized, double-blind, placebo-controlled trial of rhGM-CSF following allogeneic bone marrow transplantation. Bone Marrow Transplant. 1995;15:949-954.
33. Rowe JM, Aandersen JW, Mazza JJ, et al. A randomized placebo controlled phase III study of granulocyte-macrophage colony-stimulating factor in adult patients (>55 to 70 years of age) with acute myelogenous leukemia: A study of the Eastern Cooperative Oncology Group (E1490). Blood. 1995;86:457-462.
34. Stone RM, Berg DT, George SL, et al. Granulocyte-macrophage colony-stimulating factor after initial chemotherapy for elderly patients with primary acute myelogenous leukemia. N Engl J Med. 1995;332:1671-1677.
35. Antman KS, Griffin JD, Elias A, et al. Effect of recombinant human granulocyte-macrophage colony-stimulating factor on chemotherapy-induced myelosuppression. N Engl J Med. 1988;319:593-598.
36. Anaissie EJ, Vartivarian S, Bodey GP, et al. Randomized comparison between antibiotics alone and antibiotics plus granulocyte-macrophage colony-stimulating factor (Escherichia coli-derived) in cancer patients with fever and neutropenia. Am J Med. 1996;100:17-23.
37. Bodey GP, Anaissie E, Gutterman J, Vadhan-Raj S. Role of granulocyte-macrophage colony-stimulating factor as adjuvant treatment in neutropenic patients with bacterial and fungal infections. Eur J Clin Microbiol Infect Dis. 1994;13(Suppl 2):S18-S22.
38. Peters BG, Adkins DR, Harrsion BR, et al. Antifungal effects of yeast-derived rhu-GM-CSF in patients receiving high-dose chemotherapy given with or without autologous stem cell transplantation: A retrospective analysis. Bone Marrow Transplant. 1996;18:93-102.
39. Angel JB, High K, Rhame F, et al. Phase III study of granulocyte-macrophage colony-stimulating factor in advanced HIV disease: Effect on infections, CD4 counts and HIV suppression. AIDS. 2000;14:387-395.
40. Scadden DT, Pickus O, Hammer SM, et al. Lack of in vivo effect of granulocyte-macrophage colony-stimulating factor on human immunodeficiency virus type 1. AIDS Res Hum Retroviruses. 1996;12:1151-1159.
41. Kedzierska K, Mak J, Mijch A, et al. Granulocyte-macrophage colony-stimulating factor augments phagocytosis of Mycobacterium avium complex by human immunodeficiency virus type 1-infected monocytes/macrophages in vitro and in vivo. J Infect Dis. 2000;181:390-394
42. Price D, Klein J, Fisher M, et al. Potential role for granulocyte-macrophage colony-stimulating factor in the treatment of HIV-associated cryptococcal meningitis. AIDS. 1997;11:693-694.
43. Vasquez JA, Gupta S, Villanueva A. Potential utility of recombinant human GM-CSF as adjunctive treatment of refractory oropharyngeal candidiasis in AIDS patients. Eur J Clin Microbiol Infect Dis. 1998;17:781-783.
44. Lieschke GJ, Cebon J, Mortsyn G. Characterization of the clinical effects after the first dose of bacterially synthesized recombinant granulocyte-macrophage colony-stimulating factor. Blood. 1989;74:2634-2643.
45. Nemunaitis J. Use of macrophage colony-stimulating factor in the treatment of fungal infections. Clin Infect Dis. 1998;26:1279-1281.
46. Nemunaitis J, Meyers JD, Buckner CD, et al. Phase I trial of recombinant macrophage colony-stimulating factor (rhM-CSF) in patients with invasive fungal infections. Blood. 1991;78:907-913.
47. Nemunaitis J, Dorcy KS, Appelbaum FR, et al. Long-term follow-up of patients with invasive fungal disease who received adjunctive therapy with recombinant human macrophage colony-stimulating factor. Blood. 1993;82:1422-1427.
48. National Institutes of Health Consensus Development Conference Statement: Management of hepatitis C: June 10-12, 2002. Hepatology. 2002;36:S3-S20.
49. Flamm SL. Chronic hepatitis C virus infection. JAMA. 2003;289:2413-2417.
50. Manns MP, McHutchinson JG, Gordon SC, et al. Peginterferon alfa-2b plus ribavirin compared with interferon alfa-2b for initial treatment of chronic hepatitis C: A randomized trial. Lancet. 2001;358:958-965.
51. Fried MW, Shiffman ML, Reddy RK, et al. Peginterferon alfa-2a plus ribavirin for chronic hepatitis C infection. N Engl J Med. 2002;347:975-982.
52. Jaeckel E, Cornberg M, Wedemeyer H, et al. Treatment of acute hepatitis C with interferon alfa-2b. N Engl J Med. 2001;345:1452-1457.
53. Poynard T, Regimbeau C, Myers RP, et al. Interferon for acute hepatitis C. Cochrane Database Syst Rev. 2002;(1):CD000369.
54. Lok AS, Heathcote EJ, Hoofnagle JH. Management of hepatitis B 2000, summary of a workshop. Gastroenterology. 2001;120:1828-1853.
55. Wong DK, Cheung AM, O'Rourke K, et al. Effect of alpha-interferon treatment in patients with hepatitis B e antigen-positive chronic hepatitis B. A meta-analysis. Ann Intern Med. 1993;119:312-323.
56. Lau DY, Everhart J, Kleiner DE, et al. Long-term follow-up of patients with chronic hepatitis treated with interferon α. Gastroenterology. 1997;113:1660-1667.
57. Niederau C, Heintges T, Lange S, et al. Long-term follow-up of HBeAg-positive patients treated with interferon alfa for chronic hepatitis B. N Engl J Med. 1996;334:1422-1427.
58. Mellerup MT, Krogsgaard K, Mathurin P, et al. Sequential combination of glucocorticosteroids and alfa interferon versus alfa interferon alone for HBeAg-positive chronic hepatitis B. Cochrane Database Syst Rev. 2002;(2):CD000345.
59. Janssen HL, Gerken G, Carreno V, et al. Interferon alfa for chronic hepatitis B infection: Increased efficacy of prolonged treatment. The European Concerted Action on Viral Hepatitis (EUROHEP). Hepatology. 1999;30:238-243.
60. Schalm SW, Heathcote J, Cianciara J, et al. Lamivudine and alpha interferon combination treatment of patients with chronic hepatitis B infection: A randomized trial. Gut. 2000;46:562-568.
61. Papatheodoridis GV, Manesis E, Hadziyannis SJ. The long-term outcome of interferon-alpha treated and untreated patients with HBeAg-negative chronic hepatitis B. J Hepatol. 2001;34:306-313.
62. Reichman RC, Oakes D, Bonnez W, et al. Treatment of condyloma acuminatum with three different alpha interferon preparations administered parenterally: A double-blind, placebo-controlled trial. J Infect Dis. 1990;162:1270-1276.
63. Leventhal BG, Kashima HK, Mounts P, et al. Long-term response of recurrent respiratory papillomatosis to treatment with lymphoblastoid interferon α-n1. N Engl J Med. 1991;325:613-617.
64. Hayden FG, Albrecht JK, Kaiser DL, et al. Prevention of natural colds by contact prophylaxis with intranasal alpha 2-interferon. N Engl J Med. 1986;314:71-75.
65. Douglas RM, Moore BW, Miles HB, et al. Prophylactic efficacy of intranasal alpha 2 interferon against rhinovirus infections in the family setting. N Engl J Med. 1986;314:65-70.
66. Birch CJ, Tyssen DP, Tachedjian G, et al. Clinical effects and in vitro studies of trifluorothymidine combined with interferon-alpha for treatment of drug-resistant and sensitive herpes simplex virus infections. J Infect Dis. 1992;166:108-112.
67. Borrego L, Castro I, Adela F, et al. Treatment of acyclovir-resistant perianal herpetic ulceration with intramuscular interferon alfa. Arch Dermatol. 1996;132:1157-1158.
68. Schnittman SM, Vogel S, Baseler M, et al. A phase I study of interferon-α2b in combination with interleukin-2 in patients with human immunodeficiency virus infection. J Infect Dis. 1994;169:981-989.
69. Giosue S, Casarini M, Alemanno L, et al. Effects of aerosolized interferon-alpha in patients with pulmonary tuberculosis. Am J Resp Crit Care Med. 1998;158:1156-1162.
70. Palmero D, Eiguchi K, Rendo P, et al. Phase II trial of recombinant interferon-alpha2 in patients with advanced intractable multidrug-resistant pulmonary tuberculosis: Long-term follow-up. Int J Tuberc Lung Dis. 1999;3:214-218.
71. Gallin JL, Farber JM, Holland SM, Nutman TB. Interferon-gamma in the management of infectious diseases. Ann Intern Med. 1995;123:216-224.
72. Dalton DK, Pitts-Meek S, Keshav S, et al. Multiple defects of immune cell function in mice with disrupted gamma-interferon genes. Science. 1993;259:1739-1743.
73. Huang S, Hendricks W, Althage A, et al. Immune response in mice that lack the interferon-gamma receptor. Science. 1993;259:1743-1745.
74. Altare F, Durandy A, Lammas D, et al. Impairment of mycobacterial immunity in human interleukin-12 receptor deficiency. Science. 1998;280:1432-1435.
75. De Jong R, Altare F, Haagen I-A, et al. Severe mycobacterial and Salmonella infections in interleukin-12 receptor-deficient patients. Science. 1998;280:1435-1438.
76. Gallin JI, Malech HL, Melnick DA, et al. A controlled trial of interferon-gamma to prevent infection in chronic granulomatous disease. The International Chronic Granulomatous Disease Cooperative Study Group. N Engl J Med. 1991;324:509-516.
77. Bemiller LS, Roberts DH, Starko KM, Curnutte JT. Safety and effectiveness of long-term interferon-gamma therapy in patients with chronic granulomatous disease. Blood Cells Mol Dis. 1995;21:239-247.
78. Grimbacher B, Holland SM, Gallin JI, et al. Hyper IgE syndrome with recurrent infections—An autosomal dominant multisystem disorder. N Engl J Med. 1999;340:692-702.
79. Borges WG, Augustine NH, Hill HR. Defective interleukin-12/interferon-gamma pathway in patients with hyperimmunoglobulinemia E syndrome. J Pediatr. 2000;136:176-180.
80. Jeppson JD, Jaffe HS, Hill HR. Use of recombinant human interferon-gamma to enhance neutrophil chemotactic responses in Job syndrome of hyper-immunoglobulin E and recurrent infections. J Pediatr. 1991;118:606-614.
81. Holland SM. Immunotherapy of mycobacterial infections. Adv Intern Med. 2000;45:431-452.
82. Badaro R, Falcoff E, Badaro FS, et al. Treatment of visceral leishmaniasis with pentavalent antimony and interferon-gamma. N Engl J Med. 1990;322:16-21.

83. Arana BA, Navim TR, Arana FE, et al. Efficacy of a short course (10 days) of high-dose meglumine antimonate with or without interferon-γ in treating cutaneous leishmaniasis in Guatemala. Clin Infect Dis. 1994;18:381-384.

84. Kaplan G. Recent advances in cytokine therapy in leprosy. J Infect Dis. 1993;17(Suppl 1):S18-S22.

85. Squires KE, Brown ST, Armstron D, et al. interferon-gamma treatment for *Mycobacterium avium-intracellulare* complex bacillemia in patients with AIDS. J Infect Dis. 1992;166:686-687.

86. Holland SM, Eisenstein E, Kuhns DB, et al. Treatment of refractory disseminated nontuberculous mycobacterial infection with interferon-gamma. N Engl J Med. 1994;330:1348-1355.

87. Condos R, Rom WN, Schluger NW. Treatment of multidrug-resistant pulmonary tuberculosis with interferon-gamma via aerosol. Lancet. 1997;349:1513-1515.

88. Chatte G, Panteux G, Perrin-Fayolle M, Pacheco Y. Aerosolized interferon-gamma for *Mycobacterium avium*-complex lung disease. Am J Respir Crit Care Med. 1995;152:1094-1096.

89. Dries DJ, Jurkovich GJ, Maier RV, et al. Effect of interferon gamma on infection-related death in patients with severe injuries: A randomized, double-blind, placebo-controlled trial. Arch Surg. 1994;129:1031-1041.

90. Wasserman D, Ioannovich JD, Hinzmann RD, et al. Interferon-gamma in the prevention of severe burn-related infections: A European phase III multicenter trial. Crit Care Med. 1998;26:434-439.

91. Kaplan G, Britton WJ, Hancock GE, et al. The systemic influence of recombinant interleukin 2 on the manifestations of lepromatous leprosy. J Exp Med. 1991;173:l993-1006.

92. Johnson BJ, Ress SR, Wilcox P, et al. Clinical and immune responses of tuberculosis patients treated with low-dose IL-2 and multidrug therapy. Cytokines Cell Mol Ther. 1995;1:185-196.

93. Johnson B, Bekker LG, Ress S, Kaplan G. Recombinant interleukin 2 adjunctive therapy in multidrug-resistant tuberculosis. Novartis Found Symp. 1998;217:99-106.

94. De Paoli P. Immunological effects of interleukin-2 therapy in human immunodeficiency virus-positive subjects. Clin Diag Lab Immunol. 2001;8:671-677.

95. Kovacs JA, Vogel S, Albert JM, et al. Controlled trial of interleukin-2 infusions in patients infected with the human immunodeficiency virus. N Engl J Med. 1996;335:1350-1356.

96. Losso MH, Belloso WH, Emery S, et al. A randomized, controlled, phase II trial comparing escalating doses of subcutaneous interleukin-2 plus antiretrovirals versus antiretrovirals alone in human immunodeficiency virus-infected patients with CD4+ cell counts >350/mm³. J Infect Dis. 2000;181:1614-1621.

97. Chun T, Davey RJ, Ostrowski M, et al. Relationship between preexisting viral reservoirs and the re-emergence of plasma viremia after discontinuation of highly active anti-retroviral therapy. Nat Med. 2000;6:757-761.

98. Angel JB, Jacobson MA, Skolnik, et al. A multicenter, randomized, double-blind, placebo-controlled trial of recombinant human interleukin-10 in HIV-infected subjects. AIDS. 2000;14:2503-2508.

99. Colombo MP, Trinchieri G. Interleukin-12 in anti-tumor immunity and immunotherapy. Cytokine Growth Fact Rev. 2002;13:155-158.

100. Fieschi C, Dupuis S, Catherinot E, et al. Low penetrance, broad resistance, and favorable outcome of interleukin 12 receptor beta1 deficiency: Medical and immunological implications. J Exp Med. 2003;197:527-535.

101. Zeuzem S, Carreno V. Interleukin-12 in the treatment of chronic hepatitis B and C. Antiviral Res. 2001;52:181-188.

102. Pockros PJ, Patel K, O'Brien C, et al. A multicenter study of recombinant human interleukin 12 for the treatment of chronic hepatitis C virus infection in patients nonresponsive to previous therapy. Hepatology. 2003;37:1368-1374.

103. Jacobson MA, Spritzler J, Landay A, et al. A phase I, placebo-controlled trial of multi-dose recombinant human interleukin-12 in patients with HIV infection. AIDS. 2002;16:1147-1154.

104. Greinert U, Ernst M, Schlaak M, Entzian P. Interleukin-12 as successful adjuvant in tuberculosis treatment. Eur Respir J. 2001;17:1049-1051.

105. Hemming VG. Use of intravenous immunoglobulins for prophylaxis or treatment of infectious diseases. Clin Diag Lab Immunol. 2001;8:859-863.

106. Bonilla FA, Geha RS. Immunologic disorders 12. Primary immunodeficiency diseases. J Allergy Clin Immunol. 2003;111:S571-S581.

107. Bjoro K, Froland SS, Yuru Z, et al. Hepatitis C infection in patients with primary hypogammaglobulinemia after treatment with contaminated immune globulin. N Engl J Med. 1994;331:1607-1611.

108. Tabor E. The epidemiology of virus transmission by plasma derivatives: Clinical studies verifying the lack of transmission of hepatitis B and C viruses and HIV-1. Transfusion. 1999;39:1160-1165.

109. Tabor E, Yu MW, Hewlitt I, et al. Summary of a workshop on the implementation of NAT to screen donors of blood and plasma for viruses. Transfusion. 2000;40:1273-1275.

110. Busse PJ, Razvi S, Cunningham-Rundles C. Efficacy of intravenous immunoglobulin in the prevention of pneumonia in patients with common variable immunodeficiency. J Allergy Clin Immunol. 2002;109:1001-1004.

111. Spector A, Gelber RD, McGrath N, et al. Controlled trial of intravenous immune globulin for the prevention of serious bacterial infections in children receiving zidovudine for advanced human immunodeficiency virus infection. N Engl J Med. 1994;331:1181-1187.

112. Stiehm ER, Lambert JS, Mofenson LM, et al. Efficacy of zidovudine and human immunodeficiency virus (HIV) hyperimmune immunoglobulin for reducing perinatal HIV transmission from HIV-infected women with advanced disease: Results of Pediatric AIDS Clinical Trials Group protocol 185. J Infect Dis. 1999;179:567-575.

113. Kiehl MG, Stoll R, Broder M, et al. A controlled trial of intravenous immune globulin for the prevention of serious infections in adults with advanced human immunodeficiency virus infection. Arch Intern Med. 1996;156:1545-1550.

114. Kurtzman GJ, Frickhofen NK, Kimball J, et al. Pure red cell aplasia of 10 years duration due to persistent parvovirus infection and its cure with immunoglobulin therapy. N Engl J Med. 1989;321:519-523.

115. Sullivan KM, Kopecky KJ, Jocom J, et al. Immunomodulatory and antimicrobial efficacy of intravenous immunoglobulin in bone marrow transplantation. N Engl J Med. 1990;323:705-712.

116. Weeks JC, Tierney MR, Weinstein MC. Cost effectiveness of prophylactic intravenous immune globulin in chronic lymphocytic leukemia. N Engl J Med. 1991;325:81-86.

117. Berkman SA, Lee ML, Gale RP. Clinical uses of intravenous immunoglobulins. Ann Intern Med. 1990;112:705-712.

118. Bass EB, Power NR, Goodman SN, et al. Efficacy of immune globulin in preventing complications of bone marrow transplantation: A meta-analysis. Bone Marrow Transplant. 1993;12:273-282.

119. Falagas ME, Snydman DR, Ruthazer R, et al. Cytomegalovirus immunoglobulin (CMVIG) prophylaxis is associated with increased survival after orthotopic liver transplantation. Clin Transplant. 1997;11:432-437.

120. Snydman DR, Werner BG, Tilney NL, et al. A final analysis of the use of cytomegalovirus disease prevention in renal transplant recipients with cytomegalovirus immune globulin: Comparison of randomized and open-label trials. Transplant Proc. 1991;23:1357-1360.

121. Reed EC, Bowden RA, Dandliker PS, et al. Treatment of cytomegalovirus pneumonia with ganciclovir and intravenous immunoglobulin in patients with bone marrow transplants. Ann Intern Med. 1988;198:783-788.

122. King SM, Superina R, Andrews W, et al. Randomized comparison of ganciclovir plus intravenous immune globulin (IVIG) with IVIG alone for prevention of primary cytomegalovirus diseases in children receiving liver transplants. Clin Infect Dis. 1997;25:1173-1179.

123. The Intravenous Immunoglobulin Collaborative Study Group. Prophylactic intravenous administration of standard immune globulin as compared with core-lipopolysaccharide immune globulin in patients at high risk of postsurgical infection. N Engl J Med. 1992;327:234-240.

124. Douzinas EE, Pitaridis MT, Louris G, et al. Prevention of infection in multiple trauma patients by high-dose intravenous immunoglobulins. Crit Care Med. 2000;28:8-15

125. Alejandra MM, Lansang MA, Dans LF, Mantaring JB. Intravenous immunoglobulin for treating sepsis and septic shock. Cochrane Database Syst Rev. 2002;(1):CD001090.

126. Sandberg K, Fasth K, Berger A, et al. Preterm infants with low immunoglobulin levels have increased risk for neonatal sepsis but do not benefit from prophylactic immunoglobulin G. J Pediatr. 2000;137:623-628.

127. Ohlsson A, Lacy JB. Intravenous immunoglobulin for preventing infection in preterm and/or low-birth-weight infants. Cochrane Database Syst Rev. 2004;(1):CD000361.

128. Schlievert PM. Use of intravenous immunoglobulin in the treatment of staphylococcal and streptococcal toxic shock syndromes and related illnesses. J Allergy Clin Immunol. 2001;108(4 Suppl):S107-S110.

129. Darenberg J, Ihendyane N, Sjolin J, et al. Intravenous immunoglobulin G therapy in streptococcal toxic shock syndrome: A European randomized, double-blind, placebo-controlled trial. Clin Infect Dis. 2003;37:333-340.

130. Bacdhot N, Revuz J, Roujeau JC. Intravenous immunoglobulin treatment for Stevens-Johnson syndrome and toxic epidermal necrolysis: A prospective noncomparative study showing no benefit on mortality or progression. Arch Dermatol. 2003;139:33-36.

131. Whiting P, Bagnall AM, Sowden AJ, et al. Interventions for the treatment and management of chronic fatigue syndrome: A systematic review. JAMA. 2001;286:1360-1368.

132. Brogan PA, Bose A, Burgner D, et al. Kawasaki disease: An evidence based approach to diagnosis, treatment, and proposals for future research. Arch Dis Child. 2002;86:286-290.

133. Sanchez PJ. Immunoprophylaxis for respiratory syncytial virus. Pediatr Infect Dis J. 2002;21:473-478.

134. IMpact-RSV Study Group. Palivizumab, a respiratory syncytial virus monoclonal antibody reduces hospitalization from respiratory virus infection in high risk infants. Pediatrics. 1998;102:1173-1179.

135. Sacher RA, IVIG Advisory Panel. Intravenous immunoglobulin consensus statement. J Allergy Clin Immunol. 2001;108(4 Suppl):S139-S146.

136. Gagnon S, Boota AM, Fischl MA, et al. Corticosteroids as adjunctive therapy for *Pneumocystis carinii* pneumonia in the acquired immunodeficiency syndrome. N Engl J Med. 1990;323:1440-1441.

137. The National Institutes of Health—University of California Expert Panel for Corticosteroids as Adjunctive Therapy for Pneumocystis Pneumonia. Consensus statement on the use of corticosteroids as adjunctive therapy for *Pneumocystis* pneumonia in the acquired immunodeficiency syndrome. N Engl J Med. 1990;323:1500-1504.

138. Bukharie H. Paradoxical response to anti-tuberculous drugs: Resolution with corticosteroid therapy. Scand J Infect Dis. 2000;32:96-97.

139. Girgis NI, Farid Z, Kilpatrick ME, et al. Dexamethasone adjunctive treatment for tuberculous meningitis. Pediatr Infect Dis J. 1991;10:179-183.

140. Molavi A, Lefrock JL. Tuberculous meningitis. Med Clin North Am. 1985;69:315-331.

141. Prasad K, Volmink J, Menon GR. Steroids for treating tuberculous meningitis. Cochrane Database Syst Rev. 2000;(3):CD002244.

142. Mayoshi BM, Ntsekhe M, Volmink JA, Commerford PJ. Interventions for treating tuberculous pericarditis. Cochrane Database Syst Rev. 2002;(4):CD000526.

143. Alrajhi AA, Halim MA, al-Hokail A, et al. Corticosteroid treatment of peritoneal tuberculosis. Clin Infect Dis. 1998;27:52-56.

144. Matchaba PT, Volmick J. Steroids for treating tuberculous pleurisy. Cochrane Database Syst Rev. 2000;(2):CD001876.

145. Smego RA, Ahmed N. A systematic review of the adjunctive use of systemic corticosteroids for pulmonary tuberculosis. Int J Tuberc Lung Dis. 2003;7:208-213.

146. Annane D, Sebille V, Charpentier C, et al. Effect of treatment with low doses of hydrocortisone and fludrocortisone on mortality in patients with septic shock. JAMA. 2002;288:862-871.

147. Hoffman SL, Punjabi NH, Kumala S, et al. Reduction of mortality in chloramphenicol-treated severe typhoid fever by high-dose dexamethasone. N Engl J Med. 1984;310:82-88.

148. Thompson BT. Glucocorticoids and acute lung injury. Crit Care Med. 2003;31(Suppl):S253-S257.

149. Cronin L, Crook DJ, Carlet J, et al. Corticosteroid treatment for sepsis: A critical appraisal and meta-analysis of the literature. Crit Care Med. 1995;23:1430-1439.

150. Meduri GU, Headley AS, Golden E, et al. Effect of prolonged methylprednisolone therapy in unresolving acute respiratory distress syndrome. JAMA. 1998;280:159-165.

151. Lebel MH, Freij BJ, Syrogiannopoulos GA, et al. Dexamethaone therapy for bacterial meningitis: Results of two double-blind, placebo-controlled trials. N Engl J Med. 1988;319:964-971.

152. Quagliarello VJ, Scheld WM. Treatment of bacterial meningitis. N Engl J Med. 1997;336:211-218.

153. De Gans J, van de Beek D, European Dexamethasone in Adulthood Bacterial Meningitis Study Investigators. Dexamethasone in adults with bacterial meningitis. N Engl J Med. 2002;347:1549-1556.

154. Tunkel AR, Scheld WM. Corticosteroids for everyone with meningitis? N Engl J Med. 2002;347:1613-1615.

155. Chotmongkol V, Sawanyawisuth K, Thavornpitak Y. Corticosteroid treatment of eosinophilic meningitis. Clin Infect Dis. 2000;31:660-662.

156. Prasad K, Garner P. Steroids for treating cerebral malaria. Cochrane Database Syst Rev. 2000;(2):CD000972.

157. Shelburne SA III, Hamill RJ, Rodriguez-Barradas MC, et al. Immune reconstitution inflammatory syndrome—Emergence of a unique syndrome during highly active antiretroviral therapy. Medicine. 2002;81:213-227.

158. McComsey GA, Whalen CC, Mawhorter SD, et al. Placebo-controlled trial of prednisone in advanced HIV-1 infection. AIDS. 2001;15:321-327.

159. Vincent J-L, Sun Q, Dubois M-J. Clinical trials of immunomodulatory therapies in severe sepsis and septic shock. Clin Infect Dis. 2002;34:1084-1093.

160. Hotchkiss RS, Karl IE. The pathophysiology and treatment of sepsis. N Engl J Med. 2003;348:138-150.

161. McCloskey RV, Straube RC, Sanders C, et al. Treatment of septic shock with human monoclonal antibody HA-1A: A randomized, double-blind, placebo-controlled trial. Ann Intern Med. 1994;121:1-5.

162. Angus DC, Birmingham MC, Balk RA, et al. E5 murine monoclonal antiendotoxin antibody in gram-negative sepsis: A randomized controlled trial. E5 Study Investigators. JAMA. 2000;283:1723-1730.

163. Fisher CJ, Agosti JM, Opal SM, et al. Treatment of septic shock with the tumor necrosis factor receptor:Fc fusion protein. N Engl J Med. 1996;334:1697-1702.

164. Abraham E, Anzueto A, Guitterez G, et al. Double-blind randomized controlled trial of monoclonal antibody to human necrosis factor in treatment of septic shock. Lancet. 1998;351:929-933.

165. Opal SM, Fisher CJ Jr, Dhainaut JF, et al. Confirmatory interleukin-1 receptor antagonist trial in severe sepsis: A phase III, randomized, double-blind, placebo-controlled, multicenter trial. Crit Care Med. 1997;25:1115-1124.

166. Dhainaut JF, Tenaillon A, Hemmer M, et al. Confirmatory platelet-activating factor receptor antagonist trial in patients with severe gram-negative bacterial sepsis: A phase II, randomized, double-blind, placebo-controlled, multicenter trial. BN 52021 Sepsis Investigator Group. Crit Care Med. 1998;26:1963-1971.

167. Fein AM, Bernard GR, Criner GJ, et al. Treatment of severe systemic inflammatory response syndrome and sepsis with a novel bradykinin antagonist, deltibant (CP-0127). JAMA. 1997;277:482-487.

168. Warren BL, Eid A, Singer P, et al. High-dose antithrombin III in severe sepsis: A randomized controlled trial. JAMA. 2001;286:1869-1878.

169. Abraham E, Reinhart K, Opal S, et al. Efficacy and safety of tifacogin (recombinant tissue factor pathway inhibitor) in severe sepsis: A randomized controlled trial. JAMA. 2003;290:238-247.

170. Bernard GR, Vincent J-L, Laterre P-F, et al. Efficacy and safety of recombinant human activated protein C for severe sepsis. N Engl J Med. 2001;344:699-709.

171. Dellinger RP. Inflammation and coagulation: Implications for the septic patient. Clin Infect Dis. 2003;36:1259-1265.

172. Warren HS, Suffredini AF, Eichacker PQ, Munford RS. Risks and benefits of activated protein C treatment for severe sepsis. N Engl J Med. 2002; 347:1027-1030.

173. Eichacker PQ, Natanson C. Recombinant human activated protein C in sepsis: Inconsistent trial results, an unclear mechanism of action, and safety concerns resulted in labeling restrictions and the need for phase IV trials. Crit Care Med. 2002;31(Suppl 1):S94-S96.

174. Banks SM, Gerstenberger E, Eichacker PQ, Natanson C. Long-term cost effectiveness of drotrecogin alfa (activated): An unanswered question. Crit Care Med. 2003;31:308-309.

175. Levin M, Quint PA, Goldstein B, et al. Recombinant bactericidal/permeability-increasing protein (rBPI21) as adjunctive treatment for children with severe meningococcal sepsis: A randomized trial. rBPI21 Meningococcal Sepsis Study Group. Lancet 2000;356:961-967.

176. Tyring S, Conant M, Marini M, et al. Imiquimod; an international update on therapeutic uses in dermatology. Int J Dermatol. 2002;41:810-816.

177. Hengge UR, Esser S, Schulewolter T, et al. Self-administered topical 5% imiquimod for the treatment of common warts and molluscum contagiosum. Br J Dermatol. 2000;143:1026-1031.

178. Looareesuwan S, Wilariatana P, Vannaphan S, et al. Pentoxifylline as an ancillary treatment for severe *falciparum* malaria in Thailand. Am J Trop Med Hyg. 1998;58:348-353.

179. Stockschlader M, Kalhs P, Peters S, et al. Intravenous pentoxifylline failed to prevent transplant-related toxicities in allogeneic bone marrow transplant recipients. Bone Marrow Transplant. 1993;12:357-362.

180. Noel C, Copin MC, Hazzan M, et al. Immunomodulatory effect of pentoxifylline during human allograft rejection: Involvement of tumor necrosis factor-alpha and adhesion molecules. Transplantation. 2000;69:1102-1107.

181. Staubach, K-H, Schroder J, Stuber F, et al. Effect of pentoxifylline in severe sepsis: Results of a randomized, double-blind, placebo-controlled study. Arch Surg. 1998;133:94-100.

182. Lauterbach R, Pawlik D, Kowalczyk D, et al. Effect of the immunomodulating agent, pentoxifylline, in the treatment of sepsis in prematurely delivered infants: A placebo-controlled, double-blind trial. Crit Care Med. 1999;27:807-814.

183. Clerici M, Ponci S, Balotta C, et al. Pentoxifylline improves cell-mediated immunity and reduces human immunodeficiency virus (HIV) plasma viremia in asymptomatic HIV-seropositive persons. J Infect Dis. 1997;175:1210-1215.

184. De Carsalade GY, Achirafi A, Flageul B. Pentoxifylline in the treatment of erythema nodosum leprosum. J Dermatol. 2003;30:64-68.

185. List AF, Maziarz R, Stiff P, et al. A randomized placebo-controlled trial of lisofylline in HLA-identical, sibling-donor, allogeneic bone marrow transplant recipients. The Lisofylline Marrow Transplant Study Group. Bone Marrow Transplant. 2000;25:283-291.

186. The ARDS Clinical Trials Network. Randomized placebo-controlled trial of lisofylline for early treatment of acute lung injury and acute respiratory distress syndrome. Crit Care Med. 2002;30:1-6.

187. Teo SK, Resztak KE, Scheffler MA, et al. Thalidomide in the treatment of leprosy. Microbes Infect. 2002;4:1193-1202.

188. Reyes-Teran G, Sierra-Madero JG, Martinez del Cerro V, et al. Effects of thalidomide on HIV-associated wasting syndrome: A randomized, double-blind, placebo-controlled clinical trial. AIDS. 1996;10:1501-1508.

189. Jacobson JM, Greenspan JS, Spritzler J, et al. Thalidomide for the treatment of oral aphthous ulcers in patients with human immunodeficiency virus infection. N Engl J Med. 1997;336:1487-1493.

190. Alexander LN, Wilcox CM. A prospective trial of thalidomide for the treatment of HIV-associated esophageal ulcers. AIDS Res Hum Retroviruses. 1997;13:301-304.

191. Cattelan AM, Trevenzoli M, Aversa SM. Recent advances in the treatment of AIDS-related Kaposi's sarcoma. Am J Clin Dermatol. 2002;3:451-462.

192. Lau GK. Use of immunomodulatory therapy (other than interferon) for the treatment of chronic hepatitis B virus infection. J Gastroenterol Hepatol. 2000;15 Suppl:E46-52.

193. Rasi G, Mutchnick MG, Di Virgilio, et al. Combination low-dose lymphoblastoid interferon and thymosin α_1 therapy in the treatment of hepatitis B. J Viral Hepat. 1996;3:191-196.

194. Lau GK, Nanji A, Hou J, et al. Thymosin-alpha 1 and famciclovir combination therapy activate T-cell response in patients with chronic hepatitis B virus infection in immune-tolerant phase. J Viral Hepat. 2002;9:280-287.

195. Sherman KE, Sjogren M, Creager RL, et al. Combination therapy with thymosin alpha1 and interferon for treatment of chronic hepatitis C infection: A randomized, placebo-controlled double-blind trial. Hepatology. 1998;27:1128-1135.

196. Ramachandran R, Katzenstein DA, Winters MA, et al. Polyethylene glycol-modified interleukin-2 and thymosin alpha 1 in human immunodeficiency virus type 1 infection. J Infect Dis. 1996;173:1005-1008.

197. Dellinger EP, Babineau TJ, Bleicher P, et al. Effect of PGG-glucan on the rate of serious postoperative infection or death observed after high-risk gastrointestinal operations. Betafectin Gastrointestinal Study Group. Arch Surg. 1999;134:977-983.

198. Breshnihan B, Cunnane G. Infection complications associated with use of biologic agents. Rheum Dis Clin North Am. 2003;29:185-202.

CHAPTER **40**

Hyperbaric Oxygen

RONALD RABINOWITZ

JEAN MARIE MULINDE

ELLIS S. CAPLAN

As defined by the Undersea and Hyperbaric Medicine Society, hyperbaric medicine is "a therapeutic technique using air or other gas mixtures at greater-than-atmospheric pressure for short intervals, over days or months, to treat various disease states." Dr. Orville Cunningham constructed a 64-foot-diameter "steel ball" chamber to treat various ailments including syphilis, cancer, and rheumatoid arthritis. His theory was that anaerobes caused a variety of diseases.[1] The American Medical Association (AMA) censored him in 1925, and his chamber

TABLE 40-1   Disorders Approved by the Hyperbaric Oxygen Committee of the Undersea and Hyperbaric Medicine Society for Hyperbaric Oxygen Therapy

Infectious Diseases	Noninfectious Diseases
Gas gangrene	Decompression sickness
Necrotizing soft tissue infections	Air or gas embolism
Osteomyelitis, refractory	Carbon monoxide and cyanide
Intracranial abscess	poisoning
	Radiation osteonecrosis
	Exceptional blood loss anemia
	Crush injury
	Selected wound problems
	Skin grafts and flaps
	Thermal burns

was destroyed. Albert Behnke, in 1939, reported the first clinical use of hyperbaric oxygen (HBO) therapy using intermittent inhalation of 100% oxygen under pressure to treat decompression sickness.[2] It was not until 1967, however, that HBO treatment of "the bends" was officially accepted, and it has since become the standard worldwide.[2] The first nondiving-related use of HBO was by Boerema in 1956,[2] when he used a large pressurized operating room to perform procedures requiring the interruption of circulation to the brain and other vital organs, operations that would otherwise have been impossible in the pre–heart-lung bypass era. A number of similar operating chambers were built in the United States and United Kingdom, but with the development of effective cardiopulmonary bypass equipment, by the mid-1970s they became obsolete for this indication.[2] In the interim, however, hyperbaric practitioners (frequently nonphysicians) began treating a wide variety of conditions with HBO, often making claims without sound scientific foundation. In 1977, in response to concerns about the misuse of HBO therapy, the Undersea and Hyperbaric Medicine Society produced a report defining those conditions for which animal experiments and clinical series showed that HBO treatment was beneficial, and these disorders became eligible for reimbursement by third-party payers. This report has been updated every 2 to 3 years and currently recognizes 13 disorders that are reimbursable for HBO treatment (http://www.uhms.org/Indications/indications.htm) (Table 40-1).[3]

EQUIPMENT

HBO can be delivered through monoplace or multiplace chambers. Monoplace chambers are essentially Plexiglas tubes that are continuously flooded with 100% oxygen at pressures up to 3 atmospheric pressures at sea level (ATA). Ports for hemodynamic monitoring, electrocardiographs, intravenous infusions, oxygen monitoring, and respirator management are available, and the controls for chamber operation are on the unit. The advantages of monoplace units are decreased expenses and a limited need for space; the disadvantages include a decreased access to the patient and an increased risk of fire in the chamber because the entire internal environment is flooded with 100% oxygen. Multiplace chambers accommodate from 2 to 14 patients and their attendants (Fig. 40-1A). A chamber pressure of up to 6 ATA is provided by air, and the patient breathes 100% oxygen via a closely fitting hood or mask or, if mechanically ventilated, through the ventilator circuit (see Fig. 40-1B). Advantages of the multiplace chamber include ready access to patients by the inside attendant and the ability to provide pressures of up to 6 ATA. Disadvantages include the large expense of such a unit and the potential for attendants to experience nitrogen-saturation illness. All medical equipment (IVs, ventilators, monitoring equipment) used in the chamber must be certified for use in pressurized situations and in increased oxygen concentrations.[4]

PHYSIOLOGY

HBO has two basic physiologic effects. The first is the reduction of bubble size; this phenomenon is governed by Boyle's law, which states that the volume of gas in an enclosed space is inversely proportional to the pressure exerted on it. It is this reduction of bubble size that is important in the treatment of iatrogenic air embolism and in nitrogen-saturation illness (the bends). The second physiologic effect of HBO is increased partial pressure of oxygen in body tissues. When air is inspired under normal pressure, 98.4% of the available oxygen is bound to hemoglobin and the remaining portion is dissolved in plasma.[5] For each increased atmosphere of pressure, an additional 2.3 VOL% of oxygen is dissolved in plasma. At 3 ATA, the most common pressure used, more than 6 VOL% of oxygen is carried by plasma. Because approximately 5 VOL% is required for adequate tissue oxygenation, inspired 100% oxygen at 3 ATA provides enough oxygen in plasma alone to support life and can raise peripheral tissue oxygen tensions measured through the skin from 40 to more than 2200 mm Hg.[5] The logistics of a "dive" involve being placed in a monoplace or multiplace chamber at between 2 and 3 atmospheres with 100% O_2 via mask or ventilator for about 2 hours. This time includes compression, dive, and decompression.

The dramatic increase in tissue oxygenation by HBO results in a number of local tissue effects. These effects include an increased ability of leukocytes to kill some bacteria[6] and exert a bacteriostatic effect on others[7-9]; the direct killing of some anaerobic bacteria[10] and the inhibition of formation of clostridial toxin[11,12]; the stimulation of fibroblast growth, which results in increased collagen formation and resultant neovascularization[13-15]; and the inhibition of neutrophil adherence to ischemic vessel walls, a reduction in postischemic vasoconstriction, and reduced lipid peroxidation (vasoconstriction and lipid peroxidation are key components of ischemic tissue injury).[16-18]

ADVERSE EFFECTS

Absolute contraindications of HBO use include untreated pneumothorax and recent chemotherapy with Adriamycin or cisplastin.[19] The most common adverse effects associated with HBO are barotrauma of the middle ear, cranial sinuses, or teeth. Auditory barotrauma occurs in less than 1% of patients and rarely permanently curtails treatment.[20] The occurrence of auditory barotrauma may be minimized by careful screening of individuals for their ability to clear their ears and may be minimized with the use of decongestants. For those who display an inability to clear their ears or for those who are obtunded, needle myringotomy or tympanotomy tube placement provides a simple solution. Lung barotrauma is a potentially more severe adverse effect of HBO. Pulmonary barotrauma is of particular concern in asthmatic patients, those with chronic obstructive lung disease, and those with lung cysts or bullae because they are at increased risk of developing a pneumothorax during decompression.[5] Although rare, oxygen toxicity is also a potential risk, occurring in 1 in 10,000 patient therapies.[3] When present, oxygen toxicity usually manifests as symptoms involving the central nervous system, which range from agitation to generalized seizures. The etiology is thought to be related to the presence of oxygen radicals.[19] The risk is minimized by adhering to well-defined guidelines for time and pressure limits. Additional adverse effects of HBO include a reversible myopia, resulting from a direct toxic effect of oxygen on the lens, and cataract formation.[21] A summary of adverse effects is presented in Table 40-2.

HYPERBARIC OXYGEN THERAPY IN INFECTIOUS DISEASES

Clostridial Myonecrosis

HBO serves a number of important functions in the treatment of clostridial myonecrosis. At 3 ATA oxygen, Van Unnik demonstrated that the production of α-toxin ceases.[11] Because α-toxin, a lecithinase C, is believed to be responsible for tissue destruction and shock, a clear theoretical benefit is evident. Van Unnik also demonstrated the arrest of clostridial growth with 3 ATA oxygen. Bacterial growth and toxin production resumed, however, on return to a normal environment. Other in vitro studies support the finding of a bacteriostatic effect by HBO but have found that the addition of blood or muscle to culture media inhibits this effect of HBO because a catalase present in blood and muscle protects the bacteria from the effects of oxy-

FIGURE 40-1. A, Hyperbaric chamber at the RA Cowley Shock Trauma Center. **B,** Patients fitted with hoods in the hyperbaric oxygen chamber.

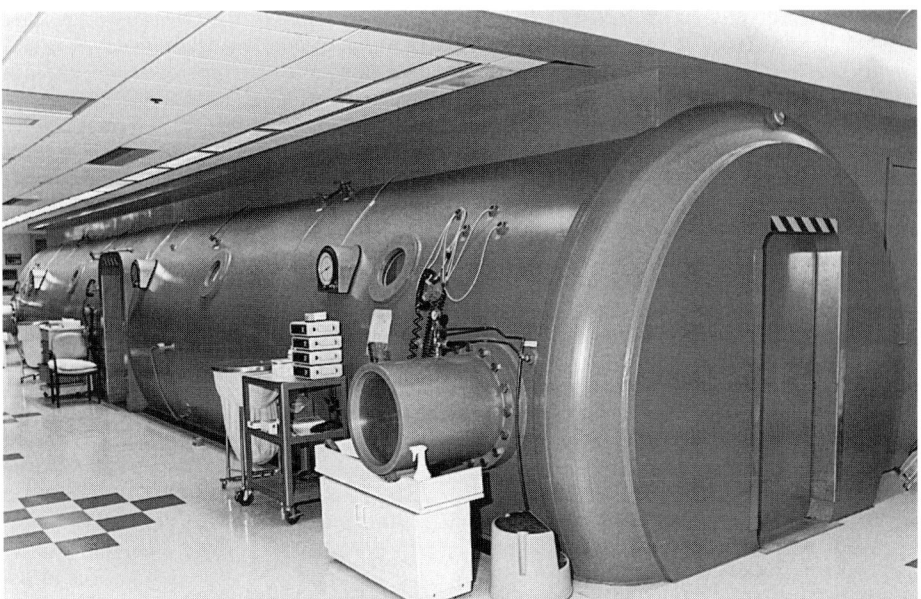

A

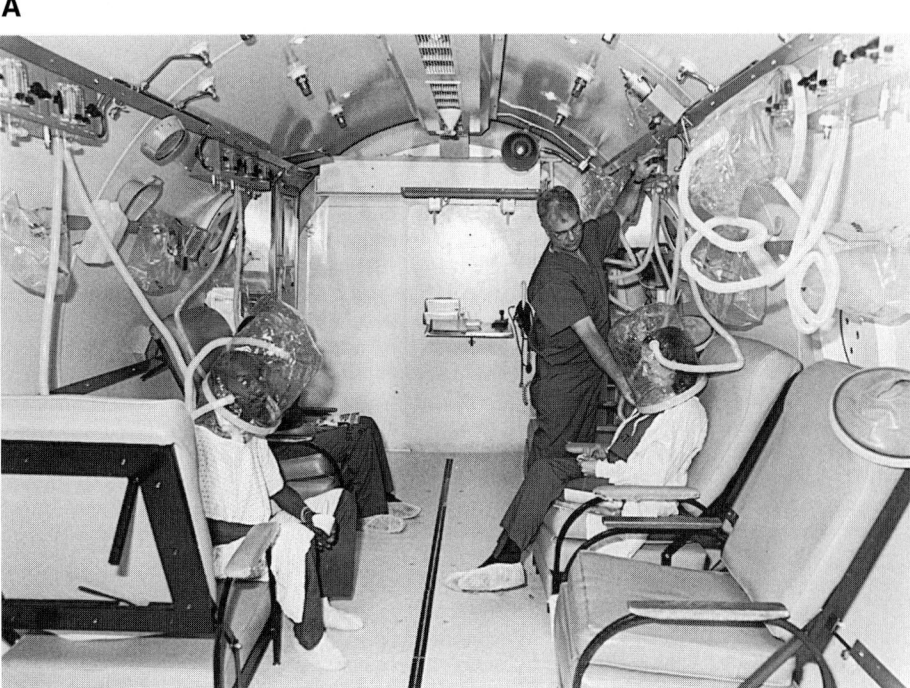

B

gen,[10,12,22-24] suggesting that for HBO therapy to provide optimal results, blood and necrotic tissue should be débrided from the wound.

Brummelkamp first reported the use of HBO for the treatment of clostridial myonecrosis in 1961.[25] He described four patients with clostridial myonecrosis whose disease was progressing despite surgery and antibiotic therapy; HBO therapy produced a rapid and dramatic improvement in their clinical condition, and all patients sur-

vived. Since 1961 there have been many reports of the treatment of clostridial myonecrosis with HBO in both experimental animal models[10,12,26-29] and human disease.[30-35] A review of 20 clinical series, including a total of more than 1200 patients in whom HBO was used, reported a cumulative mortality of 23%.[32] Although there has never been a controlled, randomized study of the use of HBO for clostridial myonecrosis in humans, historical data suggest a mortality of 45% without HBO.[36] A recent study reviewed data that captured greater than 650 additional patients in nonrandomized studies and case series concluded a beneficial effect and a decrease in mortality with the use of HBO.[37] In perhaps the most well-designed in vivo study to date, Demello and colleagues reported on the use of HBO in the treatment of gas gangrene in a dog model.[27] They showed that survival increased from 70% in animals treated with surgery and antibiotics alone to 95% with the addition of HBO to surgery and antimicrobial therapy.

TABLE 40-2 Complications and Side Effects of Hyperbaric Oxygen Treatment

Barotrauma to the ear	Seizures
Sinus pain	Numb fingers
Visual refractive changes	Pulmonary oxygen toxicity
Pneumothorax	Chamber fire

The timing of HBO in the treatment of clostridial myonecrosis is somewhat controversial. If readily available, an initial treatment before surgery may help to delineate the surviving tissue and decrease the production of α-toxin, resulting in a patient who is more hemodynamically stable. If HBO therapy cannot be administered within 24 hours of the onset of disease, initial surgical débridement should be performed with subsequent transfer of the patient to a facility providing HBO. The recommended HBO treatment protocol for clostridial myonecrosis is 100% oxygen at 3 ATA for 90 minutes (with appropriate air breaks), two or three times daily, for 5 to 7 days.[38] In addition to HBO and surgical débridement, appropriate antibiotic therapy is essential. Antimicrobials recommended for the treatment of clostridial myonecrosis include penicillin G, clindamycin, and metronidazole. It has been our clinical experience at the RA Cowley Shock Trauma Center that these infections frequently also involve aerobic gram-negative rods and that additional gram-negative coverage is appropriate pending culture data. Combination drugs may be useful if culture data suggest multiple pathogens. Ampicillin/sulbactam can be used if the preponderance of organisms is gram-positive. Piperacillin/tazobactam can be used if there is a preponderance of gram-negative rods.

Necrotizing Fasciitis, Fournier's Gangrene, and Other Progressive Necrotizing Infections

Necrotizing fasciitis is a rapidly progressing infection of the skin, underlying subcutaneous soft tissues, and fascia without muscle involvement. Other eponyms include Meleney's progressive synergistic gangrene, and when the external genitourinary (GU) tract is involved, Fournier's gangrene. Bacteriologically these infections may be divided into two groups: those caused by a single aerobic species such as *Streptococcus pyogenes* and more commonly those that are polymicrobial, involving both anaerobes and aerobes. Although fluid resuscitation, surgical débridement, and antibiotic therapy are considered the mainstays of therapy for necrotizing fasciitis, HBO therapy can be used as adjunctive therapy. The rationale for the use of HBO includes the reversal of tissue hypoxia, enhanced neutrophil function, a direct toxic effect on selected bacteria, and enhanced activity of certain antimicrobial agents.[39,40]

Although carefully controlled trials of HBO for the treatment of necrotizing fasciitis in humans have not been performed and some authors refute the role of HBO for the treatment of necrotizing fasciitis,[41] studies in animals[17,40,42-45] and other retrospective clinical studies have reported efficacy, whereas others have not.[40,42,46] Risenman and associates retrospectively described 29 adults with necrotizing fasciitis.[46] Those patients receiving HBO, despite being more seriously ill at the time of presentation, had a lower mortality rate (23% versus 66% in those not receiving HBO) and required fewer surgical débridements (1.16 versus 3.25 in those not receiving HBO).[46] Brown in a retrospective review of 54 patients showed no significant differences in outcomes of patients who received HBO.[47] If utilized, it is recommended that HBO begin after the first surgical débridement and that three sessions be given within the first 24 hours, consisting of 3 ATA 100% oxygen for 90 minutes (with appropriate air breaks) followed by twice-daily sessions until granulation is obtained.[48] Traditional treatment should not be delayed pending initiation of HBO.

Refractory Osteomyelitis

Mader and coworkers, in a rabbit model of *Staphylococcus aureus* osteomyelitis, showed the oxygen tension in osteomyelitic bone to be markedly reduced at 23 mm Hg.[6] At 23 mm Hg, there was a reduced ability of phagocytes to kill bacteria compared with killing in normal bone at an oxygen tension of 45 mm Hg. When the rabbits were subjected to 100% oxygen at 2 ATA, the oxygen tension in osteomyelitic bone increased to 109 mm Hg and phagocytic killing of *S. aureus* was restored. Thus, Mader concluded that for osteomyelitic bone, HBO therapy allows the return of intramedullary oxygen tensions to normal or supranormal levels, resulting in normalization of phagocytic killing. Work by other authors suggests that similarly enhanced phagocytic killing may also be the

mechanism by which HBO is beneficial in *Staphylococcus epidermidis*, *Pseudomonas aeruginosa*, and *Escherichia coli* osteomyelitis.[49] In addition, increased oxygen tension can promote osteogenesis and neovascularization. HBO can also increase osteoclastic activity, which can increase the removal of bony debris.[50] HBO for refractory osteomyelitis is an approved Medicare indication.

HBO therapy should be viewed as adjunctive therapy to surgical débridement and antibiotic therapy in patients with refractory osteomyelitis (defined as failure after standard surgical débridement and at least 6 weeks of appropriate antibiotic therapy). Although there has not been a placebo-controlled, double-blind study of the use of HBO in osteomyelitis, animal data[51] and clinical experience[52-54] suggest benefit. Davis studied 38 patients with refractory osteomyelitis treated with débridement, antimicrobial therapy, and adjunctive HBO; this combination therapy was successful in 34 patients.[54] In another study, no benefit of HBO was found when patients treated with surgical débridement and antibiotics were compared with those with surgical débridement, antibiotics, and HBO.[55] New areas of investigation include spine infections, craniotomy flaps, and sternal infections.[56-58] However, because more than 90% of patients in the control group were cured, there is some question as to whether these patients truly had refractory osteomyelitis.[21] The recommended protocol for adjunctive HBO therapy for refractory osteomyelitis is 2.4 ATA for 95 minutes with appropriate air breaks. Sessions are usually once daily for at least 15 days.[49]

Mucormycosis

Traditional therapy for mucormycosis includes control of underlying predisposing conditions, aggressive surgical débridement, and administration of high-dose amphotericin B. Adjunctive HBO therapy may offer additional benefit. Oxygen-based free radicals are believed to be responsible for the fungistatic and fungicidal effects of HBO.[39] HBO may potentiate the antifungal effect of amphotericin B by reversing tissue hypoxia, which protects fungal proteoplasts from lysis.[39,59] Tissue hypoxia is secondary to vascular invasion of organisms. In a review of 145 cases of rhino-orbital-cerebral mucormycosis, 24 patients with bilateral disease (a situation associated with increased mortality) were identified.[60] In 18 patients who received standard treatment with amphotericin B, surgery, or both, the mortality was 78%, whereas the mortality in 6 patients treated with standard therapy in addition to HBO was 17%. A recent animal model of mucor failed to show a benefit, but the HBO protocol used was lower than normal.[61] Although there have been multiple case reports of the benefits of HBO in the treatment of mucormycosis,[62-65] the exact role of HBO in the treatment of mucormycosis remains uncertain.

MISCELLANEOUS CONDITIONS

In 1993, Reillo published a study that looked at the effect of HBO on debilitating fatigue and decreased immunologic function related to human immunodeficiency virus (HIV)–acquired immunodeficiency diseases.[66] Twenty-five patients positive for HIV and with CD4 counts of 500 mm[3] or less and Karnofsky performance scales of 75% or less were studied. Reillo stated that "all patients had significant improvements in energy levels, as measured by the Karnofsky Performance Scale." Sixty percent of the patients had a decrease in the total CD8 count and stabilization or improvement in CD4/CD8 ratios (only 20% of patients were reported to be receiving antiretroviral therapy). Weight rose or stabilized in all patients. Although HBO therapy cannot be recommended for HIV-acquired immunodeficiency disease based on the limited data presented by Reillo, further investigation may be warranted. There are some theoretical antiviral properties of HBO by producing reactive oxygen intermediaries that are virucidal to enveloped viruses.[67]

Intracranial abscesses are another potential diagnosis in which HBO may play a role. Conservative management with computed tomography (CT) diagnosis and appropriate antibiotic has been the mainstay of therapy. In patients with multiple abscesses, immunosuppression, failure of standard treatment, or surgical contraindication, HBO may play a role. HBO treatment may inhibit anaerobes found in abscesses. There are preliminary data on the use of HBO in intracranial abscesses that have shown a favorable outcome.[68,69]

SUMMARY

HBO therapy has been used to treat hundreds of conditions ranging from skin wrinkles and baldness to impotence.[2] There are, however, only 12 indications recognized by the Undersea and Hyperbaric Medicine Society and third-party payers as legitimate uses supported by sound scientific data. The recognized infectious disease-associated uses include the treatment of clostridial gangrene, necrotizing fasciitis, and refractory osteomyelitis. Other areas in which HBO may be useful include the treatment of mucormycosis, intracranial abscesses, and HIV-associated fatigue. However, further well-designed studies are needed before recommending HBO as a standard therapy in these disorders.

REFERENCES

1. Cunningham OJ. Oxygen therapy by means of compressed air. Anesth Analg. 1927;6:64.
2. Kindwall EP. Uses of hyperbaric oxygen therapy in the 1990s. Clev Clin J Med. 1992;59:517-528.
3. Thom SR. Hyperbaric Oxygen Therapy: A Committee Report. Bethesda, Md: Undersea and Hyperbaric Medicine Society; 1994.
4. Sheridan RL, Shank ES. Hyperbaric oxygen treatment: A brief overview of a controversial topic. J Trauma. 1999; 426-35.
5. Tabrah FI, Tanner R, Vega R, Batkin S. Baromedicine today—Rational uses of hyperbaric oxygen therapy. Hawaii Med J. 1994;53:112-119.
6. Mader TJ, Brown GL, Guckian JC, et al. A mechanism for the amelioration by hyperbaric oxygen of experimental staphylococcal osteomyelitis in rabbits. J Infect Dis. 1980;142:915-922.
7. Boehme DE. Oxygen and toxicity inhibition of amino acid biosynthesis. Nature. 1976;262:418-420.
8. Brown OR. Reversible inhibition of *Escherichia coli* by hyperoxia. Microbiology. 1972;5:7-16.
9. Park MK, Muhvich KH, Myers RAM, Marzella L. Hyperoxia prolongs the aminoglycoside-induced postantibiotic effect in *Pseudomonas aeruginosa*. Antimicrob Agents Chemother. 1991;35:691-695.
10. Hill GB, Osterhout S. Experimental effects of hyperbaric oxygen on selected clostridial species. I. In vitro studies. J Infect Dis. 1972;125;17-25.
11. Van Unnik AJM. Inhibition of toxin production in *Clostridium perfringens* in vitro by hyperbaric oxygen. Antonie Van Leeuwenhoek. 1965;31:181-186.
12. Kaye D. Effect of hyperbaric oxygen on clostridia in vitro and in vivo. Proc Soc Exp Biol Med. 1967;124:360-366.
13. Prockop DJ, Kivirikko KI, Tuderman L, Guzman NA. The biosynthesis of collagen and its disorders. N Engl J Med. 1979;301:13-23.
14. Hunt TK. The physiology of wound healing. Ann Emerg Med. 1988;17:1265-1273.
15. Hunt TK, Pai MP. The effect of varying ambient oxygen tensions on wound metabolism and collagen synthesis. Surg Gynecol Obstet. 1972;135:561-567.
16. Zamboni WA, Roth AC, Russell RC, et al. The effect of acute hyperbaric oxygen therapy on axial pattern skin flap survival when administered during and after total ischemia. J Reconstr Microsurg. 1989;5:343-347.
17. Thom SR. Leukocytes in carbon monoxide-mediated brain oxidative injury. Toxicol Appl Pharmacol. 1993;123:234-247.
18. Zamboni WA, Roth AC, Russell RC, et al. Morphologic analysis of the microcirculation during perfusion of ischemic skeletal muscle and the effect of hyperbaric oxygen. Plast Reconstr Surg. 1993;91:1110-1123.
19. Korhonen K. Hyperbaric oxygen therapy in acute necrotizing infections. With a special reference to the effects on tissue gas tensions. Ann Chir Gyn Suppl. 2000;214:10-36.
20. Thom SR. Hyperbaric oxygen therapy. J Intensive Care Med. 1989;4:58-74.
21. Tibbles PM, Edelsberg JS. Hyperbaric-oxygen therapy. N Engl J Med. 1996;334:1642-1648.
22. Brown IW, Cox BG, eds. In Vitro and In Vivo Experimental Effects of Hyperbaric Oxygen on *Clostridium perfringens*. Washington DC: National Academy of Science, National Research Council Publication 1404. 1966:538-543.
23. Wada J, Iwa T, eds. The Effect of Hyperbaric Oxygen on the Germination and Toxin Production of *Clostridium perfringens* Spores. Baltimore: Williams & Wilkins; 1969:276-281.
24. Nuckolls JG, Osterhout SS. The effect of hyperbaric oxygen on anaerobic bacteria. Clin Res. 1964;12:244.
25. Brummelkamp WH, Hogendijk J, Boerema I. Treatment of anaerobic infections (clostridial myositis) by drenching the tissues with oxygen under high atmospheric pressure. Surgery. 1961;49:299-302.
26. Glover JL, Mendelson J, Heitkamp DH. Effects of hyperbaric oxygenation on rabbits with *Clostridium perfringens* infection. J Trauma. 1964;4:642-651.
27. Demello FJ, Haglin JJ, Hitchcock CR. Comparative study of experimental *Clostridium perfringens* infection in dogs treated with antibiotics, surgery, and hyperbaric oxygen. Surgery. 1973;73:936-941.
28. Muhvich KH, Anderson LH, Mehm WJ. Evaluation of antimicrobials combined with hyperbaric oxygen in a mouse model of clostridial myonecrosis. J Trauma. 1994;36:7-10.
29. Stevens DL, Bryant AE, Adams K, et al. Evaluation of therapy with hyperbaric oxygen for experimental infection with *Clostridium perfringens*. Clin Infect Dis. 1993;17:231-237.
30. Unsworth IP, Shap PA. Gas gangrene. An 11-year review of 73 cases managed with hyperbaric oxygen. Med J Aust. 1984;1430:256-259.
31. Darke SG, King AM, Slack WK. Gas gangrene and related infection: Classification, clinical features and etiology, managements and mortality. A report of 88 cases. Br J Surg. 1977;64:104-112.
32. Rudge FW. The role of hyperbaric oxygenation in the treatment of clostridial myonecrosis. Mil Med. 1993;158:80-83.
33. Keogh G, Unsworth I, Vowels M, et al. Spontaneous *Clostridium septicum* myonecrosis in congenital neutropenia. Aust N Z J Surg. 1994;64:574-575.
34. Bush GW, Clements RH, Phillips M, et al. *Clostridium perfringens* sepsis with intravascular hemolysis following laparoscopic cholecystectomy: A newly reported complication. Am Surg. 1996;62:326-327.
35. Rich RS, Salluzzo RF. Spontaneous clostridial myonecrosis with abdominal involvement in a nonimmunocompromised patient. Ann Emerg Med. 1993;22:1477-1480.
36. Hitchock CR, Demello FJ, Haglin JJ. Gangrene infection. New approaches to an old disease. Surg Clin North Am. 1975;55:1403-1410.
37. Wang C, Schwaitzberg S, Berliner E, et al. Hyperbaric oxygen for treating wounds. Arch Surg. 2003;138:272-279.
38. Brown RB, Sands M. Infectious disease indications for hyperbaric oxygen therapy. Compr Ther. 1995;21:663-667.
39. Park MK, Muhvich KH, Myers RAM, et al. Effects of hyperbaric oxygen in infectious diseases: Basic mechanisms. In: Kindwall EP, ed. Hyperbaric Medicine Practice. Flagstaff, Ariz: Best; 1994:141-172.
40. Zamboni WA, Mazolewski PJ, Erdmann D, et al. Evaluation of penicillin and hyperbaric oxygen in the treatment of streptococcal myositis. Ann Plast Surg. 1997;39:131-136.
41. Shupack A, Shoshani O, Goldenberg I, et al. Necrotizing fasciitis: An indication for hyperbaric oxygenation therapy? Surgery. 1995;118:873-878.
42. Thom SR, Lauerman MW, Hart GW. Intermittent hyperbaric oxygen therapy for reduction of mortality in experimental polymicrobial sepsis. J Infect Dis. 1986;154:504-510.
43. Park MK, Myers RAM, Marzella L. Oxygen tensions and infection: Modulation of microbial growth, activity of antimicrobial agents, and immunologic responses. Clin Infect Dis. 1992;14:720-740.
44. Hirn M, Niinikoski J, Lehtonen OP. Effect of hyperbaric oxygen and surgery on experimental gas gangrene. Eur Surg Res 1992;24:356-362.
45. Stevens DL, Bryant AE, Adams K, et al. Evaluation of therapy with hyperbaric oxygen for experimental infection with *Clostridium perfringens*. Clin Infect Dis. 1993;17:231-237.
46. Risenman JA, Zamboni WA, Curtis A, et al. Hyperbaric oxygen therapy for necrotizing fasciitis reduced mortality and the need for debridements. Surgery. 1990;108:847-850.
47. Brown DR, Davis Nl. Lepawksy M, et al. A multicenter review of the treatment of major truncal necrotizing infections with and without hyperbaric oxygen therapy. Am J Surg. 1994;167:485-489.
48. Baker DJ. Selected aerobic and anaerobic soft tissue infections-diagnosis and the use of hyperbaric oxygen as an adjunct. In: Kindwall EP, ed. Hyperbaric Medicine Practice. Flagstaff, Ariz: Best; 1994:395-418.
49. Britt M, Calhoun J, Mader TJ, et al. The use of hyperbaric oxygen in the treatment of osteomyelitis. In: Kindwall EP, ed. Hyperbaric Medicine Practice. Flagstaff, Ariz: Best; 1994:419-427.
50. Hampson NB, chairman and editor. Hyperbaric oxygen therapy: 1999 committee report. Kensington, Md: Undersea and Hyperbaric Medical Society; 1999:4.
51. Mader TJ, Guckian JC, Glass DL, et al. Therapy with hyperbaric oxygen for experimental osteomyelitis due to *Staphylococcus aureus* in rabbits. J Infect Dis. 1978;138:312-318.
52. Depenbusch FL, Thompson RE, Hart GB. The use of hyperbaric oxygen in the treatment of refractory osteomyelitis: A preliminary report. J Trauma. 1972;12:807-812.
53. Morrey BF, Dunn JM, Heimback RD, et al. Hypberbaric oxygen and chronic osteomyelitis. Clin Orthop. 1979;144:121-127.
54. Davis JC, Heckman JD, DeLee JC, et al. Chronic non-hematogenous osteomyelitis treated with adjuvant hyperbaric oxygen. J Bone Joint Surg Am. 1986;68:1210-1217.
55. Esterhai JL, Pisarello J, Brighton CT, et al. Adjunctive hyperbaric oxygen therapy in the treatment of chronic refractory osteomyelitis. J Trauma. 1987;27:763-768.
56. Martinez RL, Falero RAP, Cardentey AL, Machin PLV. Contemporary management of spinal osteomyelitis. Neurosurgery. 2000; 46:1024.
57. Petzold, T, Feindt P, Ulrich C, Gams E.: Hyperbaric oxygen therapy in deep sternal wound infection after heart transplantation. Chest. 1999;115(5):1455-1458.
58. Larsson A, Engstrom M, Uusijarvi J, et al. Hyperbaric oxygen treatment of postoperative neurosurgical infections. Neurosurgery. 2002;287-296.
59. Sokol-Anderson ML, Brajtburg J, Medoff G. Amphotherecin-B induced oxidative damage and killing of *Candida albicans*. J Infect Dis. 1986;154:76.
60. Yohai RA, Bullock JD, Aziz AA, et al. Survival factors in rhino-orbital-cerebral mucormycosis. Surv Ophthalmol. 1994;39:3-22.
61. Barratt DM, Meter KV, Asmar P, et al. Hyperbaric oxygen as an adjunct in zygomycosis: Randomized controlled trial in a murine model. Antimicrob Agents Chemo. 2001;45:3601-3602.

62. Bentur Y, Shupak A, Ramon Y, et al. Hyperbaric oxygen therapy for cutaneous/soft-tissue zygomycosis complicating diabetes mellitus. Plast Reconstr Surg. 1998;102:822-824.

63. Garcia-Covarrubias, L, Bartlett R, Barratt DM, Wasserman RJ. Rhino-orbitocerebral mucormycosis attributable to *Apophysomyces elegans* in an immunocompetent individual: Case report and review in the literature. J Trauma Injury Infect Crit Care. 2000;50(2):353-357.

64. Ferguson BJ, Mitchell TG, Moon R, et al. Adjunctive hyperbaric oxygen for treatment of rhinocerebral mucormycosis. Rev Infec Dis. 1988;10(3):551-559.

65. Bell S, Mahoney L. Mucormycosis: A case study. Crit Care Nurse. 2000;20(1):18-23.

66. Reillo MR. Hyperbaric oxygen therapy for the treatment of debilitating fatigue associated with HIV/AIDS. J Assoc Nurses AIDS Care. 1993;4:33-38.

67. Baugh MA. HIV: Reactive oxygen species, enveloped viruses and hyperbaric oxygen. Med Hypotheses. 2000;55(3):232-238.

68. Lampl L, Frey G, Bock KH. Hyperbaric oxygen in intracranial abscesses—Update of a series of 13 patients. Undersea Biomed Res. 1992;19(Suppl):83.

69. Lampl L, Ruhr P, Junz U, et al. Brain abscess management by adjuvant HBO in a pediatric patient—A case report. In: Marroni A, Oriani G, Wattel F, eds. Proceedings of the International Joint Meeting on Hyperbaric and Underwater Medicine (EUBS, ECHM, ICHM, DAN). Milano, Italy: 1996: 401-406.

CHAPTER **41**

Agents Active against Parasites and *Pneumocystis*

RICHARD D. PEARSON

A comprehensive discussion of antiparasitic chemotherapy must take into account the large number of parasites that can infect humans, the complexity of their life cycles, differences in their metabolism, and the wide array of drugs that have been developed to treat them.[1-4]

Taxonomically, parasites are divided into protozoa and helminths. The protozoa are unicellular. Helminths are multicellular and have highly developed neuromuscular systems, digestive tracts, reproductive organs, and integuments. *Pneumocystis jirovecii* is now classified as a fungus, but so many antiparasitic drugs are also useful against it that treatment of pneumocystosis is included in this chapter instead of in the chapter on antifungal agents.

The susceptibility of the parasites to chemotherapeutic agents correlates to some degree with their taxonomy and metabolism (Table 41-1). The parasites can be grouped along those parameters. Protozoa that inhabit the gastrointestinal lumen and vagina form one group. Although they arise from several taxonomic classes, they share a common microenvironment and in many instances have similar metabolic adaptations. Included in this group are amebae of the superclass Rhizopodia, the luminal flagellates of the class Zoomastigophorea, and ciliates of the class Kinetofragminophorea. The second major group includes members of the phylum Apicomplexa. These protozoa are important causes of morbidity and mortality worldwide. They include *Plasmodium* species, which cause malaria; *Babesia* species and the coccidians *Toxoplasma gondii, Cyclospora* species, *Isospora belli,* and *Cryptosporidium parvum;* and the microsporidia *Encephalitozoon intestinalis, Enterocytozoon bieneusi,* and others. The coccidians have emerged as important pathogens in persons with the acquired immunodeficiency syndrome (AIDS). The third group of protozoal pathogens includes flagellates of the class Zoomastigophorea, family Trypanosomatidae. They are arthropod-borne and cause leishmaniasis, Chagas' disease, and human African trypanosomiasis (sleeping sickness).

The susceptibility of helminths also correlates with their taxonomy. The helminths can be divided into nematodes (roundworms), which can be subdivided into those that live in the lumen of the intestine and those that reside in tissue; trematodes (flukes); and cestodes (tapeworms). Chemotherapeutic agents are often active against multiple genera within these groups.

The discussion of antiparasitic drugs that follows is arranged according to these taxonomic groups. Some drugs are active against pathogens in more than one group. This is particularly true for praziquantel, which is active against a broad spectrum of trematodes and

TABLE 41-1 Spectrum of Activity of the Major Antiparasitic and Antipneumocystis Drugs

Drug	*Indications*
***Amoebae, Intestinal and Vaginal Flagellates, and* Balantidium coli**	
Metronidazole	*Entamoeba histolytica* (invasive disease)
	Entamoeba polecki
	Trichomonas vaginalis
	Blastocystis hominis
	Giardia lamblia
	Balantidium coli (alternative)
Tinidazole[†]	*Entamoeba histolytica* (invasive disease)
	Entamoeba polecki
	Trichomonas vaginalis
	Blastocystis hominis
	Giardia lamblia
	Balantidium coli (alternative)
Iodoquinol	*E. histolytica* (luminal infection)
	Dientamoeba fragilis
	B. hominis
	B. coli (alternative)
Nitazoxanide	*Cryptosporidium parvum*
	Giardia lamblia
	Other protozoa and helminths
Diloxanide furoate[†]	*E. histolytica* (asymptomatic and luminal infection)
Paromomycin	*E. histolytica* (asymptomatic and luminal infection)
	D. fragilis
	G. lamblia (alternative)
Furazolidone	*G. lamblia* (alternative)

Drugs without asterisk or dagger are licensed for use in the United States and are available from the manufacturer.
[*]Available from the CDC Drug Service, Centers for Disease Control and Prevention.
[†]Not currently available in the United States.

TABLE 41-1 Spectrum of Activity of the Major Antiparasitic and Antipneumocystis Drugs—cont'd

Drug	Indications
Amoebae, Intestinal and Vaginal Flagellates, and* Balantidium coli, *cont'd	
Tetracycline	*B. coli* *D. fragilis*
Amphotericin B	*Naegleria* spp. (used with miconazole and rifampin) *Leishmania* spp. (liposome-encapsulated amphotericin B is approved for the treatment of visceral leishmaniasis)
Plasmodium spp. (Malaria)	
Chloroquine	Suppressive prophylaxis and treatment of the asexual erythrocytic phase of susceptible *Plasmodium vivax, Plasmodium ovale, Plasmodium malariae,* and susceptible *Plasmodium falciparum*
Primaquine	Radical cure of the exoerythrocytic hypnozoites of *P. vivax* and *P. ovale;* prophylaxis for all *Plasmodium* spp. under special circumstances
Quinine	Treatment of chloroquine-resistant *P. falciparum;* effective against asexual erythrocytic phase of other *Plasmodium* spp.
Quinidine	Treatment of chloroquine-resistant *P. falciparum* when parenteral therapy is required; effective against asexual erythrocytic phase
Mefloquine	Prophylaxis and occasionally treatment of chloroquine-resistant *P. falciparum;* effective against asexual erythrocytic phase of other *Plasmodium* spp.
Atovaquone/proguanil	Used for suppressive prophylaxis and treatment of chloroquine-resistant *P. falciparum* and other *Plasmodium* spp.
Doxycycline	Used alone for suppressive and treatment prophylaxis or with quinine for treatment of chloroquine-resistant *P. falciparum*
Artemisinin derivatives (Qinghaosu)[†]	Treatment of *Plasmodium* spp. in the asexual erythrocytic phase, including chloroquine-resistant *P. falciparum*
Other Apicomplexa (Toxoplasmosis, Isosporiasis, Cyclosporiasis)	
Pyrimethamine plus sulfadiazine	*Toxoplasma gondii*
Trimethoprim-sulfamethoxazole (cotrimoxazole)	*Isospora belli, Pneumocystis jirovecii* *Cyclospora cayatanensis*
Clindamycin	Used with steroids for treatment of ocular *T. gondii* in immunocompetent hosts; used with pyrimethamine for *T. gondii* encephalitis in persons with AIDS who cannot tolerate sulfonamides Used with quinine for treatment of *Babesia* spp. Used with quinine for *P. falciparum* (alternative)
Spiramycin[*]	*T. gondii* during pregnancy and in the neonate
Atovaquone	Used with azithromycin for babesiosis
Pneumocystis jirovecii	
Atovaquone	*P. jirovecii*—treatment of mild to moderate disease (alternative)
Dapsone	*P. jirovecii*—with trimethoprim for treatment of mild to moderate disease (alternative); with or without trimethoprim for prophylaxis Also used for *T. gondii* (with pyrimethamine) and *Mycobacterium leprae*
Trimethoprim-sulfamethoxazole	*P. jirovecii*—treatment or prophylaxis
Pentamadine isethionate	*P. jirovecii*—treatment, IV (alternative); prophylaxis, aerosolized (alternative)
Primaquine and clindamycin	*P. jirovecii*—treatment of mild to moderate disease (alternative)
Members of the Family Trypanosomatidae (Leishmaniasis, Chagas' Disease, African Trypanosomiasis)	
Eflornithine[*]	*Trypanosoma brucei gambiense* (hemolymphatic and late disease with nervous system involvement)
Suramin[*]	*T. b. gambiense* and *Trypanosoma brucei rhodesiense* (hemolymphatic stage)
Melarsoprol B[*]	*T. b. gambiense* and *T. b. rhodesiense* (late disease with central nervous system involvement)
Nifurtimox[*]	*Trypanosoma cruzi*
Benznidazole[†]	*T. cruzi*
Stibogluconate sodium[*]	*Leishmania* spp.
Meglumine antimonate[†]	*Leishmania* spp.
Miltefosine[†]	*Leishmania* spp.
Amphotericin B deoxycholate	*Leishmania* spp. (alternative)
Liposome-encapsulated amphotericin B	Visceral leishmaniasis
Pentamidine isethionate	*T. b. gambiense* and *T. b. rhodesiense* (alternative for use in the hemolymphatic stage) *Leishmania* spp. (alternative)
Helminthic Diseases: Nematodes (Roundworms)	
Albendazole	*Ascaris lumbricoides* *Ancylostoma duodenale* *Necator americanus* *Enterobius vermicularis* *Trichuris trichiura* (alternative) Cutaneous larva migrans Visceral larva migrans (alternative) *Gnathostoma spinigerum* *Trichostrongylus* spp. (alternative) *Capillaria philippinensis* (alternative)

Continued

TABLE 41-1 Spectrum of Activity of the Major Antiparasitic and Antipneumocystis Drugs—cont'd

Drug	*Indications*
Helminthic Diseases: Nematodes (Roundworms), cont'd	
Mebendazole	*A. lumbricoides*
	A. duodenale
	N. americanus
	T. trichiura
	E. vermicularis
	C. philippinensis
	Moniliformis moniliformis (alternative)
	Mansonella perstans
	Angiostrongylus cantonensis
	Trichostrongylus spp. (alternative)
	Trichinella spiralis (recommended by some; used with steroids)
	Visceral larva migrans (alternative)
Pyrantel pamoate	*E. vermicularis*
	A. lumbricoides
	A. duodenale
	N. americanus
	Trichostrongylus spp.
Diethylcarbamazine	*Wuchereria bancrofti*
	Brugia malayi
	Mansonella streptocerca
	Loa loa
	Tropical eosinophilia
	Visceral larva migrans
Ivermectin	*Onchocerca volvulus*
	Strongyloides stercoralis
	Cutaneous larva migrans
	M. streptocerca
	Mansonella ozzardi
	Scabies
Metronidazole	*Dracunculus medinensis*
Nitazoxanide	Preliminary data suggest activity against a number of intestinal nematodis
Helminthic Diseases: Trematodes (Flukes) and Cestodes (Tapeworms)	
Praziquantel	*Schistosoma* spp.
	Clonorchis sinensis
	Opisthorchis viverrini
	Paragonimus westermani
	Fasciolopsis buski
	Heterophyes heterophyes
	Metagonimus yokogawai
	Metorchis conjunctus
	Nanophyetus salmincola
	Taenia solium (adult worm and cysticercosis)
	Taenia saginata
	Diphyllobothrium latum
	Hymenolepis nana
	Dipylidium caninum
Bithionol	*Fasciola hepatica*
	P. westermani (alternative), other *Paragonimus* spp.
Niclosamide[†]	*D. latum*
	T. saginata
	T. solium (adult stage, alternative)
	Hymenolepis nana (alternative)
	D. caninum
Albendazole	Cysticercosis
	Echinococcus granulosus
	Echinococcus multilocularis
	C. sinensis
Nitazoxanide	Preliminary data suggest activity against some cestodes

Drugs without asterisk or dagger are licensed for use in the United States and are available from the manufacturer.
[*]Available from the CDC Drug Service, Centers for Disease Control and Prevention.
[†]Not currently available in the United States.

cestodes; albendazole, with activity against nematodes and larval cestodes; ivermectin, with activity against many nematodes as well as blood-sucking arthropods; and nitazoxanide, which is active against a number of protozoa and helminthes that reside in the gastrointestinal tract. Drugs that have a broad spectrum of activity are discussed in the context of their primary indications.

The dosage and duration of therapy for specific parasitic diseases as recommended by the *Medical Letter on Drugs and Therapeutics*[5]

and adverse effects of some antiparasitic drugs are provided in Tables 41-2 and 41-3, respectively. Not all of these drugs are licensed or available through pharmacies in the United States. Some (marked with an asterisk) can be obtained only from the manufacturer or from the Drug Service at the Centers for Disease Control and Prevention (CDC), Atlanta, Georgia. Others (marked with a dagger) are not available in the United States but are discussed because they are used elsewhere in the world or hold promise for the future.

Text continues on page 582

TABLE 41-2 Drugs for Treatment of Parasitic Infections and Pneumocystosis

Infection	Drug	Adult Dosage	Pediatric Dosage
Acanthamoeba *keratitis*			
Drug of choice:	See footnote 1		
AMEBIASIS *(Entamoeba histolytica)*			
		Asymptomatic	
Drug of choice:	Iodoquinol	650 mg tid × 20 days	30-40 mg/kg/day (max. 2 g) in 3 doses × 20 days
OR	Paromomycin	25-35 mg/kg/day in 3 doses × 7 days	25-35 mg/kg/day in 3 doses × 7 days
Alternative:	Diloxanide furoate[2]	500 mg tid × 10 days	20 mg/kg/day in 3 doses × 10 days
Mild to moderate intestinal disease[3]			
Drug of choice:[4,**]	Metronidazole	500-750 mg tid × 7-10 days	35-50 mg/kg/day in 3 doses × 7-10 days
OR	Tinidazole[5]	2 g/day divided tid × 3 days	50 mg/kg (max. 2 g) qd × 3 days
Severe intestinal and extraintestinal disease[3]			
Drug of choice:	Metronidazole	750 mg tid × 7-10 days	35-50 mg/kg/day in 3 doses × 7-10 days
OR	Tinidazole[5,*]	800 mg tid × 5 days	60 mg/kg/day (max. 2 g) × 5 days
AMEBIC MENINGOENCEPHALITIS, PRIMARY			
Naegleria			
Drug of choice:	Amphotericin B[6,7]	1 mg/kg/day IV, uncertain duration	1 mg/kg/day IV, uncertain duration
Acanthamoeba			
Drug of choice:	See footnote 8		
Balamuthia mandrillaris			
Drug of choice:	See footnote 9		
Sappinia diploidea			
Drug of choice:	See footnote 10		
***ANCYLOSTOMA** caninum (Eosinophilic enterocolitis)*			
Drug of choice:	Albendazole[7]	400 mg once	400 mg once
OR	Mebendazole	100 mg bid × 3 days	100 mg bid × 3 days
OR	Pyrantel pamoate[7]	11 mg/kg (max. 1 g) × 3 days	11 mg/kg (max. 1 g) × 3 days
Ancylostoma duodenale, see **HOOKWORM**			
ANGIOSTRONGYLIASIS			
Angiostrongylus cantonensis			
Drug of choice:	See footnote 11		
Angiostrongylus costaricensis			
Drug of choice:	See footnote 12		
ANISAKIASIS *(Anisakis)*			
Treatment of choice:	Surgical or endoscopic removal		
ASCARIASIS *(Ascaris lumbricoides,* **roundworm***)*			
Drug of choice:	Albendazole[7]	400 mg once	400 mg once
OR	Mebendazole	100 mg bid × 3 days or 500 mg once	100 mg bid × 3 days or 500 mg once
OR	Pyrantel pamoate[7]	11 mg/kg once (max. 1 g)	11 mg/kg once (max. 1 g)
BABESIOSIS *(Babesia microti)*			
Drugs of choice:[13]	Clindamycin[7]	1.2 g bid IV or 600 mg tid PO × 7-10 days	20-40 mg/kg/day PO in 3 doses × 7 days
	plus quinine	650 mg tid PO × 7 days	25 mg/kg/day PO in 3 doses × 7 days
OR	Atovaquone[7]	750 mg bid × 7-10 days	20 mg/kg bid × 7-10 days
	plus azithromycin[7]	600 mg PO daily × 7-10 days	12 mg/kg daily × 7-10 days
Balamuthia mandrillaris, see **AMEBIC MENINGOENCEPHALITIS, PRIMARY**			
BALANTIDIASIS *(Balantidium coli)*			
Drug of choice:	Tetracycline[7,14]	500 mg qid × 10 days	40 mg/kg/day (max. 2 g) in 4 doses × 10 days
Alternative:	Metronidazole[7]	750 mg tid × 5 days	35-50 mg/kg/day in 3 doses × 5 days
OR	Iodoquinol[7]	650 mg tid × 20 days	40 mg/kg/day in 3 doses × 20 days
BAYLISASCARIASIS *(Baylisascaris procyonis)*			
Drug of choice:	See footnote 15		
***BLASTOCYSTIS** hominis infection*			
Drug of choice:	See footnote 16		
CAPILLARIASIS *(Capillaria philippinensis)*			
Drug of choice:	Mebendazole[7]	200 mg bid × 20 days	200 mg bid × 20 days
Alternatives:	Albendazole[7]	400 mg daily × 10 days	400 mg daily × 10 days
Chagas' disease, see **TRYPANOSOMIASIS**			
Clonorchis sinensis, see **FLUKE infection**			
CRYPTOSPORIDIOSIS *(Cryptosporidium)*			
Drug of choice:	Nitazoxanide[17,**]	500 mg bid × 3 days	Ages 1-3 yr: 100 mg bid × 3 days Ages 4-11 yr: 200 mg bid × 3 days
CUTANEOUS LARVA MIGRANS *(creeping eruption, dog and cat hookworm)*			
Drug of choice:[18]	Albendazole[7]	400 mg daily × 3 days	400 mg daily × 3 days
OR	Ivermectin[7]	200 µg/kg daily × 1-2 days	200 µg/kg daily × 1-2 days
OR	Thiabendazole	Topically	Topically

*Availability problems. See Table 41-3.

**Recommendations modified from Med Lett Drugs Ther 2002, on the basis of recent information.

Continued

TABLE 41-2 Drugs for Treatment of Parasitic Infections and Pneumocystosis—cont'd

Infection	Drug	Adult Dosage	Pediatric Dosage
CYCLOSPORA infection			
Drug of choice:[19]	Trimethoprim (TMP)-sulfamethoxazole (SMX)[7]	TMP 160 mg, SMX 800 mg bid × 7-10 days	TMP 5 mg/kg, SMX 25 mg/kg bid × 7-10 days
CYSTICERCOSIS, see TAPEWORM infection			
DIENTAMOEBA fragilis infection			
Drug of choice:	Iodoquinol	650 mg tid × 20 days	30-40 mg/kg/days (max. 2 g) in 3 doses × 20 days
OR	Paromomycin[7]	25-35 mg/kg/day in 3 doses × 7 days	25-35 mg/kg/days in 3 doses × 7 days
OR	Tetracycline[7,14]	500 mg qid × 10 days	40 mg/kg/days (max. 2 g) in 4 doses × 10 days
OR	Metronidazole	500-750 mg tid × 10 days	20-40 mg/kg/days in 3 doses × 10 days
Diphyllobothrium latum, see TAPEWORM infection			
DRACUNCULUS medinensis (guinea worm) infection			
Drug of choice:	Metronidazole[7,20]	250 mg tid × 10 days	25 mg/kg/days (max. 750 mg) in 3 doses × 10 days
Echinococcus, see TAPEWORM infection			
Entamoeba histolytica, see AMEBIASIS			
ENTAMOEBA polecki infection			
Drug of choice:	Metronidazole[7]	750 mg tid × 10 days	35-50 mg/kg/day in 3 doses × 10 days
ENTEROBIUS vermicularis (pinworm) infection			
Drug of choice:[21]	Pyrantel pamoate	11 mg/kg base once (max. 1 g); repeat in 2 wk	11 mg/kg base once (max. 1 g); repeat in 2 wk
OR	Mebendazole	100 mg once; repeat in 2 wk	100 mg once; repeat in 2 wk
OR	Albendazole[7]	400 mg once; repeat in 2 wk	400 mg once; repeat in 2 wk
Fasciola hepatica, see FLUKE infection			
FILARIASIS[22]			
Wuchereria bancrofti, Brugia malayi, Brugia timori			
Drug of choice:[23,24]	Diethyl-carbamazine[25,*]	Day 1: 50 mg, PC Day 2: 50 mg tid Day 3: 100 mg tid Days 4 through 14: 6 mg/kg/day in 3 doses	Day 1: 1 mg/kg PC Day 2: 1 mg/kg tid Day 3: 1-2 mg/kg tid Days 4 through 14: 6 mg/kg/day in 3 doses
Loa loa			
Drug of choice:[24,26]	Diethyl-carbamazine[25,*]	Day 1: 50 mg PC Day 2: 50 mg tid Day 3: 100 mg tid Days 4 through 21: 9 mg/kg/day in 3 doses	Day 1: 1 mg/kg PC Day 2: 1 mg/kg tid Day 3: 1-2 mg/kg tid Days 4 through 21: 9 mg/kg/day in 3 doses
Mansonella ozzardi			
Drug of choice:[24]	See footnote 27		
Mansonella perstans			
Drug of choice:[24]	Mebendazole[7]	100 mg bid × 30 days	100 mg bid × 30 days
OR	Albendazole[7]	400 mg bid × 10 days	400 mg bid × 10 days
Mansonella streptocerca			
Drug of choice:[24,28]	Diethylcarbamazine*	6 mg/kg/day × 14 days	6 mg/kg/day × 14 days
OR	Ivermectin[7]	150 µg/kg once	150 µg/kg once
Tropical pulmonary eosinophilia (TPE)			
Drug of choice:	Diethylcarbamazine*	6 mg/kg/day in 3 doses × 21 days	6 mg/kg/day in 3 doses × 21 days
Onchocerca volvulus (River blindness)			
Drug of choice:	Ivermectin[29]	150 µg/kg once, repeated every 6 to 12 mo until asymptomatic	150 µg/kg once, repeated every 6 to 12 mo until asymptomatic
FLUKE, hermaphroditic, infection			
Clonorchis sinensis (Chinese liver fluke)			
Drug of choice:	Praziquantel	75 mg/kg/day in 3 doses × 1 day	75 mg/kg/day in 3 doses × 1 day
OR	Albendazole[7]	10 mg/kg × 7 days	10 mg/kg × 7 days
Fasciola hepatica (sheep liver fluke)			
Drug of choice:[30]	Triclabendazole*	10 mg/kg once	10 mg/kg once
Alternative:	Bithionol*	30-50 mg/kg on alternate days × 10-15 doses	30-50 mg/kg on alternate days × 10-15 doses
Fasciolopsis buski, Heterophyes heterophyes, Metagonimus yokogawai (intestinal flukes)			
Drug of choice:	Praziquantel[7]	75 mg/kg/day in 3 doses × 1 day	75 mg/kg/day in 3 doses × 1 day
Metorchis conjunctus (North American liver fluke)[31]			
Drug of choice:	Praziquantel[7]	75 mg/kg/day in 3 doses × 1 day	75 mg/kg/day in 3 doses × 1 day
Nanophyetus salmincola			
Drug of choice:	Praziquantel[7]	60 mg/kg/day in 3 doses × 1 day	60 mg/kg/day in 3 doses × 1 day
Opisthorchis viverrini (Southeast Asian liver fluke)			
Drug of choice:	Praziquantel	75 mg/kg/day in 3 doses × 1 day	75 mg/kg/day in 3 doses × 1 day
Paragonimus westermani (lung fluke)			
Drug of choice:	Praziquantel[7]	75 mg/kg/day in 3 doses × 2 days	75 mg/kg/day in 3 doses × 2 days
Alternative:[32]	Bithionol*	30-50 mg/kg on alternate days × 10-15 doses	30-50 mg/kg on alternate days × 10-15 doses

*Availability problems. See Table 41-3.

**Recommendations modified from Med Lett Drugs Ther 2002, on the basis of recent information.

TABLE 41-2 Drugs for Treatment of Parasitic Infections and Pneumocystosis—cont'd

Infection	Drug	Adult Dosage	Pediatric Dosage
GIARDIASIS (*Giardia lamblia*)			
Drug of choice:	Metronidazole[7]	250 mg tid × 5 days	15 mg/kg/day in 3 doses × 5 days
Alternatives:[33]	Quinacrine[2]	100 mg tid × 5 days (max. 300 mg/day)	2 mg/kg tid × 5 days (max. 300 mg/day)
OR	Tinidazole[5]	2 g once	50 mg/kg once (max. 2 g)
OR	Furazolidone	100 mg qid × 7-10 days	6 mg/kg/day in 4 doses × 7-10 days
OR	Paromomycin[7,34]	25-35 mg/kg/day in 3 doses × 7 days	25-35 mg/kg/day in 3 doses × 7 days
OR	Nitazoxanide[17,**]	500 mg bid × 3 days	Ages 1-3 yr: 100 mg bid × 3 days
			Ages 4-11 yr: 200 mg bid × 3 days
GNATHOSTOMIASIS (*Gnathostoma spinigerum*)			
Treatment of choice:[35]	Albendazole[7]	400 mg bid × 21 days	400 mg bid × 21 days
OR	Ivermectin[7]	200 μg/kg/day × 2 days	200 μg/kg/day × 2 days
OR	Surgical removal		
GONGYLONEMIASIS (*Gongylonema* spp.)			
Treatment of choice:	Surgical removal		
OR	Albendazole[7,36]	10 mg/kg/day × 3 days	10 mg/kg/day × 3 days
HOOKWORM infection (*Ancylostoma duodenale, Necator americanus*)			
Drug of choice:	Albendazole[7]	400 mg once	400 mg once
OR	Mebendazole	100 mg bid × 3 days or 500 mg once	100 mg bid × 3 days or 500 mg once
OR	Pyrantel pamoate[7]	11 mg/kg (max. 1 g) × 3 days	11 mg/kg (max. 1 g) × 3 days
Hydatid cyst, see TAPEWORM infection			
***Hymenolepis nana,* see TAPEWORM infection**			
ISOSPORIASIS (*Isospora belli*)			
Drug of choice:[37]	Trimethoprim-sulfamethoxazole[7]	TMP 160 mg, SMX 800 mg bid × 10 days	TMP 5 mg/kg, SMX 25 mg/kg bid × 10 days
LEISHMANIASIS[38]			
Drug of choice:[39]	Liposomal amphotericin B[39]	3 mg/kg/day on days 1-5, 14, 21[40]	3 mg/kg/day on days 1-5, 14, 21[40]
OR	Sodium stibogluconate*	20 mg Sb/kg/day IV or IM × 20-28 days[41]	20 mg Sb/kg/day IV or IM × 20-28 days[41]
OR	Meglumine antimoniate*	20 mg Sb/kg/day IV or IM × 20-28 days[41]	20 mg Sb/kg/day IV or IM × 20-28 days[41]
OR	Amphotericin B[7]	0.5 to 1 mg/kg IV daily or every 2 days for up to 8 wk	0.5 to 1 mg/kg IV daily or every 2 days for up to 8 wk
OR	Miltefosine[42,**]	100 mg/day for 4 wk	Ages 2-11 yrs: 2.5 mg/kg/day for 4 wk
Alternative:	Pentamidine	2-4 mg/kg daily or every 2 days IV or IM for up to 15 doses[43]	2-4 mg/kg daily or every 2 days IV or IM for up to 15 doses[43]
OR	Paromomycin[44,*]	Topically 2×/day × 10-20 days	Topically bid × 10-20 days
LICE infestation (*Pediculus humanus, Pediculus capitis, Phthirus pubis*)[45]			
Drug of choice:	1% Permethrin[46]	Topically	Topically
OR	0.5% Malathion[47]	Topically	Topically
Alternatives:	Pyrethrins with piperonyl butoxide[46]	Topically	Topically
OR	Ivermectin[7,48]	200 μg/kg once	200 μg/kg once
***Loa loa,* see FILARIASIS**			
MALARIA, Treatment of (*Plasmodium falciparum, Plasmodium ovale, Plasmodium vivax*, and *Plasmodium malariae*)			
Chloroquine-resistant *P. falciparum*[49]			
		ORAL	
Drugs of choice:	Quinine sulfate	650 mg q8h × 3-7 days[50]	25 mg/kg/day in 3 doses × 3-7 days[50]
	plus doxycycline[7,14]	100 mg bid × 7 days	2 mg/kg/day × 7 days
	or plus tetracycline[7,14]	250 mg qid × 7 days	6.25 mg/kg qid × 7 days
	or plus pyrimethamine-sulfadoxine[51]	3 tablets at once on last day of quinine	On last days of quinine: <1 yr: ¼ tablet 1-3 yrs: ½ tablet 4-8 yrs: 1 tablet 9-14 yrs: 2 tablets
	or plus clindamycin[7,52]	900 mg tid × 5 days	20-40 mg/kg/day in 3 doses × 5 days
OR	Atovaquone/proguanil[53]	4 adult tablets/day × 3 days	11-20 kg: 1 adult tablet/day × 3 days 21-30 kg: 2 adult tablets/day × 3 days 31-40 kg: 3 adult tablets/day × 3 days >40 kg: 4 adult tablets/day × 3 days
Alternatives:[54]	Mefloquine[55,56]	750 mg followed by 500 mg 12 hr later	<45 kg: 15 mg/kg PO followed by 10 mg/kg PO 8-12 hr later
OR	Halofantrine[57*,58**]		
OR	Artesunate[59*]	4 mg/kg/day × 3 days	—
	plus mefloquine[55,56]	750 mg followed by 500 mg 12 hr later	15 mg/kg followed by 10 mg/kg 8-12 hr later
Chloroquine-resistant *P. vivax*[60]			
Drugs of choice:	Quinine sulfate	650 mg q8h × 3-7 days[50]	25 mg/kg/day in 3 doses × 3-7 days[50]
	plus doxycycline[7,14]	100 mg bid × 7 days	2 mg/kg/day × 7 days
OR	Mefloquine[55,56]	750 mg followed by 500 mg 12 hr later	15 mg/kg followed by 10 mg/kg 8-12 hr later
Alternatives:	Halofantrine[57,61,*,**]		
OR	Chloroquine	25 mg base/kg in 3 doses over 48 hr	—
	plus primaquine[62]	2.5 mg base/kg in 3 doses over 48 hr	—

*Availability problems. See Table 41-3.
**Recommendations modified from Med Lett Drugs Ther 2002, on the basis of recent information.

Continued

TABLE 41-2   Drugs for Treatment of Parasitic Infections and Pneumocystosis—cont'd

Infection	Drug	Adult Dosage	Pediatric Dosage
MALARIA, treatment of, cont'd			
All *Plasmodium* except chloroquine-resistant *P. falciparum*[49] and chloroquine-resistant *P. vivax*[60]			
Drug of choice:	Chloroquine phosphate[63]	1 g (600 mg base), then 500 mg (300 mg base) 6 hr later, then 500 mg (300 mg base) at 24 and 48 hr	10 mg base/kg (max. 600 mg base), then 5 mg base/kg 6 hr later, then 5 mg base/kg at 24 and 48 hr
All *Plasmodium* PARENTERAL			
Drug of choice:[64]	Quinidine gluconate[65]	10 mg/kg loading dose (max. 600 mg) in normal saline slowly over 1-2 hr, followed by continuous infusion of 0.02 mg/kg/min until oral therapy can be started	10 mg/kg loading dose (max. 600 mg) in normal saline slowly over 1-2 hr, followed by continuous infusion of 0.02 mg/kg/min until oral therapy can be started
OR	Quinine dihydrochloride[65]	20 mg/kg loading dose IV in 5% dextrose over 4 hr, followed by 10 mg/kg over 2-4 hr q8h (max. 1800 mg/day) until oral therapy can be started	20 mg/kg loading dose IV in 5% dextrose over 4 hr, followed by 10 mg/kg over 2-4 hr q8h (max. 1800 mg/day) until oral therapy can be started
Alternative:	Artemether[66,*]	3.2 mg/kg IM, then 1.6 mg/kg daily × 5-7 days	3.2 mg/kg IM, then 1.6 mg/kg daily × 5-7 days
Prevention of relapses: *P. vivax* and *P. ovale* only			
Drug of choice:	Primaquine phosphate[62,67]	26.3 mg (15 mg base)/day × 14 days or 79 mg (45 mg base)/wk × 8 wk	0.3 mg base/kg/day × 14 days
MALARIA, Prevention of[68]			
Chloroquine-sensitive areas[49]			
Drug of choice:	Chloroquine phosphate[69,70]	500 mg (300 mg base) once/wk[71]	5 mg/kg base once/wk, up to adult dose of 300 mg base[71]
Chloroquine-resistant areas[49]			
Drug of choice:	Mefloquine[56,70,72]	250 mg once/wk[71]	Once/wk: <15 kg: 5 mg/kg[71] 15-19 kg: ¼ tablet[71] 20-30 kg: ½ tablet[71] 31-45 kg: ¾ tablet[71] >45 kg: 1 tablet[71]
OR	Doxycycline[7,70]	100 mg daily[73]	2 mg/kg/days, up to 100 mg/day[73]
OR	Atovaquone/ proguanil[53,70]	250 mg/100 mg (1 adult tablet) daily[74]	*Daily:* 11-20 kg: 62.5 mg/25 mg[53,74] 21-30 kg: 125 mg/50 mg[53,74] 31-40 kg: 187.5 mg/75 mg[53,74] >40 kg: 250 mg/100 mg[53,74]
Alternatives:	Primaquine[7,62,75]	30 mg base daily	0.5 mg/kg base daily
OR	Chloroquine phosphate	500 mg (300 mg base) once/wk[71]	5 mg/kg base once/wk, up to adult dose of 300 mg base[71]
plus proguanil[76]		200 mg once/day	<2 yrs: 50 mg once/day 2-6 yrs: 100 mg once/day 7-10 yrs: 150 mg once/day >10 yrs: 200 mg once/day
Presumptive treatment			
Drug of choice:	Atovaquone/ proguanil[53]	4 adult tablets/day × 3 days[74]	11-20 kg: 1 adult tablet/day × 3 days[74] 21-30 kg: 2 adult tablets/day × 3 days[74] 31-40 kg: 3 adult tablets/day × 3 days[74] 4 adult tablets/day × 3 days[74]
OR	Pyrimethamine-sulfadoxine[51]	Carry a single dose (3 tablets) for self treatment of febrile illness when medical care is not immediately available	<1 yr: ¼ tablet 1-3 yrs: ½ tablet 4-8 yrs: 1 tablet 9-14 yrs: 2 tablets
MICROSPORIDIOSIS			
Ocular (*Encephalitozoon hellem, Encephalitozoon cuniculi, Vittaforma corneae [Nosema corneum]*)			
Drugs of choice:	Albendazole[7]	400 mg bid	—
plus	Fumagillin[77,*]	—	—
Intestinal (*Enterocytozoon bieneusi, Encephalitozoon [Septata] intestinalis*)			
E. bieneusi[78]			
Drug of choice:	Fumagillin*	60 mg/day PO × 14 days	—
E. intestinalis			
Drug of choice:	Albendazole[7]	400 mg bid × 21 days	—
Disseminated (*E. hellem, E. cuniculi, E. intestinalis, Pleistophora* sp., *Trachipleistophora* spp., and *Brachiola vesicularum*)			
Drug of choice:[79]	Albendazole[7]	400 mg bid	
Mites, see SCABIES			
MONILIFORMIS moniliformis infection			
Drug of choice:	Pyrantel pamoate[7]	11 mg/kg once, repeat twice, 2 wk apart	11 mg/kg once, repeat twice, 2 wk apart

*Availability problems. See Table 41-3.
**Recommendations modified from Med Lett Drugs Ther 2002, on the basis of recent information.

TABLE 41-2 Drugs for Treatment of Parasitic Infections and Pneumocystosis—cont'd

Infection	Drug	Adult Dosage	Pediatric Dosage
Naegleria species, see AMEBIC MENINGOENCEPHALITIS, PRIMARY			
Necator americanus, see HOOKWORM infection			
OESOPHAGOSTOMUM bifurcum			
Drug of choice:	See footnote 80		
Onchocerca volvulus, see FILARIASIS			
Opisthorchis viverrini, see FLUKE infection			
Paragonimus westermani, see FLUKE infection			
Pediculus capitis, P. humanus, Phthirus pubis, see LICE			
Pinworm, see *ENTEROBIUS*			
PNEUMOCYSTIS jirovecii pneumonia (PCP)[81]			
Drug of choice:	Trimethoprim-sulfamethoxazole	TMP 15 mg/kg/day, SMX 75 mg/kg/day, oral or IV in 3 or 4 doses × 14-21 days	TMP 15 mg/kg/day, SMX 75 mg/kg/day, oral or IV in 3 or 4 doses × 14-21 days
Alternatives:	Primaquine[7,62]	30 mg base PO daily × 21 days	—
	plus clindamycin[7]	600 mg IV q6h × 21 days, or 300-450 mg PO q6h × 21 days	—
OR	Trimethoprim[7]	5 mg/kg PO tid × 21 days	—
	plus dapsone[7]	100 mg PO daily × 21 days	—
OR	Pentamidine	3-4 mg/kg IV daily × 14-21 days	3-4 mg/kg IV daily × 14-21 days
OR	Atovaquone	750 mg bid PO × 21 days	
Primary and secondary prophylaxis[82]			
Drug of choice:	Trimethoprim-sulfamethoxazole	1 tablet (single or double strength) daily	TMP 150 mg/m², SMX 750 mg/m² in 2 doses on 3 consecutive days per wk
Alternatives:[83]	Dapsone[7]	50 mg bid or 100 mg daily	2 mg/kg (max. 100 mg) daily or 4 mg/kg (max. 200) mg each wk
OR	Dapsone[7]	50 mg daily or 200 mg each wk	—
	plus pyrimethamine[84]	50 mg or 75 mg each wk	—
OR	Pentamidine aerosol	300 mg inhaled monthly via Respirgard II nebulizer	≥5 yrs: 300 mg inhaled monthly via Respirgard II nebulizer
OR	Atovaquone[7]	1500 mg daily	—
Roundworm, see ASCARIASIS			
Sappinia diploidea, See AMEBIC MENINGOENCEPHALITIS, PRIMARY			
SCABIES *(Sarcoptes scabiei)*			
Drug of choice:	5% Permethrin	Topically	Topically
Alternatives:	Ivermectin[7,85]	200 μg/kg PO once	200 μg/kg PO once
OR	10% Crotamiton	Topically once/days × 2 days	Topically once/day × 2 days
SCHISTOSOMIASIS (Bilharziasis)			
Schistosoma haematobium			
Drug of choice:	Praziquantel	40 mg/kg/day in 2 doses × 1 day	40 mg/kg/day in 2 doses × 1 day
S. japonicum			
Drug of choice:	Praziquantel	60 mg/kg/day in 3 doses × 1 day	60 mg/kg/day in 3 doses × 1 day
S. mansoni			
Drug of choice:	Praziquantel	40 mg/kg/day in 2 doses × 1 day	40 mg/kg/day in 2 doses × 1 day
Alternative:	Oxamniquine[86]	15 mg/kg once[87]	20 mg/kg/day in 2 doses × 1 day[87]
S. mekongi			
Drug of choice:	Praziquantel	60 mg/kg/day in 3 doses × 1 day	60 mg/kg/day in 3 doses × 1 day
Sleeping sickness, see TRYPANOSOMIASIS			
STRONGYLOIDIASIS *(Strongyloides stercoralis)*			
Drug of choice:[88]	Ivermectin 200 μg/kg/day × 1-2 days	200 μg/kg/day × 1-2 days	200 μg/kg/day × 1-2 days
Alternative:	Thiabendazole	50 mg/kg/day in 2 doses (max. 3 g/day) × 2 days[89]	50 mg/kg/day in 2 doses (max. 3 g/day) × 2 days[89]
TAPEWORM infection			
Adult (intestinal stage)			
Diphyllobothrium latum (fish), *Taenia saginata* (beef), *Taenia solium* (pork), *Dipylidium caninum* (dog)			
Drug of choice:	Praziquantel[7]	5-10 mg/kg once	5-10 mg/kg once
Alternative:	Niclosamide	2 g once	50 mg/kg once
Hymenolepis nana (dwarf tapeworm)			
Drug of choice:	Praziquantel[7]	25 mg/kg once	25 mg/kg once
Larval (tissue stage)			
Echinococcus granulosus (hydatid cyst)			
Drug of choice:[90]	Albendazole	400 mg bid × 1-6 mo	15 mg/kg/day (max. 800 mg) × 1-6 mo
Echinococcus multilocularis			
Treatment of choice:	See footnote 91		
Cysticercus cellulosae (cysticercosis)			
Treatment of choice:	See footnote 92		
Alternatives:	Albendazole	400 mg bid × 8-30 days; can be repeated as necessary	15 mg/kg/day (max. 800 mg) in 2 doses × 8-30 days; can be repeated as necessary
OR	Praziquantel[7]	50-100 mg/kg/day in 3 doses × 30 days	50-100 mg/kg/day in 3 doses × 30 days

*Availability problems. See Table 41-3.

**Recommendations modified from Med Lett Drugs Ther 2002, on the basis of recent information.

Continued

TABLE 41-2 Drugs for Treatment of Parasitic Infections and Pneumocystosis—cont'd

Infection	Drug	Adult Dosage	Pediatric Dosage
Toxocariasis, see VISCERAL LARVA MIGRANS			
TOXOPLASMOSIS (Toxoplasma gondii)[93]			
Drugs of choice:[94]	Pyrimethamine[95]	25-100 mg/day × 3-4 wk	2 mg/kg/day × 3 days (max. 25 mg/days) × 4 wk[96]
	plus sulfadiazine	1-1.5 g qid × 3-4 wk	100-200 mg/kg/day × 3-4 wk
Alternative:[97]	Spiramycin*	3-4 g/day × 3-4 wk	50-100 mg/kg/day × 3-4 wk
TRICHINOSIS (Trichinella spiralis)			
Drugs of choice:	Steroids for severe symptoms		
	plus mebendazole[7]	200-400 mg tid × 3 days, then 400-500 mg tid × 10 days	200-400 mg tid × 3 days, then 400-500 mg tid × 10 days
Alternative:	Albendazole[7]	400 mg bid × 8-14 days	400 mg bid × 8-14 days
TRICHOMONIASIS (Trichomonas vaginalis)			
Drug of choice:[98]	Metronidazole	2 g once or 500 mg bid × 7 days	15 mg/kg/day orally in 3 doses × 7 days
OR	Tinidazole[5,*]	2 g once	50 mg/kg once (max. 2 g)
TRICHOSTRONGYLUS infection			
Drug of choice:	Pyrantel pamoate[7]	11 mg/kg base once (max. 1 g)	11 mg/kg once (max. 1 g)
Alternatives:	Mebendazole[7]	100 mg bid × 3 days	100 mg bid × 3 days
OR	Albendazole[7]	400 mg once	400 mg once
TRICHURIASIS (Trichuris trichiura, whipworm)			
Drug of choice:	Mebendazole	100 mg bid × 3 days or 500 mg once	100 mg bid × 3 days or 500 mg once
Alternative:	Albendazole[7]	400 mg × 3 days	400 mg × 3 days
TRYPANOSOMIASIS			
Trypanosoma cruzi **(American trypanosomiasis, Chagas' disease)**			
Drug of choice:	Benznidazole*	5-7 mg/kg/day in 2 divided doses × 30-90 days	Up to 12 yrs: 10 mg/kg/day in 2 doses × 30-90 days
OR	Nifurtimox[99,*]	8-10 mg/kg/day in 3-4 doses × 90-120 days	1-10 yrs: 15-20 mg/kg/day in 4 doses × 90 days; 11-16 yrs: 12.5-15 mg/kg/day in 4 doses × 90 days
T. brucei gambiense **(West African trypanosomiasis, sleeping sickness)**			
Hemolymphatic stage			
Drug of choice:[100]	Pentamidine isethionate[7]	4 mg/kg/day IM × 10 days	4 mg/kg/day IM × 10 days
Alternatives:	Suramin*	100-200 mg (test dose) IV, then 1 g IV on days 1, 3, 7, 14, and 21	20 mg/kg on days 1, 3, 7, 14, and 21
OR	Eflornithine*	See footnote 101	
T. b. rhodesiense **(East African trypanosomiasis, sleeping sickness)**			
Hemolymphatic stage			
Drug of choice:	Suramin*	100-200 mg (test dose) IV, then 1 g IV on days 1, 3, 7, 14, and 21	20 mg/kg on days 1, 3, 7, 14, and 21
Late-stage disease with CNS involvement (T.b. gambiense or T.b. rhodesiense)			
Drug of choice:	Melarsoprol[102,*]	2-3.6 mg/kg/day IV × 3 days; after 1 wk, 3.6 mg/kg/day IV × 3 days; repeat again after 10-21 days	18-25 mg/kg total over 1 mo; initial dose of 0.36 mg/kg IV, increasing gradually to max. 3.6 mg/kg at intervals of 1-5 days for total of 9-10 doses
OR	Eflornithine	See footnote 101	
VISCERAL LARVA MIGRANS[103] (Toxocariasis)			
Drug of choice:	Albendazole[7]	400 mg bid × 5 days	400 mg bid × 5 days
OR	Mebendazole[7]	100-200 mg bid × 5 days	100-200 mg bid × 5 days
Whipworm, see TRICHURIASIS			
***Wuchereria bancrofti*, see FILARIASIS**			

*Availability problems. See Table 41-3.

**Recommendations modified from Med Lett Drugs Ther 2002, on the basis of recent information.

1. For treatment of keratitis caused by *Acanthamoeba,* concurrent topical use of 0.1% propamidine isethionate (Brolene) plus neomycin–polymyxin B–gramicidin ophthalmic solution has been successful (Hargrave SL, McCulley JP, Husseini Z. Results of a trial of combined propamidine isethionate and neomycin therapy for *Acanthamoeba* keratitis. Brolene Study Group. Ophthalmology. 1999;106:952). In addition, 0.02% topical polyhexamethylene biguanide (PHMB) and/or chlorhexadine has been used successfully in a large number of patients (Tabin G, Taylor H, Snibson G, et al. Atypical presentation of *Acanthamoeba* keratitis. Cornea. 2001;20:757; Wysenbeek YS, Blank-Porat D, Harizman N, et al. The reculture technique: Individualizing the treatment of *Acanthamoeba* keratitis. Cornea. 2000;19:464). PHMB is available from Leiters Park Avenue Pharmacy, San Jose, Calif. (800-292-6773).

2. The drug is not available commercially, but as a service it can be compounded by Medical Center Pharmacy, New Haven, Conn. (203-688-6816) or Panorama Compounding Pharmacy, 6744 Balboa Blvd, Van Nuys, Calif. 91406 (800-247-9767).

3. Treatment should be followed by a course of iodoquinol or paromomycin in the dosage used to treat asymptomatic amebiasis.

4. Nitazoxanide 500 mg bid × 3 days for adults is also effective for treatment of amebiasis (JF Rossignol, Ayoub A, Ayers MS. Treatment of diarrhea caused by *Giardia intestinalis* and *Entamoeba histolytica* or *E. dispar*: A randomized, double-blind, placebo-controlled study of nitazoxanide. J Infect Dis. 2001;184:381).**

5. A nitroimidazole similar to metronidazole, tinidazole appears to be at least as effective as metronidazole and better tolerated. Ornidazole, a similar drug, is also used outside the United States.

6. A *Naegleria* infection was treated successfully with intravenous and intrathecal use of both amphotericin B and miconazole, plus rifampin (Seidel JS, Harmatz P, Visvesvara GS, et al. Successful treatment of primary amebic meningoencephalitis. N Engl J Med. 1982;306:346). Other reports of successful therapy are questionable.

7. An approved drug but considered investigational for this condition by the FDA.

8. Strains of *Acanthamoeba* isolated from fatal granulomatous amebic encephalitis are usually susceptible in vitro to pentamidine, ketoconazole (Nizoral), flucytosine (Ancobon), and (less so) to amphotericin B. Chronic *Acanthamoeba* meningitis has been successfully treated in two children with a combination of oral TMP-SMX, rifampin, and ketoconazole (Singhal T, Bajpai A, Kalra V, et al. Successful treatment of *Acanthamoeba* meningitis with combination oral antimicrobials. Pediatr Infect Dis J. 2001;20:623), and, in a patient with AIDS, with fluconazole and sulfadiazine combined with surgical resection of the CNS le-

TABLE 41-2 Drugs for Treatment of Parasitic Infections and Pneumocystosis—cont'd

sion (Seijo Martinez M, Gonzalez-Mediero G, Santiago P, et al. Granulomatous amebic encephalitis in a patient with AIDS: Isolation of *Acanthamoeba* sp. group II from brain tissue and successful treatment with sulfadiazine and fluconazole. J Clin Microbiol. 2000;38:3892). Disseminated cutaneous infection in an immunocompromised patient has been treated successfully with IV pentamidine isethionate, topical chlorhexidine, and 2% ketoconazole cream, followed by oral itraconazole (Sporanox) (Slater CA, Sickel JZ, Visvesvara GS, et al. Brief report: Successful treatment of disseminated *Acanthamoeba* infection in an immunocompromised patient. N Engl J Med. 1994;331:85).

9. A free-living leptomyxid ameba that causes subacute to chronic granulomatous CNS disease. In vitro pentamidine isethionate 10 μg/mL is amebastatic (Denney CF, Iragui VJ, Uber-Zak LD, et al. Amebic meningoencephalitis caused by *Balamuthia mandrillaris:* Case report and review. Clin Infect Dis. 1997;25:1354). One patient, according to *Medical Letter* consultants, was successfully treated with clarithromycin (Biaxin) 500 mg tid, fluconazole (Diflucan) 400 mg once daily, sulfadiazine 1.5 g q6h, and flucytosine (Ancobon) 1.5 g q6h.

10. A recently described free-living ameba not previously known to be pathogenic to humans. It was successfully treated with azithromycin, IV pentamidine, itraconazole, and flucytosine (Gelman BB, Rauf SJ, Nader R, et al. Amoebic encephalitis due to *Sappinia diploidea*. JAMA. 2001;285:2450).

11. Most patients have a self-limited course and recover completely. Analgesics, corticosteroids, and careful removal of CSF at frequent intervals can relieve symptoms (Pien FD, Pien BC. *Angiostrongylus cantonensis* eosinophilic meningitis. Int J Infect Dis. 1999;3:161; Lo Re V 3rd, Gluckman SJ. Eosinophilic meningitis due to *Angiostrongylus cantonensis* in a returned traveler: Case report and review of the literature. Clin Infect Dis. 2001;33:e112). In a recent report, mebendazole and a glucocorticosteroid appeared to shorten the course of infection (Tsai HC, Liu YC, Kunin CM, et al. Eosinophilic meningitis caused by *Angiostrongylus cantonensis:* Report of 17 cases. Am J Med. 2001;111:109). No drug is proven to be effective and some patients have worsened when given thiabendazole, albendazole, mebendazole, or ivermectin.

12. Mebendazole has been used in experimental animals.

13. Exchange transfusion has been used in severely ill patients and those with high (>10%) parasitemia (Hatcher JC, Greenberg PD, Antique J, Jimenez-Lucho VE. Severe babesiosis in Long Island: Review of 34 cases and their complications. Clin Infect Dis. 2001;32:1117). Combination therapy with atovaquone and azithromycin is as effective as clindamycin/quinine and may be better tolerated (Krause PJ, Lepore T, Sikand VK, et al. Atovaquone and azithromycin for the treatment of babesiosis. N Engl J Med. 2000;343:1454). Concurrent use of pentamidine and TMP-SMX has been reported to cure an infection with *B. divergens,* the most common *Babesia* species in Europe (Raoult D, Soulayrol L, Toga B, et al. Babesiosis, pentamidine, and cotrimoxazole. Ann Intern Med. 1987;107:944).

14. Use of tetracyclines is contraindicated in pregnancy and in children younger than 8 years.

15. No drugs have been demonstrated to be effective. Albendazole 25 mg/kg/day × 10 days started up to 3 days after possible infection might prevent clinical disease and is recommended for children with known exposure (ingestion of raccoon stool or contaminated soil) (Raccoon roundworm encephalitis: Chicago, Illinois, and Los Angeles, California, 2000. MMWR Morb Mortal Wkly Rep. 2002;50:1153). Mebendazole, thiabendazole, levamisole (Ergamisol), and ivermectin could also be tried. Steroid therapy may be helpful, especially in eye and CNS infections. Ocular baylisascariasis has been treated successfully using laser photocoagulation therapy to destroy the intraretinal larvae.

16. Clinical significance of these organisms is controversial, but metronidazole 750 mg tid × 10 days or iodoquinol 650 mg tid × 20 days has been reported to be effective (Stenzel DJ, Boreham PF. Clin Microbiol Rev. *Blastocystis hominis* revisited. 1996;9:563). Metronidazole resistance may be common (Haresh K, Suresh K, Khairul Anus A, Saminathan S. Isolate resistance of *Blastocystis hominis* to metronidazole. Trop Med Int Health. 1999;4:274). TMP-SMX is an alternative regimen (Ok UZ, Girginkardesler N, Balcioglu C, et al. Effect of trimethoprim-sulfamethoxazole in *Blastocystis hominis* infection. Am J Gastroenterol. 1999;94:3245).

17. Nitazoxanide is licensed for treating giardiasis and cryptosporidial diarrhea in immunocompetent children ages 1 to 11 years. It is available in a liquid preparation.[**]

18. G Albanese, Venturi C, Galbiati G. Treatment of larva migrans cutanea (creeping eruption): A comparison between albendazole and traditional therapy. Int J Dermatol. 2001;40:67.

19. HIV-infected patients may need a higher dosage and long-term maintenance. In cases of cotrimoxazole intolerance, ciprofloxacin 500 mg bid × 7 days has been effective (Verdier RI, Fitzgerald DW, Johnson WD Jr, Pape JW. Trimethoprim-sulfamethoxazole compared with ciprofloxacin for treatment and prophylaxis of *Isospora belli* and *Cyclospora cayetanensis* infection in HIV-infected patients: A randomized, controlled trial. Ann Intern Med. 2000;132:885).

20. Not curative, but decreases inflammation and facilitates removing the worm. Mebendazole 400 to 800 mg/day for 6 days has been reported to kill the worm directly.

21. Because all family members are usually affected, treatment of the entire household is recommended.

22. Endosymbiotic *Wolbachia* bacteria may have a role in filarial development and host response and may represent a new target for therapy (Cross HF, Haarbrink M, Egerton G, et al. Severe reactions to filarial chemotherapy and release of *Wolbachia* endosymbionts into blood. Lancet. 2001;358:1873). Doxycycline 100 mg daily × 6 weeks has eradicated *Wolbachia* and led to sterility of adult worms in onchocerciasis (Hoerauf A, Volkmann L, Hamelmann C, et al. Endosymbiotic bacteria in worms as targets for a novel chemotherapy in filariasis. Lancet. 2000;355:1242).

23. Most symptoms caused by the adult worm. Single-dose combination of albendazole (400 mg) with either ivermectin (200 μg/kg) or diethylcarbamazine (6 mg/kg) is effective for reduction or suppression of *W. bancrofti* microfilaremia (Ismail MM, Jayakody RL, Weil GJ, et al. Long-term efficacy of single-dose combinations of albendazole, ivermectin and diethylcarbamazine for the treatment of bancroftian filariasis.Trans R Soc Trop Med Hyg. 2001;95:332; Nutman TB. Lymphatic filariasis: New insights and prospects for control. Curr Opin Infect Dis. 2001;14:539).

24. Antihistamines or corticosteroids may be required to decrease allergic reactions due to disintegration of microfilariae in treatment of filarial infections, especially those caused by *Loa loa.*

25. For patients with no microfilariae in the blood, full doses can be given from day 1.

26. In heavy infections with *Loa loa,* rapid killing of microfilariae can provoke an encephalopathy. Apheresis has been reported to be effective in lowering microfilarial counts in patients heavily infected with *Loa loa* (Ottesen EA. Filarial infections. Infect Dis Clin North Am. 1993;7:619). Albendazole and ivermectin have also been used to reduce microfilaremia; albendazole is preferred because of its slower onset of action (Klion AD, Massougbodji A, Horton J, et al. Albendazole in human loiasis: Results of a double-blind, placebo-controlled trial. J Infect Dis. 1993;168:202; Kombila M, Duong TH, Ferrer A, et al. Short- and long-term action of multiple doses of ivermectin on loiasis microfilaremia. Am J Trop Med Hyg. 1998;58:458). Albendazole may be useful for treatment of loiasis when diethylcarbamazine is ineffective or cannot be used but repeated courses may be necessary (Klion AD, Horton J, Nutman TB. Albendazole therapy for loiasis refractory to diethylcarbamazine treatment. Clin Infect Dis. 1999;29:680). Diethylcarbamazine, 300 mg once weekly, has been recommended for prevention of loiasis (Nutman TB, Miller KD, Mulligan M, et al. Diethylcarbamazine prophylaxis for human loiasis: Results of a double-blind study. N Engl J Med. 1988;319:752).

27. Diethylcarbamazine has no effect. Ivermectin, 200 μg/kg once, has been effective.

28. Diethylcarbamazine is potentially curative due to activity against both adult worms and microfilariae. Ivermectin is active against only microfilariae.

29. Annual treatment with ivermectin 150 μg/kg can prevent blindness caused by ocular onchocerciasis (Mabey D, Whitworth JA, Eckstein M, et al. The effects of multiple doses of ivermectin on ocular onchocerciasis: A six-year follow-up. Ophthalmology. 1996;103:1001).

30. Unlike infections with other flukes, *Fasciola hepatica* infections may not respond to praziquantel. Triclabendazole, a veterinary fasciolide, may be safe and effective but data are limited (Graham CS, Brodie SB, Weller PF. Imported *Fasciola hepatica* infection in the United States and treatment with triclabendazole. Clin Infect Dis. 2001;33:1). It should be given with food for better absorption.

31. MacLean JD, Arthur JR, Ward BJ, et al. Common-source outbreak of acute infection due to the North American liver fluke *Metorchis conjunctus*. Lancet. 1996;347:154.

32. Triclabendazole may be effective in a dosage of 5 mg/kg once daily for 3 days or 10 mg/kg twice in 1 day (Calvopiña M, Guderian RH, Paredes W, et al. Treatment of human pulmonary paragonimiasis with triclabendazole: Clinical tolerance and drug efficacy. Trans R Soc Trop Med Hyg. 1998;92:566). See footnote 30.

33. In one study, nitazoxanide (see footnote 4) was as effective as metronidazole and has been used successfully in high doses to treat a case of *Giardia* resistant

Continued

TABLE 41-2   Drugs for Treatment of Parasitic Infections and Pneumocystosis—cont'd

to metronidazole and albendazole (Ortiz JJ, Ayoub A, Gargala G, et al. Randomized clinical study of nitazoxanide compared to metronidazole in the treatment of symptomatic giardiasis in children from Northern Peru. Aliment Pharmacol Ther. 2001;15:1409; Abboud P, Lemee V, Gargala G, et al. Successful treatment of metronidazole- and albendazole-resistant giardiasis with nitazoxanide in a patient with acquired immunodeficiency syndrome. Clin Infect Dis. 2001;32:1792). Albendazole 400 mg daily × 5 days may be effective (Hall A, Nahar Q. Albendazole as a treatment for infections with *Giardia duodenalis* in children in Bangladesh. Trans R Soc Trop Med Hyg. 1993;87:84; Dutta AK, Phadke MA, Bagade AC, et al. A randomised multicentre study to compare the safety and efficacy of albendazole and metronidazole in the treatment of giardiasis in children. Indian J Pediatr. 1994;61:689). Bacitracin zinc or bacitracin 120,000 U bid for 10 days may also be effective (Andrews BJ, Panitescu D, Jipa GH, et al. Chemotherapy for giardiasis: Randomized clinical trial of bacitracin, bacitracin zinc, and a combination of bacitracin zinc with neomycin. Am J Trop Med Hyg. 1995;52:318). Combination treatment with standard doses of metronidazole and quinacrine given for 3 weeks has been effective for a small number of refractory infections (Nash TE, Ohl CA, Thomas E, et al. Treatment of patients with refractory giardiasis. Clin Infect Dis. 2001;33:22).

34. Not absorbed; may be useful for treatment of giardiasis in pregnancy.
35. Chappuis F, Farinelli T, Loutan L. Ivermectin treatment of a traveler who returned from Peru with cutaneous gnathostomiasis. Clin Infect Dis. 2001;33:e17; Nontasut P, Bussaratid V, Chullawichit S, et al. Comparison of ivermectin and albendazole treatment for gnathostomiasis. Southeast Asian J Trop Med Public Health. 2000;31:374.
36. One patient has been successfully treated with albendazole (Eberhard ML, Busillo C. Human *Gongylonema* infection in a resident of New York City. Am J Trop Med Hyg. 1999;61:51).
37. Immunosuppressed patients: TMP-SMX qid × 10 days followed by bid × 3 wk. In sulfonamide-sensitive patients, pyrimethamine 50 to 75 mg daily in divided doses has been effective. HIV-infected patients may need long-term maintenance. Ciprofloxacin 500 mg bid × 7 days has also been effective (Verdier RI, Fitzgerald DW, Johnson WD Jr, Pape JW. Trimethoprim-sulfamethoxazole compared with ciprofloxacin for treatment and prophylaxis of *Isospora belli* and *Cyclospora cayetanensis* infection in HIV-infected patients: A randomized, controlled trial. Ann Intern Med. 2000;132:885).
38. Treatment dosage and duration vary on the basis of disease symptoms, host immune status, species, and the area of the world where infection was acquired. Cutaneous infection is caused by *Leishmania mexicana, L. tropica, L. major, L. braziliensis;* mucocutaneous infection is mainly caused by *L. braziliensis,* and visceral infection is caused by *L. donovani* (kala-azar), *L. infantum,* and *L. chagasi.* Dosage range listed includes many but not all possibilities.
39. Three preparations of lipid-encapsulated amphotericin B have been used for treatment of visceral leishmaniasis. Largely on the basis of clinical trials in patients infected with *L. infantum,* the FDA approved liposomal amphotericin B (AmBisome) for treatment of visceral leishmaniasis (Meyerhoff A. U.S. Food and Drug Administration approval of AmBisome (liposomal amphotericin B) for treatment of visceral leishmaniasis. Clin Infect Dis. 1999;28:42; Berman JD. U.S Food and Drug Administration approval of AmBisome (liposomal amphotericin B) for treatment of visceral leishmaniasis. Clin Infect Dis. 1999;28:49). Amphotericin B lipid complex (Abelcet) and amphotericin B cholesteryl sulfate (Amphotec) have also been used with good results. Limited data in a few patients suggest that liposomal amphotericin B may also be effective for mucocutaneous disease (Amato VS, Nicodemo AC, Amato JG, et al. Mucocutaneous leishmaniasis associated with HIV infection treated successfully with liposomal amphotericin B (AmBisome). J Antimicrob Chemother. 2000;46:341; Sampaio RNR, Marsden PD. Mucosal leishmaniasis unresponsive to glucantime therapy successfully treated with AmBisome. Trans R Soc Trop Med Hyg. 1997;91:77). Some studies indicate that *L. donovani* resistant to pentavalent antimonial agents may respond to lipid-encapsulated amphotericin B (Sundar S, Goyal AK, More DK, et al. Treatment of antimony-unresponsive Indian visceral leishmaniasis with ultra-short courses of amphotericin-B-lipid complex. Ann Trop Med Parasitol. 1998;92:755).
40. The dose for immunocompromised patients with HIV is 4 mg/kg/day (days 1 to 5) and 4 mg/kg/day on days 10, 17, 24, 31, and 38. The relapse rate is high, suggesting that maintenance therapy may be indicated.
41. May be repeated or continued. A longer duration may be needed for some forms of visceral leishmaniasis (Herwaldt BL. Leishmaniasis. Lancet. 1999;354:1191).
42. Miltefosine is the drug of choice for treating pentavalent antimony–resistant *Leishmania donovani* in India.** For treatment of kala-azar, oral miltefosine 100 mg daily for 4 wk is 97% effective after 6 months. Gastrointestinal adverse effects are common and the drug is contraindicated in pregnancy (Jha TK, Sundar S, Thakur CP, et al. Miltefosine, an oral agent, for the treatment of Indian visceral leishmaniasis. N Engl J Med. 1999;341:1795). In an uncontrolled trial, oral miltefosine was effective for the treatment of American cutaneous leishmaniasis at a dosage of about 2.25 mg/kg/day for 3 to 4 wks. "Motion sickness" was the most frequent adverse effect (Soto J, Toledo J, Gutierrez P, et al. Treatment of American cutaneous leishmaniasis with miltefosine, an oral agent. Clin Infect Dis. 2001;33:e57).
43. For *L. donovani:* 4 mg/kg once/day × 15 doses; for cutaneous disease: 2 mg/kg once/day × 7, or 3 mg/kg once/day × 4 doses.
44. Topical paromomycin can be used only in geographic regions where cutaneous leishmaniasis species have low potential for mucosal spread. A formulation of 15% paromomycin and 12% methylbenzethonium chloride (Leshcutan) in soft white paraffin for topical use, has been reported to be effective in some patients against cutaneous leishmaniasis due to *L. major* (Ozgoztasi O, Baydar I. A randomized clinical trial of topical paromomycin versus oral ketoconazole for treating cutaneous leishmaniasis in Turkey. Int J Dermatol. 1997;36:61; Arana BA, Mendoza CE, Rizzo NR, Kroeger A. Randomized, controlled, double-blind trial of topical treatment of cutaneous leishmaniasis with paromomycin plus methylbenzethonium chloride ointment in Guatemala. Am J Trop Med Hyg. 2001;65:466).
45. For infestation of eyelashes with crab lice, use petrolatum. For pubic lice, treat with 5% permethrin or ivermectin as for scabies (see Scabies, later).
46. A second application is recommended 1 week later to kill hatching progeny. Some lice are resistant to pyrethrins and permethrin (Pollack RJ, Kiszewski A, Armstrong P, et al. Differential permethrin susceptibility of head lice sampled in the United States and Borneo. Arch Pediatr Adolesc Med. 1999;153:969).
47. Roberts RJ, Casey D, Morgan DA, Petrovic M. Comparison of wet combing with malathion for treatment of head lice in the UK: a pragmatic randomised controlled trial. Lancet. 2000;356:540.
48. Ivermectin is effective against adult lice but has no effect on nits (TA Bell. Treatment of *Pediculus humanus* var. *capitis* infestation in Cowlitz County, Washington, with ivermectin and the LiceMeister comb. Pediatr Infect Dis J. 1998;17:923).
49. Chloroquine-resistant *P. falciparum* occur in all malarious areas except Central America west of the Panama Canal Zone, Mexico, Haiti, the Dominican Republic, and most of the Middle East (chloroquine resistance has been reported in Yemen, Oman, Saudi Arabia, and Iran).
50. In Southeast Asia, relative resistance to quinine has increased and the treatment should be continued for 7 days.
51. Fansidar tablets contain 25 mg of pyrimethamine and 500 mg of sulfadoxine. Resistance to pyrimethamine-sulfadoxine has been reported from Southeast Asia, the Amazon basin, sub-Saharan Africa, Bangladesh, and Oceania.
52. For use in pregnancy.
53. Atovaquone plus proguanil is available as a fixed-dose combination tablet: adult tablets (250 mg atovaquone/100 mg proguanil, Malarone) and pediatric tablets (62.5 mg atovaquone/25 mg proguanil, Malarone Pediatric). To enhance absorption, it should be taken within 45 minutes after eating (Looareesuwan S, Chulay JD, Canfield CJ, Hutchinson DB. Malarone [atovaquone and proguanil hydrochloride]: A review of its clinical development for treatment of malaria. Malarone Clinical Trials Study Group. Am J Trop Med Hyg. 1999;60:533). Although approved for once-daily dosing, to decrease nausea and vomiting the dose for treatment may be divided in two.
54. For treatment of multidrug-resistant *P. falciparum* in Southeast Asia, especially Thailand, where resistance to mefloquine and halofantrine is frequent, a 7-day course of quinine and tetracycline is recommended (Watt G, Loesuttivibool L, Shanks GD, et al. Quinine with tetracycline for the treatment of drug-resistant falciparum malaria in Thailand. Am J Trop Med Hyg. 1992;47:108). Artesunate plus mefloquine (Luxemburger C, ter Kuile FO, Nosten F, et al. Single day mefloquine-artesunate combination in the treatment of multi-drug resistant falciparum malaria. Trans R Soc Trop Med Hyg. 1994;88:213), artemether plus mefloquine (Karbwang J, Na-Bangchang K, Thanavibul A, et al. A comparative clinical trial of two different regimens of artemether plus mefloquine in multidrug resistant falciparum malaria. Trans R Soc Trop Med Hyg. 1995;89:296), mefloquine plus doxycycline or atovaquone/proguanil may also be used to treat multidrug-resistant *P. falciparum*.
55. At this dosage, adverse effects including nausea, vomiting, diarrhea, dizziness, disturbed sense of balance, toxic psychosis, and seizures can occur. Mefloquine is teratogenic in animals and should not be used for treatment of malaria in pregnancy. It should not be given together with quinine, quinidine or halofantrine, and caution is required in using quinine, quinidine, or halofantrine to treat patients with malaria who have taken mefloquine for prophylaxis. The pediatric dosage has not been approved by the FDA. Resistance to mefloquine has been reported in some areas, such as the Thailand-Myanmar and -Cambodia borders and in the Amazon basin, where 25 mg/kg should be used.
56. In the United States, a 250-mg tablet of mefloquine contains 228 mg mefloquine base. Outside the United States, each 275-mg tablet contains 250 mg base.

TABLE 41-2 Drugs for Treatment of Parasitic Infections and Pneumocystosis—cont'd

57. May be effective in multidrug-resistant *P. falciparum* malaria, but treatment failures and resistance have been reported, and the drug has caused lengthening of the PR and QTc intervals and fatal cardiac arrhythmias. It should not be used for patients with cardiac conduction defects or with other drugs that may affect the QT interval, such as quinine, quinidine and mefloquine. Cardiac monitoring is recommended. Variability in absorption is a problem; halofantrine should not be taken 1 hour before to 2 hours after meals because food increases its absorption. It should not be used in pregnancy.

58. A single 250-mg dose can be used for repeat treatment in mild to moderate infections (Touze JE, Perret JL, Nicolas X, et al. Efficacy of low-dose halofantrine for second treatment of uncomplicated falciparum malaria. Lancet. 1997;349:255).

59. Na-Bangchang K, Tippanangkosol P, Ubalee R, et al. Comparative clinical trial of four regimens of dihydroartemisinin-mefloquine in multidrug-resistant falciparum malaria. Trop Med Int Health. 1999;4:602.

60. *P. vivax* with decreased susceptibility to chloroquine is a significant problem in Papua New Guinea and Indonesia. There are also a few reports of resistance from Myanmar, India, Thailand, the Solomon Islands, Vanuatu, Guyana, Brazil, Colombia, and Peru.

61. Baird JK, Basri H, Subianto B, el al. Treatment of chloroquine-resistant *Plasmodium vivax* with chloroquine and primaquine or halofantrine. J Infect Dis. 1995;171:1678.

62. Primaquine phosphate can cause hemolytic anemia, especially in patients whose red cells are deficient in glucose-6-phosphate dehydrogenase. This deficiency is most common in African, Asian, and Mediterranean peoples. Patients should be screened for G-6-PD deficiency before treatment. Primaquine should not be used during pregnancy.

63. If chloroquine phosphate is not available, hydroxychloroquine sulfate is as effective; 400 mg of hydroxychloroquine sulfate is equivalent to 500 mg of chloroquine phosphate.

64. Exchange transfusion has been helpful for some patients with high-density (>10%) parasitemia, altered mental status, pulmonary edema, or renal complications (Miller KD, Greenberg AE, Campbell CC. Treatment of severe malaria in the United States with a continuous infusion of quinidine gluconate and exchange transfusion. N Engl J Med. 1989;321:65).

65. Continuous EKG, blood pressure, and glucose monitoring are recommended, especially in pregnant women and young children. For problems with quinidine availability, call the manufacturer (Eli Lilly, 800-821-0538) or the CDC Malaria Hotline (1-877-394-8747). Quinidine may have greater antimalarial activity than quinine. The loading dose should be decreased or omitted in those patients who have received quinine or mefloquine. If more than 48 hours of parenteral treatment is required, the quinine or quinidine dose should be reduced by one third to one half.

66. Artemether-Quinine Meta-Analysis Study Group. A meta-analysis using individual patient data of trials comparing artemether with quinine in the treatment of severe falciparum malaria. Trans R Soc Trop Med Hyg. 2001;95:637. Not available in the United States.

67. Relapses have been reported with this regimen, and should be treated with a second 14-day course of 30 mg base/day. In Southeast Asia and Somalia, the higher dose (30 mg base/day) should be used initially.

68. No drug regimen guarantees protection against malaria. If fever develops within a year (particularly within the first 2 months) after travel to malarious areas, travelers should be advised to seek medical attention. Insect repellents, insecticide-impregnated bed nets, and proper clothing are important adjuncts for malaria prophylaxis.

69. In pregnancy, chloroquine prophylaxis has been used extensively and safely.

70. For prevention of attack after departure from areas where *P. vivax* and *P. ovale* are endemic, which includes almost all areas where malaria is found (except Haiti), some experts prescribe in addition primaquine phosphate 26.3 mg (15 mg base)/day or, for children, 0.3 mg base/kg/day during the last 2 weeks of prophylaxis. Others prefer to avoid the toxicity of primaquine and rely on surveillance to detect cases when they occur, particularly when exposure was limited or doubtful. See also footnotes 62 and 67.

71. Beginning 1 to 2 weeks before travel and continuing weekly for the duration of stay and for 4 weeks after leaving.

72. **Mefloquine has not been approved for use during pregnancy. However, it has been reported to be safe for prophylactic use during the second or third trimester of pregnancy and possibly during early pregnancy as well (CDC Health Information for International Travel, 2003-2004, page 234; Smoak BL, Writer JV, Keep LW, et al. The effects of inadvertent exposure of mefloquine chemoprophylaxis on pregnancy outcomes and infants of US Army servicewomen. J Infect Dis. 1997;176:831). Mefloquine is not recommended for patients with cardiac conduction abnormalities. Patients with a history of seizures or psychiatric disorders should avoid mefloquine (Medical Letter. 1990;32:13). Resistance to mefloquine has been reported in some areas, such as Thailand; in these areas, doxycycline or malarone** can be used for prophylaxis.

73. Beginning 1 to 2 days before travel and continuing for the duration of stay and for 4 weeks after leaving. Use of tetracyclines is contraindicated in pregnancy and in children less than 8 years old. Doxycycline can cause gastrointestinal disturbances, vaginal moniliasis, pseudomembranous colitis,** and photosensitivity reactions.

74. Shanks GE, Gordon D, Klotz F, et al. Efficacy and safety of atovaquone/proguanil as suppressive prophylaxis for *Plasmodium falciparum* malaria. Clin Infect Dis. 1998;27:494; Lell B, Luckner D, Ndjave M, et al. Randomised placebo-controlled study of atovaquone plus proguanil for malaria prophylaxis in children. Lancet. 1998;351:709. Begin 1 to 2 days before travel and continue for the duration of stay and for 1 week after leaving. Atovaquone/proguanil is better tolerated than mefloquine in nonimmune travelers (Overbosch D, Schilthuis H, Bienzle U, et al. Atovaquone-proguanil versus mefloquine for malaria prophylaxis in nonimmune travelers: Results from a randomized, double-blind study. Clin Infect Dis. 2001;33:1015).

75. Several studies have shown that daily primaquine beginning 1 day before departure and continued until 7 days after leaving the malaria area provides effective prophylaxis against chloroquine-resistant *P. falciparum* (Baird JK, Lacy MD, Basri H, et al. Randomized, parallel placebo-controlled trial of primaquine for malaria prophylaxis in Papua, Indonesia. Clin Infect Dis. 2001;33:1990). Some studies have shown less efficacy against *P. vivax*. Nausea and abdominal pain can be diminished by taking with food.

76. Proguanil (Paludrine: Wyeth Ayerst, Canada; AstraZeneca, United Kingdom), which is not available alone in the United States but is widely available in Canada and Europe, is recommended mainly for use in Africa south of the Sahara. Prophylaxis is recommended during exposure and for 4 weeks afterward. Proguanil has been used in pregnancy without evidence of toxicity (Phillips-Howard PA, Wood D. The safety of antimalarial drugs in pregnancy. Drug Saf. 1996;14:131).

77. Ocular lesions due to *E. hellem* in HIV-infected patients have responded to fumagillin eye drops prepared from Fumidil-B, a commercial product (Mid-Continent Agrimarketing, Inc., Olathe, Kan., 800-547-1392) used to control a microsporidial disease of honey bees (Diesenhouse MC, Wilson LA, Corrent GF, et al. Treatment of microsporidial keratoconjunctivitis with topical fumagillin. Am J Ophthalmol. 1993;115:293). For lesions due to *V. corneae*, topical therapy is generally not effective and keratoplasty may be required (Davis RM, Font RL, Keisler MS, Shadduck JA. Corneal microsporidiosis: A case report including ultrastructural observations. Ophthalmology. 1990;97:953).

78. Oral fumagillin (see footnote 77, Sanofi Recherche, Gentilly, France) has been effective in treating *E. bieneusi* (Molina JM, Goguel J, Sarfati C, et al. Trial of oral fumagillin for the treatment of intestinal microsporidiosis in patients with HIV infection. ANRS 054 Study Group. Agence Nationale de Recherche sur le SIDA. AIDS. 2000;14:1341) but has been associated with thrombocytopenia. Highly active antiretroviral therapy (HAART) may lead to microbiologic and clinical response in HIV-infected patients with microsporidial diarrhea (Foudraine NA, Weverling GJ, van Gool T, et al. Improvement of chronic diarrhoea in patients with advanced HIV-1 infection during potent antiretroviral therapy. AIDS 1998;12:35; Carr A, Marriott D, Field A, et al. Treatment of HIV-1-associated microsporidiosis and cryptosporidiosis with combination antiretroviral therapy. Lancet. 1998;351:256). Octreotide (Sandostatin) has provided symptomatic relief in some patients with large volume diarrhea.

79. Molina JM, Oksenhendler E, Beauvais B, et al. Disseminated microsporidiosis due to *Septata intestinalis* in patients with AIDS: Clinical features and response to albendazole therapy. J Infect Dis. 1995;171:245. There is no established treatment for *Pleistophora* infection.

80. Albendazole or pyrantel pamoate may be effective (Krepel HP, Haring T, Baeta S, Polderman AM. Treatment of mixed *Oesophagostomum* and hookworm infection: Effect of albendazole, pyrantel pamoate, levamisole and thiabendazole. Trans R Soc Trop Med Hyg. 1993;87:87).

81. In severe disease with room air PO2 ≤70 mm Hg or Aa gradient ≥35 mm Hg, prednisone should also be used (Gagnon S, Boota AM, Fischl MA, et al. Corticosteroids as adjunctive therapy for severe *Pneumocystis carinii* pneumonia in the acquired immunodeficiency syndrome: A double-blind, placebo-controlled trial. N Engl J Med. 1990;323:1444; Caumes E, Roudier C, Rogeaux O,et al. Effect of corticosteroids on the incidence of adverse cutaneous reactions to trimethoprim-sulfamethoxazole during treatment of AIDS-associated *Pneumocystis carinii* pneumonia. Clin Infect Dis. 1994;18:319).

82. Primary/secondary prophylaxis in patients with HIV can be discontinued after CD4 count increases to greater than 200 × 10⁶/L for more than 3 months (HIV/AIDS Treatment Information Service, U.S. Department of Health and Human Services, 2001; www.hivatis.org).

83. An alternative TMP-SMX regimen is one DS tablet 3 × /week. Weekly therapy with sulfadoxine 500 mg/pyrimethamine 25 mg/leucovorin 25 mg was ef-

Continued

TABLE 41-2   Drugs for Treatment of Parasitic Infections and Pneumocystosis—cont'd

fective PCP prophylaxis in liver transplant recipients (Torre-Cisneros J, De la Mata M, Pozo JC, et al. Randomized trial of weekly sulfadoxine/pyrimethamine vs. daily low-dose trimethoprim-sulfamethoxazole for the prophylaxis of *Pneumocystis carinii* pneumonia after liver transplantation. Clin Infect Dis. 1999;29:771).

84. Plus leucovorin 25 mg with each dose of pyrimethamine.

85. Effective for crusted scabies in immunocompromised patients (Larralde M, Mijelshon LM, Gonzalez A, et al. Ivermectin-responsive crusted scabies in four patients. Pediatr Dermatol. 1999;16:69; Patel A, Hogan P, Walder B. Crusted scabies in two immunocompromised children: Successful treatment with oral ivermectin. Australas J Dermatol. 1999;40:37; Chosidow O. Scabies and pediculosis. Lancet. 2000;355:819).

86. Oxamniquine has been effective in some areas in which praziquantel is less effective (Stelma FF, Sall S, Daff B,et al. Oxamniquine cures *Schistosoma mansoni* infection in a focus in which cure rates with praziquantel are unusually low. J Infect Dis. 1997;176:304). Oxamniquine is contraindicated in pregnancy.

87. In East Africa, the dose should be increased to 30 mg/kg, and in Egypt and South Africa to 30 mg/kg/day × 2 days. Some experts recommend 40 to 60 mg/kg over 2 to 3 days in all of Africa (Shekhar KC. Schistosomiasis drug therapy and treatment considerations. Drugs. 1991;42:379).

88. In immunocompromised patients or disseminated disease, it may be necessary to prolong or repeat therapy or use other agents. A veterinary parenteral formulation of ivermectin was used in one patient (Chiodini PL, Reid AJ, Wiselka MJ, et al. Parenteral ivermectin in *Strongyloides* hyperinfection. Lancet. 2000;355:43).

89. This dose is likely to be toxic and may have to be decreased.

90. Patients may benefit from or require surgical resection of cysts. Praziquantel is useful preoperatively or in case of spill during surgery. Percutaneous drainage with ultrasound guidance plus albendazole therapy has been effective for management of hepatic hydatid cyst disease (Khuroo MS, Wani NA, Javid G, et al. Percutaneous drainage compared with surgery for hepatic hydatid cysts. N Engl J Med. 1997;337:881; Akhan O, Ozman M. Percutaneous treatment of liver hydatid cysts. Eur J Radiol. 1999;32:76).

91. Surgical excision or the PAIR (Puncture, Aspirate, Inject, Re-aspirate) technique is the only reliable means of cure. Reports have suggested that in nonresectable cases, use of albendazole or mebendazole can stabilize and sometimes cure infection (Wen H, Zou PF, Wang WG, et al. Albendazole chemotherapy for human cystic and alveolar echinococcosis in Northwestern China. Trans R Soc Trop Med Hyg. 1994;88:340; WHO Group, Bull WHO 1996;74:231).

92. Initial therapy of parenchymal disease with seizures should focus on symptomatic treatment with anticonvulsant drugs. Treatment of parenchymal disease with albendazole and praziquantel is controversial and randomized trials have not been conclusive. Obstructive hydrocephalus is treated with surgical removal of the obstructing cyst or CSF diversion. Prednisone 40 mg daily may be given in conjunction with surgery. Arachnoiditis, vasculitis, or cerebral edema is treated with prednisone 60 mg daily or dexamethasone 4 to 16 mg/day combined with albendazole or praziquantel (White AC Jr. Neurocysticercosis: Updates on epidemiology, pathogenesis, diagnosis, and management. Annu Rev Med. 2000;51:187). Patients with subarachnoid cysts or giant cysts in the fissures should receive albendazole for at least 30 days (Proano JV, Madrazo I, Avelar F, et al. Medical treatment for neurocysticercosis characterized by giant subarachnoid cysts. N Engl J Med. 2001;345:879). Any cysticercocidal drug may cause irreparable damage when used to treat ocular or spinal cysts, even when corticosteroids are used. An ophthalmic examination should always be done before treatment to rule out intraocular cysts.

93. In ocular toxoplasmosis with macular involvement, corticosteroids are recommended for an anti-inflammatory effect on the eyes.

94. To treat CNS toxoplasmosis in HIV-infected patients, some clinicians have used pyrimethamine 50 to 100 mg daily (after a loading dose of 200 mg) with sulfadiazine and, when sulfonamide sensitivity developed, have given clindamycin 1.8 to 2.4 g/day in divided doses instead of the sulfonamide (JS Remington JS, Vilde JL. Clindamycin for toxoplasma encephalitis in AIDS. Lancet. 1991;338:1142; Luft BJ, Hafner R, Korzun AH, et al. Toxoplasmic encephalitis in patients with the acquired immunodeficiency syndrome. Members of the ACTG 077p/ANRS 009 Study Team. N Engl J Med. 1993;329:995). Atovaquone plus pyrimethamine appears to be an effective alternative in sulfa-intolerant patients (Kovacs JA. Efficacy of atovaquone in treatment of toxoplasmosis in patients with AIDS. The NIAID-Clinical Center Intramural AIDS Program. Lancet. 1992;340:637). Treatment is followed by chronic suppression with lower dosage regimens of the same drugs. For primary prophylaxis in HIV-infected patients with less than 100 CD4 cells, either TMP-SMX, pyrimethamine with dapsone, or atovaquone with or without pyrimethamine can be used. Primary/secondary prophylaxis may be discontinued when the CD4 count increases to greater than 200 × 10⁶/L for more than 3 months (HIV/AIDS Treatment Information Service U.S. Department of Health and Human Services, 2001; www.hivatis.org). See also footnote 95.

95. Plus leucovorin 10 to 25 mg with each dose of pyrimethamine.

96. Congenitally infected newborns should be treated with pyrimethamine every 2 or 3 days and a sulfonamide daily for about 1 year (Remington JS, Desmonts G. Toxoplasmosis. In: Remington JS, Klein JO, eds. Infectious Disease of the Fetus and Newborn Infant, 5th ed. Philadelphia: Saunders; 2001:290).

97. For prophylactic use during pregnancy. If it is determined that transmission has occurred in utero, therapy with pyrimethamine and sulfadiazine should be started. Pyrimethamine is a potential teratogen and should be used only after the first trimester.

98. Sexual partners should be treated simultaneously. Metronidazole-resistant strains have been reported and should be treated with metronidazole 2 to 4 g/day × 7 to 14 days. Desensitization has been recommended for patients allergic to metronidazole (Pearlman MD, Yashar C, Ernst S, Solomon W. An incremental dosing protocol for women with severe vaginal trichomoniasis and adverse reaction to metronidazole. Am J Obstet Gynecol. 1996;174:934). High-dose tinidazole has also been used for the treatment of metronidazole-resistant trichomoniasis (Sobel JD, Nyirjesy P, Brown W. Tinidazole therapy for metronidazole-resistant vaginal trichomoniasis. Clin Infect Dis. 2001;33:1341).

99. Available from the CDC. The addition of interferon-γ to nifurtimox for 20 days in a limited number of patients and in experimental animals appears to have shortened the acute phase of Chagas' disease (McCabe RE, Meagher SG, Mullins BT. Endogenous interferon-gamma, macrophage activation, and murine host defense against acute infection with *Trypanosoma cruzi*. J Infect Dis. 1991;163:912).

100. For treatment of *T.b. gambiense,* pentamidine and suramin have equal efficacy but pentamidine is better tolerated.

101. Eflornithine is highly effective in *T.b. gambiense* and variably effective in *T.b. rhodesiense* infections. It is available in limited supply only from the WHO, and is given at 400 mg/kg/day IV in 4 divided doses for 14 days.

102. In frail patients, begin with as little as 18 mg and increase the dose progressively. Pretreatment with suramin has been advocated for debilitated patients. Corticosteroids have been used to prevent arsenical encephalopathy (Pepin J, Milord F, Khonde AN, et al. Risk factors for encephalopathy and mortality during melarsoprol treatment of *Trypanosoma brucei gambiense* sleeping sickness. Trans R Soc Trop Med Hyg. 1995;89:92). Up to 20% of patients with *T. b. gambiense* fail to respond to melarsoprol (Barrett MP. The fall and rise of sleeping sickness. Lancet. 1999;353:1113). A shortened course consisting of 10 daily injections of 2.2 mg/kg gave a similar outcome to the usual 26-treatment schedule (Burri C, Nkunku S, Merolle A, et al. Efficacy of new, concise schedule for melarsoprol in treatment of sleeping sickness caused by *Trypanosoma brucei gambiense:* A randomised trial. Lancet. 2000;355:1419).

103. Optimal duration of therapy is not known; some *Medical Letter* consultants would treat for up to 20 days. For severe symptoms or eye involvement, corticosteroids can be used in addition.

Abbreviations: AIDS, acquired immunodeficiency syndrome; CDC, Centers for Disease Control and Prevention; CNS, central nervous system; CSF, cerebrospinal fluid; EKG, electrocardiogram; FDA, U.S. Food and Drug Administration; HIV, human immunodeficiency virus; IM, intramuscularly; IV, intravenously; PC, after food; PO, by mouth; PCP, *Pneumocystis jirovecii* pneumonia; TMP-SMX, trimethoprim-sulfamethoxazole.

Adapted from The Medical Letter on Drugs and Therapeutics, April 2002:1-11 (available at www.medletter.com), and used with permission.

TABLE 41-3 Manufacturers and Adverse Effects of Some Antiparasitic Drugs*

Albendazole—Albenza (GlaxoSmithKline)
Occasional: abdominal pain; reversible alopecia; increased serum transaminase activity; migration of *Ascaris* through mouth and nose
Rare: leukopenia; rash; renal toxicity
†Artemether—Artenam (Arenco, Belgium)
Occasional: neurologic toxicity; possible increase in length of coma in patients with cerebral malaria; increased convulsions; prolongation of QTc interval
†Artesunate—(Guilin No. 1 Factory, People's Republic of China)
Occasional: ataxia; slurred speech; neurologic toxicity; possible increase in length of coma in patients with cerebral malaria; increased convulsions; prolongation of QTc interval
Atovaquone—Mepron (GlaxoSmithKline); with proguanil, Malarone (GlaxoSmithKline)
Frequent: Rash; nausea (in patients with HIV)
Occasional: diarrhea, abdominal pain, nausea
†Benznidazole—Rochagan (Roche, Brazil)
Frequent: allergic rash; dose-dependent polyneuropathy; GI disturbances; psychic disturbances
‡Bithionol—Bitin (Tanabe, Japan)
Frequent: photosensitivity reactions; vomiting; diarrhea; abdominal pain; urticaria
Rare: leukopenia; toxic hepatitis
Chloroquine HCl and chloroquine phosphate—Aralen (Sanofi), others
Occasional: pruritus; vomiting; headache; confusion; depigmentation of hair; skin eruptions; corneal opacity; weight loss; partial alopecia; extraocular muscle palsies; exacerbation of psoriasis; eczema, and other exfoliative dermatoses; myalgias; photophobia
Rare: irreversible retinal injury (especially when total dosage exceeds 100 g); discoloration of nails and mucous membranes; nerve-type deafness; peripheral neuropathy and myopathy; heart block; blood dyscrasias; hematemesis
Crotamiton—Eurax (Westwood-Squibb)
Occasional: rash; conjunctivitis
Dapsone—(Jacobus)
Frequent: rash; transient headache; GI irritation; anorexia; infectious mononucleosis–like syndrome
Occasional: cyanosis due to methemoglobinemia; other blood dyscrasias, including hemolytic anemia; nephrotic syndrome; liver damage; peripheral neuropathy; hypersensitivity reactions; increased risk of lepra reactions; insomnia; irritability; uncoordinated speech; agitation; acute psychosis
Rare: renal papillary necrosis; severe hypoalbuminemia; epidermal necrolysis; optic atrophy; agranulocytosis; neonatal hyperbilirubinemia after use in pregnancy
‡Diethylcarbamazine citrate USP (University of Iowa School of Pharmacy)
Frequent: severe allergic or febrile reactions in patients with microfilariae in the blood or the skin; GI disturbances
Rare: encephalopathy
†Diloxanide furoate—Furamide (Boots, United Kingdom)
Frequent: flatulence
Occasional: nausea; vomiting; diarrhea
Rare: diplopia, dizziness; urticaria; pruritus
‡Eflornithine (Difluoromethylornithine, DFMO)—Ornidyl (Aventis)
Frequent: anemia, leukopenia
Occasional: diarrhea; thrombocytopenia; seizures
Rare: hearing loss
Furazolidone—Furoxone (Roberts)
Frequent: nausea; vomiting
Occasional: allergic reactions; including pulmonary infiltration, hypotension, urticaria, fever, vesicular rash; hypoglycemia; headache
Rare: hemolytic anemia in G6PD deficiency and neonates; disulfiram-like reaction with alcohol; MAO-inhibitor interactions; polyneuritis
†Halofantrine—Halfan (GlaxoSmithKline)
Occasional: diarrhea; abdominal pain, pruritus; serious prolongation of QTc and PR interval
Rare: Sudden death
Iodoquinol—Yodoxin (Glenwood), others
Occasional: rash; acne; slight enlargement of the thyroid gland; nausea; diarrhea; cramps; anal pruritus
Rare: optic neuritis; optic atrophy, loss of vision, peripheral neuropathy after prolonged use (for months) at high dosage; iodine sensitivity

Ivermectin—Stromectol (Merck)
Occasional: Mazzotti-type reaction seen in onchocerciasis, including fever, pruritus, tender lymph nodes, and joint and bone pain
Rare: hypotension
†Malathion—Ovide (Medicis)
Occasional: local irritation
Mebendazole—Vermox (McNeil)
Occasional: diarrhea; abdominal pain; migration of *Ascaris* through mouth and nose
Rare: leukopenia; agranulocytosis; hypospermia
Mefloquine—Lariam (Roche)
Frequent: vertigo; lightheadedness; nausea; other GI disturbances; nightmares; visual disturbances; headache; insomnia
Occasional: confusion
Rare: psychosis; hypotension; convulsions; coma; paresthesias
†Meglumine antimonate—Glucantime (Aventis, France)
Similar to sodium stibogluconate
‡Melarsoprol—Mel-B (Specia)
Frequent: myocardial damage; albuminuria; hypertension; colic; Herxheimer-type reaction; encephalopathy; vomiting; peripheral neuropathy
Rare: shock
Metronidazole—Flagyl (Searle), others
Frequent: nausea; headache; anorexia; metallic taste
Occasional: vomiting; diarrhea; insomnia; weakness; dry mouth; stomatitis; vertigo; tinnitus; paresthesias; rash; dark urine; urethral burning; disulfiram-like reaction with alcohol; candidiasis
Rare: seizures; pseudomembranous colitis; ataxia; leukopenia; peripheral neuropathy; pancreatitis; encephalopathy
†Miltefosine—(Zentaris/ASTA Medica, Germany)
Frequent: nausea; diarrhea and motion sickness (high doses)
Occasional: elevated liver enzymes
‡Nifurtimox—Lampit (Bayer, Germany)
Frequent: anorexia; vomiting; weight loss; loss of memory; sleep disorders; tremors; paresthesias; weakness; polyneuritis
Rare: convulsions; fever; pulmonary infiltrates and pleural effusion
Nitazoxanide—Alinia (Romark Labs)
Occasional: vomiting; diarrhea; abdominal pain and headache
Rare: yellow sclerae (resolves with discontinuation of drug)
†Ornidazole—Tiberal (Hoffman-LaRoche, Switzerland)
Occasional: dizziness; headache; GI disturbances
Rare: reversible peripheral neuropathy
Paromomycin—Humatin (Monarch); aminosidine (topical and parenteral formulations not available in United States)
Frequent: GI disturbances with oral use
Occasional: 8th-nerve damage (mainly auditory) and renal damage when aminosidine is given IV; vertigo; pancreatitis
Pentamidine isethionate—Pentam 300, NebuPent (Fujisawa)
Frequent: hypotension; hypoglycemia often followed by diabetes mellitus; vomiting; blood dyscrasias; renal damage; pain at injection site; GI disturbances
Occasional: may aggravate diabetes; shock; hypoglycemia; liver damage; cardiotoxicity; delirium; rash
Rare: Herxheimer-type reaction; anaphylaxis; acute pancreatitis; hyperkalemia; ventricular arrhythmias
Permethrin—Nix (GlaxoSmithKline), Elimite (Allergan)
Occasional: burning; stinging; numbness; increased pruritus; pain; edema; erythema; rash
Praziquantel—Biltricide (Bayer)
Frequent: abdominal pain; diarrhea; malaise; headache; dizziness
Occasional: sedation; fever; sweating; nausea; eosinophilia
Rare: rash; edema; hiccup
Primaquine phosphate USP
Frequent: hemolytic anemia in G6PD deficiency
Occasional: neutropenia; GI disturbances; methemoglobinemia
Rare: CNS symptoms; hypertension; arrhythmias
Proguanil—Paludrine (Wyeth Ayerst, Canada; AstraZeneca, United Kingdom); with atovaquone as Malarone (GlaxoSmithKline)
Occasional: nausea; vomiting; rash
Rare: hematuria (with large doses); vomiting; abdominal pain; diarrhea (with large doses); thrombocytopenia

*Drug interactions are generally not included here; see the current edition of *The Medical Letter Handbook of Adverse Drug Reactions.*
†Not available in the United States.
‡Available from the CDC Drug Service, Centers for Disease Control and Prevention, Atlanta, Ga 30333; 404-639-3670 (evenings, weekends, or holidays: 404-639-2888).
§Available in the United States only from the manufacturer.
CNS, central nervous system; G6PD, glucose-6-phosphate dehydrogenase; GI, gastrointestinal; IV, intravenously; MAO, monoamine oxidase.
Modified from Drugs for parasitic infections. Med Lett Drugs Ther. 1998;40:1-12, and Drugs for parasitic infections. Med Lett Drugs Ther. April 2002:1-11 (available at www.medletter.com), and used with permission.

Continued

TABLE 41-3   Manufacturers and Adverse Effects of Some Antiparasitic Drugs*—cont'd

Pyrantel pamoate—Antiminth (Pfizer)
    Occasional: GI disturbances; headache; dizziness; rash; fever
Pyrethrins and piperonyl butoxide –RID (Pfizer), others
    Occasional: allergic reactions
Pyrimethamine USP—Daraprim (GlaxoSmithKline)
    Occasional: blood dyscrasias; folic acid deficiency
    Rare: rash; vomiting; convulsions; shock; possibly pulmonary eosinophilia; fatal cutaneous reactions with pyrimethamine-sulfadoxine (Fansidar)
Quinine sulfate—many manufacturers
    Frequent: cinchonism (tinnitus, headache, nausea, abdominal pain, visual disturbance)
    Occasional: deafness; hemolytic anemia; other blood dyscrasias; photosensitivity reactions; hypoglycemia; arrhythmias; hypotension; drug fever
    Rare: blindness; sudden death if injected too rapidly

‡Sodium stibogluconate—Pentostam (GlaxoSmithKline, United Kingdom)
    Frequent: muscle and joint pain; fatigue; nausea; transaminase elevations; T-wave flattening or inversion; pancreatitis
    Occasional: weakness; abdominal pain; liver damage; bradycardia; leucopenia; thrombocytopenia; rash; vomiting
    Rare: diarrhea; pruritus; myocardial damage; hemolytic anemia; renal damage; shock; sudden death
§Spiramycin—Rovamycine (Aventis)
    Occasional: GI disturbances
    Rare: allergic reactions
‡Suramin sodium—(Bayer, Germany)
    Frequent: vomiting; pruritus; urticaria; paresthesias; hyperesthesias of hands and feet; photophobia; peripheral neuropathy
    Occasional: kidney damage; blood dyscrasias; shock; optic atrophy
†Tinidazole—Fasigyn (Pfizer, Presutti Laboratories)
    Occasional: metallic taste; nausea; vomiting; rash

*Drug interactions are generally not included here; see the current edition of *The Medical Letter Handbook of Adverse Drug Reactions.*
†Not available in the United States.
‡Available from the CDC Drug Service, Centers for Disease Control and Prevention, Atlanta, Ga 30333; 404-639-3670 (evenings, weekends, or holidays: 404-639-2888).
§Available in the United States only from the manufacturer.
CNS, central nervous system; G6PD, glucose-6-phosphate dehydrogenase; GI, gastrointestinal; IV, intravenously; MAO, monoamine oxidase.
Modified from Drugs for parasitic infections. Med Lett Drugs Ther. 1998;40:1-12, and Drugs for parasitic infections. Med Lett Drugs Ther. April 2002:1-11 (available at www.medletter.com), and used with permission.

DRUGS ACTIVE AGAINST LUMINAL PROTOZOA: AMEBAE, INTESTINAL AND VAGINAL FLAGELLATES, AND CILIATES

Metronidazole and Tinidazole

Metronidazole (Fig. 41-1) and tinidazole† have selective activity against numerous anaerobic protozoa and bacteria. Metronidazole, 2-methyl-5-nitroimidazole-1-ethanol, is used for the treatment of invasive enterocolitis and liver abscess due to *Entamoeba histolytica*[6-8] and *Entamoeba polecki* infections.[9,10] Metronidazole kills the trophozoites of *E. histolytica* in the intestine and in tissue, but it does not invariably eradicate the cysts.[6-8] A luminally active agent is required for that purpose and to treat asymptomatic cyst passers. Metronidazole is also the treatment of choice for vaginitis due to *Trichomonas vaginalis*,[11] but resistance has been well documented in some isolates.[12]

Although metronidazole has the approval of the U.S. Food and Drug Administration (FDA) only for the treatment of amebiasis and trichomoniasis, this does not prevent physicians from using it off label for other diseases, such as giardiasis, for which data support its efficacy.[13,14] Metronidazole is considered an alternative drug for the treatment of enterocolitis associated with *Blastocystis hominis*,[15] the pathogenicity of which has been debated, and *Balantidium coli*.[16] Finally, metronidazole is used for the treatment of the guinea worm, *Dracunculus medinensis*,[17,18] but its clinical activity does not appear to be related to a direct effect on the worm. The use of metronidazole for the treatment of anaerobic bacterial infections is discussed in Chapter 27.

Metronidazole is available for oral and parenteral administration. When it is administered orally, 90% to 95% is absorbed[19,20]; peak serum levels are reached within 1 hour. Metronidazole has limited plasma protein binding. It is widely distributed throughout the body and penetrates well into tissues, abscesses, fluid compartments, vaginal secretions, bone, central nervous system, and breast milk.[21,22] The elimination half-life is 6.2 to 11.5 hours. Metronidazole is extensively metabolized in the liver. The principal metabolites result from oxidation of side chains and glucuronide formation and are excreted via the kidney. Although renal failure prolongs the half-life of these metabolites, the hepatic metabolism is such that the drug dosage need not be modified during renal failure; however, it should be adjusted in liver failure and in persons with severe malnutrition.[23]

Metronidazole is activated in anaerobic organisms by reduction of the 5-nitro group through a sequence of intermediate steps involving microbial electron transport proteins of low redox potential.[24] This results in a concentration gradient across the membrane of the parasite and permits accumulation of high concentrations of the reduced compound within the cell. Metronidazole acts as an electron sink, depriving the anaerobe of reducing equivalents. Furthermore, the reduced form of metronidazole causes loss of the helical structure of DNA, strand breakage, and impaired template function.[25,26]

Gastrointestinal side effects include nausea, vomiting, diarrhea, and a metallic aftertaste. They are less common with the low doses (250 mg three times daily) recommended for giardiasis than with the high doses (750 mg three times daily) used for amebiasis. Other, less frequent side effects include headache, dizziness, dry mouth, stomatitis, rash, urethral burning, vaginal or oral candidiasis, and reversible neutropenia.[27] Side effects are seldom severe enough to cause discontinuation of the drug. The urine of some persons may become red or brown because of the presence of metabolites. Metronidazole can potentiate the anticoagulant effects of warfarin.[28] Rarely, patients treated with metronidazole experience peripheral neuropathy, paresthesia, tinnitus, vertigo, seizures, ataxia, psychotic disorders, or encephalopathy.[29] Acute pancreatitis has been reported.[30] Alcohol in beverages or elixirs must be avoided because of the disulfiram (Antabuse)-like effects of metronidazole and the potential of a life-threatening reaction if alcohol is ingested.[31]

The potential role of metronidazole in human carcinogenesis and birth defects has been debated.[32] Although metronidazole is mutagenic and causes DNA strand fragmentation in bacteria,[33] and human urine contains metabolites that are carcinogenic in rodents,[34] long-term follow-up studies of persons who have been treated with metronidazole have failed to demonstrate an increased prevalence of cancer.[35] Although it is not approved or recommended for use during pregnancy, treatment with oral metronidazole during pregnancy has not been associated with birth defects.[36]

Tinidazole† and ornidazole,† two other 5-nitroimidazole derivatives, have amebicidal, giardiacidal, and trichomonicidal activity similar to that of metronidazole.[5,37-40] Tinidazole has activity against some but not all strains of metronidazole-resistant *T. vaginalis*.[40,41] A single 2-g dose of tinidazole is effective for the treatment of giardiasis.[42] Both tinidazole and ornidazole are well absorbed orally, have good tissue penetration, and are widely distributed in the body. Tinidazole and ornidazole have half-lives of 14 and 12 to 13 hours, respectively.[43,44] They are excreted primarily in urine, 50% of tinidazole and 96% of ornidazole in the form of metabolites. These drugs have a favorable side effect profile when compared with metronidazole. Reported side effects include nausea, vomiting, anorexia, and a metallic or bitter taste. Tinidazole has recently been approved for use in the United States.

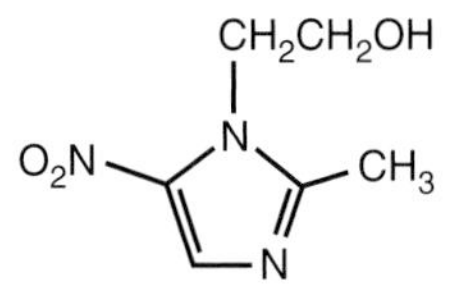

CH₂CH₂OH

O₂N — [imidazole ring] — CH₃

FIGURE 41-1. Metronidazole.

Nitazoxanide

Nitazoxanide is a 5-nitrothiazole-salicylamide derivative with a broad spectrum of antiprotozoal and anthelmintic activity.[45-49] It was approved by the FDA in 2003 for the treatment of diarrhea caused by *Cryptosporidium parvum* and *Giardia lamblia*.[45,46] It is the first drug to be licensed for cryptosporidiosis, and it has advantages over metronidazole, quinacrine, and paromomycin in the treatment of giardiasis. Unfortunately, nitazoxanide failures are common in patients with AIDS and cryptosporidiosis.[47] Its broad spectrum of activity includes other enteric protozoa such as *Entamoeba histolytica/dispar* and *Isospora belli;* two of the major intestinal roundworms, *Ascaris lumbricoides* and *Trichuris trichiura;* the tapeworms *Taenia saginata* and *Hymenolepis nana;* and variable activity against the liver fluke *Fasciola hepatica*.

Nitazoxanide is available in liquid form, making it ideal for the treatment of children as young as 12 months. Its mechanism of action is unknown, but has been postulated to relate to inhibition of pyruvate-ferredoxin oxidoreductase enzyme-dependent electron transfer reactions that are essential to the metabolism of anaerobic organisms.[46] In general, nitazoxanide is well tolerated. In a pooled analysis of pediatric patients who were negative for human immunodeficiency virus (HIV) infection, adverse events occurred with a frequency similar to that observed with the placebo.[46] They included abdominal pain, diarrhea, vomiting, and headache. Yellow sclerae occur rarely because of deposition of the drug in the sclera, but this effect resolves after discontinuation.

Intestinal parasites are prevalent in developing areas of the world where sanitation is poor. Children are often infected with multiple parasitic pathogens. Nitazoxanide may eventually be shown to have a role in the empiric treatment of children with diarrhea or other clinical syndromes in areas where pathogenic intestinal protozoa and helminths are prevalent and diagnostic tests are not available or too costly, and possibly even in community- or school-based mass treatment programs,[48,49] but further studies are needed before such recommendations can be made.

Paromomycin (Aminosidine, Humatin)

Paromomycin, like other aminoglycoside antibiotics, is poorly absorbed after oral administration and reaches high concentrations in the lumen of the colon. It is used for the treatment of asymptomatic intestinal amebiasis, for the eradication of *E. histolytica* cysts in persons with intestinal or extraintestinal amebiasis who are treated with metronidazole,[50,51] and for treatment of *Dientamoeba fragilis* infection.[52] Administration of paromomycin was initially reported to improve diarrhea in some persons with HIV infection and cryptosporidiosis,[53] but other studies have shown no effect.[54] Paromomycin has been used topically to treat metronidazole-resistant trichomoniasis, but this has been associated with local side effects[55,56] It has been applied topically in the treatment of cutaneous leishmaniasis caused by *Leishmania major*,[57,58] and it has been administered systemically to a limited number of persons to treat visceral leishmaniasis.[59,60]

Paromomycin is administered orally to treat enteric infections. Like other aminoglycoside antibiotics, it binds to 30S ribosomal RNA in the aminoacyl-tRNA site, resulting in inhibition of protein synthesis. Side effects are primarily gastrointestinal and include nausea, vomiting, abdominal cramps, and diarrhea in some patients. Paromomycin is potentially ototoxic and nephrotoxic when adminis-

tered parenterally. Although little is absorbed from the gastrointestinal tract, oral paromomycin is contraindicated in persons with renal failure. Pancreatitis was reported in a patient with AIDS and cryptosporidiosis who received paromomycin.[61]

Iodoquinol

Iodoquinol (diiodohydroxyquin), a halogenated oxyquinoline (5,7-diiodo-8-quinolinol), is a luminally active agent used to eradicate cysts in persons with asymptomatic *E. histolytica* infection or after metronidazole administration in persons with invasive intestinal or extraintestinal disease. Iodoquinol is also recommended for the treatment of *D. fragilis* and *B. hominis*, and it is used as an alternative drug for the treatment of *B. coli*.[5,62]

Iodoquinol is administered orally. It is poorly absorbed and best tolerated if given with meals. The mechanism of action is not known. Side effects include headache, diarrhea, nausea, vomiting and abdominal pain, fever, itching, seizures, and encephalopathy.[63,64] The high iodine content (63%) can interfere with the results of thyroid function tests for months after completion of therapy. Occasionally, the drug is associated with iodine dermatitis (iodine toxicoderma). Iodoquinol is contraindicated in persons with iodine intolerance. A related compound, iodochlorhydroxyquin, gained notoriety as a cause of subacute myelo-optic neuropathy and was discontinued. Optic nerve damage or inflammation and peripheral neuropathy may occur with prolonged or high doses of iodoquinol as well. The dosage regimen recommended for amebic disease (see Table 41-2) avoids these complications, but the recommended doses and duration of therapy should never be exceeded.[5]

Diloxanide Furoate

Diloxanide furoate,† a substituted acetanilide, 4-(*N*-methyl-2,2-dichloroacetamido)phenyl-2-furoate, is a luminally active agent used for the treatment of asymptomatic *E. histolytica* infection[50,65,66] and to eradicate cysts after treatment of invasive disease with metronidazole, but it is less effective than paromomycin.[50] It is not effective in the treatment of invasive or extraintestinal amebiasis. Diloxanide furoate is hydrolyzed by intestinal esterases, releasing diloxanide, which is absorbed. Delayed or reduced absorption of the ester results in higher concentrations in the large intestine and the desired luminal effect.

Diloxanide furoate is formulated in tablets. In experimental animals, 60% to 90% of the drug is excreted in the urine within 48 hours.[69] Excretion in the feces accounts for 4% to 9%. Diloxanide is amebicidal at low concentrations, but the mechanism of action is unknown. There are rarely serious side effects at the recommended dosage. The most common untoward effect is flatulence.[67] Mild gastrointestinal complaints may also occur.

Furazolidone

Furazolidone, 3-([5-nitro-2-furanyl]methylene-amino)-2-oxazolidinone, is a nitrofuran derivative. Like other nitrofurans, it acts by damaging DNA. It is available as a liquid and has been used for the treatment of giardiasis in children who are unable to take metronidazole tablets.[68,69] Furazolidone also has activity against *Helicobacter pylori* and a variety of enteropathogenic bacteria. Although not curative, it has been shown to provide symptomatic relief in patients with AIDS who have diarrhea and are infected with *E. bieneusi*.[70]

Furazolidone is well absorbed; more than 65% is recovered in the urine in the form of metabolites.[67] Common side effects include nausea, vomiting, diarrhea, and fever.[68] Some of the metabolites are brown and may discolor the urine. Rare side effects include hypotension, urticaria, serum sickness, hypersensitivity reactions, and mood disorders.[67,71] Mild to moderate hemolysis may occur in patients with glucose-6-phosphate dehydrogenase (G6PD) deficiency. As with metronidazole, alcohol should not be ingested because furazolidone has disulfiram-like activity. It is also a monoamine oxidase inhibitor. Furazolidone should not be administered to mothers who are breast-feeding or to neonates, because hemolytic anemia due to glutathione instability may occur.

DRUGS USED AGAINST MALARIA, TOXOPLASMOSIS, CRYPTOSPORIDIOSIS, CYCLOSPORIASIS, AND PNEUMOCYSTOSIS

Malaria and related coccidian diseases are important causes of morbidity and mortality worldwide. The four *Plasmodium* species that infect humans are responsible for an estimated 300 to 500 million new cases of malaria annually, and between 1.5 and 3.0 million deaths, most of which are due to *Plasmodium falciparum* (see Chapter 272).[72] Countries in tropical Africa account for more than 90% of the total cases and mortality. As travel has increased, so has the exposure of nonimmune hosts to malaria. For example, every year more than 1 million Americans visit tropical or subtropical areas, where they are potentially exposed. At least 10,000 cases of acute malaria are estimated to occur among international travelers from the United States and other industrialized countries each year.[72] The erythrocytic stage of *Plasmodium* species is the most susceptible to chemotherapy and prophylaxis.[73] A limited number of drugs are active against the exoerythrocytic stages in the liver. Sporozoites, which are inoculated by mosquitoes, are resistant to all currently available drugs. The resistance of *P. falciparum* and, more recently, *Plasmodium vivax* to antimalarials has complicated prophylaxis and treatment.[72,73] *P. ovale* and *P. malariae* have remained susceptible to chloroquine. The CDC provides updated information on susceptibility by geographic region.[74]

T. gondii is ubiquitous throughout the world. Acquired infection is usually asymptomatic or mild, but acute infection during pregnancy can result in severe birth defects. *T. gondii* is an important cause of encephalitis in persons with AIDS and other immunocompromising conditions. *Cryptosporidium parvum* and *I. belli* can cause sporadic and epidemic diarrhea in immunocompetent hosts, and, along with the microsporidia, are important enteric pathogens in persons with AIDS. *Cyclospora cayetanensis* has been associated with diarrhea in residents of developing areas, travelers, and North Americans who have eaten imported raspberries from Central America.

Drugs used for the treatment and prevention of malaria as well as toxoplasmosis, and those used to treat *I. belli* and *C. cayetanensis* are described in detail under the following headings. Nitazoxanide, the only drug licensed for treatment of cryptosporidiosis, was reviewed earlier. As mentioned earlier, *Pneumocystis jirovecii* is now classified as a fungus, but it is susceptible to many of the drugs used to treat malaria and related protozoa. Drugs used to treat pneumocystosis are therefore included in this section.

Aminoquinolines Used for the Prophylaxis and Treatment of Malaria

Chloroquine. Chloroquine (Fig. 41-2), 7-chloro-4-(4-diethylamino-1-methylbutylamino)-quinoline, the best known of the 4-aminoquinolines, is active against the erythrocytic stages of susceptible *Plasmodium* species. It was once the mainstay of antimalarial chemotherapy and prophylaxis, but the widespread emergence of chloroquine-resistant *P. falciparum* throughout the world has limited its use. Only Central America west of the Panama Canal, Haiti, the Dominican Republic, and some areas of the Middle East can be considered free of chloroquine-resistant *P. falciparum*.[74] Although still geographically restricted, chloroquine-resistant *P. vivax* has been identified in Papua New Guinea, India, Irian Jaya, the Solomon Islands, Indonesia, Myanmar, Guyana, and the Brazilian Amazon region.[75-80] *P. ovale* and *P. malariae* have remained susceptible to chloroquine. Chloroquine has also been used for the treatment of rheumatoid arthritis and systemic lupus erythematosus. Hydroxychloroquine has a spectrum of antimalarial activity similar to that of chloroquine and has been used for prophylaxis.

Chloroquine phosphate is available as a bitter white medication, which is dispensed in tablets containing 250 or 500 mg of the salt (150- and 300-mg base, respectively). Prescriptions should clearly indicate whether chloroquine is being ordered as the salt or as the base to avoid confusion. Chloroquine is rapidly absorbed after oral ingestion and is slowly excreted.[81] The therapeutic blood concentration is reached within 2 or 3 hours. Chloroquine is widely distributed

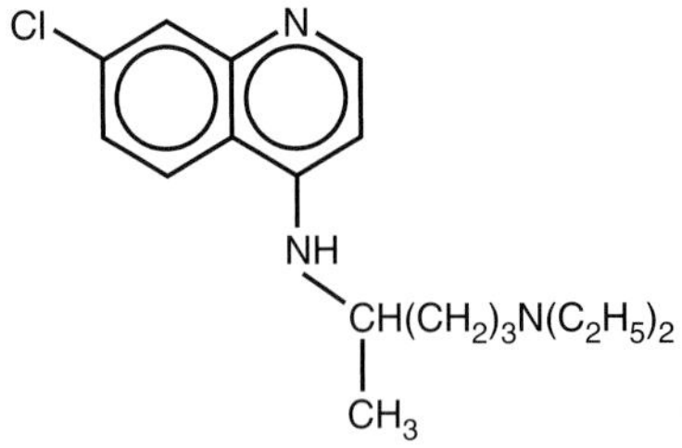

FIGURE 41-2. Chloroquine.

throughout the body and is relatively concentrated in the liver, spleen, kidneys, and erythrocytes. It is metabolized by alkylation in the liver, but approximately 50% of the parent drug is excreted in the urine. The half-life is 4 days, which allows once-weekly administration for prophylaxis.[82,83] Approximately 50% of chloroquine is protein bound. The renal status of the patient does not affect the amount used for acute malaria, but prophylactic doses should be reduced for those with reduced renal function.[83]

Chloroquine is a dibasic compound. It is concentrated in the acidic vacuoles of intraerythrocytic parasites.[84,85] The concentration in parasitized erythrocytes is 100-fold higher than in nonparasitized ones.[84] In erythrocytes with schizonts, the concentration of chloroquine is 600-fold higher than in plasma. Chloroquine has a marked and rapid effect on the hemoglobin-containing digestive vesicles of asexual erythrocytic parasites.

Ferriprotoporphyrin IX, a product of hemoglobin degradation by the parasite, damages membranes and inhibits a variety of parasitic enzymes in its soluble form. *Plasmodium* species protect themselves from the toxic effects of this molecule by the activity of a heme polymerase that incorporates ferriprotoporphyrin IX into an insoluble, nontoxic crystalline material. Chloroquine and hydroxychloroquine inhibit this enzyme.[86]

Chloroquine-resistant plasmodia transport chloroquine out of intraparasitic compartments more rapidly than susceptible strains and maintain lower chloroquine concentrations in their acid vesicles.[87] There is experimental evidence that this situation can be reversed by drugs that block calcium channels,[88,89] but the high concentrations required in vivo have prevented such a treatment from being used clinically.

Chloroquine is relatively well tolerated when used at the recommended doses for chemoprophylaxis or treatment of susceptible *Plasmodium* species. Oral administration is preferred. Temporary side effects include headache, nausea, vomiting, blurred vision, dizziness, fatigue, and confusion.[81,83] Some Africans experience pruritus, which responds to an antihistamine. Rare side effects include depigmentation of hair, corneal opacities, weight loss, insomnia, leukopenia, myalgias, exacerbation of psoriasis, and exfoliative dermatoses. Extremely rare reactions include blood dyscrasias, peripheral neuropathy, nerve deafness, myopathy, arrhythmia, heart block, toxic psychosis, and photophobia. Permanent retinal damage has occurred with long-term, high-dose therapy administered to persons with collagen vascular diseases[90] but not with long-term weekly doses for malaria prophylaxis. Chloroquine is relatively contraindicated in persons with retinal disease, psoriasis, or porphyria.

Chloroquine can also be given by intravenous infusion, but it must be administered slowly and with great caution.[83,91] Respiratory depression, hypotension, cardiovascular collapse, and seizures can follow excessively rapid parenteral administration. Heart block and cardiac arrest are thought to be caused by a direct toxic effect on the myocardium of high plasma chloroquine concentrations. It is recommended that oral administration be substituted for parenteral administration as soon as possible. In the United States, quinidine is used when parenteral therapy is necessary for acute malaria.

Deaths from chloroquine toxicity have followed accidental ingestion by children and have occurred in adults who habitually self-medicate and in persons attempting suicide. The ingestion of as little as 5 g of

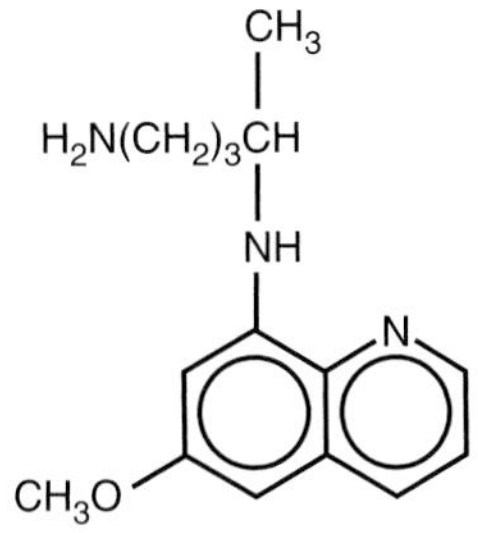

FIGURE 41-3. Primaquine.

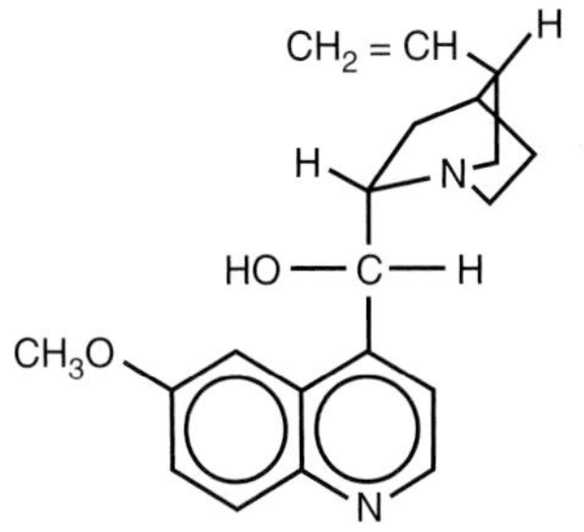

FIGURE 41-4. Quinine.

chloroquine can be fatal. Therapy includes mechanical ventilation and other supportive measures. Although diazepam has been recommended, its efficacy in this setting has not been documented.[92] Chloroquine was implicated in severe cochleovestibular abnormalities in the fetus of a mother taking high doses for the treatment of systemic lupus erythematosus.[93] There does not appear to be an association between chloroquine administered in antimalarial doses and fetal abnormalities.[83]

Primaquine. Primaquine (Fig. 41-3), an 8-aminoquinoline, 8-(4-amino-1-methylbutylamino)-6-methoxyquinoline, is the only drug available that has activity against the exoerythrocytic, hypnozoite forms of *P. vivax* and *Plasmodium ovale* that reside in the liver. It is administered after chloroquine treatment of acute *P. vivax* or *P. ovale* infection and after prophylaxis with chloroquine or other drugs in persons who have had substantial exposure to *P. vivax* or *P. ovale*.[5,72-74] Relapses occur in a variable percentage of persons after primaquine therapy at the recommended dose of 26.3 mg (salt) daily for 14 days. This was initially reported from the Western Pacific; more recent reports have suggested decreased sensitivity to primaquine in areas of Southeast Asia, Africa, and Latin America. Relapses after conventional primaquine therapy can be treated with higher doses or for longer periods of time.[94-98] Primaquine and a related 8-aminoquinoline, tafenoquine, have been used effectively as prophylaxis against *P. falciparum* in controlled clinical trials,[99,100] but the risk of hemolysis in persons with G6PD deficiency and in fetuses has limited enthusiasm for their use in prophylaxis. Primaquine has gametocytocidal activity against all four *Plasmodium* species that infect humans, but it is not of clinical significance. Primaquine in combination with clindamycin has been used for the treatment of mild to moderately severe *Pneumocystis carinii* pneumonia.[101] The combination has also been used for prophylaxis against *P. carinii*, but it was less effective than trimethoprim-sulfamethoxazole or dapsone in the doses studied.[102]

Primaquine phosphate is supplied in tablets containing 26.3 mg of the salt, which is equivalent to 15 mg of the base. The therapeutic dosage is usually expressed in terms of the base and should be clearly indicated on prescriptions. It has a bitter taste. Tablets may be crushed and added to sweet liquid or fruit to make it more palatable for children. Primaquine is readily absorbed when taken orally. Plasma concentrations reach a peak at 6 hours and decline to undetectable levels by 24 hours.

The mechanism of action is uncertain, but primaquine is fully active only after metabolism by the host. The nature of the active metabolites is not clear. Based on studies with pamaquine,† the first in this series of drugs, primaquine is thought to affect both the mitochondrial electron transport chain and pyrimidine synthesis.[103] Primaquine also selectively inhibits the formation of functional cellular transport vesicles in vitro.[104]

The major toxicity with primaquine is hemolysis in persons with G6PD deficiency.[105,106] Approximately 1% of males in the Middle East, 5% of Chinese males, and 10% of black males are deficient. G6PD deficiency is rare in whites, but it is recommended that all persons be tested for G6PD deficiency before primaquine is prescribed. Primaquine is contraindicated during pregnancy because of the risk of hemolysis if the fetus is G6PD deficient. Administration of primaquine should be discontinued if signs of hemolysis (darkening of the urine or a fall in hematocrit) are noted. For persons with the more mild African

form of G6PD deficiency, a dose of 45 mg (base) weekly for 8 weeks has been used.[73,74] Because hypnozoites of *P. vivax* and *P. ovale* have finite life spans, long-term suppression with chloroquine or another agent active against intraerythrocytic parasites is an alternative in patients with G6PD deficiency.

Apart from the potential for hemolysis, primaquine is usually well tolerated. Abdominal cramps, epigastric distress, and nausea occur in some patients. Mild anemia, cyanosis, methemoglobinemia, with primaquine alone or in combination with dapsone,[108] or leukocytosis is observed in some persons given higher doses. Rare complications include granulocytopenia or agranulocytosis, hypertension, and arrhythmias.

Cinchona Alkaloids: Quinine and Quinidine

Quinine. Quinine (Fig. 41-4), a cinchona alkaloid, is the oldest of the antimalarial drugs, dating to the use of cinchona bark by South American Indians for febrile illnesses.[83] It acts rapidly against asexual erythrocytic stages of all four *Plasmodium* species that infect humans. After the introduction of chloroquine, the use of quinine diminished, but with the widespread emergence of chloroquine-resistant *P. falciparum*, its use increased dramatically. Decreasing sensitivity to quinine has been documented in isolates of *P. falciparum* in Southeast Asia,[74] and there have been reports of decreased sensitivity in West Africa as well.[109,110]

Quinine sulfate is available for oral use, but it has a bitter taste. It is rapidly absorbed from the gastrointestinal tract and reaches peak levels in 1 to 3 hours. Peak serum concentrations after the recommended dose of 10 mg/kg are 7 to 17 µg/mL; side effects can be seen at concentrations greater than 10 µg/mL.[83] Quinine is formulated for parenteral use as quinine dihydrochloride. The parenteral preparation is no longer available in the United States. Intravenous quinidine, its dextrostereoisomer, is used in the United States and some other industrialized countries.[5]

Quinine is metabolized in the liver and excreted in the urine, mainly as metabolites. Only 20% of the drug is excreted unchanged.[111] It is not as avidly bound to tissues as chloroquine and has a shorter half-life of 5 to 15 hours. Malaria is associated with a reduction in the systemic clearance of quinine that is proportional to the severity of disease. The elimination half-life is prolonged by approximately 50% in persons with malaria.[112] Monitoring of blood levels is recommended for persons with impaired renal or hepatic function, and dose reduction is necessary in those with severe renal impairment.[113]

The exact mechanism of action of quinine as an antimalarial is unknown, but, like chloroquine, it may act at the level of the hemoglobin-containing digestive vesicles of intraerythrocytic parasites. Quinine and other quinolinemethanols bind to high-density lipoproteins in the serum and may be transported into plasmodium-infected erythrocytes via a pathway for the uptake of exogenous phospholipids.[114] There is speculation that they may act on specific parasite proteins. Quinine can intercalate into DNA, but this does not appear to be its primary mode of action.

Quinine has the poorest therapeutic-to-toxic ratio of all of the antimalarial drugs. The side effects are collectively referred to as *cinchonism* and include tinnitus, temporary hearing loss, headache, dysphoria, nausea, vomiting, and mild visual disturbances.[83] These alterations are dose related and reversible. Other, less common side effects include rash, urticaria, angioedema of the face, pruritus, agranulocytosis, hepatitis, and, rarely, massive hemolysis in persons with falciparum malaria (blackwater fever). Quinine has a curare-like effect on skeletal muscle and was used for the treatment of nocturnal leg cramps. It can result in respiratory depression in patients with myasthenia gravis.

An important adverse effect in patients with severe *P. falciparum* malaria is hypoglycemia, which is caused in part by the parasites' consumption of glucose and in part by the release of insulin from the pancreas by quinine.[115] It can be treated and prevented by the administration of intravenous glucose.

Quinine can cause hemolysis in patients with G6PD deficiency. It can stimulate uterine contractions and may produce abortion if given in high doses. However, quinine has been used successfully to treat seriously ill women with malaria during the third trimester of pregnancy.[116] Quinine must be used cautiously if administered by the intravenous route, because rapid infusion may cause shock as a result of myocardial depression and peripheral vasodilatation. Overdoses are associated with convulsions, coma, delirium, depressed respiration, circulatory collapse, and death.

Quinidine. Quinidine, the dextrostereoisomer of quinine, is used in the United States and elsewhere for persons requiring parenteral treatment of falciparum malaria.[117-120] An advantage of parenteral quinidine over parenteral quinine has been its usefulness in the treatment of cardiac arrhythmias, but its availability has diminished in recent years as less toxic cardiotropic drugs have taken its place for this purpose.[121]

Quinidine gluconate is available for intravenous administration. The half-life is 12.8 hours. Electrocardiographic changes including prolonged QTc intervals are common, but life-threatening arrhythmias are rare if proper doses are used. Hypotension may occur if the infusion is too rapid. The rate of infusion, blood pressure, and electrocardiograms of persons receiving intravenous quinidine should be monitored closely in an intensive care setting.[121]

4-Quinoline-Carbinolamines (Quinolinemethanols): Mefloquine

Mefloquine (Fig. 41-5) is a quinolinemethanol derived chemically from quinine. Like quinine and chloroquine, mefloquine is a blood schizonticidal drug and has no effect on exoerythrocytic schizonts or gametocytes. Used in a single weekly dose, it is effective in prophylaxis against all four *Plasmodium* species that infect humans, including chloroquine-resistant isolates of *P. falciparum*. Mefloquine was once widely used for prophylaxis against chloroquine-resistant *P. falciparum*, but it has come under increasing scrutiny because of its association with severe neuropsychiatric side effects in a small proportion of recipients. The FDA now requires that all persons who receive mefloquine for prophylaxis receive a printed drug information sheet describing its potential neuropsychiatric effects and other toxicities. Mefloquine administered at a higher dosage can be used to treat acute chloroquine-resistant falciparum malaria, but toxicity is common. Resistance to mefloquine is prevalent in Thailand and some other areas of Southeast Asia, and it has been reported from West Africa and South America.[122-127]

Mefloquine is available only for oral administration. It is slowly and incompletely absorbed.[128] It is widely distributed in the body; 99% of the drug is protein bound. It has a long (but variable) half-life in humans, ranging from 6 to 23 days, with a mean of 14 days. Mefloquine is given weekly at an adult dose of 250 mg for malaria prophylaxis. When used for the treatment of acute malaria, it can be administered as a single dose of 1250 mg or in divided doses of 750 mg followed in 12 hours by 500 mg, but toxicity is common. It is extensively metabolized and excreted through bile and feces. Mefloquine concentrates in red blood cell membranes and seems to interfere with the food vacuoles of *Plasmodium* species in a manner similar to that of quinine.[129]

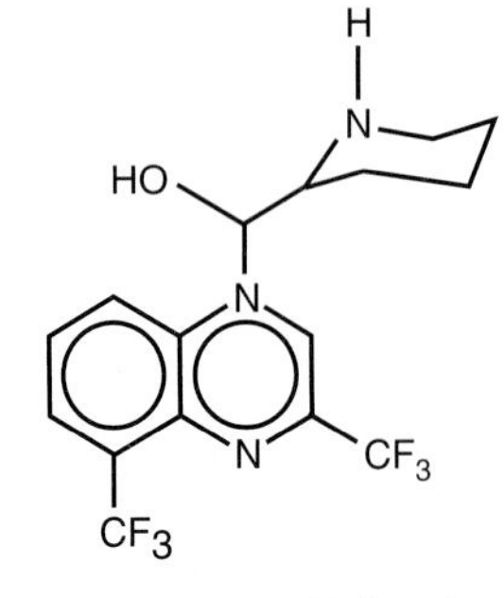

Mild side effects with mefloquine, such as nausea, dizziness, and vivid dreams, are relatively common. More severe neuropsychiatric reactions such as seizures, acute psychosis, anxiety neurosis, and disturbances of the sleep-wake cycle have been estimated to occur in 0.5% of users after treatment dosages.[130] They are less common with prophylactic dosages, but serious psychiatric syndromes occur and have sparked debate over the risk-benefit ratio of mefloquine for prophylaxis.[131,132] Treatment doses of mefloquine have been associated with vertigo, nausea, and headache in the majority of recipients, often requiring bed rest for days.[133]

Mefloquine can cause alterations in cardiac conduction. Sinus bradycardia and sinus arrhythmia are common during therapy, but in the absence of other cardiac medications, these changes are transient and benign. Mefloquine is contraindicated in persons with cardiac abnormalities who are taking drugs that alter cardiac conduction, such as β-blockers, and in persons with a history of epilepsy and psychiatric disorders. It is also contraindicated during pregnancy.

Rare adverse effects with mefloquine include exfoliative dermatitis and the Stevens-Johnson syndrome, agranulocytosis, cutaneous vasculitis, and paresthesias.[134-138] Mefloquine has antibiotic activity and kills the live *Salmonella typhi* (Ty21a) oral vaccine at concentrations achieved enterally. Consequently, administration of that vaccine should be separated in time from administration of mefloquine.[139] Mefloquine has not been observed to cause birth defects in humans,[140] but it is teratogenic in animals at high doses. It is advisable for women to avoid taking the drug while pregnant unless the benefit is deemed to outweigh the risk. Because of its long half-life, women should be advised to use contraceptive measures for 3 months after the last dose of mefloquine. Despite initial concerns, mefloquine does not appear to adversely affect fine motor coordination or spatial discrimination and can be prescribed for persons whose activities involve those skills.[141]

Halofantrine

Halofantrine** is a 9-phenanthrenemethanol with activity against chloroquine-sensitive and chloroquine-resistant *P. falciparum* and *P. vivax*. It is a blood schizonticide with activity against the intraerythrocytic stages of *Plasmodium* species. Although not available in the United States, halofantrine is used for the treatment of falciparum malaria in residents and travelers to areas where chloroquine and sulfonamide-pyrimethamine resistance are prevalent. Cross-resistance between halofantrine and mefloquine has been documented, although some patients who have failed to respond to mefloquine have responded to halofantrine. The use of halofantrine has been associated with infrequent but potentially life-threatening cardiac effects, including prolongation of the QTc interval, torsades de pointes, and fatal arrhythmias.[142,143] Whenever possible, alternative forms of treatment should be used.

Artemisinin Derivatives (Qinghaosu)

Artemisinin and its derivatives, artemether, artesunate, and arteether, are sesquiterpene lactones derived from the wormwood plant *Artemisia annua*. Qinghaosu, an extract of the plant, has been used for centuries as a traditional Chinese medication for febrile illnesses and is known to have activity against *Plasmodium* species, the free-living ameba *Naegleria fowleri*, and the trematodes *Schistosoma japonicum, Schistosoma mansoni*, and *Clonorchis sinensis*. Artemisinin and its derivatives represent an exciting breakthrough in the treatment of multidrug-resistant falciparum malaria.[144-147] They result in more rapid parasitologic clearance than the aminoquinoline antimalarials and have comparable efficacy against susceptible strains. They are relatively cheap to produce and are well tolerated. They have short half-

FIGURE 41-5. Mefloquine.

lives, however, which limits their potential for prophylaxis. To date, the lack of detailed data on their pharmacology and toxicity have precluded approval by Western regulatory agencies.

Artemisinin and its derivatives are endoperoxide-containing compounds. Although their mode of action is not fully understood, it is thought that they are converted to free radicals and other intermediates in the presence of intraparasitic iron, which alkylate malarial proteins or damage membranes.[148] They act rapidly, arresting parasite development and preventing cytoadherence and rosetting, both thought to be important pathophysiologic mechanisms in severe falciparum malaria.

Depending on the derivative, the compounds are available for enteral, intravenous, or intramuscular administration.[148,149] They are cleared rapidly from the circulation. Delivery of artemisinin by suppository allows treatment of severe malaria in patients who cannot take oral medications and in settings where injections cannot be given.[146] Artemisinin derivatives are frequently administered with mefloquine or other antimalarial drugs to prevent relapse.

Experience to date suggests that the artemisinin derivatives are much better tolerated than quinine or treatment doses of mefloquine in patients with acute falciparum malaria. Adverse effects have been infrequent and mild.[144-147] They have included decreases in reticulocyte and neutrophil counts, elevated liver transaminases, abdominal pain, diarrhea, and drug fever. Contact dermatitis is well documented with sesquiterpene lactones,[150] and cerebellar dysfunction has been reported in association with artesunate.[151] Neuropathic effects have been reported in dogs given chronic, high-dose therapy.[152] To date, similar neuropathic effects have not been documented in humans.[153] Clinical isolates resistant to artemisinin derivatives have been reported from Africa.[154]

Atovaquone

Hydroxynaphthoquinones have been known to have antimalarial activity since World War II, but problems with poor absorption and rapid metabolism limited their use.[155] Atovaquone, a newer member of the class, is an exception (Fig. 41-6). Atovaquone has activity against *Plasmodium* species, but early studies suggested that there was a high relapse rate when it was used alone.[156] The fixed combination of atovaquone and proguanil (Malarone; see later) has proven to be as effective as mefloquine for the prophylaxis of chloroquine-resistant *falciparum* malaria but has fewer side effects.[157-162] Resistance has been documented in a limited number of cases.[163]

Atovaquone is also an alternative to trimethoprim-sulfamethoxazole for the treatment of mild to moderately severe *Pneumocystis* pneumonia.[155,164] It can be used for prophylaxis in immunocompromised patients intolerant of sulfonamides.[165,166] The combination of atovaquone and pyrimethamine has also been used to treat toxoplasmosis and for long-term suppression of *T. gondii* in persons with AIDS who cannot tolerate sulfonamides.[155,167,168]

Atovaquone is available in tablets or oral suspension. The bioavailability is low after oral administration, but it can be enhanced by administration with a fatty meal. Atovaquone is highly lipophilic and protein bound. The half-life is 2.2 to 3.2 days. More than 90% of the drug is eliminated in the feces. Rifampin reduces atovaquone serum concentrations by 50%, whereas either fluconazole or prednisolone raises steady-state atovaquone concentrations by 20%. Atovaquone is generally well tolerated. Side effects include fever,

FIGURE 41-6. Atovaquone.

skin rash, cough, nausea, vomiting, diarrhea, headache, and insomnia. The Stevens-Johnson syndrome has been associated with the use of atovaquone-proguanil.[169]

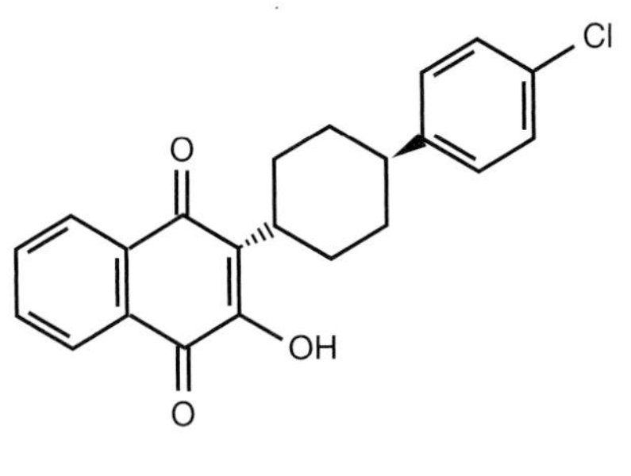

Dihydrofolate Reductase Inhibitors, Sulfonamides, and Sulfones

Proguanil. Also known as chloroguanide, this was the first agent found to inhibit plasmodial dihydrofolate reductase through the action of its metabolite, cycloguanil. The elucidation of its mechanism of action led to the synthesis of the diaminopyrimidines pyrimethamine and trimethoprim.[170] Daily proguanil has been used with weekly chloroquine as prophylaxis against *P. falciparum,* but failures were common in East Africa, and other drugs are now recommended.[171] More recently, proguanil has been used successfully in fixed combination with atovaquone (Malarone) for prophylaxis against *P. falciparum* malaria (as discussed later).

Proguanil reaches peak serum concentrations 2 to 4 hours after ingestion. The serum levels decline to practically zero by 24 hours. It must be taken daily to provide effective malaria prophylaxis. The concentration of proguanil in erythrocytes is six times that in plasma. Approximately 40% to 60% is excreted in the urine and 10% in the feces. It is the metabolite, cycloguanil, that inhibits plasmodial dihydrofolate reductase. Proguanil is generally well tolerated at doses used for malaria prophylaxis, but hematologic effects have been reported on rare occasion.[172] At higher levels, proguanil can produce nausea, vomiting, abdominal pain, and diarrhea. Excessive amounts have been associated with hematuria, proteinuria, and renal casts.

Atovaquone Plus Proguanil (Malarone). The fixed combination of atovaquone plus proguanil (Malarone) is effective for both prophylaxis and treatment of uncomplicated *P. falciparum* malaria and has a favorable toxicity profile.[157-162] For prophylaxis, a traveler takes the drug daily beginning 2 to 3 days prior to departure, while being exposed, and for 7 days after leaving the malaria-endemic area, because atovaquone-proguanil has activity against developing exoerythrocytic parasites. The combination has also been used effectively for the treatment of acute, uncomplicated malaria. Treatment of *P. vivax* and *P. ovale* with atovaquone-proguanil should be followed by a course of primaquine to prevent late relapse.[73,74] Although resistance to the combination is not currently widespread, cases have been reported and point mutations leading to resistance may become more common.[163]

For adults, each tablet of Malarone contains 250 mg atovaquone and 100 mg proguanil. Pediatric tablets are one quarter of the adult size. Atovaquone acts by selectively inhibiting electron transport in the cytochrome bc_1 complex in *Plasmodium*. Proguanil enhances the ability of atovaquone to collapse the mitochondrial potential, and its metabolite, cycloguanil, inhibits plasmodial dihydrofolate reductase thymidylate synthetase. Nausea, headache, and dizziness can occur, but Malarone is generally well tolerated.

Pyrimethamine and Trimethoprim. Studies of the mechanism of action of proguanil led to the synthesis of the diaminopyrimidines pyrimethamine and trimethoprim.[170] These dihydrofolate reductase inhibitors have been used alone and, more commonly, in conjunction with sulfonamides to treat a number of protozoal infections. Sensitive *Plasmodium* species, and presumably other susceptible parasites, are dependent on de novo pyrimidine synthesis. Folic acid derivatives are essential cofactors. Unlike mammalian cells, these parasites cannot use preformed pyrimidines obtained through salvage pathways. Dihydrofolate reductase inhibitors and sulfonamides act at sequential steps in the folic acid cycle.

Pyrimethamine is more active than trimethoprim in inhibiting the dihydrofolate reductases of *Plasmodium* species and *T. gondii*. In contrast, trimethoprim has greater activity against bacteria. Both of these drugs have some inhibitory effect on mammalian dihydrofolate reductase. This is more of a problem with pyrimethamine than with trimethoprim. Trimetrexate,[†] a low-molecular-weight, lipid-soluble dihydrofolate reductase inhibitor, has been used for treatment of pneumocystosis and toxoplasmosis.[173] To prevent potentially fatal bone marrow toxicity, leucovorin must be administered concurrently and patients monitored closely for hematologic toxicity with trimetrexate.

Pyrimethamine. Pyrimethamine (Fig. 41-7), a 2,4-diaminopyrimidine, has been used alone and in combination with sulfadoxine, a long-acting sulfonamide, for the prevention and treatment of chloroquine-resistant falciparum malaria (each tablet of Fansidar[†] contains 25 mg pyrimethamine and 500 mg sulfadoxine). However, resistance is now common, and furthermore sulfadoxine was associated with severe, life-threatening hypersensitivity reactions in 1 in 11,000 to 26,000 recipients.[174]

Pyrimethamine also has activity against *T. gondii*[175-178] and *P. jirovecii*[179,180] and is currently recommended for the treatment of toxoplasmosis. The majority of immunocompetent persons who acquire *T. gondii* have mild or asymptomatic, self-limited infections and do not require treatment. For those with syndromes that require treatment, a combination of pyrimethamine and sulfadiazine is the treatment of choice.[5] In immunocompromised persons, including those with AIDS, *Toxoplasma* encephalitis can be life-threatening, and therapy with pyrimethamine and sulfonamides for prolonged periods is recommended.[175-178] Untoward side effects are encountered in more than half of persons with AIDS and *Toxoplasma* encephalitis who receive sulfonamides and pyrimethamine. They include fever, skin rash, bone marrow suppression, and hepatotoxicity. In persons who cannot tolerate sulfonamides, clindamycin[178] or atovaquone[167,168] is used as an alternative with pyrimethamine. Pyrimethamine can also be used with a short-acting sulfonamide or dapsone for primary prophylaxis against *T. gondii* in HIV-infected patients with low CD4 T-lymphocyte counts (lower than 100 cells/mm³), but trimethoprim-sulfamethoxazole is better tolerated and provides protection against *Pneumocystis* pneumonia as well.[179,180] The optimal treatment for prenatal toxoplasmosis during pregnancy is uncertain[181]; pyrimethamine is contraindicated, at least for the first trimester, and sulfonamides cannot be used close to the time of delivery because they displace bilirubin from binding sites on albumin. Spiramycin, a macrolide, is an alternative, but it has not been licensed for use in the United States. The combination of pyrimethamine and sulfadoxine (Fansidar, described earlier) is effective against *P. jirovecii,* but allergic reactions are prevalent and may be severe.[182] Pyrimethamine and sulfonamides also have activity against *I. belli,*[183] but trimethoprim-sulfamethoxazole is the combination of choice.[5]

Pyrimethamine is well absorbed orally; the half-life is 4 to 6 days.[184] It is extensively metabolized; less than 3% of the drug is excreted unchanged in the urine in 24 hours. Pyrimethamine is approximately 1000-fold more active against the parasite's dihydrofolate reductase than against the human enzyme, but it does affect the human enzyme.[185] It can produce bone marrow suppression with neutropenia, anemia, and thrombocytopenia with the daily doses used for the treatment of acute toxoplasmosis (50 to 100 mg/day). Concurrent administration of folinic acid (10 to 25 mg daily) usually prevents these complications, but careful follow-up is necessary. Pyrimethamine is teratogenic in animals[186,187] and is contraindicated during the first 16 weeks of pregnancy. It has been used to treat pregnant women with primary toxoplasmosis after this period, but concern remains about its safety.[188,189] Blood dyscrasias, rash, vomiting, seizures, and shock are rare side effects.

Sulfonamides. Sulfonamides decrease the activity of dihydropteroate synthetase and reduce the binding of *p*-aminobenzoic acid to this enzyme in bacteria and in a number of protozoa. They are frequently used concurrently with pyrimethamine or trimethoprim. The

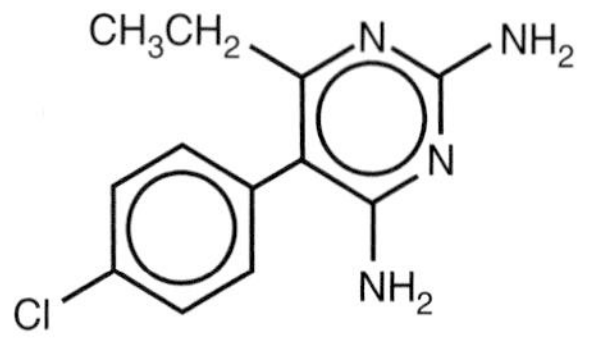

pharmacology and adverse effects of sulfonamides are described in detail in Chapter 32.

Sulfonamides are well absorbed orally. Their most common untoward effects are allergic reactions and gastrointestinal side effects. Allergic reactions, including fever and rash, occur in immunocompetent persons and are common in those infected with HIV. Severe reactions, including toxic epidermal necrolysis, erythema multiforme, Stevens-Johnson syndrome, hepatitis, pneumonitis, bone marrow depression, and serum sickness, may occur.

Trimethoprim-Sulfamethoxazole. The combination trimethoprim-sulfamethoxazole (co-trimoxazole) has been widely used for the treatment of bacterial infections and *P. jirovecii* pneumonia (see Chapter 268).[5] It is also effective for several parasitic diseases. Prophylactic administration of trimethoprim-sulfamethoxazole in persons with AIDS and low CD4+ T-cell counts has been shown to protect against the development of *T. gondii* encephalitis as well as *P. jirovecii* pneumonia.[178,180] Trimethoprim-sulfamethoxazole is also the treatment of choice for gastroenteritis caused by *I. belli*[183] and cyclosporiasis.[190]

Both trimethoprim and sulfamethoxazole are well absorbed when administered orally (Chapter 32). Peak blood levels are reached in 1 to 4 hours. The half-lives are similar: 10 to 12 hours for trimethoprim and 9 to 11 hours for sulfamethoxazole. Excretion is through the kidney; renal failure prolongs the half-lives of both drugs. Trimethoprim has greater lipid solubility than sulfamethoxazole, and its apparent volume of distribution is five to six times greater. As a result, the drugs are formulated at a trimethoprim-to-sulfamethoxazole ratio of 1:5. The combination is also available in suspension for oral use and for intravenous use.

The most common untoward effects are allergic reactions and gastrointestinal side effects,[191] which are more prevalent and often more serious in persons infected with HIV.[192] Malnourished persons receiving prolonged therapy may require concomitant therapy with folinic acid to prevent megaloblastic anemia. The drug combination is not recommended during pregnancy.

Dapsone. Dapsone, a sulfone that has been widely used in the treatment of leprosy, is also active in the prevention of pneumocystosis in HIV-infected and other immunocompromised persons who are intolerant of trimethoprim-sulfamethoxazole.[193,194] It is substantially cheaper than atovaquone.[195] Dapsone has been used with trimethoprim as an alternative to trimethoprim-sulfamethoxazole for the treatment of mild to moderate *P. jirovecii* pneumonia.[196] It has also been combined with pyrimethamine as prophylaxis against *T. gondii* in patients infected with HIV.[196] Finally, it was used in combination with pyrimethamine (Maloprim,[†] a combination of 25 mg pyrimethamine and 100 mg dapsone) for prophylaxis against malaria, but resistance and side effects limited its use.

Like the sulfonamides, dapsone interferes with folic acid metabolism by competitively inhibiting dihydropteroate synthetase. Dapsone is well absorbed after oral administration and is widely distributed in tissues. About 70% to 80% of the drug is bound to plasma proteins. After acetylation and deacetylation, the drug is excreted in the urine as glucuronide or sulfate conjugates. The half-life is variable but averages 25 to 27 hours.

Side effects of dapsone include fever, hemolytic anemia, methemoglobinemia, and bone marrow suppression. Dapsone is contraindicated in patients with G6PD deficiency. Complete blood counts should be performed periodically for patients receiving dapsone and pyrimethamine. Uncommon side effects include skin rash, exfoliative dermatitis, lymphadenopathy, anorexia, vomiting, vertigo, blurred vision, tinnitus, headache, peripheral neuropathy, pruritus, psychosis, hematuria, and agranulocytosis.[197,198]

Other Antibacterial Drugs with Activity against Plasmodium and Other Parasites

Doxycycline and Tetracycline. Tetracycline and doxycycline (see Chapter 25 for discussion of their antibacterial activity and pharmacology) play an important role in prophylaxis and treatment of falciparum malaria acquired in areas where *P. falciparum* is resistant to

FIGURE 41-7. Pyrimethamine.

chloroquine and other antimalarial drugs.[73,74] The tetracyclines act too slow to be used alone for the treatment of acute malaria, but they are often administered with quinine to prevent relapses. Daily doses of doxycycline have been used prophylactically as an alternative to weekly chloroquine or mefloquine in areas where there is chloroquine- or mefloquine-resistant *P. falciparum.* Prophylactic doxycycline is given daily starting 2 days before anticipated exposure, during exposure, and for 4 weeks after leaving the endemic area.[73,74]

In recent years, studies have linked tetracycline treatment of filaria-infected persons with reduced adult filarial burdens and decreased microfilaremia.[200] These observations have been attributable to clearance of *Wolbachia,* an intracellular rickettsia-like organism found within filarial nematodes. Further studies are needed to determine whether tetracyclines will play a role in the treatment of filarial diseases.

Tetracyclines are well absorbed orally. It is likely that their inhibition of protein synthesis in *Plasmodium* is similar to their action in bacteria. Their most common untoward effects are gastrointestinal. Photosensitivity occurs in a small percentage of recipients and can be an important problem for travelers exposed to the sun in the tropics. *Candida* vaginitis can complicate tetracycline use in women, and pseudomembranous colitis caused by *Clostridium difficile* can develop, particularly in older adults. The tetracyclines are concentrated in bone and teeth and may cause dental staining, hypoplasia of dental enamel, and impaired bone growth in a fetus or young child, and they are therefore contraindicated during pregnancy and for children younger than 8 years.

Clindamycin. Clindamycin has activity against several protozoa. The combination of clindamycin plus pyrimethamine can be used for treatment or suppression of toxoplasmosis in persons who cannot tolerate the standard regimen of pyrimethamine plus sulfadiazine.[201] Clindamycin is also used along with prednisone for the treatment of ocular toxoplasmosis in immunocompetent patients.[202,203] It has relatively good penetration into the eye and inhibits replication of *T. gondii.* Although the outcome of therapy has been good, there are no prospective, double-blind studies comparing the efficacy of clindamycin with the combination of pyrimethamine and a sulfonamide. Clindamycin has been used with quinine for the treatment of chloroquine-resistant falciparum malaria and for babesiosis.[204] Finally, clindamycin with primaquine has been used as an alternative to trimethoprim-sulfamethoxazole for the treatment of *P. carinii* pneumonia in persons who do not tolerate the latter. The pharmacokinetics and untoward effects of clindamycin are discussed in Chapter 28. The major concern is the development of pseudomembranous colitis, a side effect that increases in incidence with the recipient's age.

Spiramycin. Spiramycin, a macrolide antibiotic, is active against *T. gondii,* but it is not licensed in the United States. It has been used to treat primary toxoplasmosis acquired during pregnancy[5,206] and congenital toxoplasmosis in newborns.[5,207] Spiramycin has also been widely used as an additive in animal feeds. One important, although rare, complication in neonates, is QTc prolongation with associated life-threatening ventricular arrhythmias.[208]

Azithromycin. Azithromycin (see Chapter 28 for details of pharmacology and adverse effects) has activity against several protozoa as well as bacteria. Azithromycin used in combination with atovaquone has become the treatment of choice for babesiosis.[209] It is as effective as quinine and clindamycin and much better tolerated. Azithromycin has been used with pyrimethamine for the treatment and suppression of *T. gondii* in a limited number of persons with AIDS, but maintenance doses used for suppression were associated with a high rate of relapse.[210,211] It has activity against *Plasmodium* species, but it is not sufficiently active to be used alone for malaria prophylaxis.[212,213]

Pentamidine. Pentamidine isethionate (Fig. 41-8), a diamidine, is active against *P. jirovecii* and a number of protozoa, but it is associated with substantial toxicity. Pentamidine is used for the treatment of *P. jirovecii* in persons with AIDS who cannot tolerate sulfonamides.[214,215] It is active when aerosolized for prophylaxis against pneumocystis pneumonia, but it is less effective than trimethoprim-sul-

famethoxazole, and its administration can result in environmental contamination.[216] Pentamidine is also effective in the treatment of the hemolymphatic stage of *Trypanosoma brucei gambiense* infection and, to a lesser degree, *Trypanosoma brucei rhodesiense* infection.[217,218] It has been used for the treatment of leishmaniasis in persons who fail to respond to pentavalent antimony,[219,220] and for secondary prophylaxis in patients who have AIDS and visceral leishmaniasis.[221,222]

Pentamidine isethionate is water soluble and available for intramuscular, intravenous, or aerosol administration. Intramuscular injections are frequently complicated by pain, swelling, and sterile abscesses at the administration site. As a consequence, pentamidine is usually given intravenously after being diluted in 100 to 250 mL of 5% dextrose in water. It must be administered slowly over 1 to 2 hours.[223] It is highly tissue bound and excreted slowly over an extended period. It does not penetrate well into the central nervous system.

The mechanism of action has not been defined.[224] Pentamidine is known to bind to DNA in a nonintercalative manner. It interacts selectively with trypanosomal kinetoplast DNA, resulting in swelling and loss of structure of the kinetoplast; it inhibits RNA polymerase ribosomal function; and it interferes with the synthesis of nucleic acids, proteins, and phospholipids. It decreases the amount of membrane phospholipids, thereby altering cytoplasmic and mitochondrial membranes.[225] It affects polyamine synthesis by decreasing the activity of ornithine decarboxylase.[226] It inhibits trypsin and related proteases. It also inhibits folic acid synthesis, but this does not appear to be its mode of action.

The administration of pentamidine isethionate by the intravenous or the intramuscular route is associated with toxicity in approximately half of the recipients. Adverse effects include tachycardia, nausea, vomiting, dizziness, rash, facial flushing, breathlessness, and a metallic taste. Severe hypotension may result after rapid intravenous infusion.[223] Hypoglycemia, which has been reported during therapy in 6% to 9% of persons treated in the United States,[227–229] can be severe and life-threatening, and it can even develop after the completion of therapy. It is probably caused by a direct toxic effect of pentamidine on pancreatic beta cells.[228,229] Hypoglycemia can be followed by the development of insulin-dependent diabetes mellitus. Severe hypoglycemia can be treated with glucose infusion and diazoxide.

Reversible renal failure occurs in approximately 25% of persons who receive pentamidine.[227] Although severe renal failure has been reported in a few patients, it was impossible to attribute the renal toxicity solely to pentamidine because of the concurrent administration of other nephrotoxic agents. Other adverse effects of pentamidine include leukopenia and thrombocytopenia, increased transaminase levels, fever, hypocalcemia, hyperkalemia, confusion, hallucinations, and, rarely, QTc prolongation and cardiac arrhythmias, particularly torsades de pointes. Rare cases of fatal pancreatitis have been reported in patients with AIDS who received pentamidine.[230,231]

Aerosolized pentamidine is better tolerated than parenterally administered pentamidine and has been used for prevention of *P. jirovecii* pneumonia in persons with AIDS.[232,233] Only a small amount of drug reaches the systemic circulation. Failures with aerosolized pentamidine are more likely in those with underlying bullous or obstructive lung disease. In addition, patients receiving prophylaxis with inhaled pentamidine are at risk for development of extrapulmonary pneumocystosis. Untoward effects include a metallic taste, pharyngeal irritation, and bronchospasm, the last occurring particularly in patients with a history of asthma or chronic obstructive pulmonary disease. Pretreatment with inhaled bronchodilators helps reduce bron-

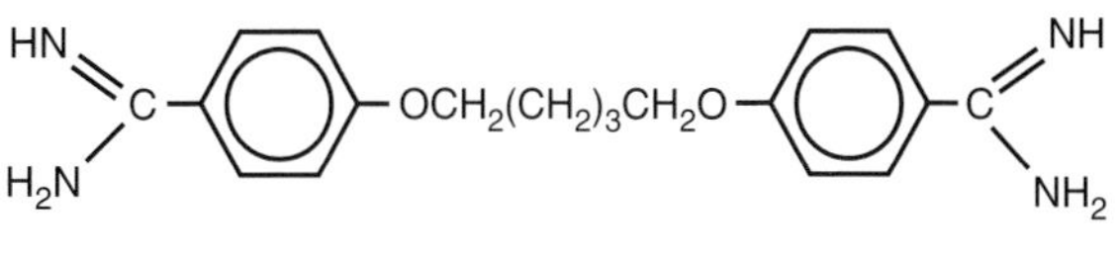

FIGURE 41-8. Pentamidine.

chospasm. The results of pulmonary function tests suggest that chronic aerosolized pentamidine is well tolerated over a 5-year period in HIV-infected patients, although there is a modest reduction in flow rate at the level of the small airways, especially in smokers.[232] Finally, aerosol pentamidine raises environmental safety concerns for health care workers, because of both exhaled drug and the potential for exposure to pathogens such as *Mycobacterium tuberculosis*.[216] All patients for whom aerosolized pentamidine is prescribed should be screened for tuberculosis before therapy begins.

DRUGS FOR TREATMENT OF HUMAN AFRICAN TRYPANOSOMIASIS, CHAGAS' DISEASE, AND LEISHMANIASIS

Members of the genera *Trypanosoma* and *Leishmania,* also known as kinetoplastids, are important causes of morbidity and mortality in the tropics. Although treatment is available for them, the drugs used are variably effective and often associated with toxicity, and a number are available only for parenteral administration. New chemotherapeutic modalities are needed for these diseases.

T. b. gambiense and *T. b. rhodesiense* cause human African trypanosomiasis (sleeping sickness). The early hemolymphatic stage of this disease has traditionally been treated with suramin* or pentamidine isethionate. Neither of these compounds reaches therapeutic levels in the central nervous system. Once central nervous system involvement is documented, melarsoprol, a toxic trivalent arsenical, is the treatment of choice. Eflornithine, an inhibitor of ornithine decarboxylase, is effective in patients with hemolymphatic and central nervous system *T. b. gambiense* infection, but it is not active against *T. b. rhodesiense.* Eflornithine is less toxic but more costly than conventional therapy, and supplies of the drug are now very limited.

Trypanosoma cruzi, the cause of Chagas' disease, is endemic in Central and South America. The drugs currently used for therapy, nifurtimox and benznidazole,[†] are variably effective and associated with substantial toxicity. They have been used for many years to treat acute infections and disseminated disease in immunocompromised patients. Recent experience suggests that as many as two thirds of persons with asymptomatic, indeterminate infection can be cured with benznidazole, possibly sparing them from the later development of chagasic cardiomyopathy or enteric megadisease. Efforts continue to identify more effective and less toxic alternative medications.

Leishmania species produce a spectrum of clinical disease including cutaneous, mucosal, and visceral leishmaniasis. Cutaneous disease is the syndrome most commonly observed in North American travelers to endemic areas. Mucosal leishmaniasis caused by *Leishmania braziliensis* and related species is endemic in Brazil and other Latin American countries. Visceral leishmaniasis poses a major heath problem in eastern India and Bangladesh, among refugees in the Sudan, in persons with concurrent AIDS in southern Europe, and in rural and periurban endemic areas of Latin America. Cases are rare among North American travelers.

For many years, the pentavalent antimonials stibogluconate* sodium and meglumine antimonate[†] were the mainstay of treatment for leishmaniasis. Although they are still used in many areas, antimony resistance is now prevalent among *Leishmania donovani* isolates in India and increasingly recognized in other areas. Conventional amphotericin B deoxycholate and pentamidine isethionate are effective but associated with untoward effects and difficult to administer. Liposome-encapsulated amphotericin B (AmBisome), which is licensed for visceral leishmaniasis, and other lipid-associated amphotericin B preparations are effective. Miltefosine,[†] a new orally administered drug, is being used for visceral leishmaniasis in India. A number of other forms of therapy have been studied. Topical paromomycin with methylbenzethonium chloride has been used successfully to treat cutaneous leishmaniasis caused by *L. major,* and the imidazole antifungals, fluconazole, ketoconazole, and itraconazole, have activity against some, but not all, *Leishmania* species.

Suramin

Suramin is a nonmetallic compound that is effective for the treatment of the hemolymphatic stage of African trypanosomiasis.[234,235] It has been used on occasion as prophylaxis against *T. b. gambiense* in persons working in highly endemic areas. Suramin also has some activity against adult *Onchocerca volvulus,* but ivermectin is the drug of choice for onchocerciasis.

Suramin sodium is a white microcrystalline powder that is soluble in water. It is available only for parenteral administration. Suramin binds to plasma proteins and persists at low levels in the serum for up to 3 months after infusion. There seems to be negligible metabolism of the drug. Suramin does not penetrate the central nervous system, which limits its usefulness to the hemolymphatic stage of human African trypanosomiasis. Its mechanism of action is uncertain, but suramin is known to inhibit many enzymes, even at low concentrations. It is polyanionic and forms firm complexes with proteins. The antitrypanosomal activity of suramin correlates with its inhibition of glycerol-3-phosphate oxidase and glycerol-3-phosphate dehydrogenase, two trypanosomal enzymes that are involved in energy metabolism.[236]

Suramin causes a variety of untoward effects.[237] Immediate reactions include nausea, vomiting, shock, loss of consciousness, and occasionally death. Fever and urticaria can also occur. Later reactions, which appear up to 24 hours after administration, include fever, papular rash, exfoliative dermatitis, stomatitis, paresthesias of the palms and soles, photophobia, lacrimation, palpebral edema, and hyperesthesia. These may be followed by renal dysfunction with albuminuria, hematuria, and renal casts. Other reactions include diarrhea and severe prostration. Jaundice, hemolytic anemia, and agranulocytosis are rare. The frequency and severity of side effects are more severe in malnourished hosts. Suramin is relatively contraindicated in persons with preexisting kidney or liver disease.

Melarsoprol

Melarsoprol, or Mel B, is a trivalent arsenical used for the treatment of central nervous system human African trypanosomiasis.[238] It is also effective in treatment of the hemolymphatic phase, but it is too toxic to be recommended in that setting. High failure rates and relapses have been reported from several foci in recent years.[238]

Melarsoprol is only slightly soluble in water, but it is readily soluble in propylene glycol, in which it is dispensed as a 3.6% weight/volume solution. Melarsoprol is administered intravenously. A small but sufficient amount of the drug penetrates the central nervous system, where it can have a lethal effect on trypanosomes. Data indicate that the drug enters the parasite via an adenosine transporter; resistant strains lack this transport system.[239] Arsenicals react avidly with sulfhydryl groups and thereby interact with and inactivate enzymes. This is the most likely mechanism of action against trypanosomes and the cause of its toxicity in humans.

Melarsoprol is a highly toxic drug. Febrile reactions are common and may be accompanied by hypertension, abdominal pain, vomiting, and arthralgia. Reactive encephalopathy, which usually appears in the first 3 or 4 days of therapy, is the most serious side effect; it has been reported to cause death in approximately 6% of recipients.[240-242] The clinical manifestations include headache, dizziness, mental dullness, confusion, and ataxia with progression to obtundation and seizures. The pathophysiology is thought to be caused at least in part by an immune response to trypanosomal antigens that are released during therapy. Data suggest that the administration of corticosteroids can reduce the incidence of encephalopathy and mortality during treatment.[241] Recently, attention has focused on the efficacy and potentially reduced toxicity of new treatment schedules using melarsoprol.[243]

Less common untoward effects include hemorrhagic encephalopathy and agranulocytosis. A Guillain-Barré–like syndrome has also been described.[244] Allergic reactions including rash may complicate subsequent courses of therapy. On occasion, the appearance of numerous casts in the urine or evidence of hepatotoxicity necessitates a modification of therapy. Severe hemolysis can occur in patients with G6PD deficiency. The gastrointestinal side effects can be reduced by administering the drug slowly to fasting patients. Melarsoprol therapy can precipitate erythema nodosum in patients who have leprosy.

Eflornithine

Eflornithine* (DL-α-difluoromethylornithine) is effective in the treatment of African sleeping sickness caused by *T. b. gambiense,* even in patients with advanced central nervous system disease.[245,246] Although it is less toxic than melarsoprol, it is more expensive and supplies are very limited.[247] Eflornithine is not effective in east African sleeping sickness caused by *T. b. rhodesiense.*[248] Although introduced as the "resurrection" drug, the amount needed for each treatment course, the very limited supplies worldwide, and the cost have severely limited its use. The development of eflornithine as a depilatory cream in industrialized countries offers hope that supplies may be available in the future.[249]

Eflornithine hydrochloride can be administered intravenously or orally; 80% of the drug is excreted unchanged in the urine.[248] Serum levels during administration of 20 g/day by intravenous infusion approach 1200 nmol/mL; oral administration of 5 g every 4 hours produces levels of approximately 500 nmol/mL. The ratio of cerebrospinal fluid (CSF) concentration to serum concentration ranges from 0.09 to 0.45. The highest CSF levels are found in persons with the most severe central nervous system involvement. Eflornithine is an enzyme-activated, irreversible inhibitor of the enzyme ornithine decarboxylase, which is involved in the first step of the polyamine pathway. Polyamines play an essential role in the growth, differentiation, and replication of the trypanosomatids.

In comparison with the other drugs used to treat African trypanosomiasis, eflornithine is well tolerated. Generally, adverse reactions to eflornithine are reversible after the end of treatment. They include convulsions, gastrointestinal symptoms (e.g., nausea, vomiting, diarrhea), bone marrow toxicity leading to anemia, leukopenia and thrombocytopenia, hearing impairment, and alopecia.[245]

Nifurtimox

Nifurtimox,* 4-([5-nitrofurfurylidene]amino)-3-methylthiomorpholine-1,1-dioxide, a nitrofuran, is available for the treatment of *T. cruzi* infection in the United States.[250] It is currently out of production, but supplies are available through the CDC. Nifurtimox treatment can reduce the duration of symptoms of acute disease, and it decreases mortality resulting from acute myocarditis and meningoencephalitis. The level and duration of parasitemia are also reduced. However, in clinical trials, substantial numbers of recipients remain parasitemic after therapy. There also seems to be geographic variation in responsiveness. Treatment has been found to be most effective in Argentina and Chile, but therapy in Brazil and in some other countries has been less successful. Prolonged therapy for 120 days is recommended, but it is not unusual for a treatment course to be terminated prematurely because of drug toxicity. High-dose nifurtimox has also been used for the treatment of arsenoresistant *T. b. gambiense* sleeping sickness.[251]

Nifurtimox is well absorbed orally, but marked first-pass metabolism results in low serum and tissue concentrations.[252] The elimination half-life is 2 to 4 hours. The trypanosomicidal activity is thought to relate to the ability of nifurtimox to form reactive oxygen radicals in the parasite.[253,254]

Toxicity occurs in 40% to 70% of persons who receive nifurtimox. This is probably caused at least in part by free radical formation and oxidative damage to host tissues.[254] Most of the symptoms are related to the gastrointestinal tract and the central and peripheral nervous systems. Nifurtimox seems to be better tolerated in children than in adults. Nausea, vomiting, abdominal pain, anorexia, and weight loss are common and may require premature termination of therapy. Neurologic sequelae include restlessness, disorientation, insomnia, twitching, paresthesias, polyneuritis, weakness, and stiffness. Convulsions may occur. Rashes, neutropenia, and decreased sperm counts have also been reported. The side effects are usually reversible with discontinuation of the drug, but they frequently pose a therapeutic dilemma given the prolonged course of therapy that is necessary.

Benznidazole

Benznidazole,† a nitroimidazole derivative, is used in Latin America for the treatment of *T. cruzi* infection.[250] It seems to be similar to nifurtimox in efficacy. Recent reports from Latin America suggest that benznidazole may be effective in eradicating *T. cruzi* in more than two thirds of patients with indeterminate or chronic infection and may consequently prevent or limit the development of late chagasic cardiomyopathy or megadisease.[255,256] Benznidazole is administered orally for 30 to 90 days. Therapy is often limited by polyneuropathy, rash, gastrointestinal disturbances, or neuropsychiatric effects.

Pentavalent Antimony: Stibogluconate Sodium and Meglumine Antimonate

Two pentavalent antimonials, stibogluconate sodium* and meglumine antimonate,† have been widely used for the treatment of leishmaniasis.[257] The compounds are of comparable efficacy and toxicity when administered on the basis of their pentavalent antimony content. Stibogluconate is the only pentavalent antimonial available in the United States. Meglumine antimonate has been widely used in Central and South America. The efficacy of the pentavalent antimonials varies with the leishmanial syndrome and the causative *Leishmania* species. Treatment failures are common in patients with visceral leishmaniasis in India and have become increasingly recognized in some other areas. Resistance appears to be acquired and can arise from subcurative therapy resulting in selection of resistant parasite strains.[258] Relapses are also common in persons with AIDS, indicating that human immune responses play a role in the clinical response.

Sodium stibogluconate is available in sterile aqueous solution for parenteral administration. The recommended dose is 20 mg of pentavalent antibody per kilogram of body weight per day. Pentostam is supplied in 10-mL bottles; each milliliter contains 330 mg of drug, which is equivalent to 100 mg of pentavalent antimony. Meglumine antimonate is available in 5-mL bottles, with 85 mg of antimony per milliliter. These drugs are prescribed on the basis of their antimony content. They can be administered intramuscularly but are usually given intravenously, either undiluted over a 5-minute period or diluted in 50 mL of 5% dextrose in water or saline and administered over 20 minutes.

The antimony concentration in blood is best described by a three-compartment model, with a short initial distribution phase followed by biexponential elimination, primarily through the kidneys.[259] The mean half-lives for the elimination phases have been reported to be 1.7 and 33 hours after intravenous administration, and 2 and 766 hours after the drug is given intramuscularly. Pentavalent antimony is concentrated in cells of reticuloendothelial origin where the parasite resides. The mechanism of action is uncertain, but pentavalent antimony appears to affect parasite metabolism.

The pentavalent antimonials have a number of adverse effects, but therapy can usually be completed.[260,261] Common adverse effects include abdominal pain, nausea, vomiting, malaise, headache, increased transaminase levels, nephrotoxicity, weakness, myalgias, arthralgias, fever, skin rash, cough, and pneumonitis, but these seldom prevent completion of the treatment course. Pancreatic enzymes are frequently elevated, and clinically significant pancreatitis occurs in some recipients, particularly those with impaired renal function.[262] Dose-related changes are observed in the electrocardiogram. The most common are nonspecific ST-T wave changes and a prolonged QTc interval. Rarer but more serious effects include atrial and ventricular arrhythmias. Sudden death has been associated with doses higher than the 20 mg/kg body weight per day that is recommended. The use of pentavalent antimony is relatively contraindicated in patients with myocarditis, hepatitis, pancreatitis, or renal failure.

Amphotericin B Deoxycholate, Liposomal Amphotericin B, Ketoconazole, and Itraconazole

The leishmania are susceptible to several traditional antifungal agents (see Chapter 37). Amphotericin B deoxycholate has been used as an alternative drug for the treatment of visceral, cutaneous, and mucosal leishmaniasis for years.[263,264] It is highly effective, but it is associated with substantial toxicity and it is difficult to administer.[265-267] Liposomal amphotericin B (AmBisome) is as effective as amphotericin B deoxycholate in the treatment of visceral leishmaniasis, and it is less toxic. It was the first drug to receive FDA approval for the treatment of visceral leishmaniasis in the United States.[265,266] Other lipid-associated preparations of amphotericin B are less well studied but appear to be effective.[268,269] Amphotericin binds to sterols and probably damages the surface membrane of *Leishmania* organisms, as it does those of susceptible fungi. Amphotericin B has also been used with miconazole and rifampin to treat amebic encephalitis caused by *Naegleria* species. The pharmacokinetics and toxicity of amphotericin are summarized in Chapter 37.

The imidazole antifungal drugs fluconazole, ketoconazole, and itraconazole (see Chapter 37) have activity against some *Leishmania* species. The results with ketoconazole[271-274] and itraconazole[275-280] used for the treatment of cutaneous and visceral leishmaniasis have been variable, depending on the infecting species of *Leishmania*, the site of infection, and the clinical syndrome.

Miltefosine

Miltefosine† (hexadecylphosphocholine) has been marketed and used successfully to treat patients with visceral leishmaniasis in India where pentavalent antimony resistance is common.[281-286] The data on its use for the cutaneous disease are promising but less substantial.[287] Miltefosine was initially developed as an antineoplastic agent.[288] The mechanism of action against leishmania has not been precisely identified, but miltefosine is known to interact with membrane constituents and can affect cell signaling pathways by inhibiting protein kinase C and phospholipase C. It also interferes with the biosynthesis of glycosylphosphatidylinositol anchors, which are important in leishmania and related kinetoplastids.

Miltefosine is administered orally and is relatively well tolerated. It has been associated with nausea, vomiting, and motion sickness in some patients, but the side effects seldom interfere with completion of therapy. Transaminase elevations and increases in blood urea nitrogen (BUN) and creatinine have been noted, but they have usually decreased with continuation of the drug. Although additional postmarketing studies are needed, miltefosine may assume an increasingly important role in the treatment of leishmaniasis in the future.[289]

DRUGS FOR TREATMENT OF INTESTINAL NEMATODES (ROUNDWORMS)

The intestinal nematodes remain prevalent in areas of the world where sanitation is poor. The pinworm, *Enterobius vermicularis,* is common in the United States. In industrialized countries, geohelminths are most likely to be encountered among immigrants from endemic areas, or occasionally in returning travelers who have had intense local exposure.

Albendazole

Albendazole (Fig. 41-9), methyl-5-*N*-propoxythio-2-benzimidazole carbamate, has an exceptionally broad spectrum of antiparasitic activity. Albendazole has been widely used throughout the world in individuals and in community-based treatment programs for intestinal nematode infections. It has the advantage of being effective when given as a single dose for the treatment of *A. lumbricoides,* the hookworms *Ancylostoma duodenale* and *Necator americanus,* and, to a lesser extent, *T. trichiura.*[290-292] Periodic treatment at 4- to 6-month intervals with albendazole has been shown to improve the nutritional status, growth, and function of malnourished children infected with multiple species of intestinal helminths.[293-295] Albendazole is also effective against *E. vermicularis.* It has been used successfully for the treatment of cutaneous[296-298] and visceral larva migrans,[299] gnathostomiasis,[300] *Capillaria philippinensis,*[301] mixed hookworm and *Oesophagostomum* infections,[302] *Trichinella spiralis,*[303] *Mansonella perstans,*[304] and *Clonorchis sinensis.*[305] Multiple doses have been used to treat *Strongyloides stercoralis,*

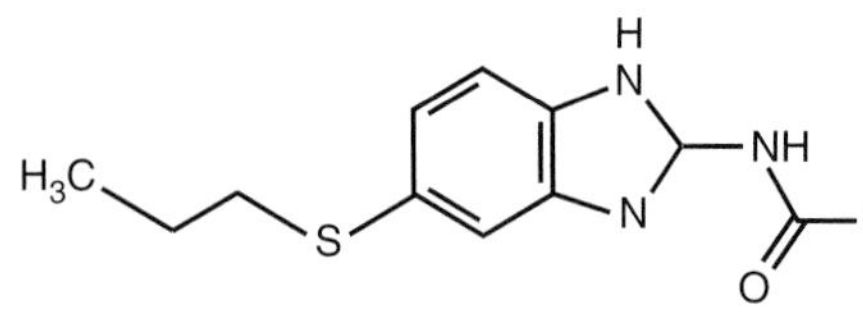

FIGURE 41-9. Albendazole.

but failures occur in more than half of the cases.[306,307] Albendazole has been used with ivermectin to treat filariasis.[308,309]

Albendazole has activity against *Giardia lamblia,*[310,311] but it is not currently recommended for the treatment of giardiasis. It has been used successfully for the treatment of intestinal and disseminated microsporidiosis caused by *Encephalitozoon* species in persons with AIDS.[312-315] Given empirically to African patients with HIV infection and persistent diarrhea of more than 3 weeks' duration, albendazole resulted in a significant reduction in days of diarrhea and led to remission in approximately a quarter of those treated.[316]

High-dose, prolonged therapy with albendazole (cycles of 400 mg twice a day for 6 months) has emerged as the best approach for the medical treatment of *Echinococcus granulosus, Echinococcus multilocularis,* and *Echinococcus vogeli.*[317-320] It is estimated that approximately one third of persons with *E. granulosus* can be cured with albendazole, and an additional 50% show improvement.[317,318] Preoperative administration of albendazole decreases the viability of liver hydatid cysts and reduces the likelihood of peritoneal implantation if cyst contents are spilled during surgery or percutaneous drainage.[321,322]

Albendazole has also been used successfully for the treatment of neurocysticercosis. Although it has not been compared with praziquantel in a double-blind, controlled manner, albendazole appears to produce higher response rates.[323-334] Corticosteroids are usually administered concurrently to control the inflammatory response elicited by the release of parasite antigens. Albendazole has been used successfully to treat some patients with subarachnoid and ventricular cysticercosis,[331-334] but not all respond. Albendazole has variable activity against adult *Taenia* species in the human gastrointestinal tract.[335,336]

Albendazole is a white, odorless powder that is dispensed as 400-mg tablets. It is practically insoluble in water; absorption is enhanced when the drug is taken with a fatty meal.[318] Albendazole undergoes extensive first-pass metabolism in the liver, and only albendazole sulfoxide, which is primarily responsible for the systemic anthelmintic effects, is detectable in serum. Sulfoxidation of albendazole also occurs in the gut.[337] Albendazole sulfoxide reaches peak levels in 2.0 to 2.4 hours and has a half-life of 10 to 15 hours.[318,338] Plasma levels of albendazole sulfoxide at steady state show great individual variability. Drug concentrations in the central nervous system are approximately 40% those in serum.[339] Concurrent administration of dexamethasone increases the levels of albendazole by approximately 50%,[340] a positive interaction for persons receiving both for neurocysticercosis. The concentration of albendazole sulfoxide in echinococcal cysts is approximately 25% of the serum concentration. The bile appears to be the major route of elimination, and enterohepatic recirculation occurs. Albendazole, like other benzimidazoles, binds to β-tubulin, inhibits its assembly into microtubules,[341] and impairs the uptake of glucose leading to the depletion of glycogen stores in helminths. It also inhibits helminth-specific fumarate reductase.[342]

Albendazole is usually well tolerated when given as a single 400-mg dose for the treatment of intestinal nematodes. Diarrhea, abdominal discomfort, rash, or migration of *Ascaris* through the nose or mouth can occur. On rare occasions it has been associated with fever, rash, the Stevens-Johnson syndrome, or pseudomembranous colitis.[318,343,344] High-dose, prolonged therapy for echinococcal disease or neurocysticercosis is occasionally complicated by serum transaminase elevation, bone marrow suppression with anemia, neutropenia or thrombocytopenia, or, less commonly, alopecia.[345,346] Liver enzymes and complete blood counts should be measured at least every 2 weeks.

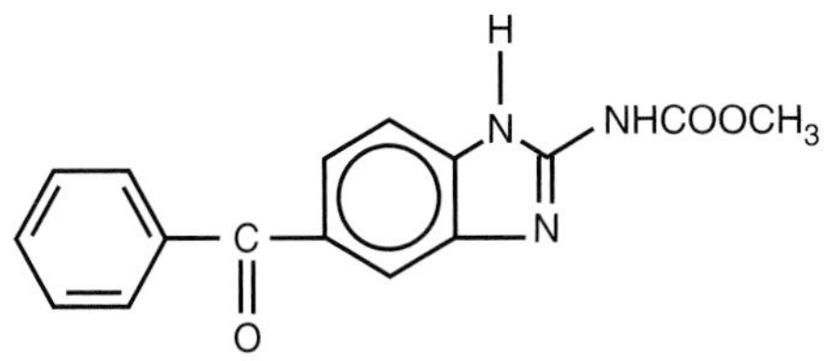

FIGURE 41-10. Mebendazole.

Liver and bone marrow toxicity are reversible with discontinuation of the drug. Occasionally, gastrointestinal disturbances, headache, or dizziness occur. In view of the potential teratogenicity of benzimidazole compounds, albendazole is contraindicated during pregnancy.

Mebendazole

Mebendazole (Fig. 41-10), a synthetic benzimidazole, methyl 5-benzoylbenzimidazole-2-carbamate, has been widely used for the treatment of intestinal nematodes.[347] It has a spectrum of activity similar to that of albendazole, but it is less well absorbed. Mebendazole is effective against *Ascaris lumbricoides, Necator americanus, Ancylostoma duodenale,* and *Trichuris trichiura.* Treatment with a single dose is effective against *A. lumbricoides,* but twice-daily administration for 3 days is recommended for the hookworms and *T. trichiura.*[347-349] Albendazole, which is more effective as a single dose, has replaced mebendazole in community treatment programs. *E. vermicularis* responds to a single dose of 100 mg with a repeat dose given after 2 weeks.[347] The effect of mebendazole on *Strongyloides stercoralis* is variable[350-352]; ivermectin is the treatment of choice. Mebendazole has been used successfully for treatment of *Capillaria philippinensis.*[347]

Mebendazole is active against adult *Trichinella spiralis* and has some activity against invading larvae.[353,354] Steroids are administered concomitantly. Mebendazole is effective in the treatment of *Mansonella perstans.*[355,356] It has some activity against *Loa loa,* but it is not recommended for it.[355,356] Mebendazole also has activity against *Taenia* species,[357] but praziquantel and niclosamide are more effective.

Mebendazole has been used at very high doses for prolonged periods to treat *Echinococcus granulosus* and *Echinococcus multilocularis,* but albendazole is better absorbed and superior.[317-321] The major anthelmintic metabolite of albendazole, albendazole sulfoxide, attains higher serum and cyst concentrations than mebendazole.[324,325]

Mebendazole is dispensed in 100-mg tablets. It is only slightly soluble in water and is poorly absorbed from the gastrointestinal tract.[347] This contributes to its low frequency of side effects but limits its usefulness in treating tissue larvae. Up to 10% of an orally administered dose of mebendazole is recovered within 48 hours in the urine. Most of the drug excreted by the kidney is the decarboxylated metabolite. Mebendazole selectively binds to helminthic β-tubulin,[358] prevents microtubule assembly in susceptible helminths, and inhibits glucose uptake. Parasite immobilization and death follow, but it can take several days for susceptible nematodes to be cleared from the gastrointestinal tract. Mebendazole also inhibits the development of the ova of hookworms and *T. trichiura.*

Side effects are uncommon when mebendazole is used at low doses (100 mg twice a day for 3 days) for the treatment of the common intestinal helminths.[347] Transient abdominal pain and diarrhea occur in a small number of persons, usually those with large parasite burdens. Migration of adult *A. lumbricoides* to the nose or mouth occurs occasionally. At the high doses used for the treatment of echinococcal cysts, systemic side effects such as alopecia, liver enzyme abnormalities, and transient bone marrow suppression with severe but reversible neutropenia have been observed.[359,360] The leukocyte count should be monitored closely after initiation of high-dose therapy; neutropenia is usually observed within the first 30 days. Accidental poisoning in one infant was associated with respiratory arrest, tachyarrhythmia, and seizures.[361] Mebendazole produces embryotoxicity and teratogenicity in animals; it is therefore contraindicated during pregnancy.

Thiabendazole

Thiabendazole,[†] 2-(4'-thiazolyl)-1H-benzimidazole, is a potent anthelmintic drug, but it frequently causes untoward effects. It is now difficult to obtain in the United States. Thiabendazole is active against a number of adult nematodes that infect the gastrointestinal tract and against larvae in tissues. The most common indication for thiabendazole has been infection with *S. stercoralis*[362] or *Strongyloides fuelleborni,*[363] but ivermectin, which is less toxic, is now recommended. Topical thiabendazole is effective in the treatment of cutaneous larva migrans.[364]

Thiabendazole is rapidly absorbed after oral administration. No parenteral preparation is available, which poses a problem for critically ill patients with disseminated *S. stercoralis* infection who cannot take oral medications. Most of the drug is excreted in urine within 24 hours as 5-hydroxythiabendazole conjugated as the glucuronide or as the sulfate. Like other benzimidazoles, thiabendazole binds to β-tubulin and is thought to prevent microtubule formation and glucose uptake.

Approximately half of the persons who receive thiabendazole experience one or more side effects, most commonly nausea, anorexia, vomiting, and dizziness. Less frequent are diarrhea, epigastric pain, pruritus, drowsiness, giddiness, and headache. Rare side effects include tinnitus, abnormal sensation in the eyes, numbness, decreased pulse and blood pressure, elevated liver enzymes, and progressive bile duct injury. Transient neutropenia has been observed in some patients. Allergic manifestations such as fever, facial flush, angioneurotic edema, lymphadenopathy, perianal rash, and skin rashes also occur; some or all of these may be caused by the release of parasite antigens. Thiabendazole can give urine an asparagus-like odor. Crystalluria has been reported. Because of the central nervous system effects, activities requiring alertness should be avoided during therapy. The drug should be used with caution in persons with hepatic disease or decreased hepatic function, and it is contraindicated during pregnancy. Thiabendazole increases the half-life of theophylline and was associated with theophylline toxicity and severe nausea and vomiting when the two were administered concurrently.[365]

Pyrantel Pamoate

Pyrantel pamoate is effective against *E. vermicularis.* It can also be used to treat *A. lumbricoides, N. americanus, A. duodenale,* and *Moniliformis moniliformis.*[366-370] Treatment with pyrantel pamoate resulted in increased appetite and growth in children infected with *A. lumbricoides.*[371] Pyrantel pamoate is an alternative to mebendazole for the treatment of *Trichostrongylus* species. It is not active against *T. trichiura,*

Pyrantel is available as a suspension. It is poorly absorbed; less than 15% is excreted in the urine as the parent drug or metabolite. Pyrantel acts as an agonist at nicotinic acetylcholine receptors of sensitive nematodes. It functions as a depolarizing neuromuscular blocking agent that results in a short period of calcium-dependent stimulation followed by irreversible paralysis of the worm.[372,373] Pyrantel also inhibits acetylcholinesterases.

Pyrantel pamoate has minimal toxicity at the oral dosages used to treat intestinal helminths. Mild, transient gastrointestinal symptoms, headache, drowsiness, insomnia, or dizziness is occasionally encountered. The metabolites of pyrantel pamoate are mutagenic in bacteria. Pyrantel pamoate has not been studied in pregnancy, and it is not recommended for pregnant women or children younger than 1 year. Pyrantel and piperazine (which produces hyperpolarization with a reduction in spike wave activity in helminthic muscle cells) appear to be mutually antagonistic and should not be used together.[369,370]

Piperazine

Piperazine[†] citrate was once widely used for the treatment of *A. lumbricoides.* It has been replaced in the United States and most other areas by mebendazole, albendazole, or pyrantel pamoate, which are less toxic. Piperazine also has activity against *E. vermicularis.* The piperazine moiety has been incorporated into a number of compounds that have a broad range of pharmacologic activity. Some substituted piperazines are central serotonin agonists; others depress monosynaptic spinal cord excitation, block chloride channels, have antioxidant effects, display antiarrhythmic activity, or act as vasodilators. One of the derivatives, diethylcarbamazine, is effective against filaria, as discussed later.

Piperazine is well absorbed orally. Some of the drug is metabolized; the remainder is excreted in the urine. Piperazine causes flaccid paralysis of susceptible intestinal helminths. It acts as a low-potency agonist at extrasynaptic γ-aminobutyric acid–gated chloride channels in nematode muscle.[374] Activation of these receptors gives rise to an increase in chloride conductance. There is hyperpolarization and suppression of spontaneous action potentials. Worms are paralyzed and excreted alive, usually without migrating.

Piperazine is generally well tolerated. On occasion, there are gastrointestinal symptoms, transient neurologic side effects, or urticarial reactions. Lethal overdoses have been associated with convulsions and respiratory depression. Epileptic activity may be exaggerated, so piperazine is contraindicated in persons with a history of seizures.[375] Neurotoxicity has also been observed in persons with impaired renal function. Visual disturbances, ataxia, and hypotonia occur rarely.[376] Piperazine has been used during pregnancy without apparent adverse effects, but it has not been thoroughly evaluated in this setting. Although adverse dermatologic reactions are rare, rashes have been reported with piperazine and compounds containing the piperazine moiety.[377]

DRUGS FOR TREATMENT OF SYSTEMIC NEMATODES

Diethylcarbamazine

Diethylcarbamazine* (Fig. 41-11) is a piperazine derivative, *N,N*-diethyl-4-methyl-1-piperazinecarboxamide dihydrogen citrate. It results in the rapid death of microfilaria of *Wuchereria bancrofti, Brugia malayi,* and *Brugia timori,* the three lymphatics-dwelling filaria that infect humans.[378-383] The annual administration of a single dose of diethylcarbamazine to persons with lymphatic filariasis reduces microfilaremia by 90%, and in combination with a single dose of ivermectin, by 99%.[380,381] A major reduction in microfilaremia has also been observed with the administration of diethylcarbamazine-medicated salt.[380,381] Field studies have confirmed that reductions in microfilarial load and prevalence can interrupt transmission. Diethylcarbamazine is variably effective against adult *W. bancrofti*[384] and, although not well documented, probably has some macrofilaricidal action against *B. malayi* and *B. timori* as well. It is currently the drug of choice for all three species. Males with hydroceles before treatment have demonstrated improvement 1 year after starting therapy,[380] but the chronic lymphatic damage that results in elephantiasis is not reversed. Recurrent bacterial lymphangitis is thought to contribute to the pathology and should be treated with antibiotics. Mass treatment campaigns with diethylcarbamazine have been associated with a decrease in the frequency of advanced hydroceles.[379]

Diethylcarbamazine has been used successfully to treat persons with pulmonary infiltrates with eosinophilia in the tropics, because this syndrome is in many instances caused by microfilaria in the lungs.[385] Diethylcarbamazine kills the microfilaria of *L. loa,* but severe adverse reactions, including encephalopathy caused by the release of parasite antigens, can occur in persons with heavy microfilarial burdens.[386] Diethylcarbamazine has no effect against *Mansonella ozzardi* or *M. perstans*[387,388]; it has been used to treat visceral larva migrans but with variable success.[389,390]

Ivermectin has replaced diethylcarbamazine for the treatment of onchocerciasis. Diethylcarbamazine rapidly kills microfilaria of *O. volvulus* in the skin and eye, but the resulting inflammatory reaction can cause severe damage.[391-393] Ocular complications, which may be permanent, include visual field constriction, optic nerve damage,

chorioretinitis, anterior uveitis, and punctate keratitis.[391-396] Diethylcarbamazine does not kill adult *O. volvulus,* and microfilaria reaccumulate after therapy.[394] Ivermectin is associated with a slower reduction of microfilaria in the eye and much less toxicity. Diethylcarbamazine is also widely used in veterinary practice to kill *Dirofilaria immitis,* the dog heartworm.

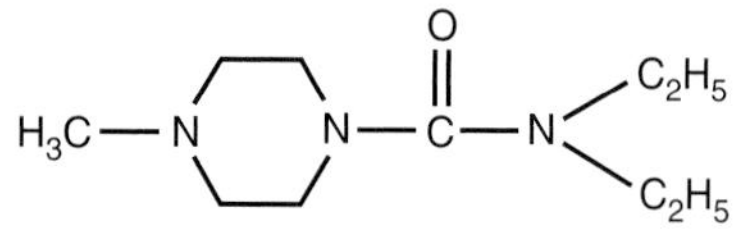

Diethylcarbamazine is readily absorbed from the gastrointestinal tract. Peak blood levels are reached in 1 to 2 hours; the serum half-life is approximately 8 hours.[397] The parent compound and its metabolites are cleared through the kidney. Diethylcarbamazine is distributed equally throughout all body compartments except adipose tissue, and there is little accumulation even after repeated doses are given.

The drug seems to affect microfilariae in multiple ways. First, it is associated with a decrease in helminthic muscle activity, which leads eventually to immobilization of the worm.[398] The piperazine moiety may result in hyperpolarization, causing the observed paralysis. Second, the drug appears to alter the surface membranes of microfilariae, resulting in enhanced killing by the host's immune system.[399,400] Diethylcarbamazine has also been shown to enhance the adherence properties of eosinophils and polymorphonuclear leukocytes,[401] and there is evidence to suggest that human platelets may contribute to the antimicrofilarial effects.[402] Diethylcarbamazine has effects on arachidonic acid metabolism and inhibits parasite eicosanoid production.[403] It also disrupts microtubules and inhibits their formation in vitro.[404]

Untoward effects include those produced directly by the drug and inflammatory reactions that follow the release of filarial antigens. Common reactions include headache, malaise, weakness, arthralgia, anorexia, nausea, and vomiting. The gastrointestinal effects are usually dose related. Acute psychotic reactions have been reported but are rare.

Systemic and ocular reactions occur when diethylcarbamazine is used to treat onchocerciasis. They include severe pruritus, edema of the skin, fever, hypotension, heightened eosinophilia, lymphadenopathy, splenomegaly, and proteinuria.[395,396] The elicitation of such reactions by even low doses of diethylcarbamazine is the basis for the Mazzotti test,[405] which has been used to diagnose onchocerciasis but is potentially dangerous. In *W. bancrofti* and *B. malayi* infections, localized swellings or nodules may develop along lymphatics, and there may be accompanying lymphadenitis.[396] Transient hydrocele formation or lymphedema may be observed. Serious reactions including encephalopathy, presumably caused by release of parasite antigens, have been observed in persons treated with diethylcarbamazine who had heavy *L. loa* burdens.[406]

Ivermectin

Ivermectin is the 22,23-dihydro derivative of ivermectin B1, a macrocyclic lactone produced by the actinomycete *Streptomyces avermitilis.*[407] It is active at low doses against a large number of nematodes and blood-sucking arthropods that parasitize humans and animals. Ivermectin is the treatment of choice for human onchocerciasis.[391-393,408-416] It kills microfilariae in the skin and produces a gradual reduction in the eye. The systemic and ocular inflammatory responses that occur after treatment are much less severe than with diethylcarbamazine. In mass community-based treatment programs, ivermectin has proved safe, acceptable to indigenous populations, and effective in reducing microfilarial loads and the prevalence of onchocerciasis. Although ivermectin does not kill adult *O. volvulus,* it inhibits oviposition. Successive annual treatments are associated with a progressive decline in the microfilarial burden.[417,418]

Ivermectin kills microfilariae of *W. bancrofti* and *B. malayi,*[419-422] but despite a profound effect on blood microfilaremia, it has no observable activity on the viability of the adult worms.[423] Diethylcarbamazine remains the treatment of choice for lymphatic filariasis. Ivermectin also kills microfilariae of *L. loa,*[424,425] but in persons with high concentrations of *L. loa,* treatment can be associated with encephalopathy, presumably because of the release of antigens in the central nervous system. Ivermectin is also active against microfilariae of *Mansonella streptocerca* and *M. ozzardi,* but not *M. perstans.*[426]

Ivermectin has activity against several intestinal nematodes.[427] It has emerged as the treatment of choice for strongyloidiasis.[428-430] It is as ef-

FIGURE 41-11. Diethylcarbamazine.

fective as thiabendazole in the treatment of uncomplicated strongyloidiasis, but it has fewer untoward effects. Failures have been reported in persons with disseminated strongyloidiasis, and multiple doses of ivermectin are recommended. Ivermectin is also effective in the treatment of cutaneous larva migrans.[431] It is active against the human intestinal pathogens *A. lumbricoides* and *E. vermicularis* and has some activity against *T. trichiura*, but it is not effective for the hookworms.[429]

Ivermectin administered orally is useful in the treatment of scabies.[430,432,433] A single dose is usually effective in immunocompetent persons, but multiple doses are often necessary in persons with HIV infection and crusted scabies. Ivermectin is widely used in veterinary practice for the treatment of helminthic and arthropod infestations.

Ivermectin is odorless and colorless and has been effective when administered as a single oral dose. Peak serum concentrations are reached 4 to 5 hours after an oral dose, and the elimination half-life is 50 to 60 hours.[434] It is highly protein bound.[435,436] It is concentrated in the liver and adipose tissues. Only a small percentage of the drug is excreted in the urine; the rest is excreted in the stool. Ivermectin activates the opening of gated chloride channels that are found only in nematodes and arthropods. The result is an influx of chloride ions leading in nematodes to paralysis of the pharyngeal pumping motion.[436]

Ivermectin is generally well tolerated. The initiation of therapy in persons with onchocerciasis can be associated with fever, pruritus, tender lymphadenopathy, headache, arthralgias, myalgia, and cutaneous edema resulting from the release of microfilarial antigens, but the side effects are less frequent and less severe than those of diethylcarbamazine.[391-393,408-416,437,438] Similar symptoms can occur during the treatment of other filarial diseases. The administration of ivermectin to patients with high burdens of *L. loa* microfilaremia has been associated with the development of encephalopathy. Cases have been reported during mass treatment programs for onchocerciasis in areas of Africa where *L. loa* is coendemic.[439,440] No teratogenicity has been reported in animals. In a study of 203 children born to women inadvertently treated during pregnancy, no increase in the rate of birth defects was observed, but ivermectin is not approved for use during pregnancy.[441]

DRUGS FOR TREATMENT OF PLATYHELMINTHS: TREMATODES (FLUKES) AND CESTODES (TAPEWORMS)

Praziquantel

Praziquantel (Fig. 41-12), 2-(cyclohexylcarbonyl-[1,2,3,6,7,11β]-hexahydro-4H-pyrazino[2,1-α]isoquinolin-4-one), is a heterocyclic prazino-isoquinoline derivative with a broad spectrum of activity against trematodes and cestodes.[442-444] Praziquantel is highly effective in the treatment of chronic schistosomiasis caused by all of the *Schistosoma* species that infect humans.[445-448] Mass treatment programs have been associated with improved physical fitness and school performance among children in endemic regions.[449,450] It has even been effective in the treatment of schistosomiasis of the central nervous system.[451,452] Praziquantel does not kill migrating schistosomula larvae, and as a consequence, it is not effective in prophylaxis after acute exposure to *Schistosoma* species.[445] The possibility of praziquantel-resistant *S. mansoni* is suggested by reports of therapeutic failures,[453,454] but to date, widespread praziquantel resistance has not emerged.

Praziquantel is also the drug of choice for the liver flukes *C. sinensis, Opisthorchis viverrini,* and *Metorchis conjunctus;* the lung flukes *Paragonimus westermani, Paragonimus kellicotti,* and other *Paragonimus* species; and the intestinal flukes *Heterophyes heterophyes, Fasciolopsis buski, Metagonimus yokogawai,* and *Nanophyetus salmincola.*[443,444,455] Only against the liver fluke, *Fasciola hepatica,* have praziquantel failures been frequent.[456,457] Bithionol or triclabendazole is recommended for the treatment of *F. hepatica* infections.

Praziquantel is also active against adult and larval forms of the cestodes. It is highly effective in the treatment of adult *Taenia solium, T. saginata, Diphyllobothrium latum, Diphyllobothrium pacificum, Hymenolepis nana,* and *Dipylidium caninum* infections in the human intestine.[442-444,458] It was the first drug to be successfully used for the treatment of parenchymal neurocysticercosis caused by *T. solium.*[459-463] Although not compared in a double-blind, controlled manner, albendazole appears to be more effective; it has more favorable pharmacokinetics and is administered over a shorter course. Praziquantel is often ineffective when there is subarachnoid involvement, cysticercal meningitis, or cysts in the ventricular system,[463,464] although it has been used successfully in some cases when albendazole has failed. Praziquantel is contraindicated in persons with intraocular cysticerci.[463,464] It is not effective in the treatment of human hydatid disease. Although it damages protoscolices in hydatids, the germinal layer is not destroyed.[466,467] Albendazole is the drug of choice when medical treatment of echinococcal disease is indicated.

Praziquantel is dispensed in tablets that contain a mixture of its two enantiomers.[468,469] The drug is crystalline, colorless, and almost insoluble in water. Variability has been reported in the bioavailability of different praziquantel preparations.[470] A peak serum concentration of 1 μm/mL is reached 1 to 2 hours after an oral dose of 50 mg/kg body weight of the standard preparation is administered.[471,472] Praziquantel is approximately 80% protein bound. There is pronounced first-pass metabolism. Approximately 80% of praziquantel is excreted in the urine in 4 days; 90% of that amount is excreted within the first 24 hours. The remainder is excreted in the feces. The pharmacokinetics of the drug are not significantly altered in patients undergoing hemodialysis. The concentration of praziquantel in the CSF is approximately 14% to 24% of the concentration of free plus protein-bound drug in the plasma.[473] Plasma levels are decreased by approximately 50% in patients with neurocysticercosis receiving corticosteroids, which is a problem because corticosteroids are typically administered with praziquantel to reduce cerebral edema.[474] In contrast, serum and CSF levels are increased when corticosteroids are administered concurrently with albendazole.

Praziquantel is rapidly taken up by susceptible flukes and tapeworms. It is uniformly distributed in these organisms and is not metabolized. It damages the integument and increases the permeability to calcium ions.[475] In adult schistosomes, an influx of calcium is followed by tetanic contraction and paralysis of the musculature.[476-478] The initial effects are rapid and associated with intense vacuolation of the tegument.[476] Adult worms are then swept to the liver, where they are attacked by phagocytes. Praziquantel results in exposure of parasite antigens, including actin, on the surface of adult schistosomes; this facilitates the host immune response.[479,480] In the tapeworm *Hymenolepis diminuta,* praziquantel causes calcium release from endogenous stores, leading to massive contraction of the worm.[481] Expulsion from the gastrointestinal tract follows. The tegument of the neck of the tapeworm develops blebs, but the scolex and proglottids appear to be unaffected.

Praziquantel is generally well tolerated.[442-444] Reactions are common, but they are usually mild and transient. They may be due in part to release of worm antigens. The most common are nausea, vomiting, abdominal pain, dizziness, headache, and lassitude. Only rarely is vomiting severe. Polyserositis with respiratory failure was reported in one patient.[482] Urticarial reactions have been observed during the treatment of paragonimiasis.[483] Intense abdominal pain and bloody diarrhea have occurred in patients with heavy *S. mansoni* infections.[484-486] Increased intracranial pressure, cerebral edema, and inflammation have been observed during the treatment of neurocysticercosis. That is why corticosteroids are usually administered concomitantly with praziquantel in this setting.[487,488] There has been no evidence of mutagenicity or teratogenicity with praziquantel in humans,[489] but the drug has not been approved for use during pregnancy or during lactation. Praziquantel is

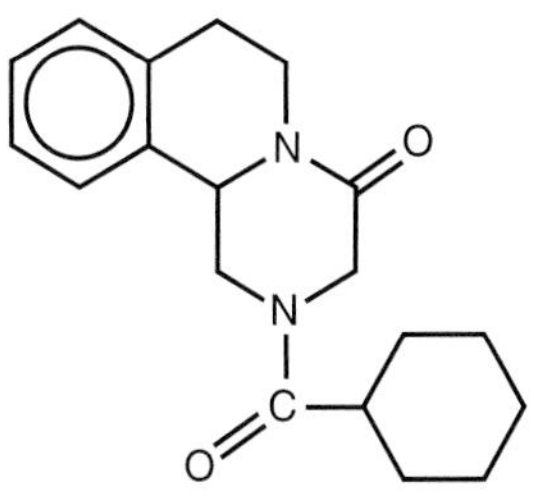

FIGURE 41-12. Praziquantel.

excreted in breast milk. Cimetidine, ketoconazole, and miconazole inhibit the metabolism of praziquantel and increase serum levels.[490]

Oxamniquine

Oxamniquine,[†] a tetrahydroquinoline, is an alternative to praziquantel for the treatment of *S. mansoni* infections.[491-493] It has been used successfully in mass treatment programs and in a focus of *S. mansoni* infection where the response to praziquantel was unusually poor.[493] The sensitivity of *S. mansoni* to oxamniquine varies in different geographic regions. Higher doses are recommended in many areas of Africa.

Oxamniquine is well absorbed orally, and the parent drug and its metabolites are excreted in the urine. Peak plasma concentrations are achieved 1 to 4 hours after dosing, and the elimination half-life is 2.2 hours.[494] It is given as a single dose. Oxamniquine produces marked tegumental alterations in treated adult schistosomes that appear 4 to 8 days after treatment.[495] The tegumental changes seen after praziquantel treatment are much more rapid. Side effects include dizziness, which occurs in 40% of the treated population, drowsiness, headache, fever, diarrhea, rash, hepatic enzyme elevations, electrocardiographic changes, electroencephalographic changes and orange-to-red discoloration of the urine. Convulsions and neuropsychiatric disturbances occur rarely. Oxamniquine should not be used in persons with epilepsy. It is contraindicated during pregnancy.

Bithionol

Bithionol[†] is used for treatment of *F. hepatica*,[496] although triclabendazole,[†] a veterinary drug, is a better choice.[496] Bithionol is also an alternative to praziquantel for the treatment of paragonimiasis.[497] It is administered orally, usually on alternate days, for 10 to 15 doses. It is frequently associated with urticaria, photosensitivity reactions, and gastrointestinal complaints, including vomiting, diarrhea, and abdominal pain. These reactions may be caused, in part or solely, by the release of worm antigens. Leukopenia and toxic hepatitis are rare complications.

Niclosamide

Niclosamide,[†] *N*-(2′-chloro-4′-nitrophenyl)-5-chloro-salicylamide (Fig. 41-13), given as a single dose, is active against a number of adult tapeworms that reside in the human gastrointestinal tract.[500] It kills *T. saginata,* the beef tapeworm; *D. latum,* the fish tapeworm; *H. nana,* the dwarf tapeworm; and *D. caninum,* the dog tapeworm. Although niclosamide also kills *T. solium,* it results in the disintegration of the tapeworm and the release of viable ova, raising the theoretical possibility of autoinfection. Praziquantel, which is active against larvae as well as the adult *T. solium,* is the treatment of choice. If niclosamide is used for *T. solium,* it is often followed by a purge to reduce the theoretical risk of autoinfection. In the case of *H. nana,* praziquantel is effective when administered as a single dose, whereas niclosamide must be administered daily for 6 days. Finally, niclosamide is a molluscicide and has been used in large-scale snail control programs.

Niclosamide is very poorly absorbed. It is supplied in tablets that should be chewed thoroughly and washed down with water. The anthelmintic mechanisms of niclosamide are not completely understood. The drug appears to uncouple oxidative phosphorylation in the scolex and proximal segments of the adult tapeworm and to stimulate adenosine triphosphatase activity of mitochondria, resulting in death of the worm and rapid disintegration of the scolex.[499] Niclosamide is relatively free of side effects except for occasional mild gastrointestinal complaints, lightheadedness, and, rarely, rash. It is not approved for use during pregnancy.

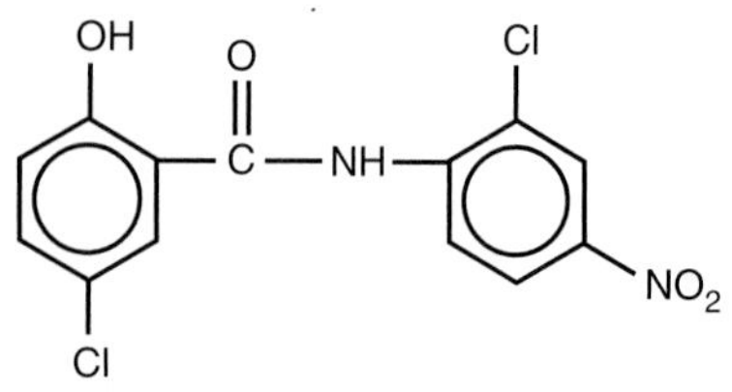

Triclabendazole

Triclabendazole,[†] a benzimidazole [6-chloro-5-(2,3-dichlorophenoxy)-2-methyl thiobenzimidazole], has been used widely in veterinary medicine for the treatment of the liver fluke *F. hepatica* in domestic animals. Although the published experience in humans is limited,

FIGURE 41-13. Niclosamide.

triclabendazole has been considered by many to be the treatment of choice for human fascioliasis based on its ease of administration, paucity of untoward effects, and efficacy.[488,499] Triclabendazole is administered to humans as a single oral dose of 10 mg/kg, or, in heavy infections, two separate doses each of 10 mg/kg with food to increase absorption. Untoward effects include mild abdominal pain, nausea, and transiently elevated liver enzymes. Resistant *F. hepatica* strains have been isolated from animals. Triclabendazole has not been approved by the U.S. FDA, and it has been difficult to obtain the drug since production of the human formulation was discontinued.

REFERENCES

1. Marr JJ, Nilsen TW, Komuniecki RW. Molecular Medical Parasitology. Amsterdam: Academic Press; 2003.
2. Gillespie SH, Pearson RD. Principles and Practice of Clinical Parasitology, Chichester, United Kingdom: Wiley; 2001.
3. Freeman DO. Immunopathogenetic Aspects of Disease Induced by Helminth Parasites. Basel: Karger; 1997.
4. Neva FA. Basic Clinical Parasitology/Franklin A. Neva, Harold W. Brown. 6th ed. Norwalk, Conn: Appleton & Lange; 1994.
5. Drugs for treatment of parasitic infections. Med Lett Drugs Ther. April 2002. Available at www.medletter.com.
6. Raether W, Hanel H. Nitroheterocyclic drugs with broad spectrum activity. Parasitol Res. 2003;90(Suppl 1):S19-39.
7. Katz DE, Taylor DN. Parasitic infections of the gastrointestinal tract. Gastroenterol Clin North Am. 2001;30:797-781.
8. Petri WA Jr, Singh U. Diagnosis and management of amebiasis. Clin Infect Dis. 1999;29:1117-1125.
9. Chacin-Bonilla L. Successful treatment of human *Entamoeba polecki* infection with metronidazole. Am J Trop Med Hyg. 1980;29:521-523.
10. Salaki JS, Shirey JL, Strickland GT. Successful treatment of symptomatic *Entamoeba polecki* infection. Am J Trop Med Hyg. 1979;28:190-193.
11. Lossick JG. Treatment of sexually transmitted vaginosis/vaginitis. Rev Infect Dis. 1990;12(Suppl 6):S665-S681.
12. Upcroft P, Upcroft JA. Drug targets and mechanisms of resistance in the anaerobic protozoa. Clin Microbiol Rev. 2001;14:150-164.
13. Wolfe MS. Giardiasis. N Engl J Med. 1978;298:319-321.
14. Lerman SJ, Walker RA. Treatment of giardiasis: Literature review and recommendations. Clin Pediatr. 1982;21:409-414.
15. Nigro L, Larocca L, Massarelli L, et al. A placebo-controlled treatment trial of *Blastocystis hominis* infection with metronidazole. J Travel Med. 2003;10:128-130.
16. Garcia-Laverde A, de Bonilla L. Clinical trials with metronidazole in human balantidiasis. Am J Trop Med Hyg. 1975;24:781-783.
17. Kale OO, Elemile T, Enahoro F. Controlled comparative trial of thiabendazole and metronidazole in the treatment of dracontiasis. Ann Trop Med Parasitol. 1983;77:1 51-157.
18. Sharma VP, Rathore HS, Sharma MM. Efficacy of metronidazole in dracunculiasis: A clinical trial. Am J Trop Med Hyg. 1979;28:658-660.
19. Houghton GW, Smith J, Thorne PS, et al. The pharmacokinetics of oral and intravenous metronidazole in man. J Antimicrob Chemother. 1979;5:621-623.
20. McGilveray IJ, Midha KK, Loo JCK, et al. The bioavailability of commercial metronidazole formulations. Int J Clin Pharmacol. 1978;16:110-115.
21. Norris SM, Ravdin JI. The pharmacology of antiamebic drugs. In: Ravdin JI, ed. Amebiasis: Human Infection by *Entamoeba histolytica.* New York: Wiley; 1988: 734-740.
22. Lau AH, Lam NP, Piscitelli SC, et al. Clinical pharmacokinetics of metronidazole and other nitroimidazole anti-infectives. Clin Pharmacokinet. 1992;23:328-364.
23. Lares-Asseff I, Cravioto J, Santiago P, et al. Pharmacokinetics of metronidazole in severely malnourished and nutritionally rehabilitated children. Clin Pharmacol Ther. 1992;51:42-50.
24. Lindmark DG, Müller M. Antitrichomonad action, mutagenicity, and reduction of metronidazole and other nitroimidazoles. Antimicrob Agents Chemother. 1976;10:476-482.
25. Knight RC, Skolimowski IM, Edwards DI. The interaction of reduced metronidazole with DNA. Biochem Pharmacol. 1978;27:2089-2093.

26. LaRusso NF, Tomasz M, Müller M, et al. Interaction of metronidazole with nucleic acids in vitro. Mol Pharmacol. 1977;13:872-882.

27. Lefebvre Y, Hesseltine HC. The peripheral white blood cells and metronidazole. JAMA. 1965;194:15-18.

28. Kazmier FJ. A significant interaction between metronidazole and warfarin. Mayo Clin Proc. 1976;51:782-784.

29. Kusumi RK, Plouffe JF, Wyatt RH, et al. Central nervous system toxicity associated with metronidazole therapy. Ann Intern Med. 1980;93:59-60.

30. Feola DJ, Thornton AC. Metronidazole-induced pancreatitis in a patient with recurrent vaginal trichomoniasis. Pharmacotherapy. 2002;22:1508-1510.

31. Cina SJ, Russell RA, Conradi SE. Sudden death due to metronidazole/ethanol interaction. Am J Forensic Med Pathol. 1996;17:343-346.

32. Bendesky A, Menendez D, Ostrosky-Wegman P. Is metronidazole carcinogenic? Mutat Res. 2002;511:133-144.

33. Sisson G, Jeong JY, Goodwin A, et al. Metronidazole activation is mutagenic and causes DNA fragmentation in *Helicobacter pylori* and in *Escherichia coli* containing a cloned *H. pylori* RdxA(+) (nitroreductase) gene. J Bacteriol. 2000;182:5091-5096.

34. Koch RL, Beaulieu BB Jr, Chrystal EJT, et al. A metronidazole metabolite in human urine and its risk. Science. 1981;211:398-400.

35. Falagas ME, Walker AM, Ruthazer R, et al. Late incidence of cancer after metronidazole use: A matched metronidazole user/nonuser study. Clin Infect Dis. 1998;26:384-388.

36. Czeizel AE, Rockenbauer M. A population based case-control teratologic study of oral metronidazole treatment during pregnancy. Br J Obstet Gynecol. 1998;105:322-327.

37. Bassily S, Farid Z, el-Masry NA, Mikhail EM. Treatment of intestinal *E. histolytica* and *G. lamblia* with metronidazole, tinidazole and ornidazole: A comparative study. J Trop Med Hyg. 1987;90:9-12.

38. Pengsaa K, Limkittikul K, Pojjaroen-anant C, et al. Single-dose therapy for giardiasis in school-age children. Southeast Asian J Trop Med Public Health. 2002;33:711-717.

39. Escobedo AA, Nunez FA, Moreira I, et al. Comparison of chloroquine, albendazole and tinidazole in the treatment of children with giardiasis. Ann Trop Med Parasitol. 2003;97:367-71.

40. Sobel JD, Nyirjesy P, Brown W. Tinidazole therapy for metronidazole-resistant vaginal trichomoniasis. Clin Infect Dis. 2001;33:1341-1346.

41. Narisi EM, Secor WE. In vitro effect of tinidazole and furazolidone on metronidazole-resistant *Trichomonas vaginalis*. Antimicrob Agents Chemother. 1996;40:1121-1125.

42. Gupta JP, Jain AK, Nanivadekar AS. Efficacy of tinidazole (Fasigyn) in giardiasis by parasitologic, biochemical, and gut transit studies. Indian J Gastroenterol. 1989;8:103-104.

43. Goldman P. The development of 5-nitroimidazoles for the treatment and prophylaxis of anaerobic bacterial infections. J Antimicrob Chemother. 1982;10(Suppl A):23-33.

44. Rossignol JF, Maisonneuve H, Cho YW. Nitroimidazoles in the treatment of trichomoniasis, giardiasis, and amebiasis. Int J Clin Pharmacol Ther Toxicol. 1984;22:63-72.

45. Anonymous. New drug for parasitic infections in children. FDA Consumer. 2003;37:4.

46. Anonymous. Nitazoxanide (Alinia): A new anti-protozoal agent. Med Lett Drugs Ther. 2003;45:29-31.

47. Amadi B, Mwiya M, Musuku J, et al. Effect of nitazoxanide on morbidity and mortality in Zambian children with cryptosporidiosis: A randomized controlled trial. Lancet. 2002;360:1375-1380.

48. White AC Jr. Nitazoxanide: An important advance in anti-parasitic therapy. Am J Trop Med Hyg. 2003;68:382-383.

49. Pearson RD. Nitazoxanide as treatment of intestinal parasites in children. Curr Infect Dis Rep. 2004;6:25-26.

50. Blessmann J, Tannich E. Treatment of asymptomatic intestinal *Entamoeba histolytica* infection. N Engl J Med. 2002;347:1384.

51. Simon M, Shookhoff HB, Terner H, et al. Paromomycin in the treatment of intestinal amebiasis: A short course of therapy. Am J Gastroenterol. 1967;48:504-511.

52. Wolfe MS. The treatment of intestinal protozoan infections. Med Clinics North Am. 1982;66:707-720.

53. White AC Jr, Chappell CL, Hayat CS, et al. Paromomycin for cryptosporidiosis in AIDS: A prospective, double-blind trial. J Infect Dis. 1994;170:419-424.

54. Hewitt RG, Yiannoutsos CT, Higgs ES, et al. Paromomycin: No more effective than placebo for treatment of cryptosporidiosis in patients with advanced human immunodeficiency virus infection. AIDS Clinical Trial Group. Clin Infect Dis. 2000;31:1084-1092.

55. Poppe WA. Nitroimidazole-resistant vaginal trichomoniasis treated with paromomycin. Eur J Obstet Gynecol Reprod Biol. 2001;96:119-120.

56. Nyirjesy P, Sobel JD, Weitz MV, et al. Difficult-to-treat trichomoniasis: Results with paromomycin cream. Clin Infect Dis. 1998;26:986-988.

57. Asilian A, Jalayer T, Nilforooshzadeh M, et al. Treatment of cutaneous leishmaniasis with aminosidine (paromomycin) ointment: Double-blind, randomized trial in the Islamic Republic of Iran. Bull World Health Organ. 2003;81:353-359.

58. el-On J, Halevy S, Grunwald MH, et al. Topical treatment of old world cutaneous leishmaniasis caused by *Leishmania major*: A double-blind control study. J Am Acad Dermatol. 1992;27:227-231.

59. Berman JD. Human leishmaniasis: Clinical, diagnostic, and chemotherapeutic developments in the last 10 years. Clin Infect Dis. 1997;24:684-703.

60. Jha TK, Olliaro P, Thakur CP, et al. Randomised controlled trial of aminosidine (paromomycin) vs sodium stibogluconate for treating visceral leishmaniasis in North Bihar, India. BMJ. 1998;316:1200-1205.

61. Tan WW, Chapnick EK, Abter EI, et al. Paromomycin-associated pancreatitis in HIV-related cryptosporidiosis. Ann Pharmacother. 1995;29:22-24.

62. McAuley JB, Juranek DD. Luminal agents in the treatment of amebiasis. Clin Infect Dis. 1992;14:1161-1162.

63. Fisher AK, Walter FG, Szabo S. Iodoquinol-associated seizures and radiopacity. J Toxicol Clin Toxicol. 1993;31:113-120.

64. Oakley GP Jr. The neurotoxicity of the halogenated hydroxyquinolines. JAMA. 1973;225:395-397.

65. Pehrson PD. Treatment of cyst passers. Clin Infect Dis. 1992;15:559.

66. Pehrson P, Bengtsson E. Treatment of non-invasive amoebiasis: A comparison between tinidazole alone and in combination with diloxanide furoate. Trans R Soc Trop Med Hyg. 1983;77:845-846.

67. Tracy JW, Webster LT Jr. Drugs used in the chemotherapy of protozoal infections: Trypanosomiasis, leishmaniasis, amebiasis, giardiasis, trichomoniasis, and other protozoal infections. In: Hardman JG, Limbird LE, eds. Goodman & Gilman's Pharmacological Basis of Therapeutics. 9th ed. New York: McGraw-Hill; 1996:987-1008.

68. Nash TE. Treatment of *Giardia lamblia* infections. Pediatr Infect Dis J. 2001;20:193-195.

69. Gardner TB, Hill DR. Treatment of giardiasis. Clin Microbiol Rev. 2001;14:114-128.

70. Dionisio D, Manneschi LI, Di Lollo S, et al. *Enterocytozoon bieneusi* in AIDS: Symptomatic relief and parasite changes after furazolidone. J Clin Pathol. 1997;50:472-476.

71. Elliott AM, Klaus BD, Morth DS, Martin HP. Furazolidone-induced mood disorder during treatment of refractory giardiasis in a patient with AIDS. Clin Infect Dis. 1998;26:1015.

72. Wellems TE, Miller LH. Two worlds of malaria. N Engl J Med. 2003;349:1496-1498.

73. Jong EC, Nothdurft HD. Current drugs for antimalarial chemoprophylaxis: A review of efficacy and safety. J Travel Med. 2001;8(Suppl 3):S48-56.

74. Health Information for International Travel, 2003-2004. Centers for Disease Control and Prevention, United States Department of Health and Human Services. Atlanta, GA. Available at www.cdc.gov/travel/yb/index.htm.

75. Whitby M. Drug-resistant *Plasmodium vivax* malaria. J Antimicrob Chemotherapy. 1997;40:749-752.

76. Collignon P. Chloroquine resistance in *Plasmodium vivax*. J Infect Dis. 1991;164:222-223.

77. Schwartz IK, Lackritz EM, Patchen LC. Chloroquine-resistant *Plasmodium vivax* from Indonesia. N Engl J Med. 1991;324:927.

78. Marlar-Than, Myat-Phone-Kyaw, Aye-Yu-Soe, et al. Development of resistance to chloroquine by *Plasmodium vivax* in Myanmar. Trans R Soc Trop Med Hyg. 1995;89:307-308.

79. Phillips EJ, Keystone JS, Kain KC. Failure of combined chloroquine and high-dose primaquine therapy for *Plasmodium vivax* malaria acquired in Guyana, South America. Clin Infect Dis. 1996;23:1171-1173.

80. Alecrim M das G. Alecrim W. Macedo V. Plasmodium vivax resistance to chloroquine (R2) and mefloquine (R3) in Brazilian Amazon region. Rev Soc Bras Med Trop. 1999;32:67-68.

81. Krogstad DJ, Herwaldt BL, Schlesinger PH. Antimalarial agents: Specific treatment regimens. Antimicrob Agents Chemother. 1988;32:957-961.

82. Brohult J, Rombo L, Sirleaf V, et al. The concentration of chloroquine in serum during short and long term malaria prophylaxis with standard and "double" dosage in non-immunes: Clinical implications. Ann Trop Med Parasitol. 1979;73:401-405.

83. Tracey JW, Webster LT Jr. Drugs used in the chemotherapy of protozoal infections: Malaria. In: Hardman JG, Limbird LE, eds. Goodman and Gilman's Pharmacological Basis of Therapeutics. 9th ed. New York: McGraw-Hill; 1996:965-985.

84. Andrews P, Haberkorn A, Thomas H. Antiparasitic drugs: Mechanisms of action, pharmacokinetics, and in vitro and in vivo assays of drug activity. In: Lorian V, ed. Antibiotics in Laboratory Medicine. 2nd ed. Baltimore: Williams & Wilkins; 1986:282-345.

85. Krogstad DJ, Schlesinger PH. Acid-vesicle function, intracellular pathogens and the action of chloroquine against *Plasmodium falciparum*. N Engl J Med. 1987;317:542-549.

86. Slater AFG, Cerami A. Inhibition by chloroquine of a novel heme polymerase enzyme activity in malaria trophozoites. Nature. 1992;355:167-169.

87. Foley M, Tilley L. Quinoline antimalarials: Mechanisms of action and resistance. Int J Parasitol. 1997;27:231-240.

88. Kyle DE, Milhous WK, Rossan RN. Reversal of *Plasmodium falciparum* resistance to chloroquine in Panamanian *Aotus* monkeys. Am J Trop Med Hyg. 1993;48:126-133.

89. Martin SK, Oduola AMJ, Milhous WK. Reversal of chloroquine resistance in *Plasmodium falciparum* by verapamil. Science. 1987;235:899-901.

90. Marks JS. Chloroquine retinopathy: Is there a safe daily dose? Ann Rheum Dis. 1982;41:52-58.

91. White NJ, Watt G, Berquist Y, et al. Parenteral chloroquine for treating falciparum malaria. J Infect Dis. 1987;155:192-201.

92. Clemessy JL, Taboulet P, Hoffman JR, et al. Treatment of acute chloroquine poisoning: A 5-year experience. Crit Care Med. 1996;24:1189-1195.

93. Hart CW, Naunton RF. The ototoxicity of chloroquine phosphate. Arch Otolaryngol. 1964;80:407-412.

94. Arias AE, Corredor AM. Low response rate of Colombian strains of *Plasmodium vivax* to classical antimalarial therapy. Trop Med Parasitol. 1989;40:21-23.

95. Luzzi GA, Warrell DA, Barnes AJ, et al. Treatment of primaquine resistant *Plasmodium vivax* malaria. Lancet. 1992;340:310.

96. Looareesuwan S, Buchachart K, Wilairatanan P, et al. Primaquine-tolerant vivax malaria in Thailand. Ann Trop Med Parasitol. 1997;91:939-943.

97. Smoak BL, DeFraites RF, Magill AJ, et al. *Plasmodium vivax* infections in U.S. Army troops: Failure of primaquine to prevent relapse in studies from Somalia. Am J Trop Med Hyg. 1997;56:231-234.

98. Collins WE, Jeffery GM. Primaquine resistance in *Plasmodium vivax*. Am J Trop Med Hyg. 1996;55:243-249.

99. Nasveld P, Kitchener S, Edstein M, Rieckmann K. Comparison of tafenoquine (WR238605) and primaquine in the post-exposure (terminal) prophylaxis of vivax malaria in Australian Defence Force personnel. Trans R Soc Trop Med Hyg. 2002;96:683-684.

100. Baird JK, Lacy MD, Basri H, et al. United States Naval Medical Research Unit 2 Clinical Trials Team. Randomized, parallel placebo-controlled trial of primaquine for malaria prophylaxis in Papua, Indonesia. Clin Infect Dis. 2001;33:1990-1997.

101. Toma E, Thorne A, Singer J, et al. Clindamycin with primaquine vs. trimethoprim-sulfamethoxazole therapy for mild and moderately severe *Pneumocystis carinii* pneumonia in patients with AIDS: A multicenter, double-blind, randomized trial (CTN 004). CTN-PCP Study Group. Clin Infect Dis. 1998;27:524-530.

102. Barber BA, Pegram PS, High KP. Clindamycin/primaquine as prophylaxis for *Pneumonocystis carinii* pneumonia. Clin Infect Dis. 1996;23:718-722.

103. Warhurst DC. Antimalarial drugs: Mode of action and resistance. J Antimicrob Chemother. 1986;18(Suppl B):51-59.

104. Hiebsch RR, Raub TJ, Wattenberg BW. Primaquine blocks transport by inhibiting the formation of functional transport vesicles. J Biol Chem. 1991;266:20323-20328.

105. Kellermeyer RW, Tarlov AR, Brewer GJ, et al. Hemolytic effect of therapeutic drugs: Clinical considerations of the primaquine-type hemolysis. JAMA. 1962;180:388-394.

106. Clyde DF. Clinical problems associated with the use of primaquine as a tissue schizontocidal and gametocytocidal drug. Bull World Health Organ. 1981;59:391-395.

107. Alving AS, Johnson CF, Tarlov AR, et al. Mitigation of the haemolytic effect of primaquine and enhancement of its action against exoerythrocytic forms of the Chesson strain of *Plasmodium vivax* by intermittent regimens of drug administration: A preliminary report. Bull World Health Organ. 1960;22:621-631.

108. Sin DD, Shafran SD. Dapsone- and primaquine-induced methemoglobinemia in HIV-infected individuals. J Acquir Immune Defic Syndr Hum Retrovirol. 1996;12:477-481.

109. Brasseur P, Kouamouo J, Moyou-Somo R, et al. Multi-drug resistant falciparum malaria in Cameroon in 1987-1988: I. Stable figures of prevalence of chloroquine- and quinine-resistant isolates in the original foci. Am J Trop Med Hyg. 1992;46:1-7.

110. Lege-Oguntoye L, Abua JU, Werblinska B, et al. Chloroquine-resistant *Plasmodium falciparum* with reduced sensitivity in vitro to mefloquine and quinine in Zaria, Northern Nigeria. J Trop Med Hyg. 1991;94:73-75.

111. White NJ, Looareesuwan S, Warrell DA, et al. Quinine pharmacokinetics and toxicity in cerebral and uncomplicated falciparum malaria. Am J Med. 1982;73:564-572.

112. Krishna S, White NJ. Pharmacokinetics of quinine, chloroquine and amodiaquine: Clinical implications. Clin Pharmacokinet. 1996;30:263-299.

113. Canfield CJ, Miller LH, Bartelloni PJ, et al. Acute renal failure in *Plasmodium falciparum* malaria. Arch Intern Med. 1968;122:199-203.

114. Foley M, Tilley L. Quinoline antimalarials: Mechanism of action and resistance. Int J Parasitol. 1997;27:231-240.

115. White NJ, Warrell DA, Chanthavanich P, et al. Severe hypoglycemia and hyperinsulinemia in falciparum malaria. N Engl J Med. 1983;309:61-66.

116. Phillips RE, Looareesuwan S, White NJ, et al. Quinine pharmacokinetics and toxicity in pregnant and lactating women with falciparum malaria. Br J Clin Pharmacol. 1986;21:677-683.

117. Phillips RE, Warrell DA, White NJ, et al. Intravenous quinidine for the treatment of severe falciparum malaria. N Engl J Med. 1985;312:1273-1278.

118. Rudnitsky G, Miller KD, Padua T, et al. Continuous-infusion quinidine gluconate for treating children with severe *Plasmodium falciparum* malaria. J Infect Dis. 1987;155:1040-1043.

119. Miller KD, Greenberg AE, Campbell CC. Treatment of severe malaria in the United States with a continuous infusion of quinidine gluconate and exchange transfusion. N Engl J Med. 1989;321:65-70.

120. Swerdlow CD, Yu JO, Jacobson E, et al. Safety and efficacy of intravenous quinidine. Am J Med. 1983;75:36-42.

121. Anonymous. Availability and use of parenteral quinidine gluconate for severe or complicated malaria. MMWR Morb Mortal Wkly Rep. 2000;49:1138-1140.

122. Wongsrichanalai C, Webster HK, Wimonwattrawatee T, et al. Emergence of multidrug-resistant *Plasmodium falciparum* in Thailand: In vitro tracking. Am J Trop Med Hyg. 1992;47:112-116.

123. Nosten F, ter Kuile F, Chongsuphajaisiddhi T, et al. Mefloquine-resistant falciparum malaria on the Thai-Burmese border. Lancet. 1991;337:1140-1143.

124. Hopperus Buma AP, van Thiel PP, Lobel HO, et al. Long-term malaria chemoprophylaxis with mefloquine in Dutch marines in Cambodia. J Infect Dis. 1996; 173:1506-1509.

125. Oduola AM, Sowunmi A, Milhous WK, et al. Innate resistance to new antimalarial drugs in *Plasmodium falciparum* from Nigeria. Trans R Soc Trop Med Hyg. 1992; 86:123-126.

126. Brasseur P, Kouamouo J, Moyou-Somo R, et al. Multi-drug resistant falciparum malaria in Cameroon in 1987-1988: II. Mefloquine resistance confirmed in vitro and in vivo and its correlation with quinine resistance. Am J Trop Med Hyg. 1992;46:8-14.

127. Oduola AM, Milhous WK, Salako LA, et al. Reduced in-vitro susceptibility to mefloquine in West African isolates of *Plasmodium falciparum*. Lancet. 1987;2:1304-1305.

128. Desjardins RE, Pamplin CL III, von Bredow J, et al. Kinetics of a new antimalarial, mefloquine. Clin Pharmacol Ther. 1979;26:372-379.

129. Jacobs GH, Aikawa M, Milhous WK, et al. An ultrastructural study of the effects of mefloquine on malaria parasites. Am J Trop Med Hyg. 1987;36:9-14.

130. Weinke T, Trautmann M, Held T, et al. Neuropsychiatric side effects after the use of mefloquine. Am J Trop Med Hyg. 1991;45:86-91.

131. Barrett PJ, Emmins PD, Clarke PD, et al. Comparison of adverse events associated with use of mefloquine and combination of chloroquine and proguanil as antimalarial prophylaxis: Postal and telephone survey of travellers. BMJ. 1996;313:525-528.

132. Croft AM, Clayton TC, World MJ. Side effects of mefloquine prophylaxis for malaria: An independent randomized controlled trial. Trans R Soc Trop Med. 1997;91:199-203.

133. Rendi-Wagner P, Noedl H, Wernsdorfer WH, et al. Unexpected frequency, duration and spectrum of adverse events after therapeutic dose of mefloquine in healthy adults. Acta Trop. 2002;81:167-173.

134. Olson PE, Kennedy CA, Morte PD. Paresthesias and mefloquine prophylaxis. Ann Intern Med. 1992;117:1058-1059.

135. Van den Enden E, Gompel AV, Colebunders R, et al. Mefloquine-induced Stevens-Johnson syndrome. Lancet. 1991;337:683.

136. Hennequin C, Bouree P, Halfon P. Agranulocytosis during treatment with mefloquine. Lancet. 1991;337:984.

137. Martin GJ, Malone JL, Ross EV. Exfoliative dermatitis during malarial prophylaxis with mefloquine. Clin Infect Dis. 1993;16:341-342.

138. White AC Jr, Gard DA, Sessoms SL. Cutaneous vasculitis associated with mefloquine. Ann Intern Med. 1995;123:894.

139. Horowitz H, Carbonaro CA. Inhibition of *Salmonella typhi* oral vaccine strain, Ty21a, by mefloquine and chloroquine. J Infect Dis. 1992;166:1462-1464.

140. Vanhauwere B, Maradit H, Kerr L. Post-marketing surveillance of prophylactic mefloquine (Lariam) use in pregnancy. Am J Trop Med Hyg. 1998;58:17-21.

141. Schlagenhauf P, Lobel H, Steffen R, et al. Tolerance of mefloquine by SwissAir trainee pilots. Am J Trop Med Hyg. 1997;56:235-240.

142. Touze JE, Fourcade L, Peyron F, et al. Is halofantrine still advisable in malaria attacks? Ann Trop Med Parasitol. 1997;91:867-873.

143. Matson PA, Luby SP, Redd SC, et al. Cardiac effects of standard-dose halofantrine therapy. Am J Trop Med Hyg. 1996;54:229-231.

144. Hien TT, White NJ. Qinghaosu. Lancet. 1993;341:603-608.

145. Newton PN, Angus BJ, Chierakul W, et al. Randomized comparison of artesunate and quinine in the treatment of severe falciparum malaria. Clin Infect Dis. 2003;37:7-16.

146. Wilairatana P, Viriyavejakul P, Looareesuwan S, et al. Artesunate suppositories: An effective treatment for severe falciparum malaria in rural areas. Ann Trop Med Parasitol. 1997;91:891-896.

147. Tran TH, Day NP, Nguyen HP, et al. A controlled trial of artemether or quinine in Vietnamese adults with severe falciparum malaria. N Engl J Med. 1996;335:76-83.

148. Meshnick SR, Taylor TE, Kamchonwongpaisan S. Artemisinin and the antimalarial endoperoxides: From herbal remedy to targeted chemotherapy. Microbiol Rev. 1996;60:301-315.

149. Batty KT, Thu LT, Davis TM, et al. A pharmacokinetic and pharmacodynamic study of intravenous vs oral artesunate in uncomplicated *falciparum* malaria. Br J Clin Pharmacol. 1998;45:123-129.

150. Warshaw EM, Zug KA. Sesquiterpene lactone allergy. Am J Contact Dermat. 1996;7:1-23.

151. Miller LG, Panosian CB. Ataxia and slurred speech after artesunate treatment for falciparum malaria. N Engl J Med. 1997;336:1328.

152. Brewer TG, Grate SJ, Peggins JO, et al. Fatal neurotoxicity of arteether and artemether. Am J Trop Med Hyg. 1994;51:251-259.

153. Hien TT, Turner GD, Mai NT, et al. Neuropathological assessment of artemether-treated severe malaria. Lancet. 2003;295-296.

154. Basko L, Le Bras J. In vitro activity of artemisinin derivatives against African isolates and clones of *Plasmodium falciparum*. Am J Trop Med Hyg. 1993;49:301-307.

155. Baggish AL, Hill DR. Antiparasitic agent atovaquone. Antimicrob Agents Chemother. 2002;46:1163-1173.

156. Chiodini PL, Conlon CP, Hutchinson DB, et al. Evaluation of atovaquone in the treatment of patients with uncomplicated *Plasmodium falciparum* malaria. J Antimicrob Chemother. 1995;36:1073-1078.

157. Marra F, Salzman JR, Ensom MH. Atovaquone-proguanil for prophylaxis and treatment of malaria. Ann Pharmacother. 2003;37:1266-1275.

158. Marra F, Salzman JR, Ensom MH. Atovaquone-proguanil for prophylaxis and treatment of malaria. Ann Pharmacother. 2003;37:1266-1275.

159. Overbosch D, Schilthuis H, Bienzle U, et al. Malarone International Study Team. Atovaquone-proguanil versus mefloquine for malaria prophylaxis in nonimmune travelers: Results from a randomized, double-blind study. Clin Infect Dis. 2001;33:1015-1021.

160. Kofoed K, Petersen E. The efficacy of chemoprophylaxis against malaria with chloroquine plus proguanil, mefloquine, and atovaquone plus proguanil in travelers from Denmark. J Travel Med. 2003;10:150-154.

161. Overbosch D. Post-marketing surveillance: Adverse events during long-term use of atovaquone/proguanil for travelers to malaria-endemic countries. J Travel Med. 2003;10(Suppl 1):S16-20.

162. Petersen E. The safety of atovaquone/proguanil in long-term malaria prophylaxis of nonimmune adults. J Travel Med. 2003;10(Suppl 1):S13-15, 21.

163. Schwartz E, Bujanover S, Kain KC. Genetic confirmation of atovaquone-proguanil-resistant *Plasmodium falciparum* malaria acquired by a nonimmune traveler to East Africa. Clin Infect Dis. 2003;37:450-451.

164. Anonymous. Atovaquone for *Pneumocystis carinii* pneumonia. Med Lett Drugs Ther. 1993;35:28-29.

165. Colby C, McAfee S, Sackstein R, et al. A prospective randomized trial comparing the toxicity and safety of atovaquone with trimethoprim/sulfamethoxazole as *Pneumocystis carinii* pneumonia prophylaxis following autologous peripheral blood stem cell transplantation. Bone Marrow Transplant. 1999;24:897-902.

166. El-Sadr WM, Murphy RL, Yurik TM, et al. Atovaquone compared with dapsone for the prevention of *Pneumocystis carinii* pneumonia in patients with HIV infection who cannot tolerate trimethoprim, sulfonamides, or both. N Engl J Med. 1998;339:1889-1895.

167. Araujo FG, Lin T, Remington JS. The activity of atovaquone (566C80) in murine toxoplasmosis is markedly augmented when used in combination with pyrimethamine or sulfadiazine. J Infect Dis. 1993;167:494-497.

168. Katlama C, Mouthon B, Gourdon D, et al. Atovaquone as long-term suppressive therapy for toxoplasmic encephalitis in patients with AIDS and multiple drug intolerance. Atovaquone Expanded Access Group. AIDS. 1996;10:1107-1112.

169. Emberger M, Lechner AM, Zelger B. Stevens-Johnson syndrome associated with Malarone antimalarial prophylaxis. Clin Infect Dis. 2003;37:5-7.

170. Rollo IM. The mode of action of sulphonamides, proguanil and pyrimethamine on *Plasmodium gallinaceum.* Br J Pharmacol Chemother. 1955;10:208-214.

171. Barnes AJ, Ong ELC, Dunbar EM, et al. Failure of chloroquine and proguanil prophylaxis in travellers to Kenya. Lancet. 1991;338:1338-1339.

172. Eriksson B, Bjorkman A, Keisu M. How safe is proguanil? A post-marketing investigation of side effects. Scand J Infect Dis. 1991;23:489-493.

173. Kovacs JA, Allegra CJ, Chabner BA, et al. Potent effect of trimetrexate, a lipid-soluble antifolate, on *Toxoplasma gondii.* J Infect Dis. 1987;155:1027-1032.

174. Miller KD, Lobel HO, Satriale RF, et al. Severe cutaneous reactions among American travelers using pyrimethamine-sulfadoxine (Fansidar) for malaria prophylaxis. Am J Trop Med Hyg. 1986;35:451-458.

175. Luft BJ, Conley F, Remington JS. Outbreak of central-nervous-system toxoplasmosis in Western Europe and North America. Lancet. 1983;1:781-784.

176. Haverkos HW. Assessment of therapy for toxoplasma encephalitis: The TE study group. Am J Med. 1987;82:907-914.

177. Luft BJ, Hafner R, Korzun AH, et al. Toxoplasmic encephalitis in patients with the acquired immunodeficiency syndrome: Members of the ACTG077p/ANRS009 Study Team. N Engl J Med. 1993;329:995-1000.

178. Anonymous. 1999 USPHS/IDSA guidelines for the prevention of opportunistic infections in persons infected with human immunodeficiency virus. USPHS/IDSA Prevention of Opportunistic Infections Working Group. Clin Infect Dis. 2000;30:S29-65.

179. Deresinski SC. Treatment of *Pneumocystis carinii* pneumonia in adults with AIDS. Semin Respir Infect. 1997;12:79-97.

180. Ioannidis JP, Cappelleri JC, Skolnik PR, et al. A meta-analysis of the relative efficacy and toxicity of *Pneumocystis carinii* prophylactic regimens. Arch Intern Med. 1996;156:177-188.

181. Daffos F, Forestier F, Capella-Pavlovsky M, et al. Prenatal management of 746 pregnancies at risk for congenital toxoplasmosis. N Engl J Med. 1988;318:271-275.

182. Navin TR, Miller KD, Satriale RF, et al. Adverse reactions associated with pyrimethamine-sulfadoxine prophylaxis for *Pneumocystis carinii* infections in AIDS. Lancet. 1985;1:1332.

183. Pape JW, Verdier RI, Johnson WD. Treatment and prophylaxis of *Isospora belli* infection in patients with the acquired immunodeficiency syndrome. N Engl J Med. 1989;320:1044-1047.

184. Weidekamm E, Plozza-Nottebrock H, Forgo I, et al. Plasma concentrations of pyrimethamine and sulfadoxine and evaluation of pharmacokinetic data by computerized curve fitting. Bull World Health Organ. 1982;60:115-122.

185. Jaffe JJ. Dihydrofolate reductase in parasitic protozoa and helminths. In: Van den Bossche H, ed. Biochemistry of Parasites. London: Academic Press; 1972:219-233.

186. Hayama T, Kokue E. Use of the Goettingen miniature pig for studying pyrimethamine teratogenesis. Crit Rev Toxicol. 1985;14:403-421.

187. Petter C, Bourbon J. Foetal red cell macrocytosis induced by pyrimethamine: Its teratogenic role. Experientia. 1975;31:369-370.

188. Anonymous. Pyrimethamine combinations in pregnancy (Editorial). Lancet. 1983;2:1005-1007.

189. Harpey JP, Darbois Y, LeFèbvre G. Teratogenicity of pyrimethamine. Lancet. 1983;2:399.

190. Herwaldt BL, Ackers ML. An outbreak in 1996 of cyclosporiasis associated with imported raspberries. The Cyclospora Working Group. N Engl J Med. 1997;336:1548-1556.

191. Jick H. Adverse reactions to trimethoprim-sulfamethoxazole in hospitalized patients. Rev Infect Dis. 1982;4:426-428.

192. Gordin FM, Simon GL, Wofsy CB, et al. Adverse reactions to trimethoprim-sulfamethoxazole in patients with the acquired immunodeficiency syndrome. Ann Intern Med. 1984;100:495-499.

193. Castro M. Treatment and prophylaxis of *Pneumocystis carinii* pneumonia. Semin Respir Infect. 1998;13:296-303.

194. Goldie SJ, Kaplan JE, Losina E, et al. Prophylaxis for human immunodeficiency virus-related *Pneumocystis carinii* pneumonia: Using simulation modeling to inform clinical guidelines. Arch Intern Med. 2002;162:921-928.

195. Horowitz HW, Wormser GP. Atovaquone compared with dapsone to prevent *Pneumocystis carinii* pneumonia. N Engl J Med. 1999;340:1512-1513.

196. Bucher HC, Griffith L, Guyatt GH, Opravil M. Meta-analysis of prophylactic treatments against *Pneumocystis carinii* pneumonia and toxoplasma encephalitis in HIV-infected patients. J Acquir Immune Defic Syndr Hum Retrovirol. 1997;15:104-114.

197. Wolf M, Matz H, Orion E, et al. Dapsone. Dermatol Online J. 2002;8:2.

198. Lee KB, Nashed TB. Dapsone-induced sulfone syndrome. Ann Pharmacother. 2003;37:1044-1046.

199. Ohrt C, Richie TL, Widjaja H, et al. Mefloquine compared with doxycycline for the prophylaxis of malaria in Indonesian soldiers: A randomized, double-blind, placebo-controlled trial. Ann Intern Med. 1997;126:963-972.

200. Smith HL, Rajan TV. Tetracycline inhibits development of the infective-stage larvae of filarial nematodes in vitro. Exp Parasitol. 2000;95:265-270.

201. Meek SR, Doberstyn EB, Gaürzère BA, et al. Treatment of falciparum malaria with quinine and tetracycline or combined mefloquine/sulfadoxine/pyrimethamine on the Thai-Kampuchean border. Am J Trop Med Hyg. 1986;35:246-250.

202. Danneman B, McCutchan A, Isrealski D, et al. Treatment of toxoplasmic encephalitis in patients with AIDS: A randomized trial comparing pyrimethamine plus clindamycin to pyrimethamine plus sulfadiazine. Ann Intern Med. 1992;116:33.

203. Lakhanpal V, Schocket SS, Nirankari VS. Clindamycin in the treatment of toxoplasmic retinochoroiditis. Am J Ophthalmol. 1983;95:605-613.

204. Ferguson JG Jr. Clindamycin therapy for toxoplasmosis. Ann Ophthalmol. 1981;13:95-100.

205. Anonymous. Clindamycin and quinine treatment for *Babesia microti* infections. MMWR Morb Mortal Wkly Rep. 1983;32:65-66.

206. Vergani P, Ghidini A, Ceruti P, et al. Congenital toxoplasmosis: Efficacy of maternal treatment with spiramycin alone. Am J Reprod Immunol. 1998;39:335-340.

207. Mombro M, Perathoner C, Leone A, et al. Congenital toxoplasmosis: 10-Year follow-up. Eur J Pediatr. 1995;154:645-649.

208. Stramba-Badiale M, Nador F, Porta N, et al. QT interval prolongation and risk of life-threatening arrhythmias during toxoplasmosis prophylaxis with spiramycin in neonates. Am Heart J. 1997;133:108-111.

209. Krause PJ, Lepore T, Sikand VK, et al. Atovaquone and azithromycin for the treatment of babesiosis. N Engl J Med. 2000;343:1454-1458.

210. Nasta P, Chiodera S. Azithromycin for relapsing cerebral toxoplasmosis in AIDS. AIDS. 1997;11:1188.

211. Jacobson JM, Hafner R, Remington J, et al. ACTG 156 Study Team. Dose-escalation, phase I/II study of azithromycin and pyrimethamine for the treatment of toxoplasmic encephalitis in AIDS. AIDS. 2001;15:583-589.

212. Anderson SL, Berman J, Kuschner R, et al. Prophylaxis of *Plasmodium falciparum* malaria with azithromycin administered to volunteers. Ann Intern Med. 1995; 123:771-773.

213. Andersen SL, Oloo AJ, Goron DM, et al. Successful double-blinded, randomized, placebo-controlled field trial of azithromycin and doxycycline as prophylaxis for malaria in western Kenya. Clin Infect Dis. 1998;26:146-150.

214. Deresinski SC. Treatment of *Pneumocystis carinii* pneumonia in adults with AIDS. Semin Respir Dis. 1997;12:79-97.

215. Bozzette SA, Finkelstein DM, Spector SA, et al. A randomized trial of three antipneumocystis agents in patients with advanced human immunodeficiency virus infection: NIAID AIDS Clinical Trials Group. N Engl J Med. 1995;332:693-699.

216. Ros JJ, Langen MC, Stallen PC, et al. Pentamidine aerosols and environmental contamination: Health-care worker risk. Pharm World Sci. 1996;18:148-152.

217. Doua F, Miezan TW, Sanon Singaro JR, et al. The efficacy of pentamidine in the treatment of early-late stage *Trypanosoma brucei gambiense* trypanosomiasis. Am J Trop Med Hyg. 1996;55:586-588.

218. Pepin J, Khonde N. Relapses following treatment of early-stage *Trypanosoma brucei gambiense* sleeping sickness with a combination of pentamidine and suramin. Trans R Soc Trop Med Hyg. 1996;90:183-186.

219. Jha TK. Evaluation of diamidine compound (pentamidine isethionate) in the treatment of resistant cases of kala-azar occurring in North Bihar, India. Trans R Soc Trop Med Hyg. 1983;77:167-170.

220. Kager PA, Rees PH, Manguyu FM, et al. Clinical, haematological and parasitological response to treatment of visceral leishmaniasis. Trop Geogr Med. 1984;36:21-35.

221. Lustig V, Karger PA, Meenhorst PL. Treatment of visceral leishmaniasis in a patient with AIDS with antimony and gamma-interferon: Remission and prevention of relapse by maintenance therapy with weekly pentamidine. Neth J Med. 1995;47:66-69.

222. Perez-Molina JA, Lopez-Velez R, Montilla P, et al. Pentamidine isethionate as secondary prophylaxis against visceral leishmaniasis in HIV-positive patients. AIDS. 1996;10:237-238.

223. Navin TR, Fontaine RE. Intravenous versus intramuscular administration of pentamidine (Letter). N Engl J Med. 1984;311:1701-1702.

224. Pearson RD, Hewlett EL. Pentamidine for the treatment of *Pneumocystis carinii* pneumonia and other protozoal diseases. Ann Intern Med. 1985;103:782-786.

225. Basselin M, Robert-Gero M. Alterations in membrane fluidity, lipid metabolism, mitochondrial activity and lipophosphoglycan expression in pentamidine-resistant *Leishmania.* Parasitol Res. 1998;84:78-83.

226. Basselin M, Badet-Denisot MA, Lawrence F, et al. Effects of pentamidine on polyamine level and biosynthesis in wild-type, pentamidine-treated, and pentamidine-resistant *Leishmania.* Exp Parasitol. 1997;85:274-282.

227. Western KA, Perera DR, Schultz MG. Pentamidine isethionate in the treatment of *Pneumocystis carinii* pneumonia. Ann Intern Med. 1970;73:695-702.

228. Assan R, Perronne C, Assan D, et al. Pentamidine-induced derangements of glucose homeostasis. Determinant roles of renal failure and drug accumulation. A study of 128 patients. Diabetes Care. 1995;18:47-55.

229. Bouchard P, Sai P, Reach G, et al. Diabetes mellitus following pentamidine-induced hypoglycemia in humans. Diabetes. 1982;31:40-45.

230. Girgis I, Gualberti J, Langan L, et al. A prospective study of the effect of I.V. pentamidine therapy on ventricular arrhythmias and QTc prolongation in HIV-infected patients. Chest. 1997;112:646-653.

231. O'Brien JG, Dong BJ, Coleman RL, et al. A 5-year retrospective review of adverse drug interactions and their risk factors in human immunodeficiency virus-infected patients who were receiving intravenous pentamidine therapy for *Pneumocystis carinii* pneumonia. Clin Infect Dis. 1997;24:854-859.

232. Obaji J, Lee-Pack LR, Gutierrez C, Chan CK. The pulmonary effects of long-term exposure to aerosol pentamidine: A 5-year surveillance study in HIV-infected patients. Chest. 2003;123:1983-1987.

233. Marras TK, Sanders K, Lipton JH, et al. Aerosolized pentamidine prophylaxis for *Pneumocystis carinii* pneumonia after allogeneic marrow transplantation. Transplant Infect Dis. 2002;4:66-74.

234. Docampo R, Moreno SN. Current chemotherapy of human African trypanosomiasis. Parasitol Res. 2003;90(Suppl 1):S10-13.

235. Nok AJ. Arsenicals (melarsoprol), pentamidine and suramin in the treatment of human African trypanosomiasis. Parasitol Res. 2003;90:71-79.
236. Fairlamb AH, Bowman IB. *Trypanosoma brucei:* Suramin and other trypanocidal compounds' effects on *sn*-glycerol-3 phosphate oxidase. Exp Parasitol. 1977;43:353-361.
237. Anderson J, Fuglsang H, de C Marshall TF. Effects of suramin on ocular onchocerciasis. Tropenmed Parasitol. 1976;27:279-296.
238. Legros D, Ollivier G, Gastellu-Etchegorry M, et al. Treatment of human African trypanosomiasis: Present situation and needs for research and development. Lancet Infect Dis. 2002;2:437-440.
239. Carter NS, Fairlamb AH. Arsenical-resistant trypanosomes lack an unusual adenosine transporter. Nature. 1993;361:173-176.
240. Arrox JO. Melarsoprol and reactive encephalopathy in *Trypanosoma brucei rhodesiense.* Trans R Soc Trop Med Hyg. 1987;81:192.
241. Pepin J, Milord F, Khonde AN, et al. Risk factors for encephalopathy and mortality during melarsoprol treatment of *Trypanosoma brucei gambiense* sleeping sickness. Trans R Soc Trop Med Hyg. 1995;89:92-97.
242. Pepin J, Milord F. African trypanosomiasis and drug-induced encephalopathy: Risk factors and pathogenesis. Trans R Soc Trop Med Hyg. 1991;85:222-224.
243. Burri C, Nkunku S, Merolle A, et al. Efficacy of new, concise schedule for melarsoprol in treatment of sleeping sickness caused by *Trypanosoma brucei gambiense:* A randomised trial. Lancet. 2000;355:1419-1425.
244. Gherardi RK, Chariot P, Vanderstigel M, et al. Organic arsenic-induced Guillain-Barré-like syndrome due to melarsoprol: A clinical, electrophysiological, and pathological study. Muscle Nerve. 1990;13:637-645.
245. Burri C, Brun R. Eflornithine for the treatment of human African trypanosomiasis. Parasitol Res. 2003;90(Suppl 1):S49-52.
246. Milord F, Pepin J, Loko L, et al. Efficacy and toxicity of eflornithine for treatment of *Trypanosoma brucei gambiense* sleeping sickness. Lancet. 1992;340:652-655.
247. Politi C, Carrin G, Evans D, et al. Cost-effectiveness analysis of alternative treatments of African gambiense trypanosomiasis in Uganda. Health Econ. 1995;4:273-287.
248. Bacchi CJ, Nathan HC, Livingston T, et al. Differential susceptibility to DL-α-difluoromethylornithine in clinical isolates of *Trypanosoma brucei rhodesiense.* Antimicrob Agents Chemother. 1990;34:1183-1188.
249. Malhotra B, Noveck R, Behr D, Palmisano M. Percutaneous absorption and pharmacokinetics of eflornithine HCl 13.9% cream in women with unwanted facial hair. J Clin Pharmacol. 2001;41:972-978.
250. Cerecetto H, Gonzalez M. Chemotherapy of Chagas' disease: Status and new developments. Curr Top Med Chem. 2002;2332:1187-1213.
251. Pepin J, Milord F, Meurice F, et al. High-dose nifurtimox for arseno-resistant *Trypanosoma brucei gambiense* sleeping sickness: An open trial in central Zaire. Trans R Soc Trop Med Hyg. 1992;86:254-256.
252. Paulos C, Paredes J, Vasquez I, et al. Pharmacokinetics of a nitrofuran compound, nifurtimox, in healthy volunteers. Int J Clin Pharmacol Ther Toxicol. 1989;27:454-457.
253. Docampo R, Morena SN. Free radical metabolites in the mode of action of chemotherapeutic agents and phagocytic cells on *Trypanosoma cruzi.* Rev Infect Dis. 1984;6:223-238.
254. Moreno SN, Palmero DJ, Eiguchi de Palmero K, et al. Stimulation of lipid peroxidation and ultrastructural alterations by nifurtimox in mammalian tissues. Medicina (B Aires). 1980;40:553-559.
255. de Andrade AL, Zicker F, de Oliveira RM, et al. Randomised trial of efficacy of benznidazole in treatment of early *Trypanosoma cruzi* infection. Lancet. 1996;348:1407-1413.
256. Coura JR, de Abreu LL, Willcox HP, et al. Comparative controlled study on the use of benznidazole, nifurtimox and placebo, in the chronic form of Chagas' disease, in a field area with interrupted transmission: I. Preliminary evaluation. Rev Soc Bras Med Trop. 1997;30:139-144.
257. Pearson RD, Navin TR, Sousa AQ, et al. Leishmaniasis. In: Kass EH, Platt R, eds. Current Therapy in Infectious Diseases. Toronto: Decker; 1990:384-389.
258. Grogl M, Thomason TN, Franke ED. Drug resistance in leishmaniasis: Its implications in systemic chemotherapy of cutaneous and mucocutaneous disease. Am J Trop Med Hyg. 1992;47:117-126.
259. Chulay JD, Fleckenstein L, Smith DH. Pharmacokinetics of antimony during treatment of visceral leishmaniasis with sodium stibogluconate or meglumine antimonate. Trans R Soc Trop Med Hyg. 1988;82:69-72.
260. Berman JD. Human leishmaniasis: Clinical, diagnostic, and chemotherapeutic developments in the last 10 years. Clin Infect Dis. 1997;24:684-703.
261. Herwaldt BL, Berman JD. Recommendations for treating leishmaniasis with sodium stibogluconate (Pentostam) and review of pertinent clinical studies. Am J Trop Med Hyg. 1992;46:296-306.
262. Donovan KL, White AD, Cooke DA, et al. Pancreatitis and palindromic arthropathy with effusions associated with sodium stibogluconate treatment in a renal transplant recipient. J Infect. 1990;21:107-110.
263. Mishra M, Biswas UK, Jha DN, et al. Amphotericin versus pentamidine in antimony-unresponsive kala-azar. Lancet. 1992;340:1256-1257.
264. Thakur CP, Sinha GP, Pandey AK, et al. Daily versus alternate-day regimen of amphotericin B in the treatment of kala-azar: A randomized comparison. Bull World Health Organ. 1994;72:931-936.
265. Berman JD. U.S. Food and Drug Administration approval of AmBisome (liposomal amphotericin B) for treatment of visceral leishmaniasis. Clin Infect Dis. 1999;28:49-51.
266. Meyerhoff A. U.S. Food and Drug Administration approval of AmBisome (liposomal amphotericin B) for treatment of visceral leishmaniasis. Clin Infect Dis. 1999;28:42-48; discussion 49-51.
267. Minodier P, Retornaz K, Horelt A, Garnier JM. Liposomal amphotericin B in the treatment of visceral leishmaniasis in immunocompetent patients. Fundam Clin Pharmacol. 2003;17:183-188.
268. Sundar S, Agrawal, NK, Sinha PR, et al. Short-course, low-dose amphotericin B lipid complex therapy for visceral leishmaniasis unresponsive to antimony. Ann Intern Med. 1997;127:133-137.
269. Berman JD, Ksionski G, Chapman WL, et al. Activity of amphotericin B cholesterol dispersion (Amphocil) in experimental visceral leishmaniasis. Antimicrob Agents Chemother. 1992;36:1978-1980.
270. Saenz RE, Paz H, Berman JD. Efficacy of ketoconazole against *Leishmania braziliensis panamensis* cutaneous leishmaniasis. Am J Med. 1990;89:147-155.
271. Navin TR, Arana BA, Arana FE, et al. Placebo-controlled clinical trial of sodium stibogluconate (Pentostam) versus ketoconazole for treating cutaneous leishmaniasis in Guatemala. J Infect Dis. 1992;165:528-534.
272. Wali JP, Aggarwal P, Gupta U, et al. Ketoconazole in the treatment of antimony- and pentamidine-resistant kala-azar. J Infect Dis. 1992;166:215-216.
273. Wali JP, Aggarwal P, Gupta U, et al. Ketoconazole in treatment of visceral leishmaniasis. Lancet. 1990;336:810-811.
274. Sundar S, Kumar K, Singh VP. Ketoconazole in visceral leishmaniasis. Lancet. 1990;336:1582-1583.
275. Pialoux G, Hennequin C, Dupont B, et al. Cutaneous leishmaniasis in an AIDS patient: Cure with itraconazole. J Infect Dis. 1990;162:1221-1222.
276. Dogra J, Aneja N, Behari Lal B, et al. Cutaneous leishmaniasis in India: Clinical experience with itraconazole (R51 211 Janssen). Int J Dermatol. 1990;29:661-662.
277. Albanese G, Giorgetti P, Santagostino L, et al. Cutaneous leishmaniasis: Treatment with itraconazole. Arch Dermatol. 1989;125:1540-1542.
278. Akuffo H, Dietz M, Teklemariam S, et al. The use of itraconazole in the treatment of leishmaniasis caused by *Leishmania aethiopica.* Trans R Soc Trop Med Hyg. 1990;84:532-534.
279. Al-Fouzan AS, Al Saleh QA, Najeem NM, et al. Cutaneous leishmaniasis in Kuwait: Clinical experience with itraconazole. Int J Dermatol. 1991;30:519-521.
280. Guderian RH, Chico ME, Rogers MD, et al. Placebo controlled treatment of Ecuadorian cutaneous leishmaniasis. Am J Trop Med Hyg. 1991;45:92-97.
281. Fischer C, Voss A, Engel J. Development status of miltefosine as first oral drug in visceral and cutaneous leishmaniasis. Med Microbiol Immunol. 2001;190:85-87.
282. Sundar S, Jha TK, Thakur CP, et al. Oral miltefosine for Indian visceral leishmaniasis. N Engl J Med. 2002;347:1739-1746.
283. Jha TK, Sundar S, Thakur CP, et al. Miltefosine, an oral agent, for the treatment of Indian visceral leishmaniasis. N Engl J Med. 1999;341:1795-1800.
284. Sundar S, Rosenkaimer F, Makharia MK, et al. Trial of oral miltefosine for visceral leishmaniasis. Lancet. 1998;352:1821-1823.
285. Sundar S, Gupta LB, Makharia MK, et al. Oral treatment of visceral leishmaniasis with miltefosine. Ann Trop Med Parasitol. 1999;93:589-597.
286. Sundar S, Makharia A, More DK, et al. Short-course oral miltefosine for treatment of visceral leishmaniasis. Clin Infect Dis. 2000;31:1110-1113.
287. Soto J, Toledo J, Gutierrez P, et al. Treatment of American cutaneous leishmaniasis with miltefosine, an oral agent. Clin Infect Dis. 2001;33:E57-61.
288. Croft SL, Neal RL, Pendergast W, Chan JH. The activity of alkyl phosphorylcholines and related derivatives against *Leishmania donovani.* Biochem Pharmacol. 1987;36:2633-2636.
289. Pearson RD. The development of miltefosine for the treatment of visceral and cutaneous leishmaniasis. Curr Infect Dis Rep. 2003;5 41-42.
290. Bassily S, El-Masry NA, Trabolsi B, et al. Treatment of ancylostomiasis and ascariasis with albendazole. Ann Trop Med Parasitol. 1984;78:81-82.
291. Jagota SC. Albendazole, a broad-spectrum anthelmintic, in the treatment of intestinal nematode and cestode infections: A multicenter study in 480 patients. Clin Ther. 1986;8:226-231.
292. Raccurt CP, Lambert MT, Bouloumie J, et al. Evaluation of the treatment of intestinal helminthiases with albendazole in Djohong (North Cameroon). Trop Med Parasitol. 1990;41:46-48.
293. Stephenson LS, Latham MC, Adams EJ, et al. Weight gain of Kenyan school children infected with hookworm, *Trichuris trichiura* and *Ascaris lumbricoides* is improved following once- or twice-yearly treatment with albendazole. J Nutr. 1993;123:656-665.
294. Stephenson LS, Latham MC, Kinoti SN, et al. Improvements in physical fitness of Kenyan schoolboys infected with hookworm, *Trichuris trichiura* and *Ascaris lumbricoides* following a single dose of albendazole. Trans R Soc Trop Med Hyg. 1990;84:277-282.
295. Albonico M, Smith PG, Ercole E, et al. Rate of reinfection with intestinal nematodes after treatment of children with mebendazole or albendazole in a highly endemic area. Trans R Soc Trop Med Hyg. 1995;89:538-541.
296. Albanese G, Venturi C, Galbiati G. Treatment of larva migrans cutanea (creeping eruption): A comparison between albendazole and traditional therapy. Int J Dermatol. 2001;40:67-71.
297. Davies HD, Sakuls P, Keystone JS. Creeping eruption. A review of clinical presentation and management of 60 cases presenting to a tropical disease unit. Arch Dermatol. 1993;129:588-591.
298. Rizzitelli G, Scarabelli G, Veraldi S. Albendazole: A new therapeutic regimen in cutaneous larva migrans. Int J Dermatol. 1997;36:700-703.
299. Sturchler D, Schubarth P, Gualzata M, et al. Thiabendazole vs. albendazole in treatment of toxocariasis: A clinical trial. Ann Trop Med Parasitol. 1989;83:473-478.
300. Kraivichian P, Kulkumthorn M, Yingyourd P, et al. Albendazole for the treatment of human gnathostomiasis. Trans R Soc Trop Med Hyg. 1992;86:418-421.
301. Chichino G, Bernuzzi AM, Bruno A, et al. Intestinal capillariasis *(Capillaria philippinensis)* acquired in Indonesia: A case report. Am J Trop Med Hyg. 1992;47:10-12.
302. Krepel HP, Haring T, Baeta S, et al. Treatment of mixed *Oesophagostomum* and hook worm infection: Effect of albendazole, pyrantel pamoate, levamisole and thiabendazole. Trans R Soc Trop Med Hyg. 1993;87:87-89.
303. Cabie A, Bouchaud O, Houze S, et al. Albendazole versus thiabendazole as therapy for trichinosis: A retrospective study. Clin Infect Dis. 1996;22:1033-1035.
304. Lipani F, Caramello P, Biglino A, Sacchi C. Albendazole for the treatment of *Mansonella perstans* filariasis. Trans R Soc Trop Med Hyg. 1997;91:221.

305. Liu YH, Wang XG, Gao P, et al. Experimental and clinical trial of albendazole in the treatment of *Clonorchiasis sinensis*. Chin Med J (Engl). 1991;104:27-31.

306. Chanthavanich P, Nontasut P, Prarinyanuparp V, et al. Repeated doses of albendazole against strongyloidiasis in Thai children. Southeast Asian J Trop Med Public Health. 1989;20:221-226.

307. Marti H, Haji HJ, Savioli L, et al. A comparative trial of a single-dose ivermectin versus three days of albendazole for treatment of *Strongyloides stercoralis* and other soil-transmitted helminth infections in children. Am J Trop Med Hyg. 1996;55:477-481.

308. Addiss DG, Beach MJ, Streit TG, et al. Randomised placebo-controlled comparison of ivermectin and albendazole alone and in combination for *Wuchereria bancrofti* microfilaraemia in Haitian children. Lancet. 1997;350:480-484.

309. Maher D, Ottesen EA. The Global Lymphatic Filariasis Initiative. Trop Doct. 2000;30:178-179.

310. Hall A, Nahar Q. Albendazole as a treatment for infections with *Giardia duodenalis* in children in Bangladesh. Trans R Soc Trop Med Hyg. 1993;87:84-86.

311. Misra PK, Kumar A, Agarwal V, et al. A comparative clinical trial of albendazole versus metronidazole in children with giardiasis. Indian Pediatr. 1995;32:779-782.

312. Blanshard C, Ellis DS, Tovey DG, et al. Treatment of intestinal microsporidiosis with albendazole in patients with AIDS. AIDS. 1992;6:311-313.

313. Molina JM, Chastang C, Goguel J, et al. Albendazole for treatment and prophylaxis of microsporidiosis due to *Encephalitozoon intestinalis* in patients with AIDS: A randomized double blind controlled trial. J Infect Dis. 1998;177:1373-1377.

314. Molina JM, Oksenhendler E, Beauvais B, et al. Disseminated microsporidiosis due to *Septata intestinalis* in patients with AIDS: Clinical features and response to albendazole therapy. J Infect Dis. 1995;171:245-249.

315. Dore GJ, Marriott DJ, Hing MC, et al. Disseminated microsporidiosis due to *Septata intestinalis* in nine patients infected with the human immunodeficiency virus: Response to therapy with albendazole. Clin Infect Dis. 1995;21:70-76.

316. Kelly P, Lungu F, Keane E, et al. Albendazole chemotherapy for treatment of diarrhoea in patients with AIDS in Zambia: A randomized double blind controlled trial. BMJ. 1996;312:1187-1191.

317. Horton RJ. Albendazole in treatment of human cystic echinococcosis: 12 years of experience. Acta Trop. 1997;64:79-93.

318. Eskazole: Clinical and technical review. SmithKline Beecham Pharmaceuticals. 1990:A1-B28.

319. Wilson JF, Rausch RL, McMahon BJ, et al. Parasiticidal effect of chemotherapy in alveolar hydatid disease: Review of experience with mebendazole and albendazole in Alaskan Eskimos. Clin Infect Dis. 1992;15:234-249.

320. Keshmiri M, Baharvahdat H, Fattahi SH, et al. Albendazole versus placebo in treatment of echinococcosis. Trans R Soc Trop Med Hyg. 2001;95:190-194.

321. Morris DL. Pre-operative albendazole therapy for hydatid cyst. Br J Surg. 1987; 74:805-806.

322. Aktan AO, Yalin R. Preoperative albendazole treatment for liver hydatid disease decreases the viability of the cyst. Eur J Gastroenterol Hepatol. 1996;8:877-879.

323. Sotelo J, del Brutto OH, Penagos P, et al. Comparison of therapeutic regimen of anticysticercal drugs for parenchymal brain cysticercosis. J Neurol. 1990;237:69-72.

324. Escobedo F, Penagos P, Rodriguez J, et al. Albendazole therapy for neurocysticercosis. Arch Intern Med. 1987;147:738-741.

325. Meneghelli UG, Martinelli AL, Bellucci AD, et al. Polycystic hydatid disease *(Echinococcus vogeli)*. Treatment with albendazole. Ann Trop Med Parasitol. 1992;86:151-156.

326. Takayanagui OM, Jardim E. Therapy for neurocysticercosis. Comparison between albendazole and praziquantel. Arch Neurol. 1992;49:290-294.

327. Sanchez M, Suastegui R, Gonzalez-Esquivel D, et al. Pharmacokinetic comparison of two albendazole dosage regimens in patients with neurocysticercosis. Clin Neuropharmacol. 1993;16:77-82.

328. Cruz M, Cruz I, Horton J. Clinical evaluation of albendazole and praziquantel in the treatment of cerebral cysticercosis. Southeast Asian J Trop Med Public Health. 1991;22(Suppl):279-283.

329. Cruz M, Cruz I, Horton J. Albendazole versus praziquantel in the treatment of cerebral cysticercosis: Clinical evaluation. Trans R Soc Trop Med Hyg. 1991;85:244-247.

330. Cruz I, Cruz ME, Carrasco F, et al. Neurocysticercosis: Optimal dose treatment with albendazole. J Neurol Sci. 1995;133:152-154.

331. del Brutto OH, Sotelo J, Aguirre R, et al. Albendazole therapy for giant subarachnoid cysticerci. Arch Neurol. 1992;49:535-538.

332. del Brutto OH, Sotelo J. Albendazole therapy for subarachnoid and ventricular cysticercosis: Case report. J Neurosurg. 1990;72:816-817.

333. del Brutto OH. Albendazole therapy for subarachnoid cysticerci: Clinical and neuroimaging analysis of 17 patients. J Neurol Neurosurg Psychiatry. 1997;62:659-661.

334. Proano JV, Madrazo I, Garcia L, et al. Albendazole and praziquantel treatment in neurocysticercosis of the fourth ventricle. J Neurosurg. 1997;87:29-33.

335. Chung WC, Fan PC, Lin CY, et al. Poor efficacy of albendazole for the treatment of human taeniasis. Int J Parasitol. 1991;21:269-270.

336. de Kaminsky RG. Albendazole treatment for human taeniasis. Trans R Soc Trop Med Hyg. 1991;85:648-650.

337. Lawrenz A, Eglit S, Kroker R. The metabolism of albendazole in the isolated perfused intestine of rats. DTW Dtsch Tierarztl Wochenschr. 1992;99:416-418.

338. Jung H, Hurtado M, Sanchez M, et al. Clinical pharmacokinetics of albendazole in patients with brain cysticercosis. J Clin Pharmacol. 1992;32:28-31.

339. Jung H, Hurtado M, Sanchez M, et al. Plasma and CSF levels of albendazole and praziquantel in patients with neurocysticercosis. Clin Neuropharmacol. 1990;13:559-564.

340. Jung H, Hurtado M, Medina MT, et al. Dexamethasone increases plasma levels of albendazole. J Neurol. 1990;237:279-280.

341. Ireland CM, Gull K, Gutteridge WE, et al. The interaction of benzimidazole carbamates with mammalian microtubule protein. Biochem Pharmacol. 1979;28: 2680-2682.

342. Barrowman MM, Marriner SE, Bogan JA. The fumarate reductase system as a site of anthelmintic attack in *Ascaris suum*. Biosci Rep. 1984;4:879-883.

343. Dewerdt S, Machet L, Jan-Lamy V, et al. Stevens-Johnson syndrome after albendazole. Acta Derma Venereol. 1997;77:411.

344. Shah V, Marino C, Altice FL. Albendazole-induced pseudomembranous colitis. Am J Gastroenterol. 1996;91:1453-1454.

345. Morris DL, Smith PG. Albendazole in hydatid disease: Hepatocellular toxicity. Trans R Soc Trop Med Hyg. 1987;81:343-344.

346. Pilar Garcia-Muret M, Sitjas D, Tuneu L, et al. Telogen effluvium associated with albendazole therapy. Int J Dermatol. 1990;29:669-670.

347. Keystone JS, Murdoch JK. Mebendazole. Ann Intern Med. 1979;91:582-586.

348. Tankhiwale SR, Kudade AL, Sarmah HC, et al. Single dose therapy of ascariasis: A randomized comparison of mebendazole and pyrantel. J Commun Dis. 1989;21:71-74.

349. Nontasut P, Singhasivanon V, Prarinyanuparp V, et al. Effect of single-dose albendazole and single-dose mebendazole on *Necator americanus*. Southeast Asian J Trop Med Public Health. 1989;20:237-242.

350. Abadi K. Single dose mebendazole therapy for soil-transmitted nematodes. Am J Trop Med Hyg. 1985;34:129-133.

351. Pelletier LL Jr, Baker CB. Treatment failures following mebendazole therapy for chronic strongyloidiasis. J Infect Dis. 1987;156:532-533.

352. Wilson KH, Kauffman CA. Persistent *Strongyloides stercoralis* in a blind loop of the bowel: Successful treatment with mebendazole. Arch Intern Med. 1983;143:357-358.

353. Levin ML. Treatment of trichinosis with mebendazole. Am J Trop Med Hyg. 1983;32:980-983.

354. Schellenberg RS, Tan BJ, Irvine JD, et al. An outbreak of trichinellosis due to consumption of bear meat infected with *Trichinella nativa,* in 2 northern Saskatchewan communities. J Infect Dis. 2003;188:835-843.

355. Van Hoegaerden M, Ivanoff B, Flocard F, et al. The use of mebendazole in the treatment of filariasis due to *Loa loa* and *Mansonella perstans*. Ann Trop Med Parasitol. 1987;81:275-282.

356. Van Hoegaerden M, Flocard F. Mebendazole treatment of loiasis (Letter). Lancet. 1985;1:1278.

357. Cruz AC. Treatment of human taeniasis in the Philippines: A review. Southeast Asian J Trop Med Public Health. 1991;22(Suppl):271-274.

358. Gill JH, Lacey E. The kinetics of mebendazole binding to *Haemonchus contortus* tubulin. Int J Parasitol. 1992;22:939-946.

359. Levin MH, Weinstein RA, Axelrod JL, et al. Severe, reversible neutropenia during high-dose mebendazole therapy for echinococcosis. JAMA. 1983;249:2929-2931.

360. Fernández-Bañares F, González-Huix F, Xiol X, et al. Marrow aplasia during high dose mebendazole treatment. Am J Trop Med Hyg. 1986;35:350-351.

361. el Kalla S, Menon NS. Mebendazole poisoning in infancy. Ann Trop Paediatr. 1990;10:313-314.

362. Berk SL, Verghese A, Alvarez S, et al. Clinical and epidemiological features of strongyloidiasis: A prospective study in rural Tennessee. Arch Intern Med. 1987;147:1257-1261.

363. Barnish G, Barker J. An intervention study using thiabendazole suspension against *Strongyloides fuelleborni*-like infections in Papua New Guinea. Trans R Soc Trop Med Hyg. 1987;81:60-63.

364. Blackwell V, Vega-Lopez F. Cutaneous larva migrans: Clinical features and management of 44 cases presenting in the returning traveller. Br J Dermatol. 2001;145:434-437.

365. Schneider D, Gannon R, Sweeney K, et al. Theophylline and antiparasitic drug interactions. A case report and study of the influence of thiabendazole and mebendazole on theophylline pharmacokinetics in adults. Chest. 1990;97:84-87.

366. Austin WC, Courtney W, Danilewicz JC, et al. Pyrantel tartrate, a new anthelmintic effective against infections of domestic animals. Nature. 1966;212:1273-1274.

367. Bumbalo TS, Figazzoto DJ, Wyzalek JV. Treatment of enterobiasis with pyrantel pamoate. Am J Trop Med Hyg. 1969;18:50-52.

368. Tankhiwale SR, Kukade AL, Sarmah HC, et al. Single dose therapy of ascariasis: A randomized comparison of mebendazole and pyrantel. J Commun Dis. 1989;21:71-74.

369. Aubry ML, Cowell P, Davey MJ, et al. Aspects of the pharmacology of a new anthelminthic: Pyrantel. Br J Pharmacol. 1970;38:332-344.

370. Eyre P. Some pharmacodynamic effects of the nematocides: Methyridine, tetramisole and pyrantel. J Pharm Pharmacol. 1970;22:26-36.

371. Hadju V, Stephenson LS, Abadi K, et al. Improvements in appetite and growth in helminth-infected schoolboys three and seven weeks after a single dose of pyrantel pamoate. Parasitology. 1996;113:497-504.

372. Ganguly B, Awasthi PK, Singhal KC. Regulation of cholinomimetic action of pyrantel pamoate by calcium channels in *Setaria cervi*. Indian J Physiol Pharmacol. 1996;40:245-248.

373. Rayes D, De Rosa MJ, Spitzmaul G, Bouzat C. The anthelmintic pyrantel acts as a low efficacious agonist and an open-channel blocker of mammalian acetylcholine receptors. Neuropharmacology. 2001;41:238-45.

374. Martin RJ. γ-Aminobutyric acid- and piperazine-activated single-channel currents from *Ascaris suum* body muscle. Br J Pharmacol. 1985;84:445-461.

375. Nickey LN. Possible precipitation of petit mal seizures with piperazine citrate. JAMA. 1966;195:1069-1070.

376. Parsons AC. Piperazine neurotoxicity: "Worm wobble." Br Med J. 1971;4:792.

377. Wright S, Harman RRM. Ethylenediamine and piperazine sensitivity. BMJ. 1983;287:463-464.

378. Ottesen EA, Duke BO, Karam M, et al. Strategies and tools for the control/elimination of lymphatic filariasis. Bull World Health Organ. 1997;75:491-503.

379. Bockarie MJ, Alexander ND, Hyun P, et al. Randomized community-based trial of annual single-dose diethylcarbamazine with or without ivermectin against *Wuchereria bancrofti* infection in human beings and mosquitoes. Lancet. 1998;351:162-168.

380. Meyrowitsch DW, Simonsen PE, Makunde WH. Mass diethylcarbamazine chemotherapy for control of bancroftian filariasis through community participation: Comparative efficacy of a low monthly dose and medicated salt. Trans R Soc Trop Med Hyg. 1996;90:74-79.

381. Reddy GS, Venkateswaralu N. Mass administration of DEC-medicated salt for filariasis control in the endemic population of Karaikal, south India: Implementation and impact assessment. Bull World Health Organ. 1996;74:85-90.

382. Hakim SL, Vythilingam I, Marzukhi MI, et al. Single-dose diethylcarbamazine in the control of periodic brugian filariasis in peninsular Malaysia. Trans R Soc Trop Med Hyg. 1995;89:686-689.

383. Partono F. Treatment of elephantiasis in a community with timorian filariasis. Trans R Soc Trop Med Hyg. 1985;79:44-46.

384. Noroes J, Dreyer G, Santos A, et al. Assessment of the efficacy of diethylcarbamazine on adult Wuchereria bancrofti in vivo. Trans R Soc Trop Med Hyg. 1997;91:78-81.

385. Ong RK, Doyle RL. Tropical pulmonary eosinophilia. Chest. 1998;113:1673-1679.

386. Hawking F. Chemotherapy of filariasis. Antimicrob Agents Chemother. 1980;30:135-162.

387. Chadee DD, Tilluckdharry CC, Rawlins SC, et al. Mass chemotherapy with diethylcarbamazine for the control of Bancroftian filariasis: A twelve-year follow-up in northern Trinidad, including observations on Mansonella ozzardi. Am J Trop Med Hyg. 1995;52:174-176.

388. Bartholomew CF, Nathan MD, Tikasingh ES. The failure of diethylcarbamazine in the treatment of Mansonella ozzardi infections. Trans R Soc Trop Med Hyg. 1978;72:423-424.

389. Wiseman RA, Woodruff AW, Pettitt LE. The treatment of toxocaral infection: Some experimental and clinical observations. Trans R Soc Trop Med Hyg. 1971;65:591-598.

390. Megnaval JF. Comparative efficacy of diethylcarbamazine and mebendazole for the treatment of human toxocariasis. Parasitology. 1995;110:529-533.

391. Taylor HR. Recent developments in the treatment of onchocerciasis. Bull World Health Organ. 1984;62:509-515.

392. Lariviere M, Vingtain P, Aziz M, et al. Double-blind study of ivermectin and diethylcarbamazine in African onchocerciasis patients with ocular involvement. Lancet. 1985;2:174-177.

393. Diallo S, Aziz MA, Lariviere M, et al. A double-blind comparison of the efficacy and safety of ivermectin and diethylcarbamazine in a placebo controlled study of Senegalese patients with onchocerciasis. Trans R Soc Trop Med Hyg. 1986;80:927-934.

394. Dadzie KY, Bird AC, Awadzi K, et al. Ocular findings in a double-blind study of ivermectin versus diethylcarbamazine versus placebo in the treatment of onchocerciasis. Br J Ophthalmol. 1987;71:78-85.

395. Greene BM, Taylor HR, Brown EJ, et al. Ocular and systemic complications of diethylcarbamazine therapy for onchocerciasis: Association with circulating immune complexes. J Infect Dis. 1983;147:890-897.

396. Ottesen EA. Description, mechanisms and control of reactions to treatment in the human filariases. Ciba Found Symp. 1987;127:265-283.

397. Rée GH, Hall AP, Hutchinson DB, et al. Plasma levels of diethylcarbamazine in man. Trans R Soc Trop Med Hyg. 1978;71:542-543.

398. Langham ME, Kramer TR. The "in vitro" effect of diethylcarbamazine on the motility and survival of Onchocerca volvulus microfilariae. Tropenmed Parasitol. 1980;31:59-66.

399. Hawking F. Diethylcarbamazine and new compounds for the treatment of filariasis. Adv Pharmacol Chemother. 1979;16:129-194.

400. Van den Bossche H. A new look at the mode of action of some old and new antifilarial compounds. Ann Soc Belg Med Trop. 1981;16:287-296.

401. King CH, Greene BM, Spagnuolo PJ. Diethylcarbamazine citrate, an antifilarial drug, stimulates human granulocyte adherence. Antimicrob Agents Chemother. 1983;24:453-456.

402. Cesbron J-V, Capron A, Vargaftig BB, et al. Platelets mediate the action of diethylcarbamazine on microfilariae. Nature. 1987;325:533-536.

403. Kanesa-thasan N, Douglas JG, Kazura JW. Diethylcarbamazine inhibits endothelial and microfilarial prostanoid metabolism in vitro. Mol Biochem Parasitol. 1991;49:11-20.

404. Fujimaki Y, Ehara M, Kimura E, et al. Diethylcarbamazine, antifilarial drug, inhibits microtubule polymerization and disrupts preformed microtubules. Biochem Pharmacol. 1990;39:851-856.

405. Francis H, Awadzi K, Ottesen EA. The Mazzotti reaction following treatment of onchocerciasis with diethylcarbamazine: Clinical severity as a function of infection intensity. Am J Trop Med Hyg. 1985;34:529-536.

406. Carme B, Boulesteix J, Boutes H, et al. Five cases of encephalitis during treatment of loaiasis with diethylcarbamazine. Am J Trop Med Hyg. 1991;44:684-690.

407. Campbell WC, Fisher MH, Stapley EO, et al. Ivermectin: A potent new antiparasitic agent. Science. 1983;221:823-828.

408. Taylor HR, Pacque M, Munoz B, et al. Impact of mass treatment of onchocerciasis with ivermectin on the transmission of infection. Science. 1990;250:116-118.

409. Dadzie KY, Remme J, De Sole G. Changes in ocular onchocerciasis after two rounds of community-based ivermectin treatment in a holo-endemic onchocerciasis focus. Trans R Soc Trop Med Hyg. 1991;85:267-271.

410. Taylor HR, Semba RD, Newland HS, et al. Ivermectin treatment of patients with severe onchocerciasis. Am J Trop Med Hyg. 1989;40:494-500.

411. Abiose A, Jones BR, Cousens SN, et al. Reduction in the incidence of optic nerve disease with annual ivermectin to control onchocerciasis. Lancet. 1993;341:130-135.

412. Pacque M, Munoz B, Greene BM. Safety of compliance with community-based ivermectin therapy. Lancet. 1990;335:1377-1380.

413. Pacque M, Munoz B, Greene BM, et al. Community-based treatment of onchocerciasis with ivermectin: Safety, efficacy, and acceptability of yearly treatment. J Infect Dis. 1991;163:381-385.

414. Somo R, Ngosso A, Dinga JS, et al. A community-based trial of ivermectin for onchocerciasis control in the forest of southwest Cameroon: Clinical and pathologic findings after three treatments. Am J Trop Med Hyg. 1993;48:9-13.

415. Collins RC, Gonzalez-Peralta C, Castro J, et al. Ivermectin: Reduction in prevalence and infection intensity of Onchocerca volvulus following biannual treatments in five Guatemalan communities. Am J Trop Med Hyg. 1992;47:156-169.

416. Pacque M, Greene BM, Munoz B, et al. Ivermectin therapy: A 5-year follow-up. J Infect Dis. 1991;164:1035-1036.

417. Duke BO, Pacque MC, Munoz B, et al. Viability of adult Onchocerca volvulus after six 2-weekly doses of ivermectin. Bull World Health Organ. 1991;69:163-168.

418. Plaisier AP, Alley ES, Boatin BA, et al. Irreversible effects of ivermectin on adult parasites in onchocerciasis patients in the Onchocerciasis Control Programme in West Africa. J Infect Dis. 1995;172:204-210.

419. Kumaraswami V, Ottesen EA, Vijayasekaran V, et al. Ivermectin for the treatment of Wuchereria bancrofti filariasis: Efficacy and adverse reactions. JAMA. 1988;259:3150-3153.

420. Ottesen EA, Vijayasekaran V, Kumaraswami V, et al. A controlled trial of ivermectin and diethylcarbamazine in lymphatic filariasis. N Engl J Med. 1990;322:1113-1117.

421. Mak JW, Navaratnam V, Grewel JS, et al. Treatment of subperiodic Brugia malayi infection with a single dose of ivermectin. Am J Trop Med Hyg. 1993;48:591-596.

422. Addiss DG, Eberhard ML, Lammie PJ, et al. Comparative efficacy of clearing-dose and single-dose ivermectin and diethylcarbamazine against Wuchereria bancrofti microfilaremia. Am J Trop Med Hyg. 1993;48:178-185.

423. Dreyer G, Addiss D, Noroes J, et al. Ultrasonographic assessment of the adulticidal efficacy of repeat high-dose ivermectin in bancroftian filariasis. Trop Med Int Health. 1996;1:427-432.

424. Kombila M, Duong TH, Ferrer A, et al. Short- and long-term action of multiple doses of ivermectin on loiasis microfilaremia. Am J Trop Med Hyg. 1998;58:258-260.

425. Gardon J, Kamgno J, Folefack G, et al. Marked decrease in Loa loa microfilaremia six and twelve months after a single dose of ivermectin. Trans R Soc Trop Med Hyg. 1997;91:593-594.

426. Fischer P, Bamuhiiga J, Buttner DW. Treatment of human Mansonella streptocerca infection with ivermectin. Trop Med Int Health. 1997;2:191-199.

427. Naquira C, Jimenez G, Guerra JG, et al. Ivermectin for human strongyloidiasis and other intestinal helminths. Am J Trop Med Hyg. 1989;40:304-309.

428. Lyagoubi M, Datry A, Mayorga R, et al. Chronic persistent strongyloidiasis cured by ivermectin. Trans R Soc Trop Med Hyg. 1992;86:541.

429. Marti H, Haji HJ, Savioli L, et al. A comparative trial of a single-dose ivermectin versus three days of albendazole for treatment of Strongyloides stercoralis and other soil-transmitted helminth infections in children. Am J Trop Med Hyg. 1996;55:477-481.

430. Ottesen EA, Campbell WC. Ivermectin in human medicine. J Antimicrob Chemother. 1994;34:195-203.

431. Bouchaud O, Houze S, Schiemann R, et al. Cutaneous larva migrans in travelers: A prospective study, with assessment of therapy with ivermectin. Clin Infect Dis. 2000;31:493-498.

432. Meinking TL, Taplin D, Hermida JL, et al. The treatment of scabies with ivermectin. N Engl J Med. 1995;333:26-30.

433. Taplin D, Meinking TL. Treatment of HIV-infected scabies with emphasis on the efficacy of ivermectin. Semin Cutan Med Surg. 1997;16:235-240.

434. Okonkwo PO, Ogbuokiri JE, Ofoegbu E, et al. Protein binding and ivermectin estimations in patients with onchocerciasis. Clin Pharmacol Ther. 1993;53:426-429.

435. Klotz U, Ogbuokiri JE, Okonkwo PO. Ivermectin binds avidly to plasma proteins. Eur J Clin Pharmacol. 1990;39:607-608.

436. Brownlee DJ, Holden-Dye L, Walker RJ. Actions of the anthelmintic ivermectin on the pharyngeal muscle of the parasite nematode, Ascaris suum. Parasitology. 1997;115:553-561.

437. Chijioke CP, Okonkwo PO. Adverse events following ivermectin therapy for onchocerciasis. Trans R Soc Trop Med Hyg. 1992;86:284-286.

438. Baraka OZ, Khier MM, Ahmed KM, et al. Community based distribution of ivermectin in eastern Sudan: Acceptability and early post-treatment reactions. Trans R Soc Trop Med Hyg. 1995;89:316-318.

439. Boussinesq M, Gardon J, Gardon-Wendel N, et al. Three probable cases of Loa loa encephalopathy following ivermectin treatment for onchocerciasis. Am J Trop Med Hyg. 1998;58:461-469.

440. Gardon J, Gardon-Wendel N, Demanga-Ngangue, et al. Serious reactions after mass treatment of onchocerciasis with ivermectin in an area endemic for Loa loa infection. Lancet. 1997;350:18-22.

441. Pacque M, Munoz B, Poetschke G, et al. Pregnancy outcome after inadvertent ivermectin treatment during community-based distribution. Lancet. 1990;336:1486-1489.

442. Cioli D, Pica-Mattoccia L. Praziquantel. Parasitol Res. 2003;90(Suppl 1):S3-9.

443. King CH, Mahmoud AA. Drugs five years later: Praziquantel. Ann Intern Med. 1989;110:290-296.

444. Pearson RD, Wilson ME. Role of praziquantel in the treatment of helminthic diseases. Int Med Specialist. 1986;7:183-204.

445. Ross AG, Bartley PB, Sleigh AC, et al. Schistosomiasis. N Engl J Med. 2002;346:1212-1220.

446. Frenzel K, Grigull L, Odongo-Aginya E, et al. Evidence for a long-term effect of a single dose of praziquantel on Schistosoma mansoni-induced hepatosplenic lesions in northern Uganda. Am J Trop Med Hyg. 1999;60:927-931.

447. Karanja DM, Boyer AE, Strand M, et al. Studies on schistosomiasis in western Kenya: II. Efficacy of praziquantel for treatment of schistosomiasis in persons coinfected with human immunodeficiency virus-1. Am J Trop Med Hyg. 1998;59:307-311.

448. Wegner DHG. The profile of the trematodicidal compound praziquantel. Arzneimittelforschung. 1984;34:1132-1136.

449. Latham MC, Stephenson LS, Kurz KM, et al. Metrifonate or praziquantel treatment improves physical fitness and appetite of Kenyan schoolboys with *Schistosoma haematobium* and hookworm infections. Am J Trop Med Hyg. 1990;43:170-179.

450. Kimura E, Moji K, Uga S, et al. Effects of *Schistosoma haematobium* infection on mental test scores of Kenyan school children. Trop Med Parasitol. 1992;43:155-158.

451. Watt G, Adapon B, Long GW, et al. Praziquantel in treatment of cerebral schistosomiasis. Lancet. 1986;2:529-532.

452. Richards F Jr, Sullivan J, Ruiz-Tiben E, et al. Effect of praziquantel on the eggs of *Schistosoma mansoni*, with a note on the implications for managing central nervous system schistosomiasis. Ann Trop Med Parasitol. 1989;83:465-472.

453. William S, Botros S, Ismail M, et al. Praziquantel-induced tegumental damage in vitro is diminished in schistosomes derived from praziquantel-resistant infections. Parasitology. 2001;122:63-66.

454. Ismail M, Botros S, Metwally A, et al. Resistance to praziquantel: Direct evidence from *Schistosoma mansoni* isolated from Egyptian villagers. Am J Trop Med Hyg. 1999;60:932-935.

455. Fritsche TR, Eastburn RL, Wiggins LH, et al. Praziquantel for treatment of human *Nanophyetus salmincola (Troglotrema salmincola)* infection. J Infect Dis. 1989; 160:896-899.

456. Farid Z, Trabolsi B, Boctor F, et al. Unsuccessful use of praziquantel to treat acute fascioliasis in children. J Infect Dis. 1986;154:920-921.

457. Farag HF, Ragab M, Salem A, et al. A short note on praziquantel in human fascioliasis. J Trop Med Hyg. 1986;89:79-80.

458. Groll E. Praziquantel for cestode infections in man. Acta Trop (Basel). 1980;37:293-296.

459. Botero D, Castano S. Treatment of cysticercosis with praziquantel in Colombia. Am J Trop Med Hyg. 1982;31:811-821.

460. De Ghetaldi LD, Norman RM, Douville AW Jr. Cerebral cysticercosis treated biphasically with dexamethasone and praziquantel. Ann Intern Med. 1983;99:179-181.

461. Sotelo J, Torres B, Rubio-Donnadieu F, et al. Praziquantel in the treatment of neurocysticercosis: Long-term follow-up. Neurology. 1985;35:752-755.

462. Norman RM, Kapadia C. Cerebral cysticercosis: Treatment with praziquantel. Pediatrics. 1986;78:291-294.

463. Vasconcelos D, Cruz-Segura H, Mateos-Gomez H, et al. Selective indications for the use of praziquantel in the treatment of brain cysticercosis. J Neurol Neurosurg Psychiatry. 1987;50:383-388.

464. Joubert J. Cysticercal meningitis: A pernicious form of neurocysticercosis which responds poorly to praziquantel. S Afr Med J. 1990;77:528-530.

465. Santos R, Chavarria M, Aguirre AE. Failure of medical treatment in two cases of intraocular cysticercosis. Am J Ophthalmol. 1984;97:249-250.

466. Heath DD, Lawrence SB. The effect of mebendazole and praziquantel on the cysts of *Echinococcus granulosus, Taenia hydatigena,* and *T. ovis* in sheep. N Z Vet J. 1978;26:11-15.

467. Marshall I, Edwards GT. The effects of sustained release praziquantel on the survival of protoscolices of *Echinococcus granulosus equinus* in laboratory mice. Ann Trop Med Parasitol. 1982;76:649-651.

468. Irie Y, Utsunomiya H, Tanaka M, et al. *Schistosoma japonicum* and *S. mansoni:* Ultrastructural damage in the tegument and reproductive organs after treatment with levo- and dextropraziquantel. Am J Trop Med Hyg. 1989;41:204-211.

469. Staudt U, Schmahl G, Blaschke G, et al. Light and scanning electron microscopy studies on the effects of the enantiomers of praziquantel and its main metabolite on *Schistosoma mansoni* in vitro. Parasitol Res. 1992;78:392-397.

470. Kaojarern S, Nathakarnkikool A, Suvanakoot U. Comparative bioavailability of praziquantel tablets. DICP. 1989;23:29-32.

471. Mandour ME, el Turabli H, Homeida MM, et al. Pharmacokinetics of praziquantel in healthy volunteers and patients with schistosomiasis. Trans R Soc Trop Med Hyg. 1990;84:389-393.

472. Leopold G, Ungethum W, Groll E, et al. Clinical pharmacology in normal volunteers of praziquantel, a new drug against schistosomes and cestodes: An example of a complex study covering both tolerance and pharmacokinetics. Eur J Clin Pharmacol. 1978;14:281-291.

473. Thomas H, Andrews P, Mehlhorn H. New results on the effect of praziquantel in experimental cysticercosis. Am J Trop Med Hyg. 1982;31:803-810.

474. Vazquez ML, Jung H, Sotelo J. Plasma levels of praziquantel decrease when dexamethasone is given simultaneously. Neurology. 1987;37:1561-1562.

475. Andrews P. Praziquantel: Mechanisms of anti-schistosomal activity. Pharmacol Ther. 1985;29:129-156.

476. Xiao S-H, Friedman PA, Catto BA, et al. Praziquantel-induced vesicle formation in the tegument of male *Schistosoma mansoni* is calcium dependent. J Parasitol. 1984;70:177-179.

477. Gardner DR, Brezden BL. The sites of action of praziquantel in smooth muscle of *Lymnaea stagnalis*. Can J Physiol Pharmacol. 1984;62:282-287.

478. Ruenwongsa P, Hutadilok N, Yuthavong Y. Stimulation of Ca²⁺ uptake in the liver fluke *Opisthorchis viverrini* by praziquantel. Life Sci. 1983;32:2529-2534.

479. Harnett W, Kusel JR. Increased exposure of parasite antigens at the surface of adult *Schistosoma mansoni* exposed to praziquantel in vitro. Parasitology. 1986;93:401-405.

480. Linder E, Thors C. *Schistosoma mansoni*: Praziquantel-induced tegumental lesion exposes actin on surface spines and allows binding of actin depolymerizing factor, gelsolin. Parasitology. 1992;105:71-79.

481. Prichard RK, Bachmann R, Hutchinson GW, et al. The effect of praziquantel on calcium in *Hymenolepis diminuta*. Mol Biochem Parasitol. 1982;5:297-308.

482. Azher M, el-Kassimi FA, Wright SG, et al. Exudative polyserositis and acute respiratory failure following praziquantel therapy. Chest. 1990;98:241-243.

483. Johnson RJ, Jong EC, Dunning SB, et al. Paragonimiasis: Diagnosis and the use of praziquantel in treatment. Rev Infect Dis. 1985;7:200-206.

484. Polderman AM, Gryseels B, Gerold JL, et al. Side effects of praziquantel in the treatment of *Schistosoma mansoni* in Maniema, Zaire. Trans R Soc Trop Med Hyg. 1984;78:752-754.

485. Farid Z, Wallace CK. Schistosomiasis and praziquantel. Ann Intern Med. 1983;99:883.

486. Watt G, Baldovino PC, Castro JT, et al. Bloody diarrhoea after praziquantel therapy. Trans R Soc Trop Med Hyg. 1986;80:345-346.

487. Markwalder K, Hess K, Valavanis A, et al. Cerebral cysticercosis: Treatment with praziquantel. Report of two cases. Am J Trop Med Hyg. 1984;33:273-280.

488. Sotelo J, Escobedo F, Rodriguez-Carbajal J, et al. Therapy of parenchymal brain cysticercosis with praziquantel. N Engl J Med. 1984;310:1001-1007.

489. Olds GR. Administration of praziquantel to pregnant and lactating women. Acta Trop. 2003;86:185-195.

490. Diekmann HW, Schneidereit M, Overbosch D. Inhibitory effects of cimetidine, ketoconazole and miconazole on the metabolism of praziquantel. Acta Leiden. 1989;57:217-228.

491. Ferrari ML, Coelho PM, Antunes CM, et al. Efficacy of oxamniquine and praziquantel in the treatment of *Schistosoma mansoni* infection: A controlled trial. Bull World Health Organ. 2003;81:190-196.

492. Gryseels B, Nkulikyinka L. Two-year follow-up of *Schistosoma mansoni* infection and morbidity after treatment with different regimens of oxamniquine and praziquantel. Trans R Soc Trop Med Hyg. 1989;83:219-228.

493. Katz N, Rocha RS, de Sousa CP, et al. Efficacy of alternating therapy with oxamniquine and praziquantel to treat *Schistosoma mansoni* in children following failure of first treatment. Am J Trop Med Hyg. 1991;44:509-512.

494. Kokwaro GO, Taylor G. Oxamniquine pharmacokinetics in healthy Kenyan African volunteers. East Afr Med J. 1991;68:359-364.

495. Fallon PG, Fookes RE, Wharton GA. Temporal differences in praziquantel and oxamniquine-induced tegumental damage in adult *Schistosoma mansoni*: Implications for drug-antibody synergy. Parasitology. 1996;112:47-58.

496. Kodama K. Human fascioliasis: Comparison of a fasciolicidal effect of bithionol and praziquantel. Kansenshogaku Zasshi (J Japan Assoc Infect Dis). 1997;71:1162-1167.

497. Kim JS. Treatment of *Paragonimus westermani* infections with bithionol. Am J Trop Med Hyg. 1970;19:940-942.

498. Apt W, Aguilera X, Vega F, et al. Treatment of human chronic fascioliasis with triclabendazole: Drug efficacy and serologic response. Am J Trop Med Hyg. 1995;52:532-535.

499. Graham CS, Brodie SB, Weller PF. Imported *Fasciola hepatica* infection in the United States and treatment with triclabendazole. Clin Infect Dis. 2001;33:1-5.

500. Apt W, Aguilera X, Vega F, et al. Treatment of human chronic fascioliasis with triclabendazole: Drug efficacy and serologic response. Am J Trop Med Hyg. 1995;52:532-535.

501. Graham CS, Brodie SB, Weller PF. Imported *Fasciola hepatica* infection in the United States and treatment with triclabendazole. Clin Infect Dis. 2001;33:1-5.

Complementary and Alternative Medicines for Infectious Diseases

JONATHAN D. BERMAN
STEPHEN E. STRAUS

Complementary and alternative medicine (CAM) consists of diverse clinical interventions that are remarkably popular yet share a lack of proof that they are safe and effective. Alternative interventions are those used in place of conventional treatments; complementary interventions are used together with conventional treatments, often without the knowledge of the patients' physicians. Of the many forms of CAM, Kessler and colleagues list approximately 20 that are commonly employed in the United States.[1] These and other CAM therapies can be conveniently grouped into five categories, or domains: biologically based therapies such as botanicals, vitamins, minerals, and amino acids; manipulative and body-based interventions such as chiropractic and massage; mind–body interventions such as meditation and prayer; therapies that involve putative or demonstrable energies such as Qi gong and exposure to magnetic fields; and entirely alternative medical systems of European origin, such as homeopathy, or of Asian origin, such as traditional Chinese medicine, which incorporates elements of the other four major CAM domains.

CAM includes many types of interventions that evolved with indigenous peoples over the millennia. Prayer must have been used to encourage healing and prevent illness since the onset of human existence. Personal effects found in melting Alpine snows alongside the well-preserved "ice man" included medicinal herbs. The body itself bore numerous tattoos, whose locations are curiously reminiscent of acupuncture needling points. Acupuncture and massage have been used for more than 2500 years.

Despite the dramatic advances in health wrought over the past 2 centuries through scientific medicine, people have not abandoned their penchant for many of these traditional and "more natural" healing approaches. In fact, rates of use by Americans have risen in recent decades. In 1997, Americans made an estimated 629 million visits to CAM practitioners and paid some $27 billion out of pocket for alternative therapies. In a 1999 survey of U.S. adults by the Centers for Disease Control and Prevention (CDC), 33% of women and 24% of men used CAM; 31% to 33% of 35- to 54-year-olds used CAM. The most commonly used modalities were prayer (used by 14% of adults), herbal medicine (10%), and chiropractic therapies (8%).[2] Using CAM to treat or prevent some infectious diseases is even more prevalent: according to some surveys, as many as 84% of patients with acquired immunodeficiency disease (AIDS) use CAM.[3]

The appeal of CAM rests in the advantages it aims to offer over conventional medicine. These include products that may be cheaper than drugs, the ability to acquire these products from health food stores and supermarkets without a prescription, and the more nurturing environment of body-based therapies and mind–body interventions. Complementary interventions are particularly attractive when conventional approaches prove limited, because they promise longer survival, improved quality of life, and palliation of side effects.[4] Their disadvantages stem from the route by which CAM modalities have entered clinical practice: a favorable therapeutic index has generally not been demonstrated, and manufacturing of the products may not be standardized. As a result, CAM interventions may not be effective, may be toxic, and may distract the patient from fully pursuing proven treatments.

Although examples of all CAM domains have been used for infectious diseases, the most prevalent approaches involve biologically based interventions. The possible mechanisms by which these and other CAM interventions could ameliorate or prevent infections include direct killing or inhibition of the pathogen, modification of host immune responses, and modification of the host's subjective response to the disease.

To simplify what could become a protracted catalogue of tried interventions, we have focused this review on CAM approaches for which there is substantial evidence, pro or con, related to clinical value, and on the mechanisms by which they may be exerting their effects. Salient data are summarized in Table 42-1.

TABLE 42-1 Efficacy of Selected CAM Agents Used to Treat or Prevent Infectious Diseases

Infection	Patients	Agent	Dose	Primary Endpoint	Efficacy vs Placebo	Reference
Malaria—treat	Severe disease	Artemether	~20 mg/kg IM	Parasite clearance time	72 hr vs 90 hr for quinine	8
					48 hr vs 60 hr for quinine	9
UTI—prevent	Older adult women	Cranberry	300 mL/day × 6 mo	Bacteriuria + pyuria for 6 mo	OR = 0.42 (0.23-0.76, 95% CI)	16
UTI—prevent	Female students	Cranberry	7.5 g/day × 6 mo	Bacteriuria over 6 mo	8/50 vs 18/50 ($P = .023$)	17
UTI—treat/prevent	Children neurogenic bladder	Cranberry	300 mL/day × 3 mo	Bacteriuric cultures	75% of cultures vs 75% of cultures	18
Pneumonia—treat	Children with measles	Vitamin A	200,000 IU twice	Pneumonia duration	6.3 days vs 12.4 days ($P < .001$)	19
Diarrhea—prevent	Children under-nourished	Zinc	5-20 mg/day × 12-54 wk	Diarrhea incidence	OR = 0.82 (0.72-0.93, 95% CI)	34
Diarrhea—treat	Children under-nourished (symptoms ≤ 4 days)	Zinc	20 mg/day	> 7 day diarrhea	RR = 0.61 (0.39-0.93, 95% CI)	36
Cold—treat	U.S. population	Zinc	13 mg 6×/day until cured	Duration of symptoms	4.5 days vs 8.1 days ($P < .01$)	42
Cold—treat	U.S. population (natural colds)	Zinc	11 mg 6×/day until cured	Duration of symptoms	5.5 days vs 5.5 days	44
	U.S. population (rhinovirus challenge)	Zinc	13 mg 6×/day until cured	Duration of symptoms	2.5 days vs 3.5 days ($P = .035$)	
Cold—treat	U.S. population	Zinc	~0.5 mg qid to nose until cured	Duration of symptoms	4.3 days vs 6.0 days ($P = 0.002$)	41
Cold—prevent	German adults	Echinacea	4 mL bid × 8 wk	% Patients with new cold	65% vs 74% (RR = 0.6-1.2)	46
Cold—prevent	U.S. students (rhinovirus challenge)	Echinacea	300 mg tid × 14 days prechallenge	% Patients with cold	50% vs 59% ($P = .8$)	47
				% Patients with infection	44% vs 57% ($P = .3$)	
Cold—treat	U.S. students	Echinacea	~1 g tid until cured	Duration of symptoms	6.3 days vs 5.8 days (−1 to +0.2)	48
Cold—treat	German adults	Echinacea	5 mL bid × 10 days	Duration of symptoms	6.0 days vs 9.0 days ($P = .01$)	49
Cold—prevent	Navajo children	Vitamin C	1 g/day × 4 mo	Episodes	133 vs 129	51
				Duration of symptoms	5.5 days vs 5.8 days	
Cold—prevent	U.S. Marines	Vitamin C	2 g/day × 8 wk	% Recruits with new colds	90% vs 90%	52
				Duration of symptoms	11.2 days vs 11.5 days	
Cold—treat	Australian adults	Vitamin C	3 g/day × 3 days	Duration of symptoms	10.4 days vs 8.5 days	53

Abbreviations: CI, confidence interval; IM, intramuscularly; OR, odds ratio; RR, relative risk.

SPECIFIC CAM APPROACHES

Artemisinins to Treat Malaria

The use of artemisinins to treat malaria (see Chapters 41 and 272) conveys in a most compelling way the promise of CAM and reveals the venerable wisdom inherent in some traditional medical systems.

Ancient Chinese physicians identified an approach to fevers that held the secret to a new class of antimalarial drugs. In AD 340, the (Chinese) Handbook of Prescriptions for Emergency Treatments recommended drinking an aqueous extract of the leaves of *Artemisia annua* for fever.[5] Pursuing this early observation, in 1971-1972, Chinese scientists found that although a hot-water extraction from the leaves failed to efficiently yield antimalarial activity, ether extraction was successful. Crystalline artemisinin is now available from Chinese *Artemisia annua,* and it is the starting material for the semisynthetic artemisinins now being employed worldwide. *Artemisia annua* also grows along the Potomac river in Washington, D.C. (Fig. 42-1), but the yield from Potomac *Artemisia annua* is 0.06%, as little as one tenth the yield from varieties grown in Sichuan province.[5] Artemisinins illustrate the general principle that local growth conditions of identical species may have a marked effect on the quality of botanical extracts.

Artemisinin (Fig. 42-2A), a sesquiterpene lactone peroxide, is poorly soluble in water.[6] Solubility is improved by the addition of a polar succinic acid group to form water-soluble artesunate, or a nonpolar methyl group to form oil-soluble artemether, both of which are essentially prodrugs of dihydroartemisinin (see Fig. 42-2A). The active moiety of all the artemisinins is the endoperoxide ring, which is thought to lead ultimately to alkylation and oxidation of essential proteins and lipids.[6] The endoperoxide group in artemisinins is unique with respect to known antimalarials and was entirely unanticipated by malariologists.

In vitro, artemisinins have direct antimicrobial effects and prevent the further development of both young and later parasite forms, whereas other antimalarials such as quinine prevent only the maturation of later forms.[7] Perhaps for this reason, clinical artemisinins are more rapidly effective than conventional antimalarials. In two trials that studied severe malaria, the times to clear 100% of the *Plasmodium* parasites from the blood were 48 and 72 hours for intramuscular (IM) artemether, but they were 60 and 90 hours, respectively, for patients given IM quinine.[8,9]

In addition to acting rapidly, artemisinins are effective against parasites that are resistant to all other antimalarial agents. The short half-lives of artemisinins have encouraged their co-administration with agents that have longer half-lives, to fully clear the few parasites remaining after artemisinin treatment. Artemether is formulated with lumefantrine ($T_{1/2}$ = approximately 6 days), and artesunate is typically administered with mefloquine ($T_{1/2}$ = approximately 3 weeks). In clinical trials in Thailand, a region with *Plasmodium falciparum* resistant to chloroquine, pyrimethamine-sulfadoxine, mefloquine, and quinine, artemether (80 mg) plus lumefantrine (480 mg) twice a day for 3 days cured 96% of 155 patients with mild-moderate malaria, and artesunate (4 mg/kg/day for 3 days) plus mefloquine (15 mg/kg on day 2 and 10 mg/kg on day 3) cured 100% of 53 patients.[10] Artesunate was compared with quinine for the treatment of severe falciparum malaria and was found to be more effective (mortality, 12% versus 22%), but the differences were not significant in this study of 113 adults.[11]

Cranberry Juice to Prevent Urinary Tract Infection

Approximately 80% of urinary tract infections (UTIs) are caused by *Escherichia coli,* and from 25% to 35% of initial urinary tract infections, including those caused by *E. coli,* recur within 6 months. *E. coli* possesses surface adhesion organelles (fimbriae) that bind to uroepithelial cell receptors. Type 1 fimbriae are expressed by virtually all *E. coli* strains and contain a mannose-specific lectin[12]; most pyelonephritogenic strains of *E. coli* also express P-fimbria, characterized by mannose-resistant adhesion molecules.

Cranberry juice, widely touted for UTI (see Chapter 66), typically contains 3% glucose and 1% fructose. Cranberry juice cocktail has added sugars and typically contains 7% glucose and 5% fructose.[12] Both pure 0.35% fructose and a dilution of cranberry juice that resulted in 0.4% fructose inhibited adherence of type 1 fimbriated *E. coli* to mannose-sensitive receptors. A variety of studies, however, showed that these sugars are not the factor that inhibits adherence of P-fimbria.[12] In vivo evidence that cranberry juice contains specific inhibitors of P-fimbria–mediated adherence was provided by a study that showed that urine from women who had consumed cranberry juice prevented adhesion of 80% of the patients' *E. coli* to P-receptor–coated resins.[13] Proanthocyanidins (see Fig. 42-2B), present at perhaps 0.01% by weight in cranberries,[14] have been identified as a cranberry constituent that inhibits binding to mannose-resistant receptors in vitro at concentrations of 10 to 50 µg/mL.[15]

Cranberry-containing beverages probably prevent the recurrence of urinary tract infections in women, but how well do they do this? Older adult women who consumed 300 mL of cranberry juice cocktail per day for 6 months had, compared with placebo juice recipients, a 58% reduction in likelihood of developing bacteriuria with pyuria.[16] This study was criticized because of possibly meaningful differences in the study groups before treatment. In another study, female students who drank 50 mL of cranberry-lingonberry juice (containing 7.5 g cranberry concentrate and 1.7 g lingonberry concentrate) daily for 6 months had a reduced risk (P = .048) of recurrent bacteriuria (defined as $>10^5$ colony-forming units [CFU]/mL) compared with placebo controls.[17] On the other hand, cranberry juice did not prevent UTIs in a blinded, controlled trial of children with neurogenic bladder. Children received the equivalent of 300 mL of cranberry juice cocktail or placebo for 3 months, then crossed over to the other beverage. There were 120 positive bacteriuric cultures (defined as $>10^4$ CFU/mL in a bladder-catheterized specimen) per 160 cultures (75% positive) when taking cranberry

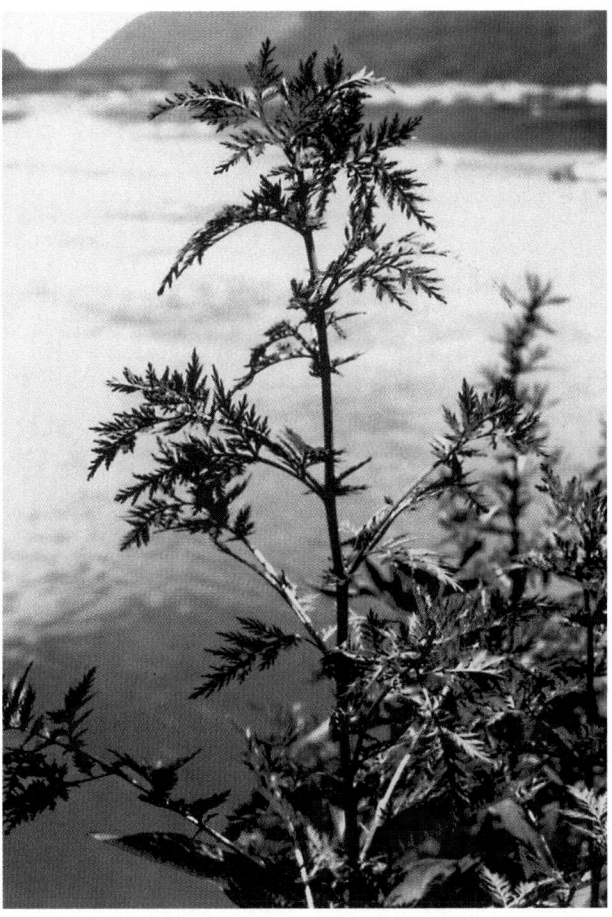

FIGURE 42-1. *Artemisia annua.*

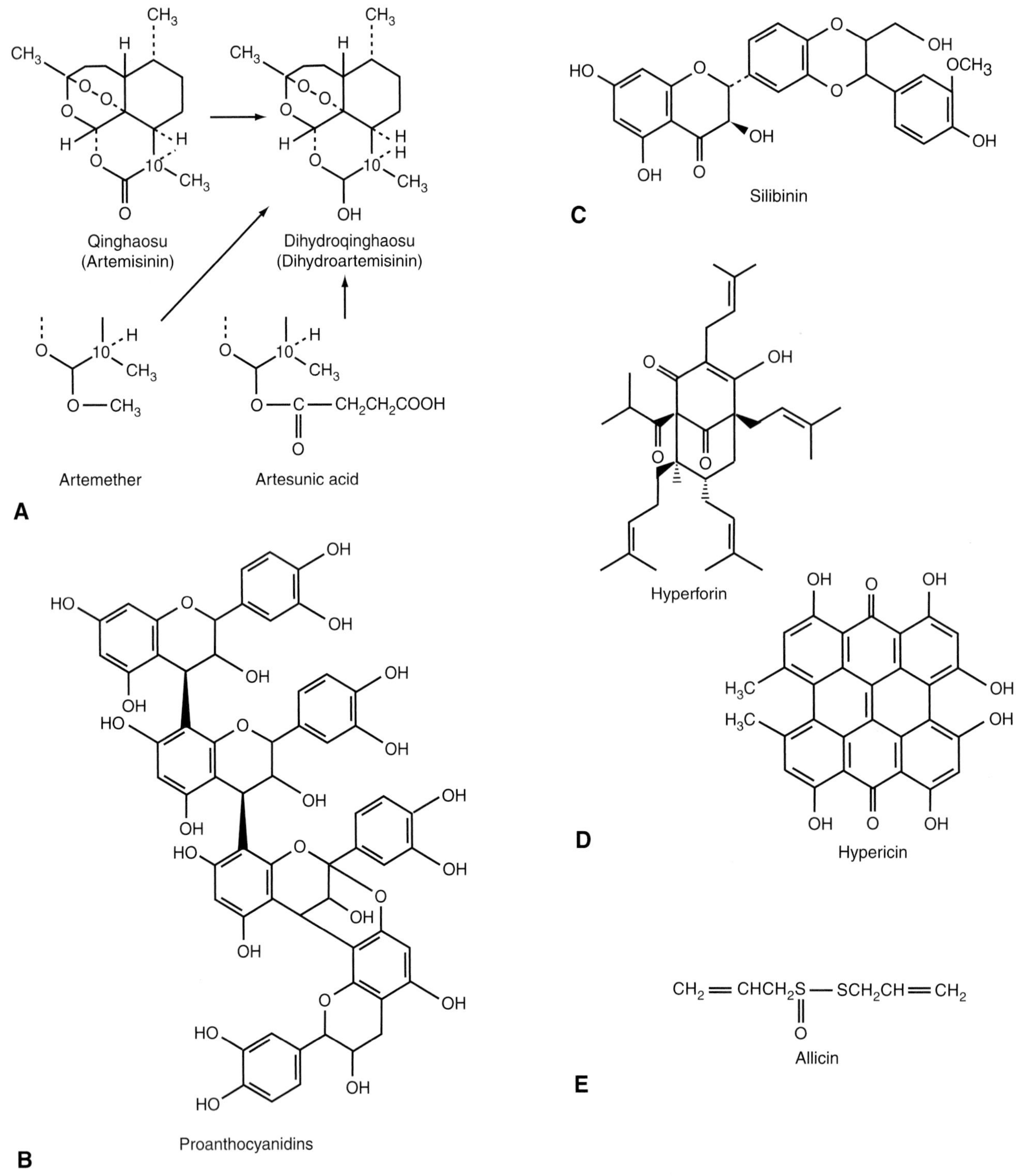

FIGURE 42-2. Structures of actual or hypothesized active moieties of botanical drugs. **A,** The artemisinins. Artemisinin; the oil-soluble derivative artemether with a methyl group in ether linkage; the water-soluble artesunic acid with a succinic acid group in ester linkage; the common metabolite dihydroartemisinin. **B,** A proanthocyanidin from cranberry. **C,** Silibinin from milk thistle. **D,** Hyperforin and hypericin from St. John's wort. **E,** Allicin from garlic.

juice, and 114 positive cultures per 151 cultures (75% positive) when taking placebo.[18]

Vitamin A for Measles Pneumonia

In children with poor nutrition who present with acute complicated measles, the death rate due to pneumonia may be close to 10%.[19] Vitamin A (retinol) and its metabolites retinaldehyde and retinoic acid are needed for vision, growth, and cell differentiation, and for normal humoral and cell-mediated immunity. The normal plasma concentration of vitamin A is 30 to 65 μg/dL. Diets that are low in dark green vegetables and dark-colored fruits, liver, and fish can result in vitamin A deficiency. This deficiency is treated with oral administration of 60 mg (200,000 international units [IU]) initially and then at 6-month intervals if needed. Ingestion of 20,000 IU by children daily for several months, however, can lead to vitamin A toxicity, characterized by increased intracranial pressure, bone pain, and fractures.

Clinical vitamin A deficiency in children is associated with increased mortality.[20] Vitamin A prophylaxis of undernourished children resulted in a statistical decrease in all-cause mortality;[21,22] a component of the decrease in mortality was related to deaths due to measles. The first major study that suggested that measles morbidity and mortality might be improved by vitamin A treatment was that of Ellison, who in the early 1930s administered vitamin A (cod liver oil) for 7 days (in mild cases) or 21 days (in complicated cases) to hospitalized children with measles and noted a reduction in mortality from 26/300 to 11/300 (odds ratio [OR] = 0.4; confidence interval = 0.19 to 0.83).[23] Deaths due to pneumonia fell from 23 to 10. In the 1980s, Barclay and colleagues reported a trend toward reduced measles mortality in vitamin A–deficient Tanzanian children treated with vitamin A supplementation (200,000 IU twice over 2 days).[24] More convincing evidence of benefit was then obtained with the subsets of children whose measles was complicated by pneumonia or diarrhea. Hussey and Klein, for example, studied 189 South African children, 92% of whom were vitamin A deficient, who presented with complicated measles, and who received vitamin A (200,000 IU twice over 2 days) or placebo.[19] The mean recovery times for pneumonia and diarrhea in the vitamin A group (6.3 days and 5.6 days, respectively) were shorter than in the placebo group (12.4 days and 8.5 days, respectively) (P < .001 for both pneumonia and diarrhea). Coutsoudis and colleagues followed with a smaller trial of 60 South African patients (total) presenting with measles pneumonia in which the duration in vitamin A–treated patients (360,000 IU thrice over 8 days) was 3.8 days, versus 5.7 days for those given placebo (P = .04).[25]

It should be noted that in contrast to these South African studies in which two doses of vitamin A reduced measles morbidity, one dose of vitamin A has not been shown to reduce morbidity. Zambian children with acute measles who developed respiratory complications were given one dose of 200,000 IU of vitamin A or placebo.[26] The vitamin A group had a smaller chance of developing pneumonia (OR = 0.73) if pneumonia was not present on admission, but they also had a greater chance of failing to recover from pneumonia (OR = 1.2) if pneumonia was present on admission.

It is even less clear whether morbidity and mortality due to other specific infectious etiologies is improved with vitamin A supplementation. Vitamin A given as prophylaxis to Indonesian children every 4 months for 2 years resulted in a rise in acute lower respiratory disease compared with placebo (rate ratio = 1.39; 95% confidence interval = 1.003 to 1.931);[27] vitamin A treatment of Peruvian children with community pneumonia resulted in a modest increase in symptoms[28]; and vitamin A supplementation in American children with confirmed respiratory syncytial virus infection resulted in slightly longer hospital stays than placebo controls (5.0 days versus 4.4 days, P = .01).[29] Brazilian children with nonmeasles pneumonia did not materially benefit from vitamin A supplementation.[30]

In 1993, the American Academy of Pediatrics viewed "the data on efficacy and safety of vitamin A in U.S. children with measles to be limited, and therefore, cautions practitioners to select patients for treatment carefully."[31]

Zinc for Diarrhea in Children of the Developing World

Zinc is a divalent cation that, compared with iron and copper, is relatively stable to oxidation and reduction. Zinc therefore is an ideal metal cofactor for enzymatic reactions that require a redox-stable cation to accept a pair of electrons.[32] It is an essential cofactor for at least one representative of each enzyme class, and hundreds of zinc metalloenzymes are known.[33] The importance of zinc is illustrated by acrodermatitis enteropathica, an autosomal recessive disorder attributed to a defect in zinc metabolism. Patients with this disorder suffer from diarrhea and immune dysfunction, including T-cell dysfunction and susceptibility to viral, bacterial, and fungal infections. The ubiquity of zinc-requiring enzymes makes it difficult to determine precisely which enzymatic deficiencies cause these symptoms.

The normal level of zinc is 65 to 140 μg/mL. Because mild deficiency can occur in breast-fed children after 6 months of age if the diet does not include animal products, attempts have been made to ameliorate diarrhea in undernourished children of the developing world via zinc supplementation. In a meta-analysis of prophylaxis trials in which 5 to 20 mg zinc per day (the U.S. recommended daily allowance of zinc is 5 to 10 mg/day) was provided to children less than 5 years old in developing countries for 12 to 54 weeks, the pooled odds ratio for diarrhea incidence (0.82) was statistically decreased with respect to controls.[34] Plasma zinc levels in the treated patients rose from a mean of 75 μg/dL before therapy to 93 μg/dL after therapy, whereas in untreated persons, zinc levels remained constant at 77 to 78 μg/dL, confirming the use and bioavailability of the prescribed zinc. A more recent report of 2400 patients from India is confirmatory. Administration of 10 to 20 mg zinc daily for 4 months increased plasma zinc levels from 62 μg/dL to 129 μg/dL in the zinc group, and the incidence of diarrhea was statistically decreased (OR = 0.88; confidence interval = 0.82 to 0.95).[35] The odds ratio was 0.92 for 1- to 6-day episodes, 0.79 for 7- to 13-day episodes, and 0.69 for episodes lasting longer than 13 days. Thus, zinc appeared most effective in preventing episodes of diarrhea that are more severe and prolonged.

Zinc is also an effective treatment for diarrhea in undernourished children in developing countries, although it may be necessary to treat patients by day 3 or 4 of symptoms to achieve statistical evidence of benefit.[36] For Indian children, the relative risk (RR) of diarrhea lasting more than 7 days was statistically reduced (RR = 0.61 [0.39 to 0.93]) in children who received zinc supplementation and who enrolled by day 4 of symptoms but not in children who enrolled after a longer period of prior diarrheal symptoms (RR = 0.87 [0.65 to 1.16]).[36] Roy and co-workers confirmed that if zinc supplementation (20 mg/day) is started in children with diarrhea of less than 3 days' duration, the time to recovery is shortened compared with controls (4.7 versus 6.2 days; P < .04).[37] A meta-analysis of three studies of acute diarrhea (defined as diarrhea present for less than 14 days prior to zinc supplementation) and four studies of persistent diarrhea (defined as diarrhea present for greater than 14 days) showed that zinc supplementation had a borderline-significant effect on the odds ratio of diarrhea continuing for a further 7 days in the acute cases (OR = 0.79 [0.61 to 1.01]) and also for the persistent cases (OR = 0.60 [0.38 to 0.93]).[38] In a recent report, administration of three times the recommended daily allowance of zinc to children with diarrhea of less than 96 hours' duration significantly reduced disease duration. For patients whose diarrhea lasted more than 3 days after starting treatment, the risk ratio for zinc patients compared with controls was 0.75 (0.61 to 0.91), and for the lesser number of cases lasting more than 7 days, the risk ratio was 0.57 (0.38 to 0.86).[39] Plasma zinc values increased by approximately 4 μmol/dL in patients who received zinc supplementation.[39]

Zinc supplementation to prevent or to treat diarrhea, however, has been associated with an increased risk of vomiting. In one recent prevention study in India, there was a small but significant increase in the mean days of vomiting in the zinc group (4.3 days) compared with the placebo group (2.6 days).[35] In the treatment study, 5% of zinc treatments were regurgitated compared with 1.3% of placebo treatments.[39]

Homeopathy for Childhood Diarrhea

Homeopathic medicine is based on the concept of "similars," namely, that symptoms of an illness will respond to administration of infinitesimal amounts of a drug that in higher concentrations would produce similar symptoms in healthy subjects; the mechanism of action is perhaps stimulation of host defense mechanisms.[40] Homeopathic medications are believed to remain active, and possibly more effective, when they are very greatly diluted, even well beyond the point at which a single molecule of the original substance has any likelihood of remaining in the solvent. That no coherent mechanism has been articulated to explain the biologic effects of such diluted products remains a central problem that discourages wider acceptance of homeopathic approaches.

Homeopathic products are prescribed for treatment or prevention of many infectious diseases. Homeopathic interventions are chosen on the basis of a patient's individual signs and symptoms. Thus, for example,

Jacobs and colleagues[40] investigated homeopathic treatment in Nepalese children with diarrhea. Patients with eight to nine unformed stools in the past 24 hours, approximately one third caused by enterotoxic *E. coli,* were randomly assigned to homeopathic treatment or placebo. On the basis of each patient's symptoms, one or more of 19 homeopathic medications were prescribed. These included arsenic trioxide, German chamomile, calcium carbonate, *Podophyllum* (Mayapple), and flowers of sulfur, each of which was "diluted 1:100 in a water/alcohol solution 30 times for a final concentration of 1×10^{-60}." Diluted arsenic was given for patients with "great anxiety and restlessness. Tossing about in bed"; chamomile was given for the qualities of "capricious; irritable; quarrelsome, nothing pleases." Kaplan-Meier plots showed an 18% greater probability that a child would be free of diarrhea by day 5 in the homeopathic group compared with the placebo group ($P = .036$). These data have not been confirmed.

Zinc for the Common Cold

Adults in temperate regions experience two to four viral colds per year (see Chapter 50). Rhinoviruses cause 30% to 50% of colds, but other viruses can also be etiologic agents. Conventional treatment is symptomatic rather than specific for the etiologic cause. Cold symptoms are most likely caused by the release of inflammatory mediators, including selected cytokines and chemokines. Several studies suggest that zinc could mitigate cold symptoms. The mechanisms postulated include a direct antiviral effect, or modulation of the inflammatory response to infection. Nonclinical reports have shown that zinc prevents formation of rhinoviral capsid proteins, binding of surface proteins to specific receptors on the respiratory epithelium,[41] and modulation of the amount or function of inflammatory mediators.[41,42]

Treatment of patients with common cold symptoms, however, has yielded contradictory results, with about as many reports indicating efficacy as not. For example, in one study, adults and students (mean age, 37 years) with less than 24 hours of cold symptoms who received one (13-mg) oral lozenge containing zinc acetate six times per day had a statistically diminished duration of cold symptoms compared with placebo recipients (4.5 days versus 8.1 days: $P < .01$).[42] There were no instances of nausea, vomiting, or abdominal pain in the zinc group, although gastrointestinal symptoms and adverse taste of the preparation did seem to unblind some of the zinc trials. Zinc intake in this study was approximately 80 mg/day and blood zinc levels increased from 14.8 µmol/L to 17.7 µmol/L. In contrast, a study of grade school children who enrolled after 24 hours of cold symptoms and received 10-mg zinc lozenges five to six times daily showed no improvement in cure times (9 days) over placebo (9 days).[43] In a study of 18- to 65-year-old persons with colds of 1 day's duration, the median duration of illness was 5.5 days in both the oral zinc acetate group (approximately 70 mg/day) and the placebo group.[44] In the latter study, the effect of zinc on colds induced by specific challenge with rhinovirus type 39 was also studied. The duration of illness was 2.5 days in a zinc gluconate group (78 mg/day) compared with 3.5 days in the placebo group ($P = .035$), but the severity of the symptoms was unaffected.

Topical zinc treatment has also been the subject of contradictory reports. On the positive side, patients within 48 hours of onset of illness received two 120-µL sprays of a nasal gel containing 33 mM zinc four times per day until symptoms resolved.[41] Their total dose was 960 µL or 2.1 mg zinc per day. The duration of symptoms was statistically shortened in the zinc group (4.3 days) compared with the placebo group (6 days) ($P = .002$). The improvement in the course of colds acquired naturally contradicted the previous data of Turner on colds induced by challenge by rhinovirus type 23.[45] In the challenge study, a slightly lower dose of zinc (120 µL of 33 mM zinc gluconate, five times per day for a total of 600 µL) was sprayed for 3 days prior to challenge and then for 6 days thereafter. The nares were lavaged with a solution of 6.5 µg/dL zinc just prior to virus challenge. In zinc recipients, the lavage fluid contained zinc 48 µg/dL; in patients receiving placebo, zinc levels in the lavage fluid remained at 6.7 µg/dL, confirming delivery of the desired preparation. Rhinovirus infection occurred in 78% of zinc-treated

volunteers and 74% of placebo-treated volunteers, and the incidence of clinical colds also did not differ between the groups (59% of the zinc group versus 54% of the placebo group). Thus, despite its prevalent use, there remains no consistent evidence that zinc (topically or orally) ameliorates or prevents viral colds.

Echinacea for the Common Cold

Extracts of the genus *Echinacea* (purple coneflower) were used by Native Americans for a wide range of diseases, including colds, arthritis, snake bite, rabies, seizures, and cancer.[46] In terms of annual sales, echinacea is hugely popular in Europe and among the top several herbal products in the United States. In 1996, there were more than 500 distinct *Echinacea*-containing products sold in Germany. Its oft-claimed power to prevent or treat upper respiratory tract infections is attributed to the immunologic activity its constituents manifest in nonclinical models. For example, purified *Echinacea* polysaccharides activate phagocytes in vitro and in animal models (reviewed in reference 46).

Despite these claims and echinacea's in vitro immunologic activity, it has been difficult to prove that *Echinacea* extracts are truly effective for either prevention or treatment of the common cold. In a prevention trial in 40-year-old adults (see Table 42-1) who received 4 mL of fresh expressed juice of whole flowering plants of *Echinacea purpurea* twice a day for 8 weeks, the incidence of natural colds was not statistically reduced (65% in the echinacea group versus 74% in the placebo group; RR, 0.88 [range, 0.6 to 1.2]).[46] Echinacea (300 mg) three times a day for 14 days prior to challenge with rhinovirus type 23 and for 5 days thereafter were also not protective compared with placebo: infection occurred in 44% and 57% of volunteers ($P = .3$), respectively, and illness occurred in 50% and 59% of volunteers, respectively, who had documented rhinovirus infection ($P = .77$).[47] In treatment trials, students with 1-day onset of a cold were administered a mixture of unrefined *Echinacea* root and herb (123 mg of *Echinacea angustifolia* root, 62 mg of *E. purpurea* root, 62 mg of *E. purpurea* herb) approximately three times a day until cold symptoms resolved. Compared with placebo, there was no difference in mean cold duration (6.3 days versus 5.8 days) or in illness severity.[48] On the other hand, in one study, adult cold sufferers with "incipient" cold symptoms who received 5 mL of pressed juice from fresh flowering *Echinacea purpurea* twice a day for 10 days demonstrated a statistically significant reduction in median time of illness (6.0 days versus 9.0 days for placebo: $P = .01$).[49] Borchers and colleagues reviewed German literature that also demonstrates a statistical improvement.[50]

Vitamin C for the Common Cold

That Linus Pauling, a polymath and twice Nobel Prize winner, proposed the broad health value of ascorbic acid lent enormous credibility to such claims. Perhaps the best known of its touted benefits is its ability to prevent or rapidly terminate viral colds. In spite of these claims and initial reports, vitamin C does not seem to be effective prophylaxis or treatment for the common cold. Daily prophylaxis with 1 to 2 g has proved ineffective in reducing the incidence of respiratory disease and colds in Navajo children[51] and in Marines[52] (see Table 42-1). In the Navajo study, plasma ascorbic acid levels were raised to 1.3 mg/dL in the treated group, compared with 1.0 mg/dL in the placebo group, yet the incidences of illness were approximately equal (133 versus 129 episodes) and the mean duration of illness was also similar (5.5 versus 5.8 days).[51] In the Marine study, whole blood ascorbic acid levels rose to 1.4 mg/dL in the vitamin C group versus 0.9 mg/dL in the placebo group, yet there were 1.8 colds lasting 11 days per recruit in each group.[52] Treatment with "mega-dose" vitamin C, 3 g daily for 3 days, or a high dose of 1 g daily for 3 days, did not reduce the severity or duration of cold symptoms when taken at the onset of cold symptoms.[53] The mean duration of symptoms was 10 days in the vitamin C 3-g and 1-g dose groups, compared with 8.5 days in the "placebo" group given a very low dose (30 mg/day) of vitamin C.

Negative data, however, have not stayed the hand of all who are tempted to use this essential and benign vitamin. Vitamin C still has its proponents and testimonials. Its adherents criticize most of the negative studies as having employed too low a dose. However, raising the dose of vitamin C does not result in increased efficacy. The recommended dietary allowance for vitamin C is approximately 75 to 90 mg/day. Audera and co-workers used a dose of 3 g/day, which did not shorten the duration or diminish the severity of disease compared with the lower dose of 1 g/day or with the very low dose of 30 mg/day.

Milk Thistle for Chronic Hepatitis

Milk thistle extracts have been used since ancient Roman days as treatment for various disorders including those of the liver, and recent studies suggest plausible mechanisms by which they could be beneficial in selected settings.[54] Milk thistle seeds contain approximately 60% silymarin, which is a mixture of four flavolignan isomers. Administration of 80 mg silibinin (an isomer that makes up about half of silymarin[55]) in commercial formulations results in maximum plasma concentrations of 200 to 700 ng/mL, and it is excreted with a half-life of approximately 6 hours. Bile concentrations of silibinin are approximately 100 times those found in serum.

Silibinin (see Fig. 42-2C) and the other flavonoids are thought to function as antioxidants. Saller and co-workers reviewed the effect of silymarin/silibinin on cellular metabolism in vitro.[55] Silibinin reacted rapidly with hydroxyl radicals but poorly with O_2 and with H_2O_2. In addition, formation of leukotriene B_4 (but not prostaglandin E_2) was inhibited with a 50% inhibitory concentration (IC_{50}) of 15 μM. Silymarin suppressed nuclear factor kappa B (NF-κB) DNA activation and binding activities. In human cells in vitro, Silymarin reduced natural killer (cell-mediated) cytotoxicity but not antigen-dependent cellular cytotoxicity. In rats, silymarin/silibinin protected liver mitochondria and microsomes from lipid peroxidation induced by several hepatotoxic agents. In all, these mechanisms could retard inflammation and fibrosis.

Recent clinical evidence, however, suggests that antioxidant or other activities of silymarin may be of only modest benefit in viral hepatitis. In a pilot study of chronic active hepatitis caused by hepatitis B or C, 10 patients who received 240 mg silibinin twice a day for 7 days demonstrated a statistically significant reduction in hepatocellular enzyme levels. Aspartate aminotransferase decreased from 88 U/L to 66 U/L in silibinin patients, whereas in placebo patients the reduction was 3 U/L.[56]

GENERAL AND SUPPORTIVE APPROACHES

Complementary Approaches in Patients with Acquired Immunodeficiency Syndrome

AIDS is a chronic, multisystem disease for which specific antiretroviral therapy has proved hugely beneficial but does not ensure cure. Retroviral agents may themselves have distressing side effects, such as lipodystrophy. In this context, complementary medicines are particularly attractive, as they offer hope, an improved quality of life, and palliation of morbidity. Of 100 patients participating in National Institutes of Health clinical protocols related to human immunodeficiency virus (HIV), 84% used a mean of 4.8 CAM therapies.[3] Biologic therapies (herbs and high-dose vitamins/antioxidants) were used by 68 persons; body-based therapies were used by 17 (acupuncture), 16 (chiropractic), and 34 (massage) patients; spirituality by 29; energy healing by 10; and homeopathy by 7.[3]

Prominent examples of CAM use for patients with AIDS are St. John's wort, L-carnitine, dehydroepiandrosterone (DHEA), garlic, and body-based therapies such as massage and acupuncture.

St. John's Wort for Depression

St. John's wort has been used for centuries for wound healing and many other clinical conditions. Its most popular use today is as a treatment for depressive disorders of varying severity. St. John's wort extracts contain naphthodianthrones such as hypericin (see Fig. 42-2D) and pseudohypericin; flavones such as hyperoside, quercitrin, and rutin; aglycones such as quercetin, kampferol, luteolin, and myricetin; and phloroglucinaols such as hyperforin (see Fig. 42-2D).[56a] Extracts of St. John's wort and pure hyperforin are potent inducers of cy-

tochrome P450 (CYP)-3A mono-oxygenase gene expression in hepatocytes in vitro. The pregnane X receptor, which regulates expression of CYP3A4, was activated sevenfold by 9 μg/mL of the Nature's Way extract of St. John's wort and by 1 μM of pure hyperforin.[57] In a phase I clinical study, St. John's wort containing 0.3% hypericin, when administered at 300 mg three times a day for 14 days, decreased the area-under-the-curve concentration of the anti-HIV drug indinavir (800 mg four times over 2 days) by a mean of 57% in normal volunteers.[58] The St. John's wort example shows that not only can botanicals interact with conventional drugs but also that this effect can be sufficient to have clinical consequences.

Dehydroepiandrosterone

In men and women with HIV infection, serum levels of cortisol are often increased, whereas the levels of DHEA, an antagonist to the immunoregulatory actions of cortisol, tend to be reduced.[59] In addition, HIV-infected men frequently exhibit reduced testosterone levels.[60] Taken together, these steroid hormone changes are thought to contribute to a shift in cytokine production from a type 1 to a type 2 pattern, leading to suppression of cell-mediated immunity and release of interleukin-2 and interferon-γ. In HIV-infected individuals, low DHEA and testosterone levels are associated with muscle wasting, lipodystrophy, and weight loss. Whether administration of DHEA or testosterone will improve immune function, reduce muscle wasting, and improve overall quality of life remains to be established. In one recent trial, for example, 32 patients were randomized between DHEA sulfate (50 mg daily for 4 months) or placebo.[61] Serum DHEA sulfate levels rose from 5 to 20 μM in the treated group. DHEA-sulfate administration did not lead to significant weight changes or side effects but may have given rise to an improvement in mental health, as assessed by a quality-of-life questionnaire.

L-Carnitine for Lipodystrophy

L-Carnitine is required for fatty acid oxidation in mitochondria, and it is being distributed by HIV buyer-clubs in the United States to reverse lipodystrophy. However, 12 consecutive patients with HIV treated with 1000 mg L-carnitine twice a day for 3 months did not report diminution in median body weight, hip circumference, or waist circumference.[62]

Garlic for Hypercholesterolemia

Garlic (*Allium sativum*) contains alliin (see Fig. 42-2E), which is converted to allicin by the enzyme alliinase, and then to further, partially identified metabolites. It is thought that garlic ingestion leads to a lowering of plasma cholesterol and that it does so via these compounds.[63] However, the data have been uninspiring. In a recent meta-analysis, there was a significantly greater reduction in cholesterol levels in the garlic groups (−0.41 mmol/L) compared with the placebo groups, but this difference was reduced to −0.11 mmol/L and became nonsignificant when controlled for diet and other methodologic factors.[64] Kannar and colleagues found a significant reduction in cholesterol (−0.36 mmol/L) in hypercholesterolemic patients given garlic supplements with 9.6 mg of allicin-releasing potential daily for 12 weeks compared with placebo subjects (+0.13 mmol/L), but the garlic group evidenced significantly decreased energy intake compared with control subjects.[63] Because garlic is commonly used by HIV patients, Piscitelli and co-workers determined the effect of garlic supplements on the pharmacokinetics of saquinavir.[65] In 10 healthy volunteers, the tested garlic formulation diminished the saquinavir area-under-the-curve concentration by 51%, probably because of decreased bioavailability of the protease inhibitor.

Body-Based and "Energy" Therapies (Massage and Acupuncture)

Massage has the potential to reduce musculoskeletal morbidity and mental stress, and it has been proposed that it affects immune function. The efficacy of massage for immune function and for overall improvement in quality of life is beginning to be examined in HIV-infected people.[66]

Acupuncture also has the potential for symptom relief and possibly even modification of immune function,[67] and it is also starting to be studied in HIV patients. Many studies suggest that acupuncture attenuates the nausea that follows chemotherapy and relieves acute postsurgical pain. In one study, acupuncture was not found to be helpful for pain related to HIV peripheral neuropathy,[68] but this study has been criticized for choosing the wrong acupuncture points.

COMMENT

The literature on the use of CAM to treat infectious diseases makes a variety of claims, some of which may be borne out. Data indicate that a biologically based alternative treatment can be effective (artemisinins for malaria), probably effective (cranberry for UTI, vitamin A for measles in vitamin A–deficient children, zinc for diarrhea in poorly nourished children), of undecided efficacy (zinc for the common cold), probably ineffective (echinacea for colds), too preliminary for conclusions to be drawn (milk thistle for hepatitis), or ineffective (vitamin C for colds). As complementary treatments, St. John's wort, L-carnitine, garlic, DHEA, massage, and acupuncture have been used, respectively, for depression, lipodystrophy, hypercholesterolemia, wasting, general well-being, and pain relief in HIV patients, without proof of efficacy.

Recommendations for clinical use, or at least concurrence with a patient's choice to engage in a CAM approach, should be based on evidence of clinical utility and lack of toxicity, but such data remain woefully limited. Conventional drug development relies on three major sets of data: (1) chemistry and manufacturing data that give confidence in the reproducible quality of the drug, (2) nonclinical data, and (3) clinical data defining the optimal dose (phase I and II studies) and verifying that dose is likely to be safe and effective for the target population (phase III studies).

Chemistry and manufacturing considerations are particularly an issue for botanical agents, which are complex mixtures of perhaps thousands of components.[69] The example of St. John's wort shows that even the list of named components can be daunting. A plant extract can be a starting point for identifying a single active compound that could then be purified and used according to the criteria for conventional drugs. This route was followed for the artemisinins. Another route is to use the whole extract for treatment, under the assumption that a number of unidentified components combine to produce the total therapeutic effect. The practical issue in using whole extract is how to reproducibly ensure the quality of the active ingredients when their identity and optimal relative concentrations are not known.

The inability to specify active ingredients in complex botanical mixtures makes it hard to correctly discern which herbal medicines are truly beneficial. This problem could, for example, underlie the disparate results for echinacea for the common cold. The manufacturing, and therefore the composition, of the product used in the referenced successful treatment trial—pressed juice from fresh flowering *Echinacea purpurea*—is totally dissimilar to the manufacturing of product for the unsuccessful treatment trials—unrefined *Echinacea* roots and herb. Borchers and colleagues pointed out that the extraction procedure—using ethanol or not—will radically affect whether any of the putatively active *Echinacea* constituents are extracted.[50]

The pharmacologic effects of St. John's wort and of garlic may also reflect the issue of botanical complexity. Even if St. John's wort and garlic are shown to be active for specific clinical indications, until active ingredients of these botanicals are identified it will be unclear whether the active ingredients also lead to induction of cytochrome P450, or whether a formulation could be made that preserves efficacy but removes induction of cytochrome P450.

Clinical trials of CAM products must proceed by the method used for conventional drugs. Eventually, large trials need to be undertaken to determine which patient populations experience efficacy, and to rule out toxicity. As De Smet stated, "Since the drug receptors in our body cannot distinguish whether a molecule comes from the plant kingdom or from the chemical laboratory, naturalness does not, by definition, guarantee harmlessness."[70]

REFERENCES

1. Kessler RC, Davis RB, Foster DF, et al. Long-term trends in the use of complementary and alternative medical therapies in the United States. Ann Intern Med. 2001;135:262-268.
2. Ni H, Simile C, Hardy AM. Utilization of complementary and alternative medicine by United States adults: Results from the 1999 National Health Interview Survey. Med Care. 2002;40:353-358.
3. Sparber A, Wootton JC, Bauer L, et al. Use of complementary medicine by adult patients participating in HIV/AIDS clinical trials. J Altern Complement Med. 2000;6:415-422.
4. Richardson MA, Straus S. Complementary and alternative medicine: opportunities and challenges for cancer management and research. Semin Oncol. 2002;29:531-545.
5. Klayman DL. Qinghaosu (artemisinin): An antimalarial drug from China. Science. 1985;228:1049-1055.
6. Hien TT, White NJ. Qinghaosu. Lancet. 1993;341:603-608.
7. Ter Kuile F, White NJ, Holloway P, et al. *P. falciparum:* In vitro studies of the pharmacodynamic properties of drugs used for the treatment of severe malaria. Exp Parasitol. 1993;76:85-95.
8. Hien TT, Day NPJ, Phu NH, et al. A controlled trial of artemether or quinine in Vietnamese adults with severe falciparum malaria. N Engl J Med. 1996;335:76-83.
9. Van Hensbroek MB, Onyioray E, Jarrar S, et al. A trial of artemether or quinine in children with cerebral malaria. N Engl J Med. 1996;335:69-75.
10. Lefevre G, Looareesuwan S, Treeprasertsuk S, et al. A clinical and pharmacokinetic trial of 6 doses of artemether-lumefantrine for multidrug-resistant *P. falciparum* malaria in Thailand. Am J Trop Med Hyg. 2001;64:247-256.
11. Newton PN, Angus BJ, Chierakul W, et al. Randomized comparison of artesunate and quinine in the treatment of severe falciparum malaria. Clin Infect Dis. 2003;37:7-16.
12. Zafriri D, Ofek I, Adar R, et al. Inhibitory activity of cranberry juice on adherence of type 1 and type P fimbriated *E. coli* to eucaryotic cells. Antimicrob Agents Chemother. 1989;33:92-98.
13. Howell AB, Foxman B. Cranberry juice and adhesion of antibiotic-resistant uropathogens (Letter). JAMA. 2002;287:3082-3083.
14. Foo LY, Lu Y, Howell AB, Vorsa N. The structure of cranberry proanthocyanidins which inhibit adherence of uropathogenic P-fimbriated *E. coli* in vitro. Phytochemistry 2000;54:173-181.
15. Howell AM, Vorsa N, Marderosian AD, Foo LY. Inhibition of the adherence of P-fimbriated *E. coli* to uroepithelial-cell surfaces by proanthocyanidin extracts from cranberries (Letter). N Engl J Med. 1998.339;1085-1086.
16. Avorn J, Monane M, Gurwitz H, et al. Reduction of bacteriuria and pyuria after ingestion of cranberry juice. JAMA. 1994;271:751-754.
17. Kontiokari T, Sundqvist K, Nuutinen M, et al. Randomized trial of cranberry-lingonberry juice and lactobacillus GG drink for the prevention of urinary tract infections in women. Br Med J. 2001;322:1-5.
18. Schlager TA, Anderson S, Trudell J, Hendley JO. Effect of cranberry juice on bacteriuria in children with neurogenic bladder receiving intermittent catherterization. J Pediatr. 1999;135:698-702.
19. Hussey GD, Klein M. A randomized, controlled trial of vitamin A in children with severe measles. N Engl J Med. 1990;323:160-164.
20. Sommer A, Hussaini G, Tarwotjo I, Susanto D. Increased mortality in children with mild vitamin A deficiency. Lancet. 1983;2:584-588.
21. Fawzi WW, Chalmers TC, Herrera MG, Mosteller F. Vitamin A supplementation and child mortality: A meta-analysis. JAMA. 1993;269:898-903.
22. Glasziou PP, Mackerras DEM. Vitamin A supplementation in infectious diseases: A meta-analysis. Br Med J. 1993;306:366-370.
23. Ellison JB. Intensive vitamin therapy in measles. Br Med J. 1932;2:708-711.
24. Barclay AJG, Foster A, Sommer A. Vitamin A supplements and mortality related to measles: A randomized clinical trial. Br Med J. 1987;294:294-296.
25. Coutsoudis A, Broughton M, Coovadia HM. Vitamin A supplementation reduces measles morbidity in young African children: A randomized, placebo-controlled, double-blind trial. Am J Clin Nutr. 1991;54:890-895.
26. Rosales FJ, Kjolhede, C, Goodman S. Efficacy of a single oral dose of 200,000 IU of oil-soluble vitamin A in measles-associated morbidity. Am J Epidemiol. 1996;143:413-422.
27. Dibley MJ, Sadjimin T, Klolhede CL, Moulton LH. Vitamin A supplementation fails to reduce incidence of acute respiratory illness and diarrhea in preschool-age Indonesian children. J Nutr. 1996;126:434-442.
28. Stephensen CB, Franchi LM, Hernandez H, et al. Adverse effects of high-dose vitamin A supplements in children hospitalized with pneumonia. Pediatrics. 1998;101:e3
29. Bresee JS, Fischer M, Dowell SF. Vitamin A therapy for children with respiratory syncytial virus infection: A multicenter trial in the United States. Pediatr Infect Dis J. 1996;15:777-782.
30. Nacul LC, Kirkwood BR, Arthur P, et al. Randomized, double-blind placebo-controlled clinical trial of efficacy of vitamin A treatment in non-measles childhood pneumonia. Br Med J. 1997;315:505-510.
31. Committee on Infectious Diseases. Vitamin A treatment of measles. Pediatrics. 1993;91:1014-1015.
32. McCall KA, Huang C-C, Fierke CA. Function and mechanism of zinc metalloenzymes. J Nutr. 2000;130:1437s-1446s.
33. Hambridge M. Human zinc deficiency. J Nutr. 2000;130;1344S-1349S.
34. Bhutta ZA, Black RE, Brown KH, et al. Prevention of diarrhea and pneumonia by zinc supplementation in children in developing countries: Pooled analysis of randomized controlled trials. J Pediatr. 1999;135:689-697.
35. Bhandari N, Baho R, Taneja S. Substantial reduction in severe diarrheal morbidity by daily zinc supplementation in young North Indian children. Pediatrics. 2002;109:e86.

36. Sazawal S, Black RE, Bhan M, et al. Zinc supplementation in young children with acute diarrhea in India. N Engl J Med. 1995;333:839-844.

37. Roy SK, Tomkins AM, Akramuzzaman SKL, et al. Randomized controlled trial of zinc supplementation in malnourished Bangladeshi children with acute diarrhoea. Arch Dis Child. 1997;77:196-200.

38. Bhutta ZA, Bird SM, Black RE, et al. Therapeutic effects of oral zinc in acute and persistent diarrhea in children in developing countries: Pooled analysis of randomized controls trials. Am J Clin Nutr. 2000;72:1516-1522.

39. Strand TA, Chandyo RK, Bahl R, et al. Effectiveness and efficacy of zinc for the treatment of acute diarrhea in young children. Pediatrics. 2002;109:898-903.

40. Jacobs J, Jimenez M, Malthouse S, et al. Homeopathic treatment of acute childhood diarrhea: Results from a clinical trial in Nepal. J Altern Complement Med. 2000;6:131-139.

41. Mossad SB. Effect of zincum gluconicum nasal gel on the duration and symptom severity of the common cold in otherwise healthy adults. QJM. 2003;96:35-43.

42. Prasad AS, Fitzgerald JT, Bao B, et al. Duration of symptoms and plasma cytokine levels in patients with the common cold treated with zinc acetate. Ann Intern Med. 2000;133:245-252.

43. Macknin ML, Piedmonte M, Calendine C, et al. Zinc gluconate lozenges for treating the common cold in children. JAMA. 1998;279:1962-1967.

44. Turner RB, Cetnarowski WE. Effect of treatment with zinc gluconate or zinc acetate on experimental and natural colds. Clin Infect Dis. 2000;31:1202-1208.

45. Turner RB. Ineffectiveness of intranasal zinc gluconate for prevention of experimental rhinovirus colds. Clin Infect Dis. 2001;33:1865-1870.

46. Grimm W, Muller H-H. A randomized controlled trial of the effect of fluid extract of *Echinacea purpurea* on the incidence and severity of colds and respiratory infections. Am J Med. 1999;106:138-143.

47. Turner RM, Riker DK, Gangemi JD. Ineffectiveness of *Echinacea* for prevention of experimental rhinovirus colds. Antimicrob Agents Chemother. 2000;44:1708-1709.

48. Barrett BP, Brown RL, Locken K, et al. Treatment of the common cold with unrefined *Echinacea*. Ann Intern Med. 2002;137:939-946.

49. Schulten B, Bulitta M, Ballering-Bruhl B, et al. Efficacy of *Echinacea purpurea* in patients with a common cold. Arzneimittelforschung. 2001;51:563-568.

50. Borchers AT, Keen CL, Stern JS, Gershwin ME. Inflammation and Native American medicine: The role of botanicals. Am J Clin Nutr. 2000;72:339-347.

51. Coulehan JL, Everhard S, Kapner L, et al. Vitamin C and acute illness in Navajo schoolchildren. N Engl J Med. 1976;295:973-977.

52. Pitt HA, Costrini AM. Vitamin C prophylaxis in marine recruits. JAMA. 1979;241:908-911.

53. Audera C, Patulny RV, Sander BH, Douglas RM. Mega-dose vitamin C in treatment of the common cold: A randomized controlled trial. Med J Aust. 2001;175:359-362.

54. Flora C, Hahn M, Rosen H, Benner K. Milk thistle *(Silybum marianum)* for the therapy of liver disease. Am J Gastroenterol. 1998;93:139-143.

55. Saller R, Meier R, Brignoli R. The use of silymarin in the treatment of liver diseases. Drugs. 2001;61:2035-2063.

56. Buzzelli G, Moscarella S, Giusti A, et al. A pilot study of the liver protective effect of silybin-phosphatidylcholine complex (IdB1016) in chronic active hepatitis. Int J Clin Pharmacol Ther Toxicol. 1993;31:456-460.

56a. Berman JD, Straus SE. Implementing a research agenda for complementary and alternative medicine. Ann Rev Med. 2004;55:239-254.

57. Moore LB, Goodwin B, Jones SA, et al. St. John's wort induces hepatic drug metabolism through activation of the pregnane X receptor. Proc Natl Acad Sci U S A. 2000;97:7500-7502.

58. Piscitelli SC, Burstein AH, Chaitt D, et al. Indinavir concentrations and St. John's wort. Lancet. 2000;355:547-548.

59. Clerici M, Galli M, Bosis S, et al. Immunoendocrinologic abnormalities in human immunodeficiency virus infection. Ann N Y Acad Sci. 2000;917:956-961.

60. Dobs AS, Few WL, Blackman MR, et al. Serum hormones in men with human immunodeficiency virus–associated wasting. J Clin Endocrinol Metab. 1996;81:4108-4112.

61. Piketty C, Jayle D, Leplege A, et al. Double-blind placebo-controlled trial of oral dehydroepiandrosterone in patients with advanced HIV disease. Clin Endocrinol (Oxf). 2001;55:325-330.

62. Mauss S, Schmutz G. L-Carnitine in the treatment of HIV-associated lipodystrophy syndrome. HIV Med. 2001;2:59-60.

63. Kannar D, Wattanapenpaiboon N, Savige GS, Wahlqvist ML. Hypocholesterolemic effect of an enteric-coated garlic supplement. J Am Coll Nutr. 2001;20:225-231.

64. Stevinson C, Pittler MH, Ernst E. Garlic for treating hypercholesterolemia: A meta-analysis of randomized clinical trials. Ann Intern Med. 2000;133:420-429.

65. Piscitelli SC, Burstein AH, Welden N, et al. The effect of garlic supplements on the pharmacokinetics of saquinavir. Clin Infect Dis. 2002;34:234-238.

66. Birk TJ, McGrady A, MacArthur RD, Khuder S. The effects of massage therapy alone and in combination with other complementary therapies on immune system measure and quality of life in HIV. J Altern Complement Med. 2000;6:405-414.

67. Beal MW, Nield-Anderson L. Acupuncture for symptom relief in HIV positive adults: Lessons learned from a pilot study. Altern Ther Health Med. 2000;6:33-42.

68. Shlay JC, Chaloner K, Max MB, et al. Acupuncture and amitriptyline for pain due to HIV-related peripheral neuropathy: A randomized controlled trial. JAMA. 1999;280:1590-1595.

69. Nahin RL, Straus SE. Research into complementary and alternative medicine: Problems and potential. Br Med J. 2001;322:161-164.

70. De Smet PA. Health risks of herbal remedies. Drug Saf. 1995;13:81-93.

Antimicrobial Management: Cost and Resistance

RONALD E. POLK

NEIL O. FISHMAN

The potential for the misuse and abuse of antibiotics was recognized shortly after their introduction into clinical use in the early 1940s. The introduction of new antibiotics during the next decade increased the inappropriate use of these agents. In his review of the subject in 1956, Jawetz was the first to recognize the problems caused by the attractiveness of new antibiotics to physicians, the exaggerated claims by the pharmaceutical industry, and the enormous impact that promotion by the drug companies had on medical practice.[1] Studies have demonstrated that at least one third of all hospitalized patients receive a course of antimicrobial therapy and that approximately 50% of this use is unnecessary or otherwise inappropriate.[2-5] These problems continue to the present.[6,7] Antibiotic expenditures can account for as much as 30% to 50% of a hospital's total drug budget.[8-10] Among the unwanted consequences of antimicrobial therapy are adverse reactions, the emergence of drug-resistant microorganisms, predisposition to secondary infections, and the increased cost of medical care.[11,12] Broad-spectrum antimicrobial therapy is held responsible, at least in part, for the rising incidence of serious nosocomial infections due to methicillin-resistant *Staphylococcus aureus*, glycopeptide-resistant *S. aureus*, vancomycin-resistant enterococci, extended-spectrum β-lactamase–producing Enterobacteriaceae, fluoroquinolone-resistant *Pseudomonas aeruginosa*, and fungi,[12-14] as well as the proliferation of penicillin-resistant pneumococci as a cause of community-acquired upper and lower respiratory tract infections. Therefore, it is not surprising that a number of methods for facilitating more appropriate use of antimicrobials have been developed, including (1) educational programs, sometimes incorporating feedback of information obtained from antimicrobial audits; (2) administrative measures, such as limiting the antimicrobials in a hospital's formulary, using standardized order forms, and requiring justification for the use of particular agents; (3) concurrent monitoring of antimicrobial usage with intervention when misuse is identified; and (4) computer-assisted selection of antibiotics.[15-17] The potential benefits of such programs are somewhat intuitive and include more discriminate use of new agents, decreased development of antimicrobial resistance, improved education of physicians, improved outcomes in patients (such as decreased drug toxicity and a decreased length of stay), increased nursing availability for direct patient care, and cost containment resulting from a decrease in both direct drug expenditures and associated costs. In this chapter we review the various antimicrobial management strategies that have been reported in the literature, summarize the clinical and institutional outcomes of these efforts, and end with recommendations for the development, implementation, and funding of a successful antimicrobial management and cost-containment program.

PHILOSOPHY OF ANTIMICROBIAL USE

To address the problem of inappropriate antimicrobial usage, we first must understand the constraints under which physicians work and the pressures that are exerted on them to prescribe drugs. The prescription of antibiotics has become more of a psychological or philosophic endeavor than a scientific exercise. Several factors have been identified that lead to inappropriate use of antimicrobial agents.[15-18] These include the following:

1. Good intentions. The physician is motivated to give the best treatment, often without regard to cost or the spectrum of activity of the chosen agent.
2. Inappropriate dosing. Some physicians believe that if a small amount of drug is effective, greater and more prolonged administration may be better.
3. Inappropriate prophylaxis. Approximately 30% of patients who receive antibiotics during a hospitalization are given the drugs for a variety of prophylactic purposes, despite limited data supporting the efficacy of such practices. In addition, antimicrobial prophylaxis is continued for greater than 48 hours in 80% of cases.[19]
4. Use of multiple antimicrobial agents or broad-spectrum combinations to cover uncommon organisms. This approach, generalized from management of the neutropenic febrile patient, is often used as a substitute for appropriate diagnostic evaluation.
5. Pressure from the patient to be treated with an antimicrobial agent (most likely in adult and pediatric outpatient settings).
6. Time constraints. It is much more time consuming for physicians to explain why they are not prescribing an antibiotic than it is simply to write the prescription.
7. Cost and availability of radiographic studies and diagnostic tests in relation to the ready solution offered by simply prescribing an antimicrobial drug. This varies with practice setting and may be more operative in community hospitals.
8. Inadequacy of the physician's knowledge of diagnostic procedures and management of patients with infectious diseases. This is becoming more important in an era of increasingly complex infectious disease issues, such as acquired immunodeficiency syndrome and infections in oncology patients, transplant recipients, and other immunocompromised hosts.[20]
9. Malpractice considerations and fear of litigation.
10. Concern about the increasing prevalence of antimicrobial resistance and the perceived need to prescribe ever more broad-spectrum antimicrobials to "cover" these pathogens.
11. Easy solutions provided by pharmaceutical manufacturers. The industry exploits the physician's fear of failure and takes advantage of the previously described concerns and problems by offering expensive and often inappropriate panaceas supported by heavy promotion.

In this environment some physicians feel that antimicrobial control programs impose unnecessary or even deleterious constraints on the practice of medicine.[20,21] Furthermore, prescribers fail to appreciate that antimicrobial use has significant microbiologic and ecologic consequences that extend beyond the individual patient under their care and can affect their entire practice population.[22] This skepticism may arise from the perception that there is a lack of documented efficacy of management programs across varied health care settings, a paucity of direct evidence demonstrating an improvement in clinical outcomes, limited physician time or incentive to pursue such efforts, and a weak causal link between the emergence of resistance and antibiotic use patterns. Although there are no large multicenter randomized controlled trials to address these questions, the preponderance of evidence supports the implementation of such efforts.

ANTIMICROBIAL MANAGEMENT STRATEGIES

As noted, a number of methodologies have been employed to address these issues in an attempt to curb soaring antimicrobial expenditures and to limit the adverse consequences of inappropriate antimicrobial therapy. The various strategies are listed in Table 43-1. In a 1983 survey of 112 hospitals associated with medical schools, Klapp and Ramphal found that 62 of 108 respondents had some form of direct control of antimicrobial usage, either through requirements for authorization by a specialist or through restriction of acceptable indications for the use of particular agents.[23] A survey of the 47 hospitals participating in phase 3 of Project ICARE (Intensive Care Antimicrobial Resistance Epidemiology) revealed that all hospitals had an antimi-

TABLE 43-1 Antimicrobial Management Strategies

Educational programs
Direct interaction
Performance evaluation
Formal seminars
Newsletters
Antimicrobial formulary restriction
Prior-approval programs
Telephone approval
Antibiotic order forms
Automatic stop orders
Simple chart entry
Therapeutic substitution and streamlining programs
Costing of items in clinical microbiology laboratory
Purchase plans
Computer-assisted management programs
Antibiotic rotation
Multidisciplinary approaches
Clinical practice guidelines

crobial formulary and 91% of hospitals also used at least one of the following three mechanisms to improve use: stop orders, antibiotic restriction, or clinical practice guidelines.[24] Nearly 500 infectious diseases physicians who participate in the Emerging Infections Network of the Infectious Diseases Society of America responded to a questionnaire that assessed their roles in antimicrobial management programs.[25] Overall, half indicated that the hospitals in which they worked required their approval before restricted antimicrobials could be dispensed, but payment for such services was rare (18%). John and Fishman published a critical review of antimicrobial management programs that summarized the results of 37 strategies and evaluated the strengths and weaknesses of each approach.[26] The emphasis of the programs that were reviewed is illustrated in Figure 43-1. We now consider the data supporting major strategies.

Educational Programs

Although education has long been considered one of the hallmarks of the activities of the infectious diseases physician, it is the least rigorously studied intervention. A variety of approaches have been used over the years, including staff conferences, lectures by visiting professors (grand rounds), clinical pharmacy consultations, drug-utilization evaluations, newsletters, and the development of clinical pathways or guidelines.[15,26,27] Inasmuch as there are significant ongoing deficiencies in physicians' knowledge concerning antibiotics and inappropriate use remains a problem,[28,29] it is reasonable to assume that education alone is not an effective method to achieve a long-term impact on prescribing practices. Educational programs are difficult to assess because of the complex nature of educational variables, the diverse nature of various efforts, the lack of standardized feedback, and the intricacy of the infectious diseases decision-making process. Nonetheless, several generalizations can be culled from the existing literature. Individual instruction by an antibiotic-utilization expert appears to be the most successful educational strategy, whereas utilization review is less useful.[15,26] Contemporaneous interventions have a greater impact than those removed from the original antibiotic order by space and time. However, in the absence of continuous reinforcement, all results extinguish rapidly.[30,31] Therefore, although education should be the cornerstone of any antimicrobial management program, this approach should not be used as the sole intervention strategy.

Antimicrobial Formulary Restriction

Limiting the availability of agents on formulary is the most direct method to influence antimicrobial utilization; it is a simple way to prohibit the use of newer more expensive antibiotics in favor of older equally effective drugs.[32] The Infectious Diseases Society of America established guidelines for an optimal antimicrobial control program in 1997 with recommendations to (1) determine which antimicrobial(s) to control, (2) develop a method to achieve usage control, (3) determine who will be responsible for maintaining control, (4) develop a method to educate and enroll prescribers in the control process, (5) de-

FIGURE 43-1. Diversity in Antimicrobial Usage. The graph illustrates the percentage of total antibacterial drug use composed of different antibacterial classes at two hospitals. Antibiotic use in hospital number two is more diverse than in hospital number one.

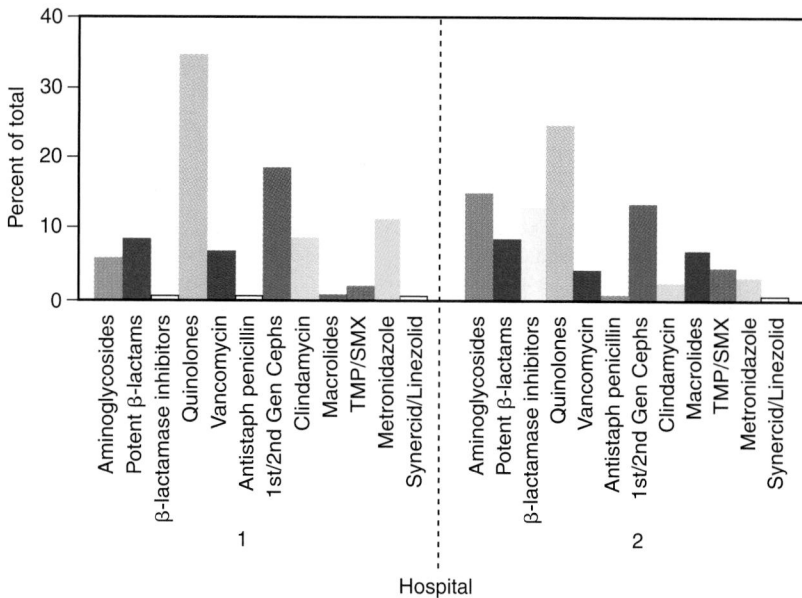

velop a system to measure use of controlled and uncontrolled antimicrobials, (6) develop a method to determine antimicrobial use per geographic area per unit time, and (7) develop a method to ensure that clinical care will not be harmed by control measures.[33]

One of the landmark studies in this area was published by Woodward and colleagues in 1987.[34] Use of a restricted formulary resulted in cost savings of $34,597 per month for restricted agents and $24,620 per month for all antibiotics ($P < 0.03$), with no adverse impact on the clinical outcomes of patients with bacteremia or a variety of other infections. Before implementation, unnecessarily expensive agents were prescribed 37% of the time, compared with just 2% of the time during the study period. Therefore, they were able to demonstrate that the restriction of certain agents could result in significant cost savings without decreasing the quality of patient care. Conversely, a study by Himmelberg and associates evaluated the impact of removing long-standing formulary restrictions at a university hospital.[35] Antimicrobial expenditures escalated by 103% during the study. Imipenem-cilastatin accounted for the greatest proportion of the increase, with costs rising from $44,423 to $126,332 annually, whereas expenditures for unrestricted drugs did not change appreciably. Although the study was not designed to test this hypothesis, the results imply that the increase was due to unnecessary use of formerly restricted agents and not substitution of drugs. Antimicrobial formulary restriction is a simple and effective means of controlling drug costs without resulting in adverse patient outcomes and should be included in most antimicrobial management schemes.

Prior-Approval Programs

Multiple innovative prior-approval or justification approaches have been designed to improve the utilization of antibiotics. These include telephone-approval mechanisms, antibiotic order forms, automatic stop orders, direct interaction with an antimicrobial management team, implementation of control categories, and simple chart entry.

McGowan and Finland were the first to use telephone calls for justification by prescribers and approval by infectious diseases physicians to limit the use of systemic antimicrobial agents.[36] Most approvals were given by telephone, and formal consultation was generally not required. Chloramphenicol prescription rates demonstrated the most dramatic results of this program, with annual usage decreasing from 20,000 to 3000 g. Recco and colleagues were the first to demonstrate the economic impact of a prior-approval program.[37] These researchers also utilized a telephone-approval mechanism, but disagreements necessitated consultation with an infectious diseases physician. A concomitant educational program was implemented as well. Antimicrobial expenditures decreased by $131,826 during the first year, and savings were sustained during the initial 3 years reported in

the study. In addition, inappropriate use of antibiotics was curtailed significantly. Antibiotic order forms also have effected similar improvements in the use of anti-infectives for empirical and prophylactic purposes.[38] However, order forms should be used in conjunction with a restricted formulary, and the forms should be reviewed regularly to document reporting accuracy.

The final landmark study in this category was conducted by Coleman and colleagues and was the first effort to critically analyze reductions in antibiotic expenditures in a long-term fashion among many different clinical syndromes.[39] They collected baseline data for 18 months before instituting four categories of restricted usage (cephalosporins, penicillins, aminoglycosides, and miscellaneous agents) and maximal dosage guidelines for seven drugs. In addition, a review of treatment plans was required before the pharmacy could distribute drugs. The program yielded savings of $7600 per month ($91,200 annually). The doses and cost of antibiotics decreased for pneumonia, urinary tract infection, and septicemia, but increased for cellulitis. The cost per treatment day, the cost per admission, and the total number of doses all differed significantly from those in the prestudy period. The length of therapy did not differ between the pre- and postrestriction intervals. The most significant decreases in use were seen with cefoxitin and clindamycin, whereas the largest increases were demonstrated with ticarcillin-clavulanate and cefotetan.

Obviously, enforcement of a prior-approval program can be difficult, and the process may be viewed as a punitive exercise. Therefore, it is important to stress that the major goal of such efforts is to improve the care of patients.[17,21] Although these strategies are the most onerous to prescribing physicians, they undoubtedly are the most effective single interventions to change or improve usage patterns and to control the antimicrobial budget.[26]

Switch Therapy and Streamlining Programs

In private practices, infectious diseases physicians are not enthusiastic about restricting antibiotics because of concerns that the policies will place them in a policing role and thereby damage their traditional referral patterns.[25] Programs to switch patients from intravenous to oral therapy (also called step-down therapy) and streamlining programs (a change from broad-spectrum and combination therapy to narrow-spectrum therapy) tend to be less onerous. The feasibility of switch therapy has been investigated primarily in the management of pulmonary infections. Early studies demonstrate significant savings in drug costs, as well as decreased lengths of stay[40] and a decreased incidence of catheter-related infections.[41]

An antibiotic optimization program at Maine Medical Center has been evaluated in a randomized controlled trial, with promising results.[42] Patients receiving 1 or more of 10 designated parenteral antibiotics for 3 days or more were randomized to either an intervention or a control group. The intervention group, consisting of an infectious diseases fellow and a clinical pharmacist, suggested changes in therapy for nearly half of the patients evaluated, and most (84%) were accepted. The majority involved a switch to oral therapy. Antibiotic charges were $400 less per patient in the intervention group, which can be extrapolated to annual savings of $390,000.

There was no difference in clinical outcomes between the two groups, and duration of hospitalization was not significantly different. The largest and most ambitious study of switch therapy produced somewhat more modest results.[43] A seven-hospital, cluster randomized trial evaluated outcomes of patients admitted for treatment of community-acquired pneumonia. The intervention was designed to switch patients to oral therapy, to discharge as early as medically feasible, and to assess medical outcomes. The physicians responsible for treatment of patients randomized to the control arm of 325 patients received only a practice guideline via the mail. The intervention arm of 283 patients received a "multifaceted guideline intervention," consisting of daily monitoring of the patients' status to meet criteria for conversion to oral therapy and early discharge. Verbal and written interventions were made daily to the responsible physician as appropriate. There were non-significant trends toward earlier conversion to oral therapy ($P = .06$) and earlier discharge ($P = .11$), but medical complications were significantly fewer in the intervention group ($P = .04$). There were no differences in morbidity or mortality between the groups.

Comprehensive antibiotic management programs at single hospitals continue to report that switch therapy is an important component of the program, especially when the switch program is expanded to patients beyond CAP.[7] This study also reported that the management program resulted in significantly earlier institution of appropriate antimicrobial therapy ($P = .003$) but that streamlining was already performed in the majority of patients and the program made no appreciable improvement.

Although streamlining is usually considered to be a change to a more narrow-spectrum agent, discontinuing therapy when none is indicated is an important goal of any management program.[44] Hecker and colleagues reviewed 1941 days of antimicrobial therapy in 129 patients and reported that 30% of the days represented unnecessary therapy, mostly related to excessive treatment duration or treatment for nonbacterial syndromes.[45] In addition, drugs with antianaerobic activity were often prescribed when an anaerobic spectrum was not indicated. The authors argued that, when indicated, streamlining to therapy with primarily aerobic activity would reduce the prevalence of VRE that is linked to antianaerobic drugs. Innovative and aggressive programs to limit the duration of therapy to 3 days in patients suspected of having ventilator-associated pneumonia, but with less severe infection scores, have been evaluated.[46] There were significantly fewer superinfections in the short-duration arm and a near-significant lower mortality ($P = .06$).

The most effective antibiotic management programs will likely have switch therapy, streamlining therapy, and early termination of inappropriate therapy as important adjuncts to the restriction and prior-approval components of their programs.

Computer-Assisted Management Programs

The computer has the potential to be the ultimate method for antibiotic stewardship and education. Computer order entry affords a unique opportunity for instantaneous feedback, education, and alteration in prescription patterns.[47] A group of researchers headed by Evans, Pestotnik, and Classen at the LDS Hospital in Salt Lake City have been the leaders in developing this field.[16,48] They developed a computerized decision-support program that is linked to computer-based patient records. The program presents epidemiological information, detailed information, and warnings and assists in the selection of anti-infective regimens and courses of therapy for patients.

The system has been prospectively studied for 1 year in a 12-bed intensive care unit.[16] When compared with the management of patients admitted to the same unit during the 2 years before the intervention period, computer-assisted antimicrobial selection led to significant reductions in orders for drugs to which the patient had reported allergies (35 versus 146; $P < 0.01$), excess drug dosages (87 versus 405; $P < 0.01$), and mismatches of antibiotic susceptibility (12 versus 206, $P < 0.01$). There were also marked reductions in the mean number of days of excessive drug dosage and in adverse events caused by antimicrobial agents. Additionally, those patients treated with regimens that were recommended by the computer program demonstrated significant reductions in anti-infective costs, total hospital costs, and the length of stay compared with the control groups. This computer-assisted management program is commercially available and is designed to be integrated into the hospital information system (www.theradoc.com).

Multidisciplinary Approaches

The review by John and Fishman readily demonstrates that multidisciplinary programs offer the best potential for sustained improvements in both clinical and economic outcomes.[26] DeLisle and Perl have described the framework needed to develop a multidisciplinary antibiotic management program.[49] Approaches that utilized four or more strategies appeared to be the most effective. For example, the Antimicrobial Management Program at Hartford Hospital emphasizes formulary streamlining reinforced by formulary restriction and review, antibiotic order forms, and educational efforts.[32] In addition, such programs tend to be more readily accepted because they involve input from a variety of hospital services, including the departments of infectious diseases, clinical pharmacy, infection control, clinical microbiology, nursing, and hospital administration. The team approach supports the implementation of multiple strategies and offers the best option for sustained success.[50]

OUTCOMES OF ANTIMICROBIAL MANAGEMENT PROGRAMS

In assessing whether comprehensive antimicrobial management programs are effective, one must consider both clinical and institutional (economic) outcomes. Although the preponderance of evidence supports the positive impact of such efforts, it is important to recognize that the literature is of "limited strength."[50] A recent systematic review of the quality of the literature describing methods to improve antibiotic use in hospitals found that only 30% of 306 papers met the minimum inclusion criteria for a Cochrane review.[51]

Clinical Outcomes

The best evidence for improved clinical outcomes resulting from an antimicrobial management strategy comes from the computerized antibiotic assistant at LDS Hospital in Salt Lake City discussed earlier.[16] Additional data come from a retrospective review before and after the initiation of a prior-approval program at Indiana University Medical Center.[51] In this review, Frank and co-workers found statistically significant decreases in the rates of enterococcal bacteremia (0.34 versus 0.16 events per 1000 patient-days), selected gram-negative bacteremias (0.26 versus 0.11), methicillin-resistant *S. aureus* colonization or infection (0.66 versus 0.20), and *Stenotrophomonas* colonization or infection (0.35 versus 0.17). The program also resulted in a decrease in antimicrobial expenditures from $2,486,902 to $1,701,522. The effort resulted in improved clinical outcomes in the form of significant decreases in rates of selected nosocomial infections due to resistant organisms coupled with substantial cost savings.

Further support can be found in the results of a randomized controlled trial designed to assess the clinical and economic outcomes of a comprehensive antimicrobial management program compared with required approval by the Infectious Disease fellow at the Hospital of the University of Pennsylvania.[52] A summary of the results of the univariate analysis is shown in Table 43-2. The program resulted in an improved cure rate, a decreased failure rate, and more appropriate use of antimicrobial agents as judged by adherence to institutional guidelines. Although a large multicenter trial of various interventions is

TABLE 43-2 Comparison of Antimicrobial Treatment Managed by an AMT or by ID Fellows

	No. Patients Whose Treatment was Managed by			
Outcome	AMT (n = 87)	ID Fellows (n = 93)	Unadjusted OR (95% CI)	P
Appropriate	76	44	7.7 (3.7-16.2)	<.001
Cure	49	35	2.4 (1.3-4.5)	.007
Failure	13	26	0.5 (0.2-0.9)	.03

AMT, Antimicrobial management team; CI, confidence interval; ID, Division of Infectious Diseases.

From Gross R, Morgan AS, Kinky DE, et al. Impact of a hospital-based antimicrobial management program on clinical and economic outcomes. Clin Infect Dis. 2001;33:289-295.

lacking, the majority of published evidence demonstrates a beneficial impact of antimicrobial management programs on patient outcomes.

Economic Outcomes

It is clear from the discussion of antimicrobial management strategies that most published reports demonstrate successful cost containment. However, if savings are calculated as a function of pharmacy expenditures, they tend to plateau over time; this likely is a function of improved antimicrobial utilization practices and sustained benefits of the program. In order to address this issue, Gross and colleagues developed a probability pathway model to calculate both the direct and the indirect cost savings of a management program.[53] In this model, total cost was defined as the sum of drug expenditures, microbiology costs, bed costs, and the costs of infectious diseases consultations; additional costs accrued if the initial antibiotic regimen failed. The median drug costs per recommendation were $50 lower for the antimicrobial management program compared with usual practice, and total costs were $379 lower per recommendation. Using the probability pathway model, this annualizes to savings of $363,000 in antibiotic expenditures and $2.7 million in total costs.

DO ANTIMICROBIAL MANAGEMENT PROGRAMS PREVENT THE EMERGENCE OF RESISTANCE?

The effectiveness of antimicrobial control as a means to prevent the emergence of resistance has been reviewed in detail.[54,55] Available studies are suggestive but not conclusive about the efficacy of this approach.[53,54] The shortcomings of published studies include the presence of selection biases, a small sample size, a limitation to single institutions, and a failure to control for confounding variables.[54] In addition, most studies utilized a "before and after" design and do not follow trends in antibiotic use or resistance for a sufficient period before and after the intervention to establish a casual relationship.[51] However, recent data suggest benefits from attention to inappropriate antimicrobial utilization.

White and colleagues instituted a prior-authorization program in response to an epidemic of multidrug-resistant *Acinetobacter* in the surgical intensive care unit of their institution that did not respond to routine infection control interventions.[56] Susceptibilities to all β-lactam and fluoroquinolone antibiotics increased, with dramatically increased susceptibilities in isolates recovered in intensive care units, increased susceptibilities in isolates recovered in other inpatient sites, and little change in susceptibilities in isolates recovered in outpatient sites.[55] These changes occurred despite a lack of change in infection control practices. In addition, antimicrobial expenditures decreased by 32%, and neither patient outcomes nor the length of hospital stay was compromised. Furthermore, when the program was administratively disbanded, antimicrobial resistance rates increased. Reimplementation of the program once again resulted in improved rates of resistance (A.C. White, personal communication).

In 1999 Landman and colleagues reported their experience at the Department of Veterans Affairs Medical Center at Brooklyn.[57] In an attempt to contain an outbreak of vancomycin-resistant enterococci

(VRE), the use of third-generation cephalosporins, vancomycin, and clindamycin required prior approval from a member of the infectious diseases division, and use of β-lactam/β-lactamase inhibitors was encouraged. Coincident with marked changes in antibiotic use, the incidence of methicillin-resistant *Staphylococcus aureus* (MRSA) and ceftazidime-resistant *Klebsiella pneumoniae* decreased significantly. Unexpectedly however, the incidence of cefotaxime-resistant *Acinetobacter* infections increased significantly, an early example of what has become known as "squeezing the balloon."[57]

Rahal and colleagues attempted to control an outbreak of extended-spectrum beta-lactamase (ESBL)–producing *Klebsiella* infections by requiring prior approval for use of most third-generation cephalosporins in 1996 at the New York Hospital Medical Center of Queens.[58] During this time imipenem use increased while cephalosporin usage declined by 80%. Coincident with these changes, there was a 44% decline in the incidence of ceftazidime-resistant *Klebsiella* colonization and infections, but there was a corresponding 69% increase in the incidence of imipenem-resistant *P. aeruginosa*. A follow-up report from these authors in 2002 emphasized that the appropriate response to emerging resistance should be individualized to the institution, depending on whether one wishes to prevent emergence of resistance or to contain and eliminate an outbreak.[59] In either case, multiple methods should be employed when appropriate, including education, infection control efforts, and antibiotic use management.

Additional support of a positive correlation between limiting antibiotic use and preventing the emergence of resistance can be found in the Finnish experience with group A streptococci.[60] In the early 1990s, there was an increase in erythromycin resistance among this organism in Finland. In response, nationwide recommendations were issued that called for reductions in the use of macrolides for respiratory and skin infections in outpatients. Consumption of macrolide antibiotics decreased from 2.40 defined daily doses per 1000 inhabitants per day in 1991 to 1.38 in 1992 ($P = 0.007$). The change in consumption was followed by a steady decrease in the frequency of erythromycin resistance among group A streptococcal isolates from throat swabs and pus samples.

Fridkin and colleagues have investigated relationships between antibiotic use in hospital intensive care units (ICUs) and resistance profiles, using the Centers for Disease Control and Prevention (CDC) database, National Nosocomial Infections Surveillance (NNIS) program, and Project ICARE.[61] When 50 ICUs from 20 hospitals each received risk-adjusted (by ICU type) measures of vancomycin use, some ICUs decreased vancomycin use over the following 2 years. The provision of relative measures of antibiotic use to an institution is often called "benchmarking," and some have postulated that once a hospital becomes aware that use of a particular antibiotic is "excessive," measures will be taken to reduce use. There was a significant association between changes in vancomycin use and changes in the prevalence of VRE in these ICUs, suggesting that benchmarking programs may be another method to change prescribing practices and impact favorably on rates of resistance.

These reports are increasing in number and are promising. They suggest that attention to antimicrobial use may produce a favorable impact on the emergence of resistance. However, the relationships between antibiotic use in the hospital and rates of resistant organisms is complex, and further work is needed to evaluate the role that infection control and community factors play in other institutions, including acute care settings and long-term care facilities.[21]

ADDITIONAL STRATEGIES

Homogeneity in Antimicrobial Prescribing

A restricted formulary—also called a "closed" formulary—tends to result in more homogeneous antimicrobial use from fewer antimicrobial classes. Clinical practice guidelines that encourage use of a specific drug or drugs for an infection also promote less variability in antimicrobial use. Several investigators have suggested that these guidelines and restrictions may actually promote resistance because bacteria are exposed to a limited number of agents.[20,46,58] The implication is that greater variability in antimicrobial use, associated with an "open" or unrestricted formulary, may be less likely to select for resistant organisms. Greater heterogeneity in use can be viewed as "random rotation" of antibiotic usage across the entire hospital. There are few experimental data to support one position or the other.[63] As hospitals adopt the electronic database it will soon be possible to routinely measure antibiotic consumption, and to determine patterns and variability in antibiotic use. Figure 43-1 illustrates antibiotic consumption by electronic capture of billing records in two hospitals. Both hospitals have restricted formularies, but antibiotic use is very different, indicating that the terms "open" and "closed" formularies are of little value in describing actual usage. Interestingly, mathematical models predict that a heterogeneous and balanced pattern of antibiotic use will result in lower rates of resistance than antibiotic cycling (see below).[62,64] Limited and preliminary data suggest that hospitals with greater diversity in antimicrobial use are associated with lower rates of resistance for selected nosocomial pathogens,[63] but much more work is needed to determine if this is a feasible strategy to delay emergence of resistance in hospitals.

Antibiotic Rotation (Cycling)

Concerns for increasing resistance in nosocomial pathogens have led to the suggestion that antibiotics be rotated or cycled in the various hospital units. The rationale behind cycling is that as bacteria in an ICU or hospital acquire new resistance genes directed against a predominant antibiotic, a new antibiotic is introduced into the environment to which the organism is susceptible. The new antibiotic will eradicate the merging pathogen and the process is then repeated throughout each cycle.[44] Guidelines for appropriate cycling investigations have been developed,[64] but there are few data available to help assess the potential impact of such schemes.

The earliest attempt to cycle antibiotics was performed by Gerding in the mid-1980s.[65,66] The dominant aminoglycoside used in a midwestern hospital cycled between gentamicin and amikacin, and the rates of aminoglycoside resistance among gram-negative bacteria during each cycle were monitored. There was a temporal association between greater gentamicin use and a greater prevalence of resistance over a number of cycles, and resistance rates decreased during the amikacin cycle. Although this investigation would not meet the current requirements for a rigorous study design, it set an optimistic stage for additional investigations.

Kollef and colleagues switched empirical therapy of suspected gram-negative infections in cardiac surgery from ceftazidime to ciprofloxacin at 6-month intervals.[67] Subsequently they demonstrated a decrease in the incidence of ventilator-associated pneumonia from 11.6% to 6.7%; pneumonia caused by antibiotic-resistant gram-negative bacilli decreased from 4% to 0.9%. Although there was a trend toward a lower incidence of bacteremia with resistant gram-negative organisms, the total incidence of bacteremia did not decline.[68] Additionally, the use of postoperative antibiotics did not decrease despite fewer suspected and proven infections during the study period; this may indicate an increase in inappropriate use. Many more questions are engendered than answered in this study.

Gruson and colleagues reported results from an antibiotic cycling investigation in a French hospital.[68] Ciprofloxacin and ceftazidime use was severely restricted, and monthly cycles of other agents including cefipime and piperacillin/tazobactam were promoted.[69] The authors reported that rates of resistance decreased for selected organisms as a result of cycling. This investigation, however, had a number of confounding variables that have made the interpretation of the results problematic, including implementation of alcohol-based hand washing during the investigation.[44,69] A CDC-sponsored multicenter 3-year trial will likely provide the most compelling evidence for or against cycling, but preliminary reports that the scheduled cycling regimen could not be given in up to 50% of patients because of allergy or other contraindications suggest that even this investigation may not be able to sort out the relevant variables.[70] One report of a beneficial effect of cycling[71] has been criticized because both an antimicrobial management team and alcohol-based hand washes were introduced during the study.[44] At least one additional report failed to exhibit any benefit of a rotation scheme.[72]

The identification of the correct antibiotics to be cycled, the duration of cycles, and the preferred order of rotation all remain unknown. In addition, there are compelling reasons to believe cycling may not be able to significantly impact on resistance, including the multidrug-resistant nature of many nosocomial pathogens.[69] At this time there is little evidence to support the routine rotation or cycling of antimicrobial agents.

Formulary Decisions and Antibiotic Resistance

The purchase cost of adding a new drug to the formulary has historically been the focus of pharmacy and therapeutics committee deliberations. Cost includes not only the purchase costs, but also costs of administration, adverse effects, and monitoring. However, as the costs of antibiotic resistance are increasingly appreciated, and as strategies are devised to accurately characterize these costs,[72] additional issues are raised.

For example, are there differences between antibiotic classes in the propensity to select for resistance? Patterson and Rice argue that third-generation cephalosporins may be most likely to result in resistance problems, and it is possible that selection of a different class of antibiotic for routine use may forestall resistance.[44] It is also possible that there are important differences in propensity to cause resistance within an antibiotic class. Arguments have been put forth that preferential use of the most potent fluoroquinolone for treatment of respiratory tract infections caused by *Streptococcus pneumoniae*, such as moxifloxacin or gatifloxacin instead of levofloxacin, will delay or prevent the emergence of resistant strains.[73] In addition to intrinsic differences in potency between agents for a particular pathogen, it is also possible that dose optimization using pharmacodynamic principles may help delay emergence of resistance during therapy for some organisms.[74] All of these issues are in early stages of investigation, and there are few experimental data to justify formulary decisions based solely on their consideration. However, as data accumulate, new strategies to effectively use antimicrobial drugs while minimizing the probability of resistance will become increasingly important.

DESIGN AND IMPLEMENTATION

A summary of guidelines for the design and implementation of a successful antimicrobial management program is listed in Table 43-3 and described in this section.[26,48,50]

1. Define the philosophy of the program. This may seem to be a trivial step, but the initial approach defined at this early time is likely to form the foundation for the success or failure of the program. Although most physicians generally understand that resistance is important, increasing in scope, and costly, they do not necessarily agree that the care of individual patients affects this issue. However, antibiotic misuse more often results from inadequate information than from inappropriate behavior.[20] Therefore, physicians are more likely to respond to a program designed to "improve" antibiotic use or patient care, rather than to an effort to "restrict" or "control" antimicrobials or solely to decrease costs. Most physicians will alter their behavior to improve the quality of patient care (JE McGowan Jr, personal communication).

TABLE 43-3 Guidelines for the Design and Implementation of an Antimicrobial Management Program

Define philosophy of program
Gather baseline data
Define structure of program
Develop budget
Meet with hospital administrators
Evaluate antimicrobial formulary for redundancy
Develop and publish guidelines for antimicrobial use
Define intervention strategies
Develop mechanisms to arbitrate disagreements
Develop innovative educational methods
Develop and maintain database
Continually reevaluate program

FIGURE 43-2. Organizational structure of a comprehensive antimicrobial management program. *(Adapted from John JF Jr, Fishman NO. Programmatic role of the infectious diseases physician in controlling antimicrobial costs in the hospitals. Clin Infect Dis. 1997;24:471.)*

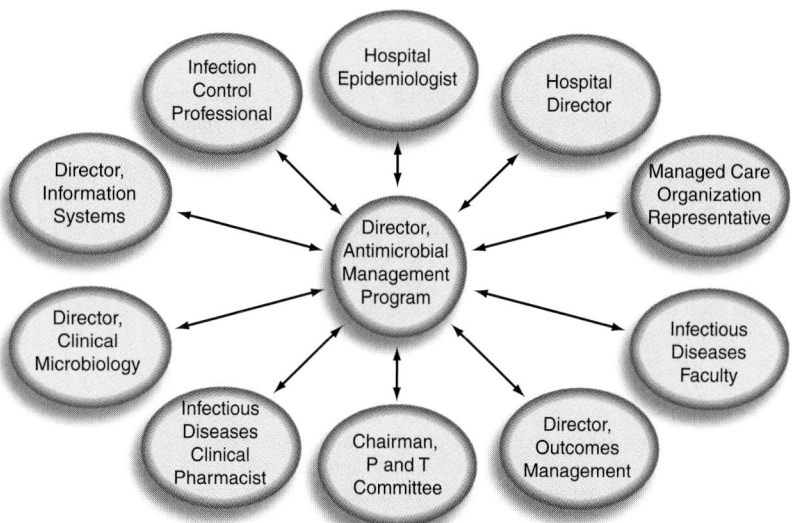

2. Gather baseline data concerning antimicrobial expenditures, antimicrobial utilization patterns, and susceptibilities of nosocomial and community pathogens. Benchmark the antimicrobial budget and antimicrobial use to equivalent institutions. The most appropriate measure of hospital antibiotic use is the defined daily dose/1000 patient-days (DDD/1000 PD).[75]

3. Define the structure of participation in the antimicrobial management program. An example of a comprehensive program is diagrammed in Figure 43-2. The minimal requirements for an effective team include an infectious diseases physician, an infectious diseases clinical pharmacist, the director of clinical microbiology, and the hospital epidemiologist.

4. Develop a budget for all official positions and operating costs.

5. Involve hospital administrators early in the design and implementation process, and clarify budgetary issues. Agree upon a formula to calculate cost savings. It may be prudent to involve managed-care organizations in these discussions if they are at risk for pharmacy costs. The support of key officials is critical to the success of the program. Physicians are more likely to comply with a health system effort rather than with an infectious diseases or pharmacy program that may be perceived to have predominantly financial motives. Maintain an open dialogue with chief administrative personnel and update them frequently concerning the progress of the program.

6. Evaluate the antimicrobial formulary for redundancy and seek competitive bidding between therapeutic equivalents.

7. Develop and publish guidelines for antibiotic use and empirical antimicrobial therapy. Recommendations should be based on local susceptibility profiles. Additionally, establish appropriate dosing and dosage intervals based on disease-state and pharmacokinetic principles. This step is critical to the success of the program. Involve key personnel from all departments when designing the guidelines in order to build consensus for the program. Be willing to compromise on certain issues, but demand that all recommendations be evidence based. It is also worthwhile to consider multimedia formats. For example, we have posted University of Pennsylvania guidelines on the Internet and have included links to relevant articles, as well as other educational materials.[76] It is also useful to publish reports of antimicrobial susceptibility and price lists along with the clinical guidelines.

8. Define the strategies that the program will use. As previously discussed, multidisciplinary efforts offer the greatest potential for sustained improvements. However, interventions must be tailored to the character of the institution. For example, telephone-approval mechanisms are less likely to be successful at a community hospital staffed by busy private practitioners. Begin with a focus on the most frequently used and most costly agents.

9. Develop mechanisms to arbitrate disagreements. A discussion between the prescriber and the director of the program is usually sufficient, if the director has administrative time to handle these issues. A mandatory infectious diseases consultation is another viable option.

10. Develop innovative educational methods. We have found the Internet to be a useful tool in this regard.[76] Information systems personnel may be helpful in incorporating guidelines, recommendations, or reminders into the hospital computer network.

11. Develop and maintain a database to follow clinical and institutional outcomes.

12. Continually reevaluate the program, paying particular attention to changes in susceptibility profiles and patterns of use. Drug-utilization evaluations should be a part of this process. Reformulate the program as indicated to address problems as they arise. This should be a dynamic process that is responsive to the needs of prescribers and their patients.

FUNDING

It is clear from the data presented previously that the cost savings from comprehensive antimicrobial management efforts can easily offset the budget of the program. Minimal requirements include support by a part-time physician and a full-time clinical pharmacist. New salary lines for antimicrobial management are beginning to emerge nationally.[26] There are three options for support: (1) defined compensation; (2) payment on a time basis for consultative services; and (3) negotiation as a percentage of the cost savings. Toward this end it is critical to gather baseline data and to define a formula to calculate cost savings before implementing a program. The method and amount of compensation will vary with the size and setting of the program. Managed-care organizations may offer additional options for funding, particularly if the program expands to the ambulatory setting or oversees devices used to treat infections.

THE FUTURE

Health care is changing. Providers are challenged to deliver high-quality care in an increasingly cost-constrained environment. This requires limiting cost-increasing technology while improving patient and population health outcomes. Although the data are limited, comprehensive antimicrobial management programs have the potential to decrease costs while improving both patient and institutional outcomes. However, further work is needed to clearly identify the relationship between antimicrobial use and the emergence of resistance in a way that colleagues will appreciate and accept.[77] Relevant studies will require sufficient statistical power to describe baseline resistance, to deal with limits of random variation, and to control for a multitude of confounding variables (J. E. McGowan Jr, personal communication). It is likely that a multicenter trial will be necessary to accomplish these tasks.

In addition, we also must begin to focus on issues of antimicrobial use and the emergence of resistance throughout the entire health care system. As these systems expand and become a prominent feature of medical practice in the United States, it is no longer sufficient to consider infection solely in the context of the acute care hospital. Rather, health care must be viewed in the larger context of acute care, extended care, and ambulatory components of the integrated delivery system.[21] Therefore, future efforts to improve the use of antimicrobial agents and studies to document efficacy must be expanded to include these arenas.

The high cost of antimicrobial drugs remains an important reason to implement management procedures as described in this chapter. However, the rising prevalence of resistance and its clinical and economic impact are increasingly noticed by all clinicians and administrators. Since few new drugs will become available for these multidrug-resistant pathogens, the therapeutic options will become increasingly limited or nonexistent. The focus on antimicrobial management strategies will continue to shift from cost containment to efforts to limit resistance. However antibiotic management is defined, measures summarized in this chapter will increasingly become the responsibility of all clinicians.

REFERENCES

1. Jawetz E. Antimicrobial chemotherapy. Annu Rev Microbiol. 1956;10:85.
2. Achong MR, Hauser BA, Krusky JL. Rational and irrational use of antibiotics in a Canadian teaching hospital. Can Med Assoc J. 1977;116:256.
3. Maki DG, Schuna AA. A study of antimicrobial misuse in a university hospital. Am J Med Sci. 1978;275:271.
4. Roberts AW, Visconti JA. The rational and irrational use of systemic antimicrobial drugs. Am J Hosp Pharm. 1972;29:828.
5. Scheckler WE, Bennett JV. Antibiotic use in seven community hospitals. JAMA. 1970;213:264.
6. Hecker MT, Aron DC, Patel NP, et al. Unnecessary use of antimicrobials in hospitalized patients. Arch Int Med. 2003;163:972-978.
7. Vogtlander NPJ, van Kasteren MEE, Natsch S, Kullberg BJ, et al. Improving the process of antibiotic therapy in daily practice: Interventions to optimize timing, dosage adjustment to renal function, and switch therapy. Arch Intern Med. 2004;164:1206-1212.
8. Col NF, O'Connor RW. Estimating world-wide current antibiotic usage; report of task force. 1. Rev Infect Dis. 1987;9(Suppl):S232.
9. Craig WA, Sarver KP. Antimicrobial usage in the USA. In: Williams JD, Geddes AM, eds. Chemotherapy, v. 4. New York: Plenum; 1976:293.
10. Craig WA, Uman SJH, Shaw WR, et al. Hospital use of antimicrobial drugs: Survey of 19 hospitals and results of antimicrobial control programs. Ann Intern Med. 1978;89:793.
11. Cosgrove S, Carmelli Y. The impact of antimicrobial resistance on health and economic outcomes. Clin Inf Dis. 2003;36:1433-1437.
12. McGowan JE Jr. Antimicrobial resistance in hospital organisms and its relation to antibiotic use. Rev Infect Dis. 1983;5:1033.
13. McGowan JE Jr. Changing etiology of nosocomial bacteremia and fungemia and other hospital-acquired infections. Rev Infect Dis. 1985;7(Suppl):S357.
14. Archibald L, Phillips L, Monnet D, et al. Antimicrobial resistance in isolates from inpatients and outpatients in the United States: Increasing importance of the intensive care unit. Clin Infect Dis. 1997;24:211.
15. Avorn J, Solomon DH. Cultural and economic factors that (mis)shape antibiotic use: The (non)pharmacologic basis of therapeutics. Ann Intern Med. 2000;133:128-135.
16. Evans RS, Pestotnik SL, Classen DC, et al. A computer-assisted management program for antibiotics and other antiinfective agents. N Engl J Med. 1998;338:232.
17. Kunin CM. Problems in antibiotic usage. In: Mandell GL, Douglas RG Jr, Bennett JE, eds. Principles and Practice of Infectious Diseases, 3rd ed. New York: Churchill Livingstone; 1990;427.
18. Centers for Disease Control and Prevention. Defining the public health impact of drug-resistant *Streptococcus pneumoniae:* Report of a working group. MMWR Morb Mortal Wkly Rep. 1996;45(RR-1):1-14.
19. Shapiro M, Townsend TR, Rosner B, Kass EH. Use of antimicrobial drugs in general hospitals: Patterns of prophylaxis. N Engl J Med. 1979;301:351.
20. Burke JP. Antibiotic resistance-squeezing the balloon? JAMA. 1998;280:1270.
21. McGowan JE Jr. Minimizing antimicrobial resistance: The key role of the infectious diseases physician. Clin Infect Dis. 2004;38:939-942.
22. Rice L. Collateral damage. Ann Int Med. 2003;139:523-524.
23. Klapp DL, Ramphal R. Antibiotic restriction in hospitals associated with medical schools. Am J Hosp Pharm. 1983;40:1957.
24. Lawton RM, Fridkin SK, Gaynes RP, McGowan JE Jr. Practices to improve antimicrobial use at 47 US hospitals: The status of the 1997 SHEA/IDSA position paper recommendations. Society for Healthcare Epidemiology of America/Infectious Diseases Society of America. Infect Control Hosp Epidemiol. 2000;21:256-259.
25. Sunenshine RH, Liedtke LA, Jernigan DB, Strausbaugh LJ, for the Infectious Diseases Society of America Emerging Infections Network. Role of infectious diseases consultants in management of antimicrobial use in hospitals. Clin Infect Dis. 2004;38:934-938.
26. John JF, Fishman NO. Programmatic role of the infectious diseases physician in controlling antimicrobial costs in the hospital. Clin Infect Dis. 1997;24:471.
27. Kunin CM, Johansen KS, Worning AM, Daschner FD. Report of a symposium on use and abuse of antibiotics worldwide. Rev Infect Dis. 1990;12:12.
28. Neu HC, Howrey SP. Testing the physician's knowledge of antibiotic use: Self-assessment and learning via videotape. N Engl J Med. 1975;293:1291.
29. Barclay LP, Hation RH, Doering PL, Shands JW. Physicians' perceptions and knowledge of drug costs: Results of a survey. Formulary. 1995;30:268.
30. Gilbert DN, Eubanks NM, Jackson JM. The effects of monitoring the use of gentamicin in a community hospital. J Med Educ. 1978;53:129.
31. Jones SR, Pannell J, Barks J, et al. The effect of an educational program upon hospital antibiotic use. Am J Med Sci. 1977;273:79.
32. Crowe HM, Quintiliani R. Antibiotic formulary selection. Med Clin North Am. 1995;79:463.
33. Shlaes DM, Gerding DN, John JF, et al. Society for Healthcare Epidemiology of America and Infectious Diseases Society of America Joint Committee on the Prevention of Antimicrobial Resistance: Guidelines for the prevention of antimicrobial resistance in hospitals. Clin Infect Dis. 1997;25:584-599.
34. Woodward RS, Medoff G, Smith MD, Gray JL III. Antibiotic cost savings from formulary restrictions and physician monitoring in a medical school–affiliated hospital. Am J Med. 1987;83:817.
35. Himmelberg CJ, Pleasants RA, Weber DJ, et al. Use of antimicrobial drugs before and after removal of a restriction policy. Am J Hosp Pharm. 1991;48:1220.
36. McGowan JE Jr, Finland M. Usage of antibiotics in a general hospital: Effect of requiring justification. J Infect Dis. 1974;130:165.
37. Recco RA, Gladstone JL, Friedman SA, Gerken EH. Antibiotic control in a municipal hospital. JAMA. 1979;241:2283.
38. Durbin WA Jr, Lapidas B, Goldmann DA. Improved antibiotic usage following introduction of a novel prescription system. JAMA. 1981;246:1796.
39. Coleman RW, Rodondi LC, Kaubisch S, et al. Cost-effectiveness of prospective and continuous parenteral antibiotic control: Experience at the Palo Alto Veterans Affairs Medical Center from 1987 to 1989. Am J Med. 1991;90:439.
40. Ehrenkranz NJ, Nerenberg DE, Shultz JM, Slater KC. Intervention to discontinue parenteral antimicrobial therapy in patients hospitalized with pulmonary infections: Effect on shortening patient stay. Infect Control Hosp Epidemiol. 1992;13:21.
41. Ramirez JA. Switch therapy in community-acquired pneumonia. Diagn Microbiol Infect Dis. 1995;22:219.
42. Fraser GL, Stogsdill P, Dickens JD Jr, et al. Antibiotic optimization: An evaluation of patient safety and economic outcomes. Arch Intern Med. 1997;157:1689.
43. Fine MJ, Stone RA, Lave JR, et al. Implementation of an evidence-based guideline to reduce duration of intravenous antibiotic therapy and length of stay for patients hospitalized with community-acquired pneumonia: A randomized controlled trial. Am J Med. 2003;115:343.
44. Patterson D, Rice L. Empirical antibiotic choice for the seriously ill patient: Are minimization of selection of resistant organisms and maximization of individual outcome mutually exclusive? Clin Infect Dis. 2003;36:1006-1012.
45. Hecker MT, Aron DC, Patel NP, et al. Unnecessary use of antimicrobials in hospitalized patients: Current patterns of misuse with an emphasis on the antianaerobic spectrum of activity. Arch Intern Med. 2003;163:972-978.
46. Singh N, Rogers P, Atwood CW, et al. Short-course empiric antibiotic therapy for patients with pulmonary infiltrates in the intensive care unit: A proposed solution for indiscriminate antibiotic prescription. Am J Respir Crit Care Med. 2000;162:505.
47. Bailey TC, McMullin ST. Using information systems technology to improve antibiotic Prescribing. Crit Care Med. 2001;29(Suppl):N87.
48. Evans RS, Classen DC, Pestotnik SL. Improving empiric antibiotic selection using computer decision support. Arch Intern Med. 1994;154:878.
49. DeLisle S, Perl TM. Antimicrobial management measures to limit resistance: A process-based conceptual framework. Crit Care Med. 2001;29(Suppl 4):N121-N127.
50. Struelens MJ. Multidisciplinary antimicrobial management teams: The way forward to control antimicrobial resistance in hospitals. Curr Opin Infect Dis. 2003;16:305-307.
51. Ramsay C, Brown E, Hartman G, Davey P. Room for improvement: A systematic review of the quality of evaluations of interventions to improve hospital antibiotic prescribing. J Antimicrob Chemother. 2003;52:764-771.
52. Frank MO, Batteiger BE, Sorensen SJ, et al. Decrease in expenditures and selected nosocomial infections following implementation of an antimicrobial-prescribing improvement program. Perform Quality Health Care. 1997;5:180.
53. Gross R, Morgan AS, Kinky DE, et al. Impact of a hospital-based antimicrobial management program on clinical and economic outcomes. Clin Infect Dis. 2001;33:289-295.
54. McGowan JE Jr. Do intensive hospital antibiotic control programs prevent the spread of antibiotic resistance? Infect Control Hosp Epidemiol. 1994;15:478.
55. McGowan JE Jr, Gerding DN. Does antibiotic restriction prevent resistance? New Horiz. 1996;4:370.
56. White AC Jr, Atmar RL, Wilson J, et al. Effects of requiring prior authorization for selected antimicrobials: Expenditures, susceptibilities, and clinical outcomes. Clin Infect Dis. 1997;25:230.
57. Landman D, Chockalingam M, Quale JM. Reduction in the incidence of methicillin-resistant *Staphylococcus aureus* and ceftazidime-resistant *Klebsiella pneumoniae* following changes in a hospital antibiotic formulary. Clin Infectious Dis. 1999;28:1062-1066
58. Rahal JJ, Urban C, Horn D, et al. Class restriction of cephalosporin use to control total cephalosporin resistance in nosocomial *Klebsiella*. JAMA. 1998;280:1233-1237.
59. Rahal JJ, Urban C, Segal-Maurer S. Nosocomial antibiotic resistance in multiple gram-negative species: Experience at one hospital with squeezing the resistance balloon at multiple sites. Clin Infectious Dis. 2002;34:499-503.
60. Seppala H, Klaukka T, Vuopio-Varkila J, et al. The effect of changes in the consumption of macrolide antibiotics on erythromycin resistance in group A streptococci in Finland. N Engl J Med. 1997;337:441.

61. Fridkin SK, Lawton R, Edwards Jr, et al. The Intensive Care Antimicrobial Resistance Epidemiology (ICARE) Project, and the National Nosocomial Infections Surveillance (NNIS) system hospitals. Monitoring antimicrobial use and resistance: Comparison with a national benchmark on reducing vancomycin use and vancomycin-resistant enterococci. Emerg Infect Dis. 2002;8:702-707.

62. Bonhoeffer S, Lipsitch M, Levin BR. Evaluating treatment protocols to prevent antibiotic resistance. Proc Natl Acad Sci U S A. 1997;94:12106-12111.

63. Polk RE, Nichols M, Johnson CK, Edmond M, Wenzel R. Hospitals with "closed" antibiotic formularies are associated with higher rates of bacterial resistance: From the SCOPE-MMIT Antimicrobial Surveillance Network (Abstract K-1352). In: Programs and abstracts of the 42nd Interscience Conference on Antimicrobial Agents and Chemotherapy. San Diego: September 27-30, American Society for Microbiology, 2002.

64. McGowan JE Jr. Strategies for study of the role of cycling on antimicrobial use and resistance. Infect Control Hosp Epidemiol. 2000;21(1 Suppl):S36-S43.

65. Gerding DN. Antimicrobial cycling: Lessons learned from the aminoglycoside experience. Infect Control Hosp Epidemiol. 2000;21(Suppl 1):S2-S7.

66. Gerding DN, Larson TA. Resistance surveillance programs and the incidence of gram-negative bacillary resistance to amikacin from 1967-1985. Am J Med. 1986;80:22-28.

67. Kollef MH, Vlasnik J, Sharpless L, et al. Scheduled change of antibiotic classes: A strategy to decrease the incidence of ventilator-associated pneumonia. Am J Crit Care Med. 1997;156:1040.

68. Gruson D, Hilbert G, Vargas F, et al. Rotation and restricted use of antibiotics in a medical intensive care unit: Impact on the incidence of ventilator-associated pneumonia caused by antibiotic-resistant gram-negative bacteria. Am J Respir Crit Care Med. 2000;162:837-843.

69. Fridkin SK. Routine cycling of antimicrobial agents as an infection-control measure. Clin Infect Dis. 2003;36:1438-1444.

70. Bochorishvili V, Madariaga M, Pur S, et al. Reasons for noncompliance with voluntary cycling of antibiotics (Abstract 109). In: Proceedings of the 40th Annual Meeting of the Infectious Diseases Society of America. Alexandria, Va: Infectious Diseases Society of America, 2002.

71. Raymond DP, Pelletier SJ, Crabtree TD, et al. Impact of a rotating empiric antibiotic schedule on infectious mortality in an intensive care unit. Crit Care Med. 2001;29:1101-1108.

72. Moss WP, Beers MC, Johnson E, et al. Pilot study of antibiotic cycling in a pediatric intensive care unit. Crit Care Med. 2002; 30:1877-1822.

73. Goldstein EJC, Garabedian-Ruffalo SM. Widespread use of fluoroquinolones versus emerging resistance in pneumococci. Clin Infect Dis. 2002;35:1505-1511.

74. Craig WA. Does the dose matter? Clin Infect Dis. 2001;33(Suppl 3):S233-7.

75. ATC/DDD Index 2004. Oslo, Norway: WHO Collaborating Centre for Drug Statistics Methodology, 2004. Available from: URL: http://www.whocc.no/atcddd/indexdatabase/ (Accessed June 21, 2004).

76. Guidelines for antimicrobial therapy at the hospital of the University of Pennsylvania. Available at http://www.uphs.upenn.edu/bugdrug (Accessed June 21, 2004).

77. Moellering RC Jr. Antibiotic resistance: Lessons for the future. Clin Infect Dis. 1998;27(Suppl):S135.

CHAPTER **44**

Interpreting the Results of Clinical Trials on Antimicrobial Agents

JOHN H. POWERS

Although evidence-based medicine has origins that extend back for centuries, the move for clinicians to base treatment decisions for patients upon evidence-based scientific information[1] recently has taken on increased prominence. The use of evidence-based medicine is important for clinicians in their care of patients but also for policy makers and in the development of treatment guidelines. The design and analysis of clinical trials also are important for regulatory agencies in order to make decisions on the licensing of new drugs or expanding the licensing of already marketed drugs. The evidence for clinical decision making may come from personal experience with patients and from various forms of research. Personal experience, however, cannot

control for various confounders that may affect outcomes. In addition, clinicians may have little personal experience with less common diseases. Therefore, the soundest evidence for clinical decision making comes from clinically relevant research, with application of those results to individual patients based on clinical expertise and personal experience. In vitro data, pharmacokinetic studies, and animal research form the building blocks for proofs of principles and important hypotheses concerning drug efficacy and safety. However, clinicians obtain the soundest and most relevant evidence on the efficacy and safety of the treatment and prevention of diseases from randomized controlled clinical trials in humans with the disease under study.[2]

Familiarity with the design and analysis of clinical trials can help clinicians quickly identify trials that may be helpful in clinical decision making. Busy clinicians often have little time to keep up with the medical literature. A comparison of the time necessary to review medical journals compared with the time available for general practitioners showed that clinicians would need to read 19 journal articles per day for 365 days a year to stay current. However, this same study showed clinicians indicated by self-reports that they had well under an hour a week to review new medical information.[1] Many clinicians also now participate in clinical trials as investigators. Familiarity with the design and analysis of trials will help clinicians decide which trials have the greatest chance of benefiting patients in their practice and the greatest potential for showing useful and important results.

The results of trials are intuitively the most interesting, but delving into the methods section of a published paper can at times seem daunting. The statistical descriptions in the methods sections seem far removed from clinical practice. Clinicians often receive little formal training on how to analyze the design and results of a clinical trial. However, it is the design of a trial that determines the applicability of the results to clinical practice.

The purpose of a clinical trial is to determine the efficacy and/or safety of a drug and to distinguish drug effects from other influences such as the natural history of the illness, placebo effect, or biased observations. The basic principle is to hold constant as many factors as possible while varying only the drug administered to the patients in each arm of the trial. In this way, one can attempt to ascribe causality of the results to the drug under study.[3] Elements such as the definition of the disease under study, definitions of the hypothesis of the study, the selection criteria for patients, and the end points examined are crucial in distinguishing the effects of a drug from other sources of bias and confounding factors.[4]

Bias is systematic error that distorts the results of the trial.[5] Random error is error that occurs by chance variation. Both kinds of error may result in conclusions that do not reflect the results that a trial would show in the population as a whole with the disease under study. In designing a trial, the goal of investigators is to minimize or eliminate most if not all biases. If biases cannot be eliminated, it is important to define them so that readers take them into consideration when drawing conclusions from the trial.

Although the results of trials should be clinically relevant, there are important differences between clinical practice and clinical trials. In clinical practice, all patients with a disease may receive treatment by clinicians, but in an effort to limit confounding factors, not all patients are eligible for enrollment in a clinical trial. Investigators commonly perform procedures in clinical trials that are not standard in clinical practice, such as obtaining multiple blood samples at scheduled times or more definitive diagnostic procedures to define the disease under study to more adequately explain the efficacy and safety of a drug.

A useful way to approach interpreting a trial is to follow the same path as a clinical researcher designing and analyzing the trial (Table 44-1). A clinical researcher first needs to define the goals of the trial, which includes the hypothesis tested and the design used in testing that hypothesis. Next, investigators must decide which patients are appropriate for inclusion or exclusion to the trial, which in turn effectively defines the disease and the patient population with the disease under study. The investigator must then decide how to appropriately divide patients into the various treatment arms of the trial and follow them

This chapter represents the opinions of the author and not necessarily those of the U.S. Food and Drug Administration.

TABLE 44-1 Points to Examine in Interpreting Clinical Trials

Define goals of study
    Treatment or prophylaxis
    Superiority or noninferiority
    Management or explanatory trial
Define disease under study by appropriate inclusion and exclusion criteria
Assignment of patients to arms of study
    Randomization
    Blinding
    Stratification
Study design considerations
    Sample size
    Assignment of types of error
    Selection of margin of superiority or noninferiority (hypothesis testing)
Potential bias during conduct of study
    Crossover
    Contamination
    Concomitant medications
    Loss to follow-up
Selection of appropriate end points
Appropriate analysis of results
Appropriate conclusions based on data presented in trial

through the course of the study while attempting to keep potential confounding factors to a minimum. Finally, the researcher must analyze the results and draw appropriate conclusions based on the available data. Each of these steps entails the potential for introduction of bias into the trial. At each step there are also mechanisms for limiting bias as much as possible.

DEFINING THE GOALS OF A STUDY

One can discern three types of goals for a clinical trial of an antimicrobial: (1) whether the clinical trial examines *prevention* or *treatment* of an infectious disease, (2) whether the trial sets out to prove the study drug is *similar* or *superior* in efficacy and/or safety to some control regimen, and (3) whether the trial is a *management* trial or an *explanatory* trial, as explained below.

In clinical trials of antimicrobials, one should distinguish between trials that examine prevention of a disease from treatment of established disease. The designs of prevention trials and treatment trials have important differences in the overall risk-benefit analysis and the selection of patient populations and end points. One should distinguish prophylaxis trials from those that examine preemptive therapy, empirical therapy, or treatment of definitive disease. The presence or absence of invasion of pathogenic organisms and the presence or absence of symptoms differentiates these entities.[6]

For the purposes of clinical trials, one can define *prophylaxis* as antimicrobials administered to patients at high risk of developing the disease under study, who are not infected at the time of study entry, and who are not manifesting symptomatic disease. One can define infection, for the purposes of such trials, as invasion of a potentially pathogenic organism measured by laboratory testing for the organism (culture, antigen testing, etc.) or the host response to that organism (serologic testing). "Infection" in this sense is not synonymous with the presence of signs and symptoms, but rather a measurement of invasion of the organism. The goal of prophylaxis is to prevent the invasion of pathogenic organisms and/or to prevent the development of symptomatic disease. A clinical trial in prophylaxis examines a specific disease caused by a specific organism or set of organisms in a specific patient population. For example, the clinical trial that resulted in U.S. Food and Drug Administration (FDA) approval of fluconazole as antifungal prophylaxis examined the prevention of *Candida* infections in the population receiving bone marrow transplantation.[7]

Authors have used the term *preemptive therapy* in a variety of ways in the medical literature. For the purposes of clinical trials, one can define preemptive therapy as the administration of antimicrobials to patients already infected, that is in whom there are markers of pathogen

invasion, but who do not yet manifest symptomatic disease. This same definition, however, is synonymous with what authors have termed *secondary prophylaxis* or *preventive therapy*. Patients who have been previously infected and experienced symptomatic disease may still harbor organisms and/or remain at risk for further episodes of symptomatic disease. For example, the administration of ganciclovir to asymptomatic solid organ transplant patients with positive tests for cytomegalovirus (CMV) antigen or CMV cultures in the blood has been called preemptive therapy.[8] Isoniazid administration to asymptomatic patients with a positive skin test after exposure to *Mycobacterium tuberculosis* is preventive therapy,[9] and administration of fluconazole to patients after recovery from cryptococcal meningitis has been called secondary prophylaxis.[10] In all these examples, the goal of administering antimicrobials is the same, namely, the prevention of symptomatic disease after the occurrence of documented infection. One then could consider the design of trials for preemptive therapy, secondary prophylaxis, and preventive therapy in a similar way. Authors have used the term *preemptive prophylaxis* to refer to prophylaxis in the setting of patients with specific risk factors for infection.[11] Study of a drug in this setting would still seem to be consistent with prophylaxis rather than preemptive therapy. It would be helpful in the future for investigators, clinicians, and regulators to clarify the terminology of preemptive therapy trials.

One can define *empirical therapy* as administration of antimicrobials to patients with signs and symptoms of disease when clinicians interpret those signs and symptoms as indicative of infection with a particular organism or set of organisms. In empirical therapy, there is no microbiologically or histologically definitive proof, at least initially, by culture or other means, of an infectious etiology. There is, however, a high suspicion that infection is the cause of the patient's symptoms. This situation is not unusual in clinical trials of infectious diseases. For instance, patients with fever, cough, sputum production, and an infiltrate on chest radiograph often are enrolled in clinical trials of community-acquired pneumonia even in the absence of positive blood or sputum cultures.[12] One should be certain, however, that the constellation of signs and symptoms in the absence of a confirmed microbiologic etiology is sufficiently specific for the disease under study. Lack of specificity could lead to enrollment of significant numbers of patients without the disease under study and resultant incorrect conclusions regarding drug efficacy.

One should determine whether a clinical trial intends to show that the test drug is similar or better in efficacy and/or safety to some control regimen.[13] Trials that attempt to show that the test drug is better than the control regimen are *superiority* trials. Trials that attempt to show that the study drug is similar to the control regimen are either *equivalence* trials or *noninferiority* trials. Equivalence trials attempt to prove that the test drug is no worse *and* no better than the control regimen by some specific margin.[14] The best examples of these trials are bioequivalence trials of a generic drug compared with the original compound where the pharmacokinetics of the generic drug should be between 80% and 120% of that of the original compound.[13] On the other hand, noninferiority trials only attempt to show that the test drug is no worse than the control regimen by some amount. Most trials in infectious diseases that attempt to show similarity of the test drug to a control regimen are noninferiority trials.

There are important differences in the design and interpretation of superiority trials compared with noninferiority trials.[15] Superiority trials provide the best evidence that a drug is more effective than placebo, either because the test drug is directly compared with placebo or a control regimen that is at least as effective as placebo. In the case of noninferiority trials, showing that two drugs have similar efficacy within some margin may mean that both drugs are effective in the disease under study, or neither drug is effective relative to placebo. This is because noninferiority trials do not directly compare the test drug to placebo. Therefore, in the context of a noninferiority trial, the efficacy of the control drug relative to placebo is assumed. Although it may seem self-evident that antimicrobials are effective in alleviating the signs and symptoms of infection, it is equally important in noninferiority trials to know the magnitude of that benefit in order to properly interpret the results of the trial, as is discussed in more detail later.

Clinical trials of antimicrobials can be *explanatory* trials or *management* (or *strategy*) trials.[4] These two types of trials determine the *efficacy* and *effectiveness*, respectively, of a study drug.[16] Explanatory trials set out to show that the drug has some clinical effect in the patients who actually have the disease under study and who take the medication as prescribed. The results of such a trial determine the efficacy of a study drug. On the other hand, management trials examine the clinical effects of a drug in those to whom it is offered. This may entail enrolling patients in whom the disease under study is not well defined or who do not take the drug exactly as detailed in the protocol. The results of management trials determine the effectiveness of the study drug. For example, a clinical trial that evaluates the safety and efficacy of an antimicrobial in patients with acute bacterial otitis media (ABOM) defined by a tympanocentesis prior to enrollment in the trial is an explanatory trial. A trial in ABOM that evaluates all children with an erythematous tympanic membrane is a management trial, as many of these patients may not have bacterial disease.

The distinction between efficacy and effectiveness is an important one.[16] Both explanatory and management trials give important information to clinicians but the interpretation of each type of trial differs. A drug that has efficacy in an explanatory trial may not show effectiveness in a management trial but this does not mean that the drug does not "work" for the infection under study. A management trial that fails to show effectiveness for the study drug may be due to lack of true efficacy of the drug in the disease under study or other factors such as inclusion of a large proportion of patients who do not have the disease under study. If a drug does show effectiveness in a management trial, the absolute magnitude of the benefit of the antimicrobial in the management trial may underestimate the true effect of the antimicrobial in an explanatory trial. However, the antimicrobial effects in an explanatory trial may overestimate the benefit in actual clinical practice. As an example of these distinctions, a recent FDA review of 14 placebo-controlled trials for acute bacterial sinusitis showed that in 12 of these trials, the effectiveness of antimicrobials was not statistically or clinically superior to placebo.[17] However, none of these trials defined patients with bacterial disease by means of sinus punctures at the time of enrollment into the trials. Therefore, these trials are management trials. Lack of effectiveness could mean that either the drugs under study were not effective for acute bacterial sinusitis or the trials enrolled large numbers of patients with viral disease. One would not expect patients with viral disease to benefit from antibacterial therapy and patients with viral disease would dilute out the treatment effects in those who did benefit from the study drugs. Therefore, it is important to be certain that a drug has efficacy in an explanatory trial in the disease under study before proceeding with an effectiveness or management trial.

INCLUSION AND EXCLUSION CRITERIA

When studying a disease, one must first define the disease and then select a subset of the population for study from the universe of patients with that disease.[18] Clear definitions of the disease under study allow (1) consistency among investigators about the types of patients they enroll in a trial, (2) generalization of the results to patients outside the trial, (3) regulatory agencies to accurately describe the intended use of the drug in prescription drug labeling, and (4) clinicians to appropriately use the information presented in the trial in clinical practice.

Infectious diseases are usually defined by a constellation of signs and symptoms in addition to confirmation of the microbiologic etiology of the disease. However, investigators may differ in their own determinations of which signs and symptoms define a given disease and their thresholds for initiating antimicrobial therapy. Therefore, a clinical trial should clearly delineate which signs and symptoms investigators used in defining the disease. The absence of a clear definition of the disease under study may result in differences in the nature of patients enrolled across arms of a clinical trial. This in turn may result in spurious differences between drugs or may obscure true differences between therapies. Although the process of randomization, discussed further below hopefully distributes differences in disease definition equally, or at least randomly, across arms of a trial, the process of randomization is not foolproof. In addition, even if patients with varying definitions of disease are randomly distributed across arms of the study, the success rate in the trial may not accurately reflect the true success rate in the disease in clinical practice. For instance, in studies of antibacterial agents, inclusion of patients with self-resolving viral illness may result in a falsely elevated success rate for that study drug compared with a trial that enrolls only patients with true bacterial disease.

Microbiologic information is often helpful in defining the infectious etiology of a given constellation of signs and symptoms. The host response to infection may mimic other diseases of noninfectious etiology. One would always prefer a diagnostic test with both high sensitivity and specificity in microbiologically defining an infection in both clinical trials and clinical practice. However, when diagnostic testing is less then optimal and one must choose between high sensitivity or high specificity, the desirable characteristics of a diagnostic test differ importantly between clinical practice and clinical trials. In clinical practice, one needs to use a diagnostic test with high sensitivity so that clinicians do not fail to diagnose patients with the disease, especially for infections with high morbidity and mortality. In the setting of a clinical trial, however, one needs to use tests with high specificity to ensure that patients enrolled in the trial actually have the disease under study. For instance, guidelines recommend treating patients with symptoms of uncomplicated urinary tract infections with colony counts as low as 10^2 CFU/mL of urine.[19] However, to increase specificity, clinical trials usually enroll only patients with at least 10^5 CFU/mL of urine to more accurately differentiate patients with true uncomplicated urinary tract infection from those with symptoms of dysuria due to other etiologies with potentially contaminated urine specimens.

Selecting the appropriate patient population often entails striking a balance between including enough different types of patients so that one may extrapolate the results of the trials to clinical practice but not being so inclusive as to blur important distinctions in drug efficacy or safety across patient subgroups. In trials of prophylaxis of infectious diseases, the inclusion criteria should select a patient population at high enough risk for disease.[20] If the patient population is at low risk it may take an extremely large sample size to show a difference between a prophylactic drug and placebo. In treatment trials, the inclusion criteria should select patients in whom one would expect similar outcomes based on host effects and the microbiology of the disease. For instance, the microbiology and the types of hosts affected with community-acquired pneumonia and nosocomial pneumonia are sufficiently different that they are usually studied in separate trials. Similarly, severely immunocompromised patients with human immunodeficiency virus (HIV) are often excluded from trials of community-acquired pneumonia because the outcome in these patients, even with similar microbiology, is often different than in nonimmunocompromised hosts. However, investigators wish to be inclusive enough so that results of the trial are useful in making treatment decisions for a broad range of patients. For instance, clinical trials often include elderly patients or patients with mild renal or hepatic insufficiency in an attempt to determine the efficacy and safety of a drug in these patient populations, even though outcomes may be different in this subset of patients.

GENERAL STUDY DESIGN CONSIDERATIONS

Randomization, Blinding, and Stratification

Once the investigator selects the population for study, he or she must allocate the patients to the various kinds of treatments, or arms, tested in the trial. Randomization is the process by which patients are assigned to the study or control regimen using no specific pattern.[21] Therefore, a process such as assigning every other patient alternately to the study drug and control arms is not randomization because this entails using a specific pattern. Investigators can use various randomization charts or computer programs to randomize patients. Trials that do not use randomization to assign patients are termed *observational* trials because they observe the behavior clinicians would use in practice.

Through the process of randomization it is equally likely that a patient will receive study medication or control.[22] The advantage of randomization is that it decreases the possible effect of investigators interjecting their own opinions into assigning patients to a particular treatment. If investigators have an opinion based on preclinical testing that one drug is more effective than the other, they may selectively enroll the sickest patients in that arm and only less ill patients in the other arm of the trial. This may result in obscuring important differences between treatments. Probably just as important, randomization also makes it equally likely that unmeasured as well as measured factors that may affect outcomes are distributed equally between arms of the trial. Unmeasured factors may be very important in some cases in which the pathophysiology of the disease or the mechanism of action of the drug is less well known.

Randomization is only a *probability* of equally distributing important variables between arms of a trial. When important variables are not equally distributed across arms of the trial randomization has not "failed" because the process of random distribution did occur as planned but without the desired result. However, unequal distribution of factors between the arms of a trial may have an impact on the interpretation of the results. The importance of unequal distribution of various factors depends not only on the statistical significance of the difference in the distribution of the factor between the study arms but also the strength of the association of the outcome with that factor. In other words, one should consider small differences in the distribution of factors between study arms as clinically significant if the factor has a known large impact on outcomes even though the differences are not statistically significant.[22] For example, factors like severity of illness may have a great effect on the results of a trial if there are differences in the distribution of more severely ill patients between arms of the trial, even if those differences between arms of the trial are not statistically significant. In addition, multiple small differences in factors that are not statistically significant or clinically important individually may influence outcomes if they are all in the same direction.

The process of randomization is most effective when the process is performed in a blinded fashion.[23] Blinding is the lack of knowledge of the identity of the trial treatment. Patients, investigators, data review committees, ancillary personnel, statisticians and monitors are all groups who may be kept blinded to study treatment. Blinding is another method that prevents the opinions of patients, investigators, or others involved in the trial from influencing the results. Studies that are not blinded are open-label trials. A study in which only patients do not know which drug they are to receive is called single-blinded. Trials are investigator-blinded when only the investigator does not know study assignment. In a double-blinded trial neither patients nor investigators are aware of which drug the patient will receive. One study that evaluated the importance of randomization and blinding showed that at least one prognostic factor was not distributed equally between arms of the trial in 14% of trials that were blinded and randomized, in 26.7% of open-label randomized trials, and in 58.1% of the open-label observational trials. The authors found statistically significant differences in case-fatality rates between the treatment and control groups in 8.8% of the blinded and randomized trials, 24.4% of the open-label, randomized studies, and 58.1% of open-label, observational trials.[24]

Given that randomization and blinding are not foolproof, it is often wise to employ other means to ensure equal distribution of patients across arms of a trial when there are factors known or expected to have an important influence on outcomes. Investigators can ensure equal distribution of important factors by a process known as stratification, also called block randomization.[16] Through the process of stratification, investigators separate patients into groups (or strata) based on some important factor. Patients are then randomized within each strata to receive the study or control regimen. For example, investigators may first separate patients into groups according to severity of disease using some measure such as an APACHE (Acute Physiology and Chronic Health Evaluation) score, and then randomize patients within each severity group to receive the study or control regimen.

Sample Size, Hypothesis Testing, and Types of Error

Investigators must also consider how many patients to enroll in a clinical trial.[25] Selecting the appropriate sample size entails choosing a number of patients large enough to show a difference between treatments should one actually exist but not so large as to incur extra time and expense, as well as exposing more patients to an experimental treatment.[26] Investigators use statistical principles such as hypothesis testing and types of error to aid in selecting the appropriate sample size.

In a clinical trial, an investigator tests a research question that the study drug is safe and effective in a selected sample of the patients with the disease under study. However, the investigator cannot determine the "absolute truth" of whether the drug is safe and effective for the disease under study without testing every single patient with the disease. Obviously this is not practical or possible. Therefore, investigators test the research question in a given representative sample of patients with the disease. Investigators then use statistical tests to determine the likelihood that the results of the trial in their sample of patients represent the safety and efficacy in the population as a whole versus a chance result that does not reflect the absolute truth.[27]

Because an investigator cannot directly determine the safety and efficacy of a study drug in the entire population with a disease, the investigator starts off with the hypothesis that the drug is *not* safe and effective and then tries to disprove this hypothesis. This is similar to assuming a defendant in a court case is innocent until proven guilty by examining evidence showing beyond a reasonable doubt that the defendant is not innocent. The hypothesis that the drug is not safe and effective is called the *null hypothesis*, termed null because the assumption is there is no effect of the drug in the disease under study.[16] The null hypothesis in a superiority trial is that the study drug is not more effective than the control regimen. In a noninferiority trial the null hypothesis is that the study drug is less effective than the control regimen by some amount. In both cases, the investigator sets out to disprove, or reject, the null hypothesis. Thus the sometimes-confusing double-negative terminology of *not* showing that a drug is *not* effective. If the investigator shows there is good evidence to reject the notion the drug is not safe and effective, then the investigator can infer, or accept, the *alternative hypothesis* as true, that is, that the drug is safe and effective in the disease under study. Note that investigators are not directly testing the alternative hypothesis but inferring it is true based on rejecting the null hypothesis. This is called proof by contradiction.

Statistical testing gives investigators and readers of clinical trials a way to express the degree of certainty that the null hypothesis is not true beyond a reasonable doubt.[28] In clinical trials, this reasonable doubt is expressed as the amount of error one is willing to accept that the results deviate from the absolute truth. There are two major types of error that investigators consider when designing a clinical trial. Type I error is the risk of accepting that the drug is safe and effective when in fact it is not, in other words, a false-positive result.[27] In the language of hypothesis testing, this is the chance of rejecting the null hypothesis when in fact the null hypothesis is true. By convention, the type I error, also called alpha (α), usually is set at 0.05 (i.e., 5% or 1 in 20). This means that there is a 5% probability that the results of the trial could have occurred by chance alone. It also means that if the investigator performed 20 similar trials, one of them would be likely to yield a false result. Type II error is the risk of determining that a drug is not safe and effective when in fact it is safe and effective, in other words, a false negative result.[29] In the language of hypothesis testing this is the chance of accepting the null hypothesis when in fact the null hypothesis is false. Type II error, also called beta (β), is usually set at 0.10 or 0.20 (i.e., 10% or 20%, or 1 in 5 or 10). This means that if the investigator performed 10 similar trials, 1 or 2 of them would reach a false conclusion. Power is related to type II error. Power is the ability to show the drug is safe and effective when in fact the drug is safe and effective in the whole population with the disease under study. Power is defined as 1 minus the type II error; therefore, most studies have an 80% to 90% chance of showing that a drug is safe and effective. In other words, 8 or 9 out of 10 similar trials would come to a correct conclusion.

Investigators use the types of error, as well as the expected magnitude of the difference between the study drug and the control drug (also called *effect size*), to select the sample size for the trial. Treatment effect is different for a superiority trial compared with a noninferiority trial.[13,27,30,31] In a superiority trial, the investigator must decide how much more effective the study drug is compared with the control regimen. In a noninferiority trial, the investigator must decide how much less effective the study drug can be than the control regimen and still consider the drugs similar in efficacy.[32] Obviously, the treatment effect is what the trial ultimately sets out to determine, so investigators often must make an educated guess as to the expected magnitude of the treatment effect, or choose a treatment effect size that is clinically relevant and/or feasible. As the magnitude of the treatment effect decreases, the sample size of the trial increases. For instance, a clinical trial that attempts to show a 5% difference between the study drug and the control regimen will require a larger sample size than a trial that attempts to show a 15% difference between the same drugs.[33]

For readers of clinical trials, knowledge of the actual method of sample size selection used by investigators is not of prime importance. However, readers should look to see that investigators have specified the values for the various types of error, specified the hypothesized magnitude of the treatment effect, and determined an appropriate sample size based on these factors prior to initiation of the trial.

SELECTING THE CONTROL REGIMEN

The most basic goal of a clinical trial of an antimicrobial is to show that the test drug is more effective than no treatment for the disease under study. However, often there are effective therapies already available for many types of infections, and clinicians also may want to know how the efficacy and safety of the study drug compare with a control drug known to be safe and effective in the disease. Differences in the end points of previous trials and changes in adjunctive therapies, ancillary care, and the epidemiology of a disease over time may make it difficult to determine an absolute success rate for a given type of infection.[34] Clinicians also wish to know how the safety of a study agent compares to other therapies for the disease in question. The use of a control regimen also allows a comparison of the results of the trial with results obtained in previous trials with the control regimen. Differing results would alert investigators to look for explanations for such differences, such as changes in study design or the outcome of the disease over time. A controlled trial also allows clinicians to see whether adverse events are related to drug therapy or to the natural history of the illness by comparing the adverse event profile of the study drug with that of the control regimen.

There are five types of controls investigators may use in a clinical trial: (1) no treatment concurrent controls, (2) placebo concurrent controls, (3) dose comparison concurrent controls, (4) historical controls, and (5) active treatment concurrent controls.[35] In a trial with a no therapy control, investigators randomize patients to study medication or to standard care with no antimicrobial therapy. Therefore, when no therapy is the control, investigators are not blinded to study treatment. In a placebo-controlled trial investigators randomize patients to receive study drug or a matching placebo. Therefore, in a placebo-controlled trial the potential for blinding still exists. Placebo-controlled trials can also compare the efficacy and safety of antimicrobial therapy plus other appropriate nonantimicrobial therapies versus other nonantimicrobial therapies plus a matching placebo to ascertain the additive benefit of antimicrobial therapies in self-resolving diseases. There are situations in infectious diseases where placebo-controlled trials are ethical and necessary.[36,37] In self-resolving diseases in which the risk of withholding antimicrobials may be a few more days of uncomfortable symptoms and the risk of serious outcomes is low, placebo-controlled trials are still useful. Clinical trials can also use the study

drug at increasing doses as its own control. Demonstrating increasing efficacy with increasing doses of a drug would demonstrate efficacy for that drug. This design often is useful when there is no available therapy for a given infection. Historical controlled trials compare the results of the study drug with a control regimen that is external to the trial, as in previous studies or results compiled over time in the medical literature on the disease under study. Historical controlled trials are not randomized and cannot control for changes in the epidemiology of the disease or advances in adjunctive therapies over time. Historical controlled trials also are less helpful when comparing the safety of the study drug to the control regimen as often safety data in the historical control are not obtained in the same fashion or as rigorously. Historical controlled trials also tend to underestimate the treatment effect in the control arm,[38,39] so a direct comparison of the study drug and the control regimen is more difficult. Given these limitations, most clinical trials of antimicrobials are active controlled concurrent trials in which investigators choose a control regimen known to be safe and effective in the disease under study. When choosing an active control, the investigator usually chooses a dose and duration of the control regimen that is optimal for the disease under study. Choosing a suboptimal dose or duration of a control agent obviously can impact the conclusions about the safety and efficacy of the study drug.

SOURCES OF BIAS DURING THE STUDY

The main principle in clinical trials is to keep as many factors constant between the arms of the trial while varying only the drugs administered to patients in each arm. Bias can occur when treatment of patients in the arms of the trial differs by factors other than the medication they receive.[23] Patients in the study drug arm may receive the control medication and vice versa, a phenomenon known as crossover. Entry into a trial may cause some patients and caregivers to alter their behavior, a process called contamination. For instance, in a prophylaxis trial, caregivers may institute more stringent infection control procedures merely because they are participating in the trial. This may alter the expected rate of infections in the study. Patients also may receive concomitant medications differently in the various arms of the trial. This is most evident when investigators prescribe concomitant medications at their own discretion, rather than by criteria specified in the study protocol.

Bias may also occur if there are systematic differences between arms of the trial in patients who do not adhere to their medication or who do not complete the trial. It is often unavoidable that some patients will be lost to follow-up during the course of a trial. However, when reporting the results of a trial, investigators should account for all randomized patients. Readers should look for systematic differences in the reasons for discontinuation of patients from the study between the arms of the trial.[40] Patients who are feeling well may not complete their medication or may not return for follow-up. Alternately, if patients continue to feel ill they may seek care elsewhere or take additional or alternative medications. Both instances may affect the interpretation of the results of the trial. The success rate in the trial may not reflect the true success rate in the population or differential rates of compliance, and loss to follow-up may influence the success rates in each arm of the trial.

One must also account for all patients who enter into a trial. Patients may not complete the trial for various reasons. Some patients may be lost to follow-up for various reasons. Some discontinue treatment due to adverse events or for other reasons.[40]

END POINTS

The interpretation of the results of a clinical trial are highly dependent upon the questions one asks prior to initiation of the trial. Perhaps this is most evident in the selection of end points. End points for trials should be clinically relevant to patients and clinicians. Patients are most concerned about the signs and symptoms of disease and whether they will survive an episode of infection. Clinical end points, then, are defined as measurements of how patients feel, function, or survive.[41] Clinical end points should measure the resolution or improvement of the same signs and symptoms that cause patients to seek medical care or clinicians to initiate antimicrobial therapy. In prophylaxis trials, patients are initially asymptomatic, so the relevant end point is the occurrence of signs and symptoms.[6]

Often, more than one manifestation of a disease is clinically relevant. In these cases, it is appropriate to evaluate all the relevant clinical signs and symptoms as well as mortality in a composite end point. The use of a composite end point often provides a more comprehensive evaluation of drug efficacy.[42] For example, in clinical trials of community-acquired pneumonia, an appropriate end point may evaluate resolution or improvement of cough, shortness of breath, and chest pain as well as mortality. Evaluation of only one of these signs and symptoms or mortality alone would not provide as clear a picture of the effects of the drug.

Clinical trials also can utilize surrogate markers other than clinical end points. A surrogate marker is any end point, either a laboratory measurement or a physical sign, used as a substitute for a clinically meaningful end point that measures how a patient feels, functions, or survives.[43,44] Microbiologic end points that measure the suppression or elimination of pathogenic organisms are surrogate end points because they do not directly measure effects on the patient. Although antimicrobials exert a direct effect on microorganisms, an improvement in a microbiologic end point should translate into clinically meaningful benefits for patients.[45] Surrogate markers are most useful when the clinical end points cannot be measured for a prolonged period of time and there is a good correlation and validation between clinical and microbiologic end points.[46] A good correlation means that the effect on the microbiologic end points should predict the clinical outcome. Outcomes include both successes and failures. Therefore, microbiologic success should predict clinical success and microbiologic failure should predict clinical failure. Surrogate end points are often measured in smaller, pilot studies attempting to demonstrate proof of principle that an antimicrobial may be effective in a given disease. Such trials are appropriate to generate hypotheses for further trials that demonstrate the clinical efficacy of the drug.

Although it may seem intuitive that suppression or elimination of pathogenic organisms should correlate with clinical outcomes, this is not always the case.[45] Antimicrobials may exert direct effects on the immune system that may affect clinical outcomes.[47,48] Antimicrobials may also have effects on organisms, such as rapid lysis with subsequent stimulation of the immune system, which also may influence clinical outcomes. The recommendation to administer steroids prior to the administration of antimicrobials in acute bacterial meningitis is based on this phenomenon.[49,50] Since these effects are the result of administration of the antimicrobial, they are not solely effects related to the host. Measuring clinical end points is the only way to capture such effects.

The use of the surrogate marker of viral load in clinical trials of HIV serves as an example of an adequate surrogate marker. The clinical end points in HIV trials, progression to opportunistic infections or death, may take months to years to measure. Therefore a reliable surrogate marker is desirable. Measurements of HIV viral load have the characteristics of a good surrogate marker. A lower viral load on therapy (a microbiologic success) predicts a clinical response of less opportunistic infections and death (a clinical success). In addition, higher viral loads on therapy (a microbiologic failure) predict more opportunistic infections and death (a clinical failure).[51] On the other hand, CD4 counts do not serve as an adequate surrogate marker because the changes in CD4 count do not correlate with clinical outcomes.[52,53]

The timing of end point measurements also is important.[54] Investigators should time the measurement of clinical end points based on the natural history of the disease. For example, placebo-controlled trials show that most cases of traveler's diarrhea will resolve spontaneously within a few days.[55] Therefore, measuring resolution of diarrhea several weeks after the start of symptoms would not allow one to differentiate the effects of antimicrobial therapy from placebo in this disease. Often, in spontaneously resolving diseases, the time to resolution of symptoms may be a more clinically meaningful end point than measurement of clinical outcomes at some fixed time point. However, in more serious diseases, a fixed time point may be more informative because whether the patient dies earlier or later in the course of illness may not be as clinically relevant. When trials use fixed end points in diseases that tend to recur, the timing of measurements of outcomes should be soon enough so that one is sure of measuring the effect of the drug on the initial episode of infection and not the natural history of the disease. The timing of measurements of microbiologic end points is also relevant. Measurements taken on therapy may represent suppression rather than elimination of organisms. The most relevant timing of the measurement of microbiologic end points is at some point after the drug has been eliminated from the body to measure true elimination of organisms versus suppression, relapse, or reinfection.

Investigators should specify the definitions of clinical success and failure used in the trial. In clinical trials of infectious disease, it is often most informative to use a global measure of success defined as resolution of signs and symptoms of infection as well as elimination of the causative pathogen. The utility of microbiologic end points, however, depends on the quality of the specimen. Cultures from sterile body sites are more informative than culture from nonsterile sites.

The tools used to measure success and failure are important as well. End points such as mortality are self-explanatory, but the measurement of clinical signs and symptoms is subjective and may vary between patients and between clinicians. Trials should use valid scales to measure resolution of signs and symptoms.[56] Use of nonvalidated scales is akin to using a noncalibrated laboratory instrument to measure blood chemistry values. Outcomes have no context in the absence of validation of the measurement tool.

The measurement of mortality can examine all causes of death or death specific to the infection under study. All-cause mortality is a relevant end point because the overall impact of curing an infection is minimal if the patient expires regardless of treatment. Also, the drug itself may result in mortality that would not be captured by examining only infection-related deaths. When measuring cause-specific mortality, investigators should be sure that the tools used to define the cause of death are sufficiently specific to rule out other causes. For instance, current diagnostic tools to diagnose fungal infections are not sufficiently sensitive or specific.[57] Patients with serious fungal infections often have multiple other co-morbid conditions, and it may be difficult to ascribe a cause of death even with autopsy data.[6]

ANALYZING THE RESULTS OF TRIALS

In analyzing results of a trial, investigators use statistical tests to evaluate the original hypotheses. Investigators use statistical tests to examine the likelihood that the results of the trial could have occurred by chance alone. If the likelihood of accepting a chance result is low, as determined by parameters set up prior to initiation of the trial, then investigators conclude that the evidence is strong enough to reject the null hypothesis that the drug is not safe and effective. They then can assume that the alternative hypothesis is likely true, that is, that the drug is safe and effective.[58]

Investigators must first decide on the population of patients in the trial that they wish to analyze. The *intention-to-treat* population assigns patients according to the group to which they were initially randomized, regardless of whether the patient actually received the drug, discontinued therapy, or switched to a different therapy.[59] In other words, investigators evaluate patients by the treatment they intended to give. Investigators often use a modified intention-to-treat population of patients who actually received at least one dose of the study medication. The *per-protocol* population (sometimes called the "clinically evaluable" population) is composed of patients who received some minimal amount of the study or control drug, followed the protocol as specified, and returned for an assessment of their outcome.

The intention-to-treat and per-protocol populations have differing strengths and limitations. The intention-to-treat population conserves the benefits of randomization. The per-protocol population does not necessarily preserve the benefits of randomization if patients who drop out of the trial systematically differ from those who complete the trial. The intention-to-treat population usually considers patients who drop out of the trial for various reasons as treatment failures. This takes into account patients who may not tolerate the drug. The intention-to-treat population, therefore, is a way of examining the effectiveness of a drug in a more realistic practice setting, taking into account both safety and efficacy. However, patients who do not complete therapy usually are not included in the per-protocol population. The per-protocol population separates considerations of the issues of the efficacy of the drug from issues related to safety and toxicity. In this way, clinicians may be able to determine that a drug has efficacy if the patient is able to tolerate it. This may be important in serious diseases in which there are few treatment options and clinicians may be willing to accept more substantial toxicities if the drug is effective.

In superiority trials, the intention-to-treat population is usually the most appropriate patient population used for analysis of the primary end point because it provides the least likelihood of coming to a false-positive conclusion.[60] However, in a noninferiority trial, the analysis of the intention-to-treat population tends to make the study and control drugs appear more similar. This may lead to a false-positive conclusion that the drugs are similar in efficacy when there may be important differences between the drugs. As the benefits of randomization may be lost in the per-protocol population, this population also may not be a reflective comparison of the true efficacy of drugs in a noninferiority trial. Given the limitations of both the intention-to-treat and the per-protocol population in noninferiority trials, it is often most informative to examine analyses of the primary end point in both populations. Differences in the comparative efficacy of the study and control drugs between the intention-to-treat and per-protocol populations in a noninferiority trial would require an examination of the reasons for such differences.

Once investigators decide which population to analyze, they calculate the *point estimate* for successful outcomes for the primary end point in the study drug and control groups.[33] The point estimate is the number of patients with successful outcomes divided by the total number of patients in the analyzed population. For instance, consider an example of a trial in which the primary analysis population contains 300 patients in each arm of the trial, where 225 and 240 patients have successful outcomes in the study drug and control drug arms, respectively. In this case the point estimates of successful outcomes are 75% (225/300) in the study drug arm and 80% (240/300) in the control arm.

The next step is to make a comparison of the outcomes of the study and the control drug. In our example, the absolute difference in outcomes between the study and control drugs is 75% minus 80% or a difference of minus 5%. One can also examine the relative outcomes of the test and control drug. In our example, the rate of unsuccessful outcomes is 25% for the study drug and 20% for the control. Therefore, the relative reduction in unsuccessful outcomes is a 20% decrease in treatment failures for the control drug relative to the study drug (1 minus 20% divided by 25%).

Investigators use statistical testing to determine the likelihood that the difference in the point estimates of the study and control drugs could have occurred by chance alone. The actual statistical tests used depend on the types of data examined in the trial. A discussion of various statistical tests and their appropriate use is beyond the scope of this chapter. Commonly, investigators use tests such as the chi squared to examine dichotomous variables (cure versus success) and Student's t-test to examine continuous variables (e.g., weight and age).[23,61] However, readers should ensure that investigators identify the statistical tests used in examining the results of a trial.

One of the most commonly used results in statistical testing is the P value.[62,63] Unfortunately, it is often misinterpreted. In one study, only about one fifth of respondents to a multiple-choice questionnaire understood the meaning of the P value.[64] If the P value is less than the specified type I error, usually set at 0.05, the result is called statistically significant. A P value of less than 0.05 means that there is a less than 5% chance that results as extreme as those observed in the trial are due to chance or random error.[65] Therefore, the P value is a measure of doubt, not a measure of clinical significance.[61] A larger treat-

ment effect, that is, the difference between the study and control drugs, is capable of demonstrating statistical significance with a smaller sample size. However, P values are a unitless measure and thus do not directly measure the magnitude of the treatment effect. Therefore, larger sample sizes may result in smaller P values but do not necessarily translate into greater clinical effects. In our example, the P value for the difference between a study drug with a success rate of 75% and a control drug with a success rate of 80% with 300 patients per arm is 0.14. If one studies 1000 patients per arm and the success rates remain at 75% and 80% for the study and control drugs, respectively, the P value decreases to 0.007, even though the difference in point estimates remains at minus 5%. However, if the study drug success rate remains at 75% and the success rate in the control increases to 85% with 300 patients per arm in the trial, the P value is 0.002.

A P value of 0.05 means that 1 in 20 comparisons made in a clinical trial may represent a false-positive result. If an investigator makes more than one comparison in a clinical trial, the chance of drawing a false conclusion increases. For five independent comparisons, the type I error increases from 5% to 20% and for 10 comparisons to 40%. For 20 comparisons the type I error increases to 64%.[66] In other words, at this level one is more likely than not to find a statistically significant result that is false. For this reason, it often is appropriate to use a lower P value to define statistical significance when making multiple comparisons, a procedure known as the Bonferroni correction.[66] One usually divides the P value by the number of comparisons to determine the corrected definition for statistical significance. Therefore, if one makes 5 comparisons the P value used to define statistical significance decreases from 0.05 to 0.01. If the comparisons are not independent, some authors feel that the Bonferroni correction is too conservative.[67] The important point for readers of clinical trials is that authors should describe what procedure they use when accounting for multiple comparisons. The most common use of multiple comparisons is in subgroup analyses.[68]

Confidence intervals are another way of analyzing trial results and provide adjunctive information to P values.[69] Confidence intervals are measured in the same units as the point estimate, for example, percentage of patients with a successful outcome. Therefore, confidence intervals can provide an estimate of the size of the treatment effect. The width of the confidence interval also provides some estimate of the uncertainty of the result. With larger sample sizes, the width of the confidence interval decreases. A 95% confidence interval indicates that the investigator can be 95% sure that the calculated interval contains the true difference between the drugs for the outcome in the population studied. In our example the difference in point estimates is minus 5%. For a trial with 300 patients in each arm, the lower bound of the 95% confidence interval is minus 11.7% and the upper bound is plus 1.7%. This means that one is 95% confident that the study drug is somewhere from 11.7% worse to 1.7% better than the control drug for the measured outcome. Increasing the sample size to 1000 patients in each arm would give greater precision to the results by narrowing the confidence interval to minus 10.0% to plus 0.002% if the success rates remained the same.

An examination of the upper and lower bounds of the confidence interval allows one to determine whether a study drug is statistically superior, inferior, or noninferior to a control drug (Fig. 44-1). A statistically superior drug has a lower bound of the 95% confidence interval that is greater than zero. A statistically inferior drug has an upper bound of the 95% confidence interval that is less than zero. To determine whether a study drug is noninferior to a control drug, one must compare the lower bound of the 95% confidence interval to some prespecified margin of noninferiority. The P value and the confidence interval are related. If the 95% confidence interval excludes zero, then the P value is less than 0.05.

Noninferiority trials attempt to show that the study drug is no worse than the control drug by some amount. That amount is called the noninferiority margin, or delta (δ).[14] This noninferiority margin is the maximum degree of inferiority of the study drug to the control drug that the clinical trial will attempt to exclude statistically. Selection of a noninferiority

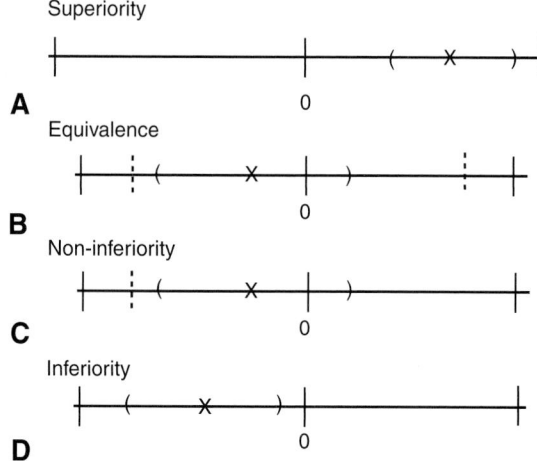

FIGURE 44-1. Interpretation of results using confidence intervals in clinical trials. X represents the difference in the point estimates of two therapies. The central zero mark indicates no difference between drugs. The brackets represent the upper and lower bounds of the 95% confidence intervals. The dotted lines are the noninferiority and equivalence margins. **A,** A study drug that demonstrated superiority over the control has a point estimate and the upper and lower bounds of the 95% confidence intervals greater than zero. **B,** A study drug that demonstrates equivalence to a control drug has upper and lower bounds of the 95% confidence intervals within a prespecified margin. The point estimate can be greater or less than zero. **C,** A study drug that demonstrates noninferiority to a control drug has a lower bound of the 95% confidence interval greater than some prespecified margin. If the lower bound is more negative than the prespecified margin, the study drug is said not to meet the definition of noninferiority. **D,** A drug that is inferior to the control drug has the upper bound of the 95% confidence interval below zero. (See text for further explanation.)

margin is based upon two factors.[70] First, one must know the margin of benefit of the active control relative to placebo. This is based on factual information from prior natural history studies or placebo-controlled trials in the disease under study. If the magnitude of the effect of the active control relative to placebo is known and sufficiently large, then the second factor for consideration is the magnitude of the potential loss of efficacy relative to the control. This second factor is based on clinical judgment. For example, consider a disease in which the benefit of the control drug over placebo is 20% based on prior randomized, placebo-controlled trials of the disease in question. A noninferiority margin of 10% would preserve a degree of benefit relative to the effect of the control drug while allowing for some margin of error. However, selection of a noninferiority margin of 10% would be inappropriate for a different disease in which the benefit of the active control over placebo is only 5%. Selection of an inappropriate noninferiority margin may lead to the conclusion that the study drug meets the statistical definition of noninferiority when the drug actually may have no benefit over placebo. In our example, the lower bound of the 95% confidence interval is minus11.7%. If the noninferiority margin selected prior to initiation of the trial was minus 15%, then one can conclude that the study drug is statistically noninferior to the control. If the prespecified noninferiority margin was minus 10%, then the study drug fails to meet the statistical definition of noninferiority.

Many clinical trials are designed to evaluate both the safety and efficacy of a study drug. Fortunately, adverse events with antimicrobials usually are relatively uncommon. As a consequence, however, clinical trials usually do not have a large enough sample size to rule out many adverse events, especially those that are rare. Absence of evidence of a difference is not the same as evidence of absence of a difference. When a clinical trial shows no cases of a particular adverse event, one can only rule out a rate of one in the number of patients examined divided by three. For example, if one sees no cases of a particular adverse event

in 300 patients, that rules out a risk of 1 in 100 or in other words, a rate of greater than 1%. If one does not see an adverse event in 3000 patients, that rules out a risk of 1 in 1000 or greater than 0.1%.

EXAMINING THE CONCLUSIONS

In the discussion section of a published clinical trial, investigators summarize the results, discuss the strengths and limitations of the data, and relate the results to other trials of the disease under study.[71] However, previous studies show that authors commonly make claims not justified by the results of the trial. A review of trials in obstetrics and pediatrics journals concluded that in only 10% of the trials were the conclusions justified by the results.[72] In another study, the authors found doubtful or invalid statements in 76% of 196 trials.[73] Authors may tend to highlight statistically significant results over other less impressive findings.[74]

Some common pitfalls readers should look for in examining the discussion section of clinical trials are summarized in Table 44-2 and include the following:

1. Concluding noninferiority from a trial designed to demonstrate superiority. Conclusions of superiority or noninferiority of the study drug should relate to the initial hypothesis. A noninferiority trial may show a superior result for one of the drugs when the results show a lower bound of the confidence interval around the difference in the point estimates that is greater than zero. However, it is difficult to claim noninferiority from a superiority trial. In most cases, investigators do not select a noninferiority margin prior to initiation of a superiority trial. This results in difficulties in interpretation of the results, as noninferiority is based upon comparison of the lower bound of the confidence interval to the prespecified noninferiority margin. In addition, the sample size of a noninferiority trial is often larger than a superiority trial; therefore, the trial may not have adequate sample size to conclude noninferiority when designed for superiority.
2. Extrapolation of results to patient groups not studied in the trial. The results of the trial are most applicable to patients who fit the definition of the disease as specified in the trial and the population studied. It is more difficult to extrapolate results to other populations, especially those that may differ in host immune function, age, and pathophysiology or severity of underlying disease.
3. Concluding lack of efficacy based on data from a management (effectiveness) trial. Data from an explanatory (efficacy) trial may not describe the effectiveness of the drug in the real world setting. Conversely, management (effectiveness) trials may not provide useful information on the efficacy of a drug when patients take the drug as prescribed. Failure to show effectiveness in a management trial may be due to selection of a patient population unlikely to benefit or to selection of patients who do not truly have the disease under study (e.g., patients with viral disease in a trial of an antibacterial agent). This does not infer that the drug would be ineffective if studied in a different population. Therefore, study of the effectiveness of a drug assumes that the efficacy of the drug is known.

TABLE 44-2 Common Issues for Readers to Examine in Conclusions of Clinical Trials

Concluding noninferiority from a trial designed to demonstrate superiority
Extrapolation of results to patient groups not studied in the trial
Concluding lack of efficacy based on data from a management (effectiveness) trial
Presenting the results in a way to make them appear more favorable
Conclusions of efficacy or safety based on results that do not achieve statistical significance
Conclusions of efficacy or safety based on subgroup analyses when results were not significant for the primary end point
Conclusions of clinical outcomes based on nonvalidated surrogate end points

4. Presenting the results in a way to make them appear more favorable. The presentation of results may influence clinicians' interpretations of trials and their application in clinical practice. One study found that nearly half of surveyed clinicians were more impressed and indicated a higher likelihood of treating their patients when investigators presented the results of trials as a relative change in outcomes (i.e., percent reduction in a undesirable outcome) rather than as an absolute change. One should examine both the relative and absolute differences in outcomes when interpreting the results of trials. Small absolute differences may translate into large relative differences that may be clinically insignificant.

5. Conclusions of efficacy or safety based on results that do not achieve statistical significance. Authors may describe results that do not achieve statistical significance as a trend toward successful outcomes. Readers should interpret such claims with care. A trend assumes that further study of similar patients would yield similar results. However, to validate this assumption requires further study. For instance, if one flips a fair coin five times and the results are four heads and one tail, this could be considered a trend. This does not mean that one would obtain the same results if one flipped the coin another five times.

6. Conclusions of efficacy based on subgroup analyses when results were not significant for the primary end point. The results of the trial are most relevant for the specified primary end point. Claims based on subgroup analyses are associated with several issues. The sample size of the trial usually is based on assumptions related to the primary end point. The sample size may be insufficient to draw adequate conclusions about subgroups. In addition, subgroups picked out after the conclusion of the trial are not randomized. As discussed previously, multiple comparisons within a trial increase the likelihood of coming to a false-positive conclusion. The more comparisons, the more likely one is to find a result related to chance alone. Therefore, using a P value of 0.05 to define statistical significance for subgroup analyses increases the risk of making false-positive conclusions. The increase in type I error is related to the number of comparisons made by the authors, not the number of comparisons presented in the publication. Therefore, readers should ensure that authors specify whether (1) they planned the subgroup analysis prior to initiation of the trial, (2) they considered the use of subgroup analysis when they planned the calculation of sample size, (3) they specified how many comparisons were made, and (4) they specified the correction for type I error. Subgroup analyses are most useful for generating hypotheses for study in future clinical trials rather than for making definitive conclusions.

7. Conclusions of clinical outcomes based on nonvalidated surrogate end points. The end points of a trial should support claims made about treatment or prophylaxis of a disease. A study that uses a decrease in colonization as the primary end point in a prophylaxis trial can claim a decrease in the incidence of the disease only if the results of the trial or previous trials also show a significant decrease in infections. This validation applies only to the population in the validation study. In treatment trials, elimination or suppression of causative pathogens is the mechanism of action of antimicrobials, but the ultimate goal of administering these drugs is the resolution or improvement in the signs and symptoms of the disease. Therefore, there should be a proven validation of microbiologic surrogate markers with clinical outcomes. A large body of literature shows that antimicrobials can have direct effects on the host immune system,[47,75] or effects on the causative organisms can result in secondary effects on the host.[48,76] One can only measure such effects by examining clinical end points. Often, authors present an association between elimination or suppression of the organism and clinical failures.[77,78] Measurement of outcomes includes both failures and successes; therefore, a correlation should show that clinical success also correlates with microbiologic success.[45] A true correlation is bidirectional. Readers should also discern that investigators perform the assessment of microbiologic end points for acute disease at a point when the drug is not likely to interfere with the assessment.[45] This is usually when the drug is cleared from the body and not on therapy. This is not the case with chronic disease such as HIV in which assessments are done on therapy.

There can be significant variation in trial results based on differing definitions of disease, outcomes, and patient populations. When making treatment decisions in clinical practice, clinicians should examine a range of trials on a given disease. Reproducible results in several trials of similar design are the strongest evidence of a true effect.[2] Also, clinicians should examine trials that show positive, negative, and neutral results for the disease under study. However, investigators are more likely to publish trials with positive results.[79,80] This publication bias can in turn affect meta-analyses and reviews. One study showed review articles tend to omit trials with negative or neutral results.[81]

Ultimately, clinicians must decide the relevance of a clinical trial to their particular practice. The distinction between clinical significance and statistical significance is an important one. Statistical significance indicates that the results of the trial are unlikely to occur by chance and that the results likely reflect the outcomes in a population similar to those studied in the trial. However, statistics do not reflect the clinical importance of the outcomes of the trial. Clinical significance reflects the clinical value of the outcome for patients.[27] A trial with a very large sample size may show that small differences in outcomes are statistically significant, but such small differences may be clinically meaningless. However, one could consider demonstration of successful clinical outcomes in well-documented cases of a disease that had previously been universally fatal and for which there was no available therapy as very important despite the fact that the result is not statistically significant. Such situations are relatively few and documentation of such cases is sometimes difficult.

Clinical trials examine the effect of a drug on a population of patients. When making individual treatment decisions, however, clinicians should examine the risks and benefits of administering the drug for a particular patient. This entails an evaluation of factors such as the patient's co-morbid illnesses, drug allergies and intolerance, concomitant medications, and the severity of the disease under treatment. Antimicrobial resistance is also an issue. Antimicrobials are the only drug class in which administration of the drug affects other patients as well as those who receive them.[82] Whereas a careful consideration of the design, analysis, and results of clinical trials helps guide clinical decision making, there is no substitute for sound clinical judgment at the bedside.

REFERENCES

1. Sackett DL, Rosenberg WM, Gray JA, et al. Evidence based medicine: What it is and what it isn't. BMJ. 1996;312(7023):71-72.
2. Ball C, Sackett DL, Phillips R, et al. Levels of evidence and grades of recommendations. Oxford Centre for Evidence Based Medicine. 2001. Available at: http://www.cebm.net/levels_of_evidence.asp
3. Elwood JM. The diagnosis of causation. In: Elwood JM, ed. Critical Appraisal of Epidemiological Studies and Clinical Trials. New York: Oxford University Press; 1998:218-246.
4. Elwood JM. Confounding. In: Elwood JM, ed. Critical Appraisal of Epidemiological Studies and Clinical Trials. New York: Oxford University Press; 1998:116-160.
5. Spilker B. Bias and confounding factors. In: Spilker B, ed. Guide to Clinical Trials. Philadelphia: Lippincott Williams and Wilkins; 2000:21-26.
6. Powers JH. Issues in clinical trials of prophylaxis of fungal infections. Clin Infect Dis. In press.
7. Goodman JL, Winston DJ, Greenfield RA, et al. A controlled trial of fluconazole to prevent fungal infections in patients undergoing bone marrow transplantation. N Engl J Med. 1992;326(13):845-851.
8. Singh N. Preemptive therapy versus universal prophylaxis with ganciclovir for cytomegalovirus in solid organ transplant recipients. Clin Infect Dis. 2001;32(5):742-751.
9. Miller B. Preventive therapy for tuberculosis. Med Clin North Am. 1993;77(6):1263-1275.
10. Vibhagool A, Sungkanuparph S, Mootsikapun P, et al. Discontinuation of secondary prophylaxis for cryptococcal meningitis in human immunodeficiency virus-infected patients treated with highly active antiretroviral therapy: A prospective, multicenter, randomized study. Clin Infect Dis. 2003;36(10):1329-1331.
11. Singh N, Paterson DL, Gayowski T, et al. Preemptive prophylaxis with a lipid preparation of amphotericin B for invasive fungal infections in liver transplant recipients requiring renal replacement therapy. Transplantation 2001;71(7):910-913.

12. File TM, Jr., Segreti J, Dunbar L, et al. A multicenter, randomized study comparing the efficacy and safety of intravenous and/or oral levofloxacin versus ceftriaxone and/or cefuroxime axetil in treatment of adults with community-acquired pneumonia. Antimicrob Agents Chemother. 1997;41(9):1965-1972.

13. Aras G. Superiority, noninferiority, equivalence and bioequivalence—Revisited. Drug Inf J. 2001;35:1157-1164.

14. Wiens BL. Choosing an equivalence limit for noninferiority or equivalence studies. Control Clin Trials. 2002;23(1):2-14.

15. Gould AL. Another view of active-controlled trials. Control Clin Trials. 1991;12(4):474-485.

16. Knapp RG, Miller MCI. Comparing therapies: The randomized controlled clinical trial. In: Knapp RG, Miller MCI, eds. Clinical Epidemiology and Biostatistics. Baltimore: Williams and Wilkins; 1992:131-139.

17. Powers, JH. Clinical trial design in acute bacterial sinusitis. Anti-infective Drugs Advisory Committee October 29, 2003, Gaithersburg, Md. Available at: http://www.fda.gov/ohrms/dockets/ac/03/transcripts/3997T2.htm.

18. Elwood JM. Selection of subjects for study. In: Elwood JM, ed. Critical Appraisal of Epidemiological Studies and Clinical Trials. New York: Oxford University Press; 1998:55-93.

19. Warren JW, Abrutyn E, Hebel JR, et al. Guidelines for antimicrobial treatment of uncomplicated acute bacterial cystitis and acute pyelonephritis in women. Infect Diseases Society of America (IDSA). Clin Infect Dis. 1999;29(4):745-758.

20. Rex JH, Sobel JD. Prophylactic antifungal therapy in the intensive care unit. Clin Infect Dis. 2001;32(8):1191-1200.

21. Spilker B. Randomization procedures. In: Spilker B, ed. Guide to Clinical Trials. Philadelphia: Lippincott Williams and Wilkins; 2000:69-73.

22. Cummings SR, Grady D, Hulley SB. Designing an experiment: clinical trials I. In: Hulley SB, Cummings SR, Browner WS, et al, eds. Designing Clinical Research. Philadelphia: Lippincott Williams and Wilkins; 2001:143-155.

23. Guyatt GH, Sackett DL, Cook DJ. Users' guides to the medical literature. II. How to use an article about therapy or prevention. A. Are the results of the study valid? Evidence-Based Medicine Working Group. JAMA. 1993;270(21):2598-2601.

24. Chalmers TC, Celano P, Sacks HS, Smith H Jr. Bias in treatment assignment in controlled clinical trials. N Engl J Med. 1983;309(22):1358-1361.

25. Makuch R, Simon R. Sample size requirements for evaluating a conservative therapy. Cancer Treat Rep. 1978;62(7):1037-1040.

26. Browner WS, Newman TB, Hearst N, Hulley SB. Getting ready to estimate sample size; hypotheses and underlying principles. In: Hulley SB, Cummings SR, Browner WS, et al, eds. Designing Clinical Research. Philadelphia: Lippincott Williams and Wilkins; 2001:51-63.

27. Redmond AC, Keenan AM. Understanding statistics. Putting p-values into perspective. J Am Podiatr Med Assoc. 2002;92(5):297-305.

28. Altman DG. Statistics in medical journals: Some recent trends. Stat Med. 2000;19(23):3275-3289.

29. Freiman JA, Chalmers TC, Smith H Jr, Kuebler RR. The importance of beta, the type II error and sample size in the design and interpretation of the randomized control trial. Survey of 71 "negative" trials. N Engl J Med. 1978;299(13):690-694.

30. Garbe E, Rohmel J, Gundert-Remy U. Clinical and statistical issues in therapeutic equivalence trials. Eur J Clin Pharmacol. 1993;45(1):1-7.

31. Williams RL, Chen ML, Hauck WW. Equivalence approaches. Clin Pharmacol Ther. 2002;72(3):229-237.

32. Wang SJ, Hung HM, Tsong Y. Utility and pitfalls of some statistical methods in active controlled clinical trials. Control Clin Trials. 2002;23(1):15-28.

33. Powers JH, Ross DB, Brittain E, et al. The United States Food and Drug Administration and noninferiority margins in clinical trials of antimicrobial agents. Clin Infect Dis. 2002;34(6):879-881.

34. Bailar JCI, Louis TA, Lavori PW, Polansky M. Studies without internal controls. In: Bailar JCI, Mosteller F, eds. Medical Uses of Statistics. Boston: NEJM Books; 1992:105-123.

35. Powers JH. Counterpoint: Alternative trial designs for antifungal drugs—Time to talk. Clin Infect Dis. 2001;33(1):107-109.

36. Temple R, Ellenberg SS. Placebo-controlled trials and active-control trials in the evaluation of new treatments. Part 1: Ethical and scientific issues. Ann Intern Med. 2000; 133(6):455-463.

37. Temple RJ, Meyer R. Continued need for placebo in many cases, even there is effective therapy. Arch Intern Med. 2003;163(3):371-373.

38. Sacks H, Chalmers TC, Smith H Jr. Randomized versus historical controls for clinical trials. Am J Med. 1982;72(2):233-240.

39. Sacks HS, Chalmers TC, Smith H Jr. Sensitivity and specificity of clinical trials. Randomized v historical controls. Arch Intern Med. 1983;143(4):753-755.

40. Sackett DL, Gent M. Controversy in counting and attributing events in clinical trials. N Engl J Med. 1979;301(26):1410-1412.

41. Temple RJ. A regulatory authority's opinion about surrogate endpoints. In: Nimmo WS, Tucker GT, eds. Clinical Measurement in Drug Evaluation. New York: John Wiley and Sons; 1995:3-22.

42. Lubsen J, Kirwan BA. Combined endpoints: Can we use them? Stat Med. 2002;21(19):2959-2970.

43. Fleming TR, DeMets DL. Surrogate end points in clinical trials: Are we being misled? Ann Intern Med. 1996;125(7):605-613.

44. Temple RJ. A regulatory authority's opinion about surrogate endpoints. In: Nimmo WS, Tucker GT, eds. Clinical Measurement in Drug Evaluation. New York: John Wiley and Sons; 1995:3-22.

45. Johann-Liang R, Zalkikar J, Powers JH. Correlation between bacteriologic and clinical endpoints in trials of acute otitis media. Pediatr Infect Dis J. 2003;22(10):936-937.

46. Prentice RL. Surrogate endpoints in clinical trials: Definition and operational criteria. Stat Med. 1989;8(4):431-440.

47. Labro MT. Interference of antibacterial agents with phagocyte functions: Immunomodulation or "immuno-fairy tales"? Clin Microbiol Rev. 2000;13(4):615-650.

48. Nau R, Eiffert H. Modulation of release of proinflammatory bacterial compounds by antibacterials: Potential impact on course of inflammation and outcome in sepsis and meningitis. Clin Microbiol Rev. 2002;15(1):95-110.

49. Lutsar I, Friedland IR, Jafri HS, et al. Factors influencing the anti-inflammatory effect of dexamethasone therapy in experimental pneumococcal meningitis. J Antimicrob Chemother. 2003;52(4):651-655.

50. McCracken GH Jr. Rich nations, poor nations, and bacterial meningitis. Lancet. 2002;360(9328):183.

51. Mellors JW, Rinaldo CR, Jr., Gupta P, et al. Prognosis in HIV-1 infection predicted by the quantity of virus in plasma. Science 1996; 272(5265):1167-1170.

52. Fleming TR. Surrogate markers in AIDS and cancer trials. Stat Med. 1994;13(13-14):1423-1435.

53. Sande MA, Carpenter CC, Cobbs CG, et al. Antiretroviral therapy for adult HIV-infected patients. Recommendations from a state-of-the-art conference. National Institute of Allergy and Infectious Diseases State-of-the-Art Panel on Anti-Retroviral Therapy for Adult HIV-Infected Patients. JAMA. 1993;270(21):2583-2589.

54. Pocock SJ, Clayton TC, Altman DG. Survival plots of time-to-event outcomes in clinical trials: Good practice and pitfalls. Lancet. 2002;359(9318):1686-1689.

55. DuPont HL, Jiang ZD, Ericsson CD, et al. Rifaximin versus ciprofloxacin for the treatment of traveler's diarrhea: A randomized, double-blind clinical trial. Clin Infect Dis. 2001;33(11):1807-1815.

56. Spilker B. Validation of clinical tests and measures. In: Spilker B, ed. Guide to Clinical Trials. Philadelphia: Lippincott Williams and Wilkins; 2000:313-319.

57. Berenguer J, Buck M, Witebsky F, et al. Lysis-centrifugation blood cultures in the detection of tissue-proven invasive candidiasis. Disseminated versus single-organ infection. Diagn Microbiol Infect Dis. 1993;17(2):103-109.

58. Moyle GJ. Truth, lies, and statistical tests. AIDS Read. 2003;13(3):117-126.

59. Lewis JA, Machin D. Intention to treat—Who should use ITT? Br J Cancer. 1993;68(4):647-650.

60. Lachin JM. Statistical considerations in the intent-to-treat principle. Control Clin Trials. 2000;21(3):167-189.

61. Friedman LM, Furberg CD, DeMets DL. Reporting and interpreting of results. In: Friedman LM, Furberg CD, DeMets DL, eds. Fundamentals of Clinical Trials. New York: Springer; 1998:333-344.

62. Wulff HR. Magic of p values. Lancet. 1988;1(8599):1398.

63. Ware JH, Mosteller F, Delgado F, et al. P values. In: Bailar JCI, Mosteller F, eds. Medical Uses of Statistics. Boston: NEJM Books; 1992:181-200.

64. Wulff HR, Andersen B, Brandenhoff P, Guttler F. What do doctors know about statistics? Stat Med. 1987;6(1):3-10.

65. Freeman PR. The role of p-values in analysing trial results. Stat Med. 1993;12(15-16):1443-1452.

66. Bland JM, Altman DG. Multiple significance tests: The Bonferroni method. BMJ 1995;310(6973):170.

67. Perneger TV. What's wrong with Bonferroni adjustments. BMJ. 1998;316 (7139):1236-1238.

68. Freemantle N. Interpreting the results of secondary end points and subgroup analyses in clinical trials: Should we lock the crazy aunt in the attic? BMJ. 2001; 322(7292):989-991.

69. Berry G. Statistical significance and confidence intervals. Med J Aust. 1986; 144(12):618-619.

70. Ebbutt AF, Frith L. Practical issues in equivalence trials. Stat Med. 1998;17(15-16):1691-1701.

71. Bucher HC, Guyatt GH, Cook DJ, et al. Users' guides to the medical literature: XIX. Applying clinical trial results. A. How to use an article measuring the effect of an intervention on surrogate end points. Evidence-Based Medicine Working Group. JAMA. 1999;282(8):771-778.

72. Altman DG. Statistics in medical journals. Stat Med. 1982;1(1):59-71.

73. Gotzsche PC. Methodology and overt and hidden bias in reports of 196 double-blind trials of nonsteroidal antiinflammatory drugs in rheumatoid arthritis. Control Clin Trials. 1989;10(1):31-56.

74. Pocock SJ, Hughes MD, Lee RJ. Statistical problems in the reporting of clinical trials. A survey of three medical journals. N Engl J Med. 1987;317(7):426-432.

75. Labro MT. Antibiotics as anti-inflammatory agents. Curr Opin Investig Drugs. 2002;3(1):61-68.

76. Azeh I, Gerber J, Wellmer A, et al. Protein synthesis inhibiting clindamycin improves outcome in a mouse model of Staphylococcus aureus sepsis compared with the cell wall active ceftriaxone. Crit Care Med. 2002;30(7):1560-1564.

77. Dagan R, Leibovitz E, Greenberg D, et al. Early eradication of pathogens from middle ear fluid during antibiotic treatment of acute otitis media is associated with improved clinical outcome. Pediatr Infect Dis J. 1998;17(9):776-782.

78. Carlin SA, Marchant CD, Shurin PA, et al. Host factors and early therapeutic response in acute otitis media. J Pediatr. 1991;118(2):178-183.

79. Dickersin K, Min YI. Publication bias: The problem that won't go away. Ann N Y Acad Sci. 1993;703:135-146; discussion 146-8:135-146.

80. Dickersin K, Chan S, Chalmers TC, et al. Publication bias and clinical trials. Control Clin Trials. 1987;8(4):343-353.

81. Gotzsche PC. Reference bias in reports of drug trials. Br Med J (Clin Res Ed). 1987;295(6599):654-656.

82. Colgan R, Powers JH. Appropriate antimicrobial prescribing: Approaches that limit antibiotic resistance. Am Fam Physician. 2001;64(6):999-1004.

Outpatient Parenteral Antimicrobial Therapy

ALAN D. TICE

Intravenous therapy was developed in hospitals and was considered an exclusively hospital procedure in the therapy of infectious diseases until 1974, when Rucker reported the outpatient treatment of respiratory infections in cystic fibrosis patients with intravenous antibiotics.[1] Since then, outpatient care has evolved to include provision of intravenous antimicrobials, parenteral nutrition, immune modulators, and chemotherapy in patients' homes, in infusion centers, and in physicians' offices.

The growth of outpatient parenteral antimicrobial therapy (OPAT) has been largely attributable to rising costs of hospitalization, which currently average $1000 per day.[2] This economic stimulus aside, however, home care offers a number of quality-of-life advantages over hospitalization, including the presence of family and friends, privacy, and home-cooked food. For children and some elderly people, the hospital can be a particularly stressful and frightening environment.

The managed care industry is very much interested in OPAT and outpatient care in general because it provides an unusual opportunity to reduce costs while improving quality of care and patient satisfaction.[3-5] However, the outpatient setting represents a challenge to today's physicians, who are no longer familiar with medical care beyond the confines of the hospital and their offices or clinics.[6] Now, as patient care is shifted more and more into the community, OPAT offers models for clinicians to consider in the treatment of their patients with serious infections who need intravenous antibiotics yet are otherwise able to be at home. Many of these patients are able to return to work or school during OPAT and hence earn as well as save money.[7,8] OPAT may also reduce the morbidity, mortality, and cost of nosocomial infections.

MODELS OF DELIVERY

There are three basic models of delivery of OPAT: the visiting nurse, the infusion center, and self-administration[9-11] (Table 45-1). The visiting nurse model is effective when there is an established home care agency that can provide medication at home under the supervision of a nurse. A visit to a patient's home may also be very revealing in regard to the underlying diseases and social problems of the patient but has become expensive compared with the other models. An infusion center can be established in almost any setting, including a physician's office, a clinic, and a hospital emergency department, or it may be freestanding. Such centers offer the ready availability of physicians and nurses as well as a supply of medications and equipment should there be a problem with vascular access or the need to change the antibiotic. The self-administration model has been made possible through the development of reliable vascular access catheters and infusion devices that can be programmed to automatically administer medications as reliably as in the hospital and for days at a time.

INFECTIONS TREATED

The list of diseases amenable to OPAT is long (Table 45-2), but the study of this form of therapy is limited.[10] As OPAT has evolved, the question of which infections can be treated has become more a matter of which cannot be. It appears that virtually every infection that requires intravenous antibiotic therapy can be treated outside the hospital for at least part of the therapeutic course. However, initial hospitalization is required or recommended for some infections.[10,11] For example, patients with bacterial meningitis, endocarditis, or possible sepsis should be hospitalized on presentation. If they have a good response to treatment, however, even they can often be discharged to complete the course of intravenous therapy as outpatients.

Central nervous system infections are of particular concern because of the potential for neurologic injury and the need for prompt, high-dose antibiotic therapy. Seizures are an added concern for patients with a brain abscess, who should receive prophylactic anticonvulsant therapy. Children with meningitis who have a good clinical response can safely complete their therapy at home if they meet specific criteria.[12,13]

Bacterial endocarditis was one of the first types of infections to be treated on an outpatient basis because of the requirement for 4 to 6 weeks of intravenous therapy. Although a number of studies have reported the safety and effectiveness of OPAT for endocarditis, some cautions and questions remain.[14-16] A number of potentially complicating factors may discourage, if not contraindicate, the use of OPAT for endocarditis; these include *Staphylococcus aureus* infection, left-sided disease, conduction abnormalities, a large thrombus with a potential for embolus, and heart failure that may require early surgical intervention.[14-18]

Osteomyelitis is another infection particularly suited for OPAT.[19-22] A prolonged course of intravenous therapy is usually recommended for patients who are otherwise well. Patients are often hospitalized initially for surgical intervention and then discharged when they respond. In many communities, however, patients may be

TABLE 45-1 Models of Outpatient Parenteral Antimicrobial Therapy

Model	Advantages	Disadvantages
Visiting nurse	Home evaluation	Cost of nurse time/travel
	Supervised drug administration	Concerns with privacy
		Safety of home
Infusion center	Medical staff present	Cost of facility
	Access to medications and devices	Patient travel to center
	Supervised administration	
Self-administration	Reduced facility cost	Patient/caregiver training
	Patient autonomy	Compliance
		Unsupervised administration

TABLE 45-2 Infections Amenable to Outpatient Parenteral Antimicrobial Therapy

Hospitalize first
Meningitis
Endocarditis
Suspected sepsis

Acute infections
Cellulitis
Wound infections
Pneumonia
Pyelonephritis

Chronic infections
Osteomyelitis
Diabetic foot infections
Sinusitis

Human immunodeficiency virus–related infections
Cytomegalovirus
Pneumocystis carinii
Chronic fungal infections

started directly on OPAT with elective admissions only if surgery is needed or the patient fails to respond to outpatient care. Although some of the new oral quinolones have replaced intravenous therapy for gram-negative osteomyelitis, bacteria resistant to oral antimicrobials and gram-positive organisms remain a challenge. Studies that equate oral and intravenous therapy for osteomyelitis are not yet convincing, particularly where *Staphylococcus aureus* is involved.[23] Methicillin-resistant *S. aureus* strains have also added a challenge that has led to an increasing use of vancomycin despite its not being as effective as β-lactam agents.[21] Oral linezolid and parenteral daptomycin and quinupristin-dalfopristin offer some hope with resistant staphylococci.[24-26] Surgical intervention is always an important consideration if there is a sequestrum, necrotic tissue, or inadequate blood supply, but it may be prudent to begin OPAT a few days before surgery in the face of an acute infection.

Infections related to implanted devices and materials are increasing.[23] These often involve coagulase-negative staphylococci, which elaborate a protective biofilm that promotes adherence to foreign bodies. Although there is some promise of effective therapy with a prolonged course of an oral quinolone plus rifampin, the organisms may well be resistant and vancomycin is again needed.[27] Prosthetic joint infections often require removal of the hardware followed by several weeks of intravenous therapy before and after a new joint is placed.[27,28] OPAT is also possible in this situation, as a person may be able to get along without a joint for a few weeks.

The epidemic of human immunodeficiency virus (HIV) infection with associated opportunistic infections has provided another impetus for home therapy. Many acquired immunodeficiency syndrome (AIDS) patients have staunchly refused hospitalization and challenged the medical community to provide therapies at home that would previously have been administered only in hospitals. These patients are often willing to take any risk to be treated at home. Thus, opportunistic infections that require intravenous therapies, such as cryptococcal meningitis and cytomegalovirus infections, have been treated for much of their course on an outpatient basis. Cytomegalovirus has responded well to intravenous ganciclovir, foscarnet, and cidofovir, which has an advantage in that it can be given intravenously every other week. However, some oral agents have become available that are effective in suppression.[29] Pentamidine has been administered in patients' homes but should be provided only according to careful and reliable protocols.[30] Prolonged courses of amphotericin B can also be given on an outpatient basis if oral antifungals are not sufficient or active; this treatment is commonly given in an infusion center three times a week rather than every day, which makes OPAT much more tolerable. Recent welcome additions to the antifungal armamentarium include intravenous caspofungin, which is well tolerated, and new oral agents that may replace intravenous therapies.[31]

Lower respiratory tract infections and even sinusitis may also benefit from intravenous antibiotic therapy. For community-acquired pneumonia, it has been common practice to admit patients for intravenous antibiotic therapy. According to recent studies, however, many of those patients do not require hospitalization, and for those who do, in-hospital days could be reduced if OPAT programs are available in the community.[32,33] Furthermore, patients with community-acquired pneumonia would prefer to be treated at home if it is safe to do so.[34,35] The risk-stratification system proposed by Fine and others[36] is useful in distinguishing patients who are sick enough to require hospitalization from those who are not. The Infectious Diseases Society of America and the American Thoracic Society have published guidelines for the management of community-acquired pneumonia that may also be useful in deciding on admission and parenteral therapies.[37,38]

Serious or complicated skin and soft tissue infections have traditionally been treated in the hospital for a few days with intravenous antibiotics, particularly if surgical débridement is necessary. However, many can be treated entirely in the outpatient setting with

a dose of intravenous antibiotics administered at the initial evaluation and a follow-up examination the next day.[39,40] There are some limitations, however, in treating one of the most challenging soft tissue infections—the diabetic foot infection. Poor outcomes are seldom due to a failure of the antibiotic but rather to other factors such as inadequate perfusion, neuropathy, hyperglycemia, and poor compliance. These patients should be offered hospitalization early and considered for OPAT only when they have been evaluated thoroughly, surgery is considered, are clinically stable, and the infection is responding to therapy.[41,42]

ANTIMICROBIAL USE

The first decision to be made regarding antimicrobial use in OPAT is whether a patient needs intravenous therapy. Although some oral antibiotics have been found equivalent to intravenous agents, good comparative studies are lacking. Moreover, there is a consistent need for some parenteral antibiotics, such as vancomycin, for which there is no oral equivalent. The antibiotics selected for use in the outpatient setting may be different from those administered to closely supervised hospital patients.[43,44] The ideal antimicrobial should be safe and well tolerated and have a long half-life. The selection should be tailored specifically to the infection, which calls for early and careful cultures with identification and antibiotic-susceptibility testing of the pathogen. Finally, the agent must be stable after mixing, a particularly important consideration for patients self-administering premixed medications over 3 to 4 days.[11]

The less often a drug needs to be administered, the more convenient it is for OPAT.

Ceftriaxone has been a very useful drug for OPAT because its 8-hour half-life makes it effective in once-daily dosing for most types of infection.[46] Ertapenem, caspofungin, and daptomycin all have the same once-daily dosing regimen.[31,47] A single daily dose is sufficient for some of the new quinolones, as well as for azithromycin, which has a tissue half-life of 30 hours.[48] Despite a relatively short half-life of 2 hours, the pharmacodynamics of the aminoglycosides also permit once-daily administration.[49]

Some antimicrobials can be dosed even less frequently than daily. The prolonged half-life of teicoplanin permits a dosing schedule of every other day, or three times a week for osteomyelitis.[50] Intravenous cidofovir appears to be useful in the treatment and suppression of cytomegalovirus infections when given only every 1 or 2 weeks.[51] Table 45-3 lists medications that can be given once a day or less frequently.

It is also important to assess organ function before initiating antimicrobial therapy. With renal failure vancomycin may need to be dosed only once per week.[52] Moreover, given the gradual decline in renal function with age, elderly patients may also do well with once-daily dosing of vancomycin.[53,54]

Once-daily administration is an obvious advantage for any of the delivery models. However, some antibiotics that have a shorter half-life but are relatively stable may be administered by a battery-powered, computer-operated portable infusion device programmed to deliver doses at selected intervals. These pumps can also be used for continuous infusion of antibiotics, which may be the most effective

TABLE 45-3 Antibiotics Suitable for Outpatient Parenteral Antimicrobial Therapy	
Once-Daily Antibiotics	*Less Than Once Daily*
Aminoglycosides	Amphotericin B
Azithromycin	Cidofovir
Caspofungin	Teicoplanin
Ceftriaxone	
Daptomycin	
Ertapemem	
Quinolones (some)	
Vancomycin (in the elderly)	

way to deliver cell wall–active antibiotics such as the penicillins and some of the cephalosporins.[55,56]

Caution is needed with the first dose of an intravenous antibiotic. With an estimated 1500 deaths from anaphylaxis due to drug administration annually in the United States,[57] there is a risk if the first dose is given in the home or outside a medical setting without ready access to medical personnel and emergency equipment. Although some nurses take epinephrine and an antihistamine kit to the home, it is recommended that the first dose of antibiotic be given in the hospital, the emergency department, or a physician's office equipped for emergencies.[10] Thereafter, the chances of a life-threatening reaction developing are much smaller, although anaphylactoid reactions have been reported to occur during the course of therapy.[58]

How long to continue parenteral therapy remains a question to be decided by the clinician. Some diseases, such as otitis media in children, gonorrhea, streptococcal pharyngitis, and potentially other infections, require only a single dose of ceftriaxone for good clinical and culture responses.[59-61] Once there is a good clinical response to parenteral therapy, some patients may be "switched" to an oral antimicrobial to complete the course of therapy.[62-64] Optimal management of antimicrobials requires close physician monitoring for clinical response as well as toxicity.

TECHNOLOGY

A variety of new devices have facilitated outpatient therapy. Because vascular access is essential for OPAT and nurses are not readily available to examine or restart intravenous infusions in patients' homes, a reliable intravenous line is essential. Plastic catheters are an improvement over steel needles in patient comfort and restarts. Central lines have made prolonged courses of intravenous therapy easier and more reliable. A variety of these lines have been developed to facilitate OPAT.[67,68] One of the most interesting and practical is the peripherally inserted central catheter (PICC), which is inserted into an antecubital vein and passed into the superior vena cava. A PICC should be considered for patients whose course of intravenous medication is planned for more than a week, particularly if the medication is likely to cause phlebitis or the patient already has poor venous access. Central lines can lead to a variety of complications, but the risk of infection seems to be lower with PICCs and comparable to that of peripheral catheters in some series.[69-72]

Infusion devices can also simplify an OPAT program. Gravity drip systems are increasingly being replaced by syringe pumps, which provide a consistent flow and require less patient training, with little added expense. Use of these pumps also reduces plastic waste, as the syringe is used to both mix and infuse the medication. Battery-driven, computer-operated pumps are advantageous for use in patients who require a prolonged course of therapy or frequent dosing, such as every-4-hour infusions, and for those who have difficulty manipulating the equipment for self-administration. The device can administer antimicrobials automatically without interfering with patients' daily routines or sleep.[68,73] Most pumps can also be programmed to administer antimicrobials via continuous infusion, which may be as or more effective than intermittent dosing for the penicillins and cephalosporins.[73] Pump-driven continuous infusion also may be less costly in terms of nursing staff time and the amount of antibiotic needed to maintain a level above the minimal inhibitory concentration of the bacteria.[74]

PATIENT SELECTION

Not every patient is a candidate for OPAT, despite increasing economic incentives for early hospital discharge or avoidance of hospitalization altogether. As these pressures mount, it is important that physicians understand the risks and limits of outpatient therapy. The responsibility to admit or discharge a patient from the hospital rests with the physician who signs the order. The ordering physician is also responsible for the quality and outcomes of the OPAT program.

However, he or she may know little of what it really means to send a patient home with a serious infection. Because physicians are far less involved in home visits and outpatient management than they were in previous generations,[6] they often rely on home infusion provider organizations, whose quality may vary significantly. Payers and insurance companies may direct patients to home health agencies based on charges alone.[75] The physician needs to know the quality of the home care program to be used and to compare its program with guidelines from the Infectious Diseases Society of America.[10] If the quality of OPAT care will not be as good as that in the hospital, the patient should remain in the hospital.

The criteria for the selection of patients should be carefully assessed[10,11,76,77] (Table 45-4). The patient must be stable in regard to his or her disease or diseases. Although it may be possible to treat the presenting infection with OPAT, the patient may have other conditions, such as diabetes, heart failure, or renal failure, that preclude outpatient care. Nursing needs are also an important consideration, particularly if there is limited home support and expertise. Patients also must be evaluated for their physical, emotional, and mental abilities to perform the procedures required for OPAT. Both patients and their families or caretakers should be informed about OPAT and assessed as to their willingness to participate. Patients should have the option of remaining hospitalized despite pressure from insurance companies for early discharge. The home situation and environment should also be considered. Patients with good family support and who live in safe environments are the best candidates. In general, a patient who does not have a social support system, a safe home environment with a telephone, and ready access to transportation should not be sent home. A skilled nursing facility might be a better alternative.

Once the physician and the infusion therapy nurse have identified a patient for OPAT, the insurance company should be approached for payment authorization and to see what restrictions it may have in terms of exclusive contracts and coverage of particular items, such as infusion devices. The payer may try to control the choice of provider, delivery model, technology, and even the drug that can be used.

If a physician is to provide outpatient intravenous therapy through his or her office, a number of factors must be considered. Although it is a time-honored tradition to administer limited courses of intramuscular antibiotics in the office, prolonged courses of intravenous antibiotics are more difficult, challenging, and expensive. There should be policies and procedures in place to ensure the quality of medications and care provided.[10] Table 45-5 lists recommendations to assess the quality of an infusion center.

Physicians who work with infusion providers outside their practices should consider a number of additional factors, as outlined in the Infectious Diseases Society of America guidelines (Table 45-6). The physician remains responsible for the patient's care, even though it

TABLE 45-4 Patient Selection Criteria	
Elements	*Considerations*
The infection	Risk of complications
	Complexity of therapy needed
	Oral therapy not reasonable
Other diseases	Clinical status
	Nursing needs
Patient assessment	Clinically stable
	Willing to participate
	Physically, and mentally able
	Vascular access status
	Substance abuse
Home situation	Family/caregiver support
	Transportation
	Emergency services available
	Telephone
	Running water
	Refrigeration
Reimbursement	Restrictions
	Patient responsibility

TABLE 45-5 Outpatient Parenteral Antimicrobial Therapy Requirements for Infusion Center Model

Health care team	Physician
	Nurse
	Pharmacist
Communications	Physician, nurse, and pharmacist always available
	System for rapid communication with patient, and among team members
Written policies and procedures	Outline of responsibilities of team members
	Patient admission information
	Patient selection criteria
	Patient education materials

Adapted from IDSA guidelines.[10]

may be outside the hospital and, in some respects, outside the physician's control. It is therefore important that the physician develop a good working relationship with the infusion provider and good lines of communication with the team members.[78] Continued quality assurance and quality improvement measures should be essential parts of the OPAT program and will be increasingly required for accreditation and compensation.[58,79]

MONITORING PATIENTS

The physician's role does not end with development of the treatment plan and discharge of the patient from the hospital. It is particularly important that the physician remains involved with the patient's care, periodically assess the patient for response to the antibiotic, and look for adverse drug reactions. Ongoing management of the patient's other medical problems, which are often present, may also be necessary. An OPAT program is not without risk and may require particular knowledge and experience to deal with the complexities involved.[80-82]

The schedule of visits to the physician and periodic laboratory studies should be established with the initial treatment plan.[10,58] The standard for monitoring by the physician is once or twice weekly, but as often as daily for patients who are unstable. Less frequent visits

TABLE 45-6 Criteria for Evaluating Outpatient Parenteral Antibiotic Therapy (OPAT) Programs

Medical director or advisor knowledgeable about infectious diseases and OPAT
Define roles for prescribing physician in relation to case management, medical director, nurse, and pharmacist
Standards for nurse, pharmacist, physician, and other patient care personnel in regard to training, experience, and licensure
Accreditation status in regard to providing OPAT
Policies regarding:
  a. Frequency of physician's and nurse's clinical assessment of the patient
  b. Staffing and on-call policies
  c. Frequency of clinical status reports to physicians
  d. Report of laboratory results to physicians within 24 hours
  e. Rapid reporting of patient problems and critical laboratory values
Willingness to share results of quality assurance and outcomes measures
Willingness to share charge information for referred patients
Information about:
  Anti-infective preparation and dispensing
  Vascular access systems and care
  Infusion device care
  Monitoring guidelines for laboratory studies
  Waste disposal
Patient education and resource materials
  Instructions for emergency situations
  Information about anti-infective use and adverse effects to watch for
  Understanding of potential risks and problems and patient responsibilities in regard to OPAT
System for ongoing quality assurance and outcome monitoring

may be reasonable for those who are stable but undergoing a prolonged course of intravenous antimicrobials such as with ganciclovir for a cytomegalovirus infection. The risk of phlebitis and central line infections is also significant, requiring close monitoring of vascular access devices.[70] Although the clinical course of patients on OPAT is usually one of improvement, the potential for drug toxicity increases with time. This seems to be true for the renal and vestibular toxicity associated with the aminoglycosides, which are most likely to develop several weeks into the course of therapy.[71] Leukopenia may also occur several weeks after initiation of therapy with penicillin, cephalosporins, or vancomycin.[69,72] Thus, even though the infection may be responding well, the potential for antibiotic toxicities requires increasing vigilance.

A reliable system for follow-up of patients started on OPAT may have additional benefits. Many patients are admitted to hospitals for 1- or 2-day courses of intravenous antimicrobial therapy. Many of these patients can be started on OPAT in the emergency department and then sent home if they can be ensured of seeing a physician the next morning and have the ability to be continued on OPAT.

FUTURE OF OUTPATIENT PARENTERAL ANTIBIOTIC THERAPY

The need for intravenous antimicrobial therapy will continue despite the availability of new and improving oral medications. New drugs are needed to face the challenges of increasing antimicrobial resistance and the challenges of pharmacology characteristics. Further investigations are needed of intramuscular versus intravenous medication and when to "switch" to oral agents. As pressures mount to treat patients with intravenous antimicrobials outside the hospital, physicians must be aware of the problems and risks that may be encountered. Knowledge and experience with OPAT plus outcomes measures to understand its limitations will be increasingly important.[58]

REFERENCES

1. Rucker RW, Harrison GM. Outpatient intravenous medications in the management of cystic fibrosis. Pediatrics. 1974;54:358-360.
2. AHA data offer insights into hospital cost, utilization trends. Capitation Rates Data. 2003;8:56-59.
3. Tice AD, Slama TG, Berman S, et al. Managed care and the infectious diseases specialist. Clin Infect Dis. 1996;23:341-368.
4. Goodfellow AF, Wai AO, Frighetto L, et al. Quality-of-life assessment in an outpatient parenteral antibiotic program. Ann Pharmacother. 2002;36:1851-1855.
5. Tice AD. Experience with a physician-directed, clinic-based program for outpatient parenteral antibiotic therapy in the USA. Eur J Clin Microbiol Infect Dis. 1995;14:655-661.
6. Meyer GS, Gibbons RV. House calls to the elderly—A vanishing practice among physicians. N Engl J Med. 1997;337:1815-1820.
7. Poretz DM, Eron LJ, Goldenberg RI, et al. Intravenous antibiotic therapy in an outpatient setting. JAMA. 1982;248:336-339.
8. Williams DN. Home intravenous anti-infective therapy (HIVAT): Do the benefits outweigh the risks? Drug Safety. 1996;14:1-7.
9. Tice AD, Nolet BR. Delivery models for outpatient parenteral antimicrobial therapy. Outpatient parenteral antimicrobial therapy: Current status (Special Report). Sci Am Med 1997;7-11.
10. Tice AD, Rohm SJ, Dolorisio JR, et al. Practice Guidelines for Outpatient Parenteral Antimicrobial Therapy. Clin Infect Dis. 2004;38:1651-1672.
11. Tice AD. Handbook of Outpatient Parenteral Therapy for Infectious Diseases. New York: Scientific American, Inc; 1997.
12. Tice AD, Strait K, Ramey R, Hoaglund PA. Outpatient parenteral antimicrobial therapy for central nervous system infections. Clin Infect Dis. 1999;29:1394-1399.
13. Bradley JS. Meningitis. Hosp Pract. 1993;28(suppl 2):15-19.
14. Rehm SJ. Outpatient intravenous antibiotic therapy for endocarditis. Infect Dis Clin North Am. 1998;12:879-901.
15. Montiero CE, Cobbs CG. Outpatient management of infective endocarditis. Curr Infect Dis Rep. 2001;3:319-327.
16. Andrews MM, von Reyn CF. Patient selection criteria and management guidelines for outpatient parenteral antibiotic therapy for native valve endocarditis. Clin Infect Dis. 2001;15:33:203-209.
17. Lopardo G. Management of endocarditis: Outpatient parenteral antibiotic treatment in Argentina. Chemotherapy. 2001;47(suppl 1):24-32.

18. Sexton DJ, Tenenbaum MJ, Wilson WR, et al. Ceftriaxone once daily for four weeks compared with ceftriaxone plus gentamicin once daily for two weeks for treatment of endocarditis due to pencillin-susceptible streptococci. Endocarditis Treatment Consortium Group. Clin Infect Dis. 1998;27:1470-1474.

19. Tice AD. Outpatient parenteral antimicrobial therapy for osteomyelitis. Infect Dis Clin North Am. 1998;12:903-919.

20. Bernard L, El-Hajj, Pron B, et al. Outpatient parenteral antimicrobial therapy (OPAT) for the treatment of osteomyelitis: Evaluation of efficacy, tolerance and cost. J Clin Pharm Ther. 2001;26:445-451.

21. Tice AD, Hoaglund PA, Shoultz DA. Risk factors and treatment outcomes in osteomyelitis. J Antimicrob Chemother. 2003;51:1261-1268.

22. Tice AD. The use of outpatient parenteral antimicrobial therapy in the management of osteomyelitis: Data from the Outpatient Parenteral Antimicrobial Therapy Outcomes Registry. Chemotherapy. 2001;47(suppl 1):5-16.

23. Lew DP, Waldvogel FA. Osteomyelitis. N Engl J Med. 1997;336:999-1007.

24. Till M, Wixson RI, Pertel PE. Linezolid treatment for osteomyelitis due to vancomycin-resistant Enterococcus faecium. Clin Infect Dis. 2002;34:1412-1414.

25. Mader JT, Adams K. Comparative evaluation of daptomycin (LY146032) and vancomycin in the treatment of experimental methicillin-resistant Staphylococcus aureus osteomyelitis in rabbits. Antimicrob Agents Chemother. 1989;33:689-692.

26. Summers M, Misenhimer GR, Amntony SJ. Vancomycin-resistant Enterococcus faecium osteomyelitis: Successful treatment with quinupristin-dalfopristin. South Med J. 2001;94:353-355.

27. Zimmerli W, Widmer AF, Blatter M, et al. Role of rifampin for treatment of orthopedic implant-related staphylococcal infections: A randomized controlled trial. JAMA. 1998;279;1575-1577.

28. Karchmer AW. Editorial Response: Salvage of infected orthopedic devices. Clin Infect Dis. 1998;27:714-716.

29. Winston DJ, Yeager AM, Chandrasekar PH, et. al. Randomized comparison of oral valacyclovir and intravenous ganciclovir for prevention of cytomegalovirus disease after allogeneic bone marrow transplantation. Clin Infect Dis. 2003;36:749-758.

30. Gross R, Graziani AL, Laufer D. Adverse effects of the use of intravenous pentamidine in the home. Infect Dis Clin Pract. 1996;5:456-458.

31. Arathoon EG, Gotuzzo E, Noriega LM, et al. Randomized, double-blind, multicenter study of caspofungin versus amphotericin B for treatment of oropharyngeal and esophageal candidiasis. Antimicrob Agent Chemother. 2002;46:451-457.

32. Fine MJ, Hough LJ, Medsger AR, et al. The hospital admission decision for patients with community-acquired pneumonia. Arch Intern Med. 1997;157:36-44.

33. Fine MJ, Medsger AR, Stone RA, et al. The hospital discharge decision for patients with community-acquired pneumonia. Arch Intern Med. 1997;157:47-56.

34. Coley CM, Li Y-H, Medsger AR, et al. Preferences for home vs hospital care among low-risk patients with community-acquired pneumonia. Arch Intern Med. 1996;156:1565-1571.

35. Strandvik B, Hjelte L, Malmborg AS, Widen B. Home intravenous antibiotic treatment of patients with cystic fibrosis. Acta Paediatr. 1992;81:340-344.

36. Fine MJ, Auble TE, Yealy DM, et al. A prediction rule to identify low-risk patients with community-acquired pneumonia. N Engl J Med. 1997;336:243-250.

37. Bartlett JG, Breiman RF, Mandell LA, File TM. Community-acquired pneumonia in adults: guidelines for management. Clin Infect Dis. 1998;26:811-838.

38. Niederman MS, Mandell LA, Anzueto A, et al. Guidelines for the management of adults with community-acquired pneumonia. Diagnosis, assessment of severity, antimicrobial therapy, and preventions. Am J Respir Crit Care Med. 2001;163:1730-1754.

39. Deery HG II. Outpatient parenteral anti-infective therapy for skin and soft-tissue infections. Infect Dis Clin North Am. 1998;12:935-949.

40. Nathwani D. The management of skin and soft tissue infections: Outpatient parenteral antibiotic therapy in the United Kingdom. Chemotherapy. 2001;47(suppl 1):17-23.

41. Eron LJ, Passos S. Early discharge of infected patients through appropriate antibiotic use. Arch Intern Med. 2001;161:61-65.

42. Fox HR, Karchmer AW. Management of diabetic foot infections, including the use of home intravenous antibiotic therapy. Clin Podiatr Med Surg. 1996;13:671-682.

43. Lipsky BA. A current approach to diabetic foot infection. Curr Infect Dis Rep. 1999;1:253-260.

44. Craig WA. Kinetics of antibiotics in relation to effective and convenient outpatient parenteral therapy. Int J Antimicrob Agents. 1995;5:19-22.

45. Slavik RS, Jewesson PJ. Selecting antibacterials for outpatient parenteral antimicrobial therapy: Pharmacokinetic-pharmacodynamic considerations. Clin Pharmacokinet. 2003;42:793-817.

46. Tice AD. Once-daily ceftriaxone outpatient therapy in adults with infections. Chemotherapy. 1991;37(suppl 3):7-10.

47. Gesser R, McCarroll K, Woods G. Outpatient use of parenteral antimicrobial therapy in a controlled trial of ertapenem vs. pipericillin-tazobactam. Poster 204. Presented at the annual meeting of Infectious Diseases Society of America, Chicago, Ill, October 2002.

48. Luke DR, Foulds G, Cohen SF, Levy B. Safety, toleration, and pharmacokinetics of intravenous azithromycin. Antimicrob Agents Chemother. 1996;40:2577-2581.

49. Fisman DN, Kaye KM. Once-daily dosing of minoglycoside antibiotics. Infect Dis Clin North Am. 2000;14:475-487.

50. Graninger W, Presterl E, Wenisch C, et al. Management of serious staphylococcal infections in the outpatient setting. Drugs. 1997;54:21-28.

51. Lea AP, Bryson HM. Cidofovir. Drugs. 1997;52:225-230.

52. Livornese LL Jr, Slavin D, Benz RL, et al. Use of antibacterial agents in renal failure. Infect Dis Clin North Am. 2001;15:983-1002.

53. Gleckman RA. Antibiotic concerns in the elderly: A clinician's perspective. Infect Dis Clin North Am. 1995;9:575-590.

54. Guay DRP, Vance-Bryan K, Gilliland SS, et al. Comparison of vancomycin pharmacokinetics in hospitalized elderly and young patients using a Bayesian forecaster. J Clin Pharmacol. 1993;33:918-922.

55. MacGowan AP, Bowker KE. Continuous infusion of beta-lactam antibiotics. Clin Pharmacokinet. 1998;35:391-402.

56. Turnidge JD. The pharmacodynamics of beta-lactams. Clin Infect Dis. 1998;27:10-22.

57. Matasar MJ, Neugut AI. Epidemiology of anaphylaxis in the United States. Curr Allergy Asthma Rep. 2003;3:30-35.

59. Tice AD. Documenting the value of OPAT: Outcomes studies and patient registries. Can J Infect Dis 2000;10:45A-48A.

58. Nathwani D, Tice AD. Ambulatory antimicrobial use: The value of an outcomes registry. J Antimicrob Chemother. 2002;49:149-154.

60. Kunkel MJ. Outcomes measurement in OPAT: Why and how. Outpatient parenteral antimicrobial therapy: Current status. Sci Am 1997;special report:50-54.

61. Pichichero ME, Cohen R. Shortened course of antibiotic therapy for acute otitis media, sinusitis and tonsillopharyngitis. Pediatr Infect Dis J. 1997;16:680-695.

62. Hoang KD, Pollack CV. Antibiotic use in the emergency department. I: Single-dose therapy and parenteral-loading dose therapy. J Emerg Med. 1996;14:619-628.

63. Powers RD. The role of the emergency department in OPAT. Outpatient parenteral antimicrobial therapy: Current status. Sci Am 1997;special report:28-31.

64. Ramirez JA, Srinath L, Ahkee S, et al. Early switch from intravenous to oral cephalosporins in the treatment of hospitalized patients with community-acquired pneumonia. Arch Intern Med. 1995;155:1273-1276.

65. Barlow GD, Nathwani D. Sequential antibiotic therapy. Curr Opin Infect Dis. 2000;13:599-607.

66. Cunha BA. Intravenous to oral antibiotic switch therapy. Drugs Today (Barc). 2001;37:311-319.

67. Gilbert DN, Dworkin R, Raber SR, Leggett JE. Outpatient parenteral antimicrobial-drug therapy. N Engl J Med. 1997;337:829-838.

68. Mortlock NJ, Schleis TG. Outpatient parenteral antimicrobial therapy technology. Infect Dis Clin North Am. 1998;12:861-878.

69. Tice AD, Kunkel MJ, Sullivan DR, OPIVITA Study Group. Complications of PICC line use in outpatient care (Abstract). Presented at the 33rd annual meeting of the Infectious Diseases Society of America, San Francisco, Calif, September 16-18, 1995.

70. Moureau N, Poole S, Murdock MA, et al. Central venous catheters in home infusion care: Outcomes analysis in 50,470 patients. J Vasc Interv Radiol. 2002;13:1009-1016.

71. Aston V. Community management of peripherally inserted central catheters. Br J Commun Nurs. 2000;5:318-325.

72. Herbst SL, Kaplan LK, McKinnon BT. Vascular access devices: Managing occlusions and related complications in home infusion. Infusion. 1998;4:1-32.

73. Schleis TG, Tice AD. Selecting infusion devices for use in ambulatory care. Am J Health Syst Pharm. 1996;53:868-877.

74. Hitt CM, Nightingale CH, Quintiliani R, Nicolau DP. Cost comparisons of single daily i.v. doses of ceftriaxone versus continuous infusion of cefotaxime. Am J Health Syst Pharm. 1997;54:1614-1618.

75. Birnbaum HG, Tang M. The home infusion therapy/relative benefit index: Summary of an analysis using insurance claims data. Med Care. 1998;36:757-765.

76. Nolet BR. Patient selection in outpatient parenteral antimicrobial therapy. Infect Dis Clin North Am. 1998;12:835-847.

77. Montalto M. An audit of patients admitted for home intravenous therapy directly from the emergency department. Int J Clin Pract. 1997;51:433-437.

78. Tice AD. The importance of teamwork for outpatient parenteral antibiotic therapy. Int J Antimicrob Agents. 1995;5:13-17.

79. Kunkel MJ. Quality assurance and outcomes in outpatient parenteral antibiotic therapy. Infect Dis Clin North Am. 1998;12:1023-1034.

80. Rehm SJ, Longworth DL. Rates of adverse events associated with community-based parenteral anti-infective therapy. J Clin Outcomes Manage. 2000;7:23-28.

81. Berman SJ, Johnson EW. Out-patient parenteral antibiotic therapy (OPAT): Clinical outcomes and adverse events. Hawaii Med J. 2001;60:31-33.

82. Ferriols-Lisart R, Alos-Alminana M. Effectiveness and safety of once-daily aminoglycosides: A meta-analysis. Am J Health Syst Pharm. 1996;53:1141-1150.

83. Koo J, Tight R, Rajkumar V, Hawa Z. Comparison of once-daily versus pharmacokinetic dosing of aminoglycosides in elderly patients. Am J Med. 1996;101:177-183.

84. Tice AD, Seibold GL, Martinelli LP. Adverse effects from intravenous antibiotics with OPAT. Presented at the 40th Annual Meeting of the Infectious Diseases Society of America, Chicago, Ill, October 2002.

85. Hoffman-Terry ML, Fraimow HS, Fox TR, et al. Adverse effects of outpatient parenteral antibiotic therapy. Am J Med. 1999;106:44-49.

CHAPTER **46**

Tables of Antimicrobial Agent Pharmacology

GUY W. AMSDEN

This chapter serves as a centralized source of pharmacologic information on anti-infective agents. Generic and trade name tables for antimicrobial agents are provided. The antimicrobial "family" classification also is included to help the reader locate specific information in subsequent tables. Tables describing existing dosage formulations also are broken down by chemical or pharmacologic class, or both.

DOSING GUIDELINES

The selection of an appropriate dose of an antimicrobial agent is based on the site of infection, the identity and known or presumed antibiotic susceptibility of the infecting organism, the dose-related drug toxicity, and the patient's ability to eliminate the drug. Generally, *dosage* selections from the upper end of the dosage range are recommended for severe, life-threatening infections (e.g., sepsis, meningitis). Known organisms with intermediate susceptibility (i.e., high minimal inhibitory concentration [MIC]) also should prompt the use of higher dosages. More recent data with various types of drugs, such as β-lactams, suggest that high doses of certain agents may be active against some "resistant" organisms. This may be true with agents that concentrate at the infection site and that concentrate in the phagocytes that clear the organisms, such as quinolones and macrolides/azalides.

The lowest dosages are used for urinary tract infections or when the isolated pathogen is extremely susceptible to the antimicrobial. A sizable range in dosing *intervals* exists for some antimicrobial agents, with longer durations between doses appropriate for less severe infections in which a critical threshold level in serum or other site of infection (e.g., central nervous system) is not mandatory or the drug concentrates significantly at the site of infection (e.g., urine, bile). Lower dosages also are appropriate when the patient has impairment in the function of excreting organs.

Dosing recommendations for all agents vary as research into them evolves. To prevent dosing errors, the recommendations discussed in this chapter should be compared against the most recent scientific literature, package labeling, and other current reference sources.

DOSAGE ADJUSTMENT FOR RENAL IMPAIRMENT

Drug half-life in *adults* with impaired renal function and changes related to dialysis procedures (hemodialysis, peritoneal dialysis) are summarized for the user. An alternative to the elongation of the interval between doses is reduction of the daily dose given at the "usual" dosing interval.[1] Antimicrobial serum levels should be determined and patient-specific dosage adjustments made on the basis of these determinations when appropriate.

BODY FLUID CONCENTRATIONS

In determining the appropriateness of a particular antibiotic for a given site of infection, the ultimate concentration of a drug at the site of infection compared with the MIC for the infecting organism is crucial. To be able to interpret this information, the clinician must know the basic pharmacokinetic and pharmacodynamic properties of each agent or type of agents. Although β-lactams and aminoglycosides have extracellular concentrations that are in relative equilibrium with serum concentrations, macrolides and quinolones concentrate in the extracellular site and phagocytic cells. Additionally, β-lactams and macrolides maximize their effects by maximizing time that infection site concentrations are above the pathogen's MIC, whereas quinolones and aminoglycosides maximize their effects by optimizing the peak infection site concentration-to-MIC ratio.

REFERENCES

1. Bennett WM, Arnoff GR, Morrison G, et al. Drug prescribing in renal failure: Dosing guidelines for adults. Am J Kidney Dis. 1983;3:155-193.
2. Amsden GW, Ballow CH, Schentag JJ. Population pharmacokinetic methods to optimize antibiotic effects. Drug Invest. 1993;5:256-268.
3. Nix DE, Goodwin SD, Peloquin CA, et al. Antibiotic tissue penetration and its relevance: Models of tissue penetration and their meaning. Antimicrob Agents Chemother. 35:1947-1952, 1991.
4. Nix DE, Goodwin SD, Peloquin CA, et al. Antibiotic tissue penetration and its relevance: Impact of tissue penetration on infection response. Antimicrob Agents Chemother. 35:1953-1959, 1991.
5. Schentag JJ. Correlation of pharmacokinetic parameters to efficacy of antibiotics: Relationships between serum concentrations, MIC values, and bacterial eradication in patients with gram negative pneumonia. Scand J Infect Dis. 1991;74(Suppl):218-234.
6. DeMaat MMR, Ekhart GC, Huitema ADR, et al. Drug interactions between antiretroviral drugs and comedicated agents. Clin Pharmacokinet. 2003:42:223-282.

TABLE 46-1 Generic and Trade Names

Generic Name	Trade Name	Class
Abacavir	Trizivir*, Ziagen, Ziagenavir	Antiretroviral
Acyclovir	Zovirax	Antiviral
Adefovir dipivoxil	Hepsera	Antiviral
Alatrofloxacin	Trovan IV	Fluoroquinolone
Albendazole	Eskazole, Zentel	Antiparasitic
Amantadine hydrochloride	Symadine, Symmetrel	Antiviral
Amdinocillin	Coactin	Penicillin
Amikacin sulfate	Amikin, Biclin, Biklin, Likacin	Aminoglycoside
Aminosalicylic acid	Paser	Antimycobacterial
Amoxicillin	Amoxil, Clamoxyl, Doxamil, Hiconcil, Polymox, Prevpac,* Trimox, Wymox	Penicillin
Amoxicillin/clavulanate potassium	Amoxiclav,* Augmentin,* Augmentin XR,* Clavepen*	Penicillin/β-lactamase inhibitor
Amphotericin B	Amphocin, Fungilin, Fungizone	Antifungal
Amphotericin B cholesteryl sulfate complex	Amphotec	Antifungal
Amphotericin B lipid complex	Abelcet	Antifungal
Amphotericin B liposomal	AmBisome	Antifungal
Ampicillin	Omnipen	Penicillin
Ampicillin sodium	Omnipen-N, Polycillin-N, Totacillin-N	Penicillin
Ampicillin trihydrate	Polycillin, Principen, Totacillin	Penicillin
Ampicillin/probenecid	Polycillin-PRB,* Probampacin*	Penicillin/tubular secretion inhibitor
Ampicillin/sulbactam	Bacimex,* Combactam,* Unasyn*	Penicillin/β-lactamase inhibitor

*A combination product.

Continued

TABLE 46-1 Generic and Trade Names—cont'd

Generic Name	Trade Name	Class
Amprenavir	Agenerase	Protease inhibitor
Artemether	Coartem, Paluther, Riamet*	Antimalarial
Artesunate	Plasmotrim	Antimalarial
Atazanavir	Reyataz	Protease inhibitor
Atovaquone	Mepron, Wellvone	Antiparasitic
Atovaquone/proguanil	Malarone*	Antimalarial
Azithromycin	Azitromax, Sumamed, Zithromax, Zithromax Tri-Pak, Zitromax, Z-Pak	Azalide
Azlocillin	Azlin, Securopen	Penicillin
Aztreonam	Azactam, Monobac, Primbactam, Urobactam	Monobactam
Bacampicillin	Ambaxin, Bacampicin, Penglobe, Spectrobid	Penicillin
Bacitracin	Baci-IM	Polypeptide
Bithionol	Bitin	Antiparasitic
Butoconazole nitrate	Femstat 3, Gynomyk, Mycelex-3	Antifungal
Capreomycin sulfate	Capastat Sulfate	Antimycobacterial
Carbenicillin indanyl sodium	Geocillin, Geopen	Penicillin
Carbol-fuchsin	Fungol	Antifungal
Caspofungin	Cancidas	Antifungal
Cefaclor	Ceclor, Ceclor CD, Distaclor, Keftid, Vercef	Cephalosporin
Cefadroxil	Baxam, Cefamox, Duracef, Duricef, Ultracef	Cephalosporin
Cefamandole nafate	Mandokef, Mandol	Cephalosporin
Cefazolin sodium	Ancef, Cefacidal, Cefamezin, Kefzol, Zolicef	Cephalosporin
Cefdinir	Cefzon, Omnicef	Cephalosporin
Cefditoren pivoxil	Spectracef	Cephalosporin
Cefepime	Maxcef, Maxipime	Cephalosporin
Cefixime	Cefspan, Denvar, Suprax	Cephalosporin
Cefmetazole sodium	Cefadel, Cefmetazon, Cemetol, Metazol	Cephalosporin
Cefonicid sodium	Monocid	Cephalosporin
Cefoperazone sodium	Cefobid, Cefodie, Cefoperazin*	Cephalosporin
Cefoperazone/sulbactam	Sulperazon*, Sulperazone*	Cephalosporin/β-lactamase inhibitor
Ceforanide	Precef	Cephalosporin
Cefotaxime sodium	Claforan	Cephalosporin
Cefotetan disodium	Cefotan	Cephalosporin
Cefoxitin sodium	Mefoxin, Mefoxitin	Cephalosporin
Cefpirome	Cedixen, Cefrom, Cefron	Cephalosporin
Cefpodoxime proxetil	Orelox, Podomexef, Vantin	Cephalosporin
Cefprozil	Cefzil, Procef	Cephalosporin
Cefsulodin	Cefomonil, Monaspor	Cephalosporin
Ceftazidime	Ceptaz, Fortam, Fortaz, Fortum, Kefadim, Tazicef, Tazidime	Cephalosporin
Ceftibuten	Cedax, Keimax	Cephalosporin
Ceftizoxime-alapivoxil	—	Cephalosporin
Ceftizoxime sodium	Cefizox	Cephalosporin
Ceftriaxone sodium	Rocephalin, Rocephin, Rocephine	Cephalosporin
Cefuroxime axetil	Ceftin, Zinnat	Cephalosporin
Cefuroxime sodium	Kefurox, Zinacef	Cephalosporin
Cephalexin	Cefanex, Ceporex, Keflet, Keflex	Cephalosporin
Cephalexin hydrochloride	Keftab	Cephalosporin
Cephalothin sodium	Ceporacin, Keflin	Cephalosporin
Cephapirin sodium	Cefadyl	Cephalosporin
Cephradine	Anspor, Lisacef, Velosef	Cephalosporin
Chloramphenicol	Chloromycetin	Chloramphenicol
Chloramphenicol palmitate	Chloromycetin Palmitate	Chloramphenicol
Chloramphenicol sodium succinate	Chloromycetin Sodium Succinate	Chloramphenicol
Chloroquine hydrochloride	Aralen Hydrochloride	Antimalarial
Chloroquine phosphate	Aralen Phosphate	Antimalarial
Ciclopirox	Loprox	Antifungal
Cidofovir	Vistide	Antiviral
Cinoxacin	Cinobac	Quinolone
Ciprofloxacin hydrochloride	Ciflox, Ciloxan, Cipro, Ciproxin	Fluoroquinolone
Ciprofloxacin lactate	Cipro IV	Fluoroquinolone
Clarithromycin	Biaxin, Biaxin XL, Biclar, Klacid, Prevpac*, Zeclar	Macrolide
Clindamycin hydrochloride	Cleocin, Dalacin C	Lincosamide
Clindamycin palmitate hydrochloride	Cleocin Pediatric	Lincosamide
Clindamycin phosphate	Cleocin Phosphate	Lincosamide
Clioquinol	Corque*, Diproform*	Antifungal
Clofazimine	Lampren, Lamprene	Antimycobacterial
Clotrimazole	Canesten, Cruex, Desenex, FemCare, Fungoid, Gyne-Lotrimin, Lotrimin, Lotrisone, Mycelex	Antifungal
Cloxacillin sodium	Bactopen, Cloxapen, Orbenin, Tegopen	Penicillin
Colistimethate sodium	Coly-Mycin M	Polymyxin
Cyclacillin	Calthor, Cyclapen	Penicillin
Cycloserine	Seromycin	Antimycobacterial
Dapsone	—	Sulfone
Daptomycin	Cidecin	Cyclic lipopeptide
Dehydroemetine	Mebadin	Amebicide
Delavirdine	Rescriptor	Antiretroviral
Demeclocycline hydrochloride	Declomycin	Tetracycline
Dicloxacillin sodium	Diclocil, Dycill, Dynapen, Pathocil	Penicillin
Didanosine	Videx, Videx EC	Antiretroviral

*A combination product.

TABLE 46-1 Generic and Trade Names—cont'd

Generic Name	Trade Name	Class
Diethylcarbamazine	Hetrazan, PEC-DEC	Antiparasitic
Diloxanide furoate	Entamizole	Antiparasitic
Dirithromycin	Dynabac, Dynabac D5-Pak	Macrolide
Doxycycline calcium	Vibramycin Calcium	Tetracycline
Doxycycline hyclate	Doryx, Doxy 100, Doxy Caps, Periostat, Vibramycin Hyclate, Vibra-Tabs	Tetracycline
Doxycycline monohydrate	Vibramycin Monohydrate, Monodox	Tetracycline
Drotrecogin alfa (activated)	Xigris	Antisepsis
Econazole nitrate	Ecostatin, Gyno-Pevaryl, Pevisone, Spectazole	Antifungal
Efavirenz	Stocrin, Sustiva	Antiretroviral
Emtricitabine	Coviracil	Antiretroviral
Enfuvirtide	Fuzeon	Fusion inhibitor
Enoxacin	Comprecin, Enoxor, Penetrex	Fluoroquinolone
Ertapenem	Invanz	Carbapenem
Erythromycin	Akne-mycin, Benzamycin*, E-Base, E-Mycin, ERYC, Ery-Tab, PCE, Robimycin	Macrolide
Erythromycin estolate	Ilosone	Macrolide
Erythromycin ethylsuccinate	E.E.S., EryPed, Eryzole*, E.S.P.*, Pediazole*, Sulfimycin*	Macrolide
Erythromycin gluceptate	Ilotycin	Macrolide
Erythromycin lactobionate	Erythrocin	Macrolide
Erythromycin stearate	Erythrocin Stearate, Wyamycin	Macrolide
Ethambutol hydrochloride	Myambutol, Servambutol	Antimycobacterial
Ethionamide	Trecator-SC	Antimycobacterial
Everninomycin	Ziracin	Oligosaccharide
Famciclovir	Famvir	Antiviral
Flomoxef	Flumarin	Cephalosporin
Flucloxacillin	Floxapen, Flucil, Flucillin, Fluclox	Penicillin
Fluconazole	Diflucan	Antifungal
Flucytosine	Ancobon, Ancotil	Antifungal
Foscarnet sodium	Foscavir	Antiviral
Fosfomycin tromethamine	Monuril, Monurol	Urinary anti-infective
Furazolidone	Furoxone	Antiprotozoal
Ganciclovir sodium	Cymevene, Cytovene, Vitrasert	Antiviral
Garenoxacin	—	Des-quinolone
Gatifloxacin	Tequin	Fluoroquinolone
Gemifloxacin	Factive	Fluoroquinolone
Gentamicin sulfate	Cidomycin, Garamycin, Genoptic, Jenamicin, Storz-G	Aminoglycoside
Gentian violet	—	Antifungal
Griseofulvin	Fulcin, Fulvicin P/G, Fulvicin U/F, Grifulvin V, Grisactin, Grisactin Ultra, Grisovin, Gris-PEG	Antifungal
Halofantrine	Halfan	Antiparasitic
Hydroxychloroquine sulfate	Plaquenil Sulfate	Antimalarial
Imipenem/cilastatin	Primaxin*, Tienam*	Carbapenem
Indinavir	Crixivan	Protease inhibitor
Interferon alfa-2a recombinant	Roferon-A	Antiviral
Interferon alfa-2b recombinant	Intron A, Rebetron*	Antiviral
Interferon alfacon-1	Infergen	Antiviral
Interferon alfa-n3	Alferon N	Antiviral
Iodoquinol	Yodoxin M/, Yodoxin	Amebicide
Isepamicin	Isepacin	Aminoglycoside
Isoniazid	Laniazid, Nydrazid, Rifamate*, Rifater*, Rifinah*, Rimactane/INH*	Antimycobacterial
Itraconazole	Sporanox	Antifungal
Ivermectin	Mectizan, Stromectol	Antiparasitic
Josamycin	Josalid	Macrolide
Kanamycin sulfate	Anamid, Kantrex	Aminoglycoside
Ketoconazole	Fungoral, Nizoral	Antifungal
Lamivudine (3TC)	Combivir*, Epivir, Epivir-HBV, Trizivir*, Zeffix	Antiretroviral
Levofloxacin	Levaquin, Tavanic	Fluoroquinolone
Lincomycin hydrochloride	Lincocin	Lincosamide
Linezolid	Zyvox, Zyvoxam	Oxazolidinone
Liposomal nystatin	Nyotran	Antifungal
Lomefloxacin hydrochloride	Maxaquin, Okacin, Uniquin	Fluoroquinolone
Lopinavir/ritonavir	Kaletra*	Antiretrovirals
Loracarbef	Lorabid	Carbacephem
Mafenide	Sulfamylon	Sulfonamide
Mebendazole	Vermox	Anthelmintic
Mefloquine	Lariam	Antimalarial
Meglumine antimonate	Glucantim, Glucantime	Antiparasitic
Melarsoprol B	—	Antiparasitic
Meropenem	Meronem, Merrem	Carbapenem
Methacycline	Rondomycin	Tetracycline
Methenamine hippurate	Hiprex, Urex	Urinary anti-infective
Methenamine mandelate	Mandelamine	Urinary anti-infective
Methicillin sodium	Celbenin, Staphcillin	Penicillin
Metronidazole	Elyzol, Flagyl, Helidac*, MetroGel, Protostat, Rozex	Nitroimidazole
Mezlocillin sodium	Baypen, Mezlin	Penicillin
Micafungin	Mycamine	Antifungal
Miconazole	Daktacort*, Daktarin, Gyno-Daktarin, Micatin, Monistat	Antifungal

Continued

TABLE 46-1   Generic and Trade Names—cont'd

Generic Name	Trade Name	Class
Minocycline hydrochloride	Dynacin, Minocin, Vectrin	Tetracycline
Moxalactam	Moxam	Cephalosporin
Moxifloxacin	Avelox	Fluoroquinolone
Mupirocin	Bactroban	Pseudomonic acid
Nafcillin sodium	Nafcil, Nallpen, Unipen	Penicillin
Naftifine	Naftin	Antifungal
Nalidixic acid	NegGram	Quinolone
Nelfinavir	Viracept	Protease inhibitor
Neomycin sulfate	Kenacomb*, Maxitrol*, Mycifradin Sulfate, Neosporin*	Aminoglycoside
Netilmicin sulfate	Netilyn, Netromycin	Aminoglycoside
Nevirapine	Viramune	Antiretroviral
Niclosamide	Niclocide, Yomesan	Anthelmintic
Nifurtimox	Bayer 2502	Antiparasitic
Nitazoxanide	Alinia	Antiprotozoal
Nitrofurantoin	Furadantin, Macrobid, Macrodantin	Urinary anti-infective
Norfloxacin	Chibroxin, Floxacin, Noroxin	Fluoroquinolone
Novobiocin sodium	Albamycin	—
Nystatin	Kenacomb*, Mycostatin, Mycostatin Filmlok, Nilstat	Antifungal
Ofloxacin	Exocin, Floxin, Tarivid	Fluoroquinolone
Oritavancin diphosphate	—	Glycopeptide
Oseltamivir phosphate	Tamiflu	Antiviral
Oxacillin sodium	Bactocill, Prostaphlin	Penicillin
Oxamniquine	Mansil	Anthelmintic
Oxiconazole nitrate	Oxistat	Antifungal
Oxolinic acid	Oribiox	Quinolone
Oxytetracycline hydrochloride	Terramycin, Uri-Tet, Urobiotic	Tetracycline
Palivizumab	Synagis	Antiviral
Paromomycin sulfate	Humatin	Amebicide
Pefloxacin	Peflacine, Peflox	Fluoroquinolone
Peginterferon alfa-2b	PEGASYS, Pegetron*, PEG-Intron	Antiviral
Penciclovir	Denavir, Vectavir	Antiviral
Penicillin G benzathine	Bicillin*, Bicillin C-R*, Bicillin L-A, Permapen	Penicillin
Penicillin G + phenoxymethyl penicillin	Kesso-pen*	Penicillin
Penicillin G potassium	Pfizerpen	Penicillin
Penicillin G procaine	Bicillin C-R*, Crysticillin AS, Pfizerpen-AS, Wycillin	Penicillin
Penicillin G sodium	—	Penicillin
Penicillin V potassium	Beepen-VK, Betapen-VK, Ledercillin VK, Pen-Vee K, Robicillin VK, V-Cillin K, Veetids	Penicillin
Pentamidine isethionate	NebuPent, Pentacarinat, Pentam	Antiprotozoal
Phenazopyridine/sulfisoxazole	Azo Gantrisin*	Symptomatic bladder therapy/ sulfonamide
Piperacillin sodium	Pipracil, Pipril	Penicillin
Piperacillin sodium/tazobactam sodium	Tazocin*, Zosyn*	Penicillin/β-lactamase inhibitor
Piperazine citrate	—	Anthelmintic
Pivmecillinam	Mecillin 200, Selexid	Penicillin
Polymyxin B sulfate	Aerosporin, Neosporin*	Polymyxin
Posaconazole	Noxafil	Antifungal
Praziquantel	Biltricide	Anthelmintic
Primaquine phosphate	—	Antimalarial
Proguanil	Paludrine	Antiparasitic
Pyrantel pamoate	Antiminth, Combantrin, Pin-X	Anthelmintic
Pyrazinamide	Rifater*, Zinamide	Antimycobacterial
Pyrimethamine	Daraprim	Antimalarial
Pyrimethamine/sulfadoxine	Fansidar*	Antimalarial
Quinacrine hydrochloride	Atabrine	Anthelmintic
Quinine sulfate	Legatrin, Quinamm	Antimalarial
Quinupristin/dalfopristin	Synercid*	Streptogramin
Ramoplanin	—	Glycolipodesipeptide
Ribavirin	Pegetron*, Rebetol, Rebetron*, Virazole	Antiviral
Rifabutin	Mycobutin	Antimycobacterial
Rifampin	Rifadin, Rifamate*, Rifinah*, Rimactane, Rimactane/INH*	Antimycobacterial
Rifapentine	Priftin	Antimycobacterial
Rifaximin	Lumenax	Rifamycin
Rimantadine	Flumadine, Roflual	Antiviral
Ritonavir	Norvir	Protease inhibitor
Roxithromycin	Rulid, Rulide, Surlid	Macrolide
Saquinavir	Fortovase, Invirase	Protease inhibitor
Silver sulfadiazine	Silvadene, Thermazene	Sulfonamide
Sodium stibogluconate	Pentostam	Antiparasitic
Sparfloxacin	Zagam, Zagam Respipac	Fluoroquinolone
Spectinomycin hydrochloride	Trobicin	Aminocyclitol
Spiramycin	Rovamycin, Rovamycine	Macrolide
Stavudine (d4T)	Zerit	Antiretroviral
Streptomycin sulfate	—	Aminoglycoside
Sulfabenzamide/sulfacetamide/sulfathiazole	Sultrin*, Triple Sulfa*	Sulfonamide
Sulfadiazine	—	Sulfonamide
Sulfamethizole	Thiosulfil Forte	Sulfonamide
Sulfamethoxazole	Azo Gantanol*, Gantanol	Sulfonamide
Sulfanilamide	AVC	Sulfonamide

TABLE 46-1 Generic and Trade Names—cont'd

Generic Name	Trade Name	Class
Sulfisoxazole	Azo-Sulfisoxazole*, Gantrisin	Sulfonamide
Sulfisoxazole acetyl	Eryzole*, Pediazole*	Sulfonamide
Suramin	Germanin	Antiparasitic
Teicoplanin	Targocid	Glycopeptide
Telithromycin	Ketek	Ketolide
Tenofovir	Viread	Antiretroviral
Terbinafine	Lamisil	Antifungal
Terconazole	Terazol	Antifungal
Tetracycline hydrochloride	Achromycin V, Helidac*, Panmycin, Robitet, Sumycin, Tetrachel, Tetralan	Tetracycline
Thiabendazole	Mintezol	Anthelmintic
Thiacetazone	—	Antimycobacterial
Ticarcillin disodium	Tarcil, Ticar	Penicillin
Ticarcillin disodium-clavulanate potassium	Timentin*	Penicillin/β-lactamase inhibitor
Tigecycline	—	Tetracycline
Tobramycin sulfate	Nebcin, Nebcina, Obracin, TobraDex*, Tobrex	Aminoglycoside
Tobramycin inhalation solution	TOBI	Aminoglycoside
Tolnaftate	Mycil*, Tinactin, Tinaderm	Antifungal
Trifluridine	Viroptic	Antiviral
Trimethoprim	Monotrim, Proloprim, Trimopan, Trimpex	Folate antagonist
Trimethoprim/sulfamethoxazole	Bactrim*, Bactrim DS*, Cotrim*, Cotrim D.S.*, Septra*, Septra DS*, Sulfatrim*, Sulfoxaprim*, Uroplus*	Folate antagonists
Trimetrexate glucuronate	NeuTrexin	Antiprotozoal
Trisulfapyrimidines	—	Sulfonamide
Troleandomycin	Tao	Macrolide
Trovafloxacin	Trovan	Fluoroquinolone
Valacyclovir	Valtrex, Zelitrex	Antiviral
Valganciclovir	Valcyte	Antiviral
Vancomycin hydrochloride	Lyphocin, Vancocin, Vancoled, Vancor	Glycopeptide
Vidarabine	Vira-MP	Antiviral
Voriconazole	VFend	Antifungal
Zalcitabine	Hivid	Antiretroviral
Zanamivir	Relenza	Antiviral
Zidovudine	Combivir*, Retrovir, Trizivir*	Antiretroviral

*A combination product.

TABLE 46-2 Trade and Generic Names

Trade Name	Generic Name	Class
Abelcet	Amphotericin B lipid complex	Antifungal
Achromycin V	Tetracycline hydrochloride	Tetracycline
Aerosporin	Polymyxin B sulfate	Polymyxin
Agenerase	Amprenavir	Protease inhibitor
Akne-mycin	Erythromycin	Macrolide
Albamycin	Novobiocin sodium	—
Alferon N	Interferon alfa-n3	Antiviral
Alinia	Nitazoxanide	Antiprotozoal
Ambaxin	Bacampicillin	Penicillin
AmBisome	Amphotericin B liposomal	Antifungal
Amikin	Amikacin sulfate	Aminoglycoside
Amoxiclav*	Amoxicillin/clavulanate potassium	Penicillin/β-lactamase inhibitor
Amoxil	Amoxicillin	Penicillin
Amphocin	Amphotericin B	Antifungal
Amphotec	Amphotericin B cholesteryl sulfate complex	Antifungal
Anamid	Kanamycin	Aminoglycoside
Ancef	Cefazolin sodium	Cephalosporin
Ancobon	Flucytosine	Antifungal
Ancotil	Flucytosine	Antifungal
Anspor	Cephradine	Cephalosporin
Antiminth	Pyrantel pamoate	Anthelmintic
Aralen Hydrochloride	Chloroquine hydrochloride	Antimalarial
Aralen Phosphate	Chloroquine phosphate	Antimalarial
Atabrine	Quinacrine hydrochloride	Anthelmintic
Augmentin*	Amoxicillin/clavulanate potassium	Penicillin/β-lactamase inhibitor
Augmentin XR*	Amoxicillin/clavulanate potassium	Penicillin/β-lactamase inhibitor
AVC	Sulfanilamide	Sulfonamide
Avelox	Moxifloxacin	Fluoroquinolone
Azactam	Aztreonam	Monobactam
Azitromax	Azithromycin	Azalide
Azlin	Azlocillin	Penicillin
Azo Gantanol*	Sulfamethoxazole	Sulfonamide
Azo-Sulfisoxazole*	Sulfisoxazole	Sulfonamide

*A combination product.

Continued

TABLE 46-2   Trade and Generic Names—cont'd

Trade Name	Generic Name	Class
Bacampicin	Bacampicillin	Penicillin
Baci-IM	Bacitracin	Polypeptide
Bacimex*	Ampicillin/sulbactam	Penicillin/β-lactamase inhibitor
Bactocill	Oxacillin sodium	Penicillin
Bactopen	Cloxacillin	Penicillin
Bactrim/Bactrim DS*	Trimethoprim/sulfamethoxazole	Folate antagonists
Bactroban	Mupirocin	Pseudomonic acid
Baxam	Cefadroxil	Cephalosporin
Bayer 2502	Nifurtimox	Antiparasitic
Baypen	Mezlocillin	Penicillin
Beepen-VK	Penicillin V potassium	Penicillin
Benzamycin*	Erythromycin/benzoyl peroxide	Macrolide/antiseptic
Betapen-VK	Penicillin V potassium	Penicillin
Biaxin/Biaxin XL	Clarithromycin	Macrolide
Bicillin C-R*	Penicillin G procaine/benzathine	Penicillin
Bicillin L-A	Penicillin G benzathine	Penicillin
Biclar	Clarithromycin	Macrolide
Biclin	Amikacin	Aminoglycoside
Biklin	Amikacin	Aminoglycoside
Biltricide	Praziquantel	Anthelmintic
Bitin	Bithionol	Antiparasitic
Calthor	Cyclacillin	Penicillin
Cancidas	Caspofungin	Antifungal
Canesten	Clotrimazole	Antifungal
Capastat Sulfate	Capreomycin sulfate	Polypeptide
Ceclor/Ceclor CD	Cefaclor	Cephalosporin
Cedax	Ceftibuten	Cephalosporin
Cedixen	Cefpirome	Cephalosporin
Cefacidal	Cefazolin	Cephalosporin
Cefadel	Cefmetazole	Cephalosporin
Cefadyl	Cephapirin sodium	Cephalosporin
Cefamezin	Cefazolin	Cephalosporin
Cefamox	Cefadroxil	Cephalosporin
Cefanex	Cephalexin	Cephalosporin
Cefizox	Ceftizoxime sodium	Cephalosporin
Cefmetazon	Cefmetazole	Cephalosporin
Cefobid	Cefoperazone	Cephalosporin
Cefodie	Cefoperazone	Cephalosporin
Cefomonil	Cefsulodin	Cephalosporin
Cefoperazin*	Cefoperazone/lidocaine	Cephalosporin
Cefotan	Cefotetan disodium	Cephalosporin
Cefrom	Cefpirome	Cephalosporin
Cefron	Cefpirome	Cephalosporin
Cefspan	Cefixime	Cephalosporin
Ceftin	Cefuroxime axetil	Cephalosporin
Cefzil	Cefprozil	Cephalosporin
Cefzon	Cefdinir	Cephalosporin
Celbenin	Methicillin	Penicillin
Cemetol	Cefmetazole	Cephalosporin
Ceporacin	Cephalothin	Cephalosporin
Ceporex	Cephalexin	Cephalosporin
Ceptaz	Ceftazidime	Cephalosporin
Chibroxin	Norfloxacin	Fluoroquinolone
Chloromycetin	Chloramphenicol	Chloramphenicol
Chloromycetin Palmitate	Chloramphenicol palmitate	Chloramphenicol
Chloromycetin Sodium Succinate	Chloramphenicol sodium succinate	Chloramphenicol
Cidecin	Daptomycin	Cyclic lipopeptide
Cidomycin	Gentamicin	Aminoglycoside
Ciflox	Ciprofloxacin hydrochloride	Fluoroquinolone
Ciloxan	Ciprofloxacin hydrochloride	Fluoroquinolone
Cinobac	Cinoxacin	Quinolone
Cipro	Ciprofloxacin hydrochloride	Fluoroquinolone
Cipro IV	Ciprofloxacin lactate	Fluoroquinolone
Ciproxin	Ciprofloxacin hydrochloride	Fluoroquinolone
Claforan	Cefotaxime sodium	Cephalosporin
Clamoxyl	Amoxicillin	Penicillin
Clavepen*	Amoxicillin/clavulanate potassium	Penicillin/β-lactamase inhibitor
Cleocin	Clindamycin hydrochloride	Lincosamide
Cleocin Pediatric	Clindamycin palmitate hydrochloride	Lincosamide
Cleocin Phosphate	Clindamycin phosphate	Lincosamide
Cloxapen	Cloxacillin sodium	Penicillin
Coactin	Amdinocillin	Penicillin
Coartem	Artemether	Antimalarial
Coly-Mycin M	Colistimethate sodium	Polymyxin
Combactam*	Ampicillin/sulbactam	Penicillin/β-lactamase inhibitor
Combantrin	Pyrantel pamoate	Anthelmintic
Combivir*	Lamivudine/zidovudine	Antiretroviral
Comprecin	Enoxacin	Fluoroquinolone
Corque*	Clioquinol/hydrocortisone	Antifungal

*A combination product.

TABLE 46-2 Trade and Generic Names—cont'd

Trade Name	Generic Name	Class
Cotrim/Cotrim D.S.*	Trimethoprim/sulfamethoxazole	Folate antagonists
Coviracil	Emtricitabine	Antiretroviral
Crixivan	Indinavir	Protease inhibitor
Cruex	Clotrimazole	Antifungal
Crysticillin	Penicillin G procaine	Penicillin
Cyclapen	Cyclacillin	Penicillin
Cymevene	Ganciclovir sodium	Antiviral
Cytovene	Ganciclovir sodium	Antiviral
Daktacort*	Miconazole/hydrocortisone	Antifungal
Daktarin	Miconazole	Antifungal
Dalacin C	Clindamycin hydrochloride	Lincosamide
Daraprim	Pyrimethamine	Antimalarial
Declomycin	Demeclocycline hydrochloride	Tetracycline
Denavir	Penciclovir	Antiviral
Denvar	Cefixime	Cephalosporin
Desenex	Clotrimazole	Antifungal
Diclocil	Dicloxacillin	Penicillin
Diflucan	Fluconazole	Antifungal
Diproform*	Clioquinol/betamethasone	Antifungal
Distaclor	Cefaclor	Cephalosporin
Doryx	Doxycycline hyclate	Tetracycline
Doxamil	Amoxicillin	Penicillin
Doxy 100	Doxycycline hyclate	Tetracycline
Doxy Caps	Doxycycline hyclate	Tetracycline
Duracef	Cefadroxil	Cephalosporin
Duricef	Cefadroxil	Cephalosporin
Dycill	Dicloxacillin sodium	Penicillin
Dynabac/Dynabac D5-Pak	Dirithromycin	Macrolide
Dynacin	Minocycline	Tetracycline
Dynapen	Dicloxacillin	Penicillin
E.E.S.	Erythromycin ethylsuccinate	Macrolide
E-Base	Erythromycin	Macrolide
Ecostatin	Econazole	Antifungal
Elyzole	Metronidazole	Nitroimidazole
E-Mycin	Erythromycin	Macrolide
Enoxor	Enoxacin	Fluoroquinolone
Entamizole	Diloxanide furoate	Antiparasitic
Epivir/Epivir-HBV	Lamivudine (3TC)	Antiretroviral
ERYC	Erythromycin	Macrolide
EryPed	Erythromycin ethylsuccinate	Macrolide
Ery-Tab	Erythromycin	Macrolide
Erythrocin	Erythromycin lactobionate	Macrolide
Erythrocin Stearate	Erythromycin stearate	Macrolide
Eryzole*	Erythromycin ethylsuccinate/sulfisoxazole	Macrolide/sulfonamide
Eskazole	Albendazole	Antiparasitic
E.S.P.*	Erythromycin ethylsuccinate/sulfisoxazole	Macrolide/sulfonamide
Exocin	Ofloxacin	Fluoroquinolone
Factive	Gemifloxacin	Fluoroquinolone
Famvir	Famciclovir	Antiviral
Fansidar*	Pyrimethamine/sulfadoxine	Antiparasitic
FemCare	Clotrimazole	Antifungal
Femstat 3	Butoconazole	Antifungal
Flagyl	Metronidazole	Nitroimidazole
Floxacin	Norfloxacin	Fluoroquinolone
Floxapen	Flucloxacillin	Penicillin
Floxin	Ofloxacin	Fluoroquinolone
Flucil	Flucloxacillin	Penicillin
Flucillin	Flucloxacillin	Penicillin
Fluclox	Flucloxacillin	Penicillin
Flumadine	Rimantadine	Antiviral
Flumarin	Flomoxef	Cephalosporin
Fortam	Ceftazidime	Cephalosporin
Fortaz	Ceftazidime	Cephalosporin
Fortovase	Saquinavir	Protease inhibitor
Fortum	Ceftazidime	Cephalosporin
Foscavir	Foscarnet sodium	Antiviral
Fulcin	Griseofulvin	Antifungal
Fulvicin P/G	Griseofulvin	Antifungal
Fulvicin-U/F	Griseofulvin	Antifungal
Fungilin	Amphotericin B	Antifungal
Fungizone	Amphotericin B	Antifungal
Fungoid	Clotrimazole	Antifungal
Fungol	Carbol-fuchsin	Antifungal
Fungoral	Ketoconazole	Antifungal
Furadantin	Nitrofurantoin	Urinary anti-infective
Furoxone	Furazolidone	Antiprotozoal
Fuzeon	Enfuvirtide	Fusion inhibitor
Gantanol	Sulfamethoxazole	Sulfonamide
Gantrisin	Sulfisoxazole	Sulfonamide

Continued

TABLE 46-2 Trade and Generic Names—cont'd

Trade Name	Generic Name	Class
Garamycin	Gentamicin	Aminoglycoside
Genoptic	Gentamicin	Aminoglycoside
Geocillin	Carbenicillin indanyl sodium	Penicillin
Geopen	Carbenicillin indanyl sodium	Penicillin
Germanin	Suramin	Antiparasitic
Glucantim	Meglumine antimonate	Antiparasitic
Glucantime	Meglumine antimonate	Antiparasitic
Grifulvin V	Griseofulvin	Antifungal
Grisactin	Griseofulvin	Antifungal
Grisactin Ultra	Griseofulvin	Antifungal
Grisovin	Griseofulvin	Antifungal
Gris-PEG	Griseofulvin	Antifungal
Gyne-Lotrimin	Clotrimazole	Antifungal
Gyno-Daktarin	Miconazole	Antifungal
Gynomyk	Butoconazole	Antifungal
Gyno-Pevaryl	Econazole	Antifungal
Halfan	Halofantrine	Antiparasitic
Helidac*	Bismuth/metronidazole/tetracycline	Anti-*Helicobacter*
Hepsera	Adefovir dipivoxil	Antiviral
Hetrazan	Diethylcarbamazine	Antiparasitic
Hiconcil	Amoxicillin	Penicillin
Hiprex	Methenamine hippurate	Urinary anti-infective
Hivid	Zalcitabine	Antiviral
Humatin	Paromomycin sulfate	Amebicide
Ilosone	Erythromycin estolate	Macrolide
Ilotycin	Erythromycin gluceptate	Macrolide
Infergen	Interferon alfacon-1	Antiviral
Intron A	Interferon alfa-2b recombinant	Antiviral
Invanz	Ertapenem	Carbapenem
Invirase	Saquinavir	Protease inhibitor
Isepacin	Isepamicin	Aminoglycoside
Jenamicin	Gentamicin sulfate	Aminoglycoside
Josalid	Josamycin	Macrolide
Kaletra*	lopinavir/ritonavir	Antiretrovirals
Kantrex	Kanamycin sulfate	Aminoglycoside
Kefadim	Ceftazidime	Cephalosporin
Keflet	Cephalexin	Cephalosporin
Keflex	Cephalexin	Cephalosporin
Keflin	Cephalothin sodium	Cephalosporin
Keftab	Cephalexin hydrochloride	Cephalosporin
Kefurox	Cefuroxime sodium	Cephalosporin
Kefzol	Cefazolin sodium	Cephalosporin
Keimax	Ceftibuten	Cephalosporin
Kenacomb*	Neomycin/nystatin	Aminoglycoside/antifungal
Kesso-pen*	Penicillin G/phenoxymethyl penicillin	Penicillins
Ketek	Telithromycin	Ketolide
Klacid	Clarithromycin	Macrolide
Lamisil	Terbinafine	Antifungal
Lampren	Clofazimine	Antimycobacterial
Lamprene	Clofazimine	Antimycobacterial
Laniazid	Isoniazid	Antimycobacterial
Lariam	Mefloquine	Antimalarial
Ledercillin VK	Penicillin V potassium	Penicillin
Legatrin	Quinine sulfate	Antimalarial
Levaquin	Levofloxacin	Fluoroquinolone
Likacin	Amikacin	Aminoglycoside
Lincocin	Lincomycin	Lincosamide
Lisacef	Cephradine	Cephalosporin
Loprox	Ciclopirox	Antifungal
Lorabid	Loracarbef	Carbacephem
Lotrimin	Clotrimazole	Antifungal
Lotrisone	Clotrimazole	Antifungal
Lumenax	Rifaximin	Rifamycin
Lyphocin	Vancomycin hydrochloride	Glycopeptide
Macrobid	Nitrofurantoin	Urinary anti-infective
Macrodantin	Nitrofurantoin	Urinary anti-infective
Malarone*	Atovaquone/proguanil	Antimalarial
Mandelamine	Methenamine mandelate	Urinary anti-infective
Mandokef	Cefamandole	Cephalosporin
Mandol	Cefamandole	Cephalosporin
Mansil	Oxamniquine	Anthelmintic
Maxaquin	Lomefloxacin	Fluoroquinolone
Maxcef	Cefepime	Cephalosporin
Maxipime	Cefepime	Cephalosporin
Maxitrol*	Dexamethasone/neomycin/polymyxin B	Antifungal/polymyxin
Mebadin	Dehydroemetine	Amebicide
Mecillin 200	Pivmecillinam	Penicillin
Mectizan	Ivermectin	Antiparasitic
Mefoxin	Cefoxitin	Cephalosporin

*A combination product.

TABLE 46-2   Trade and Generic Names—cont'd

Trade Name	Generic Name	Class
Mefoxitin	Cefoxitin	Cephalosporin
Mepron	Atovaquone	Antiparasitic
Meronem	Meropenem	Carbapenem
Merrem	Meropenem	Carbapenem
Metazol	Cefmetazole sodium	Cephalosporin
MetroGel	Metronidazole	Nitroimidazole
Mezlin	Mezlocillin sodium	Penicillin
Micatin	Miconazole	Antifungal
Minocin	Minocycline hydrochloride	Tetracycline
Mintezol	Thiabendazole	Anthelmintic
Monaspor	Cefsulodin	Cephalosporin
Monistat	Miconazole	Antifungal
Monobac	Aztreonam	Monobactam
Monocid	Cefonicid sodium	Cephalosporin
Monodox	Doxycycline monohydrate	Tetracycline
Monotrim	Trimethoprim	Folate antagonist
Monuril	Fosfomycin tromethamine	Urinary anti-infective
Monurol	Fosfomycin tromethamine	Urinary anti-infective
Moxam	Moxalactam	Cephalosporin
Myambutol	Ethambutol hydrochloride	Antimycobacterial
Mycamine	Micafungin	Antifungal
Mycelex	Clotrimazole	Antifungal
Mycelex-3	Butoconazole	Antifungal
Mycifradin Sulfate	Neomycin sulfate	Aminoglycoside
Mycil*	Tolnaftate	Antifungal
Mycobutin	Rifabutin	Antimycobacterial
Mycostatin (Filmlok)	Nystatin	Antifungal
Nafcil	Nafcillin sodium	Penicillin
Naftin	Naftifine	Antifungal
Nallpen	Nafcillin sodium	Penicillin
Nebcin	Tobramycin	Aminoglycoside
Nebcina	Tobramycin	Aminoglycoside
NebuPent	Pentamidine isethionate	Antiprotozoal
NegGram	Nalidixic acid	Quinolone
Neosporin*	Neomycin/polymyxin B	Aminoglycoside/polymyxin
Netilyn	Netilmicin	Aminoglycoside
Netromycin	Netilmicin	Aminoglycoside
NeuTrexin	Trimetrexate	Antiprotozoal
Niclocide	Niclosamide	Anthelmintic
Nilstat	Nystatin	Antifungal
Nizoral	Ketoconazole	Antifungal
Noroxin	Norfloxacin	Fluoroquinolone
Norvir	Ritonavir	Protease inhibitor
Noxafil	Posaconazole	Antifungal
Nydrazid	Isoniazid	Antimycobacterial
Nyotran	Liposomal nystatin	Antifungal
Obracin	Tobramycin	Aminoglycoside
Okacin	Lomefloxacin	Fluoroquinolone
Omnicef	Cefdinir	Cephalosporin
Omnipen	Ampicillin	Penicillin
Omnipen-N	Ampicillin sodium	Penicillin
Orbenin	Cloxacillin	Penicillin
Orelox	Cefpodoxime proxetil	Cephalosporin
Oribiox	Oxolinic acid	Quinolone
Oxistat	Oxiconazole nitrate	Antifungal
Paludrine	Proguanil	Antiparasitic
Paluther	Artemether	Antimalarial
Panmycin	Tetracycline hydrochloride	Tetracycline
Paser	Aminosalicylic acid	Antimycobacterial
Pathocil	Dicloxacillin sodium	Penicillin
PCE	Erythromycin	Macrolide
PEC-DEC	Diethylcarbamazine	Antiparasitic
Pediazole*	Erythromycin ethylsuccinate/sulfisoxazole	Macrolide/sulfonamide
Peflacine	Pefloxacin	Fluoroquinolone
Peflox	Pefloxacin	Fluoroquinolone
PEGASYS	Peginterferon alfa-2b	Antiviral
Pegetron*	Peginterferon alfa-2b/ribavirin	Antivirals
PEG-Intron	Peginterferon alfa-2b	Antiviral
Penetrex	Enoxacin	Fluoroquinolone
Penglobe	Bacampicillin	Penicillin
Pentacarinat	Pentamidine isethionate	Antiprotozoal
Pentam	Pentamidine isethionate	Antiprotozoal
Pentostam	Sodium stibogluconate	Antiparasitic
Pen-Vee K	Penicillin V potassium	Penicillin
Periostat	Doxycycline	Tetracycline
Permapen	Penicillin G benzathine	Penicillin
Pevisone	Econazole	Antifungal
Pfizerpen	Penicillin G potassium	Penicillin
Pfizerpen-AS	Penicillin G procaine	Penicillin

Continued

TABLE 46-2   Trade and Generic Names—cont'd

Trade Name	Generic Name	Class
Pin-X	Pyrantel pamoate	Anthelmintic
Pipracil	Piperacillin	Penicillin
Pipril	Piperacillin	Penicillin
Plaquenil Sulfate	Hydroxychloroquine sulfate	Antimalarial
Plasmotrim	Artesunate	Antimalarial
Podomexef	Cefpodoxime proxetil	Cephalosporin
Polycillin	Ampicillin trihydrate	Penicillin
Polycillin-N	Ampicillin sodium	Penicillin
Polycillin-PRB*	Ampicillin/probenecid	Penicillin/tubular secretion inhibitor
Polymox	Amoxicillin	Penicillin
Precef	Ceforanide	Cephalosporin
Prevpac*	Amoxicillin/clarithromycin/lansoprazole	Anti-*Helicobacter*
Priftin	Rifapentine	Antimycobacterial
Primaxin*	Imipenem/cilastatin	Carbapenem
Primbactam	Aztreonam	Monobactam
Principen	Ampicillin trihydrate	Penicillin
Probampacin*	Ampicillin/probenecid	Penicillin/tubular secretion inhibitor
Procef	Cefprozil	Cephalosporin
Proloprim	Trimethoprim	Folate antagonist
Prostaphlin	Oxacillin sodium	Penicillin
Protostat	Metronidazole	Nitroimidazole
Quinamm	Quinine sulfate	Antimalarial
Rebetol	Ribavirin	Antiviral
Rebetron*	Interferon alfa-2b recombinant/ribavirin	Antiviral
Relenza	Zanamivir	Antiviral
Rescriptor	Delavirdine	Antiretroviral
Retrovir	Zidovudine	Antiviral
Reyataz	Atazanavir	Protease inhibitor
Riamet*	Artemether/lumefantrine	Antimalarial
Rifadin	Rifampin	Antimycobacterial
Rifamate*	Rifampin/isoniazid	Antimycobacterial
Rifater*	Rifampin/pyrazinamide	Antimycobacterial
Rifinah*	Rifampin/isoniazid	Antimycobacterial
Rimactane	Rifampin	Antimycobacterial
Rimactane/INH*	Rifampin/isoniazid	Antimycobacterial
Robicillin VK	Penicillin V potassium	Penicillin
Robimycin	Erythromycin	Macrolide
Robitet	Tetracycline hydrochloride	Tetracycline
Rocephalin	Ceftriaxone	Cephalosporin
Rocephin	Ceftriaxone	Cephalosporin
Rocephine	Ceftriaxone	Cephalosporin
Roferon-A	Interferon alfa-2a recombinant	Antiviral
Roflual	Rimantadine	Antiviral
Rondomycin	Methacycline	Tetracycline
Rovamycin	Spiramycin	Macrolide
Rovamycine	Spiramycin	Macrolide
Rozex	Metronidazole	Nitroimidazole
Rulid	Roxithromycin	Macrolide
Rulide	Roxithromycin	Macrolide
Securopen	Azlocillin	Penicillin
Selexid	Pivmecillinam	Penicillin
Septra/Septra DS*	Trimethoprim/sulfamethoxazole	Folate antagonists
Seromycin	Cycloserine	Antimycobacterial
Servambutol	Ethambutol	Antimycobacterial
Silvadene	Silver sulfadiazine	Sulfonamide
Spectazole	Econazole nitrate	Antifungal
Spectracef	Cefditoren pivoxil	Cephalosporin
Spectrobid	Bacampicillin hydrochloride	Penicillin
Sporanox	Itraconazole	Antifungal
Staphcillin	Methicillin sodium	Penicillin
Stocrin	Efavirenz	Antiretroviral
Storz-G	Gentamicin sulfate	Aminoglycoside
Stromectol	Ivermectin	Antiparasitic
Sulfamylon	Mafenide	Sulfonamide
Sulfatrim*	Trimethoprim/sulfamethoxazole	Folate antagonists
Sulfoxaprim*	Trimethoprim/sulfamethoxazole	Folate antagonists
Sulperazon*	Cefoperazone/sulbactam	Cephalosporin/β-lactamase inhibitor
Sulperazone*	Cefoperazone/sulbactam	Cephalosporin/β-lactamase inhibitor
Sultrin Triple Sulfa*	Sulfabenzamide/sulfacetamide/sulfathiazole	Sulfonamide
Sumamed	Azithromycin	Azalide
Sumycin	Tetracycline hydrochloride	Tetracycline
Suprax	Cefixime	Cephalosporin
Surlid	Roxithromycin	Macrolide
Sustiva	Efavirenz	Antiretroviral
Symadine	Amantadine hydrochloride	Antiviral
Symmetrel	Amantadine hydrochloride	Antiviral
Synagis	Palivizumab	Antiviral
Synercid*	Quinupristin/dalfopristin	Streptogramin
Tamiflu	Oseltamivir	Antiviral

*A combination product.

TABLE 46-2 Trade and Generic Names—cont'd

Trade Name	Generic Name	Class
Tao	Troleandomycin	Macrolide
Tarcil	Ticarcillin disodium	Penicillin
Targocid	Teicoplanin	Glycopeptide
Tarivid	Ofloxacin	Fluoroquinolone
Tavanic	Levofloxacin	Fluoroquinolone
Tazicef	Ceftazidime	Cephalosporin
Tazidime	Ceftazidime	Cephalosporin
Tazocin*	Piperacillin/tazobactam	Penicillin/β-lactamase inhibitor
Tegopen	Cloxacillin sodium	Penicillin
Tequin	Gatifloxacin	Fluoroquinolone
Terazol	Terconazole	Antifungal
Terramycin	Oxytetracycline	Tetracycline
Tetrachel	Tetracycline hydrochloride	Tetracycline
Tetralan	Tetracycline hydrochloride	Tetracycline
Thermazene	Silver sulfadiazene	Sulfonamide
Thiosulfil Forte	Sulfamethizole	Sulfonamide
Ticar	Ticarcillin disodium	Penicillin
Tienam*	Imipenem/cilastatin	Carbapenem
Timentin*	Ticarcillin disodium/clavulanate potassium	Penicillin/β-lactamase inhibitor
Tinactin	Tolnaftate	Antifungal
Tinaderm	Tolnaftate	Antifungal
TOBI	Tobramycin inhalation solution	Aminoglycoside
TobraDex*	Tobramycin/dexamethasone	Aminoglycoside/corticosteroid
Tobrex	Tobramycin	Aminoglycoside
Totacillin	Ampicillin trihydrate	Penicillin
Totacillin-N	Ampicillin sodium	Penicillin
Trecator-SC	Ethionamide	Antimycobacterial
Trimopan	Trimethoprim	Folate antagonist
Trimox	Amoxicillin	Penicillin
Trimpex	Trimethoprim	Folate antagonist
Triple Sulfa*	Sulfabenzamide/sulfacetamide/sulfathiazole	Sulfonamide
Trizivir*	Abacavir/lamivudine/zidovudine	Antiretroviral
Trobicin	Spectinomycin hydrochloride	Aminocyclitol
Trovan	Trovafloxacin	Fluoroquinolone
Trovan IV	Alatrofloxacin	Fluoroquinolone
Ultracef	Cefadroxil	Cephalosporin
Unasyn*	Ampicillin/sulbactam	Penicillin/β-lactamase inhibitor
Unipen	Nafcillin sodium	Penicillin
Uniquin	Lomefloxacin	Fluoroquinolone
Urex	Methenamine hippurate	Urinary anti-infective
Uri-Tet	Oxytetracycline hydrochloride	Tetracycline
Urobactam	Aztreonam	Monobactam
Urobiotic	Oxytetracycline hydrochloride	Tetracycline
Uroplus*	Trimethoprim/sulfamethoxazole	Folate antagonists
Valcyte	Valganciclovir	Antiviral
Valtrex	Valacyclovir	Antiviral
Vancocin	Vancomycin hydrochloride	Glycopeptide
Vancoled	Vancomycin hydrochloride	Glycopeptide
Vancor	Vancomycin hydrochloride	Glycopeptide
Vantin	Cefpodoxime proxetil	Cephalosporin
V-Cillin K	Penicillin V potassium	Penicillin
Vectavir	Penciclovir	Antiviral
Vectrin	Minocycline	Tetracycline
Veetids	Penicillin V potassium	Penicillin
Velosef	Cephradine	Cephalosporin
Vercef	Cefaclor	Cephalosporin
Vermox	Mebendazole	Anthelmintic
VFend	Voriconazole	Antifungal
Vibramycin Calcium	Doxycycline calcium	Tetracycline
Vibramycin Hyclate	Doxycycline hyclate	Tetracycline
Vibramycin Monohydrate	Doxycycline monohydrate	Tetracycline
Vibra-Tabs	Doxycycline hyclate	Tetracycline
Videx	Didanosine	Antiretroviral
Videx EC	Didanosine	Antiretroviral
Vira-MP	Vidarabine	Antiviral
Viracept	Nelfinavir	Protease inhibitor
Viramune	Nevirapine	Antiretroviral
Virazole	Ribavirin	Antiviral
Viread	Tenofovir	Antiretroviral
Viroptic	Trifluridine	Antiviral
Vistide	Cidofovir	Antiviral
Vitrasert	Ganciclovir	Antiviral
Wellvone	Atovaquone	Antiparasitic
Wyamycin	Erythromycin stearate	Macrolide
Wycillin	Penicillin G procaine	Penicillin
Wymox	Amoxicillin	Penicillin
Xigris	Drotrecogin alfa (activated)	Antisepsis
Yodoxin	Iodoquinol	Amebicide
Yodoxin M/	Iodoquinol	Amebicide

Continued

TABLE 46-2 Trade and Generic Names—cont'd

Trade Name	Generic Name	Class
Yomesan	Niclosamide	Anthelmintic
Zagam	Sparfloxacin	Fluoroquinolone
Zagam Respipac	Sparfloxacin	Fluoroquinolone
Zeclar	Clarithromycin	Macrolide
Zeffix	Lamivudine	Antiretroviral
Zelitrex	Valacyclovir	Antiviral
Zentel	Albendazole	Antiparasitic
Zerit	Stavudine (d4T)	Antiretroviral
Ziagen	Abacavir	Antiretroviral
Ziagenavir	Abacavir	Antiretroviral
Zinacef	Cefuroxime sodium	Cephalosporin
Zinamide	Pyrazinamide	Antimycobacterial
Zinnat	Cefuroxime axetil	Cephalosporin
Ziracin	Everninomycin	Oligosaccharide
Zithromax	Azithromycin	Azalide
Zithromax Tri-Pak	Azithromycin	Azalide
Zitromax	Azithromycin	Azalide
Zolicef	Cefazolin sodium	Cephalosporin
Zosyn*	Piperacillin/tazobactam	Penicillin/β-lactamase inhibitor
Zovirax	Acyclovir	Antiviral
Z-PAK	Azithromycin	Azalide
Zyvox	Linezolid	Oxazolidinone
Zyvoxam	Linezolid	Oxazolidinone

*A combination product.

TABLE 46-3 Penicillin Dosage Forms

	Formulations		
	Oral		
Generic Name	Tablets/Capsules (mg)	Liquid (mg/mL)	Parenteral (g)
Amoxicillin	125*, 250*, 400*, 250, 500, 875, 1000, 3000	50/1, 125/5, 250/5, 400/5, 500/5	0.25, 0.5, 1
Amoxicillin/clavulanate‡	125, 125*, 200*, 250*, 375, 400* 250, 500, 875, 1000†	125/5, 200/5, 250/5, 400/5	0.5, 1
Ampicillin	125*, 250, 500, 1000	100/1, 125/1.25, 125/5, 250/5, 500/5	0.1, 0.125, 0.25, 0.5, 1, 2, 10
Ampicillin/sulbactam	375		1.5, 3
Azlocillin			0.5, 1, 2, 3, 4
Bacampicillin	400, 800	125/5	
Carbenicillin			1, 5
Carbenicillin indanyl sodium	382, 500		
Cloxacillin	250, 500	125/5	0.25, 0.5, 1, 2
Cyclacillin	250, 500	125/5, 250/5	
Dicloxacillin	125, 250, 500	62.5/5	
Flucloxacillin	250, 500	125/5, 250/5	0.25, 0.5, 1
Methicillin			1, 2, 4, 6, 10
Mezlocillin			0.5, 1, 2, 3, 4, 5
Nafcillin	250, 500	250/5	0.5, 1, 2, 4, 10
Oxacillin	250, 500	250/5	0.25, 0.5, 1, 2, 4, 10
Penicillin G§	0.1 MU, 0.2 MU, 0.25 MU, 0.4 MU, 0.5 MU, 0.8 MU, 4 MU	0.2 MU/5, 0.25 MU/5, 0.5 MU/5	0.3 MU, 0.5 MU, 1 MU, 5 MU, 10 MU, 20 MU
Penicillin G benzathine			0.3 MU, 0.6 MU, 1.2 MU, 2.4 MU
Penicillin G procaine			0.3 MU, 0.6 MU, 1.2 MU, 2.4 MU
Penicillin V potassium	125*, 250, 300, 312.5, 500, 625, 937.5	125/5, 180/5, 250/5, 300/5	
Piperacillin			1, 2, 3, 4, 40
Piperacillin/tazobactam			2.25, 3.375, 4.5
Pivmecillinam	200		
Ticarcillin			1, 3, 6, 20, 30
Ticarcillin/clavulanate			3.1, 31

*Chewable.
†Extended release.
‡Doses based on amoxicillin content.
§400,000 IU = 0.4 MU = 250 mg.

TABLE 46-4 Cephalosporin Dosage Forms

	Formulations		
	Oral		
Generic Name	Tablets/Capsules (mg)	Liquid (mg/mL)	Parenteral (g)
First Generation			
Cefadroxil	250, 500, 1000	125/5, 250/5, 500/5, 500/10	
Cefazolin			0.25, 0.5, 1, 2, 5, 10, 20
Cephalexin	250, 500, 1000	100/1, 125/1.25, 125/5, 250/5, 375/5, 500/5	
Cephalothin			1, 2, 4, 20
Cephapirin			0.5, 1, 2, 4, 20
Cephradine	250, 500, 1000	125/5, 250/5	0.25, 0.5, 1, 2
Second Generation			
Cefaclor	250, 375*, 500, 500*	125/5, 187/5, 250/5, 375/5	
Cefamandole			0.5, 1, 2, 10
Cefmetazole			0.25, 0.5, 1, 2
Cefonicid			0.5, 1
Cefotetan			0.5, 1, 2, 10
Cefoxitin			0.5, 1, 2, 10
Cefprozil	250, 500	125/5, 250/5	
Cefuroxime	125, 250, 500	125/5, 250/5	0.25, 0.75, 1.5, 7.5
Third Generation			
Cefdinir	300	125/5	
Cefditoren pivoxil	200		
Cefixime	50, 100, 200, 400	100/5	
Cefoperazone			0.25, 0.5, 1, 2, 10
Cefotaxime			0.5, 1, 2, 10, 20
Cefpodoxime	100, 200	50/5, 100/5	
Cefsulodin			0.5, 1, 2
Ceftazidime			0.25, 0.5, 1, 2, 6, 10
Ceftibuten	218, 400, 435	90/5, 98/5, 196/5	
Ceftizoxime sodium			0.5, 1, 2
Ceftriaxone			0.25, 0.5, 1, 2, 10
Moxalactam			0.25, 0.5, 1, 2, 10
Fourth Generation			
Cefepime			0.5, 1, 2

*Sustained release.

TABLE 46-5 Aminoglycoside Dosage Forms

	Formulations		
	Oral		
Generic Name	Tablets/Capsules (mg)	Liquid (mg/mL)	Parenteral (g)
Amikacin			0.1, 0.25, 0.35, 0.5, 0.75, 1
Gentamicin			0.01, 0.02, 0.04, 0.08, 0.8
Kanamycin	500		0.075, 0.5, 1
Neomycin	350, 500	125/5	0.5
Netilmicin			0.05, 0.1, 0.15, 0.2, 2
Streptomycin			1
Tobramycin	300*		0.02, 0.04, 0.06, 0.08, 0.3, 1.2, 2

*For inhalation.

TABLE 46-6 Tetracycline Dosage Forms

	Formulations		
	Oral		
Generic Name	Tablets/Capsules (mg)	Liquid (mg/mL)	Parenteral (g)
Demeclocycline	75, 150, 300		
Doxycycline	20, 50, 100, 100*	25/5, 50/5	0.1, 0.2
Methacycline	150, 300	75/5	
Minocycline	50, 75, 100	50/5	0.1
Oxytetracycline	125, 250	100/1, 125/5	0.05, 0.25
Tetracycline	50, 100, 250, 500	125/5	0.1, 0.25, 0.5

*Sustained release.

TABLE 46-7 Macrolide, Azalide, Lincosamide, Chloramphenicol, and Metronidazole Dosage Forms

Generic Name	Formulations		Parenteral (g)
	Oral		
	Tablets/Capsules (mg)	Liquid (mg/mL)	
Azithromycin	250, 500, 600, 1000	100/5, 200/5	0.5
Clarithromycin	250, 500, 500*	125/5, 125/15, 187.5/5, 250/5	
Dirithromycin	250		
Erythromycin base	250, 250*, 333, 333*, 500, 500*		
Erythromycin stearate	100, 250, 500	100/2.5, 125/5, 200/5, 250/5	
Erythromycin ethyl succinate	200†, 400, 600	100/2.5, 125/5, 200/5, 400/5	
Erythromycin lactobionate			0.5, 1
Erythromycin gluceptate			0.5, 1
Erythromycin estolate	125, 125†, 250†, 250, 500	100/1, 125/1, 125/5, 250/1, 250/5	
Roxithromycin	150, 300		
Telithromycin	800		
Clindamycin	75, 150, 300	75/5	0.3, 0.6, 0.9
Lincomycin	250, 500	50/1, 250/5	0.3, 0.6
Chloramphenicol	250	30/1, 125/5	1
Metronidazole	200, 250, 375, 400, 500, 500‡, 750*, 1000‡	200/5	0.5

*Sustained release.
†Chewable.
‡Vaginal suppository.

TABLE 46-8 Miscellaneous Agent Dosage Forms

Generic Name	Formulations		Parenteral (g)
	Oral		
	Tablets/ Capsules (mg)	Liquid (mg/mL)	
Aztreonam			0.5, 1, 2
Colistimethate		25/5	0.15
Ertapenem			1
Fusidic acid	250	246/5	
Imipenem			0.25, 0.5, 0.75
Linezolid	400, 600	100/5	0.2, 0.4, 0.6
Loracarbef	200, 400	100/5, 200/5	
Meropenem			0.25, 0.5, 1
Quinupristin/dalfopristin			0.15/0.35
Vancomycin	125, 250		0.5, 1, 5, 10

TABLE 46-9 Folate Antagonist Dosage Forms

Generic Name	Formulations		Parenteral (g)
	Oral		
	Tablets/ Capsules (mg)	Liquid (mg/mL)	
Trimethoprim-sulfamethoxazole	20/100, 80/400, 160/800	8/40/1, 40/200/5, 80/400/5	0.080/0.400, 0.160/0.800
Trimethoprim	100, 200, 300	50/5	0.020/1 mL
Sulfisoxazole	500	500/5	
Sulfamethoxazole	500, 1000	500/5	
Sulfamethizole	500, 1000	100/5	
Sulfadiazine	500		
Sulfadoxine*	500		
Dapsone	25, 100		
Trimetrexate			0.040

*With pyrimethamine.

TABLE 46-10 Quinolone and Urinary Anti-infective Dosage Forms

Generic Name	Formulations		Parenteral (g)
	Oral		
	Tablets/ Capsules (mg)	Liquid (mg/mL)	
Quinolones			
Cinoxacin	250, 500		
Ciprofloxacin	100, 200, 250, 500, 750	50/1, 100/1, 250/5, 500/5	0.2, 0.4
Enoxacin	200, 400		
Gatifloxacin	200, 400		0.2, 0.4
Gemifloxacin	320		
Levofloxacin	250, 500, 750		0.25, 0.5, 0.75
Lomefloxacin	400		
Moxifloxacin	400		0.4
Nalidixic acid	250, 500, 1000	50/1, 250/5	
Norfloxacin	100, 400		
Ofloxacin	100, 200, 300, 400		0.1, 0.2, 0.4
Sparfloxacin	200		
Trovafloxacin	100, 200		0.1, 0.2, 0.3
Urinary Anti-infectives			
Fosfomycin	3000		
Methenamine mandelate	250, 500, 1000	250/5, 500/5	
Nitrofurantoin	25, 50, 100	25/5	

TABLE 46-11 Antimycobacterial Dosage Forms

	Formulations		
	Oral		
Generic Name	Tablets/ Capsules (mg)	Liquid (mg/mL)	Parenteral (g)
Aminosalicylic acid	4000		
Capreomycin			1
Clofazimine	50, 100		
Cycloserine	250		
Ethambutol	100, 400		
Ethionamide	125, 250		
Isoniazid	50, 100, 300	10/1, 50/5	0.1
Pyrazinamide	500		
Rifabutin	150		
Rifampin	150, 300, 450, 600	100/5	0.6
Rifapentine	150		
Streptomycin			1

TABLE 46-13 Antiviral Dosage Forms

	Formulations		
	Oral		
Generic Name	Tablets/ Capsules (mg)	Liquid (mg/mL)	Parenteral (g)
Acyclovir	200, 400, 800	200/5	0.1, 0.5, 1
Adefovir	10		
Amantadine	50, 100	50/5	
Cidofovir			0.375
Famciclovir	125, 250, 500		
Foscarnet			6, 12
Ganciclovir	250, 500		0.5
Interferon alfa-2a			3 MIU, 4.5 MIU, 6 MIU, 9 MIU, 18 MIU, 36 MIU
Interferon alfa-2b			1 MIU, 3 MIU, 3.5 MIU, 5 MIU, 10 MIU, 18 MIU, 35 MIU, 30 MIU, 50 MIU
Interferon alfacon-1			9 μg, 15 μg, 30 μg
Interferon alfa-n3			5 MIU
Oseltamivir	75	12/1	
Palivizumab			0.1
Peginterferon alfa-2b			74 μg, 118.4 μg, 177.6 μg, 222 μg
Peginterferon alfa-2b/ribavirin			50 μg/200 mg, 80 μg/200 mg, 100 μg/200 mg, 120 μg/200 mg, 150 μg/200 mg
Ribavirin			6*
Rimantadine	100, 200, 400	50/5	
Valacyclovir	500, 556, 1000		
Valganciclovir	450		
Zanamivir	5*		

*For inhalation.

TABLE 46-12 Antifungal Dosage Forms

	Formulations		
	Oral		
Generic Name	Tablets/ Capsules (mg)	Liquid (mg/mL)	Parenteral (g)
Amphotericin B	10, 100	100/1	0.05
Amphotericin B cholesteryl sulfate complex			0.05, 0.1
Amphotericin B lipid complex			0.1
Amphotericin B liposomal			0.05
Caspofungin			0.05, 0.07
Clotrimazole	10, 100*, 200*, 500*		
Econazole	50*, 150*		
Fluconazole	50, 100, 150, 200	10/1, 40/1, 50/5, 200/5	0.2, 0.4
Flucytosine	200, 250, 500		2.5
Griseofulvin	125, 165, 250, 330, 500	125/5	
Itraconazole	100	10/1	0.25
Ketoconazole	200, 400*	20/1, 100/5	
Miconazole	100*, 200*, 250, 400*		0.01
Nystatin	100,000 U, 100,000 U*, 200,000 U, 500,000 U	100,000 U/1, 500,000 U/5	
Terbinafine	125, 250		
Terconazole	80*, 240*		
Voriconazole	50, 200		0.2

*Vaginal tablet/ovule/suppository form.

TABLE 46-14 Antiretroviral Dosage Forms

	Formulations		
	Oral		
Generic Name	Tablets/ Capsules (mg)	Liquid (mg/mL)	Parenteral (g)
Abacavir	300	20/1	
Amprenavir	50, 150	15/1	
Delavirdine	100, 200		
Didanosine	25, 50, 100, 125*, 150, 200, 200*, 250*, 400*		
Enfuvirtide			0.09
Indinavir	100, 200, 300, 333, 400		
Lamivudine	150, 300	10/1	
Lopinavir/ritonavir	133/33.3	80/20/1	
Nelfinavir	250		
Nevirapine	200	50/5	
Ritonavir	100	80/1	
Saquinavir	200		
Stavudine	5, 15, 20, 30, 40		
Tenofovir	300		
Zalcitabine	0.375, 0.75		
Zidovudine	100, 300	50/5	0.2

*Extended release.

TABLE 46-15 Antimicrobial Agent Pharmacology: Penicillins

Drug (Oral Absorption, %)	Serum and Urine Concentration; Selected Doses			Dosage Recommendations						
	Dose (g)	Peak Serum (µg/mL)	Peak or Range, Urine (µg/mL)	Adults			Children: Dose/Interval		Newborn (Parenteral): Dose/Interval	
				Dose (g)/Interval		Serious Infection Daily Dose (g)				
				Oral	Parenteral		Oral	Parenteral	Up to 1 wk	1-4 wk
Amdinocillin	10 mg/kg	50	1260		10 mg/kg q4-6h			10 mg/kg q4-6h (not approved)		
Amoxicillin[1] (74-92)	0.25 PO[2] 0.5 PO[2]	3.5-5 5.5-11		0.25-2 q8h		4	20-90 mg/kg/day in 3 doses[3]			
Amoxicillin/ clavulanate	0.25 PO 0.5 PO 0.875 PO	3.7-4.8 6-9.7 11.6	381	0.25-2 q8-12h		4	20-90 mg/kg/day in 3 doses[4]			
Ampicillin[1] (30-55)	0.25 PO[2] 0.5 PO[2] 2 IV	1.8-2.9 3-6 47.6		0.25-0.5 q6h	0.5-2 q4-6h	4 PO/12 IV	6.25-25[5] mg/kg q6h	6.25-25 mg/kg q6h[6]	25 mg/kg q12h	25 mg/kg q8h
Ampicillin/ sulbactam	1.5 IV 3 IV	40-71 109-150			1.5-3 q6h	4		25-50 mg/kg q6h		
Azlocillin (minimal)	2 IV[7] 3 IV[7]	165 214	2200-8100		2-4 q4-6h	24		75 mg/kg q6h (not approved)[6]	Not recommended	
Bacampicillin[9] (80-98)	0.4 PO 0.8 PO 1.6 PO	5.8-8.3 12.0-15.9 18.6-20.1		0.4-1.6 q12h		1.6	12.5-25 mg/kg q12h			
Carbenicillin	1 IV 3 IV[10]	45-71 278	1000 4165		5-6 q4h	30		25-100 mg/kg q4-6h	66.7-100 mg/kg q8h	400 mg/kg/day q6-8h
Carbenicillin indanyl sodium (30-40)	0.382 PO	6.5	0.576-1.13[11]	0.382-0.764 q6h		3				
Cloxacillin[1] (37-60)	0.5 PO	6.9-15		0.25-1 q6h		2	12.5-25 mg/kg q6h			
Cyclacillin	0.25 PO 0.5 PO	6-7 11-12		0.25-0.5 q6h		2	12.5-25 mg/kg q6h			
Dicloxacillin[1] (35-76)	0.5 PO	10-18		0.125-0.5 q6h		2	3.125-6.25[5] mg/kg q6h			
Flucloxacillin[1] (50-70)	0.25 PO 0.50 PO	6-9 11-20		0.25 q6h	0.25 q6h	8	62.5-125 mg q6h	62.5-250 mg q6h		

[1]Decreased rate and/or extent of absorption when given with food.
[2]Fasting.
[3]Children <20-27 kg.
[4]Children <40 kg should not receive the 250-mg film-coated tablet.
[5]Children <40-50 kg.
[6]16.7-33.3 mg/kg q4h for meningitis.
[7]Infusion over 15-30 minutes.
[8]Mean concentration.
[9]100% of bacampicillin is metabolized to ampicillin.
[10]IV push (over 2-10 minutes).
[11]Over 3 hours.
[12]Depending on severity of infection.
[13]q6h if >2 kg; q8h if <2 kg.
[14]q8h if >2 kg; q12h if <2 kg.
[15]Higher when given with probenecid.
[16]Dosage should not exceed adult dosage.

Serum Half-life (h)		With Dialysis		Standard Dose with Dosing Intervals in Renal Impairment					Dosage with Dialysis		Body Fluid Concentrations				
With Normal and Anuric Cl_{Cr} Values (mL/min)				Usual Adult Dose	For Cl_{Cr} Ranges (mL/min)										
>80	<10	HD	PD		>80	80-50	50-10	<10 (anuric)	After HD[a]	During PD (daily dose)	CSF/Serum (%)[b]	Newborn Serum/Maternal Serum (%)	Breast Milk/Maternal Serum (%)	Bile/Serum (%)	Aqueous Humor/Serum (%)
0.8-1	3.4-5.6	1.8		10 mg/kg	4	4	6-8	8	10 mg/kg					400	
0.7-1.4	7.4-21			0.25-0.5	8	8	8-12	12-16	0.25-0.5		5-10	25-33	5	100-3000	Negligible
1.1-1.3	7.5			0.25-2.0	8-12	8-12	0.25-0.5 q12h	0.25-0.5 q24h	0.25-0.5	0.25 q12h	6		Low	1100	
0.7-1.4	7.4-21			0.5-2	4-6	4-6	8	12	0.5-2	1-4		100	11	100-3000	2-8
1	9			1.5-3.0	6-8	6-8	8-12	24							
1	5	1.5-2.6		2-4	4-6	4-6	8	12	3		13.3[8]				
0.7-1.4	7.4-21			0.4-1.6	12	12	12					65-75	1.7-3.6	17	
0.78-1	9.4-23.4	6	4.2-7.4	5-6	4	4	2-3 q6h	Avoid	0.75-2	2 q6-12h	9.4[9]	50-100	0.4	50-75	Up to 3
0.78-1	9.4-23.4														
0.4-0.8	0.8-2.3			0.5-1	6	6	6	6	Usual regimen	Usual regimen					
				0.25-0.5	6	6	12-24	24							
0.6-0.8	1-2.2	1-2.2	1-2.2	0.125-0.5	6	6	6	6	Usual regimen	Usual regimen	Minimal	0-10		5-8	
0.75-1.5	0.75-1.5	0.75-1.5	0.75-1.5	0.25	6-8	6-8	6-8	6-8	Usual regimen	Usual regimen					

[a]Specified dose is supplemental to that after hemodialysis.
[b]Inflamed meninges.

Continued

TABLE 46-15 Antimicrobial Agent Pharmacology: Penicillins—cont'd

Drug (Oral Absorption, %)	Serum and Urine Concentration; Selected Doses			Dosage Recommendations						
				Adults			Children: Dose/Interval		Newborn (Parenteral): Dose/Interval	
	Dose (g)	Peak Serum (µg/mL)	Peak or Range, Urine (µg/mL)	Dose (g)/Interval		Serious Infection Daily Dose (g)	Oral	Parenteral	Up to 1 wk	1-4 wk
				Oral	Parenteral					
Methicillin	1 IV[10] 1 IM 2 IM	59.8 9-18 13.8			1-2 q4-6h	12		25-100 mg/kg q4-6h[12]	25-50 mg/kg q12h	25-50 mg/kg q8h
Mezlocillin	1 IV[10] 2 IV[10] 5 IV[10]	64-143 161-364 199-597	4000		3-4 q4-6h	24		50-75 mg/kg q4h	75 mg/kg q12h	75 mg/kg q6-8h[13]
Nafcillin[1] (36)	1 PO 1 IM 0.5 IV[10]	7.7 7.6 40		0.5-1 q6h	0.5-2 q4-6h	2 PO/9 IV	12.5-25 mg/kg q6h[5]	12.5-25 mg/kg q6h[5]	25 mg/kg q8-12h[14]	25 mg/kg q6-8h[13]
Oxacillin[1] (30-35)	0.25 PO 0.5 PO 0.5 IV	1.65 2.6-3.9 52-63		0.5-1 q4-6h	0.5-2 q4-6h	4 PO/12 IV	12.5-25 mg/kg q6h[5]	12.5-50 mg/kg q6h[5]	25-50 mg/kg q8-12h[14]	25-50 mg/kg q6-8h[13]
Penicillin G[1] (15-30)	400,000 U PO 2 mU q2h IV	0.5 U/mL[15] 20		0.5-1 q6h	1-4 mU q4-6h	4 PO/24 mU IV	25,000-90,000 U/kg/day in 3-6 doses	25,000-400,000 U/kg/day q4-6h[16]	50,000-150,000 U/kg/day q8-12h[14]	75,000-200,000 U/kg/day q6-8h[13]
Penicillin G benzathine	1.2 mU IM	0.15 U/mL			0.6-1.2 mU IM × 1	2.4 mU		0.6 mU IM × 1[3]		50,000 U/kg IM × 1
Penicillin G procaine	0.6 mU IM 1.2 mU IM	1.6 1.95			0.6-1.2 mU IM q12h	4.8 mU		25,000-50,000 U/kg/day IM[16]		50,000 U/kg/day IM
Penicillin V potassium[1] (60-73)	0.25 PO 0.5 PO	2.3-2.7 4.9-6.3		0.25-0.5 q6h		2	25000-100,000 U/kg/day in 3-6 doses			
Piperacillin	2 IV[10] 4 IV[10] 6 IV[10]	159-615 389-484 695-849	8500 14,100		3-4 q4-6h	18		50 mg/kg q4h[16]		
Piperacillin/tazobactam	3.375 IV[7] 4.5 IV[7]	209 224			3.375-4.5 q6-8h	13.5				
Ticarcillin	1 IV[10] 2 IV[10] 3 IV[10]	70-100 200-218 257	650-2500[11]		3 q4-6h	18		200-300 mg/kg/day q4-6h[5]	75 mg/kg q8-12h[14]	75 mg/kg q8h if <2 kg; 100 mg/kg q8h if >2 kg
Ticarcillin/clavulanate	3.1 IV	324	1500		3.1 q4-8h	18.6		50 mg/kg q4-6h		

[1]Decreased rate and/or extent of absorption when given with food.
[2]Fasting.
[3]Children <20-27 kg.
[4]Children <40 kg should not receive the 250-mg film-coated tablet.
[5]Children <40-50 kg.
[6]16.7-33.3 mg/kg q4h for meningitis.
[7]Infusion over 15-30 minutes.
[8]Mean concentration.
[9]100% of bacampicillin is metabolized to ampicillin.
[10]IV push (over 2-10 minutes).
[11]Over 3 hours.
[12]Depending on severity of infection.
[13]q6h if >2 kg; q8h if <2 kg.
[14]q8h if >2 kg; q12h if <2 kg.
[15]Higher when given with probenecid.
[16]Dosage should not exceed adult dosage.

| Serum Half-life (h) | | | | Standard Dose with Dosing Intervals in Renal Impairment | | | | | | | Body Fluid Concentrations | | | | |
| With Normal and Anuric Cl_{Cr} Values (mL/min) | | With Dialysis | | | For Cl_{Cr} Ranges (mL/min) | | | | Dosage with Dialysis | | | | | | |
>80	<10	HD	PD	Usual Adult Dose	>80	80-50	50-10	<10 (anuric)	After HD[a]	During PD (daily dose)	CSF/ Serum (%)[b]	Newborn Serum/ Maternal Serum (%)	Breast Milk/ Maternal Serum (%)	Bile/ Serum (%)	Aqueous Humor/ Serum (%)
0.4-0.5	4-6	4-6	4-6	1-2	4-6	6	8	12			10	50-100		≥100	Negligible
0.71-1.3	1.6-14		1.6-14	3-4	4-6	4-6	8	2 g q8h	2-3	3 g q12h	1.2-11.7[9]	70-500	Low	1000	
0.5-1.5	1.8-2.8	1.8-2.8	1.8-2.8	0.5-2	4-6	4-6	4-6	4-6	Usual regimen	Usual regimen	9-20	10-15		≥100	Negligible
0.3-0.8	0.5-2	0.5-2	0.5-2	0.5-2	4-6	4-6	4-6	4-6	Usual regimen	Usual regimen		10-15	≤3.5	20-30	0
0.4-0.9	6-20		6-20	1-4 mU	4-6	4-6	4-6	.5-2 mU q4-6	500,000 U		0-10	100	6	200-800	
Days											Minimal				
24				0.6-1.2 mU	12	12	12	12							
0.5	7-10			0.25-0.5	6	6	6	6	0.25						
0.6-1.3	2.1-6		2.1-6	3-4	4-6	4-6	8	12	1 g post then 2 g q8h				1	3000-6000	
0.7-1.1	1.9-3.5			2.5-4.5	6-8	6-8								>100	
0.93-1.3	13.5-16.2			3	4-6	4-6	6-8	2 g q12h	3 g post then 2 g q12h	3 g q12h	39				
1.1-1.5	8.5			3.1	4-6	4-6	2-3.1 g q6-h	2 g q12h	3.1	3.1 q12h			Low		

[a]Specified dose is supplemental to that after hemodialysis.
[b]Inflamed meninges.

TABLE 46-16 Antimicrobial Agent Pharmacology: Cephalosporins

Drug (Oral Absorption, %)	Serum and Urine Concentration; Selected Doses			Dosage Recommendations						
				Adults			Children: Dose/Interval		Newborn (Parenteral): Dose/Interval	
	Dose (g)	Peak Serum (µg/mL)	Peak or Range, Urine (µg/mL)	Dose (g)/Interval		Serious Infection Daily Dose (g)	Oral	Parenteral	Up to 1 wk	1-4 wk
				Oral	Parenteral					
First Generation Cefadroxil (100)	0.5 PO 1 PO	10-18 24-35	1800	0.5-1 q12-24h		2	30 mg/kg/day q12h			
Cefazolin	1 IV 1 IM	188 64-76	4000		0.5-2 q8h	6		25-100 mg/kg/day q6-8h		
Cephalexin (100)	0.25 PO 0.5 PO	9 15-18	2000	0.25-1 q6h		2	25-100 mg/kg/day in 4 doses			
Cephalothin	1 IM 1 IV	15-21 30	2500		0.5-2 q4-6h	12		80-160 mg/kg/day q6h		
Cephapirin	1 IV	67	2560		0.5-2 q4-6h	12		40-80 mg/kg/day q6h		
Cephradine[1] (>90)	0.25 PO 0.5 PO 1 IV	9 15-18 86	1600 3200	0.25-1 q6h	0.5-2 q4-6h	2 PO/8 IV	25-100 mg/kg/day q6 or 12h	50-100 mg/kg/day q6h		
Second Generation Cefaclor[1] (>52)	0.25 PO 0.5 PO	5-7 13-15	600 900	0.25-0.5 q8h		1.5	20-40 mg/kg/day q8h[2]			
Cefamandole	1 IV[3] 2 IV[3] 3 IV[3]	139 214 534	750 1400		0.5-2 q4-8h	8		50-150 mg/kg/day q4-8h[4]		
Cefmetazole					2 q6-12h	8				
Cefonicid	7.5 mg/kg IV[3] 0.5 IV 1 IV	95-156 91 221	1020		0.5-2 q24h	2				
Cefotetan	1 IV[3] 2 IV[3]	142-179.6 237	1400-2000 3500-4000		1-2 q12h	4		40-60 mg/kg/day q12h (not approved)		

[1]Decreased rate and/or extent of absorption when given with food.
[2]Should not exceed 1 g.
[3]IV push (over 2-10 minutes).
[4]Dosage should not exceed adult dosage.
[5]Should not exceed 12 g.
[6]52% after food.
[7]Infusion over 15-30 minutes.
[8]0.125 g q12h for children <2 yr.
[9]200-240 mg/kg/day q6-8h for meningitis.
[10]Microbiologic activity in hepatic bile/microbiologic activity serum.
[11]Should be given with food to increase absorption.

[12]No more than 400 mg/day for otitis or 100 mg/day for pharyngitis/tonsillitis.
[13]Creatinine clearance <30 ml/min.
[14]Arginine component not approved for children <12 yr.
[15]30-50 mg/kg q12h for <2 kg; 30 mg/kg q8h for >2 kg.
[16]2g q24h at steady-state.
[17]750 mg/kg/day for <2 kg; 50-75 mg/kg/day for >2 kg.
[18]Bleeding time should be monitored in patients receiving more than 4 g/day for more than 3 days. Prophylactic vitamin K, 10 mg/week, should be given to patients treated with moxalactam.
[19]For gram-negative meningitis in children, the manufacturer recommends an initial loading dose of 100 mg/kg.

| Serum Half-life (h) | | | | Standard Dose with Dosing Intervals in Renal Impairment | | | | | | | Body Fluid Concentrations | | | | |
| With Normal and Anuric Cl_Cr Values (mL/min) | | With Dialysis | | | For Cl_Cr Ranges (mL/min) | | | | Dosage with Dialysis | | | | | | |
>80	<10	HD	PD	Usual Adult Dose	>80	80-50	50-10	<10 (anuric)	After HD[a]	During PD (daily dose)	CSF/Serum (%)[b]	Newborn Serum/Maternal Serum (%)	Breast Milk/Maternal Serum (%)	Bile/Serum (%)	Aqueous Humor/Serum (%)
1.1-2	20-25			0.5-1	12-24	12-24	0.5 q12-24	0.5 q36	0.5-1			50	0.9-1.9	22	
1.2-2.2	18-36			0.5-2	8	8	0.5-1 q8-12	0.5-1 q18-24	0.25-0.5		1-4	35-69	3	29-300	<1.7
0.5-1.2	5-30			0.25-1	6	6	8-12	24-48	0.25-1		Minimal	60	2	216	11
0.5-0.9	3-8			0.5-2	4-6	4-6	1-1.5 q6h	0.5 q8h	0.5-2	≤6 mg/L/dialysate	1.2-5.6	16-41		22-172	4
0.6-0.9	2.4			0.5-2	4-6	6	8	12	7.5-15 mg/kg before, then q12 post			60	7		
0.7-2	8-15			0.25-1.0	6	6	0.5 q6h	0.25 q12h	0.25 pre then 12 and 36-48 hr later	0.5 q6h	≤1	9-22	14-20	10-400	5-9
0.5-1	2.8			0.25-0.5	8	8	8	8	0.25-0.5				2	≥60	1-3
0.5-2.1	12.3-18			0.5-2	4-8	6	8	0.5-1 q12h	0.5-1		2		2.4	300-400	1.5
1.2				1-2	6-12	12	16-24	48							
3.5-5.8	50-60			0.5-2	24	8-25 mg/kg q24	4-15 mg/kg q24-48	3-15 mg/kg q3-5 day	None				<1	<10	0.2
2.8-4.6	12-30			1-2	12	12	24	48	25% non-dialysis days, 50% dialysis days				2.3	2-21	

[a]Specified dose is supplemental to that after hemodialysis.
[b]Inflamed meninges.

Continued

TABLE 46-16   Antimicrobial Agent Pharmacology: Cephalosporins—cont'd

Drug (Oral Absorption, %)	Serum and Urine Concentration; Selected Doses			Dosage Recommendations						
				Adults			Children: Dose/Interval		Newborn (Parenteral): Dose/Interval	
	Dose (g)	Peak Serum (µg/mL)	Peak or Range, Urine (µg/mL)	Dose (g)/Interval		Serious Infection Daily Dose (g)				
				Oral	Parenteral		Oral	Parenteral	Up to 1 wk	1-4 wk
Second Generation, cont'd Cefoxitin	1 IM 1 IV[3] 2 IV[3]	22-24 110-125 221	3000		1-2 q6-8h	8		80-160 mg/kg/day q4-8h[5]		
Cefprozil (95)	0.25 PO 0.5 PO 1 PO	5.6-6.8 8.2-10.4 15.5-19.9	250 1000 2900	0.25-0.5 q12-24h		1	15 mg/kg q12h			
Cefuroxime (37-52)[6]	0.5 PO 0.75 IV[7]	7 51.1	1150	0.125-0.5 q12h	0.75-1.5 q8h	1 PO/4.5 IV	0.125-0.25 q12h[8]	50-100 mg/kg/day q6-8h[9]		10 mg/kg q12h (not approved)
Third Generation Cefdinir[1] (36)	0.2 PO 0.6 PO	0.7-1.7 2.4		0.3-0.6 q12-24h		0.6	14 mg/kg/day			
Cefditoren (14-16)	0.2 0.4	2.5-3 4.4-4.6		0.2-0.4 q12h		0.8	3-6 mg/kg q8h			
Cefixime[1] (30-50)	0.4 PO tabs 0.4 PO susp	3.7 4.6	15.7-305 15.7-305	0.4 q24h		0.4	8 mg/kg/day q24h			
Cefoperazone	1 IV[7] 2 IV[7]	153 253	2200		1-2 q6-12h	12		25-100 mg/kg q12h (not approved)		25-100 mg/kg q12h (not approved)
Cefotaxime	0.5 IM 1 IV[3] 2 IV[3]	11.7-11.9 102.4 214.1	90-3261		0.5-2 q8-12h	12		50-200 mg/kg/day q4-8h	50 mg/kg q12h	50 mg/kg q6-8h
Cefpodoxime[11] (50)	0.1 PO 0.2 PO 0.4 PO	1.4 2.3 3.9	60	0.1-0.4 q12h		0.8	5 mg/kg q12h[12]			
Cefsulodin (85 IM)	1 IV	65			0.5-2 q6-8h	12		60-200 mg/kg/day in 3-4 doses		
Ceftazidime[14]	0.5 IV[7] 1 IV[7] 2 IV[7]	42 69 159-185.5			1-2 q8-12h	6		25-50 mg/kg q8h	30-50 mg/kg q8h[15]	30 mg/kg q8h

[1]Decreased rate and/or extent of absorption when given with food.
[2]Should not exceed 1 g.
[3]IV push (over 2-10 minutes).
[4]Dosage should not exceed adult dosage.
[5]Should not exceed 12 g.
[6]52% after food.
[7]Infusion over 15-30 minutes.
[8]0.125 g q12h for children <2 yr.
[9]200-240 mg/kg/day q6-8h for meningitis.
[10]Microbiologic activity in hepatic bile/microbiologic activity serum.
[11]Should be given with food to increase absorption.

[12]No more than 400 mg/day for otitis or 100 mg/day for pharyngitis/tonsillitis.
[13]Creatinine clearance <30 ml/min.
[14]Arginine component not approved for children <12 yr.
[15]30-50 mg/kg q12h for <2 kg; 30 mg/kg q8h for >2 kg.
[16]2g q24h at steady-state.
[17]50 mg/kg/day for <2 kg; 50-75 mg/kg/day for >2 kg.
[18]Bleeding time should be monitored in patients receiving more than 4 g/day for more than 3 days. Prophylactic vitamin K, 10 mg/week, should be given to patients treated with moxalactam.
[19]For gram-negative meningitis in children, the manufacturer recommends an initial loading dose of 100 mg/kg.

Serum Half-life (h)				Standard Dose with Dosing Intervals in Renal Impairment					Dosage with Dialysis		Body Fluid Concentrations				
With Normal and Anuric Cl_{Cr} Values (mL/min)		With Dialysis			For Cl_{Cr} Ranges (mL/min)										
>80	<10	HD	PD	Usual Adult Dose	>80	80-50	50-10	<10 (anuric)	After HD[a]	During PD (daily dose)	CSF/ Serum (%)[b]	Newborn Serum/ Maternal Serum (%)	Breast Milk/ Maternal Serum (%)	Bile/ Serum (%)	Aqueous Humor/ Serum (%)
0.7-1.1	13-22			1-2	6-8	8-12	12-24	0.5-1 g q12-48	1-2		2.8	100	≤3	280	4-7
0.9-1.5	5.9			0.25-0.5	12-24	12-24	50% q12-24	50% q12-24							
1-2	20			.125-0.5 PO / .75-1.5 IV	12 / 8	12 / 8	12 / 8-12	.25 g q24 / .75 g q24	0.75	15 mg/kg post-dialysis	17-88	20-33	≤3	35-80	10-14
1.1-4.4				0.3-0.6	12-24										
1.3-2	4.7			0.2-0.4	12	12	0.2 q12-24h							>100	
2.4-4	11.5	7		0.4	24	24	0.3 q24	48	None				15-50		
1.6-2.6	2-2.5			1-2	6-12	6-12	6-12	6-12	Dose after dialysis		1.8-3.1	20-50	≤1.5	800-1200	1-6
0.9-1.7				0.5-2	8-12	8-12	12-24	24	0.5-2		27		Up to 3-8	15-75[10]	0.5-4
1.9-3.2	9.8			0.1-0.4	12	12	24[13]	24	Usual dose 3 ×/wk					102-127	
1.6-1.9	13	2.1-2.6	8.9	0.5-2	6-8	6-8	0.25-1 q6-12h	0.5-2 q24h	60% of usual dose	1 q24h	<10				Minimal
1.4-2	11.9-35			1-2	8-12	8-12	12-24	0.5 g q24-48	1 g load then 1 g post-dialysis	0.5 g q24h or 250 mg/2 L dialysate	20-40		7	13-54	3-12

[a]Specified dose is supplemental to that after hemodialysis.
[b]Inflamed meninges.

Continued

TABLE 46-16   Antimicrobial Agent Pharmacology: Cephalosporins—cont'd

Drug (Oral Absorption, %)	Serum and Urine Concentration; Selected Doses			Dosage Recommendations						
				Adults			Children: Dose/Interval		Newborn (Parenteral): Dose/Interval	
	Dose (g)	Peak Serum (µg/mL)	Peak or Range, Urine (µg/mL)	Dose (g)/Interval		Serious Infection Daily Dose (g)	Oral	Parenteral	Up to 1 wk	1-4 wk
				Oral	Parenteral					
Third Generation, cont'd Ceftibuten (80)	0.4 PO	15		0.2-0.4 q12-24h		0.6	9 mg/kg/day			
Ceftizoxime	1 IV[7] 2 IV 3 IV 0.1 PO	84.4 131.8 221.1 1.5	>6000	0.1 q12h?	1-3 q6-8h	12		33-50 mg/kg q6-8h[5]		
Ceftriaxone	1 IV[7] 2 IV[7] 2 IV[16]	123.2-150.7 223-276 216-281	504-995		0.5-2 q12-24h	4		50-100 mg/kg/day q12-24h	50 mg/kg q24h	50-75 mg/kg q24h[17]
Moxalactam	1 IV[7] 2 IV[3]	60-100 150-200	2100 4200		0.5-4 q8-12h[18]	12[18]		50 mg/kg q6-8h[18,19]	50 mg/kg q12h[18,19]	50 mg/kg q8h[18,19]
Fourth Generation Cefepime	1 IV 2 IV	81.7 163.9			0.5-2 q8-12h	6		50 mg/kg q8-12h		

[1]Denotes decreased rate and/or extent of absorption when given with food.
[2]Should not exceed 1 g.
[3]IV push (over 2-10 minutes).
[4]Dosage should not exceed adult dosage.
[5]Should not exceed 12 g.
[6]52% after food.
[7]Infusion over 15-30 minutes.
[8]0.125 g q12h for children <2 yr.
[9]200-240 mg/kg/day q6-8h for meningitis.
[10]Microbiologic activity in hepatic bile/microbiologic activity serum.
[11]Should be given with food to increase absorption.

[12]No more than 400 mg/day for otitis or 100 mg/day for pharyngitis/tonsillitis.
[13]Creatinine clearance <30 ml/min.
[14]Arginine component not approved for children <12 yr.
[15]30-50 mg/kg q12h for <2 kg; 30 mg/kg q8h for >2 kg.
[16]2g q24h at steady-state.
[17]50 mg/kg/day for <2 kg; 50-75 mg/kg/day for >2 kg.
[18]Bleeding time should be monitored in patients receiving more than 4 g/day for more than 3 days. Prophylactic vitamin K, 10 mg/week, should be given to patients treated with moxalactam.
[19]For gram-negative meningitis in children, the manufacturer recommends an initial loading dose of 100 mg/kg.

TABLE 46-17   Antimicrobial Agent Pharmacology: Miscellaneous β-Lactams

Drug (Oral Absorption, %)	Serum and Urine Concentration; Selected Doses			Dosage Recommendations						
				Adults			Children: Dose/Interval		Newborn (Parenteral): Dose/Interval	
	Dose (g)	Peak Serum (µg/mL)	Peak or Range, Urine (µg/mL)	Dose (g)/Interval		Serious Infection Daily Dose (g)	Oral	Parenteral	Up to 1 wk	1-4 wk
				Oral	Parenteral					
Aztreonam	1 IV[2] 2 IV[2]	90-164 204-255	3000-3500 5600-6600		1-2 q6h	6		30-50 mg/kg q6-8h		30-50 mg/kg q8-12h
Ertapenem (90 IM)	1 IV[2]	155			1-2 q24h	2				
Imipenem	0.25 IV[2] 0.5 IV[2] 1 IV[2]	14-24 21-58 41-83	50 100 ≥100		0.5-1 q6h	2		15-25 mg/kg q6h	25 mg/kg q12h	25 mg/kg q8h
Loracarbef[1] (90)	0.2 PO cap 0.4 PO cap 0.4 PO ssp.	8 14 17		0.20-0.40 q12-24h		0.8	15-30 mg/kg/day q12h			
Meropenem	0.5 IV[2] 1 IV[2]	26 55-62			0.5-2 q8-12h	6		20-40 mg/kg q8h		

[1]Decreased rate and/or extent of absorption when given with food.
[2]IV infusion over 15-30 minutes.
[3]2.7 hours during dialysis/7-9 hours between dialysis sessions.

| Serum Half-life (h) | | | | Standard Dose with Dosing Intervals in Renal Impairment | | | | | Dosage with Dialysis | | Body Fluid Concentrations | | | | |
| With Normal and Anuric Cl_cr Values (mL/min) | | With Dialysis | | | For Cl_cr Ranges (mL/min) | | | | | | | | | | |
>80	<10	HD	PD	Usual Adult Dose	>80	80-50	50-10	<10 (anuric)	After HD[a]	During PD (daily dose)	CSF/Serum (%)[b]	Newborn Serum/Maternal Serum (%)	Breast Milk/Maternal Serum (%)	Bile/Serum (%)	Aqueous Humor/Serum (%)
1.5-2.9	18-29		16	0.2-0.4	12-24	12-24	24	0.1 q24h	0.4	0.2 q24h			Negligible		
1.4-1.8	25-35			1-3	6-8	0.5-1.5 g q8h	0.25-1 q12h	0.5 q24h	Dose post-dialysis	3 g q48h	22.5	28-33	1-6	34-82	3.6-6
5.4-10.9	12.2-18.2	12.2-18.2	12.2-18.2	0.5-2	12-24	12-24	12-24	12-24	None		16-32	18-25	3-4	200-500	
2	20	4	16.7	0.5-4	8-12	3 g q8h	2-3 g q12h	1 g q12-24h	1-2 g post-dialysis	0.5 g q18-24h	4-55	30-40	2.7	152-224	1-16
2	13.5	13.5	19	0.5-2	8-12	12-24	24	0.25-0.5 q24h	0.25	1-2 q48h			0.5 mg/1 L milk		

[a]Specified dose is supplemental to that in hemodialysis.
[b]Inflamed meninges.

| Serum Half-life (h) | | | | Standard Dose with Dosing Intervals in Renal Impairment | | | | | Dosage with Dialysis | | Body Fluid Concentrations | | | | |
| With Normal and Anuric Cl_cr Values (mL/min) | | With Dialysis | | | For Cl_cr Ranges (mL/min) | | | | | | | | | | |
>80	<10	HD	PD	Usual Adult Dose	>80	80-50	50-10	<10 (anuric)	After HD[a]	During PD (daily dose)	CSF/Serum (%)[b]	Newborn Serum/Maternal Serum (%)	Breast Milk/Maternal Serum (%)	Bile/Serum (%)	Aqueous Humor/Serum (%)
1.3-2.2	6-9	2.7 7.9[3]		1-2	6	8-12	12-18	24	1/8 init. dose post-dialysis	us. ld., then 1/4 us. dose @ us. int.	3-52		0.1-0.6	115-405	5-14
4	14			1-2	24	24	0.5-2 q24h	0.5 q24h	0.15				Minimal		
0.8-1	3.5			0.5-1	6	0.5 g q6-8h	0.5 g q8-12h	0.25-0.5 g q12h	0.25-0.5 post HD then q12h		1-10			Minimal	3
1	32	4		0.2-0.4	12-24	12-24	24-48	3-5 days	0.2-0.4 post HD						
0.8-1	6-20			0.5-2	8-12	8-12	0.5-1 q12h	0.5 q24h	0.5		12			40	

[a]Specified dose is supplemental to that in hemodialysis.
[b]Inflamed meninges.

TABLE 46-18 Antimicrobial Agent Pharmacology: Aminoglycosides

Drug (Oral Absorption, %)	Serum and Urine Concentration; Selected Doses			Dosage Recommendations						
	Dose (g)	Peak Serum (μg/mL)	Peak or Range, Urine (μg/mL)	Adults		Serious Infection Daily Dose (g)	Children: Dose/Interval		Newborn (Parenteral): Dose/Interval	
				Dose (g)/Interval						
				Oral	Parenteral		Oral	Parenteral	Up to 1 wk	1-4 wk
Amikacin[1]	0.500 IM 7.5 mg/kg IV[2]	38	832		15 mg/kg/day q8-12h[3]	15 mg/kg		15 mg/kg/day q8-12h[3]	Not approved	Not approved
Gentamicin[5]	1 mg/kg IM 1 mg/kg IV[6]	4-7.6 4-7.6	113-423		3-5 mg/kg/day q8h[3]	3-5 mg/kg		3-7.5 mg/kg/day q8h[3]	2.5 mg/kg q12h[3]	7.5 mg/kg/day q8h[3]
Isepamicin	15 mg/kg IV[2] 1 IM	51 38			8-15 mg/kg q24h	15 mg/kg			7.5 mg/kg/24 hr[7]	7.5 mg/kg q12h[7]
Kanamycin[1] (1)	7.5 mg/kg IM 7.5 mg/kg IV[2]	22 22			15 mg/kg/day q8-12[3]	1.5		15 mg/kg/day q8-12h[3]	15-20 mg/kg/day q12h[3,8]	15 mg/kg/day q8-12h[3]
Neomycin[9] (3)	4 g PO	2.5-6.1		50 mg/kg/day q6h		3 PO				
Netilmicin[10]	2 mg/kg IV[2] 2 mg/kg IM	16.6 7			4-6.5 mg/kg/day q8-12h[3]	3.9 mg/kg		3-7.5 mg/kg/day q8-12h[3]	4-6.5 mg/kg/day q12h[3,8]	4-6.5 mg/kg/day q12h[3,11]
Spectinomycin	2 g IM	100			2 g day IM	2		Not approved	Not approved	Not approved
Streptomycin[12]	0.5 IM 1 IM	5-12 25-50	400 ≥1000		0.5-1 g q12h	1		20-40 mg/kg/day q6-12h		
Tobramycin[5]	1 mg/kg IM 1 mg/kg IV[2]	4-6 4-6	75-100		3-5 mg/kg/day q8h[3]	3-5 mg/kg		3-6 mg/kg/day q8h[3]	≤4 mg/kg/day q12h[3]	3-5 mg/kg/day q8h[3]

[1]Desired concentrations: peak 15-30 μg/mL; trough <5-10 μg/mL.

[2]Infused over 30-60 minutes.

[3]The dosing strategy for aminoglycosides involves the use of ideal (lean) body weight (IBW) for dosage calculation. In obese patients, this approach would result in serum aminoglycoside concentrations less than expected. Alternative dosing recommendations have been proposed that account for the change in drug distribution volume with obesity: (1) IBW + 40% of excess weight, defined as total body weight (TBW) minus IBW (J Infect Dis 1978;138:499-505); (2) IBW + 58% of excess weight (TBW − IBW) (Clin Pharmacol Ther. 1979; 26:508); (3) IBW + 38% of excess weight (TBW − IBW) (Am J Hosp Pharm 1980; 37:519-22).

[4]Dosing at creatinine clearance ≤ 10 mL/min should be assisted with serum concentrations.

[5]Desired concentrations: peak 4-10 μg/mL; trough <2 μg/mL.

[6]Infused over 2 hours.

[7]q24h for infants <16 days old; q12h for ≥16 days old.

[8]15 mg/kg/day q12h for ≤2 kg; 20 mg/kg/day q12h for >2 kg.

[9]Parenteral administration of neomycin is no longer recommended.

[10]Desired concentrations: peak 6-12 μg/mL; trough <2 μg/mL.

[11]For premature or full-term infants <6 weeks.

[12]Desired concentrations: peak 5-25 μg/mL; trough <5 μg/mL.

Serum Half-life (h)				Standard Dose with Dosing Intervals in Renal Impairment					Dosage with Dialysis		Body Fluid Concentrations				
With Normal and Anuric Cl_Cr Values (mL/min)		With Dialysis			For Cl_Cr Ranges (mL/min)										
>80	<10	HD	PD	Usual Adult Dose	>80	80-50	50-10	<10 (anuric)	After HD[a]	During PD (daily dose)	CSF/Serum (%)[b]	Newborn Serum/Maternal Serum (%)	Breast Milk/Maternal Serum (%)	Bile/Serum (%)	Aqueous Humor/Serum (%)
2-3	30-86			5-7.5 mg/kg	8	8-12	12-48	≥48[4]	2.5-3.75 mg/kg post	2.5 mg/kg/day	15-24	20		30	Minimal
2-3	24-60			1-1.7 mg/kg	8	8-12	12-48	≥48[4]	1.0-1.7 mg/kg post HD	1 mg/2 L dialysate removed	10-30	30-40		30-60	Minimal
2-2.5				8 mg/kg	24	24	48-72	96							
2-4	27-80			7.5 mg/kg	8-12	8-12	12-48	≥48[4]	4-5 mg/kg post HD	3.75 mg/kg/day	43	50	35		Minimal
2-3	12-24														Minimal
2-2.5	30			2-2.2 mg/kg	8	8-12	12-48	≥48[4]	2 mg/kg post HD		21-26				Minimal
1.2-2.8				2 g	24	24	24	24							Minimal
2-3	Up to 110			0.5-1	12	7.5 mg/kg q24h	7.5 mg/kg q24-72h	7.5 mg/kg q72-96h	0.5 g post HD		20	10-40	<25	40-300	Minimal
2-3	5-70			1-1.7 mg/kg	8	8-12	12-48	≥48	1 mg/kg post HD	1 mg/2 L dialysate removed	14-23	50		10-20	18

[a]Specified dose is supplemental to that in hemodialysis.
[b]Inflamed meninges.

TABLE 46-19 Antimicrobial Agent Pharmacology: Tetracyclines[1]

	Serum and Urine Concentration; Selected Doses			Dosage Recommendations							
				Adults			Children: Dose/Interval		Newborn (Parenteral): Dose/Interval	
Drug (Oral Absorption, %)	Dose (g)	Peak Serum (μg/mL)	Peak or Range, Urine (μg/mL)	Dose (g)/Interval		Serious Infection Daily Dose (g)				
				Oral	Parenteral		Oral	Parenteral	Up to 1 wk	1-4 wk
Demeclocycline[2] (60-80)	0.15 PO 0.3 PO	0.9-1.2 1.5-1.7		0.6/day q6-12h		0.6	6.6-13.2 mg/kg/ day q6-12h		Not recommended	
Doxycycline (90-100)	0.1 PO 0.1 IV[3]	1.5-2.1 2.5		0.1 q12h	0.1 q12h	0.2	2.2 mg/kg q12-24h	2.2 mg/kg q12-24h	Not recommended	
Methacycline[2] (58)	0.15 PO 0.3 PO	1.3 2.4		0.15 q6h or 0.3 q12h		1.2	6.6-13.2 mg/kg/day q6-12h		Not recommended	
Minocycline (90-100)	0.2 PO	2-3.5		0.1 q12h	0.1 q12h	0.2	2 mg/kg q12h	2 mg/kg q12h	Not recommended	
Oxytetracycline[2] (60)	0.25 PO 0.5 PO	1.3-1.4 4-4.2		1-2/day q6h	0.25 IM q24h	2	25-50 mg /kg/day q6h	15-25 mg/ kg/ day q8-12h[4]	Not recommended	
Tetracycline[2] (75-80)	0.25 PO 0.5 PO 0.5 PO[5]	1.5-2.2 3-4.3 2-5		0.25-0.5 q6h		2	25-50 mg/ kg/day q6-12h		Not recommended	

[1]The tetracyclines cause a brown discoloration of the teeth and may retard the growth of bone in the human fetus and children. The American Academy of Pediatrics recommends that tetracyclines be used in children who are 9 years of age or older.

[2]All tetracyclines should be given 1 hour before or 2 hours after meals.

[3]Infused over 60 minutes.

[4]No more than 250 mg/day.

[5]At steady state.

With Normal and Anuric Cl_Cr Values (mL/min)		With Dialysis		Usual Adult Dose	For Cl_Cr Ranges (mL/min)				After HD[a]	During PD (daily dose)	CSF/ Serum (%)[b]	Newborn Serum/ Maternal Serum (%)	Breast Milk/ Maternal Serum (%)	Bile/ Serum (%)	Aqueous Humor/ Serum (%)
>80	<10	HD	PD		>80	80-50	50-10	<10 (anuric)							
10-17	42-68			0.15-0.3	6-12	Not recommended					Minimal		70	200-3200	10-30
14-24	18-30	18-30		0.1	12	12	12	12	0.1 g q12h	0.1 g q12h	26		30-40	200-3200	10-13
7-15	Up to 44			0.15-0.3	6-12	Not recommended									
11-26	12-30			0.1	12	12	12	12	0.1 g q12h	0.1 g q12h		77	8-26	200-3200	17
6-10	47-66			0.25-0.5 PO .25 IM	6 24	6 24	Use doxycycline				Minimal		20-140	200-3200	
6-12	57-120			0.25-0.5	6	6	Use doxycycline				7	60-70	25-150	200-3200	9-11

[a]Specified dose is supplemental to that in hemodialysis.
[b]Inflamed meninges.

TABLE 46-20　Antimicrobial Agent Pharmacology: Azalides, Macrolides, Ketolides, Lincosamides, Chloramphenicol, and Metronidazole

Drug (Oral Absorption, %)	Serum and Urine Concentration; Selected Doses			Dosage Recommendations						
	Dose (g)	Peak Serum (µg/mL)	Peak or Range, Urine (µg/mL)	Adults			Children: Dose/Interval		Newborn (Parenteral): Dose/Interval	
				Dose (g)/Interval		Serious Infection Daily Doe (g)	Oral	Parenteral	Up to 1 wk	1-4 wk
				Oral	Parenteral					
Azithromycin[1] (35-40)	0.5 PO 0.5 IV	0.09-0.44 3.63	8.64-26.8	0.5 q24h × 3 days	0.5 q24h	0.5	5-12 mg/kg/day	10-12 mg/kg/day[2]		
Clarithromycin (50-55)	0.25 PO[3] 0.5 PO[3] 0.5 PO[3]	1 2-3 1[4]		0.25-0.5 q12h		1	7.5 mg/kg q12h			
Dirithromycin[5] (6-14)	0.5 PO	0.3-0.4	Minimal	0.5 q24h		0.5	0.5 q24h[6]			
Erythromycin base[7,8]	0.25 PO	0.1-2		0.25-0.5 q6h		2	30-50 mg/kg/day q6h			
Erythromycin stearate[8]	0.25 PO	0.1-2		0.25-0.5 q6h		2	30-50 mg/kg/day q6h			
Erythromycin ethyl-succinate[8]	0.4 PO	0.1-2		0.4 q6h		2	30-50 mg/kg/day q6h			
Erythromycin lacto-bionate[9,10]	0.2 IV	3-4			0.5-1 q6h	4		15-20 mg/kg/day q6h		
Erythromycin gluceptate[9]	0.2 IV	3-4			15-20 mg/kg/day q6h	4		15-20 mg/kg/day q6h		
Erythromycin etolate[8]	0.25 PO	0.1-2[11]		0.25-0.5 q6h		2	30-50 mg/kg/day q6h			
Josamycn (>90)	0.5 PO 0.5 PO[3]	0.65 1.64	200-400	0.5-1 q8-12h		3	30-75 mg/kg/day q6-12h			
Roxithromycin	0.15 PO 0.3 PO	6 10		0.15-0.3 q12-24h		0.3	5-7.5 mg/kg/day q12h			
Spiramycin (33-40)	1 PO 2 PO 0.5 IV	0.96 1.65 2.28		1 q6-12h	0.5-1 q8h	4-5				
Telithromycin	0.8 PO	1.4-2.4		0.8 q24h		0.8				

[1]Decreased extent of absorption of capsule formulation only when given with food.
[2]No studies to support; extrapolated from adult conversion.
[3]At steady state.
[4]Of 14-hydroxyclarithromycin (active metabolite).
[5]Must be given with food.
[6]Not approved for children <12 years of age.
[7]Denotes decreased rate and/or extent of absorption when given with food.
[8]Erythromycin and its derivatives have varying degrees of bioavailability (18%-45%).
[9]Oral erythromycin therapy should replace IV therapy as soon as possible.
[10]Due to the local irritative effects, the drug must not be administered rapidly by direct IV injection (IV push).
[11]Higher serum concentrations have been reported in patients taking erythromycin estolate versus other derivatives.
[12]Over 20 minutes.
[13]When IV clindamycin is given to neonates and infants, organ system functions should be monitored.
[14]When given over 2 hours.
[15]Chloramphenicol dosage should be administered to maintain plasma concentrations of 10-25 mg/L for peak and 5-10 mg/L for trough.
[16]<2 weeks.
[17]>2 weeks.

| Serum Half-life (h) | | | | Standard Dose with Dosing Intervals in Renal Impairment | | | | | Dosage with Dialysis | | Body Fluid Concentrations | | | | |
| With Normal and Anuric Cl_{Cr} Values (mL/min) | | With Dialysis | | | For Cl_{Cr} Ranges (mL/min) | | | | | | | | | | |
>80	<10	HD	PD	Usual Adult Dose	>80	80-50	50-10	<10 (anuric)	After HD[a]	During PD (daily dose)	CSF/ Serum (%)[b]	Newborn Serum/ Maternal Serum (%)	Breast Milk/ Maternal Serum (%)	Bile/ Serum (%)	Aqueous Humor/ Serum (%)
68	68	68	68	0.5	24	24	24	24	24	24			>100		
5-7				0.25-0.5	12	12	12-24	24			Minimal		30	7000	
20-50	20-50	20-50		0.5	24	24	24	24	Usual regimen	Usual regimen					
1.5-2	6			0.25-0.5	6	6	6	6	Usual regimen	Usual regimen	2-13	5-20	50		
1.5-2	6			0.25-0.5	6	6	6	6	Usual regimen	Usual regimen	2-13	5-20	50		
1.5-2	6			0.4	6	6	6	6	Usual regimen	Usual regimen	2-13	5-20	50		
1.5-2	6			0.5-1	6	6	6	6	Usual regimen	Usual regimen	2-13	5-20	50		
1.5-2	6			15-20 mg/kg/day	6	6	6	6	Usual regimen	Usual regimen	2-13	5-20	50		
1.5-2	6			0.25-0.5	6	6	6	6	Usual regimen	Usual regimen	2-13	5-20	50		
0.9-2				0.5-1	6-12	6-12									
12	~12			0.15-0.3	12-24	12-24	12-24	24-48				30-40	0.05		50-200
5-6				0.5-1	6-12									>100	
10-13				0.8	24	24	24								

[a]Specified dose is supplemental to that in hemodialysis.
[b]Inflamed meninges.

Continued

TABLE 46-20 Antimicrobial Agent Pharmacology: Azalides, Macrolides, Ketolides, Lincosamides, Chloramphenicol, and Metronidazole—cont'd

	Serum and Urine Concentration; Selected Doses			Dosage Recommendations							
				Adults			Children: Dose/Interval		Newborn (Parenteral): Dose/Interval		
Drug (Oral Absorption, %)	Dose (g)	Peak Serum (µg/mL)	Peak or Range, Urine (µg/mL)	Dose (g)/Interval		Serious Infection Daily Dose (g)				Up to 1 wk	1-4 wk
				Oral	Parenteral		Oral	Parenteral			
Clindamycin[7] (90)	0.15 PO 0.6 IV[12]	1.9-3.9 10		0.15-0.3 q6h	0.3-0.9 q6-8h	1.2 PO/ 2.7 IV	8-25 mg/ kg/day q6-8h	15-40 mg/kg/day q6-8h		15 mg/kg/ day q6-8h[13]	15-20 mg/ kg/day q6-8h[13]
Lincomycin[7] (20-30)	0.5 PO 0.6 IM 0.6 IV[14]	1.8-5.3 9.3-18.5 15.9-20.9		0.5 q6-8h	0.6-1 q8-12h	8	30-60 mg/ kg/day q6-8h	10-20 mg/ kg/day q8-12h		Not indicated	
Chloramphenicol[15] (75-90)	1 PO 1 PO[3] 1 IV	11 18 4.9-12		0.25-0.75 q6h	0.25-1 q6h	4	50-100 mg/kg/ day q6h	50-100 mg/ kg/day q6h		25 mg/ kg/day q24h[16]	50 mg/kg/day q12-24h[17]
Metronidazole[7] (80)	0.25 PO 7.5 mg/kg[3]	4.6-6.5 26		0.25-7.5 q8h	0.5 q6h	30 mg/kg					

[1]Decreased extent of absorption of capsule formulation only when given with food.
[2]No studies to support; extrapolated from adult conversion.
[3]At steady state.
[4]Of 14-hydroxyclarithromycin (active metabolite).
[5]Must be given with food.
[6]Not approved for children <12 years of age.
[7]Denotes decreased rate and/or extent of absorption when given with food.
[8]Erythromycin and its derivatives have varying degrees of bioavailability (18%-45%).
[9]Oral erythromycin therapy should replace IV therapy as soon as possible.
[10]Due to the local irritative effects, the drug must not be administered rapidly by direct IV injection (IV push).
[11]Higher serum concentrations have been reported in patients taking erythromycin estolate versus other derivatives.
[12]Over 20 minutes.
[13]When IV clindamycin is given to neonates and infants, organ system functions should be monitored.
[14]When given over 2 hours.
[15]Chloramphenicol dosage should be administered to maintain plasma concentrations of 10-25 mg/L for peak and 5-10 mg/L for trough.
[16]<2 weeks.
[17]>2 weeks.

Serum Half-life (h)				Standard Dose with Dosing Intervals in Renal Impairment					Dosage with Dialysis		Body Fluid Concentrations				
With Normal and Anuric Cl_{Cr} Values (mL/min)		With Dialysis			For Cl_{Cr} Ranges (mL/min)										
>80	<10	HD	PD	Usual Adult Dose	>80	80-50	50-10	<10 (anuric)	After HD[a]	During PD (daily dose)	CSF/ Serum (%)[b]	Newborn Serum/ Maternal Serum (%)	Breast Milk/ Maternal Serum (%)	Bile/ Serum (%)	Aqueous Humor/ Serum (%)
2-3	2-3.5			0.15-0.3 PO 0.3-0.9 IV	6 6-8	6 6-8	6 6-8	6 6-8	Usual regimen	Usual regimen	Minimal	46	38-50	250-300	
4-6.4	10			0.5 PO 0.6-1 IV	6-8 8-12	6-8 8-12	6-8 8-12	24 24-36			18	25	13	250-400	8.75
1.5-4.1	3-7		3-7	0.25-0.75 PO 0.25-1 IV	6 6	6 6	6 6	6 6	Schedule dose post HD	Usual regimen	45-89	30-80	100		
6-14	8-15		8-15	0.25-7.5 PO 0.5 IV	8 6	8 6	8 6	8 6	Usual regimen	Usual regimen	≥100	97	100	100	33-50

[a]Specified dose is supplemental to that in hemodialysis.
[b]Inflamed meninges.

TABLE 46-21 Antimicrobial Agent Pharmacology: Miscellaneous Gram-Positive Agents and Polymyxins/Fusidic Acid

Drug (Oral Absorption, %)	Serum and Urine Concentration; Selected Doses			Dosage Recommendations						
				Adults			Children: Dose/Interval		Newborn (Parenteral): Dose/Interval	
	Dose (g)	Peak Serum (μg/mL)	Peak or Range, Urine (μg/mL)	Dose (g)/Interval		Serious Infection Daily Dose (g)	Oral	Parenteral	Up to 1 wk	1-4 wk
				Oral	Parenteral					
Colistimethate[1]	0.15 IM	5-7.5	200-270	5-15 mg/kg/day q8h[2]	2.5-5 mg/kg/day q6-12h	5 mg/kg	5-15 mg/kg/day q8h[2]	2.5-5 mg/kg/day q6-12h	Not recommended	
Polymyxin B[3]	20,000-40,000 U/kg/IM	1-8			15,000-25,000 U/kg/day q12h			15,000-25,000 U/kg/day q12h	Not recommended	
Vancomycin (minimal)	1 IV	25		0.5-2 g/day q6-8h	1g q12h	1 PO/2 IV	40 mg/kg/day q6-8h[5]	40 mg/kg/day q6-12h	15 mg/kg load, then 10 mg/kg q12h	10 mg/kg q8h
Teicoplanin	3 mg/kg IV[6] 6 mg/kg IV[6]	53 112			0.2-0.4 q24h			10 mg/kg q24h	6 mg/kg q24h (preliminary)	6 mg/kg q24h (preliminary)
Fusidic acid	0.5 PO	14-38[7]	<1	0.5-1 q8h	0.58 q8h[8]		6.6-16.6 mg/kg q8h	6.6 mg/kg q8-12h		
Quinupristin-dalfopristin	7 mg/kg IV	5			7.5 mg/kg q8-12h	22.5 mg/kg/day		7.5 mg/kg q8h		
Evernimicin	6 mg/kg IV	49-55			1-12 mg/kg/day[9]					
Linezolid (100)	0.4 PO 0.6 PO 0.6 IV	8.1 12.7 15.1		0.4-0.6 q12h	0.4-0.6 q12h	1.2	10 mg/kg q8h	10 mg/kg q8h	10 mg/kg q8h	10 mg/kg q8h

[1]Colistimethate is the sulfamethyl derivative of colistin; colistin is absorbed to some extent in infants.
[2]Of colistin.
[3]Bioavailability can be 10% in infants.
[4]For creatinine clearance 5-20 mL/min, dose should be 7500-12,500 U/kg/day q12h.
[5]Not to exceed 2 g/day.
[6]5-Minute infusion.
[7]Accumulation occurs with multiple doses of 0.5 g given q8h; a mean serum concentration of 71 μg/mL has been reported after 96 hours of therapy.
[8]Diethanolamine fusidate, 580 mg = 500 mg sodium fusidate.
[9]Based on early phase I studies.

Serum Half-life (h)				Standard Dose with Dosing Intervals in Renal Impairment					Dosage with Dialysis		Body Fluid Concentrations				
With Normal and Anuric Cl_{Cr} Values (mL/min)		With Dialysis			For Cl_{Cr} Ranges (mL/min)										
>80	<10	HD	PD	Usual Adult Dose	>80	80-50	50-10	<10 (anuric)	After HD[a]	During PD (daily dose)	CSF/ Serum (%)[b]	Newborn Serum/ Maternal Serum (%)	Breast Milk/ Maternal Serum (%)	Bile/ Serum (%)	Aqueous Humor/ Serum (%)
1.5-8	48-72			2.5-5 mg/kg/ day IV	6-12	2.5-3.8 mg/ kg/day q12h	2.5 mg/ kg/day q12-24h	1.5 mg/ kg q36h			Minimal	50	18		25-30
4.3-6	48-72			15,000-25,000 U/kg/ day	12	12	12[4]	2250-3750 U/kg /day q12h			Minimal				
4-6	44.1-406.4			15 mg/kg	12	See the nomogram, Chapter 29, or Antimicrob Agents Chemother 1984; 25:433			1 g/wk	0.5-1 g/wk	7.21			50	Minimal
40-70	125	163		0.4	24	48	48	72							
				0.5-1 PO	8	8	8	8							
1.3-1.5				7.5 mg/kg	8-12	8-12	8-12	8-12		10-20 mg/ kg/day q12h					
8.6				1-12 g mg/kg[9]	24	24									
5.5				0.4-0.6	12	12	12	12	30% of dose		20				

[a]Specified dose is supplemental to that in hemodialysis.
[b]Inflamed meninges.

TABLE 46-22 Antimicrobial Agent Pharmacology: Sulfonamides and Trimethoprim

Drug (Oral Absorption, %)	Serum and Urine Concentration; Selected Doses			Dosage Recommendations						
				Adults			Children: Dose/Interval		Newborn (Parenteral): Dose/Interval	
	Dose (g)	Peak Serum (μg/mL)	Peak or Range, Urine (μg/mL)	Dose (g)/Interval		Serious Infection Daily (g)				
				Oral	Parenteral		Oral	Parenteral	Up to 1 wk	1-4 wk
Trimethoprim-sulfamethoxazole[1] (85-90)	0.16/0.8 PO 0.16/ 0.8 IV	1-2/40-60[2] 9/105[2]		0.16/0.8 q12-24h	3-5 mg/ kg q6-8h[3]	1.2 IV[3]	6-12 mg/ kg /day q6-12h[3]	6-12 mg/ kg/ day q6-12h[3]	Not recommended	
Trimethoprim (80)	0.1 PO 0.2 PO	1 2	30-60	0.1 q12h		0.2	4 mg/kg/day q12h[6]			
Sulfisoxazole[1] (70-90)	2-4 PO 2-4 IM	11.2-25 11.2-25		0.5-1 q6h	25 mg/kg q6h	4	120-150 mg/ kg/day q4-6h		Not recommended	
Sulfamethoxazole[1] (70-90)	2 PO	50-120		1 q8-12h		2	50-60 mg/ kg/day q12h		Not recommended	
Sulfamethizole[1] (70-90)	2 PO	60		0.5-1 q6-8h		6	30-45 mg/ kg/day q6h		Not recommended	
Sulfadiazine[1] (70-90)	3 PO	50		2-4 g/day q4-8h		4	120-150 mg/kg/ day q4-6h	100 mg/kg/ day q6-8h	Not recommended	
Sulfadoxine[1,7] (70-90)	0.5 PO[8]	51-76		1 tablet qwk or 2 tablets qowk		1.5	By age[9]		Not recommended	
Dapsone	0.2 PO	0.1-7[2]		0.05-0.1 q24h		0.1	1-2 mg/ kg/day q24h			

[1]Decreased rate and/or extent of absorption when given with food.
[2]At steady state.
[3]Based on the trimethoprim component.
[4]Uninflamed meninges.
[5]Amniotic fluid concentrations (μg/mL).
[6]Not approved for children <12 years.
[7]For malaria prophylaxis. The first dose should be given 1-2 days before departure to an endemic area and the course continued throughout the stay and 4-6 weeks thereafter.
[8]One tablet = 500 mg sulfadoxine and 25 mg pyrimethamine.
[9]<4 years, $^1/_4$ tablet weekly or $^1/_2$ tablet every other week; 4-8 years, $^1/_2$ tablet weekly or 1 tablet every other week; 9-14 years, $^3/_4$ tablet weekly or $1^1/_2$ tablets every other week.
qowk, every other week; qwk, every week.

| Serum Half-life (h) | | | | Standard Dose with Dosing Intervals in Renal Impairment | | | | | | | | Body Fluid Concentrations | | | | |
| With Normal and Anuric Cl_Cr Values (mL/min) | | With Dialysis | | | For Cl_Cr Ranges (mL/min) | | | | Dosage with Dialysis | | | | | | | |
>80	<10	HD	PD	Usual Adult Dose	>80	80-50	50-10	<10 (anuric)	After HD[a]	During PD (daily dose)	CSF/Serum (%)[b]	Newborn Serum/Maternal Serum (%)	Breast Milk/Maternal Serum (%)	Bile/Serum (%)	Aqueous Humor/Serum (%)
8-15/7-12	24/22-50			3-5 mg/kg IV[3]	6-12	18	24	Avoid	4-5 mg/kg/post HD[3]	0.16/0.8 q48h	50/40[4]	80/50[5]	125/10	100-200/40-70	10-45/20-30
8-15	24			0.1	12	12	18-24	Avoid			30-50	70-100	100	100	10
3-7	6-12			1-2	6	6	1 q8-12h	1 q12-24h			8-57[4]	≥50	10	40-70	20-30
7-12	22-50			1	8-12						25-30	≥50			
4-8	58			0.5-1	6-8							≥50			
17	34			0.5-1	4-6						50-80	≥50			
100-231				0.5 PO 1 PO	qwk qowk							≥50			
20-30				0.05-0.1	24	24	24							69	

[a]Specified dose is supplemental to that in hemodialysis.
[b]Inflamed meninges.

TABLE 46-23 Antimicrobial Agent Pharmacology: Quinolones and Urinary Anti-infectives

| Drug (Oral Absorption, %) | Serum and Urine Concentration; Selected Doses | | | Dosage Recommendations | | | | | | |
| | | | | Adults | | | Children: Dose/Interval | | Newborn (Parenteral): Dose/Interval | |
	Dose (g)	Peak Serum (μg/mL)	Peak or Range, Urine (μg/mL)	Dose (g)/Interval Oral	Dose (g)/Interval Parenteral	Serious Infection Daily (g)	Oral	Parenteral	Up to 1 wk	1-4 wk
Quinolones Cinoxacin (97)	0.25 PO 0.5 PO	8 16	400	0.25 q6h or 0.5 q12h[2]		1				
Ciprofloxacin[1] (50-85)	0.5 PO 0.75 PO 0.4 IV[5]	1.6-2.9 2.5-4.3 4.6	350	0.25-0.75 q12h	0.2-0.4 q8-12h	1.5 PO/ 1.2 IV	25 mg/kg/ day q12h	3.2-12.5 mg/kg/day q12h		
Enoxacin[1] (80-90)	0.4 PO 0.6 PO 0.2 IV	2.8-3.6 4 1.8	250-300 337	0.4 q12h	0.4 q12h	0.8				
Garenoxacin[1]	0.4 PO	5.9		0.4-0.6 q24h		0.6				
Gatifloxacin	0.4 PO 0.6 PO	4.2 5.7		0.4-0.6 q24h		0.6				
Gemifloxacin	0.32 PO	1.48		0.32 q24h		0.32				
Levofloxacin (99)	0.5 PO 0.5 IV[5] 0.75 PO	5.7 6.2 7.1		0.25-0.75 q24h	0.25-0.75 q24h	1				
Lomefloxacin (>95)	0.2 PO 0.4 PO	2.1 3-4.7	170	0.4 q24h		0.4				
Moxifloxacin (90)	0.4 PO 0.4 IV	3.1 3.9		0.4 q24h	0.4 q24h	0.4				
Nalidixic acid[1] (100)	1 PO	20-40		1q6h		4				
Norfloxacin[1] (30-50)	0.4 PO	1.3-1.9	≥ 200	0.4 q12h		0.8				
Ofloxacin[1] (85-100)	0.4 PO 0.2 PO 0.4 IV[5]	2.9-5.6 1.5-2.7 4	200	0.2-0.4 q12h	0.2-0.4 q12h	0.8				
Oxolinic acid (poor)	0.75 PO	0.9-3.6	45-100	0.75 q12h[2]		2				

[1]Decreased rate and/or extent of absorption when given with food.

[2]Use primarily for the treatment of urinary tract infections.

[3]Use during pregnancy not recommended.

[4]Animal pharmacology studies indicate the presence of drug in the milk of lactating rats receiving oral doses of cinoxacin. Human data are not currently available.

[5]Infused over 60 minutes.

[6]3.2 hours during dialysis/5.8 hours in between sessions.

[7]Case report.

[8]For creatinine clearance <30 mL/min; for >30 mL/min use normal dose.

[9]12-24 hours after dose.

[10]Ineffective urinary concentrations expected with compromised renal function.

[11]8-12 hours during dialysis/13-48 hours in between sessions.

[12]Usually coadministered with an acidifying agent to convert the methenamine salts in urine to ammonia and bactericidal formaldehyde (pH ≤ 5.5). Mandelic acid and hippuric acid are mildly antiseptic and contribute to urine acidification.

[13]Methenamine penetrates many body fluids, including bile and cerebrospinal fluid. This penetration proves clinically inconsequential because negligible amounts of formaldehyde are generated at physiologic pH.

[14]Nitrofurantoin accumulates in the serum of patients with a creatine clearance <60 mL/min, which leads to systemic toxicity.

[15]Although only small amounts of nitrofurantoin have been detected in breast milk, the drug could cause hemolytic anemia in a glucose-6-phosphate dehydrogenase-deficient infant exposed in this manner.

| Serum Half-life (h) | | | | Standard Dose with Dosing Intervals in Renal Impairment | | | | | Dosage with Dialysis | | Body Fluid Concentrations | | | | |
| With Normal and Anuric Cl_{Cr} Values (mL/min) | | With Dialysis | | | For Cl_{Cr} Ranges (mL/min) | | | | | | | | | | |
>80	<10	HD	PD	Usual Adult Dose	>80	80-50	50-10	<10 (anuric)	After HD[a]	During PD (daily dose)	CSF/ Serum (%)[b]	Newborn Serum/ Maternal Serum (%)	Breast Milk/ Maternal Serum (%)	Bile/ Serum (%)	Aqueous Humor/ Serum (%)
1.5	8.4	3-4.4		0.25-0.5	6-12	0.25 q8h	0.25 q12-24h	Not recommended				Avoid[3]	<100 (18-78)[4]		
3-5	5-10	3.2/ 5.8[6]		0.25-0.75 PO 0.2-0.4 IV	12 8-12	12 8-12	.25-.5 q12h 12-24	0.25-0.5 q18h 0.2-0.4 q18-24h	0.25-0.5 q24h post HD	0.25-0.5 q24h	11-46		400	2800-4500	3-22
5-7	40	9.8		0.2-0.4	12	12	0.1-02 ql2h[8]	0.1-0.2 q12h			67			900	
14				0.4-0.6	24	24							35-44		
7-14				0.2-0.4	24	24	0.4 then 0.2 q24h	0.4 then 0.2 q24h	0.4 then 0.2 q24h	0.4 then 0.2 q24h					
6.65				0.32	24	24									
6-8				0.25-0.75	24	24	24-48	0.25 q48h	0.25 q48h	0.25 q48h	15		100		
7-8.5	21			0.4	24	24	0.2 q24h	0.2 q24h	0.4 lod then 0.2 q24h					700	
9-16				0.4	24	24	24	24							
1.1-2.5	21			1	6	6	6	Avoid[10]			Minimal				
2.3-4	7.6			0.4	12	12	24	24						1000	
4-8	16.9-28.4	8-12/ 13-48[11]		0.2-0.4 PO/ IV	12	12	24	0.1-0.2 q24h	0.2 load then 0.1 q24h		28-87		96-112	210-1886	
6-7				0.75	12		Not recommended	Not recommended[10]						200-300	

[a]Specified dose is supplemental to that in hemodialysis.
[b]Inflamed meninges.

Continued

TABLE 46-23   Antimicrobial Agent Pharmacology: Quinolones and Urinary Anti-infectives—cont'd

Drug (Oral Absorption, %)	Serum and Urine Concentration; Selected Doses			Dosage Recommendations						
	Dose (g)	Peak Serum (µg/mL)	Peak or Range, Urine (µg/mL)	Adults		Serious Infection Daily (g)	Children: Dose/Interval		Newborn (Parenteral): Dose/Interval	
				Dose (g)/Interval						
				Oral	Parenteral		Oral	Parenteral	Up to 1 wk	1-4 wk
Quinolones, cont'd										
Pefloxacin (98)	0.4 PO 0.4 IV[5]	3.8-5.6 5.8	100-115	0.4 q12-24h						
Sparfloxacin (92)	0.4 PO	1-2		0.4 day 1, then 0.2 q24h		0.4				
Trovafloxacin (88-90)	0.2 PO 0.3 PO 0.3 IV[5]	2.3 2.9 3.6		0.1-0.2 q24h	0.2-0.3 q24h	0.3	3 mg/kg q24h	3 mg/kg q24h		
Urinary Anti-infectives										
Methenamine hippurate[12]	1 PO		40 (formaldehyde)	1 q6h[2]		4	12.5-18.75 mg/kg q6h[2]		Not recommended	
Methenamine mandelate[12]	1 PO	70-100 µmol/L	Approx. 50 (formaldehyde)	1 q12h[2]		2	12.5-25 mg/kg q12h[2]		Not recommended	
Nitrofurantoin (good but variable)	0.1 PO	<2	50-150	0.05-0.1 q6-8h		0.4	5-7 mg/kg/day q6h		Not recommended	

[1]Decreased rate and/or extent of absorption when given with food.
[2]Use primarily for the treatment of urinary tract infections.
[3]Use during pregnancy not recommended.
[4]Animal pharmacology studies indicate the presence of drug in the milk of lactating rats receiving oral doses of cinoxacin. Human data are not currently available.
[5]Infused over 60 minutes.
[6]3.2 hours during dialysis/5.8 hours in between sessions.
[7]Case report.
[8]For creatinine clearance <30 mL/min; for >30 mL/min use normal dose.
[9]12-24 hours after dose.
[10]Ineffective urinary concentrations expected with compromised renal function.
[11]8-12 hours during dialysis/13-48 hours in between sessions.
[12]Usually coadministered with an acidifying agent to convert the methanimine salts in urine to ammonia and bactericidal formaldehyde (pH ≤ 5.5). Mandelic acid and hippuric acid are mildly antiseptic and contribute to urine acidification.
[13]Methenamine penetrates many body fluids, including bile and cerebrospinal fluid. This penetration proves clinically inconsequential because negligible amounts of formaldehyde are generated at physiologic pH.
[14]Nitrofurantoin accumulates in the serum of patients with a creatine clearance <60 mL/min, which leads to systemic toxicity.
[15]Although only small amounts of nitrofurantoin have been detected in breast milk, the drug could cause hemolytic anemia in a glucose-6-phosphate dehydrogenase-deficient infant exposed in this manner.

Serum Half-life (h)				Standard Dose with Dosing Intervals in Renal Impairment					Dosage with Dialysis		Body Fluid Concentrations				
With Normal and Anuric Cl_{Cr} Values (mL/min)		With Dialysis			For Cl_{Cr} Ranges (mL/min)										
>80	<10	HD	PD	Usual Adult Dose	>80	80-50	50-10	<10 (anuric)	After HD[a]	During PD (daily dose)	CSF/ Serum (%)[b]	Newborn Serum/ Maternal Serum (%)	Breast Milk/ Maternal Serum (%)	Bile/ Serum (%)	Aqueous Humor/ Serum (%)
8-12	11-15										52-58			200-600	
16-30				0.4 load then 0.2	24	24	48	48							
9-13	9-13	9-13		0.1-0.3	24	24	24	24			25			1540	
3-6				1		6	6	Avoid[10]			13			13	13
3-6				1		12	12	Avoid[10]			13	50	70-100	13	13
0.3	1			0.05-0.1		6	6	Avoid[10,14]				100	<25[15]	200-400	

[a]Specified dose is supplemental to that in hemodialysis.
[b]Inflamed meninges.

TABLE 46-24 Antimicrobial Agent Pharmacology: Antimycobacterials

Drug (Oral Absorption, %)	Serum and Urine Concentration; Selected Doses			Dosage Recommendations						
				Adults			Children: Dose/Interval		Newborn (Parenteral): Dose/Interval	
	Dose (g)	Peak Serum (µg/mL)	Peak or Range, Urine (µg/mL)	Dose (g)/Interval		Serious Infection Daily Dose (g)	Oral	Parenteral	Up to 1 wk	1-4 wk
				Oral	Parenteral					
Aminosali-cylic acid	4 PO	76-104		150 mg/kg/day q6-12h		12	150-360 mg/kg/day q6-8h			
Capreomycin[3]	1 IM	20-47			1 g IM q24h[4]	1		10-20 mg/kg/day q24h (not approved)		10-20 mg/kg/day q24h (not approved)
Clofazimine[1] (45-70)	0.1 PO[5]	0.7[6]		0.1 q24h		0.1				
Cycloserine[8] (70-90)	0.25 PO	10		0.25-0.5 q12h		1	10-20 mg/kg/day q12h (not approved)			
Ethambutol (75-80)	25 mg/kg PO	2-5		15 mg/kg q24h		15 mg/kg	10-15 mg/kg q24h (not recommended)			
Ethionamide (80)	1 PO	20		0.25-0.5 q12h		1	15-20 mg/day[9] q24h (not approved)			
Isoniazid[2,10]	7 mg/kg PO	4.5/1[11]		0.3 q24h	0.3 IM q24h	0.3	10-20 mg/kg/day q12-24h	10-20mg/kg/day q12-24h		
Pyrazinamide	0.5 PO	9-12		15-30 mg/kg q24h		2	30 mg/kg/day q12-24h (not approved)			
Rifabutin (≥20)	0.3 PO	0.375		0.3 q24h		0.3	4-18.5 mg/kg q24h[12]			
Rifampin (100)	0.6 PO 0.6 IV[13]	7 17.5		0.6 q24h	0.6 q24h	0.6	10-20 mg/kg/day q12-24h			
Streptomycin	1 IM	25-50	≥ 1000		1 IM q24h	1		20-40 mg/kg/day q24h		

[1]Should be taken with food.
[2]Decreased rate and/or extent of absorption when given with food.
[3]Pharmacokinetics similar to streptomycin.
[4]Administer for 60-120 days followed by 1q 2-3×/wk.
[5]In leprosy patients.
[6]At steady state.
[7]8-Day serum half-life/70-day tissue half-life.
[8]Dosage should be adjusted to maintain plasma concentrations <30 µg/mL.
[9]Limited evidence suggests that 20 mg/kg daily given as a single dose in children is more likely to produce cerebrospinal fluid concentrations exceeding the minimal inhibitory concentration of 2.5 µg/mL for *M. tuberculosis.*

[10]To minimize risk of polyneuritis from isoniazid-induced pyridoxine deficiency, pyridoxine (15-50 mg) is often given concurrently.
[11]4.5 µg/mL in slow inactivators/1.0 µg/mL in rapid inactivators.
[12]Dose varies significantly by age group; see manufacturer's recommendations before prescribing.
[13]Infused over 30 minutes.
[14]Desirable serum concentrations: peak 5-25 µg/mL; trough <5 µg/mL.

| Serum Half-life (h) | | | | Standard Dose with Dosing Intervals in Renal Impairment | | | | | Dosage with Dialysis | | Body Fluid Concentrations | | | | |
| With Normal and Anuric Cl_{Cr} Values (mL/min) | | With Dialysis | | | For Cl_{Cr} Ranges (mL/min) | | | | | | | | | | |
>80	<10	HD	PD	Usual Adult Dose	>80	80-50	50-10	<10 (anuric)	After HD[a]	During PD (daily dose)	CSF/Serum (%)[b]	Newborn Serum/Maternal Serum (%)	Breast Milk/Maternal Serum (%)	Bile/Serum (%)	Aqueous Humor/Serum (%)
1	23			150 mg/kg/day	6-12						10-50				
4-6	29.4-55.5			1	24	24	7.5 mg/kg q24-48h	7.5 mg/kg 2× wk						Minimal	
8 day/70 day[7]				0.1	8	8	8	8							
10				0.25-0.5	12	12	24	0.25 q24h			80-100	100	72		
3.3	≥7			15-25 mg/kg	24	15 mg/kg q24h	15 mg/kg q24-36h	15 mg/kg q48h	15 mg/kg/day post HD	15 mg/kg/day	25-50	~100			
3	9			0.25-0.5	12	12	12	5 mg/kg q24h			100				
0.5-4	2-10			0.3 PO/IM	24	24	24	½ dose in slow acetylators	5 mg/kg post HD	Daily dose post dialysis	100	High	100		
10-16				15-30 mg/kg	24	24	24	12-20 mg/kg q24h			100				
16-69				0.3	24	24									
2-5	2-5	Minimal change		0.6	24	24	24	24			10-20	33	20-60	10,000	
2-3	Up to 110			1[14]	24	7.5 mg/kg/day q24h	7.5 mg/kg/day q24-72h	7.5 mg/kg/day q72-96h	0.5 post HD		20	10-40	<25	40-300	

[a]Specified dose is supplemental to that in hemodialysis.
[b]Inflamed meninges.

TABLE 46-25 Antimicrobial Agent Pharmacology: Antifungal Agents

Drug (Oral Absorption, %)	Serum and Urine Concentration; Selected Doses			Dosage Recommendations							
				Adults			Children: Dose/Interval		Newborn (Parenteral): Dose/Interval	
	Dose (g)	Peak Serum (µg/mL)	Peak or Range, Urine (µg/mL)	Dose (g)/Interval		Serious Infection Daily Dose (g)	Oral	Parenteral	Up to 1 wk	1-4 wk
				Oral	Parenteral					
Amphotericin B (poor)	0.03 IV[2] 0.05 IV[2]	1 2			0.25-1 mg/kg q24h[3,4]	1 mg/kg[5]		0.25-1 mg/kg q24-48h[3]	0.1-1 mg/kg/day[3]	0.1-1 mg/kg/day[3]
Caspofungin					0.07 load, then 0.05 q24h	0.07				
Fluconazole (≥90)	0.4 PO 0.1 IV[6]	6.72 3.86-4.96		0.05-0.4 q24h	0.05-0.4 q24h	0.4	3-12 mg/kg q24h	3-12 mg/kg q24h		
Flucytosine[1,7] (75-90)	2 PO	30-45		50-150 mg/kg/day q6h		150 mg/kg	50-150 mg/kg/day q6h			
Griseofulvin (50/>50)[8]	0.5/0.25 PO	0.4-2/0.4-2		0.5-1 g24h/ 0.33-0.66 q24h		1	15 mg/kg/day q24h			
Itraconazole (99.8)[9,10]	0.2 PO[11]	2.3/3.5[12]		0.2-0.4 q24h	0.2 q24h	0.4	3-5 mg/kg q24h			
Ketoconazole[10]	0.2 PO	4.2		0.2-0.4 q12-24h		0.8	5-10 mg/kg/day q12-24h			
Micafungin	0.1 IV	8.17			0.0125-0.15 q24h	0.15		4 mg/kg q24h		
Miconazole (50)	0.522 IV[14]	6			0.4-1.2 q8h	3.6		20-40 mg/kg/day q8h		
Nystatin (minimal)	All doses	Not detectable		0.4-1 mU q8h		2 mU	0.4-0.6 mU q6h		0.1 mU q6h	0.1 mU q6h
Terbinafine (80)	0.25 PO	1		0.125-0.5 q12-24h		0.5	0.062-0.25 q24h			
Voriconazole[1] (96)	0.2 PO[16] 3 mg/kg IV[16]	2.08 3.06		0.1-0.2 q12h	6 mg/kg q12h × 1 day, then 4 mg/kg q12h	4 mg/kg	0.1-0.2 q12h[17]	6 mg/kg q12h × 1 day, then 4 mg/kg q12h[17]		

[1]Decreased rate and/or extent of absorption when given with food.
[2]Infused over several hours.
[3]A test dose of 1 mg infused over 15 minutes is often given to assess febrile reactions before proceeding to higher doses.
[4]Should be administered by slow infusion; rapid IV infusion should be avoided because potentially serious adverse effects (e.g., hypotension, hypokalemia, arrhythmias, shock) may occur.
[5]Or 1.5 mg/kg every other day.
[6]Infused over 30 minutes; ascertained on days 6-7.
[7]Peak concentrations should be 25 µg/mL to avoid development of resistance but should not exceed 100-120 µg/mL to avoid side effects.
[8]Microsize/ultramicrosize.
[9]When given with meals.
[10]Gastric acid–suppressing agents decrease bioavailability to <5%.
[11]Taken 2× day for 15 days.
[12]Parent drug/active metabolite (hydroxyitraconazole).
[13]Half-life extends as dosing continues.
[14]Infused over 15 minutes.
[15]Triphasic elimination: α = 0.4 hours; β = 2.1 hours; γ = 24.1 hours.
[16]Administered q12h × 10 days after day 1 loading doses.
[17]≥12 years.

Serum Half-life (h)				Standard Dose with Dosing Intervals in Renal Impairment								Body Fluid Concentrations				
With Normal and Anuric Cl_{Cr} Values (mL/min)		With Dialysis			For Cl_{Cr} Ranges (mL/min)				Dosage with Dialysis							
>80	<10	HD	PD	Usual Adult Dose	>80	80-50	50-10	<10 (anuric)	After HD	During PD (daily dose)	CSF/ Serum (%)	Newborn Serum/ Maternal Serum (%)	Breast Milk/ Maternal Serum (%)	Bile/ Serum (%)	Aqueous Humor/ Serum (%)
24 or more	24 or more			0.25-1 mg/kg	24	24	24	24	Usual regimen	Usual regimen	3	50			25
9-11	9-11	9-11		0.05	24	24	24	24	Usual regimen						
20-50	48		71	0.05-0.4	24	24	50% of dose	25% of dose	Usual dose after		50-94		85		
3-6	30-250			37 mg/kg	6	6	12-24	15-25 mg/kg q24h	20-37.5 mg/kg post HD		60-100				
24	24			0.5-1/ 0.33-0.66	24/24	24/24	24/24	24/24					80		
21-60[13]				0.2-0.4	24	24					<10				
8	8			0.2-0.4	12-24	12-24	12-24	12-24	Usual regimen	Usual regimen	Minimal			Minimal	~10
15	15			0.0125-0.15	24	24	24	24			Undetectable				Low
0.4-24.1[15]	0.4-24.1[15]			0.4-1.2	8	8	8	8	<3-48						
				0.4-1 mU	8	8	8	8							
22-30				0.125-0.25	12-24	12-24							Unsafe		
6				4 mg/kg	12	12	12	Try to avoid			42-67				

TABLE 46-26 Antimicrobial Agent Pharmacology: Antiviral Agents

Drug (Oral Absorption, %)	Serum and Urine Concentration; Selected Doses			Dosage Recommendations					Newborn (Parenteral): Dose/Interval	
				Adults			Children: Dose/Interval			
	Dose (g)	Peak Serum (µg/mL)	Peak or Range, Urine (µg/mL)	Dose (g)/Interval		Serious Infection Daily Dose (g)	Oral	Parenteral	Up to 1 wk	1-4 wk
				Oral	Parenteral					
Acyclovir (15-30)[2]	0.2 PO[3] 0.8 PO[3] 5 mg/kg IV[4]	0.83 1.61 7.7		0.2-0.8 2-5 days	5-12 mg/kg q8h	4 PO/30 mg/kg IV	0.2 5 days	25-50 mg/kg/day q8h		
Adefovir (59)	0.01 PO	0.018		0.01-0.12 q24h		0.12				
Amantadine (85-90)	0.1 PO[3]	0.302		0.1 q12h		0.2	5-8 mg/kg/day q12h			
Cidofovir	10 mg/kg IV	24			5 mg/kg qwk[5]	5 mg/kg				
Famciclovir (75-77)	0.5 PO 0.75 PO	4 5.1-5.3		0.125-0.75 q8-12h		2.25				
Foscarnet	0.09 IV[3]	218[6]			60 mg/kg q8h[7]	120-180 mg/kg				
Ganciclovir (5)	5 mg/kg IV[4] 1.0 PO	9 0.98		1.0 q8h	5 mg/kg q12h[8]	5 mg/kg maint.	30 mg/kg q8h	5 mg/kg q12h[8]		
Interferon alfa-2a (80 IM, 90 SC)					3-6 MU 3×/wk					
Interferon alfa-2b (80 IM, 90 SC)					3-5 MU q24h-3×/wk[9]			3-6 MU/m² 3×/wk		
Interferon alfa-2b/ ribavirin[10] (33-69-ribavirin)				1-1.2 q24h	3-5 MU 3×/wk		0.2-0.4 q12h	3 MU/m² 3×/wk		

[1]Decreased rate and/or extent of absorption when given with food.
[2]Bioavailability decreases as dosage is increased.
[3]At steady state.
[4]Infused over 1 hour.
[5]qwk × 2 wk then qowk.
[6]µmol/L.
[7]For 14-21 days as initial induction therapy, then 90 mg/kg q24h as maintenance.
[8]For 14-21 days as induction therapy; then 5 mg/kg q24h.
[9]3 MU 3×/wk for hepatitis C; 5 MU q24h for hepatitis B.
[10]PO doses are ribavirin; parenteral doses are interferon.
[11]Based on weight.
[12]Inhaled over 5 hours each day for 3 days.
[13]Inhaled over 8 hours each day for 3 days.
[14]Mist of 190 µg/L via SPAG-2 aerosol generator; rate of 12.5 L mist/min × 16-18 h/day 1 of influenza A or B infection, then × 12 h/day on days 2 and 3; then × 4 hours on day 4 (not approved in United States).
[15]Mist of 190 µg/L via SPAG-2 aerosol generator; rate of 12.5 L mist/min × 12-18 h/day for 3-7 days.
[16]After administration for 4-7 wk in acquired immunodeficiency syndrome (AIDS) or AIDS-related complex patients.
[17]Half-life of valacyclovir is <30 minutes but its metabolite acyclovir has a half-life of 2.5-3.6 hours.
[18]Should be taken with food.
[19]Vidarabine/ara-hypoxanthine (less active metabolite).
[20]With normal meninges.
qowk, every other week; qwk, every week.

| Serum Half-life (h) | | | | Standard Dose with Dosing Intervals in Renal Impairment | | | | | Dosage with Dialysis | | Body Fluid Concentrations | | | | |
| With Normal and Anuric Cl_{Cr} Values (mL/min) | | With Dialysis | | | For Cl_{Cr} Ranges (mL/min) | | | | | | | | | | |
>80	<10	HD	PD	Usual Adult Dose	>80	80-50	50-10	<10 (anuric)	After HD	During PD (daily dose)	CSF/ Serum (%)	Newborn Serum/ Maternal Serum (%)	Breast Milk/ Maternal Serum (%)	Bile/ Serum (%)	Aqueous Humor/ Serum (%)
2.1-3.5	19.5		Minimal change	0.2-0.8 PO 5-12 mg/kg IV	2-5× /day 8	2-5× /day 8	2-5× /day 12-24	0.2-0.8 q24h 2.5-6 mg/ kg q24h	0.5 post HD	2.5 mg/kg/ day	50		≥100		37
7.5				0.01	24	24	48-72		0.01 qwk						
10-14	170	7-10.3 days		0.1	12	24	0.1-0.2 2- 3×/ wk	0.1-0.2 qwk	0.2 qwk		50				
2.5				5 mg/kg	qwk	qwk	Do not use	Do not use	Do not use	Do not use					
2-2.3				0.125-0.75	8-12	8-12	0.125-0.5 q12-24h	0.125-0.25 q24h	0.125-0.25 post HD						
0.1-17				60 mg/ kg	8	12	24		45-60 mg/kg		13-103				
2.5-5	10			5 mg/kg	12	2.5 mg/ kg q12h	2.5 mg/ kg q24h	1.25 mg/ kg q24h	1.25 mg/kg 3×/wk post HD		24-68				40
3.7-8.5				3-6 MU	3×/wk	3×/wk	3×/wk	3×/wk	3×/wk	3×/wk					
2-3				3-5 MU	q24h; 3× /wk	q24h; 3× /wk	q24h; 3× /wk	q24h; 3× /wk							
6.5/298				3-5 MU; 1-1.2	3× /wk; q24h	3×/wk; q24h	Not to be used	Not to be used							

Continued

TABLE 46-26 Antimicrobial Agent Pharmacology: Antiviral Agents—cont'd

Drug (Oral Absorption, %)	Serum and Urine Concentration; Selected Doses			Dosage Recommendations				Children: Dose/Interval		Newborn (Parenteral): Dose/Interval	
				Adults							
	Dose (g)	Peak Serum (µg/mL)	Peak or Range, Urine (µg/mL)	Dose (g)/Interval		Serious Infection Daily Dose (g)					
				Oral	Parenteral		Oral	Parenteral	Up to 1 wk	1-4 wk
Interferon-alfa-n3					3 MU 3×/wk						
Interferon alfacon-1 (80)					9 µg 3×/wk						
Oseltamivir (75)	0.075 PO	0.0652		0.075 q12-24h		0.15	0.03-0.075 q12-24h				
Palivizumab	15 mg/kg IV	313							15 mg/kg qmonth	15 mg/kg qmonth	
Peginterferon alfa-2b											
Ribavirin	0.82 mg/kg/hr[12] 0.82 mg/kg/hr[13]	0.275 1.1		0.4-0.6 q12h [14]	40-150 µg qwk	1.2 PO	[15]				
Rimantadine (100)	0.2	0.05-0.086		0.1 q12h		0.2 PO	5 mg/kg/day q12-24h				
Valacyclovir (55)	2 PO[3]	8.49		0.5-2 q8-24h		4					
Valganciclovir[18] (60)	0.45 PO	3.1		0.9 q12-24h		1.8 PO					
Vidarabine	10 mg/kg IV	0.2-0.4/ 3-6[19]			10-15 mg/kg/day over 12h	15 mg/kg		10-15 mg/kg/day over 12h	15-30 mg/kg/day over 12h	15-30 mg/kg/day over 12h	
Zanamivir (2)	0.01 PO	0.017-0.142		10 mg q12h			10 mg q12h				

[1]Decreased rate and/or extent of absorption when given with food.
[2]Bioavailability decreases as dosage is increased.
[3]At steady state.
[4]Infused over 1 hour.
[5]qwk × 2 wk then qowk.
[6]µmol/L.
[7]For 14-21 days as initial induction therapy, then 90 mg/kg q24h as maintenance.
[8]For 14-21 days as induction therapy; then 5 mg/kg q24h.
[9]3 MU 3×/wk for hepatitis C; 5 MU q24h for hepatitis B.
[10]PO doses are ribavirin; parenteral doses are interferon.
[11]Based on weight.
[12]Inhaled over 5 hours each day for 3 days.
[13]Inhaled over 8 hours each day for 3 days.
[14]Mist of 190 µg/L via SPAG-2 aerosol generator; rate of 12.5 L mist/min × 16-18 h/day 1 of influenza A or B infection, then × 12 h/day on days 2 and 3; then × 4 hour on day 4 (not approved in United States).
[15]Mist of 190 µg/L via SPAG-2 aerosol generator; rate of 12.5 L mist/min × 12-18 h/day for 3-7 days.
[16]After administration for 4-7 wk in acquired immunodeficiency syndrome (AIDS) or AIDS-related complex patients.
[17]Half-life of valacyclovir is <30 minutes but its metabolite acyclovir has a half-life of 2.5-3.6 hours.
[18]Should be taken with food.
[19]Vidarabine/ara-hypoxanthine (less active metabolite).
[20]With normal meninges.
qowk, every other week; qwk, every week.

| Serum Half-life (h) | | | | Standard Dose with Dosing Intervals in Renal Impairment | | | | | Dosage with Dialysis | | Body Fluid Concentrations | | | | |
| With Normal and Anuric Cl_{Cr} Values (mL/min) | | With Dialysis | | | For Cl_{Cr} Ranges (mL/min) | | | | | | | | | | |
>80	<10	HD	PD	Usual Adult Dose	>80	80-50	50-10	<10 (anuric)	After HD	During PD (daily dose)	CSF/Serum (%)	Newborn Serum/Maternal Serum (%)	Breast Milk/Maternal Serum (%)	Bile/Serum (%)	Aqueous Humor/Serum (%)
4.43-6.76				3 MU	3×/wk	3×/wk	3×/wk	3×/wk							
0.5-7				9 µg	3×/wk	3×/wk									
6-10				0.075	12-24	12-24	24-48								
13-27 days															
22-60				40-150 µg	qwk	qwk									
24-36							Not to be used	Not to be used	None		70[16]				
19.8-36.5				0.1	12	12	12	24					Not to be used		
2.5-3.6[17]	20			0.5-1	8-12	8-12	12-24	24	0.5-1	Normal		170			
3.7-4.6				0.9	12-14	12-24									
1.5/3.3				15 mg/kg/day	Over 12	Over 12	Over 12	10 mg/kg/day over 12 h	Schedule post HD		33-35[20]				
1.6-5.1				10 mg	12	12	12	12	12	12					

TABLE 46-27 Antimicrobial Agent Pharmacology: Antiretroviral Agents

| Drug (Oral Absorption, %) | Serum and Urine Concentration; Selected Doses | | | Dosage Recommendations | | | | | | |
| | | | | Adults | | | Children: Dose/Interval | | Newborn (Parenteral): Dose/Interval | |
	Dose (g)	Peak Serum (µg/mL)	Peak or Range, Urine (µg/mL)	Dose (g)/Interval Oral	Parenteral	Serious Infection Daily Dose (g)	Oral	Parenteral	Up to 1 wk	1-4 wk
Abacavir (83)	0.3 PO	3.3		0.3 q12h		0.6	8 mg/kg q12h			
Amprenavir[2]	1.2 PO	7.66		1.2-1.4 q12h[3]		2.8 PO	15-22.5 mg/kg q8-12h			
Atazanavir[4]	0.4 PO	5.226		0.4 q24h		0.4				
Delavirdine (60-100)	0.4 PO[5]	35[6]		0.4 q8h		1.2	0.4 q8h[7]			
Didanosine[1] (21-43)[8,9]	33 mg/kg	29.8[6]		0.125-0.25 q12h		12 mg/kg/day	120 mg/m^2 q12h			100 mg/m^2 q12h PO
Efavirenz	0.6 PO[5]	4.5		0.6 q24h		0.6	0.2-0.6 q24h[10]			
Emtricitabine	0.2 PO	2.1		0.2 q24h		0.2 PO				
Enfuvirtide					0.1 q12h	0.2				
Indinavir[1] (30)	0.8 PO[5,9]	251-12, 617[11]		0.8 q8h		2.4	350 mg/m^2 q8h			
Lamivudine (82-87)	2-8 mg/kg PO	1.725-5.815		0.1-0.3 q12-24h		0.6	3-4 mg/kg q12h[12]			
Lopinavir/ritonavir[4]	0.4/0.05 PO	6 (lopinavir)		0.4/0.1 q12h[13]		0.8/0.2	10-12/2.5-3 mg/kg q12h			
Nelfinavir[4]	0.75 PO[5]	2.9		0.75-1.25 q8-12h[4]		2.5	20-30 mg/kg q8h[4]			
Nevirapine (>90)	0.4 PO	2.9-3.4		0.2 q12h maint.		0.4	4 mg/kg q12h maint.[14]			
Ritonavir[15] (80)	0.6 PO 1.2 PO	5 11.2		0.6 q12h		1.2	400 mg/m^2 q12h			
Saquinavir[4]	0.6 PO	0.066		0.6-1.2 q8h[16,17]		7.2				
Stavudine (80)	4 mg/kg PO	4.2		0.03-0.04 q12h		2 mg/kg/day	2 mg/kg/day[18]		0.5 mg/kg q12h PO	1 mg/kg q12h PO
Tenofovir[4] (40)	0.3 PO	0.296		0.3 q24h		0.3 PO				
Zalcitabine[1] (80-88)[9]	0.0005 PO 0.005 PO	0.0076 0.079		0.75 mg q8h[19]		2.25 mg	0.015-0.04 mg/kg q6h			
Zidovudine (50-76)[20]				0.2-0.3 q8-12h	1 mg/kg q4h[21]	0.6	160 mg/m^2 q8h			

[1]Decreased rate and/or extent of absorption when given with food.
[2]Okay to be given with food, just not high-fat meal.
[3]Doses vary due to inequality of capsule and solution dosage forms.
[4]Give with food.
[5]At steady state.
[6]µmol/L.
[7]For children ≥13 years old.
[8]Bioavailability decreases as dosage is increased.
[9]In human immunodeficiency virus–positive patients.
[10]Based on weight.
[11]nmol.
[12]>12 years of age 150 mg q12h.

[13]Needs dosage adjustment if given with nevirapine or efavirenz in treatment-experienced patients when reduced susceptibility to lopinavir is suspected.
[14]>9 years 120 mg/m^2.
[15]In animals.
[16]Lower dose for saquinavir mesylate.
[17]600 mg q8h for saquinavir mesylate and 1200 mg q8h for plain saquinavir (Fortovase).
[18]Children >30 kg should receive adult dosage.
[19]Should be coadministered with zidovudine 200 mg q8h.
[20]Reaches systemic circulation as unchanged drug.
[21]An IV dose of 1 mg/kg q4h is equivalent to an oral dose of 100 mg q4h.

| Serum Half-life (h) | | | | Standard Dose with Dosing Intervals in Renal Impairment | | | | | | | Body Fluid Concentrations | | | | |
| With Normal and Anuric Cl_{cr} Values (mL/min) | | With Dialysis | | | For Cl_{cr} Ranges (mL/min) | | | | Dosage with Dialysis | | | | | | |
>80	<10	HD	PD	Usual Adult Dose	>80	80-50	50-10	<10 (anuric)	After HD	During PD (daily dose)	CSF/ Serum (%)	Newborn Serum/ Maternal Serum (%)	Breast Milk/ Maternal Serum (%)	Bile/ Serum (%)	Aqueous Humor/ Serum (%)
1.2	1.2			0.3	12	12	12				18-33				
7-10				1.2-1.4	12	12	Use with caution	Do not use							
5-8				0.4	24	24									
2-11				0.4	8						0.4				
1.3-1.6	4.5			0.125-0.4	12-24	12-24	0.1-0.2 q24h	0.075-0.125 q24h	25% usual dose daily		21-46				
40-55		10		0.6	24	24	24	24	0.6 q24h	0.6 q24h	1.19				
2.5-7				0.2	24	24									
				0.1	12	12									
1.5-2	1.5-2			0.8	8	8	8	8	Usual regimen		5-9		Unsafe		
3-7				0.15-0.3	12-24	12-24	0.05-0.15 q24h	0.025 q24h	0.025 q24h		6-11	~100	~100		
5-6				0.4/0.1	12	12									
3.5-5	3.5-5	3.5-5	3.5-5	0.75-1.25	8-12	8-12	8-12	8-12	None	Normal	0				
25-30	25-30			0.2	12	12	12	12	Usual regimen	Usual regimen			60		
3-3.5	3-3.5			0.6	12	12	12		None		0.2				
13	13			0.6 or 1.2[17]	8	8	8	8	None		0.2				
0.9-1.6	5.7	5.3		0.04	12	12	0.02 q12-24	0.02 q24	0.015-0.02 q24h		24-94				
4-8				0.3	24	24									
0.5-3	8.5			0.75	8	8	12	24			9-37				
0.5-3	1.4			0.2-0.3	8-12	8-12	8-12		0.1 q6-8h	0.1 q6-8h	50-70	100	100		

TABLE 46-28 Adverse Drug Interactions Involving Antimicrobial Agents

Interacting Drugs	Adverse Effect	Probable Mechanism
Abacavir with		
Amprenavir	Increased amprenavir effect/toxicity	Increased bioavailability
Methadone	Decreased methadone effect	Mechanism not established
Ribavirin	Increased risk of lactic acidosis	Mechanism not established
Acyclovir/Valacyclovir with		
Aminoglycosides	Increased nephrotoxicity and/or neurotoxicity	Mechanism not established
Cimetidine	Increased acyclovir toxicity	Mechanism not established
Cyclosporine	Increased risk of nephrotoxicity	Mechanism not established
Narcotics	Increased meperidine effect	Decreased renal excretion
Phenytoin	Decreased phenytoin effect	Altered gastrointestinal transit/pH
Probenecid	Possible increased acyclovir toxicity	Decreased renal excretion
Valproic acid	Decreased valproic acid effect	Altered gastrointestinal (GI) transit/pH
Zidovudine	Increased neurotoxicity (profound drowsiness and lethargy)	Additive toxicity
Amantadine with		
Anticholinergics	Hallucinations, confusion, nightmares	Mechanism not established
Antihistamines	Increased CNS adverse reactions	Additive anticholinergic effects
Bupropion	Increased adverse events	Mechanism not established
Central nervous system (CNS) stimulants	Additive CNS stimulant effects	Mechanism not established
Dopamine agonists	Decreased amantadine effect	Antagonism
Triamterene	CNS toxicity	Decreased renal clearance
Trimethoprim	CNS toxicity	Decreased renal clearance
Aminoglycoside Antibiotics with		
Acyclovir	Increased nephrotoxicity and/or neurotoxicity	Additive toxicity
Amphotericin B	Nephrotoxicity	Synergism
Anticoagulants, oral	Potentiation of anticoagulation effects	Decreased GI absorption or synthesis of vitamin K
Bacitracin	Increased nephrotoxicity	Additive toxicity
Bumetanide	Increased ototoxicity	Additive toxicity
Capreomycin	Increased nephrotoxicity and/or neurotoxicity	Additive toxicity
Carboplatin	Increased ototoxicity	Additive toxicity
Cephalosporins	Increased nephrotoxicity	Mechanism not established
Cidofovir	Increased nephrotoxicity	Additive toxicity
Cisplatin	Increased nephrotoxicity	Mechanism not established
Colistimethate	Increased nephrotoxicity and/or neurotoxicity	Additive toxicity
Cyclosporine	Increased renal toxicity	Possibly additive or synergistic
Digoxin	Probable decreased digoxin effect with oral gentamicin or neomycin	Decreased absorption
Ethancrynic acid	Increased ototoxicity	Additive toxicity
Furosemide	Increased ototoxicity and nephrotoxicity	Additive toxicity
Magnesium sulfate	Increased neuromuscular blockade	Additive toxicity
Methotrexate	Possible increased methotrexate toxicity with kanamycin	Mechanism not established
	Possible decreased methotrexate effect with oral aminoglycosides	Decreased absorption
Methoxyflurane	Increased nephrotoxicity	Additive toxicity
Miconazole	Possible decreased tobramycin concentration	Mechanism not established
Neuromuscular blocking agents	Neuromuscular blockade	Additive toxicity
Nonsteroidal anti-inflammatory drugs (NSAIDs)	Possible aminoglycoside toxicity in preterm infants with indomethacin given for patent ductus closure	Decreased renal clearance
Penicillins	Decreased aminoglycoside effect with high concentrations of carbenicillin or ticarcillin	Inactivation
Polymyxins	Falsely low aminoglycoside levels	In vitro inactivation
	Increased nephrotoxicity; neuromuscular blockade	Additive toxicity
Tacrolimus	Increased nephrotoxicity	Additive toxicity
Vancomycin	Possible increased nephrotoxicity and ototoxicity	Additive toxicity
Aminosalicylic Acid (PAS) with		
Anticoagulants, oral	Enhanced hypoprothrombinemic effects	Mechanism not established
Ammonium chloride	Increased probability of crystalluria	Acidification of urine
Bacille Calmette-Guérin (BCG) vaccine	Negates BCG effect	Negates immune response
Digoxin	Decreased digoxin effect	Decreased absorption with time
Diphenhydramine	Decreased effect of PAS	Decreases GI absorption
Ethionamide	GI distress/hepatotoxicity	Additive
Isoniazid	Increased INH serum concentrations	Decreased metabolism
Probenecid	Increased PAS toxicity	Decreased renal excretion
Rifampin	Rifampin effectiveness may be decreased; separate doses by 8-12 h	Decreased GI absorption due to excipient bentonite
Amphotericin B with		
Aminoglycoside antibiotics	Nephrotoxicity	Synergism
Antineoplastics	Possible increased renal toxicity, bronchospasm, and hypotension	Mechanism not established
Capreomycin	Increased nephrotoxicity	Additive toxicity
Cidofovir	Increased nephrotoxicity	Additive toxicity
Cisplatin	Increased nephrotoxicity	Additive toxicity
Colistin	Increased nephrotoxicity	Additive toxicity
Corticosteroids	Increased hypokalemia	Additive toxicity
Cyclosporine	Increased renal toxicity	Possible synergism
Digitalis glycosides	Increased digitalis toxicity	Hypokalemia
Imidazole antifungals	Possible antagonism in animal models	Mechanism not established

TABLE 46-28 Adverse Drug Interactions Involving Antimicrobial Agents—cont'd

Interacting Drugs	Adverse Effect	Probable Mechanism
Amphotericin B with—cont'd		
Methoxyflurane	Increased nephrotoxicity	Additive toxicity
Neuromuscular blocking agents	Increased neuromuscular blocking effects	Hypokalemia
Pentamidine	Increased nephrotoxicity	Additive toxicity
Polymyxins	Increased nephrotoxicity	Additive toxicity
Tacrolimus	Increased nephrotoxicity	Additive toxicity
Vancomycin	Increased nephrotoxicity	Additive toxicity
Zidovudine	Potential for increased myelotoxicity and nephrotoxicity	Mechanism not established
Azithromycin with		
Aluminum/magnesium antacids	Decreased peak; no effect on overall exposure	Mechanism not established
Cyclosporine	Possible increased cyclosporine effect/toxicity	Mechanism not established
Digoxin	Increased digoxin concentrations	Destruction of intestinal *Eubacterium lentum* in 10% of digoxin patients
Nelfinavir	Increased azithromycin exposure	P-glycoprotein competition
Warfarin	Possible increased warfarin effect/toxicity	Decreased vitamin K–producing gut flora
Aztreonam with		
Chloramphenicol	Possible in vitro antagonism. Administer a few hours apart	Mechanism not established
Bacitracin with		
Aminoglycosides	Increased nephrotoxicity	Additive toxicity
Anesthetics	Potentiation of neuromuscular blocking effects	Additive toxicity
Neuromuscular blocking drugs	Potentiation of neuromuscular blocking effects	Additive toxicity
Polymyxins	Increased nephrotoxicity	Additive toxicity
Capreomycin with		
Aminoglycosides	Increased nephrotoxicity and/or ototoxicity	Additive toxicity
BCG vaccine	Negates BCG effect	Negates immune response
Colistin	Increased nephrotoxicity	Additive toxicity
Polymyxin B	Increased nephrotoxicity	Additive toxicity
Vancomycin	Increased nephrotoxicity and/or ototoxicity	Additive toxicity
Caspofungin with		
Carbamazepine	Decreased caspofungin effect	Increased metabolism
Cyclosporine	Increased caspofungin effect/toxicity	Mechanism not established
Dexamethasone	Decreased caspofungin effect	Increased metabolism
Efavirenz	Decreased caspofungin effect	Increased metabolism
Nelfinavir	Decreased caspofungin effect	Increased metabolism
Nevirapine	Decreased caspofungin effect	Increased metabolism
Phenytoin	Decreased caspofungin effect	Increased metabolism
Rifamycins	Decreased caspofungin effect	Increased metabolism
Tacrolimus	Decreased tacrolimus effect	Mechanism not established
Cefditoren with		
Antacids	Decreased cefditoren effect	Decreased bioavailability
H₂ receptor antagonists	Decreased cefditoren effect	Decreased bioavailability
Proton pump inhibitors	Decreased cefditoren effect	Decreased bioavailability
Cephalosporins with		
Alcohol	Disulfiram-like effect with cefamandole, cefmetazole, cefotetan, cefoperazone, and moxalactam. Cefonicid also in animals, but not shown in humans	Inhibition of intermediary metabolism of alcohol
Aminoglycoside antibiotics	Increased nephrotoxicity	Mechanism not established
Ampicillin	In vitro antagonism with ceftazidime versus group B streptococci and *Listeria*	Mechanism not established
Anticoagulants, oral	Possible increased anticoagulant effect with moxalactam, cefamandole, cefmetazole, or cefoperazone	Mechanism not established
Aspirin	Possible increased bleeding risk with moxalactam	Additive toxicity
Chloramphenicol	In vitro antagonism	Mechanism not established
Colistin	Increased nephrotoxicity	Additive toxicity
Diuretics	Increased nephrotoxicity with some cephalosporins	Mechanism not established
Ethacrynic acid	Increased nephrotoxicity	Mechanism not established
Furosemide	Increased nephrotoxicity	Mechanism not established
Heparin	Possible increased bleeding risk with moxalactam	Additive toxicity
Penicillins	Possible increased cefotaxime toxicity with azlocillin in patients with renal impairment	Decreased excretion
Polymyxins	Increased nephrotoxicity	Additive toxicity
Probenecid	Higher and prolonged cephalosporin concentrations	Competitive inhibition of tubular secretion
Salicylates	Decreased cefixime concentration and area under the serum antimicrobial concentration curve (AUC)	Displacement from protein binding sites
Vancomycin	Increased nephrotoxicity	Additive toxicity
Chloramphenicol with		
Acetaminophen	Possible decreased chloramphenicol effect	Increased metabolism
Anticoagulants (oral)	Increased dicumarol effect	Decreased metabolism
Aminoglycosides	In vitro antagonism; not seen in vivo	Mechanism not established
Aztreonam	Antagonism; administer chloramphenicol separately a few hours later	Mechanism not established
Barbiturates	Increased barbiturate effect; decreased chloramphenicol effect	Decreased/increased metabolism
Cephalosporins	Antagonism	Mechanism not established
Cimetidine	Aplastic anemia	Possibly additive or synergistic
Cyclophosphamide	Decreased cyclophosphamide effect	Decreased clearance

Continued

TABLE 46-28 Adverse Drug Interactions Involving Antimicrobial Agents—cont'd

Interacting Drugs	Adverse Effect	Probable Mechanism
Chloramphenicol with—cont'd		
Etomidate	Prolonged anesthesia	Decreased metabolism
Folic acid	Delayed response to folic acid	Mechanism not established
Hypoglycemics, sulfonylurea	Increased hypoglycemic effect	Mechanism not established
Iron	Delayed response to iron	Mechanism not established
Lincomycin	Decreased lincomycin effect	Target site antagonism
Penicillins	In vitro antagonism; not seen in vivo	Mechanism not established
Phenytoin/fosphenytoin	Increased phenytoin toxicity	Decreased metabolism
	Possible increased chloramphenicol toxicity	Mechanism not established
Rifampin/rifabutin	Decreased chloramphenicol effect	Increased metabolism
Vitamin B_{12}	Delayed response to vitamin B_{12}	Mechanism not established
Chloroquine with		
Ampicillin	Decreased ampicillin effect	Decreased bioavailability
Aurothioglucose	Blood dyscrasias	Additive toxicity
Cholestyramine	Decreased effect	Decreased bioavailability
Cimetidine	Increased toxicity	Decreased clearance
Cyclosporine	Increased cyclosporine toxicity	Decreased clearance
Magnesium antacids	Decreased efficacy	Decreased bioavailability
Methotrexate (MTX)	Decreased MTX efficacy	Increased clearance
Rabies vaccine	Decreased vaccine effect	Interference with the antibody response
Ritonavir	Increased chloroquine toxicity	Decreased metabolism
Succinylcholine	Increased neuromuscular blockade	Decreased clearance
Cidofovir with		
Aminoglycosides	Increased risk of nephrotoxicity	Additive toxicity
Foscarnet	Increased risk of nephrotoxicity	Additive toxicity
Pentamidine	Increased risk of nephrotoxicity	Additive toxicity
Clarithromycin with		
Astemizole	Increased risk of cardiotoxicity	Decreased metabolism
Benzodiazepines (BZDs)	Increased CNS toxicity	Decreased metabolism
Carbamazepine (CBZ)	Increased CBZ toxicity	Decreased metabolism
Cimetidine	Decreased clarithromycin concentrations	Prolonged absorption
Cisapride	Increased cisapride effect/toxicity	Decreased metabolism
Clindamycin	In vitro antagonism; not documented clinically	Mechanism not established
Corticosteroids	Increased steroid effect/toxicity	Decreased excretion
Coumarin derivatives	Increased coumarin effect/toxicity	Decreased metabolism
Cyclosporine	Increased cyclosporine toxicity	Decreased metabolism
Delavirdine	Increased clarithromycin toxicity	Decreased metabolism
Digoxin	Increased digoxin effect	Decreased gut metabolism/increased absorption
Disopyramide	Increased disopyramide effect/toxicity	Mechanism not established
Ergot alkaloids	Increased ergot effect/toxicity	Mechanism not established
Fluoxetine	Increased fluoxetine effect/toxicity	Decreased metabolism
Hydroxymethylglutaryl–coenzyme A (HMG-CoA) reductase inhibitors	Increased risk of rhabdomyolosis	Decreased metabolism
Loratadine	Increased loratadine exposure/toxicity(?)	Decreased metabolism
Omeprazole	Increased omeprazole effect/toxicity; increased clarithromycin gastric tissue exposure	Decreased metabolism; mechanism not established
Phenytoin	Possible increased or decreased effect	Altered metabolism
Pimozide	Increased pimozide effect/toxicity	Decreased metabolism
Rifamycins	Decreased clarithromycin concentrations/increased rifamycin toxicity	Increased/decreased metabolism
Ritonavir	Increased clarithromycin effect/toxicity	Decreased metabolism
Saquinavir	Increased saquinavir effect/toxicity	Decreased metabolism
Sildenafil	Increased sildenafil effect/toxicity	Decreased metabolism
Tacrolimus	Increased tacrolimus effect/toxicity	Decreased metabolism
Terfenadine	Increased risk of cardiotoxicity	Decreased metabolism
Theophylline	Increased theophylline effect/toxicity	Decreased metabolism
Zidovudine	Decreased zidovudine effect	Mechanism not established
Clindamycin with		
Neuromuscular blocking agents	Increased neuromuscular blockade	Additive toxicity
Saquinavir	Increased clindamycin toxicity	Decreased metabolism
Clofazimine with		
Dapsone	Possible decrease or nullification of clofazimine's anti-inflammatory activity	Opposing effects on neutrophil motility and lymphocyte transformation
Isoniazid	Increased clofazimine serum and urine concentrations and decreased skin concentrations	Mechanism not established
Phenytoin	Decreased efficacy	Increased phenytoin clearance
Rifampin	Decreased rate of absorption, time to reach peak, and AUC of rifampin	Mechanism not established
Colistimethate		
Same as polymyxin B		
Cycloserine with		
Alcohol	Increased alcohol effect or convulsions	Mechanism not established
Anticoagulants, oral	Increased effect	Mechanism not established
Ethionamide	Increased neurotoxicity	Additive toxicity
Isoniazid	CNS effects, dizziness, drowsiness; increased neurotoxicity	Mechanism not established/additive toxicity
Phenytoin	Increased phenytoin effect/toxicity	Decreased metabolism

TABLE 46-28 Adverse Drug Interactions Involving Antimicrobial Agents—cont'd

Interacting Drugs	*Adverse Effect*	*Probable Mechanism*
Dapsone with		
Aniline	Increased risk of hemolysis in glucose-6-phospahte dehydro-genase (G6PD) deficiency	Additive toxicity
Clofazimine	Decreased or nullification of clofazimine's anti-inflammatory effects	Opposing effects on neutrophil motility and lymphocyte transformation in vitro
Delavirdine	Increased dapsone toxicity	Decreased metabolism
Didanosine	Increased incidence of *Pneumocystis carinii* pneumonia recurrence	Mechanism not established
Folic acid antagonists	Increased risk of hematologic toxicity	Additive toxicity
Naphthalene	Increased risk of hemolysis in G6PD deficiency	Additive toxicity
Niridazole	Increased risk of hemolysis in G6PD deficiency	Additive toxicity
Nitrite	Increased risk of hemolysis in G6PD deficiency	Additive toxicity
Nitrofurantoin	Increased risk of hemolysis in G6PD deficiency	Additive toxicity
Phenylhydrazine	Increased risk of hemolysis in G6PD deficiency	Additive toxicity
Primaquine	Increased risk of hemolysis in G6PD deficiency	Additive toxicity
Pyrimethamine	Increased risk of hematologic toxicity	Additive toxicity
Rifampin/rifabutin	Decreased dapsone serum concentrations	Hepatic enzyme induction
Saquinavir	Increased dapsone toxicity	Decreased metabolism
Trimethoprim	Increased dapsone serum concentrations; increased risk of adverse effects	Mechanism not established
Zidovudine	Increased risk of hematologic toxicity	Additive toxicity
Delavirdine with		
Acenocoumarol	Increased acenocoumarol effect/toxicity	Decreased metabolism
Alfentanil	Increased alfentanil effect/toxicity	Decreased metabolism
Amiodarone	Increased amiodarone effect/toxicity	Decreased metabolism
Amprenavir	Decreased amprenavir clearance; increased delavirdine clearance	Cytochrome P-450 (CYP) 3A4 interaction
Antacids	Decreased delavirdine effect	Decreased bioavailability
Astemizole	Increased risk of cardiotoxicity	Decreased metabolism
Atorvastatin	Increased exposure and statin side effects	Decreased metabolism
Barbiturates	Increased barbiturate effect/toxicity; decreased delavirdine effect	Decreased/increased metabolism
Bepridil	Increased bepridil effect/toxicity	Decreased metabolism
BZDs	Increased BZD effect/toxicity	Decreased metabolism
Calcium channel blockers	Increased calcium blocker effect/toxicity	Decreased metabolism
CBZ	Increased CBZ toxicity; decreased delavirdine effect	Decreased/increased metabolism
Cisapride	Increased cisapride effect/toxicity	Decreased metabolism
Clarithromycin	Increased clarithromycin/delavirdine effect/toxicity	Decreased metabolism
Clindamycin	Increased clindamycin effect/toxicity	Decreased metabolism
Corticosteroids	Increased steroid effect/toxicity	Decreased metabolism
Cyclosporine	Increased cyclosporine effect/toxicity	Decreased metabolism
Cyclophosphamide	Increased cyclophosphamide toxicity; decreased delavirdine effect	Decreased/increased metabolism
Dapsone	Increased dapsone effect/toxicity	Decreased metabolism
Daunorubicin	Increased daunorubicin effect/toxicity	Decreased metabolism
Doxorubicin	Increased doxorubicin effect/toxicity	Decreased metabolism
Ergot derivatives	Increase ergot effect/toxicity	Decreased metabolism
Erythromycin	Increased erythromycin/delavirdine effect/toxicity	Decreased metabolism
Fluoxetine	Increased delavirdine effect/toxicity	Decreased metabolism
Fluvastatin	Increased exposure and statin side effects	Decreased metabolism
Garlic supplements	Decreased delavirdine effect	Increased metabolism
Glimepiride	Increased glimepiride exposure/effects	Decreased metabolism
Glipizide	Increased glipizide exposure/effects	Decreased metabolism
Glyburide	Increased glyburide exposure/effects	Decreased metabolism
H₂ receptor antagonists	Decreased delavirdine effect	Decreased bioavailability
Ifosfamide	Increased ifosfamide effect/toxicity	Decreased metabolism
Itraconazole	Increased itraconazole effect/toxicity	Decreased metabolism
Ketoconazole	Increased delavirdine effect/toxicity	Decreased metabolism
Lidocaine	Increased lidocaine effect/toxicity	Decreased metabolism
Lovastatin	Increased exposure and statin side effects	Decreased metabolism
Metronidazole	Increased metronidazole effect/toxicity	Decreased metabolism
Nefazodone	Increased nefazodone effect/toxicity	Decreased metabolism
Paclitaxel	Increased paclitaxel toxicity	Decreased metabolism
Phenytoin	Increased phenytoin effect/toxicity; decreased delavirdine effect	Decreased/increased metabolism
Pimozide	Increased pimozide effect/toxicity	Decreased metabolism
Pioglitazone	Possible increased pioglitazone exposure/effects; possible decreased delavirdine exposure	CYP inhibition; CYP induction
Proton pump inhibitors	Decreased delavirdine effect	Decreased bioavailability
Quinidine	Increased quinidine effect/toxicity	Decreased metabolism
Repaglinide	Increased repaglinide exposure/effects	Decreased metabolism
Rifamycins	Increased rifamycin effect/toxicity; decreased delavirdine effect	Decreased/increased metabolism
Sildenafil	Increased sildenafil effect/toxicity	Decreased metabolism
Simvastatin	Increased exposure and statin side effects	Decreased metabolism
Sirolimus	Increased sirolimus effect/toxicity	Decreased metabolism
St. John's wort	Decreased delavirdine effect	Increased metabolism
Tacrolimus	Increased tacrolimus effect/toxicity	Decreased metabolism
Terfenadine	Increased risk of cardiotoxicity	Decreased metabolism
Tolbutamide	Increased tolbutamide exposure/effects	Decreased metabolism
Warfarin	Increased warfarin effect/toxicity	Decreased metabolism
Zolpidem	Increased zolpidem effect/toxicity	Decreased metabolism
Didanosine (DDI) with		
Allopurinol	Increased DDI effect/toxicity	Decreased DDI clearance
Antacids	Increased toxicity due to ingredients in both	Additive toxicity
Aurothioglucose	Increased peripheral neuropathy	Additive toxicity

Continued

TABLE 46-28 Adverse Drug Interactions Involving Antimicrobial Agents—cont'd

Interacting Drugs	Adverse Effect	Probable Mechanism
Didanosine (DDI) with—cont'd		
Benzodiazepines	Increased confusion	Mechanism not established
Bisphosphonates	Decreased effect of bisphosphonates	Decreased bioavailability
Chloramphenicol	Increased peripheral neuropathy	Additive toxicity
Cisplatin	Increased peripheral neuropathy	Additive toxicity
Dapsone	Decreased dapsone effect/increased peripheral neuropathy	Decreased dapsone bioavailability/additive toxicity
Delavirdine	Decreased delavirdine/DDI effect	Mechanism not established
Disulfiram	Increased peripheral neuropathy	Additive toxicity
Ethambutol	Increased peripheral neuropathy/ocular toxicity	Additive toxicity
Ethionamide	Increased peripheral neuropathy	Additive toxicity
Fluoroquinolones	Decreased fluoroquinolone/DDI effects	Decreased bioavailability
Ganciclovir	Increased peripheral neuropathy/pancreatitis	Altered bioavailability of both
Glutethimide	Increased peripheral neuropathy	Additive toxicity
Hydralazine	Increased peripheral neuropathy	Additive toxicity
Indinavir	Decreased indinavir effect	Decreased bioavailability
Iodoquinol	Increased peripheral neuropathy	Additive toxicity
Isoniazid	Increased peripheral neuropathy	Additive toxicity
Itraconazole	Decreased itraconazole effect	Decreased bioavailability
Ketoconazole	Decreased ketoconazole effect	Decreased bioavailability
Methadone	Decreased DDI effect	Decreased bioavailability
Metronidazole	Increased peripheral neuropathy	Additive toxicity
Nitrofurantoin	Increased peripheral neuropathy	Additive toxicity
Pentamidine	Increased risk of pancreatitis	Additive toxicity
Phenytoin	Increased peripheral neuropathy	Additive toxicity
Ribavirin	Increased risk of toxicity	Additive toxicity
Tetracyclines	Decreased tetracycline effect	Decreased bioavailability
Trimethoprim-sulfamethoxazole	Increased pancreatitis	Additive toxicity
Vincristine	Increased peripheral neuropathy	Additive toxicity
Zalcitabine	Increased neurotoxicity	Additive toxicity
Dirithromycin with		
Digoxin	Increased digoxin effect/toxicity	Change in GI flora
Warfarin	Increased warfarin effect/toxicity	Change in GI flora
Efavirenz with		
Acenocoumarol	Decreased acenocoumarol effect	Increased metabolism
Amiodarone	Decreased amiodarone effect	Increased metabolism
Astemizole	Increased risk of cardiotoxicity	Decreased metabolism
Barbiturates	Decreased barbiturate/efavirenz effects	Increased metabolism
Bupropion	Decreased bupropion effect	Increased metabolism
BZDs	Decreased BZI effect	Increased metabolism
CBZ	Decreased CBZ/efavirenz effects	Increased metabolism
Cisapride	Increased cisapride effect/toxicity	Decreased metabolism
Clarithromycin	Increased efavirenz effect/toxicity	Decreased metabolism
Corticosteroids	Decreased efavirenz/steroid effects	Increased metabolism
Cyclosporine	Decreased cyclosporine effect; increased efavirenz effect/toxicity	Increased/decreased metabolism
Ergot alkaloids	Increased ergot effect/toxicity	Decreased metabolism
Erythromycin	Increased efavirenz effect/toxicity	Decreased metabolism
Fluconazole	Increased efavirenz effect/toxicity	Decreased metabolism
Fluoxetine	Increased risk of serotonin syndrome	Decreased metabolism
Garlic supplements	Decreased efavirenz effect	Increased metabolism
Indinavir	Decreased indinavir concentrations	Increased metabolism
Itraconazole	Decreased itraconazole effect; increased efavirenz effect/toxicity	Increased/decreased metabolism
Ketoconazole	Decreased ketoconazole effect; increased efavirenz effect/toxicity	Increased/decreased metabolism
Methadone	Decreased methadone effect; withdrawal	Increased metabolism
Oral contraceptives	Decreased contraceptive effect	Increased metabolism
Paclitaxel	Decreased paclitaxel effect	Increased metabolism
Phenytoin	Decreased phenytoin/efavirenz effects	Increased metabolism
Repaglinide	Decreased repaglinide effect	Increased metabolism
Rifamycins	Decreased efavirenz effect	Increased metabolism
Ritonavir	Decreased ritonavir concentrations	Increased metabolism
St. John's wort	Decreased efavirenz effect	Increased metabolism
Terfenadine	Increased risk of cardiotoxicity	Decreased metabolism
Warfarin	Decreased warfarin effect	Increased metabolism
Zidovudine	Decreased zidovudine concentrations	Increased metabolism
Ertapenem with		
Probenecid	Increased ertapenem effect/toxicity	Decreased tubular secretion
Erythromycin with		
Alfentanil	Increased alfentanil toxicity	Decreased metabolism
Bromocriptine	Increased BZD toxicity	Decreased metabolism
BZDs	Increased toxicity	Increased bioavailability
CBZ	Increased CBZ toxicity	Decreased metabolism
Cisapride	Cardiotoxicity	Decreased metabolism
Clindamycin	Antagonism	Target site competition
Clozapine	Increased clozapine toxicity	Decreased metabolism
Corticosteroids	Increased steroid effect/toxicity	Decreased excretion
Coumarin derivatives	Increased coumarin effect/toxicity	Decreased metabolism

TABLE 46-28 Adverse Drug Interactions Involving Antimicrobial Agents—cont'd

Interacting Drugs	Adverse Effect	Probable Mechanism
Erythromycin with—cont'd		
Cyclosporine	Increased cyclosporine toxicity	Decreased metabolism
Digoxin	Increased digoxin effect	Decreased GI metabolism and increased absorption
Disopyramide	Cardiac arrhythmias	Decreased metabolism
Ergot alkaloids	Increased ergot toxicity	Mechanism not established
Felodipine	Increased toxicity	Decreased metabolism
HMG-CoA reductase inhibitors	Increased risk of rhabdomyolysis	Decreased clearance
Loratadine	Increased loratadine exposure/toxicity	Decreased metabolism
Lidocaine	Decreased clearance; increased monoethylglycinexylidide concentrations (MEGX)	Decreased metabolism
Phenytoin	Possible increased or decreased effect	Altered metabolism
Quinidine	Increased quinidine effect/toxicity	Decreased metabolism
Ritonavir	Increased erythromycin toxicity	Decreased metabolism
Sildenafil	Increased sildenafil effect/toxicity	Decreased metabolism
Tacrolimus	Increased tacrolimus toxicity	Decreased metabolism
Theophylline	Increased theophylline effect and possible toxicity	Decreased metabolism
Trimetrexate	Increased trimetrexate toxicity	Decreased metabolism
Valproic acid	Increased toxicity	Decreased metabolism
Vinblastine	Increased vinblastine toxicity	Decreased metabolism
Zafirlukast	Decreased zafirlukast effect	Mechanism not established
Ethionamide with		
Aminosalicylic acid	Increased GI distress/hepatotoxicity	Mechanism not established
BCG vaccine	Negates BCG effect	Negates immune response
Cycloserine	Increased neurotoxicity	Additive toxicity
Ethambutol	Increased ethambutol toxicity	Mechanism not established
Isoniazid	Increased neurotoxicity	Additive toxicity
Pyrazinamide	Increased hepatotoxicity	Additive toxicity
Rifampin/rifabutin	Increased hepatotoxicity	Additive toxicity
Fluconazole with		
Amitriptyline	Increased amitriptyline toxicity	Decreased metabolism
Amphotericin B	Possible antagonism in animal models	Mechanism not established
Astemizole	Increased risk of cardiotoxicity	Decreased metabolism
BZDs	Increased CNS toxicity	Decreased metabolism
Cimetidine	Decreased fluconazole effect	Decreased bioavailability
Cisapride	Increased risk of cardiotoxicity	Decreased metabolism
Coumarin anticoagulants	Increased prothrombin times	Mechanism not established
Cyclosporine	Increased cyclosporine concentrations	Mechanism not established
Dihydropyridines	Increased dihydropyridine toxicity	Decreased metabolism
HMG-CoA reductase inhibitors	Increased risk of rhabdomyolysis	Mechanism not established
Phenytoin	Increased phenytoin concentrations	Decreased metabolism
Quetiapine	Possible increased quetiapine concentrations	Decreased metabolism
Rifampin/rifabutin	Decreased fluconazole concentrations	Mechanism not established
Sulfonylureas	Increased plasma concentrations and decreased metabolism of tolbutamide, glyburide, and glipizide	Mechanism not established
Tacrolimus	Increased tacrolimus toxicity	Decreased metabolism
Terfenadine	Increased risk of cardiotoxicity	Decreased metabolism
Thiazides	Increased fluconazole concentrations and AUC of fluconazole	Decreased renal clearance
Zidovudine	Increased zidovudine concentrations	Decreased metabolism
Fluoroquinolones with		
Antacids	Decreased fluoroquinolone effect with aluminum or magnesium antacids	Decreased absorption
Anticoagulants, oral	Prolonged prothrombin times	Mechanism not established
BCG vaccine	Negates BCG effect	Negates immune response
Chloramphenicol	Inhibition in vitro of norfloxacin bactericidal activity	Mechanism not established
Cyclosporine	Increased risk of nephrotoxicity; increased serum cyclosporine concentrations	Mechanism not established
DDI	Decreased fluoroquinolone effect	Decreased GI absorption
Iron	Decreased serum fluoroquinolone concentrations	Decreased GI absorption
Mineral fortified foods	Decreased fluoroquinolone concentrations	Decreased GI absorption
Nitrofurantoin	Decreased norfloxacin activity	In vitro antagonism
NSAIDs	Possible increased risk of CNS stimulation	Mechanism not established
Oral contraceptives	Possible decreased effect of trovafloxacin/moxifloxacin	Increased metabolism of quinolones
Oral hypoglycemics	Increased incidence/severity of hypoglycemia	Unknown mechanism with gatifloxacin
Pirenzepine	Decreased rate of fluoroquinolone absorption	Mechanism not established
Probenecid	Increased serum concentrations; prolonged AUCs	Decreased tubular secretion
Rifampin/rifabutin	Inhibition in vitro of norfloxacin bactericidal activity	Mechanism not established
Riluzole	Increased risk of riluzole toxicity	Decreased elimination
Ropivacaine	Increased risk of ropivacaine toxicity	Decreased metabolism
Scopolamine	Decreased rate of fluoroquinolone absorption	Mechanism not established
Sucralfate	Decreased serum fluoroquinolone concentrations	Decreased GI absorption
Tetracycline	Inhibition in vitro of norfloxacin bactericidal activity	Mechanism not established
Theophylline	Possible theophylline toxicity	Decreased metabolism
Zinc	Decreased serum fluoroquinolone concentrations	Decreased GI absorption
Foscarnet with		
Acyclovir	Increased nephrotoxicity	Additive toxicity
Cidofovir	Increased nephrotoxicity	Additive toxicity

Continued

TABLE 46-28 Adverse Drug Interactions Involving Antimicrobial Agents—cont'd

Interacting Drugs	Adverse Effect	Probable Mechanism
Foscarnet with—cont'd	**Foscarnet with**	**Foscarnet with**
Co-trimoxazole	Increased nephrotoxicity	Additive toxicity
Pentamidine	Increased nephrotoxicity; increased hypocalcemia	Additive toxicity
Probenecid	Increased foscarnet serum concentrations; increased possibility of adverse effects	Decreased tubular secretion
Suramin	Increased nephrotoxicity	Additive toxicity
Furazolidone with		
Alcohol	Disulfiram-like effect	Either inhibition of aldehyde dehydrogenase or inhibition of monoamine oxidase
Antidepressants	Increased adverse effects	Additive
Sympathomimetics	Hypertensive crisis	Increased norepinephrine availability
Ganciclovir/Valganciclovir with		
Aminoglycosides	Increased nephrotoxicity	Additive toxicity
Amphotericin B	Increased nephrotoxicity; replication inhibition of rapidly dividing host cells	Additive toxicity; additive
Co-trimoxazole	Replication inhibition of rapidly dividing host cells	Additive
Cyclosporine	Increased nephrotoxicity	Additive toxicity
Cytotoxic antineoplastics	Replication inhibition of rapidly dividing host cells	Additive
Dapsone	Replication inhibition of rapidly dividing host cells	Additive
DDI	Increased DDI effect/toxicity	Increased bioavailability
Flucytosine	Replication inhibition of rapidly dividing host cells	Additive
Imipenem	Generalized seizures	Mechanism not established
Immunosuppressives	Increased suppression of bone marrow and immune system	Additive toxicity
Nucleoside analogues	Replication inhibition of rapidly dividing host cells	Additive
Pentamidine	Replication inhibition of rapidly dividing host cells	Additive
Probenecid	Increased ganciclovir concentrations; prolonged AUC	Decrease in tubular secretion
Pyrimethamine	Replication inhibition of rapidly dividing host cells	Additive
Tacrolimus	Increased risk of nephrotoxicity	Additive toxicity
Zidovudine	In vitro antiretroviral antagonism; increased risk of hematologic toxicity	Mechanism not established; additive toxicity
Griseofulvin with		
Alcohol	Increased alcohol effects, tachycardia and flushing	Mechanism not established
Anticoagulants, oral	Decreased anticoagulant effect	Mechanism not established
Contraceptives, oral	Decreased contraceptive effect	Increased metabolism
Phenobarbital	Decreased griseofulvin concentrations	Decreased absorption or hepatic enzyme induction
Halofantrine with		
Grapefruit juice	Increased Q-T interval prolongation	Decreased metabolism
Hydroxychloroquine with		
Digoxin	Increased digoxin effect	Mechanism not established
Imipenem with		
Aztreonam	Antagonism	β-Lactamase induction
Cephalosporins	Antagonism	β-Lactamase induction
Chloramphenicol	Antagonism; administer a few hours after imipenem	Mechanism not established
Extended-spectrum penicillins	Antagonism	β-Lactamase induction
Ganciclovir	Generalized seizures	Mechanism not established
Interferon alfa with		
Captopril	Increased hematologic toxicity	Mechanism not established
Colchicine	Decreased interferon alfa-2a effect	Mechanism not established
Enalapril	Increased hematologic toxicity	Mechanism not established
Theophylline	Increased theophylline effect/toxicity	Mechanism not established
Zidovudine	Increased risk of hematologic toxicity	Additive toxicity
Isoniazid (INH) with		
Alcohol	Increased incidence of hepatitis	Mechanism not established
	Decreased INH effect in some alcoholic patients	Increased metabolism
Aluminum antacids	Decreased INH effect	Decreased absorption
Aminosalicylic acid	Increased INH concentrations	Reduced acetylation
Anticoagulants, oral	Possible increased anticoagulant effect	Decreased metabolism
BCG vaccine	Vaccine may be ineffective	INH inhibits multiplication of BCG
BZDs	Pharmacologic effects of BZDs may be increased; documented with diazepam and triazolam	Decreased metabolism
CBZ	Increased toxicity of both drugs	Altered metabolism
Cycloserine	CNS effects, dizziness, drowsiness	Mechanism not established
Disulfiram	Psychotic episodes, ataxia	Altered dopamine metabolism
Enflurane	Possible nephrotoxicity	Increased metabolism of enflurane caused increased fluoride concentration
Ethionamide	Increased CNS adverse effects	Additive
Itraconazole	Decreased itraconazole activity	Increased metabolism
Ketoconazole	Decreased ketoconazole effect	Decreased concentration
Meperidine	Increased risk of serotonin syndrome	Additive toxicity
Phenytoin/fosphenytoin	Increased phenytoin toxicity	Decreased metabolism
Rifampin/rifabutin	Possible increased INH hepatotoxicity	Possible increased toxic metabolites
Selective serotonin reuptake inhibitor (SSRI) antidepressants	Increased risk of serotonin syndrome	Additive toxicity

TABLE 46-28 Adverse Drug Interactions Involving Antimicrobial Agents—cont'd

Interacting Drugs	Adverse Effect	Probable Mechanism
Itraconazole with		
Amphotericin B	In vitro antagonism	Mechanism not established
Antacids	Possible decreased itraconazole bioavailability	Mechanism not established
Anticoagulants, oral	Increased anticoagulant effect	Decreased metabolism
Astemizole	Increased risk of cardiotoxicity	Decreased metabolism
Barbiturates	Decreased itraconazole effect	Increased metabolism
BZDs	Increased CNS effects	Decreased metabolism
CBZ	Decreased itraconazole effect	Increased metabolism
Celiprolol	Increased celiprolol effect	Increased absorption via PGP
Cisapride	Increased risk of cardiotoxicity	Decreased metabolism
Cyclosporine	Possible increased cyclosporine concentrations	Mechanism not established
DDI	Decreased itraconazole effect	Decreased bioavailability
Digoxin	Increased digoxin toxicity	Decreased metabolism
Dihydropyridines	Increased dihydropyridine effect	Decreased metabolism
Dofetilide	Increased dofetilide effect/toxicity	Decreased metabolism
H₂ receptor antagonists	Decreased itraconazole bioavailability	Decreased gastric acidity
HMG-CoA reductase inhibitors	Increased risk of rhabdomyolosis	Decreased metabolism
Omeprazole/lansoprazole	Decreased itraconazole bioavailability	Decreased gastric acidity
Phenytoin	Decreased itraconazole effect	Increased metabolism
Pimozide	Increased pimozide effect/toxicity	Decreased metabolism
Quinidine	Increased quinidine effect/toxicity	Decreased metabolism
Rifampin/rifabutin	Decreased systemic bioavailability of itraconazole	Hepatic enzyme induction
Tacrolimus	Increased tacrolimus toxicity	Decreased metabolism
Terfenadine	Increased risk of cardiotoxicity	Decreased metabolism
Ketoconazole with		
Alcohol	Possible disulfiram-like reaction	Mechanism not established
Antacids	Decreased ketoconazole effect	Decreased absorption
Anticoagulants, oral	Increased anticoagulant effect	Mechanism not established
Astemizole	Increased risk of cardiotoxicity	Decreased metabolism
BZDs	Increased CNS toxicity	Decreased metabolism
CBZ	Increased CBZ toxicity	Decreased metabolism
Cisapride	Increased risk of cardiotoxicity	Decreased metabolism
Corticosteroids	Increased methylprednisolone effect	Decreased metabolism
Cyclosporine	Increased concentration of cyclosporine in blood	Mechanism not established
Delavirdine	Increased delavirdine concentrations	Mechanism not established
DDI	Decreased ketoconazole effect	Decreased absorption
Dihydropyridines	Increased dihydropyridine effect	Decreased metabolism
Donepezil	Increased cholinomimetic effects	Decreased metabolism
H₂ receptor antagonists	Possible decreased antifungal effect	Decreased absorption
Hepatotoxic agents	Increased hepatotoxicity	Additive toxicity
HMG-CoA reductase inhibitors	Increased risk of rhabdomyolosis	Decreased metabolism
Indinavir	Increased indinavir toxicity	Decreased metabolism
INH	Decreased ketoconazole effect	Decreased blood concentrations
Loratadine	Increased loratadine concentrations	Decreased metabolism
Omeprazole/lansoprazole	Decreased ketoconazole bioavailability	Decreased gastric acidity
Phenytoin	Altered effects of one or both drugs	Altered metabolism
Quetiapine	Increased risk of quetiapine toxicity	Decreased metabolism
Rifampin/rifabutin	Decreased rifampin and ketoconazole effects	Decreased blood concentrations
Ritonavir	Increased ketoconazole concentrations	Decreased metabolism
Saquinavir	Increased saquinavir concentrations	Decreased metabolism
Tacrolimus	Increased tacrolimus toxicity	Decreased metabolism
Terfenadine	Increased risk of cardiotoxicity	Decreased metabolism
Theophylline	Decreased theophylline concentrations	Mechanism not established
Lamivudine with		
Nelfinavir	Increased lamivudine concentrations	Decreased clearance
Pentamidine	Increased risk of pancreatitis	Additive toxicity profiles
Sulfonamides	Increased lamivudine concentrations	Decreased clearance
Trimethoprim	Increased lamivudine concentrations	Decreased clearance
Trimethoprim-sulfamethoxazole	Increased risk of pancreatitis	Additive toxicity profiles
Zidovudine	Increased zidovudine concentrations	Mechanism not established
Linezolid with		
SSRI antidepressants	Increased risk of serotonin syndrome	Decreased serotonin degradation
Mebendazole with		
CBZ	Decreased mebendazole concentrations	Hepatic microsomal enzyme induction
Phenytoin	Decreased mebendazole concentrations	Hepatic microsomal enzyme induction
Meropenem with		
Probenecid	Increased meropenem effect/toxicity	Decreased tubular secretion
Methenamine with		
Sulfonamides	Increased risk of crystalluria; precipitate formation between formaldehyde and sulfamethizole	Acidification of the urine
Metronidazole with		
Alcohol	Mild disulfiram-like symptoms	Possible inhibition of intermediary metabolism of alcohol
Anticoagulants, oral	Increased anticoagulant effect	Decreased metabolism
Azathioprine	Transient neutropenia	Mechanism not established
Barbiturates	Decreased metronidazole effect with phenobarbital	Probably increased metabolism

Continued

TABLE 46-28 Adverse Drug Interactions Involving Antimicrobial Agents—cont'd

Interacting Drugs	Adverse Effect	Probable Mechanism
Metronidazole with—cont'd		
CBZ	Increased CBZ toxicity	Decreased metabolism
Cimetidine	Possible increased metronidazole toxicity	Decreased metabolism
Disulfiram	Organic brain syndrome	Mechanism not established
Fluorouracil	Transient neutropenia	Mechanism not established
Lithium	Lithium toxicity	Mechanism not established
Miconazole with		
Aminoglycosides	Possible decreased tobramycin concentration	Mechanism not established
Amphotericin B	Possible antagonism in in vitro studies	Mechanism not established
Anticoagulants, oral	Increased anticoagulant effect	Mechanism not established
Astemizole	Increased risk of cardiotoxicity	Decreased metabolism
Cisapride	Increased cardiotoxicity	Decreased metabolism
Cyclosporine	Increased nephrotoxicity	Decreased metabolism
Hypoglycemics, sulfonylurea	Severe hypoglycemia	Mechanism not established
Phenytoin	Increased phenytoin toxicity	Decreased metabolism
Terfenadine	Increased risk of cardiotoxicity	Decreased metabolism
Nalidixic Acid with		
Antacids	Decreased nalidixic acid effect	Decreased bioavailability
Anticoagulants, oral	Increased anticoagulant effect	Displacement from binding sites
Nevirapine with		
Acenocoumarol	Decreased acenocoumarol effect	Increased metabolism
Amiodarone	Decreased amiodarone effect	Increased metabolism
Barbiturates	Decreased barbiturate/nevirapine effects	Increased metabolism
Bupropion	Decreased bupropion effect	Increased metabolism
BZDs	Decreased BZD effect	Increased metabolism
CBZ	Decreased CBZ/nevirapine effects	Increased metabolism
Cimetidine	Increased nevirapine effect/toxicity	Decreased metabolism
Clarithromycin	Increased nevirapine effect/toxicity	Decreased metabolism
Corticosteroids	Decreased nevirapine/steroid effects	Increased metabolism
Cyclosporine	Decreased cyclosporine effect; increased nevirapine effect/toxicity	Increased/decreased metabolism
Erythromycin	Increased nevirapine effect/toxicity	Decreased metabolism
Garlic supplements	Decreased nevirapine effect	Increased metabolism
Indinavir	Decreased indinavir concentrations	Increased metabolism
Itraconazole	Decreased itraconazole effect; increased nevirapine effect/toxicity	Increased/decreased metabolism
Ketoconazole	Decreased ketoconazole effect; increased nevirapine effect/toxicity	Increased/decreased metabolism
Methadone	Decreased methadone effect; withdrawal	Increased metabolism
Oral contraceptives	Decreased contraceptive effect	Increased metabolism
Paclitaxel	Decreased paclitaxel effect	Increased metabolism
Phenytoin	Decreased phenytoin/nevirapine effects	Increased metabolism
Repaglinide	Decreased repaglinide effect	Increased metabolism
Rifamycins	Decreased nevirapine effect	Increased metabolism
Ritonavir	Decreased ritonavir concentrations	Increased metabolism
St. John's wort	Decreased nevirapine effect	Increased metabolism
Warfarin	Decreased warfarin effect	Increased metabolism
Zidovudine	Decreased zidovudine concentrations	Increased metabolism
Nitrofurantoin with		
Antacids	Possible decreased nitrofurantoin effect	Decreased absorption
Fluoroquinolones	In vitro antagonism of quinolone activity	Mechanism not established
Probenecid	Increased nitrofurantoin serum concentrations	Inhibition of renal excretion
Sulfinpyrazone	Increased nitrofurantoin serum concentrations	Inhibition of renal excretion
Pentamidine with		
Aminoglycosides	Increased nephrotoxicity	Additive toxicity
Amphotericin B	Increased nephrotoxicity	Additive toxicity
Capreomycin	Increased nephrotoxicity	Additive toxicity
Cidofovir	Increased nephrotoxicity	Additive toxicity
Colistin	Increased nephrotoxicity	Additive toxicity
Cisplatin	Increased nephrotoxicity	Additive toxicity
Foscarnet	Hypocalcemia	Mechanism not established
Grepafloxacin	Increased cardiotoxicity	Additive toxicity
Methoxyflurane	Increased nephrotoxicity	Additive toxicity
Polymyxins	Increased nephrotoxicity	Additive toxicity
Sparfloxacin	Increased cardiotoxicity	Additive toxicity
Vancomycin	Increased nephrotoxicity	Additive toxicity
Piperazine with		
Chlorpromazine	Seizures	Mechanism not established
Pyrantel pamoate	Decreased piperazine and pyrantel pamoate activity	Antagonism
Polymyxin B with		
Aminoglycoside antibiotics	Increased nephrotoxicity; increased neuromuscular blockade	Additive toxicity
Neuromuscular blocking agents	Increased neuromuscular blockade	Additive toxicity
Parenteral quinidine	Increased neurotoxicity	Additive toxicity
Parenteral quinine	Increased neurotoxicity	Additive toxicity
Vancomycin	Increased nephrotoxicity	Additive toxicity
Primaquine with		
Aurothioglucose	Increased blood dyscrasias	Additive
Quinacrine	Increased toxicity to the antimalarial	Additive
Ritonavir	Increased primaquine concentrations	Decreased metabolism

TABLE 46-28 Adverse Drug Interactions Involving Antimicrobial Agents—cont'd

Interacting Drugs	Adverse Effect	Probable Mechanism
Protease Inhibitors (Except Ritonavir) with		
Alfentanil	Increased alfentanil effects/toxicity	Decreased metabolism
Amiodarone	Increased amiodarone toxicity	Decreased metabolism
Antacids	Decreased efficacy of amprenavir/indinavir	Decreased bioavailability
Astemizole	Increased cardiotoxicity	Decreased metabolism
Atorvastatin	Increased AUC and statin side effects	Decreased metabolism
Azithromycin	Possible decreased nelfinavir efficacy	PGP interaction
Barbiturates	Decreased protease effect/increased barbiturate effect/toxicity	Increased/decreased metabolism
Bepridil	Increased bepridil effects/toxicity	Decreased metabolism
Bupropion	Possible increased bupropion toxicity	Decreased metabolism
BZDs	Increased CNS BZD toxicity	Decreased metabolism
Calcium channel antagonists	Increased calcium channel blocker effects	Decreased metabolism
CBZ	Decreased protease effect/increased CBZ effect	Increased/decreased metabolism
Cisapride	Increased cardiotoxicity	Decreased metabolism
Clarithromycin	Increased protease toxicity	Decreased metabolism
Clindamycin	Increased clindamycin toxicity	Decreased metabolism
Corticosteroids	Increased risk of hypercorticism	Decreased metabolism
Coumarin derivatives	Increased coumarin derivative toxicity	Decreased metabolism
Cyclophosphamide	Increased cyclophosphamide toxicity/decreased protease effect	Decreased/increased metabolism
Cyclosporine	Increased protease/cyclosporine toxicity	Decreased metabolism
Dapsone	Increased dapsone toxicity with saquinavir	Decreased metabolism
Daunorubicin	Increased risk of cardiotoxicity	Decreased metabolism
Delavirdine	Increased protease toxicity, increased hepatotoxicity, decreased delavirdine effect	Decreased metabolism
Desipramine	Increased desipramine effect/toxicity	Decreased metabolism
Diltiazem	Increased diltiazem effect/toxicity	Decreased metabolism
Dihydropyridines	Increased dihydropyridine toxicity	Decreased clearance
Doxorubicin	Increased risk of cardiotoxicity	Decreased metabolism
Ergot derivatives	Increased ergot toxicity	Decreased metabolism
Erythromycin	Increased erythromycin/protease effect/toxicity	Decreased metabolism
Fluconazole	Possible decreased effect indinavir/increased effect nelfinavir	Increased/decreased metabolism
Fusidic acid	Increased saquinavir/fusidic acid toxicity	Decreased metabolism
Garlic supplements	Decreased protease effect	Increased metabolism
Gamma hydroxybutyrate (GHB)	Increased GHB toxicity	Decreased metabolism
Grapefruit juice	Decreased indinavir effect/increased saquinavir effect	Increased/decreased metabolism
H₂ receptor antagonists	Decreased indinavir effect	Decreased bioavailability
Ifosfamide	Increased ifosfamide toxicity	Decreased metabolism
Interferon alfa-2	Increased indinavir toxicity	Decreased metabolism
Isotretinoin	Increased isotretinoin effect/toxicity	Decreased metabolism
Itraconazole	Increased itraconazole/protease effect/toxicity	Decreased metabolism
Ketoconazole	Increased ketoconazole/protease effect/toxicity	Decreased metabolism
Levodopa	Increased levodopa effect/toxicity	Decreased metabolism
Lidocaine	Increased risk of lidocaine toxicity	Decreased metabolism
Loperamide	Decreased saquinavir efficacy	Decreased bioavailability
Lovastatin	Increased AUC and statin side effects	Decreased metabolism
Methadone	Decreased methadone/protease effect	Increased metabolism
Metronidazole	Increased metronidazole effect/toxicity	Decreased metabolism
Nefazodone	Increased nefazodone effect/toxicity	Decreased metabolism
Oral contraceptives	Altered efficacy of birth control possible	Increased/decreased metabolism
Paclitaxel	Increased effect/toxicity of paclitaxel	Decreased metabolism
Phenytoin	Decreased protease/increased phenytoin effects	Increased/decreased metabolism
Pimozide	Increased pimozide toxicity	Decreased metabolism
Pravastatin	Decreased pravastatin effect or nothing	Possible increased metabolism
Primidone	Decreased protease effect	Increased metabolism
Proton-pump inhibitors	Decreased effect of indinavir	Decreased bioavailability
Quinidine	Increased quinidine effect/toxicity	Decreased metabolism
Raloxifene	Possible decreased raloxifene effect with nelfinavir	Increased metabolism
Repaglinide	Increased repaglinide exposure/effects	Decreased metabolism
Rifampin/rifabutin	Decreased protease effect/increased rifamycin toxicity	Increased/decreased metabolism
Risperidone	Increased risperidone toxicity	Decreased metabolism
Ritonavir	Increased protease toxicity	Decreased metabolism
Sildenafil	Increased sildenafil effect/toxicity	Decreased metabolism
Simvastatin	Increased AUC and statin toxicity	Decreased metabolism
Sirolimus	Increased sirolimus effect/toxicity	Decreased metabolism
SSRI antidepressants	Increased SSRI effect/toxicity	Decreased metabolism
St. John's wort	Decreased protease effect	Increased metabolism
Tacrolimus	Increased tacrolimus effect/toxicity	Decreased metabolism
Terfenadine	Increased risk of cardiotoxicity	Decreased metabolism
Verapamil	Increased verapamil effect/toxicity	Decreased metabolism
Zolpidem	Increased zolpidem effect/toxicity	Decreased metabolism
Pyrantel pamoate with		
Piperazine	Decreased pyrantel pamoate and piperazine activities	Antagonism
Theophylline	Increased theophylline toxicity	Decreased metabolism
Quinacrine with		
Alcohol	Possible disulfiram-like reaction	Accumulation of acetaldehyde
Aurothioglucose	Increased blood dyscrasias	Additive
Hepatotoxic agents	Possible increased hepatotoxicity	Additive
Primaquine	Increased primaquine toxicity	Release from tissue binding sites causing marked increase in primaquine concentrations

Continued

TABLE 46-28   Adverse Drug Interactions Involving Antimicrobial Agents—cont'd

Interacting Drugs	Adverse Effect	Probable Mechanism
Quinine with		
Acetazolamide	Increased quinine serum concentrations; increased toxicity	Decreased clearance from increased urinary pH
Aluminum antacids	Decreased quinine serum concentrations	Decreased absorption
Anticoagulants, oral	Potentiation of hypoprothrombinemic effects	Hepatic suppression of synthesis of vitamin K–dependent clotting factors
Astemizole	Increased cardiotoxicity	Decreased metabolism
Aurothioglucose	Increased blood dyscrasias	Additive
Cimetidine	Decreased quinine clearance; prolonged AUCs	Hepatic enzyme inhibition
Digoxin/digitoxin	Increased digoxin/digitoxin concentrations	Mechanism not established
Flecainide	Increased flecainide toxicity	Decreased metabolism
Heparin	Decreased anticoagulant effect	Mechanism not established
Mefloquine	Increased cardiac events	Additive
Neuromuscular blocking agents	Potentiation of neuromuscular blocking effects	Additive
Ritonavir	Increased quinine toxicity	Decreased metabolism
Sodium bicarbonate	Increased quinine serum concentrations; increased toxicity	Decreased clearance from increased urinary pH
Ribavirin with		
Abacavir	Increased risk of lactic acidosis	Mechanism not established
DDI	Increased risk of lactic acidosis	Mechanism not established
Lamivudine	Increased risk of lactic acidosis	Mechanism not established
Stavudine	Increased risk of lactic acidosis	Mechanism not established
Zalcitabine	Increased risk of lactic acidosis; in vitro retroviral antagonism	Mechanism not established; decreased phosphorylation
Zidovudine	Increased risk of lactic acidosis; in vitro retroviral antagonism	Mechanism not established; decreased phosphorylation
Rifamycins with		
Analgesics	Possible decreased analgesic effect	Increased metabolism
Anticoagulants, oral	Possible decreased oral anticoagulant effect	Increased metabolism
Anticonvulsants	Possible decreased anticonvulsant effect	Increased metabolism
Atovaquone	Decreased atovaquone effect	Increased metabolism
Barbiturates	Possible decreased barbiturate effect	Increased metabolism
BCG vaccine	Negates BCG effect	Negates immune response
β-Blockers	Possible decreased β-blocker effect	Increased metabolism
Cardiac glycosides	Possible decreased cardiac glycoside effect	Increased metabolism
Chloramphenicol	Possible decreased chloramphenicol effect	Increased metabolism
Clarithromycin	Decreased clarithromycin concentrations/increased rifamycin toxicity	Increased/decreased metabolism
Clofibrate	Possible decreased clofibrate effect	Increased metabolism
Contraceptives, oral	Possible decreased oral contraceptive effect	Increased metabolism
Corticosteroids	Possible decreased corticosteroid effect	Increased metabolism
Cyclosporine	Possible decreased cyclosporine effect	Increased metabolism
Dapsone	Possible decreased dapsone effect	Increased metabolism
Delavirdine	Decreased delavirdine concentrations/increased rifamycin toxicity	Increased/decreased metabolism
Diazepam	Possible decreased diazepam effect	Increased metabolism
Digitalis	Decreased digitoxin and digoxin effects	Increased metabolism
Dihydropyridines	Decreased dihydropyridine effect	Increased metabolism
Disopyramide	Possible decreased disopyramide effect	Increased metabolism
Doxycycline	Decreased doxycycline effect	Increased metabolism
Estrogens	Decreased estrogen concentrations	Hepatic enzyme induction
Ethionamide	Increased hepatotoxicity	Additive
Fluconazole	Decreased fluconazole effect	Increased metabolism
HMG-CoA inhibitors	Decreased HMG effect	Increased metabolism
Hypoglycemics, oral	Possible decreased oral hypoglycemic effect	Increased metabolism
Indinavir	Decreased indinavir effect; increased rifamycin exposure	Increased metabolism; decreased metabolism
Isoniazid	Possible increased hepatotoxicity	Possible increased toxic metabolites
Itraconazole	Decreased itraconazole effect	Increased metabolism
Ketoconazole	Possible decreased ketaconazole effect	Increased metabolism
Mexiletine	Possible decreased mexiletine effect	Increased metabolism
Narcotics	Possible decreased narcotic effect	Increased metabolism
Nelfinavir	Decreased nelfinavir effect	Increased metabolism
Nevirapine	Decreased nevirapine effect	Increased metabolism
Praziquantel	Decreased praziquantel effect	Increased metabolism
Progestins	Possible decreased progestin effect	Increased metabolism
Quinidine	Possible decreased quinidine effect	Increased metabolism
Ritonavir	Decreased ritonavir effect/increased rifamycin toxicity	Increased/decreased metabolism
Saquinavir	Decreased saquinavir effect/increased rifamycin toxicity	Increased/decreased metabolism
Tacrolimus	Decreased tacrolimus effect	Increased metabolism
Terbinafine	Decreased terbinafine effect	Increased metabolism
Theophylline	Possible decreased theophylline effect	Increased metabolism
Verapamil	Possible decreased verapamil effect	Increased metabolism
Zidovudine	Decreased zidovudine concentrations/AUCs	Mechanism not established
Ritonavir, Lopinavir/Ritonavir with		
All with protease inhibitors *plus*		
Albendazole	Altered albendazole efficacy	Increased or decreased metabolism
Alimemazine	Increased alimemazine/ritonavir effect/toxicity	Decreased metabolism
Astemizole	Increased risk of cardiotoxicity	Decreased metabolism
Atovaquone	Decreased atovaquone effect	Increased phase II metabolism

TABLE 46-28   **Adverse Drug Interactions Involving Antimicrobial Agents—cont'd**

Interacting Drugs	*Adverse Effect*	*Probable Mechanism*
Ritonavir, Lopinavir/Ritonavir *with—cont'd*		
All with protease inhibitors *plus—cont'd*		
Chlorpromazine	Increased ritonavir/chlorpromazine effect/toxicity	Decreased metabolism
Clozapine	Decreased clozapine effect	Increased metabolism
Codeine	Decreased analgesic effect	Decreased metabolism
Dextropropoxyphene	Increased dextropropoxyphene effect/toxicity	Decreased metabolism
Digoxin	Increased digoxin effect/toxicity	Decreased clearance
Disopyramide	Increased disopyramide effect/toxicity	Decreased metabolism
Disulfiram	Disulfiram-like reactions	Alcohol in protease dosage forms
Encainide	Increased encainide effect/toxicity	Decreased metabolism
Ethosuximide	Increased ethosuximide effect/toxicity	Decreased metabolism
Fentanyl	Increased fentanyl effect/toxicity	Decreased metabolism
Flecainide	Increased flecainide effect/toxicity	Decreased metabolism
Fusidic acid	Increased ritonavir/fusidic effect/toxicity	Decreased metabolism
Gemfibrozil	Increased ritonavir effect/toxicity	Mechanism not established
Haloperidol	Increased haloperidol effect/toxicity	Decreased metabolism
Loratadine	Increased risk of loratadine toxicity	Decreased metabolism
Meperidine	Increased risk of normeperidine toxicity	Increased metabolism of parent
Methadone	Decreased methadone effect	Increased metabolism
MDMA	Increased MDMA toxicity	Decreased metabolism
Metoprolol	Increased metoprolol effect/toxicity	Decreased metabolism
Metronidazole	Disulfiram-like reactions	Alcohol in protease dosage forms
Mexiletine	Increased mexiletine effect/toxicity	Decreased metabolism
Morphine	Decreased morphine effect	Increased metabolism
Olanzapine	Decreased olanzapine effect	Increased metabolism
Perphenazine	Increased perphenazine/ritonavir effect/toxicity	Decreased metabolism
Prochlorperazine	Increased prochlorperazine/ritonavir effect/toxicity	Decreased metabolism
Promethazine	Increased promethazine/ritonavir effect/toxicity	Decreased metabolism
Propafenone	Increased propafenone effect/toxicity	Decreased metabolism
Quinine	Increased quinine effect/toxicity	Decreased metabolism
Tamoxifen	Increased tamoxifen effect/toxicity	Decreased metabolism
Terfenadine	Increased risk of cardiotoxicity	Decreased metabolism
Thalidomide	Increased thalidomide effect/toxicity	Decreased metabolism
Theophylline	Decreased theophylline effect	Increased metabolism
Thioridazine	Increased thioridazine/ritonavir effect/toxicity	Decreased metabolism
Timolol	Increased timolol effect/toxicity	Decreased metabolism
Tramadol	Increased tramadol effect/toxicity	Decreased metabolism
Tricyclic antidepressants	Increased tricyclic effect/toxicity	Decreased metabolism
Trifluoperazine	Increased trifluoperazine/ritonavir effect/toxicity	Decreased metabolism
Triflupromazine	Increased triflupromazine/ritonavir effect/toxicity	Decreased metabolism
Roxithromycin *with*		
Digoxin	Increased digoxin effect/toxicity	Change in gut flora
Warfarin	Increased warfarin effect/toxicity	Change in gut flora
Spectinomycin *with*		
Lithium	Increased lithium toxicity	Decreased renal excretion
Stavudine (D4T) *with*		
Aurothioglucose	Increased peripheral neuropathy	Additive toxicity
Chloramphenicol	Increased peripheral neuropathy	Additive toxicity
Cisplatin	Increased peripheral neuropathy	Additive toxicity
Clarithromycin	Possible decreased stavudine effect	Decreased bioavailability(?)
Dapsone	Increased peripheral neuropathy	Additive toxicity
Disulfiram	Increased peripheral neuropathy	Additive toxicity
Ethionamide	Increased peripheral neuropathy	Additive toxicity
Fluconazole	Possible decreased stavudine effect	Decreased bioavailability(?)
Glutethimide	Increased peripheral neuropathy	Additive toxicity
Hydralazine	Increased peripheral neuropathy	Additive toxicity
INH	Increased peripheral neuropathy	Additive toxicity
Iodoquinol	Increased peripheral neuropathy	Additive toxicity
Methadone	Decreased stavudine effect	Decreased bioavailability
Metronidazole	Increased peripheral neuropathy	Additive toxicity
Nitrofurantoin	Increased peripheral neuropathy	Additive toxicity
Pentamidine	Increased pancreatitis	Additive toxicity
Phenytoin	Increased peripheral neuropathy	Additive toxicity
Ribavirin	Increased peripheral neuropathy	Additive toxicity
Rifabutin	Decreased stavudine effect	Decreased bioavailability(?)
Trimethoprim-sulfamethoxazole	Increased pancreatitis	Additive toxicity
Vincristine	Increased peripheral neuropathy	Additive toxicity
Sulfadoxine/Pyrimethamine *with*		
Aurothioglucose	Increased hematologic toxicity	Additive toxicity
Lorazepam	Mild hepatotoxicity	Mechanism not established
Para-aminobenzoic acid	Decreased pyrimethamine effect	Interference with pyrimethamine action
Sulfonamides	Increased toxicity	Additive toxicity
Trimethoprim	Increased toxicity	Additive toxicity
Sulfonamides *with*		
Antibiotics	Altered action of sulfasalazine	Alteration of intestinal flora
Anticoagulants, oral	Increased anticoagulant effect	Decreased metabolism and displacement from binding sites

Continued

TABLE 46-28   Adverse Drug Interactions Involving Antimicrobial Agents—cont'd

Interacting Drugs	Adverse Effect	Probable Mechanism
Sulfonamides with—cont'd		
Barbiturates	Increased thiopental effect	Decreased albumin binding
Chloroprocaine	Possible antagonism of sulfonamide action	Competition for PABA site
Cyclosporine	Decreased cyclosporine effect with sulfamethazine	Possible increased metabolism
Digoxin	Possible decreased digoxin effect with sulfasalazine	Decreased digoxin absorption
Folic acid	Decreased absorption, metabolism, and concentrations with sulfasalazine	Inhibition of hepatic folate metabolism, intestinal transport of folic acid, and jejunal brush-border folate conjugase
Hypoglycemics, sulfonylurea	Increased hypoglycemic effect	Mechanism not established
Iron	Decreased sulfasalazine serum concentrations	Chelation
Lamivudine	Increased lamivudine toxicity	Competition for renal clearance
Methenamine	Crystallization of sulfonamides in the urine; precipitate of formaldehyde/sulfamethizole	Acidification of the urine
Methotrexate	Possible increased methotrexate toxicity	Decreased renal clearance and displacement from binding
Monoamine oxidase inhibitors	Possible increased phenelzine toxicity with sulfisoxazole	Decreased metabolism
PABA	Possible antagonism of sulfonamide action	Competition for PABA site
Paraldehyde	Crystallization of sulfonamides in the urine	Acidification of the urine
Phenytoin	Increased phenytoin effect, except possibly with sulfisoxazole	Decreased metabolism
Piperocaine	Possible antagonism of sulfonamide action	Competition for PABA site
Procaine	Possible antagonism of sulfonamide action	Competition for PABA site
Propoxycaine	Possible antagonism of sulfonamide action	Competition for PABA site
Sulfinpyrazone	Increased serum sulfonamide concentrations	Displacement from protein binding sites and inhibition of tubular secretion
Tetracaine	Possible antagonism of sulfonamide action	Competition for PABA site
Thiopental	Increased thiopental effect; decreased dose necessary when given with sulfisoxazole	Plasma protein binding competition
Telithromycin with		
Benzodiazepines	Increased benzodiazepine effect/toxicity	Decreased metabolism
Cisapride	Increased cisapride effect/toxicity	Decreased metabolism
Coumarin derivatives	Increased coumarin effect/toxicity	Change in GI flora
Digoxin	Increased digoxin effect/toxicity	Change in GI flora
HMG-CoA reductase inhibitors	Increased risk of rhabdomyolosis	Decreased metabolism
Itraconazole	Increased telithromycin effect/toxicity	Decreased metabolism
Ketoconazole	Increased telithromycin effect/toxicity	Decreased metabolism
Theophylline	Increased theophylline effect/toxicity	Decreased metabolism
Tenofovir with		
DDI	Increased DDI effect/toxicity	Mechanism not established
Tetracyclines with		
Alcohol	Decreased doxycycline effect in alcoholics	Increased metabolism
Aminoglycosides	In vitro antagonism; no in vivo support	Mechanism not established
Antacids, oral	Decreased oral tetracycline effects	Decreased tetracycline absorption
Anticoagulants, oral	Increased anticoagulant effect	Mechanism not established
Antidepressants, tricyclic	Localized hemosiderosis with amitriptyline and minocycline	Possible synergism
Barbiturates	Decreased doxycycline effect	Increased metabolism
Bismuth subsalicylate	Decreased tetracycline effect	Decreased absorption
CBZ	Decreased doxycycline effect	Increased metabolism
Contraceptives, oral	Decreased contraceptive effect	Possible decreased enterohepatic circulation of estrogen
Digoxin	Increased digoxin effect	Decreased gut metabolism and increased absorption
Iron, oral	Decreased tetracycline effect, but not with doxycycline; decreased iron effect	Decreased absorption
Kaolin/pectin	Decreased concentrations of tetracyclines	Decreased absorption
Lithium	Increased lithium toxicity	Decreased renal excretion
Methotrexate	Possible increased toxicity	Mechanism not established
Methoxyflurane	Increased nephrotoxicity	Displacement from binding
Molindone	Decreased tetracycline effect	Calcium as an excipient inhibits absorption
Penicillins	In vitro antagonism; rare in vivo support for this	Mechanism not established
Phenformin	Increased lactic acidosis	Possible decreased phenformin excretion
Phenytoin	Decreased doxycycline effect	Increased metabolism
Rifampin/rifabutin	Possible decreased doxycycline effect	Increased metabolism
Theophylline	Possible theophylline toxicity	Mechanism not established
Zinc sulfate	Decreased tetracycline effect	Decreased absorption
Thiabendazole with		
Theophylline	Increased theophylline toxicity	Decreased metabolism
Trimethoprim with		
Angiotensin-converting enzyme inhibitors	Hyperkalemia	Reduced potassium clearance
Amiloride	Trimethoprim may potentiate hyponatremia caused by the concomitant use of amiloride with thiazide diuretics	Additive toxicity
Azathioprine	Leukopenia	Mechanism not established
Cerivastatin	Increased risk of statin toxicity	Inhibition of CYP2C8 metabolism
Cyclosporine	Increased nephrotoxicity	Synergism
Dapsone	Increased dapsone toxicity	Altered clearance
Digoxin	Possible increased digoxin effect	Decreased renal excretion and possibly decreased metabolism

TABLE 46-28 Adverse Drug Interactions Involving Antimicrobial Agents—cont'd

Interacting Drugs	Adverse Effect	Probable Mechanism
Trimethoprim with—cont'd		
MTX	Increased MTX toxicity	Decreased clearance
Phenytoin	Increased phenytoin serum concentrations—increased risk of phenytoin toxicity; increased risk of folate deficiency	Decreased metabolism; additive toxicity
Thiazide diuretics	Trimethoprim may potentiate hyponatremia caused by the concomitant use of amiloride with thiazide diuretics	Additive toxicity
Vancomycin with		
Aminoglycosides	Possible increased nephrotoxicity and ototoxicity	Possibly additive toxicity
Amphotericin B	Increased nephrotoxicity	Additive toxicity
Bacitracin	Increased nephrotoxicity	Additive toxicity
Cephalosporins	Increased nephrotoxicity	Additive toxicity
Cisplatin	Increased nephrotoxicity	Additive toxicity
Colistin	Increased nephrotoxicity	Additive toxicity
Digoxin	Possible decreased digoxin effect	Possibly decreased absorption
Paromomycin	Increased nephrotoxicity	Additive toxicity
Polymyxins	Increased nephrotoxicity	Additive toxicity
Warfarin	Increased risk of bleeding	Mechanism not established
Vidarabine with		
Allopurinol	Increased nephrotoxicity	Decreased metabolism
Theophylline	Increased theophylline effect	Decreased metabolism
Voriconazole with		
Amprenavir	Increased amprenavir/voriconazole effect/toxicity	Decreased metabolism
Astemizole	Increased risk of cardiotoxicity	Decreased metabolism
Atorvastatin	Increased atorvastatin effect/toxicity	Decreased metabolism
Barbiturates	Decreased voriconazole effect	Increased metabolism
BZDs	Increased BZD effect/toxicity	Decreased metabolism
Calcium channel antagonists	Increased calcium channel antagonist effect/toxicity	Decreased metabolism
CBZ	Decreased voriconazole effect	Increased metabolism
Cerivastatin	Increased cerivastatin effect/toxicity	Decreased metabolism
Cisapride	Increased cisapride effect/toxicity	Decreased metabolism
Coumarin derivatives	Increased coumarin effect/toxicity	Decreased metabolism
Ergot alkaloids	Increased ergot effect/toxicity	Decreased metabolism
Fosphenytoin/phenytoin	Increased phenytoin effect/toxicity; decreased voriconazole effect	Decreased/increased metabolism
Lovastatin	Increased lovastatin effect/toxicity	Decreased metabolism
Nelfinavir	Increased nelfinavir/voriconazole effect/toxicity	Decreased metabolism
Non-nucleoside reverse transcriptase inhibitors (NNRTIs)	Increased NNRTI effect/toxicity	Decreased metabolism
Omeprazole	Increased omeprazole effect/toxicity	Decreased metabolism
Pimozide	Increased pimozide effect/toxicity	Decreased metabolism
Quinidine	Increased quinidine effect/toxicity	Decreased metabolism
Rifamycins	Increased rifamycin effect/toxicity; decreased voriconazole effect	Decreased/increased metabolism
Ritonavir	Increased ritonavir/voriconazole effect/toxicity	Decreased metabolism
Saquinavir	Increased saquinavir/voriconazole effect/toxicity	Decreased metabolism
Simvastatin	Increased simvastatin effect/toxicity	Decreased metabolism
Sirolimus	Increased sirolimus effect/toxicity	Decreased metabolism
Sulfonylureas	Increased sulfonylurea effect/toxicity	Decreased metabolism
Tacrolimus	Increased tacrolimus effect/toxicity	Decreased metabolism
Terfenadine	Increased risk of cardiotoxicity	Decreased metabolism
Vinca alkaloids	Increased vinca effect/toxicity	Decreased metabolism
Zalcitabine with		
Aminoglycosides	Increased risk of peripheral neuropathy	Decreased zalcitabine clearance
Amphotericin B	Increased risk of peripheral neuropathy	Decreased zalcitabine clearance
Antacids	Decreased zalcitabine effect	Decreased bioavailability
Aurothioglucose	Increased peripheral toxicity	Additive toxicity
Chloramphenicol	Increased peripheral neuropathy	Additive toxicity
Cimetidine	Increased peripheral neuropathy	Decreased zalcitabine clearance
Cisplatin	Increased peripheral neuropathy	Additive toxicity
Dapsone	Increased peripheral neuropathy	Additive toxicity
DDI	Increased peripheral neuropathy	Additive toxicity
Disulfiram	Increased peripheral neuropathy	Additive toxicity
Ethionamide	Increased peripheral neuropathy	Additive toxicity
Foscarnet	Increased peripheral neuropathy	Decreased zalcitabine clearance
Ganciclovir	Increased hematologic toxicity	Increased bioavailability
Glutethimide	Increased peripheral neuropathy	Additive toxicity
Hydralazine	Increased peripheral neuropathy	Additive toxicity
Iodoquinol	Increased peripheral neuropathy	Additive toxicity
INH	Increased peripheral neuropathy	Additive toxicity
Metronidazole	Increased peripheral neuropathy	Additive toxicity
Nitrofurantoin	Increased peripheral neuropathy	Additive toxicity
Pentamidine	Increased pancreatitis	Additive toxicity
Phenytoin	Increased peripheral neuropathy	Additive toxicity
Probenecid	Increased peripheral neuropathy	Decreased zalcitabine clearance
Ribavirin	Increased peripheral neuropathy; in vitro antiretroviral antagonism	Additive; mechanism not established
Trimethoprim	Increased peripheral neuropathy	Decreased zalcitabine clearance
Trimethoprim-sulfamethoxazole	Increased pancreatitis	Additive toxicity
Vincristine	Increased peripheral neuropathy	Additive toxicity

Continued

TABLE 46-28 Adverse Drug Interactions Involving Antimicrobial Agents—cont'd

Interacting Drugs	Adverse Effect	Probable Mechanism
Zidovudine (ZDV) with		
Acetaminophen	Granulocytopenia	Mechanism not established
Acyclovir	Neurotoxicity	Mechanism not established
Amphotericin B	Increased risk of nephrotoxicity/hematologic toxicity	Additive toxicity
Antimycobacterials	Possible increased risk of hematologic toxicity	Decreased phase II ZDV metabolism
Aspirin	Possible increased risk of hematologic toxicity	Decreased phase II ZDV metabolism
Atovaquone	Possible increased risk of hematologic toxicity	Decreased phase II ZDV metabolism
Chloramphenicol	Possible increased risk of hematologic toxicity	Decreased phase II ZDV metabolism
Cimetidine	Possible increased risk of hematologic toxicity	Decreased phase II ZDV metabolism
Clarithromycin	Decreased ZDV concentrations and AUCs	Mechanism not established
Cytotoxic/myelosuppressive agents	Increased risk of hematologic toxicity	Additive toxicity
Dapsone	Increased neutropenia	Additive toxicity
Fluconazole	Increased risk of hematologic toxicity	Decreased phase I metabolism
Flucytosine	Increased hematologic toxicity	Additive toxicity
Ganciclovir	Decreased ZDV effect; hematologic toxicity	Increased clearance; additive toxicity
Hydroxycarbamide	Increased hematologic toxicity	Additive toxicity
Indomethacin	Possible increased risk of hematologic toxicity	Mechanism not established; additive
Interferon alfa	Increased hematologic toxicity	Additive toxicity
Interferon beta	Increased hematologic toxicity	Additive toxicity
Methadone	Increased risk of hematologic toxicity	Decreased phase II ZDV metabolism
Nephrotoxic agents	Increased risk of toxicity	Increased serum concentrations; decreased clearance
Nucleoside analogues	Increased risk of hematologic toxicity	Additive toxicity
Oral contraceptives	Increased risk of hematologic toxicity	Decreased phase II ZDV metabolism
Oxazepam	Possible increased risk of hematologic toxicity	Decreased phase II ZDV metabolism
Phenytoin	Increased risk of hematologic toxicity	Decreased clearance
Primaquine	Increased risk of peripheral neuropathy	Additive toxicity
Probenecid	Increased risk of hematologic toxicity	Decreased clearance/phase II metabolism
Pyrazinamide	Decreased effect of pyrazinamide	Mechanism not established
Pyrimethamine	Increased hematologic toxicity	Additive toxicity
Ribavirin	In vitro antiretroviral antagonism	Decreased phosphorylation of ZDV
Rifabutin	Increased hematologic toxicity	Additive toxicity
Rifamycins	Decreased ZDV effect	Increased phase II ZDV metabolism
Sulfadiazine	Increased hematologic toxicity	Additive toxicity
Trimethoprim	Increased risk of hematologic toxicity	Decreased ZDV clearance
Trimethoprim-sulfamethoxazole	Increased hematologic toxicity	Additive toxicity
Valproic acid	Increased ZDV effect/toxicity	Decreased phase II ZDV metabolism

PART II

MAJOR CLINICAL

SYNDROMES

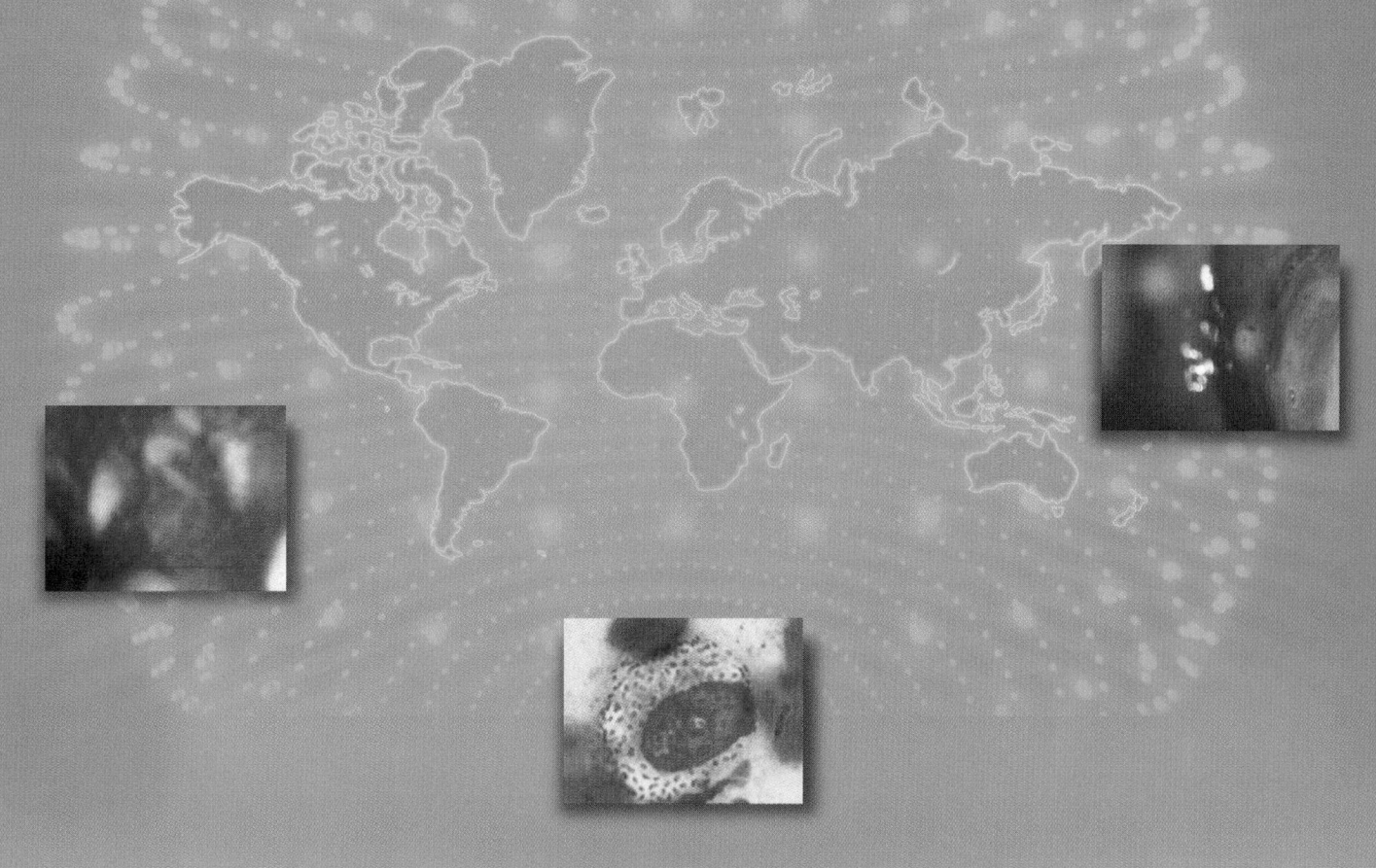

CHAPTER **47**

Temperature Regulation and the Pathogenesis of Fever

PHILIP A. MACKOWIAK

The oldest known written reference to fever exists in Akkadian cuneiform inscriptions from the 6th century BC, most likely derived from an ancient Sumerian pictogram of a flaming brazier used to symbolize both fever and the local warmth of inflammation.[1] Theoretical constructs of the pathogenesis of fever did not emerge until several centuries later, when hippocratic physicians proposed that body temperature, and physiologic harmony in general, involved a delicate balance between four corporal humors, blood, phlegm, black bile, and yellow bile.[2] Fever was then believed to result from an excess of yellow bile, a concept in concert with the fact that many infections of that era caused both fever and jaundice. During the Middle Ages, demonic possession was added to the list of mechanisms thought to be responsible for fever. By the 18th century, Harvey's discovery of the circulation of blood and the birth of clinical chemistry led iatrophysicists and iatrochemists to hypothesize alternatively that body heat and fever resulted from friction associated with the flow of blood through the vascular system and that they resulted from fermentation and putrefaction occurring in the blood and intestines.[3] Ultimately, as a result of the work of Claude Bernard, the metabolic processes occurring within the body came to be recognized as the true source of body heat. Subsequent work established that body temperature is tightly controlled within a narrow range by mechanisms regulating the rate at which such heat is allowed to dissipate from the body.

The origin of the practice of monitoring body temperature as an aid to diagnosis is uncertain. The oldest known references to devices used to measure temperature date to the 1st or 2nd century BC, when Philo of Byzantium and Hero of Alexandria are believed to have invented several such devices.[4] It is reasonably certain that Galileo manufactured a primitive (air) thermometer at about the time he assumed the chair in mathematics at Padua in 1592.[5] However, thermometry was not fully assimilated into medical practice until 1868, when Carl Reinhold August Wunderlich published a magnum opus entitled *Das Verhalten der Eigenwärme in Krankenheiten (The Course of Temperature in Diseases)*.[6]

Through *Das Verhalten der Eigenwärme in Krankenheiten,* Wunderlich gave 37° C (98.6° F) special significance with respect to normal body temperature.[7] He described the diurnal variation of body temperature and, in the process, alerted clinicians to the fact that "normal body temperature" is actually a temperature range, rather than a specific temperature. In an analysis of a series of clinical thermometric measurements, the size of which has never been equaled (estimated to have included some 1 million observations in as many as 25,000 subjects), Wunderlich posited 38° C (100.4° F) as the upper limit of the normal range and in so doing, proffered one of the first quantitative definitions of fever.

In spite of the fact that Wunderlich's work was published over a century ago and was based primarily on axillary measurements generally taken no more often than twice daily, it has survived almost verbatim in modern concepts of clinical thermometry. Interestingly, recent tests conducted with one of Wunderlich's thermometers suggest that his instruments may have been calibrated by as much as 1.4° to 2.2° C (2.6° to 4.0° F) higher than today's instruments.[7] As a result, at least some of Wunderlich's cherished dictums regarding body temperature (e.g., the special significance of 37° C [98.6° F]) have had to be revised.[8]

TERMINOLOGY

Of the many definitions of fever promulgated over the centuries, the one proposed by the International Union of Physiological Sciences Commission for Thermal Physiology in 2001[9] is the one most consistent with current concepts. It defines *fever* as "a state of elevated core temperature, which is often, but not necessarily, part of the defensive responses of multicellular organisms (host) to the invasion of live (microorganisms) or inanimate matter recognized as pathogenic or alien by the host." The *febrile response* (of which the temperature rise is a component) is a complex physiologic reaction to disease, involving not only a cytokine-mediated rise in core temperature but also the generation of acute-phase reactants, and the activation of numerous physiologic, endocrinologic, and immunologic systems. The rise in temperature during fever is to be distinguished from that occurring during episodes of hyperthermia. Unlike fever, *hyperthermia* involves an unregulated rise in body temperature, in which pyrogenic cytokines are not directly involved and against which standard antipyretics are generally ineffective. Only in the most extreme cases, complicated by gut-derived endotoxemia, do pyrogenic cytokines appear to play a role. In contrast to fever, hyperthermia represents a failure of thermoregulatory homeostasis, in which there is either uncontrolled heat production, inadequate heat dissipation, or defective thermoregulation.

In the clinical setting, fever is typically defined as a pyrogen-mediated rise in body temperature above the normal range. Although consistent with the public's perception of fever, the definition ignores the fact that a rise in body temperature is but one component of this multifaceted response. This standard clinical definition is further flawed, because it implies that "body temperature" is a single entity when, in fact, it is a pastiche of many different temperatures, each representative of a particular body part, and each varying throughout the day in response to both activities of daily living and the influence of endogenous diurnal rhythms.

CLINICAL THERMOMETRY

For over a century, the thermometer has been preeminent among clinical instruments used to distinguish health from disease and to monitor the course of illness. Unfortunately, thermometric measurements are influenced by a host of variables, all too frequently ignored when interpreting the significance of clinical temperature readings.

Observer Variability

Thermometric measurements are generally simple to perform but involve a number of technical details that, if not attended to, can invalidate estimates of body temperature. Few physicians, for example, ever take the time to ensure the reliability or proper calibration of thermometers used in clinical examinations. And yet Abbey and colleagues[10] found that a quarter of mercury-in-glass thermometers obtained from four different manufacturers were inaccurate after 8 months of use or storage.

Likewise, proper positioning of the temperature probe at the anatomic site employed is all too often given less than careful attention. Erickson has reported that oral thermometric readings vary by as much as 0.95° C (1.7° F) from the rear sublingual pocket to the area beneath the frenum in the anterior floor of the mouth.[11] Interestingly, regional differences in readings obtained within the oral cavity were more pronounced with electronic than with mercury thermometers, perhaps because of differences in the dwell times required when taking measurements with the two types of thermometers. It is also pertinent, in this regard, that studies performed earlier in the 20th century indicated that from the anus inward, the temperature gradually rises, reaching its zenith at a depth of approximately 2.5 inches (6.4 cm), and then gradually falls as the probe is advanced beyond 6 inches (15.2 cm).[12] More recent studies, however, found no significant differences between temperature readings obtained with rectal probes inserted to depths of 5, 9, and 13 cm.[13]

With today's electronic thermometers, equilibration times are relatively brief and, hence, thought not to influence the results of clinical thermometric measurements. As noted earlier, this conclusion is not necessarily justified. With mercury thermometers, opinions regarding proper placement times have varied from 2 to 12 minutes for axillary recordings and 1 to 9 minutes for rectal readings.[14,15] In a series of studies, Nichols and Kucha determined that 1 to 12 minutes are required for equilibration of mercury-in-glass thermometers during measurements of oral temperature.[16] In these studies, only 13% of the temperature readings reached their maximum after 3 minutes, whereas 90% did so after 8 minutes.

Anatomic Variability

Although clinicians frequently regard temperature readings from various anatomic sites as equivalent approximations of "body temperature,"[1] no one temperature characterizes the thermal status of the human body. This is because the body has many different temperatures, each representative of a particular body part. Nevertheless, within the body, there are two basic thermal compartments worthy of special consideration—the core and the shell.

The *shell,* which consists of skin and subcutaneous fat, insulates the core from the external environment. The *core,* of which the viscera and muscles are major components, although insulated by the shell, has temperature gradients of its own, resulting from differences in the metabolic rates and blood flow patterns of the various organs contained therein. Even during baseline conditions, organs with higher metabolic rates have slightly higher temperatures than those with lower metabolic rates; in general, tissues close to the skin have lower temperatures than those at deeper locations.[17] Although such differences are normally small, during vigorous exercise, muscle temperatures rise markedly in comparison with those of less metabolically active organs. During shock and under extreme environmental conditions, regional anatomic variations in temperature may also be exaggerated.

Rectal measurements have long been regarded as the most practical and accurate means of obtaining routine estimates of core temperature. Benzinger and Benzinger, however, have pointed out that no known thermoregulatory system exists at this particular anatomic site.[17] Rectal temperature readings are consistently higher than those obtained at other sites (even pulmonary artery blood), which some authorities have suggested might be due to heat generated as a result of the metabolic activity of fecal bacteria.[18] However, an early study showed no significant decrease in the rectal temperature after a reduction in the colonic bacterial content.[18] There is also concern that stool in the rectum acts as a heat sink to delay or mitigate changes in the rectal temperature, particularly so if the thermometer is inserted directly into stool.[19] During shock, perfusion of the rectum may be markedly impaired, causing the rectal temperature to lag significantly behind a rapidly rising or falling core temperature.[20] For this reason, Houdas and Ring have concluded that the rectal temperature provides a reliable approximation of the core temperature only if the patient is in thermal balance.[21] In neonates, even in the absence of shock, the rectal temperature (measured by standard technique) has been reported to correlate poorly with the core temperature (as measured by a deep rectal probe).[22] Although generally safe, such measurements are associated with a small risk for rectal perforation—especially in neonates and very young infants[23,24]—and if proper infection control measures are not followed, may be a source of nosocomial infection.[25]

Of the three sites most commonly used for clinical thermometric measurement (rectum, mouth, and tympanic membrane), the *mouth* is usually preferred, because it is accessible, responds promptly to changes in the core temperature, and has a long tradition of use in monitoring body temperature in clinical practice. The temperature of the sublingual pocket may be especially relevant clinically, because its main artery is a branch of the external carotid artery and, like its parent artery, responds quickly to changes in the core temperature.[18] However, because oral temperature measurements require the cooperation of the subject being examined, not all patients (e.g., young children, uncooperative adults, and intubated individuals) are amenable to such measurements.

It has long been suspected that the ingestion of hot or cold food or beverages and smoking influence oral temperature readings. In a study of 22 healthy young adults, Rabinowitz and associates showed that mastication and smoking cause both significant and persistent increases in the oral temperature, whereas drinking ice water causes a significant but much more transient decrease in the oral temperature.[26]

There is controversy regarding the effect of tachypnea on the accuracy of oral thermometric readings. In studies employing electronic thermometers, Tandberg and Sklar obtained average rectal temperature readings that were 0.96° F (0.6° C) higher than simultaneous oral temperatures in patients with respiratory rates of 20 per minute or less, compared with 1.67° F (1.0° C) higher in patients with respiratory rates of greater than 20 per minute.[27] A more recent study of 78 subjects by Neff and co-workers that controlled for open- and closed-mouth breathing and used tympanic rather than rectal temperature as a reference concluded that sublingual temperature changes do not correlate with the respiratory rate or depth but do depend on whether the mouth is open or closed.[28] As noted earlier, the probe location and equilibration time are two additional variables that can alter the results of oral temperature measurements.

The right atrium is the ideal site for measuring core temperature, because it is the nexus at which venous blood from all anatomic regions joins. However, because it is relatively inaccessible, the temperatures of other sites are more often used as approximations of core temperature. The *tympanic membrane* (TM) temperature is felt by some to be particularly useful in this regard, because the TM is perfused by a tributary of the artery that supplies the body's thermoregulatory center.[29] This fact, and the ease with which TM measurements can be obtained using modern infrared TM thermometers, have made these instruments the thermometers of choice in many clinics and intensive care units. There are two basic types of infrared TM thermometers. One type detects radiant energy emitted from the TM and portions of the ear canal, processes the information, and then displays a value representing tissue temperature in the ear canal (unadjusted mode).[30] The other displays an (adjusted) estimate of the core temperature (e.g., pulmonary arterial blood temperature) based on comparison data obtained from selected study samples. Readings obtained using the former type of TM thermometer tend to be lower than simultaneously obtained oral readings, whereas those obtained with the latter type are generally higher.[29] Unfortunately, numerous studies of many different TM thermometers have shown that although convenient, such instruments tend to give highly variable readings that correlate poorly with simultaneously obtained oral or rectal readings.[26,30-33]

Although Wunderlich's monumental treatise on clinical thermometry was based primarily on *axillary measurements,* recent experience indicates that although the axillary temperature provides a reasonable approximation of body temperature in the neonate, it does not in the older child or adult. In studies of core (deep rectal), anus, axillary, and skin temperature measurements in the newborn, Mayfield and associates observed that axillary measurements obtained with a mercury thermometer are as reliable as rectal temperature measurements.[22] Buntain and colleagues have also reported that in the neonate, axillary temperature measurements are sufficiently accurate to replace rectal measurements if a mercury-in-glass thermometer is used with an axillary dwell time of 5 minutes or more.[34] Schiffman has shown a similarly good correlation between axillary and rectal temperature measurements taken with mercury thermometers.[35]

Loudon, on the other hand, has shown that in older children, axillary temperature measurements with mercury thermometers vary from 1.6° C (2.6° F) lower to 0.6° C (1° F) higher than simultaneous oral measurements.[36] Nichols and colleagues have reported that in adults, even with 12-minute dwell times, axillary temperatures exhibit differences of 0° to 2.5° C (0° to 4.2° F) compared with oral temperature readings.[37] Furthermore, they noted that whereas 90% of rectal temperature readings reached their zenith at 4 minutes and 28% of oral readings reached their zenith at 5 minutes, only 18% of axillary readings reached a maximum at 5 minutes. Following a similar experience in children, Ogren has concluded that axillary temperature readings may be misleading and should be abandoned in the outpatient setting.[38]

Several studies have shown that monitoring the *skin temperature* using temperature-sensitive crystals incorporated into plastic strips placed on the forehead is an insensitive technique for detecting elevations in the core temperature.[39,40] The detection of fever by palpation is similarly insensitive. Bergeson and Stienfeld found that 42% of 138 febrile children (as defined by a "body temperature" of 38° C or greater) were judged to be afebrile by nurse assistants using palpation to detect fever.[41] Only 1.8% of over 1000 afebrile children were judged to be febrile using this same technique. In an evaluation of a mother's ability to assess the temperature of her child by palpation, Banco and Veltri found mothers to have a sensitivity of 73.9% and a specificity of 85.6% for detecting fever of greater than 38° C (100.4° F).[42] Thus, palpation by mothers was more sensitive than that by nurse assistants but was less specific for detecting the febrile state. Finally, Bonadio and co-workers have reported that among infants younger than 2 months of age presenting to the emergency room with a history of fever, those in whom fever had been documented at home by rectal thermometer were twice as likely to be febrile on presentation or during hospitalization than those whose fever had been documented by palpation alone (92% versus 46%; $P < .001$).[43]

Because the temperature of the rectum, mouth, and tympanic membrane are related but not identical, it would be useful to have a reliable formula for converting data from one site to that of another. In a study of healthy young adults, Rabinowitz and associates determined that on average, rectal readings exceed concurrent oral readings by 0.4° C (0.8° F) and exceed TM readings (obtained with the IVAC Core) by 0.8° C (1.6° F).[26] However, these relationships were extremely variable. Their findings concerning the relationship between rectal and oral readings were in agreement with those of several earlier investigations.[44,45] Their findings with respect to the relationship between oral and TM readings, however, differed from earlier reports,[19] which had generally shown TM readings to be higher than simultaneously obtained oral measurements. This discrepancy most likely reflected the fact that unadjusted-mode TM thermometers—for example, the IVAC Core—generally give lower readings than adjusted-mode TM thermometers, such as those used in earlier studies.[30]

Togawa has reported that on average, in a resting healthy adult, the core temperature (pulmonary artery) is 0.4° C (0.7° F) higher than the oral temperature and 0.2° C (0.4° F) lower than the rectal temperature—however, again with considerable individual variability.[46] Anagnostakis and co-workers have concluded in studies comparing rectal and axillary temperatures in infants that because of a similarly high degree of variability, no standard factor can be developed for converting axillary to rectal temperatures.[47] Thus, using a temperature reading from one anatomic site to predict the temperature at another must be done with caution.

Physiologic Variables

Wunderlich and Seguin[48] believed that "old" people have lower body temperatures than younger persons, and their views in this regard were corroborated by Howell in a report published in *Lancet* in 1948.[49] There is also a substantial body of data suggesting that thermoregulation is impaired in older persons because of various effects of aging on the autonomic nervous system.[50] Nevertheless, more recent work has not shown lower average core temperatures among healthy older subjects (mean age, 80.3 years; range, 62 to 99 years) than among healthy younger subjects.[51] Comparisons of simultaneous oral, axillary, and rectal temperature readings from such subjects have shown lower average oral and axillary readings in older persons but comparable average rectal temperatures in older and young subjects.

It has long been known that women exhibit increases in body temperature of about 0.5° C (0.9° F) at the time of ovulation.[21] Wunderlich and Seguin also maintained that women have slightly higher normal temperatures than men overall and often show greater and more sudden changes in temperature.[48] Two more recent studies have corroborated Wunderlich and Seguin's former but not latter observation.[8,52]

Body temperature, like most physiologic functions, exhibits circadian rhythmicity that is linked to the sleep-wake cycle.[53] During normal sleep-wake cycles (i.e., asleep during the night and awake during the day), the core temperature reaches its zenith in the late afternoon or early evening and its nadir in the early morning.[8] Adaptation to night-shift work causes a reversal of this pattern. Thermoregulation has also been reported to be altered in patients with neuropsychiatric disorders such as chronic depression.[54] Therefore, when interpreting clinical thermometric measurements, it is important to consider not only the time of the measurement and the site at which the temperature was taken, but also the sleep-wake cycle and mental health of the subject being studied.

In addition to these physiologic variables, exercise, digestion, and underlying disorders such as chronic renal failure, shock, and local inflammation at the site of the thermometric measurement (e.g., proctitis, external otitis, or stomatitis) may alter thermoregulatory responses or local temperatures, or both. It has, for example, been shown that the core temperature varies by as much as 3° C (36° to 39° C) in states ranging from sleep to moderately high levels of sustained exercise, and this continuum of body temperature is related to a continuum of activity.[55] Ambient temperature and humidity have been shown experimentally to affect both human sleep stages and body temperature,[56] suggesting that body temperature might also vary according to the time of year and local climate. It is pertinent in this regard that Cheng and Partridge have shown that bundling and warm environments can elevate rectal temperatures of newborns to the febrile range.[57]

Normal "Body" Temperature

A survey of physicians' perceptions of body temperature published in 1995 indicated widespread confusion regarding key features of the human body temperature.[58] Seventy-five percent of 268 physicians and medical students surveyed gave 37° C (98.6° F) as their definition of *normal body temperature*. An additional 13% defined the normal temperature as a narrow range of temperatures about a mean of 37° C (98.6° F). Only 10 (4%) subjects in the group as a whole specified a particular body site (e.g., oral or rectal) for temperature measurements in their definition. Ninety-eight percent believed that the normal temperature varies during the day, with quantitative estimates of such diurnal variability ranging from 0.2° C (0.4° F) to 2.8° C (5° F) (mean ± SD, 0.8° ± 0.4° C [1.6° ± 0.8° F]). Estimates of the lower and upper ends of the normal temperature range varied between 32.8° C (91° F) and 37.2° C (99° F) and between 36.7° C (98.0° F) and 39° C (102.2° F), respectively. Temperatures used to define fever (i.e., the lower end of the febrile range) varied between 36.9° C (98.5° F) and 40° C (104° F). Seventy-nine percent of the subjects believed that body temperature normally reaches its zenith in the evening and its nadir in the morning. However, fewer medical students (72%) than graduate physicians (85%) believed this to be the case ($P = .01$).

The origin of these perceptions of body temperature is uncertain, but in all likelihood it lies in Carl Wunderlich's 1868 book on clinical thermometry (mentioned previously), which many regard to this day as the definitive work on the subject.[6] Unfortunately, several of Wunderlich's dictums concerning body temperature, like the perceptions of modern-day physicians, appear to be in error.

A 1992 descriptive analysis of 700 baseline oral temperature observations from 148 healthy men and women found a range of 35.6° C (96.0° F) to 38.2° C (100.8° F), an overall mean of 36.8° ±0.4° C (98.2° [±0.7° F], a median of 36.8° C (98.2° F), and a mode of 36.7° C (98.0° F); 37° C (98.6° F) accounted for only 56 (8%) of the 700 oral temperature observations recorded (Fig. 47-1).[8] The mean temperature varied diurnally, with a 6 AM nadir and a 4 to 6 PM peak (Fig. 47-2). The maximal temperature (as reflected by the 99th percentile) varied from

FIGURE 47-1. Frequency distribution of 700 baseline oral temperatures obtained during 2 consecutive days of observation in 148 healthy young volunteers. *Arrow* indicates location of 98.6° F (37° C). *(From Mackowiak PA, Wasserman SS, Levine MM. A critical appraisal of 98.6°F, the upper limit of the normal body temperature, and other legacies of Carl Reinhold August Wunderlich. JAMA. 1992;268: 1578-1580.)*

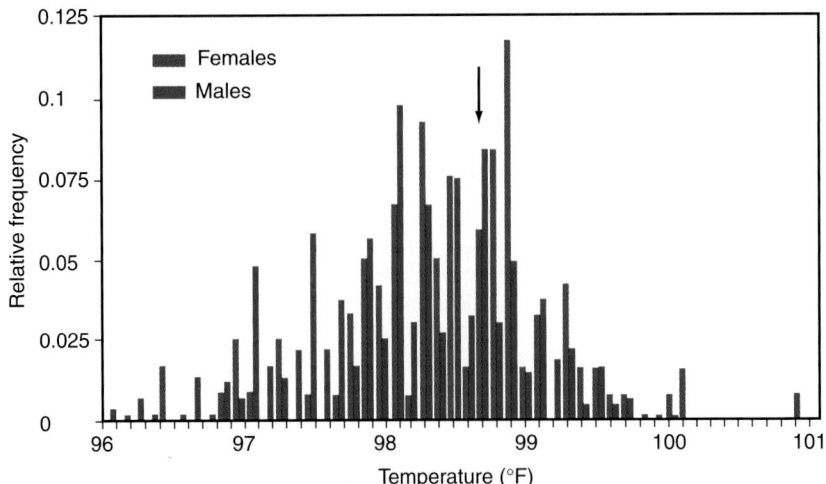

a low of 37.2° C (98.9° F) at 6 AM to a high of 37.7° C (99.9° F) at 4 PM. Comparison of initial temperature recordings obtained on admission to the research ward in which these observations were recorded, with ones obtained the same hour the day *after* admission revealed no significant difference in variability (F tests for individual studies, $P \geq .12$). Age did not significantly influence temperature within the age range studied (18 to 40 years) (linear regression, $P = .99$).

Women had a slightly higher average oral temperature than men (36.9° C [98.4° F] versus 36.7° C [98.1° F]; *t* test, $P < .001$, $df = 698$) but did not exhibit greater average diurnal temperature oscillations than male counterparts (0.56° C [1.0° F] versus 0.54° C [0.97° F]). Black subjects exhibited a slightly higher mean temperature and slightly lower average diurnal temperature oscillations than white subjects (36.8° C [98.2° F] versus 36.7° C [98.1° F] and 0.51° C [0.93° F] versus 0.61° C [1.09° F], respectively); these differences approached, but did not quite reach, statistical significance (*t* test, $P = .06$, $df = 98$). Oral temperature recordings of smokers did not differ significantly from those of nonsmokers. There was a statistically significant linear relationship between temperature and pulse rate (regression analysis, $P < .001$), with an average increase in heart rate of 4.4 beats per minute for each 1° C (2.44 beats/minute for each 1° F) rise in temperature over the range of temperatures examined (96.0° to 100.8° F).

According to Wunderlich and Seguin, "When the organism (man) is in a normal condition, the general temperature of the body maintains itself at the physiologic point: 37° C = 98.6° F."[48] Although several subsequent investigations have recorded mean temperatures of normal adult populations closer to 36.6° C (98.0° F),[59] Wunderlich's intimation that 37° C (98.6° F) is the most normal of temperatures[60] persists to this day in lay thinking, although to a lessening extent in the thinking of health care workers. The special significance formerly accorded 37° C (98.6° F) is perhaps best illustrated by the 1990 edition of *Stedman's Medical Dictionary,* which defines fever as "a body temperature above the normal of 37° C (98.6° F)."[61] In the 2000 edition, fever is defined as "A complex physiologic response to disease mediated by pyrogenic cytokines and characterized by a rise in core temperature, generation of acute-phase reactants and activation of immunological systems."[62]

The data reviewed earlier suggest that 37° C (98.6° F) has no special significance vis-à-vis body temperature in healthy young adults when such temperature is measured orally using modern thermometers. In the population examined, 37° C (98.6° F) was not the overall mean temperature, the mean temperature of any of the time periods studied, the median temperature, or the single most frequent temperature recorded. Furthermore, it did not fall within the 99.9% confidence limits for the sample mean (36.7° to 36.8° C; 98.1° to 98.2° F).

Wunderlich identified 38.0° C (100.4° F) as the upper limit of normal body temperature in his patient population and, therefore, regarded any temperature greater than 38.0° C (100.4° F) as fever.[48] However, the upper limit of normal body temperature varies among individuals, thereby limiting the applicability of mean values derived from population studies (even those as large as Wunderlich's) to individual subjects. However, the maximal temperature, like the mean

FIGURE 47-2. Mean oral temperatures and temperature ranges in 148 healthy young volunteers according to time of day. The four temperatures shown at each sample time are the 99th percentile *(top),* the 95th percentile *(second),* the mean *(third),* and the fifth percentile *(bottom)* for each sample set. (The numbers in parentheses are the temperatures in degrees Fahrenheit.) The numbers in parentheses on the x-axis indicate the number of observations analyzed at each sample time. *(From Mackowiak PA, Wasserman SS, Levine MM. A critical appraisal of 98.6°F, the upper limit of the normal body temperature, and other legacies of Carl Reinhold August Wunderlich. JAMA. 1992;268:1578-1580.)*

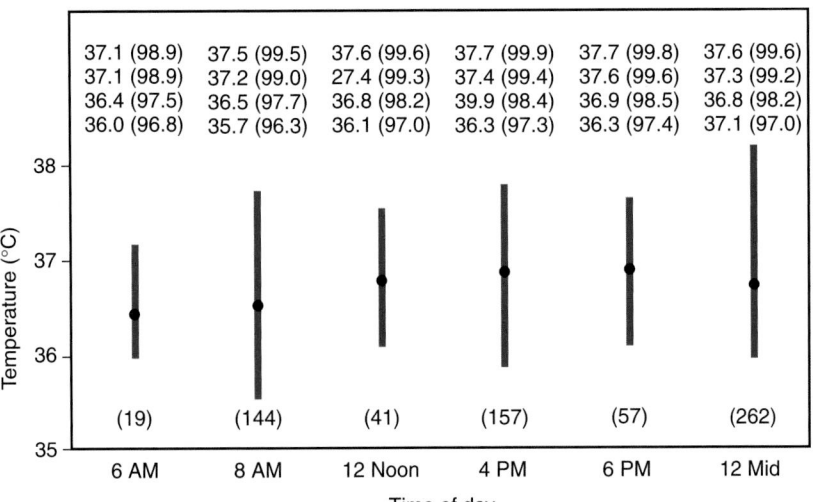

temperature, exhibited by a population varies according to the time of day and the site at which temperature measurements are taken. Because of such variability, no single temperature can be designated as the upper limit of normal. In the study population considered earlier, 37.2° C (98.9° F) was the maximal oral temperature (i.e., the 99th percentile) recorded at 6 AM, whereas at 4 PM, the maximal oral temperature observed reached 37.7° C (99.9° F). Thus, these data suggest that when modern thermometers are used to monitor oral temperature in young or middle-aged adults, fever is roughly defined as an early-morning temperature of 37.2° C (99.0° F) or greater or a temperature of 37.8° C (100° F) or greater at any time during the day.

Wunderlich wrote in 1868 that "[temperature] oscillates even in healthy persons according to time of day by 0.5° C = 0.9° F." The next year, Wunderlich and Reeve wrote, "The lowest point is reached in the morning hours between two and eight, and the highest in the afternoon between four and nine."[63] Modern authorities have generally concurred with these observations. However, Tauber has suggested that the amplitude of diurnal variation might be as high as 1° C (1.8° F).[64] The data described earlier are more consistent with the views of Wunderlich and colleagues. Nevertheless, the subjects examined in that study exhibited considerable individual variability, some having daily temperature oscillations as wide as 1.3° C (2.4° F) and others having oscillations as narrow as 0.1° C (0.2° F).

According to Wunderlich and Seguin, women have slightly higher normal temperatures than men and often show greater and more sudden changes of temperature.[48] In a study of nine healthy young adults (six male and three female), Dinarello and Wolff corroborated both observations.[52] The investigation described earlier, which did not control for the effects of ovulation on thermal observations, was able to corroborate only the former observation of Wunderlich and Seguin.[8]

It has been maintained for over a century that older persons have lower body temperatures than younger persons.[48] Howell's 1948 study (mentioned previously) seemed to substantiate this belief.[49] Although there are considerable data suggesting that thermoregulation is impaired in older persons because of various effects of aging on the autonomic system,[50] as noted previously, more recent investigation has not shown lower average core temperatures among healthy older persons than among healthy young people.[51]

Some authors believe that the first temperature reading obtained on admission to a hospital can be falsely elevated, because stress, in the broadest sense, has the capacity to elevate body temperature.[48,65] The study by Mackowiak and colleagues described previously did not find evidence that the first temperature reading obtained after admission to a research study unit was any more likely to be elevated than measurements obtained at later times.[8] The Maryland investigators, however, could not be certain that stress levels at the time of admission to their unit were comparable to levels of stress experienced by patients at the time of admission to a hospital.

As a result of work conducted earlier this century,[45,66] it is widely believed that the heart rate increases 10 beats per minute for each 1° F rise in body temperature. More recent data (presented earlier) indicate that the heart rate increases only 2.44 beats per minute for each 1° F rise in temperature.[8] The difference between the earlier and more recent investigations most likely reflects the fact that in the latter instance, subjects were afebrile and were examined seated, whereas those examined in earlier investigations were mostly febrile and rested reclining on a couch for 20 minutes before examination.

The normal range of body temperature in children is not well delineated. Lorin has written that the range is higher in children than in adults and that a decrease toward adult levels begins at about 1 year of age, continues through puberty, and stabilizes at 13 to 14 years of age in girls and at 17 to 18 years of age in boys.[67] He offers as documentation of his views on the matter a 1937 publication by Bayley and Stolz.[68] Unfortunately, these early investigators did not control for variables such as the time of day, bundling, and the thermometer dwell time, each of which might have significantly affected the results of their survey. It has also been maintained that the circadian rhythm that characterizes body temperature in the adult is less evident in the first

few months of life, is well established by the second birthday, and tends to be more pronounced during childhood than during adulthood.[67] This concept, like many concerned with the normal temperature of children, is difficult to substantiate with published data.

THERMOREGULATION

Heat is derived from biochemical reactions occurring in all living cells.[69] At the mitochondrial level, energy derived from the catabolism of metabolites such as glucose is used in oxidative phosphorylation to convert adenosine diphosphate to adenosine triphosphate (ATP). At rest, more than half of the body's heat is generated as a result of the inefficiency of the biochemical processes that convert food energy into the free energy pool (e.g., ATP). Even if no external work is being performed, heat is generated as a result of both internal work (e.g., peristalsis, myocardial contractions, and the circulation of blood) and biochemical reactions involved in maintaining the structural and functional integrity of the various organ systems (i.e., the utilization and resynthesis of ATP). When external work is performed, additional heat is generated as a byproduct of skeletal muscle contractions.

In adult humans and most other large mammals, shivering is the primary means by which heat production is enhanced. Nonshivering thermogenesis is more important in smaller mammals, newborns (including humans), and cold-acclimated mammals.[69,70] Although several tissues (e.g., the heart, respiratory muscles, and adipose tissue) contribute to the process, brown adipose tissue has been most closely associated with nonshivering thermogenesis. This highly specialized form of adipose tissue located near the shoulder blades, neck, adrenals, and deep blood vessels (adjacent to vital organs) is characterized by its brownish color, a profuse vascular system, and an abundance of mitochondria.[69,71]

Heat generated primarily in vital organs lying deep within the body core, is distributed throughout the body via the circulatory system. In response to input from the nervous system, the circulatory system determines both the temperature of the various body parts and the rate at which heat is lost from body surfaces to the environment (by conduction, convection, radiation, and evaporation).[72] In a warm environment, or in response to an elevation in the core temperature resulting from exercise, cutaneous blood flow increases so that heat is transported from the core to be dissipated at the skin surface. Simultaneous activation of sweating enhances such heat loss via evaporation. In anesthetized animals, increases in cutaneous blood flow in response to hypothalamic warming are offset by concomitant reductions in gastrointestinal blood flow.[73] In a cold environment or in response to a reduction in core temperature, cutaneous blood flow normally decreases as a means of conserving heat within the body core.

Thermoregulation is a process that involves a continuum of neural structures and connections extending to and from the hypothalamus and limbic system through the lower brain stem and reticular formation to the spinal cord and sympathetic ganglia (Fig. 47-3).[69] Nevertheless, an area of the brain located in and near the rostral hypothalamus appears to be especially important to the process of thermoregulation. Although generally referred to as the "preoptic area," it actually includes the medial and lateral aspects of the preoptic area, anterior hypothalamus, and septum. Numerous studies extending over 60 years have established that neurons located in this area are thermosensitive and exert at least partial control over physiologic and behavioral thermoregulatory responses.[72,74]

Many, although not all, thermophysiologists believe that the temperature-sensitive preoptic area "regulates" body temperature by integrating thermal input signals from thermosensors in the skin and core areas (including the central nervous system).[75] One of the more widely held theories is that such integration involves a designated thermal setpoint for the preoptic area that is maintained by a negative feedback system. According to this theory, if the preoptic temperature rises above its setpoint, for whatever reason (e.g., during exercise), heat-loss responses are activated to lower the body temperature and return the temperature of the preoptic area to the thermal setpoint (e.g., 37° C).[76]

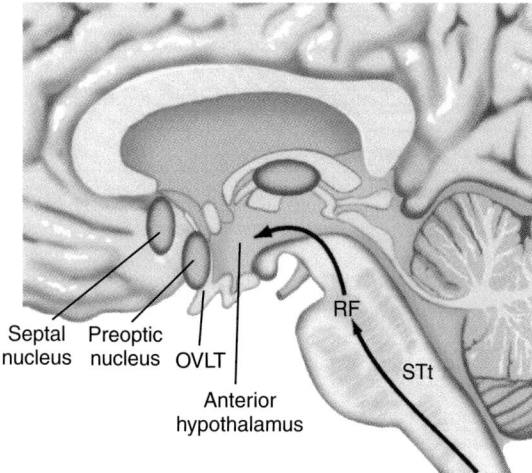

FIGURE 47-3. Sagittal view of the brain and upper spinal cord showing the multisynaptic pathway of skin and spinal thermoreceptors through the spinothalamic tract (STt) and reticular formation (RF) to the anterior hypothalamus, preoptic region, and the septum. OVLT, organum vasculosum of the lamina terminalis. *(From Mackowiak PA. Concepts of fever. Arch Intern Med. 1998;158:1870-1881.)*

The thermal setpoint of a particular heat-loss response is thus the maximal temperature tolerated by the preoptic area before the heat-loss response is evoked. If, on the other hand, the preoptic temperature falls below its thermal setpoint (e.g., as a result of cold exposure), various heat-retention and heat-production responses are activated to raise body temperature, and with it, the temperature of the preoptic area, to its thermal setpoint. The thermal setpoint of a particular heat-production response is thus the minimal temperature tolerated by the preoptic area before the response is evoked.

Although a convenient explanation of the means by which temperature elevations are coordinated during fever, the concept of a single, central setpoint temperature is regarded by many thermophysiologists as oversimplified. At least some physiologists prefer to think of body temperature as regulated within a narrow range of temperatures by a composite setpoint of several thermosensitive areas and several different thermoregulatory responses.[77-79]

A variety of endogenous substances and drugs appear to affect temperature regulation by altering the activity of hypothalamic neurons. Perhaps the best examples of such substances are the pyrogenic cytokines discussed later. These are released by mononuclear phagocytes in response to a wide array of stimuli and have the capacity to raise the thermoregulatory center's thermal setpoint. Whether they cross the blood-brain barrier to do so[80,81] or act by evoking the release of other mediators (e.g., prostaglandin E_2 [PGE_2]) in circumventricular organs, such as the organum vasculosum laminae terminalis,[80] is uncertain. Whatever the precise endogenous mediators of fever, their primary effect appears to be to decrease the firing rate of preoptic warm-sensitive neurons, leading to the activation of responses designed to decrease heat loss and increase heat production.

ENDOGENOUS PYROGENS

Pyrogens have traditionally been divided into two general categories: those that originate outside the body (exogenous pyrogens) and those that are derived from host cells (endogenous pyrogens). Exogenous pyrogens are, for the most part, microorganisms and toxins or other products of microbial origin, whereas endogenous pyrogens are host cell–derived (pyrogenic) cytokines that are the principal central mediators of the febrile response.[82] According to traditional concepts, exogenous pyrogens, regardless of their physicochemical structure, initiate fever by inducing host cells (primarily macrophages) to produce

endogenous pyrogens. Such concepts notwithstanding, certain endogenous molecules also have the capacity to induce endogenous pyrogens. These include, among others, antigen-antibody complexes in the presence of complement,[83,84] certain androgenic steroid metabolites,[85-87] inflammatory bile acids,[88] complement,[89] and various lymphocyte-derived molecules.[90,91] Likewise, data recently obtained in studies employing guinea pigs suggest that bacterial lipopolysaccharide (LPS) induces fever directly (rather than indirectly through the induction of pyrogenic cytokines) by interacting with Kupffer's cells, thereby initiating pyrogenic signals that are transmitted to the preoptic area of the hypothalamus via the hepatic branch of the vagus nerve.[92] Thus, the distinction between endogenous and exogenous pyrogens is artificial at best.

Complete understanding of the function of individual pyrogenic cytokines has been hampered by the fact that one cytokine often influences the expression of other cytokines or their receptors, or both, and may also induce more distal co-mediators of cytokine-related bioactivities (e.g., prostaglandins and platelet-activating factor).[93] In short, cytokines function within a complex regulatory network in which information is conveyed to cells by combinations, and perhaps by sequences, of a host of cytokines and other hormones.[94] Like the words of human communication, individual cytokines are basic units of information. On occasion, a single cytokine, like a single word, may communicate a complete message. More often, however, complete messages received by cells probably resemble sentences, in which combinations and sequences of cytokines convey information. Because of such interactions, it has been difficult to ascertain the direct in vivo bioactivities of particular cytokines. Nevertheless, several cytokines have in common the capacity to induce fever. On the basis of this characteristic, they have been codified together as so-called pyrogenic cytokines.

The list of currently recognized pyrogenic cytokines includes, among others, interleukin-1 (IL-1 [IL-1α and IL-β]), tumor necrosis factor-α (TNF-α), IL-6, ciliary neurotropic factor (CNF), and interferon (IFN).[95-103] Even among these few cytokines, complex relationships exist, with certain members upregulating the expression of other members or their receptors in certain situations and downregulating them in others.[93] The four major pyrogenic cytokines have monomeric molecular masses that range from 17 to 30 kDa. Undetectable under basal conditions in healthy subjects, they are produced by many different tissues in response to appropriate stimuli. Once released, pyrogenic cytokines have short intravascular half-lives. They are pleiotropic, in that they interact with receptors present on many different host cells. They are active in picomolar quantities, induce maximal cellular responses even at low receptor occupancy, and exert local (autocrine-paracrine) as well as systemic (endocrine) effects.[93]

It has long been suspected that interactions between pyrogenic cytokines and their receptors in the preoptic region of the anterior hypothalamus activate phospholipase A_2, liberating plasma membrane arachidonic acid as a substrate for the cyclooxygenase pathway. Some cytokines appear to do so by increasing cyclooxygenase expression directly, causing liberation of the arachidonate metabolite PGE_2. Because this small lipid molecule easily diffuses across the blood-brain barrier, it is thought by some to be the local mediator that actually activates thermosensitive neurons. Although it is not yet widely accepted, additional studies indicate that the C5a component of the complement cascade is integral to LPS-induced fever[104] and that in some situations, thermal information involved in the febrile response is transmitted from the periphery to the thermoregulatory center via vagal pathways (see earlier).[105]

Figure 47-4 depicts the modern, hypothetical model for the febrile response,[106] in which pyrogenic cytokines released by phagocytic leukocytes into the blood stream in response to exogenous pyrogens find their way to the organum vasculosum of the lamina terminalis (OVLT), where they induce synthesis of prostaglandins mediating the febrile response. The model has several shortcomings that have caused thermophysiologists to suspect that multiple pathways might be involved in the induction of fever (e.g., the vagal pathways referred to

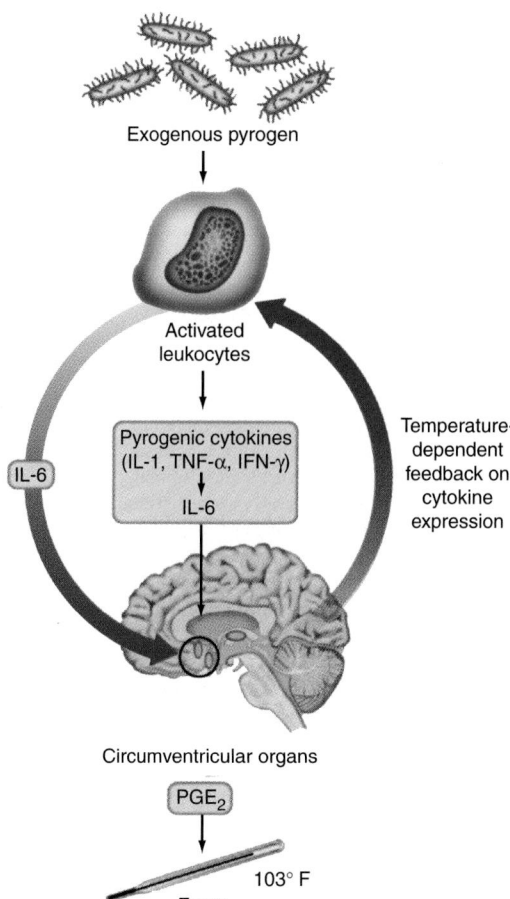

FIGURE 47-4. Hypothetical model for the febrile response. *(From Mackowiak PA. Concepts of fever. Arch Intern Med. 1998;158: 1870-1881.)*

Neuroendocrine Changes
Fever, somnolence, and anorexia
Increased secretion of corticotropin-releasing hormone, corticotropin, and
   cortisol
Increased secretion of arginine vasopressin
Decreased production of insulin-like growth factor I
Increased adrenal secretion of catecholamines

Hematopoietic Changes
Anemia of chronic disease
Leukocytosis
Thrombocytosis

Metabolic Changes
Loss of muscle and negative nitrogen balance
Decreased gluconeogenesis
Osteoporosis
Increased hepatic lipogenesis
Increased lipolysis in adipose tissue
Decreased lipoprotein lipase activity in muscle and adipose tissue
Cachexia

Hepatic Changes
Increased metallothionein, inducible nitric oxide synthase, heme
   oxygenase, manganese superoxide dismutase, and tissue inhibitor
   of metalloproteinase-1
Decreased phosphoenolpyruvate carboxykinase activity

Changes in Nonprotein Plasma Constituents
Hypozincemia, hypoferremia, and hypercupremia
Decreased plasma retinol concentrations
Increased plasma glutathione concentrations

From Gabay C, Kushner I. Acute-phase proteins and other systemic responses to inflammation. N Engl J Med. 1999;340:448-454. Copyright © 1999 Massachusetts Medical Society. All rights reserved.

---

earlier, local production of pyrogenic cytokines in the hypothalamus itself, and participation of membrane-bound cytokines as mediators), with different pathways or combinations of pathways being responsible for fever in different situations.[105,107] All of the models proposed to date have been concerned with mechanisms responsible for the induction phase of fever. None have considered the plateau or ascending phases of fever or explained why a disorder such as endocarditis, in which exogenous pyrogens (i.e., bacteria) are present continuously in the blood, is associated with a remittent rather than a continuous fever pattern. As a consequence, our understanding of the febrile response remains incomplete and largely speculative. As indicated previously, it is not yet clear whether circulating cytokines cross the blood-brain barrier or have to be produced within the central nervous system in order to activate thermosensitive neurons; or if each of the pyrogenic cytokines is capable of raising the thermoregulatory setpoint independently or must exert this effect through some final, common pathway (see Fig. 47-4); or if PGE$_2$ or other local mediators are a sine qua non of the febrile response; or what determines the magnitude of expression of individual cytokines in response to various stimuli; or how the upper limit of the febrile range is set.[93]

ACUTE-PHASE RESPONSE

As noted previously, a cytokine-mediated rise in the core temperature is but one of many features of the febrile response. Numerous other physiologic reactions, collectively referred to as the *acute-phase response,* are mediated by members of the same group of pyrogenic cytokines that activate the thermal response of fever. Such reactions include a host of behavioral, physiologic, biochemical, and nutritional

alterations (Table 47-1).[108] Stimuli capable of inducing an acute-phase response include bacterial and (to a lesser extent) viral infections, trauma, malignant neoplasms, burns, tissue infarction, immunologically mediated and crystal-induced inflammatory states, strenuous exercise, and childbirth.[94,109] There is also evidence that major depression,[110] schizophrenia,[111] and psychological stress[112] are capable of inducing an acute-phase response.

Traditionally, the phrase *acute-phase response* has been used to denote changes in plasma concentrations of a number of secretory proteins derived from hepatocytes. *Acute-phase proteins,* of which there are many (Table 47-2),[108] exhibit either increased synthesis (*positive* acute-phase proteins) or decreased synthesis (*negative* acute-phase proteins) during the acute-phase response. IL-6 is the chief stimulator of the production of most acute-phase proteins. Other pyrogenic cytokines, however, also influence the production of various subgroups of such proteins.[108]

Many of the acute-phase proteins are believed to modulate inflammation and tissue repair.[113] A major function of C-reactive protein (CRP), for example, is presumed to involve binding of phosphocholine on pathogenic microorganisms, as well as phospholipid constituents on damaged or necrotic host cells. Through such binding, CRP might both activate the complement system and promote phagocyte adherence, thereby initiating the process by which pathogenic microbes or necrotic cells are cleared from the host. Such activities are most likely potentiated by CRP-induced production of inflammatory cytokines[114] and tissue factor[115] by monocytes. Nevertheless, the ultimate function of CRP is uncertain, in that several in vivo studies have shown it to have anti-inflammatory properties.[116-118]

Another major human acute-phase protein, serum amyloid A, has been reported to potentiate adhesiveness and chemotaxis of phagocytic cells and lymphocytes.[119] There is also evidence that macrophages bear specific binding sites for serum amyloid A, that serum amyloid A–rich, high-density lipoproteins mediate the transfer of cholesterol to macrophages at sites of inflammation,[120] and that serum amyloid A enhances low-density lipoprotein oxidation in arterial walls.[121]

TABLE 47-2 Human Acute-Phase Proteins

Proteins Whose Plasma Concentrations Increase
Complement system
  C3
  C4
  C5
  C9
  MAC
  Factor B
  C1 inhibitor
  C4b-binding protein
  Mannose-binding lectin
Coagulation and fibrinolytic system
  Fibrinogen
  Plasminogen
  Tissue plasminogen activator
  Urokinase
  Protein S
  Vitronectin
  Plasminogen-activator inhibitor I
  Kininogen
Antiproteases
  α_1-Protease inhibitor
  α_1-Antichymotrypsin
  Pancreatic secretory trypsin inhibitor
  Inter-α-trypsin inhibitors
Transport proteins
  Ceruloplasmin
  Haptoglobin
  Hemopexin
Participants in inflammatory responses
  Secreted phospholipase A_2
  Lipopolysaccharide-binding protein
  Interleukin-1 receptor antagonist
  Granulocyte colony-stimulating factor
Others
  C-reactive protein
  Serum amyloid A
  α_1-Acid glycoprotein
  Fibronectin
  Ferritin
  Angiotensinogen

Proteins Whose Plasma Concentrations Decrease
  Albumin
  Transferrin
  Transthyretin
  α_2-HS glycoprotein
  Alpha-fetoprotein
  Thyroxine-binding globulin
  Insulin-like growth factor I
  Factor XII
  Retinol-binding protein

Adapted from Gabay C, Kushner I. Acute-phase proteins and other systemic responses to inflammation. N Engl J Med. 1999;340:448-454. Copyright © 1999 Massachusetts Medical Society. All rights reserved.

Complement components, many of which are acute-phase reactants, induce pyrogenic cytokines and PGE_2; modulate chemotaxis, opsonization, vascular permeability, and vascular dilation; and have cytotoxic effects as well.[108] Haptoglobin, hemopexin, and ceruloplasmin are all antioxidants. It is, therefore, reasonable to assume that, like the antiproteases α_1-antichymotrypsin and C1-esterase inhibitor, they play important roles in modulating inflammation. However, the functional capacity of such proteins is broad. There is also a growing literature concerned with the acute-phase protein LPS-binding protein, which appears both to enhance and to neutralize the biologic activity of LPS (through its interaction with the CD14 receptor on macrophages).[122]

Although closely associated with fever, the acute-phase response is not an invariable component of the febrile response.[108] Some febrile patients (e.g., those with certain viral infections) have normal blood levels of CRP. Moreover, patients with elevated blood levels of CRP are not always febrile. The acute-phase response, like the febrile response, is a complex response consisting of numerous integrated, though separately regulated, components. The particular components

expressed in response to a given disease process more than likely reflect the specific cytokines induced by the disease.

ENDOGENOUS CRYOGENS

Hippocrates maintained that "heat is the immortal substance of life endowed with intelligence. . . . However, heat must also be refrigerated by respiration and kept within bounds if the source or principle of life is to persist; for if refrigeration is not provided, the heat will consume itself."[123] Modern-day clinicians also generally subscribe to the notion that the febrile range has an upper limit but do not agree on a precise temperature defining this limit.[57] The lack of a consensus in this regard is understandable, because "body" temperature profiles exhibit considerable individual, anatomic, and diurnal variability. For this reason, the upper limit of the febrile range cannot be defined as a single temperature applicable to all body sites of all people at all times during the day. Nevertheless, the febrile response is a regulated physiologic response, in which the temperature is maintained within a specific range, the upper limit of which virtually never exceeds 41° C in adult humans, regardless of the cause of the fever or the site at which the temperature measurements are taken.[124] The physiologic necessity of this upper limit is supported by considerable experimental data demonstrating adverse physiologic consequences of core temperatures of greater than 41° to 42° C (107.6° F).[125]

The mechanisms regulating fever's upper limit have yet to be fully elucidated. They could lie with the intrinsic properties of the neurons themselves or involve the release of endogenous antipyretic substances that antagonize the effects of pyrogens on thermosensitive neurons. With regard to the former possibility, plots of the firing rates of neurons coordinating thermoregulatory responses and heat production tend to converge at 42° C (107.6° F) (Fig. 47-5).[125] At this temperature, the sustained firing rates of warm-sensitive neurons reach their zenith and cannot be increased further in response to higher temperatures. Similarly, the firing rates of cold-sensitive neurons reach their nadir at 42° C (107.6° F) and cannot decrease further, even if the temperature continues to increase. Thus, regardless of the pyrogen concentration, thermosensitive neurons appear to be incapable of providing additional thermoregulatory signals once the temperature reaches 42° C (107.6° F).

These same thermosensitive neurons are influenced by a variety of endogenous substances, at least some of which appear to function as endogenous cryogens.[125] One such substance is arginine vasopressin. Studies from several laboratories employing a variety of animal models have established that arginine vasopressin is present in the fibers and terminals of the ventral septal area of the hypothalamus, is released into the ventral septal area during fever, reduces fever by its action at type 1 vasopressin receptors when introduced into the ventral septal area, and, when inhibited, prolongs fever.[126-128]

α-Melanocyte-stimulating hormone (α-MSH) is another neuropeptide exhibiting endogenous antipyretic activity.[129] Unlike some of the other antipyretic peptides, α-MSH has not been identified in fibers projecting into the dorsolateral septal area.[130] It does, nevertheless, reduce pyrogen-induced fever when administered to experimental animals in doses below those affecting the basal body temperature.[131-135] When given centrally, α-MSH is more than 25,000 times more potent as an antipyretic than acetaminophen.[129] Repeated central administration of α-MSH does not induce tolerance to its antipyretic effect.[136] In addition, injection of anti-α-MSH antiserum into the cerebral ventricles augments the febrile response of experimental animals to IL-1.[137]

Glucocorticoids and their inducers (corticotropin-releasing hormone and corticotropin) inhibit the synthesis of pyrogenic cytokines such as IL-6 and TNF-α.[138-140] Through such effects, they are believed to exert inhibitory feedback on LPS-induced fever.[141] Lipocortin-1, a putative mediator of glucocorticoid function, has also been shown to inhibit the pyrogenic actions of IL-1 and IFN.[142] Injection of corticotropin-releasing hormone (CRH) into the third ventricle of experimental animals produces similar antipyretic effects.[143]

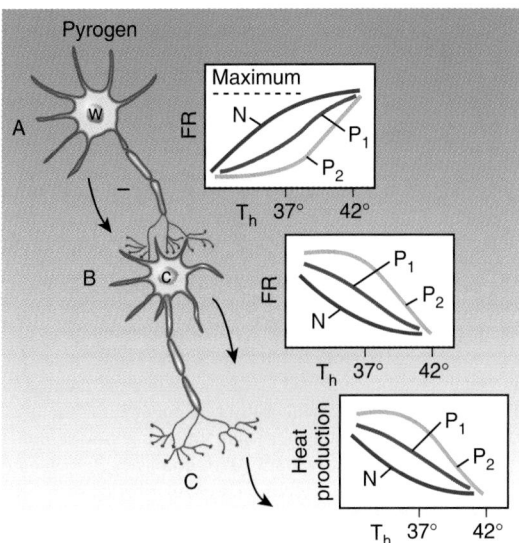

FIGURE 47-5. Model showing responses (**A** and **B**) of neuronal firing rates (FR) in the preoptic region and anterior hypothalamus and whole-body metabolic heat production (**C**) during changes in hypothalamic temperature (T_h). Thermosensitivity is reflected by the slope of each plot. The letters inside the cells indicate a warm-sensitive (w) neuron and a cold-sensitive (c) neuron. With increases in T_h, warm-sensitive neurons raise their FRs, and heat production decreases. Pyrogens inhibit (−) the FRs of warm-sensitive neurons, thereby resulting in accelerated FRs of cold-sensitive neurons and increased heat production. The plots show FR and heat production responses during normal conditions in the absence of pyrogens (N) and in the presence of low concentrations (P_1) and high concentrations (P_2) of pyrogens. *(From Mackowiak PA, Boulant JA. Fever's glass ceiling. Clin Infect Dis. 1996;22:525-536.)*

Thyrotropin-releasing hormone,[144] gastric-inhibitory peptide,[145] neuropeptide Y,[146] nitric oxide,[147] carbon monoxide,[148] and bombesin[149] likewise exhibit cryogenic properties under certain conditions. Of these, bombesin has exhibited the highest potency, in that it consistently produces hypothermia associated with changes in heat dissipation and heat production when injected into the preoptic area or anterior hypothalamus of conscious goats and rabbits.[149-151] Bombesin is believed to exert its hypothermic effect by decreasing the sensitivity of warm-sensitive neurons.[151]

Pyrogenic cytokines, the mediators of the febrile response, might themselves have a role in determining fever's upper limit. There is, for instance, experimental evidence indicating that under certain conditions (e.g., with intracerebral injection of recombinant human TNF-α in Zucker rats), TNF-α acts to lower, rather than to raise, body temperature,[152,153] although only in the presence of LPS. Thus, it is possible that at certain concentrations or in the appropriate physiologic milieu, pyrogenic cytokines function paradoxically as endogenous cryogens.

A growing body of literature indicates that the release of pyrogenic cytokines such as IL-1 is followed by increased shedding of soluble receptors for such cytokines, which function as endogenous scavengers of these pyrogens.[154] In the case of IL-1, a 22- to 25-kDa molecule identified in supernates of human monocytes blocks binding of IL-1 to its receptors.[155] The IL-1 receptor antagonist is structurally related to IL-1α and IL-1β[156] and binds to both type I and type II receptors on various target cells without inducing a specific biologic response.[157,158] Shedding of soluble receptors of TNF-α that bind to circulating TNF-α and thereby inhibit binding to cell-associated receptors has also been described.[159-163] The precise biologic function of such circulating receptor antagonists and soluble receptors is not known. However, it is possible that one function is to serve as a natural braking system for the febrile response.

RISK-TO-BENEFIT CONSIDERATIONS

Questions concerning fever's risk-to-benefit quotient have generated considerable controversy.[164] The controversy arises because of data indicating both potentiating and inhibitory effects of the response on resistance to infection. As a result, there is as yet no consensus as to the appropriate clinical situations (if any) in which fever or its mediators should be suppressed.

Data illustrating fever's beneficial effects originate from several sources. Studies of the phylogeny of fever have shown the response to be widespread within the animal kingdom.[165] With few exceptions, mammals, reptiles, amphibians, and fish, as well as several invertebrate species, have been shown to elevate the core temperature in response to a challenge with microorganisms or other known pyrogens (Fig. 47-6). It has been assumed, although not established conclusively, that such elevations in temperature are the poikilothermic corollary of fever. The prevalence of such "febrile responses" has been offered as some of the strongest evidence that fever is an adaptive response, on the basis of the argument that the metabolically expensive increase in body temperature that accompanies the febrile response would not have evolved and been so faithfully preserved in the animal kingdom unless fever had some net benefit to the host.

Further evidence of fever's beneficial effects can be found in numerous investigations demonstrating enhanced resistance of animals to infection with increases in body temperature within the physiologic range.[165] In classic studies involving experimental infection of the reptile *Dipsosaurus dorsalis* with *Aeromonas hydrophila,* Kluger and associates demonstrated a direct correlation between body temperature and survival.[166,167] They also showed in their model that suppression of the febrile response with sodium salicylate is associated with a substantial increase in mortality.[167] Covert and Reynolds corroborated these findings in an experimental model involving goldfish.[168]

In mammalian experimental models, increasing the body temperature by artificial means has been reported to enhance the resistance of mice to herpes simplex virus,[169] poliovirus,[170] Coxsackie B virus,[171] rabies virus,[172] and *Cryptococcus neoformans*[173] but to decrease resistance to *Streptococcus pneumoniae*.[174] Increased resistance of rabbits to *S. pneumoniae*[175] and *C. neoformans,*[176] dogs to herpesvirus,[177] piglets to gastroenteritis virus,[178] and ferrets to influenza virus[179] has also been observed after the induction of artificial fever. Unfortunately, because raising the body temperature by artificial means does not duplicate the physiologic alterations that occur during fever in homeotherms (and, indeed, entails a number of opposite physiologic responses[180]), data obtained using mammalian experimental models must be interpreted with caution when used to understand the febrile response.

Clinical data supporting an adaptive role for fever have accumulated slowly. Like animal data, clinical data include evidence of both beneficial effects of fever and adverse effects of antipyretics on the outcome of infections. In a retrospective analysis of 218 patients with gram-negative bacteremia, Bryant and associates reported a positive correlation between maximal temperature on the day bacteremia was diagnosed and survival.[181] A similar relationship has been observed in patients with polymicrobial sepsis and mild (but not severe) underlying diseases.[182] In an examination of factors influencing the prognosis of spontaneous bacterial peritonitis, Weinstein and co-workers identified a positive correlation between a temperature reading of greater than 38° C (100.4° F) and survival.[183]

It has been reported that children with chickenpox who are treated with acetaminophen have a longer time to total crusting of lesions than placebo-treated controls.[184] Stanley and colleagues have reported that adults infected with rhinovirus exhibit more nasal viral shedding when they receive aspirin than when given placebo.[185] Furthermore, Graham and colleagues have reported a trend toward a longer duration of rhinovirus shedding in association with antipyretic therapy and have shown that the use of aspirin or acetaminophen is associated with suppression of the serum neutralizing antibody response and with increased nasal symptoms and signs.[186] A more recent, retrospective, observational

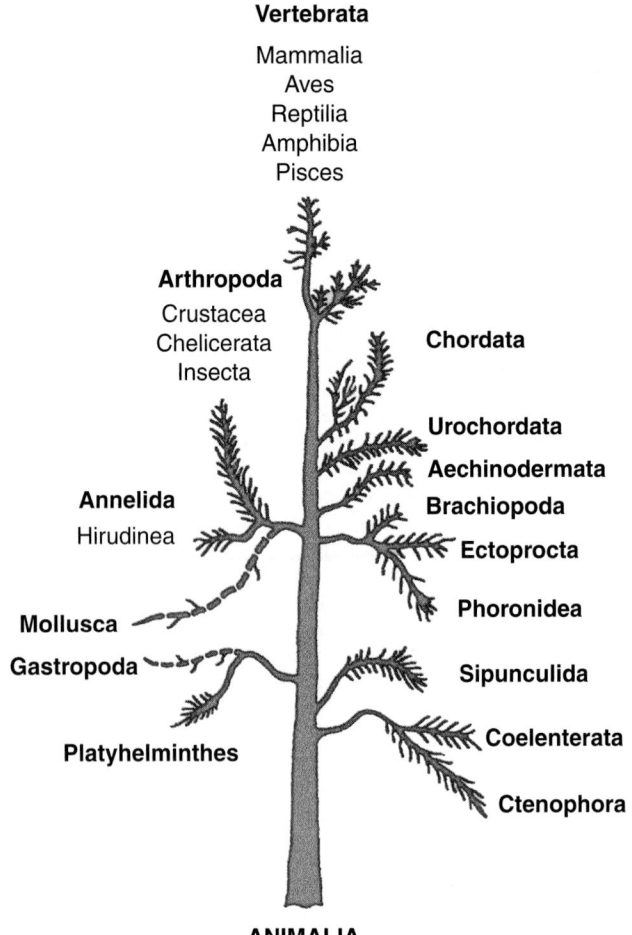

Vertebrata

Mammalia
Aves
Reptilia
Amphibia
Pisces

Arthropoda
Crustacea
Chelicerata
Insecta

Chordata

Urochordata

Aechinodermata

Annelida
Hirudinea

Brachiopoda

Ectoprocta

Phoronidea

Mollusca

Gastropoda

Sipunculida

Coelenterata

Platyhelminthes

Ctenophora

ANIMALIA

FIGURE 47-6. Evolutionary tree of animals. A febrile response has been documented in the Vertebrata, Arthropoda, and Annelida. These observations suggest that the febrile response evolved more than 400,000,000 years ago at about the time evolutionary lines leading to arthropods and annelids diverged.

analysis of studies of human volunteers infected with influenza A found a relationship between antipyretic therapy and prolonged illness.[187] These data, like those reviewed in the preceding paragraph, are subject to several interpretations and do not prove a causal relationship between fever and improved prognosis during infection. Nevertheless, they are consistent with such a relationship and when considered in concert with the phylogeny of the febrile response and the animal data summarized earlier, constitute strong circumstantial evidence that fever is an adaptive response in most situations.

Whereas many of the foregoing investigations examined the relationship between the elevation of the core temperature and the outcome of infection, others have considered the endogenous mediators of the febrile response. In such studies, all of the principal pyrogenic cytokines have been shown to have immune-potentiating capabilities, which might theoretically enhance resistance to infection.[93,188] In vitro and in vivo investigations of these cytokines have provided evidence of a protective effect of IFN, TNF-α, or IL-1, or all of these, against *Plasmodium*,[189-191] *Toxoplasma gondii*,[192] *Leishmania major*,[193] *Trypanosoma cruzi*,[194] and *Cryptosporidium*.[195]

Several reports have also shown enhancement of resistance to viral[196-198] and bacterial infections[199,200] by pyrogenic cytokines. Treatment of normal and granulocytopenic animals with IL-1 has been shown to prevent death in some gram-positive and gram-negative bacterial infections.[200] However, IL-1 is effective only if administered an

appreciable time (e.g., 24 hours) before the initiation of infections having rapidly fatal courses. In less acute infections, IL-1 administration can be delayed until shortly after the infectious challenge. Such observations suggest that those physiologic effects of the febrile response that enhance resistance to infection might be limited to localized infections or systemic infections of only mild to moderate severity.

The febrile response's potential for harm is reflected in a recent flurry of reports suggesting that IL-1, TNF-α, IL-6, and IFN mediate the physiologic abnormalities of certain infections. Although proof of an adverse effect of fever on the clinical outcome of these infections has yet to be established, the implication is that if pyrogenic cytokines contribute to the pathophysiologic burden of infections, both the mediators themselves and the febrile response are potentially deleterious.

The most persuasive evidence in this regard derives from studies of gram-negative bacterial sepsis.[201] It has long been suspected that bacterial LPS is involved in the pathophysiology of the syndrome. Purified LPS induces a spectrum of physiologic abnormalities that are similar to those occurring in patients with gram-negative bacterial sepsis. In experimental animals, challenge with LPS causes TNF-α and IL-1 to be released into the blood stream coincident with the appearance of signs of sepsis.[202] Furthermore, patients with the septic syndrome have detectable levels of circulatory TNF-α, IL-1, and IL-6 independent of culture-documented infection, and such levels correlate inversely with survival.[203] IL-1, alone or in combination with other cytokines, induces many of the same physiologic abnormalities (e.g., fever, hypoglycemia, shock, and death) seen after the administration of purified LPS.[204] In a murine experimental model for septic shock, IFN administered before or as long as 4 hours after LPS challenge increases mortality, whereas pretreatment with anti-IFN antibody significantly reduces mortality.[205] In several investigations, the adverse effects of gram-negative bacterial sepsis or LPS injections, or both, have been attenuated by pretreating experimental animals with IL-1 antagonists[206,207] and monoclonal antibodies directed against TNF-α.[208,209] Furthermore, animals rendered tolerant to TNF-α by repeated injections of the recombinant cytokine are protected against the hypotension, hypothermia, and lethality of gram-negative bacterial sepsis.[210]

The theory derived from these observations, that death from sepsis is the consequence of cytokine-mediated overstimulation of the immune system, unfortunately correlates only loosely with the clinical picture in humans, most likely because the studies cited here used large doses of endotoxin or bacteria that induced levels of circulating pyrogenic cytokines exponentially higher than those detected in patients with sepsis.[211] Thus, the "cytokine storm" created in such animals most likely has only limited relevance for human sepsis. This perhaps explains why in clinical trials, inhibition of pyrogenic cytokines in septic patients has had only modest success, improving outcome in patients with a high risk for death but not those with a low risk.[212]

ANTIPYRETIC THERAPY

Although clinicians have long had at their disposal effective means of lowering the core temperature in febrile patients, the actual benefit of such reductions in temperature is still uncertain. Moreover, it has yet to be shown in humans that increases in the core temperature encountered during fever are harmful per se. Certainly, during the course of heat stroke and other forms of hyperthermia, the core temperature can, and frequently does, rise to levels that are inherently harmful.[213] However, as discussed previously, such levels are almost never reached during fever's regulated rise in temperature, which probably never exceeds 41° C (105.8° F) in humans.[125] Nevertheless, whereas healthy volunteers have been reported to withstand core temperatures of 42° C (107.6° F) for periods of as long as 4 hours without apparent ill effect,[214] the possibility remains that in certain patients, even the relatively modest increases in core temperature encountered during fever are deleterious and should therefore be suppressed.

One such category of patients includes children—primarily between the ages of 3 months and 5 years. In such children, seizures have been reported to occur during episodes of fever at a frequency of as high as 14% in selected populations.[215] Although most children with febrile seizures have temperatures of 39° C (102.2° F) or more at the time of their seizure,[216] many tolerate even higher fevers at later dates without convulsing.[217] Unfortunately, antipyretic therapy has not been shown to protect against recurrences of febrile seizures in the few controlled trials conducted thus far (see later).[218]

It has also been suggested that patients with underlying cardiovascular or pulmonary disorders might be especially susceptible to the adverse effects of fever, because of metabolic demands imposed by the elevated temperature.[219] Such demands are particularly high during the chill phase if shivering is present, as evidenced by increases in the sympathetic tone,[180] oxygen consumption, respiratory minute volume, and respiratory quotient.[220] As a result of the associated increase in metabolic demand, the chill phase of fever might be expected to add to the burden of cardiac or pulmonary disorders. Although this possibility has been offered as justification for antipyretic therapy in patients with these disorders, the risk-to-benefit ratio of such therapy has yet to be determined.

Antipyretic therapy might also be justified, at least in theory, if fever's metabolic cost exceeded its physiologic benefit, if the treatment provided symptomatic relief without adversely affecting the course of the febrile illness, or if the toxicologic costs (side effects) of the antipyretic regimen were appreciably lower than its beneficial effects. Unfortunately, although clinicians have long argued the validity of each of these propositions as justification for antipyretic therapy, few scientific data exist to support any of these arguments.

Antipyretic drugs can be grouped into three general categories on the basis of their mechanisms of action. These include corticosteroids, aspirin and the other nonsteroidal anti-inflammatory drugs (NSAIDs), and acetaminophen. Each exerts its effects at different points in the febrile response pathway.

Although not generally used for antipyresis, corticosteroids suppress fever through both direct and indirect mechanisms. They block the transcription of pyrogenic cytokines and inducible cyclooxygenase via interactions involving the glucocorticoid receptor.[82,221] They downregulate the synthesis of cytokine receptors,[211] and by inducing lipocortin-1, they secondarily inhibit the activity of phospholipase A_2, a critical enzyme in the prostaglandin synthetic pathway.[221]

Acetaminophen and aspirin and the other NSAIDs all block the conversion of arachidonic acid to prostaglandins such as PGE_2 by inhibiting cyclooxygenase (COX, also known as prostaglandin GH synthetase).[221] This effect is thought to be critical to their antipyretic activity, in that production of PGE_2 at key sites within the hypothalamus is widely regarded as a crucial step in the process by which the physiologic cascade responsible for raising the core temperature during the febrile response is activated (see Fig. 47-4).[222] Cyclooxygenase has at least two distinct isoforms: a constitutive isoform, COX-1, and a predominantly inducible isoform, COX-2, which is undetectable in most resting cells. A third isoform, COX-3, has recently been identified.[223] It is a COX-1 variant selectively inhibited by antipyretic drugs such as acetaminophen, phenacetin, antipyrine, and dipyrone. Although it has been suggested that COX-3 could be the primary site of action of these drugs, their inhibitory effect is both nonspecific and weak.[224] COX-1 initiates production of prostacyclin, which has both antithrombogenic and cytoprotective properties, whereas COX-2 is a principal mediator of fever and the inflammatory response. The anti-inflammatory action of NSAIDs is believed to result from inhibition of COX-2, and the unwanted adverse effects, such as gastric irritation, from inhibition of COX-1.[225]

The structure and catalytic activity of the COX-1 and -2 isoforms are similar, with approximately 600 amino acids, of which 63% are in identical sequence, and active sites located at the apex of a long, narrow, hydrophobic channel. The amino acids forming the channel, as well as catalytic sites and neighboring residues, are identical in the two isoforms with two exceptions. Valine in COX-1 is substituted for isoleucine at positions 434 and 523 in COX-2. Aspirin acetylates serine 530 of both isoforms. In COX-1, this blocks access of arachidonic acid to the catalytic site, causing irreversible inhibition of the enzyme.

Because of the wider hydrophobic channel of COX-2, access of arachidonic acid to the active site persists after acetylation of serine 530 by aspirin.[225]

Physical Methods of Antipyresis

A variety of physical techniques are used to cool febrile patients. These include sponging with various solutions (e.g., tepid water or alcohol), the application of ice packs or cooling blankets, and exposure to circulating fans (most often in conjunction with sponging). With the latter method, helox (80% helium, 20% oxygen) has been shown to be superior to air in lowering core temperature, at least in experimental animals, because of the greater thermal conductivity of helium compared with that of nitrogen.[226] In contrast to antipyretic drugs, external cooling lowers the temperature of febrile patients by overwhelming effector mechanisms that have been evoked by an elevated thermoregulatory setpoint, rather than by lowering that setpoint. Therefore, unless concomitant antipyretic agents are used, or shivering is inhibited by other pharmacologic means, external cooling is vigorously opposed in the febrile patient by thermoregulatory mechanisms endeavoring to maintain the elevated body temperature.

Physical methods of antipyresis promote heat loss by conduction, convection, and evaporation. Evaporative methods have traditionally been touted as the most effective physical means of promoting heat loss in febrile patients, because such methods are deemed to be least likely to induce shivering.[227] However, carefully designed comparative trials have not yet established any one physical method of antipyresis as superior.

Direct comparisons of pharmacologic and physical methods of antipyresis are, likewise, all but nonexistent. In the only extant controlled study, Wenzel and Werner reported that salicylates reduced the second phase of endotoxin-induced fever in rabbits, whereas abdominal cooling increased heat production and did not lower the core temperature unless the animals were simultaneously exposed to environmental hyperthermia.[228] Neither antipyretic modality abolished the initial febrile response.

The few available clinical studies of the efficacy of physical methods of antipyresis have differed in their conclusions. Interpretation of the results of these studies has been difficult, because pharmacologic agents have almost invariably been administered concomitantly with external cooling. Steele and co-workers found acetaminophen (in age-adjusted dosages ranging from 80 to 320 mg) and sponging to be equally effective in lowering fever in children admitted to a pediatric hospital because of fever.[229] However, when combined, the two modalities produced more rapid cooling than either alone. By contrast, Newman found that tepid-water sponging in combination with acetaminophen (5 to 10 mg/kg) was no more effective than acetaminophen alone in lowering the temperature of febrile children.[230] O'Donnell and colleagues have concluded that in adults, although hypothermia blanket therapy adds little to the action of pharmacologic agents in lowering temperature, it induces wider temperature fluctuations and more episodes of rebound hyperthermia.[227]

Diagnostic Considerations

Numerous investigators have observed a direct correlation between the height of fevers and the rate of serious bacterial infections in children, with the maximal incidence of such infections at temperatures in excess of 40° C (104° F).[231-234] It has also been suggested that the response of a fever to antipyretic therapy might have diagnostic implications, in that a drop in temperature or improvement in the appearance of a febrile child, or both, generally indicates that the fever is not the result of a serious illness.[235] This conclusion, however, is not supported by numerous investigations comparing the temperature response of bacteremic and nonbacteremic infections to antipyretic therapy in children.[236-241]

Several studies have suggested that an antipyretic response to NSAIDs can distinguish fevers of infectious origin from those due to cancer by virtue of the fact that the latter fevers are more readily suppressed by such agents. Naproxen was the first such agent to be studied in this regard.[242] Subsequent randomized comparisons have shown naproxen, indomethacin, and diclofenac to be equally effective in inhibiting cancer-induced fever,[243] although the sensitivity and specificity of the "naproxen test" for differentiating neoplastic from infectious fevers are not yet known. Moreover, there is no physiologic rationale to explain why NSAIDs might be more effective in reducing fever due to cancer than that due to infection.

Benefits versus Risks

Two critical assumptions are made when prescribing antipyretic therapy. One is that fever is, at least in part, noxious, and the other is that suppressing fever will reduce if not eliminate fever's noxious effects. Neither assumption has been validated experimentally. In fact, there is considerable evidence that fever is an important defense mechanism that contributes to the host's ability to resist infection.[244] However, even if fever (or its mediators) does adversely affect the course of certain disorders, as for example bacterial sepsis,[164] it does not necessarily follow that inhibiting fever using current modes of antipyretic therapy will obviate this effect, especially if such therapy has intrinsic toxicity of its own.

One of the reasons commonly given to justify suppressing fever is that the metabolic cost of fever exceeds its clinical benefit. In fact, the metabolic cost of fever is substantial, especially during the chill phase of the response with its shivering-induced increase in metabolic rate, norepinephrine-mediated peripheral vasoconstriction, and increased arterial blood pressure.[180] Because of the potential adverse consequences of these metabolic effects on cardiovascular and pulmonary function, fever has been attacked with particular vigor in patients with underlying cardiovascular and pulmonary diseases.[245] Although antipyretic therapy has theoretical merit in this regard (if it does not induce shivering[246]), the detrimental effects of fever and the salutary effects of antipyretic therapy have yet to be critically evaluated.

External cooling, which is widely used in critically ill patients to suppress fevers unresponsive to antipyretic drugs, has been shown to decrease oxygen consumption by as much as 20% if shivering is prevented by therapeutic paralysis.[246] If shivering is not inhibited, external cooling causes a rise, rather than a fall, in oxygen consumption.[246] Perhaps more important to febrile patients with underlying cardiovascular disease, external cooling has the capacity to cause vasospasm of diseased coronary arteries by inducing a cold pressor response.[247,248] For all these reasons, it has been suggested that a more rational strategy for treating fevers unresponsive to antipyretic drugs is to *warm* rather than to *cool* selected skin surfaces, thereby reducing the vasoconstriction and shivering thresholds dictated by the elevated hypothalamic thermal setpoint and, in turn, effecting a decrease in the core temperature.[249]

Unfortunately, certain antipyretic drugs also appear to cause coronary vasoconstriction in patients with coronary artery disease. Friedman and associates observed significant increases in the mean arterial pressure, coronary vascular resistance, and myocardial arteriovenous oxygen difference after intravenous indomethacin (0.5 mg/kg) in such patients.[250] Coronary blood flow decreased simultaneously from 181 ± 29 to 111 ± 14 mL/min ($P < .05$). Thus, in this investigation, myocardial oxygen demand increased in the face of a fall in coronary blood flow after indomethacin administration. The authors believe that indomethacin's vasoconstrictor effect most likely derives from to its capacity to block the synthesis of vasodilatory prostaglandins. Perhaps even more disturbing are recent reports suggesting that compared to other nonsteroidal anti-inflammatory drugs, COX-2–selective NSAIDS seem to increase the risk for cardiovascular thrombotic events in patients not taking aspirin.[251]

Antipyretic therapy is also commonly administered to enhance patient comfort.[245] General experience with antipyretic drugs, which are for the most part also analgesic agents, seems to support this contention. However, carefully controlled efficacy studies have not yet established the validity of this contention. Moreover, the relative cost of such symptomatic relief, in terms of drug toxicity and adverse effects of antipyretic agents on the course of the illness responsible for the fever, have never been determined. The importance of such information is underscored by reports that acetaminophen prolongs the time to crusting of lesions in children with chickenpox,[184] that both acetaminophen and aspirin increase viral shedding and nasal signs and symptoms while suppressing the serum neutralizing antibody response in adults with rhinovirus infections,[185,186] and that antipyretic drugs might prolong the course of influenza A infections.[187]

Antipyretic therapy is also occasionally given to prevent febrile seizures in children, and to prevent or to reverse fever-induced mental dysfunction in frail older patients. Beisel and co-workers have shown that aspirin (in combination with propoxyphene) ameliorates fever-induced decrements in mental work performance in young volunteers infected with sand fly fever virus, even in the face of only partial relief of either the fever or other symptoms of the illness.[252] In view of these observations, antipyretic therapy might be expected to have a beneficial effect on fever-induced mental dysfunction in frail older patients. However, studies designed to test this hypothesis have not yet been reported.

Unfortunately, antipyretic therapy does not appear to be effective in preventing febrile seizures.[218] Camfield and colleagues conducted a randomized double-blind study comparing single-daily-dose phenobarbital plus antipyretic instruction to placebo plus antipyretic instruction to prevent recurrent seizure after an initial simple febrile seizure.[253] In children treated with both phenobarbital and antipyretics, the febrile seizure recurrence rate was 5%, whereas in those given placebo with antipyretics, the rate was 25%, suggesting that a single daily 5 mg/kg dose of phenobarbital is more effective than counseling parents about antipyretic therapy in preventing recurrent febrile seizures. More recently, acetaminophen has been given to children with fever as prophylaxis against febrile seizure recurrences. Whether given in moderate dosage (10 mg/kg dose four times a day)[254] or in relatively high doses (15 to 20 mg/kg dose every 4 hours),[255] acetaminophen failed to reduce the rate of febrile seizure recurrence.

Finally, there has been mounting interest in the use of certain antipyretic drugs to modulate the activity of pyrogenic cytokines during bacterial sepsis.[256] In some animal models of sepsis, antipyretic drugs that inhibit cyclooxygenase confer protection when given soon after bacterial challenge, presumably by blunting the adverse effects of TNF-α and IL-1. In a large clinical trial, Bernard and associates reported that 48 hours of intravenous therapy with the cyclooxygenase inhibitor ibuprofen lowered the core temperature, heart rate, oxygen consumption, and lactic acid blood levels but did not decrease the incidence of organ failure or mortality at 30 days.[257] In a more recent retrospective analysis of sepsis trials, Eichacker and co-workers could find evidence of a beneficial effect of antipyretic agents only in septic patients with a high risk for death (see above).[212] Thus, in spite of promising results obtained in some experimental models, antipyretic agents have been shown to be of only limited value clinically in the treatment of bacterial sepsis.

Indications

Although clinicians have resorted to various forms of antipyretic therapy since time immemorial, there is a dearth of scientific data concerning the actual benefits and relative risks of such treatments.[258] Nevertheless, several tentative conclusions regarding antipyretic therapy seem warranted in light of the limited data available. It is clear, for instance, that short courses of approved doses of standard antipyretic drugs carry a low risk for toxicity. Most of these drugs have analgesic as well as antipyretic properties. Therefore, if not otherwise contraindicated (e.g., aspirin in young children because of the risk for Reye's syndrome), such drugs can be prescribed to provide symptomatic relief in febrile patients, to reduce the metabolic demands of fever in patients with underlying cardiovascular and pulmonary disorders, and, possibly, to prevent or alleviate fever-induced mental dysfunction in older patients. To minimize antipyretic-induced fluctuations in temperature (as well as the risk for recurrent shivering with its associated increased metabolic demands), antipyretic agents should be administered to febrile patients at regular intervals that preclude abrupt recurrences of fever, rather than as needed for temperatures above some arbitrary level. Whenever such medications are prescribed, it should also be recognized that each carries its own risk for toxicity and might prolong the course of the illness responsible for the fever while reducing the intensity of its symptoms.

In view of the capacity of external cooling measures to induce a cold pressor response, it is questionable whether this form of antipyretic therapy should ever be administered to febrile patients (much less to intensive care unit patients for whom it is so frequently prescribed). If external cooling is used to treat fever, care must be taken to prevent shivering, because of its associated increased oxygen consumption. Unfortunately, even if shivering is prevented, there is no guarantee that a cold pressor response will be averted. In view of indomethacin's capacity to cause coronary vasoconstriction in patients with coronary artery disease and the possible increased risk for cardiovascular thrombotic events associated with COX-2–selective NSAIDs should be used cautiously to suppress fever in such patients.

REFERENCES

1. Majno G. The Healing Hand: Man and Wound in the Ancient World. Cambridge, MA: Harvard University Press; 1975:57.
2. Galen. Opera omnia. In: Siegel RE, ed. Galen's System of Physiology and Medicine, v. 11. New York: Krager; 1968.
3. Atkins E. Fever: Its history, cause and function. Yale J Biol Med. 1982;55:283-287.
4. Berger RL, Clem TR, Harden VA, Mangum BW. Historical development and newer means of temperature measurements in biochemistry. Methods Biochem Anal. 1984;30:269-331.
5. Bolton HC. Evolution of the Thermometer 1592-1743. Easton, PA: Chemical; 1900:18, 98.
6. Wunderlich C. Das Verhalten der Eigenwärme in Krankenheiten. Leipzig: Otto Wigard; 1868.
7. Mackowiak PA, Worden G. Carl Reinhold August Wunderlich and the evolution of clinical thermometry. Clin Infect Dis. 1994;18:458-467.
8. Mackowiak PA, Wasserman SS, Levine MM. A critical appraisal of 98.6° F, the upper limit of the normal body temperature, and other legacies of Carl Reinhold August Wunderlich. JAMA. 1992;268:1578-1580.
9. IUPS Commission for Thermal Physiology. Glossary of terms for thermal physiology. 3rd ed. Japanese J Physiol. 2001;51:245-280.
10. Abbey JC, Anderson AS, Close EL, et al. How long is that thermometer accurate? Am J Nurs. 1978;78:1375-1376.
11. Erickson RS. Thermometer placement for oral temperature measurement in febrile adults. Int J Nurs Stud. 1976;13:199-208.
12. Mead J, Bonmarito L. Reliability of rectal temperatures as an index of internal body temperature. J Appl Physiol. 1949;2:97-109.
13. Abrams RM, Royston JP. Some properties of rectum and vagina as sites for basal body temperature measurement. Fertil Steril. 1981;35:313-316.
14. Middleton D. Nursing 1. Oxford: Blackwell Scientific; 1983:43-45.
15. Nichols GA, Ruskin MM, Glor BAK, Kelly WH. Oral, axillary and rectal temperature determinations and relationships. Nurs Res. 1966;15:307-310.
16. Nichols GA, Kucha DH. Oral measurements. Am J Nurs. 1972;72:1091-1093.
17. Benzinger M, Benzinger TH. National Bureau of Standards Fifth Symposium on Temperature. Pittsburgh, PA: Instrument Society of America; 1971:2080-2102.
18. Blainey CG. Site selection in taking body temperature. Am J Nurs. 1974;74:1859-1861.
19. Lorin MI. Measurement of body temperature. Semin Pediatr Infect Dis. 1993;4:4-8.
20. Buck SH, Zaritsky AL. Occult core hyperthermia complicating cardiogenic shock. Pediatrics. 1989;83:782-783.
21. Houdas Y, Ring EFJ. Human body temperature. New York: Plenum; 1982:57-141.
22. Mayfield SR, Bhatia J, Nakamura KT, et al. Temperature measurement in term and preterm neonates. J Pediatr. 1984;104:271-275.
23. Fonkalsrud E, Clathworthy HW. Accidental perforation of the colon and rectum in newborn infants. N Engl J Med. 1965;272:1097-1100.
24. Horwitz MA, Bennett JV. Nursery outbreak of peritonitis with pneumoperitonium probably caused by thermometer induced perforation. Am J Epidemiol. 1976;104:632-644.
25. McAllister TA, Roud JA, Marshall A, et al. Outbreak of *Salmonella eimsbuettel* in newborn infants spread by rectal thermometers. Lancet. 1986;1:1262-1264.
26. Rabinowitz RP, Cookson ST, Wasserman SS, Mackowiak PA. Effects of anatomic site, oral stimulation and body position on estimates of body temperature. Arch Intern Med. 1996;156:777-780.
27. Tandberg D, Sklar D. Effect of tachypnea on the estimation of body temperature by an oral thermometer. N Engl J Med. 1983;308:945-946.
28. Neff J, Ayoub J, Longman A, Noyes A. Effect of respiratory rate, respiratory depth, and open versus closed mouth breathing on sublingual temperature. Res Nurs Health. 1989;12:195-202.
29. Klein DG, Mitchell C, Petrinec A, et al. A comparison of pulmonary artery, rectal, and tympanic membrane temperature measurements in the ICU. Heart Lung. 1993;22:435-441.
30. Erickson RA, Kirklin SK. Comparison of ear-based, bladder, oral and axillary methods for core temperature measurement. Crit Care Med. 1993;21:1528-1534.
31. Giuliano KK, Scott SS, Elliot S, Giuliano AJ. Temperature measurements in critically ill orally intubated adults: A comparison of pulmonary artery core, tympanic, and oral methods. Crit Care Med. 1999;27:2188-2193.
32. Modell JG, Katnoli CR, Kumaramanmgalam SM, et al. Unreliability of the infrared tympanic thermometer in clinical practice: A comparative study with oral mercury and oral electronic thermometers. South Med J. 1998;91:649-654.
33. Peterson-Smith A, Barber N, Coody DK, et al. Comparison of aural infrared with traditional rectal temperatures in children from birth to age three years. J Pediatr. 1994;125:83-85.
34. Buntain WI, Pregler M, O'Brien PC, et al. Axillary versus rectal temperature: A comparative study. J Louisiana State Med Soc. 1977;129:5-8.
35. Schiffman RF. Temperature monitoring in the neonate: A comparison of axillary and rectal temperatures. Nurs Res. 1982;31:274-277.
36. Loudon ISL. On taking the temperature in the mouth and axilla. Lancet. 1957;268:233-235.
37. Nichols GA, Kulvi RL, Life HR, et al. Measuring oral and rectal temperatures of febrile children. Nurs Res. 1972;21:261-264.
38. Ogren JM. The inaccuracy of axillary temperatures measured with an electronic thermometer. Am J Dis Child. 1990;144:109-111.
39. Reisinger KS, Kao J, Grant DM. Inaccuracy of the Clinitemp skin thermometer. Pediatrics. 1979;64:4-6.
40. Scholefield JH, Gerber MA, Dwyer P. Liquid crystal forehead temperature strips. Am J Dis Child. 1982;136:198-201.
41. Bergeson PS, Stienfeld HJ. How dependable is palpation as a screening method for fever? Clin Pediatr. 1974;13:350-351.
42. Banco L, Veltri D. Ability of mothers to subjectively assess the presence of fever in their children. Am J Dis Child. 1984;138:976-978.
43. Bonadio WA, Hegenbarth M, Zachariason M. Correlating reported fever in young infants with subsequent temperature patterns and rate of serious bacterial infections. Pediatr Infect Dis J. 1990;9:158-160.
44. Linder FE, Carmichael HY. A biometric study of the relation between oral and rectal temperatures in normal and schizophrenic subjects. Hum Biol. 1935;7:24-46.
45. Tanner JM. The relationship between the frequency of the heart, oral temperature and rectal temperature in man at rest. J Physiol. 1951;115:391-409.
46. Togawa T. Body temperature measurement. Clin Phys Physiol Meas. 1985;6:83-108.
47. Anagnostakis D, Matsaniotis N, Grafakos S, Sarafidou E. Rectal-axillary temperature difference in febrile and afebrile infants and children. Clin Pediatr. 1993;32:268-272.
48. Wunderlich KRA, Seguin E. Medical Thermometry and Human Temperature. New York: William Wood; 1871.
49. Howell TH. Normal temperature in old age. Lancet. 1948;1:517-518.
50. Weitzman ED, Moline ML, Czeisler CA, Zimmerman JC. Chronobiology of aging: Temperature, sleep-wake rhythms, and entrainment. Neurobiol Aging. 1982;3:299-309.
51. Jones SR. Fever in the elderly. In: Mackowiak PA, ed. Fever: Basic Mechanisms and Management. New York: Raven Press; 1991:233-242.
52. Dinarello CA, Wolff SM. Pathogenesis of fever in man. N Engl J Med. 1978;298:607-612.
53. Stephenson LA. Circadian timekeeping. In: Mackowiak PA, ed. Fever, Basic Mechanisms and Management. 2nd ed. Philadelphia: Lippincott-Raven; 1997:59-77.
54. Avery DH, Shah SH, Eder DN, Wildschiodtz G. Nocturnal sweating and temperature in depression. Acta Psychiatric Scand. 199;100:295-301.
55. Webb P. Daily activity and body temperature. Eur J Appl Physiol. 1993;66:174-177.
56. Okamoto-Mizuno K, Mizuno K, Michie S, et al. Effects of humid heat exposure on human sleep stages and body temperature. Sleep. 1999;22:767-773.
57. Cheng TL, Partridge JC. Effect of bundling and high environmental temperature on neonatal body temperature. Pediatrics. 1993;92:238-240.
58. Mackowiak PA, Wasserman SS. A study of physicians' perceptions of body temperature in health and disease. South Med J. 1995;88:934-938.
59. Horvath SM, Menduke H, Piersol GM. Oral and rectal temperatures of man. JAMA. 1950;144:1562-1565.
60. Wunderlich CA, Woodman WB. On the temperature in diseases: A manual of medical thermometry. London, England: New Sydenham Society; 1871:71.
61. Hensyl WR, ed. Stedman's Medical Dictionary. 25th ed. Baltimore: Williams & Wilkins; 1990:574.
62. Stedman's Medical Dictionary. 27th ed. Philadelphia: Lippincott Williams & Wilkins; 2000:658.
63. Wunderlich CA, Reeve JC. The course of the temperature in diseases: A guide to clinical thermometry. Am J Med Sci. 1869;57:425-447.
64. Tauber MG. Fever of unknown origin. In: Stein JH, ed. Internal Medicine. 3rd ed. Boston: Little Brown; 1990:1240-1246.
65. Dominguez EA, Musher DM. Clinical thermometry. In: Mackowiak PA, ed. Fever: Basic Mechanisms and Management. New York: Raven Press; 1991:71-81.
66. Lyon DM. The relation of pulse-rate to temperature in febrile conditions. Q J Med. 1927;20:205-218.
67. Lorin MI. Fever: Pathogenesis and treatment. In: Feigin RD, Cherry JD, eds. Textbook of Pediatric Infectious Diseases. 4th ed. Philadelphia: Saunders; 1998:89.
68. Bayley N, Stolz HR. Maturational changes in rectal temperatures of 61 infants from 1 to 36 months. Child Dev. 1937;8:195-206.
69. Boulant JA. Thermoregulation. In: Mackowiak PA, ed. Fever. Basic Mechanisms and Management. 2nd ed. Philadelphia: Lippincott-Raven; 1997:35-58.
70. Bruck K. Heat balance and the regulation of body temperature. In: Schmidt RF, Thews G, eds. Human Physiology. Berlin: Springer-Verlag; 1983:531-547.
71. Stanier MW, Mount LE, Bligh J. Energy Balance and Temperature Regulation. Cambridge: Cambridge University Press, 1984.
72. Boulant JA. Hypothalamic control of thermoregulation: Neurophysiological basis. In: Morgane PJ, Pankepp J, eds. Handbook of the Hypothalamus, v. 3, pt A. New York: Marcel Dekker; 1980:1-82.

73. Schonung W, Wagner H, Jessen C, Simon E. Differentiation of cutaneous and intestinal blood flow during hypothalamic heating and cooling in anesthetized dogs. Pflugers Arch. 1971;328:145-154.

74. Boulant JA. Hypothalamic neurons regulating body temperature. In: Fregly MJ, Blatteis CM, eds. APS Handbook of Physiology, sect. 4: Environmental Physiology. New York: Oxford University Press; 1996:105-126.

75. Hammel HT, Jackson DC, Stolwijk JAJ, et al. Temperature regulation by hypothalamic proportional control with an adjustable set point. J Appl Physiol. 1963;18:1146-1154.

76. Hammel HT. Neurons and temperature regulation. In: Yamamoto WS, Brobeck JR, eds. Physiological Controls and Regulations. Philadelphia:WB Saunders; 1965:71-97.

77. Sawka MN, Wenger CB. Physiological responses to acute exercise-heat stress. In: Pandolf KB, Sawka MN, Gonzalez RR, eds. Human Performance Physiology and Environmental Medicine at Terrestrial Extremes. Indianapolis: Benchmark; 1988:97-151.

78. Bligh J. Temperature Regulation in Mammals and Other Vertebrates. Amsterdam, North Holland; 1973.

79. Benzinger TH, Kitzinger C, Pratt AW. The human thermostat. In: Hardy JD, ed. Temperature—Its Measurement and Control in Science and Industry, v. 3, pt. 5: Biology and Medicine. New York: Reinhold; 1963:637-665.

80. Stitt JT. Prostaglandin E as the mediator of the febrile response. Yale J Biol Med. 1986;59:137-149.

81. Mitchell D, Laburn HP, Cooper KE, et al. Is prostaglandin E the neural mediator of the febrile response? The case against a proven obligatory role. Yale J Biol Med. 1986;59:159-168.

82. Dinarello CA. Cytokines as endogenous pyrogens. In: Mackowiak PA, ed. Fever: Basic Mechanisms and Management. 2nd ed. Philadelphia: Lippincott-Raven; 1997:87-116.

83. Mickenberg ID, Snyderman R, Root RK, et al. The relationship of complement consumption to immune fever. J Immunol. 1971;107:1466-1476.

84. Arend WP, Joslin FG, Massoni RJ. Effects of immune complexes on production by human monocytes of interleukin 1 or an interleukin 1 inhibitor. J Immunol. 1985; 134:3868-3875.

85. Dillard GM, Bodel P. Studies on steroid fever. II. Pyrogenic and anti-pyrogenic activity in vitro of some endogenous steroids of man. J Clin Invest. 1970;49:2418-2426.

86. Kappas A, Hellman L, Fukushima DK, Gallagher TF. The pyrogenic effect of etiocholanolone (Letter). J Clin Endocrinol Metab. 1957;17:451-453.

87. Wolff SM, Kimball HR, Perry S, et al. The biological properties of etiocholanolone. Ann Intern Med. 1967;67:1268-1295.

88. Bondy PK, Bodel P. Mechanism of action of pyrogenic and antipyretic steroids in vitro. In: Wolstenholme GEW, Birch J, eds. Pyrogens and Fever. Edinburgh: Churchill Livingstone; 1971:101-113.

89. Goodman MG, Chenoweth DE, Weigle WO. Induction of interleukin 1 secretion and enhancement of humoral immunity by binding of human C5a to macrophage surface C5a receptors. J Exp Med. 1982;156:912-917.

90. Bernheim HA, Block LH, Francis L, Atkins E. Release of endogenous pyrogen-activating factor from concanavalin A-stimulated human lymphocytes. J Exp Med. 1980;152:1811-1816.

91. Dinarello CA. Demonstration of a human pyrogen-inducing factor during mixed leukocyte reactions. J Exp Med. 1981;153:1215-1224.

92. Li Z, Blatteis CM. Fever onset is linked to the appearance of lipopolysaccharide in the liver. J Endotoxin Res. 2004;10:39-53.

93. Mackowiak PA, Barlett JG, Borden EC, et al. Fever: Recent advances and lingering dogma (Symposium Summary). Clin Infect Dis. 1997;25:119-138.

94. Kushner I, Rzewnicki DL. The acute phase response. In: Mackowiak PA, ed. Fever, Basic Mechanisms and Management. 2nd ed. Philadelphia: Lippincott-Raven; 1997;165-176.

95. Dinarello CA, Wolff SM. The role of interleukin-1 in disease. N Engl J Med. 1993;328:106-113.

96. Dinarello C. The interleukin-1 family: 10 years of discovery. FASEB J. 1994;8: 1314-1325.

97. Dinarello C. Interleukin-1. Adv Pharmacol. 1994;25:21-51.

98. Fiers W. Tumor necrosis factor: Characterization at the molecular, cellular and in vivo level. FEBS Lett. 1991;285:199-212.

99. Vassalli P. The pathophysiology of tumor necrosis factors. Annu Rev Immunol. 1992;10:411-452.

100. Tracey K, Cerami A. Tumor necrosis factor: A pleiotropic cytokine and therapeutic target. Annu Rev Med. 1994;45:491-503.

101. Brach M, Herrman F. Interleukin 6: Presence and future. Int J Clin Lab Res. 1992;22:143-151.

102. Lotz M. Interleukin-6. Cancer Invest. 1993;11:731-742.

103. Jones T. Interleukin-6, an endocrine cytokine. Clin Endocrinol. 1994;40:703-713.

104. Li S, Holers VM, Boackle SA, Blatteis CM. Modulation of mouse endotoxic fever by complement. Infect Immun. 2002;70:2519-2525.

105. Szekely M, Romanovsky AA. Pyretic and antipyretic signals within and without fever: A possible interplay. Med Hypotheses. 1998;50:213-218.

106. Mackowiak PA. Concepts of fever. Arch Intern Med. 1998;158:1870-1881.

107. Netea MG, Kullberg BJ, Van der Meer JWM. Do only circulating pyrogenic cytokines act as mediators in the febrile response? A hypothesis. Euro J Clin Invest. 199;29:351-356.

108. Gabay C, Kushner I. Acute-phase proteins and other systemic responses to inflammation. N Engl J Med. 1999;340:448-454.

109. Ernst E, Saradeth T, Achhammer G. ω-3 Fatty acids and acute-phase proteins. Eur J Clin Invest. 1991;21:77-82.

110. Joyce PR, Hawes CR, Mulder RT, et al. Elevated levels of acute phase plasma proteins in major depression. Biol Psychiatry. 1992;32:1035-1041.

111. Ganguli R, Yang Z, Shurin G, et al. Serum interleukin-6 concentration in schizophrenia: Elevation associated with duration of illness. Psychiatry Res. 1994;51:1-10.

112. LeMay LG, Vander AJ, Kluger MJ. The effects of psychological stress on plasma interleukin-6 activity in rats. Phys Behav. 1990;47:957-961.

113. Volanakis JE. Acute phase proteins. In: McCarty DJ, Koopman WJ, eds. Arthritis and Allied Conditions: A Textbook of Rheumatology. Malvern, PA: Lea & Febiger; 1993:469-477.

114. Ballou SP, Lozanski G. Induction of inflammatory cytokines release from cultured human monocytes by C-reactive protein. Cytokine. 1992;4:361-368.

115. Cermak J, Key NS, Bach RR, et al. C-reactive protein induces human peripheral blood monocytes to synthesize tissue factor. Blood. 1993;82:513-520.

116. Tilg H, Vannier E, Vachine G, et al. Antiinflammatory properties of hepatic acute phase proteins: Preferential induction of interleukin 1 (IL-1) receptor antagonist over IL-1β synthesis by human peripheral blood mononuclear cells. J Exp Med. 1993;178:1629-1636.

117. Dobrinich R, Spagnuolo PJ. Binding of C-reactive protein to human neutrophils: Inhibition of respiratory burst activity. Arthritis Rheum. 1991;34:1031-1038.

118. Ahmed N, Thorley R, Xia D, et al. Transgenic mice expressing rabbit C-reactive protein exhibit diminished chemotactic factor-induced alveolitis. Am J Respir Crit Care Med. 1996;153:1141-1147.

119. Xu L, Badolato R, Murphy WJ, et al. A novel biologic function of serum amyloid A-induction of T lymphocyte migration and adhesion. J Immunol. 1995;155:1184-1190.

120. Kisilevsky R, Subrahmanyan L. Serum amyloid A changes high density lipoprotein's cellular affinity. Lab Invest. 1992;66:778.

121. Berliner JA, Navab M, Fogelman AM, et al. Atherosclerosis: Basic mechanisms-oxidation, inflammation, and genetics. Circulation. 1995;91:2488-2496.

122. Wurfel MM, Monks BG, Ingalls RR, et al. Targeted deletion of the lipopolysaccharide (LPS)-binding protein gene leads to profound suppression of LPS responses ex vivo, whereas in vivo responses remain intact. J Exp Med. 1997;186:2051-2056.

123. May MT. Galen on the Usefulness of the Parts of the Body. Ithaca, NY: Cornell University Press; 1968:50-53.

124. DuBois EF. Why are fever temperatures over 106°F rare? Am J Med Sci. 1949;217:361-368.

125. Mackowiak PA, Boulant JA. Fever's glass ceiling. Clin Infect Dis. 1996;22:525-536.

126. Pittman QJ, Wilkinson MF. Central arginine vasopressin and endogenous antipyresis. Can J Physiol Pharmacol. 1992;70:786-790.

127. Pittman QJ, Poulin P, Wilkinson, MF. Role of neurohypophysial hormones in temperature regulation. Ann N Y Acad Sci. 1993;689:375-381.

128. Kasting N. Criteria for establishing a physiological role for brain peptides. A case in point: The role of vasopressin in thermoregulation during fever and antipyresis. Brain Res Rev. 1989;14:143-153.

129. Lipton JM. Disorders of temperature control. In: Rieder P, Kopp N, Pearson J. An Introduction to Neurotransmission in Health and Disease. Oxford, England: Oxford University Press; 1990:119-123.

130. Zeisberger E. The role of septal peptides in thermoregulation and fever. In: Bligh J, Voigt K, eds. Thermoreception and Temperature Regulation. Berlin: Springer-Verlag; 1990:273-283.

131. Glyn JR, Lipton JM. Hypothermic and antipyretic effects of centrally administered ACTH (−24) and α-melanotropin. Peptides. 1981;2:177-187.

132. Glyn-Ballinger JR, Bernardini GL, Lipton JM. α-MSH injected into the septal region reduces fever in rabbits. Peptides. 1983;4:199-203.

133. Lipton JM, Whisenant JD, Gean JT. Hypothermia produced by peripheral and central injections of chlorpromazine in aged rabbits. Brain Res Bull. 1979;4:297-300.

134. Murphy MT, Lipton JM. Peripheral administration of α-MSH reduces fever in older and younger rabbits. Peptides. 1982;13:775-779.

135. Murphy MT, Richard DB, Lipton JM. Antipyretic potency of centrally administered α-melanocyte stimulating hormone. Science. 1983;221:192-193.

136. Deeter LB, Martin LW, Lipton JM. Antipyretic effect of central alpha-MSH summates with that of acetaminophen or ibuprofen. Brain Res Bull. 1989;23:573-575.

137. Shih ST, Lipton JM, McCann SM. Central administration of α-MSH antiserum augments fever in the rabbit. Am J Physiol. 1986;250:R803-R808.

138. Morrow LE, McClellan JL, Conn CA, Kluger MJ. Glucocorticoids alter fever and IL-6 responses to psychological stress and to lipopolysaccharide. Am J Physiol. 1993;225:R151-R156.

139. Luedke CE, Cerami A. Interferon-gamma overcomes glucocorticoid suppression of cachectin/tumor necrosis factor biosynthesis by murine macrophages. J Clin Invest. 1990;86:1234-1240.

140. Nakano T, Ohara O, Teraoka H, Arita H. Glucocorticoids suppress group II phospholipase A₂ production by blocking mRNA synthesis and post-transcriptional expression. J Biol Chem. 1990;265:12745-12748.

141. Alexander DP, Bashore RA, Britton HG, Forsling MA. Maternal and fetal arginine vasopressin in the chronically catheterised sheep. Biol Neonate. 1974;25:242-248.

142. Carey F, Forder M, Edge D, et al. Lipocortin 1 fragment modifies pyrogenic actions of cytokines in rats. Am J Physiol. 1990;259:R266-R269.

143. Bernadini GL, Lipton JM, Clark WG. Intracerebroventricular and septal injections of arginine vasopressin are not antipyretic in the rabbit. Peptides. 1983;4:195-198.

144. Riedel W. Role of thyroid-stimulating hormone (TSH) in endogenous antipyresis and evidence of extrahypothalamic thyroid-stimulating neurons (TSN) in rabbits. Pflugers Arch 1987;408(Suppl):R49.

145. Bahendeka SK, Moor RE, Tomkin GH, Buchanan KD. Gastric inhibitory polypeptide, dietary-induced thermogenesis and obesity. Can J Physiol Pharmacol. 1987;65:1242-1247.

146. Stanley BG, Leibowitz SF. Neuropeptide Y. Stimulation of feeding and drinking by injection into the paraventricular nucleus. Life Sci. 1984;35:2635-2642.

147. Steiner AA, Colombari E, Branco LGS. Carbon monoxide as a novel mediator of the febrile response in the central nervous system. Am J Physiol. 1998;277:R499-R508.

148. Steiner AA, Branco LGS. Nitric acid in the regulation of body temperature and fever. J Therm Biol. 2001;26:325-330.

149. Jansky L, Vybiral S, Moravec J, et al. Neuropeptides and temperature regulation. J Therm Biol. 1986;11:79-83.

150. Schmid H, Pierau Fr-K. Long-term modulation of hypothalamic neurons by neuropeptides. In: Bligh J, Voigt K, eds. Thermoregulation and Temperature Regulation. Berlin, Germany: Springer-Verlag; 1990:53-63.

151. Gale CC, McCreery BR. Mechanism of bombesin hypothermia. Fed Proc. 1979;38:997.

152. Holt SJ, Grimble RF, York DA. Tumor necrosis factor-α and lymphotoxin have opposite effects on sympathetic efferent nerves to brown adipose tissue by direct action in the central nervous system. Brain Res. 1989;497:183-186.

153. Shih ST, Khorram O, Lipton JM, McCann SM. Central administration of α-MSH antiserum augments fever in the rabbit. Am J Physiol. 1986;250:R803-R806.

154. Sivo J, Salkowski CA, Politis AD, Vogel SN. Differential regulation of LPS-induced IL-1β and IL-1 receptor antagonist mRNA by IFNα and IFNγ in murine peritoneal macrophages. J Endotox Res. 1994;1:30-36.

155. Seckinger P, Lowenthal JW, Williamson K, et al. A urine inhibitor of interleukin-1 activity that blocks ligand binding. J Immunol. 1987;139:1546-1549.

156. Eisenberg SP, Brewer MT, Verderber E, et al. Interleukin-1 receptor antagonist is a member of the interleukin-1 gene family: Evolution of a cytokine control mechanism. Proc Natl Acad Sci U S A. 1991;88:5232-5236.

157. Dripps DJ, Brandhuber BJ, Thompson RC, Eisenberg SP. Interleukin-1 (IL-1) receptor antagonist binds to the 80-kDa IL-receptor but does not initiate IL-1 signal transduction. J Biol Chem. 1991;266:10331-10336.

158. Dripps DJ, Verderber E, Ng RK, et al. Interleukin-1 receptor antagonist binds to the type II interleukin-1 receptor on B cells and neutrophils. J Biol Chem. 1991;266:20311-20315.

159. Engelmann H, Aderka D, Rubinstein M, et al. A tumor necrosis factor binding protein purified to homogeneity from human urine protects cells from tumor necrosis factor toxicity. J Biol Chem. 1989;264:11974-11980.

160. Olsson I, Lantx M, Nilsson E, et al. Isolation and characterization of a tumor necrosis factor binding protein from urine. Eur J Haematol. 1989;42:270-275.

161. Engleman H, Novick D, Wallach D. Two tumor necrosis factor-binding proteins from human urine. J Biol Chem. 1990;265:1531-1536.

162. Brockhaus M, Schoenfeld HJ, Schlaeger EJ, et al. Identification of two types of tumor necrosis factor receptors on human cell lines by monoclonal antibodies. Proc Natl Acad Sci U S A. 1990;87:3127-3131.

163. Porteu F, Nathan C. Shedding of tumor necrosis factor receptors by activated human neutrophils. J Exp Med. 1990;172:599-607.

164. Mackowiak PA. Fever: Blessing or curse? A unifying hypothesis. Ann Intern Med. 1994;120:1037-1040.

165. Kluger MJ, Kozat W, Conn CA, et al. The adaptive value of fever. In: Mackowiak PA, ed. Fever: Basic Mechanisms and Management. 2nd ed. Philadelphia: Lippincott-Raven; 1997:255-266.

166. Kluger MJ, Ringler DH, Anver MR. Fever and survival. Science. 1975;188:166-168.

167. Bernheim HA, Kluger MJ. Fever: Effect of drug-induced antipyresis on survival. Science. 1976;193:237-239.

168. Covert JR, Reynolds WW. Survival value of fever in fish. Nature. 1977;267:43-45.

169. Schmidt JR, Rasmussen AF Jr. The influence of environmental temperature on the course of experimental herpes simplex infection. J Infect Dis. 1960;107:356-360.

170. Lwoff A. Factors influencing the evolution of viral diseases at the cellular level and in the organism. Bacteriol Rev. 1959;23:109-124.

171. Walker DL, Boring WD. Factors influencing host-virus interactions: III. Further studies on the alteration of Coxsackie virus infection in adult mice by environmental temperature. J Immunol. 1958;80:39-44.

172. Bell JF, Moore GJ. Effects of high ambient temperature on various stages of rabies virus infection in mice. Infect Immun. 1974;10:510-515.

173. Kuhn LR. Effect of elevated body temperature on Cryptococcus in mice. Proc Soc Exp Biol Med. 1949;71:341-343.

174. Eiseman B, Mallette WG, Wotkyns RS, et al. Prolonged hypothermia in experimental pneumococcal peritonitis. J Clin Invest. 1956;35:940-946.

175. Rich AR, McKee CM. The mechanism of a hitherto unexplained form of native immunity to the type III pneumococcus. Bull Johns Hopkins Hosp. 1936;59:171-207.

176. Kuhn LR. Growth and viability of Cryptococcus hominis at mouse and rabbit body temperatures. Proc Soc Exp Biol Med. 1939;41:573-574.

177. Carmichael LE, Barnes FD. Effect of temperature on growth of canine herpes virus in canine kidney cell and macrophage cultures. J Infect Dis. 1969;120:664-668.

178. Furuchi S, Shimizu Y. Effect of ambient temperatures on multiplication of attenuated transmissible gastroenteritis virus in the bodies of newborn piglets. Infect Immun. 1976;13:990-992.

179. Toms GL, Davies JA, Woodward CG, et al. The relation of pyrexia and nasal inflammatory response to virus levels in nasal washings of ferrets infected with influenza viruses of differing virulence. Br J Exp Pathol. 1977;588:444-458.

180. Greisman SE. Cardiovascular alterations during fever. In: Mackowiak PA, ed. Fever: Basic Mechanisms and Management. New York: Raven Press; 1991:143-165.

181. Bryant RE, Hood AF, Hood CE, Koenig MG. Factors affecting mortality of gram-negative rod bacteremia. Arch Intern Med. 1971;127:120-128.

182. Mackowiak PA, Browne RH, Southern PM Jr, Smith JW. Polymicrobial sepsis: Analysis of 184 cases using log linear models. J Med Sci. 1980;280:73-80.

183. Weinstein MR, Iannini PB, Staton CW, Eichoff TC. Spontaneous bacterial peritonitis: A review of 28 cases with emphasis on improved survival and factors influencing prognosis. Am J Med. 1978;64:592-598.

184. Dorn TF, DeAngelis C, Baumgardner RA, et al. Acetaminophen: More harm than good for chicken pox? J Pediatr. 1989;114:1045-1048.

185. Stanley ED, Jackson GG, Panusarn C, et al. Increased viral shedding with aspirin treatment of rhinovirus infection. JAMA. 1975;231:1248-1251.

186. Graham MH, Burrell CJ, Douglas RM, et al. Adverse effects of aspirin, acetaminophen, and ibuprofen on immune function, viral shedding, and clinical status in rhinovirus-infected volunteers. J Infect Dis. 1990;162:1277-1282.

187. Plaisance KI, Kudaravalli S, Wasserman SS, et al. Effect of antipyretic therapy on the duration of illness in experimental influenza A, Shigella sonnei, and Rickettsia rickettsii infections. Pharmacotherapy. 2000;20:1417-1422.

188. Dinarello CA. Endogenous pyrogens: The role of cytokines in the pathogenesis of fever. In: Mackowiak PA, ed. Fever: Basic Mechanisms and Management. New York: Raven Press; 1991:23-47.

189. Mellouk S, Green SJ, Nacy CA, Hoffman SL. IFN-γ inhibits development of Plasmodium berghei exoerythrocytic stages in hepatocytes by an L-arginine-dependent effector mechanism. J Immunol. 1991;146:3971-3976.

190. Naotunne TDS, Karunaweera ND, Del Giudice G, et al. Cytokines kill malaria parasites during infection crisis: Extracellular complementary factors are essential. J Exp Med. 1991;173:523-529.

191. Curfs JHAJ, Van Der Meer JWM, Sauerwein RW, Eling WMC. Low dosages of interleukin 1 protect mice against lethal cerebral malaria. J Exp Med. 1990;172:1287-1291.

192. Woodman JP, Dimier IH, Bout DT. Human endothelial cells are activated by IFN-α to inhibit Toxoplasmosis gondii replication: Inhibition is due to a different mechanism from that existing in mouse macrophages and human fibroblasts. J Immunol. 1991;147:2019-2023.

193. Liew FY, Li Y, Millott S. Tumor necrosis factor α synergizes with IFN-γ in mediating killing of Leishmania major through the induction of nitric oxide. J Immunol. 1990;145:4306-4310.

194. Torrico F, Heremans H, Rivera MT, et al. Endogenous IFN-γ is required for resistance to acute Trypanosoma cruzi infection in mice. J Immunol. 1991;146:3626-3632.

195. Ungar BVP, Kao T-C, Burris JA, Finkelman FD. Cryptosporidium infection in an adult mouse model: Independent roles for IFN-γ and CD4+ T lymphocytes in protective immunity. J Immunol. 1991;147:1014-1022.

196. Sambhi SK, Kohonen-Corish MRJ, Ramshaw IA. Local production of tumor necrosis factor encoded by recombinant vaccinia virus is effective in controlling viral replication in vivo. Proc Natl Acad Sci U S A. 1991;88:4025-4029.

197. Feduchi E, Carrasco L. Mechanism of inhibition of HSV-1 replication by tumor necrosis factor and interferon. Virology. 1991;180:822-825.

198. Strijp HAG, Van Der Tol ME, Miltenburgh LAM, et al. Tumor necrosis factor triggers granulocytes to internalize complement-coated virus particles. Immunology. 1991;73:77-82.

199. Hedges S, Anderson P, Lidin-Janson G, et al. Interleukin-6 response to deliberate colonization of the human urinary tract with gram-negative bacteria. Infect Immun. 1991;59:421-427.

200. Vogels MTE, Vander Meer JWM. Use of immune modulators in nonspecific therapy of bacterial infections. Antimicrob Agents Chemother. 1992;36:1-5.

201. Bernheim HA, Bodel T, Askenase PW, Atkins E. Effects of fever on host defense mechanisms after injection of the lizard Dipsosaurus dorsalis. Br J Exp Pathol. 1978;59:76-84.

202. Dinarello CA. The proinflammatory cytokines interleukin-1 and tumor necrosis factor and treatment of the septic shock syndrome. J Infect Dis. 1991;163:1177-1184.

203. Casey LC, Balk RA, Bone RC. Plasma cytokine and endotoxin levels correlate with survival in patients with the sepsis syndrome. Ann Intern Med. 1993;119:771-778.

204. Johnson J, Brigham KL, Jesmok G, Meyrick B. Morphologic changes in lungs of anesthetized sheep following intravenous infusion of recombinant tumor necrosis factor alpha. Am Rev Respir Dis. 1991;144:179-186.

205. Heinzel FP. The role of IFN-γ in the pathology of experimental endotoxemia. J Immunol. 1990;145:2920-2924.

206. Henricson BE, Neta R, Vogel SN. An interleukin-1 receptor antagonist blocks lipopolysaccharide-induced colony-stimulating factor production and early endotoxin tolerance. Infect Immun. 1991;59:1188-1191.

207. Ohlsson K, Björk P, Bergenfeldt M, et al. Interleukin-1 receptor antagonist reduces mortality from endotoxin shock. Nature. 1990;348:550-552.

208. Opal SM, Cross AS, Sadoff JC, et al. Efficacy of antilipopolysaccharide and anti-tumor necrosis factor monoclonal antibodies in a neutropenic rat model of Pseudomonas sepsis. J Clin Invest. 1991;88:885-890.

209. Overbeek BP, Veringa EM. Role of antibodies and antibiotics in aerobic gram-negative septicemia: Possible synergism between antimicrobial treatment and immunotherapy. Rev Infect Dis. 1991;13:751-760.

210. Alexander HR, Sheppard BC, Jensen JC, et al. Treatment with recombinant tumor necrosis factor-alpha protects rats against lethality, hypotension, and hypothermia of gram-negative sepsis. J Clin Invest. 1991;88:34-39.

211. Hotchkiss RS, Karl IE. The pathophysiology and treatment of sepsis. N Engl J Med. 2003;348:138-150.

212. Eichacker PQ, Parent C, Kalil A, et al. Risk and efficacy of antiinflammatory agents. Retrospective and confirmatory studies of sepsis. Am J Respir Crit Care Med. 2002;166:1197-1205.

213. Mackowiak PA. Editorial response: Assaulting a physiological response. Clin Infect Dis. 1997;24:1214-1216.

214. Neymann CA, Osborne SL. Artificial fever. Am J Syphilis Neurol. 1934;18-34.

215. Lessell S, Torres JM, Kurland LT. Seizure disorders in a Guamanian village. Arch Neurol. 1962;7:37-44.

216. Aicardi J. Febrile convulsions. In: Aicardi J, ed. Epilepsy in Children. 2nd ed. New York: Raven Press; 1994:253-275.

217. Lennox-Buchthal MA. Febrile Convulsions—A Reappraisal. Amsterdam: Elsevier; 1973:1-138.
218. Rosman NP. Febrile convulsions. In: Mackowiak PA, ed. Fever: Basic Mechanisms and Management. 2nd ed. Philadelphia: Lippincott-Raven; 1997:267-277.
219. Styrt B, Sugarman B. Antipyresis and fever. Arch Intern Med. 1990;150:1589-1597.
220. Horwath SM, Spurr GB, Hutt BK, Hamilton LH. Metabolic cost of shivering. J Appl Physiol. 1956;8:595-602.
221. Vane JR, Botting RM. New insights into the mode of action of anti-inflammatory drugs. Inflamm Res. 1995;44:1-10.
222. Blatteis CM, Sehic E. Prostaglandin E₂: A putative fever mediator. In: Mackowiak PA, ed. Fever: Basic mechanisms and Management. 2nd ed. Philadelphia: Lippincott-Raven; 1997:17-145.
223. Chandrasekharan NV, Dai H, Roos KL, et al. COX-3, a cyclooxygenase-1 variant inhibited by acetaminophen and other analgesic/antipyretic drugs: Cloning, structure, and expression. Proc Natl Acad Sci U S A. 2002;99:13926-13931.
224. Schwab JM, Schluesener HJ, Laufer S. COX-3: Just another COX or the solitary elusive target of paracetamol? Lancet 2003;361:981-982.
225. Plaisance KI, Mackowiak PA. Antipyretic therapy: Physiologic rationale, diagnostic implications, and clinical consequences. Arch Intern Med. 2000;160:449-456.
226. Blatteis CM. Antipyretic therapy with helium-oxygen. In: Thermoregulatory Mechanisms and Their Therapeutic Implications. Fourth International Symposium on the Pharmacology of Thermoregulation, Oxford 1979. Bosel: Karger; 1980:238-241.
227. O'Donnell J, Axelrod P, Fisher C, Lorber B. Use and effectiveness of hypothermia blankets for febrile patients in the intensive care unit. Clin Infect Dis. 1997;24:1208-1213.
228. Wenzel C, Werner J. Physical versus pharmacological counter-measures. Eur J Appl Physiol. 1988;57:81-88.
229. Steele RW, Tanaka PT, Lara RP, Bass JW. Evaluation of sponging and of oral antipyretic therapy to reduce fever. J Pediatr. 1970;77:824-829.
230. Newman J. Evaluation of sponging to reduce body temperature in febrile children. Can Med Assoc J. 1985;132:641-642.
231. McCarthy PL, Grundy GW, Spiesel SZ, Dolan TF. Bacteremia in children: An outpatient clinical review. Pediatrics. 1976;57:861-868.
232. McGowan JE, Bratton L, Klein JO, Finland M. Bacteremia in febrile children seen in a "walk-in" pediatric clinic. N Engl J Med. 1973;288:1309-1312.
233. Teele DW, Pelton SI, Grant MJ, et al. Bacteremia in febrile children under 2 years of age: Results of cultures of blood of 600 consecutive febrile children seen in a "walk-in" clinic. J Pediatr. 1975;87:227-230.
234. Bonadio WA, Romine K, Gyuro J. Relationship of fever magnitude to rate of serious bacterial infections in neonates. J Pediatr. 1990;116:733-735.
235. McCarthy PL. Fever in infants and children. In: Mackowiak PA, ed. Fever: Basic Mechanisms and Management, 2nd ed. Philadelphia: Lippincott-Raven; 1997: 351-362.
236. Toney SB, Henretig F, Fleisher G, et al. Temperature response to antipyretic therapy in children: Relationship to occult bacteremia. Am J Emerg Med. 1985;3:190-192.
237. Baker MD, Fosarelli PD, Carpenter RO. Childhood fever: Correlation of diagnosis with temperature response to acetaminophen. Pediatrics. 1987;80:315-318.
238. Yamamoto LT, Wigder HN, Fligner DJ, et al. Relationship of bacteremia to antipyretic therapy in febrile children. Pediatr Emerg Care. 1987;3:223-227.
239. Weisse ME, Miller G, Brien JH. Fever response to acetaminophen in viral vs. bacterial infections. Pediatr Infect Dis J. 1987;6:1091-1094.
240. Baker RC, Tiller T, Bausher JC, et al. Severity of disease correlated with fever reduction in febrile infants. Pediatrics. 1989;83:1016-1019.
241. Mazur LJ, Jones TM, Kozinetz CA. Temperature response to acetaminophen and risk of occult bacteremia: A case-control study. J Pediatr. 1989;115:888-891.
242. Chang JC, Gross HM. Utility of naproxen in the differential diagnosis of fever of undetermined origin in patients with cancer. Am J Med. 1984;76:597-603.
243. Tsavaris N, Zinelis A, Karabelis A, et al. A randomized trial of the effect of three nonsteroidal antiinflammatory agents in ameliorating cancer-induced fever. J Intern Med. 1990;228:451-455.
244. Kluger MJ, Kozak W, Conn CA, et al. The adaptive value of fever. In: Mackowiak PA, ed. Fever: Basic Mechanisms and Management. Philadelphia: Lippincott-Raven; 1997:255-266.
245. Isaacs SN, Axelrod PI, Lorber B. Antipyretic orders in a university hospital. Am J Med. 1990;88:31-35.
246. Manthous CA, Hall JB, Olson D, et al. Effect of cooling on oxygen consumption in febrile critically ill patients. Am J Respir Crit Care Med. 1995;151:10-14.
247. Raizner AE, Chahine RA, Ishimori T, et al. Provocation of coronary artery spasm by the cold pressor test: Hemodynamic, arteriographic and quantitative arteriographic observations. Circulation. 1980;62:925-932.
248. Nobel EG, Gang P, Gordon JB, et al. Dilation of normal and construction of atherosclerotic coronary arteries caused by the cold pressor test. Circulation. 1987;77: 43-52.
249. Lenhardt R, Kurz A, Sessler DI. Thermoregulation and hyperthermia. Acta Anaesthesiol Scand Suppl. 1996;109:34-38.
250. Friedman PL, Brown EJ Jr, Gunther S, et al. Coronary vasoconstrictor effect of indomethacin in patients with coronary artery disease. N Engl J Med. 1981;305: 1171-1175.
251. Mukherjee D, Nissen SE, Topol EJ. Risk of cardiovascular events associated with COX-2 inhibitors. JAMA. 2001;286:954-959.
252. Beisel WR, Morgan BB Jr, Bartelloni PJ, et al. Symptomatic therapy in viral illness: A controlled study of effects on work performance. JAMA. 1974;228:581-584.
253. Camfield PR, Camfield CS, Shapiro SH, et al. The first febrile seizure-antipyretic instruction plus either phenobarbital or placebo to prevent recurrence. J Pediatr. 1980;5:719-737.
254. Uhari M, Rantala H, Vainionpää L, et al. Effect of acetaminophen and of low intermittent doses of diazepam on prevention of recurrences of febrile seizures. J Pediatr. 1995;126:991-995.
255. Schnaiderman D, Lahat E, Sheefer T, et al. Antipyretic effectiveness of acetaminophen in febrile seizures: Ongoing prophylaxis versus sporadic usage. Eur J Pediatr. 1993;152:747-749.
256. Warren HS. Strategies for the treatment of sepsis. N Engl J Med. 1997;336:952-953.
257. Bernard GR, Wheeler AP, Russell JA, et al. The effects of ibuprofen on the physiology and survival of patients with sepsis. N Engl J Med. 1997;336:912-918.
258. Mackowiak PA, Plaisance KI. The benefits and risks of antipyretic therapy. Ann N Y Acad Sci. 1998;856:214-223.

CHAPTER **48**

Fever of Unknown Origin

PHILIP A. MACKOWIAK

DAVID T. DURACK

Most fevers are short lived and do not require diagnostic investigation or specific therapy. Some are manifestations of more serious illnesses, most of which can be readily diagnosed and effectively treated. A small but important subgroup of fevers are both persistent and difficult to diagnose. Such fevers have fascinated and frustrated clinicians since the earliest days of clinical thermometry.[1] They have generated a welter of publications over the years, the two most important of which, from a historical perspective, were the classic treatises *Prolonged and Perplexing Fevers,* by Keefer and Leard in 1955,[2] and *Fever of Unknown Origin: Report on 100 Cases,* by Petersdorf and Beeson in 1961.[3]

TERMINOLOGY

In the United States, the term *fever of unknown origin* (FUO) has generally been used to describe this special group of fevers.[4] In other countries, *pyrexia of unknown origin* (PUO) is more commonly used.[5]

The first formal definition of FUO to gain broad acceptance was proposed by Petersdorf and Beeson four decades ago: "fever higher than 38.3° C (101° F) on several occasions, persisting without diagnosis for at least 3 weeks in spite of at least 1 week's investigation in hospital."[3] Later investigators have modified and extended this classic definition to reflect evolutionary changes in clinical practice.[6,7] Such changes have included the mounting emphasis on the use of the outpatient setting for diagnostic investigations, the increasing number of immunocompromised patients (especially those with neutropenia), a proliferation of increasingly complex surgical and intensive care protocols, and the advent of human immunodeficiency virus (HIV) infection and the acquired immunodeficiency syndrome (AIDS). In response to this new evolving environment, cases of FUO are currently codified into four distinct subclasses of the disorder: classic FUO, nosocomial FUO, immune-deficient FUO, and HIV-related FUO (Table 48-1).

CLASSIC FEVER OF UNKNOWN ORIGIN

Classic FUO refers to the type of FUO defined by Petersdorf and Beeson in 1961.[3] The only alteration to their definition required to conform to modern medical practice is to incorporate the outpatient setting, which today has become the preferred venue for evaluation and treatment. Most patients with classic FUO have subacute or chronic symptoms and therefore can be safely managed as outpatients. In a series of 53 such patients, for example, the median duration of fever before diagnosis was 40 days.[1] Even though the tempo and accuracy of clinical investigation have improved in recent years, many

TABLE 48-1 Summary of Definitions and Major Features of the Four Subtypes of Fever of Unknown Origin (FUO)

	Classic FUO	Nosocomial FUO	Immune-Deficient FUO	HIV-Related FUO
Definition	>38.0° C, >3 wk, >2 visits or 3 d in hospital	>38.0° C, 3 d, not present or incubating on admission	>38.0° C, >3 d, negative cultures after 48 h	38.0° C, >3 wk for outpatients, >3 d for inpatients, HIV infection confirmed
Patient location	Community, clinic, or hospital	Acute care hospital	Hospital or clinic	Community, clinic, or hospital
Leading causes	Cancer, infections, inflammatory conditions, undiagnosed, habitual hyperthermia	Nosocomial infections, postoperative complications, drug fever	Majority due to infections, but cause documented in only 40–60%	HIV (primary infection), typical and atypical mycobacteria, CMV, lymphomas, toxoplasmosis, cryptococcosis
History emphasis	Travel, contacts, animal and insect exposure, medications, immunizations, family history, cardiac valve disorder	Operations and procedures, devices, anatomic considerations, drug treatment	Stage of chemotherapy, drugs administered, underlying immunosuppressive disorder	Drugs, exposures, risk factors, travel, contacts, stage of HIV infection
Examination emphasis	Fundi, oropharynx, temporal artery, abdomen, lymph nodes, spleen, joints, skin, nails, genitalia, rectum or prostate, lower limb deep veins	Wounds, drains, devices, sinuses, urine	Skin folds, IV sites, lungs, perianal area	Mouth, sinuses, skin, lymph nodes, eyes, lungs, perianal area
Investigation emphasis	Imaging, biopsies, sedimentation rate, skin tests	Imaging, bacterial cultures	CXR, bacterial cultures	Blood and lymphocyte count; serologic tests; CXR; stool examination; biopsies of lung, bone marrow, and liver for cultures and cytologic tests; brain imaging
Management	Observation, outpatient temperature chart, investigations, avoidance of empirical drug treatments	Depends on situation	Antimicrobial treatment protocols	Antiviral and antimicrobial protocols, vaccines, revision of treatment regimens, good nutrition
Time course of disease	Months	Weeks	Days	Weeks to months
Tempo of investigation	Weeks	Days	Hours	Days to weeks

CMV, cytomegalovirus; CXR, chest radiograph; HIV, human immunodeficiency virus; IV, intravenous.

Adapted from Durack DT. Fever of unknown origin. In: Mackowiak PA, ed. Fever. Basic Mechanisms and Management. 2nd ed. Philadelphia: Lippincott-Raven; 1997:237-249.

cases of classic FUO continue to elude diagnosis for extended periods, as reflected in the findings of a Japanese survey from 1982 to 1992, in which an average of 49 days (range 8 to 217 days) was required to complete the diagnostic evaluation.[8]

Of the many publications concerned with the etiology of FUO,[3,9-15] most have dealt with classic FUO rather than with the other subclasses as defined above.[7] Over the years a recurrent theme has been become clear: of the myriad disorders causing classic FUO, almost all belong to one of five general categories of diseases, namely, infections, neoplasms, connective tissue diseases, miscellaneous other disorders, and undiagnosed illnesses. The relative frequencies of diagnoses within these five categories vary from series to series, depending on the geographic region, ages of the patients, type of hospital, and other factors (Fig. 48-1). In most series, infection has been the commonest diagnosis overall, accounting for 25% to 50% of cases. However, in patients older than 65 years, infections have decreased in frequency to become the second or even the third most common cause of classic FUO.[8,9] In the series of Knockaert and associates[9] infection was the cause of FUO in only 25% of cases 65 years of age or older; temporal arteritis and various connective tissue diseases accounted for 31% of cases, and tumors for 12%. Only 8% of cases went undiagnosed—a percentage substantially lower than that reported in surveys involving younger adults, in which as many as 30% of cases remain undiagnosed.[16] The longer the duration of fever before medical consultation, the less likely that a final diagnosis will be made.[17]

Among the infections responsible for classic FUO, abscesses, endocarditis, tuberculosis, and complicated urinary tract infections have consistently been among the most important. These tend to vary in incidence according to locale. Visceral leishmaniasis, for example, although absent from most series of classic FUO, accounted for 8% of

cases in a study reported in 1997 from Spain.[18] Other examples of causes of classic FUO with distinctive geographic distributions include melioidosis in Southeast Asia and northern Australia[19]; Kikuchi-Fujimoto disease, an unusual form of necrotizing lymphadenitis seen primarily in Japan[20]; and familial Hibernian fever, an inherited periodic fever syndrome described only in Ireland.[21] The miscellaneous category contains both varied and individually rare causes of classical FUO (Table 48-2).

Of the connective tissue diseases responsible for classical FUO, Still's disease (juvenile rheumatoid arthritis), other variants of rheumatoid arthritis, and systemic lupus erythematosus, predominate in younger patients, whereas temporal arteritis and polymyalgia rheumatica syndromes are more common in elderly patients.

Malignant neoplasms, another important cause of FUO, can induce fever directly through the production and release of pyrogenic cytokines, as in the case of certain lymphomas. They can also generate fevers indirectly by undergoing spontaneous or induced necrosis or by creating conditions conducive to secondary infections, such as postobstructive pneumonia.[22] Although hypernephromas have traditionally been touted as an important cause of FUO,[3,23] in reality this tumor only rarely presents with fever.[24]

The relative frequency with which the major diagnostic categories are represented in series of classic FUO varies according to both the era in which the series was published[6,13] and its country of origin (see Fig. 48-1).[8,15,25,26] Since the mid-1900s, the frequency with which infections and malignant neoplasms have been identified as causes of classic FUO has fallen steadily, whereas the proportion of miscellaneous causes and undiagnosed conditions has risen.[25] However, in developing countries, the frequency with which infections are diagnosed has changed little.[15] Consequently, in these countries malignant neo-

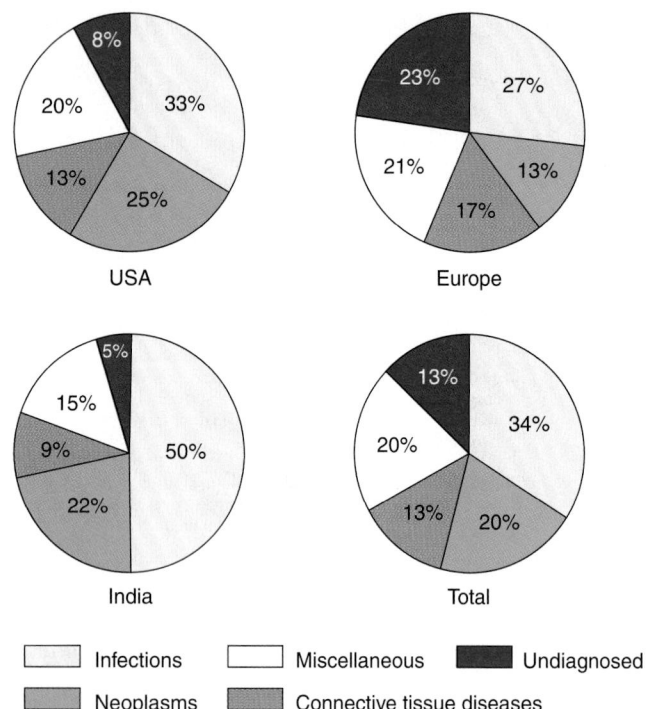

USA

Europe

India

Total

Infections   Miscellaneous   Undiagnosed

Neoplasms   Connective tissue diseases

FIGURE 48-1. The five main etiologic categories of fever of unknown origin, comparing their frequency in series from three geographic regions. *(Redrawn from Durack DT. Fever of unknown origin. In: Mackowiak PA, ed. Fever. Basic Mechanisms and Management. 2nd ed. Philadelphia: Lippincott-Raven; 1997:237-249.)*

plasms and connective tissue disorders are comparatively less important as causes of classic FUO than in developed countries (see Fig. 48-1).[15]

Infants and Children

The diseases responsible for classic FUO in infants differ from those in older children and adults. Respiratory infections cause classic FUO in infants more often than in children older than 12 months, or in adults.[10] The relative frequency of infections as the cause of FUO in infants is high, owing to the fact that connective tissue diseases and cancers are rare in this age group. Kawasaki disease is predominantly a problem of children younger than 5 years, less so of older children. Whereas connective tissue diseases are rarely seen in children younger than 12 months, Still's disease is a leading cause of FUO in older children and young adults. Joint involvement in children with FUO usually signifies a serious underlying disorder, such as a connective tissue disease, endocarditis, or leukemia.[10]

In a series of 146 pediatric cases of FUO, Jacobs and Schutze established a diagnosis in only 84 (57.5%).[27] Of these, 64 (43.8%) had infections, 11 (7.5%) autoimmune disorders, 4 (2.7%) malignant neoplasms, and 5 (3.4%) a variety of other disorders, such as drug-induced fever, sarcoidosis, and mercury poisoning. The most common infectious diseases diagnosed in their series were Epstein-Barr virus infection (15%), osteomyelitis (10%), bartonellosis (5%), and urinary tract infections (4%).

Elderly Persons

One of the most striking features of classic FUO in patients older than 65 years is the relatively high frequency with which connective tissue diseases are identified as the cause of the illness (Table 48-3).[28,29] In developed countries, connective tissue diseases surpass even infections as the leading cause of classic FUO in the elderly.[8,9] This is primarily because the temporal arteritis and polymyalgia rheumatica syndromes are common in this setting.[8,30,31] Unfortunately these diagnoses are fre-

TABLE 48-2 Examples of Rare Miscellaneous Causes of Fever

Alcoholic hepatitis	Inflammatory bowel disease
Allergic alveolitis	Kikuchi-Fujimoto disease
Aortic dissection	Lymphomatoid granulomatosis
Aortitis	Metal fume fever
Atrial myxoma	Myeloproliferative syndromes
Behçet's syndrome	Pancreatitis
Carcinomatous meningitis	Paroxysmal hemoglobinurias
Castleman's disease	Pericarditis
Chronic meningitis	Periodic fever
Cirrhotic fever	Pheochromocytoma
Cyclic neutropenia	Postpericardiotomy syndrome
Drug fever and other	Pulmonary emboli
hypersensitivities	Retroperitoneal fibrosis
Erythema multiforme	Rosai-Dorfman disease
Fabry's disease	Sarcoidosis
Factitious fever	Schnitzler's syndrome
Familial Hibernian fever	Serum sickness
Familial Mediterranean fever	Sjögren's syndrome
Granulomatous hepatitis	Subacute necrotizing lymphadenitis
Granulomatous peritonitis	Thrombotic thrombocytopenic
Hemoglobinopathies	purpura
Hemolytic anemias	Thyroiditis and thyrotoxicosis
Hemophagocytic syndrome	Veno-occlusive disease
Histiocytosis X	Vitamin B_{12} deficiency
Hypereosinophilic syndrome	Wegener's granulomatosis
Immunoblastic lymphadenopathy	Whipple's disease

Adapted from Durack DT. Fever of unknown origin. In: Mackowiak PA, ed. Fever. Basic Mechanisms and Management. 2nd ed. Philadelphia: Lippincott-Raven; 1997:237–249.

quently missed or delayed because associated symptoms are subacute and nonspecific. In elderly patients in whom infections are identified as the cause of FUO, intra-abdominal abscesses, complicated urinary tract infections, tuberculosis, and endocarditis have predominated.[9,14] For unclear reasons, factitious fever is a vary rare cause of FUO in the older compared with young adults. Relatively few cases of FUO go undiagnosed in elderly patients (see Table 48-3), yet elderly FUO patients have a distinctly poorer prognosis than their younger counterparts because of the relatively high incidence of malignancies.

Returned Travelers

Fever in returned travelers (see Chapter 329) is most often due to common infections such as malaria and respiratory or urinary tract infections.[32] However, exotic causes of fever such as amebic liver abscess or dengue are occasionally diagnosed, especially among international

TABLE 48-3 Final Diagnosis in Elderly Compared with Younger Patients with Fever of Unknown Origin

Diagnosis	<65 Years n = 152 (%)	>65 Years n = 201 (%)
Infections	33 (21%)	72 (35%)
Abscess	6	25
Endocarditis	2	14
Tuberculosis	4	20
Viral infections	8	1
Other	13	12
Tumors	8 (5%)	37 (19%)
Hematologic	3	19
Solid	5	18
Multisystem diseases[*]	27 (17%)	57 (28%)
Miscellaneous[†]	39 (26%)	17 (8%)
No diagnosis	45 (29%)	18 (9%)

[*]Rheumatic diseases, connective tissue disorders, vasculitis (including temporal arteritis), polymyalgia rheumatica, and sarcoidosis.

[†]Includes factitious fever (seven cases), habitual hyperthermia (five cases), and drug-induced fever (three cases).

Adapted from Iikuni Y, Okada J, Kondo H, et al. Current fever of unknown origin 1982-1992. Intern Med. 1994; 33:67-73; and Knockaert DC, Vanneste LJ, Bobbaers HJ. Fever of unknown origin in elderly patients. J Am Geriatr Soc. 1993; 41:1187-1192.

TABLE 48-4 Causes of Fever in the Returned Traveler*

Diagnosis	MacLean et al[118] (n = 587)	Doherty et al[119] (n = 195)
Malaria	32	42
Hepatitis	6	3
Respiratory infection[†]	11	2.6
Urinary tract infection/pyelonephritis	4	2.6
Dysentery	4.5	5.1
Dengue fever	2	6.2
Enteric fever	2	1.5
Tuberculosis	1	2
Rickettsial infection	1	0.5
Acute HIV infection	0.3	1.0
Amebic liver abscess	1	0
Other miscellaneous infections	4.3	9.2
Miscellaneous noninfectious causes	6	1
Undiagnosed	25	24.6

*Values listed are percentages.
†Includes upper respiratory tract infection, pneumonia, and bronchitis.
HIV, human immunodeficiency virus.
From Suh KN, Kozavsky PE, Keystone JS. Evaluation of fever in the returned traveler. Travel Med. 1999;83:997-1017.

travelers returning from developing countries in the tropics. Of the many febrile conditions encountered among returning travelers (Table 48-4), malaria, typhoid fever, and acute HIV infection are the ones most likely to manifest as FUO.

NOSOCOMIAL FEVER OF UNKNOWN ORIGIN

Nosocomial FUO, as the name implies, is a hospital-associated disorder in which patients first manifest fever after having been hospitalized for at least 3 days. Such FUO cases, as might be expected, are frequently attributable to risk factors encountered in the hospital environment, including surgical procedures, urinary and respiratory tract instrumentation, intravascular devices, drug therapy, and immobilization. Because acute febrile disorders are well-recognized consequences of exposure to such risk factors, it has been assumed that these same acute disorders also occasionally manifest as FUOs. Examples of such disorders commonly offered, but not yet verified in actual surveys of nosocomial FUO, include septic thrombophlebitis, recurrent pulmonary emboli, *Clostridium difficile* colitis, and drug fever.[7,33]

Postoperative Patients

Several reports have highlighted the fact that it is often difficult to identify the precise cause of postoperative fevers. In a series of 537 consecutive patients undergoing major gynecologic surgery, 211 (39%) developed postoperative fever.[34] Of 77 blood cultures performed on these patients, none was positive. Although 11 of 106 (10%) urine cultures were positive and 5 of 54 (9%) chest radiographs were abnormal, a pathologic process was detected in only 8% of febrile patients. In a study of postoperative fever following tonsillectomy in children, Anand and colleagues[35] found no association between cultures of blood, or the core or surface of tonsils, and the incidence or severity of fever, and concluded that postoperative fever, at least in the 24 hours following tonsillectomy, is rarely the result of infection.

In another series concerned with the etiology of persistent postoperative fever in patients undergoing total joint arthroplasty, few definitive diagnoses were established, causing the authors to conclude that postoperative fever is a normal component of the inflammatory response to this type of major surgery.[36]

Intensive Care Unit Patients

Fever is common in intensive care units, most often developing early after admission to the unit, in which case it tends to be of noninfective origin and carries a favorable prognosis.[37] Prolonged fever, however, is associated with a worse prognosis. Nosocomial sinusitis, a complication of mechanical ventilation arising from supine positioning and the use of

endotracheal, gastric, and feeding tubes is common[38] and should be vigorously pursued when evaluating FUO in intensive care unit patients.

Stroke Patients

In patients with acute stroke, fever is usually the result of an infection, most commonly a urinary tract infection related to urinary catheterization. However, in some cases, a focus of infection cannot be identified and when the fever does not respond to empiric antibiotic treatment, it is presumed to be due to the stroke itself. In a study of 330 patients hospitalized for acute stroke, Georgilis and associates[39] observed that noninfective fevers were most often associated with intracranial mass effects and tended to occur earlier after the onset of stroke than fevers due to infection.

IMMUNE-DEFICIENT FEVER OF UNKNOWN ORIGIN

Obviously various forms of immunosuppression predispose more or less strongly to a wide variety of infectious complications. Thus, it is not surprising that immunosuppressed patients have perhaps the highest incidence of FUO of any group of patients. In a recent series of 116 hematology-oncology patients, for example, Engelhart and associates[40] observed 33 FUOs in 28 patients, for an overall rate of 8.2 episodes per 1000 patient days. Because of impaired immune responses, signs of inflammation other than fever are notoriously absent or diminished in such patients, leading to atypical clinical manifestations and absence of radiologic abnormalities in what otherwise would be readily diagnosed infections.

In patients with impaired cell-mediated immunity, FUO is often due to conditions other than pyogenic bacterial infections, as illustrated in a recent survey of transplant recipients by Chang and coworkers.[42] In that series, infections were the cause of 7 of the 12 (58%) episodes of fever in which a diagnosis could not be established during 3 days of intensive investigation; these included 5 cases of human herpesvirus 6 infection, 1 of varicella-zoster virus infection with atypical skin lesions, and one of pneumonia due to *Serratia marcescens* (in which the pulmonary infiltrate was initially inapparent radiographically). Three (25%) cases were due to noninfectious conditions: malignant neoplasm, drug-induced fever, and adrenal insufficiency. In two (17%) cases, the cause of the fever could not be determined.

Neutropenic Fever of Unknown Origin

The number of patients with episodes of neutropenia resulting from cytotoxic therapy or hematologic malignant neoplasms is rising, even as the average duration of neutropenia in such patients is falling owing to the increasing therapeutic application of colony-stimulating factors. Many episodes of fever in neutropenic patients are short lived because they either respond quickly to treatment or are manifestations of rapidly fatal infections.

Episodes of fever are very common in patients with neutropenia. Because bacteremia and sepsis are frequent causes, empiric broad-spectrum antibiotics are typically administered immediately when fever develops in such patients. However, only about 35% of prolonged episodes of febrile neutropenia respond to broad-spectrum antibiotic therapy. Although practitioners often assume that if fever does not respond promptly to antibacterial therapy, fungal infection must be responsible, other causes are equally likely to be identified (Table 48-5).[41]

HUMAN IMMUNODEFICIENCY VIRUS–RELATED FEVER OF UNKNOWN ORIGIN

Episodes of fever are commonplace in patients infected with HIV—a special subgroup of immunodeficient patients.[43-45] The primary phase of the HIV infection itself is characterized by a mononucleosis-like illness in which fever is a prominent feature. All too often, primary HIV infection eludes diagnosis because the illness is nonspecific and precedes seroconversion. For this reason it represents an important cause of HIV-associated FUO. Once symptoms of the primary phase of the HIV infection resolve, HIV-infected patients are afebrile or exhibit only trivial elevations in oral temperature as a result of their persistent retroviral

TABLE 48-5 Possible Causes of Fever in Neutropenic Patients Not Responding to Broad-Spectrum Antibiotics

Causes	Approximate Frequency in High-Risk Patients (%)
Fungal infections susceptible to empirical therapy	40
Fungal infections resistant to empirical antifungal therapy	5
Bacterial infections (with cryptic foci and resistant organisms)	10
Toxoplasma gondii, mycobacteria, or fastidious pathogens (legionella, mycoplasma, *Chlamydophila pneumoniae*, bartonella)	5
Viral infections (herpesviruses, cytomegalovirus, Epstein-Barr virus, human herpesvirus 6, varicella-zoster virus, herpes simplex virus, parainfluenza virus, respiratory syncytial virus, influenza viruses)	5
Graft-versus-host disease after hematopoietic stem-cell transplantation	10
Undefined (e.g., drug fever, toxic effects of chemotherapy, antitumor responses, undefined pathogens)	25

From Corey L, Boeckh M. Persistent fever in patients with neutropenia. N Engl J Med. 2002;346:222-224. Copyright © 2002 Massachusetts Medical Society. All rights reserved.

infection.[46] However, in the later phases of HIV infection, fever usually signifies some superimposed illness. Many of these are potentially devastating opportunistic infections, which tend to present in atypical fashion owing to the tendency of both the disordered immune response and prior prophylactic antimicrobial therapy[47] to distort their clinical manifestations.

The frequency of FUO in HIV-infected patients has been reported to be 0.6% in those receiving highly active antiretroviral therapy

TABLE 48-6 Diseases Established as the Etiology of Fever 72 Times in 70 Cases of HIV-Associated Fever of Unknown Origin

Etiology	No. (%) of Times Diagnosis Was Established
Infection	
DMAC	22 (31)
PCP	10 (13)
CMV	8 (11)
Histoplasmosis	5 (7)
Viral (not CMV)*	5 (7)
Bacterial	4 (5)
Mycobacterium tuberculosis	4 (5)
Fungal (not histoplasmosis)†	2 (3)
Parasitic‡	2 (3)
Mycobacterium genavense	1 (1)
Total	63 (88)
Neoplasia	
Lymphoma	5 (7)
Kaposi's sarcoma	1 (1)
Total	6 (8)
Miscellaneous	
Drug fever	2 (3)
Castleman's disease	1 (1)
Total	3 (4)

*Includes hepatitis C, hepatitis B, adenovirus pneumonia, herpes simplex esophagitis, and varicella-zoster encephalitis (one case each).
†Includes disseminated crytpococcosis and pulmonary aspergillosis (one case each).
‡Includes cerebral toxoplasmosis and disseminated cryptosporidiosis (one case each).
CMV, cytomegalovirus; DMAC, disseminated *Mycobacterium avium* complex; HIV, human immunodeficiency virus; PCP, *Pneumocystis carinii* pneumonia.
From Armstrong WS, Katz JT, Kazanjian PH. Human immunodeficiency virus–associated fever of unknown origin: A study of 70 patients in the United States and review. Clin Infect Dis. 1999;28:341-345.

(HAART) and 3% in those not receiving therapy.[48] Mycobacterial infections have been the commonest cause of FUO in such patients; collagen-vascular diseases have been distinctly uncommon.[49] In a recent series reported by Armstrong and colleagues,[50] the etiology of the FUO was identified in 56 of 70 (80%) patients. A single etiology was identified in 43; 3 distinct causes of FUO were identified in 3 cases, and 2 causes in 10 others. The 72 causes of FUO in 56 patients in whom the etiology was determined are listed in Table 48-6.

CLINICAL EVALUATION OF FEVER OF UNKNOWN ORIGIN

The evaluation of a patient with FUO typically includes a comprehensive history, verification that the patient actually has fever and consideration of the fever pattern, repeated physical examinations, a host of laboratory investigations, key imaging studies, and invasive diagnostic procedures (Table 48-7).

History

It is axiomatic that a comprehensive history is a cornerstone of the evaluation of any complex illness such as FUO. The history can be especially important in determining the choice of the initial laboratory investigations. Particular attention should be given to recent travel, exposure to pets and other animals, the work environment, and recent contact with people exhibiting similar symptoms. The family history should be carefully scrutinized for possible hereditary causes of fever, for example, familial Mediterranean fever. Likewise, the past medical history must be examined for previously diagnosed conditions such as lymphoma, rheumatic fever, or intra-abdominal disorders, complications or reactivation of which might account for the source of fever. Finally, a complete list of the patient's medications must be obtained, so that each may be evaluated as a potential source of drug-induced fever.

Verification of Fever and Fever Pattern

The next step in the evaluation of the patient with FUO is to verify the presence of fever. The importance of this step should be self-evident, yet it is often overlooked. In fact, in a series of 347 patients admitted to the National Institutes of Health for prolonged fever, 35% were ultimately determined either not to have significant fever at all, or to have fever of factitious origin.[51]

Clinicians have endeavored to diagnose particular diseases by analyzing fever patterns since the earliest days of clinical thermometry.[55] These efforts have given rise to an extensive and frequently arcane terminology, including descriptors such as *remittent, intermittent, hectic, quotidian, picket fence, sustained, quartan,* and *saddleback.* Such terms have been used to codify fever patterns into general categories

TABLE 48-7 General Diagnostic Evaluation of Patients with Fever of Unknown Origin

Comprehensive history
Repeated physical examinations
Complete blood count
Routine blood chemistry determinations
Urinalysis, including microscopic examination
Chest radiograph
Erythrocyte sedimentation rate
Antinuclear antibodies
Rheumatoid factor
Blood cultures: three or more separate specimens obtained in absence of antimicrobial therapy
Cytomegalovirus IgM antibodies or viral detection in blood
Heterophile antibody test in children and young adults
Tuberculin skin test
Computed tomography of abdomen, pelvis, or other sites
Radionuclide scans
Human immunodeficiency virus antibodies or viral detection assay
Further evaluation of any abnormality detected by above tests
Venous duplex imaging of lower limbs

Adapted from Arrow PM, Flaherty JP. Fever of unknown origin. Lancet. 1997;350:575-580, with permission from Elsevier.

in an attempt to enhance their diagnostic utility. A few, such as the Pel-Ebstein pattern of Hodgkin's disease, the typhus inversus (i.e., reversal of the normal diurnal pattern) of disseminated tuberculosis, and the pulse-temperature disassociation of typhoid fever have been posited as having especially high specificity (Fig. 48-2). Unfortunately, with the possible exception of the tertian and quartan patterns of malaria, these fever patterns are neither sensitive nor specific enough to be considered diagnostic of any disease.

Today, fever patterns per se are rarely diagnostic, but they occasionally offer useful information[52] and therefore should be considered carefully. In the context of other signs, symptoms, and laboratory data, distinctive fever patterns can suggest specific diagnoses to the alert clinician. Likewise, as noted later, the resolution of fever after the institution of disease-specific therapy is occasionally the most compelling, if not the only, evidence of the cause of a febrile illness.

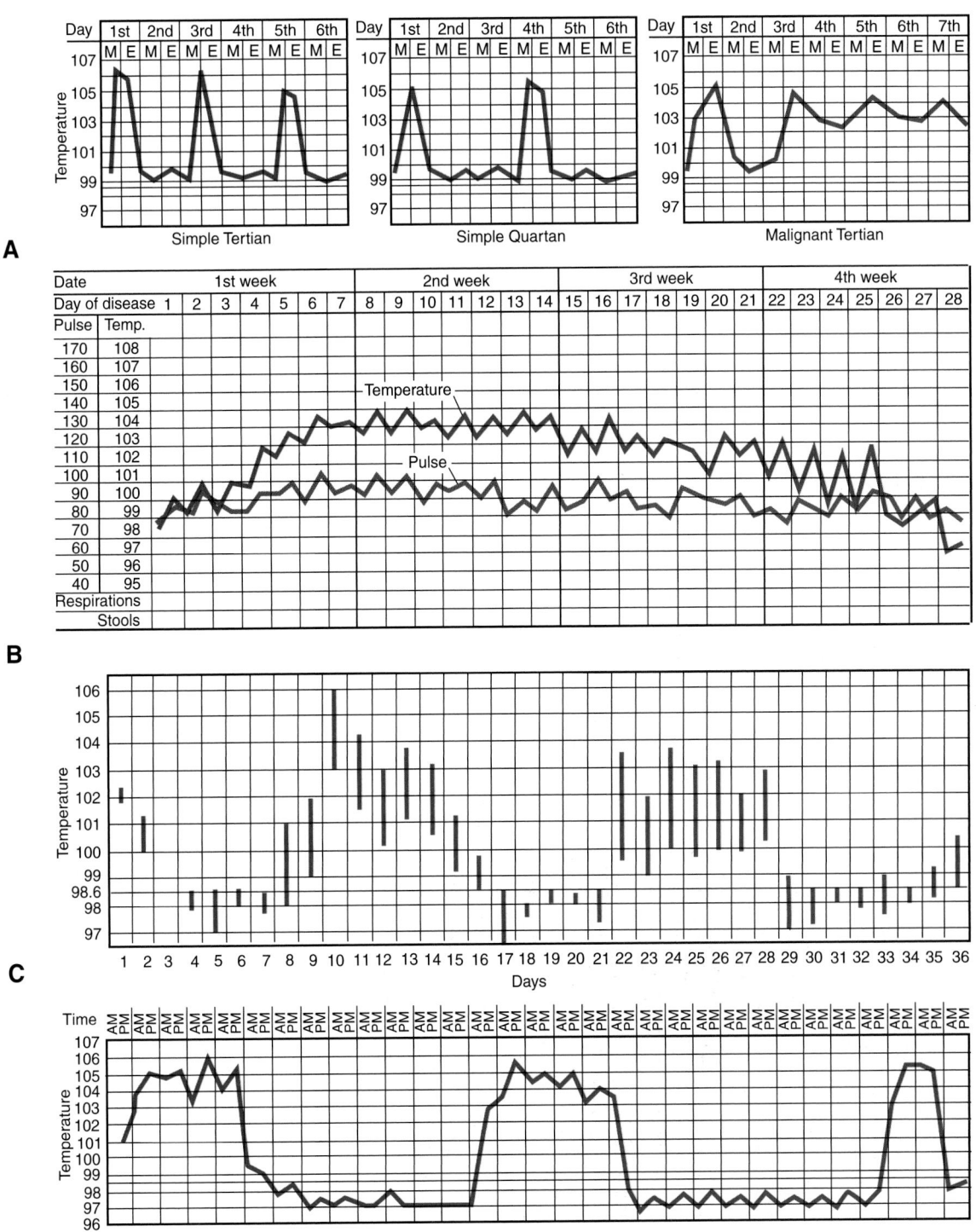

FIGURE 48-2. Distinctive fever patterns. **A,** Malaria. **B,** Typhoid fever (demonstrating relative bradycardia). **C,** Hodgkin's disease (Pel-Ebstein pattern). **D,** Borreliosis (relapsing fever pattern). *(From Woodward TE. The fever pattern as a clinical diagnostic aid. In: Mackowiak PA, ed. Fever. Basic Mechanisms and Management. 2nd ed. Philadelphia: Lippincott-Raven; 1997:215-236.)*

In pediatric populations, the height of a fever correlates roughly with the likelihood of bacteremia. McCarthy and co-workers have reported that in young children with febrile illnesses, the likelihood of bacteremia is 7% in children with temperatures of 40° C or less, 13% with temperatures of 40.5° C to 41° C, and 26% with temperatures of 41.1° C or greater.[53,54] Although there is a general perception that a similar relationship exists between the height of a fever and the likelihood of bacteremia in adults, this belief has not been substantiated. Moreover, the relationship is at best a relatively loose one even in children, with numerous examples of bacteremia in which there is little or no fever and nonbacteremic conditions, such as drug-induced fever, thrombophlebitis, and recurrent pulmonary emboli, in which extremely high fevers are encountered. Thus, although the height of fever might be useful in predicting bacteremia in febrile populations, the relationship should be invoked with caution in individual patients.

Physical Examination

In the investigation of FUO, several aspects of the physical examination should be accorded closer scrutiny than generally given during the evaluation of other illnesses (Table 48-8). Frequently, key physical abnormalities in patients with FUO are so subtle as to require repeated examinations to be appreciated. Examples include the nodular or weakly pulsatile temporal artery of temporal arteritis, the telltale oral ulcer of disseminated histoplasmosis or Behçet's syndrome, the choroid granuloma or epididymal nodule of extrapulmonary tuberculosis, the testicular nodule of polyarteritis nodosa, and the vague rectal fluctuance of a perirectal abscess. The diagnostic yield of the physical examination alone in the evaluation of FUO has not been studied directly. Nevertheless, in two pediatric series, abnormal physical findings were reported to have contributed to the diagnosis in 60% of cases of FUO.[56,57] In half of these, the abnormalities were detected only after repeated examinations. A vigorous search for lymphadenopathy is generally recommended in patients with FUO. When enlarged lymph nodes are detected in a patient with FUO, lymph node biopsy is often indicated. However, with the exception of the lymphomas, the diagnostic yield of lymph node biopsy in FUO is disappointingly low.[56,58]

Laboratory Investigations

The literature is replete with algorithms indicating which laboratory tests should be performed to evaluate FUO.[59-65] Although useful as general guides, blind application of such algorithms may result in an excessive number of tests. They should be selectively applied using clues to diagnosis gleaned from the history and physical examination. When formulating a diagnostic plan for FUO patients, the clinician should remember that the cause is more often a common disease presenting in atypical fashion, than a rare disease presenting in typical fashion.

In most series, noninvasive laboratory tests have yielded the diagnosis in approximately a quarter of the cases.[9,25,26] The most useful of these have been serologic tests for microbial pathogens and for various rheumatologic disorders. Examination of blood smears is occasionally diagnostic, especially in patients with rat-bite fever caused by *Spirillum minus*, relapsing fever caused by *Spirochaeta recurrentis*, and ehrlichiosis. Paradoxically, the advent of enhanced microbial culture systems has had less of an impact on the diagnosis of FUO than might have been anticipated. This is because such systems have become so proficient at recovering fastidious bacteria, mycobacteria, and fungi that if such microbes are present in the blood they provide the diagnosis promptly, before the time required to meet the definitions of FUO has elapsed. Bone marrow examination should be considered to rule out granulomatous diseases (e.g., tuberculosis, histoplasmosis, and sarcoidosis), carcinomatosis and hemophagocytic syndrome, especially in patients with abnormal complete blood counts (CBCs).[66] In transplant patients, procalcitonin levels may be of use in differentiating infection from acute rejection, in that elevated levels are seen in the former but not the latter condition.[67]

Imaging Studies

Imaging studies have been used primarily to localize abnormalities as a preamble to more definitive invasive tests. Computed tomography (CT) of the abdomen has been especially effective in this regard.[68] Structures appearing abnormal on CT are almost always confirmed as such on laparotomy or biopsy.[69] As a result, abdominal CT and, to a lesser extent, ultrasound imaging of the gallbladder and hepatobiliary system have been used extensively to evaluate cases of FUO. In one series, more than three CT or ultrasound examinations, or both, were performed for each FUO patient evaluated.[70] Nevertheless, the diagnostic yield per test performed is low—about 10%. False-negative CT studies have occasionally been encountered, even in cases of abscesses in solid organs, as a result of distortions of normal anatomy, small abscess size, or failure to use both oral and intravenous contrast agents.[71] Magnetic resonance imaging (MRI) is especially useful for evaluation of the central nervous system and in the abdomen for evaluation of the spleen and lymph nodes.

Scanning with labeled autologous leukocytes has been used for evaluating cases in which infections and malignant neoplasms are the cause of FUO. In such patients, labeled leukocyte scans have generally provided a higher yield overall than that obtained by either CT or ultrasound scanning.[72,73] When contemplating the use of such scans in the investigation of undiagnosed fever, one must choose between indium 111 (^{111}In)–labeled mixed leukocytes, ^{111}In-labeled pure granulocytes, and technetium 99m–labeled leukocytes.[74,75] The choice depends upon local resources and theoretical considerations. Although one might expect pure granulocytes to perform better than mixed

---

TABLE 48-8 Examples of Subtle Physical Findings Having Special Significance in Patients with Fever of Unknown Origin

Body Site	Physical Finding	Diagnosis
Head	Sinus tenderness	Sinusitis
Temporal artery	Nodules, reduced pulsations	Temporal arteritis
Oropharynx	Ulceration	Disseminated histoplasmosis
	Tender tooth	Periapical abscess
Fundi or conjunctivae	Choroid tubercle	Disseminated granulomatosis*
	Petechiae, Roth's spot	Endocarditis
Thyroid	Enlargement, tenderness	Thyroiditis
Heart	Murmur	Infective or marantic endocarditis
Abdomen	Enlarged iliac crest lymph nodes, splenomegaly	Lymphoma,† endocarditis, disseminated granulomatosis*
Rectum	Perirectal fluctuance, tenderness	Abscess
	Prostatic tenderness, fluctuance	Abscess
Genitalia	Testicular nodule	Periarteritis nodosa
	Epididymal nodule	Disseminated granulomatosis
Lower extremities	Deep venous tenderness	Thrombosis or thrombophlebitis
Skin and nails	Petechiae, splinter hemorrhages, subcutaneous nodules, clubbing	Vasculitis, endocarditis

*Includes tuberculosis, histoplasmosis, coccidioidomycosis, sarcoidosis, and syphilis.
†See text for note on the nonspecificity of lymphadenopathy identified on physical examination.

leukocytes in patients with FUO, because a greater fraction of the injected label associates with migrating cells, the literature suggests that both preparations perform equally well in practice.[74]

Another technique for evaluating undiagnosed fever, especially FUO, is gallium-67 (^{67}Ga) scanning. Its ability to image inflammation was first described by Lavender and colleagues.[76] Shortly thereafter, Hilson and Maisey reported positive results by ^{67}Ga scanning in 50 of 67 patients with FUO, of which 32 had abscesses.[77] The ^{67}Ga scan is particularly effective in visualizing chronic infections and lymphomas. In a study by Sfakianakis and co-workers, five false-negative ^{67}Ga scans and seven false-negative ^{111}In-leukocyte scans were recorded in 32 febrile patients with 26 sites of proven infection.[78] The former studies were obtained in patients with fever of less than 1 week's duration, whereas the latter came from patients who had been febrile for longer than 2 weeks. These findings suggest that if fever due to infection has been present for longer than 2 weeks, ^{67}Ga scanning is the imaging technique most likely to visualize the infectious focus.

Positron emission tomography (PET) using the positron-emitting glucose analogue, ^{18}F-fluor-2-deoxy-D-glucose (FDG), has also been shown to be useful in the evaluation of FUO, and in some studies has been more effective than ^{67}Ga scintigraphy.[79-81] In a prospective comparison of the two diagnostic modalities, Meller and colleagues[79] reported a sensitivity of 81% and a specificity of 86% for FDG imaging in detecting the focus of the fever, as compared with 67% and 78%, respectively, for ^{67}Ga scintigraphy. In another series of patients with FUO reported by Lorenzen and associates,[81] no patient with a negative FDG PET had a localizable source of fever identified by any other imaging study.

When labeled human polyclonal immunoglobulin G (IgG) was introduced as an imaging agent to detect foci of inflammation, hopes were raised that it would be both sensitive and specific for infection on the basis of binding of the Fc portion of the IgG molecule to local Fc receptors at sites of inflammation.[82,83] Although this turned out not to be the case, interest in human polyclonal IgG has persisted, owing to the publication of several articles showing human polyclonal IgG and ^{111}In-leukocyte scanning to be equally effective in visualizing infectious foci.[84,85]

The role of venous duplex imaging of the lower extremities in the evaluation of FUO is uncertain. In a survey of 89 patients with FUO, AbuRahma and colleagues identified lower extremity venous thrombosis as the probable cause of fever in 6% of the cases studied by using venous duplex imaging.[86] Their findings, which need to be corroborated by other investigators, suggest that in a small percentage of FUO patients, venous duplex imaging can establish the correct diagnosis.

Invasive Diagnostic Procedures

Histopathologic examination of tissues obtained by excisional biopsy, needle biopsy, or laparotomy provides a diagnosis in some cases, but in most published series of FUO patients, biopsy was the definitive diagnostic procedure in less than half.[71] The majority of patients with FUO undergo at least one such procedure, even though the diagnostic yield is only fair, with an average of 2.8 to 4.6 biopsies required to establish a final diagnosis.[13,87] The diagnostic yield of operative and CT-guided biopsies is higher than that of bedside biopsy procedures.[13] For this reason, bedside biopsies should rarely be performed unless guided by localizing information gained from imaging studies. An important exception to the injunction against blind biopsies concerns the temporal artery, which may merit biopsy in an elderly FUO patient with an erythrocyte sedimentation rate greater than 50 mm/hour, even in the absence of localizing signs.[9]

Exploratory laparotomy is rarely performed today unless localized findings are present. This is because few anatomic abnormalities are currently missed by CT scanning, leaving only rare cases of vasculitis, polyarteritis nodosa, granulomatous disease, and chronic cholecystitis to be diagnosed by laparotomy.[69] Laparoscopy, including laparoscopic liver biopsy, has helped further obviate the need for laparotomy.[88] Blind liver biopsy, even in patients with known liver abnormalities detected by laboratory tests or imaging, is less accurate than laparoscopic liver biopsy.[89]

Therapeutic Trials

In the past, empirical therapy with anti-inflammatory agents such as corticosteroids, aspirin, or antimicrobial agents was often given with the intent of providing an indirect diagnostic test in patients with unexplained FUO.[1] In rare cases, even antineoplastic drugs were used for this purpose. Today such trials are seldom indicated. However, in carefully selected cases, therapeutic trials employing agents with limited spectrums of activity (e.g., antimycobacterial drugs) continue to be an acceptable means of diagnosing FUO when all other means have failed.

The limitations and risks of empirical therapeutic trials are obvious. Underlying diseases may remit spontaneously during the course of ineffective therapy, giving the false impression of success. Furthermore, empirical treatment is rarely specific. Rifampin, for example, is likely to be included in empirical therapeutic regimens for tuberculosis, but is highly active against numerous bacterial species other than *Mycobacterium tuberculosis*. Similarly, fevers caused by malignant neoplasms have been reported to respond better to nonsteroidal anti-inflammatory agents such as naproxen than fevers of infectious origin,[90] but the action of naproxen is nonspecific; the ability of the so-called "naproxen test" to differentiate malignant from nonmalignant causes of FUO remains unvalidated. For these reasons, therapeutic trials, even when successful in reducing fever, may delay both the correct diagnosis and the appropriate treatment of FUO. Therefore, empirical therapeutic trials should be reserved for those very few patients in whom all other approaches have failed, and/or those so seriously ill that therapy cannot be withheld for a further period of observation.

Management

A fundamental principle in the management of classic FUO is that therapy should be withheld, whenever possible, until the cause of the fever has been determined, so that it can be tailored to a specific diagnosis.[1] This approach is based upon the oft-repeated observation that nonspecific treatment rarely cures FUO, and has the potential to delay specific diagnosis. This ideal is, however, frequently ignored in clinical practice because the road to diagnosis of FUO is, by definition, long and often frustrating. As a result, clinicians may feel compelled to treat symptoms empirically, even though the agents used may obscure the very signs and symptoms upon which the diagnosis depends. An important exception is that empirical treatment with corticosteroids may be appropriate in patients with suspected temporal arteritis, in order to prevent vascular complications such as blindness or stroke. Primary care physicians, who have learned from experience that the most cost-effective approach to many acute febrile illnesses is to try empirical antimicrobial therapy before undertaking expensive diagnostic exercises, must recognize that this approach is less likely to succeed in patients with FUO.

In neutropenic FUO, the principles of treatment are entirely different. Because of the relatively high prevalence of serious bacterial infections responsible for these fevers, febrile neutropenic patients should generally receive broad-spectrum antimicrobial therapy immediately after samples for appropriate cultures have been obtained.[91] Treatment regimens can be adjusted later, according to the results of cultures and the clinical response. Prompt antibiotic treatment is also frequently indicated in patients with nosocomial FUO, especially when such patients have severe underlying diseases or appear toxic.

Prognosis

The prognosis of FUO is determined by the cause of the fever, and by the nature of any underlying disease or diseases. The time required to establish the diagnosis is less important. Elderly patients and those with malignant neoplasms have the poorest prognosis.[1] Diagnostic delay affects the prognosis adversely in intra-abdominal infections, miliary tuberculosis, disseminated fungal infections, and recurrent pulmonary emboli.[71]

Patients in whom FUO remains undiagnosed after extensive evaluation generally have a favorable outcome, characteristically with resolution of their fever in 4 or more weeks without sequelae.[3,8,87,92] In a study of 61 patients followed long term for undiagnosed FUO,

Knockaert and associates were largely unsuccessful in identifying specific etiologies.[92] Most cases resolved spontaneously, generally obviating the need for corticosteroid therapy. Some patients, however, required nonsteroidal anti-inflammatory drugs for symptomatic relief. In this series, the 5-year mortality rate for undiagnosed FUO was only 3.2%.

SELECTED CAUSES OF FEVER OF UNKNOWN ORIGIN

The following conditions are discussed briefly because they represent some of the more important causes of FUO.

Disseminated Granulomatoses

Tuberculosis, histoplasmosis, coccidioidomycosis, blastomycosis, and sarcoidosis are all potential causes of FUO. The diagnosis of these diseases can be difficult, especially when the condition is disseminated but does not show a classic miliary pattern or other abnormalities on chest radiographs. An epididymal nodule or an oral mucosal ulcer in patients with FUO may be the only clues to disseminated tuberculosis and disseminated histoplasmosis, respectively, and should be diligently sought when performing the physical examination in FUO patients.

The disseminated granulomatoses, although potentially fatal, are among the most readily treatable causes of FUO, therefore meriting careful diagnostic attention.[71] Serial chest radiographs may demonstrate subtle infiltrates that increase gradually over time. The erythrocyte sedimentation rate is usually raised, and anemia is common. The tuberculin skin test has been reported to be nonreactive in as many as half of patients with disseminated tuberculosis, and sputum smears reveal acid-fast bacilli in only one fourth to one half of cases. Biopsies of the lung and liver each demonstrate granulomas in 80% to 90% of cases of miliary tuberculosis. Bone marrow biopsy demonstrates granulomas in only half of the patients, unless anemia, leukopenia, or monocytosis is present, in which case the likelihood of finding granulomas exceeds 80%. Bronchoalveolar lavage fluid is often culture positive, but rarely reveals acid-fast bacilli on microscopic examination. Tests based upon nucleic acid amplification can provide earlier detection of *M. tuberculosis.*

Lymphoma

Fever is a well-recognized manifestation of some malignant neoplasms, especially those originating in the hematopoietic system and those with metastases to the liver.[3,14,90,93] A number of mechanisms have been postulated for such fevers, including necrosis or inflammation in or around the tumor, and heat generated by highly metabolically active tumor cells themselves.[90] Current evidence, however, indicates that tumor-associated fever most often results from the production of pyrogenic cytokines, such as tumor necrosis factor-α and interleukin-1, either by the tumor cells themselves or by mononuclear cells that have infiltrated the tumors.[94-96]

Numerous studies have identified lymphomas as the neoplasms that most commonly cause FUO in adults.[3,13,14,29,97] Periodic (Pel-Ebstein) fevers have been reported to be characteristic of fever associated with lymphomas, especially Hodgkin's disease.[98] However, such periodic fevers are rarely reported in current reviews of FUO.

Thromboembolic Disease

Thromboembolic disease has only occasionally been reported as a cause of FUO. However, a series by AbuRahma and co-workers suggests that in contrast to the findings of earlier surveys, lower extremity venous thrombosis and recurrent occult pulmonary embolism may be responsible for as many as 6% of today's cases of FUO.[86] Thromboembolic disease is important as a cause of FUO despite its relatively low incidence because it is potentially fatal and can be effectively treated. This diagnosis is most likely to be overlooked as the cause of FUO when emboli are unaccompanied by pulmonary abnormalities, and when the attending physician fails to recognize that thrombophlebitis (even in the absence of focal signs of inflammation) and pulmonary emboli (even in the absence of radiologically apparent pulmonary infiltrates) is capable of inducing high fevers of long duration.

Endocarditis

Microorganisms causing endocarditis are generally easily identified, because in many cases they circulate continuously in the blood stream, and because today's blood culture techniques are highly efficient in isolating the bacterial species most often responsible for the infection. For these reasons, endocarditis is less common as a cause of FUO today than in earlier times. Those few cases that remain in the category of FUO belong to the special subgroup comprising culture-negative endocarditis.

The reported incidence of culture-negative endocarditis has varied widely, between 2.5% and 31% of cases of infective endocarditis.[99] The high rates of negative blood cultures reported in some previous case studies most likely reflect the use of less effective culture techniques and less rigidly defined criteria for the diagnosis of endocarditis than those employed in more recent series. Today, culture-negative cases comprise 8% to 15% of the total. The most common cause of negative blood cultures in infective endocarditis is prior antibiotic therapy; if such cases are excluded, less than 5% of cases of infective endocarditis should exhibit negative blood cultures.[100]

Some species of microorganisms that cause endocarditis are difficult to isolate using standard blood-culture techniques.[99,101,102] Most, including the HACEK group of fastidious gram-negative bacilli (*Haemophilus* spp., *Actinobacillus actinomycetemcomitans, Cardiobacterium* spp., *Eikenella* spp., and *Kingella* spp.), *Brucella, Francisella,* and strains of nutritionally variant streptococci, can be isolated within 5 to 7 days using modern blood-culture media.[103] However, a few species, for example, *Bartonella* spp., may require prolonged incubation for 2 to 3 weeks, or special culture media. If blood cultures remain sterile after 5 to 7 days in cases in which a diagnosis of endocarditis seems likely, blind subculture from liquid onto solid media may shorten the time required to isolate the etiologic microorganism. Bacteria with deficient cell walls (L-forms) are no longer believed to be a cause of culture-negative endocarditis. Therefore, special hypertonic culture media, which in the past were recommended for the isolation of L-forms, are not currently indicated in the evaluation of culture-negative endocarditis.

When infective endocarditis is caused by yeasts (most often *Candida* spp.), blood cultures will be positive in about 80% of cases. In sharp contrast, blood cultures are usually sterile in cases of endocarditis caused by filamentous fungi. Both yeasts and filamentous fungi (especially *Aspergillus* spp.) should be considered as a cause of endocarditis causing FUO in intravenous drug users, patients with prosthetic heart valves, and patients who have received prolonged intravenous antibiotic therapy.[104] In some cases of fungal endocarditis, the yield from blood cultures can be increased by using the lysis-centrifugation culture method.[99]

Serologic studies, and nucleic acid amplification tests performed on vegetations or emboli, may be helpful in diagnosing rare cases of endocarditis due to *Coxiella, Bartonella, Legionella,* and *Tropheryma whipplei.* These rare diagnoses should be considered in patients with suspected endocarditis in whom blood cultures are sterile.[105]

Temporal Arteritis and Polymyalgia Rheumatica

Temporal arteritis, also known as giant cell arteritis, and polymyalgia rheumatica are diseases with protean manifestations.[106] No single clinical symptom, sign, or noninvasive laboratory test can be relied on to establish the diagnosis. More often than not, physical findings indicative of active arteritis are absent, and a history consistent with arteritis is obtained only after careful questioning by a clinician fully versed in the varied symptoms and signs of the disorder.[106] In geriatric patients, temporal arteritis may manifest itself only through unexplained fever, or prolonged malaise, depression, or anemia.

The erythrocyte sedimentation rate is usually markedly elevated, usually more than 80 to 100 mm/hour, during active arteritis and is thus both useful as an aid to diagnosis and a clinical marker of disease activity. Rarely, the erythrocyte sedimentation rate is normal during active arteritis. For this reason, symptoms or signs, or both, consistent with the disease should be pursued even if the sedimentation rate is normal.

Nodules or diminished temporal artery pulsations need not be present for an arterial biopsy to reveal active temporal arteritis. Because pathologic abnormalities may be confined to short segments of the artery, extensive (bilateral) segments of the temporal artery may need to be examined to establish the diagnosis. Blindness, the most feared complication of temporal arteritis, can generally be averted through the use of timely corticosteroid therapy.

Adult Still's Disease (Juvenile Rheumatoid Arthritis)

Still's disease is a diagnosis based solely on clinical findings, because definitive serologic markers and other diagnostic tests for the disorder do not exist.[107] Its clinical features include high spiking fever, arthralgias or arthritis, a transient maculopapular rash, lymphadenopathy, hepatosplenomegaly, serositis, and sore throat. Leukocytosis is generally marked, and rheumatoid factor and antinuclear antibody tests are negative.

The fever of Still's disease is characteristically high and spiking, with temperatures reaching as high as 41.6° C. The fever pattern may be either intermittent (quotidian) or remittent. Although most patients seek medical attention within 2 weeks of the onset of symptoms, some 25% suffer for more than 4 weeks before doing so. A distinctive, evanescent, salmon-pink macular or maculopapular rash is typically present during the early course of the illness.

Hepatomegaly or abnormal liver function tests, or both, are common in Still's disease. Severe liver failure, however, is seen almost exclusively in conjunction with aspirin or other nonsteroidal anti-inflammatory drug therapy. In a third of patients, the disease has a self-limited course, in a quarter an intermittent course, and in a third a chronic course. In occasional patients, Still's disease has a fatal outcome.[107] Three predictors of an unfavorable outcome include root joint (shoulder and hip) arthritis on presentation, polyarthritis, and rash. No other clinical or laboratory manifestations, including human leukocyte antigen (HLA) tests, predict the outcome.[107]

Drug Fever

Fever may be the sole or most prominent feature of an adverse drug reaction.[108] This disorder is generally not accompanied by other signs of drug allergy, notwithstanding statements to the contrary in numerous textbooks and review articles. Although occasionally present, neither rash nor eosinophilia is common. Relative bradycardia is, likewise, uncommon. Several authors have suggested that there might be a characteristic drug-induced fever pattern. However, no such pattern has yet emerged, perhaps because antipyretics and external cooling measures are so frequently used to treat drug-induced fever. Considerable variability has been reported in the length of time between the onset of treatment with a drug therapy and the onset of drug-related fever. Therefore, clinicians must not assume that because a patient has been taking a certain medication for a long time, it cannot be the cause of FUO. Contrary to some early reports, there does not appear to be any clear associations between drug fever and systemic lupus erythematosus, atopy, female sex, or advanced age.[108]

Factitious Fever

Although in most series factitious fever is a relatively uncommon cause of FUO, in one report it was diagnosed in 9% of cases of prolonged FUO, suggesting that it might be more common than generally appreciated.[109] It has two forms—a fraudulent form and a self-induced form.[110] In the former, deceit is used to create the appearance of fever, whereas in the latter, genuine fever is induced by the injection or ingestion of pyrogenic materials. Fraudulent fever is most commonly created by means of thermometer manipulation involving the use of external heat sources, or substitute thermometers. Data falsification has also been used to create fraudulent fever.[111] "Fraudulent fever by proxy" refers to falsification of fever by one individual in another, usually a child.[112] Rumans and Vosti[113] reported two such cases in children, in whom the mother was believed to have manipulated thermometer readings to create the impression of fever in her children. She had previously been suspected of having orchestrated her own fraudulent fever.

Patients with self-induced fever may also cause real fevers through the self-administration of pyrogenic substances, most often bacterial suspensions.

Patients with factitious fever are generally young women, approximately 50% of whom have had training in some aspect of health care, often as nurses. Physicians have rarely been diagnosed with the disorder. In the rare male patient who manifests factitious fever, the fraudulent variety is most frequent. In women, the self-induced variety predominates. In fact, all 12 of 12 cases of self-induced infection reported by Reich and Gottfried occurred among women.[114] Factitious fever, especially the fraudulent variety, appears to be increasing somewhat in frequency among older patients.[115,116]

Obviously, factitious fever must have some psychogenic basis. However, a survey of 41 cases of factitious disorders by Reich and Gottfried found no evidence of major psychiatric diagnoses among patients with either self-induced infection or simulated illnesses.[114] Nor did these investigators find evidence of psychosis on projective testing among the few patients who underwent detailed psychological analysis.

Periodic Fevers

Many of the diseases mentioned above can cause periodic fevers, including juvenile rheumatoid arthritis, adult-onset Still's disease, Crohn's disease, and Behçet's syndrome. There are also several rare, hereditary periodic fever syndromes included on the long list of causes of FUO.[117] These include familial Mediterranean fever, hyper-IgD syndrome, and tumor necrosis factor (TNF) receptor–associated periodic syndrome. Although genetic defects responsible for these three types of hereditary periodic fever have been identified, the striking periodicity of the clinical attacks remains unexplained. They should be suspected in cases of FUO in which the fever is recurrent (i.e., febrile periods separated by symptom-free intervals of variable duration), persists for more than 2 years, and in which there is a family history of similar attacks.

REFERENCES

1. Durack DT. Fever of unknown origin. In: Mackowiak PA, ed. Fever. Basic Mechanisms and Management. 2nd ed. Philadelphia: Lippincott-Raven; 1997:237-249.
2. Keefer CS, Leard SE. Prolonged and Perplexing Fevers. Boston: Little Brown; 1955:1-248.
3. Petersdorf RG, Beeson PB. Fever of unexplained origin: Report on 100 cases. Medicine. 1961;40:1-30.
4. Alt HL, Barker MH. Fever of unknown origin. JAMA. 1930;94:1457-1461.
5. Wong SY, Lam M. Pyrexia of unknown origin—approach to management. Singapore Med J. 1995;36:204-208.
6. Smith JW. Fever of undetermined origin: Not what it used to be. Am J Med Sci. 1986;292:56-64.
7. Durack DT, Street AC. Fever of unknown origin reexamined and redefined. Curr Clin Top Infect Dis. 1991;11:35-51.
8. Iikuni Y, Okada J, Kondo H, et al. Current fever of unknown origin 1982-1992. Intern Med. 1994;33:67-73.
9. Knockaert DC, Vanneste LJ, Bobbaers HJ. Fever of unknown origin in elderly patients. J Am Geriatric Soc. 1993;41:1187-1192.
10. Chantada G, Casak S, Daza Plata J, et al. Children with fever of unknown origin in Argentina: An analysis of 113 cases. Pediatr Infect Dis J. 1994;13:260-263.
11. Knockaert DC, Vanneste LJ, Laurent J, et al. Recurrent or episodic fever of unknown origin: Review of 45 cases and survey of the literature. Medicine. 1993;72:184-196.
12. Knockaert DC. Diagnostic strategy for fever of unknown origin in the ultrasonography and computed tomography era. Acta Clin Belg. 1992;47.2:100-116.
13. Kazanjian PH. Fever of unknown origin: Review of 86 patients treated in community hospitals. Clin Infect Dis. 1992;15:968-973.
14. Larson EB, Featherstone HJ, Petersdorf RG. Fever of undetermined origin: Diagnosis and follow-up of 105 cases, 1970-1980. Medicine. 1982;61:269-292.
15. Sharma BK, Kumari S, Varma SC, et al. Prolonged undiagnosed fever in Northern India. Trop Geogr Med. 1992;44:32-36.
16. De Kleijn EMHA, Vandenbroucke JP, van der Meer, et al. Fever of unknown origin (FUO). I. A prospective multicenter study of 167 patients with FUO, using fixed epidemiologic entry criteria. Medicine. 1997;76:392-400.
17. Barbado FJ, Vazquez JJ, Pena JM, et al. Fever of unknown origin: A survey on 133 patients. J Med. 1984;15:185-192.
18. Benito N, Nunez A, de Gorgolas M, et al. Bone marrow biopsy in the diagnosis of fever of unknown origin in patients with acquired immunodeficiency syndrome. Arch Intern Med. 1997;157:1577-1580.
19. Handa R, Bhatia S, Wali JP. Meliodosis: A rare but not forgotten cause of fever of unknown origin. Br J Clin Pathol. 1996;50:116-117.

20. Norris AH, Krasinskas AM, Salhany KE, Glickman SJ. Kikuchi-Fujimoto disease: A benign cause of fever and lymphadenopathy. Am J Med. 1996;101:401-405.
21. McDermott EM, Smillie DM, Powell RJ. Clinical spectrum of familial Hibernian fever: A 14-year follow-up study of the index case and extended family. Mayo Clin Proc. 1997;72:806-817.
22. Klastersky J, Weerts D, Hensgens C, et al. Fever of unexplained origin in patients with cancer. Eur J Cancer. 1973;9:649-656.
23. Hamman L, Wainwright CW. The diagnosis of obscure fever. II. The diagnosis of unexplained high fever. Johns Hopkins Hosp Bull. 1936;58:307-331.
24. Berger L, Sinkoff MW. Systemic manifestations of hypernephroma: A review of 273 cases. Am J Med. 1957;22:791-796.
25. Shoji S, Imamura A, Imai Y, et al. Fever of unknown origin: A review of 80 patients from the Shin'etsu area of Japan from 1986-1992. Intern Med. 1994;33:74-76.
26. Saxe SE, Gardner P. The returning traveler with fever. Infect Dis Clin North Am. 1992;6:427-439.
27. Jacobs RF, Schutze GE: *Bartonella henselae* as a cause of prolonged fever and fever of unknown origin in children. Clin Infect Dis. 1998;26:80-84.
28. Gleckman RA, Esposito AL. Fever of unknown origin in the elderly: Diagnosis and treatment. Geriatrics. 1986;41:45-52.
29. Kauffman CA, Jones PG. Diagnosing fever of unknown origin in older patients. Geriatrics. 1984;39:46-51.
30. Ghose MK, Shensa S, Lerner PI. Arteritis of the aged (giant cell arteritis) and fever of unexplained origin. Am J Med. 1976;60:429-436.
31. Tal S, Guller V, Gurevich A, Levi S. Fever of unknown origin in the elderly. J Intern Med. 2002; 252:295-304.
32. Suh KN, Kozavsky PE, Keystone JS. Evaluation of fever in the returned traveler. Travel Med. 1999;83:997-1017.
33. Konecny P, Davidson RN. Pyrexia of unknown origin in the 1990s: Time to redefine. Br J Hosp Med. 1996;56:21-24.
34. Neuhoff FJ, Brewer JE, Castaneda T, et al. Frequency and yield of postoperative fever evaluation. Infect Dis Obstet Gynecol. 1998;6:252-255.
35. Anand VT, Phillipps JJ, Allen D, et al. A study of postoperative fever following paediatric tonsillectomy. Clin Otolaryngol Allied Sci. 1999;24;360-364.
36. Shaw JA, Chung R. Febrile response after knee and hip arthroplasty. Clin Orthoped Related Res. 1999;367:181-189.
37. Circiumaru B, Baldock G, Cohen J. A prospective study of fever in the intensive care unit. Intensive Care Med. 1999;25:668-673.
38. Hall J. Assessment of fever in the intensive care unit. Is the answer just beyond the tip of our nose? Am J Respir Crit Care Med. 1999;159:693-694.
39. Georgilis K, Plomaritoglou A, Dafni U, et al. Aetiology of fever in patients with acute stroke. J Intern Med. 1999;246:203-209.
40. Engelhart S, Glasmacher A, Exner M, Kramer MH. Surveillance for nosocomial infections and fever of unknown origin among adult hematology-oncology patients. Infect Control Hosp Epidemiol. 2002;23:244-248.
41. Corey L, Boeckh M. Persistent fever in patients with neutropenia. N Engl J Med. 2002;346:222-224.
42. Chang FY, Singh N, Gayowski T, et al. Fever in liver transplant recipients: Changing spectrum of etiologic agents. Clin Infect Dis. 1998;26:59-65.
43. Regnery RL, Anderson BE, Clarridge JE III, et al. Characterization of a novel *Rochalimaea* species, *R. henselae* sp nov, isolated from blood of a febrile, human immunodeficiency virus positive patient. J Clin Microbiol. 1992;30:265-274.
44. Miralles P, Moreno S, Perez-Tascon M, et al. Fever of uncertain origin in patients infected with the human immunodeficiency virus. Clin Infect Dis. 1995;20:872-875.
45. Bissuel F, Leport C, Perrone C, et al. Fever of unknown origin in HIV-infected patients: A critical analysis of a retrospective series of 57 cases. J Intern Med. 1994;236:529-535.
46. Wheeler DA, Call SC, Wasserman SS, et al. Relationship between basal body temperature and stage of disease in asymptomatic HIV-infected men. Infect Dis Clin Pract. 1997;6:47-50.
47. Sepkowitz KA. Effect of prophylaxis on the clinical manifestations of AIDS-related opportunistic infections. Clin Infect Dis. 1998;26:806-810.
48. Lozano F, Torre-Cisneros J, Santos J, et al. Impact of highly active antiretroviral therapy on fever of unknown origin in HIV-infected patients. Eur J Clin Microbiol Infect Dis. 2002;21:132-139.
49. Barbado FJ, Gomez-Cerezo J, Pena JM, et al. Fever of unknown origin: Classic and associated with human immunodeficiency virus infection. A comparable study. J Med. 2001;32:152-162.
50. Armstrong WS, Katz JT, Kazanjian PH. Human immunodeficiency virus-associated fever of unknown origin: A study of 70 patients in the United States and review. Clin Infect Dis. 1999;28:341-345.
51. Aduan RP, Fauci AS, Dale DC, Wolff SM. Prolonged fever of unknown origin (FUO): A prospective study of 347 patients. Clin Res. 1978;26:558A.
52. Mackowiak PA. Commentary: Fever patterns. Infect Dis Clin Pract. 1997;6:308-309.
53. McCarthy PL, Dolan TF. Hyperpyrexia in children. Am J Dis Child. 1976;130:849-851.
54. McCarthy PL, Jekel JF, Dolan TF. Temperature greater than or equal to 40°C in children less than 24 months of age: A prospective study. Pediatrics. 1977;59:663-668.
55. Woodward TE. The fever pattern as diagnostic aid. In: Mackowiak PA, ed. Fever: Basic Mechanisms and Management. 2nd ed. Philadelphia: Lippincott-Raven; 1997;215-235.
56. Pizzo PA, Lovejoy FH, Smith DH: Prolonged fever in children: Review of 100 cases. Pediatrics. 1975;55:468-473.
57. Lohr JA, Hendley JO. Prolonged fever of unknown origin: A record of experiences with 54 childhood patients. Clin Pediatr. 1977;16:768-773.
58. Sheon RP, Van Ommeu RA. Fever of obscure origin: Diagnosis and treatment based on a series of sixty cases. Am J Med. 1963;34:486-499.
59. Vickery DM, Quinnell RK. Fever of unknown origin. An algorithmic approach. JAMA. 1977;238:2183-2188.
60. Esposito AL, Gleckman RA. A diagnostic approach to the adult with fever of unknown origin. Arch Intern Med. 1979;139:575-579.
61. Hurley DL. Fever in adults. What to do when the cause is not obvious? Postgrad Med. 1983;74:232-244.
62. Gries E, Hoensch H, Ohnhaus EE. Differential Diagnose bei bisher ungeklärtem Fieber: Bedeutung klinischer Begleir Symptome. Klin Wochenschr. 1986;64:307-313.
63. Nolan SM, Fitzgerald FT. Fever of unknown origin: The general internist's approach. Postgrad Med. 1987;81:190-205.
64. Koch H, Jenke V. Fever unklarer Ursache-ein diagnostisches Basisprogramm. Z Gesamte Inn Med. 1990;1890:560-562.
65. Fischer JL, Henselmann L. Stufendiagnostik des Fieber unbekannter Ursache. Med Klin. 1987;82:229-235.
66. Palazzi DL, McClain KL, Kaplan SL. Hemophagocytic syndrome in children: An important diagnostic consideration in fever of unknown origin. Clin Infect Dis. 2003;36:306-312.
67. Kuse ER, Langefeld I, Jaeger K, Kulpmann WR. Procalcitonin in fever of unknown origin after liver transplantation: A variable to differentiate acute rejection from infection. Crit Care Med. 2000;28:555-559.
68. Rowland MD, Del Bene VE. Use of body computed tomography to evaluate fever of unknown origin. J Infect Dis. 1987;156:408-409.
69. Quinn MJ, Sheedy PF II, Stephen DH, Hattery RR. Computed tomography of the abdomen in evaluation of patients with fever of unknown origin. Radiology. 1980;136:407-411.
70. Knockaert DC, Vanneste LJ, Vanneste SB, Bobbaers HJ. Fever of unknown origin in the 1980s: An update of the diagnostic spectrum. Arch Intern Med. 1992;152:51-55.
71. Arnow PM, Flaherty JP. Fever of unknown origin. Lancet. 1997;350:575-580.
72. Knockaert DC, Mortelmans LA, De Roo MC, Bobbaers HJ. Clinical value of gallium-67 scintigraphy in evaluation of fever of unknown origin. Clin Infect Dis. 1994;18:601-605.
73. Syrjala MT, Valtonen V, Liewendahl K, Myllylä G. Diagnostic significance of indium-111 granulocyte scintigraphy in febrile patients. J Nucl Med. 1987;28:155-160.
74. Peters AM. Localizing the cause of undiagnosed fever. Eur J Nucl Med. 1996;23:239-242.
75. Kjaer A, Lebech A-M. Diagnostic value of ^{111}In-granulocyte scintigraphy in patients with fever of unknown origin. J Nucl Med. 2002;43:140-144.
76. Lavender JP, Lowe J, Barker JR. Ga-67 citrate scanning in neoplastic and inflammatory lesions. Br J Radiol. 1971;44:361-366.
77. Hilson AJW, Maisey MN. Gallium-67 scanning in pyrexia of unknown origin. BMJ. 1979;II:1330-1331.
78. Sfakianakis GN, Al-Sheikh W, Heal A, et al. Comparison of scintigraphy with ^{111}In leukocytes and ^{67}Ga in the diagnosis of occult sepsis. J Nucl Med. 1982;23:618-626.
79. Meller J, Altenvoerde G, Munsel U, et al. Fever of unknown origin: Prospective comparison of [^{18}F] FDG imaging with a double-bead coincidence camera and gallium-67 citrate SPECT. Eur J Nucl Med. 2000;7:1617-1625.
80. Blockmans D, Knockaert D, Maes A, et al. Clinical value of [^{18}F] fluro-deoxyglucose positron emission tomography for patients with fever of unknown origin. Clin Infect Dis. 2001;32:191-196.
81. Lorenzen J, Buchert R, Bohuslavizki KH. Value of FDG PET in patients with fever of unknown origin. Nucl Med Comm. 2001;22:779-783.
82. Rubin RH, Young LS, Hansen WP, et al. Specific and non-specific imaging of localized Fisher immunotype 1 *Pseudomonas aeruginosa* infection with radiolabeled monoclonal antibody. J Nucl Med. 1988;29:651-656.
83. Lind P, Langsteger W, Kotringer P, et al. Immunoscintigraphy of inflammatory processes with a technetium-99m-labeled monoclonal antigranulocyte antibody (Mab BW 250/183). J Nucl Med. 1990;31:417-423.
84. Oyen WJG, Claessens RAMJ, van der Meer JWM, et al. Detection of subacute infectious foci with In-111-labelled autologous leukocytes and In-111-labelled human nonspecific immunoglobulin G: A prospective comparative study. J Nucl Med. 1991;32:1854-1860.
85. Datz FL, Anderson CE, Ahluwalia R, et al. The efficacy of indium-111-polyclonal IgG for the detection of infection and inflammation. J Nucl Med. 1994;35:74-83.
86. AbuRahma AF, Saiedy S, Robinson PA, et al. Role of venous duplex imaging of the lower extremities in patients with fever of unknown origin. Surgery. 1997;121:366-371.
87. Larson EB, Featherstone HJ, Petersdorf RG. Fever of undetermined origin: Diagnosis and follow-up of 105 cases, 1970-1980. Medicine. 1982;61:269-292.
88. Solis-Herruzo JA, Benita V, Morillas JD. Laparoscopy in fever of unknown origin—Study of seventy cases. Endoscopy. 1981;13:207-210.
89. Mitchell DP, Hanes TE, Hoyumpa AM Jr, Schenker S. Fever of unknown origin—Assessment of the value of percutaneous liver biopsy. Arch Intern Med. 1977;137:1001-1004.
90. Chang JC, Hawley BH. Neutropenic fever of undetermined origin (N-FUO): Why not use the naproxen test? Cancer Invest. 1995;13:448-450.
91. Hughes WT, Armstrong D, Bodey GP, et al. Guidelines for the use of antimicrobial agents in neutropenic patients with unexplained fever. J Infect Dis. 1990;161:381-396.
92. Knockaert DC, Dujardin KS, Bobbaers HJ. Long-term follow-up of patients with undiagnosed fever of unknown origin. Arch Intern Med. 1996;156:618-620.
93. Bodel P. Tumors and fever. Ann N Y Acad Sci. 1974;230:6-13.
94. Bodel P, Ralph P, Wenc K, Long JC. Endogenous pyrogen production by Hodgkin's disease and human histiocytic lymphoma cell lines *in vitro*. J Clin Invest. 1980;65:514-518.
95. Dinarello CA. Interleukin-1. Rev Infect Dis. 1984;6:51-95.
96. Lachman LB, Moore JO, Metzger RS. Preparation and characterization of LAF from acute monocytic and myelomonocytic leukemic cells. Cell Immunol. 1978;41:189-206.
97. Esposito AL, Gleckman R. Fever of unknown origin in the elderly. J Am Geriatr Soc. 1978;26:498-505.

98. Reimann HA. Periodic (Pel-Ebstein) fever of lymphomas. Ann Clin Lab Sci. 1977;7:1-5.
99. Cannady PB Jr, Sanford JP. Negative blood cultures in infective endocarditis: A review. South Med J. 1976;69:1420-1424.
100. Von Reyn CF, Levy BS, Arbeit RD, et al. Infective endocarditis: An analysis based on strict case definitions. Ann Intern Med. 1981;94:505-518.
101. Van Scoy RE. Culture-negative endocarditis. Mayo Clin Proc. 1982;57:149-154.
102. Washington JA II. The role of the microbiology laboratory in the diagnosis and antimicrobial treatment of infective endocarditis. Mayo Clin Proc. 1982;57:22-32.
103. O'Grady NP, Barie PS, Bartlett JC, et al. Practice guidelines for evaluating new fever in critically ill adult patients. Clin Infect Dis. 1998;26:1042-1059.
104. Rubinstein E, Noriega ER, Simberkoff MS, et al. Fungal endocarditis: Analysis of 24 cases and review of the literature. Medicine (Baltimore). 1975;54:331-334.
105. Tompkins LS, Roessler BJ, Redd SC, et al. *Legionella* prosthetic-value endocarditis. N Engl J Med. 1988;318:530-535.
106. Goodman BW. Temporal arteritis. Am J Med. 1979;67:839-852.
107. Pouchot J, Sampalis JS, Beaudet F, et al. Adult Still's disease: Manifestations, disease course, and outcome in 62 patients. Medicine. 1991;70:118-136.
108. Mackowiak PA, LeMaistre CF. Drug fever: A critical appraisal of conventional concepts. Ann Intern Med. 1987;106:728-733.
109. Aduan RP, Fauci AS, Dale DC, et al. Factitious fever and self-induced infection, a report of 32 cases and review of the literature. Ann Intern Med. 1979;90:230-242.
110. Sarwari AR, Mackowiak PA. Factitious fever. Curr Clin Topics Infect Dis. 1997;17:88-94.
111. Petersdorf RG, Bennet IL. Factitious fever. Ann Intern Med. 1957;46:1039-1062.
112. Rosenberg DA. Web of deceit: A literature review of Munchausen syndrome by proxy. Child Abuse Negl. 1987;11:547-563.
113. Rumans LW, Vosti KL. Factitious and fraudulent fever. Am J Med. 1978;65:745-755.
114. Reich D, Gottfried LA. Factitious disorders in a teaching hospital. Ann Intern Med. 1983;99:240-247.
115. Potin M, Regamey C, Glauser MP. Factitious fever as a cause of prolonged fevers (in French). J Suisse Med. 1983;113:1534-1539.
116. Marcus EL, Van Dijk JM. Fever of unknown origin (Letter). J Am Geriatr Soc. 1991;36:637-638.
117. Drenth JPH, van der Meer JWM. Hereditary periodic fever. N Engl J Med. 2001;345:1748-1757.
118. MacLean JD, Lalonde RG, Ward B. Fever from the tropics. Trav Med Advisor. 1994;5:27.
119. Doherty JF, Grant AD, Bryceson ADM. Fever as the presenting complaint of travellers returning from the tropics. Quarterly J Med. 1995;88:277.

CHAPTER **49**

The Acutely Ill Patient with Fever and Rash

DAVID J. WEBER

MYRON S. COHEN

WILLIAM A. RUTALA

A recognizable rash can lead to immediate diagnosis and appropriate therapy. Material isolated from involved skin, when properly handled, can confirm a specific diagnosis. Unfortunately, rashes often present a bewildering array of diagnostic possibilities. Dermatologists, who are generally more comfortable with evaluation of the skin, are not always available for immediate consultation. Furthermore, dermatologists and infectious disease specialists frequently differ in their approach to the patient with a rash.

This chapter provides a framework for investigation of the cause of rash, with emphasis on the following: (1) a diagnostic approach to patients with fever and rash, (2) categories of skin lesions, and (3) brief descriptions of the most important febrile illnesses characterized by a rash.

APPROACH TO THE PATIENT

In the initial evaluation of a patient with fever and rash, four concerns must be addressed immediately. The first is whether the patient is well enough to provide further history, or whether cardiorespiratory support is urgently required. The second is whether the nature of the rash, in the context of presentation, demands institution of isolation precautions. Isolation is required primarily for patients whose illnesses allow droplet or airborne spread of the pathogen and includes both viral and bacterial disease. If deemed necessary, isolation practices should be scrupulously used. Health care workers should exercise caution in all interactions with patients with undiagnosed infectious diseases, and they should use standard precautions including the avoidance of intimate contact with secretions.[1-5] Although the vast majority of skin eruptions are noninfectious in origin, gloves should always be worn during the examination of the skin whenever an infectious cause is being considered, because some infections (e.g., syphilis, herpes simplex virus [HSV]) may be acquired via direct skin contact. In the event of potential exposure to a pathogen, health care workers should be evaluated by their occupational health service for postexposure prophylaxis or the need for work restrictions.[6] The third concern is whether the skin lesions are consistent with meningococcal disease (see later); such cases require immediate institution of antibacterial therapy.[7] Similar urgency may be warranted when lesions suggest bacterial septic shock, staphylococcal or streptococcal toxic shock, necrotizing fasciitis, or Rocky Mountain spotted fever, because appropriate use of antibiotics may improve survival.[8] Finally, consideration must be given to the possibility that the patient has an exotic disease acquired as a result of travel or the intentional release of an agent of bioterrorism.[9] Bioterrorist agents that may be acquired via person-to-person transmission and characteristically cause a generalized rash include smallpox[10] and the viral hemorrhagic fevers[11] (i.e., Ebola, Lassa fever, Marburg, Congo-Crimean fever, Bolivian hemorrhagic fever, and Argentinean hemorrhagic fever). Plague[12] and anthrax[13] may present with localized skin lesions. Patients with plague should be placed on droplet precautions (gown, gloves, and eye protection) until pneumonia is excluded or until the patient has been on appropriate therapy for 48 hours.[12] Nonprotected contact with cutaneous anthrax has rarely led to person-to-person transmission, and patients with cutaneous anthrax lesions should be placed on contact precautions.[14]

The history obtained from the patient should elicit the following information:

1. Drug ingestion within the past 30 days
2. Travel outside the local area
3. Occupational exposure
4. Sun exposure
5. Immunizations
6. Sexually transmitted disease exposure, including risk factors for infection with human immunodeficiency virus (HIV)
7. Factors affecting immunologic status, including chemotherapy, steroid use, hematologic malignancy, solid organ or bone marrow transplantation, and functional or anatomic asplenia
8. Valvular heart disease
9. Prior illnesses, including a history of drug or antibiotic allergies
10. Exposure to febrile or ill persons within the recent past
11. Exposure to wild or rural habitats, insects, arthropods, and wild animals
12. Pets and habits

The clinician should pay particular attention to the season of the year, which dramatically affects the epidemiology of febrile rashes of infectious origin.

Physical examination should focus on the following:

1. Vital signs
2. General appearance
3. Signs of toxicity
4. Presence and location of adenopathy
5. Presence and morphology of genital, mucosal, or conjunctival lesions
6. Detection of hepatosplenomegaly
7. Presence of arthritis
8. Signs of nuchal rigidity, meningismus, or neurologic dysfunction

Key ingredients in arriving at a correct diagnosis, or at least a useful, limited, "working" list of likely diagnoses, include determination of (1) the primary type(s) of skin lesions present, (2) the distribution of the eruption, (3) the pattern of progression of the rash, and (4) the timing of the onset of the rash relative to the onset of fever and other signs of systemic illness.[15-21] Although histologic findings from lesional skin biopsies may help to confirm some diagnoses,[22] the patterns observed are frequently not specific for a single organism, the presence of infectious agents may not always be detectable, and laboratory studies often require at least 24 hours to complete. Thus, the clinician must attempt to use other diagnostic skills during the early evaluation of a patient with fever and rash. As discussed elsewhere, specific types of primary skin lesions frequently suggest different infectious disorders in patients with fever and rash. For example, palpable purpura, the hallmark feature of leukoclastic vasculitis, is the prototypic early finding in meningococcemia and Rocky Mountain spotted fever, whereas rapidly enlarging but asymptomatic red dermal nodules instead suggest candidemia in the appropriate host. Skin nodules noted on very deep palpation are probably located within the subcutaneous fat, suggesting one of several types of panniculitis, including erythema nodosum, a disorder caused by many different types of inflammatory or infectious processes, and erythema induratum, which is a classic tuberculoid reaction.

Examples of differences in the types of primary skin lesions present in the setting of underlying systemic infectious diseases are summarized (Table 49-1), although it should be clear that such a classification, by itself, rarely ever suggests only a single diagnosis. On the other hand, the presence of other, more specific lesions, most notably "target" or "iris" lesions (as in erythema multiforme), may suggest a single diagnosis, implicating a limited group of underlying infectious diseases as possible causes. Similarly, the presence of some lesions in the setting of fever may immediately exclude an infectious disorder as the cause of rash. For example, high fever accompanying a paucity of tender, red to violaceous, peripherally mamilled plaques suggests Sweet's syndrome (a rare hypersensitivity reaction frequently associated with selected underlying malignancies)[23] or neutrophilic eccrine hidradenitis, a rare neutrophilic dermatosis most commonly found in patients treated with chemotherapy for malignancies.[24]

Distribution or direction of spread of an eruption may be highly informative. The rash of Rocky Mountain spotted fever and acute meningococcal infection, for example, most often begins on the lower extremities and then spreads centrally (i.e., centripetally), whereas most drug- and viral infection–associated eruptions (with the exception of those caused by echoviruses and coxsackieviruses) begin on the face or trunk and spread outward (centrifugally). "Streaky" facial involvement, usually without other skin findings, is characteristic of infection due to parvovirus B19 (fifth disease, erythema infectiosum).

The number of lesions can also provide useful insight. For example, "rose spots" (see later), the hallmark cutaneous feature of *Salmonella* infection, are characteristically present in much greater numbers in patients who have paratyphoid fever than in those who have typhoid fever.

TABLE 49-1 Systemic Infections with Prominent Cutaneous Manifestations

Organism/Disease	Macules, Papules	Vesicles, Bullae	Petechiae, Purpura	Organism/Disease	Macules, Papules	Vesicles, Bullae	Petechiae, Purpura
Viruses				**Bacteria, cont'd**			
Human immunodeficiency virus type 1	X			*Bartonella henselae*	X		
Echoviruses	X	X	X	*Bartonella quintana*	X		
Coxsackieviruses	X	X	X	*Salmonella typhi*	X		
Rubeola (measles)	X			*Francisella tularensis*	X		
Atypical measles	X		X	*Streptobacillus moniliformis* (rat-bite fever)	X		X
Adenovirus	X		X	*Treponema pallidum* (secondary syphilis)	X		
Lymphocytic chorio-meningitis	X			*Mycobacterium haemophilum*	X		
Dengue	X		X	*Neisseria gonorrhoeae*	X		X
Viral hemorrhagic fevers			X	*Neisseria meningitidis*			X
Rubella (German measles)	X		X	*Leptospira* spp.	X		
Colorado tick fever	X			*Listeria monocytogenes*		X (rare)	
Yellow fever			X	*Bartonella bacilliformis*	X		
Varicella-zoster (disseminated)		X		*Borrelia* spp. (relapsing fever)	X		X
Herpes simplex (disseminated)		X		*Borrelia burgdorferi* (Lyme disease)	X (annular)		
Varicella (chickenpox)		X		*Pseudomonas aeruginosa*	X		
Vaccinia		X		*Spirillum minus* (rat-bite fever)	X		X
Variola		X	X	*Staphylococcus aureus*	X		X
Cytomegalovirus	X			Streptococci— group A (scarlet fever)	X		
Congenital cytomegalovirus			X	*Capnocytophaga canimorsus*			X
Epstein-Barr	X		X	*Vibrio vulnificus*		X	
Hepatitis B	X		X (as palpable purpura)	**Fungi (disseminated infection)**			
Monkeypox	X			*Candida* spp.	X		
Parvovirus B19 (erythema infectiosum)	X			*Cryptococcus neoformans*	X		
Human herpesvirus 6	X			*Histoplasma capsulatum*	X		
Human herpesvirus 7	X			*Blastomyces dermatitidis*	X		
Bacteria				*Coccidioides immitis*	X		
Chlamydophila psittaci	X	X		*Fusarium* spp. (agents of mucormycosis)	X		
Mycoplasma pneumoniae	X			**Protozoa**			
Ehrlichia spp.	X			*Plasmodium falciparum* (malaria)			X
Rickettsiae							
Rickettsia rickettsii (RMSF)	X		X				
Rickettsia akari (rickettsialpox)	X	X					
Rickettsia prowazekii (epidemic/louse-borne typhus)	X		X				
Rickettsia typhi (endemic/murine typhus)	X						
Rickettsia tsutsugamushi (scrub typhus)	X						

In contrast, brucellosis may be associated with only one or a few clinically subtle skin lesions, as seen in a fixed drug eruption.

Finally, timing of the rash may be particularly helpful in allowing the clinician to exclude reactions due to certain drugs as the underlying cause. With the exception of urticarial eruptions, which usually occur within a few minutes to a few hours of the administration of a systemic agent, the more typical generalized maculopapular or morbilliform drug eruption typically occurs within the first 7 to 14 days of the first dose of the offending agent, suggesting the need for a very careful drug history (including start and stop dates for all medications taken within 30 days of the onset of eruption).

It must be emphasized that noninfectious processes often include skin rash and fever and should be among the diagnostic considerations in the initial evaluation.[25] As noted previously, the presence of some highly specific morphologic types or patterns of skin lesions may quickly suggest a noninfectious cause to the astute clinician, thereby obviating the need to pursue a more extensive clinical and laboratory evaluation.

About 5% of all patients to whom a drug is administered experience an adverse reaction. Adverse cutaneous reactions to drugs are frequent, affecting 2% to 3% of all hospitalized patients[26-28] and 0% to 8% of all patients placed on medications.[29] The rate of cutaneous reactions to drugs is highest for antibiotics (1% to 8% depending on the class of antibiotic).[29] Therefore, a drug reaction must be considered in any patient with a generalized maculopapular rash, especially if associated with palmoplantar involvement. Severe cutaneous reactions often induced by drugs include Stevens-Johnson syndrome (SJS), toxic epidermal necrolysis (TEN), hypersensitivity syndrome, small-vessel vasculitis, serum sickness, anticoagulant-induced necrosis, and angioedema.[28,30] As with other rashes, a morphologic approach to drug eruptions should be used in evaluating the patient.[30]

Rashes associated with occupational exposures,[31-33] athletics,[34-36] animal exposures,[37] and international travel[38-42] have been reviewed elsewhere.

PATHOGENESIS OF SKIN RASH

Skin rash with fever can result from a local infectious process due to virtually any class of microbe that has been allowed to penetrate the stratum corneum and multiply locally. A typical example is streptococcal cellulitis. In rare cases, such localized inoculations result in more generalized eruptions, and the diagnosis is then relatively straightforward. However, eruptions that begin as generalized exanthems are the "rashes" that constitute the focus of this chapter.

An *exanthem* is a cutaneous eruption due to the systemic effects of a microorganism infecting the skin. An *enanthem* is an eruption caused in similar fashion but involving the mucous membranes. Microorganisms may produce eruptions through (1) multiplication in the skin (e.g., HSV), (2) release of toxins that act on skin structures (e.g., in scarlet fever, infections due to *Pseudomonas aeruginosa*, toxic shock syndrome [TSS], staphylococcal scalded skin syndrome [SSSS]), (3) evoking an inflammatory response involving phagocytes and lymphocytes, in which the microbicidal/tumoricidal metabolism of host defense cells is directed at the skin, and (4) via effects on vasculature, including vaso-occlusion and necrosis or vasodilation with edema and hyperemia. Obviously, for many eruptions, several concurrent mechanisms can play a role.

DIFFERENTIAL DIAGNOSIS IN SKIN RASH

There are two ways to approach the investigation of infectious rash: either by the type of lesion visualized or by knowledge of individual pathogens and the rashes they produce (Table 49-2). Unfortunately, neither system alone serves both to generate a complete list of diagnostic possibilities to rule out disorders as appropriate. Accordingly, both approaches should be incorporated into evaluation of the patient with skin rash and fever.

Characteristics of the Lesion

Morphologic types of primary skin lesions include macules, papules, nodules, vesicles, bullae, pustules, and plaques. *Macules* are flat, nonpalpable lesions in the plane of the skin. *Papules* are small, solid, palpable lesions elevated above the plane of the skin. Large papules are referred to as *nodules*. *Vesicles* and *bullae* are small and large blisters, respectively, and *pustules* are usually small, palpable lesions filled with pus. *Plaques* are large, flat lesions, usually greater than 1 cm in diameter, that are palpable. In addition to morphology, lesions are characterized by their color and, particularly in the setting of a systemically ill-appearing patient, by the presence or absence of hemorrhage, which hemorrhagic lesions being termed *purpura* or *petechiae*. Lesions may be skin-colored, hyperpigmented or hypopigmented, or any of several other colors, of which red is the most common; the presence of such reddening is *erythema*. Blanching erythematous

				Time to Appearance
TABLE 49-2 Skin Lesions and Systemic Infections				
Lesion	*Common Pathogens*	*Histologic Findings*	*Smears Positive for Pathogens*	*(after onset of illness)*
Symmetric peripheral gangrene, purpura fulminans, acrocyanosis	Noninfectious or gram-negative bacteria, *Capnocytophaga canimorsus*	Bleeding in the skin, vascular thrombosis, perivascular infiltration	No	12-36 hr
Multiple purpuric lesions in severely ill patients	*Neisseria meningitidis, Capnocytophaga canimorsus, Rickettsia* spp., other gram-negative bacteria	Vascular thrombosis, perivascular hemorrhage	Yes*	12-36 hr†
Ecthyma gangrenosum, other bullous lesions	*Pseudomonas,* gram-negative bacteria, *Vibrio vulnificus*	Veins, mainly involved, intima spared, inflammatory reaction	Yes	Several days
Macronodular lesions	*Candida, Cryptococcus neoformans, Histoplasma capsulatum, Fusarium*	Hyphae, mononuclear perivascular reaction	No	Several days
Delayed-onset rash with nonsymmetric, scattered maculopapular or vesicular lesions	*Neisseria gonorrhoeae, N. meningitidis* (chronic)	Perivascular mononuclear infiltrate, immune complex	Occasionally (few bacteria only)	3-10 days
Rose spots	*Salmonella* spp.	Perivascular mononuclear infiltrate, or leukoclastic vasculitis	No	5-10 days
"Toxic erythema"	*Staphylococcus aureus* (SSS)	Dilatation and perivascular edema	No	At presentation

*Except for Rocky Mountain spotted fever, in which therapy biopsy and immunofluorescent staining may aid early diagnosis.
†In Rocky Mountain spotted fever, 1-7 days.
Adapted from Kingston ME, Mackey D. Skin clues in the diagnosis of life-threatening infections. Rev Infect Dis. 1986;8:1-11.

lesions are those in which erythema is due to vasodilatation, whereas nonblanching erythema may be due to extravasation of blood. As noted, purpuric lesions are those in which there is hemorrhage into the skin and may be small (petechial) or large (ecchymotic). For purposes of the following discussion, it is useful to divide eruptions into those that are maculopapular (characterized by both flat and elevated lesions), nodular, vesiculobullous, erythematous, and purpuric.

Maculopapular Rash

Maculopapular rashes are usually seen in viral illnesses, drug eruptions, and immune complex–mediated syndromes. Potentially responsible viral disorders include the classic childhood viral diseases such as measles, rubella, erythema infectiosum, and roseola.[43-48] Other viral agents that occasionally produce a maculopapular rash are coxsackieviruses, echoviruses, cytomegalovirus, and hepatitis B virus. Nineteen percent of patients with West Nile fever, an emerging infectious disease in the United States, have been reported to have a rash described as an erythematous macular, papular, or morbilliform eruption involving some combination of the neck, the trunk, and the arms and legs.[49]

Erythema multiforme and its variants may be considered a special category of maculopapular rash. The erythema multiforme group of diseases encompasses a number of acute self-limited exanthematic intolerance reactions that share at least two characteristic features: target lesions (stable circular erythemas or urticarial plaques with areas of blistering, necrosis, and /or resolution in a concentric array) and histologically satellite-cell (or more widespread) necrosis of the epidermis.[50] These disorders result from a cytotoxic immunologic attack on keratinocytes expressing nonself antigens. The antigens are predominately microbes (viruses) or drugs. The spectrum of disease may be divided into two main groups: (1) erythema multiforme, a common, usually mild and relapsing eruption and (2) the SJS-TEN complex, an infrequent severe mucocutaneous intolerance reaction.[50] The spectrum of disorders included in group 2 has been further divided into five subgroups depending on the pattern of lesions distribution and extent of blisters or detachment: erythema multiforme majus (localized, <10% blisters per detachment), SJS (widespread, <10% blisters per detachment), overlap SJS-TEN (widespread, 10% to 29% blisters per detachment), TEN with "spots" (widespread, <30% blisters per detachment), and TEN without "spots" (widespread, >10% blisters per detachment).[51]

Erythema multiforme is an acute self-limited exanthem that is usually mild and relapsing. Lesions of erythema multiforme usually begin as round to oval macules and papules that range in size from less than 1 cm up to 1 to 2 cm in diameter. The most characteristic lesions of erythema multiforme have central erythema surrounded by a narrow ring of normal-appearing skin that is in turn surrounded by another thin ring of erythema to form so-called target lesions (iris or "bull's-eye" lesions). The central area may be dark red, blue, or dusky gray in color and may develop into a blister. Lesions are generally symmetrically distributed on the trunk and extremities and may show a predilection for knees, elbows, palms, and soles. Nikolsky's sign is absent. Mucosal involvement is usually present but mild, and usually involves only oral mucosa. Constitutional symptoms are absent to moderate. The course of illness is typically 1 to 3 weeks. Lesions heal without scarring and complications are absent. HSV (HSV-1 and HSV-2) infection is the dominant causative factor of erythema multiforme, both in adults and in children.[52-54] Many other agents have been linked to erythema multiforme, including hepatitis B, hepatitis C, other viruses, progesterone, and other drugs.[51] In recurrent erythema multiforme, continuous therapy with an antiviral drug active against HSV (i.e., acyclovir, valacyclovir) for a 6-month period is highly effective in preventing episodes of both HSV and erythema multiforme, even in patients in whom HSV was not the obvious precipitating factor.[53] More atypical rashes that may be initially suggestive of erythema multiforme can occur in chronic meningococcemia, bacterial endocarditis, secondary syphilis, SSSS, Kawasaki disease, TSS, Rocky Mountain spotted fever, collagen vascular disease, and a variety of viral disorders. A clue useful in differentiating these disorders from erythema multiforme is the lack of target lesions.

SJS and TEN are severe, episodic, acute mucocutaneous reactions. Most cases of SJS-TEN in children follow an infectious process, especially *Mycoplasma pneumoniae*.[54] In adults, drugs are the major precipitating factor.[50,55] The antimicrobials most common associated with SJS-TEN include sulfadiazine (and other sulfa-based antibiotics), co-trimoxazole, and aminopenicillins. Other antimicrobials associated with SJS-TEN include cephalosporins, fluoroquinolones, vancomycin, rifampin, ethambutol, and thiabendazole. The two syndromes are closely related or identical, differing only in the extent of the amount of body surface area involved (i.e., <30% or >30%, respectively). In most cases SJS-TEN occurs as a single event, but after reexposure to the precipitating factor (usually a drug), it takes a more severe course. The incidence is increased up to 1000-fold in the HIV-infected population.[56] Both SJS and TEN are characterized by rapidly expanding, often irregular macules ("atypical target lesions"), and involvement of more than one mucosal site (oral, conjunctival, and anogenital). Untreated, TEN rapidly progresses to widespread full-thickness necrosis of the epidermis, resulting in separation of large sheets of epidermis from the underlying dermis either spontaneously or following the application of minimal lateral traction or pressure to the skin. Constitutional symptoms and internal organ involvement occur often and may be severe. Treatments used for SJS-TEN have included intravenous immunoglobulin, systemic corticosteroids, cyclosporin A, and thalidomide.[57,58] Thalidomide has been associated with a significantly higher mortality than placebo.[59] The other interventions have not been assessed in randomized clinical trials and their efficacy remains unproven. The mortality rate for SJS is 1% to 5%, and for TEN, 30% to 40%, with sepsis and gram-negative pneumonia the leading causes of death. Management includes appropriate supportive care (e.g., intravenous fluid replacement), prompt recognition, and withdrawal of all potentially causative drugs.[60] Treatment of patients with TEN in a burn center has been associated with reduced mortality rates.[61]

Human parvovirus B19 infection, the cause of erythema infectiosum (fifth disease), is manifested as a common exanthem in childhood and as a polyarthropathy syndrome in adults.[62-66] Symptoms associated with infection include fever, coryza, headache, and gastrointestinal distress (abdominal discomfort, nausea, vomiting). Other important disease syndromes include transient aplastic crisis in patients with hemoglobinopathies (e.g., sickle cell anemia), hydrops fetalis and intraurine fetal,[67] chronic infection in immunocompromised hosts, persistent or recurrent arthritis, myocarditis, hepatitis, and neurologic disease. Erythema infectiosum is characterized by a three-stage rash. The initial stage is that of an erythematous, warm but nontender "slapped cheek" or streaked facial rash. Simultaneously or up to 4 days later, a more variable rash appears, most often on the upper extremities, that may have a morbilliform, confluent, lacelike ("reticulate"), or even annular appearance. Later the rash may remit, but it may recur with stress, exercise, exposure to sunlight, or bathing. The rash usually disappears within 1 to 2 weeks. Because by the time this rash has appeared in immunocompetent patients, viremia can no longer be detected, such patients are infective only before the appearance of the rash.[68] Rarely (approximately 25 cases reported), parvovirus B19 may cause the "papular-purpuric gloves and socks syndrome" (PPGSS), which is characterized by a rapidly progressive painful and highly pruritic, symmetric swelling and erythema of the distal hands and feet.[69] Confluent papular, purpuric lesions then develop that involve the dorsal and palmar surfaces of the hands and feet, with sharp margins at the wrists and ankles. Subsequently, most patients develop a polymorphous enanthem involving the hard and soft palates, buccal mucosa, and lips. This syndrome generally clears spontaneously within 1 to 2 weeks. The differential diagnosis includes serum sickness, erythema multiforme, hand-foot-mouth disease, Gianotti-Crosti syndrome, Kawasaki disease, and Rocky Mountain spotted fever.[70]

In several life-threatening infections, the presenting manifestations may include blanching erythematous maculopapular lesions that later evolve into petechiae, making initial diagnosis difficult on the basis of lesion morphology alone. These infections include acute meningococcemia, Rocky Mountain spotted fever, and viral hemorrhagic fevers such as dengue. Although a diagnostic feature of rheumatic fever is an annular or a polycyclic, migrating (or expanding) erythema known as *erythema marginatum,* this disease may also be associated with the presence of a maculopapular eruption and subcutaneous nodules. Patients with enteric fever due to *Salmonella* may develop "rose spots," a transient scattering of rose-colored macules over the abdomen. Typically, the rose spots of typhoid fever are pale pink, oval or circular, completely blanchable, few in number, moderately sized (up to 0.5 to 1.0 cm in diameter), and usually present on the abdomen or trunk.[71] In contrast, rose spots of paratyphoid fever are typically smaller and more numerous.[72]

Physicians should be familiar with the cutaneous manifestations of syphilis, because primary and secondary syphilis and congenital syphilis continue to occur in the United States, especially in the South Atlantic states.[73,74] The primary skin lesion (chancre) typically develops about 21 days after exposure. Secondary syphilis is often accompanied by a rash with highly variable morphology. Lesions may be macular, papular, maculopapular, papulosquamous, or pustular. Occasionally, all types of lesions may be present in the same patient. A characteristic presentation of secondary syphilis is that of a pityriasis rosea–like eruption, appearing as numerous, tan to reddish-brown, scaly macules, usually distributed along skin tension lines on the trunk and, to a lesser extent, other body sites. Typically, no herald patch (a hallmark feature of pityriasis rosea) is present when this eruption is caused by syphilis, and usually the patient with secondary syphilis lacks associated pruritus and may have concurrent "copper penny" macules or plaques on the palms or soles. Condylomata lata, which are grayish, raised, broad, flat-appearing papular lesions, may occur in skinfolds or apposed skin in moist areas, such as the anus, vulva, and scrotum.

Nodular Lesions

A nodule is a palpable, solid, round or ellipsoidal lesion, usually resulting from disease in the dermis. Nodules may contain various inflammatory cells (as part of a hypersensitivity phenomenon), organisms (most notably fungi, as in septic emboli), or tumor cells (from metastatic cancer, lymphoma, or leukemia cutis). In the appropriate clinical setting, sudden development of dermal nodules may suggest candidal sepsis (see later), but other fungal diseases including blastomycosis, histoplasmosis, coccidioidomycosis, and sporotrichosis may produce skin nodules. Bacteria such as *Nocardia* and atypical mycobacteria (especially *Mycobacterium marinum*) may also cause nodular lesions (which typically later ulcerate).[75,76] Lesions consistent with ecthyma gangrenosum, typified by the presence of deep, "punched-out" ulcerations with overlying black eschar and peripheral erythema, suggest *Pseudomonas* sepsis. A skin biopsy specimen with appropriate stains and cultures defines the diagnosis.

Subcutaneous nodules pose a real diagnostic challenge, because they may reflect the presence of a variety of underlying disorders, including hypersensitivity reactions to systemic infection. The lesions of erythema nodosum are characterized by tender, erythematous nodules that range in diameter from less than a centimeter to several centimeters.[77,78] They are usually multiple and occur on the anterior portions of the legs but may be solitary and occur on other parts of the body. They typically do not suppurate. These lesions often develop in crops and usually heal in days to a few weeks without scarring. Infectious agents are a prominent cause of this lesion (Table 49-3). In contrast, erythema induratum, a known tuberculoid reaction, typically presents as painful, red, subcutaneous nodules over the posterior ankles. These lesions tend to suppurate, distinguishing them morphologically from erythema nodosum and most other types of panniculitis. Furthermore, erythema induratum can usually be easily differentiated from erythema nodosum on histologic examination of a wedge biopsy specimen: inflammation can be seen within subcutaneous fat lobules in the former, rather than within septal connective tissue as classically seen in erythema nodosum. Acid-fast bacilli are rarely visible within the lesions of erythema induratum, because this condition typically represents reactivation of long-standing infection with, or hypersensitivity to, the tuberculosis bacilli that are present at distant sites.

Diffuse Erythema

Diffuse erythema, especially if desquamation or peeling is present, should lead to consideration of scarlet fever, TSSs, mucocutaneous lymph node syndrome (Kawasaki disease), SSSS, SJS, and TEN. Desquamation may occur late in all of these syndromes, and its absence early in the clinical course should not be considered a reason for excluding any disease process. Most of these disorders can be easily diagnosed on the basis of the patient's history and appropriate tests.

Vesiculobullous Eruptions

A vesicle is a circumscribed, elevated lesion containing free fluid. A vesicular lesion larger than 0.5 cm is termed a *bulla.* Most vesiculobullous eruptions are immunologic in origin; few are associated with infectious systemic infections. Infectious diseases to be considered include varicella, disseminated herpes simplex, eczema herpeticum (herpes simplex superinfection of atopic eczema), and infections due to echoviruses and coxsackieviruses (including coxsackievirus A16, a cause of hand-foot-and-mouth disease). In addition, other poxvirus infections

---

TABLE 49-3 Known Causes of Erythema Nodosum

Noninfectious
Systemic lupus erythematosus
Sarcoidosis
Ulcerative colitis
Crohn's disease
Malignancies (Hodgkin's and non-Hodgkin's lymphoma, leukemia, renal cell carcinoma)
Behcet's disease
Drugs (especially oral contraceptives, sulfonamides)
Pregnancy

Infectious

Viral
 Hepatitis B virus
 Hepatitis C virus
 Herpes simplex virus
 Human immunodeficiency virus
 Epstein-Barr virus
 Measles
 Parvovirus B19
 Varicella

Bacterial
 Bartonella henselae (cat scratch disease)
 Brucella spp. (brucellosis)
 Campylobacter spp. (campylobacteriosis)
 Chlamydia trachomatis (lymphogranuloma venereum)
 Chlamydophila psittaci (psittacosis)
 Corynebacterium diphtheriae (diphtheria)
 Coxiella burnetii (Q fever)
 Franciscella tularensis (tularemia)
 Haemophilus ducreyi (chancroid)
 Mycoplasma pneumoniae
 Mycobacterium tuberculosis (tuberculosis)
 Mycobacterium leprae (leprosy)
 Mycobacterium marinum (atypical mycobacteriosis)
 Neisseria gonorrhoeae (gonorrhea)
 Neisseria meningitidis (meningitis)
 Salmonella spp. (salmonellosis)
 Shigella spp. (shigellosis)
 Streptococcus pyogenes (respiratory tract infection)
 Treponema pallidum (syphilis)
 Yersinia spp. (gastroenteritis)

Fungal
 Aspergillus spp. (aspergillosis)
 Cryptococcus neoformans (cryptococcosis)
 Blastomycosis dermatitidis (blastomycosis)
 Histoplasma capsulatum (histoplasmosis)
 Coccidioides immitis (coccidioidomycosis)
 Sporothrix schenckii (sporotrichosis)

Protozoal/helminths
 Ascaris lumbricoides (ascariasis)
 Giardia lamblia (giardiasis)
 Toxoplasma gondii (toxoplasmosis)
 Wuchereria bancrofti (filariasis)

such monkeypox, smallpox, and generalized vaccinia need to be considered (see later). HSV infection, the most common of these infection causing vesiculobullous lesions, is characterized by a grouped clustering of vesicles on an erythematous base that progresses to mucocutaneous ulceration.[79,80] Viral culture of a scraping from a blister may allow determination of a herpes infection. In addition, the demonstration of multinucleated giant cells in a scraping (Tzanck preparation) of the base of a vesicle indicates infection with HSV or varicella-zoster virus. Older vesicles can be easily confused with pustules. A *pustule* is an elevation of the skin enclosing a purulent exudate. Vesicular lesions may at times become pustules, as can occur with HSV or varicella-zoster lesions. Diffuse pustular diseases usually represent a noninfectious dermatologic illness (e.g., pustular psoriasis) or a cutaneous infection (e.g., pustular *Pseudomonas* lesions developing after the use of contaminated hot tubs or staphylococcal folliculitis). Pustular skin lesions associated with arthralgias should lead to a consideration of gonococcemia, *Moraxella* bacteremia, chronic meningococcemia, subacute bacterial endocarditis, coxsackievirus infection, and Behçet's syndrome.

Bullous skin lesions with sepsis are suggestive of the following infections: group A streptococcal erysipelas with necrotizing fasciitis (gangrenous erysipelas), ecthyma gangrenosum (due to *Pseudomonas aeruginosa* or *Aeromonas* spp.), *Vibrio* infections (especially those due to *Vibrio vulnificus*), staphyloccocal cellulitis or impetigo, and streptococcal cellulitis. Rarely, in immunocompromised patients the initial manifestation of gram-negative sepsis may be the appearance of a solitary hemorrhagic blister. *V. vulnificus* infection should be strongly considered in patients with preexisting liver disease, or other immunocompromising states, who have recently ingested raw seafood, especially oysters.[81,82] *V. vulnificus* sepsis may also occur in persons with open wounds exposed to a marine environment. Vesicopustular eruptions in the neonate may be due to both noninfectious and infectious causes. Potential infectious causes include congenital and neonatal candidiasis, staphylococcal infections, streptococcal infections, *Listeria monocytogenes* infection, HSV, neonatal varicella, and bacterial sepsis (due to various organisms).[83]

Petechial and Purpuric Eruptions

Petechiae are lesions less than 3 mm in diameter that contain extravasated red blood cells or hemoglobin. Larger lesions are termed *ecchymoses* or *purpura*. Diffuse petechial lesions should always prompt urgent investigation. In critically ill patients, these lesions are often associated with symmetric peripheral gangrene (purpura fulminans), consumptive coagulopathy, and shock. The most common infectious agents include gram-negative organisms, especially *Neisseria meningitidis*, and rickettsiae. Less commonly, *L. monocytogenes* or staphylococci may be associated with a similar clinical picture. Asplenic patients are at an increased risk of overwhelming sepsis (lifetime risk of approximately 5%), which may be accompanied by symmetric peripheral gangrene.[84-87] The lifetime risk of sepsis in asplenic hosts has been reported to range from 3% to 5%. *Streptococcus pneumoniae* is responsible for the 50% to 90% of infections in the asplenic patients and has a mortality rate of approximately 50%. Other important pathogens include *Haemophilus influenzae*, *N. meningitidis*, and *Capnocyphaga canimorsus*. Additional occasional pathogens include *Staphylococcus aureus*, group B streptococci, *Escherichia coli* and other Enterobacteriaceae, *Salmonella*, *Campylobacter*, *Bacteroides*, and *Pseudomonas*. Asplenic patients should receive the pneumococcal and meningococcal vaccines and be considered for immunization with *H. influenzae* vaccine. Pneumococcal vaccination significantly reduces the risk of pneumococcal sepsis.[88]

Viral illnesses associated with petechial rashes include infections due to coxsackievirus A9, echovirus 9, Epstein-Barr virus, or cytomegalovirus; atypical measles; and the viral hemorrhagic fevers (see Chapter 159). Although children with coxsackievirus and echovirus infections are usually nontoxic in appearance, some may appear very ill. In these patients, differential diagnosis from acute meningococcemia is difficult. However, in a series of children presenting with fever and petechiae, only 8% had meningococcal infections and 4% had bacterial sepsis secondary to other disorders.[89,90]

A diffuse rash is often a prominent characteristic of the tick-borne diseases found in the United States. (i.e., infections caused by *Rickettsia*, *Ehrlichia*, *Borrelia*, and *Coxiella*), with the exception of tularemia.[91] The frequency of a diffuse rash has been reported as follows: *Rickettsia rickettsii* (Rocky Mountain spotted fever), 99%; *Ehrlichia chaffeensis* (ehrlichiosis), 36%; *Anaplasma phagocytophilia* (ehrlichiosis), 2% to 11%; *Borrelia* spp. (relapsing fever), 28%; and *Coxiella burnetii* (Q fever), 5% to 21%.[91] Although Lyme arthritis is characterized by erythema migrans (EM), a diffuse rash may occur at the time of disseminated infection. Lesions caused by rickettsiae are usually generalized and symmetric. An eschar *(tache noire)* characteristically develops at the site of inoculation in the following rickettsial infections (infecting species): African tick bite fever *(R. africae)*, Mediterranean spotted fever *(R. conorii)*, North Asian tick typhus *(R. sibirica)*, Queensland tick typhus *(R. australis)*, rickettsialpox (due to *R. akari*), and scrub- or chigger-borne typhus *(R. tsutsugamushi)*. New rickettsioses continue to be recognized worldwide that are characterized by generalized skin lesions, often with *tache noire* lesions such as Japanese or Oriental spotted fever *(R. japonica)*, Flinders Island spotted fever *(R. honei)*, and Astrakhan fever *(R. conorii* Astrakhan).[91]

In patients with an appropriate travel history, infection with *Plasmodium falciparum* must be considered.[92] In addition, clinicians should be aware that malaria may occasionally be acquired in the United States.[93] Heavy parasitization may lead to severe hemolysis, renal failure, central nervous system abnormalities, and petechiae secondary to thrombocytopenia (rash is present in about 5% of affected patients).

The most important causes of noninfectious petechiae are thrombocytopenia, large and small vessel necrotizing vasculitis (usually presenting as palpable purpura), and the pigmented purpuric eruptions (which usually represent capillaritis).

Enanthems

In attempting to classify the exanthem, it is essential that a thorough search of the mucous membranes (including the mouth, conjunctiva, and occasionally also the vagina, rectum, and glans penis) be made for the presence of enanthems. In many allergic reactions, the mucous membranes are frequently involved. Koplik spots, diagnostic of rubeola, are tiny, white or blue-gray specks superimposed on an erythematous base, located on the buccal mucosa, most prominently on that adjacent to the molars. A "strawberry tongue" suggests the possibility of Kawasaki disease, TSS, or scarlet fever. Petechiae of the palate are common in scarlet fever and some vasculitides and with thrombocytopenia. In infectious mononucleosis, petechiae of both the hard palate and soft palate are common. Oral ulcers occur in a variety of noninfectious immunologic diseases and also with coxsackievirus A16 infection.

SWEET'S SYNDROME: A DERMATOLOGIC CONDITION ASSOCIATED WITH FEVER AND FREQUENTLY CONFUSED WITH AN INFECTIOUS PROCESS

Sweet's syndrome, also known as febrile neutrophilic dermatosis, is an unusual hypersensitivity phenomenon characterized by the presence of an angiocentric, vessel-based primary neutrophilic inflammatory cell infiltrate.[23,94] The syndrome is more frequent in women between the ages of 30 and 70 years. The disease is often preceded by symptoms suggestive of an upper respiratory tract infection. The skin demonstrates one or more tender, red, edematous, urticarial plaques or large papules. Often the border of each plaque is studded with papules (or, infrequently, with vesicles or pustules), giving an irregularly contoured, mamillated appearance reminiscent of that of the aureoles of the breast. If solitary and large, such lesions may be confused with those caused by a variety of infectious processes, including primary HSV infection or streptococcal cellulitis. When solitary and present on the dorsum of the hand, a lesion of Sweet's syndrome may mimic erysipeloid or a severe reaction to an arthropod bite. Occasionally, these plaques become dusky in color and frankly hemorrhagic, suggesting instead erythema multiforme or leukocytoclastic vasculitis. Some lesions may also become bullous, suggesting bullous erythema multiforme or fixed drug eruption. Rare bullous lesions may erode or ulcerate, mimicking pyoderma gangrenosum. Mucosal surfaces may rarely be involved. Characteristically, patients with Sweet's syndrome have associated fever; other findings may include leukocytosis, malaise, arthralgias, myalgias, conjunctivitis, and episcleritis.

The diagnosis of Sweet's syndrome is one of exclusion. Infections, neoplasia, vasculitis, and factitial disease must be excluded. Sweet's syndrome responds rapidly to high-dose systemic corticosteroids, but relapse is frequent if tapering is too rapid. Although at times idiopathic, this disorder may be a marker for underlying leukemia (especially acute myelogenous leukemia), as well as other internal malignancies.

PATHOGENS OR INFECTIOUS CONDITIONS STRONGLY ASSOCIATED WITH RASH

As noted previously, the investigation of infectious rash requires consideration of not only the characteristics of the skin lesions but also the pathogens and infectious processes strongly associated with rash. The following discussion reviews the various skin manifestations of these pathologic processes.

Sepsis

In 1992, the American College of Chest Physicians/Society of Critical Care Medicine Consensus Panel defined the severe inflammatory response syndrome (SIRS), sepsis, severe sepsis, and septic shock.[95,96] SIRS is associated with a variety of pathophysiologic insults, including infection, trauma, burns, and pancreatitis. Sepsis has been defined as "the clinical syndrome defined by the presence of both infection and a systemic inflammatory response."[97] The diagnoses of sepsis, severe sepsis, and septic shock are clinical diagnoses and do not require positive culture results. However, in a large study, the incidence of positive blood cultures increased along the continuum from 17% with sepsis to 69% with septic shock.[98] The mortality rate within a category was not influenced by the culture results. In an analysis of sepsis in the United States from 1979 through 2000, it was found that incidence of sepsis increased 8.7%.[99] Among the organisms reported to have caused sepsis in 2000, gram-positive bacteria accounted for 52.1%, gram-negative bacteria for 37.6%, polymicrobial infections accounted for 37.6%, anaerobes for 1.0%, and fungi for 4.6%.

Kingston and Mackey[22] classified the skin lesions associated with sepsis into five pathogenic processes (major categories of infectious causes): (1) disseminated intravascular coagulation (DIC) and coagulopathy (due to *N. meningitidis,* streptococci, enteric gram-negative bacilli); (2) direct vascular invasion and occlusion by bacteria and fungi (*N. meningitidis, P. aeruginosa, Aspergillus* spp., agents of mucormycosis, *Rickettsia* spp.); (3) immune vasculitis and immune complex formation (associated with infection due to *N. meningitidis, Neisseria gonorrhoeae, Salmonella typhi*); (4) formation of emboli in endocarditis (due to *S. aureus,* streptococci); and (5) vascular effects of toxins (in SSSS, TSS, scarlet fever). Various systemic bacterial infections may spread to the skin, generally producing discrete lesions from which the organisms can be isolated or recognized on biopsy with special stains. Cutaneous manifestations of DIC include symmetric peripheral gangrene, purpura fulminans, localized gangrene, acrocyanosis, other types of purpura, ecchymoses, bleeding from wound and venipuncture sites, and subcutaneous hematomas.[100] *Symmetric peripheral gangrene* is defined as ischemic necrosis simultaneously involving the distal portions of two or more extremities without proximal arterial obstruction.[101] Potential causative disorders include cardiogenic shock and other low-flow states, disorders that induce severe vasospasm such as ergot poisoning and Raynaud syndrome, disorders that lead to obstruction of small blood vessels such as cold agglutinin disease/syndrome or primary polycythemia, snake bites, and infections. Acute infectious purpura fulminans is a rare complication of septic shock.[102,103] *N. meningitidis* is the organism most commonly re-

sponsible for symmetric peripheral gangrene, but this disorder may also be due to *S. pneumoniae* and other streptococcal species, *H. influenzae, S. aureus, E. coli, Klebsiella* spp., *Proteus* spp., *Aeromonas hydrophila, Aspergillus,* and other gram-negative organisms. Symmetric peripheral gangrene is preceded by bleeding into the skin, ecchymosis, purpura, and acrocyanosis (a grayish cyanosis that does not blanch on pressure and occurs on the lips, legs, nose, ear lobes, and genitalia). Subsequently, the ecchymotic lesions become confluent, blister, undergo necrosis and ulceration, and develop overlying eschars. Histologic examination reveals a Shwartzman-like reaction in the skin characterized by diffuse and extensive hemorrhages, perivascular cuffing, and intravascular thrombosis. Bacteria are usually absent from smears of the lesions. Shock rather than DIC appears to be the major factor in the pathogenesis of symmetric peripheral gangrene.

The term *purpura fulminans* has been used synonymously with *symmetric peripheral gangrene* and in a more restricted sense to describe symmetric bleeding into the skin and subsequent necrosis after a benign infection. This latter syndrome, although most commonly reported in children, may affect adults as well and usually follows pharyngitis or a viral exanthem by several days. Common preceding illnesses include scarlet fever, streptococcal pharyngitis, staphylococcal bacteremia, varicella, and measles. Histologically, it resembles an Arthus reaction or localized Shwartzman reaction with deposition of antigen-antibody complexes in tissues. The pathogenesis of purpura fulminans appears to be related to an acquired or transient deficiency of protein C or protein S, or of both, because identical lesions have been seen in infants with homozygous protein C deficiency and in patients with heterozygous deficiency of protein C or S during the initial phase of warfarin sodium (Coumadin) therapy.[104]

Infections Due to *Neisseria* Species

Neisseria meningitidis Infection

N. meningitidis is the second most common cause of bacterial meningitis in the United States; for children and young adults, it is the leading cause of bacterial meningitis.[105] Skin hemorrhages are the hallmark of invasive meningococcal disease.[106,107] Of children presenting with fever and petechiae, *N. meningitidis* has been cultured from 0.5%,[108] 5.5%,[109] 11.1%,[110] and 27.5%.[111] Conversely, purpuric skin lesions have been noted in 50% to 90% of patients with fulminant meningococcemia.[112,113] The lesions characteristically are petechial but may be noted to blanch with pressure early in the course of infection, thus resembling a viral exanthem. The petechiae are irregular and small and are often accompanied by palpable purpuric lesions, some of which may have pale centers. Coalescing lesions, often macular, may have a characteristic gun metal–gray color centrally, consistent with epidermal necrosis. Lesions most commonly occur on the extremities and trunk but may also be found on the head, palms and soles, and mucous membranes. Symmetric peripheral gangrene may rapidly develop, often in association with DIC. Histologic examination reveals diffuse endothelial damage, fibrin thrombi, necrosis of the vessel walls, and perivascular hemorrhage in the involved skin. Gram staining of aspirates of the involved areas frequently reveals the presence of organisms.[114] In addition to the direct involvement of skin vessels by meningococci, many of the cutaneous hemorrhagic lesions may be due directly to the effects of lipo-oligosaccharide (LOS) endotoxin or indirectly to the stimulation of host cytokines.[115] Skin lesions and bacteremia are rarely findings in patients with meningococcal syndromes such as pneumonia.[116]

Chronic meningococcemia is a rare disease. The classic clinical constellation of symptoms includes intermittent or sustained fevers; recurring maculopapular, nodular, pustular, or petechial eruptions; and migratory arthritis or arthralgias with little systemic toxicity.[117-119] In one large series comprising 148 patients, skin lesions were noted to occur in 93%.[118] A variety of skin lesions may occur in chronic meningococcemia, the most frequently reported being pale to pink-colored macules and papules, seen in over 40% of cases. Nodular lesions may occur, mostly on the lower extremities. Petechiae of variable size may be seen, with superimposed vesicles or pustules centrally. Small, irregularly round, subcutaneous hemorrhages with a bluish-gray center containing pus cells are a distinctive lesion of this syndrome. Ecchymotic areas or hemorrhagic, tender nodules that are located deep in the dermis may also occur. Lesions associated with chronic meningococcemia tend to appear in showers in association with the onset of fever. In contrast to the lesions associated with fulminant meningococcemia, those of chronic meningococcemia rarely include organisms demonstrable on Gram-stained smear or biopsy specimen.[120] In addition, purpura fulminans is not a typical finding in chronic meningococcemia. A number of diseases with periodic fever, skin lesions, and joint involvement may resemble chronic meningococcemia including subacute bacterial endocarditis, acute rheumatic fever, Henoch-Schönlein purpura, rat-bite fever, erythema multiforme, and chronic gonococcemia.

Neisseria gonorrhoeae Infection

Disseminated gonococcal infection (DGI) follows untreated mucosal infection with *N. gonorrhoeae* in 1.0% to 3% of patients.[121-124] Skin lesions are the most common manifestation of DGI and occur in 50% to 70% of patients.[125] The eruption typically appears during the first day of symptoms and may recur with each bout of fever.[126] The skin lesions associated with DGI begin as tiny red papules or petechiae 1 to 5 mm in diameter, many of which evolve rapidly through vesicular or pustular stages to develop a gray necrotic center, often on a hemorrhagic base.[126,127] Papules, bullae, pustules, and hemorrhagic lesions all may be present simultaneously. The lesions tend to be scanty but widely distributed. The distal portions of the extremities are most commonly involved (at times associated with tenosynovitis), with sparing of the scalp, face, trunk, and oral mucous membranes. Histologic examination reveals leukocytoclastic vasculitis with fibrin thrombi.[128] Gram-stained smears of material from skin lesions infrequently contain organisms, although most smears are positive for gonococci when examined by immunofluorescence techniques. Circulating immune complexes may play a role in the pathogenesis of DGI-associated skin lesions and arthritis/tenosynovitis.[129]

Pseudomonas Infection

Pseudomonas spp. are ubiquitous environmental organisms that are important pathogens in the hospital and in patients with certain underlying host defense abnormalities (e.g., cystic fibrosis). They may also cause infection in normal hosts, especially when the skin has been moistened. Thus, superficial infection with *P. aeruginosa* (pseudomonal folliculitis) has followed bathing in contaminated whirlpools, hot tubs, and swimming pools.[130] The lesions appear as large, follicular-based, tender, red papules. They are present only in areas exposed to *Pseudomonas*-contaminated waters. Skin lesions have been reported to accompany *P. aeruginosa* sepsis in 13% to 39% of patients.[131-133] The dermatologic manifestations of *P. aeruginosa* sepsis consist of four types of lesions. First, vesicles and bullae that may occur singly or in clusters and frequently are spread in random fashion over the skin. They may become hemorrhagic as they evolve. Second, gangrenous cellulitis that may present as a sharply demarcated, superficial, painless, necrotic lesion. It may also begin abruptly as an acute infection with local pain, swelling, erythema, and involving deep tissue and fascia. Third, macular or popular nodular lesions located predominately over the trunk; the lesions are small, oval, and painless. These lesions may resemble the rose spots of typhoid fever. Finally, ecthyma gangrenosum, a lesion characteristic but not pathognomonic of *P. aeruginosa* sepsis. Ecthyma gangrenosum has generally been reported to occur in 1.3% to 2.8% of septic patients,[131,134,135] but one report noted ecythyma gangrenosum in 28% of patients with *Pseudomonas* bacteremia.[133]

Ecthyma gangrenosum lesions begin as painless, round, erythematous macules, with or without adherent vesicles, that soon become indurated and progress to hemorrhagic bluish bullae. Later, the lesion sloughs to form a deep gangrenous ulcer with a gray-black eschar and a surrounding erythematous halo. The process evolves rapidly over a period of 12 to 24 hours. Lesions may be discrete or multiple and are usually found in the groin, axilla, or perianal areas but may occur anywhere on the body. Although most commonly associated with *P. aeruginosa* sepsis, ecthyma

gangrenosum-like lesions have also been reported in sepsis associated with other pseudomonal species,[136] *A. hydrophila*,[137,138] *Candida* spp,[139] *Serratia marcescen*,[140] *S. aureus*,[140] *Aspergillus* spp.,[140] *Morganella morganii*,[141] *Klebsiella pneumoniae*,[142] and *Mucor* spp.[143] It may also result from vasculitis or malignant infiltration.[144] Rarely, ecthyma gangrenosum due to *P. aeruginosa* may occur in the absence of sepsis.[145-148]

Histologically, ecthyma gangrenosum is characterized by three features: bacterial invasion of the media and adventitia of vein walls deep in the dermis, sparing of the intima and lumen, and minimal inflammation.[144] Bacterial invasion results in marked fibrin exudation and frank hemorrhage, followed by bulla formation. Finally, necrosis of the dermis occurs. Bacteria are readily visible in biopsy samples and can be demonstrated in Gram-stained material scraped from the base of the lesion.

Subcutaneous nodules may also result from *P. aeruginosa* bacteremia. Characteristically, the nodules are erythematous and warm, may be either fluctuant or nonfluctuant, and may be tender. Despite prolonged antibiotic therapy, these lesions may contain viable bacteria weeks after the blood has been cleared of infection. The absence of fluctuance may be due to either the lack of pus in neutropenic patients or the deep location of the abscess, or both. Although successful treatment may require incision and drainage,[149,150] prolonged antibiotic therapy without drainage may result in a cure.[151,152]

Bacterial Endocarditis

Skin lesions have been reported to accompany bacterial endocarditis in 15% to 50% of cases.[153-156] The cutaneous manifestations of bacterial endocarditis are important clues to the diagnosis, although they occur less frequently than in the preantibiotic era.[157] They include Osler's nodes, Janeway lesions, subungual splinter hemorrhages, cutaneous purpura and petechiae, and conjunctival petechiae (Roth's spots). The prevalence of embolic and hypersensitivity lesions in skin and mucous membranes (50%) in heroin-associated infective endocarditis is similar to that described in patients with non–heroin-associated infective endocarditis.[158]

Petechiae are the most common skin and mucous membrane lesions observed in endocarditis, occurring in about 20% to 40% of patients. The lesions are small, flat, reddish-brown lesions that do not blanch on pressure. The petechiae may be observed on the skin, especially on the heels, shoulders, and legs. Mucous membrane (oral and conjunctiva) involvement is common. Petechiae frequently occur in small crops. Lesions usually are transient.

Osler's nodes occur in about 5% to 15% of patients with subacute bacterial endocarditis. These lesions are tender, indurated, erythematous nodules, with a pale center about 1.0 to 1.5 mm in diameter.[159,160] Osler's nodes most commonly occur on the pads of the fingers or toes but may also occur on the thenar and hypothenar eminences and over the arms. Pain may be elicited by palpating the tips of the digits. Osler's nodes tend to occur in crops, are rarely numerous, and tend to be transient. The lesions usually resolve without necrosis or suppuration 1 to 3 days after antibiotic therapy is initiated. Histologically, Osler's nodes show microabscesses with microemboli in adjacent arterioles. Osler's nodes are most commonly associated with subacute bacterial endocarditis due to infection with streptococci but may occur in endocarditis due to infection with fungi or gram-negative bacilli[160] or in systemic lupus erythematosus, typhoid fever, and gonococcemia.[25] Osler's nodes probably represent the sequelae of vascular occlusion by microemboli leading to localized vasculitis.[161]

Janeway lesions consist of small erythematous macules or, less commonly, small nodular hemorrhages in the palms and soles. Although they may be seen in subacute bacterial endocarditis, they are more common in acute endocarditis, especially that due to *S. aureus*. Unlike Osler's nodes, Janeway lesions are painless. Histologically, they show microabscesses with neutrophil infiltration of capillaries.

Infections Due to *Staphylococcus aureus* and *Streptococcus pyogenes*

Most commonly, *S. aureus* and *Streptococcus pyogenes* cause local skin infections, including cellulitis and folliculitis (see Chapter 86). Both pathogens may produce serious local infection including abscesses, myositis, and fasciitis. *S. aureus* is responsible for a variety of infectious syndromes that may produce local or diffuse skin lesions.[162-167] Skin lesions arise from (1) production of toxins,[167-170] (2) shock, and (3) vascular invasion, often in association with endocarditis. Staphylococcal toxins linked to disease syndromes include TSS toxin-1, Panton-Valentine leukocidin (community-acquired skin infections and pneumonia), epidermolysins or exfoliative toxins (SSSS), and paired enterotoxin A and LukE-LukD (antibiotic-associated diarrhea).

In recent years, there has been growing concern regarding reports of infections with community-acquired methicillin-resistant *S. aureus* (CA-MRSA).[171-173] Strains of CA-MRSA have been found to be polyclonal and demonstrate differences from the typical health care–associated strains of MRSA. Many of the CA-MRSA strains carry a novel genetic element, staphylococcal cassette chromosome (SCCmec) type IV, that includes the mecA gene. Many of the CA-MRSA strains are devoid of other antibiotic resistance genes (e.g., clindamycin) and produce Panton-Valentine leukocidin. Case series of children with CA-MRSA have reported that skin and soft tissue infections accounted for 74% to 89% of infections.[174,175] Skin infections included cellulitis, abscesses, and deep-seated infections such as pyomyositis.

Staphylococcal Scalded Skin Syndrome

SSSS describes a spectrum of superficial blistering skin disorders caused by the exfoliative toxins (also known as epidermolytic toxins, epidermolysins, and exfoliatins) of *S. aureus*.[168,176-180] Its severity varies from localized blisters to generalized exfoliation affecting the entire body surface. Although mortality in appropriately treated children is less than 4%, in adults it can reach almost 60%. Approximately 5% of all *S. aureus* produce exfoliative toxins; two serotypes have been identified at affecting humans, ETA and ETB.

Bullous impetigo, a disorder usually confined to children that results from toxin-producing strains of *S. aureus*, is characterized by discrete, flaccid bullae containing clear or cloudy yellow fluid. Lesions are frequently localized to the umbilicus, groin, or axillae. The surrounding skin may appear normal or mildly erythematous. The bullae rapidly rupture, leaving raw, denuded erosions that reepithelialize in 5 to 7 days. Affected infants are usually afebrile and lack constitutional signs.

SSSS (Ritter's disease) usually occurs in neonates or young children but may affect older children or, rarely, adults. Most cases in adults occur in association with renal impairment, lymphoma, or immunosuppression.[181-187] A well-characterized animal model exists for SSSS. Unlike in bullous impetigo, in which the staphylococcal infection is in the skin at the site of the lesion, in SSSS the infection begins abruptly with a diffuse, blanchable erythema in association with marked skin tenderness, fever, and irritability. Light stroking of the ill-defined bullae causes rupture and separation of the upper portion of the epidermis (Nikolsky's sign). Generalized desquamation usually occurs. Unless secondary infection intervenes, the skin heals within 10 to 14 days. A skin biopsy specimen (or a frozen section of an induced peel for more rapid diagnosis) may be studied to distinguish between SSSS and TEN. In SSSS, the cleavage plane of the early intraepidermal bulla is just beneath the granular cell layer, whereas in TEN, the bulla is subepidermal and associated with full-thickness necrosis of the epidermis. Early distinction between these two diseases is important because the therapy for SSSS includes antistaphylococcal antibiotics, whereas in TEN discontinuation of treatment with the offending drug and initiation of aggressive burn unit intervention may be lifesaving. SSSS due to MRSA has been reported.[188,189]

A mild form of SSSS is characterized by a generalized scarlatiniform eruption with exfoliation ("staphylococcal scarlet fever"). The skin has a sandpaper roughness, and Pastia's lines are present, as in streptococcal scarlet fever, but the strawberry tongue and palatal enanthem of streptococcal scarlet fever are absent.

Staphylococcal Toxic Shock Syndrome

TSS is an acute febrile illness characterized by a generalized erythematous eruption that is due to in vivo production of a toxin at the site of localized, often relatively asymptomatic or unnoticed infection by *S. au-*

reus strains capable of toxin production.[167,169,190] The multisystem effects observed in TSS patients are induced by TSS toxin-1 (TSST-1). TTST-1 has been shown to act as a superantigen that stimulates T cells to proliferate nonspecifically through interaction with class II major histocompatibility complex products on antigen-presenting cells and then with variable regions on the Vβ-chain of the T-cell receptor complex.[169] The superantigen family includes TSST-1; the SE serotypes A, B, Cn, D, E, G, H, I, J, K, L, and P; and the SPE serotypes A, C, G, H, and J; as well as streptococcal superantigen and multiple variants of streptococcal mitogenic exotoxin Z.[169] All of these toxins share the ability to cause symptoms via release of immune cytokines, leading to high fever and enhanced host susceptibility to lethal endotoxin shock. Although TSS has been mostly commonly linked to *S. aureus*, TSST-1–producing coagulase-negative staphylococci have also been described.[191]

In the early 1980s, most cases of TSS occurred in menstruating females, often in association with tampon use.[192,193] In recent years, less than 150 cases of TSS have reported each year for an incidence rate of approximately 0.05:100,000 population. Less than 60% of TSS cases currently reported are associated with menstruation.[194] Nonmenstrual TSS has been associated with a variety of infections, including postoperative wounds, cutaneous infections, burn wounds, postpartum complications, and *S. aureus* respiratory infections, often after viral influenza.[195-201] Recurrent nonmenstrual toxic shock has been described.[202]

TSS may range in severity from a relatively mild disease, often misdiagnosed as a viral syndrome, to a severe life-threatening illness. The most common symptoms include a temperature greater than 104° F (40° C), hypotension, and diffuse erythroderma with desquamation 1 to 2 weeks after the onset of illness. Additional early features include conjunctival, oropharyngeal, and vaginal hyperemia; vomiting and diarrhea; and myalgias.[202-205] Most patients have abnormalities in three or more organ systems: (1) muscular-rhabdomyolysis; (2) central nervous system–toxic encephalopathy; (3) renal-azotemia; (4) liver-abnormal transaminases; and (5) hematologic-thrombocytopenia. The rash of TSS is almost always noted within the first 24 hours of illness. Desquamation occurs after 7 to 10 days, most prominently on the hands and feet. Histologically, the epidermis exhibits cleavage in the basilar layers, which differentiates TSS from SSSS and from viral and drug eruptions.[206] *S. aureus* septicemia may be associated with erythematous, petechial, or pustular lesions.[207] In addition, lesions associated with endocarditis such as Osler's nodes, Janeway lesions, and splinter hemorrhages may occur. Such skin lesions have been reported in 10% to 64% of patients with staphylococcal septicemia.[208] Purpuric lesions may in some cases be so extensive as to suggest meningococcemia or Rocky Mountain spotted fever.[209-212] Gram-stained smears of the material in these lesions usually demonstrate gram-positive cocci.

Streptococcal Infections

The group A streptococci *(S. pyogenes)* cause a wide variety of local (e.g., impetigo, erysipelas, cellulitis, lymphangitis) and invasive syndrome (e.g., bacteremia, necrotizing soft-tissue infections, streptococcal TSS) associated with cutaneous manifestations.[213,214] These manifestations of streptococcal infection occur via three distinct mechanisms[215]: (1) direct infection of the skin, (2) immunologically mediated disease, and (3) toxin-mediated disease. Rheumatic fever affects up to 3% of people with untreated group A hemolytic streptococcal infections of the nasopharynx. Cutaneous manifestations include erythema marginatum (occurring in 10% to 20% of cases), subcutaneous nodules (in up to 30%), and erythema papulatum (rare).

Scarlet fever is a diffuse erythematous eruption that results from the production of pyrogenic exotoxin (erthrogenic toxin) produced by *S. pyogenes*, most commonly in the setting of pharyngitis. There appear to be three distinct exotoxins (types A, B, and C) produced by approximately 90% of group A strains. The rash of scarlet fever requires both the presence of pyrogenic exotoxin and the existence of delayed-type skin reactivity to streptococcal products. The latter requires prior exposure to organism. The pharynx is usually beefy red with edema involving the tonsillar area extending anteriorly to the soft palate and uvula. The rash of scarlet fever usually starts on the head and neck and then rapidly expands to cover the trunk and finally the extremities. The palms and soles are usually spared. The rash is a diffuse erythema, blanching on pressure, with numerous small (1 to 2 mm) popular elevations, giving a "sandpaper" quality to the skin. The rash is most marked in the skin folds of the inguinal, axillary, antecubital, and abdominal areas and about pressure points (e.g., buttocks). The rash often exhibits a linear petechial character in the antecubital fossae and axillary folds (Pastia's lines).

Over the past decade, the incidence of severe disease as a result of infection with *S. pyogenes* has increased dramatically.[216,217] The term *streptococcal toxic shock syndrome* has been suggested to those patients with hypotension and multiorgan failure, as occurs in staphylococcal TSS[218-221] (Table 49-4). Many, but not all, patients have a rash at the time of presentation. Skin manifestations include generalized erythroderma with desquamation and localized cellulitis with vesiculation or bulla formation.[219] Unlike in TSS, a focus of pyogenic inflammation is usually present, and a large proportion of the patients have documented bacteremia.[215] Commonly the local focus of infection results in necrotizing fasciitis manifest by diffuse swelling and tenderness, a peau d'orange appearance, and erythema with subsequent formation of bullae. Later the skin color changes from red to purple or black as the skin becomes necrotic. However, initially the clinical symptom of the local site of infection often is only severe pain, with tenderness and other physical findings appearing later. As with staphylococcal TSS, streptococcal TSS has been associated with the production of superantigens by the infecting pathogen.[222] Rarely, group G streptococci have been reported to cause myositis with TSS.[223]

Rickettsial Infections

Rickettsiae are obligate intracellular parasites whose primary target in humans appears to be the endothelial cell.[91] After parasitization of the endothelial cell, necrosis of the media and intima results in thrombosis, formation of microinfarcts, and extravasation of blood. The end result is increased vascular permeability and vasculitis.

Rash is a hallmark of Rocky Mountain spotted fever,[224-229] the most common rickettsial disease in the United States. Initially, a maculopapular rash develops. Subsequently, the rash becomes more petechial. Characteristically, the rash appears between the second and sixth days of illness (average, 4 days). However, the rash may be absent in 5% to 17% of patients, and in up to 50% it may not appear within the first 3 days of illness.[224,225,227,230,231] Failure to initiate proper therapy within 5 days of onset of symptoms[232] and failure to use a tetracycline[229] have been associated with an increased mortality rate. Independent predictors of failure by the physician to initiate therapy the first time a patient was seen include absence of a rash, presentation between August 1 and April 30, and presentation within 3 days of illness. Most commonly, the rash begins on the extremities, often around the wrists and ankles, and spreads centripetally to the trunk, with relative sparing of the face. However, the rash may begin on the trunk (10%) and spread centrifugally or may have a diffuse distribution at the time of onset (10%). Characteristically, the rash involves the palms and/or soles in the later

TABLE 49-4 Staphylococcal versus Streptococcal Toxic Shock Syndrome

Feature	Staphylococcal	Streptococcal
Age	Primarily 15-35 yr	Primarily 20-50 yr
Gender	Higher frequency in women	Men and women equally affected
Severe pain	Rare	Common
Hypotension	100%	100%
Erythroderma rash	Very common	Less common
Renal failure	Common	Common
Bacteremia	Low frequency	60%
Tissue necrosis	Rare	Common
Predisposing factors	Tampons, surgery	Cuts, burns, varicella
Thrombocytopenia	Common	Common
Motality rare	<3%	30-70%

Adapted for Stevens DL. The toxic shock syndromes. Infect Dis Clin North Am. 1996;10:727-746.

stages of infection. Over time, the rash, which begins as maculopapular lesions, may progress to become petechial or ecchymotic. Rarely, gangrene or skin necrosis that requires amputation occurs.[233] The rash may rarely be urticarial or pruritic. Because the mortality rate for infection may be decreased from 15% to 3% with appropriate treatment, institution of antibiotic therapy should never be delayed in the absence of rash. Signs and symptoms similar to those of Rocky Mountain spotted fever may occur with ehrlichiosis (see later).[234]

Capnocytophaga canimorsus Infection

Capnocytophaga canimorsus (dysgonic fermenter-2 [DF-2]) is a fastidious, gram-negative, opportunistic pathogen that can cause serious multiorgan disease in humans. The organism is found worldwide. Studies suggest that it is part of the normal gingival flora of cats and dogs.

More than 100 cases of infection due to *C. canimorsus* have been described.[235-243] Although infected patients have ranged in age from 5 months to 77 years, most infections have been reported in adults over 40 years of age. Approximately 80% of patients described in the literature have a predisposing condition, most commonly surgical asplenia. Other predisposing factors have included Hodgkin's disease, trauma, idiopathic thrombocytopenic purpura, alcohol abuse, steroid therapy, and chronic lung disease.

Infection is strongly associated with dog bites, with more than 50% of patients reporting dog bites before clinical evidence of infection. Infections have also followed cat bites or scratches,[244] scratches from dogs, and contact with wild animals. An additional 20% of patients have reported exposure to dogs without a history of an actual bite or scratch. The clinical syndrome in humans is characterized by fever, DIC, cellular necrosis in certain organs such as kidneys and adrenal glands, thrombocytopenia, hypotension, and renal failure with oliguria and anuria. Dermatologic lesions occur in about 50% of patients and may include petechiae, a macular or papular eruption, eschar formation, or painful erythema. Patients frequently develop a hemorrhagic diathesis with purpuric skin lesions and petechiae that may progress to cutaneous gangrene.

The case-fatality rate is approximately 25%. Death has not been confined to immunocompromised patients. Infection with *C. canimorsus* should be considered in patients who have a compatible clinical syndrome coupled with a history of a dog bite or animal exposure. Definitive diagnosis requires isolation of the organism from blood or other body fluids or tissues. Empirical therapy based on the clinical presentation should be given. In patients who show high-grade bacteremia, the organism has been demonstrated in peripheral blood smears. Therefore, in all patients suspected of having *C. canimorsus* sepsis, especially splenectomized patients, Gram staining of the buffy coat should be performed.

Borrelia burgdorferi Infection

Lyme disease is a tick-borne borreliosis with broad distribution and myriad manifestations.[245,246] Skin lesions are prominent clinical manifestations of all stages of Lyme disease.[247-251] Clinically, the disease is divided into three stages of illness: early localized disease, early disseminated disease, and persisting late disease. The most common manifestation of early localized Lyme disease is EM that usually appear at the site of the tick bite with 7 to 10 days (range, 3 to 30 days). Approximately, 70 to 80% of infected patients will demonstrate EM.[252] EM initially begins as a red macule or papule that is usually homogeneous in its redness and may remain so until it heals. More commonly, the lesion partly or totally clears centrally, leaving an annular erythema that spreads centrifugally. EM may develop anywhere, but the most frequently located around the knees, axilla, and in the groin. Although the lesion may last from a few days to about 1 year, it usually disappears within a few weeks to months. In about half of the patients, itching, dysesthesia/hyperesthesia, or sensations of heat may develop at the site of erythema. Many patients who develop early disseminated disease exhibit EM-like lesions. The disseminated lesions are usually smaller than the primary lesion and often multiple. These lesions may be ring shaped but are often homogeneous and nonmigrating.

Acrodermatitis chronica atrophicans (ACA) has been more commonly described in Europe but may rarely occur in the United States and is a manifestation of persistent infection with *Borrelia afzelii*. ACA begins with an inflammatory phase with a bluish-red erythema, usually on the distal lower leg or foot. The course is chronic, with persistence of inflammatory lesions for years and gradual conversion to markedly atrophic skin.

Candidiasis

The incidence and relative frequency of infections due to *Candida* as a nosocomial pathogen appear to be increasing.[253-254] Disseminated candidiasis is frequently fatal and is a major cause of death in immunocompromised patients.[255,256] Predisposing factors are malignancy with cytotoxic therapy, neutropenia, antimicrobial therapy, hyperalimentation, severe burn injuries, very low birth weight, use of intravenous catheters, systemic administration of adrenocortical steroids, and gastrointestinal surgery.[255,256]

Disseminated candidiasis may be accompanied by a characteristic macronodular skin rash in up to 13% of patients.[256] The lesions are discrete, firm, nontender, subcutaneous raised erythematous papules or nodules.[257-260] Nodules may sometimes have a pale center, and some may become hemorrhagic. Often the lesions are diffuse, but they may be localized to a small area. The face is usually spared.

Many other fungi produce nodular lesions identical to those caused by *Candida* and must be considered as possible pathogens in immunocompromised patients. In patients with acquired immunodeficiency syndrome (AIDS), cryptococci may cause umbilicated nodules that mimic the lesions of molluscum contagiosum.

NEW AND EMERGING INFECTIOUS DISEASES

The Institute of Medicine defines *new and emerging diseases* as "new, reemerging or drug-resistant infections whose incidence in humans has increased within the past two decades or whose incidence threatens to increase in the near future."[261] To this definition we suggest the addition of infections whose geographic range is increasing. The factors leading to the development of new and emerging diseases have been reviewed in the literature.[262-264] It is important for infectious disease clinicians to realize that international travel has dramatically increased; accordingly, patients may present with diseases only rarely seen in the United States.[263] Many of these diseases may be associated with either local or generalized skin lesions, including dengue fever, yellow fever, viral hemorrhagic fevers, malaria, and leptospirosis.[263]

Infections Due to New Herpesviruses

In recent years, the number of human viruses in the herpesvirus family has increased from five to eight.[265] Human herpesvirus 6 (HHV-6) is now recognized as the cause of exanthem subitum in infants and other febrile diseases in children.[266] HHV-6 infection, a worldwide disease, is normally acquired at a very early age. Classically, patients with exanthem subitum present with a high fever that lasts from 3 to 5 days.[266] As the temperature normalizes, a macular or maculopapular rash develops, generally beginning on the trunk, with later spread to the extremities and often to the neck and face. Typical dermal lesions are 2 to 3 mm in diameter and blanch with pressure. In one study of Japanese children, about half had a morbilliform rash and half had a rubella-like rash.[267] However, a study of febrile children seen in an emergency department in the United States reported the following data on the frequency of rash in those children diagnosed as having HHV-6 infection: rash at presentation, 18% (described as macular or maculopapular); rash within 1 week of presentation, 18% (described as variable); and classic roseola-like rash after fever subsided, 9%.[268] In children, HHV-6 infection may be manifested as fever without a rash, rash without a fever, infectious mononucleosis–like illness, or, rarely, a vesicular rash.[269] Cases clinically identified as either measles or rubella can be due to primary HHV-6 infection.[269,270] In adults, HHV-6 produces an infectious mononucleosis–like illness either occurring without a rash[271] or associated with erythematous macules and papules[272] or erythroderma.[273] Human herpesvirus 7 (HHV-7) has not been as firmly linked to human illness; it likely is a less important cause of exanthem subitum.[274] However, some investigators suggest that this association is related to the ability of HHV-7 to reactivate HHV-6 from latency.[275] Human herpesvirus 8 (HHV-8) has now been firmly linked to Kaposi's sarcoma.[276-278]

Viral Hemorrhagic Fever

Hemorrhagic fever may be caused by viruses belonging to several families including Arenaviridae (e.g., Argentine hemorrhagic fever, Lassa fever, Venezuelan hemorrhagic fever), Bunyaviridae (e.g., hantavirus pulmonary syndrome), Filoviridae (Ebola virus disease), and Flaviviridae (yellow fever, dengue fever, Omsk hemorrhagic fever).[279]

Hantaviruses are RNA viruses that belong to the family Bunyaviridae and include Hantaan, Seoul, Puumala, Dobrava, Sin Nombre, Bayou, Black Creek Canal, and New York viruses.[280] Hemorrhagic fever with renal syndrome (HFRS) may be caused by Hantaan, Seoul, Dobrava, and Puumala viruses. Severe forms of HFRS have characteristic phases that may not be seen with milder disease. After an incubation period of 2 to 3 weeks, patients present with abrupt onset of fever in association with malaise, headache, myalgias, back pain, abdominal pain, nausea, and vomiting. Conjunctival injection or hemorrhage with palatal and upper torso petechiae is commonly seen on physical examination.[280] During this phase, a characteristic erythematous flush that blanches with pressure may be observed, usually affecting the face, neck, and upper torso.[281] After the 3- to 7-day febrile phase, a period of hypotension and severe shock ensues that is characterized by hemorrhagic manifestations. Overall, about 20% of the patients manifest severe disease, with death from shock and renal failure in 5% to 10% of cases. The hantavirus pulmonary syndrome caused by the Sin Nombre virus is not associated with facial flushing, petechiae, or conjunctival injection.

Filoviruses include the agents that cause Marburg and Ebola hemorrhagic fever.[282-286] Ebola virus is more virulent than Marburg virus and causes more severe clinical disease, with an accelerated course and high morbidity and mortality rates. Patients present with an acute onset of fever, severe frontal headache, anorexia, malaise, and myalgias. These signs and symptoms are followed 2 to 3 days later by clinical deterioration heralded by pharyngitis, conjunctivitis, severe nausea and vomiting, abdominal pain, and watery diarrhea. Five days later, patients develop a maculopapular rash on the trunk and back that is followed by the appearance of petechiae, ecchymoses, subconjunctival hemorrhages, epistaxis, hemoptysis, hematemesis, and melena. Hemorrhagic shock may progress to death. Patients with Marburg virus infection may develop a scarlatiniform rash rather than a maculopapular rash. Considerations in the differential diagnosis of African hemorrhagic fevers also include yellow fever and Lassa fever, but these illnesses are not accompanied by a rash.

The etiologic agents of dengue fever are four serologically related RNA viruses belonging to the family Flaviviridae.[287,288] Classic dengue fever begins after an incubation period of 3 to 15 days (average, 5 to 8 days) with an abrupt onset of fever that may be accompanied by chills, headache, and general malaise. The fever usually lasts 3 to 7 days and may be biphasic. Erythema may appear shortly before the onset of fever, concurrently with fever onset, or 24 to 48 hours later. This rash may be noted as a flushing or erythematous mottling beginning on the trunk and spreading centrifugally to the face, neck, and extremities. Flushing may disappear after 1 or 2 days or may blend into an erythematous macular or maculopapular rash that develops anytime during the course of illness. Pruritus and desquamation, especially on the palms and soles, may follow termination of the eruption. Dengue hemorrhagic fever/dengue shock syndrome is a more severe disease whose skin manifestations may include petechiae, purpura, ecchymoses, epistaxis, and gum bleeding.

Bacterial Diseases Due to *Bartonella* Species

Bartonella and *Afipia* are closely related genera. *Afipia* spp. differ from *Bartonella* spp. in that they are urease and oxidase positive. Eight species of *Bartonella* have been demonstrated to be pathogenic for humans. Clinical syndromes caused by these bacteria (etiologic agents) include Oroya fever and verruga peruana (*B. bacilliformis*), bacteremia and endocarditis (*B. quintana, B. henselae*), bacillary angiomatosis and peliosis (*B. quintana, B. henselae*), HIV-associated neurologic syndromes (*B. quintana*), and cat scratch disease (CSD) (*B. henselae, B. clarridgeiae*, and *Afipia felis*).[289-296] *B. henselae* is considered the primary agent of CSD.

Infection with *B. henselae* results in disease syndromes of variable severity, ranging from lymphadenopathy to systemic disease. CSD occurs primarily in children and young adults and is generally a benign self-limited disease. Characteristically, it presents as lymphadenopathy, usually preceded by an erythematous papule at the inoculation site. About 30% of the patients have low-grade fever and malaise. Less common clinical findings include rash, hepatosplenomegaly, lytic bone lesions, granulomatous conjunctivitis, pneumonitis, and central nervous system involvement.[297] Uncomplicated CSD-mediated lymphadenopathy usually resolves spontaneously in 2 to 6 months. The differential diagnosis includes other causes of regional or generalized lymphadenopathy, other pyogenic infections, tularemia, infection with nontuberculous mycobacteria, and lymphoma.

As noted by Anderson and Neuman,[294] the severity and presentation of infection due to *B. henselae* are related to immune status. In general (excluding *B. bacilliformis*), immunocompetent patients who are otherwise healthy tend to present with classic CSD when infected with *B. henselae*. Patients who are immunocompromised by having AIDS, chronic alcoholism, immunosuppression, or other serious health problems tend to have systemic disease. However, there have been rare reports of systemic disease, including bacillary angiomatosis, in immunocompetent persons.[298] Both *B. henselae* and *B. quintana* (the agent of trench fever) have been identified as causative agents of bacillary angiomatosis and bacillary peliosis.

Manifestations of *Bartonella* infection in the immunocompromised patient include cutaneous bacillary angiomatosis (BA), extracutaneous lesions, bacillary peliosis hepatitis, and fever with bacteremia.[299-309] BA is the most common clinical manifestation of *Bartonella* infection in the immunocompromised person. The clinical constellation of BA in AIDS patients includes fever, a low CD4 lymphocyte count, cutaneous or subcutaneous vascular lesions, lymphadopathy, and often abdominal symptoms. Several different skin lesions have been described in BA, including elevated, friable, firm, bright red papules (in approximately 67% of cases), subcutaneous nodules (in approximately 50%), and cellulitic plaques (in 5% to 10%). Lesions may be located anywhere on the body, and patients may have several forms of lesions at the same time or sequentially. The lesions of BA may be clinically and histologically similar to Kaposi's sarcoma; therefore, biopsy specimens and special stains may be required to confirm the diagnosis. Cutaneous BA may also have extracutaneous manifestations ranging from subclinical to life-threatening infection.[294] *Bartonella* infection may be associated with local or generalized complications[308,309] or may manifest as overwhelming disseminated infection.[289] In addition to extracutaneous lesions, multiple cutaneous lesions may develop.[310] Visceral lesions may involve the respiratory or gastrointestinal mucosa, heart, liver, spleen, bone marrow, muscles, or lymph nodes. *B. quintana* and *B. henselae* have been successfully cultured from the blood or from cutaneous lesions of patients with BA.

Arthropod-Borne Bacterial Diseases Due to *Ehrlichia* Species

Arthropod-borne diseases that occur in the United States include Rocky Mountain spotted fever, murine typhus, rickettsialpox, sylvatic typhus, Lyme disease, tick-borne relapsing fever, Colorado tick fever, and tularemia. Recently, *Ehrlichia* spp. have emerged as important and potentially life-threatening pathogens.[311-317] Currently, three different ehrlichiae are known to be pathogenic for humans: *E. chaffeensis,* the agent of human monocytic ehrlichiosis (HME); HGE agent (closely related to *E. equi* and *E. phagocytophila*, pathogens of horses and ruminants, respectively), the cause of human granulocytic ehrlichiosis (HGE); and *E. ewingi*, a less-described cause of ehrlichiosis.[91] The severity of HME and HGE ranges from subclinical to fatal. There are no clinical features that consistently distinguish HME from HGE. The onset of symptoms generally occurs about 1 week after tick exposure

(range, 0 to 34 days). Patients with ehrlichiosis characteristically present with abrupt onset of fever, headache, myalgia, and shaking chills. Less common signs and symptoms include nausea, vomiting, diarrhea, abdominal pain, cough, and confusion. A rash has been reported to accompany HME in about 35% and HGE in 2% to 11%[91] and may be more common in children.[313] Rashes may not develop until several days into the illness, are short-lived, and are generally found on the trunk. The exanthems reported in patients with ehrlichiosis have been highly variable and have been described as macular, maculopapular, petechial, and even vesicular. Other less common skin symptoms reported include conjunctival injection, palatal petechiae, and acral edema with desquamation.

Involvement of the palms and soles is unusual, having been reported in less than 5% of patients. Several forms of rash may be present in the same patient. The clinical features of ehrlichiosis may mimic those of Rocky Mountain spotted fever, Kawasaki disease, meningococcemia, enterovirus and cytomegalovirus infections, infectious mononucleosis, leptospirosis, and babesiosis. The overall mortality rate has ranged from 2% to 5% for HME and from 7% to 10% for HGE, but these estimates are probably inflated, as severe cases are overrepresented in the literature.

Orthopoxviruses

The genus of orthopoxviruses contains four species that infect humans: variola, monkeypox, vaccinia, and cowpox. Variola and monkeypox are often life-threatening diseases, whereas vaccinia and cowpox generally are associated with local lesions. The eradication of smallpox represents one of the greatest public health achievements of the 20th century. After the successful eradication of smallpox, the routine use of vaccinia vaccine was discontinued. However, the threat of bioterrorism raises the prospect for an intentional use of smallpox.[318-322] As a result of this threat, vaccinia immunization of selected health care workers has been advised.[323] Recently, the first outbreak of monkeypox was reported in the United States.[324] Thus, the clinician is now confronted with having to distinguish the skin lesions of several possible poxvirus infections, including smallpox, complications of vaccinia (i.e., generalized or progressive vaccinia, eczema vaccinatum), and monkeypox. These lesions must be distinguished from varicella, disseminated herpes simplex, and other disorders characterized by a similar eruption, including meningococcal septicemia, coagulation disorders, and typhus.

After a 12- to 14-day incubation period (range, 7 to 17 days) , the patient with smallpox typically develops high fever, malaise, and prostration with headache and backache.[10,325,326] A maculopapular rash then appears on the mucosa of the mouth and pharynx, face, and forearms and spreads to the trunk and legs. Within 1 to 2 days, the rash becomes vesicular and later pustular. The pustules are characteristically round, firm, and deeply embedded in the skin. Crusts begin to form after 7 to 9 days; the scabs later separate, leaving pits and scars. Bacterial superinfection of skin lesions may complicate smallpox. The rash of variola differs from that of varicella in several ways. First, the lesions of variola appear during a 1- to 2-day period and evolve at the same time, whereas the lesions of varicella demonstrate different stages of maturation and generally appear in crops every few days. Second, the lesions of variola tend to involve the extremities and face, whereas the lesions of varicella have a centripetal predilection with a greater concentration of lesions on the trunk than on the face and extremities. Also, varicella lesions are almost never found on the palms and soles. Finally, the lesions of variola are much more deeply embedded than the rash of varicilla, where the lesions are more superficial. The rash of smallpox may be confused with the SJS, measles, and coxsackie infections.

Vaccinia vaccine has been recommended for selected health care workers and the military.[323] Recognition and management of the complications of vaccinia vaccination have been summarized.[327] Vaccinia vaccination leads to the local lesion at the site of immunization. Local complications include satellite lesions, lymphangitis, secondary bacterial infections, lesions from inadvertent remote inoculation, and progressive vaccinia at the site of the vaccination most commonly in immune suppressed persons. Disseminated lesions characterize generalized vaccinia and eczema vaccinatum. *Generalized vaccinia* refers to a benign generalized eruption in which each lesion is identical to its primary smallpox vaccination. The incidence has been reported to range from 23 to 242 per 1 million first-time vaccinees. During the vaccinia campaign of 2003, the incidence (per 1 million vaccinees) of generalized vaccinia (suspect, probable, and confirmed) among civilians[328] was 79.3, and among the military,[329] it was 79.9. Severe complications can be treated with variola immune globulin (VIG), cidofovir, or both. After vaccinia vaccination, patients also may develop a generalized erythema multiforme–like rash. This is a benign condition and does not require therapy.

Eczema vaccinatum occurs in persons with a history of eczema or atopic dermatitis regardless of disease activity or severity. It has also been reported in persons without a history of dermatologic conditions. Eczema vaccinatum is characterized by high fever and generalized lymphadenopathy with an extensive vesicular and pustular eruption. The syndrome begins concurrently or shortly after the onset of local vaccinial lesions in the vaccinee. It may also occur in contacts 5 to 19 days after exposure. There is a significant risk for secondary bacterial or fungal infections. This adverse reaction is associated with a poor prognosis and high mortality. Therapy consists of multiple doses of VIG, hemodynamic support, and treatment of secondary infections. Cidofovir might be useful for therapy, but there are no published clinical data on its efficacy. Historically, the rate of eczema vaccinatum per 1 million vaccinees was reported as 10.4 to 41.5. During the vaccinia campaign of 2003, no cases of eczema vaccinatum were reported among either civilians[328] or the military.[329]

Monkeypox is enzootic in squirrels and monkeys in the rain forests of western and central Africa. The disease appears to be endemic in these regions of Africa, but multiple outbreaks have been described.[330,331] Clinical signs of monkeypox include respiratory distress, lymphadenopathy, and a centrifugally distributed vesiculopustular rash. The case-fatality rate has been reported to be approximately 10% in persons not vaccinated against smallpox. A recent multistate outbreak in humans in the United States was traced to infected prairie dogs that had acquired disease from a shipment of Gambian giant rats from Ghana.[324] Fortunately, none of 71 patients died.

Skin Lesions in Immunocompromised Patients

The diagnosis of skin lesions in the immunocompromised patient is complex because of the wide range of potential microbial pathogens that may cause disease in patients with abnormal immune responses[332-338] (Table 49-5). In addition, in immunocompromised persons, common infections may have unusual manifestations. Johnson and Sober[338] recommend the following approach to cutaneous lesions suspected to be infectious. First, the most rapid and sensitive methods for detecting microbes both histologically and immunologically should be used. Second, appropriate cultures and stains should be obtained to optimize the chance for identifying the pathogen. A 6- or 8-mm punch biopsy is usually adequate. Half of the tissue is sent for histopathologic evaluation by routine methods and by special stains for fungi, mycobacteria, and bacteria. The other half is sent to the microbiology laboratory for culture of aerobic and anaerobic bacteria, mycobacteria, and fungi (at 25° C and 37° C) and for Gram stain, acid-fast, modified acid-fast, and direct fungal stains of touch preparations or ground tissue. Recommendations for processing specimens have been published.[337]

Solid organ transplant recipients are at high risk for disease due to opportunistic bacterial, viral, and fungal pathogens. The risk of infection and the most likely infecting pathogen depend on the type of transplant, type and dose of immunosuppressive medications, time since transplant, presence of coexisting diseases including viral infections, and epidemiologic exposures.

Johnson and Sober[338] categorized cutaneous infections in immunocompromised persons into four groups based on pathophysiology: (1) infection originating in skin that is typical of those occurring in immunocompetent persons, albeit with the potential for more serious illness; (2) extensive cutaneous involvement with pathogens that normally produce trivial or well-localized disease in immunocompetent patients; (3) infection originating from a cutaneous source that is caused by opportunistic pathogens that rarely cause disease in immunocompetent patients but may cause either localized or widespread disease in immunocompromised patients; and (4) cutaneous or subcutaneous infection that represents metastatic spread from a noncutaneous site. Only life-threatening infections with cutaneous manifestations are discussed further here. In general, most cases of skin infection result from secondary dissemination after initial infection of the lungs or other organ systems. Primary cutaneous infection resulting from

TABLE 45-5 Types of Skin Infections in Immune Compromised Hosts by Pathophysiologic Events

Type of Infection	Pathogen	Site of Infection	Healthy Host	Compromised Host
Primary skin infections with common pathogens	*Staphylococcus aureus,* group A	Epidermis, hair follicles	Impetigo, ecythma, folliculitis	Soft tissue infection, necrotizing
Septicemia	*Streptococcus*	Dermis	Abscesses, intertrigo	Soft tissue infection
Unusually widespread cutaneous infection	Dematophytes, *Candida* spp.	Epidermis, intertriginous sites, hair follicles	Dermatophytosis; epidermal (limited), folliculitis	Dermatophytosis; epidermal (extensive), folliculitis
	Candida spp.	Oropharynx, esophagus, genitalia	Candidiasis; intertrigo, genital	Candidiasis; intertrigo, folliculitis, mucosal
	HSV		Localized herpes, resolves spontaneously	Chronic herpetic ulcers
	VZV		Herpes zoster (mild)	Herpes zoster (extensive)
	EBV			Hairy leukoplakia
	MCV		MCV (localized, nonfacial)	Widespread MC, resistant to therapy
	HPV		Common and mucosal warts	Widespread warts; squamous cell carcinoma in situ
Opportunistic primary cutaneous infection	NTM	Dermis, hypodermis	Swimming pool granuloma	Soft tissue infection ± necrosis
	Nocardia			Infection ± necrosis
	Molds			Septicemia
	Prototheca			
Systemic infection metastatic to cutaneous and subcutaneous sites	Bacteria		Soft tissue	
	Fungal pneumonitis with fungemia	Dermis, hypodermis	Infection ± necrosis	Soft tissue infection ± necrosis
			Nodules	Nodules

EBV, Epstein-Barr virus; HPV, human papillomavirus; HSV, herpes simplex virus; MCV, molluscum contagiosum virus; NTM, nontuberculous mycobacteria; VZV, varicella-zoster virus.

Adapted from Johnson RA. Semin Cutaneous Med Surg. 2000;19:19-61.

direct inoculation is less common. In transplant patients, infections with viruses and fungi are probably more common than skin infections caused by bacteria.

Immunocompromised patients are at increased risk for the development of cellulitis due to *S. pyogenes* and *S. aureus*. Neutropenic patients are also susceptible to more unusual pathogens such as members of the family Enterobacteriaceae and *Pseudomonas* spp. Patients with leukemia or impaired cell-mediated immunity may develop erysipelas-like lesions due to *Candida* spp. or *Cryptococcus neoformans*. Both local and diffuse skin infections with herpesviruses, especially herpes simplex and varicella-zoster, are very common. Cutaneous cytomegalovirus infection has a highly variable appearance that may include nodules, ulcers, indurated plaques, maculopapular eruptions, vesicles, and petechiae.

Johnson and Sober[338] noted that in immunocompromised patients, cutaneous lesions resulting from hematogenous spread of infection are caused by three classes of organisms: (1) *P. aeruginosa* and other bacteria; (2) the endemic systemic mycoses caused by *Histoplasma capsulatum*, *Coccidioides* spp., and, rarely, *Blastomyces dermatitidis*; and (3) the opportunistic organisms *Aspergillus*, *C. neoformans*, *Candida*, *Rhizopus*, and *Nocardia*. *P. aeruginosa* may cause either cellulitis or ecthyma gangrenosum, which may develop in the absence of bacteremia. Patients with malignancy may develop sepsis associated with a variety of uncommon bacteria that are also associated with skin lesions (e.g., *A. hydrophila*, *C. canimorsus*, *Clostridium septicum*, mycobacteria, and *Salmonella enteritidis* serotype Typhimurium).[335] Most commonly, *H. capsulatum* causes cellulitis, but it may also cause papules, nodules, pustules, and hemorrhagic lesions. Metastatic spread to the skin from noncutaneous sites of infection most commonly occurs with *Aspergillus* spp., *C. neoformans*, *Candida* spp., *Rhizopus* spp., and *Nocardia*. With the exception of *Candida*, the initial portal of entry is the respiratory tract. However, the respiratory tract infection may be asymptomatic, with the initial signs of illness seen in the skin. In neutropenic patients, cutaneous lesions due to *Aspergillus* spp. are often found in association with the sino-orbital form of disease.[334] Neutropenic patients may also develop disseminated infection with other fungi such as *Fusarium* spp. and *Trichosporon beigelii*.

Human Immunodeficiency Virus Infection

HIV infection commonly results in dermatologic disorders in both adults and children.[339-341] Clinically, the skin lesions associated with HIV infection may be classified by morphologic appearance, stage of HIV infection, pathophysiology (infectious, neoplastic, vascular, miscellaneous), and, for infectious diseases, etiologic agent.

Skin disorders are related to the stage of HIV infection. Primary HIV infection is characterized by fever, lymphadenopathy, sore throat, myalgias and arthralgias, diarrhea, headache, nausea and vomiting, and weight loss. Skin eruptions are observed in more than 50% of patients, generally developing on day 1 to 5 of the acute illness.[342] The rash characteristically consists of 10 to hundreds of 5- to 10-mm, oval or round, pink to deep red macules or slightly raised papules. Other skin manifestations have included diffuse urticaria, vesicular and pustular exanthema, desquamation of palms and soles, and alopecia.[342]

Like other immunocompromised patients, persons with AIDS develop infections with opportunistic pathogens that rarely, if ever, cause infection in immunocompetent people. Furthermore, infections due to common pathogens may have clinical manifestations that are unusual, more severe, more prolonged, or poorly responsive to therapy. Skin lesions often yield multiple pathogens. Several common pathogens may cause disease with unusual presenting manifestations. Severe, chronic herpes simplex lesions have been reported. These ulcers are frequently perianal in homosexual men but may also involve the lips and perioral area. Severe herpetic whitlow may be confused with osteomyelitis or other chronic ulcerative conditions. Herpes zoster occurs with a higher-than-expected frequency in HIV-infected persons. Chronic varicella-zoster infection has been reported and may lead to severe scarring. Molluscum contagiosum may involve both the genital area and the face. The number and size of the lesions and their response to therapy tend to correlate with the degree of immunosuppression.

S. aureus is the most common cutaneous bacterial pathogen in HIV-infected persons. Infection usually presents as folliculitis of the face, trunk, or groin. Cutaneous staphylococcal infections may progress to botryomycosis, a rare condition characterized by aggregates of bacteria in skin. Syphilis is common in HIV-infected persons. Primary infection is manifested by a chancre. Secondary syphilis may manifest as a generalized maculopapular eruption with or without scaling; palmoplantar vesicles, papules, or macules; hypopigmented axillary macules; and oral lesions.[291] Unusual patterns of syphilis have been reported in the HIV-infected person, including coexistent lesions of secondary syphilis and tertiary gummas and noduloulcerative lesions with lymphadenopathy in precocious tertiary syphilis. In patients with AIDS, typical serologic tests (i.e., Venereal Disease Research Laboratory [VDRL] and fluorescent treponemal antibody absorption [FTA-ABS] tests) for syphilis may be unreliable, and a biopsy of the skin with silver staining to show the spirochetes may be required for diagnosis. Scabies may be widespread and be manifested as an erythematous papulosquamous eruption in which numerous mites can easily be found in the skin scraping. Less commonly, classic Norwegian scabies with marked hyperkeratosis may occur.

Unusual pathogens that may involve the skin include cytomegalovirus, nontuberculous mycobacteria (*M. avium* complex, *Mycobacterium haemophilum*, *Mycobacterium fortuitum*), *Candida* spp. (disseminated candidiasis), *Acanthamoeba castellani*, *Pneumocystis carinii*, and *Toxoplasma gondii*. Dissemination to the skin may occur with histoplasmosis, cryptococcosis, and coccidioidomycosis. Cutaneous histoplasmosis may be manifested as slightly pinkish to red papules with little or no induration or inflammation, a cellulitis-like eruption, and ulcerations and acneiform papules and pustules. The most common cutaneous presentation of cutaneous cryptococcosis is that of widespread dome-shaped papules with slight central umbilication and waxy translucence. Because these may mimic the papules of molluscum contagiosum, biopsy should be considered for diagnosis.

Papulopustular lesions may be the presenting sign of disseminated coccidioidomycosis. Gradon and colleagues[343] have classified the unusual skin and soft tissue manifestations of opportunistic infections in AIDS as follows: nodular lesions, *Sporothrix schenckii*, *Mycobacterium tuberculosis*, *Corynebacterium jekeium*, *Demodex* mites, and *Sarcoptes scabiei*; ulcerating lesions, *M. haemophilum*, herpesviruses including herpes simplex virus and cytomegalovirus; scalded skin syndrome, *S. aureus*; and pyomyositis, *S. aureus* and group C streptococci.

Well-described primary dermatologic disorders not associated with fever but associated with HIV infection include psoriasis, seborrheic dermatitis, papular eruptions, ichthyosis, infectious eczemoid dermatitis, yellow nail syndrome, vitiligo, telangiectasias of the anterior portion of the chest, and alopecia. Many of these diseases are more severe in patients with HIV infection, and their presence in undiagnosed patients should lead to consideration of HIV infection. Several patients have developed an eosinophilic pustular rash ("eosinophilic folliculitis"), responsive to ultraviolet therapy.

Drug reactions are common in patients with AIDS. Up to 50% of HIV-infected patients who receive trimethoprim-sulfamethoxazole develop a rash, usually an erythematous, maculopapular rash involving the entire body that is commonly associated with fever. SJS may develop. Rash may also accompany pentamidine therapy or treatment with dapsone-trimethoprim. A variety of cutaneous eruptions may occur as a consequence of antiretroviral therapy.[344,345]

REFERENCES

1. Garner JS. Guideline for isolation precautions in hospitals. Infect Control Hosp Epidemiol. 1996;17:53-80.
2. Centers for Disease Control and Prevention. Management of patients with suspected viral hemorrhagic fever. MMWR Morb Mortal Wkly Rep. 1988;37(suppl 3):1-16.
3. Centers for Disease Control and Prevention. Risks associated with human parvovirus B19 infection. MMWR Morb Mortal Wkly Rep. 1989;38:8188, 8193-8197.
4. Centers for Disease Control and Prevention. Recommendations for using smallpox vaccine in a pre-event vaccination program. MMWR Morb Mortal Wkly Rep. 2003;52(RR-7):1-16.

5. Centers for Disease Control and Prevention. Updated interim infection control and exposure management guidance in the health-care and community setting for patients with possible monkeypox virus infection. Available at www.cdc.gov/ncidod/monkeypox/pdf/mpoxinfectioncontrol.pdf. Accessed October 1, 2003.

6. Bolyard EA, Tablan OC, Williams WW, et al. Guideline for infection control in health care personnel, 1998. Am J Infect Control. 1998;26:289-354.

7. Yung AP, McDonald M. Early clinical clues in meningococcaemia. Med J Austral. 2003;178:124-137.

8. Kollef MH, Sherman G, Ward S, Fraser VJ. Inadequate antimicrobial treatment of infections: A risk factor for hospital mortality among critically ill patients. Chest. 1999;11:462-474.

9. Weber DJ, Rutala WA. Risks and prevention of nosocomial transmission of rare zoonotic diseases. Clin Infect Dis. 2001;32:446-456.

10. Henderson DA, Inglesby TV, Bartlett JG, et al. Smallpox as a biological weapon. JAMA. 1999;281:2127-2137.

11. Borio L, Inglesby T, Peters CJ, et al. Hemorrhagic fever viruses as biological weapons. JAMA. 2002;287:2391-2405.

12. Inglesby TV, Dennis DT, Henderson DA, et al. Plague as a biological weapon. JAMA. 2000;283:2281-2290.

13. Inglesby TV, O'Toole T, Henderson DA, et al. Anthrax as a biological weapon, 2002. JAMA. 2002;287:2236-2252.

14. Weber DJ, Rutala WA. Cutaneous anthrax infection (Letter). N Engl J Med. 2002;346:944.

15. Valman HB. Common rashes. BMJ. 1981;283:970-971.

16. Corey L, Kirby P. Rash and fever. In: Braunwald E, Isselbacher KJ, Petersdorf RG, et al, eds. Harrison's Principles of Internal Medicine. 11th ed. New York: McGraw-Hill; 1987:240-244.

17. Kline PP. Fever and rash. Emerg Decis. 1988;April:27-37.

18. Habif TP. Clinical Dermatology. St Louis: Mosby; 1996.

19. McKinnon HD, Howard T. Evaluating the febrile patient with a rash. Am Family Phys. 2000;62:804-816.

20. Drago F, Rampini P, Rampini E, Rebora A. Atypical exanthems: Morphology and laboratory investigations may lead to an aetiological diagnosis in about 70% of cases. Br J Dermatol. 2002;147:255-260.

21. Stewart MI, Bernhard JD, Cropley T, Fitzpatrick TB. The structure of skin lesions and fundamentals of diagnosis. In: Freedberg IM, Eisen AZ, Wolff K, et al, eds. Dermatology in General Medicine. 6th ed. New York: McGraw-Hill; 2003:11-29.

22. Kingston ME, Mackey D. Skin clues in the diagnosis of life-threatening infections. Rev Infect Dis. 1986;8:1-11.

23. Cohen PR, Kurzrock R. Sweet's syndrome: A neutrophilic dermatosis classically associated with acute onset and fever. Clin Dermatol. 2000;18:265-282.

24. Bachmeyer C, Aractingi S. Neutrophilic eccrine hedradenitis. Clin Dermatol. 2000;18:319-330.

25. Lazar AP. Cutaneous manifestations of systemic diseases. Compr Ther. 1992;18:5-9.

26. Manders SM. Serious and life-threatening drug eruptions. Am Fam Physician. 1995;51:1865-1872.

27. Roujeau JC, Sterm RS. Severe adverse cutaneous reactions to drugs. N Engl J Med. 1994;331:1272-1285.

28. Wolkenstein P, Revuz J. Drug-induced severe skin reactions. Drug Safety. 1995;13:56-68.

29. Bigby M. Rates of cutaneous reactions to drugs. Arch Dermatol. 2001;137:765-770.

30. Nigen S, Knowles SR, Shear NH. Drug eruptions: Approaching the diagnosis of drug-induced skin diseases. J Drugs Dermatol. 2003;2:278-299.

31. Veraldi S, Rizzitelli G, Schianchi-Veraldi R. Occupational cutaneous infections. Clin Dermatol. 1992;10:225-230.

32. Taylor JS. Occupational dermatoses. Dermatol Clin. 1994;12:461-610.

33. Lushniak BD. Occupational skin disease. Prim Care. 2000;27:895-915.

34. Helm TN, Bergfeld WF. Sports dermatology. Clin Dermatol. 1998;16:159-165.

35. Adams BB. Transmission of cutaneous infections in athletes. Br J Sports Med. 2000;34:413-414.

36. Halstead ME, Bernhardt DT. Common infections in the young athlete. Pediatr Ann. 2002;31:42-48.

37. Thomsett L. Zoonotic skin diseases. Practitioner. 1990;234:52-55.

38. Lucchina LC, Wilson ME, Drake LA. Dermatology and the recently returned traveler: Infectious diseases with dermatologic manifestations. Int J Dermatol. 1997;36:167-181.

39. Tornieporth NG, Johnson WD. Infectious considerations in the world traveler. Dermatol Clin. 1997;15:285-293.

40. Wilson ME. Skin problems in the traveler. Infect Dis Clin North Am. 1998;12:471-488.

41. James WD. Imported skin diseases in dermatology. J Dermatol. 2001;28:663-666.

42. Joyce MP. Skin diseases of travelers. Prim Care Clin Office Prac. 2002;29:971-981.

43. Frieden IJ. Childhood exanthems. Curr Opin Pediatr. 1995;7:411-414.

44. Resnick SD. New aspects of exanthematous diseases of childhood. Dermatol Clin. 1997;15:257-265.

45. Mancini AJ. Exanthems in childhood: An update. Pediatr Ann. 1998;27:163-170.

46. Gable EK, Liu G, Morrell DS. Pediatric exanthems. Primary Care. 2000;27:353-369.

47. Mancini AJ. Childhood exanthems: A primer and update for the dermatologist. Adv Dermatol. 2000;16:3-37.

48. Scott LA, Stone MS. Viral exanthams. Dermatol Online J. 2003;9:4.

49. Nash D, Mostashari F, Fine A, et al. The outbreak of West Nile virus infection in the New York City area in 1999. N Engl J Med. 2001;344:1807-1814.

50. Fritsch PO, Ruiz-Maldonado R. Erythema multiforme, Stevens-Johnson syndrome, and toxic epidermal necrolysis. In: Freedberg IM, Eisen AZ, Wolff K, et al, eds. Dermatology in General Medicine. 6th ed. New York: McGraw-Hill; 2003:543-557.

51. Auquier-Dunant A, Mockenhaupt M, Naldi L, et al. Correlations between clinical patterns and causes of erythema multiforme majus, Stevens-Johnson syndrome, and toxic epidermal necrolysis. Arch Dermatol. 2002;138:1019-1024.

52. Huff JC. Erythema multiforme and latent herpes simplex infection. Semin Dermatol. 1992;11:207-210.

53. Schofield JK, Tatnall FM, Leigh IM. Recurrent erythema multiforme: Clinical features and treatment in a large series of patients. Br J Dermatol. 1993;128:542-545.

54. Leaute-Labreze C, Lamireau T, Chawki D, et al. Diagnosis, classification, and management of erythema multiforme and Stevens-Johnson syndrome. Arch Dis Child. 2000;83:347-352.

55. Wolkenstein P, Revuz J. Toxic epidermal necrolysis. Dermatol Clin. 2000;18:485-495.

56. Rzany B, Mockenhaupt M, Stocker U, et al. Incidence of Stevens-Johnson syndrome and toxic epidermal necrolysis in patients with the acquired immunodeficiency syndrome in Germany. Arch Dermatol. 1993;129:1059.

57. Fine J-D. Management of acquired bullous skin diseases. N Engl J Med. 1995;333:1475-1484.

58. Mockenhaupt MS, Roujeau J-C, Townshend A. Interventions for toxic epidermal necrolysis. Cochrane Database Syst Rev. 2002.

59. Wolkenstein P, Latarjet J, Roujeau J-C, et al. Randomized comparison of thalidomide versus placebo in toxic epidermal necrolysis. Lancet. 1998;352:1586-1589.

60. Ghislain P-D, Roujeau J-C. Treatment of severe drug reactions: Stevens-Johnson syndrome, toxic epidermal necrolysis and hypersensitivity syndrome. Dermatol Online J. 2002;8:5

61. Palmieri TL, Greenhalgh DG, Saffle JR, et al. A multicenter review of toxic epidermal necrolysis treated in U.S. burn centers at the end of the twentieth century. J Burn Care Rehabil. 2002;23:87-96.

62. van Elsacker-Niele AMW, Kroes ACM. Human parvovirus B19: Relevance in internal medicine. Neth J Med. 1999;54:221-230.

63. Brown KE. Haematological consequences of parvovirus B19 infection. Ballieres Clin Heamatol. 2000;13:245-259.

64. Bultmann BD, Klingel K, Sotlar K, et al. Parvovirus B19: A pathogen responsible for more than hematologic disorders. Virchows Arch. 2003;442:8-17.

65. Katta R. Parvovirus B19: A review. Dermatol Clin. 2002;20:333-342.

66. Heegaard ED,Brown KE. Human parvovirus B19. Clin Microbiol Rev. 2002;15:485-505.

67. Markenson GR, Yancey MK. Parvovirus B19 infections in pregnancy. Semin Perinatol. 1998;22:309-317.

68. Anderson LJ. Human parvoviruses. J Infect Dis. 1990;161:603-608.

69. Smith PT, Landry ML, Carey H, et al. Papular-purpuric gloves and socks syndrome associated with acute parvovirus B19 infection: Case report and review. Clin Infect Dis. 1998;27:164-168.

70. Nelson JS, Stone MS. Update on selected viral exanthams. Curr Opin Pediatr. 2000;12:359-364.

71. Crum NF. Current trends in typhoid fever. Curr Gastroenterol Rep. 2003;5:279-286.

72. Nishie H, Imayama S, Fukrue M. Non-typhoid Salmonella infection associated with 'rose spots.' Br J Dermatol. 1999;140:558-560.

73. Hook EW, Marra CM. Acquired syphilis in adults. N Engl J Med. 1992;326:1060-1069.

74. Centers for Disease Control and Prevention. Summary of notifiable diseases, United States, 2001. MMWR Morb Mortal Wkly Rep. 2001;50:1-108.

75. Palenque E. Skin disease and nontuberculous atypical mycobacteria. Int J Dermatol. 2000;39:659-666.

76. Weitzul S, Eichhron PJ, Pandya AB. Nontuberculous mycobacterial infections of the skin. Dermatol Clin. 2000;18:358-377.

77. Brodell RT, Mehrabi D. Underlying causes of erythema nodosum. Postgrad Med. 2000;108:147-149.

78. Requena L, Requena C. Erythema nodosum. Dermatol Online J. 2002;8:4

79. Whitely RJ, Roizman B. Herpes simplex virus infections. Lancet. 2001;357:1513-1518.

80. Yeung-Yue KA, Brentjens MH, Lee PC, Tyring SK. Herpes simplex viruses 1 and 2. Dermatol Clin. 2003;20:249-266.

81. Borenstein M, Kerdel F. Infections with *Vibrio vulnificus*. Dermatol Clin. 2003;21:245-248.

82. Chiang SR, Chuang YC. *Vibrio vulnificus* infection: Clinical manifestations, pathogenesis, and antimicrobial therapy. J Microbiol Immunol Infect. 2003;36:81-88.

83. Esterly NB. Vesicopustular eruptions in the neonate. Australas J Dermatol. 1991;32:1-12.

84. Lynch AM, Kapila R. Overwhelming postsplenectomy infection. Infect Dis Clin North Am. 1996;10:693-707.

85. Bisharat N, Omari H. Lavi I, Raz R. Risk of infection and death among post-splenectomy patients. J Infect Dis. 2001;43:182-186.

86. Sumarajo V, Smith LG, Smith SM. Infectious complications in asplenic hosts. Infect Dis Clin North Am. 2001;15:551-565.

87. Lutwick LI. Life threatening infections in the asplenic or hyposplenic individual. In: Remington JS, Swatz MN, eds. Current Topics in Infectious Diseases. Boston: Blackwell; 2002:78-96.

88. Ejstrud P, Kristensen B, Hansen JB, et al. Risk and patterns of bacteraemia after splenectomy: A population-based study. Scand J Infect Dis. 2000;32:521-525.

89. Baker RC, Seguin JH, Gilchrist MJ, Myers MG. Fever and petechiae in children. Pediatrics. 1989;84:1051-1055.

90. Van Nguyen Q, Nguyen EA, Weiner LB. Incidence of invasive bacterial disease in children with fever and petechiae. Pediatrics. 1984;74:77-80.

91. Parola P, Raoult D. Ticks and tickborne bacterial diseases in humans: An emerging disease threat. Clin Infect Dis. 2001;32:897-928.

92. Murphy GS, Oldfield EC. Falciparum malaria. Infect Dis Clin North Am. 1996;10:747-775.

93. Zucker JR. Changing patterns of autochthonous malaria transmission in the United States: A review of recent outbreaks. Emerg Infect Dis. 1996;2:37-43.

94. Callen JP. Neutrophilic dermatoses. Dermatol Clin. 2002;20:409-419.

95. Anonymous. American College of Chest Physicians/Society of Critical Care Medicine Consensus Conference: Definitions for sepsis and organ failure and guidelines for the use of innovative therapies in sepsis. Crit Care Med. 1992;20:864-874.

96. Bone RC, Balk RA, Cerra FB, et al. Definitions for sepsis and organ failure and guidelines for the use of innovative therapies in sepsis. Chest. 1992;101:1644-1655.

97. Levy MM, Fink MP, Marshall JC, et al. 2001 SCCM/ESICM/ACCP/ATS/SIS International Sepsis Definitions Conference. Crit Care Med. 2003;31:1250-1256.

98. Rangel-Frausto MS, Pitter D, Costigan M, et al. The natural history of the systemic inflammatory response syndrome (SIRS). JAMA. 1995;273:117-123.

99. Martin GS, Mannino DM, Eaton S, Moss M. The epidemiology of sepsis in the United States from 1979 through 2000. N Engl J Med. 2003;348:1546-1554.

100. Robboy SJ, Mihm MC, Colman RW, et al. The skin in disseminated intravascular coagulation. Prospective analysis of thirty-six cases. Br J Dermatol. 1973;88:221-229.

101. Goodwin JN, Berne TV. Symmetrical peripheral gangrene. Arch Surg. 1974;108:780-784.

102. Warner PM Kagan RJ, Yakuboff KP, et al. Current management of purpura fulminans: A multicenter study. J Burn Care Rehabil. 2003;24:119-126.

103. Childer BJ, Cobanov B. Acute infectiouis purpura fulminans: A 15-year retrospective review of 28 consecutive cases. Am Surg. 2003;69:86-90.

104. Faust SN, Levin M, Harrison OB, et al. Dysfunction of endothelial protein C activation in severe meningococcal sepsis. N Engl J Med. 2001;345:408-416.

105. Schuchat A, Robinson K, Wenger JD, et al. Bacterial meningitis in the United States in 1995. N Engl J Med. 1997;337:970-976.

106. Rosenstein NE, Perkins BA, Stephens DS, et al. Menigoccoccal disease. N Engl J Med. 2001;344:1378-1388.

107. van Deuren M, Brandtzaeg P, van der Meer JWM. Update on meningococcal disease with emphasis on pathogenesis and clinical management. Clin Microbiol Rev. 2000;13:144-146.

108. Dagan R, Powell KR, Hall CB, Menegus MA. Identification of infants unlikely to have serious bacterial infection although hospitalized for suspected sepsis. J Pediatr. 1985;107:855-860.

109. Brogan PA, Raffles A. The management of fever and petechiae: Making sense of rash decisions. Arch Dis Child. 2000;83:506-507.

110. van Nguyen Q, Nguyen EA, Weiner LB. Incidence of invasive disease in children with fever and petechiae. Pediatrics. 1984;74:77-80.

111. Benerjee I, Roberts R, Looker N. Incidence of meningococcal infection in children with fever and non-blanching rash. J Infect. 2001;45:275-277.

112. DeVoe IW. The meningococcus and mechanisms of pathogenicity. Microbiol Rev. 1982;46:162-190.

113. Salzman MB, Runin LG. Meningococcemia. Infect Dis Clin North Am. 1996;10:709-725.

114. van Deuren M, van Dijke BJ, Koopman RJ, et al. Rapid diagnosis of acute meningococcal infections by needle aspiration or biopsy or skin lesions. BMJ. 1993;306:1229-1232.

115. Hackett SJ, Thomson AP, Hart CA. Cytokines, chemokines and other effctor molecules involved in meningococcal disease. J Med Microbiol. 2001;50:847-859.

116. Koppes GM, Ellenbogen C, Gebhart RJ. Group Y meningococcal disease in United States Air Force recruits. Am J Med. 1977;62:661-666.

117. Leibel RL, Fangman JJ. Chronic meningococcemia in childhood. Am J Dis Child. 1974;127:94-98.

118. Benoit FL. Chronic meningococcemia. Am J Med. 1963;35:103-112.

119. Ploysangam T, Sheth AP. Chronic meningococcemia in childhood: Case report and review of literature. Pediatr Dermatol. 1996;13:483-487.

120. Ognibene AJ, Dito WR. Chronic meningococcemia. Arch Intern Med. 1964;114:29-32.

121. Barr J, Danielsson D. Septic gonococcal dermatitis. BMJ. 1971;1:482-485.

122. Holmes KK, Weisner PJ, Pederson AHB, et al. The gonococcal arthritis-dermatitis syndrome. Ann Intern Med. 1971;75:470-471.

123. Kerle K, Mascola JR, Miller TA. Disseminated gonococcal infection. Am Fam Physician. 1992;45:209-214.

124. Buntin DM, Rosen T, Lesher JL, et al. Sexually transmitted diseases: Bacterial infections. J Am Acad Dermatol. 1991;25:287-299.

125. Handsfield HH. Disseminated gonococcal infection. Clin Obstet Gynecol. 1975;18:131-142.

126. Abu-Nassar H, Hill N, Fred HL, et al. Cutaneous manifestations of gonococcemia. Arch Intern Med. 1963;112:731-737.

127. Holmes KK, Counts GW, Beaty HN. Disseminated gonococcal infection. Ann Intern Med. 1971;74:979-993.

128. Tronca E, Handsfield HH, Wiesner PJ, et al. Demonstration of Neisseria gonorrhoeae with fluorescent antibody in patients with disseminated gonococcal infection. J Infect Dis. 1974;129:583-586.

129. Walker LC, Ahlin TD, Tung KSK, et al. Circulating immune complexes in disseminated gonorrheal infection. Ann Intern Med. 1978;89:28-33.

130. Ratnam S, Hogan K, March SB, Butler RW. Whirlpool-associated folliculitis caused by Pseudomonas aeruginosa: Report of an outbreak and review. J Clin Microbiol. 1986;23:655-659.

131. Flick MR, Cluff LE. Pseudomonas bacteremia. Am J Med. 1976;60:501-508.

132. Forkner CE, Frei E, Edgcomb JH, et al. Pseudomonas septicemia. Am J Med. 1958;25:877-889.

133. Whitecar JP, Luna M, Bodey GP. Pseudomonas bacteremia in patients with malignant diseases. Am J Med Sci. 1970;260:216-223.

134. Baltch AL, Griffin PE. Pseudomonas aeruginosa bacteremia: A clinical study of 75 patients. Am J Med Sci. 1977;274:119-129.

135. Bodey GP, Jadeja L, Elting L. Pseudomonas bacteremia. Arch Intern Med. 1985;145:1621-1629.

136. Mandell IN, Feiner HD, Price NM, et al. Pseudomonas cepacia endocarditis and ecthyma gangrenosum. Arch Dermatol. 1977;113:199-202.

137. Ketover BP, Young LS, Armstrong D. Septicemia due to Aeromonas hydrophila: Clinical and immunologic aspects. J Infect Dis. 1973;127:284-290.

138. Shackelford PG, Ratzan SA, Shearer WT. Ecthyma gangrenosum produced by Aeromonas hydrophila. J Pediatr. 1973;83:100-101.

139. Fine JD, Miller JA, Harrist TJ, et al. Cutaneous lesions in disseminated candidiasis mimicking ecthyma gangrenosum. Am J Med. 1981;70:1133-1135.

140. Bodey GP, Boliva R, Fainstein V, et al. Infections caused by Pseudomonas aeruginosa. Rev Infect Dis. 1983;5:279-313.

141. Del Pozo J, Garcia-Silva J, Almagro M, et al. Ecthyma gansgrenosum-like eruption associated with Morganella morganii infection. Br J Dermatol. 1998;139:520-521.

142. Rodot S, Lacour JP, van Elsande L, et al. Ecthyma gangrenosum caused by Klebsiella pneumoniae. Int J Dermatol. 1995;34:216-217.

143. Anderson MG. Pseudomonas septicaemia and ecthyma gangrenosum. S Afr Med J. 1979;55:504-509.

144. Musher DM. Cutaneous and soft-tissue manifestations of sepsis due to gram-negative enteric bacilli. Rev Infect Dis. 1980;2:854-866.

145. El Baze P, Ortonne J-P. Ecthyma gangrenosum. J Am Acad Dermatol. 1985;13:299-300.

146. Huminer D, Siegman-Igra Y, Morduchowicz G, et al. Ecthyma gangrenosum without bacteremia. Arch Intern Med. 1987;147:299-310.

147. Gucluer H, Ergun T, Demircay Z. Ecthyma gangrenosum. Int J Dermatol. 1999;38:298-305.

148. Song WK, Kim YC, Park HJ, Cinn YW. Ecthyma gangrenosum without bacterium in a leukaemic patient. Clin Exp Dermatol. 2001;26:395-396.

149. Picou KA, Jarratt MT. Persistent subcutaneous abscesses following Pseudomonas sepsis. Arch Dermatol. 1979;115:459-460.

150. Reed RK, Larter WE, Sieber OF, et al. Peripheral nodular lesions in Pseudomonas sepsis: The importance of incisions and drainage. J Pediatr. 1976;88:977-979.

151. Bagel J, Grossman ME. Subcutaneous nodules in Pseudomonas sepsis. Am J Med. 1986;80:528-529.

152. Schlossberg D. Multiple erythematous nodules as a manifestation of Pseudomonas aeruginosa septicemia. Arch Dermatol. 1980;116:446-447.

153. Von Reyn CF, Levy BS, Arbeit RD, et al. Infective endocarditis: An analysis based on strict case definitions. Ann Intern Med. 1981;94:505-518.

154. Venezio FR, Westenfelder GO, Cook FV, et al. Infective endocarditis in a community hospital. Arch Intern Med. 1982;142:789-792.

155. Terpenning MS, Buggy BP, Kauffman CA. Infective endocarditis: Clinical features in young and elderly patients. Am J Med. 1987;83:626-634.

156. King K, Harnkess JL. Infective endocarditis in the 1980s. Part 1. Aetiology and diagnosis. Med J Aust. 1986;144:536-540.

157. Mylonakis E, Calderwood SB. Infective endocarditis in adults. N Engl J Med. 2001;345:1318-1330.

158. Dreyer NP, Fields BN. Heroin-associated endocarditis. Ann Intern Med. 1973;78:699-702.

159. Alpert JS, Krous HF, Dalen JE, et al. Pathogenesis of Osler's nodes. Ann Intern Med. 1976;85:471-473.

160. Yee J, McAllister CK. Osler's nodes and the recognition of infective endocarditis: A lesion of diagnostic importance. South Med J. 1987;80:753-757.

161. Cardullo AC, Silvers DN, Grossman ME. Janeway lesions and Osler's nodes: A review of histopathologic findings. J Am Acad Dermatol. 1990;22:1088-1090.

162. Sheagren JN. Staphylococcus aureus. The persistent pathogen (first of two parts). N Engl J Med. 1984;310:1368-1373.

163. Sheagren JN. Staphylococcus aureus. The persistent pathogen (second of two parts). N Engl J Med. 1984;310:1437-1442.

164. Williams RE, MacKie RM. The staphylococci. Dermatol Clin. 1993;11:201-206.

165. Aly R. The pathogenic staphylococci. Semin Dermatol. 1990;9:292-299.

166. Weems JJ. The many faces of Staphylococcus aureus infection. Postgrad Med. 2001;110:24-6,29-31,35-36.

167. Lowy FD. Staphylococcus aureus infections. N Engl J Med. 1998;339:520-532.

168. Prevost G, Couppie P, Monteil H. Staphylococcal epidermolysins. Curr Opin Infect Dis. 2003;16:71-76.

169. McCormick JK, Yarwood JM, Schlievert PM. Toxic shock syndrome and bacterial superantigens: An update. Annu Rev Microbiol. 2001;55:77-104.

170. Alouf JE, Muller-Alouf H. Staphylococcal and streptococcal superantigens: Molecular, biological and clinical aspects. Int J Med Microbiol. 2003;292:429-440.

171. Eady EA, Cove JH. Staphylococcal resistance revisited: Community-acquired methicillin resistant Staphylococcus aureus—An emerging problem for the management of skin and soft tissue infections. Curr Opin Infect Dis. 2003;16:103-124.

172. Marcinak JF, Frank AL. Treatment of community-acquired methicillin resistant Staphylococcus aureus in children. Curr Opin Infect Dis. 2003;16:265-269.

173. Denise B. Community-acquired methicillin resistant Staphylococcus aureus in the community. Pediatr Infect Dis J. 2001;20:1167-1168.

174. Frank AL, Marcinak JF, Mangat PD, et al. Clindamycin treatment of community-acquired methicillin resistant Staphylococcus aureus infections in children. Pediatr Infect Dis J. 2002;21:530-534.

175. Sattler CA, Mason EO, Kaplan SL. Prospective comparison of risk factors and demographic and clinical characteristics of community-acquired methicillin resistant Staphylococcus aureus versus methicillin-susceptible Staphylococcus aureus infection in children. Pediatr Infect Dis J. 2002;21910-21916.

176. Ladhani S. Recent developments in staphylococcal scalded skin syndrome. Clin Microbiol Infect. 2001;7:301-307.

177. Patel GK, Finley AY. Staphylococcal scalded skin sydrome: Diagnosis and management. Am J Clin Dermatol. 2003;4:165-175.

178. Ladhani S, Evans RW. Staphylococcal scalded skin sydrome. Arch Dis Child. 1998;78:85-88.

179. Ladhani S, Joannou CJ. Difficulties in diagnosis and management of the staphylococcal scalded skin sydrome. Pediatr Infect Dis J. 2000;19:819-821.

180. Farrell AM. Staphylococcal scalded skin sydrome. Lancet. 1999;354:880-881.

181. Melish ME, Glasggow LA. Staphylococcal scalded skin syndrome: The expanded clinical syndrome. J Pediatr. 1971;78:958-967.

182. Borchers SL, Gomez EC, Isseroff RR. Generalized staphylococcal scalded skin syndrome in anephric boy undergoing hemodialysis. Arch Dermatol. 1984;120:912-918.

183. O'Keefe R, Dagg JH, MacKie RM. The staphylococcal scalded skin syndrome in two elderly immunocompromised patients. BMJ. 1987;295:179-180.

184. Richard M, Mathieu-Serra A. Staphylococcal scalded skin syndrome in a homosexual adult. J Am Acad Dermatol. 1986;15:385-389.

185. Beers B, Wilson B. Adult staphylococcal scalded skin syndrome. Int J Dermatol. 1990;29:428-429.

186. Donohue D, Robinson B, Goldbert NS. Staphylococcal scalded skin syndrome in a woman with chronic renal failure exposed to human immunodeficiency virus. Cutis. 1991;47:317-318.

187. Prabhash K, Babu KG, Ravi S, et al. Staphylococcal scalded skin syndrome. Lancet Infect Dis. 2003;3:442.

188. Ito K, Funabashi YM, Toda K, et al. Staphylococcal scalded skin syndrome in an adult due to methicillin-resistant *Staphylococcus aureus*. J Infect Chemother. 2002;8:256-261.

189. Acland KM, Darvay A, Griffin C, et al. Staphylococcal scalded skin syndrome in an adult associated with methicillin-resistant *Staphylococcus aureus*. Br J Dermatol. 1999;140:518-520.

190. Issa NC, Thompson RL. Staphylococcal toxic shock syndrome. Postgrad Med. 2001;110:55-56, 59-62.

191. Crass BA, Bergdoll MS. Involvement of coagulase-negative staphylococci in toxic shock syndrome. J Clin Microbiol. 1986;23:43-45.

192. Davis JP, Chesney PJ, Wand PJ, et al. Toxic shock syndrome. Epidemiologic features, recurrence, risk factors, and prevention. N Engl J Med. 1980;303:1429-1435.

193. Fisher RF, Goodpasture HC, Peterie JD, et al. Toxic shock syndrome in menstruating women. Ann Intern Med. 1981;94:156-163.

194. Hajjeh RA, Reingold A, Weil A, et al. Toxic shock syndrome in the United States: Surveillance update, 1979-1996. Emerg Infect Dis. 1999;5:807-810.

195. Holt PA, Armstrong AM, Norfolk GA, et al. Toxic-shock syndrome due to staphylococcal infection of a burn. Br J Clin Pract. 1987;41:582-583.

196. Reingold AL, Dan BB, Shands KN, et al. Toxic-shock syndrome not associated with menstruation. Lancet. 1982;1:1-4.

197. Reingold AL, Hargrett NT, Dan BB, et al. Nonmenstrual toxic shock syndrome. A review of 130 cases. Ann Intern Med. 1982;96:871-874.

198. Bates I. Characteristic rash associated with staphylococcal pneumonia. Lancet. 1987;2:1026-1027.

199. Center for Disease Control and Prevention. Toxic shock syndrome associated with influenza—Minnesota. MMWR Morb Mortal Wkly Rep. 1986;35:143-144.

200. Center for Disease Control and Prevention. Toxic shock syndrome following influenza-Oregon; update on influenza activity—United States. MMWR Morb Mortal Wkly Rep. 1987;36:64-65.

201. Wilkins EGL, Ney F, Roberts C, et al. Probable toxic shock syndrome with primary staphylococcal pneumonia. J Infect. 1985;11:231-232.

202. Andrews M-M, Parent EM, Barry M, Parsonnet J. Recurrent nonmenstrual toxic shock syndrome: Clinical manifestations, diagnosis, and treatment. Clin Infect Dis. 2001;32:1470-1479.

203. Finch R, Whitby M: Toxic shock syndrome. J R Coll Phys Lond. 1985;19:219-223.

204. Tofte RW, Williams DN. Clinical and laboratory manifestations of toxic shock syndrome. Ann Intern Med. 1982;96:843-847.

205. Tofte RW, Williams DN. Toxic shock syndrome: Clinical and laboratory features in 15 patients. Ann Intern Med. 1981;94:149-156.

206. Todd J, Fishuat M, Kapral F, et al. Toxic-shock syndrome associated with phage-group-1 staphylococci. Lancet. 1978;2:1116-1117.

207. Plaut MD. Staphylococcal septicemia and pustular purpura. Arch Dermatol. 1969;99:82-85.

208. Musher DM, McKenzie SO. Infections due to *Staphylococcus aureus*. Medicine (Baltimore). 1977;56:383-409.

209. Aach R, Kissane J, eds. A thirty-eight year old woman with overwhelming sepsis. Am J Med. 1972;53:233-241.

210. Murray HW, Tuazon CU, Sheagren JN. Staphylococcal septicemia and disseminated intravascular coagulation. Arch Intern Med. 1977;137:844-847.

211. Milunski MR, Gallis HA, Fulkerson WJ. *Staphylococcus aureus* septicemia mimicking fulminant Rocky Mountain spotted fever. Am J Med. 1987;83:801-803.

212. Rahal JJ, MacMahon E, Weinstein L. Thrombocytopenia and symmetrical peripheral gangrene associated with staphylococcal and streptococcal bacteremia. Ann Intern Med. 1968;69:35-43.

213. Bisno AL, Brito MO, Collins CM. Molecular basis of group A streptococcal virulence. Lancet Infect Dis. 2003;3:191-200.

214. Stevens SL. Invasive streptococcal infections. J Infect Chemother. 2001;7:69-80.

215. Bryan BO, Frieden I. Streptococcal skin disease in children. Semin Dermatol. 1992;11:3-10.

216. Low DE, Schwartz B, McGeer A. The reemergence of severe group A streptococcal disease: An evolutionary perspective. In: Scheld WM, Armstrong D, Hughes JM, eds. Emerging Infections, v. 1. Washington, DC: ASM Press; 1998.

217. Musser JM, Krause RM. The revival of group A streptococcal diseases, with a commentary on staphylococcal toxic shock syndrome. In: Krause RM, ed. Emerging Infections. London: Academic Press; 1998.

218. Stevens DL. The toxic shock syndromes. Infect Dis Clin North Am. 1996;10:727-746.

219. Stevens DL, Tanner MH, Winship J, et al. Severe group A streptococcal infections associated with toxic shock-like syndrome and scarlet fever toxin A. N Engl J Med. 1989;321:1-7.

220. Stevens SL. Streptococcal toxic-shock syndrome: Spectrum of disease, pathogenesis, and new concepts in treatment. Emerg Infect Dis. 1995;1:69-78.

221. Baxter F, McChesney J. Severe group A streptococcal infection and streptococcal toxic shock syndrome. Can J Anaesth. 2000;47:1129-1140.

222. Profit T, Sriskandan S, Yang L, Fraser JD. Superantigens and streptococcal toxic shock syndrome. Emerg Infect Dis. 2003;9:1211-1218.

223. Wagner JG, Schlievert PM, Assimacopoulos AP, et al. Acute group G streptococcal myositis associated with streptococcal toxic shock syndrome: Case report and review. Clin Infect Dis. 1996;23:1159-1161.

224. Kirk JL, Fine DP, Sexton DJ, Muchmore HG. Rocky Mountain spotted fever: A clinical review based on 48 confirmed cases, 1943-1986. Medicine. 1990;69:35-45.

225. Helmick CG, Bernard KW, D'Angelo LJ. Rocky Mountain spotted fever: Clinical, laboratory, and epidemiological features of 262 cases. J Infect Dis. 1984;150:480-488.

226. Hazard GW, Ganz RN, Nevin RW, et al. Rocky Mountain spotted fever in the Eastern United States. N Engl J Med. 1969;280:57-62.

227. Kaplowitz LG, Fischer JJ, Sparling PF. Rocky Mountain spotted fever: A clinical dilemma. In: Remington JS, Swartz MN, eds. Current Clinical Topics in Infectious Diseases. New York: McGraw-Hill; 1981:89-108.

228. Sexton DJ, Burgdorder W. Clinical and epidemiologic features of Rocky Mountain spotted fever in Mississippi, 1933-1973. South Med J. 1975;68:1529-1535.

229. Holman RC, Paddock CD, Curns AT, et al. Analysis of risk factors for fatal Rocky Mountain spotted fever: Evidence for superiority of tetracyclines for therapy. J Infect Dis. 2001;184:1437-1444.

230. Cohen JI, Corson AP, Corey GR. Late appearance of skin rash in Rocky Mountain spotted fever. South Med J. 1983;76:1457-1458.

231. Ramsey PG, Press OW. Successful treatment of Rocky Mountain "spotless" fever. West J Med. 1984;140:94-96.

232. Kirkland KB, Wilkinson E, Sexton DJ. Therapeutic delay and mortality in cases of Rocky Mountain spotted fever. Clin Infect Dis. 1995;20:1118-1121.

233. Kirkland KB, Marcom PK, Sexton DJ, et al. Rocky Mountain spotted fever complicated by gangrene: Report of six cases and review. Clin Infect Dis. 1993;16:629-634.

234. Harkess JR. Ehrlichiosis. Infect Dis Clin North Am. 1991;5:37-52.

235. Hicklin H, Verghese A, Alvarez S. Dysgonic fermenter 2 septicemia. Rev Infect Dis. 1987;9:884-890.

236. Zumla A, Lipscomb G, Corbett M, et al. Dysgonic fermenter-type 2: An emerging zoonosis: Report of two cases and review. Q J Med. 1988;257:741-752.

237. Job L, Horman JT, Grigor JK, Israel E. Dysgonic fermenter-2: A clinico-epidemiologic review. J Emerg Med. 1989;7:185-191.

238. Krol-van Staaten MJ, Landheer JE, de Maat CEM. *Capnocytophaga canimorsus* (formerly DF-2) infections: Review of the literature. Neth J Med. 1990;36:304-309.

239. Kullberg B-J, Westendorp RGJ, van't Wout JW, Meinders AE. Purpura fulminans and symmetrical peripheral gangrene caused by *Capnocytophaga canimorsus* (formerly DF-2) septicemia—A complication of dog bite. Medicine. 1991;70:287-292.

240. Bilgrami S, Bergstrom SK, Peterson DE, et al. *Capnocytophaga* bacteremia in a patient with Hodgkin's disease following bone marrow transplantation: Case report and review. Clin Infect Dis. 1992;14:1045-1049.

241. Pers C, Gahrn-Hansen B, Frederiksen W. *Capnocytophaga canimorsus* septicemia in Denmark, 1982-1995: Review of 39 cases. Clin Infect Dis. 1996;23:71-75.

242. Lion C, Escande F, Burdin JC. *Capnocytophaga canimorsus* infections in human: Review of the literature and cases report. Eur J Epidemiol. 1996;12:521-533.

243. Hovenga S, Tulleken JE, Moller LV, et al. Dog-bite induced sepsis: A report of four cases. Intens Care Med. 1997;23:1179-1180.

244. Mahrer S, Raik E. *Capnocytophaga canimorsus* septicemia associated with cat scratch. Pathology. 1992;24:194-196.

245. Steere AC. Lyme disease. N Engl J Med. 2001;345:115-125.

246. Hengge UR, Tannapfel A, Tyring SK, et al. Lyme borreliosis. Lancet Infect Dis. 2003;3:489-500.

247. Trevisan G, Cinco M. Lyme disease. Int J Dermatol. 1990;29:1-8.

248. Thyresson N. Historical notes on skin manifestations of Lyme borreliosis. Scand J Infect Dis. 1991;77:9-13.

249. Hercogova J, Tomankova M, Bartak P. Contributions to the treatment of dermatologic manifestations of Lyme borreliosis. Cutis. 1992;49:409-411.

250. Asbrink E. Cutaneous manifestations of Lyme borreliosis. Scand J Infect Dis. 1991;77(suppl):44-50.

251. Asbrink E, Hovmark A. Lyme borreliosis: Aspects of tick-borne *Borrelia burgdorferi* infection from a dermatologic viewpoint. Semin Dermatol. 1990;9:277-291.

252. Steere AC, Sikand VK. The presenting manifestations of Lyme disease and the outcomes of treatment. N Engl J Med. 2003;3438:2472-2474.

253. Syndman DR. Shifting patterns in the epidemiology of nosocomial Candida infections. Chest. 2003;123(suppl):500s-503s.

254. Singh N. Changing patterns of invasive candidiasis and its therapeutic implications. Clin Microbiol Infect. 2001;7(suppl 2);1-7.

255. Bodey GP. Fungal infection and fever of unknown origin in neutropenic patients. Am J Med. 1986;80:112-119.

256. Maksymiuk AW, Thongprasert S, Hopfer R, et al. Systemic candidiasis in cancer patients. Am J Med. 1984;77(suppl):20-27.

257. Bodey GP. Candidiasis in cancer patients. Am J Med. 1984;77(suppl):13-19.

258. Balandran L, Rothschild H, Pugh N, et al. A cutaneous manifestation of systemic candidiasis. Ann Intern Med. 1973;78:400-403.

259. Jacobs MI, Magid MS, Jarowski CI. Disseminated candidiasis. Arch Dermatol. 1980;116:1277-1279.

260. Kirkpatrick CH. Host factors in defense against fungal infections. Am J Med. 1984;77(suppl):1-12.

261. Lederberg J, Shope RE, Oaks SC. Emerging Infections: Microbial Threats to Health in the United States. Institute of Medicine. Washington, DC: National Academies Press; 1992.

262. Morse SS. Factors in the emergence of infectious diseases. Emerg Infect Dis. 1995;1:7-15.

263. Ostroff SM, Kozarsky P. Emerging infectious diseases and travel medicine. Infect Dis Clin North Am. 1998;12:231-241.

264. Smolinski MS, Hamburg MA, Lederberg J. Microbial Threats to Health. Institute of Medicine. Washington, DC: National Academies Press; 2003.

265. Levy JA. Three new human herpesviruses (HHV6, 7, and 8). Lancet. 1997;349:558-563.

266. Braun DK, Dominguez G, Pellett P. Human herpesvirus 6. Clin Microbiol Rev. 1997;10:521-567.

267. Asano Y, Nakashima T, Yoshikawa T, et al. Severity of human herpesvirus-6 viremia and clinical findings in infants with exanthem subitum. J Pediatr. 1991;118:891-895.

268. Pruksananonda P, Hall CB, Insel R, et al. Primary human herpesvirus 6 infection in young children. N Engl J Med. 1992;326:1445-1450.

269. Black JB, Durigon E, Kite-Powell K, et al. Seroconversion to human herpesvirus 6 and human herpesvirus 7 among Brazilian children with clinical diagnoses of measles and rubella. Clin Infect Dis. 1996;23:1156-1158.

270. Tait DR, Ward KN, Brown DWG, Miller E. Measles and rubella misdiagnosed in infants as exanthem subitum (roseola infantum). BMJ. 1996;312:101-102.

271. Steeper TA, Horwitz CA, Ablashi D, et al. The spectrum of clinical and laboratory findings resulting from the human herpesvirus-6 (HHV-6) in patients with mononucleosis-like illnesses not resulting from Epstein-Barr virus or cytomegalovirus. Am J Clin Pathol. 1990;93:776-783.

272. Akashit K, Eizuru Y, Sumiyoshi Y, et al. Brief report: Severe infectious mononucleosis-like syndrome and primary herpesvirus 6 infection in an adult. N Engl J Med. 1993;329:168-171.

273. Sumiyoshi Y, Akashi K, Kikichi M. Detection of human herpes virus (HHV 6) in the skin of a patient with primary HHV 6 infection and erythroderma. J Clin Pathol. 1994;47:762-763.

274. Ablashi DV, Berneman ZN, Kramarsky B, et al. Human herpes virus-7 (HHV-7): Current status. Clin Diagn Virol. 1995;4:1-13.

275. Katsafanas GC, Schirmer EC, Wyatt LS, Frenkel N. In vitro activation of human herpesviruses 6 and 7 from latency. Proc Natl Acad Sci U S A. 1996;93:9788-9792.

276. Martinelli PT, Tyring SK. Human herpesvirus 8. Dermatol Clin. 2002;20:307-314.

277. Jenson HB. Human herpesvirus 8 infection. Curr Opin Pediatr. 2003;15:85-91.

278. Dukers NHTM, Rezza G. Human herpesvirus 8 epidemiology: What we do and do not know. AIDS. 2003;17:1717-1730.

279. Melnick JL. Taxonomy of viruses. In: Murray PR, ed. Manual of Clinical Microbiology. 6th ed. Washington, DC: ASM Press; 1995.

280. Mertz GJ, Hjelle BL, Bryan RT. Hantavirus infection. Dis Mon. 1998;44:87-138.

281. Schmaljohn C, Hjelle B. Hantaviruses: A global disease problem. Emerg Infect Dis. 1997;3:95-103.

282. Gill MV, Cunha BA. Ebola hemorrhagic fever. Infect Dis Pract. 1995;19:37-41.

283. Klenk HD, Feldmann H. Marbug and Ebola viruses. Adv Virus Res. 1996;47:1-52.

284. Feldmann H, Slenczka W, Klenk HD. Emerging and reemerging of filoviruses. Arch Virol. 1996;11(suppl):77-100.

285. Sodhi A. Ebola virus disease: Recognizing the face of a rare killer. Postgrad Med. 1996;99:75-76, 78.

286. Borio L, Inglesby T, Peters CJl, et al. Hemorrhagic fever viruses as biological weapons. JAMA. 2002;287:2391-2405.

287. Ramirez-Ronda CH, Garcia CD. Dengue in the Western Hemisphere. Infect Dis Clin North Am. 1994;8:107

288. Rigau-Perez JG. Clinical manifestations of dengue hemorrhagic fever in Puerto Rico, 1990-1991. Rev Panam Salud Publica. 1997;1:381-387.

289. Adal KA, Cockerell CJ, Petri WA. Cat scratch disease, bacillary angiomatosis, and other infections due to Rochalimaea. N Engl J Med. 1994;330:1509-1515.

290. Midani S, Ayoub EM, Anderson B. Cat-scratch disease. Adv Pediatr. 1996;43:397-422.

291. Maurin M, Raoult D. Bartonella (Rochalimaea) quintana infections. Clin Microbiol Rev. 1996;9:273-292.

292. Koehler JE. Bartonella infections. Adv Pediatr Infect Dis. 1996;11:1-27.

293. Williams A, Sheldon CD, Riordan T. Cat scratch disease. BMJ. 2002;324:1199-1200.

294. Anderson BE, Neuman MA. Bartonella spp. as emerging human pathogens. Clin Microbiol Rev. 1997;10:203-219.

295. Spach DH, Koehler JE. Bartonella-associated infections. Infect Dis Clin North Am. 1998;12:137-155.

296. Koehler JE. Bartonella: An emerging human pathogen. In: Scheld WM, Armstrong D, Hughes JM, eds. Emerging Infections I. Washington, DC: ASM Press; 1998.

297. Margileth AM, Wear DJ, English CK. Systemic cat scratch disease: Report of 23 patients with prolonged or recurrent severe bacterial infection. J Infect Dis. 1987;155:390-402.

298. Tappero JW, Koehler JE, Berger TM, et al. Bacillary angiomatosis and bacillary splenitis in immunocompetent adults. Ann Intern Med. 1993;118:363-365.

299. Jimenez-Acosta F, Pardo RJ, Cohen RJ, et al. Bacillary angiomatosis and acquired immunodeficiency syndrome: Case report and literature review. J Am Acad Dermatol. 1990;22:525-529.

300. Schwartzman WA, Marchevsky A, Meyer RD. Epithelioid angiomatosis or cat scratch disease with splenic and hepatic abnormalities in AIDS: Case report and review of the literature. Scand J Infect Dis. 1990;22:121-133.

301. Schwartzman WA. Infections due to Rochalimaea: The expanding spectrum clinical spectrum. Clin Infect Dis. 1992;15:893-902.

302. Mohle-Boetani JC, Koehler JE, Berger TG, et al. Bacillary angiomatosis and bacillary peliosis in patients infected with human immunodeficiency virus: Clinical characteristics in a case-control study. Clin Infect Dis. 1996;22:794-800.

303. Manders SM. Bacillary angiomatosis. Clin Dermatol. 1996;14:295-299.

304. Chomel BB. Cat-scratch disease and Bacillary angiomatosis. Rev Sci Techn. 1996;15:1061-1073.

305. Nosal JM. Bacillary angiomatosis, cat-scratch disease, and bartonellosis: What's the connection? Int J Dermatol. 1997;36:405-411.

306. Wong R, Tappero J, Cockrell CJ. Bacillary angiomatosis and other Bartonella species infections. Semin Cutan Med Surg. 1997;16:188-199.

307. Gasquet S, Maurin M, Brouqui P, et al. Bacillary angiomatosis in immunocompromised patients. AIDS. 1998;12:1793-1803.

308. Santos R, Cardoso O, Rodriques P, et al. Bacillary angiomatosis by Bartonella quintana in an HIV-infected patient. J Am Acad Dermatol. 2000;42:299-301.

309. Plattenberg A, Lorenzen T, Burtsche BT, et al. Bacillary angiomatosis in HIV-infected patients—An epidemiological and clinical study. Dermatology. 2000;201:326-331.

310. Miam MW, Balerdi MJ, Toney JF, et al. Epithelioid angiomatosis secondary to disseminated cat scratch disease involving the bone marrow and skin in a patient with acquired immunodeficiency syndrome: A case report. Am J Med. 1990;88:180-183.

311. Walker DH, Dumler JS. Emergence of the ehrlichiosis as human health problems. Emerg Infect Dis. 1996;2:18-27.

312. Walker DH. Emerging human ehrlichiosis: Recently recognized, widely distributed, life-threatening tick-borne disease. In: Scheld WM, Armstrong D, Hughes JM, eds. Emerging Infections I. Washington, DC: ASM Press; 1998.

313. Fritz CL, Glaser CA. Ehrlichiosis. Infect Dis Clin North Am. 1998;12:123-136.

314. McQuiston J, Paddock CD, Holman RC, Childs JE. Emerg Infect Dis. 1999;5:635-642.

315. Bakken JS, Dumler JS. Human granulocytic ehrlichiosis. Clin Infect Dis. 2000;31:554-560.

316. Lantos P, Krause PJ. Ehrlichiosis in children. Semin Pediatr Infect Dis. 2002;13:249-256.

317. Olano JP, Walker DH. Human ehrlichiosis. Med Clin North Am. 2002;86:375-392.

318. Atlas RM. The medical threat of biological weapons. Crit Rev Microbiol. 1998;24:157-168.

319. Centers for Disease Control and Prevention. Biological and chemical terrorism: Strategic plan for preparedness and response. MMWR Morb Mortal Wkly Rep. 2000;49(RR-4).

320. Franz DR, Jahrling PB, McClain DJ, et al. Clinical recognition and management of patients exposed to biological warfare agents. Clin Lab Med. 2001;21:435-473.

321. Bronze MS, Huycke MM, Machado LJ, et al. Viral agents as biological weapons and agents of bioterrorism. Am J Med Sci. 2002;323:316-325.

322. Darling RG, Catlett CL, Huebner KD, Jarrett DG. Threats in bioterrorism. I: CDC category A agents. Emerg Med Clin North Am. 2002;20:273-309.

323. Centers for Disease Control and Prevention. Recommendations for using smallpox vaccine in a pre-event vaccination program. MMWR Morb Mortal Wkly Rep. 2003;52(RR-7):1-15.

324. Centers for Disease Control and Prevention. Update: Multistate outbreak of monkeypox—Illinois, Indiana, Kansas, Missouri, Ohio, and Wisconsin, 2003. MMWR Morb Mortal Wkly Rep. 2003;52:642-646.

325. Breman JG, Henderson DA. Diagnosis and management of smallpox. N Engl J Med. 2002;346:1300-1308.

326. Kawalek A, Rudikoff D. A spotlight on smallpox. Clin Dermatol. 2002;20:376-387.

327. Centers for Disease Control and Prevention. Smallpox vaccination and adverse reactions. MMWR Morb Mortal Wkly Rep. 2003;52(RR-4):1-28.

328. Centers for Disease Control and Prevention. Update: Cardiac and other adverse events following civilian smallpox vaccination—United States, 2003. MMWR Morb Mortal Wkly Rep. 2003;52:639-642.

329. Grabenstein JD, Winkenwerder W. US military smallpox vaccination program experience. JAMA. 2003;289:3278-3282.

330. Bregman JG, Henderson DA. Poxvirus dilemmas—Monkeypox, smallpox, and biologic terrorism. N Engl J Med. 1998;339:556-559.

331. Hutin YJF, Williams RJ, Malfait P, et al. Outbreak human monkeypox, Democratic Republic of Congo, 1996-1997. Emerg Infect Dis. 2001;7:434-438.

332. Johnson RA. The immune compromised host in the twenty-first century: Management of mucocutaneous infections. Sem Cutaneous Med Surg. 2000;19:19-61.

333. Gentry LO, Zeluff B, Kielhofner MA. Dermatologic manifestations of infectious diseases in cardiac transplant patients. Infect Dis Clin North Am. 1994;8:637-654.

334. Bodey GP. Dermatologic manifestations of infections in neutropenic patients. Infect Dis Clin North Am. 1994;8:655-675.

335. Beebe JL, Koneman EW. Recovery of uncommon bacteria from blood: Association with neoplastic disease. Clin Rev Microbiol. 1995;8:336-356.

336. LaRocco MT, Burgert SJ. Infection in the bone marrow transplant recipient and role of the microbiology laboratory in clinical transplantation. Clin Rev Microbiol. 1997;10:277-297.

337. Lopez FA, Sanders CV. Dermatologic infections in the immunocompromised (non-HIV) host. Infect Dis Clin North Am. 2001;15:671-702.

338. Johnson RA, Sober AJ. Mucocutaneous infections in the in the compromised host. In: Rubin RH, Young LS, eds. Clinical Approach to Infection in the Compromised Host. 4th ed. New York: Plenum; 2002:49-110.

339. Tschachler E, Bergstresser PR, Stingl G. HIV-related skin diseases. Lancet. 1996;348:659-663.

340. Berger TG. Dermatologic care of the AIDS patients. In: Sande MA, Verberding PA, eds. The Medical Management of AIDS. 6th ed. Philadelphia: WB Saunders; 1999:185-194.

341. Stefanaki C, Stratigos AJ, Stratigos JD. Skin manifestations of HIV-1 infection in children. Clin Dermatol. 2002;20:74-86.

342. Lapkins J, Gaines H, Lindback S, et al. Skin and mucosal characteristics of symptomatic primary HIV-1 infection. AIDS Patient Care Stds. 1997;11:67-70.

343. Gradon JD, Timpone JG, Schnittman SM. Emergence of unusual opportunistic pathogens in AIDS: A review. Clin Infect Dis. 1992;15:134-157.

344. Heller HM. Adverse cutaneous drug reactions in patients with human immunodeficiency virus-1 infection. Clin Dermatol. 2000;18:485-489.

345. Ward HA, Russo GG, Shrum J. Cutaneous manifestation of antiretroviral therapy. J Am Acad Dermatol. 2002;46:284-293.

SECTION B

UPPER RESPIRATORY TRACT INFECTIONS

TABLE 50-1　Viruses Associated with the Common Cold

Virus Group	Antigenic Types	Percentage of Cases*
Rhinoviruses	100 types and 1 subtype	30-40
Coronavirus	3 or more types	10-15
Parainfluenza virus	4 types	5
Respiratory syncytial virus	2 types	5
Influenza virus	3 types	25-30
Adenovirus	47 types	5-10
Other viruses (human meta- pneumovirus, enteroviruses, rubeola, rubella, varicella)		
Presumed undiscovered viruses		
Group A β-hemolytic streptococci†		

*Estimated percentage of colds annually.
†Included because differentiation of streptococcal and viral pharyngitis is not possible by clinical means.

CHAPTER 50

The Common Cold

JACK M. GWALTNEY, JR.

Common cold is the traditional term used by both physicians and laypersons for the syndrome of acute upper respiratory tract illness. The existence of a single entity, as implied by the term, is incorrect. Instead, the "common cold" is a group of diseases caused, for the most part, by members of five families of viruses. The viruses in these families have distinctive biochemical properties that govern their differing pathogenic and epidemiologic behaviors. In addition, the immunotypes found in the various viral families have antigenic variations that are of biologic importance to the immune system of their human host. The problem of controlling acute respiratory disease presents a complex challenge that requires approaches suitable for the properties of the individual virus groups. Therefore, the hope for development of a single "cure" for the "common cold" is an unrealistic expectation that has led to the diversion of resources into attempts at simplistic and unrealistic solutions to the problem.

As a clinical entity, the common cold results from inflammation of the nasal passages and pharynx and usually or often of the paranasal sinuses, middle ear, and tracheobronchial tree. It is the leading cause of acute morbidity and of visits to physicians in the United States. It is also a major cause of industrial and school absenteeism.[1] It has been estimated that the total economic impact of the common cold in the United States approaches $40 billion annually.[2] A small proportion of colds is complicated by bacterial infections of the paranasal sinuses and the middle ear, and these require antimicrobial therapy.

Based on early observations of their contagious nature, colds have long been thought to be caused by infectious agents. However, it was not until the isolation of a number of new respiratory viruses in cell culture in the 1950s that the specific cause of colds was known. The first of these, a parainfluenza virus, was discovered in 1955.[3] In 1956, rhinoviruses were isolated from adults with common colds.[4,5] The following year, respiratory syncytial virus (RSV) was associated with acute respiratory illness in infants,[6] and in 1958 one of the enteroviruses, coxsackievirus A21, was recovered from military recruits with mild respiratory disease.[7] Another important group of common cold viruses, the coronavirus, was first reported in the 1960s.[8,9] Most recent was the discovery of human metapneumovirus.[10] The microbial etiology of some colds remains unknown. Other respiratory viruses, such as influenza virus and adenovirus, produce the common cold syndrome but are characteristically associated with a more severe illness, which often involves the lower respiratory tract.

ETIOLOGY

The major respiratory viruses causing colds and similar upper respiratory tract illnesses are found in the myxovirus, paramyxovirus, adenovirus, picornavirus, and coronavirus groups (Table 50-1).[11-14] Within these groups of viruses are many different antigenic types. The rhinovirus group, which accounts for more than 50% of colds in adults, has 100 immunotypes. The proportion of colds caused by the coronavirus

group and the number of immunotypes of this virus have not been fully determined, but with the use of new methods such as reverse transcriptase–polymerase chain reaction (RT-PCR), this percentage continues to increase.[15,16] The parainfluenza viruses and RSV each account for a small proportion of colds on an annual basis. Influenza virus and adenovirus produce a spectrum of illness that overlaps the common cold syndrome. Some of the enteroviruses produce coryza,[17] as do some viruses that usually produce other characteristic findings, such as exanthems. Because mild streptococcal pharyngitis cannot be differentiated from viral pharyngitis on clinical grounds, it also is included as a cause of "colds." With the use of currently available methods of detection, the cause of approximately one third to one fourth of colds in adults remains unknown.[18] Some illnesses may be undiagnosed because of the insensitivity of methods currently used for detection of known viruses, and others may be caused by undiscovered agents. Colds in children are caused by the same viruses in roughly the same proportion, but the total number of colds that can be diagnosed in children is usually lower.

Colds are frequent because of the large number of different causative viruses and also because reinfections may occur with the same virus type. Second infections probably occur with members of all the viral groups; with some, such as coronavirus, reinfections appear to be particularly common. Up to 80% of people infected with coronavirus OC43 have prior neutralizing antibody to the virus.[19]

SEASONAL INCIDENCE

The respiratory viruses have a worldwide distribution. Annual epidemics of upper respiratory tract disease occur in the colder months in temperate areas and during the rainy season in the tropics. In the United States the respiratory disease season begins in late August to mid-September.[20,21] Respiratory illness rates rise sharply for a few weeks and then remain elevated until spring. During March, April, and May, rates decline to the low summer level.

The events controlling the seasonal variation in attack rates of acute respiratory disease are not well understood. Adding to the complexity of the problem has been the discovery that some of the virus groups have their own seasonal pattern within the overall respiratory disease season. Rhinovirus outbreaks typically occur in the early fall and in middle to late spring,[21] and coronaviruses are most prominent in the winter.[19] Studies with a specific virus, rhinovirus type 15, showed that chilling of volunteers did not increase their susceptibility to infection and illness.[22] Therefore, the effect of thermal cold per se on the host does not appear to explain the seasonal outbreaks of colds.

Undoubtedly, among the responsible variables for seasonal fluctuations in colds are the bringing together of children during school terms and the increased crowding indoors of populations during colder months.[23] Also, seasonal changes in relative humidity may be an important variable that controls the prevalence of the different virus families because of the effect of relative humidity on virus survival. In general, enveloped viruses survive better under conditions of low relative humidity, as found in colder months of the year, and the converse is true for the nonenveloped viruses.

ATTACK RATES

During peak months in the respiratory disease season in the United States, adults average six to eight colds per 1000 persons per day.[21] In the summer, rates fall to two or three colds per 1000 per day. Overall, adults in the United States average two to four colds per year, and children average six to eight.[20,21] In one 10-year study of illness in families, young children in nursery school averaged up to nine colds for the period of September through May. Annual illness rates decline in older children and reach adult levels in adolescence. Boys have slightly more colds than girls until adolescence, but after that the incidence is slightly higher in women, perhaps reflecting their greater exposure to young children.[14] Adults with children in the home have more colds than those without this exposure.[20,24] Tonsillectomy does not reduce the incidence of colds.[20] Cigarette smokers have the same incidence of colds as nonsmokers, but the severity of their illnesses is greater.[21,25]

TRANSMISSION

The main reservoir of respiratory viruses is in the upper airway in young children. Spread of colds takes place most commonly in the home,[20,24] in schools,[26] and in daycare centers.[27] Children acquire new viral strains from their schoolmates, which they then bring home and pass to other family members. Intervals of 1 to 5 days occur between cases. Secondary attack rates of family members vary depending on age, position in the family, and prior immunity to the virus. Age and immunity are related risk factors. Young children and mothers have high secondary attack rates as a result of close and prolonged exposure to schoolchildren in the family. The secondary attack rate of fathers is relatively low.

The mechanisms for the spread of cold viruses have not been well established. Possible means of transmission include (1) direct contact with infectious secretions on skin and environmental surfaces, (2) large particles of respiratory secretions that are briefly transported in air, (3) infectious droplet nuclei suspended in air, and (4) combinations of these methods.[28] For some viruses, such as rhinovirus, close physical contact appears to be necessary for efficient spread. Rhinovirus is produced primarily in the nose and is shed in highest concentrations in nasal secretions. Peak viral titers in nasal mucus occur on the second to fourth days of experimental infection and coincide with the period of maximum communicability.[28] A high proportion of people with natural and experimental rhinovirus colds have virus on their hands. Virus also contaminates objects in the environment of cold sufferers. With experimental rhinovirus infection, brief hand contact permits ready transfer of virus-contaminated nasal secretions from the hands of infected subjects to the hands of susceptible subjects. When the contaminated fingers of the susceptible subjects are then placed in contact with nasal and conjunctival mucosa, infection results in a high percentage of cases.[29] In one study conducted in the home setting, treatment of fingers with a virucidal solution reduced the rate of infection in mothers exposed to other family members with fresh colds.[30] This study provides direct evidence of the mechanisms of common cold transmission under natural conditions and suggests that a proportion of colds are spread by hand contamination and self-inoculation.

Another rhinovirus transmission model has been developed in which virus is transmitted through the air in large- and/or small-particle aerosol.[31] This model demonstrates the feasibility of the aerosol route of spread but does not prove that it occurs under natural conditions. Studies conducted in the field with intervention techniques specific for aerosol transmission are needed to address this question. There is epidemiologic evidence that influenza and adenovirus may be spread, at least in part, by small airborne droplets. All respiratory viruses may

not behave in the same way, and further studies are necessary to determine which routes of transmission are important in the natural dissemination of these viruses.

PATHOGENESIS

Viral invasion of the upper respiratory tract is the basic mechanism in the pathogenesis of colds, but the specific events leading to clinical illness are not fully understood. Infection with common cold viruses is characteristically of short duration and self-limited. For example, rhinovirus shedding lasts 3 weeks or less in young adults with experimental colds,[32,33] and coronavirus excretion has been detected for up to 14 days.[19,34] Cold viruses are not usually present in asymptomatic persons,[34,35] although subclinical infections do occur, and viral carriage may be somewhat prolonged in children.[36] Rhinovirus is produced primarily in nasal cells, but has also been recovered from sinus[37] and middle ear[38,39] aspirates. Recently, rhinovirus replicative-strand ribonucleic acid (RNA) has been demonstrated in bronchial epithelial cells.[40]

Characteristic changes have been described in sloughed columnar epithelial cells in nasal secretions of persons with natural colds of unknown cause.[41] Cells with persistent ciliary activity have been found in nasal secretions on days 1 through 3 of illness. Also, some exfoliated cells show degenerative changes characterized by progressive nuclear pyknosis and the formation of apparent inclusion bodies. Ciliated epithelial cells containing viral antigen have been found in the nasal mucus of volunteers with experimental rhinovirus colds.[42]

Attempts to demonstrate specific histopathologic changes in nasal biopsy specimens of volunteers with rhinovirus colds have not been successful.[43,44] Examination by light and electron microscopy of nasal biopsy specimens from young adults with natural colds also confirmed the absence of destruction of the nasal epithelium.[45] In this study there was a significant increase in the number of neutrophils in the epithelium and in the lamina propria. The number of epithelial mast cells was not increased. The findings with rhinovirus contrast with the destructive changes to the respiratory epithelium that are seen with influenza virus and adenovirus infections.

With rhinovirus colds, the period of maximum viral excretion in nasal secretions coincides with the peak of clinical illness[46] and the appearance of ciliated epithelial cells in nasal mucus.[42] At that time, large quantities of protein, including immunoglobulins and cross-linked fibrin,[47] are present in nasal secretions. In addition to any direct destructive effect that the virus may have on the respiratory mucous membrane, there is increasing evidence that chemical mediators and neurologic reflexes play a role in the pathogenesis of the common cold. Bradykinin,[48,49] prostaglandin,[49,50] histamine,[49,51] interleukin-1,[52] interleukin-6,[53] and interleukin-8[54,55] have been associated with rhinovirus pathogenesis and with parasympathetic[56] and α-adrenergic nerve pathways.[57] Pathogenic mechanisms for the various respiratory viruses are undoubtedly somewhat different.

A self-limited cold virus infection may lead to changes that affect the resident bacterial flora of the upper respiratory tract and result in secondary bacterial infection. Bacteria reach the sinuses and middle ear, which are normally sterile, and establish infection. An important mechanism for these events may be nose blowing during colds. A recent study showed that nose blowing, but not coughing or sneezing, generates pressures of up to 60 to 80 mm Hg in the nasal passages.[58] The study also showed that nose blowing propels contrast medium from the pharynx into the sinuses and middle ear. During colds, nasal fluid contains viruses, bacteria, and inflammatory mediators, all or any of which are capable of producing inflammation. Experimental and natural colds routinely lead to acute, reversible anatomic and physiologic abnormalities of the ostiomeatal area and sinus cavities.[59,60] It is unknown whether direct viral invasion of the sinuses and middle ear is necessary for disease to occur at these sites during colds. However, respiratory viruses have been recovered from sinus[61] and middle ear[11,62] aspirates obtained by direct puncture from patients with inflammation at these sites. Abnormalities in eustachian tube function and middle ear pressures have been observed in volunteers with experimental rhinovirus infection.[63] During colds, increases have also been noted in titers of resident bacterial populations of the upper airways, but the significance of this is unknown.[64,65]

CLINICAL CHARACTERISTICS

The incubation period of the common cold varies somewhat with the different viruses but is usually between 12 and 72 hours. The symptoms of experimental rhinovirus colds have an onset 8 to 16 hours after viral inoculation into the nose.[48,66] The cardinal symptoms are nasal discharge, nasal obstruction, sneezing, sore or "scratchy" throat, and cough.[20,25] Slight fever may be found, but a temperature elevation of more than 1° F is distinctly uncommon in adults. Infants and young children more frequently have temperature elevation. The early symptoms may be minimal, with only scratchy throat, mild malaise, and nasal complaints. With rhinovirus infection, sneezing, nasal discharge, and nasal obstruction usually begin simultaneously on the first day of illness and rapidly increase to maximum severity by the second or third day. Paralleling the nasal symptoms is a sore, dry, or scratchy throat. Cough may begin early in the course of illness but tends to persist or increase in severity during the first week of symptoms, by which time nasal and pharyngeal complaints are subsiding. Limited information is available, suggesting that symptom patterns are similar with coronavirus colds (see Chapter 152).[19]

The median duration of rhinovirus colds is 1 week, but in approximately one fourth of cases the illness lasts up to 2 weeks. In cigarette smokers with rhinovirus colds, cough is increased and prolonged. Other complaints may include mild burning of the eyes, but true conjunctivitis is not seen except in some adenovirus and enterovirus infections. There may also be loss of the senses of smell and taste and a feeling of facial pressure and fullness in the ears. The voice may have a nasal quality. Painful maceration of the skin around the nostrils is often bothersome when rhinorrhea has been profuse and persistent.

On physical examination, the findings are often minimal despite the subjective discomfort of the patient. A red nose and a dripping nasal discharge are the characteristic features of the patient with a cold, but many patients lack these outward manifestations of the infection. The nasal mucous membrane may have a glassy appearance owing to the exudation of serum proteins and increased mucus secretions. It is difficult to accurately detect the presence of increased erythema of the mucous membrane of the nose and throat because of normal variations in the color of these structures. Marked pharyngeal erythema and exudate are not seen with rhinovirus and coronavirus infections, but they do occur with pharyngoconjunctival fever of adenovirus infection and with primary herpes simplex pharyngitis. Examination of the chest may reveal the presence of rhonchi.

The clinical picture of the common cold is similar in children and in adults. However, in young children, parainfluenza virus and RSV infections may lead to viral pneumonia, croup, and bronchiolitis, whereas in normal adults these viruses usually cause only colds. In both adults and children the upper airway manifestations of rhinovirus, coronavirus, parainfluenza virus, and RSV infections are indistinguishable in the individual patient.

DIAGNOSIS

The manifestations of the common cold are so typical and familiar that self-diagnosis by the patient is usually correct. Hay fever and vasomotor rhinitis may result in similar nasal symptoms, but the recurrent and chronic nature of these diseases is recognized by the patient and diagnosed by the physician from the patient's history of seasonality and exposure to allergens. Diagnosis of the specific virus involved is usually not possible on the basis of clinical observation. Some acute respiratory infections, such as influenza and pharyngoconjunctival fever, when seen in a typical epidemiologic setting, can be recognized without benefit of viral culture or serologic tests. Knowledge of the characteristic seasonal patterns for the different virus groups may also suggest a particular virus.

The main challenge to the physician is to distinguish the uncomplicated cold from cases of streptococcal pharyngitis and secondary bacterial sinusitis (0.5%-2% of colds)[20,67] and otitis media (2%).[20] The latter is not easy because of the lack of inexpensive and noninvasive diagnostic tests for this purpose. A complete physical examination should be performed on the pharynx, nasal cavity, ears, and sinuses. In the pharynx, marked erythema or exudate should raise suspicion of streptococcal or adenovirus infection, herpes simplex pharyngitis, Vincent's angina, mononucleosis, or diphtheria. Occasionally, patients have small vesicles on the palate as a result of coxsackievirus A infections. The presence of nasal polyps is suggestive of an underlying allergy problem. In children, a foreign body may lead to persistent nasal discharge. Examination of the ears is directed at finding changes in the appearance of the tympanum, indicating infection (see Chapter 54). The use of the pneumatic otoscope is helpful in determining whether fluid is present behind the ear drum. There may be sinus tenderness or swelling and erythema over the area of a sinus, but these findings are uncommon. Most colds are over or better by 7 to 10 days, and a history of an illness that has not improved or has worsened by that time suggests development of a secondary bacterial sinusitis.

Sinus computed tomography (CT) scans are sensitive for detecting abnormalities in the sinuses of patients with cold symptoms[60]; however, their cost precludes their use in routine practice. More important, sinus CT scans do not reliably distinguish between viral and bacterial infections of the sinus. The most valuable laboratory test in patients with prominent pharyngeal complaints is rapid antigen detection for group A β-hemolytic streptococci, with throat culture when indicated (see Chapter 51). Many of the respiratory viruses can be isolated in cell culture or identified by RT-PCR, although specific virologic diagnosis is often not available in clinical practice. Rhinoviruses grow in human embryonic lung cells, myxoviruses and paramyxoviruses in primary rhesus monkey kidney cells, and RSV in Hep2 cells. Isolation of common cold–associated coronaviruses in cell culture has proved difficult with currently available techniques, although the severe acute respiratory syndrome (SARS)–associated coronavirus grows well in VERO cells (see Chapter 152).

Serologic diagnostic analyses for influenza virus, parainfluenza virus, RSV, and adenovirus infection are available in some state health department laboratories. Serum specimens should be obtained in the acute phase of illness and again approximately 3 weeks later and tested simultaneously. A rise of fourfold or greater in antibody titer is indicative of infection. Serologic diagnosis of rhinovirus infection is not practical because of the many different antigenic types. Rapid techniques using fluorescent antibody, other immunodiagnostic procedures, and nucleic acid probes are being used in clinical laboratories for the diagnosis of influenza virus, parainfluenza virus, RSV, and adenovirus (see Chapters 2, 139, 153, 155, 162). Of most importance is the diagnosis of influenza by clinical or laboratory means because of the availability of effective antiviral treatment.

TREATMENT

Although a "cure" for the common cold remains elusive, some commercial remedies provide good symptomatic relief. Leading the list of effective cold treatments are the first-generation antihistamines and the nonsteroidal anti-inflammatory drugs (NSAIDs). Antihistamines provide good relief in adults for sneezing, rhinorrhea, nasal mucus weights, and, with one of the drugs, cough.[68-70] The newer, nonsedating antihistamines do not have the same effectiveness as the first-generation compounds in treating sneezing, possibly because of differences in crossing the blood-brain barrier.[71]

NSAIDs sulindac,[72] indomethacin,[73] and naproxen[50,74] have shown effectiveness in reducing cough, presumably through blocking prostaglandin action.[49] These compounds also are useful for treating headaches, malaise, and other systemic complaints.

The combination of a first-generation antihistamine and an NSAID provides good relief of cold symptoms. In volunteers with experimental rhinovirus colds, chlorpheniramine (12 mg, extended release) and ibuprofen (400 mg) given on an every-12-hour schedule resulted in clinically relevant reductions in sneezing, rhinorrhea, nasal mucus weights, nasal tissue use, cough, and headache.[75] Treatment was begun 24 hours after viral challenge, during early symptomatic infection, and continued regularly for 5 days. It is recommended that this, or a similar combination of a first-generation antihistamine and an NSAID, be started at the first symptom of a suspected cold and continued on a regular 12-hour dosing schedule until cold symptoms subside or it is determined that the initial symptom was not due to a cold. First-generation antihistamines cause clinically important drowsiness in 10% to 15% of patients, and NSAIDs can result in gastric irritation.

Because this combined antihistamine-NSAID therapy provides some relief of nasal obstruction, decongestant therapy may not be necessary. When required, oral decongestants are recommended to avoid the rebound nasal obstruction and pharyngeal irritation associated with topical preparations such as phenylephrine and oxymetazoline. Oral decongestants have been shown to be safe in patients with hypertension on therapy.[76] Dextromethorphan and codeine have been used successfully in practice for cough suppression, although their effectiveness has been difficult to demonstrate in controlled clinical trials in patients with colds.[77]

Sore throat can be relieved with warm saline gargles or lozenges containing a topical anesthetic. The regular application of an ointment containing a petrolatum base is useful in controlling painful maceration of the nares. The patient's activities should be restricted during the height of the illness, when the patient is most contagious to others. Regular hand washing and care to avoid contamination of the environment with nasal secretions may also help to prevent spread of infection.

Antibiotics have no place in the treatment of uncomplicated colds. Until specific treatment becomes available, there will continue to be fads in the use of "alternative" cold remedies. The ingestion of large doses of vitamin C has been widely used as a preventive or therapeutic measure for colds. Controlled studies have shown a modest therapeutic benefit of vitamin C for colds but have failed to show any usefulness in preventing cold.[78,79] Vitamin C has mild anticholinergic activity.

Three properly designed clinical trials failed to show a beneficial effect of zinc for treatment of colds,[80-82] and positive studies probably reflected poor masking of subjects and other problems with experimental design.[83] Echinacea, an herbal medicine, has received testing in only one properly designed study in which no benefit was observed.[84] Echinacea has potential side effects because of reported CD4+ T-lymphocyte suppression.[85,86]

PROSPECTS FOR VACCINES, NEW TREATMENTS, AND INTERRUPTION OF TRANSMISSION

Vaccine development for the common cold has reached an impasse because of the discovery of the many different cold viruses, particularly the 100 different serotypes of rhinoviruses. Unless ways are found to combine large numbers of viral antigens effectively or take advantage of minor antigenic cross-relationships that exist, prospects for common cold vaccines are not good. A number of chemical compounds have inhibitory activity against respiratory viruses in tissue culture systems, and attempts are being made to develop antiviral agents for clinical use. The activity of such compounds tends to be relatively group specific, but some, such as the capsid binders, which block viral attachment and uncoating, have activity against most of the rhinoviruses.

Intranasal recombinant human interferon-alfa-2b has effective prophylactic activity against experimental rhinovirus infection.[87-89] When given therapeutically intranasally, interferon reduces viral excretion, but its effect on illness has been of only minimal benefit.[90] In addition, chronic application of intranasal interferon is associated with local side effects such as nasal stuffiness, dryness, discomfort, and pinpoint areas of ulceration.[91,92] Short-term contact prophylaxis with intranasal interferon by family members exposed to individuals with colds of recent onset reduced the incidence of total colds by 40% and virtually

eliminated rhinovirus-specific infections.[93,94] Side effects of interferon were avoided by the short duration of the course of prophylaxis.

Pleconaril, an orally active antipicornavirus agent that inhibits rhinovirus replication by binding into the hydrophobic pockets of the capsid surface, was evaluated in two double-blind controlled trials in the early treatment of colds.[95] A mild effect on duration of colds (1 day more rapid alleviation of illness) was seen, along with a slight increase in nausea and vomiting. A U.S. Food and Drug Administration (FDA) advisory committee recommended against approval of the drug for that indication.

The failure to observe worthwhile clinical benefits with the use of potent antivirals such as interferon-alfa-2b[90] and the capsid binders[95] suggests that treatment with antiviral compounds alone will not be useful in clinical practice. The failure of this approach may be the result of the inflammatory events accompanying the infection, which would not be expected to respond to an antiviral. To test this hypothesis, an experimental treatment has been developed that combines a compound with antiviral activity with other compounds that block selected pathways of inflammation. Promising results were obtained in two controlled clinical trials, one in which volunteers with early rhinovirus colds were given interferon-alfa-2b and ipratropium topically into the nose plus oral naproxen,[74] and another in which intranasal interferon was combined with oral chlorpheniramine and ibuprofen.[75]

Another approach to control of colds is to interrupt the person-to-person transmission of the viruses. A virucidal hand treatment used in the home by mothers exposed to children with new colds reduced the mothers' incidence of total colds by 60% and eliminated laboratory-proven rhinovirus colds.[30] In another study, children trained to avoid self-inoculatory behavior had reduced cold-associated asthmatic attacks and laboratory-proven respiratory virus infections.[96] These studies suggest that spread of cold viruses occurs in part by direct hand contact and self-inoculation. Hand washing and avoidance of finger-nose and finger-eye contact should be practiced, particularly when there is exposure to someone with a cold. Also, covering of coughs and sneezes with disposable nasal tissues is recommended as a means of controlling aerosol transmission.

REFERENCES

1. Rice DP, Feldman JJ, White KL. The current burden of illness in the United States. Occasional Papers of the Institute of Medicine. Washington, DC: National Academy of Science; 1976:1.
2. Fendrick AM, Monto AS, Nightengale B, Sarnes, M. The economic burden of non-influenza-related viral respiratory tract infection in the United States. Arch Intern Med. 2003;163:487-494.
3. Chanock RM. Association of a new type of cytopathogenic myxovirus with infantile croup. J Exp Med. 1956;104:55.
4. Pelon W, Mogabgab WJ, Phillips IA, et al. A cytopathogenic agent isolated from naval recruits with mild respiratory illness. Proc Soc Exp Biol Med. 1957;94:262.
5. Price WH. The isolation of a new virus associated with respiratory clinical disease in humans. Proc Natl Acad Sci U S A. 1956;43:892.
6. Chanock RM, Roizman B, Myers R. Recovery from infants with respiratory illness of a virus related to chimpanzee coryza agent (CCA): I. Isolation, properties, and characterization. Am J Hyg. 1957;66:281.
7. Lennette EH, Fox VL, Schmidt NJ, et al. The COE virus: An apparently new virus recovered from patients with mild respiratory disease. Am J Hyg. 1958;68:272.
8. Tyrrell DAJ, Bynoe ML. Cultivation of a novel type of common-cold virus in organ cultures. BMJ. 1965;1:1467.
9. Hamre D, Procknow JJ. A new virus isolated from the human respiratory tract. Proc Soc Exp Biol Med. 1966;121:190.
10. Boivin G, Abed Y, Pelletier G, et al. Virological features and clinical manifestations associated with human metapneumovirus: A new paramyxovirus responsible for acute respiratory tract infections in all age groups. J Infect Dis. 2002;186:1330-1334.
11. Gwaltney JM Jr. Virology of middle ear. Ann Otol Rhinol Laryngol. 1971;80:365.
12. Stuart-Harris CH, Andrewes C, Andrews BE, et al. A collaborative study of the aetiology of acute respiratory infection in Britain 1961-4: A report of the Medical Research Council working party on acute respiratory virus infections. BMJ. 1965;2:319.
13. Hamre D, Connelly AP Jr, Procknow JJ. Virologic studies of acute respiratory disease in young adults: IV. Virus isolations during four years of surveillance. Am J Epidemiol. 1966;83:238.
14. Monto AS, Bryan ER, Ohmit S. Rhinovirus infections in Tecumseh, Michigan: Frequency of illness and number of serotypes. J Infect Dis. 1987;156:43-49.
15. Falsey AR, McCann RM, Hall WJ, et al. The "common cold" in frail older persons: Impact of rhinovirus and coronavirus in a senior daycare center. J Am Geriatr Soc. 1997;45:706-711.

16. Vabret A, Mourez T, Gouarin S, et al. An outbreak of coronavirus OC43 respiratory infection in Normandy, France. Clin Infect Dis. 2003;36:985-989.

17. Kepfer PD, Hable KA, Smith TF. Viral isolation rates during summer from children with acute upper respiratory tract disease and healthy children. AJCP. 1974;16:1-5.

18. Makela MJ, Puhakka T, Ruuskanen O, et al. Viruses and bacteria in the etiology of the common cold. J Clin Microbiol. 1998;36(2):539-542.

19. Monto AS. Coronaviruses. In: Evans AS, ed. Viral Infections of Humans: Epidemiology and Control. 4th ed. New York: Plenum; 1997:211-227.

20. Dingle JH, Badger GF, Jordan WS Jr. Illness in the Home: Study of 25,000 Illnesses in a Group of Cleveland Families. Cleveland: The Press of Western Reserve University; 1964:1.

21. Gwaltney JM Jr, Hendley JO, Simon G, et al. Rhinovirus infections in an industrial population: I. The occurrence of illness. N Engl J Med. 1966;275:1261.

22. Douglas RG Jr, Lindgren KM, Couch RB. Exposure to cold environment and rhinovirus common cold: Failure to demonstrate effect. N Engl J Med. 1968;279:743.

23. Gwaltney JM Jr. The Jeremiah Metzger lecture: Climatology and the common cold. Trans Am Clin Climatol Assoc. 1984;96:159.

24. Hendley JO, Gwaltney JM Jr, Jordan WS Jr. Rhinovirus infections in an industrial population: IV. Infections within families of employees during two fall peaks of respiratory illness. Am J Epidemiol. 1969;89:184.

25. Gwaltney JM Jr, Hendley JO, Simon G, et al. Rhinovirus infections in an industrial population: II. Characteristics of illness and antibody response. JAMA. 1967;202:494.

26. Beem MO. Acute respiratory illness in nursery school children: A longitudinal study of the occurrence of illness and respiratory viruses. Am J Epidemiol. 1969;90:30.

27. Frenck RW, Glezen WP. Respiratory tract infections in children in day care. Semin Pediatr Infect Dis. 1990;1:234-244.

28. Gwaltney JM Jr. Epidemiology of the common cold. Ann N Y Acad Sci. 1980;353:54.

29. Gwaltney JM Jr, Moskalski PB, Hendley JO. Hand-to-hand transmission of rhinovirus colds. Ann Intern Med. 1978;88:463.

30. Hendley JO, Gwaltney JM Jr. Mechanisms of transmission of rhinovirus infections. Epidemiol Rev. 1988;10:242.

31. Dick EC, Jennings LC, Mink KA, et al. Aerosol transmission of rhinovirus colds. J Infect Dis. 1987;156:442.

32. Cate TR, Couch RB, Johnson KM. Studies with rhinoviruses in volunteers: Production of illness, effect of naturally acquired antibody, and demonstration of a protective effect not associated with serum antibody. J Clin Invest. 1964;43:56.

33. Winther B, Gwaltney JM Jr, Mygind N, et al. Sites of rhinovirus recovery after point inoculation of the upper airway. JAMA. 1986;256:1763.

34. van Elden LJR, van Loon AM, van Alphen F, et al. Frequent detection of human coronaviruses in clinical specimens of patients with respiratory tract infection by use of a novel real-time reverse-transcriptase polymerase chain reaction. J Infect Dis. 2004;189:652-657.

35. Hamre D, Rhinoviruses. In: Melnick JL, ed. Monographs in Virology 1. Basel: Karger; 1968:1.

36. Frank AL, Taber LH, Wells CR, et al. Patterns of shedding of myxoviruses in children. J Infect Dis. 1981;144:433.

37. Hamory BH, Sande MA, Sydnor A Jr, et al. Etiology and antimicrobial therapy of acute maxillary sinusitis. J Infect Dis. 1979;139:197-202.

38. Gwaltney JM Jr. Viral vaccines in the control of otitis media. Pediatr Infect Dis J. 1989;8:S78-S79.

39. Pitkaranta A, Arruda E, Virolainen A, Hayden FG. Polymerase chain reaction-based detection of rhinovirus, respiratory syncytial virus, and coronavirus in otitis media with effusion. J Pediatr. 1998;133:390-394.

40. Papadopoulos NG, Bates PJ, Bardin PG, et al. Rhinoviruses infect the lower airway. J Infect Dis. 2000;181:1875-1884.

41. Bryan WTK, Bryan MP, Smith CA. Human ciliated epithelial cells in nasal secretions. Transactions of the 85th Annual Meeting of the American Laryngological Association, San Francisco, California, April 10-11, 1964, p. 145.

42. Turner RB, Hendley JO, Gwaltney JM Jr. Shedding of infected ciliated epithelial cells in rhinovirus colds. J Infect Dis. 1982;145:849.

43. Douglas RG Jr, Alford BR, Couch RB. Atraumatic nasal biopsy for studies of respiratory virus infection in volunteers. Antimicrob Agents Chemother. 1968;8:340.

44. Winther B, Farr B, Turner RB, et al. Histopathologic examination and enumeration of polymorphonuclear leukocytes in the nasal mucosa during experimental rhinovirus colds. Acta Otolaryngol (Stockh). 1984;413(Suppl):19-24.

45. Winther B, Brofeldt S, Christensen B, et al. Light and scanning electron microscopy of nasal biopsies from patients with naturally acquired common colds. Acta Otalaryngol. 1984;97:309.

46. Douglas RG Jr, Cate TR, Gerone PJ, et al. Quantitative rhinovirus shedding patterns in volunteers. Am Rev Respir Dis. 1966;94:159.

47. Winther B, Gwaltney JM Jr, Humphries JE, Hendley JO. Cross-linked fibrin in the nasal fluid of patients with the common cold. Clin Infect Dis. 2002;34:708-710.

48. Naclerio RM, Proud D, Lichtenstein LM, et al. Kinins are generated during experimental rhinovirus colds. J Infect Dis. 1988;157:133.

49. Doyle WJ, Boehm S, Skoner DP. Physiologic responses to intranasal dose-response challenges with histamine, methacholine, bradykinin, and prostaglandin in adult volunteers with and without nasal allergy. J Allergy Clin Immunol. 1990;86:924-935.

50. Sperber SJ, Hendley JO, Hayden FG, et al. Effects of naproxen on experimental rhinovirus colds: A randomized, double-blind, controlled trial. Ann Intern Med. 1992;117:37-41.

51. Doyle WJ, McBride TP, Skoner DP, et al. A double-blind, placebo-controlled clinical trial of the effect of chlorpheniramine on the response of the nasal airway, middle ear and eustachian tube to provocative rhinovirus challenge. Pediatr Infect Dis J. 1988;7:229-238.

52. Proud D, Gwaltney JM Jr, Hendley JO, et al. Increased levels of interleukin-1 are detected in nasal secretions of volunteers during experimental rhinovirus colds. J Infect Dis. 1994;169:1007-1013.

53. Zhu Z, Tang W, Ray A, et al. Rhinovirus stimulation of interleukin-6 in vivo and in vitro: Evidence for NFκjkB-dependent transcriptional activation. J Clin Invest. 1966;97:421-430.

54. Zhu Z, Tang W, Gwaltney JM Jr, et al. Rhinovirus stimulation of interleukin-8 in vivo and in vitro: Role of NFκjkB. Am J Physiol. (Lung Cell Mol Physiol) 1997;17:L814-L824.

55. Turner RB, Weingand K, Yeh CH, et al. Association between interleukin-8 concentration in nasal secretions and severity of symptoms of experimental rhinovirus colds. Clin Infect Dis. 1988;26:840-846.

56. Gaffey MJ, Hayden FG, Boyd JC, et al. Ipratropium bromide treatment of experimental rhinovirus infection. Antimicrob Agents Chemother. 1988;32:1644-1647.

57. Sperber SJ, Sorrentino JV, Riker DK, et al. Evaluation of an alpha agonist alone and in combination with a nonsteroidal anti-inflammatory agent in the treatment of experimental rhinovirus colds. Bull N Y Acad Med. 1989;65:145-160.

58. Gwaltney JM Jr, Hendley JO, Phillips CD, et al. Nose blowing propels nasal fluid into the paranasal sinuses. Clin Infect Dis. 2000;30:387-391.

59. Turner BW, Cail WS, Hendley JO, et al. Physiologic abnormalities in the paranasal sinuses during experimental rhinovirus colds. J Allergy Clin Immunol. 1992;90:474-478.

60. Gwaltney JM Jr, Phillips CD, Miller RD, et al. Computed tomographic study of the common cold. N Engl J Med. 1994;330:25-30.

61. Evans FO Jr, Sydnor JB, Moore WEC, et al. Sinusitis of the maxillary antrum. N Engl J Med. 1975;293:735.

62. Arola M, Ruuskanen O, Ziegler T, et al. Clinical role of respiratory virus infection in acute otitis media. Pediatrics. 1990;86:848-855.

63. Doyle WJ, McBride TP, Skoner DP. A double blind placebo-controlled clinical trial of the effect of chlorpheniramine on the response of the nasal airway, middle ear and eustachian tube to provocative rhinovirus challenge. Pediatr Infect Dis J. 1988;7:222-229.

64. Straker E, Hill AB, Lovell RA. A study of the nasopharyngeal bacterial flora of different groups of persons observed in London and south-east England during the years 1930 to 1937. Reports on Public Health and Medical Subjects, no. 90. London: His Majesty's Stationery Office; 1939;7.

65. Brimblecombe FSW, Cruickshank R, Master P, et al. Family studies of respiratory infections. BMJ. 1958;1:119.

66. Harris JM II, Gwaltney JM Jr. The incubation periods of experimental rhinovirus infection and illness. Clin Infect Dis. 1996;23:1286-1290.

67. Berg O, Carenfelt C, Rystedt G, et al. Occurrence of asymptomatic sinusitis in common cold and other acute ENT-infections. Rhinology. 1986; 24:223-225.

68. Gwaltney JM Jr, Park J, Paul RA, et al. Randomized controlled trial of clemastine fumarate for treatment of experimental rhinovirus colds. Clin Infect Dis. 1996;22:656-662.

69. Turner RB, Sperber SJ, Sorrentino JV, et al. Effectiveness of clemastine fumarate for treatment of rhinorrhea and sneezing associated with the common cold. Clin Infect Dis. 1997;25:824-830.

70. Gwaltney JM Jr, Druce HM. Efficacy of brompheniramine maleate treatment for rhinovirus colds. Clin Infect Dis. 1997;25:1188-1194.

71. Muether PS, Gwaltney JM Jr. Variant effect of first- and second-generation antihistamines as clues to their mechanism of action on the sneeze reflex in the common cold. Clin Infect Dis. 2001;33:1483-1488.

72. Nozhat JRM, Choudry B, Fuller RW. The effect of sulindac on the abnormal cough reflex associated with dry cough. J Pharmacol Exper Ther. 1990;255:161-164.

73. Fogari R, Zoppi A, Tettamanti F, et al. Effects of nifedipine and indomethacin on cough induced by angiotensin-converting enzyme inhibitors: A double-blind, randomized, cross-over study. J Cardiovasc Pharmacol. 1992;19:670-673.

74. Gwaltney JM Jr. Combined antiviral and antimediator treatment of rhinovirus colds. J Infect Dis. 1992;166:776-782.

75. Gwaltney JM Jr, Winther B, Patrie JT, Hendley JO. Combined antiviral-antimediator treatment for the common cold. J Infect Dis, 2002;186:147-154.

76. Coates ML, Rembold CM, Farr BM. Does pseudoephedrine increase blood pressure in patients with controlled hypertension? J Fam Pract. 1995;40:22-26.

77. Freestone C, Eccles R. Assessment of the antitussive efficacy of codeine in cough associated with common cold. J Pharm Pharmacol. 1997;49:1045-1049.

78. Walker GH, Bynoe ML, Tyrrell DAJ. Trial of ascorbic acid in prevention of colds. BMJ. 1967;1:603.

79. Schwartz AR, Togo Y, Hornick RB, et al. Evaluation of the efficacy of ascorbic acid in prophylaxis of induced rhinovirus 44 infection in man. J Infect Dis. 1973;128:500.

80. Farr BM, Gwaltney JM Jr. The problems of taste in placebo matching: An evaluation of zinc gluconate for the common cold. J Chronic Dis. 1987;40:875-879.

81. Farr BM, Conner EM, Betts FR, et al. Two randomized controlled trials of zinc gluconate lozenge therapy of experimentally induced rhinovirus colds. Antimicrob Agents Chemother. 1987;31:1183-1187.

82. Smith DS, Helzner EC, Nuttall CE Jr, et al. Failure of zinc gluconate in treatment of acute upper respiratory tract infections. Antimicrob Agents Chemother. 1989;33:646-648.

83. Farr BM, Hayden FG, Gwaltney J Jr. Zinc gluconate lozenges for treating the common cold (Letter). Ann Intern Med. 1997;126:738.

84. Barrett BP, Brown RL, Locken K, et al. Treatment of the common cold with unrefined Echinacea. Ann Intern Med. 2002;137:939-946.

85. Gaisbauer M, Zimmermann W, Schleich T. Nat Med. 1986;3:6-10.

86. Coeugniet EG, Elek E. Immunomodulation with *Viscum album* and *Echinacea purpurea* extracts. Onkologie. 1987:10(Suppl):27-33.

87. Scott GM, Phillpotts RJ, Wallace J, et al. Purified interferon as protection against rhinovirus infections. BMJ. 1982;284:1822.

88. Hayden FG, Gwaltney JM Jr. Intranasal interferon-alpha$_2$ for prevention of rhinovirus infection and illness. J Infect Dis. 1983;148:543.

89. Samo T-C, Greenberg SB, Couch RB Jr, et al. Evaluations of efficacy and tolerance to intranasally applied recombinant leukocyte A interferon in normal volunteers. J Infect Dis. 1983;148:535.

90. Hayden FG, Gwaltney JM Jr. Intranasal interferon-α_2 treatment of experimental rhinoviral colds. J Infect Dis. 1984;150:174.

91. Douglas RM, Albrecht JK, Miles HB, et al. Intranasal interferon-α_2 prophylaxis of natural respiratory virus infection. J Infect Dis. 1985;151:731.

92. Hayden FG, Gwaltney JM Jr, Johnson ME. Prophylactic efficacy and tolerance of low-dose intranasal interferon-alpha$_2$ in natural respiratory viral infections. Antiviral Res. 1985;5:11.

93. Hayden FG, Albrecht JK, Kaiser DL, et al. Prevention of natural colds by contact prophylaxis with intranasal alpha$_2$-interferon. N Engl J Med. 1986;314:71.

94. Douglas RM, Moore BW, Miles HB, et al. Prophylactic efficacy of intranasal alpha$_2$-interferon against rhinovirus infections in the family setting. N Engl J Med. 1986; 314:65.

95. Hayden FG, Herrington DT, Coats TL, et al. Efficacy and safety of oral pleconaril for treatment of colds due to picornaviruses in adults: Results of 2 double-blind, randomized, placebo-controlled trials. Clin Infect Dis. 2003;36:1523-1532.

96. Corley DL, Gevirtz R, Nideffer R, Cummins L. Prevention of postinfectious asthma in children by reducing self-inoculatory behavior. J Pediatr Psychol. 1987;12:242-258.

CHAPTER **51**

Pharyngitis

ALAN L. BISNO

Acute pharyngitis is one of the commonest illnesses for which patients visit primary care physicians. According to the National Ambulatory Medical Care Survey, upper respiratory infections, including acute pharyngitis, are responsible for 200 visits per 1000 population annually to physicians' offices in the United States.[1] This is more than double the rate for any other infectious disease category.

Although acute pharyngitis is more common in children, there were an estimated 6.7 million visits to primary-care office-based physicians by adults between 1989 and 1999 with the chief complaint of sore throat.[2]

Acute pharyngitis is an inflammatory syndrome of the pharynx caused by several different groups of microorganisms. Most cases are of viral etiology and occur as part of common colds and influenzal syndromes. The most important of the bacterial infections is that caused by group A beta-hemolytic streptococci (*Streptococcus pyogenes*). It is important to differentiate streptococcal from viral pharyngitis because of the response of streptococcal infection to antimicrobial therapy and the ineffectiveness of antibiotic therapy in viral infections. Also, streptococcal pharyngitis may be complicated by acute rheumatic fever and acute glomerulonephritis. There are other uncommon or rare types of pharyngitis, and, for some of these, treatment is also available.

ETIOLOGY

The known microbial causes of pharyngitis are listed in Table 51-1, which shows the syndromes of respiratory illness caused by the various agents[3-6] and their estimated contribution to all cases of pharyngitis.[7,8] The relative importance of the different agents is not fully defined, and it is still not possible to determine the cause in a sizable proportion of cases. The results of epidemiologic investigations are influenced by the season of the year, the age of the population, the severity of illness, and the diagnostic methods used to detect cases. A large proportion of mild cases of pharyngitis are associated with rhinovirus[9] and coronavirus colds. Adenovirus and herpes simplex virus pharyngitis, although less common, are important because of their clinical severity. Others of the known respiratory viruses each account for a small proportion of cases. The acute retroviral syndrome caused by human immunodeficiency virus-1 (HIV-1) has joined the list of viral infections associated with acute pharyngitis.[10]

Approximately 15% to 30% of all cases of pharyngitis in children and 10% in adults are due to *S. pyogenes*. In children with sore throat,

TABLE 51-1 **Microbial Causes of Acute Pharyngitis**

Pathogen	Syndrome/Disease	Estimated Importance*
Viral		
Rhinovirus (100 types and 1 subtype)	Common cold	20
Coronavirus (3 or more types)	Common cold, SARS	≥5
Adenovirus (types 3, 4, 7, 14, 21)	Pharyngoconjunctival fever, ARD	5
Herpes simplex virus (types 1 and 2)	Gingivitis, stomatitis, pharyngitis	4
Parainfluenza virus (types 1-4)	Common cold, croup	2
Influenza virus (types A and B)	Influenza	2
Coxsackievirus A (types 2, 4-6, 8, 10)	Herpangina	<1
Epstein-Barr virus	Infectious mononucleosis	<1
Cytomegalovirus	Infectious mononucleosis	<1
HIV-1	Primary HIV infection	<1
Bacterial		
Streptococcus pyogenes (group A β-hemolytic streptococci)	Pharyngitis/tonsillitis, scarlet fever	15-30
Group C and G β-hemolytic streptococci	Pharyngitis/tonsillitis	5-10
Mixed aerobic/anaerobic infection	Gingivitis (Vincent's angina)	<1
	Peritonsillitis/peritonsillar abscess (quinsy)	<1
Neisseria gonorrhoeae	Pharyngitis	<1
Corynebacterium diphtheriae	Diphtheria	≥1
Corynebacterium ulcerans	Pharyngitis, diphtheria	<1
Arcanobacterium haemolyticum (*Corynebacterium haemolyticum*)	Pharyngitis, scarlatiniform rash	<1
Yersinia enterocolitica	Pharyngitis, enterocolitis	<1
Treponema pallidum	Secondary syphilis	<1
Francisella tularensis	Oropharyngeal tularemia	
Chlamydial		
Chlamydophila pneumoniae	Pneumonia/bronchitis/pharyngitis	Unknown
Mycoplasmal		
Mycoplasma pneumoniae	Pneumonia/bronchitis/pharyngitis	<1
Mycoplasma hominis (type 1)	Pharyngitis in volunteers	Unknown
Unknown		30

*Estimated percentage of cases of pharyngitis due to indicated organism in persons of all ages.
ARD, Acute respiratory disease; HIV, human immunodeficiency virus; SARS, severe acute respiratory syndrome.
Data from refs. 1-6.

S. pyogenes may cause up to half of the cases during some periods. The importance of non–group A beta-hemolytic streptococci as a cause of pharyngitis is not entirely clear. Beta-hemolytic streptococci of groups C and G have long been associated with foodborne outbreaks of pharyngitis.[11-14] Group C streptococci have also been associated with endemic pharyngitis in college students[15] and other adult populations.[16] Group G streptococci have been implicated in one community outbreak.[17] Other non–group A beta-hemolytic streptococci have not been definitely implicated as a cause of endemic pharyngitis.[18-21] Mixed anaerobic bacterial infections (Vincent's angina) cause occasional cases of acute pharyngitis, as do *Corynebacterium diphtheriae, Arcanobacterium hemolyticum, Yersinia enterocolitica, Francisella tularensis,* and *Neisseria gonorrhoeae. Mycoplasma pneumoniae* has been associated with pharyngitis since the late 1950s, but in epidemiologic studies of unselected patients, *M. pneumoniae* has not been an important cause of the disease.[9,22] The recognition of the role of *Chlamydiophila pneumoniae* in acute respiratory disease[23] has added another agent to the list of those causing pharyngitis, but its relative importance has yet to be determined.[24]

EPIDEMIOLOGY

Most cases of pharyngitis occur during the colder months of the year, during the respiratory disease season. Viral agents such as rhinoviruses tend to have annual periods of peak prevalence in the fall and spring; coronaviruses have been found most often in the winter. Influenza appears in epidemics, which in the United States usually occur between December and April. In military recruits, adenoviruses cause an influenza-like syndrome during the colder months (see Chapter 139). This has been termed acute respiratory disease (ARD). In civilians, wintertime ARD occurs, as do epidemics of pharyngoconjunctival fever in the summer. Streptococcal pharyngitis occurs during the respiratory disease season, with peak rates of infection in winter and early spring. Spread among family members in the home is a prominent feature of the epidemiologic behavior of most of these agents, with children being the major reservoir of infection. For details on the epidemiologic behavior of these organisms, the reader is referred to the chapters dealing with each.

PATHOGENESIS

Symptoms of sore or scratchy throat occur in approximately 50% of people with rhinovirus colds[9,25] and in 20% to 70% of people with colds due to conventional coronaviruses (see Chapter 152).[26,27] Pharyngeal complaints are present in up to 80% of people with parainfluenza virus illness[28] and in approximately 50% of people with type A influenza or adenovirus illness.[28] Other viral respiratory illnesses with pharyngitis occur with coxsackievirus A21, echoviruses 6 and 20, herpes simplex virus,[29] Epstein-Barr virus (EBV), and cytomegalovirus infections.

The pathogenic mechanisms are different for the various organisms. Nasal epithelial biopsies obtained from volunteers with experimental rhinovirus infections have shown little or no evidence of viral cytopathic effect.[30,31] However, it has been noted that bradykinin and lysylbradykinin are generated in the nasal passages of persons with experimental and natural rhinovirus colds.[32,33] These inflammatory mediators are potent stimulators of pain nerve endings. Also, volunteers given experimental intranasal challenge with bradykinin have developed symptoms of sore throat.[34] With other respiratory virus infections, such as those caused by adenovirus and coxsackievirus, there is evidence that direct invasion of pharyngeal mucosa occurs.

The events leading to invasive streptococcal infection of the pharynx and tonsil are also not well understood. Pharyngeal carriage of *S. pyogenes* is commonly observed in asymptomatic people. Factors that influence the balance between colonization and invasive infection may include natural and acquired host immunity, and interference among the bacteria present in the oropharynx. *S. pyogenes* elaborates a number of extracellular factors, including pyrogenic exotoxins,

hemolysins, streptokinase, deoxyribonucleases, proteinase, and hyaluronidase, which are of known or possible pathogenic importance.[35] Complications of acute streptococcal pharyngitis may include acute rheumatic fever, acute glomerulonephritis, and invasive infection. There is a general association of specific M serotypes or genotypes with these complications.[36] It is likely, however, that strain-related virulence factors rather than M serotype per se are the major determinants of disease expression.

The usual pathologic changes occurring in viral pharyngitis are edema and hyperemia of the tonsils and the pharyngeal mucous membrane. An inflammatory exudate may be present with adenovirus and EBV infections; with the latter, nasopharyngeal lymphoid hyperplasia also occurs. Vesiculation and mucosal ulceration may occur with herpes simplex virus and some coxsackievirus A infections. With streptococcal tonsillopharyngitis, there is an intense inflammatory response characterized by marked erythema and edema of the fauces and uvula, and frequently by a grayish-yellow tonsillar exudate. With diphtheria, a fibrous pseudomembrane containing necrotic epithelium, leukocytes, and bacterial colonies develops on the epithelial surface. For a more detailed discussion of the pathogenic events associated with infection by the wide variety of microorganisms that cause pharyngitis, the reader is referred to the chapters describing the individual agents.

CLINICAL PRESENTATION

Pharyngitis with the Common Cold

Mild to moderate pharyngeal discomfort is frequently present during a cold but is usually not the primary complaint. The symptom is characterized as soreness, scratchiness, or irritation. Severe pharyngeal pain and odynophagia are not characteristic of this type of pharyngitis. Nasal signs and symptoms and cough are also usually present. Systemic complaints of fever, chills, and myalgia are not prominent. In older children and adults, a temperature elevation, if it occurs, is modest. On examination, the pharynx may appear normal or show a mild amount of edema and erythema. Rhinorrhea and postnasal discharge are usually present. Pharyngeal and tonsillar exudates and painful lymphadenopathy are not seen. Pharyngeal complaints usually subside over 3 or 4 days, and most patients have recovered by the end of a week (see Chapter 50).

Human Immunodeficiency Virus Infection

Febrile pharyngitis is a characteristic feature of primary infection with HIV.[37,38] Following an incubation period of 3 to 5 weeks, patients develop fever and pharyngitis associated with varying amounts of myalgia, arthralgia, lethargy, and in some cases a nonpruritic maculopapular rash. This has been followed in approximately 1 week by the development of lymphadenopathy. Pharyngeal hyperemia, sometimes marked, has been noted, as have mucosal ulcerations, but exudate has not been described (see Chapter 117).

Streptococcal Pharyngitis

The severity of illness associated with *S. pyogenes* infection of the pharynx varies greatly.[18] In severe cases, there is marked pharyngeal pain, odynophagia, and a temperature of 39.4° C or greater. Headache, chills, and abdominal pain may occur. The pharyngeal membrane is a fiery red, and a patchy, grayish-yellow exudate is present on the tonsils. Edema of the uvula is often pronounced. Tender, enlarged cervical nodes and a leukocyte count of over 12,000/mm³ complete the picture of an acute suppurative bacterial infection. At the other extreme are those streptococcal infections that are quite mild or may even go unrecognized by the patient. Infection with strains of *S. pyogenes* that produce pyrogenic exotoxins may result in the characteristic erythematous rash of scarlet fever, which is followed by desquamation. The tongue is red, and the papillae are enlarged (strawberry tongue). Rarely, noninvasive pharyngitis due to *S. pyogenes* may be the cause of streptococcal toxic shock syndrome (see Chapter 195).[39,40]

The clinical features of pharyngeal infection with strains of group C and group G streptococci are similar to those of *S. pyogenes*, including the occurrence of purulent exudates, fever, and anterior cervical adenopathy.[15] In group C–associated pharyngitis, the signs and symptoms on average are less severe than in group A pharyngitis but more so than in patients with negative bacterial cultures. Cases of group C and group G pharyngitis are often recognized in the setting of a common-source foodborne outbreak; milk, egg salad, and chicken salad have been recognized as vehicles.

Vincent's and Ludwig's Angina, Lemierre Disease, and Peritonsillar Abscess (Quinsy)

Vincent's angina, also called *acute necrotizing ulcerative gingivitis* or *trench mouth,* is a mixed bacterial-spirochetal infection of the gingival margin, usually in patients with poor dental hygiene. Inflamed and painful gingiva, ulcerations on the interdental papillae, and halitosis may be accompanied by purulent debris in the gingival clefts. Ludwig's angina is an acute cellulitis of dental origin, extending into the submaxillary and sublingual space (see Chapter 57). Neither Vincent's nor Ludwig's angina is associated with pharyngitis. Lemierre disease begins as pharyngitis, usually due to *Fusobacterium necrophorum,*[41] but presents as acute septicemia and findings consistent with jugular vein thrombosis (Fig. 51-1). There may be pain, edema, and tenderness in the anterior cervical triangle. Exudative tonsillitis is present early in the disease but may subside spontaneously despite progression of the infection elsewhere. Septic emboli to the lung may lead to pulmonary abscesses and empyema.

Peritonsillar abscess (quinsy) may be a suppurative complication of group A streptococcal pharyngitis, but oral anaerobes are frequently involved. Pharyngeal pain is usually severe, and dysphagia is common. On examination, there is inflammation and swelling of the peritonsillar area with medial displacement of the tonsil, and patients speak with a "hot potato" voice (see Chapter 57).

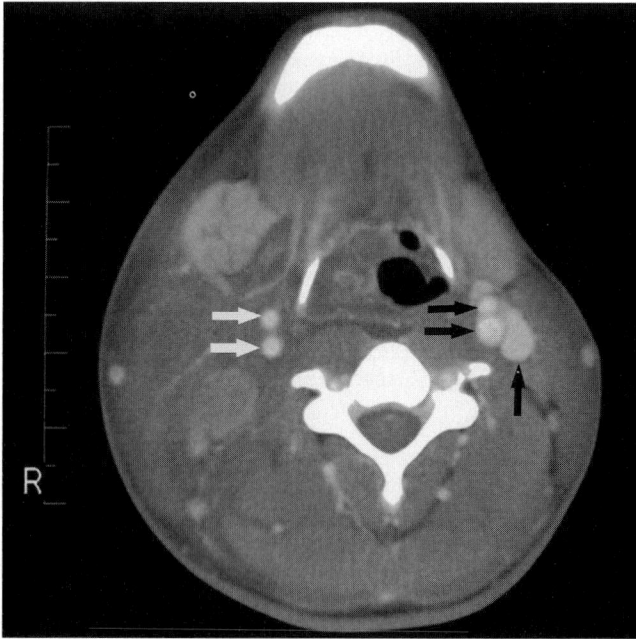

FIGURE 51-1. Postanginal septicemia (Lemierre syndrome). Computed tomographic scan of the neck with intravenous contrast at the level of the hyoid bone. Note the normal enhancement of the lumen of the internal jugular vein (*vertical black arrow*) and the internal and external carotid arteries (*horizontal black arrows*) on the left. The internal and external carotid arteries are observed on the right side (*horizontal white arrows*) but the thrombosed left internal jugular vein is not. There is also diffuse soft-tissue edema of the right side of the neck with stranding of subcutaneous fat planes. *(Courtesy of J. Chirinos.)*

Gonococcal Pharyngitis

Most oral gonorrheal infections are asymptomatic, but gonorrheal infection may be responsible for an occasional case of mild pharyngitis (see Chapter 209).[42] A recent study from a San Francisco sexually transmitted disease clinic found the prevalence of gonococcal pharyngeal colonization in homosexual men performing fellatio during the preceding 2 weeks to be 6% by culture and 11% by DNA amplification techniques.[43] Such colonization may be associated with disseminated disease.[44]

Pharyngitis with Influenza

Sore throat is a major complaint in some patients with influenza. It is usually associated with other manifestations of the disease, such as myalgia, headache, and cough.[18,28] Coryzal symptoms and hoarseness may also be present. Temperature elevations are common in both adults and children, to levels of 38.3° C or higher. Edema and erythema of the pharyngeal mucosa may be present but are not marked. Pharyngeal exudates and painful cervical adenopathy are not part of influenzal pharyngitis. Defervescence occurs in 3 to 4 days on the average, but in some uncomplicated cases fever may last up to 1 week (see Chapter 162).

Pharyngoconjunctival Fever

The clinical presentation of adenoviral pharyngitis is usually more severe than pharyngitis associated with the common cold. Malaise, myalgia, headache, chills, and dizziness often accompany adenovirus infections. Temperature elevations persist for 5 to 6 days in studies of recognized cases. Sore throat is often marked. On examination, pharyngeal erythema and exudate may be present, mimicking streptococcal pharyngitis. A distinguishing feature of adenovirus pharyngitis, when present, is conjunctivitis, which occurs in one third to one half of cases. The conjunctivitis is of the follicular type and is bilateral in about one fourth of affected patients. Cough, hoarseness, and substernal pain occur in ARD in military recruits but are usually not prominent features of pharyngoconjunctival fever in civilian populations (see Chapter 139).

Acute Herpetic Pharyngitis

Primary infection with herpes simplex virus may present as an acute pharyngitis. Mild cases are indistinguishable from those caused by other respiratory viruses. In severe cases of herpetic pharyngitis, the presence of inflammation and exudate may mimic full-blown streptococcal pharyngitis. Vesicles and shallow ulcers of the palate are characteristic of herpetic infection and when present are helpful in the differential diagnosis. Tender cervical adenopathy and fever are noted in some cases. Vesicles or ulcers are present on the labial and buccal mucosa when there is an associated gingivostomatitis. Acute primary herpetic infection should be distinguished from chronic mucocutaneous infection of the oropharynx due to herpes simplex virus. The chronic form of the disease is seen exclusively in patients with impaired immunity and is characterized by large, shallow, painful ulcers that slowly progress unless the patient's immune status improves or antiviral therapy is given (see Chapter 132). Recurrent painful small ulcers of the tonsil, palate, tongue or buccal mucosa are rarely due to herpes simplex but more likely to aphthous ulcers, a condition of unknown etiology. Painful oral ulcers also occur in Behçet's disease. Syphilitic chancre may present as an oropharyngeal ulcer following orogenital sex, though the chancre is not painful.

Herpangina

Herpangina is an uncommon type of pharyngitis caused by coxsackieviruses and is distinguished by the presence of small vesicles (1 to 2 mm across) on the soft palate, uvula, and anterior tonsillar pillars. The lesions rupture to become small white ulcers. Herpangina has been recognized primarily in children, in whom it may be manifested as a severe febrile illness with marked sore throat and dysphagia. In some cases anorexia and abdominal pain mimic acute appendicitis (see Chapter 169).

Infectious Mononucleosis

Pharyngitis, often exudative, occurs in approximately 85% of the cases of infectious mononucleosis caused by EBV. Fever and cervical adenopathy are characteristically present. The pharyngeal complaints of mononucleosis are usually associated with other features of the disease, such as headache and persistent malaise and fatigue. Posterior and anterior cervical adenopathy is most prominent, but axillary and inguinal nodes are also frequently enlarged, and there is enlargement of the spleen in approximately half the cases. Approximately 5% of patients have a rash of variable morphology, but the administration of ampicillin will provoke a pruritic maculopapular eruption in nearly all patients. The mononucleosis syndrome is also associated with cytomegalovirus infection. Some patients with cytomegalovirus mononucleosis have pharyngeal soreness, but on examination, the pharynx usually appears unremarkable (see Chapters 134 and 135).

Diphtheria

Although quite rare in the United States today, diphtheria still occurs among unimmunized or underimmunized members of socioeconomically disadvantaged populations.[45] The disease characteristically has a slow onset, and pharyngeal discomfort is usually not marked. Temperature elevation is present but is low grade. The characteristic tonsillar or pharyngeal membrane varies in color from light to dark gray, is firmly adherent to the tonsil and pharyngeal mucosa, and dislodgement provokes bleeding. Human infection with *Corynebacterium ulcerans* is a rare cause of pharyngitis associated with the consumption of raw milk (see Chapter 202).[46]

Arcanobacterial Pharyngitis

A. hemolyticum has been increasingly identified as a cause of exudative pharyngitis, clinically similar to that caused by β-hemolytic streptococci.[47-50] Characteristically, the infection has been recognized in children, adolescents, and young adults and is associated with a diffuse, sometimes pruritic, erythematous maculopapular skin rash on the extremities and trunk. In a 2-year study conducted in Ottawa, Canada, *A. hemolyticum* was isolated from 0.36% of throat swabs from sore throat patients and from none of over 2000 controls. Pharyngeal exudates were present in 54% of patients, cervical lymphadenopathy in 41%, and rash in 44%.[51] Cases of *A. hemolyticum* infection with membranous pharyngitis that mimics diphtheria[52] and with peritonsillar abscess[53] have also been reported.

Yersinial Pharyngitis

Y. enterocolitica causes exudative pharyngitis, which is associated with ingestion of contaminated food and drink and in adults may occur without the typical enterocolitis seen in children. Fever, prominent cervical lymphadenopathy, and abdominal pain with or without diarrhea have been reported.[54,55] A fulminant course with high mortality has been associated with reported cases of yersinial pharyngitis, making recognition important (see Chapter 226).

Chlamydophila Pharyngitis

C. pneumoniae has been established as an etiologic agent of acute infections of the respiratory tract, some of which have pharyngeal manifestations.[24] Pharyngitis with or without fever has occurred as a separate illness and also in association with pneumonia or bronchitis.[56] Distinguishing clinical features of the pharyngitis have not been described, but chronicity of infection despite antimicrobial therapy has been noted (see Chapter 179).

Mycoplasmal Pharyngitis

Epidemiologic studies of pharyngitis have associated some cases with *M. pneumoniae* infection. The illnesses observed have been relatively mild and have had no distinguishing clinical features. *M. pneumoniae* characteristically causes bronchitis and pneumonia (see Chapter 181).

Noninfectious Pharyngitis

Occasional cases presenting as an inflammatory pharyngitis may have noninfectious causes. These include conditions such as bullous pemphigoid, systemic lupus erythematosus, Behçet's disease, staphylococcal toxic shock syndrome, Stevens-Johnson syndrome, and paraquat ingestion. Kawasaki disease may manifest as a febrile sore throat without exudate. It occurs in children and is associated with characteristic lesions on the lips, tongue, and skin.

DIAGNOSIS

The primary objectives in the diagnosis of acute pharyngitis are to distinguish cases of common viral etiology, which predominate and do not require antimicrobial therapy, from those due to *S. pyogenes,* and to detect and identify the occasional case caused by an unusual organism for which treatment is available.[57] This distinction is critical, because the majority of patients seeing primary care physicians continue to receive unnecessary antimicrobials, and an increasing percentage of these prescriptions are for expensive, broad-spectrum agents.[2,58,59]

In the majority of cases, an etiologic diagnosis is not possible on clinical grounds alone. The presence of pharyngeal or tonsillar exudates, tender adenopathy, skin rash, or conjunctivitis aids in the differential diagnosis, but these findings are not entirely specific and are not present with sufficient frequency to be helpful in most cases. The list of etiologic agents associated with the presence of pharyngeal exudates includes group A, group C, and group G streptococci; *C. diphtheriae*; *A. hemolyticum*; *Y. enterocolitica*; adenovirus; herpes simplex virus; and EBV. However, pharyngeal exudate is not always present with infections due to these infections, so that its absence does not exclude them from consideration. On the other hand, exudate is rarely if ever seen in the large group of cases of pharyngitis due to the common cold viruses and influenza virus. The presence of skin rash suggests the possibility of infection with *S. pyogenes*, *A. hemolyticum*, HIV, and, rarely, EBV. Toxic shock syndrome should also be considered. The presence of conjunctivitis suggests infection with adenovirus and some types of enteroviruses.

The development of rapid antigen detection tests, using a specimen collected by throat swab, has made possible early microbiologic confirmation of the diagnosis of streptococcal pharyngitis. When such tests are used in clinical practice, the reported specificity has been over 90%, but the sensitivity has been quite variable, depending in part on the sensitivity of the culture method with which it is compared.[60-63] For a detailed discussion of currently recommended strategies for diagnosis of streptococcal pharyngitis see Chapter 195.

The patient's history and a consideration of epidemiologic factors may be helpful in suggesting a specific etiologic diagnosis in cases in which results of throat cultures or rapid antigen tests are negative for group A streptococci. Other family members frequently have common colds and influenzal illnesses. The season of the year and the occurrence of known epidemics may provide clues to the diagnosis. Rhinovirus infections predominate in the fall and spring and coronavirus infections in the winter. The occurrence of an influenza epidemic in the community is usually known to the physician. Patients with pharyngoconjunctival fever, a summer illness, may give a history of swimming, and they or a family member may have conjunctivitis. The diagnosis of infectious mononucleosis, primary HIV infection, and diphtheria may be suggested by the nonpharyngeal manifestations of these infections.

Examination of the structures of the pharynx should be thorough and should include inspection of the nasopharynx and larynx when diphtheria is suspected. In children under the age of 3 years, the presence of an exudate is a less reliable indicator of streptococcal infection than it is in older children and adults. Diphtheria produces a pseudomembrane that may be mistaken for an exudate. The presence of small vesicles or ulcers suggests herpes simplex virus infection or herpangina. The mucosal lesions of herpangina are less numerous and more confined to the area of the palate than are those of herpes simplex virus, which may involve the entire oropharynx. Aphthous stomatitis, a benign condition of unknown cause, produces small painful mucosal ulcers that are sometimes confused with those of herpetic infection. Aphthosis tends to be recurrent, in contrast to acute herpetic pharyngitis, and with the usual case of aphthosis there are fewer lesions, which are usually located in the anterior part of the mouth.

Medial displacement of one or both tonsils is seen with peritonsillitis or peritonsillar abscess, and dysphagia may be present. Patients with postanginal septicemia with jugular vein thrombophlebitis have malaise, fever, and chills, suggestive of serious illness; also, pain, tenderness, and swelling at the angle of the jaw are characteristic, but these findings may be subtle. Patients with infectious mononucleosis usually have generalized adenopathy and may have enlargement of the spleen. Severe sore throat and odynophagia in an adult in the absence of findings in the pharynx should suggest epiglottitis (see Chapter 56).

Laboratory tests are available to help in the diagnosis of some of the aforementioned infections. *N. gonorrhoeae* may be isolated on Thayer-Martin medium. DNA amplification techniques may be more sensitive[43] but are not yet widely available. Vincent's angina is diagnosed by a crystal violet-stained smear of the pharyngeal or tonsillar exudate showing numerous fusobacteria and spirochetes. Blood cultures should be obtained in cases of suspected postanginal septicemia, and radiographic examination of the lungs, bones, and large joints may detect metastatic infection. A throat swab for culture using Loeffler's or tellurite selective medium should be obtained in all suspected cases of diphtheria (see Chapter 202). The hemolysis associated with *A. hemolyticum* becomes maximal at 48 to 72 hours and is more prominent on rabbit and human blood agar than sheep blood agar; thus, this organism may be missed on standard throat culture.[48,50] The diagnosis of infectious mononucleosis can be supported by the hematologic findings and confirmed by spot or slide tests for heterophile antibodies or by specific serologic tests (see Chapter 135). In a patient with compatible clinical findings, primary HIV infection can be confirmed by the demonstration of a high viral load or positive p24 antigen and a negative test for HIV antibodies.[37] Cultures and rapid diagnostic tests for influenza virus, adenovirus, herpes simplex virus, cytomegalovirus, and *M. pneumoniae* are now available in many laboratories. Acute and convalescent (3-week) serum specimens are necessary for serologic tests for these agents. Laboratory tests for the common cold viruses are not readily available. Serologic tests for antibodies to *C. pneumoniae* are commercially available, although experience with such tests is limited at present.

Pharyngitis due to noninfectious causes may sometimes present a diagnostic problem. Pemphigus, bullous pemphigoid, and systemic lupus erythematosus are among the diseases that can cause pharyngeal inflammation and discomfort. Also, drug reactions are sometimes manifested by pharyngeal soreness, as is agranulocytosis. The presence of other manifestations of these diseases, particularly involvement of the skin, is helpful in leading to the diagnosis.

TREATMENT AND PREVENTION

Antimicrobial Therapy

Streptococcal Pharyngitis

Patients with pharyngitis due to *S. pyogenes* should receive a 10-day course of penicillin[64-66] or an equivalent antibiotic if they are allergic to penicillin (see Chapter 195, on *Streptococcus pyogenes*, for dosage schedule). An injection of long-acting benzathine penicillin is an excellent although painful form of therapy because it does not require patient compliance. The adult dose of benzathine penicillin is 1.2 million units. In patients who are allergic to penicillin, a 10-day course of erythromycin is recommended. The prevalence of macrolide resistance has remained below 5% in the United States as a whole, but increased levels of resistance have been reported in certain areas.[67] With the increasing use of newer macrolides

(azithromycin and clarithromycin) for treatment of upper respiratory tract infections in primary care practice,[68] it may be anticipated that macrolide resistance will likely increase. First-generation cephalosporins such as cephalexin and cefadroxil and a second-generation cephalosporin such as cefuroxime axetil are also suitable for treating streptococcal pharyngitis in patients whose penicillin hypersensitivity is not of the immediate type. Although a number of newer antimicrobial drugs have activity against *S. pyogenes*, they offer no advantage over penicillin, erythromycin, or the cephalosporins mentioned above. Although the incidence of acute rheumatic fever had declined to a low level in the United States, the resurgence of rheumatic fever in some areas of the United States during the 1980s and 1990s[69-71] and its continuing prevalence in other areas of the world are sufficient reasons not to abandon the general policy of using antimicrobials in the treatment of streptococcal pharyngitis. In addition to prevention of nonsuppurative sequelae, such treatment, if initiated early in the course of the disease,[72-74] can speed clinical recovery and is important for limiting transmission to school and household contacts and for prevention of suppurative complications of streptococcal pharyngitis, which include peritonsillar abscess, suppurative cervical adenitis and, rarely, sinusitis, otitis media, mastoiditis, bacteremia, and pneumonia.

Vincent's and Ludwig's Angina, Lemierre Disease, and Peritonsillar Abscess

Vincent's angina responds to an oral penicillin, such as amoxicillin, plus metronidazole or clindamycin or amoxicillin-clavulanate. Ludwig's angina requires emergent safeguarding the airway, antibiotics and possibly surgical drainage, as described in Chapter 57. Peritonsillar abscess can be treated by needle aspiration, or incision and drainage, and parenteral antibiotics, such as penicillin or clindamycin, active against aerobic and anaerobic oral flora. Possible regimens for adults with Lemierre disease would include clindamycin 600 mg IV q8h, ampicillin-sulbactam 3 g q6h or penicillin G 2 mu q4h plus metronidazole 500 mg q6h. Surgical ligation of the jugular vein is rarely indicated.

Diphtheria

The treatment of diphtheria, which requires both antimicrobials and hyperimmune diphtheria antitoxin, is described in Chapter 202.

Arcanobacterial Pharyngitis

Arcanobacterium haemolyticum is susceptible in vitro to penicillin, cephalosporins, macrolides, clindamycin, ciprofloxacin, and vancomycin but not to trimethoprim-sulfamethoxazole.[75] Some strains are resistant to tetracyclines.[76] There are no controlled trials of therapy of pharyngitis due to this organism. Reports on the efficacy of penicillin are contradictory, however, and tolerance to penicillin has been described.[77,78]

Yersinial Pharyngitis

Y. enterocolitica is usually susceptible to aminoglycosides, trimethoprim-sulfamethoxazole, and third-generation cephalosporins but resistant to penicillin (see Chapter 226).

Gonococcal Pharyngitis

The treatment of gonococcal infections is described in Chapter 209.

Mycoplasmal Pharyngitis

The treatment of *M. pneumoniae* infection is described in Chapter 181.

Viral Pharyngitis

When administered within 2 days of onset of illness, amantadine or rimantadine can reduce the duration of symptoms in uncomplicated influenza A, and the neuraminidase inhibitors, zanamivir and oseltamivir, have a similar effect on uncomplicated influenza A and B (see Chapter 160).[79] Acyclovir, valacyclovir, famciclovir, and foscarnet are available for the treatment of ulcerative oropharyngeal herpes simplex virus infection in immunosuppressed patients (see Chapter 38).

Symptomatic Therapy

Treatment is directed at relieving pharyngeal discomfort and associated systemic or respiratory symptoms. Warm saline gargles and supportive measures such as rest, analgesics, and liquids are sufficient in most cases of viral pharyngitis. Ibuprofen was found to be superior to acetaminophen in relieving throat pain associated with tonsillitis and pharyngitis in 6- to 12-year-old children.[80] Symptomatic therapy is also helpful in relieving symptoms of streptococcal pharyngitis. Patients with severe streptococcal pharyngitis or peritonsillitis may be in extreme discomfort and require liberal use of analgesics during the early course of illness. Hospitalization is necessary with some types of pharyngitis that are associated with systemic illness or that have serious or life-threatening complications.

Prevention

Tonsillectomy has been shown to reduce for at least 2 years the incidence of throat infections in children who experience extremely frequent recurrences of acute pharyngitis.[81] However, it is not recommended as a routine practice.[82] The risks, morbidity, and cost of the operation are clearly not justified in less severely affected children.[83] Continuous antimicrobial prophylaxis for *S. pyogenes* infection is required for patients at risk of recurrent rheumatic fever (see Chapter 196). Active immunization is available for type A and type B influenza and for diphtheria (see Chapters 162 and 319). The prophylactic administration of amantadine or rimantadine is also effective against type A influenza. Zanamivir and oseltamivir are similarly effective in preventing febrile, laboratory-confirmed influenza, but only the latter has been approved for this indication at this writing.[79] Prophylactic intravenous and oral regimens of acyclovir are effective in preventing mucocutaneous herpes simplex virus infection in immunosuppressed patients (see Chapter 38). Live adenovirus vaccines have been used successfully in military populations but are not available for civilian use (see Chapter 139). There has been work on experimental vaccines for a number of the agents that cause pharyngitis, including *S. pyogenes*,[84] but these vaccines are still in the experimental stage of development.

REFERENCES

1. Armstrong GL, Pinner RW. Outpatient visits for infectious diseases in the United States, 1980 through 1996. Arch Intern Med. 1999;159:2531-2536.
2. Linder JA, Stafford RS. Antibiotic treatment of adults with sore throat by community primary care physicians: A national survey, 1989-1999. JAMA. 2001;286:1181-1186.
3. Stuart-Harris CH, Andrewes C, Andrews BE, et al. A collaborative study of the aetiology of acute respiratory infection in Britain 1961-4. A report of the Medical Research Council working party on acute respiratory virus infections. Br Med J. 1965;2:319-326.
4. Gwaltney JM Jr. Virology of middle ear. Ann Otol Rhinol Laryngol. 1971;80:365-370.
5. Hamre D, Connelly AP Jr, Procknow JJ. Virologic studies of acute respiratory disease in young adults. IV. Virus isolations during four years of surveillance. Am J Epidemiol. 1966;83:238-249.
6. Monto AS, Ullman BM. Acute respiratory illness in an American community. The Tecumseh study. JAMA. 1974;227:164-169.
7. Evans AS, Dick EC. Acute pharyngitis and tonsillitis in University of Wisconsin students. JAMA. 1964;190:699-708.
8. Glezen WP, Clyde WAJ, Senior RJ, et al. Group A streptococci, mycoplasmas, and viruses associated with acute pharyngitis. JAMA. 1967;202:455-460.
9. Gwaltney JM. Clinical significance and pathogenesis of viral respiratory infections. Am J Med. 2002;112(Suppl 6A):13S-18S.
10. Hare CB, Kahn JO. Primary HIV infection. Curr Infect Dis Rep. 2004;6:65-71.
11. Stryker WS, Fraser DW, Facklam RR. Foodborne outbreak of group G streptococcal pharyngitis. Am J Epidemiol. 1982;116:533-540.
12. Cohen D, Ferne M, Rouach T, et al. Food-borne outbreak of group G streptococcal sore throat in an Israeli military base. Epidemiol Infect. 1987;99:249-255.
13. Duca E, Teodorovici GR, Radu C, et al. A new nephritogenic streptococcus. J Hyg (Lond). 1969;67:691-698.
14. Bisno AL. Acute pharyngitis: Etiology and diagnosis. Pediatrics. 1996;97:949-954.
15. Turner JC, Hayden GF, Kiselica D, et al. Association of group C beta-hemolytic streptococci with endemic pharyngitis among college students. JAMA. 1990; 264:2644-2647.
16. Meier FA, Centor RM, Graham L Jr, Dalton HP. Clinical and microbiological evidence for endemic pharyngitis among adults due to group C streptococci. Arch Intern Med. 1990;150:825-829.
17. Gerber MA, Randolph MF, Martin NJ, et al. Community-wide outbreak of group G streptococcal pharyngitis. Pediatrics. 1991;87:598-603.
18. McMillan JA, Sandstrom C, Weiner LB, et al. Viral and bacterial organisms associated with acute pharyngitis in a school-aged population. J Pediatr. 1986;109:747-752.
19. Reed BD, Huck W, Lutz LJ, Zazove P. Prevalence of *Chlamydia trachomatis* and *Mycoplasma pneumoniae* in children with and without pharyngitis. J Fam Pract. 1988;26:387-392.
20. Hofkosh D, Wald ER, Chiponis DM. Prevalence of non–group-A beta-hemolytic streptococci in childhood pharyngitis. South Med J. 1988;81:329-331.
21. Gaviria JM, Bisno AL. Group C and G streptococci. In: Kaplan EL, Stevens DL, eds. Streptococcal Infections. New York: Oxford University Press; 2000:238-254.
22. Gwaltney JM Jr, Hendley JO, Simon G, Jordan WS Jr. Rhinovirus infections in an industrial population. I. The occurrence of illness. N Engl J Med. 1966;275:1261-1268.
23. Grayston JT, Kuo CC, Wang SP, Altman J. A new *Chlamydia psittaci* strain, TWAR, isolated in acute respiratory tract infections. N Engl J Med. 1986;315:161-168.
24. Grayston JT. Infections caused by *Chlamydia pneumoniae* strain TWAR. Clin Infect Dis. 1992;15:757-563.
25. Gwaltney JM Jr. Rhinoviruses. In: Evans AS, ed. Viral Infections of Humans: Epidemiology and Control. New York: Plenum; 1989:593-611.
26. Hendley JO, Fishburne HB, Gwaltney JM Jr. Coronavirus infections in working adults. Eight-year study with 229 E and OC 43. Am Rev Respir Dis. 1972;105:805-811.
27. Wenzel RP, Hendley JO, Davies JA, Gwaltney JM Jr. Coronavirus infections in military recruits. Three-year study with coronavirus strains OC43 and 229E. Am Rev Respir Dis. 1974;109:621-624.
28. Tyrrell DAJ. Common Colds and Related Diseases. Baltimore: Williams & Wilkins; 1965.
29. Glezen WP, Fernald GW, Lohr JA. Acute respiratory disease of university students with special reference to the etiologic role of *Herpesvirus hominis*. Am J Epidemiol. 1975;101:111-121.
30. Douglas RG Jr, Alford BR, Couch RB. Atraumatic nasal biopsy for studies of respiratory virus infection in humans. Antimicrobial Agents Chemother. 1968;8:340-343.
31. Winther B, Farr B, Turner RB, et al. Histopathologic examination and enumeration of polymorphonuclear leukocytes in the nasal mucosa during experimental rhinovirus colds. Acta Otolaryngol Suppl. 1984;413:19-24.
32. Naclerio RM, Proud D, Lichtenstein LM, et al. Kinins are generated during experimental rhinovirus colds. J Infect Dis. 1988;157:133-142.
33. Proud D, Naclerio RM, Gwaltney JM, Hendley JO. Kinins are generated in nasal secretions during natural rhinovirus colds. J Infect Dis. 1990;161:120-123.
34. Proud D, Reynolds CJ, Lacapra S, et al. Nasal provocation with bradykinin induces symptoms of rhinitis and a sore throat. Am Rev Respir Dis. 1988;137:613-616.
35. Bisno AL, Brito MO, Collins CM. Molecular basis of group A streptococcal virulence. Lancet Infect Dis. 2003;3:191-200.
36. Johnson DR, Stevens DL, Kaplan EL. Epidemiologic analysis of group A streptococcal serotypes associated with severe systemic infections, rheumatic fever, or uncomplicated pharyngitis. J Infect Dis. 1992;166:374-382.
37. Kahn JO, Walker BD. Acute human immunodeficiency virus type 1 infection. N Engl J Med. 1998;339:33-39.
38. Kessler HA, Blaauw B, Spear J, et al. Diagnosis of human immunodeficiency virus infection in seronegative homosexuals presenting with an acute viral syndrome. JAMA. 1987;258:1196-1199.
39. Herold AH. Group A beta-hemolytic streptococcal toxic shock from a mild pharyngitis. J Fam Pract. 1990;31:549-551.
40. Chapnick EK, Gradon JD, Lutwick LI, et al. Streptococcal toxic shock syndrome due to noninvasive pharyngitis. Clin Infect Dis. 1992;14:1074-1077.
41. Chirinos JA, Lichtstein DM, Garcia J, Tamariz LJ. The evolution of Lemierre syndrome: Report of 2 cases and review of the literature. Medicine (Baltimore). 2002; 81:458-465.
42. Hutt DM, Judson FN. Epidemiology and treatment of oropharyngeal gonorrhea. Ann Intern Med. 1986;104:655-658.
43. Page-Shafer K, Graves A, Kent C, et al. Increased sensitivity of DNA amplification testing for the detection of pharyngeal gonorrhea in men who have sex with men. Clin Infect Dis. 2002;34:173-176.
44. Wiesner PJ, Tronca E, Bonin P, et al. Clinical spectrum of pharyngeal gonococcal infection. N Engl J Med. 1973;288:181-185.
45. Bisgard KM, Hardy IR, Popovic T. Respiratory diphtheria in the United States, 1980-1995. Am J Public Health. 1998;88:787-791.
46. Hart RJ. *Corynebacterium ulcerans* in humans and cattle in North Devon. J Hyg (Lond). 1984;92:161-164.
47. Banck G, Nyman M. Tonsillitis and rash associated with *Corynebacterium haemolyticum*. J Infect Dis. 1986;154:1037-1040.
48. Miller RA, Brancato F, Holmes KK. *Corynebacterium hemolyticum* as a cause of pharyngitis and scarlatiniform rash in young adults. Ann Intern Med. 1986;105:867-872.
49. Greenman JL. *Corynebacterium hemolyticum* and pharyngitis. Ann Intern Med. 1987;106:633.
50. Karpathios T, Drakonaki S, Zervoudaki A, et al. *Arcanobacterium haemolyticum* in children with presumed streptococcal pharyngotonsillitis or scarlet fever. J Pediatr. 1992;121:735-737.
51. Mackenzie A, Fuite LA, Chan FT, et al. Incidence and pathogenicity of *Arcanobacterium haemolyticum* during a 2-year study in Ottawa. Clin Infect Dis. 1995;21:177-181.

52. Green SL, LaPeter KS. Pseudodiphtheritic membranous pharyngitis caused by *Corynebacterium haemolyticum*. JAMA. 1981;245:2330-2331.

53. Kovatch AL, Schuit KE, Michaels RH. *Corynebacterium hemolyticum* peritonsillar abscess mimicking diphtheria. JAMA. 1983;249:1757-1758.

54. Rose FB, Camp CJ, Antes EJ. Family outbreak of fatal *Yersinia enterocolitica* pharyngitis. Am J Med. 1987;82:636-637.

55. Cover TL, Aber RC. Yersinia enterocolitica. N Engl J Med. 1989;321:16-24.

56. Hammerschlag MR, Chirgwin K, Roblin PM, et al. Persistent infection with *Chlamydia pneumoniae* following acute respiratory illness. Clin Infect Dis. 1992;14:178-182.

57. Bisno AL. Acute pharyngitis. N Engl J Med. 2001;344:205-211.

58. Steinman MA, Gonzales R, Linder JA, Landefeld CS. Changing use of antibiotics in community-based outpatient practice, 1991-1999. Ann Intern Med. 2003;138:525-533.

59. Gonzales R, Malone DC, Maselli JH, Sande MA. Excessive antibiotic use for acute respiratory infections in the United States. Clin Infect Dis. 2001;33:757-762.

60. Gieseker KE, Mackenzie T, Roe MH, Todd JK. Comparison of two rapid *Streptococcus pyogenes* diagnostic tests with a rigorous culture standard. Pediatr Infect Dis J. 2002;21:922-927.

61. Roosevelt GE, Kulkarni MS, Shulman ST. Critical evaluation of a CLIA-waived streptococcal antigen detection test in the emergency department. Ann Emerg Med. 2001;37:377-381.

62. Joslyn SA, Hoekstra GL, Sutherland JE. Rapid antigen detection testing in diagnosing group A beta-hemolytic streptococcal pharyngitis. J Am Board Fam Pract. 1995;8:177-182.

63. Baker DM, Cooper RM, Rhodes C, et al. Superiority of conventional culture technique over rapid detection of group A *Streptococcus* by optical immunoassay. Diagn Microbiol Infect Dis. 1995;21:61-64.

64. Dajani A, Taubert K, Ferrieri P, et al. Treatment of acute streptococcal pharyngitis and prevention of rheumatic fever: A statement for health professionals. Committee on Rheumatic Fever, Endocarditis, and Kawasaki Disease of the Council on Cardiovascular Disease in the Young, the American Heart Association. Pediatrics. 1995;96:758-764.

65. Bisno AL, Gerber MA, Gwaltney JM Jr, et al. Practice guidelines for the diagnosis and management of group A streptococcal pharyngitis. Infectious Diseases Society of America. Clin Infect Dis. 2002;35:113-125.

66. Committee on Infectious Diseases. Group A streptococcal infections. In: Pickering LK, ed. 2003 Red Book. Elk Grove Village, IL: American Academy of Pediatrics; 2003:573-584.

67. Martin JM, Green M, Barbadora KA, Wald ER. Erythromycin-resistant group A streptococci in schoolchildren in Pittsburgh. N Engl J Med. 2002;346:1200-1206.

68. Steinman MA, Landefeld CS, Gonzales R. Predictors of broad-spectrum antibiotic prescribing for acute respiratory tract infections in adult primary care. JAMA. 2003;289:719-725.

69. Wald ER, Dashefsky B, Feidt C, et al. Acute rheumatic fever in western Pennsylvania and the tristate area. Pediatrics. 1987;80:371-374.

70. Veasy LG, Tani LY, Hill HR. Persistence of acute rheumatic fever in the intermountain area of the United States. J Pediatr. 1994;124:9-16.

71. Wallace MR, Garst PD, Papadimos TJ, Oldfield EC. The return of acute rheumatic fever in young adults. JAMA. 1989;262:2557-2561.

72. Randolph MF, Gerber MA, DeMeo KK, Wright L. Effect of antibiotic therapy on the clinical course of streptococcal pharyngitis. J Pediatr. 1985;106:870-875.

73. Krober MS, Bass JW, Michels GN. Streptococcal pharyngitis: Placebo-controlled double-blind evaluation of clinical response to penicillin therapy. JAMA. 1985;253:1271-1274.

74. Nelson JD. The effect of penicillin therapy on the symptoms and signs of streptococcal pharyngitis. Pediatr Infect Dis J. 1984;3:10-13.

75. Carlson P, Korpela J, Walder M, Nyman M. Antimicrobial susceptibilities and biotypes of *Arcanobacterium haemolyticum* blood isolates. Eur J Clin Microbiol Infect Dis. 1999;18:915-917.

76. Almuzara MN, de Mier C, Barberis CM, et al. *Arcanobacterium hemolyticum*: Identification and susceptibility to nine antimicrobial agents. Clin Microbiol Infect. 2002;8:828-829.

77. Nyman M, Banck G, Thore M. Penicillin tolerance in *Arcanobacterium haemolyticum*. J Infect Dis. 1990;161:261-265.

78. Carlson P, Kontianinen S, Renkonen OV, et al. *Arcanobacterium haemolyticum* and streptococcal pharyngitis in army conscripts. Scand J Infect Dis. 1995;27:17-18.

79. Prevention and control of influenza: Recommendations of the Advisory Committee on Immunization Practices (ACIP). MMWR Morb Mortal Wkly Rep. 2003;52(RR-8):1.

80. Bertin L, Pons G, d'Athis P, et al. Randomized, double-blind, multicenter, controlled trial of ibuprofen versus acetaminophen (paracetamol) and placebo for treatment of symptoms of tonsillitis and pharyngitis in children. J Pediatr. 1991;119:811-814.

81. Paradise JL, Bluestone CD, Bachman RZ, et al. Efficacy of tonsillectomy for recurrent throat infection in severely affected children: Results of parallel randomized and nonrandomized clinical trials. N Engl J Med. 1984;310:674-683.

82. Hendley JO. Tonsillectomy: Justified but not mandated in special patients. N Engl J Med. 1984;310:717-718.

83. Paradise JL, Bluestone CD, Colborn DK, et al. Tonsillectomy and adenotonsillectomy for recurrent throat infection in moderately affected children. Pediatrics. 2002;110:7-15.

84. Hu MC, Walls MA, Stroop SD, et al. Immunogenicity of a 26-valent group A streptococcal vaccine. Infect Immun. 2002;70:2171-2177.

CHAPTER **52**

Acute Laryngitis

MARY T. CASERTA

Acute laryngitis is a common clinical syndrome encountered by primary care physicians. The symptoms are often described as the recent onset of hoarseness or a husky voice with a high pitch often associated with a dry cough.[1] There may be voice breaks or episodes of aphonia, which frequently occur in the context of an upper respiratory tract infection with rhinorrhea and sore throat. The duration of symptoms is difficult to discern from the literature; however, in a study of 100 adults with the common cold, hoarseness was reported for a median of 3 days, and 8 days represented the 75th percentile.[2] Although most reports describe acute laryngitis as a mild and self-limited syndrome, a survey of intercollegiate athletes found substantial morbidity associated with laryngitis.[3] Students reported laryngitis significantly more often as a cause of missed practice compared with cough, nasal discharge, or myalgia, and as an adverse effect on their athletic performance.

The incidence of acute laryngitis reported in the literature is variable and highly dependent on the study methods used. In a report by Higgins of more than 3900 patients older than 5 years of age with acute respiratory infections, only 2% were given a primary diagnosis of laryngitis.[4] However, in other studies, 38% of patients with pneumonia reported hoarseness as a symptom, as did 33% of adults with colds.[5,6] Laryngitis has also been noted in approximately 22% of adolescents or school-aged children with nonstreptococcal sore throat, and in 70% of children with acute respiratory symptoms during a croup epidemic.[7,8] Despite this demonstration that laryngitis is a problem at all ages, a recent report of more than 800 patients seen in an ear, nose, and throat clinic showed that the majority of patients with acute laryngitis presenting for care were young women with a mean age of 38 years.[9] In addition, the study demonstrated that the frequency of laryngitis during the winter months was almost double that observed in the warmer half of the year.

All of the major respiratory viruses have been etiologically associated with laryngitis. In the study by Higgins of patients older than 5 years of age with a primary diagnosis of laryngitis, 21% had infection with parainfluenza virus, 15% had rhinovirus, 3% had influenza virus, and 3% had adenovirus.[4] Only 18% of patients with laryngitis in this study had a viral pathogen recovered from the respiratory tract. Also, the pattern of infection was age dependent, with only parainfluenza virus identified in children 5 to 15 years of age. The risk of developing laryngitis with a particular type of respiratory infection is summarized in Table 52-1. McMillan and colleagues reported that laryngitis and cough were noted significantly more often among patients with influenza (29%) than among those with group A β-hemolytic streptococcal infection (2.3%).[7] In a retrospective review of an epidemic of influenza in the United Kingdom, the rate of laryngitis or tracheitis reported by general practitioners peaked at approximately 100 per 100,000 population, coincident with the peak of influenza illness.[10] Younger patients were significantly more likely to report hoarsness than elderly subjects in a recent study of human metapneumovirus (hMPV) infection.[11] This study also reported hoarseness in 91% of young adults with hMPV infection compared with 42% of similarly aged subjects with respiratory syncytial virus (RSV) infection. Hoarseness has also been reported to be a prominent manifestation of infection with coronavirus and parainfluenza virus, identified in up to 63% and 90% of cases, respectively, in children and young adults.[8,12] Among older adults admitted to the hospital for respiratory disorders, hoarseness was reported by 25% of subjects with illness due to rhinovirus or coronavirus.[13] Hoarseness or laryngitis has not been reported as a symptom in patients with severe acute respiratory syndrome (SARS) due to the newly recognized human pneumonia–associated coronavirus.[14]

TABLE 52-1   Frequency of Laryngitis Associated with Common Respiratory Pathogens

Rhinovirus	25%-29%	(13, 26)[*]
Influenza	28%-35%	(7, 13, 26)
Parainfluenza	8.5%-90%	(8, 27)
Adenovirus	22%-35%	(28)
Coronavirus	25%-63%	(12, 13)
Mycoplasma pneumoniae	3%-37%	(5, 29)
Chlamydophila pneumoniae	30%	(29)
Group A β-hemolytic streptococcus	2.3%-19%	(7, 26)
Human metapneumovirus	4%-91%	(11, 30)

[*]Numbers in parentheses refer to reference number.

Bacterial respiratory infections have also been associated with acute laryngitis. Several authors have noted the presence of hoarseness in patients with acute streptococcal pharyngitis, as noted in Table 52-1. Laryngitis due to diphtheria has been virtually eliminated in the United States, although diphtheria continues to be an important cause of laryngeal disease worldwide. The possible etiologic role of *Moraxella (Branhamella) catarrhalis* in adults with acute laryngitis was investigated in several reports from Sweden. In a case-control study of 40 adults with hoarseness and symptoms of upper respiratory tract infection, 55% of the patients and 14% of controls had *M. catarrhalis* isolated from a nasopharyngeal culture.[15] *Haemophilus influenzae* was the second most frequently recovered bacterial pathogen from patients with laryngitis (8%-20%), which suggests that that organism may also play a role in this condition. However, treatment of patients with *M. catarrhalis* with oral penicillin or erythromycin for 5 days failed to show any objective clinical benefit over placebo, despite a significant rate of bacteriologic eradication, casting doubt on the significance of the association.[16,17]

Uncommon causes of acute laryngitis include herpesviruses, candida, *Coccidioides immitis*, *Cryptococcus neoformans*, and group G β-hemolytic streptococci in both normal and immunocompromised patients.[18-21] Clinical findings in patients with laryngitis due to herpes simplex virus 1 or 2 (HSV-1, HSV-2), varicella-zoster virus (VZV), or cytomegalovirus (CMV) include edema and inflammation of the glottic or supraglottic region with vesicles or ulcerative lesions with or without vocal cord paralysis.[18] Laryngitis due to tuberculosis and blastomycosis is usually a complication of pulmonary infection.[19,22] Although in the past laryngeal tuberculosis was frequently detected in young patients with recognized pulmonary tuberculosis (TB), more recent reports have described changes in the epidemiology and clinical features of TB of the larynx. In a study of 31 patients with biopsy-confirmed laryngeal TB, only 55% were referrred because of a previous diagnosis of pulmonary TB, whereas 33% had odynophagia or a suspicion of carcinoma.[23] The mean age of patients with laryngeal TB was 60 years in a case series reported by Kandiloros and colleagues.[24] Historically, patients with laryngeal TB had a large burden or organisms in their sputum. However, in a recent study from India, patients with laryngeal TB were no more likely to have positive sputum results than patients with pulmonary TB without laryngeal disease.[22] Clinical findings reported in laryngeal TB range from the classic description of cranial nerve palsies with ulcerative lesions of the posterior larynx to anterior tumor-like masses. Given this changing clinical picture, a high degree of diagnostic suspicion is warranted to make a diagnosis of laryngeal TB.

Laryngeal histoplasmosis is a complication of disseminated infection and manifests as hoarseness of indolent onset without cough. Blastomycosis and histoplasmosis of the larynx can be mistaken for squamous carcinoma by the indolent onset, gross appearance on laryngoscopy, and pseudoepitheliomatous hyperplasia on biopsy. Fever is low grade or absent. Diagnosis depends on demonstration of the fungi in the submucosa. Hoarseness may also be noted as a component of other laryngeal infections, such as croup, acute epiglottitis or supraglottitis, and bacterial tracheitis. These conditions are discussed separately (in Chapters 53 and 56). Other noninfectious causes of acute laryngitis include voice abuse, gastroesophageal reflux disease, and laryngeal malignancy.

The diagnosis of acute laryngitis caused by an upper respiratory infection can often be made by history alone. Examination of the larynx reveals hyperemic and erythematous vocal folds resulting from edema and vascular engorgement of the mucous membranes.[25] Treatment needs to be directed at the underlying infectious cause of hoarseness, but in general is symptomatic in nature, with voice rest and humidification.[25] As noted, studies evaluating the use of antibiotics for patients with acute laryngitis have not shown objective benefit, and they are not routinely recommended.

REFERENCES

1. Banfield G, Tandon G, Solomons N. Hoarse voice: An early symptom of many conditions. Practitioner. 2000;244:267.
2. Mossad SB, Macknin ML, Medendorp SV, et al. Zinc gluconate lozenges for treating the common cold: A randomized, double-blind, placebo-controlled study. Ann Intern Med. 1996;125:81.
3. Weidner TG. Reporting behaviors and activity levels of intercollegiate athletes with an URI. Med Sci Sports Exerc. 1994;26:22.
4. Higgins PG. Viruses associated with acute respiratory infections 1961-71. J Hyg Camb. 1974;72:425.
5. Foy HM, Kenney GE, McMahan R, et al. *Mycoplasma pneumoniae* pneumonia in an urban area: Five years of surveillance. JAMA. 1970;214:1666.
6. Tarlo S, Broder I, Spence L. A prospective study of respiratory infection in adult asthmatics and their normal spouses. Clin Allergy. 1979;9:293.
7. McMillan JA, Sandstrom C, Weiner LB, et al. Viral and bacterial organisms associated with acute pharyngitis in a school-aged population. J Pediatr. 1986;109:747.
8. Hall CB, Geiman JM, Breese BB, Douglas RG Jr. Parainfluenza viral infections in children: Correlation of shedding with clinical manifestations. J Pediatr. 1977;91:194.
9. Danielides V, Nousia CS, Patrikakos G, et al. Effect of meterological parameters on acute laryngitis in adults. Acta Otolaryngol. 2002;122:655.
10. Miller DL, Lee JA. Influenza in Britain 1967-68. J Hyg Camb. 1969;67:559.
11. Falsey AR, Erdman D, Anderson LJ, et al. Human metapneumovirus infections in young and elderly adults. J Infect Dis. 2003; 187:785.
12. Wenzel RP, Hendley JO, Davies JA, et al. Coronavirus infections in military recruits: Three-year study with coronavirus strains OC43 and 229E. Am Rev Respir Dis. 1974; 109:621.
13. Falsey AR, Walsh EE, Hayden FG. Rhinovirus and coronavirus infection-associated hospitalizations among older adults. J Infect Dis. 2002;185:1338.
14. Peiris JS, Lai ST, Poon LLM, et al. Coronavirus as a possible cause of severe acute respiratory sydrome. Lancet. 2003;361:1319.
15. Schaleæn L, Christensen P, Kamme C, et al. High isolation rate of *Branhamella catarrhalis* from the nasopharynx in adults with acute laryngitis. Scand J Infect Dis. 1980;12:277.
16. Schaleæn L, Fex S, Christensen P, et al. Inefficacy of penicillin V in acute laryngitis in adults: Evaluation from results of double-blind study. Ann Otol Rhinol Laryngol. 1985;94:14.
17. Schaleæn L, Kamme C, Eliasson I, et al. Erythromycin in acute laryngitis in adults. Ann Otol Rhinol Laryngol. 1993;102:209.
18. Vrabec JT, Molina CP, West B. Herpes simplex laryngitis. Ann Otol Rhinol Laryngol 2000;109:611.
19. Vrabec DP. Fungal infections of the larynx. Otolaryngol Clin North Am. 1993; 26:1091.
20. Browning DG, Schwartz DA, Jurado RL. Cryptococcosis of the larynx in a patient with AIDS: An unusual cause of fungal laryngitis. South Med J. 1992;85:762.
21. Nasri S, True LD, Abemayor E. Upper airway obstruction caused by Group G streptococcal laryngitis. Am J Otolaryngol. 1995;16:53.
22. Kulkarni N, Gopal GS, Ghaisas SG, et al. Epidemiologic considerations and clinical features of ENT tuberculosis. J Laryngol Otol. 2001;115:555.
23. Agarwal P, Bais AS. A clinical and videostroboscopic evaluation of laryngeal tuberculosis. J Laryngol Otol. 1998; 112:45.
24. Kandiloros DC, Nikolopoulos TP, Ferekidis EA, et al. Laryngeal tuberculosis at the end of the 20th century. J Laryngol Otol. 1997;111:619.
25. Vaughan CW. Current concepts in otolaryngology: Diagnosis and treatment of organic voice disorders. N Engl J Med. 1982;307:863.
26. Gwaltney JM Jr. Rhinoviruses. In: Evans AS, Kaslow RA, eds. Viral Infections of Humans, Epidemiology and Control. 4th ed. New York: Plenum Medical Book Company; 1997:815.
27. Knott AM, Long CE, Hall CB. Parainfluenza viral infections in pediatric outpatients: Seasonal patterns and clinical characteristics. Pediatr Infect Dis J. 1994;13:269.
28. McNamara MJ, Pierce WE, Crawford YE, et al. Patterns of adenovirus infection in the respiratory diseases of naval recruits: A longitudinal study of two companies of naval recruits. Am Rev Respir Dis. 1962;86:485.
29. Thom DH, Grayston JT, Wang S-P, et al. *Chlamydia pneumoniae* strain twar, *Mycoplasma pneumoniae*, and viral infections in acute respiratory disease in a university student health clinic population. Am J Epidemiol. 1990;132:248.
30. Freymuth F, Vabret A, Legrand L, et al. Presence of the new human metapneumovirus in French children with bronchiolitis. Pediatr Infect Dis J. 2003;22:92.

CHAPTER 53

Acute Laryngotracheobronchitis (Croup)

CAROLINE BREESE HALL

JOHN T. McBRIDE

. . . the sharp stridulous voice which I can resemble to nothing more nearly than the crowing of a cock . . . is the true diagnostic sign of the disease.

—Francis Home, 1765[1]

Croup, or acute laryngotracheobronchitis, is an age-specific viral infection of the upper and lower respiratory tracts that produces inflammation in the subglottic area and results in a striking picture of dyspnea accompanied on inspiration by the characteristic stridulous notes of croup. Croup perhaps best demonstrates the piquant interaction of host and microorganism. Age, sex, an undefined predisposition of the child, and type of virus all appear to influence the susceptibility and severity of the infection.

Francis Home of Edinburgh first introduced the word *croup* in his treatise, "An Inquiry into the Nature, Causes and Cure of the Croup," in which he describes 12 patients with croup.[1] The term *croup* has been traced to an Anglo-Saxon word *Kropan*[2] or the old Scottish term *roup*, which meant "to cry out in a shrill voice."

For the next century the term *croup* was applied to a number of disease entities, including diphtheria. John Cheyne, however, appeared to describe not only diphtheria, "cynache trachealis," but also the disease entity that appears to be similar to the viral laryngotracheobronchitis of today.[3] Bretonneau, in 1859, argued that diphtheria was a separate and specific disease.[4] However, the confusion between "membranous" or "true" croup and "spasmodic" or "false" croup continued. Differentiation awaited Klebs's discovery of *Corynebacterium diphtheriae* in 1883. In 1948, Rabe[5] classified the forms of infectious croup according to etiology—bacterial or nonbacterial—and suggested that the latter, larger group was viral in origin. In only 15% of his 347 patients was he able to identify a pathogen, namely, *C. diphtheriae* or *Haemophilus influenzae* type B.

The term *croup* now generally refers to an acute laryngotracheitis or laryngotracheobronchitis caused by a viral infection. Many children develop croup only once during childhood despite multiple infections with the viruses that are the prime etiologic agents. In some children, however, such viral infections cause repeated episodes of croup in early childhood. In such children the illness is often called "spasmodic croup." Some also have applied this appellation of "spasmodic" to those episodes of croup that are particularly abrupt in onset. Spasmodic croup in general, however, cannot be differentiated from a single episode of the usual type of croup in its clinical manifestations, or in its etiology, which is usually viral.[6]

INCIDENCE

Croup is a relatively common illness in young children, accounting for about 10% to 15% of lower respiratory tract disease. In Hoekelman's prospective study[7] of infectious diseases occurring in the first year of life, 1.2% of infants studied had croup. The peak occurrence is in the second year of life, with most cases occurring between 3 months and 3 years of age.[6,8-13] In a Seattle prepaid group practice, the annual incidence of croup was 7 per 1000 for all children younger than 6 years of age. In the first 6 months of life, the rate was 5.2 per 1000, and in the second 6 months, it was 11.[8] The peak incidence was 14.9 in the second year of life and fell to half that rate in the third year. In a group practice in North Carolina, the overall incidence was three to five times higher, with a peak of 47 annual episodes per 1000 children in the second year of life.[11] Even in the first 6 months of life the incidence was 24, and after 6 years of age it was 4.6. In series of hospitalized or outpatient cases of croup, boys have predominated, although the attack rates of upper respiratory tract illnesses by these same viral agents show no sex preference.[8,10-17]

ETIOLOGY

Acute laryngotracheobronchitis may be caused by a variety of viral agents and occasionally by *Mycoplasma pneumoniae*.[8,9,11,14-16,18-20] Parainfluenza type 1 virus is the most common cause of croup in the United States and Great Britain (Table 53-1). Parainfluenza type 3 virus is usually the second most frequently associated agent. In infants, parainfluenza type 3 virus causes bronchiolitis and pneumonia, but croup is the more usual manifestation in children 2 to 3 years of age, and tracheobronchitis in older children.[14,21]

Croup is the characteristic manifestation of parainfluenza type 2 viral infection. However, the total proportion of croup cases produced by parainfluenza type 2 virus is less than that associated with types 1 and 3.[21] The seasonal pattern of parainfluenza type 2 virus also is less predictable, and sizable outbreaks of infection with

TABLE 53-1 Percentage of Croup Cases Associated with Various Agents

Agent	Cramblett et al, 1977[18] (%)	Parrott et al, 1962[19] (%)	Loda et al, 1968[20] (%)	Glezen et al, 1971[14] (%)	Foy et al, 73[8] (%)		Buchan et al, 1974[16] (%)	Downham et al, 1974[9] (%)	Denny et al, 1983[11] (%)
Parainfluenza virus									
Type 1	8	21	39	21	13	6.4†	25	26	18
Type 2	6	8	1.6	4	*	7.3	1.7	6	3
Type 3	14	10	1.6	9	1.4	13	8	10	6.6
Influenza A virus	6	8	—	2	3	3.7	10	6	1.4
Influenza B virus	—		—	1	1	2	—	—	1.2
Respiratory syncytial virus	—	8	11.4	6	1	9	1.7	6	3.8
Adenovirus	4	9	3	1	1	4.6	1.7	3	—
Rhinovirus	—	—	—	0.6	4	—	1	6	—
Enterovirus	12	—	—	1	2	—	1	—	—
Other viruses	—	—	—	—	1	—	5	—	2
Mycoplasma pneumoniae	—	—	5	1.4	0.5	2	—	1	1.4
Total percentage of cases with identified agent	50	64	62	47	56		54	64	37.6

*Identified by isolation of agent.
†Identified by serology.

parainfluenza type 2 virus are unusual in comparison to outbreaks with type 1.[10,11,14,21]

Outbreaks with influenza A and B viruses, especially the former, may result in appreciable numbers of croup cases. Influenza, because of its unpredictable nature and fluctuating seasonal occurrence, may be a less common instigator of croup than the parainfluenza viruses, but some studies have reported it to be more severe,[22-24] although others have not.[11] Influenza A virus may produce croup in a broader age range of children and sometimes with a higher frequency of hospitalization. In Washington, D.C., between 1957 and 1976, 14.3% of the patients with croup had influenza A or B viral infection.[24] The frequency of croup cases was related to the type of influenza (A more than B) and to the strain, especially H3N2.

Only a small proportion (approximately 5%) of respiratory syncytial viral infections result in croup, but of all reported cases of croup, 1% to 11% have been associated with respiratory syncytial virus (see Table 53-1). The mean age of croup cases associated with respiratory syncytial virus tends to be younger, less than 1 year of age, especially in hospitalized cases, and the course may be more severe and prolonged.

Outbreaks of measles in the United States or elsewhere serve as a reminder that rubeola in the prevaccine era often resulted in severe and complicated croup. During the 1989-1991 upsurge of measles cases in the United States, laryngotracheobronchitis complicated approximately 20% of the cases of measles in hospitalized patients in Los Angeles and Houston.[25,26] Children with croup as a complication of measles tended to be younger and had a more severe course, and 17% to 22% required intubation. In some, the outcome was fatal.

Adenoviral infection infrequently results in croup, although laryngitis is a relatively common manifestation of adenoviral infection. Rhinoviruses, enteroviruses, herpes simplex virus, and *M. pneumoniae* all contribute to a small but variable percentage of cases.[12,13,17]

The proportion of croup cases caused by the different agents varies somewhat according to age. The parainfluenza viruses remain the major agents at all ages, but in the first few months of life respiratory syncytial virus ascends in importance, and the influenza viruses and *M. pneumoniae* predominantly cause croup in children older than 5 years of age.[11] Of these agents, only the parainfluenza viruses and influenza viruses occur in epidemics and have a great enough of a predilection for causing croup to produce during their outbreaks an appreciable rise in the number of croup cases in the community.[8,11,16,24,27]

EPIDEMIOLOGY

The epidemiologic patterns of croup reflect mainly the seasonal personalities of the major agents. The major peak of croup cases coincides with the height of activity of parainfluenza type 1 virus, which in recent years has been every other year in the fall.[10,11,14,21] Parainfluenza type 2 virus also may contribute to outbreaks of croup occurring in the fall, whereas those in the winter to early spring are more apt to be related to parainfluenza virus type 3, influenza A and B viruses, and respiratory syncytial virus.[9-11,14-16,21,27] Sporadic cases of croup also are commonly associated with parainfluenza type 3 virus. This virus tends to be present through much of the year, with swells of activity during the spring to summer and into the fall if no outbreak of parainfluenza virus type 1 occurs.[9,11,14] Sporadic cases of croup may also be caused by any of the less commonly associated agents, such as the adenoviruses, rhinoviruses, and *M. pneumoniae*, all of which may be prevalent through many months of the year. Croup caused by enteroviruses, although uncommon, tends to occur in the summer and early fall.

PATHOPHYSIOLOGY

The viral infection initially affects the upper respiratory tract, and usually produces inflammation of the nasal passages and nasopharynx. Subsequently, in the primary infection, the lower respiratory tract also

becomes involved. However, the classic signs of croup—stridor, hoarseness, and cough—arise mostly from the inflammation that occurs in the larynx and trachea. The inflammation and obstruction are greatest at the subglottic level. This is the least distensible part of the airway because it is encircled by the cricoid cartilage, with the narrow anterior ring and the larger posterior quadrangular lamina, forming a "signet ring."

Inflammation at the subglottic level results in the characteristic obstruction observed in viral croup. The impeded flow of air through this narrowed area produces the classic high-pitched vibratory sounds, or stridor. This is most apparent on inspiration because the negative intraluminal pressure tends to narrow the extrathoracic airway further, much as sucking on a partially occluded paper straw causes it to collapse inwardly. This effect is enhanced in young children because their airway walls are relatively compliant.[28]

In 1836, Ley[29] descriptively expressed the characteristic findings of croup as follows:

"The shrill sonorous inspiration so characteristic of this complaint, marks very unequivocally its seat. . . . From some cause there is an unusual approximation of the sides of the glottis . . . the influence being very analogous to that produced by too strong compression of the reed against the mouthpiece of the clarinet by the lips of one who has made no great proficiency in that instrument, when a harsh, squeaking sound is produced abundantly discordant and grating to the ear."

In histologic sections, inflammatory changes may be seen in the epithelium, mucosa, and submucosa of the larynx, in the trachea, and the linings of the bronchi, bronchioles, and sometimes the alveoli.[30] Small areas of atelectasis may also be present.

Why children in the second year of life are particularly likely to develop croup is not entirely clear. Most of these children are experiencing primary infection with the viral agent, which is more likely to result in spread of the virus to involve the larynx and the lower respiratory tract. The anatomy of the young child also may be important in the age predilection. The diameters of the larynx and glottis are relatively small in the young child, and inflammation of the membranes lining these passages causes an appreciably greater degree of obstruction. Airway resistance is highly sensitive to even small changes in the diameter of the airway because the resistance to airflow is inversely related to the fourth power of the radius of the airway. The mucous membrane is also relatively looser and more vascular, and the cartilage ring is less rigid. Furthermore, nasal obstruction and crying can aggravate the dynamic narrowing of the child's airway.

Immunologic mechanisms also have been postulated to contribute to the pathogenesis of croup.[31-33] Greater concentrations of immunoglobulin E (IgE) antibody to parainfluenza viral antigen and histamine have been detected in children with parainfluenza viral infections whose illness was manifested as croup, wheezing, or both, compared with those with only upper respiratory tract illness.[32] The lymphoproliferative responses of peripheral blood lymphocytes from children with parainfluenza viral croup were demonstrated to be significantly greater than those from children with upper respiratory tract illnesses, and their histamine-induced suppression of the lymphoproliferative response was diminished.[33] From these findings, Welliver and colleagues[32,33] suggested that a defect in the regulation of the immune response, similar to that found in atopic subjects, contributes to the pathogenesis of croup.

Physiologic Correlations

When the infection produces obstruction at the subglottic level, the child's tidal volume initially declines. This is compensated by an increase in the respiratory rate to maintain adequate alveolar ventilation (Fig. 53-1). If the degree of obstruction worsens, the work of breathing may increase such that the child tires and can no longer maintain the necessary compensatory respiratory effort. The tidal volume may

FIGURE 53-1. Physiologic abnormalities in croup.

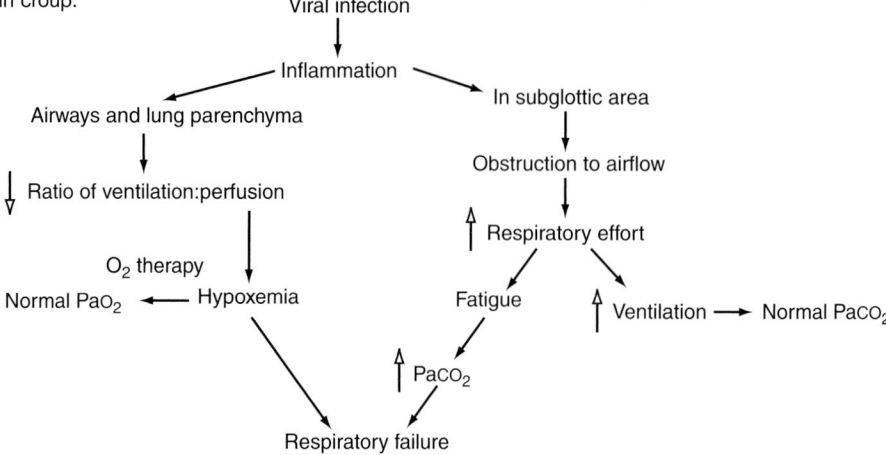

then further decrease, and, as the respiratory rate declines, hypercarbia and secondary hypoxemia ensue.

The occurrence of hypoxemia in children hospitalized with croup may not be suspected and may seem surprising because upper airway obstruction that does not disrupt the distribution of ventilation and perfusion in the lung should not cause hypoxemia. The inflammation in the lung parenchyma, however, results in areas of abnormally low ventilation-perfusion ratio and increased alveolar-to-arterial oxygen gradient (see Fig. 53-1). In some children, hypoxemia may result from transient airway hyperreactivity or from pulmonary edema caused by the marked negative intrathoracic pressures exerted during inspiration in an attempt to compensate for the obstruction of the upper airway. In those few patients who require intubation, the abrupt relief of the negative mean intrathoracic pressure can also be associated with acute onset of pulmonary edema.

CLINICAL MANIFESTATIONS

The disease generally comes on in the evening after the little patient has been exposed to the weather during the day and often after a slight catarrh of some days' standing. At first his voice is observed to be hoarse and pulling . . . he awakens with a most unusual cough, rough, and stridulous. And now his breathing is laborious, each inspiration being accompanied by a harsh, shrill noise.

—John Cheyne, 1814[2]

Most children with croup have a history of an upper respiratory tract infection for one to several days previously. Commonly, the child has had rhinorrhea, a sore throat, and a mild cough. Most children have fever, either initially during the upper respiratory tract infection or at the onset of croup. Children with croup caused by influenza or parainfluenza viruses commonly have fevers with temperatures ranging from 38° C to 40° C.[34] Fever with respiratory syncytial viral infection tends not to be as high or may even be absent.

The onset of croup often is heralded by hoarseness and a deepening cough. The cough usually is not productive but has the striking brassy tone that has earned it the sobriquet "seal's bark." The child may awaken at night with this distinctive cough, tachypnea, and the characteristic inspiratory stridor. In 1836, Ley[29] described the stridor as *"the crowing of a cock, the yelping of a fox, the barking of a dog, the braying of an ass, or a ringing sound, as if the voice came from a brazen tube."* The child may sit forward in bed and appear apprehensive. Often accompanying the stridor are retractions of the chest wall, usually most marked in the supraclavicular and suprasternal areas.

In children who are more severely affected, auscultation of the chest may reveal both inspiratory and expiratory stridor, as well as crackles and wheezing. The respiratory rate is commonly elevated to 35 to 45 per minute, but rates above 50 per minute are unusual in children with croup, in contrast to the marked tachypnea that is often evident in bronchiolitis. With progression of the disease, auscultation of the chest may reveal poor exchange of air with diminished breath sounds.

One of the hallmarks of croup is its fluctuating course. A child may appear clinically to worsen or improve within an hour. In milder cases of croup, children commonly improve in the morning, only to worsen again at night. In most children the course of croup is 3 to 4 days, although the cough may persist for a longer period.

ROENTGENOGRAPHIC FINDINGS

The characteristic manifestations of viral laryngotracheobronchitis in an anterior-posterior radiograph at the neck is a 5- to 10-mm narrowed shadow of the trachea in the subglottic area. This is often described as the "hourglass" or "steeple" sign (Fig. 53-2).[35] The lateral view of the neck may show an increased width of the air space in the hypopharyngeal area; increased respiratory drive resulting from the tracheal obstruction leads to active dilation of the pharyngeal airway.

The diagnostic value of these roentgenographic findings is questionable, as well as controversial.[36-38] They are not consistently observed in all cases of viral laryngotracheobronchitis, and some studies have shown them to be of low specificity and sensitivity for confirming or ruling out viral croup.

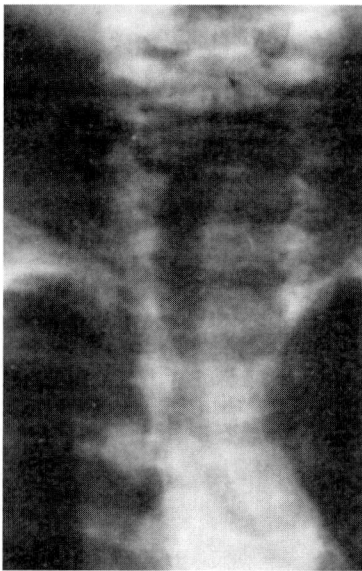

FIGURE 53-2. Roentgenogram of the neck of a child with viral croup that shows the characteristic narrowing of the air shadow of the trachea in the subglottic area.

LABORATORY FINDINGS

In most cases of croup, the leukocyte and differential counts are not particularly abnormal or helpful. In the more severely stressed child, the leukocyte count may be somewhat elevated, and an increase in the proportion of immature polymorphonuclear cells may be observed.

Hypoxemia and hypercapnea may be present in hospitalized children.[39] Pulmonary function testing has shown an increased functional residual capacity, but few pulmonary function studies have been obtained in children with croup.[40]

DIAGNOSIS

Identification of the specific viral agent of laryngotracheobronchitis may be accomplished by isolation in tissue culture or by one of the newer techniques of rapid antigen diagnosis.[41,42] In most reported series of cases, the cause was determined in approximately one third to two thirds of the patients with croup (see Table 53-1), which is higher than that generally reported for other respiratory tract syndromes. Isolation and identification of parainfluenza and influenza virus from a nasopharyngeal swab, or in older children, a nasopharyngeal wash, are available in 24 to 48 hours by use of shell vial spin amplification culture (see Chapter 15). Rapid tests for influenza virus A and B antigens in respiratory specimens are commercially available and are particularly useful during peak winter months.[43]

Rapid techniques may be used to identify the viral antigens in the respiratory secretions, including immunofluorescent assays and enzyme immunoassays (EIA) or to detect viral ribonucleic acid (RNA), as by reverse transcriptase–polymerase chain reaction (RT-PCR).[44,45] The RT-PCR has generally appeared to be the most sensitive technique, but it has been primarily used in research laboratories.[46-48]

Serologic diagnosis is generally made only retrospectively, and for some of the major agents of croup, serologic rises are variable and unreliable. Heterotypic antibody rises are frequent among the various types of the parainfluenza viruses and related viruses such as mumps.[49] Furthermore, during initial and repeated infections, diagnostic homotypic antibody responses for diagnosis may not occur.

DIFFERENTIAL DIAGNOSIS

Although in most cases of croup the clinical and epidemiologic presentation makes the diagnosis of viral laryngotracheobronchitis evident, other entities should be considered as possible causes of the stridor in atypical cases. Among these are bacterial entities, including bacterial epiglottitis or supraglottitis, bacterial tracheitis (discussed separately below), and noninfectious causes of obstruction.

Cases of bacterial epiglottitis are rarely seen since widespread immunization of infants and children for *H. influenzae* type B, which was the major cause of epiglottitis previously. Differentiation of epiglottitis usually can be made on the basis of the history, the striking rapidity of the onset of severe respiratory distress, and sometimes anterior-posterior and lateral roentgenograms of the neck (see Chapter 56).[35,50] Affected children tend to be slightly older (usually 2 to 4 years of age) than those with viral croup. Characteristically the course of epiglottitis is much more rapidly progressive, and the children appear markedly toxic. The history of an upper respiratory tract infection with rhinorrhea and laryngitis usually is not present in epiglottitis. The absence of the distinctive cough or seal's bark, the presence of a muffled voice, and marked dysphagia with drooling are some of the more helpful differentiating clinical signs. In contrast to viral laryngotracheobronchitis, the lateral neck view in epiglottitis may show an edematous epiglottis without subglottic narrowing. The roentgenographic picture, however, may not always be diagnostic for croup or epiglottitis, and conflicting data exist about its reliability and usefulness in the acute situation.[36-38]

Other non-viral infectious causes of stridor now rarely seen in the United States and other developed countries include *C. diphtheriae* and *Mycobacterium tuberculosis*. *M. pneumoniae*, *Candida albicans*, and *Cryptosporidium* have also occasionally been associated with stridor.[11,51,52]

Noninfectious causes of obstruction include aspiration of a foreign body, which is relatively common in the same age group as that of viral croup, trauma to the upper airway as from toxic ingestions, and angioneurotic edema. Anatomic abnormalities, such as vocal cord paralysis and anomalies, which impinge upon the laryngeal tracheal area, may cause stridor, especially when a respiratory infection augments the obstruction to airflow. Occasionally recurrent episodes of stridor may be related to gastrointestinal reflux or hypocalcemia.

THERAPY

Despite a plethora of home therapies for croup, none has proved consistently effective. The natural fluctuations in the course of croup make evaluation of many therapies difficult. Vaporizers and other means of producing mist in the home have long been advised. In the past century, steaming tea kettles were an integral, if not primary, mode of therapy.[53] Nevertheless, the beneficial effects of mist have not been proved, and hot water humidification devices carry the risk to cause burns.[12,13,54] These methods provide humidification of the upper airway, but the droplet size produced is generally too large to reach the lower respiratory tract. The advantages of such home humidification devices must be balanced against the discomfort or fear they may produce in the child.[55] Crying and lack of rest may worsen the condition.

Humidification of the airway at home has usually been administered by small cool mist devices. In the hospital, an ultrasonic nebulizer fitted to a mask or an oxygen tent may be used. Although humidification may aid the upper airway secretions, a beneficial effect on the subglottic swelling and on the lower parenchymal abnormalities has not been shown, and few controlled studies have examined this therapy.[56] In one small controlled trial of 16 children, humidification did not result in discernible improvement.[12,54] In another study, nebulized water administered to five children did not produce a change in the measured total respiratory resistance.[57]

In a dog model of croup, cold-dry, cold-moist, and dry air were more effective than warm-moist air in decreasing airway resistance.[58] All of these types of air contain little humidification compared with warm-moist air. These findings correlate with the clinical observation that some children with croup improve when taken out into cold night air, which would contain little moisture.

In hospitalized patients, the essence of successful management is close observation and good supportive care based on a thorough understanding of the physiologic changes associated with croup. Clinical estimation of the severity of croup is difficult. Cyanosis may not be present despite compromising degrees of hypoxemia.[59] An increase in the work of breathing may indicate progressive subglottic obstruction and hypoxemia. Oximetry offers a simple, noninvasive means of monitoring the child's arterial oxygen saturation.[60] In the more severely ill child, the Pco_2 also may need to be assessed. In most cases, however, blood drawing and other frightening procedures should be kept to a minimum to avoid compounding the dyspnea and respiratory obstruction. Inspirations that are rapid and shallow, such as commonly accompany anxiety and crying, aggravate the narrowing of the airway and further increase the metabolic demand for gas exchange. Most children with hypoxemia who are not hypercarbic respond to relatively low concentrations of supplemental oxygen, because the hypoxemia results primarily from areas of lung with an abnormal ratio of ventilation to perfusion (see Fig. 53-1).[61]

A variety of pharmacologic agents have been evaluated in the treatment of croup, including nebulized adrenaline and systemic and nebulized corticosteroids. Most studies accessing these therapies have been done in hospitalized patients or in facilities for evaluation of acute illnesses, such as emergency departments. Few have been performed in private practice offices. In general, trials have contained few numbers of cases or were not well designed, which makes the interpretation of the benefit of these agents difficult to assess.

Nebulized epinephrine or adrenaline has been one of the most frequently and long-term agents used in the treatment of viral croup.[6,12,13,17,56,62] Epinephrine, by stimulus of both α- and β-adrenergic receptors, results in a decreased blood flow to capillary beds, especially to skin and mucosal surfaces. This diminished blood flow to the tissues of the upper respiratory tract shrinks the mucosa and reduces the edema. Racemic epinephrine with both D- and L-isomers has been used preferentially in the past over the L-form, which was believed to have caused more cardiovascular adverse effects.

In general, recent randomized, controlled trials of nebulized adrenaline have shown benefit in relieving the symptoms of viral laryngotracheobronchitis, but the effect has been transient.[12,13,17] Of four randomized and controlled trials comparing nebulized epinephrine to placebo, three showed clinical improvement lasting for about 2 hours, and two small trials were unable to show significant difference.[63-67] Nebulized epinephrine in comparison with nebulized corticosteroids has not been adequately studied, although some have suggested that the two therapies may have an additive effect.

Therapy with systemic or nebulized corticosteroids has become a mainstay in moderately to severely ill children with viral croup. In general, in comparison to children receiving placebo, nebulized or systemic corticosteroid therapy has resulted in significant improvement in acute symptoms and significant reduction in hospitalization and follow-up visits.[12,13,17,68-77] Systemic corticosteroid therapy has usually resulted in clinical benefit by 12 hours and has allowed earlier discharge in hospitalized children. Intramuscular or oral dexamethasone has been used most commonly at 0.3 to 0.6 mg/kg, administered as a single dose or repeatedly over 1 to 2 days. The lower dose of oral dexamethasone (0.3 mg/kg) appears to be as effective as the higher dose of 0.6 mg/kg. Placebo-controlled studies of nebulized corticosteroids found similar benefits of more rapid improvement, earlier discharge, and fewer follow-up visits. Adverse effects from these short course regimens with either epinephrine or corticosteroids have been uncommon.[56]

Despite the general acknowledgment that viruses are the perpetrators of croup, antibiotics are frequently used.[78,79] Bacterial infection superimposed on or occurring after croup is uncommon, and administration of antibiotics to children with croup prophylactically or without evidence of concomitant bacterial infection is not warranted.

OUTCOME

The outcome for children with viral laryngotracheobronchitis is generally excellent with available modern technical and pharmacologic modalities. The rates of hospitalization have generally been less than 2%.[11,80] Of those hospitalized, up to 2% have required nasotracheal intubation, but currently this is rarely needed.

The secondary bacterial infections in the normal child with acute laryngotracheobronchitis also appear rare. Such a complication is often suspected, but rarely confirmed. Among the 130 children reported in controlled and randomized studies evaluating therapy with systemic corticosteroids, 9 developed a secondary bacterial complication with a relative risk of 0.94 for treatment with systemic corticosteroids compared with placebo.[74,81,82]

Repeated episodes of croup have been reported as sequelae in some children. In a retrospective study, recurrent croup was reported to occur in 5% of children 5 to 8 years of age.[83] John Cheyne[3] noted that "the first attack establishes a predisposition to the disease. I have observed, that after the first attack, a slighter cause will produce Croup a second time than is required originally." Some such children have been diagnosed as having spasmodic croup. An allergic diathesis or hyperreactivity of the airway may contribute to the illness in these children; positive intradermal skin tests and family members with allergy have been reported as being more frequent in children with recurrent versus single episodes of croup.[84,85]

Mortality associated with croup is currently rare. One review of deaths associated with croup over a 10-year period showed two deaths in 208 children who required intubation.[86] A more recent review of more than 1000 children with croup showed no associated deaths and few complications.[56]

PREVENTION

Preventing acute laryngotracheobronchitis is unlikely in the near future considering the multiple infectious etiologies and mechanisms of pathogenesis. However, immunization against some of the most common viral agents may significantly diminish the burden to health care from this entity. Immunization against influenza virus is available both via the killed vaccine and recently with a live intranasal vaccine. However, this is unlikely to diminish significantly the occurrence of croup cases because influenza is not the major cause, the killed vaccine has been rarely used in children in this age group, and the new live vaccine is currently not approved for children in the prime age group for developing croup. No parainfluenza viral vaccine has thus far been approved, but promising candidates are under investigation.

BACTERIAL TRACHEITIS

An atypical form of croup with a clinical picture more similar to epiglottitis than to the usual case of laryngotracheobronchitis has been described and designated *bacterial tracheitis*.[87-89] Although this entity appears to have been described before 1940, it received little attention until it was rediscovered toward the end of the 1970s. This relatively uncommon disease tends to affect somewhat older children but may affect those of any age. Its onset is acute and dramatic, marked by high fever, stridor, and dyspnea with copious amounts of purulent sputum. The clinical picture may progress rapidly, within minutes to hours. It is unresponsive to therapy with nebulized epinephrine or corticosteroids and requires endotracheal intubation. Suspected cases should be managed as a medical emergency.

The primary area of inflammation and obstruction is subglottic. The subglottis is covered with a thick exudate, but the epiglottis and supraglottic structures tend to be minimally inflamed. A lateral soft tissue roentgenogram of the neck characteristically reveals a normal epiglottis with subglottic narrowing within which a shaggy membrane may sometimes be visible.

The organisms most commonly recovered from this exudate are *Staphylococcus aureus*, group A β-hemolytic streptococci, and, before widespread immunization became available, *H. influenzae* type B.[88,89] The pathogenesis of this entity, nevertheless, is not clear. The syndrome appears to develop in children who are predisposed by previous conditions, especially those associated with injury to the trachea. Children who have been intubated recently and sometimes those with a preceding viral infection causing acute laryngotracheobronchitis appear to be at greater risk. This suggests that mucosal damage or impairment of local immune mechanisms may predispose to invasive infections with common pyogenic organisms.

The rapidly progressive course of this disease demands its prompt diagnosis and differentiation from viral croup by its clinical picture, which may be aided by roentgenographic findings. Direct laryngoscopy can confirm the diagnosis and provide specimens of the localized exudate for culture. Initial antibiotic therapy should be broad enough to cover the associated major pathogens.

REFERENCES

1. Home F. An Inquiry into the Nature, Cause and Cure of Croup. Kincaid A and Bell JS, eds. Edinburgh, ed, 1765.
2. Cherry J. Croup. In: Kiple KS, eds. Cambridge History and Geography of Human Disease Project, ed. Bowling Green, OH: University of Cambridge Press; 1990:654-657.
3. Cheyne J. Essays on the Diseases of Children, with Cases and Dissections. Philadelphia: Anthony Finley Merritt; 1814:20.
4. Semple R. Memoirs on diphtheria. From the Writings of Bretonneau, Guersant, Trousseau, Bouchut, Empis, Daviot 1859. London: New Sydenham Society Publications; 5.
5. Rabe E. Infectious croup: I. Etiology. Pediatrics. 1948;2:255-265.
6. Ewig J. Croup. Pediatr Ann. 2002;31:125-130.
7. Hoekelman R. Infectious illness during the first year of life. Pediatrics. 1977;59:119-121.
8. Foy H, Cooney M, Maletzky A, et al. Incidence and etiology of pneumonia, croup, and bronchiolitis in preschool children belonging to a prepaid medical care group over a four-year period. Am J Epidemiol. 1973;97:80-92.

9. Downham M, McQuillan J, Gardner P. Diagnosis and clinical significance of parainfluenza virus infections in children. Arch Dis Child. 1974;49:8-15.
10. Glezen W, Denny F. Epidemiology of acute lower respiratory disease in children. N Engl J Med. 1973;288:498-505.
11. Denny F, Murphy T, Clyde WJ, et al. Croup: An 11 year study in a pediatric practice. Pediatrics. 1983;71:871-876.
12. Geelhoed G. Croup. Pediatr Pulmonol. 1997;23:370-374.
13. Klassen T. Croup. A current perspective. Pediatr Clin North Am. 1999;46:1167-1178.
14. Glezen W, Loda F, Clyde WJ, et al. Epidemiologic patterns of acute lower respiratory disease of children in a pediatric group practice. J Pediatr. 1971;78:397-406.
15. Loda F, Glezen W, Clyde WJ. Respiratory disease in group day care. Pediatrics. 1972;49:428-437.
16. Buchan K, Marten K, Kennedy D. Aetiology and epidemiology of viral croup in Glasgow, 1966-72. J Hyg (Camb). 1974;73:143-150.
17. Kaditis A, Wald E. Viral croup: Current diagnosis and treatment. Pediatr Infect Dis J. 1998;17:827-834.
18. Cramblett H. Croup (epiglottitis, laryngitis, laryngotracheobronchitis). In: Kendig EJ, Chernick VS, eds. Disorders of the Respiratory Tract in Children. 3rd ed. Philadelphia: WB Saunders; 1977:353.
19. Parrott R, Vargosko A, Kim H, et al. Acute respiratory diseases of viral etiology. III. Myxoviruses: Parainfluenza. Am J Public Health. 1962;52:907-917.
20. Loda F, Clyde W, Glezen W, et al. Studies of the role of viruses, bacteria, and *M. pneumoniae* as causes of lower respiratory tract infections in children. J Pediatr. 1968;72:161-176.
21. Knott A, Long C, Hall C. Parainfluenza viral infections in pediatric outpatients: Seasonal patterns and clinical characteristics. Pediatr Infect Dis J. 1994;13:269-273.
22. Howard J, McCracken GJ, Luby J. Influenza A 2 virus as a cause of croup requiring tracheotomy. J Pediatr. 1972;81:1148-1150.
23. Eller J, Fulginiti V, Plunkett D, et al. Attack rates for hospitalized croup in children in a military population: Importance of A2 influenza infection. Pediatr Res. 1972;6:126.
24. Kim H, Brandt C, Chanock R, et al. Influenza A and B virus infection in infants and young children during the years 1957-1976. Am J Epidemiol. 1979;109:464-479.
25. Ross L, Mason W, Lanson J, et al. Severe laryngotracheobronchitis as a complication of measles during an urban epidemic. J Pediatr. 1992;121:511-515.
26. Fortenberry J, Mariscalco M, Louis P, et al. Severe laryngotracheobronchitis complicating measles. Am J Dis Child. 1992;146:1040-1043.
27. Hall C, Douglas RJ. Respiratory syncytial virus and influenza: Practical community surveillance. Am J Dis Child. 1976;130:615-620.
28. McBride J. Stridor in childhood. J Fam Prac 1984;19:782-790.
29. Ley H. An essay on the Laryngismus Stridulus or Croup-like Inspiration of Infants. London: Churchill; 1836:6.
30. Szpunar J, Glowacki J, Laskowski A, et al. Fibrinous laryngotracheobronchitis in children. Arch Otolaryngol. 1971;93:173-178.
31. Urquhart G, Kennedy D, Ariyawansa J. Croup associated with parainfluenza type 1 virus: Two subpopulations. BMJ. 1979;1:1604.
32. Welliver R, Wong D, Middleton EJ, et al. Role of parainfluenza virus-specific IgE in pathogenesis of croup and wheezing subsequent to infection. J Pediatr. 1982;101:889-896.
33. Welliver R, Sun M, Rinaldo D. Defective regulation of immune responses in croup due to parainfluenza virus. Pediatr Res. 1985;19:716-720.
34. Hall C, Geiman J, Breese B, et al. Parainfluenza viral infections in children: Correlation of shedding with clinical manifestations. J Pediatr. 1977;91:194-198.
35. Rapkin R. The diagnosis of epiglottitis: Simplicity and reliability of radiographs of the neck in the differential diagnosis of the croup syndrome. J Pediatr. 1972;80:96-98.
36. Jones J. False positives in lateral neck radiographs used to diagnose epiglottitis. Ann Emerg Med. 1983;12:797.
37. Currarino G, Williams B. Lateral inspiration and expiration radiographs of the neck in children with laryngotracheobronchitis (croup). Radiology. 1982;195:365-366.
38. Stankiewicz J, Bowes A. Croup and epiglottitis: A radiologic study. Laryngoscope. 1985;95:1159-1160.
39. Newth C, Levison H, Bryan A. The respiratory status of children with croup. J Pediatr. 1972;81:1068-1073.
40. Loughlin G, Taussig L. Pulmonary function in children with a history of laryngotracheobronchitis. J Pediatr. 1979;94:365-369.
41. Miller M, Cherry J. Use of diagnostic virology laboratory. In: Feigin R, Cherry JS, eds. Textbook of Pediatric Infectious Diseases. 4th ed. Philadelphia: WB Saunders; 1998:2873-2891.
42. Storch G. Respiratory infections. In: Storch GS, ed. Essentials of Diagnostic Virology. 1st ed. St. Louis: Churchill Livingstone; 2000:59-78.
43. Olsen M, Shuck K, Sambol A. Isolation of seven respiratory viruses in shell vials: A practical and highly sensitive method. J Clin Microbiol. 1993;31:422-425.
44. Karron R, Froehlich P, Bobo L, et al. Rapid detection of parainfluenza virus type 3 RNA in respiratory specimens: Use of reverse transcription-PCR-enzyme immunoassay. J Clin Microbiol. 1994;32:484-488.
45. Freymuth F, Vabret A, Galateau-Salle F, et al. Detection of respiratory syncytial virus, parainfluenzavirus 3, adenovirus and rhinovirus sequences in respiratory tract of infants by polymerase chain reaction and hybridization. Clin Diagn Virol. 1997;8:31-40.
46. Weinberg G, Erdman D, Edwards K, et al. Viral diagnosis by polymerase chain reaction (PCR) is superior to that by cell culture in prospective, population-based study of pediatric acute respiratory infections (ARI). Presented at the IDSA 40th Annual Meeting, Chicago, Ill, October 24-27, 2002.
47. Abels S, Nadal D, Stroehle A, et al. Reliable detection of respiratory syncytial virus infection in children for adequate hospital infection control management. J Clin Microbiol. 2001;39:3135-3139.

48. Kehl S, Henrickson K, Hua W, et al. Evaluation of the Hexaplex assay for detection of respiratory viruses in children. J Clin Microbiol. 2001;39:1696-1701.
49. Hodinka R, Moshal K. Childhood infections. In: Storch GS, ed. Essentials of Diagnostic Virology. 1st ed. St. Louis: Churchill Livingstone; 2000:167-186.
50. Wildin S, Chonmaitree T, Swischuk L. Roentgenographic features of common pediatric viral respiratory tract infections. Am J Dis Child. 1988;142:43-46.
51. Denny F, Clyde W, Glezen W. *Mycoplasma pneumoniae* disease: Clinical spectrum, pathophysiology, epidemiology, and control. J Infect Dis. 1971;123:74-92.
52. Harari M, West B, Dwyer B. *Cryptosporidium* as cause of laryngotracheitis in an infant. Lancet. 1986;1:1207.
53. Baugh R, Gilmore B. Infectious croup: A critical review. Otolaryngol Head Neck Surg. 1986;95:40-46.
54. Bourchier D, Dawson K, Fergusson D. Humidification in viral croup: A controlled trial. Aust Paediatr J. 1984;20:289-291.
55. Henry R. Moist air in the treatment of laryngotracheitis. Arch Dis Child. 1983;58:577.
56. Osmond M. Croup. Clin Evid. 2002;June:297-306.
57. Lenney W, Milner A. Treatment of acute viral croup. Arch Dis Child. 1978;53:704-706.
58. Wolfsdorf J, Swift D. An animal model simulating acute infective upper airway obstruction of childhood and its use in the investigation of croup therapy. Pediatr Res. 1978;12:1062-1065.
59. Hall C, Hall W, Speers D. Clinical and physiological manifestations of bronchiolitis and pneumonia: Outcome of respiratory syncytial virus. Am J Dis Child. 1979;133:798-802.
60. Gussack G, Tacchi E. Pulse oximetry in the management of pediatric airway disorders. South Med J. 1987;80:1381-1384.
61. Newth C, Levison H. Upper airway obstruction in pediatric patients: Diagnosing and managing croup and epiglottitis. J Respir Dis. 1981;2:22-41.
62. Wright R, Pomerantz W, Luria J. New approaches to respiratory infections in children: Bronchiolitis and croup. Emerg Med Clin North Am. 2002;20:93-114.
63. Kristjansson S, Berg-Kelly K, Winso E. Inhalation of racemic adrenaline in the treatment of mild and moderately severe croup. Clinical symptom score and oxygen saturation measurements for evaluation of treatment effects. Acta Paediatr. 1994;83:1156-1160.
64. Gardner H, Powell K, Roden V, et al. The evaluation of racemic epinephrine in the treatment of infectious croup. Pediatrics. 1973;52:52-55.
65. Taussig L, Castro O, Beaudry P, et al. Treatment of laryngotracheobronchitis (croup). Use of intermittent positive-pressure breathing and racemic epinephrine. Am J Dis Child. 1975;129:790-793.
66. Waisman Y, Klein B, Boenning D, et al. Prospective randomized double-blind study comparing L-epinephrine and racemic epinephrine aerosols in the treatment of laryngotracheitis (croup). Pediatrics. 1992;89:302-306.
67. Westley C, Cotton E, Brooks J. Nebulized racemic epinephrine by IPPB for the treatment of croup: A double-blind study. Am J Dis Child. 1978;132:484-487.
68. Johnson D, Jacobson S, Edney P, et al. A comparison of nebulized budesonide, intramuscular dexamethasone, and placebo for moderately severe croup. N Eng J Med. 1998;339:498-503.
69. Geelhoed G, Turner J, Macdonald W. Efficacy of a small single dose of oral dexamethasone for outpatient croup: A double blind placebo controlled clinical trial. BMJ. 1996;313:140-142.
70. Cruz M, Stewart G, Rosenberg N. Use of dexamethasone in the outpatient management of acute laryngotracheitis. Pediatrics. 1995;96:220-223.
71. Ausejo M, Saenz A, Pham B, et al. The effectiveness of glucocorticoids in treating croup: Meta-analysis. BMJ. 1999;319:595-600.
72. Geelhoed G, Macdonald W. Oral dexamethasone in the treatment of croup: 0.15 mg/kg versus 0.3 mg/kg versus 0.6 mg/kg. Pediatr Pulmonol. 1996;20:362-368.
73. Kairys S, Olmstead E, O'Connor G. Steroid treatment of laryngotracheitis: A meta-analysis of the evidence from randomized trials. Pediatrics. 1989;83:683-693.
74. Sumboonnanonda A, Suwanjutha S, Sirinavin S. Randomized controlled trial of dexamethasone in infectious croup. J Med Assoc Thai. 1997;80:262-265.
75. Husby S, Agertoft L, Mortensen S, et al. Treatment of croup with nebulised steroid (budesonide): A double blind, placebo controlled study. Arch Dis Child. 1993;68:352-355.
76. Godden C, Campbell M, Hussey M, et al. Double blind placebo controlled trial of nebulised budesonide for croup. Arch Dis Child. 1997;76:155-158.
77. Roberts G, Master V, Staugas R, et al. Repeated dose inhaled budesonide versus placebo in the treatment of croup. J Paediatr Child Health. 1999;35:170-174.
78. Skolnik N. Treatment of croup. Am J Dis Child. 1989;143:1045-1049.
79. Pianosi P, Feldman W, Robson M, et al. Inappropriate use of antibiotics in croup at three types of hospital. Can Med Assoc J. 1986;134:357-359.
80. Phelan P, Landau L, Olinsily A. Respiratory illness in children. 2nd ed. Oxford: Blackwell Science; 1982:32-33.
81. Super D, Cartelli N, Brooks L, et al. A prospective randomized double-blind study to evaluate the effect of dexamethasone in acute laryngotracheitis. J Pediatr. 1989;115:323-329.
82. Kuusela A-L, Vesikari T. A randomized double-blind, placebo-controlled trial of dexamethasone and racemic epinephrine in the treatment of croup. Acta Paediatr Scand. 1988;77:99-104.
83. van Bever H, Wieringa M, Weyler J, et al. Croup and recurrent croup: Their association with asthma and allergy. An epidemiological study on 5-8-year-old children. Eur J Pediatr. 1999;158:253-257.

84. Hide D, Guyer B. Recurrent croup. Arch Dis Child. 1985;60:585-586.
85. Laufer P. The relationship of respiratory allergies to croup. J Asthma. 1986;23:9-10.
86. McEniery J, Gillis J, Kilham H, et al. Review of intubation in severe laryngotracheo-bronchitis. Pediatrics. 1991;87:847-853.
87. Jones R, Santos J, Overall J. Bacterial tracheitis. JAMA. 1979;242:721-726.
88. Donnelly B, McMillan J, Weiner L. Bacterial tracheitis: Report of eight new cases and review. Rev Infect Dis. 1990;12:729-735.
89. Long S. Bacterial tracheitis. Report on pediatric infectious diseases. 1992;2:29-31.

CHAPTER **54**

Otitis Externa, Otitis Media, and Mastoiditis

JEROME O. KLEIN

OTITIS EXTERNA

Infection of the external auditory canal (otitis externa) is similar to infection of skin and soft tissue elsewhere. Unique problems occur because the canal is narrow and tortuous; fluid and foreign objects enter, are trapped, and cause irritation and maceration of the superficial tissues. The pain and itching that result may be severe because of the limited space for expansion of the inflamed tissue. Infections of the external canal may be subdivided into four categories: acute localized otitis externa, acute diffuse otitis externa, chronic otitis externa, and malignant otitis externa. Reviews by Senturia and colleagues,[1] Hirsch,[2] and Rubin and Yu[3] provide more complete information.

Pathogenesis

The external auditory canal is approximately 2.5 cm long from the concha of the auricle to the tympanic membrane. The lateral half of the canal is cartilaginous; the medial half tunnels through the temporal bone. A constriction, the isthmus, present at the juncture of the osseous and cartilaginous portions, limits the entry of wax and foreign bodies to the area near the tympanic membrane. The skin of the canal is thicker in the cartilaginous portion and includes a well-developed dermis and subcutaneous layer. The skin lining the osseous portion is thinner and firmly attached to the periosteum and lacks a subcutaneous layer. Hair follicles are numerous in the outer third and sparse in the inner two thirds of the canal.

The microbial flora of the external canal is similar to the flora of skin elsewhere. There is a predominance of *Staphylococcus epidermidis, Staphylococcus aureus, Corynebacteria*, and, to a lesser extent, anaerobic bacteria such as *Propionibacterium acnes*.[4-6] Pathogens responsible for infection of the middle ear (*Streptococcus pneumoniae, Haemophilus influenzae*, or *Moraxella catarrhalis*) are uncommonly found in cultures of the external auditory canal when the tympanic membrane is intact.

The epithelium absorbs moisture from the environment. Desquamation and denuding of the superficial layers of the epithelium may follow. In this warm, moist environment, the organisms in the canal may flourish and invade the macerated skin. Inflammation and suppuration follow. Invasive organisms include those of the normal skin flora and gram-negative bacilli, particularly *Pseudomonas aeruginosa*. Invasive otitis media is a necrotizing infection frequently associated with *P. aeruginosa*. The organism gains access to the deeper tissues of the ear canal and causes a localized vasculitis, thrombosis, and necrosis of tissues. Diabetic microangiopathy of the skin overlying the temporal bone results in poor local perfusion and a milieu for invasion by *P. aeruginosa*.

Clinical Manifestations and Management

Acute localized *otitis externa* may occur as a pustule or furuncle associated with hair follicles; it is due to *S. aureus*. Erysipelas caused by group A *Streptococcus* may involve the concha and the canal. Pain may be severe. Bluish-red hemorrhagic bullae may be present on the osseous canal walls and also on the tympanic membrane. Adenopathy in the lymphatic drainage areas is often present. Local heat and systemic antibiotics are usually curative. Incision and drainage may be necessary to relieve severe pain.

Acute diffuse otitis externa (swimmer's ear) occurs mainly in hot, humid weather. The ear itches and becomes increasingly painful. The skin of the canal is edematous and red. Gram-negative bacilli, mainly *P. aeruginosa*, may play a significant role. A severe hemorrhagic external otitis due to *P. aeruginosa* was associated with mobile redwood hot tub systems.[7] Gentle cleansing to remove debris including irrigation with hypertonic saline (3%) and cleansing with mixtures of alcohol (70% to 95%) and acetic acid should be used initially. Hydrophilic solutions such as 50% Burrow's solutions may be used for 1 to 2 days to reduce inflammation. A 10-day regimen of a fluoroquinolone otic solution such as ofloxacin or ciprofloxacin-dexamethasone otic or ear drops of neomycin alone or with polymyxin combined with hydrocortisone are effective in reducing local inflammation and infection.[8]

Chronic otitis externa is due to irritation from drainage through a perforated tympanic membrane. The underlying cause is chronic suppurative otitis media. Itching may be severe. Management is directed to treatment of the middle ear disorder. Rare causes of chronic otitis externa include tuberculosis, syphilis, yaws, leprosy, and sarcoidosis.

Invasive ("malignant") otitis externa is a severe, necrotizing infection that spreads from the squamous epithelium of the ear canal to adjacent areas of soft tissue, blood vessels, cartilage, and bone.[3,9] Severe pain and tenderness of the tissues around the ear and mastoid are accompanied by the drainage of pus from the canal. Elderly, diabetic, immunocompromised, and debilitated patients are at particular risk. Life-threatening disease may result from spread to the temporal bone and then on to the sigmoid sinus, jugular bulb, base of the skull, meninges, and brain. Permanent facial paralysis is frequent, and cranial nerves 9, 10, and 12 may also be affected.[10] *Pseudomonas aeruginosa* is almost always the causative agent (see Chapter 216). The extent of damage to soft tissue and bone may be identified and monitored by the use of computed tomography and magnetic resonance imaging.[3] Diagnostic tests for underlying disease should be instituted. The canal should be cleansed, devitalized tissue removed, and ear drops with antipseudomonal antibiotics combined with steroid instilled into the external auditory canal. Systemic therapy with regimens including activity for *Pseudomonas* spp. should be used for 4 to 6 weeks. The combination of ceftazidime, cefepime, or piperacillin with an aminoglycoside (gentamicin or tobramycin) should be considered. Oral quinolones with activity against *Pseudomonas* spp., such as ciprofloxacin, have been effective therapy early in the course of invasive external otitis.[11]

Fungal otitis may be part of a general or local fungal infection. *Aspergillus* spp. are responsible for most cases of fungal otitis.[12] *Candida albicans* is a frequent cause of external otitis in children with chronic mucocutaneous candidiasis.

OTITIS MEDIA

Otitis media, or inflammation of the middle ear, is defined by the presence of fluid in the middle ear accompanied by signs or symptoms of acute illness. In 1990, there were an estimated 24.5 million visits made to offices of physicians in the United States at which the principal diagnosis was otitis media. For children younger than 15 years, otitis media was the most frequent diagnosis in physicians' office practices. Office visits with a principal diagnosis of otitis media increased from 9.9 million visits in 1975 to 24.5 million visits in 1990.[13] The peak incidence occurs in the first 3 years of life. The disease is less common in the school-aged child, adolescents, and adults. Nevertheless, infection of the middle ear may be the cause of fever, significant pain, and impaired hearing in these age groups. In addition, adults suffer from the sequelae of otitis media of childhood: hearing loss, cholesteatoma, adhesive otitis media, and chronic perforation of the tympanic membrane. A comprehensive review of otitis media is included in the text *Otitis Media in Infants and Children*.[14]

Epidemiology

By 3 years of age, more than two thirds of children have had one or more episodes of acute otitis media, and one third have had three or more episodes.[15] The highest incidence of acute otitis media occurs between 6 and 24 months of age. Subsequently, the incidence declines with age except for a limited reversal of the downward trend between 5 and 6 years of age, the time of school entry. Otitis media is infrequent in adults, but the bacteriology and therapy are similar to those in children.[16,17]

Longitudinal studies have provided information about the characteristics of children who have recurrent and severe episodes of acute otitis media. The vast majority of children have no obvious defect responsible for severe and recurrent otitis media, but a small number have anatomic changes (cleft palate, cleft uvula, submucous cleft), alteration of normal physiologic defenses (patulous eustachian tube), or congenital or acquired immunologic deficiencies. Children with acquired immunodeficiency syndrome have a higher age-specific incidence of otitis media, beginning at 6 months of age, than uninfected children or children who initially were positive for human immunodeficiency virus antibody but who seroreverted.[18]

As is true for most infectious diseases of childhood, acute otitis media occurs more often in males than in females. Correlation of the index child with severe or recurrent acute otitis media in a sibling or parent identifies a likely genetic susceptibility. The age at the time of the first episode of acute otitis media appears to be among the most powerful predictors of recurrent middle ear infections. Breast-feeding for 3 or more months is associated with a decreased risk of acute otitis media in the first year of life.[15] Race and ethnicity provide additional data suggesting a genetic basis for recurrent middle ear infections; Native Americans, Alaskan and Canadian Eskimos, and Australian aborigines have an extraordinary incidence and severity of otitis media.

The role of increased exposure to infectious agents and the importance of environmental pollutants are identified in studies of the incidence of infection in group daycare and the effects of passive smoking on children. The introduction of infants into large daycare groups increases the incidence of respiratory infections, including otitis media. The daycare risk of infection is associated with the number of children in the facility. Almost one episode of respiratory tract infections a month occurs during the first year of life, and acute otitis media is a complication of about one third to one half of the respiratory tract infections.[19] Passive smoking documented by a biochemical marker, the serum nicotine level, increased the incidence of new episodes of otitis media with effusion and the duration of effusion.[20] Kim and colleagues identified an association of invasive pneumococcal disease and otitis media with atmospheric conditions, air pollution, and the isolation of respiratory viruses.[21] The study documented an association between pneumococcal infection and levels of sulfur dioxide as a marker for air pollution.

Pathogenesis

The middle ear is part of a continuous system that includes the nares, nasopharynx, and eustachian tube medially and anteriorly, and the mastoid air cells posteriorly. These structures are lined with a respiratory epithelium that contains ciliated cells, mucus-secreting goblet cells, and cells capable of secreting local immunoglobulins.

Anatomic or physiologic dysfunction of the eustachian tube appears to play a critical role in the development of otitis media. The eustachian tube has at least three physiologic functions with respect to the middle ear: protection of the ear from nasopharyngeal secretions, drainage into the nasopharynx of secretions produced within the middle ear, and ventilation of the middle ear to equilibrate air pressure

with that in the external ear canal. When one or more of these functions is compromised, the results may be the development of fluid and infection in the middle ear. Congestion of the mucosa of the eustachian tube may result in obstruction. Secretions that are constantly formed by the mucosa of the middle ear accumulate behind the obstruction, and if a bacterial pathogen is present, a suppurative otitis media may result.

Microbiology

Bacteria

The bacteriology of otitis media has been documented by appropriate cultures of middle ear effusions obtained by needle aspiration. Many studies of the bacteriology of acute otitis media have been performed. The results are remarkably consistent in demonstrating the importance of *S. pneumoniae* and *H. influenzae* in all age groups (Table 54-1).[22,23]

S. pneumoniae is the most important bacterial cause of otitis media. Relatively few types are responsible for most disease. The most common types in order of decreasing frequencies are 19, 23, 6, 14, 3, and 18.[24-26] A 7 valent pneumococcal conjugate polysaccharide vaccine introduced in 2000 contains serotypes 4, 6B, 9V, 14, 18C, 19F, and 23F, which represent about 70% of serotypes responsible for acute otitis media.[27]

Otitis media due to *H. influenzae* is associated with nontypable strains in the vast majority of patients. In approximately 10%, the otitis is due to type B and should be preventable by immunization. Some of these patients appear to be in a very toxic state, and about one quarter have concomitant bacteremia or meningitis.[28] Nontypable strains of *H. influenzae* are a significant cause of otitis media in older children, adolescents, and adults.[16,17]

In 12 reports from the United States, Finland, and Canada, *M. catarrhalis* was isolated from a mean of 10% of children with acute otitis media (range 2% to 15%).[22,29,30] Before 1970, almost all strains of *M. catarrhalis* were sensitive to penicillin. Today most strains produce β-lactamase and are resistant to penicillin G, ampicillin, and amoxicillin.

Viruses

Virologic and epidemiologic data suggest that viral infection is frequently associated with acute otitis media.[31-33] In a study of children attending a daycare program, isolation of viruses from the upper respiratory tract was correlated with a clinical diagnosis of otitis media. Virus outbreaks coincided with epidemics of otitis media. Recent studies identify respiratory viruses[31] or viral antigens[32] in approximately one quarter of middle ear fluids of children with acute otitis media. Respiratory syncytial virus, influenza virus, enteroviruses, and rhinoviruses were the most common viruses found in middle ear fluids. Many patients with

TABLE 54-1 **Bacterial Pathogens Isolated from Middle Ear Fluid in Children with Acute Otitis Media, 1985-1992***

	Percentage[†] of Children with Pathogen	
Bacterial Pathogen	*Mean*	*Range*
Streptococcus pneumoniae	38	27-52
Haemophilus influenzae	27	16-52
Moraxella catarrhalis	10	2-15
Streptococcus, group A	3	0-11
Staphylococcus aureus	2	0-16
Miscellaneous bacteria	8	0-24
None or nonpathogens	28	12-35

*Data from twelve reports from the United States, Canada, Colombia, and Finland, 1985 to 1992: Harrison et al, 1985; Odoi et al, 1985; Rodriguez et al, 1985; Kaleida et al, 1986, 1987; Karma et al, 1986; Marchant et al, 1986; Bergeron et al, 1987; Carlin et al, 1987; Kenna et al, 1987; Trujillo et al, 1989; Del Beccaro et al, 1992.
[†]Total percentages are greater than 100% because of multiple pathogens per middle-ear effusion.
Modified from Bluestone CD, Klein JO. Microbiology. In: Otitis Media in Infants and Children, 3rd ed. Philadelphia: W.B. Saunders; 2001:79.

virus in middle ear fluid have a mixed viral-bacterial infection. It may be assumed that middle ear infection may occur with any respiratory virus that causes common cold signs, including the group of viruses of recent interest, the coronaviruses.[34] Respiratory signs may be prolonged in children with dual bacterial and viral infection.[35,36]

Mycoplasma, Chlamydia, and Unusual Organisms

Mycoplasma pneumoniae was responsible for hemorrhagic bullous myringitis in a study of nonimmune volunteers inoculated with the organism.[37] However, the middle ear fluid of a large number of patients (771) has been studied, and *M. pneumoniae* was isolated in only 1 case.[38,39] Although mycoplasmas do not appear to play a significant role in acute otitis media, some patients with lower respiratory tract disease due to *M. pneumoniae* may have concomitant otitis media.

Chlamydia trachomatis is associated with acute respiratory infections in infants younger than 6 months and is a cause of acute infection of the middle ear in this age group. The organism has been isolated from middle ear fluid of infants with acute infection.[40]

Uncommon forms of otitis include diphtheritic otitis, tuberculous otitis, otogenous tetanus, otitis due to *Mycobacterium chelonae*,[41] and otitis due to *Ascaris lumbricoides* or Wegener's granulomatosis.

Immunology

The middle ear is the site of a secretory immune system similar to those of other areas of the respiratory tract. Local and systemic immune responses occur in patients with acute or chronic otitis media with effusion. In the middle ear, immunologically active antigen interacts with immunocompetent cells in the lamina propria to produce a local immune response. The middle ear effusion that results from acute or chronic infection contains all the major classes of immunoglobulins, complement, cells, immune complexes of antigen and antibody, and various chemical mediators of inflammation. The role of these substances in the course of otitis media is uncertain. The immune response to various antigens may prevent subsequent infection, assist in clearance of fluid during the acute episode, or contribute to the accumulation and persistence of fluid in the middle ear cavity, which becomes the culture medium for the next infection.

Diagnosis and Clinical Course

Acute otitis media is defined by the presence of fluid in the middle ear along with signs or symptoms of acute illness. Signs and symptoms may be specific, such as ear pain, ear drainage, or hearing loss, or may be nonspecific, such as fever, lethargy, or irritability. Vertigo, nystagmus, and tinnitus may occur. Redness of the tympanic membrane is an early sign of otitis media, but erythema alone is not diagnostic of middle ear infection since it may be caused by inflammation of the mucosa throughout the upper respiratory tract.

The presence of fluid in the middle ear is determined by the use of pneumatic otoscopy, a technique that permits an assessment of the mobility of the tympanic membrane. The motion of the tympanic membrane is proportional to the pressure applied by gently squeezing and then releasing the rubber bulb attached to the head of the otoscope. Normal mobility is apparent when positive pressure is applied and the tympanic membrane moves rapidly inward; with release of the bulb and the resulting negative pressure, the membrane moves outward. Fluid or high negative pressure in the middle ear dampens the mobility of the tympanic membrane. Adjunctive techniques are available to confirm the results of otoscopic examinations and assist in the accuracy of diagnosis. Tympanometry uses an electroacoustic impedance bridge to record compliance of the tympanic membrane and middle ear pressure. This technique presents objective evidence of the status of the middle ear and the presence or absence of fluid.[42] Acoustic reflectometry measures sound reflectivity from the middle ear and is able to distinguish an air- or fluid-filled space. Spatial-gradient analysis is correlated with the probability of middle ear effusion in children.[43] In addition to a professional model, a consumer model (MDI Instruments) is available that permits home monitoring of the development or persistence of middle ear fluid.

Fluid persists in the middle ear for prolonged periods after the onset of acute otitis media even though symptoms usually resolve within a few days after the initiation of antimicrobial therapy. About 70% of children with otitis media have fluid in the middle ear 2 weeks after the onset of disease, 40% still have fluid 1 month after the onset, and 10% still have fluid 3 months after the first signs of middle ear infection.[14]

Patients with middle ear effusion suffer from hearing loss of variable severity. On average, a patient with fluid in the middle ear has a 25-dB (pure-tone average) loss.[44] Since development of speech, language, and cognitive skills is dynamic during infancy when the incidence of acute otitis media is highest, there is concern that any impediment to reception or interpretation of auditory stimuli might have an adverse effect. Children with histories of recurrent episodes of acute otitis media score lower in tests of speech, language, and cognitive abilities than do their disease-free peers.[45,46]

The results of microbiologic studies of middle ear effusions in patients with acute otitis media are so consistent that the choice of antimicrobial agents may be based on knowledge of the bacteriologic characteristics of otitis media acquired from the many investigations rather than the results of cultures from other sites such as the throat or nasopharynx (see Table 54-1). If the patient is toxic or has focal infection elsewhere, cultures of samples of the blood and of the focal infection are warranted. Needle aspiration of the middle ear effusion (tympanocentesis) to define the microbiological characteristics of the infection should be considered in selected patients: the patient who is critically ill at the onset, the patient who has not responded to initial antimicrobial therapy in 48 to 72 hours and is toxic, and the patient with altered host defenses (e.g., an immunologic defect, including the newborn infant).

Management

Acute Otitis Media

Antimicrobial Agents. The preferred antimicrobial agent for the patient with otitis media must be active against *S. pneumoniae*, *H. influenzae*, and *M. catarrhalis*. Group A streptococci and *S. aureus* are infrequent causes of acute otitis media and need not be considered in initial therapeutic decisions. Gram-negative enteric bacilli must be considered when otitis media occurs in the newborn infant, in the patient with a depressed immune response, and in the patient with suppurative complications of chronic otitis media. The antimicrobial agent should achieve concentrations in middle ear fluid above the expected minimal inhibitory concentration of the likely pathogens. Craig and Andes examined the relationship between bacteriologic cure in otitis media and serum and middle ear fluid concentrations for various antimicrobial agents.[47] They found that a bacteriologic cure required the presence of serum concentrations above the minimal inhibitory concentration for at least 70% of the dosing interval.

There are now 19 antimicrobial agents approved by the Food and Drug Administration for acute otitis media. Amoxicillin remains the drug of choice for initial treatment because of its 25-year record of clinical success, acceptability, limited side effects, and relatively low cost. The drug is ineffective against β-lactamase–producing strains of *H. influenzae* and *M. catarrhalis*. The current incidence of ampicillin-resistant *H. influenzae* and *M. catarrhalis* is not high enough to require a change in the initial therapy.

The recent recommendation of doubling the dose of amoxicillin to 80 mg/kg/day will achieve higher concentrations in middle ear fluid and further reduce the number of children in whom amoxicillin therapy will fail because of resistant pneumococci.[48] *H. influenzae* and *M. catarrhalis* are responsible for about 30% and 10% of acute otitis media cases, respectively. If 30% of the former and 75% of the latter are β-lactamase producing, then 16% of acute otitis media cases are caused by β-lactamase–producing organisms. If 50% improve spontaneously or despite β-lactamase activity, then less than 10% of the failures could be anticipated to be due to failure of amoxicillin to be active against β-lactamase–producing organisms. Alternatives to amoxicillin include amoxicillin-clavulanate, three sulfa- or trimethoprim-containing preparations (erythromycin plus sulfisoxazole, trimethoprim and trimethoprim-sulfamethoxazole), two macrolides (azithromycin and clarithromycin), nine oral cephalosporins (cephalexin, cefaclor, cefixime, ceftibuten, cefprozil, cefpodoxime, cefuroxime axetil, cefprozil, and cefdinir), one parenteral cephalosporin (ceftriaxone) and topical fluoroquinolones, and ciprofloxacin-dexamethasone otic, which are effective in children who have tympanostomy tubes and suffer acute otorrhea. An expert panel convened by the Centers for Disease Control and Prevention suggested amoxicillin in standard (40 mg/kg/day) or high dose (80 mg/kg/day) as the drug of choice. If the patient fails amoxicillin therapy, preferred regimens including an increased dosage schedule of amoxicillin clavulanate (80 to 90 mg/kg/day in two doses), cefuroxime axetil (cefdinir may be preferred by some children because of better taste), or intramuscular ceftriaxone. For children with severe and recurrent disease, the use of tympanocentesis to identify the bacterial pathogen and the susceptibility pattern may be necessary for choosing the most effective drug.[48] For children with known and severe allergy to beta-lactam antibiotics, a macrolide (erythromycin plus sulfisoxazole, azithromycin or clarithromycin) is the preferred drug but trimethoprim-sulfamethoxazole may be useful in regions where pneumococcal resistance to this combination is not a concern. The recommendations for antibiotics for acute otitis media have been revised in guidelines presented by the American Academy of Family Physicians in 2004.[67]

Some children with acute otitis media due to a bacterial pathogen improve without the use of antimicrobial agents.[49,50] Howie and Ploussard performed dual aspirates of middle ear fluid in children with acute otitis media 2 to 7 days apart with placebo given instead of an antibacterial drug: 19% of middle ear fluids infected initially with pneumococci became sterile; 48% of middle ear fluids infected initially with *H. influenzae* became sterile.[51] The discrepancy between the proportion of infections sterilized with the two bacterial species indicates that a simple mechanical effect (drainage of the infected fluid via a patent eustachian tube or a perforated tympanic membrane) was unlikely to be responsible for the microbiologic effect. A host mechanism (likely based on humoral or cellular immunity) acted preferentially to rid the ear of *H. influenzae* more frequently than of *S. pneumoniae*. The microbiologic results indicating that approximately one quarter of children have acute otitis media due to a viral pathogen and that some of the episodes of bacterial otitis media resolve without antibacterial drugs prompted some European physicians to withhold antibiotic therapy from children with ear infections.[52,53] Because physicians cannot distinguish children who may benefit from antimicrobial therapy from those who respond without treatment, representatives of the Centers for Disease Control and Prevention and the American Academy of Pediatrics concluded that physicians should continue to treat all patients with a diagnosis of acute otitis media.[54] An option of observation of children rather than initial antimicrobial therapy is practiced extensively in Western Europe.[55] A similar protocol for children with mild to moderate disease and/or "uncertain diagnosis" has been suggested in guidelines prepared by the American Academy of Pediatrics and American Academy of Family Physicians that were published in 2004. The recommendation to withhold antimicrobial agents from selected infants and children with acute otitis media will be controversial. Wald[56] pointed out that the evidence is not sufficient to conclude that the role of antibiotics is minimal in most cases of acute otitis media. Although the intent of those who encourage initial observation of acute otitis media is to curb overuse of the drug and decrease the resultant pressure for selection of resistant pathogens in the upper respiratory tract, overuse of antimicrobial agents for acute otitis media is due most frequently to misdiagnosis of middle ear effusion and inappropriate treatment of viral upper respiratory tract infections.

With appropriate antimicrobial therapy, most children with acute otitis media are significantly improved within 48 to 72 hours. If there is no improvement, the patient should be reexamined. Toxicity with persistent or recurrent fever or otalgia should prompt reevaluation of the patient. The child may have developed a new focus of infection or have received inadequate therapy.

Decongestants, Antihistamines, and Corticosteroids. Nasal and oral decongestants, administered either alone or in combination with an antihistamine, are used extensively for the treatment of otitis media with effusion. The use of the drugs is based on the consideration that they reduce congestion of the respiratory mucosa and relieve the obstruction of the eustachian tube that results from inflammation caused by respiratory infection. The results of clinical trials, however, indicate no significant evidence of efficacy of any of these preparations, used alone or in combination, for relief of signs of disease or a decrease in the time spent with middle ear effusion.[57,58] Although there are data suggesting efficacy of systemic corticosteroid therapy for the treatment of persistent middle ear effusion, particularly when combined with an antibiotic,[59] there are no studies of the use of corticosteroids alone or in combination with antimicrobial agents for amelioration or prevention of acute otitis media.

Prevention of Acute Otitis Media

Prevention of severe and recurrent episodes of acute otitis media includes chemoprophylaxis; the use of innovative substances such as oligosaccharides and xylitol; use of bacterial and viral vaccines; and surgery.

Chemoprophylaxis

Chemoprophylaxis has been shown to be of value for the prevention of acute illness in children who have suffered from recurrences of middle ear infections. A variety of studies including various antimicrobial agents and a placebo have documented the efficacy of an antimicrobial agent in modified dosage in reducing the number of episodes of acute febrile illnesses due to otitis media.[60-62] However, a modified dosage form of an antimicrobial agent may select resistant strains in the nasopharynx, and chemoprophylaxis should be considered only in children with severe and recurrent infections. On the basis of available information,[51] a protocol has been suggested that uses a once-a-day regimen of amoxicillin or sulfisoxazole during winter and spring, the periods of high incidence of infections of the respiratory tract. Children should be considered for prophylaxis if they have had two episodes of acute otitis media in the first 6 months of life or, in older children, three episodes in 6 months or four episodes in 1 year. Amoxicillin, 20-40 mg/kg, or sulfisoxazole, 50 mg/kg, may be administered once a day. Chemoprophylaxis may suppress symptoms of otitis media, but middle ear effusion may persist (though without apparent symptoms). The physician who chooses to use chemoprophylaxis to prevent acute recurrent disease must examine the patient at approximately 1-month intervals for middle ear effusion. Because of concerns for the development of resistance, the physician should be certain that the episodes of acute otitis media are well documented and that the chemoprophylaxis is warranted.[54]

Oligosaccharides

The concerns about antibiotic resistance have led to innovative approaches to chemoprophylaxis including the use of oligosaccharides to prevent adhesion of bacterial pathogens to respiratory mucosa and the use of xylitol to inhibit bacterial colonization. Carbohydrates or homologues have been suggested as materials that might interfere with bacterial attachment to respiratory mucosa. Oligosaccharides interfere with the establishment and progression of experimental pneumococcal pneumonia.[63] However, the only clinical trial of an oligosaccharide for prevention of acute otitis media failed to prevent new episodes.[64]

Xylitol

Xylitol is a polyol sugar alcohol produced from birch trees, strawberries, and other fruits that is effective in reducing dental caries, presumably because it inhibits the growth of *Streptococcus mutans*. Uhari and colleagues demonstrated in vitro reduction of growth of *S. pneumoniae* and a reduction in the number of episodes of acute otitis media in children who used daily xylitol chewing gum contrasted with those who used sucrose chewing gum.[65,66]

Xylitol administered during respiratory infections failed to prevent acute otitis media.

Pneumococcal Vaccines

Polysaccharide pneumococcal vaccines have been evaluated for the prevention of recurrences of acute otitis media in children.[68-70] As in previous studies, children younger than 2 years had unsatisfactory responses to single-dose regimens. A 7-valent conjugate pneumococcal polysaccharide vaccine employing CRM 197 as the protein carrier (Prevnar, Wyeth Lederle Vaccines) was approved by the FDA in February 2000. The vaccine (PCV 7) combined pneumococcal serotypes 4, 6B, 9V, 18C, 19F, and 23F and was demonstrated to be immunogenic in children as young as 2 months of age.[71] Antibody titers that were protective for prevention of invasive disease were achieved after doses administered at 2, 4, and 6 months but waned during the following 6 months, requiring a booster between the ages of 12 and 15 months.

PCV 7 was effective in preventing vaccine-type invasive disease (97.4% efficacy in children immunized per protocol)[71] and pneumonia (18% decrease for radiographically identifiable disease) but the results were more modest for prevention of acute otitis media.[27] The vaccine reduced the number of episodes of acute otitis media by 7% and reduced the number of procedures for placement of ventilating tubes by 23% (as a reflection of recurrent episodes requiring placement of tubes). Bacteriologic efficacy of PCV 7 was evaluated for prevention of acute otitis media in Finnish infants.[72] Bacteriologic diagnosis was based on aspiration of middle ear fluids in patients with acute otitis media who had completed the infant three dose schedule (Table 54-2). Similar to the study in Northern California, the vaccine reduced the incidence of acute otitis media by 6%. The reduction in number of episodes of pneumococcal acute otitis media was 34% but the reduction in episodes due to vaccine serotype disease was 57%. Of concern were increases in number of episodes of acute otitis media due to non-vaccine organisms in children who received PCV 7: a 33% increase in non-vaccine serotype pneumococcal acute otitis media; and an 11% increase in episodes due *to H. influenzae*. These data suggested that the vaccine was successful in reducing carriage of vaccine serotypes but that pneumococcal carriage was replenished with non-vaccine serotypes which subsequently spread from the upper respiratory tract to the middle ear to cause acute otitis media.

Respiratory Virus Vaccines

Because of the importance of respiratory viruses in the pathogenesis of acute otitis media, viral vaccines could be of preventive value. Inactivated parenteral influenza virus vaccines have been documented to decrease the incidence of acute otitis media in children in daycare

TABLE 54-2 Efficacy Of PCV7 in Finnish Children with Acute Otitis Media (AOM)

End Point	AOM Episodes		Vaccine Efficacy (%) Point Estimate
	PCV7 (N = 831)	Control* (N = 831)	
Any AOM	1251	1345	6
Pneumococcal AOM	271	414	34
Vaccine serotypes	107	250	57
Cross-reactive serotypes	41	84	51
Nonvaccine serotypes	125	95	−33
Haemophilus influenzae AOM	315	287	−11
Moraxella catarrhalis AOM	379	381	−1

*Hepatitis B vaccine.

Data from Eskola J, Kilpi T, Palmu A, et al. Efficacy of a pneumococcal conjugate vaccine against acute otitis media. N Engl J Med 2001;344(6): 403-409.

in Finland[73] and North Carolina.[74] A reduction of 30% of episodes of febrile otitis media was also reported in children after administration of live, attenuated intranasal influenza vaccine[75] Immunoprophylaxis against respiratory syncytial virus disease has progressed with use of high-titered RSV immune globulin[76] and the introduction of palivizumab, an RSV monoclonal antibody immune globulin with high titers of neutralizing RSV antibody.[77] The RSV immune globulin but not the monoclonal antibody was effective in reducing the number of episodes of acute otitis media.

Surgical Management

Surgical management of recurrent episodes of acute otitis media and persistent effusion of the middle ear includes use of myringotomy, adenoidectomy, and the placement of tympanostomy tubes. Myringotomy, or incision of the tympanic membrane, is a method of draining middle ear fluid. Before the introduction of antimicrobial agents, myringotomy was the major method of managing suppurative otitis media. Today, the use of myringotomy is limited to the relief of intractable ear pain, hastening resolution of mastoid infection, and drainage of persistent middle ear effusion that is unresponsive to medical therapy.

Enlarged adenoids may obstruct the orifice of the eustachian tube in the posterior portion of the nasopharynx and interfere with adequate ventilation and drainage of the middle ear. Studies of the use of adenoidectomy in children with prolonged effusions in the middle ear identify in selected children a beneficial effect in reducing the time spent with effusion.[78,79]

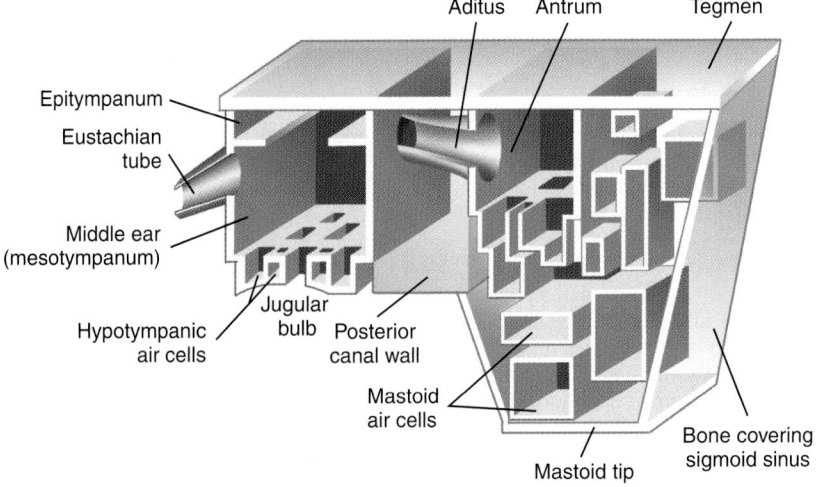

FIGURE 54-1. Diagrammatic representation of the anatomy of the middle and mastoid air cell system showing the narrow connection (aditus and antrum) between the two.

Tympanostomy tubes resemble small collar buttons. They are placed through an incision in the tympanic membrane to provide drainage of fluid and ventilation of the middle ear. The placement of these tubes is now one of the most common surgical procedures in children. The criteria for the placement of tubes include persistent middle ear effusions unresponsive to adequate medical treatment over a period of 3 months and persistent negative pressure. Hearing improves dramatically after placement of the ventilating tubes. The tubes have also been of value in patients who have difficulty maintaining ambient pressure in the middle ear such as would occur due to barotrauma in airline personnel. The liabilities of the placement of tubes include those of anesthesia associated with the procedure, persistent perforation, scarring of the tympanic membrane, the development of cholesteatoma, and otitis media caused by swimming with ventilating tubes in place, but these occur infrequently.

MASTOIDITIS

The proximity of the mastoid to the middle ear cleft suggests that most cases of suppurative otitis media are associated with inflammation of the mastoid air cells (Fig. 54-1). The incidence of clinically significant mastoiditis, however, is low since the introduction of antimicrobial agents. Nevertheless, acute and chronic disease still occur and may be responsible for significant morbidity and life-threatening disease.

Pathogenesis

At birth, the mastoid consists of a single cell, the antrum, connected to the middle ear by a small channel. Pneumatization of the mastoid bone takes place soon after birth and is extensive by 2 years of age. The clinical importance of the mastoid is related to contiguous structures including the posterior cranial fossa, the middle cranial fossa, the sigmoid and lateral sinuses, the canal of the facial nerve, the semicircular canals, and the petrous tip of the temporal bone. The mastoid air cells are lined with modified respiratory mucosa, and all are connected with the antrum.

Infection in the mastoid follows middle ear infection. Initially, there is hyperemia and edema of the mucosal lining of the air cells. Serous, then purulent exudate collects in the cells. Necrosis of bone due to pressure of the purulent exudate on the thin bony septa follows. Coalescence of pus in contiguous areas results in abscess cavities.

Clinical Manifestations

Acute mastoiditis is usually accompanied by acute infection in the middle ear. During early stages, the signs are those of acute otitis media with hearing loss, otalgia, and fever. Subsequently, swelling, redness, and tenderness are present over the mastoid bone. The pinna is displaced outward and downward. A purulent discharge may emerge through a perforation in the tympanic membrane.

Chronic otitis media with mastoiditis can erode through the roof of the antrum, causing temporal lobe abscess, or extend posteriorly, causing septic thrombosis of the lateral sinus.

Diagnosis

Radiographs of the mastoid area may show a loss of sharpness of the shadows of cellular walls due to demineralization of bony septa and cloudiness of areas of pneumatization due to inflammatory swelling of the air cells. Computed tomography is very helpful in delineating the extent of disease.

Cultures for bacteria from ear drainage fluid must be taken with care to distinguish fresh drainage fluid from material in the external canal. The canal must be cleaned and fresh pus obtained as it exudes from the tympanic membrane. If the tympanic membrane is not perforated, tympanocentesis should be performed to obtain material from the middle ear.

Management

The antimicrobial drugs of choice for acute infection are similar to those for acute otitis media: antibiotics with activity against *S. pneu-*

moniae and *H. influenzae.* If the disease in the mastoid has had a prolonged course, coverage for *S. aureus* and gram-negative enteric bacilli may be considered for initial therapy until the results of cultures become available.

A mastoidectomy is performed when an abscess has formed in the mastoid bone. The procedure should be performed at a time when antimicrobial agents have controlled sepsis.

REFERENCES

1. Senturia BH, Marcus MD, Lucente FE. Diseases of the External Ear. An Otologic Dermatologic Manual. 2nd ed. New York: Grune & Stratton; 1980.
2. Hirsch BE. Disease of the external ear. In: Bluestone CD, Stool SE, eds. Pediatric Otolaryngology. 3rd ed. Philadelphia: WB Saunders; 1996:378-387.
3. Rubin J, Yu VL. Malignant external otitis: Insights into pathogenesis, clinical manifestations, diagnosis, and therapy. Am J Med. 1988;85:391-398.
4. Riding KH, Bluestone CD, Michaels RH, et al. Microbiology of recurrent and chronic otitis media with effusion. J Pediatr. 1978;93:739-743.
5. Pelton SI, Teele DW, Shurin PA, et al. Disparate cultures of middle ear fluids. Am J Dis Child. 1980;134:951-953.
6. Brook I, Schwartz R. Anaerobic bacteria in acute otitis media. Acta Otolaryngol. 1981;91:111-114.
7. Centers for Disease Control and Prevention. Otitis due to *Pseudomonas aeruginosa* serotype 0:10 associated with mobile redwood hot tub systems—North Carolina. MMWR Morb Mortal Wkly Rep. 1982;31:541-542.
8. Myer CM III. Historical perspective on the use of otic antimicrobial agents. Pediatr Infect Dis J. 2001;20:98-101.
9. Doroghazi RM, Nadol JB, Hyslop NE, et al. Invasive external otitis. Am J Med. 1981;71:603-613.
10. Johnson MP, Ramphal R. Malignant external otitis: Report on therapy with ceftazidime and review of therapy and prognosis. Rev Infect Dis. 1990;12:173-180.
11. Rapoport Y, Shalit I, Redianu C, Himmelfarb MZ. Oral ofloxacin therapy for invasive external otitis. Ann Otol Rhinol Laryngol. 1991;100:632-637.
12. Phillips P, Bryce G, Shepherd J. Invasive external otitis caused by *Aspergillus.* Rev Infect Dis. 1990;12:277-281.
13. Schappert SM. Office visits for otitis media: United States, 1975-90. In: Vital and Health Statistics of the Centers for Disease Control/National Centers for Health Statistics. Atlanta: Centers for Disease Control and Prevention; 1992:214:3-18.
14. Bluestone CD, Klein JO. Otitis Media in Infants and Children. 3rd ed. Philadelphia: WB Saunders; 2001.
15. Teele DW, Klein JO, Rosner B. Epidemiology of otitis media during the first seven years of life in children in greater Boston: A prospective, cohort study. J Infect Dis. 1989;160:83-94.
16. Celin S, Bluestone C, Stephenson J, et al. Bacteriology of acute otitis media in adults. JAMA. 1991;266:2249-2252.
17. Schwartz LE, Brown RB. Purulent otitis media in adults. Arch Intern Med. 1992;152:2301-2304.
18. Barnett ED, Klein JO, Pelton SI, Luginbuhl LM. Otitis media in children born to human immunodeficiency virus–infected mothers. Pediatr Infect Dis J. 1992;11:360-364.
19. Schwartz B, Giebink GS, Henderson GW, et al. Respiratory infections in day care. Pediatrics. 1994;94:1018-1020.
20. Etzel RA, Pattishall EN, Haley NJ, et al. Passive smoking and middle ear effusion among children in day care. Pediatrics. 1992;90:228-232.
21. Kim PE, Musher DM, Glezen WP, et al. Association of invasive pneumococcal disease with season, atmospheric condition, air pollution, and the isolation of respiratory viruses. Clin Infect Dis. 1996;22:100-106.
22. Bluestone CD, Klein JO. Otitis media, atelectasis, and eustachian tube dysfunction. In: Bluestone CD, Stool SE, eds. Pediatric Otolaryngology. 3rd ed. Philadelphia: WB Saunders; 1996:388-582.
23. Del Baccaro MA, Mendelman PM, Inglis AF, et al. Bacteriology of acute otitis media: A new perspective. J Pediatr. 1992;120:81-84.
24. Kamme C, Ageberg M, Lundgren K. Distribution of *Diplococcus pneumoniae* types in acute otitis media in children and influence of the types on the clinical course in penicillin V therapy. Scand J Infect Dis. 1970;2:183-190.
25. Austrian R, Howie VM, Ploussard JH. The bacteriology of pneumococcal otitis media. Johns Hopkins Med J. 1977;141:104-111.
26. Gray BM, Converse GM, Dillion HC. Serotypes of *Streptococcus pneumoniae* causing disease. J Infect Dis. 1979;140:979-983.
27. Fireman B, Black SB, Shinefield HR, et al. Impact of the pneumococcal conjugate vaccine on otitis media. Pediatr Infect Dis J. 2003;22:10-16.
28. Harding AL, Anderson P, Howie VM, et al. *Haemophilus influenzae* isolated from children with otitis media. In: Sell SHW, Karzon DT, eds. *Haemophilus influenzae.* Nashville: Vanderbilt University Press; 1973:21.
29. Van Hare GF, Shurin PA, Marchant CD, et al. Acute otitis media caused by *Branhamella catarrhalis*: Biology and therapy. Rev Infect Dis. 1987;9:16-27.
30. Kovatch AL, Wald ER, Michaels RH. β-Lactamase–producing *Branhamella catarrhalis* causing otitis media in children. J Pediatr. 1983;102:261-264.
31. Chonmaitree T, Howie VM, Truant AL. Presence of respiratory viruses in middle ear fluids and nasal wash specimens from children with acute otitis media. Pediatrics. 1986;77:698-702.

32. Klein BS, Dallette ER, Volken RH. The role of respiratory syncytial virus and other viral pathogens in acute otitis media. J Pediatr. 1982;101:16-20.
33. Henderson FW, Collier AM, Sanyal MA, et al. A longitudinal study of respiratory viruses and bacteria in the etiology of acute otitis media with effusion. N Engl J Med. 1982;306:1377-1383.
34. Vabert A, Mourezz T, Gouarin S, et.al. An outbreak of coronavirus OC43 respiratory infection in Normandy, France. Clin Infect Dis. 2003;36:985-989.
35. Arola M, Ziegler T, Ruuskanen O. Respiratory virus infection as a cause of prolonged symptoms in acute otitis media. J Pediatr. 1990;116:697-701.
36. Chonmaitree T, Owen MJ, Patel JA, et al. Effect of viral respiratory tract infection on outcome of acute otitis media. J Pediatr. 1992;120:856-862.
37. Rifkind DR, Chanock RM, Kravetz H, et al. Ear involvement (myringitis) and primary atypical pneumonia following inoculation of volunteers with Eaton agent. Am Rev Respir Dis. 1962;85:479-489.
38. Klein JO, Teele DW. Isolation of viruses and mycoplasma from middle ear effusions: A review. Ann Otol Rhinol Laryngol. 1976;85:140-144.
39. Sobeslavsky O, Syrucek L, Bruckoya M, et al. The etiological role of *Mycoplasma pneumoniae* in otitis media in children. Pediatrics. 1965;35:652-657.
40. Tipple MA, Beem MO, Saxon EM. Clinical characteristics of the afebrile pneumonia associated with *Chlamydia trachomatis* infection in infants less than 6 months of age. Pediatrics. 1979;63:192-197.
41. Lowry PW, Jarvis WR, Oberle AD, et al. *Mycobacterium chelonae* causing otitis media in an ear-nose-and-throat practice. N Engl J Med. 1988;391:978-982.
42. Brookhouser PE. Use of tympanometry in office practice for diagnosis otitis media. Pediatr Infect Dis J. 1998;17:544-551.
43. Kimball S. Acoustic reflectometry: Spectral gradient analysis for improved detection of middle ear effusion in children. Pediatr Infect Dis J. 1998;17:522-555.
44. Fria TJ, Cantekin EI, Eichler JA. Hearing acuity of children with effusion. Arch Otolaryngol. 1985;111:10-16.
45. Holm VA, Kunze LH. Effects of chronic otitis media on language and speech development. Pediatrics. 1969;43:833-839.
46. Teele DW, Klein JO, Chase C, et al. Otitis media in infancy and intellectual ability, school achievement, speech and language at age 7 years. J Infect Dis. 1990;162:685-694.
47. Craig WA, Andes D. Pharmacokinetics and pharmacodynamics of antibiotics in otitis media. Pediatr Infect Dis J. 1996;15:255-259.
48. Dowell SF, Butler J, Giebink FS, et al. Acute otitis media: Management and surveillance in an era of pneumococcal resistance—A report from the Drug-resistant *Streptococcus pneumoniae* Therapeutic Working Group. Pediatr Infect Dis J. 1999;18:1-9.
49. Kaleida PH, Casselbrant ML, Rockette HE, et al. Amoxicillin or myringotomy or both for acute otitis media: Results of a randomized clinical trial. Pediatrics. 1991;87:466-474.
50. Marchant CD, Carlin SA, Johnson CE, Shurin PA. Measuring the comparative efficacy of antibacterial agents for acute otitis media: The "Pollyanna phenomenon." J Pediatr. 1992;120:72-77.
51. Howie VM, Ploussard JH. The "in-vivo sensitivity test": Bacteriology of middle ear exudate during antimicrobial therapy in otitis media. Pediatrics. 1969;44:940-944.
52. Van Buchem FL, Dunk JH, van't Hof MA. Therapy of acute otitis media: Myringotomy, antibiotics or neither? A double-blind study in children. Lancet. 1981:2:883-887.
53. Browning GG. Childhood otalgia: Acute otitis media. BMJ. 1990;300:1005-1007.
54. Dowell SF, Marcy SM, Phillips WR, et al. Otitis media: Principles of judicious use of antimicrobial agents. Pediatrics. 1998;101:165-171.
55. van Buchem FL, Peeters MF, van't Hof MA. Acute otitis media: A new treatment strategy. Br Med J 1985;290:1033-1037.
56. Wald ER. Acute otitis media: More trouble with the evidence. Pediatr Infect Dis J. 2003;22:103-104.
57. Cantekin EI, Mandel EM, Bluestone CD. Lack of efficacy of a decongestant-antihistamine combination for otitis media with effusion ("secretory" otitis media) in children. N Engl J Med. 1983;308:297-301.
58. Bluestone CD, Connell JT, Doyle WJ, et al. Symposium: Questioning the efficacy and safety of antihistamines in the treatment of upper respiratory infection. Pediatr Infect Dis J. 1988;7:15-42.
59. Berman S. Medical management of children with otitis media with effusion. In: The Report on Pediatric Infectious Diseases. New York: Churchill Livingstone; 1993:37-38.
60. Perrin JM, Charney E, MacWhinney JB, et al. Sulfisoxazole as chemoprophylaxis for recurrent otitis media: A double-blind crossover study in pediatric practice. N Engl J Med. 1974;291:664-667.
61. Maynard JE, Fleshman JK, Tschopp CF. Otitis media in Alaskan Eskimo children: Prospective evaluation of chemoprophylaxis. JAMA. 1972;219:597-599.
62. Klein JO, Bluestone CD. Acute otitis media: Management of pediatric infectious diseases in office practice. Pediatr Infect Dis J. 1982;1:66-73.
63. Idänpään-Heikkilä I, Simon PM, Zopf D, et al. Oligosaccharides interfere with the establishment and progression of experimental pneumococcal pneumonia. J Infect Dis. 1997;176:704-712.
64. Ukkonen P, Varis K, Jernfors M, et al. Treatment of acute otitis media with an antiadhesive oligosaccharide: A randomized, double-blind, placebo controlled trial. Lancet. 2000;356:1398-1402.
65. Uhari M, Kontiokari T, Koskela M, Niemelä M. Xylitol chewing gum in prevention of acute otitis media: Double blind randomized trial. BMJ. 1996;313:1180-1184.
66. Uhari M, Kontiokari T, Niemela M. A novel use of xylitol sugar in preventing acute otitis media. Pediatrics. 1998;102:879-884.
67. Subcommittee on Management of Acute Otitis Media: American Academy of Pediatrics, American Academy of Family Physicians. Clinical Practice Guideline. Diagnosis and Management of Acute Otitis Media. Pediatrics. (In press.)
68. Teele DW, Klein JO, the Greater Boston Collaborative Study Group. Use of pneumococcal vaccine for prevention of recurrent acute otitis media in infants in Boston. Rev Infect Dis. 1981;3(Suppl):S113-S118.
69. Sloyer JL, Ploussard JH, Howie VM. Efficacy of pneumococcal polysaccharide vaccine in preventing acute otitis media in infants in Huntsville, Alabama. Rev Infect Dis. 1981;3(Suppl):S119-S123.
70. Makela PH, Leinonen M, Pukander J, et al. A study of the pneumococcal vaccine in prevention of clinically acute attacks of recurrent otitis media. Rev Infect Dis. 1981;3(Suppl):S124-S132.
71. Black S, Shinefield H, Fireman B, et al. Efficacy, safety and immunogenicity of heptavalent pneumococcal conjugate vaccine in children. Pediatr Infect Dis J. 2000; 19:187-195.
72. Eskola J, Kilpi T, Palmu A, et al. Efficacy of a pneumococcal conjugate vaccine against acute otitis media. N Engl J Med. 2001;344:403-409.
73. Heikkinen T, Ruuskanen O, Waris M, et al. Influenza vaccination in the prevention of acute otitis media in children. Am J Dis Child. 1991;145:445-448.
74. Clements DA, Langdon L, Bland C, et al. Influenza A vaccine decreases the incidence of otitis media in 6 to 30 month old children in day care. Arch Pediatr Adolesc Med. 1995;149:1113-1117.
75. Belshe RB, Mendelman PM, Treanor J, et al. The efficacy of live attenuated, cold-adapted, trivalent, intranasal influenza virus vaccine in children. N Engl J Med. 1998;338:1459-1461.
76. Simoes EA, Groothuis JR, Tristram DA, et al. Respiratory syncytial virus–enriched globulin for the prevention of acute otitis media in high risk children. J Pediatr. 1996;129:214-219.
77. Impact-RSV Study Group. Palivizumab, a humanized respiratory syncytial virus monoclonal antibody, reduces hospitalization from respiratory syncytial virus infection in high-risk infants. Pediatrics. 1998;102:531-537.
78. Paradise JL, Bluestone CD, Rogers KD, et al. Efficacy of adenoidectomy in recurrent otitis media: Historical overview and preliminary results from a randomized, controlled trial. Ann Otol Rhinol Laryngol. 1980;89:319-321.
79. Gates GA, Avery CA, Prihoda TJ, et al. Effectiveness of adenoidectomy and tympanostomy tubes in the treatment of chronic otitis media with effusion. N Engl J Med. 1987;317:1444-1451.

CHAPTER **55**

Sinusitis

JACK M. GWALTNEY, JR.

ACUTE

Sinusitis is an inflammatory condition of one or more of the paranasal sinuses. Most acute cases result from infection, although other causes including allergy may be responsible. Acute infectious sinusitis can be classified into various categories on the basis of several characteristics including its occurrence in the community or hospital setting, the immune status of the patient, and its viral, bacterial, or fungal etiology (Table 55-1). Recognizing these categories and using precise terminology are important to understand the pathogenesis and clinical characteristics and to optimize the approach to diagnosis and treatment of the disease.

Managing cases of acute community-acquired sinusitis is a challenge for physicians because of the difficulty to make an etiologic diagnosis with accuracy and to evaluate the effectiveness of treatment with precision. These problems would not exist if the paranasal sinuses were accessible to direct examination and to noninvasive sampling for microbial culture. Because they are not, physicians have traditionally relied on clinical findings that are either insensitive or nonspecific to diagnosis of the condition.[1] Adding further complexity to the problem was the discovery that sinus disease is an inherent part of the common cold syndrome, and that a high proportion of patients with colds have viral sinusitis.[2] Thus, the common cold is in reality a viral rhinosinusitis (VRS), not simply a rhinitis as traditionally held. An unawareness of the existence of viral sinusitis led to confusion in the past because all *acute sinusitis* was considered to be of bacterial etiology. Cases of viral etiology were misdiagnosed in clinical practice

TABLE 55-1 Classification of Acute Sinusitis

Patient with Normal Immunity

Infectious
Community-acquired
   Viral
   Viral-bacterial
   Bacterial
   Fungal (noninvasive)
   Nonallergic
   Allergic
   Fungus ball
Nosocomial
   Bacterial
   Fungal

Noninfectious
Allergic
Toxic

Immunocompromised Patient
Viral
Bacterial
Fungal (invasive)

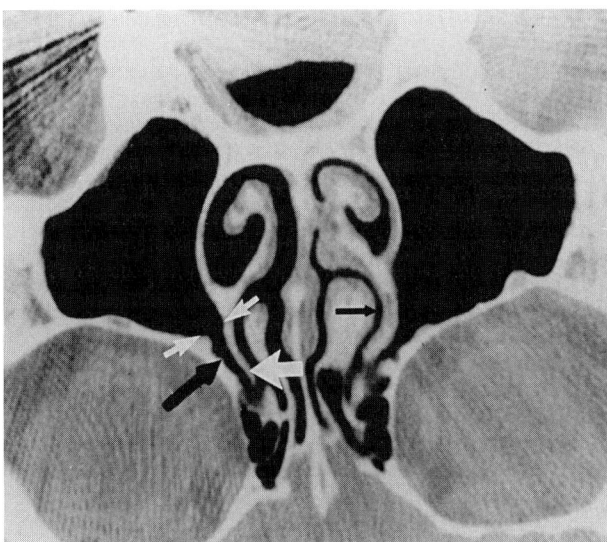

FIGURE 55-1. Selected features of the anatomy of the drainage system of the maxillary sinus shown on computed tomography scan. The ostium is located between the two *small white arrows*. The ostium opens into a tubular structure, the infundibulum, shown by the *large black arrow*. The *large white arrow* indicates the upper part of the uncinate process, which forms the inferior portion of the infundibulum. The infundibulum empties into the middle meatus. The *small black arrow* indicates the contralateral middle meatus, which is narrowed as a result of turbinal distention from the normal nasal cycle.

and misclassified in clinical trials.[3] It is still true that without the benefit of sinus aspirate culture, a distinction between acute viral sinusitis and acute community-acquired bacterial sinusitis (ACABS) cannot be made with assurance.

Anatomy and Physiology

Paranasal pneumaticity, the antorbital cavity, originated in animals somewhat earlier than the common ancestor of the dinosaurs.[4] A similar structure, the maxillary sinus, arose in the evolutionary line leading to humans. The ethmoid, frontal, and sphenoid sinuses are of more recent origin and have been described as characteristic of conventional mammals.[5] The function of the paranasal sinuses remains somewhat in doubt. It has been proposed that sinuses reduce the bony mass and weight of the skull, participate in warming and humidification of inspired air, and add resonance to the voice.

The maxillary sinus has a pyramidal shape, with the base of the pyramid formed by the lateral wall of the nasal cavity, and the apex extending toward the zygomatic process (Fig. 55-1). In the adult, the maxillary sinus cavity has a volume of 15 to 30 mL. The sinus is lined with ciliated pseudostratified epithelium and is covered with a mucous blanket. The epithelium is well supplied with goblet cells (Table 55-2).[6,7] In contrast, seromucous gland densities in the sinus cavity are low compared with those in the nasal passages.[8]

The maxillary ostium is located on the highest part of the medial wall of the sinus cavity (see Fig. 55-1). It is connected to the nasal cavity by a small tubular passage, the infundibulum, which is encased in bone and lies directly under the lamina papyracea of the orbit. The infundibulum leads to the hiatus semilunaris of the middle meatus, which is posterolateral to the uncinate process in a shielded location. The anterior ethmoid and frontal sinuses also empty into the middle meatus. This area and the region of the anterior ethmoid are described together as the ostiomeatal complex.

The infundibulum is approximately 6 mm in length and has an average diameter of 3 mm, which is of adequate size to drain 30 mL (the maxillary sinus volume) of water by gravity in approximately 11 seconds. Mucus and other fluids produced in the maxillary sinus cavity are transported by ciliary action in a spiral direction up to and through the infundibulum and delivered into the hiatus semilunaris of the middle meatus.[9,10] Mucociliary transit times of 4.6 to 12.3 mm/minute have been measured in the nose[11] and are presumably similar in the sinus. The mucous blanket changes two to three times each hour,[12] and normally, mucus does not accumulate in the sinus cavity.

In 10% to 30% of adults, the maxillary sinus cavity is connected to the nasal passage by one or more accessory ostia that are located infe-

riorly to the infundibulum in the area of the anterior and posterior nasal fontanelles. The fontanelles are areas of very thin bone or membrane located in the lateral nasal wall at the level of the middle meatus and lie anteriorly and posteriorly to the uncinate process. Accessory ostia are created when fontanelles rupture.

The paranasal sinuses, although directly connected to the nasal passages, which are colonized with bacteria,[13] are themselves sterile under normal conditions.[14-17] Sterility is maintained in the sinus by mechanisms that are not fully understood but are believed to include mucociliary clearance, the immune system, and possibly antibacterial concentrations of nitric oxide gas in the sinus cavity.[18]

Epidemiology

In the United States, the incidence of the common cold (VRS) in children is six to eight and in adults two to three episodes per person per year.[19] VRS rates follow a well-established seasonal pattern with annual epidemics in the fall, winter, and spring and periods of relative inactivity during the summer. The periods of high prevalence for rhinovirus are early fall and late spring, and for coronavirus, respiratory

TABLE 55-2 Density (per mm²) of Mucus-Producing Structures in the Nasal Passages and Paranasal Sinuses

Site	No. of Goblet Cells*	No. of Seromucous Glands†
Nasal passages	5700-11,000	8
Sinuses		
Maxillary	9700	0.2
Ethmoid	6500	0.5
Frontal	5900	0.08
Sphenoid	6200	0.05

*Data from Morgensen C, Tos M. Density of goblet cells in the normal adult human nasal septum. Anat Anz. 1977;141:237-247.

†Data from Morgensen C, Tos M. Quantitative histology of the maxillary sinus. Rhinology. 1977;55:129-140; and Morgensen C, Tos M. Quantitative histology of the normal sphenoid sinus. Rhinology. 1978;56:203-213.

syncytial virus, and influenza, winter and early spring. A small proportion of VRS episodes are, in turn, complicated by an acute bacterial infection of the sinus. This has been reported to occur in 0.5% to 2% of cases.[20,21] The seasonal trends in the incidence of presumed bacterial sinusitis have been shown to correlate with those of VRS.[22] In addition to VRS-related cases, ACABS occurs throughout the year, and is associated with allergy, swimming, and nasal obstruction due to polyps, foreign bodies, and tumors. Other less common risk factors are immune deficiencies such as agammaglobulinemia and acquired immunodeficiency syndrome; abnormalities of white cell function as found in chronic granulomatous disease; structural defects, especially cleft palate; and disorders of mucociliary clearance including cilial dysfunction and cystic fibrosis. Based on epidemiologic studies, approximately 1 billion cases of VRS can be expected to occur annually in the United States (260 million people [adults and children] × 4 acute respiratory illnesses = 1 billion cases or more of VRS annually), and these, in turn, can be expected to be complicated by 20 million cases of ACABS, assuming a 2% complication rate.

Pathogenesis

Viral

A central feature of rhinovirus pathogenesis is the virus's ability to evade the host's protective defenses in the upper airway. The vulnerability of the nose to rhinovirus is shown by the fact that intranasal inoculation of virus in nonimmune volunteers routinely leads to a 90% or greater infection rate.[23] After infection, however, only three quarters of persons develop symptoms of a cold, and the rest have an inapparent infection. Viral deposition in the nose is followed by transport to the posterior nasopharynx[24] and attachment to the rhinovirus receptor, intercellular adhesion molecule 1 (ICAM-1).[25] In posterior pharyngeal biopsies, ICAM-1 has been located on M (membranous) cells present in the adenoid crypts, but not on adjacent ciliated epithelial cells.[26,27] Nucleic acid probe studies have shown only sparse and scattered foci of rhinovirus infection in biopsies of nasal turbinates of experimentally infected volunteers.[28] Infection leads to the activation of several inflammatory pathways and of the parasympathetic nervous system, causing engorgement of the capacitance vessels in the venous erectile tissue of the nasal turbinates, intercellular leakage of plasma into the nose and presumably sinuses, discharge of seromucous glands and goblet cells, and stimulation of pain nerve and sneeze and cough reflexes.[29]

Reversible sinus cavity abnormalities were observed on CT scan in 87% of adults with early natural colds and included all the sinuses (Table 55-3).[2] Also, the infundibulum was occluded in 77% of patients, and the ostiomeatal complex was also frequently congested. In a recent study of children with colds of an average duration of 6 days, reversible abnormalities in the sinus cavity were observed with MRI in 88% of cases.[30] Another study of adults with colds of 1 week duration using sinus x-rays found sinus cavity abnormalities in 39% of the patients.[31] The presence of air bubbles in the material seen on computed tomography (CT) and the irregular distribution of the material

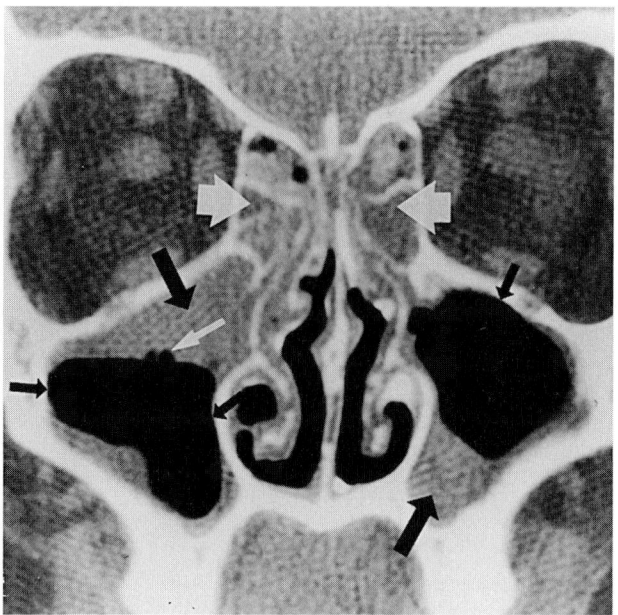

FIGURE 55-2. Sinus computed tomography scan from an adult with a common cold of 4 days' duration shows abnormalities of the roof and floor of the maxillary sinuses (*large black arrows*). Gaseous bubbles in the material (*small white arrow*) and its irregular distribution along the walls of the sinus cavity suggest that it is thick exudate adherent to the sinus wall and not mucosal swelling. The *small black arrows* show portions of the air-bone interfaces of the sinus wall, which are normal. The uneven distribution of the abnormalities is not compatible with mucosal swelling, which would be expected to be more uniform. Bilateral disease of the ethmoid sinuses is also present (*large white arrows*).

on the walls of the sinus suggest the presence of a highly viscous exudate that is adherent to the floor, sides, and, in some cases, ceiling of the sinus cavity (Fig. 55-2).

The source and composition of the material in the sinus cavity are unknown. A recent study suggests that during colds, nose blowing may propel nasal fluid into the site.[32] In that study, nose blowing, but not sneezing or coughing, elevated intranasal pressures, which transiently reached levels of 60 to 80 mm of mercury (Fig. 55-3). Also nose blowing, but not sneezing or coughing, propelled contrast medium from the nasopharynx into the sinus cavity. If nose blowing during colds is responsible for propelling nasal fluid into the sinus cavity, it could explain the appearance of the viscous exudates observed on CT scan. During colds, nasal fluid contains viruses, bacteria, and inflammatory mediators that are capable of producing infection and/or inflammation in the sinus cavity. The high concentration of goblet cells in the sinus epithelium[6-8] provides a ready source of mucus when stimulated. Also, it has recently been demonstrated that as a result of transudation of plasma, cross-linked fibrin is present in the nasal fluid of patients with colds and presumably also in sinus fluid at the same time.[33] If so, there may, at times, be the formation of an actual clot that would further enhance the viscosity of the sinus cavity exudates. Sequential sinus CT scans in patients with VRS showed a failure of the cilia to move deposits of the material toward the ostium over a period of hours (Fig. 55-4).[34] Thus, malfunction of mucociliary clearance, because of the presence of viscous exudate, has as important a role in the pathogenesis of acute sinus disease as does infundibular occlusion. Viruses have been recovered from sinus cavity aspirates taken from patients with acute community-acquired sinusitis,[35] but it is not clear if viral infection of the cavity is necessary to cause the disease. The erratic distribution of the abnormalities seen in different sinuses of the same patient is compatible with the hypothesis that nasal fluid pro-

TABLE 55-3 Frequency of Sinus Imaging Abnormalities in Adults and Children with Common Colds

Abnormality	Adults* (CT, %)	Children† (MRI, %)
Occlusion of infundibulum	77	NR‡
Abnormality of sinus cavity		
Maxillary	87	75
Ethmoid	65	83
Frontal	32	28
Sphenoid	39	45

*ref 2
†ref 30
‡Not reported.

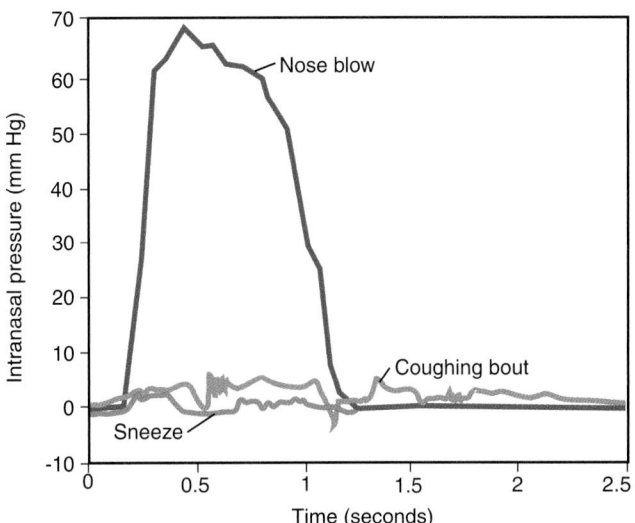

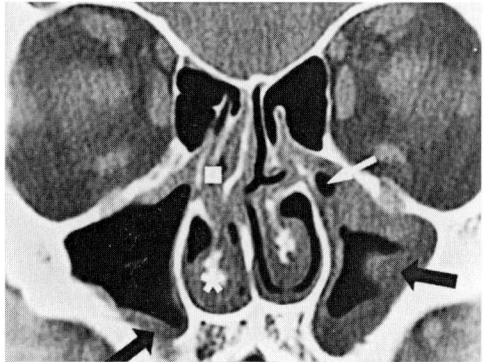

A

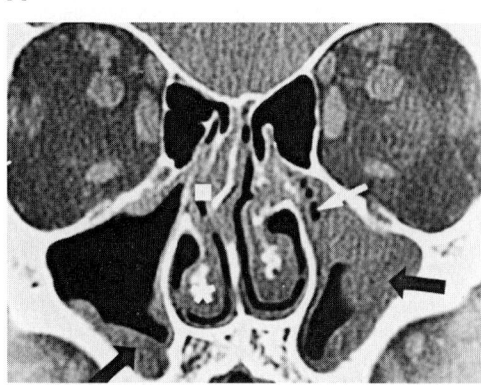

B

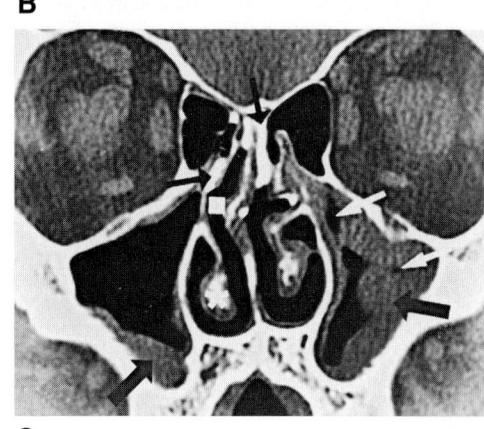

C

FIGURE 55-3.   Intranasal pressure (mm Hg) over time (in seconds) for a representative nose blow, coughing bout, and sneeze shown on the same scale for comparison (*dashed line*, nose blow; *solid line*; coughing bout; *dotted line*, sneeze).

pelled into the sinuses by nose blowing is responsible for the process since this would be expected to occur in a random fashion.

Bacterial

The nasal passages and nasopharynx are colonized with the same bacterial species that cause ACABS,[13] and, undoubtedly, the bacteria in these areas serve as the reservoir for this infection. As discussed above, nose blowing creates intranasal pressures that deposit nasal fluid containing these bacteria into the sinus cavity.[32] In a rabbit model, the introduction of *Streptococcus pneumoniae* or *Haemophilus influenzae* into an acutely obstructed maxillary sinus led to infection and disease, whereas obstruction of the sinus ostium without bacterial instillation did not.[36,37] Once bacteria are deposited into the cavity of an obstructed sinus, growth conditions are favorable, as indicated by the high titers attained, which are present in sinus aspirates at concentrations of up to 10^7 colony-forming units per milliliter.[15] Cases of ACABS were also associated with a leukocytosis of 10,000 or more white blood cells per millimeter[3] in sinus aspirates. Granulocyte phagocytosis may be impaired by the reduced oxygen tension present in an obstructed sinus.

Although experimental sinus infection in the rabbit model leads to marked destruction of ciliated epithelial cells,[37-39] in humans, the histopathologic changes of acute bacterial sinusitis have been observed in the lamina propria.[40] These changes include edema, massive infiltration of neutrophils, increases in lymphocytes and plasma cells, microabscesses, and, in severe cases, thrombosed blood vessels and necrotic foci. Acute bacterial sinusitis in humans is a process of sufficient severity to require several weeks to heal. Studies using serial sinus imaging have shown resolving cavitary abnormalities that persist after clinical complaints have resolved.[15,41,42] In a study of 13 adults, serial sinus MRI examinations showed a rapid increase in the mean aeration of the sinus cavity during the first 10 days of observation, but this was then followed by a slow resolution for up to day 56, the last day of observation.[42] The mean aeration had only approached 80% when observations were discontinued.

FIGURE 55-4.   Serial sinus computed tomography scan from an adult with a common cold of 4 days' duration. **A,** Scan taken at 2:00 PM. There are abnormalities in both maxillary sinuses (*black arrows*). A gaseous bubble is present on the right (*white arrow*), indicating that the material causing the abnormality is thick fluid. The nasal turbinates are engorged (*asterisk*), and the middle meatus is congested (*square*). Immediately after the scan was obtained, the patient was given 60 mg of pseudoephedrine orally. **B,** Scan taken at 4:00 PM on the same day. The material in the maxillary sinuses (*black arrows*) has not moved, and the findings are essentially unchanged after treatment with pseudoephedrine. The turbinates remain engorged (*asterisk*) and the middle meatus congested (*square*). Immediately after the scan was obtained, the patient was given two intranasal sprays of .05% oxymetazoline. **C,** Scan taken 10 minutes after oxymetazoline administration, showing shrinkage of the turbinates (*asterisk*) and decongestion of the middle meatus (*square*). Omnipaque dye was given intranasally immediately before the scan with the patient supine and is present in the middle meatus and olfactory recess (*small black arrows*). The location of the material in the maxillary sinus cavities (*large black arrows*) has not changed.

Microbial Cause

Specimen Collection

The method of specimen collection is critical to determine the accuracy of sinus culture results. Unless sinus cavity specimens are collected without contamination by nasal secretions, there is always the danger that the specimens will yield bacteria that are growing in the nose instead of the sinus. For this reason, sinus cavity culture obtained by puncture and aspiration has been the gold standard for microbial diagnosis (Table 55-4). Sinus puncture is a relatively painless and safe procedure when performed by an experienced operator, although it is not appropriate for routine clinical use. The bacteria recovered from sinus aspirates in experimental studies have been associated with findings including high titers, correlation with Gram stain, and association with leukocytosis which confirm their pathogenic role.[15]

It is not possible to enter the sinus cavities with an endoscope by way of the natural ostia. With the maxillary sinus, the sheltered location of the hiatus semilunaris, behind the turbinate and uncinate process, and the small diameter of the infundibulum and its acute angle relative to the lower nasal passage make it physically impossible to pass an endoscope into the cavity (see Fig. 55-1).[43] It may be possible to enter the maxillary sinus cavity in some of the 10% to 30% of persons with accessory ostia, but to do so without contaminating the specimen with nasal secretions is difficult or impossible. Therefore, the endoscopic approach is actually directed at sampling secretions in the middle meatus. It is not clear whether the middle meatus is normally sterile or is colonized or contaminated with nasopharyngeal bacteria. In patients with acute viral upper respiratory infection who have excessive secretions in the nasal passages, the possibility of contamination appears great. In a study of 47 patients with ACABS, endoscopic sampling had a sensitivity of 65% and a specificity of 40% compared with sampling by sinus aspiration.[44] The sensitivity (79%) and specificity (85%) were improved when the data were analyzed for only *S. pneumoniae*, *H. influenzae*, and *Moraxella catarrhalis*, but this ignores other relevant pathogens including beta hemolytic streptococci, pus-forming alpha hemolytic streptococci, anaerobic bacteria, and *Staphylococcus aureus*. The information available on the direct comparison of sinus aspiration and endoscopic sampling in the same patient does not permit replacement of aspirate cultures as the gold standard for microbiologic diagnosis.

Viral

Only a limited number of sinus aspirates from patients with acute sinusitis have been tested for the presence of virus (Table 55-5). In one study, viruses were recovered from 11 (16%) of 70 positive aspirates.[35] Most of these specimens were collected after the first 3 days of illness when the chances of viral recovery declines. Rhinovirus, parainfluenza virus, and influenza virus were identified, which support the role of viruses in the pathogenesis of sinusitis.

Bacterial

Acute Community-Acquired. The etiology of ACABS has been well defined by puncture studies going back to the late 1940s and 1950s.[14,15,45-54] There has been good agreement among the results. *S. pneumoniae* and *H. influenzae* have been the most important

pathogens, and together account for more than 50% of cases (see Table 55-5). Other streptococcal species including *Streptococcus intermedius*, *Streptococcus pyogenes*, and other α-hemolytic streptococci; *M. catarrhalis*; *S. aureus*; and anaerobic bacteria each account for an additional proportion of cases. *M. catarrhalis* is more prevalent in children than in adults, whereas anaerobic infections are infrequent in children.[51] Most sinusitis due to anaerobic bacteria arises from infection of the roots of the premolar teeth, and thus represents a pure bacterial infection. Some of the anaerobic infections have included up to six different species of microaerophilic and anaerobic bacteria. Viruses and bacteria have been recovered simultaneously from the same sinus aspirate, confirming the dual nature of the infection.

The relative importance of the different bacteria has not changed in the last half century, but there have been important changes in their antimicrobial susceptibilities. The appearance of penicillin resistance in *S. aureus* was followed by the emergence of β-lactam–resistant strains of *H. influenzae* and *M. catarrhalis*. The most recent and serious event has been the emergence of strains of *S. pneumoniae* that are resistant to multiple antibiotics.

Only approximately 60% of sinus aspirates in suspected cases of ACABS yield bacteria.[55] The cause of the culture-negative cases is not clear, but undoubtedly, many have a viral cause. *Chlamydia pneumoniae* has been identified in patients with respiratory illness that includes features of sinusitis.[56] However, until *C. pneumoniae* has been repeatedly identified in sinus aspirates, its role as a cause of sinusitis will remain unclear. Also, *M. pneumoniae* has been suggested as a cause of ACABS, but there are no reports of attempts to isolate it from sinus aspirates. Atypical pneumonia and bronchitis are the characteristic syndromes associated with *M. pneumoniae* infection. The clinical features of sinusitis have not been described with that infection.

Nosocomial. Nosocomial sinusitis is a major complication of critically ill, mechanically ventilated patients and those undergoing nasal intubation for other purposes. Radiographic evidence of sinus abnormalities had been observed in 25% to 75% of critically ill patients and in 18% to 32% of those with endotracheal intubation.[57] Nasal colonization with enteric gram negative bacilli is a risk factor for nosocomial sinusitis.[58] This type of sinusitis has been most often associated with *S. aureus*, *Pseudomonas aeruginosa*, *Serratia marcescens*,

---

TABLE 55-4   Method of Sinus Puncture and Aspiration for Specimen Collection

Disinfect the anterior nares and the area below the inferior turbinate (puncture site).
Anesthetize the puncture site with a topical anesthetic.
Puncture the medial wall of the antrum with a 12-gauge needle (or spring-loaded puncture device).
Aspirate the sinus contents into a syringe; if necessary, add 1 to 2 mL of sterile normal saline (without preservatives) to obtain a specimen.
Cap the syringe and transport the specimen in the syringe to the laboratory.
Obtain quantitative bacterial cultures if possible.

TABLE 55-5   Viral and Bacterial Cause of Acute Community-Acquired Maxillary Sinusitis

Organism	Mean Percentage of Cases (Range)	
	Adults	Children
Viruses*		
Rhinovirus	15	—
Influenza virus	5	—
Parainfluenza virus	3	2
Adenovirus	—	2
Bacteria†		
Streptococcus pneumoniae	31 (20-35)	36
Haemophilus influenzae (unencapsulated)	21 (6-26)	23
S. pneumoniae and *H. influenzae*	5 (1-9)	—
α-Streptococci	9 (3-19)	—
Moraxella catarrhalis	8 (2-10)	19
Anaerobic bacteria	6 (0-10)	—
(*Prevotella, Bacteroides, Peptostreptococcus, Fusobacterium* spp., and so forth)		
Staphylococcus aureus	4 (0-8)	—
Streptococcus pyogenes	2 (1-3)	2
Gram-negative bacteria‡	9 (0-24)	2

*Data from Hamory BH, Sande MA, Sydnor A Jr, et al. Etiology and antimicrobial therapy of acute maxillary sinusitis. J Infect Dis. 1979;139: 197-202.

†Data from references 15, 45-54.

‡One study had 24% isolation of gram-negative bacteria, but in four other studies the recovery rate was not over 5%. Gram-negative bacteria recovered included *Pseudomonas aeruginosa, Klebsiella pneumoniae,* and *Escherichia coli.*

Klebsiella pneumoniae, *Enterobacter* spp., and *Proteus mirabilis*, and is often polymicrobic.[59-64] *Pseudomonas aeruginosa* is the most frequent isolate in sinus aspirates from patients with cystic fibrosis.[65] *Legionella pneumophila* was identified in sinus tissue from a patient with acquired immunodeficiency syndrome.[66]

Fungal

Fungi are a well-established cause of occasional cases of acute community-acquired sinusitis. Also, fungal infections occur in hospitalized patients and those with other diseases such as diabetes mellitus. In such patients, fungi may be the cause of serious life-threatening infections. An increasing number of fungal groups have been associated with sinus infection (Table 55-6).[15,67-81]

Clinical Features

Viral

Viral sinusitis (viral rhinosinusitis) is the same disease as the common cold or the "flulike" illness associated with more invasive respiratory viruses. The clinical characteristics of the common cold are described elsewhere (see Chapter 50).

Bacterial

Bacterial sinusitis acquired in the community is usually superimposed on preexisting VRS; therefore, the clinical features of the illness reflect the dual nature of the infection. In most cases, it is not possible to separate the clinical features of VRS from those of ACABS. Sneezing, nasal discharge, rhinorrhea, nasal obstruction, facial pressure, and headache commonly occur with both conditions. The more classic features of ACABS: temperatures of 38° C or more, facial pain, and erythema occur in some cases but are relatively uncommon. Purulence or a colored nasal discharge, which is commonly considered a sign of ACABS, also occurs in cases of VRS. Cough has been noted as a characteristic of ACABS in children[51] and is also a common complaint in adults with the disease. Hyposmia may also be present. When the sinusitis follows dental infection, molar pain and a foul odor to the breath are characteristic features.

Patients with bacterial infection of the sphenoid sinus present with severe frontal, temporal, or retro-orbital headache that radiates to the occipital region, and may also have hypesthesia or hyperesthesia of the ophthalmic or maxillary dermatomes of the fifth cranial nerve.[82] Lethargy and the clinical findings of cavernous sinus or cortical vein thrombosis may also be present as well as signs of orbital cellulitis and abscess. With severe frontal sinusitis, pus may collect under the periosteum of the frontal bone, causing swelling and edema of the forehead, which is known as *Pott puffy tumor*.[83]

Nosocomial

Nosocomial sinusitis of bacterial origin typically presents as a fever of obscure origin in the critically ill patient undergoing prolonged mechanical ventilation by nasotracheal intubation or receiving other forms of nasal intubation. Risk factors for the disease also include sedation and a Glasgow coma score of less than 7.[58] It has been suggested that nosocomial sinusitis is a risk factor for ventilator-associated pneumonia[84]; however, this relationship is still open to question.[85]

Fungal

Patients with community-acquired fungal sinusitis usually present with masses, proptosis, and bony erosion due to pressure effects. The invasive form of fungal sinusitis typically presents as a rapidly progressive infection (see Chapters 256 and 257).

Diagnosis

Viral

The diagnosis of viral rhinosinusitis is based on the presence of the typical signs and symptoms of the common cold which include sneezing, rhinorrhea, nasal obstruction, sore/scratchy throat, cough, headache, and malaise (see Chapter 50). The majority of colds have improved by 7 to 10 days of onset,[86] and this characteristic of the illness is an important feature for distinguishing VRS from ACABS, as discussed below.

Bacterial

Diagnostic evaluation should include a history and an examination of the pharynx, nose, ears, sinuses, teeth, and chest. Information should be obtained about coryzal and influenzal illnesses, respiratory allergies, toothache, and other dental complaints. An initial distinction must be made between infectious and allergic or other noninfectious sinusitis syndromes. Differentiation must then be made between viral, combined viral-bacterial, or pure bacterial causes. It is desirable to determine the specific microbial cause, but this is not usually possible in the clinical setting. An allergic cause can usually be established by a history of paroxysmal sneezing, itching eyes, allergen exposure, and similar prior episodes.

Separating viral from viral-bacterial or bacterial infections is a difficult problem. None of the signs and symptoms with which patients present are both sensitive and specific for this purpose (Table 55-7),[1] and none have been compared to sinus aspirate culture, the gold standard.[3] One study examined adults with paranasal symptoms and pus observed coming from the middle meatus, using a purulent sinus aspirate (without bacterial culture) as the comparison standard.[87] The presence of two of the three findings of local pain with unilateral predominance, unilateral purulent rhinorrhea, and an erythrocyte sedimentation rate of more than 12 had a sensitivity of 79% and a specificity of 83%. In another study of adults in general practice using purulent maxillary sinus aspirate as the criterion standard, an elevated C-reactive protein concentration (>10 mg/L) combined with an elevated erythrocyte sedimentation rate (10 mm/hour for men, 20 mm/hour for women) had a sensitivity of 82% and a specificity of 57%.[88] Other standard laboratory tests such as white blood cell and differential counts are not useful because of lack of sensitivity and specificity.

As an aid to diagnosis, three categories of ACABS can be recognized (Table 55-8). The first presentation, which is rare, is that in which sinusitis has been complicated by meningitis, brain abscess, or orbital infection. In these cases, the clinical features of the sinus infection are overshadowed by the more serious illness. The second presentation is that in which the classic and relatively specific features of ACABS are present. These include fever of 38° C or higher and facial pain, marked tenderness, erythema, or swelling. Also in this category are patients with molar pain or other evidence of an odontogenic cause of the infection. The third presentation, which is most common, is that of a patient with VRS or an influenza-like illness in which symptoms have not improved or worsened after 7 10 days of illness. Colored nasal discharge, nasal obstruction, facial pressure, and sometimes cough are characteristically present. Uncomplicated rhinovirus colds have a median duration of 1 week,[86,89] and most patients with colds are improved by that time. Continuing without improvement or worsening raises the suspicion of a bacterial complication such as

TABLE 55-6 Fungal Cause of Paranasal Sinusitis		
	Community Acquired	*Impaired Host*
Aspergillus (*A. fumigatus*, *A. flavus*, *A. niger*, *A. oryzae*, *A. nidulans*)	Yes	Yes
Pseudallescheria (*P. boydii*)	Yes	Yes
Holobasidiomycetes (*Schizophyllum commune*)	Yes	Yes
Phaeohyphomycetes (*Bipolaris hawaiiensis*, *Bipolaris spicifera*, *Exserohilum rostratum*, *Exserohilum mcginnisii*, *Alternaria alternata*, *Curvularia lunata*)	Yes	Yes
Zygomycefes (*Mucor* spp., *Rhizopus* spp., *Cunninghamella bertholetiae*, *Rhizomucor* spp., *Conidiobolus coronatus*, *Scedosporium prolificans*)	Yes	Yes

TABLE 55-7 Sensitivity and Specificity of Clinical Findings in Adults with Acute Community-Acquired Sinusitis

Population	Criterion Standard	Finding	Sensitivity (%)	Specificity (%)
Males with nasal discharge*	Positive sinus radiologic examination	History of colored nasal discharge	72	52
		Cough	70	44
		Sneezing	70	34
		Poor response to decongestants	41	80
		Maxillary toothache	18	93
		Purulent secretion	51	76
		Sinus tenderness	48	65
		Temperature >38° C	16	85
Emergency ward patients with paranasal symptoms†	Purulent sinus aspirate‡	Purulent rhinorrhea, unilateral	48	—
		Pain, unilateral	37	—
		Purulent rhinorrhea, bilateral	35	—
		Sinus tenderness on percussion	43	—
		Pus in nasal cavity	41	—

*Data from Williams JW Jr, Simel DL, Roberts L, Samsa GP. Clinical evaluation for sinusitis. Making the diagnosis by history and physical examination. Ann Intern Med. 1992;117:705-710.
†Data from Killingsworth SM, Wetmore SJ. *Curvularia/Drechslera* sinusitis. Laryngoscope. 1990;100:932-937.
‡Bacterial culture was not performed.

ACABS. Also, sinus puncture studies have shown that approximately 60% of patients with an initial presentation of VRS who are no better after 1 week have a positive bacterial culture from a sinus aspirate specimen.[55] This diagnostic criterion, based on duration of illness without improvement, has been adopted by several expert groups.[90-92]

Sinus imaging is not recommended for the routine diagnosis of VRS or ACABS, but is reserved for cases of unusual severity or those with suspected CNS or orbital extension. CT scanning, because of its superior sensitivity, has largely supplanted conventional radiography as the imaging method of choice. The cost of a CT scan limited to the sinuses is comparable to that of a plain sinus radiograph in many clinics and hospitals. MRI is often preferred in patients with suspected intracranial extension of infection including epidural abscess or cavernous sinus thrombosis. Patients with VRS have sinus CT scan abnormalities that usually cannot be distinguished from those associated with ACABS.[2] However, the presence of a classic air-fluid level with a flat meniscus (indicating thin fluid in the cavity) correlates well with positive bacterial aspirate culture. In adults, an air-fluid level on a conventional sinus radiograph had a specificity of 89% when compared with positive aspirate culture, although the finding was present in only 37.5% of 48 patients with positive cultures.[35]

Dental infection as a cause of sinusitis may go undiagnosed because the dental condition is unrecognized by the patient. Previous or current toothache and other dental complaints are important features of the history. A foul odor may be detected on examination of the pharynx. Panorex examination of the teeth is indicated in these cases.

Nosocomial

Nosocomial sinusitis should be suspected in critically ill patients with fever and an indwelling nasal tube. Other positive findings suggesting the diagnosis are feeding via nasoenteric tube, sedation, and a Glasgow coma score of less than 7.[58] Nosocomial sinusitis presents most often during the second week of hospitalization. CT scan is recommended for the radiologic diagnosis of sinusitis in a critically ill patient.[57] Microbiologic diagnosis can only be established by sinus aspirate culture.[57] Careful disinfection of the puncture site is necessary because the nasal passages of ICU patients are colonized with potentially pathogenic organisms.

Fungal

Acute fungal sinusitis occurs in patients with serious underlying diseases and has a marked propensity for invading through contiguous bone into the orbit, brain, and hard palate (see Chapters 256 and 257). Fungal sinusitis also presents subacutely as a mass in the sinus cavity with ultimate bone erosion and pressure symptoms that depend on the site of involvement. Chronic fungal sinusitis has three forms: invasive sinusitis, fungus ball of the sinus, and allergic fungal sinusitis. Invasive infection resembles squamous carcinoma, Wegener's granulomatosis, and midline granuloma. Fungus ball of the sinus is a benign mass of hyphae, usually *Aspergillus*. Allergic fungal sinusitis presents as chronic sinus pain and an expansile mass of inspissated mucus, eosinophils, and hyphae that can deform the bony wall between the ethmoid sinus and the orbit or between the maxillary sinus and the nasal cavity. Patients usually have a history of allergic rhinitis and nasal polyps.

Noninfectious

Noninfectious causes of sinus disease include chemical irritation, nasal and sinus tumors, foreign bodies, Wegener's granulomatosis, and midline granuloma.

Complications

ACABS may lead to intracranial, orbital, and respiratory complications. The intracranial complications include meningitis, brain abscess, subdural empyema, and cavernous sinus and cortical vein thrombosis. Orbital complications are most common in young children and include

TABLE 55-8 Categories of Severity and Management Plans for Suspected Acute Community-Acquired Bacterial Sinusitis*

Category	Features	Management Plan
Emergent	Signs and symptoms suggesting intracranial (meningitis, brain abscess) or orbital extension	Emergency diagnostic measures; head computed tomography, lumbar puncture, surgical consultation. Intravenous antimicrobial therapy (vancomycin and a third-generation cephalosporin) while awaiting culture and susceptibility results
Urgent	Fever (temperature of ≥ 38° C), facial pain, edema, and erythema; maxillary toothache; classic air-fluid level	Oral antimicrobial therapy effective against sinus pathogenesis plus a decongestant, first-generation antihistamine, and mucoevacuant
Elective	Cold or "flulike" illness that has persisted for 8 to 10 d or more with no improvement or with worsening	Antimicrobial and supportive treatment (as for urgent cases)

*In the setting of an illness beginning as a common cold, "flulike" illness, or allergic rhinitis or associated with swimming or other risk factors.

orbital cellulitis, subperiosteal abscess, and orbital abscess. Sinusitis is also associated with the onset or exacerbation of asthma and bronchitis. Sinopulmonary disease is a well-recognized combination, especially when the condition has become chronic.

Whether the usual type of ACABS can lead to chronic sinus disease is unknown. Certain specific microorganisms might predispose to chronic sinus disease, or the development of chronic sinus disease may be related to problems with host immunity, including allergy. Little work has been done on this important question.

Therapy

Antimicrobial

General Considerations. The recommendation for treating ACABS patients with antimicrobials is based on published evidence of bacteriologic and clinical improvement.[93] Studies using pre- and post-treatment sinus aspirate cultures have shown that antimicrobials with appropriate spectra given in adequate doses and duration are effective in eradicating or substantially reducing bacterial titers in the sinus cavity compared with treatment in which the drug spectrum or the dose is inadequate (Table 55-9).[35,49,55,94] Since the early 1970s, a number of antimicrobials have been tested in patients with ACABS using pre- and post-therapy aspirate cultures. With a 10-day course of an antimicrobial with an appropriate spectrum used at the correct dose, bacteriologic cure rates of 90% or higher have been routinely obtained.[55]

In clinical trials of antimicrobial therapy for ACABS, pretreatment bacterial aspirate culture is necessary to exclude cases of uncomplicated VRS, which invariably confound the patient sample if inclusion criteria are based solely on clinical and imaging parameters.[3] Post-treatment aspirate culture is also necessary to determine the effectiveness of bacterial eradication. Currently, the Food and Drug Administration does not require post-treatment aspirate cultures for approval of a sinusitis treatment indication. In the literature, there are reports of "bacteriologic cures" in which post-therapy aspirate cultures were not performed, and "bacteriologic cure" was based on clinical response and not on the results of aspirate cultures.

Evidence for clinical improvement after antimicrobial therapy in ACABS may be found in a double-blind controlled trial of antimicrobial therapy in adults.[95] A significant difference in the duration of illness favoring antimicrobial therapy appeared by the third day of treatment and continued throughout the 30-day observation period (Fig. 55-5). By day 10, 86% of antimicrobial-treated patients recovered or were much better compared with 57% of those on placebo. By day 10, 86% of pa-

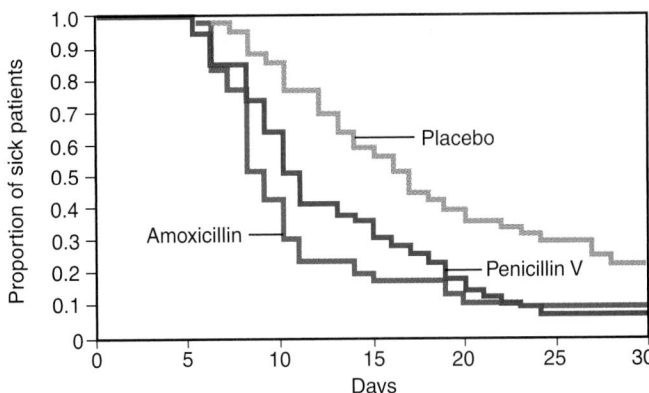

FIGURE 55-5. Duration of illness in adults with acute community-acquired sinusitis in a randomized double-blind clinical trial of antimicrobial treatment. (penicillin V, *n* = 39; amoxicillin, *n* = 44; placebo, *n* = 44). *(From Lindbaek M, Hjortdahl P, Johnsen U. Randomised, double-blind, placebo-controlled trial of penicillin V and amoxycillin in treatment of acute sinus infections in adults. BMJ. 1996;313:325-329.)*

tients on treatment also showed sinus CT scan improvement compared with 66% on placebo. After 30 days, 25% of patients receiving placebo judged themselves to be still sick compared with 10% of those on antimicrobial treatment.

Recommendations for antimicrobial treatment have changed as the sensitivities of the causative bacteria have evolved. The emergence of penicillin- and methicillin-resistant *S. aureus* was not a major problem because of its relative infrequency as a cause of ACABS. The subsequent emergence of β-lactamase–producing strains of *H. influenzae* and *M. catarrhalis* reduced the usefulness of ampicillin, but a number of more expensive antimicrobials were still available.[55] The emergence of intermediate- and high-level resistant strains of *Strep. pneumoniae* is a much more serious problem. A number of antimicrobials that were previously useful in the treatment of ACABS now have MIC_{90}s against intermediately resistant pneumococci that are not achievable.[96]

Current Recommendations. Antimicrobial therapy is usually selected on an empirical basis because sinus aspirate culture results are not available in the usual clinical setting. Treatment should be directed against the known sinus pathogens (see Table 55-5). The oral β-lactam antimicrobials that continue to show the best activity against intermediately resistant strains of pneumococci and are also effective against β-lactamase–producing *H. influenzae* and *M. catarrhalis* are amoxicillin-clavulanate, cefpodoxime, cefdinir, and cefuroxime. Also, the new quinolones provide excellent activity against pneumococci and other sinusitis pathogens. Of these drugs, amoxicillin-clavulanate, cefdinir, cefuroxime, and levofloxacin have been shown to be effective in 10-day courses in pre- and post-therapy sinus puncture clinical trials in patients with ACABS.[53-55] A 10-day course of treatment with one of these antimicrobials is recommended

TABLE 55-9 Comparative Bacteriologic Cure Rates (Determined by Sinus Puncture) in Patients with Acute Community-Acquired Bacterial Sinusitis

	No. Bacteriologic Cures/No. Cases
C Carenfelt et al[49]	
Antibiotic concentration ≥ MIC of causative bacteria*	19/21 (90%)
Antibiotic concentration < MIC of causative bacteria	15/33 (45%)
BH Hamory et al[35]	
Appropriate antimicrobial and dose	47/49 (96%)
Inappropriate antimicrobial†	0/6 (0%)
C Carenfelt et al[94]	
Appropriate antimicrobial and dose	105/115 (91%)
Suboptimal dose‡	37/50 (74%)
JM Gwaltney Jr et al[55]	
Appropriate antimicrobial and dose	126/136 (93%)
Suboptimal dose‡	1/5 (20%)
Suboptimal dose§	15/21 (71%)

*Antibiotic concentration in sinus aspirate after 2 to 3 days of treatment.
†Clindamycin for *Haemophilus influenzae.*
‡Cefaclor 500 mg bid.
§Cefaclor 500 mg tid.
MIC, minimal inhibitory concentration.

TABLE 55-10 Antimicrobial Treatment of Acute Community-Acquired Bacterial Sinusitis in Adults

Amoxicillin-clavulanate*	875-125 mg q12h
Cefdinir*	600 mg qd
Cefpodoxime proxetil*	200 mg q12h
Cefuroxime axetil*	250 mg q12h
Levofloxacin*	500 mg qd
Moxifloxacin	400 mg qd

*Have been found effective in pre- and post-treatment sinus aspirate culture studies.

for patients with ACABS (Table 55-10). There are no pre- and post-sinus aspirate culture data on the effectiveness of longer or shorter courses of treatment for ACABS, and these other regimens are not recommended. Also, the use of an inexpensive antimicrobial that does not have an optimum antibacterial spectrum may prolong infection and morbidity and put the patient at risk of complications.

The symptoms of acute community-acquired sinusitis usually improve after 2 or 3 days of treatment and are generally resolved by 10 to 14 days.[42,95] *However, it is important to be aware that patients with acute sinusitis may have symptomatic improvement despite the persistence in the sinus of purulent material containing high titers of bacteria.*[15] In one clinical trial, 38% of patients on placebo reported improvement by the third day of observation.[95] In patients with evidence of severe infection or in whom intracranial or orbital extension of infection is suspected, intravenous therapy should be started with vancomycin and ceftriaxone or cefotaxime until the results of culture and sensitivity testing are available for directing treatment. These patients should have emergency evaluations by CT or MRI, and may also require diagnostic lumbar puncture or surgical decompression and drainage, or both. Antimicrobial treatment of patients with nosocomial sinusitis should be directed by culture and sensitivity information when available, or, when empirical, should cover the usual pathogens responsible for these infections.

Fungal

Community-acquired fungal sinusitis in persons with normal immunity is usually effectively treated with surgical débridement of the affected sinus cavities. Complicated cases and patients with immunodeficiencies suspected of having invasive infection should be evaluated on an individual basis for appropriate surgical and antifungal therapy (see Chapters 256 and 257).

Ancillary

Most patients with ACABS are successfully treated as outpatients. Patients with severe infection, especially those in whom intracranial or orbital extension is suspected, require hospitalization. In the usual case, ancillary treatment should be directed at drainage of the nasal passages and sinuses and the relief of sneezing, coughing, and systemic complaints.[97] Topical decongestants are rapidly effective in shrinking the erectile vascular tissue of the turbinates and, thus, helping relieve ostiomeatal and nasal obstruction (see Fig. 55-4).[34] However, sequential CT scans have shown that decongestants are not effective in opening the infundibulum and draining the sinus cavity itself. The exudate in the sinus cavity is often too viscous to be moved by ciliary action. The action of oral decongestants is less immediate, but theses drugs avoid rebound vasodilatation and pharyngeal irritation. Oral decongestants have been shown to be safe in patients with stable hypertension on antihypertensive treatment.[98]

Topical steroids have not been rigorously evaluated in treating patients with ACABS,[97] add unnecessary expense, and are not recommended. The value of mucoevacuants, such as guaifenesin, is also not established, but they are used on theoretical grounds. Nonsteroidal anti-inflammatory drugs are useful in treating systemic complaints such as fever and malaise and may be helpful in reducing cough.[99-101] Other cough suppressants such as dextromethorphan and codeine may be needed for cough control.

First-generation antihistamines have not been recommended in the past for treating VRS or ACABS because of their anticholinergic activity and the possibility of drying secretions. Although this is a reasonable theoretical consideration, actual testing of these drugs under randomized controlled blinded conditions has shown a 50% or greater reduction in sneezing and a 30% reduction in rhinorrhea and nasal mucus weights in volunteers with experimental rhinovirus VRS.[101-103] Also, there was no evidence for worsening of other symptoms or prolongation of the overall illness. By reducing sneezing and nose blowing, antihistamines may reduce the frequency of viral and bacterial dissemination in the nasal passages and into the sinus cavities.[32] Experimental upper airway challenge with histamine in volunteers

stimulates the release of secretions with an increased sulfate concentration characteristic of mucus, suggesting that histamine stimulates goblet cell exocytosis.[104] Thus, antihistamine therapy may reduce the amount of mucus that accumulates in the sinus cavity.

In patients with ACABS who do not respond to an initial course of appropriate antimicrobial therapy, sinus puncture and lavage, repeatedly if necessary, is highly recommended. This more invasive form of treatment is justified because once sinus disease has progressed to a chronic state, the prognosis for eventual recovery is reduced considerably.

Prevention

Preventing colds may be possible to some extent by avoiding contact with cold sufferers and by hygienic measures such as hand washing when contact occurs between infected and noninfected persons. Also, covering coughs and sneezes with disposable nasal tissues is desirable. Vaccine is effective in preventing influenza as is the prophylactic use of antivirals during periods of epidemic influenza. There are no proven measures for preventing secondary bacterial infection of the sinuses, although reducing nose blowing may be of value.[32] Also, the promotion of decongestion and drainage is possible in the lower nasal passages and ostiomeatal area but, as discussed previously, its value in clearing the sinus cavity is problematic. *Prophylactic antimicrobial administration to prevent recurrent ACABS is not recommended. The practice of using antimicrobials to treat such a common illness as VRS leads to the emergence of bacteria with new patterns of antibiotic resistance.* Better treatments for colds may be available in the future, and these, when given early in the course of the illness, may modify the viral sinusitis and, in turn, lower the incidence of secondary bacterial sinusitis.

Avoiding nasal intubation has been shown to be effective in reducing the incidence of nosocomial sinusitis.[64]

CHRONIC SINUS DISEASE

Chronic sinus disease (CSD) remains a largely neglected area of study. Published sinus aspirate culture data on specimens obtained from intact sinuses of CSD patients are very limited. Understanding of the etiology and pathogenesis of CSD remains poor, and except for surgery, treatment modalities are inadequate. The disease is best classified into pre- and postsurgical categories because patients in these categories present different problems in management.

Presurgical Cases

Etiology and Pathogenesis

Approximately 5% to 10% of cases of ACABS fail to show bacteriologic cure by sinus aspirate culture after a course of antimicrobial therapy.[55] In a clinical trial of adults with acute community-acquired sinusitis, 25% of the patients who received placebo were still symptomatic after 1 month.[95] It is reasonable to speculate that most cases of CSD arise from patients with typical ACABS who are nonresponders to treatment or who have not received treatment, but evidence for this hypothesis is lacking. Anecdotal evidence from clinical practice indicates that some cases of ACABS do not resolve despite repeated courses of more than adequate antimicrobial treatment. Posttherapy sinus aspirate cultures of these patients are often nonrevealing. This suggests that at least some or many cases of CSD do not evolve from typical ACABS but may represent a separate and distinct entity of undetermined cause. However, somewhat paradoxically, two small studies have recovered *S. pneumoniae*, *H. influenzae*, and other streptococcal species from aspirate cultures obtained from the intact sinuses of CSD patients.[105,106]

Persistent sinus disease can result from certain conditions including obstruction of sinus drainage, abnormalities in mucociliary clearance, severe immunoglobulin deficiency, granulocyte dysfunction, and acquired immunodeficiency syndrome, but most CSD patients do not have these problems. Anecdotal evidence may be accumulating that less severe immune problems such as deficiencies in immunoglobulin subtypes may play a role in the pathogenesis of CSD, but this is not well established. Also, there is a subset of patients with CSD associated with aspirin sensitivity, nasal polyposis, and asthma.

It has recently been hypothesized that a large proportion of cases of CSD are the result of immune system response to fungal infection (colonization) of the sinus cavity. This suggestion is based on a study in which 31 different species of fungi were cultured from the sinuses of CSD patients.[107] However, interpretation of this finding is difficult because, in the same study, a similar finding was observed in control patients. Also, convincing evidence that antifungal therapy results in sustained improvement in CSD patients has, so far, not been reported.

Management

In patients with ACABS in whom an initial course of antimicrobial therapy fails, the usual practice is to give an additional course(s) of antimicrobials, sometimes guided by aspirate culture results; prescribe intranasal and sometimes oral steroids; and evaluate the patient for allergic and immune deficiency states. Sinus lavage was used in the pre-antibiotic era, and it still is an effective form of treatment that is currently neglected or underused. When comprehensive medical management, including the previously mentioned therapies, has failed and there is sinus CT scan evidence of persistent disease, the patient should be evaluated as a candidate for sinus surgery.

Prolonged noncurative medical management is not recommended because of the risk that sinus inflammation may become so well established that the chances of success with sinus surgery may be lessened. In patients with prolonged CSD, remodeling of the facial bones is often seen on CT scan (Fig. 55-6), and evidence of osteomyelitis has been demonstrated in specimens from such patients (Fig. 55-7).[108] Also, there is the possibility that irreversible mucosal damage may occur.

Modern endoscopic surgery is reported to result in "marked" short-term improvement in approximately 85% of patients.[109] In the standard procedure, the ostiomeatal area is opened, antrostomies are created, and ethmoid partitions are removed. A portion of the anterior wall of the sphenoid sinus may be removed, but the frontal sinuses are usually not opened in the initial procedure.

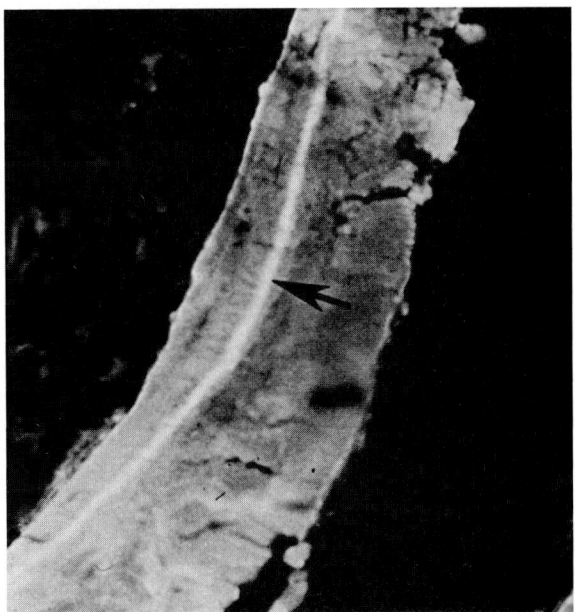

A

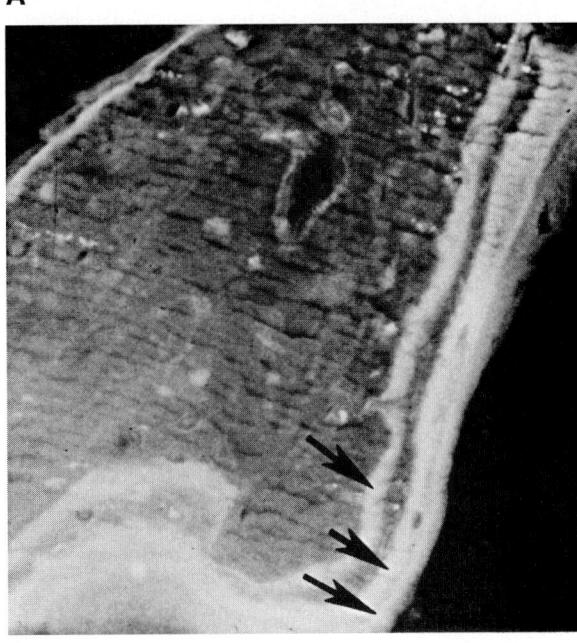

B

FIGURE 55-7. Tetracycline labeling of ethmoid bone removed from a normal control with a single area of neogenesis (*arrow*) (**A**) and a patient with chronic sinus disease with multiple areas of neogenesis (*arrows*) (**B**).

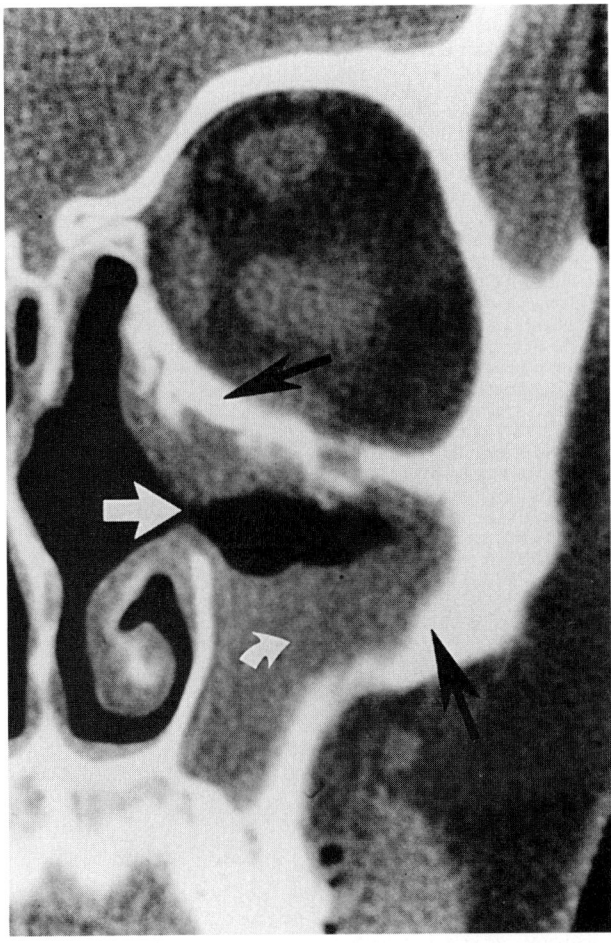

FIGURE 55-6. Bone remodeling (*black arrows*) in a 60-year-old diabetic with chronic sinus disease of 8 years' duration. Despite a widely patent surgical antrostomy (*large white arrow*), exudate (*small curved arrow*) is present in the sinus cavity. A highly viscous exudate that grew a strain of *Pseudomonas aeruginosa* was removed by endoscopy.

TABLE 55-11 Bacterial Culture Categories in Patients with Chronic Sinus Disease

Category 1: *Streptococcus pneumoniae, Haemophilus influenzae, Moraxella catarrhalis*, other species of *Streptococcus (intermedius*, etc.)
  Setting: recovered in sinus aspirates; in high titers
  Interpretation: cause of acute exacerbations or possibly of ongoing disease
Category 2: *Staphylococcus aureus* and/or *Pseudomonas aeruginosa* (and other *Pseudomonas* species)
  Setting: recovered in sinus aspirates in cystic fibrosis; postoperative sinus cavity exudates; persistent infection
  Interpretation: cause of disease (crusts, thick and/or "concretized" secretions)
Category 3: *Staphylococcus epidermidis* (other coagulase-negative staphylococci), *Corynebacterium* spp., anaerobes, gram-negative bacteria
  Setting: recovered from tissue and swab specimens collected at time of surgery, in nasal and sinus swabs; low titers
  Interpretation: role in pathogenesis unclear or suspect

Postsurgical Cases

Pathogenesis

Patients in whom initial sinus surgery fails and who continue to have chronic purulent nasal discharge, nasal crusting, anosmia, facial pain, headache, cough, and fatigue represent a very difficult management problem. When the condition is fully developed, it is the cause of serious morbidity and typically continues for years. Bacterial cultures obtained from the nasal passages and sinus cavities are usually positive but may be difficult to interpret (Table 55-11). Serial cultures are most often positive for *S. aureus, Pseudomonas* spp., *S. marcescens, Stenotrophomonas maltophilia*, and other gram-negative bacteria. These organisms appear to play a role in the ongoing disease, although it is unlikely that they are responsible for the original development of CSD. The reason that sinus surgery fails remains obscure, but as with presurgical CSD, host immune factors may play a role. As described previously, bony involvement is often identified.[108] Microbial factors such as the presence of small-colony bacterial variants[110] and allergy to the presence of fungii[107] have also been suggested as having a role in the condition.

Management

The management of CSD patients in whom surgery has failed is a difficult and frustrating challenge. Surgery is recommended on unopened areas of the sinus that show continuing disease by CT scan examination. The most frequent targets for this are isolated ethmoid air cells and the sphenoid and frontal sinuses. Antimicrobial treatment should be based on serial culture and sensitivity results and coordinated with surgery. A course of antimicrobial therapy directed at possible low-grade osteomyelitis seems reasonable, but experience with this approach is limited and results with individual patients are not encouraging. Patients so treated may have improvement, but relapses are usually seen when antimicrobials are discontinued. Some physicians have observed sustained improvement with immunoglobulin replacement therapy, but evaluation of this form of treatment has not been subjected to controlled evaluation. Less aggressive management relies on short-term courses of antimicrobials during periods of unusually severe exacerbation combined with daily nasal irrigations and removal of crusts when necessary. Irrigating fluids and devices should be maintained under sterile conditions, and unsterilized tap water lavages are not recommended.

REFERENCES

1. Williams JW Jr, Simel DL, Roberts L, Samsa GP. Clinical evaluation for sinusitis. Making the diagnosis by history and physical examination. Ann Intern Med. 1992;117:705-710.
2. Gwaltney JM Jr, Phillips CD, Miller RD, Riker DK. Computed tomographic study of the common cold. N Engl J Med. 1994;330:25-30.
3. Gwaltney JM Jr, Wiesinger BA, Patrie JT. Acute community-acquired bacterial sinusitis: The value of antimicrobial treatment and the natural history. Clin Infect Dis. 2004;38:227-233.
4. Witmer LM. Homology of facial structures in extant archosaurs (birds and crocodilians), with special reference to paranasal pneumaticity and nasal conchae. J Morphol. 1995;225:269-327.
5. Rowe T. Definition, diagnosis, and the origin of Mammalia. J Vert Paleontol. 1988;8:241-264.
6. Mogensen C, Tos M. Quantitative histology of the maxillary sinus. Rhinology. 1977;55:129-140.
7. Mogensen C, Tos M. Quantitative histology of the normal sphenoid sinus. Rhinology. 1978;56:203-213.
8. Mogensen C, Tos M. Density of goblet cells in the normal adult human nasal septum. Anat Anz. 1977;141:237-247.
9. Hilding A. The physiology of drainage of nasal mucus. III. Experimental work on the accessory sinuses. Am J Rhinol. 1932;May:664-670.
10. Messerklinger W. Über die Drainage der menschlichen Nasennebenhöhlen unter normalen und pathologischen Bedingungen 1. Monatsschr Ohrenheilkd Laryngorhinol. 1966;100:56-58.
11. Deitmer T. Physiology and pathology of the mucociliary system. In: Pfaltz CR, ed. Advances in Oto-Rhino-Laryngology, v. 43. Basel: Karger; 1989:28.
12. Maran AGD, Lund VJ. Nasal physiology. In: Clinical Rhinology. New York, Thieme Medical; 1990:37.
13. Gwaltney JM Jr, Hayden FG. The nose and infection. In: Proctor DF, Andersen I, eds. The Nose. Upper Airway Physiology and the Atmospheric Environment. Amsterdam: Elsevier Biomedical; 1982:399-422.
14. Björkwall T. Bacteriological examinations in maxillary sinusitis: Bacterial flora of the maxillary antrum. Acta Otolaryngol Suppl (Stockh). 1950;83:33-58.
15. Evans FO Jr, Sydnor JB, Moore WEC, et al. Sinusitis of the maxillary antrum. N Engl J Med. 1975;293:735-739.
16. Bjuggren G, Kraepelien S, Lind J. Sinusitis in children at home and in day-nurseries. Ann Paediatr. 1949;173:205-221.
17. Shapiero ED, Wald ER, Doyle WJ, Rohm DD. Bacteriology of maxillary sinuses of the rhesus monkey. Ann Otol Rhinol Laryngol. 1982;91:150-151.
18. Runer T. Studies of Mucociliary Activity and Blood Flow in the Upper Airways, with Special Reference to Endothelins and Nitric Oxide. PhD thesis. Department of Oto-Rhino-Laryngology, Head and Neck Surgery, University of Lund, Sweden, 1996.
19. Gwaltney JM Jr. Rhinoviruses. In: Evans AS, Kaslow RA, eds. Viral Infections of Humans: Epidemiology and Control. 4th ed. New York: Plenum; 1997:815-838.
20. Dingle JH, Badger GF, Jordan WS Jr. Illness in the Home. A Study of 25,000 Illnesses in a Group of Cleveland Families. Cleveland: The Press of Western Reserve University; 1964:347.
21. Berg O, Carenfelt C, Rystedt G, Ånggård A. Occurrence of asymptomatic sinusitis in common cold and other acute ENT-infections. Rhinology. 1986;24:223-225.
22. Gable CA, Jones JK, Floor M, et al. Chronic sinusitis: Relation to upper respiratory infections and allergic rhinitis. Pharmacoepidemiol Drug Saf. 1994;3:337-349.
23. Gwaltney JM Jr, Hayden FG. Response to psychological stress and susceptibility to the common cold (Letter). N Engl J Med. 1992;326:644-645.
24. Winther B, Gwaltney JM Jr, Mygind N, et al. Sites of recovery after point inoculation of the upper airway. JAMA. 1986;256:1763-1767.
25. Greve JM, Davis G, Meyer AM, et al. The major human rhinovirus receptor is ICAM-1. Cell. 1989;56:839-847.
26. Winther B, Innes DJ. The human adenoid. A morphologic study. Arch Otolaryngol Head Neck Surg. 1994;120:144-149.
27. Winther B, Innes DJ, Hendley JO, et al. Distribution of the human rhinovirus receptor, ICAM-1, on epithelium of the upper airways (Abstract 100). J Jpn Rhinol Soc. 1991;100.
28. Arruda E, Boyle TR, Winther B, et al. Localization of human rhinovirus replication in the upper respiratory tract by in situ hybridization. J Infect Dis. 1995;171:1329-1333.
29. Gwaltney JM Jr, Heinz BA. Rhinovirus. In: Richman DD, Whitley RJ, Hayden FG, eds. Clinical Virology. Washington, DC: ASM Press; 2002:995-1018.
30. Kristo A, Uhari M, Luotonen J, et al. Paranasal sinus findings in children during respiratory infection evaluated with magnetic resonance imaging. Pediatrics. 2003;111:586-589.
31. Puhakka T, Mäkelä MJ, Alanen A, et al. Sinusitis in the common cold. J Allergy Clin Immunol. 1998;102:403-408.
32. Gwaltney JM Jr, Hendley JO, Phillips CD, et al. Nose blowing propels nasal fluid into the paranasal sinuses. Clin Infect Dis. 2000;30:387-391.
33. Winther B, Gwaltney JM Jr, Humphries JE, Hendley JO. Cross-linked fibrin in the nasal fluid of patients with the common cold. Clin Infect Dis. 2002;34:708-710.
34. Gwaltney JM Jr. State-of-the-art. Acute community-acquired sinusitis. Clin Infect Dis. 1996;23:1209-1223.
35. Hamory BH, Sande MA, Sydnor A Jr, et al. Etiology and antimicrobial therapy of acute maxillary sinusitis. J Infect Dis. 1979;139:197-202.
36. Hinni ML, McCaffrey TV, Kasperbauer JL. Early mucosal changes in experimental sinusitis. Otolaryngol Head Neck Surg. 1992;107:537-548.
37. Fukami M, Norlander T, Stierna P, et al. Mucosal pathology of the nose and sinuses: A study in experimental maxillary sinusitis in rabbits induced by *Streptococcus pneumoniae, Bacteroides fragilis*, and *Staphylococcus aureus*. Am J Rhinol. 1993;7:125-132.
38. Westrin KM, Stierna P, Carlsöö B, Nord CE. Mucosubstance histochemistry of the maxillary sinus mucosa in experimental sinusitis: A model study on rabbits. ORL J Otolaryngol Relat Spec. 1991;53:508-513.

39. Fukami M, Norlander T, Stierna P, et al. Mucosal pathology of the nose and sinuses: A study in experimental maxillary sinusitis in rabbits induced by *Streptococcus pneumoniae*, *Bacteroides fragilis*, and *Staphylococcus aureus*. Am J Rhinol. 1993;7:125-132.

40. Berger G, Kattan A, Bernheim J, et al. A histopathological and immunohistochemical study. Laryngoscope. 2000;110:2089-2094.

41. Axelsson A, Runze U. Comparison of subjective and radiological findings during the course of acute maxillary sinusitis. Ann Otol Rhinol Laryngol. 1983;92:75-77.

42. Leopold DA, Stafford CT, Sod EW, et al. Clinical course of acute maxillary sinusitis documented by sequential MRI scanning. Am J Rhinol. 1994;8:19-28.

43. Yanagisawa E, Yanagisawa K. Endoscopic view of maxillary sinus ostia. Ear Nose Throat J. 1993;72:518-519.

44. Talbot G, Kennedy D, Scheld M, et al. Utility of sinus endoscopy versus sinus aspiration for microbiologic documentation of acute maxillary sinusitis (AMS). Abstract D42. Presented at the Thirty-fifth Interscience Conference of Antimicrobial Agents and Chemotherapy, San Francisco, September 17-20, 1995.

45. Urdal K, Berdal P. The microbial flora in 81 cases of maxillary sinusitis. Acta Otolaryngol (Stockh). 1949;37:20-25.

46. Lystad A, Berdal P, Lund-Iverson L. The bacterial flora of sinusitis with an in vitro study of the bacterial resistance to antibiotics. Acta Otolaryngol Suppl (Stockh). 1964;188:390-399.

47. Rantanen T, Arvilommi H. Double-blind trial of doxycycline in acute maxillary sinusitis: A clinical and bacteriological study. Acta Otolaryngol (Stockh). 1973;76:58-62.

48. Axelsson A, Brorson JE. The correlation between bacteriological findings in the nose and maxillary sinus in acute maxillary sinusitis. Laryngoscope. 1973;83:2003-2011.

49. Carenfelt C, Eneroth C-M, Lundberg C, Wretlind B. Evaluation of the antibiotic effect of treatment of maxillary sinusitis. Scand J Infect Dis. 1975;7:259-264.

50. Sydnor A Jr, Gwaltney JM Jr, Cocchetto DM, Scheld WM. Comparative evaluation of cefuroxime axetil and cefaclor for therapy of acute bacterial maxillary sinusitis. Arch Otolarngol Head Neck Surg. 1989;115:1054-1059.

51. Wald ER, Milmoe GJ, Bowen A, et al. Acute maxillary sinusitis in children. N Engl J Med. 1981;304:749-754.

52. Sydnor TA Jr, Scheld WM, Gwaltney J Jr, et al. Loracarbef (LY163892) vs amoxicillin/clavulanate in bacterial maxillary sinusitis. Ear Nose Throat J. 1992;71:225-232.

53. Gwaltney JM Jr, Savolainen S, Rivas P, et al. Comparative effectiveness and safety of cefdinir and amoxicillin-clavulanate in treatment of acute community-acquired bacterial sinusitis. Antimicrob Agents Chemother. 1997;41:1517-1520.

54. Sydnor A, Scheld WM, Gwaltney JM. A noncomparative study to evaluate the safety and efficacy of levofloxacin in the treatment of acute bacterial sinusitis in adults. Data on file. The Robert Wood Johnson Pharmaceutical Institute/Ortho-McNeil Pharmaceutical, Raritan, NJ, 1995.

55. Gwaltney JM Jr, Scheld WM, Sande MA, Sydnor A. The microbial etiology and antimicrobial therapy of adults with acute community-acquired sinusitis: A fifteen-year experience at the University of Virginia and review of other selected studies. J Allergy Clin Immunol. 1992;90:457-462.

56. Hahn DL, Dodge RW, Golubjantnikov R. Association of *Chlamydia pneumoniae* (strain TWAR) infection with wheezing, asthmatic bronchitis, and adult-onset asthma. JAMA. 1991;266:225-230.

57. Talmor M, Li P, Barie PS. Acute paranasal sinusitis in critically ill patients: Guidelines for prevention, diagnosis, and treatment. Clin Infect Dis. 1997;25:1441-1442.

58. George DL, Falk PS, Meduri GU, et al. Nosocomial sinusitis in patients in the medical intensive care unit: A prospective epidemiological study. Clin Infect Dis. 1998;27:463-470.

59. Pope TL, Stelling CB, Leitner YB. Maxillary sinusitis after nasotracheal intubation. South Med J. 1981;74:610-612.

60. Via-Reque E, Rattenborg CC. Prolonged oro- or nasotracheal intubation. Crit Care Med. 1981;9:637-639.

61. Caplan ES, Hoyt NJ. Nosocomial sinusitis. JAMA. 1982;247:639-641.

62. Deutschman CS, Wilton PB, Sinow J, et al. Paranasal sinusitis: A common complication of nasotracheal intubation in neurosurgical patients. Neurosurgery. 1985;17:296-299.

63. Linden BE, Aguilar EA, Allen SJ. Sinusitis in the nasotracheally intubated patient. Arch Otolaryngol Head Neck Surg. 1988;114:860-861.

64. Rouby J-J, Laurent P, Gosnach M, et al. Risk factors and clinical relevance of nosocomial maxillary sinusitis in the critically ill. Am J Respir Crit Care Med. 1994;150:776-783.

65. Shapiro ED, Milmoe GJ, Wald ER, et al. Bacteriology of the maxillary sinuses in patients with cystic fibrosis. J Infect Dis. 1982;146:589-593.

66. Schlanger G, Lutwick LI, Kurzman M, et al. Sinusitis caused by *Legionella pneumophila* in a patient with the acquired immune deficiency syndrome. Am J Med. 1984;77:957-960.

67. Morriss FH Jr, Spock A. Intracranial aneurysm secondary to mycotic orbital and sinus infection. Report of a case implicating *Penicillium* as an opportunistic fungus. Am J Dis Child. 1970;119:357-362.

68. McGuirt WF, Harril JA. Paranasal sinus aspergillosis. Laryngoscope. 1979;89:1563-1570.

69. Stevens MH. Primary fungal infections of the paranasal sinuses. Am J Otolaryngol. 1981;2:348-357.

70. Romett J, Newman R. Aspergillosis of the nose and paranasal sinuses. Laryngoscope. 1982;92:764-766.

71. Rinaldi MG. Invasive aspergillosis. Rev Infect Dis. 1983;5:1061-1077.

72. Morgan MA, Wilson WR, Neel B III, Roberts GD. Fungal sinusitis in healthy and immunocompromised individuals. Am J Clin Pathol. 1984;82:597-601.

73. Parfrey NA. Improved diagnosis and prognosis of mucormycosis. A clinico-pathologic study of 33 cases. Medicine (Baltimore). 1986;65:113-120.

74. Kern ME, Uecker FA. Maxillary sinus infection caused by the homobasidio-mycetous fungus *Schizophyllum commune*. J Clin Microbiol. 1986;23:1001-1005.

75. MacMillan RH III, Cooper PH, Body BA, Mills AS. Allergic fungal sinusitis due to *Curvularia lunata*. Hum Pathol. 1987;18:960-964.

76. Washburn RG, Kennedy AW, Begley MG, et al. Chronic fungal sinusitis in apparently normal hosts. Medicine (Baltimore). 1988;67:231-247.

77. Killingsworth SM, Wetmore SJ. *Curvularia/Drechslera* sinusitis. Laryngoscope. 1990;100:932-937.

78. Zieske LA, Kipke RD, Hamill R. Dematiaceous fungal sinusitis. Otolaryngol Head Neck Surg. 1991;105:567-577.

79. Morrison VA, Weisdorf DJ. *Alternaria*: A sinonasal pathogen of immunocompromised hosts. Clin Infect Dis. 1993;16:265-270.

80. Fothergill AW. Identification of dematiaceous fungi and their role in human disease. Clin Infect Dis. 1996;22(Suppl 2):S179-S184.

81. Iwen PC, Rupp ME, Hinrichs SH. Invasive mold sinusitis: 17 cases in immunocompromised patients and review of the literature. Clin Infect Dis. 1997;24:1178-1184.

82. Lew D, Southwick FS, Montgomery WW, et al. Sphenoid sinusitis. A review of 30 cases. N Engl J Med. 1983;309:1149-1154.

83. Wells RC, Sty JR, Landers AD. Radiological evaluation of Pott puffy tumor. JAMA. 1986;255:1331-1333.

84. Holzapfel L, Chastang C, Demingeon G, et al. A randomized study assessing the systematic search for maxillary sinusitis in nasotracheally mechanically ventilated patients. Am J Respir Crit Care Med. 1999;159:695-701.

85. Hall J. Assessment of fever in the intensive care unit. Is the answer just beyond the tip of our nose? Am J Respir Crit Care Med. 1999;159:693-694.

86. Gwaltney JM Jr, Hendley JO, Simon G, Jordan WS Jr. Rhinovirus infections in an industrial population. II. Characteristics of illness and antibody response. JAMA. 1967;202:494-500.

87. Berg O, Carenfelt C. Analysis of symptoms and clinical signs in the maxillary sinus empyema. Acta Otolaryngol (Stockh). 1988;105:343-349.

88. Hansen JG, Schmidt H, Rosborg J, Lund E. Predicting acute maxillary sinusitis in a general practice population. BMJ. 1995;311:233-236.

89. Gwaltney JM Jr, Buier RM, Rogers JL. The influence of signal variation, bias, noise, and effect size on statistical significance in treatment studies of the common cold. Antiviral Res. 1996;29:287-295.

90. Snow V, Mottur-Pilson C, Hickner JM. Principles of appropriate antibiotic use for acute sinusitis in adults. Ann Intern Med. 2001;134:495-497.

91. American Academy of Pediatrics. Subcommittee on Management of Sinusitis and Committee on Quality Improvement. Clinical practice guideline: Management of sinusitis. Pediatrics. 2001;108:798-808.

92. Sinus and Allergy Health Partnership. Antimicrobial treatment guidelines for acute bacterial rhinosinusitis. Otolaryng Head Neck Surg. 2000;123(Suppl):S1-S32.

93. Gwaltney JM Jr. Acute community-acquired bacterial sinusitis: To treat or not to treat. Can Respir J. 1999;6(Suppl A):46A-50A.

94. Carenfelt C, Melen I, Ödkvist L, et al. Treatment of sinus empyema in adults. A co-ordinated Nordic multicenter trial of cefixime vs. cefaclor. Acta Otolaryngol (Stockh). 1990;110:128-135.

95. Lindbæk M, Hjortdahl P, Johnsen U. Randomised, double-blind, placebo controlled trial of penicillin V and amoxycillin in treatment of acute sinus infections in adults. BMJ. 1996;313:325-329.

96. Doern GV, Brueggemann A, Holley HP Jr, Rauch AM. Antimicrobial resistance of *Streptococcus pneumoniae* recovered from outpatients in the United States during the winter months of 1994 to 1995: Results of a 30-center national surveillance study. Antimicrob Agents Chemother. 1996;40:1208-1213.

97. Zeiger RS. Prospects for ancillary treatment of sinusitis in the 1990s. J Allergy Clin Immunol. 1992;90:478-495.

98. Coates ML, Rembold CM, Farr BM. Does pseudoephedrine increase blood pressure in patients with controlled hypertension? J Fam Pract. 1995;40:22-26.

99. Sperber SJ, Hendley JO, Hayden FG, et al. Effects of naproxen on experimental rhinovirus colds. A randomized, double-blind, controlled trial. Ann Intern Med. 1992;117:37-41.

100. Gwaltney JM Jr. Combined antiviral and antimediator treatment of rhinovirus colds. J Infect Dis. 1992;166:776-782.

101. Gwaltney JM Jr, Winther B, Patrie JT, Hendley JO. Combined antiviral-antimediator treatment for the common cold. J Infect Dis. 2002;186:147-154.

102. Gwaltney JM Jr, Park J, Paul RA, et al. A randomized controlled trial of clemastine fumarate in experimental rhinovirus colds. Clin Infect Dis. 1996;22:656-662.

103. Gwaltney JM Jr, Druce HM. Efficacy of brompheniramine maleate treatment for rhinovirus colds. Clin Infect Dis. 1997;25:1188-1194.

104. Brofeldt S, Mygind N, Srrensen GH, et al. Biochemical analysis of nasal secretions induced by methacholine, histamine, and allergen provocations. Am Rev Respir Dis. 1986;133:1138-1142.

105. Wald E. Microbiology of acute and chronic sinusitis. In: Lusk RP, ed. Pediatric Sinusitis. New York: Raven Press; 1992:43-47.

106. Winther B, Vickery CL, Gross CW, Hendley JO. Microbiology of the maxillary sinus in adults with chronic sinus disease. Am J Rhinol. 1996;10:347-350.

107. Ponikau JU, Sherris DA, Kern EB, et al. The diagnosis and incidence of allergic fungal sinusitis. Mayo Clin Proc. 1999;74:877-884.

108. Kennedy DW, Senior BA, Gannon FH, et al. Histology and histomorphometry of ethmoid bone in chronic rhinosinusitis. Laryngoscope. 1998;108:502-507.

109. Kennedy D. Prognostic factors, outcomes and staging in ethmoid sinus surgery. Laryngoscope. 1992;102:1-18.

110. Proctor RA, Balwit JM, Vesga O. Variant subpopulations of *Staphylococcus aureus* as cause of persistent and recurrent infections. Infect Agents Dis. 1994;3:302-312.

CHAPTER 56

Epiglottitis

JAMES E. BURNS

J. OWEN HENDLEY

Acute epiglottitis (supraglottitis) is a cellulitis of the epiglottis and adjacent structures that has the potential for causing abrupt, complete airway obstruction.

The typical patient has been a 2- to 4-year-old boy having a 6- to 12-hour history of fever, irritability, dysphonia, and dysphagia, which can occur at any time of year. However, as the use of *Haemophilus influenzae* type B conjugated vaccine increases, the typical patient is becoming an adult with a sore throat. At the time medical attention is sought, varied degrees of respiratory distress may be evident. The pediatric patient usually prefers to sit leaning forward while drooling oral secretions. Respirations tend to be tentative and careful without marked tachypnea. Tachycardia is usually commensurate with fever but may be related to hypoxia and be out of proportion to fever.[1] Inspiratory stridor and hoarseness may occur, but the barking cough and aphonia typical in croup syndrome are rare. The diagnosis is established by visualizing an edematous "cherry red" epiglottis (Figs. 56-1 and 56-2). The course of acute epiglottitis may be fulminating, as emphasized by the report of a patient who progressed from being completely asymptomatic to having complete airway obstruction in 30 minutes.[2]

Laboratory data may include moderate leukocytosis with a "shift to the left," positive cultures of blood and epiglottis, and evidence of pneumonia on chest radiographs in up to 25% of cases.[3] A radiograph of the lateral neck may show an enlarged epiglottis, ballooning of the hypopharynx, and normal subglottic structures.[4] However, the use of radiographs in the diagnosis of epiglottitis is questionable because of both the delay in securing an airway while the films are being obtained and the variable sensitivity (as low as 3%) and false-positive rates (as high as 30%) of this procedure.[1,5,6] Although careful analysis of the films may be able to improve their diagnostic efficiency, their clinical usefulness is limited.[7] The epiglottis should be visualized directly, even if the radiograph is negative, in those patients in whom there is a suspicion of epiglottitis. This examination should be performed only

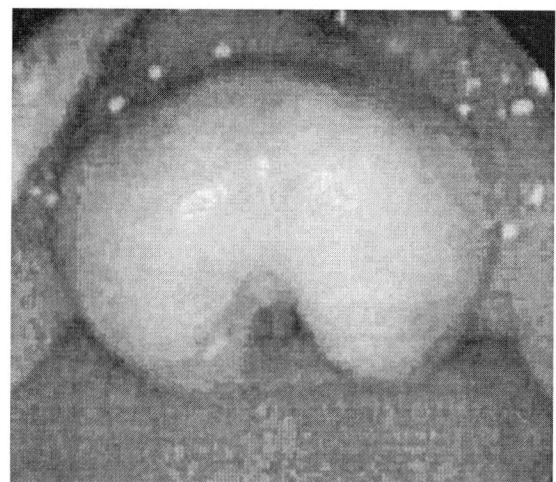

FIGURE 56-2. Epiglottitis showing a markedly enlarged epiglottis obscuring the adjacent structures. *(Courtesy of Dr. Carlos Nunez, University of Miami, Miami, Fla.)*

when one is prepared to immediately secure the airway. *H. influenzae* type B is isolated from cultures of blood or epiglottis, or both, in most pediatric patients and in up to 26% of adult patients with epiglottitis.[8] Other agents occasionally implicated include pneumococci, staphylococci, and streptococci.[2,8,9] Establishing the etiologic role of rarer agents is difficult because of the small number of cases and the frequent lack of recovery of the same organism from both the epiglottis and the blood. Organisms can be incidentally cultured from the surface of the epiglottis or from blood without being etiologic. However, a large number of etiologic agents have been reported in association with epiglottitis (Table 56-1).[10] The role of viruses in epiglottitis, other than possible rare herpes simplex infections, has not been established.[10,11] Patients with underlying diseases or immune system compromise appear more likely to have atypical causes.[10,11]

H. influenzae bacteremia occurs in up to 100% of children with epiglottitis.[1] Significantly, this bacteremia has been associated with only a small number of metastatic infections such as meningitis and arthritis.[1,2,12]

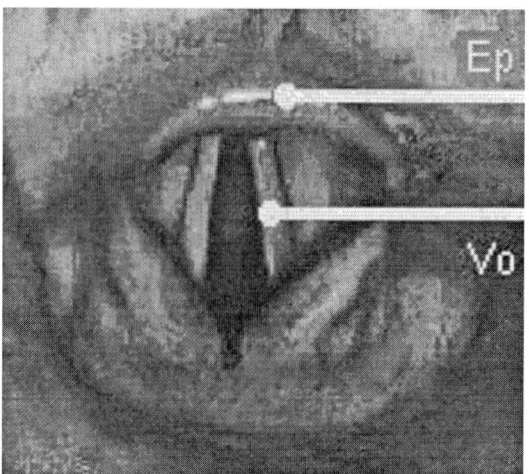

FIGURE 56-1. Normal epiglottis (Ep) and adjacent structures. Vo, vocal cords.

TABLE 56-1 Etiologic Agents That Have Been Associated with Epiglottitis

Infectious agents	*Propionibacterium*
Aspergillus	*Pseudomonas aeruginosa*
Bacteroides melaninogenicus	*Serratia marcescens*
β-Hemolytic streptococcus	*Staphylococcus aureus*
Branhamella catarrhalis	*Streptococus milleri*
Candida albicans	*Streptococcus pneumoniae*
Citrobacter diversus	*Streptococcus pyogenes*
Cytomegalovirus	*Streptococcus viridans*
Enterobacter cloacae	Varicella-zoster virus
Epstein-Barr virus	*Vibrio vulnificus*
Escherichia coli	**Chemical agents**
Fusobacterium	Caustic ingestion
Haemophilus influenzae	Gastroesophageal reflux
Haemophilus parainfluenzae	**Physical causes**
Herpes simplex	Hot water ingestion or inhalation
Kingella kingae	Smoking illicit drugs
Klebsiella pneumoniae	Blind finger sweep
Mycobacterium tuberculosis	Laryngeal mask
Neisseria meningitidis	Tonsillectomy complication
Pasteurella multocida	**Other**
Peptostreptococcus	Allergic reactions

EPIGLOTTITIS IN ADULTS

Epiglottitis in adults manifests as a sore throat with odynophagia. There is a 2:1 male predominance and variable seasonality. Most patients are in good health before the onset, but underlying conditions compromising immunity may be a factor in some patients. Up to 29% of adults at the time of diagnosis of epiglottitis had been previously seen for the same illness without the diagnosis being made, and 44% had an abnormal oropharyngeal examination without examination of the epiglottis. This emphasizes the need for a complete examination in adults with severe sore throats, which would include the epiglottis.[9] Predictors of airway compromise include sitting erect, stridor, high white blood cell counts, blood cultures positive for *H. influenzae,* dyspnea, and pneumonia on chest radiographs. Although the disease is generally milder in adults, Mayo-Smith and associates found the death rate for adults (3.2%) higher than that for children (2.2%).[13] In the same study, 3.7% of adults, compared with 4.5% of children, had airway obstruction on presentation. They speculated that there are two forms of disease in adults: a severe form caused by *H. influenzae* and a milder form caused by other organisms.

DIFFERENTIAL DIAGNOSIS

The croup syndrome is the most frequent differential consideration in pediatric epiglottitis. Although the barking cough typical of croup is an infrequent feature of epiglottitis, differentiation from croup is sometimes difficult unless the epiglottis is visualized. In contrast to epiglottitis, croup is frequently preceded by an upper respiratory infection, has a more gradual onset, involves somewhat younger children (ages 3 months to 3 years), and may last up to a week. The cause is usually viral, and the area of obstruction is subglottic, whereas the epiglottis is normal. Children with croup are more likely to prefer to lie supine and do not have the dysphagia and drooling that are characteristic of epiglottitis. In croup, radiographs of the lateral neck may show the airway narrowed in the subglottic region and are likely to reveal a normal epiglottis.[4] However, such films may be falsely read as suggesting epiglottitis in up to 27% of patients.[5]

Diphtheria can be differentiated from epiglottitis by the presence of a pseudomembrane in the respiratory tract and the presence of typical organisms on direct smear and culture of the membrane. Allergic laryngeal edema (angioneurotic edema) and foreign body aspiration lack the toxic manifestations of epiglottitis and often have a history that is helpful in suspecting the correct diagnosis. Retropharyngeal abscess, peritonsillar abscess, bacterial tracheitis, epiglottic hemangioma, toxic epidermal necrolysis, and lingual tonsillitis are other rare causes of upper airway obstruction; these can usually be differentiated from epiglottitis on physical examination. Abscess formation may complicate epiglottitis.[14]

IMMUNOCOMPROMISED HOSTS

Epiglottitis may present a somewhat different clinical picture in patients with human immunodeficiency virus (HIV) infection.[15] It may rarely be part of the initial presentation of HIV infection, the epiglottitis may be "pale and floppy," the patient may not demonstrate leukocytosis, and the course may be more fulminant than in the immunocompetent host.[16] HIV infection may also be associated with unique causes such as Kaposi's sarcoma[17] and organisms that are rare at this site such as *Candida.*[19]

Epiglottitis caused by rare organisms may be associated with other conditions that compromise immunity. Examples of these associations include single-case reports of polyarteritis nodosa and *Candida,* testicular cancer and *Kingella kingae,* thalassemia and *Vibrio vulnificus,* and various neoplasms and *Candida.* Necrotizing epiglottitis has been reported in leukemia with *Aspergillus* and in drug-induced neutropenia with *Escherichia coli.*[10,17] Recurrent epiglottitis in adults may result from impaired humoral immunity.[18]

THERAPY

Maintenance of an adequate airway should be the primary concern as soon as the diagnosis of epiglottitis is even suspected in a child or an adult. Appropriate management of the pediatric patient with epiglottitis requires the immediate insertion of an endotracheal tube. Observation of a child with epiglottitis for signs of airway obstruction cannot be recommended because the mortality is up to 25% in those observed and 80% in those in whom obstruction occurs.[2,20]

Many more adults than children have been managed with observation and no artificial airway. There have been no reported cases of airway compromise precipitated by examination in adults, so all adults presenting with a severe sore throat and odynophagia should have their epiglottis examined by direct or indirect laryngoscopy.[3,9,13,21] If laryngoscopy cannot be performed, a lateral neck radiograph may be obtained, but it will not always be positive in epiglottitis. A computed tomography scan may also be useful. Observation of an adult with epiglottitis can be dangerous.[3] Mayo-Smith and colleagues reported that only 7 of 220 adults managed with observation required an artificial airway, but 3 of these 7 died.[13] With careful observation and the ability to immediately secure an artificial airway, observation of adults without signs of airway compromise (stridor, dyspnea) may be relatively safe. Patients with higher temperatures and higher peripheral white blood cell counts warrant closer observation. Patients with dyspnea should be very carefully observed and may benefit from early intubation.[22]

Pediatric patients even suspected of having acute epiglottitis should be handled as a medical emergency because of the potential for rapid deterioration to complete respiratory obstruction. Painful or anxiety-provoking procedures should be minimized until the airway is secured or the diagnosis has been eliminated. Patients should be allowed to maintain the posture that is most comfortable for them; separation from caregivers should be minimized. Patients being transported between medical facilities and within such facilities must be accompanied by personnel capable of securing the airway should obstruction occur.

The epiglottis can be visualized in many patients by inspection alone and in most patients by depressing the tongue with a depressor placed as far posteriorly as the tonsillar pillars. However, it may be unwise to examine the epiglottis of a pediatric patient suspected of having epiglottitis because of the possibility of precipitating complete airway obstruction or a vagally mediated cardiopulmonary arrest. This caution may, however, be more anecdotal than absolute.[3,23] It is also unwise to restrain pediatric patients in the supine position because this also may lead to airway obstruction.[2] As a consequence, it is safer to transfer a pediatric patient thought to have epiglottitis to an operating room and to visualize the epiglottis with a laryngoscope or bronchoscope after the induction of anesthesia and after all is in readiness for the insertion of an artificial airway under controlled conditions. As soon as the diagnosis is made by visualization of the cherry red epiglottis, an uncuffed endotracheal tube should be inserted. In spite of theoretical difficulties with the insertion of an endotracheal tube through the region of the inflamed epiglottis, this has generally not proved to be a problem. In rare circumstances in which difficulty is encountered, a bronchoscope may be used to secure and dilate the airway before insertion of the tube.[3,24] If the epiglottis is normal, the patient may be managed in a manner appropriate for croup or laryngotracheobronchitis. If difficulty is encountered or if obstruction occurs while transporting the patient or while trying to establish the airway, the possibility of ventilating the apneic patient by bag and mask or mouth-to-mouth ventilation should not be overlooked.[25,26] If these attempts are unsuccessful, a needle cricothyrotomy should be performed before a more stable airway is established.

Contrary to common belief, the sudden obstruction of the airway that can occur in epiglottitis is not due to the abrupt impaction of the edematous epiglottis into the laryngeal inlet. Instead, cellulitis of the supraglottic structures progressively narrows the airway. Airflow in the upper airways is turbulent,[27] and resistance is inversely proportional to the fifth power of the diameter.[28,29] Therefore, reducing the airway diameter by half increases airflow resistance by 32 times. The potential abrupt airway obstruction in epiglottitis is a functional rather than a complete physical obstruction (although virtually complete physical obstruction can occur with severe edema). The airway resistance can simply exceed the patient's ability to overcome it, and this leads to respiratory failure.

After the establishment of an airway, blood and the surface of the epiglottis should be cultured, and the pediatric patient should be given intravenous antibiotic therapy directed at *H. influenzae*. In view of the risk of infection with ampicillin-resistant *H. influenzae*,[30] cefotaxime (50-180 mg/kg/day in four divided doses), ceftriaxone (80-100 mg/kg/day in two divided doses), or ampicillin-sulbactam (200-300 mg of ampicillin/kg/day in four divided doses) should be given as initial therapy. Adults should receive ceftriaxone 1 to 2 g intravenously daily or cefotaxime 2 g intravenously every 6 hours as initial therapy.

Pediatric patients with acute epiglottitis usually improve 12 to 48 hours after the initiation of appropriate antibiotic therapy. Depending on the patient's progress, the artificial airway can usually be removed within this period.[3,31] Before extubation, the patient should be clinically improved, afebrile, and alert. The decision to extubate may be based on the clinical condition of the patient, evidence of resolution by direct visualization with a fiber-optic laryngoscope, or the presence of an air leak around the endotracheal tube. Antibiotics should be continued for 7 to 10 days for adult and pediatric patients. The clinical response and status of the patient should dictate the route by which the antibiotic is administered after extubation.

A small number of patients experiencing severe respiratory distress or arrest before intubation develop pulmonary edema. The cause of this complication is not known.[31,32]

Nebulized epinephrine or steroids, or both, appear to be ineffective in epiglottitis.[9]

If the patient with *H. influenzae* epiglottitis has unvaccinated household contacts who are younger than 4 years, rifampin prophylaxis given once daily for 4 days in a dose of 20 mg/kg/day (maximum of 600 mg/day) is recommended for all household contacts, regardless of immunization status.[33] In addition, the patient should receive rifampin in the same dosage before discharge to eliminate carriage and to prevent reintroduction of the organism into the household (see Chapter 222).

IMMUNITY

An episode of *H. influenzae* epiglottis usually results in high levels of serum antibody to capsular polysaccharide.[34] This response appears to provide immunity, because second cases of epiglottitis are extremely rare. However, when epiglottitis occurs in children younger than 24 months, an age-appropriate immunization series should be completed, ignoring previously administered vaccine.[33] The presence of maternally derived serum antibody at birth explains the infrequent occurrence of *H. influenzae* infections in infants. After disappearance of this maternal antibody, there is an inverse relationship between rising naturally acquired antibody and the declining incidence of epiglottitis in unvaccinated populations.[35]

Widespread use of *H. influenzae* type B polysaccharide vaccine has dramatically decreased the incidence of invasive *H. influenzae* disease[36,37] and epiglottitis.[38] In the United States, *H. influenzae* type B invasive disease decreased greater than 99% from the prevaccine era to 2000.[38] Childhood vaccination will probably have little effect on the 2 in 100,000 incidence of disease in adults.[8,9,13] Vaccination will also not decrease *H. influenzae* disease due to types other than B.

REFERENCES

1. Sendi K, Crysdale WS. Acute epiglottitis: Decade of change—A 10-year experience with 242 children. J Otolaryngol. 1987;16:196.
2. Bass JW, Steele RW, Wiebe RA. Acute epiglottitis: A surgical emergency. JAMA. 1974;229:671.
3. Andreassen UK, Baer S, Nielsen TG, et al. Acute epiglottitis—25 years' experience with nasotracheal intubation, current management policy, and future needs. J Laryngol Otol. 1992;106:1072.
4. Podgore JK, Bass JW. The "thumb sign" and "little finger sign" in acute epiglottitis. J Pediatr. 1976;88:154.
5. Stankiewicz JA, Bowes AK. Croup and epiglottitis: A radiologic study. Laryngoscope. 1985;95:1159.
6. Jones JL, Holland P. False positives in lateral neck radiographs used to diagnose epiglottitis. Ann Emerg Med. 1983;12:797.
7. Rothrock SG, Pignatiello GA, Howard RM. Radiologic diagnosis of epiglottitis: Objective criteria for all ages. Ann Emerg Med. 1990;19:978.
8. Trollfors B, Nylén O, Strangert K. Acute epiglottitis in children and adults in Sweden 1981-3. Arch Dis Child. 1990;65:491.
9. Frantz TD, Rasgon BM, Quesenberry CP. Acute epiglottitis in adults: Analysis of 129 cases. JAMA. 1994;272:1358.
10. Carey MJ. Epiglottitis in adults. Am J Emerg Med. 1996;14:421.
11. D'Angelo AJ Jr, Zweillenberg S, Oleskszyk JP, et al. Adult supraglottitis due to herpes simplex virus. J Otolaryngol. 1990;19:179.
12. Dajani AS, Asmar BI, Thirumoorthi MC. Systemic *Haemophilus influenzae* disease: An overview. J Pediatr. 1979;94:355.
13. Mayo-Smith MF, Spinale JW, Donskey CJ, et al. Acute epiglottitis: An 18-year experience in Rhode Island. Chest. 1995;108:1640.
14. Torkkeli T, Ruoppi P, Nuutinen J, Kari A. Changed clinical course and current treatment of acute epiglottitis in adults: A 12-year experience. Laryngoscope. 1994;104:1503.
15. Pedersen BK, Pedersen C. Epiglottitis as a manifestation of acute HIV infection. J Acquir Immune Defic Syndr. 1994;7:1210.
16. Rothstein SG, Persky MS, Edelman BA, et al: Epiglottitis in AIDS patients. Laryngoscope. 1989;99:389.
17. Laing RBS, Wadrop PJC, Welsby PD, Brettle RP. Stridor in patients with HIV infection. J Otolaryngol. 1995;109:1197.
18. Gagnon R, Bédard P, Côté L, et al. Recurrent acute epiglottitis in adults: Defective antibody response. Ann Allergy Asthma Immunol. 2002;88:513.
19. Israel L, Sadigh M. *Candida* epiglottitis in an adult with acquired immunodeficiency syndrome treated with oral fluconazole. J Laryngol Otol. 1995;109:337.
20. Rapkin RH. Tracheostomy in epiglottitis. Pediatrics. 1973;52:426.
21. Dort JC, Frohlich AM, Tate RB. Acute epiglottitis in adults: Diagnosis and treatment in 43 patients. J Otolaryngol. 1994;23:281.
22. Hébert PC, Ducic Y, Boisvert D, Lamothe A. Adult epiglottitis in a Canadian setting. Laryngoscope. 1998;108:64.
23. Mauro RD, Poole SR, Lockhart CH. Differentiation of epiglottitis from laryngotracheitis in the child with stridor. Am J Dis Child. 1988;142:679.
24. Walker P, Crysdale WS. Croup, epiglottitis, retropharyngeal abscess, and bacterial tracheitis: Evolving patterns of occurrence and care. Int Anesthesiol Clin. 1992; 30:57.
25. Adair JC, Ring WH. Management of epiglottitis in children. Anesth Analg. 1975;54:622.
26. Blanc VF, Weber ML, Ludec C, et al. Acute epiglottitis in children: Management of 27 consecutive cases with nasotracheal intubation with special emphasis on anaesthetic considerations. Can Anaesth Soc J. 1977;24:1.
27. West JB. Respiratory Physiology—The Essentials. 5th ed. Baltimore: Williams & Wilkins; 1995:103.
28. Glauser SC, Glauser EM, Rusy BF. Influence of gas density and viscosity on the work of breathing. Arch Environ Health. 1969;19:654.
29. Watts AMI, McCallum MID. Acute airway obstruction following facial scalding: Differential diagnosis between a thermal and infective cause. Burns. 1996;22:570.
30. Kessler A, Wetmore RF, Marsh RR. Childhood epiglottitis in recent years. Int J Pediatr Otorhinolaryngol. 1993;25:155.
31. Butt W. Shann F, Walker C, et al. Acute epiglottitis: A different approach to management. Crit Care Med. 1988;16:43.
32. Bonadio WA, Losek JD. The characteristics of children with epiglottitis who develop the complication of pulmonary edema. Arch Otolaryngol Head Neck Surg. 1991;117:205.
33. Committee on Infectious Diseases, American Academy of Pediatrics. Report of the Committee on Infectious Diseases. 24th ed. Evanston, Ill: American Academy of Pediatrics; 1994.
34. Whisnant JK, Rogentine GN, Gralnick MA, et al. Host factors and antibody response in *Haemophilus influenzae* type b meningitis and epiglottitis. J Infect Dis. 1976;133:448.
35. Schneerson R, Rodrigues LP, Parke JC Jr, Robbins JB. Immunity to disease caused by *Hemophilus influenzae* type b. J Immunol. 1971;107:1081.
36. Centers for Disease Control and Prevention. Progress toward elimination of *Haemophilus influenzae* type b disease among infants and children. United States, 1987-1995, MMWR Morb Mortal Wkly Rep. 1996;45:901.
37. Adams WG, Deaver KA, Cochi SL, et al. Decline of childhood *Haemophilus influenzae* type b (Hib) disease in the Hib vaccine era. JAMA. 1993;269:221.
38. Centers for Disease Control and Prevention. Progress Toward Elimination of *Haemophilus influenzae* Type b Invasive Disease Among Infants and Children— United States, 1998-2000. MMWR Morb Mortal Wkly Rep. 2002;51;234.

Infections of the Oral Cavity, Neck, and Head

ANTHONY W. CHOW

Infections of the oral cavity most commonly are odontogenic in origin. Odontogenic orofacial infections include dental caries, pulpitis, periapical abscess, gingivitis, and periodontal and deep fascial space infections. Although rare, such life-threatening complications as intracranial, retropharyngeal, or pleuropulmonary extension and hematogenous dissemination to heart valves, prosthetic devices, and other metastatic foci clearly indicate the potentially serious nature of these infections. Nonodontogenic infections of the oral cavity include ulcerative and gangrenous stomatitis and infection of the major salivary glands. Suppurative orofacial infections can also arise from the middle ear, oronasopharynx, and mastoids and paranasal sinuses; these are discussed in Chapters 54 and 55, respectively.

Infections of the neck and head in the adult most commonly result from human or animal bites, trauma, irradiation, and surgical procedures. In children, cervical adenitis or thyroiditis due to bacterial or viral causes are more common. Rarely do embryologic cysts in the neck region become secondarily infected. These are considered separately from oral infections, since they frequently involve a different microflora and require alternative approaches to diagnosis and therapy.

OROFACIAL ODONTOGENIC INFECTIONS

Microbiologic Considerations

The microbiota associated with odontogenic infections is complex and generally reflects the indigenous oral flora. Such infections are typically polymicrobial, and invasiveness is often influenced by synergistic interactions of multiple microbial species. Moreover, certain species or combinations may be more invasive or more resistant to therapy than others.[1-3] Despite this complexity, recent evidence strongly supports a causative role of specific microorganisms in different forms of odontogenic infections.[1] Since the microflora associated with these infections is typically polymicrobial, it does not necessarily follow that each component of this complex flora has equal pathogenic potential or that the numerically predominant cultivatable microflora are the most important. Furthermore, it may not be necessary to eradicate the complete microflora for effective therapy. In addition, recent surveys using molecular tools indicate a level of diversity in the human subgingival microflora that cannot be recognized by conventional culture techniques.[4] In most instances, the cultivable microflora likely represent less than one percent of the total extant population as estimated by microscopy or other means.[4] Nevertheless, an appreciation of the indigenous oral flora and the host factors that may modify its composition, and knowledge of the specific microorganisms implicated in different odontogenic infections should greatly provide a more rational approach to such infections arising from the oral cavity.[5]

Indigenous Oral Flora

The oral cavity cannot be regarded as a single, uniform environment. Although representative species of microorganisms can be isolated from most areas of the mouth, certain sites such as the tongue, tooth surface, gingival crevice, and saliva tend to favor colonization by specific organisms (Table 57-1).[6-8] Quantitative studies indicate that obligate anaerobes constitute a large and important part of the residential oral flora. In the gingival crevice of healthy adults, for example, the total microscopic counts averaged 2.7×10^{11} microorganisms/g wet weight.[9] The total cultivatable anaerobic bacteria averaged 1.8×10^{11} microorganisms/g, whereas facultative bacteria averaged 2.2×10^{10} microorganisms/g, which is an eightfold difference. Overall, *Streptococcus*, *Peptostreptococcus*, *Veillonella*, *Lactobacillus*, *Corynebacterium*, and *Actinomyces* account for more than 80% of the total cultivatable oral flora. Facultative gram-negative rods are uncommon in healthy adults but may be more prominent in seriously ill, hospitalized, and elderly patients.[5,10] Unique ecologic niches are observed.[10] For example, *Streptococcus sanguis*, *Streptococcus mutans*, and *Streptococcus mitis* as well as *Actinomyces viscosus* preferentially colonize the tooth surface.[11] In contrast, *Streptococcus salivarius* and *Veillonella* spp. have a predilection for the tongue and buccal mucosa.[10] *Fusobacterium*, *Porphyromonas*, *Prevotella*, and anaerobic spirochetes appear concentrated in the gingival crevice. Factors that appear to govern these localization patterns include selective adherence characteristics of certain bacteria for various types of cells, local environmental conditions such as oxygen tension, oxidation-reduction potential (Eh) and pH, interbacterial coaggregation, and microbial inhibition.[5,7,10,12,13] Apart from anatomic considerations, numerous factors such as age, diet and nutrition, eruption of deciduous dentition, oral hygiene, smoking

TABLE 57-1 Predominant Cultivatable Bacteria from Various Sites of the Oral Cavity

Type	Predominant Genus or Family	Total Viable Count (Mean %)			
		Gingival Crevice	Dental Plaque	Tongue	Saliva
Facultative					
Gram-positive cocci	*Streptococcus*	28.8	28.2	44.8	46.2
	S. mutans group	(0-30)	(0-50)	(0-1)	(0-1)
	S. sanguis	(10-20)	(40-60)	(10-20)	(10-30)
	S. mitis	(10-30)	(20-40)	(10-30)	(30-50)
	S. salivarius group	(0-1)	(0-1)	(40-60)	(40-60)
Gram-positive rods	*Lactobacillus*	15.3	23.8	13.0	11.8
Gram-negative cocci	*Moraxella*	0.4	0.4	3.4	1.2
Gram-negative rods	Enterobacteriaceae	1.2	ND	3.2	2.3
Anaerobic					
Gram-positive cocci	*Peptostreptococcus*	7.4	12.6	4.2	13.0
Gram-positive rods	*Actinomyces, Eubacterium, Leptotrichia*	20.2	18.4	8.2	4.8
Gram-negative cocci	*Veillonella*	10.7	6.4	16.0	15.9
Gram-negative rods		16.1	10.4	8.2	4.8
	Fusobacterium	1.9	4.1	0.7	0.3
	Prevotella or *Porphyromonas*	4.7	ND	0.2	ND

ND, Not detected.
Data from references 1-3

habits, the presence of dental caries or periodontal disease, antimicrobial therapy, hospitalization, pregnancy, and genetic and racial factors may influence the composition of the oral flora.[7,12,14]

Microbial Specificity in Odontogenic Infections

Although it had been recognized for some time that odontogenic infections are initiated by microorganisms through the establishment of dental plaques, the microbial specificity of these infections was not fully appreciated until recently.[1] This breakthrough was brought about by technologic advances in sampling and anaerobic culture of specimens as well as by improved methods for species identification and taxonomy.[15,16] Important differences in bacterial compositions have been noted for dental caries, gingivitis, and different forms of periodontitis when compared with cultures from healthy tissues.[17,18] An etiologic association of *S. mutans* in dental caries has been firmly established.[19,20] *S. mutans* is the only organism consistently isolated from all decayed dental fissures and is the only organism consistently found in greater numbers in carious compared with noncarious teeth. The infectious and transmissible nature of this organism in dental caries has been demonstrated in both experimental animals and longitudinal studies in humans.

Similarly, in gingivitis and periodontitis, a unique and specific bacterial composition of the subgingival plaque has been identified. In the healthy periodontium, the microflora is sparse and consists mainly of gram-positive organisms such as *Streptococcus oralis*, *S. sanguis*, and *Actinomyces* spp. In the presence of gingivitis, the predominant subgingival flora shifts to a greater proportion of anaerobic gram-negative rods, and *Prevotella intermedia* (formerly *Bacteroides intermedius*), *Capnocytophaga* spp., and *Peptostreptococcus* spp. are most commonly isolated.[16,21] With established periodontitis, the flora further increases in complexity, with a preponderance of anaerobic gram-negative and motile organisms and spirochetes (*Treponema denticola*).[22,23] *Porphyromonas gingivalis* (formerly *Bacteroides gingivalis*), *Actinobacillus actinomycetemcomitans*, *Bacteroides forsythus*, *P. intermedia*, and *T. denticola* are most commonly isolated.[24,25] In juvenile periodontitis, a clinical variant seen primarily in adolescents, the subgingival plaque mainly consists of saccharolytic organisms, with *A. actinomycetemcomitans* and *Capnocytophaga* spp. as the most common identifiable species. *P. gingivalis* is rarely found in this condition.[26] In suppurative odontogenic infections such as periapical abscesses or deep fascial space infections, a polymicrobial flora is usually present, with *Fusobacterium nucleatum*, pigmented *Bacteroides*, *Peptostreptococcus*, *Actinomyces*, and *Streptococcus* as the most predominant isolates.[1,27,28] Except in selected patients with serious underlying illnesses, facultative gram-negative bacilli and *Staphylococcus aureus* are uncommonly isolated.[29]

This microbial specificity demonstrated for different odontogenic infections probably reflects the acquisition of a unique microflora during the development of a supragingival dental plaque and its progression to a subgingival dental plaque.[30,31] Plaques that accumulate above the gingival margin are composed mainly of gram-positive facultative and microaerophilic cocci and rods; plaques that accumulate below the gingival margin are composed mainly of gram-negative anaerobic rods and motile forms including spirochetes (Fig. 57-1).[32] Microorganisms residing within the supragingival plaque are characterized by their ability to adhere to the tooth surface and by their saccharolytic activity.[33] Microorganisms in the subgingival plaque are frequently asaccharolytic and need not be adherent.

Pathogenetic Mechanisms

The mechanisms by which pathogenic microorganisms in the oral cavity can cause disease are varied. To some extent, these microbes must be able to adhere to mucosal or tooth surfaces, resist elimination by mechanical means such as flushing by oral fluids, compete for space and nutrients with other resident flora, evade host defenses, and penetrate host tissues.[5] The ability to attach to mucosal and tooth surfaces appears important for both commensal and pathogenic microbes.[33] For example, a 36-kDa fimbrial protein has been identified in *Streptococcus sanguis* and *S. parasanguis* that allows these organisms to bind to hydroxyapatite on the tooth surface, and is apparently an important virulence factor for infective endocarditis.[34,35] In the case of *Porphyromonas gingivalis*, various proteases as well as collagenase and hyaluronidase may enhance binding to fibroblasts and matrix proteins by degrading host proteins, thus exposing cryptic receptors for the microorganisms.[36]

Suppurative orofacial infections are usually preceded by dental caries or periodontal disease. The pathogenetic mechanisms of cariogenesis remain poorly defined.[37] The most universally accepted theory is that originated by W. D. Miller in 1882, which proposes that bacterial

FIGURE 57-1. Microbial specificity in odontogenic infections. A unifying hypothesis demonstrating a microbial shift from a plaque-free tooth surface and progression to supragingival and subgingival plaque organisms. *(Modified from Chow AW. Odontogenic infections. In: Schlossberg D, ed. Infections of the Head and Neck. New York: Springer; 1987:148.)*

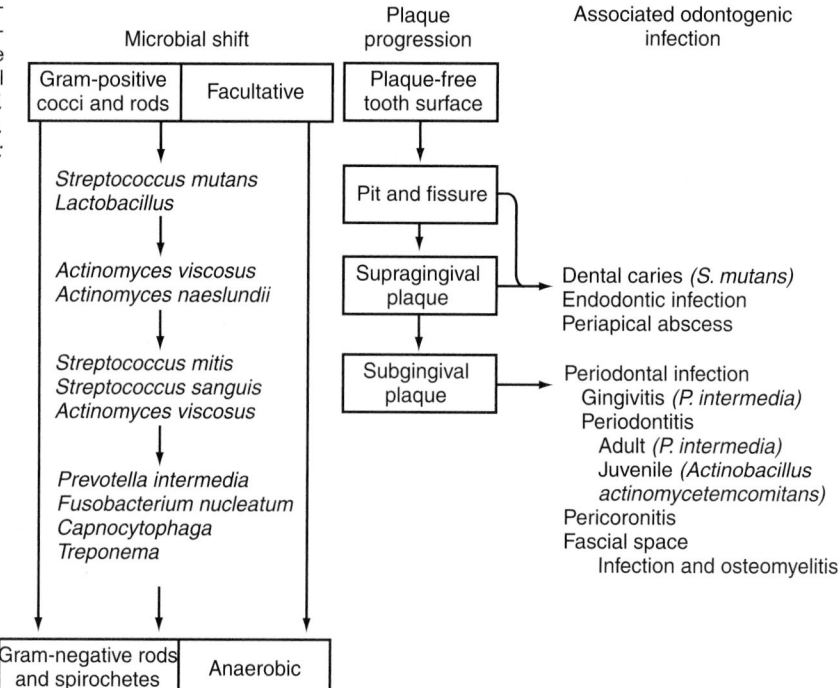

action on carbohydrates produces acidic substances that cause demineralization and dissolution of the hard tissues of the tooth.[20,32] In order for dental caries to develop, three factors need to be present: (1) a susceptible tooth surface (host factors), (2) acidogenic (acid-producing) and aciduric (able to grow at low pH) bacteria within a dental plaque (microbial factors), and (3) simple sugars and other carbohydrates (dietary factors). In the healthy host, at least three mechanisms protect the tooth from carious decay: (1) the cleaning action of the tongue and buccal membranes, which removes any food particles from the proximity of the tooth; (2) the buffering effect of saliva, which has a neutral pH, washes away bacterial acids, and provides essential substrates for remineralization and repair of damaged tooth surfaces; and (3) the protective effect of an acellular bacteria-free coating of salivary origin on the tooth surface, known as the *acquired pellicle*, which acts as a surface barrier to most dietary and bacterial acids and other proteolytic substances. In the absence of tooth brushing and flossing, the acquired pellicle becomes rapidly colonized and is replaced by the bacterial plaque. It is not surprising, therefore, that carious lesions occur most often in areas inaccessible to the self-cleaning mechanisms of the mouth and on the occlusal surfaces and sites that are protected from the reaches of the toothbrush.

Unlike its effect on dental caries, diet does not appear to have a significant role in the pathogenesis of periodontal disease. The periodontal microflora associated with the subgingival plaque have the ability to penetrate the gingival epithelium and elicit an inflammatory host response that ultimately results in destruction of the periodontium.[2,17,38-40] Two major predisposing factors are poor oral hygiene and increasing age.[41] Other factors include hormonal effects, with exacerbation of disease activity during puberty, menstruation, and pregnancy.[42] Diabetes mellitus causes an increased incidence, particularly in juvenile diabetic patients. Finally, various genetic disorders are associated with an increased incidence of periodontal disease.[43] In particular, those with neutrophil defects (such as Chédiak-Higashi syndrome, agranulocytosis, and cyclic neutropenia) have a higher incidence of periodontal disease.[44]

It is a tribute to the local defenses in the healthy host that infections within the oral cavity are not more common. The establishment of the normal resident flora appears to be particularly important in providing a strong mucosal defense against colonization and invasion by potential pathogens (*colonization resistance*).[45] Other nonspecific local defenses include the continuous cell shedding and turnover of the mucosal epithelium and the constant flow of saliva containing lysozyme, lactoferrin, β-lysin, lactoperoxidase, and other antimicrobial systems.[45] Various salivary glycoproteins and histidine-rich polypeptides have been reported to inhibit bacteria and fungi and may prevent infection by the inhibition of microbial attachment to oral epithelium by way of competition for cellular receptor sites or clumping of microorganisms. The epithelial barrier may be affected by radiation therapy, cancer chemotherapy, or trauma. A reduced turnover rate of the epithelial cells allows retention of adherent organisms. A reduction in saliva volume also has significant effects on the oral environment and predisposes to microbial invasion.

In addition to nonspecific host defenses, specific humoral and cellular immune mechanisms are also important. Specific antibodies are present in saliva, with secretory immunoglobulin A (IgA) as the predominant immunoglobulin. Salivary antibodies may affect the oral flora by the aggregation of organisms and the prevention of their attachment to mucosal epithelium.[46,47] Cell-mediated immunity is important in oral defense against intracellular pathogens, including viruses, fungi, and bacteria. In the severely immunocompromised patient, a reactivation of viral infection involving the oral cavity is common, often with potentially life-threatening complications.[48]

In addition to humoral and cellular immunity, various phagocytic cells in the oral mucosa also appear important. Phagocytic cells such as lymphocytes, granulocytes, and macrophages are abundant in the lamina propria and presumably contribute to the removal of foreign matter that has breached the epithelial barrier. Unique defects in host defenses have been identified in periodontal infections. For example, impairment of neutrophil chemotaxis has been demonstrated in patients with

juvenile periodontitis.[49] As well, several oral microorganisms associated with periodontitis, including *Actinobacillus actinomycetemcomitans*, produce a leukotoxin that destroys polymorphonuclear leukocytes and macrophages and is believed to be a key virulence factor.[50] A number of oral anaerobes and streptococci implicated in periodontitis including *P. gingivalis*, *P. intermedia*, *Prevotella melaninogenica*, *Capnocytophaga* spp., *S. sanguis*, and *S. mitis* are found to secrete IgA proteases.[51,52] The pathogenic significance of this finding is uncertain at present; but it has been suggested that cleavage of IgA by microbial IgA proteases may impair local mucosal immunity of the host. It remains to be seen if similar or other defects of host resistance can be identified in different forms of destructive odontogenic infections. On the other hand, excessive inflammatory host responses to commensal oral microflora or failure to down-regulate this immune response may also be important in some patients with destructive forms of periodontal disease.[39,40] Thus, host-mediated tissue injury as a consequence of microbial infection rather than the infection itself has become a major focus in the pathogenesis of periodontitis and its possible link to coronary atherosclerosis and heart disease.[53]

Anatomic Considerations

Soft tissue infections of odontogenic origin tend to spread along planes of least resistance from the supporting structures of the affected tooth to various potential spaces in the vicinity. Accumulated pus, therefore, must generally perforate bone at the site where it is thinnest and weakest before it extends into the periapical areas or deeper fascial spaces. In the mandible, this is usually in the region of the molar teeth on the lingual aspect and more anterior on the buccal aspect.[54] In the maxilla, the bone is weakest on the buccal aspect throughout and relatively thicker on the palatal aspect. If pus perforates through either the maxillary or the mandibular buccal plate, it presents intraorally if inside the attachment of the buccinator muscle to the maxilla or mandible and extraorally if outside this muscle attachment (Fig. 57-2).[6] When a

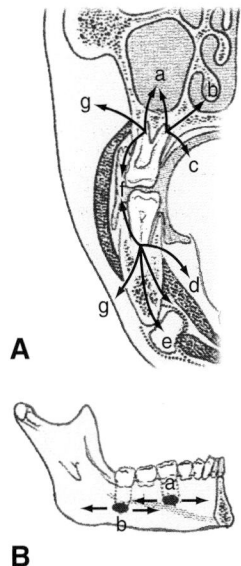

FIGURE 57-2. Routes of spread of odontogenic orofacial infections along planes of least resistance. **A,** Coronal section in the region of the first molar teeth: a, maxillary antrum; b, nasal cavity; c, palatal plate; d, sublingual space (above the mylohyoid muscle); e, submandibular space (below the mylohyoid muscle); f, intraoral presentation with infection spreading through the buccal plates inside the attachment of the buccinator muscle; g, extraoral presentation to buccal space with infection spreading through the buccal plates outside the attachment of the buccinator muscle. **B,** Lingual aspect of the mandible: a, apices of the involved tooth above the mylohyoid muscle, with spread of infection to the sublingual space; b, apices of involved tooth below the mylohyoid muscle, with spread of infection into the submandibular space. *(From Chow AW, Roser SM, Brady FA. Orofacial odontogenic infections. Ann Intern Med. 1978;88:392-402.)*

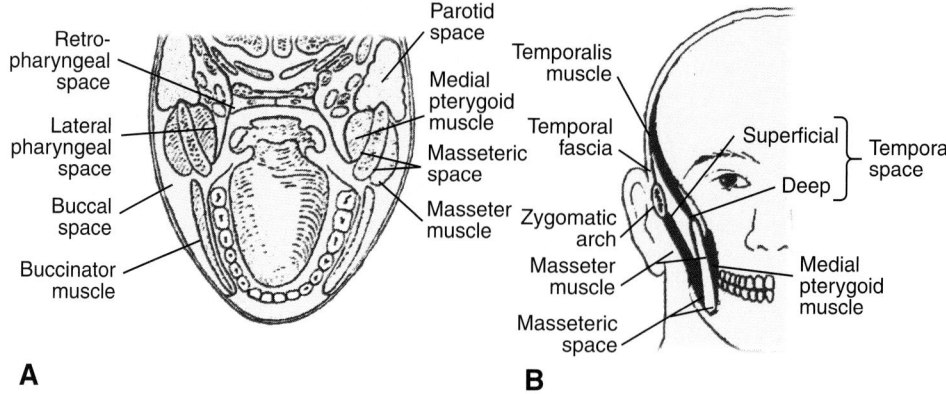

FIGURE 57-3. Fascial spaces around the mouth and face. **A,** Horizontal section at the level of the occlusal surface of the mandibular teeth. **B,** Frontal view of the face. (*From Chow AW, Roser SM, Brady FA. Orofacial odontogenic infections. Ann Intern Med. 1978;88:392-402.*)

mandibular infection perforates lingually, it presents in the sublingual space if the apices of the involved teeth lie above the attachment of the mylohyoid muscle (e.g., mandibular incisor, canines, premolars, and first molars) and in the submandibular space if below the attachment of this muscle (e.g., second and third molars) (see Fig. 57-2). Thus, these local anatomic barriers of bone, muscle, and fascia predetermine the routes of spread, extent, and clinical manifestations of many orofacial infections of odontogenic origin. The clinically important "fascial spaces" most often involved are illustrated in Figures 57-3 and 57-4. These are potential spaces between layers of fascia normally bound together by loose connective tissue. The breakdown of these attachments by a spreading infective process results in a fascial space infection. These spaces intercommunicate with one another to varied degrees, and the potential pathways of extension from one space to another are illustrated in Figure 57-5. A thorough understanding of the potential *anatomic routes* of infection not only provides valuable information on the nature and extent of infection but also suggests the optimal surgical approach for effective drainage.

Clinical Presentations

Odontogenic infections originate in either the dental pulp or the periodontium. The most common site is the dental pulp and results in dentoalveolar infections.

Dentoalveolar Infections

Pulpal infection most frequently results from carious exposure, rarely from physical or chemical injury. The carious process most frequently begins in pits and fissures on the occlusal surfaces of molars and premolars, which encourage food retention. Interproximal sites and the gingival margin are the next most common. Demineralization of the enamel results in discoloration, the first visible evidence of carious involvement. Destruction of the enamel and dentin and invasion of the pulp produce either a localized or a generalized pulpitis. If drainage from the pulp is obstructed, a rapid progression with pulpal necrosis and proliferation of endodontic microorganisms leads to invasion of the periapical areas (periapical abscess) and alveolar bone (acute alveolar abscess).[2]

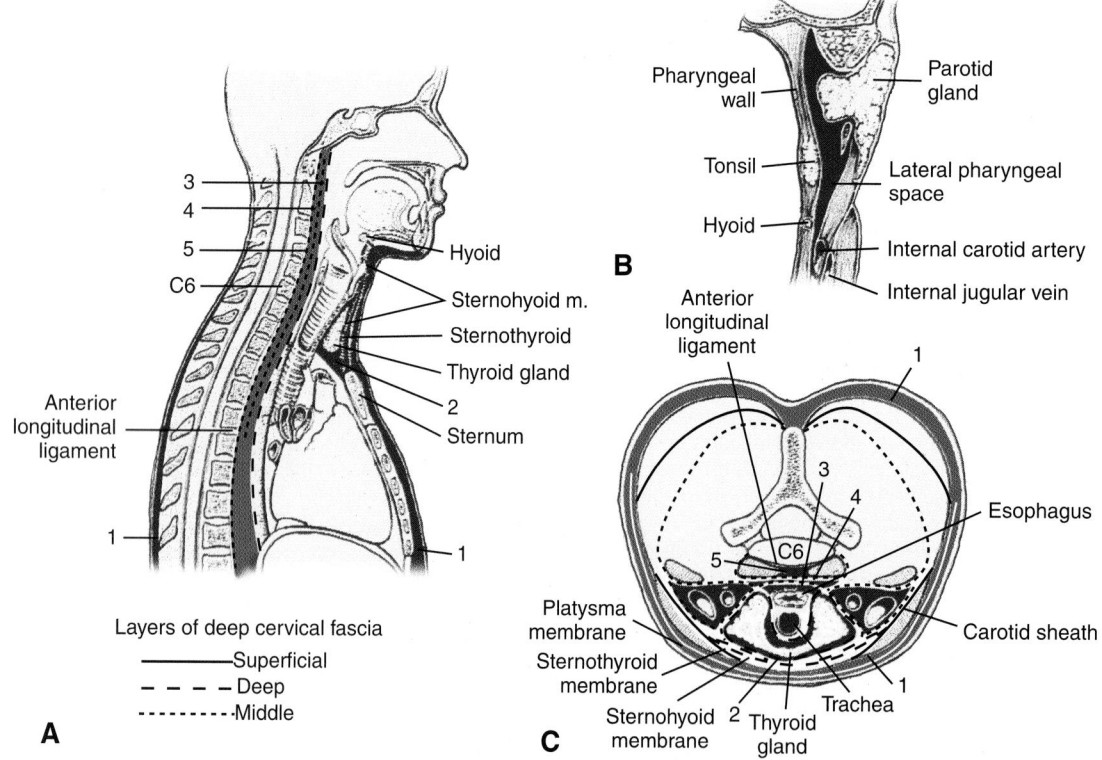

FIGURE 57-4. Relation of lateral pharyngeal, retropharyngeal, and prevertebral spaces to the posterior and anterior layers of the deep cervical fascia. 1, Superficial space; 2, pretracheal space; 3, retropharyngeal space; 4, "danger" space; 5, prevertebral space. **A,** Midsagittal section of the head and neck. **B,** Coronal section in the suprahyoid region of the neck. **C,** Cross-section of the neck at the level of the thyroid isthmus.

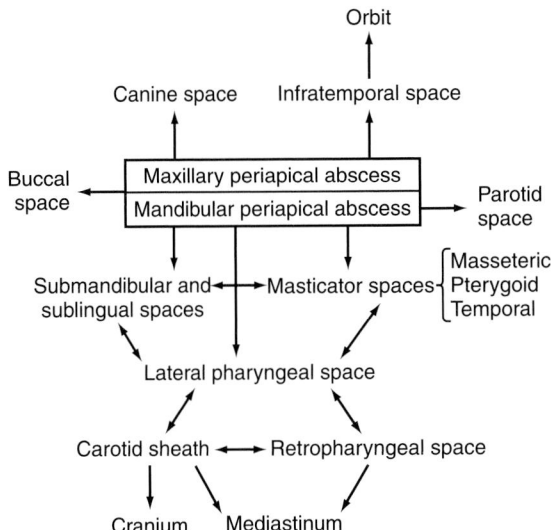

Orbit

Canine space   Infratemporal space

Buccal space ← Maxillary periapical abscess
              Mandibular periapical abscess → Parotid space

Submandibular and sublingual spaces ← → Masticator spaces { Masseteric, Pterygoid, Temporal

Lateral pharyngeal space

Carotid sheath ← → Retropharyngeal space

Cranium   Mediastinum

FIGURE 57-5. Potential pathways of extension in deep fascial space infections.

Clinically, the tooth is sensitive to percussion and to both heat and cold during early or reversible pulpitis, although the painful response stops abruptly when the stimulus is withdrawn. During late or irreversible pulpitis, the tooth is exquisitely painful to a hot stimulus, with prompt relief by the application of cold. If drainage is established through the tooth before extension into the periapical region, chronic irritation from the necrotic pulp may result in periapical granuloma or cyst formation that may be relatively asymptomatic. Dental radiographs are particularly helpful for the detection of silent lesions, particularly those caused by interproximal caries, which are difficult to detect clinically.

The principles of treatment in dentoalveolar infections include prompt elimination of the infected pulp, deep periodontal scaling, or extraction of the affected tooth.[1] Dentoalveolar abscess should be surgically drained at the same time. Other supportive measures include hydration, a soft diet, analgesics, and oral hygiene. Antibiotic therapy is indicated primarily if drainage cannot be adequately established or when infection has perforated the cortex and spread into surrounding soft tissue.

Gingivitis and Periodontal Infections

Periodontal disease is a general term that refers to all diseases involving the supporting structures of the teeth (periodontium), including the gingiva, periodontal ligament, alveolar bone, and cementum. In the early phase of periodontal disease, infection is confined to the gingiva (gingivitis). Later, the underlying supporting tissues are affected (periodontitis), ultimately leading to complete destruction of the periodontium and a permanent loss of teeth. Periodontal infections tend to localize in intraoral soft tissues and seldom spread into deeper structures of the face or neck.

Gingivitis. Acute and chronic inflammation of the gingiva is initiated by local irritation and microbial invasion.[22,25] Subgingival plaque is always present. In simple gingivitis, there is a bluish-red discoloration, with swelling and thickening of the free gingival margin. A tendency for bleeding of the gums after eating or toothbrushing may be one of the earliest findings. There is usually no pain, but a mild fetor oris may be noticed. In acute necrotizing ulcerative gingivitis (Vincent's disease, or trench mouth), the patient typically experiences a sudden onset of pain in the gingiva that interferes with normal mastication. Necrosis of the gingiva occurs mainly in the interdental papilla and results in a marginated, punched-out, and eroded appearance. A superficial grayish pseudomembrane is formed, and a characteristic halitosis with altered taste sensation is present. There is usually

associated fever, malaise, and regional lymphadenopathy. Treatment includes local débridement and lavage with oxidizing agents, which usually brings relief from pain within 24 hours. Antibiotic therapy with penicillin or metronidazole is indicated and is highly effective during the acute phase of infection.[55,56]

Periodontitis. Chronic inflammation of the periodontium is the major cause of tooth loss in adults. The destructive process proceeds insidiously, usually beginning in early adulthood. Subgingival plaque is always present, and both supragingival and subgingival calculi are usually abundant. Unlike pulpal infection in which drainage is frequently obstructed, periodontal infections drain freely, and patients experience little or no discomfort. Associated sensations include pressure and an itchy feeling in the gums and between the teeth, a bad taste in the mouth, hot and cold sensitivity, and vague pains in the jaws. The gingiva is inflamed and discolored, bleeds readily, and presents as periodontal pockets around the affected teeth. Frank pus can be readily expressed by digital pressure or may exude freely from the pockets. As periodontitis advances, the supporting tissues are destroyed, ultimately leading to loosening and exfoliation of teeth. Localized juvenile periodontitis is a particularly destructive form of periodontitis seen in adolescents and is characterized by rapid vertical bone loss affecting the first molar and incisor teeth. Plaque is usually minimal, and calculus is absent. Recent experience suggests excellent therapeutic results with systemic tetracycline or metronidazole therapy combined with local periodontal treatment involving root débridement and surgical resection of inflamed periodontal tissues.[57,58] An effective plaque control program with root débridement may be necessary for long-term maintenance of the diseased periodontium.[57]

Periodontal Abscess. Periodontal abscesses may be focal or diffuse and present as red, fluctuant swelling of the gingiva, which is extremely tender to palpation. These abscesses are always in communication with a periodontal pocket from which pus can be readily expressed after probing. Treatment is surgical and aimed at drainage of loculated pus. After abscess resolution, endodontic or periodontal infections should continue to be treated by removing necrotic infected pulpal tissues or by subgingival scaling and root planing. Apical surgery may sometimes be necessary to reach the apical part of the root for débridement.[1]

Pericoronitis. Pericoronitis is an acute localized infection associated with gum flaps overlying a partially erupted or impacted wisdom tooth. Food debris and microorganisms become entrapped under the affected gingival tissues. If drainage is interrupted due to sudden swelling or trauma, infection extends along fascial planes of least resistance into adjacent soft tissues. The underlying alveolar bone is usually not involved. Clinically, the pericoronal tissues are erythematous and swollen. Digital pressure produces a small amount of exudate from under the infected flap. Since the masticator spaces are often involved, marked trismus secondary to irritation of the masseter or medial pterygoid muscle is a prominent presenting feature. Treatment of pericoronitis includes incision of the lesion and irrigation of the pericoronitis pouch with antiseptics. Systemic antibiotics may be necessary if cellulitis of fascial planes occurs. Excision of the operculum or extraction of the involved tooth may also be considered.

Deep Fascial Space Infections

Infections of either odontogenic or oropharyngeal origin may extend to potential fascial spaces of the lower part of the head and upper portion of the neck. These "space infections" can be conveniently divided into those around the face (masticator, buccal, canine, and parotid spaces), those in the suprahyoid region (submandibular, sublingual, and lateral pharyngeal spaces), and those involving the infrahyoid region or the total neck (retropharyngeal, "danger," and pretracheal spaces).[27,29]

Masticator Spaces. Masticator spaces consist of the masseteric, pterygoid, and temporal spaces, all of which are well differentiated but intercommunicate with each other, as well as with the buccal, submandibular, and lateral pharyngeal spaces (see Fig. 57-3). Infection of the masticator spaces occurs most frequently from molar teeth, particularly the third molars (wisdom teeth). Clinically, the hallmark of masticator space infection is trismus and pain in the area of the body or ramus of the mandible. Swelling may not be a prominent finding, especially in the masseteric compartment, since infection exists deep in large muscle masses, which obscures or prevents clinically apparent swelling. When present, swelling tends to be brawny and indurated, which suggests the possibility of cervicofacial actinomycosis or mandibular osteomyelitis. If infection extends internally, it can involve an area close to the lateral pharyngeal wall and result in dysphagia. A true lateral pharyngeal space infection, however, is accompanied by displacement of the lateral pharyngeal wall toward the midline, a finding not present in masticator space infections. Infection of the deep temporal space usually originates from involvement of the posterior maxillary molar teeth. Very little external swelling is observed early in the course; if present, it usually affects the preauricular region and an area over the zygomatic arch. As infection progresses, the cheek, eyelids, and whole side of the face may be involved (Fig. 57-6).[6] Infection may extend directly into the orbit via the inferior orbital fissure and produce proptosis, optic neuritis, and abducens nerve palsy.

Buccal, Canine, and Parotid Spaces. As noted previously, infections arising from mandibular or maxillary bicuspid and molar teeth tend to extend in a lateral or buccal direction. The relation of the root apices to the origins of the buccinator muscle determines whether infection will exit intraorally into the buccal vestibule or extraorally into the buccal space (see Fig. 57-2). Infection of the buccal space is readily diagnosed because of marked cheek swelling with minimal trismus and systemic symptoms. There is a great tendency to resolution with antibiotic therapy alone. Drainage, if required, is superficial and should be performed extraorally. Involvement of the maxillary incisors and canines may result in a canine space infection, which presents as dramatic swelling of the upper lip, canine fossa, and frequently the periorbital tissues. Pain is usually moderate, and systemic signs are minimal. Occasionally, a purulent maxillary sinusitis may result due to direct extension of infection into the adjoining antrum. Treatment consists of antibiotics and drainage, which can be accomplished intraorally. Parotid space infection from an odontogenic cause generally represents secondary spread from a masseteric space infection in the area of the ramus of the mandible (see Fig. 57-3). There is marked swelling of the angle of the jaw without associated trismus. Pain may be intense and accompanied by high fever and chills. Because of its close relationship with the posterior aspect of the lateral pharyngeal space, a parotid space infection carries the potential risk of direct extension into the danger and visceral spaces and hence to the posterior mediastinum (see Fig.57-4).

Submandibular and Sublingual Spaces. These two spaces are separated by the mylohyoid muscle (see Fig. 57-2), and the submandibular space is further divided into the submaxillary and submental spaces. Infection in these spaces usually arises from the second and third mandibular molar teeth since their root apices lie inferior to the mylohyoid muscle. There is typical swelling, although much less trismus, in contradistinction to masseteric space infection, since the major muscles of mastication are usually not involved. Submandibular odontogenic infection should be distinguished from submandibular sialadenitis and lymphadenitis that are due to other causes. Therapy includes antibiotics, dental extraction, and extraoral surgical drainage. Infection of the sublingual space generally arises from mandibular incisors, since their root apices lie above the mylohyoid muscle. Clinically, this space infection presents as a brawny, erythematous, tender swelling of the floor of the mouth that begins close to the mandible and spreads toward the midline or beyond. Some elevation of the tongue may be noted in late states. Surgical drainage of the sublingual space should be performed intraorally by an incision through the mucosa parallel to Wharton's duct. If the submandibular space is also to be drained, both spaces can be reached through a submandibular approach.

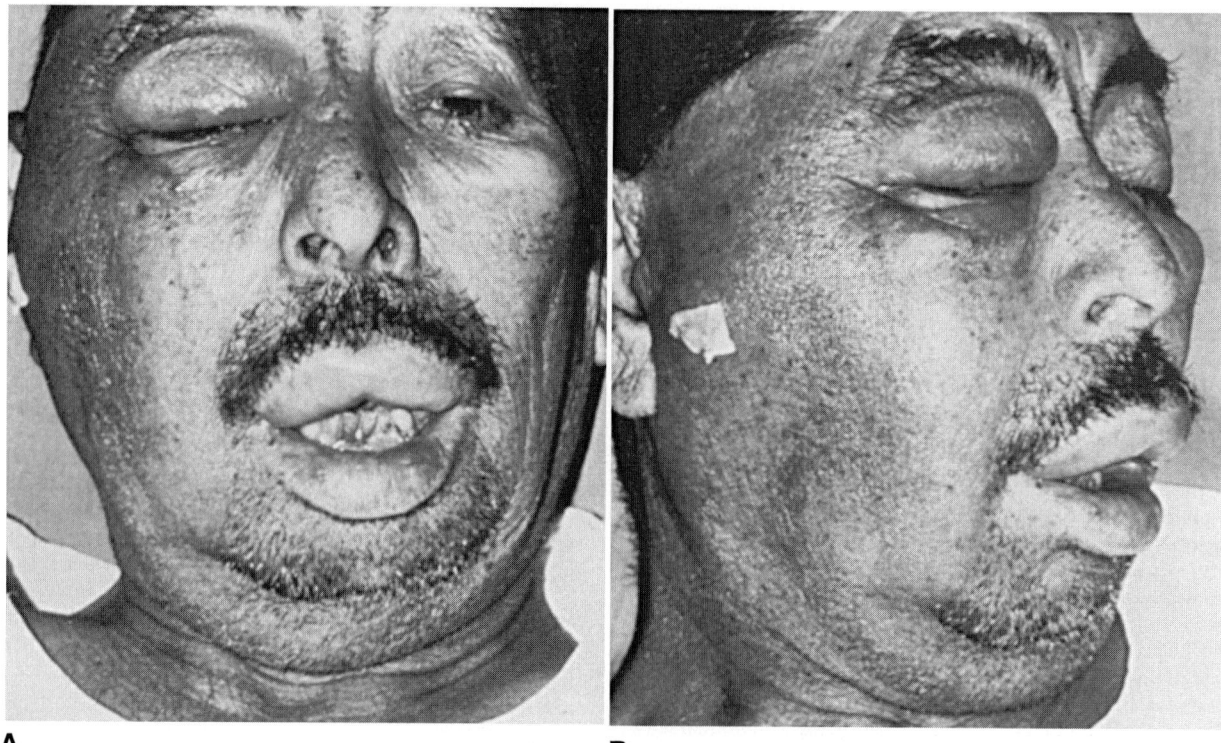

A **B**

FIGURE 57-6. Deep temporal space infection with spread to the right parotid space and the orbit. This patient developed right optic neuritis with permanent loss of vision in that eye. **A,** Frontal view. **B,** Lateral view. *(From Chow AW, Roser SM, Brady FA. Orofacial odontogenic infections. Ann Intern Med. 1978; 88:392-402.)*

Ludwig's Angina. The term *Ludwig's angina* has been loosely applied to a heterogeneous array of infections involving the sublingual, submaxillary, and submandibular spaces.[59] However, for therapeutic and prognostic purposes, it is desirable to restrict this diagnosis to cases that conform to the following classic description: (1) the infection is always bilateral, (2) both the submandibular and sublingual spaces are involved, (3) the infection is a rapidly spreading indurated cellulitis without abscess formation or lymphatic involvement, and (4) the infection begins in the floor of the mouth. A dental source of infection has been found in 50% to 90% of reported cases. The second and third mandibular molars are most commonly involved. Clinically, patients present with a brawny boardlike swelling in the submandibular spaces that does not pit on pressure (Fig. 57-7). The mouth is usually held open and the floor elevated, which pushes the tongue to the roof of the mouth. Eating and swallowing are difficult, and respiration may be impaired by obstruction from the tongue. A rapid progression of the infection results in edema of the neck and glottis and may precipitate asphyxiation. Fever and systemic toxicity are usually present and may be severe. Treatment requires high doses of parenteral antibiotics such as ampicillin-sulbactam or penicillin G plus metronidazole, airway monitoring, early intubation or tracheostomy when required, soft tissue decompression, and surgical drainage. Systemic antibiotics combined with aggressive surgical intervention have lowered the mortality rate for Ludwig's angina dramatically from over 50% in the preantibiotic era to 0% to 4% currently.[60]

Lateral Pharyngeal Space. The lateral pharyngeal space (also known as the pharyngomaxillary space) in the lateral aspect of the neck is shaped like an inverted cone, with its base at the skull and its apex at the hyoid bone (see Fig. 57-4). Its medial wall is contiguous

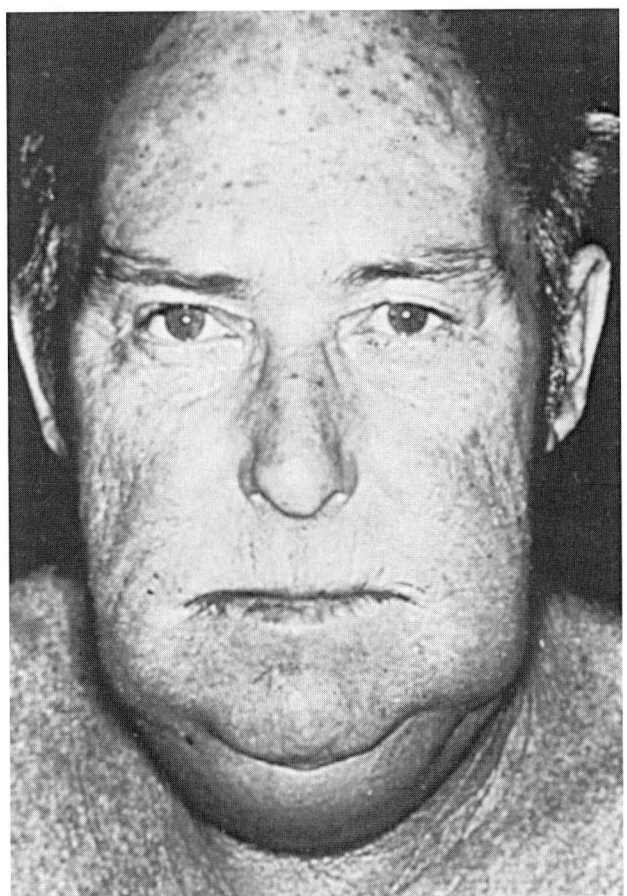

FIGURE 57-7. Early appearance of a patient with Ludwig's angina with a brawny, boardlike swelling in the submandibular spaces. *(From Chow AW, Roser SM, Brady FA. Orofacial odontogenic infections. Ann Intern Med. 1978; 88:392-402.)*

with the carotid sheath, which contains several vital structures including the common carotid artery, the internal jugular vein, and the vagus nerve, and lies deep to the pharyngeal constrictor muscle. Infection of the lateral pharyngeal space may result from pharyngitis, tonsillitis, parotitis, otitis, or mastoiditis, as well as odontogenic infection, especially if the masticator spaces are primarily involved. The source of infection is best investigated by computed tomography (CT) or magnetic resonance imaging (MRI). If the anterior compartment is infected, the patient exhibits fever, chills, marked pain, trismus, swelling below the angle of the mandible, dysphagia, and medial displacement of the lateral pharyngeal wall. The contiguous parotid gland is usually swollen. Although not prominent, dyspnea can occur. Posterior compartment infection is potentially life-threatening because of the carotid sheath, and is characterized by septicemia with little pain or trismus. Swelling is usually internal and deep and can often be missed because it is behind the palatopharyngeal arch. Complications include respiratory obstruction from edema of the larynx, thrombosis of the internal jugular vein, and erosion of the internal carotid artery. Suppuration may advance rapidly to other spaces, particularly the retropharyngeal and danger spaces, thus reaching directly to the mediastinum inferiorly or the base of the skull superiorly (see Fig. 57-4). Because respiratory obstruction from laryngeal edema can occur suddenly, the patient must be closely observed, and prophylactic tracheostomy may be required. Treatment includes high levels of antibiotics and surgical drainage. It is usually prudent to wait for the infection to localize before drainage is attempted unless respiratory obstruction or hemorrhage necessitates early surgical intervention.

Retropharyngeal, Danger, and Pretracheal Spaces. The retropharyngeal space comprises the posterior part of the visceral compartment in which the esophagus, trachea, and thyroid glands are enclosed by the middle layer of deep cervical fascia (see Fig. 57-4). It lies behind the hypopharynx and the esophagus and extends inferiorly into the superior mediastinum to about the level from T1 to T2. Posterior to this compartment lies the danger space, which descends directly into the posterior mediastinum to the level of the diaphragm. Infection of the retropharyngeal space may result from contiguous infection of the lateral pharyngeal space or from lymphatic spread from more distant sites to involve the retropharyngeal lymph nodes. Dysphagia, dyspnea, nuchal rigidity, and esophageal regurgitation, as well as high fever and chills, may be present. Bulging of the posterior pharyngeal wall may be observed. Lateral soft tissue radiographs of the neck may reveal marked widening of the retropharyngeal space. Infection of the retropharyngeal space is potentially life-threatening and requires prompt surgical drainage. Complications include hemorrhage and spontaneous rupture into the airway with asphyxiation, laryngeal spasm, bronchial erosion, and thrombosis of the jugular vein. The pretracheal space comprises the anterior portion of the visceral compartment and completely surrounds the trachea. Most commonly, infections reach this space through perforations of the anterior esophageal wall, occasionally through contiguous extension from a retropharyngeal space infection. The clinical presentation is characterized by severe dyspnea, but hoarseness may be the first complaint. Swallowing is difficult, and regurgitation of fluids through the nose may occur. A pretracheal space infection is always serious because of possible extension into the mediastinum, and prompt surgical drainage is critically important.

Complications of Odontogenic Infections

Complications of odontogenic infections can occur either by hematogenous spread or by direct extension. Transient bacteremia is common during or after various dental procedures, especially the extraction of infected teeth.[34,61] The temporal relationship between these procedures and subsequent bacterial endocarditis and cardiovascular prosthetic infections is well documented.[62] Reports of infected total hip replacements after dental procedures add further concern.[34,63] Prophylactic antibiotic treatment during dental procedures, although frequently used, remains a controversial issue, especially in the absence of preexisting valvular heart disease.[62,64] Complications of odontogenic infections secondary to direct extension include mediastinal spread,[65-67] intracranial suppuration (especially cavernous sinus thrombosis),[68] suppurative jugular thrombophlebitis, carotid artery erosion,[69] maxillary sinusitis,[70] and osteomyelitis.[71] Acute mediastinitis and intracranial suppuration secondary to odontogenic infections are relatively uncommon in the antibiotic era.

Suppurative Jugular Thrombophlebitis (Lemierre Syndrome) and Carotid Artery Erosion

These are uncommon complications of oropharyngeal or odontogenic infections in the postantibiotic era. Extension of infection to the carotid sheath, which encloses both the internal jugular vein and the internal carotid artery, usually arises from the lateral pharyngeal space.[69] Since the carotid sheath space in this area is relatively compact with little areolar connective tissue, there is little tendency of spread up and down this vascular sheath, with the exception of possible retrograde thrombophlebitis and intracranial extension. The major concern is protracted septicemia and erosion of the carotid artery or one of its branches.

The onset of suppurative jugular thrombophlebitis (also known as Lemierre syndrome or postanginal sepsis) is acute, with shaking chills, spiking fevers, and profound prostration.[72] Localizing signs of pain and swelling at the angle of the jaw, tenderness and induration along the sternocleidomastoid muscle, and swelling of the lateral pharyngeal wall with dysphagia and neck rigidity are usually present. However, these findings may be subtle, and their clinical significance may not be fully recognized until postmortem examination. Dysphagia and dysphonia may also occur. Ipsilateral vocal cord paralysis or other neurologic signs representing lower cranial nerve involvement may be present. Systemic evidence of infection such as septic pulmonary emboli and metastatic abscesses to the brain, lungs, kidneys, and joints is not infrequent. Empyema may also occur. Contrast-enhanced CT may show the normal carotid artery and an enlarged jugular venous wall surrounding a more lucent intraluminal clot (Fig. 57-8). Thrombosis of the jugular vein can also be demonstrated by magnetic resonance angiography.

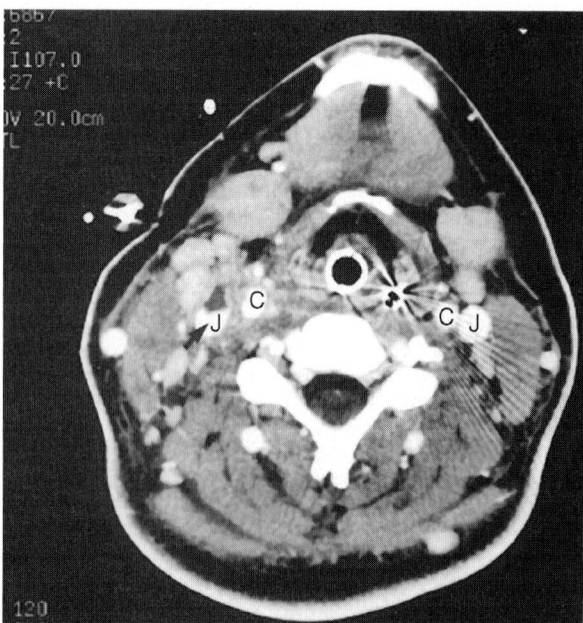

FIGURE 57-8. Jugular venous thrombosis associated with a right peritonsillar abscess in a young adult. Contrast-enhanced axial CT scan showing a normal right common carotid (C) artery but an enlarged right internal jugular vein (J) (*arrow*) with a dense or enhancing wall that surrounds the more lucent intraluminal clot. (*From Chow AW. Head and neck infections. In: Baddour L, Gorbach SL, eds. Therapy of Infectious Diseases. Philadelphia: WB Saunders; 2003:37.*)

The organisms most frequently involved are anaerobic streptococci and *Bacteroides* (now including *Prevotella*) species and *Fusobacterium necrophorum*.[73] Most cases of suppurative jugular thrombophlebitis can be managed medically without the need for ligation or surgical resection of the infected vein. Prolonged courses of intravenous antibiotics (3 to 6 weeks) will be required. Anticoagulants have sometimes been used in this setting, but efficacy is unconfirmed. Surgical ligation of the internal jugular vein, the only available therapeutic option in the preantibiotic era, is now required only in the rare patient who fails to respond to antibiotic treatment alone.[74]

Erosion of the carotid artery is a rare complication following odontogenic infection involving the carotid sheath.[75] Infection may arise by spread from the lateral pharyngeal space, Ludwig's angina, or suppuration of deep cervical lymph nodes.[76] The initial pathology is an arteritis caused by contiguous inflammation that eventually forms a false aneurysm. The patient presents in a toxic or insidious condition with a fever of undetermined origin. Trismus is absent, and signs of local suppuration may be subtle because of the tight connective tissue around and within the carotid sheath. Rupture of the carotid artery may be heralded by recurrent minor hemorrhages from the nose, mouth, or ear ("herald bleeds"). This is followed by hematoma formation in the surrounding tissues of the neck, a protracted clinical course, and eventually shock due to exsanguinations. Emergency ligation of the carotid artery may be necessary in cases of major hemorrhage, but the risk of stroke is significant.[77] The mortality ranges from 20% to 40% irrespective of treatment.[69]

Septic Cavernous Sinus Thrombosis

This dreaded complication is fortunately rare in the antibiotic era. Facial furuncles and purulent paranasal sinusitis were the major predisposing conditions. Infection of the maxillary teeth was the most common dental cause. Eagleton described six criteria for the diagnosis of septic cavernous sinus thrombosis to help distinguish it from other less lethal infections, particularly those of the ethmoid sinus and the orbit: (1) a known site of infection; (2) evidence of blood-stream invasion; (3) early signs of venous obstruction in the retina, conjunctiva, and eyelid; (4) paresis of the third, fourth, and sixth cranial nerves resulting from inflammatory edema; (5) abscess formation in neighboring soft tissue; and (6) evidence of meningeal irritation.[78] Clinically, there is an abrupt onset with diplopia, photophobia, orbital edema, and progressive exophthalmos. Involvement of the cranial nerves III, IV, V, and VI produces ophthalmoplegia, a midposition fixed pupil, loss of corneal reflex, and diminished sensation over the upper face. Obstruction of venous return from the retina results in papilledema, retinal hemorrhage, and visual loss. Contrast-enhanced CT (Fig. 57-9) and MRI are the imaging modalities of choice. Treatment requires early recognition, high-dose intravenous antibiotics, and surgical decompression of the underlying predisposing infection. Anticoagulation and steroid therapy are not indicated. Mortality remains high, approximately 15% to 30%.[79-81]

Maxillary Sinusitis

In many people, the roots of the maxillary molars lie proximate to the maxillary antrum. At times, congenital bony defects occur, with the root adjacent to the sinus membrane. In these cases, sinusitis can result from direct extension of an odontogenic infection or from perforation of the sinus floor during extraction of a maxillary tooth.[70] The clinical presentation of secondary sinus involvement is similar to that of primary sinus disease.

Osteomyelitis of the Jaws

The mandible is much more susceptible to osteomyelitis than is the maxilla, mainly because the cortical plates of the mandible are thin and its medullary tissues are relatively poor in vascular supply.[71] In view of the large number of odontogenic infections and the intimate relationship of teeth to the medullary cavity, it is surprising that osteomyelitis of the jaws is not more frequent. When osteomyelitis occurs, there is usually a predisposing condition that affects host resistance such as a compound fracture, previous irradiation, osteopetrosis, Paget's disease, diabetes mellitus, or steroid therapy. With the initiation of infection, the intramedullary pressure markedly increases, further compromising blood supply and leading to bone necrosis. Pus travels through the haversian and perforating canals, accumulates beneath the periosteum, and elevates it from the cortex. If pus continues to accumulate, the periosteum is eventually penetrated, and mucosal and cutaneous abscesses and fistulas may develop. As the inflammatory process becomes more chronic, granulation tissue is formed. Spicules of necrotic and nonviable bone may become either totally isolated (sequestrum) or encased in a sheath of new bone (involucrum).

Severe mandibular pain is a common symptom and may be accompanied by anesthesia or hypoesthesia on the affected side. In protracted cases, mandibular trismus may develop. A clinical variant is chronic sclerosing osteomyelitis associated with a proliferative periostitis. Clinically, it is characterized by a localized, hard, nontender swelling over the mandible. Actinomycosis and radiation necrosis are two common causes of this form of osteomyelitis of the jaws. Actinomycosis may be associated with obvious or occult dental disease, usually progresses slowly, and is manifested by rock-hard induration that can drain spontaneously through the skin. Prolonged antibiotic treatment is usually required (see Chapter 253).

Diagnostic Approaches

Specimen Collection and Processing

For closed-space infections, it is imperative that the normal resident oral flora be excluded during specimen collection in order that the culture results be appropriately interpreted. Needle aspiration of loculated pus by an extraoral approach is desirable, and specimens should be transported immediately to the laboratory under anaerobic conditions. For intraoral lesions, direct microscopic examination of stained smears often provides more useful information than do culture results from surface swabs. Gram and acid-fast stains for bacteria and potassium hydroxide preparations for fungi should be routinely performed. Tissue biopsy specimens should be routinely examined for histopathologic evidence of acute or chronic inflammation and infection. The presence of

specific microbial agents can be detected by immunofluorescence or polymerase chain reaction for certain suspected bacterial, mycobacterial, fungal, and viral infections. In chronic osteomyelitis, soft tissue swelling and draining fistulas are frequently present. Aspirates from the adjacent soft tissue swellings may be valuable, but cultures from the sinus tracts may be misleading, because these sinus tracts are often colonized by organisms that do not reflect what is actually occurring within the infected bone.[82] Bone biopsies for histopathologic examination and culture are often required for a definitive diagnosis.

Imaging Techniques for the Localization of Infection

Pantomography (orthopantomograph) may reveal the true extent of advanced periodontitis or the presence of periapical abscess. Ultrasonography, radionuclide scanning, CT, and MRI are particularly useful for the localization of deep fascial space infections of the head and neck.[83,84] Since CT can both localize a process and define its extent, particularly invasion into the cranial vault, mediastinum, or the bone, it is an invaluable tool for guiding needle aspiration or open drainage. A lateral radiograph of the neck may demonstrate compression or deviation of the tracheal air column or the presence of gas within necrotic soft tissues.[85] The soft tissues of the posterior wall of the hypopharynx are approximately 5 mm deep, less than one third the diameter of the fourth cervical vertebra (C4). The retropharyngeal soft tissues should be approximately two thirds the width of C4, and the retropharyngeal space slightly less (Fig. 57-10).[86] A lateral radiograph of the cervical spine or a CT scan can determine if the soft tissue swelling or an abscess originated from the retropharyngeal space or the prevertebral space. The former suggests an odontogenic source, whereas the latter likely indicates involvement of the cervical spine.[87] Technetium bone scanning, used in combination with gallium- or indium-labeled white blood cells, is particularly useful for the diagnosis of acute or chronic osteomyelitis. In acute osteomyelitis, both the bone scan and the gallium scan are likely to have positive findings. In chronic osteomyelitis, the gallium or indium scans may be negative, but the technetium scan may be positive. MRI is more sensitive than CT, and probably more accurate than bone scan in detecting bone involvement.[88] T2-weighted images may identify and localize areas of pus for drainage or aspiration. Gadolinium enhancement is important to accurately define the soft tissue component. Finally, MRI is useful for imaging vascular lesions, such as jugular thrombophlebitis.[89]

Therapeutic Considerations

Dental Caries and Periodontitis

For both caries prevention and the treatment of periodontitis, the most important strategy is the effective control of the supragingival and subgingival plaques through active promotion of and meticulous attention to oral hygiene. The diet should be scrutinized to eliminate or discourage frequent snacking on carbohydrate-rich foods or the intake of sugar-containing beverages. Fluoride-containing dentifrices and rinses (e.g., sodium fluoride 1.1% or stannous fluoride 0.4%) and dental flossing should be encouraged after each meal. Fluoride forms a complex with the apatite crystals in dentin by replacing the hydroxyl group, thereby lending strength to the entire structure. Further, fluoride promotes remineralization of the carious lesions and also exerts a bacteriostatic effect. Oral antimicrobial rinses with 0.12% chlorhexidine are also effective for the control of dental plaque bacteria that lead to gingivitis and periodontitis (Table 57-2).[90] Chlorhexidine acts as a cationic detergent that kills a wide range of bacteria and is retained on the oral surfaces for prolonged periods to prevent plaque advancement.[91] Despite this beneficial effect, it has a bitter taste and stains the enamel and tongue. Prolonged application may also promote the emergence of resistant microorganisms. Among topical antibiotics, although both penicillin and tetracycline have cariostatic effects in animal models, only the topical application of vancomycin has been shown to reduce dental caries with some degree of success in humans.[16] Although none of these measures is routinely applied in clinical practice, they are useful for the control of dental plaques in selected patients with rampant caries. With the development of improved

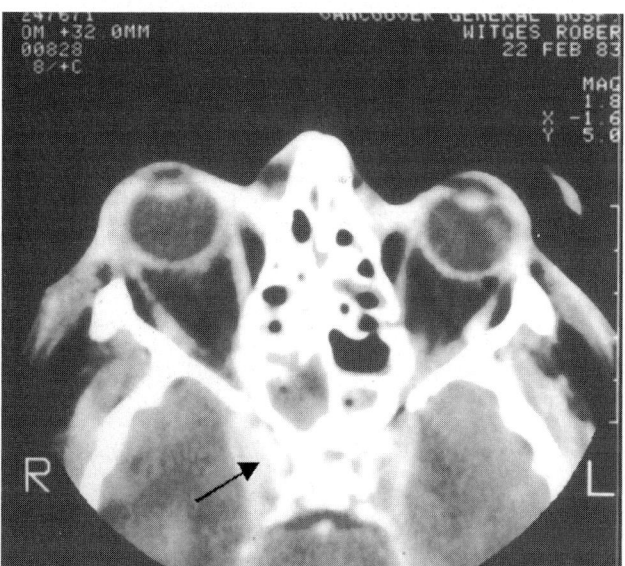

FIGURE 57-9. Cavernous sinus thrombosis associated with pansinusitis in a young adult. Contrast-enhanced axial CT showing opacification of the sphenoid and ethmoid sinuses, and thrombus in the right cavernous sinus (arrow). (From Chow AW: Life-threatening infections of the head, neck, and upper respiratory tract. In: Hall JB, Schmidt GA, Wood LH, eds. Principles of Critical Care. 2nd ed. New York: McGraw-Hill; 1998:899.)

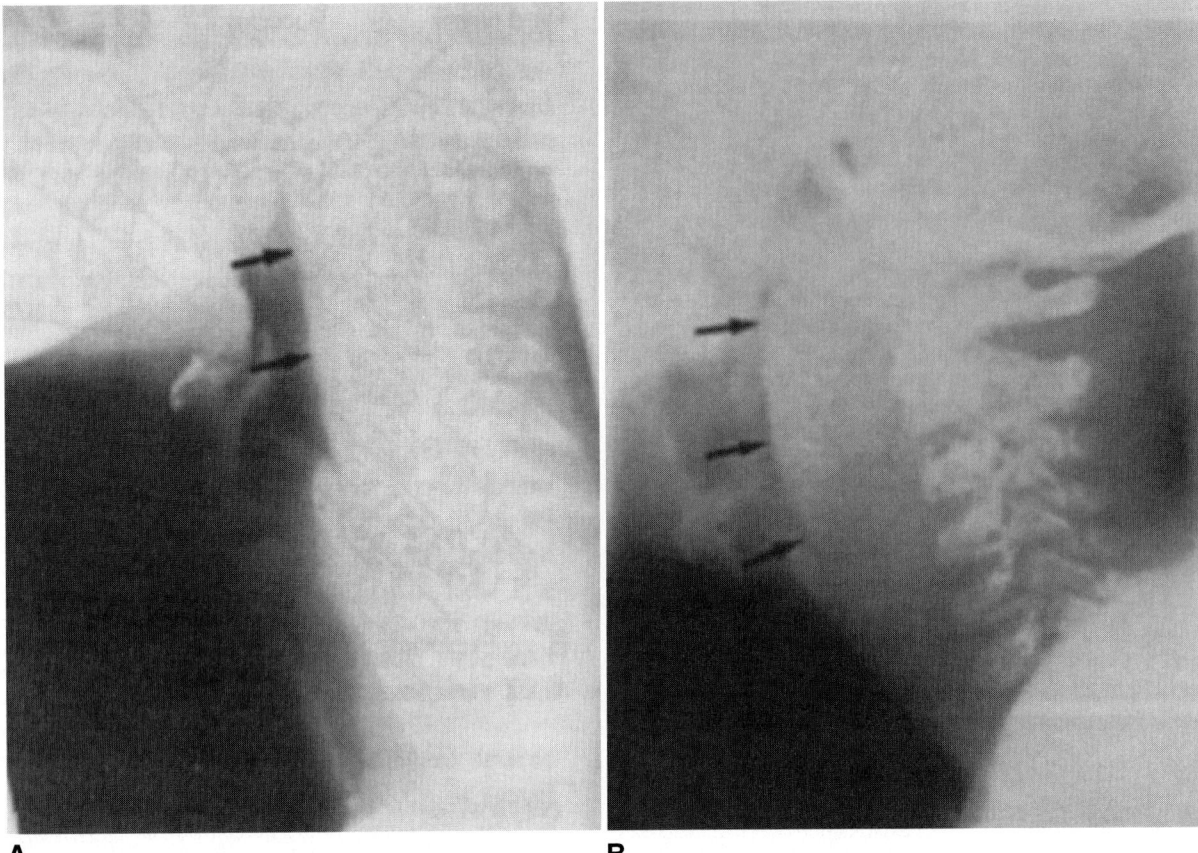

A   **B**

FIGURE 57-10.   Lateral radiograph of the neck. **A,** Normal lateral cervical view. **B,** Expansion of the retropharyngeal soft tissues. *(From Chow AW. Head and neck infections. In: Baddour L, Gorbach SL, eds. Therapy of Infectious Diseases. Philadelphia: WB Saunders; 2003:5.)*

restorative dental care and dental restorative materials, such as bonding and fluoride-releasing agents, the need for dental extractions has become much less frequent than in the past.[92,93]

Acute necrotizing ulcerative gingivitis should be treated with systemic antimicrobials such as metronidazole or penicillin (see Table 57-2).[55] Certain types of severe periodontitis are amenable to systemic antimicrobial therapy in conjunction with mechanical débridement (scaling and root planing).[58] This has often obviated the need for radical surgical resection of periodontal tissues. In double-blind clinical studies of advanced periodontitis, systemic metronidazole (500 mg PO three times daily) or doxycycline (200 mg PO twice daily) for 1 or 2 weeks in conjunction with rigorous mechanical débridement of the root surfaces was found to reduce the need for radical surgery by 80% compared with débridement plus placebo.[94] A topical antibiotic approach is also feasible. The United States Food and Drug Administration recently approved Arestin, a powder containing minocycline microspheres that release controlled amounts of the antibiotics beneath the gum for use in conjunction with scaling and root planing to reduce pocket depth in adult periodontitis. In localized juvenile periodontitis, systemic tetracycline therapy directed against *A. actinomycetemcomitans*, combined with local periodontal treatment, has yielded excellent results.[58] Unfortunately, the administration of tetracycline to children younger than 9 years can cause staining of the permanent dentition and is not generally recommended. Furthermore, tetracycline resistance among periodontal pathogens has been increasingly recognized.[95] The routine use of systemic antimicrobials prophylactically during oral or periodontal surgery in a healthy host is unwarranted, because the risk of postoperative infections following periodontal surgery is less than 1%.[96]

TABLE 57-2   Antimicrobial Regimens in Dental Caries and Different Clinical Forms of Periodontal Disease

Clinical Entity	Unique Microbial Species	Antimicrobial Regimens
Supragingival dental plaque and dental caries	*Streptococcus mutans,* other streptococci, *Actinomyces* spp.	Fluoride-containing dentifrices or oral rinses (e.g., sodium fluoride 1.1% or stannous fluoride 0.4%)
Subgingival dental plaque and simple gingivitis Acute necrotizing ulcerative gingivitis	Streptococci, *Actinomyces* spp., spirochetes *Prevotella intermedia, Fusobacterium* spp., spirochetes	Chlorhexidine 0.12% oral rinses Penicillin G 1-4 MU IV q4-6h Ampicillin-sulbactam 1.5-3 g IV q6h Metronidazole 500 mg PO or IV q8h Clindamycin 450 mg PO q6h or 600 mg IV q6-8h
Periodontitis, juvenile Periodontitis, adult	*Actinobacillus actinomycetemcomitans* Spirochetes, black-pigmented *Bacteroides* (*Porphyromonas gingivalis* and *Prevotella melaninogenica*), *A. actinomycetemcomitans*	Tetracycline 500 mg PO q6h or 1 g IV q12h Doxycycline 200 mg PO or IV q12h Metronidazole 500 mg PO or IV q8h Topical application of minocycline microspheres (Aristin)

The need for definitive restoration or extraction of the infected tooth, the primary source of an odontogenic infection, is readily apparent. Deep periodontal scaling and endodontic treatment with root fillings are required in most instances. The key for the prevention and control of dental caries and advanced periodontitis is the active promotion of oral hygiene, including the following:

1. Rigorous brushing and dental flossing after each meal
2. Dietary counseling to reduce the ingestion of carbohydrate-rich foods or beverages
3. Use of topical fluorides and oral antimicrobial rinses such as chlorhexidine for high-risk patients
4. Behavioral modification of risk factors such as tobacco smoking
5. Overcoming the reluctance for regular visits to dental professionals

Vaccines based upon various immunogens derived from *S. mutans*, the principal bacterial agent associated with dental caries, have been explored.[97,98] However, the availability of an effective and safe vaccine for clinical application is unlikely in the near future.[99]

Suppurative Odontogenic Infections

The most important therapeutic modality for pyogenic odontogenic infections is surgical drainage and the removal of necrotic tissue. Needle aspiration by the extraoral route can be particularly helpful both for microbiologic sampling and for evacuation of pus. Effective surgical management requires a thorough understanding of the most likely anatomic routes of spread. The neighboring potential fascial spaces should be carefully and systematically surveyed. For effective drainage, the incision site should be in the most dependent location. It is equally important that the timing for incision and drainage is optimum. Premature incision into an area of poorly localized cellulitis in an ill-conceived search for pus can disrupt the normal physiologic barrier and cause further spread of infection.

Antibiotic therapy is important in halting the local spread of infection and in preventing hematogenous dissemination. Antimicrobial agents are generally indicated if fever and regional lymphadenitis are present or when infection has perforated the bony cortex and spread into surrounding soft tissue. Severely immunocompromised patients are particularly at risk for rapidly advancing orofacial infections, and empirical broad-spectrum antimicrobial therapy in these patients is warranted. The initial choice of specific antibiotics is based more upon knowledge of the indigenous organisms that colonize the teeth, gums, and mucous membranes than on the results of culture and sensitivity testing (Table 57-3).[28] Most organisms, including both anaerobes and aerobes, are sensitive to penicillin.[100] Thus, penicillin monotherapy in doses appropriate for the severity of infection remains a good choice. Penicillin-allergic patients can be treated usually with clindamycin (450 mg PO four times daily or 600 mg IV every 6 to 8 hours). Cefoxitin, cefotetan, or ceftizoxime are alternative choices. Erythromycin and tetracycline are not recommended because of increasing resistance among some strains of streptococci and their lack of optimal anaerobic activity.[95]

The problem of β-lactamase production and penicillin resistance among *Bacteroides* species and *Prevotella* melaninogenica has been increasingly recognized, and treatment failure with penicillin in

TABLE 57-3 Initial Empirical Antimicrobial Regimens for Suppurative Infections of the Head and Neck

Infection	*Usual Causative Organisms*	*Antibiotic Regimens, Normal Host*[*]
Suppurative orofacial odontogenic infections including Ludwig's angina	Viridans and other streptococci, *Peptostreptococcus* spp., *Bacteroides* spp., and other oral anaerobes	Penicillin G 2-4 MU IV q4-6h, *plus* Metronidazole 0.5 g IV q6h *or* Ampicillin-sulbactam 2 g IV q4h *or* Clindamycin 600 mg IV q6h *or* Doxycycline 200 mg IV q12h *or* Cefoxitin 1-2 g IV q6h *or* Cefotetan 2 g IV q12h
Lateral pharyngeal or retropharyngeal space infections		
Odontogenic	Viridans and other streptococci, *Staphylococcus* spp, *Peptostreptococcus* spp., *Bacteroides* spp., and other oral anaerobes	Penicillin G 2-4 MU IV q4-6h, *plus* Metronidazole 0.5 g IV q6h *or* Ampicillin-sulbactam 2 g IV q4h *or* Clindamycin 600 mg IV q6h
Rhinogenic	*Streptococcus pneumoniae, Haemophilus influenzae,* viridans and other streptococci, *Bacteroides* spp., *Peptostreptococcus* spp., and other oral anaerobes	Penicillin G 2-4 MU IV q4-6h *or* Levofloxacin 500 mg IV q24h, *plus* Metronidazole 0.5 g IV q6h *or* Clindamycin 600 mg IV q6h; *or* Gatifloxacin 400 mg IV q24h *or* Moxifloxacin 400 mg IV q24h
Otogenic	Same as for rhinogenic space infections	Same as for rhinogenic space infections
Cervicofacial actinomycosis	*Actinomyces israelii, Arachnia propionica, Actinobacillus actinomycetemcomitans*	Penicillin G 2-4 MU IV q4-6h, *or* Doxycycline 200 mg PO q12h or IV q12h, *or* Clindamycin 450 mg PO q6h or 600 mg IV q6h
Suppurative jugular thrombophlebitis (Lemierre syndrome)	*Fusobacterium necrophorum;* same as for odontogenic space infections	Same as for odontogenic space infections
Suppurative cavernous sinus thrombosis	Same as for odontogenic, rhinogenic, or otogenic space infections	Same as for odontogenic, rhinogenic, or otogenic space infections
Mandibular osteomyelitis	Same as for odontogenic space infections	Clindamycin 600 mg IV q6h *or* Gatifloxacin 400 mg IV q24h *or* Moxifloxacin 400 mg IV q24h
Extension of osteomyelitis from prevertebral space infection	*Staphylococcus aureus,*[†] facultative gram-negative bacilli	Nafcillin 2 g IV q4h, *plus* Tobramycin 1.7 mg/kg IV q8h *or* Ciprofloxacin 400mg IV q12h
Sialadenitis and suppurative parotitis	*Staphylococcus aureus,*[†] viridans and other streptococci, *Bacteroides* spp., *Peptostreptococcus* spp., and other oral anaerobes	Nafcillin 2 g IV q4h *plus* Metronidazole 0.5 g IV q6h *or* Clindamycin 600 mg IV q6h

[*]For compromised hosts can consider replacing penicillin G with either cefotaxime 2 g IV q4h *or* ceftriaxone 1 g IV q12h. Other regimens to consider are piperacillin/tazobactam 3.375 g IV q6h *or* imipenem 500 mg IV q6h *or* meropenem 1 g IV q8h *or* gatifloxacin 400 mg IV q24h *or* moxifloxacin 400 mg IV q24h.

[†]For *S. aureus* infections in which MRSA is suspected, replace nafcillin with vancomycin, 0.5 g IV q6h, and in immunosuppressed hosts can add cefotaxime or ceftriaxone or imipenem as above.

odontogenic infections because of such β-lactamase–producing strains has been reported.[101-103] Therefore in patients with life-threatening, deep fascial space infections and in patients who have had an unfavorable or delayed response to penicillin, alternative therapy with a broader spectrum against anaerobes as well as facultative gram-negative bacilli may be considered (see Table 57-3). Ambulatory patients with less serious odontogenic infections can be treated with amoxicillin with or without a β-lactamase inhibitor, or with penicillin in combination with metronidazole. Metronidazole, although highly active against anaerobic gram-negative bacilli and spirochetes, is only moderately active against *Peptostreptococcus* species and is not active against aerobes, including streptococci.[104] Except in acute necrotizing gingivitis and in advanced periodontitis, it should not be used as a single agent in odontogenic infections.

In the compromised host such as the patient with leukemia and severe neutropenia after chemotherapy, it is prudent to cover for facultative gram-negative bacilli as well, and agents with broad-spectrum activity against both aerobes and anaerobes are desirable (see Table 57-3).

Osteomyelitis

Treatment of osteomyelitis of the jaws is complicated by the presence of teeth and persistent exposure to the oral environment. Antibiotic therapy needs to be prolonged, often for weeks to months. Adjuvant therapy with hyperbaric oxygen may prove beneficial in hastening the healing process, but its overall efficacy remains controversial.[71] In one study of 33 patients with early chronic osteomyelitis of the jaw, 79% were free of symptoms 10 to 34 months after hyperbaric therapy combined with surgical débridement.[105] Surgical management, including sequestrectomy, saucerization, decortication, and closed-wound suction irrigation, occasionally may be necessary. Rarely, in advanced cases, the entire segment of the infected jaw may have to be resected.

OROFACIAL NONODONTOGENIC INFECTIONS

Nonodontogenic infections of the oral cavity most frequently occur secondary to chemical, thermal, or traumatic injury. Virtually all infectious microorganisms can present with intraoral manifestations, particularly sexually transmitted agents and childhood viral enanthems. Cancer patients with mucositis from cytotoxic drugs and HIV-infected individuals are especially susceptible to acute and chronic opportunistic infections of the oral cavity, particularly candidiasis, aspergillosis, mucormycosis, herpetic gingivostomatitis, and mixed gram-negative infections.[106,107] In this section, some of the conditions affecting primarily the oral mucosa and salivary glands, in which an infectious cause is either proved or suspected, are briefly discussed.

Infections of the Oral Mucosa

Noma, or Gangrenous Stomatitis

Noma, or gangrenous stomatitis, also known as cancrum oris, is an acute, fulminating, and gangrenous infection of the oral and facial tissues. It usually occurs in the presence of severe debilitation and malnutrition, and children are most often affected.[108,109] The earliest lesion is a small, painful, red spot or vesicle on the attached gingiva in the premolar or molar region of the mandible. A necrotic ulcer rapidly develops and undermines the deeper tissue. Painful cellulitis of the lips and cheeks is observed as the lesion extends outward in a conelike fashion. Within a short period, sloughing of necrotic soft tissues occurs and exposes underlying bone, teeth, and deeper tissues.

Noma is thought to be an infectious disease, but its cause remains unknown. Fusospirochetal organisms such as *Borrelia vincentii* and *F. nucleatum* are consistently cultured from noma lesions.[110,111] *Prevotella melaninogenica* may also be present. Biopsy specimens of tissue from the advancing lesion shows a mat of predominantly gram-negative threadlike bacteria that cannot be positively identified.[110,112] Thus, this lesion bears a similarity to acute necrotizing ulcerative gingivitis in several respects but appears to be more focal and destructive, involving deeper tissues beyond the gingiva. Treatment of noma

requires high doses of intravenous penicillin. Every effort should be directed to correct the dehydration and underlying malnutrition and debility. Loose teeth and sequestra may be removed, but saucerization should be avoided. Healing is by secondary intention. Serious mutilation and facial deformity may require subsequent cosmetic surgery.[113]

Aphthous Stomatitis

Aphthous ulcers are the most common causes of recurrent oral lesions and must be distinguished from other conditions such as those caused by herpes simplex virus or coxsackievirus infections, agranulocytosis, and Behçet's syndrome. The cause of aphthous ulcers remains uncertain, although a number of infectious agents including viruses have been implicated. The most prevailing hypothesis suggests that the mechanism causing the ulceration is autoimmune.[114,115] Cross-reactivity between the 60 kDa heat shock protein (hsp60) of oral streptococci (*Streptococcus sanguis*) and oral mucosal hsp60 has been demonstrated.[115] It is postulated that the *S. sanguis* hsp60 may initiate an affector response resulting in a cytotoxic T lymphocyte reaction directed at human mitochndrial hsp60, thus causing mucosal damage. Reactivity to hsp-derived peptides has been observed in gamma-delta T cells and cytotoxic CD8+ lymphocytes, with the lymphoproliferative response particularly marked in the ulcerative phase as compared to the healing phase.[116] The elevated cytotoxicity of lymphocytes for epithelium suggests a strong role for these cells in the pathogenesis of recurrent aphthous stomatitis.[117]

Three major clinical variants are recognized: (1) minor aphthous ulcers, (2) major aphthous ulcers, and (3) herpetiform aphthous ulcers. In their most characteristic form, minor aphthous ulcers appear as a number of small ulcers on the buccal and labial mucosa, the floor of the mouth, or the tongue. The palatal soft tissues are rarely involved. Moreover, the ulcers are concentrated in the anterior part of the oral cavity, whereas the pharynx and tonsillar fauces are rarely implicated. A prodromal stage is usually present. The ulcers appear gray-yellow, often with a raised and erythematous margin, and are exquisitely painful. Lymph node enlargement is seen only with secondary bacterial infection. The course of ulceration varies from a few days to a little over 2 weeks and is followed by spontaneous healing. Major aphthous ulcers are more protracted and last up to several months. All areas of the oral cavity including the soft palate and tonsillar areas may be involved. Long periods of remission may be followed by intervals of intense ulcer activity. Herpetiform aphthous ulcers are small and multiple and characteristically affect the lateral margins and tip of the tongue. The ulcers are gray, without a delineating erythematous border, and are extremely painful, which makes eating and speaking difficult. Despite its name, there is little clinical resemblance to an acute herpetic gingivostomatitis. Although intranuclear inclusions have been demonstrated in herpetiform aphthous ulcers, there is no evidence to suggest that these inclusions bear any relationship to the presence of viruses.

The treatment of aphthous ulcers is primarily symptomatic. Strict oral hygiene should be maintained, and the use of antiseptic mouthwashes may be helpful in temporarily reducing secondary infection. Local anesthetic lozenges or gels may be used as a last resort for brief periods of pain relief. Topical or systemic steroids may be beneficial in selected people with extensive disease, but caution must be exercised in their administration. Thalidomide (100 to 200 mg/day orally for 2 to 6 weeks) has been reported to be effective for the treatment of large aphthous lesions in patients with acquired immunodeficiency syndrome.[118-120]

Mucositis and Stomatitis in the Severely Immunocompromised Person

Much of what is known about the management of oromucosal infections has been studied in cancer patients being treated with radiotherapy, chemotherapy, and bone marrow transplantation.[121] Mucositis involving the nonkeratinized oral epithelium is a frequent complication following irradiation or during chemotherapy for acute leukemia. Other patient groups that develop oromucosal complications include those undergoing solid organ transplantation, patients with acquired immunodeficiency syndrome,[107,115] and those with autoimmune diseases associated with xerostomia and systemic immunosuppression. The underlying mechanism appears to be a breakdown of the mucosal epithelium that leads to mucositis and secondary bacterial or fungal infection, or reactivation of latent viral infection. Oral candidiasis, herpes simplex, varicella-zoster, and cytomegalovirus infections may occur concomitantly. Four stages of disease progression are described: (1) inflammatory or vascular phase; (2) epithelial phase; (3) ulcerative/bacteriologic phase; and (4) healing phase.[122] Ulceration and pseudomembrane formation are evident usually between 4 and 7 days after the initiation of chemotherapy, and commonly involve the buccal and labial mucosa, soft palate, oropharynx, floor of the mouth, and the ventral and lateral surfaces of the tongue. The clinical manifestations may be quite variable. The lesions are often protracted in duration and may not be associated with an obvious inflammatory reaction. Pain or tenderness may be the only abnormal finding.

Management of oral mucositis remains controversial and is primarily directed at symptomatic relief. Various intervention strategies have been attempted, but none has been shown to be superior to others.[123,124] Frequent saline rinses may reduce mucosal irritation, remove thickened secretions or debris, and increase moisture in the mouth. Coating agents such as milk of magnesia or aluminum hydroxide gel (Amphojel) have been useful for the symptomatic relief of painful oral lesions. Topical antiseptic (e.g., chlorhexidine) and anesthetic (e.g., benzydamine or viscous lidocaine) applications are usually prescribed.[106] Topical or oral cytoprotective agents (e.g., sucralfate) or nonsteroidal anti-inflammatory analgesics (e.g., benzydamine or salicylates) may provide additional benefit, but further controlled clinical trials are required to assess their efficacy and appropriate indications.[125,126] Since secondary infection is common but the etiologic agents cannot be readily predicted on clinical grounds alone in such patients, specific microbiologic diagnosis by culture, histopathologic examination, or antigen detection techniques may be necessary to guide appropriate antimicrobial treatment. However, a meta-analysis of the published literature on the usefulness of antimicrobial agents to ameliorate the signs and symptoms of oral mucositis failed to demonstrate a clear benefit for the use of antimicrobial agents in the management of oral mucositis, mainly because of the generally poor quality of published studies and numerous confounding variables among this patient population.[122] Meticulous oral and dental hygiene, effective management of xerostomia, selective suppression of oropharyngeal microbial colonization, and early control of reactivation by latent viral infections appear to be the key for prevention and reduction of the overall morbidity of oromucosal infections in the severely immunocompromised.[106]

Infections of the Salivary Gland

Sialadenitis, or infection of salivary tissue, is a relatively common disease. Sialolithiasis in elderly patients (particularly calculi in Wharton's duct) often leads to ductal obstruction and secondary infection. Other predisposing factors for ductal occlusion include dehydration, sialogogic drugs, general debility, and trauma.

Suppurative Parotitis

Acute bacterial parotitis is a specific clinical entity primarily affecting the elderly, malnourished, dehydrated, or postoperative patient.[127,128] Clinically, there is a sudden onset of firm, erythematous swelling of the pre- and postauricular areas that extends to the angle of the mandible. This is associated with exquisite local pain and tenderness. Systemic findings of high fevers, chills, and marked toxicity are generally present. Progression of the infection may lead to massive swelling of the neck, respiratory obstruction, septicemia, and osteomyelitis of the adjacent facial bones. Staphylococci have been the predominant isolates, and antibiotic therapy should include an antistaphylococcal agent.[128] Enterobacteriaceae, other gram-negative

bacilli, and anaerobes have also been reported to cause parotitis. Early surgical drainage and decompression of the gland are generally required because spontaneous drainage is uncommon.[129]

Chronic Bacterial Parotitis

In this condition, parotitis is recurrent with intermittent acute exacerbations. There is chronic, low-grade, bacterial infection resulting in functional destruction of the salivary gland. Pus, when obtained directly from the gland, usually reveals the growth of staphylococci or mixed oral aerobes and anaerobes. Sialography during remission may reveal a sialectatic pattern of pooling of contrast medium that suggests multiple cystic cavities in place of the normal acinar pattern. Chronic parotitis may be confused with Sjögren syndrome, a noninfectious illness characterized by the triad of xerostomia, keratoconjunctivitis, and systemic autoimmune disease such as rheumatoid arthritis, lupus erythematosus, scleroderma, periarteritis nodosa, and polymyositis. The presence of associated temporomandibular arthritis or arthralgia should strongly suggest Sjögren syndrome rather than chronic bacterial parotitis.

Therapy for chronic parotitis should initially be conservative and consists of systemic antibiotics and ductal saline or antibiotic irrigations. Parotidectomy may eventually be required for people with long-standing infection.

Viral Parotitis

Mumps parotitis is characterized by the rapid, painful swelling of one or both parotid glands within 2 to 3 weeks after exposure. A prodromal phase of preauricular pain, fever, chills, and headache may be present (see Chapter 154). Other viral causes of parotitis include influenza and enteroviruses, and virus cultures or serologic examinations may be required for distinguishing these from true mumps. Mumps parotitis usually resolves spontaneously in 5 to 10 days. Symptomatic relief of pain and fever is necessary, and prevention of dehydration and secondary bacterial infection is essential.

MISCELLANEOUS INFECTIONS OF THE NECK AND HEAD

In the antibiotic era, dental causes have surpassed oropharyngeal and tonsillar sources of deep neck infections.[27,130] Other miscellaneous infections of the neck and head include suppurative cervical adenitis, infected embryologic cysts of the neck, various infections secondary to human and animal bites, maxillofacial trauma, irradiation, and surgical procedures of the head and neck.

Cervical Adenitis

The cervical lymph nodes comprise six groups (occipital, mastoid, parotid, facial, submandibular, and submental) that form a collar at the junction of the head and neck. Within this collar near the base of the tongue lie the sublingual and retropharyngeal nodes. The anterior and lateral cervical nodes form a chain along the front and side of the neck, respectively. The lateral cervical chain serves as a common root for drainage. The final conduit from all lymphatics in the head and neck is the large deep chain situated along the carotid sheath. Cervical adenitis that arises unilaterally is usually due to pyogenic bacterial infections. Its anatomic location in relationship to major cervical landmarks provides the clinical clues to the primary source of infection.[131] Bilateral acute cervical adenitis generally suggests a nonspecific or viral cause, toxoplasmosis, or group A streptococcal infection. A more chronic or recurrent cervical adenitis should suggest the possibility of typical or atypical mycobacteria, human immunodeficiency virus infection, Epstein-Barr virus or cytomegalovirus mononucleosis, cat-scratch fever, actinomycosis, sarcoidosis, or lymphoproliferative and neoplastic disorders.

Infected Embryologic Cysts

Three distinct embryologic abnormalities can present with infection in the neck. They are (1) cystic hygroma or lymphangioma, (2) pharyngeal and bronchial cleft cysts, and (3) thyroglossal duct cysts.

Cystic hygroma is associated with a diffuse tumor mass usually evident within the first 2 years of life. It commonly involves the lower aspect of the neck, but it can appear anywhere in the cervical region. It is probably an abnormal development of lymphatic vessels from the jugular lymphatic sacs. Sudden enlargement by infection or hemorrhage into a lymphangioma may cause obstruction of the upper airways. Pharyngeal cleft cysts can develop from the first, second, or third pharyngeal clefts, although the second is most common. They usually present in childhood as fistulas or masses just posterior to the angle of the mandible along the anterior border of the sternocleidomastoid muscle. The mass can fluctuate in size, and enlargement can be associated with upper respiratory infection. Thyroglossal duct cysts originate from the foramen cecum of the tongue and descend through the body of the hyoid bone into the anterior portion of the neck. Any residual secretory lining may give rise to a thyroglossal duct cyst that is midline. It can cause respiratory obstruction or fistula formation if secondarily infected. Treatment of these congenital abnormalities during secondary bacterial infection requires broad-spectrum antibiotics such as a cephalosporin. Definitive surgical excision to prevent recurrence should be performed after complete resolution of the acute process.

Suppurative Thyroiditis

Although infections of the thyroid gland are rare, they are potentially life-threatening. Such infections may arise by a variety of pathways, including hematogenous dissemination, direct spread from an adjacent deep fascial space infection, an infected thyroglossal fistula, or anterior perforation of the esophagus. Preexisting diseases of the thyroid gland such as a goiter or adenoma are frequently present.[131,132] Acute suppurative thyroiditis is characterized by fever, local pain, tenderness, warmth, erythema, and symptoms of dysphagia, dysphonia, hoarseness, or pharyngitis. The infection may involve single or both lobes, and fluctuance may not be apparent until late in the course. Subacute thyroiditis may have similar local findings, but systemic manifestations are not as severe and tend to be more self-limiting. Laboratory investigation of thyroid infections should include ultrasonography, radionuclide scanning, and lateral radiographs or computed tomographic scanning of the neck for evidence of peritracheal extension; thyroid function tests; and diagnostic needle aspiration for microbiologic diagnosis. *Staphylococcus aureus*, *Streptococcus pyogenes*, and *Streptococcus pneumoniae* are most frequently isolated. Other pathogens include *Haemophilus influenzae*, viridans streptococci, *Eikenella corrodens*, and *Bacteroides*, *Peptostreptococcus*, and *Actinomyces* spp. Treatment requires specific antimicrobial agents and appropriate surgical drainage.

Infections from Bites, Maxillofacial Trauma, Irradiation, and Surgical Wounds

Human and Animal Bites

Human and animal bite wounds to the head and neck are relatively common. Although they may look innocuous initially, serious complications can occur (also see Chapter 318). For this reason, empirical antibiotic therapy is recommended when the bite wound involves the face, head, or neck. Studies that used adequate anaerobic culture techniques indicate indigenous oral flora rather than the skin flora to be the major source of bite wound infections.[133] Streptococci, *E. corrodens*, and *S. aureus* are the most prevalent facultative organisms, and *Bacteroides* and *Peptostreptococcus* are the most common anaerobic isolates. Penicillin-resistant gram-negative rods are infrequent. *Eikenella corrodens* is unique in that it is susceptible to penicillin and ampicillin but resistant to oxacillin, methicillin, nafcillin, and clindamycin.[134] In animal bite wounds, *Pasteurella multocida* has been a common cause of infection.[135] It is susceptible to penicillin and cefoxitin, but resistant to clindamycin and erythromycin. In view of these findings, amoxicillin-clavulanate, amoxicillin, or penicillin are reasonable antibiotic choices for initial therapy for either human or animal bite wounds.

Maxillofacial Trauma

Automobile and motorcycle accidents cause the most severe maxillofacial trauma. Particular attention should be paid to fractures that may traverse sinus cavities and tooth-bearing areas of the maxilla or mandible, since secondary infection rates at these sites are particularly high. Treatment is aimed not only at correcting the fracture but also at the prevention of infection and subsequent osteomyelitis. Early stabilization of the fracture and the jaws is generally required to protect the airway. Tracheostomy with the use of inflated, cuffed endotracheal tubes may prevent aspiration of blood and other foreign materials. The occurrence of otorrhea or rhinorrhea with a persistent cerebrospinal fluid leak should be carefully observed.

Irradiation and Postsurgical Wounds

Malignancies of the head and neck are frequently treated with a combination of irradiation, chemotherapeutic agents, and surgical resection. Infectious complications are particularly common after such procedures. Pharyngocutaneous fistulas, osteonecrosis of the mandible, or radionecrosis of the laryngeal cartilage may occur. *S. aureus* and *Pseudomonas aeruginosa* are frequent pathogens.[136] Prolonged courses of intravenous antibiotics selected according to culture and sensitivity data as well as frequent wound débridement and cleansing are indicated. Although some controversy still exists, immunocompromised patients undergoing oropharyngeal surgery for cancer should receive perioperative antibiotics as they are at particular high risk for infection. A broad-spectrum antibiotic such as cefazolin, cefuroxime, cefoxitin, or ceftizoxime appears appropriate in this setting.[96,137,138]

REFERENCES

1. Dahlen G. Microbiology and treatment of dental abscesses and periodontal-endodontic lesions. Periodontol 2000. 2002;28:206-239.
2. Zehnder M, Gold SI, Hasselgren G. Pathologic interactions in pulpal and periodontal tissues. J Clin Periodontol. 2002;29:663-671.
3. Colombo AP, Haffajee AD, Dewhirst FE, et al. Clinical and microbiological features of refractory periodontitis subjects. J Clin Periodontol. 1998;25:169-180.
4. Kroes I, Lepp PW, Relman DA. Bacterial diversity within the human subgingival crevice. Proc Natl Acad Sci USA. 1999;96:14547-14552.
5. Schuster GS. Oral flora and pathogenic organisms. Infect Dis Clin North Am. 1999;13:757-774.
6. Chow AW, Roser SM, Brady FA. Orofacial odontogenic infections. Ann Intern Med. 1978;88:392-402.
7. Miller CH. The oral microbial flora. In: Schuster GS, ed. Oral Microbiology and Infectious Disease. Philadelphia: BC Decker; 1990:441.
8. Hamada S, Slade HD. Biology, immunology and carcinogenicity of *Streptococcus mutans*. Microbiol Rev. 1980;44:331-384.
9. Gordon DF, Stutman M, Loesche WJ. Improved isolation of anaerobic bacteria from the gingival crevice area of man. Appl Microbiol. 1971;21:1046-1050.
10. Miller CH. Microbial ecology of the oral cavity. In: Schuster GS, ed. Oral Microbiology and Infectious Disease. Philadelphia: BC Decker; 1990:465.
11. Schuster GS. The microbiology of oral and maxillofacial infections. In: Topazian RG, Goldberg MH, eds. Oral and Maxillofacial Infections. Philadelphia: WB Saunders; 1987:33.
12. Kononen E. Development of oral bacterial flora in young children. Ann Med. 2000;32:107-112.
13. Preston AJ, Gosney MA, Noon S, et al. Oral flora of elderly patients following acute medical admission. Gerontology. 1999;45:49-52.
14. Yao ES, Lamont RJ, Leu SP, et al. Interbacterial binding among strains of pathogenic and commensal oral bacterial species. Oral Microbiol Immunol. 1996;11:35-41.
15. Maiden MFJ, Macuch PJ, Murray L, et al. "Checkerboard" DNA-probe analysis and anaerobic culture of initial periodontal lesions. Clin Infect Dis. 1997;25(Suppl 2):S230-S232.
16. Moore WEC, Moore LVH. The bacteria of periodontal diseases. Periodontol 2000. 1994;5:66-77.
17. Darveau RJP, Tanner A, Page RC. The microbial challenge in periodontitis. Periodontol 2000. 1997;14:202-215.
18. Tanner A, Stillman N. Oral and dental infections with anaerobic bacteria: Clinical features, predominant pathogens, and treatment. Clin Infect Dis. 1993;16(Suppl 4):S304-S309.
19. Whiley RA, Beighton D. Current classification of the oral streptococci. Oral Microbiol Immunol. 1998;13:195-216.
20. Shaw JH. Causes and control of dental caries. N Engl J Med. 1987;317:996-1004.
21. Johnson TC, Reinhardt RA, Payne JB, et al. Experimental gingivitis in periodontitis-susceptible subjects. J Clin Periodontol. 1997;24:618-625.
22. Rams TE, Flynn MJ, Slots J. Subgingival microbial associations in severe human periodontitis. Clin Infect Dis. 1997;25(Suppl 2):S224-S226.

23. Haffajee AD, Cugini MA, Tanner A, et al. Subgingival microbiota in healthy, well-maintained elder and periodontitis subjects. J Clin Periodontol. 1998;25:346-353.

24. Socransky SS, Haffajee AD, Cugini MA, et al. Microbial complexes in subgingival plaque. J Clin Periodontol. 1998;25:134-144.

25. Tanner A, Maiden MF, Macuch PJ, et al. Microbiota of health, gingivitis, and initial periodontitis. J Clin Periodontol. 1998;25:85-98.

26. Matto J, Asikainen S, Vaisanen ML, et al. Role of *Porphyromonas gingivalis*, *Prevotella intermedia*, and *Prevotella nigrescens* in extraoral and some odontogenic infections. Clin Infect Dis. 1997;25(Suppl 2):S194-S198.

27. Chow AW. Life-threatening infections of the head and neck. Clin Infect Dis. 1992;14:991-1004.

28. Peterson LR, Thomson RB Jr. Use of the clinical microbiology laboratory for the diagnosis and management of infectious diseases related to the oral cavity. Infect Dis Clin North Am. 1999;13:775-795.

29. Baker AS, Montgomery WW. Oropharyngeal space infections. Curr Clin Top Infect Dis. 1987;8:227-265.

30. Loesche WJ, Grossman NS. Periodontal disease as a specific, albeit chronic, infection: Diagnosis and treatment. Clin Microbiol Rev. 2001;14:727-752, table.

31. Waki MY, Jolkovsky DL, Otomo-Corgel J, et al. Effects of subgingival irrigation on bacteremia following scaling and root planing. J Periodontol. 1990;61:405-411.

32. Chow AW. Odontogenic infections. In: Schlossberg D, ed. Infections of the Head and Neck. New York: Springer-Verlag; 1987:148-160.

33. Hamada S, Amano A, Kimura S, et al. The importance of fimbriae in the virulence and ecology of some oral bacteria. Oral Microbiol Immunol. 1998;13:129-138.

34. Lockhart PB, Durack DT. Oral microflora as a cause of endocarditis and other distant site infections. Infect Dis Clin North Am. 1999;13:833-850, vi.

35. Viscount HB, Munro CL, Burnette-Curley D, et al. Immunization with FimA protects against *Streptococcus parasanguis* endocarditis in rats. Infect Immun. 1997;65:994-1002.

36. Gibbons RJ, Hay DI, Childs WC III, et al. Role of cryptic receptors (cryptitopes) in bacterial adhesion to oral surfaces. Arch Oral Biol. 1990;35(Suppl):107S-114S.

37. Milgrom P, Riedy CA, Weinstein P, et al. Dental caries and its relationship to bacterial infection, hypoplasia, diet, and oral hygiene in 6- to 36-month-old children. Community Dent Oral Epidemiol. 2000;28:295-306.

38. Ishikawa I, Nakashima K, Koseki T, et al. Induction of the immune response to periodontopathic bacteria and its role in the pathogenesis of periodontitis. Periodontol 2000. 1997;14:79-111.

39. Van Dyke TE, Serhan CN. Resolution of inflammation: A new paradigm for the pathogenesis of periodontal diseases. J Dent Res. 2003;82:82-90.

40. Kantarci A, Van Dyke TE. Neutrophil-mediated host response to *Porphyromonas gingivalis*. J Int Acad Periodontol. 2002;4:119-125.

41. Slots J, Kamma JJ. General health risk of periodontal disease. Int Dent J. 2001;51:417-427.

42. Salvi SE, Lawrence HP, Offenbacher S, et al. Influence of risk factors in the pathogenesis of periodontitis. Periodontol 2000. 1997;14:173-201.

43. Hart TC, Korman KS. Genetic factors in the pathogenesis of periodontitis. Periodontol 2000. 1997;14:202-215.

44. Kureishi K, Chow AW. The tender tooth—Dentoalveolar, pericoronal, and periodontal infections. Infect Dis Clin North Am. 1988;2:163-182.

45. Roscoe DL, Chow AW. Normal flora and mucosal immunity of the head and neck. Infect Dis Clin North Am. 1988;2:1-19.

46. McGhee JR, Michalek SM. Immunobiology of dental caries—Microbial aspects and local immunity. Annu Rev Microbiol. 1981;35:595-638.

47. Ogawa T, Kusumoto Y, Hamada S, et al. *Bacteroides gingivalis*–specific serum IgG and IgA subclass antibodies in periodontal diseases. Clin Exp Immunol. 1990;82:318-325.

48. Raber-Durlacher JE, Epstein JB, Raber J, et al. Periodontal infection in cancer patients treated with high-dose chemotherapy. Support Care Cancer. 2002;10:466-473.

49. Van Dyke TE, Horoszewicz HU, Cianciola LJ, et al. Neutrophil chemotaxis dysfunction in human periodontitis. Infect Immun. 1980;27:124-132.

50. Fives-Taylor PM, Meyer DH, Mintz KP, et al. Virulence factors of *Actinobacillus actinomycetemcomitans*. Periodontol 2000. 1999;20:136-167.

51. Kilian M. Degradation of immunoglobulins A1, A2, and G by suspected principal periodontal pathogens. Infect Immun. 1981;34:757-765.

52. Gronbaek Frandsen EV. Bacterial degradation of immunoglobulin A1 in relation to periodontal diseases. APMIS Suppl. 1999;87:1-54.

53. De Nardin E. The role of inflammatory and immunological mediators in periodontitis and cardiovascular disease. Ann Periodontol. 2001;6:30-40.

54. Thadepalli H, Mandal AK. Anatomic basis of head and neck infections. Infect Dis Clin North Am. 1988;2:21-34.

55. Shinn DLS, Squires S, McFadzean JA. The treatment of Vincent's disease with metronidazole. Dent Pract. 1965;15:275-280.

56. Stephen KW, McLatchie MF, Mason DK, et al. Treatment of acute ulcerative gingivitis (Vincent's type). Br Dent J. 1966;121:313-322.

57. Research, Science and Therapy Committee of the American Academy of Periodontology. Treatment of plaque-induced gingivitis, chronic periodontitis, and other clinical conditions. J Periodontol. 2001;72:1790-1800.

58. Fine DH, Hammond BF, Loesche WJ. Clinical use of antibiotics in dental practice. Int J Antimicrob Agents. 1998;9:235-238.

59. Kurien M, Mathew J, Job A, et al. Ludwig's angina. Clin Otolaryngol. 1997;22:263-265.

60. Busch RF. Ludwig angina: Early aggressive therapy. Arch Otolaryngol Head Neck Surg. 1999;125:1283-1284.

61. Crawford JJ, Sconyers JR, Moriarty JD, et al. Bacteremia after tooth extractions studied with the aid of prereduced anaerobically sterilized culture media. Appl Microbiol. 1974;27:927-932.

62. Hall G, Hedstrom SA, Heimdahl A, et al. Prophylactic administration of penicillins for endocarditis does not reduce the incidence of postextraction bacteremia. Clin Infect Dis. 1993;17:188-194.

63. Bartzokas CA, Johnson R, Jane M, et al. Relation between mouth and haematogenous infection in total joint replacements. BMJ. 1994;309:506-508.

64. Lockhart PB, Brennan MT, Fox PC, et al. Decision-making on the use of antimicrobial prophylaxis for dental procedures: A survey of infectious disease consultants and review. Clin Infect Dis. 2002;34:1621-1626.

65. Furst IM, Ersil P, Caminiti M. A rare complication of tooth abscess—Ludwig's angina and mediastinitis. J Can Dent Assoc. 2001;67:324-327.

66. Zeitoun IM, Dhanarajani PJ. Cervical cellulitis and mediastinitis caused by odontogenic infections: Report of two cases and review of literature. J Oral Maxillofac Surg. 1995;53:203-208.

67. Takao M, Ido M, Hamaguchi K, et al. Descending necrotizing mediastinitis secondary to retropharyngeal abscess. Eur Respir J. 1994;7:1716-1718.

68. Yoshikawa TT, Quinn W. The aching head—Intracranial suppuration due to head and neck infections. Infect Dis Clin North Am. 1988;2:265-277.

69. Blomquist IK, Bayer AS. Life-threatening deep fascial space infections of the head and neck. Infect Dis Clin North Am. 1988;2:237-264.

70. Chow AW. Acute sinusitis: Current status of etiologies, diagnosis, and treatment. Curr Clin Top Infect Dis. 2001;21:31-63.

71. Topazian RG. Osteomyelitis of the jaws. In: Topazian RG, Goldberg MH, eds. Oral and Maxillofacial Infections. Philadelphia: WB Saunders; 1987:204-238.

72. Armstrong AW, Spooner K, Sanders JW. Lemierre's syndrome. Curr Infect Dis Rep. 2000;2:168-173.

73. Sinave CP, Hardy GJ, Fardy PW. The Lemierre syndrome—Suppurative thrombophlebitis of the internal jugular vein secondary to oropharyngeal infection. Medicine (Baltimore). 1989;68:85-94.

74. Singhal A, Kerstein MD. Lemierre's syndrome. South Med J. 2001;94:886-887.

75. Knouse MC, Madeira RG, Celani VJ. *Pseudomonas aeruginosa* causing a right carotid artery mycotic aneurysm after a dental extraction procedure. Mayo Clin Proc. 2002;77:1125-1130.

76. Alexander DW, Leonard JR, Trail ML. Vascular complications of deep neck abscesses. Laryngoscope. 1968;78:361-370.

77. Kono T, Kohno A, Kuwashima S, et al. CT findings of descending necrotising mediastinitis via the carotid space ('Lincoln Highway'). Pediatr Radiol. 2001;31:84-86.

78. Eagleton WP. Cavernous sinus thrombophlebitis and allied septic and traumatic lesions of the basal venous sinuses. A clinical study of blood stream infection. New York: Macmillan;1926;1-196.

79. Bhatia K, Jones NS. Septic cavernous sinus thrombosis secondary to sinusitis: Are anticoagulants indicated? A review of the literature. J Laryngol Otol. 2002;116:667-676.

80. Ferrera PC, Busino LJ, Snyder HS. Uncommon complications of odontogenic infections. Am J Emerg Med. 1996;14:317-322.

81. Harbour RC, Trobe JD, Ballinger WE. Septic cavernous sinus thrombosis associated with gingivitis and parapharyngeal abscess. Arch Ophthalmol. 1984;102:94-97.

82. Mackowiak PA, Jones SR, Smith JW. Diagnostic value of sinus-tract cultures in chronic osteomyelitis. JAMA. 1978;239:2772-2775.

83. Salit IE. Diagnostic approaches to head and neck infections. Infect Dis Clin North Am. 1988;2:35-55.

84. Holt GR, McManus K, Newman RK, et al. Computed tomography in the diagnosis of deep-neck infections. Arch Otolaryngol. 1982;108:693-696.

85. Wholey MH, Bruwer AJ, Baker HL. The lateral roentgenogram of the neck. Radiology. 1958;71:350.

86. Chow AW. Head and neck infections. In: Baddour L, Gorbach SL, eds. Therapy of Infectious Diseases. Philadelphia: WB Saunders; 2003:25-39.

87. Bryan CS, King BGJ, Bryant RE. Retropharyngeal infection in adults. Arch Intern Med. 1974;134:127-130.

88. Chong VF, Fan YF. Comparison of CT and MRI features in sinusitis. Eur J Radiol. 1998;29:47-54.

89. Latchaw RE, Hirsch WL Jr, Yock DH Jr. Imaging of intracranial infection. Neurosurg Clin North Am. 1992;3:303-322.

90. Achong RA, Briskie DM, Hildebrandt GH, et al. Effect of chlorhexidine varnish mouthguards on the levels of selected oral microorganisms in pediatric patients. Pediatr Dent. 1999;21:169-175.

91. Offenbacher S. Periodontal diseases: Pathogenesis. Ann Periodontol. 1996;1:821-878.

92. Chow AW. Odontogenic infections in the elderly. Inf Dis Clin Pract. 1998;6:587-596.

93. Ewoldsen N, Herwig L. Decay-inhibiting restorative materials: Past and present. Compend Contin Educ Dent. 1998;19:981-984, 986, 988.

94. Loesche WJ. Antimicrobials in dentistry: With knowledge comes responsibility. J Dent Res. 1996;75:1432-1433.

95. Olsvik B, Tenover FC. Tetracycline resistance in periodontal pathogens. Clin Infect Dis. 1993;16(Suppl 4):S310-S313.

96. Rikhotso E, Ferretti C. Prophylactic antibiotic use in oral surgery—A review of current concepts. SADJ. 2002;57:408-413.

97. Gregory RL, Filler SJ. Protective secretory immunoglobulin A antibodies in humans following oral immunization with *Streptococcus mutans*. Infect Immun. 1987;55:2409-2415.

98. Taubman MA, Holmberg CJ, Smith DJ. Immunization of rats with synthetic peptide constructs from the glucan-binding or catalytic region of mutans streptococcal glucosyltransferase protects against dental caries. Infect Immun. 1995;63:3088-3089.

99. Bowen WH. Vaccine against dental caries—A personal view. J Dent Res. 1996;75:1530-1533.

100. Peterson LJ. Contemporary management of deep infections of the neck. J Oral Maxillofac Surg. 1993;51:226-231.

101. Heimdahl A, von Konow L, Nord CE. Isolation of β-lactamase–producing *Bacteroides* strains associated with clinical failures with penicillin treatment of human orofacial infections. Arch Oral Biol. 1980;25:689-692.

102. Lewis MA, Parkhurst CL, Douglas CW, et al. Prevalence of penicillin resistant bacteria in acute suppurative oral infection. J Antimicrob Chemother. 1995;35:785-791.

103. Brook I. Antibiotic resistance of oral anaerobic bacteria and their effect on the management of upper respiratory tract and head and neck infections. Semin Respir Infect. 2002;17:195-203.

104. Hood FJC. The place of metronidazole in the treatment of acute orofacial infection. Antimicrob Agents Chemother. 1978;15:71-73.

105. Aitasalo K, Niinikoski J, Granman R, et al. A modified protocol for early treatment of osteomyelitis and osteoradionecrosis of the mandible. Head Neck. 1998;20:411-417.

106. Epstein JB, Chow AW. Oral complications associated with immunosuppression and cancer therapies. Infect Dis Clin North Am 1999;13:901-923.

107. Patton LL, Phelan JA, Ramos-Gomez FJ, et al. Prevalence and classification of HIV-associated oral lesions. Oral Dis. 2002;8(Suppl 2):98-109.

108. Enwonwu CO, Falkler WA, Idigbe EO. Oro-facial gangrene (noma/cancrum oris): Pathogenetic mechanisms. Crit Rev Oral Biol Med. 2000;11:159-171.

109. Baratti-Mayer D, Pittet B, Montandon D, et al. Noma: An "infectious" disease of unknown aetiology. Lancet Infect Dis. 2003;3:419-431.

110. Paster BJ, Falkler JW Jr, Enwonwu CO, et al. Prevalent bacterial species and novel phylotypes in advanced noma lesions. J Clin Microbiol. 2002;40:2187-2191.

111. Falkler WA Jr, Enwonwu CO, Idigbe EO. Microbiological understandings and mysteries of noma (cancrum oris). Oral Dis. 1999;5:150-155.

112. Topazian RG. Uncommon infections of the oral and maxillofacial regions. In: Topazian RG, Goldberg MH, eds. Oral and Maxillofacial Infections. Philadelphia: WBSaunders; 1987:317-338.

113. Marck KW, de Bruijn HP. Surgical treatment of noma. Oral Dis. 1999;5:167-171.

114. Scully C, Gorsky M, Lozada-Nur F. The diagnosis and management of recurrent aphthous stomatitis: A consensus approach. J Am Dent Assoc. 2003;134:200-207.

115. Williams DW, Leigh J, Ramirez-Amador V, et al. Host pathogen interaction and the development of oral lesions. Oral Dis. 2002;8(Suppl 2):120-125.

116. Direskeneli H, Eksioglu-Demiralp E, Kibaroglu A, et al. Oligoclonal T cell expansions in patients with Behçet's disease. Clin Exp Immunol. 1999;117:166-170.

117. Hasan A, Childerstone A, Pervin K, et al. Recognition of a unique peptide epitope of the mycobacterial and human heat shock protein 65-60 antigen by T cells of patients with recurrent oral ulcers. Clin Exp Immunol. 1995;99:392-397.

118. Barrons RW. Treatment strategies for recurrent oral aphthous ulcers. Am J Health Syst Pharm. 2001;58:41-50.

119. Shek LP, Lim DL. Thalidomide in Behçet's disease. Biomed Pharmacother. 2002;56:31-35.

120. Jacobson JM, Greenspan JS, Spritzler J, et al. Thalidomide for the treatment of oral aphthous ulcers in patients with human immunodeficiency virus infection: National Institute of Allergy and Infectious Diseases. AIDS Clinical Trials Group. N Engl J Med 1997;336:1487-1493.

121. Epstein JB, Schubert MM. Oral mucositis in myelosuppressive cancer therapy. Oral Surg Oral Med Oral Pathol Oral Radiol Endod. 1999;88:273-276.

122. Donnelly JP, Belim LA, Epstein JB, et al. Antimicrobial therapy to prevent or treat oral mucositis. Lancet Infect Dis. 2003;3:405-412.

123. Worthington HV, Clarkson JE, Eden OB. Interventions for treating oral mucositis for patients with cancer receiving treatment. Cochrane Database Syst Rev. 2002;CD001973.

124. Biron P, Sebban C, Gourmet R, et al. Research controversies in management of oral mucositis. Support Care Cancer. 2000;8:68-71.

125. Epstein JB, Stevenson-Moore PB. Benzydamine hydrochloride in prevention and management of pain in oral mucositis associated with radiation therapy. Oral Surg. 1986;62:145-148.

126. Adams S, Toth B, Dudley BS. Evaluation of sucralfate as a compounded oral suspension for the treatment of stomatitis. Clin Pharmacol Ther. 1985;2:178.

127. Brook I. Acute bacterial suppurative parotitis: Microbiology and management. J Craniofac Surg. 2003;14:37-40.

128. Bradley PJ. Microbiology and management of sialadenitis. Curr Infect Dis Rep. 2002;4:217-224.

129. Fattahi TT, Lyu PE, Van Sickels JE. Management of acute suppurative parotitis. J Oral Maxillofac Surg. 2002;60:446-448.

130. Chow AW. Life-threatening infections of the head, neck, and upper respiratory tract. In: Hall JB, Schmidt GA, Wood LDH, eds. Principles of Critical Care. New York: McGraw-Hill; 1998:887-902.

131. Brook I. The swollen neck—Cervical lymphadenitis, parotitis, thyroiditis and infected cysts. Infect Dis Clin North Am. 1988;2:221-236.

132. Berger SA, Zonszein J, Villanema P, et al. Infectious diseases of the thyroid gland. Rev Infect Dis. 1983;5:108-122.

133. Goldstein EJC, Citron DW, Wield B, et al. Bacteriology of human and animal bite wounds. J Clin Microbiol. 1978;8:667-672.

134. Tami TA, Parker GS. *Eikenella corrodens*—An emerging pathogen in head and neck infections. Arch Otolaryngol. 1984;110:752-754.

135. Weber DJ, Hansen AR. Infections resulting from animal bites. Infect Dis Clin North Am. 1991;5:663-680.

136. Brook I, Hirokawa R. Microbiology of wound infection after head and neck cancer surgery. Ann Otol Rhinol Laryngol. 1989;98:323-325.

137. Gerard M, Meunier F, Dor P, et al. Antimicrobial prophylaxis for major head and neck surgery in cancer patients. Antimicrob Agents Chemother. 1988;32:1557-1559.

138. Heit JM, Stevens MR, Jeffords K. Comparison of ceftriaxone with penicillin for antibiotic prophylaxis for compound mandible fractures. Oral Surg Oral Med Oral Pathol Oral Radiol Endod. 1997;83:423-426.

CHAPTER **58**

Acute Bronchitis

JACK M. GWALTNEY, JR.

Acute bronchitis is a self-limited inflammatory syndrome of the tracheobronchial tree that is most commonly the result of an acute respiratory infection. It occurs most often during the winter months when acute respiratory tract infections are prevalent. Patients seen in general practices in Great Britain had annual attack rates of acute bronchitis that varied between 40 and 54 per 100,000.[1] Weekly attack rates peaked (117 to 171 per 100,000) in January and February and fell to trough levels (26 to 42 per 100,000) in August. The diagnosis was made most often in children younger than 5 years.

Acute bronchitis can be divided into cases of short duration in which the bronchitic symptoms are part of the common cold syndrome, and cases of longer duration, here termed *infectious bronchitis* or *postinfectious bronchitis*. The latter syndrome is associated with more severe infection of the lower respiratory tract such as occurs with influenza and adenovirus and persists after the infection is over. Nonviral causes of the more prolonged syndrome include *Bordetella pertussis, Mycoplasma pneumoniae,* and *Chlamydophila pneumoniae.* In healthy individuals there is no evidence to support a primary or secondary invasion of the tracheobronchial tree by the common respiratory bacteria such as *Streptococcus pneumoniae* and *Haemophilus influenzae.*

MICROBIAL ETIOLOGY

Cough occurs in approximately 50% of the cases of common respiratory illness in people of all ages.[2] Cough is the localizing symptom in the respiratory tract that is most frequently associated with fever and is also highly associated with the occurrence of hoarseness. Infection with members of all the major respiratory virus groups causes cough (Table 58-1).[2-10] Cases of acute bronchitis are particularly common during influenza epidemics. Although rhinovirus infections do not produce as severe and extensive an involvement of the tracheobronchial tree as influenza, rhinovirus infections, because of their frequency, are an important cause of acute bronchitis. In populations of military recruits, adenovirus infections are a major cause of acute bronchitis. Among the other respiratory viruses that cause acute bronchitis, measles virus has

TABLE 58-1 Cough Associated with Acute Viral Infections of the Respiratory Tract

Virus	Percentage of Cases with Cough (References)
Influenza virus	75-93[2,3]
Adenovirus	45-90[4,6]
Rhinovirus	32-60[3,5]
Coronavirus	10-50[7,8]
Parainfluenza virus	2-45[5]
Respiratory syncytial virus	−61[9]
Human metapneumovirus	−75[10]
Coxsackievirus A21	−26[5]
Miscellaneous (rubeola, rubella, etc.)	—

been recognized as causing a particularly severe form of the disease, which may be seen in unvaccinated populations.

A small proportion of all cases of acute bronchitis have a nonviral cause. However, in the group with the more prolonged course, termed *infectious bronchitis,* *M. pneumoniae* and *B. pertussis* play a more prominent role. In adolescents and adults with prolonged cough, *B. pertussis* has been associated with 12% to 32% of cases.[11] *C. pneumoniae* strain TWAR[12] respiratory tract infections have also included cases with the clinical features of acute bronchitis.[13-17]

An etiologic role in acute bronchitis for common respiratory bacteria such as *S. pneumoniae* and *H. influenzae* has not been established.

PATHOGENESIS

The pathogenesis of acute bronchitis appears to be a mixture of viral cytopathic events and host-related inflammatory responses. It has long been known that some respiratory viruses such as influenza infect the lower respiratory tract, but solid evidence for rhinovirus infection of the lower airway in the form of replicative-strand viral ribonucleic acid (RNA) in bronchial epithelial cells is of recent origin.[18] During acute bronchial infection the mucous membrane of the tracheobronchial tree is traditionally described as hyperemic and edematous, and there are increased bronchial secretions. Destruction of respiratory epithelium may be extensive in some infections, such as influenza[19,20] but appears to be minimal in others, such as rhinovirus colds.[21,22] In cultured human bronchial epithelial cells infected with rhinovirus, significant increases have been observed in the production of interleukin-6 (IL-6), IL-8, IL-16, and RANTES.[18] Bronchial mucociliary function may be diminished in infections in which overt mucosal damage is limited.[23] Much remains to be learned about the complexities of the pathogenesis of the different respiratory viruses. With *M. pneumoniae* infection, the pathogenesis is similar to that of *B. pertussis,* in that the organism attaches to the bronchial mucosa between the cilia of the epithelial cells.[24] (For more on pathogenesis, see *M. pneumoniae,* Chapter 181; *B. pertussis,* Chapter 227; and *C. pneumoniae,* Chapter 179.)

It is also possible that the severity of attacks of acute bronchitis may be increased by exposure to cigarette smoke and air pollutants. These substances, in association with recurrent acute bronchial infection, may result in permanent injury to the bronchi. Epidemiologic studies support the idea that acute respiratory infections play a role in the pathogenesis of chronic obstructive lung disease.[25,26] Also studies of pulmonary function in adults with acute bronchitis have shown abnormalities in airway resistance and reactivity.[27-29]

The relationship between acute bronchitis and heightened airway reactivity has been investigated. Mild bronchial asthma was found to be increased in patients with a history of recurrent acute bronchitis over that seen in the general population.[30] Also, in a case-control study, patients with acute bronchitis were more likely to have a previous history of asthma and a history or diagnosis of atopic disease.[31] These findings suggest that transient bronchial hyper-responsiveness is an important mechanism in the persistent cough of infectious bronchitis.[29]

CLINICAL PRESENTATION

Although cough may begin early in the course of acute respiratory infections, it tends to become more prominent as the illness progresses. Of the different respiratory viruses, influenza virus, which routinely invades the lower airway, is the most important cause of cough. In a 6-year study of a group of young adults in which daily records of respiratory symptoms including cough were kept, the highest incidence of cough occurred in patients with influenza, reaching 70% on day 3 of the illness (Fig. 58-1).[32] By comparison, in patients with rhinovirus colds, the incidence of cough remained at approximately 35% over the 7-day period of illness. Two syndromes, the common cold and what is called here *infectious bronchitis,* account for the overwhelming majority of cases of self-limited cough.[24] Although often caused by the same agents and showing overlap in clinical characteristics, the common cold and infectious bronchitis represent two somewhat different

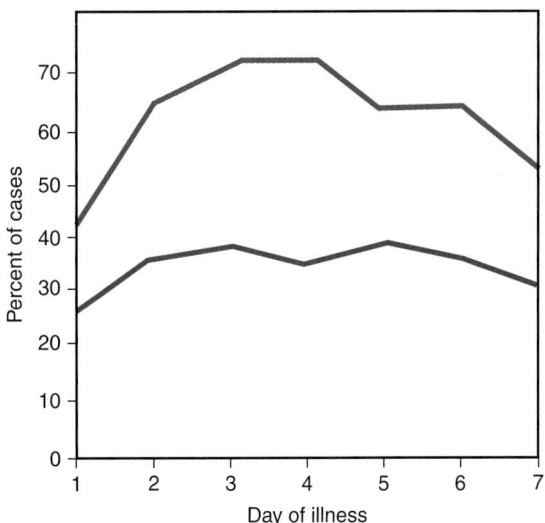

FIGURE 58-1. Occurrence of cough in rhinovirus colds (139 cases) *(red line)* and type A2 influenza (33 cases) *(blue line)* in young adults. *(Modified from Gwaltney JM Jr. Rhinoviruses. In: Evans AS, ed. Viral Infections of Humans: Epidemiology and Control. 3rd ed. New York: Plenum; 1989:593-615.)*

clinical syndromes (Table 58-2). In the typical common cold, cough is only one of several symptoms, is not unusually severe or predominant, and subsides along with the other complaints, although often lasting a few days longer. In rhinovirus colds, nasal and pharyngeal complaints on average improve after 4 or 5 days, whereas cough severity reaches a maximum.[32] Also, 30% of adults still have cough at day 9 of illness.

With infectious bronchitis, cough is, or becomes, the predominant symptom and may last for several weeks. Patients with infectious bronchitis often present in the second or third week of illness, complaining of prolonged cough. They represent a small subset of all patients with acute respiratory infection. The episode may last up to a month or longer before eventually subsiding. Some cases with this syndrome progress into adult-onset asthma. In one prospective study of acute respiratory disease, 45% of patients were still coughing 2 weeks after presentation and 25% were still coughing after 3 weeks.[32] With a variety of different respiratory virus infections, sputum production was reported in approximately one half of the cases in which cough occurred.[4,5] Initially the cough of a cold results in mucoid sputum, which may become more purulent in character in the later stages of illness. A study of natural rhinovirus infections in young adults has shown that the frequency and duration of cough are prolonged in cigarette smokers.[32] The prolonged cough of infectious bronchitis is typically nonproductive.

With severe tracheal involvement there may be burning substernal pain associated with respiration and coughing. Dyspnea and cyanosis are not seen in adults unless the patient has underlying chronic obstructive pulmonary disease or other conditions that impair lung function. Rhonchi and coarse rales may be heard on ex-amination of the chest. Signs of consolidation and alveolar involvement are not present in uncomplicated bronchitis. The frequency with which fever occurs depends on the specific infectious agent involved and the age of the patient. In adults, influenza virus, adenovirus, and *M. pneumoniae* infections are commonly associated with temperature elevations. Fever is unusual in adults with bronchitis associated with cold viruses, such as rhinovirus and coronavirus with the unusual exception of severe acute respiratory syndrome (SARS) coronavirus infection in which fever is a presenting symptom[33] (see Chapter 152).

DIAGNOSIS

Bronchitis may be suspected in the patient with an acute respiratory infection with cough, but because a large variety of more serious diseases of the lower respiratory tract cause cough, bronchitis must be considered as a diagnosis of exclusion. A complete history should be obtained, including information on travel, exposure to toxic substances, and cigarette use. Complaints involving other organ systems should be sought. Epidemiologic considerations and a vaccination history may aid in the diagnosis of specific causes of bronchitis, such as influenza, *M. pneumoniae* infection, and whooping cough.

After every influenza epidemic, there is a small percentage of patients with influenza who, for unknown reasons, develop persistent bronchitis. Another important cause of persistent bronchitis that is receiving increasing attention is pertussis infection (whooping cough). The epidemiology of pertussis has changed due to widespread pertussis vaccination of children. A major reservoir of *B. pertussis* is now in adults who were immunized as children but no longer have immunity. These individuals present with a severe bronchitis that is clinically indistinguishable from that of other infectious causes. Pertussis has often been unrecognized, but recent studies have shown that 12% to 32% of adolescents and adults with episodes of acute, severe persistent cough have pertussis.[34] The serologic diagnosis of *B. pertussis* may be complicated by the presence of cross-reacting antibodies to other respiratory pathogens and/or the occurrence of mixed infections with other agents.[34,35]

Included in a complete physical examination should be a careful evaluation of the chest for evidence of pneumonia and signs of cardiovascular and thromboembolic diseases. Radiologic examination of the chest may be required in patients in whom the question of parenchymal disease of the lung remains after the physical examination. Respiratory secretions should be examined by culture or rapid diagnostic tests for influenza virus, *M. pneumoniae,* and *B. pertussis* when these agents are suspected. Cultures or rapid diagnostic tests for the other respiratory viruses are available in many clinical microbiology laboratories. Culture methods and a microimmunofluorescence test have been developed for the laboratory diagnosis of *C. pneumoniae.*[12] The use of an immunoglobulin M (IgM)–specific conjugate helps detect current infections. Routine bacterial cultures of expectorated sputum are not helpful. Patients in whom cough persists beyond the expected duration of the acute illness should have further diagnostic examinations, including chest radiographs, sputum cytologic examination, and bronchoscopy to

TABLE 58-2 The Two Major Syndromes of Acute Self-Limited Cough		
Syndrome	*Clinical Features*	*Cause*
Common cold	Cough is one of several symptoms Cough is not usually predominant symptom Cough usually subsides in 7-10 days	Rhinovirus Coronavirus Parainfluenza virus Respiratory syncytial virus Influenza virus
Acute infectious bronchitis	May begin as severe cold or "flulike" illness Cough is severe and becomes predominant complaint Cough persists for a month or longer May progress into adult-onset asthma	Influenza virus Adenovirus *Bordetella pertussis* (*B. parapertussis*) *Mycoplasma pneumoniae* *Chlamydophila pneumoniae*

exclude foreign body aspiration, tuberculosis, tumors, and other chronic diseases of the tracheobronchial tree and lungs. The diagnosis of cough-variant asthma should also be considered.[36]

TREATMENT

Symptomatic Treatment

Treatment of most cases of acute bronchitis is symptomatic and is directed primarily at the control of cough. Otherwise, healthy patients do not require hospitalization except in cases of unusual severity. Patients with underlying chronic cardiopulmonary diseases who contract influenzal or other severe forms of bronchitis may develop serious ventilatory abnormalities that require hospitalization with ventilatory assistance and oxygen therapy. Narcotic cough suppressants such as codeine and dextromethorphan have been the mainstay of treatment for cough associated with colds. Although clinical experience suggests that these drugs are useful, the results of placebo-controlled clinical trials have not supported their effectiveness in patients with upper respiratory tract infection.[37]

Placebo-controlled clinical trials have shown that nonsteroidal anti-inflammatory drugs are effective in cough control in patients with common colds. In two studies, naproxen at doses of 250 to 500 mg three times daily reduced cough severity in volunteers with experimental rhinovirus colds.[24] In a large placebo-controlled clinical trial, the first-generation antihistamine brompheniramine (12 mg every 12 hours) also reduced cough severity in volunteers with experimental rhinovirus colds.[38] In a more recent study, early and regular (every 12 hours) administration of combined therapy with chlorpheniramine and ibuprofen (400 mg) reduced cough in subjects with experimental rhinovirus colds.[39] The use of a nonsteroidal anti-inflammatory compound with or without the addition of a first-generation antihistamine may prove to be a more effective treatment than narcotics for cough associated with the common cold, but there have been no direct comparisons of the two treatments.

For symptomatic treatment of cough in cases of *postinfectious* bronchitis, studies have appeared that provide some support for the use of a β-agonist such as albuterol or fenoterol to treat a bronchospastic component of the illness.[40-43] However, further clinical trials are needed to define the value of this form of treatment. Oral or inhaled steroids have also been used in clinical practice but are not recommended. In one small controlled trial of oral dexamethasone in children with whooping cough, the results were not impressive.[44] The value of expectorants is not well established,[45] and in patients with a good cough reflex, maintaining hydration is probably the most effective way to prevent the drying of bronchial secretions. Aspirin or acetaminophen and bed rest are beneficial in influenzal syndromes in which malaise and fever are prominent.

Antimicrobial Treatment

Antimicrobial treatment is not recommended for cases of acute bronchitis in otherwise healthy patients unless there is evidence to support a diagnosis of *B. pertussis* infection or of influenzal, mycoplasmal, or chlamydial bronchitis. Two reviews and three meta-analyses have concluded that antimicrobial treatment is not warranted in unselected cases of acute bronchitis, although small reductions in duration of cough were reported in two of the meta-analyses.[46-50] The reason for these positive findings are unknown and, if not real, could be the result of reporting bias, misclassification of cases, or placebo effect related to the recognition of antimicrobial side effects.

Perhaps the most clinical benefit in treating acute bronchitis can be gained by the proper management of influenza. Effective antivirals are available to treat influenza but are underutilized. The drugs are the older compounds, amantadine and rimantadine and the newer neuraminidase inhibitors, zanamivir, and oseltamivir. Amantadine and rimantadine are inexpensive but have the disadvantages that they only inhibit influenza virus type A and that resistance may develop. The neuraminidase inhibitors are active against both type A and B viruses, and development of resistance has not been a major problem. Early institution of treatment (within 48 hours) is necessary for these drugs to be effective. Annual immunization with influenza vaccine and consideration of prophylaxis with an antiviral as needed is recommended, especially for patients with chronic cardiopulmonary disease (see Chapter 162).

M. pneumoniae infection should be treated with erythromycin or tetracycline (see Chapter 181), *B. pertussis* infection with erythromycin (see Chapter 227), and *C. pneumoniae* infection with tetracycline, erythromycin, or one of the newer macrolide or azalide antibiotics (see Chapter 179). Children should receive pertussis vaccine as part of their routine immunizations. It is particularly important to discourage cigarette smoking in patients in whom acute respiratory tract infections are associated with protracted cough and sputum production.

REFERENCES

1. Ayres JG. Seasonal pattern of acute bronchitis in general practice in the United Kingdom 1976-83. Thorax. 1986;41:107-110.
2. Dingle JH, Badger GF, Jordon WS Jr. Illness in the Home: A Study of 25,000 Illnesses in a Group of Cleveland Families. Cleveland, Ohio: The Press of Western Reserve University; 1964:68.
3. Gwaltney JM Jr. Rhinoviruses. In: Evans AS, ed. Viral Infections of Humans: Epidemiology and Control. 3rd ed. New York: Plenum; 1989:593-615.
4. Dascomb HE, Hilleman MR. Clinical laboratory studies in patients with respiratory disease caused by adenovirus (RI-APC-ARD agents). Am J Med. 1956;21:161.
5. Tyrrell DAJ. Common Colds and Related Diseases. Baltimore: Williams & Wilkins; 1965.
6. Bloom HH, Forsyth BR, Johnson KM, et al. Patterns of adenovirus infections in Marine Corps personnel. I. A 42-month survey in recruit and nonrecruit populations. Am J Hyg. 1964;80:328.
7. Kaye HS, Marsh HB, Dowdle WR. Seroepidemiologic survey of coronavirus (strain OC43) related infections in a children's population. Am J Epidemiol. 1971;94:43.
8. Hendley JO, Fishburne HB, Gwaltney JM Jr. Coronavirus infections in working adults. Eight-year study with 229E and OC43. Am Rev Respir Dis. 1972;105:805.
9. Knight V, Kapikian AZ, Kravetz MH, et al. Ecology of a newly recognized common respiratory agent RS-virus. Ann Intern Med. 1961;55:507.
10. Boivin G, Abed Y, Pelletier G, et al. Virological features and clinical manifestations associated with human metapneumovirus: A new paramyxovirus responsible for acute respiratory-tract infections in all age groups. J Infect Dis. 2002;186:1330-1334.
11. Cherry JD. Epidemiological, clinical, and laboratory aspects of pertussis in adults. Clin Infect Dis 1999; 28(Suppl 2):S112-S117.
12. Grayston JT. Infections caused by *Chlamydia pneumoniae* strain TWAR. Clin Infect Dis. 1992;16:757-763.
13. Grayston JT, Kuo C-C, Wang S-P, et al. A new *Chlamydia psittaci* strain, TWAR, isolated in acute respiratory tract infections. N Engl J Med. 1986;315:161-168.
14. Grayston JT, Kuo C-C, Wang S-P, et al. Clinical findings in TWAR respiratory tract infections. In: Oriel JD, Ridgway G, Schacter J, et al, eds. Chlamydial Infections. Cambridge: Cambridge University Press; 1986:337-340.
15. Hahn DL, Dodge RW, Golubjatnikov R. Association of *Chlamydia pneumoniae* (strain TWAR) infection with wheezing, asthmatic bronchitis, and adult-onset asthma. JAMA. 1991;266:225-230.
16. Hammerschlag MR, Chirgwin K, Roblin PM, et al. Persistent infection with *Chlamydia pneumoniae* following acute respiratory illness. Clin Infect Dis. 1992; 14:178-182.
17. Falck G. Heyman L, Gnarpe J, Gnarpe H. *Chlamydia pneumoniae* (TWAR): A common agent in acute bronchitis. Scand J Infect Dis. 1994;26:179-187.
18. Papadopoulos NG, Bates PJ, Bardin PG, et al. Rhinoviruses infect the lower airways. J Infect Dis. 2000;181:1875-1884.
19. Loosli CG, Stinson SF, Ryan DP, et al. The destruction of type 2 pneumocytes by airborne influenza PR8-A virus: Its effect on surfactant and lecithin content of the pneumonic lesions of mice. Chest. 1975;67(Suppl):7S.
20. Mulder J, Hers JFPh. Influenza. Groningen, The Netherlands: Wolters-Noordhoff; 1972;1-300.
21. Douglas RG Jr, Alford BR, Cough RB: Atraumatic nasal biopsy for studies of respiratory virus infection in volunteers. Antimicrob Agents Chemother. 1968;8:340.
22. Winther B, Farr B, Turner RB, et al. Histopathologic examination and enumeration of polymorphonuclear leukocytes in the nasal mucosa during experimental rhinovirus colds. Acta Otolaryngol Suppl (Stockh). 1984;413:19-24.
23. Sasaki Y, Togo Y, Wagner NH Jr, et al. Mucociliary function during experimentally induced rhinovirus infection in man. Ann Otol. 1973;82:203.
24. Gwaltney J Jr. Clinical and mechanistic perspectives on acute self-limited cough. Symposium Report from the World Congress of Pharmacy and Pharmaceutical Sciences. Int Pharm J. 1997;11:5-7.
25. Lebowitz MD, Burrows B. The relationship of acute respiratory illness history to the prevalence and incidence of obstructive lung disorders. Am J Epidemiol. 1977;105:544.
26. Monto AS, Ross HW. The Tecumseh study of respiratory illness. X. Relation of acute infections to smoking, lung function and chronic symptoms. Am J Epidemiol. 1978;107:57.

27. Hall WJ, Hall CB, Speers DM. Respiratory syncytial virus infection in adults. Clinical, virologic, and serial pulmonary function studies. Ann Intern Med. 1978;88:203.

28. Boldy DAR, Skidmore SJ, Ayres JG. Acute bronchitis in the community: Clinical features, infective factors, changes in pulmonary function and bronchial reactivity to histamine. Respir Med. 1990;84:377-385.

29. Gonzales R, Sande MA. Uncomplicated acute bronchitis. Ann Intern Med. 2000;133:981-991.

30. Hallett JS, Jacobs RL. Recurrent acute bronchitis: The association with undiagnosed bronchial asthma. Ann Allergy. 1985;55:568-570.

31. Williamson HA, Jr, Schultz P. An association between acute bronchitis and asthma. J Fam Pract. 1987;24:35-38.

32. Gwaltney JM Jr, Hendley JO, Simon G, et al. Rhinovirus infections in an industrial population. II. Characteristics of illness and antibody response. JAMA. 1967; 202:494.

33. Ksuazek TC, Erdman D, Goldsmith CS, et al. A novel coronavirus associated with severe acute respiratory syndrome. N Engl J Med. 2003;348-1953-1966.

34. Jackson LA, Cherry JD, Wang S-P, et al. Frequency of serological evidence of *Bordetella* infections and mixed infections with other respiratory pathogens in university students with cough illness. Clin Infect Dis. 2000; 31:3-6.

35. Vincent JM, Cherry JD, Nauschuetz WF, et al. Prolonged afebrile nonproductive cough illnesses in American soldiers in Korea: A serological search for causation. Clin Infect Dis. 2000;30:534-539.

36. Pender ES, Pollack CV Jr. Cough-variant asthma in children and adults: Case reports and review. J Emerg Med. 1990;8:727-731.

37. Freestone C, Eccles R. Assessment of the antitussive efficacy of codeine in cough associated with common cold. J Pharm Pharmacol. 1997;49:1045-1049.

38. Gwaltney JM Jr, Druce HM. Efficacy of brompheniramine maleate treatment for rhinovirus colds. Clin Infect Dis. 1997;25:1188-1194.

39. Gwaltney JM Jr, Winther B, Patrie JT, Hendley JO. Combined antiviral-antimediator treatment for the common cold. J Infect Dis, 2002;186:147-154.

40. Melbye H, Aasebo U, Straume B. Symptomatic effect of inhaled fenoterol in acute bronchitis: A placebo-controlled double-blind study. Fam Pract. 1991;8:216-222.

41. Hueston WJ. A comparison of albuterol and erythromycin for the treatment of acute bronchitis. J Fam Pract. 1991;33:476-480.

42. Littenberg B, Wheeler M, Smith DS. A randomized controlled trial of oral albuterol in acute cough. J Fam Pract. 1996;42:49-53.

43. Hueston WJ. Albuterol delivered by metered-dose inhaler to treat acute bronchitis. J Fam Pract. 1994;39:437-440.

44. Roberts I, Gavin R, Lennon D. Randomized controlled trial of steroids in pertussis (Letter). Pediatr Infect Dis J. 1992;11:982-983.

45. Kuhn JJ, Hendley JO, Adams KF, et al. Antitussive effect of guaifenesin in young adults with natural colds. Objective and subjective assessment. Chest. 1982;82:713.

46. Orr PH, Scherer K, Macdonald A, et al. Randomized placebo-controlled trials of antibiotics for acute bronchitis: A critical review of the literature. J Fam Pract. 1993;36:505-512.

47. McKay DN. Treatment of acute bronchitis in adults without underlying lung disease. J Gen Intern Med. 1996;11:557-562.

48. Fahey T, Stocks N, Thomas T. Quantitative systematic review of randomised controlled trials comparing antibiotic with placebo for acute cough in adults. BMJ. 1998;316:906-910.

49. Smucny JJ, Becker LA, Glazier RH, et al. Are antibiotics effective treatment for acute bronchitis? A meta-analysis. J Fam Pract. 1998;47:453-460.

50. Bent S, Saint S, Vittinghoff E, et al. Antibiotics in acute bronchitis: A meta-analysis. Am J Med. 199;107:62-67.

CHAPTER **59**

Chronic Obstructive Pulmonary Disease, Chronic Bronchitis, and Acute Exacerbations

HERBERT Y. REYNOLDS

Chronic obstructive pulmonary disease (COPD) is characterized as airflow limitation on spirometric measurement that is not fully reversible.[1] Asthma[2,3] is excluded because atopy and allergic immunopathogenic mechanisms are different from those of COPD. Chronic bronchitis no longer is mentioned specifically in some expert group guidelines[1] except that the diagnosis of COPD should be considered in any person with cough, sputum production, or dyspnea and exposure to appropriate risk factors.[1] Chronic bronchitis might coexist and can cause an exacerbation of stable COPD. Overlap of clinical descriptions continues, and more recent patient research still may refer to chronic bronchitis. Future patient trials will need to define diagnoses more specifically. Because there may be clinical confusion or at least uncertainty, some historical perspective is necessary to provide semantic context for what COPD now is intended to include.[4-6]

Based on clinical and functional manifestations, the presence of chronic bronchitis was defined for a person having a productive cough from bronchial hypersecretion of mucus causing expectoration of phlegm on most days during at least 3 consecutive months for more than 2 successive years.[4] Implicit was the exclusion of other causes of expectoration, such as localized lung disease from bronchiectasis or tuberculosis, generalized lung disease from interstitial pneumonitis/fibrosis, and cardiac or renal disease that might cause pulmonary edema, although these conditions could coexist with chronic bronchitis. Included within chronic bronchitis were three subsets, two of which were based on the visual appearance of the sputum: (1) an increased volume of mucoid bronchial secretions causing expectoration (simple) and (2) mucopurulent sputum produced intermittently or persistently a part of every day for at least 1 year. Finally, chronic bronchitis could cause widespread narrowing of intrapulmonary airways, resulting in increased resistance to airflow, as measured by forced expiratory volume in 1 second (FEV_1) or peak expiratory flow; this was defined as *chronic obstructive bronchitis*.[4] This entity has been a source of confusion because it could include emphysema and asthma as well, although asthma usually shows some reversibility in obstructive airway function. Separating these overlapping conditions[5] can be problematic, although new technology is helpful, such as high-resolution computed lung tomography, to reveal the anatomic changes required to delineate emphysema.[7,8] Use of terms such as *asthmatic bronchitis* or *hyperactive airways disease* persist, but these should be avoided; when chronic bronchitis and asthma coexist, the term *chronic bronchitis with asthma* has been suggested.[4]

Because the inclusive term *COPD*[6,9] has continued to include patients with chronic obstructive bronchitis, emphysema, mucus plugging,[2] and chronic bronchitis, and perhaps asthma, syndromes can overlap or coexist in patients and be difficult to separate clinically. Another approach has been to lump them together as done by Dutch and European investigators as *chronic nonspecific lung diseases*.[10] This is referred to as the *Dutch hypothesis*,[9,11] which contrasts with a splitting approach now favored in the United States.[1] A careful attempt to separate asthma from COPD was made,[6] based on the different immunopathogenic mechanisms known to be involved with asthma[3,12,13] and the characteristic reversibility of airflow obstruction,[6] but with qualifications. Patients with asthma whose airflow obstruction was completely reversible were not considered to have COPD (subset 9 in Venn diagram in reference 6); however, patients with unremitting asthma were classified as having COPD (subsets 6, 7, and 8). This schema recognized that it is difficult to separate patients with chronic bronchitis and emphysema who have airway hyperactivity and partially reversible airflow obstruction from patients with asthma whose airflow obstruction does not remit completely.[6] A critical review[2] has stated that most patients with COPD have all three pathologic conditions—chronic obstructive bronchitis, emphysema, and mucus plugging—variably contributing to airflow limitation. Intriguing now is the coalescence of observations from murine models of inflammation to simulate asthma and to create proteolysis and apoptosis required for emphysema that pathways seem intertwined with unexpected findings.[14] Overlapping nonspecific airways disease may reinforce the Dutch hypothesis.[9-11]

The broadly inclusive workshop[1] on the global initiative to address diagnosis, management, and prevention of COPD, or the GOLD standard,[15] was precise in defining COPD as a disease state characterized by airflow limitation that is not fully reversible.[1] This diagnosis in a patient can be considered if symptoms of cough, sputum production, or dyspnea occur with or without a history of exposure to relevant risk factors, notably tobacco smoke, and exposure to occupational dusts and chemicals or to air pollution. Spirometry confirms the diagnosis, if the postbronchodilator FEV_1 is less than 80% of the predicted value in combination with an FEV_1/forced vital capacity ratio less than 70%, which confirms that the airflow limitation present is not fully reversible.[1] Flares of COPD result from infection of the tracheo-bronchial tree and air pollution, but the cause of approximately one third of severe exacerbations cannot be identified.[1] It is hoped that the implications from this more precise identification of COPD will be more accuracy in judging clinically when an exacerbation has occurred and development of better parameters to assess outcome.

PREVALENCE AND IMPACT OF CHRONIC OBSTRUCTIVE PULMONARY DISEASE

Over the past several decades, the prevalence of COPD has increased worldwide, especially in industrialized countries and among women. COPD is the only leading cause of death that is increasing in prevalence worldwide[16] and is ranked fourth as a cause of death in the United States.[1] A dramatic increase in the prevalence of COPD is expected to continue[1,2,17-19]; by 2020, COPD is expected to rank fifth as a worldwide burden of disease.[19] This apparent epidemic of COPD reflects not only reduced mortality from cardiovascular diseases in industrialized countries, but also increased cigarette smoking, environmental pollution, and infectious diseases occurring in developing countries.[2]

ETIOLOGY AND AIRWAY PATHOLOGY

Multiple factors can cause COPD and the chronic bronchitis often associated, but tobacco smoking is considered the major culprit in industrialized countries and probably worldwide in all societies now.[1,2] Development of significant airflow obstruction occurs in only a few cigarette smokers, however, about 15% of white male smokers and less among other groups.[20] In one study, the prevalence of COPD for populations of smokers, age 45 years and older, in eight countries of Europe and North America[18] was about 4% (range 3.2% to 5.4%). Among adult French smokers, prevalence of chronic bronchitis was 4.1% to 6.9%.[21] Undoubtedly, genes and other susceptibility factors help determine which smokers develop disease.

In patients with COPD or bronchitis without obvious risk factors, it is appropriate to consider in a differential diagnosis if a subtle defect in pulmonary host defense exists or an immunodeficiency syndrome is present.[22,23] This possibility first may become evident in teenagers or young adults and not just in young children as generally expected. Evaluation for cystic fibrosis, caused by a gene defect in the transmembrane conductance regulator of the chloride channel in epithelial cells[24]; an immunoglobulin deficiency involving IgA or selective IgG subclasses, or both[25,26]; a structural or acquired defect in cilia on epithelial cells impairing clearance of mucosal secretions[27]; and, rarely, abnormal polymorphonuclear granulocyte function all should be considered. Early onset of COPD, especially in a smoker, raises the possibility of a deficiency of the protease inhibitor, α_1-antitrypsin, which also can occur in a nonsmoker with signs of emphysema at an early age.[28]

Airway Pathology and Inflammatory Changes

COPD and chronic bronchitis feature pathologic changes induced by a combination of airway irritants, microbial infections, inflammation, and possibly defective regulation of innate and adaptive immunity components, all of which cause widespread degenerative changes and reflect imperfect repair attempts by the host, leading to abnormal structural remodeling in all tissue sites at all respiratory levels—central and peripheral airways, lung parenchyma, and pulmonary vasculature.

CLINICAL PRESENTATION

Because manifestations of COPD variously reflect the overlap between chronic bronchitis, emphysema, and often asthma or hyperreactive airways, causing intermittent wheezing with flares, interplay among the entities can vary for a particular patient, creating subsets of COPD patients with different symptoms.[9] Initial descriptions of COPD patients with so-called American emphysema versus British bronchitis[29] defined radiographic groups of emphysematous, inflammatory, and unclassified patients who also had distinguishing symptoms and cardiopulmonary physiology.[30] The major groups, types A and B, descriptively evolved as "pink puffers" and "blue bloaters."

Clinically, this classification is an oversimplification because of "type X," or indeterminate patients with a mixture of features. Nevertheless, for patients with COPD, separating the extreme forms as predominantly emphysema or predominantly bronchitis, based on clinical and physiologic criteria, still remains helpful. Briefly the emphysema-predominant patient typically has more dyspnea, less sputum, and fewer respiratory infections. The patient is more likely to be of thin habitus with a barrel chest, has diminished breath sounds but clear lungs on auscultation, maintains reasonably normal arterial blood gas levels, and has an hyperexpanded appearance of the lung fields on chest films. In contrast, the bronchitis-predominant patient has more productive coughing, is prone to infections, maintains body weight or is obese, has lung crackles and wheezing, and perhaps has right heart failure and pedal edema. Lethargy or somnolence can develop. Also, acrocyanosis, polycythemia, and arterial blood gas levels that feature hypoxemia, carbon dioxide retention, and acidemia often are present. Digital clubbing is not a finding in a patient with uncomplicated COPD and bronchitis.

Frequent coughing interrupts the life of most patients with advanced COPD and bronchitis, causing them to clear their throats frequently and expectorate sputum throughout the day. Many patients cough up the largest amount in the morning on arising. Sputum may be tenacious and sticky and obviously purulent. Nasal or sinus congestion and a postnasal drip often are associated. Many patients with chronic bronchitis are not especially incapacitated, unless an acute infection or another comorbid illness occurs. Some degree of expiratory airflow limitation is present, however, that defines the illness as COPD. Several situations must be considered in diagnosing patients. At-risk individuals may be unaware that their lung function has some airflow obstruction consistent with mild COPD,[1] especially if cough and sputum production are not prominent, and have unrecognized illness and undiagnosed airway obstruction. Mild COPD and chronic bronchitis can occur in nonsmokers, so other contributing factors may need assessment. Among elderly people who are asymptomatic and nonsmokers or ex-smokers, some may be overdiagnosed with COPD because age-specific criteria for spirometry values are not considered.[30a] Other details about clinical presentation can affect how patients are managed when stable and are discussed further.

DEFINING AN EXACERBATION OF CHRONIC OBSTRUCTIVE PULMONARY DISEASE OR CHRONIC BRONCHITIS

Using the more precise definition and diagnosis for COPD that includes patient symptoms of cough, sputum production, or dyspnea and documented airflow limitation that is not fully reversible,[1] asthma is excluded and chronic bronchitis is not mentioned specifically, although chronic cough and sputum production suggest that chronic airway inflammation exists. Overlap of conditions associated with poorly reversible airflow limitation is acknowledged so that bronchiectasis, tuberculosis, and asthma must be considered when appropriate. Prior guidelines and clinical literature[31,32] have defined an acute exacerbation of chronic bronchitis.

The initial attempt by a workshop group to define a COPD exacerbation[51] produced "a sustained worsening of the patient's condition, from the stable state and beyond normal day-to-day variations, that is acute in onset and necessitates a change in regular medications in a patient with underlying COPD." The group[33] amplified several concepts, as follows: "Sustained" is worsening for at least 24 hours; "worsening of condition" can include symptoms of increased sputum purulence or volume or both, dyspnea or wheeze, chest tightness, and retention of fluid; as stable disease has daily fluctuations, beyond normal variations have occurred; acute onset; and regular medications are not effective, especially a short-acting β_2-agonist bronchodilator. In addition, gradations of exacerbation are given as *mild*; *moderate*, requiring additional medical assistance; and *severe*, leading to hospitalization. Managing exacerbations and assessing severity also were presented in the GOLD workshop summary.[1] Other more recent analyses[34,35] of a definition for COPD exacerbations and therapeutic intervention are helpful.

Implication of an Exacerbation

For patients with moderate-to-severe COPD, the median occurrence for exacerbations is documented to be almost 3 times per year (2.7 to 2.9 times per year), although patients self-report only about half of these.[31,36] Symptoms did not differentiate between reported and unreported exacerbations, and the decrease in peak expiratory flow did not affect reporting. Because patients with COPD experience frequent changes of symptoms, they tend to underreport exacerbations to physicians.[36] The cause of a flare often is elusive, and a cause is not found for a large percentage of severe exacerbations, perhaps for about one third[1] to possibly half of cases. Most commonly, infection of the tracheobronchial tree is the cause, but other causes, such as exposures to air pollution and temperature fluctuations and cardiac failure, can be contributory. Continued cigarette smoking or exposure to second-hand smoke is frequent for many patients with COPD, and occupational exposure to dusts and chemicals still might be relevant for patients continuing to work.

As expected, quality of life is affected adversely for patients with frequent exacerbations.[36] Of patients who have an exacerbation of COPD, 3% to 16% are hospitalized,[34,37] with a subsequent mortality rate of 3% to 10%. Mortality is greater if an intensive care admission has been necessary (15% to 24%); this rate approaches 30% for older patients. Subsequent mortality after hospitalization for an acute exacerbation of COPD is striking. Mortality rates at 6 months, 1 year, and 2 years were recorded as approximately 13%, 22%, and 36%.[38] The economic burden of health care costs is great with a recognized impact of sizable hospital costs for medical care expenditures for COPD and for managing an exacerbation in the ambulatory setting.[37] Finding ways to prevent a stable COPD patient from experiencing an exacerbation, which has a mean recovery time of 6 days for return to baseline of the morning peak expiratory flow rate and about 7 days for the total symptom score to revert, is important; however, in about 25% of exacerbations, recovery of peak expiratory flow rate requires 48 days, and for about 7%, the recovery time is 3 months.[31] Preventing a more severe flare that requires hospitalization is a high priority of management.

RELATIONSHIP OF INFECTION TO ACUTE EXACERBATIONS OF CHRONIC OBSTRUCTIVE PULMONARY DISEASE AND CHRONIC BRONCHITIS

COPD features pathologic changes in all tissues[1] of the lung—airways, parenchyma, and vasculature—and its pathogenesis represents a complex interaction of host risk factors. Rarely, hereditary deficiencies; environmental exposures, especially components in cigarette smoke and ambient air and occupational pollutants; and microbial agents can contribute to the widespread inflammation and resultant destructive changes produced. The role of infection is important but vigorously debated.[39-42] Although assessment of the evidence that microbial infection causes acute respiratory illness in patients with stable COPD or exacerbates chronic bronchitis continues,[32,35,43-45] this idea seems less controversial now that 50% to 80% of exacerbations can be associated with recovery of relevant microorganisms.[44] Use of better analytical methods now can identify new strains of bacteria[46] appearing among species already colonizing the airways. New strains can be responsible for flares of infection and stimulating the host's inflammatory response.

Three classes of pathogens infecting the lower respiratory tract have been implicated as causing acute exacerbations of COPD: (1) respiratory viruses, (2) atypical bacteria, and (3) gram-positive and gram-negative aerobic bacteria.[44] Each of these classes is reviewed, after examining what microbial flora may exist in the healthy lung and with chronic lung disease.

Microbial Flora in Normal Lungs

Although a variety of bacteria and perhaps protozoa inhabit the nasooropharynx, these microbes were not listed in the lower airways.[47] The lower airways have been considered sterile.[48,49] Although aspiration of upper airway secretions does occur in normal persons during sleep,[50] host defenses, such as mucociliary clearance and cough, clear microbes and debris quickly.[51] Because samples of bronchoalveolar lavage (BAL) fluid probably are contaminated by microbes pushed down into the bronchi by passage of the bronchoscope,[52] specimens obtained with protected brush specimen catheters (PBC) provide a more accurate analysis.[53-55] The results have varied, however. In 25 healthy volunteers, smoking status not given, 21 of 25 subjects (84%) from 38 of 52 lower lung sampling sites (73%), using a plugged telescoping double-catheter system, yielded specimens that were contaminated with oropharyngeal organisms.[53] Another study of eight healthy nonsmokers,[54] comparing PBC and BAL fluid samples and using quantitative bacterial cultures, found seven of eight BAL fluid cultures positive for oropharyngeal flora, but seven of eight PBC specimens sterile. Quantitative bacteriology cultures have been suggested for separating contaminants from pathogenic organisms; lidocaine, used for topical anesthesia, at the concentration found in specimens was not sufficient to affect recovery of bacteria. Another study[55] in 16 healthy nonsmoker volunteers, comparing BAL fluid and PBC samples and using quantitative cultures, found 14 of 16 (88%) PBC samples to be negative (sterile or $<10^2$ colony-forming units [CFU]/mL) and 13 of 15 BAL fluids to be negative (6 sterile and 7 with $<10^2$ to 10^3 CFU/mL). Generally, healthy lower airways of nonsmokers are sterile or have minimal bacterial counts, possibly consistent with some low-level colonization with nonpathogens that perhaps is transient.

Bacteria in Stable Chronic Obstructive Pulmonary Disease and Chronic Bronchitis

Many patients with chronic bronchitis can have *Streptococcus pneumoniae, Haemophilus influenzae,* and oropharyngeal commensal bacteria cultured from bronchial secretions.[56] Comparing transtracheal aspiration, area sampling for oropharyngeal secetions, and, after endotracheal intubation, fiberoptic bronchoscopic bronchial aspirates, the predominant organisms found in 24 patients with chronic bronchitis[57] were unencapsulated or nontypable strains of *H. influenzae* (58%), *S. pneumoniae* (38%), and anaerobic bacteria (17% [4 of 24 patients]). In 18 patients with stable COPD,[55] PBC cultures were positive from 83% (15 of 18 patients) with several species of potentially pathogenic bacteria in 5 patients (*H. influenzae* or *S. pneumoniae*, 2 of each, and *Staphylococcus aureus*, 1). A mixture of nonpathogens was cultured, including *Streptococcus viridans, Neisseria* spp., *Corynebacterium* spp., and *Candida* spp. Also, in 33 patients evaluated for bronchogenic carcinoma, of whom 31 had concomitant COPD, 42% were determined to be colonized with similar potentially pathogenic bacteria based on PBC and BAL fluid culture results.[55]

Viruses in Stable Chronic Obstructive Pulmonary Disease

Respiratory viruses have been associated with acute exacerbations of COPD,[58] but these are not considered to persist, and patients do not become carriers of a virus. This relationship has been reexamined,[59] however, in stable COPD for the presence of respiratory viruses.[60,61] Viruses were found in 16.2% of nasal aspirates from 68 patients during a stable phase of COPD and included rhinovirus, coronaviruses, respiratory syncytial virus, and parainfluenza virus. Patients who had viruses detected in their aspirates gave a history of more frequent exacerbations, however, than patients who had no viruses recovered.[60] Because respiratory syncytial virus was detected in 23.5% of 68 stable COPD patients, this virus might represent asymptomatic infection or prolonged shedding of virus from a previous symptomatic infection.[60,61]

Atypical Bacteria

Atypical bacteria considered important for respiratory illness include *Chlamydophila* (formerly *Chlamydia*) *pneumoniae* and *Mycoplasma pneumoniae*[61]; both have been implicated in a few COPD exacerbations, about 4%[62] and 1%.[63] In stable COPD, almost no isolates were detected of either microbe in nasal aspirates.[60] In another study[63] of patients with steady-state chronic bronchitis, sputum colonization with *C. pneumoniae* was found for 38% of patients (16 of 42), who also tended to have more severe airflow impairment (FEV$_1$ ≤35%), and for 43% in a larger group of similar patients (61 of 141) when a polymerase chain reaction method was used to detect *C. pneumoniae* DNA in peripheral blood mononuclear cells. There is some discrepancy reported for baseline colonization with this intracellular bacterium, which might be methodologic.[64] Because *C. pneumoniae* has emerged as a cause of chronic inflammatory illness in several organs, its persistence in lung tissue needs further investigation.[23]

MICROBES IMPLICATED IN AN ACUTE EXACERBATION OF CHRONIC OBSTRUCTIVE PULMONARY DISEASE

As a baseline in patients with stable COPD or chronic bronchitis based on microbial culture results obtained from mucous membranes of the nasopharynx,[60,61] by transtracheal aspiration[58] and quantitative cultures of bronchoscopic PBC or BAL fluid,[55] 58% to 83% of patients had bacterial bronchial airway colonization, most often with nonpotential pathogens, such as viridans group streptococci, *Neisseria* spp., and *Corynebacterium* spp., and with potential pathogens, including *H. influenzae* and *S. pneumoniae*. Of patients, 16% to 23.5% had viruses, including respiratory syncytial virus, rhinoviruses, coronaviruses, and parainfluenza. *C. pneumoniae* may colonize about 40% of patients.[62,63]

An exacerbation of stable COPD or chronic bronchitis[1,2] is signaled clinically by an increased volume of more purulent sputum, worsening cough, perhaps dyspnea, and need for some adjustment of medications. Many patients (21% to 49%) may not recognize the flare, however, which would go unreported in clinical trials. By objective assessment, patients have about three exacerbations yearly that affect their quality of life.[36] Microbial persistence in the nasopharynx and lower airways is relevant in two situations:[63] (1) Colonizing microbes, especially potentially pathogenic ones, may create more inflammation and trigger an exacerbation, or (2) colonizing microbes may cause an ongoing, smoldering inflammatory milieu in the bronchial mucosa that might facilitate entry and survival of other microbes that possibly could exert immunosuppressive effects.[65,66] Host defense factors that control growth of the microbial flora on the mucous membranes lining the naso-oropharynx, trachea, and bronchi are poorly understood[67] still after 2 decades of research, as is the regulation of innate and adaptive immunity responses in the respiratory tract.[23] Because bacteria can be isolated during an exacerbation, and antibiotic therapy is effective,[32] infection presumably has a causative role. Distinguishing between microbes that just irritate and create mucositis versus microbes that can exploit the ciliated epithelial airway surface to create an added or synergistic inflammatory effect seems important. Also, bacteria may be secondary invaders after viral infections[60]; mixed viral/bacterial infections of the respiratory tract may be important in COPD patients.[68,69] Determining precisely the particular infectious cause of a COPD exacerbation can be difficult.[70]

Although respiratory viruses have been associated with asthmatic exacerbations, less emphasis was given to their role in COPD[43,58] until more recently.[59-61,68] Previously, it was reported that 18% of acute respiratory illnesses in patients with COPD were attributed to viruses, but about 6% of similarly acute infections occurred during illness-free intervals or were not realized or were unreported by the patients.[58] Gump and colleagues[43] followed 25 patients with defined chronic bronchitis for 4 years; all were immunized against influenza A and B each year. One third of the 116 exacerbations of chronic bronchitis were related to viral infections and just one to *M. pneumoniae*.[43] Among COPD patients, who were about 90% vaccinated annually against influenza virus,[68] 19% had a documented acute respiratory tract viral infection. The most commonly identified viruses were picornaviruses (primarily rhinoviruses), parainfluenza viruses, and coronaviruses.[68] Aaron and co-workers[70] conclusively showed an acute viral infection in 14% of patients (2 of 14) with COPD. About 20% on average (range 14% to 33%) of flares of COPD or chronic bronchitis are caused by viral respiratory infections.

Seemungal and colleagues[60] prospectively studied the association between viral infections and exacerbations of COPD with polymerase chain reaction methods in addition to usual viral cultures and serology, so detection or evidence of viruses was more sensitive. About 40% of exacerbations were virus associated.[60] Several other findings help to dissect the relationship between stable COPD and a preceding viral infection triggering the exacerbation. Of the 83 patients, 74% had yearly immunization against influenza. Forty-eight percent of exacerbations were not reported by patients. Among the 168 reported exacerbations

in these 83 stable COPD patients, 51% were preceded by colds, 18% by sore throat, and 76% by increased dyspnea. Two thirds of exacerbations could be associated with a cold 18 days before the onset. Viral-detected exacerbations, which occurred in 40%, also were accompanied by total daily symptom count that was higher, plus the recovery time from the illness was longer, a median of 13 days rather than 6 days for a nonviral exacerbation. Patients in whom viruses were detected gave a history of more frequent exacerbations than patients without virus detection—4 versus 2.5. Viral-associated exacerbations in patients with stable COPD occurred in about 40%; resulting illness was more severe with a higher daily symptom score, and a longer time to recover or resolve symptoms was required by many patients.[61]

At the severe end of the spectrum, when an exacerbation of COPD led to acute respiratory failure and admission to an intensive care unit for mechanical ventilation,[71] initial cultures, obtained in several ways, contained potentially pathogenic bacterial species in more than 40% of cases (50 patients in study) and nonpathogenic bacteria in about 20% of cultures. As diagnosed by serologic titers, 40% (15 of 38 cases) initially had viruses, mostly influenza virus, or atypical bacteria, with 7 or 18% considered to be *C. pneumoniae*. A cold previously may initiate the flare. Perhaps a viral respiratory infection often predisposes to a flare with the existing bacteria that are colonizing the airways. Alternatively, viruses might suppress temporarily ongoing innate immunity that is holding proliferation of colonizing bacteria in check, or this creates an opportunity for new microbes or new strains of existing ones to emerge.

With an exacerbation of stable COPD or chronic bronchitis, bacteria can be recovered in cultures of sputum in about half the cases, and the predominant species isolated are the potential pathogens—nontypable *H. influenzae*, *S. pneumoniae*, and *Moraxella catarrhalis*. Assessing the host's immune response against pathogenic or any persistent microbes may indicate preparedness, particularly if this is being enhanced with good or increasing levels of antibody titers. A preliminary study of pre-exacerbation and postexacerbation paired sera for strain-specific, bactericidal antibodies against nontypable *H. influenzae* in two patients[72] indicated that new, strain-specific antibodies could develop toward the homologous infecting strain.

A more detailed study of 81 patients with moderate-to-severe COPD who were followed for more than 4 years[46] found that at 374 clinic visits for exacerbations (18.9%), in almost 40% of sputum cultures performed, pathogenic bacteria were recovered, if the patient had not received antibiotic treatment within the prior 48 hours. If an antibiotic had been received, pathogen isolation was slightly less (31%). Most isolates contained *H. influenzae*, *M. catarrhalis*, *S. pneumoniae*, and *Pseudomonas aeruginosa*. New strains of the bacterial species were isolated for 33% of the associated exacerbations, in contrast to 15.4% for which no new strains were found. Molecular typing to detect newly acquired strains was done for *H. influenzae*, *M. catarrhalis*, and *S. pneumoniae*. This study[46] emphasizes several concepts, as follows: (1) There is increasing evidence that bacteria cause many of the exacerbations of COPD, about 40% in the present study; (2) other new strains of the same bacterial species are associated in one third of the symptomatic exacerbations; and (3) perhaps 15% or more of flares occur without development of a new strain, allowing perhaps for an antecedent viral or atypical bacterial infection contributing to a flare.[44,60,61] Viruses were not identified in this study.[46] Finally, a plausible mechanism to help explain recurrent bacterial exacerbations in COPD has been advanced that strain-specific protective immunity develops subsequent to an exacerbation, leaving the patient susceptible again to infection by another strain of the same bacterium.

OVERALL MANAGEMENT

For patients with stable COPD or chronic bronchitis, acute flares of illness can be expected to occur about two to three times per year, but with almost half the episodes being unrecognized and not reported by patients. Overall management should address four areas: (1) maintenance therapy during quiescent intervals designed to optimize daily activity, enhance exercise tolerance, and keep secretions, cough, and wheezing minimal (Tables 59-1 and 59-2); (2) prevention of respiratory infections; (3) more intensive treatment when exacerbations occur;

TABLE 59-1 General Medical Measures

Have patient discontinue cigarette smoking, using cessation course and/or nicotine replacement medication to minimize withdrawal (gum, transdermal patch, and nasal spray or inhaler forms); bupropion, an antidepressant, may be helpful. If cessation is unsuccessful, at least attempt to reduce the amount of daily smoking.

Assess for any concomitant allergic disease—rhinitis, asthma, and sulfite sensitivity.

Judge involvement of sinus disease and/or nasal obstruction with baseline sinus CT scan; obtain otolaryngology consultation to evaluate possible obstruction from nasal polyps or septal deviation. Exclude gastroesophageal reflux, which can contribute to cough and other symptoms.[95,96]

Review for any potential host factor or hereditary illness causing recurrent sinopulmonary infections (e.g., immunoglobulin deficiency, cystic fibrosis, ciliary defect).

Obtain nutritional counseling to reduce weight if obese; use dietary supplementation if patient is malnourished or experiencing early satiety or may benefit from antioxidant-rich foods and cereal fiber.[76] Peripheral muscle wasting or myopathy may represent cachexia in COPD, causing altered metabolism because of systemic inflammation.[97-99]

Minimize contact with environmental irritants. Arrange for periodic cancer screening, as risk of lung cancer is usually increased.

Obtain pulmonary spirometry tests and oximetry for oxygen saturation on room air with a 6-minute walk test (baseline arterial blood gas levels are advised).

Record daily peak-flow-meter readings (keep a patient log).

Encourage pulmonary rehabilitation program or daily exercise routine, especially respiratory muscle training,[101] using upper body and arm strengthening, as tiredness in COPD patients comes with upper limb use.[102] Also, exercise may improve cognitive function.[103] Prescribe use of supplemental oxygen as dictated by oxygen desaturation with exercise, arterial blood gas values, and degree of pulmonary hypertension.

In addition to spirometry to document airflow obstruction, consider cardiopulmonary exercise testing to better assess patient's functional impairment.[104] Echocardiography will estimate pulmonary artery pressure and right heart involvement.[105,106]

Give preventive immunizations—pneumococcal vaccine[107] and yearly influenza vaccine.

If sputum production is copious, use flutter valve tube and perform postural drainage to help mobilize secretions.

Assess for clinical depression, which is common with most chronic diseases.

COPD, chronic obstructive pulmonary disease; CT, computed tomography.

and (4) selection of antibiotic therapy. Recommendations reflect suggestions from several general sources that can be consulted for more details.[1,2,73-79]

Prophylactic antibiotic therapy may have some usefulness in highly selected patients who experience frequent exacerbations (four

TABLE 59-2 Maintenance Therapy—Bronchodilator, Anti-inflammatory Medications, and Perhaps Antibiotics[*] (representative drugs given)

Salmeterol inhalation aerosol or powder, 25 μg or 50 μg, 2 puffs at bedtime; this may decrease awakening with symptoms during the night.

Ipratropium inhalational aerosol, 18 μg/activation, 2 puffs qid.

Combination inhaler of albuterol-ipratropium, 2 puffs qid.

Oral theophylline (for patients with suboptimal response to above bronchodilators); e.g., Theo-Dur 200 or 300 mg bid or tid (dose of theophylline must be individualized based on peak serum concentration).

Orally inhaled aerosol corticosteroids, such as fluticasone, available in various doses calculated from the activator as 44 μg, 110 μg, or 220 μg; 2 puffs bid. An inhalational powder form is available also.

Powder disc combination containing fluticasone at various doses, and salmeterol can be prescribed bid.

Oral prednisone, dose 20-30 mg/day initially, with a tapering schedule and switching to an alternate-day regimen of about 10 and 5 mg/day on alternate days, if possible.

Cough suppressant (example, benzonatate 100 mg bid).

For more severe asthma or to spare amount of corticosteroids, use inhibitor of cysteinyl leukotrienes (example—montelukast 10-mg tablet/day or zafirlukast 20 mg tablet bid).

Mucolytic agents usually are not very effective.

Prophylactic antibiotic—rotating schedule with oral, broad-spectrum antibiotic is suggested (see text); requirement for continuous antibiotic is unusual.

[*]Use of a spacer with an inhaler is recommended if patient has difficulty coordinating use.

or more per year). The realization that perhaps one third of acute flares are preceded by viral respiratory infections has an impact on this decision. Several antibiotics can be used based on considerations of microbial sensitivity, the patient's tolerance, the dosing interval, and the cost. Several strategies seem to be effective. Patients may receive antibiotics daily or 4 days per week during the winter or a 7-day course at the first sign of a "chest cold."

ANTIMICROBIAL THERAPY

Although there is no consistently used definition[33,34,80] in clinical practice for an acute flare of COPD or chronic bronchitis, a combination of worsening symptoms, such as dyspnea, more cough, and increased volume or the purulent appearance of sputum, may prompt a patient to call the health care provider about medications and advice about an outpatient or emergency service visit. Airway infection often is contributory, but other factors also have to be assessed, especially comorbid illnesses, medication compliance, allergens, air pollution, and other environmental exposures. The role of infection has many components, including underlying airway microbial colonization, antecedent viral infection, subsequent secondary bacterial infection, or the emergence of a new strain of an existing bacterial species. Greater airway inflammation from any microbial cause may create more sputum purulence, giving a yellowish or greenish color representing myeloperoxidase from azurophil granules in polymorphonuclear granulocytes,[81] which frequently would yield a positive bacterial culture (84%) compared with fewer positive cultures from mucoid sputum (38%). Another measurement of inflammation might be determination of endogenously exhaled gaseous mediators such as nitric oxide[70,82,83] to correlate sputum findings in a clinical study or use of positron emission imaging to assess inflammatory cell activity.[84] Along with any adjustment of medications to treat the flare, an oral antibiotic usually is started promptly. Even if other noninfectious causes contribute to the flare, antibiotics usually are not withheld.[85] A spontaneously coughed or an induced sputum specimen may not be obtained for cellular analysis, Gram stain, and routine microbial culture, unless a research therapy protocol exists, or the patient has not responded well to a prior antibiotic course.

In general, antibiotic treatment improves clinical outcome and hastens recovery based on reviews of many antibiotic trials.[32,77,78,85-89] Also, keeping the airway bacterial load low helps to decrease the decline in FEV_1. COPD patients who had an increase in sputum bacterial growth or had changes in colonizing species of bacteria had greater airway inflammation and accelerated decline in FEV_1.[90] The usual strategy is to begin oral antimicrobial therapy for 5 to 10 days or parenterally if hospitalization occurs; an objective end point for success usually is lacking. Many acute exacerbations probably are due to viral infections, and for these, antimicrobial therapy would not be beneficial. The clinician usually is unable to determine, however, when exacerbations are due to bacterial infection versus viral infection.

There are many considerations in selecting an appropriate antibiotic, as outlined by Schentag and Tillotson,[91] including the spectrum of activity, mode of action, tissue penetration, tolerance of the drug by the patient, frequency of administration, modification of dose based on the mechanism of excretion or inactivation, and cost. The array of acceptable antibiotics is large, and new agents are being introduced. Antimicrobial choices must be made in the context of present or emerging antibiotic-resistant patterns or rates to the advanced-generation macrolides and fluoroquinolone agents (Table 59-3).[92-94] Currently, most patients in an outpatient setting with putatively acute bacterial exacerbations of COPD and chronic bronchitis receive a short course of one of three commonly used antibiotics—amoxicillin-clavulanate, azithromycin, or levofloxacin. Effectiveness and safety among these agents is comparable, as are the eradication rates of usual respiratory bacterial pathogens isolated in sputum cultures.

Acknowledgment

The author appreciates Mrs. Susan K. Crawford's preparation of the manuscript.

TABLE 59-3 Oral Antibiotics for Common Agents Associated with an Exacerbation of COPD and Chronic Bronchitis

Antibiotic	Usual Oral Dosage	Streptococcus pneumoniae*	Haemophilus pneumoniae*	Moraxella catarrhalis	Mycoplasma pneumoniae	Chlamydia pneumoniae
Ampicillin	250 mg qid	±	−	−	−	−
Amoxicillin	250-500 mg tid	±	±	−	−	−
Amoxicillin-clavulanate	250-mg tablet tid	+	+	+	−	−
Doxycycline	200 mg first day, then 100 mg/day	−	±	±	+	+
Azithromycin	500 mg/day, then 250 mg/day	±	+	+	+	+
Trimethoprim-sulfamethoxazole (Bactrim DS)	160-800 mg (IDS/day)	±	+	+	−	−
Cefuroxime axetil	250-500 mg bid	±	+	+	−	−
Levofloxacin†	500 mg/day	+	+	+	+	+

*Antibiotic resistance can occur with some strains, designated as ±. Antibiotic susceptibility testing is required.
†Selected as a representative of fluoroquinolones.

REFERENCES

1. Pauwels RA, Buist AS, Calverley PMA, et al. Global strategy for the diagnosis, management, and prevention of chronic obstructive pulmonary disease. NHLBI/WHO Global Initiative for Chronic Obstructive Lung Disease (COLD) Workshop Summary. Am J Respir Crit Care Med. 2001;163:1256-1276.
2. Barnes PJ. Chronic obstructive pulmonary disease-medical progress. N Engl J Med. 2000;343:269-280.
3. Barnes PJ. Mechanisms in COPD—differences from asthma. Chest. 2000;117:10S-14S.
4. Stuart-Harris CH, Crofton J, Gilson JC, et al (Committee for the Medical Research Council). Definition and classification of chronic bronchitis for clinical and epidemiological purposes. Lancet. 1965;1:775-779.
5. Wilson R, Wilson CB. Defining subsets of patients with chronic bronchitis. Chest. 1997;112:303S-309S.
6. Celli BR, Snider GL, Heffner J, et al. American Thoracic Society Statement. Standards for the diagnosis and care of patients with chronic obstructive pulmonary disease: Definitions, epidemiology, pathophysiology, diagnosis, and staging. Am J Respir Crit Care Med. 1995;152:S77-S120.
7. Clark KD, Wardobe-Wong N, Elliott JJ, et al. Patterns of lung disease in a "normal" smoking population: Are emphysema and airflow obstruction found together? Chest. 2001;120:743-747.
8. Satoh K, Kobayashi T, Misao T, et al. CT assessment of subtypes of pulmonary emphysema in smokers. Chest. 2001;120:725-729.
9. Rennard SI. COPD: Overview of definitions, epidemiology, and factors influencing its development. Chest. 1998;113:235S-241S.
10. Brand PLP, Kerstjens HAM, Postma DS, et al. Long-term multicentre trial in chronic nonspecific lung disease: Methodology and baseline assessment in adult patients. Eur Respir J. 1992;5:21-31.
11. Hahn DL. Chlamydia pneumoniae and the "Dutch hypothesis." Chest. 2002; 122: 1510-1512.
12. Elias JA, Lee CG, Zheng T, et al. New insights into the pathogenesis of asthma. J Clin Invest. 2003;111:291-297.
13. Davies DE, Wicks J, Powell RM, et al. Airway remodeling in asthma: New insights. J Allergy Clin Immunol. 2003;111:215-225.
14. Tuder RM, Petrache I, Elias JA, et al. Apoptosis and emphysema—the missing link (a perspective). Am J Respir Cell Mol Biol. 2003;28:551-554.
15. Gross NJ. The GOLD standard for chronic obstructive pulmonary disease (Editorial). Am J Respir Crit Care Med. 2001;163:1047-1048.
16. Hurd SS. The impact of COPD on lung health worldwide-epidemiology and incidence. Chest. 2000;117:1S-4S.
17. Coultas DB, Mapel DW. Undiagnosed airflow obstruction: Prevalence and implications. Curr Opin Pulm Med. 2003;9:96-103.
18. Rennard S, Decramer M, Calverley PMA, et al. Impact of COPD in North America and Europe in 2000: Subjects' perspective of confronting COPD international survey. Eur Respir J. 2002;20:799-805.
19. Lenfant C. Preface in Reference 1, pp 1256-1257.
20. Centers for Disease Control and Prevention. Current Estimates from the National Health Interview Survey, 1995. Vital and Health Statistics. DHHS Publication No. (PHS) 96-1527. Washington, DC: Government Printing Office; 1996.
21. Huchon GJ, Vergnenègre A, Neukirch F, et al. Chronic bronchitis among French adults: High prevalence and underdiagnosis. Eur Respir J. 2002;20:806-812.
22. Reynolds HY. Host defense mechanisms of the lung. In: Davis GS, Marcy TW, Seward EA, eds. Medical Management of Pulmonary Disease. New York: Marcel Dekker; 1999:65-78.
23. Reynolds HY. Modulating airway defenses against microbes. Curr Opin Pulm Med. 2002;8:154-165.
24. Ratjen F, Döring G. Cystic fibrosis. Lancet. 2003;361:681-689.
25. Pilette C, Ouadrhiri Y, Godding V, et al. Lung mucosal immunity: Immunoglobulin-A revisited. Eur Respir J. 2001;18:571-588.
26. Reynolds HY. Immunoglobulin G and its function in the human respiratory tract. Mayo Clin Proc. 1988;63:161-174.
27. Ho JC, Chan KN, Hu WH, et al. The effect of aging on nasal mucociliary clearance, beat frequency, and ultrastructure of respiratory cilia. Am J Respir Crit Care Med. 2001;163: 983-988.
28. Lee P, Gildea TR, Stoller JK. Emphysema in non-smokers: Alpha 1 antitrypsin deficiency and other causes. Cleve Clin J Med. 2002;69:928-929, 933, 936.
29. Fletcher CM, Jones NL, Burrows B, Niden AH. American emphysema and British bronchitis. Am Rev Respir Dis. 1964;90:1-13.
30. Burrows B, Niden AH, Fletcher CM, Jones NL. Clinical types of chronic obstructive lung disease in London and Chicago. Am Rev Respir Dis. 1964;90:14-27.
30a. Hardie JA, Buist AS, Vollmer WM, et al. Risk of over-diagnosis of COPD in asymptomatic elderly never-smokers. Eur Respir J. 2002;20:1117-1122.
31. Seemungal TAR, Donaldson GC, Bhowmik A, et al. Time course and recovery of exacerbations in patients with chronic obstructive pulmonary disease. Am J Respir Crit Care Med. 2000;161:1608-1613.
32. Anthonisen NR, Manfreda J, Warren CPW, et al. Antibiotic therapy in exacerbations of chronic obstructive pulmonary disease. Ann Intern Med. 1987;106:196-204.
33. Rodriguez-Roisin R. Toward a consensus definition for COPD exacerbations. Chest. 2000;117:398S-401S.
34. Soto FJ, Varkey B. Evidence-based approach to acute exacerbations of COPD. Curr Opin Pulm Med. 2003;9:117-124.
35. Sohy C, Pilette C, Niederman MS, Sibille Y. Acute exacerbation of chronic obstructive pulmonary disease and antibiotics: What studies are still needed? Eur Respir J. 2002;19: 966-975.
36. Seemungal TAR, Donaldson GC, Paul EA, et al. Effect of exacerbation on quality of life in patients with chronic obstructive pulmonary disease. Am J Respir Crit Care Med. 1998;157:1418-1422.
37. Miravitlles M, Murio C, Guerrero T, et al. Pharmacoeconomic evaluation of acute exacerbations of chronic bronchitis and COPD. Chest. 2002;121:1449-1455.
38. Almagro P, Calbo E, Ochoa de Echagüen A, et al. Mortality after hospitalization for COPD. Chest. 2002;121:1441-1448.
39. Leeder SR. Role of infection in the cause and course of chronic bronchitis and emphysema. J Infect Dis. 1975;131:731-742.
40. Tager I, Speizer FE. Role of infection in chronic bronchitis. N Engl J Med. 1975; 292: 563-571.
41. Wilson R. The role of infection in COPD. Chest. 1998;113:242S-248S.
42. Murphy TF, Sethi S. Bacterial infection in chronic obstructive pulmonary disease—state of the art. Am Rev Respir Dis. 1992;146:1067-1083.
43. Gump DW, Phillips CA, Forsyth BR, et al. Role of infection in chronic bronchitis. Am Rev Respir Dis. 1976;113:465-474.
44. Sethi S. Infectious etiology of acute exacerbations of chronic bronchitis. Chest. 2000; 117:380S-385S.
45. Anthonisen NR. Bacteria and exacerbations of chronic obstructive pulmonary disease (Editorial). N Engl J Med. 2002;347:526-527.
46. Sethi S, Evans N, Grant BJB, Murphy TF. New strains of bacteria and exacerbations of chronic obstructive pulmonary disease. N Engl J Med. 2002;347:465-471.
47. Mackowiak PA. The normal microbial flora—medical progress. N Engl J Med. 1982; 307:83-93.
48. Laurenzi GG, Potter RT, Kass EH. Bacterial flora of the lower respiratory tract. N Engl J Med. 1961;265:1273-1278.
49. Potter RT, Rotman F, Fernandez F, et al. The bacteriology of the lower respiratory tract: Bronchoscopic study of 100 clinical cases. Am Rev Respir Dis. 1968;97:1051-1061.
50. Huxley EJ, Viroslav J, Gray WR, Pierce AK. Pharyngeal aspiration in normal adults and patients with depressed consciousness. Am J Med. 1978;64:564-568.
51. Reynolds HY. Defense mechanisms against lung infections. Curr Opin Pulm Med. 1999;5:136-142.
52. Reynolds HY, Newball HH. Analysis of proteins and respiratory cells obtained from human lungs by bronchial lavage. J Lab Clin Med. 1974;84:559-573.
53. Halperin SA, Suratt PM, Gwaltney JM Jr, et al. Bacterial cultures of the lower respiratory tract in normal volunteers with and without experimental rhinovirus infection using a plugged double catheter system. Am Rev Respir Dis. 1982;125:678-680.
54. Kirkpatrick MB, Bass JB Jr. Quantitative bacterial cultures of bronchoalveolar lavage fluids and protective brush catheter specimens from normal subjects. Am Rev Respir Dis. 1986;139:546-548.
55. Cabello H, Torres A, Celis R, et al. Bacterial colonization of distal airways in healthy subjects and chronic lung disease: A bronchoscopic study. Eur Respir J. 1997;10:1137-1144.
56. Lees AW, McNaught W. Bacteriology of lower-respiratory-tract secretions, sputum, and upper-respiratory-tract secretions in "normals" and chronic bronchitics. Lancet. 1959; 2: 1112-1115.
57. Hass H, Morris JF, Samson S, et al. Bacterial flora of the respiratory tract in chronic bronchitis: Comparisons of transtracheal, fiber-bronchoscopic and oropharyngeal sampling methods. Am Rev Respir Dis. 1977;116:41-47.
58. Smith CB, Golden CA, Canner RE, Renzetti AD. Association of viral and Mycoplasma pneumoniae infections with acute respiratory illness in patients with chronic obstructive pulmonary disease. Am Rev Respir Dis. 1980;121:225-232.
59. Hogg JC. Viral infection and exacerbations of chronic obstructive pulmonary disease. Am J Respir Crit Care Med. 2001;164:1555-1556.
60. Seemungal TAR, Harper-Owen R, Bhowmik A, et al. Respiratory viruses, symptoms, inflammatory markers in acute exacerbations and stable chronic obstructive pulmonary disease. Am J Respir Crit Care Med. 2001;164:1618-1623.

61. Seemungal TAR, Wedzicha JA. Viral infections in obstructive airway diseases. Curr Opin Pulm Med. 2003;9:111-116.
62. Blasi F, Legnani D, Lombardo VM, et al. *Chlamydia pneumoniae* infection in acute exacerbations of COPD. Eur Respir J. 1993;6:19-22.
63. Blasi F, Damato S, Cosentini R, et al. *Chlamydia pneumoniae* and chronic bronchitis: Association with severity and bacterial clearance following treatment. Thorax. 2002;57:6 72-676.
64. Seemungal TAR, Wedzicha JA, MacCallum PK, et al. Authors and reply: Blasi F, Allegra L, Damato S, et al. *Chlamydia pneumoniae* and COPD exacerbation. Thorax. 2002;57: 1087-1089.
65. Atabani SF, Byrnes AA, Jaye A, et al. Natural measles causes prolonged suppression of interleukin-12 production. J Infect Dis. 2001;184:1-9.
66. Slifka MK, Homann D, Tishon A, et al. Measles virus infection results in suppression of both innate and adaptive immune responses to secondary bacterial infection. J Clin Invest. 2003;111:805-810.
67. Bates JH. The role of infection during exacerbations of chronic bronchitis. Ann Intern Med. 1982;97:130-132.
68. Greenberg SB, Allen M, Wilson J, Atmar RL. Respiratory viral infections in adults with and without chronic obstructive pulmonary disease. Am J Respir Crit Care Med. 2000;162: 167-173.
69. Greenberg SB. Respiratory consequences of rhinovirus infection. Arch Intern Med. 2003;163:278-284.
70. Aaron SD, Angel JB, Lunau M, et al. Granulocyte inflammatory markers and airway infection during acute exacerbation of chronic obstructive pulmonary disease. Am J Respir Crit Car Med. 2001;163:349-355.
71. Soler N, Torres A, Ewig S, et al. Bronchial microbial patterns in severe exacerbations of chronic obstructive pulmonary disease (COPD) requiring mechanical ventilation. Am J Respir Crit Care Med. 1998;157:1498-1505.
72. Yi K, Sethi S, Murphy T. Human immune response to nontypeable *Haemophilus influenzae* in chronic bronchitis. J Infect Dis. 1997;176:1247-1252.
73. Ferguson GT, Cherniack RM. Management of chronic obstructive pulmonary disease. N Engl J Med. 1993;328:1017-1022.
74. Manda W, Rennard SI. Taking pharmacologic management of COPD into the future. J Crit Illness. 2003;18:33-42.
75. Altose MD. Approaches to slowing the progression of COPD. Curr Opin Pulm Med. 2003;9:125-130.
76. Mozaffarian D, Kumanyika SK, Lemaitre RN, et al. Cereal, fruit, and vegetable fiber intake and the risk of cardiovascular disease in elderly individuals. JAMA. 2003;289:1659-1666.
77. McCrory DC, Brown C, Gelfand SE, Bach PB. Management of acute exacerbations of COPD—a summary and appraisal of published evidence. Chest. 2001;119:1190-1209.
78. Stoller JK. Acute exacerbations of chronic obstructive pulmonary disease. N Engl J Med. 2002;346:988-994.
79. Neuzil KM, O'Connor TZ, Gorse GJ, Nichol K. Recognizing influenza in older patients with chronic obstructive pulmonary disease who have received influenza vaccine. Clin Infect Dis. 2003;36:169-174.
80. White AJ, Gompertz S, Stockley RA. Chronic obstructive pulmonary disease 6: The aetiology of exacerbations of chronic obstructive pulmonary disease. Thorax. 2003;58: 73-80.
81. Stockley RA, O'Brien C, Pye A, Hill SL. Relationship of sputum color to nature and outpatient management of acute exacerbations of COPD. Chest. 2000;117: 1638-1645.
82. Corradi M, Rubinstein I, Andreoli R, et al. Aldehydes in exhaled breath condensate of patients with chronic obstructive pulmonary disease. Am J Respir Crit Care Med. 2003;167:1380-1386.
83. Silkoff PE, Martin D, Pak J, et al. Exhaled nitric oxide correlated with induced sputum findings in COPD. Chest. 2001;119:1049-1055.
84. Jones HA, Marino PS, Shakur BH, Morrell NW. In vivo assessment of lung inflammatory cell activity in patients with COPD and asthma. Eur Respir J. 2003;21:567-573.
85. Amsden GW, Baird IM, Simon S, Treadway G. Efficacy and safety of azithromycin vs levofloxacin in the outpatient treatment of acute bacterial exacerbations of chronic bronchitis. Chest. 2003;123:772-777.
86. Saint S, Brent S, Vittinghoff E, Grady D. Antibiotics in chronic obstructive pulmonary disease exacerbations: A meta-analysis. JAMA. 1995;273:957-960.
87. Chodosh S, McCarty J, Farkas S, et al. Randomized, double-blind study of ciprofloxacin and cefuroxime axetil for treatment of acute bacterial exacerbations of chronic bronchitis. Clin Infect Dis. 1998;27:722-729.
88. Chodosh S, Schreurs A, Siami G, et al. Efficacy of oral ciprofloxacin vs clarithromycin for treatment of acute bacterial exacerbations of chronic bronchitis. Clin Infect Dis. 1998;27:730-738.
89. Grossman RF. The value of antibiotics and the outcomes of antibiotic therapy in exacerbations of COPD. Chest. 1998;113:249S-255S.
90. Wilkinson TMA, Patel IS, Wilks M, et al. Airway bacterial load and FEV1 decline in patients with chronic obstructive pulmonary disease. Am J Respir Crit Care Med. 2003;167:1090-1095.
91. Schentag JJ, Tillotson GS. Antibiotic selection and dosing for the treatment of acute exacerbations of COPD. Chest. 1997;112:314S-319S.
92. Bartlett JG, Dowell SF, Mandell LA, et al. Practice guidelines for the management of community-acquired pneumonia in adults: Guidelines from the Infectious Diseases Society of America. Clin Infect Dis. 2000;31:811-838.
93. Urban C, Rahman N, Zhao X, et al. Fluoroquinolone-resistant *Streptococcus pneumoniae* associated with levofloxacin therapy. J Infect Dis. 2001;184:794-798.
94. Klugman KP. The role of clonality in the global spread of fluoroquinolone-resistant bacteria. Clin Infect Dis. 2003;36:783-785.
95. Mokhlesi B, Morris AL, Huang CF, et al. Increased prevalence of gastroesophageal reflux symptoms in patients with COPD. Chest. 2001;119:1043-1048.
96. Poe RH, Kallay MC. Chronic cough and gastroesophageal reflux disease—experience with specific therapy for diagnosis and treatment. Chest. 2003;123:679-684.
97. Agusti AGN, Noguera A, Sauleda J, et al. Systemic effects of chronic obstructive pulmonary disease (review). Eur Respir J. 2003;21:347-360.
98. Debigaré R, Côté CH, Maltais F. Peripheral muscle wasting in chronic obstructive pulmonary disease—clinical relevance and mechanisms. Am J Respir Crit Care Med. 2001;164:1712-1717.
99. Couillard A, Koechlin C, Cristol JP, et al. Evidence of local exercise-induced systemic oxidative stress in chronic obstructive pulmonary disease patients. Eur Respir J. 2002;20: 1123-1129.
100. Poulain M, Durand F, Palomba B, et al. Six-minute walk testing is more sensitive than maximal incremental cycle testing for detecting oxygen desaturation in patients with COPD. Chest. 2003;123:1401-1407.
101. Sturdy G, Hillman D, Green D, et al. Feasibility of high-intensity, interval-based respiratory muscle training in COPD. Chest. 2003;123:142-150.
102. Velloso M, Stella SG, Cendon S, et al. Metabolic and ventilatory parameters of four activities of daily living accomplished with arms in COPD patients. Chest. 2003;123:1047-1053.
103. Emery CF, Honn VJ, Frid DJ, et al. Acute effects of exercise on cognition in patients with chronic obstructive pulmonary disease. Am J Respir Crit Care Med. 2001;164:1624-1627.
104. O'Donnell DE, Vodue N. Should your COPD patients have cardiopulmonary exercise testing? J Respir Dis. 2003;24:106-118.
105. Presberg KW, Dincer HE. Pathophysiology of pulmonary hypertension due to lung disease. Curr Opin Pulm Med. 2003;9:131-138.
106. Maloney JP. Advances in the treatment of secondary pulmonry hypertension. Curr Opin Pulm Med. 2003;9:139-143.
107. Sisk JE, Whang W, Butler JC, et al. Cost-effectiveness of vaccination against invasive pneumococcal disease among people 50-64 years of age: Role of comorbid conditions and race. Ann Intern Med. 2003;138:960-968.

CHAPTER **60**

Bronchiolitis

CAROLINE BREESE HALL

JOHN T. McBRIDE

*In bronchiolitis we must now contend
with both the disease of the "now" and the "then";
For many such infants a mold has been cast,
perhaps by their unborn and unknown past,
which destines that they shall in time wheeze again.
For them this disease
is the distant, boding knell
of vulnerable lungs
to a microbe's mystic spell.*

C.B.H.

Bronchiolitis is an acute viral lower respiratory tract illness that occurs during the first 2 years of life. The illness also has been called "wheezy bronchitis" and "asthmatic bronchitis." Whatever term is applied, the syndrome is caused primarily by viral infections. The characteristic clinical manifestations include an acute onset of wheezing and hyperinflation, most commonly associated with cough, rhinorrhea, tachypnea, and respiratory distress.

The term *bronchiolitis* appears to have been born from a long lineage of confusing sobriquets, including "acute catarrhal bronchitis," "interstitial bronchopneumonia," "spastic bronchopneumonia," "capillary or obstructive bronchiolitis," and "asthmatic bronchiolitis."[1] Bronchiolitis, however, did not become recognized as a distinct entity until the 1940s.[1-5]

ETIOLOGY

Although bronchiolitis was initially thought to be caused by bacteria, viruses and occasionally *Mycoplasma pneumoniae* are now known to be the instigators. Respiratory syncytial virus (RSV) is clearly the major pathogen, and the parainfluenza viruses are the second most commonly isolated agents, with parainfluenza type 3 predominating (Table 60-1 and Fig. 60-1).[6-8] The recently discovered human metapneumovirus also produces bronchiolitis and appears to have clinical and epidemiologic characteristics similar to those of RSV.[9-12] The role of human metapneumovirus in causing respiratory illness in young children awaits further study, but information thus far suggests its contribution may be appreciable but secondary to that of RSV.

A long-term study of respiratory illnesses associated with wheezing in children from a private practice in Chapel Hill, North Carolina,

TABLE 60-1 Agents Causing Bronchiolitis

Agent	Cases (% of Total)	Epidemiologic Occurrence
Respiratory syncytial virus	40-80	Yearly epidemics, winter to spring
Parainfluenza viruses		
Type 3	8-15	Predominantly spring to fall
Type 1	5-12	Epidemics in fall every other year
Type 2	1-5	Fall
Rhinoviruses	3-8	Endemic, all seasons
Adenoviruses	3-10	Endemic, all seasons
Influenza viruses	6-8	Endemic, winter to spring
Mycoplasma pneumoniae	1-7	Endemic, all seasons
Enteroviruses	1-5	Summer to fall
Human metapneumovirus	Unknown	Predominately winter in some areas

showed that RSV, parainfluenza 1 and 3 viruses, adenoviruses, rhinoviruses, and *M. pneumoniae* make up 87% of the isolates obtained from children of all ages.[6] Within the first 2 years of life, RSV accounted for 44% of the isolates, with parainfluenza 1 and 3 viruses and adenoviruses each accounting for about 13%. Similarly, RSV constituted 60% of the isolates obtained from children with bronchiolitis from two group practices in Rochester, New York, over an 11-year period.[13] The second most frequently identified agent was parainfluenza 3 virus, which accounted for 12% of the cases. The relative proportions of these agents may change depending on the population and

whether the cases occur as part of an outbreak. However, RSV remains the prime identified cause of bronchiolitis in most ambulatory patients and especially in hospitalized cases, and even in all lower respiratory tract admissions of young infants.[1,4,14-17]

EPIDEMIOLOGY

Bronchiolitis shows a definite seasonal pattern in temperate climates, with a yearly upsurge in the number of cases during winter to early spring.[6,8,13,18] This pattern mirrors that of its prime agent, RSV (see Fig. 60-1). Lesser swells of activity are seen during the fall and spring, when parainfluenza viruses are active.

Bronchiolitis is a common illness during the first year of life, with the peak attack rate generally occurring between 1 and 10 months of age and between 5 weeks and 6 months in hospitalized cases.[5,6,8,14,16,18,19] In outpatients studied in Chapel Hill, the incidence of bronchiolitis was about 11 cases per 100 children for both the first and second 6 months of life.[6,18] In the second year of life, the incidence fell to approximately half that. Among children in the first year of life enrolled in a health maintenance organization in Tucson, Arizona, the rate of occurrence of lower respiratory tract illness was 32.9 cases per 100 children, and 60% of these cases were bronchiolitis.[8]

An appreciable proportion of hospital admissions for infants within the first year of life results from bronchiolitis, especially from RSV. In a review by Breese and colleagues, bronchiolitis was the reason for admission in 4% of their group-practice patients of all ages who required hospitalization for medical illnesses.[19] In a Seattle prepaid medical care group, the rate of hospitalization among infants with bronchiolitis

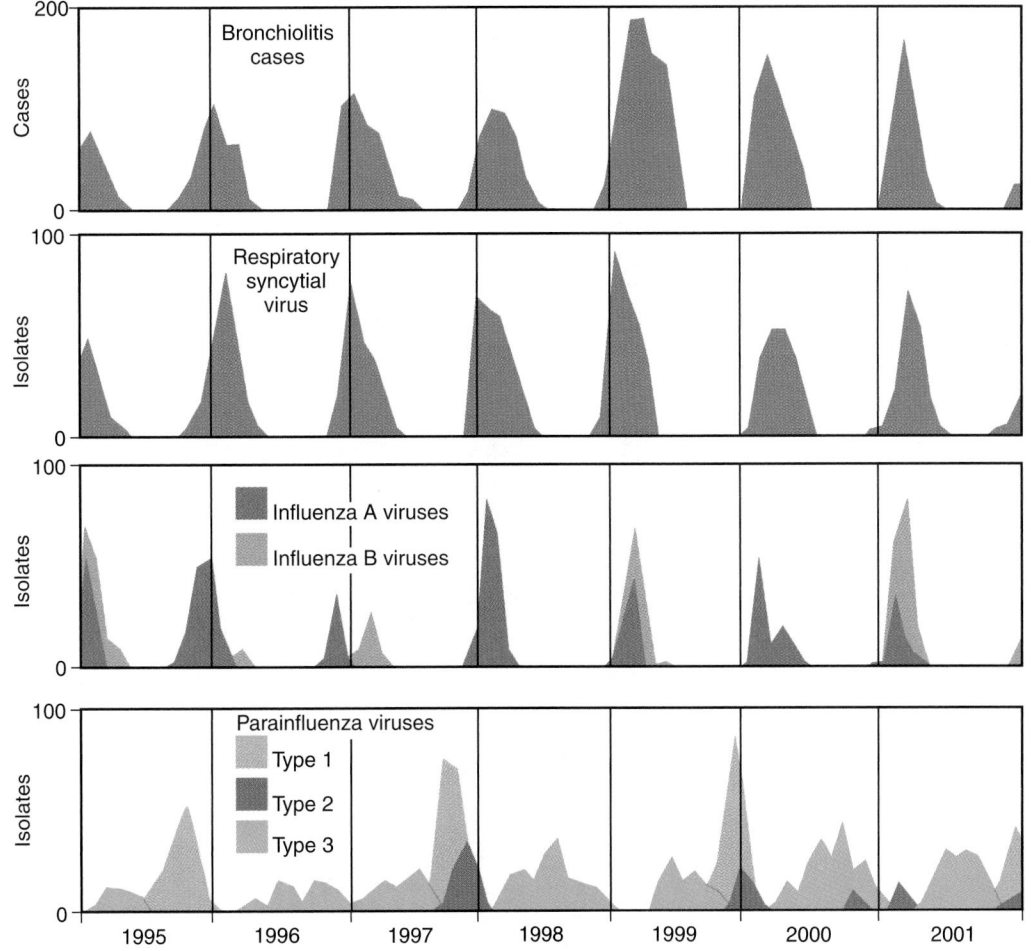

FIGURE 60-1. Patterns of reported cases of bronchiolitis shown in relation to the activity of the major respiratory viruses in Monroe County, New York. Data are obtained from a weekly community surveillance program for infectious disease.

during the first 6 months of life was 6 per 1000 children per year.[5] More recent studies using hospital discharge diagnoses have estimated that RSV caused 50% to 80% of hospitalizations of infants under 1 year of age with bronchiolitis, resulting in 73,400 to 126,300 admissions each year.[16] In this same age group, the RSV hospitalization rate has been estimated to be 25 to 41 per 1000 children.[14,20] RSV hospitalizations for all children under 5 years of age have been judged to be 110,000 each year, resulting in hospital costs of up to $750 million.[21,22] Studies from the Centers for Disease Control and Prevention have estimated the associated mortality for bronchiolitis between 1979 and 1997 was 95 cases (range, 66 to 127) annually for children under 5 years of age, and in infants in the first year of life it was 2.0 per 100,000 live births from 1996 through 1998[23-25]; 55% of these deaths occurred in infants 1 to 3 months of age.

Bronchiolitis is more common in boys, especially among children requiring hospitalization, with a sex ratio of about 1.5 to 1.[6] Other factors described as increasing the chances of hospitalization for bronchiolitis in otherwise normal children include young age, being less than 6 months of age prior to onset of RSV season, young maternal age, lower cord blood antibody titers to RSV, lower socioeconomic status, tobacco smoke exposure, living in crowded surroundings, having older siblings, daycare attendance, lack of breast-feeding, a predisposition to atopy or hyperreactivity of the airway, and illness caused by RSV.[3,6,26-28] Infants at risk for most severe disease, however, are those with underlying conditions, especially cardiopulmonary disease, and preterm gestation.[24] In addition, certain ethnic groups of infants have higher rates of hospitalization for bronchiolitis. Native American and Native Alaskan children have been estimated to have two to three times higher rates than those for all infants in the United States.[25,29]

PATHOPHYSIOLOGY

The term *bronchiolitis* was first used by Engle and Newns in 1940 for the lower respiratory tract disease they observed in young infants that tended to be severe, often fatal, and that was probably viral in origin.[1,2] They carefully described the pathologic findings in these infants dying of bronchiolitis, which over the subsequent half century have been confirmed and expanded.[30]

The pathologic findings in bronchiolitis are characteristically focused on the respiratory epithelium with generalized involvement. The virus initially replicates in the epithelium of the upper respiratory tract, but in the young infant it tends to spread rapidly to the lower tract airways. Early inflammation of the bronchial and bronchiolar epithelium progresses rapidly to necrosis. Subsequently, the epithelium may proliferate and demonstrate cuboidal cells without cilia. Peribronchiolar infiltration, mostly with mononuclear cells, and edema of the submucosa and adventitia occur, and these progress to the observed necrosis and sloughing of the bronchiolar epithelium (Figs. 60-2 and 60-3).

Inflammatory changes of variable severity are observed in most small bronchi and bronchioles. Because resistance to the flow of air is related inversely to the cube of the radius of the airway, the inflammation and edema make the small-lumen airways in infants particularly vulnerable to obstruction. Plugs of necrotic material and fibrin may completely or partially obstruct the small airways.

Smooth muscle constriction does not appear to be important in the obstruction. In areas peripheral to sites of partial obstruction, air becomes trapped by a process similar to a ball-valve mechanism. The negative intrapleural pressure exerted during inspiration allows air to flow beyond the point of partial obstruction. However, on expiration, the size of the lumen decreases with the positive pressure, thereby resulting in increased obstruction and hyperinflation. Thus, although airflow is impeded during both inspiration and expiration, the latter is more affected and prolonged. In areas peripheral to complete obstruction, the trapped air eventually becomes absorbed, which results in multiple areas of atelectasis. This absorptive atelectasis is greatly accelerated when the child is breathing high concentrations of oxygen. The degree of atelectasis or hyperinflation that develops may be greater in infants because collateral channels that maintain alveolar expansion in the presence of airway obstruction are not well developed early in life.

The physiologic correlates of this resistance to airflow are dyspnea, tachypnea, a diminished tidal volume, and a markedly altered distribution of ventilation. In significant areas of lung parenchyma, the ratio of ventilation to perfusion is low, and this produces arterial hypoxemia. When an infant is no longer able to compensate for the disordered gas exchange by increasing ventilation, hypercarbia may ensue. The pathologic process may progress to involve the alveolar walls and spaces, producing an interstitial pneumonitis. Recovery tends to be slow and requires several weeks.

Experimental and clinical studies have suggested that the development of wheezing and the pathogenesis of bronchiolitis in some children, and their risk for subsequent wheezing and pulmonary function abnormalities, are related to the type of inflammatory response initiated by RSV or other viruses and to a predisposition of the host (see Chapter 155). In particular, hypersensitivity responses characterized

FIGURE 60-2. Inflammation and necrosis in bronchiolitis, resulting in obliteration of the bronchiolar lumen.

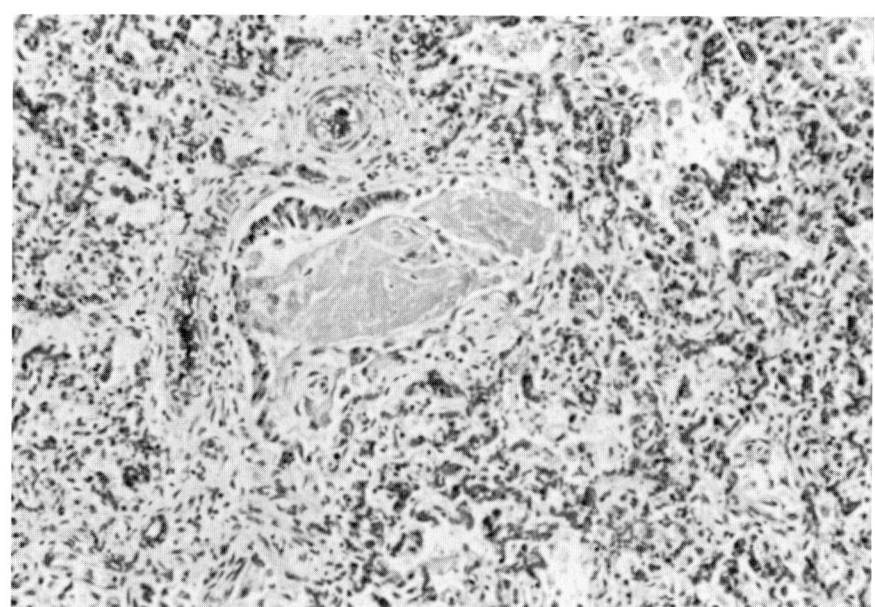

by increased levels of virus-specific IgE antibody and certain cellular inflammatory mediators have been related to the development and severity of wheezing in infants and the risk of recurrent wheezing.[31-33] Studies detecting cytokines and chemokines in respiratory secretions of children with bronchiolitis and with recurrent wheezing have suggested the expression of interferon-γ, interleukin (IL)-8, IL-10, and cytokines produced by helper T (Th)1 and Th2 lymphocytes are important in the pathogenesis of bronchiolitis and subsequent recurrent episodes of wheezing.[31-38]

Clarifying the relationship between bronchiolitis and subsequent asthma is complicated by confusion about the pathophysiology of asthma itself.[39] Asthma is a heterogeneous group of disorders engendered by multiple factors, both genetic and environmental. These include not only an atopic predisposition and the environmental risk factors noted earlier but also specific genetic polymorphisms.[3,40-44] Studies on twins have demonstrated that 70% of the risk of developing asthma in early childhood is related to genetic factors,[45] and many of the specific linkages identified to date are related to inflammation. Nevertheless, the disorders in this heterogeneous group share, in various combinations, wheezing, reversible airway obstruction, airway inflammation, and structural airway wall remodeling. Many distinct asthma phenotypes exist, and the following are examples of only three: (1) Some children wheeze repeatedly with respiratory viral infections in the first 5 years of life but have few problems thereafter.[46] (2) Other children with atopy and allergies develop wheezing beyond 5 years of age. Many of these have fewer problems when they become teenagers and adults. (3) Other individuals with adult-onset wheezing are at increased risk of developing irreversible airway obstruction.

Much of asthma, therefore, seems to be related to a dysregulation of airway inflammation. Inherited traits that do not involve the inflammatory response may also be important in some individuals, such as variations in the beta adrenergic receptor or in airway geometry (e.g., size). Any traits that contribute to the dysregulation of airway inflammation or airway dysfunction in asthma may also contribute to the same processes with respiratory viral infections. Thus, the increased incidence of wheezing with subsequent respiratory viral infections among children with a history of bronchiolitis in infancy is not surprising. Nevertheless, the association between bronchiolitis and asthma is not straightforward. Several investigators have demonstrated that children with bronchiolitis in infancy have no increased risk for asthma or abnormal pulmonary function by the time they reach early adolescence.[47]

CLINICAL MANIFESTATIONS

Bronchiolitis may have a variety of appellations, including wheezing, bronchiolitis, infectious asthma, and asthmatic bronchitis, but all refer to the clinical syndrome in young children presenting with wheezing and hyperinflation of the lungs often accompanied by tachypnea. The onset of bronchiolitis, however, consists of upper respiratory tract signs, especially coryza and cough. Commonly, a prodromal period of 1 to 7 days occurs and is marked by fever, which is usually mild, especially with RSV. Sometimes the initial presentation is apnea. Apnea usually appears after 1 to 3 days of upper respiratory signs that are so mild as to go unnoticed and before lower respiratory tract disease is evident. Manifestations of lower respiratory tract involvement become evident after the several days of the prodromal upper respiratory tract signs. The progression of the disease may be reflected initially in the development of a prominent cough, and subsequently by an increase in the respiratory rate and in nonspecific systemic symptoms such as irritability, lethargy, and anorexia. With progression, tachypnea and tachycardia may be marked, although fever may no longer be present. Retractions of the chest wall, flaring of the nasal alae, and grunting are evidence of the increased work of breathing. Cyanosis is rarely observed, even though moderate to severe hypoxemia may be present.[48] Auscultatory findings, which may vary from hour to hour, include wheezing with or without crackles. Increasing dyspnea with decreasing lung sounds on auscultation and diminished movement of air may indicate progressive obstruction and impending respiratory failure.

Dehydration is a common accompaniment of bronchiolitis and results from paroxysms of coughing, which may trigger vomiting, and from a poor oral intake related to the respiratory distress and lethargy. Tachypnea further increases the fluid requirement. Otitis media occurs in 10% to 30% of infants, and mild conjunctivitis and occasionally diarrhea may also be present.

The acute course typically lasts 3 to 7 days. Most infants show improvement within 3 to 4 days and gradually recover over 1 to 2 weeks, but the cough may persist for longer. One study, examining the duration of illness in ambulatory children diagnosed with bronchiolitis, found that the median duration of symptoms was 12 days. After 3 weeks, 18% remained symptomatic, and after 4 weeks, 9% continued to be ill.[49] No factor—sex, age, weight, or respiratory rate—appeared to be predictive of longer illness. The viral etiology was not examined.

FIGURE 60-3. Inflammation of the bronchiole with regenerating epithelium.

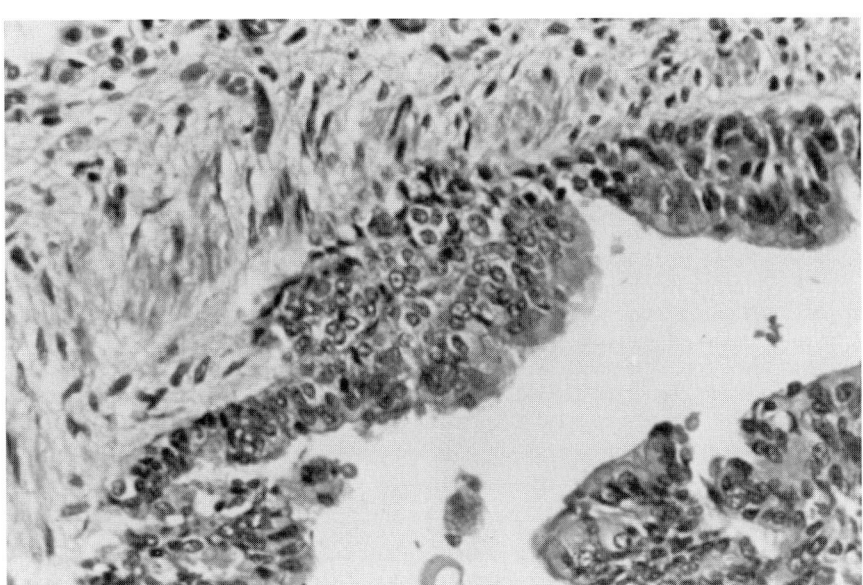

COMPLICATIONS

Almost all children recover from bronchiolitis without difficulty.[3,49] Complications from bronchiolitis are relatively rare, especially in normal children. A number of studies have attempted to predict by epidemiologic and clinical characteristics which children with acute bronchiolitis are most likely to have complicated or severe courses. Infants with underlying diseases, especially cardiac, pulmonary, and immunodeficiency diseases, and those who were premature are most at risk for prolonged or complicated illness.[24,27,50,51] Clinical characteristics at the onset of the acute illness, such as respiratory rate or auscultatory findings, have not been of consistent prognostic value. Diminished arterial oxygen saturation, however, has been associated with complicated illness.[3,50,52] Progression to respiratory failure and prolonged hypoxemia are uncommon with currently available technical and pharmacologic methods of management. If such complications occur, they are most likely to be in infants with compromising underlying conditions and in very young infants.

Cardiovascular abnormalities have been occasionally reported to occur during bronchiolitis in children with no underlying cardiac disease.[53,54] In one study, 2% of infants with bronchiolitis had mild electrocardiographic abnormalities.[54] In a small group of infants with bronchiolitis from RSV or parainfluenza virus, about half were demonstrated to have some transient tricuspid valve regurgitation during the most acute phase of the illness.[53]

Aspiration has also been demonstrated to be a relatively frequent complication in infants with RSV bronchiolitis.[55,56] Infants who received no therapy for aspiration were much more likely to develop reactive airway disease subsequently.

The sequelae of bronchiolitis that occur frequently and are of major concern are recurrent episodes of reactive airway disease, which are accompanied by pulmonary function abnormalities in some children. As discussed previously (see "Pathophysiology"), the link between this and bronchiolitis in infancy is unclear. Nevertheless, the prognosis for most children with subsequent episodes of wheezing during early childhood is good. Some follow-up studies of children who had bronchiolitis diagnosed in infancy have shown that these children at school age had no greater occurrence of reactive airway disease than those without an early history of bronchiolitis.[57,58] The mortality associated with bronchiolitis has been markedly reduced with the advancement in the technology of supportive care. Overall, the mortality in hospitalized infants has been estimated to be less than 1%.[59,60] The mortality rate, however, increases significantly in those children with underlying compromising conditions and is estimated at 3% to 5%.[23,59] In these children, the greatest proportion of bronchiolitis-associated deaths has occurred in infants of low birth weight (<2500 g), especially in those with very low birth weight (<1500 g).[24] Nevertheless, the majority (63%) of all bronchiolitis-associated deaths in children under 1 year of age occurs in those with a normal birth weight.[24]

LABORATORY FINDINGS

The total white blood cell count in children with bronchiolitis is usually within the normal range or slightly elevated.[3,48] In hospitalized infants who are more seriously ill and hypoxemic, the white blood cell count may be elevated, and the differential count may show a leftward shift. Most infants requiring hospitalization will have some degree of hypoxemia on measurement of the arterial oxygen saturation levels. Clinically, this is difficult to assess, because the degree of wheezing and retractions correlates poorly with the level of oxygenation. Only the most severely ill children develop hypercarbia, as most are able to compensate for the compromised gas exchange by increasing the minute ventilation despite the increased work of breathing.[1]

DIAGNOSIS

The diagnosis of bronchiolitis is made most frequently on the basis of the characteristic clinical and epidemiologic findings. However, considerable confusion exists over the exact definition of bronchiolitis.[61]

A variety of entities may cause a similar picture of dyspnea and wheezing in the infant. Asthma is not easily differentiated, particularly if it is the infant's first episode. Furthermore, the two diseases may be combined. An appreciable proportion of wheezing episodes occurring in a child with an atopic diathesis may arise from viral infections.[62] RSV in particular has a propensity to induce wheezing in young children. Even in adults with acute RSV infection that is clinically manifested as an upper respiratory tract infection, hyperreactivity of the airways can be detected by pulmonary function testing and may last for 1 or 2 months.[63]

Specific laboratory and radiologic tests are not required for most cases of bronchiolitis.[64] In hospitalized infants, determination of the viral etiology may be helpful for infection control procedures, including cohorting, and when specific antiviral therapy, as for influenza or RSV, is being considered.[51]

Identification of the specific agent of acute bronchiolitis can be made in an appreciable proportion of infants by viral isolation from respiratory secretions, preferably from a nasal wash.[6,65] In most cases, the viruses associated with bronchiolitis may be identified in tissue culture within 3 to 7 days. More commonly used are the rapid viral diagnostic techniques, especially for RSV and influenza A and B viruses, which allow identification of the viral antigen in the respiratory secretions within hours.[66,67] The sensitivity of these assays is variable, and the positive predictive value significantly diminishes when RSV infection or the influenza viruses are not epidemic in the community. The use of culture in addition to the screening rapid antigen detection assay may be of particular benefit when the suspected viral agent is not highly prevalent in the community, and when results of the screening rapid-technique tests are negative. Viral isolation procedures and rapid antigen tests that include multiple viral antigens offer the further advantage of detecting other agents that may be the cause of the illness or that are concurrently present. The sensitivity of detecting the viral etiology appears to be markedly enhanced by the use of reverse transcriptase–polymerase chain reaction (RT-PCR).[67-69] Serologic tests to determine the etiologic agent are rarely helpful in clinical management and may be difficult to interpret, because the young infant has maternally acquired antibody to many of the viral agents of bronchiolitis.

A chest radiograph is not routinely recommended for first-time wheezers in the first year of life if there are no complications or underlying disease.[3] If a chest roentgenogram is obtained, the hallmarks of acute bronchiolitis are hyperinflation with associated depressed diaphragms, hyperlucency of the parenchyma, and decreased costophrenic angles.[70-73] The bronchovascular markings are usually prominent, with linear densities radiating from the hila. Multiple areas of atelectasis of variable degree are also commonly present and difficult to differentiate from the infiltrates of pneumonia. Indeed, both bronchiolitis and pneumonia may be concurrently present, especially with RSV infection.

The abnormalities observed on the chest roentgenogram in acute bronchiolitis often do not correlate with the degree of clinical illness; the child may be severely ill despite minimal findings on the chest roentgenogram. Furthermore, considerable intraobserver and interobserver variation has been observed to occur among radiologists in their assessment of roentgenographic findings for the diagnosis of lower respiratory tract disease in infants, especially those with bronchiolitis.[73]

The differential diagnosis of wheezing in an infant is broad and requires a careful history and examination.[61] Gastric reflux and aspiration may produce a picture that is indistinguishable clinically from acute bronchiolitis. Other considerations include obstruction of the airway by a foreign body, vascular rings, retropharyngeal abscess, and even enlarged adenoids. Wheezing may also be associated with cystic fibrosis, immunodeficiency, and congestive heart failure in young infants.

THERAPY

Supportive care is the mainstay of therapy in both outpatient and inpatient cases. At home, care is aimed primarily at comfort, maintaining adequate hydration, and treating fever if necessary. Antibiotics are not routinely recommended and should be reserved for cases in which proven coinfection with bacteria exists.[3,64]

Hospitalization is necessary for those infants unable to maintain adequate hydration and for those infants with evidence of increasing lethargy and respiratory distress. This may be signaled by increasing retractions of the chest wall and by tachypnea. However, determination of the respiratory rate in young infants is often confounded by crying and fever, and the normal respiratory rate according to age must be considered.[3]

More than two decades ago, Reynolds and Cook noted for hospitalized infants that "oxygen is vitally important in bronchiolitis, and there is little convincing evidence that any other therapy is consistently or even occasionally useful."[74] Today, the mainstay of therapy for the hospitalized child remains supportive care with oxygen administration to maintain an adequate oxygen saturation level (usually at 92% or greater).[1,3,64,75] Although mist therapy is also commonly employed, its use has not been proven beneficial, and chest physiotherapy has been shown to be of no help.[76,77]

The only specific therapy currently available for hospitalized cases of bronchiolitis caused by RSV is inhaled ribavirin (1-β-D-ribofuranosyl-1,2,4-triazole-3-carboxamide), a synthetic nucleoside (see Chapter 155). Ribavirin should be considered for therapy only for those infants who have or are at risk of developing severe or complicated RSV infection, such as those with underlying predisposing conditions, especially prematurity and cardiopulmonary disease.[51] The drug is expensive and the relative benefit to cost must be considered on the basis of the individual patient.

Medical therapy commonly includes bronchodilators, corticosteroids, and antibiotics. Evidence for use of any of these has been confusing, contrasting, or incomplete.[64,78] A recent review by the Agency for Healthcare Research and Quality[64] of the efficacy of these therapies in managing bronchiolitis concluded that no single agent could be routinely recommended for the management of bronchiolitis. Convincing evidence for the use of these or other agents was not identified, and some had adverse effects, including budesonide and interferon-alfa-2. The agency's review suggested that several agents should be further studied in correctly designed trials, including nebulized epinephrine, nebulized salbutamol plus ipratropium bromide, nebulized ipratropium bromide, oral or parental corticosteroids (preferably dexamethasone), and inhaled corticosteroids. Despite this lack of evidence of efficacy, these agents, including antibiotics, are used in the majority of infants hospitalized with bronchiolitis and with bronchiolitis identified as caused by RSV.[79,80]

One meta-analysis of bronchodilating agents concluded that no recommendation could be made because determination of their benefit was confounded by the various methods and populations included in the available studies.[81] However, a recent multicenter, randomized, double-blind, controlled study of infants less than 12 months of age with acute bronchiolitis demonstrated that therapy with nebulized epinephrine did not significantly shorten the duration of hospitalization, or the number of days until the infant was ready for discharge.[78] Furthermore, in the cohort of infants who required supplemental oxygen and intravenous fluids, the time until an infant was ready to be discharged was significantly longer for those who received nebulized epinephrine than for those who received placebo. These agents, therefore, are not routinely recommended for infants.[3,64,82] A carefully monitored trial of nebulized bronchodilators in individual cases has been recommended by some. The response should be objectively documented by diminished respiratory distress and improved oxygen saturation. An initial beneficial response, however, may not be seen when bronchodilators are again used later. Repeated use of inhaled bronchodilators in the absence of a positive clinical response is inappropriate.

Studies examining the benefit of corticosteroid therapy have included infants with a clinical diagnosis of bronchiolitis but without a determination of specific viral etiology. The results have been conflicting; most corticosteroids have shown no benefit, and their use is not routinely recommended.[3,64,75] A meta-analysis of therapy with systemic corticosteroids employed in six trials concluded that the duration of hospitalization and symptoms was shortened by 0.43 days.[83]

However, two of the six trials included infants with a history of previous wheezing. If these two studies were eliminated from the analysis, the remaining four studies with only first-time wheezers showed that corticosteroids had no significant benefit. Patients with underlying asthma or chronic lung disease (bronchopulmonary dysplasia) who have bronchiolitis related to a lower respiratory viral infection are much more likely to benefit from bronchodilator therapy or a brief course of corticosteroids than are previously well infants. Therefore, such therapy should be considered for infants with bronchiolitis who have bronchopulmonary dysplasia or chronic lung disease, a history of previous wheezing, or a strong family history of asthma.

PREVENTION

Prevention of the clinical entity of bronchiolitis is very difficult because of its multiple etiologies and varying pathogenesis. For bronchiolitis associated with primary RSV infection, antibody preparations, including intravenous immunoglobulin and intravenous immunoglobulin with high titers of neutralizing antibody to RSV (RSV-IVIgG), and more recently monoclonal antibody directed against the F protein of RSV (palivizumab), have been examined for use therapeutically and prophylactically.[51] None of these preparations has shown any benefit in therapy. In high-risk infants, controlled trials have shown a significant reduction in hospitalization for RSV infection when RSV-IVIgG or palivizumab is given on a monthly basis over the 5-month period of RSV activity in the community.[51] Whether infants with high-risk conditions would derive significant benefit compared to the cost remains controversial and in general should be determined on the basis of each infant's circumstances and estimated risk.

BRONCHIOLITIS OBLITERANS

A rare, chronic type of bronchiolitis termed bronchiolitis obliterans has been reported in both adults and children.[84,85] Bronchiolitis obliterans has been cited as an uncommon complication of viral infections, usually viral bronchiolitis, lung transplantation, connective tissue diseases, and inhalation of toxic substances. Often, no cause is identified.[85,86]

In infants, especially those with certain undefined genetic predispositions, the major association has been with adenovirus infection.[87] The disease appears to be particularly prevalent among Native American populations in central Canada and among Polynesians in New Zealand. In some geographic areas, the frequency or clustering of bronchiolitis obliterans cases has been correlated with the occurrence of adenoviral infection in the community.

Pathogenesis

Bronchiolitis obliterans is believed to result from an injury to the bronchioles and smaller airways. The healing process produces large amounts of inflammatory cells, mucoid tissue, granulation tissue, and thickening of the airway walls with connective tissue. This subsequently produces obstruction, bronchiectasis, and even obliteration of the airways.[88,89]

Clinical Findings

The respiratory illness in children initially appears similar to other viral lower respiratory tract illnesses, characterized by cough and lower respiratory tract signs. An interim period of improvement may occur, followed by progressive symptoms of respiratory distress, productive cough, and wheezing. The obstructive respiratory symptoms progress and persist, and the child becomes chronically ill. Many develop bronchiectasis, cor pulmonale, and dependence on oxygen.

Diagnosis

A nodular, diffuse picture, similar to that for miliary tuberculosis, is present on chest roentgenogram. Some patients may also develop Swyer-James syndrome, characterized by a decrease in pulmonary vascular markings and unilateral hyperlucency. Computed tomography reveals bronchiectasis, and bronchography shows that the contrast does not reach the peripheral areas of the lung because of the obstruction.

Pulmonary function tests indicate hyperinflation, and irreversible obstructive and restrictive airway disease.[84,88] Definitive diagnosis may be made by lung biopsy.[84]

Therapy

No specific treatment currently exists. Corticosteroid treatment has been tried, particularly in adults, but controlled trials are not available.

REFERENCES

1. Wohl M. Bronchiolitis. In: Chernick V, Kendig EJ, eds. Disorders of the Respiratory Tract in Children. 6th ed. Philadelphia: Saunders; 1998:473-485.
2. Engle S, Newns G. Proliferative mural bronchiolitis. Arch Dis Child. 1940;15:219-229.
3. Clineanswers, Hall CB. Bronchiolitis. Los Angeles: Wolters Kluwer Clineguide; 2002.
4. Selwyn B. The epidemiology of acute respiratory tract infection in young children: Comparison of findings from several developing countries. Coordinated Data Group of BOSTID Researchers. Rev Infect Dis. 1990;12:S870-S888.
5. Foy H, Cooney M, Maletzky A, et al. Incidence and etiology of pneumonia, croup, and bronchiolitis in preschool children belonging to a prepaid medical care group over a four-year period. Am J Epidemiol. 1973;97:80-92.
6. Henderson F, Clyde WJ, Collier A, et al. The etiologic and epidemiologic spectrum of bronchiolitis in pediatric practice. J Pediatr. 1979;95:183-190.
7. Glezen W, Loda F, Clyde WJ, et al. Epidemiologic patterns of acute lower respiratory disease of children in a pediatric group practice. J Pediatr. 1971;78:397-406.
8. Wright A, Taussig L, Ray C, et al. The Tucson Children's respiratory study: II. Lower respiratory illness in the first year of life. Am J Epidemiol. 1989;129:1232-1246.
9. Boivin G, De Serres G, Cote S, et al. Human metapneumovirus infections in hospitalized children. Emerg Infect Dis. 2003;9:634-640.
10. Boivin G, Abed Y, Pelletier G, et al. Virological features and clinical manifestations associated with human metapneumovirus: A new paramyxovirus responsible for acute respiratory-tract infections in all age groups. J Infect Dis. 2002;186:1330-1334.
11. Stockton J, Stephenson I, Fleming D, et al. Human metapneumovirus as a cause of community-acquired respiratory illness. Emerg Infect Dis. 2002;8:897.
12. van den Hoogen B, de Jong J, Groen J, et al. A newly discovered human pneumovirus isolated from young children with respiratory tract disease. Nature Med. 2001;7:719-724.
13. Hall C. Infect Dis Newslett Commun Surveill. 1982-93;29-51:1.
14. Leader S, Kohlhase K. Respiratory syncytial virus-coded pediatric hospitalizations, 1997-1999. Pediatr Infect Dis J. 2002;21:629-632.
15. Muller-Pebody B, Edmunds W, Zambon M, et al. Contribution of RSV to bronchiolitis and pneumonia-associated hospitalizations in English children, April 1995-March 1998. Epidemiol Infect. 2002;129:99-106.
16. Shay D, Holman R, Newman R, et al. Bronchiolitis-associated hospitalizations among US children, 1980-1996. JAMA. 1999;282:1440-1446.
17. Stensballe L, Devasundaram J, Simoes E. Respiratory syncytial virus epidemics: The ups and downs of a seasonal virus. Pediatr Infect Dis J. 2003;22:S21-S32.
18. Denny F, Clyde WJ. Acute lower respiratory tract infections in nonhospitalized children. J Pediatr. 1986;108:635-646.
19. Breese B, Disney F, Talpey W. The nature of a small pediatric group practice: Part I. Pediatrics. 1966;38:264-277.
20. Boyce T, Mellen B, Mitchel EJ, et al. Rates of hospitalization for respiratory syncytial virus infection among children in Medicaid. J Pediatr. 2000;137:865-870.
21. Stang P, Brandenburg N, Carter B. The economic burden of respiratory syncytial virus-associated bronchiolitis hospitalizations. Arch Pediatr Adolesc Med. 2001;155:95-96.
22. Howard T, Hoffman L, Stang P, et al. Respiratory syncytial virus pneumonia in the hospital setting: Length of stay, charges, and mortality. J Pediatr. 2000;137:227-232.
23. Shay D, Holman R, Roosevelt G, et al. Bronchiolitis-associated mortality and estimates of respiratory syncytial virus-associated deaths among US children, 1979-1997. J Infect Dis. 2001;183:16-22.
24. Holman R, Shay D, Curns A, et al. Risk factors for bronchiolitis-associated deaths among infants in the United States. Pediatr Infect Dis J. 2003;22:483-490.
25. Lowther S, Shay D, Holman R, et al. Bronchiolitis-associated hospitalizations among American Indian and Alaska Native children. Pediatr Infect Dis J. 2000;19:11-17.
26. Carlsen K-H, Larsen L, Bjerve O, et al. Acute bronchiolitis: Predisposing factors and characterizations of infants at risk. Pediatr Pulmonol. 1987;3:153-160.
27. Holberg C, Wright A, Martinez F, et al. Risk factors for respiratory syncytial virus-associated lower respiratory illnesses in the first year of life. Am J Epidemiol. 1991;133:1135-1151.
28. Martinez FD, Morgan WJ, Wright AL, et al. Initial airway function is a risk factor for recurrent wheezing respiratory illnesses during the first three years of life. Am Rev Respir Dis. 1991;143:312-316.
29. Liu L, Stout J, Sullivan M, et al. Asthma and bronchiolitis hospitalizations among American Indian children. Arch Pediatr Adolesc Med. 2000;154:991-996.
30. Aherne W, Bird T, Court S, et al. Pathological changes in virus infections of the lower respiratory tract in children. J Clin Pathol. 1970;23:7-18.
31. Welliver R. Immunology of respiratory syncytial virus infection: Eosinophils, cytokines, chemokines, and asthma. Pediatr Infect Dis J. 2000;19:780-783.
32. Welliver R. Respiratory syncytial virus and other respiratory viruses. Pediatr Infect Dis J. 2003;22:S6-S12.
33. Martinez F. Respiratory syncytial virus bronchiolitis and the pathogenesis of childhood asthma. Pediatr Infect Dis J. 2003;22:S76-S82.
34. Noah T, Ivins S, Murphy P, et al. Chemokines and inflammation in the nasal passages of infants with respiratory syncytial virus bronchiolitis. Clin Immunol. 2002;104:86-95.
35. Wang S, Forsyth K. The interaction of neutrophils with respiratory epithelial cells in viral infection. Respirology. 2000;5:1-10.
36. Bont L, Heijnen C, Kavelaara A, et al. Monocyte IL-10 production during respiratory syncytial virus bronchiolitis is associated with recurrent wheezing in a one-year follow-up study. Am J Respir Crit Care Med. 2000;161:1518-1523.
37. Bont L, Kavelaars A, Heijnen C, et al. Monocyte interleukin-12 production is inversely related to duration of respiratory failure in respiratory syncytial virus bronchiolitis. J Infect Dis. 2000;181:1772-1775.
38. Garofalo R, Patti J, Hintz K, et al. Macrophage inflammatory protein-1a (not T helper type 2 cytokines) is associated with severe forms of respiratory syncytial virus bronchiolitis. J Infect Dis. 2001;184:393-399.
39. Martinez F, Helms P. Types of asthma and wheezing. Eur Respir J. 1998;27:3s-8s.
40. Crowe J, Williams J. Immunology of viral respiratory tract infection in infancy. Paediatr Respir Rev. 2003;4:112-119.
41. Hoebee B, Rietveld E, Bont L, et al. Association of severe respiratory syncytial virus bronchiolitis with interleukin-4 and interleukin-4 receptor a polymorphisms. J Infect Dis. 2003;187:2-11.
42. Choi E, Lee H, Yoo T, et al. A common haplotype of interleukin-4 gene IL4 is associated with severe respiratory syncytial virus disease in Korean children. J Infect Dis. 2002;186:1207-1211.
43. Hull J, Thomson A, Kwiatkowski D. Association of respiratory syncytial virus bronchiolitis with the interleukin 8 gene region in UK families. Thorax. 2000;55:1023-1027.
44. Martinello R, Chen M, Weibel C, et al. Correlation between respiratory syncytial genotype and severity of illness. J Infect Dis. 2002;186:839-842.
45. Koeppen-Schomerus G, Stevenson J, Plomin R. Genes and environment in asthma: A study of 4 year old twins. Arch Dis Child. 2001;85:398-400.
46. ten Brinke A, Zwinderman A, Sterk P, et al. Factors associated with persistent airflow limitation in severe asthma. Am J Crit Care Med. 2001;164:744-748.
47. Ober C, Moffatt M. Contributing factors to the pathobiology: The genetics of asthma. Clin Chest Med. 2000;21:245-261.
48. Hall C, Hall W, Speers D. Clinical and physiological manifestations of bronchiolitis and pneumonia: Outcome of respiratory syncytial virus. Am J Dis Child. 1979;133:798-802.
49. Swingler G, Hussey G, Zwarenstein M. Duration of illness in ambulatory children diagnosed with bronchiolitis. Arch Pediatr Adolesc Med. 2000;154:997-1000.
50. Shaw K, Bell L, Sherman N. Outpatient assessment of infants with bronchiolitis. Am J Dis Child. 1991;145:151-155.
51. Meissner H. Selected populations at increased risk from respiratory syncytial virus infection. Pediatr Infect Dis J. 2003;22:S40-S45.
52. Mulholland E, Olinsky A, Shann F. Clinical findings and severity of acute bronchiolitis. Lancet. 1990;335:1259-1261.
53. Sreeran N, Watson J, Hunter S. Cardiovascular effects of acute bronchiolitis. Acta Paediatr Scand. 1991;80:133-136.
54. Scott L, Gutelius M, Parrott R. Children with acute respiratory tract infections: An electrocardiographic survey. Am J Dis Child. 1970;119:111-113.
55. Khoshoo V, Ross G, Kelly B, et al. Benefits of thickened feeds in previously healthy infants with respiratory syncytial virus bronchiolitis. Pediatr Pulmonol. 2001;31:301-302.
56. Hernandez E, Khoshoo V, Thoppil D, et al. Aspiration: A factor in rapidly deteriorating bronchiolitis in previously healthy infants? Pediatr Pulmonol. 2002;33:30-31.
57. Stein R, Sherrill D, Morgan W, et al. Respiratory syncytial virus in early life and risk of wheeze and allergy by age 13 years. Lancet. 1999;354:541-545.
58. Henderson F, Stewart P, Burchinal M, et al. Respiratory allergy and the relationship between early childhood lower respiratory illness and subsequent lung function. Am Rev Respir Dis. 1992;145:283-290.
59. Navas L, Wang E, de Carvalho V, et al. Improved outcome of respiratory syncytial virus infection in a high-risk hospitalized population of Canadian children. J Pediatr. 1992;121:348-354.
60. Clarke S, Gardner P, Poole P, et al. Respiratory syncytial virus infection: Admissions to hospital in industrial, urban, and rural areas. Br Med J. 1978;2:796-798.
61. Mahesh V, Taussig L. When an infant wheezes: Clues to the differential. J Respir Dis. 1990;11:739-750.
62. Lemanske R. Viruses and asthma: Inception, exacerbation, and possible prevention. J Pediatr. 2003;142:S3-S8.
63. Hall W, Hall C, Speers D. Respiratory syncytial virus infections in adults: Clinical, virologic, and serial pulmonary function studies. Ann Intern Med. 1978;88:203-205.
64. AHRQ. Management of bronchiolitis in infants and children. Agency for Healthcare Research and Quality: Evidence Report/Technology Assessment. 2003;03-E009:1-5.
65. Hall C, Douglas RJ. Clinically useful method for the isolation of respiratory syncytial virus. J Infect Dis. 1975;131:1-5.
66. Kellogg J. Culture vs direct antigen assays for detection of microbial pathogens from lower respiratory tract specimens suspected of containing the respiratory syncytial virus. Arch Pathol Lab Med. 1991;115:451-458.
67. Abels S, Nadal D, Stroehle A, et al. Reliable detection of respiratory syncytial virus infection in children for adequate hospital infection control management. J Clin Microbiol. 2001;39:3135-3139.
68. Kehl S, Henrickson K, Hua W, et al. Evaluation of the Hexaplex assay for detection of respiratory viruses in children. J Clin Microbiol. 2001;39:1696-1701.
69. Weinberg G, Erdman D, Edwards K, et al. Viral diagnosis by polymerase chain reaction (PCR) is superior to that by cell culture in prospective, population-based study of pediatric acute respiratory infections (ARI). In: Infectious Disease Society of America, 40th Annual Meeting. Chicago; 2002.

70. Khamapirad T, Glezen W. Clinical and radiographic assessment of acute lower respiratory tract disease in infants and children. Semin Respir Infect. 1987;2:130-144.
71. Wildin S, Chonmaitree T, Swischuk L. Roentgenographic features of common pediatric viral respiratory tract infections. Am J Dis Child. 1988;142:43-46.
72. Friis B, Eiken M, Hornsleth A, et al. Chest x-ray appearances in pneumonia and bronchiolitis. Acta Paediatr Scand. 1990;79:219-225.
73. Davies H, Wang E, Manson D, et al. Reliability of the chest radiograph in the diagnosis of lower respiratory infections in young children. Pediatr Infect Dis J. 1996;15:600-604.
74. Reynolds E, Cook C. The treatment of bronchiolitis. J Pediatr. 1963;63:1205-1207.
75. Panitch H. Respiratory syncytial virus bronchiolitis: Supportive care and therapies designed to overcome airway obstruction. Pediatr Infect Dis J. 2003;22:S83-S88.
76. Taussig L. Mists and aerosols: New studies, new thoughts (Editorial). J Pediatr. 1974;84:619-622.
77. Webb M, Martin G, Cartlidge P, et al. Chest physiotherapy in acute bronchiolitis. Arch Dis Child. 1985;60:1078-1079.
78. Wainwright C, Altamirano L, Cheney M, et al. A multicenter, randomized, double-blind, controlled trial of nebulized epinephrine in infants with acute bronchiolitis. N Engl J Med. 2003;349:27-35.
79. Kimpen J, Schaad U. Treatment of respiratory syncytial virus bronchiolitis: 1995 poll of members of the European Society for Paediatric Infectious Diseases. Pediatr Infect Dis J. 1997;16:479-481.
80. Behrendt C, Decker M, Burch D, et al. Internation variation in the management of infants hospitalized with respiratory syncytial virus. Eur J Pediatr. 1998;157:215-220.
81. Kellner J, Ohlsson A, Gadomski A, et al. Efficacy of bronchodilator therapy in bronchiolitis: A meta-analysis. Arch Pediatr Adolesc Med. 1996;150:1166-1172.
82. Kellner J, Ohlsson A, Gadomski A, et al. Bronchodilators for bronchiolitis. Cochrane Database Syst Rev. 2000;2:CD001266.
83. Garrison M, Christakis D, Harvey E, et al. Systemic corticosteroids in infant bronchiolitis: A meta-analysis. Pediatrics. 2000;105:e44.
84. Kim C, Kim S, Kim J, et al. Bronchiolitis obliterans in the 1990s in Korea and the United States. Chest. 2001;120:1101-1106.
85. Fischer G, Teper A, Colom A. Acute viral bronchiolitis and its sequelae in developing countries. Paediatr Respir Rev. 2002;3:298-302.
86. Vilchez R, Dauber J, McCurry K, et al. Parainfluenza virus infection in adult lung transplant recipients: An emergent clinical syndrome with implications on allograft function. Am J Transplant. 2003;3:116-120.
87. Chuang Y, Chiu C, Wong K, et al. Severe adenovirus infection in children. J Microbiol Immunol Infect. 2003;36:37-40.
88. Mauad T, Dolhnikoff M, Sao Paulo Bronchiolitis Obliterans Study Group. Histology of childhood bronchiolitis obliterans. Pediatr Pulmonol 2002;33:466-474.
89. Schlesinger C, Koss MN. Bronchiolitis: Update 2001. Curr Opin Pulm Med. 2002;8:112-116.

CHAPTER **61**

Acute Pneumonia

GERALD R. DONOWITZ

GERALD L. MANDELL

In 1901, Sir William Osler noted in the fourth edition of his book *The Principles and Practice of Medicine* that "the most widespread and fatal of all acute diseases, pneumonia, is now Captain of the Men of Death."[1] Over a century later, the prominence of pneumonia as a clinical entity remains. It is the sixth most common cause of death in the United States and the most common cause of infection-related mortality.[2] A wide array of microbial agents can cause acute pneumonia (Table 61-1), and no single antimicrobial regimen can be expected to cover all the possibilities. Because a specific etiologic diagnosis is often not possible at the time initial treatment is begun, the clinician must decide what empirical therapy is most appropriate. The increasing prevalence of antibiotic resistance among many of the most common pathogens has made this challenge more difficult. An understanding of the pathogenesis of the disease, evaluation of

TABLE 61-1 Causative Agents of Acute Pneumonia

Bacterial	Fungal	Viral
Common	Aspergillus spp.	**CHILDREN**
Streptococcus pneumoniae	*Candida* spp.	**Common**
Staphylococcus aureus	*Coccidioides immitis*	Respiratory syncytial virus
Haemophilus influenzae	*Cryptococcus neoformans*	Parainfluenza virus types 1, 2, 3
Mixed anaerobic bacteria (aspiration)	*Histoplasma capsulatum*	Influenza A virus
Bacteroides spp.	Agents of mucormycosis	**Uncommon**
Fusobacterium spp.	*Rhizopus* spp.	Adenovirus types 1, 2, 3, 5
Peptostreptococcus spp.	*Absidia* spp.	Influenza B virus
Peptococcus spp.	*Mucor* spp.	Rhinovirus
Prevotella spp.	*Cunninghamella* spp.	Coxsackievirus
Enterobacteriaceae	**Rickettsial**	Echovirus
Escherichia coli	*Coxiella burnetii*	Measles virus
Klebsiella pneumoniae	*Rickettsia rickettsiae*	Hantavirus
Enterobacter spp.	**Mycoplasma and Chlamydia**	**ADULTS**
Serratia spp.	*Mycoplasma pneumoniae*	**Common**
Pseudomonas aeruginosa	*Chlamydophila psittaci*	Influenza A virus
Legionella spp. (including *L. pneumophila and L. micdadei*)	*Chlamydia trachomatis*	Influenza B virus
Uncommon	*Chlamydophila pneumoniae* (TWAR)	Adenovirus types 4 and 7 (in military recruits)
Acinetobacter var. anitratus	**Mycobacterial**	**Uncommon**
Actinomyces and *Arachnia* spp.	*Mycobacterium tuberculosis*	Rhinovirus
Aeromonas hydrophilia	Nontuberculous mycobacteria	Adenovirus types 1, 2, 3, 5
Bacillus spp.	**Parasitic**	Enteroviruses
Moraxella catarrhalis	*Ascaris lumbricoides*	Echovirus
Campylobacter fetus	*Pneumocystis carinii*	Coxsackievirus
Eikenella corrodens	*Strongyloides stercoralis*	Poliovirus
Francisella tularensis	*Toxoplasma gondii*	Epstein-Barr virus
Neisseria meningitidis	*Paragonimus westermani*	Cytomegalovirus
Nocardia spp.		Respiratory syncytial virus
Pasteurella multocida		Varicella-zoster virus
Proteus spp.		Parainfluenza virus
Pseudomonas pseudomallei		Measles virus
Salmonella spp.		Herpes simplex virus
Enterococcus faecalis		Hantavirus
Streptococcus pyogenes		Human herpesvirus 6
		Metapneumovirus
		Coronavirus (SARS)

SARS, severe acute respiratory syndrome.

relevant data from a careful history and physical examination, recognition of common clinical patterns of infection, and information from the microbiology laboratory all aid in narrowing down the possible etiologic agents of pneumonia, thereby allowing reasonable therapy to be selected empirically.

HOST DEFENSES AND PATHOGENESIS

The lung is constantly exposed to the mixture of gases, particulate material, and microbes that constitute inspired air. In addition, organisms from oral secretions are frequently seeping down from the upper airways as a consequence of microaspiration. Yet, the lower airways usually remain sterile because of the defense mechanisms of the respiratory tract. The development of acute pulmonary infection indicates either a defect in host defenses, exposure to a particularly virulent microorganism, or an overwhelming inoculum. Infectious agents gain entry to the lower respiratory tract through aspiration of upper airway resident flora, inhalation of aerosolized material, and, less frequently, metastatic seeding of the lung from blood.

Pulmonary Defense Systems

The pulmonary defense system includes anatomic and mechanical barriers, humoral immunity, cell-mediated immunity, and phagocyte activity (Table 61-2).[3-11] The upper airways, including the nasopharynx, oropharynx, and larynx, are the sites first exposed to inhaled microorganisms. Particles greater than 10 μm in size are efficiently filtered by the hair in the anterior nares or impact onto mucosal surfaces because of the configuration of the upper airways and the nasal turbinates. The nasal mucosa contains ciliated epithelium and mucus-producing cells. Mechanical clearance of entrapped organisms occurs through the nasopharynx via expulsion or swallowing. In the oropharynx, the flow of saliva, sloughing of epithelial cells, local production of complement, and bacterial interference from resident flora serve as important factors in local host defense. Secretory immunoglobulin A (IgA) is the major immunoglobulin produced in the upper airways and accounts for 10% of the total protein of nasal secretions.[7] It possesses antibacterial and antiviral activity despite being a relatively poor opsonin. Low IgA levels have been associated with increased bacterial infection.[12] IgG and IgM enter the airways predominantly via transudation from the blood. Their roles in bacterial opsonization, complement

activation, agglutination, and neutralization activity are similar to those noted in serum.

Adherence of microorganisms to epithelial surfaces of the upper airways is a critical initial step in colonization and subsequent infection. Changes in fibronectin secretion and in binding characteristics of epithelium for various lectins occur as a response to underlying diseases. This may help to explain why colonization occurs in some clinical settings and not in others.[13] Microbes possess surface adhesions, pili, exotoxins, and proteolytic enzymes that can degrade IgA, which serves to overcome host defenses and allow colonization.[8]

The cough and epiglottic reflexes keep most large particulate matter from reaching the central airways. The trachea and conducting airways of the transbronchial tree are usually effective in entrapping particles from 2 to 10 μm in size. The sharp angles at which the central airways branch cause particles to impact on mucosal surfaces, where they are entrapped by endobronchial mucus. Once entrapped, particles are removed by ciliated epithelium to the oropharynx.

Epithelial cells, which line the conducting airways, submucosal glands, and alveoli, produce airway surface liquid—a complex mixture of proteins and peptides mixed with plasma transudate.[9,10] Airway surface liquid contains lysozyme, lactoferrin, and secretory leukocyte proteinase inhibitor, all of which possess microbicidal activity. Respiratory epithelial cells produce other potent antimicrobial peptides including cathelicidins and β-defensins. These peptides possess individual antimicrobial activity as well as synergistic antimicrobial activity with each other.[10] In addition, the β-defensins may act as chemokines for memory T cells and dendritic cells, thereby serving as a link between nonspecific immune lung host defenses (innate defense) and specific immune lung host responses (adaptive defense).

Most bacteria are 0.5 to 2 μm in size. This size particle may reach the terminal airways and alveoli. No mucociliary apparatus exists at this level, yet a variety of humoral and cell-mediated host defenses function here. The alveolar-lining fluid contains surfactant, fibronectin, IgG, and complement, all of which are effective opsonins. Surfactant is composed of several components (SP-A, SP-B, SP-C, SP-D) that serve to increase the microbicidal capacity of macrophages. These compounds may also affect free-radical production and lymphocyte activity.[14] SP-A and SP-D are collectins—a family of collagenous carbohydrate-binding proteins. These proteins bind a variety of organisms, including viruses, gram-negative and gram-positive bacteria, mycobacteria, and fungi, which may decrease their virulence or enhance phagocytosis by neutrophils and alveolar macrophages.[15] Free fatty acids, lysozyme, iron-binding proteins, and defensins are also present and may be directly microbicidal.

Phagocytic cells play a major role in pulmonary host defense. Four distinct populations of macrophages exist in the lung and vary in their location and function.[16] The alveolar macrophage is located in the alveolar-lining fluid at the interphase between air and lung tissue. It serves as the resident phagocytic cell in the lower airway and is the first phagocyte encountered by inert particles and potential pathogens entering the lung via inspired air. Alveolar macrophages play several critical roles.[5] As phagocytic cells, they can eliminate certain organisms. If the numbers of organisms increase beyond the macrophages' capability to handle them or if the organisms involved are particularly virulent (e.g., *Pseudomonas aeruginosa*), the macrophage becomes a mediator of an inflammatory response by producing cytokines that recruit neutrophils into the lung.[17,18] Interstitial macrophages are located in the lung connective tissue and serve both as phagocytic cells and antigen-processing cells. Animal models suggest that interstitial macrophages, although equal to alveolar macrophages in Fc-receptor–dependent phagocytosis, are less active in demonstrating Fc-receptor–independent phagocytosis, cytokine production, and oxygen radical production. On the other hand, their class II antigen expression is superior to that of the alveolar macrophage.[16] Dendritic cells derive from monocytes and are located within the epithelium of the trachea, conducting airways, terminal airways, alveolar septa, pulmonary vasculature, and visceral pleura. These cells are therefore positioned to interact with antigens in inhaled air. Dendritic cells possess an enhanced capacity to capture,

TABLE 61-2	**Pulmonary Host Defenses**
Location	*Host Defense Mechanism*
Upper Airways	
Nasopharynx	Nasal hair
	Turbinates
	Anatomy of upper airways
	Mucociliary apparatus
	IgA secretion
Oropharynx	Saliva
	Sloughing of epithelial cells
	Bacterial interference
	Complement production
Conducting Airways	
Trachea, bronchi	Cough, epiglottic reflexes
	Sharp-angled branching of airways
	Mucociliary apparatus
	Immunoglobulin production (IgG, IgM, IgA)
	Airway surface liquid (lysozyme, lactoferrin, secretory leukocyte proteinase inhibitor)
Lower Respiratory Tract	
Terminal airways, alveoli	Alveolar lining fluid (surfactant, fibronectin, immunoglobulin, complement, free fatty acid, iron-binding proteins)
	Cytokines (TNF, IL-1, IL-8, and others)
	Alveolar macrophages
	Polymorphonuclear leukocytes
	Cell-mediated immunity

IL, interleukin; TNF, tumor necrosis factor.

process, and present class II antigens. They can migrate to lymphoid tissue, where they can stimulate T-cell immune responses. Dendritic cells can also produce a variety of cytokines and chemokines including interleukin (IL)-12, which serves to stimulate B-cell immune function.[19] The intravascular macrophage is located in the capillary endothelial cells. These cells are actively phagocytic and remove foreign or damaged material entering the lungs via the blood stream.

Neutrophil recruitment is central to the inflammatory response in the lung and is mediated by a variety of cytokines.[20,21] These mediators are involved in both attracting and maintaining adequate numbers of neutrophils in areas of lung damage as well as in regulating the extent of inflammation. IL-1, tumor necrosis factor-α (TNF-α), colony-stimulating factor, interferon-γ, IL-10, IL-12, and certain α-chemokines are important mediators in this regard.[22] Although TNF-α and IL-I are not thought to have chemotactic activity, they induce the production of IL-8, which is a potent neutrophil chemoattractant. In addition, the fifth component of complement (C5), leukotriene B$_4$, and formylmethionyl peptides of bacterial cell walls may be present in the lower airways and help recruit neutrophils into areas of inflammation as well. Recent data suggest that neutrophils themselves may secrete cytokines with anti-inflammatory effects that modulate the inflammatory response.[23]

Other lung parenchymal cells may also help regulate the inflammatory response.[24,25] In addition to epithelial cells, interstitial macrophages, and dendritic cells, endothelial cells, pulmonary smooth muscle cells, and fibroblasts produce both proinflammatory (e.g., colony-stimulating factors, chemokines) and anti-inflammatory (IL-10) factors.

Cell-mediated immunity in the lung is especially important against certain pathogens, including viruses and intracellular parasites, that can survive within pulmonary macrophages (e.g., *Mycobacterium, Legionella*). The lung has lymphoid tissue where homing and differentiation of previously uncommitted cells to memory T and B cells occur.[26] Most of the organized lymphoid tissue in the lung is located in follicles along the bronchial tree in bronchus-associated lymphoid tissues (BALT). The lymphoid centers are morphologically similar to Peyer's patches in the intestine and are similarly associated with mucosal epithelium. Inhaled antigens therefore are able to cross the epithelial surface and immediately encounter cells involved with antigen processing. Once these antigens are processed and presented, it is in the BALT that B and T lymphocytes localize and are stimulated to become memory cells and effector cells.

Normal lung parenchyma usually contains few lymphoid cells, which represent only 5% to 10% of the total cell population. The lymphocytes present are memory cells located in the submucosa and lamina propria; effector cells located between epithelial cells and in the interstitium; and cells thought to be "preactivated," awaiting stimulation by inhaled antigens in the alveolus. The majority of lymphocytes are T cells, with 35% to 45% representing a CD$_4$ (helper, inducer) phenotype, and 18% to 32% representing a CD$_8$ (suppressor) phenotype.[27]

Antigens inhaled into the alveolus and captured by antigen-presenting cells, subsequently activate intra-alveolar lymphoid cells. These cells can stimulate the migration of memory lymphocytes into the area, leading to a localized accumulation of antigen-specific T and B lymphocytes, many of which possess effector cell function. As is true in other anatomic areas, binding of T cells to endothelium is a critical first step in the inflammatory process and is mediated by the interaction of leukocyte function-associated antigen (LFA)-1 integrins on the lymphocyte cell surface with ligands exposed by endothelium in areas of inflammation (intercellular adhesion molecules 1 and 2 and vascular cell adhesion molecule 1). Expression of these ligands on pulmonary endothelium is upregulated by inflammatory mediators such as IL-1, interferon-γ, and TNF-α as well as by bacterial lipopolysaccharides.

Pulmonary lymphocytes are thought to shuttle between two functionally distinct lymphoid areas, the BALT, which can be viewed as the afferent limb where antigens first stimulate an immune response, and the lung parenchyma, where differentiated T and B cells participate in the inflammatory response, which can be viewed as the efferent limb.

The increase in numbers of memory T cells after antigenic stimulation may occur as a result of local proliferation or via migration of cells from BALT.

Lymphocytes in the lung have three major roles[28]: (1) the production of antibody, (2) cytotoxic activity, and (3) production of inflammatory mediators. The lung contains a variety of cytotoxic T cells including natural killer cells (antigen nonrestricted), antibody-dependent cytotoxic cells, and antigen-restricted cytotoxic cells. Pulmonary T cells produce a large number of cytokines. Mouse models suggest that unstimulated T cells produce mainly IL-2. After stimulation and conversion to memory T cells, two distinct groupings of cytokines are produced. The helper T-cell 1 (Th1) and Th2 pattern of cytokine production noted in murine models occurs in humans, although it appears to be less restrictive. Th1 cells produce interferon-γ, IL-2, IL-6, and IL-10 and contribute to cell-mediated immunity, whereas Th2 cells produce IL-4, IL-5, and IL-10 and contribute to humoral immune function. Furthermore, IL-3, TNF-α, granulocyte-macrophage colony-stimulating factor, and chemokines are secreted by both Th1 and Th2 phenotypes. Th1 cells are involved in cell-mediated inflammatory reactions, whereas Th2 cells stimulate antibody production, especially IgE, and stimulate eosinophil activity.

Impairment of Pulmonary Defenses

The defenses of the lung, when it is functioning normally, are extremely efficient in maintaining sterility of the lower airways. However, a number of factors are known to interfere with these defenses and predispose the host to infection.[3] Alterations in the level of consciousness from any cause (stroke, seizures, drug intoxication, anesthesia, alcohol abuse, and even normal sleep) can compromise epiglottic closure and lead to aspiration of oropharyngeal flora into the lower respiratory tract.[29] Cigarette smoke, perhaps the most common agent involved in compromising natural pulmonary defense mechanisms, disrupts both mucociliary function and macrophage activity.[30]

Alcohol not only impairs the cough and epiglottic reflexes but also has been associated with increased colonization of the oropharynx with aerobic gram-negative bacilli, decreased mobilization of neutrophils,[31] abnormal phagocyte oxidative metabolism, and abnormal chemotaxis.[32] Alcohol effectively blocks the TNF response to endotoxin, with decreased recruitment of neutrophils to the lung. Furthermore, alcohol enhances monocyte production of 1L-10, a cytokine with anti-inflammatory properties.[33]

Infections with *Mycoplasma pneumoniae* or *Haemophilus influenzae* may interfere with normal ciliary function.[34] Viruses may actually destroy respiratory epithelium and may disrupt normal ciliary activity.[11,12] Neutrophil function, including chemotaxis, phagocytosis, and stimulation of oxidative metabolism and alveolar macrophage function, may also be inhibited by certain viral infections.[35] Sepsis associated with extrapulmonary infections may undermine lung defense mechanisms. In animal models, exposure to lipopolysaccharide or endotoxin decreases lung clearance of a bacterial challenge.[36] Infection with human immunodeficiency virus (HIV) undermines many of the components of pulmonary host defense. Quantitative defects involve the naive CD$_4$ T cells initially, and the memory CD$_4$ T cells are depleted more rapidly later in infection. Functional defects caused by the virus include impaired response to remote recall antigens, inhibited response to soluble antigen followed in time by decreased T-cell response to alloantigens and mitogens, impaired IL-2 and interferon-γ production, and decreased immunoglobulin production.[37] In BALT, destruction of dendritic cells and degeneration of lymphoid follicles have been noted. Defective antigen presentation by dendritic cells has also been observed. Abnormal chemotaxis, phagocytosis, and oxidative metabolism in neutrophils of patients with acquired immunodeficiency syndrome (AIDS) have been described.

Iatrogenic manipulations that bypass or interfere with the usual host defenses of the upper airways (endotracheal tubes, nasogastric tubes, and respiratory therapy machinery) all predispose to infection.[38] A variety of commonly prescribed drugs have been shown to inhibit host defenses in vitro or in models, but the clinical significance of this is uncertain. These agents include aspirin,[39] erythromycin,[40] and aminophylline.[41] Other factors that impair pulmonary host defenses include hypoxemia, acidosis, toxic inhalations,[42] pulmonary edema,[43] uremia, malnutrition, immunosuppressive agents,[44] and mechanical obstruction.[4] The outbreak of severe acute respiratory syndrome (SARS) showed that hospitals can be a major location for the transmission of respiratory viruses to hospital staff, visitors, and other patients. Triage in emergency departments and isolation precautions need major changes in the face of such epidemics (see Chapter 152).

Older adults are at increased risk for the development of pneumonia (see Chapter 314). Although a variety of factors play an important role in this regard, including an increased number and increased severity of underlying diseases and an increased number of hospitalizations, there are age-related impairments in host defenses.[45,46] Less effective mucociliary clearance and abnormal elastic recoil may lead to less effective coughing and clearing of the upper airways. Changes in humoral immunity and cell-mediated immune function have been documented in older persons.

Recurrent episodes of bacterial pneumonia suggest the presence of specific predisposing factors.[47,48] In children and young adults, recurrent pneumonia is associated with defects in host defenses, including leukocyte function[49] and immunoglobulin production.[49-52] Congenital defects in ciliary activity including the immotile cilia syndrome,[53] Kartagener's syndrome (ciliary dysfunction, situs inversus, sinusitis, bronchiectasis),[54] Young's syndrome (azoospermia, sinusitis, pneumonia),[55] and cystic fibrosis are other clinical entities associated with recurrent pneumonia in young persons. Structural lung abnormalities such as bronchiectasis and pulmonary sequestration[56] are also important predisposing factors for both younger and older patient populations.

Although most congenital defects in host defenses appear in childhood, common variable hypogammaglobulinemia may first appear in adulthood with recurrent pneumonia. Acquired host defense defects are more varied and include malignancies (lymphoma, chronic lymphocytic leukemia, myeloma), infection (AIDS), and iatrogenic causes (immune suppression associated with solid organ or marrow transplantation or cancer chemotherapy). Underlying respiratory tract disorders such as chronic obstructive pulmonary disease (COPD), bronchiectasis, adult-onset cystic fibrosis, bronchopulmonary sequestration, and tracheobronchiomegaly may present with pneumonia. Bronchial obstruction due to intrinsic compression (adenocarcinoma) or extrinsic compression (lymphadenopathy due to sarcoid or malignancy) has also been associated with recurrent episodes of pneumonia. Underlying diseases that predispose to aspiration lead to an increased incidence of pneumonia. These may be associated with gastrointestinal diseases (tracheoesophageal fistula, esophageal diverticula, esophageal reflux, esophageal stricture), neuromuscular disorders (myasthenia gravis, dementia, amyotrophic lateral sclerosis), and cancer of the head and neck. Some systemic illnesses, including Weber-Christian disease, chronic renal failure, diabetes, and sickle cell disease, have been associated with pneumonia.

CLINICAL EVALUATION

History

The history should attempt to define (1) symptoms consistent with the diagnosis of pneumonia, (2) the clinical setting in which the pneumonia takes place, (3) defects in host defense that could predispose to the development of pneumonia, and (4) possible exposures to specific pathogens.

Respiratory symptoms are commonly encountered in primary care practices but are usually not associated with pneumonia. In 1994, over 10 million visits were associated with a chief complaint of cough; only 4% to 6% of these visits involved pneumonia.[57,58] Although the prevalence of pneumonia may vary depending on the age of the patient population and the presence of comorbid diseases, pneumonia remains only one of many possible explanations for the clinical presentation. Therefore, a serious effort should be made to differentiate pneumonia from other diagnostic possibilities with which it may be confused. Although the clinical findings of pneumonia related to the respiratory

tract should be sought, including cough, sputum production, dyspnea, and fever, it should be recognized that nonrespiratory symptoms are commonly present. These include fatigue, sweats, headache, nausea, and myalgia.[59,60] With increasing age, both respiratory and nonrespiratory symptoms of pneumonia become less frequent. Unfortunately, symptoms at presentation elucidated by a careful history will not always be able to distinguish pneumonia from other respiratory problems.[61]

Specific etiologic agents of pneumonia have been associated with certain underlying diseases and patient populations. Mycoplasmal pneumonia occurs more often in younger people,[62] but it may be a cause of pneumonia in older patients and require hospitalization.[63] Gram-negative pneumonia tends to occur in older adults, especially those who are debilitated with comorbid diseases.[64] Tuberculosis should be suspected in the homeless, those infected with HIV, those who come from developing countries where tuberculosis is prevalent, and those who have been exposed to others with the disease.[65] Staphylococcal pneumonia has been noted during epidemics of influenza, and SARS, recently defined as being caused by a coronavirus, has been associated with travel to China, Taiwan, Hong Kong, Singapore, Vietnam, and Toronto, Canada.[66] Unusually severe pneumonia in a previously normal host or a cluster of unusual cases should warrant consideration of a bioterrorist attack, and the local health department should be immediately notified.

Pneumonia has been noted to occur with increased frequency in patients with a variety of underlying disorders such as congestive heart failure, diabetes, alcoholism, and COPD.[64,67] In one series of 292 patients with pneumonia, only 18% were found to have no underlying disease.[64] A history of antecedent upper respiratory tract infection has been elicited in 36% to 50% of patients with acute pneumonia, especially in those with pneumococcal disease.[68] Recent dental manipulations, sedative overdoses, seizures, alcoholism, or loss of consciousness for any reason should raise the suspicion of anaerobic infection caused by aspiration of oral contents.[29]

Special note needs to be made of the relationship between pneumonia and patients with COPD.[69] Although well-controlled studies are lacking, it does appear that patients with COPD have an increased incidence of pneumonia. However, because the tracheobronchial tree is often colonized with *Streptococcus pneumoniae* and *H. influenzae,* it has been difficult to distinguish clearly between colonization and infection in many studies. Although these organisms play an important role as etiologic agents of pneumonia in this patient population, most of the clinical studies were carried out before it was recognized that other, less common pathogens also play a significant role in causing disease. The roles of *Moraxella catarrhalis, Legionella, Chlamydophila,* and aerobic gram-negative rods including *P. aeruginosa* have been established.[69-72] Cystic fibrosis is associated with *Pseudomonas* and staphylococcal pulmonary infections.[73] Pulmonary alveolar proteinosis is associated with *Nocardia* infection.

Patients infected with HIV are at high risk for the development of pulmonary infections.[74,75] Although *Pneumocystis* pneumonia remains an important clinical entity in this patient population, prophylaxis has reduced its incidence and importance as a cause of death.[76,77] In considering the nature of pulmonary infection in patients infected with HIV, geographic exposures, demographic characteristics of the patient, and the degree of immune suppression need to be considered.[74,75] *Pneumocystis* infection is relatively uncommon in Africa but more frequent in Europe and the United States. *Mycobacterium tuberculosis* is more common in the northeastern United States than in other parts of the country.[78] Because fungal infections play a major role in this patient population, exposure in endemic areas of histoplasmosis, blastomycosis, and coccidioidomycosis needs to be considered. The overall incidence of bacterial pneumonia in patients with HIV is five times higher than in non–HIV-infected populations, and the greatest risk appears to be associated with intravenous and inhaled drug use.[74,79,80] Common pulmonary pathogens such as *S. pneumoniae, H. influenzae,* and *Staphylococcus aureus* play an important role.[75] The incidence of invasive pneumococcal pneumonia is 100 to 300 times higher in HIV-infected patients,[81,82] and the incidence of *H. influenzae* infection may be up to 100-fold higher in this population.[83] *P. aeruginosa* pneumonia is often associated with bacteremia or cavitary lung disease and is a later complication of HIV infection occurring with CD_4 counts of less than 25/μL. The infection is associated with the presence of central venous catheters, urinary catheters, and the use of steroids.[84,85] Bacterial agents such as *Legionella, Nocardia,* aerobic gram-negative bacilli, and *Rhodococcus equi* are important causes of pneumonia.

In patients infected with HIV, the relationship between the degree of immune suppression using the CD_4 count as a marker and the specific etiology of pneumonia deserves emphasis. Bacterial pneumonia and tuberculosis usually occur when the CD_4 count is less than 400/μL.[80,86] *Pneumocystis* and disseminated tuberculosis are associated with CD_4 counts below 200/μL, and disseminated nontuberculous mycobacterial infections and disseminated fungal infection occur with CD_4 counts less than 50 to 100/μL.[86] Pulmonary infections in HIV-infected patients are discussed in more detail in Chapter 118.

Pneumonia developing in hospitalized patients often involves Enterobacteriaceae, *P. aeruginosa,* and *S. aureus,* organisms that are unusual in community-acquired disease.[87] Pneumonia in older adults, especially those who are bedridden or who have chronic diseases, is more often associated with gram-negative bacilli than is pneumonia in younger populations.[88] However, lack of clear definition between colonization and true infection has made the actual role of gram-negative organisms unclear in this regard. In general, *S. pneumoniae,* nontypable strains of *H. influenzae,* and *M. catarrhalis* are important pathogens in older adults.

Important aspects of a patient's history that may suggest specific potential infectious agents include occupation, exposure to animals, travel, and sexual history (Table 61-3). The presence of noninfectious pulmonary disease, such as tumors or pulmonary emboli, which may masquerade as pneumonia, may also be suggested by a careful history.

TABLE 61-3 Pneumonia Agent Suggested by Environmental History

Infectious Agent	Environmental History
Anthrax	Exposure to cattle, swine, horses, goat hair, raw wool, animal hides. (Possible agent of bioterrorism)
Brucellosis	Exposure to cattle, goats, pigs; ingestion of unpasteurized dairy products; employment as abattoir worker or veterinarian
Melioidosis	Travel to West Indies, Australia, Guam, Southeast Asia, South and Central America
Plague	Exposure to ground squirrels, chipmunks, rabbits, prairie dogs, rats. (Possible agent of bioterrorism)
Tularemia	Exposure to tissue or body fluids of infected animals during trapping, hunting, or skinning (rabbits, hares, foxes, squirrels) or to bites of an infected arthropod (flies, ticks) Handling or ingesting poorly cooked meat from an infected animal (Possible agent of bioterrorism)
Psittacosis	Exposure to birds (parrots, budgerigars, cockatoos, pigeons, turkeys)
Leptospirosis	Exposure to wild rodents, dogs, cats, pigs, cattle, or horses, or exposure to water contaminated with animal urine
Coccidioidomycosis	Residence in or travel to San Joaquin Valley, southern California, southwestern Texas, southern Arizona, New Mexico
Histoplasmosis	Exposure to bat droppings or dust from soil enriched with bird droppings
Q fever	Exposure to infected goats, cattle, sheep, domestic animals, and their secretions (milk, amniotic fluid, placenta, feces)
Legionnaires' disease	Exposure to contaminated aerosols (e.g., air coolers, hospital water supply)
Pasteurella multocida	Exposure to infected dogs and cats
Hantavirus	Exposure to rodent droppings, urine, saliva
SARS	Travel to area of outbreaks

SARS, severe acute respiratory syndrome.

Physical Examination

Fever is reported to be present in 65% to 90% of patients with pneumonia. It may be sustained, remittent, or at times hectic. Fever patterns per se, however, are not useful for establishing a specific diagnosis. The temperature should be taken rectally to reduce error caused by rapid mouth breathing. Recording of postural changes in blood pressure and pulse rate is useful in assessing hydration and intravascular fluid volume. The pulse usually increases by 10 beats per minute for every degree (centigrade) of temperature elevation. A pulse–temperature deficit (e.g., a relative bradycardia for the amount of fever) should suggest viral infection, mycoplasmal infection, chlamydial infection, tularemia, or infection with *Legionella.* Cyanosis, a rapid respiratory rate, the use of accessory muscles of respiration, sternal retraction, and nasal flaring suggest serious respiratory compromise.

Furuncles are rarely secondary to staphylococcal pneumonia acquired by the respiratory route, but they may signal a source of bacteremia with subsequent pneumonia via hematogenous spread, although this is uncommon. Herpes labialis is seen in up to 40% of patients with pneumococcal pneumonia.[89] Bullous myringitis is an infrequent but significant finding in mycoplasmal pneumonia.[62] The presence of poor dentition should suggest a mixed infection due to aspiration of anaerobes and aerobes that colonize the oropharynx. Although edentulous people may develop anaerobic pneumonia as a result of aspiration, it is uncommon.[90]

Examination of the thorax may reveal "splinting," or an inspiratory lag on the side of the lesion, that is suggestive of bacterial pneumonia. Early in the disease process, definite signs of pulmonary involvement may be lacking or may be manifest only as fine rales. Chest examination may reveal these early signs of pneumonia even though the chest film is normal. Evidence of consolidation (dullness on percussion, bronchial breath sounds, and E to A changes) is highly suggestive of bacterial infection but may be absent in two thirds of patients ill enough to be hospitalized and may be absent more often in patients treated as outpatients.[91] Patients with mycoplasmal or viral infection may exhibit few abnormalities on physical examination despite the presence of impressive infiltrates on the chest film.

The overall usefulness of the history and physical examination to detect the presence of pneumonia has been questioned.[61,92,93] A great deal of interobserver variation exists in detecting the signs and symptoms.[61] In one series, three examiners seeing the same patients could not consistently agree on the physical examination findings. The diagnosis of pneumonia could be made with a sensitivity of only 47% to 69% and with a specificity of 50% to 75%.[94] Rare findings such as egobronchophony and asymmetric chest movements have a high predictive value for pneumonia. Other findings are usually not helpful. The absence of any vital sign abnormalities (i.e., respiratory rate >20 breaths/minute, heart rate >100 beats/minute, and temperature >37.8° C) has been associated with a less than 1% chance of a patient's having pneumonia, assuming a pneumonia prevalence of 5% in the population under study.[92] Others have questioned the importance of any of these specific findings on detecting the presence of pneumonia.[61] The probability of detecting pneumonia varies with the patient population, the prevalence of pneumonia in that population, the threshold values for defining a vital sign as abnormal, and the ability of the clinician to detect abnormal physical findings. No single physical finding is particularly helpful in making a definite diagnosis. However, a constellation of cough, fever, tachycardia, and crackles raises the possibility of pneumonia being present to 18% to 42%. Therefore, although variable and nondefinitive, a complete history and physical examination may be extremely helpful in guiding the workup of pneumonia.

Sputum Examination

Microscopic examination and culture of expectorated sputum remain the mainstays of the laboratory evaluation of pneumonia despite ongoing controversy concerning their sensitivity and specificity.[95-101]

In the guidelines for the management of community-acquired pneumonia developed by the Infectious Disease Society of America, the sputum Gram stain is viewed as a simple, quick, inexpensive procedure that

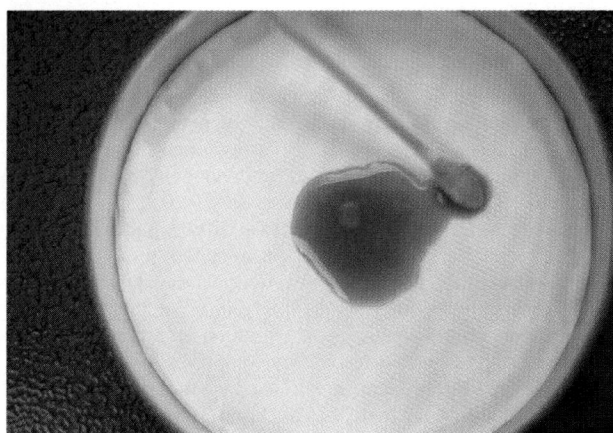

FIGURE 61-1. "Currant-jelly" sputum associated with *Klebsiella pneumoniae* pneumonia.

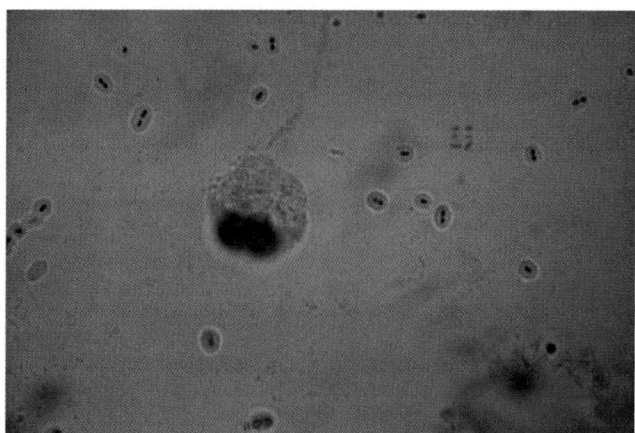

FIGURE 61-3. Expectorated sputum demonstrating a positive quellung reaction in a patient with pneumococcal pneumonia.

may serve as a guide to initial antibiotic therapy.[98] The overall helpfulness of the procedure for aiding in the etiologic diagnosis of pneumonia is unclear.[99] This partly because there is no gold standard for the "true" cause of pneumonia, partly because there is interobserver variability, and partly because 30% to 40% of patients fail to produce sputum.[99] Increased accuracy appears to be associated with experience—laboratory technicians have greater accuracy than house staff.[102] However, despite the pitfalls, the procurement of expectorated sputum is a noninvasive technique that can be carried out at no risk to the patient and may allow the clinician to make a presumptive diagnosis.

Examination of the sputum should include observation of the color, amount, consistency, and odor of the specimen. Mucopurulent sputum is most commonly found with bacterial pneumonia or bronchitis. However, sputum of a similar nature has been described in one third to one half of patients with mycoplasma[62] or adenovirus infections.[103] Scant or watery sputum is more often noted with these and other atypical pneumonias. "Rusty" sputum suggests alveolar involvement and has been most commonly (although not solely) associated with pneumococcal pneumonia.[104] Dark red, mucoid sputum (currant-jelly sputum) suggests Friedlander's pneumonia caused by encapsulated *Klebsiella pneumoniae* (Fig. 61-1).[105] Foul-smelling sputum is associated with mixed anaerobic infections most commonly seen with aspiration.[90] The utility of the sputum Gram stain remains an area of controversy—most infectious disease specialists feel that it is useful, whereas their colleagues in pulmonary medicine feel that it usually is not.

Where possible, frankly purulent material should be selected for microscopic examination and Gram stain. To maximize the diagnostic yield of the sputum examination, only samples with minimal oropharyngeal contamination should be reviewed. As a guide, the number of neutrophils and epithelial cells should be quantitated under low power ($\times 100$), with further examination reserved for samples containing 25 or more neutrophils and 10 or fewer epithelial cells.[106] Samples with more epithelial cells and fewer neutrophils are usually nondiagnostic and should be discarded. The morphologic and staining characteristics of any bacteria seen should be recorded and an estimate made of the predominant organisms (Figs. 61-2 through 61-6). When no bacterial predominance exists, this should be noted as well.

In the appropriate clinical setting, a predominance of gram-positive, lancet-shaped diplococci should suggest pneumococcal infection (see Fig. 61-2). When strict criteria for Gram stain positivity are used (predominant flora or more than 10 gram-positive, lancet-shaped diplococci per oil immersion field [$\times 1000$], or both), the specificity of the Gram stain for identifying pneumococci has been shown to be 85%, with a sensitivity of 62%.[107] The diagnostic yield of the sputum examination for pneumococci can be maximized by the use of the quellung reaction (see Fig. 61-3). Anticapsular antiserum reacts with capsular polysaccharide, and this may be seen as a distinctly outlined capsule. Rare false-positive results may occur with α-hemolytic streptococci. Occasional false-negative results may occur as well. An 89% correlation between pneumococcal isolation by culture and a positive sputum quellung test has been demonstrated.[96]

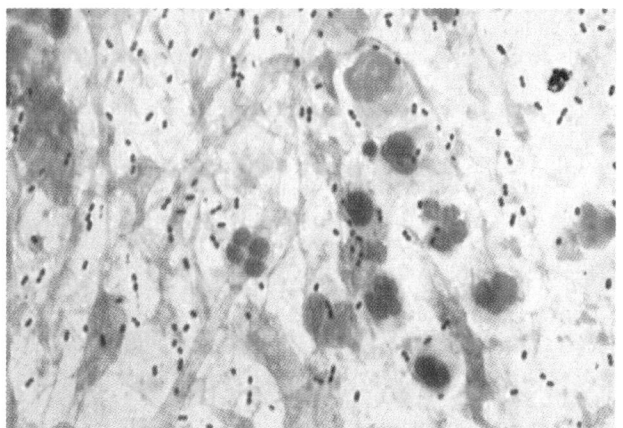

FIGURE 61-2. Expectorated sputum with gram-positive, lancet-shaped diplococci from a patient with pneumococcal pneumonia.

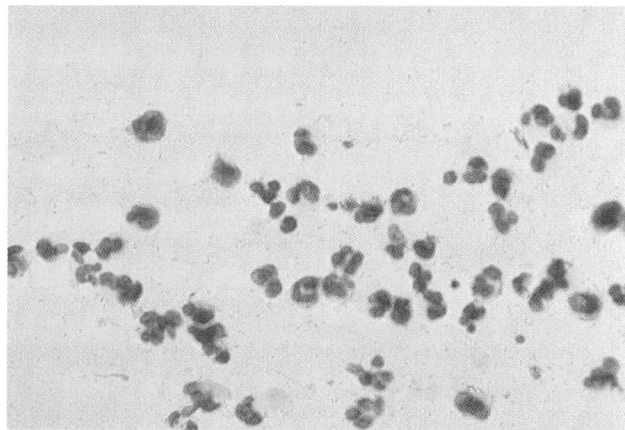

FIGURE 61-4. Expectorated sputum with gram-negative coccobacillary forms from a patient with *Haemophilus influenzae* pneumonia.

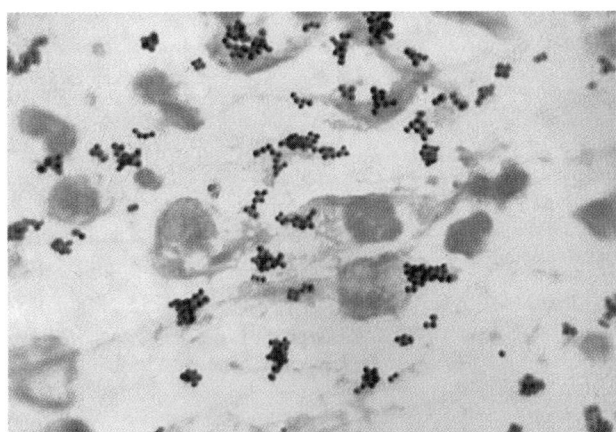

FIGURE 61-5. Expectorated sputum with clusters of gram-positive cocci in a patient with *Staphylococcus aureus* pneumonia.

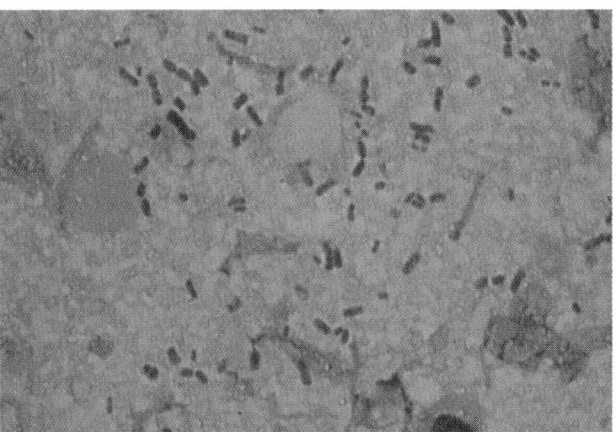

FIGURE 61-6. Expectorated sputum with gram-negative rods in a patient with *Klebsiella pneumoniae* pneumonia.

Because pneumococci may be part of the nasopharyngeal flora in 10% to 50% of healthy adults and often colonize the lower airways in patients with chronic bronchitis, identification of the organism does not mean that it is the cause of disease.[108,109] However, it is our experience that the large number of pneumococci necessary to produce a positive Gram stain or quellung reaction is unusual in carriers. The Gram stain may reveal large numbers of organisms in patients with bronchitis.

The sputum Gram stain is helpful to identify organisms other than pneumococci. Small gram-negative coccobacillary organisms are characteristic of *H. influenzae* (see Fig. 61-4). However, the sensitivity of the sputum Gram stain for detecting *H. influenzae* is usually less than that for *S. pneumoniae* and has been reported to be 40% to 80%.[100,102] Staphylococci appear as gram-positive cocci in tetrads and grapelike clusters (see Fig. 61-5). Organisms of mixed morphology are characteristic of anaerobic infection. Few bacteria are seen with legionnaires' disease, mycoplasma pneumonia, and viral pneumonia. When the criteria of more than 25 neutrophils and fewer than 10 squamous epithelial cells per low-power ($\times$100) magnification are met, and when a predominant morphology is observed, the sensitivity of the sputum Gram stain in matching organisms found in the blood was reported to be 85% in patients with community-acquired pneumonia. In contrast, sputum cultures positive for pneumococci are found in only 50% to 60% of patients with pneumonia and pneumococcal bacteremia.[110] Sputum examination has been a useful means of diagnosing *Pneumocystis* pneumonia in patients with AIDS. The use of commercially available monoclonal antibodies or Giemsa's, Gomori's methenamine silver, or toluidine blue O stain has led to a diagnosis in more than 50% of cases, making more aggressive diagnostic procedures unnecessary.[111] Special sputum staining techniques are important in identifying other organisms such as mycobacteria (Fig. 61-7).

Sputum culture as a means of diagnosing pneumonia is as controversial as the sputum Gram stain. Only 60% of patients with pneumonia may produce sputum. As noted previously, patients with bacteremic pneumococcal pneumonia have been reported to have negative sputum cultures in 45% to 50% of cases, even when large numbers of organisms have been noted on a Gram stain.[110] Similarly, 34% to 47% of sputum cultures are negative with proven *H. influenzae* pneumonia.[112,113] Furthermore, sputum cultures have frequently been shown to yield more bacterial species than more invasive methods of obtaining respiratory tract secretions.[114] Contamination with gram-negative bacilli from the oropharynx has been noted in 32% of sputum cultures. A lack of correlation between findings from sputum culture and findings from blood cultures and serologic studies has been observed.

Several key parameters have been identified in efforts to maximize the diagnostic yield from sputum culture. Procurement of adequate sputum samples is an essential first step. When fewer than 10 epithelial cells and more than 25 neutrophils per low-power field are noted, oropharyngeal contamination is minimal and sputum samples are comparable to transtracheal aspirates in terms of the number of bacterial species isolated.[106] With increasing numbers of epithelial cells and decreasing numbers of neutrophils, an increased amount of oropharyngeal contamination is present, as indicated by the isolation of more bacterial species.

The presence of alveolar macrophages does not alter the bacteriologic findings when substantial numbers of epithelial cells are present, indicating that otherwise adequate samples of sputum can be contaminated with oropharyngeal contents and thereby rendered nondiagnostic. This type of initial screening has proved helpful in differentiating adequate sputum samples from saliva, thereby increasing the diagnostic yield of sputum culture. When organisms such as *M. tuberculosis* (see Fig. 61-7), *Legionella,* and *Pneumocystis* are found in sputum, clinical infection is indicated regardless of the sputum quality because these organisms are not normal flora.

When culture of sputum is delayed, the isolation of pneumococci is less likely because of overgrowth by oropharyngeal flora. Rapid processing of samples is therefore another important factor leading to higher diagnostic yield.

Laboratory techniques for maximizing the useful information from sputum cultures have included quantitative cultures, washing of samples to remove contaminating mouth flora, and the use of mucolytic agents. However, the results have not warranted the increased efforts. Furthermore, washing samples does not guarantee that adequate samples of lower respiratory tract secretions are

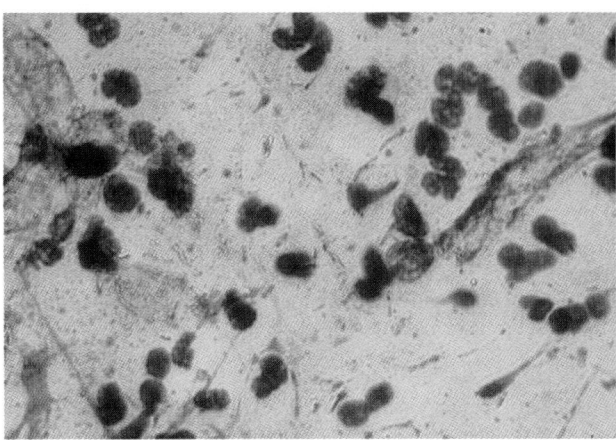

FIGURE 61-7. Expectorated sputum with acid-fast bacilli in a patient with *Mycobacterium tuberculosis.*

present. Some reports suggest that with adequate sputum samples and prompt culture of specimens, the diagnostic yield of the sputum culture may be improved.[95]

Antigen detection in respiratory secretions has been used for over 2 decades to try to maximize the diagnostic yield of sputum, especially for infections caused by *S. pneumoniae, Pneumocystis, Legionella pneumophila*, and a variety of respiratory viruses.[115] In addition to the quelling reaction, counterimmunoelectrophoresis (CIE), coagglutination, and enzyme-linked immunosorbent assay (ELISA) have been used to detect pneumococcal polysaccharide with 70% to 90% sensitivity and a specificity of 80%. However, with these assays, colonization may be confused with infection, cross-reactivity with oral streptococci may occur, and prior therapy with antibiotics may lower overall sensitivity. Direct fluorescent antibody assays may detect *L. pneumophila* with a specificity of over 90%. Sensitivity ranges from 25% to 75% and non-*pneumophila* strains of *Legionella* may be missed.[116,117] Lipopolysaccharide detection with enzyme immunoassay has been used to detect both *Chlamydia trachomatis* and *Chlamydophila pneumoniae* in respiratory tract secretions. However, cross-reactivity with normal oral flora, the relatively low amount of lipopolysaccharide in respiratory secretions, and the inability to distinguish one species of *Chlamydia* from another are persistent problems.

Although direct fluorescent antibody tests have been used to detect *C. trachomatis,* the assay is insufficiently sensitive (varying between 20% and 60%) for detection of *C. pneumoniae*.[115] On the other hand, direct fluorescent antibody assays are over 80% sensitive and 90% specific when used for the detection of *Pneumocystis*.[118,119]

Detection of microbial nucleic acid in respiratory tract secretions remains an area of ongoing study.[120-122] Initially, nucleic acid hybridization techniques were used to detect herpes simplex virus, cytomegalovirus, *M. pneumoniae, Legionella* species, and mycobacteria. Nucleic acid amplification using the polymerase chain reaction (PCR) has received the most recent attention.[122] The technique represents a rapid and relatively simple means of identifying organisms with potentially high specificity and sensitivity and has been applied to organisms that are otherwise cumbersome to identify using usual microbiologic techniques; these organisms include *L. pneumophila, M. pneumoniae, C. pneumoniae,* cytomegalovirus, and *Pneumocystis,* as well as more common bacterial pathogens including *S. pneumoniae*.[123] Although the majority of studies have involved sputum, PCR of throat swabs has been shown (in small numbers of patients) to be a rapid way of diagnosing *L. pneumophila, M. pneumoniae,* and *C. pneumoniae* infections. PCR offers the potential advantage of high sensitivity even early in the course of infection, with little loss of sensitivity due to prior antibiotic usage. Furthermore, the assay does not depend on a normal host response to infection. Differentiation between infection and colonization and between active infection, latent infection, and past infection remains a problem. False-negative results may occur because of the presence of natural inhibitors. Furthermore, the technique has not yet been standardized. PCR techniques have been used to identify DNA from *M. tuberculosis* in both sputum and lavage fluid. Sensitivities of 83.5% and specificities as high as 99% have been noted. Sensitivities of 63% have been reported in patients who were smear negative but culture positive.[124] However, PCR has been reported to be positive in 70% of people with prior exposure to tuberculosis but no active disease. This problem of false-positive results remains.

Antibody coating of bacteria in respiratory secretions has been used as a means of differentiating infection from colonization in intubated patients.[125] Although the assay has been reported as specific for the presence of lower respiratory infection, the sensitivity is only 46%, and it cannot clearly differentiate purulent bronchitis from pneumonia. It, too, remains experimental.

Transtracheal Aspiration

Although the sputum examination should always be included in the initial evaluation of patients with pneumonia, it may be inadequate for a presumptive diagnosis. In cases in which (1) no sputum is produced, (2) no clear predominance of a potential pathogen exists on sputum Gram stain or culture, (3) there has been a poor response to antibiotics chosen on the basis of expectorated sputum, (4) gram-negative rods or yeast forms are found in the sputum, or (5) the possibility of superinfection exists, a more direct method of obtaining lower respiratory tract secretions may be necessary.

In the past, transtracheal aspiration has been used as a means of obtaining lower respiratory tract secretions with minimal oropharyngeal contamination. However, because of the fear of adverse reactions, most clinicians now use other methods to obtain lower respiratory tract secretions.

Fiberoptic Bronchoscopy

Initial studies concerning the usefulness of fiberoptic bronchoscopy for the diagnosis of bacterial pneumonia demonstrated that the procedure was limited by contamination of specimens by oropharyngeal flora. Cultures obtained via the bronchoscope averaged two to three more bacterial isolates than samples from paired transtracheal aspirates.[126] In patients without lower respiratory tract infections, cultures of aspirates obtained at bronchoscopy produced an average of five different bacterial species. The development of the protected brush catheter (a brush within two catheters sealed at the end with a polyethylene glycol plug) decreased but did not eliminate this problem. Quantitative culturing has been used to differentiate contaminants from true infecting agents.

Approximately 10^6 to 10^8 organisms per milliliter are present in lung tissue involved with pneumonia. Accounting for dilution of samples, a bacterial count of more than 10^3 to 10^4 has been used as a breakpoint for determining the clinical significance of an isolate.

Studies employing the protected brush catheter have proved experimentally and clinically to be both sensitive (70% to 97%) and specific (95% to 100%) for the diagnosis of bacterial pneumonia.[127] However, not all series using this technique have produced impressive results,[128-130] and in some patient groups this technique is not useful. These include patients who have already received antibiotics, patients with purulent bronchitis in whom bacterial counts greater than 10^3 are noted, and patients with underlying structural disease in whom over 50% of bronchoscopic specimens yield significant numbers of organisms even in the absence of pneumonia.[127] Detection of the antibody coating of organisms found at bronchoscopy has been used in an attempt to differentiate colonization from true infection. Experience has been limited and results have been mixed, with a high false-positive rate noted in patients with chronic bronchitis. Gram stain of specimens obtained from fiberoptic bronchoscopy has been used as a guide to empirical therapy while cultures are pending.[131,132] A positive Gram stain predicts growth of more than 10^3 colony-forming units (CFU)/mL with up to 78% sensitivity.

In practice, however, fiberoptic bronchoscopy is usually not performed on patients with community-acquired pneumonia unless severe pneumonia, unresolving pneumonia, or a clear failure of antibiotic therapy is encountered.[133,134] The procedure may be useful in defining the cause of ventilator-associated pneumonia. Bronchoscopy with a protected specimen brush has been shown to have a sensitivity of 82% to 100%, a specificity of 60% to 77%, a positive predictive value of 43% to 74%, and a negative predictive value of 85% to 100% when compared with quantitative cultures of infected lung.[135-138] Not all studies have shown such good results; a sensitivity of 36%, a specificity of 50%, and positive and negative predictive values of 43% have also been reported.[139,140] Differences in exclusion and inclusion criteria, different definitions of pneumonia, and the acceptance or rejection of patients with recent antibiotic changes may explain the different results. The use of antibiotics markedly diminishes the diagnostic yield of the procedure.[141,142] Most bacterial species initially found by a protected specimen brush are undetectable after 72 hours of antibiotic therapy, and the majority of organisms found are resistant to the antibiotics given. These may have no role in the infection. However, in a patient with ongoing pneumonia despite antibiotic therapy, bronchoscopy with a protected specimen brush should pick up resistant organisms that may be playing a role in infection.[136]

False-negative findings are seen in up to 30% to 40% of patients, which may reflect the fact that bacterial counts may differ by 50-fold in areas of infected lung versus noninfected adjacent areas, making the sampling site an important consideration.[128] Other possible explanations include prior antibiotic use, technique problems, and in some cases an early stage of pneumonia where bacterial numbers are not yet high enough to reach the breakpoint of the procedure.[143]

Bronchoalveolar Lavage

Bronchoalveolar lavage (BAL), in which a segment of the lung is washed with sterile fluid, has been used for determining the cause of pneumonia. Approximately 100 million alveoli are sampled, and consequently a larger area of lung is evaluated than with the protected specimen brush. A diagnostic threshold of 10^4 CFU/mL is utilized with lavage since the procedure recovers 5 to 10 times more organisms than brushing. The most consistent results have been seen in the diagnosis of *Pneumocystis* pneumonia in patients with AIDS. Diagnostic yields of 89% to 98% have been reported.[144,145] Excellent yields have been noted in detecting cytomegalovirus in patients with AIDS as well as in bone marrow and solid organ transplant recipients.[146,147] The isolation of the organism does not prove that it is the cause of the pneumonia. By using immunofluorescent monoclonal antibodies to viral antigens or centrifuging lavage material into tissue culture preparations, the identification of cytomegalovirus can be made within hours rather than days to weeks.[148]

BAL has proved especially useful for diagnosing pneumonia caused by *M. tuberculosis*.[149,150] Culture of BAL material has a sensitivity of 85%, even in the presence of negative cultures of expectorated sputum and gastric aspirate. In patients with miliary tuberculosis in whom sputum culture yields are low (25%), culture of *M. tuberculosis* from BAL fluid approximates 100%. In addition to culture and staining, adenosine deaminase levels and ELISA for antibodies to *M. tuberculosis* have been studied.[151-154] BAL has also been used for the diagnosis of atypical pneumonias, including those caused by *Legionella* species and *Mycoplasma pneumoniae*.[151]

BAL has been used as a means of diagnosing ventilator-associated pneumonia. When compared with quantitative cultures of infected lung, sensitivities of up to 91%, specificities of 78% to 100%, positive predictive values of 83%, and negative predictive values of 87% have been noted.[192] Microscopic examination of cells from lavage has also been used to diagnose pneumonia. When greater than 5% of cells from BAL contain bacteria, pneumonia has been diagnosed with sensitivities of up to 90% and specificities of 89% to 100%.[136,155] Similar values have been noted when more than 2%, or more than 7% of cells with intracellular bacteria have been used as the threshold for diagnosing pneumonia.[156,157] The procedure appears to be repeatable and may yield results even if antibiotics are present, especially if no recent changes in antibiotics have occurred.[142,158] Studies vary as to threshold levels of bacteria, patient selection, and standards for determining the presence of pneumonia. Consequently, sensitivity, specificity, and predictive values vary. Overall, however, despite the inconsistencies of study design, bronchoalveolar lavage appears similar in efficacy to the protected specimen brush as a means of diagnosing the cause of ventilator-associated pneumonia.[159]

The use of BAL for the diagnosis of pneumonia in other clinical settings and with other pathogens is less well defined. By using cytologic screening, quantitative cultures of BAL fluid, or Gram stain criteria, bacterial pneumonia has been identified in non-AIDS immunosuppressed patients, patients with severe community-acquired pneumonia, and patients with nonresolving pneumonia.[134] In addition to quantitative culture and Gram stain of BAL fluid, quantitation of endotoxin has been used to detect the presence of gram-negative pneumonia.[160]

Although the risks of bronchoscopy are relatively small, hypoxia occurs in 13% to 28% of patients on ventilators undergoing BAL.[132,161] In patients with gram-negative pneumonia, the procedure may be followed by a sepsis-like picture with increased temperature and decreased mean arterial pressure.[162]

Other Techniques

A variety of less invasive techniques have been used in attempts to determine the cause of pneumonia without resorting to bronchoscopy. Blind endotracheal suctioning with quantitative cultures has compared favorably with bronchoscopic procedures in some studies.[163,164] With a threshold of greater than 10^5 CFU/mL, the sensitivity for predicting ventilator-associated pneumonia was comparable to that of lavage or protected brush procedures, although the specificity was somewhat lower.[164] Furthermore, no differences in mortality, the length of stay in the intensive care unit, or the duration of mechanical ventilation were noted when quantitative endotracheal cultures were used as the sole means of diagnosis compared to bronchoalveolar lavage and to protected specimen brush.[165] Others have reported false-negative rates of over 30% and many more organisms isolated by endotracheal suctioning than by brushing.[166] At present, this procedure is best used when bronchoscopy cannot be done.

The blind protected specimen brush has compared favorably with bronchoscopically guided procedures, with 86% agreement.[165,167] Nonbronchoscopic bronchioloalveolar lavage has been obtained in some cases by a protected catheter to minimize contamination. Sensitivities of 70% to 80% and a specificity of 66% to 96% have been noted.[168-170] Mortality from ventilator-associated pneumonia is unchanged independent of whether bronchoscopic or nonbronchoscopic procedures are used for diagnosis.[171]

Lung Biopsy

Direct means of obtaining diagnostic material in patients with pneumonia include percutaneous lung aspiration, transbronchial lung biopsy, thoracoscopy, and open lung biopsy.[172] These procedures are usually reserved for cases of pneumonia in impaired hosts and in pediatric populations, in whom sputum is not routinely available.

Biopsy procedures are rarely indicated in the previously well patient with acute pneumonia. The indications and usefulness of these invasive procedures remain controversial. Lung aspiration has provided a diagnostic yield of 30% to 82% in adults and children, although false-negative rates of up to 18% have been reported.[173,174] Bleeding and pneumothorax have been reported as major complications in 5% to 39% of procedures.[174] The use of transbronchial biopsy in the diagnosis of pneumonia has been reviewed, revealing similar diagnostic yields although somewhat lower complication rates.[175]

Thoracoscopy, in which the pleura and underlying lung are visualized before biopsy, has been used in several series of children and adults with pneumonia. Despite a diagnostic yield of over 90% and low complication rates,[176,177] there has not been extensive experience with this procedure.

Open lung biopsy remains the definitive invasive procedure for making an etiologic diagnosis of pneumonia in immunosuppressed patients, with diagnostic yields of 60% to 100%.[175,178] The incidence of pneumothorax and bleeding is usually less than 10%, even in patients who are thrombocytopenic.[175] However, some have questioned whether open lung biopsy provides meaningful information that significantly affects patients' clinical outcome.

Examination of Pleural Effusions

The characteristics of pleural effusions and their importance in the differential diagnosis of pulmonary disease are discussed in Chapter 62. It should be noted that the incidence of pleural effusions associated with pneumonia varies with the etiologic agent, from approximately 10% with pneumococci, to 50% to 70% with gram-negative bacilli, to up to 95% with group A streptococci.[104,179,180] Pleural fluid cultures, when positive, are specific for the organism causing the underlying pneumonia. Furthermore, analysis of pleural fluid may play a major role in differentiating other causes of pulmonary infiltrates that may mimic pneumonia, including tuberculosis, tumors, pulmonary emboli, and collagen vascular diseases.[181] Pleural biopsy specimens from patients with acute bacterial pneumonia are nonspecific and are therefore of little use in the differential diagnosis. Analysis of pleural fluid may be of prognostic significance.

A pleural fluid pH of less than 7.2 has been associated with the presence of a complicated parapneumonic effusion and the need for a tube thoracostomy.[182] Although the determination of glucose and lactate dehydrogenase levels has been suggested by some to discriminate between complicated and uncomplicated parapneumonic effusions, they do not appear to be as accurate as pH in this regard. PCR technology has been useful in detecting *M. tuberculosis* in effusions with a sensitivity of approximately 70% and specificity of 100%.[183] Adenosine deaminase, an enzyme associated with lymphocytes, may also be used to detect *M. tuberculosis,* with sensitivity and specificity of 93%.[184] Detection of the lymphocyte-related cytokine soluble IL-2 receptor may also be useful.[185]

Blood Culture, Serologic Studies, and Urine Studies, Including Antigen Detection and DNA Amplification

Blood cultures are positive in only 1% to 16% of patients hospitalized with community-acquired pneumonia, and their usefulness and cost effectiveness have been questioned.[186] However, the presence of positive blood cultures is highly specific, helps identify a patient population with a greater mortality rate, and may be of use in narrowing antibiotic alternatives. In addition, patients with HIV infection, those with underlying malignancy, those receiving immunosuppressive agents, and those residing in nursing homes have an increased risk for bacteremia. Finally, unusual organisms may be identified that may not be adequately treated by routine empirical coverage.[187] Therefore, blood cultures should be obtained from all patients suspected of having bacterial pneumonia who are ill enough to be hospitalized.

Serologic assays have been used for decades to try to identify potential etiologies of pneumonia. Success in this regard has been limited, although recent improvements have been made. Serum antibody assays for diagnosis of the *M. pneumoniae* and *Chlamydophila pneumoniae* have been widely utilized. The Centers for Disease Control and Prevention (CDC) and the Laboratory Centre for Disease Control (LCDC) have established diagnostic standards. Microimmunofluorescence (MIF) for serum chlamydophilal antigens has been recommended, and an IgM titer of greater than 1:16 or a fourfold rise in IgG value is used to define positivity. Use of a single IgG value is not viewed as a definitive test. Because the present assays show day-to-day variation, it has been suggested that acute and convalescent titers be assayed at the same time.[188] A fourfold rise in IgG rather than a single clinical titer is accepted as a positive test for *M. pneumoniae.* Although an elevated IgM titer suggests a recent infection, reinfection with mycoplasma occurs frequently and a rise of IgM may not always be seen.[189] Cold agglutinins may be elevated in infections with *M. pneumoniae* among others. Titers greater than or equal to 1:4 are suggestive of *M. pneumoniae* infection.

S. pneumoniae produces a variety of antigens and surface markers that are type- or species-specific.[190] Since the demonstration by Dorff and associates that pneumococcal-related antigens could be detected by CIE,[191] a variety of techniques have been used to attempt to identify pneumococci. Antigen detection in serum with these methods has not proven clinically useful. Serologic assays have been used to detect antibodies against pneumococcal antigens, including pneumococcal C polysaccharide, capsular polysaccharide, phosphorylcholine, pneumolysin, and pneumococcal surface adhesin A. Antibody detection against the capsular polysaccharide and C polysaccharide have reported sensitivities of 97% and 89%, respectively.[192] Similar sensitivities have been reported with detection of antibodies to surface adhesin A. Overall, lack of uniform testing criteria, lack of clear controls in some series, and positive results in patients without evidence of pneumococcal disease have made the role of antibody detection in diagnosing pneumococcal pneumonia unclear. CIE and latex agglutination techniques have been used for the detection of *H. influenzae* and pneumococcal antigens in patients with pneumonia, although clinical experience has been limited and the results have been inconsistent.[193]

A variety of assays have been utilized to detect pathogens that have been difficult to isolate using routine culture techniques. Serologic assays have been used to diagnose infections caused by *Legionella* species, *M. pneumoniae, Chlamydophila* species, and *Coxiella burnetii.*[194] The sensitivity and specificity of the assays vary, and their usefulness in making a rapid diagnosis is limited.

PCR techniques for the detection of microbial DNA continue to be developed. *S. pneumoniae* may be detected in the blood of bacteremic patients with a sensitivity as high as 100% and a specificity of 94%.[195] The highest diagnostic yields have been associated with phenol extraction of DNA to remove serum inhibitors, a technique that is labor intensive and therefore not suited to most clinical labs. Moreover, only pneumonia associated with bacteremia would be expected to be detected. PCR has also been used to detect DNA from *Pneumocystis* in blood from patients with AIDS[196] and in BAL fluid.[123] Diagnostic efficacy has essentially been equal to that of immunofluorescence staining.

PCR techniques have also been used for detection of *Legionella,* but the assay remains experimental. DNA probes have been used to successfully identify *M. tuberculosis, Mycobacterium avium intracellulare, Mycobacterium kansasii,* and *Mycobacterium gordonae* from colonies growing in solid and liquid medium. This has reduced the time of identification from 59 days to between 17 and 31 days.

Recent evidence suggests that cytokine responses may be a useful adjunct in diagnosing pneumonia.[197,198] C-reactive protein is an acute-phase reactant produced in the liver as a response to a variety of stimuli, including infection. Elevated C-reactive protein levels have been observed in patients with community-acquired pneumonia and appear to be a potential means of distinguishing pneumonia from purulent bronchitis and noninfectious conditions. Normal values of less than 10 mg/L are unusual in patients with pneumonia and can be used to exclude the diagnosis. Levels of 100 mg/L or greater suggests the diagnosis of pneumonia but may be seen in noninfective processes such as pulmonary infarction and neoplasia. Other cytokines studied include IL-6 and TNF-α, but their correlations with pneumonia appear less consistent.

Antigen detection in urine rather than blood or sputum has become a successful means of detecting some important pulmonary pathogens. Soluble *L. pneumophila* antigen can be detected in urine using a radioimmunoassay, although it is useful for detecting only *L. pneumophila* serogroup 1.[199] This assay offers the advantage of being noninvasive, and it has a sensitivity of 80% to 95% and a specificity estimated to be 99%. An ELISA is also available. Although test results may be available on the day of testing, antigenuria may persist for weeks to months after therapy.[199] Recently, an immunochromatographic membrane test has been developed to detect in urine the C polysaccharide cell wall antigen found in all *S. pneumoniae.*[200] Using a variety of standard diagnostic tests as controls, overall sensitivities of approximately 70% to 80%, specificities of approximately 77% to 97%, and positive predictors of 62% have been noted.[201,202] Sensitivities have, in general, been high in bacteremia episodes, with the yields increased slightly by concentrating the urine. The assay in children has a decreased specificity, as false-positive tests occur with nasopharyngeal carriage alone without documented pneumonia.[203]

Radiologic Examination

Chest radiography plays a critical role in the diagnosis of pneumonia, and for many it represents the gold standard of making a clinical diagnosis. The differential diagnosis of respiratory complaints and abnormal physical findings includes upper and lower respiratory tract infection as well as an array of noninfectious entities.[204] Demonstration of an abnormal chest radiograph consistent with pneumonia differentiates a patient population that may benefit from antibiotic therapy from the populations that will not. Because overuse of antibiotics for therapy of upper respiratory infections has been documented and may contribute to the growing problem of antibiotic resistance, identifying patients who really should be receiving antibiotic therapy is clearly of importance. The chest radiograph is readily available, is reasonably reliable (despite interobserver variability),[205] and should be obtained in most patients suspected of having pneumonia.[205,206] The extent and nature of radiographic abnormalities may define patients who are more seriously ill and may need close monitoring.[207]

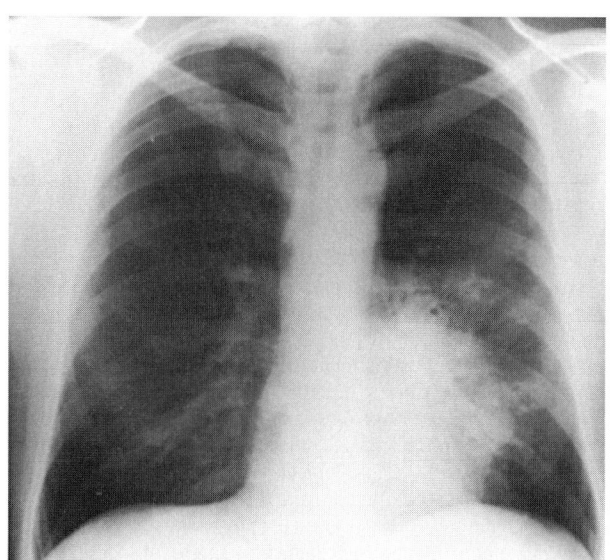

FIGURE 61-8. Patchy infiltrate representing bronchopneumonia in a patient with *Streptococcus pneumoniae* infection.

However, the chest film usually does not show an infiltrate pattern that is very helpful in making a specific etiologic diagnosis (Fig. 61-8). Certain features may be of some diagnostic aid. Lobar consolidation, cavitation, and large pleural effusions support a bacterial cause (Fig. 61-9). Most lobar pneumonias are pneumococcal, whereas most pneumococcal pneumonias are not lobar. When bilateral diffuse involvement is noted, *Pneumocystis* pneumonia, *Legionella* pneumonia, or a

primary viral pneumonia should be suspected. Staphylococcal pneumonia may result from infection metastasizing from a primary focus unrelated to the lung. In these cases, multiple nodular infiltrates throughout the lung may be seen. Staphylococci may cause marked necrosis of lung tissue with ill-defined thin-walled cavities (pneumatoceles), bronchopleural fistulas, and empyema, especially in children (Fig. 61-10). Although pneumatoceles are diagnostically significant findings in staphylococcal pneumonia, they may be seen in pneumonias with other causes, including *K. pneumoniae, H. influenzae, S. pneumoniae,* and, more rarely, *Pneumocystis.*[208] Pulmonary infections due to *Pseudomonas* may cavitate. *Pseudomonas* and other gram-negative bacilli most commonly cause lower lobe pneumonia.

Aspiration pneumonia should be considered along with gram-negative and staphylococcal pneumonias as a source of necrotizing pneumonia, cavitation, and empyema. Aspiration pneumonia commonly involves either the superior segment or the basilar segment of either lower lobe, or the posterior segment of the upper lobes, depending on whether aspiration occurred in the dependent or the upright position.[209] Chronic aspiration most commonly results in a bilateral lower lobe pneumonia, although it may involve one side more than the other.

Viral infection of the lower airway involves respiratory epithelium and parenchyma adjacent to terminal respiratory bronchioles. Diffuse hemorrhagic congestion of alveolar septa may occur as well.[210] The radiographic concomitants of these pathologic findings usually involve patchy areas of peribronchial ground-glass opacity, air-space consolidation, and poorly defined small nodules. Diffuse and localized involvement with both interstitial and alveolar patterns has been noted (Fig. 61-11).[210] There is little radiologic distinction between the various viral etiologies of pneumonia. Influenza pneumonia is associated with poorly defined, patchy air-space consolidation with rapid confluence. Varicella pneumonia usually involves peribronchial involvement with nodular infiltrates. Adenovirus may be associated with diffuse

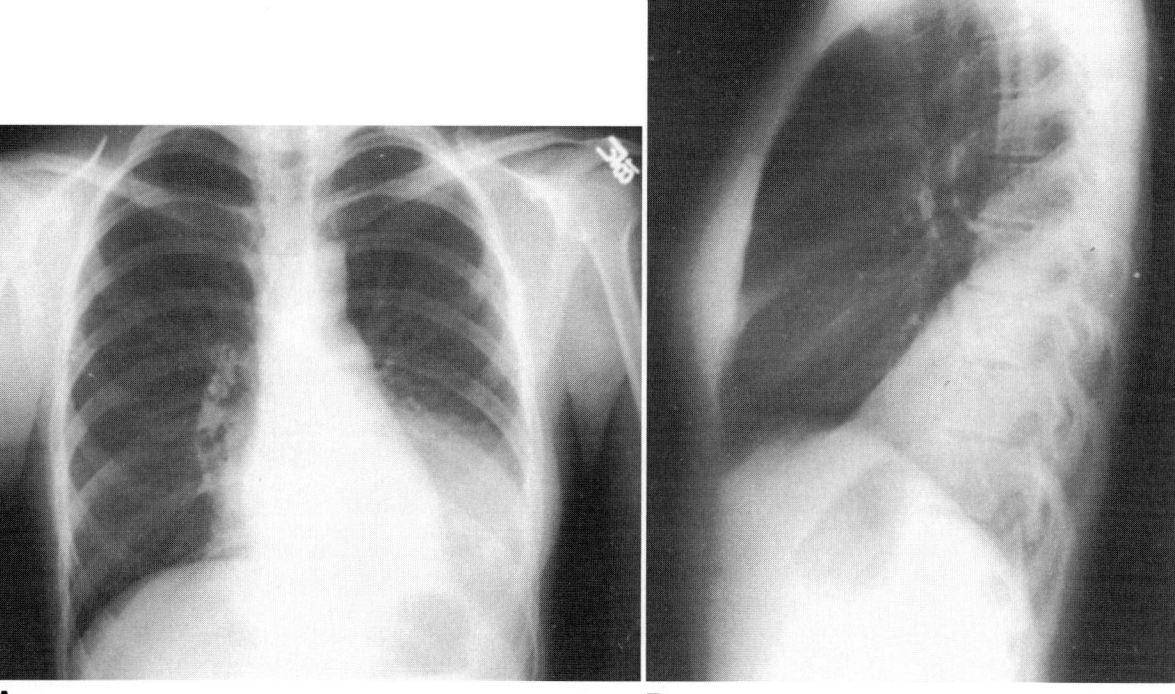

A   **B**

FIGURE 61-9. A, Posteroanterior film showing dense left lower consolidation consistent with bacterial pneumonia, in this case caused by *Streptococcus pneumoniae.* **B,** Lateral film of a patient with left lower lobe pneumococcal pneumonia.

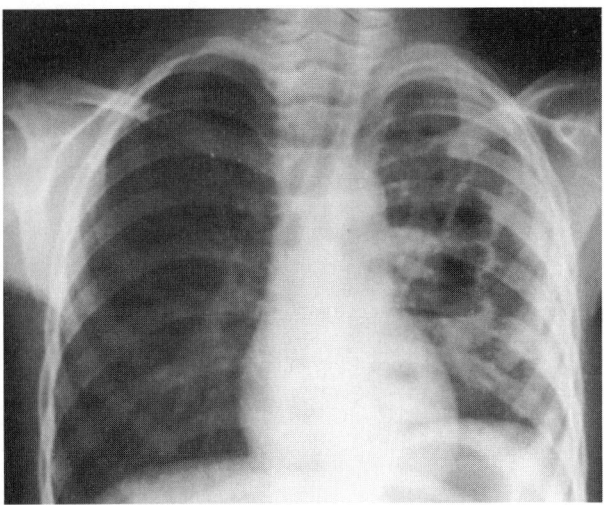

FIGURE 61-10. Pneumatocele formation in the left upper lobe of a patient with staphylococcal pneumonia.

bilateral bronchopneumonia, areas of overinflation, and atelectasis. Lobar or subsegmental consolidation mimicking bacterial pneumonia may also be seen. Hantavirus pneumonia usually presents with interstitial edema, which may progress to consolidation representing a pulmonary capillary leak syndrome. Bilateral involvement and pleural effusion are common.[210] The most recently described viral cause of pneumonia is the coronavirus associated with SARS. The majority of cases manifest with bilateral basilar infiltrates primarily involving an interstitial pattern. Progression with symmetric air-space disease has been commonly described.[211,212]

Mycoplasmal pneumonia often manifests with an interstitial pattern in a peribronchial distribution. As more edema fluid is elaborated, there may be rapid progression to lobar or sublobar consolidation. Once this consolidation stage is reached, radiologic differentiation between bacterial and mycoplasmal pneumonia is difficult. *Mycoplasma* is usually associated with lower lobe disease. Cavitation is rare, although pleural effusion may be seen in 20% of the cases.[213]

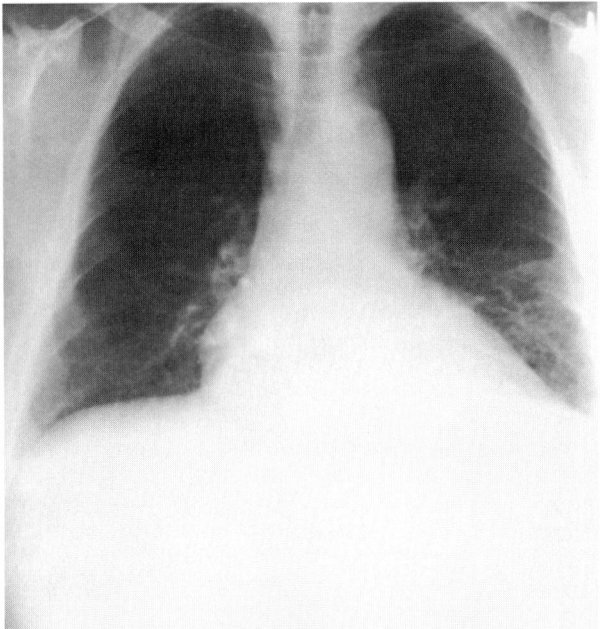

FIGURE 61-11. Bilateral involvement with a mixed interstitial-alveolar pattern in a patient with viral pneumonia.

Legionnaires' disease may initially present with a radiographic picture similar to that of mycoplasmal pneumonia. A patchy interstitial or finely nodular pattern is seen in the lower lobe.[214] However, unlike the situation with mycoplasmal pneumonia, pneumonia with more than two-lobe involvement is commonly seen. Rapid progression and pleural effusions are also common. Pneumonia caused by *Legionella micdadei* may present with pulmonary nodules, either single or multiple, as well as with segmental infiltrates. As in pneumonia caused by *L. pneumophila,* rapid radiologic progression of the disease is characteristic.[215]

Chest radiographs are most helpful in conjunction with the clinical history and physical examination, but, as noted previously, are often not helpful in making a specific etiologic diagnosis. This point was clearly shown by Tew and associates, who evaluated readings of radiographs of patients with pneumonia made without clinical information.[216] Pneumonia was correctly identified as bacterial only 67% of the time and as viral only 65% of the time. Mycoplasmal pneumonia was incorrectly identified as bacterial 81% of the time.

The usefulness of computed tomography (CT) in managing chest infections, including pneumonia, has been reviewed.[217-219] In the immunocompetent host, chest CT is most helpful in evaluating recurrent pneumonia or infections unresponsive to therapy. Pneumonia developing behind an obstruction caused by tumors or other masses and lung abscess may also be better defined by CT than by routine chest radiographs. High-resolution CT has been shown to improve radiographic characterization of lung infection.[217-219] Compared with a routine chest radiograph, high-resolution CT detects lung abnormalities more often and does a better job in defining disease in the upper and lower lobes and in the lingula.[218] However, exposure to more radiation (the radiation from one CT scan equals that from six to seven chest radiographs) and the increased expense (approximately seven times the cost of a chest radiograph) has limited its use as the initial radiographic procedure. Furthermore, it is unclear if all abnormalities found on the chest CT scan truly represent pneumonia. In the immunocompromised host in whom infection is only one of the possible causes of abnormal chest radiographs, chest CT or one of its variations, such as spiral CT or high-resolution CT, may aid in better defining a "questionable" chest radiograph and may be helpful in localizing involved areas of lung as a guide to biopsy procedures.[218] Certain infections, such as those caused by *Aspergillus, M. tuberculosis,* and *Pneumocystis,* have characteristic appearances on CT that in the correct clinical setting may make invasive procedures unnecessary. Newer techniques such as perfusion magnetic resonance imagery have been shown to be able to differentiate pneumonia from COPD and pulmonary emboli. The overall clinical utility of these techniques remains to be proven.[220]

Nuclear medicine procedures have been used to detect pneumonia. These procedures include gallium-67 citrate scans, indium 111–labeled granulocyte scans, and technetium-99 diethylenetriamine penta-acetic acid aerosol clearance.[221] In general, these procedures have been used in patients with AIDS to define the presence of lung infection in the absence of abnormal chest radiographs. In patients with AIDS, diffuse uptake of gallium is usually seen with *Pneumocystis* infection but may also be seen with infection caused by *Mycobacterium avium* complex, cytomegalovirus, and *Cryptococcus neoformans,* and in patients with lymphoma. Localized uptake may be associated with bacterial disease. Focal uptake corresponding to lymph node areas has been associated with *M. avium* complex, *M. tuberculosis,* and lymphoma.

PNEUMONIA SYNDROMES

Acute Community-Acquired Pneumonia

A long list of bacterial, fungal, viral, and protozoal agents may cause pneumonia. Because initial evaluation rarely results in a specific etiologic diagnosis, antibiotic therapy is usually begun empirically. Defining pneumonia syndromes on the basis of clinical, epidemiologic, radiographic, and laboratory parameters, with a limited number of organisms commonly associated with each syndrome, has helped the clinician to select rational empirical therapy for the most likely organisms involved. Many of the syndromes have overlapping signs and symptoms, which at times makes clear identification of a specific syndrome in an individual impossible.[222,223] Furthermore, the characteristics of the syndrome of acute community-acquired pneumonia as defined almost 30 years ago[64,67] are changing.[223-231] The patient population is aging and includes more patients with significant coexistent diseases and more patients who are immunosuppressed. Microbial agents now recognized as potential causes of community-acquired pneumonia were not previously recognized.[223-228]

The American Thoracic Society, in consensus statements in 1993 and 2001, developed four subgroupings of community-acquired pneumonia based on the age of the patient, the need for hospitalization, the severity of illness, and the presence of coexisting disease.[230] This "splitting" of the syndrome of acute community-acquired pneumonia recognized the diversity of the patient population and of the organisms potentially involved. It grouped together bacterial causes usually involved in acute community-acquired pneumonia and those involved in atypical pneumonia syndromes, including *M. pneumoniae, Chlamydophila* species, respiratory viruses, and *Legionella* species. Treatment recommendations were made for each subgroup. The Infectious Disease Society of America developed similar guidelines in 1998 and 2000, with an update in December 2003.[232] These guidelines based the criteria for antibiotic selection on the severity of illness, comorbidity, exposure, and the epidemiologic setting.[98] The distinction between acute bacterial community-acquired pneumonia and atypical pneumonia became blurred even further. However, defining pneumonia syndromes as they have classically been described is a reasonable first step in making clinical decisions.

Patients with acute community-acquired pneumonia are usually in their mid-fifties to late sixties.[186,226,227] Although peak incidences of disease in midwinter and early spring have been described, there is no "pneumonia season," and disease takes place throughout the year.[228] Most patients (58% to 89%) have one or more chronic underlying diseases, including COPD, cardiovascular disease, neurologic disease, diabetes, or alcohol abuse.[186,223,227,232,233] Immunosuppression related to malignancy, neutropenia, the chronic use of steroids or myelosuppressive agents, or HIV infection may be present in up to 57% of patients.[100,223,234]

Classically, community-acquired pneumonia presents with a sudden onset of a chill followed by fever, pleuritic chest pain, and cough that produces mucopurulent sputum. The signs, symptoms, and physical findings vary according to the age of the patient, therapy with antibiotics before presentation, and the severity of illness. These classic findings in some combination are present in approximately 81% of patients with community-acquired pneumonia. Patients usually present after having been ill for a mean of 6 days. Cough is noted in greater than 80% to 90% of patients and is productive in 60% to 80%.[60,223,228-231] Chest pain is present in 30% to 46% of cases, chills in 40 to 70%, and true rigors in 15%.[59,60,223,227,228]

A variety of nonrespiratory symptoms are associated with pneumonia, including fatigue (91%), anorexia (71%), sweats (69%), and nausea (41%).[59] Both respiratory and nonrespiratory findings occur less frequently in older age groups.[59]

Physical examination reveals fever in 68% to 78% of patients but may be seen less commonly in older populations. Tachypnea (respiratory rate greater than 24 to 30 breaths per minute) is noted in 45% to 69% of patients and may be more frequently seen in older age groups.[59] Tachycardia (pulse rate greater than 100 beats per minute) is noted in 45%. Rales are noted in 78% of patients, and signs of consolidation are noted in 29%.

Most commonly, the white blood cell count is in the range of 15,000 to 35,000/mm³, and the differential cell count reveals an increased number of juvenile forms. Leukopenia may be noted and is a poor prognostic sign.[235] The hematocrit and the red blood cell indices are usually normal. Elevation of C-reactive protein (as noted earlier) to 50 to 100 mg/L is usually found in patients with pneumonia, with a sensitivity of up to 100%.[61] Sputum is thick and purulent and may be rust colored. The sputum Gram stain reveals numerous neutrophils and bacteria, often with a single organism predominating. Chest films show areas of parenchymal involvement, usually with an alveolar-

filling process. There is moderate hypoxemia due to ventilation perfusion abnormalities. Even with rigorous laboratory evaluation and using definitions of *definite, probable,* and *possible* causes, a microbiologic diagnosis may be made in only 20% to 70% of cases of community-acquired pneumonia.[63,100,186,207,223,228,232]

In the past, 50% to 90% of cases of acute community-acquired pneumonia were caused by *S. pneumoniae.*[57] More recently, some published reports have indicated that the relative importance of the pneumococcus has varied, showing this range to be from 16% to 60%.[86,224-229] However, the pneumococcus remains the leading cause of the syndrome of acute community-acquired pneumonia in most series.

Advanced age, cigarette smoking, congestive heart failure, institutionalization, dementia, seizures, diabetes mellitus, malnutrition, and the presence of chronic illnesses such as COPD, chronic liver and kidney diseases, AIDS, malignancy, and cerebrovascular disease have been identified as significant risk factors for the development of pneumococcal pneumonia.[236] Severe pneumococcal infections, including pneumonia, have been associated with prior splenectomy due either to trauma or to staging for Hodgkin's disease,[237,238] abnormal immunoglobulin responses (myeloma, lymphoma, HIV infection),[239] and functional asplenia due to systemic lupus erythematosus or marrow transplant.

An estimated 3% to 38% of cases of acute community-acquired pneumonia are caused by *H. influenzae.*[64,67,100,240,241] The true incidence of this organism is obscured by the difficulty of isolating it from sputum and identifying it in sputum Gram stain, and by the difficulty of distinguishing colonization from infection. The age of patients, presence of underlying disease, and presentation are all similar to those of pneumococcal disease.

S. aureus accounts for 2% to 5% of acute community-acquired pneumonia cases[100,242] and takes on increased importance as a cause of pneumonia in older adults, and in those with influenza.[243] Patients who develop postinfluenza pneumonia are usually younger and have less underlying disease than most other patients with community-acquired pneumonia. Clinical signs and symptoms of influenza are present but appear to resolve over several days. After a variable period of time ranging from 2 to 14 days, symptoms suddenly reappear, with the onset of shaking chills, pleuritic chest pain, and cough that produces purulent sputum. An elevated white blood cell count with a shift to the left, physical signs of pulmonary consolidation, and radiographic evidence of focal parenchymal disease appear. The sputum Gram stain is consistent with bacterial pneumonia. Although the pneumococcus still represents the most common etiologic agent, staphylococcal disease occurs with a higher frequency than that noted in non–influenza-related, community-acquired pneumonia.[243]

Aerobic gram-negative bacteria, exclusive of *H. influenzae,* and mixed aerobic and anaerobic infections cause most of the remaining cases of acute community-acquired pneumonia. Gram-negative rods may cause anywhere from 7% to 18% of pneumonia cases. Half of these cases will be caused by *Pseudomonas aeruginosa.*[100] Gram-negative bacilli are particularly important pathogens in older adults, especially those with chronic underlying disease and those who are bedridden and recently hospitalized. *Pseudomonas* infection should be suspected in patients with pulmonary comorbidities and recent hospital stays.

The importance of *Legionella* species in causing pneumonia varies greatly in different geographic areas. Although incidences as high as 17% to 30% have been reported,[244] some centers report significantly lower rates of 2% to 8%.[100,223,228] No clinical features reliably distinguish *Legionella* species pneumonia from that caused by other bacteria. However, the presence of a high fever (>40° C), male sex, previous β-lactam therapy, multilobar involvement, rapid progression of radiographic abnormalities, a need for intensive care, gastrointestinal and neurologic abnormalities, elevated liver enzyme levels, and increased creatinine levels have all been associated with *Legionella* pneumonia.[223,244,245] Scoring systems have been developed using these criteria to differentiate *Legionella* pneumonia from pneumococcal pneumonia, but sensitivities and specificities have remained unacceptably low.[246,247]

Moraxella catarrhalis has also been identified as a cause of pneumonia.[248] The overall incidence of disease caused by this bacterium is low, but it is an important pathogen in older adults with COPD and various forms of immunosuppression.

Mild Community-Acquired Pneumonia

Most of the information concerning the cause of community-acquired pneumonia has been gathered from series of hospitalized patients. However, approximately 50% to 80% of episodes of community-acquired pneumonia are treated in the outpatient setting, and the relative importance of various etiologic agents has not been well characterized in this patient population. *S. pneumoniae* has been implicated in 9% to 36% of outpatient community-acquired pneumonias. The relative importance of *H. influenzae* appears similar to that noted in inpatients, although an increased incidence of *H. influenzae* pneumonia was observed in a recent series.[249] In the outpatient setting, the percentage cases of pneumonia involving *S. aureus* appears lower (0% to 1%) and those involving *M. pneumoniae* higher (up to 37%). Approximately 8% to 14% of mild pneumonias are viral in origin. Influenzae A and B, parainfluenza virus, adenovirus, and respiratory syncytial virus are the important agents involved.[250]

Community-Acquired Pneumonia in the Older Adult

Pneumonia is the third most common reason for hospitalization in those 65 and older and represents a major cause of morbidity and mortality. In some series, pneumonia represents the leading cause of death in this population (see Chapter 314).[251] For those over the age of 60, pneumonia is a predictor of increased mortality after the specific episode has resolved and for several years thereafter.[252]

The clinical presentation of pneumonia in older adults (especially those over 80) may be more subtle than in younger populations, with more gradual onset of symptoms and fever and the classic signs of pneumonia.[59,223,253-255] Fever occurs less commonly in older adults, and temperature elevation is muted.[59,223,255] The classic findings of cough, fever, and dyspnea may be absent in over half of older adults.[253,256,257] Chills and rigors may be less frequently seen as well.[59,223,253,254] Tachypnea (respiratory rate of greater than 24 to 30 per minute) is a more frequent finding in older adults and has been observed in up to 69% of patients. Rales are common and are noted in 78% to 84% of patients, although signs of true consolidation are found in only 29%. Nonrespiratory symptoms may be the major presenting feature. The initial presentation of older adults with pneumonia may include decline in functional status, weakness, subtle changes in mental status, and anorexia or abdominal pain. It has been suggested that the nonspecific presentation of pneumonia in older adults may result in great part from the prevalence of dementia in this population.[256] Bacteremia, metastatic foci of infection, and death are more frequent in older populations.[64,88,233,235]

Specific etiologic diagnoses are made less frequently in older adults, with approximately 20% to 50% of patients having an etiologic agent defined.[253,255,258,259] The absence of productive cough and common prior use of antibiotics may explain this observation. Etiologies have varied in different series depending on the means of diagnosis, the patient population studied (outpatient versus institutionalized older adults), and the geographic location.[253] In general, the cause of community-acquired pneumonia in the older population follows the general trend of infection in younger populations. *S. pneumoniae* remains the predominant organism, accounting for 20% to 60% of cases.[253] *Haemophilus influenzae*, usually a nontypable strain, is frequently the second most common agent, accounting for 7% to 11% of episodes.[260] The importance of other aerobic gram-negative bacilli in causing pneumonia in older adults remains a question in part because the criteria for diagnosis of true pneumonia versus colonization varies. In recent studies, 1% to 3% of pneumonia may be caused by non-*Haemophilus* gram-negative bacilli.[255] Although increased oropharyngeal colonization with aerobic gram-negative bacilli has been documented in the older population and is thought to be a predisposition to development of pneumonia caused by these organisms, colonization appears to be related to debility of the patient rather than age.[261] Other factors associated with increasing colonization with gram-negative organisms include prior use of antibiotics, decreased activity, diabetes, alcoholism, and incontinence.[254] Older adults are at greater risk for infection with group B streptococci, *M. catarrhalis,* and *Legionella* species, although the overall incidence of these agents in the older population is relatively low.[248] Polymicrobial infections and pneumonia due to aspiration have both been noted to occur more frequently in older adults.[88,262,263]

It is unclear which agents cause atypical pneumonia in the older population. Most series suggest that *M. pneumoniae* pneumonia is unusual, although it has been documented by other investigators to be a significant cause of pneumonia leading to hospitalization in older adults.[63,264] *Chlamydophila* infections appear commonly in the older population and may cause up to 21% of pneumonias.[265]

Viral agents may also play an important role in causing pneumonia in the older population. In one series, both respiratory syncytial virus and influenza A caused infection in 10% to 11% of the patients studied. Forty-eight percent of those infected with respiratory syncytial virus and 30% of those infected with influenza virus had pneumonia.[266] As in younger populations, dyspnea, wheezing, and sputum production are hallmarks of disease with those agents, with bronchospasm appearing more frequently with respiratory syncytial virus.[267] Coinfection with bacteria was noted in over 17% of cases, making the role of the viruses in causing the presenting symptoms of pneumonia somewhat unclear. Rhinovirus also appears to be an important cause of respiratory infection in older adults, with 24% of some populations infected. Although about two thirds of those infected have lower respiratory tract symptoms, the role of rhinovirus as a cause of pneumonia is unclear.[268]

Residents of nursing homes represent an important subpopulation of older adults at risk for pneumonia.[269] Pneumonia is the second most frequent infection in this setting and carries the highest mortality of any infection. Silent aspiration[270] is a major risk factor, as are poor functional status, nasogastric feeding, swallowing difficulties, confusion, the presence of obstructive lung disease, the presence of a tracheostomy, and advancing age. The subtle presentation noted in other older adult populations occurs in those in a nursing home setting.[271] *Streptococcus pneumoniae* remains the predominant cause, followed by nontypable strains of *H. influenzae* and *M. catarrhalis.* Other organisms such as *Chlamydophila, Mycoplasma pneumoniae, Legionella,* and aerobic gram-negative bacilli including *P. aeruginosa,* are infrequent causes. Outbreaks of pneumonia have occurred in nursing homes and have involved *Legionella, Chlamydophila, influenza, parainfluenza,* and respiratory syncytial virus.[258]

Community-Acquired Pneumonia in Patients with AIDS

The cause of community-acquired pneumonia in patients with AIDS has changed significantly since the beginning of the epidemic. Before the development of effective prophylactic regimens, *Pneumocystis* pneumonia occurred in approximately 85% of these patients, with a mortality rate in 1987 of 32.5%.[272,273] The incidence of *Pneumocystis* disease was halved and mortality rates dropped to 13.8% in 1992.[77,274] In patients who refuse prophylaxis or who have advanced untreated HIV infection, *Pneumocystis* infection remains a significant problem. Furthermore, even with prophylaxis, *Pneumocystis* infection may develop in the setting of severe immune deficiency.[77,275] Recent data suggest that *Pneumocystis* still accounts for over one third of episodes of pneumonia in HIV-positive populations.[276] Bacterial pneumonia remains a major source of morbidity and mortality in HIV-infected patients. The rate of invasive pneumococcal disease can be 100 to 300 times greater in HIV-infected patients than in non–HIV-infected controls.[276,277] *H. influenzae* and *S. aureus* are also important pathogens.[75,81,82,274,277,278] A variety of other bacteria have been implicated, including *Rhodococcus equi* and *P. aeruginosa,* the latter being associated with late stages of disease, the presence of central venous catheters, the presence of urinary catheters, and the use of steroids. *Mycobacterium tuberculosis,* nontuberculous mycobacteria, *Cryptococcus neoformans,* and cytomegalovirus also play important roles as etiologic agents.[75] The incidence of pneumonia reported to be caused by atypical agents is low.[276] Even with careful study, up to one third of HIV-infected patients with pneumonia may have an infection without a proven etiology.

Severe Community-Acquired Pneumonia

Approximately 10% of community-acquired pneumonia cases are severe enough to require intensive care and/or mechanical ventilation.[227,279-281] Advanced age, presence of significant comorbid diseases including pulmonary disease and congestive heart failure, inadequate or delayed antibiotic therapy, and genetic predisposition have all been thought to be associated with the development of severe community-acquired pneumonia.[282] *S. pneumoniae* and *L. pneumophila* are the organisms most commonly involved. Gram-negative bacilli, especially *Klebsiella* species, must be considered in patients who have significant underlying disease such as COPD, diabetes, and alcohol abuse.[279] In some series, *M. pneumoniae* is involved in up to 11% of community-acquired pneumonia patients requiring intensive care.

In 1993, the American Thoracic Society developed a series of parameters, any one of which would define severe pneumonia.[283] These included the following:

1. Greater than 30 breaths per minute on admission
2. A ratio of arterial oxygen tension to fractional inspired oxygen, or PaO$_2$/FIO$_2$, of less than 250
3. The need for mechanical ventilation
4. Bilateral or multilobar involvement on chest radiograph
5. An increase in the size of the pulmonary infiltrate of up to 50% in the first 48 hours
6. Systolic blood pressure less than 90 mm Hg
7. Diastolic blood pressure less than 60 mm Hg
8. The need for vasopressors for more than 4 hours
9. A urine output of less than 20 mL/hour or total output of less than 80 mL over 4 hours
10. Acute renal failure

Although the majority of these parameters have been associated with mortality, a validation of this definition of severe pneumonia found a high sensitivity but a low specificity.[284]

A means of predicting mortality in patients with community-acquired pneumonia requiring mechanical ventilation has been attempted on the basis of parameters collected over the first 24 hours of admission.[285] Advanced age (>80), medical comorbidities with a survival expectancy of less than 5 years, organ failure, immune suppression, and a hypoxemic index measuring lung damage helped predict hospital mortality.

Mortality rates in patients with severe pneumonia have ranged from 20% to 53%, which is higher than the 2% to 30% noted in all community-acquired pneumonias.[63,100,227,279-282,286,287] Tachypnea (>30 breaths per minute), diastolic blood pressure less than 60 mm Hg, and blood urea nitrogen levels above 7 mmol/L have been shown to be independently associated with death from pneumonia.[288-290] Other parameters identified with increased mortality include severe underlying disease, underlying neoplastic disease, age greater than 60 years, absence of pleuritic chest pain, a change in mental status, acute respiratory failure requiring ventilatory support, bilateral pulmonary involvement, bacteremia, a neutrophil count under 3500, a total serum protein level less than 45 g/L, a serum creatinine level greater than 15 mg/L, the presence of shock, inadequate initial antibiotic therapy, radiographic evidence of spreading disease, and pneumonia caused by *S. aureus* or gram-negative bacilli.[290,291]

Slowly Resolving Community-Acquired Pneumonia

The natural history of adequately treated community-acquired pneumonia is usually that of prompt resolution.[292] In healthy young military personnel recovering from pneumococcal pneumonia, fever resolved after 2.5 days, cough after 7.9 days, and "crackles" on physical examination of the chest by 8 days.[293] Normalization of the white blood cell count occurred by day 4. Similar results are found in more

"typical" patients with community-acquired pneumonia, who were older with more comorbid illnesses.[294] Vital sign stabilization usually occurred in 2 to 6 days, depending on the definition of normalization. Radiographic abnormalities may take 4 to 10 weeks to normalize, with younger (<50 years of age) patients resolving more quickly.[295,296] Patients who fail to resolve their radiographic abnormalities by day 30, despite clearing of signs and symptoms, usually have significant underlying pulmonary disease such as emphysema, chronic bronchitis, pneumoconiosis, or asthma.

Slowly resolving pneumonia has been defined as less than 50% clearing of radiographic abnormalities at 2 weeks and less than complete clearing of abnormalities by 4 weeks.[296] Host factors such as age greater than 50 years, a history of alcoholism, and the presence of significant underlying diseases (COPD, diabetes, congestive heart failure, asthma, malignancy) have been found to be associated with slow resolution of pneumonia. Rate of resolution may also depend on the etiologic agent, with *S. pneumoniae* usually requiring up to 6 weeks, *Legionella* usually requiring 2 to 6 months, and *Mycoplasma* usually requiring several weeks.[296,297]

When pneumonia appears to be slowly resolving, several explanations must be explored. The organism under treatment may have developed resistance, the wrong organism may have been treated, or pneumonia may be the incorrect diagnosis. A variety of clinical entities may mimic pneumonia, including bronchiolitis obliterans organizing pneumonia (BOOP), neoplasms, vasculitis, pulmonary hemorrhage, and eosinophilic pneumonia.

Atypical Pneumonia Syndrome

By the late 1930s, most of the main bacterial causes of pneumonia had been defined. In 1938, Hobart Reiman described a small number of patients with a clinical picture that was atypical in that episodes began as a mild respiratory tract illness that was followed by pneumonia with dyspnea and cough without sputum.[298] *M. pneumoniae*, *Chlamydophila pneumoniae* (formerly known as *Chlamydia pneumoniae*), and *L. pneumophila* are the most significant causes of atypical pneumonia. Other agents such as *Chlamydophila psittaci* (formerly *Chlamydia psittaci*), *Francisella tularensis*, *M. tuberculosis*, *Coxiella burnetii*, and a variety of respiratory viruses may also cause atypical pneumonia. In AIDS patients, *Pneumocystis* and nontuberculous mycobacteria should also be included. Although some series report that almost 50% of patients with community-acquired pneumonia demonstrate serologic evidence of mycoplasmal or chlamydial pneumonia, or both, other series suggest an incidence of 7% to 28%.[63,222,299] The overall frequency of atypical pneumonia varies depending on the means of diagnosis. A single IgG elevation, which is commonly used for diagnosis, may not be as specific as a fourfold rise in antibody, thereby falsely increasing the reported incidence of disease. As noted previously (see "Blood Culture, Serologic Studies, and Urine Studies"), a more standardized means of diagnosing *C. pneumoniae* infection has been suggested by the CDC and the LCDC. Cultures, although technically more difficult, have also been viewed as a definitive means of diagnosis, as has PCR on respiratory tract secretions. Other variables that play a role in the incidence of infection include the geographic location, the age of the patients, and the presence or absence of an epidemic during the study period.[299,300] Furthermore, dual infections, usually with a "typical" bacterial pathogen, may occur in up to two thirds of patients with suspected mycoplasmal or chlamydial infection, which raises the question as to the true role of atypical agents.[301,302]

In the past, the epidemiology and clinical features of the atypical pneumonias were thought to be distinct enough to clearly differentiate them from other causes of community-acquired pneumonia. However, it is now clear that differentiation between atypical agents and typical bacterial causes of community-acquired pneumonia is imprecise.[223]

Mycoplasma pneumoniae infection is most likely to occur in the older child (older than 5 years), the adolescent, and the young adult. The majority of cases occur in those less than 40 years of age. Data suggest that *M. pneumoniae* is an etiologic agent of pneumonia leading to hospitalization in older patients as well, although the incidence of mycoplasma in the older population varies from less than 1% to 5%.[63,264] Overall, this agent accounts for 1% to 20% of cases of community-acquired pneumonia, with the highest percentages noted in patients who remain ambulatory.[63,98,100,222] As noted earlier, the lack of a definitive means to diagnose the infection early makes a discussion of epidemiology tentative. An increased incidence of disease and true epidemics has been documented in relatively enclosed populations of young adults at military bases, colleges, and boarding schools. Mycoplasmal infection occurs throughout the year, although a relative increase in incidence is noted in the late summer and fall. In contrast, adenovirus infection, another cause of atypical pneumonia, most commonly occurs between January and April, and these outbreaks occur primarily in military recruit camps.

The course of *M. pneumoniae* is characterized by up to 10 days of symptoms before presentation, as is true with many of the other agents involved in atypical pneumonia. In its classic form, mycoplasmal infection presents with constitutional symptoms and a progression from the upper to the lower respiratory tract. Sore throat is often the initial finding. Bullous myringitis is seen in only about 5% of cases but when present is suggestive of mycoplasmal infection. Fever, malaise, coryza, headache, and cough represent the major clinical findings. Pleuritic chest pain, splinting, and respiratory distress are not usually seen. Moist or crepitant rales may be heard. Sputum production is variable, and the sputum is purulent in one third to one half of the cases. Gram stain and culture of sputum usually reveal mouth flora. White blood cell counts greater than 10,000/mm³ are uncommon, occurring in approximately 20% of the patients.[103] An elevated sedimentation rate is noted in about 25% of the cases. Pulmonary involvement seen on radiographs is commonly more extensive than the physical examination would indicate. Unilateral or bilateral patchy infiltrates in one or more segments, usually in the lower lobes, are noted in a bronchial or peribronchial distribution. Upper lobe involvement and pleural effusions are rare. Progression of the radiographic picture, despite a stable clinical picture, may be seen. The overall clinical course in most cases is benign. Disappearance of constitutional symptoms is usually noted in the first and second weeks, although cough and radiographic changes may persist for several weeks. Occasionally, *M. pneumoniae* infection presents as severe community-acquired pneumonia requiring intensive care.[227] A large number of extrapulmonary manifestations may occur with *M. pneumoniae,* including involvement of skin, central nervous system, blood, and kidneys (see Chapter 181).

Chlamydophila pneumoniae has emerged as an important cause of atypical pneumonia and may account for approximately 6% to 12% of community-acquired pneumonia cases.[63,98,100,222,303,304] It has also been postulated to be an important copathogen, most often associated with *S. pneumoniae*.[305] Although disease is uncommon in those younger than 5 years, serologic evidence of infection has been noted in over 50% of adults.[306] Disease usually occurs sporadically, although epidemics have been well documented. The majority of infections are either asymptomatic or produce mild symptoms. As with mycoplasmal infection, sore throat and hoarseness herald the onset of pneumonia, although the progression of symptoms appears slower than that noted with mycoplasma or viral pneumonia.[306,307] Cough may begin after several days to weeks, suggesting a biphasic illness. Hoarseness and sinus tenderness appear more commonly than in patients infected with *Mycoplasma* or viruses.[306] The white blood cell count is rarely elevated. Pneumonia with *C. pneumoniae* is usually mild, although complete recovery may be slow. Cough and malaise may persist for weeks to months. Reinfection occurs and appears to be milder than primary infection and is usually not associated with pneumonia. Chronic and latent infections have also been described. Infection with *C. pneumoniae* has been associated with exacerbations of COPD and asthma.[308] In general, few features distinguish chlamydial pneumonia from infection caused by other atypical agents or other bacteria.[309] *C. pneumoniae* infections have been associated with extrapulmonary manifestations, including otitis, sinusitis, pericarditis, myocarditis, and endocarditis.[310] It has also been associated with coronary artery disease, although the definite relationship remains unclear (see Chapter 179).

Chlamydia trachomatis may be a pulmonary pathogen in immunocompromised and in healthy hosts.[311,312] Productive cough, myalgias, and fever associated with diffuse nonsegmental infiltrates appear most commonly. The agent has also been associated with chronic pneumonia in neonates and infants. Onset occurs at 2 to 3 weeks of age and is associated with tachypnea, a staccato cough with periods of cyanosis and emesis, a lack of fever, and diffuse interstitial and patchy alveolar infiltrates on chest radiographs. Elevated IgG and IgM levels and absolute eosinophilia have also been noted.

Of the viral agents associated with atypical pneumonia in adults, influenza A and B, adenovirus types 3, 4, and 7 (especially in military recruits), parainfluenza virus,[313] and respiratory syncytial virus (especially in older adult and immune-suppressed patients) are the most common.[314-316] Data suggest that respiratory syncytial virus may cause pneumonia in 1% to 5% of immunocompetent adults. Wheezing by history and rhonchi on physical examination are characteristic. Reports of other viral agents causing pneumonia are scant but have included rhinovirus,[192] enterovirus, coronavirus, the herpesviruses, hantavirus,[317,318] and the newly described human metapneumovirus. A coronavirus has been shown to be the agent involved in SARS (see Chapter 152).[319]

Legionella is now recognized as an important cause of the atypical pneumonia syndrome, although patients infected with *Legionella* may also present with acute bacterial community-acquired pneumonia. It accounts for 2% to 8% of cases involving hospitalization.[63,98] *Legionella* species are among the top three to four organisms causing pneumonia that requires intensive care unit monitoring.[287,320,321] *L. pneumophila* causes over 80% of cases of *Legionella* pneumonia, with approximately 50% of cases caused by serogroup 1.[299,322] Inhalation of aerosolized organisms after exposure to environmental reservoirs, such as fresh water and moist soil, has been the usual means of acquiring the organism, although aspiration is now thought to be an alternate route of infection.[323] An increased incidence during summer months has been observed.

Cigarette smoking, chronic lung disease, and immunosuppression are consistently noted risk factors for the development of disease. *Legionella* pneumonia may present as either a typical acute community-acquired pneumonia or as an atypical pneumonia. Although early symptoms of malaise, muscle aches, headaches, and nonproductive cough resemble the onset of a viral syndrome, the rapid progression of pulmonary symptoms and relatively high fever, often exceeding 40° C, is noteworthy.[323]

Legionella pneumophila pneumonia is associated with a variety of extrapulmonary findings and laboratory abnormalities, including mental status changes, abdominal complaints (loose stools or diarrhea), headache, bradycardia, elevation of hepatic enzyme levels, hypophosphatemia, hyponatremia, elevated serum lactate dehydrogenase levels, and elevated serum creatinine levels. No single finding or laboratory test can distinguish *L. pneumophila* pneumonia from pneumonias of other causes. As noted earlier, scoring systems have been developed that may help identify *Legionella,* but the systems have not been validated in large prospective series.[245-247] Extrapulmonary infection is unusual, but when it does occur, it usually involves the heart with myocarditis, pericarditis, and postcardiotomy-like syndrome.[323] Unfortunately, none of these findings distinguishes between *L. pneumophila* pneumonia, pneumonia caused by other atypical agents, and pneumonia caused by more typical bacterial pathogens.[324] Similarly, radiographic manifestations do not distinguish *Legionella* infections from those of other causes. Patchy interstitial infiltrates, or nodular infiltrates that may progress rapidly even with adequate therapy, are characteristic. Pleural effusions may be noted in up to one third of patients.

Pneumonia in the Setting of Aspiration

The clinical setting in which aspiration occurs includes any disease state in which consciousness is altered and the normal gag and swallowing reflexes are abnormal. Older adult patients; patients in chronic care facilities, especially those who are neurologically impaired;

patients during the acute phase of stroke; bedridden patients receiving tube feedings; and patients with dementia fit into the category of individuals susceptible to aspiration.[262,263,325,326]

The pathogenesis of lung injury due to acid aspiration has been delineated.[327] The presence of acidic contents in the lung induces the release of proinflammatory cytokines including TNF-α and IL-8. These and other cytokines recruit neutrophils into the lung. Activated neutrophils appear to be the key mediators of acute lung injury after acid aspiration, although a role for complement has also been demonstrated.[328]

Although aspiration may be a witnessed event, the majority of episodes are silent and are brought to medical attention by their sequelae.[326] Three major syndromes are recognized as a consequence of aspiration: chemical pneumonitis, bronchial obstruction secondary to aspiration of particulate matter, and bacterial aspiration pneumonia.[329,330] Aspiration may be associated with the acute respiratory distress syndrome, atelectasis, bronchial hyperreactivity, and fibrosis. Bacterial aspiration pneumonia occurs in more than 60% of cases of chemical aspiration.[262] Although chemical pneumonitis and mechanical obstruction usually cause acute symptoms, aspiration pneumonia is more insidious, with symptoms usually occurring gradually several days after the initial episode of aspiration. Pneumonitis, necrotizing pneumonia, abscess, and empyema are common. Symptoms often include fever, weight loss, and productive cough. Putrid sputum is produced in 50% of the cases.[90,218] Anemia and an elevated white blood cell count are frequently associated findings. The bacteriologic findings in aspiration pneumonia reflect the flora of the oropharynx, and the importance of periodontal disease in this regard has been noted. Studies have documented anaerobic involvement alone in 45% to 58% of cases[331,332] or in combination with aerobes in 22% to 46% of cases.[90,333] *Bacteroides* species, *Porphyromonas* species, *Prevotella melaninogenica, Fusobacterium* species, and anaerobic gram-positive cocci are the predominant anaerobes isolated. In community-acquired aspiration pneumonia, *Streptococcus* species and *H. influenzae* are the most common aerobic isolates.[331,334,335] *M. catarrhalis* and *Eikenella corrodens* may also be involved.[334] In contrast, gram-negative bacilli (including *P. aeruginosa*) and *S. aureus* are the most commonly isolated aerobes from nosocomial aspiration pneumonia including ventilator-associated pneumonia.[331,335]

Pulmonary Infiltrates with Eosinophilia

Pulmonary infiltrates with eosinophilia (PIE) is a syndrome associated with a variety of clinical entities, only some of which have an infectious cause.[336] Pulmonary eosinophilia with transient, peripheral pulmonary infiltrates and minimal symptoms has been associated with *Ascaris* and *Strongyloides* infections. *Ascaris* is probably the leading parasitic cause of the syndrome worldwide. Prolonged pulmonary eosinophilia associated with weight loss, fever, cough, and dyspnea may be due to tuberculosis, brucellosis, psittacosis, coccidioidomycosis, histoplasmosis, and parasitic infections including ascariasis, strongyloidiasis, paragonimiasis, echinococcosis, visceral larva migrans, cutaneous larva migrans, and infections with *Schistosoma, Dirofilaria immitis,* and *Ancylostoma* species. Noninfectious causes include drug allergy, sarcoidosis, eosinophilic leukemia, Hodgkin's disease, and hypersensitivity pneumonitis (e.g., pigeon breeders' disease).[337] A PIE syndrome has been associated with *Pneumocystis* pneumonia in AIDS patients.[338]

Acute eosinophilic pneumonia is a distinct clinical entity occurring in younger (20- to 30-year-old) otherwise healthy individuals. It is marked by the acute onset of dyspnea, nonproductive cough, fever, hypoxia, and chest pain.[339] Although leukocytosis is common, peripheral eosinophilia is usually absent. Bilateral, diffuse pulmonary infiltrates are commonly seen. Radiographic abnormalities usually begin as interstitial infiltrates that progress to alveolar infiltrates. Chest CT reveals a "ground glass" opacification with interlobular septal thickening.[339] BAL yields marked (25% to 62%) eosinophilia, which is the diagnostic feature of the disease. Although most patients have received antibiotics, rapid stabilization occurs with steroid use.

It has been suggested that chronic eosinophilic pneumonia may represent a unique clinical entity that is a form of collagen-vascular disease or an infection in a hyperimmune patient.[340-342] A subacute onset of cough, dyspnea, fever, and weight loss associated with peripheral eosinophilia are the common features. Unlike the situation in acute eosinophilic pneumonia, respiratory failure is rare. Peripheral infiltrates are usually seen on radiographs. Focal interstitial fibrosis, bronchiolitis obliterans, microabscesses, and sarcoid-like granulomas are characteristic pathologic features. A rapid response to steroids has been reported.[341]

Tropical eosinophilia consists of myalgia, fatigue, weight loss, and anorexia associated with cough, frequently with nocturnal exacerbations, wheezing, dyspnea, and marked peripheral eosinophilia in patients who have lived in or visited the tropics.[343] Radiographic changes are distinctive and include increased interstitial markings with 2- to 4-mm nodules throughout the lungs with preferential involvement of the bases. Most cases are thought to represent immunologic hyperresponsiveness to microfilarial infection and can be treated with diethylcarbamazine.

Other causes of PIE syndrome include bronchopulmonary *Aspergillus,* which should be suspected when a patient with PIE presents with asthma and pulmonary vasculitis. Patients with the Churg-Strauss syndrome frequently have eosinophilia along with allergic angiitis and granulomatosis and present with asthma, diffuse pulmonary infiltrates, and multiorgan involvement. Hypereosinophilic syndrome, eosinophilic granuloma (also known as primary pulmonary Langerhans' cell histiocytosis), BOOP, Sjögren's syndrome, and postradiation pneumonitis are unusual cases of pulmonary infiltrates with eosinophilia.

Nosocomial Pneumonia and Pneumonia in the Immunosuppressed Host

Nosocomial pneumonia is the second leading type of nosocomial infection and accounts for 13% to 18% of all such infections. It is the leading cause of infection-related deaths in hospitalized patients with an attributable mortality of 33% to 50%.[344-347] Higher mortality rates have been observed when patients are bacteremic or have pneumonia caused by *P. aeruginosa* or *Acinetobacter* species. The morbidity associated with nosocomial pneumonia includes longer hospital stays (an average of 7 to 9 days) and higher costs for health care (an estimated $2 billion annually).[348]

Risk factors for the development of nosocomial pneumonia have been categorized as patient related, infection-control related, or intervention related.[347] Patient-related risk factors include age greater than 70 years, severe underlying disease, malnutrition, coma, metabolic acidosis, and the presence of any of a number of comorbid illnesses (COPD, alcoholism, azotemia, central nervous system dysfunction). An association has been made between the presence of sinusitis and the subsequent development of pneumonia, although it remains unclear whether the relationship is causal.[349] Infection-control–related risk factors include a lack of hand hygiene and glove-use practices and the use of contaminated respiratory equipment. Intervention-related risk factors involve those procedures and therapies that undermine normal host defenses or allow the host to be exposed to large inocula of bacteria. Sedatives and narcotics may lead to aspiration; corticosteroids and cytotoxic agents blunt the normal host response to infection; and the prolonged use of antibiotics engenders resistance. Surgical procedures, especially involving the chest and abdomen, are associated with changes in host defenses that predispose to pneumonia. The use of ventilatory support is perhaps the greatest risk factor for the development of nosocomial pneumonia, presenting a risk over 20 times that of unventilated patients.[350,351] Data suggest that there is a 1% to 3% per day risk for developing pneumonia while on a ventilator.[350] Because of this preeminence as a risk factor, the term *ventilator-associated pneumonia* (VAP) has been accepted as an important subcategory of nosocomial pneumonia.

The use of antacids and histamine type 2 blockers that raise the gastric pH has been shown to increase stomach colonization with aerobic gram-negative rods. Whether this leads to an increase in nosocomial pneumonia remains controversial.[352-354] Demonstration that gastric colonization precedes tracheal colonization has been inconsistent: colonization has been noted in only 9% to 32% of patients observed. Furthermore, the percentage of patients with VAP caused by organisms initially found in the stomach ranges from 0% to 55%.[355]

Approximately 60% of cases of nosocomial pneumonia are caused by aerobic gram-negative bacilli, with members of the family Enterobacteriaceae (*K. pneumoniae, Escherichia coli, Serratia marcescens, Enterobacter* species) and *Pseudomonas* species accounting for the majority of these. *S. aureus* causes 13% to 40% of nosocomial pneumonia and appears to be more common in burn units, in patients with wound infections, and in patients recently ventilated after neurosurgery or head trauma.[351,356] In contrast to its prominent role in community-acquired pneumonia, *S. pneumoniae* causes only 3% to 20% of nosocomial pneumonias in most studies and is associated with infection developing early in the hospital course.[87,357] Anaerobic bacteria have been isolated in up to 35% of cases of nosocomial pneumonia, although usually less than 5% of infections are thought to be caused by these organisms.[358,359] They play a role when aspiration is likely to have occurred. Pneumonia caused by *Legionella* species may occur sporadically or as part of outbreaks. As many as 60% of patients with nosocomial *Legionella* pneumonia are immunosuppressed. Inhalation of organisms from environmental sources has been suspected as the primary route of entry, although aspiration has been suspected as well.[360] Twenty-five percent to 46% of VAP may be polymicrobial.[350] Nosocomial viral infections have been recognized in children and adults. Respiratory syncytial virus, influenza, and parainfluenza make up the majority of viral causes.[361,362]

Nosocomial pneumonia has been characterized as early, occurring within the first 4 days of hospitalization, or late, occurring after this time. Early-onset pneumonia usually involves organisms associated with community-acquired pneumonia including the pneumococcus, *H. influenzae*, and *M. catarrhalis*. Late-onset pneumonia is more often associated with enteric gram-negative bacilli (*E. coli, Enterobacter* species, *Serratia* species), *P. aeruginosa*, and *S. aureus*.

The clinical features of nosocomial pneumonia are nonspecific, and a variety of noninfectious diseases may be responsible for fever, changing chest radiographs, purulent sputum, and an elevated white blood cell count in a critically ill patient. Using clinical criteria alone, the presence of nosocomial pneumonia may be missed 20% to 30% of the time and therapeutic decisions may be ineffective in two thirds of patients.[363,364] The role of invasive procedures in diagnosing nosocomial pneumonia, especially VAP, remains controversial.[365,366] Although both bronchoscopic and nonbronchoscopic samplings of lower respiratory tract secretions have been used to successfully diagnose VAP, differences in patient populations examined, different results from different centers, a lack of agreement on quantitative breakpoints for a positive study, and lack of a clear gold standard have prevented meaningful comparisons of procedures. An in-depth discussion of nosocomial pneumonia can be found in Chapter 301.

Pneumonia in the immunocompromised host is perhaps the most complex of all the pneumonia syndromes, as it represents the interaction of host defense defects engendered by the underlying disease as well as the chemotherapy of that disease, exposure to potential pathogens in the community and within the hospital setting, and reactivation of infectious processes that had previously been dormant. Community-acquired pneumonia, atypical pneumonia, aspiration pneumonia, and nosocomial pneumonia all take place in the compromised host. A large number of bacterial, fungal, viral, and noninfectious etiologies must be considered.[367] A review of the topic is found in Chapters 304, 306 to 308, and 310 to 312.

CLINICAL EVALUATION AND THERAPY FOR PNEUMONIA

The first decision confronting the clinician is whether the patient presenting with respiratory symptoms in fact has pneumonia. The difficulties in establishing a diagnosis on clinical grounds and the potential problem of overprescribing empirical antibiotics for all patients with respiratory findings have been reviewed. A chest radiograph is usually necessary to establish a diagnosis of pneumonia.

The next decision is whether the patient is to be hospitalized, as will be the case approximately 18% to 30% of the time.[349,368,369] Over a dozen series have examined prognostic features and predictors of the clinical outcome for patients with community-acquired pneumonia that are useful to address this issue. Most use a combination of clinical, epidemiologic, laboratory, and radiographic parameters.[61,368-370]

The most widely used prediction system (the PORT study) was generated by analyzing over 14,000 hospitalized patients and applying it to over 40,000 patients in both an inpatient and an outpatient setting.[371] In non–HIV-positive patients, the 30-day mortality was lowest (0.1%) in patients younger than 50 years with no coexisting condition (neoplasia, heart failure, cerebral vascular disease, renal disease, or liver disease) and normal physical findings (including normal mental status, pulse <125 beats per minute, respiratory rate <30/minute, systolic blood pressure >90 mm Hg, and temperature >35° C and <40° C). For patients demonstrating some abnormalities, these and seven further laboratory and radiographic parameters were used to develop a pneumonia severity index. On the basis of the scoring, patients were placed in one of five risk groups with varying mortalities. In general, the older the patient, the greater the physiologic impairment, and the greater the severity index, the higher was the associated mortality. Those with the lowest scores had the lowest risk for death and could therefore be safely considered for outpatient therapy.

Subsequent trials have documented that this index works efficiently and safely to reduce hospitalization for low-risk patients with community-acquired pneumonia.[372,373] Limitations of this type of severity index exist in part because risk for death is not the sole reason for hospitalization. Stability of the home situation, ability to take oral medications, reliability in taking medication, likelihood of returning for follow-up, and likelihood of calling for help when needed all play a role in deciding where a patient should be treated.

It has been suggested that a three-step appraisal be utilized to decide where a patient should be treated. The first step identifies any adverse contraindications to care outside the hospital (e.g., hypoxia, social instability, emotional or psychological instability). The second step involves calculating the pneumonia severity index and assigning the patient to a risk group. The final step is using clinical judgment to be sure the decision to treat a patient at home is consistent with the information gleaned from the history and physical examination. Clinical indices serve only as guidelines and are not meant to be substituted for clinical judgment. Strict reliance on severity indices has failed to predict complex outcomes in up to 39% of patients thought to be well enough to be treated as outpatients.[374]

The next problem is determining the most likely cause of the pneumonia. If diagnostic studies, as described previously, yield a likely cause, then specific therapy should be initiated. Most patients fall into a group in which a specific diagnosis cannot be established with certainty prior to the onset of therapy.

Empirical Therapy of Community-Acquired Pneumonia

Selecting an empirical antibiotic regimen is a continuing clinical challenge. The choice of antibiotic is complicated by the increasing incidence of drug resistance in pneumococci, the potential need to cover both typical and atypical pathogens in certain patient populations, and data suggesting the advantages of combination therapy.

Although it was known that penicillin resistance could be induced in the pneumococcus in 1943,[375] it was not until the late 1960s and the 1970s that penicillin nonsusceptibility was encountered clinically in Australia, Papua New Guinea, and South Africa.[376] In the United States, the incidence of penicillin nonsusceptibility has increased dramatically since the 1970s. Surveillance studies between 1979 and 1987 showed a 4% to 5% incidence of penicillin nonsusceptibility among pneumococci.[377] By the early 1990s, the incidence had increased to 20%, and by the winter of 1999-2000, 34.1% of pneumococcal strains were nonsusceptible and 16.0% were penicillin resistant (minimal inhibitory concentration [MIC] >2 µg/mL).[378,379] Of note, large regional differences in resistance rates were observed, with high rates in the South Atlantic area (24.8%) compared with those in New England (8.3%). Data for the 2001-2002 season suggest that resistance rates have plateaued, with overall nonsusceptibility rates of 33.9% and with 18.4% of strains being overtly resistant to penicillin.

The therapeutic importance of penicillin resistance remains controversial. Several studies have suggested that the presence of a high level of penicillin resistance is associated with an increased mortality in patients with pneumococcal pneumonia.[380,381] However, a recent large prospective study and other older studies could not detect an effect of penicillin resistance on therapy.[380,382-384] Differences in the findings remain unexplained, and for now, most authors feel that the penicillins still have an important role in therapy of community-acquired pneumonia.[385]

An explanation for why penicillins should be effective against relatively penicillin-resistant pneumococci comes from animal data that suggest that clinical success or failure is related to the amount of time serum antibiotic levels remain above the MIC for the infecting organism.[386] Maximal efficiency is achieved when drug levels are above the MIC for at least 40% of the dosage interval. With regard to nonsusceptible *S. pneumoniae,* using higher doses of antibiotic or shorter dosage intervals may provide effective therapy for relatively resistant organisms. Oral penicillins such as amoxicillin and amoxicillin-clavulanic acid can provide this degree of activity even for some organisms that are penicillin resistant. Among the oral cephalosporins, cefuroxime appears to be the most potentially useful, but only for penicillin-intermediate strains of pneumococci. High-dose parenteral penicillin and third-generation cephalosporins such as ceftriaxone and cefotaxime provide consistent coverage even for resistant strains. Other agents, such as ceftazidime and ceftizoxime, appear less potent.[387]

Pneumococcal resistance to penicillin has been paralleled by resistance to other agents frequently used in the therapy of pneumonia. Up to 25.5% of pneumococci resistant to penicillin are resistant to other antibiotics.[388] Resistance patterns of penicillin-resistant pneumococci (as well as sensitive and intermediate strains) to other clinically important antibiotics are shown in Table 61-4.[378,386,389-392] Not enough data have been gathered to reasonably predict what level of resistance will yield clinical failures.

It is important to note that as with penicillins, in vitro susceptibility to other agents does not always predict clinical efficacy. Resistance of *S. pneumoniae* to macrolides and azalides occurs either because of a blockage of the ribosomal binding area encoded by the *erm* (B) gene or because of an efflux pump mechanism encoded by the *nef* (A) gene that removes drug from the cell's interior. The latter usually leads to low-level resistance that may be overcome by higher dosages. The former mechanism is usually associated with high-level resistance that cannot be overcome by higher dosages. Clinical failure has been described even with low-level resistance, making the empirical use of azalides and macrolides problematic.[393-395]

A number of "respiratory tract quinolones" (levofloxacin, moxifloxacin, gemifloxacin, gatifloxacin) are licensed for use in the United States as therapy for respiratory infections. These agents possess activity against the majority of bacterial and atypical agents involved in lower respiratory infections, and their potency is not significantly affected by the presence of penicillin resistance. Interestingly, when these agents are compared clinically with β-lactam antibiotics with various activities against nonsusceptible strains of pneumococci and no real activity against atypical agents, the overall outcomes have, in general, been equivalent. No clear clinical difference in efficacy in therapy for any respiratory tract quinolone over any other has been consistently demonstrated. Resistance to the respiratory tract quinolones by pneumococcal strains has already been reported. Overall resistance rates are 0.2% to 0.9%, but rates may be significantly higher in certain geographic areas. Failure of quinolone therapy for *S. pneumoniae* infection due to resistance is very uncommon.[396]

The question of empirical therapy has been made even more confusing by what appears to be a synergy between β-lactam antibiotics and macrolides, especially azithromycin. Combination therapy with these antibiotics has been associated with decreased mortality and decreased length of hospital stay in older adult patients with community-acquired pneumonia and patients with proven pneumococcal pneumonia, including those with bacteremia.[397-399] Although many of the studies were retrospective, could not identify the etiology of pneumonia in up to 60% to 90% of cases, and did not always control for confounding variables, the possibility that this synergy is clinically significant cannot be discounted.[397-401] It is unclear whether these observations are the result of the activity of macrolide/azalide compounds against agents of

TABLE 61-4 Percentage of Penicillin-Sensitive, -Intermediate, and -Resistant Strains of *Streptococcus pneumoniae* That Show Resistance to Other Antibiotics[*]

Other Antibiotics	*Penicillin Sensitive (MIC ≤ 0.06 µg/mL)*	*Penicillin Intermediate (MIC = 0.12-1 µg/mL)*	*Penicillin Resistant (MIC ≥ 2 µg/mL)*
Amoxicillin-clavulanic acid	0	0	47.4
Cefuroxime	0.1	32-48.9	99-100
Ceftriaxone	0	0.3	9.1-65.7[†]
Trimethoprim-sulfamethoxazole	6.3-11.7	39-60.7	87-96.4
Erythromycin	3.2-5.6	35-44.7	61-77.8
Azithromycin	5.7	43-51	77
Clarithromycin	5.3	41.8	78.1
Tetracycline	1.3	19.1	25.5
Imipenem	0	0	>60%
Meropenem	0	0.8-19	52-96.8[†]
Respiratory tract quinolones[§] (levofloxacin, trovafloxacin, sparfloxacin, grepafloxacin)	0.1-0.4	0.3-1.2	0-1.7
Quinupristin/dalfopristin	0	0.6	0.2
Linezolid	0	0	0
Telithromycin	0	0	0

MIC, minimal inhibitory concentration.

[*]Data are presented as percentages of strains showing resistance based on MIC breakpoint data.
Not all drugs were compared in all studies. The percentage of resistance varies between studies.
Values of MICs may not predict clinical outcomes

[†]Large differences noted in different series may reflect the change in resistance breakpoints occurring in 2000 and 2002 for various agents. Other differences between series are unexplained.

[§]Averages for the group.
Data from references 232, 379, 387, 390, and 391-393.

atypical pneumonia that may be coinfecting agents.[401,402] Other potential explanations include synergistic antimicrobial activity provided by both agents, and macrolide-related anti-inflammatory effects.

Because of the problem of increasing drug resistance, new agents are continually being evaluated. Telithromycin is the first member of the ketolide class of antibiotics to be studied clinically and has good activity against susceptible and penicillin-resistant strains of *S. pneumoniae*, *H. influenzae*, and *Moraxella* species. It is also active against macrolide-resistant strains of *S. pneumoniae*. Early clinical tests suggests that it may play a role in empirical therapy of community-acquired pneumonia.[403]

Guidelines have been developed by the American Thoracic Society, the Infectious Diseases Society of America (IDSA; see update of IDSA guidelines in Table 61-5), and the Canadian Infectious Disease Society.[232] In general, patients are stratified into outpatient versus inpatient treatment. Categories used in analyses are age, severity of illness defined by level of physiologic abnormalities, and

comorbidities as determined by analysis similar to that of the PORT study described earlier. Recognition of the most likely etiologic agent in any given clinical situation and recognition of the organisms most likely to cause morbidity and mortality are emphasized. Finally, prevalence of common antibiotic resistance patterns and risks of acquisition are recognized.[98,101,230]

For a patient who does not require hospitalization and for whom no clear distinction between typical (e.g., pneumococcal) and atypical (mycoplasmal, chlamydial) pneumonia can be made, both types of organisms should be covered. Risks for the presence of drug-resistant *S. pneumoniae* should be assessed. Use of previous antibiotics, especially a β-lactam or macrolide, is most predictive of the presence of resistance. Age alone, in general, should not influence drug choice. Where risk of drug-resistant *S. pneumoniae* is low, oral β-lactam agents (amoxicillin-clavulanic acid, cefuroxime axetil), azalides/macrolides (azithromycin, clarithromycin, or erythromycin), or respiratory tract quinolones (levofloxacin, gemifloxacin, gatifloxacin,

TABLE 61-5 Guide to Empirical Choice of Antimicrobial Agent for Treating Patients with Community-Acquired Pneumonia (CAP)

Patient Variable	Preferred Treatment Options
Outpatient	
Previously Healthy	
No recent antibiotic therapy	A macrolide[a] or doxycycline
Recent antibiotic therapy[b]	A respiratory fluoroquinolone[c] alone, an advanced macrolide[d] plus high-dose amoxicillin,[e] or an advanced macrolide plus high-dose amoxicillin-clavulanate[f]
Comorbidities (COPD, Diabetes, Renal or Congestive Heart Failure, or Malignancy)	
No recent antibiotic therapy	An advanced macrolide[d] or a respiratory fluoroquinolone
Recent antibiotic therapy	A respiratory fluoroquinolone[c] alone or an advanced marcolide plus a β-lactam[g]
Suspected aspiration with infection	Amoxicillin-clavulanate or clindamycin
Influenza with bacterial superinfection	A β-lactam[g] or a respiratory fluoroquinolone
Inpatient	
Medical Ward	
No recent antibiotic therapy	A respiratory fluoroquinolone alone or an advanced macrolide plus a β-lactam[h]
Recent antibiotic therapy	An advanced macrolide plus a β-lactam or a respiratory fluoroquinolone alone (regimen selected will depend on nature of recent antibiotic therapy)
Intensive Care Unit (ICU)	
Pseudomonas infection is not an issue	A β-lactam[h] plus either an advanced macrolide or a respiratory fluoroquinolone
Pseudomonas infection is not an issue but patient has a β-lactam allergy	A respiratory fluoroquinolone, with or without clindamycin
Pseudomonas infection is an issue[i]	Either (1) an antipseudomonal agent[j] plus ciprofloxacin, or (2) an antipseudomonal agent plus an aminoglycoside[k] plus a respiratory fluoroquinolone or a macrolide
Pseudomonas infection is an issue but the patient has a β-lactam allergy	Either (1) aztreonam plus levofloxacin[l] or (2) aztreonam plus moxifloxacin or gatifloxacin, with or without an aminoglycoside
Nursing Home	
Receiving treatment in nursing home	A respiratory fluoroquinolone alone or amoxicillin-clavulanate plus an advanced macrolide
Hospitalized	Same as for medical ward and ICU

COPD, chronic obstructive pulmonary disease.

[a] Erythromycin, azithromycin, or clarithromycin.

[b] That is, the patient was given a course of antibiotic(s) for treatment of any infection within the past 3 months, excluding the current episode of infection. Such treatment is a risk factor for drug-resistant *Streptococcus pneumoniae* and possibly for infection with gram-negative bacilli. Depending on the class of antibiotics recently given, one or another of the suggested options may be selected. Recent use of a fluoroquinolone should dictate selection of a nonfluoroquinolone regimen, and vice versa.

[c] Moxifloxacin , gatifloxacin, levofloxacin, or gemifloxacin (oral gemifloxacin only, which was approved by the U.S. Food and Drug Administration on 4 April 2003 and which is the only fluoroquinolone approved for multidrug-resistant *S. pneumoniae;* not yet marketed).

[d] Azithromycin or clarithromycin.

[e] Dosage, 1 g PO tid.

[f] Dosage, 2 g PO bid.

[g] High-dose amoxicillin, high-dose amoxicillin-clavulanate, cefpodoxime, cefprozil, or cefuroxime.

[h] Cefotaxime, ceftriaxone, ampicillin-sulbactam, or ertapenem; ertapenem was recently approved for such use (in once-daily parenteral treatment), but there is little experience thus far.

[i] The antipseudomonal agents chosen reflect this concern. Risk factors for *Pseudomonas* infection include severe structural lung disease (e.g., bronchiectasis) and recent antibiotic therapy or stay in hospital (especially in the ICU). For patients with CAP in the ICU, coverage for *S. pneumoniae* and *Legionella* species must always be assured. Piperacillin-tazobactam, imipenem, meropenem, and cefepime are excellent β-lactams and are adequate for most *S. pneumoniae* and *Haemophilus influenzae* infections. They may be preferred when there is concern for relatively unusual CAP pathogens, such as *Pseudomonas aeruginosa, Klebsiella* species, and other gram-negative bacteria.

[j] Piperacillin, piperacillin-tazobactam, imipenem, meropenem, or cefepime.

[k] Data suggest that older adults receiving aminoglycosides have worse outcomes.

[l] Dosage for hospitalized patients, 750 mg qd.

Data from Mandell LA, Bartlett JG, Dowell SF, et al. Update of practice guidelines for the management of community-acquired pneumonia in immunocompetent adults. Clin Infect Dis. 2003;37:1405-1433.

moxifloxacin) are all adequate choices. Doxycycline (a preferred treatment option in the IDSA guideline) and trimethoprim-sulfamethoxazole may be used but are less favored because of decreasing activity against strains of pneumococci.

In some centers, erythromycin (despite poor activity against *H. influenzae*) is used for therapy.[404] Decreased activity against penicillin-resistant strains of pneumococci and gastrointestinal intolerance have made this a less attractive choice than the newer azalides/macrolides. Azithromycin or clarithromycin has been favored by some because of a spectrum of activity more directed toward the major respiratory tract pathogens and a satisfactory safety profile. However, increased resistance in strains of pneumococci is a problem because therapeutic failures have been noted, with strains of *S. pneumoniae* showing in vitro resistance.

For patients with an increased risk for poor outcome because of age or underlying disease, or where the risk for infection with resistant pneumococci exists, the respiratory tract quinolones are the agents most likely to be effective. They have activity against all strains of *S. pneumoniae* including penicillin-resistant strains, and they have the added benefit of activity against atypical agents. Although resistance is a potential problem of increased use of quinolones, it has not yet emerged as a significant problem.

Regardless of the initial choice of antibiotic, once an organism is isolated, coverage should be narrowed down, if possible, on the basis of susceptibility.

Patients who are ill enough to require hospitalization should be treated with parenteral agents that cover the likely pathogens. Our choice would be a respiratory tract quinolone, or ceftriaxone plus azithromycin. Of course, if there are factors that suggest a specific etiology, or a Gram stain is revealing, specific antibiotic coverage should be used.

Although these regimens represent the basic course of therapy, specific clinical circumstances may warrant variation. For example, *S. aureus* pneumonia should be considered during an influenza outbreak even though *S. pneumoniae* is still the major etiologic agent. Although the regimens just listed should be effective, agents with activity against methicillin-resistant *S. aureus* (MRSA) may be utilized if there is reason to suspect MRSA, until culture results are available. Vancomycin, linezolid, and quinupristin/dalfopristin are considerations. Where aspiration pneumonia is a possibility, agents with activity against oral anaerobes are needed, including ampicillin-sulbactam or clindamycin. Seven percent to 18% of community-acquired pneumonia cases are caused by aerobic gram-negative bacilli, including *P. aeruginosa*. Risk factors previously noted for gram-negative pneumonia should therefore be sought. Where gram-negative bacilli are suspected, infection with *P. aeruginosa* should be a concern, and therapy with an antipseudomonal β-lactam compound (e.g., cefepime, piperacillin-tazobactam, imipenem, or meropenem) is a reasonable choice. Where *Pseudomonas* involvement can be excluded, agents such as cefotaxime, ceftriaxone, or ertapenem could be considered. Debate exists as to whether agents such as aminoglycosides or quinolones need to be added to a β-lactam therapy for gram-negative pneumonia. Data exist to support both sides of the controversy.[405-407] We favor combination therapy for patients who are severely ill, at least until culture results from sputum and blood are available. In patients who are allergic to penicillin, aztreonam with a respiratory tract quinolone, with or without an aminoglycoside, could be used.

In the patient admitted to an intensive care unit, therapy should be directed against *S. pneumoniae,* penicillin-resistant strains, *Legionella* species, gram-negative rods, and *M. pneumoniae*. If infection with *P. aeruginosa* is unlikely (no recent hospitalization, no recent antibiotic use, no pulmonary comorbidities, no gram-negative rods on Gram stain), a β-lactam plus either an azalide/macrolide or a respiratory tract quinolone would be therapies of first choice. Ceftriaxone or cefotaxime would be reasonable choices for the β-lactam. Where *Pseudomonas* infection cannot be excluded, an antipseudomonal β-lactam (cefepime, imipenem, meropenem, or piperacillin-tazobactam)

plus a respiratory tract quinolone or azalide/macrolide could be used. We favor cefepime or piperacillin-tazobactam plus a respiratory tract quinolone. An aminoglycoside could be added as a third agent for synergy against *Pseudomonas*. Evidence in the literature favoring one regimen over any other is lacking.

Duration and Route of Therapy

Prompt initiation of therapy is important. Initiation of antibiotic therapy within 4 hours of presentation has been associated with a shorter hospital stay independent of clinical or demographic parameters.[408] Not surprisingly, appropriate antibiotic selection was found to have a similar effect.[409] Clinical stability is defined as normalization of previously abnormal physiologic parameters, including heart rate, respiratory rate, oxygenation, blood pressure, mental state, and ability to care for oneself.[410] Most physiologic abnormalities will correct in 2 to 3 days. Normalization of all physiologic abnormalities may take 5 to 7 days. Patients who score higher on the severity scale take longer to stabilize than patients who score lower. By day 3, relapses of previously corrected physiologic abnormalities occur only 4% to 6% of the time.

Oral antibiotic therapy is safe after clinical stability has been reached.[411-414] There is no clear usefulness of observing a patient within the hospital after a switch to oral therapy.[415] However, it is important to recognize that discharging patients before stability has been reached may lead to increased rehospitalization and mortality.[416] Using the same definitions of clinical stability, it has been shown that the greater the number of factors remaining abnormal at discharge, the greater is the chance of readmission or death.

Once discharged, outpatient follow-up may be required, as greater than 64% of patients with community-acquired pneumonia will have some related residual symptoms, including fever, cough, shortness of breath, chest pain, sputum production, fatigue, or gastrointestinal symptoms. In younger patients without underlying pulmonary disease, these findings are more likely to resolve earlier.

There is no evidence-based data on the optimal course of antibiotic therapy for pneumonia. Historically, the course of therapy for pneumonia has been 10 to 14 days, depending on whether the patient was ill enough to be hospitalized, on the virulence of the etiologic agent, on the presence of comorbidities, and on the rate of response. Azalides, ketolides, and quinolones have been used in high-dose and/or short-duration therapies of 5 to 7 days with initial success.[417-419] At present, 10- to 14-day therapy for hospitalized patients seems most appropriate.[419]

Aspiration pneumonia and lung abscess are discussed in Chapter 63. Therapy and nosocomial pneumonia is discussed in Chapter 301.

PNEUMONIA PREVENTION

Vaccination against influenza and *S. pneumoniae* are important interventions in preventing pneumonia. In older adults, influenza vaccine may decrease the incidence of pneumonia by 53%.[420,421] Influenza vaccine is suggested for any person 6 months of age or older, who, because of age or underlying disease, is at risk for influenza-related complications. This includes persons older than 50 years; nursing home residents; people with chronic pulmonary or cardiac disease, or with chronic diseases such as diabetes, renal failure, or hematologic disorders; patients who are immunosuppressed; those taking chronic salicylate therapy; and women in their second or third trimester of pregnancy. Health care workers, workers in nursing homes, and those who provide care to older adults or debilitated persons should also be targeted for influenza vaccination.[422]

The role of pneumococcal polysaccharide vaccine continues to be somewhat controversial. The incidence of bacteremia may be reduced, but the incidence of pneumonia appears unchanged.[423] Although a protein polysaccharide vaccine is available, it is for pediatric use only. Pneumococcal vaccine is recommended for patients older than 65 and those who have recovered from community-acquired pneumonia (see Chapter 197).

REFERENCES

1. Osler W. The Principles and Practice of Medicine. 4th ed. New York: Appleton; 1901:108.
2. Advanced Report of Final Mortality Statistics, v. 42. Hyattsville, Md: National Center for Health Statistics; 1992.
3. Johanson WG Jr, Gould KG Jr. Lung defense mechanisms. Basics RD. 1977;6:1-6.
4. Green G. In defense of the lung. Am Rev Respir Dis. 1970;102:691-703.
5. Sibille Y, Reynolds HY. Macrophage and polymorphonuclear neutrophils in lung defense and injury. Am Rev Respir Dis. 1990;141:471-501.
6. Reynolds HY. Pulmonary host defenses. Chest. 1989;95(Suppl):223S-230S.
7. Reynolds H. Normal and defective respiratory host defense. In: Pennington JE, ed. Respiratory Infections: Diagnosis and Management. 2nd ed. New York: Raven; 1988:1-33.
8. Coonrod J. The role of extracellular bactericidal factors in pulmonary host defense. Semin Respir Infect. 1986;1:118-129.
9. Twigg HL III. Pulmonary host defenses. J Thorac Imaging. 1998;13:221-233.
10. Schutte BC, McCray PB. β-Defensins in lung host defense. Ann Rev Physiol. 2002;64:709-748.
11. Busse WW. Pathogenesis and sequelae of respiratory infections. Rev Infect Dis. 1991;13(Suppl 6):S477-S485.
12. Niederman MS, Merrill WW, Polonski LM, et al. Influence of sputum IgA and elastase on tracheal cell bacterial adherence. Am Rev Respir Dis. 1981;133:255-260.
13. Niederman MS, Merrill WW, Ferrante RD, et al. Nutritional status and bacterial binding in the lower respiratory tract in patients with chronic tracheostomy. Ann Intern Med. 1984;100:795-800.
14. Wright JR. Immunomodulatory functions of surfactant. Physiol Rev. 1997;77:931-962.
15. Zhang P, Summer WR, Bagby GJ, Nelson S. Innate immunity and pulmonary host defense. Immunol Rev. 2000;173:39-51.
16. Lohmann-Matthes ML, Steinmüller C, Franke-Ullman G. Pulmonary macrophages. Eur Respir J. 1994;7:1678-1689.
17. Lipscomb MF, Onofrio JM, Nash EJ, et al. A morphological study of the role of phagocytes in the clearance of Staphylococcus aureus from the lung. J Reticuloendothel Soc. 1983;33:429-442.
18. MacNee W, Selby C. Neutrophil kinetics in the lung. Clin Sci. 1990;79:97-107.
19. Reynolds HY. Advances in understanding pulmonary host defense mechanisms: Dendritic cell function and immunomodulation. Curr Opin Pulm Med. 2000;6:209-216.
20. Strieter RM, Standiford TJ, Huffnagle GB, et al. The good, the bad, and the ugly: The role of chemokines in models of human disease. J Immunol. 1996;196:3583-3586.
21. Standiford TJ, Huffnagle GB. Cytokines in host defense against pneumonia. J Investig Med. 1997;45:335-343.
22. Luster AD. Chemokines. Chemotactic cytokines that mediate inflammation. N Engl J Med. 1998;338:436-445.
23. Kolling UK, Hansen F, Braun J, et al. Leucocyte response and anti-inflammatory cytokines in community acquired pneumonia. Thorax. 2001;56:121-125.
24. Standiford TJ, Kunkel SL, Basha MA, et al. Interleukin-8 gene expression by a pulmonary epithelial cell line-a model for cytokine networks in the lung. J Clin Invest. 1990;86:1945-1953.
25. Strieter RM, Kunkel S, Showell H, et al. Endothelial cell gene expression of a neutrophil chemotactic factor by TNF-α, LPS, and IL-β. Science. 1989;243:1467-1469.
26. Agostini C, Chilosi M, Zambello R, et al. Pulmonary immune cells in health and disease. Lymphocytes. 1993;6:1378-1401.
27. Fishman AP, Reynolds HY, Elias JA, et al. Pulmonary defense mechanisms against infection. In: Fishman AP, ed. Fishman's Pulmonary Diseases and Disorders. 3rd ed. New York: McGraw Hill; 1998:265-274.
28. Mosmann TR, Sad S. The expanding universe of T-cell subsets: Th1, Th2 and more. Immunol Today. 1995;17:138-146.
29. Huxley EJ, Viroslav J, Gray WR, et al. Pharyngeal aspiration in normal adults and patients with depressed consciousness. Am J Med. 1978;64:564-568.
30. Green GM, Carolin D. The depressant effect of cigarette smoke on the in vitro antibacterial activity of alveolar macrophages. N Engl J Med. 1967;276:421-427.
31. MacGregor RR. Alcohol and immune defense. JAMA. 1986;256:1474-1479.
32. Schopf RE, Trompter M, Bork K, et al. Effects of ethanol and acetaldehyde on phagocytic function. Arch Dermatol Rev. 1985;277:131-137.
33. Zhang P, Bagby GJ, Happel KI, et al. Pulmonary host defenses and alcohol. Front Biosci. 2002;7:1314-1330.
34. Nelson S, Mason LM, Kolls J, Summer WR. Pathophysiology of pneumonia. Clin Chest Med. 1995;16:1-12.
35. Warshauer D, Goldstein E, Akers T, et al. Effect of influenza viral infection on the ingestion and killing of bacteria by alveolar macrophages. Am Rev Respir Dis. 1977;115:269-277.
36. Nelson S, Chidiac C, Bagby G, et al. Endotoxin-induced suppression of lung host defenses. J Med. 1990;21:85-103.
37. Phair J, Palella FJ Jr. Host impairments associated with human immunodeficiency virus infection. In: Niederman MS, Sarosi GA, Glassroth J, eds. Resp Infections. 2nd ed. Philadelphia: Lippincott, Williams & Wilkins; 2001:59-66.
38. Mason CM. The pathogenesis and presentation of nosocomial pneumonia. Crit Care Rev. 1991;2:145-155.
39. Espesito AL. Aspirin impairs antibacterial mechanisms in experimental pneumococcal pneumonia. Am Rev Respir Dis. 1984;130:857-862.
40. Nelson S, Summer WR, Terry PB, et al. Erythromycin-induced suppression of pulmonary antibacterial defenses: A potential mechanism of superinfection in the lung. Am Rev Respir Dis. 1987;136:1207-1212.
41. Nelson S, Summer WR, Jakab EJ. Aminophylline-induced suppression of pulmonary antibacterial defenses. Am Rev Respir Dis. 1985;131:923-927.
42. Ehrlich R, Henry MC. Chronic toxicity of nitrogen dioxide: 1. Effect on resistance to bacterial pneumonia. Arch Environ Health. 1968;17:860-865.
43. LaForce FM, Mullane JF, Boehme RF, et al. The effect of pulmonary edema on antibacterial defenses of the lung. J Lab Clin Med. 1973;82:634-648.
44. Huber GL, LaForce FM, Mason RJ, et al. Impairment of pulmonary bacterial defense mechanisms by immunosuppressive agents. Surg Forum. 1970;21:285-286.
45. Gyetko MR, Toews GB. Immunology of the aging lung. Clin Chest Med. 1993;14:379-391.
46. Granton JT, Grossman RF. Community-acquired pneumonia in the elderly patient. Clin Chest Med. 1993;14:537-553.
47. Ekdahl K, Braconier JH, Rollof J. Recurrent pneumonia: A review of 90 adult patients. Scand J Infect Dis. 1992;24:71-76.
48. Geppert EF. Chronic recurrent pneumonia. Semin Respir Infect. 1992;7:282-288.
49. Donowitz GR, Mandell GL. Clinical presentation and unusual infections. In: Gallin JI, Fauci AS, eds. Advances in Host Defense Mechanisms, v. 3. New York: Raven Press; 1983:55-75.
50. Donabedian H, Gallin JI. The hyperimmunoglobulin E recurrent infection (Jobs) syndrome. Medicine (Baltimore). 1983;62:195-208.
51. Beck S, Heiner DC. Selective immunoglobulin G₄ deficiency and recurrent infections of the respiratory tract. Am Rev Respir Dis. 1981;124:94-96.
52. Ammann AJ, Hong R. Selective IgA deficiency: Presentation of 30 cases and a review of the literature. Medicine (Baltimore). 1971;50:223-236.
53. Eliasson R, Mossberg B, Camner P, et al. The immotile-cilia syndrome. N Engl J Med. 1977;297:1-6.
54. Kartagener M. Zur Pathologie der Bronchiektasien: Bronchiektasien bei Situs Inversus. Beitr Klin Tuberk. 1933;83:489-501.
55. Handelsman DJ, Conway AJ, Boylan LM, et al. Young's syndrome: Obstructive azoospermia and chronic sinopulmonary infections. N Engl J Med. 1984;310:3-9.
56. Savic B, Birtel FJ, Tholen W, et al. Lung sequestration: Report of seven cases and review of 540 published cases. Thorax. 1979;34:96-101.
57. Metlay JP, Stafford RS, Singer DE. National trends in the use of antibiotics by primary care physicians for adult patients with cough. Arch Intern Med. 1998;158:1813-1818.
58. Emerman CL, Dawson N, Speroff T, et al. Comparison of physician judgment and decision aids for ordering chest radiographs for pneumonia in outpatients. Ann Emerg Med. 1991;20:1215-1219.
59. Metlay JP, Schulz R, Li YH, et al. Influence of age on symptoms at presentation in patients with community-acquired pneumonia. Arch Intern Med. 1997;157:1453-1459.
60. Halm EA, Teirstein AS. Management of community-acquired pneumonia. N Engl J Med. 2002;347:2039-2045.
61. Metlay JP, Fine MJ. Testing strategies in the initial management of patients with community acquired pneumonia. Ann Intern Med. 2003;138:109-118.
62. Murray HW, Masur H, Senterfit L, et al. The protean manifestations of Mycoplasma pneumoniae infection in adults. Am J Med. 1975;58:229-242.
63. Marston BJ, Plouffe JF, File TM, et al. Incidence of community-acquired pneumonia requiring hospitalization: Results of a population-based active surveillance study in Ohio. Arch Intern Med. 1997;157:1709-1718.
64. Dorff GJ, Rytel MW, Farmer SG, et al. Etiologies and characteristic features of pneumonias in a municipal hospital. Am J Med Sci. 1973;266:349-358.
65. Braun MM, Coté TR, Rabkin CS. Trends in death with tuberculosis during the AIDS era. JAMA. 1993;269:2865-2868.
66. Franklin B. SARS: 1918 Revisited? The urgent need for global collaboration in public health. Mayo Clinic Proc. 2003;78:813-816.
67. Sullivan RJ, Dowdle WR, Marine WM, et al. Adult pneumonia in a general hospital: Etiology and host risk factors. Arch Intern Med. 1972;129:935-942.
68. Lepow ML, Balassanian N, Emmerich J, et al. Interrelationships of viral, mycoplasmal and bacterial agents in uncomplicated pneumonia. Am Rev Respir Dis. 1968;97:533-545.
69. Griffith DE, Mazurek GH. Pneumonia in chronic obstructive lung disease. Infect Dis Clin North Am. 1991;5:467-484.
70. Wright PW, Wallace RJ, Shepard JR. A descriptive study of 42 cases of Branhamella catarrhalis pneumonia. Am J Med. 1990;88(Suppl 5A):SA25-75.
71. Torres A, Dorca J, Zalacain R, et al. Community-acquired pneumonia in chronic obstructive pulmonary disease: A Spanish multicenter study. Am J Respir Crit Care Med. 1996;154:1456-1461.
72. Pietila MP, Thomas CF. Inflammation and infection in exacerbations of chronic obstructive pulmonary disease. Semin Resp Infect. 2003;18:9-16.
73. Hoiby N. Epidemiological investigations of the respiratory tract bacteriology in patients with cystic fibrosis. Acta Pathol Microbiol Scand B. 1974;82:541-550.
74. Wallace JM, Rao AV, Glassroth J, et al. Respiratory illness in person with acquired immunodeficiency virus infection. Am Rev Respir Dis. 1993;148:1523.
75. Rosen MJ. Overview of pulmonary complications. Clin Chest Med. 1996;17:621.
76. Hoover DR, Saah AJ, Bacellar H, Phair J. Clinical manifestations of AIDS in the era of pneumocystis prophylaxis. N Engl J Med. 1993;329:1922.
77. Selik RM, Chu SY, Ward JW. Trends in infectious diseases and cancers among persons dying of HIV infection in the United States from 1987-1992. Ann Intern Med. 1995;123:933.
78. Chan ISF, Neaton JD, Sarvolatz LD, et al. Frequencies of opportunistic diseases prior to death among HIV-infected persons. AIDS. 1995;98:1145-1151.
79. Caiaffa WT, Vlahov D, Graham NMH, et al. Drug smoking, Pneumocystis carinii pneumonia, and immune suppression, increase risk of bacterial pneumonia in human immunodeficiency virus-seropositive infection drug users. Am J Respir Crit Care Med. 1994;150:1493-1498.
80. Hirschtick RE, Glassroth J, Jordan MC, et al. Bacterial pneumonia in persons infected with the human immunodeficiency virus. N Engl J Med. 1995;333:845-851.

81. Schuchat A, Brown CV, Hightoner A, et al. Use of surveillance for invasive pneumococcal disease to estimate the size of the immunosuppressed HIV-infected population. JAMA. 1991;265:3275-3279.

82. Redd SC, Rutherford GW III, Sande MA, et al. The role of human immunodeficiency virus infection in pneumococcal bacterium in San Francisco residents. J Infect Dis. 1990;162:1012-1017.

83. Steinhart R, Reingold AL, Taylor F, et al. Invasive *Haemophilus influenzae* infection in men with HIV infection. JAMA. 1992;268:3350-3352.

84. Baron AD, Hollander H. *Pseudomonas aeruginosa* bronchopulmonary infection in late human immunodeficiency virus disease. Am Rev Respir Dis. 1993;148:992-996.

85. Dropulic LK, Leslie JM, Eldred LJ, et al. Clinical manifestations and risk factors of *Pseudomonas aeruginosa* infection in patients with AIDS. J Infect Dis. 1995; 171:930-937.

86. Hanson DL, Chusy SY, Farizo KM, et al. Distribution of CD_4 T lymphocytes at diagnosis of acquired immunodeficiency syndrome-defining and other human immunodeficiency virus-related illness. Arch Intern Med. 1995;155:1537.

87. Gross PA. Epidemiology of hospital-acquired pneumonia. Semin Respir Infect. 1987;2:2-7.

88. Marrie TJ, Haldane EV, Faulkner RS, et al. Community acquired pneumonia requiring hospitalization: Is it different in the elderly? J Am Geriatr Soc. 1985;33:671-680.

89. Heffron R. Pneumonia. New York: Commonwealth Fund; 1939:505.

90. Bartlett JG, Finegold SM. Anaerobic infections of the lung and pleural space. Am Rev Respir Dis. 1974;110:56-77.

91. Woodhead M. Management of pneumonia in the outpatient setting. Semin Respir Infect. 1998;13:848.

92. Metlay JP, Kapoor WN, Fine MJ. Does this patient have community-acquired pneumonia? JAMA. 1997;278:1440.

93. Gennis P, Gallagher J, Falvo C, et al. Clinical criteria for the detection of pneumonia in adults: Guidelines for ordering chest roentgenograms in the emergency department. J Emerg Med. 1989;7:263-268.

94. Wipf JE, Lipsky BA, Hirschmann JV, et al. Diagnosing pneumonia by physical examination: Relevant or relic? Arch Intern Med. 1999;159:1082-1087.

95. Thorsteinsson SB, Musher DM, Fagan T. The diagnostic value of sputum culture in acute pneumonia. JAMA. 1975;233:894-895.

96. Merrill C, Gwaltney JM, Hendley JO, et al. Rapid identification of pneumococci. N Engl J Med. 1973;288:510-512.

97. Drew WL. Value of sputum culture in diagnosis of pneumococcal pneumonia. J Clin Microbiol. 1977;6:62-65.

98. Bartlett JG, Dowell SF, Mandell LA, et al. Practice guidelines for management of community-acquired pneumonia in adults. Clin Infect Dis. 2000;31:347-382.

99. Reed WW, Byrd GS, Gates RH Jr, et al. Sputum Gram's stain in community-acquired pneumococcal pneumonia: A meta analysis. West J Med. 1996;165:197-204.

100. Bartlett JG, Mundy LM. Community-acquired pneumonia. N Engl J Med. 1995; 333:1618-1624.

101. Niederman MS, Bass JB Jr, Campbell GD, et al. Guidelines for the initial management of adults with community-acquired pneumonia: Diagnosis, assessment of severity and initial antimicrobial therapy. Am Rev Respir Dis. 1993;148:1418-1426.

102. Fine MJ, Orloff JJ, Rihs JD, et al. Evaluation of housestaff physicians' preparation and interpretation of sputum Gram stains for community-acquired pneumonia. J Gen Intern Med. 1991;6:189-198.

103. Goerge RB, Ziskind MM, Rasch JR, et al. Mycoplasma and adenovirus pneumonias: Comparison with other atypical pneumonias in a military population. Ann Intern Med. 1966;65:931-942.

104. Reimann H. The Pneumonias. Philadelphia: Saunders; 1938:67.

105. Solomon S. Primary Friedlander pneumonia. JAMA. 1937;108:937-947.

106. Murray PR, Washington JA III. Microscopic and bacteriologic analysis of expectorated sputum. Mayo Clin Proc. 1975;50:339-344.

107. Rein MF, Gwaltney JM, O'Brien WM, et al. Accuracy of the Gram's stain in identifying pneumococci in sputum. JAMA. 1978;239:2671-2673.

108. Hendley JO, Sande MA, Stewart PM, et al. Spread of *Streptococcus pneumoniae* in families: I. Carriage rates and distribution of types. J Infect Dis. 1975;132:55-61.

109. Lees AW, McNaught W. Bacteriology of lower-respiratory tract secretions, sputum and upper-respiratory tract secretions in "normals" and "chronic bronchitis." Lancet. 1959;2:1112-1115.

110. Barrett-Connor E. The non-value of sputum culture in the diagnosis of pneumococcal pneumonia. Am Rev Respir Dis. 1971;103:845-848.

111. Zaman MK, Wooten OH, Suprahmonya B, et al. Rapid non-invasive diagnosing of *Pneumocystis carinii* from induced liquefied sputum. Ann Intern Med. 1988;109:7-10.

112. Wallace RJ, Musher DM, Martin RR. *Haemophilus influenzae* pneumonia in adults. Am J Med. 1978;64:87-93.

113. Levin D, Schwarz M, Matthay R, et al. Bacteremic *Haemophilus influenzae* pneumonia in adults: A report of 24 cases and a review of the literature. Am J Med. 1977; 62:219-224.

114. Davidson M, Tempest B, Palmer DL. Bacteriologic diagnosis of acute pneumonia: Comparison of sputum, transtracheal aspirates, and lung aspirates. JAMA. 1976; 235:158-163.

115. Skerrett SJ. Diagnostic testing to establish a microbial cause is helpful in the management of community-acquired pneumonia. Semin Respir Infect. 1997;12:308-321.

116. Edelstein PH. Legionnaires' disease. Clin Infect Dis. 1993;16:741-749.

117. Roig J, Domingo C, Morera J. Legionnaires' disease. Chest. 1994;105:1817-1825.

118. Ng VL, Virani NA, Chaisson RE, et al. Rapid detection of *Pneumocystis carinii* using a direct fluorescent monoclonal antibody stain. J Clin Microbiol. 1990;28:2228-2233.

119. Willocks L, Burns S, Cossar R, Brettle R. Diagnosis of *Pneumocystis carinii* pneumonia in a population of HIV-positive drug users with particular reference to sputum induction and fluorescent antibody techniques. J Infect Dis. 1993;26:257-264.

120. Menéndez R, Córdoba J, de la Cuadra P, et al. Value of the polymerase chain reaction assay in noninvasive respiratory samples for diagnosis of community-acquired pneumonia. Am J Respir Crit Care Med. 1999;159:1868-1873.

121. Tong CY, Donnelly C, Harvey G, Sillis M. Multiplex polymerase chain reaction for the simultaneous detection of *Mycoplasma pneumoniae, Chlamydia pneumoniae,* and *Chlamydia psittaci* in respiratory samples. J Clin Pathol. 1999;52:257-263.

122. Murdoch DR. Nucleic acid amplification tests for the diagnosis of pneumonia. Clin Infect Dis. 2003;36:1162-1170.

123. Schluger NW, Rom WN. The polymerase chain reaction in the diagnosis and evaluation of pulmonary infections. Am J Respir Crit Care Med. 1995;152:11-16.

124. Clarridge JE III, Shawar RM, Shinnick TM, Plikaytis BB. Large-scale use of polymerase chain reaction for detecting *Mycobacterium tuberculosis* in a routine mycobacteriology laboratory. J Clin Microbiol. 1993;31:2049-2051.

125. Wonderink RG, Russell GB, Mezger E, et al. The diagnostic utility of the antibody-coated bacteria test in intubated patients. Chest. 1991;99:84-88.

126. Jordan GW, Wong GA, Hoeprich PD. Bacteriology of the lower respiratory tract as determined by fiber-optic bronchoscopy and transtracheal aspiration. J Infect Dis. 1976;134:428-435.

127. Pollock HM, Hawkins EL, Bonner JR, et al. Diagnosis of bacterial pulmonary infections with quantitative protected catheter cultures obtained during bronchoscopy. J Clin Microbiol. 1983;17:255-259.

128. Halperin SA, Suratt PM, Gwaltney JM, et al. Bacterial cultures of the lower respiratory tract in normal volunteers with and without experimental rhinovirus infection using a plugged double catheter system. Am Rev Respir Dis. 1982;125:678-680.

129. Bordelon JY Jr, Legrand P, Gewin WL, et al. The telescoping plugged catheter in suspected anaerobic infections: A controlled series. Am Rev Respir Dis. 1983;128:465-468.

130. Wimberly NW, Bass JR Jr, Boyd DW, et al. Bronchial brush specimens from patients with stable chronic bronchitis. Chest. 1986;90:534-536.

131. Bass JB, Hawkins EL, Bonner JR, et al. Use of bronchoscopy protected catheter technique in the clinical evaluation of a new antibiotic. Diagn Microbiol Infect Dis. 1983;1:95-106.

132. Guerra LF, Baughman RP. Use of bronchoalveolar lavage to diagnose bacterial pneumonia in mechanically ventilated patients. Crit Care Med. 1990;18:169-173.

133. Ortquist A, Kalin M, Lejdeborn L, et al. Diagnostic fiberoptic bronchoscopy and protected brush culture in patients with community-acquired pneumonia. Chest. 1990; 97:576-582.

134. Feinsilver SH, Fein AM, Niederman MS, et al. Utility of fiberoptic bronchoscopy in nonresolving pneumonia. Chest. 1990;98:1322-1326.

135. Chastre J, Viau F, Brun P, et al. Prospective evaluation of the protected specimen brush for the diagnosis of pulmonary infections in ventilated patients. Am Rev Respir Dis. 1994;130:924-925.

136. Chastre J, Fagon J, Barnet-Lesco M, et al. Evaluation of bronchoscopic techniques for the diagnosis of nosocomial pneumonia. Am J Respir Crit Care Med. 1995;152:231-240.

137. Mortos JA, Ferrer M, Torres A, et al. Specificity of quantitative cultures of protected specimen brush and bronchoalveolar lavage in mechanically ventilated patients. Am Rev Respir Dis. 1990;161:A276.

138. Broughton WA, Middleton RM, Kirkpatrick MB, et al. Bronchoscopic protected specimen brush and bronchoalveolar lavage in the diagnosis of bacterial pneumonia. Infect Dis Clin North Am. 1991;5:432-452.

139. Torres A, El-Ebiary M, Padro L, et al. Validation of different techniques for the diagnosis of ventilator-associated pneumonia: Comparison with immediate postmortem pulmonary biopsy. Am J Respir Crit Care Med. 1994;149:324-331.

140. Marquette CH, Copin M, Wallet F, et al. Diagnostic tests for pneumonia in ventilated patients: Prospective evaluation of diagnostic accuracy using histology as a diagnostic gold standard. Am J Respir Crit Care Med. 1995;151:1878-1888.

141. Montravers P, Fagon J, Chastre J, et al. Follow-up protected specimen brushes to assess treatment in nosocomial pneumonia. Am Rev Respir Dis. 1993;147:38-44.

142. Timsit J, Misset B, Renard B, et al. Effect of previous antimicrobial therapy on the accuracy of the main procedure used to diagnose nosocomial pneumonia in patients who are using ventilation. Chest. 1995;108:1036-1040.

143. Torres A, El-Ebiary M. Invasive diagnostic techniques for pneumonia: Protected specimen brush, bronchoalveolar lavage and lung biopsy methods. Infect Dis Clin North Am. 1998;12:701-722.

144. Broaddus C, Dake MD, Stulburg MS, et al. Bronchoalveolar lavage and transbronchial biopsy for the diagnosis of pulmonary infections in the acquired immunodeficiency syndrome. Ann Intern Med. 1986;102:747-752.

145. Jules-Elysee KM, Stover DE, Zaman MB, et al. Aerosolized pentamidine: Effect on diagnosis and presentation of *Pneumocystis carinii* pneumonia. Ann Intern Med. 1990;112:750-787.

146. Crawford SW, Bowden RA, Hackman RC, et al. Rapid detection of cytomegalovirus pulmonary infection by bronchoalveolar lavage and centrifugation culture. Ann Intern Med. 1988;108:180-185.

147. Pisani RJ, Wright AJ. Clinical utility of bronchoalveolar lavage in immunocompromised hosts. Mayo Clin Proc. 1992;67:221-227.

148. Crawford SW, Bowden RA, Hackman RC, et al. Rapid detection of cytomegalovirus pulmonary infection by bronchoalveolar lavage and centrifugation culture. Ann Intern Med. 1988;108:180-185.

149. Xavier R, Henn L, Costa R. Bronchoalveolar lavage in pulmonary tuberculosis. Chest. 1990;98:975.

150. Baughman RP, Dohn MN, Loudon RG, et al. Bronchoscopy with bronchoalveolar lavage in tuberculosis and fungal infection. Chest. 1991;99:92-97.

151. Meduri GH, Baselski V. The role of bronchoalveolar lavage in diagnosing nonopportunistic bacterial pneumonia. Chest. 1991;100:179-190.

152. Bovornkittz S, Pushpakom R. Adenosine deaminase in bronchoalveolar lavage fluid. Chest. 1988;94:1113.

153. Levy H, Wadee AA, Feldman C, et al. Enzyme-linked immunosorbent assay for detection of antibodies against *Mycobacterium tuberculosis* in bronchial washings and serum. Chest. 1988;93:762-766.

154. Raja A, Baughman RP, Daniel TM. The detection by immune assay of antibody to mycobacterial antigens in bronchoalveolar lavage fluid from patients with tuberculosis and control subjects. Chest. 1988;94:133-137.

155. Torres A, El-Ebiary M, Fabregos N, et al. Value of intracellular bacteria detection in the diagnosis of ventilator associated pneumonia. Thorax. 1996;51:378-384.

156. Chastre J, Fagon JY, Soler P, et al. Quantification of BAL cells containing intracellular bacteria rapidly identifies ventilated patients with nosocomial pneumonia. Chest. 1989;15:190s-192.

157. Allaouchiche B, Jaumain H, Dumontet C, et al. Early diagnosis of ventilator associated pneumonia: Is it possible to define a cutoff value of infected cells in BAL fluid? Chest. 1996;110:1558-1565.

158. Gerbeaux P, Ledoray V, Boussuges A, et al. Diagnosis of nosocomial pneumonia in mechanically ventilated patients. Am J Respir Crit Care Med. 1998;157:76-80.

159. Jourdain B, Joly-Guillou ML, Dombret MC, et al. Usefulness of quantitative cultures of BAL fluid for diagnosing nosocomial pneumonia in ventilated patients. Chest. 1997;111:411-418.

160. Pugin J, Auckenthaler R, Delaspre O, et al. Rapid diagnosis of gram-negative pneumonia by assay of endotoxin in bronchoalveolar lavage fluid. Thorax. 1992;47:547-549.

161. Trouillet JL, Guiguet M, Gibert L, et al. Fiberoptic bronchoscopy in ventilated patients: Evaluation of cardiopulmonary risk under midazolam sedation. Chest. 1990;97:927-933.

162. Pugin J, Suter PM. Diagnostic bronchoalveolar lavage in patients with pneumonia produces sepsis-like systemic effects. Intensive Care Med. 1992;18:6-10.

163. Prokop A, Gawenda M, Krüger I, Pichlmaier H. Value of bronchoscopic pneumonia diagnosis: Prospective study. World J Surg. 1996;29:22-26.

164. El-Ebiary M, Torres A, Gonzalez J, et al. Quantitative cultures of endotracheal aspirates for the diagnosis of ventilator-associated pneumonia. Am Rev Respir Dis. 1993;148:1552-1557.

165. Sanchez-Nieto JM, Torres A, Garcia-Cordoba F, et al. Impact of invasive and noninvasive quantitative culture sampling on outcome of ventilator-associated pneumonia: A pilot study. Am J Respir Crit Care Med. 1998;157:371-376.

166. Jourdain B, Novora A, Joly-Guillou ML, et al. Role of quantitative values of endotracheal aspirate in the diagnosis of nosocomial pneumonia. Am J Respir Crit Care Med. 1995;152:241-246.

167. Marik PE, Brown WJ. A comparison of bronchoscopic vs blind protected specimen brush sampling in patients with suspected ventilator-associated pneumonia. Chest. 1995;108:203-207.

168. Meduri GU, Beals D, Maijub G, et al. Protected bronchoalveolar lavage, a new bronchoscopic technique to retrieve uncontaminated distal airway secretion. Am Rev Respir Dis. 1991;143:855-864.

169. Pugin J, Auckenthaler R, Mili N, et al. Diagnosis of ventilator-associated pneumonia by bacteriologic analysis of bronchoscopic and non-bronchoscopic "blind" bronchoalveolar lavage fluid. Am Rev Respir Dis. 1991;143:1121-1129.

170. Kollef MH, Bock KR, Richards RD, Hearns ML. The safety and diagnostic accuracy of minibronchoalveolar lavage in patients with suspected ventilator-associated pneumonia. Ann Intern Med. 1995;122:743-748.

171. Bregeon F, Papazian L, Visconti A, et al. Relationship of microbiologic diagnostic criteria to morbidity and mortality in patients with ventilator-associated pneumonia. JAMA. 1997;277:655-662.

172. Busk MF, Rosenow EC III, Wilson WR. Invasive procedures in the diagnosis of pneumonia. Semin Respir Infect. 1988;3:113-122.

173. Bartlett JG. Invasive diagnostic techniques in respiratory infections. In: Pennington JE, ed. Respiratory Infections: Diagnosis and Management. New York: Raven Press; 1983:55-77.

174. Torres A, Jimenez P, de la Bellacasa JP, et al. Diagnostic value of nonfluoroscopic percutaneous lung needle aspiration in patients with pneumonia. Chest. 1990;98:840-844.

175. Cockerill FR III, Wilson WR, Carpenter HA, et al. Open lung biopsy in immunocompromised patients. Arch Intern Med. 1985;145:1398-1404.

176. Dijkman JH, van der Meer JWM, Bakker W, et al. Transpleural lung biopsy by the thoracoscopic route in patients with diffuse interstitial pulmonary disease. Chest. 1982;82:76-83.

177. Rodgers BM. Thoracoscopy in children. Poumon Coeur. 1981;37:301-306.

178. Springmeyer SC, Silvestri RC, Sale GE, et al. The role of transbronchial biopsy for the diagnosis of diffuse pneumonias in immunocompromised marrow transplant recipients. Am Rev Respir Dis. 1982;116:763-765.

179. Lowell JR. Pleural Effusions: A Comprehensive Review. Baltimore: University Park Press; 1977:96.

180. Unger JD, Rose HD, Unger GF. Gram-negative pneumonia. Diagn Radiol. 1973;107:283-291.

181. Light RW. Pleural effusion. N Engl J Med. 2002;346:1971-1977.

182. Heffner JE, Brown LK, Barbieri L, DeLeo JM. Pleural fluid chemical analysis in para-pneumonia effusions: A meta analysis. Am J Respir Crit Care Med. 1995;151:1700-1708.

183. Nagesh BS, Sehgol S, Jindd SK, Arora SK. Evaluation of polymerase chain reaction for detection of Mycobacterium tuberculosis in pleural fluid. Chest. 2001;119:1737-1741.

184. Greco S, Girardi E, Masciangelo R, et al. Adenosine deaminase and interferon gamma measurements for the diagnosis of tuberculous pleurisy: A meta-analysis. Int J Tuberc Lung Dis. 2003;7:777-786.

185. Poral JM, Gasquez I, Vives M, Perez B. Diagnosis of tuberculosis pleuritis by the measurement of soluble interleukin 2 receptor in pleural fluid. Int J Tuberc Lung Dis. 2000;4:975-979.

186. Bohte R, van Furth R, van den Broek PJ. Aetiology of community-acquired pneumonia: A prospective study among adults requiring admission to hospital. Thorax. 1995;50:543-547.

187. Berk SL. Justifying the use of blood cultures when diagnosing community-acquired pneumonia. Chest. 1995;108:891-892.

188. Dowell SF, Peeling RW, Boman J, et al. Standardizing *Chlamydia pneumoniae* assays: Recommendations from the Centers for Disease Control and Prevention (USA) and the Laboratory Centre for Disease Control (Canada). Clin Infect Dis. 2001;33:492-503.

189. Sillis M. The limitation of IgM assays in the serologic diagnosis of *Mycoplasma pneumoniae* infections. J Med Microbiol. 1990;33:253-258.

190. Venkatesan P, MacFarlane JT. Role of pneumococcal antigen in the diagnosis of pneumococcal pneumonia (Editorial). Thorax. 1992;47:329-331.

191. Dorff GJ, Coonrod JD, Rytel MW. Detection of immunoelectrophoresis of antigen in sera of patients with pneumococcal bacteremia. Lancet. 1971;1:578-579.

192. Burman LA, Trollfors B, Andersson B, et al. Diagnosis of pneumonia by cultures, bacterial and viral antigen detective tests and serology with special reference to antibodies against pneumococcal antigens. J Infect Dis. 1991;163:1087-1095.

193. Martin SJ, Hogansan DA, Thomas ET. Detection of *Streptococcus pneumoniae* and *Haemophilus influenzae* type B antigens in acute nonbacteremic pneumonia. J Clin Microbiol. 1987;25:248-250.

194. Campbell JF, Spika JS. The serodiagnosis of nonpneumococcal bacterial pneumonia. Semin Respir Infect. 1988;3:123-130.

195. Salo P, Örtquist Ä, Leinonen M. Diagnosis of bacteremic pneumococcal pneumonia by amplification of pneumolysin gene fragments in serum. J Infect Dis. 1995;171:479-482.

196. Schlager N, Godwin K, Sepkowitz D, et al. Application of the polymerase chain reaction in *Pneumocystis carinii* and frequent detection of *Pneumocystis carinii* in serum of patients with pneumocystis pneumonia. J Exp Med. 1992;176:1327-1333.

197. Smith RP, Lipworth BJ, Cree IA, et al. C-reactive protein: A clinical marker in community-acquired pneumonia. Chest. 1995;108:1288-1291.

198. Örtquist Ä, Hedlund J, Wretlind B, et al. Diagnostic and prognostic value of interleukin 6 and C-reactive protein in community-acquired pneumonia. Scan J Infect Dis. 1995;27:457-462.

199. Ruf B, Schurmann D, Horbach I, et al. Frequency and diagnosis of *Legionella pneumophila*: A 3-year prospective study with emphasis on application of urinary antigen detection. J Infect Dis. 1990;162:1341-1347.

200. Domínguez J, Galí N, Blanco S, et al. Detection of *Streptococcus pneumoniae* antigen by a rapid immunochromatographic assay in urine samples. Chest. 2001;119:243-249.

201. Murdoch DR, Laing RTR, Mills GD, et al. Evaluation of a rapid immunochromatographic test for detection of *Streptococcus pneumoniae* antigen in urine samples from adults with community-acquired pneumonia. J Clin Microbiol. 2001;39:3495-3498.

202. Gutiérrez F, Masiá M, Rodríguez JC, et al. Evaluation of the immunochromatographic Binax NOW assay for detection of *Streptococcus pneumoniae* urinary antigen in a prospective study of community-acquired pneumonia in Spain. Clin Infect Dis. 2003;36:286-292.

203. Dowell SF, Garman RL, Liu G, et al. Evaluation of Binax NOW, an assay for the detection of pneumococcal antigen in urine samples performed among pediatric patients. Clin Infect Dis. 2001;32:824-825.

204. Woodhead M. Management of pneumonia in the outpatient setting. Semin Respir Infect. 1998;13:8-16.

205. Albaum MN, Hill LC, Murphy M, et al. Interobserver reliability of the chest radiograph in community-acquired pneumonia. Chest. 1996;110:343-350.

206. Gonzales R, Steiner JF, Sande MA. Antibiotic prescribing for adults with colds, upper respiratory tract infections and bronchitis by ambulatory care physicians. JAMA. 1997;278:901-904.

207. Hasley PB, Albaum MN, Li Y-H, et al. Do pulmonary radiographic findings at presentation predict mortality in patients with community-acquired pneumonia? Ann Intern Med. 1996;156:2206-2212.

208. Dines DE. Diagnostic significance of pneumatocoeles of the lung. JAMA. 1968;204:1169-1172.

209. Bartlett JG, Finegold SM. Anaerobic pleuropulmonary infections. Medicine (Baltimore). 1972;51:413-450.

210. Kim EA, Soo Lee K, Primack SL, et al. Viral pneumonias in adults: Radiologic and pathologic findings. Radiographics. 2002;22:S137-149.

211. Poutanen SM, Low DE, Henry B, et al. Identification of severe acute respiratory syndrome in Canada. N Engl J Med. 2003;348:1995-2005.

212. Wong KT, Antonio GE, Hui DS, et al. Severe acute respiratory syndrome: Radiographic appearances and pattern of progression in 138 patients. Radiology. 2003;228:401-406.

213. Fine NL, Smith LR, Sheedy PF. Frequency of pleural effusions of mycoplasma and viral pneumonias. N Engl J Med. 1970;283:790-793.

214. Fraser DW, Tsai TR, Orenstein W, et al. Legionnaires' disease: Description of an epidemic of pneumonia. N Engl J Med. 1977;297:1189-1197.

215. Pope TL Jr, Armstrong P, Thompson R, Donowitz GR. Pittsburgh pneumonia agent chest film manifestations. AJR Am J Roentgenol. 1982;138:237-241.

216. Tew J, Calenoff L, Berlin BS. Bacterial or nonbacterial pneumonia: Accuracy of radiographic diagnosis. Radiology. 1977;124:607-612.

217. Wheeler JH, Fishman EK. Computed tomography in the management of chest infections: Current status. Clin Infect Dis. 1996;23:232-240.

218. Primack SL, Müller NL. High resolution computed tomography in acute diffuse lung disease in the immunocompromised patient. Radiol Clin North Am. 1994;32:731-744.

219. Syrjälä H, Broas M, Suramo I, et al. High resolution computed tomography for the diagnosis of community-acquired pneumonia. Clin Infect Dis. 1998;27:358-363.

220. Amundsen T, Torheim G, Waage A, et al. Perfusion magnetic resonance imaging of the lung: Characterization of pneumonia and chronic obstructive pulmonary disease—A feasibility study. J Magn Reson Imaging. 2000;12:224-231.

221. Kramer EL, Chaitanya RD. Pulmonary applications of nuclear medicine. Clin Chest Med. 1991;12:55-75.

222. Marrie TJ, Peeling RW, Fine MJ, et al. Ambulatory patients with community-acquired pneumonia: The frequency of atypical agents and clinical course. Am J Med. 1996; 101:508-515.

223. Fang GD, Fine M, Orloff J, et al. New and emerging etiologies for community-acquired pneumonia with implications for therapy: A prospective multicenter study of 359 cases. Medicine (Baltimore). 1990;69:307-316.

224. Pennington JE. Community-Acquired Pneumonia and Acute Bronchitis in Respiratory Infections: Diagnosis and Management. New York: Raven Press; 1994.

225. Gleckman R, DeVita J, Hibert D, et al. Sputum Gram stain assessment in community-acquired bacteremic pneumonia. J Clin Microbiol. 1988;26:846-849.

226. Woodhead MA, Arrowsmith J, Chamberlain-Webber R, et al. The value of routine microbial investigation in community-acquired pneumonia. Respir Med. 1991;85:313-317.

227. The British Thoracic Society Research Committee and the Public Health Laboratory Service. The aetiology, management and outcome of severe community-acquired pneumonia on the intensive care unit. Respir Med. 1992;86:7-13.

228. Marrie TJ, Durant H, Yates L. Community-acquired pneumonia requiring hospitalization: Five year prospective study. Rev Infect Dis. 1989;11:586-599.

229. Fine M, Smith D, Singer DE. Hospitalization decision in patients with community-acquired pneumonia: A prospective chart review. Am J Med. 1990;89:713-714.

230. American Thoracic Society. Guidelines for the management of adults with community-acquired pneumonia: Diagnosis, assessment of severity, antimicrobial therapy, and prevention. Am J Respir Crit Care Med. 2001;163:1730-1754.

231. Marrie TJ. Community-acquired pneumonia. Clin Infect Dis. 1994;18:501-515.

232. Mandell LA, Bartlett JG, Dowell SF, et al. Update of practice guidelines for the management of community-acquired pneumonia in immunocompetent adults. Clin Infect Dis. 2003;37:1405-1433.

233. Musher DM, Alexandraki I, Graviss EA, et al. Bacteremic and nonbacteremic pneumococcal pneumonia: A prospective study. Medicine (Baltimore). 2000;79:210-221.

234. Mundy LM, Auwaerter PG, Oldach D, et al. Community-acquired pneumonia: Impact on immune status. Am J Respir Crit Care Med. 1995;152:1309-1315.

235. Austrian R, Gold J. Pneumococcal bacteremia with especial reference to bacteremic pneumococcal pneumonia. Ann Intern Med. 1964;60:759-776.

236. Lipsky BA, Boyko EJ, Inui TS, et al. Risk factors for acquiring pneumococcal infections. Arch Intern Med. 1986;146:2179-2185.

237. Rosner F, Zarrabi MH. Late infections following splenectomy in Hodgkin's disease. Cancer Invest. 1983;1:57-65.

238. Zarrabi MH, Rosner F. Serious infections in adults following splenectomy for trauma. Arch Intern Med. 1984;144:1421-1424.

239. Musher DM. Infections caused by Streptococcus pneumoniae: Clinical spectrum, pathogenesis, immunity and treatment. Clin Infect Dis. 1992;14:801-809.

240. Hirschmann JV, Everett ED. Haemophilus influenzae infections in adults: Report of nine cases and a review of literature. Medicine (Baltimore). 1979;58:80-94.

241. Gotfried MH. Epidemiology of clinically diagnosed community-acquired pneumonia in the primary care setting: Results from the 1999-2000 respiratory surveillance program. Am J Med. 2001;111(9A):25S-29S.

242. Hausmann W, Karlish AJ. Staphylococcal pneumonia in adults. Br Med J. 1956;2: 845-847.

243. Schwarzmann SW, Adler JL, Sullivan RJ, et al. Bacterial pneumonia during the Hong Kong influenza epidemic of 1968-1969: Experience in a city-county hospital. Arch Intern Med. 1971;127:1037-1041.

244. Yu VL, Kroboth FJ, Shonnard J, et al. Legionnaires' disease: New clinical perspective from a prospective pneumonia study. Am J Med. 1982;73:357-361.

245. Cunha BA. Clinical features of legionnaires' disease. Semin Respir Infect. 1998;13: 116-127.

246. Fernández-Sabé N, Rosón B, Carratalà J, et al. Clinical diagnosis of Legionella pneumonia revisited: Evaluation of the community-based pneumonia incidence study group scoring system. Clin Infect Dis. 2003;37:483-489.

247. Gupta SK, Imperiale TF, Sarosi GA. Evaluation of the Winthrop University Hospital criteria to identify Legionella pneumonia. Chest. 2001;120:1064-1071.

248. Nicotra B, Rivera M, Luman I, et al. Branhamella catarrhalis as a lower respiratory tract pathogen in patients with chronic lung disease. Arch Intern Med. 1986;146:890-893.

249. Pfaller MA, Ehrhardt AF, Jones RN. Frequency of pathogen occurrence and antimicrobial susceptibility among community-acquired respiratory tract infections in the respiratory surveillance program study: Microbiology from the medical office practice environment. Am J Med. 2001;111(9A):4S-12S.

250. Marrie TJ. Epidemiology of mild pneumonia. Semin Respir Infect. 1998;13:3-7.

251. Gross JS, Neufeld RR, Libon LS, et al. Autopsy study of the elderly institutionalized patients: Review of 234 autopsies. Arch Intern Med. 1988;148:173-176.

252. Koivula I, Stén M, Mäkelä PH. Prognosis after community-acquired pneumonia in the elderly. Arch Intern Med. 1999;159:1550-1555.

253. Granton JT, Grossman RF. Community-acquired pneumonia in the elderly patient. Clin Chest Med. 1993;14:537-553.

254. Musgrave T, Verghese A. Clinical features of pneumonia in the elderly. Semin Respir Infect. 1990;5:269-275.

255. Fernández-Sabé N, Carratalà J, Rosón B, et al. Community-acquired pneumonia in very elderly patients: Causative organisms, clinical characteristics, and outcomes. Medicine (Baltimore). 2003;82:159-169.

256. Johnson JC, Jayadevappa R, Baccash PD, Taylor L. Nonspecific presentation of pneumonia in hospitalized older people: Age effect or dementia? J Am Geriatr Soc. 2000;48:1316-1320.

257. Houston MS, Silverstein MD, Suman VJ. Community-acquired lower respiratory tract infection in the elderly: A community-based study of incidence and outcome. J Am Board Fam Pract. 1995;8:347-356.

258. Marrie TJ. Community-acquired pneumonia in the elderly. Clin Infect Dis. 2000;31:1066-1078.

259. Feldman C. Pneumonia in the elderly. Med Clin North Am. 2001;85:1441-1459.

260. Berk SL, Holtsclaw SA, Wiener SL, Smith JK. Nontypeable Haemophilus influenzae in the elderly. Arch Intern Med. 1982;142:532-539.

261. Valenti WM, Trudell RG, Bentley DW. Factors predisposing to oropharyngeal colonization with gram-negative bacilli in the aged. N Engl J Med. 1978;298:1108-1111.

262. Kidd D, Lawson J, Nesbitt R, MacMahon J. The natural history and clinical consequences of aspiration in acute stroke. Q J Med. 1995;88:409-413.

263. Pick N, McDonald A, Bennett N, et al. Pulmonary aspiration in a long-term care setting: Clinical and laboratory observation and an analysis of risk factors. J Am Geriatr Soc. 1996;44:763-768.

264. Marrie TJ. Mycoplasma pneumoniae requiring hospitalization with emphasis on infection in the elderly. Arch Intern Med. 1993;153:488-494.

265. Orr PH, Peeling RW, Fast M, et al. Serologic study of responses to selected pathogens causing respiratory tract infection in the institutionalized elderly. Clin Infect Dis. 1996;23:1240-1245.

266. Falsey AR, Cunningham CK, Barber WH, et al. Respiratory syncytial virus and influenza A infections in the hospitalized elderly. J Infect Dis. 1995;172:389-394.

267. Dowell SF, Anderson LJ, Gary HE Jr, et al. Respiratory syncytial virus is an important cause of community-acquired lower respiratory infection among hospitalized adults. J Infect Dis. 1996;174:456-462.

268. Nicholson KG, Kent J, Hammersley V, Cancio E. Risk factors for lower respiratory complications of rhinovirus infections in elderly people living in the community: Prospective cohort study. BMJ. 1996;313:1119-1123.

269. Mylotte JM. Nursing home-acquired pneumonia. Clin Infect Dis. 2002;35:1205-1211.

270. Yamaya M, Yanai M, Ohrui T, et al. Interventions to prevent pneumonia among older adults. J Am Geriatr Soc. 2001;49:85-90.

271. Mehr DR, Binder EF, Kruse RL, et al. Clinical findings associated with radiographic pneumonia in nursing home residents. J Fam Pract. 2001;50:931-937.

272. Murray JF, Felton CP, Garay SM, et al. Pulmonary complications of the acquired immunodeficiency syndrome: Report of a National Heart, Lung and Blood Institute Workshop. N Engl J Med. 1984;310:1682-1688.

273. Stover DE, White DA, Romano PA, et al. Spectrum of pulmonary diseases associated with the acquired immune deficiency syndrome. Am J Med. 1985;78:429-437.

274. Murray JF. Pulmonary complications of HIV infection. Annu Rev Med. 1996;47:117-126.

275. Saah AJ, Hoover DR, Pengy Phair JP, et al. Predictors for failure of Pneumocystis carinii pneumonia prophylaxis multicenter AIDS cohort study. JAMA. 1995;273:1197-1202.

276. Rimland D, Navin TR, Lennox JL, et al. Prospective study of etiologic agents of community-acquired pneumonia in patients with HIV infection. AIDS. 2002;16:85-95.

277. Baril L, Astagneau P, Nguyen J, et al. Pyogenic bacterial pneumonia in human immunodeficiency virus-infected inpatients: A clinical, radiological, microbiological, and epidemiological study. Clin Infect Dis. 1998;26:964-971.

278. Pulmonary Complications of HIV Infection Study Group: Design of a prospective study of the pulmonary complications of human immunodeficiency virus infection. J Clin Epidemiol. 1993;46:497.

279. Pachon J, Prados D, Capote F, et al. Severe community-acquired pneumonia: Etiology, prognosis, treatment. Am Rev Respir Dis. 1990;142:369-373.

280. Potgieter PD, Hammond JMJ. Etiology and diagnosis of pneumonia requiring ICU admission: A discussion. Chest. 1992;101:199-203.

281. Leroy O, Santre C, Beuscart C, et al. A five-year study of severe community-acquired pneumonia with emphasis on prognosis in patients admitted to an intensive care unit. Intensive Care Med. 1995;21:44-51.

282. Neuhaus T, Ewig S. Defining severe community-acquired pneumonia. Med Clinic North Am. 2001;85:1413-1425.

283. Niederman MS, Mandell LA, Anzueto A, et al. Guidelines for the management adults with community-acquired pneumonia: Diagnosis, assessment of severity, and antimicrobial therapy and prevention. Am J Resp Crit Care Med. 1993;148:1418-1426.

284. Ewig S, Ruiz M, Mensa J, et al. Severe community-acquired pneumonia: Assessment of severity criteria. Am J Resp Crit Care Med. 1998;158:1102-1108.

285. Pascual FE, Matthay MA, Bacchetti P, Wachter RM. Assessment of prognosis in patients with community-acquired pneumonia who require mechanical ventilation. Chest. 2000;117:503-512.

286. Leeper KV Jr, Torres A. Community-acquired pneumonia in the intensive care unit. Clin Chest Med. 1995;16:155-178.

287. Leeper KV Jr. Severe community-acquired pneumonia. Semin Respir Infect. 1996;11:96-108.

288. Farr BM, Sloman AJ, Fisch MJ. Predicting death in patients hospitalized for community-acquired pneumonia. Ann Intern Med. 1991;115:428-436.

289. The British Thoracic Society Research Committee and the Public Health Laboratory Service. Community-acquired pneumonia in adults in British hospitals in 1982-1983: A survey of aetiology, mortality, prognostic factors and outcome. Q J Med. 1987;62:195-220.

290. Fine MJ, Orloff JJ, Arisumi D, et al. Prognosis of patients hospitalized with community-acquired pneumonia. Am J Med. 1990;88:S1N-S8N.

291. Leroy O, Santre L, Beuscart L. A five-year old study of severe community-acquired pneumonia with emphasis on prognosis in patients admitted to an intensive care unit. Intensive Care Med. 1995;21:24-31.

292. Marrie TJ. Normal resolution of community-acquired pneumonia. Semin Respir Infect. 1992;7:256-270.

293. Lehtomaki K. Clinical diagnosis of pneumococcal adenoviral, mycoplasmal and viral pneumonia in young men. Eur Respir J. 1988;1:324-329.

294. Halm EA, Fine MJ, Marrie TJ, et al. Time to clinical stability in patients hospitalized with community-acquired pneumonia: Implications for practice guidelines. JAMA. 1998;279:1452-1457.

295. Jay SJ, Johnson WG Jr, Pierce WK. The radiographic resolution of *Streptococcus pneumoniae* pneumonia. N Engl J Med. 1991;293:798-801.

296. Corley DE, Winterbauer RH. Infectious diseases that result in slowly resolving and chronic pneumonia. Semin Respir Med. 1993;8:3-13.

297. Rome L, Murali G, Lippmann M. Nonresolving pneumonia and mimics of pneumonia. Med Clinic North Am. 2001;85:1511-1530.

298. Reiman HA. An acute infection of the respiratory tract with atypical pneumonia. JAMA. 1938;111:2377-2384.

299. File TM, Tan JS, Plouffe JF. The role of atypical pathogens: *Mycoplasma pneumoniae, Chlamydia pneumoniae* and *Legionella pneumophila* in respiratory infection. Infect Dis Clin North Am. 1998;12:509-592.

300. File TM Jr, Tan JS, Plouffe TF. Community-acquired pneumonia: What's needed for accurate diagnosis. Postgrad Med. 1996;99:95-107.

301. Gaydos CA, Eiden JJ, Oldach D, et al. Diagnosis of *Chlamydia pneumoniae* infection in patients with community-acquired pneumonia by polymerase chain reaction enzyme immunoassay. Clin Infect Dis. 1994;19:157-160.

302. Lieberman D, Schlaeffer F, Lieberman D, et al. *Mycoplasma pneumoniae* community-acquired pneumonia: A review of 101 hospitalized adult patients. Respiration. 1996;63:261-266.

303. Grayston JT, Diwan VK, Cooney M, et al. Community and hospital acquired pneumonia associated with chlamydia TWAR infection demonstrated serologically. Arch Intern Med. 1989;149:169-173.

304. Thorn DH, Grayston JT. Infections with *Chlamydia pneumoniae* strain TWAR. Clin Chest Med. 1991;12:245-256.

305. Kauppinen M, Saikku P. Pneumonia due to *Chlamydia pneumoniae:* Prevalence, clinical features, diagnosis, and treatment. Clin Infect Dis. 1995;21(Suppl 3):S244-S252.

306. Grayston JT, Campbell LA, Kuo CC, et al. A new respiratory tract pathogen: *Chlamydia pneumoniae* strain TWAR. J Infect Dis. 1990;161:618-625.

307. Kleemola M, Saikku P, Viskorpi R, et al. Epidemics of pneumonia caused by TWAR, a new *Chlamydia* organism in military trainees in Finland. J Infect Dis. 1988;157:230-236.

308. Von Hurtzen L, Alakarppa H, Koskinen R, et al. *Chlamydia pneumoniae* infection in patients with chronic obstructive pulmonary disease. Epidemiol Infect. 1997;118:155-164.

309. Kauppinen MT, Saikku P, Kujala P, et al. Clinical picture of community-acquired *Chlamydia pneumoniae* pneumonia requiring hospital treatment: A comparison between chlamydial and pneumococcal pneumonia. Thorax. 1996;51:185-190.

310. Grayston JT. Infection caused by *Chlamydia pneumoniae* strain TWAR. Clin Infect Dis. 1992;15:757-763.

311. Tack KJ, Peterson PK, Rasp FL, et al. Isolation of *Chlamydia trachomatis* from the lower respiratory tracts of adults. Lancet. 1980;1:116-120.

312. Komaroff AL, Aronson MD, Schachter J. *Chlamydia trachomatis* infections in adults with community acquired pneumonia. JAMA. 1981;245:1319-1322.

313. Wenzel RP, McCormick DP, Beam WE Jr. Parainfluenza pneumonia in adults. JAMA. 1972;221:294-295.

314. Falsey AR, Cunningham CK, Baber WH, et al. Respiratory syncytial virus and influenza A infections in the hospitalized elderly. J Infect Dis. 1995;172:389-394.

315. Englund JA, Sullivan CJ, Jordan MC, et al. Respiratory syncytial virus infections in immunocompromised adults. Ann Intern Med. 1988;109:203-208.

316. Harrington RD, Hooton TM, Hackman RC, et al. An outbreak of respiratory syncytial virus in a bone marrow transplant center. J Infect Dis. 1992;165:987-993.

317. Duchin JS, Koster FT, Peters CJ, et al. Hantavirus pulmonary syndrome: A clinical description of 17 patients with a newly recognized disease. N Engl J Med. 1994;330:949-955.

318. Jenison S, Hjelle BM, Simpson S, et al. Hantavirus pulmonary syndrome: Clinical, diagnostic and virologic aspects. Semin Respir Infect. 1995;10:259-269.

319. Ksiazek TG, Erdman D, Goldsmith CS, et al. A novel coronavirus associated with severe acute respiratory syndrome. N Engl J Med. 2003;348:1953-1966.

320. Rello J, Quintana E, Ausiner V, et al. A three-year study of severe community-acquired pneumonia with emphasis on outcome. Chest. 1993;103:232-235.

321. Leeper KV Jr, Torres A. Community-acquired pneumonia in the intensive care unit. Clin Chest Med. 1995;16:155-171.

322. Waterer GW, Baselski VS, Wunderink RG. Legionella and community-acquired pneumonia: A review of current diagnostic tests from a clinician's viewpoint. Am J Med. 2001;110:41-48.

323. Stout JE, Yu VL. Legionellosis. N Engl J Med. 1997;337:682-687.

324. Sopena N, Sabria-Leal M, Pedro-Botet ML, et al. Comparative study of the clinical presentation of *Legionella* pneumonia and other community-acquired pneumonias. Chest. 1998;113:1195-1200.

325. Nakajoh K, Nakagawa T, Sekizawa K, et al. Relation between incidence of pneumonia and protective reflexes in post-stroke patients with oral or tube feeding. J Intern Med. 2000;247:39-42.

326. Perry L, Love CP. Screening for dysphagia and aspiration in acute stroke: A systematic review. Dysphagia. 2001;16:7-18.

327. Matthay MA, Rosen GD. Acid aspiration induced lung injury: New insights and therapeutic options. Am J Respir Crit Care Med. 1996;154:277-278.

328. Robinovici R, Neville LF, Abdullah F, et al. Aspiration-induced lung injury: Role of complement. Crit Care Med. 1995;23:1405-1411.

329. Bartlett JG, Gorbach SL. The triple threat of aspiration pneumonia. Chest. 1979;68:560-566.

330. Marik PE. Aspiration pneumonitis and aspiration pneumonia. N Engl J Med. 2001;344:665-671.

331. Marik PE, Careau P. The role of anaerobes in patients with ventilator-associated pneumonia and aspiration pneumonia. Chest. 1999;115:178-183.

332. Dreyfuss D, Mier L. Aspiration pneumonia (Correspondence). N Engl J Med. 2001;344:1868-1870.

333. Hammond JMJ, Potgieter PD, Hanslo D, et al. The etiology and antimicrobial susceptibility patterns of microorganisms in acute community-acquired lung abscess. Chest. 1995;108:937-941.

334. Finegold SM. Aspiration pneumonia. Rev Infect Dis. 1991;13(Suppl 9):S737-S742.

335. Lorber B, Swenson RM. Bacteriology of aspiration pneumonia: A prospective study of community and hospital-acquired cases. Ann Intern Med. 1974;81:329-331.

336. Allen JN, Davis WB. What is eosinophilic pneumonia? Arch Intern Med. 1992;152:1765-1766.

337. Schatz M, Wasserman S, Patterson R. Eosinophils and immunologic lung disease. Med Clin North Am. 1981;65:1055-1071.

338. Fleury-Feith J, Van Nhieu JT, Picard L, et al. Bronchoalveolar lavage eosinophilia associated with *Pneumocystis carinii* pneumonitis in AIDS patients. Chest. 1989;95:1198-1201.

339. Pope-Harman AL, Davis WB, Allen ED. Acute eosinophilic pneumonia: A summary of 15 cases and a review of the literature. Medicine (Baltimore). 1996;75:334-342.

340. Liebow AA, Carrington CB. The eosinophilic pneumonias. Medicine (Baltimore). 1969;48:251-285.

341. Jederlinic PJ, Sicilian L, Graensler EA. Chronic eosinophilic pneumonia. Medicine (Baltimore). 1988;67:154-162.

342. Marchand E, Reynand-Gaubert M, Lauque D, et al. Idiopathic chronic eosinophilic pneumonia. Medicine (Baltimore). 1998;77:299-312.

343. Marshall BG, Wilkinson RJ, Davidson RN. Pathogenesis of tropical pulmonary eosinophilia, parasitic alveolitis, and parallels with asthma. Respir Med. 1998;92:1-3.

344. Haley RW, Culver DH, White JW, et al. The nationwide nosocomial infection rate: A new need for vital statistics. Am J Epidemiol. 1985;121:159-167.

345. Simmons BP, Wong ES. CDC guidelines for the prevention and control of nosocomial infections: Guideline for prevention of nosocomial pneumonia. Am J Infect Control. 1983;11:230-233.

346. McEachern R, Campbell GD Jr. Hospital-acquired pneumonia: Epidemiology, etiology, and treatment. Infect Dis Clin North Am. 1998;12:761-779.

347. American Thoracic Society. Hospital-acquired pneumonia in adults: Diagnosis, assessment of severity, initial antimicrobial therapy, and prevention strategies. Am J Respir Crit Care Med. 1996;153:1711-1725.

348. Wenzel RP. Hospital-acquired pneumonia: An overview of the current state of the art for prevention and control. Eur J Clin Microbiol Infect Dis. 1989;8:56-60.

349. Rouby JL, Laurent P, Gosnach M, et al. Risk factors and clinical relevance of nosocomial maxillary sinusitis in the critically ill. Am J Respir Crit Care Med. 1994;150:776-783.

350. George DL. Epidemiology of nosocomial pneumonia in intensive care unit patients. Clin Chest Med. 1995;16:29-44.

351. Craven DE, Steger KA. Epidemiology of nosocomial pneumonia: New perspectives on an old disease. Chest. 1995;108(2 Suppl):1S-16S.

352. Donowitz LG, Page MC, Mileur BL, et al. Alteration of normal gastric flora in critical care patients receiving antacid and cimetidine therapy. Infect Control. 1986;7:23-26.

353. Craven DE, Steger KA, Barber TW. Preventing nosocomial pneumonia: State of the art and perspective for the 1990s. Am J Med. 1991;91(Suppl 3B):44S-53S.

354. Simms HH, DeMoria E, McDonald L, et al. Role of gastric colonization in the development of pneumonia in critically ill trauma patients: Results of a prospective randomized trial. J Trauma. 1991;31:531-537.

355. Bonten MJM, Gaillard CA, deLeeuw PW, Stobberingh EE. Role of colonization of the upper intestinal tract in the pathogenesis of ventilator-associated pneumonia. Clin Infect Dis. 1997;24:309-319.

356. Rello J, Ausina V, Castella J, et al. Incidence, etiology and outcome of nosocomial pneumonia in mechanically ventilated patients. Chest. 1991;100:439-444.

357. Septimus EJ. Nosocomial bacterial pneumonia. Semin Respir Infect. 1989;4:245-252.

358. A'Court C, Garrard CS. Nosocomial pneumonia in the intensive care unit: Mechanism and significance. Thorax. 1992;47:465-473.

359. Bartlett JG, O'Keefe P, Tally FP, et al. Bacteriology of hospital-acquired pneumonia. Arch Intern Med. 1986;146:868-871.

360. Carratala J, Guidol F, Pallares J, et al. Risk factors for nosocomial *Legionella pneumophila* pneumonia. Am J Respir Crit Care Med. 1994;149:625-629.

361. Graman PS, Hall CB. Nosocomial viral respiratory infections. Semin Respir Infect. 1989;4:253-260.

362. Holladay RC, Campbell GD Jr. Nosocomial viral pneumonia in the intensive care unit. Clin Chest Med. 1995;16:121-133.

363. Fagon JY, Chastre J, Hance AJ, et al. Evaluation of clinical judgment in the identification and treatment of nosocomial pneumonia in ventilated patients. Chest. 1993;103:547-553.

364. Wunderink RG. Clinical criteria in the diagnosis of ventilator-associated pneumonia. Chest. 2000;117:191S-194S.

365. Grossman RF. Evidence-based assessment of diagnostic tests for ventilator-associated pneumonia. Chest. 2000;117:177S-181S.

366. Rello J, Paiva JA, Baraibor J, et al. International conference for the development of consensus on the diagnosis and treatment of ventilator-associated pneumonia. Chest. 2001;120:955-970.

367. Cunha BA. Pneumonia in the compromised host. Infect Dis Clin North Am. 2001;15:591-612.

368. Niederman MS, Peters SP. Update in pulmonary medicine. Ann Intern Med. 1998;128:208-215.

369. Black ER, Mushlin AI, Griner PF, et al. Predicting the need for hospitalization of ambulatory patients with pneumonia. J Gen Intern Med. 1991;6:394-400.

370. Fine MJ, Smith DN, Singer DE. Hospitalization decision on patients with community-acquired pneumonia: A prospective cohort study. Am J Med. 1990;89:713-721.

371. Fine MJ, Auble TE, Yealy DM, et al. A prediction rule to identify low risk patients with community-acquired pneumonia. N Engl J Med. 1997;336:1248-1250.

372. Marrie TJ, Lau CY, Wheeler SL, et al. A controlled trial of a critical pathway for treatment of community-acquired pneumonia. JAMA. 2000;283:749-755.

373. Atlas SJ, Benzer TI, Borowsky LH, et al. Safely increasing the proportion of patients with community-acquired pneumonia treated as outpatients: An interventional trial. Arch Intern Med. 1998;158:1350-1356.

374. Porath A, Schlaeffer F, Lieberman D. Appropriateness of hospitalization of patients with community-acquired pneumonia. Ann Emerg Med. 1996;27:176-183.

375. Schmidt LN, Sesler CL. Development of resistance to penicillin by pneumococci. Proc Soc Exp Biol Med. 1943;52:353-357.

376. Klugman PK. Pneumococcal resistance to antibiotics. Clin Microbiol Rev. 1990; 3:171-176.

377. Spika JS, Facklam RR, Rlikaytis BD, et al. Antimicrobial resistance to *Streptococcus pneumoniae* in the United States: 1979-1987. J Infect Dis. 1991;163:1273-1278.

378. Doern GV, Heilmann KP, Huynh HK, et al. Antimicrobial resistance among clinical isolates of *Streptococcus pneumoniae* in the United States during 1999-2000 including a comparison of resistance rates since 1994-1995. Antimicrob Agents Chemother. 2001;45:1721-1729.

379. Karlowsky JA, Thornsberry C, Jones ME, et al. Factors associated with relative rates of antimicrobial resistance among *Streptococcus pneumoniae* in the United States: Results from the TRUST Surveillance Program (1998-2002). Clin Infect Dis. 2003;36:963-970.

380. Feikin DR, Schuchat A, Kolczak M, et al. Mortality from invasive pneumococcal pneumonia in the era of antibiotic resistance 1995-1997. Am J Public Health. 2000;90:223-229.

381. Turett GS, Blum S, Fazal B, et al. Penicillin resistance and other predictors of mortality in pneumococcal bacteremia in a population with high human immunodeficiency virus seroprevalence. Clin Inf Dis. 1999;29:321-327.

382. Klugman KP, Feldman C. The clinical relevance of antibiotic resistance in the management of pneumococcal pneumonia. Infect Dis Clin Pract. 1998;7:180-184.

383. Yu VL, Chiou CC, Feldman C, et al. An international prospective study of pneumococcal bacteremia: Correlation with in vitro resistance, antibiotics administered, and clinical outcome. Clin Infec Dis. 2003;37:230-237.

384. Pallares R, Liñares J, Vadillo M, et al. Resistance to penicillin and cephalosporin and mortality from severe pneumococcal pneumonia in Barcelona, Spain. N Engl J Med. 1995;333:474-480.

385. Mandell LA. Relationship of penicillin resistance to mortality in pneumococcal pneumonia. Curr Infect Dis Rep. 2001;3:9-12.

386. Craig WA. Antimicrobial resistance issues of the future. Diagn Microbiol Infect Dis. 1996;25:213-217.

387. Liñares J, Alonso T, Perez JL. Decreased susceptibility of penicillin-resistant pneumococci to twenty-four β-lactam antibiotics. J Antimicrob Chemother. 1992;30:279-288.

388. Butler JC, Hofmann J, Cetron MS, et al. The continued emergence of drug-resistant *Streptococcus pneumoniae* in the United States: An update from the Centers for Disease Control and Prevention's Pneumococcal Sentinel Surveillance System. J Infect Dis. 1996;174:986-993.

389. Simor AE, Louie M, Low DE. The Canadian Bacterial Surveillance Network: Canadian national survey of prevalence of antimicrobial resistance among clinical isolates of *Streptococcus pneumoniae*. Antimicrob Agents Chemother. 1996;40:2190-2193.

390. Thornburn CE, Knott SJ, Edwards DI. In vitro activities of oral β-lactams at concentrations achieved in humans against penicillin-susceptible and resistant pneumococci and potential to select resistance. Antimicrob Agents Chemother. 1998;42:1973-1979.

391. Whitney CG, Farley MM, Hadler J, et al. Increasing prevalence of multidrug-resistant *Streptococcus pneumoniae* in the United States. N Engl J Med. 2000;343:1917-1924.

392. Thornsberry C, Sahm DF, Kelly LJ, et al. Regional trends in antimicrobial resistance among clinical isolates of *Streptococcus pneumoniae, Haemophilus influenzae,* and *Moraxella catarrhalis* in the United States: Results from the TRUST Surveillance Program, 1999-2000. Clin Infect Dis. 2002;34(Suppl 1):S4-16.

393. Jacobs MR. In vivo veritas: In vitro macrolide resistance in systemic *Streptococcus pneumoniae* infections does result in clinical failure. Clin Infect Dis. 2002;35: 565-569.

394. Kelley MA, Weber DJ, Gilligan P, Cohen MS. Breakthrough pneumococcal bacteremia in patients being treated with azithromycin and clarithromycin. Clin Infect Dis. 2000;31:1008-1011.

395. Lonks JR, Garau J, Gomez L, et al. Failure of macrolide antibiotic treatment in patients with bacteremia due to erythromycin-resistant *Streptococcus pneumoniae*. Clin Infect Dis. 2002;35:556-564.

396. Davidson R, Cavalconti R, Brunton JL, et al. Resistance to levofloxacin and failure of treatment of Pneumococcal pneumonia. N Engl J Med. 2002;346:747-750.

397. Waterer GW, Somes GW, Wunderink RG. Monotherapy may be suboptimal for severe bacteremic pneumococcal pneumonia. Arch Intern Med. 2001;161:1837-1842.

398. Gleason PP, Meehan TP, Fine JM, et al. Associations between initial antimicrobial therapy and medical outcomes for hospitalized elderly patients with pneumonia. Arch Intern Med. 1999;159:2562-2572.

399. Stahl JE, Barza M, DesJardin J, et al. Effect of macrolides as part of initial empiric therapy on length of stay in patients hospitalized with community-acquired pneumonia. Arch Intern Med. 1999;159:2576-2580.

400. Martínez JA, Horcajada JP, Almela M, et al. Addition of a macrolide to a β-lactam-based empirical antibiotic regimen is associated with lower in-hospital mortality for patients with bacteremic pneumococcal pneumonia. Clin Infect Dis. 2003;36:389-395.

401. File TM, Mandell LA. What is optimal antimicrobial therapy for bacteremic pneumococcal pneumonia? Clin Infect Dis. 2003;36:396-398.

402. Waterer GW. Combination antibiotic therapy with macrolides in community-acquired pneumonia: More smoke but is there any fire? Chest. 2003;123:1328-1329.

403. Clark JP, Langston E. Ketolides: A new class of antibacterial agents for treatment of community-acquired respiratory tract infections in a primary care setting. Mayo Clin Proc. 2003;78:1113-1124.

404. Gleason PP, Kapoor WN, Stone RA, et al. Medical outcomes and antimicrobial costs with the use of the American Thoracic Society guidelines for outpatients with community-acquired pneumonia. JAMA. 1997;278:32-39.

405. Craig WA, Andes D. Aminoglycosides are useful for severe respiratory tract infections. Semin Respir Infect. 1997;12:271-277.

406. Schentag JJ, Birmingham MC, Paladins JA, et al. Nosocomial pneumonia, optimizing antibiotics other than aminoglycosides is a more important determinant of successful clinical outcome and a better means of avoiding resistance. Semin Respir Infect. 1997;12:278-293.

407. Arancibia F, Bauer TT, Ewig S, et al. Community-acquired pneumonia due to gram-negative bacteria and *Pseudomonas aeruginosa:* Incidence, risk, and prognosis. Arch Intern Med. 2002;162:1849-1858.

408. Battleman DS, Callahan M, Thaler HT. Rapid antibiotic delivery and appropriate antibiotic selection reduce length of hospital stay of patients with community-acquired pneumonia. Arch Intern Med. 2002;162:682-688.

409. Brown RB, Iannini P, Gross P, Kunkel M. Impact of initial antibiotic choice on clinical outcomes in community-acquired pneumonia. Chest. 2003;123:1503-1511.

410. Halm EA, Fine MJ, Marrie TJ, et al. Time to clinical stability in patients hospitalized with community-acquired pneumonia: Implication for practice guidelines. JAMA. 1998;279:1452-1457.

411. Rhew DC, Weingarten SR. Achieving a safe and early discharge for patients with community-acquired pneumonia. Med Clin North Am. 2001;85:1427-1440.

412. Castro-Guardiola A, Viejo-Rodríguez AL, Soler-Simon S, et al. Efficacy and safety of oral and early-switch therapy for community-acquired pneumonia: A randomized controlled trial. Am J Med. 2001;111:367-374.

413. Ramirez JA. Managing antiinfective therapy of community-acquired pneumonia in the hospital setting: focus on switch therapy. Pharmacotherapy. 2001;21:79S-82S.

414. Hitt CM, Nightingale CH, Quintiianc R, Nicolau DP. Streamlining antimicrobial therapy for lower respiratory tract infections. Clin Infect Dis. 1997;24(Suppl 2):S231-S237.

415. Beaumont M, Shuster MG. Is an observation period necessary after intravenous antibiotics are changed to oral administration? Am J Med. 1999;106:114-116.

416. Halm EA, Fine MJ, Kapoor WN, et al. Instability on hospital discharge and the risk of adverse outcomes in patients with pneumonia. Arch Intern Med. 2002;162: 1278-1284.

417. Chan R, Hemeryck L, O'Regan M, et al. Oral versus intravenous antibiotics for community-acquired lower respiratory tract infection in a general hospital, open, randomized controlled trial. BMJ. 1995;310:1360-1362.

418. Dunbar LM, Wunderink RG, Habib MP, et al. High-dose, short course levofloxacin for community-acquired pneumonia: A new treatment paradigm. Clin Infect Dis. 2003;37:752-760.

419. Mandell L, File TM Jr. Short course treatment of community-acquired pneumonia. Clin Infect Dis. 2003;37:761-763.

420. Gross PA, Hermogenes AW, Sacks HS, et al. The efficacy of influenza vaccine in elderly patients: A meta-analysis and review of the literature. Ann Intern Med. 1995;123:518-527.

421. Nichol KL, Nordin J, Mullooly J, et al. Influenza vaccination and reduction in hospitalizations for cardiac disease and stroke among the elderly. N Engl J Med. 2003;348:1322-1332.

422. Advisory Committee on Immunization Practices (ACIP) on the use of influenza vaccine and antiviral agents. MMWR Morb Mortal Wkly Rep. 2003;52:1-44.

423. Jackson LA, Neuzil KM, Yu O, et al. Effectiveness of pneumococcal polysaccharide vaccine in older adults. N Engl J Med. 2003;348:1747-1755.

CHAPTER **62**

Pleural Effusion and Empyema

EDWARD SEPTIMUS

Despite newer antimicrobial agents and improved diagnostic imaging, infections of the pleural space remain an important cause of morbidity and mortality around the world. Delay in diagnosis, failure to institute appropriate antimicrobial therapy, and inadequate drainage contribute to increased morbidity and mortality.[1-3]

Infections of the pleural space most commonly follow pneumonia, accounting for 40% to 60% of all empyemas. Thoracotomy is the next most common precursor of empyema, accounting for 20%, and trauma accounts for 4% to 10%. Less commonly, empyema can develop as a result of esophageal rupture and subdiaphragmatic spread. Other uncommon causes include hematogenous seeding of an existing pleural effusion and direct extension from head and neck infections.[4-7]

PATHOPHYSIOLOGY

When pleural effusions develop without pleural inflammation, factors that can be identified include increased hydrostatic pressure, decreased oncotic pressure, and alteration in lymphatic drainage.[8] In the noninflamed state, the pleural space contains a small amount of transudative pleural fluid with a low concentration of protein and 1000 to 5000 cells per cubic millimeter, primarily lymphocytes, macrophages, and mesothelial cells. Neutrophils are usually absent.[8] In addition, infected pleural fluid is deficient in the opsonins and complement necessary for optimal phagocytic function, and the low pH and hypoxia in infected pleural fluid further impair neutrophil function.[9-10]

With pleural inflammation, the interaction of bacteria, lipopolysaccharide (LPS), cytokines, and chemokines lead to changes in pleural permeability. The initial events during pleural inflammation are mediated via responses of stimulated pleural mesothelial cells (PMCs). Bacterial cell wall products bind to PMCs and stimulate production of interleukin (IL)-1, IL-8, epithelial neutrophil-activating protein (ENA)-78, tumor necrosis factor (TNF)-α, and platelet-activating factor. In vitro, IL-1, TNF-α, and LPS have been shown to release IL-8, although levels of TNF-α and IL-1 in pleural fluid did not correlate with IL-8 production.[11]

The primary role of PMCs is coordinating and facilitating the permeability and recruitment of neutrophils and mononuclear phagocytes. PMCs are also capable of phagocytosis and release of nitric oxide (NO). Owens and Grisham demonstrated that PMC could be induced to produce large amounts of NO in response to specific combinations of proinflammatory cytokines and LPS.[12] NO can play a role in bacterial killing.

Jonjic and colleagues studied the capacity of PMC to express adhesion molecules and chemoattractant cytokines, two basic mechanisms in the regulation of neutrophil recruitment.[13] PMCs were able to express the chemotactic cytokines IL-8 and monocyte chemoattractant protein 1 at the mRNA and protein levels. Their results also indicated that PMCs can express a set of adhesion molecules, intercellular adhesion molecule 1 (ICAM-1) and vascular cell adhesion molecule 1 (VCAM-1), and that these are functionally important in interacting with mononuclear phagocytes. The regulated expression of adhesion molecules and chemotactic cytokines by PMCs is important in inflammation and immune mediation. The interaction between CD11/CD18 integrins expressed on neutrophils and ICAM-1 can lead to adherence of neutrophils to the surface of the implicated cell. Expression of these adhesive glycoproteins by PMCs enhances the recruitment of neutrophils and mononuclear cells into the pleural space.[13]

Pleural fluid from patients who develop parapneumonic effusions has been found to be chemotactic to neutrophils when compared with pleural fluid collected from patients with other diagnoses.[14] Studies have found a positive correlation between IL-8 levels and the number of neutrophils in pleural fluid. Broaddus and co-workers reported that anti-IL-8 antibodies decreased chemotactic activity in empyema fluid.[14] Antony and co-workers showed elevated IL-8 levels in both parapneumonic effusions and empyema fluid when compared with pleural effusions secondary to other diseases. IL-8 levels were higher in empyema fluid than in parapneumonic effusions. They also found a significant correlation between IL-8 levels and the total number of neutrophils in pleural fluid. Chemotactic activity for neutrophils was increased in empyema fluid but was decreased with the addition of IL-8 neutralizing serum.[15]

ENA-78 is a CXC chemokine that has been shown to be present in high amounts in parapneumonic effusions. For early parapneumonic effusions, ENA-78 is the dominant chemokine responsible for neutrophil chemotaxis. In the later stages of the development of empyema, IL-8 becomes the dominant chemokine.[15,16] Parapneumonic pleural fluid has also been shown to have increased procoagulant activity and also depressed fibrinolytic activity that favors fibrin deposition in the pleural space. The deposition of fibrin and the increased activity of fibroblasts leads to a thick pleural peel characteristic of the later stages seen in empyema.[17] However, if pneumonia associated with a parapneumonic effusion is treated promptly with an appropriate antimicrobial agent, the cellular and cytokine mediators of inflammation are aborted. Resolution of uncomplicated parapneumonic effusions leaves the pleura essentially normal without clinically significant fibrosis.[18]

MICROBIOLOGY

The microbiology of empyema has changed dramatically in the last 50 years. In the preantibiotic era, *Streptococcus pneumoniae* accounted for 60% to 70% of cases, *Streptococcus pyogenes* for 10% to 15% of cases, and *Staphylococcus aureus* for 5% to 10% of cases.[19] *S. pneumoniae* now accounts for only 5% to 10% of cases, and many infections are mixed, with anaerobes present in 25% to 76% of empyemas either as sole organisms or in combination with other aerobic or facultative organisms.[20] Bartlett and Finegold found that pleural empyema was caused by aerobic bacteria in 24%, anaerobic bacteria in 35%, and both aerobic and anaerobic bacteria in 41% of 83 medical service patients without prior antibiotic therapy or surgical procedures.[21] The most common anaerobes isolated include the *Bacteroides fragilis* group, *Prevotella* species, *Fusobacterium nucleatum*, and *Peptostreptococcus*. A 1990 study suggests that anaerobic infection may occur in 25% to 33% of children with empyema.[22] Pleural infection secondary to subdiaphragmatic disease is often polymicrobial and anaerobic in origin.[23]

Predisposing factors are most important in predicting the most likely pathogens. Pneumonia continues to be the most frequent predisposing factor in the development of empyemas.[3-7] In otherwise healthy adults with pneumonia, the most common bacteria causing pleural empyema are *S. aureus*, *S. pneumoniae*, or *S. pyogenes*.[1,19,24] The incidence of a parapneumonic effusion in hospitalized patients is estimated to be 40%.[25] Although *S. pneumoniae* is the most common cause of community-acquired pneumonia, empyema has occurred in only 1% to 2% of cases of pneumococcal pneumonia compared with 10% to 18% in the preantibiotic era.[26] Empyema caused by *S. aureus*, *S. pneumoniae*, or *Haemophilus influenzae* has been common in children.[27] The *H. influenzae* conjugate vaccine has dramatically reduced the frequency of suppurative complications caused by *H. influenzae* infection in children. The use of the pneumococcal conjugate vaccine has reduced the incidence of invasive disease caused by *S. pneumoniae* in young children and may prevent invasive disease in adults as well.[28] Buckingham and colleagues recently published their experience on complicated parapneumonic effusions in children.[29] They found that the incidence of these effusions in children with community-acquired pneumonia increased from 1996 to 1999 and then declined with the introduction of the pneumococcal conjugate vaccine. Although cases caused by *S. pneumoniae* decreased, community-onset methicillin-resistant *S. aureus* emerged as a significant cause of pneumonia and complicated parapneumonic effusions in children.[29]

Most cases of *S. aureus* empyema result from *S. aureus* pneumonia,[30] which is most often seen in older hospitalized patients with underlying medical problems. *S. aureus* is an uncommon cause of pneumonia in otherwise healthy adults except during an influenza outbreak.[31] *S. aureus* has a tendency to cause cavitation, with resultant secondary lung abscesses. Empyema can be seen in 10% to 24% of adults with *S. aureus* pneumonia.[24,30] In children, multiple thin-walled cavities or abscesses, or pneumatoceles, develop with *S. aureus* pneumonia. Empyema can develop in as many as 50% of children.[29]

S. pyogenes was a common cause of pneumonia in the preantibiotic era, but cases are uncommon today. *S. pyogenes* pneumonia can be seen in military recruits or as a sequela of a viral respiratory infection.

Empyema occurs in 30% to 40% of cases and tends to develop early in the course of infection.[32,33]

Factors predisposing to aspiration, such as altered mental status, alcoholism, and periodontal disease, are common in patients with anaerobic infections of the pleura. Many of these cases tend to be polymicrobial. In addition to anaerobes, viridans streptococci, aerobic gram-negative bacilli, and occasionally *S. aureus* have been recovered.

Viridans streptococci are normally found in the mouth and in the gastrointestinal tract. A study of pulmonary infections caused by viridans streptococci found that the majority (68%) of the isolates belonged to the *Streptococcus anginosus (Streptococcus milleri)* group.[34] Many of the *S. anginosus* group isolates, particularly those of *Streptococcus intermedius,* are nonhemolytic, but some are α- or β-hemolytic, and most carry Lancefield group F antigen.[35] Isolates in the *S. anginosus* group are known by their propensity for an invasive pyogenic process that results in abscess formation; this is attributed to their ability to produce hydrolytic enzymes that facilitate the spread and liquefaction of pus.[36]

Pleuropulmonary actinomycosis can result from aspiration. These patients exhibit a chronic pulmonary infection with chest wall involvement or draining sinus tracts with sulfur granules, or both. Up to 50% of pulmonary actinomycoses have pleural involvement.[37] Isolation of *Actinomyces* confirms the diagnosis.

Legionella can be isolated from parapneumonic effusions. These effusions tend to be small and usually do not progress to empyema.[38] Mycoplasmal and viral infections can also produce small effusions that usually resolve spontaneously.

In many parts of the world, tuberculous effusions are common,[39] and they can be either secondary to a primary infection or a reactivation tuberculosis.[40] In most instances, tuberculous effusions resolve spontaneously; however, up to 50% of patients not treated with appropriate antituberculous medication will develop active tuberculous within 5 years.[41,42]

There is a high frequency of *S. aureus* and aerobic gram-negative bacillary infection in patients with empyema after trauma or surgery.[43,44] Empyema complicating hemothorax is often staphylococcal, whereas that associated with pneumothorax or hematogenous seeding of a serous effusion is often caused by aerobic gram-negative bacilli. Several studies have indicated an increased risk of post-traumatic empyema associated with retained hemothorax and significant pulmonary contusion.[45,46]

Mixed oropharyngeal organisms and occasionally *Candida* species are the organisms most frequently cultured from pleural fluid after esophageal rupture. Cultures obtained after subdiaphragmatic extension of an intra-abdominal infection usually show mixed enteric gram-negative bacilli, anaerobes, and *Candida.*

Although fungal infections of the pleural space are uncommon in the normal host, there has been an increase in fungal empyemas, and the majority are caused by *Candida* species. Candida empyema has been reported as a complication of surgery, as a result of esophageal rupture, as a subdiaphragmatic infection, and as being spread hematogenously. Many of these infections are polymicrobial.[47]

Amebic liver abscess is associated with pleural involvement in up to 15% to 20% of cases. Two mechanisms have been identified. First, an amebic liver abscess can irritate the diaphragm, producing a sympathetic pleural effusion. Second, a complex pleural effusion can develop when the amebic liver abscess ruptures into the pleural space through the diaphragm.[48]

Immunocompromised patients have a higher frequency of empyema caused by fungi and gram-negative bacilli.[6,44,49] Organ transplant recipients and patients with acquired immunodeficiency syndrome (AIDS) may reactivate pleural foci of mycobacterial or fungal infection, but they rarely present with empyema without disseminated disease. Unsuccessful resection of cavitary coccidioidomycosis or aspergillosis may be complicated by empyema and bronchopleural fistula from that organism.[50] Nocardia infections occur more frequently in patients with underlying conditions, such as organ transplantation, malignancy, diabetes mellitus, AIDS, and long-term use of steroids. Pleural effusions can develop in up to 50% of patients with nocardiosis.[51]

Several noninfectious etiologies should be considered in the differential diagnosis in patients who present with pleural effusions and fever. Pulmonary embolism is commonly overlooked as a cause of pleural effusion. It is estimated that between 30% and 50% of patients with pulmonary emboli have an associated pleural effusion.[52] Patients with acute pancreatitis frequently have associated pleural effusions. Patients with acute pancreatitis who develop a pleural effusion tend to have more severe disease.[53] Approximately 5% of patients with rheumatoid arthritis have a pleural effusion, and 20% present with pleuritic chest pain.[54,55] Forty percent of patients with systemic lupus erythematosus develop a pleural effusion at some point in the course of their disease.[56] Finally, after pericardiectomy[57] or myocardial infarction,[58] patients may present with pericarditis and pleural disease. The syndrome typically appears about 3 weeks after the injury and is characterized by fever and chest pains. Pleural fluid can be demonstrated in greater than 50% of cases.[59]

CLINICAL MANIFESTATIONS

The pleural response to microbial invasion can be divided into three stages. The initial, or exudative, stage is characterized by a collection of thin, free-flowing fluid with low numbers of neutrophils, pH higher than 7.2, lactate dehydrogenase (LDH) levels less than 1000 IU/L, glucose levels higher than 60 mg/dL, and negative cultures. The second, or fibropurulent, stage is characterized by increasing numbers of neutrophils and fibrin deposition over the pleura, with a tendency to loculate. Pleural glucose levels and pH fall and the LDH level increases. In the final, or organizing, stage, fibroblast formation and scarring produce a pleural peel that encases and traps the lung.[60] The clinical presentation varies with the underlying disease process, the microbiology, and host factors.

Patients with bacterial pneumonia usually present with fever, shortness of breath, productive cough, and chest pain. Patients with anaerobic pleuropulmonary infection exhibit a more indolent course and present with weight loss, fever, and chronic cough. A history of aspiration is often obtained and poor oral hygiene is often evident.[20]

Esophageal rupture or perforation, and subdiaphragmatic rupture of a liver abscess or subphrenic abscess frequently present with acute pain, fever, and respiratory distress.

The physical exam reveals decreased breath sounds, dullness to percussion, and crackles over the affected area. Chronic empyemas may erode the chest wall and present with a spontaneous draining abscess termed empyema necessitatis. Anemia and leukocytosis are nonspecific findings.

IMAGING STUDIES

The standard plain radiograph is still the initial approach in detecting and evaluating pleural effusions (Fig. 62-1). Up to 200 to 500 mL of pleural fluid is required to cause blunting of the costophrenic angle.[61] The lateral decubitus chest film can detect as little as 5 mL of free pleural fluid.[62] With extensive adjacent pulmonary consolidation and intrapleural loculations, the radiographic assessment of pleural collections becomes more difficult.

Ultrasound is widely available, and it enables bedside studies, is fast, and costs less than computed tomography (CT) or magnetic resonance imaging (MRI). Ultrasound is particularly useful for detecting small amounts of pleural fluid, for guiding diagnostic thoracentesis, and for pleural drainage. A recent study found that ultrasound evaluation was more accurate in estimating pleural fluid volume than plain decubitus radiographs.[63] The use of ultrasound has also been shown to significantly reduce the incidence of pneumothorax after thoracentesis.[64] The appearance of pleural collections varies from echo free to very echogenic. Highly echogenic empyemas may mimic consolidated lung or pulmonary abscess.[65] Ultrasonography can distinguish solid from liquid pleural abnormalities with 92% accuracy, compared with 68% accuracy of chest radiography. When ultrasonography and the chest radiograph are used together, their combined accuracy rises to

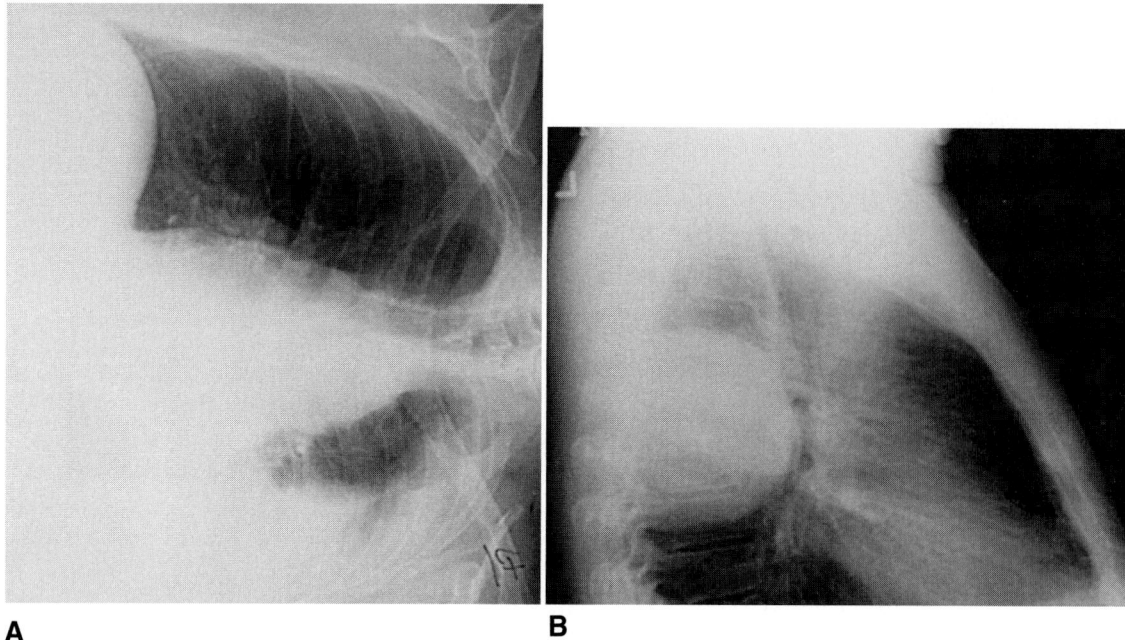

A   **B**

FIGURE 62-1.   A, Empyema fluid is seen layering out along the dependent chest wall of a patient with left lower lobe pneumonia (left lateral decubitus film). **B,** D-shaped mass representing a loculated empyema at the site of a former right upper lobectomy.

98%.[66] Unlike consolidated lung or abscess, pleural fluid varies in sonographic configuration during the respiratory cycle. Septation can be found by ultrasonography in up to 74% of intrapleural exudates even when not seen by chest CT.[67] The presence of septation has prognostic significance because loculated pleural collections require drainage and are usually larger than unloculated collections.[68]

In patients with complex fluid collections, the chest CT has emerged as the imaging study of choice. It is more accurate in distinguishing lung abscess from empyema than the conventional chest radiograph. Stark and co-workers reported pleural separation, adjacent lung compression, and wall characteristics to be the most reliable signs for distinguishing empyema from lung abscess.[69] The walls of empyemas were generally smooth in contrast to lung abscesses, which tended to have irregular walls (Fig. 62-2) Chest CT

with contrast may also differentiate transudates from exudates. Parietal pleural thickening and enhancement is usually seen only with exudative effusions. The margins formed by the inflamed and thickened visceral and parietal layers enhance with intravenous contrast material and are separated by the interposed empyema fluid, giving rise to the *split pleura sign* of empyema.[69,70] Pleural thickening and attenuation of extrapleural or subcostal fat can be defined accurately, increasing the accuracy of the diagnosis of empyema (Fig. 62-3). Plain radiography cannot distinguish this fatty hyperplasia from pleural thickening or effusion. Despite advances in technology, a recent study of the role of CT and ultrasound in adult patients with parapneumonic effusions and empyema concluded that neither technique could reliably identify the stage of pleural disease or predict those who required surgery.[71]

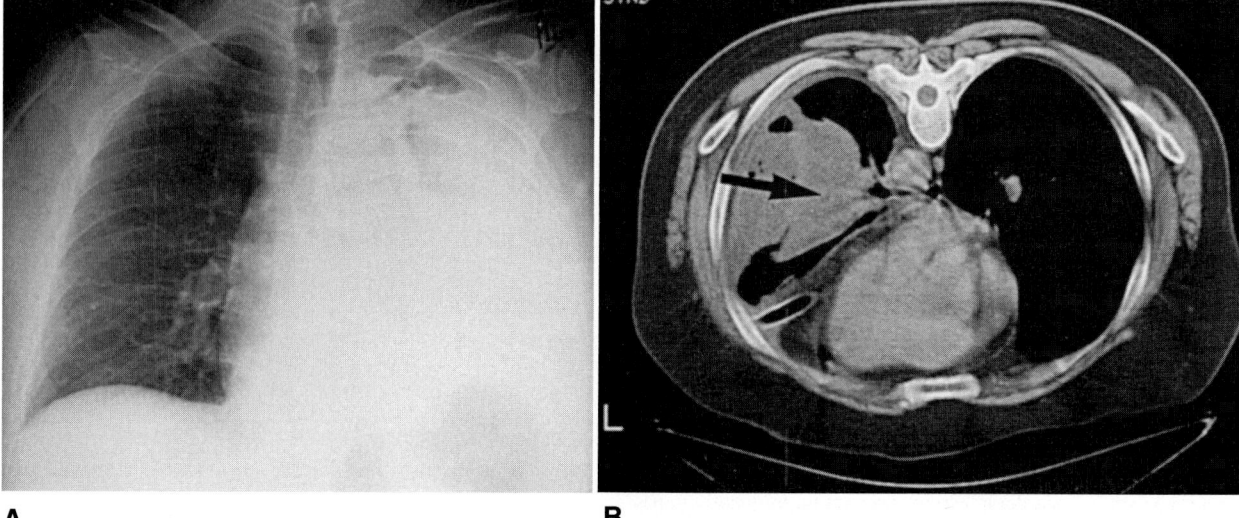

A   **B**

FIGURE 62-2.   A, The patient's empyema progressed despite percutaneous drainage and appropriate antibiotic therapy. **B,** Computed tomography showed malposition of chest tubes, and all attempts at tube drainage failed. The *arrow* indicates the loculated empyema. The patient responded promptly to surgical decortication.

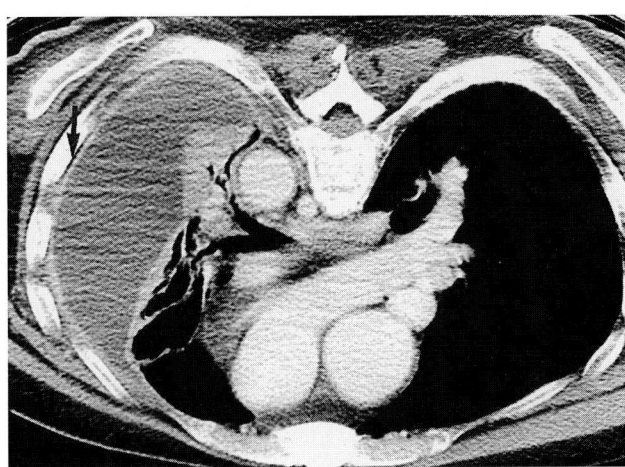

FIGURE 62-3. The *arrow* points to the "clear" area of fat hypertrophy between the pleural peel and the inner margin of the rib.

The role of MRI in the evaluation of pleural infection is limited. It may be a useful alternative when the intravenous contrast required to complete the CT imaging is contraindicated for the patient. MRI can detect pleural effusions, pleural tumors, and chest wall invasion. In some cases, it may be useful for distinguishing hemorrhagic effusions from other causes.[72] Fresh blood has a low signal on T1-weighted sequences and a high signal on T2-weighted sequences, whereas blood that is several days to weeks old gives a high signal on T1-weighted sequences and a low signal on T2-weighted sequences. It may also be possible to differentiate transudates and exudates with the use of triple echo pulse sequence or the use of gadolinium-enhanced MRI.[73,74] Exudative effusions showed an increased signal intensity within the pleural space on post–gadolinium-enhanced T1-weighted sequences.

LABORATORY DIAGNOSIS

In general, an effusion should be sampled if the fluid is free flowing, is greater than 10 mm on a lateral decubitus film, or is loculated. The first step is to determine whether an effusion is transudative or exudative by applying Light's criteria (Table 62-1).[75] Fluid obtained by thoracentesis should be examined with a differential cell count and analyzed for glucose, protein, LDH, and pH. Fluid should also be sent to the microbiology laboratory for a Gram stain and for both aerobic and anaerobic cultures. Special studies for mycobacteria, fungi, and other organisms should be done if clinically indicated. Cytologic studies may be indicated if an infected malignant effusion is suspected. Preservative-free heparin may need to be added to prevent clotting.

A predominance of leukocytes indicates an acute process in the pleural space. Unfortunately, the concentration of leukocytes in pleural fluid can be misleading because of lysis of leukocytes in pleural fluid.[76] A predominance of mononuclear cells usually indicates a most indolent process such as tuberculosis or fungal infection.[77] Pleural fluid eosinophilia (>10%) is found in up to two thirds of cases and is caused by blood or air in the pleural space.[78,79] Other, less common causes of eosinophilic pleural effusions may be fungal, parasitic, or drug induced.[79]

Most experts recommend drainage of the pleural space for a positive pleural fluid culture or Gram stain. However, only 61% of patients with established empyemas have a positive Gram stain.[7] Although most patients with empyemas have a positive culture, the absence of growth does not mean that a pleural effusion does not require drainage.[7]

The effect of a pleural infection on metabolic processes in the pleural space depends on its duration and extent. Extensive pleural space infection decreases pH, lowers the glucose level, and raises the LDH level in the pleural fluid.[2] A low pleural fluid glucose level (<60 mg/dL) is consistent with a complicated parapneumonic effusion or a malignancy.[80] The level of LDH correlates with the degree of pleural inflammation.[75] Empyema fluid characteristically has a pH of less than 7.2, a glucose level of less than 40 mg/dL, and LDH activity of at least 1000 IU/L. A recent meta-analysis found pleural fluid pH to have the best diagnostic accuracy in identifying parapneumonic effusions that require drainage. A pleural fluid pH below 7.2 indicates the need for drainage.[81,82] Pleural fluid pH less than 6 suggests esophageal rupture.[83,84] At the other extreme, frankly purulent empyema fluid can have a high pH when infection is caused by urea-splitting *Proteus* species, but these infections are rare.[85]

Pleural tuberculosis can be diagnosed by stains of pleural fluid in only 18% to 23% of patients, but cultures of pleural fluid and histologic examination of pleural biopsy specimens permit the diagnosis in up to 95% of patients.[86] Liquid culture media are preferable to solid culture media.[87] Radiometric culture may increase the speed of diagnosis in patients with pleural tuberculosis. Three other diagnostic tests are now available to help establish the diagnosis of tuberculous pleural disease: tests for adenosine deaminase (ADA) and interferon-γ, and the polymerase chain reaction (PCR). In one study, pleural fluid adenosine deaminase levels above 40 U/L were found in 99.6% of patients with tuberculous pleurisy.[88] Villena and colleagues found that an elevated level of interferon-γ of 140 pg/mL was comparable to an elevated level of adenosine deaminase for diagnosing tuberculous pleurisy.[89] The results of using PCR to detect *M. tuberculosis* DNA in pleural fluid have varied. In one study, PCR was as sensitive as the ADA test,[90] but in another study, the sensitivity of PCR was only 42%.[89] Two tests for *M. tuberculosis* nucleic acid are commercially available and, although approved only for respiratory specimens, can be used on nonrespiratory specimens such as pleural fluid (see Chapter 15). Increased risk of exposure to tuberculosis, host defense defects favoring reactivation, skin test conversion, or symptoms of weight loss, night sweats, and fever are helpful clues to the diagnosis of tuberculosis.

The diagnosis of amebic abscess with subdiaphragmatic rupture is suggested by the anchovy paste or chocolate appearance of pleural fluid. Approximately 98% of patients with pleural or pulmonary amebiasis have positive serologic tests for *Entamoeba histolytica*.[48,91]

The best screening test for pulmonary embolus is the level of D-dimer in the blood.[92] Spiral CT of the chest and perfusion scanning of the lungs can also be used to establish the diagnosis.

The pleural fluid of patients with rheumatoid arthritis, pancreatitis, malignancy, or postpericardiotomy syndrome occasionally has features suggestive of empyema.[1] Exudates of rheumatoid or pancreatic origin only rarely have a pH of less than 7.2 and these two sources can be identified by serologic tests or increased pleural fluid amylase levels, respectively. Pleural fluid from patients with lupus erythematosus or rheumatoid pleuritis characteristically demonstrates titers of antinuclear antibody of at least 1:160 or rheumatoid factor of at least 1:320, respectively, with values exceeding those found in serum.[93,94] Pleural fluid from patients with rheumatoid disease frequently has a glucose level of less than 30 mg/dL. The rare malignant effusion with a pH of less than 7 is readily diagnosed by cytologic examination and is associated with a worse prognosis than that of alkaline malignant effusion.[84]

The pleural fluid in patients with postpericardiotomy or postmyocardial infarction syndrome tends to be exudative, with glucose levels greater than 60 mg/dL and a pH usually above 7.40. The fluid is

TABLE 62-1 Features Differentiating Exudative from Transudative Pleural Effusion		
	Transudate	*Exudate*
Appearance	Serous	Cloudy
Leukocyte count	<10,000/mm³	>50,000/mm³
pH	>7.2	<7.2
Protein	<3.0 g/dL	>3.0 g/dL
Ratio of pleural fluid protein to serum	<0.5	>0.5
Lactate dehydrogenase (LDH)	<200 IU/L	>200 IU/L
Ratio of pleural fluid LDH to serum	<0.6	>0.6
Glucose	≥60 mg/dL	<60 mg/dL

frequently serosanguineous, with a pleural fluid differential cell count that demonstrates either neutrophils or mononuclear cells.[59]

TREATMENT

Therapeutic options for a pleural effusion depend on the type or stage of the effusion. Light and Rodriguez proposed a classification and treatment scheme for parapneumonic effusions and empyema.[95] It is based on the amount of fluid, the gross and biochemical characteristics of the pleural fluid, and whether or not the fluid was loculated. Recently, the American College of Chest Physicians published an evidence-based consensus guideline on the medical and surgical treatment of parapneumonic effusions (Table 62-2).[82] Three variables, pleural space anatomy, pleural fluid microbiology, and pleural fluid chemistries, were used to categorize patients into four risk levels for poor outcome: categories 1 (very low risk), 2 (low risk), 3 (moderate risk), and 4 (high risk). The panel grouped management of pleural effusions into six categories: no drainage, therapeutic thoracentesis, tube thoracostomy, fibrinolytic therapy, video-assisted thoracoscopic surgery (VATS), and open surgery. The fibrinolytic approach requires tube thoracostomy for administration of drug, and VATS requires tube thoracostomy after the procedure.

Uncomplicated effusions (category 1 or 2) generally resolve with antibiotics alone. Drainage is recommended for management of patients in category 3 or 4. On the basis of a literature review, therapeutic thoracentesis and tube thoracostomy appear to be insufficient for managing most patients in category 3 or 4. Fibrinolytic drugs, VATS, and surgery are better choices for these patients.

Antimicrobial Therapy

In most cases with complicated pleural space infection, antimicrobial therapy and appropriate drainage of the pleural space play complementary roles. Many antimicrobial agents are able to adequately penetrate into infected pleural fluid to exceed the minimal inhibitory concentration of most common organisms; these include penicillins, cephalosporins, clindamycin, metronidazole, vancomycin, and quinolones.[2,96] Aminoglycosides are less capable of entering the pleural space and have decreased activity in an acid anaerobic environment.[97,98] However, aminoglycosides may be combined with β-lactam antibiotics to achieve a synergistic activity against empyema caused by *Pseudomonas aeruginosa, Enterobacter cloacae, Acinetobacter calcoaceticus,* or *Serratia marcescens.*[99]

Initial empiric antimicrobial therapy should be based on the most likely pathogens, local antimicrobial susceptibility patterns, and all available results including Gram stains. There are many choices including a combination of a β-lactam and a β-lactamase inhibitor (amoxicillin/clavulanate, a ampicillin/sulbactam, or piperacillin/tazobactam), a carbapenem (imipenem, ertapenem, or meropenem), or combination therapy with a third-generation cephalosporin (cefotaxime, ceftriaxone, or cefepime) and either clindamycin or metronidazole. These choices cover the most common pathogens associated with pleural empyema,

including anaerobic organisms. If *S. aureus* is suspected, vancomycin should be administered along with metronidazole and a third-generation cephalosporin because of increased community-onset and health care associated methicillin-resistant *S. aureus.*[100,101]

Unfortunately, there are no conclusive studies on duration of therapy for most bacterial pleural space infections. Patients with uncomplicated simple parapneumonic effusions can be treated for the same duration that is indicated for the underlying pneumonia. For patients with complicated parapneumonic effusions and empyema, the duration of treatment should be dictated by the clinical response to drainage and antimicrobial therapy. Prolonged antimicrobial therapy (3 weeks or more) may be necessary. Patients with pulmonary actinomycosis or nocardiosis may require 6 to 12 months of antimicrobial treatment.[102,103] Penicillin or amoxicillin is the preferred drug for actinomycosis, and a sulfonamide is the preferred drug for nocardiosis. Patients with tuberculous pleural disease should be treated with the same regimen and for the same duration as those with pulmonary tuberculosis.[104] Patients infected with a *Candida* should receive an appropriate antifungal drug (fluconazole, caspofungin, or amphotericin B) for 2 weeks after the resolution of signs and symptoms of infection.[105,106] Most patients with amebic disease respond to pleural drainage and an appropriate antimicrobial agent.[107] Metronidazole is considered the drug of choice and is administered for 10 days.

Drainage

In addition to antimicrobial therapy to control infection, drainage of the pleural space and expansion of the lung are essential for a good outcome. Clinical patterns that indicate that drainage is necessary include persistent fever and chills despite appropriate antimicrobial therapy, anaerobic infection, isolation of organisms such as *S. pyogenes* or *S. aureus*, an air-fluid level in the pleural space, and the presence of loculations or a large effusion. Ferguson and colleagues found that only 24% of patients with a parapneumonic effusion greater than 40% of a hemithorax responded to antimicrobial agents alone, compared with an 81% response if the effusion was less than 20% of the hemithorax.[108] The success rate with effusions occupying 20% to 40% of the hemithorax was 50%. Larger pleural effusions tended to be multiloculated. Several studies have also suggested that early drainage improves outcomes in patients with pneumonia. Ashbaugh reported that mortality increased from 3.4% to 16% in patients when drainage was delayed longer than 3 days.[109] Heffner and colleagues found that patients undergoing thoracentesis within 2 days of radiographic signs of a significant parapneumonic effusion had shorter hospital stays than patients with delayed drainage.[110]

Repeated thoracentesis is infrequently adequate unless the empyema fluid is quite thin and present in a small volume. To be successful, thoracentesis needs to completely evacuate all pleural fluid. Recurrence of pleural fluid indicates a need for a more aggressive approach. When used as the initial mode of drainage, repeat thoracentesis was successful in only 36% of cases.[4]

TABLE 62-2 Categorizing Risk of Poor Outcome in Patients with Parapneumonic Effusion

Pleural Space Anatomy		Pleural Fluid Microbiology	Pleural Fluid Chemistry*	Category	Risk of Poor Outcome	Perform Drainage
Minimal, free-flowing effusion (<10 mm on lateral decubitus film)	AND	Culture and Gram stain results unknown	pH unknown	1	Very low	No
Small to moderate, free-flowing effusion (<½ hemithorax)	AND	Negative culture and Gram stain	pH ≥ 7.20	2	Low	No
Large, free-flowing effusion (≥½ hemithorax); loculated or thickened pleura	OR	Positive culture or Gram stain	pH < 7.20	3	Moderate	Yes
		Pus	—	4	High	Yes

*pH is the preferred pleural fluid chemistry value and must be determined by blood gas analyzer. If blood gas analyzer is not available, pleural fluid glucose level should be used (glucose ≥60 mg/dL is equivalent to pH ≥7.20; glucose <60 mg/dL is equivalent to pH <7.20).
Modified from Colice GL, Curtis A, Deslauriers J, et al. Chest. 2000;118:1158-1171.

Closed chest tube drainage without fibrinolytic therapy is successful in up to two thirds of patients.[111,112] The most common reason for closed chest tube failure is pleural adhesions and intrapleural loculations that do not communicate with the chest tubes. When patients do not respond to a short course of chest tube drainage, a more definitive approach is needed.[113] Closed chest tubes should be reserved for patients in the early fibrinopurulent stage of empyema.

Several reports support an expanded role for the interventional radiologist in the management of thoracic empyema.[114-118] Image-guided percutaneous chest tubes have been suggested to address the problem of tube placement in patients with intrapleural loculations. The use of CT or ultrasound makes it relatively easy to place one or more catheters in specific locations. The catheters used are smaller, ranging from 8 to 16 French instead of 28 to 36 French, and better tolerated. The success rates of guided tube placement range from 67% to 80%.[119]

Fibrinolytic Therapy

Recent reports on the efficacy of fibrinolytic therapy are promising, with success rates in the range of 70% to 90%. Patients with a bronchopleural fistula are not candidates for this procedure because of the possibility of enzyme entering the bronchial tree. Davies and colleagues published a randomized trial of 24 patients with a parapneumonic effusion who received either intrapleural streptokinase (SK) 250,000 IU once a day for 3 days or normal saline as control.[120] The SK group showed significant benefit in the volume of pleural drainage ($P < .01$) and chest radiograph improvement ($P < .05$). The study did not have sufficient power to detect differences in mortality and the need for surgery. A second randomized trial involving 31 patients with multiloculated pleural effusions compared urokinase (UK) 100,000 IU/day for 3 days versus saline placebo.[120] The UK-treated group drained more pleural fluid ($P < .001$), had decreased time to defervescence ($P < .01$), and had decreased hospital days ($P < .01$). Pleural fluid drainage was complete in 86.5% in the UK group but in only 25% in the saline group. Treatment failure occurred in 2 of 15 (13.5%) in the UK group versus 12 of 16 (75%) in the control group. Bouros and co-workers published a double-blind, randomized, controlled study comparing SK versus UK in 50 consecutive patients with complicated parapneumonic effusions or empyema.[121] Clinical and radiographic improvement was seen in all but two patients in each group. Two patients were switched from SK to UK because of high fever after the first dose. The total cost of treating the UK group was twice that of the SK group. In summary, although the side-effect profile slightly favored UK and the cost analysis favored SK, the study established that SK and UK could be used with equal efficacy.

In a multicenter trial, fibrinolytic therapy with SK was a viable therapeutic option for patients with loculated effusions less than 12 days.[122] In another study, the success rate of fibrinolytic therapy decreased to 61% if the empyema was greater than 20 days old.[123] Based on this limited experience, fibrinolytic therapy alone may not be as successful if symptoms of empyema exceed 3 to 4 weeks. For these patients, a surgical approach is preferred. The sole randomized trial of fibrinolysis in pediatrics studied 60 children from 10 centers who were randomized to receive either UK or saline.[124] Treatment with UK resulted in a significantly decreased length of stay ($P < .03$). There were no differences in other clinical outcomes in the children. The advantages of fibrinolysis may be confined to adults.

Surgical Intervention

Surgical options include thoracoscopy usually by VATS or full thoracotomy with decortication. VATS is most commonly employed to improve drainage of a multiloculated complex effusion or empyema as an alternative to fibrinolytic therapy. The results of the only prospective, randomized, controlled study comparing early VATS to SK suggest that early VATS significantly reduced the number of hospital days and had a higher success rate than SK ($P < .05$).[125] The mortalities were similar, but the number of patients studied was small. A nonrandomized, prospective study of 82 patients compared tube thoracostomy (T) alone, versus T plus SK (T/SK), versus T with initial SK followed by early surgical intervention with either VATS or thoracotomy (SK/OP).[126] This study demonstrated significantly decreased length of hospital stay in the SK/OP group compared with the T and T/SK groups ($P < .01$), and reduced mortality in the SK/OP group compared with the T group ($P < .01$) but not compared with the T/SK group. This study suggests that surgical intervention is preferred when fibrinolytic therapy is delayed or if initial fibrinolytic therapy is not successful. Cassina and colleagues published a prospective series of 45 patients who underwent VATS after chest tube drainage and antibiotics had failed.[127] In 37 patients (82%), VATS was successful. In eight cases, decortication by open thoracotomy was necessary. The authors concluded that VATS was a suitable treatment option for fibrinopurulent empyema when tube drainage and fibrinolytic therapy had failed. For empyema in a later, organized stage, full thoracotomy with decortication may be the surgical treatment of choice. Landreneau and associates reported that 46% of patients with an empyema known to be greater than 3 weeks old required full thoracotomy with decortication after failing VATS.[128] Surgical intervention is needed less frequently in children.[1]

PERSPECTIVE

Several key principles guide the successful treatment of patients with pleural space infections: (1) early detection of a significant pleural effusion, (2) appropriate antimicrobial therapy based on the most likely organism(s) and guided by local susceptibility patterns, (3) accurate staging of the pleural effusion on the basis of pleural space anatomy, biochemical characteristics, and microbiology, and (4) effective and complete drainage of complex pleural effusions or empyemas.

REFERENCES

1. Light RW. Parapneumonic effusions and empyema. In: Light RW, ed. Pleural Diseases. 3rd ed. Baltimore: Williams & Wilkins; 1995:129-153.
2. Sahn SA. Management of complicated parapneumonic effusions. Rev Respir Dis. 1993;148:813-817.
3. Bryant RE, Salmon CJ. Pleural empyema. Clin Infect Dis. 1996;22:747-764.
4. Lemmer JH, Botham MJ, Orringer MB. Modern management of adult thoracic empyema. J Thorac Cardiovasc Surg. 1985;90:849-855.
5. Ali I, Unruh H. Management of empyema thoracis. Ann Thorac Surg. 1990;50:355-359.
6. Smith JA, Mullerworth MH, Westlake GW, Tatoulis J. Empyema thoracis: A 14-year experience in a teaching center. Ann Thorac Surg. 1991;51:39-42.
7. Alfageme I, Munoz F, Pena N, et al. Empyema of the thorax in adults: Etiology, microbiologic findings and management. Chest. 1993;103:839-843.
8. Sahn SA. State of the art: The pleura. Am Rev Respir Dis. 1988;138:184-234.
9. Lew Z, Zubler R, Vaudaux P. Decreased heat-labile opsonic activity and complement levels associated with evidence of C3 breakdown products in infected pleural effusions. J Clin Invest. 1979;63:326-334.
10. Bryant RE. Pus: Friend or foe? In: Root RK, Trunkey DD, Sande MA, eds. Contemporary Issues in Infectious Diseases, v. 6. New Surgical and Medical Approaches. New York: Churchill Livingstone; 1987:31-48.
11. Miller EJ, Idell S. Interleukin-8: An important neutrophil chemotaxin in some cases of exudative pleural effusions. Exp Lung Res. 1993;19:589-601.
12. Owens MW, Grisham MB. Nitric oxide synthesis by rat pleural mesothelial cells: Induction by cytokines and lipopolysaccharide. Am J Physiol. 1993;265:L110-116.
13. Jonjic N, Peri G, Bernasconi S, et al. Expression of adhesion molecules and chemotactic cytokines in cultured human mesothelial cells. J Exp Med. 1992;176:1165-1174.
14. Broaddus VC, Hebert CA, Vitangcol RV, et al. Interleukin-8 is a major neutrophil chemotactic factor in pleural liquid of patients with empyema. Am Rev Respir Dis. 1992;146:825-830.
15. Antony VB, Godbey SW, Kunkel SL, et al. Recruitment of inflammatory cells to the pleural space: Chemotactic cytokines, IL-8 and monocyte chemotactic peptide-I in human pleural fluids. J Immunol. 1993;151:7216-7223.
16. Antony VB, Hott JW, Kunkel SL, et al. Pleural mesothelial cell expression of C-C (monocyte chemotactic peptide) and C-X-C (interleukin 8) chemokines. Am J Respir Cell Mol Biol. 1995;12:581-588.
17. Antony VB, Godbey SW, Sparks JA, et al. Pleural mesothelial cells release a growth factor for fibroblasts. Eur Respir Rev. 1993;3:156-158.
18. Hott JW, Sparkes JA, Godbey JW, et al. Mesothelial cell response to pleural injury: Thrombin induced proliferation and chemotaxis of rat pleural mesothelial cell. Am J Respir Cell Mol Biol. 1992;6:421-425.
19. Finland M, Barnes MW: Changing ecology of acute bacterial empyema: Occurrence and mortality at Boston City Hospital during 12 selected years from 1935-1972. J Infect Dis. 1978;137:274-291.
20. Civens R, Jousimies-Somer H, Marina M, et al. A retrospective review of cases of anaerobic empyema and update of bacteriology. Clin Infect Dis. 1995;20:S224-229.

21. Bartlett JG, Finegold SM. Anaerobic infections of the lung and pleural space. Am Rev Respir Dis. 1974;110:56-77.
22. Brook I. Microbiology of empyema in children. Pediatrics. 1990;85:722-726.
23. Ballantyne KC, Sethia B, Reece IJ, et al. Empyema following intra-abdominal sepsis. Br J Surg. 1984;71:723-725.
24. Kelly JW, Morris MJ. Empyema thoracis: Medical aspects of evaluation and treatment. South Med J. 1994;87:1103-1110.
25. Light RW, Girard WM, Jenkinson SG, et al. Parapneumonic effusions. Am J Med. 1980;69:507-512.
26. Taryle DA, Potts DE, Sahn SA. The incidence and clinical correlates of parapneumonic effusions in pneumococcal pneumonia. Chest. 1978;74:170-173.
27. Freij BJ, Kusmiesz H, Nelson JD, McCracken GH. Parapneumonic effusions and empyema in hospitalized children: A retrospective review of 227 cases. Pediatr Infect Dis. 1984;3:578-591.
28. Whitney CG, Farley MM, Hadler J, et al. Decline in invasive pneumococcal disease after the introduction of protein-polysaccharide conjugated vaccine. N Engl J Med. 2003;348:1737-1746.
29. Buckingham SC, King MD, Miller ML. Incidence and etiology of complicated parapneumonic effusions in children, 1996 to 2001. Pediatr Infect Dis J. 2003;22:499-504.
30. Kaye MG, Fox MJ, Bartlett JG, et al. The clinical spectrum of *Staphylococcus aureus* pulmonary infection. Chest. 1990;97:788-792.
31. Schwarzmann SW, Adler JL, Sullivan RFJ, Marine WM. Bacterial pneumonia during the Hong Kong influenza epidemic of 1968-1969. Arch Intern Med. 1971;127:1037-1041.
32. Welch CC, Tombridge TL, Baker WJ, Kinney RJ. Beta-hemolytic streptococcal pneumonia: Report of an outbreak in a military population. Am J Med Sci. 1961;242:157-165.
33. Braman SS, Donat WE. Explosive pleuritis: manifestation of group A beta-hemolytic streptococcal infection. Am J Med. 1986;81:723-726.
34. Jerng JS, Hsueh PR, Teng LJ, et al. Empyema thoracis and lung abscesses caused by viridans streptococci. Am J Respir Crit Care Med. 1997;156:1508-1514.
35. Ruoff KL, Kunz LJ, Ferraro MJ. Occurrence of *Streptococcus milleri* among beta-hemolytic streptococci isolated from clinical specimens. J Clin Microbiol. 1985;22:149-151.
36. Takao A, Nagashima H, Usui H, et al. Hyaluronidase activity in human pus from which *Streptococcus intermedius* was isolated. Microbiol Immunol. 1997;41:795-798.
37. Flynn MW, Felson B. The roentgen manifestations of thoracic actinomycosis. Am J Roentgenol Radium Ther Nucl Med. 1970;110:707-716.
38. Muder RR, Yu VL, Parry MF. The radiographic manifestations of *Legionella* pneumonia. Semin Respir Infect. 1987;2:242-254.
39. Mlika-Cabanne N, Brauner M, Mugusi F, et al. Radiographic abnormalities in tuberculosis and risk of coexisting human immunodeficiency virus infection. Am J Respir Crit Care Med. 1995;152:786-793.
40. Moudgil H, Sridhar G, Leitch AG. Reactivation disease: The commonest form of tuberculous pleural effusion in Edinburgh, 1980-1991. Respir Med. 1994;88:301-304.
41. Roper WH, Waring JJ. Primary serofibrinous pleural effusion in military personnel. Am Rev Respir Dis. 1955;71:616-634.
42. Antoniskis D, Amin K, Barnes PF. Pleuritis as a manifestation of reactivation tuberculosis. Am J Med. 1990;89:447-450.
43. Caplan ES, Hoyt NJ, Rodriguez A, et al. Empyema occurring in the multiply traumatized patient. J Trauma. 1984;24:785-798.
44. Vianna NJ. Nontuberculous bacterial empyema in patients with and without underlying disease. JAMA. 1971;215:69-71.
45. Aguilar MM, Battistella FD, Owings JT, Su T. Post traumatic empyema: Risk factor analysis. Arch Surg. 1997;132:647-651.
46. Helling TS, Gyles NR III, Eisenstein CL, Soracco CA. Complications following blunt and penetrating injuries in 216 victims of chest trauma requiring tube thoracostomy. J Trauma. 1989;29:1367-1370.
47. Ko SC, Chen KY, Hsueh PR, et al. Fungal empyema thoracis: An emerging entity. Chest. 2000;117:1672-1678.
48. Reed SI. Amebiasis: An update. Clin Infect Dis. 1992;15:385-393.
49. Varkey B, Rose HD, Kutty CPK, Politis J. Empyema thoracis during a ten-year period: Analysis of 72 cases and comparison to a previous study (1952 to 1967). Arch Intern Med. 1981;141:1771-1776.
50. Wex P, Utta E, Drozdz W. Surgical treatment of pulmonary and pleuropulmonary *Aspergillus* disease. Thorac Cardiovasc Surg. 1993;41:64-70.
51. Lerner PI. Nocardiosis. Clin Infect Dis. 1996;22:891-905.
52. Stein PD, Henry JW. Clinical characteristics of patients with acute pulmonary embolism stratified according to their presenting syndromes. Chest. 1997;112:974-979.
53. Lankisch PG, Droge M, Becher R. Pleural effusions: A new negative prognostic parameter for acute pancreatitis. Am J Gastroenterol. 1994;89:1849-1851.
54. Horler AR, Thompson M. The pleural and pulmonary complications of rheumatoid arthritis. Ann Intern Med. 1959;51:1179-1203.
55. Walker WC, Wright V. Rheumatoid pleuritis. Ann Rheum Dis. 1967;26:467-474.
56. Good JT, King TE, Antony VB, et al. Lupus pleuritis: Clinical features and pleural fluid characteristics with special reference to pleural fluid antinuclear antibodies. Chest. 1983;84:714-718.
57. Light RW, Rogers JT, Cheng D-S, et al. Large pleural effusions occurring after coronary artery bypass grafting. Ann Intern Med. 1999;130:891-896.
58. Dressler W. The post-myocardial infarction syndrome. Arch Intern Med. 1959;103:28-42.
59. Stelzner TJ, King TE Jr, Antony VB, et al. The pleuropulmonary manifestations of postcardiac injury syndrome. Chest. 1983;84:383-387.
60. Andrews NC, Parker EF, Shaw RP, et al. Management of nontuberculous empyema. Am Rev Respir Dis. 1962;85:935-936.
61. Blackmore CC, Black WC, Dallas RV, et al. Pleural fluid volume estimation: A chest radiograph prediction rule. Acad Radiol. 1996;3:103-109.
62. Moskowitz H, Platt RT, Schachar R, Mellins H. Roentgen visualization of minute pleural effusion: An experimental study to determine the minimum amount of pleural fluid visible on a radiograph. Radiology. 1973;109:33-35.
63. Eibenberger KL, Dock WI, Ammann ME, et al. Quantification of pleural effusions: Sonography vs. radiography. Radiology. 1994;191:681-684.
64. Raptopoulos V, Davis LM, Lee G, et al. Factors affecting the development of pneumothorax associated with thoracentesis. AJR Am J Roentgenol. 1991;156:917-920.
65. Landay MJ, Conrad MR. Lung abscess mimicking empyema on ultrasonography. AJR Am J Roentgenol. 1979;133:731-734.
66. Lipscombe DJ, Flower CDR, Hadfield JW. Ultrasound of the pleura: An assessment of its clinical value. Clin Radiol. 1981;32:289-290.
67. Hirsch JH, Rogers JV, Mack LA. Real-time sonography of pleural opacities. AJR Am J Roentgenol. 1981;136:297-301.
68. Lee MJ, Saini S, Brink JA, et al. Interventional radiology of the pleural space: Management of thoracic empyema with image-guided catheter drainage. Semin Intervent Radiol. 1991;8:29-35.
69. Stark DD, Federle MP, Goodman PC, et al. Differentiating lung abscess and empyema: Radiography and computed tomography. AJR Am J Roentgenol. 1983;141:163-167.
70. Hanna JW, Reed JC, Choplin RH. Pleural infections: A clinical-radiologic review. J Thorac Imaging. 1991;6:68-79.
71. Kearney SE, Davies CW, Davies RJ, et al. Computed tomography and ultrasound in parapneumonic effusions and empyema. Clin Radiol. 2000;55:542-547.
72. Gamsu G, Sostman D. Magnetic resonance imaging of the thorax. Am Rev Respir Dis. 1989;139:254-274.
73. Davis SK, Henschke CI, Yankelevitz, et al. MR imaging of pleural effusions. J Comput Assist Tomogr. 1990;14:192-198.
74. Frola C, Cantoni S, Turtulici I, et al. Transudative vs. exudative pleural effusions: Differentiating using Gd-DTPA-enhanced MRI. Eur Radiol. 1997;7:860-864.
75. Light RW. Pleural effusion. N Engl J Med. 2002;346:1971-1977.
76. Heffner JE. Indications for draining a parapneumonic effusion: Evidence-based approach. Semin Respir Infect. 1999;14:48-58.
77. Yam LT. Diagnostic significance of lymphocytes in pleural effusions. Ann Intern Med. 1967;66:972-982.
78. Adelman M, Albelda SM, Gottlieb J, Haponik EF. Diagnostic utility of pleural fluid eosinophilia. Am J Med. 1984;77:915-920.
79. Kalomenidis I, Light RW. How to approach a patient with an eosinophilic pleural effusion. J Respir Dis. 2002;24:247-253.
80. Light RW, Ball WC Jr. Glucose and amylase in pleural effusions. JAMA. 1973;225:257-259.
81. Heffner JE, Brown LK, Barbieri C, et al. Pleural fluid chemical analysis in parapneumonic effusions: A meta-analysis. Am J Respir Crit Care Med. 1995;151:1700-1708.
82. Colice GL, Curtis A, Deslauriers J, et al. Medical and surgical treatment of parapneumonic effusions: An evidence-based guideline. Chest. 2000;118:1158-1171.
83. Light RW. Management of empyema. Semin Respir Med. 1992;13:167-176.
84. Good JT Jr, Taryle DA, Maulitz RM, et al. The diagnostic value of pleural fluid pH. Chest. 1980;78:55-59.
85. Pine JR, Hollman JL. Elevated pleural fluid pH in *Proteus mirabilis* empyema. Chest. 1983;84:109-111.
86. Levine H, Metzger W, Lacera D, et al. Diagnosis of tuberculous pleurisy by culture of pleural biopsy specimen. Arch Intern Med. 1970;126:269-271.
87. Wichelhausen RH, McLean RL, Lowrey FB. Reinforcement of diagnostic value of pleural biopsy by culture in liquid medium. Am Rev Respir Dis. 1996;92:288-290.
88. Lee YCG, Rogers JT, Rodriguez RM, et al. Adenosine deaminase levels in nontuberculous lymphocytic pleural effusions. Chest. 2001;120:356-361.
89. Villena V, Lopez-Encuentra A, Echave-Sustaeta J, et al. Interferon-gamma in 388 immunocompromised and immunocompetent patients for diagnosing pleural tuberculosis. Eur Respir J. 1996;9:2635-2639.
90. Querol JM, Minguez J, Garcia-Sanchez E, et al. Rapid diagnosis of pleural tuberculosis by polymerase chain reaction. Am J Respir Crit Care Med. 1995;152:1977-1981.
91. Adams EB, MacLeod IN. Invasive amebiasis: I. Amebic dysentery and its complications. Medicine (Baltimore). 1977;56:315-323.
92. Ahearn GS, Bounameaux H. The role of the D-dimer in the diagnosis of venous thromboembolism. Semin Respir Crit Care Med. 2000;21:521-536.
93. Halla JT, Schrohenloher RE, Valanakis JE, et al. Immune complexes and other features of pleural effusions. Ann Intern Med. 1980;92:748-752.
94. Good JT Jr, King TE, Antony VB, et al. Lupus pleuritis: Clinical features and pleural fluid characteristics with special reference to pleural fluid antinuclear antibodies. Chest. 1983;84:714-718.
95. Light RW, Rodriguez RM. Management of parapneumonic effusions. Clin Chest Med. 1998;19:373-382.
96. Teixeira LR Antibiotic levels in empyema pleural fluid. Chest. 2000;117:1734-1739.
97. Thys JP, Vanderhoeft P, Herchuelz A, et al. Penetration of aminoglycosides in uninfected pleural exudates and in pleural empyema. Chest. 1988;93:530-532.
98. Vandeauz P, Waldvogel FA. Gentamicin inactivation in purulent exudates: The role of cell lysis. J Infect Dis. 1980;142:586-593.
99. Bryant RE, Fox KE, Oh G, Morthland VH. β-Lactam enhancement of aminoglycoside activity under conditions of reduced pH and oxygen tension that may exist in infected tissues. J Infect Dis. 1992;165:676-682.
100. Chambers HF. The changing epidemiology of *Staphylococcus aureus*. Emerg Infect Dis. 2001;7:178-182.
101. Stevens DL, Herr D, Lampiris H, et al. Linezolid versus vancomycin of the treatment of methicillin-resistant *Staphylococcus aureus* infections. Clin Infect Dis. 2002;34:1481-1490.

102. Wallace RJ Jr, Septimus EJ, Williams TW Jr, et al. Use of trimethoprim-sulfamethoxazole for the treatment of infections due to *Nocardia*. Rev Infect Dis. 1982;4:315-325.

103. Peabody JW, Seabury JH. Actinomycosis and nocardiosis: A review of basic differences in therapy. Am J Med. 1960;60:99-115.

104. Small PM, Fujiwara PI. Management of tuberculosis in the United States. N Engl J Med. 2001;345:189-200.

105. Rex JH, Walsh TJ, Sobel JD, et al. Practice guidelines for the treatment of candidiasis. Clin Infect Dis. 2000;30:662-678.

106. Mora-Duarte J, Betts R, Rotstein C, et al. Comparison of caspofungin and amphotericin B for invasive candidiasis. N Engl J Med. 2002;347:2020-2029.

107. Baijal SS, Agarwal DK, Roy S, et al. Complex ruptured amebic liver abscesses: The role of percutaneous catheter drainage. Eur J Radiol. 1995;20:65-67.

108. Ferguson AD, Prescott RJ, Selkon JB, et al. The clinical course and management of thoracic empyema. Q J Med. 1996;89:285-289.

109. Ashbaugh DG. Empyema thoracis: Factors influencing morbidity and mortality. Chest. 1991;99:1162-1165.

110. Heffner JE, McDonald J, Barbieri C, et al. Management of parapneumonic effusions: An analysis of physician practice patterns. Arch Surg. 1995;130:433-438.

111. Miller KS, Sahn SA. Chest tubes. Chest. 1987;91:258-264.

112. Hutter JA, Harari D, Braimbridge MV. The management of empyema thoracis by thoracoscopy and irrigation. Ann Thorac Surg. 1985;39:517-520.

113. Pothula V, Krellenstein DJ. Early aggressive surgical management of parapneumonic empyema. Chest. 1994;105:832-836.

114. Merriam MA, Cronan JJ, Dorgman GS, et al. Radiographically guided percutaneous catheter drainage of pleural fluid collections. AJR Am J Roentgenol. 1988;151:1113-1116.

115. Goldberg MA, Mueller PR, Saini S, et al. Importance of daily rounds by the radiologist after interventional procedures of the abdomen and chest. Radiology. 1991;180:767-770.

116. Stavas J, van Sonneberg E, Casola G, Wittich GR. Percutaneous drainage of infected and noninfected thoracic fluid collections. J Thorac Imaging. 1987;2:80-87.

117. Silverman SG, Mueller PR, Saini S, et al. Thoracic empyema: Management with image-guided catheter drainage. Radiology. 1988;169:5-9.

118. Moulton JS. Image-guided drainage techniques. Semin Respir Infect. 1999;14:59-72.

119. Moulton JS. Image-guided management of complicated pleural fluid collections. Radiol Clin North Am. 2000;38:345-374.

120. Davies RJO, Traill ZC, Gleeson FV. Randomized controlled trial of intrapleural streptokinase in community acquired pleural infection. Thorax. 1997;52:416-421.

121. Bouros D, Schiza S, Patsourakis G, et al. Intrapleural streptokinase versus urokinase in the treatment of complicated parapneumonic effusions. Am J Respir Crit Care Med. 1997;155:291-295.

122. Jerjes-Sanchez C, Ramirez-Rivera A, Elizalde JJ, et al. Intrapleural fibrinolytics with streptokinase as an adjunctive treatment in hemothorax and empyema. Chest. 1996;109:1514-1519.

123. Temes RT, Folles F, Kessler RM, et al. Intrapleural fibrinolytics in management of empyema thoracis. Chest. 1996;110:102-106.

124. Thomson AH, Hull J, Kumar MR, et al. Randomized trial of intrapleural urokinase in the treatment of childhood empyema. Thorax. 2002;57:343-347.

125. Wait MA, Sharma S, Hohn J, Nogare AD. A randomized trial of empyema therapy. Chest. 1997;111:1548-1551.

126. Lim TK, Chin NK. Empiric treatment with fibrinolysis and early surgery reduces the duration of hospitalization in pleural sepsis. Eur Respir J. 1999;13:514-518.

127. Cassina PC, Hauser M, Hillejan L, et al. Video-assisted thoracoscopy in the treatment of pleural empyema: Stage-based management and outcome. J Thorac Cardiovasc Surg. 1999;117:234-238.

128. Landreneau RJ, Keenan RJ, Hazelrigg SR, et al. Thoracoscopy for empyema and hemothorax. Chest. 1995;109:18-24.

CHAPTER **63**

Lung Abscess

BENNETT LORBER

Lung abscess results when microbial infection causes necrosis of the lung parenchyma producing one or more cavities. These cavities often communicate with large airways resulting in cough with purulent sputum and the presence of air-fluid levels on lung imaging studies. There may be more than one cavity, but usually one is large and dominant. The term *necrotizing pneumonia* often is used to describe a similar pathologic process with multiple small (<2 cm in diameter) cavities in contiguous areas of the lung. Although many organisms may produce lung abscess, most cases are due to anaerobic mouth flora bacteria and follow aspiration. Lung abscess was much more common in the preantibiotic era when, owing to lack of treatment, bacterial pneumonia sometimes progressed to abscess formation, with or without empyema. Reduction in incidence also occurred in the late 1940s and 1950s, when it became clear that performing oral surgery and tonsillectomy in the sitting position was a risk factor for lung abscess, and this practice was discontinued.[1] The incidence of and mortality rate from lung abscess have decreased considerably during the past several decades.

CLASSIFICATION

Before the wide availability of reliable methods for growing anaerobic bacteria, many patients with lung abscesses had no pathogen recovered from coughed sputum. These patients were said to have a "nonspecific lung abscess." It is now clear that, in almost all instances, anaerobic bacteria caused these infections.

Abscesses of the lung are classified variously by (1) the causative organism (e.g., anaerobic lung abscess or staphylococcal lung abscess); (2) the presence of a foul odor to expectorated sputum (putrid lung abscess); (3) the duration of symptoms before diagnosis (acute, symptoms present <1 month; chronic, symptoms present >1 month); or (4) the presence or absence of associated conditions (lung cancer, acquired immunodeficiency syndrome [AIDS], immunosuppression). The term *primary lung abscess* generally is used when an abscess develops in individuals prone to aspiration or individuals in relatively good health. Secondary lung abscess indicates an obstructing airway neoplasm, a complication of intrathoracic surgery, or a systemic condition or treatment that compromises host defense mechanisms, such as human immunodeficiency virus infection or transplant immunosuppressive therapy. Approximately 80% of lung abscesses are primary, and roughly half of these are associated with putrid sputum.

PATHOPHYSIOLOGY

Most lung abscesses occur as a complication of aspiration pneumonia and are polymicrobial infections due to anaerobic bacteria that are normally present in the mouth. The bacteria that cause aspiration pneumonia[2,3] and the bacteria responsible for lung abscess in aspiration-prone persons are virtually identical, attesting to the role of antecedent aspiration in the pathogenesis of most lung abscesses. The initial aspiration lung insult may be due to direct chemical injury from aspirated stomach acid or to areas of obstruction due to aspirated particulate matter, such as food; secondary bacterial infection then may supervene. If the aspirated bacterial inoculum is sufficiently large or virulent, or if lung defense mechanisms are compromised, infection can occur without prior insult to the lung. Studies of animal models and patients in whom a specific time of aspiration is known show that tissue necrosis with lung abscess formation takes, at minimum, 1 week and usually 2 weeks to develop.[4,5]

The typical patient with a lung abscess has a predisposition to aspiration due to altered consciousness. Common causes for altered consciousness in these patients include alcoholism, seizures, stroke, drug overdose, and general anesthesia. Other causes for aspiration include dysphagia due to neurologic or esophageal disease; respiratory muscle dysfunction due to amyotrophic lateral sclerosis, Parkinson's disease, or stroke; tooth extraction; and mechanical interference with anatomic and physiologic barriers to aspiration (e.g., nasogastric tubes and endotracheal intubation). Characteristically, patients with lung abscess have poor dentition with gingivitis resulting in an unusually high density of oral anaerobic organisms, particularly in the gingival crevices. Lung abscess is rare in an edentulous person, and this association should raise the possibility of an airway obstruction, often due to bronchogenic carcinoma. In some studies, almost 50% of lung abscesses in adults older than age 50 years are associated with carcinoma of the lung, either due to infection behind an obstructing tumor or infection within the necrotic tumor itself. Other, less common causes of airway obstruction that may lead to lung abscess include foreign bodies and extrinsic compression from an enlarged lymph node.

A study that employed an isotope tracer technique to detect aspiration showed that 45% of healthy individuals aspirated during sleep, as did 70% of patients with altered consciousness secondary to disease.[6] Considering that 1 mL of saliva contains 10^9 or more live bacteria, the infrequency of aspiration pneumonia provides strong evidence for the efficacy of the normal intrinsic lung clearance and defense mechanisms. These mechanisms may fail, and pneumonia (and later abscess) ensues, when the aspirated inoculum is large, the organisms are particularly virulent, or the defense mechanisms (e.g., mucociliary apparatus, alveolar macrophages) are impaired due to intoxication or disease.

Other processes that may result in lung abscess or necrotizing pneumonia or both include bronchiectasis, secondary infection of bland infarction from pulmonary embolism, and septic embolization from tricuspid valve endocarditis or suppurative phlebitis. Septic phlebitis of the neck veins due to *Fusobacterium necrophorum* with embolic infection in the lung (Lemierre syndrome) may complicate an oropharyngeal infection, such as peritonsillar abscess. This syndrome is less likely to present with cavitary lung lesions than in the preantibiotic era.[7] A distinguishing characteristic of abscesses due to septic embolization is the involvement of multiple, noncontiguous areas of the lung.[8]

Aspirated bacteria are carried by gravity to dependent portions of the lung, and aspiration usually occurs with the patient in a reclining or supine position. Additionally, the right main stem bronchus is larger in diameter, shorter, and less angulated from the trachea than is the left main stem bronchus. Lung abscesses occur most frequently in the posterior segment of the right upper lobe followed by the same segment on the left, then by the superior segments of the lower lobes. Spread of pulmonary parenchymal infection to the pleural space by direct extension results in empyema in one third of patients. Amebic lung abscess typically occurs in the right lower lobe, arising by direct extension of a liver abscess through the diaphragm.

MICROBIOLOGY

Some microorganisms capable of producing lung abscess or necrotizing pneumonia are listed in Table 63-1. The predominant organisms responsible for lung abscess are bacteria, specifically mouth anaerobes that are normal flora in the gingival crevices.[5] In the presence of periodontal disease, the gingival crevice deepens and fills with anaerobic gram-negative organisms that can reach truly astronomical numbers (10^{12} colony-forming units/g of scraped gingival contents).[9] Studies employing sample collection techniques that avoid contamination with oral flora combined with good anaerobic culture methods showed that anaerobes are found in about 90% of lung abscesses and are the only organisms present in about half of cases.[10] The most frequently isolated anaerobes are *Peptostreptococcus* spp., *Fusobacterium nucleatum,* and *Prevotella melaninogenica.*[11,12] Abscesses usually contain multiple anaerobe species, usually three to four per culture specimen; microaerophilic streptococci and viridans streptococci often are present as well.

Monomicrobial lung abscess occasionally may be caused by bacteria including *Staphylococcus aureus,* enteric gram-negative rods such as *Klebsiella* spp., *Pseudomonas aeruginosa, Burkholderia pseudomallei* (melioidosis), *Pasteurella multocida,* group A streptococcus, *Haemophilus influenzae* types b and c, *Legionella* spp., *Rhodococcus equi, Actinomyces* spp., and *Nocardia* spp. *Streptococcus pneumoniae,* particularly type 3, has been reported to cause lung abscess, but cavitation in the setting of pneumococcal pneumonia may be due to concomitant infection with anaerobes.[13] Other organisms that can cause lung abscess include many fungi, mycobacterial species, and parasites (e.g., *Paragonimus westermani, Entamoeba histolytica*).

Oropharyngeal colonization with *P. aeruginosa,* other aerobic gram-negative rods, and, less often, *S. aureus* is a common event in hospitalized patients, particularly patients who receive ventilatory support. These bacteria are important pathogens when lung abscess or

necrotizing pneumonia develops during hospitalization and may produce infection as the sole pathogen or as one component of a mixed-flora infection involving other aspirated oropharyngeal organisms.

In patients with impaired cell-mediated immunity (AIDS, transplant immunosuppression), opportunistic pathogens, such as mycobacteria, *Nocardia, Aspergillus,* and *Rhodococcus,* are important causes of cavitary lung lesions. In patients with impaired host defenses due to granulocytopenia (leukemia, chemotherapy), aerobic bacteria (*P. aeruginosa, S. aureus*) and fungi, including *Aspergillus* and Zygomycetes, are important pathogens.

CLINICAL MANIFESTATIONS

Primary lung abscess due to mouth flora anaerobic bacteria usually presents in a subacute or indolent fashion with symptoms present for several weeks or longer.[5,10,14] Fever, malaise, night sweats, and cough with purulent sputum usually are present; pleuritic pain is common. Weight loss may be profound even in the absence of underlying malignancy. Shaking chills almost never are reported. Patients often seek medical attention when the sputum production becomes copious or they develop pleuritic pain. The sputum has a putrid smell in about 50% of cases, and the patients, or their close contacts, may complain of the foul sputum smell or of the patient's bad breath.[15] Hemoptysis occurs in some instances. There is often a history of antecedent loss of consciousness due to seizure or intoxication. Physical examination findings include fever, poor dentition and gingival disease, and abnormal lung findings consistent with parenchymal infection or pleural fluid or both. Amphoric or cavernous breath sounds may be heard. Clubbing of the digits may be seen. The gag reflex, a physiologic defense against large-volume aspiration, may be absent. Anemia of

---

TABLE 63-1 Differential Diagnosis of a Cavitary Lesion on Chest Radiograph

Infections*

Bacteria
 Usually: mouth flora anaerobes
 Less commonly: *Staphylococcus aureus, Pseudomonas aeruginosa,* enteric gram-negative rods, *Pasteurella multocida, Burkholderia, Haemophilus influenzae* types b and c, *Legionella,* group A streptococcus, *Streptococcus pneumoniae* (?), *Streptococcus milleri* group, *Nocardia, Rhodococcus, Corynebacterium pseudodiphtheriticum, Actinomyces*

Mycobacteria
 Tuberculosis and nontuberculous pathogens

Fungi
 Including endemic mycoses (*Histoplasma, Coccidioides, Blastomyces*) and opportunistic pathogens (*Aspergillus, Cryptococcus,* Zygomycetes, *Pneumocystis*)

Parasites
 Paragonimus westermani, Entamoeba histolytica, Echinococcus

Noninfectious Causes

Neoplasms
 Primary lung cancer, metastatic carcinoma, lymphoma

Pulmonary infarction
 Due to bland embolus (may be secondarily infected)

Septic embolism
 Tricuspid endocarditis due to *S. aureus* and others, jugular venous septic phlebitis due to *Fusobacterium necrophorum* (Lemierre syndrome)

Vasculitis
 Wegener's granulomatosis, rheumatoid lung nodule

Airway disease
 Bullae, blebs, or cystic bronchiectasis

Developmental
 Pulmonary sequestration

Other
 Sarcoidosis, transdiaphragmatic bowel herniation giving appearance of cavity with air-fluid level

*Empyema with an air-fluid level may be mistaken for lung abscess on chest radiograph; computed tomography is useful in distinguishing abscess from empyema.

FIGURE 63-1. A, Admission chest radiograph from a 61-year-old man with fever, cough, and putrid sputum of 4 weeks' duration and a 12-lb weight loss. A large infiltrate is seen in the right lung without obvious cavitation. **B,** A repeat radiograph on day 6 of hospitalization, after the patient began to produce copious sputum, shows a large, thick-walled cavity with an air-fluid level. Because the patient was a heavy smoker and had no aspiration risk and excellent oral hygiene, a bronchoscopy was performed, which showed a partially obstructing carcinoma.

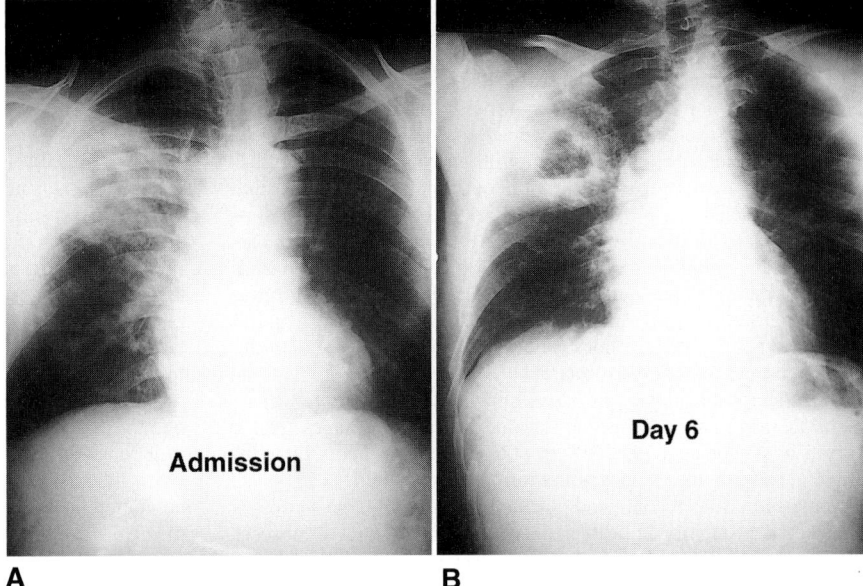

A   B

chronic disease and leukocytosis with approximately 15,000 white blood cells/mm³ usually are present. Associated empyema is present in about one third of cases and may be seen with or without bronchopleural fistula.

Necrotizing pneumonia occasionally presents with a more rapid course, often presenting within 1 week of symptom onset.[14] Early extension to other lobes and to the pleural space, high fever, and pronounced leukocytosis (>20,000/mm³) are common. Rapidly progressive necrotizing pneumonia has been referred to as *pulmonary gangrene.*

DIAGNOSIS

The diagnosis usually is made by chest radiography showing a lung cavity with an air-fluid level (Fig. 63-1). Typically the cavity wall is thick and irregular, and a surrounding pulmonary infiltrate often is present. The infiltrate usually is localized to one pulmonary segment or lobe, and hilar adenopathy is not prominent. Multilobar involvement suggests an underlying impairment in host defense mechanisms.[16] Computed tomography (CT) is more sensitive than chest radiograph and is useful to detect small cavities, provide evidence for obstructing endobronchial lesions, and distinguish lung abscesses from air-fluid levels in the pleural space.[17]

In the typical aspiration-prone patient with gingival disease, a subacute illness, and foul-smelling sputum, a putative diagnosis can be made, polymicrobial anaerobic infection can be assumed, and therapy can be instituted without microbiologic studies. Sputum Gram stains in these patients show many neutrophils and mixed flora with many morphologically different bacteria; routine cultures usually grow "normal respiratory flora." The physician should smell expectorated sputum and aspirated pleural fluid from patients with lung abscess to detect the presence of a putrid odor, considered pathognomonic of anaerobic infection. Because expectorated sputum is contaminated by oral flora containing large numbers of anaerobes, special techniques for obtaining lower tract specimens are necessary to confirm the role of anaerobes. These techniques include transtracheal aspiration, transthoracic aspiration, protected-brush fiberoptic bronchoscopy, bronchoalveolar lavage with quantitative cultures,[18] and empyema fluid obtained by thoracentesis. Blood cultures are rarely positive in anaerobic lung abscess. Patients without the classic presentation and patients with secondary lung abscess should have stains and cultures of expectorated sputum for aerobic bacteria, mycobacteria, fungi, and, in some instances, parasites.

DIFFERENTIAL DIAGNOSIS

The infectious and noninfectious causes of an apparent cavitary lesion on a chest radiograph are listed in Table 63-1. Hospitalized patients routinely become colonized in the oropharynx with gram-negative rods[3,19]; nosocomial lung infections, whether after aspiration or intrathoracic surgery, commonly involve virulent aerobic pathogens, such as *Klebsiella* spp. and *Pseudomonas* spp. If a specific diagnosis is not clear (e.g., putrid sputum indicating anaerobic infection), patients may need to be placed in appropriate isolation until the possibility of tuberculosis is eliminated. Lung cancer masses may develop cavitation even without secondary infection; more commonly, infection occurs behind a tumor-obstructed airway or within a large necrotic tumor mass. Fewer than 5% of pulmonary infarcts due to bland embolism become secondarily infected; infection should be suspected when fever persists for more than a few days, temperature is elevated (>103° F), or the leukocyte count is >20,000/mm³. Metastatic lung abscesses that occur by hematogenous dissemination from septic phlebitis or tricuspid valve endocarditis typically are distinguished by being multiple, bilateral, peripheral, and found in multiple lung fields; blood cultures are characteristically positive, a rare finding in abscesses secondary to aspiration. Lung nodules in patients with Wegener's granulomatosis and rheumatoid arthritis may cavitate and be mistaken for abscesses, but the systemic features of these illnesses usually are apparent. Bullae and blebs are characteristically thin-walled and without surrounding infiltrates.

TREATMENT

Antimicrobial Therapy

A major advance in the treatment of primary lung abscess attended the widespread use of penicillin. Although sulfonamides, the first widely used antimicrobials, had shown no impact on morbidity or mortality, high-dose oral penicillin was proved to be highly efficacious, even in patients showing delayed closure of the abscess cavity. For many years, penicillin was considered the drug of choice for anaerobic infections "above the diaphragm." In recent decades, however, many mouth flora anaerobes, including fusobacteria, *Prevotella* spp., and non-*fragilis Bacteroides* spp., have been shown to produce penicillinase.[20] Also, two prospective studies[21,22] have shown superiority of clindamycin over penicillin in the treatment of anaerobic lung abscess, as judged by time to defervescence, time to resolution of putrid sputum, and relapse rates. Metronidazole, used as monotherapy, has been disappointing and is inferior to clindamycin.[23] Although highly active against most anaerobes, metronidazole is not active against the microaerophilic streptococci and some anaerobic cocci that are typical constituents of anaerobic lung infection. These bacteria are susceptible to penicillin, and the combination of penicillin and metronidazole is inexpensive, is generally well tolerated, and has yielded favorable results. Metronidazole must be used with caution in alcoholics because of the potential for a disulfiram-like reaction. Other agents that could be predicted to have utility in the treatment of lung abscess include combinations of a penicillin with a β-lactamase inhibitor, carbapenems, and quinolones with good anaerobic activity (moxifloxacin and gatifloxacin).[24] One study[25] showed excellent results using intravenous followed by oral amoxicillin-clavulanate (oral dose, 1 g/125 mg every 8 hours). Tetracyclines should not be used because of widespread resistance across many anaerobe species.

Oral therapy for lung abscess was shown to be equivalent to parenteral therapy many years ago.[26] Recommended oral dosages are 1 g every 8 hours for penicillin, 300 to 600 mg every 8 hours for clindamycin, and 500 mg every 8 hours for metronidazole.

Some authorities recommend placing patients with large abscesses and excessive coughing in a lateral decubitus position with the abscess side down to avoid sudden discharge of abscess contents causing asphyxiation or spread of infection to healthy lung segments.[12] If coughing is excessive and associated with even scant hemoptysis, cough suppressants may be useful, but, as a general principle in lung abscess management, sedation should be minimized.

Aspiration is the usual antecedent occurrence that eventuates in lung abscess. Occasionally, patients are observed to aspirate oral or gastric contents. There is no evidence that administering antibiotics to patients with observed aspiration prevents lung infection.

Duration of Therapy

There is no generally agreed-on duration for the treatment of lung abscess. Patients often are treated for 6 to 8 weeks or more. One study using clindamycin to treat anaerobic lung abscess showed excellent efficacy with no advantage of 6 weeks over 3 weeks of therapy.[21] Many authorities recommend following weekly or biweekly chest radiographs in patients showing clinical improvement, with discontinuation of therapy when the radiograph is clear or there is a small, stable, residual lesion.

Bronchoscopy

Although bronchoscopy or physical therapy may improve drainage, studies in the preantibiotic era showed no advantage for bronchoscopic or postural drainage of abscesses compared with conservative management or surgery. Attempts to drain large abscesses may result in rapid unloading of the pus and necrotic material from the abscess into other lung segments and may produce acute asphyxiation or adult respiratory distress syndrome. Bronchoscopy should be reserved for patients who do not respond to medical management and patients in whom an endobronchial tumor is suspected. Clinical features associated with an underlying malignancy and indications for early bronchoscopy to help diagnose a tumor include location of the abscess in an anterior lobar segment, lack of aspiration risk, edentulous patient, age older than 50 combined with a strong smoking history, and lack of systemic symptoms.

Surgical Intervention

Previously, resectional surgery was the treatment for lung abscess. Today, almost all patients respond to appropriate antimicrobial therapy, and surgery is reserved for the 10% to 15% of patients who do not improve with appropriate medical management. Drainage is the most important step in the management of abscesses regardless of location. Lung abscesses, in contrast to other visceral abscesses, usually drain themselves, through communication with large airways. This drainage is indicated by the presence of air-fluid levels.

Causes of medical treatment failure and indications for consideration of lobectomy or pneumonectomy include large cavities (>8 cm),

abscesses due to resistant organisms such as *P. aeruginosa,* obstructing neoplasm, and massive hemorrhage (rare). More recently, CT-guided percutaneous drainage has been used safely and successfully in patients who were not responding to antimicrobial treatment.[27]

Response to Therapy

Patients typically have diminished fever and a subjective sense of a change for the better within a few days of beginning antimicrobial therapy. Defervescence can be expected in 7 to 10 days. Persistence of fever beyond 2 weeks should lead to diagnostic tests to rule out complications or obstructions or both (CT scan, bronchoscopy), along with cultures for unusual pathogens, such as fungi and mycobacteria. When medical management fails, it most often is secondary to undrained pleural collections, endobronchial obstruction due to a neoplasm or foreign body, resistant organisms, or large cavity size (>8 cm in diameter).

Chest radiographs commonly show worsening in approximately one third of patients during the first week of treatment.[28] The median time to cavity closure is 4 weeks, and surrounding infiltrates may take twice that time to resolve. Radiographic improvement may lag well behind clinical cure. In some patients with a clear clinical response to medical treatment, cavities resolve slowly and may take many weeks or months to disappear radiographically; a small percentage of patients are left with a residual cavity.

PROGNOSIS

In the preantibiotic era, more than 45% of patients with lung abscess underwent surgery, and one third died. In more recent years, less than 15% of patients have undergone surgery, and the overall mortality rate is approximately 10%. Death in patients with primary lung abscess or community-acquired abscesses is infrequent (approximately 2%); but a fatal outcome is seen in more than 65% of cases associated with obstructing airway lesions, impaired host defenses, or nosocomial acquisition.[29]

REFERENCES

1. Schweppe HI, Knowles JH, Kane L. Lung abscess: An analysis of the Massachusetts General Hospital cases from 1943 through 1956. N Engl J Med. 1961;265:1039-1043.
2. Bartlett JG, Gorbach SL, Finegold SM. The bacteriology of aspiration pneumonia. Am J Med. 1974;56:202-207.
3. Lorber B, Swenson RM. Bacteriology of aspiration pneumonia: A prospective study of community- and hospital-acquired cases. Ann Intern Med. 1974;81:329-331.
4. Smith DT. Experimental aspiratory abscess. Arch Surg. 1927;14:231-239.
5. Bartlett JG. Anaerobic bacterial infections of the lung and pleural space. Clin Infect Dis. 1993;16(Suppl 4):S248-S255.
6. Huxley EJ, Viroslav J, Gray WR, et al. Pharyngeal aspiration in normal adults and patients with depressed consciousness. Am J Med. 1978;64:564-568.
7. Chirinos JA, Lichstein DM, Garcia J, et al. The evolution of Lemierre syndrome: Report of 2 cases and review of the literature. Medicine. 2002;81:458-465.
8. Alcantara AL, Tucker RB, McCarroll KA. Radiologic study of injection drug use complications. Infect Dis Clin N Am. 2002;16:713-743.
9. Slots J. Subgingival microflora and periodontal disease. J Clin Periodont. 1979;6:351-382.
10. Bartlett JG, Gorbach SL, Tally FP, et al. Bacteriology and treatment of primary lung abscess. Am Rev Respir Dis. 1974;109:510-518.
11. Marina M, Strong CA, Civen R, et al. Bacteriology of anaerobic pleuropulmonary infections: Preliminary report. Clin Infect Dis. 1993;16(Suppl 4):S256-S262.
12. Davis B, Systrom DM. Lung abscess: Pathogenesis, diagnosis and treatment. Curr Clin Top Infect Dis. 1998;18:252-273.
13. Leatherman JW, Iber C, Davies SF. Cavitation in bacteremic pneumococcal pneumonia: Causal role of mixed infection with anerobic bacteria. Am Rev Respir Dis. 1984;129:317-321.
14. Bartlett JG, Finegold SM. Anaerobic infections of the lung and pleural space. Am Rev Respir Dis. 1974;110:56-77.
15. Lorber B. "Bad breath": Presenting manifestation of anaerobic pulmonary infection. Am Rev Respir Dis. 1975;112:875-877.
16. Mansharamani N, Balachandran D, Delaney D, et al. Lung abscess in adults: Clinical comparison of immunocompromised to non-immunocompromised patients. Respir Med. 2002;96:178-185.
17. Stark DD, Federle MP, Goodman PC, et al. Differentiating lung abscess from empyema: Radiography and computed tomography. AJR Am J Roentgenol. 1983;141:163-168.
18. Henriquez AH, Mendoza J, Gonzalez PC. Quantitative culture of bronchoalveolar lavage from patients with anaerobic lung abscesses. J Infect Dis. 1991;164:414-417.
19. Johanson WG, Pierce AK, Sanford JP. Changing pharyngeal bacterial flora of hospitalized patients: Emergence of gram-negative bacilli. N Engl J Med. 1969;281:1137-1140.

20. Kononen E, Saarela M, Kanervo A, et al. Beta-lactamase production and penicillin susceptibility among different ribotypes of Prevotella melaninogenica simultaneously colonizing the oral cavity. Clin Infect Dis. 1995;20(Suppl 2):S364-S366.
21. Levison ME, Mangura CT, Lorber B, et al. Clindamycin compared with penicillin for the treatment of anaerobic lung abscess. Ann Intern Med. 1983;98:466-471.
22. Guidol F, Manresa F, Pallares R, et al. Clindamycin vs. penicillin for anaerobic lung infections: High rate of penicillin failures associated with penicillin-resistant Bacteroides melaninogenicus. Arch Intern Med. 1990;150:2525-2529.
23. Perlino CA. Metronidazole vs. clindamycin treatment of anaerobic pulmonary infection: Failure of metronidazole therapy. Arch Intern Med. 1981;141:1424-1427.
24. Levison ME. Anaerobic pleuropulmonary infection. Curr Opin Infect Dis. 2001;14:187-191.
25. Fernandez-Sabe N, Carratala J, Dorca J, et al. Efficacy and safety of sequential amoxicillin-clavulanate in the treatment of anaerobic lung infections. Eur J Clin Microbiol Infect Dis. 2003;22:185-187.
26. Weiss W, Cherniack NS. Acute nonspecific lung abscess: A controlled study comparing orally and parenterally administered penicillin G. Chest. 1974;66:348-351.
27. Wali SO, Shugaeri A, Samman YS, et al. Percutaneous drainage of pyogenic lung abscess. Scand J Infect Dis. 2002;34:673-679.
28. Landay MJ, Christensen EE, Bynum LJ, et al. Anaerobic pleural and pulmonary infections. Am J Radiol. 1980;134:233-240.
29. Perlman LV, Lerner E, D'Esposo N. Clinical classification and analysis of 97 cases of lung abscess. Am Rev Respir Dis. 1969;99:390-398.

CHAPTER **64**

Chronic Pneumonia

PETER G. PAPPAS

WILLIAM E. DISMUKES

Chronic pneumonia syndrome is a pulmonary parenchymal process that may have an infectious or a noninfectious etiology, that has been present for weeks to months rather than for days, and that is manifested by abnormal chest radiographic findings and by chronic or progressive pulmonary symptoms. The abnormal chest radiograph, which may reveal any of several radiologic patterns, is probably the most important consideration in the diagnosis of chronic pneumonia. Indeed, in many patients, the diagnosis is based more on the pulmonary radiographic findings than on the pulmonary symptoms. However, asymptomatic patients who have abnormal findings such as solitary or multiple nodules on routine roentgenographic evaluation should not be considered to have chronic pneumonia.

The emphasis in this chapter is on the chronic pneumonias caused by infectious agents. However, it is important to recognize the importance of noninfectious causes of chronic pneumonia, including vasculitides,[1-5] neoplasia,[6-8] drugs,[9] radiation, amyloidosis,[10] sarcoidosis,[11-13] alveolar phospholipoproteinosis,[14] bronchiolitis obliterans with organizing pneumonia,[15-17] and other, idiopathic causes.[18-20]

ETIOLOGY

The infectious causes of chronic pneumonia can be divided into two main groups: (1) agents that typically cause acute pneumonia and are unusual causes of chronic pneumonia, and (2) infectious agents that typically cause chronic pneumonia. Among those agents that typically cause acute pneumonia, anaerobic bacteria, Staphylococcus aureus, Haemophilus influenzae, the Enterobacteriaceae, and Pseudomonas aeruginosa are the organisms most likely to produce a persistent chronic pneumonia. This is usually a chronic necrotizing process that most commonly occurs in patients with significant underlying disease (such as alcoholism, diabetes mellitus, intrathoracic malignancy, and chronic obstructive lung disease), hospitalized patients, individuals requiring long-term ventilatory assistance, patients with chronic swallowing and reflux disorders, and others at risk for recurrent aspiration, such as patients with Parkinson's disease.[21-24] Acute pneumonias caused by most viruses or by Streptococcus pneumoniae, Mycoplasma

pneumoniae, Legionella species, Coxiella burnetii, or Chlamydia pneumoniae[25-27] rarely progress to a chronic pulmonary illness.

Table 64-1 lists the most common infectious and noninfectious causes of chronic pneumonia. In the otherwise healthy host, the most common considerations are tuberculosis[28,29] and mycobacterial infections other than tuberculosis (MOTT),[30-32] the endemic fungal infections

TABLE 64-1 Etiology of Chronic Pneumonia Syndrome

Infectious Agents That Typically Cause Chronic Pneumonia

Bacteria and Actinomycetes
Mixed aerobic and anaerobic bacteria
Actinomyces spp.
Propionibacterium propionicum
Nocardia spp.
Rhodococcus equi
Burkholderia pseudomallei

Mycobacteria
Mycobacterium tuberculosis
Mycobacterium kansasii
Mycobacterium avium complex

Fungi
Aspergillus spp.
Blastomyces dermatitidis
Coccidioides spp.
Cryptococcus neoformans
Emmonsia
Histoplasma capsulatum
Sporothrix schenckii
Paracoccidioides brasiliensis

Worms
Dirofilaria
Echinococcus granulosus
Filaria (tropical pulmonary eosinophilia)
Paragonimus westermani

Noninfectious Causes of Pneumonia
Neoplasia
  Carcinoma (primary or metastatic)
  Lymphoma
Cystic fibrosis
Sarcoidosis
Amyloidosis
Vasculitis (autoimmune diseases)
  Systemic lupus erythematosus
  Polyarteritis nodosa
  Allergic angiitis and granulomatosis (Churg-Strauss syndrome)
  Progressive systemic sclerosis
  Rheumatoid arthritis
  Mixed connective tissue syndrome (overlap syndrome)
  Wegener's granulomatosis
  Lymphomatoid granulomatosis
Chemicals, drugs
Radiation
Recurrent pulmonary emboli
Bronchial obstruction with atelectasis (e.g., tumor, foreign body)
Pulmonary infiltration with eosinophilia syndrome
  Loeffler syndrome—usually transient
  Pneumonia plus asthma (e.g., allergic bronchopulmonary aspergillosis)
  Bronchocentric granulomatosis
  Eosinophilic pneumonia—chronic
Pneumoconiosis: asbestosis, berylliosis, silicosis, anthracosilicosis
Chronic form of extrinsic allergic alveolitis (hypersensitivity pneumonitis)

Other Lung Diseases—Cause Unknown
Bronchiolitis obliterans organizing pneumonia
Chronic interstitial pneumonia (fibrosing alveolitis, idiopathic pulmonary fibrosis)
  Usual interstitial pneumonia (UIP)
  Desquamative interstitial pneumonia (DIP)
  Lymphocytic interstitial pneumonia (LIP)
  Giant cell interstitial pneumonia (GIP)
Eosinophilic granuloma (histiocytosis X)
Lymphangioleiomyomatosis
Goodpasture's syndrome
Pulmonary alveolar proteinosis
Pulmonary alveolar microlithiasis
Idiopathic pulmonary hemosiderosis
Angiocentric immunoproliferative lesions

(including histoplasmosis,[33,34] coccidioidomycosis,[35,36] blastomycosis,[37,38] and paracoccidioidomycosis,[39] in their appropriate geographic areas), other mycoses (e.g., cryptococcosis),[40,41] mixed aerobic and anaerobic bacterial infection,[21-23] and actinomycosis.[42] Pseudallescheriasis (scedosporiosis),[43,44] sporotrichosis,[45] and adiaspiromycosis (caused by *Emmonsia* species)[46-48] are rare causes of chronic fungal pneumonia in the normal host. In the immunocompromised host, mycobacteria, especially *M. tuberculosis*, remain common causes of chronic pneumonia.[49,50] Classic opportunistic infections including nocardiosis,[51] cryptococcosis,[41] aspergillosis,[52] and infections caused by other molds such as the Zygomycetes are also important in this population. In the appropriate geographic areas, coccidioidomycosis, histoplasmosis, and blastomycosis are also important considerations among immunocompromised hosts.[34-36,53] In persons with acquired immunodeficiency syndrome (AIDS), these same infections are frequently seen.[34-36,53-59] Furthermore, in these patients, chronic pneumonia may be caused by *Rhodococcus equi, Penicillium marneffei, Pneumocystis jirovecii* (formerly *P. carinii*), or cytomegalovirus, or by such noninfectious disorders as Kaposi's sarcoma, lymphoma, radiation therapy, and nonspecific interstitial pneumonitis.[60-64] The protozoa and worms listed in Table 64-1 are uncommon causes of chronic pneumonia syndrome among persons living in industrialized countries, but they are important considerations for those who live in or have traveled to areas in which these agents are endemic.

There have been no large-series studies that address the frequencies of the various causes of chronic pneumonia. This lack of perspective on the incidence of the causes of chronic pneumonia contrasts with our better understanding of the *acute* pneumonia syndrome. In addition, since the introduction of antibiotics in the 1940s, the overall spectrum of pneumonia has changed significantly; new pathogens have emerged, organisms that were once considered to be harmless commensals are now recognized as pathogens, and powerful immunosuppressive therapies render some patients more susceptible to certain microorganisms. Consequently, in considering the differential diagnosis of chronic pneumonia in an individual patient, emphasis on specific entities usually must be based less on statistical likelihood and more on a thorough and methodical analysis of all available clinical, epidemiologic, and laboratory data.

EPIDEMIOLOGY

Age, Sex, Race

In the United States over the past quarter century, pulmonary tuberculosis has become a disease of the homeless, alcoholic, older adult, human immunodeficiency virus (HIV)-infected, and immigrant population groups. (An exception is pulmonary lymphangioleiomyomatosis, a neoplastic disorder that occurs almost exclusively in adolescent and young adult women.[65]) The significance of age and sex for patients with chronic pneumonia from other causes also usually relates, indirectly, to associated epidemiologic factors. For example, an older adult is at higher risk of having a cerebrovascular accident, which in turn might predispose this patient to an aspiration episode and subsequent chronic bacterial pneumonia and abscess. Older, debilitated patients are at higher risk for development of chronic necrotizing pneumonia caused by aerobic gram-negative bacteria. Similarly, the sex of a given patient is likely to affect or determine occupation and hobbies and therefore the likelihood of exposure to certain infectious agents or other etiologic vehicles. Racial and genetic characteristics are increasingly recognized as predisposing factors to severe disease manifestations from a variety of pathogens.[66] For example, pulmonary tuberculosis should be the presumptive diagnosis in a black individual with bilateral upper lobe cavitary disease; coccidioidomycosis is much more likely to be severe in darker-skinned persons, including blacks and Asians, among certain human leukocyte antigen (HLA) types, and among persons with O blood type who have lived in or have traveled to an area endemic for *Coccidioides immitis* or *Coccidioides posadasii*.[35,36,67,68] Conversely, chronic cavitary histoplasmosis is much more likely to occur in the older white male population with a history

of chronic lung disease.[33,34] Fungus ball of the lung occurs in a previously existing apical cavity in patients with prior sarcoidosis, histoplasmosis, tuberculosis, or other fibrocavitary lung disease.

Occupation and Hobbies

Certain occupations and hobbies should arouse suspicion of particular diseases. Occupational exposure to plant materials predisposes an individual to cutaneous sporotrichosis and, according to some authorities, to pulmonary involvement. Some classic examples of conditions linked to occupational and recreational behavior include the following: tuberculosis among health care workers; coccidioidomycosis among rock collectors, archeologists conducting excavations, construction workers, and others exposed to desert dust in the endemic area; histoplasmosis among persons who are exposed to pigeon or starling roosts, who clean out old chicken houses with dirt floors, who cut and clear hollow trees, or who explore old buildings or caves inhabited by bats; blastomycosis among forestry workers, earth-moving and heavy equipment operators, and hunters. In contrast to the previous examples, cryptococcosis has *not* been strongly linked to occupational or recreational behavior,[69] perhaps reflecting the fact that *Cryptococcus neoformans* is a ubiquitous pathogen that is not geographically restricted. Moreover, there has been no strong association between exposure to pigeon droppings and development of disease. Other associations include echinococcosis among sheep herders; berylliosis among workers in the aircraft, electronics, and nuclear industries; the pneumoconioses (e.g., silicosis, asbestosis) among sandblasters and shipyard workers; and both chronic and acute pulmonary disease from repeated occupational or environmental exposure to the aerosolized organic antigens associated with extrinsic allergic alveolitis (hypersensitivity pneumonitis)[70] or to irritant gases such as phosgene, ammonia, ozone, and nitrogen dioxide.

Travel

Because the initial exposure to the microbiologic agents of many chronic or indolent infectious diseases may have occurred months or years before the disease appears, a detailed travel history is essential in any patient with chronic pneumonia. For example, a patient with bilateral upper lobe infiltrates, with or without cavitation, who has never traveled to or lived in Central America, Mexico, South America, or west of the Mississippi River is unlikely to have coccidioidomycosis. On the other hand, if the patient has lived in the eastern half of the United States, especially the mid-central area, chronic pulmonary histoplasmosis and blastomycosis should be considered, because the etiologic agents are endemic to that area. Similarly, paracoccidioidomycosis should be considered only for patients who have lived in Mexico, Central America, or the endemic regions of South America.

In addition to identifying regions visited, there may be a need for detailed questioning about rural or urban exposure, type of lodging, sources of drinking water, exposure to local foods, working environment, and other activities such as swimming and hiking. For example, if a person who has lived or traveled extensively in Southeast Asia, particularly in low-lying or rice-growing areas, subsequently manifests chronic pneumonia with pulmonary roentgenographic abnormalities resembling those of tuberculosis or a pulmonary mycosis, melioidosis due to *Burkholderia pseudomallei* should be suspected.[71] Similarly, pulmonary paragonimiasis should be suspected in the visitor to Japan, Southeastern Asia, or the Philippines, who consumes raw or partly cooked shellfish, and who has chronic pulmonary symptoms plus dense, nodular lung opacities and ring shadows on the chest roentgenogram.[72]

Contacts, Habits, and Drugs

In patients and health care workers in whom tuberculosis is suspected, contacts among companions, relatives, or patients with tuberculosis should be sought. In addition, tuberculosis should be suspected in persons living or working in closed environments such as jails and prisons, schools, daycare centers, and nursing homes. Inquiry should be made into the patient's smoking and drinking history and other personal habits. The likelihood of cancer of the lung in a patient with coal worker's pneumoconiosis is greater in a smoker than in a nonsmoker. Aspiration pneumonia, chronic gram-negative bacillary pneumonia, tuberculosis, and pulmonary sporotrichosis are more likely to occur in an alcoholic than in a nondrinker. Intravenous drug users who inject heroin or other illicit agents are at risk not only for infection with HIV and subsequent development of AIDS but also for septic pulmonary emboli associated with tricuspid or pulmonic valve infective endocarditis, necrotizing pneumonia, single or multiple lung abscesses, or an interstitial granulomatous reaction to the injected material resulting in pulmonary hypertension. Similarly, frequent use of free-base cocaine has been reported to cause bronchiolitis obliterans with organizing pneumonia, eosinophilic lung disease, interstitial pneumonitis, and pulmonary hemorrhage or infarction.[73]

More than 100 different drugs have been reported to cause acute and chronic pulmonary symptoms with radiographic abnormalities.[9,74] Early in the course of drug-induced pulmonary disease, the chest roentgenogram findings may be normal; later, an interstitial, nodular, or alveolar pattern (or a combination of these) may be present. Still later, the chest radiograph may reveal only a fibrotic pulmonary process. The drugs that are most likely to cause chronic pulmonary disease include cytotoxic agents such as bleomycin, busulfan, cyclophosphamide, methotrexate, nitrosoureas and noncytotoxic agents such as amiodarone, gold salts, nitrofurantoin, and penicillamine. Because drug-induced pulmonary disease may develop after drug therapy has been discontinued, the physician should inquire not only about all drugs the patient is presently taking but also about those taken in the recent past.

Questions about previous or current antimicrobial therapy are important. Did the antimicrobial therapy result in roentgenographic or clinical improvement? If not, was the antimicrobial drug used in sufficient quantity and duration to cure the suspected process or alter its course? Was the appropriate agent used? What effect did the antimicrobial agent have on the results of cultures? Does the report of "normal flora" from the sputum culture merely reflect the elimination of a specific pathogen by antimicrobial therapy?

Underlying Disease

Pulmonary complications, including both acute and chronic or refractory pneumonia, are especially common among persons with AIDS[53-64] and other immunocompromising conditions, such as high-dose corticosteroid therapy, cytotoxic therapy, hematopoietic stem cell and organ transplantation, and chronic granulomatous disease.[49,50,75-77] Patients with diabetes mellitus or preexisting chronic obstructive pulmonary disease are at higher risk for development of chronic or persistent bacterial pneumonia. Similarly, chronic obstructive lung disease commonly precedes fibrocavitary histoplasmosis or *Mycobacterium avium* complex infection. Structural lung disease, such as preexisting bullae, bronchiectasis, and endobronchial lesions, may also predispose to chronic pneumonia. For example, recurrent or persistent pneumonia in the same area of the lung raises the suspicion of a local endobronchial lesion that may not be apparent on routine chest radiographs. Because aspiration may predispose to chronic pneumonia, inquiry should be made into a history of recent dental problems or manipulation, sinusitis with chronic nasal congestion, disorders of swallowing resulting from neurologic or esophageal disease, seizure disorders, recent anesthesia, quantity and frequency of alcohol consumption, or any illness leading to an unconscious state. Finally, it should be determined whether the chronic pneumonia is most likely community- or hospital-acquired.

CLINICAL FEATURES

Symptoms

There are many causes of chronic pneumonia, and no single symptom complex is common to all causes. Often, nonspecific and constitutional symptoms including fever, chills, and malaise are present initially. A history of progressive anorexia and weight loss usually indicates chronic illness. Pulmonary symptoms may be present early but frequently appear later in the course of the illness. Any patient with a prolonged illness and nonspecific constitutional complaints plus pulmonary symptoms—including a new or persistent cough, sputum production, hemoptysis, chest pain (especially pleuritic pain), or dyspnea—deserves medical evaluation, including a chest roentgenogram and, when findings on routine chest radiograph are nonspecific and suggestive of a chronic parenchymal process, a computed tomographic examination of the chest (chest CT).

Evidence of extrapulmonary involvement should be explored with each patient. For example, chronic pneumonia with skin lesions should suggest coccidioidomycosis, blastomycosis, or, in the right epidemiologic setting, paracoccidioidomycosis. Similarly, cryptococcosis, nocardiosis, and Kaposi's sarcoma should be important considerations for patients with AIDS or other conditions associated with significant impairment of cell-mediated immune function. Mucous membrane lesions might suggest histoplasmosis, paracoccidioidomycosis, Wegener's granulomatosis, or Kaposi's sarcoma. Monoarticular or polyarticular arthritis, polyarthralgia, or localized bone tenderness or pain may indicate a systemic vasculitis. A history of chronic pneumonia with persistent headache and abnormal cerebrospinal fluid should raise the suspicion of tuberculosis, cryptococcosis, or coccidioidomycosis involving both the lungs and the central nervous system. The presence of focal neurologic symptoms and signs is strong clinical evidence for a space-occupying lesion in the central nervous system; such findings in a patient with a cavitary infiltrate seen on a chest radiograph suggest the possibility of a brain abscess associated with chronic suppurative lung disease due to microaerophilic or anaerobic bacteria, or nocardiosis.[51] Similarly, the triad of skin nodules, pulmonary nodules, and central nervous system abnormalities suggests lymphomatoid granulomatosis.[5]

Signs

Although the findings on physical examination of the chest are usually not helpful in differentiating specific causes of chronic pneumonia, the presence of generalized wheezing or other signs of bronchospasm, in the absence of underlying lung disease, indicates an asthmatic component to the pulmonary illness and raises the possibility of a disorder causing both pneumonia and asthma, such as extrinsic allergic alveolitis, allergic bronchopulmonary aspergillosis, or allergic angiitis and granulomatosis (Churg-Strauss syndrome).[4] Similarly, localized wheezing suggests the presence of an endobronchial obstructing lesion. The findings of tachycardia, cardiomegaly, gallop rhythm, and ankle edema provide evidence of cardiac disease and suggest that the pulmonary symptoms and signs result at least in part from cardiovascular causes. The presence of skin lesions, clubbing, cyanosis, or phlebitis is not specific for any single pulmonary disorder but may help to narrow the differential diagnosis, especially when considered along with other clinical and epidemiologic information. Similarly, the finding of jaundice, adenopathy, hepatomegaly, splenomegaly, or ascites suggests that a systemic disorder involving multiple organs is the cause.

DIAGNOSTIC PROCEDURES

Initial Laboratory Studies

Routine laboratory studies often provide some important clues to diagnosis. Pancytopenia may suggest miliary tuberculosis, disseminated histoplasmosis, or a myelophthisic disorder such as metastatic tumor involving the bone marrow. Anemia alone is commonly associated with most of these disorders and is not particularly helpful in discerning an etiology. A normal leukocyte count does not exclude infection. In particular, chronic fungal pneumonia is usually associated with a normal or minimally elevated leukocyte count. Leukopenia or lymphopenia should raise the suspicion of an HIV infection. In addition, leukopenia should suggest sarcoidosis, systemic lupus erythematosus, tuberculosis, histoplasmosis, or neoplasia. A leukemoid reaction is nonspecific and may be seen in disseminated mycobacteriosis and mycoses. Leukocytosis with a polymorphonuclear cell predominance is suggestive of, but not specific for, a bacterial cause, including actinomycosis.

Routine laboratory tests that measure the function of other organs may provide more helpful information. Liver function studies, including bilirubin, alkaline phosphatase, and serum aspartate aminotransferase determinations and prothrombin time, should be obtained for most patients. Urinalysis, with particular attention to the urinary sediment, plus tests of renal function including measurement of blood urea nitrogen and creatinine, should also be done. Abnormalities of liver function (especially elevated enzyme levels), kidney function, or both should raise the suspicion of disorders that are not limited to the lung but are known to involve multiple other organs including the liver and kidney. Such disorders include disseminated histoplasmosis and disseminated mycobacteriosis as well as the vasculitides, sarcoidosis, and certain neoplastic diseases, especially the lymphoproliferative disorders.

In a patient with an abnormally low serum globulin level, a quantitative serum immunoglobulin determination should be obtained to evaluate for hypogammaglobulinemia. Studies that should be performed in patients with suspected vasculitis include serologic tests for antinuclear antibodies, rheumatoid factor, antineutrophil cytoplasmic autoantibodies (C-ANCA), C-reactive protein, and erythrocyte sedimentation rate. In addition, measurement of serum angiotensin-converting enzyme may be useful, although it is a nonspecific test for which levels are increased among patients with a number of granulomatous disorders, including 30% to 80% of patients with sarcoidosis.[11]

Additional Studies

There are basic core studies that should usually be performed on all patients with chronic pneumonia, regardless of the suspected cause, but there should be flexibility in choosing additional tests or procedures to confirm a specific diagnosis. The orderly sequence of diagnostic studies described in the following paragraphs necessarily results in oversimplification and consequently overlooks the unique aspects of a given patient's illness.

Chest Radiographic Studies. The chest radiograph, including a posteroanterior and a lateral film, is a reasonable screening procedure, but high-resolution CT (HRCT)[78,79] provides invaluable information. Occasionally, magnetic resonance imaging or fluorodeoxyglucose

positron-emission tomography[80] is helpful, particularly in the evaluation of the noninfectious causes of chronic pneumonia. In Table 64-2, disorders are grouped according to the type of radiologic abnormality that is characteristic of the disease. In some disorders, there is a spectrum of radiologic manifestations, and these disorders appear more than once in the table. Typical radiographic findings may provide clues to specific diagnoses. For example, demonstration of anterior mediastinal involvement argues strongly in favor of neoplasia, including lymphoma and metastatic carcinoma, as the cause of chronic pneumonia syndrome and argues against an infectious cause.

Tuberculosis and nontuberculous mycobacterial diseases, histoplasmosis, coccidioidomycosis, sporotrichosis, paragonimiasis, and the pneumoconioses, especially silicosis, characteristically produce fibrocavitary disease—a contracted area of lung with linear fibrosis, nodular or rounded densities, and cavitation. In addition, mycobacterial diseases, histoplasmosis, and silicosis characteristically involve the upper lobes. Many experts believe that anterior segment upper lobe involvement argues strongly against tuberculosis as an etiology. A thin-walled cavity is suggestive of coccidioidomycosis, sporotrichosis, or paragonimiasis, whereas a thick-walled cavity surrounded by an area of pneumonitis is more typical of tuberculosis, other mycobacterial infection, histoplasmosis, aspergillosis, melioidosis, nocardiosis, actinomycosis, pyogenic lung abscess, and lung disease caused by *Rhodococcus equi*. Cavitation is seen but is less common in blastomycosis and cryptococcosis. Calcification is typical of tuberculosis, histoplasmosis, and coccidioidomycosis but is rare in actinomycosis, nocardiosis, blastomycosis, and cryptococcosis. Abscess of the chest wall or osteomyelitis of a rib adjacent to the pneumonia or pleural effusion may be seen in actinomycosis, nocardiosis, and tuberculosis. Although these radiographic manifestations of selected pulmonary diseases are typical in the majority of patients, experience during the AIDS pandemic has shown that pulmonary diseases in these patients may be highly atypical in radiographic appearance and clinical course.[34,36,53-61] Representative radiographs are shown in Figures 64-1 through 64-14.

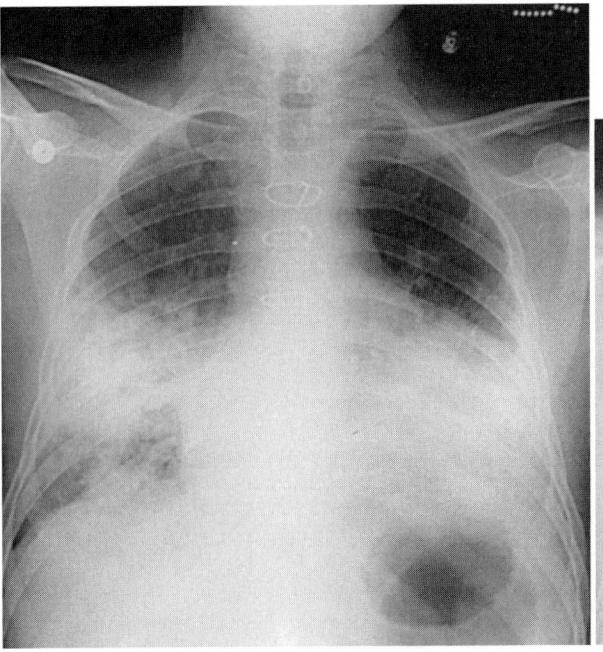
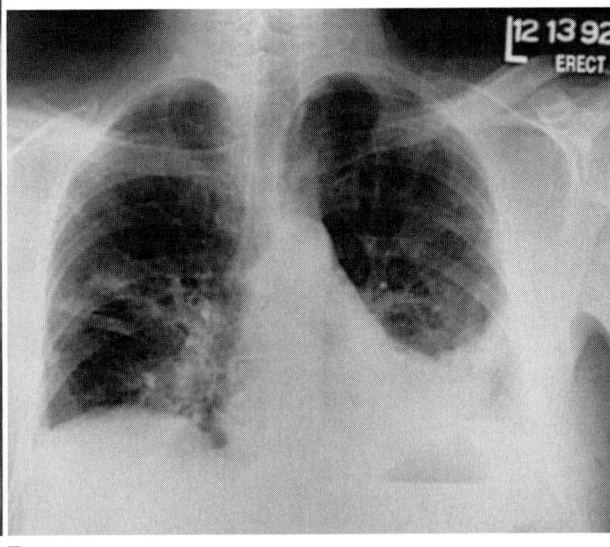

A   **B**

FIGURE 64-1. A, Bronchiolitis obliterans organizing pneumonia (BOOP) in a 32-year-old man who developed progressive chronic pneumonia several weeks after an open pericardiectomy to relieve cardiac tamponade associated with renal failure. Note the bilateral airspace consolidation. Bronchoscopy with transbronchial biopsy was nondiagnostic. The diagnosis of BOOP was established from tissue obtained at open lung biopsy. Corticosteroid therapy was dramatically beneficial. **B,** BOOP in a 60-year-old man with a 1-month illness manifested by fever, malaise, weight loss, nonproductive cough, dyspnea, and bilateral subpleural nodular opacities. Both symptoms and radiographic abnormalities progressed during antibiotic therapy. A bronchoscopy with transthoracic biopsy was nondiagnostic. The diagnosis of BOOP was made from tissue obtained at open lung biopsy. Corticosteroid therapy was beneficial.

Diseases That Cause Patchy Infiltrates and/or Bronchopneumonia or Lobar Consolidation

Infectious Processes

Aspiration pneumonia secondary to mixed aerobic and anaerobic infection	Usually dependent portions; superior or basilar segments of lower lobes, or posterior segments of upper lobes; pleural involvement with empyema common
Necrotizing pneumonia secondary to infection by Enterobacteriaceae, *Pseudomonas aeruginosa, Staphylococcus aureus,* or *Nocardia*	Any lobe or segment
Actinomycosis	Commonly involves lower lobes; cavitation frequently present; pleural involvement with empyema common
Tuberculous exudative pneumonia	Not restricted to upper lobes; often bilateral with perihilar distribution
Blastomycosis	Often a dense area of lobar or segmental consolidation; calcification and pleural disease infrequent
Cryptococcosis	Single or multiple infiltrates, often with sharp border, rarely cavitary or calcified; pleural effusions in presence of parenchymal disease
Paracoccidioidomycosis	Asymptomatic bilateral fluffy infiltrates; may be extremely indolent and asymptomatic at presentation

Noninfectious Processes

Chronic eosinophilic pneumonia	Rapidly progressive, dense infiltrates; usually peripheral (pattern is the reverse of pulmonary edema)
Bronchiolitis obliterans organizing pneumonia	Patchy nonsegmental areas of consolidation, often subpleural and bilateral; large irregular nodules

Diseases That Cause Pulmonary Cavitation

Infectious Processes

Pyogenic lung abscess complicating aspiration pneumonia	Usually single cavity; location same as aspiration pneumonia; air-fluid level common
Complicating necrotizing pneumonia	May involve any lobe; often multiple and bilateral, depending on route of acquisition of pneumonia
Tuberculosis-reactivation or adult type	Usually upper lobes; often bilateral; may be multiple; fibrosis and calcification common
Atypical mycobacterial disease	Radiologically indistinguishable from tuberculosis, except that cavitation may be more frequent
Melioidosis	May be acute or chronic and involve any lobe
Rhodococcal lung disease	Simulates tuberculosis or nocardiosis; cavitation common
Histoplasmosis, chronic cavitary	Mimics tuberculosis; upper lobes frequently involved but any lobe can be involved; unilateral or bilateral
Coccidioidomycosis	Usually a single, thin-walled cavity with minimal involvement of surrounding lung; occasionally a thick-walled cavity surrounded by extensive parenchymal disease
Sporotrichosis	May mimic tuberculosis but can involve any lobe; cavitation is frequent
Aspergillosis	Single or multiple areas of pneumonia with or without central cavitation; not to be confused with fungus ball of the lung
Paragonimiasis	Cystlike lesions as well as cavities, usually associated with linear or patchy infiltrates, fibrosis, and/or calcification
Echinococcosis	Single or multiple discrete, sharply defined, round lesions (cysts) with little surrounding inflammatory response; cavitation and/or calcification may occur

Noninfectious Processes

Wegener's granulomatosis and lymphomatoid granulomatosis	Often multiple nodules with cavitation; may be unilateral or bilateral granulomatosis
Silicosis	Associated with conglomerate nodular densities, frequently in upper lobes; usually superimposed on background of diffuse nodulation; rarely, eggshell calcification of hilar nodes
Bronchogenic carcinoma	Eccentric cavitation more common in squamous cell type
Lymphoma, especially Hodgkin's disease	Cavitation may occur in peripheral parenchymal nodules
Kaposi's sarcoma	Small or large nodules associated with peribronchial cuffing and tram track opacities

Diseases That Cause One or More Dense, Well-Circumscribed Nodules

Dirofilariasis (usually single)	—
Histoplasmosis (histoplasmoma)	May have calcification in center or in hilar nodes
Coccidioides spp. (coccidioidoma)	May have calcification in center or in hilar nodes
Tuberculosis (tuberculoma)	May have calcification in center or in hilar nodes
Malignancy	—
Fungus ball of the lung: *Aspergillus,* rarely *Scedosporium* or other molds	Mass forms in previously existing apical cavity; adjacent pleura thickened

Infectious and Noninfectious Diseases That Cause Chronic Diffuse Pulmonary Infiltration and Fibrosis

Alveolar Pattern
Bronchioloalveolar carcinoma
Intrapulmonary bleeding (e.g., Goodpasture's syndrome)
Pulmonary alveolar proteinosis

Ground Glass Pattern
Sarcoidosis
Early asbestosis or berylliosis
Bronchiolitis obliterans organizing pneumonia

Nodular Interstitial Pattern, Including Miliary Spherical Nodules
Granulomatous infectious diseases (e.g., miliary tuberculosis, disseminated histoplasmosis)
Sarcoidosis
Lymphangitic carcinomatosis
Wegener's granulomatosis
Lymphomatoid granulomatosis
Allergic angiitis and granulomatosis
Rheumatoid lung disease
Pneumoconiosis (including asbestosis, silicosis, and berylliosis)

Linear Interstitial Pattern, Including Fine Reticular Markings and Dense Fibrosis
Chronic form of hypersensitivity pneumonitis
Idiopathic pulmonary hemosiderosis
Radiation injury—chronic
Progressive systemic sclerosis
Sarcoidosis

Honeycombing (Coarse Reticular Pattern with Cystic Air Spaces)
Advanced form of fibrosing alveolitis
Bronchiectasis
Eosinophilic granuloma (histiocytosis X)
Sarcoidosis

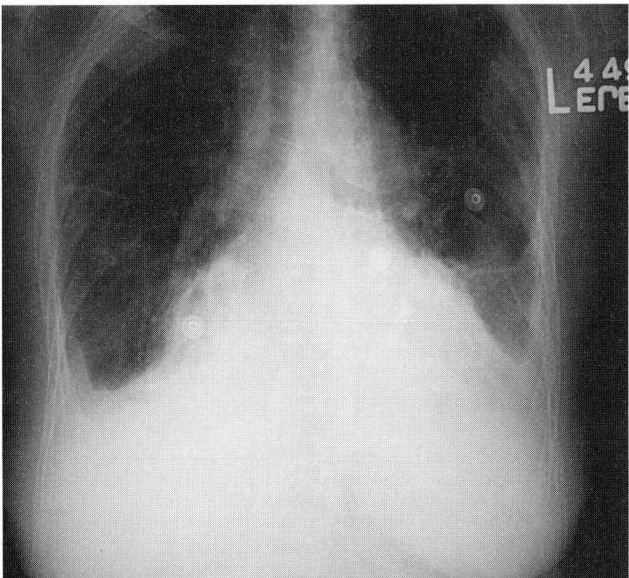

FIGURE 64-2. Systemic lupus erythematosus in a previously healthy 66-year-old woman with a 5-month illness characterized by fever, nonproductive cough, shortness of breath, pleuritic chest pain, polyarthralgia, weakness, and proteinuria. Note the cardiomegaly, bilateral pleural effusions, and lower lobe pneumonitis. Cardiac echocardiogram showed a large pericardial effusion. Test results for antinuclear antibody and antibodies to double-stranded DNA were positive.

Studies in Patients with Radiographic Evidence of Localized Infiltrates or Cavitation. In all patients with radiographic evidence of localized infiltrates or cavitation, examination of the sputum is essential. This is in striking contrast to the questionable value of sputum in the setting of acute community-acquired pneumonia.[81,82] The specimen of sputum must be a representative sample—that is, a deep, coughed specimen. If the expectorated sputum is of adequate volume and is acceptable after cytologic screening, other procedures to obtain

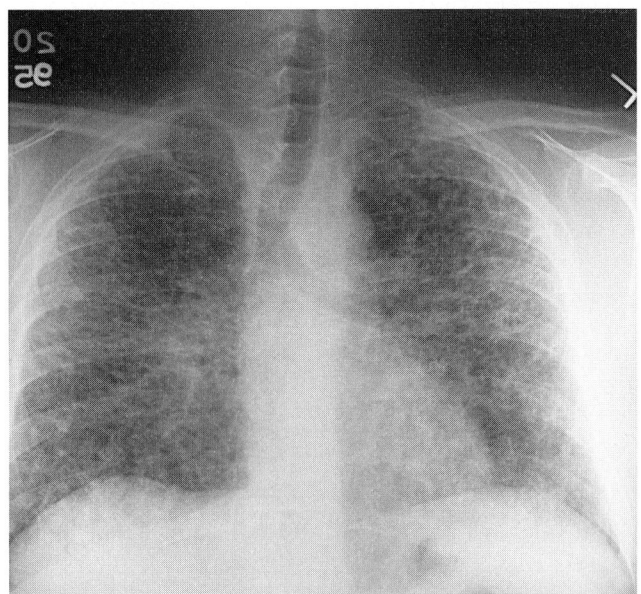

FIGURE 64-3. Pulmonary sarcoidosis in a 42-year-old man with a 6-month illness characterized by low-grade fever, intermittent night sweats, nonproductive cough, and progressive dyspnea. Note the bilateral panlobar reticulonodular pattern. A pathologic diagnosis was made from lung tissue obtained by transbronchial biopsy.

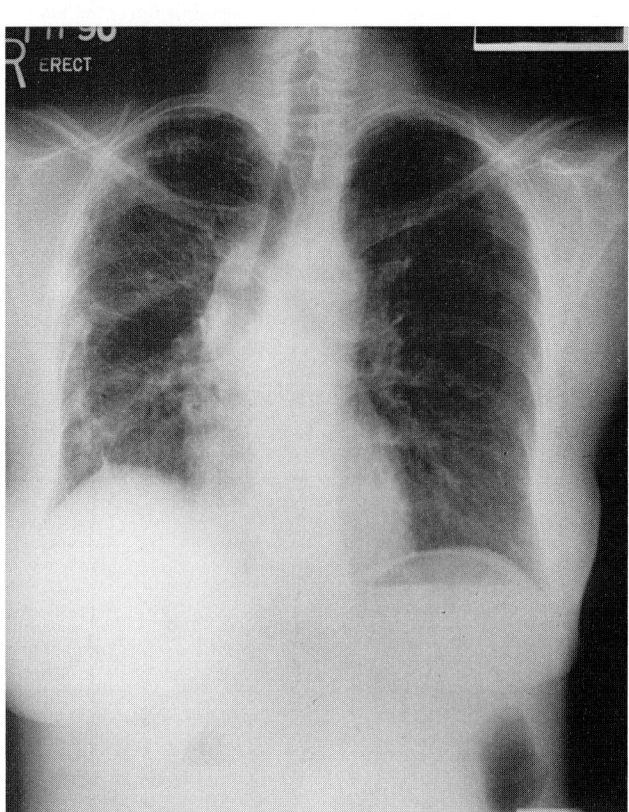

FIGURE 64-4. Drug-induced lung disease secondary to bleomycin in a 50-year-old woman receiving chemotherapy for Hodgkin's disease. She had noted fever, dyspnea, and nonproductive cough over the preceding 5-week period. Note the bilateral reticulonodular infiltrates, most prominent in the right middle and lower lung fields.

sputum may not be necessary. Microscopic examination of sputum should include the following:

1. Gram staining for bacteria and actinomycetes
2. Acid-fast staining for mycobacteria and modified acid-fast staining for *Nocardia*
3. Wet mount for fungi and eggs of *Paragonimus* (calcofluor white–potassium hydroxide preparation with phase contrast may enhance detection of fungi)
4. Gomori methenamine silver stain or the periodic acid–Schiff stain for fungi
5. Cytologic preparations for neoplastic cells, eosinophils, and fungi

Generous volumes of expectorated sputum should also be sent to the microbiology laboratory for culture of bacteria, fungi, and mycobacteria. In addition, contacting the microbiology laboratory personnel directly to alert them to specific etiologic considerations is often helpful in confirming a suspected diagnosis. In this way, specimens can be inoculated on the most appropriate media, and the microbiologists can be made more aware of the likely pathogens. With appropriate communication, the newer diagnostic techniques (e.g., rapid culture techniques, molecular probes, polymerase chain reaction [PCR] techniques, and antigen detection assays and the enzyme-linked immunosorbent assay [ELISA]) can be used in a rational and thoughtful manner to facilitate laboratory diagnosis.[83,84]

When an infectious cause is being considered, cultures from other appropriate sources should be obtained. These sources may include blood, urine, and pleural fluid in all patients with pleural effusion (pleural tissue should also be obtained for culture); cerebrospinal fluid in all patients with central nervous system symptoms or signs; synovial fluid in all patients with joint effusion; and samples of skin, mucous membrane, or any tissue obtained at biopsy.

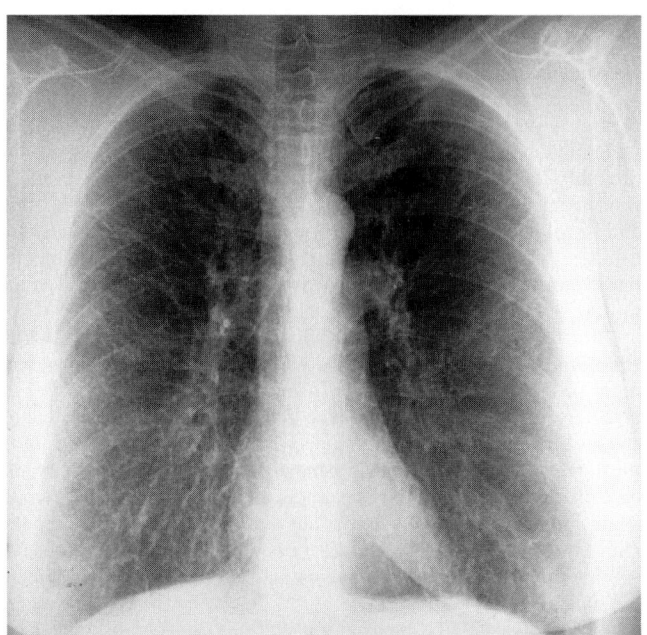

FIGURE 64-5. Lymphangioleiomyomatosis in a 42-year-old woman with a 6-month history of progressive dyspnea and intermittent blood-streaked sputum. She denied fever or history of pneumothorax. Note the diffuse reticular pattern with areas of cystic dilation and enlarged lung volumes. A pathologic diagnosis was made from lung tissue obtained by transbronchial biopsy.

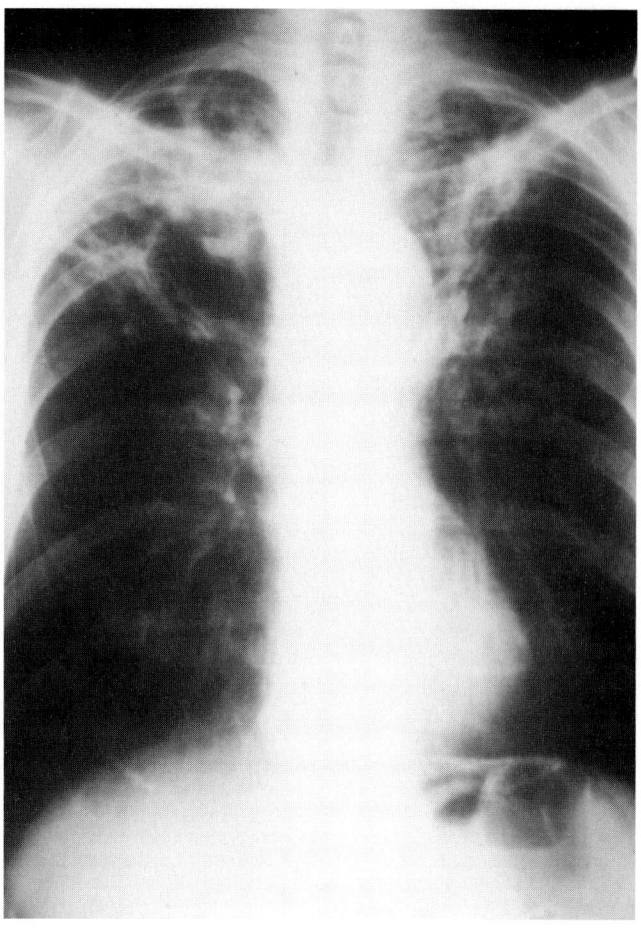

FIGURE 64-6. Chronic fibrocavitary pulmonary histoplasmosis in a 60-year-old Caucasian man with chronic obstructive pulmonary disease, a long smoking history, and a 9 month history of progressive weight loss, fever, cough and occasional hemoptysis. There is prominent biapical involvement and marked hilar retraction resembling pulmonary tuberculosis.

To obtain sputum, if adequate sputum cannot be readily produced via spontaneous expectoration by the patient, consider these methods: (1) sputum induction by hypertonic aerosol and ultrasonic nebulization, hydration, chest physiotherapy, or postural drainage, and (2) bronchoscopy for bronchial brushing, transbronchial biopsy, bronchoalveolar lavage, or protected specimen brush sampling of lower respiratory tract secretions.[85-87]

Skin tests should be administered whenever an infectious cause is being considered. The tuberculin skin test with purified protein derivative (PPD) is the single most important test. Skin test antigens for the detection of infection with atypical mycobacteria are not commercially available. Skin tests of the tuberculin type are no longer available for patients with suspected histoplasmosis or coccidioidomycosis.

Serologic tests for HIV should be performed for all patients with unexplained chronic pneumonia. In addition, serologic tests may be helpful when other infectious causes, especially fungi, are considered. However, there may be problems with certain of these tests, including delays in obtaining results, and limited sensitivity and specificity. Complement fixation tests for antibody to *Coccidioides* species are very helpful in patients with disseminated or fibrocavitary coccidioidomycosis but usually not above background positivity in patients with a solitary pulmonary cavity. Serum capsular antigen may be detectable in cryptococcosis patients with extensive lung disease or extension beyond the lung. *Histoplasma* antigen in serum or urine is helpful in disseminated histoplasmosis but uncommonly positive in infection confined to the lung. Acute and convalescent antibody can help confirm the diagnosis of acute pulmonary histoplasmosis or coccidioidomycosis. Serologic tests for paracoccidioidomycosis are available in the endemic area and useful. The recently licensed Platelia ELISA assay for early diagnosis of acute invasive aspergillosis has proven useful in severely immunocompromised patients, but its utility in facilitating a diagnosis of pulmonary aspergillosis in other groups is unproven.[88,89] If hypersensitivity pneumonitis is suspected, serum should be examined for precipitating antibodies to various inhalant antigens, and, if allergic bronchopulmonary aspergillosis is suspected,

total serum immunoglobulin E and serum IgG anti-*Aspergillus* antibody should be measured. Finally, serologic tests for less common causes of chronic pneumonia, such as *Legionella* species, *Chlamydophila pneumoniae,* and *Coxiella burnetii,* should be considered in selected patients.

Invasive Procedures. Certain clinical situations dictate a more aggressive diagnostic approach. In patients who are unable to raise sputum spontaneously and in whom attempts to induce sputum production are unsuccessful, invasive procedures may be necessary. Fiberoptic bronchoscopy is usually the initial procedure. It is diagnostically helpful when it is accompanied by bronchial washings and transbronchial biopsy with appropriate microbiologic and histologic studies.[83,85-87] Analysis of bronchoalveolar lavage fluid may increase the diagnostic yield of bronchoscopy, especially in immunocompromised persons such as patients with AIDS and suspected opportunistic infections or patients with suspected noninfectious causes of chronic pneumonia.[18,87] In a patient with extensive pleural involvement, thoracentesis and pleural biopsy (or rigid thoracoscopy in selected situations) may be more helpful diagnostically than bronchoscopy.[90] In some institutions, open lung biopsy is the procedure of choice for patients with interstitial lung disease and for many immunosuppressed patients with pulmonary disease because of the relatively large piece of tissue obtained, the expediency of diagnosis, and the safety of the procedure.[18,91,92] In contrast, in other institutions with seasoned operators, transthoracic needle aspiration of the lung[93,94] or

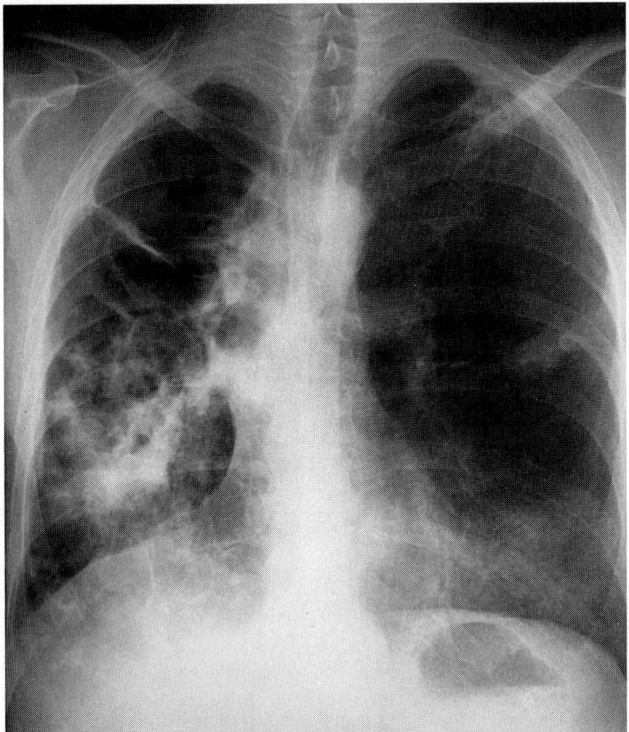

FIGURE 64-7. Atypical tuberculosis caused by *Mycobacterium avium* complex in a 52-year-old man with chronic obstructive pulmonary disease and an 18-month history of fever, weight loss, cough, intermittent hemoptysis, and progressive dyspnea associated with persistently positive acid-fast smears and cultures of expectorated sputum and worsening chest films despite appropriate antimycobacterial therapy. Note the bilateral lower lobe fibronodular disease, worse in the right lung, associated with cavitation.

video-assisted thoracoscopy[90,95] is preferred to open lung biopsy and is associated with a low risk of complications and a high sensitivity.

All specimens, regardless of source, should be submitted for microscopic examination and culture, as described earlier. Any lung or pleural tissue should also be submitted for histopathologic studies, including special stains. When there is extrapulmonary disease that probably has the same cause as the chronic pneumonia, tissue or fluid from the extrapulmonary sites should be obtained for culture and histologic studies. In such patients, consider the following procedures: arthrocentesis, abdominal paracentesis, lumbar puncture, bone marrow biopsy, liver biopsy, lymph node biopsy, and skin and muscle biopsy.

Studies in Patients with Radiographic Evidence of Diffuse Pulmonary Infiltration and Fibrosis. In patients whose chest radiographs show a predominantly diffuse infiltrative pattern of either the alveolar or the interstitial type (see Table 64-2), pulmonary function studies may be of greater importance. These studies not only quantify the degree of pulmonary insufficiency but may help delineate the disease processes by virtue of the patterns of pulmonary function impairment. Pulmonary function studies are particularly useful in characterizing those diseases that impair gas transfer and predispose to ventilation-perfusion inequalities, such as sarcoidosis or other interstitial lung diseases.[20]

Studies that may be especially useful in this group of patients include the following:

1. Arterial blood gas studies and exercise oximetry
2. Tests of pulmonary function, including spirometric measurements, measurements of lung volume, and measurement of pulmonary diffusing capacity
3. Studies on sputum as previously outlined (cytologic examination is especially important)
4. Lung biopsy—the procedure of choice to make an accurate morphologic diagnosis (transbronchial biopsy via the fiberoptic bronchoscope, open lung biopsy, or video-assisted thoracoscopy)[15,59,64]

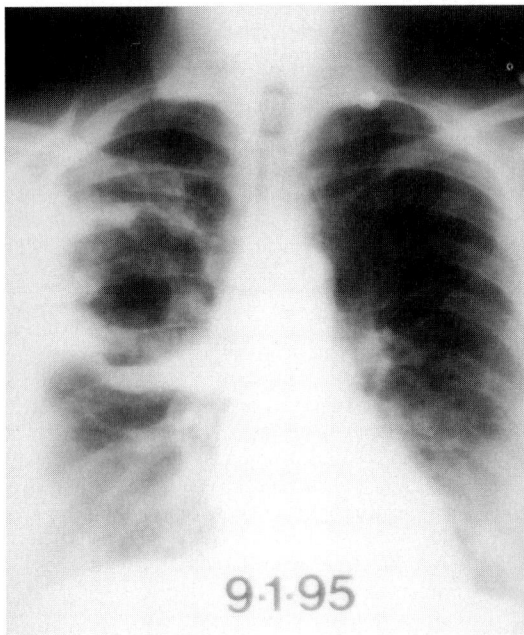

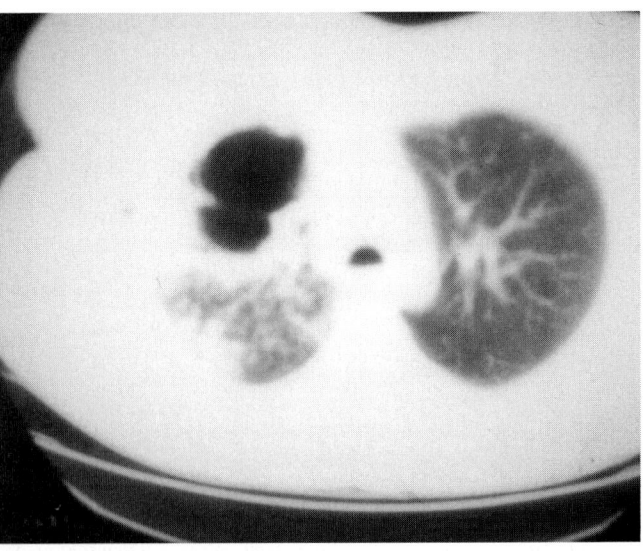

A   **B**

FIGURE 64-8. A, Chronic fibrocavitary coccidioidomycosis in a 47-year-old woman who had lived in Arizona in the early 1970s and was diagnosed with chronic pulmonary coccidioidomycosis in 1975. She received prolonged courses of antifungal therapy over the next 2 decades, with periods of alternating remission and relapse. She presented 20 years after the original diagnosis with progressive cough, weight loss, dyspnea, and low-grade fever. Sputum cultures were positive for *Coccidioides immitis*. **B,** A chest CT obtained at the same time reveals extensive fibrocavitary disease and a nodular parenchymal infiltrate involving the right lung.

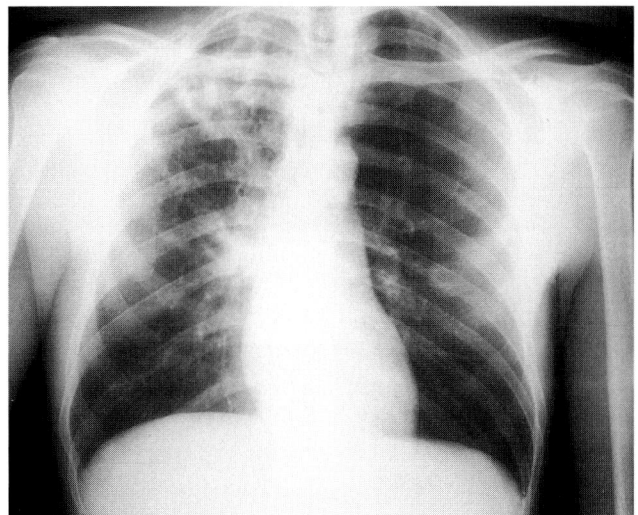

FIGURE 64-9. Pulmonary tuberculosis in a 38-year-old man with a 3-month history of cough, hemoptysis, and fever, and a 30-pound weight loss. He was recently incarcerated for 6 months. He is human immunodeficiency virus (HIV) negative. Sputum smears were positive for acid-fast bacilli and cultures were positive for *Mycobacterium tuberculosis*. Note the right upper lobe cavitary lesions associated with hilar adenopathy.

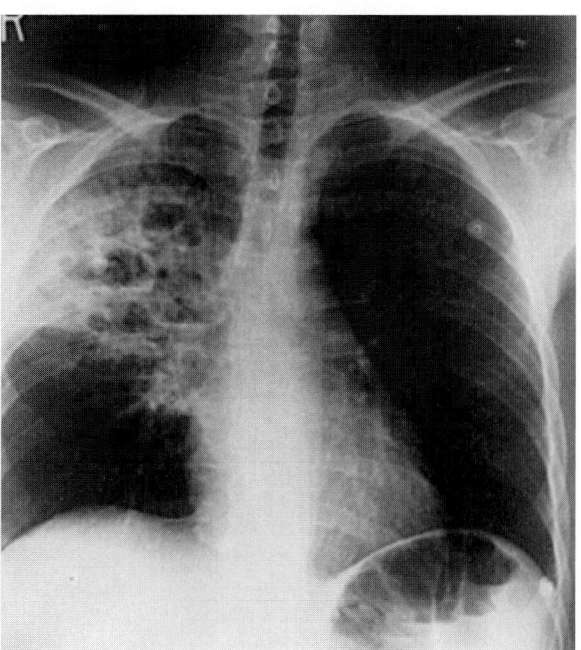

A

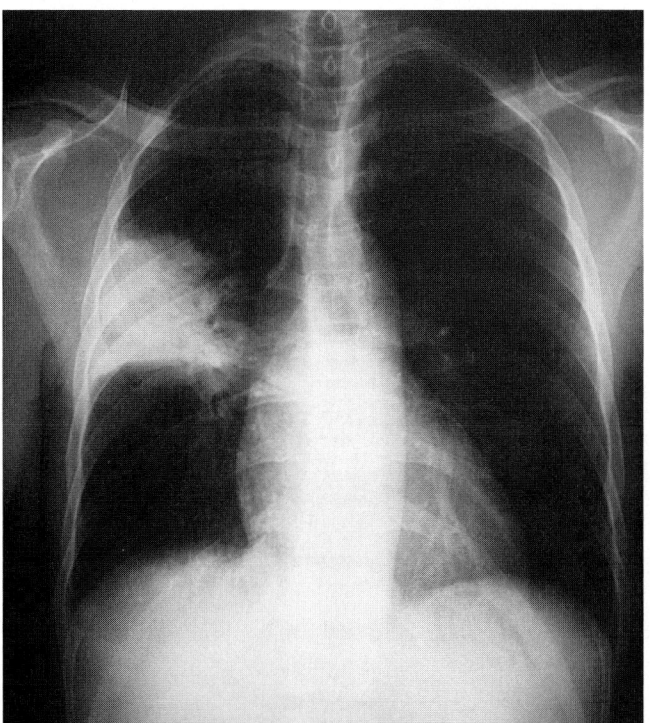

FIGURE 64-10. Pulmonary nocardiosis in a 40-year-old man with advanced acquired immunodeficiency syndrome (CD4+ cell count 51/mm³ and plasma human immunodeficiency virus RNA 72,000 copies/mL) and a 6-week illness consisting of fever, cough, pleuritic chest pain, shortness of breath, and nonresponsiveness to two courses of oral antibiotics. Note the pleura-based right upper lobe segmental bronchopneumonia. Microbiologic diagnosis was made from stains and cultures of bronchial washings obtained at bronchoscopy.

B

FIGURE 64-11. A, *Rhodococcus equi* pneumonia in a patient with acquired immunodeficiency syndrome (AIDS) who had a 2-month progressive illness characterized by fever, night sweats, weight loss, and nonproductive cough. Note the necrotizing, cavitary infiltrate involving the right upper lobe. The microbiologic diagnosis was made from washings and tissue obtained at bronchoscopy. **B,** *R. equi* pneumonia in a patient with AIDS and a 6-week history of fever, weight loss, and right-sided pleuritic pain. Note the pleura-based, well-circumscribed mass lesion. The microbiologic diagnosis was made from tissue obtained at open lung biopsy.

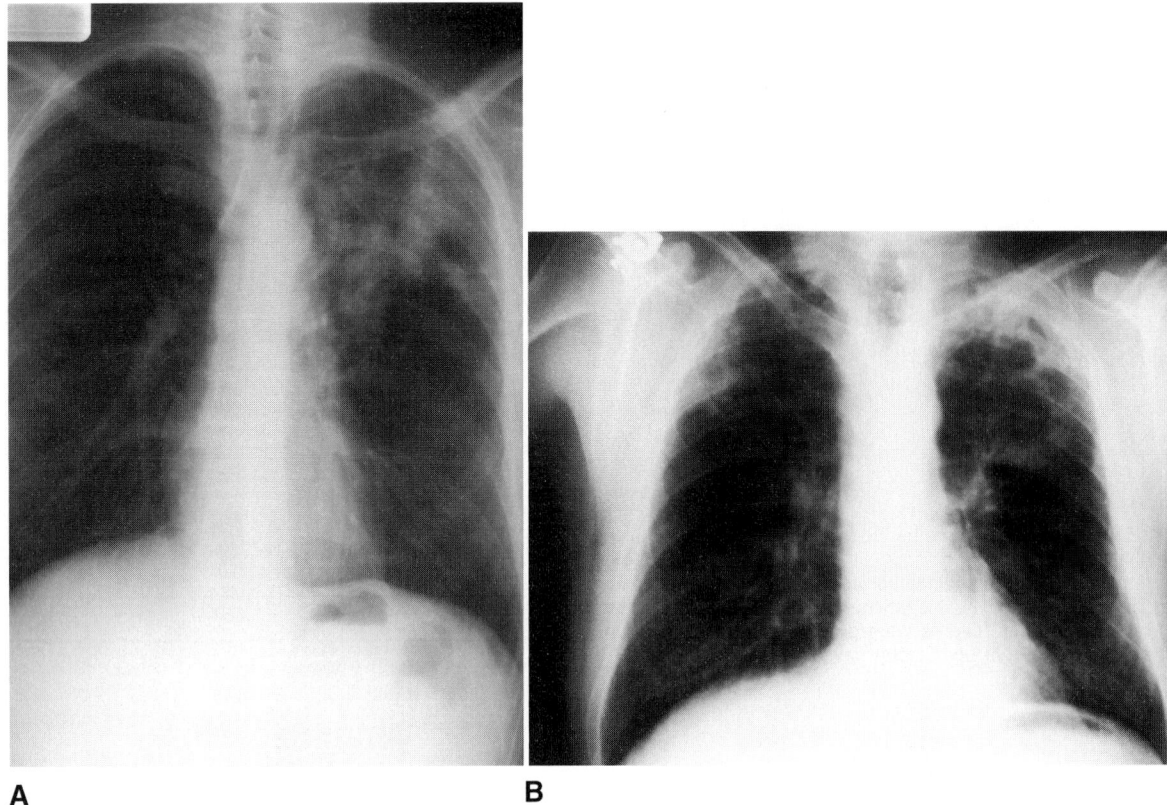

A   B

FIGURE 64-12. **A,** Chronic necrotizing pulmonary aspergillosis in an otherwise normal 56-year-old man with chronic cough, scant sputum production, moderate weight loss, and an abnormal plain chest radiograph. Sputum samples were repeatedly positive for *Aspergillus terreus;* a transbronchial biopsy reveals invasive disease. Note the dense infiltrate and multiple cavitary lesions in the left upper lobe. **B,** Chronic necrotizing pulmonary aspergillosis in a 63-year-old man with significant chronic obstructive pulmonary disease. Sputum cultures were positive for *Aspergillus fumigatus;* transbronchial biopsy revealed invasive disease. This patient also had 35% peripheral eosinophilia. Note the bilateral upper lobe cavitary lesions.

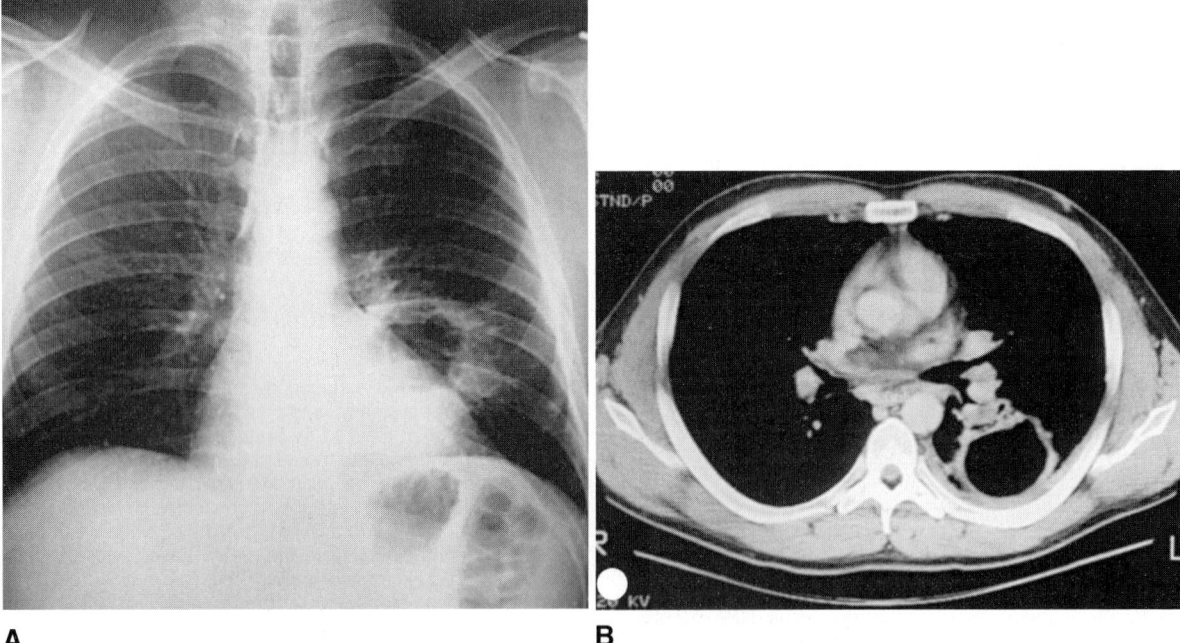

A   B

FIGURE 64-13. **A,** Wegener's granulomatosis in a 35-year-old cattle farmer with a 2-month illness manifested by fever, malaise, weight loss, pleurisy, polyarthralgia, and palpable purpura of the lower extremities. Laboratory studies included a markedly elevated erythrocyte sedimentation rate, a positive test result for antineutrophil cytoplasmic autoantibody, and an abnormal urine sediment. Note the large cavitary mass lesion of the left lower lobe. **B,** A chest computed tomography scan demonstrates the lower lobe cavitary lesion and a small pleural effusion but no other pulmonary parenchymal abnormalities.

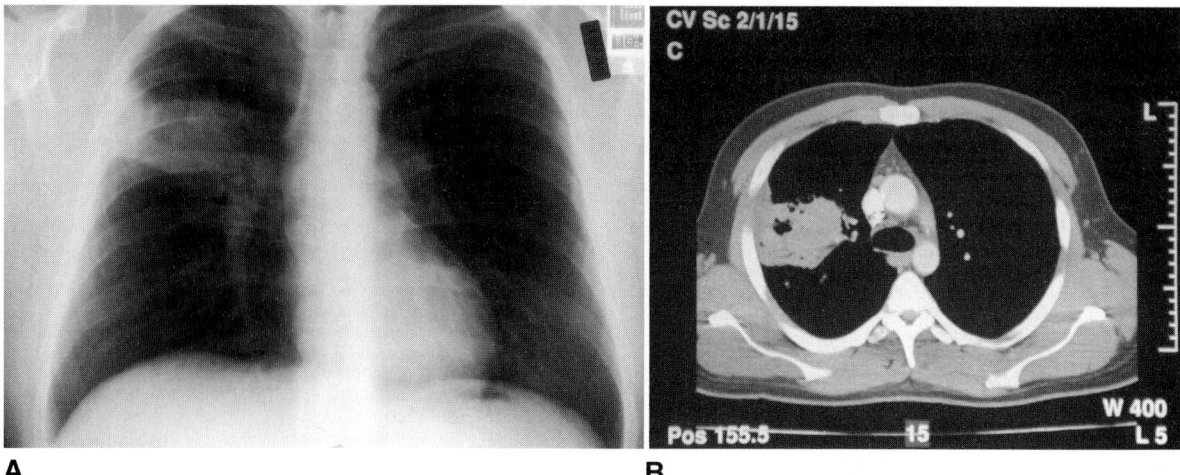

FIGURE 64-14. A, Pulmonary blastomycosis in a 24-year-old man who works as a heavy equipment operator. He is also an avid hunter. He reports fever, night sweats, and a productive cough for 6 weeks unresponsive to outpatient antibacterial therapy. He has lost 25 pounds during this time. He denies skin lesions or bone pain. Note the right upper lobe infiltrate on plain chest film. **B,** Chest CT scan shows a dense right upper lobe infiltrate with a central cavity not seen on plain films. Diagnosis was established by visually assisted thoracoscopy (VATS) biopsy. Histopathology revealed broad-based budding yeasts, and cultures were positive for *Blastomyces dermatitidis.*

THERAPY

Antimicrobial Agents

In many patients, no etiologic agent is identified on the basis of the initial stains and cultures, and a definitive diagnosis must await the completion of serologic, histologic, and bacteriologic studies as well as other diagnostic tests. In such situations, if immediate empirical therapy is advisable, the choice of antimicrobial agents must be based on the available epidemiologic, clinical, and microbiologic data. For example, if an otherwise healthy young patient has been ill for a relatively short period (2 to 3 weeks), the chest radiograph shows a lobar or patchy pneumonia (especially in the lower lobes), the Gram stain of the sputum reveals few to a moderate number of polymorphonuclear leukocytes and organisms resembling normal flora, and the infection was acquired in the community setting, the patient may have persistent or chronic pneumonia as a complication of one or more common acute pneumonia syndromes, namely, pneumococcal pneumonia, *Mycoplasma* pneumonia, *Chlamydophila* pneumonia, or legionnaires' disease. Reasonable empirical therapy in such a patient is one of the newer fluoroquinolones (gatifloxacin, moxifloxacin, or levofloxacin), because these drugs in general provide effective treatment of these common pneumonias. If, on the other hand, a patient has chronic pneumonia after thoracotomy or has been chronically intubated in an intensive care unit, initial antimicrobial therapy should provide broad-spectrum coverage against hospital-acquired flora, including anaerobes, *Staphylococcus aureus,* and aerobic gram-negative bacteria. In both of the cases described, once the pathogen or pathogens have been identified and sensitivity testing has been completed, appropriate changes in the antibiotic regimen should be made.

If a patient has a more chronic, indolent illness, is stable, and does not require immediate empirical therapy, a methodic and thorough diagnostic evaluation is the initial priority. In a patient with bilateral upper lobe cavitary disease in whom the initial microscopic examinations are nonrevealing, the leading considerations include tuberculosis, histoplasmosis, and coccidioidomycosis. If such a patient has a positive tuberculin skin response, tuberculosis should be presumed to be the diagnosis until proven otherwise, and antituberculosis therapy should be initiated and continued for at least 6 weeks, pending the results of the mycobacterial cultures. Disseminated tuberculosis should be strongly suspected in any patient with unexplained fever and a chest radiograph showing a nodular interstitial pattern; prompt institution of antituberculosis therapy may be lifesaving in this otherwise fatal condition. Similarly, empirical antifungal therapy, usually with an amphotericin B formulation (or voriconazole if invasive mold disease is suspected), may be indicated in an HIV-infected or other immunocompromised patient with chronic pneumonia, because fungal pulmonary diseases in this setting can be particularly severe and rapidly progressive.

Corticosteroids

The use of treatment with glucocorticosteroids in the treatment of a patient with chronic pneumonia is controversial. If the cause of the illness is an infectious agent, particularly a bacterium or a fungus, steroids are usually not indicated. However, some experts advocate a short course of glucocorticosteroid therapy for patients with advanced pulmonary tuberculosis and severe inanition. Generally, corticosteroids are beneficial in chronic pneumonia from noninfectious causes, such as the vasculitides,[1-5] sarcoidosis,[11,12] chronic eosinophilic pneumonia,[96] radiation injury, bronchiolitis obliterans organizing pneumonia,[15-17] and many of the fibrotic lung diseases including chronic hypersensitivity pneumonitis (along with avoidance of exposure to the offending antigen).[70] Other immunosuppressive drugs, such as cyclophosphamide and azathioprine, may also be effective in some patients, especially those with pulmonary vasculitis.

Bronchoscopy and Surgery

Bronchoscopy is frequently used as a therapeutic adjunct, especially for patients who have thick, tenacious secretions that cannot be raised by noninvasive techniques. In other patients, mucus plugs or foreign bodies may predispose to atelectasis and chronic pneumonia, and therapeutic bronchoscopy may be necessary to expand the collapsed lung.

Surgery plays a limited role in the treatment of chronic pneumonia. Lobectomy or pneumonectomy should be considered in a patient with chronic destructive pneumonia, multiple macroabscesses or microabscesses involving an entire lobe or lung, and a ventilation-perfusion scan indicating nonfunction of the involved lung (e.g., pulmonary gangrene).[97] Thoracotomy may also be indicated to decorticate the pleura in patients with significant pleural reaction and resultant restrictive lung disease.

REFERENCES

1. Fauci AS, Haynes BF, Costa J, et al. Lymphomatoid granulomatosis: Prospective clinical and therapeutic experience over 10 years. N Engl J Med. 1982;306:69-74.
2. Langford CA, Hoffman GS. Wegener's granulomatosis. Thorax. 1999;54:629-637.
3. Hoffman GS, Kerr GS, Leavitt RY, et al. Wegener granulomatosis: An analysis of 158 patients. Ann Intern Med. 1992;116:488-498.
4. Hoffman GS, Kerr GS, Leavitt RY, et al. Systemic vasculitis with asthma and eosinophilia: a clinical approach to the Churg-Strauss syndrome. Medicine (Baltimore). 1984;63:65-80.
5. Fauci AS, Haynes BF, Costa J, et al. Lymphomatoid granulomatosis: Prospective clinical and therapeutic experience over 10 years. N Engl J Med. 1982;306:69-74.
6. Hill CA. Bronchioloalveolar carcinoma: A review. Radiology. 1984;150:15-20.
7. Cordier JF, Chailleux E, Lauque D, et al. Primary pulmonary lymphomas: A clinical study of 70 cases in nonimmunocompromised patients. Chest. 1993;103:201-208.
8. Casey KR. Neoplastic mimics of pneumonia. Semin Respir Infect. 1995;10:131-142.
9. Cooper JA Jr. Drug-induced lung disease. Adv Intern Med. 1997;42:231-268.
10. Cordier JF, Loire R, Brune J. Amyloidosis of the lower respiratory tract: Clinical and pathologic features in a series of 21 patients. Chest. 1986;90:827-831.
11. Lynch JP, Kazerooni EA, Gay SE. Pulmonary sarcoidosis. Clin Chest Med. 1997;18:755-785.
12. Nagai S, Shigematsu M, Hamada K, Izumi T. Clinical courses and prognoses of pulmonary sarcoidosis. Curr Opin Pulm Med. 1999;5:293-298.
13. Chiles C. Imaging features of thoracic sarcoidosis. Semin Roentgenol. 2002;37:82-93.
14. Prakash UB, Barham SS, Carpenter HA, et al. Pulmonary alveolar phospholipoproteinosis: Experience with 34 cases and a review. Mayo Clin Proc. 1987;62:499-518.
15. Epler GR. Bronchiolitis obliterans organizing pneumonia. Semin Respir Infect. 1995;10:65-77.
16. Lohr RH, Boland BJ, Douglas WW, et al. Organizing pneumonia: Features and prognosis of cryptogenic, secondary and focal variants. Arch Intern Med. 1997;157:1323-1329.
17. Afessa B, Litzow MR, Tefferi A. Bronchiolitis obliterans and other late onset noninfectious pulmonary complications in hematopoietic stem cell transplantation. Bone Marrow Transplant. 2001;28:425-434.
18. Crystal RG, Bitterman PB, Rennard SI, et al. Interstitial lung diseases of unknown cause: Disorders characterized by chronic inflammation of the lower respiratory tract: Parts 1 and 2. N Engl J Med. 1984;310:154-166, 235-244.
19. Schwartz MI. Clinical overview of interstitial lung disease. In: Schwarz MI, King TE Jr, eds. Interstitial Lung Disease. 2nd ed. St. Louis: Mosby-Yearbook; 1994:1-22.
20. Green FH. Overview of pulmonary fibrosis. Chest. 2002;122(Suppl 6):334s-339s.
21. Bartlett JG. Anaerobic bacterial infections of the lung. Chest. 1987;91:901-909.
22. Eisenstadt J, Crane LR. Gram-negative bacillary pneumonias. In: Pennington JE, ed. Respiratory Infections: Diagnosis and Management. 3rd ed. New York: Raven Press; 1994:369-406.
23. Kirtland SH, Winterbauer RH, Dreis DF, et al. A clinical profile of chronic bacterial pneumonia: Report of 115 cases. Chest. 1994;106:15-22.
24. Close LG. Laryngopharyngeal manifestations of reflux: Diagnosis and therapy. Eur J Gastroenterol Hepatol. 2002;14(Suppl 1):S23-S27.
25. Bartlett JG, Dowell SF, Mandell LA, et al. Practice guidelines for the management of community-acquired pneumonia. Clin Infect Dis. 2000;31:347-382.
26. Mandell LA, Marrie TJ, Grossman RF, et al., and the Canadian Community-Acquired Pneumonia Working Group. Clin Infect Dis. 2000;31:383-421.
27. American Thoracic Society. Guidelines for the management of adults with community-acquired pneumonia: Diagnosis, assessment of severity, antimicrobial therapy, and prevention. Am J Respir Crit Care Med. 2001;163:1730-1745.
28. Case records of the Massachusetts General Hospital. Case 8-1994. N Engl J Med. 1994;330:557-564.
29. Khan MA, Kovnat DM, Bachus B, et al. Clinical and roentgenographic spectrum of pulmonary tuberculosis in the adult. Am J Med. 1977;62:31-38.
30. Case records of the Massachusetts General Hospital. Case 48-1990. N Engl J Med. 1990;323:1546-1555.
31. Prince DS, Peterson DD, Steiner RM, et al. Infection with Mycobacterium avium complex in patients without predisposing conditions. N Engl J Med. 1989;321:863-868.
32. Patz EF Jr, Swensen SJ, Erasmus J. Pulmonary manifestations of nontuberculous Mycobacteria. Radiol Clin North Am. 1995;33:719-729.
33. Goodwin RA, Owens FT, Snell JD, et al. Chronic cavitary histoplasmosis. Medicine (Baltimore). 1976;55:413-452.
34. Wheat JL, Kauffman CA. Histoplasmosis. Infect Dis Clin North Am. 2003;17:1-19.
35. Galgiani JN. Coccidioidomycosis. West J Med. 1993;159:153-171.
36. Chiller TM, Galgiani JN, Stevens DA. Coccidioidomycosis. Infect Dis Clin North Am. 2003;17:41-57.
37. Davies SF, Sarosi GA. Epidemiological and clinical features of pulmonary blastomycosis. Semin Respir Infect. 1997;12:206-218.
38. Bradsher RW, Chapman SW, Pappas PG. Blastomycosis 2003;17:21-40.
39. Restreppo A, Robledo M, Giraldo H, et al. The gamut of paracoccidioidomycosis. Am J Med. 1976;61:33-42.
40. Balmes JR, Hawkins JG. Pulmonary cryptococcosis. Semin Respir Med. 1987;9:180-186.
41. Aberg JA, Mundy LM, Powderly WG. Pulmonary cryptococcosis in patients without HIV infection. Chest. 1999;115:734-740.
42. Hsieh MI, Liu HP, Chang JP, et al. Thoracic actinomycosis. Chest. 1993;104:366-370.
43. Saadah HA, Dixon T. Petriellidium boydii (Allescheria boydii) necrotizing pneumonia in a normal host. JAMA. 1981;245:605-606.
44. Castiglioni B, Sutton DA, Rinaldi MG, et al. Pseudallescheria boydii (Anamorph Scedosporium apiospermum): Infection in solid organ transplant recipients in a tertiary medical center and review of the literature. Medicine (Baltimore). 2002;81:333-348.
45. Plus JL, Opal SM. Pulmonary sporotrichosis: Review of treatment and outcome. Medicine (Baltimore). 1986;65:143-153.
46. Watts JC, Callaway CS, Chandler FW, et al. Human pulmonary adiaspiromycosis. Arch Pathol. 1975;99:11-15.
47. dos Santos VM, Fatureto MC, Saldanha JC, Adad SJ. Pulmonary adiaspiromycosis: Report of two cases. Rev Soc Bras Med Trop. 2000;33:483-488.
48. Turner D, Burke M, Bashe E, et al. Pulmonary adiaspiromycosis in a patient with acquired immunodeficiency syndrome. Eur J Clin Microbiol Infect Dis. 1999;18:893-895.
49. Shelhamer JH, Toews GB, Masur H, et al. Respiratory disease in the immunosuppressed patient. Ann Intern Med. 1992;117:415-431.
50. Rivera MP, Jules-Elysee KM, Stover DE. Immunocompromised patients: Nontransplant chemotherapy immunosuppression. In: Niederman MS, Sarosi GA, Glassroth J, eds. Respiratory Infections. Philadelphia: Saunders; 1994:163-181.
51. Lerner PI. Nocardiosis. Clin Infect Dis. 1996;22:891-905.
52. Denning DW. Invasive aspergillosis. Clin Infect Dis. 1998;26:781-805.
53. Pappas PG, Threlkeld MG, Bedsole GD, et al. Blastomycosis in immunocompromised patients. Medicine (Baltimore). 1993;72:311-325.
54. Barnes PF, Block AB, Davidson PT, et al. Tuberculosis in patients with human immunodeficiency virus infection. N Engl J Med. 1991;324:1644-1650.
55. Murray JF. Pulmonary complications of HIV infection. Ann Rev Med. 1996;47:117-126.
56. Cameron ML, Bartlett JA, Gallis HA, et al. Manifestations of pulmonary cryptococcosis in patients with acquired immunodeficiency syndrome. Rev Infect Dis. 1991;13:64-67.
57. Wheat LJ, Connolly-Stringfield PA, Baker RL, et al. Disseminated histoplasmosis in the acquired immunodeficiency syndrome: Clinical findings, diagnosis and treatment, and review of literature. Medicine (Baltimore). 1990;69:361-374.
58. Gallant JE, Ko AH. Cavitary pulmonary lesions in patients infected with human immunodeficiency virus. Clin Infect Dis. 1996;22:671-682.
59. Kalavjiian RC, Toossi Z, Tomashefski JR Jr, et al. Pulmonary disease due to infection by Mycobacterium avium complex in patients with AIDS. Clin Infect Dis. 1995;20:1186-1194.
60. Mutaner L, Leyes M, Payeras A, et al. Radiologic features of Rhodococcus equi pneumonia in AIDS. Eur J Radiol. 1997;24:66-70.
61. Supparatpinyo K, Chiewchanvir S, Hirunsri P, et al. Penicillium marneffei infection in patients with human immunodeficiency virus. Clin Infect Dis. 1992;14:871-874.
62. Gruden JF, Huang L, Webb WR, et al. AIDS-related Kaposi sarcoma of the lung: Radiographic findings and staging system with bronchoscopic correlation. Radiology. 1995;195:545-552.
63. Suffredini AF, Ognibene FP, Lack EE, et al. Nonspecific interstitial pneumonitis: A common cause of pulmonary disease in the acquired immunodeficiency syndrome. Ann Intern Med. 1987;107:7-13.
64. Decker CF, Masur H. Pneumocystosis. In: Dismukes WE, Pappas PG, Sobel JD, eds. Clinical Mycology. 1st ed. New York: Oxford University Press; 2003:407-419.
65. Kitaichi M, Nishimura K, Itoh H, et al. Pulmonary lymphangioleiomyomatosis: A report of 46 patients including a clinicopathologic study of prognostic factors. Am J Respir Crit Care Med. 1995;151:527-533.
66. Taylor JG, Choi EH, Foster CB, Chanock SJ. Using genetic variation to study human disease. Trends Mol Med. 2001;7:507-512.
67. Deresinski SC, Pappagianis D, Stevens DA. Association of ABO blood group and outcome of coccidioidal infections. Sabouraudia. 1979;17:261-264.
68. Louie L, Ng S, Hajjeh R, et al. Influence of host genetics on the severity of coccidioidomycosis. Emerg Infect Dis. 1999;5:672-680.
69. Hajjeh RA, Conn LA, Stephens DS, et al., and the Cryptococcal Active Surveillance Group. Cryptococcosis: Population-based multistate active surveillance and risk factors in human immunodeficiency virus-infected persons. J Infect Dis. 1999;179:449-464.
70. Sharma OP, Fujimura N. Hypersensitivity pneumonitis: A noninfectious granulomatosis. Semin Respir Infect. 1995;10:96-106.
71. Leelarasamee A, Bovornkitti S. Melioidosis: Review and update. Rev Infect Dis. 1989;11:413-425.
72. Im IG, Whang HY, Kim WS, et al. Pleuropulmonary paragonimiasis: Radiologic findings in 71 patients. AJR Am J Roentgenol. 1992;159:39-43.
73. Haim DY, Lippman ML, Goldberg SK, et al. The pulmonary complications of crack cocaine: A comprehensive review. Chest. 1995;107:233-240.
74. Carmus PH, Foucher P, Bonniaud PH, Ask K. Drug-induced infiltrative lung disease. Eur Respir J. 2001;32(Suppl 6):93s-100s.
75. Winkelstein JA, Marino MC, Johnston RB, et al. Chronic granulomatous disease. Report on a national registry of 368 patients. Medicine (Baltimore). 2000;79:155-169.
76. Patel R, Paya CV. Infections in solid organ transplant recipients. Clin Micro Rev. 1997;10:86-124.
77. Cunha BA. Pneumonias in the compromised host. Infect Dis Clin North Am. 2001;15(2):591-612.
78. Grenier P, Valeyre D, Cluzel P, et al. Chronic diffuse interstitial disease: Diagnostic value of chest radiography and high-resolution CT. Radiology. 1991;179:123-132.
79. Lynch DA, Gamsu G. Newer imaging techniques in the assessment of interstitial lung disease. In: Schwarz MI, King TE Jr, eds. Interstitial Lung Disease. 2nd ed. St. Louis: Mosby-Year Book; 1993:91-118.
80. Bury T, Dowlati A, Paulus P, et al. Evaluation of the solitary pulmonary nodule by positron emission tomography imaging. Eur Respir J. 1996;9:410-414.

81. Bartlett-Connor E. The nonvalue of sputum culture in the diagnosis of pneumococcal pneumonia. Am Rev Respir Dis. 1971;103:845-848.
82. Davidson M, Tempest B, Palmer DL. Bacteriologic diagnosis of acute pneumonia. JAMA. 1976;235:158-163.
83. Shelhamer JH, Gill VJ, Quinn TC, et al. The laboratory evaluation of opportunistic pulmonary infections. Ann Intern Med. 1996;124:585-589.
84. Saubolle MA, McKellar PP. Laboratory diagnosis of community-acquired lower respiratory tract infection. Infect Dis Clin North Am. 2001;15:1025-1045.
85. Feinsilver SH, Fein AM, Niederman MS, et al. Utility of fiberoptic bronchoscopy in non-resolving pneumonia. Chest. 1990;98:1322-1326.
86. Cazzadori A, DiPein G, Todeschini G, et al. Transbronchial biopsy in the diagnosis of pulmonary infiltrates in immunocompromised patients. Chest. 1995;107:96-100.
87. Pisani RJ, Wright AJ. Clinical utility of bronchoalveolar lavage in immunocompromised hosts. Mayo Clin Proc. 1992;67:221-227.
88. Maertens J, Verhaegen J, Lagrou K, et al. Screening for circulating galactomannan as a noninvasive diagnostic tool for invasive aspergillosis in prolonged neutropenic patients and stem cell transplantation recipients: A prospective validation. Blood. 2001;97:1604-1610.
89. Maertens J, Van Eldere J, Verhaegan J, et al. Use of circulating galactomannan screening for early diagnosis of invasive aspergillosis in allogeneic stem cell transplant recipients. J Infect Dis. 2002;186:1297-1306.
90. Harris RJ, Kavuru MS, Rice TW, et al. The diagnostic and therapeutic utility of thoracoscopy: A review. Chest. 1995;108:828-841.
91. Cockerill FR III, Wilson WR, Carpenter HA, et al. Open lung biopsy in immunocompromised patients. Arch Intern Med. 1985;145:1398-1404.
92. Cheson BD, Samlowski WE, Tang TT, et al. Value of open-lung biopsy in 87 immunocompromised patients with pulmonary infiltrates. Cancer. 1985;55:543-549.
93. Sokolowski JW Jr, Burgher LW, Jones FL Jr, et al. Guidelines for percutaneous transthoracic needle biopsy: Position paper of the American Thoracic Society. Am Rev Respir Dis. 1989;140:255-256.
94. Zalacain R, Llorente JL, Gazfelurrutia L, et al. Influence of three factors on the diagnostic effectiveness of transthoracic needle aspiration in pneumonia. Chest. 1995;107:96-100.
95. Bensard DD, McIntyre RC Jr, Waring BJ, et al. Comparison of video thoracoscopic lung biopsy to open lung biopsy in the diagnosis of interstitial lung diseases. Chest. 1993;103:765-770.
96. Jederline PJ, Sicilian L, Gaensler EA. Chronic eosinophilic pneumonia: A report of 19 cases and a review of the literature. Medicine (Baltimore). 1988;67:154-162.
97. Penner C, Maycher B, Long R. Pulmonary gangrene: A complication of bacterial pneumonia. Chest. 1994;105:567-573.

CHAPTER 65

Cystic Fibrosis

MICHAEL R. KNOWLES
PETER H. GILLIGAN
RICHARD C. BOUCHER

A clearer understanding of the recessive genetic disorder cystic fibrosis (CF) has evolved since identification of the *CFTR* gene in 1989.[1] The molecular and cellular pathogenesis of the organ-level disease are complex, but unifying theories have emerged.[2,3] The clinical syndrome is variable.[4] Currently, nearly 40% of identified patients with CF are adults, and treatment programs for adults have emerged.[5,6] Clinical manifestations include chronic obstructive lung disease, with characteristic sputum microbiologic flora that typically includes *Staphylococcus aureus* and mucoid *Pseudomonas aeruginosa.* Pancreatic exocrine insufficiency occurs in 90% of patients. The clinical diagnosis is usually supported by the hallmark laboratory abnormality, an elevated sweat chloride concentration, and/or by identification of a CF mutation on each allele of the *CFTR* gene.[7,4] The upper limit of normal for sweat chloride concentrations measured by pilocarpine iontophoresis is higher for adults than for children; measured Cl^- concentrations must be less than 40 mEq/L to be clearly normal in children, whereas healthy adults may have Cl^- concentrations of up to 70 mEg/L.[3]

CLINICAL MANIFESTATIONS

The clinical manifestations of CF reflect obstruction of organs by viscous secretions and chronic bacterial infection in the lung. Although multiple organ systems are involved, chronic suppurative airway disease is present in more than 98% of adults who have CF, and greater than 90% of CF deaths are related to progressive pulmonary insufficiency. Most respiratory bacterial infections in affected adults are caused by *S. aureus, P. aeruginosa,* and *Burkholderia cepacia* complex, whereas the incidence of infections with most other infectious agents (e.g., *Mycoplasma pneumoniae,* viruses) is believed to be similar to that in the general population.[8] It has been recently noted that up to 20% of adults in some CF centers may harbor nontuberculous mycobacteria (NTM) in respiratory secretions.[9] In general, the pathogenic effect of these organisms is not clearly defined in CF, although some patients have well-established pathogenic infection.[10-12]

The clinical picture of CF is dominated by a chronic cough punctuated by episodes of clinical deterioration characterized by an increased volume and purulence of sputum, dyspnea, and sometimes anorexia and weight loss.[13,14] Although adults with CF may exhibit low-grade fever with these exacerbations, high fever is unusual, and sepsis or bacteremia is uncommon despite the large number of bacteria in the airways (10^8 organisms per milliliter of sputum). Clinical exacerbations are associated with modest elevations in the white blood cell count and worsening spirometric values. The chest radiograph typically shows diffuse shadowing that reflects airway wall thickening and retained secretions and also cystic bronchiectatic changes. In many adult patients with CF, these roentgenographic abnormalities are seen predominantly in upper lung zones, which may initially suggest tuberculosis. Significant gas exchange abnormalities usually occur only in the later stages of the disease, and hypoxemia and carbon dioxide retention are uncommon during acute exacerbations until the forced expiratory volume in 1 second (FEV_1) is less than 40% of the predicted value.[13,14]

Adults with CF have frequent complications of hemoptysis and pneumothorax.[15] Minor hemoptysis is common, and massive hemoptysis occurs in about 1% of these patients each year. Fortunately, medical (nonsurgical) intervention is usually sufficient for the treatment of pulmonary hemorrhage.[15,16] Epithelial dysfunction in the nasal sinus of patients with CF and the frequent occurrence of nasal polyps make subacute or chronic sinusitis a major problem in many adult patients.[17] The microbiology of sinusitis is not always reflected by the flora identified in expectorated sputum.

Because most patients with CF have progressive destruction of the pancreas and loss of endocrine function, the prevalence of diabetes mellitus increases with age and may be as high as 35% by the age of 25 years.[18,19] The presence of glucose intolerance may add further difficulty to the treatment of pulmonary infection.

PATHOGENESIS

The clinical syndrome of CF reflects a genetic disorder inherited in autosomal recessive fashion. The CF gene was identified in 1989 and is located on the long arm of chromosome 7.[1] It is a relatively large gene consisting of 27 exons and codes for a 1480–amino acid polypeptide known as cystic fibrosis transmembrane regulator (CFTR). More than 1200 different mutations have been identified in the CF gene. The most common mutation is a three–base-pair deletion that leads to the absence of a phenylalanine in the CFTR protein at position 508 (ΔF508).[3]

The molecular pathogenesis of CF is complex and varies with the type of CF gene mutation. The CFTR protein resides in the plasma membrane, typically in the apical domain of polarized epithelial cells. Molecular modeling predicts that the polypeptide contains, in sequence, a six-transmembrane-spanning region, a nucleotide (adenosine triphosphate [ATP])-binding fold that is the site of the ΔF508 mutation, a large hydrophilic domain that is the site of kinase-phosphatase regulation (the R domain), another six-transmembrane-spanning region, and another nucleotide-binding fold.[1] The full spectrum of functions of the CFTR protein is still emerging. CFTR functions as the cyclic adenosine monophosphate (cAMP)-regulated Cl⁻ channel in the plasma membrane.[20,21] However, it also appears to regulate the activity of other ion channels in the plasma membrane as well.[22,23] The most common CF mutation, ΔF508, leads to abnormal folding of the CFTR polypeptide in the endoplasmic reticulum and degradation of the protein by intracellular "editing."[24] Thus, the molecular pathogenesis of the ΔF508 mutation reflects the absence of protein at the relevant cellular site (i.e., the plasma membrane). Other, less common *CFTR* mutations appear to allow the transport of CFTR to the plasma membrane but lead to abnormal Cl⁻ channel regulation or abnormal Cl⁻ ion permeation, or both.[3]

Two general features characterize the pathogenesis of CF at the cellular level: (1) the affected cells in target organs are epithelial cells, and (2) the abnormality in epithelial cells involves regulation of ion transport. The most prevalent defect is abnormal function of the cAMP-dependent plasma membrane Cl⁻ (CFTR) channels. Defective CFTR Cl⁻ function has been detected in the airways,[25,26] sweat ducts,[27] and small intestine[28] of patients with CF. A second major defect in ion transport has been detected in CF airway epithelia: the rate of absorption of Na⁺ ions from the airway lumen to the interstitium is raised threefold over that in non-CF epithelia.[29,30] The molecular mechanisms that confer regulation of Na⁺ transport by CFTR are still unknown, but they probably involve a cascade of protein-protein interactions.

The linkage between CF-specific ion transport defects and the pathogenesis of CF lung disease is becoming more clear.[31] The ion transport abnormalities that characterize CF airways appear to deplete the amount of water on airway surfaces. Water is organized into two compartments on airway surfaces and both are affected in CF.[32] First, the periciliary liquid layer is depleted of water, which leads to a failure of cilia-dependent mucus clearance and, perhaps more importantly, removes the lubricant that prevents the mucus layer from adhering to the airway surface. Second, the mucins in the mucus layer are concentrated because of the water depletion. Concentrated mucus becomes more tacky, so that it adheres more tenaciously to airway surfaces, which accounts for the failure to clear mucus by cough mechanisms. The thickened, adherent mucus plaques and plugs are the nidi for the initial airway infections that characterize CF lung disease. The thickened mucus masses also promote chronic infection by exerting a pressure for biofilm formation by *P. aeruginosa* and reducing the efficiency of secondary host defense mechanisms (e.g., neutrophil-mediated bacterial killing and the activity of lactoferrin and lysozyme).

Whether reduced clearance of thickened secretions from airways is sufficient alone to lead to selection for and persistence of staphylococcal and pseudomonal infection is not yet clear. Studies of bacterial competition within immobilized, thickened plaques have not been performed, nor has a role for the mucus hypoxia that results from abnormal CF ion transport in bacterial selection been established.[33] A role for increased bacterial adherence to epithelia and to mucus, particularly after the epithelium has been injured by the initial infection, has recently been postulated to contribute to disease pathogenesis, but the role in selection of specific bacteria is unknown.[34,35]

An advance in the understanding of the CF airway microenvironment relevant to bacterial growth and pathogenesis has recently emerged. Studies of infected CF airway mucus plugs in vivo have revealed that they are markedly hypoxic (i.e., Po₂ = 2 torr).[33] Subsequent in vitro studies revealed that *P. aeruginosa* grows well in an O₂-deprived environment in the presence of nitrate, and indeed, restricted O₂ environments may predispose to a form of biofilm growth.[36] Studies of material isolated from these plugs have revealed bacterial proteins that are selectively expressed under anaerobic conditions, and patients with CF have antibodies to these proteins.[36] Thus, it appears likely that most CF bacterial pathogens reside in an O₂-restricted environment in the CF lung. This finding will be likely to have major effects on the strategies for antimicrobial sensitivity testing (see later) and perhaps for identification of novel targets for antimicrobial drug development.

The development of persistent bacterial infection generates a complex series of events that lead to airway wall damage and ultimately to destroyed or bronchiectatic airways. Bacterial exoproducts from both *S. aureus* and *P. aeruginosa* have been implicated in airway destruction. In adults, lipopolysaccharides, exotoxin A, and a cell wall–associated rhamnolipid from *P. aeruginosa* have been implicated as important bacterial toxins.[37] The host inflammatory response is in part mediated by Toll receptors expressed in airway epithelia and inflammatory cells and appears intact in CF. The vigorous host response, which is ineffective in clearing the persistent bacterial infection of airway mucus, may actually contribute to airway damage.[38] For example, chemotactic agents, both bacterial and locally derived (e.g., arachidonic acid metabolites from airway epithelia), attract inflammatory cells into the airway lumen. Polymorphonuclear cell–derived enzymes (e.g., elastase) damage airway wall structures, and they cleave immune receptors on neutrophils and bacteria,[39] impairing immune function. In addition, the chronic antigenic stimulus of persistent airway infection generates immunologically mediated airway wall destruction.[38] Large amounts of neutrophil-derived DNA further thicken and impair clearance of airway secretions.[3,13] Eventually, the combination of retained secretions and airway damage deranges gas exchange, perturbs cardiac function, and leads to death.

MICROBIOLOGY

S. aureus and *P. aeruginosa* are the primary etiologic agents of pulmonary infection in patients with CF. *S. aureus* often colonizes the respiratory tract in the first 2 years of life and can be found in approximately 30% of patients with CF in the United States. Before the advent of effective antistaphylococcal therapy, lung infection due to this organism was the leading cause of death. Antistaphylococcal penicillins such as oxacillin control infections with this organism. Ominously, resistance to these agents is increasing in patients with CF; in some centers, 10% to 20% of these patients are infected with methicillin-resistant *S. aureus* (MRSA). Person-to-person spread of MRSA has been documented in patients with CF, with transmission from persons both with and without CF.[40-42] Interestingly, a case-control study suggests that patients with CF and infected with MRSA do not have worsening lung function, although they do require more frequent administration of antimicrobials.[43] A further problem in patients with CF and MRSA is the emergence of strains with reduced vancomycin susceptibility.[44]

Small-colony variants of *S. aureus* are being recognized with increasing frequency in patients with CF. These auxotrophic, slow-growing, antimicrobial-resistant organisms were first recognized in patients receiving long-term (for >3 months) prophylactic trimethoprim-sulfamethoxazole therapy and were referred to as thymidine-dependent *S. aureus*.[45,46] Approximately half of patients with CF infected with *S. aureus* harbor small-colony variants.[45] It is speculated that these small-colony variants evolve in the CF airway and play a role in the persistence of *S. aureus,* in part because they are more resistant to antibiotics than their parent strains.[47] Because *S. aureus* small-colony variants grow poorly on most commonly used isolation media but grow well on mannitol salts agar, this agar should be used to ensure reliable recovery of *S. aureus*.[45]

In childhood or early adolescence, patients with CF become chronically infected with *P. aeruginosa*. Most patients become infected by environmental strains, but it is now recognized that cross-infection among patients with CF as well as transmission to and from patients without CF can also occur.[48] Up to 80% of adolescent and adult patients with CF are infected with this organism.[3] As this chronic infective state evolves, isolates of *P. aeruginosa* from these patients may produce large amounts of an extracellular mucoid polysaccharide called alginate.[49] A large number of different *P. aeruginosa* strains are capable of producing this virulence factor.[50,51] Mucoid colonies that result from alginate production are predominant in infected patients with CF but are rarely seen in patients with other chronic airway diseases, except older adults with primary ciliary dyskinesia.[52] Currently, it is believed that a thickened mucus coat overlying the CF airway epithelium contains hypoxic/anaerobic regions (see earlier). Within these seemingly metabolically hostile regions, motile *P. aeruginosa* bacteria undergo adaptation to nonmotile, anaerobically respiring, mucoid variants growing as a biofilm.[33,36] These mucoid variants form microcolonies in the airway mucus and are resistant to both mechanical and immunologic clearance.[33] The exuberant immune response to these microcolonies is believed to be responsible, in part, for the progressive deterioration in pulmonary function that is the hallmark of this disease.[38]

Current theory of the pathogenesis of chronic *P. aeruginosa* infection in patients with CF requires a reexamination of how susceptibility testing of these isolates is performed and interpreted. In the early stage of CF infection, planktonically growing *P. aeruginosa* are typically seen.[53] These isolates are usually susceptible to all antipseudomonal β-lactams, imipenem, quinolones, and aminoglycosides. With increasing antimicrobial pressure due to repeated antibiotic treatment of pulmonary exacerbations and the emergence of chronic mucoid strains, antibiotic resistance increases. Determining the degree to which this resistance has developed is difficult because currently used susceptibility testing does not take into account two factors: (1) growth as a biofilm, and (2) growth under anaerobic conditions. Studies have shown that *P. aeruginosa* growing as a biofilm is much more resistant to antimicrobials than planktonically growing cells.[53] In addition, aminoglycosides, one of the cornerstones of *P. aeruginosa* therapy in patients with CF, are not active under anaerobic conditions.[54] For now, conventionally performed susceptibility testing done by preferred methods of either disk diffusion or E-test[55] may underestimate the drug resistance of mucoid *P. aeruginosa*. This may result in poor correlation between in vitro susceptibility results and the clinical efficacy of selected antimicrobials such as aminoglycosides.

As life expectancy has increased in patients with CF, *Burkholderia cepacia* has emerged as an important pathogen, and it is being recovered from approximately 10% of adults with CF.[56] Some patients with CF and infected with *B. cepacia* develop what has been characterized as the *cepacia* syndrome.[57] In this syndrome, adolescent and young adult patients with CF and with relatively mild pulmonary disease become infected, have rapid deterioration of pulmonary function, may develop bacteremia, and die within 6 months. Other patients with CF may be infected with *B. cepacia* without a corresponding decline in clinical status.

Recent taxonomic and molecular studies of *B. cepacia* have led to a better understanding of the biology and the epidemiology of the organism (see Chapter 217).[58-65] Intimate social contact appears to be the major mode of spread.[63] Segregation of *B. cepacia*–infected patients has been used successfully in some CF centers to prevent spread of *B. cepacia* to noninfected patients with CF.[66] Because *B. cenocepacia* can replace *B. multivorans*, patients with this more virulent and transmissible organism should be segregated from patients with other organisms belonging to the *B. cepacia* complex.[56] Patient-to-patient transmission of *B. multivorans* has also been documented.[60]

B. cepacia is a cause for concern in patients with CF who undergo double lung transplantation. The transplanted lungs of these patients frequently become reinfected with organisms that infected the native lungs and are still present in the sinuses or trachea of the recipient. CF lung transplant recipients who are infected with *B. cepacia* complex have a significantly poorer 5-year survival rate than those infected with *P. aeruginosa*.[67,68] This poorer outcome can be attributed in part to deaths due to sepsis caused by *B. cenocepacia* in the immediate post-transplant period. Although the numbers are still too small to be convincing, patients infected with *B. multivorans* appear to have a much better post-transplant survival rate than those infected with *B. cenocepacia*.[68] A multicenter study examining the outcome of CF lung transplant based on the species of the *B. cepacia* complex causing post-transplant infections is needed to determine whether patients with *B. cenocepacia*, but not those with *B. multivorans*, should be excluded from transplantation because of the likelihood of a poor outcome.

A significant problem in managing *B. cepacia*–infected patients is the organism's resistance to antimicrobials. *B. cepacia* is intrinsically resistant to aminoglycosides and the polymyxins. On initial isolation,

the organism may be susceptible to trimethoprim-sulfamethoxazole and antipseudomonal β-lactams. However, under antimicrobial pressure, resistance quickly develops, and the clinician is frequently faced with the challenge of managing a patient infected with an organism resistant to all available antimicrobials.[57]

To accurately detect the presence of *B. cepacia* complex in the respiratory tract of patients with CF, selective media specifically designed for the recovery of this group of organisms should be used, because several studies have shown that they enhance the recovery of organisms in this complex.[57] The use of *B. cepacia*–selective agar, coupled with relentless antimicrobial pressure and expanding life span, has resulted in the recovery of a number of novel organisms from this patient population that are phenotypically similar to members of the *B. cepacia* complex. Using a polyphasic identification approach for many of these species, isolates of *Burkholderia gladioli, Ralstonia pickettii, Ralstonia mannitolytica, Ralstonia gilardii,* members of the genus *Pandoraea, Inquilinus limosus, Comamonas testeroni,* and *Chryseobacterium* species have been recovered from a small number of patients with CF.[69,70] Although none have been clearly associated with CF lung disease, they can be misidentified by commonly used commercial identification systems as members of *B. cepacia* complex. Such misclassification may result in the patient receiving improper antimicrobial treatment, being placed on isolation precaution, and segregated socially from other patients with CF, and in the worst-case scenario, being excluded from consideration for lung transplant. To avoid this misclassification, the identity of all isolates determined by phenotypic means as a member of the *B. cepacia* complex should be confirmed using molecular methods.[69,70] Other bacteria such as *Haemophilus influenzae, Moraxella catarrhalis, Stenotrophomonas maltophilia, Alcaligenes xylosoxidans, Burkholderia pseudomallei,* and members of the family Enterobacteriaceae are recovered from the respiratory tract of patients with CF and may play a role in their pulmonary disease.

As CF life expectancy increases and more patients with CF survive into adulthood, the multidrug-resistant organisms *S. maltophilia* and *A. xylosoxidans* are being seen with increasing frequency. This results from the selective pressure of repeated courses of antipseudomonal antimicrobials given to these patients, to which these organisms are frequently resistant.[71] The role of these two species in CF lung disease is currently undefined.[56] The finding of *B. pseudomallei* in patients with CF in northern Australia, where the organism is endemic, is not surprising. On the basis of a small number of patients, the organism appears to respond to antimicrobial therapy in this patient population. Whether it will cause chronic infection in patients with CF, as *B. cepacia* complex does, is unknown.[72]

The role of mycobacteria in the lung disease of patients with cystic fibrosis has recently come under scrutiny. A recently completed multicenter prevalence study has shown that 13% of approximately 1000 patients with CF older than 10 years have nontuberculous mycobacterium recovered from their sputum. Of the NTM recovered, 72% were *Mycobacterium avium* complex (MAC) organisms and 18% were *Mycobacterium abscessus*.[9] In a nested cohort study of this patient population, patients with multiple positive cultures had changes on high-resolution computed tomography of the lungs indicating disease progression, although there were no changes in pulmonary function in the short-term (15-month) follow-up.[10] A case report of fatal *M. abscessus* infection[12] coupled with the findings of this study suggests that patients with CF repeatedly positive for NTM should be carefully assessed and should be considered for antimycobacterial therapy. As for *B. cepacia*, special culture techniques are required to reliably prevent overgrowth of mucoid *P. aeruginosa* and to allow recovery of NTM from CF respiratory secretions.[73] *M. tuberculosis* is rarely recovered in this patient population.

Aspergillus fumigatus may be cultured from specimens from patients with CF.[57] However, the clinical diagnosis of allergic bronchopulmonary aspergillosis (ABPA) should be based on rigorous criteria, because many patients with CF but without the clinical syndrome of ABPA have positive results on immediate hypersensitivity skin testing and an assay for serum-precipitating antibodies to

Aspergillus.[74-76] *Scedosporium apiospermum* is a mold that is being recovered from patients with CF with increased frequency. The role of this mold in pulmonary exacerbation in patients with CF is unknown, although fatal infection with this organism has been reported in a lung transplant recipient.[56]

There are limited data on the role of viruses in CF lung disease, and the data that do exist are found primarily in children.[77,78] The viruses seen in patients with CF are similar to those in patients without CF, with respiratory syncytial virus and parainfluenza virus being most common. Rhinovirus and influenza virus infections may also occur. Children with CF tend to have a more severe disease course with respiratory syncytial virus, as evidenced by more episodes of lower respiratory tract infections requiring hospitalization and a marked inflammatory response during infection.[78]

TREATMENT

The goal of therapy is to retard progressive lung damage by removing viscous and purulent airway secretions, by controlling bacterial infection with antibiotics, and by providing proper nutrition for host defense.[13,14,79] Because person-to-person spread of drug-resistant organisms has been frequently noted in CF,[41,48,60] recent efforts have focused on limiting the transmission through rigorous infection control practices.[56]

The presence of a large bacterial burden in the bronchiectatic airways of patients dictates that airway clearance techniques be combined with antibacterial therapy to achieve optimal results. Chest percussion with postural drainage is the time-honored method, but deep breathing and voluntary coughing, exercise, and other maneuvers are also effective.[14,80] Aerosolized recombinant DNase I improves clearance of purulent airway secretions and offers another modality for treatment in some patients with DNA-laden secretions.[81] Anti-inflammatory agents may be useful in reducing the severity of mucosal edema and assisting in airway clearance. Oral administration of high-dose ibuprofen retards the decline in lung function in children with mild to moderate disease, but benefit has not been demonstrated in adults.[14,82] The indications for systemic steroids are poorly defined,[14] and long-term usage of systemic steroids is associated with adverse side effects.[83,84] The use of topical (inhaled) steroids is common, but benefit has not been established in clinical trials.[85,86] Bronchodilators may assist in clearing retained secretions in some patients, but the finding of a paradoxical reduction in airflow in some patients,[87] coupled with potential acceleration of abnormal Na+ transport,[29] suggests that these agents should be used intermittently and with caution in adult patients with CF. There is little role for the use of inhaled mucolytic agents or bronchial lavage.[14]

Antibiotics have played a key role in improved survival.[88] Oral antibiotics (amoxicillin, cephalexin, dicloxacillin, tetracycline, trimethoprim-sulfamethoxazole) can provide useful therapy for subacute pulmonary exacerbations, despite the presence of *P. aeruginosa* organisms that are resistant to these agents by standard testing. The clinical benefit may reflect antibiotic activity against pathogens that are difficult to culture in the presence of mucoid *P. aeruginosa* (e.g., *S. aureus*, *H. influenzae*), or in airway infection with high concentrations of bacteria ($>10^5$ organisms per milliliter) that are not typical pathogens,[89] or against bacteria growing in a biofilm or under anaerobic conditions,[33,54] or it may be due to inhibition of the release of toxic bacterial exoproducts in the absence of bacterial killing.[57,90] High doses and prolonged therapy (2 to 4 weeks) with oral agents are recommended for treatment of acute illnesses (exacerbations). Certain quinolones (ciprofloxacin, moxifloxacin, and gatifloxacin) have antipseudomonal activity and are useful for intermittent therapy. The emergence of bacterial resistance during monotherapy with these drugs limits usefulness for long-term treatment, and the duration of periodic treatment should be limited to 2 to 4 weeks.[91] Oral antibiotics are also of benefit in chronic bacterial sinusitis, which results from pathogens that are frequently sensitive to broad-spectrum antimicrobials.[17] The use of nonmacrolide oral antibiotics for prophylactic (maintenance) therapy is controversial but appears to have a useful role in some patients.

Chronic oral administration of macrolides has been recently shown to reduce the frequency of clinical exacerbations and improve lung function in patients with CF and *P. aeruginosa*.[92-94] The mechanism of action is undefined, but it is speculated to be through an anti-inflammatory effect, or through antimicrobial actions against *P. aeruginosa* under biofilm or hypoxic conditions. For adults, the dosage is 500 mg of azithromycin three times per week. Patients must be screened for acid-fast bacilli in sputum to ensure that they do not have infection with NTM, before chronic monotherapy with macrolides is initiated.

Aerosolized antibiotics, usually coupled to an oral agent, can be used for subacute pulmonary exacerbations. However, the most beneficial use of chronically inhaled antibiotics is to assist in the maintenance of stable clinical status. Large studies have demonstrated improved lung function and reduced episodes of respiratory illness with chronic use of aerosolized tobramycin (TOBI) in clinically stable patients.[14,95] Colistin is a useful alternative agent for inhalation therapy, because the rare development of bacterial resistance during prolonged aerosol therapy with colistin does not change the bacterial sensitivity to parenteral aminoglycosides.[96,97]

Aggressive parenteral therapy is indicated for clinical exacerbations that do not respond to oral and aerosolized antimicrobials.[13,14] Although sterilization of airway secretions rarely occurs and is not the goal of parenteral therapy, the bacterial burden in conducting airways can be reduced[79,98] and irreversible lung damage presumably retarded. Parenteral therapy should be guided by results of sputum bacteriologic and drug sensitivity studies, although treatment in adult patients with CF is usually directed at *P. aeruginosa*. A combination of antibiotics is indicated to treat infection caused by *P. aeruginosa* because thickened airway secretions prevent drug penetration, aminoglycoside activity is reduced by suppurative secretions, and a combination protects against the emergence of resistant strains.[99] The pharmacologic regimen usually includes an aminoglycoside (gentamicin, tobramycin, amikacin) plus another agent effective against *P. aeruginosa*, such as a cephalosporin (e.g., ceftazidime, cefepime), an antipseudomonal penicillin, or imipenem. If *S. aureus* is clinically suspected or cultured from sputum, addition of a specific antistaphylococcal agent should be considered if the antipseudomonal drug regimen is not adequate for treatment of *S. aureus* infection.

Increased plasma clearance of almost all effective antibiotics in patients with CF dictates the use of large, frequent doses of antimicrobials.[100] For example, adults with CF require 6 to 15 mg/kg/day of tobramycin to achieve desired peak serum levels of 10 μg/mL in an every-8-to-12-hour dosing regimen. Aminoglycoside renal toxicity is uncommon in patients with CF, but trough serum levels should be monitored. Aminoglycoside ototoxicity is becoming more prevalent in adults with CF, as it is related to cumulative total dose and probably to peak concentration; therefore, most recommend against every-24-hour dosing of aminoglycosides in these patients.[101] Parenteral therapy should be continued for a minimum of 10 to 14 days or longer, if necessary, to achieve full clinical and pulmonary functional response. Effective parenteral antibiotic therapy can be administered on an outpatient basis.[102]

Despite intensive antibiotic exposure, symptomatic disease due to *Clostridium difficile* is uncommon in patients with CF, despite the presence of the organism in fecal samples.[103] The asymptomatic carriage of *C. difficile* may reflect the inability of the CF intestinal epithelium to respond to *C. difficile*–derived secretory toxins.[28,104] There are a few case reports of severe or lethal pseudomembranous colitis in patients with CF.[105]

Chronic malabsorption, coupled with increased caloric requirements because of chronic infection and increased respiratory activity, can induce malnutrition and impaired host defense mechanisms in patients with CF. It is very clear that pulmonary outcome is related, in part, to nutritional status. Osteoporosis is common in adults with CF, which reflects several factors, including abnormal absorption.[14,106,107] High caloric intake with supplemental pancreatic digestive enzymes and appropriate fat-soluble vitamins (A, D, E, K) is standard treatment in these patients.

Although *Aspergillus* organisms are frequently cultured from the sputum of adults with CF, treatment is not indicated unless the syndrome of ABPA is established.[74-76] Treatment with systemic corticosteroids is usually sufficient, but antifungal agents may be useful for adjunctive therapy in some patients.[108] Treatment guidelines for ABPA in patients with cystic fibrosis have recently been published.[109] The Cystic Fibrosis Foundation Consensus Conference recommends that in the setting of "slow or poor response to corticosteroids, relapse, corticosteroid dependence or corticosteroid toxicity," itraconazole be added. The itraconazole dosage is 5 mg/kg/day, with a maximum of 400 mg/day PO unless itraconazole levels are determined; twice-a-day dosing is required when the daily dose exceeds 200 mg. The increasing number of adults in the CF patient population is associated with increasing recovery of NTM from sputum cultures.[9] Although as many as 20% of adult patients with CF have NTM in respiratory secretions, the pathogenesis is not clearly defined, and clinical and radiologic studies should be monitored for evidence of pathogenic mycobacterial activity[10,11] before therapy is initiated. *M. abscessus* appears to be more frequently pathogenic than MAC, although both can cause significant disease.[9-12]

Annual influenza vaccinations are recommended, but pneumococcal vaccine is not routinely indicated because of the relative absence of *Streptococcus pneumoniae* as a pathogen, although some consultants recommend its use.

Lung transplantation is a viable therapeutic option for patients with end-stage lung disease. In general, patients with *B. cepacia* have a poorer 5-year survival, and better guidelines are needed to identify specific risk factors (see comments under "Microbiology").[67,68] In experienced lung transplant centers, the 1-year survival rate is 80% to 90%, and the 5-year survival rate may be as high as 50%.[110-112]

Recent progress in defining the organ-level and molecular pathogenesis of CF has led to the development of new therapeutic approaches.[113] Novel anti-inflammatory agents are currently undergoing Phase I and II trials. New approaches with aerosolized antibiotics are underway for treatment of secondary manifestations of the lung disease. Correction of abnormal airway epithelial ion transport, targeting defective Cl⁻ secretion, offers the possibility of long-term "preventive" therapy that might impede the development of airway disease. Studies of other pharmacotherapies to enhance the cellular processing or function of CFTR are also underway.[113] Finally, gene transfer of a normal *CFTR* cDNA to airway cells offers the promise of treatment at the molecular level. Although the technique is some distance from clinical practice, several studies of gene transfer with adeno-associated virus vectors and liposome-DNA complexes are under development.[113]

REFERENCES

1. Riordan JR, Rommens JM, Kerem B-T, et al. Identification of the cystic fibrosis gene: Cloning and characterization of complementary DNA. Science. 1989;245:1066.
2. Boucher RC. An overview of the pathogenesis of cystic fibrosis lung disease. Adv Drug Deliv Rev. 2002;54.
3. Welsh MJ, Ramsey BW, Accurso FJ, Cutting GR. Cystic fibrosis. In: Scriver CR, Beaudet AL, Sly WS, Valle D, eds. The Metabolic and Molecular Bases of Inherited Disease. 8th ed. New York: McGraw-Hill; 2001:5121-5188.
4. Stern RC. The diagnosis of cystic fibrosis. N Engl J Med. 1997;336:487.
5. Yankaskas JR, Marshall BC, Sufian B, et al. Cystic fibrosis adult care: Consensus conference report. Chest. 2004;125(Suppl 1):1S-39S.
6. Yankaskas JR, Knowles MR, eds. Cystic Fibrosis in Adults. Philadelphia: Lippincott-Raven; 1999.
7. Rosenstein BJ, Cutting GR. The diagnosis of cystic fibrosis: A consensus statement. Cystic Fibrosis Foundation Consensus Panel. J Pediatr. 1998;132:589.
8. Gilligan PH. Microbiology of cystic fibrosis lung disease. In: Yankaskas JR, Knowles MR, eds. Cystic Fibrosis in Adults. Philadelphia: Lippincott-Raven; 1999:93-114.
9. Olivier KN, Weber DJ, Wallace RJ Jr, et al. Nontuberculous mycobacteria in cystic fibrosis: I. Multicenter prevalence study of a potential pathogen in a susceptible population. Am J Respir Crit Care Med. 2003;167:835.
10. Olivier KN, Weber DJ, Lee JH, et al. Nontuberculous Mycobacteria in Cystic Fibrosis Study Group. Nontuberculous mycobacteria: II. Nested cohort study of impact on cystic fibrosis lung disease. Am J Respir Crit Care Med. 2003;167:835.
11. Olivier KN, Yankaskas JR, Knowles MR. Nontuberculous mycobacterial pulmonary disease in cystic fibrosis. Semin Respir Infect. 1996;11:272.
12. Sanguinetti M, Ardito F, Fiscarelli E, et al. Fatal pulmonary infection due to multidrug-resistant *Mycobacterium abscessus* in a patient with cystic fibrosis. J Clin Microbiol. 2001;39:816.
13. Davis PB, Drumm M, Konstan MW. Cystic fibrosis. Am J Respir Crit Care Med. 1996;154:1229.
14. Noone PG, Knowles MR. Standard therapy of cystic fibrosis lung disease. In: Yankaskas JR, Knowles MR, eds. Cystic Fibrosis in Adults. Philadelphia: Lippincott-Raven; 1999:145.
15. Schidlow DV, Taussig LM, Knowles MR. Cystic Fibrosis Foundation Consensus Conference Report on pulmonary complications of cystic fibrosis. Pediatr Pulmonol. 1993;15:187.
16. Brinson GM, Noone PG, Mauro MA, et al. Bronchial artery embolization for the treatment of hemoptysis in patients with cystic fibrosis. Am J Respir Crit Care Med. 1998;157:1951.
17. Stern RC, Jones K. Nasal and sinus disease. In: Yankaskas JR, Knowles MR, eds. Cystic Fibrosis in Adults. Philadelphia: Lippincott-Raven; 1999:221.
18. Lanng S. Glucose intolerance in cystic fibrosis patients. Paediatr Respir Rev. 2001;2:253.
19. Moran A, Hardin D, Rodman D, et al. Diagnosis, screening and management of cystic fibrosis related diabetes mellitus: A consensus conference report. Diabetes Res Clin Pract. 1999;45:61-73.
20. Anderson MP, Rich DP, Gregory RJ, et al. Generation of cAMP-activated chloride currents by expression of CFTR. Science. 1991;251:679.
21. Kartner N, Hanrahan JW, Jensen TJ, et al. Expression of the cystic fibrosis gene in non-epithelial invertebrate cells produces a regulated anion conductance. Cell. 1991;64:681.
22. Gabriel SE, Clarke LL, Boucher RC, Stutts MJ. CFTR and outward rectifying chloride channels are distinct proteins with a regulatory relationship. Nature. 1993;363:263.
23. Stutts MJ, Canessa CM, Olsen JC, et al. CFTR as a cAMP-dependent regulator of sodium channels. Science. 1995;269:847.
24. Cheng SH, Gregory RJ, Marshall J, et al. Defective intracellular transport and processing of CFTR is the molecular basis of most cystic fibrosis. Cell. 1990;63:827.
25. Knowles MR, Stutts MJ, Spock A, et al. Abnormal ion permeation through cystic fibrosis respiratory epithelium. Science. 1983;221:1067.
26. Knowles M, Gatzy J, Boucher R. Relative ion permeability of normal and cystic fibrosis nasal epithelium. J Clin Invest. 1983;71:1410.
27. Quinton PM. Chloride impermeability in cystic fibrosis. Nature. 1983;301:421.
28. Berschneider HM, Knowles MR, Azizkhan RG, et al. Altered intestinal chloride transport in cystic fibrosis. FASEB J. 1988;2:2625.
29. Boucher RC, Stutts MJ, Knowles MR, et al. Na⁺ transport in cystic fibrosis respiratory epithelia: Abnormal basal rate and response to adenylate cyclase activation. J Clin Invest. 1986;78:1245.
30. Knowles M, Gatzy J, Boucher R. Increased bioelectric potential difference across respiratory epithelia in cystic fibrosis. N Engl J Med. 1981;305:1489.
31. Knowles MR, Boucher RC. Mucus clearance as a primary innate defense mechanism for mammalian airways (Perspective). J Clin Invest. 2002;109:571.
32. Matsui H, Grubb BR, Tarran R, et al. Evidence for periciliary liquid layer depletion, not abnormal ion composition, in the pathogenesis of cystic fibrosis airways disease. Cell. 1998;95:1005.
33. Worlitzsch D, Tarran R, Ulrich M, et al. Effects of reduced mucus oxygen concentration in airway *Pseudomonas* infections of cystic fibrosis patients. J Clin Invest. 2002;109:317.
34. de Bentzmann S, Plotkowski C, Puchelle E. Receptors in the *Pseudomonas aeruginosa* adherence to injured and repairing airway epithelium. Am J Respir Crit Care Med. 1996;154:S155.
35. Imundo L, Barasch J, Prince A, Al-Awqati Q. Cystic fibrosis epithelial cells have a receptor for pathogenic bacteria on their apical surface. Proc Natl Acad Sci U S A. 1995;92:3019.
36. Yoon SS, Hennigan RF, Hilliard GM, et al. *Pseudomonas aeruginosa* anaerobic respiration in biofilms: Relationships to cystic fibrosis pathogenesis. Dev Cell. 2002; 3:593.
37. Stutts MJ, Schwab JH, Chen MG, et al. Effects of *Pseudomonas aeruginosa* on bronchial epithelial ion transport. Am Rev Respir Dis. 1986;134:17.
38. Konstan MW, Berger M. Current understanding of the inflammatory process in cystic fibrosis: Onset and etiology. Pediatr Pulmonol. 1997;24:137.
39. Tosi MF, Zakem H, Berger M. Neutrophil elastase cleaves C3bi on opsonized *Pseudomonas* as well as CR1 on neutrophils to create a functionally important opsonin receptor mismatch. J Clin Invest. 1990;86:300.
40. Gilligan P, Jordan M, Wait K, et al. Oxacillin-resistant *Staphylococcus aureus* in patients with cystic fibrosis (CF). Pediatr Pulmonol. 1996;Suppl 13:297.
41. Givney R, Vickery A, Pegler M, Benn R. Methicillin-resistant *Staphylococcus aureus* in a cystic fibrosis unit. J Hosp Infect. 1997;35:27.
42. Goerke C, Kraning K, Stern M, et al. Molecular epidemiology of community-acquired *Staphylococcus aureus* in families with and without cystic fibrosis patients. J Infect Dis. 2000;181:984.
43. Miall LS, McGinley NT, Brownlee KG, Conway SP. Methicillin resistant *Staphylococcus aureus* (MRSA) infection in cystic fibrosis. Arch Dis Child. 2001; 84:160.
44. Denis O, Nonhoff C, Byl B, et al. Emergence of vancomycin-intermediate *Staphylococcus aureus* in a Belgian hospital. J Antimicrob Chemother. 2002;50:383.
45. Gilligan PH, Gage PA, Welch DF, Muszynski MJ, Wait KR. Prevalence of thymidine-dependent *Staphylococcus aureus* in patients with cystic fibrosis. J Clin Microbiol. 1987;25:1258.
46. Kahl B, Herrmann M, Everding AS, et al. Persistent infection with small colony variant strains of *Staphylococcus aureus* in patients with cystic fibrosis. J Infect Dis. 1998;177:1023.

47. Proctor RA, Peters G. Small colony variants in staphylococcal infections: Diagnostic and therapeutic implications. Clin Infect Dis. 1998;27:419.

48. McCallum SJ, Corkill J, Gallagher M, et al. Superinfection with a transmissible strain of *Pseudomonas aeruginosa* in adults with cystic fibrosis chronically colonised by *P. aeruginosa*. Lancet. 2001;358:558.

49. Govan JRW, Deretic V. Microbial pathogenesis in cystic fibrosis: Mucoid *Pseudomonas aeruginosa* and *Burkholderia cepacia*. Microbiol Rev. 1996;60:539.

50. Boukadida J, De Montalembert M, Lenoir G, et al. Molecular epidemiology of chronic colonisation by *Pseudomonas aeruginosa* in cystic fibrosis. J Med Microbiol. 1993;38:29.

51. Romling U, Grothues D, Koopmann U, et al. Pulsed-field gel electrophoresis analysis of a *Pseudomonas aeruginosa* pathovar. Electrophoresis. 1992;13:646.

52. Noone PG. Primary ciliary dyskinesia. Pediatr Pulmonol. 2001;Suppl. 22:132.

53. Aaron SD, Ferris W, Ramotar K, et al. Single and combination antibiotic susceptibilities of planktonic, adherent, and biofilm-grown *Pseudomonas aeruginosa* isolates cultured from sputa of adults with cystic fibrosis. J Clin Microbiol. 2002;40:4172.

54. Hassett DJ, Cuppoletti J, Trapnell B, et al. Anaerobic metabolism and quorum sensing by *Pseudomonas aeruginosa* biofilms in chronically infected cystic fibrosis airways: Rethinking antibiotic treatment strategies and drug targets. Adv Drug Deliv Rev. 2002;54:1425.

55. Burns JL, Saiman L, Whittier S, et al. Comparison of agar diffusion methodologies for antimicrobial susceptibility testing of *Pseudomonas aeruginosa* isolates from cystic fibrosis patients. J Clin Microbiol. 2000;38:1818.

56. Saiman L, Siegel J. Infection control recommendations for patients with cystic fibrosis: Microbiology, important pathogens, and infection control practices to prevent patient-to-patient transmission. Am J Infect Control. 2003;31:S1.

57. Miller MB, Gilligan PH. Laboratory aspects of management of chronic pulmonary infections in patients with cystic fibrosis. J Clin Microbiol. 2003;41:4009.

58. Vandamme P, Holmes B, Coenye T, et al. *Burkholderia cenocepacia* sp. nov.—a new twist to an old story. Res Microbiol. 2003;154:91.

59. LiPuma JJ, Spilker T, Gill LH, et al. Disproportionate distribution of *Burkholderia cepacia* complex species and transmissibility markers in cystic fibrosis. Am J Respir Crit Care Med. 2001;164:92.

60. Heath DG, Hohneker K, Carriker C, et al. Six-year molecular analysis of *Burkholderia cepacia* complex isolates among cystic fibrosis patients at a referral center for lung transplantation. J Clin Microbiol. 2002;40:1188.

61. Mahenthiralingam E, Vandamme P, Campbell ME, et al. Infection with *Burkholderia cepacia* complex genomovars in patients with cystic fibrosis: Virulent transmissible strains of genomovar III can replace *Burkholderia multivorans*. Clin Infect Dis. 2001;33:1469.

62. Coenye T, LiPuma JJ. Population structure analysis of *Burkholderia cepacia* genomovar III: Varying degrees of genetic recombination characterize major clonal complexes. Microbiology. 2003;149:77.

63. Govan JRW, Brown PH, Maddison J, et al. Evidence for transmission of *Pseudomonas cepacia* by social contact in cystic fibrosis. Lancet. 1993;342:15.

64. Sun L, Jiang RZ, Steinbach S, et al. The emergence of a highly transmissible lineage of *cbl+ Pseudomonas (Burkholderia) cepacia* causing CF centre epidemics in North America and Britain. Nat Med. 1995;1:661.

65. Goldstein R, Sun L, Jiang RZ, et al. Structurally variant classes of pilus appendage fibers coexpressed from *Burkholderia (Pseudomonas) cepacia*. J Bacteriol. 1995; 177:1039.

66. Smith DL, Smith EG, Gumery LB, Stableforth DE. *Pseudomonas cepacia* infection in cystic fibrosis. Lancet. 1992;339:252.

67. Chaparro C, Maurer J, Gutierrez C, et al. Infection with *Burkholderia cepacia* in cystic fibrosis: Outcome following lung transplantation. Am J Respir Crit Care Med. 2001;163:43.

68. Aris RM, Routh JC, LiPuma JJ, et al. Lung transplantation for cystic fibrosis patients with *Burkholderia cepacia* complex: Survival linked to genomovar type. Am J Respir Crit Care Med. 2001;164:2102.

69. Coenye T, Goris J, Spilker T, et al. Characterization of unusual bacteria isolated from respiratory secretions of cystic fibrosis patients and description of *Inquilinus limosus* gen. nov., sp. nov. J Clin Microbiol. 2002;40:2062.

70. Segonds C, Paute S, Chabanon G. Use of amplified ribosomal DNA restriction analysis for identification of *Ralstonia* and *Pandoraea* species: Interest in determination of the respiratory bacterial flora in patients with cystic fibrosis. J Clin Microbiol. 2003;41:3415.

71. Denton M, Todd NJ, Littlewood JM. Role of anti-pseudomonal antibiotics in the emergence of *Stenotrophomonas maltophilia* in cystic fibrosis patients. Eur J Clin Microbiol Infect Dis. 1996;15:402.

72. Holland DJ, Wesley A, Drinkovic D, Currie BJ. Cystic fibrosis and *Burkholderia pseudomallei* infection: An emerging problem? Clin Infect Dis. 2002;35:e138.

73. Whittier S, Hopfer RL, Knowles MR, Gilligan PH. Improved recovery of *Mycobacteria* from respiratory secretions of patients with cystic fibrosis. J Clin Microbiol. 1993;31:861.

74. Moss RB. Allergic bronchopulmonary aspergillosis. Clin Rev Allergy Immunol. 2002;23:87.

75. Maiz L, Cuevas M, Quirce S, et al. Serologic IgE immune responses against *Aspergillus fumigatus* and *Candida albicans* in patients with cystic fibrosis. Chest. 2002;121:782.

76. Nikolaizik WH, Weichel M, Blaser K, Crameri R. Intracutaneous tests with recombinant allergens in cystic fibrosis patients with allergic bronchopulmonary aspergillosis and *Aspergillus* allergy. Am J Respir Crit Care Med. 2002;165:916.

77. Hiatt PW, Grace SC, Kozinetz CA, et al. Effects of viral lower respiratory tract infection on lung function in infants with cystic fibrosis. Pediatrics. 1999;103:619.

78. Armstrong D, Grimwood K, Carlin JB, et al. Severe viral respiratory infections in infants with cystic fibrosis. Pediatr Pulmonol. 1998;26:371.

79. Ramsey BW. Management of pulmonary disease in patients with cystic fibrosis. N Engl J Med. 1996;335:179.

80. Wagener JS, Headley AA. Cystic fibrosis: Current trends in respiratory care. Respir Care. 2003;48:234.

81. Fuchs HJ, Borowitz DS, Christiansen DH, et al. Effect of aerosolized recombinant human DNase on exacerbations of respiratory symptoms and on pulmonary function in patients with cystic fibrosis. The Pulmozyme Study Group. N Engl J Med. 1994;331:637.

82. Konstan MW, Byard PJ, Hoppel CL, Davis PB. Effect of high-dose ibuprofen in patients with cystic fibrosis. N Engl J Med. 1995;332:848.

83. Conway SP, Morton AM, Oldroyd B, et al. Osteoporosis and osteopenia in adults and adolescents with cystic fibrosis: Prevalence and associated factors. Thorax. 2000;55:798.

84. Rosenstein BJ, Eigen H. Risks of alternate-day prednisone in patients with cystic fibrosis. Pediatrics. 1991;87:245.

85. Bisgaard H, Pedersen SS, Nielsen KG, et al. Controlled trial of inhaled budesonide in patients with cystic fibrosis and chronic bronchopulmonary *Pseudomonas aeruginosa* infection. Am J Respir Crit Care Med. 1997;156:1190.

86. Dezateux C, Walters S, Balfour-Lynn I. Inhaled corticosteroids for cystic fibrosis. Cochrane Database Syst Rev. 2000;2:CD001915.

87. Shapiro GG, Bamman J, Kanerek P, Bierman CW. The paradoxical effect of adrenergic and methylxanthine drugs in cystic fibrosis. Pediatrics. 1976;58:740.

88. Michel BC. Antibacterial therapy in cystic fibrosis: A review of the literature published between 1980 and 1987. Chest. 1988;94:129S.

89. Myers MG, Koontz FP, Weinberger M. Lower respiratory infections in patients with cystic fibrosis. In: Lloyd-Still JD, ed. Textbook of Cystic Fibrosis. Boston: Wright PSG; 1983:91.

90. Grimwood K, To M, Rabin HR, Woods DE. Subinhibitory antibiotics reduce *Pseudomonas aeruginosa* tissue injury in the rat lung model. J Antimicrob Chemother. 1989;24:937.

91. Schaad UB, Wedgwood J, Ruedeberg A, et al. Ciprofloxacin as antipseudomonal treatment in patients with cystic fibrosis. Pediatr Infect Dis J. 1997;16:106.

92. Wolter J, Seeney S, Bell S, et al. Effect of long term treatment with azithromycin on disease parameters in cystic fibrosis: A randomised trial. Thorax. 2002;57:212.

93. Equi A, Balfour-Lynn IM, Bush A, Rosenthal M. Long term azithromycin in children with cystic fibrosis: A randomised, placebo-controlled crossover trial. Lancet. 2002; 360:978.

94. Saiman L. What have we learned from further analysis of the U.S. macrolide trial? Subgroup Analysis of Azithromycin Trial. Pediatr Pulmonol. 2003; Suppl 25:165-167.

95. Ramsey BW, Pepe MS, Quan JM, et al. Intermittent administration of inhaled tobramycin in patients with cystic fibrosis. The Cystic Fibrosis Inhaled Tobramycin Study Group. N Engl J Med. 1999;340:23.

96. Jensen T, Pedersen SS, Garne S, et al. Colistin inhalation therapy in cystic fibrosis patients with chronic *Pseudomonas aeruginosa* lung infection. J Antimicrob Chemother. 1987;19:831.

97. Diot P, Gagnadoux F, Martin C, et al. Nebulization and anti-*Pseudomonas aeruginosa* activity of colistin. Eur Respir J. 1997;10:1995.

98. Smith AL, Redding G, Doershuk C, et al. Sputum changes associated with therapy for endobronchial exacerbation in cystic fibrosis. J Pediatr. 1988;112:547.

99. Mendelman PM, Smith AL, Levy J, et al. Aminoglycoside penetration, inactivation, and efficacy in cystic fibrosis sputum. Am Rev Respir Dis. 1985;132:761.

100. Smith A, Cohen M, Ramsey B. Pharmacotherapy. In: Yankaskas JR, Knowles MR, eds. Philadelphia: Lippincott-Raven; 1999:345.

101. Stavroulaki P, Vossinakis IC, Dinopoulou D, et al. Otoacoustic emissions for monitoring aminoglycoside-induced ototoxicity in children with cystic fibrosis. Arch Otolaryngol Head Neck Surg. 2002;128:150.

102. Donati MA, Guenette G, Auerbach H. Prospective controlled study of home and hospital therapy of cystic fibrosis pulmonary disease. J Pediatr. 1987;111:28.

103. Welkon CJ, Long SS, Thompson CM Jr, Gilligan PH. *Clostridium difficile* in patients with cystic fibrosis. Am J Dis Child. 1987;139:805.

104. Gabriel SE, Brigman KN, Koller BH, et al. Cystic fibrosis heterozygote resistance to cholera toxin in the cystic fibrosis mouse model. Science. 1994;266:107.

105. Chaun H. Colonic disorders in adult cystic fibrosis. Can J Gastroenterol. 2001;15:586.

106. Greer RM, Buntain HM, Potter JM, et al. Abnormalities of the PTH-vitamin D axis and bone turnover markers in children, adolescents and adults with cystic fibrosis: Comparison with healthy controls. Osteoporos Int. 2003;14:404.

107. Aris RM, Lester GE, Dingman S, Ontjes DA. Altered calcium homeostasis in adults with cystic fibrosis. Osteoporos Int. 1999;10:102.

108. Skov M, Hoiby N, Koch C. Itraconazole treatment of allergic bronchopulmonary aspergillosis in patients with cystic fibrosis. Allergy. 2002;57:723.

109. Stevens DA, Moss RB, Kurup VP, et al. Allergic bronchopulmonary aspergillosis in cystic fibrosis: State of the art. Cystic Fibrosis Foundation Consensus Conference. Clin Infect Dis. 2003;37(Suppl 3):S225-264.

110. Egan TM, Detterbeck FC, Mill MR, et al. Long term results of lung transplantation for cystic fibrosis. Eur J Cardiothorac Surg. 2002;22:602.

111. Zuckerman JB and Kotloff RM. Lung transplantation for cystic fibrosis. Clin Chest Med. 1998;19:535.

112. Huddleston CB, Bloch JB, Sweet SC, et al. Lung transplantation in children. Ann Surg. 2002;236:270.

113. Johnson LG, Knowles MR. New therapeutic strategies for cystic fibrosis lung disease. In: Yankaskas JR, Knowles MR, eds. Cystic Fibrosis in Adults. Philadelphia: Lippincott-Raven; 1999:233.

CHAPTER **66**

Urinary
Tract Infections

JACK D. SOBEL
DONALD KAYE

Bacteriuria is a frequently used term meaning bacteria in the urine. The probability of the presence of infected urine in the bladder can be ascertained by quantifying the bacteria in voided urine or in urine obtained via urethral catheterization. The term *significant bacteriuria* indicates that the number of bacteria in the voided urine exceeds the number that can be expected from contamination from the anterior urethra (i.e., $\geq 10^5$ bacteria/mL). The implication is that in the presence of at least 10^5 bacteria/mL of urine, infection must be seriously considered. *Asymptomatic bacteriuria* refers to significant bacteriuria in a patient without symptoms.

Urinary tract infection may involve only the lower urinary tract or may involve both the upper and the lower tracts. The term *cystitis* has been used to describe the syndrome involving dysuria, frequency, urgency, and occasionally suprapubic tenderness. However, these symptoms may be related to lower tract inflammation without bacterial infection and can be caused by urethritis (for example, gonorrheal or chlamydial urethritis). Furthermore, the presence of symptoms of lower tract infection without upper tract symptoms by no means excludes upper tract infection, which is also often present.

Acute pyelonephritis describes the clinical syndrome characterized by flank pain or tenderness, or both, and fever, often associated with dysuria, urgency, and frequency. However, these symptoms can occur in the absence of infection (for example, in renal infarction or renal calculus). A more rigorous definition of acute pyelonephritis is the previously described syndrome accompanied by significant bacteriuria and acute infection in the kidney.

Uncomplicated urinary tract infection refers to infection in a structurally and neurologically normal urinary tract. *Complicated urinary tract infection* refers to infection in a urinary tract with functional or structural abnormalities (including indwelling catheters and calculi). In general, infection in men, pregnant women, children, and patients who are hospitalized or in health care–associated settings may be considered complicated. In the patient with complicated infection, infecting microorganisms are more likely to be resistant to antimicrobial agents. Some consider upper tract infection to be complicated.[1,2] Recurrences of urinary tract infection may be either *relapses* or *reinfections*. Relapse of bacteriuria refers to a recurrence of bacteriuria with the same infecting microorganism that was present before therapy was started. This is due to persistence of the organism in the urinary tract. Reinfection is a recurrence of bacteriuria with a microorganism different from the original infecting bacterium. It is a new infection. Reinfection may also occur with the same microorganism, which may have persisted in the vagina or feces. This can be mistaken for a relapse.

Urosepsis is commonly used to describe the sepsis syndrome due to urinary tract infection. It includes clinical evidence of urinary tract infection plus two or more of the following: (1) temperature greater than 38° C or less than 36° C; (2) heart rate greater than 90 beats per minute; (3) respiratory rate greater than 20/minute, or Pa_{CO_2} less than 32 mm Hg; (4) white blood count greater than 12,000/mm³, less than 4000/mm³, or greater than 10% band forms.

The term *chronic urinary tract infection* has little meaning in many patients. True chronic infection should really mean persistence of the same organism for months or years with relapses after treatment. Reinfections do not mean chronicity any more than repeated episodes of pneumonia indicate chronic pneumonia.

The term *chronic pyelonephritis* means different things to different authors. To some, chronic pyelonephritis refers to pathologic changes in the kidney due to infection only. However, identical pathologic alterations are found in several other entities, such as chronic urinary tract obstruction, analgesic nephropathy, hypokalemic nephropathy, vascular disease, and uric acid nephropathy. Pathologic descriptions do not (and cannot) differentiate between the changes produced by infection versus those produced by these other entities.

Papillary necrosis from infection is an acute complication of pyelonephritis, usually in the presence of diabetes mellitus, urinary tract obstruction, sickle cell disease, or analgesic abuse. Papillary necrosis can occur in the absence of infection in some of these conditions. The necrotic renal papillae may slough and cause unilateral or bilateral ureteral obstruction. *Intrarenal abscess* may result from bacteremia or may be a complication of severe pyelonephritis. *Perinephric abscess* occurs when microorganisms from either the renal parenchyma or blood are deposited in the soft tissues surrounding the kidneys.

PATHOLOGIC CHARACTERISTICS

For further details on pathologic characteristics, consult reference 3.

Acute Pyelonephritis

In severe pyelonephritis, the kidney is somewhat enlarged, and discrete, yellowish, raised abscesses are apparent on the surface. The pathognomonic histologic feature is suppurative necrosis or abscess formation within the renal substance.

Chronic Pyelonephritis (Chronic Interstitial Nephritis)

In chronic pyelonephritis, one or both kidneys contain gross scars, but even when involvement is bilateral, the kidneys are not equally damaged. This uneven scarring is useful in differentiating chronic pyelonephritis from diseases that cause symmetric contracted kidneys—for example, chronic glomerulonephritis. There are inflammatory changes in the pelvic wall with papillary atrophy and blunting. The parenchyma shows interstitial fibrosis with an inflammatory infiltrate of lymphocytes, plasma cells, and occasionally neutrophils (Fig. 66-1). The tubules are dilated or contracted with atrophy of the lining

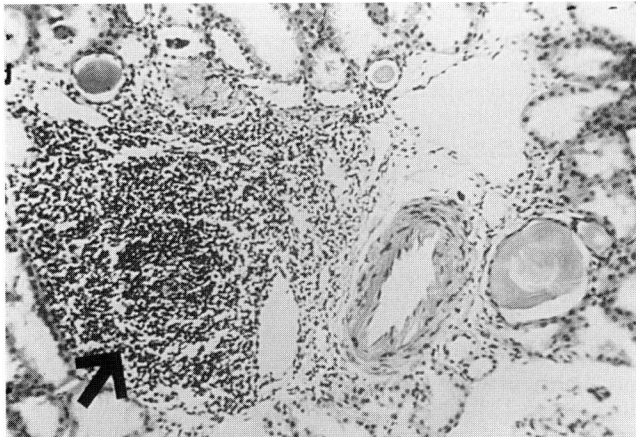

FIGURE 66-1. Chronic pyelonephritis. Tubules are filled with eosinophilic casts and surrounded by a dense infiltrate of lymphocytes and plasma cells *(arrow)*.

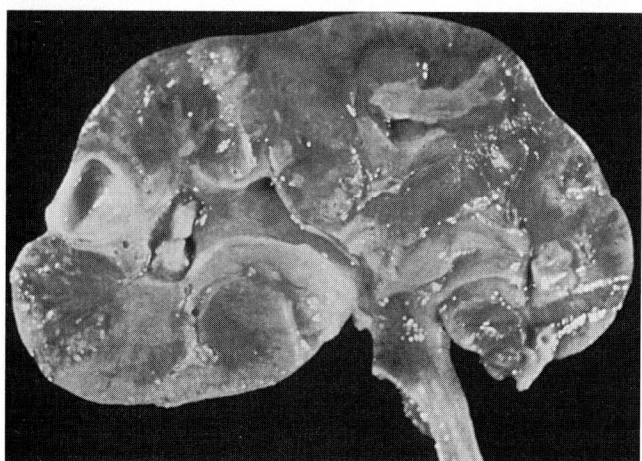

FIGURE 66-2. Necrotizing papillitis (papillary necrosis) complicating acute pyelonephritis in a diabetic patient. The pelvis is hemorrhagic. Note large and irregular defects. *(Courtesy of M. Bergeron, M.D.)*

epithelium. Many of the dilated tubules contain colloid casts, which suggest the appearance of thyroid tissue ("thyroidization" of the kidney). There is also concentric fibrosis about the parietal layer of Bowman's capsule (termed *periglomerular fibrosis*) and vascular changes similar to those of benign or malignant arteriolar sclerosis.

Several studies have found little correlation between these pathologic findings and evidence for past or present urinary tract infection.[4-6] Clearly, a better term for this pathologic entity would be *chronic interstitial nephritis* to encompass all the clinical states that can cause these changes. To incriminate infection as the sole cause of chronic interstitial nephritis, one needs evidence of past or present urinary tract infection and the absence of any other condition that can cause the pathologic picture of chronic interstitial nephritis. These criteria are seldom met, and even if they are, it is frequently impossible to establish whether infection is complicating interstitial nephritis from some unrecognized cause.

Papillary Necrosis Caused by Infection

Frequently both kidneys are affected, and one or more pyramids may be involved (Fig. 66-2). The pyramids are replaced by wedge-shaped areas of yellow necrotic tissue with the base located at the corticomedullary junction. As the lesion progresses, a portion of the necrotic papilla may break off, producing a calyceal deformity that results in a recognizable radiologic filling defect. The sloughed portion may be voided and in some instances can be recovered from the urine. Microscopically, edema is initially seen in the interstitium. Eventually, the lesion resembles an infarct with coagulation necrosis involving the entire pyramid. The collecting tubules are filled with bacteria and polymorphonuclear leukocytes.

PATHOGENESIS OF URINARY TRACT INFECTION

Urinary infections occur as a result of the interaction between bacterial virulence and host biologic and behavioral factors as opposed to highly efficient host defense mechanisms. There are three possible routes by which bacteria can invade and spread within the urinary tract: the ascending, hematogenous, and lymphatic pathways.

Ascending Route

The urethra is usually colonized with bacteria. Studies using suprapubic puncture techniques have revealed the occasional presence of small numbers of microorganisms in the urine of uninfected persons. Massage of the urethra in women and sexual intercourse[7-12] can force bacteria into the female bladder. Condom use may heighten the trau-

matic effects.[13] Furthermore, just one catheterization of the bladder results in urinary tract infection in about 1% of ambulatory patients,[14] and infection develops within 3 or 4 days in essentially all patients with indwelling catheters with open drainage systems. (For a discussion of catheter-associated urinary tract infection, see Chapter 302.) Both the diaphragm with nonoxynol-9 contraceptive jelly in women and the condom catheter in men have been shown to predispose to infection.[11,12,15-19] Studies have implicated the spermicide rather than the diaphragm. Spermicides increase colonization of the vagina with uropathogens.[20] Although the dominant *Lactobacillus* vaginal flora is more sensitive to nonoxynol-9 than *Escherichia coli*, it has not been proved that the high coliform presence in nonoxynol-9 users is the result of a loss of lactobacilli. Spermicide use also increases adherence of *E. coli* to vaginal epithelial cells.[19] Estrogen deficiency is now recognized as a predisposing factor to recurrent UTIs in postmenopausal women because of consequent vaginal flora changes, with protective lactobacilli being replaced by coliforms and other uropathogens.[21,22] Uropathogenic *E. coli* are not infrequently shared between heterosexual sex partners.

The fact that urinary tract infection is much more common in women than in men gives support to the importance of the ascending route of infection. The female urethra is short and is in proximity to the warm moist vulvar and perianal areas, making contamination likely. It has been shown that the organisms that cause urinary tract infection in women colonize the vaginal introitus and the periurethral area before urinary infection results.[23] Once within the bladder, bacteria may multiply and then pass up the ureters, especially if vesicoureteral reflux is present, to the renal pelvis and parenchyma. Animal studies have also confirmed the importance of ascending infection. If bladder bacteriuria is established after unilateral ureteral ligation, only the unligated kidney develops pyelonephritis. Finally, studies have correlated intestinal carriage of urovirulent *E. coli* and susceptibility to urinary tract infections in children.[24]

Hematogenous Route

Infection of the renal parenchyma by blood-borne organisms clearly occurs in humans. The kidney is frequently the site of abscesses in patients with *Staphylococcus aureus* bacteremia or endocarditis, or both. Experimental pyelonephritis can be produced by the intravenous injection of several species of bacteria and *Candida*.[25] However, producing experimental pyelonephritis by the intravenous route with gram-negative enteric bacilli, the common pathogens in urinary tract infection, is difficult. Additional manipulations, such as creating ureteral obstruction, are often necessary.[25] It appears that in humans, infection of the kidney with gram-negative bacilli rarely occurs by the hematogenous route.

Lymphatic Route

Evidence for a significant role for renal lymphatics in the pathogenesis of pyelonephritis is unimpressive and consists of the demonstration of lymphatic connections between the ureters and kidneys in animals and the fact that increased pressure in the bladder can cause lymphatic flow to be directed toward the kidney. Thus, it would seem that the ascending pathway of infection is the most important.

Host-Parasite Interaction

Organism

Although urinary tract infections are caused by many species of microorganisms, most are caused by *E. coli*. However, only a few serogroups of *E. coli*, O1, O2, O4, O6, O7, O8, O75, O150, and O18ab, cause a high proportion of infections.[26] This has led to the concept of uropathogenic *E. coli* clones, or lineages, to differentiate pathogenic populations from commensals. Certain O, K, and H serotypes also correlate with clinical severity, especially pyelonephritis. Accordingly, certain strains of *E. coli* are selected from the fecal flora

TABLE 66-1 Uropathogenic *Escherichia coli* Adhesins and Corresponding Epithelial Receptors

Adhesin	Genetic Sequence	Receptor	Comments
Type 1 fimbriae (MS)	*Pil, fimH*	Mannosylated proteins on epithelial cells (uroplakin Ia) and PMNs	Bind to Tamm-Horsfall protein (THP) and SIgA
P fimbriae (MR)	*pap*G (class Ia) ($papG_{J96}$)	Gal-α 1-4 (P blood group antigen)	Rare
	*pap*GAP (class II) ($papG_{IA2}$)		Strongly associated with pyelonephritis and bacteremia
	*pap*G (class III) ($prsG_{J96}$)		Cystitis predominates among patients with urinary tract abnormalities
S/F1C fimbriae (MR)	*Sfa/fac*	Sialyl-(α-2-3) galactoside	Adherence inhibited by THP
Type 1C (MR)	*Fac*	Undetermined	Possibly associated with pyelonephritis
G fimbriae (MR)	—	Terminal *N*-acetyl-D-glucosamine	
M fimbriae (MR)	—	Galactose-*N*-acetyl-galactosamine Blood group M (glycophorin A)	—
Dr family (fimbriated and nonfimbriated)	*Drb* operon Adhesin (E gene) *Afa* E1-5 *Afa* F	Dr blood group antigen component of DAF (decay accelerating factor) and type IV collagen	16% of first-time cystitis isolates

PMN, polymorphonuclear neutrophil; MR, mannose resistant; MS, mannose sensitive. SIgA, secretory immunoglobulin A.

by the presence of virulence factors that enhance both colonization and invasion of the urinary tract and the capacity to produce disease. Cystitis and pyelonephritic *E. coli* isolates are genetically distinct, exhibiting differences in O, K, and H antigens. Genetic differences among uropathogens may be responsible for different clinical outcomes. Johnson and colleagues confirmed that certain O, K, and H serotypes are associated with urovirulence and with the presence and expression of multiple chromosomal virulence factor determinants.[27,28] Recognized virulence factors include increased adherence to vaginal and uroepithelial cells,[29] resistance to serum bactericidal activity, a higher quantity of K antigen (K1, K5, K12) in capsules, the presence of aerobactin, cytotoxic necrotizing factor type 1, and hemolysin production.[29] Recently, autotransported proteolytic toxin Sat, encoded in the *sat* gene, has been described and the importance of extracellular polysaccharide as a virulence factor suggested.[30,31] Genes for the various urovirulence factors are often duplicated in uropathogens and also frequently linked as large multigene chromosomal segments called *pathogenicity islands* and are absent in coliforms found in normal fecal flora.[32] Recently described putative virulence genes for *E. coli* urinary tract infection include *usp* coding, a uropathogenic specific protein, and *iro*N$_{Ecoli}$ coding, a catechol siderophore receptor homologue.[33] All uropathogens are able to use urine as a growth medium. Urine is, however, an incomplete growth medium; hence, the synthesis of one or more nutritional factors by uropathogenic *E. coli* is essential. Bacterial synthesis of guanine, arginine, and glutamine is required for optimal growth in urine.[34]

In particular, adhesive properties of the organism are involved in the selection of bacteria capable of colonizing the colon[24] and reaching and colonizing the normal urinary tract, and they influence the anatomic level of infection in the urinary tract (Table 66-1).[35] Accordingly, bacteria with enhanced adherence to vaginal and periurethral cells would be selected to colonize the anatomic regions adjacent to the urethral orifice. Human studies and the mouse model of nonobstructive ascending pyelonephritis have confirmed the significance of the adhesive capacity of the urinary pathogen in causing lower and upper tract infection.[36] *E. coli* pyelonephritis isolates adhere better than *E. coli* cystitis isolates, and urinary isolates tend to adhere more strongly to uroepithelial cells than do random fecal *E. coli* isolates. The adhesins of uropathogenic *E. coli* exist either as filamentous surface organelles termed *pili* or *fimbriae* or as nonfilamentous proteins in the outer membrane. The fimbrial structure consists of helically arranged protein units. Genes encoding the expression of fimbriae on uropathogenic *E. coli* have been found in the chromosomes, as opposed to the plasmid-encoded adhesins of enterotoxigenic *E. coli*. Methods such as electron microscopy and erythrocyte agglutination have been used to characterize fimbriae, and several

specific morphologic and functional types have been identified. Numerous uropathogenic strains adhere in the absence of fimbriae. The binding of *E. coli* to epithelial cell receptors containing globoseries glycosphingolipid accounts for the attachment of most strains that cause kidney infection and is not inhibited by mannose (this binding is called MR for mannose resistant).[37] Fimbriae attaching to globoseries receptors are termed *P fimbriae* because the receptor is a constituent of the P blood group antigen complex present in human erythrocytes and uroepithelial cells.[37] The glycosphingolipids, synthesized by specific glycosyltransferases, are components of the glycocalyx that surrounds epithelial cells; they consist of an oligosaccharide moiety on the cell surface covalently linked to a lipid position embedded in the outer leaflet of the plasma membrane. Glycosphingolipases are highly specific to a given host and play an important role both in determining tissue tropism for microbial pathogens and in an individual host's susceptibility to urinary tract infection. The globoseries glycosphingolipid receptors (gal-gal) are distributed throughout the urinary tract, particularly in the kidney.[37]

P fimbriae are frequently present in uropathogens. P fimbriae augment the virulence of uropathogenic *E. coli* at different stages of infection, including remaining longer in the intestinal tract and spreading more efficiently to the urinary tract for purposes of both colonizing and producing ascending infection.[24,38] Once in the urinary tract, P-fimbriated strains adhere, persist, and, despite enhancing epithelial cytokine response, invade the kidney and induce bacteremia.[38] The main subunit Pap A of P fimbriae gives rise in its polymerized form to fibrillin, the structural protein of the fimbriae, and the carrier molecule for the G adhesin (Pap G) at the tip of the fimbriae. A chromosomal gene cluster (genes *pap*A through I) code for different Pap proteins and for expression of the highly specific complex adhesion molecule.[29] P fimbriae reveal considerable antigenic variation, giving rise to multiple subgroups. Pap G tip adhesin of P fimbriae is essential in the pathogenesis of pyelonephritis. The *pap* gene EFG sequences encode the adhesin complex. Three molecular variants of Pap G adhesin, encoded by Pap G alleles I through IV, exhibit subtle receptor-binding preferences that influence clinical outcome. Allele II predominates among strains causing pyelonephritis and bacteremia, and class III allele is more commonly found in children and women with cystitis.[39-41] P fimbriae also appear to confer enhanced ability of *E. coli* uropathogenic clones to colonize the colon and spread to the perineum. Although relatively resistant to phagocytosis by neutrophils, *E. coli* with P fimbriae paradoxically enhance the host inflammatory response by inducing the elaboration of proinflammatory cytokines.[42] Neutrophils, however, lack receptors for P fimbriae. P-fimbriated *E. coli* dominate as a cause of pyelonephritis and urosepsis, and they especially dominate among blood isolates; nevertheless, downregulation of P-fimbriae expression may occur in the bacteria when they are within the kidney, and this would facilitate parenchymal persistence. There are limited studies that indicate that there is a potential for the development of P-fimbriae–containing vaccines. In the mouse model of pyelonephritis, antibodies directed against P fimbriae that block bacterial adherence to uroepithelial cells in vitro, prevent upper tract infection in vivo. With the same model, a vaccine utilizing P fimbriae has shown some encouraging results.

Binding of *E. coli* to mannose-containing host epithelial receptor glycoproteins uroplakin I and II occurs with most uropathogenic strains.[43] In fact, strains from cystitis patients are more likely to bind than those from pyelonephritis patients.[36] Fimbriae attaching to mannosylated proteins via FimH subunits are the common type 1 fimbriae (pili), and attachment is inhibited in the presence of mannose (MS, for mannose sensitive). Type 1 fimbriae bind mannose epitopes on secreted glycoproteins such as secretory immunoglobulin A (IgA) and urinary mucus, Tamm-Horsfall protein (THP), bladder uroplakin protein, and fibronectin.[44] Type 1 fimbriae are encoded by the *pil* or *fim* gene cluster, which includes nine genes that encode structural and regulatory proteins.[45] The gene *fim*A encodes the fimbrial subunit protein, which can be expressed independently of the *fim*H-encoded adhesin protein.[46] The *fim* DNA sequences encoding type 1 fimbriae occur in most clinical isolates; consequently, epidemiologic evidence of an association between type 1 fimbriae and the site or severity of infection is more difficult to obtain. Expression of type 1 fimbriae is not especially prevalent among pyelonephritogenic strains. Almost all cystitis-causing strains of *E. coli* express type 1 fimbriae. Experimental animal studies have correlated type 1 fimbriae with persistence of *E. coli* in the urinary tract, and the use of a *fim*H null mutant of a type 1–positive *E. coli* isolate resulted in rapid elimination of the mutant from the urinary tract. Similarly, clinical correlations in childhood urinary infections suggest that type 1 fimbriae contribute to virulence in the urinary tract when expressed in the background of a fully virulent uropathogen. Paradoxically, *fim*H also promotes adhesion to phagocytic cells that should presumably result in early bacterial clearance due to enhanced intracellular killing. In fact, antibody-opsonized and internalized type 1 fimbriae–bearing *E. coli* are rapidly killed. This is likely to occur within renal parenchyma, and hence type 1–fimbriated *E. coli* are programmed to shed their fimbriae upon reaching the renal pelvis. In contrast, *E. coli* internalized only by a type 1 fimbrial mechanism survive intracellularly within the phagocyte because the organism can attenuate, resulting in parasitism. Once inside the macrophage, the bacterium is safe from antibiotic assault, only to emerge later and possibly contribute to the relapse of bacteriuria.[47] Bacterial adherence to urinary catheters is also type 1 fimbriae dependent. Type 1 fimbriae–mediated attachment to mast cells and lymphocytes results in further release of cytokines, causing cell proliferation and secretion of antibodies.

In addition to type 1 and P fimbriae, a variety of adhesins, including S (7% of uropathogenic strains), type 1c, G, Dr fimbriae, and M and X adhesins[48] (with different molecular binding specificities and serologic properties), have been identified on uropathogenic strains of *E. coli* and are expressed in vivo in urine (see Table 66-1). The Dr hemagglutinin family includes both fimbrial and nonfimbrial adhesins. Four genes (*dra*A, B, C, D) that encode the structural proteins and adhesins of the fimbriae have been identified. The adhesins bind to the Dr blood group antigen component of decay-accelerating factor, which is widely distributed along the urinary tract. Dr-expressing uropathogens have a relatively low invasive potential and demonstrate low multiplication rates; however, Dr-positive *E. coli* persist in renal infections and may play a role in chronic pyelonephritis and interstitial nephritis.[48] Adherent bacteria not only persist within the urinary tract but have growth advantages and enhanced toxicity.[49] Type 1 pili and the Dr adhesin have been linked to bladder epithelial cell invasion and intracellular persistence by uropathogenic *E. coli*. A significant number of recurrent urinary tract infections are caused by the same bacterial strain as that isolated from the original infection, suggesting

possible reemergence of intracellular *E. coli* from the underlying bladder epithelium.[50] A possible correlation exists between the presence of bacterial adhesin and the difficulty in eradicating organisms with short-course antibiotic therapy.

Studies with other species of bacterial uropathogens, for example, *Proteus mirabilis* and *Klebsiella* species, have similarly demonstrated the significance of adherence in the pathogenesis of urinary infections.[51] *S. aureus* uncommonly causes cystitis and ascending pyelonephritis; in contrast, *Staphylococcus saprophyticus* is a frequent cause of lower urinary tract infections. *S. saprophyticus* adheres significantly better to uroepithelial cells than do *S. aureus* or *Staphylococcus epidermidis*.

Evaluation of urinary isolates for virulence characteristics in the presence of underlying structural abnormalities (e.g., severe reflux) frequently fails to demonstrate the typical bacterial virulence factors.[36] Similarly, *E. coli* blood isolates obtained from patients with urosepsis after bladder instrumentation lack virulence factors.[52] Virulence determinants are more frequently expressed by urinary isolates of *E. coli* obtained from women with cystitis than by fecal isolates from healthy women.[53] No difference in the prevalence of *E. coli* virulence determinants was found between the subjects with first-time cystitis and those with recurrent cystitis, suggesting that host rather than bacterial factors determine the risk for recurrent infection.[13] Stapleton and associates observed that *E. coli* isolates that caused cystitis in women using diaphragms with spermicides had fewer virulence determinants than those of nonusers,[53] suggesting that the use of diaphragms with spermicides may allow infection with less virulent *E. coli*. Recently, evidence has accumulated that quinolone-resistant uropathogenic *E. coli* are less virulent and have decreased invasive capacity.[54] Resistant organisms have been shown to have reduced type 1 fimbriae expression and proteolytic toxin Sat elaboration.[55] Trimethoprim-sulfamethoxazole, extensively used to prevent urinary infection, reduces the synthesis, expression, and adhesive function of type 1 fimbriae at concentrations well below the minimal inhibitory concentration.

The evaluation of the importance of adherence as a virulence factor is not complete without consideration of the role of the host. A difference in receptor density linked to a difference in genetic susceptibility to infection has been proposed. In women and children with recurrent urinary tract infection, an increased avidity of bacterial attachment to vaginal, periurethral, and uroepithelial[56] cells has been found. However, some authors have failed to corroborate these findings.[57]

Certain other characteristics of bacteria may be important in the production of upper tract infection. Motile bacteria can ascend in the ureter against the flow of urine, and the endotoxins of gram-negative bacilli have been shown to decrease ureteral peristalsis and to possibly contribute to the renal parenchymal inflammatory response by phagocytic cell activation.[58] In *Proteus* species, the production of urease by infecting microorganisms has been correlated with the ability to cause pyelonephritis. The presence of K capsular antigen protects bacteria from leukocyte phagocytosis. Most uropathogenic strains produce hemolysin, which facilitates tissue invasion and causes renal tubular epithelial and parenchymal cell damage, possibly making iron available to invading *E. coli*. The hemolysin gene is frequently located adjacent to genes encoding for serum resistance and sialic acid–specific (S) fimbriae, but the pathogenic role of hemolysis in pyelonephritis remains controversial.[59] Aerobactin, an iron-scavenging protein, or siderophore, is present with increased frequency in uropathogenic strains of *E. coli*.[29] Genes have now been identified that encode for their virulence factors; *hly*A (encoding hemolysin), *cnf*1 (encoding cytotoxic necrotizing factor 1), and *iut*A (encoding aerobactin receptor).

The greater the number of organisms delivered to the kidneys, the greater is the chance of producing infection. The kidney itself is not uniformly susceptible to infection—very few organisms are needed to infect the medulla, whereas 10,000 times as many are needed to infect the cortex.[60] The greater susceptibility of the medulla may be due to its high concentration of ammonia, which may inactivate complement, and to poor chemotaxis of polymorphonuclear neutrophils (PMNs) in an area of high osmolality, low pH, and low blood flow.[61]

Host

With the exception of urethral mucosa, the normal urinary tract is resistant to colonization by bacteria and for the most part efficiently and rapidly eliminates both pathogenic and nonpathogenic microorganisms that gain access to the bladder. This is achieved by the presence of several lower urinary tract antibacterial defense mechanisms (Table 66-2).

Uropathogenic clones elicit an inflammatory response at all levels in the urinary tract by stimulating uroepithelial and other cells to produce cytokines and other proinflammatory factors. The intensity and efficiency of a host response is genetically regulated and is a critical factor for the host-organism interaction in the urinary tract.[62] Systemic elaboration of interleukin 1β (IL-1β) and IL-6 may lead to fever and activation of the acute-phase response. Urine and serum IL-6 concentrations reflect the severity of infection, with the highest levels in pyelonephritis and bacteremia.[63] The chemotactic cytokine IL-8 is released at the mucosal site recruiting PMNs, resulting in pyuria and contributing to the eradication of bacteriuria. IL-8 receptor deficiency confers susceptibility to acute pyelonephritis.[64] Cytokine elaboration is a consequence of bacterial adherence to epithelial cells and to a lesser extent a consequence of bacterial lipopolysaccharide.

Direct contact between adherent bacteria and uroepithelial cells may also result in bacterial growth suppression. This antibacterial epithelial defense function is activated by transmembranous signals from bacteria attached to the host cell surface and involves adenylate cyclase activity.

Although urine is generally considered to be a good culture medium for most bacteria, it does possess antibacterial activity. Anaerobic bacteria and other fastidious organisms that make up most of the urethral flora generally do not multiply in urine. It has been shown that extremes of osmolality, a high urea concentration, and low pH levels are inhibitory for the growth of some of the bacteria that cause urinary tract infection.[65,66] Furthermore, the pH and osmolality of urine from pregnant women tend to be more suitable for bacterial growth than those of nonpregnant women, and these in turn are more suitable for bacterial growth than those of urine from men. The presence of glucose makes urine a better culture medium, whereas the addition of prostatic fluid to urine inhibits bacterial growth.[67] Furthermore, urine has been shown to inhibit the migrating, adhering, aggregating, and killing functions of PMNs.

The epithelial surface of the urinary tract is covered by a thin layer of both urine and fluid secreted by the epithelial cells. The epithelial secretions possess antimicrobial properties, mainly the product of neutrophils providing a surveillance function. Neutrophil defensins are 3- to 5-kDa disulfide cationic peptides; their presence on epithelial surfaces may play a role in clearance of adherent bacteria.

By means of its mannose-containing side chains, THP, secreted by cells of the ascending loop of Henle, binds strongly to *E. coli* that express type 1 and S fimbriae.[68] THP is the most abundant protein of renal origin in urine and may function as a urinary antibacterial defense mechanism by binding to mannose-sensitive (MS) strains of *E. coli,* preventing them from attaching to epithelial cell receptors (Fig. 66-3).[68] Significantly reduced levels of THP in older adults occur during episodes of urinary tract infection.

The flushing mechanism of the bladder exerts a major protective effect. When bacteria are introduced into the bladders of humans, there is a tendency for spontaneous clearance. Because flushing alone would probably not completely clear the bacteria, there must be additional protective factors. Certain host factors including bladder catheterization increase the susceptibility of uroepithelial cells to attachment by uropathogens, and this in turn increases susceptibility to bacteriuria.[69]

In a study of bladder defense mechanisms in dogs, Parsons and colleagues demonstrated an active antiadherence mechanism of bladder mucosa.[70] Pretreatment of the bladder with acid was shown to increase bacterial adherence 20- to 50-fold. The increased adherence was independent of the bacterial species employed. Histochemical studies revealed that bacterial adherence was increased by the removal of a surface mucopolysaccharide, glycosaminoglycan, which seems to be responsible for the natural resistance to adherence. Thus, normally small inocula of bacteria are probably unable to adhere, and they remain suspended in urine and are removed by voiding. In the presence of a larger inoculum of bacteria to the bladder, especially with good adhesive qualities, the primary defense of antiadherence may be overcome, colonization can occur, and subsequent bladder infection may result. After bladder infection, secondary defense mechanisms such as mobilization of leukocytes, phagocytosis, and bacterial destruction

TABLE 66-2 Antibacterial Host Defenses in the Urinary Tract

Urine (osmolality, pH, organic acids)
Urine flow and micturition
Urinary tract mucosa (bactericidal activity, cytokines)
Urinary inhibitors of bacterial adherence
   Tamm-Horsfall protein
   Bladder mucopolysaccharide
   Low-molecular-weight oligosaccharides
   Secretory immunoglobulin A (SIgA)
   Lactoferrin
Inflammatory response
   Polymorphonuclear neutrophils (PMNs)
   Cytokines
Immune system
   Humoral immunity
   Cell-mediated immunity
   Miscellaneous
      Prostatic secretions

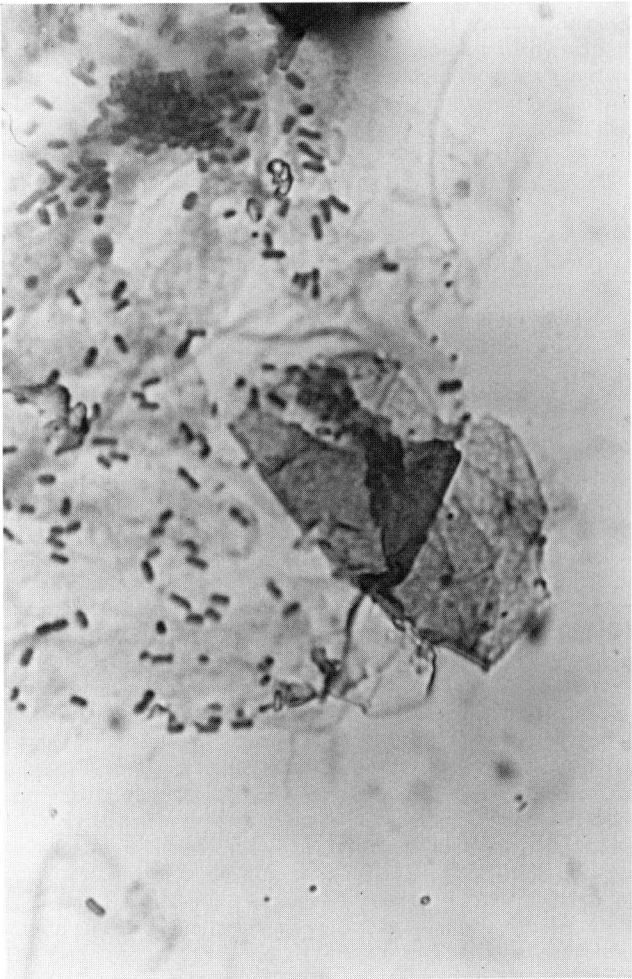

FIGURE 66-3. Light-microscopic specimen of urine showing uromucoid (Tamm-Horsfall protein) with large numbers of adherent uropathogenic bacteria.

remove bacteria. Bacteria stimulate PMNs to secrete IL-8, IL-1β, and tumor necrosis factor, and they stimulate lymphocytes to elaborate immunoregulatory cytokines ultimately resulting in immunoglobulin synthesis and modifying epithelial cell responses to bacteria. Epithelial cells participate in PMN recruitment by secreting neutrophil chemoattractants (e.g., IL-8) and by the expression of adhesion molecules involved in PMN transmigration (e.g., intercellular adhesion molecule 1).[64]

In women, colonization of the vaginal introitus and periurethral region by Enterobacteriaceae is critical in the pathogenesis of urinary tract infections.[23] Periurethral colonization with the same organism almost invariably precedes episodes of significant bacteriuria.[23,71,72] Microbiologic studies have demonstrated that the urethra, periurethral region, and vaginal vestibule of women with recurrent urinary tract infections tend to be more commonly colonized with coliform bacteria.[71,73] Stamey has postulated that such colonization is often the prelude to new infection and that women with recurrent urinary tract infection have a biologic predisposition to infection.[73] In a series of studies, the effects of several factors in vaginal secretions on colonization were examined. A low vaginal pH level was the most important factor related to a lack of colonization. Furthermore, serogroups of uropathogenic *E. coli* were more resistant to low pH levels. It was also found in these studies that *E. coli* was less susceptible to the inhibitory effects of vaginal fluid than *P. mirabilis* or *Pseudomonas aeruginosa*. Finally, it was noted by others that *E. coli* adhered more avidly to vaginal epithelial cells of women and young girls with recurrent urinary tract infection.[56] These observations, together with experimental studies using inbred mice, suggest predisposition of some women to urinary tract infection due to genetically determined host cell receptors for uropathogenic *E. coli*. This is supported by several epidemiologic studies demonstrating that women who are epithelial antigen and receptor nonsecretors have an increased risk for urinary tract infection, and their uroepithelial cells bind *E. coli* more avidly than do cells from secretors.[74] The secretor gene *Se* encodes a glycosyltransferase that transfers a fucose residue to specific acceptor molecules, resulting in detectable blood group antigens in secretions of people carrying the gene.[75] The Lewis gene acts on the same acceptor molecules, and Lewis blood type reflects the synthesis of ABH blood group antigens. Nonsecretors, who appear to have an increased susceptibility to urinary infections, express two unique globoseries glycosphingolipids present on vaginal and uroepithelial cells that preferentially bind uropathogenic *E. coli* that express class II *pap*-encoded adhesin. Other endogenous factors, such as estrogenic hormones, may influence bacterial attachment to uroepithelial cells and affect the risk for urinary tract infection.[76] From an acquired or behavioral point of view, both colonization of the vaginal introitus and bacteriuria due to *E. coli* have been strongly associated with diaphragm and spermicide use, which may contribute to the increased risk for urinary tract infection associated with sexual activity.[11,12] The dominant pathogenic mechanism is probably related to the differential antibacterial effect of nonoxynol-9, whereby more susceptible lactobacilli are replaced by coliform uropathogens.

Not all authors agree that periurethral colonization is the most important factor in the pathogenesis of recurrent urinary tract infection.[77] They point out that vestibular colonization with Enterobacteriaceae is as common in women not prone to infection. Furthermore, Parsons and Schmidt found no enhanced bacterial adherence to vaginal epithelial cells in women with recurrent urinary tract infection,[57] and Kurdydyk and co-workers studied IgG and IgA levels in cervicovaginal washings and found no difference between washings from women prone to infection and those from women with no past history of urinary tract infection.[78] Kunin and associates stated that all women who do not have a structural or neurologic problem in the voiding mechanism are approximately at the same risk for having a first urinary tract infection.[71] There exists the view that once established, each infection sets the stage for the next episode, because infection, and the antibiotic treatment thereof, may lead to colonization unless vaginal and periurethral colonization is eradicated by therapy. Antibiotics, especially β-lactams, promote vestibular colonization with *E. coli*. The longer the interval between infections, the less likelihood there is for recurrences. The antagonists to Stamey's hypothesis have concluded that the decisive factor is not the colonization of the periurethral area per se but rather the ability of these organisms to ascend the urethra, including the ability of infecting organisms to adhere to mucosal cells and withstand normal host defense mechanisms.

The role of humoral immunity in the host's defense against infection of the urinary tract, although extensively studied, is poorly understood.[79] During acute pyelonephritis, there is a systemic antibody response. Antibodies against the O antigen and occasionally the K antigen of the infecting strain have been found, and antibodies to type 1 and P fimbriae were described.[80] IgM antibodies dominate in the response to the first upper tract infection but not to subsequent episodes. High levels of IgG antibodies to lipid A correlate with the severity of renal infection and the progression of renal parenchymal destruction. An antibody response consisting of IgG and secretory IgA antibodies can be detected in the urine. In contrast to upper tract infection, lower urinary infection is usually associated with a reduced or nondetectable serologic response, reflecting the superficial nature of the infection. Macrophages are well distributed in the submucosa throughout the urinary tract, and Ia-expressing cells, analogous to Langerhans cells, have been identified in the urinary mucosa, including among renal tubular cells.[81] IgA-producing lymphocytes are found in the submucosa of infected rat bladders. Similarly, Christmas observed high numbers of IgA-producing plasma cells in the bladder submucosa of patients with bacterial cystitis in comparison with healthy controls.[82] Finally, in animal models, antibody-secreting cells and B lymphocytes migrate to kidney and urinary tract submucosa during urinary tract infections. The reduced immunologic response to the infecting organism in cystitis may explain reinfection with the same strain. Hopkins and associates, however, using a monkey model, reported the production of systemic and urinary IgG and IgA that accompanied experimental cystitis.[83]

In particular, antifimbrial antibodies are absent in the urine in lower tract infection. At least one third of women with a second urinary tract infection have an identical strain isolated, indicating incomplete or inadequate immunity with a single episode of infection.[84] Local coating of bacteria with antibodies within the kidney (and prostate) has formed the basis of localization techniques that clarified modern approaches to therapy.

In spite of the impressive systemic and local urinary antibody production that follows acute pyelonephritis, the protective role of these antibodies is unclear. When bacteria persist in the kidney for several months, antigenic drift may occur. Antibodies against several bacterial structures, including O and K antigen and more recently fimbrial antigens, have been found to protect against hematogenous or ascending pyelonephritis in experimental animals. Animal recipients of vaccines based on Pap A fimbriae were protected against experimental pyelonephritis caused by homologous and heterologous Gal-Gal–binding uropathogenic *E. coli* strains. Militating against an important role for urinary and systemic antibodies are experimental studies with mice exhibiting profound B-cell immunodeficiency and a normal capacity to clear experimental ascending urinary tract infection.

Antibodies may be of value in limiting the damage incurred within the kidney or preventing colonization preceding recurrence. Svanborg-Eden and Svennerholm reported that the urine of patients with pyelonephritis inhibited the adherence of *E. coli* to uroepithelial cells and that this activity was removed by absorption with O antigen.[85] Antibodies have not been shown to protect against bladder infection. Cell-mediated immunity has not been shown to play a major role in host defenses against urinary tract infection. Urinary tract mucosa contains few T lymphocytes, although both CD4+ and CD8+ T cells can be found in the submucosa and lamina propria; however, they generally lack γδ T cells.[86] Experimental studies in athymic mice showed similar resistance to intravesical infections when compared with normal controls. Similarly, clinical experience in human immunodeficiency virus (HIV)-infected women with severe defects in cell-mediated immunity, including low CD4 lymphocyte counts, does not indicate increased susceptibility to or severity of urinary infection.[87] Nevertheless, a useful role for cell-mediated immunity may still exist in that T-cell–derived proinflammatory cytokines (e.g., interferon-γ) stimulate epithelial cells to produce IL-6 in a similar manner to helper T cell (Th2) lymphocyte responses involving IL-4, IL-5, IL-10, and IL-13.[42] Thus, urinary tract T cells producing immunoregulatory cytokines may influence the mucosal epithelial cell response to bacterial adherence and invasion. The IL-6 secreted by renal tubular epithelial cells[42] may contribute to mucosal antibacterial activity by increasing IgA secretion by committed B cells.

During pyelonephritis, an acute inflammatory exudate consisting predominantly of PMNs is present. Although the inflammatory reaction is directed at limiting bacterial spread and persistence within the kidney, infiltrating phagocytic cells may contribute to tissue damage[62] and renal scarring, as evidenced by reduced parenchymal kidney destruction in experimental neutropenia. It has been suggested that chronic pyelonephritis and persistent renal damage may develop after successful eradication of bacterial pyelonephritis with antimicrobial therapy. According to these concepts, bacterial remnants or antigen or THP persistence induces a chronic humoral immunologic response resulting in cryptogenic renal scarring.

The binding capacity of vaginal fluid from women colonized with *E. coli* is greater than that from noncolonized women, and it correlates with susceptibility to urinary tract infection. Secretory IgA is one of three glycoproteins that bind type 1 *E. coli* and could affect vaginal colonization.[88]

Several abnormalities of the urinary tract interfere with its natural resistance to infection. Obstruction to urine flow is the most important of these. Extrarenal obstruction can result from congenital anomalies of the ureter or urethra, such as valves, stenosis, or bands; calculi; extrinsic ureteral compression from a variety of causes; and benign prostatic hypertrophy. Intrarenal obstruction may be produced by entities such as nephrocalcinosis, uric acid nephropathy, analgesic nephropathy, polycystic kidney disease, hypokalemic nephropathy, and the renal lesions of sickle cell trait or disease. Obstruction inhibits the normal flow of urine, and the resulting stasis is important in increasing susceptibility to infection.

In animals, obstruction of a ureter markedly increases susceptibility to hematogenous infection. Intrarenal obstruction, experimentally produced by scars in a variety of ways, also increases the susceptibility of the kidney to infection. Medullary scars, which produce greater amounts of obstruction than cortical scars, increase the susceptibility of animals to infection more than cortical scars.[89] Furthermore, the intravenous injection of *E. coli* in animals with renal scars from prior staphylococcal pyelonephritis produces pyelonephritis in the regions of intrarenal hydronephrosis caused by the old scars.[90] Men of any age and pregnant women are the most prone to lesions that result in obstruction to the free flow of urine.

Calculi may increase susceptibility to urinary tract infection by producing obstruction (Fig. 66-4). However, not all stones obstruct, and local irritative phenomena may also be important. Furthermore, calculi may develop secondary to infection. It has been observed clinically and experimentally that *Proteus* species and other urea-splitting organisms are most likely to produce calculi. Furthermore, bacteria survive deep within the calculi and are extremely difficult to eradicate even by artificial means, such as by incubating in solutions containing antibiotics or iodine and alcohol. This may account for the well-known difficulties encountered clinically in trying to cure urinary tract infection in the presence of stones.

Vesicoureteral reflux and urinary tract infection are also intricately related. Reflux due to a congenital abnormality, to bladder overdistention, or to unknown causes probably contributes to upper tract infection via the ascending route. On the other hand, clinical observations have demonstrated that infection may, in fact, produce reflux, especially in children.[91] Reflux tends to perpetuate infection by maintaining a residual pool of infected urine in the bladder after voiding. It is probable that reflux, especially in young children, plays an important role in the production of upper tract infection and subsequent scarring. Patients with

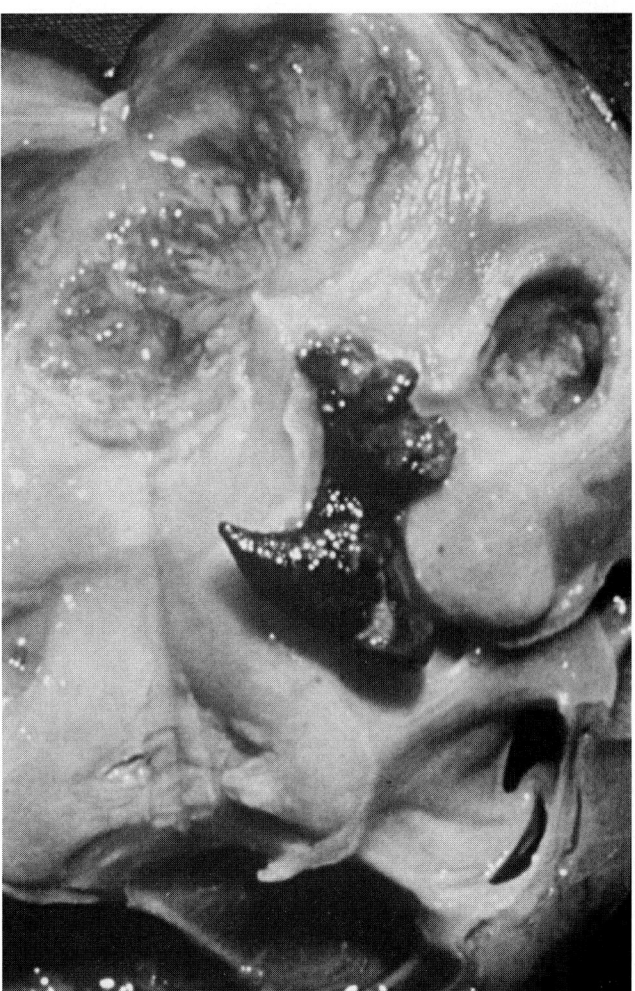

FIGURE 66-4. Staghorn calculus visible in the dilated pelvis of a hydronephrotic kidney. *(Courtesy of M. Bergeron, M.D.)*

incomplete emptying of the bladder for either mechanical reasons (bladder neck obstruction, urethral valves, urethral strictures, prostatic hypertrophy) or neurogenic malfunction (poliomyelitis, tabes dorsalis, diabetic neuropathy, cord injuries) are prone to frequent urinary tract infections. These patients are subject to bladder overdistention, which may interfere with local defense mechanisms, and, most importantly, frequent instrumentation of the urinary tract.

EPIDEMIOLOGY OF URINARY TRACT INFECTION

Infecting Organisms

More than 95% of urinary tract infections are caused by a single bacterial species. There is a great difference between the bacterial flora of the urine in patients with an initial episode of urinary tract infection and the flora from those with frequent recurrences of infection. *E. coli* is by far the most frequent infecting organism in acute infection.[92,93] In recurrent urinary tract infections, especially in the presence of structural abnormalities of the urinary tract (such as obstructive uropathy, congenital anomalies, neurogenic bladder, and fistulous communication involving the urinary tract), the relative frequency of infection caused by *Proteus, Pseudomonas, Klebsiella,* and *Enterobacter* species and by enterococci and staphylococci increases greatly. In the presence of structural abnormalities, it is also relatively common to isolate multiple organisms from the urine. Because instrumentation and repeated courses of antimicrobial therapy are common in these patients, antibiotic-resistant isolates might be expected.

The hospital environment is an important determinant of the nature of the bacterial flora in urinary tract infection. *Proteus, Klebsiella, Enterobacter,* and *Pseudomonas* species and staphylococci and enterococci are more often isolated from inpatients, whereas there is a greater preponderance of *E. coli* in an outpatient population.[94] Cross-infections are important in the pathogenesis of hospital-related urinary tract infections, especially with indwelling catheters.[95] *Corynebacterium urealyticum (Corynebacterium* group D2) has been recognized as an important nosocomial pathogen.[96] This gram-positive, urea-splitting, slow-growing bacillus may cause infected mucosal encrustations of the bladder and urinary collecting system, especially in immunosuppressed patients and in particular in renal transplant recipients. It is highly resistant to antimicrobial agents, although it is usually sensitive to vancomycin.[97] It should be considered in the presence of high urine pH, urologic problems, previous urinary tract infection, and recent antibiotic treatment.

Anaerobic organisms are rarely pathogens in the urinary tract. A variety of bacteria may be found in the urine in specific clinical settings. Fungi (particularly *Candida* species) occur in patients with indwelling catheters who are receiving antimicrobial therapy.[98] Coagulase-negative staphylococci are a common cause of urinary tract infection in some reports.[99] *S. saprophyticus* tends to cause infection in young women of a sexually active age,[100] accounting for 5% to 15% of acute cystitis episodes in the United States. Coagulase-positive staphylococci most often invade the kidney from the hematogenous route, resulting in intrarenal or perinephric abscesses. DNA typing of *E. coli* has substantially aided in the epidemiologic study of urinary tract infection.

Adenoviruses (particularly type 11) have been strongly implicated as causative agents in hemorrhagic cystitis in pediatric patients, especially boys, and in allogeneic bone marrow transplant recipients.[101,102] Cell wall–deficient bacteria have been demonstrated in urine from patients with pyelonephritis, particularly in association with therapy using cell wall–active antibiotics. However, these forms have not been consistently isolated from either urine or renal tissue despite the use of adequate techniques and are probably not of major importance.

Although various investigators, using special media, have isolated fastidious organisms from women with lower tract symptoms, the causal role of these organisms is controversial. Similarly, *Gardnerella vaginalis* is frequently isolated from the urine of women with and without urinary tract symptoms, but its pathogenic role is unclear. *Ureaplasma urealyticum* and *Mycoplasma hominis* are possible but unproven causes of pyelonephritis and cystourethritis.

One group has reported nanobacteria as tiny (0.05 to 0.5 mm) cell wall–possessing bacteria that are associated with renal stones.[103] In vitro, the organisms produce carbonate apatite that can fix calcium. In clinical material, all 30 kidney stones were positive for a nanobacteria-specific protein epitope, and organisms were seen in all 30 specimens examined by immunofluorescence microscopy. Others have been unable to reproduce these results.

Bacteriuria in Children

The problem of urinary tract infection spans all age-groups, beginning with neonates.[104] The frequency of urinary tract infection in infants is about 1% to 2%. It is much more common in boys during the first 3 months and thereafter occurs more often in girls. Bacteremia is common in association with urinary tract infection in male newborns. Autopsy series of infants with pyelonephritis have revealed a predominance of infant boys with pyelonephritis. A lack of circumcision predisposes to urinary tract infection in infants and young boys.[105,106]

During the preschool years, urinary tract infection is more common in girls than in boys. When infection occurs in preschool boys, it is frequently associated with serious congenital abnormalities. With repeated study over a period of 1 year, the period prevalence of significant bacteriuria in this age group is 4.5% for girls and about 0.5% for boys. Infections during this period often are symptomatic, and it is believed that much of the renal damage that occurs in association with urinary tract infection takes place at this time (Fig. 66-5).[107]

Much information on the natural history and epidemiology of urinary tract infection has been gleaned from the studies of Kunin and associates[108,109] with schoolchildren from central Virginia. It was found that bacteriuria is common in girls in this population, is often asymptomatic, and frequently recurs. For example, the prevalence of bacteriuria among schoolgirls was about 1.2%, and about 5% of the girls had significant bacteriuria at some time before leaving high school. About one third of these patients had some symptom referable to the urinary tract when the bacteriuria was first detected. It was shown that

FIGURE 66-5. Vesicoureteral reflux in a young girl with recurrent urinary tract infections. A, Right kidney demonstrates grade II reflux. **B,** Left kidney shows dilatation of the ureter, grade III reflux, and calyceal clubbing. *(Courtesy of T. Slovis, M.D.)*

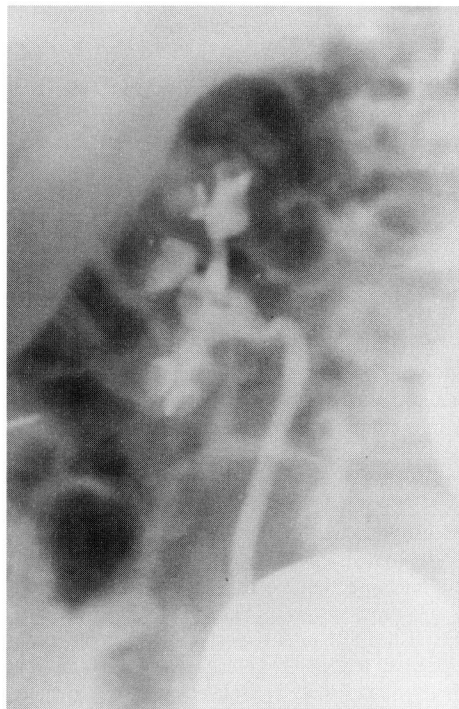

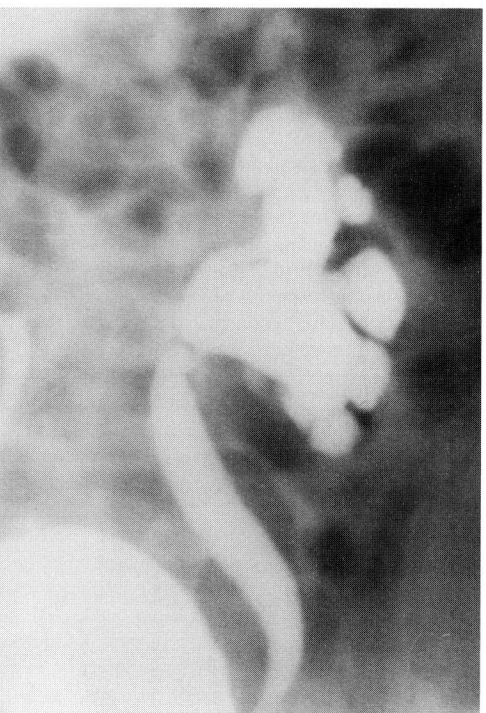

A

B

each year about 0.3% to 0.4% of the female population (25% of those infected) was cured either spontaneously or with antimicrobial agents, and an equal number of girls developed new cases of bacteriuria. Bacteriuria was rare in schoolboys (prevalence, 0.03%).

These studies also provided an opportunity to treat the patients and follow their clinical course. Patients were initially treated for 10 days to 2 weeks. Girls with frequent infections were given longer courses of therapy (1 to 3 months). White girls tended to have frequent reinfections, whereas black girls became reinfected less frequently. With each course of therapy, about 20% of white girls went into long-term remission. However, when many of these girls were married or became pregnant, bacteriuria recurred at a rate far above that expected for the general population. Over 50% developed bacteriuria within 3 months after marriage. Thus, the presence of bacteriuria in childhood defines a population at higher risk for the development of bacteriuria in adulthood.

Bacteriuria in Adults

Once adulthood is reached, the prevalence of asymptomatic bacteriuria increases in the female population. The prevalence of bacteriuria in young nonpregnant women is about 1% to 3%.[110] Each year, about 25% of bacteriuric women clear their bacteriuria, and an equal number become infected (often women who have had urinary infection previously). Up to 40% to 50% of the female population will experience a symptomatic urinary tract infection at some time during their life.[111] Frequent sexual intercourse, diaphragm use (especially with use of a spermicide), lack of urination after intercourse, and a history of recurrent infections are risk factors for urinary infection in women.[1,111,112] The diaphragm can cause urinary obstruction in some women, but its main effect is probably a change in vaginal flora due to the spermicide.[111] The risk for a second urinary tract infection in young women is greater than that for the first, with at least 20% developing a recurrent infection by the 6-month follow-up.[111] *E. coli* causing urinary tract infection may be transmitted between sexual partners, as the same strains have been found in the urine of men who are sexual partners of women with urinary tract infection.[113]

The prevalence of bacteriuria in adult men is low (0.1% or less) until the later years, when it rises. The increase in bacteriuria in older men is probably in part related to prostatic disease and the resultant instrumentation. Men with bacteriuria frequently have anatomic abnormalities of the urinary tract. In young men, a lack of circumcision increases the risk for urinary tract infection caused by uropathogenic strains of *E. coli*, including the development of symptomatic urethritis.[114] Male homosexuality is a risk factor, probably related to rectal insertive intercourse.

Bacteriuria in the Older Adult Population

At least 10% of men and 20% of women older than 65 years have asymptomatic bacteriuria. In contrast to young adults, among whom bacteriuria is 30 times more frequent in women than in men, in those older than 65 years the ratio alters dramatically, with a progressive decrease in the female-to-male ratio.[115,116] In both sexes, the prevalence of bacteriuria rises substantially. Possible reasons for the high frequency of urinary tract infections in older adults include obstructive uropathy from the prostate and loss of the bactericidal activity of prostatic secretions in men, poor emptying of the bladder due to prolapse in women, soiling of the perineum from fecal incontinence in demented women, and neuromuscular diseases and increased instrumentation and bladder catheter usage in both sexes.[116] There is a high rate of spontaneous cure and reinfection in both women and men.[116] The spectrum of microorganisms is unaltered in older adults. Asymptomatic bacteriuria is much more frequent than symptomatic urinary tract infection.

Bacteriuria in Patients with Other Conditions

There is a higher prevalence of bacteriuria in hospitalized patients than in outpatients. The general ill health of hospitalized patients and the higher probability of urinary tract instrumentation are probably the major contributors to these differences.

A single catheterization causes urinary tract infection in only about 1% of ambulatory persons.[14] However, after catheterization of hospitalized patients, infection occurs in at least 10%. Race apparently does not appreciably affect the prevalence of bacteriuria. However, socioeconomic status is important, with pregnant women from lower socioeconomic groups having a higher prevalence of bacteriuria.[117]

Various underlying diseases have also been associated with an increased frequency of urinary tract infection. Diabetic women but not men have been found to have a higher prevalence of asymptomatic bacteriuria than nondiabetic patients.[118,119]

Black women with sickle cell trait have a higher prevalence of bacteriuria during pregnancy than black women without the sickle trait.[120] Other conditions stated to be associated with urinary tract infection (but without documentation) include chronic potassium deficiency, gout, hypertension, and other conditions causing interstitial renal disease. There is an increased frequency and severity (more sepsis) of urinary tract infection in men with HIV infection and CD4 counts below 200.[121] There is no evidence for an increase in frequency or severity in women with HIV infection. However, one recent study found an association in women with increased viral loads but not decreased CD4 counts.[87]

At least 50% of renal transplant patients develop urinary tract infection in the early postoperative period, with about a 40% incidence of bacteremia.[122,123] Some centers advocate routine use of antibacterial prophylaxis to prevent urinary tract infection after renal transplantation. Regardless of whether prophylaxis is given, early diagnosis and therapy of urinary tract infection is important in these patients.

Table 66-3 lists risk factors for urinary tract infections.

TABLE 66-3 Risk Factors for Urinary Tract Infection		
	Female	*Male*
All Ages	Previous urinary tract infection	Lack of circumcision (children and young adults)
	Urologic instrumentation or surgery	Urologic instrumentation or surgery
	Urethral catheterization	Urethral catheterization
	Urinary tract obstruction, including calculi	Urinary tract obstruction including calculi
	Neurogenic bladder	Neurogenic bladder
	Renal transplantation	Renal transplantation
Adults	Sexual intercourse	Insertive rectal intercourse
	Lack of urination after intercourse	
	Spermicidal contraceptive jellies	
	Diaphragm use	
	Pregnancy	
	Lower socioeconomic group	
	Diabetes	
	Sickle cell trait in pregnancy	
	Human immunodeficiency virus with high viral load	
Older Age	Functional or mental impairment	Functional or mental impairment
	Estrogen deficiency (loss of vaginal lactobacilli)	Prostatic enlargement
	Bladder prolapse	Condom catheter drainage

CLINICAL MANIFESTATIONS

Symptoms

Urinary tract infection in children tends to manifest with different symptoms depending on the age of the child. Symptoms in neonates and children younger than 2 years are nonspecific.[104,106] Failure to thrive, vomiting, and fever seem to be the major manifestations. When children older than 2 years (and more consistently, older than 5 years) develop infection, they are more likely to display localized symptoms such as frequency, dysuria, and abdominal or flank pain.

The manifestations of urinary tract infection in adults are usually easy to recognize. The lower tract symptoms result from bacteria producing irritation of urethral and vesical mucosa, causing frequent and painful urination of small amounts of turbid urine. Patients sometimes complain of suprapubic heaviness or pain. Occasionally, the urine is grossly bloody or shows a bloody tinge at the end of micturition. Fever tends to be absent in infection limited to the lower tract.

The classic clinical manifestation of upper urinary tract infection includes fever (sometimes with chills), flank pain, and frequently lower tract symptoms (e.g., frequency, urgency, and dysuria). At times, the lower tract symptoms antedate the appearance of fever and upper tract symptoms by 1 or 2 days. It should be recognized that the symptoms described, although classic, may vary greatly. In fact, pyelonephritis may show protean clinical manifestations in adults as well as in children. Flank tenderness or discomfort is frequent in upper tract infection in adults and is more intense when there is obstructive disease. Severe pain with radiation into the groin is rare in acute pyelonephritis per se and suggests the presence of a renal calculus. The pain from the kidney is occasionally felt in or near the epigastrium and may radiate to one of the lower quadrants. These manifestations may offer difficulties in differential diagnosis and suggest gallbladder disease or appendicitis.

The vast majority of older adult patients with urinary infection are asymptomatic.[115,116] Symptoms, when present, are often not diagnostic, because noninfected older adults often experience frequency, dysuria, hesitancy, and incontinence. Furthermore, symptoms of upper tract infection are often atypical, suggesting processes other than in the urinary tract (e.g., abdominal pain, change in mental status). Nevertheless, typical symptoms may occur. Gleckman and associates found a much higher frequency of bacteremia (61%) associated with pyelonephritis in older adult patients than is found in young patients, and shock commonly supervened.[124] Most of the patients had significant urologic abnormalities. The effect of asymptomatic bacteriuria on the general sense of well-being, appetite, and urinary continence has been studied, and no association could be demonstrated.[115,125,126]

The clinical manifestations of recurrent or persistent urinary tract infection are more difficult to define. Patients with lower urinary tract involvement tend to have repeated bouts of transient symptomatic or asymptomatic infection. Patients with upper tract infection may have episodes of fever, pain in the renal regions, and dysuria during acute exacerbations or new bouts of infection. However, upper tract infection may result in only lower tract symptoms or no symptoms at all. Patients with urinary tract infection in the presence of an indwelling urinary catheter usually have no lower tract symptoms, but flank pain or fever may occur. Urinary tract infection is the most common source of bacteremia produced by gram-negative bacilli. Bacteremia may occur with no urinary symptoms, especially in the presence of an indwelling catheter.

Because symptoms of urinary tract infection are often difficult to elicit in older adults because of the presence of dementia, indwelling urinary catheters, and the atypical symptoms often seen in this population, a diagnosis of urosepsis may be made erroneously in the absence of urinary symptoms because of the presence of bacteriuria (which is often present in this population).

Alterations in Renal Function

In experimentally produced pyelonephritis, the only consistent abnormality of renal function is the inability to concentrate the urine maximally.[127,128] The mechanism of the concentrating defect is not clear but seems to be related in experimental animals to inflammation and perhaps to the increased production of prostaglandins.[128] The concentrating defect occurs early in the course of experimental infection and is rapidly reversible with antimicrobial therapy and with the administration of prostaglandin inhibitors. The same phenomenon occurs in humans.

Progressive destruction of the kidney (particularly in the presence of obstruction) may occur and give rise to clinical manifestations of renal insufficiency. Bilateral papillary necrosis can occasionally lead to rapidly progressive renal failure.

DIAGNOSIS

Presumptive Diagnosis of Urinary Tract Infection

Microscopic examination of the urine is the first step in the laboratory diagnosis of urinary tract infection. Using the preferred definition of pyuria, which is at least 10 leukocytes/mm^3 of midstream urine by counting chamber, the vast majority of patients with either symptomatic or asymptomatic bacteriuria have pyuria. In fact, with symptomatic infection most have hundreds of leukocytes per cubic millimeter. A less reliable method is to obtain a clean-catch midstream urine specimen, centrifuge it for 5 minutes at 2000 rpm, and then examine the sediment under high power. With this method, 5 to 10 leukocytes per high-power field in the sediment is the upper limit of normal. It should be emphasized that the finding of pyuria is nonspecific, and patients with pyuria may or may not have infection.[129] However, pyuria without infection remains common.[130]

The dipstick leukocyte esterase test is a rapid screening test for detecting pyuria. Although the sensitivity and specificity are high for detecting more than 10 white blood cells/mm^3 of urine (75% to 96% and 94% to 98%, respectively), patients with a negative leukocyte esterase test and urinary tract infection symptoms should have a urine microscopic examination for pyuria or a urine culture.[131-133]

Microscopic or sometimes gross hematuria is occasionally seen in patients with urinary tract infection (i.e., hemorrhagic cystitis). However, red blood cells may be indicative of other disorders such as calculi, tumor, vasculitis, glomerulonephritis, and renal tuberculosis. White cell casts in the presence of an acute infectious process are strong evidence for pyelonephritis, but the absence of white cell casts does not rule out upper tract infection. White cell casts can also be seen in renal disease in the absence of infection.

Proteinuria is a common but not universal finding in urinary tract infection. Most patients with urinary tract infection excrete less than 2 g of protein in 24 hours; excretion of 3 g or more suggests glomerular disease.

One of the most useful tests for the presumptive diagnosis of urinary tract infection is the microscopic examination of a specimen for bacteria. The ability to identify bacteria in the urine depends on whether the specimen has been centrifuged and on whether it has been stained with Gram or methylene blue stain (Table 66-4). Smaller numbers of bacteria can be detected microscopically in a stained than in an unstained specimen, and smaller numbers can be detected in centrifuged urine sediment than in uncentrifuged urine. The presence of at least one bacterium per oil immersion field in a midstream, clean-catch, Gram-stained, uncentrifuged urine correlates with 10^5 bacteria or more per milliliter of urine. As this titer is regarded to represent significant bacteriuria, Gram staining of an uncentrifuged specimen is an easy, rapid, and relatively reliable way to detect significant numbers of organisms. The absence of bacteria in several fields in a stained sedimented specimen indicates the probability of fewer than 10^4 bacteria/mL.

TABLE 66-4 Bacterial Count by Direct Examination of Urine: CFU/mL Extrapolated from the Finding of One Bacterium per Microscopic Field

	Unstained (×400)	Stained (×1000)
Uncentrifuged sample	≥10^6	≥10^5
Centrifuged sample	≥10^5	≥10^4

CFU, colony-forming units.

A number of rapid indirect methods have been devised to detect bacteriuria for presumptive diagnosis. Most common are tests that detect the presence of urine nitrite, which is formed when bacteria reduce the nitrate that is normally present.[131,132] False-negative tests are common, especially in the detection of low-count bacteriuria (10^2 to 10^3/mL and with certain bacterial species) but false-positive results are unusual. Automated rapid screening tests have become available that may be cost-effective for processing large numbers of samples.

Diagnosis of Urinary Tract Infection by Culture

General

Urine in the bladder is normally sterile. Because the urethra and periurethral areas are very difficult to sterilize, even the most carefully collected specimens (including those obtained by catheterization) are frequently contaminated. By quantitating bacteria in midstream, clean-voided urine, it is possible statistically to separate contamination from urinary tract infection. Patients with infection usually have at least 10^5 bacteria/mL in urine in the bladder, and therefore voided urine usually contains at least 10^5 bacteria/mL. Patients without infection have sterile bladder urine, and with proper collection, voided urine usually contains less than 10^4 bacteria/mL. However, it is important to remember that about one third of young women with symptomatic lower tract infection have fewer than 10^5 bacteria/mL of urine (see "Urinary Tract Infection with Low Numbers of Organisms," later). It is likely that a significant proportion of other patients with both symptomatic and asymptomatic infection have fewer than 10^5 bacteria/mL of urine. The Infectious Diseases Society of America consensus definition of cystitis for use in antibiotic treatment studies is 10^3 colony-forming units (CFU)/mL or more of a uropathogen (sensitivity 80% and specificity 90%) and for pyelonephritis 10^4 CFU/mL or more (sensitivity 90% and specificity 95%).[134] In more recent practice guidelines, 10^2 CFU/mL or more of a uropathogen was used to define cystitis.[135] These concentrations of microorganisms can be identified by standard microbiologic techniques in most clinical laboratories.

Calibrated loops serve as a simple inexpensive way to examine quantitatively the bacteriologic characteristics of urine specimens. Platinum loops that deliver 0.01 mL and 0.001 mL are used to streak urine onto agar plates. After incubation at 37° C for 24 hours, the number of CFUs is counted, and the total number of organisms originally present in 1 mL of the specimen is estimated by multiplying the colony count by 10^2 or 10^3, respectively. A further refinement of the technique involves the use of differential agars to allow isolation from mixed cultures and more rapid identification. Other methods such as the dip inoculum method, in which an agar-coated glass slide is dipped into urine, have excellent correlations with calibrated-loop techniques and are available inexpensively for office use.

Acceptable methods for urine collection include (1) midstream clean catch, (2) catheterization, and (3) suprapubic aspiration. The clean-catch method is preferred for the routine collection of urine for culture. It avoids the risk for infection inherent in catheterization. The patient must be instructed in the proper technique of obtaining the urine; this is especially important in women. The woman should wash her hands, straddle the commode (facing the back of the commode), wash the vulva from front to back four times with four different sterile gauze pads soaked in green soap or another appropriate cleansing agent, and then rinse with two more sponges soaked in sterile distilled water. She should then spread the labia and void, discarding the first portion of urine and collecting the second. The urine should be processed immediately, or if refrigerated at 4° C, it can be cultured within 24 hours.

A recent study, which requires validation, has challenged the need for cleansing or for using a midstream specimen from women in collecting urine for culture. The investigators found that contamination rates were similar when midstream urine was collected after cleansing and when it was collected without cleansing.[136]

In men, the prepuce should be retracted, and thereafter the technique is similar to that for women. In infants and small children, sterile bags have been used for the collection of urine, but contamination is common.[137]

In patients unable to cooperate, such as those with an altered sensorium or those who are unable to void for neurologic or urologic reasons, catheterization may be necessary. When catheterization is performed, scrupulous aseptic technique should be observed.

The suprapubic aspiration method has been established as a safe technique in premature infants, neonates, children, adults, and even pregnant patients,[106,120,137] but it is rarely used. With this method, the bladder must be full. The patient refrains from voiding until the bladder can be percussed above the symphysis pubis, and suprapubic pressure causes the urge to void. After preparation of the skin, the bladder is then punctured above the symphysis pubis with a 22-gauge needle on a syringe (local anesthesia is not required). After the procedure, self-limited hematuria may be observed. Suprapubic aspiration may be indicated in special clinical situations such as in pediatric practice when urine is difficult to obtain. Another situation is the rare case of an adult in whom infection is suspected, results obtained from more routine procedures have been confusing or equivocal, and diagnosis is critical.

If there are more than 10^5 bacteria/mL in a clean-catch urine specimen from an asymptomatic woman, there is an 80% probability that this represents true bacteriuria. If two different specimens demonstrate at least 10^5 of the same bacterium per milliliter, the probability increases to 95%. Thus, two clean-catch specimens should be obtained in an asymptomatic woman to confirm the diagnosis. When the number of bacteria per milliliter is between 10^4 and 10^5 in an asymptomatic woman, a confirmatory second specimen will contain 10^5 or more bacteria/mL in only 5% of instances. Thus, in asymptomatic women, 95% of the time, 10^4 to 10^5 bacteria/mL represents contamination, with occasional infection manifested by fewer than 10^5 bacteria/mL of urine. In men, in whom contamination is less likely, 10^3 or more organisms per milliliter is suggestive of infection. False-positive cultures are caused by contamination or incubation of urine before processing. False-negative cultures may be the result of the use of antimicrobial agents, soap from the preparation falling into the urine, total obstruction below the infection, infection with a fastidious organism, renal tuberculosis, and diuresis.

These criteria apply only to the Enterobacteriaceae. Gram-positive organisms, fungi, and bacteria with fastidious growth requirements may not reach titers of 10^5/mL in patients with infection and may be in the 10^4 to 10^5/mL range. The organism recovered often helps to distinguish contamination from true bacteriuria. Samples with counts of less than 10^4 organisms/mL often contain saprophytic skin organisms such as diphtheroids, *Neisseria,* and staphylococci. Pure growth of Enterobacteriaceae is uncommonly found in low-titer specimens but is present in over 90% of the urine samples containing more than 10^5 bacteria/mL. High colony counts containing more than one species of bacteria from urine of asymptomatic persons often represent contamination but may be more significant in the presence of symptoms. Mixed infection occurs in about 5% of cases.

In patients with symptoms of urinary tract infection, one titer of 10^5 or more bacteria/mL of urine carries a 95% probability of true bacteriuria. With titers below 10^5/mL but in the presence of frequency, urgency, and dysuria, women have a 33% chance of having bacterial infection (see "Urinary Tract Infection with Low Numbers of Organisms"). The presence of low numbers of Enterobacteriaceae (i.e., 10^2 to 10^5/mL) in such women correlates highly with infection. The presence of fewer than 10^2 Enterobacteriaceae per milliliter is evidence against urinary tract infection.

Samples obtained by catheterization from noninfected patients are less likely to become contaminated enough to demonstrate 10^5 bacteria/mL. For example, in an asymptomatic patient, one catheterized specimen that contains 10^5 or more organisms per milliliter has a 95% chance of indicating infection, and counts between 10^4 and 10^5 per milliliter (which are uncommon) are significant at least 50% of the time. The contamination is presumably from the urethra. Bladder urine obtained by suprapubic aspiration is either sterile or contains significant growth even if bacterial numbers are below 10^5 per milliliter. The practice of forcing fluids before the procedure tends to reduce numbers of organisms. In fact, almost 50% of suprapubic aspirates from infected patients contain fewer than 10^5 organisms/mL. However, small numbers of bacteria may be found in aspirated urine from presumably noninfected persons. This suggests that bladder urine may be occasionally contaminated from the urethra.

Urinary Tract Infection with Low Numbers of Organisms

Most women with an acute onset of frequency, urgency, or dysuria, or all of these, have urinary tract infection with 10^5 or more bacteria per milliliter of urine (Fig. 66-6). However, up to half are found to have fewer than 10^5 bacteria/mL of urine, and the term *urethral syndrome* has been used to refer to this entity. Stamm and associates have demonstrated that many of these women have urinary tract infection but with low numbers of organisms.[138-141] Using suprapubic bladder aspirates compared with voided midstream urine in acutely dysuric women, they found that 10^2 or more coliforms per milliliter in midstream urine had a sensitivity and specificity of 95% and 85%, respectively, for urinary tract infection. These women have urinary infections mainly restricted to the lower tract. Furthermore, about one fourth to one third of young women with symptomatic infection localized to the lower urinary tract have fewer than 10^5 bacteria/mL in urine.

Kunin and colleagues, in a study of women coming to a university health clinic for any reason, demonstrated that stepwise increases in bacterial counts from 10^2 to 10^5 CFU/mL were significantly associated with an increased incidence of symptoms and pyuria. They postulated that low-count bacteriuria represents an early phase of urinary infection.[142] This hypothesis appears to have been supported in a clinical study in which 21 women with low-count bacteriuria (10^2 to less than 10^5 CFU/mL) had therapy delayed for 2 days, and reculture showed that 10 of 21 (48%) developed concentrations of, or more than, 10^5 CFU/mL.[143]

The remaining women with the urethral syndrome (after excluding those with bacteria in the bladder and those with genital herpes infection or vaginitis) can be divided into two groups: (1) those with pyuria from urethritis due to *Chlamydia trachomatis, Neisseria gonorrhoeae,* or *Mycoplasma genitalium* infection, and (2) those without pyuria, in whom all bacterial cultures are negative. The pathogenesis of this latter symptom complex is unknown, but various fastidious microorganisms as well as noninfectious factors (traumatic, psychological, allergic, and chemical) have been suggested as causes. Patients with *C. trachomatis, N. gonorrhoeae,* and *M. genitalium* urethritis respond to antibacterial therapy. Komaroff and co-workers reported that vaginitis is a common cause of dysuria, and, accordingly, patients should be questioned regarding vaginal symptoms, particularly if the complaint of burning is external, such as pain felt in the inflamed labia during micturition.[144] If vaginitis is suspected, a pelvic examination should be performed. Dysuria has also been described in 10% of women with initial genital herpes infection.

Although symptoms and the clinical settings cannot reliably distinguish between the causes of dysuria in women, they can be suggestive.[133] Bacterial urinary tract infections tend to have a sudden onset of severe dysuria with frequency and urgency; suprapubic pain or hematuria or both may be present; there is pyuria. Clinical clues to urethritis (chlamydial, gonococcal, or mycoplasmal) include a patient with a gradual onset of milder dysuria with or without frequency and urgency, who is sexually active with a recent new sexual partner; hematuria is absent but vaginal discharge or bleeding may be present from chlamydial or gonococcal cervicitis; pyuria is present. With herpes, there are usually lesions in the periurethral area. The diagnosis of urethral chlamydial or gonococcal infection may be confirmed by nucleic acid amplification tests on urine.[145] With vaginitis, the dysuria tends to be mild with gradual onset and is felt externally; frequency and urgency are absent; there is often a vaginal discharge; and pyuria is usually absent in a midstream specimen.

Localization of Site of Infection

Localization of the site of infection to the kidney versus the bladder is not important in any given patient but has been useful in understanding the epidemiology and response to therapy of urinary tract infection.

Direct ureteral catheterization with quantitative cultures is an accurate but invasive method of localization. The Fairley bladder-washout technique, which involves bladder catheterization, is less invasive and less accurate.[146] Many other techniques such as measuring the urinary concentrating ability, urinary levels of various enzymes, urinary β_2-microglobulin levels, and serum antibody levels have been evaluated but are not reliable.

The antibody-coated bacteria test has fallen out of favor because of concerns about its reliability.[147,148]

The outcome of therapy can also be used in a crude but useful manner to separate those with upper and lower tract infection. Virtually all patients with infection restricted to the lower tract can be cured with a short course of antimicrobial therapy.[149] However, the relapse rate with upper tract infection is appreciable, even with 7 to 10 days of therapy.

NATURAL HISTORY OF URINARY TRACT INFECTION

Children

In general, children with urinary tract infections without obstruction or vesicoureteral reflux have a very good prognosis.[104,107,150] In the presence of obstruction (e.g., at the urethral valves), severe destruction of renal parenchyma can occur.

Reflux is found in 30% to 50% of the children with symptomatic bacteriuria (see Fig. 66-5).[151] Reflux can be caused by obstruction with increased pressure in the bladder, delayed development of the vesicoureteral junction, a short intravesical ureter, or inflammation of the vesicoureteral junction, or all of these. Reflux in the presence of infection is associated with the development of scarring detected by intravenous pyelography.[107,137] Infants and young children (preschool age group) are at the highest risk for the development of progressive renal scarring. These children frequently have severe degrees of reflux with repeated infections, and some develop end-stage renal disease and hypertension. Obstruction (most commonly in infant boys with congenital anomalies) is likely to be associated with marked reflux.

It should be emphasized that the contribution of reflux alone compared with reflux plus infection in the progression of renal scarring has not been clearly delineated. Reflux alone can apparently lead to renal damage and insufficiency.[152] Studies in uninfected animals[153] have demonstrated that reflux alone and in particular *intrarenal reflux* can produce "pyelonephritic" scars. It has also been shown that the immature kidneys of infants are more prone to intrarenal reflux.[154] The term *reflux nephropathy,* infected or uninfected, has been suggested to emphasize the primary role of reflux in scarring. However, it is probable

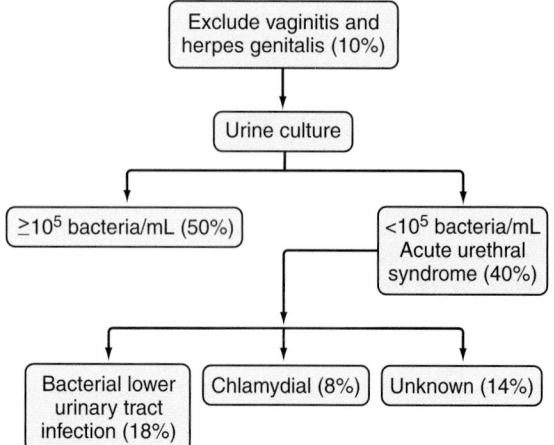

FIGURE 66-6. Relative frequencies of causes of acute onset of frequency or dysuria, or both, in young women. *(Adapted from data published in Stamm WE, Wagner KF, Amsel R, et al. Causes of acute urethral syndrome in women. N Engl J Med. 1980;303:409-415.)*

that reflux is more likely to lead to severe damage and scarring when infection is also present.[153] It is also clear that infection tends to produce reflux or at least to make it more severe.

After the age of 5 years, children (predominantly girls) with bacteriuria frequently have renal scars presumably acquired during the preschool years. Many of these children also have reflux. Reflux tends to decrease with the elimination of bacteriuria. In addition, mild to moderate degrees of reflux are likely to disappear with the passage of time, probably in relation to maturation of the vesicoureteral junction.[155] Progression of scars already present or the development of new ones is uncommon after the age of 5 years.[6,155] In fact, some investigators have questioned the need for detecting and treating bacteriuria in school-aged children (or, for that matter, in any asymptomatic children including infants).[104,156] Furthermore, screening of children for asymptomatic bacteriuria is not cost-effective.[156] However, it is clear that progression does occur in some of these children, especially in the presence of severe reflux.[155]

Adults

Urinary tract infections are much more common in women than in men. Many of these patients previously had urinary tract infections as children and continue to have infections as adults.[6,104] Once a woman develops infection, she is more likely to develop subsequent infections than a patient who has had no previous infections.

The courses of women with symptomatic recurrent urinary tract infections were described by Kraft and Stamey.[157] However, it was not defined whether these recurrences were reinfections or relapses. Twenty-three patients were followed over a total of 800 patient-months, and each episode of urinary tract infection was treated. The overall attack rate was about 0.2 infections per month. Even in these women (i.e., those with recurrent urinary tract infections), significant bacteriuria (i.e., 10^5 or greater bacteria/mL urine) was present in only 70% of symptomatic episodes. Infections tended to occur in clusters with an increased attack rate of 0.5% per month. These periods of more frequent infection were followed by a remission or infection-free interval that averaged about 13 months. However, most remissions were followed by further clusters of infection. Thus, in many women it is more correct to use the term *remission* rather than *cure* of urinary tract infection. It may be a simple matter to cure an individual episode, but recurrence, most often reinfection, is common.

It is clear that urinary tract infection in adults can lead to progressive renal damage in the presence of obstruction. However, recurrent infection in adults in the absence of obstruction rarely, if ever, leads to renal failure.[110]

Autopsy studies have shown that it is difficult to implicate infection per se (i.e., in the absence of other renal abnormalities) as an important pathogenic factor in the production of severe renal disease in adults.[6] One exception might be severe papillary necrosis secondary to infection. In fact, one group of investigators was unable to find any case of uncomplicated pyelonephritis that progressed to end-stage renal disease among 173 patients admitted to dialysis programs.[158] In prospective studies, hundreds of patients with persistent or recurrent infections have been followed for years without documenting the progression of renal disease from infection alone.[104,107,109,159,160]

The role of infection in the progression of clinically or radiographically diagnosed interstitial renal disease has also been examined.[107,110,161] In general, these studies indicate that infection is rarely, if ever, the major factor leading to further renal decompensation. However, infection may occasionally accelerate the progression of the primary underlying disease process. In summary, except perhaps for rare instances, there is no evidence to indicate that uncomplicated urinary tract infection alone produces renal failure in adults.

Some studies had demonstrated decreased survival among older adults with bacteriuria.[162] However, more recent studies have not confirmed this association.[163,164] At present, it seems unlikely that asymptomatic bacteriuria in older adults has any deleterious effects. Furthermore, there is no evidence to suggest that treatment of asymptomatic bacteriuria in older patients has any beneficial effects.[165]

Therefore, routine treatment of asymptomatic bacteriuria in older adults is not indicated.[115,166]

Diabetic women have an increased frequency of asymptomatic urinary tract infection and probably symptomatic disease. Diabetics also have a higher incidence of severe infection including severe pyelonephritis and uncommon complications such as emphysematous pyelonephritis and perinephric abscess. However, a recent study that followed diabetic women for up to 3 years found no advantage in screening for and treating asymptomatic urinary tract infection; it concluded that diabetes per se should not be an indication for screening for or treatment of asymptomatic bacteriuria.[167]

Hypertension

It is clear that severe renal disease may cause hypertension. The entity of chronic interstitial renal disease (not necessarily related to infection) has also been related to hypertension. It has been suggested that patients with bacteriuria in the absence of other renal disease are more likely to have hypertension, but the data have not shown a clear-cut relationship. No definite cause-and-effect relationships have been documented.

MANAGEMENT OF URINARY TRACT INFECTION

General Considerations

All symptomatic urinary tract infection should be treated. The diagnosis of infection in the asymptomatic patient should be made on no fewer than two cultures of clean-voided, midstream urine in which the same microorganism is present in significant titers. If the patient is symptomatic, one specimen suffices.

There has been much controversy about how vigorously chemotherapy should be pursued in the patient with asymptomatic bacteriuria. A rational approach to the treatment of urinary tract infection depends on an appreciation of the prognosis of the untreated infection and the long-term results to be expected from therapy. The side effects, cost, and inconvenience of different therapeutic regimens must also be considered. As the prognosis of urinary tract infection in nonpregnant adult women seems to be quite good and reinfection is common, therapy of asymptomatic bacteriuria makes little sense in this group.

Although asymptomatic bacteriuria in older adults is associated with degenerative and debilitating diseases and in some reports with mortality, there is no convincing evidence for a cause-and-effect relationship.[116,163,165,168] There certainly is no evidence that treatment of the urinary tract infection alters the patient's course. Urinary tract infection serves as a marker for debilitating diseases, which in turn may contribute to mortality. In addition, urinary tract infection is very common in the older adult population, and many of these patients become reinfected or relapse after antimicrobial therapy. Furthermore, a higher frequency of side effects from chemotherapy would be expected in an older age group because of preexisting renal, auditory, and other diseases. Considering the large numbers of patients involved, antimicrobial therapy may lead to an unwarranted financial burden and the danger of drug toxicity and thus may do more harm than good in older adult patients. Treatment is not indicated for asymptomatic bacteriuria in older adults.[115]

In contrast, bacteriuria in preschool children with vesicoureteral reflux (especially if congenital anomalies are present) can result in stunted growth of the kidney, scar formation, and, rarely, renal failure. Bacteriuria in pregnancy may also have serious implications. Treatment of children and pregnant women with asymptomatic bacteriuria is most likely to be beneficial. Furthermore, it is feasible to treat all these patients, as the prevalence of bacteriuria is relatively low in these groups.

Hospitalized patients with bacteriuria have higher mortality rates than those without bacteriuria.[169] This observation may be related to deaths from bacteremia in patients with indwelling urinary catheters.

It is usually necessary to treat all symptomatic patients regardless of age, even when infection is likely to recur. Some patients have such frequent symptomatic episodes (either relapses or reinfections) that they are almost chronically incapacitated. In these patients, it may be necessary to give prolonged therapy or prophylaxis to prevent recurrent symptoms.

In males with urinary tract infection, the possibility of a correctable obstructive lesion must arise. At a minimum, a postvoiding ultrasound of the the urinary tract should be obtained to evaluate bladder emptying.

Nonspecific Therapy

Hydration

Forcing fluids has been advocated in the therapy of urinary tract infection. There is some theoretical support for this method of treatment. Hydration produces rapid dilution of the bacteria and removal of infected urine by frequent bladder emptying, which in the presence of minimal residual volume may offset the logarithmic growth of gram-negative bacilli. Forcing fluids usually results in a rapid reduction of bacterial counts. Permanent loss of bacteriuria has been reported in a few patients with rapid hydration, but in most patients bacterial counts return to the original levels when hydration is stopped (e.g., overnight when the urine flow rate and frequency of micturition are reduced).

Medullary hypertonicity tends to inhibit leukocyte migration into the renal medulla, and the high concentration of ammonia tends to inactivate complement. Abolition of medullary hypertonicity by diuresis would be expected to reverse these effects. In addition, a reduction in bacterial counts in the urine by hydration would enhance the effect of factors otherwise overwhelmed by large numbers of bacteria (e.g., bladder mucosal defenses or the effect of relatively low concentrations of antimicrobial drugs).

Hydration may also have some disadvantages. Increased fluid intake could theoretically result in increased vesicoureteral reflux and possibly cause acute urinary retention in the partially obstructed bladder. The larger urine output results in dilution of antibacterial substances normally present in the urine as well as lower urinary concentrations of antimicrobial agents. Water diuresis also decreases urinary acidification, which enhances the antibacterial activity of urine and certain antimicrobial agents.

As there is no evidence that hydration improves the results of appropriate antimicrobial therapy, and because continuous hydration is inconvenient, we are not in favor of this approach.

Urinary pH

The antibacterial activity of urine results mainly from a high urea concentration and osmolality, and it is pH-dependent, being greater at a lower pH.[66] The pH-dependent activity may be related to a high concentration of various weakly ionizable organic acids, such as hippuric and β-hydroxybutyric acids. The antibacterial activity of these organic acids is related to the concentration of the undissociated molecule, which probably penetrates better than the ionized form into the bacterial cell. As these organic acids have a relatively low pK_a (the pH at which 50% of the molecules are undissociated), the lower the urinary pH, the greater is the concentration of undissociated molecules and the greater is the antibacterial activity of the organic acid.

Hippuric acid is a common constituent of urine, being the glycine conjugate of dietary benzoic acid, and is bacteriostatic in proportion to the concentration of undissociated molecules. The production of antibacterial activity in urine by the ingestion of large volumes of cranberry juice (if the urinary pH level is kept low) results from the appearance in the urine of high concentrations of hippuric acid derived from precursors in the berry. The successful use of mandelic acid, another organic acid, is also dependent on the maintenance of a low urinary pH level.

The urinary pH level affects the antibacterial activity of many chemotherapeutic agents used in the treatment of urinary tract infections. The activity of methenamine results from the release of formaldehyde as the urinary pH level is decreased below 5.5. Clinically, methenamine is used in the form of its mandelic acid salt (methenamine mandelate) or its hippuric acid salt (methenamine hippurate). The

antibacterial activity of these salts is related to the formation of the un-ionized organic acid and formaldehyde, which is highly dependent on the maintenance of a urinary pH of 5.5 or less. The effectiveness of nitrofurantoin (pK_a 7.2) is also greater at a low urinary pH level. In contrast, the aminoglycoside antibiotics such as gentamicin, tobramycin, and amikacin are more effective in alkaline urine.

Although different antimicrobial agents have maximal effectiveness at different pH levels, most agents exhibit adequate antibacterial activity at usual urinary pH levels. The maintenance of urine at the low pH level required for effective antibacterial activity of organic acids and methenamine can be accomplished by the administration of ascorbic acid or methionine. Acidification of the urine can result in precipitation of urate stones, and, because oxalate is a metabolite of ascorbic acid, large doses of ascorbic acid can cause the formation of oxalate stones.

To acidify the urine, it is often necessary to modify the diet by restriction of agents that tend to alkalinize the urine—for example, milk, fruit juices (except cranberry juice), and sodium bicarbonate. Another major problem with acidification is that patients with renal insufficiency are unable to excrete an acid load and may become systemically acidotic when urinary acidification is attempted. It may be impossible to acidify urine infected with urea-splitting organisms such as *Proteus* because of the production of ammonia from urea. Acidification for long-term antimicrobial therapy should be used only with the concomitant use of organic acids or methenamine. Urinary acidification is frequently difficult to achieve and is rarely if ever necessary.

Analgesics

Urinary analgesics such as phenazopyridine hydrochloride (Pyridium) have little place in the routine management of symptomatic infections. The dysuria of urinary tract infection usually responds rapidly to antibacterial therapy and requires no local analgesia. If flank pain or dysuria is severe, systemic analgesics can be used. Analgesics such as phenazopyridine hydrochloride may be useful in the management of certain patients with dysuria but without infection.

Principles of Antimicrobial Therapy

In most cases, any of many available agents are satisfactory for treatment of urinary tract infection. Given two or more drugs with good activity against the probable infecting microorganism, the agent chosen should be the one with the least toxicity and the least likelihood of affecting the normal flora of the vagina and gastrointestinal tract.

There is no evidence to support any superiority of bactericidal drugs over bacteriostatic agents in urinary tract infection. However, there may be theoretical reasons for using bactericidal drugs in the treatment of relapsing urinary tract infection.

Serum, Tissue, and Urine Concentrations of Antimicrobial Agents

A poor correlation exists between the response of bacteriuria and blood levels of antimicrobial agents.[170] In the dosages commonly used for urinary tract infection, some oral antimicrobial agents do not achieve serum levels above the minimal inhibitory concentration for most urinary pathogens.

The disappearance of bacteriuria is closely correlated with the sensitivity of the microorganism to the concentration of the antimicrobial agent achieved in the urine.[170] Urinary concentrations that are inhibitory for sensitive microorganisms are achieved after oral administration of essentially all commonly used antimicrobial agents. Although blood levels do not seem to be important in the treatment of urinary tract infection, they may be critical in patients with bacteremia and may be important in the cure of patients with renal parenchymal infection who relapse.

In patients with renal insufficiency, dosage modifications are necessary for agents that are excreted primarily by the kidneys and cannot be cleared by any other mechanism. In renal failure, the kidney may not be able to concentrate an antimicrobial agent in the urine, and difficulty in eradicating bacteriuria may occur. This may be an

important factor in the failure of therapy for urinary tract infection with aminoglycosides.

In addition, high concentrations of magnesium and calcium as well as a low pH level can raise the minimal inhibitory concentration of aminoglycosides for gram-negative bacilli to levels above those achievable in the urine of patients with renal failure. In general, the penicillins, cephalosporins, and many fluoroquinolones attain adequate urine concentrations despite severely impaired renal function. From the point of view of safety, the penicillins and cephalosporins should be considered the agents of first choice in treatment of urinary tract infection in patients with renal insufficiency.

Response to Therapy

There are four patterns of response of bacteriuria to antimicrobial therapy: cure, persistence, relapse, and reinfection. Quantitative bacterial counts in urine should decrease within 48 hours after the initiation of an antimicrobial agent to which the microorganism is sensitive in vitro. If titers do not decrease within this time, the therapy being given will almost invariably be unsuccessful. However, it is important to recognize that symptoms of urinary tract infection are self-limited and will eventually abate even when therapy is ineffective or not given.

Bacteriologic cure is defined as negative urine cultures on chemotherapy and during the follow-up period (usually 1 to 2 weeks). However, it must be understood that many of these patients will develop reinfection at a later time.

Bacteriologic persistence has been used in two ways to describe a response to therapy: (1) persistence of significant bacteriuria after 48 hours of treatment, and (2) persistence of the infecting organism in low numbers in urine after 48 hours. Significant bacteriuria usually persists only if the urinary levels of the antimicrobial agent are below the concentration of the drug needed to inhibit the microorganism. This can occur when the infecting strain is resistant to the urinary levels usually attained (i.e., a resistant organism) or because the urinary levels of the drug are inordinately low (i.e., from not taking the agent, insufficient dosage, poor intestinal absorption, or poor renal excretion as in renal insufficiency). Persistence of the infecting microorganism in low titers in voided urine may mean persistence in the urinary tract or contamination from the urethra or vagina. Bladder-puncture cultures would be needed to evaluate the significance of low titers of bacteria obtained when the patient is receiving therapy, and this procedure is rarely indicated. Bacteria may persist within the urinary tract during therapy without excretion of organisms in the urine. Sites of persistence within the urinary tract are the renal parenchyma, calculi, and the prostate. The simplest way of determining the significance of persistence of the organism in low titers in the urine is to obtain follow-up urine cultures after therapy has been stopped. Prompt relapse of significant bacteriuria usually follows persistence of the organism in the urinary tract.

Bacteriologic relapse usually occurs within 1 to 2 weeks after the cessation of chemotherapy and is often associated with renal infection, with structural abnormalities of the urinary tract, or with chronic bacterial prostatitis. Relapse indicates that the infecting microorganism has persisted in the urinary tract during therapy. However, an apparent relapse can be related to reinfection (new infection) with the same microorganism. In spite of eradication from the urinary tract, the original infecting organism may still be present in the periurethral area, the vagina, or the intestine and then may cause a new infection. Delayed relapses (more than 1 to 2 weeks after stopping therapy) are much more likely due to this phenomenon or to chronic bacterial prostatitis than to true relapse. Relapses occurring within 1 week are usually true relapses (i.e., from within the urinary tract).

After initial sterilization of the urine, *reinfection* may occur during the administration of chemotherapy (also called *superinfection*) or at any time thereafter. Reinfection is easy to identify when there is a change in bacterial species. However, there may be reinfection with a different serotype of the same species (usually *E. coli*) or even the same serotype.

Classification and Antimicrobial Therapy for Different Groups

Acute Pyelonephritis

Patients who are severely ill with pyelonephritis should be hospitalized. Although mild to moderate illness responds well to orally administered antimicrobial agents, nausea and vomiting may preclude oral treatment, necessitating parenteral therapy. The patient who is reliable, compliant, and tolerates oral therapy may be treated with a variety of oral antimicrobial agents. At the time of antibiotic selection, a Gram stain of the urine should have indicated the morphology of the infecting organism (e.g., gram-negative bacillus, gram-positive coccus), but the precise identity and antimicrobial susceptibility are usually unknown. Therefore, the selection of antimicrobial therapy is usually empirical. When gram-positive cocci in chains are seen, ampicillin or amoxicillin is probably the agent of choice. When staphylococci are implicated on Gram stain, cephalosporins (such as cephalexin) are appropriate agents.

Although amoxicillin and first-generation cephalosporins have been mainstays of oral therapy for gram-negative bacillus infection for many years, these agents can no longer be recommended as reliable agents, because at least 35% of isolates from community-acquired urinary tract infection are now resistant to these agents.[171,172] The oral antimicrobial agents currently advocated by most experts for gram-negative bacillus infection of the upper urinary tract include trimethoprim (100 mg twice a day), trimethoprim-sulfamethoxazole (one double-strength tablet twice a day), and the fluoroquinolones (e.g., ciprofloxacin 500 mg twice a day). A caveat is that resistance of *E. coli* to trimethoprim-sulfamethoxazole is approaching 20% in the United States and has exceeded this level in some areas.[171-174] Clinical and microbiologic failure is more likely to occur when trimethoprim-sulfamethoxazole is used in these patients.[175] For this reason, we no longer consider trimethoprim-sulfamethoxazole to be appropriate for initial empirical therapy for acute pyelonephritis. Our preference is for a fluoroquinolone. There is increasing evidence that cell wall–active agents (e.g., penicillins and cephalosporins) are not as effective in eradicating infection in the kidneys, or for that matter anywhere in the urinary tract, as trimethoprim-sulfamethoxazole, fluoroquinolones, or aminoglycosides.[1,135,176] In all patients with symptoms of upper tract infection, therapy should be preceded by culture of a clean-catch midstream urine sample.

In hospitalized patients, particularly those with suspected gram-negative bacillary bacteremia complicating pyelonephritis (high fever, shaking chills, hypotension), parenteral therapy should be used and is directed at the life-threatening bacteremia. In these seriously ill patients, the spectrum of antibacterial activity of the initial agents should include all potential pathogens. In seriously ill patients with community-acquired acute pyelonephritis, when the Gram stain reveals gram-negative bacilli, empirical therapy includes a wide selection of antimicrobial agents: aminoglycosides (such as gentamicin, 3 to 5 mg/kg/day); aztreonam, 3 to 6 g/day; piperacillin-tazobactam (as 18 g of piperacillin per day); ampicillin-sulbactam (as 12 g of ampicillin per day); third-generation cephalosporins (e.g., cefotaxime or ceftriaxone); or a parenteral fluoroquinolone. In patients with hospital-acquired gram-negative bacillary infection, particularly in those seriously ill, the initial selection of antibiotics should not leave any hiatus in the spectrum of activity and should anticipate the possibility of resistant microorganisms. Under these circumstances, ceftazidime (3 to 6 g/day), cefepime (2 to 4 g/day), piperacillin-tazobactam (as 18 g of piperacillin per day); aztreonam (3 to 6 g/day), imipenem (2 g/day), meropenem (1.5 to 3 g/day), or ertapenem (1g/day), often used in combination with aminoglycosides or a parenteral fluoroquinolone, can be recommended. When the susceptibility pattern of the infecting organism is known, therapy can be altered to less expensive single-agent therapy, and oral treatment can be used once a response has occurred.

Effective therapy results in a marked decrease in bacterial titers in the urine within 48 hours after the onset of treatment. Antimicrobial agents are sometimes effective in vivo even when disk sensitivity tests indicate drug resistance, because most antimicrobials are excreted in the urine in concentrations much higher than those tested for by disk sensitivity testing.

If a bacteriologic response does not occur by 48 hours, there is no point in continuing the same regimen. Therapy is then changed to an alternative drug on the basis of susceptibility tests (e.g., from the initial isolate). The finding of continuing positive blood cultures or persistent high fever and toxicity past the first 3 days suggests the need for investigation to exclude urinary obstruction or intrarenal or perinephric abscess formation. Investigation should include renal ultrasonography, computed tomography (CT) or magnetic resonance imaging (MRI) scan, and, depending on the findings, perhaps an intravenous pyelography (IVP) examination. The availability of sensitive noninvasive studies has resulted in early diagnosis of intrarenal or perinephric abscess formation that may respond to antibiotic therapy alone. In uncomplicated pyelonephritis, after a clinical response and defervescence occur, oral therapy is initiated and classically has been continued to complete a course of 14 days of antimicrobial therapy.[177] A recent study demonstrated that 7 days of ciprofloxacin was at least as effective as 14 days of trimethoprim-sulfamethoxazole for therapy of uncomplicated pyelonephritis.[175] However, until there is much more experience with such short courses, 14 days should remain the standard. When upper tract infection is complicated by abscesses, more prolonged therapy and perhaps drainage is indicated (see "Perinephric Abscess" and "Intrarenal Abscess," later). Routine imaging studies are not indicated in women with acute uncomplicated pyelonephritis. Follow-up urine cultures are mandatory within 1 to 2 weeks of completion of therapy in pregnant women, children, and patients with recurrent symptomatic pyelonephritis in whom suppressive maintenance therapy is being contemplated. In the majority of nonpregnant adults who remain asymptomatic, follow-up cultures are optional.

Renal infection is a special problem in adults with hereditary polycystic disease. Although parenchymal infections respond well to appropriate antibiotics, cyst infections frequently fail to improve and may require antibiotics that diffuse into these closed sites (e.g., trimethoprim-sulfamethoxazole or a fluoroquinolone) or surgical aspiration or drainage. Emphysematous pyelonephritis is most often seen in older adult female diabetic patients with chronic urinary infections and renal vascular disease (Fig. 66-7). Because of the extraordinarily high mortality rate of 70% in spite of appropriate antibiotics and supportive therapy, immediate nephrectomy is almost always indicated for this condition.[178] However, some cases have been cured with antibiotic therapy plus percutaneous drainage.[179]

Lower Urinary Tract Infection

Conventional Therapy. In the past, 7 to 10 days of therapy were routinely recommended for patients with lower tract symptoms. However, in recent years it has become apparent that most women with lower tract infection have only a superficial mucosal infection and can be cured with much shorter courses of therapy and in fact with only a single dose of an antimicrobial agent.

Short-Course Therapy. Short-course therapy is defined as 3 or fewer days of treatment. The advantages of short-course therapy include a lesser expense, better compliance, fewer side effects, and perhaps less intensive selective pressure for the emergence of resistant organisms in gut, urethral, or vaginal flora. Possible deleterious effects include a poorer outcome of infections that are actually in the upper tract.

Single-dose therapy with certain agents achieves high urinary concentrations that are prolonged for at least 12 to 24 hours, and it eliminates infection when it is confined to the bladder. The most widely used regimens have been oral doses of 3 g of amoxicillin or one to two double-strength tablets of trimethoprim-sulfamethoxazole.[180] Other regimens have included sulfonamides, aminoglycosides, tetracycline, trimethoprim, nitrofurantoin, fosfomycin, cephalosporins, and fluoroquinolones. Cure rates have ranged from 65% to 100%. It should not be assumed that every antibiotic administered as a single dose will be effective even with regard to susceptible organisms. Results depend on

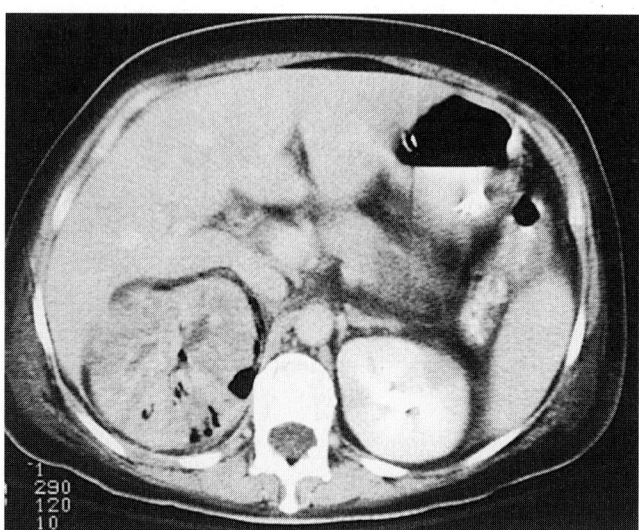

FIGURE 66-7. Emphysematous pyelonephritis in a patient with diabetes. The computed tomographic scan shows an enlarged, inflamed right kidney with air within the parenchyma and subcapsular space. *(Courtesy of M. Bergeron, M.D.)*

high sustained urinary concentrations of the antimicrobial agent. For example, a 2-g oral dose of cefaclor resulted in a 57% failure rate.[181]

A byproduct of single-dose therapy is that a failure to eradicate a urinary tract infection after a single dose of an appropriate agent may indicate a patient in whom further investigation should be considered, and it is suggestive of upper tract infection. Response to single-dose therapy appears comparable with the antibody-coated bacteria test in localizing the site of infection.

Multiple reviews have concluded that 3 days of therapy are superior to single-dose therapy.[135] It is our preference and that of the Guidelines from the Infectious Diseases Society of America[135] to use 3 days of therapy with standard doses for treatment of uncomplicated lower tract infection in women. It seems clear that with either a single dose or 3 days of therapy, trimethoprim-sulfamethoxazole and probably fluoroquinolones are superior to β-lactam antibiotics in terms of avoiding both early (i.e., <2 weeks) and late (i.e., >2 weeks) reinfection.[135] Some of the preferred agents for 3 days of therapy have been trimethoprim-sulfamethoxazole (one double-strength tablet twice a day), trimethoprim (100 mg twice a day), ciprofloxacin (500 mg twice a day), and other fluoroquinolones. Because of increased resistance of E. coli to trimethoprim-sulfamethoxazole (greater than 20% in some parts of the United States), it is our preference to use a fluoroquinolone as the drug of choice for short-course therapy.[171-174] In an attempt to minimize toxicity, we would advocate low doses, such as 250 mg ciprofloxacin twice a day.

Because of the higher cost of the fluoroquinolones and the concern over more rapid emergence of bacterial resistance with their widespread use, some may prefer to use trimethoprim-sulfamethoxazole. If this is the case, we would recommend that it be used only in patients who have not received recent antimicrobial therapy and are therefore more likely to have a susceptible infecting organism. Other agents that have been used with varying degrees of success for treatment of lower tract infection are nitrofurantoin, amoxicillin-clavulanic acid, cephalosporins, tetracyclines, and fosfomycin. Sulfonamides, ampicillin, and amoxicillin probably should not be used, unless the infecting organism is known to be susceptible, because of the relatively high frequency of E. coli resistant to these agents among community-acquired urinary tract infections.

The approach to the management of lower urinary tract infection has evolved to the point where 3 days of therapy should be the standard for most female patients with suspected lower tract infection.

Studies in pediatric populations have shown similarly good results with 3 days of therapy.[182,183] Short-course therapy has not been adequately evaluated in men and is not recommended at present. Short-course therapy is not appropriate for women who have a history of previous urinary infection caused by antibiotic-resistant organisms or more than 7 days of symptoms.[184] In these patients (who have an increased likelihood of upper tract infection) and in men, 7 to 10 days of therapy are recommended.

If symptoms do not respond or if they recur, a urine culture should be obtained. In pregnant women, children, and patients at high risk for renal damage who remain asymptomatic, follow-up cultures should be obtained 1 to 2 weeks after discontinuation of therapy to detect relapses.

Office Strategy for Frequency, Urgency, and Dysuria Syndrome

When a woman is first seen with onset of classic acute lower urinary tract infection (frequency, urgency, and dysuria), urine culture is not mandatory, and the therapeutic decision is based on the clinical presentation and the presence or absence of pyuria. If pyuria (defined as at least 10 leukocytes/mm^3) is present, antimicrobial therapy is warranted for urinary tract infection. Dipstick methods of measuring pyuria are sufficiently accurate to be used. Short-course therapy is a reasonable first approach in women except in settings in which occult pyelonephritis is more likely, as described previously. An agent likely to be effective against most pathogens (e.g., a fluoroquinolone, or, if a fluoroquinolone cannot be used, trimethoprim or trimethoprim-sulfamethoxazole or amoxicillin-clavulanic acid) should be used. If a clinical response does not occur, a culture should be obtained (for the possibility of a resistant organism), and therapy should be changed. The possibility of urethritis rather than urinary tract infection should also be considered.

A symptomatic response followed by recurrence after therapy is discontinued indicates the probability of upper tract infection and the need for a culture and 2 weeks of therapy. Men and children should have a urine culture, and males should receive 7 to 10 days of treatment. In males, obstructive uropathy must be considered.

Asymptomatic Bacteriuria

Most patients with asymptomatic bacteriuria are women and are in the older age groups. Although cure may result after treatment, relapse and especially reinfection are common. The approach to asymptomatic bacteriuria depends on the age of the patient. In children, therapy should be given as described for symptomatic infection. In contrast, therapy for asymptomatic bacteriuria in the adult, including diabetic women, is rarely indicated in the absence of obstruction except during pregnancy.[115,166,167] If therapy is indicated in a patient with asymptomatic bacteriuria, there is no urgency to treat. Therapy should be delayed until two cultures have been obtained for confirmation of the presence of bacteriuria. By that time, the identity and antimicrobial susceptibility pattern of the infecting organism will have been determined. In males, obstructive uropathy must be considered.

Relapsing Urinary Tract Infection

If the patient relapses after therapy for symptomatic urinary tract infection or for asymptomatic bacteriuria, the most likely possibilities are that the patient has (1) renal involvement, (2) a structural abnormality of the urinary tract (e.g., calculi), or (3) chronic bacterial prostatitis. As there is no demonstrated value in treating an asymptomatic relapse in the nonpregnant adult without obstructive uropathy, we do not advocate taking urine cultures to look for relapses in these asymptomatic patients, nor do we advocate treatment if infection is found.

Relapses, especially in the absence of structural abnormalities, may be related to renal infection that may require a longer duration of therapy. Patients who relapse after a short course or 7 to 10 days of therapy should be considered for a 2-week course. Turck and colleagues demonstrated that a 6-week course of therapy resulted in a higher cure rate than a 2-week course in patients who relapsed after 2 weeks of therapy.[185]

Structural abnormalities of the urinary tract predispose to relapse. Urinary tract infection in the presence of obstruction is likely to be associated with renal involvement, a tendency for renal functional impairment, and bacteremia. Obstructive lesions can be corrected surgically and should be sought in the evaluation of patients with relapsing infection. Calculi may be a cause of relapse of urinary tract infection. The ultimate success of chemotherapy is dependent on the removal of stones.

Some patients continue to relapse despite surgical correction of urologic abnormalities. In others, surgical correction may not be indicated or feasible, or no abnormalities may be found. In those patients who relapse after 2 weeks of chemotherapy, a repeat course of 2 weeks should be considered in the presence of obstruction. After another relapse, a 4- to 6-week course should be considered. In men, chronic bacterial prostatitis should first be ruled out. Only carefully selected patients, such as children, adults who have continuous symptoms, or adults who are at high risk for developing progressive renal damage (e.g., those with obstruction not amenable to surgery), should be considered for 4-week or longer courses of therapy. Some of the agents that can be used for long-term therapy are amoxicillin (250 mg three times a day), cephalexin, trimethoprim-sulfamethoxazole, trimethoprim, and ciprofloxacin, in usual doses and nitrofurantoin in full dosage for 1 week and then half the usual dosage.

An antimicrobial agent being used for long-term therapy is continued only as long as significant bacteriuria is absent. If bacteriuria persists or relapses during chemotherapy (indicating that the infecting organism is now resistant to that agent), the agent is altered. The aim is to achieve continuous suppression of bacteriuria for the entire course of therapy. If relapse occurs after discontinuation of the antimicrobial agent, therapy is reinstituted with the same or another drug. If deemed necessary, the agent can administered for a more prolonged period of time. All patients are followed with urine cultures at least monthly while on therapy.

A creatinine clearance determination and imaging studies of the kidneys initially and yearly (or at least every 2 years) should be obtained on patients receiving long-term therapy to determine the glomerular filtration rate and structural changes in the kidneys. Blood counts, urinalyses, and liver chemistry tests (when indicated) are also obtained periodically as tests for drug toxicity.

Reinfection of the Urinary Tract

Patients with reinfection can generally be divided into two groups: (1) those who have relatively infrequent reinfections, perhaps only once every 2 or 3 years to several times a year, and (2) those who develop frequent reinfections. An extreme example of the latter group is the patient who becomes reinfected during or shortly after each course of antimicrobial therapy. With infrequent reinfections, each episode can be approached with therapy (or without therapy) as if it were a new episode of either symptomatic or asymptomatic infection. Short-course therapy should be used in women with lower tract symptoms. Women with reinfections associated with lower tract symptoms can be managed with self-administration of short-course therapy with the onset of symptoms.[186] In the absence of obstructive uropathy and pregnancy, asymptomatic reinfections should not be treated in adults.

Occasionally, patients of any age develop symptomatic reinfection so frequently that they can be incapacitated. In some women, these symptomatic reinfections are associated with sexual activity. Voiding immediately after intercourse may help prevent reinfection. However, single-dose prophylactic chemotherapy taken after sexual intercourse (e.g., a single-strength trimethoprim-sulfamethoxazole tablet, 100 mg of nitrofurantoin, or 100 mg of ciprofloxacin) is a more effective method of decreasing these episodes.[187,188]

In other patients with frequent symptomatic reinfections, no precipitating event is apparent; in these patients, when symptoms are severe, long-term chemoprophylaxis may be instituted. Although these courses seem to decrease the frequency of reinfections and symptoms in most patients, it is impossible to completely prevent reinfection in many patients. If reinfection occurs when the patient is receiving therapy, the prophylactic agent must be changed.

Long-term chemoprophylaxis should be considered for asymptomatic patients who reinfect frequently and are at risk for developing renal parenchymal damage with each reinfection (e.g., young children with vesicoureteral reflux and children and adults with obstructive uropathy). In these groups, keeping the patient abacteriuric may help to protect the kidneys. Several studies in patients with frequent reinfections indicate that such prolonged chemotherapy reduces the frequency of reinfections. Chemoprophylaxis should be considered in all renal transplant patients to prevent infection of the graft.[122,123]

Long-term prophylactic antimicrobial agents have reduced the frequency of symptomatic infections of the urinary tract in older men, women, and children.[189,190] Before prophylaxis is initiated, the patient should receive a course of therapy with an appropriate antimicrobial agent. Used alone, trimethoprim-sulfamethoxazole, nitrofurantoin, and trimethoprim are particularly useful for long-term prophylaxis, because these drugs are inexpensive.

Full antimicrobial dosage is not necessary for successful prophylaxis. One 50-mg capsule of nitrofurantoin or one half-tablet of trimethoprim-sulfamethoxazole (40 mg of trimethoprim, 200 mg of sulfamethoxazole) nightly suffices. Fluoroquinolones and other agents have been used with good results.[191]

Patients receiving long-term prophylaxis should be followed with urine cultures monthly or more often if interim symptomatic episodes develop. Therapy is continued with the same agent as long as the patient remains abacteriuric. If bacteriuria persists or recurs during the administration of an antimicrobial agent, therapy is altered using the response of bacteriuria as a parameter of the adequacy of therapy. Long-term prophylaxis can be undertaken only if urine cultures are obtained periodically, and therapy is altered if bacteriuria recurs.

A recent investigational approach to preventing reinfections in postmenopausal women with frequent recurrent urinary tract infections is the use of oral or intravaginal estrogens.[192] The use of estrogens in these women has resulted in a decrease in the number of episodes of urinary tract infection, presumably by decreasing the vaginal pH, increasing colonization of the vagina with lactobacilli, and decreasing colonization with Enterobacteriaceae. Other experimental approaches include daily ingestion of cranberry juice, exogenously applied or orally taken lactobacilli, and attempts at use of vaginal mucosal immunization with a mixture of uropathogens.[193-195] Although some of these may have merit, much more evaluation is needed before they can be recommended.

Fungal Infections

Most *Candida* urinary tract infections occur in patients with indwelling catheters. Removal of the catheter may result in cure of 30% to 40% of patients with candiduria.[196] Continuous amphotericin B bladder irrigation or oral fluconazole 200 mg per day for 7 days in association with removing (if possible) or replacing the catheter may be effective in the short term in eliminating candiduria.[98] However, with longer follow-up, oral fluconazole is no more effective than no therapy.[196] There is no demonstrated benefit in the treatment of asymptomatic infection, and therefore therapy is not recommended. Exceptions include renal transplant patients and patients who are to undergo elective urinary tract surgery. In these instances, attempts should be made to eliminate or at least suppress the candiduria. Occasionally, ascending infection resulting in pyelonephritis occurs, especially in patients with diabetes or obstruction. This clearly requires systemic antifungal therapy.

URINARY TRACT INFECTION IN PREGNANCY

Physiologic Alterations in the Urinary Tract

During pregnancy, there is dilatation of the ureters and renal pelvis, with markedly decreased ureteral peristalsis. These changes begin as early as the 7th week of gestation and progress to term.[117] The bladder also decreases in tone, so that late in gestation it can contain twice its normal contents without causing discomfort. These changes vary from patient to patient. They are more marked on the right side and are more likely to occur during the first pregnancy or when pregnancies occur in rapid succession. The urinary tract tends to revert to normal by the 2nd month after delivery.[117] The urinary tract alterations may be at least in part related to hyperestrogenism.[117] Other possible explanations for the alterations are obstruction of the ureters by the gravid uterus and hypertrophy of muscle bundles at the lower end of the ureter.[117] To investigate the effects of estrogens on these changes, Andriole and Cohn treated nonpregnant female and male rats with estrogens and obtained intravenous pyelograms before and during treatment.[197] Hydroureter and a markedly increased susceptibility to E. coli pyelonephritis were observed in both male and female animals. In addition to host factors, unique gestational bacterial virulence factors are now recognized for a narrow group of genetically related *E. coli*.[198] Each trimester appears to be associated with specific DNA fingerprints and serotypes of *E. coli* as well as trimester-specific virulence patterns.

Epidemiology

The microbiologic picture of bacteriuria during gestation is similar to that seen in nonpregnant women. The prevalence of asymptomatic bacteriuria in pregnancy ranges from 4% to 7%.[199] However, recurrent episodes are more common in pregnant women who had bacteriuria documented at their initial prenatal visit. Although anecdotal cases of clinical disease are reported, it is unclear if *U. urealyticum* and *G. vaginalis*, reported by some to be in bladder urine of an additional 10% to 15% of pregnant women, play a significant pathogenic role.[117] Pregnant women of higher socioeconomic status have a lower frequency of bacteriuria of pregnancy than women of lower socioeconomic status.[117] The prevalence of bacteriuria also rises with parity, age, and sexual activity, in diabetes mellitus, in women with sickle cell trait, and in women with a past history of urinary tract infection.[199,200] For example, in low-income populations, the prevalence of bacteriuria is about 2% in primiparas younger than 21 years, compared with 8% to 10% in grand-multiparas older than 35 years. Most women who develop bacteriuria during pregnancy have infection at the first prenatal visit. However, 1% to 1.5% of pregnant women or about 25% of those with bacteriuria of pregnancy develop infection in the later trimesters.[117,201] The development of symptomatic pyelonephritis late in pregnancy is usually an expression of asymptomatic bacteriuria that was present earlier in the pregnancy. The marked dilatation of the ureters during the later stages apparently allows bacteria in the bladder to reach the upper tract and to produce symptomatic pyelonephritis.

About 20% to 40% of the patients with untreated bacteriuria early in gestation develop acute symptomatic pyelonephritis later in pregnancy.[117] In contrast, less than 1% of patients whose urine is uninfected early in gestation develop acute infection. Therefore, most of the cases of acute pyelonephritis can be prevented by eliminating asymptomatic bacteriuria in the early stages of pregnancy.[117,200,202] It has also been noted that those whose bacteriuria fails to respond to treatment are at the highest risk for developing symptomatic infection.[203] A lack of cure is probably an indication of upper versus lower tract infection.

An association between acute pyelonephritis of pregnancy and premature delivery was well known in the preantibiotic era.[117] The rate of prematurity can be as high as 20% to 50%. In 1959, Kass reported that there was an association between asymptomatic bacteriuria and prematurity and that the eradication of bacteriuria significantly reduced the rate of premature delivery.[204] Since then, conflicting studies have both supported and denied these observations.[117,205,206] It seems that prematurity and low birth weight[202,207] are increased in patients with asymptomatic bacteriuria, primarily in those women with renal involvement. However, it does not necessarily follow that asymptomatic bacteriuria is a cause of prematurity. It is possible that certain patients are predisposed both to bacteriuria and to delivering premature infants. Some investigators have reported that the elimination of bacteriuria decreases the frequency of prematurity.[117,205] However, other studies have failed to show a decrease in prematurity or fetal wastage with the elimination of asymptomatic bacteriuria.[117] Neonates of patients refractory to multiple courses of therapy have been reported to have a

significantly lower birth weight than infants of those who respond; this phenomenon may be related to the presence of upper tract infection in these patients.[207] There have been several studies that have attempted to relate asymptomatic bacteriuria to the development of hypertension in pregnancy, but the results have been unclear.

Even though the data relating asymptomatic bacteriuria of pregnancy to prematurity are not clear-cut, the relationship of asymptomatic bacteriuria to the later development of acute pyelonephritis is indisputable. Acute pyelonephritis has possible serious consequences for both the mother and the fetus. Accordingly, screening for and treatment of bacteriuria of pregnancy seems justified. Quantitative urine cultures should be obtained in all pregnant patients at the initial prenatal visit because treatment given at that time would provide the greatest number of bacteriuria-free gestational weeks.

Postpartum studies of patients with bacteriuria of pregnancy demonstrate a high frequency of bacteriuria even with treatment during the pregnancy. Postpartum intravenous pyelography of these patients has shown that 10% to 30% have radiologic changes of "chronic pyelonephritis" and other abnormalities.[208] These abnormalities are most common in patients in whom renal bacteriuria has been demonstrated or in whom bacteriuria during pregnancy was difficult to eradicate with antimicrobial therapy.[117] However, pyelographic abnormalities should not necessarily be attributed to the infection that occurred during the pregnancy. In fact, these abnormalities probably antedate the pregnancy and in most cases are related to childhood infection. Treatment of bacteriuria of pregnancy has little effect on the long-term course of the patient. When patients who had bacteriuria of pregnancy were studied 10 to 14 years later, there were no differences between those who were treated and those who were not. About 25% of the women in each group had bacteriuria at the time of follow-up.[117]

Management of Bacteriuria of Pregnancy

Because screening and treatment of asymptomatic bacteriuria has been shown to prevent pyelonephritis,[200] treatment with an appropriate antimicrobial agent is recommended for all pregnant patients found to have significant bacteriuria.[117,205] Ideally, all women should be screened in the first and third trimesters of pregnancy. The goal of therapy is to maintain sterile urine throughout gestation and thereby to avoid the complications associated with urinary tract infection during pregnancy. The administration of a relatively nontoxic drug for 7 days (e.g., a sulfonamide, amoxicillin, amoxicillin-clavulanate, cephalexin, nitrofurantoin) eradicates bacteriuria in 70% to 80% of patients.[117] As in nongravid women, increased ampicillin-resistant *E. coli* causing gestational cystitis and pyelonephritis has been reported.[209] Failure of treatment is most commonly seen in patients with renal infection or radiologic abnormalities of the urinary tract.[117] Sulfonamides should not be administered in the last few weeks of gestation because they may contribute to hyperbilirubinemia and kernicterus in the newborn. Tetracyclines and quinolones should be avoided during pregnancy.

Relatively few studies have evaluated the efficacy of single-dose or 3-day antimicrobial therapy for asymptomatic bacteriuria during pregnancy. In general, results of single-dose therapy appear to be inferior to those of conventional therapy.[117,210] However, 3 days of therapy has now emerged as the first option in both symptomatic and asymptomatic infection in an attempt to decrease drug administration in pregnancy. Acute pyelonephritis in pregnancy is treated vigorously with parenteral antibiotics as in the nongravid state, but mild episodes may respond to outpatient management.

Urine cultures should be obtained 1 to 2 weeks after discontinuing therapy and at regular intervals (e.g., monthly) for the remainder of gestation. If bacteriuria recurs, therapy should be given for relapse or reinfection, as already discussed. Catheterization should be avoided at the time of delivery. If relapses or multiple reinfections occurred during pregnancy, an imaging evaluation should be considered postpartum. Effective prophylaxis for recurrent urinary infection in pregnancy can be achieved by postcoital prophylaxis consisting of a single oral dose of either cephalexin (250 mg) or nitrofurantoin macrocrystals (50 mg).[188]

PROSTATITIS

Bacterial prostatitis can manifest as either an acute or a chronic disease. Although the manner by which bacteria reach the prostate is unknown,[211,212] possibilities include the hematogenous route, ascending infection from the urethra, and lymphatic spread from the rectum. Reflux of infected urine may also play a role in the pathogenesis of bacterial prostatitis.[213] Urethral instrumentation and prostatic surgery are known causes of prostatitis, but many patients have no history of a precipitating event.

Stamey has noted that male sex partners of women with vaginal colonization by gram-negative bacilli may develop transient urethral colonization with the same organisms.[214] He postulated that sexual intercourse might play an important role in infection of the prostate. Prostatic fluid constituents, notably zinc, normally have substantial antibacterial properties.[67,215] However, the prostatic secretions of some patients with chronic bacterial prostatitis have been shown to lack such activity.[215,216] Bacterial prostatitis infrequently develops after transurethral prostatectomy in men who have infected urine.[212] A bacterial cause is easily demonstrated in less than 10% of cases of prostatitis; these respond symptomatically to conventional antimicrobial treatment.

The syndromes of acute and chronic bacterial prostatitis are distinctly different. Acute prostatitis does not usually result in chronic prostatitis, and chronic bacterial prostatitis is not usually antedated by acute prostatitis. Acute prostatitis is similar to an acute localized infection in any other organ, producing local heat, tenderness, and fever. In contrast, chronic bacterial prostatitis often produces few or no symptoms related to the prostate, which just serves as a nidus of low-grade infection. Symptoms of acute cystitis or pyelonephritis occur when the bacteria that are repeatedly invading the bladder overcome the defense mechanisms of the bladder.

After acute bacterial prostatitis, a serum and local immune response is elicited, with the presence of IgA and IgG bacteria-specific immunoglobulins being detected in prostatic secretions. More prolonged prostatic secretion of antigen-specific IgG and IgA is observed in chronic bacterial prostatitis.[217]

The standard classification of prostatitis (i.e., acute bacterial prostatitis, chronic bacterial prostatitis, nonbacterial prostatitis, and prostadynia) has recently been replaced because it was recognized that few practitioners still utilize the Meares and Stamey localization procedure (see "Type II Prostatitis," later).[218] The new National Institutes of Health (NIH) classification system emphasizes the importance of pain in patients with chronic bacterial prostatitis and prostadynia (Table 66-5). The new classification further recognizes the significance of inflammatory cells in a variety of prostate-specific specimens, such as expressed prostatic secretion (EPS), and it has defined a new entity of asymptomatic prostatitis.[219]

Type I Prostatitis (Acute Bacterial Prostatitis)

Most cases of acute bacterial prostatitis in the preantibiotic era were caused by *N. gonorrhoeae*. Gram-negative enteric organisms, most commonly *E. coli,* are now the most frequent pathogens.[211,212] *N. gonorrhoeae* is currently an unusual cause. Rarely, hematogenous *S. aureus* abscess formation has been reported.

TABLE 66-5 The National Institutes of Health Prostatitis Classification System[219]

Category	Inflammatory Type
I	Acute bacterial prostatitis
II	Chronic bacterial prostatitis
III	Chronic pelvic pain syndrome (CPPS) (chronic nonbacterial prostatitis)
IIIA	Inflammatory
IIIB	Noninflammatory
IV	Asymptomatic inflammatory prostatitis

Pathologically, acute bacterial prostatitis is characterized by inflammation of part or all of the gland, with marked cellular infiltrate (predominantly PMNs), diffuse edema, and hyperemia of the stroma. Microabscesses may occur and may be followed by large, clinically apparent collections of pus. Transrectal ultrasonography is the study of choice to demonstrate the presence of an abscess. If ultrasonography is not available, a CT or an MRI scan of the pelvis may be useful.

Acute bacterial prostatitis is characterized by high fever, chills, perineal and back pain, and by symptoms of urinary tract infection such as frequency, urgency, and dysuria.[212] The patient may have urinary retention due to bladder outlet obstruction. The prostate gland is warm, swollen, and extremely tender on rectal examination. Expressed prostatic fluid contains many PMNs, and the infecting organism can frequently be seen on Gram stain. However, massage of the acutely infected prostate gland can precipitate bacteremia and should be discouraged. Since most patients also have bacteriuria, the infecting organism can usually be isolated by midstream urine culture. Many antibiotics diffuse well into the acutely inflamed prostate, and acute bacterial prostatitis responds well to appropriate antimicrobial therapy. Complications such as bacteremia, prostatic abscess (Fig. 66-8), epididymitis, seminal vesiculitis, and pyelonephritis may occur.

Type II Prostatitis (Chronic Bacterial Prostatitis)

Chronic bacterial prostatitis is most commonly caused by *E. coli* (80%), but *Klebsiella, Enterobacter* species, *P. mirabilis,* and enterococci are also common causes.[212] Although *S. epidermidis, S. aureus,* and diphtheroids have been frequent isolates in some series,[216] there is considerable doubt as to their real pathogenic role, and most gram-positive bacteria cultured in association with prostatitis represent urethral commensals.[212] Reported rare causes of prostatitis include *Candida* species, *Blastomyces dermatitidis, Histoplasma capsulatum, Mycobacterium tuberculosis,* and nontuberculous mycobacteria. The prostate gland has been identified as an important subclinical focus of *Cryptococcus neoformans* infection. Occasionally, histologic specimens of prostatic tissue reveal granulomatous prostatitis of unknown cause.

The histologic findings of chronic bacterial prostatitis are focal, nonacute inflammation. Similar findings may be noted in patients without evidence of bacterial infection and are therefore not diagnostic of bacterial prostatitis.

Many men with chronic infection of the prostate are totally asymptomatic. However, some have perineal discomfort, low back pain, frequency, or dysuria. Symptoms of acute urinary tract infection may appear periodically. In fact, chronic bacterial prostatitis is probably the most common cause of relapsing urinary tract infection in men. Fever, if present, tends to be low grade unless pyelonephritis occurs. The results of rectal examination and imaging studies are unremarkable

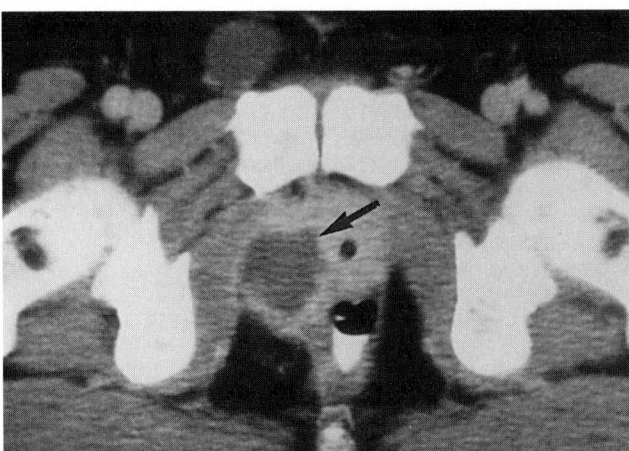

FIGURE 66-8. Computed tomogram demonstrating a large prostatic abscess *(arrow)* adjacent and lateral to the urethra. The rectum contains contrast material.

unless the patient also has an enlarged prostate gland from benign prostatic hypertrophy or carcinoma. In the absence of characteristic findings on physical examination, the hallmark of chronic bacterial prostatitis is bacterial persistence in repeated urine cultures yielding the same microorganisms.

Because of the focal nature of chronic bacterial prostatitis, needle biopsy of the prostate gland for culture of tissue is unreliable.[220] Demonstration of leukocytes in prostatic fluid is not specific for bacterial prostatitis. Most clinicians agree that more than 15 leukocytes per high-power field represents an abnormal number of leukocytes in prostatic fluid.[212] Provided that simultaneous urethral and midstream specimens show insignificant pyuria, this finding would indicate prostatic inflammation irrespective of the cause.

Meares and Stamey described a quantitative localization technique for making the bacteriologic diagnosis.[218] Because bacteria present in the urethra can contaminate prostatic secretions obtained by prostatic massage, accurate diagnosis requires simultaneous quantitative cultures of (1) urethral urine (VB_1), (2) midstream urine (VB_2), (3) prostatic secretions expressed by massage (EPS), and (4) the urine voided after massage (VB_3). The specimens must be cultured immediately after collection, and methods of quantitating small numbers of bacteria must be used. The study should be done at a time that the patient does not have significant bacteriuria. If bacteriuria is present, ampicillin, cephalexin, or nitrofurantoin should be given for 2 to 3 days to sterilize the urine; these agents will not affect bacterial counts in the prostate in chronic bacterial prostatitis. If chronic bacterial prostatitis is present, the number of bacteria in EPS or ejaculate will exceed those in VB_1 or VB_2 urine by at least 10-fold. If no EPS or ejaculate can be obtained, the bacterial counts in the VB_3 specimen should be at least 10-fold higher than the VB_1 or VB_2 samples.

Chronic bacterial prostatitis is very difficult to cure because few antimicrobial agents penetrate well into the noninflamed prostate. Furthermore, the nidus of infection in some patients may be small prostatic calculi or abscesses that presumably are difficult to sterilize. Transrectal ultrasonography will demonstrate prostatic calculi in many patients with chronic bacterial prostatitis.[211] Chronic bacterial prostatitis is therefore likely to persist and cause relapsing urinary tract infection. Unlike classic urinary tract infection, relapses may occur after long periods (e.g., months) without bacteriuria. Management may be difficult (see "Therapy," later).

Type III Prostatitis: Chronic Pelvic Pain Syndrome (Nonbacterial Prostatitis)

Nonbacterial prostatitis is the most common type of prostatitis (90%) and represents an inflammatory or noninflammatory condition of unknown cause.[212] Symptoms are perineal pressure, dysuria, urgency, or low back pain, but all of these symptoms can also be caused by chronic bacterial prostatitis. However, bacterial pathogens cannot be demonstrated using sequential quantitative cultures. Urinary tract infection does not occur, although prostatic secretions contain excessive numbers of leukocytes and fat-laden macrophages. Although *Chlamydia* and *Ureaplasma* species have been implicated as causes of nonbacterial prostatitis, supporting evidence is not convincing.[211,212,221] Recent techniques identifying bacterial DNA in prostatic tissue in chronic nonbacterial prostatitis sufferers suggest a microbial etiology in some cases.[222] The term *prostadynia* or *prostatosis* refers to a similar clinical syndrome in the absence of any objective signs of prostatic inflammation. Some think that the symptoms may be caused by spasm of the pelvic floor musculature.[211,223,224] Others say that there may be a major psychological component. Because the cause of both entities is unknown, therapy is difficult.

Therapy

A dog model has been used to measure the diffusion of antimicrobial agents into the noninflamed prostate.[225] In this system, antimicrobial agents were infused, giving high and constant plasma levels, and prostatic secretions are simultaneously collected. Although the basic macrolides such as erythromycin penetrated well into prostatic secretions,

penicillins, cephalosporins, tetracyclines, nitrofurantoin, and vancomycin did not. The explanation given was that only lipid-soluble and basic compounds are capable of entering the acid milieu of the prostate gland. Trimethroprim[226] and the fluoroquinolones diffuse into prostatic fluid in high concentrations.[211,224,227]

Acute bacterial prostatitis frequently responds dramatically to antibacterial therapy. It is thought that the intense diffuse inflammatory reaction of acute bacterial prostatitis allows the passage of antimicrobial agents from plasma into the prostate.[212] Therefore, in the management of acute prostatitis, antimicrobial agents should be given to the patient in doses that achieve therapeutic concentrations in the blood. Appropriate treatment of coliform infections includes trimethoprim-sulfamethoxazole, cephalosporins, amoxicillin, or any of the fluoroquinolones. Ciprofloxacin, 500 mg twice daily, is suitable for the occasional episodes caused by *P. aeruginosa*. Rarely, parenteral antibiotics are required. After a favorable clinical response, antimicrobial therapy should be continued for a minimum of 4 weeks. Measures such as hydration, analgesics, bed rest, and stool softeners may be helpful. Urethral instrumentation should be avoided. If acute urinary retention occurs, drainage of urine through a suprapubic catheter is required. Prostatic abscess is rarely cured by antimicrobial agents alone and requires surgical drainage. Drainage can often be achieved by an ultrasound-guided needle.

Chronic bacterial prostatitis is very difficult to cure. Although it is not widely accepted, some urologists recommend transurethral resection to unroof and remove calculi. Partial transurethral prostatectomy is curative only if all the infected tissue is removed; about one third of the patients are cured by this procedure.[212] However, a higher percentage are cured if a radical transurethral prostatectomy is performed.[212] Complete prostatectomy is contraindicated because of the complications of sexual impotence and incontinence.

The primary approach to chronic bacterial prostatitis is an attempt at cure with antimicrobial therapy. Although occasional cures have been achieved with penicillins, cephalosporins, tetracyclines, or aminoglycosides, the focus of infection in the prostate has usually persisted, resulting in relapse after therapy is discontinued. Better results have been reported in limited trials with trimethoprim-sulfamethoxazole (one double-strength tablet twice a day). Cure rates have varied from one third to most of the patients treated for several months. The sulfonamide component of trimethoprim-sulfamethoxazole probably contributes little, and rifampin may be more suitable than sulfamethoxazole as a partner for trimethoprim.[228] Although prospective comparative studies are needed, clinical series indicate that fluoroquinolones (e.g., ciprofloxacin 500 mg twice a day for 30 days) achieve comparable if not superior results to trimethoprim-sulfamethoxazole.[211,212,224,227,229] At present, the initial regimen of choice is trimethoprim-sulfamethoxazole or a quinolone. Long-term cure rates of 60% to 70% are obtained with antibiotics prescribed for 6 to 12 weeks. If therapy fails with these regimens, the patient should be managed either with treatment of acute exacerbations of urinary tract infection or with chronic suppressive therapy to prevent urinary tract infections using low daily doses (e.g., half-normal doses) of an antimicrobial agent. Nonbacterial prostatitis, both inflammatory and noninflammatory, can be treated empirically with a macrolide or a tetracycline, relying on the clinical response to justify a further trial of therapy; a positive response occurs in about 40% of patients. Reassurance is important. Other treatment options include nonsteroidal anti-inflammatory drugs, α-blockers, pelvic floor physiotherapy, and amitriptyline.[230]

PERINEPHRIC ABSCESS AND INTRARENAL ABSCESS

Perinephric Abscess

Perinephric abscess is an uncommon complication of urinary tract infection.[231] The most common predisposing factors are urinary tract calculi and diabetes mellitus. It usually occurs secondary to obstruction of an infected kidney or calyx or occasionally secondary to bacteremia. It may occur insidiously, and up to one third of cases may not be diagnosed until autopsy. The infecting bacteria are usually gram-negative enteric bacilli and occasionally gram-positive cocci when the infection is of hematogenous origin. Multiple bacterial species are present in about 25% of cases, and occasionally fungi, especially *Candida* species, can be cultured from the abscess. The abscess is usually confined by Gerota's fascia to the perinephric space but may extend throughout the retroperitoneum to affect adjacent structures.[232]

The patients have a syndrome suggestive of acute pyelonephritis, with fever, abdominal and flank pain (usually unilateral), and often symptoms of lower tract infection. However, presenting symptoms are often nonspecific. The patient has often been ill for 2 or more weeks. The diagnosis should be strongly considered in any patient with a febrile illness and unilateral flank pain who does not respond to therapy for acute pyelonephritis. A palpable mass may or may not be present. About one half of the patients have an abnormal plain film of the abdomen (e.g., an abdominal mass, an enlarged kidney with indistinct outlines, a loss of the psoas margin, a calculus, a poorly defined renal shadow). Pyuria and proteinuria are frequently found, but about 30% of patients have a normal urinalysis, and about 40% have sterile urine cultures.[232]

Intrarenal Abscess

Intrarenal abscess may occur as a consequence of bacteremia (often caused by coagulase-positive staphylococci). Hematogenous lesions are usually unilateral, single, and located in the cortex. However, these focal suppurative lesions are being recognized with increasing frequency as a complication of classic acute pyelonephritis and are located in the cortex or the medulla, or both. The clinical setting is usually that of acute pyelonephritis with high fever, with severe flank pain and tenderness, but with no response or very slow response to appropriate antimicrobial therapy. Contrast-enhanced CT may detect intense parenchymatous inflammation and necrosis in a lobe of the kidney, termed *lobar nephronia* or *acute focal bacterial nephritis*. Although antibiotics may arrest progression at this stage, coalescence of microabscesses (multifocal bacterial nephritis) can lead to intrarenal abscess. Emphysematous pyelonephritis is an uncommon, severe, necrotizing form of acute multifocal bacterial nephritis in which retroperitoneal, extraluminal gas is seen in the renal parenchyma and perirenal space on an abdominal radiograph. The presence of gas suggests a gas-forming, gram-negative, facultative anaerobic uropathogen. *E. coli* is the most common organism associated with this complication, but *Klebsiella* species, *P. mirabilis,* and *Citrobacter* species may be involved. This condition occurs most commonly in diabetic patients with or without urinary obstruction.[233] The mortality rate is 70% in spite of antibiotic therapy, and immediate nephrectomy is almost always necessary.[178]

Xanthogranulomatous pyelonephritis is an uncommon but severe focal or diffuse chronic infection of the renal parenchyma. Destroyed tissue is replaced by granulomatous tissue containing lipid-laden macrophages (foam cells). Predisposing factors include renal calculi, urinary obstruction, lymphatic obstruction, renal ischemia and secondary metabolic alterations in lipid metabolism, an abnormal host immune response, and diabetes mellitus.[234]

Diagnosis and Therapy

Urinalysis is abnormal in 70% of patients with a corticomedullary abscess, whereas it is usually normal in the patient with a hematogenous cortical or perinephric abscess. Confirmation of the diagnosis requires imaging techniques.

The introduction of renal ultrasonography and in particular CT scans has added a new dimension of sensitivity and specificity, permitting the early diagnosis of intrarenal and perinephric abscesses (Figs. 66-9 through 66-11).[235-237] The most common CT findings include thickening of Gerota's fascia, renal enlargement, focal parenchymal decreased attenuation, and fluid or gas, or both, in and around the kidney.[235,236]

In patients with a clinical or radiographic suspicion of perinephric abscess, diagnostic needle aspiration can be safely performed by using ultrasonography or CT guidance. When an abscess is confirmed,

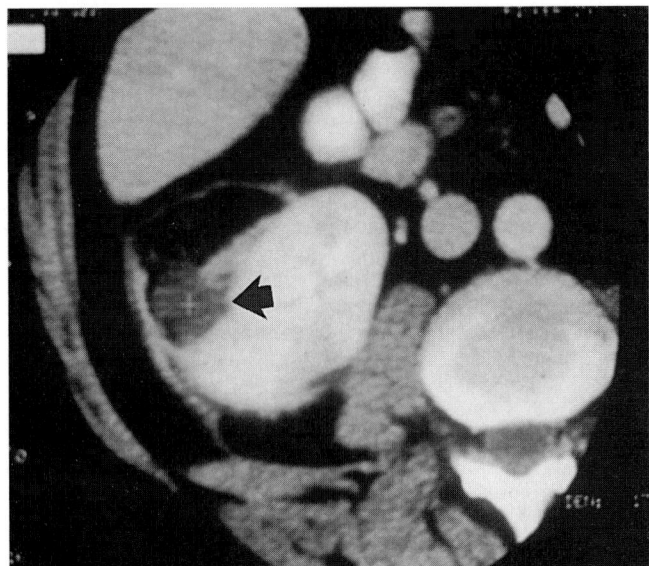

FIGURE 66-9. On computed tomography, an intrarenal abscess, evident as a well-delineated hypodense lesion *(arrow),* is seen extending into the intrarenal space. *(Courtesy of M. Bergeron, M.D.)*

small catheters can be introduced percutaneously to provide immediate decompression as well as continuous and definitive drainage without the need for surgery.[237,238] Advantages to guided percutaneous drainage compared with open surgical drainage include earlier diagnosis and treatment, the avoidance of general anesthesia and surgery, less expensive therapy, easier nursing care, and greater patient acceptance of closed drainage. Accordingly, it is now recommended that after antimicrobial therapy directed against the most likely pathogens is started, a trial of percutaneous drainage should be the initial mode of therapy for perinephric abscess. Surgical intervention should be undertaken only when percutaneous drainage fails or is contraindicated. Although parenteral antimicrobial therapy directed against the infecting organism isolated from blood or urine should be initiated before drainage, additional organisms may be isolated at the time of drainage, and then treatment directed against these organisms must be added. Therapy must also be used for the underlying disease (e.g., obstructive uropathy).

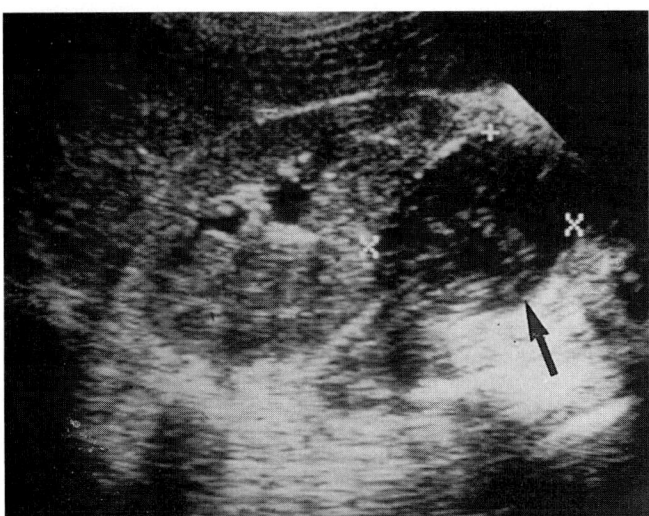

FIGURE 66-10. Ultrasound examination revealing a perinephric abscess *(arrow).* *(Courtesy of M. Bergeron, M.D.)*

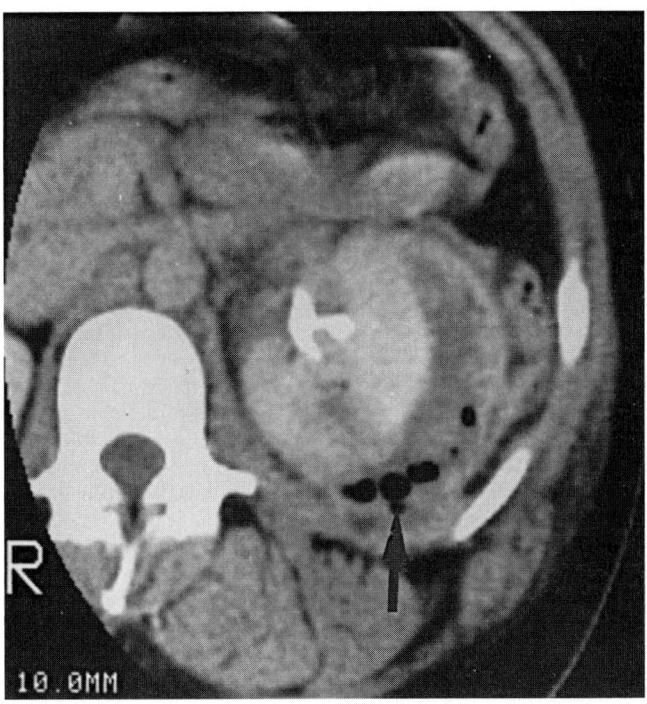

FIGURE 66-11. Computed tomography with contrast material demonstrating a large left perinephric abscess containing gas *(arrow).*

When antimicrobial therapy with appropriate agents fails with infected renal cysts or abscesses, percutaneous drainage should be tried. Agents that diffuse into these closed sites, such as trimethoprim-sulfamethoxazole and fluoroquinolones, may have an advantage.[239,240] Percutaneous drainage often avoids the previous approach of open surgical drainage or nephrectomy.[237,238,241]

Successful percutaneous treatment has been reported in 90% of patients with renal or perinephric abscess formation.[241] In the past, delay and missed diagnosis resulted in mortality rates of 20% to 50% in patients with perinephric abscess, with approximately one third of cases diagnosed only postmortem. Today, with early recognition utilizing modern imaging techniques, together with prompt drainage and antibiotic therapy, the mortality is extremely low. Most patients with intrarenal abscess respond, although slowly, to antimicrobial therapy, but fever and severe flank pain may persist for days. Siegel and coworkers reported that virtually all intrarenal abscesses less than 3 cm in diameter resolved on antibiotic therapy alone, as did 92% of those 3 to 5 cm in diameter, whereas larger abscesses (>5 cm) often required percutaneous (33%) or open (37%) surgical drainage.[242] Nephrectomy is reserved for emphysematous pyelonephritis, patients with diffusely damaged renal parenchyma, or older adults with septicemia requiring urgent intervention for survival.

IMAGING EVALUATION OF PATIENTS WITH URINARY TRACT INFECTION

Imaging procedures play an important role in the diagnosis and management of patients with urinary tract infection,[236] both in the control of complicated episodes of acute pyelonephritis and in the investigation of patients of all ages in whom the clinician suspects the presence of underlying structural abnormalities that may be surgically correctable. In adults, uncomplicated acute renal infections do not require an imaging workup. Studies are useful when the diagnosis is in doubt, in severely ill or immunocompromised patients, in those patients with pyelonephritis who fail to improve after 72 hours of appropriate antibiotic therapy, or when complications are suspected. Imaging may also be indicated when

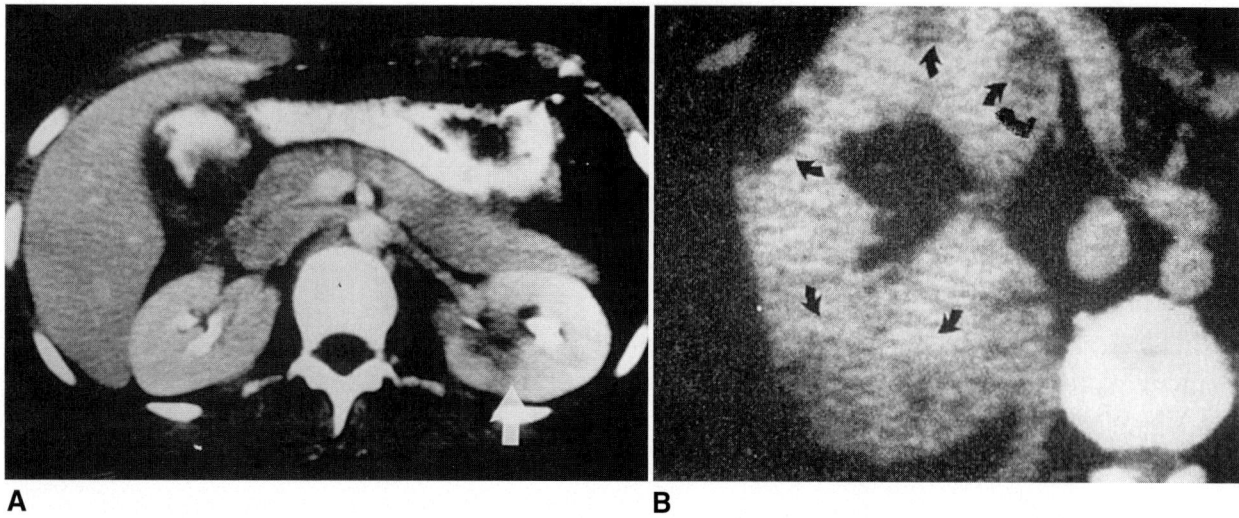

A   **B**

FIGURE 66-12. Computed tomography in acute pyelonephritis. The masslike lesion of pyelonephritis is often well defined because it is less dense than the cortex. **A,** It can be irregular with a nonhomogeneous center *(arrow),* as seen in the left kidney. The contralateral kidney is normal. **B,** Acute pyelonephritis can appear as multifocal with diffuse masslike lesions *(arrows). (Courtesy of Huang, M.D.)*

certain bacterial species such as *C. urealyticum* are isolated, as infection with these organisms may be a clue to renal stones.

Imaging assessment should commence with a plain film of the abdomen for the detection of urinary tract calculi, calcification, soft tissue masses, and abnormal gas collections. In the past, excretory urography in the form of IVP was the initial and definitive investigatory study, but this has been largely replaced by both ultrasonography and CT scans (Figs. 66-12 and 66-13). In general, sonography serves as a rapid, noninvasive, and relatively inexpensive means of evaluating the renal collecting system, parenchyma, and surrounding retroperitoneum.[238] Ultrasonography is more sensitive than IVP for detecting parenchymal changes associated with renal infection.

Johnson and associates confirmed that ultrasonographically demonstrable renal swelling characteristically occurs in almost all women with acute pyelonephritis.[243] Enlargement may be unilateral or bilateral and correlates with protracted pretreatment symptoms, leukocytosis, high fever, focal suppurative complications, and prolonged hospitalization. They also indicated that the frequency of underlying abnormalities and focal complications is low.[243] Several large studies have now confirmed that ultrasonography, especially when combined with a plain film of the abdomen, has become the radiologic investigation of choice in young women with urinary tract infection,[244,245] replacing excretory urography.

CT is the most sensitive technique of all, and guidelines issued by the American College of Radiology recommend contrast-enhanced CT as the study of choice.[246] Nevertheless, compared with CT, sonography offers several advantages, including no irradiation, portability, relative accessibility, and the fact that contrast material does not have to be administered.[244] The increased sensitivity of contrast-enhanced CT, especially helical CT, is particularly apparent in identifying renal parenchymal abnormalities in all but the mildest cases of acute pyelonephritis. Newer ultrasound techniques, such as Doppler, power Doppler, and pulse inversion harmonic imaging, are currently under investigation to overcome its lack of sensitivity. Sonography is normal in most uncomplicated cases with acute pyelonephritis. A common CT finding is decreased opacification of the affected renal parenchyma, usually in a patchy, wedge-shaped, or linear pattern. Different patterns may coexist, and abnormalities vary in size. Non–contrast-enhanced CT is often normal but may show focal areas of decreased attenuation. Areas of markedly decreased attenuation should raise a suspicion of abscess formation, and then contrast material should, if possible, be administered. Other CT findings in pyelonephritis include diffuse or focal kidney enlargement, perinephric stranding, and mild collecting system dilatation. In moderate and severe cases of acute pyelonephritis, CT-scan abnormalities

usually persist for several weeks, well after clinical symptoms and laboratory findings have returned to normal.[247] After adequate therapy, most cases eventually demonstrate complete resolution of imaging abnormalities. In recurrent infection associated with chronic reflux, the affected renal lobes develop changes of reflux nephropathy. Recurrent infection results in deformity and dilatation of calyces and focal cortical loss, with upper and lower poles severely affected.

Both CT and ultrasonography are sensitive in diagnosing intrarenal and perirenal suppuration. On contrast-enhanced CT, the hallmark of an abscess is a focal area that fails to enhance, indicating an avascular state. Abscesses are typically sharply demarcated and round or ovoid and contain a low-density center. The abscess wall enhances after contrast injection, resulting in the "rind sign" owing to the presence of inflamed dilated vessels.[237] When detected, gas within a low-density mass is pathognomonic for abscess formation. In contradistinction to pyelonephritis, intrarenal abscesses reaching 2 to 3 cm are well evaluated by ultrasonography, showing sharp demarcation and the presence of liquefaction.[233] Ultrasonography demonstrates a well-marginated, hypoechoic mass with good through transmission, an irregular interior wall margin, and scattered echogenic foci within the mass representing debris. Gas formation is highly echogenic. Both these procedures may be used for the guidance of percutaneous needle aspiration.

Neither the CT scan nor ultrasonography reliably distinguishes an uninfected obstructed renal collection system (hydronephrosis) from pyonephrosis. Suggestive findings on CT scan include an increased thickness of the renal pelvis wall and the presence of increased density within the renal pelvis indicative of pus or debris. The strongest indication of pyonephrosis on CT is the presence of gas within the collecting system, but this is uncommon. Sonography may identify echogenic contents or debris (Fig. 66-14).

Gas formation within the renal parenchyma as a consequence of severe infection by facultative anaerobes or *Candida* species is termed *emphysematous pyelonephritis.* Although gas may be seen on plain radiographs, it is often mistaken for bowel gas. CT is exquisitely sensitive in the detection of gas, which appears as small bubbles or as linear streaks. Gas often collects in a subcapsular location, forming a sharp line around the margin of the kidney, or it may be seen within the renal collecting system.

IVP remains useful for detecting lesions of the collecting system and ureters. Contrast-enhanced CT provides physiologic information similar to that obtained with IVP, with much better parenchymal delineation but less-than-optimal delineation of the collecting system.[235] When renal calculi may be present, the CT study should also include

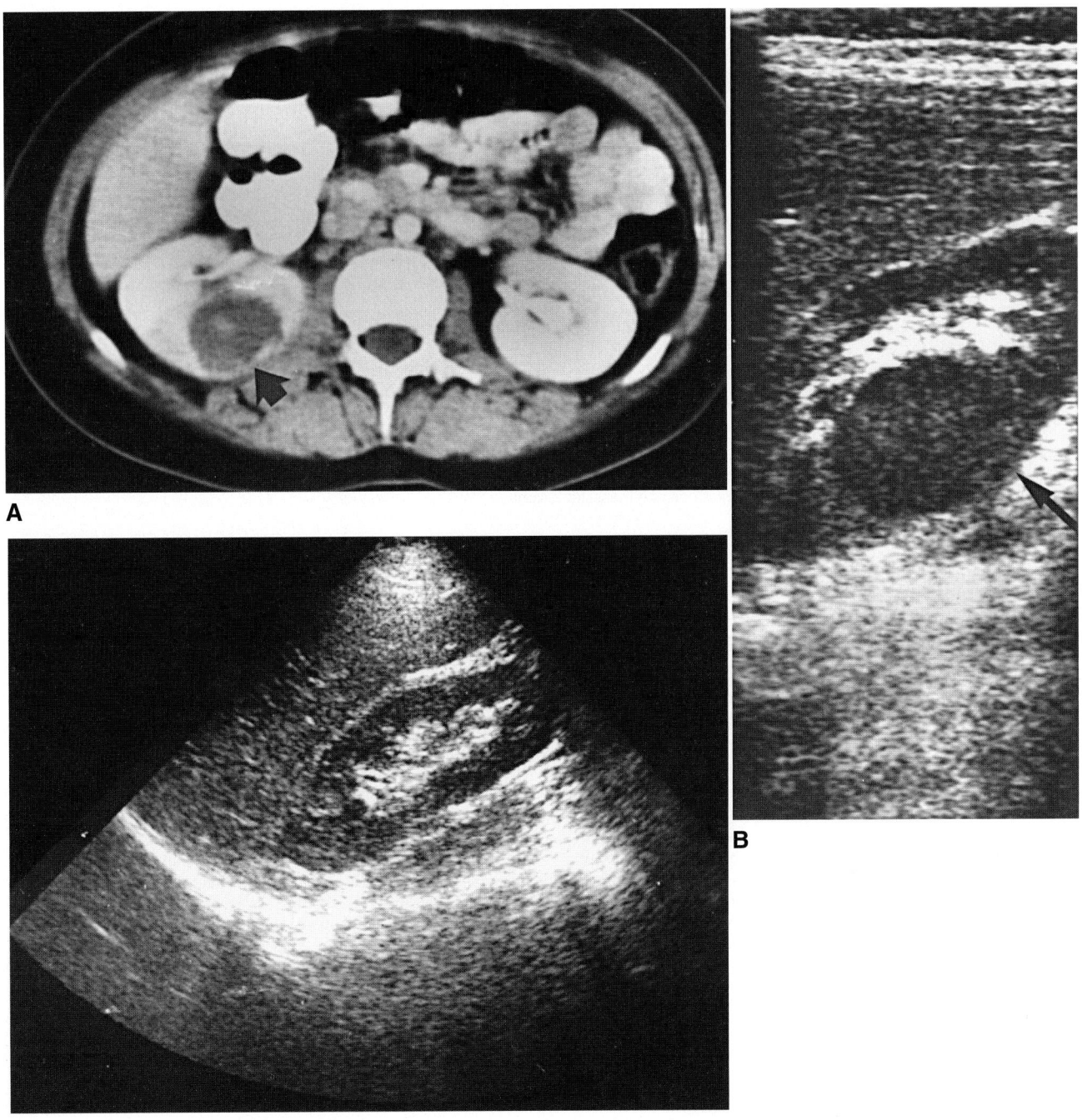

FIGURE 66-13. A, On a computed tomography scan, acute pyelonephritis with a masslike lesion is evident in the right kidney *(arrow)*. **B,** Ultrasound examination of the same right kidney. **C,** The mass has resolved on the follow-up ultrasound study performed 2 months later. *(Courtesy of T. Slovis, M.D.)*

noncontrast images through the kidney. Helical CT without contrast material is a highly effective means to confirm or exclude the presence of obstructing ureteral calculi.[248]

All studies requiring the parenteral administration of contrast material are associated with some risk for allergy or contrast-induced renal insufficiency. Predisposing factors for renal insufficiency include myeloma, diabetes mellitus, preexisting renal failure, severe intravascular volume depletion, and the recent administration of large doses of iodinated contrast material. MRI offers no advantage over CT in the diagnosis of intrarenal or perinephric abscess but may be considered as an alternative to contrast-enhanced CT in patients with a contraindication to iodinated contrast administration.

Radioisotope studies play only a small role in the investigation of the urinary tract. Gallium-67 citrate scanning, indium-111–labeled white blood cell studies, and renal scintigraphy utilizing technetium-99m (^{99m}Tc) dimercaptosuccinic acid (DMSA) occasionally prove useful in localizing inflammation or infection to the kidneys in patients with fever of unknown origin, especially those patients with spinal cord injuries (Fig. 66-15). Radionuclide scanning may be of value, after ultrasonography or CT scans have identified a solid renal mass, in suggesting the inflammatory nature of the lesion. Neither of these radionuclide studies distinguishes pyelonephritis from abscess.

Another important contribution provided by these imaging modalities is the detection of surgically correctable abnormalities of the urinary

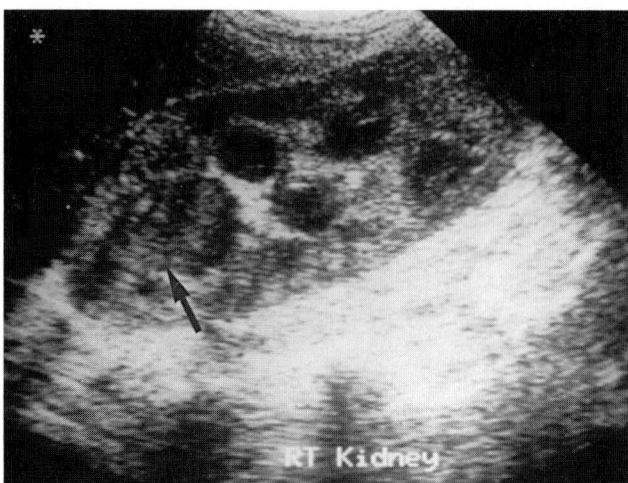

FIGURE 66-14. Ultrasound study demonstrating pyonephrosis (i.e., hydronephrosis) and echogenic content of the collecting system *(arrow)*.

tract. Investigation should be considered in patients at the greatest risk for having surgically correctable abnormalities. Persons with urinary tract infection included in this higher-risk category are all children, men of any age, patients who relapse after therapy, and patients whose infection has been complicated by bacteremia. In the past, excretory urography was indicated for all these categories and for adult women only after multiple episodes of urinary tract infection. As mentioned

previously, given the value of ultrasonography, its availability, and its safety, it might be reasonable to study all patients with upper tract infection by this method.[245] However, as indicated by Johnson and co-workers and now supported by the American College of Radiology, the routine use of noninvasive renal ultrasonography in women with acute uncomplicated pyelonephritis appears excessive because focal complications are rare and underlying structural abnormalities occur in only about 5% of cases.[243,246] Women with bacteriuria of pregnancy in whom eradication of infection is difficult should be evaluated. Whereas ultrasonography can be safely performed during pregnancy, accurate delineation of the urinary tract should be delayed until at least 2 months after delivery, by which time the physiologic alterations to the urinary tract that occur during pregnancy should be reversed.[117,208] Ultrasound examination is also useful in diagnosing lower urinary tract obstruction and detecting residual urine in the bladder. A radionuclide diethylenetriaminepentaacetic acid (DPTA) scan with furosemide to increase urine flow is useful in determining if there is structural as opposed to functional ureteropelvic junction obstruction.

In addition to delineating lesions amenable to surgical correction, imaging frequently provides information previously unknown to the patient or physician. For example, unsuspected renal scarring may be seen, suggesting the presence of undiagnosed urinary tract infection in childhood. Occasionally, an unusual or unsuspected type of renal infection such as tuberculosis, papillary necrosis, or xanthogranulomatous pyelonephritis may be discovered.[236] Two major radiologic patterns of xanthogranulomatous pyelonephritis are seen: that of a localized mass and that of diffuse nodularity (Fig. 66-16). When a mass lesion is present, differentiation from pyogenic abscess, tuberculous abscess, or avascular carcinoma may not be possible. Additional findings include nephromegaly, thickening of Gerota's fascia, and infiltration into the perinephric space and surrounding retroperitoneal tissues.

Children with urinary tract infection are evaluated with imaging studies to identify those who may be at risk for chronic renal damage and to identify children who require corrective surgery to preserve renal function (Fig. 66-17).

Although controversial, ultrasonography and voiding cystourethrography are recommended in all boys after the first episode of urinary infection and in preschool girls at least after the second infection.[249-251] Investigation is indicated because the incidence of vesicoureteral reflux in this population has been reported to be 20% to 50%, and obstruction is not uncommon in boys. Reflux is associated

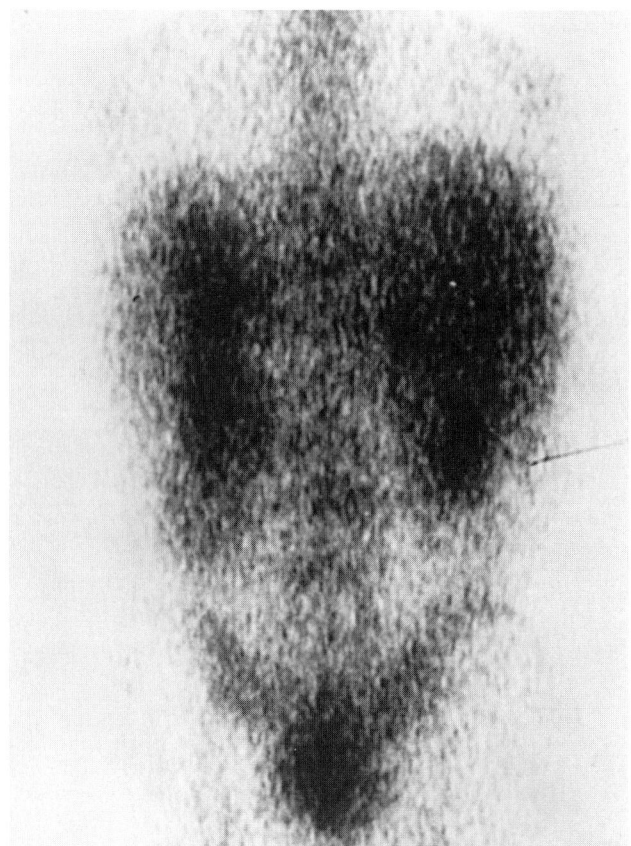

FIGURE 66-15. Renal gallium-67 scan in a young girl with bilateral acute pyelonephritis and increased uptake in both kidneys due to inflammation. *(Courtesy of M. Bergeron, M.D.)*

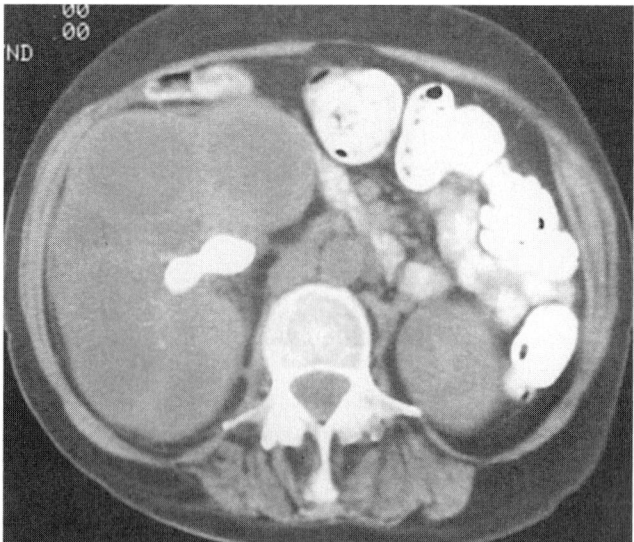

FIGURE 66-16. Computed tomography scan of a patient with right-sided xanthogranulomatous pyelonephritis. A huge multilobulated inflammatory mass replaces the right kidney. *Proteus mirabilis* was grown from the urine. *(Courtesy of L. E. Nicolle, M.D.)*

FIGURE 66-17. Voiding cystourethrogram. A, Posterior urethral valve on computed tomography scan. Note the discrepancy in size of the anterior *(arrow)* and the posterior urethra. **B,** There is irregular trabeculation of the bladder with right ureteric reflux. *(Courtesy of T. Slovis, M.D.)*

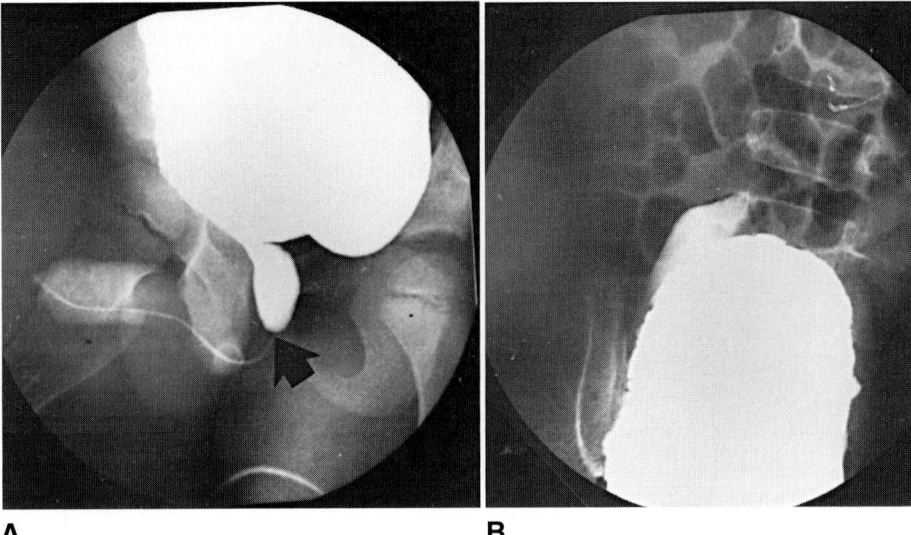

A   **B**

with renal scar formation, and surgery may be indicated in some of these children and infants. Several investigators consider that renal cortical scintigraphy is superior to renal ultrasonography and IVP in detecting evidence of both acute pyelonephritis and renal scarring.[249,252] Performing both renal cortical scintigraphy and ultrasonography appears unnecessary, and both have largely eliminated the need for IVP in children.[253] Radionuclide scanning with either ^{99m}Tc-glucoheptonate or ^{99m}Tc-DMSA has been shown to be a sensitive means of identifying not only renal scars but acute and chronic renal infection and upper urinary tract involvement (Fig. 66-18). These scans are utilized in identifying those children in whom lower urinary tract investigation is indicated to detect reflux, obstruction, or other congenital anomalies. DMSA abnormalities tend to resolve with time; however, an abnormal DMSA study at the time of urinary tract infection identifies most children with significant reflux.[254]

As an elective procedure for the detection and evaluation of vesicoureteral reflux, either conventional cystourethrography or high-resolution radionuclide voiding cystography is still required, especially because reflux with urinary tract dilatation is frequently undetected by ultrasonography and IVP (Fig. 66-19). The use of radionuclide cystography involves less irradiation and is better tolerated than conventional contrast material introduced by bladder catheterization. Recently, Hoberman and colleagues compared voiding cystourethrogram and renal ultrasound with renal DMSA scanning in

children (1 to 24 months old) and questioned the value of these procedures in facilitating the management of such children, especially because intervention options are limited and the efficacy of antimicrobial prophylaxis is not substantiated.[255] The authors recommended limiting urinary tract imaging after a first urinary tract infection to voiding cystourethrography.[255] They emphasized the importance of close follow-up, including urinalysis and urine culture, in planning additional imaging studies. Cystourethrography should be avoided in older children unless renal imaging shows evidence of renal scars. However, even with scars, if serial urographic evaluation demonstrates stability of upper tract lesions, the need for studying the lower tract is questionable unless the child experiences recurrent symptomatic infections. When reflux is found, it should be graded as minimal (grade I) to severe (grade IV), so progression or improvement can be quantitated and decisions about surgery can be made.[256,257]

SURGICAL MANAGEMENT

Surgical therapy in the management of urinary tract infection consists of the elimination of obstructive lesions or calculi and the reimplantation of ureters in the bladder for reflux. An obstruction may be intrinsic (such as renal cysts), or it may be extrinsic anywhere along the urinary conduit from the ureteropelvic junction to the external urethral meatus. Surgical therapy should be directed toward eliminating the

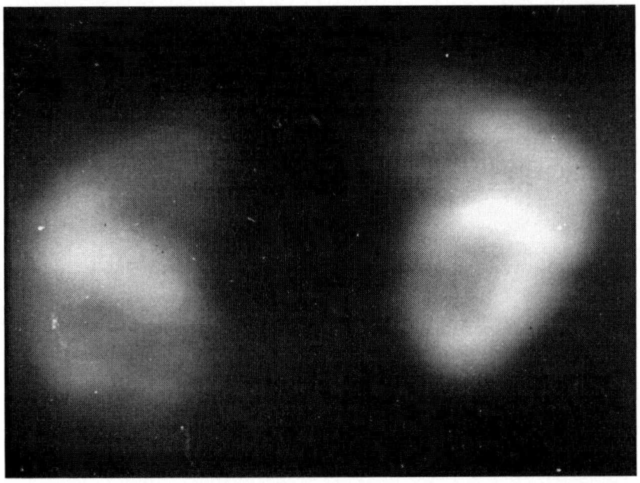

FIGURE 66-18. Acute pyelonephritis. A technetium-99m glucoheptonate, single photon-emission computed tomography scan with markedly decreased visualization of the upper and lower poles of the right kidney. The midportions are normal. *(Courtesy of T. Slovis, M.D.)*

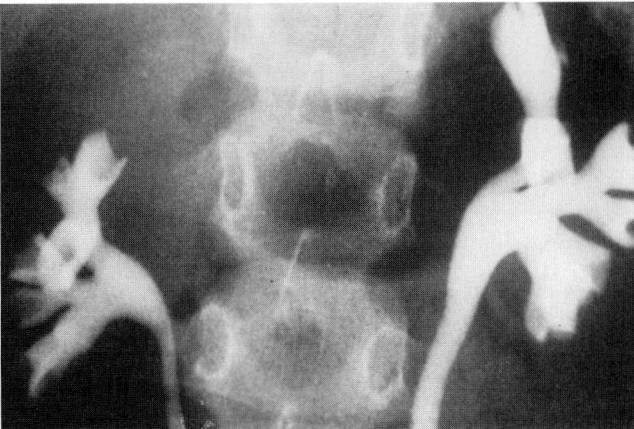

FIGURE 66-19. Grades II and III reflux in a voiding cystourethrographic study from a young boy who presented with recurrent urinary tract infection. Note early clubbing of the calyces and dilatation of the ureter on the left side. *(Courtesy of L. E. Nicolle, M.D.)*

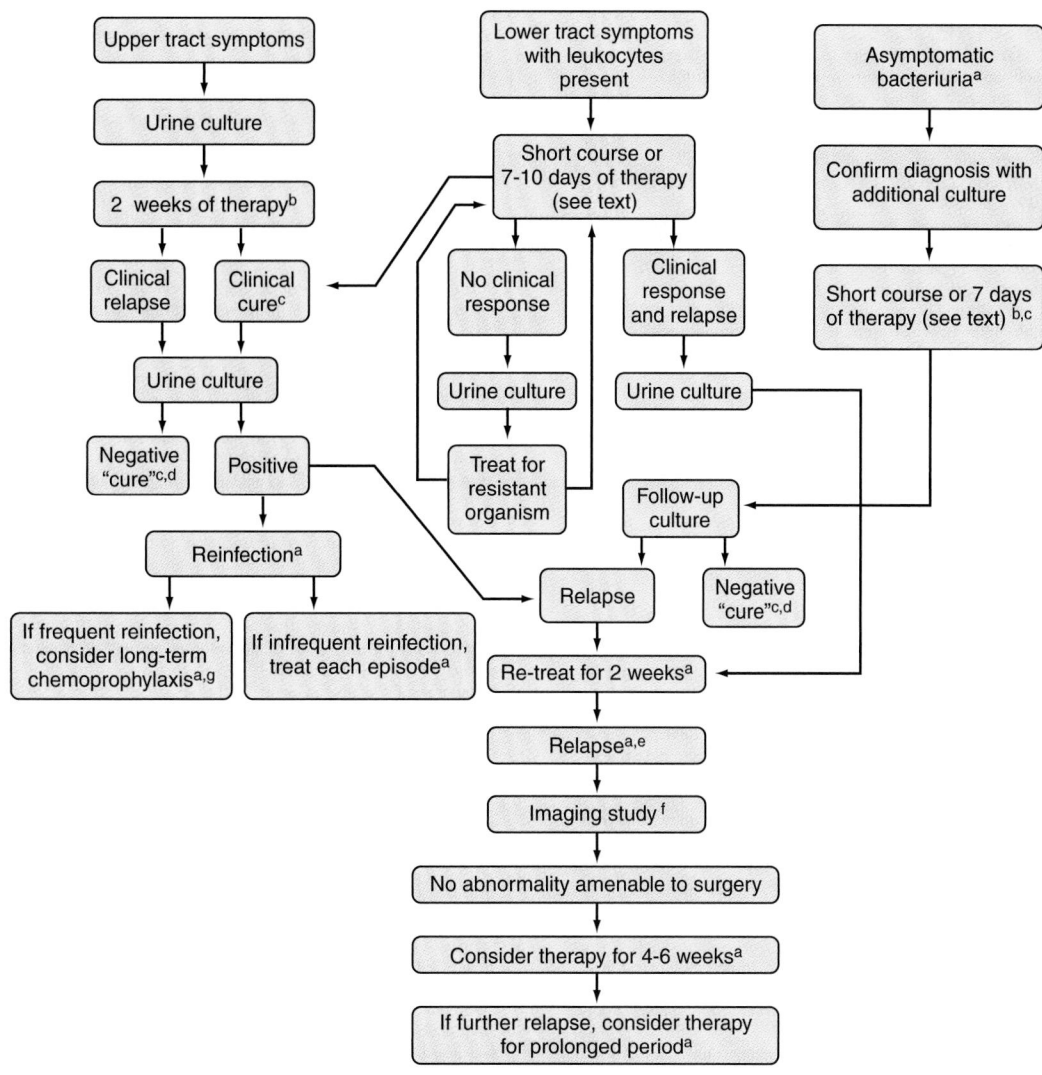

FIGURE 66-20. Approach to the management of urinary tract infection.
[a]Consider no therapy in nonpregnant adults without obstructive uropathy or symptoms of urinary tract infection.
[b]Consider imaging studies in all children and men with correction of significant lesions.
[c]Follow-up culture is required only in pregnancy, in children, and in adults with obstructive uropathy.
[d]Obtain follow-up cultures monthly in pregnant women and at 6 weeks and 6 months in children.
[e]Evaluate men for chronic bacterial prostatitis.
[f]Delay until 2 months postpartum in pregnant women.
[g]Consider imaging studies after three to four reinfections in women.

obstruction and preserving renal function. After the obstruction is eliminated, the patient should be followed with urine cultures. Urinary tract infection should be treated before surgery to render the urine sterile at the time of surgery; this decreases the possibility of bacteremia occurring in association with the surgery. Figure 66-20 summarizes the approach to the management of urinary tract infection. For management of perinephric or intrarenal abscess, see "Perinephric Abscess" or "Intrarenal Abscess," earlier.

REFERENCES

1. Hooton TM, Stamm WE. Diagnosis and treatment of uncomplicated urinary tract infection. Infect Dis Clin North Am. 1997;11:551-581.
2. Ronald AR, Harding GK. Complicated urinary tract infections. Infect Dis Clin North Am. 1997;11:583-592.
3. Cotran R, Kumar V, Collins T. Robbins Pathologic Basis of Disease. 6th ed. Philadelphia: Saunders; 1999.
4. Freedman LR. Chronic pyelonephritis at autopsy. Ann Intern Med. 1967;66:697-710.
5. Huland H, Busch R. Chronic pyelonephritis as a cause of end stage renal disease. J Urol. 1982;127:642-643.
6. Kunin CM. Natural history of "lower" urinary tract infections. Infection. 1990;18(Suppl 2):S44-49.
7. Buckley RM Jr, McGuckin M, MacGregor RR. Urine bacterial counts after sexual intercourse. N Engl J Med. 1978;298:321-324.
8. Kelsey MC, Mead MG, Gruneberg RN, et al. Relationship between sexual intercourse and urinary-tract infection in women attending a clinic for sexually transmitted diseases. J Med Microbiol. 1979;12:511-512.
9. Nicolle LE, Harding GK, Preiksaitis J, et al. The association of urinary tract infection with sexual intercourse. J Infect Dis. 1982;146:579-583.
10. Bran JL, Levison ME, Kaye D. Entrance of bacteria into the female urinary bladder. N Engl J Med. 1972;286:626-629.
11. Strom BL, Collins M, West SL, et al. Sexual activity, contraceptive use, and other risk factors for symptomatic and asymptomatic bacteriuria: A case-control study. Ann Intern Med. 1987;107:816-823.
12. Foxman B, Frerichs RR. Epidemiology of urinary tract infection: I. Diaphragm use and sexual intercourse. Am J Public Health. 1985;75:1308-1313.
13. Foxman B, Geiger AM, Palin K, et al. First-time urinary tract infection and sexual behavior. Epidemiology. 1995;6:162-168.
14. Turck M, Goffe B, Petersdorf RG. The urethral catheter and urinary tract infection. J Urol. 1962;88:834-837.
15. Gillespie L. The diaphragm: An accomplice in recurrent urinary tract infections. Urology. 1984;24:25-30.

16. Fihn SD, Latham RH, Roberts P, et al. Association between diaphragm use and urinary tract infection. JAMA. 1985;254:240-245.

17. Fihn SD, Johnson C, Pinkstaff C, et al. Diaphragm use and urinary tract infections: Analysis of urodynamic and microbiological factors. J Urol. 1986;136:853-856.

18. Johnson ET. The condom catheter: Urinary tract infection and other complications. South Med J. 1983;76:579-582.

19. Hooton TM, Scholes D, Hughes JP, et al. A prospective study of risk factors for symptomatic urinary tract infection in young women. N Engl J Med. 1996;335:468-474.

20. Hooton TM, Hillier S, Johnson C, et al. *Escherichia coli* bacteriuria and contraceptive method. JAMA. 1991;265:64-69.

21. Raz R, Gennesin Y, Wasser J, et al. Recurrent urinary tract infections in postmenopausal women. Clin Infect Dis. 2000;30:152-156.

22. Eriksen B. A randomized, open, parallel-group study on the preventive effect of an estradiol-releasing vaginal ring (Estring) on recurrent urinary tract infections in postmenopausal women. Am J Obstet Gynecol. 1999;180:1072-1079.

23. Stamey TA, Timothy M, Millar M, et al. Recurrent urinary infections in adult women: The role of introital enterobacteria. Calif Med. 1971;115:1-19.

24. Plos K, Connell H, Jodal U, et al. Intestinal carriage of P fimbriated *Escherichia coli* and the susceptibility to urinary tract infection in young children. J Infect Dis. 1995; 171:625-631.

25. Measley RE Jr, Levison ME. Host defense mechanisms in the pathogenesis of urinary tract infection. Med Clin North Am. 1991;75:275-286.

26. Roberts AP, Phillips R. Bacteria causing symptomatic urinary tract infection or asymptomatic bacteriuria. J Clin Pathol. 1979;32:492-496.

27. Johnson JR, Orskov I, Orskov F, et al. O, K, and H antigens predict virulence factors, carboxylesterase B pattern, antimicrobial resistance, and host compromise among *Escherichia coli* strains causing urosepsis. J Infect Dis. 1994;169:119-126.

28. Johnson JR, Weissman SJ, Stell AL, et al. Clonal and pathotypic analysis of archetypal *Escherichia coli* cystitis isolate NU14. J Infect Dis. 2001;184:1556-1565.

29. Dennenberg MS, Welsh RA. Virulence determinants of uropathogenic *Escherichia coli*. In: Mobley HLT, Warren JW, eds. Urinary Tract Infections: Molecular Pathogenesis and Clinical Management, v. 5. Washington, DC: American Society for Microbiology; 1996:80-128.

30. Guyer DM, Henderson IR, Nataro JP, et al. Identification of sat, an autotransporter toxin produced by uropathogenic *Escherichia coli*. Mol Microbiol. 2000;38:53-66.

31. Bahrani-Mougeot FK, Buckles EL, Lockatell CV, et al. Type 1 fimbriae and extracellular polysaccharides are preeminent uropathogenic *Escherichia coli* virulence determinants in the murine urinary tract. Mol Microbiol. 2002;45:1079-1093.

32. Hacker J, Kaper JB. Pathogenicity islands and the evolution of microbes. Annu Rev Microbiol. 2000;54:641-679.

33. Bauer RJ, Zhang L, Foxman B, et al. Molecular epidemiology of 3 putative virulence genes for *Escherichia coli* urinary tract infection—*usp, iha,* and *iro*N(*E. coli*). J Infect Dis. 2002;185:1521-1524.

34. Hull RA, Hull SI. Nutritional requirements for growth of uropathogenic *Escherichia coli* in human urine. Infect Immun. 1997;65:1960-1961.

35. Svanborg-Eden C, Gotschlich EC, Korhonen TK, et al. Aspects on structure and function of pili on uropathogenic *Escherichia coli*. Prog Allergy. 1983;33:189-202.

36. Eden CS, Eriksson B, Hanson LA. Adhesion of *Escherichia coli* to human uroepithelial cells in vitro. Infect Immun. 1977;18:767-774.

37. Leffler H, Svanborg-Eden C. Glycolipid receptors for uropathogenic *Escherichia coli* on human erythrocytes and uroepithelial cells. Infect Immun. 1981;34:920-929.

38. Wullt B, Bergsten G, Samuelsson M, et al. The role of P fimbriae for colonization and host response induction in the human urinary tract. J Infect Dis. 2001;183(Suppl 1):S43-46.

39. Otto G, Magnusson M, Svensson M, et al. *pap* genotype and P-fimbrial expression in *Escherichia coli* causing bacteremic and nonbacteremic febrile urinary tract infection. Clin Infect Dis. 2001;32:1523-1531.

40. Tseng CC, Wu JJ, Liu HL, et al. Roles of host and bacterial virulence factors in the development of upper urinary tract infection caused by *Escherichia coli*. Am J Kidney Dis. 2002;39:744-752.

41. Johnson JR, Russo TA, Brown JJ, et al. *pap*G alleles of *Escherichia coli* strains causing first-episode or recurrent acute cystitis in adult women. J Infect Dis. 1998;177:97-101.

42. Hedges SR, Agace WW, Svanborg C. Epithelial cytokine responses and mucosal cytokine networks. Trends Microbiol. 1995;3:266-270.

43. Wu XR, Sun TT, Medina JJ. In vitro binding of type 1-fimbriated *Escherichia coli* to uroplakins Ia and Ib: Relation to urinary tract infections. Proc Natl Acad Sci U S A. 1996;93:9630-9635.

44. Zhou G, Mo WJ, Sebbel P, et al. Uroplakin Ia is the urothelial receptor for uropathogenic *Escherichia coli*: Evidence from in vitro FimH binding. J Cell Sci. 2001; 114:4095-4103.

45. Sokurenko EV, Chesnokova V, Dykhuizen DE, et al. Pathogenic adaptation of *Escherichia coli* by natural variation of the FimH adhesin. Proc Natl Acad Sci U S A. 1998;95:8922-8926.

46. Schembri MA, Hasman H, Klemm P. Expression and purification of the mannose recognition domain of the FimH adhesin. FEMS Microbiol Lett. 2000;188:147-151.

47. Baorto DM, Gao Z, Malaviya R, et al. Survival of FimH-expressing enterobacteria in macrophages relies on glycolipid traffic. Nature. 1997;389:636-639.

48. Nowicki B, Selvarangan R, Nowicki S. Family of *Escherichia coli* Dr adhesins: Decay-accelerating factor receptor recognition and invasiveness. J Infect Dis. 2001; 183(Suppl 1):S24-27.

49. Zafriri D, Oron Y, Eisenstein BI, et al. Growth advantage and enhanced toxicity of *Escherichia coli* adherent to tissue culture cells due to restricted diffusion of products secreted by the cells. J Clin Invest. 1987;79:1210-1216.

50. Schilling JD, Mulvey MA, Hultgren SJ. Structure and function of *Escherichia coli* type 1 pili: New insight into the pathogenesis of urinary tract infections. J Infect Dis. 2001;183(Suppl 1):S36-40.

51. Mobley HL, Belas R, Lockatell V, et al. Construction of a flagellum-negative mutant of *Proteus mirabilis*: Effect on internalization by human renal epithelial cells and virulence in a mouse model of ascending urinary tract infection. Infect Immun. 1996; 64:5332-5340.

52. Johnson JR, Roberts PL, Stamm WE. P fimbriae and other virulence factors in *Escherichia coli* urosepsis: Association with patients' characteristics. J Infect Dis. 1987;156:225-229.

53. Stapleton A, Moseley S, Stamm WE. Urovirulence determinants in *Escherichia coli* isolates causing first-episode and recurrent cystitis in women. J Infect Dis. 1991;163:773-779.

54. Velasco M, Horcajada JP, Mensa J, et al. Decreased invasive capacity of quinolone-resistant *Escherichia coli* in patients with urinary tract infections. Clin Infect Dis. 2001;33:1682-1686.

55. Vila J, Simon K, Ruiz J, et al. Are quinolone-resistant uropathogenic *Escherichia coli* less virulent? J Infect Dis. 2002;186:1039-1042.

56. Kallenius G, Winberg J. Bacterial adherence to periurethral epithelial cells in girls prone to urinary-tract infections. Lancet. 1978;2:540-543.

57. Parsons CL, Schmidt JD. In vitro bacterial adherence to vaginal cells of normal and cystitis-prone women. J Urol. 1980;123:184-187.

58. Svanborg-Eden C, Hagberg L, Hull R, et al. Bacterial virulence versus host resistance in the urinary tracts of mice. Infect Immun. 1987;55:1224-1232.

59. Connell H, de Man P, Jodal U, et al. Lack of association between hemolysin production and acute inflammation in human urinary tract infection. Microb Pathog. 1993; 14:463-472.

60. Freedman LR, Beeson PB. Experimental pyelonephritis: IV. Observations on infections resulting from direct inoculation of bacteria in different zones of the kidney. Yale J Biol Med. 1958;30:406-414.

61. Rocha H, Fekety FR. Acute inflammation in the renal cortex and medulla following thermal injury. J Exp Med. 1964;119:131-138.

62. Svanborg C, Frendeus B, Godaly G, et al. Toll-like receptor signaling and chemokine receptor expression influence the severity of urinary tract infection. J Infect Dis. 2001;183(Suppl 1):S61-65.

63. Otto G, Braconier J, Andreasson A, et al. Interleukin-6 and disease severity in patients with bacteremic and nonbacteremic febrile urinary tract infection. J Infect Dis. 1999;179:172-179.

64. Godaly G, Hang L, Frendeus B, et al. Transepithelial neutrophil migration is CXCR1 dependent in vitro and is defective in IL-8 receptor knockout mice. J Immunol. 2000;165:5287-5294.

65. Asscher AW, Sussman M, Weiser R. Bacterial growth in human urine. In: O'Grady F, Brumfitt W, eds. Urinary Tract Infection. London: Oxford University Press; 1968:3-13.

66. Kaye D. Antibacterial activity of human urine. J Clin Invest. 1968;47:2374-2390.

67. Stamey TA, Fair WR, Timothy MM, et al. Antibacterial nature of prostatic fluid. Nature. 1968;218:444-447.

68. Reinhart HH, Obedeanu N, Robinson R, et al. Urinary excretion of Tamm-Horsfall protein in elderly women. J Urol. 1991;146:806-808.

69. Daifuku R, Stamm WE. Bacterial adherence to bladder uroepithelial cells in catheter-associated urinary tract infection. N Engl J Med. 1986;314:1208-1213.

70. Parsons CL, Mulholland SG, Anwar H. Antibacterial activity of bladder surface mucin duplicated by exogenous glycosaminoglycan (heparin). Infect Immun. 1979; 24:552-557.

71. Kunin CM, Polyak F, Postel E. Periurethral bacterial flora in women: Prolonged intermittent colonization with *Escherichia coli*. JAMA. 1980;243:134-139.

72. Stamey TA, Timothy MM. Studies of introital colonization in women with recurrent urinary infections: I. The role of vaginal pH. J Urol. 1975;114:261-263.

73. Stamey TA. The role of introital enterobacteria in recurrent urinary infections. J Urol. 1973;109:467-472.

74. Scholes D, Hooton TM, Roberts PL, et al. Risk factors for recurrent urinary tract infection in young women. J Infect Dis. 2000;182:1177-1182.

75. Stapleton A. Host factors in susceptibility to urinary tract infections. Adv Exp Med Biol. 1999;462:351-358.

76. McGroarty FA, Chong S, Reid G. Influence of the spermicidal compound nonoxynol-9 on the growth and adhesion of urogenital bacteria in vitro. Curr Microbiol. 1990; 21:219-223.

77. Cattell WR, McSherry MA, Northeast A, et al. Periurethral enterobacterial carriage in pathogenesis of recurrent urinary infection. Br Med J. 1974;4:136-139.

78. Kurdydyk LM, Kelly K, Harding GK, et al. Role of cervicovaginal antibody in the pathogenesis of recurrent urinary tract infection in women. Infect Immun. 1980; 29:76-82.

79. Hanson LA, Ahlstedt S, Fasth A, et al. Antigens of *Escherichia coli,* human immune response, and the pathogenesis of urinary tract infections. J Infect Dis. 1977; 136(Suppl):S144-149.

80. de Ree JM, van den Bosch JF. Serological response to the P fimbriae of uropathogenic *Escherichia coli* in pyelonephritis. Infect Immun. 1987;55:2204-2207.

81. Kantele A, Papunen R, Virtanen E, et al. Antibody-secreting cells in acute urinary tract infection as indicators of local immune response. J Infect Dis. 1994;169: 1023-1028.

82. Christmas TJ. Lymphocyte sub-populations in the bladder wall in normal bladder, bacterial cystitis and interstitial cystitis. Br J Urol. 1994;73:508-515.

83. Hopkins WJ, Uehling DT, Balish E. Local and systemic antibody responses accompany spontaneous resolution of experimental cystitis in cynomolgus monkeys. Infect Immun. 1987;55:1951-1956.

84. Foxman B, Gillespie B, Koopman J, et al. Risk factors for second urinary tract infection among college women. Am J Epidemiol. 2000;151:1194-1205.

85. Svanborg-Eden C, Svennerholm AM. Secretory immunoglobulin A and G antibodies prevent adhesion of *Escherichia coli* to human urinary tract epithelial cells. Infect Immun. 1978;22:790-797.

86. Vroom TM, Scholte G, Ossendorp F, et al. Tissue distribution of human gamma delta T cells: No evidence for general epithelial tropism. J Clin Pathol. 1991;44:1012-1017.

87. Park JC, Buono D, Smith DK, et al. Urinary tract infections in women with or at risk for human immunodeficiency virus infection. Am J Obstet Gynecol. 2002;187: 581-588.

88. Rajan N, Cao Q, Anderson BE, et al. Roles of glycoproteins and oligosaccharides found in human vaginal fluid in bacterial adherence. Infect Immun. 1999;67: 5027-5032.

89. Rocha H, Guze LB, Freedman LR. Experimental pyelonephritis: III. The influence of localized injury in different parts of the kidney on susceptibility to bacillary infection. Yale J Biol Med. 1958;30:341-354.

90. DeNavasquez SJ. Further studies in experimental pyelonephritis produced by various bacteria, with special reference to renal scarring as a factor in pathogenesis. J Pathol Bacteriol. 1956;71:27-32.

91. Smellie JM, Normand IC. Bacteriuria, reflux, and renal scarring. Arch Dis Child. 1975;50:581-585.

92. Jellheden B, Norrby RS, Sandberg T. Symptomatic urinary tract infection in women in primary health care: Bacteriological, clinical and diagnostic aspects in relation to host response to infection. Scand J Prim Health Care. 1996;14:122-128.

93. Ronald A. The etiology of urinary tract infection: Traditional and emerging pathogens. Am J Med. 2002;113(Suppl 1A):14S-19S.

94. Bronsema DA, Adams JR, Pallares R, et al. Secular trends in rates and etiology of nosocomial urinary tract infections at a university hospital. J Urol. 1993;150:414-416.

95. Wagenlehner FM, Krcmery S, Held C, et al. Epidemiological analysis of the spread of pathogens from a urological ward using genotypic, phenotypic and clinical parameters. Int J Antimicrob Agents. 2002;19:583-591.

96. Soriano F, Aguado JM, Ponte C, et al. Urinary tract infection caused by *Corynebacterium* group D2: Report of 82 cases and review. Rev Infect Dis. 1990; 12:1019-1034.

97. Meria P, Desgrippes A, Arfi C, et al. Encrusted cystitis and pyelitis. J Urol. 1998; 160:3-9.

98. Jacobs LG. Fungal urinary tract infections in the elderly: Treatment guidelines. Drugs Aging. 1996;8:89-96.

99. Pead L, Crump J, Maskell R. Staphylococci as urinary pathogens. J Clin Pathol. 1977;30:427-431.

100. Schneider PF, Riley TV. *Staphylococcus saprophyticus* urinary tract infections: Epidemiological data from Western Australia. Eur J Epidemiol. 1996;12:51-54.

101. Numazaki Y, Kumasaka T, Yano N, et al. Further study on acute hemorrhagic cystitis due to adenovirus type 11. N Engl J Med. 1973;289:344-347.

102. Akiyama H, Kurosu T, Sakashita C, et al. Adenovirus is a key pathogen in hemorrhagic cystitis associated with bone marrow transplantation. Clin Infect Dis. 2001; 32:1325-1330.

103. Kajander EO, Ciftcioglu N. Nanobacteria: An alternative mechanism for pathogenic intra- and extracellular calcification and stone formation. Proc Natl Acad Sci U S A. 1998;95:8274-8279.

104. Hansson S, Martinell J, Stokland E, et al. The natural history of bacteriuria in childhood. Infect Dis Clin North Am. 1997;11:499-512.

105. Craig JC, Knight JF, Sureshkumar P, et al. Effect of circumcision on incidence of urinary tract infection in preschool boys. J Pediatr. 1996;128:23-27.

106. Practice parameter: The diagnosis, treatment, and evaluation of the initial urinary tract infection in febrile infants and young children. American Academy of Pediatrics Committee on Quality Improvement, Subcommittee on Urinary Tract Infection. Pediatrics. 1999;103:843-852.

107. Smellie JM, Prescod NP, Shaw PJ, et al. Childhood reflux and urinary infection: A follow-up of 10-41 years in 226 adults. Pediatr Nephrol. 1998;12:727-736.

108. Kunin CM. Urinary tract infections in children. Hosp Pract. 1976;11:91-98.

109. Gillenwater JY, Harrison RB, Kunin CM. Natural history of bacteriuria in schoolgirls: A long-term case-control study. N Engl J Med. 1979;301:396-399.

110. Ronald AR, Pattullo AL. The natural history of urinary infection in adults. Med Clin North Am. 1991;75:299-312.

111. Foxman B. Epidemiology of urinary tract infections: Incidence, morbidity, and economic costs. Am J Med. 2002;113(Suppl 1A):5S-13S.

112. Hooton TM. Pathogenesis of urinary tract infections: An update. J Antimicrob Chemother. 2000;46(Suppl A):1-7.

113. Foxman B, Zhang L, Tallman P, et al. Transmission of uropathogens between sex partners. J Infect Dis. 1997;175:989-992.

114. Spach DH, Stapleton AE, Stamm WE. Lack of circumcision increases the risk of urinary tract infection in young men. JAMA. 1992;267:679-681.

115. Nicolle LE. Urinary tract infections in long-term-care facilities. Infect Control Hosp Epidemiol. 2001;22:167-175.

116. Baldassarre JS, Kaye D. Special problems of urinary tract infection in the elderly. Med Clin North Am. 1991;75:375-390.

117. Patterson TF, Andriole VT. Detection, significance, and therapy of bacteriuria in pregnancy: Update in the managed health care era. Infect Dis Clin North Am. 1997;11:593-608.

118. Patterson JE, Andriole VT. Bacterial urinary tract infections in diabetes. Infect Dis Clin North Am. 1997;11:735-750.

119. Stapleton A. Urinary tract infections in patients with diabetes. Am J Med. 2002; 113(Suppl 1A):80S-84S.

120. Andriole VT, Patterson TF. Epidemiology, natural history, and management of urinary tract infections in pregnancy. Med Clin North Am. 1991;75:359-373.

121. De Pinho AM, Lopes GS, Ramos-Filho CF, et al. Urinary tract infection in men with AIDS. Genitourin Med. 1994;70:30-34.

122. Brown PD. Urinary tract infections in renal transplant recipients. Curr Infect Dis Rep. 2002;4:525-528.

123. Schmaldienst S, Dittrich E, Horl WH. Urinary tract infections after renal transplantation. Curr Opin Urol. 2002;12:125-130.

124. Gleckman R, Blagg N, Hibert D, et al. Acute pyelonephritis in the elderly. South Med J. 1982;75:551-554.

125. Boscia JA, Kobasa WD, Abrutyn E, et al. Lack of association between bacteriuria and symptoms in the elderly. Am J Med. 1986;81:979-982.

126. Ouslander JG, Schapira M, Schnelle JF, et al. Does eradicating bacteriuria affect the severity of chronic urinary incontinence in nursing home residents? Ann Intern Med. 1995;122:749-754.

127. Kaye D, Rocha H. Urinary concentrating ability in early experimental pyelonephritis. J Clin Invest. 1970;49:1427-1437.

128. Levison SP, Levison ME. Effect of indomethacin and sodium meclofenamate on the renal concentrating defect in experimental enterococcal pyelonephritis in rats. J Lab Clin Med. 1976;88:958-964.

129. Thysell H. Evaluation of chemical and microscopical methods for mass detection of bacteriuria. Acta Med Scand. 1969;185:393-400.

130. Boscia JA, Abrutyn E, Levison ME, et al. Pyuria and asymptomatic bacteriuria in elderly ambulatory women. Ann Intern Med. 1989;110:404-405.

131. Winkens RA, Leffers P, Trienekens TA, et al. The validity of urine examination for urinary tract infections in daily practice. Fam Pract. 1995;12:290-293.

132. Pappas PG. Laboratory in the diagnosis and management of urinary tract infections. Med Clin North Am. 1991;75:313-325.

133. Bent S, Saint S. The optimal use of diagnostic testing in women with acute uncomplicated cystitis. Am J Med. 2002;113(Suppl 1A):20S-28S.

134. Rubin RH, Shapiro ED, Andriole VT, et al. Evaluation of new anti-infective drugs for the treatment of urinary tract infection. Infectious Diseases Society of America and the Food and Drug Administration. Clin Infect Dis. 1992;15(Suppl 1):S216-227.

135. Warren JW, Abrutyn E, Hebel JR, et al. Guidelines for antimicrobial treatment of uncomplicated acute bacterial cystitis and acute pyelonephritis in women. Infectious Diseases Society of America (IDSA). Clin Infect Dis. 1999;29:745-758.

136. Lifshitz E, Kramer L. Outpatient urine culture: Does collection technique matter? Arch Intern Med. 2000;160:2537-2540.

137. Leung AK, Robson WL. Urinary tract infection in infancy and childhood. Adv Pediatr. 1991;38:257-285.

138. Stamm WE, Wagner KF, Amsel R, et al. Causes of acute urethral syndrome in women. N Engl J Med. 1980;303:409-415.

139. Stamm WE, Running K, McKevitt M, et al. Treatment of the acute urethral syndrome. N Engl J Med. 1981;304:956-958.

140. Stamm WE. Quantitative urine cultures revisited. Eur J Clin Microbiol. 1984;3:279-281.

141. Stamm WE, Counts GW, Running KR, et al. Diagnosis of coliform infection in acutely dysuric women. N Engl J Med. 1982;307:463-468.

142. Kunin CM, White LV, Hua TH. A reassessment of the importance of "low-count" bacteriuria in young women with acute urinary symptoms. Ann Intern Med. 1993; 119:454-460.

143. Arav-Boger R, Leibovici L, Danon YL. Urinary tract infections with low and high colony counts in young women: Spontaneous remission and single-dose vs multiple-day treatment. Arch Intern Med. 1994;154:300-304.

144. Komaroff AL, Pass TM, McCue JD, et al. Management strategies for urinary and vaginal infections. Arch Intern Med. 1978;138:1069-1073.

145. Johnson RE, Newhall WJ, Papp JR, et al. Screening tests to detect *Chlamydia trachomatis* and *Neisseria gonorrhoeae* infections: 2002. MMWR Recomm Rep. 2002;51 (RR-15):1-38.

146. Fairley KF, Carson NE, Gutch RC, et al. Site of infection in acute urinary-tract infection in general practice. Lancet. 1971;2:615-618.

147. Thomas VL, Forland M. Antibody-coated bacteria in urinary tract infections. Kidney Int. 1982;21:1-7.

148. Merritt JL, Keys TF. Limitations of the antibody-coated bacteria test in patients with neurogenic bladders. JAMA. 1982;247:1723-1725.

149. Ronald AR, Conway B, Zhanel GG. The value of single-dose therapy to diagnose the site of urinary infection. Chemotherapy. 1990;36(Suppl 1):2-9.

150. Martinell J, Lidin-Janson G, Jagenburg R, et al. Girls prone to urinary infections followed into adulthood: Indices of renal disease. Pediatr Nephrol. 1996;10:139-142.

151. Olbing H, Hirche H, Koskimies O, et al. Renal growth in children with severe vesicoureteral reflux: 10-year prospective study of medical and surgical treatment: The International Reflux Study in Children (European branch). Radiology. 2000;216:731-737.

152. Andriole VT. Advances in the treatment of urinary infections. J Antimicrob Chemother. 1982;9(Suppl A):163-172.

153. Hodson J, Maling TM, McManamon PJ, et al. Reflux nephropathy. Kidney Int Suppl. 1975;4:S50-58.

154. Rolleston GL, Maling TM, Hodson CJ. Intrarenal reflux and the scarred kidney. Arch Dis Child. 1974;49:531-539.

155. Edwards D, Normand IC, Prescod N, et al. Disappearance of vesicoureteric reflux during long-term prophylaxis of urinary tract infection in children. Br Med J. 1977;2:285-288.

156. Kemper KJ, Avner ED. The case against screening urinalyses for asymptomatic bacteriuria in children. Am J Dis Child. 1992;146:343-346.

157. Kraft JK, Stamey TA. The natural history of symptomatic recurrent bacteriuria in women. Medicine (Baltimore). 1977;56:55-60.

158. Schechter H, Leonard CD, Scribner BH. Chronic pyelonephritis as a cause of renal failure in dialysis candidates: Analysis of 173 patients. JAMA. 1971;216:514-517.

159. Gaches CG, Miller KW, Roberts JB, et al. The Bristol Pyelonephritis Registry: 10 years on. Br J Urol. 1975;47:721-725.

160. Zinner SH, Kass EH. Long-term (10 to 14 years) follow-up of bacteriuria of pregnancy. N Engl J Med. 1971;285:820-824.

161. Murray T, Goldberg M. Chronic interstitial nephritis: Etiologic factors. Ann Intern Med. 1975;82:453-459.

162. Dontas AS, Kasviki-Charvati P, Papanayiotou PC, et al. Bacteriuria and survival in old age. N Engl J Med. 1981;304:939-943.

163. Boscia JA, Abrutyn E, Kaye D. Asymptomatic bacteriuria in elderly persons: Treat or do not treat? Ann Intern Med. 1987;106:764-766.

164. Nordenstam GR, Brandberg CA, Oden AS, et al. Bacteriuria and mortality in an elderly population. N Engl J Med. 1986;314:1152-1156.

165. Abrutyn E, Mossey J, Berlin JA, et al. Does asymptomatic bacteriuria predict mortality and does antimicrobial treatment reduce mortality in elderly ambulatory women? Ann Intern Med. 1994;120:827-833.

166. Nicolle LE. Urinary tract infection in geriatric and institutionalized patients. Curr Opin Urol. 2002;12:51-55.

167. Harding GK, Zhanel GG, Nicolle LE, et al. Antimicrobial treatment in diabetic women with asymptomatic bacteriuria. N Engl J Med. 2002;347:1576-1583.

168. Boscia JA, Kaye D. Asymptomatic bacteriuria in the elderly. Infect Dis Clin North Am. 1987;1:893-905.

169. Platt R. Adverse consequences of asymptomatic urinary tract infections in adults. Am J Med. 1987;82:47-52.

170. Stamey TA, Fair WR, Timothy MM, et al. Serum versus urinary antimicrobial concentrations in cure of urinary-tract infections. N Engl J Med. 1974;291:1159-1163.

171. Prais D, Straussberg R, Avitzur Y, et al. Bacterial susceptibility to oral antibiotics in community acquired urinary tract infection. Arch Dis Child. 2003;88:215-218.

172. Karlowsky JA, Kelly LJ, Thornsberry C, et al. Trends in antimicrobial resistance among urinary tract infection isolates of *Escherichia coli* from female outpatients in the United States. Antimicrob Agents Chemother. 2002;46:2540-2545.

173. Karlowsky JA, Thornsberry C, Jones ME, et al. Susceptibility of antimicrobial-resistant urinary *Escherichia coli* isolates to fluoroquinolones and nitrofurantoin. Clin Infect Dis. 2003;36:183-187.

174. Gupta K, Sahm DF, Mayfield D, et al. Antimicrobial resistance among uropathogens that cause community-acquired urinary tract infections in women: A nationwide analysis. Clin Infect Dis. 2001;33:89-94.

175. Talan DA, Stamm WE, Hooton TM, et al. Comparison of ciprofloxacin (7 days) and trimethoprim-sulfamethoxazole (14 days) for acute uncomplicated pyelonephritis in women: A randomized trial. JAMA. 2000;283:1583-1590.

176. Nicolle LE. A practical guide to the management of complicated urinary tract infection. Drugs. 1997;53:583-592.

177. Stamm WE, McKevitt M, Counts GW. Acute renal infection in women: Treatment with trimethoprim-sulfamethoxazole or ampicillin for two or six weeks—A randomized trial. Ann Intern Med. 1987;106:341-345.

178. Shokeir AA, El-Azab M, Mohsen T, et al. Emphysematous pyelonephritis: A 15-year experience with 20 cases. Urology. 1997;49:343-346.

179. Mallet M, Knockaert DC, Oyen RH, et al. Emphysematous pyelonephritis: No longer a surgical disease? Eur J Emerg Med. 2002;9:266-269.

180. Norrby SR. Short-term treatment of uncomplicated lower urinary tract infections in women. Rev Infect Dis. 1990;12:458-467.

181. Greenberg RN, Sanders CV, Lewis AC, et al. Single-dose cefaclor therapy of urinary tract infection: Evaluation of antibody-coated bacteria test and C-reactive protein assay as predictors of cure. Am J Med. 1981;71:841-845.

182. Tran D, Muchant DG, Aronoff SC. Short-course versus conventional length antimicrobial therapy for uncomplicated lower urinary tract infections in children: A meta-analysis of 1279 patients. J Pediatr. 2001;139:93-99.

183. Michael M, Hodson EM, Craig JC, et al. Short compared with standard duration of antibiotic treatment for urinary tract infection: A systematic review of randomised controlled trials. Arch Dis Child. 2002;87:118-123.

184. Johnson JR, Stamm WE. Diagnosis and treatment of acute urinary tract infections. Infect Dis Clin North Am. 1987;1:773-791.

185. Turck M, Ronald AR, Petersdorf RG. Relapse and reinfection in chronic bacteriuria: II. The correlation between site of infection and pattern of recurrence in chronic bacteriuria. N Engl J Med. 1968;278:422-427.

186. Gupta K, Hooton TM, Roberts PL, et al. Patient-initiated treatment of uncomplicated recurrent urinary tract infections in young women. Ann Intern Med. 2001;135:9-16.

187. Melekos MD, Asbach HW, Gerharz E, et al. Post-intercourse versus daily ciprofloxacin prophylaxis for recurrent urinary tract infections in premenopausal women. J Urol. 1997;157:935-939.

188. Pfau A, Sacks TG. Effective postcoital quinolone prophylaxis of recurrent urinary tract infections in women. J Urol. 1994;152:136-138.

189. Nicolle LE, Ronald AR. Recurrent urinary tract infection in adult women: Diagnosis and treatment. Infect Dis Clin North Am. 1987;1:793-806.

190. Mangiarotti P, Pizzini C, Fanos V. Antibiotic prophylaxis in children with relapsing urinary tract infections: Review. J Chemother. 2000;12:115-123.

191. Brumfitt W, Hamilton-Miller JM. Efficacy and safety profile of long-term nitrofurantoin in urinary infections: 18 years' experience. J Antimicrob Chemother. 1998;42:363-371.

192. Cardozo L, Lose G, McClish D, et al. A systematic review of estrogens for recurrent urinary tract infections: Third report of the hormones and urogenital therapy (HUT) committee. Int Urogynecol J Pelvic Floor Dysfunct. 2001;12:15-20.

193. Uehling DT, Hopkins WJ, Balish E, et al. Vaginal mucosal immunization for recurrent urinary tract infection: Phase II clinical trial. J Urol. 1997;157:2049-2052.

194. Reid G. The role of cranberry and probiotics in intestinal and urogenital tract health. Crit Rev Food Sci Nutr. 2002;42:293-300.

195. Miller JL, Krieger JN. Urinary tract infections, cranberry juice, underwear, and probiotics in the 21st century. Urol Clin North Am. 2002;29:695-699.

196. Sobel JD, Kauffman CA, McKinsey D, et al. Candiduria: A randomized, double-blind study of treatment with fluconazole and placebo. The National Institute of Allergy and Infectious Diseases (NIAID) Mycoses Study Group. Clin Infect Dis. 2000;30:19-24.

197. Andriole VT, Cohn GL. The effect of diethylstilbestrol on the susceptibility of rats to hematogenous pyelonephritis. J Clin Invest. 1973;43:1136-1145.

198. Nowicki B. Urinary tract infection in pregnant women: Old dogmas and current concepts regarding pathogenesis. Curr Infect Dis Rep. 2002;4:529-535.

199. Golan A, Wexler S, Amit A, et al. Asymptomatic bacteriuria in normal and high-risk pregnancy. Eur J Obstet Gynecol Reprod Biol. 1989;33:101-108.

200. Gratacos E, Torres PJ, Vila J, et al. Screening and treatment of asymptomatic bacteriuria in pregnancy prevent pyelonephritis. J Infect Dis. 1994;169:1390-1392.

201. Norden CW, Kass EH. Bacteriuria of pregnancy: A critical appraisal. Annu Rev Med. 1968;19:431-470.

202. Schieve LA, Handler A, Hershow R, et al. Urinary tract infection during pregnancy: Its association with maternal morbidity and perinatal outcome. Am J Public Health. 1994;84:405-410.

203. Condie AP, Williams JD, Reeves DS. Complications of bacteriuria in pregnancy. In: Brumfitt W, ed. Urinary Tract Infections. London: Oxford; 1968:148-159.

204. Kass EH. Bacteriuria and pyelonephritis of pregnancy. Trans Assoc Am Physicians. 1959;72:257-264.

205. Miller LK, Cox SM. Urinary tract infections complicating pregnancy. Infect Dis Clin North Am. 1997;11:13-26.

206. Meis PJ, Michielutte R, Peters TJ, et al. Factors associated with preterm birth in Cardiff, Wales: II. Indicated and spontaneous preterm birth. Am J Obstet Gynecol. 1995;173:597-602.

207. Schultz R, Read AW, Straton JA, et al. Genitourinary tract infections in pregnancy and low birth weight: Case-control study in Australian aboriginal women. BMJ. 1991;303:1369-1373.

208. Leigh DA, Gruneberg RN, Brumfitt W. Long-term follow-up of bacteriuria in pregnancy. Lancet. 1968;1:603-605.

209. Hart A, Nowicki BJ, Reisner B, et al. Ampicillin-resistant *Escherichia coli* in gestational pyelonephritis: Increased occurrence and association with the colonization factor Dr adhesin. J Infect Dis. 2001;183:1526-1529.

210. Adelson MD, Graves WL, Osborne NG. Treatment of urinary infections in pregnancy using single versus 10-day dosing. J Natl Med Assoc. 1992;84:73-75.

211. Roberts RO, Lieber MM, Bostwick DG, et al. A review of clinical and pathological prostatitis syndromes. Urology. 1997;49:809-821.

212. Meares EM Jr. Prostatitis. Med Clin North Am. 1991;75:405-424.

213. Kirby RS, Lowe D, Bultitude MI, et al. Intra-prostatic urinary reflux: An aetiological factor in abacterial prostatitis. Br J Urol. 1982;54:729-731.

214. Stamey TA. Urinary infections in males. In: Pathogenesis and Treatment of Urinary Tract Infections. Baltimore: Williams & Wilkins; 1980:342-429.

215. Fair WR, Couch J, Wehner N. The purification and assay of the prostatic antibacterial factor (PAF). Biochem Med. 1973;8:329-339.

216. Drach GW. Prostatitis: Man's hidden infection. Urol Clin North Am. 1975;2:499-520.

217. Shortliffe LM, Wehner N. The characterization of bacterial and nonbacterial prostatitis by prostatic immunoglobulins. Medicine (Baltimore). 1986;65:399-414.

218. Meares EM, Stamey TA. Bacteriologic localization patterns in bacterial prostatitis and urethritis. Invest Urol. 1968;5:492-518.

219. Krieger JN, Nyberg L Jr, Nickel JC. NIH consensus definition and classification of prostatitis. JAMA. 1999;282:236-237.

220. Kohnen PW, Drach GW. Patterns of inflammation in prostatic hyperplasia: A histologic and bacteriologic study. J Urol. 1979;121:755-760.

221. Abdelatif OM, Chandler FW, McGuire BS Jr. *Chlamydia trachomatis* in chronic abacterial prostatitis: Demonstration by colorimetric in situ hybridization. Hum Pathol. 1991;22:41-44.

222. Krieger JN, Riley DE, Vesella RL, et al. Bacterial DNA sequences in prostate tissue from patients with prostate cancer and chronic prostatitis. J Urol. 2000;164:1221-1228.

223. Segura JW, Opitz JL, Greene LF. Prostatosis, prostatitis or pelvic floor tension myalgia? J Urol. 1979;122:168-169.

224. Moul JW. Prostatitis: Sorting out the different causes. Postgrad Med. 1993;94:191-194.

225. Winningham DG, Nemoy NJ, Stamey TA. Diffusion of antibiotics from plasma into prostatic fluid. Nature. 1968;219:139-143.

226. Stamey TA, Bushby SR, Bragonje J. The concentration of trimethoprim in prostatic fluid: Nonionic diffusion or active transport? J Infect Dis. 1973;128(Suppl):686-692.

227. Naber KG. The role of quinolones in the treatment of chronic bacterial prostatitis. Infection. 1991;19(Suppl 3):S170-177.

228. Giamarellou H, Kosmidis J, Leonidas M, et al. A study of the effectiveness of rifaprim in chronic prostatitis caused mainly by *Staphylococcus aureus*. J Urol. 1982;128:321-324.

229. Weidner W, Schiefer HG, Brahler E. Refractory chronic bacterial prostatitis: A re-evaluation of ciprofloxacin treatment after a median followup of 30 months. J Urol. 1991;146:350-352.

230. McNaughton Collins M, MacDonald R, Wilt TJ. Diagnosis and treatment of chronic abacterial prostatitis: A systematic review. Ann Intern Med. 2000;133:367-381.

231. Thorley JD, Jones SR, Sanford JP. Perinephric abscess. Medicine (Baltimore). 1974;53:441-451.

232. Sheinfeld J, Erturk E, Spataro RF, et al. Perinephric abscess: Current concepts. J Urol. 1987;137:191-194.

233. Patel NP, Lavengood RW, Fernandes M, et al. Gas-forming infections in genitourinary tract. Urology. 1992;39:341-345.

234. Brown PS Jr, Dodson M, Weintrub PS. Xanthogranulomatous pyelonephritis: Report of nonsurgical management of a case and review of the literature. Clin Infect Dis. 1996;22:308-314.

235. Bova JG, Potter JL, Arevalos E, et al. Renal and perirenal infection: The role of computerized tomography. J Urol. 1985;133:375-378.

236. Kaplan DM, Rosenfield AT, Smith RC. Advances in the imaging of renal infection: Helical CT and modern coordinated imaging. Infect Dis Clin North Am. 1997;11:681-705.

237. Gerzof SG, Gale ME. Computed tomography and ultrasonography for diagnosis and treatment of renal and retroperitoneal abscesses. Urol Clin North Am. 1982;9:185-193.

238. Huligowska E, Newman B, White S. Interventional ultrasound in detection and treatment of renal inflammatory disease. Radiology. 1983;147:521-526.

239. Bergeron MG. Treatment of pyelonephritis in adults. Med Clin North Am. 1995;79:619-649.

240. Schwab SJ, Bander SJ, Klahr S. Renal infection in autosomal dominant polycystic kidney disease. Am J Med. 1987;82:714-718.

241. Finn DJ, Palestrant AM, DeWolf WC. Successful percutaneous management of renal abscess. J Urol. 1982;127:425-426.

242. Siegel JF, Smith A, Moldwin R. Minimally invasive treatment of renal abscess. J Urol. 1996;155:52-55.

243. Johnson JR, Vincent LM, Wang K, et al. Renal ultrasonographic correlates of acute pyelonephritis. Clin Infect Dis. 1992;14:15-22.

244. McNicholas MM, Griffin JF, Cantwell DF. Ultrasound of the pelvis and renal tract combined with a plain film of abdomen in young women with urinary tract infection: Can it replace intravenous urography? A prospective study. Br J Radiol. 1991;64:221-224.

245. Spencer J, Lindsell D, Mastorakou I. Ultrasonography compared with intravenous urography in investigation of urinary tract infection in adults. BMJ. 1990;301:221-224.

246. Sandler CM, Amis ES Jr, Bigongiari LR, et al. Imaging in acute pyelonephritis. American College of Radiology. ACR Appropriateness Criteria. Radiology. 2000;215(Suppl):677-681.

247. Papanicolaou N, Pfister RC. Acute renal infections. Radiol Clin North Am. 1996;34:965-995.

248. Smith RC, Verga M, McCarthy S, et al. Diagnosis of acute flank pain: Value of unenhanced helical CT. AJR Am J Roentgenol. 1996;166:97-101.

249. Sreenarasimhaiah V, Alon US. Uroradiologic evaluation of children with urinary tract infection: Are both ultrasonography and renal cortical scintigraphy necessary? J Pediatr. 1995;127:373-377.

250. Koff SA. A practical approach to evaluating urinary tract infection in children. Pediatr Nephrol. 1991;5:398-400.

251. Hanbury DC, Whitaker RH, Sherwood T, et al. Ultrasound and plain x-ray screening in childhood urinary tract infection. Br J Urol. 1989;64:638-640.

252. Preston AA. Imaging strategies and discussion of vesicoureteric reflux as a risk factor in the evaluation of urinary tract infection in children. Curr Opin Pediatr. 1994;6:178-182.

253. Honkinen O, Ruuskanen O, Rikalainen H, et al. Ultrasonography as a screening procedure in children with urinary tract infection. Pediatr Infect Dis. 1986;5:633-635.

254. Rosenberg AR, Rossleigh MA, Brydon MP, et al. Evaluation of acute urinary tract infection in children by dimercaptosuccinic acid scintigraphy: A prospective study. J Urol. 1992;148:1746-1749.

255. Hoberman A, Charron M, Hickey RW, et al. Imaging studies after a first febrile urinary tract infection in young children. N Engl J Med. 2003;348:195-202.

256. Smellie JM. Reflections on 30 years of treating children with urinary tract infections. J Urol. 1991;146:665-668.

257. Gordon I. Vesico-ureteric reflux, urinary-tract infection, and renal damage in children. Lancet. 1995;346:489-490.

CHAPTER **67**

Sepsis, Severe Sepsis, and Septic Shock

ROBERT S. MUNFORD

Sepsis, severe sepsis, and septic shock are terms used to describe the body's systemic responses to infection. Lacking precise biochemical characterization of the syndromes or a certain understanding of their causation, experts have defined them by applying clinical and laboratory findings to a likely framework of pathogenesis. One widely used set of definitions (Table 67-1) was developed by a consensus committee of American experts in 1992.[1] These experts assumed that even the early systemic responses to infection, such as tachycardia, leukocytosis, and fever, are inflammatory, and they used them to define a systemic inflammatory response syndrome (SIRS). "We characterize SIRS as an abnormal generalized inflammatory reaction in organs remote from the initial insult."[2] When it occurs in a patient with proven or suspected infection, they recommended that SIRS be called "sepsis." If sepsis is associated with hypotension or with dysfunction of organs distant from the site of

infection, it becomes "severe sepsis." "Septic shock" is sepsis-associated hypotension that is associated with lactic acidosis or organ hypoperfusion and cannot be reversed by the administration of intravenous fluids.

Many authors have criticized these definitions,[3-5] noting that the criteria for SIRS are both nonspecific (many nonseptic patients have similar findings) and insensitive (in the intensive care unit [ICU], infected patients who do and those who do not meet SIRS criteria have similar risks of dying[4]). The fact that the consensus definitions are still commonly used after more than a decade reflects several points: they seem to describe a clinically observable continuum,[6,7] they are easy to use, and, perhaps most important, a more precise or clinically helpful set of definitions has not evolved.[8] In particular, there are still no reliable biochemical (laboratory-based) definitions for the different stages of the systemic response to infection. Another conference was convened in 2001 to reconsider definitions for sepsis and related conditions; this international group endorsed the 1992 definitions and proposed a new system for staging sepsis based on predisposition, insult infection, response, and organ dysfunction (resulting in the acronym PIRO).[8] For simplicity and convenience, the 1992 consensus definitions will be used in this chapter. For intelligent discussions of this nomenclature, see references 4, 5, 8, and 9.

It is possible that the fundamental assumption of 1992 was incorrect. It is hard to imagine how systemic inflammation would have had survival value at any stage of animal evolution. To the contrary, advantageous adaptations should have helped animals destroy microbial invaders without doing harm to themselves. At least in theory, these goals (defense without self-destruction) would be accomplished most economically by confining infection, and the inflammatory reaction to it, to the tissue site or sites where microbial invasion occurs.[10] The systemic response should support local defenses while it prevents infection and inflammation in uninvolved tissues; local and systemic responses should be integrated via the blood and the nervous system. Many recent observations are consistent with these ideas, which form the conceptual foundation for this chapter.

TABLE 67-1 Definitions

Term	Definition	Comment
Infection	Presence of microorganisms in a normally sterile site	May be confused with "colonization," which is the presence of microorganisms on an epithelial surface
Bacteremia	Cultivatable bacteria in the blood stream	May be transient and inconsequential; inconsistent correlation with severe sepsis
Systemic inflammatory response syndrome (SIRS)	The systemic response to a wide range of stresses. Currently used criteria include two or more of the following: Temperature >38° C or <36° C Heart rate >90 beats/min Respiratory rate >20 breaths/min, or $PaCO_2$ <32 mm Hg WBC >12,000 cells/mm³ or <4000 cells/mm³, or >10% immature (band) forms	A potentially misleading term. The evidence that the body's early responses to infection cause systemic inflammation is controversial. See "Pathogenesis" in text.
Sepsis	The systemic response to infection. If associated with proven or clinically suspected infection, SIRS is called "sepsis" in the American consensus scheme.[1]	With the exceptions of leukopenia and hypothermia, these changes are among the body's normal systemic responses to infection and do not necessarily imply a poor prognosis. In clinical parlance, the term *septic* is often used informally to describe patients with severe sepsis or septic shock.
Hypotension	A systolic blood pressure of <90 mm Hg, MAP <70 mm Hg, or a reduction of >40 mm Hg from baseline	To be considered sepsis related, hypotension must have no other cause.
Severe sepsis	Sepsis associated with dysfunction of organ(s) distant from the site of infection, hypoperfusion, or hypotension. The term *sepsis syndrome* had a similar definition.[3]	Abnormalities may include lactic acidosis, oliguria, acutely altered mental status, and acute lung injury.[8] To be considered *severe sepsis*, hypotension must be reversible by the administration of fluids. Organ dysfunction can be defined according to Marshall et al.[307] or the SOFA score.[308]
Septic shock	Sepsis with hypotension that, despite adequate fluid resuscitation, requires pressor therapy. In addition, there are perfusion abnormalities that may include lactic acidosis, oliguria, altered mental status, and acute lung injury.	If septic shock lasts for >1 hr and does not respond to pressor administration, the term *refractory* septic shock is often used.

MAP, mean arterial pressure; SOFA, sequential organ failure assessment; WBC, white blood cell count.

EPIDEMIOLOGY

Estimates of the incidence of sepsis, severe sepsis, and septic shock are compromised by the absence of both standardized definitions and population-based prospective cohort studies.[5] Most of the available estimates are based on hospital discharge diagnoses, which do not use the definitions just described. In a survey of hospital discharge records from seven large states in 1995, Angus and colleagues estimated the annual incidence of severe sepsis, defined as documented infection and acute organ dysfunction, to be 300 cases per 100,000 population.[11] The estimated mortality was 28%; this extrapolated to 215,000 deaths nationally, or 9.3% of all deaths in the United States in 1995. A more recent review of data in the National Hospital Discharge Survey (U.S.) found that the incidence of sepsis increased by almost fourfold during the interval from 1979 to 2000, to 240 cases per 100,000 population per year (approximately 660,000 cases/year).[12] Incidence was higher in men than in women and in nonwhite persons than in white persons. Over the same period, the in-hospital mortality rate for patients with a sepsis-related diagnosis fell from 28% to 18%.

Although the median age for patients with a sepsis-related hospital discharge diagnosis is approximately 60 years, the attack rate is very high among infants (over 500 cases/100,000 population per year), with low-birth-weight newborns experiencing particularly high risk.[13] Sepsis incidence and sepsis-related mortality decrease after the first year of life and then increase steadily with increasing age.

In surveys performed in ICUs in the United States and Europe during the 1990s, approximately 80% of the cases of severe sepsis in adults occurred in individuals who were already hospitalized for another reason.[4,14] In 30% to 50% of the cases in these and other series, a definite microbial etiology was not found.[6,14,15] Moreover, the microorganism cultured from blood or an infected local site was often one that does not usually cause disease in otherwise healthy people (in most cases, a commensal),[14,15] and in many patients more than one isolate was found (polymicrobial infection). Severe sepsis due to classic bacterial pathogens, such as *Neisseria meningitidis* and *Streptococcus pyogenes*, is much less frequently encountered nowadays than is sepsis triggered by commensal microbes that infect individuals whose epithelial barriers and other antimicrobial defenses have been compromised by injury or illness. Although for many years gram-negative bacteria were isolated from the majority of bacteremic patients with severe sepsis, the fraction of cases associated with gram-positive bacteria has steadily increased over the last 2 decades, and now *Staphylococcus aureus*, coagulase-negative staphylococci, and enterococci account for approximately 30% to 50% of the cases in most clinical series. Another recent trend is the emergence of fungi (in particular, *Candida* species) as etiologic agents of severe sepsis; in some recent series, *Candida* species have caused 5% to 12% of the microbiologically documented cases.[4,14]

In a prospective cohort study performed by Rangel-Frausto and others at the University of Iowa Hospitals,[6] 68% of the 3708 patients admitted to three general wards and three ICUs developed SIRS; of these, 26% developed evidence of sepsis, 18% developed severe sepsis, and 4% developed septic shock. The rates were higher for patients in the surgical and medical ICUs than for those in the medical or surgical wards. In a study of 1101 patients admitted to 99 Italian ICUs, Salvo and co-workers found SIRS in 58%, sepsis in 16%, severe sepsis in 5%, and septic shock in 6%.[7] Both of these prospective studies provided evidence that patients can progress along a continuum from sepsis to septic shock.

PATHOGENESIS

Normal Host Responses to Infection

Local Defenses: Walling Off and Killing Invading Microbes. When a bacterium breaches an epithelial barrier and enters the underlying tissue, it quickly encounters tissue-resident macrophages, mast cells, and dendritic cells. These cells sense the invader and react to it by secreting mediators that mobilize the local inflammatory response. Their sensory ability is conferred by host proteins that bind to highly conserved microbial molecules, usually lipids or sugars, and then take these molecules to the sentinel cells. The best understood system is the one for recognizing bacterial lipopolysaccharide (LPS), but others exist for sensing the presence of bacterial peptidoglycan, DNA, lipopeptides, flagella, viral double-stranded RNA, and other conserved microbial molecules.[16,17] In the case of LPS, a 60-kDa protein (LPS-binding protein [LBP]) can transfer LPS from bacterial membranes to another host protein, CD14, which is expressed on the surfaces of phagocytes. CD14 then passes the LPS to a signaling complex that has two members: an extracellular protein called MD-2 and the transmembrane receptor element, Toll-like receptor 4 (TLR4). TLR4 transmits the LPS recognition signal to the interior of the cell, where signal transduction and gene transcription pathways promote the production and/or secretion of numerous molecules that mediate the inflammatory response (Fig. 67-1). These mediators include cytokines (in particular, tumor necrosis factor [TNF], interleukin [IL]-1β, IL-12), chemokines (IL-8, macrophage inflammatory

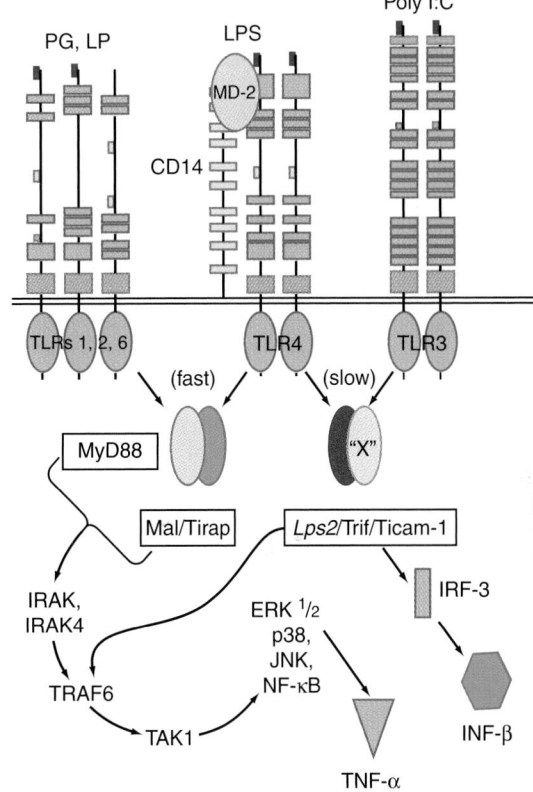

FIGURE 67-1. Toll-like receptor signaling pathways. Lipopolysaccharide (LPS)-binding protein (not shown) transfers LPS to CD14, which in turn passes it to MD-2 and Toll-like receptor 4 (TLR4). Via its cytosolic domain, TLR4 initiates transmembrane signaling through two pathways, the MyD88-dependent path via IRAK and TRAF6 that leads to production of tumor necrosis factor (TNF), and the slower MyD88-independent, LPS2/Trif-dependent pathway that increases interferon-β synthesis.[310] Peptidoglycan (PG) and bacterial lipoproteins (LP) interact with TLR2, which oligomerizes with TLR6 and TLR1 to form a signaling complex that uses the MyD88-dependent pathway. TLR3, which recognizes double-stranded RNA (poly I:C), signals via LPS2/Trif to induce interferon (IFN)-β production but also can elicit TNF via TRAF6. Not shown is the interleukin (IL)-1 receptor, which also signals via IRAK and TRAF6. The members of the TLR family of transmembrane proteins thus sense invading microbes by recognizing diverse microbial molecules and use both combinatorial interactions and different yet overlapping downstream pathways to activate the inflammatory response. (*Diagram by Bruce Beutler, with minor modifications by the author.*)

protein [MIP]-1α), lipid mediators (prostaglandins, leukotrienes), and others, and they result in the familiar elements of local inflammation, such as increased capillary permeability and blood flow, infiltration of neutrophils, and pain. In addition, local deposition of fibrin, initiated by the expression of tissue factor on activated macrophages and endothelial cells, helps wall off the infected tissue and provides an important impediment to blood-stream invasion.

Although neutrophils circulate in the blood stream, they carry out phagocytosis largely in tissue spaces, where they can attach to extracellular matrix, spread out, get traction, and ingest. (In the sinusoids of the liver, bacteria may bind to Kupffer cells and then be ingested and killed by neutrophils, which are then phagocytosed by the Kupffer cells.[18]) Because phagocytes may regurgitate the contents of their lysosomes as they eat, limiting this activity to local tissues minimizes the release of digestive enzymes and oxidants into the circulating blood. The major inherited mechanisms for killing microbes in the blood are soluble molecules—the mannose-binding lectin and C-reactive protein (CRP) pathways for activating complement, the alternative complement pathway, and natural IgM antibodies. Increased capillary permeability allows these molecules to diffuse into tissues where local inflammation is present.

In most instances, invading microbes are eliminated by phagocytes, complement, and perhaps natural antibodies, and the invaded tissue returns to normal. These rapidly activatable, broadly applicable host defenses are hardwired in the genome. Shaped by evolution, they normally provide effective protection from the host's commensal flora. Human pathogens, in contrast, have mechanisms that allow them to avoid or overcome these defenses, or they invade individuals who have inherited one or more defects in innate immunity genes. The inherited host defense mechanisms have recently been called innate immunity to distinguish them from the acquired immune mechanisms that develop more slowly and employ gene rearrangements to achieve exquisite specificity in the recognition of foreign molecules (Table 67-2).[16,19]

Systemic Responses: Keeping Infection and Inflammation Localized. Much evidence now supports the notion that the body's systemic responses to injury, infection, and other stresses generally suppress inflammation within the blood stream.[10] Preventing systemic inflammation supports local defenses by providing antimicrobial molecules (Table 67-3) and effector leukocytes (neutrophils, natural killer [NK] cells), and it prevents systemic damage by minimizing leukocyte–endothelial adhesion in uninvolved tissues and neutralizing chemical mediators that enter the blood from inflamed sites.

The systemic responses are controlled principally by the brain and the liver. Their regulation has much in common with that of the body's systemic flight-or-fight reaction to noninfectious stresses.

Central Nervous System Regulation of Systemic Responses. The central nervous system (CNS) receives news about microbial invasion via two routes. First, afferent impulses along nociceptive and vagal nerves rapidly transmit signals from infected or inflamed local tissues to the hypothalamus and brainstem, where they can activate the hypothalamic-pituitary-adrenal (HPA) axis, the autonomic nervous system, and the hypothalamic thermoregulatory center. Second, blood-borne mediators (IL-1β, TNF, IL-6, interferons, prostaglandin E₂) can cross the blood-brain barrier or be transported passively through the fenestrated capillaries in the circumventricular organs to reach the hypothalamus.[20] Remarkably, the output of three major CNS efferent pathways (the HPA and the sympathetic and parasympathetic nervous systems) inhibits inflammation within the circulating blood (see later and Table 67-3), and the thermoregulatory center may enhance antimicrobial activity by elevating body temperature.[21,22]

The Liver and Spleen: Essential Roles in Systemic Responses to Infection. The liver is anatomically situated to remove microorganisms that translocate across the gut mucosa and enter the portal circulation, whereas the spleen is the major filter for opsonized microorganisms. Impairment of the hepatic filter (e.g., by cirrhosis) predisposes to bacteremic infections with *Vibrio vulnificus* and certain other gut bacteria, and individuals with hyposplenism may experience overwhelming blood-stream infections, usually with encapsulated bacteria (e.g., *Streptococcus pneumoniae*). Circulating TNF, IL-1β, IL-6, and other cytokines may act on hepatocytes to induce many of the body's acute phase and metabolic responses to injury and infection (see later). IL-6, which is produced by many types of cells in response to injury or other stimuli, is the major trigger for most elements of the acute phase response; IL-1β may also be an important stimulus.[23]

The liver also seems to play a key role in the sensory system that informs the CNS that microbes have invaded. In rodents, the ability of low doses of endotoxin or IL-1β to induce fever and activate the HPA axis can be blocked by cutting or poisoning the hepatic branches of the vagus nerve.[24] Activation of vagal afferents by pyrogens is thought to involve prostaglandin E₂.[24] Conversely, stimulation of vagus nerve efferents suppresses endotoxin-induced TNF production in rats via a cholinergic anti-inflammatory pathway that involves inhibition of macrophage-cytokine synthesis by acetylcholine.[25] Because much of the TNF produced in response to intravenous challenge with endotoxin arises from the splanchnic bed,[26] vagal efferent activity may be very important for regulating systemic responses to microbial agonists within the blood stream.

The liver is thus a key element of innate immunity—as a blood filter that collects and kills blood-borne microbes, as a "listening station" that senses low concentrations of circulating cytokines and transmits this information to the CNS, as a factory for the production of many (acute-phase) elements of the systemic response, and as a major site of infection-associated metabolic adaptations.[27]

Acute-Phase Responses. It is useful to think of the acute systemic responses to injury, infection, and other stresses in five categories (see Table 67-2): anti-infective, anti-inflammatory, procoagulant, metabolic, and thermoregulatory. The scavenging and wound-healing responses will not be discussed here.

Anti-infective Responses. Acute *leukocytosis*, which largely reflects the demargination of neutrophils, is brought about by epinephrine, by cortisol, and possibly by IL-10 and other mediators. Mobilization of marrow neutrophils by granulocyte colony-stimulating factor (G-CSF) and other cytokines also plays an important role. Circulating neutrophils go to a site of infection where they can adhere to inflammation-activated endothelium and move by diapedesis into the infected tissue. Enhanced surface expression of CD11b/CD18 on neutrophils[28] may promote their adhesion to intercellular adhesion molecule (ICAM)-1 on the surfaces of activated endothelial cells. In addition to mobilizing neutrophils into the circulation and delivering them to sites of infection, the acute-phase response also involves increased production of several proteins that bind conserved microbial molecules and assist in recognizing and killing microbes (LBP, mannose-binding lectin, CRP, CD14, bactericidal perme-

---

TABLE 67-2 Innate and Acquired Immunity

Innate Immunity
- Senses microbes through proteins that bind highly conserved microbial molecules (e.g., lipopolysaccharide [LPS], peptidoglycan)
- "Hard-wired"—that is, inherited in the genome; shaped by evolution
- Responds rapidly to microbial invasion
- Elements: mannose-binding lectin, alternative complement pathway, "natural" antibodies, pattern-recognition proteins (e.g., LBP, MBP), the "professional" phagocytes, mast cells, natural killer (NK) cells

Acquired Immunity
- Recognizes microbial epitopes using T-cell and B-cell receptors → cellular and humoral immunity
- Requires gene rearrangements during the life of the individual
- Develops slowly after microbial invasion
- Protects the body from subsequent exposure to same and some related (cross-reactive) microbes
- Is the basis for vaccine-induced immunity
- Elements: antibodies, cytotoxic and helper T cells

LBP, LPS-binding protein; MBP, mannose-binding protein.

ability-increasing protein [BPI], and complement components [C3, C4b]). Release of lactoferrin promotes sequestration of iron in the reticuloendothelial system, and zinc is retained within cells by binding to metallothionein.

Anti-inflammatory Responses. The mechanisms that induce neutrophils to demarginate also seem to inhibit their ability to adhere to uninflamed vascular endothelium, thereby preventing unnecessary accumulation of neutrophils in uninfected tissues. Other responses that may prevent inflammation within the systemic compartment include increases in the blood levels of cytokine antagonists (IL-1Ra, soluble TNF receptors), other anti-inflammatory mediators (epinephrine, cortisol, α-melanocyte-stimulating hormone [α-MSH], adrenocorticotropic hormone [ACTH], IL-4, IL-6, IL-10, IL-13, transforming growth factor [TGF]-β, CRP), protease inhibitors, and antioxidants.

In an important experiment, van der Poll and colleagues showed how systemic responses may be modulated by the sympathetic nervous system during periods of stress.[29] They infused a bolus of endotoxin into volunteers and then measured blood levels of TNF and IL-10 over several hours. Another group of volunteers received an infusion of epinephrine for 3 hours prior to the endotoxin bolus. Epinephrine dramatically shifted the response from proinflammatory (TNF >> IL-10) to anti-inflammatory (IL-10 >> TNF). Epinephrine-induced reprogramming of cellular responses to endotoxin, damping the production of TNF while increasing or maintaining production of IL-10, can also be demonstrated in whole blood ex vivo; similar reprogramming can be caused by histamine, prostaglandin E₂, and other agonists that raise intracellular cAMP. Infusing hydrocortisone also has dramatic (though somewhat less predictable) effects on the cytokine response to an endotoxin bolus.[30] A similar reprogramming of circulating blood cells seems to occur in vivo in response to relatively minor stresses.[31]

Recent evidence suggests that the body's inflammatory responses to infection and other stresses are compartmentalized. In patients with pancreatitis, for example, Dugernier and co-workers found that the concentrations of pro- and anti-inflammatory cytokines decreased from the peritoneal fluid to the lymph to the blood, yet net anti-inflammatory activity was measured in virtually all lymph and blood samples whereas net proinflammatory activity was detected only in ascites.[32] Similarly, in patients with acute appendicitis, TNF and interferon (IFN)-γ were found in peritoneal fluid but not in plasma,

whereas high concentrations of IL-10 and IL-4 were found in plasma, which inhibited the ability of LPS to stimulate monocytes ex vivo.[33] Studies performed in rabbits suggest that, with low bacterial inocula, the proinflammatory cytokine responses to infection are compartmentalized to the lung[34] or peritoneum,[35] depending on the site of inoculation.

Metabolic Responses. Several mechanisms maintain euglycemia in the face of stress. Epinephrine, cortisol, and other counter-regulatory hormones increase insulin release from pancreatic beta cells and stimulate glycogenolysis and gluconeogenesis in the liver. Insulin resistance reduces glucose uptake by muscle and contributes to muscle catabolism.[36] The counter-regulatory hormones also induce lipolysis (so blood levels of free fatty acids and glycerol increase) and muscle proteolysis. Lipolysis, which occurs principally in adipocytes, involves activation of hormone-sensitive lipase; lipoprotein lipase is inhibited, accounting in part for the increase in circulating triglycerides that often occurs. Muscle proteolysis releases amino acids (alanine, glutamine, and others) that are used for hepatic gluconeogenesis and for producing acute-phase proteins.

A long-accepted rationale for the changes in glucose metabolism is the requirement to maintain blood glucose levels at concentrations that can supply the brain and immune cells until levels of ketone bodies, which can also be used by the CNS, rise later in the course of starvation.[37] Treatment of critically ill patients with intravenous glucose solutions and parenteral or enteral feeding has largely supplanted the body's need to maintain euglycemia through insulin resistance and other adaptive mechanisms, and it may help induce hyperglycemia in many individuals.

It is important to note that the body's systemic anti-inflammatory and metabolic responses to injury and infection are regulated by many of the same molecules—most prominently, catecholamines and glucocorticoids. The effects of cortisol on metabolism—promoting gluconeogenesis, glycogenolysis, insulin resistance, and lipolysis—are dose related in a monogenic fashion. In contrast, its effects on various aspects of inflammation may be permissive (allowing acute-phase protein synthesis) at normal concentrations and either suppressive (inhibiting cytokine and acute-phase protein production) or stimulatory (increasing IL-10 production) at high concentrations within the physiologic concentration range.[38] It is also important that the regulated mechanisms that diminish the impact of glucocorticoids (e.g., receptor downregulation, the actions of macrophage migration–inhibiting fac-

TABLE 67-3 Normal Systemic Responses to Infection and Injury: Presumed Contributions to Host Defense

Leukocytosis	Mobilizes neutrophils into the circulation
Tachycardia	Increases cardiac output, blood flow to injured tissue
Fever	Raises core temperature; peripheral vasoconstriction shunts blood flow to injured tissue. Occurs much more often when infection is the trigger for systemic responses
Acute-Phase Responses (categorized according to possible roles in defense)	
Anti-infective	Increases synthesis of complement factors, microbe pattern–recognition molecules (mannose-binding lectin, LBP, CRP, CD14, others) Sequesters iron (lactoferrin) and zinc (metallothionein)
Anti-inflammatory	Releases anti-inflammatory neuroendocrine hormones (cortisol, ACTH, epinephrine, α-MSH) Increases synthesis of proteins that help prevent inflammation within the systemic compartment • Cytokine antagonists (IL-1Ra, sTNF-Rs) • Anti-inflammatory mediators (e.g., IL-4, IL-6,IL-6R, IL-10, IL-13, TGF-β) • Protease inhibitors (e.g., α1-antiprotease) • Antioxidants (haptoglobin) Reprograms circulating leukocytes (epinephrine, cortisol, PGE₂, ? other)
Procoagulant	Walls off infection, prevents systemic spread • Increases synthesis or release of fibrinogen, PAI-1, C4b • Decreases synthesis of protein C, anti-thrombin III
Metabolic	Preserves euglycemia, mobilizes fatty acids, amino acids • Epinephrine, cortisol, glucagon, cytokines
Thermoregulatory	Inhibits microbial growth • Fever

*At the present time, the evidence for this pathway is limited to rodents.

ACTH, adrenocorticotropic hormone; CRP, C-reactive protein; IL, interleukin; LBP, lipopolysaccharide-binding protein; MSH, melanocyte-stimulating hormone; PAI, plasminogen activator inhibitor; sTNF-R, soluble tumor necrosis factor receptor; TGF, transforming growth factor.

tor [MIF]) affect both immune and nonimmune cells. In a similar way, the tachyphylaxis or desensitization that reduces responses to catecholamines affects both vascular smooth muscle and inflammatory cells.[29,39,40] It is thus possible that mechanisms that may have evolved to prevent stress-induced hypertension and damp systemic anti-inflammation also contribute to the pathogenesis of severe sepsis and septic shock.

Procoagulant Responses. Inflammation and coagulation are closely linked.[41,42] Clotting is perhaps the oldest host defense mechanism, as it preceded complement and the acquired immune system during the evolution of animals. Inflammation-induced procoagulant responses contribute to abscess formation and delayed hypersensitivity reactions in humans.

In individuals who have sustained physical trauma, activation of coagulation and inhibition of fibrinolysis occur roughly in proportion to the severity of injury.[43] Briefly, inflammation-induced expression of tissue factor on the surfaces of monocytes and endothelial cells is thought to initiate the production of thrombin via factors VIIa and Xa, whereas increased production of plasminogen activator inhibitor-1 (PAI-1) inhibits fibrinolysis (Fig. 67-2).[44,45]

Much recent attention has focused on protein C, which can be converted to its activated form (aPC) when thrombin binds thrombomodulin, an endothelial cell surface protein. Activated protein C then dissociates from its own receptor, endothelial protein C receptor (EPCR), before binding soluble protein S to produce a complex that inactivates factors Va and VIIIa, thereby blocking the activation of thrombin.[46] During acute-phase responses, depletion of protein C and antithrombin III parallels the fall in serum albumin concentration, because these anticoagulants are also negative acute-phase reactants.[47] The available molecules of a third natural anticoagulant, protein S, decrease as it binds to its circulating partner, C4b, a positive acute-phase reactant. Paradoxically, generation of low amounts of thrombin may inhibit clotting by activating protein C.[45]

Thermoregulatory Responses. The adaptations to stress just described often occur in the absence of fever; in fact, there is evidence that fever and the other elements of the acute-phase response are independently regulated.[21] Because TNF, IL-6, and other putative pyrogens can be found in the blood in the absence of fever, and because the evidence that endogenous pyrogens circulate in human blood is surprisingly weak,[20,48] it is possible that infection-related thermogenesis is induced when local inflammation activates neural afferent signals to the thermoregulatory center, either via local nerves[49] or the vagus.[24]

The physiologic responses that increase body temperature include shivering (rhythmic contractions of skeletal muscles) and redirection of blood flow from the skin and extremities to internal organs by means of vasoconstriction.

An increase in body temperature may favor host survival in several ways.[21] It may help inhibit bacterial growth and increase the bactericidal activities of neutrophils and macrophages,[22] for example, and the redistribution of blood flow that occurs during thermogenesis may increase blood delivery to infected tissues.

Summary. There is considerable overlap between the body's acute systemic responses to infection, injury, and many other stresses. Indeed, many of the same responses occur after strenuous exercise and during periods of psychological stress. As shown best in studies performed in patients who have sustained trauma, the intensity of the response generally increases with increasing stimulus severity,[50] and there is individual variability in the expression of its different elements. The evidence that normal systemic responses can be immunosuppressive, increasing one's risk for acquiring viral as well as bacterial infections, is intriguing but still largely circumstantial (see references cited in reference 10). This phenomenon may account, in part, for the increased susceptibility to infection experienced by patients who have sustained major trauma or are experiencing critical illness.[51-53]

In most patients in whom severe sepsis occurs today, many of the acute-phase responses discussed here would probably have been activated by injury or illness prior to the onset of infection. Local infection or inflammation would provide a further stimulus to these responses, broadening and intensifying their expression. If uncontrolled infection then induces severe sepsis and septic shock, it does so when anti-inflammatory influences may dominate in the peripheral blood; as will be discussed later, a net anti-inflammatory balance seems to be maintained during severe sepsis, and immunosuppression becomes even more prominent.

Pathologic Host Responses to Infection

Sepsis. *Sepsis* is perhaps the most confusing term in the lexicon of this controversial field, because although it has recently been used (see Table 67-1) to describe the body's early systemic responses to infection (leukocytosis, tachycardia, tachypnea, fever), to many clinicians it implies a more serious, life-threatening state. Moreover, Alberti and colleagues recently found that the outcomes of ICU patients seem to be unaffected by the number of systemic response (SIRS) criteria that were present when infection was diagnosed.[4]

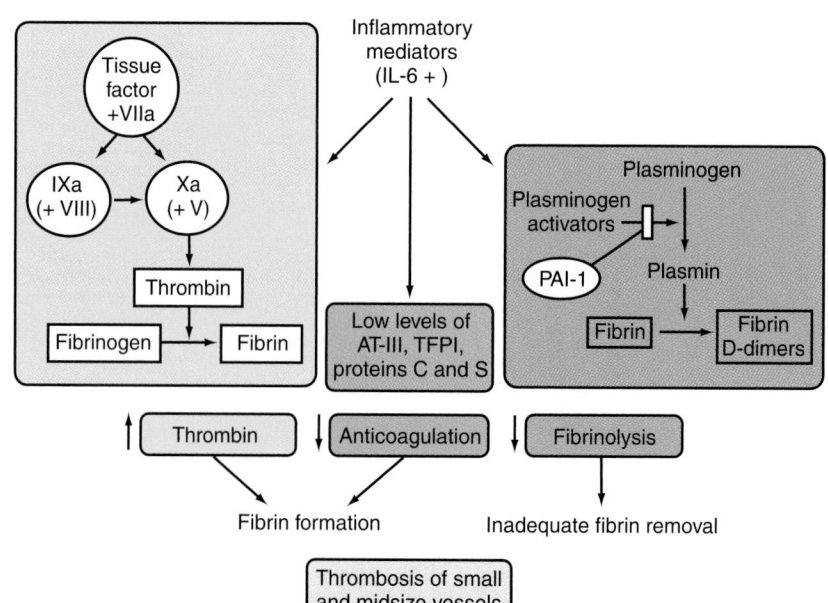

FIGURE 67-2. Inflammation-activated coagulation. Inflammation-associated coagulation begins when cytokines, Toll-like receptor (TLR) agonists, or other stimuli induce tissue factor expression on the surfaces of monocytes and vascular endothelial cells. Increased concentrations of plasminogen activator inhibitor (PAI)-1 prevent the formation of plasmin, decreasing fibrinolysis. Tissue factor pathway inhibitor (TFPI) modulates thrombin activation by blocking the activity of the tissue factor/factor VIIa/factor Xa complex. Hepatic synthesis of protein C and antithrombin III (AT-III) decreases during the acute phase response, whereas an increase in the plasma concentration of complement factor C4b binds more of the available protein S, reducing its ability to inhibit clotting. Factors may also be consumed during clot formation. Despite these procoagulant and antifibrinolytic changes, intravascular thrombosis is unusual. *(Modified from Levi M, ten Cate H. Disseminated intravascular coagulation. N Engl J Med. 1999;341: 586-592. Copyright © 1999 Massachusetts Medical Society. All rights reserved.)*

Patients with infection but with no evident systemic response were just as likely to die in the ICU as were patients with infection who met SIRS criteria and would thus have been considered "septic." As these authors concluded, "Refinement of risk stratification of patients presenting with infection and no organ dysfunction is needed."[4] Their observation also suggests that there is still much to be learned about the body's early responses to infection.

Severe Sepsis. Sepsis-associated organ dysfunction and hypotension are often reversible. Moreover, there is often little or no detectable evidence for cell death in the microscopic appearance of tissues of patients who die from severe sepsis.[54-57] Pathologists have found apoptosis of cells in the spleen and intestine,[55] myopathic changes in skeletal muscle,[58] and changes in blood vessel morphology (in meningococcal disease, for example[46]), but significant necrosis does not seem to occur in the major organs,[55] which argues against a prominent general role for thrombosis or necrotic cell death in the pathogenesis of organ dysfunction. On the other hand, much evidence points to a prominent role for microcirculatory dysfunction and abnormal oxygen utilization.

Microcirculatory Dysfunction. Two groups have reported their findings using orthogonal polarization spectral imaging of the most accessible muscle, the tongue, in patients with severe sepsis. When they were compared with controls, patients with severe sepsis had significantly reduced vessel density and the proportion of perfused small vessels was also below normal.[59,60] Mechanisms often invoked to account for changes in the microcirculation include reduced deformability of erythrocytes and activated neutrophils, neutrophil aggregation, and microthrombosis.[61] There is little evidence that any of these phenomena alters microcirculatory function in humans, however, and the aforementioned changes noted by spectral imaging were reversible by the application of acetylcholine[59] or nitroprusside,[60] indicating that they have a chemical basis and are not anatomically fixed.

Maldistribution of blood flow at the level of the microcirculation is thought to contribute to low oxygen utilization by affected tissues. One attractive theory is *cytopathic hypoxia,* a term proposed by Fink to denote "diminished production of ATP despite normal (or even supranormal) Po_2 values in the vicinity of mitochondria within cells."[62] Several phenomena might contribute, including diminished entry of pyruvate into the tricarboxylic acid cycle, activation of poly-(ADP-ribose) polymerase (PARP), or uncoupling of oxidation from phosphorylation due to collapse of the proton gradient across the mitochondrial membrane. Much attention has been focused on the ability of peroxynitrite and nitric oxide to activate PARP, which rapidly polymerizes cellular ADP and thus robs the cell of ATP.[63] Dysfunction of mitochondria in muscle[64] and peripheral blood monocytes[65] has correlated with sepsis severity in clinical studies.

Activation or Injury of the Vascular Endothelium. Many experts consider diffuse endothelial injury to be the central abnormality that leads to severe sepsis and septic shock. Indeed, the vascular endothelium is involved in three processes that play major roles in sepsis pathophysiology: vascular tone, vascular permeability, and coagulation. The evidence that endothelial activation or injury contributes to the observed abnormalities in blood pressure, fluid extravasation, and coagulation is almost entirely derived from studies in endotoxin-challenged animals or from in vitro investigations, however.[66,67] In humans, there is ample clinical evidence that capillary permeability increases in the dysfunctional organs of patients with severe sepsis; it is most obvious in patients with acute lung injury (see later) or peripheral edema. Similarly, a role for endothelial activation in the initiation or propagation of intravascular coagulopathy seems likely, although direct evidence for this in humans is limited almost entirely to patients with fulminant meningococcemia.[46] Mutunga and co-workers found that patients with severe sepsis and septic shock had higher concentrations of von Willebrand factor–positive (endothelial) cells in their plasma than did healthy human controls, suggesting that endothelial damage occurs in human sepsis.[68] Although the source of these circulating endothelial cells was not determined, others have found both high circulating levels of immunoreactive von Willebrand factor and decreased von Willebrand factor staining in dermal vessels of patients with SIRS, suggesting a generalized endothelial response to inflammation.[69] In one study of muscle biopsies from patients with severe sepsis, endothelial activation was suggested by increased expression of ICAM-1 and by an increased proportion of capillaries expressing P-selectin and E-selectin.[58] On the other hand, others have found that the skin microcirculation of patients with septic shock has normal endothelium-dependent responses to vasodilators,[70] and that circulating levels of soluble adhesion molecules do not correlate well with endothelial activation in skin biopsies.[71] More information is needed before the role of endothelial activation in the pathogenesis of severe sepsis in humans can be accurately assessed. Recent findings indicate that there is considerable heterogeneity in the structure and function of endothelial cells in different tissue beds,[72] so it is quite possible that the changes noted in the tissues that are most accessible to examination (skin, skeletal muscle, tongue) are not representative of those in the organs that are affected most significantly during severe sepsis (lungs, kidneys, liver, brain).

Cytokines and Other Mediators. The discovery of the major proinflammatory cytokines (TNF and IL-1β) was quickly followed by evidence that these proteins, individually or in combination, can induce severe sepsis and septic shock in experimental animals. Moreover, higher than normal levels of these cytokines were found in the blood of many septic patients, and, in some studies, these levels correlated with risk of dying. During the 1990s, however, investigators found that the blood of severely septic patients contains not only these and other proinflammatory mediators (e.g., IL-12, platelet activating factor [PAF]) but also a broad array of anti-inflammatory molecules (e.g., IL-4, IL-10, IL-1Ra, soluble TNF receptors). Remarkably, all attempts to define the dominant molecules in the plasma of septic patients have concluded that the anti-inflammatory cytokines (in particular, IL-10 and IL-4) are most active.[73-75] A similar trend has been found in studies of peripheral blood monocytes from patients with severe sepsis: they respond to LPS and other agonists ex vivo by producing lower than normal amounts of TNF, IL-12, and IFN-γ yet normal or high amounts of IL-1Ra and IL-10.[76-79] There may also be a marked elevation in circulating CD4+ CD25+ regulatory T cells.[80] A minor population of circulating monocytes (CD14+CD16+DR++) seems to account for most of the TNF produced by circulating cells.[81]

It has been especially challenging to understand the role of IL-6.[82] Although early studies suggested that this abundant cytokine is proinflammatory, more recent evidence suggests that it is an SOS signal that can be produced by most cells in response to injury. Indeed, epinephrine induces IL-6 production in vivo, whereas IL-6 infusion enhances blood levels of IL-1Ra, IL-10, and cortisol.[83] Experiments in genetically manipulated mice suggest that IL-6 is the most important activator of the HPA axis in response to stress,[84] for example, and IL-6–deficient mice have exaggerated inflammatory responses to bacterial infections.[85,86] Studies in volunteers and in chimpanzees suggest that IL-6 is the major procoagulant cytokine. More than any other cytokine, IL-6 thus seems to direct the body's systemic acute-phase responses.[82,87]

Two proinflammatory mediators may become very important late in the course of the response to severe infection. Macrophage MIF is a product of T lymphocytes and macrophages that is induced by, and opposes the actions of, glucocorticoids.[88] Although MIF normally circulates at a low basal level, its plasma concentration increases during infection and stress, and very high levels have been found in the plasma of patients with severe sepsis.[89,90] The role played by MIF in endotoxin-induced sepsis is disputed, however.[89,91] A second "late" proinflammatory molecule is a transcription factor, high-mobility group box (HMGB)-1, that appears in the blood several hours after infection begins, stimulates monocyte/macrophages to produce proinflammatory cytokines,[92] increases gut permeability, and contributes to death in a mouse endotoxin challenge model.[93] The only interventions shown to rescue experimental animals from established endotoxic shock or septic peritonitis are antibodies to MIF[89] or HMGB-1[93] or an infusion of ethyl pyruvate, which decreases HMGB-1 production.[94] (To be effective, other interventions must be given before, or with, the challenge.)

For many years, it has seemed that TNF and other proinflammatory mediators are produced at a local site of infection, diffuse into the blood stream, initiate systemic inflammation, and are then opposed by a counter-regulatory anti-inflammatory response. An imbalance in these opposing forces ("immune dissonance"[95]) was thought to cause severe sepsis. This view found support in the results of numerous studies that measured the cytokine responses of healthy subjects to a bolus injection of endotoxin, as well as in observations made in patients with fulminant meningococcemia. On the other hand, it is difficult to envision the same sequence of events in patients who, as a consequence of trauma or illness, are already experiencing acute-phase systemic responses at the time that a sepsis-triggering infection begins. In such patients, anti-inflammatory mechanisms seem to dominate in the blood throughout the clinical course. In others, an early anti-inflammatory systemic response, as reflected in a high ratio of IL-10 to TNF in plasma at the time of hospital admission, has been associated with a poor outcome.[96,97] No theory proposed to date adequately accounts for the transition from sepsis to severe sepsis to septic shock, however. Prospective studies that combine clinical observation with serial measurements of mediator biosynthesis and cellular responsiveness in patients at risk (e.g., previously healthy young individuals who sustain major trauma) could provide the information needed to produce an accurate account.

Complement Activation. The ability of normal human serum to kill bacteria is largely conferred by the complement system, which can be activated by antigen–antibody complexes or CRP (classical pathway), certain bacterial surface sugars (mannose-binding lectin pathway), or (lipo)polysaccharides (alternative pathway). There is evidence that each of these pathways can be activated in the serum of patients with sepsis,[98-100] and at least two of the complement proteins may contribute to the septic response. Activation of both the complement and the contact systems is regulated by C1-esterase inhibitor, which undergoes proteolytic inactivation in patients with severe sepsis[100]; administration of the inhibitor had only modest effects on the outcome of severe sepsis in a nonhuman primate model, however.[101] Factor C5a is a potent chemoattractant that also can induce vasodilatation, increase vascular permeability, and augment the release of granule enzymes from phagocytes.[102] The blood neutrophils of humans with early sepsis may lose responsiveness to C5a. Studies in septic rodents suggest that antibody-mediated neutralization of C5a or its receptor may prevent death.[102]

Coagulopathy. Although coagulopathy is commonly seen in patients with severe sepsis, the factors that provoke it are not well understood. In most patients it may simply be an extension of the normal acute-phase response to infection (see earlier), but in others it might be triggered by vascular endothelial injury or dysfunction either at a local site of infection or more diffusely. The extent to which coagulopathy contributes to organ dysfunction in septic humans is also controversial. Although there is a strong experimental basis for suspecting that microthrombi form in a generalized fashion when patients develop disseminated intravascular coagulation (DIC), autopsy studies have not found a convincing link between fibrin deposition and organ failure.[57,103] Moreover, the administration of two different anticoagulant drugs (tissue factor pathway inhibitor, antithrombin III) did not improve organ function or survival in patients with severe sepsis.[104,105] Although a 4-day intravenous infusion of a third anticoagulant, recombinant activated protein C, did improve survival during the second phase of its clinical trial (see "Therapy," later), its apparent efficacy was not attributed to its anticoagulant properties.[106] As noted by Levi and ten Cate, "It remains uncertain to what extent intravascular fibrin or coagulation proteases are the critical factors in determining the clinical course, rather than just the consequences of a more severe systemic inflammatory response."[44]

The best-documented exception to this conclusion is fulminant meningococcemia. Autopsy studies have found meningococci within the lumina of dermal vessels, as well as in endothelial cells, and thrombi have been noted in small vessels of many tissues, most notably the adrenal glands.[107,108] In patients with viral hemorrhagic fevers (e.g., Ebola virus), in contrast, DIC typically occurs late in the course, and the clotting factor abnormalities, triggered in part by expression of tissue factor on infected monocytes, may be surprisingly modest; mucosal hemorrhage may be largely a consequence of platelet dysfunction,[109] and there is little evidence that DIC contributes to organ dysfunction.

Immunosuppression. Patients with severe sepsis are usually profoundly immunosuppressed.[110] They often lose their ability to exhibit cutaneous delayed hypersensitivity to recall antigens, becoming anergic[111]; this is associated with decreased surface expression of class II (human leukocyte antigen [HLA]-DR) and costimulatory[112] molecules on circulating monocytes. When compared with monocytes from normal controls, peripheral blood monocytes from septic patients produce less TNF, but unchanged or increased amounts of IL-1Ra and IL-10, when stimulated ex vivo with LPS[73,75,77]; there is evidence that IL-10 both inhibits TNF production[77] and promotes intracellular sequestration of HLA-DR.[113] These changes normalize as patients recover.[76] Neutrophils obtained from severely septic patients show reduced IL-1β and IL-8[114,115] production when stimulated with LPS or streptococci; similar behavior can be induced in normal neutrophils by treatment with IL-10.[115]

Hotchkiss and colleagues have noted extensive apoptosis of CD4+ lymphocytes, dendritic cells, and B cells in the spleens of patients with severe sepsis.[116,117] Intestinal epithelial cells may also undergo apoptosis,[55] yet NK cells and CD8+ lymphocytes are not affected. These changes were not noted in critically ill but nonseptic patients, suggesting that they do not contribute to the immunosuppressive state that follows injury and other stresses.[55] Studies of inflammation-associated apoptosis in experimental animals suggest that glucocorticoids are more important inducers of apoptosis than are TNF or Fas ligand (FasL).[118] Hyperactivation of splenic sympathetic input may also play a role. How loss of these cells contributes to the pathogenesis of severe sepsis is uncertain, however. Remarkably, in the murine model of septic peritonitis, death can be prevented by administering a caspase inhibitor or overexpressing Bcl-2, an antiapoptotic protein, in lymphocytes.[119]

In contrast to these observations on lymphocytes, the life span of neutrophils is prolonged by proinflammatory mediators, such as TNF and G-CSF, and shortened by IL-10, which promotes neutrophil apoptosis.[120]

Septic Shock. Septic shock may have two distinguishable phases. Vasoconstrictive (cold) shock, characterized by low cardiac output and high peripheral resistance, occurs in patients who are hypovolemic[121]; factors that contribute to decreased effective intravascular volume include redistribution of blood flow, venous pooling, increased capillary permeability, increased insensible losses, and poor fluid intake. During this phase, the blood pressure is supported by peripheral vasoconstriction. Restoration of effective intravascular volume by the administration of fluids is usually followed by vasodilation. Vasodilation is not often seen with acute hemorrhagic shock and almost never seen with cardiogenic shock, and it does not usually occur in patients with shock due to viral hemorrhagic fever or Hantavirus infections, which cause myocardial dysfunction and profound increases in capillary permeability.[122] The clinical hallmarks of vasodilation are decreased systemic vascular resistance and high cardiac output. The following factors may contribute to inflammation-induced vasodilation:

- Tachyphylaxis to catecholamines, which diminishes the sensitivity of vascular smooth muscle to catecholamines as pressors[39]
- The underproduction or ineffectiveness of glucocorticoids, which upregulate adrenergic receptors[39]
- The production of adrenomedullin, which has vasodilatory actions, increases renal blood flow, and inhibits aldosterone secretion[123]
- The release of nitric oxide from sites of inflammation[124] and/or distant vascular endothelium
- The absence of the normal baroreflex response that increases circulating vasopressin levels (and depletion of neurohypophyseal vasopressin stores)[125]
- The release of PAF
- The activation of K_{ATP} channels in arteriolar smooth muscle cells by hypoxia and lactate[126]
- The generation of bradykinin, a vasodilator that also increases capillary permeability[127]

Remarkably, inflammation-induced vasodilation can occur when there are very high blood levels of several vasoconstrictor hormones (norepinephrine, epinephrine, endothelin-1, and angiotensin II). The best clues to its pathogenesis may be the ability of treatment with hydrocortisone or vasopressin to improve the pressor potency of catecholamines in many patients (see "Therapy," later).

Influence of Gene Polymorphisms on Infection Susceptibility and Outcome

A major obstacle to understanding the pathogenesis of severe sepsis is the striking heterogeneity of the patient population that experiences the syndrome. Patients differ in age, sex, ethnic group, underlying disease, inciting microbe, medications, and numerous other variables. Despite this heterogeneity, several groups of investigators have found single nucleotide polymorphism (SNP)-outcome associations in small groups of critically ill patients. Although there has been significant variability in the results of these studies, some SNPs do seem to have associations with susceptibility to bacterial infection or with risk for developing severe sepsis or dying, at least in some ethnic groups.

Phagocytes express FcγRIIA, the major Fc receptor for binding molecules of IgG$_2$, the most abundant antibodies to polysaccharide antigens. A common polymorphism changes the amino acid at position 131 in the peptide; the arginine (R) allele is associated with less effective phagocytosis than is the histidine (H) allele. In studies from several locations, R/R homozygosity has been associated with increased severity of meningococcal[128] and pneumococcal[129] disease. More severe meningococcal disease has also been associated with polymorphisms in the genes that encode PAI-1, TNF, IL-1β and angiotensin-converting enzyme.[130-132]

Gene polymorphisms that have been associated with increased risk for bacterial infection include mannose-binding lectin and TLR4 (for gram-negative infections).[133,134] Polymorphisms in these genes have also been associated with increased risk for septic shock due to gram-negative infection.[135] Polymorphisms associated with increased risk for severe sepsis in critically ill patients include TNF-308 (in France,[136] Taiwan,[137] and the United States,[138] but not in Germany[139]) and TNF-B2 (in Germany[139] but not in the United States or France). German workers have also found an association between the -174 allelic polymorphism of IL-6 and the outcome of sepsis.[140]

These associations must be confirmed in larger populations and others must be sought. Because some of the implicated polymorphisms may not alter gene function,[141,142] understanding the basis for their apparent association with infection risk or sepsis susceptibility may provide new insights into pathogenesis. The hope is that certain SNPs can be used to identify individuals at increased risk for immunosuppression, nosocomial infection, or an adverse outcome. A patient's genetic profile may someday be useful for guiding specific preventive or therapeutic interventions.

Microbial Triggers for Severe Sepsis

The most commonly identified sites of primary infection in patients with severe sepsis are the lungs and the abdomen (Fig. 67-3). No obvious source of infection can be found in approximately one third to one half of the cases in most series.[6,104,106] Culture-negative and culture-positive cases have had similar morbidity and mortality rates.[6]

In keeping with the recent discovery that conserved gram-positive (peptidoglycan, lipoteichoic acid) and gram-negative (LPS) bacterial molecules are recognized by distinct TLRs on leukocytes, with distinct yet overlapping downstream signaling pathways (see Fig. 67-1), patients with severe sepsis due to gram-positive and gram-negative bacteria may have somewhat different cytokine responses. In one study, IL-1β, IL-6, and IL-18 concentrations were higher in the plasma of patients with sepsis due to gram-positive bacteria[143]; another found higher levels of TNF in the plasma of patients with severe sepsis due to a gram-negative bacterial infection.[144] Microarray analysis of mRNA from macrophages and whole blood stimulated ex vivo has also identified numerous differences in gene expression in response to gram-positive compared with gram-negative stimuli.[143,145-147] Although

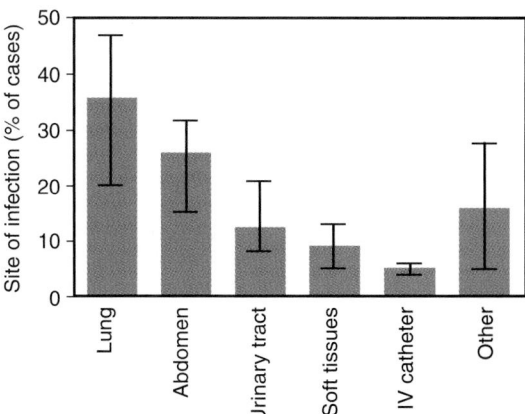

FIGURE 67-3. Presumed sites of infection in patients with culture-positive severe sepsis. *Bars* show the means of data from four studies.[15,224,311,312] *Brackets* show the minimum and maximum values reported. Note that the lung and abdomen are the most common primary sites.

the clinical features of severe sepsis caused by different microbes are indistinguishable, it is possible that these new molecular signatures will provide new insights into pathogenesis and be useful for diagnosis as well as for directing therapy.

Bacteremia. How local infection leads to multiorgan dysfunction and hypotension is uncertain. One long-favored hypothesis is that uncontrolled local infection eventuates in bacteremia or toxemia; circulating bacteria, or their products, stimulate inflammatory reactions within the vasculature and distant organs, and this leads to organ dysfunction and hypotension. Given the long history of this idea, it is surprising that strong evidence for it is actually limited to a few special situations. The most prominent example is fulminant meningococcemia, when *N. meningitidis* bacteria grow in the blood, release their endotoxin, and rapidly induce DIC, severe sepsis, and shock. Other examples are the neutropenic or splenectomized individuals who develop overwhelming bacteremia[148] and patients with *Yersinia pestis,*[149] *Burkholderia pseudomallei,*[150] or *Capnocytophaga canimorsus* bacteremia.

These examples are special because they are uncommon and because the responsible bacteria are usually human pathogens. In contrast, the great majority of the cases of severe sepsis that occur today are associated with bacterial or fungal microorganisms that are members of the patient's own microbial flora.[151] These commensal microbes—enteric gram-negative bacilli, coagulase-negative staphylococci, enterococci, *Candida* species, and others—rarely cause disease in humans who have normal innate immune defenses. Individuals who develop serious disease due to a commensal bacterium generally have a significant immune defect—most often, epithelial barrier disruption (e.g., catheters, bites, cuts) or immunosuppression.

The evidence that circulating commensal bacteria stimulate inflammation within the blood stream is limited to a few circumstantial observations. Blood cultures are positive more commonly in patients who have severe sepsis than in those with sepsis,[6] for example, and the fraction of patients who have a positive culture is even greater among those with septic shock.[6,14] In patients with severe sepsis and documented infection, moreover, bacteremia has been associated with early mortality.[15] Blood-stream infection with certain microorganisms, such as *Candida albicans,*[152] methicillin-resistant *S. aureus,*[153] and vancomycin-resistant *Enterococcus faecium,*[154] has also been associated with significant attributable mortality (an often-used but imperfect surrogate outcome for severe sepsis/septic shock).

In contrast, other lines of evidence suggest that circulating commensal bacteria usually do not directly trigger severe sepsis or septic shock. First, bacteremia is usually low grade and transient, even in the absence of antimicrobial chemotherapy, provided that reseeding of the blood stream does not occur.[155,156] The body's innate immune mechanisms for clearing commensal bacteria and fungi from the blood stream are evidently very effective.[155] Second, with some exceptions (such as *S. aureus* bacteremia and septicemic melioidosis[150]), the risk for developing severe sepsis has not correlated directly with the density of cultivatable bacteria in the blood.[157,158] Third, bacteremia has no distinctive clinical features—at the bedside, bacteremic patients with severe sepsis are indistinguishable from those whose cultures are negative.[159,160] Finally, the case-fatality rates for culture-positive and culture-negative patients with severe sepsis and septic shock are very similar,[6,15,161] suggesting that bacteremia may contribute little to outcome. In keeping with this idea, little or no excess mortality could be attributed to bacteremia associated with indwelling vascular catheters,[162-164] antibiotic-resistant nosocomial bacteria,[165] transfusion-related *Serratia*,[166] nosocomial *Enterobacter*,[167] or bacteremia that occurred in a tertiary hospital population.[168]

A second hypothesis may be more likely to account for the occurrence of severe sepsis in patients who have primary extravascular infections with commensal organisms. This is that inflammatory mediators produced in the infected tissue enter the blood stream, where they then stimulate either intravascular cells or cells in distant organs. In such patients, circulating bacteria would be a marker for uncontrolled local infection, not the direct trigger for severe sepsis. It has been known for many years that the outcome of bacteremia is strongly related to the site of the local infection (i.e., the source),[169] with higher case-fatality rates occurring in bacteremic patients with pulmonary or abdominal infections than in those with urinary tract infections.[170] Secondary bacteremia (from an infected tissue) is much more likely to have a fatal outcome than is bacteremia from a vascular catheter.[164,169] Similarly, among bacteremic patients, the risk for developing severe sepsis is strongly related to the site of the primary infection. In a large series of patients with positive blood cultures, Brun-Buisson and co-workers found that the relative risk for developing severe sepsis was almost 10-fold higher for patients with intra-abdominal infection than it was for those with urinary tract infection.[171] Direct introduction of bacteria into the blood stream (as from an infected vascular catheter) was much less likely to induce septic shock than was secondary bacteremia.[164,171] In their multivariate analysis, age and the site of infection were the only variables that correlated with risk for developing severe sepsis; the nature of the offending bacterium was not important.

Remarkably clear evidence for the role of local cytokine production in inducing septic shock has been published by Kurahashi and colleagues.[34] These workers were unable to induce shock when they continuously infused rabbits with a virulent strain of *Pseudomonas aeruginosa*. In contrast, when they introduced the same strain into the lungs, pneumonia developed and shock occurred well before bacteremia could be detected. A mutant that did not disrupt alveolar epithelial integrity was able to cause pneumonia, but it did not induce shock, nor did it promote movement of radiolabeled TNF from the lungs into the circulation. Shock induced by the virulent strain could be prevented by intravenous administration of an anti-TNF monoclonal antibody or by administering IL-10. Kurahashi and co-workers concluded from these observations that the virulent strain caused sufficient alveolar epithelial cell injury to allow TNF to escape into the circulation, where it induced shock. In a different experimental model, Martin and colleagues found that bacteremia was insufficient to produce pulmonary inflammation in rabbits with bacterial peritonitis; only when the abdominal infection was uncontrolled did inflammation occur in the lung.[35] These findings again point to compartmentalization of the inflammatory response and suggest that bacteremia may not be as important for the pathogenesis of severe sepsis as is the elaboration of inflammatory mediators at a site of uncontrolled local infection.

In the case of *N. meningitidis* and a few other intravascular pathogens, the circulating bacteria seem to be directly responsible for initiating inflammation within the vasculature. Bacteremia may have a similar importance in patients whose local defenses are compromised by neutropenia. In most other instances, however, the presence of cultivatable bacteria in the peripheral blood may be a marker for severe infection/inflammation in a local tissue. A positive blood culture

should alert the clinician to look for an uncontrolled local infection. The conclusion reached by Felty and Keefer in their 1924 review of patients with *Escherichia coli* bacteremia seems valid for many patients today: "We are inclined toward the view not only that the symptoms of the generalized infection are difficult to differentiate from those of the local process, but also that the prognosis depends largely on the character of the primary focus. In short, the essential feature is the extent, severity and amenability to treatment, of the local process rather than the sepsis itself."[172]

Endotoxemia. It is widely held that bacterial endotoxin, when it enters the blood stream, triggers systemic inflammation. Fulminant meningococcemia has provided the most striking evidence for this idea, because the high levels of circulating endotoxin found in patients with this syndrome have correlated directly with plasma TNF levels and the risk of dying.[173,174] Infusing endotoxin directly into the blood stream of healthy volunteers readily confirms the ability of this substance to induce dramatic changes in circulating mediator concentrations and to cause symptoms.[175]

Fulminant meningococcemia is a very distinctive syndrome, however, in which a pathogenic bacterium invades a healthy individual and grows within the blood stream before the victim can mount an effective defense. In most instances, there is no local (i.e., nasopharyngeal) inflammation to impede bacterial invasion or induce systemic responses. Moreover, meningococci shed membrane blebs that contain endotoxin and other molecules; these particles may serve as surfaces for activating complement and coagulation within the blood stream. Meningococcemia may thus be a poor model for the typical case of gram-negative bacteremia, in which a commensal bacterium such as *E. coli* or *Klebsiella* invades an already-sick patient, triggers inflammation in a local tissue, and transiently invades the blood stream. The endotoxin infusion model resembles meningococcemia in important ways (healthy subjects, acute exposure to endotoxin, no local infection/inflammation), and its usefulness for studying sepsis pathogenesis is limited for similar reasons.

For over 3 decades, the *Limulus* amebocyte lysate (LAL) assay has been used to measure endotoxin in plasma. This method and a newer antibody-based assay[176] measure both active endotoxin and endotoxin that may circulate in plasma in an inactive form.[177,178] It is thus uncertain that the plasma endotoxin detected using these assays is truly able to induce inflammation in vivo. Moreover, several endotoxin-neutralizing mechanisms are more active in the plasma of sick humans.[179-181] The factors that promote the binding of endotoxin to plasma lipoproteins are more effective,[181] for example, and blood levels of BPI, a neutrophil-derived, endotoxin-neutralizing protein, increase.[182] The low amounts of endotoxin that circulate in septic patients may thus be unable to stimulate cells within the systemic compartment. In addition, even relatively mild stress induces changes in circulating monocytes that "reprogram" them to produce less TNF when they are stimulated by endotoxin.[31] This is similar to the ability of epinephrine infusion to alter the response of the systemic compartment to a bolus injection of endotoxin.[29] Finally, the high concentrations of LBP that prevail in plasma, particularly during the systemic response to infection, may inhibit the ability of LPS to activate monocytes, possibly by preventing the transfer of LPS from CD14 to MD-2-TLR4.[183,184]

It is thus not surprising that the correlation between endotoxemia, gram-negative bacteremia, and severe sepsis has been inconsistent and often weak.[185-187] This does not mean that endotoxin contributes little or nothing to the pathogenesis of severe sepsis, however. In most patients who develop severe sepsis due to a commensal gram-negative bacterium, the major site for the stimulatory action of endotoxin may be in an infected extravascular tissue, not the circulating blood. It is also possible that endotoxin is more active in the blood of acutely infected, previously healthy patients, in whom the enhanced endotoxin-inactivating mechanisms cited previously have yet to be induced and in whom circulating endotoxin has been associated with poor outcome.[174,185]

Other Bacterial Toxins. Staphylococcal and streptococcal toxic shock syndrome toxins (TSST-1, streptococcal pyrogenic exotoxins, streptococcal mitogenic exotoxin Z[188]) are superantigens that can activate large numbers of circulating T cells to release cytokines. They do so by cross-linking major histocompatibility complex (MHC) class II molecules on antigen-presenting cells with T-cell receptor Vβ domains, thus triggering the T cell to release proinflammatory cytokines.[189] Although there is strong circumstantial evidence that these toxins play a central role in producing the gram-positive bacterial toxic shock syndromes, proof of causation has not been attained.[190] There is also evidence that bacterial cell wall lipoproteins, which can signal cells via TLR2, may circulate in the blood of septic animals and provoke inflammation.[191]

Summary

The evidence reviewed here suggests that severe sepsis is a heterogeneous disorder of tissue metabolism in which an altered microcirculation plays a major role. Because tissue metabolism and the microcirculation are normally regulated via peripheral nerves and circulating hormones, it seems likely that neuroendocrine derangements are closely tied to organ dysfunction and septic shock. The most proximal causes remain unknown, however, and how the phenomena discussed here (e.g., complement activation, coagulopathy, mediator action or desensitization thereto, endothelial injury) interact to produce the syndromes is uncertain. On the other hand, one may draw tentative conclusions regarding the interactions between certain microbial triggers and the human host. Three plausible scenarios illustrate the spectrum:

1. Bacterial pathogens often invade previously healthy individuals, whereas most commensal bacteria invade across disrupted epithelia, usually into hosts in whom acute-phase responses are already occurring. The invaders typically initiate an extravascular tissue infection that activates local inflammation and may enhance systemic antiinflammatory responses. They invade the blood stream when local defenses are unable to kill or contain them; bacteremia, when it occurs, is often transient and may be less important than locally produced mediators as a trigger for severe sepsis and septic shock. DIC predisposes to hemorrhage, but its role in the pathogenesis of organ injury is uncertain. Outcome is strongly related to the patient's underlying physiologic state. In the acute management of these patients, a diligent search for the primary focus of infection is essential.
2. At the other end of the spectrum are microbes that can invade healthy people and enter the blood stream without eliciting extravascular inflammation; in essence, they invade below the radar of the local innate immune defenses. If their growth is not controlled by circulating antibody or complement, these invaders may infect vascular endothelial cells or circulating blood cells, or both, releasing (endo)toxins or other molecules that stimulate inflammation within the blood and various organs. The circulating microbes provoke both shock and profound coagulopathy that not uncommonly results in hemorrhage or arterial thrombosis, or both. Examples include *N. meningitidis*, *Rickettsia rickettsii*, and probably *V. vulnificus* and *C. canimorsus*. With some of these pathogens, the absence of an early proinflammatory host defense may be an important key to their pathogenesis. Certain viruses may also be in this category; there is evidence that symptomatic infection with filoviruses (e.g., Ebola), for example, which invade without provoking local inflammation and infect monocyte-macrophages in many tissues, may be prevented by an early proinflammatory systemic response.[192]
3. Other stimuli, such as gram-positive bacterial superantigens, may diffuse into the blood or be released into it by circulating bacteria. They activate T lymphocytes in the blood and tissues to release cytokines; in poorly understood ways, these cytokines induce organ dysfunction and cause shock.

Although each of these microbe–host interactions leads to the syndromes known now as severe sepsis and septic shock, they are sufficiently different from one another that they force the question, Is the apparent continuum from sepsis to septic shock truly a single process, a "final common path" that can be induced by many different initiating events? Or do different microbe–host interactions produce severe sepsis and septic shock in different ways? If the latter, which are the most important determinants: susceptibility alleles, underlying disease, age, physiologic state at the time infection occurs, primary extravascular versus intravascular infection, infection with commensal versus pathogen, or others? Answers to these questions will become possible when a quantitative description of the underlying biochemical mechanisms of severe sepsis and septic shock is achieved.

CLINICAL MANIFESTATIONS

Patients with severe sepsis and septic shock experience derangements in both of the body's major communication networks, the nervous system and the blood. The function of every organ may be affected.

The Nervous and Neuroendocrine Systems

Cerebral Function. Individuals who experience relatively mild infectious illnesses may exhibit subtle abnormalities in cognitive performance.[193] It is therefore not surprising that confusion and other alterations in higher cerebral function are often early manifestations of severe sepsis, particularly in older adult patients. Focal signs, seizures, and cranial nerve palsies are rare,[194] however, and the brain is anatomically normal when studied by computed tomography or magnetic resonance imaging. Although cerebral function returns to normal when patients recover from sepsis, encephalopathy may be associated with a poor prognosis: in one clinical trial, septic patients who were not competent to give informed consent experienced significantly higher mortality than did those who were able to understand and sign the consent form.[195]

The Hypothalamic-Pituitary-Adrenal Axis. The normally pulsatile pattern of pituitary hormone release (growth hormone, ACTH, prolactin) is often blunted in critically ill patients, as is normal circadian variability in levels of cortisol, leptin, IL-6, and other hormones. As many patients develop septic shock, high plasma concentrations of vasopressin are followed by relatively low levels, probably reflecting both loss of baroreflex feedback regulation and vasopressin depletion from the posterior pituitary.[125,196,197]

Adrenal Insufficiency. Rarely, infectious agents cause absolute adrenal insufficiency by directly inducing adrenal hemorrhage or necrosis. The most frequently implicated microbes are *N. meningitidis*, *Mycobacterium tuberculosis*, cytomegalovirus, and *Histoplasma capsulatum*. Cytomegalovirus (CMV)-related adrenalitis is common in patients with end-stage human immunodeficiency virus (HIV) infection, but its significance is usually uncertain. Secondary adrenal insufficiency, due to pituitary infection or apoplexy, is quite rare.

Inadequate adrenal reserve has often been diagnosed in patients with septic shock, but the diagnostic criteria are controversial. Septic shock is assumed to stimulate adrenal glucocorticoid release, raising the basal level that characterizes normal function. Using a moderately stringent diagnostic cutoff (a basal cortisol level of 20 μg/dL or less), the percentage of septic shock patients with relative adrenal insufficiency has ranged from 9%[198] to 37%[199]; using as a cutoff a basal level of 25 μg/dL, another study found 61% of the patients to have insufficiency.[200] Although one would expect the cortisol response to a large dose of ACTH to vary inversely with the basal cortisol level, this has not always been observed,[199,201] and some authors have found that a response of less than 9 μg/dL to a 250-μg bolus of ACTH identifies patients who are likely to die.[202] In another recent study, the cortisol response to ACTH was inversely related to mortality.[203] Whereas the aldosterone response to exogenous ACTH seems to be maintained in most patients with severe sepsis,[203] a state of hyperreninemic hypoaldosteronism has been described in critically ill individuals, most of whom have been hypotensive.[204,205]

Among the factors that may contribute to hypoadrenalism in septic patients are anatomic damage to the adrenals or pituitary, hypoperfusion, cytokine-induced dysfunction of the adrenals, drug-induced steroid hypermetabolism (rifampin, phenytoin) or inhibition of steroidogenesis (ketoconazole), and desensitization to glucocorticoid responsiveness at the cellular level.[206,207] Adrenal responsiveness to ACTH infusion typically returns to normal in patients who recover from septic shock.[208]

The textbook manifestations of adrenal insufficiency (hyponatremia with hyperkalemia, hypothermia, eosinophilia, hyperpigmentation, nausea, vomiting) are not often attributable to adrenal dysfunction in septic patients. Hypotension and hypoglycemia may be the most commonly recognized manifestations.

Autonomic Dysfunction. Heart rate variability (HRV)[209] is influenced by the balance of vagal and sympathetic inputs to the sinoatrial node. Autonomic reflexes can modulate these inputs, as can the central (vasomotor and respiratory centers) and peripheral (arterial pressure and respiratory movements) oscillators. Several studies have found that abnormalities in heart rate characteristics, measured using spectral analysis, precede (in neonates[210-212]) or coincide with (in adults[213]) the onset of septic shock. Although the precise basis for these changes is uncertain, in general they seem to reflect a decrease in sympathetic input to the cardiac pacemaker. They may reflect an uncoupling of the biologic oscillations in heart rate, blood pressure, respiration, and other functions that are normally connected through neural networks.[214,215]

Peripheral Nerves, Muscles. Critical illness polyneuropathy and myopathy may occur in patients who have been ill for a week or more.[194] The clinical features include difficulty in weaning from a ventilator, generalized wasting of the limbs, and diffuse weakness (tetraparesis). The diagnosis is usually made when electromyographic examination reveals denervation potentials compatible with axonal polyneuropathy, predominantly of distal motor fibers. A muscle biopsy may show edema, atrophy, and necrosis; a mononuclear cell infiltrate may be present.[216] Sedatives, glucocorticoids, and neuromuscular blocking agents may confuse the clinical picture.

The Blood Stream

The Heart. A pattern of sepsis-associated myocardial dysfunction was recognized during the 1980s. It includes reduced left and right ventricular ejection fractions, increased left and right ventricular end-diastolic volumes, and an elevated heart rate and cardiac output.[217] This pattern typically follows fluid resuscitation, occurs 24 to 48 hours after the onset of severe sepsis, and is reversible in patients who survive 5 to 10 days after its onset. It does not usually require inotropic therapy. In some patients, myocardial dysfunction may persist and be a major contributing factor to septic shock.

Blood Cells. The composition of the circulating blood has usually been viewed through a limited window, the peripheral vein. A neutrophilic leukocytosis is the normal response to bacterial or fungal infection. It is produced by mobilizing neutrophils from the marginal pool as well as the marrow (see acute-phase and anti-infective responses under "Pathogenesis"). Failure to mount a neutrophilic leukocytosis has been associated with a poor outcome.

The number of circulating NK cells is usually greatly reduced in patients with severe sepsis, as are the numbers of CD4$^+$ and CD8$^+$ T lymphocytes. At least in part, the reduction in circulating CD4$^+$ cells may be due to apoptosis.[116] In contrast, the numbers of circulating B lymphocytes may increase[218] despite apoptotic cell death. During sepsis, cytokine production by circulating T cells often has a helper T-cell 2 (Th2) predominance.[110]

Thrombocytopenia is a frequent finding in patients with severe sepsis. In one recent clinical trial, for example, approximately 40% of the patients with severe sepsis had platelet counts of less than 80,000/mm^3 at entry into the study.[106] Although thrombocytopenia often accompanies DIC (see later), it may be the only routinely measured clotting parameter that is abnormal; on the other hand, many patients with low-grade DIC do not have thrombocytopenia. The basis for isolated thrombocytopenia in septic patients is probably multifactorial, with peripheral nonimmune destruction[219] and marrow suppression playing significant roles.

Plasma. Abnormal concentrations of more than 50 molecules have been found in the venous plasma of patients with severe sepsis. On balance, this rich soup seems to have an anti-inflammatory impact when it is incubated with reporter cells ex vivo; in some cases, removing IL-10 and IL-4 or TGF-β from the plasma has restored the ability of reporter cells to respond to LPS.[73,220]

Lipids. Striking changes occur in the circulating lipids and lipoproteins.[221] High-density lipoprotein (HDL) and low-density lipoprotein (LDL) levels decrease, whereas triglyceride, free fatty acid, and very low density lipoprotein (VLDL) levels increase. The decrease in serum cholesterol is almost entirely accounted for by lower concentrations of cholesterol esters in circulating HDL and LDL (due to inhibition of lecithin cholesterol acyltransferase [LCAT]).[181]

Glucose. Hypoglycemia is a relatively uncommon manifestation of sepsis. Although many of the reported cases have occurred in patients with hepatic or renal disease or malnutrition, hypoglycemia has also been observed in patients with no definable cause other than sepsis.[222] Its pathogenesis is not well understood, but adrenal insufficiency should be considered in such patients. The body's acute metabolic responses to infection maintain the blood sugar concentration through gluconeogenesis, glycogenolysis, and insulin resistance (see acute-phase and metabolic responses under "Pathogenesis," earlier); hyperglycemia may result, especially in diabetics or when glucose-containing fluids are administered.

Lactate. Increased blood lactate concentrations and an increased lactate-to-pyruvate ratio are often seen in patients with severe sepsis, even in the absence of shock. Contrary to long-standing dogma, the accumulation of lactate and pyruvate in the blood is not simply a consequence of limited tissue oxygenation; rather, there is evidence that it results from marked increases in pyruvate production,[223] most likely from increased glycolysis. Other mechanisms also seem to contribute, including impaired hepatic lactate clearance and mitochondrial dysfunction. The ability of ibuprofen to decrease blood lactate in septic patients points to a role for arachidonic acid metabolites in lactate production.[224] Correction of hypotension with vasopressors does not always correct lactic acidosis, possibly because tissue perfusion remains compromised by vasoconstriction or by abnormal microcirculatory vasoregulation.

Coagulopathy. The prevalence of DIC increases as the inflammatory response intensifies,[6] reaching approximately 30% to 50% in patients with severe sepsis. Commonly used diagnostic criteria for DIC include (1) a platelet count of less than 100,000/mm^3 or a rapid decrease in the platelet count, (2) the presence of fibrin degradation products (or D-dimers) in plasma, (3) prolongation of the prothrombin time or the activated partial thromboplastin time (to >1.2 times the upper limit of normal), and (4) low plasma levels of coagulation inhibitors, such as antithrombin III.[44,225] The use of low levels of antithrombin and protein C for the diagnosis of DIC was recently challenged by Asakura and colleagues, who found no differences in the plasma activity of antithrombin and protein C between septic and control patients after stratification for plasma albumin levels.[47]

The most common adverse consequence of DIC is hemorrhage. Hemorrhage is most often apparent as oozing from wounds or as gastrointestinal (GI) bleeding. Thrombosis of large and small vessels may also occur, usually in relationship to local tissue infection.[56,57] Although thrombosis of small arterioles or arteries might in theory contribute to multiorgan dysfunction, the histopathologic evidence for this connection is limited to patients with fulminant meningococcemia.[56,57,103,107,108] In general, thrombosis-induced tissue injury is most apparent when there is cutaneous necrosis[103] and, especially, when blood flow to a distal structure (finger, toe, hand, foot, tip of the nose) is interrupted. There is evidence that vasoconstriction contributes to the pathogenesis of arterial thrombosis[226]; most attempts to restore blood flow have involved interfering with the sympathetic nerve supply to the affected extremity.[227] In one instructive case, a young boy with purpura fulminans developed gangrene of three extremities; in the spared limb, vasoconstriction was impaired due to a brachial plexus injury acquired at birth.[226]

Septic Shock. In prospective studies of the natural history of critical illness,[6,7] patients have progressed from sepsis to severe sepsis to septic shock, suggesting that these syndromes are part of a continuum. In the study of Rangel-Frausto and co-workers, 71% of the patients who developed septic shock had been previously classified as having severe sepsis, sepsis, or SIRS.[6]

Hypovolemic shock can usually be reversed by administering intravenous fluids. In the normovolemic patients with vasodilatory (warm, hyperdynamic) shock studied prospectively by Abraham and colleagues,[228,229] the first noticeable change was a fall in oxygen consumption, which was followed by compensatory increases in cardiac output and oxygen delivery; peripheral vascular resistance decreased progressively over the 24-hour period prior to the onset of overt hypotension. The lowest blood pressure was recorded when the cardiac output failed to compensate for low vascular resistance.

Dysfunction of Other Organs

Patients entered into studies of severe sepsis must have evidence for one or more dysfunctional organ systems. As is shown in Figure 67-4, hypotension is the most commonly noted abnormality; the frequency with which other organ systems are affected ranges from 5% to 50%. There is thus considerable patient-to-patient variability in the manifestations of severe sepsis.

Acute Lung Injury. Hyperventilation, with respiratory alkalosis, can be one of the earliest manifestations of sepsis. Similarly, pulmonary dysfunction typically occurs early in the course of severe sepsis. The clinical diagnosis of acute lung injury (ALI) is made when there is a combination of arterial hypoxemia ($PaO_2/FIO_2 < 300$) and bilateral pulmonary infiltrates on the chest radiograph, in the absence of pneumonia or heart failure.[230] With more severe hypoxemia ($PaO_2/FIO_2 < 200$), the diagnosis becomes acute respiratory distress syndrome (ARDS). The underlying pathology is diffuse alveolar epithelial injury, with increased barrier permeability and exudation of protein-rich fluid into the interstitial and airspace compartments. Neutrophils and monocytes accumulate in the lungs and may form cellular aggregates in pulmonary vessels.[41] Significant right-to-left shunting occurs. Dead space volume increases and compliance decreases, augmenting the work of breathing and often necessitating mechanical ventilation. Indeed, a common indication for mechanical ventilation is respiratory muscle fatigue; in patients who are obtunded or have impaired gag reflexes, intubation may also be used to prevent aspiration of oropharyngeal or gastric contents.

Patients who recover from ARDS may have significant functional impairment related to the healing process, which can produce restrictive defects and diminish diffusing capacity.

Renal Dysfunction. Severe sepsis is often accompanied by azotemia and oliguria. The renal abnormalities range from minimal proteinuria to profound renal failure. The pathogenetic mechanisms include hypovolemia, hypotension, renal vasoconstriction, and toxic drugs (in particular, aminoglycosides). Oliguria often follows the onset of hypotension and may resolve with fluid resuscitation. If urine flow ceases abruptly, obstruction must be excluded. Although drugs that interfere with prostaglandin synthesis should theoretically be avoided, ibuprofen administration for 48 hours was not associated with significant impairment of renal function.[224] Sepsis-induced renal insufficiency is usually reversible.

Gastrointestinal Tract Injury. Peripheral vasodilation redistributes the cardiac output so that visceral organs are underperfused; the morbidity and mortality of septic shock have correlated with the degree of tissue (e.g., gastric) hypoperfusion. The barrier function of the gut may be impaired, allowing translocation of bacteria into the lymph and blood streams. One study of critically ill patients in an ICU found that increased GI permeability preceded the onset of multiple organ dysfunction.[231]

In addition, aspiration of the microbial and chemical contents of the upper GI tract into the tracheobronchial tree may initiate nosocomial pneumonia. Small erosions of the gastric and duodenal mucosa predispose to upper GI bleeding. Ileus, a common feature of septic shock, may persist for a day or two after shock resolves.

Hepatic Dysfunction. The principal sepsis-associated abnormality is cholestatic jaundice, characterized by elevations in conjugated and unconjugated bilirubin (<10 mg/dL). These changes occur in patients with and without preexisting liver disease and may precede recognition of infection.[232] In patients with severe sepsis, elevated alkaline phosphatase, bilirubin, and aminotransferase levels are common, but frank hepatic failure ("shock liver") is unusual.

Immune Dysfunction. Reactivation of latent herpes simplex and CMV infections occurs in approximately 35% of critically ill surgical patients,[233] and CMV viremia has been described in a similar fraction of patients with severe sepsis.[234] The extent to which CMV contributes to immunosuppression in these patients is not known. Although clinical experience suggests that patients with severe sepsis are at increased risk for secondary infections, documentation of this risk has not been published.

Cutaneous Manifestations. A wide range of skin lesions may occur in patients with severe sepsis. They include the cutaneous reaction at a local inoculation site (pustule, eschar), lesions that appear at sites of hematogenous seeding of the skin or underlying soft tissue (petechiae, pustules, ecthyma gangrenosum, cellulitis), diffuse eruptions caused by blood-borne toxins (TSS), and hemorrhagic or necrotic lesions. Recognition of certain characteristic lesions can greatly assist etiologic diagnosis.

Musher distinguished three patterns of tissue involvement by gram-negative enteric bacilli.[235]

1. Cellulitis and thrombophlebitis are associated with intense local inflammation. Bacteria implicated in case reports include *Campylobacter fetus, Vibrio* species, and *Aeromonas hydrophila*. Only a few bacteria are present in the affected tissues, however.
2. When the inflammatory response is impaired, usually by neutropenia, ecthyma gangrenosum or bullous lesions may occur (see later); *P. aeruginosa* is the most commonly isolated microorganism.
3. In symmetrical peripheral gangrene associated with DIC, fibrin thrombi are seen in small vessels, but neither inflammatory cells nor bacteria are found.

Palpable petechiae or purpura suggests leukocytoclastic vasculitis, which may be caused by *N. meningitidis, R. rickettsii,* and occasionally *S. aureus*. Pustules often contain *S. aureus* or *C. albicans*. Cellulitis is most often caused by *S. pyogenes* but may, in unusual settings, reflect bacteremia due to clostridial species or one of the gram-negative bacilli mentioned earlier.

The term *ecthyma gangrenosum* ("necrotic blister") is used for lesions that begin as papules surrounded by erythema and edema and evolve into hemorrhagic, necrotic ulcers. They typically appear between the umbilicus and the knees. Although often considered pathognomonic for *P. aeruginosa* bacteremia, ecthyma gangrenosum has also

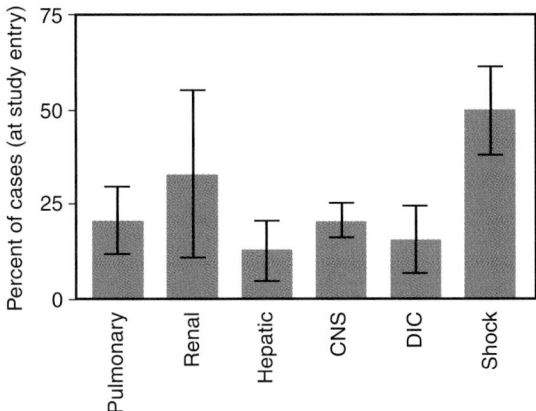

FIGURE 67-4. Organ dysfunction at entry into studies of severe sepsis. *Bars* show means of data from six representative studies.[14,224,311,313-315] *Brackets* show the minimal and maximal values reported. The definitions used to diagnose organ dysfunction varied somewhat from study to study. Renal dysfunction was uncommon in some series and very common in others.

been observed in patients whose blood cultures grew *Klebsiella, Serratia, A. hydrophila,* or *E. coli.* Pathologic examination reveals direct invasion of venules by bacteria, and local thrombosis. Almost all patients with ecthyma gangrenosum are neutropenic at the time the lesions develop.

Diffuse erythema (erythroderma) is a characteristic finding in TSS caused by either *S. aureus* or *S. pyogenes.* Desquamation of the skin of the distal extremities does not usually occur until the second week of illness.

Ischemic changes (dusky or pallid color, coldness, loss of pulses) usually occur in the hands and feet, where they may follow thrombosis of small to middle-size arteries. Inflammation-induced coagulopathy and vasoconstriction both contribute to their pathogenesis, as noted earlier.

DIAGNOSIS

No bedside or laboratory test provides a definitive diagnosis. There is also considerable interindividual and time-dependent variability in the expression of the body's responses to infection, so a diagnostically useful profile of laboratory tests is not possible. On the other hand, certain findings are sufficiently suggestive that they should prompt further evaluation. In addition to the findings used to diagnose SIRS (tachycardia, tachypnea, leukocytosis or leukopenia, and fever or hypothermia [see Table 67-1]), altered mental status, unexplained hyperbilirubinemia, metabolic acidosis, and thrombocytopenia can be useful clues. The appearance of new lesions on the skin or mucosae may also be helpful.

One of the body's normal responses to infection is a neutrophilic leukocytosis in the peripheral blood. In patients with typhoid fever or brucellosis, on the other hand, a slight leukopenia is the typical response. Other infections that are typically associated with peripheral blood leukopenia include Rocky Mountain spotted fever, Colorado tick fever, and ehrlichiosis. In individuals with severe sepsis induced by bacteria, leukopenia is more common among children than adults.[219] Fever is also a normal response to infection, and an increase in body temperature above a certain level (usually 38.0° or 38.3° C) is often the trigger for initiating a diagnostic evaluation. Some septic patients may be euthermic or hypothermic, however. These include older adults, patients with open wounds or large burns, and patients taking anti-inflammatory or antipyretic drugs.

Differential Diagnosis

Numerous noninfectious conditions can mimic sepsis. They include burns, trauma, adrenal insufficiency, pancreatitis, pulmonary embolism, dissecting or ruptured aortic aneurysm, myocardial infarction, occult hemorrhage, cardiac tamponade, and drug overdose. Fever and hypotension can also be caused by a number of noninfectious processes, including adrenal insufficiency, thyroid storm, pancreatitis, drug hypersensitivity reactions, malignant hyperthermia, and heatstroke. Vasodilatory shock can be a manifestation of anaphylaxis. A sepsis-like syndrome may follow cardiopulmonary bypass; there is circumstantial evidence that the trigger is pump trauma to circulating leukocytes or bacterial endotoxin absorbed from the gut.

Cultures

Cultures are useful for identifying the likely microbial invaders and ascertaining antimicrobial susceptibility patterns. For optimal sensitivity and specificity, blood cultures (aerobic and anaerobic bottles) should be drawn from two or three different venipuncture sites.[236] In patients with indwelling vascular catheters, the rate of microbial growth in a culture of blood drawn through the catheter may be compared with that of blood drawn from a peripheral vein to assess the likelihood of catheter infection; a difference in the "time to positivity" of 2 or more hours suggests catheter infection.[237] Careful preparation of the skin with either 10% povidone iodine or 1% to 2% tincture of iodine prior to obtaining blood for culture can reduce the incidence of false-positive results, which greatly increase costs and waste resources.[238]

Cultures and microscopic examination of urine, sputum (including tracheal aspirate if done within a few hours of intubation), likely in-

fected fluids, purulent wound drainage, and skin lesions should also be obtained. A Gram stain of material obtained from biopsies or needle aspirates of petechial lesions can provide a rapid diagnosis in patients with meningococcemia.[239]

Cytokine Levels

Although there have been many attempts to identify a cytokine profile that would distinguish infected patients from those with systemic responses to other stimuli, none has been very successful. Perhaps the most promising indicator to date is the plasma procalcitonin level, which in one study had a sensitivity of 97% and a specificity of 78% for differentiating patients with SIRS from those with sepsis[240]; a second group found that daily measurements of procalcitonin was superior to CRP for identifying patients who had become infected.[241] At present, no laboratory test result is sufficiently reliable to warrant delaying the institution of antimicrobial therapy in a patient who, on clinical grounds, may have sepsis.

Adrenal Insufficiency in Patients with Septic Shock

The clinical and laboratory diagnoses of sepsis-associated relative adrenal insufficiency are inexact and controversial (see adrenal insufficiency under "Clinical Manifestations"). The most useful definition of relative adrenal insufficiency may be based on the response to hydrocortisone administration. The presence of "pressor-dependent hypotension that responds to the administration of 50 to 100 mg hydrocortisone every 6 hours" would strongly support the diagnosis.[200] A low basal level of plasma cortisol (e.g., <15 µg/dL) or a low response to the administration of 250 µg of synthetic ACTH (<9 µg/dL increase above basal) would be supportive.

THERAPY

Sepsis, severe sepsis, and septic shock are medical emergencies. As summarized by L. Young, "Early clinical suspicion, rigorous diagnostic measures, aggressive initiation of appropriate antimicrobial therapy, comprehensive supportive care, and measures aimed at reversing predisposing causes are the cornerstones of successful management."[242]

Antimicrobial Drugs

Numerous analyses have concluded that early treatment of bacteremic patients with an appropriate antimicrobial drug improves survival.[161,243-249] In most of these studies, a drug was considered appropriate if it was able to inhibit the patient's microbial isolate(s) in vitro and was administered within 24 to 48 hours of the onset of bacteremia or severe sepsis. In one study of patients in a university-affiliated teaching hospital, inappropriate antimicrobial treatment was most common (45%) in patients with nosocomial infections that developed after treatment for a community-acquired infection.[244]

Patients with severe sepsis should thus receive a broad-spectrum, intravenous regimen that is effective for both gram-negative and gram-positive bacteria. The choice of drugs should be modified according to the patient's own microbiologic culture data and the resistance patterns prevalent in the patient's community or hospital. Under some circumstances, such as when a patient develops severe sepsis after having received a broad-spectrum regimen for another infection, empirical antifungal therapy may be warranted (*Candida* species now account for 10% or more of the cases of severe sepsis in such patients). Specific recommendations are provided in Table 67-4.

With the possible exception of neutropenic patients, there is little evidence to support the use of combination therapy using an aminoglycoside, over monotherapy with a broad-spectrum drug such as a carbapenem.[249] Many experts also consider an extended-spectrum penicillin, combined with a β-lactamase inhibitor, to be effective empirical therapy for most patients. In centers with a high prevalence of methicillin-resistant *S. aureus* (MRSA) infections, adding a glycopeptide (vancomycin) is appropriate in patients who have an indwelling vascular catheter and develop severe sepsis. If a vancomycin-resistant

TABLE 67-4 Empirical Antibiotic Options for Patients with Severe Sepsis or Septic Shock

| | Suspected Source | | | | |
	Lung	Abdomen	Skin/Soft Tissue	Urinary Tract	Meninges
Major community-acquired pathogens	*Streptococcus pneumoniae* *Haemophilus influenzae* *Legionella* *Chlamydophila pneumoniae*	*Escherichia coli* *Bacteroides fragilis*	*Streptococcus pyogenes* *Staphylococcus aureus* Polymicrobial	*E. coli* *Klebsiella* species *Enterobacter* species *Proteus* species Enterococci	*S. pneumoniae* *Neisseria meningitidis* *Listeria monocytogenes* *H. influenzae*
Empirical antibiotic therapy	Moxifloxacin *or* gatifloxacin *or* azithromycin *plus either* cefotaxime *or* ceftazidime	Imipenem-cilastatin *or* meropenem *or* piperacillin-tazobactam ± aminoglycoside	Vancomycin *plus either* imipenem *or* meropenem *or* piperacillin-tazobactam	Ciprofloxacin *or* levofloxacin (If gram-positive cocci, use ampicillin plus gentamicin)	Vancomycin *plus either* ceftriaxone *or* cefepime
Major commensal or nosocomial microorganisms	Aerobic gram-negative bacilli	Aerobic gram-negative rods Anaerobes *Candida* species	*Staphylococcus aureus* (? MRSA) Aerobic gram-negative rods	Aerobic gram-negative rods Enterococci	Aerobic gram-negative rods Staphylococci
Empirical antibiotic therapy	Imipenem-cilastatin *or* meropenem *or* cefepime	Imipenem *or* meropenem *or* piperacillin-tazobactam ± aminoglycoside (Consider amphotericin B)	Vancomycin *plus* cefepime	Vancomycin *plus* cefepime	Cefepime *plus* vancomycin

Dosages for intravenous administration (normal renal function):
Imipenem-cilastatin, 0.5 g q6h
Meropenem, 1.0 g q8h
Piperacillin-tazobactam, 3.375 g q4h or 4.5 g q6h
Vancomycin 15 mg/kg q12h (if meningitis, 25 mg/kg q12h)
Cefepime 1-2 g q8h
Ciprofloxacin, 400 mg q12h, Gatifloxacin, 400 mg qd, Moxifloxacin 400 mg qd
Ceftriaxone, 2.0 gm q24h
Levofloxacin 500 mg qd
MRSA, methicillin-resistant *S. aureus*.
Format adapted from Simon D, Trenholme G. Antibiotic selection for patients with septic shock. Crit Care Clin. 2000;16:215-230.

enterococcus (VRE) is the likely trigger for severe sepsis, linezolid should be included.

Although there are few data on the use of once-daily dosing of aminoglycosides in critically ill patients, the available evidence suggests that this administration method is safe.[250] The volume of distribution of both tobramycin and gentamicin is higher in critically ill patients with septic shock than in those without shock. A once-daily dosage of 7 mg/kg produced maximal peak concentration (C_{max}) to minimal inhibitory concentration (MIC) ratios in most patients.[250] Therapeutic drug monitoring is warranted, and more than one drug level may be needed to determine the appropriate dosing interval.

Antimicrobial Chemotherapy for Specific Etiologies of Severe Sepsis. In patients with suspected or proven streptococcal myositis/fasciitis or TSS, clindamycin should be given in addition to penicillin G. In patients who may have eaten raw oysters and acquired *V. vulnificus* bacteremia, intravenous doxycycline or a quinolone should be used. Severe sepsis that follows a dog bite may be caused by *C. canimorsus,* which is usually susceptible to cephalosporins and quinolones but resistant to trimethoprim-sulfamethoxazole and aminoglycosides. Cefotaxime or ceftriaxone is preferred for asplenic patients, who may have overwhelming bacteremia with *S. pneumoniae, N. meningitidis, Haemophilus influenzae,* or *C. canimorsus.*

Surgical Drainage

Recovery from severe sepsis or septic shock is unlikely, even with appropriate antimicrobial therapy and diligent ICU care, if the patient has an undrained abscess or an obstructed viscus.[169] An excellent discussion of surgical and nonsurgical source-control measures was published by Jimenez and Marshall.[251] In patients with community-acquired infections, the most common occult sources are in the lungs and the urinary tract. Intra-abdominal infections (e.g., diverticulitis, cholecystitis, pylephlebitis), septic arthritis, endocarditis, and osteomyelitis should also be sought. Nosocomial infections often arise at sites of epithelial barrier disruption and thus frequently involve intravascular catheters, endotracheal tubes (pneumonia, and paranasal sinusitis), urinary catheters, and operative wounds or other sites of traumatic injury.

In general, when a patient develops severe sepsis, all intravascular and bladder catheters should be removed, with reinsertion at new sites as needed. It is not often necessary to do surgical exploration of an infected thrombus, because medical management usually suffices.[252]

Intravenous Fluids, Blood Transfusion, Pressor Drugs

Fluid resuscitation is the mainstay of hemodynamic support in patients with septic shock. Crystalloid is generally preferred over colloid.[253,254] A reasonable goal is maintenance of mean arterial pressure (MAP) above 60 mm Hg. In most patients, 4 to 6 L of fluid is required. Although a pulmonary artery (PA) or central venous catheter may be useful for monitoring volume status, the overall benefit of right heart catheterization is disputed.[255] High filling pressures (PA occlusion pressure > 16 mm Hg) may presage the onset of pulmonary edema.

A central venous or PA catheter may also facilitate measurement of cardiac output, mixed venous oxygen saturation (Svo_2), filling pressures, and systemic vascular resistance. Svo_2 can be used to assess the adequacy of oxygen delivery; values less than 70% suggest decreased systemic perfusion. A recent study found that patients in whom initial fluid, blood transfusion, and pressor therapy were promptly and aggressively titrated to maintain SvO_2 greater than 70% had significantly better survival than did patients who received "conventional" resuscitation in an ICU.[256] Many experts feel that the rapidity with which the patients in the treatment group were resuscitated was the key element of the successful regimen.

Another placebo-controlled clinical trial found that mortality was lower in patients with ARDS who received low tidal volume ventilation (6 mL/kg) with limited plateau pressure (<30 cm H_2O).[257] The trial was criticized for using, as the comparison group, patients who may have received a higher tidal volume than that currently used in most ICUs.[258]

The optimal threshold for administering erythrocytes to septic patients is uncertain. The Transfusion Requirements in Critical Care (TRICC) trial found that a transfusion threshold (trigger) of 7.0 μg/dL and maintenance of hemoglobin concentrations between 7.0 and 9.0 μg/dL was at least equivalent to, and possibly superior to, the more liberal use of red cells.[259] Although only one third of the patients in this trial had severe sepsis, its investigators argued that the results should be applicable to almost all critically ill patients. There is currently no clear indication for using erythropoietin in critically ill patients.[260]

For many years, dopamine was considered the drug of choice for restoring normotension in patients with septic shock. When used at low doses (<5 μg/kg/min), its preferential interaction with dopaminergic receptors was thought to produce renal and splanchnic vasodilation. This notion has been challenged by recent studies and analyses.[261] In particular, a randomized controlled clinical trial found that low-dose dopamine infusion did not improve survival or prevent renal failure in critically ill patients at risk for renal dysfunction,[262] and a similar conclusion was reached by a retrospective analysis of patients with septic shock in a large clinical trial.[263] Nevertheless, many experts continue to use dopamine as the initial pressor agent in septic patients, adding norepinephrine cautiously as needed. Although others favor using norepinephrine over dopamine, a recent comparison study concluded that the two drugs had similar hemodynamic effects.[264]

Other Therapies

Hydrocortisone. Many patients with septic shock exhibit a rightward shift in the dose–response relationship between blood pressure and catecholamines. Annane and co-workers found that this occurs most often in patients with impaired adrenal function and that, in such patients, administration of hydrocortisone can return the dose–response curve to normal.[39] In a more recent study, the same investigators found that hydrocortisone restored the dose–response curve with respect to phenylephrine in septic patients without affecting baroreflex sensitivity.[265] Several factors probably contribute to reduced sensitivity to catecholamines, including downregulation of adrenoreceptors and nitric oxide (NO)-induced vasopressor resistance. Hydrocortisone increases adrenoreceptor expression.

Numerous recent studies attest to the safety and potential benefit of a trial of hydrocortisone (50 or 100 mg every 6 to 8 hours intravenously) in pressor-dependent patients with septic shock.[198,201,266-268] In patients with a positive response (cessation of the need for pressor infusion to maintain a mean arterial pressure >65 mm Hg within 24 hours of the first dose of hydrocortisone[200]), the hydrocortisone regimen would be continued for 7 days.

The impact of hydrocortisone administration on the long-term outcome of patients with septic shock has been evaluated in only one randomized, placebo-controlled clinical trial. Annane and colleagues found that a 7-day regimen that included both hydrocortisone (50 mg intravenous bolus every 6 hours) and an oral mineralocorticoid (fludrocortisone, 50 μg daily) significantly improved the 28-day survival in patients with septic shock who had absolute or relative adrenal insufficiency.[269] Patients who did not meet the authors' criteria for adrenal insufficiency were not benefited by this regimen, however (there was a statistically nonsignificant trend toward harm).

In a double-blind, placebo-controlled, randomized crossover study, Keh and co-workers found that hydrocortisone (100 mg loading dose, then 10 mg/hr until day 3) rapidly induced an increase in MAP and

systemic vascular resistance in patients with septic shock.[266] During the hydrocortisone infusion, plasma levels of anti-inflammatory mediators (IL-10, soluble TNF receptors, IL-1Ra) decreased, as did plasma nitrite/nitrate levels and indices of neutrophil chemotaxis and endothelial adhesion (plasma IL-8 and E-selectin concentrations, neutrophil CD11b expression). In contrast, plasma levels of IFN-γ and IL-12 p70 were unaffected, suggesting that hydrocortisone therapy did not diminish the proinflammatory response to infection. Abrupt cessation of hydrocortisone infusion was followed by rebound changes in many of these parameters; the authors recommended tapering the hydrocortisone dose over several days.

Vasopressin. Vasopressin levels initially rise as patients develop shock, then they fall with more prolonged hypotension. Continuous infusion of arginine vasopressin (AVP) may restore normotension in patients with catecholamine-resistant vasodilatory shock. The doses of vasopressin that increase blood pressure in septic patients are lower than those required in normal individuals. Landry and Oliver speculate that the increase in vasopressor potency may be caused by unoccupied vascular receptors for vasopressin, the coexistence of autonomic failure (which potentiates vasopressin action), or vasopressin's ability to enhance the vasoconstrictor effect of norepinephrine, which is present in markedly elevated concentrations in patients with septic shock.[126] Vasopressin also directly inactivates K_{ATP} channels in vascular smooth muscle and inhibits the inducible form of NO synthase.

A prospective controlled trial recently found that patients randomized to receive a combined infusion of AVP (4 U/hr) and norepinephrine had significantly improved cardiovascular function when compared to patients who received norepinephrine infusion alone.[270] GI perfusion, as assessed by gastric tonometry, was also improved in the AVP-treated group. On the other hand, the patients who received AVP had significant elevations in transaminases and bilirubin; although these were well tolerated, they probably reflected AVP-induced hepatic dysfunction. The impact of AVP infusion on long-term outcome has not been studied in a randomized, placebo-controlled trial.

Anti-inflammatory Drugs. During the 1990s, clinical trials were performed to test the ability of numerous immunomodulatory drugs to improve survival in patients with severe sepsis.[102,271,272] They included large doses of glucocorticoids; antiendotoxin antibodies and bactericidal permeability-increasing protein, which neutralizes endotoxin; antibodies to TNF and TNF-immunoglobulin fusion proteins that trap TNF; IL-1 receptor antagonist; and antagonists to PAF, bradykinin, phospholipase A_2, NO synthase, cyclooxygenase, bradykinin, and others. Although many of these agents appeared promising in preliminary trials, none reproducibly improved 28-day all-cause survival. Explanations offered for the failure of this approach have included using the wrong drugs, doses, or duration of therapy; administration of the drug too late in the clinical course; heterogeneity in the clinical population treated; and ineffectiveness of single interventions.

A meta-regression analysis of 23 of these trials recently concluded that the efficacy of anti-inflammatory drugs in patients with severe sepsis depends on the risk of dying.[273] Although many of the agents studied work through different biologic mechanisms, their efficacy was consistently greater in patients with a high risk of dying, whereas they were ineffective or harmful in those with low mortality risk. Studies in experimental animal models showed similar trends.[273] Some of the same drugs have been very effective in the treatment of rheumatoid arthritis and other rheumatologic diseases, yet they have also predisposed patients to reactivation of tuberculosis and other infections. By analogy with this experience, perhaps interfering with the proinflammatory response impairs antimicrobial defenses in patients with less severe sepsis (in whom systemic anti-inflammation may already be dominant), whereas some benefit can be derived from blocking even a single proinflammatory mediator in patients at the more severe end of the spectrum. There is clearly much more to be learned.

Several studies have found that patients with severe sepsis who are hypothermic (< 35.5° C or 96° F) have almost twice the risk of dying as patients with normal or elevated body temperature.[169,274,275] In a randomized, controlled clinical trial, the administration of ibuprofen (10 mg/kg IV every 6 hours for 48 hours) was associated with a significant reduction in mortality in patients who were hypothermic at the time treatment was initiated (90% versus 54%, $P = .02$).[224] Although ibuprofen did not prevent death in patients who were not hypothermic, it was administered for only 48 hours; during this period, there were dramatic improvements in several parameters, including lactic acidosis. A specific inhibitor of the inducible form of cyclooxygenase (COX-2) has not been tested in septic patients, nor has longer therapy with ibuprofen.

Anticoagulants. Three recombinant anticoagulant drugs were recently tested for their ability to increase the survival of patients with severe sepsis or septic shock. Whereas neither tissue factor pathway inhibitor (TFPI; tifacogin) nor antithrombin III significantly improved outcome,[104,105] aPC (drotrecogin alfa [Xigris]) reduced mortality from 31% (placebo control) to 25% (treatment group) ($P < .005$).[106] The basis for the apparent impact of aPC on sepsis survival is uncertain; its clinical efficacy did not correlate with preinfusion levels of aPC, and its putative anti-inflammatory effects have not been apparent in studies of volunteers infused with aPC prior to a bolus injection of endotoxin. Xigris infusion was also associated with a small but statistically significant increase in the incidence of severe bleeding, including intracranial hemorrhage.

The U.S. Food and Drug Administration approved Xigris for the treatment of severe sepsis in patients with more than one organ dysfunction and/or an APACHE II (Acute Physiology and Chronic Health Evaluation) score greater than 25.[276] The drug performed quite differently during the two halves of its pivotal trial (see later), however, prompting a request for a confirmatory trial.[277] Until the efficacy and safety of Xigris can be confirmed, use of the drug should be limited to patients who meet both the entry criteria used for the pivotal trial and the severity criterion noted earlier. Perhaps most important, the clinical trial did not enroll patients who had experienced sepsis-induced organ failure for more than 24 hours. The drug should also not be used in patients with severe liver disease, a platelet count of less than 30,000/mm³, prothrombin time–International Normalized Ratio (INR) greater than 3.0, recent bleeding (including hemorrhagic stroke) or known bleeding diathesis, or recent surgery. The clinical trial also did not include patients who were pregnant or younger than 18 years of age, obese patients (>135 kg), or patients with acute pancreatitis, chronic renal failure requiring dialysis, or HIV with CD4 count less than 50/mm³. Although meningitis is currently not a formal contraindication, anecdotal experience suggests that patients with meningitis may be at increased risk for intracranial hemorrhage as a complication of Xigris infusion.

Two unanticipated features of the anticoagulant trials deserve further comment. First, analysis of the first 722 patients in the TFPI trial showed a highly significant difference in mortality that favored the TFPI group (38.9% for placebo versus 29.1% for TFPI, $P = .006$), yet this trend reversed when an additional 1032 patients were enrolled; at the end of the trial, mortality was higher in the patients that received TFPI.[104] In the case of Xigris, there was a nonsignificant difference between drug (28% mortality) and placebo (30% mortality; $P = .57$) in the first 720 patients studied, whereas a strikingly beneficial trend favoring the drug ($P = .001$) was seen in the 712 patients entered during the second half of the trial.[277] These contrasting experiences illustrate how difficult it can be to get reproducible results when studying sepsis therapeutics, even within the same clinical trial; basing therapeutic recommendations on the results of a single phase III trial seems very premature, especially when the drug may have significant toxicity.[277,278] It is also noteworthy that, in each of the three recent trials of anticoagulant drugs, administration of heparin in a nonrandomized fashion to patients in the placebo group was associated with a reduction in mortality. The basis for these unexpected results is not clear; because most ICU patients receive low-dose heparin as prophylaxis for deep venous thrombosis unless there is a contraindication to its use, it is possible that the observed outcome difference simply reflects selection bias. Although heparin is the most widely available and least expensive anticoagulant (and, quite possibly, the safest), it has not been tested rigorously for its ability to benefit patients with severe sepsis.

Summary. Progress during the last 5 years has made it possible to recommend a trial of hydrocortisone and a mineralocorticoid in patients with pressor-dependent septic shock, and favorable results with other interventions (aPC, vasopressin, ibuprofen, and an inhibitory lipid A analog[279]) should encourage further clinical testing. Drugs in early development include inhibitors of HMGB-1 and MIF. Aggressive management to reverse hypotension and maintain adequate venous oxygen saturation may also improve survival.[256] In addition, there is now evidence (see "Prevention," later) that avoiding hyperglycemia may prevent infection and sepsis in critically ill patients. Although improvements in clinical trial design have reduced the impact of patient heterogeneity by using more restrictive entry criteria and enrolling larger numbers of patients, the nonreproducibility of clinical trial results remains a major problem. Using all-cause, 28-day mortality as the primary end point may have obscured the benefit of some drugs. Combined therapy using drugs with different mechanisms of action has not been attempted.[280]

Nutrition and Other Supportive Measures

Much evidence now supports the use of enteral, instead of intravenous, nutrition in critically ill patients. Prophylaxis for GI bleeding, deep venous thrombosis, and decubitus ulcers should be routine. Bedsores may be prevented by avoiding prolonged skin exposure to stool and urine, by frequent repositioning, and by adequate nutrition. Patients with low bleeding risk should receive low doses of heparin, whereas intermittent compression devices should be applied to the lower extremities of those at risk for bleeding. H_2-receptor antagonists are superior to sucralfate or antacids for preventing GI bleeding[281]; proton pump inhibitors would be expected to be similarly effective.

Preventing Secondary Infections

Because patients with severe sepsis are immunosuppressed and subjected to invasive procedures, they may be at risk for secondary infections. These arise most often from the patient's own microbial flora. Measures that decrease acquisition of hospital-associated microorganisms include hand washing[282] and the use of barrier precautions when examining patients colonized with resistant bacteria. The Centers for Disease Control and Prevention issued guidelines for preventing intravascular catheter infections in 2002.[283]

The risk for nosocomial pneumonia is greatest in patients who receive mechanical ventilation for longer than 1 week. Randomized trials have shown that the semirecumbent body position reduces the risk for nosocomial pneumonia, especially in patients who receive enteral nutrition.[284] Maintaining an adequate intracuff pressure and effective aspiration of subglottic secretions is also important.[285] Avoiding nasal tubes decreases the risk for developing sinusitis. A closed urinary drainage system is essential.

PREVENTION

Prevention of Hyperglycemia

Van den Berghe and colleagues tested the effects of administering intensive insulin therapy to critically ill patients, most of whom had recently undergone cardiac surgery.[286] When compared with patients who received conventional insulin treatment (to achieve blood glucose levels between 180 and 200 mg/dL), patients who received intensive insulin therapy (maintaining blood glucose between 80 and 100 mg/dL) were significantly less likely to develop bacteremia, acute renal insufficiency, or critical illness polyneuropathy, less likely to require red blood cell transfusion, and less likely to die in the hospital. The reduction in in-hospital mortality was striking (34%); most of the deaths were from "multiple-organ failure with a septic focus." Multivariate logistic regression analysis revealed that a low blood glucose level, rather than the insulin dose, correlated with these beneficial effects.[287]

The often-stated rationale for stress-induced hyperglycemia is preservation of fuel for the brain until starvation-induced ketone body production provides an alternative energy substrate.[37]

Prolonged hyperglycemia, in contrast, seems to be harmful. Although hyperglycemia has been associated with increased infection risk in other clinical studies,[288-290] its immunosuppressive mechanism is not well established or understood beyond its ability to inhibit phagocytosis. There is evidence that insulin treatment can improve neutrophil function and prevent postoperative infection in diabetics,[289,290] however, and numerous studies in experimental models suggest that it may reduce several aspects of the acute-phase response.[291-293]

Fortunately, preventing hyperglycemia is unlikely to harm patients whose nutritional needs are supported in the ICU, provided that hypoglycemia (<80 mg/dL) does not occur. Until the findings of van den Berghe and co-workers can be confirmed, limiting glucose infusions to 50 g/day and administering insulin as needed to keep the blood glucose level between 100 and 140 mg/dL are reasonable goals for critically ill patients. Frequent monitoring may be necessary to avoid hypoglycemia.

Augmentation of Host Defenses

During the 1990s, several studies addressed the ability of recombinant IFN-γ to prevent severe sepsis in patients who had recently undergone major surgery or sustained major trauma. Unfortunately, prophylactic administration of IFN-γ did not significantly reduce the incidence of nosocomial infection and severe sepsis,[294,295] even though an impact of the drug on monocyte function was observed.[296] The goal of this approach is to prevent immunosuppression by providing a proinflammatory (Th1) cytokine; if proinflammatory molecules could be provided at the local site of infection, rather than systemically, they might be safer and more efficacious.

One retrospective analysis found that patients who developed bacteremia while taking a statin were significantly less likely to die than non–statin-users.[297] Although statins may have anti-inflammatory actions, a mechanistic basis for this unconfirmed report is not obvious, and further studies are needed. Although there is evidence that both passive[298] and active[299] immunization can benefit patients at risk for hospital-acquired infection, neither of these approaches can be recommended for general clinical use. Preventing perioperative hypothermia may reduce the incidence of surgical wound infections[300]; the authors of the study attributed this result to the beneficial effect of euthermia on phagocytosis.

PROGNOSIS

Severe sepsis and septic shock are associated with case-fatality ratios of approximately 30% and 50%, respectively. As initially noted by McCabe and Jackson,[301] outcome is significantly (and most profoundly) influenced by the patient's underlying disease.[168,302] Bacteremia with certain microbes (e.g., *S. aureus*) may also be independently related to mortality in multivariate analyses.[171] Of the many studied biologic markers, plasma IL-6 levels and a high IL-10/TNF ratio[96,303] may correlate best with risk of dying. None of these measurements warrants routine use. Prognostic scores based on bedside evaluations such as the APACHE II and the sequential organ failure assessments (SOFA) are more appropriate in the usual ICU setting.[304,305]

Although most clinical trials of sepsis therapies have used 28-day, all-cause mortality as the outcome variable, Perl and colleagues found that the median day of death was 30.5 days after the onset of sepsis.[302] Another study concluded that patients who survive an episode of severe sepsis, when compared with controls matched for age and underlying disease, have significantly decreased life expectancy over the ensuing 5 years. Experiencing severe sepsis may also diminish an individual's subsequent quality of life.[302,306]

REFERENCES

1. American College of Chest Physicians/Society of Critical Care Medicine Consensus Conference Committee. Definitions for sepsis and organ failure and guidelines for the use of innovative therapies in sepsis. Crit Care Med. 1992;20:864-874.
2. Bone RC, Grodzin CJ, Balk RA. Sepsis: A new hypothesis for pathogenesis of the disease process. Chest. 1997;112:235-243.
3. Vincent J-L. Sepsis: The magnitude of the problem. In: Vincent J-L, Carlet J, Opal SM, eds. The Sepsis Text. Boston: Kluwer Academic; 2002:1-10.
4. Alberti C, Brun-Buisson C, Goodman SV, et al. Influence of systemic inflammatory response syndrome and sepsis on outcome of critically ill infected patients. Am J Respir Crit Care Med. 2003;168:77-84.
5. Angus DC, Wax RS. Epidemiology of sepsis: An update. Crit Care Med. 2001; 29:S109-S116.
6. Rangel-Frausto MS, Pittet D, Costigan M, et al. The natural history of the systemic inflammatory response syndrome (SIRS). JAMA. 1995;273:117-123.
7. Salvo I, de Cian W, Musicco M, et al. The Italian SEPSIS study: Preliminary results on the incidence and evolution of SIRS, sepsis, severe sepsis, and septic shock. Intensive Care Med. 1995;21:S244-S249.
8. Levy MM, Fink MP, Marshall JC, et al. 2001 SCCM/ESICM/ACCP/ATS/SIS International Sepsis Definitions Conference. Crit Care Med. 2003;31:1250-1256.
9. Vincent J-L. Dear SIRS, I'm sorry to say that I don't like you. . . . Crit Care Med. 1997;25:372-374.
10. Munford RS, Pugin J. Normal responses to injury prevent systemic inflammation and can be immunosuppressive. Am J Respir Crit Care Med. 2001;163:316-321.
11. Angus DC, Linde-Zwirble WT, Lidicker J, et al. Epidemiology of severe sepsis in the United States: Analysis of incidence, outcome, and associated costs of care. Crit Care Med. 2001;29:1303-1310.
12. Martin GS, Mannino DM, Eaton S, et al. The epidemiology of sepsis in the United States from 1979 through 2000. N Engl J Med. 2003;348:1546-1554.
13. Watson RS, Carcillo JA, Linde-Zwirble WT, et al. The epidemiology of severe sepsis in children in the United States. Am J Respir Crit Care Med. 2003;167:695-701.
14. Sands KE, Bates DW, Lanken PN, et al. Epidemiology of sepsis syndrome in 8 academic medical centers. JAMA. 1997;278:234-240.
15. Brun-Buisson C, Doyon F, Carlet J, et al. Incidence, risk factors, and outcome of severe sepsis and septic shock in adults: A multicenter prospective study in intensive care units. JAMA. 1995;274:968-974.
16. Medzhitov R, Janeway CA Jr. Decoding the patterns of self and nonself by the innate immune system. Science. 2002;296:298-300.
17. Takeda K, Kaisho T, Akira S. Toll-like receptors. Annu Rev Immunol. 2003;21:335-376.
18. Gregory SH, Wing EJ. Neutrophil-Kupffer cell interaction: A critical component of host defenses to systemic bacterial infections. J Leukoc Biol. 2002;72:239-248.
19. Janeway CA Jr. Approaching the asymptote? Evolution and revolution in immunology. Cold Spring Harbor Symp Quant Biol. 1989;54:1-13.
20. Netea MG, Kullberg B-J, Van der Meer JWM. Circulating cytokines as mediators of fever. Clin Infect Dis. 2000;31:S178-S184.
21. Mackowiak PA, Bartlett JG, Borden EC, et al. Concepts of fever: Recent advances and lingering dogma. Clin Infect Dis. 1997;25:119-138.
22. Rosenspire AJ, Kindzelskii AL, Petty HR. Cutting edge: Fever-associated temperatures enhance neutrophil responses to lipopolysaccharide: A potential mechanism involving cell metabolism. J Immunol. 2002;169:5396-5400.
23. Leon LR, Kozak W, Peschon J, et al. Altered acute phase responses to inflammation in IL-1 and TNF receptor knockout mice. Ann N Y Acad Sci. 1997;813:244-254.
24. Romanovsky AA, Ivanov AI, Székely M. Neural route of pyrogen signaling to the brain. Clin Infect Dis. 2000;31:S162-S167.
25. Borovikova LV, Ivanova S, Zhang M, et al. Vagus nerve stimulation attenuates the systemic inflammatory response to endotoxin. Nature. 2000;405:458-462.
26. Fong Y, Marano MA, Moldawer LL, et al. The acute splanchnic and peripheral tissue metabolic response to endotoxin in humans. J Clin Invest. 1990;85:1896-1904.
27. Munford RS, Pugin J. The crucial role of systemic responses in the innate (non-adaptive) host defense. J Endotoxin Res. 2001;7:327-332.
28. Davis HM, Carpenter DC, Stahl JM, et al. Human granulocyte CD11b expression as a pharmacodynamic biomarker of inflammation. J Immunol Methods. 2000;240:125-132.
29. van der Poll T, Coyle SM, Barbosa K, et al. Epinephrine inhibits tumor necrosis factor-α and potentiates interleukin 10 production during human endotoxemia. J Clin Invest. 1996;97:713-719.
30. Barber AE, Coyle SM, Marano MA, et al. Glucocorticoid therapy alters hormonal and cytokine responses to endotoxin in man. J Immunol. 1993;150:1999-2006.
31. Lemaire LC, van der Poll T, Van Lanschot JB, et al. Minimally invasive surgery induces endotoxin-tolerance in the absence of detectable endotoxemia. J Clin Immunol. 1998;18:414-420.
32. Dugernier TL, Laterre PF, Wittebole X, et al. Compartmentalization of the inflammatory response during acute pancreatitis: Correlation with local and systemic complications. Am J Respir Crit Care Med. 2003;168:148-157.
33. Rivera-Chavez FA, Wheeler H, Lindberg G, et al. Regional and systemic cytokine responses to acute inflammation of the vermiform appendix. Ann Surg. 2003;237:408-416.
34. Kurahashi K, Kajikawa O, Sawa T, et al. Pathogenesis of septic shock in *Pseudomonas aeruginosa* pneumonia. J Clin Invest. 1999;104:743-750.
35. Matute-Bello G, Frevert CW, Kajikawa O, et al. Septic shock and acute lung injury in rabbits with peritonitis: Failure of the neutrophil response to localized infection. Am J Respir Crit Care Med. 2001;163:234-243.
36. Gore DC, Wolf SE, Herndon DN, et al. Relative influence of glucose and insulin on peripheral amino acid metabolism in severely burned patients. JPEN J Parenter Enteral Nutr. 2002;26:271-277.
37. Foster DW, McGarry JD. Glucose, lipid and protein metabolism. In: Griffin JE, Ojeda SR, eds. Textbook of Endocrine Physiology. New York: Oxford University Press; 2000:393-420.
38. Sapolsky RM, Romero LM, Munck AU. How do glucocorticoids influence stress responses? Integrating permissive, suppressive, stimulatory, and preparative actions. Endocr Rev. 2000;21:55-89.
39. Annane D, Bellisant E, Sebille V, et al. Impaired pressor sensitivity to noradrenaline in septic shock patients with and without impaired adrenal function reserve. Br J Clin Pharmacol. 1998;46:589-597.

40. Bernardin G, Strosberg AD, Bernard A, et al. Beta-adrenergic receptor-dependent and -independent stimulation of adenylate cyclase is impaired during severe sepsis in humans. Intensive Care Med. 1998;24:1315-1322.
41. Zimmerman GA, Albertine KH, McIntyre TM. Pathogenesis of sepsis and septic-induced lung injury. In: Matthay MA, ed. Acute Respiratory Distress Syndrome. New York: Marcel Dekker; 2003:245-287.
42. Altieri D. Inflammatory cell participation in coagulation. Semin Cell Biol. 1995;6:269-274.
43. Gando S, Kameue T, Nanzaki S, et al. Participation of tissue factor and thrombin in posttraumatic systemic inflammatory syndrome. Crit Care Med. 1997;25:1820-1826.
44. Levi M, ten Cate H. Disseminated intravascular coagulation. N Engl J Med. 1999; 341:586-592.
45. Hack C. The coagulation system in sepsis. In: Vincent J-L, Carlet J, Opal SM, eds. The Sepsis Text. Boston: Kluwer; 2003:687-704.
46. Faust SN, Levin M, Harrison OB, et al. Dysfunction of endothelial protein C activation in severe meningococcal sepsis. N Engl J Med. 2001;345:408-416.
47. Asakura H, Ontachi Y, Mizutani T, et al. Decreased plasma activity of antithrombin or protein C is not due to consumption coagulopathy in septic patients with disseminated intravascular coagulation. Eur J Haematol. 2001;67:170-175.
48. Greisman SE, Hornick RB. On the demonstration of circulating human endogenous pyrogen. Proc Soc Exp Biol Med. 1972;139:690-697.
49. Ross G, Roth J, Störr B, et al. Afferent nerves are involved in the febrile response to injection of LPS into artificial subcutaneous chambers in guinea pigs. Physiol Behav. 2000;71:305-313.
50. Majetschak M, Flach R, Kreuzfelder E, et al. The extent of traumatic damage determines a graded depression of the endotoxin responsiveness of peripheral blood mononuclear cells from patients with blunt injuries. Crit Care Med. 1999;27:313-318.
51. Hershman MJ, Cheadle WG, Wellhausen SR, et al. Monocyte HLA-DR antigen expression characterizes clinical outcome in the trauma patient. Br J Surg. 1990;77:204-207.
52. Taylor JV, Gordon LE, Polk HC. Early decrease in surface expression of HLA-DQ predicts the development of infection in trauma patients. Clin Exp Immunol. 2000;122:308-311.
53. Volk H-D, Reinke P, Döcke WD. Clinical aspects: From systemic inflammation to "immunoparalysis." In: Jack RS, ed. CD14 in the Inflammatory Response. Basel: Karger; 1999:162-177.
54. Hotchkiss RS, Karl IE. Medical progress: The pathophysiology and treatment of sepsis. N Engl J Med. 2003;348:138-150.
55. Hotchkiss RS, Swanson PE, Freeman BD, et al. Apoptotic cell death in patients with sepsis, shock, and multiple organ dysfunction [see comments]. Crit Care Med. 1999;27:1230-1251.
56. Mant MJ, King EG. Severe, acute disseminated intravascular coagulation: A reappraisal of its pathophysiology, clinical significance and therapy based on 47 patients. Am J Med. 1979;67:557-563.
57. Robboy SJ, Major MC, Colman RW, et al. Pathology of disseminated intravascular coagulation (DIC): Analysis of 26 cases. Hum Pathol. 1972;3:327-343.
58. Helliwell TR, Wilkinson A, Griffiths RD, et al. Microvascular endothelial activation in the skeletal muscles of patients with multiple organ failure. J Neurol Sci. 1998;154:26-34.
59. De Backer D, Creteur J, Preiser JC, et al. Microvascular blood flow is altered in patients with sepsis. Am J Respir Crit Care Med. 2002;166:98-104.
60. Spronk PE, Ince C, Gardien MJ, et al. Nitroglycerin in septic shock after intravascular volume resuscitation. Lancet. 2002;360:1395-1396.
61. Lehr HA, Bittinger F, Kirkpatrick CJ. Microcirculatory dysfunction in sepsis: A pathogenetic basis for therapy? J Pathol. 2000;190:373-386.
62. Fink M. Cytopathic hypoxia in sepsis. Acta Anaesthesiol Scand. 1997;110:87-95.
63. Liaudet L. Poly(adenosine 5′-diphosphate) ribose polymerase activation as a cause of metabolic dysfunction in critical illness. Curr Opin Clin Nutr Metab Care. 2002;5:175-184.
64. Brealey D, Brand M, Hargreaves I, et al. Association between mitochondrial dysfunction and severity and outcome of septic shock. Lancet. 2002;360:219-223.
65. Adrie C, Bachelet M, Vayssier-Taussat M, et al. Mitochondrial membrane potential and apoptosis peripheral blood monocytes in severe human sepsis. Am J Respir Crit Care Med. 2001;164:389-395.
66. Bannerman DD, Goldblum SE. Mechanisms of bacterial lipopolysaccharide-induced endothelial apoptosis. Am J Physiol Lung Cell Mol Physiol. 2003;284:L899-L914.
67. Aird WC. The role of the endothelium in severe sepsis and multiple organ dysfunction syndrome. Blood. 2003;101:3765-3777.
68. Mutunga M, Fulton B, Bullock R, et al. Circulating endothelial cells in patients with septic shock. Am J Respir Crit Care Med. 2001;163:195-200.
69. McGill SN, Ahmed NA, Christou NV. Increased plasma von Willebrand factor in the systemic inflammatory response syndrome is derived from generalized endothelial cell activation. Crit Care Med. 1998;26:296-300.
70. Kubli S, Boegli Y, Ave AD, et al. Endothelium-dependent vasodilation in the skin microcirculation of patients with septic shock. Shock. 2003;19:274-280.
71. Leone M, Boutiere B, Camoin-Jau L, et al. Systemic endothelial activation is greater in septic than in traumatic-hemorrhagic shock but does not correlate with endothelial activation in skin biopsies. Crit Care Med. 2002;30:808-814.
72. Aird WC. Endothelial cell heterogeneity. Crit Care Med. 2003;31:S221-S230.
73. Brandtzaeg P, Osnes L, Ovstebo R, et al. Net inflammatory capacity of human septic shock plasma evaluated by a monocyte-based target cell assay: Identification of interleukin-10 as a major functional deactivator of human monocytes. J Exp Med. 1996;184:51-60.
74. Ertel W, Kremer J-P, Kenney J, et al. Downregulation of proinflammatory cytokine release in whole blood from septic patients. Blood. 1995;85:1341-1347.
75. Randow F, Syrbe U, Meisel C, et al. Mechanism of endotoxin desensitization: Involvement of interleukin 10 and transforming growth factor beta. J Exp Med. 1995;181:1887-1892.
76. Munoz C, Carlet J, Fitting C, et al. Dysregulation of in vitro cytokine production by monocytes during sepsis. J Clin Invest. 1991;88:1747-1754.
77. Sfeir T, Saha DC, Astiz M, et al. Role of interleukin-10 in monocyte hyporesponsiveness associated with septic shock. Crit Care Med. 2001;29:129-133.
78. Spolarics Z, Siddiqi M, Siegel JH, et al. Depressed interleukin-12-producing activity by monocytes correlates with adverse clinical course and a shift toward Th2-type lymphocyte pattern in severely injured male trauma patients. Crit Care Med. 2003;31:1722-1729.
79. Ertel W, Keel M, Neidhardt R, et al. Inhibition of the defense system stimulating interleukin-12 interferon-gamma pathway during critical illness. Blood. 1997;89:1612-1620.
80. Monneret G, Debard AL, Venet F, et al. Marked elevation of human circulating CD4+CD25+ regulatory T cells in sepsis-induced immunoparalysis. Crit Care Med. 2003;31:2068-2071.
81. Belge KU, Dayyani F, Horelt A, et al. The proinflammatory CD14+CD16+DR++ monocytes are a major source of TNF. J Immunol. 2002;168:3536-3542.
82. Tilg H, Dinarello CA, Mier JW. IL-6 and APPs: Anti-inflammatory and immunosuppressive mediators. Immunol Today. 1997;9:428-432.
83. Steensberg A, Fischer CP, Keller C, et al. IL-6 enhances plasma IL-1ra, IL-10, and cortisol in humans. Am J Physiol Endocrinol Metab. 2003;285:E433-E437.
84. Bethin KE, Vogt SK, Muglia LJ. Interleukin-6 is an essential, corticotropin-releasing hormone-independent stimulator of the adrenal axis during immune system activation. Proc Natl Acad Sci U S A. 2000;97:9317-9322.
85. van der Poll T, Keogh CV, Guirao X, et al. Interleukin-6 gene-deficient mice show impaired defense against pneumococcal pneumonia. J Infect Dis. 1997;176:439-444.
86. Xing Z, Gauldie J, Cox G, et al. IL-6 is an antiinflammatory cytokine required for controlling local or systemic acute inflammatory responses. J Clin Invest. 1998; 101:311-320.
87. Kopf M, Baumann H, Freer G, et al. Impaired immune and acute-phase responses in interleukin-6-deficient mice. Nature. 1994;368:339-342.
88. Bucala R. MIF rediscovered: Cytokine, pituitary hormone, and glucocorticoid-induced regulator of the immune response. FASEB J. 1996;10:1607-1613.
89. Calandra T, Echtenacher B, Le Roy D, et al. Protection from septic shock by neutralization of macrophage migration inhibitory factor. Nature Med. 2000;6:164-170.
90. Calandra T, Froidevaux W, Martin C, et al. Macrophage migration inhibitory factor and host innate immune defenses against bacterial sepsis. J Infect Dis. 2003; 187:S385-S390.
91. Honma N, Koseki H, Akasaka T, et al. Deficiency of the macrophage migration inhibitory factor gene has no significant effect on endotoxaemia. Immunology. 2000;100:84-90.
92. Andersson U, Wang H, Palmblad K, et al. High mobility group 1 protein (HMG-1) stimulates proinflammatory cytokine synthesis in human monocytes. J Exp Med. 2000;192:565-570.
93. Wang H, Bloom O, Zhang M, et al. HMG-1 as a late mediator of endotoxin lethality in mice. Science. 1999;285:248-251.
94. Ulloa L, Ochani M, Yang H, et al. Ethyl pyruvate prevents lethality in mice with established lethal sepsis and systemic inflammation. Proc Natl Acad Sci U S A. 2002; 99:12351-12356.
95. Bone RC. Immunologic dissonance: A continuing evolution in our understanding of the systemic inflammatory response syndrome (SIRS) and the multiple organ dysfunction syndrome (MODS). Ann Intern Med. 1996;125:680-687.
96. Van Dissel JT, van Langevelde P, Westendorp RG, et al. Anti-inflammatory cytokine profile and mortality in febrile patients. Lancet. 1998;351:950-953.
97. Baize S, Leroy EM, Georges AJ, et al. Inflammatory responses in Ebola virus-infected patients. Clin Exp Immunol. 2002;128:163-168.
98. Wolbink GJ, Bossink AW, Groeneveld AB, et al. Complement activation in patients with sepsis is in part mediated by C-reactive protein. J Infect Dis. 1998;177:81-87.
99. Brandtzaeg P, Hogasen K, Kierulf P, et al. The excessive complement activation in fulminant meningococcal septicemia is predominantly caused by alternative pathway activation. J Infect Dis. 1996;173:647-655.
100. Nuijens JH, Eerenberg-Belmer AJM, Huijbregts CCM, et al. Proteolytic inactivation of plasma C1 inhibitor in sepsis. J Clin Invest. 1989;84:443-450.
101. Jansen PM, Eisele B, De Jong IW, et al. Effect of C1 inhibitor on inflammatory and physiologic response patterns in primates suffering from lethal septic shock. J Immunol. 1998;160:475-484.
102. Riedemann NC, Guo RF, Ward PA. Novel strategies for the treatment of sepsis. Nat Med. 2003;9:517-524.
103. Robboy SJ, Mihm MC, Colman RW, et al. The skin in disseminated intravascular coagulation. Br J Dermatol. 1973;88:221-229.
104. Abraham E, Reinhart K, Opal S, et al. Efficacy and safety of tifacogin (recombinant tissue factor pathway inhibitor) in severe sepsis: A randomized controlled trial. JAMA. 2003;290:238-247.
105. Warren BL, Eid A, Singer P, et al. Caring for the critically ill patient. High-dose antithrombin III in severe sepsis: A randomized controlled trial. JAMA. 2001;286: 1869-1878.
106. Bernard GR, Vincent JL, Laterre P, et al. Efficacy and safety of recombinant human activated protein C for severe sepsis. N Engl J Med. 2001;344:699-709.
107. Evans RW, Glick B, Kimball F, et al. Fatal intravascular consumption coagulopathy in meningococcal sepsis. Am J Med. 1969;46:910-918.
108. McGehee WG, Rapaport SI, Hjort PF. Intravascular coagulation in fulminant meningococcemia. Ann Intern Med. 1967;67:250-260.
109. Fisher-Hoch SP, Platt GS, Neild GH, et al. Pathophysiology of shock and hemorrhage in a fulminating viral infection (Ebola). J Infect Dis. 1985;152:887-894.

110. Reddy RC, Chen GH, Tekchandani PK, et al. Sepsis-induced immunosuppression: From bad to worse. Immunol Res. 2001;24:273-287.

111. Christou NV, Meakins JL, Gordon J, et al. The delayed hypersensitivity response and host resistance in surgical patients: 20 years later. Ann Surg. 1995;222:534-548.

112. Manjuck J, Saha DC, Astiz M, et al. Decreased response to recall antigens is associated with depressed costimulatory receptor expression in septic critically ill patients. J Lab Clin Med. 2000;135:153-160.

113. Fumeaux T, Pugin J. Role of interleukin-10 in the intracellular sequestration of human leukocyte antigen-DR in monocytes during septic shock. Am J Respir Crit Care Med. 2002;166:1475-1482.

114. McCall CE, Grosso-Wilmoth LM, LaRue K, et al. Tolerance to endotoxin-induced expression of the interleukin-1β gene in blood neutrophils of humans with the sepsis syndrome. J Clin Invest. 1993;91:853-861.

115. Marie C, Muret J, Fitting C, et al. Reduced ex vivo interleukin-8 production by neutrophils in septic and nonseptic systemic inflammatory response syndrome. Blood. 1998;91:3439-3446.

116. Hotchkiss RS, Tinsley KW, Swanson PE, et al. Sepsis-induced apoptosis causes progressive profound depletion of B and CD4+ T lymphocytes in humans. J Immunol. 2001;166:6952-6963.

117. Hotchkiss RS, Tinsley KW, Swanson PE, et al. Depletion of dendritic cells, but not macrophages, in patients with sepsis. J Immunol. 2002;168:2493-2500.

118. Oberholzer C, Oberholzer A, Clare-Salzler M, et al. Apoptosis in sepsis: A new target for therapeutic exploration. FASEB J. 2001;15:879-892.

119. Hotchkiss RS, Tinsley KW, Swanson PE, et al. Prevention of lymphocyte cell death in sepsis improves survival in mice. Proc Natl Acad Sci U S A. 1999;96:14541-14546.

120. Keel M, Ungethüm U, Steckholzer U, et al. Interleukin-10 counterregulates proinflammatory cytokine-induced inhibition of neutrophil apoptosis during severe sepsis. Blood. 1997;90:3356-3363.

121. MacLean LD, Mulligan WG, McLean AP, et al. Patterns of septic shock in man: A detailed study of 56 patients. Ann Surg. 1967;166:543-562.

122. Hallin GW, Simpson SQ, Crowell RE, et al. Cardiopulmonary manifestations of Hantavirus pulmonary syndrome. Crit Care Med. 1996;24:252-258.

123. Nishio K, Akai Y, Murao Y, et al. Increased plasma concentrations of adrenomedullin correlate with relaxation of vascular tone in patients with septic shock. Crit Care Med. 1997;25:953-957.

124. Annane D, Sanquer S, Sébille V, et al. Compartmentalised inducible nitric-oxide synthase activity in septic shock. Lancet. 2000;355:1143-1148.

125. Holmes CL, Patel BM, Russell JA, et al. Physiology of vasopressin relevant to management of septic shock. Chest. 2001;120:989-1002.

126. Landry DW, Oliver JA. The pathogenesis of vasodilatory shock. N Engl J Med. 2001;345:588-595.

127. Fein AM, Bernard GR, Criner GJ, et al. Treatment of severe systemic inflammatory response syndrome and sepsis with a novel bradykinin antagonist, Deltibant (CP-0127). JAMA. 1997;277:482-487.

128. Domingo P, Muñiz-Diaz E, Baraldès MA, et al. Associations between Fc gamma receptor IIA polymorphisms and the risk and prognosis of meningococcal disease. Am J Med. 2002;112:19-25.

129. Yee AM, Phan HM, Zuniga R, et al. Association between Fc gammaRIIA-R131 allotype and bacteremic pneumococcal pneumonia. Clin Infect Dis. 2000;30:25-28.

130. Westendorp RGJ, Hottenga JJ, Slagboom PE. Variation in plasminogen-activator-inhibitor-1 gene and risk of meningococcal septic shock. Lancet. 1999;354:561-563.

131. Read RC, Camp NJ, Di Giovine FS, et al. An interleukin-1 genotype is associated with fatal outcome of meningococcal disease. J Infect Dis. 2000;182:1557-1560.

132. Nadel S, Newport MJ, Booy R, et al. Variation in the tumor necrosis factor-α gene promoter region may be associated with death from meningococcal disease. J Infect Dis. 1996;174:878-880.

133. Agnese DM, Calvano JE, Hahm SJ, et al. Human toll-like receptor 4 mutations but not CD14 polymorphisms are associated with an increased risk of gram-negative infections. J Infect Dis. 2002;186:1522-1525.

134. Smirnova I, Mann N, Dols A, et al. Assay of locus-specific genetic load implicates rare Toll-like receptor 4 mutations in meningococcal susceptibility. Proc Natl Acad Sci U S A. 2003;100:6075-6080.

135. Lorenz E, Mira JP, Frees KL, et al. Relevance of mutations in the TLR4 receptor in patients with gram-negative septic shock. Arch Intern Med. 2002;162:1028-1032.

136. Mira JP, Cariou A, Grall F, et al. Association of TNF2, a TNF-α promoter polymorphism, with septic shock susceptibility and mortality. JAMA. 1999;282:561-568.

137. Tang GJ, Huang SL, Yien HW, et al. Tumor necrosis factor gene polymorphism and septic shock in surgical infection. Crit Care Med. 2000;28:3090-3091.

138. O'Keefe GE, Hybki DL, Munford RS. The G→A single nucleotide polymorphism at the −308 position in the tumor necrosis factor-alpha promoter increases the risk for severe sepsis. J Trauma 2002;52:817-826.

139. Stuber F, Petersen M, Bokelmann F, et al. A genomic polymorphism within the tumor necrosis factor locus influences plasma tumor necrosis factor-alpha concentrations and outcome of patients with severe sepsis. Crit Care Med. 1996;24:381-384.

140. Schlüter B, Raufhake C, Erren M, et al. Effect of the interleukin-6 promoter polymorphism (−174 G/C) on the incidence and outcome of sepsis. Crit Care Med. 2002;30:32-37.

141. Erridge C, Stewart J, Poxton IR. Monocytes heterozygous for the Asp299Gly and Thr399Ile mutations in the toll-like receptor 4 gene show no deficit in lipopolysaccharide signaling. J Exp Med. 2003;197:1787-1791.

142. Feterowski C, Emmanuilidis K, Miethke T, et al. Effects of functional Toll-like receptor-4 mutations on the immune response to human and experimental sepsis. Immunology. 2003;109:426-431.

143. Feezor RJ, Oberholzer C, Baker HV, et al. Molecular characterization of the acute inflammatory response to infections with gram-negative versus gram-positive bacteria. Infect Immun. 2003;71:5803-5813.

144. Cohen J, Abraham E. Microbiologic findings and correlations with serum tumor necrosis factor-alpha in patients with severe sepsis and septic shock. J Infect Dis. 1999;180:116-121.

145. Nau GJ, Richmond JF, Schlesinger A, et al. Human macrophage activation programs induced by bacterial pathogens. Proc Natl Acad Sci U S A. 2002;99:1503-1508.

146. Wang ZM, Liu C, Dziarski R. Chemokines are the main proinflammatory mediators in human monocytes activated by Staphylococcus aureus, peptidoglycan, and endotoxin. J Biol Chem. 2000;275:20260-20267.

147. Boldrick JC, Alizadeh AA, Diehn M, et al. Stereotyped and specific gene expression programs in human innate immune responses to bacteria. Proc Natl Acad Sci U S A. 2002;99:972-977.

148. Shenep JL, Flynn PM, Barrett FF, et al. Serial quantitation of endotoxemia and bacteremia during therapy for gram-negative bacterial sepsis. J Infect Dis. 1988;157:565-568.

149. Butler T, Levin J, Linh NN, et al. Yersinia pestis infection in Vietnam: II. Quantitative blood cultures and detection of endotoxin in the cerebrospinal fluid of patients with meningitis. J Infect Dis. 1976;133:493-499.

150. Walsh AL, Smith MD, Wuthiekanun V, et al. Prognostic significance of quantitative bacteremia in septicemic melioidosis. Clin Infect Dis. 1995;21:1498-1500.

151. Murono K, Hirano Y, Koyano S, et al. Molecular comparison of bacterial isolates from blood with strains colonizing pharynx and intestine in immunocompromised patients with sepsis. J Med Microbiol. 2003;52:527-530.

152. Wenzel RP. Nosocomial candidemia: Risk factors and attributable mortality. Clin Infect Dis. 1995;20:1531-1534.

153. Blot SI, Vandewoude KH, Hoste EA, et al. Outcome and attributable mortality in critically ill patients with bacteremia involving methicillin-susceptible and methicillin-resistant Staphylococcus aureus. Arch Intern Med. 2002;162:2229-2235.

154. Linden PK, Pasculle AW, Manez R, et al. Differences in outcomes for patients with bacteremia due to vancomycin-resistant Enterococcus faecium or vancomycin-susceptible E. faecium. Clin Infect Dis. 1996;22:663-670.

155. Rogers DE. Host mechanisms which act to remove bacteria from the blood stream. Bacteriol Rev. 1960;24:50-66.

156. Harris JA, Cobb CG. Persistent gram-negative bacteremia: Observations in twenty patients. Am J Surg. 1973;125:705-717.

157. DuPont HL, Spink WW. Infections due to gram-negative organisms: An analysis of 860 patients with bacteremia at the University of Minnesota Medical Center, 1958-1966. Medicine. 1969;48:307-332.

158. Sullivan TD, LaScolea LJ. Neisseria meningitidis bacteremia in children: Quantitation of bacteremia and spontaneous clinical recovery without antibiotic therapy. Pediatrics. 1987;80:63-67.

159. Schwenzer KJ, Gist A, Durbin CG. Can bacteremia be predicted in surgical intensive care unit patients? Intensive Care Med. 1994;20:425-430.

160. Bates DW, Sands K, Miller E, et al. Predicting bacteremia in patients with sepsis syndrome. J Infect Dis. 1997;176:1538-1551.

161. Jones GR, Lowes JA. The systemic inflammatory response syndrome as a predictor of bacteraemia and outcome from sepsis. Q J Med. 1996;89:515-522.

162. DiGiovine B, Chenoweth C, Watts C, et al. The attributable mortality and costs of primary nosocomial bloodstream infections in the intensive care unit. Am J Respir Crit Care Med. 1999;160:976-981.

163. Rello J, Ochagavia A, Sabanes E, et al. Evaluation of outcome of intravenous catheter-related infections in critically ill patients. Am J Respir Crit Care Med. 2000;162:1027-1030.

164. Renaud B, Brun-Buisson C. Outcomes of primary and catheter-related bacteremia: A cohort and case-control study in critically ill patients. Am J Respir Crit Care Med. 2001;163:1584-1590.

165. Blot S, Vandewoude K, De Bacquer D, et al. Nosocomial bacteremia caused by antibiotic-resistant gram-negative bacteria in critically ill patients: Clinical outcome and length of hospitalization. Clin Infect Dis. 2002;34:1600-1606.

166. Roth VR, Arduino MJ, Nobiletti J, et al. Transfusion-related sepsis due to Serratia liquefaciens in the United States. Transfusion. 2000;40:931-935.

167. Blot SI, Vandewoude KH, Colardyn FA. Evaluation of outcome in critically ill patients with nosocomial Enterobacter bacteremia: Results of a matched cohort study. Chest. 2003;123:1208-1213.

168. Bates DW, Pruess KE, Lee TH. How bad are bacteremia and sepsis? Outcomes in a cohort with suspected bacteremia. Arch Intern Med. 1995;155:593-598.

169. Weinstein MP, Murphy JR, Reller LB, et al. The clinical significance of positive blood cultures: A comprehensive analysis of 500 episodes of bacteremia and fungemia in adults—II. Clinical observations, with special reference to factors influencing prognosis. Rev Infect Dis. 1983;5:54-70.

170. Knaus WA, Sun X, Nystrom P-O, et al. Evaluation of definitions for sepsis. Chest. 1992;101:1656-1662.

171. Brun-Buisson C, Doyon F, Carlet J, et al. Bacteremia and severe sepsis in adults: A multicenter prospective survey in ICUs and wards of 24 hospitals. Am J Respir Crit Care Med. 1996;154:617-624.

172. Felty AR, Keefer CS. Bacillus coli sepsis. JAMA. 1924;82:1430-1433.

173. Waage A, Halstensen A, Espevik T. Association between tumour necrosis factor in serum and fatal outcome in patients with meningococcal disease. Lancet. 1987;1:355-357.

174. Brandtzaeg P, Kierulf P, Gaustad P, et al. Plasma endotoxin as a predictor of multiple organ failure and death in systemic meningococcal disease. J Infect Dis. 1989;159:195-204.

175. Burrell R. Human responses to bacterial endotoxin. Circ Shock. 1994;43:137-153.

176. Romaschin AD, Harris DM, Ribeiro MB, et al. A rapid assay of endotoxin in whole blood using autologous neutrophil dependent chemiluminescence. J Immunol Methods. 1998;212:169-185.

177. Warren HS, Novitsky TJ, Ketchum PA, et al. Neutralization of bacterial lipopolysaccharides by human plasma. J Clin Microbiol. 1985;22:590-595.

178. Braun JM, Blackwell CC, Poxton IR, et al. Proinflammatory responses to lipo-oligosaccharide of *Neisseria meningitidis* immunotype strains in relation to virulence and disease. J Infect Dis. 2002;185:1431-1438.
179. Kitchens RL, Thompson PA, Viriyakosol S, et al. Plasma CD14 decreases monocyte responses to LPS by promoting the transfer of cell-bound LPS to plasma lipoproteins. J Clin Invest. 2001;108:485-493.
180. Levels JH, Lemaire LC, van den Ende AE, et al. Lipid composition and lipopolysaccharide binding capacity of lipoproteins in plasma and lymph of patients with systemic inflammatory response syndrome and multiple organ failure. Crit Care Med. 2003;31:1647-1653.
181. Kitchens RL, Thompson PA, Munford RS, O'Keefe GE. Acute inflammation and infection maintain circulating phospholipid levels and enhance lipopolysaccharide binding to plasma lipoproteins. J Lipid Res. 2003;44:2339-2348.
182. Froon AHM, Dentener MA, Greve JWM, et al. Lipopolysaccharide toxicity-regulating proteins in bacteremia. J Infect Dis. 1995;171:1250-1257.
183. Zweigner J, Gramm HJ, Singer OC, et al. High concentrations of lipopolysaccharide-binding protein in serum of patients with severe sepsis or septic shock inhibit the lipopolysaccharide response in human monocytes. Blood. 2001;98:3800-3808.
184. Thompson PA, Tobias PS, Viriyakosol S, et al. Lipopolysaccharide (LPS)-binding protein inhibits responses to cell-bound LPS. J Biol Chem. 2003;278:28367-28371.
185. van Langevelde P, Joop K, Van Loon J, et al. Endotoxin, cytokines, and procalcitonin in febrile patients admitted to the hospital: Identification of subjects at high risk of mortality. Clin Infect Dis. 2000;31:1343-1348.
186. Hurley JC. Concordance of endotoxemia with gram-negative bacteremia: A meta-analysis using receiver operating characteristic curves. Arch Pathol Lab Med. 2000;124:1157-1164.
187. Hurley JC. Reappraisal with meta-analysis of bacteremia, endotoxemia, and mortality in gram-negative sepsis. J Clin Microbiol. 1995;33:1278-1282.
188. Unnikrishnan M, Altmann DM, Proft T, et al. The bacterial superantigen streptococcal mitogenic exotoxin Z is the major immunoactive agent of *Streptococcus pyogenes*. J Immunol. 2002;169:2561-2569.
189. Kotb M. Bacterial pyrogenic exotoxins as superantigens. Clin Microbiol Rev. 1995;8:411-426.
190. Cohen J. The immunopathogenesis of sepsis. Nature. 2002;420:885-891.
191. Hellman J, Roberts JD Jr, Tehan MM, et al. Bacterial peptidoglycan-associated lipoprotein is released into the bloodstream in gram-negative sepsis and causes inflammation and death in mice. J Biol Chem. 2002;277:14274-14280.
192. Leroy EM, Baize S, Volchkov VE, et al. Human asymptomatic Ebola infection and strong inflammatory response. Lancet. 2000;355:2210-2215.
193. Alluisi EA, Beisel WR, Bartelloni PJ, et al. Behavioral effects of tularemia and sandfly fever in man. J Infect Dis. 1973;128:710-717.
194. Bolton CF, Young GB, Zochodne DW. The neurological complications of sepsis. Ann Neurol. 1993;33:94-100.
195. Sprung CL, Peduzzi PN, Shatney CH, et al. Impact of encephalopathy on mortality in the sepsis syndrome. Crit Care Med. 1990;18:801-805.
196. Sharshar T, Blanchard A, Paillard M, et al. Circulating vasopressin levels in septic shock. Crit Care Med. 2003;31:1752-1758.
197. Sharshar T, Carlier R, Blanchard A, et al. Depletion of neurohypophyseal content of vasopressin in septic shock. Crit Care Med. 2002;30:497-500.
198. Rivers EP, Gaspari M, Saad GA, et al. Adrenal insufficiency in high-risk surgical ICU patients. Chest. 2001;119:889-896.
199. Rothwell PM, Udwadia ZF, Lawler PG. Cortisol response to corticotropin and survival in septic shock. Lancet. 1991;337:582-583.
200. Marik PE, Zaloga GP. Adrenal insufficiency during septic shock. Crit Care Med. 2003;31:141-145.
201. Bollaert PE, Fieux F, Charpentier C, et al. Baseline cortisol levels, cortisol response to corticotropin, and prognosis in late septic shock. Shock. 2003;19:13-15.
202. Annane D, Sébille V, Troché T, et al. A 3-level prognostic classification in septic shock based on cortisol levels and cortisol response to corticotropin. JAMA. 2000;283:1038-1045.
203. Manglik S, Flores E, Lubarsky L, et al. Glucocorticoid insufficiency in patients who present to the hospital with severe sepsis: A prospective clinical trial. Crit Care Med. 2003;31:1668-1675.
204. Zipser RD, Davenport MW, Martin KL, et al. Hyperreninemic hypoaldosteronism in the critically ill: A new entity. J Clin Endocrinol Metab. 1981;53:867-873.
205. Findling JW, Waters VO, Raff H. The dissociation of renin and aldosterone during critical illness. J Clin Endocrinol Metab. 1987;64:592-595.
206. Lamberts SWJ, Bruining HA, de Jong FH. Corticosteroid therapy in severe illness. N Engl J Med. 1997;337:1285-1292.
207. Shenker Y, Skatrud JB. Adrenal insufficiency in critically ill patients. Am J Respir Crit Care Med. 2001;163:1520-1523.
208. Briegel J, Schelling G, Haller M, et al. A comparison of the adrenocortical response during septic shock and after complete recovery. Intensive Care Med. 1996;22:894-899.
209. Task Force of the European Society of Cardiology and the North American Society of Pacing and Electrophysiology. Heart rate variability: Standards of measurement, physiological interpretation, and clinical use. Eur Heart J. 1996;17:354-381.
210. Griffin MP, Moorman JR. Toward the early diagnosis of neonatal sepsis and sepsis-like illness using novel heart rate analysis. Pediatrics. 2001;107:97-104.
211. Lake DE, Richman JS, Griffin MP, et al. Sample entropy analysis of neonatal heart rate variability. Am J Physiol Regul Integr Comp Physiol. 2002;283:R789-R797.
212. Griffin MP, O'Shea TM, Bissonette EA, et al. Abnormal heart rate characteristics preceding neonatal sepsis and sepsis-like illness. Pediatr Res. 2003;53:920-926.
213. Annane D, Trabold F, Sharshar T, et al. Inappropriate sympathetic activation at onset of septic shock. Am J Respir Crit Care Med. 1999;160:458-465.
214. Seely AJE, Christou NV. Multiple organ dysfunction syndrome: Exploring the paradigm of complex nonlinear systems. Crit Care Med. 2000;28:2193-2200.
215. Godin PJ, Buchman TG. Uncoupling of biological oscillators: A complementary hypothesis concerning the pathogenesis of multiple organ dysfunction syndrome. Crit Care Med. 1996;24:1107-1116.
216. Diaz NL, Finol HJ, Torres SH, et al. Histochemical and ultrastructural study of skeletal muscle in patients with sepsis and multiple organ failure syndrome (MOFS). Histol Histopathol. 1998;13:121-128.
217. Parillo JE. Septic shock in humans: Advances in the understanding of pathogenesis, cardiovascular dysfunction, and therapy. Ann Intern Med. 1990;113:227-242.
218. Holub M, Kluckova Z, Helcl M, et al. Lymphocyte subset numbers depend on the bacterial origin of sepsis. Clin Microbiol Infect. 2003;9:202-211.
219. Aird WC. The hematologic system as a marker of organ dysfunction in sepsis. Mayo Clin Proc. 2003;78:869-881.
220. Randow F, Syrbe U, Meisel C, et al. Mechanism of endotoxin desensitization: Involvement of interleukin 10 and transforming growth factor beta. J Exp Med. 1995;181:1887-1892.
221. Khovidhunkit W, Memon RA, Feingold KR, et al. Infection and inflammation-induced proatherogenic changes of lipoproteins. J Infect Dis. 2000;181:S462-S472.
222. Harris RL, Musher DM, Bloom K, et al. Manifestations of sepsis. Arch Intern Med. 1987;147:1895-1906.
223. Gore DC, Jahoor F, Hibbert JM, et al. Lactic acidosis during sepsis is related to increased pyruvate production, not deficits in tissue oxygen availability. Ann Surg. 1996;224:97-102.
224. Bernard GR, Wheeler AP, Russell JA, et al. The effects of ibuprofen on the physiology and survival of patients with sepsis. N Engl J Med. 1997;336:912-918.
225. Bick RL. Disseminated intravascular coagulation: Pathophysiological mechanisms and manifestations. Semin Thromb Hemost. 1998;24:3-18.
226. Willis TMS, Hopp RJ, Romero JR, et al. The protective effect of brachial plexus palsy in purpura fulminans. Pediatr Neurol. 2001;24:379-381.
227. Chandler WL. Treatment of thrombosis associated with septic shock. J Lab Clin Med. 1991;118:513-514.
228. Abraham E, Shoemaker WD, Bland RD, et al. Sequential cardiorespiratory patterns in septic shock. Crit Care Med. 1983;11:799-803.
229. Shoemaker WC, Appel PL, Kram HB, et al. Temporal hemodynamic and oxygen transport patterns in medical patients: Septic shock. Chest. 1993;104:1529-1536.
230. Matthay MA, Zimmerman GA, Esmon C, et al. Future research directions in acute lung injury: Summary of a National Heart, Lung, and Blood Institute working group. Am J Respir Crit Care Med. 2003;167:1027-1035.
231. Doig CJ, Sutherland LR, Sandham JD, et al. Increased intestinal permeability is associated with the development of multiple organ dysfunction syndrome in critically ill ICU patients. Am J Respir Crit Care Med. 1998;158:444-451.
232. Franson TR, Hierholzer WJ Jr, LaBrecque DR. Frequency and characteristics of hyperbilirubinemia associated with bacteremia. Rev Infect Dis. 1985;7:1-9.
233. Cook CH, Martin LC, Yenchar JK, et al. Occult herpes family viral infections are endemic in critically ill surgical patients. Crit Care Med. 2003;31:1923-1929.
234. Kutza AS, Muhl E, Hackstein H, et al. High incidence of active cytomegalovirus infection among septic patients. Clin Infect Dis. 1998;26:1076-1082.
235. Musher D. Cutaneous and soft-tissue manifestations of sepsis due to gram-negative enteric bacilli. Rev Infect Dis. 1980;2:854-866.
236. Lamy B, Roy P, Carret G, et al. What is the relevance of obtaining multiple blood samples for culture? A comprehensive model to optimize the strategy for diagnosing bacteremia. Clin Infect Dis. 2002;35:842-850.
237. Gaur AH, Flynn PM, Giannini MA, et al. Difference in time to detection: A simple method to differentiate catheter-related from non-catheter-related bloodstream infection in immunocompromised pediatric patients. Clin Infect Dis. 2003;37:469-475.
238. Bates DW, Goldman L, Lee TH. Contaminant blood cultures and resource utilization: The true consequences of false-positive results. JAMA. 1991;265:365-369.
239. Van Deuren M, van Dijke BJ, Koopman RJ, et al. Rapid diagnosis of acute meningococcal infections by needle aspiration or biopsy of skin lesions. BMJ. 1993;306:1229-1232.
240. Harbarth S, Holeckova K, Froidevaux C, et al. Diagnostic value of procalcitonin, interleukin-6, and interleukin-8 in critically ill patients admitted with suspected sepsis. Am J Respir Crit Care Med. 2001;164:396-402.
241. Luzzani A, Polati E, Dorizzi R, et al. Comparison of procalcitonin and C-reactive protein as markers of sepsis. Crit Care Med. 2003;31:1737-1741.
242. Young LS. Sepsis syndrome. In: Mandell GL, Bennett JE, Dolin R, eds. Principles and Practice of Infectious Diseases. Philadelphia: Churchill Livingstone; 2000:806-819.
243. Bryan CS, Reynolds KL, Brenner ER. Analysis of 1,186 episodes of gram-negative bacteremia in non-university hospitals: The effects of antimicrobial therapy. Rev Infect Dis. 1983;4:629-638.
244. Kollef MH, Sherman G, Ward S, et al. Inadequate antimicrobial treatment of infections: A risk factor for hospital mortality among critically ill patients. Chest. 1999;115:462-474.
245. Kreger BE, Craven DE, McCabe WR. Gram-negative bacteremia: IV. Re-evaluation of clinical features and treatment in 612 patients. Am J Med. 1980;68:344-355.
246. Leibovici L, Paul M, Poznanski O, et al. Monotherapy versus beta-lactam-aminoglycoside combination treatment for gram-negative bacteremia: A prospective, observational study. Antimicrob Agents Chemother. 1997;41:1127-1133.
247. Leibovici L, Shraga I, Drucker M, et al. The benefit of appropriate empirical antibiotic treatment in patients with bloodstream infection. J Intern Med. 1998;244:379-386.
248. Ibrahim EH, Sherman G, Ward S, et al. The influence of inadequate antimicrobial treatment of bloodstream infections on patient outcomes in the ICU setting. Chest. 2000;118:146-155.
249. Bochud PY, Glauser MP, Carlet J, Calandra T. Empirical antibiotic therapy for patients with severe sepsis and septic shock. In: Vincent J-L, Carlet J, Opal SM, eds. The Sepsis Text. Boston: Kluwer; 2002:539-558.

250. Buijk SE, Mouton JW, Gyssens IC, et al. Experience with a once-daily dosing program of aminoglycosides in critically ill patients. Intensive Care Med. 2002;28: 936-942.

251. Jimenez MF, Marshall JC. Source control in the management of sepsis. Intensive Care Med. 2001;27(Suppl 1):S49-S62.

252. O'Grady NP, Barie PS, Bartlett JG, et al. Practice guidelines for evaluating new fever in critically ill adult patients. Task Force of the Society of Critical Care Medicine and the Infectious Diseases Society of America. Clin Infect Dis. 1998;26:1042-1059.

253. Schierhout G, Roberts I. Fluid resuscitation with colloid or crystalloid solutions in critically ill patients: A systematic review of randomised trials. BMJ. 1998;316: 961-964.

254. Choi PT-L, Yip G, Quinonez LG, et al. Crystalloids vs. colloids in fluid resuscitation: A systematic review. Crit Care Med. 1999;27:200-210.

255. Connors AF Jr, Speroff T, Dawson NV, et al. The effectiveness of right heart catheterization in the initial care of critically ill patients. SUPPORT Investigators. JAMA. 1996;276:889-897.

256. Rivers E, Nguyen B, Havstad S, et al. Early goal-directed therapy in the treatment of severe sepsis and septic shock. N Engl J Med. 2001;345:1368-1377.

257. The ARDS Network. Ventilation with lower tidal volumes as compared with traditional tidal volumes for acute lung injury and the acute respiratory distress syndrome. N Engl J Med. 2003;342:1301-1308.

258. Eichacker PQ, Gerstenberger EP, Banks SM, et al. Meta-analysis of acute lung injury and acute respiratory distress syndrome trials testing low tidal volumes. Am J Respir Crit Care Med. 2002;166:1510-1514.

259. Hebert PC, Fergusson DA. Red blood cell transfusions in critically ill patients. JAMA. 2002;288:1525-1526.

260. Corwin HL, Gettinger A, Pearl RG, et al. Efficacy of recombinant human erythropoietin in critically ill patients: A randomized controlled trial. JAMA. 2002;288:2827-2835.

261. Holmes CL, Walley KR. Bad medicine: Low-dose dopamine in the ICU. Chest. 2003;123:1266-1275.

262. Australian and New Zealand Intensive Care Society (ANZICS) Clinical Trials Group. Low-dose dopamine in patients with early renal dysfunction: A placebo-controlled randomized trial. Lancet. 2000;356:2139-2143.

263. Marik PE, Iglesias J, NORASEPT II Study Investigators. Low-dose dopamine does not prevent acute renal failure in patients with septic shock and oliguria. Am J Med. 1999;107:387-390.

264. De Backer D, Creteur J, Silva E, et al. Effects of dopamine, norepinephrine, and epinephrine on the splanchnic circulation in septic shock: Which is best? Crit Care Med. 2003;31:1659-1667.

265. Bellissant E, Annane D. Effect of hydrocortisone on phenylephrine-mean arterial pressure dose-response relationship in septic shock. Clin Pharmacol Ther. 2000; 68:293-303.

266. Keh D, Boehnke T, Weber-Cartens S, et al. Immunologic and hemodynamic effects of "low-dose" hydrocortisone in septic shock: A double-blind, randomized, placebo-controlled, crossover study. Am J Respir Crit Care Med. 2003;167:512-520.

267. Oppert M, Reinicke A, Gräf K-J, et al. Plasma cortisol levels before and during "low-dose" hydrocortisone therapy and their relationship to hemodynamic improvement in patients with septic shock. Intensive Care Med. 2000;26:1747-1755.

268. Bollaert PE, Charpentier C, Levy B, et al. Reversal of late septic shock with supra-physiologic doses of hydrocortisone. Crit Care Med. 1998;26:645-650.

269. Annane D, Sébille V, Charpentier C, et al. Effect of treatment with low doses of hydrocortisone and fludrocortisone on mortality in patients with septic shock. JAMA. 2002;288:862-871.

270. Dünser MW, Mayr AJ, Ulmer H, et al. Arginine vasopressin in advanced vasodilatory shock: A prospective, randomized, controlled study. Circulation. 2003;107:2313-2319.

271. Vincent JL, Sun QH, Dubois MJ. Clinical trials of immunomodulatory therapies in severe sepsis and septic shock. Clin Infect Dis. 2002;34:1084-1093.

272. Marshall JC. Such stuff as dreams are made on: Mediator-directed therapy in sepsis. Nat Rev Drug Discov. 2003;2:391-405.

273. Eichacker PQ, Parent C, Kalil A, et al. Risk and the efficacy of antiinflammatory agents: Retrospective and confirmatory studies of sepsis. Am J Respir Crit Care Med. 2002;166:1197-1205.

274. Arons MM, Wheeler AP, Bernard GR, et al. Effects of ibuprofen on the physiology and survival of hypothermic sepsis. Crit Care Med. 1999;27:699-707.

275. Pittet D, Thiévent B, Wenzel RP, et al. Bedside prediction of mortality from bacteremic sepsis: A dynamic analysis of ICU patients. Am J Respir Crit Care Med. 1996;153:684-693.

276. Siegel JP. Assessing the use of activated protein c in the treatment of severe sepsis. N Engl J Med. 2002;347:1030-1034.

277. Warren HS, Suffredini AF, Eichacker PQ, et al. Risks and benefits of activated protein C treatment for severe sepsis. N Engl J Med. 2002;347:1027-1030.

278. Warren HS, Danner RL, Munford RS. Anti-endotoxin monoclonal antibodies. N Engl J Med. 1992;326:1153-1157.

279. Lynn M, Rossignol DP, Wheeler JL, et al. Blocking of responses to endotoxin by E5564 in healthy volunteers with experimental endotoxemia. J Infect Dis. 2003; 187:631-639.

280. Cross AS, Opal SM. A new paradigm for the treatment of sepsis: Is it time to consider combination therapy? Ann Intern Med. 2003;138:502-505.

281. Cook D, Guyatt G, Marshall J, et al. A comparison of sucralfate and ranitidine for the prevention of upper gastrointestinal bleeding in patients requiring mechanical ventilation. Canadian Critical Care Trials Group. N Engl J Med. 1998;338:791-797.

282. Doebbeling BN, Stanley GL, Sheetz CT, et al. Comparative efficacy of alternative hand-washing agents in reducing nosocomial infections in intensive care units. N Engl J Med. 1992;327:88-93.

283. O'Grady NP, Alexander M, Dellinger EP, et al. Guidelines for the Prevention of Intravascular Catheter-Related Infections. MMWR Recomm Rep. 2002;51(RR-10):1-29.

284. Drakulovic MB, Torres A, Bauer TT, et al. Supine body position as a risk factor for nosocomial pneumonia in mechanically ventilated patients: A randomised trial. Lancet. 1999;354:1851-1858.

285. Rello J, Sonora R, Jubert P, et al. Pneumonia in intubated patients: Role of respiratory airway care. Am J Respir Crit Care Med. 1996;154:111-115.

286. Van den Berghe G, Wouters P, Weekers F, et al. Intensive insulin therapy in critically ill patients. N Engl J Med. 2001;345:1359-1367.

287. Van den Berghe G, Wouters PJ, Bouillon R, et al. Outcome benefit of intensive insulin therapy in the critically ill: Insulin dose versus glycemic control. Crit Care Med. 2003;31:359-366.

288. Gore DC, Chinkes D, Heggers J, et al. Association of hyperglycemia with increased mortality after severe burn injury. J Trauma. 2001;51:540-544.

289. Zerr KJ, Furnary AP, Grunkemeier GL, et al. Glucose control lowers the risk of wound infection in diabetics after open heart operations. Ann Thorac Surg. 1997; 63:356-361.

290. Rassias AJ, Givan AL, Marrin CA, et al. Insulin increases neutrophil count and phagocytic capacity after cardiac surgery. Anesth Analg. 2002;94:1113-1119.

291. Das UN. Is insulin an antiinflammatory molecule? Nutrition. 2001;17:409-413.

292. Dandona P, Aljada A, Mohanty P, et al. Insulin inhibits intranuclear nuclear factor kappaB and stimulates IkappaB in mononuclear cells in obese subjects: Evidence for an anti-inflammatory effect? J Clin Endocrinol Metab. 2001;86:3257-3265.

293. Hansen TK, Thiel S, Wouters PJ, et al. Intensive insulin therapy exerts antiinflammatory effects in critically ill patients and counteracts the adverse effect of low mannose-binding lectin levels. J Clin Endocrinol Metab. 2003;88:1082-1088.

294. Wasserman D, Ioannovich JD, Hinzmann RD, et al. Interferon-gamma in the prevention of severe burn-related infections: A European phase III multicenter trial. Crit Care Med. 1998;26:434-349.

295. Dries DJ. Interferon-gamma therapy for infectious complications of injury: A called third strike? Crit Care Med. 1998;26:419-420.

296. Hershman MJ, Appel SH, Wellhausen SR, et al. Interferon-gamma treatment increases HLA-DR expression on monocytes in severely injured patients. Clin Exp Immunol. 1989;77:67-70.

297. Liappis AP, Kan VL, Rochester CG, et al. The effect of statins on mortality in patients with bacteremia. Clin Infect Dis. 2001;33:1352-1357.

298. Zanetti G, Glauser MP, Baumgartner JD. Use of immunoglobulins in prevention and treatment of infection in critically ill patients: Review and critique. Rev Infect Dis. 1991;13:985-992.

299. Campbell WN, Hendrix E, Cryz S Jr, et al. Immunogenicity of a 24-valent Klebsiella capsular polysaccharide vaccine and an eight-valent Pseudomonas O-polysaccharide conjugate vaccine administered to victims of acute trauma. Clin Infect Dis. 1996;23:179-181.

300. Kurz A, Sessler DI, Lenhardt R, et al. Perioperative normothermia to reduce the incidence of surgical wound infection and shorten hospitalization. N Engl J Med. 1996;334:1209-1215.

301. McCabe WR, Jackson GG. Gram-negative bacteremia: I. Etiology and ecology. Arch Intern Med. 1962;110:83-91.

302. Perl TM, Dvorak L, Hwang T, et al. Long-term survival and function after suspected gram-negative sepsis. JAMA. 1995;274:338-345.

303. Gogos CA, Drosou E, Bassaris HP, et al. Pro- versus anti-inflammatory cytokine profile in patients with severe sepsis: A marker for prognosis and future therapeutic options. J Infect Dis. 2000;181:176-180.

304. Friedland JS, Porter JC, Daryanani S, et al. Plasma proinflammatory cytokine concentrations, Acute Physiology and Chronic Health Evaluation (APACHE) III scores and survival in patients in an intensive care unit. Crit Care Med. 1996;24:1775-1781.

305. Vincent JL, de Mendonca A, Cantraine F, et al. Use of the SOFA score to assess the incidence of organ dysfunction/failure in intensive care units: Results of a multicenter, prospective study. Working group on "sepsis-related problems" of the European Society of Intensive Care Medicine. Crit Care Med. 1998;26:1793-1800.

306. Quartin AA, Schein RMH, Kett DH, et al. Magnitude and duration of the effect of sepsis on survival. JAMA. 1997;277:1058-1063.

307. Marshall JC, Cook DJ, Christou NV, et al. Multiple organ dysfunction score: A reliable descriptor of a complex clinical outcome. Crit Care Med. 1995;23:1638-1652.

308. Ferreira FL, Bota DP, Bross A, et al. Serial evaluation of the SOFA score to predict outcome in critically ill patients. JAMA. 2001;286:1754-1758.

309. Simon D, Trenholme G. Antibiotic selection for patients with septic shock. Crit Care Clin. 2000;16:215-230.

310. Hoebe K, Du X, Georgel P, et al. Identification of Lps2 as a key transducer of MyD88-independent TIR signalling. Nature. 2003;424:743-748.

311. Angus DC, Birmingham MC, Balk RA, et al. E5 murine monoclonal antiendotoxin antibody in gram-negative sepsis: A randomized controlled trial. JAMA. 2000; 283:1723-1730.

312. Fisher CJ Jr, Dhainaut J-FA, Opal SM, et al. Recombinant human interleukin 1 receptor antagonist in the treatment of patients with sepsis syndrome: Results from a randomized, double-blind, placebo-controlled trial. JAMA. 1994;271:1836-1843.

313. Abraham E, Glauser MP, Butler T, et al. p55 tumor necrosis factor receptor fusion protein in the treatment of patients with severe sepsis and septic shock: A randomized controlled multicenter trial. JAMA. 1997;277:1531-1538.

314. Kieft H, Hoepelman AIM, Zhou W, et al. The sepsis syndrome in a Dutch university hospital: Clinical observations. Arch Intern Med. 1993;153:2241-2247.

315. Fisher CJ, Agosti JM, Opal SM, et al. Treatment of septic shock with the tumor necrosis factor receptor:Fc fusion protein. N Engl J Med. 1996;334:1697-1702.

CHAPTER **68**

Peritonitis and Intraperitoneal Abscesses

MATTHEW E. LEVISON

LARRY M. BUSH

Intra-abdominal infection can take several forms. Infection may be in the retroperitoneal space or within the peritoneal cavity. Intraperitoneal infection may be diffuse or localized into one or more abscesses. Intraperitoneal abscesses may form in dependent recesses, such as the pelvic space or Morrison's pouch; in the various perihepatic spaces; within the lesser sac; or along the major routes of communication between intraperitoneal recesses, such as the right paracolic gutter. In addition, infection may be contained within the intraabdominal viscera, as in hepatic, pancreatic, splenic, tubo-ovarian, or renal abscesses. Abscesses also frequently form about diseased viscera (pericholecystic, periappendiceal, pericolic, and tubo-ovarian) and between adjacent loops of bowel (i.e., interloop abscesses).

ANATOMY

The anatomic relationships within the abdomen are important in determining possible sources and routes of spread of infection. The peritoneal cavity extends from the undersurface of the diaphragm to the floor of the pelvis. In men, the peritoneal cavity is a closed space. In women, the peritoneal cavity is perforated by the free ends of the fallopian tubes. The stomach, jejunum, ileum, cecum, appendix, transverse and sigmoid colons, liver, gallbladder, and spleen lie within the peritoneal cavity, some being suspended by a mesentery.

The peritoneal reflections and mesenteric attachments compartmentalize the intraperitoneal space and route, spreading exudate to sites that often are distant from the source (Fig. 68-1). The transverse mesocolon divides the peritoneal cavity horizontally into an upper and a lower space. The greater omentum, extending from the transverse mesocolon and lower border of the stomach, covers the lower peritoneal cavity and further separates the upper from the lower peritoneal cavity (Fig. 68-2). The small bowel mesentery divides the lower peritoneal space.

The peritoneal cavity has several recesses into which exudate may become loculated. The most dependent recess of the peritoneal cavity in the supine position is in the pelvis. Between the rectum and bladder in men is a pouch of peritoneal cavity that extends slightly below the level of the seminal vesicles. In women, the uterus and fallopian tubes project into the pelvic recess. Between the rectum and the body of the uterus is the pouch of Douglas, which lies above the posterior fornix of the vagina. On either side of the rectum and bladder are the pararectal and paravesical fossae. The pelvic recess is continuous with the right and the left paracolic gutters.

The phrenicocolic ligament, which fixes the splenic flexure of the colon to the diaphragm, partially bridges the junction between the left paracolic gutter and the left perihepatic space. In contrast, the right paracolic gutter is continuous with the right subhepatic space and the right subphrenic space. A posterior superior extension of the right subhepatic space, Morrison's pouch, is the most dependent portion in the

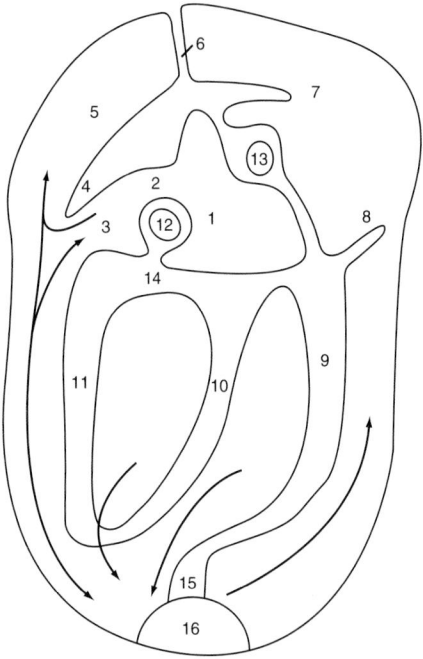

FIGURE 68-1. Schema of the posterior peritoneal reflections and recesses of the peritoneal cavity. *1,* Lesser sac; *2,* foramen of Winslow; *3,* Morrison's pouch; *4,* right triangular ligament; *5,* right subphrenic spaces; *6,* falciform ligament; *7,* left subphrenic space; *8,* phrenocolic ligament; *9,* bare area of the descending colon; *10,* root of the small bowel mesentery; *11,* bare area of the ascending colon; *12,* duodenum; *13,* esophagus; *14,* root of the transverse mesocolon; *15,* bare area of rectum; *16,* bladder.

supine position of the right paravertebral groove and lies just above the beginning of the transverse mesocolon. The horizontal posterior reflection of the serosal surface of the liver onto the diaphragm (the right triangular and coronary ligaments) and the vertical reflection (falciform ligament) divide the right perihepatic space into right subphrenic and right subhepatic spaces (see Figs. 68-1 and 68-2A). The left subphrenic and subhepatic spaces communicate freely around the smaller left lobe of the liver and its more superiorly placed left triangular ligament (see Figs. 68-1 and 68-2B).[1,2] The right and left subphrenic spaces are separated by the falciform ligament, which probably prevents the

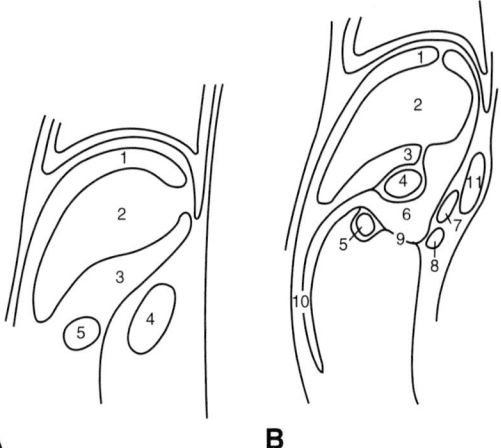

A   **B**

FIGURE 68-2. Schema of a sagittal section of the peritoneal cavity. **A,** Right upper quadrant. *1,* Subphrenic space; *2,* liver; *3,* subhepatic space; *4,* right kidney; *5,* transverse colon. **B,** Left upper quadrant. *1,* Subphrenic space; *2,* liver, left lobe; *3,* subhepatic space; *4,* stomach; *5,* transverse colon; *6,* lesser sac; *7,* pancreas; *8,* duodenum; *9,* transverse mesocolon; *10,* omemtum; *11,* left kidney.

spread of pus to the opposite side and explains why only about 5% to 15% of subphrenic abscesses are bilateral.[2] The left subhepatic space is divided by the gastrohepatic omentum into an anterior space and the lesser sac (see Fig. 68-2B). Abscesses within the perihepatic spaces become localized by pyogenic membranes. In the right subphrenic space, abscesses lie anteriorly or posteriorly and in the subhepatic space superiorly or inferiorly.[1,2] Abscesses of the left perihepatic space are either in the single left subphrenic space or in the lesser sac.[1,2]

The lesser sac, the largest recess of the peritoneal cavity, is connected to the main peritoneal space by the foramen of Winslow, an opening situated between the free border of the gastrohepatic omentum and the posterior parietal peritoneum. The lesser sac is surrounded posteriorly by the pancreas and kidneys, anteriorly by the stomach, and laterally by the liver and spleen. It also may extend to a variable extent between the folds of the greater omentum. Because of the limited communication from the lesser sac to the major cavity via the foramen of Winslow, suppuration in the lesser sac may exist with little or no involvement of the major cavity. Abscesses in the lesser sac lie between the stomach and the pancreas but may spread to the right and lie anterior to the right kidney and inferior to the liver.

After intraperitoneal injection of water-soluble contrast material selectively into various intraperitoneal spaces, Myers[3] showed that the right paracolic gutter is the main communication between the upper and the lower peritoneal cavities. Fluid introduced into the right upper peritoneal space gravitates toward Morrison's pouch, then into the right subphrenic space and along the right paracolic gutter into the pelvic recess (Fig. 68-3). Flow of fluid in the left upper peritoneal space is mainly into the left subphrenic space. The phrenicocolic ligament limits flow inferiorly into the left paracolic gutter. Fluid introduced into the lower peritoneal cavity first gravitates to the pelvic recess, then ascends, whether in the supine or erect position, along the

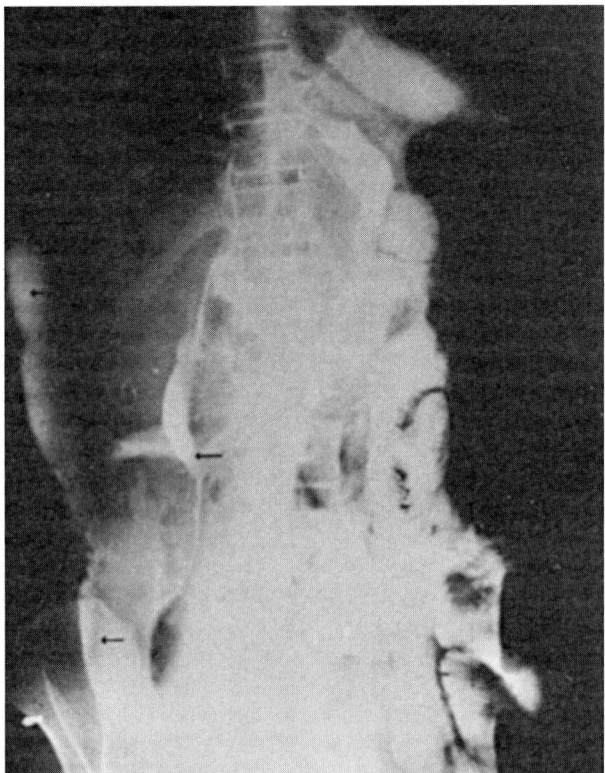

FIGURE 68-3. Abdominal radiograph (right decubitus) after oral administration of radiopaque contrast medium (Gastrografin) to a patient with dehiscence of an esophageal-gastric anastomosis. Radiopaque Gastrografin (*arrows*) can be seen in the subhepatic space, right paracolic gutter, and right subphrenic space and within the lumen of the intestinal tract.

right paracolic gutter into the right subhepatic space, especially into Morrison's pouch, and into the right subphrenic space. Ascension of fluid from the pelvic space along the left paracolic gutter is minimal and is limited by the phrenicocolic ligament. Although gravity would account for the pooling of fluid in the dependent peritoneal recesses, such as the pelvic recess and Morrison's pouch, ascension of fluid from the pelvis to the subphrenic space probably is caused by hydrostatic pressure differences between the upper and the lower peritoneal cavities created by diaphragmatic motion. Normal intestinal and abdominal wall motion also would account for some spread of intraperitoneal fluid.

The retroperitoneal space lies between the posterior peritoneal membrane and the transversalis fascia, extending from the diaphragm to the pelvic brim. In the anterior retroperitoneal space between the peritoneum and anterior renal fascia lie the ascending and descending colons, duodenum, and pancreas. The kidneys and ureters lie within the posterior retroperitoneal (perinephric) space, between the anterior and posterior renal fasciae. The renal fascia encloses the kidneys and adrenals superiorly and laterally, but not inferiorly, favoring spread of infection in this space inferiorly.[4]

The parietal peritoneum, mainly the anterior portion, is well supplied by somatic afferent nerves and is sensitive to all forms of stimuli. The ability of the anterior parietal peritoneum to sense sharp, well-localized pain in response to local inflammation is crucial in diagnosing abdominal infection and may be associated with involuntary abdominal muscle contraction, tenderness, and rebound tenderness. Irritation of the peripheral diaphragmatic peritoneum is felt as pain near the adjacent body wall, and irritation of the central portion is felt as pain referred to the shoulder. Stimulation of the visceral peritoneum, usually by distention of an organ, causes poorly localized, dull pain.

The peritoneal cavity is lined by a serous membrane. The surface area of this membrane approximates that of the skin. The membrane consists of a monolayer of flat polygonal cells, beneath which are lymphatics, blood vessels, and nerve endings. Normally the peritoneal space contains only sufficient fluid to maintain moistness of the surface, facilitating movements of the viscera. Noninflamed serous fluid is clear yellow with a low specific gravity (<1.016) and low protein content (usually <3 g/dL). The protein is predominantly albumin. Fibrinogen is not present, and serous fluid does not clot. Solute concentrations are almost identical to concentrations in plasma. A few leukocytes (<250/mm^3), mostly mononuclear cells, and desquamated serosal cells may be found.

The peritoneal membrane is highly permeable. Bidirectional transfer of substances across this membrane is rapid and, because of the large surface area involved, potentially great in quantity. The peritoneal surface has been used extensively as a dialyzing membrane for the treatment of uremia and has been used for the administration of fluid, electrolytes, antibiotics, and blood. The effective serum oncotic pressure and the hydrostatic pressure in the portal veins and lymphatics are major determinants of the rate and direction of fluid movement. The rate of movement of water and solutes between blood and peritoneal fluid also depends on concentration gradients between these compartments and has been studied in detail.[5,6] Water and solutes diffuse via blood capillaries and to a lesser extent through the lymphatics. Lymphatics are involved primarily in removal of nonirritating colloids and particles into the blood stream. Absorption into lymphatics of particulate matter is thought to occur mostly from the diaphragmatic surface and is aided by the pumping action of diaphragmatic motion.[7] After infusion of radioactive sodium chromate–labeled red blood cells into the peritoneal cavity of dogs, Rochlin and associates[8] reported absorption of about 70% of the labeled cells by 48 to 96 hours. This absorption occurred mostly through the lymphatics. In humans, two thirds of intraperitoneally injected red blood cells in anticoagulated blood have been found in the circulation 8 to 12 days after infusion.[9] The quantity of resorbed cells was less when no anticoagulant was used with the transfused cells, presumably because of trapping of red blood cells in intraperitoneal clots.[9] Transport of other particulate matter, such as intraperitoneal bacteria, may be similarly impeded because of trapping in fibrinous intraperitoneal exudate.[10]

In addition, there are communications between the peritoneal and pleural cavities that are independent of the blood stream. In patients with Meigs' syndrome, radioactive colloidal gold instilled into the peritoneal cavity appears in the pleural space, probably as a result of transdiaphragmatic lymphatic transport.[11]

PERITONITIS

Inflammation of the peritoneum may be the result of contamination of the peritoneal cavity with microorganisms, irritating chemicals, or both. Infective peritonitis has been categorized as primary, secondary, or tertiary. Peritonitis complicating peritoneal dialysis can be considered as an additional category. In the primary variety, the peritoneal infection is not related directly to other intra-abdominal abnormalities. In the secondary variety, an intra-abdominal process, such as a ruptured appendix or a perforated peptic ulcer, is evident. Tertiary peritonitis has been conceived as a later stage of the disease, when clinical peritonitis and signs of sepsis and multiorgan failure persist or recur after treatment for secondary peritonitis, and no pathogens or only low-grade pathogens (e.g., coagulase-negative staphylococci) or nosocomial, frequently multiple drug–resistant, pathogens (e.g., enterococci, *Candida,* and *Enterobacter* spp.) are isolated from the peritoneal exudate.[12,13]

Primary Peritonitis

Etiology

Primary peritonitis, sometimes referred to as *spontaneous bacterial peritonitis,* is probably not a specific entity with a common cause but represents a group of diseases with different causes having in common only infection of the peritoneal cavity without an evident source. Primary peritonitis occurs at all ages. The prevalence of primary peritonitis in children apparently has been decreasing.[14] In the preantibiotic era, primary peritonitis occurred in about 10% of all pediatric abdominal emergencies; it now accounts for less than 1% to 2%.[15,16] The decline has been attributed to widespread use of antibiotics for minor upper respiratory tract illness. Although primary peritonitis may occur in children without predisposing disease,[14] it is known to occur particularly in children with postnecrotic cirrhosis[15,17] and in 2% of children with the nephrotic syndrome.[14,18] In one study, it also frequently was associated with urinary tract infections.[15] In some nephrotic children, repeated episodes of peritonitis occur, and peritonitis may precede other manifestations of nephrosis.[14]

In adults, primary peritonitis usually has been reported in patients with cirrhosis and ascites. The prevalence of primary peritonitis in hospitalized patients with cirrhosis and ascites has been estimated at 10% to 30%.[19] Primary peritonitis occurs in patients with alcoholic cirrhosis,[20-27] postnecrotic cirrhosis,[17] chronic active hepatitis,[28] acute viral hepatitis,[29] congestive heart failure,[30] metastatic malignant disease,[31] systemic lupus erythematosus,[32] or lymphedema[33] and, rarely, in patients with no underlying disease.[34] The presence of ascites seems to be the common link among these various conditions. The risk of developing primary peritonitis is greater in patients with a coexisting gastrointestinal bleed, a previous episode of primary peritonitis, or a low ascitic fluid protein concentration.[19]

Bacteriologic Characteristics

Several decades ago, the organisms reported to cause primary peritonitis in children were *Streptococcus pneumoniae* and group A streptococci.[14-16] By the 1970s, the number of nephrotic children with streptococcal peritonitis had declined, and the relative frequency of peritonitis caused by gram-negative enteric bacilli[15,16,18] and by staphylococci[14,16] apparently had increased.

In cirrhotic patients, microorganisms presumably of enteric origin account for 69% of the pathogens.[35] *Escherichia coli* is the most frequently recovered pathogen, followed by *Klebsiella pneumoniae,* *S. pneumoniae,* and other streptococcal species, including enterococci.[20,23,35-37] *Staphylococcus aureus* is an unusual isolate in primary peritonitis, accounting for 2% to 4% of cases in most series, and it has been noted to occur in patients with an erosion of an umbilical hernia.[36] Anaerobes and microaerophilic organisms are reported infrequently.[23,27] Possible explanations include the intrinsic bacteriostatic activity of ascites against *Bacteroides* spp.,[38] the relatively high partial pressure of oxygen of ascitic fluid,[39] and the lack of optimal anaerobic bacteriologic techniques to study patients with primary peritonitis in the past. In a review of 126 cases of primary peritonitis in cirrhotic patients recorded in the literature, only 8 patients (6%) had disease caused by anaerobic or microaerophilic bacteria, including *Bacteroides* spp., *Bacteroides fragilis, Clostridium perfringens, Peptostreptococcus* spp., *Peptococcus* spp., and *Campylobacter fetus.*[23] Polymicrobial infection was present in four of these eight cirrhotic patients with peritonitis caused by anaerobes, in contrast to the relatively low frequency of polymicrobial infection (only 10 of 118 cases of peritonitis) when aerobes alone were involved.

Ascitic fluid with positive cultures but few leukocytes, termed *bacterascites,* in patients without clinical findings of peritonitis has been noted.[37] This condition may represent early colonization before a host response.[27] Patients with a low leukocyte response have the same mortality rate as patients with a greater response, however.[26] Conversely, several series have identified cases of primary peritonitis with negative ascitic fluid cultures.[20,27] In one series, sterile cultures occurred in 35% of patients with clinical findings consistent with primary peritonitis, ascitic fluid leukocyte counts greater than 500/mm^3, and no evident source of intra-abdominal infection.[40] Blood cultures were positive in one third of these patients.[40] The frequency of culture-negative ascitic fluid may be decreased by inoculating blood-cultured bottles with ascitic fluid at the bedside.[41]

Bacteremia is present in 75% of patients with primary peritonitis caused by aerobic bacteria,[35] but it rarely is found in patients with peritonitis caused by anaerobes.[23] Usually the same organisms isolated from the peritoneal fluid are recovered from the blood.[20,23] Occasionally, peritonitis may result from infection with *Mycobacterium tuberculosis, Neisseriae gonorrhoeae, Chlamydia trachomatis,* or *Coccidioides immitis,* but this is usually the result of disseminated infection or sometimes spread from adjacent foci of infection (see "Pathogenesis").

Pathogenesis

The route of infection in primary peritonitis usually is not apparent, and often it is presumed to be hematogenous, lymphogenous, or transmural migration through an intact gut wall from the intestinal lumen or, in women, from the vagina via the fallopian tubes. Enteric bacteria have been postulated to migrate from the bowel lumen into mesenteric lymph and to enter the systemic circulation via the thoracic duct, a process termed *bacterial translocation.*[42] Enteric bacteria also could enter the systemic circulation from the portal vein by passage through the liver or by portosystemic shunts in patients with portal hypertension.[20] The hepatic reticuloendothelial system is known to be a major site for removal of bacteria from blood.[43] Conn and Fessel[20] postulated that organisms removed from the systemic circulation by the liver contaminate hepatic lymph and pass through the permeable lymphatic walls into the ascitic fluid. Animal studies have suggested, however, that destruction of blood-borne bacteria by the reticuloendothelial system is impaired in experimental cirrhosis[44] and in alcoholic liver disease.[45] Infection of ascitic fluid would be facilitated by impaired reticuloendothelial clearance of bacteria from the blood stream, which would tend to perpetuate bacteremia and increase the opportunity to cause metastatic infection at susceptible sites, such as the ascitic collection. Primary bacteremia, usually caused by coliforms, is a common complication in cirrhosis,[46] and metastatic infection in the pleural space has been reported in cirrhotic patients.[47] An increased frequency of gram-negative endocarditis also has been noted in cirrhotics.[48]

Additionally, alcohol abuse and cirrhosis have been reported to be associated with impaired intracellular killing by monocytes and neutrophils[49] and with impaired opsonization[50] and low levels of serum complement.[51] The decrease in phagocytic activity seen in alcoholic cirrhosis is proportional to the severity of the liver disease.[52] Impaired local defenses in the peritoneal cavity also facilitate infection of ascites. Opsonic activity, as reflected by low levels of complement and immunoglobulins, is reduced in the ascitic fluid of patients with the nephrotic syndrome and cirrhosis.[53,54]

Enteric bacteria also may gain access to the peritoneal cavity by directly traversing the intact intestinal wall. This activity has been shown in animals. Schweinburg and coworkers[55] showed in dogs that radioactive carbon–labeled *E. coli* passed from the bowel into the peritoneal cavity after the introduction of hypertonic solutions into the peritoneum. A similar mechanism may explain the enteric bacterial peritonitis that frequently complicates peritoneal dialysis.[56] The infrequent occurrence of bacteremia and the multiplicity of species in peritoneal fluid when anaerobic bacteria are involved suggest that transmural migration of bacteria is the probable route of infection of ascitic fluid in most of these patients.[23] In addition, the occurrence of polymicrobial anaerobic peritonitis in two patients after infusion of vasopressin into the superior mesenteric or gastroduodenal arteries suggested that arterial vasoconstriction decreased the intestinal mucosal barrier and permitted transmural migration of enteric organisms.[22] Colonic microorganisms have been reported to colonize the upper small bowel in cirrhotic patients.[57]

The simultaneous presence of pneumococci in vaginal secretions and peritoneal fluid in prepubertal girls[58] makes an ascending infection of genital origin likely in these patients. The alkaline vaginal secretions of prepubertal girls may be less inhibitory to bacterial growth than the acidic secretions of postpubertal women. Transfallopian spread also is suggested by the development of peritonitis in women with intrauterine devices.[59,60] The route of spread in women with gonococcal or chlamydial perihepatitis (Fitz-Hugh-Curtis syndrome) is presumably from the fallopian tubes and paracolic gutters to the subphrenic space, but it also may be hematogenous. In the one man with this syndrome, *N. gonorrhoeae* was recovered from a liver biopsy specimen, and the route of spread presumably was via bacteremia.[61]

Although tuberculous peritonitis may result from direct entry into the peritoneal cavity of tubercle bacilli (from the lymph nodes, intestine, or genital tract in patients with active disease of these organs), it is more likely to result from hematogenous dissemination from remote foci of tuberculosis, most commonly in the lung. Tuberculous peritonitis can become clinically evident after the initial focus has healed completely.

Infection of ascites stimulates a dramatic increase in proinflammatory cytokines, such as tumor necrosis factor (TNF)-α and interleukin (IL)-6, and soluble adhesion molecules in the ascitic fluid and serum,[62,63] which may lead to further reduction of effective arterial blood volume, as indicated by an increase in plasma renin activity and the development of renal insufficiency. Approximately 30% of patients with primary peritonitis develop renal insufficiency, which has been found to be the most sensitive predictor of in-hospital mortality.

Clinical Manifestations

Primary peritonitis is an acute febrile illness often confused with acute appendicitis in children. Fever, abdominal pain, nausea, vomiting, and diarrhea usually are present with diffuse abdominal tenderness, rebound tenderness, and hypoactive or absent bowel sounds. In cirrhotic patients with primary peritonitis, preexisting ascites is present. In some patients, the clinical manifestations are atypical. The onset may be insidious, and findings of peritoneal irritation may be absent in an abdomen distended with ascites. Fever (>37.8° C [>100° F]) is the most common presenting sign, occurring in 50% to 80% of cases,[20,26] and may be present without abdominal signs or symptoms, or the process may be completely silent. Primary peritonitis in cirrhotic patients generally is associated with other features of end-stage liver disease (hepatorenal syndrome,[64] progressive encephalopathy, and

variceal bleeding). Primary peritonitis always should be considered in the differential diagnosis of decompensation of previously stable chronic liver disease.

Gonococcal perihepatitis (Fitz-Hugh-Curtis syndrome) most often occurs in women. It manifests with sudden onset of pain in the right upper quadrant of the abdomen, at times referred to the right shoulder. There may be low-grade fever, right upper quadrant tenderness, guarding, and a friction rub over the liver.[65] Gonococcal cervicitis or salpingitis may or may not be clinically evident. Chlamydial perihepatitis and gonococcal perihepatitis are clinically indistinguishable.

Primary tuberculous peritonitis usually is gradual in onset, with fever, weight loss, malaise, night sweats, and abdominal distention. The abdomen may not be rigid and often is characterized as being "doughy" on palpation. The findings at operation or laparoscopy consist of multiple nodules scattered over the peritoneal surface and omentum. Adhesions and a variable amount of peritoneal fluid usually are present. Similarly, *C. immitis* can cause a granulomatous peritonitis with a variable clinical manifestation.[66]

Laboratory Findings

Fluid obtained by paracentesis should be examined for cell count, differential count, and protein concentration, and a Gram stain and culture of the fluid should be obtained.[67] A polymorphonuclear leukocyte count in peritoneal fluid greater than 250 cells/mm³ is considered diagnostic of primary peritonitis, even when culture of ascitic fluid is negative.[19] An increase in the leukocyte count in ascitic fluid has been noted, however, during diuresis in patients with chronic liver disease.[68] Gram staining of the sediment, when positive, is diagnostic, but it is negative in 60% to 80% of patients with primary peritonitis.[20,25] Culture of ascitic fluid may be negative in 40% of patients with a clinical picture of primary peritonitis and an elevated ascitic fluid polymorphonuclear leukocyte count.[19,24] The ascitic fluid protein concentration may be low[20] perhaps because of (1) hypoalbuminemia[69] or (2) dilution of ascitic fluid with transudate from the portal system when there is cirrhosis or the portal vein is obstructed.[70] Other parameters of ascitic fluid that might help in diagnosing primary bacterial peritonitis are lactate concentration greater than 25 mg/dL and pH less than 7.35.[71-73] Ascitic fluid in tuberculous peritonitis may have an elevated protein concentration (>3 g/dL) and a lymphocytic pleocytosis, but neither may be present, especially in cirrhotic patients.[74]

Diagnosis

The diagnosis of primary peritonitis is one of exclusion of a primary intra-abdominal source of infection. Oral and intravenous contrast material with computed tomography (CT) has enhanced greatly detection of intra-abdominal sources of peritonitis. Surgery often can be directed toward a potential source of infection identified on the basis of CT findings, rather than the approach of a full exploratory laparotomy, which was used more commonly before the availability of CT in this setting and was associated with high mortality in certain groups of patients, such as cirrhotics.[75] Patients with primary peritonitis usually respond within 48 to 72 hours to appropriate antimicrobial therapy.[76] The observation of an exponential rate of decline in the number of ascitic fluid leukocytes after the initiation of antimicrobial therapy for primary peritonitis also has been found to help differentiate primary from secondary bacterial peritonitis.[77]

Recovery of pneumococci from peritoneal fluid may not indicate primary peritonitis, as illustrated by a case report of appendicitis and secondary peritonitis due to pneumococci.[78] For this reason, some surgeons have considered the differential diagnosis in children between appendicitis and primary peritonitis too difficult to make without operative examination, even when gram-positive bacteria are identified in peritoneal fluid.[16] Paracentesis for smear and culture is indicated in all cirrhotic patients with ascites and in children with gross proteinuria and abdominal pain, whether or not the diagnosis of nephrotic syndrome has been established. Paracentesis is not without hazard, however, especially in patients with hemorrhagic tendencies and bowel distention. In a retrospective analysis of 242 consecutive diagnostic abdominal paracenteses in patients with liver disease and ascites, major complications were reported in 7, including perforation of the bowel with generalized peritonitis or abdominal wall abscess and serious hemorrhage.[79]

The diagnosis of tuberculous peritonitis usually can be made at operation or laparoscopy and confirmed by the histologic characteristics of the peritoneal biopsy specimen[80] and by bacteriologic examination of the peritoneal biopsy specimen and fluid.[81] The diagnosis of *C. immitis* peritonitis is made best by culture of ascitic fluid.[66] The laboratory should be apprised of this diagnostic possibility because isolation of the fungus is a biohazard.

Prognosis

The treatment of primary peritonitis has been reported to be successful in more than half of cirrhotic patients, but because of the frequency of accompanying end-stage cirrhosis, the overall mortality rate in cirrhotic adults has been 95%.[20] More recent studies have reported lower mortality rates of 70% and 57%, however, with 28% and 40%, respectively, dying from the primary peritonitis.[25,26] Patients with the poorest prognosis were found to have renal insufficiency,[64] hypothermia, hyperbilirubinemia, and hypoalbuminemia. The lower mortality rates in these later series perhaps can be explained by the less frequent occurrence of hepatic encephalopathy. The lowest hospitalization mortality and infection-related mortality rates (37.8% and 2.2), reported more recently, were attributed to early diagnosis and treatment.[76] Treatment of peritonitis caused by gram-positive organisms and of early infections has been more frequently successful than treatment of gram-negative or late infections. In nephrotic patients with gram-positive infections and patients who do not have a preterminal underlying illness, the survival rate is higher than 90%.[14]

Treatment

Because the Gram stain frequently is negative in primary bacterial peritonitis, the initial choice of antimicrobial drug often is empirical, based on the most likely pathogens. The antimicrobial regimen can be modified when the results of the culture and susceptibility tests are available. Some third-generation cephalosporin antibiotics have been shown to be as efficacious as the combination of ampicillin plus an aminoglycoside for empirical therapy in primary bacterial peritonitis.[82] The third-generation cephalosporins also avoid the risk of nephrotoxicity, which is sufficiently common in this group of patients to warrant the avoidance of aminoglycosides if an equally effective alternative antimicrobial regimen can be used.[26,83] In addition, these extended-spectrum cephalosporins may be effective in treating patients who are suspected of being infected with a fluoroquinolone-resistant pathogen as a consequence of their having taken oral fluoroquinolone prophylaxis.[84] Other antimicrobial agents, such as broad-spectrum penicillins (e.g., ticarcillin and piperacillin), carbapenems (e.g., imipenem, meropenem, and ertapenem), β-lactam/β-lactamase combinations (e.g., piperacillin-tazobactam, ticarcillin-clavulanate, and ampicillin-sulbactam), and the newer fluoroquinolones (e.g., levofloxacin, gatifloxacin, and moxifloxacin), are potential alternatives.[19] Although intravenous antimicrobial therapy may be preferred, oral administration of antibiotics, such as amoxicillin-clavulanate or fluoroquinolones, may be equally efficacious in uncomplicated patients.[19]

Primary bacterial peritonitis caused by either *S. pneumoniae* or group A streptococci is treated best with high-dose penicillin, ceftriaxone, or cefotaxime. If the pneumococcal strain is highly resistant to these drugs, vancomycin is the preferred drug, and it may be prudent to include vancomycin until sensitivities of pneumococci are ascertained. Peritonitis suspected of being caused by methicillin-sensitive *S. aureus* should be treated with a penicillinase-resistant penicillin (e.g., nafcillin) or with a first-generation cephalosporin (e.g., cefazolin); if the strain is methicillin resistant or the patient is allergic to penicillin, vancomycin can be used. If *Pseudomonas aeruginosa* is isolated, an antipseudomonal penicillin, ceftazidime, cefepime, aztreonam, a carbapenem (e.g., imipenem, meropenem), or a fluoroquinolone with good antipseudomonal activity (e.g.,

ciprofloxacin) combined with another antipseudomonal antibiotic[85] should be used, although use of aminoglycosides is discouraged because of nephrotoxicity.[86]

In cases in which there is a strong clinical suspicion of primary bacterial peritonitis but all cultures are sterile, antimicrobial therapy should be continued. Clinical improvement together with a significant decline in the ascitic fluid leukocyte count of greater than 25% should occur after 24 to 48 hours of antimicrobial therapy if the diagnosis is correct.[76,77,87] Lack of the expected clinical response or persistence of an elevated ascitic fluid leukocyte count should make other diagnoses a consideration. Antimicrobial therapy should be continued for 10 to 14 days if improvement is noted; however, shorter course (5-day) therapy has been shown to be as efficacious.[76] The administration of intraperitoneal antimicrobials is not necessary. Antibiotic therapy has been supplemented effectively by intravenous albumin infusion to prevent renal insufficiency, which occurs in about one third of patients with primary peritonitis as a consequence of further reduction in effective arterial blood volume with a resultant increased renin-angiotensin-aldosterone system activity in one study.[86]

Prevention

Patients who have survived one episode of primary peritonitis have an increased 1-year probability of another episode.[88] Selective decontamination of the bowel with oral norfloxacin (400 mg daily)[89] or trimethoprim-sulfamethoxazole (one double-strength dose given once daily for 5 days each week) has been shown to decrease the frequency of spontaneous bacterial peritonitis and may be an option in patients awaiting liver transplantation, but it has not been shown otherwise to confer a survival advantage.[90]

Secondary Peritonitis

Etiology

Secondary intra-abdominal infection usually is caused by spillage of gastrointestinal or genitourinary microorganisms into the peritoneal cavity secondary to loss of the integrity of the mucosal barrier. The primary intra-abdominal processes that can give rise to secondary peritonitis are numerous and include diseases or injuries of the gastrointestinal or genitourinary tracts (e.g., perforation of a peptic ulcer; traumatic perforation of the uterus, urinary bladder, stomach, or small or large bowel; spontaneous perforation associated with typhoid, tuberculous,[91] amebic, *Strongyloides* or cytomegalovirus ulcers in immunocompromised persons; appendicitis, diverticulitis, or intestinal neoplasms; gangrene of the bowel from strangulation, bowel obstruction, or mesenteric vascular obstruction; suppurative cholecystitis; bile peritonitis; pancreatitis; operative contamination of the peritoneum or disruption of a surgical anastomosis site; septic abortion, puerperal sepsis, postoperative uterine infection, or endometritis complicating an intrauterine device[92]; gonococcal salpingitis or gonococcal vulvo-vaginitis in children; suppurative prostatitis; and rupture of an intraperitoneal or visceral abscess, such as renal or perinephric, tubo-ovarian, liver, splenic, or pancreatic abscess). Peritonitis is a major hazard of chronic ambulatory peritoneal dialysis (CAPD) used in the management of renal failure, fluid and electrolytic imbalance, and certain intoxications.[56] Bacterial peritonitis commonly occurs secondary to the use of peritoneovenous and ventriculoperitoneal shunts.[93,94]

Microbiologic Characteristics

Infrequently, exogenous microorganisms, such as *S. aureus, N. gonorrhoeae,* or *M. tuberculosis,* which cause infection in intra-abdominal or adjacent viscera and spread to involve the peritoneum, cause secondary peritonitis. Most cases of secondary peritonitis are endogenous in origin, however, and are caused by the large number and variety of microorganisms that normally colonize mucous membranes lining certain viscera within the abdominal cavity. Although forming a continuous surface, the mucous membranes of the stomach, upper small bowel, lower small bowel, and large bowel each have a characteristic microflora in terms of type of microbial species, total number of different species, and microbial density. The vagina also has a distinct microflora. Normally, invasive activities of indigenous bacteria are controlled by the intact mucosa of the gastrointestinal tract and vagina. Disturbances in this mucosal barrier can occur as a result of spontaneous disease, trauma, or surgical operations that permit escape of indigenous bacteria and cause an infection of the peritoneum, the abdominal viscera, or the retroperitoneal space. The frequency with which various indigenous organisms are recovered from intra-abdominal infections varies according to the site of the primary process and whether the primary process is associated with an alteration of the indigenous microflora.[95]

The stomach normally contains 10^3 colony-forming units (CFU) of microorganisms per milliliter in the fasting state. If bacteria are present, they are mostly facultative, gram-positive, salivary microorganisms, such as *Candida*, lactobacilli, and streptococci. The numbers of these organisms in stomach contents transiently increase after a meal.[96] Gastric flora is more numerous and may be composed of different organisms when there is achlorhydria (e.g., from cimetidine) or blood in the stomach.[96,97] The flora of the upper small intestine is normally sparse and consists of salivary microorganisms.[98] In the presence of achlorhydria,[96] intestinal obstruction, or other processes affecting intestinal motility or absorption, however, the flora of the small intestine is more profuse and varied. Conditions that favor small bowel stasis include scleroderma, regional enteritis, small bowel strictures, nontropical sprue, tropical sprue, duodenal and jejunal diverticula, presence of an afferent loop of the Billroth II gastrojejunostomy, and intestinal pseudo-obstruction.[99] Large bowel flora has been found in the proximal small bowel of cirrhotic patients.[57] The ileum normally contains *E. coli*, enterococci, and an equal number of microorganisms that are obligately anaerobic, such as *B. fragilis*.[98] It is the colon, however, in which a profuse microflora exists in concentrations of about 10^{11} bacteria per milliliter of feces, a wet sludge of practically pure bacteria.[100] The colonic flora is composed predominantly of the obligate anaerobes *B. fragilis* and *Bifidobacterium* spp., which outnumber facultative microorganisms, primarily *E. coli*, by 10^3:1 to 10^4:1. Other colonic bacteria are viridans streptococci, enterococci, *Eubacterium* spp., *Klebsiella* spp., *Proteus* spp., *Enterobacter* spp., and *C. perfringens*. The large bowel flora is relatively stable[100] but may be altered significantly by antibiotic therapy.[101]

With loss of the integrity of the mucosal barrier at some point along the gastrointestinal tract, a variable number of bacteria (in terms of bacterial density and number of different species) is found in the peritoneal cavity, depending on the level of the mucosal defect and comorbid conditions. With perforation of the colon, initially a total of more than 10^{11} CFU/mL of hundreds of different species spills into the peritoneal cavity. A simplification of the microflora occurs so that when peritoneal infection is established, only about five species are isolated from peritoneal exudate, usually three anaerobic and two aerobic species, even when care is exercised to ensure recovery of the obligate anaerobes. The obligate anaerobes isolated from clinical specimens have been found to be more oxygen tolerant and to have identifiable virulence factors compared with the rest of the anaerobic microflora in the gut. The facultative anaerobes isolated also have virulence factors. *B. fragilis* is the most frequently isolated obligate anaerobe after colonic perforation, and *E. coli* is the most frequently isolated facultative anaerobe.

As would be anticipated from the nature of the gastrointestinal flora, Altemeier[102] reported anaerobes in 96% of 100 cases of peritonitis secondary to acute appendicitis with perforation. *Prevotella melaninogenica* and anaerobic gram-positive cocci were the most frequent isolates. Studies of the bacteriologic characteristics of intra-abdominal infections,[103-105] using modern bacteriologic techniques that provide an anaerobic environment during collection, transport, and incubation, have confirmed the findings of Altemeier that anaerobes play a major role. Finegold[103] reported that in a series of 73 intra-abdominal infections, including 16 cases of peritonitis, there were an average of 4.5 isolates per case (range 1 to 12 organisms), with 2.5 anaerobes and 2 aerobes or facultative organisms. The most common isolate was

E. coli, followed by *B. fragilis* (the most common anaerobic isolate), enterococci, other *Bacteroides* spp., *Fusobacterium*, *C. perfringens*, other clostridia, *Peptococcus*, *Peptostreptococcus*, and *Eubacterium*. Similar findings were reported by Gorbach and coworkers[104] in a series of 43 patients, including 10 with peritonitis, in 93% of whom anaerobes or a mixture of anaerobes and facultative organisms were recovered, and by Swenson and colleagues[106] in a series of 64 patients, including 26 with peritonitis, in 81% of whom anaerobes were recovered. In these series, bacteremia was reported in 20% to 30% of patients. Organisms recovered from blood frequently included *B. fragilis* or *E. coli*. In a series of patients with *Bacteroides* bacteremia, 14% to 62% had a gastrointestinal source.[107-110]

In a study of perforated appendicitis in which careful anaerobic culture techniques were used, an average of 9.4 species of anaerobes were isolated from each patient.[111] *Bilophila wadsworthia*, a more recently recognized anaerobic gram-negative bacillus, was the fourth most common obligate anaerobe recovered and was found in one third of patients with gangrenous appendicitis and half of patients with perforated appendicitis.[112]

Relatively antibiotic-resistant organisms, such as *Candida*, enterococci, *Enterobacter*, *Serratia*, *Acinetobacter*, and *P. aeruginosa*, are isolated more frequently from patients whose intra-abdominal infection developed while they were in the hospital, after they received broad-spectrum antimicrobial agents.[113,114] Several studies have found, however, that *P. aeruginosa* makes up a more significant portion of the aerobic isolates in community-acquired intra-abdominal infections[115-118] than had been noted previously.[119] Monomicrobial infections with microorganisms that have relatively low pathogenicity, such as *Candida*, enterococci, or coagulase-negative staphylococci, also have been observed in what was thought to be new-onset peritonitis in patients with severely impaired defenses.[120] Penetrating injuries to the liver and spleen rarely are followed by infection because of the usual sterility of these organs.[121]

Quantitative studies[122-124] of sexually active women of childbearing age have revealed that the predominant vaginal microflora is composed of five to seven different microorganisms and that anaerobes are approximately 10 times more numerous than facultative organisms. There are about 10^8 to 10^9 CFU of anaerobes and about 10^7 to 10^8 CFU of facultative organisms per milliliter of vaginal secretions. The most frequent isolates in titers of 10^5 per milliliter or more are obligate or facultative anaerobic lactobacilli, nonenterococcal streptococci, anaerobic gram-positive cocci, Bacteroidaceae other than *B. fragilis* (e.g., *P. melaninogenica*, *Prevotella bivia*, *Prevotella ruminicola*), and a group of unidentified catalase-negative facultative bacilli. Diphtheroids and *S. epidermidis* also have been reported to be frequent vaginal isolates.[124] When specifically looked for, *Gardnerella vaginalis* in high counts also has been found to be only slightly less common than lactobacilli in the vaginal secretions of healthy women.[122,123]

Colonic organisms, such as *B. fragilis*, Enterobacteriaceae, and enterococci, are found rarely as predominant components of the normal vaginal flora and probably proliferate at this site only under exceptional circumstances. These organisms have been reported to appear in vaginal secretions in the immediate postoperative period after vaginal operations,[125] and *C. perfringens* has been reported more frequently in vaginal secretions after difficult labor or abortion.[126] Hite and colleagues[127] noted the relative infrequency of *Bacteroides* and anaerobic gram-positive cocci in the vagina of healthy prenatal women, whereas during the puerperium, in women with postpartum endometritis and noninfected women, these organisms were found to be more prevalent.[127,128] Factors favoring colonization by these anaerobes after surgery and in the puerperium are unknown but possibly are related to blood or necrotic tissue, which provides the reduced, enriched environment required by these anaerobes.

Sequential sampling of vaginal secretions during the menstrual cycle has been reported to show constant levels of anaerobes, although recovery of specific organisms varied from specimen to specimen in each woman.[124] In contrast, levels of facultative organisms decrease 100-fold in the premenstrual week.[124] This variation in microflora may reflect cyclic fluctuation in the vaginal environment caused by changes in hormonal activity during the menstrual cycle. Because the vaginal flora varies under certain conditions, and members of this flora have differing pathogenicity, the frequency of endogenous intra-abdominal infections of gynecologic origin and the types of pathogens involved vary accordingly. The frequency of vaginal colonization with group B streptococci increases during pregnancy, and infections caused by these organisms are relatively common in the postpartum period.[129] In addition, in women with trichomoniasis, *Bacteroides* spp. may be found more often in vaginal secretions.[123,127] Postpartum infection, presumably caused by anaerobes, has been reported to be more common in women who have trichomoniasis during pregnancy.[130]

The bacteriologic characteristics of intra-abdominal infections that complicate female genital tract infections are similar to those of secondary peritonitis from a gastrointestinal source except for the occurrence of *N. gonorrhoeae* in cul-de-sac aspirates.[131] According to data compiled by Swenson,[132] Thadepalli,[133] and Chow[134] and their colleagues, anaerobes were found in 72% of 200 gynecologic infections. Anaerobes were especially frequent (92%) in closed-space infections, such as tubo-ovarian and pelvic abscesses. *Bacteroides* spp., in particular *B. fragilis* and *P. melaninogenica,* and anaerobic gram-positive cocci were the most frequently isolated anaerobes. *E. coli* and streptococci were the most prevalent facultative organisms. Bacteriologic studies have shown in most patients, even patients with acute salpingitis, the presence of anaerobes, usually gram-positive cocci in cul-de-sac aspirates, despite the recovery of gonococci from the endocervix.[135-137] The data are interpreted as supporting the concept of superinfection with anaerobes late in the course of this disease, after initial infection with *N. gonorrhoeae.*[138] In children, gonococcal peritonitis has been reported rarely with gonococcal vulvovaginitis.[139,140]

Intraperitoneal rupture has been reported in 10% of cases of amebic liver abscess, and it may cause acute generalized peritonitis or, less commonly, a localized intraperitoneal abscess, with a mortality rate of about 18%.[141] Perforation of the colon with bacterial peritonitis due to fulminant amebic colitis also is unusual but often fatal.[142] Similarly, *Strongyloides stercoralis* infestation of the small bowel rarely may cause fatal peritonitis, with or without concurrent bacterial contamination.[143] Intestinal perforation complicating penetrating cytomegalovirus enterocolitis has been described as a cause of acute abdomen in these patients. *Candida* has been isolated from the abdominal fluid of patients undergoing peritoneal dialysis, as has *S. aureus,* Enterobacteriaceae, and *P. aeruginosa.*[144] *Candida* peritonitis also has been observed as a complication of gastrointestinal surgery or in perforation of a viscus,[145,146] and its occurrence is related to numerous factors that increase the rate of *Candida* colonization in the gastrointestinal tract. These factors include immunosuppression, prolonged hospitalization, and antimicrobial or antacid therapy. *Candida* most commonly is isolated from the peritoneum after perforation of a gastric or duodenal peptic ulcer or after spillage of colonic contents into the peritoneum as a result of trauma, mesenteric artery occlusion, or dehiscence of a surgical anastomosis.

Pathogenesis

The virulence of the bacteria that cause peritonitis is enhanced when certain microorganisms either are combined intraperitoneally with substances such as mucus, enzymes, or hemoglobin or are combined with certain other microorganisms. Chemical peritonitis can be produced by escape of bile or of gastric or pancreatic secretions into the peritoneal cavity. When gastric acid escapes into the peritoneal cavity, there is an outpouring of serum protein and electrolytes from the blood into the peritoneal cavity. The acidity is neutralized quickly by these buffers and by diffusion of hydrogen ions into the body fluids.[147,148] Widespread necrosis may result from enzymatic digestion after intraperitoneal spillage of potent pancreatic enzymes. Escape of bile into the peritoneal cavity generally is considered to be a grave, often fatal situation.[149,150] The severity of peritonitis after escape of these intestinal secretions results in subsequent bacterial peritonitis. In a dog model with experimentally produced partial biliary diversion into the

peritoneal cavity, fatal effects were reduced by oral nonabsorbable or parenteral antibiotics.[151] Bacteria may enter the peritoneal cavity with contaminated intestinal secretions through perforations in the gastrointestinal wall or by migration through the wall of the intact gastrointestinal tract in response to the irritation of bile and possibly other intestinal tract secretions on the serosal surface.[55]

Nemir and associates[152,153] showed that after experimental strangulation obstruction of a loop of bowel in a dog model, the animal usually died within 36 hours, and the peritoneal fluid at first was light pink and eventually became black. When this black fluid was removed and injected into the peritoneal cavity of a healthy animal, the recipient also developed a similar fatal peritonitis, but the early peritoneal fluid was nontoxic.[152-154] The toxicity largely could be counteracted by instilling antibiotics into the obstructed loop of intestine or by giving antibiotics simultaneously when the fluid was injected into healthy animals.[155,156] Many workers previously showed that intraperitoneal injection of large numbers of organisms in pure culture is incapable of producing peritonitis unless some additional factor is present, such as gum tragacanth, talc, mucin, turpentine, or another irritant. It seemed unlikely that the toxicity of strangulation obstruction fluid was caused by its bacterial content alone. It has been reported that viable bacteria in addition to the presence of free hemoglobin in the peritoneal fluid are necessary to account for the lethality of bowel strangulation and of the fluid that collects in the peritoneal cavity after bowel strangulation.[157-159] The mechanism by which free hemoglobin enhances peritoneal infection is unknown but perhaps is related to free iron. Iron is required for bacterial metabolism and, in amounts that leave an excess of free iron after having saturated transferrin, may enhance greatly infections caused by certain microorganisms, such as Enterobacteriaceae and *C. perfringens.*[160] Hau and colleagues[161] showed that intraperitoneal hemoglobin depresses the influx of granulocytes into the peritoneal cavity in response to intraperitoneal bacteria, and hemoglobin depresses in vitro the chemotactic response of granulocytes and monocytes.

Intraperitoneal fluid and fibrin that enter the peritoneal cavity as a result of the increased vascular permeability caused by local trauma or bacterial infection are important components of the inflammatory response and play adjuvant roles. Low numbers of *E. coli* in small volumes of saline infused intraperitoneally are innocuous, but these numbers can become lethal in direct proportion to the increase in the volume of saline infused; this is thought to be related to dilution of opsonic proteins.[162] Trapping of bacteria beneath layers of fibrin may limit their spread but also may lead to abscess formation and isolation of bacteria from host defense mechanisms.[163-165]

Many other substances, such as hog gastric mucin, bile salts,[166] and barium sulfate,[167,168] have been used as adjuvants in producing lethal intraperitoneal infections. The mechanisms of their effects have been the subject of numerous studies. It has been postulated that hog gastric mucin coats bacteria, protecting them from intraperitoneal phagocytosis.[169]

Cuevas and Fine[170] attributed the lethality of bowel strangulation and infectious or chemical irritation of the serosal surface of the bowel to endotoxemia. Endotoxin was thought to escape from the gut lumen, cross the intact bowel wall into the peritoneal cavity, and become absorbed into the systemic circulation. Within minutes after experimental superior mesenteric artery occlusion, endotoxin was detected in the systemic circulation before its appearance in the portal vein.[170] Similarly, endotoxin levels were reported to be increased in plasma or peritoneal fluid of patients with severe intra-abdominal infection, but this parameter was not of prognostic significance.[171]

Secondary peritonitis usually is a mixed infection involving predominantly obligate and facultative anaerobes. Obligate anaerobes are sensitive to oxygen in the molecular form and to bound oxygen, as in organic peroxides. Survival and growth of anaerobes also depend on the oxidation-reduction potential (i.e., the oxidizing capacity of the environment). Most pathogenic anaerobes require a negative potential of at least -150 mV. Low oxidation-reduction potentials are thought to occur in many abscesses,[172] and oxidation-reduction potentials of -150 mV or less are measured in abscesses from which anaerobes are recovered.[173] Some anaerobic organisms have additional requirements, such as vitamin K, arginine, serum, blood pigments, or bile, before growth is obtained. Establishment of an anaerobic infection requires an environment in which the oxygen tension is low, the oxidation-reduction potential is low, and abundant nutrients are available to support anaerobic metabolism. These requirements usually are met by devitalized tissue as a consequence of ischemia, trauma, or neoplastic growth. When proper conditions are obtained, anaerobic organisms can achieve doubling rates equivalent to rates seen with aerobic enteric bacilli. In vivo, the rapidly expanding bacterial and inflammatory cell mass, frequently accompanied by gas production, can interrupt the blood supply to the immediately surrounding tissue and cause further tissue necrosis.

Gram-negative anaerobic cocci and bacilli (including *B. fragilis* and *P. melaninogenica*) possess endotoxins with much weaker biologic activity compared with endotoxins extracted from their aerobic counterparts, and they have low or absent 2-keto-3-deoxyoctanoate content.[174] In addition, certain anaerobes elaborate collagenase,[175] other proteolytic enzymes, and deoxyribonuclease.[176] Certain Bacteroidaceae are capable of degrading heparin,[177] a capability that may be responsible for the suppurative thrombophlebitis frequently seen in infections caused by these microorganisms.[178] These factors tend to provide more areas well adapted to the growth requirements of the anaerobe, with the result that the infection progresses.

In addition, anaerobes may be resistant to host defenses. Although leukocytes have been shown to have bactericidal activity under aerobic and anaerobic conditions against several anaerobic species, including *B. fragilis,* presumably by mechanisms other than those dependent on the superoxide anion O_2^- or H_2O_2,[179] Keusch and Douglas[180] found that granulocytic killing of *C. perfringens* was impaired under anaerobic conditions. Also, a capsule has been demonstrated on *B. fragilis*[181] and *Porphyromonas asaccharolytica* (formerly *B. melaninogenicus* spp. *asaccharolyticus*),[182] which might protect the organisms from phagocytosis and favor abscess formation.[183-185] Some anaerobes, especially *B. fragilis,* may be resistant to the normal bactericidal activity of serum.[179]

Many anaerobic infections seem to be synergistic. Although it is probable that most bacteria isolated in mixed infections are nonpathogenic by themselves, their presence nevertheless may be essential for the pathogenicity of the bacterial mixture. These examples of bacterial synergism in infection were shown in periodontal infection by Socransky and Gibbons[186] and in peritonitis by Altemeier.[187]

Facultative organisms in mixed infections may be essential by providing a sufficiently reduced environment for the growth of obligate anaerobic organisms. Another mechanism of bacterial synergy is the generation of a substance by one organism that is essential for the growth of another (e.g., the production of vitamin K, a required growth factor for *P. melaninogenica,* by diphtheroids). Anaerobes such as *Bacteroides* spp. also have shown the ability to protect aerobic bacteria from phagocytic killing[188,189] and from otherwise effective antibiotic therapy (e.g., via β-lactamase production).[190]

In addition, each component of the pathogenic mixture may contribute in different ways to the clinical picture. In a series of experiments, Weinstein and coworkers[191] clarified the sequence of events that occurs after contamination of the peritoneum with fecal flora. In this model, after implantation of fecal contents intraperitoneally into rats, Onderdonk and associates[192] observed that *E. coli* initially predominated in the peritoneal exudate. Bacteremia, caused by *E. coli* during this phase, was uniformly present and frequently fatal. In rats that survived, indolent intra-abdominal abscesses developed in which *B. fragilis* predominated. Elimination of *E. coli* by early administration of gentamicin reduced early mortality but did not prevent late intra-abdominal abscess caused by obligate anaerobes; elimination of obligate anaerobes with clindamycin did not prevent early mortality from *E. coli* bacteremia, but it did reduce late abscess formation in survivors. These findings indicate that although *E. coli* is responsible for early mortality, *B. fragilis,* in concert with *E. coli* and perhaps other microorganisms (e.g., enterococci),[193,194] is responsible for late intraperitoneal abscess formation. This synergy between obligate and facultative anaerobes has long been recognized in mixed infections.[195] Studies in animal models of intraperitoneal infection also have shown that bacterial interactions with host components, specifically activation of IL-17 producing CD4+ T lymphocytes by constituents of abscess-inducing bacteria such as *B. fragilis,* are necessary for abscess formation.[196]

Pathophysiologic Responses

Whatever the initiating cause of peritonitis, a similar series of reactions takes place locally and systemically.

Local Response. The local inflammatory response of the peritoneum is similar to that in other tissues, but the peritoneal lining presents a large exudative and absorptive surface. At sites of irritation, there is an outpouring of fluid into the peritoneal cavity that, in contrast to normal serous fluid, has a high protein content (>3 g/dL) and many cells, primarily granulocytes, that phagocytose and kill organisms. The exudate contains fibrinogen that polymerizes, and plaques of fibrinous exudate form on the inflamed peritoneal surfaces. This exudate glues together adjacent bowel, mesentery, and particularly omentum. Localization is aided further by inhibition of motility in involved intestinal loops. Experimentally, radiopaque medium injected intraperitoneally at one locus can be shown to have spread over much of the greater peritoneal sac within a short time. The extent and rate of intraperitoneal spread of contamination depend on the volume and nature of the exudate[10] and on the effectiveness of the localizing processes.

If peritoneal defenses aided by appropriate supportive measures control the inflammatory process, the disease may resolve spontaneously. A second possible outcome is a confined abscess. A third course results when the peritoneal and systemic defense mechanisms are unable to localize the inflammation, which progresses to spreading diffuse peritonitis. Factors favoring spread of the inflammatory process are (1) greater virulence of bacteria, (2) greater extent and duration of contamination, and (3) impaired host defenses.

The cytokine response in peritonitis has been the subject of an excellent review.[197] Many of the local abdominal and systemic manifestations of peritonitis undoubtedly are mediated by cytokines, including TNF, IL-1, IL-6, and interferon-γ. Cytokines appear in the peritoneal exudate to a much greater extent than in systemic circulation of patients with peritonitis.[198] These cytokines are produced by macrophages and other host cells in response to bacteria or bacterial products, such as endotoxin,[199] and by tissues traumatized during abdominal operative procedures.[200]

Cytokine responses have been studied in the peritoneal exudate in experimental animal models of peritonitis,[201-204] in patients with spontaneous bacterial peritonitis,[205,206] in patients undergoing CAPD,[207-209] and in patients with severe secondary bacterial peritonitis who were undergoing planned relaparotomy.[210] Anti-TNF antibody failed to afford protection against death[211] and failed to reduce serum levels of IL-1 and IL-6 in an experimental model of peritonitis.[201,204,212] In contrast, in this model, antiendotoxin antibodies were found to prevent death[213] and to reduce bacterial numbers in the peritoneal exudates and serum levels of TNF, IL-1, and IL-6. Anti–interferon-γ antibodies also afforded a protective effect in this model of experimental peritonitis and after intravenous injection of endotoxin.[214]

Systemic Response. Peritonitis leads to changes not only locally in the peritoneal cavity, but also throughout the body.

Gastrointestinal. Initially in peritonitis there is hypermotility, followed by paralysis of the bowel. Accumulation of fluid and electrolytes in the lumen of the adynamic bowel continues until distention is sufficient to inhibit capillary inflow and secretion ceases.

Cardiovascular. Because of the large surface area of the peritoneum, shifts of fluid into the peritoneal cavity, combined with fluid shifts into the bowel lumen, can produce a profound decrease in circulating blood volume and elevation of the hematocrit.[215,216] Fluid and electrolyte loss is exaggerated further by coexistent fever, vomiting, diarrhea, and loss of aspirated gastrointestinal fluid. As the process continues, the decreased venous return to the right side of the heart results in a decrease in cardiac output, with resulting hypotension.[216] Usually there is evidence of increased adrenergic activity, such as sweating, tachycardia, and cutaneous vasoconstriction (i.e., cold moist skin, mottled and cyanotic extremities).

With adequate replacement of blood volume, cardiac output may be maintained above normal.[216] Cardiac output of two or three times normal may be required to satisfy the increased metabolic needs of the body in the presence of infection. Failure to sustain increased cardiac output results in progressive lactic acidosis, oliguria, hypotension, and ultimately death if the infection cannot be controlled.

Respiratory. The intraperitoneal inflammation results in relatively high and fixed diaphragms and considerable pain on respiration. This condition results in basilar atelectasis with intrapulmonary shunting of blood. Satisfactory compensation is possible only if the increase in energy demands does not exceed the respiratory reserve. Heavy cigarette smoking, chronic bronchitis, emphysema, and obesity compound the problem. With decompensation in respiratory function, hypoxemia is accompanied first by hypocapnia (respiratory alkalosis) and later by hypercapnia (respiratory acidosis). In some patients, pulmonary edema develops, not because of left ventricular failure, but perhaps because of increased pulmonary capillary leakage as a consequence of hypoalbuminemia or direct effects of bacterial toxins (adult respiratory distress syndrome). In these patients, progressive hypoxemia develops with decreasing pulmonary compliance. This condition requires volume-cycled ventilatory assistance with increasingly higher concentrations of inspired oxygen and positive end-expiratory pressure.

Renal. Low renal perfusion may be followed by acute tubular necrosis and progressive azotemia.

Metabolic. The excretion of cortisol is increased during the first few days and subsequently returns to normal.[217] The increased energy demands of infection rapidly deplete body stores of glycogen; this leads to catabolism of protein (muscle) and fat, accounting for the rapid weight loss of severely infected patients. Prolonged intra-abdominal infection is associated with extreme wasting. Heat production eventually may fail, then body temperature decreases. Exhaustion and death may ensue.

Clinical Manifestations

Symptoms. The early manifestations of peritonitis that results from disease of abdominal viscera are frequently those of the primary disease process. Moderately severe abdominal pain is almost always the predominant symptom. Any motion, even respiration, aggravates the pain. The progression of abdominal pain is a function of the rate of dissemination of the material producing the pain stimulus. Rupture of a peptic ulcer with massive spillage of gastric contents produces severe epigastric pain that, within minutes, may spread to involve the entire abdomen. In contrast, the spread of pain from a lesion such as a ruptured appendix is much more gradual. Decreased intensity and extent of pain with time usually suggest localization of the inflammatory process.

Anorexia, nausea, and vomiting commonly accompany abdominal pain. Patients also may complain of feverishness, sometimes with chill, thirst, scanty urination, inability to pass feces or flatus, and abdominal distention.

The formation and progression of an intraperitoneal abscess often are gradual. The patient who seemed to be recovering from peritonitis or an abdominal operation stops improving, fever returns, and localizing symptoms may develop.

Physical Findings. Patients with peritonitis characteristically lie quietly in bed, supine, with the knees flexed and with frequent limited intercostal respirations because any motion intensifies the abdominal pain. The patient is alert, restless, and irritable early in the course but later may become apathetic or delirious.

Body temperatures may reach 42° C. Subnormal temperatures in the range of 35° C often are seen in the early stages of chemical peritonitis. They are a grave sign late in the course in patients with continuing intra-abdominal sepsis or septic shock.

Increasing tachycardia with weak, thready peripheral pulses reflects decreased effective blood volume. The blood pressure is maintained within normal limits early in the disease process. As peritonitis progresses, the blood pressure decreases to shock levels. Respiration is increasingly rapid and shallow.

Marked abdominal tenderness to palpation is present, usually maximally over the organ in which the process originated. Direct and referred rebound tenderness signifies parietal peritoneal irritation. This finding sometimes is more accurate than direct palpation in locating the point of maximal tenderness and delineating the extent of peritoneal irritation.

Muscular rigidity of the abdominal wall is produced by voluntary guarding and reflex muscular spasm. Hyperresonance due to gaseous intestinal distention usually can be shown by percussion. Pneumoperitoneum from a ruptured hollow viscus may produce decreased liver dullness to percussion. Bowel sounds, initially hypoactive, later disappear. Rectal and vaginal examination may reveal tenderness and the presence of a pelvic abscess and may indicate a primary focus in the female pelvic organs.

Abdominal pain and muscle spasm may be deceptively absent in some patients. Patients with lax abdominal musculature (e.g., patients in the postpartum period, patients with ascites due to cirrhosis, patients with marked cachexia) may not have abdominal rigidity. Similarly, patients who are in shock, who are receiving glucocorticosteroid therapy, or in whom loculated intra-abdominal abscesses are not in contact with the anterior abdominal wall (e.g., subphrenic, lesser sac, pelvic) may not exhibit marked abdominal pain and spasm. Absent bowel sounds may be the only manifestation of peritonitis in these patients, and a high index of suspicion is necessary.

Diagnostic Studies

The differential diagnosis in patients with symptoms and signs of peritonitis includes pneumonia, sickle cell anemia, herpes zoster, diabetic ketoacidosis, tabes dorsalis, porphyria, familial Mediterranean fever, plumbism, lupus erythematosus, and uremia. A peripheral blood leukocyte count of 17,000 to 25,000 cells/mm^3 is usual in acute peritonitis, the differential count showing polymorphonuclear predominance and a moderate-to-marked shift to the left. Reliance on the significance of the total leukocyte count may be misleading, however. Massive peritoneal inflammation can mobilize leukocytes into the diseased area; there may be fewer than 5000 leukocytes per milliliter in the circulating blood, but the differential smear in this situation may show an extreme shift to immature polymorphonuclear forms.

Hemoconcentration and dehydration are reflected by increased hematocrit and blood urea nitrogen values. Hyperglycemia and glycosuria usually are not present in peritonitis but may be seen in diabetic acidosis and acute pancreatitis, which can manifest with signs suggesting peritonitis. Hematuria and pyuria without bacteriuria may reflect intra-abdominal inflammatory disease, such as appendicitis adjacent to the urinary tract. Elevated serum amylase levels may be seen in peritonitis from almost any cause, but very high levels are seen only in acute pancreatitis. Hyponatremia may be seen in patients given water to replace isotonic fluid losses, but it also is characteristic of porphyria. Metabolic and respiratory acidosis is present in severe and late peritonitis.

Supine, upright, and lateral decubitus radiographs of the abdomen may reveal distention of the small intestine and the colon, with adynamic loops of bowel or features of mechanical intestinal obstruction, volvulus, intussusception, or vascular occlusion. Inflammatory exudate and edema of the intestinal wall produces a widening of the space between adjacent loops. Peritoneal fat lines and psoas shadows may be obliterated. Free air may be visible if there is a ruptured viscus. Chest radiographs always should be obtained to rule out a pulmonary or thoracic problem as the cause of abdominal distress. The presence of air beneath the diaphragm may be defined best in these pictures. Trapped gas with a fluid level or mottling due to gas also may be visible in intraperitoneal or visceral abscesses. Calcification in the gallbladder or other organs also may be noted on radiographs.

Ultrasonography frequently is the initial step in evaluating intra-abdominal sepsis, especially for detecting processes in the right upper quadrant, retroperitoneum, and pelvis. Dilated air-filled loops of bowel, obesity, overlying lungs, bandages, wounds, drains, and ostomies can interfere with the quality of ultrasound images. CT of the entire abdomen and pelvis with oral and intravenous contrast agents has become invaluable for evaluating patients with a suspected intra-abdominal infection. CT frequently has replaced exploratory laparotomy for this purpose. CT can facilitate detection of lesions outside the suspected area on the basis of clinical findings and guidance of percutaneous drainage of peritoneal fluid or abscesses. Although CT is more costly than ultrasound, it is the preferred initial study except when the lesion is suspected to be in the right upper quadrant, retroperitoneum, or pelvis.[218-220] Ultrasound also is more operator dependent than CT, and abdominal tenderness may preclude the use of the desired amount of external pressure to visualize the intra-abdominal contents adequately. Laparoscopic evaluation of patients with suspected secondary peritonitis also has been reported to be useful.[221]

Needle aspiration of the peritoneal cavity is often helpful. If no fluid can be aspirated, peritoneal lavage with Ringer's lactate solution should be done to obtain fluid for examination. In performing a paracentesis, the region of abdominal scars, where bowel may be adherent to the underside of the scar, should be avoided. The aspirate is examined grossly for content of blood, pus, bile, or digested fat; chemically for amylase content; and microscopically, with Gram staining, for bacteria. A positive paracentesis is meaningful; a dry or negative paracentesis is of little significance. Guidance for the paracentesis may be obtained by ultrasound or CT.

Prognosis

Survival of a patient with secondary peritonitis depends on many factors, including the age of the patient, comorbid conditions, the duration of peritoneal contamination, the presence of foreign material (e.g., bile or pancreatic secretions, barium), the primary intra-abdominal process, and the microorganisms involved.[222,223] Altemeier[102] showed that the more organisms present in peritoneal exudate, the worse the prognosis, although there was no correlation between severity of infection and the presence of any particular organism. Mortality increases with more distal gastrointestinal sources of contamination.[224] In a very young patient, because of the relatively small omentum, the walling-off process is less effective, and diffuse peritonitis occurs more frequently than in an adult. In elderly patients, preexisting conditions, such as emphysema, diabetes, or cardiovascular disease, reduce the capacity of the patient to meet the demands on the cardiovascular, respiratory, and renal systems during this period of intense metabolic activity.[222] Mortality rates range from 3.5% in patients with early infection caused by penetrating abdominal trauma to more than 60% in patients with established intra-abdominal infection and secondary organ failure.[225] Persistent peritoneal contamination; leakage of pancreatic enzymes; septicemia; fluid and electrolyte abnormalities; pneumonia[226]; and cardiovascular, renal, and respiratory failure[227] are the principal causes of death.

With a disease process that has widely varying mortality rates, the ability to predict outcome and stratify severity of disease is important for clinical decision making and for ensuring comparability in trials that evaluate different management strategies with surgical protocols or antimicrobial agents.[228] Outcome has been found to be related mainly to host-related factors (e.g., preoperative nutritional status, organ impairment, severity of the patient's systemic response, and the patient's premorbid physiologic reserves, as predicted by the Acute Physiologic and Chronic Health Evaluation II [APACHE II] scoring system),[229] rather than type and source of the infection.[230,231]

Death from intra-abdominal infection, especially when the tertiary phase is reached, is thought to result from an exaggerated, uncontrolled cytokine release that is unresponsive to all therapeutic attempts.[232] This cytokine release has led to the use of endotoxin and cytokine levels in circulation to predict outcome. The magnitude of levels of TNF-α and IL-6 in circulation in patients with peritonitis has

not been related invariably to prognosis, however.[233-237] Determination of cytokine levels in the peritoneal exudate, rather than in blood, has been suggested to reflect better the severity of the compartmentalized peritoneal infection and to predict outcome.[210]

Treatment

Antimicrobial Therapy. Medical management includes use of antimicrobial therapy and supportive measures to maintain vital functions (e.g., improve or maintain circulation, nutrition, and oxygenation to vital organs). As yet the clinical efficacy of immunomodulators, such as anti-TNF antibodies, antiendotoxin antibodies, and IL-1 receptor antagonists, is unproven.

Secondary peritonitis typically is polymicrobial, and the pathogens in most cases are derived from the gastrointestinal tract, even in patients with a primary gynecologic process. Typically the facultative microorganisms are *E. coli*, *Klebsiella/Enterobacter* spp., *Proteus* spp., and enterococci, and the obligate anaerobes are *B. fragilis*, *P. melaninogenica*, *Peptococcus*, *Peptostreptococcus*, *Fusobacterium*, *Eubacterium lentum*, and *Clostridium*. Other, less commonly isolated pathogens include *S. aureus*, *P. aeruginosa*, and *Candida*.

The role of antimicrobial therapy in the outcome of infection caused by anaerobes or by a mixture of anaerobes and facultative microorganisms is extremely difficult to assess. Often dramatic response to surgical drainage and débridement alone occurs when there is localized infection. Nevertheless, appropriate antimicrobial therapy has been shown to reduce mortality significantly among patients with bacteremic infections caused by Bacteroidaceae or Enterobacteriaceae.[110,238,239] Antimicrobial drugs are expected to control bacteremia and early metastatic foci of infection, to reduce suppurative complications if given early, and to prevent local spread of existing infection. When suppuration has occurred, it may be difficult to cure the infection if antimicrobial drugs are used without drainage; also, antimicrobial drugs used alone may mask some of the clinical manifestations of abscess formation. Some intra-abdominal abscesses can be treated successfully, however, with antibiotics alone.[240,241]

Antimicrobial agents must penetrate to the site of infection in concentrations that are sufficient to overcome the effects of a high bacterial density, the metabolic inactivity and slow growth rate of probably more than 90% of the bacterial inoculum, low pH, low redox potential, necrotic tissue, and bacterial products that may lower the drug's activity. Aminoglycosides and clindamycin are less active at acid pH, aminoglycosides are less active at low redox potentials, and β-lactams are less active against high bacterial densities.

Although the results of many antimicrobial trials for the treatment of intra-abdominal infections have been published, caution must be exercised when interpreting these studies because of the possibility of inadequate study design and analysis of data.[242] Some of the variables that must be considered are differences in patient populations, types and severity of underlying illnesses, community-acquired versus hospital-acquired infection, and the pathogens isolated. Table 68-1 lists many of the antimicrobial regimens that have been found to be efficacious for the treatment of intra-abdominal infections in clinical trials.

Antimicrobial therapy should be started immediately after appropriate specimens (blood and, if possible, peritoneal fluid) are obtained for culture. Antimicrobial therapy often is started before the completion of in vitro antimicrobial sensitivity testing of the specific facultative pathogens. In addition, rapid isolation, identification, and in vitro sensitivity testing of anaerobes, in contrast to testing of facultative bacteria, are not possible in many community hospitals. Several factors account for the delay in obtaining anaerobic bacteriologic results. Infections caused by anaerobes frequently involve mixtures of five or more microorganisms, and cultures require long periods for growth and isolation. In addition, in vitro sensitivity testing by the conventional disk diffusion technique has not been standardized for anaerobes.[173] These tests are influenced to a large extent by the growth rate of the bacteria, inoculum size, pH and type of medium, duration of incubation, and carbon dioxide concentration in the atmosphere.[243,244] In vitro studies of the stability of the β-lactam antibiotics

TABLE 68-1   Comparative Antimicrobial Trials for Treatment of Intra-abdominal Infections

Regimen	Reference
Cefoxitin ± aminoglycoside vs clindamycin + aminoglycoside	448-450
Ticarcillin + aminoglycoside vs clindamycin + aminoglycoside	451
Piperacillin vs cefoxitin	452
Ampicillin-sulbactam vs clindamycin + aminoglycoside	453
Imipenem vs clindamycin + aminoglycoside	251, 454-456
Aztreonam + clindamycin vs clindamycin + aminoglycoside	457
Trovafloxacin vs imipenem	458

when exposed to reducing agents such as mercaptoamines (cysteine), which frequently are incorporated in media used for the growth of anaerobes, have shown that these compounds are able to open the β-lactam ring and to inactivate penicillins.[245] Susceptibility of anaerobic organisms can be determined reliably, however, by the broth or agar dilution technique with the use of appropriate media.[246] Because these tests generally are performed by research laboratories, knowledge of the antimicrobial susceptibility of anaerobes is gained from periodically published reports on anaerobic isolates by centers that specialize in performing these tests. Initial chemotherapy usually is empirical, based on the most reliable and least toxic antimicrobial agents for the most probable anaerobic and facultative pathogens. In vitro sensitivity reports (usually reliable only for the facultative or aerobic organisms) allow subsequent adjustment of the initial regimen to more specific therapy.

Because these infections commonly are polymicrobial, a broad spectrum of antimicrobial activity is required. Data suggest that survival in patients with intra-abdominal infection is diminished if initial therapy is inadequate, regardless of the adequacy of subsequent treatment.[247] The ideal regimen remains controversial. The animal model of intra-abdominal sepsis showed the necessity of treating the facultative enteric gram-negative bacilli—*E. coli*—and the anaerobic gram-negative bacilli—*B. fragilis*. Empirical use of an antimicrobial regimen active against *E. coli* and *B. fragilis* has been well established. The need for intraoperative cultures to document the etiologic microorganisms and their antimicrobial susceptibilities has been controversial because postoperative changes based on results of intraoperative cultures may not improve outcome.[248-250]

Drugs active against anaerobic bacteria may be inactive against the accompanying aerobic or facultative pathogens in the mixed infections and vice versa. For this reason, combinations of usually two or three drugs are used. These combinations of antimicrobial agents are selected for their activity against most of the more virulent pathogens in the infective mixture (e.g., the Enterobacteriaceae, *B. fragilis*), although monotherapy for polymicrobial intra-abdominal infection now is possible because of the availability of broad-spectrum agents with activity against aerobes and anaerobes.[251]

Antibiotics need not be active against every pathogen isolated. It is apparent that if only some of the organisms can be eliminated, the synergistic effect may be removed, and the patient's defenses may be able to eradicate the remaining organisms. Clindamycin alone (which has no activity against Enterobacteriaceae or enterococci) has been reported to be sufficient treatment for some patients with infections resulting from a mixture of Enterobacteriaceae, enterococci, and anaerobes.[252]

Although enterococci are found in about 20% of intra-abdominal infections, the exact role they play in polymicrobial intra-abdominal infection and the need for an antimicrobial regimen specific for these organisms are controversial.[253] In several studies, patients were treated successfully with clindamycin and gentamicin despite absence of activity of this therapeutic regimen against enterococci.[254,255] Selective therapy against *E. coli* and *B. fragilis* that has no or borderline in vitro antimicrobial activity against enterococci has been found to be sufficient to reduce enterococcal counts.[256] Nevertheless, in animal models

of experimental polymicrobial intra-abdominal infection, enterococci have been found to be a significant component of the inoculum; as such, they enhance abscess formation, weight loss, bacteremia with *B. fragilis* and *E. coli*, and mortality.[256,257] Similarly, clinical reports have emphasized the importance of enterococci in intra-abdominal infection[258] and noted the emergence of enterococcal abscesses and bacteremia supervening after treatment of intra-abdominal sepsis with antimicrobial agents that lack significant in vitro enterococcal activity.[259-269] Enterococci have emerged as major nosocomial pathogens, undoubtedly as a result of their inherent resistance to many commonly used antimicrobial agents and their recent acquisition of resistance to previous standard therapy (i.e., ampicillin, aminoglycosides, and the glycopeptides, vancomycin and teicoplanin).[270-273] Only clinically unproven older antimicrobial agents (e.g., doxycycline and chloramphenicol) and a few new antimicrobial agents (e.g., a combination of two streptogramin antibiotics [quinupristin/dalfopristin] and linezolid) are available as potential therapy for infections caused by these multiple-drug–resistant strains of enterococci. Daptomycin is an investigational drug that has activity in vitro against vancomycin-resistant enterococci. The efficacy of agents with antienterococcal activity for primary empirical therapy to prevent emergence of enterococcal superinfection is unknown. A multicenter study of intra-abdominal infection[274,275] found that the presence of enterococci in the initial culture, independently from the APACHE II score, predicted treatment failure with broad-spectrum antimicrobial regimens that lacked specific enterococcal activity. APACHE II score, age, length of preinfection hospital stay, and postoperative infections predicted the presence of enterococci. It is unknown whether inclusion of antienterococcal therapy would improve outcome in these high-risk patients, although one study suggested that postoperative addition of antienterococcal antimicrobial therapy after results of intraoperative peritoneal cultures did not improve the mortality rate.[276]

Treatment of *Candida* in polymicrobial infections also is controversial.[277,278] Isolation of this microorganism from blood cultures, as the sole organism within residual or recurrent intra-abdominal infection, or as the predominant organism on Gram staining of peritoneal exudate, represents an indication for specific antifungal therapy plus drainage of abscesses, if present.[145,279,280] Amphotericin B is standard therapy for invasive *Candida* infection, although lipid-associated amphotericin and caspofungin may be efficacious, less nephrotoxic, but more expensive alternatives. Azoles also are less toxic, although no comparative trials in *Candida* peritonitis exist. *Candida krusei* and *Torulopsis glabrata* are inherently more resistant to azoles, and resistance to azoles among previously sensitive *Candida* spp. is increasing.

When combinations of antibiotics are used, synergism or antagonism may occur. Chloramphenicol has been shown to impair early bactericidal activity of gentamicin in vitro, and antagonism was shown in mice with experimental *Proteus mirabilis* infection when phagocytic function was impaired (i.e., in neutropenic mice).[281] Two studies suggested that clindamycin inhibits early in vitro killing of *E. coli* and *K. pneumoniae* by gentamicin.[282] In an in vivo study of aminoglycoside therapy of *E. coli* peritonitis and bacteremia in healthy and neutropenic mice, however, prior or simultaneous administration of clindamycin with the aminoglycoside did not inhibit the therapeutic effect of the aminoglycoside.[283] Clindamycin combined in vitro with gentamicin has been reported to have indifferent or synergistic activity against Enterobacteriaceae after 18 hours of incubation.[284] The activities of various antimicrobial agents against the usual peritoneal pathogens and the results of clinical trials are discussed in the following sections.

Chloramphenicol. At a concentration of 16 μg/mL, chloramphenicol has activity against more than 99% of the anaerobic pathogens involved in intra-abdominal infections, especially *B. fragilis*.[285] The availability of equally effective and potentially less toxic antimicrobial agents to treat anaerobic infections (e.g., clindamycin, metronidazole, imipenem) has all but eliminated the need for chloramphenicol,[281] however, except perhaps for significant infection caused by strains of enterococci that are resistant to all other antimicrobial agents.

Clindamycin. Clindamycin has been reported to inhibit more than 95% of the anaerobes, including *B. fragilis*, at a concentration of 8 μg/mL,[286] and early clinical trials established the efficacy of clindamycin plus aminoglycoside.[287,288] About 15% of the strains of *Clostridium* spp. other than *C. perfringens*, *Peptococcus* spp., and rare strains of *Fusobacterium* spp. have been reported to be resistant to clindamycin. Most strains of *B. fragilis* have remained highly susceptible to clindamycin since the 1990s.[289,290] Plasmid-mediated, transferable clindamycin resistance in *B. fragilis* has been shown,[289] and clindamycin resistance among *B. fragilis* has become a problem at certain medical centers. Clindamycin is active against certain facultative gram-positive cocci, such as *S. aureus* and *Streptococcus pyogenes*, but not enterococci, and it has virtually no activity against Enterobacteriaceae.

Diarrhea is reported to be the most common side effect of clindamycin therapy, occurring at an incidence of 2% to 20%.[291] The severity of the diarrhea varies, but it may be associated with pseudomembranous colitis in half of patients with diarrhea, as reported in one study.[292] Toxic megacolon, colonic perforation, and death rarely have been reported and attributed to an exotoxin produced by clindamycin-resistant strains of *C. difficile*.[291]

Metronidazole. Metronidazole is active against strict anaerobes; inhibits most *B. fragilis* strains, *Fusobacterium* spp., and *Clostridium* spp.; and has a unique bactericidal action against *B. fragilis* and *C. perfringens*.[293] Resistance among *B. fragilis* to metronidazole is rare. The in vitro activity of metronidazole is poor, however, against aerobes, microaerophiles, and anaerobes that may become aerotolerant on subculture (i.e., certain anaerobic gram-positive cocci and sporeless gram-positive rods),[285, 294] although there is some in vivo evidence in animal models and humans that metronidazole has activity against *E. coli* and other aerobes in mixed aerobic-anaerobic infections.[295,296] The mechanism for this is poorly understood but may be related to the conversion by *B. fragilis* of metronidazole into metabolites with activity against *E. coli* and other aerobes.[295] Nonetheless, because facultative gram-negative bacilli and microaerophilic gram-positive cocci, which are frequent copathogens in polymicrobial anaerobic infection, are resistant to metronidazole, the drug should be used in combination with another agent that is active against these pathogens to compensate for these defects in its spectrum.

The relative incidence of *C. difficile*–associated diarrhea and colonization was found to be less after use of metronidazole than after clindamycin in a retrospective study.[297] Metronidazole is the drug of choice for treatment of this disease.

Tetracyclines. The large number of resistant anaerobes, especially *B. fragilis*, precludes the use of tetracyclines[298,299] except perhaps for infection caused by strains of enterococci that are resistant to all other antimicrobial agents.

Cephalosporins. *B. fragilis* and other *Bacteroides* spp. usually are resistant to the first-generation cephalosporins (e.g., cefazolin) and to some second-generation cephalosporins (e.g., cefuroxime). Cefoxitin is distinctly more active than any of the other second-generation cephalosporins against *Bacteroides* spp.,[285,300,301] but cefoxitin resistance has become a problem at certain medical centers.[290] Cefotetan has activity similar to that of cefoxitin except that it is less active against the *B. fragilis* group (not including *B. fragilis*).[300,301] These first-generation and second-generation cephalosporins also are active against most strains of *E. coli*, *P. mirabilis*, and *K. pneumoniae*. The third-generation cephalosporins (cefotaxime, ceftizoxime, cefoperazone, ceftriaxone, and ceftazidime) and cefepime have shown significantly better activity against the Enterobacteriaceae. Only ceftazidime and cefepime, and to a lesser extent cefoperazone, have activity against *P. aeruginosa*. With a few exceptions, the third-generation cephalosporins have relatively poor activity against *B. fragilis* and other *Bacteroides* spp.[302] Ceftizoxime was reported to have good in vitro activity against *B. fragilis* and other *Bacteroides* spp. in some studies[301,303] but was inadequate against *Bacteroides* spp., including *B. fragilis*, in other in vitro studies.[300,304] Because the activity of ceftizoxime is affected greatly by the inoculum of

Bacteroides in in vitro studies,[285] this antibiotic most likely would be inadequate to treat severe intra-abdominal infections in which the inoculum of organisms is great.[305,306]

Regimens in which a third-generation cephalosporin is substituted for the aminoglycoside compare favorably with clindamycin plus aminoglycoside. Resistance emerges readily, however, under selective pressure of antimicrobial therapy with third-generation cephalosporins among certain gram-negative bacilli that produce chromosomal-encoded inducible β-lactamases, such as *Enterobacter, Serratia, Citrobacter, Morganella, Acinetobacter,* and *P. aeruginosa*. These organisms have a high spontaneous mutation rate for constitutive production of large amounts of these β-lactamases, which confer resistance to all β-lactams except imipenem, meropenem, and cefepime and are poorly antagonized by the clinically available β-lactamase inhibitors, sulbactam, clavulanic acid, and tazobactam. Patients who are likely to be infected with these organisms (patients with prolonged hospital stays, prior antibiotic treatment, postoperative peritonitis, or tertiary peritonitis) are treated best with imipenem, meropenem, cefepime, a fluoroquinolone, or an aminoglycoside.

Strains of *K. pneumoniae* and, to a lesser extent, *E. coli* have acquired plasmid-encoded, extended-spectrum β-lactamases that inactivate all third-generation cephalosporins, especially ceftazidime, extended-spectrum penicillins, and aztreonam. These strains also frequently are resistant to the fluoroquinolones. These β-lactamases may be inactivated to some extent by sulbactam, clavulanic acid, and tazobactam, which confer activity to the β-lactam/β-lactamase inhibitor combinations containing these agents. Imipenem, meropenem, and, to a lesser degree, cefepime are most active against these strains.

Penicillins. Penicillin G and ampicillin have excellent activity against anaerobes, with the exception of β-lactamase–producing anaerobic gram-negative bacilli, such as *Bacteroides* spp. (especially *B. fragilis*) and *Prevotella* spp. Ampicillin also is active against 70% to 80% of the strains of *E. coli* and almost all *P. mirabilis*. There is some evidence to suggest that penicillin G may fail to achieve inhibitory concentrations at sites of *B. fragilis* infection because of a reduction in penetration of penicillin into infected sites and inactivation of the drug by *B. fragilis*.[307] Therapeutic failures despite high doses of penicillin for *B. fragilis* bacteremia have been well documented.[107]

About 80% to 90% of strains of *B. fragilis* may be sensitive to high concentrations (minimal inhibitory concentration [MIC] ≤125 (g/mL) of the extended-spectrum penicillins, piperacillin, ticarcillin, mezlocillin, and azlocillin,[308-310] and the clinical experience with these drugs in polymicrobial anaerobic infections has been favorable.[311-313] The spectrum of these penicillins also includes most aerobic enteric gram-negative bacilli and *P. aeruginosa*, but is not likely to include *K. pneumoniae* and some strains of *E. coli* as a consequence of β-lactamase production. The combination of ticarcillin or piperacillin with the β-lactamase inhibitors, clavulanic acid or tazobactam, confers activity against almost all β-lactamase–producing strains of anaerobic gram-negative bacilli, *E. coli,* and *K. pneumoniae*,[314-316] but does not confer activity against the chromosomal-encoded, inducible, β-lactamase–producing strains of *Serratia, Enterobacter, P. aeruginosa, Citrobacter, Acinetobacter,* and *Morganella*.[317] In addition, ticarcillin is inherently much less active against enterococci than piperacillin is. Ampicillin-sulbactam is active against many community-acquired, β-lactamase–producing bacteria that are resistant to ampicillin, including *E. coli, Klebsiella,* and *Bacteroides*,[318,319] but inactive against nosocomial pathogens, such as *Enterobacter, Serratia,* and *P. aeruginosa*. Monotherapy for polymicrobial anaerobic intra-abdominal infection is possible with β-lactam/β-lactamase combinations, such as ampicillin-sulbactam, ticarcillin-clavulanate, and piperacillin-tazobactam, because of their broad spectrum of activity against aerobes and anaerobes.

Other β-Lactams. The carbapenem antibiotics, imipenem and meropenem, have a broad antimicrobial spectrum,[320] with activity against almost all aerobic and anaerobic pathogens, although *E. faecium* are resistant. Meropenem is slightly more active than imipenem against gram-negative bacilli and slightly less active against gram-positive cocci. The activity of ertapenem, a new carbapenem, is similar to the other carbapenems, but ertapenem is not active against enterococci and is not reliably active against *P. aeruginosa*. The carbapenems are resistant to most β-lactamases, including chromosomal, inducible β-lactamases produced by bacteria, such as *Enterobacter, Serratia,* and *P. aeruginosa*,[321] and the plasmid-encoded, extended-spectrum β-lactamases produced by *K. pneumoniae* and *E. coli.* The carbapenems are susceptible, however, to metallo-β-lactamases produced by rare strains of *B. fragilis*[322] and *Stenotrophomonas maltophilia.* Monotherapy for polymicrobial anaerobic intra-abdominal infection is possible with the carbapenems because of their broad spectrum of activity against aerobes and anaerobes.

Aztreonam, a monobactam antibiotic, has a spectrum of activity limited to aerobic gram-negative bacilli.[323] It would be necessary to use an antibiotic with activity against anaerobes and microaerophilic and aerobic gram-positive cocci—clindamycin[324-326]—rather than metronidazole, which has poor activity against these common pathogens, along with aztreonam in the treatment of secondary intra-abdominal infections.

Aminoglycosides. Aminoglycosides are active against many gram-negative aerobic bacilli. Over the decades of aminoglycoside usage, aminoglycoside resistance has increased, however, and other antibiotic classes with predictable activity against gram-negative aerobic bacilli have become available. Amikacin, which is less susceptible to some gentamicin-modifying and tobramycin-modifying enzymes, nevertheless may be active against gentamicin-resistant or tobramycin-resistant pathogens. In some medical facilities, many gram-negative bacilli currently are found to be resistant to aminoglycosides, however, and the MICs of sensitive pathogens have increased steadily close to breakpoint concentrations. Pharmacodynamic effects of aminoglycoside antibiotics favor peak serum levels that are at least 10 times the MIC for the pathogen to maximize efficacy. Persistent inhibition of growth of the pathogen after brief exposure to an aminoglycoside (the postantibiotic effect) allows the serum levels of aminoglycosides to decline to less than the MIC of the pathogen during the dosing interval without loss of efficacy. Because aminoglycoside nephrotoxicity and perhaps ototoxicity are time dependent, not concentration dependent, high peak serum levels to maximize efficacy can be achieved without excess toxicity if the dosing interval is lengthened. This is the rationale for giving the total daily aminoglycoside dose as a single dose every 24 hours in patients with normal renal function, rather than giving the daily dose in two (amikacin) or three (gentamicin or tobramycin) equally divided doses every 24 hours. Single daily dosing of the aminoglycoside may be required to achieve serum levels that are at least 10 times the MIC of sensitive pathogens that are close to breakpoint concentrations. The serum concentrations of gentamicin are unpredictable after a dose based on the body weight, so peak and trough serum levels must be confirmed by any of the various assay methods available.[327] The numbers of severely ill patients with intra-abdominal sepsis studied are too limited, however, to recommend general use of single daily dosing of these drugs.

Aminoglycosides are inactive against obligate anaerobes, and their activity against sensitive pathogens is antagonized by an anaerobic environment[328] and by reducing substances, such as sulfhydryl compounds. Aminoglycosides also are not active in acidic conditions. Anaerobic and acidic conditions frequently are present in intra-abdominal abscesses. In contrast, the β-lactams are relatively nontoxic, can be used in concentrations that are many times higher than the MIC for the pathogen, and are active under anaerobic or acidic conditions. For these reasons, the efficacy of aminoglycosides in intra-abdominal infection has been questioned.[329] The β-lactams are probably more reliable antibiotics than the aminoglycosides against sensitive pathogens. If indicated on the basis of in vitro sensitivity testing, β-lactams should be used in preference to aminoglycosides. An aminoglycoside usually is included with a β-lactam antibiotic in the initial antimicrobial regimen for patients who are critically ill or in whom a resistant pathogen (e.g., *P. aeruginosa*) is suspected.

Fluoroquinolones. The fluoroquinolones (norfloxacin, ciprofloxacin, ofloxacin, levofloxacin, moxifloxacin, gatifloxacin, and trovafloxacin) are active against almost all aerobic gram-negative bacilli.[330] Ciprofloxacin remains the most potent fluoroquinolone against *P. aeruginosa.* Levofloxacin, moxifloxacin, gatifloxacin, and trovafloxacin are more active than the older fluoroquinolones[331] against gram-positive cocci, although enterococci and methicillin-resistant *S. aureus* tend to be less susceptible than other gram-positive cocci. In addition, moxifloxacin, gatifloxacin, and trovafloxacin are active against obligate anaerobes, in contrast to other fluoroquinolones[332,333] (although data for moxifloxacin and gatifloxacin are limited to oral anaerobes). Their ability to kill bacteria in the exponential and the stationary phases of growth, along with the lack of development of plasmid-mediated resistance, makes the fluoroquinolones valuable antimicrobial agents for the treatment of intra-abdominal infections, including abscesses.

Currently, six fluoroquinolones (ciprofloxacin, ofloxacin, levofloxacin, moxifloxacin, gatifloxacin, and trovafloxacin) are available for parenteral administration. These six agents also are well absorbed after oral administration and are concentrated in tissues so that tissue levels are well in excess of the MICs of many sensitive pathogens. Toxicity has limited significantly the usefulness of trovafloxacin, however. With current fluoroquinolone dosing regimens, serum levels may be inadequate to treat susceptible pathogens with relatively high MICs (e.g., >0.5 μg/mL of ciprofloxacin), which include some strains of *P. aeruginosa,* enterococci, and *S. aureus,* especially the methicillin-resistant strains.[334] If such organisms can be anticipated (e.g., in nosocomial infections), additional antimicrobial agents may be necessary to broaden the spectrum of an empirical regimen. The addition of an antimicrobial agent active against anaerobic bacteria and aerobic or microaerophilic gram-positive cocci (e.g., clindamycin, ampicillin-sulbactam, amoxicillin-clavulanic acid) would be required if the use of ciprofloxacin were considered for secondary intra-abdominal infection. The absence of data on in vitro susceptibility against intestinal anaerobes and clinical trials in intra-abdominal sepsis for moxifloxacin and gatifloxacin and the toxicity of trovafloxacin do not favor use of these agents as monotherapy for polymicrobial intra-abdominal infection.

Duration of Antimicrobial Therapy. Antibiotic therapy should be given before, during, and after surgery to ensure tissue and blood levels of the antibiotic that can combat local and metastatic spread of the infection. The duration of antimicrobial therapy after adequate surgery is usually 5 to 7 days and depends on severity of infection, clinical response, and normalization of the leukocyte count.[287,335,336] Only a short course of antimicrobial therapy (24 hours) is required for sterile peritonitis that occurs in the peritoneal space about an infected, but resectable intra-abdominal organ, such as appendix or gallbladder, after resection of the organ. Similarly, contamination of the peritoneum with bacteria from a defect in the intestinal wall (e.g., immediately following penetrating abdominal trauma) also may require only operative intervention to remove the diseased organ and to stop continued peritoneal contamination and a brief course of antimicrobial therapy.[287,335,336] Persistent sepsis suggests formation of an intra-abdominal abscess requiring drainage, continued contamination of the peritoneum from an inadequately controlled source, superimposed nosocomial infection with a resistant pathogen, or tertiary peritonitis.

The antibiotic regimen should be adjusted to include the most efficacious, least toxic, and least expensive agents, when cultures have been finalized, with the proviso that therapy must have activity against anaerobes even when they are not isolated because anaerobic bacteriologic techniques frequently are inadequate.

In patients able to tolerate oral intake, conversion to oral therapy after an initial response to intravenous therapy is possible.[275] Oral therapy allows earlier discharge in some patients and reduces costs and risks of infusion-related complications. When ileus no longer prohibits oral intake, efficacy of oral therapy depends on the adequacy of absorption after oral administration of the antimicrobial agents, the availability of potent oral agents against the significant pathogens (i.e., *E. coli* and *B. fragilis*), and the effects of oral versus intravenous administration of these agents on bowel flora. Potential oral agents include clindamycin, metronidazole, amoxicillin-clavulanic acid, trimethoprim-sulfamethoxazole, trovafloxacin, and ciprofloxacin.

The addition of antibiotics or antiseptics to intraperitoneal lavage fluid continues to be debated,[337-340] and its efficacy intraoperatively[287] or by continuous peritoneal lavage postoperatively[340] remains unclear. One study showed that irrigation of the peritoneal cavity with povidone-iodine decreased the frequency of intra-abdominal abscess formation compared with saline irrigation.[341] Povidone-iodine has been shown to be a potent inactivator of neutrophil functions such as chemotaxis and phagocytosis, however, and may have a detrimental effect.[342]

Hyperbaric Oxygen. The increased oxygen tension attainable with hyperbaric oxygen therapy inhibits and kills *C. perfringens*[343] and reduces the production of *C. perfringens* α-toxin. Hyperbaric oxygenation has been used clinically and experimentally for clostridial myonecrosis, with some reported success.[344] *C. perfringens* is a relatively oxygen-tolerant pathogen compared with other obligate anaerobes, and it is reasonable to assume that hyperbaric oxygen therapy would be at least equally efficacious with anaerobic infections caused by these more oxygen-sensitive anaerobes. Except for a few reports,[345] however, almost no clinical or experimental data are available. Hill[346] reported suppression of experimental liver abscesses due to anaerobes in mice after treatment with hyperbaric oxygen therapy alone. In one study, it seemed that the use of hyperbaric oxygen therapy favorably affected the outcome of experimental sepsis in a rat model, perhaps by enhancing host defense mechanisms.[347] Consideration also should be given to the hazards of hyperbaric oxygen therapy. See Chapter 40 for a more detailed discussion.

Gastrointestinal Drainage. In the presence of peritonitis, the patient should receive nothing by mouth. If no distention is present when treatment is instituted, continuous gastric suction usually is sufficient. For patients who are distended when treatment is started and for patients who become distended despite gastric drainage, intubation of the small intestine should be instituted.

Water and Electrolyte Administration. The type of fluid replacement is determined in large part by the chemical abnormalities found. In general, hypovolemia, dehydration, and metabolic acidosis predominate, so plasma or albumin, Ringer's lactate solution, and 5% dextrose in water usually suffice. The amount to be given in the 2 to 4 hours before anticipated surgery is determined by watching vital signs, hematocrit values, hourly urinary output, and central venous pressure.

Blood and Plasma Transfusion. Although many patients recover from an illness satisfactorily with a hemoglobin of 8 or 10 g/dL, some surgeons recommend that the patient be transfused to maintain levels of 12 to 13 g/dL to provide a margin of safety should some complication, such as septic shock or upper gastrointestinal hemorrhage, supervene.

Respiratory Support. Fluid sequestered in the abdomen and loops of bowel distended by gas may elevate the diaphragm. Inflammation of the parietal peritoneum, including the diaphragmatic surface, leads to guarding and splinting of the muscular wall, which interferes with deep breathing and coughing. A subphrenic abscess may be responsible for splinting of the diaphragm. Retained bronchial secretions may lead to atelectasis and subsequent pneumonitis. These factors impair the ability to augment respiratory exchange in the face of the increased expenditure of energy required by the inflammatory process and produce hypoxemia and respiratory alkalosis. When the patient tires, the combination of metabolic and respiratory acidosis may develop and prove fatal.

Arterial blood gas studies are necessary to detect and quantitate respiratory decompensation. Measures aimed primarily at gastrointestinal decompression, elevation of the head of the bed, and control of the inflammation may improve respiration sufficiently. Administration of oxygen may improve arterial oxygen saturation. If these measures are inadequate, endotracheal intubation or tracheostomy should be performed without delay. A volume-cycled respirator should be used and adjusted to give a partial pressure of oxygen of 80 to 100 mm Hg and a normal pH. If the partial pressure of carbon dioxide is not normal then, metabolic acidosis or alkalosis

may need to be treated. As the intra-abdominal process subsides, the patient may be able to breathe spontaneously again and may be weaned from the ventilator. In certain severe cases, positive end-expiratory pressure also may be necessary.

Operative Approach. Surgical intervention is aimed at controlling the source of peritoneal contamination and débridement of necrotic tissue and foreign intraperitoneal matter. Optimal management includes the following: (1) bowel decompression (e.g., by proximal colostomy for perforation, diverticulitis, or colonic carcinoma); (2) closure of traumatic perforations and resection of a diseased, perforated viscus to stop continued peritoneal contamination with bacteria and adjuvants; and (3) drainage of any purulent collections, which reduces the bacterial inoculum, removes excessive levels of proinflammatory cytokines and adjuvants (e.g., fecal matter, food, blood, bile, barium) that would enhance the virulence of peritoneal infection, and eliminates anaerobic conditions. In the absence of perforation, when the disease process (e.g., acute appendicitis, necrotic bowel) is anticipated to progress, the involved organ is resected. Acute increase in intra-abdominal pressure, which itself can lead to multiorgan dysfunction (e.g., acute pulmonary and renal failure, shock), requires decompression laparotomy and, if necessary, leaving the abdomen open and covered with a protective dressing.[348-350] Operative intervention generally is not indicated for patients with primary peritonitis; in patients in whom the disease process subsides and localizes while the patient is being prepared for surgery; in moribund patients; or in patients with pelvic peritonitis caused by pelvic inflammatory disease, which usually responds to medical management.

Intraoperative peritoneal lavage with saline, after drainage of purulent peritoneal exudates, fecal matter, food, and other foreign debris, is standard procedure during laparotomy for peritonitis. Continuous postoperative peritoneal lavage for 48 to 72 hours or until the fluid is clear, using large volumes of fluid to ensure dispersion of the fluid and to prevent loculations, has not been effective, however.[340,351,352] Radical peritoneal débridement of all fibrinous deposits on peritoneal surfaces likewise no longer is thought to be effective.[353,354]

Initial reports were favorable for planned reexplorations in which a commitment is made at the first operation to perform laparotomies at frequent intervals until the abdomen is macroscopically clean, regardless of the patient's condition, with additional surgical procedures (e.g., resections) performed as necessary.[355,356] The abdominal fascia is left open between laparotomies, with the abdominal wall defect bridged by saline-soaked gauze or by a temporary abdominal closure device, such as mesh. On resolution of the septic process and establishment of granulation, the mesh is removed, and a skin graft is applied to the granulating bed. These demanding and costly procedures have been complicated by multiple fistulas, wound contamination, incisional hernias, and secondary peritonitis with organisms such as enterococci or *Candida*.[356-359] Repeated entry into the inflamed peritoneum may escalate the cascade further.[360] A review concluded that, in the absence of randomized, controlled prospective trials with appropriate stratification of patients by severity of illness, insufficient evidence now exists to determine whether these procedures improve outcome in severe diffuse peritonitis, but nevertheless they may be lifesaving in some patients.[359,361-363] In localized infection, local drainage alone is adequate because the risk of disseminating infection outweighs any possible benefit of removing foreign material that may have escaped mechanical removal.

Use of multiple drains for drainage of the general peritoneal cavity is physically impossible because exudate and adhesions rapidly isolate and occlude the drains and may increase secondary infections.[364] Drains often are placed, however, in a dependent point to which fluid can be expected to gravitate or in an area of devitalized tissue that cannot be removed.

Prevention

Prevention of postoperative peritonitis requires avoiding contamination of the peritoneum with gastrointestinal or vaginal secretions. In addition to using good surgical technique, avoidance of contamination can be accomplished by early treatment of an intra-abdominal infection. Leigh and coworkers[365] noted that the rate of wound infection in patients with perforated appendix was greater than 50% if no antimicrobial therapy was used but only 15% in the group given appropriate therapy. Similarly, two studies showed the efficacy of early use of antibiotics in penetrating wounds of the abdomen, especially wounds involving the colon.[366,367] Surgeons also have used various means to reduce the complex gastrointestinal or vaginal flora before performing clean, contaminated surgery. Mechanical cleansing of the bowel with a low-residue diet followed by a liquid diet, cathartics, and enemas can reduce the total fecal mass and coliform count in the colon, although not the predominant anaerobic flora.[368] The use of oral antibiotics preoperatively to reduce bowel flora is well accepted. *E. coli* in the colonic flora is sensitive to oral neomycin or kanamycin, whereas *B. fragilis* frequently is sensitive to erythromycin or metronidazole. Combinations such as neomycin and erythromycin base have been shown to be effective in reducing total bowel flora preoperatively and decreasing the incidence of postoperative infection.[369]

Parenteral antibiotics also have been used in gastrointestinal and vaginal surgery prophylactically when there is a chance of contamination with normal microflora at the operative site (clean, contaminated surgery). Of these types of operations, 30% may be complicated by infections. These procedures involve cutting through the large bowel without significant spillage, compromising the blood supply of the large bowel, cutting through the stomach or small bowel when there is anticipated intraluminal bacterial overgrowth, appendectomy for appendicitis without rupture, penetrating wounds of the abdomen, gallbladder surgery in an elderly patient, cesarean section after rupture of the membranes and labor, vaginal hysterectomy in a premenopausal woman, and radical pelvic surgery for gynecologic malignancy.[370] Several studies have shown significant reduction in the frequency of postoperative infection, from about 20% to 30% to about 4% to 8% after prophylactic antibiotic use in clean, contaminated surgery.[371,372] The basic principle of antibiotic prophylaxis is to provide adequate tissue levels at the site of contamination and adequate blood levels during the procedure and for 24 hours after the procedure. See Chapter 316 for a more detailed discussion.

Peritonitis during Peritoneal Dialysis

Long-Term Peritoneal Dialysis

Peritoneal dialysis has been used successfully to treat uremia in patients with end-stage renal disease since the mid-1940s. Peritonitis was a frequently associated side effect that hindered the acceptance of chronic peritoneal dialysis until an improved access catheter was developed by Tenckhoff in 1968. This catheter significantly decreased the incidence of peritonitis, but initial reports of patients undergoing CAPD with this catheter indicated peritonitis rates of more than six episodes per patient-year.[373,374] This rate has appeared to decline with the introduction of collapsible plastic bags, improved adapters, and better techniques. Peritonitis remains the major complication of CAPD today, however.[375] It occurs at a rate of about one episode per patient-year (range <0.5 to ≥ 3). Of patients, 45% experience peritonitis at least once during their initial 6 months of CAPD treatment. This rate increases to 60% to 70% during the first year.[376-378] Recurrent peritonitis occurs in 20% to 30% of patients and is one of the most common reasons for discontinuation of CAPD.[379] A small proportion of patients seem to have an unusually high frequency of peritonitis.[380] This disparity has been attributed partly to faulty sterile technique on the part of patients during self-administration of CAPD.

The origin of infection in most cases seems to be contamination of the catheter by common skin organisms.[374] Alterations of skin flora in CAPD patients[381] may lead to peritoneal contamination with enteric pathogens. A higher incidence of peritonitis has been reported in dialysis patients who are nasal carriers of *S. aureus*.[382] Pathogens also may contaminate the peritoneum from exit-site and subcutaneous-tunnel infections, transient bacteremia, and contamination of the dialysate

delivery system during bag exchanges. As mentioned previously, enteric bacteria also may gain access to the peritoneal cavity by transmural migration through an intact intestinal wall after the introduction of hypertonic solutions into the peritoneum.[55] This mechanism may account for enteric bacterial peritonitis in dialysis patients.[56] Polymicrobial infection with fecal organisms suggests perforation of the bowel as a complication of catheter placement.

Alterations in peritoneal defenses may increase the risk of peritonitis in CAPD patients. The antimicrobial function of peritoneal macrophages and polymorphonuclear cells generally requires the presence of opsonins. A reduction in the levels of IgG and C3 has been noted in peritoneal dialysis effluents compared with serum, and the concentrations of these crucial opsonizing agents are related inversely to the frequency of peritonitis.[383] The addition of IgG to peritoneal dialysis fluid has been found to have a prophylactic effect.[384] Other important factors that impair host defense mechanisms are the low pH and high osmolality of peritoneal dialysis fluid, both of which can impair polymorphonuclear function and antibiotic efficacy.[385]

Gram-positive organisms constitute 60% to 80% of isolates, most commonly *S. epidermidis*, followed by *S. aureus*, *Streptococcus* spp., and diphtheroids. Staphylococcal isolates have been noted to grow on polymer surfaces and frequently produce an extracellular slime substance or biofilm that may protect these bacteria from host defenses.[386] Gram-negative organisms are obtained from 15% to 30% of isolates. *E. coli* is the most common, followed by *Klebsiella/Enterobacter, Proteus,* and *Pseudomonas* spp. Less common pathogens include *Acinetobacter* spp., *Candida albicans,* and anaerobic bacteria. Rare isolates include atypical mycobacteria (usually *Mycobacterium chelonei* or *Mycobacterium fortuitum*), *M. tuberculosis, Candida parapsilosis, Aspergillus fumigatus, Nocardia asteroides,* and *Fusarium* spp.[380,387-389] Polymicrobial peritonitis in peritoneal dialysis patients usually is assumed to be secondary to a primary intestinal process (e.g., bowel perforation) and requires surgical exploration, although this has been questioned.[390]

Diagnosis of peritonitis is made when microorganisms and an increased number of leukocytes are present in the dialysate combined with a constellation of clinical findings that include abdominal pain and tenderness (60% to 80% of patients), nausea and vomiting (30%), fever (10% to 20%), and diarrhea (10%).[374,380,388,389] Not all these criteria need to be met, however, to fulfill the diagnosis.

The dialysate almost always is cloudy, and microscopic examination reveals a leukocyte count greater than 100 cells/mm³, approximately 85% being more than 500/mm³, with neutrophils predominating.[380] A preponderance of eosinophils in the peritoneal fluid is seen in a self-limited condition called *eosinophilic peritonitis* that often follows placement of the Tenckhoff catheter and may represent allergy to the tubing.[391,392] Peritoneal eosinophilia also is seen in fungal peritonitis. Gram staining of the fluid reveals organisms in 9% to 50% of cases.[374,380] Peripheral leukocytosis has been reported to be a poor indicator for peritonitis in this group of patients.[388] Blood cultures are rarely positive, in contrast to the 30% to 50% positive rate in other types of intra-abdominal infection.

Peritonitis with negative cultures occurs in 5% to 10% of cases. Constant flow of dialysis fluid into and out of the peritoneal cavity dilutes the microbial density and may lower falsely the rate of positive dialysate culture results. Negative cultures also may result from infection with fastidious organisms, previous antimicrobial treatment, or inadequate culture techniques. One method that has been used to improve the yield of dialysate cultures is the filtration method. A 100-mL aliquot of peritoneal fluid is filtered through a 0.45-μm filter. Then the filter is washed with sterile saline and incubated in thioglycolate broth.[388] Rubin and colleagues[374] compared the filtration method with direct inoculation of blood culture bottles and found no significant difference in positive culture rates. Other investigators found the inoculation of 2 to 3 mL of dialysate into thioglycolate broth to be the most sensitive culture technique.[388] A study comparing direct inoculation of dialysate into a biphasic blood culture system, direct inoculation of dialysate into routine blood culture bottles, and centrifugation of 50 mL of dialysate and culture of the sediment failed to show a significant difference among these methods in the recovery of a pathogen.[393] All cultures should be performed aerobically. Fungal, mycobacterial, and anaerobic cultures should be performed if clinically indicated (e.g., negative aerobic cultures).

The prognosis of peritonitis in dialysis patients is generally favorable. One large series reported less than 1% mortality attributed directly to infection.[380] The duration of illness and positive peritoneal fluid cultures after institution of antimicrobial therapy is usually 1 to 4 days. Some infections, especially infections caused by *S. aureus, Pseudomonas,* or fungus, resolve more slowly, however, and may cause relapse more frequently.[388]

Adequate levels of antimicrobial agents necessary to treat peritonitis successfully can be obtained in the peritoneal fluid by either the systemic or the intraperitoneal route.[380,387,388,394] Because CAPD peritonitis is a localized infection, however, the intraperitoneal route is preferred, as no therapeutic advantage of intravenously administered antibiotic has been shown.[395] The increased use of intraperitoneal antibiotic therapy for peritonitis has allowed most patients to be treated on an ambulatory basis. Hospitalization is indicated for patients who are severely ill or who are unable to manage the administration of intraperitoneal antibiotics at home. Although a variety of doses can be found in the literature, the initial doses recommended in Table 68-2 for intraperitoneal administration result in effective peritoneal fluid drug concentrations. Subsequent dosing is used to maintain these levels. The aim of the dosing regimen is to maintain a concentration of the drug in the peritoneal cavity fluid greater than the MIC of the offending pathogen for most if not the entire dosing interval. Caution must be exercised when reviewing the MIC and minimal bactericidal concentration data because these concentrations have been markedly increased when peritoneal dialysis effluent is used as the in vitro growth medium.[396]

Because of the lack of comparative, prospective clinical trials, no one antimicrobial regimen can be called superior to another. After cultures are obtained, initial antimicrobial therapy should be based on the results of Gram staining or on the most likely pathogens if the Gram stain is not helpful. A reasonable initial empirical regimen would be vancomycin in combination with an aminoglycoside. Vancomycin is preferable to a cephalosporin because of the frequency of β-lactam resistance (i.e., methicillin resistance) in staphylococci, which predicts resistance to cephalosporins as well. Initial antibiotic choices should be modified, if necessary, after culture results are obtained. Because *P. aeruginosa* peritonitis is associated with high failure rates and relapses, it is treated best with a combination of agents active against the infecting strain, in addition to catheter removal. The minimal length of therapy needed for dialysis-related peritonitis has not been determined, but the usual duration ranges from 10 days to 3 weeks. Most patients with CAPD peritonitis show clinical improvement within 48 to 96 hours after initiation of antimicrobial therapy. If the signs and symptoms of peritonitis persist after 96 hours of therapy, reevaluation is warranted, with consideration given to the possibilities of resistant pathogens, unusual organisms (e.g., mycobacterial, fungal), and other intra-abdominal processes, as recommended by Keane and colleagues.[395]

Fungal peritonitis, usually caused by *C. albicans,* should be treated with amphotericin B.[397-399] Some molds, including *Fusarium* spp., may be resistant to amphotericin, however. If CAPD is continued, amphotericin B should be given intraperitoneally, but it can cause appreciable abdominal pain when given by this route. Most patients with fungal CAPD infection fail to respond unless the catheter is removed, after which amphotericin B should be given intravenously (0.4 to 1.0 mg/kg IV q24-48h for 10 days after catheter removal). Oral or intravenous fluconazole penetrates adequately into the peritoneal fluid to treat peritonitis in CAPD patients after the catheter has been removed. Flucytosine is not recommended in azotemic patients because of potentially lethal toxicity to the colon and bone marrow. Ketoconazole rarely is indicated.

Removal of the catheter is necessary in 10% to 20% of patients. The indications for catheter removal include persistent skin exit-site or tunnel infection; fungal, fecal, or mycobacterial peritonitis; *P. aeruginosa* peritonitis; persistent peritonitis; recurrent peritonitis with the same organism; and catheter malfunction (e.g., poor flow). The catheter also should be removed in patients with intraperitoneal abscess. Use of oral or intraperitoneal antibiotics has not been shown to be effective in preventing peritonitis during peritoneal dialysis.[55,400] In addition, topical mupirocin has been used to eliminate nasal carriage with *S. aureus* but has yet to be shown to reduce significantly the incidence of CAPD-related peritonitis.[401] Advances in CAPD instrumentation, such as titanium adapters, connector systems with disinfectant, and in-line filters, may decrease the frequency of peritonitis but add to the overall cost of CAPD.

Acute Peritoneal Dialysis

The incidence of peritonitis during acute peritoneal dialysis has remained stable since the 1980s. Innovations in technique, which began during the 1960s, reduced the rate of peritonitis from 50% to acceptably low levels. These innovations included closed-drainage systems, small-bore catheters, limitation of dialysis to no longer than 48 to 72 hours, incorporation of a millipore filter into the tubing, and development of closed automatic systems. Also the use of dry-heat incubators to warm the dialysate decreases the risk of contamination that may occur when water baths are used for this purpose.[402]

Some authorities have recommended that cultures of dialysate be obtained every 8 to 24 hours during acute peritoneal dialysis and at its termination. Culture of dialysate from the last exchange is more useful than culture of the catheter tip at the end of dialysis because of the frequent contamination of the catheter tip at the time of its removal. Results of theses routine cultures, in the absence of symptoms or cloudy fluid, provide a guide of doubtful value for initiation of therapy. More importantly, dialysate samples should be cultured and examined microscopically (cell count, Gram stain) if the dialysate becomes cloudy or the patient develops signs or symptoms of peritonitis (e.g., fever, abdominal pain). Cultures are obtained best by syringe from the port closest to the catheter.

Antibiotic-resistant, hospital-acquired, gram-negative bacilli and staphylococci frequently cause peritonitis during acute peritoneal dialysis. It is recommended that therapy be initiated with intraperitoneal vancomycin and gentamicin (or tobramycin), with or without concurrent or subsequent addition of the same antibiotics parenterally, depending on the severity of the illness and the response to initial therapy (see Table 68-2 for dosages). Modification of the antibiotic regimen should be made when the culture results become available. The clinical manifestations, prognosis, and response to therapy are

TABLE 68-2   Antibiotic Dosage for Peritonitis during Peritoneal Dialysis

Drug	Initial Intraperitoneal Dosage (mg/L dialysate)*	Intraperitoneal Maintenance Dosage (mg/L dialysate)*
Amphotericin B	1.5	1.5
Ampicillin	500	125
Ampicillin/Sulbactam	1000	100
Cefazolin	500	125
Ceftazidime	250	125
Ciprofloxacin	50	25
Clindamycin	300	150
Fluconazole	200	200 IP or PO qd
Gentamicin	8	8
Piperacillin	4000 IV	250
Trimethoprim-sulfamethoxazole	320/1600 PO	80/400 PO qd
Vancomycin	30-50	30-50

*Unless otherwise specified.

Adapted from Keane WF, Bailie GR, Boeschoten E. Adult peritoneal dialysis–related peritonitis treatment recommendations: 2000 update. Perit Dial Intern. 2000;20:396-411.

similar to those described previously for peritonitis associated with chronic peritoneal dialysis.

INTRAPERITONEAL ABSCESSES

Etiology

Intraperitoneal abscess can complicate either primary or secondary peritonitis.[403,404] Diseases causing secondary intraperitoneal abscesses include appendicitis, diverticulitis, biliary tract lesions, pancreatitis, perforated peptic ulcers, inflammatory bowel disease, trauma, and abdominal surgery. The relative frequency of abscess formation associated with appendicitis may be declining, and the frequency of trauma and diverticulitis may be increasing.[404,405] The location of an abscess generally is related to the site of primary disease and the direction of dependent peritoneal drainage. Appendicitis has been reported to be associated most commonly with right lower quadrant and pelvic abscesses; colonic diverticulitis with left lower quadrant and pelvic abscesses; and pancreatitis with lesser sac abscesses.[403] In one large series[403] of 194 intraperitoneal abscesses, about 44% were in the right lower quadrant, 14% in the left lower quadrant, and 14% in the pelvis, whereas 20% were perihepatic. In a series reported by Saini and associates,[404] the frequency of various abscess locations had changed, perhaps reflecting the change in the relative frequency of the various etiologic diseases.

Of the various perihepatic (right subphrenic, right subhepatic, left perihepatic, and lesser sac) abscesses, the most common is in the right subphrenic space, but the difference in numbers between the right and left sides has been decreasing. In one large series of 267 cases of intra-abdominal abscesses, about half were in the subphrenic space, 60% of which were noted in the left perihepatic space.[406] This increased frequency of left perihepatic space abscess also was noted by Ozeran,[407] Sherman and associates,[408] and Sanders.[409] This finding is in contrast to the series of Ochsner and DeBakey in 1939,[410] when right subphrenic abscesses were most common, owing to the numerous ruptured appendices.

In children, appendicitis still is responsible for more than 50% of the cases of subphrenic abscess.[411] In adults, perihepatic abscesses currently are seen mainly as postoperative complications,[407-409,412] rather than in neglected primary intra-abdominal infections, such as appendicitis or perforated peptic ulcer. This fact may explain the increasing frequency of subphrenic abscess, especially on the left, compared with other intraperitoneal sites.[406] Usually the surgery has been in the gastroduodenal and biliary tracts. One group of investigators[413] noted that abscesses that occurred after gastric operations were left subphrenic if incidental splenectomy had been performed but right subhepatic if splenectomy had not been done. The subhepatic space is involved less frequently than the subphrenic spaces. Lesser sac abscesses usually follow pancreatitis or perforation of the stomach or duodenum. Multiple perihepatic space abscesses have been reported in 5% to 26% of the patients.[407-409,412,413]

Bacteriologic Findings

These infections typically are polymicrobial. In studies in which bacteriologic techniques permitted isolation of anaerobes, anaerobes were found in 60% to 70% of cases.[403,404,412,414] In one study,[412] anaerobes were recovered in 20 of 24 subphrenic abscesses, and *B. fragilis* was the most common pathogen, with anaerobic cocci and clostridia found in 50% of the patients. Other bacteria frequently recovered are *E. coli*, *Klebsiella/Enterobacter* group, *Proteus* spp., *P. aeruginosa*, *S. aureus*, and enterococci.[403,407,408,412]

Pathogenesis

Intraperitoneal abscesses develop as a result of localization of diffuse peritonitis, usually in the pelvis, perihepatic spaces, and paracolic gutters. In addition, abscess may develop about diseased organs (e.g., periappendiceal or pericholecystic abscesses) or after a penetrating wound (stab, gunshot, auto accident, or other trauma) or surgical procedure. These abscesses are termed *secondary* and

account for most of these cases. In contrast, the pathogenesis of primary abscesses is unknown and is presumably similar to that of primary peritonitis.

Clinical Manifestations

An acute course, with a high intermittent fever, shaking chills, abdominal pain, and tenderness over the involved area, is characteristic. The clinical pattern may be that of an acute secondary illness occurring after surgery for primary abdominal disease or prolonged recuperative course in a patient who has been receiving antibiotics after abdominal surgery. Various authors[408-413] have emphasized the occasional chronicity of subphrenic abscesses and have speculated that the course often is modified by antibiotics. Subphrenic abscesses have been described with 6 months or more of an indolent illness.[415]

Local symptoms and signs vary widely with the location and source of the abscess. Subphrenic abscesses usually are accompanied by chest findings with costal tenderness and pleural or pulmonary involvement, whereas subhepatic abscesses have more dominant signs of upper abdominal or subcostal involvement and fewer pulmonary changes.

Diagnosis

Noninvasive diagnostic procedures, including ultrasonography and CT, have provided greater sensitivity and specificity than routine radiography and radionuclide scanning.[416,417] These latter techniques may be useful occasionally, however, and sometimes a combination of diagnostic tests is the optimal approach to confirm the diagnosis of intra-abdominal abscess.[418]

Plain radiographs of the abdomen can suggest the location of abscesses in 50% of patients.[419] Radiologic findings associated with a subphrenic abscess may include pleural effusion, elevation of the hemidiaphragm, or loss of diaphragmatic movement on fluoroscopy. Routine radiography also may reveal displacement of viscera by an abscess. These findings can be enhanced by contrast radiology. The stomach may be outlined with barium or air to indicate displacement caused by a left perihepatic or lesser sac abscess. The presence of gas, either as a single air-fluid level or as mottling within the abscess, may aid localization on routine abdominal radiography.

Leukocytes tagged with gallium-67 and indium-111 are used in radionuclide scans, which at times may be helpful in detecting intra-abdominal abscesses, although they have been largely supplanted by CT and magnetic resonance imaging (MRI). In contrast to the technetium-99m sulfur colloid liver-spleen scan, which visualizes the entire organ and delineates abnormal areas as "cold" spots caused by decreased uptake of the isotope, ^{67}Ga-tagged and ^{111}In-tagged leukocytes accumulate in areas of inflammation, such as abscesses, and appear as areas of increased radioactivity or "hot" spots (Fig. 68-4).[420-423] Gallium is excreted into the intestinal tract and can accumulate in any inflammatory process and in certain neoplasms. For these reasons, false-positive scan readings can occur when radioactivity within the lumen of the bowel, within the wall of an inflamed bowel, or within a noninfected operative site in the process of healing is misinterpreted as an intra-abdominal abscess.

[111]In-tagged leukocyte scans are as sensitive as but more specific than ^{67}Ga-tagged scans. The labeled leukocytes tend to concentrate only in areas of inflammation because, in contrast to ^{67}Ga, ^{111}In is not secreted into the bowel.[424,425] Abscesses in the liver and spleen may be difficult to detect solely on ^{67}Ga-tagged or ^{111}In-tagged leukocyte images because normal accumulation of activity in these organs may mask an adjacent inflammatory focus. This problem can be overcome by comparing ^{67}Ga or ^{111}In images with technetium-99m scans.

Ultrasonography is a noninvasive technique that is helpful in the determination of the size, shape, consistency, and anatomic relationships of an intra-abdominal mass.[426,427] A pulsed, focused beam of high-frequency sound is directed into the suspect area of the patient's body by means of a transducer. Echoes are received by the same transducer from skin and tissue planes. The echo pattern is displayed on an oscilloscope as the transducer is moved along the surface of the body. The appearance of abscesses may vary widely from echo-free lesions

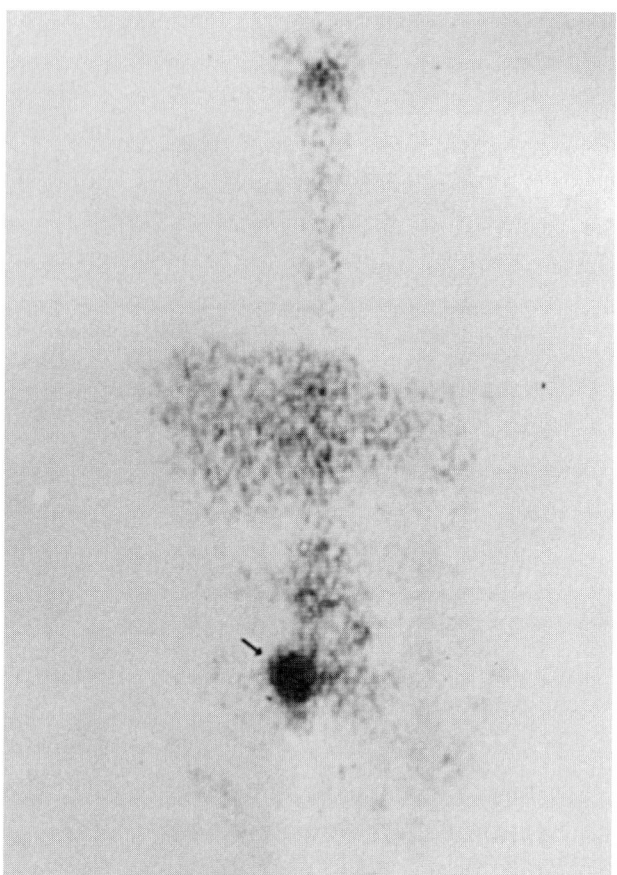

FIGURE 68-4. Gallium 67 scan in a patient with regional enteritis and signs of an intra-abdominal abscess. Note the area of increased radioactivity on the right lower quadrant *(arrow)*.

Prognosis

The period of morbidity is unusually prolonged in patients with intraperitoneal abscesses. Altemeier and colleagues[403] reported average hospital stays of 21 to 47 days. The presence of residual recurrent infection due to inadequate surgical drainage, more common in patients with multiple or bilateral abscesses, is associated with significantly greater mortality.

Treatment

The main therapy for any intraperitoneal abscess is drainage. Effective management depends on accurate localization of the abscess, discrimination between single and multiple abscesses, and early and adequate drainage. Conventional therapy for intraperitoneal abscesses usually has included surgical drainage. In recent years, successful therapy has been accomplished using percutaneous catheter drainage as an alternative to surgery.[437-439] This method has become possible with the use of refined imaging techniques, especially ultrasonography and CT.[440-442]

The general requirements for CT-guided or ultrasound-guided percutaneous catheter drainage include (1) an abscess that can be approached adequately via a safe percutaneous route; (2) an abscess that is unilocular; (3) an abscess that is not vascular, and the patient has no coagulopathy; (4) joint radiologic and surgical evaluation, with surgical backup for any complication or failure; and (5) the possibility of dependent drainage via the percutaneously placed catheter. CT also allows detection of an unsuspected additional intra-abdominal problem that otherwise would require surgical intervention. Percutaneous catheter drainage can be used as an initial approach in a patient too unstable to withstand immediate surgery. Definitive surgery can be postponed until the patient is in better condition. Percutaneous drainage of peridiverticular or appendiceal abscesses may permit a subsequent one-stage procedure of primary resection and immediate anastomosis, rather than the more costly and complicated multistage procedure.[443,444] After percutaneous placement of the catheter with CT or ultrasound guidance and aspiration of the abscess cavity, the catheter is placed for drainage by gravity or low suction until the daily drainage volume is minimal. Clinical response and collapse of the abscess cavity on repeat scanning should follow successful drainage. Some patients with percutaneous catheter drainage can be managed at home with their catheters in place. Of the patients who fit these criteria, percutaneous drainage has been successful in 80% to 90%.[439,445] Attempts at drainage of loculated, poorly organized, multiple, or extensive collections are less successful. In most series, the frequency of complications ranges from 5% to 15%,[437,446] including septicemia, hemorrhage, peritoneal spillage, and fistula formation. In addition, failure may occur because of undrained abscesses or pus too viscid to drain via the catheter. Reports indicate that the morbidity and mortality associated with percutaneous drainage may be less than with surgical treatment.[438,447]

Antimicrobial therapy should be started immediately after appropriate specimens (e.g., blood) are obtained for culture; usually this occurs before drainage. Because the pathogens usually are similar to those involved in secondary peritonitis, initial antibiotic therapy is directed similarly at the anaerobes, especially *B. fragilis* and the Enterobacteriaceae. The antimicrobial regimens discussed in the section on treatment of secondary peritonitis should be appropriate initial therapy. This antibiotic regimen should be adjusted to conform to results of in vitro testing of the infecting organisms isolated from blood or from purulent material obtained at surgery or catheter drainage. During the course of a prolonged illness, repeated cultures of blood and purulent collections, when clinically indicated, should provide a basis for change in antimicrobial therapy.

to highly echogenic masses, but they typically appear as a fluid collection with an irregular wall and the presence of a few internal echoes. Ultrasound images may be obscured by overlying gas-filled viscera and by postoperative wounds and drains.

CT has proved especially well suited for the diagnosis of intra-abdominal abscess.[428-433] Definition is unimpeded by intraluminal gas and postoperative changes except in the presence of surgical metallic clips or residual barium that may disrupt the image. Observed findings consistent with abscess include a low-density tissue mass and a definable capsule. CT can detect extraluminal gas, a finding highly suggestive of abscess.[417] Contrast material commonly is administered orally and intravenously when attempting to diagnose intra-abdominal abscess. The intraluminal contrast material helps to distinguish loops of bowel from abscess cavities, and the parenteral contrast material may enhance a surrounding capsule, allowing for easier identification.

MRI has the potential to display normal anatomy and to show abnormal conditions in many of the body's organ systems and anatomic regions.[434,435] Only a few trials have compared MRI with older radiologic procedures. In one study, MRI showed a clearer delineation of the extent of inflammatory changes than did CT, and it distinguished the abscess better from the surrounding structures.[436] In addition, the use of MRI does not require the administration of contrast medium and eliminates exposure to radiation, but it may be more costly than radiologic techniques.

Arteriographic localization also has been helpful. Overreliance on any one of these techniques is dangerous, and results should be confirmed by other methods and by the clinical findings.

REFERENCES

1. Whalen JP, Bierny JP. Classification of perihepatic abscesses. Radiology. 1969;92:1427-1437.
2. Sanders RC, James AE Jr, Fischer K. Correlation of liver scans and images with abdominal radiographs in perihepatic sepsis. Am J Surg. 1972;124:346-352.
3. Myers MA. The spread and localization of acute intraperitoneal effusions. Radiology. 1970;95:547-554.

4. Altemeier WA, Culbertson WR, Fullen WD, et al. Intra-abdominal abscesses. Am J Surg. 1973;125:70-79.
5. Shear L, Swartz C, Shinaberger JA, et al. Kinetics of peritoneal fluid absorption in adult men. N Engl J Med. 1965;272:123-127.
6. Boen ST. Kinetics of peritoneal dialysis: A comparison with artificial kidney. Medicine (Baltimore). 1961;40:243-287.
7. Tsilibury EC, Wissig SL. Absorption from the peritoneal cavity: SEM study of the mesothelium covering the peritoneal surface of the muscular portion of the diaphragm. Am J Anat. 1977;149:127-133.
8. Rochlin DB, Zill H, Blakemore WS. Studies of the resorption of chromium-51 tagged erythrocytes from the peritoneal cavity: The absorption of fluids and particulate matter from the peritoneal cavity. Int Abstr Surg. 1958;107:1-14.
9. Pritchard JA, Adams RH. The fate of blood in the peritoneal cavity. Surg Gynecol Obstet. 1957;105:621-629.
10. Zinsser HH, Pryde AW. Experimental study of physical factors, including fibrin formation, influencing the spread of fluids and small particles within and from the peritoneal cavity of the dog. Ann Surg. 1952;136:818-827.
11. Macbeth RA, Mackenzie WC. The abdominal wall, umbilicus, peritoneum, mesenteries, and retroperitoneum. In: Sabiston DC Jr, ed. Davis-Christopher Textbook of Surgery. 10th ed. Philadelphia: WB Saunders; 1972:773-795.
12. Nathens AB, Rotstein OD, Marshall JC. Tertiary peritonitis: Clinical features of a complex nosocomial infection. World J Surg. 1998;22:158-163.
13. Malangione MA. Evaluation and management of tertiary peritonitis. Am Surg. 2000;66:157-161.
14. Nohr CW, Marshall DG. Primary peritonitis in children. Can J Surg. 1984;27:179-181.
15. McDougal WS, Izant RJ, Zollinger RM Jr. Primary peritonitis in infancy and childhood. Ann Surg. 1975;181:310-313.
16. Golden GT, Shaw A. Primary peritonitis. Surg Gynecol Obstet. 1972;135:513-516.
17. Epstein M, Calia FM, Gabuzda GJ. Pneumococcal peritonitis in patients with postnecrotic cirrhosis. N Engl J Med. 1968;278:69-71.
18. Speck WT, Dresdale SS, McMillan RW. Primary peritonitis and the nephrotic syndrome. Am J Surg. 1974;127:267-269.
19. Mowat C, Stanley AJ. Spontaneous bacterial peritonitis—diagnosis, treatment and prevention. Aliment Pharmacol Therap. 2001;15:1851-1859.
20. Conn HO, Fessel JM. Spontaneous bacterial peritonitis in cirrhosis: Variations on a theme. Medicine (Baltimore). 1971;50:161-197.
21. Conn HO. Spontaneous bacterial peritonitis, multiple revisitations. Gastroenterology. 1976;70:455-457.
22. Bar-Meir S, Conn HO. Spontaneous bacterial peritonitis induced by intra-arterial vasopressin therapy. Gastroenterology. 1976;70:418-421.
23. Targan SR, Chow AW, Guze LB. Role of anaerobic bacteria in spontaneous peritonitis of cirrhosis: Report of two cases and review of the literature. Am J Med. 1977; 62:397-403.
24. Kline MM, McCallum RW, Guth PH. The clinical value of ascitic fluid culture and leukocyte count studies in alcoholic cirrhosis. Gastroenterology. 1976;70:408-412.
25. Weinstein MP, Iannini PB, Stratton CW, et al. Spontaneous bacterial peritonitis: A review of 28 cases with emphasis on improved survival and factors influencing prognosis. Am J Med. 1978;64:592-598.
26. Hoefs JC, Canawati HN, Sapico FL, et al. Spontaneous bacterial peritonitis. Hepatology. 1982;2:399-407.
27. Pinzello G, Simonetti R, Craxi A, et al. Spontaneous bacterial peritonitis: A prospective investigation in predominantly nonalcoholic cirrhotic patients. Hepatology. 1983;3:545-549.
28. Conn HO. Cirrhosis. In: Schiff L, Schiff ER, eds. Diseases of the Liver. 5th ed. Philadelphia: JB Lippincott; 1982:847-977.
29. Thomas FB, Fromkes JJ. Spontaneous bacterial peritonitis associated with acute viral hepatitis. J Clin Gastroenterol. 1982;4:259-262.
30. Runyon BA. Spontaneous bacterial peritonitis with cardiac ascites. Am J Gastroenterol. 1984;79:796.
31. Isner J, MacDonald JS, Schein PS. Spontaneous Streptococcus pneumoniae peritonitis in a patient with metastatic gastric cancer. Cancer. 1977;39:2306-2309.
32. Shesol BF, Rosato EF, Rosato FE. Concomitant acute lupus erythematosus and primary pneumococcal peritonitis. Am J Gastroenterol. 1975;63:324-326.
33. Friedland JA, Harris MN. Primary pneumococcal peritonitis in a young adult. Am J Surg. 1970;119:737-739.
34. Golden GT, Stevenson TR, Ritchie WP Jr. Primary peritonitis in adults. South Med J. 1975;68:413-414.
35. Wilcox CM, Dismukes WE. Spontaneous bacterial peritonitis: A review of pathogenesis, diagnosis and treatment. Medicine (Baltimore). 1987;66:447-456.
36. Correia JP, Conn HO. Spontaneous bacterial peritonitis in cirrhosis: Endemic or epidemic? Med Clin North Am. 1975;59:963-981.
37. Hoefs JC, Runyon BA. Spontaneous bacterial peritonitis. Dis Mon. 1985;31:1-48.
38. Fromkes JJ, Thomas FB, Mekhjian HS, et al. Antimicrobial activity of human ascitic fluid. Gastroenterology. 1977;73:668-672.
39. Scheckman P, Onderdonk AB, Bartlett JG. Anaerobes in spontaneous peritonitis. Lancet. 1977;2:1223.
40. Runyon BA, Hoefs JC. Culture-negative neutrocytic ascites: A variant of spontaneous peritonitis. Hepatology. 1984;4:1209-1211.
41. Runyon BA, Umland ET, Merlin T. Inoculation of blood culture bottles with ascitic fluid: Improved detection of spontaneous bacterial peritonitis. Arch Intern Med. 1987;147:73-75.
42. Runyon BA, Squier S, Borzio M. Translocation of gut bacteria in rats with cirrhosis to mesenteric lymph nodes partially explains the pathogenesis of spontaneous bacterial peritonitis. J Hepatol. 1994;21:792-796.
43. Beeson PB, Brannon ES, Warren JU. Observations on the sites of removal of bacteria from the blood in patients with bacterial endocarditis. J Exp Med. 1945;81:9-23.
44. Rutenburg AM, Sonnenblick F, Koven I, et al. Comparative response of normal and cirrhotic rats to intravenously injected bacteria. Proc Soc Exp Biol Med. 1959;101:279-281.
45. Lahnborg G, Friman L, Berghem L. Reticuloendothelial function in patients with alcoholic liver disease. Scand J Gastroenterol. 1981;16:481-489.
46. Whipple RL Jr, Harris JF. E. coli septicemia in Laennec's cirrhosis of the liver. Ann Intern Med. 1950;33:462-469.
47. Murray HW, Marks SJ. Spontaneous bacterial empyema, pericarditis and peritonitis in cirrhosis. Gastroenterology. 1977;72:772-773.
48. Snyder N, Atterbury CE, Correia JP, et al. Increased concurrence of cirrhosis and bacterial endocarditis. Gastroenterology. 1977;73:1107-1113.
49. Rajkovic IA, Williams R. Abnormalities of neutrophilic phagocytosis, intracellular killing and metabolic activity in alcoholic cirrhosis and hepatitis. Hepatology. 1986;6:252-262.
50. Wyke RJ, Rajkovic IA, Eddleston WF, et al. Defective serum opsonization in patients with chronic liver disease (Abstract). Gut. 1979;20:A931.
51. Yousif-Kadura AGM, Rajkovic IA, Wyke RJ, et al. Defects in serum attractant activity in different types of chronic liver disease. Gut. 1984;25:79-84.
52. Rimola A, Soto R, Bory F, et al. Reticuloendothelial system phagocytic activity in cirrhosis and its relation to bacterial infections and prognosis. Hepatology. 1984;4:53-58.
53. Simberkoff MS, Moldover NH, Weiss G. Bactericidal and opsonic activity of cirrhotic ascites and nonascitic peritoneal fluid. J Lab Clin Med. 1978;91:831-839.
54. Runyon BA, Hoefs JC. Ascitic fluid analyis in the differentiation of spontaneous bacterial peritonitis from gastrointestinal perforation into ascitic fluid. Hepatology. 1984;4:447-450.
55. Schweinburg FB, Seligman AM, Fine J. Transmural migration of intestinal bacteria: A study based on the use of radioactive Escherichia coli. N Engl J Med. 1950; 242:747-751.
56. Schwartz FD, Kallmeyer J, Durea G, et al. Prevention of infection during peritoneal dialysis. JAMA. 1967;199:79-81.
57. Gorbach SL, Lai D, Levitan R. Intestinal microflora in Laennec's cirrhosis (Abstract). J Clin Invest. 1970;49:36A.
58. McCartney JE, Fraser J. Pneumococcal peritonitis. Br J Surg. 1922;9:479-489.
59. Herbert TJ, Mortimer PP. Recurrent pneumococcal peritonitis associated with an intrauterine contraceptive device. Br J Surg. 1974;61:901-902.
60. Brinson RR, Kolts BE, Monif GRG. Spontaneous bacterial peritonitis associated with an intrauterine device. J Clin Gastroenterol. 1986;8:82-84.
61. Kimball MW, Knee S. Gonococcal perihepatitis in a male: The Fitz-Hugh-Curtis syndrome. N Engl J Med. 1970;282:1082-1084.
62. Navasa M, Follo A, Filella X, et al. Tumor necrosis factor and interleukin-6 in spontaneous bacterial peritonitis in cirrhosis: Relationship with the development of renal impairment and mortality. Hepatology. 1998;27:1227-1232.
63. Giron-Gonzalez JA, Rodriquez-Ramos C, Elvira J, et al. Serial analysis of serum and ascitic fluid levels of soluble adhesion molecules and chemokines in patients with SBP. Clin Exp Immunol. 2001;123:56-61.
64. Follo A, Llovet JM, Navasa M, et al. Renal impairment after spontaneous bacterial peritonitis in patients with cirrhosis: Incidence, clinical course, predictive factors and prognosis. Hepatology. 1994;20:1495-1501.
65. Vickers FN, Maloney PJ. Gonococcal perihepatitis: Reports of three cases with comments on diagnosis and treatment. Arch Intern Med. 1964;114:120-123.
66. Saw EC, Shields SJ, Comer TP, et al. Granulomatous peritonitis due to Coccidioides immitis. Arch Surg. 1974;108:369-371.
67. Hoefs JC. Diagnostic paracentesis: A potent clinical tool. Gastroenterology. 1990;98:230-236.
68. Hoefs JC. Increase in ascites white blood cell and protein concentrations during diuresis in patients with chronic liver disease. Hepatology. 1981;1:249-254.
69. Luetscher JA Jr. Electrophoretic analysis of the proteins of plasma and serous effusions. J Clin Invest. 1941;20:99-106.
70. Witte MH, Witte CL, Davis WM, et al. Peritoneal transudate: A diagnostic clue to portal system obstruction in patients with intra-abdominal neoplasms or peritonitis. JAMA. 1972;221:1380-1383.
71. Stassen WN, McCullough AJ, Bacon BR, et al. Immediate diagnostic criteria for bacterial infection of ascitic fluid: Evaluation of ascitic fluid polymorphonuclear leukocyte count, pH, and lactate concentration, alone and in combination. Gastroenterology. 1986;90:1247-1254.
72. Garcia-Tsao G, Conn HO, Lerner E. The diagnosis of bacterial peritonitis: Comparison of pH, lactate concentration and leukocyte count. Hepatology. 1985; 5:91-96.
73. Yang C-Y, Liaw F, Chu E-M, et al. White count, pH and lactate in ascites in the diagnosis of spontaneous bacterial peritonitis. Hepatology. 1985;5:85-90.
74. Burack WR, Hollister RM. Tuberculous peritonitis: A study of forty-seven proved cases encountered by a general medical unit in twenty-five years. Am J Med. 1960;28:510-523.
75. Harrison RN, Cryer HM, Howard DA, et al. Clarification of risk factors for abdominal operations in patients with hepatic cirrhosis. Ann Surg. 1984;199:648-665.
76. Runyon BA, McHutchison JG, Antillon MR, et al. Short-course versus long-course antibiotic treatment of spontaneous bacterial peritonitis: A randomized controlled study of 108 patients. Gastroenterology. 1991;100:1737-1742.
77. Runyon BA, Hoefs JC. Spontaneous vs. secondary bacterial peritonitis: Differentiation by response of ascitic fluid neutrophil count to antimicrobial therapy. Arch Intern Med. 1986;146:1563-1565.
78. Dimond M, Proctor HJ. Concomitant pneumococcal appendicitis, peritonitis and meningitis. Arch Surg. 1976;111:888-889.

79. Mallory A, Schaefer JW. Complications of diagnostic paracentesis in patients with liver disease. JAMA. 1978;239:628-630.

80. Levine H. Needle biopsy of peritoneum in exudative ascites. Arch Intern Med. 1967;120:542-545.

81. Dineen P, Homan WP, Grafe WR. Tuberculous peritonitis: 43 years experience in diagnosis and treatment. Ann Surg. 1976;184:717-722.

82. Felisart J, Rimona A, Arroyo V, et al. Cefotaxime is more effective than is ampicillin-tobramycin in cirrhotics with severe infections. Hepatology. 1985;5:457-462.

83. Cabrera J, Arroyo V, Ballesta AM, et al. Aminoglycoside nephrotoxicity in cirrhosis: Value of urinary β_2-microglobulin to discriminate functional renal failure from acute tubular damage. Gastroenterology. 1982;82:97-105.

84. Llovet JM, Rodriguez-Iglesias P, Moitinho E, et al. Spontaneous bacterial peritonitis in patients with cirrhosis undergoing selective intestinal decontamination. J Hepatol. 1997;26:88-95.

85. Forrest A, Nix DE, Ballow CH, et al. Pharmacodynamics of intravenous ciprofloxacin in seriously ill patients. Antimicrob Agents Chemother. 1993;37:1073-1081.

86. Sort P, Navasa M, Arroyo V, et al. Effect of intravenous albumin on renal impairment and mortality in patients with cirrhosis and spontaneous bacterial peritonitis. N Engl J Med. 1999;341:403-409.

87. Runyon BA, Hoefs JC. Ascitic fluid chemical analysis before, during and after spontaneous bacterial peritonitis. Hepatology. 1985;5:257-259.

88. Tito L, Rimola A, Gines P, at el. Recurrence of spontaneous bacterial peritonitis in cirrhosis: Frequency and predictive factors. Hepatology. 1988;8:27-31.

89. Gines P, Rimola A, Planas R, et al. Norfloxacin prevents spontaneous bacterial peritonitis recurrence in cirrhosis: Results of a double-blind, placebo-controlled trial. Hepatology. 1990;12:716-724.

90. Singh N, Gayowski T, Yu VL. Trimethoprim/sulfamethoxazole for the prevention of spontaneous bacterial peritonitis in cirrhosis: A randomized trial. Ann Intern Med. 1995;122:595-598.

91. Porter JM, Snowe RJ, Silver D. Tuberculous enteritis with perforation and abscess formation in childhood. Surgery. 1972;71:254-257.

92. Rowland TC Jr. Severe peritonitis complicating an intrauterine contraceptive device. Am J Obstet Gynecol. 1971;110:786-787.

93. Prokesch RC, Rimland D. Infectious complications of the peritoneovenous shunt. Am J Gastroenterol. 1983;78:235-240.

94. Reynold M, Sherman JO, Mclone DG. Ventriculoperitoneal shunt infections masquerading as an acute abdomen. J Pediatr Surg. 1983;18:951-954.

95. Nichols RL. Intra-abdominal infections: An overview. Rev Infect Dis. 1985;7(Suppl 4):S709-S715.

96. Drasar BS, Shiner M, McLeod GM. Studies on the intestinal flora: I. The bacterial flora of the gastrointestinal tract in healthy and achlorhydric persons. Gastroenterology. 1969;56:71-79.

97. Nichols RL, Smith JW. Intragastric microbial colonization in common disease states of the stomach and duodenum. Ann Surg. 1975;182:557-561.

98. Gorbach SL, Plaut AG, Nahas L, et al. Studies of intestinal microflora: II. Microorganisms of the small intestine and their relations to oral and fecal flora. Gastroenterology. 1967;53:856-867.

99. Drasar BS, Shiner M. Studies on the intestinal flora: Part II. Bacterial flora of the small intestine in patients with gastrointestinal disorders. Gut. 1969;10:812-819.

100. Gorbach SL, Nahas L, Lerner PI, et al. Studies of intestinal microflora: I. Effects of diet, age, and periodic sampling of numbers of fecal microorganisms in man. Gastroenterology. 1967;53:845-855.

101. Finegold SM. Interaction of antimicrobial therapy and intestinal flora. Am J Clin Nutr. 1970;23:1466-1471.

102. Altemeier WA. The bacterial flora of acute perforated appendicitis with peritonitis. Ann Surg. 1938;107:517-528.

103. Finegold SM. Abdominal and perineal infections. In: Finegold SM, ed. Anaerobic Bacteria in Human Disease. New York: Academic Press; 1977:257-313.

104. Gorbach SL, Thadepalli H, Norsen J. Anaerobic microorganisms in intra-abdominal infections. In: Balows A, de Haan RM, Dowell VR Jr, et al, eds. Anaerobic Bacteria: Role in Disease. Springfield, IL: Charles C Thomas; 1974:399-407.

105. Lorber B, Swenson RM. The bacteriology of intra-abdominal infections. Surg Clin North Am. 1975;55:1349-1354.

106. Swenson RM, Lorber B, Michaelson TC, et al. The bacteriology of intra-abdominal infections. Arch Surg. 1974;109:398-399.

107. Bodner SJ, Koenig MG, Goodman JS. Bacteremic *Bacteroides* infections. Ann Intern Med. 1970;73:537-544.

108. Gelb EF, Seligman SJ. Bacteroidaceae bacteremia: Effect of age and focus of infection upon clinical course. JAMA. 1970;212:1038-1041.

109. Fry DE, Garrison RN, Polk HC Jr. Clinical implications in *Bacteroides* bacteremia. Surg Gynecol Obstet. 1979;149:189-192.

110. Chow AW, Guze LB. Bacteroidaceae bacteremia: Clinical experience with 112 patients. Medicine (Baltimore). 1974;53:93-126.

111. Bennion RS, Thompson JL, Baron EL, et al. Gangrenous and perforated appendicitis with peritonitis: Treatment and bacteriology. Clin Ther. 1990;12(Suppl C):31-44.

112. Bennion RS, Thompson JL, Baron EL, et al. The bacteriology of gangrenous and perforated appendicitis—revisited. Ann Surg. 1990;211:165-167.

113. Tally FP, McGowan K, Kellum JM, et al. A randomized comparison of cefoxitin with or without amikacin and clindamycin plus amikacin in surgical sepsis. Ann Surg. 1981;193:318-323.

114. Rotstein OD, Pruett TL, Simmons RL. Microbiologic features and treatment of persistent peritonitis in patients in the intensive care unit. Can J Surg. 1986;29:247-250.

115. Aronoff SC, Olson MM, Gaudierer MWL, et al. *Pseudomonas aeruginosa* as a primary pathogen in children with bacterial peritonitis. J Pediatr Surg. 1987;22:861-864.

116. Heseltine PNR, Yellin AE, Applebaum MD, et al. Perforated and gangrenous appendicitis: An analysis of antibiotic failures. J Infect Dis.1983;148:322-329.

117. Bower RJ, Bell MJ, Ternberg JL. Controversial aspects of appendicitis management in children. Arch Surg. 1981;116:885-887.

118. Yellin AE, Heseltine PNR, Berne TV, et al. The role of *Pseudomonas* species in patients treated with ampicillin and sulbactam for gangrenous and perforated appendicitis. Surg Obstet Gynecol. 1985;161:303-307.

119. Dunn DL, Simmons RL. The role of anaerobic bacteria in intra-abdominal infections. Rev Infect Dis. 1984;6(Suppl 1):S139-S146.

120. Sawyer RG, Rosenlof LK, Adams RB, et al. Peritonitis in the 1990's: Changing pathogens and changing strategies in the critically ill. Am Surg. 1992;58:82-87.

121. Nichols RL, Smith JW, Klein DB, et al. Risk of infection after penetrating abdominal trauma. N Engl J Med. 1984;311:1065-1070.

122. Levison ME, Korman LC, Carrington ER, et al. Quantitative microflora of the vagina. Am J Obstet Gynecol. 1977;127:80-85.

123. Levison ME, Trestman I, Quach R, et al. Quantitative bacteriology of the vaginal flora in vaginitis. Am J Obstet Gynecol. 1979;133:139-144.

124. Bartlett JG, Onderdonk AB, Drude E, et al. Quantitative bacteriology of the vaginal flora. J Infect Dis. 1977;136:271-277.

125. Ohm M, Galask RP. The effect of antibiotic prophylaxis on patients undergoing vaginal operations: II. Alteration of microbial flora. Am J Obstet Gynecol. 1975;123:597-604.

126. Ramsay AM. The significance of *C. welchii* in the cervical swab and blood serum in postpartum and postabortum sepsis. J Obstet Gynecol. 1949;56:247-258.

127. Hite KE, Hesseltine HC, Goldstein L. A study of the bacterial flora of the normal and pathologic vagina and uterus. Am J Obstet Gynecol. 1947;53:233-240.

128. Gibbs RS, O'Dell TN, MacGregor RR, et al. Puerperal endometritis: A prospective microbiologic study. Am J Obstet Gynecol. 1975;121:919-925.

129. Baker CJ, Barrett FF, Yow MD. The influence of advancing gestation on group B streptococcal colonization in pregnant women. Am J Obstet Gynecol. 1975;122:820-823.

130. Penza JF. Moniliasis and trichomoniasis. In: Charles D, Finland M, eds. Obstetric and Perinatal Infections. Philadelphia: Lea & Febiger; 1973:209.

131. Finegold SM. Female genital tract infections. In: Finegold SM, ed. Anaerobic Bacteria in Human Disease. New York: Academic Press; 1977:350-385.

132. Swenson RM, Michaelson TC, Daly MJ, et al. Anaerobic bacterial infections of the female genital tract. Obstet Gynecol. 1973;42:538-541.

133. Thadepalli H, Gorbach SL, Keith L. Anaerobic infections of the female genital tract: Bacteriologic and therapeutic aspects. Am J Obstet Gynecol. 1973;117:1034-1040.

134. Chow AW, Marshall JR, Guze LB. Anaerobic infections of the female genital tract: Prospects and perspectives. Obstet Gynecol Surg. 1975;30:477-494.

135. Chow AW, Malkasian KI, Marshall JR, et al. The bacteriology of acute pelvic inflammatory disease: Value of cul-de-sac cultures and relative importance of gonococcal and other aerobic and anaerobic bacteria. Am J Obstet Gynecol. 1975;122:876-879.

136. Eschenbach DA, Buchanon TM, Pollock HM, et al. Polymicrobial etiology of acute pelvic inflammatory disease. N Engl J Med. 1975;293:166-171.

137. Wasserheit JN, Bell TA, Kiviat NB, et al. Microbial causes of proven pelvic inflammatory disease and efficacy of clindamycin and tobramycin. Ann Intern Med. 1986;104:187-193.

138. Monif GRG, Welkos SI, Baer H, et al. Cul-de-sac isolates from patients with endometritis-salpingitis-peritonitis and gonococcal endocervicitis. Am J Obstet Gynecol. 1976;126:158-161.

139. Burry VF. Gonococcal vulvovaginitis and possible peritonitis in prepubertal girls. Am J Dis Child. 1971;121:536-537.

140. Fuld GL. Gonococcal peritonitis in a prepubertal child. Am J Dis Child. 1968;115:621-622.

141. Adams EB, MacLeod IN. Invasive amebiasis: II. Amebic liver abscess and its complications. Medicine (Baltimore). 1977;56:325-334.

142. Turner GR, Millikan M, Carter E, et al. Surgical significance of fulminating amebic colitis: Report of perforation of the colon with peritonitis. Am Surg. 1965;31:759-763.

143. Lintermans JP. Fatal peritonitis, an unusual complication of *Strongyloides stercoralis* infestation. Clin Pediatr. 1975;14:974-975.

144. Eisenberg ES, Leviton I, Soeiro R. Fungal peritonitis in patients receiving peritoneal dialysis: Experience with 11 patients and review of the literature. Rev Infect Dis. 1986;3:309-321.

145. Bayer AS, Blumenkrantz MJ, Montgomerie JZ, et al. Candida peritonitis: Report of 22 cases and review of the English literature. Am J Med. 1976;61:832-840.

146. Solomkin JS, Flohr AB, Quie PG, et al. The role of *Candida* in intraperitoneal infections. Surgery. 1980;88:524-530.

147. Howard JM, Singh LM. Peritoneal fluid pH after perforation of peptic ulcers. Arch Surg. 1963;87:483-484.

148. Mortez WH, Erickson WG. Neutralization of hydrochloric acid in the peritoneal cavity. Arch Surg. 1957;75:834-837.

149. Santschi DR, Huizenga KA, Scudamore HH, et al. Bile ascites. Arch Surg. 1963;87:851-856.

150. Diamonon JS, Barnes JP. Choleperitoneum. Am Surg. 1964;30:331-334.

151. Cohn I, Coltar AM, Atik M, et al. Bile peritonitis. Ann Surg. 1960;152:827-835.

152. Nemir P Jr, Hawthorne HR, Cohn I, et al. I. The cause of death in strangulation obstruction: An experimental study. Ann Surg. 1949;130:857-873.

153. Nemir P Jr, Hawthorne HR, Cohn I, et al. II. The lethal action of the peritoneal fluid. Ann Surg. 1949;130:874-875.

154. Barnett WO, Hardy JD. Observations concerning the peritoneal fluid in experimental strangulated intestinal obstruction: The effects of removal from the peritoneal cavity. Surgery. 1958;43:440-444.

155. Barnett WO, Doyle RS. The effects of neomycin upon the toxicity of peritoneal fluid resulting from strangulation obstruction. Surgery. 1958;44:442-446.

156. Barnett WO, Messina AJ. The influence of massive antibiotics in experimental strangulation obstruction. Gastroenterology. 1959;36:534-536.

157. Davis JH, Yull AB. A possible toxic factor in abdominal surgery. J Trauma. 1962;2:291-300.

158. Filler RM, Sleeman HK, Hendry WS, et al. Lethal factors in experimental peritonitis. Surgery. 1966;60:671-678.

159. Lee JT, Ahrenholz DN, Nelson RD, et al. Mechanisms of the adjuvant effect of hemoglobin in experimental peritonitis: V. The significance of the coordinated iron component. Surgery. 1979;86:41-48.

160. Weingerg ED. Roles of iron in host-parasite interactions. J Infect Dis. 1971;124:401-410.

161. Hau T, Nelson RD, Fiegel VD, et al. Mechanisms of the adjuvant action of hemoglobin in experimental peritonitis: 2. Influence of hemoglobin on human leukocyte chemotaxis in vitro. J Surg Res. 1977;22:174-180.

162. Dunn DL, Barke RA, Ahrenholz DH, et al. The adjuvant effect of peritoneal fluid in experimental peritonitis. Ann Surg. 1984;199:37-43.

163. Rotstein OD, Pruett TL, Simmons RD. Fibrin in peritonitis: V. Fibrin inhibits phagocytic killing of *Escherichia coli* by human polymorphonuclear leukocytes. Ann Surg. 1986;203:413-419.

164. McRitchie DI, Girotti MJ, Glynn MF, et al. Effect of systemic fibrinogen depletion on intraabdominal abscess formation. J Lab Clin Med. 1991;118:48-55.

165. Dubrow T, Schwartz RJ, Kissock J, et al. Effect of aerosolized fibrin solution in intraperitoneal contamination. Arch Surg. 1991;126:80-83.

166. Schneierson SS, Amsterdam D, Perlman L. Enhancement of intraperitoneal staphylococcal virulence for mice with different bile salts. Nature. 1961;190:829-830.

167. Sisel RJ, Donovan AJ, Yellin AE. Experimental fecal peritonitis: Influence of barium sulfate or water-soluble radiographic contrast material on survival. Arch Surg. 1972;104:765-768.

168. Westfall RH, Nelson RH, Musselman MM. Barium peritonitis. Am J Surg. 1966;112:760-763.

169. Olitzki L. Mucin as a resistance-lowering substance. Bacteriol Rev. 1948;12:149-172.

170. Cuevas P, Fine J. Role of intraintestinal endotoxin in death from peritonitis. Surg Gynecol Obstet. 1972;134:953-957.

171. Fugger R, Hamilton G, Rogy M, et al. Prognostic significance of endotoxin determination in patients with severe intraabdominal infection. J Infect Dis. 1990;161:1314-1315.

172. Bieluch VM, Tally FP. Pathophysiology of abscess formation. Clin Obstet Gynecol. 1983;10:93-103.

173. Gorbach SL, Bartlett JG. Anaerobic infections (third of three parts). N Engl J Med. 1974;290:1289-1294.

174. Hofstad T. Endotoxins of anaerobic gram-negative microorganisms. In: Balows A, de Haan RM, Dowell VR Jr, et al, eds. Anaerobic Bacteria: Role in Disease. Springfield, IL: Charles C Thomas; 1974:295.

175. Gibbons RJ, MacDonald JB. Degradation of collagenous substrates by *Bacteroides melaninogenicus*. J Bacteriol. 1961;81:614-621.

176. Bjornson HS. Enzymes associated with the survival and virulence of gram-negative anaerobes. Rev Infect Dis. 1984;6(Suppl 1):S21-S24.

177. Gesner BM, Jenkin CR. Production of heparinase by bacteroides. J Bacteriol. 1961;81:595-604.

178. Bjornson H, Hill EO. Bacteroidaceae in thromboembolic disease: Effects of cell wall components on blood coagulation in vivo and in vitro. Infect Immun. 1974;9:337-341.

179. Casciato DA, Rosenblatt JE, Goldberg LS, et al. In vitro interaction of *Bacteroides fragilis* with polymorphonuclear leukocytes and serum factors. Infect Immun. 1975;11:337-342.

180. Keusch GT, Douglas SD. Intraleukocytic survival of anaerobic bacteria. Clin Res. 1974;22:445A.

181. Kasper DL. The polysaccharide capsule of *Bacteroides fragilis* subspecies fragilis: Immunochemical and morphologic definition. J Infect Dis. 1976;133:79-87.

182. Mansheim BJ, Orderdonk AB, Kasper DL. Immunochemical characterization of surface antigens of *Bacteroides melaninogenicus*. Rev Infect Dis. 1979;1:263-277.

183. Onderdonk AB, Kasper DL, Cisneros RL, et al. The capsular polysaccharide of *Bacteroides fragilis* as a virulence factor: Comparison of the pathogenic potential of encapsulated and unencapsulated strains. J Infect Dis. 1977;136:82-89.

184. Ingham HR, Tharagonnet D, Sisson PR, et al. Inhibition of phagocytosis in vitro by obligate anaerobes. Lancet. 1977;2:1252-1254.

185. Simon GL, Klempner MS, Kasper DL, et al. Alterations in opsonophagocytic killing by neutrophils of *Bacteroides fragilis* associated with animal and laboratory passage: Effect of capsular polysaccharide. J Infect Dis. 1982;145:72-77.

186. Socransky SS, Gibbons RJ. Required role of *Bacteroides melaninogenicus* in mixed anaerobic infections. J Infect Dis. 1965;115:247-253.

187. Altemeier WA. The pathogenicity of the bacteria of appendicitis peritonitis. Surgery. 1942;11:374-384.

188. Namavar FA, Verweij MJ, Bal M, et al. Effects of anaerobic bacteria on killing of *Proteus mirabilis* by human polymorphonuclear leukocytes. Infect Immun. 1983;40:930-935.

189. Rotstein OD, Nasmith PE, Grinstein S. The bacteroides by-product succinic acid inhibits neutrophil respiratory burst by reducing intracellular pH. Infect Immun. 1987;55:864-870.

190. Brook I. Anaerobic infections in childhood. Rev Infect Dis. 1984;6(Suppl 1):S187-S192.

191. Weinstein WN, Onderdonk AB, Bartlett JG, et al. Experimental intra-abdominal abscesses in rats: Development of an experimental model. Infect Immun. 1974;10:1250-1255.

192. Onderdonk AB, Weinstein WN, Sullivan NM, et al. Experimental intra-abdominal abscess in rats: Quantitative bacteriology of infected animals. Infect Immun. 1974;10:1256-1259.

193. Weinstein WM, Onderdonk AB, Bartlett JG, et al. Antimicrobial therapy of experimental intraabdominal sepsis. J Infect Dis. 1975;132:282-286.

194. Onderdonk AB, Bartlett JG, Louie T, et al. Microbial synergy in experimental intra-abdominal abscess. Infect Immun. 1976;13:22-26.

195. Rotstein OD, Pruett TL, Simmons RL. Mechanisms of microbial synergy in polymicrobial surgical infections. Rev Infect Dis. 1985;7:151-170.

196. Chung DR, Kasper DL, Panzo RJ, et al. CD4+ T cells mediate abscess formation in intra-abdominal sepsis by an IL-17-dependent mechanism. J Immunol. 2003;170:1958-1963.

197. Schein M, Wittmann DH, Holzheimer R, et al. Hypothesis: Compartmentalization of cytokines in intraabdominal infection. Surgery. 1996;119:694-700.

198. Holzheimer R, Schein M, Wittmann DH. Inflammatory response in peritoneal exudate and plasma of patients undergoing planned relaparotomy for severe secondary peritonitis. Arch Surg. 1995;130:1314-1319.

199. Giroir BP. Mediators of septic shock: New approaches for interrupting the endogenous inflammatory cascade. Crit Care Med. 1993;21:780-789.

200. Baigrie RJ, Lamont PM, Kwiatowski D, et al. Systemic cytokine response after major surgery. Br J Surg. 1992;79:757-760.

201. Bagby GJ, Plessala KJ, Wilson LA, et al. Divergent efficacy of antibody to tumor necrosis factor-δ in intravascular and peritonitis models of sepsis. J Infect Dis. 1991;163:83-88.

202. Asitz ME, Saha DC, Carpati CM, et al. Induction of endotoxin tolerance with monophosphoryl lipid A in peritonitis: Importance of localized therapy. J Lab Clin Med. 1994;123:89-93.

203. McMaster KM, Cheadle WG. Regulation of macrophage TNF-alpha, IL-1 beta and 1a (1a-alpha) mRNA expression during peritonitis is site dependent. J Surg Res. 1993;54:426-430.

204. Zannetti G, Heumann D, Gerain J, et al. Cytokine production after intravenous or peritoneal gram-negative bacterial challenge in mice. J Immunol. 1992;148:1890-1897.

205. Propst T, Propst A, Herold M, et al. Spontaneous bacterial peritonitis is associated with high levels of interleukin-6 and its secondary mediators in ascitic fluid. Eur J Clin Invest. 1993;23:823-836.

206. Zeni F, Tardy B, Vindimian M, et al. High levels of tumor necrosis factor-alpha and interleukin-6 in the ascitic fluid of cirrhotic patients with spontaneous bacterial peritonitis. Clin Infect Dis. 1993;17:218-223.

207. Nakahama H, Tanaka Y, Shirai D, et al. Plasma interleukin-6 levels in continuous ambulatory peritoneal dialysis and hemodialysis patients. Nephron. 1992;61:132-134.

208. Zemel D, Krediet RT, Koomen GC, et al. Interleukin-8 during peritonitis in patients treated with CAPD: An in-vivo model of acute inflammation. Nephrol Dial Transplant. 1994;9:169-176.

209. Zemel D, Koomen GC, Hart AA, et al. Relationship of TNF-alpha, interleukin-6, and prostaglandins to peritoneal permeability for macromolecules during longitudinal follow-up of peritonitis in continuous ambulatory peritoneal dialysis. J Lab Clin Med. 1993;22:686-696.

210. Holzheimer R, Schein M, Wittmann DH. Inflammatory response in peritoneal exudate and plasma of patients undergoing planned relaparotomy for severe secondary peritonitis. Arch Surg. 1995;130:1314-1320.

211. Slack AM, Saladino RA, Thompson C, et al. Failure of prophylactic and therapeutic use of murine anti-tumor necrosis factor monoclonal antibody in *Escherichia coli* sepsis in the rabbit. Crit Care Med. 1995;23:1512-1518.

212. Echtenacher B, Falk W, Mannel DN, et al. Requirement of endogenous tumor necrosis factor/cachectin for recovery from experimental peritonitis. J Immunol. 1990;145:3762.

213. Battafarano RJ, Burd RS, Kurrelmeyer KM, et al. Inhibition of splenic macrophage tumor necrosis factor alpha secretion in vivo by antilipopolysaccharide monoclonal antibodies. Arch Surg. 1994;129:179-181.

214. Kohler J, Heumann D, Garotta G, et al. IFN-gamma involvement in the severity of gram-negative infections in mice. J Immunol. 1993;151:916-921.

215. Rosoff L, Weil M, Bradely EC, et al. Hemodynamic and metabolic changes associated with bacterial peritonitis. Am J Surg. 1967;114:180-189.

216. MacLean LD, Mulugan WG, McLean APH, et al. Patterns of septic shock in man: A detailed study of 56 patients. Ann Surg. 1967;166:543-562.

217. Davis JH. Current concepts of peritonitis. Am Surg. 1967;33:673-681.

218. Debrin PB, Gully PH, Greenlee HB, et al. Radiographic diagnosis of an intra-abdominal abscess: Do multiple tests help? Arch Surg. 1986;121:41-46.

219. Gerzof SG, Johnson WC. Radiologic aspects of diagnosis and treatment of abdominal abscesses. Surg Clin North Am. 1984;54:53-65.

220. Haaga JR. Imaging intraabdominal abscesses and non-operative drainage procedures. World J Surg. 1990;14:204-209.

221. Sanna A, Adani GL, Anani G, Donini A. The role of laparoscopy in patients with suspected peritonitis: Experience of a single institution. L Laparoendosc Adv Surg Tech A. 2003;13:17-19.

222. Pine RW, Wertz MJ, Lennard ES, et al. Determinants of organ malfunction or death in patients with intra-abdominal sepsis. Arch Surg. 1983;118:242-249.

223. Nystrom PO, Bax R, Dellinger EP, et al. Proposed definitions for diagnosis, severity scoring, stratification, and outcome for trials on intraabdominal infection: Joint Working Party of SIS North America and Europe. World J Surg. 1990;14:148-158.

224. Dellinger EP, Wertz MJ, Meakins JL, et al. Surgical infection stratification system for intra-abdominal infection. Arch Surg. 1985;120:21-29.

225. Meakins JL, Solomkin JS, Allo MD, et al. A proposed classification of intra-abdominal infections: Stratification of etiology and risk for future therapeutic trials. Arch Surg. 1984;119:1372-1378.

226. Mustard RA, Bohnen JM, Rosati C, et al. Pneumonia complicating abdominal sepsis: An independent risk factor for mortality. Arch Surg. 1991;126:170-175.

227. Runcie C, Ramsey G. Intra-abdominal infection: Pulmonary failure. World J Surg. 1990;14:196-203.

228. Nystrom PO, Bax R, Dellinger EP, et al. Proposed definitions for diagnosis, severity scoring, stratification, and outcome for trials on intra-abdominal infection. World J Surg. 1990;14:148-158.

229. Knaus WA, Draper EA, Wagner DP, et al. APACHE II: A severity of disease classification. Crit Care Med. 1985;13:818-829.

230. Pacelli F, Doglietto GB, Alfiere S, et al. Prognosis in intraabdominal infections: Multivariate analysis on 604 patients. Arch Surg. 1996;131:641-645, 665.

231. Christon NV, Barie PS, Dellinger EP, et al. Intra-abdominal study. Arch Surg. 1993;128:193-199.

232. Goris RJA, teBoekhorst, TPA, Nuytinck JKS, et al. Multiple-organ failure: Generalized autodestructive inflammation? Arch Surg. 1985;120:1109-1115.

233. Damas P, Ledoux D, Nys M, et al. Cytokine serum level severe sepsis in human: IL-6 as a marker of severity. Ann Surg. 1992;215:356-362.

234. Fugger R, Zadrobilek E, Gotzinger P, et al. Perioperative TNF-alpha and IL-6 concentrations correlate with septic state, organ dysfunction, and APACHE II scores in intra-abdominal infection. Eur J Surg. 1993;159:525-529.

235. Patel RT, Deen KI, Youngs J, et al. Interleukin 6 is a prognostic indicator of outcome in severe intra-abdominal sepsis. Br J Surg. 1994;81:1306-1308.

236. Hamilton G, Hofbauer S, Hamilton B. Endotoxin, TNF-alpha, interleukin-6 and parameters of cellular immune system in patients with intraabdominal sepsis. Scand J Infect Dis. 1992;24:361-368.

237. Barriere SL. An overview of mortality risk prediction in sepsis. Crit Care Med. 1995;23:376-393.

238. Nobles ER Jr. Bacteroides infections. Ann Surg. 1973;177:601-606.

239. Young LS, Martin WJ, Meyer RD, et al. Gram-negative rod bacteremia: Microbiologic, immunologic and therapeutic considerations. Ann Intern Med. 1977;86:456-471.

240. Maier JA Jr, Reynolds TB, Yellin AE. Successful medical treatment of pyogenic liver abscess. Gastroenterology. 1979;77:618-622.

241. Herbert DA, Fogel DA, Rothman J, et al. Pyogenic liver abscesses: Successful nonsurgical therapy. Lancet. 1982;1:134-136.

242. Solomkin JS, Meakins JC, Allo MD, et al. Antibiotic trials in intra-abdominal infections: A critical evaluation of study design and outcome reporting. Ann Surg. 1984;200:29-39.

243. Stalons DR, Thonsberry C, Dawell VR. Effect of culture medium and carbon dioxide concentration of growth of anaerobic bacteria commonly encountered in clinical specimens. Appl Microbiol. 1974;27:1098-1104.

244. Rosenblatt JE, Schoenknecht F. Effect of several components of anaerobic incubation on antibiotic susceptibility test results. Antimicrob Agents Chemother. 1972;1:437-440.

245. Wagoner ES, Gorman M. The reaction of cysteine and related compounds with penicillins and cephalosporins. J Antibiot (Tokyo). 1971;24:647-658.

246. Wilkins TD, Chalgren S. Medium for use in antibiotic susceptibility testing of anaerobic bacteria. Antimicrob Agents Chemother. 1976;10:926-928.

247. Mosdell DM, Morris DM, Voltura A, et al. Antibiotic treatment for surgical peritonitis. Ann Surg. 1991;214:543-549.

248. Nathens AB. Relevance and utility of peritoneal cultures in patients with peritonitis. Surg Infect (Larchmt). 2001;2:153-160.

249. Wittmann DH, Bergstein JM, Franzides CT. Calculated empiric antimicrobial therapy for mixed surgical infections. Infection. 1991;19(Suppl 6):345-350.

250. Finegold SM, Wexler HM. Therapeutic implications of bacteriologic findings in mixed aerobic-anaerobic infections. Antimicrob Agents Chemother. 1988;32:611-616.

251. Solomkin JS, Dellinger EP, Christou NV, et al. Results of a multicenter trial comparing imipenem cilastatin to tobramycin-clindamycin for intra-abdominal infections. Ann Surg. 1990;212:581-591.

252. Gorbach SL, Thadepalli H. Clindamycin in pure and mixed anaerobic infections. Arch Intern Med. 1974;134:87-92.

253. Bartlett JG, Louie TJ, Gorbach SL, et al. Therapeutic efficacy of 29 antimicrobial regimens in experimental intraabdominal sepsis. Rev Infect Dis. 1981;3:535-542.

254. Fass RJ, Scholand JF, Hodges GR, et al. Clindamycin in the treatment of serious anaerobic infections. Ann Intern Med. 1973;78:853-859.

255. Levison ME, Santoro J, Bran JL, et al. In vitro activity and clinical efficacy of clindamycin in the treatment of infections due to anaerobic bacteria. J Infect Dis. 1977;135:S49-S53.

256. Montravers P, Andremont A, Massias L, et al. Investigation of the potential role of Enterococcus faecalis in the pathophysiology of experimental peritonitis. J Infect Dis. 1994;169:821-830.

257. Matlow AG, Bohnen JMA, Nohr C, et al. Pathogenicity of entercocci in a rat model of fecal peritonitis. J Infect Dis. 1989;160:142-145.

258. Doughtery SH. Role of enterococcus in intra-abdominal sepsis. Am J Surg. 1984;148:303-312.

259. Weinstein MP, Reller LB, Murphy J, et al. The clinical significance of positive blood cultures: A comprehensive analysis of 500 episodes of bacteremia and fungemia in adults: I. Laboratory and epidemiologic observations. Rev Infect Dis. 1983;5:35-53.

260. Shlaes DM, Levy J, Wolinksy E. Enterococcal bacteremia without endocarditis. Arch Intern Med. 1981;141:578-581.

261. Doughtery SH, Flohr AB, Simmons RL. Breakthrough enterococcal septicemia in surgical patients. Arch Surg. 1983;118:232-238.

262. Salzer W, Pegram PS, McCan CE. Clinical evaluation of moxalactam: Evidence of decreased efficacy in gram-positive aerobic infection. Antimicrob Agents Chemother. 1983;23:565-570.

263. Doughtery SH, Flohr AB, Simmons RL. "Breakthrough" entercoccal septicemia in surgical patients. Arch Surg. 1983;118:232-238.

264. Murphy TF, Barza M. Treatment of intraabdominal infection with moxalactam. Rev Infect Dis. 1982;4:670-675.

265. Stellato TA, Danziger LH, Hau T, et al. Moxalactam vs. tobramycin-clindamycin: A randomized trial in secondary peritonitis. Arch Surg. 1988;123:714-717.

266. Yu VL. Enterococcal superinfection and colonization after therapy with moxalactam, a new broad-spectrum antibiotic. Ann Intern Med. 1981;94:784-785.

267. Jones RN. Gram-positive superinfection following beta-lactam chemotherapy: The significance of the enterococcus. Infection. 1985;13(Suppl 1):S81-S88.

268. Barrall DT, Kenney PR, Slotman GJ, et al. Enterococcal bacteremia in surgical patients. Arch Surg. 1985;120:57-63.

269. Weigelt JA, Easley SM, Thal ER, et al. Abdominal surgical wound infection is lowered with improved enterococcus and bacteroides therapy. J Trauma. 1993;34:579-585.

270. Livornese LL Jr, Dias S, Samel C, et al. Hospital-acquired infection with vancomycin-resistant Enterococcus faecium transmitted by electronic thermometers. Ann Intern Med. 1992;117:112-116.

271. Murray BE. The life and times of the enterococci. Clin Microbiol Rev. 1990;3:46-65.

272. Courvalin P. Resistance of enterococci to glycopeptides. Antimicrob Agents Chemother. 1990;34:2291-2296.

273. Moellering RC. Emergence of enterococci as a significant pathogen. Clin Infect Dis. 1992;14:1173-1178.

274. Burnett RJ, Haverstock DC, Dellinger EP, et al. Definition of the role of enterococcus in intraabdominal infection: Analysis of a prospective randomized trial. Surgery. 1995;188:716-721.

275. Solomkin JS, Reinhart HH, Dellinger EP, et al. Results of a randomized trial comparing sequential intravenous/oral treatment with ciprofloxacin plus metronidazole to imipenem/cilastatin for intra-abdominal infections. Ann Surg. 1996;223:303-313.

276. Sotto A, Lefrant JY, Fabbro-Peray P, et al. Evaluation of antimicrobial therapy management of 120 consecutive patients with secondary peritonitis. J Antimicrob Chemother. 2002;50:569-576.

277. Peoples JB. Candida and perforated peptic ulcers. Surgery. 1986;100:758-764.

278. Rutledge R, Mandel SR, Wilde RE. Candida species: Insignificant contaminant or pathogenic species? Am Surg. 1986;52:299-302.

279. Marsh PK, Tally FP, Kellum J, et al. Candida infections in surgical patients. Ann Surg. 1983;198:42-47.

280. Sobel JD. Candida infections in the intensive care unit. Crit Care Clin North Am. 1988;4:325-344.

281. Sande MA, Overton JW. In vivo antagonism between gentamicin and chloramphenicol in neutropenic mice. J Infect Dis. 1973;128:247-250.

282. Zinner SH, Provonchee RB, Elias KS. Effect of clindamycin on the in vitro activity of amikacin and gentamicin against gram negative bacilli. Antimicrob Agents Chemother. 1976;9:661-666.

283. Ekwo E, Peter G. Effect of clindamycin on aminoglycoside activity in murine model of Escherichia coli infection. Antimicrob Agents Chemother. 1976;10:893-898.

284. Fass RJ, Rotilie CA, Prior RB. Interaction of clindamycin and gentamicin in vitro. Antimicrob Agents Chemother. 1974;6:582-587.

285. Cuchural GJ Jr, Tally FB, Jacobus NV, et al. Susceptibility of the Bactroides fragilis group in the United States: Analysis by site of isolation. Antimicrob Agents Chemother. 1988;32:717-722.

286. Van Scoy RE, Wilkowske CJ, O'Fallon WM, et al. Clindamycin versus chloramphenicol in treatment of anaerobic infections: A prospective, randomized double-blind study. Mayo Clin Proc. 1984; 59:842-846.

287. Bohnen JMA, Solomkin JS, Dellinger EP, et al. Guidelines for clinical care: Anti-infective agents for intra-abdominal infection: A Surgical Infection Society policy statement. Arch Surg. 1992;127:83-89.

288. Shands JW Jr. Empiric antibiotic therapy of abdominal sepsis and serious perioperative infections. Surg Clin North Am. 1993;73:291-306.

289. Tally FB, Sosa A, Jacobus NV, et al. Clindamycin resistance in Bacteroides fragilis. J Antimicrob Chemother. 1981;8(Suppl):43-48.

290. Tally FP, Cuchural GH Jr, Jacobus NV, et al. Nationwide study of the susceptibility of the Bacteroides fragilis group in the United States. Antimicrob Agents Chemother. 1985;28:675-677.

291. Wilson WR, Cockerill FR III. Tetracyclines, chloramphenicol, erythromycin and clindamycin. Mayo Clin Proc. 1987;62:906-915.

292. Tedesco FJ, Barton RW, Alpers DH. Clindamycin associated colitis: A prospective study. Ann Intern Med. 1974;81:429-433.

293. Ralph ED, Kirby WMM. Unique bactericidal action against Bacteroides fragilis and Clostridium perfringens. Antimicrob Agents Chemother. 1975;8:409-414.

294. Chow AW, Patten V, Guze LB. Susceptibility of anaerobic bacteria to metronidazole: Relative resistance of non-spore-forming gram-positive bacilli. J Infect Dis. 1975;131:182-185.

295. Onderdonk AB, Louie TJ, Tally FP, et al. Activity of metronidazole against Escherichia coli in experimental intra-abdominal sepsis. J Antimicrob Chemother. 1979;5:201-210.

296. Bartlett JG, Louie TJ, Gorbach SL, et al. Therapeutic efficacy of 29 antimicrobial regimens in experimental intra-abdominal sepsis. Rev Infect Dis. 1981;3:535-542.

297. Gerding DN, Olson MM, Johnson S, et al. Clostridium difficile diarrhea and colonization after treatment with abdominal infection regimens containing clindamycin or metronidazole. Am J Surg. 1990;159:212.

298. Sutter VL, Kwoh Y-Y, Finegold SM. Standardized antimicrobial disc susceptibility testing of anaerobic bacteria: I. Susceptibility of Bacteroides fragilis to tetracyclines. Appl Microbiol. 1972;23:268-275.

299. Sutter VL, Finegold SM. Susceptibility of anaerobic bacteria to 23 antimicrobial agents. Antimicrob Agents Chemother. 1976;10:736-752.

300. Wexler HM, Finegold SM. In vitro activity of cefotetan compared with that of other antimicrobial agents against anaerobic bacteria. Antimicrob Agents Chemother. 1988;32:601-604.

301. O'Keefe JP, Vlenezio FR, Divincenzo CA, et al. Activity of newer beta-lactam agents against clinical isolates of Bacteroides fragilis and other Bacteroides species. Antimicrob Agents Chemother. 1987;31:2002-2004.

302. Rolfe RD, Finegold SM. Comparative in vitro activity of new beta-lactam antibiotics against anaerobic bacteria. Antimicrob Agents Chemother. 1981;200:600-609.

303. Aldridge KE. Comparison of the activities of penicillin G and new beta-lactam antibiotics against clinical isolates of *Bacteroides* species. Antimicrob Agents Chemother. 1984;26:410-413.

304. Chow AW, Finegold SM. In vitro activity of ceftizoxime against anaerobic bacteria and comparison with other cephalosporins. J Antimicrob Chemother. 1982;10(Suppl C):45-50.

305. Harding GJ, Vincelette A, Rachlis I, et al. A preliminary report on the use of ceftizoxime vs clindamycin/tobramycin for the therapy of intra-abdominal and pelvic infections. J Antimicrob Chemother. 1982;10(Suppl C):191-192.

306. Lou MA, Chen DF, Bansal M, et al. Evaluation of ceftizoxime in acute peritonitis. J Antimicrob Chemother. 1982;10(Suppl C):183-189.

307. O'Keefe JP, Tally FP, Barza M, et al. Inactivation of penicillin G during experimental infection with *Bacteroides fragilis*. J Infect Dis. 1978;137:437-442.

308. Schoutens E, Yourassowsky E. Speed of bactericidal action of penicillin G, ampicillin and carbenicillin on *Bacteroides fragilis*. Antimicrob Agents Chemother. 1974;6:227-231.

309. Trestman I, Kaye D, Levison ME. Activity of semisynthetic penicillins and synergism with mecillinam against *Bacteroides* species. Antimicrob Agents Chemother. 1979;16:283-286.

310. Levison ME, Trestman I, Egert J, et al. Evaluation of ticarcillin in anaerobic infections (Abstract 176). Presented at 17th Interscience Conference on Antimicrobial Agents and Chemotherapy, New York, October 12-14, 1977.

311. Swenson RM, Lorber B. Clindamycin and carbenicillin in treatment of patients with intra-abdominal and female genital tract infections. J Infect Dis. 1977;135:S40-S45.

312. Winston DJ, Murphy W, Young LS, et al. Piperacillin therapy for serious bacterial infections. Am J Med. 1980;69:255-261.

313. Harding GKM, Buckwalk FJ, Ronald AR, et al. Prospective, randomized comparative study of clindamycin, chloramphenicol, and ticarcillin, each in combination with gentamicin, for therapy of intra-abdominal and female genital tract sepsis. J Infect Dis. 1980;142:384-393.

314. Gould IM, Wise R. Beta-lactamase inhibitors. In: Peterson PK, Verhoef J, eds. The Antimicrobial Agents Annual. 2nd ed. New York: Elsevier; 1987:58-69.

315. Wise R, Andrews JM, Bedford KA. Clavulanic acid and CP-45, 899: A comparison of their in vitro activity in combination with penicillins. J Antimicrob Chemother. 1980;6:197-206.

316. Donowitz GR, Mandell GL. Beta-lactam antibiotics (first of two parts). N Engl J Med. 1988;318:419-426.

317. Bansal MB, Chuah SK, Thadepalli H. In vitro activity and in vivo evaluation of ticarcillin plus clavulanic acid against aerobic and anaerobic bacteria. Am J Med. 1985;79(Suppl 5B):33-38.

318. Retsema JA, English AR, Girard A, et al. Sulbactam/ampicillin: In vitro spectrum, potency and activity in models of acute infection. Rev Infect Dis. 1986;8(Suppl 5):S528-S542.

319. Reinhardt JF, Johnston L, Ruane P, et al. A randomized double blind comparison of sulbactam/ampicillin and clindamycin for the treatment of aerobic-anaerobic infections. Rev Infect Dis. 1986;8(Suppl 5):S569-S575.

320. Jones RN. Review of the in vitro spectrum of activity of imipenem. Am J Med. 1985;78(Suppl 6A):22-32.

321. Sanders CC, Sanders WE Jr. Clinical significance of inducible beta-lactamase in gram-negative bacteria. Eur J Clin Microbiol. 1987;6:435.

322. Yotsuji A, Minami S, Inoue M, et al. Properties of a novel beta-lactamase produced by *Bacteroides fragilis*. Antimicrob Agents Chemother. 1983;24:925-929.

323. Jacobus NV, Ferreira MC, Barza M. In vitro activity of aztreonam, a monobactam antibiotic. Antimicrob Agents Chemother. 1982;22:832-838.

324. Williams RR, Hotchkin D. Aztreonam plus clindamycin versus tobramycin plus clindamycin in the treatment of intraabdominal infections. Rev Infect Dis. 1991;13(Suppl 7):S629-S633.

325. Berne TV, Yellin AE, Appleman MD, et al. Surgically treated gangrenous or perforated appendicitis: A comparison of aztreonam and clindamycin versus gentamicin and clindamycin. Ann Surg. 1987;205:133-137.

326. Birolini D, Morales MF, deSouza OS. Aztreonam plus clindamycin vs. tobramycin plus clindamycin for the treatment of intraabdominal infections. Rev Infect Dis. 1985;7(Suppl 4):S724-S729.

327. Kaye D, Levison ME, Labovitz ED. The unpredictability of serum concentrations of gentamicin: Pharmacokinetics of gentamicin in patients with normal and abnormal renal function. J Infect Dis. 1974;130:150-154.

328. Verklin RM Jr, Mandell GL. Alteration of effectiveness of antibiotics by anaerobiosis. J Lab Clin Med. 1977;89:65-71.

329. Ho JL, Barza M. Minireview: Role of aminoglycoside antibiotics in the treatment of intra-abdominal infection. Antimicrob Agents Chemother. 1987;31:485-491.

330. Wolfson JS, Hooper DC. The fluoroquinolones: Structures, mechanisms of action and resistance, and spectra of activity in vitro. Antimicrob Agents Chemother. 1985;28:581-586.

331. Neu HE. New antibiotics: Areas of appropriate use. J Infect Dis. 1987;155:403-417.

332. Wexler HM, Molitoris E, Molitoris D, et al. In vitro activities of trovafloxacin against 557 strains of anaerobic bacteria. Antimicrob Agents Chemother. 1996;40:2232-2235.

333. Citron DM, Appleman MA. Comparative activities of trovafloxacin (CP-99, 219) against 221 aerobic and 217 anaerobic bacteria isolated from patients with intra-abdominal infections. Antimicrob Agents Chemother. 1997;41:2312-2316.

334. Forrest A, Nix DE, Ballow CH, et al. Phamacodynamics of intravenous ciprofloxacin in seriously ill patients. Antimicrob Agents Chemother. 1993;37:1073-1081.

335. Lennard ES, Derllinger EP, Wertz MJ, et al. Implications of leukocytosis and fever at the conclusion of antibiotic therapy for intra-abdominal sepsis. Ann Surg. 1982;195:19-24.

336. Stone HH, Bourneuf AA, Stinson LD. Reliability of criteria for predicting persistent or recurrent sepsis. Arch Surg. 1985;120:17-20.

337. Hau T, Nishilawa R, Phuangsab A. Irrigation of the peritoneal cavity and antibiotics in the treatment of peritonitis. Surg Gynecol Obstet. 1983;156:25-30.

338. Rambo WM. Irrigation of the peritoneal cavity with cephalothin. Am J Surg. 1972;123:192-195.

339. Nichols RL. Management of intra-abdominal sepsis. Am J Med. 1985;80(Suppl 6B):204-209.

340. Leiboff AR, Soroff HS. The treatment of generalized peritonitis by closed postoperative peritoneal lavage: A critical review of the literature. Arch Surg. 1987;122:1005-1010.

341. Sindelar WF, Mason GR. Intraperitoneal irrrigation with povidone-iodine solution for the prevention of intra-abdominal abscess in the bacterially contaminated abdomen. Surg Gynecol Obstet. 1979;148:409-411.

342. Ahrenholz DH, Simmons RL. Povidone-iodine in peritonitis: I. Adverse effects of local instillation in experimental *E. coli* peritonitis. J Surg Res. 1979;26:458-463.

343. Hill GB, Osterhout S. Experimental effects of hyperbaric oxygen on selected clostridial species: In vitro studies. J Infect Dis. 1972;125:17-25.

344. Holland JA, Hill GB, Wolfe WG, et al. Experimental and clinical experience with hyperbaric oxygen in the treatment of clostridial myonecrosis. Surgery. 1975;77:75-85.

345. Schreiner A, Tonjum S, Digranes A. Hyperbaric oxygen therapy in bacteroides infections. Acta Chir Scand. 1974;140:73-76.

346. Hill GB. Hyperbaric oxygen exposures for intrahepatic abscesses produced in mice by non-spore-forming anaerobic bacteria. Antimicrob Agents Chemother. 1976;9:312-317.

347. Thom SR, Lavermann MW, Hart GB. Intermittent hyperbaric oxygen therapy for reduction of mortality in experimental polymicrobial sepsis. J Infect Dis. 1986;154:504-510.

348. Sugarman HJ, Bloomfield GL, Saggi BW. Multisystem organ failure secondary to increased intraabdominal pressure. Infection. 1999;27:61-66.

349. Garcia C, Parramon F, Delas F, et al. Abdominal compartment syndrome in non-injured patients. Rev Esp Anestesiol Reanim. 2000;47:126-129.

350. Beck B, Halberthal M, Zunis Z, et al. Abdominal compartment syndrome in children. Pediatr Crit Care Med. 2001;2:51-56.

351. Bhushan C, Mital VK, Elhence IP. Continuous postoperative peritoneal lavage in diffuse peritonitis using balanced saline antibiotic solution. Int Surg. 1975;60:526-528.

352. Hallerback B, Anderson C, Englund N, et al. A prospective randomized study of continuous peritoneal lavage postoperatively in the treatment of purulent peritonitis. Surg Gynecol Obstet. 1986;163:433-436.

353. Hudspeth AS. Radical surgical debridement in the treatment of advanced generalized bacterial peritonitis. Arch Surg. 1975;110:1233-1236.

354. Polk HC, Fry DE. Radical peritoneal debridement for established peritonitis: The result of a prospective randomized clinical trial. Ann Surg. 1980;192:350-355.

355. Aprahamian C, Wittman DH. Operative management of intraabdominal infection. Infection. 1991;19:453-455.

356. Wittman D, Aprahamian C, Bergstein J. Etappenlavage: Advance diffuse peritonitis managed by planned multiple laparotomies utilizing zippers, slide fastener, and Velcro analogue for temporary abdominal closure. World J Surg. 1990;14:218-226.

357. Teichmann W, Wittman DH, Andreone PA. Scheduled reoperations (etappenlavage) for diffuse peritonitis. Arch Surg. 1986;121:147-152.

358. Cuesta MA, Doblas M, Castaneda L, et al. Sequential abdominal reexploration with the zipper technique. World J Surg. 1991;15:74-80.

359. Schein M, Hirshberg A, Hashmonai M. Current surgical management of severe intraabdominal infection. Surgery. 1992;112:489.

360. Zugel N, Siebeck M, Geissler B, et al. Circulating mediators and organ function in patients undergoing planned relaparotomy vs conventional surgical therapy in severe secondary peritonitis. Arch Surg. 2002;137:590-599.

361. Jiminez MF, Marshall JC. Source control in the management of sepsis. Intensive Care Med. 2001;27(Suppl 1):S49-62.

362. Schein M. Surgical management of intra-abdominal infection: Is there any evidence? Langenbecks Arch Surg. 2002;387:1-7.

363. Holzheimer RG, Gathof B. Re-operation for complicated secondary peritonitis how to identify patients at risk for peritoneal sepsis. Eur J Med Res. 2003;8:125-134.

364. Haller JA Jr, Shaker IJ, Donahoo JS, et al. Peritoneal drainage versus non-drainage for generalized peritonitis from ruptured appendicitis in children: A prospective study. Ann Surg. 1973;177:595-600.

365. Leigh DA, Simmons K, Norman E. Bacterial flora of the appendix fossa in appendicitis and postoperative wound infection. J Clin Pathol. 1974;27:997-1000.

366. Follen WD, Hunt J, Altemeier WA. Prophylactic antibiotics in penetrating wounds of the abdomen. J Trauma. 1972;12:282-288.

367. Fabian TC, Boldreghini SJ. Antibiotics in penetrating abdominal trauma: Comparison of ticarcillin plus clavulanic acid with gentamicin plus clindamycin. Am J Med. 1985;79(Suppl 5B):157-160.

368. Nichols RL, Gorbach SL, Condon RE. Alteration of intestinal microflora following preoperative mechanical preparation of the colon. Dis Colon Rectum. 1971;14:123-127.

369. Condon RE, Bartlett JG, Greenlee H, et al. Efficacy of oral and systemic antibiotic prophylaxis in colorectal operations. Arch Surg. 1983;118:496-502.

370. Kaiser AB. Antibiotic prophylaxis in surgery. N Engl J Med. 1986;315:1129-1138.

371. Baum ML, Anish DS, Chalmers TC, et al. A survey of clinical trials of antibiotic prophylaxis in colon surgery: Evidence against further use of nontreatment controls. N Engl J Med. 1981;305:795-799.

372. Guglielmo BJ, Hohn DC, Koo PJ, et al. Antibiotic prophylaxis in surgical procedures: A critical analysis of the literature. Arch Surg. 1983;118:943-955.

373. Holph KD, Sorkin M, Rubin J, et al. Continuous ambulatory peritoneal dialysis: Three-year experience at one center. Ann Intern Med. 1980;92:609-613.

374. Rubin J, Rogers WA, Taylor HM, et al. Peritonitis during continuous ambulatory peritoneal dialysis. Ann Intern Med. 1980;92:7-13.

375. Fenton SSA, Pei Y, Delmore T, et al. The CAPD peritonitis rate is not improving with time. Trans Am Soc Artif Intern Organs. 1986;32:546-549.

376. Peterson PK, Matzke GR, Keane WF. Current concepts in the management of peritonitis in continuous ambulatory peritoneal dialysis patients. Rev Infect Dis. 1987;9:604-612.

377. Vas SL. 2. Peritonitis of peritoneal dialysis patients: Pathogenesis and treatment. Med Microbiol. 1986;5:21-63.

378. Everett ED. Diagnosis, prevention and treatment of peritonitis. Perit Dial Bull. 1984;4(Suppl):139-142.

379. Steinberg SM, Cutler SJ, Novak JK, et al. Report of the National CAPD Registry of the National Institutes of Health: Characteristics of participants and selected outcome measures for the period January 1, 1981 through August 31, 1984. In: National CAPD Registry of the National Institute of Arthritis, Diabetes, and Digestive and Kidney Diseases. Washington, DC: U.S. Public Health Services; 1985.

380. Kraus ES, Spector DA. Characteristics and sequelae of peritonitis in diabetics and non-diabetics receiving chronic intermittent peritoneal dialysis. Medicine (Baltimore). 1983;62:52-57.

381. Fenton S, Wu G, Cattran D, et al. Clinical aspects of peritonitis in patients on CAPD. Perit Dial Bull. 1981;1(Suppl):4-8.

382. Sewell CM, Clarridge J, Lacke C, et al. Staphylococcal nasal carriage and subsequent infection in peritoneal dialysis patients. JAMA 1982;248:1493-1495.

383. Keane WJ, Comty CM, Verbrugh HA, et al. Opsonic deficiency of peritoneal dialysis effluent in CAPD. Kidney Int. 1984;25:539-543.

384. Lamperi S, Carozzi S, Nasini MG. Intraperitoneal immunoglobulin treatment in prophylaxis of bacterial peritonitis in CAPD. In: Khanna R, Nolph KD, Provant B, et al, eds. Advances in CAPD. Toronto: University of Toronto Press;1986:110.

385. Duwe AK, Vas SI, Weatherhead IW. Effects of composition of peritoneal dialysis fluid on chemiluminescence, phagocytosis and bacterial activity in vitro. Infect Immun. 1981;33:130-135.

386. Marrie TJ, Noble MA, Costerton JW. Examination of the morphology of bacteria adhering to peritoneal dialysis catheters by scanning and transmission electron microscopy. J Clin Microbiol. 1983;18:1388-1398.

387. Arfania D, Everett ED, Nolph KD, et al. Uncommon causes of peritonitis in patients undergoing peritoneal dialysis. Arch Intern Med. 1981;141:61-64.

388. Vas SI. Microbiologic aspects of chronic ambulatory dialysis. Kidney Int. 1983;23:83-92.

389. Peterson PK, Keane WF. Infections in chronic peritoneal dialysis patients. In: Remington JS, Swartz MN, eds. Current Clinical Topics in Infectious Diseases. New York: McGraw-Hill; 1985:239-260.

390. Szeto CC, Chow KM, Wong TY, et al. Conservative management of polymicrobial peritonitis complicating peritoneal dialysis-a series of 140 consecutive cases. Am J Med. 2002;113:728-733.

391. Digenis GE, Khanna K, Panatlony D. Eosinophilia after implantation of the peritoneal catheter. Perit Dial Bull. 1982;2:98-99.

392. Gokal R, Ramos JM, Ward MK, et al. "Eosinophilic" peritonitis in continuous ambulatory peritoneal dialysis (CAPD). Clin Nephrol. 1981;15:328-330.

393. Woods GL, Washington JA II. Comparison of methods for processing dialysate in suspected continuous ambulatory peritoneal dialysis–associated peritonitis. Diagn Microbiol Infect Dis. 1987;7:155-157.

394. Gokal R, Ramos JM, Francis DM, et al. Peritonitis in continuous ambulatory peritoneal dialysis: Laboratory and clinical studies. Lancet. 1982;2:1388-1391.

395. Keane WF, Alexander SR, Bailie GR, et al. Peritoneal dialysis–related peritonitis treatment recommendations: 1996 update. Perit Dial Intern. 1996;16:557-573.

396. Verbrogh HA, Keane WF, Conroy WE, et al. Bacterial growth and killing in chronic ambulatory peritoneal dialysis fluids. J Clin Microbiol. 1984;20:199-203.

397. Eisenberg ES, Leviton I, Soeiro R. Fungal peritonitis in patients receiving peritoneal dialysis: Experience with 11 patients and review of the literature. Rev Infect Dis. 1986;8:309-321.

398. Rubin J, Kirchner K, Walsh D, et al. Fungal peritonitis during continuous ambulatory peritoneal dialysis: A report of 12 cases. Am J Kidney Dis. 1987;10:361-368.

399. Vargemezis V, Papadopoulov ZL, Llamos H, et al. Management of fungal peritonitis during continuous ambulatory peritoneal dialysis (CAPD). Perit Dial Bull. 1986;6:17-20.

400. Axelrod J, Meyers BR, Hirschman SZ, et al. Prophylaxis with cephalothin in peritoneal dialysis. Arch Intern Med. 1973;132:368-371.

401. Perez-Fontan M, Rosales M, Rodriguez-Carmona A, et al. Treatment of *Staphylococcus aureus* nasal carriers in CAPD with mupirocin. Adv Perit Dial. 1992;8:242-245.

402. Abrutyn E, Goodhart GL, Ries K, et al. *Acinetobacter calcoaeticus* outbreak associated with peritoneal dialysis. Am J Epidemiol. 1978;107:328-335.

403. Altemeir WA, Culbertson WR, Fullen WD, et al. Intra-abdominal abscesses. Am J Surg. 1973;125:70-79.

404. Saini S, Kellum JM, O'Leary MP, et al. Improved localization and survival in patients with intra-abdominal abscesses. Am J Surg. 1983;145:136-142.

405. Gibson DM, Feliciano DV, Mattox KL, et al. Intra-abdominal abscess after penetrating abdominal trauma. Am J Surg. 1981;142:699-703.

406. Patterson HC. Left subphrenic abscess. Am Surg. 1977;43:430-433.

407. Ozeran RS. Subdiaphragmatic abscess: Diagnosis and treatment. Am Surg. 1967;33:64-67.

408. Sherman NJ, Davis JR, Jesseph JE. Subphrenic abscess: A continuing hazard. Am J Surg. 1969;117:117-123.

409. Sanders RC. The changing epidemiology of subphrenic abscess and its clinical and radiological consequences. Br J Surg. 1970;57:449-455.

410. Ochsner A, DeBakey M. Subphrenic abscess: Collective review of 3608 collected and personal cases. Surg Gynecol Obstet. 1939;66:426.

411. Mackenzie M, Fordyle J, Young DG. Subphrenic abscess in children. Br J Surg. 1975;62:305-308.

412. Wang SMS, Wilson SE. Subphrenic abscess: The new epidemiology. Arch Surg. 1977;112:934-936.

413. DeCosse JJ, Poulin TL, Fox PS, et al. Subphrenic abscess. Surg Gynecol Obstet. 1974;138:841-846.

414. Gorbach SL. Treatment of intra-abdominal infection. Am J Med. 1984;76 (Suppl5A):107-110.

415. Milne GAC, Geere IW. Chronic subphrenic abscess: The missed diagnosis. Can J Surg. 1977;20:162-165.

416. Mueller PR, Simeone JF. Intra-abdominal abscesses: Diagnosis by sonography and computed tomography. Radiol Clin North Am. 1983;21:425-443.

417. Ferrucci JT Jr, Van Sonnenberg E. Role of ultrasound and computed tomography in the diagnosis and treatment of intraabdominal abscess. In: Remington JS, Swartz MN, eds. Current Clinical Topics in Infectious Diseases. New York: McGraw-Hill; 1982:136-159.

418. Kerlan RK Jr, Pogany AC, Jeffrey RB, et al. Radiologic management of abdominal abscesses. AJR Am J Roentgenol. 1985;144:145-149.

419. Connell TR, Stephens DH, Carlson HC, et al. Upper abdominal abscess: A continuing and deadly problem. AJR Am J Roentgenol. 1980;134:759-765.

420. Caffee HH, Watts G, Mena I. Gallium 67 citrate scanning in the diagnosis of intra-abdominal abscess. Am J Surg. 1977;133:665-669.

421. Tsan M. Mechanism of gallium 67 accumulation in inflammatory lesions. J Nucl Med. 1985;26:88-92.

422. Disbro M, Datz F, Cook P, et al. Indium-111 labeled leukocytes: Clinical utility and accuracy. Clin Nucl Med. 1982;7:44-46.

423. Froelich JW, Krasicky GA. Radionuclide imaging of abdominal infections. Curr Concepts Diagn Nucl Med. 1985;2:12-16.

424. Coleman RE, Brack RE, Welch DM, et al. Indium-111 labeled leukocytes in the evaluation of suspected abdominal abscess. Am J Surg. 1980;139:99-104.

425. Sfakianakis GN, Al-Sheikh W, Heal A, et al. Comparisons of scintigraphy with In-111 leukocytes and Ga^{67} in the diagnosis of occult sepsis. J Nucl Med. 1982;23:618-626.

426. Hill BA, Yamaguchi K, Flynn JJ, et al. Diagnostic sonography in general surgery. Arch Surg. 1975;110:1089-1094.

427. Goudie E, Andrew WK. The role of diagnostic ultrasound in the assessment of masses in the left upper quadrant of the abdomen. S Afr Med J. 1976;50:1391-1394.

428. Knochel JQ, Koehler PR, Lee TG, et al. Diagnosis of abdominal abscesses with computed tomography, ultrasound and ^{111}In leukocyte scans. Radiology. 1980;137:425-432.

429. Koehler PR, Moss AA. Diagnosis of intraabdominal and pelvic abscesses by computerized tomography. JAMA. 1980;224:49-52.

430. Gisi P, Graham DB. Splenic abscess: Two case reports. S D J Med. 1992;45:37-40.

431. Ooi LL, Nambiar R, Rauff A, et al. Splenic abscess. Aust N Z J Surg. 1992;62:780-784.

432. Balthazar EJ, Robinson DL, Megibow AJ, et al. Acute pancreatitis: Value of CT in establishing diagnosis. Radiology. 1990;174:331-336.

433. Brock JS, Pachter HL, Schreiber J, et al. Surgical diseases of the falciform ligament. Am J Gastroenterol. 1992;87:757-758.

434. Baker HL Jr, Berquist TN, Kispert DB, et al. Magnetic resonance imaging in a routine clinical setting. Mayo Clin Proc. 1985;60:75-90.

435. Cammoun D, Hendee WR, Davis KA. Clinical applications of magnetic resonance imaging: Current status. West J Med. 1985;143:793-803.

436. Wall SD, Fisher MR, Amparo EG, et al. Magnetic resonance imaging in the evaluation of abscesses. AJR Am J Roentgenol. 1985;144:1217-1221.

437. Gerzof SG, Robbins AH, Johnson WC, et al. Percutaneous catheter drainage of abdominal abscesses. N Engl J Med. 1981;305:653-657.

438. Mandel SR, Boyd D, Jaques PF, et al. Drainage of hepatic, intra-abdominal and mediastinal abscesses guided by computerized axial tomography: Successful alternative to open drainage. Am J Surg. 1983;145:120-125.

439. Pruett TL, Simmons RL. Status of percutaneous catheter drainage of abscesses. Surg Clin North Am. 1988;68:89-105.

440. Jaques P, Mauro M, Safrit H, et al. CT features of intraabdominal abscesses: Prediction of successful percutaneous drainage. Am J Radiol. 1986;146:1041-1045.

441. Malangioni MA. Pathogenesis and treatment of intraabdominal infection. Surg Gynecol Obstet. 1990;171:31-34.

442. Fornari F, Buscarini L. Ultrasonically guided fine-needle biopsy of gastrointestinal organs: Indications, results and complications. Dig Dis. 1992;10:121-133.

443. Flancbaum L, Nosh JL, Brolin RE. Percutaneous catheter drainage of abdominal abscesses associated with perforated viscus. Am J Surg. 1990;56:52-56.

444. Boulos PB. Complicated diverticulosis. Best Pract Res Clin Gastroenterol. 2002;16:649-662.

445. Brolin RE, Nosher JL, Leiman S, et al. Percutaneous catheter versus open surgical drainage in the treatment of abdominal abscesses. Am Surg. 1984;50:102-108.

446. Van Sonnenberg E, Ferruci JT Jr, Mueller PR, et al. Percutaneous drainage of abscesses and fluid collections: Technique, results and applications. Radiology. 1982;142:1-10.

447. Olak J, Christov NV, Stein LA, et al. Operative vs percutaneous drainage of intra-abdominal abscesses. Arch Surg. 1986;121:141-146.

448. Drusano GL, Warren WJ, Saah AJ, et al. A prospective randomized controlled trial of cefoxitin versus clindamycin-aminoglycoside in mixed aerobic-anaerobic infections. Surg Gynecol Obstet. 1982;154:715-720.

449. Tally FP, McGowan K, Kellum JM, et al. A randomized comparison of cefoxitin with or without amikacin and clindamycin plus amikacin in surgical sepsis. Ann Surg. 1981;193:318-323.

450. Nichols RL, Smith JW, Klein DB, et al. Risk of infection after penetrating abdominal trauma. N Engl J Med. 1984;311:1065-1070.
451. Tally FP, Kellum JM, Ho TF, et al. Randomized prospective study comparing moxalactam and cefoxitin with or without tobramycin for treatment of serious surgical infections. Antimicrob Agents Chemother. 1986;29:244-249.
452. Najem AZ, Kaminski CR, Spiller CR, et al. Comparative study of parenteral piperacillin and cefoxitin in the treatment of surgical infections of the abdomen. Surgery. 1983;157:423-425.
453. Study Group of Intra-Abdominal Infections. A randomized controlled trial of ampicillin plus sulbactam vs gentamicin plus clindamycin in the treatment of intra-abdominal infections. Rev Infect Dis. 1986;8(Suppl 5):S533-S588.
454. Scandinavian Study Group. Imipenem-cilastatin versus gentamicin-clindamycin for treatment of serious bacterial infections. Lancet. 1983;1:868-871.
455. Solomkin JS, Fant WK, Rivera JO, et al. Randomized trial of imipenem-cilastatin versus gentamicin and clindamycin in mixed flora infections. Am J Med. 1985;78 (Suppl 6A):85-91.
456. Guerra JG, Casaline GE, Plomina JC, et al. Imipenem-cilastatin versus gentamicin-clindamycin for treatment of moderate to severe infections in hospitalized patients. Rev Infect Dis. 1985;7(Suppl 3):463-470.
457. Birolini D, Moraes MF, Soare de Souza O. Aztreonam plus clindamycin vs tobramycin plus clindamycin for the treatment of intra-abdominal infections. Rev Infect Dis. 1985;7(Suppl 4):S724-S728.
458. Donahue PE, Smith DL, Yellin AE, et al. Trovafloxacin in the treatment of intra-abdominal infections: Results of a double-blind, multicenter comparison with imipenem/cilastatin. Am J Surg. 1998;176(Suppl 6A):53S-61S.

CHAPTER **69**

Infections of the Liver and Biliary System

ERIC C. JOHANNSEN
LAWRENCE C. MADOFF

LIVER ABSCESS

Liver abscesses fall broadly into two categories: amebic and pyogenic. Amebic liver abscess represents a distinct clinical entity caused by invasive *Entamoeba histolytica* infection. It has a distinct pathogenesis, characterized by the specific induction of hepatocyte apoptosis by the organism. Pyogenic liver abscess, by contrast, does not represent a specific liver disease, but is the end result of a number of pathologic processes that cause a suppurative infection of the liver parenchyma.

Epidemiology/Etiology

Amebic Liver Abscess

In the United States, amebic liver abscess has become a rare disease that is found almost exclusively in travelers and immigrants. In 1994, the last year in which incidence data were collected, there were only 2983 cases of amebiasis; the percentage of cases complicated by abscess is unknown, but it is probably well under 10%, roughly 1 case per million persons per year.[1] Worldwide, contamination of food and drinking water has maintained *E. histolytica* infection second only to malaria as a cause of death from parasitic disease. The epidemiology of this disease has been greatly informed by the appreciation that a closely related nonpathogenic species, *Entamoeba dispar*, colonizes between 5% and 25% of persons.[2,3] *E. dispar* has no apparent propensity for invasive disease, even among patients with acquired immunodeficiency syndrome (AIDS). In industrialized countries, most asymptomatic individuals with *Entamoeba* in their stool are colonized with *E. dispar*, whereas in highly endemic regions, asymptomatic infection with *E. histolytica*

may exceed the rate of *E. dispar* colonization.[4-11] Because these species are indistinguishable by light microscopy, the presence of *Entamoeba* in the stool is not sufficient to establish the cause of a liver abscess. Men and women experience equivalent rates of *E. histolytica* infection, but adult men are at 10-fold higher risk for invasive disease (colitis or extracolonic disease) than other populations.[12] Although environmental factors and genetic factors have been proposed, this gender bias remains unexplained.

Pyogenic Liver Abscess

The incidence of pyogenic liver abscess is about 10 to 20 cases per 100,000 hospital admissions, or 11 cases per million persons per year.[13,14] This incidence has been relatively stable, with a slight increasing trend in more recent case series that may reflect changes in the true incidence, improved detection, or changed admission practices. Pyogenic liver abscess is a disease of middle-aged persons, with a peak incidence in the fifth and sixth decades of life; this pattern mirrors the prevalence in the population of biliary disease, which is now the major cause of pyogenic liver abscess. No significant sex, ethnic, or geographic differences seem to exist in disease frequency, in contrast to the epidemiology of amebic liver abscess. About one half of patients have a solitary abscess. Right-sided abscesses are most common, followed by left-sided abscesses and then abscesses involving the caudate lobe. This distribution probably reflects the relative mass of each lobe, although more complicated explanations, such as patterns of hepatic blood flow, have been proposed.

Pathogenesis and Pathophysiology

Amebic Liver Abscess

Infection with *E. histolytica* results from ingestion of cysts in fecally contaminated food or water. Excystation occurs in the intestinal lumen and trophozoites migrate to the colon, where they adhere by means of a lectin that specifically binds galactose *N*-acetyl-D-galactosamine (Gal/GalNAc lectin) on colonic epithelium and multiply by binary fission.[15,16] At high densities, trophozoite encystation is initiated, and newly formed cysts are released into the stool to complete the life cycle. Most individuals experience asymptomatic infection, but approximately 10% develop symptomatic colitis when invasion of the colonic mucosa occurs. Spread to the liver via the portal system occurs in fewer than 1% of cases.[2] A number of virulence factors have been identified, including small proteins (amoebapores) that punch holes in lipid bilayers of target cells, cysteine proteases, and the Gal/GalNAc lectin.[17-19] *E. histolytica* induces apoptosis in hepatocytes and neutrophils, forming large, nonpurulent, "anchovy paste" abscesses that grow inexorably without treatment.[20,21] The mechanism by which *E. histolytica* induces apoptosis is unknown, but its importance is underscored by the resistance of caspase-3-deficient mice to amebic liver abscess formation.[22,23]

Pyogenic Liver Abscess

Pyogenic liver abscess does not represent a distinct pathophysiologic process but occurs whenever the initial inflammatory response fails to clear an infectious insult from the liver. Pyogenic liver abscesses are usually classified by presumed route of hepatic invasion: (1) biliary tree, (2) portal vein, (3) hepatic artery, (4) direct extension from contiguous focus of infection, and (5) penetrating trauma. Ideally, this approach defines the microbiology of the abscess and therefore guides empiric antibiotic choice, but it is limited by the high frequency of cryptogenic abscesses. The frequencies of the presumed routes of hepatic invasion are presented in Table 69-1.

1. Biliary tree. Cholangitis (discussed later) is now the major identifiable cause of pyogenic liver abscess. In such cases, multiple abscesses are usually present and anaerobes are infrequent. The underlying biliary obstruction is usually a result of gall stone disease, but it can also be caused by an obstructing tumor, an occluded stent, or *Ascaris lumbricoides* migration into the biliary tree.

TABLE 69-1 Frequency of Route of Infection in Hepatic Abscess

Route of Infection	Frequency (%)
Biliary tree	40-50
Hepatic artery	5-10
Portal vein	5-15
Direct extension	5-10
Trauma	0-5
Cryptogenic	20-40

Derived from references 14 and 24-46.

TABLE 69-2 Microbiology of Liver Abscess

Type of Organism	Common (>10%)	Uncommon (1-10%)
Gram-negative	*Escherichia coli* *Klebsiella* spp.	*Pseudomonas* *Proteus* *Enterobacter* *Citrobacter* *Serratia*
Gram-positive	*Streptococcus* (anginosus group) *Enterococcus* spp. Other viridans streptococci	*Staphylococcus aureus* β-Hemolytic streptococci
Anaerobic	*Bacteroides* spp.	*Fusobacterium* Anaerobic streptococci *Clostridium* spp. Lactobacilli

2. **Hepatic artery.** Any systemic bacteremia (e.g., endocarditis, line sepsis) can spread to liver via this route. Patients who die of overwhelming sepsis frequently have extensive microabscess formation in their livers at autopsy, but macroscopic liver abscess formation in patients who recover from septic shock is uncommon, underscoring the capacity of the liver to clear even large insults.

3. **Portal vein.** The portal venous system drains almost all of the abdominal viscera. Pylephlebitis from diverticulitis, pancreatitis, omphalitis, inflammatory bowel disease, or postoperative infection can result in pyogenic liver abscess. Untreated appendicitis was historically a major cause in this category but was greatly diminished in importance with the introduction of antibiotics.

4. **Direct extension** from a contiguous focus of infection. This may occur with cholecystitis, subphrenic abscess, or perinephric abscess.

5. **Trauma.** Any penetrating trauma to the liver, even as subtle as ingestion of a toothpick, can result in abscess formation. Blunt trauma can also predispose to pyogenic liver abscess formation, presumably because of hepatic hematoma formation and subsequent increased risk of seeding by bacteria. Similarly, hepatic destruction from sickle cell disease, tumor necrosis (including iatrogenic embolization), or cirrhosis can predispose to abscess formation.

Host factors that predispose to abscess formation from "routine" hepatic bacterial insults may be present in many cryptogenic abscesses. Systemic illness such as diabetes mellitus, cardiopulmonary disease, malignancy, and cirrhosis are common in patients with liver abscesses and may be predisposing factors. Moreover, neutrophil defects such as chronic granulomatous disease or Job's syndrome are associated with a marked predisposition for abscesses of the liver and elsewhere. Finally, hemachromatosis conveys a particular susceptibility to abscesses caused by *Yersinia enterocolitica*.[47]

Microbiology

Pyogenic Liver Abscess

In light of the diverse pathologic processes that have been discussed, it is understandable that sweeping generalizations about the microbiology of pyogenic liver abscess are difficult. The picture is further complicated because abscess material is rarely obtained before the administration of antibiotics. Even in the preantibiotic era, a high rate of sterile cultures was seen, probably reflecting inadequate culture techniques. Despite these difficulties, abscess cultures are positive in 80% to 90% of cases. The demonstration of anaerobic organisms in 45% of pyogenic liver abscess by Sabbaj and colleagues[48] in 1972 led to an increased awareness of fastidious pathogens, and in recent case series anaerobes were recovered 15% to 30% of the time.[14,34-36,39,42,45,46] Some of this decrease in the isolation of anaerobic organisms is probably attributable to the emergence of biliary tract disease as the major underlying cause of pyogenic liver abscess, but because of the difficulty in obtaining adequate culture data, these should be viewed as minimum estimates. There has also been an increased appreciation that many liver abscesses are polymicrobial, with estimates ranging from 20% to 50%, depending on the case series. If the source of the abscess is considered, abscesses with a biliary source are most likely to be polymi-

crobial, and crytpogenic abscesses are most frequently monomicrobial.[39] Some observers have noted that solitary abscesses are more likely to be polymicrobial than are multiple ones.[32,33] Although this has not been universally observed[39] and the small size of these studies prevents conclusive statements, it does suggest two alternative mechanisms for abscess formation. In the first, a synergistic combination of organisms converges by chance to form a single abscess; in the second, a highly pathogenic organism forms abscesses wherever it was seeded.

In terms of specific pathogens (Table 69-2), *Escherichia coli* and *Klebsiella pneumoniae* are by far the most common isolates. The latter is frequently associated with gas-forming abscesses. Enterococci and viridans streptococci are also common, primarily in polymicrobial abscesses. *Staphylococcus aureus,* by contrast, is more commonly associated with monomicrobial abscesses. Although pyogenic liver abscesses due to fungi, particularly *Candida* species, have been reported, they are comparatively rare and are excluded from most case series.

Clinical Presentation

Amebic Liver Abscess

Patients with amebic liver abscess typically present with fever and a dull, aching pain localizing to the right upper quadrant, but jaundice is rare. Only 15% to 35% of patients present with concurrent gastrointestinal symptoms, including nausea, vomiting, abdominal cramping, or diarrhea (Table 69-3). Symptoms are acute (of less than 2 weeks' duration) in about two thirds of cases but can develop months to years after travel to an endemic area.[2,3] The presentation is indistinguishable

TABLE 69-3 Signs and Symptoms of Liver Abscess

Feature	Amebic Liver Abscess[49-54]	Pyogenic Liver Abscess[14,24-46]
Epidemiology		
Male/female ratio	5-18	1.0-2.4
Age (yr)	30-40	50-60
Duration (days)	<14 (≈75% of cases)	5-26
Mortality (%)	10-25	0-5
Symptoms and Signs (approx. % of cases)		
Fever	80	80
Weight loss	40	30
Abdominal pain	80	55
Diarrhea	15-35	10-20
Cough	10	5-10
Jaundice	10-15	10-25
Right upper quadrant tenderness	75	55
Laboratory Tests (approx. % of cases)		
Leukocytosis	80	75
Elevated alkaline phosphatase	80	65
Solitary lesion	70	70

from pyogenic liver abscess on clinical grounds, and a careful search for epidemiologic risk factors is of paramount importance. Corticosteroid use and male sex are well-established risk factors for invasive amebic disease.[12,49]

Pyogenic Liver Abscess

Only 1 patient in 10 presents with the classic triad of fever, jaundice, and right upper quadrant tenderness. Fever is common, often without localizing signs but only a general failure to thrive, including malaise, fatigue, anorexia, or weight loss (see Table 69-3). When present, localizing symptoms such as vomiting or abdominal pain are not specific. The duration of symptoms before presentation varied widely in most case series, and there was seldom agreement on an average duration. Butler and McCarthy[26] attempted to address this issue by stratifying according to acute and chronic presentations. They found the former to be typically associated with acute, identifiable abdominal pathology such as cholangitis or appendicitis, whereas abscesses that presented chronically were often cryptogenic. Other series support an association between etiology and chronicity. For example, Seeto and Rockey[39] found that hematogenous liver abscesses presented most acutely (3 days), and those secondary to pylephlebitis had the longest duration of symptoms (42 days).

Diagnosis

The diagnosis of liver abscess should be suspected in all patients with fever, leukocytosis, and a space-occupying liver lesion. Because of the nonspecific symptoms on presentation, the initial clinical impression is frequently wrong and may include cholangitis, pneumonia, intraabdominal catastrophe, or pneumonia.[28] Before the widespread use of noninvasive imaging, liver abscess was among the most frequently identifiable causes of fever of unknown origin. Leukocytosis is present in most patients; two recent studies[45,46] reported leukocytosis in 84% to 88% of their patients, with mean white blood cell counts of 17,000/mm^3. An elevated alkaline phosphatase concentration is the most frequently abnormal liver function test, occurring in about two thirds of patients with liver abscess, but a normal value does not exclude the diagnosis. Abnormalities of alanine aminotransferase (ALT), aspartate aminotransferase (AST), and bilirubin are generally small, although may be more pronounced in some patients with biliary disease. Albumin concentration and prothrombin time tend to be normal or nearly so. Chest radiographs are abnormal about half of the time but are of no real value in making the diagnosis Therefore, although laboratory studies may suggest liver abnormalities, they are of no use in making the diagnosis of pyogenic liver abscess, and a high index of suspicion is required if the diagnosis is to be made in a timely fashion. Laboratory abnormalities may be of prognostic significance, most likely as markers of comorbidities: a multivariate analysis of risk factors found that a hemoglobin concentration of less than 10g/dL and a blood urea nitrogen (BUN) concentration greater than 28 mg/dL were independent predictors of mortality in patients found to have pyogenic liver abscess (odds ratios of 13 and 14, respectively).[43]

Once the diagnosis is suspected, radiographic imaging studies are essential to diagnose pyogenic liver abscess. Ultrasonography and computed tomographic (CT) scanning have proved particularly useful for demonstration and drainage of abscesses. Ultrasonography is the study of choice in patients with suspected biliary disease and in those who must avoid intravenous contrast or radiation exposure; it has a sensitivity of 70% to 90%. Contrast-enhanced CT scanning has improved sensitivity (approximately 95%) and is superior for guiding complex drainage procedures. Intravenous contrast is required for optimal imaging in two thirds of patients.[55] Magnetic resonance imaging (MRI) studies are seldom required, but they may be better at distinguishing abscesses from noninfectious liver lesions such as neoplasia. Fine-needle aspiration is the definitive diagnostic procedure, and MRI is a cumbersome tool for guiding drainage procedures.

In patients with pyogenic liver abscess, blood cultures are positive about half of the time. It is imperative that multiple sets of anaerobic and aerobic cultures be obtained, because these are frequently the only cultures obtained before antibiotic administration, and in about 7% of cases they are the only positive culture data obtained.[32,39] The diagnosis ultimately rests on obtaining purulent material from an aspiration of the abscess cavity, usually under radiographic guidance. Failure to obtain the expected pus should prompt a reevaluation of the differential diagnosis, considering liver cyst, malignancy, and amebic liver abscess. Purulent material should always be sent for Gram stain, which may provide the only clue to a mixed infection in patients heavily treated with antibiotics. The importance of prompt delivery of anaerobic specimens under proper conditions cannot be stressed enough.

Patients with amebic liver abscess classically present with a single large abscess in the right lobe of the liver, but the abscess can be anywhere, and multiple lesions are not infrequent. Moreover, there is near-complete overlap in the symptomatology of the two diseases (see Table 69-3). Therefore, distinguishing amebic from pyogenic liver abscess is not possible with the use of clinical criteria; however, a presumptive diagnosis of amebic liver abscess can be made in a patient with positive serology and a space-occupying liver lesion on CT or ultrasonography. Amebic serology (antiamebic antibodies) has a sensitivity of about 95% and is highly specific for *E. histolytica* infection; although the test can be negative in a minority of acute presentations (symptom duration less than 2 weeks), a repeat serology determination is usually positive.[56-59] *E. histolytica* antigen is detectable in almost 100% of serum samples and 40% of stool samples from patients with amebic liver abscess. Examination of the stool for cysts is of little value, because *E. histolytica* cannot be distinguished from *E. dispar*. It should be remembered that a positive serology result only confirms present or prior *E. histolytica* infection and cannot distinguish colitis from extraintestinal disease. Some investigators have argued that, in areas of low endemicity, suspected amebic liver abscess should be aspirated to exclude pyogenic liver abscess. Certainly, if there is no response to initial therapy, the abscess should be aspirated to confirm the diagnosis and to exclude pyogenic liver abscess. Bacterial superinfection of amebic liver abscess has been described in about 1% to 5% of cases, frequently as a complication of drainage procedures.[60]

Echinococcal cysts of the liver are distinguishable from amebic and pyogenic abscesses by CT but require separate consideration for aspiration (see Chapter 288).

Treatment

Amebic Liver Abscess

Amebic liver abscess can almost always be treated with medical therapy alone. Metronidazole (750 mg three times daily) is typically given for 7 to 10 days.[2,3] Nitroimidazoles with longer half-lives, such as tinidazole, secnidazole, and ornidazole, are also effective but are not currently available in the United States. Decreased fever and abdominal pain usually are observed within 3 to 5 days after initiation of therapy. Patients frequently remain colonized with *E. histolytica* despite nitroimidazole treatment and should be treated with paromomycin, a nonabsorbable aminoglycoside with *E. histolytica* activity to eliminate this condition. It is generally accepted that uncomplicated amebic liver abscess does not require drainage. Percutaneous image-guided aspiration has replaced surgical drainage and should be employed if there is no response to appropriate therapy or the diagnosis is uncertain, to exclude pyogenic liver abscess and bacterial superinfection. Drainage should also be considered for large lesions at risk for rupture, particularly left-sided abscesses that can rupture into the pericardium. Percutaneous drainage has not been demonstrated to shorten hospital stay or to hasten clinical improvement, with the exception of one randomized control trial that found a salutary effect in patients with large abscesses (greater than 300 mL).[50,61-64]

Pyogenic Liver Abscess

Unlike amebic liver abscess, pyogenic liver abscesses usually require drainage in addition to antibiotic therapy. Surgical drainage was traditionally the treatment of choice and, in the preantibiotic era, the only hope for cure. As early as 1953, McFadzean and associates[65] reported the use of percutaneous drainage with antibiotic therapy to treat 14 patients with liver abscess. After ultrasonography and CT became widely available, multiple studies confirmed this approach and made image-guided drainage procedures the preferred primary therapy, although some still advocate surgical drainage (Fig. 69-1). Surgical intervention should be considered if percutaneous drainage fails or management of concurrent intra-abdominal disease is required, and also for some patients with multiple large or loculated abscesses. Percutaneous catheter drainage is successful in 69% to 90% of cases; the procedure is generally well tolerated and usually can be performed at the time of radiographic diagnosis.[38-40,42,66,67] Aspirated material should be sent for Gram stain and cultured for aerobic and anaerobic bacteria. Meticulous handling of the specimen and rapid transportation to a qualified laboratory are essential for efficient recovery of anaerobes. Histopathologic biopsy specimens should also be obtained if possible. Depending on host and epidemiologic factors, microbiologic evaluation for fungi, mycobacteria, and *E. histolytica* should be considered. The catheter usually is left in place until drainage becomes minimal, typically 5 to 7 days. Percutaneous aspiration without catheter placement has received recent attention, with several studies reporting success rates between 58% and 88%, similar to those observed with catheter placement.[39,40,42,67,68] Success rates of 94% to 98% were reported in two studies in which percutaneous aspiration without catheter placement was followed by close clinical monitoring and serial ultrasound studies as indicated. Both investigations found that reaspiration was required in about 50% of cases, and a minority of patients required three or more aspiration procedures.[69,70] Therefore, catheter placement may not be required in some patients, but prospective randomized control trials are needed to clarify the role of aspiration alone versus catheter placement in the management of hepatic abscess.

Attempts to treat pyogenic liver abscess with antibiotics but no drainage have met with some success. Two early studies with a combined total of 25 patients found cure rates of 87% to 90%.[71,72] These studies have been criticized because 68% of the patients underwent diagnostic aspiration and therefore had at least partial drainage. Moreover, this success rate was substantially higher than the conventional experience at the time, when undrained abscesses carried a mortality rate of 60% to 100%. The results may be subject to selection bias: most patients did not have drainage because they were deemed to be poor surgical candidates. Even severely debilitated patients can tolerate percutaneous drainage, but the procedure may not always be required for cure: Success rates of 75% and 85% with medical therapy alone were reported in two studies, of 20 and 13 patients, respectively.[39,68] Until criteria for patient selection are better defined, medical management of pyogenic liver abscess should be reserved for patients with small abscesses not amenable to drainage and those patients in whom the risk of drainage is unacceptably high.

Treatment with empiric antibiotics should begin as soon as the diagnosis of pyogenic liver abscess is suspected. Multiple blood cultures should be sent before antibiotic initiation, but delaying antibiotic therapy until abscess material is obtained is not necessary and is potentially dangerous. Antibiotic choice should be guided by the suspected source of the abscess (Table 69-4). Abscesses arising from a biliary source frequently involve enterococci and aerobic gram-negative bacilli, whereas abscesses from a colonic or pelvic source are more commonly caused by aerobic gram-negative bacilli and anaerobes. Metronidazole at appropriately high doses should be included if amebic liver abscess is a consideration. Fluoroquinolones may be substituted for gentamicin, but this may not be advisable in cases complicated by enterococcal bacteremia. If a hematogenous (hepatic artery) source is suspected, coverage should include an antibiotic with activity against *S. aureus*.

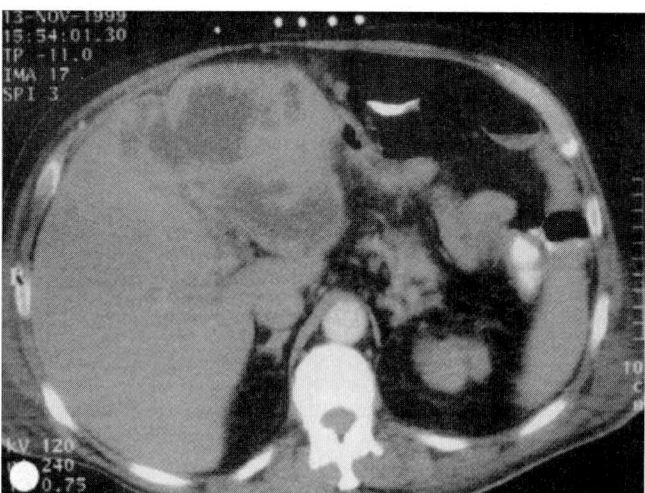

A

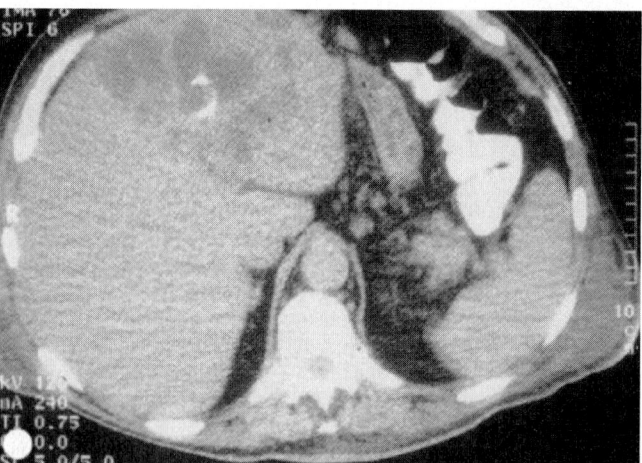

B

FIGURE 69-1. Drainage of liver abscesses by percutaneous aspiration guided by computed tomography (CT). A 67-year-old man with a history of diabetes mellitus and rheumatoid arthritis and a distant history of a Billroth II gastric resection, recently diagnosed with adenocarcinoma of the stomach, presented with fever. A blood culture grew *Escherichia coli*. The liver was imaged by CT (**A**), revealing multiple hypodense lesions in the right hepatic lobe. The lesion was aspirated under radiologic guidance, and more than 500 mL of frank pus was drained. Cultures produced *E. coli* and several anaerobic bacterial species. Cytologic findings were consistent with metastatic adenocarcinoma. A radiodense percutaneous drainage catheter was left in place (**B**), and the patient was treated with intravenous antibiotics and continued drainage. Note the position of the catheter and the decrease in size of the abscess. (*Photographs courtesy of Lindsey Baden, MD, Brigham and Women's Hospital, Boston, Massachusetts. From Johannsen EC, Sifri CD, Madoff LC. Pyogenic liver abscesses. Infect Dis Clin North Am. 2000;14:547-563, vii.*)

TABLE 69-4 Antibiotic Therapy for Hepatic Abscess

Suspected Source	Primary Therapy	Alternative
Biliary	Ampicillin + gentamicin* ± metronidazole	Vancomycin + gentamicin* ± metronidazole
		Imipenem or meropenem†
Colonic	Third-generation cephalosporin + metronidazole	Imipenem or meropenem†
		Antipseudomonal penicillin with β-lactamase inhibitor†
		Gentamicin* + metronidazole

*Fluoroquinolones may be substituted for gentamicin, especially in patients at risk for nephrotoxicity or if oral therapy is desired.
†Metronidazole should be included for presumptive therapy of amebic abscess if suspected.

Pyogenic liver abscesses are usually treated parenterally for 2 to 3 weeks, the 4- to 6-week total course being completed with oral agents. Some have reported successful treatment with less than 2 weeks of antibiotic therapy. The patient's clinical response and follow-up imaging should be monitored to judge response to therapy for considerations of antibiotic duration and the need for further aspiration. Abscess cavities usually resolve completely after therapy, but occasionally they persist despite prolonged courses of antibiotics. In such cases, patients should be observed closely. Recurrent symptoms such as fever or abdominal pain should prompt repeat imaging and possible re-aspiration.

INFECTION OF THE BILIARY SYSTEM

Infections of the biliary tract, including the common bile duct and gallbladder, are most often associated with obstruction to the flow of bile. In the United States and many developed countries, gall stones are very common and most often asymptomatic. In the United States, for example, it is estimated that 25 million adults have gall stones.[73] In a small percentage of cases, gall stones may obstruct the cystic or common bile ducts, resulting in inflammation. Approximately 600,000 cholecystectomies are performed every year in the United States, most commonly for acute cholecystitis secondary to impacted gall stones. Other causes of biliary obstruction include tumors of the biliary tree or adjacent structures, strictures secondary to surgery or other injury (including prior infection), and, in many geographic areas, infection by parasites including *Ascaris* and *Clonorchis*. Stasis of bile, inflammation, and loss of mechanical barriers can lead to bacterial infection of the bile, which can result in severe morbidity and death.

Pathogenesis

Cholecystitis

Only about 20% of patients with gall stones experience biliary colic, typified by right upper quadrant pain after a fatty meal when the contracting gallbladder is prevented from emptying by an obstructing stone. Biliary colic must be distinguished from the far more serious acute cholecystitis, which occurs in 1% to 3% of persons with symptomatic gall stones. In this disease, biliary obstruction is accompanied by an intense inflammatory reaction. Obstruction is thought to lead to increased intraluminal pressure; may lead to compromised blood supply and lymphatic drainage; and, in the setting of supersaturated bile, leads to acute inflammation. This process is mediated, at least in part, by prostaglandins, particularly prostaglandins I_2 and E_2 (Fig. 69-2).[74] Infection is not thought to precipitate acute cholecystitis, but it may complicate 20% to 50% of

cases. In a microbiologic study of biliary tract processes, 24 (46%) of 52 patients presenting with acute cholecystitis had positive bile cultures, compared with 0 of 42 normal controls and 49 (22%) of 221 patients with symptomatic gall stones but no evidence of acute cholecystitis.[75] Untreated cholecystitis may abate spontaneously; however, serious complications also occur at a high rate. Once infection is established, complications include emphysematous cholecystitis, gallbladder empyema, pyogenic liver abscess (see earlier discussion), and bacteremia.

Acalculous Cholecystitis

In 2% to 15% of cases, cholecystitis occurs in the absence of gall stones, although usually in the presence of other predisposing conditions. These include critical illnesses such as trauma, burns, and sepsis, as well as human immunodeficiency virus (HIV) infection, immunosuppression, diabetes, nonbiliary surgery, and childbirth.[76] Some of these conditions predispose to ischemia in the gallbladder wall or stasis of bile (or both) resulting in concentration of bile salts and leading to inflammation and necrosis of the gallbladder wall.

Cholangitis

Cholangitis refers to inflammation or infection of the common bile duct. The normally sterile bile may become infected because of the loss of protective factors, including the flow of bile. Obstruction of the common bile duct leads to stasis, which favors the growth of bacteria; increased pressure predisposes to bacteremia. Other factors may involve the loss of antibacterial activity of bile on the proximal small intestine, allowing for greater growth of bacteria. Bacteria may then ascend to the biliary tract (hence, the terms "ascending" and "suppurative" cholangitis) Other routes of infection have been proposed, including via the portal system or from the lymphatics. Primary sclerosing cholangitis is a disease of immunologic origin and is not covered here. AIDS cholangiopathy, which has many features of acute cholangitis, is discussed later in this chapter.

Clinical Presentation

Patients with biliary tract disease most often present with pain in the right upper quadrant of the abdomen, although occasionally localizing findings are absent. The pain may radiate to the infrascapular region. Cholecystitis and cholangitis are distinguished from simple biliary colic by the continuous nature of the pain. The finding of tenderness in the right upper quadrant on physical examination and the presence of Murphy's sign (inhibition of inspiration by pain when the area of the gallbladder fossa is palpated), with or without a mass, are highly suggestive of biliary tract disease. Fever and tachycardia are frequent findings. Complications of acute cholecystitis, which occur in 10% to 15%

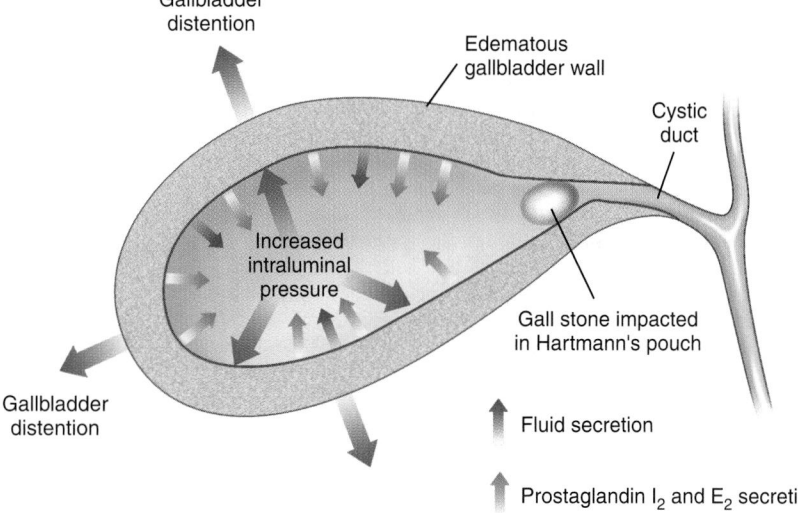

FIGURE 69-2. Pathogenesis of acute cholecystitis. Impaction of a gall stone leads to obstruction of the cystic duct and increased intraluminal pressure. An acute inflammatory response is in part mediated by prostaglandins. Infection may then result from biliary stasis. *(From Indar AA, Beckingham IJ. Acute cholecystitis. BMJ. 2002;325:639-643.)*

Gallbladder distention

Edematous gallbladder wall

Cystic duct

Increased intraluminal pressure

Gall stone impacted in Hartmann's pouch

Gallbladder distention

Fluid secretion

Prostaglandin I_2 and E_2 secretion

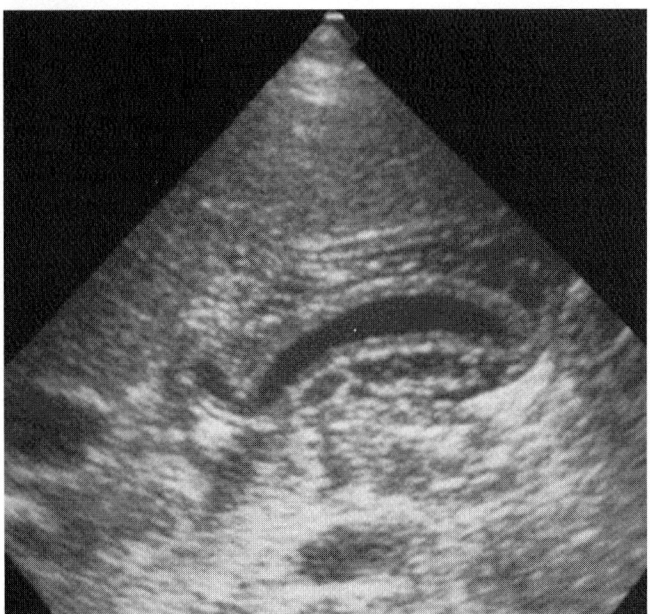

FIGURE 69-3. Ultrasonographic visualization of the gallbladder (sagittal view) in a case of acalculous cholecystitis, demonstrating mural thickening and hypoechoic regions within the gallbladder wall. *(From Gore RM, Yaghmai V, Newmark GM, et al. Imaging benign and malignant disease of the gallbladder. Radiol Clin North Am. 2002;40:1307-1323, vi.)*

of cases, include hepatic or intra-abdominal abscess, necrosis or gangrene of the gallbladder, and perforation, which in turn leads to sepsis and peritonitis.

Acalculous cholecystitis, particularly in a critically ill patient who is unresponsive, may produce very subtle findings, such as unexplained fever or vague abdominal pain.[77] A high index of suspicion is required, because serious complications such as gangrenous gallbladder and perforation frequently occur.

Acute or ascending cholangitis is suggested by Charcot's triad of right upper quadrant pain, fever and chills, and jaundice, reported in 50% to 100% of patients. The additional, less frequent signs of hypotension and altered mental status, in combination with Charcot's triad, constitute Reynold's pentad, which is reportedly seen in fewer than 14% of patients with ascending cholangitis.[78] Symptoms and signs of an inflammatory response usually are present and are reflected in the presence of fever, leukocytosis, and other markers.

Diagnosis

Leukocytosis with a left shift is the most frequent laboratory abnormality in acute cholecystitis. Alkaline phosphatase and bilirubin are not usually elevated unless the common bile duct is involved. However, in one study of 217 patients with acute cholecystitis, 25% of patients without obstruction of the common bile duct had elevated bilirubin.[79] Several also had elevations in amylase. The mechanism underlying these abnormalities is unclear but may be the passage of small stones or sludge through the common bile duct.

Acute cholangitis results in presentation with the clinical findings mentioned earlier. Abnormalities suggestive of sepsis syndrome, including leukocytosis, are frequently observed. Additional laboratory abnormalities include cholestatic liver function tests with elevations in alkaline phosphatase and bilirubin, particularly conjugated bilirubin. Elevations in γ-glutamyl transpeptidase are often seen as well. Abnormal amylase may suggest an associated pancreatitis, and elevations in transaminases may indicate associated inflammation or infection of the liver parenchyma (or both). Blood cultures are positive in 30% to 40% of patients.[80]

Imaging Studies

Ultrasonography can frequently establish the diagnosis of cholecystitis and is usually the first study obtained. A sonographic Murphy's sign (i.e., pain when the ultrasound transducer probes the gallbladder) is a useful diagnostic clue. In addition, the testing may be done at the bedside of critically ill patients, is relatively inexpensive, and can directly visualize stones, particularly in the gallbladder. Abnormalities such as gallbladder wall thickening of greater than 2 mm, pericholecystic fluid, and intramural gas or ductal dilation are suggestive of cholecystitis (Fig. 69-3). The combination of stones and either wall thickening or a sonographic Murphy's sign in the appropriate clinical picture were shown to have positive and negative predictive values exceeding 90%.[81]

Radionuclide cholescintigraphy (hepato-iminodiacetic acid [HIDA] scanning) may be used if ultrasound fails to ascertain a diagnosis. A technetium 99m (^{99m}Tc)-labeled derivative of acetanilide iminodiacetic acid is injected intravenously and is secreted into the bile. It is taken up by the gallbladder, which can then be visualized. Failure of the gallbladder to accumulate the marker is highly suggestive of acute cholecystitis due to obstruction of the cystic duct. Normally, visualization of the common bile duct and small bowel occurs within 30 to 60 minutes; failure to visualize these structures indicates obstruction within the common bile duct or at the ampulla. In one study of cholescintigraphy in the diagnosis of acalculous cholecystitis in 62 critically ill patients, ultrasonography had a sensitivity of only 30%, whereas HIDA scanning had a sensitivity of 100% and a specificity of 88%.[82]

CT is not commonly used for the initial evaluation of cholecystitis, and its sensitivity and specificity for detection of this condition are not known.[83,84] CT findings associated with acute cholecystitis include gall stones, particularly within the cystic duct, gallbladder distention and mural thickening, and enhancement of the liver adjacent to the gallbladder, which is the CT equivalent of the scintigraphic "rim sign."

Magnetic resonance (MR) cholangiography is a noninvasive technique that has been used to visualize the bile ducts. In one study of 35 patients comparing ultrasonography with MR cholangiography, the latter modality showed 100% sensitivity for the presence of stones but was less sensitive than ultrasound in the detection of gallbladder wall thickening (69% versus 96%). In a recent meta-analysis of 67 studies of MR cholangiography, the technique was highly sensitive (99%) for the detection of biliary obstruction, and 92% sensitive for the detection of stones.[85]

Microbiology

The constituents of the normal intestinal flora are commonly isolated from the bile and surgical sites of patients with acute cholecystitis and acute cholangitis. These include gram-negative bacilli such as *E. coli*, *Klebsiella* spp., and *Enterobacter* spp. Anaerobes, most frequently *Bacteroides* spp., *Fusobacterium* spp., and clostridia, are recovered less frequently but are isolated more often from patients with prior biliary tract surgical procedures and those with biliary-intestinal anastomoses. Finally, enterococci are not uncommonly found in infected bile, usually in association with other organisms.[86]

Parasites that infect the biliary tree include *Clonorchis sinensis*, *Opisthorchis felineus*, *Opisthorchis viverrini*, and *Fasciola hepatica*.[87] These organisms are prevalent in regions of Asia and can cause acute and relapsing cholangitis with associated stricture and stone formation. *Clonorchis* and *Opisthorchis* infection can lead to the development of carcinoma of the biliary tract. *Ascaris lumbricoides*, a more cosmopolitan parasite, occasionally obstructs the biliary tree, resulting in acute cholangitis.[88] Echinococcal disease can cause biliary obstruction due to mass effect. Parasites that complicate HIV disease may also invade the biliary tree (see later discussion).

AIDS Cholangiopathy (AIDS-Related Sclerosing Cholangitis)

Biliary tract disease is a complication of late HIV infection[89] (discussed in Chapter 119). Although it is possible that this entity is caused by infection of the biliary tract with HIV per se, more likely it results from opportunistic infection of the biliary system. The pathologic findings of AIDS cholangiopathy include stenosis of the distal common bile duct and irregularities of the intrahepatic and extrahepatic bile ducts.[90] The most common pathogen associated with cholangitis in HIV is *Cryptosporidium.* After an outbreak of cryptosporidiosis in Milwaukee, Wisconsin, in 1995, 29% of patients with HIV infection and intestinal cryptosporidiosis developed cholangiopathy as well. Cytomegalovirus is also a major cause of AIDS-related cholangitis, having been described in as many as 42% of patients. Other pathogens associated with AIDS cholangiopathy include *Enterocytozoon bieneusi, Isospora belli,* and *Mycobacterium avium intracellulare.* The clinical manifestations of biliary tract disease do not differ markedly from those in non-HIV infected individuals and include right upper quadrant pain and fever. Diagnosis is usually made by characteristic findings on ultrasound, with dilatation of the common bile duct observed in approximately two thirds of cases. Endoscopic retrograde cholangiopancreatography (ERCP) demonstrates dilatation and irregularities of the ducts and has become the gold standard for the diagnosis.[91] It is also useful in treatment: sphincterotomy provides symptomatic benefit for many patients.

Treatment

Because biliary disease results most commonly from obstruction of the bile ducts, definitive treatment involves removal of the obstruction or the infected material. This can be accomplished surgically, percutaneously, or endoscopically (i.e., by ERCP). Antibiotics and other supportive measures must be considered temporizing.

The role of antibiotics in acute cholecystitis has not been well established. Studies of patients with uncomplicated cholecystitis have failed to demonstrate a reduction in complications such as pericholic abscess or perforation with antibiotic administration.[92] Indeed, many cases of acute cholecystitis remit spontaneously. Antibiotics are clearly indicated for patients with complications of cholecystitis such as emphysematous or gangrenous cholecystitis or perforation. Antibiotics directed against the enteric flora (as described earlier) should be given to patients who are debilitated, severely ill, elderly, immunocompromised, or jaundiced. A combination of ampicillin and gentamicin or piperacillin/tazobactam are reasonable empiric therapy for acute cholecystitis. Alternatively, a third- or fourth-generation cephalosporin may be used despite the lack of activity against enterococci. In one study, a cephalosporin (cefepime) was as effective as a combination that covered enterococci (mezlocillin and gentamicin), despite the presence of enterococci in bile cultures of 6 of 56 cefepime-treated patients. This finding may be a result of the low pathogenic potential of enterococci in this setting; elimination of other pathogens effectively treats the infection even in the setting of persistent enterococcal contamination. As enterococcal resistance to many antibiotics increases, the difficulty in directing therapy to these pathogens makes attempts at empiric coverage more difficult. Many authorities also recommend the use of an agent active against gram-negative anaerobes, such as metronidazole. This is particularly important in settings in which anaerobes are more likely to be present, such as prior biliary tract surgery or enterocholedochal fistula.

In the presence of suspected gangrene or perforation, immediate surgery is indicated. Ideally, this includes cholecystectomy with intraoperative cholangiogram. Alternatively, in unstable patients, cholecystotomy (percutaneous drainage of the biliary system with removal of obstructing stones) may be performed as a temporizing measure.[93] This procedure can be performed under local anesthesia and at the bedside in critically ill patients and can be lifesaving. In some circumstances, further surgery may not be required.

In the absence of severe complications, the timing of definitive surgical intervention in the management of acute cholecystitis is the subject of some debate. Traditionally, in the group of patients who are stable and respond to conservative management, surgery has been delayed for 6 to 12 weeks. However, several studies have shown that patients who undergo early surgical intervention (most often laparoscopic cholecystectomy) have a lower complication rate, a shorter hospital stay, and, if laparoscopic cholecystectomy is performed, a lower requirement for conversion to an open procedure, compared with patients undergoing delayed surgery.[94,95] For patients with high surgical risk and those who are unstable, delayed surgery may still be preferable.

Acute Cholangitis

Acute cholangitis remains a disease with substantial mortality, and therapy should include antibiotics and supportive measures along with decompression/drainage of the biliary system for cases that do not respond promptly to conservative therapy. A variety of antibiotic regimens have been used in the management of acute cholangitis.[78] Empiric coverage should be directed against enteric gram-negative bacilli. The combination of an extended-spectrum penicillin such as ampicillin or piperacillin with an aminoglycoside is appropriate initial empiric therapy and provides coverage for many enterococci.[96] Cephalosporins, carbapenems (imipenem or meropenem), and fluoroquinolones have also proved efficacious.[78,80] Although anaerobes are only infrequently cultured from bile in acute cholangitis, the addition of metronidazole to the noncarbapenem regimens is often advocated, or piperacillin/tazobactam can be used to provide anaerobic coverage.

Drainage of the biliary tract may be accomplished surgically, endoscopically, or percutaneously. ERCP has, to a large extent, supplanted open surgical procedures in the management of acute cholangitis and is successful in more than 90% of cases.[97,98] (Paradoxically, ERCP is not infrequently the cause of acute cholangitis when it is used in an attempt to decompress an obstructed but not frankly infected bile duct.[99]) ERCP is generally though to have a lower morbidity rate than open surgery, and it is more likely to offer definitive treatment (e.g., by removal of an impacted gall stone) than percutaneous biliary drainage.

Treatment of parasitic infections affecting the biliary tree is covered in Chapters 285, 287, and 288.

REFERENCES

1. Summary of notifiable diseases, United States. MMWR Morb Mortal Wkly Rep. 1994;43:800.
2. Haque R, Huston CD, Hughes M, et al. Amebiasis. N Engl J Med. 2003;348:1565-1573.
3. Stanley SL Jr. Amoebiasis. Lancet 2003;361:1025-1034.
4. Haque R, Ali IM, Petri WA Jr. Prevalence and immune response to *Entamoeba histolytica* infection in preschool children in Bangladesh. Am J Trop Med Hyg. 1999;60:1031-1034.
5. Haque R, Faruque AS, Hahn P, et al. *Entamoeba histolytica* and *Entamoeba dispar* infection in children in Bangladesh. J Infect Dis. 1997;175:734-736.
6. Braga LL, Mendonca Y, Paiva CA, et al. Seropositivity for and intestinal colonization with *Entamoeba histolytica* and *Entamoeba dispar* in individuals in northeastern Brazil. J Clin Microbiol. 1998;36:3044-3045.
7. Rivera WL, Tachibana H, Kanbara H. Field study on the distribution of *Entamoeba histolytica* and *Entamoeba dispar* in the northern Philippines as detected by the polymerase chain reaction. Am J Trop Med Hyg 1998;59:916-921.
8. Gathiram V, Jackson TF. A longitudinal study of asymptomatic carriers of pathogenic zymodemes of *Entamoeba histolytica.* S Afr Med J. 1987;72:669-672.
9. Abd-Alla MD, Wahib AA, Ravdin JI. Comparison of antigen-capture ELISA to stool-culture methods for the detection of asymptomatic *Entamoeba* species infection in Kafer Daoud, Egypt. Am J Trop Med Hyg. 2000;62:579-582.
10. Abd-Alla MD, Ravdin JI. Diagnosis of amoebic colitis by antigen capture ELISA in patients presenting with acute diarrhoea in Cairo, Egypt. Trop Med Int Health. 2002;7:365-370.
11. Evangelopoulos A, Legakis N, Vakalis N. Microscopy, PCR and ELISA applied to the epidemiology of amoebiasis in Greece. Parasitol Int. 2001;50:185-189.
12. Acuna-Soto R, Maguire JH, Wirth DF. Gender distribution in asymptomatic and invasive amebiasis. Am J Gastroenterol. 2000;95:1277-1283.
13. Johannsen EC, Sifri CD, Madoff LC. Pyogenic liver abscesses. Infect Dis Clin North Am. 2000;14:547-563, vii.
14. Hansen PS, Schonheyder HC. Pyogenic hepatic abscess: A 10-year population-based retrospective study. APMIS. 1998;106:396-402.
15. Mann BJ. Structure and function of the *Entamoeba histolytica* Gal/GalNAc lectin. Int Rev Cytol. 2002;216:59-80.
16. Petri WA Jr, Haque R, Mann BJ. The bittersweet interface of parasite and host: Lectin-carbohydrate interactions during human invasion by the parasite *Entamoeba histolytica.* Annu Rev Microbiol. 2002;56:39-64.
17. Braga LL, Ninomiya H, McCoy JJ, et al. Inhibition of the complement membrane attack complex by the galactose-specific adhesion of *Entamoeba histolytica.* J Clin Invest. 1992;90:1131-1137.
18. Leippe M. Antimicrobial and cytolytic polypeptides of amoeboid protozoa: Effector molecules of primitive phagocytes. Dev Comp Immunol. 1999;23:267-279.

19. Que X, Reed SL. Cysteine proteinases and the pathogenesis of amebiasis. Clin Microbiol Rev. 2000;13:196-206.
20. Ragland BD, Ashley LS, Vaux DL, Petri WA Jr. *Entamoeba histolytica:* Target cells killed by trophozoites undergo DNA fragmentation which is not blocked by Bcl-2. Exp Parasitol. 1994;79:460-467.
21. Seydel KB, Stanley SL Jr. *Entamoeba histolytica* induces host cell death in amebic liver abscess by a non-Fas-dependent, non-tumor necrosis factor alpha-dependent pathway of apoptosis. Infect Immun. 1998;66:2980-2983.
22. Huston CD, Houpt ER, Mann BJ, et al. Caspase 3-dependent killing of host cells by the parasite *Entamoeba histolytica.* Cell Microbiol. 2000;2:617-625.
23. Yan L, Stanley SL Jr. Blockade of capsaises inhibits amebic liver abscess formation in a mouse model of disease. Infect Immun. 2001;69:7911-7914.
24. Ochsner A, DeBakey M, Murray S. Pyogenic abscess of the liver. Am J Surg. 1938;40:292-353.
25. Joseph WL, Kahn AM, Longmire WP Jr. Pyogenic liver abscess: Changing patterns in approach. Am J Surg. 1968;115:63-68.
26. Butler TJ, McCarthy CF. Pyogenic liver abscess. Gut 1969;10:389-399.
27. Lazarchick J, De Souza e Silva NA, Nichols DR, Washington JA 2nd. Pyogenic liver abscess. Mayo Clin Proc. 1973;48:349-355.
28. Rubin RH, Swartz MN, Malt R. Hepatic abscess: Changes in clinical, bacteriologic and therapeutic aspects. Am J Med. 1974;57:601-610.
29. Pitt HA, Zuidema GD. Factors influencing mortality in the treatment of pyogenic hepatic abscess. Surg Gynecol Obstet. 1975;140:228-234.
30. Miedema BW, Dineen P. The diagnosis and treatment of pyogenic liver abscesses. Ann Surg. 1984;200:328-335.
31. Greenstein AJ, Lowenthal D, Hammer GS, et al. Continuing changing patterns of disease in pyogenic liver abscess: A study of 38 patients. Am J Gastroenterol. 1984;79:217-226.
32. McDonald MI, Corey GR, Gallis HA, Durack DT. Single and multiple pyogenic liver abscesses: Natural history, diagnosis and treatment, with emphasis on percutaneous drainage. Medicine (Baltimore). 1984;63:291-302.
33. Branum GD, Tyson GS, Branum MA, Meyers WC. Hepatic abscess: Changes in etiology, diagnosis, and management. Ann Surg. 1990;212:655-662.
34. Yoo HM, Kim WH, Shin SK, et al. The changing patterns of liver abscess during the past. 20 years: A study of 482 cases. Yonsei Med J. 1993;34:340-351.
35. Mischinger HJ, Hauser H, Rabl H, et al. Pyogenic liver abscess: Studies of therapy and analysis of risk factors. World J Surg. 1994;18:852-857; discussion, 858.
36. Hashimoto L, Hermann R, Grundfest-Broniatowski S. Pyogenic hepatic abscess: Results of current management. Am Surg. 1995;61:407-411.
37. Chou FF, Sheen-Chen SM, Chen YS, Lee TY. The comparison of clinical course and results of treatment between gas-forming and non-gas-forming pyogenic liver abscess. Arch Surg. 1995;130:401-405; discussion, 406.
38. Huang CJ, Pitt HA, Lipsett PA, et al. Pyogenic hepatic abscess: Changing trends over 42 years. Ann Surg. 1996;223:600-607; discussion, 607-609.
39. Seeto RK, Rockey DC. Pyogenic liver abscess: Changes in etiology, management, and outcome. Medicine (Baltimore). 1996;75:99-113.
40. Chu KM, Fan ST, Lai EC, et al. Pyogenic liver abscess: An audit of experience over the past decade. Arch Surg. 1996;131:148-152.
41. Tazawa J, Sakai Y, Maekawa S, et al. Solitary and multiple pyogenic liver abscesses: Characteristics of the patients and efficacy of percutaneous drainage. Am J Gastroenterol. 1997;92:271-274.
42. Chou FF, Sheen-Chen SM, Chen YS, Chen MC. Single and multiple pyogenic liver abscesses: Clinical course, etiology, and results of treatment. World J Surg. 1997;21:384-388; discussion, 388-389.
43. Alvarez Perez JA, Gonzalez JJ, Baldonedo RF, et al. Clinical course, treatment, and multivariate analysis of risk factors for pyogenic liver abscess. Am J Surg. 2001;181:177-186.
44. Petri A, Hohn J, Hodi Z, et al. Pyogenic liver abscess—20 years' experience: Comparison of results of treatment in two periods. Langenbecks Arch Surg. 2002;387:27-31.
45. Mohsen AH, Green ST, Read RC, McKendrick MW. Liver abscess in adults: Ten years experience in a UK centre. QJM. 2002;95:797-802.
46. Wong WM, Wong BC, Hui CK, et al. Pyogenic liver abscess: Retrospective analysis of 80 cases over a 10-year period. J Gastroenterol Hepatol. 2002;17:1001-1007.
47. Vadillo M, Corbella X, Pac V, et al. Multiple liver abscesses due to *Yersinia enterocolitica* discloses primary hemochromatosis: Three case reports and review. Clin Infect Dis. 1994;18:938-941.
48. Sabbaj J, Sutter VL, Finegold SM. Anaerobic pyogenic liver abscess. Ann Intern Med. 1972;77:627-638.
49. el-Hennawy M, Abd-Rabbo H. Hazards of cortisone therapy in hepatic amoebiasis. J Trop Med Hyg. 1978;81:71-73.
50. Barnes PF, De Cock KM, Reynolds TN, Ralls PW. A comparison of amebic and pyogenic abscess of the liver. Medicine (Baltimore). 1987;66:472-483.
51. Thompson JE Jr, Forlenza S, Verma R. Amebic liver abscess: A therapeutic approach. Rev Infect Dis. 1985;7:171-179.
52. Adams EB, MacLeod IN. Invasive amebiasis: II. Amebic liver abscess and its complications. Medicine (Baltimore). 1977;56:325-334.
53. Shandera WX, Bollam P, Hashmey RH, et al. Hepatic amebiasis among patients in a public teaching hospital. South Med J. 1998;91:829-837.
54. Abuabara SF, Barrett JA, Hau T, Jonasson O. Amebic liver abscess. Arch Surg. 1982;117:239-244.
55. Ralls PW. Focal inflammatory disease of the liver. Radiol Clin North Am. 1998;36:377-389.
56. Haque R, Ali IK, Akther S, Petri WA Jr. Comparison of PCR, isoenzyme analysis, and antigen detection for diagnosis of *Entamoeba histolytica* infection. J Clin Microbiol. 1998;36:449-452.
57. Krogstad DJ, Spencer HC Jr, Healy GR, et al. Amebiasis: Epidemiologic studies in the United States, 1971-1974. Ann Intern Med. 1978;88:89-97.
58. Krupp IM, Powell SJ. Comparative study of the antibody response in amebiasis: Persistence after successful treatment. Am J Trop Med Hyg. 1971;20:421-424.
59. Pillai DR, Keystone JS, Sheppard DC, et al. *Entamoeba histolytica* and *Entamoeba dispar:* Epidemiology and comparison of diagnostic methods in a setting of nonendemicity. Clin Infect Dis. 1999;29:1315-1318.
60. Katzenstein D, Rickerson V, Braude A. New concepts of amebic liver abscess derived from hepatic imaging, serodiagnosis, and hepatic enzymes in 67 consecutive cases in San Diego. Medicine (Baltimore). 1982;61:237-246.
61. Sharma MP, Rai RR, Acharya SK, et al. Needle aspiration of amoebic liver abscess. BMJ. 1989;299:1308-1309.
62. Van Allan RJ, Katz MD, Johnson MB, et al. Uncomplicated amebic liver abscess: Prospective evaluation of percutaneous therapeutic aspiration. Radiology. 1992;183:827-830.
63. Weinke T, Grobusch MP, Guthoff W. Amebic liver abscess: Rare need for percutaneous treatment modalities. Eur J Med Res. 2002;7:25-29.
64. Zafar A, Ahmed S. Amoebic liver abscess: A comparative study of needle aspiration versus conservative treatment. J Ayub Med Coll Abbottabad. 2002;14:10-12.
65. Mc FA, Chang KP, Wong CC. Solitary pyogenic abscess of the liver treated by closed aspiration and antibiotics: A report of 14 consecutive cases with recovery. Br J Surg. 1953;41:141-152.
66. Bertel CK, van Heerden JA, Sheedy PF 2nd. Treatment of pyogenic hepatic abscesses: Surgical vs percutaneous drainage. Arch Surg. 1986;121:554-558.
67. Stain SC, Yellin AE, Donovan AJ, Brien HW. Pyogenic liver abscess: Modern treatment. Arch Surg. 1991;126:991-996.
68. Barakate MS, Stephen MS, Waugh RC, et al. Pyogenic liver abscess: A review of 10 years' experience in management. Aust N Z J Surg. 1999;69:205-209.
69. Ch Yu S, Hg Lo R, Kan PS, Metreweli C. Pyogenic liver abscess: Treatment with needle aspiration. Clin Radiol. 1997;52:912-916.
70. Giorgio A, Tarantino L, Mariniello N, et al. Pyogenic liver abscesses: 13 years of experience in percutaneous needle aspiration with US guidance. Radiology. 1995;195:122-124.
71. Reynolds TB. Medical treatment of pyogenic liver abscess. Ann Intern Med. 1982;96:373-374.
72. Herbert DA, Fogel DA, Rothman J, et al. Pyogenic liver abscesses: Successful nonsurgical therapy. Lancet. 1982;1:134-136.
73. Everhart JE, Khare M, Hill M, Maurer KR. Prevalence and ethnic differences in gallbladder disease in the United States. Gastroenterology. 1999;117:632-639.
74. Indar AA, Beckingham IJ. Acute cholecystitis. BMJ. 2002;325:639-643.
75. Csendes A, Burdiles P, Maluenda F, et al. Simultaneous bacteriologic assessment of bile from gallbladder and common bile duct in control subjects and patients with gallstones and common duct stones. Arch Surg. 1996;131:389-394.
76. Shapiro MJ, Luchtefeld WB, Kurzweil S, et al. Acute acalculous cholecystitis in the critically ill. Am Surg. 1994;60:335-339.
77. Ko CW, Lee SP. Gastrointestinal disorders of the critically ill: Biliary sludge and cholecystitis. Best Pract Res Clin Gastroenterol. 2003;17:383-396.
78. Hanau LH, Steigbigel NH. Acute (ascending) cholangitis. Infect Dis Clin North Am. 2000;14:521-546.
79. Kurzweil SM, Shapiro MJ, Andrus CH, et al. Hyperbilirubinemia without common bile duct abnormalities and hyperamylasemia without pancreatitis in patients with gallbladder disease. Arch Surg. 1994;129:829-833.
80. Sung JJ, Lyon DJ, Suen R, et al. Intravenous ciprofloxacin as treatment for patients with acute suppurative cholangitis: A randomized, controlled clinical trial. J Antimicrob Chemother. 1995;35:855-864.
81. Ralls PW, Colletti PM, Lapin SA, et al. Real-time sonography in suspected acute cholecystitis: Prospective evaluation of primary and secondary signs. Radiology. 1985;155:767-771.
82. Puc MM, Tran HS, Wry PW, Ross SE. Ultrasound is not a useful screening tool for acute acalculous cholecystitis in critically ill trauma patients. Am Surg. 2002;68:65-69.
83. Bennett GL, Rusinek H, Lisi V, et al. CT findings in acute gangrenous cholecystitis. AJR Am J Roentgenol. 2002;178:275-281.
84. Gore RM, Yaghmai V, Newmark GM, et al. Imaging benign and malignant disease of the gallbladder. Radiol Clin North Am. 2002;40:1307-1323, vi.
85. Romagnuolo J, Bardou M, Rahme E, et al. Magnetic resonance cholangiopancreatography: A meta-analysis of test performance in suspected biliary disease. Ann Intern Med. 2003;139:547-557.
86. Yellin AE, Berne TV, Appleman MD, et al. A randomized study of cefepime versus the combination of gentamicin and mezlocillin as an adjunct to surgical treatment in patients with acute cholecystitis. Surg Gynecol Obstet. 1993;177(Suppl):23-29; discussion, 35-40.
87. Liu LX, Harinasuta KT. Liver and intestinal flukes. Gastroenterol Clin North Am. 1996;25:627-636.
88. Sandouk F, Haffar S, Zada MM, et al. Pancreatic-biliary ascariasis: Experience of 300 cases. Am J Gastroenterol. 1997;92:2264-2267.
89. Nash JA, Cohen SA. Gallbladder and biliary tract disease in AIDS. Gastroenterol Clin North Am. 1997;26:323-335.
90. Margulis SJ, Honig CL, Soave R, et al. Biliary tract obstruction in the acquired immunodeficiency syndrome. Ann Intern Med. 1986;105:207-210.
91. Ducreux M, Buffet C, Lamy P, et al. Diagnosis and prognosis of AIDS-related cholangitis. AIDS. 1995;9:875-880.
92. Kune GA, Burdon JG. Are antibiotics necessary in acute cholecystitis? Med J Aust. 1975;2:627-630.
93. Berger H, Pratschke E, Arbogast H, Stabler A. Percutaneous cholecystostomy in acute acalculous cholecystitis. Hepatogastroenterology. 1989;36:346-348.

94. Lo CM, Liu CL, Fan ST, et al. Prospective randomized study of early versus delayed laparoscopic cholecystectomy for acute cholecystitis. Ann Surg. 1998;227:461-467.
95. Lai PB, Kwong KH, Leung KL, et al. Randomized trial of early versus delayed laparoscopic cholecystectomy for acute cholecystitis. Br J Surg. 1998;85:764-767.
96. Afdhal N. Acute cholangitis. In: Rose B, ed. Wellesley, MA: UpToDate (electronic publication), 2003.
97. Lai EC, Mok FP, Tan ES, et al. Endoscopic biliary drainage for severe acute cholangitis. N Engl J Med. 1992;326:1582-1586.
98. Sharma BC, Agarwal DK, Baijal SS, et al. Endoscopic management of acute calculous cholangitis. J Gastroenterol Hepatol. 1997;12:874-876.
99. Deviere J, Motte S, Dumonceau JM, et al. Septicemia after endoscopic retrograde cholangiopancreatography. Endoscopy. 1990;22:72-75.

CHAPTER **70**

Pancreatic Infections

MIRIAM J. BARON
LAWRENCE C. MADOFF

Clinically, pancreatic tissue inflammation commonly manifests as severe acute upper abdominal pain and elevated serum levels of pancreatic enzymes. Most episodes of acute pancreatitis (AP) are associated with gall stones or alcohol. Other causes of AP are hypercalcemia, hypertriglyceridemia, anatomic abnormalities, familial syndromes, autoimmune disease, ischemia, pancreatic carcinoma, trauma, endoscopic retrograde cholangiopancreatography (ERCP), and drugs, among which are antimicrobial agents such as tetracycline, pentamidine, sulfonamides, didanosine, erythromycin, nitrofurantoin, and metronidazole (Box 70-1).[1] Infection of damaged pancreatic tissue may complicate disease initiated by any of these mechanisms and confers significant morbidity and mortality risks. Less commonly, many different microorganisms may infect the pancreas directly, with or without inciting a syndrome of AP. This chapter reviews the infectious agents associated with primary pancreatic infection before focusing on infectious complications of AP. Issues of nonpancreatic infection related to gall stones are addressed in Chapter 69.

INFECTIOUS CAUSES OF ACUTE PANCREATITIS

Many organisms have been reported to cause pancreatic disease. The human case reports in this area have been reviewed and assessed for documentation of pancreatitis and infection (Box 70-2).[2] In this series, "definite" pancreatitis required either the presence of pancreatitis at surgery or autopsy or radiographic evidence, and "definite" infection required identification of an organism in the pancreas or pancreatic duct by stain or culture. The criteria for "probable" pancreatitis included a threefold increase in amylase or lipase or both, as well as characteristic symptoms; "probable" infection required either culture of the organism from blood or pancreatic juice or serologic diagnosis in a characteristic clinical or epidemiologic setting. Using these definitions, the reports of "definite" or "probable" association with pancreatitis described patients with coxsackieviruses, cytomegalovirus (CMV), varicella-zoster virus (VZV), herpes simplex virus type 2 (HSV-2), mumps, hepatitis B, *Mycoplasma*, *Leptospira*, *Legionella*, *Salmonella typhi*, *Aspergillus*, *Toxoplasma*, *Cryptosporidium*, and *Ascaris*.

Among these, ascariasis causes pancreatic-biliary disease commonly in countries with high infection rates; in some tropical areas, ascariasis ranks second to gall stones as a cause of pancreatitis.[3] After hatching in the duodenum, *Ascaris* larvae penetrate the small bowel mucosa, enter the venous circulation, and arrive in the lungs, where they enter the alveoli, ascend the bronchial tree, and are swallowed. In the gastrointestinal tract, they mature into adult worms and then may cause clinical and pathologic AP by migrating across the ampulla of Vater to obstruct the common bile duct or the pancreatic duct. One study documented an increased risk for pancreatic-biliary ascariasis among Syrian women who had prior unrelated endoscopic sphincterotomy, with particularly high frequency of illness during the fasting period of Ramadan.[4]

Another group of organisms causes pancreatic infection, forming microabscesses or macroabscesses but without inducing the signs, symptoms, or pathology of AP. This group includes *Mycobacterium tuberculosis*, *Mycobacterium avium*, *Nocardia asteroides*, *Cryptococcus*

BOX 70-1

Drugs That Can Cause Acute Pancreatitis

Azathioprine	Erythromycin
6-Mercaptopurine	α-Methyldopa
Valproic acid	Nitrofurantoin
Estrogens	Acetaminophen (overdose)
Tetracycline	Aminosalicylic acid
Thiazide diuretics	Cimetidine
Furosemide	Ranitidine
Cytarabine	Steroids
L-Asparaginase	Sulfasalazine
Pentamidine	Procainamide
Sulfonamides	Metronidazole
Didanosine	Nonsteroidal anti-inflammatory drugs

Modified from Sakorafas GH, Tsiotou AG. Etiology and pathogenesis of acute pancreatitis. J Clin Gastroenterol. 2000;30:343-356.

BOX 70-2

Infectious Causes of Pancreatic Disease

Definite Pancreatitis
Mumps
Coxsackievirus B, B3, B4
Hepatitis B virus
Cytomegalovirus
Herpes simplex virus type 2
Varicella-zoster virus
Mycoplasma
Salmonella typhi
Leptospira
Legionella
Toxoplasma
Cryptosporidium
Ascaris

Pancreatic Infection without Acute Pancreatitis
Aspergillus
Mycobacterium tuberculosis
Mycobacterium avium
Actinomyces
Nocardia asteroides
Cryptococcus neoformans
Coccidioides immitis
Paracoccidioides brasiliensis
Histoplasma capsulatum
Candida spp.
Zygomycetes
Pneumocystis jirovecii
Leishmania donovani
Entamoeba histolytica
Strongyloides stercoralis
Schistosoma haematobium
Paragonimus westermani
Clonorchis sinensis
Echinococcus granulosus

From Parenti DM, Steinberg W, Kang P. Infectious causes of acute pancreatitis. Pancreas. 1996;13:356-371.

neoformans, Coccidioides immitis, Paracoccidioides brasiliensis, Histoplasma capsulatum, Candida spp., Phycomycetes, *Pneumocystis jirovecii, Leishmania donovani, Entamoeba histolytica, Strongyloides stercoralis, Schistosoma haematobium, Paragonimus westermani, Clonorchis sinensis,* and *Echinococcus granulosus.*[2]

Other organisms, including Epstein-Barr virus (EBV), vaccinia, rubella, adenovirus, and rubeola, have been cited as causes of pancreatic infection in case reports but without adequately rigorous investigation to qualify for "definite" or "probable" association with pancreatitis.[2]

Therefore, pathologic or radiographic evidence of pancreatitis associated with well-documented infection has been noted with viruses (mumps, coxsackieviruses, hepatitis B, CMV, VZV, HSV), bacteria (*Mycoplasma, Legionella, Leptospira, Salmonella*), fungi (*Aspergillus*), and parasites (*Toxoplasma, Cryptosporidium, Ascaris*). However, the frequencies with which these organisms contribute to idiopathic pancreatitis remain unclear.

PANCREATITIS AND HUMAN IMMUNODEFICIENCY VIRUS INFECTION

Although the human immunodeficiency virus (HIV) itself has not been identified in pancreatic tissue by molecular methods, HIV infection has been associated with an increased risk of clinical pancreatitis. One study reported a 14% incidence of mild to moderately severe AP among patients with HIV in 1993-1994, with an inverse correlation between serum pancreatic enzyme level and number of CD4+ T-lymphocytes.[5] Causes of pancreatitis specific to HIV-infected patients include drugs (e.g., pentamidine, didanosine, trimethoprim/sulfamethoxazole) and opportunistic infections (e.g., CMV, HSV, others listed earlier). For the most part, however, the infections in these reports (microabscesses or macroabscesses) were noted incidentally at autopsy, without prior associated symptoms or pathologic evidence of AP. In addition, advanced HIV infection is associated with an increased risk of pancreatic malignancies, including Kaposi's sarcoma and lymphoma, which may lead to signs, symptoms, or laboratory abnormalities suggesting pancreatitis. Finally, isolated pancreatic enzyme elevations have been noted in patients with HIV infection who lack other signs or symptoms of pancreatitis.[6] In the study discussed earlier,[5] the most frequent causes of pancreatitis were gall stones, abuse of alcohol or intravenous drug use, pentamidine intake, and infections with *P. jirovecii* and *Mycobacterium avium-intracellulare.* Of note, no pancreatic tissue sampling was performed to document the presence of these microorganisms.

INFECTION COMPLICATING ACUTE PANCREATITIS

Background

Most pancreatic infections occur as complications of AP initiated by noninfectious causes. Regardless of the inciting event, the pathogenesis of AP involves activation and release of toxic materials, including pancreatic proteolytic enzymes and vasoactive substances that injure pancreatic cells and blood vessels: trypsin, cathepsin B, phospholipase, chymotrypsin, elastase, cytokines, and the kallikrein-kinin, coagulation, and fibrinolysis cascades. Such damage increases vascular permeability and leads to pancreatic swelling, a condition described clinically as edematous/interstitial pancreatitis. This disorder accounts for 80% of AP cases[7] and usually responds well to supportive care. In more severe disease, liberation of these toxic materials into the surrounding retroperitoneal spaces, lesser sac, and peritoneal cavity causes chemical irritation and contributes to third-space losses of protein-rich fluid, leading to hypovolemia and hypotension. In 20% of AP cases,[8] hypoxia, free radicals, and ongoing release of pancreatic enzymes cause disruption of the pancreatic microcirculation, which leads to more severe pancreatic tissue injury and ultimately to pancreatic necrosis. In addition, recruited inflammatory cells release substances such as phospholipase A_2, polymorphonuclear cell elastase, interleukins, leukotrienes, and complement factors which contribute to a systemic inflammatory response syndrome (SIRS) that may include fever, acute respiratory distress syndrome (ARDS), pleural effusions, renal failure, shock, myocardial depression, and metabolic abnormalities.[9] Necrotizing pancreatitis is associated with mortality rates of 30% to 40%.[10] Twenty percent of the deaths occur during the first week of illness, in the setting of this inflammatory milieu and associated multiple organ failure. The remaining 80% of deaths from AP occur later, often in association with local and systemic infectious complications.[11,12]

Significance of Infection in Acute Pancreatitis

Some reports suggest that infection increases the mortality rate. In one series of 114 patients with pancreatic necrosis, intestinal microorganisms were cultured from the necrotic tissue in 39.4% of cases. Mortality rates in patients with less than 50% gland necrosis rose from 12.9% to 38.9% if the necrotic tissue was infected, whereas mortality rates in patients with greater than 50% necrosis rose from 14.3% to 66.7% in the presence of infection.[13] Of note, other studies have reported equal mortality rates among patients with severe sterile necrosis and those with infected necrosis.[14] Nonetheless, the association of mortality with infection in AP in some studies suggests that prevention, identification, and treatment of infections may decrease the risks of adverse outcomes.

Although infection is rare in mild pancreatitis, severe pancreatitis is associated with infection rates as high as 70%.[13,15-18] This difference in infection risk has driven extensive efforts to identify patients with severe pancreatitis early in the course of illness. Multiple criteria have been suggested. There is some consensus that severe AP is characterized by abnormalities in physiology, manifested by an Acute Physiology and Chronic Health Evaluation (APACHE II) score greater than 8 (or equivalent on other scoring systems) in conjunction with computed tomographic (CT) evidence of greater than 30% pancreatic necrosis, chest radiographic evidence of pleural effusions, and a C-reactive peptide (CRP) value greater than 150 mg/L.[19] Importantly, the risk of infection increases with the extent of necrosis.[13,20]

Defining Pancreatic Infections

Pancreatic infection nomenclature, derived by consensus at the International Symposium on Acute Pancreatitis in Atlanta in 1992,[21] is summarized in Table 70-1. In early AP (the first 3 weeks),[14] local infection may arise in necrotic pancreatic and peripancreatic tissue without significant pus collections.[22] The incidence of infection increases with the extent of necrosis and with time.[23] In one study, 49% of infections in necrotizing pancreatitis developed within the first 2 weeks of illness, and 71% within the first 3 weeks of illness.[14] Another group documented contamination rates of 25% at 1 week, 45% at 2 weeks, and 60% at 3 weeks of illness.[24] A third group reported that the incidence of infection was highest among patients undergoing surgery 15 to 21 days into their illness.[13] The contamination rate was 24% within the first week after onset of symptoms and rose to 36% within 2 weeks and 71% within 3 weeks.

Later in the course of AP (weeks 4-7), after the serum markers of pancreatitis resolve, pancreatic necrosis liquefies into fluid collections. Sterile necrosis therefore develops into pancreatic pseudocysts, whereas infected necrosis matures into pancreatic abscesses in about 3% of patients with necrotizing pancreatitis.[13,16] Pseudocysts may subsequently become superinfected and develop into abscesses as well. Pancreatic abscess typically manifests with fever, abdominal pain, and leukocytosis in patients recovering from recognized pancreatic disease. In general, the rates of systemic toxicity and mortality are higher with infected necrosis than with pancreatic abscess. Specifically, one group reported mortality rates of 26% for infected necrosis and 12% for abscess,[14] and another described 32.1% mortality for infected necrosis versus 22.2% for abscess.[22]

Diagnosis of Pancreatic Infection

Identification of infection in AP can be difficult, because patients with extensive necrosis of pancreatic and peripancreatic tissue frequently display a sepsis-like syndrome without a septic focus. Such patients

TABLE 70-1 Definitions Derived from the International Symposium on Acute Pancreatitis, 1992*

Acute pancreatitis (AP)	Acute inflammatory process of the pancreas with variable involvement of other regional tissues or remote organ systems
Severe AP	Association with organ failure and/or local complications, such as necrosis, abscess, or pseudocyst
Acute fluid collection	Occurs early in the course of AP, located in or near the pancreas, always lacking a wall of granulation or fibrous tissue; bacteria variably present; occurs in 30% to 50% of severe AP cases; most acute fluid collections regress, but some progress to pseudocyst or abscess
Pancreatic necrosis	One or more focal or diffuse areas of nonviable pancreatic parenchyma, typically associated with peripancreatic fat necrosis, diagnosed by computed tomography scan with intravenous contrast enhancement
Acute pseudocyst	Collection of pancreatic juice enclosed by a wall of fibrous or granulation tissue, which arises as a consequence of AP, pancreatic trauma, or chronic pancreatitis; formation requires ≥4 weeks from onset of AP
Pancreatic abscess	Circumscribed intra-abdominal collection of pus, usually in or near the pancreas, containing little or no pancreatic necrosis, which arises as a consequence of AP or pancreatic trauma

*The use of terms such as phlegmon, infected pseudocyst, hemorrhagic pancreatitis, and persistent acute pancreatitis is explicitly discouraged.

From Bradley EL. A clinically based classification system for acute pancreatitis. Arch Surg. 1993;128:586-590.

may develop physiologic abnormalities indistinguishable from those associated with infection, including systemic organ failure syndrome involving the lungs, kidneys, liver, and cardiovascular systems. In one study,[25] 60% of AP patients developed fever; in 22% the fever was related to pancreatitis per se; in 33% it was attributed to extrapancreatic infection; and in 45% it was caused by infected pancreatic necrosis. Imaging by CT can aid in the diagnosis of infected pancreatic necrosis only if gas is seen in and around areas of pancreatic necrosis. Several laboratory parameters have been evaluated as markers of pancreatic infection, the most promising of which is procalcitonin, a 116-amino-acid propeptide of calcitonin, but more data from larger studies must be obtained.[26,27] Therefore, tissue sampling must be undertaken in order to detect infection. Gram staining and culture of pancreatic tissue sampled by CT-guided fine-needle aspiration (FNA) provides high diagnostic sensitivity and specificity with minimal risk of introducing infection or disseminating organisms by intestinal puncture.[14] This procedure is recommended for patients with necrotizing AP and persistent systemic toxicity or organ failure in the first 7 to 14 days. Similarly, culture of material retrieved by FNA of collections seen by CT or ultrasound imaging allows diagnosis of pancreatic abscess. Such collections may spread from the pancreas into the retroperitoneum, mesentery, mediastinum, and elsewhere, through tissue damaged by activated proteases, vasoactive substances, and inflammatory mediators.[28]

The Flora of Pancreatic Infection

Pancreatic superinfection (both infected necrosis and abscess) usually involves gastrointestinal flora, including aerobes and anaerobes. Historically, both gram-negative bacteria (most commonly *Escherichia coli* and *Klebsiella* spp., less commonly *Enterobacter*, *Pseudomonas*, *Proteus*, and others) and gram-positive bacteria (enterococcal, streptococcal, and staphylococcal species) participate, and infections may be monomicrobial or polymicrobial. In a collected series of 45 articles representing more than 1100 cases of secondary pancreatic infections,[29] the responsible organisms were *E. coli* in 35%, *Klebsiella pneumoniae* in 24%, *Enterococcus* spp. in 24%, *Staphylococcus* spp. in 14%, and *Pseudomonas* spp. in 11%.

One group[30] reported finding different microbiology of infected pancreatic necrosis in patients with alcoholic versus biliary pancreatitis among 70 patients with similar degrees of necrosis who underwent surgery for pancreatitis. The authors noted a higher rate of infection overall and a preponderance of gram-negative organisms in the patients with biliary disease, compared with a tendency toward more gram-positive pancreatic infections in the alcoholic group. A higher number of patients in the biliary disease group had received presurgical antibiotic therapy (83% versus 74%), but the duration and spectrum of preoperative therapy were similar, and the authors included culture data only from an initial surgical procedure. No patients had undergone prior procedures that could introduce pancreatic infection. The authors hypothesized that the differences in patterns of infection could be explained by a biliary origin of pancreatic infection among patients with biliary disease and a hematogenous origin of infection from catheter contamination in the alcoholic population. Other work has shown that mortality from pancreatitis is related to the severity of the attack and not to the underlying etiology.[31]

Earlier exposure to broadly active antimicrobial therapy changes the flora that cause infections,[32] and increasingly resistant bacterial and fungal infections have become more common.[33] The literature contains inconsistent reports of the impact of fungal infection in the setting of pancreatitis. One group reported no correlation of fungal infection with negative outcomes,[34] but other studies suggest otherwise. One report[35] included prospective data on 57 patients with infected necrotizing AP between 1983 and 1995, of whom 7 patients (12%) developed either pure fungal infection or mixed fungal/bacterial infection; isolates were *Candida albicans* and *Candida glabrata*, detected at an average of 36 days (range, 18-80 days) after onset of pancreatitis. Four of these seven patients had "primary" fungal infection that developed in the absence of prior operative interventions. Fungal infection was associated with ERCP as the cause of AP (*P* = .02) and with exposure to parenteral nutrition and broad-spectrum antibiotics. Treatment included amphotericin B in five patients, two of whom received antifungal therapy only after developing candidemia 35 and 67 days after diagnosis of pancreatic fungal infection, respectively; two additional patients did not receive antifungal therapy at all because of concerns about toxicity. There was a trend toward a higher mortality rate among patients with fungal isolates (three of seven patients, or 43%) compared with patients with bacterial infection (24%). Two of the five patients receiving antifungal therapy died, as did one of the two untreated patients; two of the deaths were associated with fungemia. Survivors underwent twice as many necrosectomies (surgical excisions of necrotic tissue) as did nonsurvivors (four versus two surgeries per patient), suggesting that aggressive surgical management of these infections is warranted. Another study reported a 41% rate of *Candida* infection in peripancreatic sepsis (7 of 17 consecutive patients treated between 1988 and 1992). The mortality rate was 0% for the 10 patients without fungal infection and 42% among the *Candida*-infected patients (*P* = .05), without apparent relationship to microbiologic cure.[36] Most recently, another group[37] reported data on 46 patients with infected necrosis over an 8-year period. Fungal infection occurred in 17 (37%) of these patients; no features were found to distinguish these patients from the uninfected subjects. There was no mortality difference attributable to fungal infection. A lower rate of fungal infection without mortality benefit was noted in a subset of 18 patients who received prophylactic antifungal treatment.

Overall the profile of organisms suggests most pancreatic infections originate in the gastrointestinal tract and seed the pancreas via the bowel, the biliary tree, the lymphatics, or the blood stream. Initially, bowel flora may translocate across a gastrointestinal mucosal barrier damaged by ischemia during the hypovolemic phase of AP.

Management of Pancreatic Infection

In most cases, treatment of pancreatic infection requires antimicrobial therapy directed at organisms identified in cultures of the infected site, in combination with mechanical removal of the infected material. Although some groups[38] have reported successful medical management of infected necrosis, most believe that thorough surgical débridement of infected necrosis and removal of all associated collections are necessary. The timing of surgery is a matter of some debate in the literature. The intended benefit from early intervention is prompt removal of the infected material, in the hope of more rapid resolution of the inflammatory processes. However, a delay in surgery may allow for a more stable patient with better-demarcated areas of necrotic tissue. No studies have evaluated the optimal timing of surgery for infected necrosis in particular, but one randomized clinical trial studying patients with severe necrotizing pancreatitis found a trend toward a higher mortality rate (58% versus 27%) in patients undergoing early surgery.[39] The details of the surgical approach (i.e., necrosectomy with continuous closed lavage, débridement with open packing, or necrosectomy and drainage with planned reoperation) have not been found to differ in efficacy.[40,41] Surgical management often requires multiple, staged operations to remove all necrotic pancreatic and peripancreatic material. For patients with infected necrosis or pancreatic abscess, percutaneous catheter drainage may be a reasonable adjunct to surgery for initial stabilization of a septic patient or for postoperative management of further abscesses. In contrast, postpancreatitis abscesses remote from the pancreas itself and superinfected pancreatic pseudocysts are unlikely to be associated with significant amounts of necrotic tissue; these conditions may be managed successfully by catheter drainage or by surgical drainage in conjunction with appropriate antimicrobial therapy.[28]

The role of surgery in the management of sterile necrosis is more controversial; some believe that a subset of patients with severe sterile necrosis that has organized over the course of a prolonged illness (4-6 weeks or longer) may benefit from surgical débridement.[42] The decision to drain sterile fluid collections is also based predominantly on symptoms.

Prevention of Pancreatic Infection

Because infection may be associated with increased mortality rates in AP despite aggressive medical and surgical therapy, major efforts have been devoted toward preventing infection. Studies have focused on maintaining the gut barrier function, on selective gut decontamination (SGD) with oral nonabsorbable antibiotics, and on early therapy with systemic antibiotics. A reasonable aim for such studies is to identify interventions that decrease the frequency of pancreatic infection, leading to fewer surgical procedures and lower mortality rates.

Early Enteral Feeding

Several groups have studied enteral feeding in AP for its ability to lower infection risk both by reducing dependence on central venous access for parenteral alimentation and by sustaining the integrity of the intestinal barrier. In animal studies of AP,[43] enteral nutrition was associated with less bacterial and endotoxin translocation into mesenteric lymph nodes but did not influence pancreatic healing or overall survival. In one human study, 38 patients with severe AP were randomly assigned to receive either parenteral nutrition (TPN) or enteral nutrition via nasojejunal tube (NJT) within the first 48 hours after admission. The NJT patients suffered fewer complications ($P < .05$) and fewer infectious complications ($P < .01$), but no significant differences were found for any particular infection site.[44] All patients in this study received imipenem from admission until clinical recovery and restoration of normal CRP concentrations. The authors speculated that enteral feeding "improves the gut immune system, restores normal gut structure and microflora, and aids the mucosa in withstanding challenges … [but] it is, in fact, still unclear whether (enteral feeding) improves the rate of septic morbidity or whether TPN itself causes an increase in septic complications." Another study of 89 patients with pancreatitis observed that enteral nutrition significantly reduced septic complications but did not affect the rates of multiple organ failure or death.[45] Beyond enteral feeding, another randomized, double-blind study showed significantly less pancreatic sepsis and fewer surgical interventions in 22 AP patients given live *Lactobacillus* for 1 week, compared with 23 control patients given heat-killed *Lactobacillus*. Both groups received early enteral feeding with oat fiber supplementation as a substrate for the lactic acid bac-

teria. The authors noted a need for further work in this field to determine the role for such therapy in the management of AP.[46]

Selective Gut Decontamination

Animal studies of SGD (reviewed by Ratschko and associates[7]) show a mortality benefit in dog, rat, and mouse models of AP. However, experimental studies in rats suggest that eliminating gram-negative bowel flora may facilitate overgrowth of *Enterococcus* spp. in the gut and increase the risk of gram-positive infections from translocation of gastrointestinal flora.[47]

Only one controlled study in human patients has evaluated the effects of SGD on infection rates.[48] In this nonblinded trial, 102 patients with severe AP (but without pancreatic necrosis on CT) were randomly assigned to receive either conventional therapy or conventional therapy plus SGD. The SGD regimen included enteral colistin, norfloxacin, and amphotericin B, given as a daily rectal enema and as a sticky paste containing 2% of these drugs smeared along the gums and at the tracheostomy (if present) every 6 hours. The SGD group also received short-term intravenous cefotaxime until aerobic gram-negative bacteria were eliminated from the oral cavity and rectum. The treatments continued until patients were able to discontinue supplemental oxygen and infusions, were ambulatory, and were taking a regular oral diet. There was no difference in mortality on an intention-to-treat basis (35% for the control group versus 22% for the treatment group, $P = .19$). However, correction for illness severity by multivariate analysis yielded a narrow survival benefit for the SGD group ($P = .048$) that was attributable to a decrease in infected necrosis (18% versus 37%, $P = .03$), with an effect on gram-negative pancreatic infection in particular (8% versus 33%, $P = .003$). Of note, the follow-up was very long (40 days) in this study. In addition, pancreatic necrosis was documented to be sterile in 11 of 16 patients who died within 2 weeks after onset (mostly from multiple organ dysfunction syndrome), suggesting that mortality was unrelated to infection. The administration of intravenous cefotaxime along with SGD obscured interpretation of the effect of SGD alone.

In a follow-up report,[49] the authors of this human SGD trial noted that, in both SGD and control groups, gram-negative infection of pancreatic necrosis was associated with a mortality rate 15-fold higher than that associated with sterile necrosis, whereas gram-positive pancreatic infection was not associated with an increased mortality rate. Furthermore, there was no significant difference in the incidence of gram-positive infected necrosis between the SGD and control groups. These issues may be related to the treatment with systemic cefotaxime, which protects against some of the more virulent gram-positive organisms—streptococci and *Staphylococcus aureus*—but not against the more virulent gram-negative organisms, such as *Pseudomonas aeruginosa*. In fact, the most frequent gram-negative isolates in this study were *P. aeruginosa* and *E. coli* (13 patients each), whereas the most frequent gram-positive isolates were enterococci and *Staphylococcus epidermidis*.

Preemptive Systemic Antibiotic Treatment

Several groups have examined the efficacy of early treatment with systemic antibiotics in diminishing the risks of infection in AP. This literature generally describes such an approach as "prophylactic" antimicrobial therapy, but the strategy might be described more accurately as "early" or "preemptive" therapy. Numerous animal pancreatitis studies have shown a benefit from early antibiotic administration (as reviewed by Ratschko and associates[7] and Powell and colleagues[50]). Among other things, the ability to administer antibiotics very early in the course of pancreatitis in such studies distinguishes these models from the treatment in human patients, who did not appear to benefit from antibiotic therapy in the initial prospective randomized studies from the 1970s.[51-53] However, the human studies enrolled patients with mild disease who were at low risk for infection; among the aggregate of 199 patients in these studies, only 1 patient died. In addition, the treatment groups received monotherapy with ampicillin, which provides suboptimal activity against the relevant organisms and also penetrates poorly into pancreatic tissue and fluid.[7]

Several groups have evaluated antimicrobial penetration into pancreatic tissue in healthy animals, in human patients with pancreatic cancer, and in human patients with acute necrotizing pancreatitis.[7] In human studies, antibiotic levels in pancreatic tissue and fluid tend to correlate with the degree of inflammation; higher levels occur in patients with pancreatitis than in controls.[7] The data from these studies vary, however, possibly because of differences in the patient populations selected and in the method and timing of pancreatic area sampling relative to systemic drug administration. In general, antimicrobials can be assigned to three categories: (1) those with poor pancreatic penetration (aminoglycosides, first-generation cephalosporins, cefoxitin, and ampicillin); (2) those with variable penetration, which reach minimum inhibitory concentrations (MIC) for some but not all relevant organisms (mezlocillin/piperacillin and cefotaxime); and (3) those with penetration reaching MIC for most relevant organisms (fluoroquinolones, imipenem, ceftazidime, cefepime, metronidazole, clindamycin, chloramphenicol, doxycycline, and fluconazole).[50,54-57] One group developed an efficacy factor that incorporated each drug's pancreatic penetration and activity against organisms typically associated with pancreatic infection, with a factor of 1.0 considered optimal.[54] The calculated factors were 0.98 for imipenem, 0.86 to 0.87 for fluoroquinolones, and 0.71 to 0.78 for piperacillin and third-generation cephalosporins. However, the relationship between antibiotic levels in pancreatic tissue or fluid and antibiotic efficacy in preventing or treating infections in necrotic pancreatic parenchyma or in the retroperitoneal fat outside the pancreas remains unclear.

Five more recent nonblinded studies[20,58-61] have addressed the efficacy of systemic antibiotics in diminishing infection in AP, focusing on patients with severe disease and employing broad-spectrum antibiotics with reasonable pancreatic penetration, as summarized in Table 70-2. The results of these studies are not definitive, however, because of problems in study design and sample size.

In one randomized, prospective (but not placebo-controlled) multicenter trial[20] of 74 patients with necrotizing pancreatitis, mostly of biliary origin, early imipenem treatment (500 mg intravenously [IV] three times daily for 14 days) reduced morbidity by decreasing the rates of tissue-confirmed pancreatic infection (from 30.3% to 12.2%, $P < .01$) and nonpancreatic sepsis (48.5% versus 14.6%, $P = .01$) but did not influence time to onset of pancreatic sepsis (1 to 3 weeks), rate of multiorgan failure, need for surgery, or survival, compared with no early antibiotic treatment. Preemptive antibiotic therapy was especially effective for patients with mild-to-moderate pancreatic necrosis; no patient in the treated group with less than 50% necrosis developed septic complications (in contrast to 29% in the control group).[20]

In another randomized (but not placebo-controlled) trial,[58] 60 patients with severe acute alcoholic pancreatitis and necrosis of at least one third of the pancreas by contrast-enhanced CT were given either no preemptive antibiotics or cefuroxime (1.5 g IV three times daily), administered until clinical recovery and normalization of CRP level. In cases of persistent CRP elevation after full clinical recovery in the antibiotic group, cefuroxime was continued by mouth for 14 days. Cefuroxime was chosen for activity against *S. aureus* (methicillin-resistant *S. aureus* was infrequent in the center performing the study) and *E. coli*. The treated group had fewer total infectious complications (30 versus 54), fewer infections per patient (1.8 versus 1.0, $P = .01$), fewer operations (8 versus 36, $P = .012$), and fewer deaths (3% versus 23%, $P = .028$). However, the difference in the rate of culture-proven sepsis was not statistically significant between groups, and only urinary tract infections were reduced significantly. The study has been criticized because of the large number of urinary tract infections[17] and the high rate of *S. epidermidis* "infections" of questionable clinical significance. In addition, 67% of the patients in the treatment group changed antibiotics after a mean of 9.2 days—3 because of strong clinical suspicion for (culture-negative) sepsis and the other 17 for unstated reasons.[7] Finally, because the timing of the deaths was not reported and two patients died with sterile cultures, it is unclear whether these deaths were related to infection. The authors acknowledged that the reasons for the mortality benefit from early cefuroxime treatment in this study were unclear, because cefuroxime would not have been expected to alleviate most of the infections in the control group.[58]

A third group performed a randomized study[59] evaluating the effects of a 10-day course of ceftazidime (2g IV every 8 hours), amikacin (7.5mg/kg IV every 12 hours), and metronidazole (500 mg IV every 8 hours) in a group of 23 patients with alcohol-induced severe AP (with pancreatic fluid collections but without pancreatic necrosis on CT). Infections occurred in none of the patients in the treatment group, compared with 58% of those in the placebo group ($P = .03$). Rates of mortality and multiple organ failure were not significantly different.[59]

A fourth study[60] (not placebo-controlled) randomly assigned 26 patients with CT-confirmed pancreatic necrosis to receive either early intravenous ofloxacin (200 mg twice daily) and metronidazole (500 mg twice daily) or no antibiotics. All patients underwent FNA on days 1, 3, 5, 7, and 10; antibiotics were administered to those control patients who showed evidence of infection. There was no difference in the incidence or timing of infected necrosis (median, 9.5 days in the treated

TABLE 70-2   Pancreatic Infection Incidence and Mortality Rate in Controlled Trials with Antibiotic Therapy

Reference	Antibiotic	No. Patients	Pancreatic Infection Rate, Control/Case (%)	Mortality Rate, Control/Case (%)	Comments
Luiten et al[48]	SGD: enteral colistin, norfloxacin, and amphotericin B until clinical recovery PLUS cefotaxime IV until gram-negative bacteria are eliminated from the oral cavity	102	38/18*	35/22	Necrosis not defined; mortality difference was statistically significant when disease severity differences between groups were taken into account
Pederzoli et al[20]	Imipenem, 14 days	74	30/12*	12/7	Nonpancreatic infections also reduced (15% vs 49%, $P < .01$)
Sainio et al[58]	Cefuroxime, until clinical recovery	60	40/30	23/3*	Reduction in total infections statistically significant
Delcenserie et al[59]	Ceftazidime, amikacin, and metronidazole, 10 days	23	58/0*	25/9	Two or more fluid collections on CT, necrosis not defined
Schwarz et al[60]	Ofloxacin and metronidazole, 10 days	26	53/61	15/0	Better clinical course in intervention group, but no effect on development of pancreatic infections
Isenmann et al[60a]	Ciprofloxacin and metronidazole	114	9/12	7/5	AP and serum CRP >150 mg/L and/or necrosis on CT
Bassi et al[33]	Pefloxacin vs imipenem, 14 days	60	Pefloxacin, 33* Imipenem, 10*	Pefloxacin, 24 Imipenem, 10	At least 50% necrosis confirmed by CT

AP, acute pancreatitis; CRP, C-reactive peptide; CT, computed tomography; SGD, selective gut decontamination.
*$P < .05$.
Modified from Toouli J, Brooke-Smith M, Bassi C, et al. Guidelines for the management of acute pancreatitis. J Gastroenterol Hepatol. 2002;17(Suppl):S15-S39.

group versus 10 days in the control group). The mortality rate trended downward from 15% to 0% in the antibiotic-treated group.[60]

The fifth study[60a] assigned 114 patients with AP and CRP >150 mg/L and/or necrosis on CT in a placebo-controlled double-blind design to receive intravenous ciprofloxacin (400 mg twice daily) and metronidazole (500 mg twice daily) or placebo. Open antibiotic treatment was started when infection, multiple organ failure sepsis, or systemic inflammatory response syndrome (SIRS) occurred. There were no differences in the rate of open antibiotic treatment versus the rate of infected pancreatic necrosis or mortality.

Therefore, of the five randomized studies comparing routine early antibiotic treatment versus no treatment in AP, three showed lower rates of sepsis, two showed reduced rates of pancreatic infection, and none showed any effect on the rate of surgical intervention. Only one study[58] showed a statistically significant reduction in mortality rate associated with preemptive antibiotic therapy, and that study found no change in the pancreatic infection rate related to antibiotic use. The inconsistencies among trials may arise from the relatively small numbers of patients, providing inadequate power to detect significant differences. Additional discrepancies may be related to differences in patient populations and in nonantibiotic management, such as rates, timing, and techniques of surgery, enteral nutrition, fluid resuscitation, and other factors.

A meta-analysis[62] of eight controlled trials,[20,48,51-53,58-60] including the trials from the 1970s, found that early antibiotic administration reduced mortality from AP, but only for patients with severe pancreatitis who received broad-spectrum antibiotics reaching therapeutic levels in pancreatic tissue. Another meta-analysis[63] included only randomized, controlled, nonblinded studies evaluating patients with necrotizing pancreatitis who received either no preemptive antibiotics or preemptive treatment with antibiotics reaching therapeutic levels in necrotic pancreatic tissue.[20,58,60] In all, 84 patients received antibiotic prophylaxis, and 76 patients did not. This meta-analysis found a nonsignificant trend toward decreased local infection in patients given early imipenem, cefuroxime, or ofloxacin; the incidence rates of sepsis and overall mortality were significantly lower for antibiotic treatment (absolute risk reductions, 21.1% and 12.3% respectively, for a relative risk reduction of 72%). On this basis, the authors recommended that "all patients with acute necrotizing pancreatitis...be given prophylaxis with an antibiotic with proven efficacy in necrotic pancreatic tissue."[62] Of note, the total of 160 patients in the pooled data set is inadequate for detection of a 50% reduction in the rate of infections.[50] In addition, the validity of meta-analysis for these studies is unclear, because the enrollment criteria, antibiotic regimens, and methods of diagnosing infections used in the trials are not uniform. Finally, one author pointed out that the absence of blinding in these studies may have encouraged clinicians to offer surgical débridement preferentially to control patients; such surgery might convert sterile necrosis to infected necrosis, which might increase mortality.[42]

Observational reports provide additional information. Two groups[14,63] have described single-institution experiences with infection rates during periods before and after routine use of early antibiotic therapy. Both noted lower rates of infected necrosis after introduction of preemptive antibiotics (decreases from 67% to 32% and from 76% to 27%, respectively). The first study[14] included 104 patients who underwent FNA between 1980 and 1995. Between the periods 1980-1987 and 1988-1995, the overall infection rate fell from 60% to 34% (P = .011), and the infected necrosis rate declined from 67% to 32% (P = .015). This difference is attributed to a change in the patterns of early administration of antibiotics. Of note, the mortality rate remained 20% during both periods of this study, despite the lower infection rates.

The other group[63] performed a retrospective cohort review evaluating three groups of patients with necrotizing pancreatitis: 50 patients from 1982-1989 who received no early antibiotics, 55 patients from 1990-1992 who received variable antibiotic regimens at the discretion of their physicians, and 75 patients from 1993-1996 who received imipenem until discharge or for up to 4 weeks, according to standard protocol, based on an APACHE score greater than 6 and the presence

of pancreatic necrosis (greater than 15% of the gland), peripancreatic necrosis, or peripancreatic collection. The frequency of pancreatic infection was significantly lower among patients receiving preemptive antibiotics: 76% in the earliest group, compared with 45% in the middle group (P = .003) and 27% in the latest group (P < .001). In addition, the difference in infection rate between the group of patients receiving nonprotocol antibiotics and the group receiving imipenem by protocol was statistically significant (P = .04). The mortality rates trended downward in the three groups, from 16% to 7% to 5%, respectively (P = .11). Mortality rates ranged from 19% to 40% for patients developing infection within the first 4 weeks, compared with 0% to 8% for those infected after 4 weeks. Time to infection, however, was the same across all groups. The authors concluded that early imipenem, or possibly ciprofloxacin, for a 4-week course, should be the standard of care for patients with severe AP. Although this study has been invoked in support of routine administration of imipenem, the results are confounded by several factors. The middle group may have received antibiotics with inadequate spectrum of coverage, later in the course of illness, or for inadequate durations. Because the causative organisms were not reported, the importance of spectrum of coverage cannot be assessed. In addition, the longitudinal retrospective design of this study impairs understanding of the effects of non–antibiotic-related changes in detection and management of severe AP that may have influenced mortality rates. Of note, lower infection rates were not associated with improved survival in either retrospective study.

Additional Data

One trial has addressed the selection of optimal antibiotic therapy.[33] This (nonblinded) study compared a 2-week course of pefloxacin (400 mg twice daily) with a 2-week course of imipenem (500 mg three times daily) in 56 patients with severe necrotizing pancreatitis. The rates of infected necrosis and extrapancreatic infection were 33% and 43%, respectively, in the pefloxacin group, compared with 10.3% and 20.6% in the imipenem group (P < .05). Rates of death, all resulting from sepsis, did not differ significantly (pefloxacin group, 17%; imipenem group, 10%).[33]

Review Article Recommendations

The literature lacks consensus about the most appropriate approach for minimizing infection in AP. One group wrote, "a general recommendation concerning the use of prophylactic antibiotics has to await the results of larger, double-blind studies."[23] Another group agreed that "the data are insufficiently strong to mandate prophylaxis or to elevate it to the standard of care" but went on to state that "although its importance is unproved, it would make sense to choose an antibiotic regimen that achieves bactericidal concentrations in pancreatic tissue against most likely pathogens.... The combination of a fluoroquinolone plus metronidazole, or monotherapy with a carbapenem antibiotic, would be appropriate choices." These authors called for multicenter, blinded, large, placebo-controlled studies to address additional questions, including the minimum degree of AP severity that might benefit from antibiotics and the most appropriate end points to be used in assessing efficacy.[13] Other groups have made more specific recommendations (Table 70-3), largely supporting use of a carbapenem alone or a quinolone plus metronidazole as first-choice therapy, with third-generation cephalosporins or ureidopenicillins as alternative aerobic coverage and clindamycin as alternative anaerobic coverage.

Most authors have recognized that optimal duration of preemptive antimicrobial therapy has not been studied, but some recommend 1 to 4 weeks, depending on the course of disease.[7] In contrast, other authors have favored minimizing exposure to antimicrobials. One group[69] described efforts to avoid imipenem and to limit the duration of empiric coverage to 14 days because of concerns about facilitating fungal superinfection. Another group[64] concluded that the risks of fungal infection warrant a policy of limiting treatment with broad-spectrum antibiotics to "as short a period as seems prudent (typically 5-7 days)."

Regarding fungal infection, some authors[35,70] have recommended low-dose prophylactic fluconazole for all patients with necrotizing

TABLE 70-3 Recommendations from Review Articles and Guidelines Supporting Early Administration of Antibiotics in Patients with Acute Pancreatitis

Reference	Year	Inclusion Criteria	Drug	Duration
Beger et al[13]	1986	Acute necrotizing AP	A drug with therapeutic levels in the inflamed pancreas	—
American College of Gastroenterology guidelines[42]	1997	Necrotizing pancreatitis associated with organ failure	Coverage of aerobes and anaerobes	—
Ho & Frey[63]	1997	Necrosis or disruption of the pancreatic ductal system/fluid collections	Ciprofloxacin or imipenem-cilastatin	4 wk
Spanish Consensus Conference[66]	1997	Necrotizing pancreatitis	Imipenem	Minimum 14 days
U.K. guidelines[65]	1998	Before ERCP or surgery; severe AP	Cefuroxime	—
Kramer & Levy[67]	1999	Ranson score[32] >2, >1 acute fluid collection, or necrosis involving at least one third of pancreas by CT	Third-generation cephalosporin or quinolone or imipenem or extended-spectrum penicillin	14 days
Ratschko et al[7]	1999	Severe AP	*First choices:* a carbapenem antibiotic or quinolone (second-generation) + metronidazole *Alternatives:* Cephalosporins (third generation) + metronidazole or clindamycin *OR* Ureidopenicillin + metronidazole *OR* Quinolone + clindamycin	Minimum 7-10 days
Santorini Consensus Conference[19]	1999	Severe AP	Broad-spectrum coverage, especially gram-negative	—
Gumaste[68]	2000	Significant necrosis or fluid collections or organ dysfunction	—	Minimum 10-14 days
Bangkok World Congress of Gastroenterology[32]	2002	Pancreatic necrosis	A carbapenem antibiotic	14 days
Yousaf et al[64]	2003	Severe AP	Broad-spectrum	5-7 days

AP, acute pancreatitis; CT, computed tomography; ERCP, endoscopic retrograde cholangiopancreatography.

pancreatitis who receive broad-spectrum antibiotics, particularly for the treatment of ERCP-induced pancreatitis. Interestingly, one group wrote that fungemic patients should receive systemic antifungal therapy but that "patients with yeast cultured from the necrotic excised pancreatic parenchyma but without fungemia may be observed, provided that optimal necrosectomy is performed with repeated operations, if necessary."[35] This recommendation contrasts with that of other groups, who believe that "all patients with isolation of fungus in the setting of acute necrotizing pancreatitis should be treated with antifungal therapy and surgical drainage and débridement regardless of previous pancreatic manipulation."[71] Others also strongly oppose routine antifungal prophylaxis, hoping instead that enteral nutrition will lower the risks of fungal infection, and in particular the risks of fluconazole-resistant fungal infection.[72]

Guidelines

Several groups have offered consensus guidelines for minimizing infections in AP. Guidelines from the Bangkok World Congress of Gastroenterology 2002 recommended CT scan evaluation at 4 to 7 days, followed by "a systemic antibiotic such as imipenem-cilastatin 500 mg three times a day for 2 weeks in patients with documented pancreatic necrosis,"[32] in the hope of decreasing the need for surgical intervention.[73]

The Santorini Consensus Conference guidelines support routine early antimicrobial therapy in severe AP, while acknowledging a lack of evidence to assist in the selection of agents, to support the use of gut decontamination, or to determine the optimal timing or duration of therapy. The group recommended that antibiotics with gram-negative activity be started "as early as possible after the identification of a severe attack."[19]

The United Kingdom guidelines specifically recommend no routine administration of antibiotics to patients with mild AP but early administration of intravenous cefuroxime to patients with severe AP, as "a reasonable balance between efficacy and cost."[65]

The Spanish Consensus Conference guidelines conclude that all patients with acute necrotizing pancreatitis should receive 2 weeks of imipenem (500 mg IV every 8 hours) on documentation of necrosis, with a longer course of therapy if clinically warranted.[66]

The American College of Gastroenterology guidelines state, "It is reasonable to initiate treatment with antibiotics with a good spectrum of activity against aerobic and anaerobic bacteria" in patients with necrotizing pancreatitis associated with organ failure.[42]

No consensus guidelines currently recommend routine antifungal prophylaxis or SGD.

General Practice

General practice varies but usually reflects a belief that early antibiotic therapy is beneficial in AP, particularly in severe AP. In the United Kingdom and Ireland, 88% of surgeons surveyed reported prescribing preemptive antibiotics in AP. Of note, 24% of the respondents reported initiating antibiotics in all cases, regardless of disease severity. The most commonly reported regimen was cefuroxime with or without metronidazole (46% of surgeons using early therapy).[74]

CONCLUSIONS

In general, mild-to-moderate AP is self-limited and is rarely complicated by infection. Severe AP is associated with significant morbidity and mortality rates that may be related to pancreatic superinfection with gastrointestinal flora. The management of such infections requires optimal diagnosis by way of imaging studies and percutaneous aspiration of necrotic pancreatic material, as well as aggressive medical and surgical care. Reducing the infection rate in AP is a worthy goal if doing so decreases morbidity and mortality, but whether this may be expected remains unclear. Human and experimental data suggest that enteral feeding prevents infection in AP. Early antibacterial treatment may reduce the risk of pancreatic infection for patients with severe AP, and a consensus favoring this practice has emerged. However, small size and design flaws render studies in this area difficult to interpret, and the optimal regimen, dose, and duration of preemptive therapy are unknown. These issues need to be addressed in large, well-designed, randomized, blinded, placebo-controlled trials. Enthusiasm for preemptive or prophylactic antibiotic treatment must be tempered by concerns about selecting for increasingly resistant organisms.

REFERENCES

1. Sakorafas GH, Tsiotou AG. Etiology and pathogenesis of acute pancreatitis. J Clin Gastroenterol. 2000;30:343-356.
2. Parenti DM, Steinberg W, Kang P. Infectious causes of acute pancreatitis. Pancreas. 1996;13:356-371.
3. Khuroo MS, Zargar SA, Yattoo GN, et al. Ascaris-induced acute pancreatitis. Br J Surg. 1992;79:1335-1338.
4. Sandouk F, Haffar S, Zada MM, et al. Pancreatic-biliary ascariasis: Experience of 300 cases. Am J Gastroenterol. 1997;92:2264-2267.
5. Dutta SK, Ting CD, Lai LL. Study of prevalence, severity, and etiological factors associated with acute pancreatitis in patients infected with human immunodeficiency virus. Am J Gastroenterol. 1997;92:2044-2048.
6. Murthy UK, DeGregorio F, Oates RP, et al. Hyperamylasemia in patients with the acquired immunodeficiency syndrome. Am J Gastroenterol. 1992;87:332-336.
7. Ratschko M, Fenner T, Lankisch PG. The role of antibiotic prophylaxis in the treatment of acute pancreatitis. Gastroenterol Clin North Am. 1999;28:641-659.
8. Bradley EL, Allen K. A prospective longitudinal study of observation versus surgical intervention in the management of necrotizing pancreatitis. Am J Surg. 1991;161:19-24.
9. Gross V, Leser H-G, Heinisch A, et al. Inflammatory mediators and cytokines: New aspects of the pathophysiology and assessment of severity of acute pancreatitis. Hepatogastroenterology. 1993;40:522-530.
10. Karimgani I, Porter K, Langevin R, et al. Prognostic factors in sterile pancreatic necrosis. Gastroenterology. 1992;103:1636-1640.
11. Renner J, Savage W, Pantoja J, et al. Death due to acute pancreatitis: A retrospective analysis of 405 autopsy cases. Dig Dis Sci. 1985;30:1005-1018.
12. Bassi C. Infected pancreatic necrosis. Int J Pancreatol. 1994;16:1-10.
13. Beger HG, Bittner R, Block S, et al. Bacterial contamination of pancreatic necrosis: A prospective clinical study. Gastroenterology. 1986;91:433-438.
14. Banks PA, Gerzof SG, Langevin RE, et al. CT-guided aspiration of suspected pancreatic infection: Bacteriology and clinical outcome. Int J Pancreatol. 1995;18:265-270.
15. Widdison AL, Karanjia ND. Pancreatic infection complicating acute pancreatitis. Br J Surg. 1993;80:148-154.
16. Gerzof SG, Banks PA, Robbins AH, et al. Early diagnosis of pancreatic infection by computed tomography–guided aspiration. Gastroenterology. 1987;93:1315-1320.
17. Wilson C, Heath DI, Imrie CW. Prediction of outcome in acute pancreatitis: A comparative study of APACHE-II clinical assessment and multiple factor scoring systems. Br J Surg. 1990;77:1260-1264.
18. Allardyce D. Incidence of necrotizing pancreatitis and factors related to mortality. Am J Surg. 1987;154:295-299.
19. Dervenis C, Johnson CD, Bassi C, et al. Diagnosis, objective assessment of severity, and management of acute pancreatitis. Int J Pancreatol. 1999;25:195-210.
20. Pederzoli P, Bassi S, Vesentini S, et al. A randomized multicenter clinical trial of antibiotic prophylaxis of septic complications in acute necrotizing pancreatitis with imipenem. Surg Gynecol Obstet. 1993;176:480-483.
21. Bradley EL 3rd. A clinically based classification system for acute pancreatitis. Arch Surg. 1993;128:586-590.
22. Bradley EL. A clinically based classification system for acute pancreatitis. Arch Surg. 1993;128:586-590.
23. Bittner R, Block S, Buchler M, et al. Pancreatic abscess and infected pancreatic necrosis: Different local septic complications in acute pancreatitis. Dig Dis Sci. 1987;32:1082-1087.
24. Isenmann R, Beger HG. Natural history of acute pancreatitis and the role of infection. Baillieres Best Pract Res Clin Gastroenterol. 1999;13:291-301.
25. Beger HG, Rau B, Mayer J, et al. Natural course of acute pancreatitis. World J Surg. 1997;21:130-135.
26. Bohidar NP, Garg PK, Khanna S, et al. Incidence, etiology, and impact of fever in patients with acute pancreatitis. Pancreatology. 2003;3:9-13.
27. Riche FC, Cholley BP, Laisne MJ, et al. Inflammatory cytokines, C reactive protein, and procalcitonin as early predictors of necrosis infection in acute necrotizing pancreatitis. Surgery. 2003;133:257-262.
28. Rau B, Steinbach G, Gansauge F, et al. The potential role of procalcitonin and interleukin 8 in the prediction of infected necrosis in acute pancreatitis. Gut. 1997;41:832-840.
29. Mithofer K, Mueller PR, Warshaw AL. Interventional and surgical treatment of pancreatic abscess. World J Surg. 1997;21:162-168.
30. Lumsden A, Bradley EL 3rd. Secondary pancreatic infections. Surg Gynecol Obstet. 1990;170:459-467.
31. Raty S, Sand J, Nordback I. Difference in microbes contaminating pancreatic necrosis in biliary and alcoholic pancreatitis. Int J Pancreatol. 1998;24:187-191.
32. Ranson JHC. Etiological and prognostic factors in human pancreatitis: A review. Am J Gastroenterol. 1982;77:633-638.
33. Toouli J, Brooke-Smith M, Bassi C, et al. Guidelines for the management of acute pancreatitis. J Gastroenterol Hepatol. 2002;17(Suppl):S15-S39.
34. Bassi C, Falconi M, Talamini G, et al. Controlled clinical trial of pefloxacin versus imipenem in severe acute pancreatitis. Gastroenterology. 1998;115:1513-1517.
35. Gloor B, Muller CA, Worni M, et al. Pancreatic infection in severe pancreatitis: The role of fungus and multiresistant organisms. Arch Surg. 2001;136:592-596.
36. Grewe M, Tsiotos GG, De-Ieon EL, et al. Fungal infection in acute necrotizing pancreatitis. J Am Coll Surg. 1999;188:408-414.
37. Aloia T, Solomkin J, Fink AS, et al. Candida in pancreatic infection: A clinical experience. Am Surg. 1994;60:793-796.
38. DeWaele JJ, Vogelaers D, Blot S, et al. Fungal infections in patients with severe acute pancreatitis and the use of prophylactic therapy. Clin Infect Dis. 2003;37:208-213.
39. Dubner H, Steinberg W, Hill M, et al. Infected pancreatic necrosis and peripancreatic fluid collections: Serendipitous response to antibiotics and medical therapy in three patients. Pancreas. 1996;12:298-302.
40. Mier J, Leon EL, Castillo A, et al. Early versus late necrosectomy in severe necrotizing pancreatitis. Am J Surg. 1997;173:71-75.
41. Farkas G, Maron J, Mandi Y, Szederkenyi E. Surgical strategy and management of infected pancreatic necrosis. Br J Surg. 1996;83:930-933.
42. McFadden W, Reber HA. Indications for surgery in severe acute pancreatitis. Int J Pancreatol. 1994;15:83-90.
43. Banks PA. Practice guidelines in acute pancreatitis. Am J Gastroenterol. 1997;92:377-386.
44. Kotani J, Usami M, Nomura H, et al. Enteral nutrition prevents bacterial translocation but does not improve survival during acute pancreatitis. Arch Surg. 1999;134:287-292.
45. Kalfarentzos F, Kehagias J, Mead N, et al. Enteral nutrition is superior to parenteral nutrition in severe acute pancreatitis: Results of a randomized prospective trial. Br J Surg. 1997;84:1665-1669.
46. Olah A, Pardavi G, Belagyi T, et al. Early nasojejunal feeding in acute pancreatitis is associated with a lower complication rate. Nutrition. 2002;18:259-262.
47. Olah A, Belagyi T, Gamal ME, et al. Randomized clinical trial of specific lactobacillus and fibre supplement to early enteral nutrition in patients with acute pancreatitis. Br J Surg. 2002;89:1103-1107.
48. Jackson RJ, Smith SD, Rowe MI. Selective bowel decontamination results in gram-positive translocation. J Surg Res. 1990;48:444-447.
49. Luiten EJ, Hop WC, Lange JF, et al. Controlled clinical trial of selective decontamination for the treatment of severe acute pancreatitis. Ann Surg. 1995;222:57-65.
50. Luiten EJ, Hop WC, Lange JF, et al. Differential prognosis of gram-negative versus gram-positive infected and sterile pancreatic necrosis: Results of a randomized trial in patients with severe acute pancreatitis treated with adjuvant selective decontamination. Clin Infect Dis. 1997;25:811-816.
51. Powell JJ, Miles R, Siriwardena AK. Antibiotic prophylaxis in the initial management of severe acute pancreatitis. Br J Surg. 1998;85:582-587.
52. Craig R, Dordal E, Myles L. The use of ampicillin in acute pancreatitis. Ann Intern Med. 1975;83:831-832.
53. Finch WT, Sawyers JL, Schenker S. A prospective study to determine the efficacy of antibiotics in acute pancreatitis. Ann Surg. 1976;183:667-671.
54. Howes R, Zuidema GD, Cameron JL. Evaluation of prophylactic antibiotics in acute pancreatitis. J Surg Res. 1975;18:197-200.
55. Buchler M, Malfertheiner P, Friess H, et al. Human pancreatic tissue concentration of bactericidal antibiotics. Gastroenterology. 1992;103:1902-1908.
56. Gloor B, Worni M, Strobel O, et al. Cefepime tissue penetration in experimental acute pancreatitis. Pancreas. 2003;26:117-121.
57. Shrikhande S, Friess H, Issenegger C, et al. Fluconazole penetration into the pancreas. Antimicrob Agents Chemother. 2000;44:2569-2571.
58. Bassi C, Pederzoli P, Vesentini S, et al. Behavior of antibiotics during human necrotizing pancreatitis. Antimicrob Agents Chemother. 1994;38:830-836.
59. Sainio V, Kemppainen E, Puolakkainen P, et al. Early antibiotic treatment in acute necrotising pancreatitis. Lancet. 1995;346:663-667.
60. Delcenserie R, Yzet T, Ducroix JP. Prophylactic antibiotics in treatment of severe acute alcoholic pancreatitis. Pancreas. 1996;13:198-201.
60a. Isenmann R, Runzi M, Kron M, et al. Prophylactic antibiotic treatment in patients with predicted severe acute pancreatitis: A placebo-controlled, double-blind trial. Gastroenterology. 204;126:997-1004.
61. Schwarz M, Isenmann R, Meyer H, et al. Antibiotic use in necrotizing pancreatitis: Results of a controlled study. Dtsch Med Wochenschr. 1997;122:356-361.
62. Golub R, Siddiqi F, Pohl D. Role of antibiotics in acute pancreatitis: A meta-analysis. J Gastrointest Surg. 1998;2:496-503.
63. Sharma VK, Howden CW. Prophylactic antibiotic administration reduces sepsis and mortality in acute necrotizing pancreatitis: A meta-analysis. Pancreas. 2001;22:28-31.
64. Ho HS, Frey CF. The role of antibiotic prophylaxis in severe acute pancreatitis. Arch Surg. 1997;132:187-192.
65. Yousaf M, McCallion K, Diamond T. Management of severe acute pancreatitis. Br J Surg. 2003;90:407-420.
66. United Kingdom guidelines for the management of acute pancreatitis. Gut. 1998;42(Suppl 2):S1-S13.
67. Martinez JF, Palazon JM, Perez-Mateo M. Prophylactic antibiotics in acute pancreatitis: Results from a consensus conference. Rev Esp Enf Digest. 1997;89:781-785.
68. Kramer KM, Levy H. Prophylactic antibiotics for severe acute pancreatitis: The beginning of an era. Pharmacotherapy. 1999;19:592-602.
69. Gumaste V. Prophylactic antibiotic therapy in the management of acute pancreatitis. J Clin Gastroenterol. 2000;31:6-10.
70. Clancy TE, Ashley SW. Current management of necrotizing pancreatitis. Adv Surg. 2002;36:103-121.
71. Laws HL, Kent RB. Acute pancreatitis: Management of complicating infection. Am Surg. 2000;66:145-152.
72. Robbins EG, Stollman NH, Bierman P, et al. Pancreatic fungal infections: A case report and review of the literature. Pancreas. 1996;12:308-312.
73. Butturini G, Salvia R, Bettini R, et al. Infection prevention in necrotizing pancreatitis: An old challenge with new perspectives. J Hosp Infect. 2001;49:4-8.
74. Nordback I, Sand J, Saaristo R, et al. Early treatment with antibiotics reduces the need for surgery in acute necrotizing pancreatitis: A single-center randomized study. J Gastrointest Surg. 2001;5:113-118.
75. Powell JJ, Campbell E, Johnson CD, et al. Survey of antibiotic prophylaxis in acute pancreatitis in the UK and Ireland. Br J Surg. 1999;86:320-322.

Splenic Abscess

LAWRENCE C. MADOFF

EPIDEMIOLOGY

The spleen is a highly vascular organ that is part of the reticuloendothelial arm of the immune system. If the spleen is surgically removed, its absence is marked by heightened susceptibility to overwhelming infection by encapsulated bacteria and intraerythrocytic parasites (see Chapter 315). Abscesses of the spleen usually result from bacteremia, particularly in the setting of abnormalities caused by trauma, embolization, or hemoglobinopathy. Immunodeficiency, such as that resulting from human immunodeficiency virus (HIV) infection, is also a risk factor.[1] Occasionally, splenic abscess results from extension of a contiguous focus of infection.

Splenic abscesses are relatively uncommon. For example, in one series of 540 intra-abdominal abscesses, none was in the spleen.[2] Autopsy series have placed the incidence of splenic abscesses at 0.2% to 0.7%.[3,4] There is a suggestion that the incidence may be rising because of improved detection, increasing use of illicit intravenous drugs, and the increased number of immunocompromised individuals.[5-7] Splenic abscess has a bimodal age distribution with peaks in the third and sixth decades of life.[7]

PATHOGENESIS

Bacteremic infection from a variety of sites is the most common cause of splenic abscess. Classically, infective endocarditis has been most strongly associated with splenic abscess, and in most series endocarditis is identified as the leading cause.[8] Other common sources of infection are the urinary tract, surgical wounds, and the gastrointestinal tract. Immunodeficiency has become a more important risk factor for the development of splenic abscess. In large reviews, 18% to 34% of patients were immunosuppressed (from disease, cancer chemotherapy, or steroid use), including as many as 9% who were infected with HIV.[9,10] Trauma to the spleen, either iatrogenic or accidental, accounts for 7% to 30% of cases, with lower numbers in more recent studies,, and contiguous spread of infection (e.g., from an adjacent intra-abdominal process) continues to account for a small percentage of cases (2% to 7%).[9] Other conditions associated with splenic abscess include splenic abnormalities such as Felty's syndrome or amyloidosis, intravenous drug use, hemoglobinopathy, and diabetes mellitus.

Complications of splenic abscess can be life-threatening and include perforation into the peritoneum, which occurred in 19 (6.6%) of 287 patients in a recent series.[9] Rupture into adjacent organs can occur, with resulting fistulas into the gastrointestinal tract, the pleural space, or lung parenchyma. Overall mortality rates of 0% to 14% have been reported with appropriate therapy (see "Therapy"), although higher rates occur among immunocompromised patients.

MICROBIOLOGY

Streptococci, staphylococci, salmonellae, and *Escherichia coli* have been the major causative agents of splenic abscess for the past century (Table 71-1). However, with the increased number of immunocompromised patients, recent series have shown greater numbers of fungal isolates, including *Candida* spp., *Aspergillus* spp., and agents of mucormycosis. Mycobacteria have also become more common. Anaerobic bacteria remain a relatively infrequent cause of splenic abscess compared with other intra-abdominal abscesses, despite improvements in culture techniques.

TABLE 71-1 Organisms Cultured from Splenic Abscesses: Comparison of Three Time Periods

Organism	% of Cultures Positive		
	1900-1977[*] (N = 129)	1977-1986[†] (N = 159)	1987-1995[‡] (N = 225)
Aerobic Bacteria			
Streptococcus spp.	21.7	6.9	10.2
Staphylococcus spp.	20.2	15.7	17.3
Salmonella spp.	10.9	10.7	16.1
Pseudomonas	0	1.3	6.3
Escherichia coli	24.1[§]	10.7	12.5
Enterococcus spp.		6.3	3.9
Klebsiella		1.9	1.9
Proteus		1.3	3.1
Other aerobes		8.2	7.1
Anaerobic bacteria	5.4	17.6	7.1
Mycobacteria			
Mycobacterium tuberculosis	0.8	0	5.5
Mycobacterium avium complex	0	0	1.9
Fungi	0.8	25.8	7.1
Sterile cultures	28.7	11.9	11.4

[*]Chun CH, Raff MJ, Contreras, L, et al. Splenic abscess. Medicine (Baltimore). 1980;59:50-65.
[†]Nelken N, Ignatius J, Skinner M, Christensen N. Changing clinical spectrum of splenic abscess: A multicenter study and review of the literature. Am J Surg. 1987;154:27-34.
[‡]Ooi LL, Leong SS. Splenic abscesses from 1987 to 1995. Am J Surg. 1997;174:87-93. Table 71-1 modified from data in Ooi et al.
[§]Total percentage for *E. coli*, *Enterococcus* spp., *Klebsiella*, *Proteus*, and other aerobes.

In HIV-infected patients, *Salmonella* spp. and *Mycobacterium tuberculosis* are common causes of splenic abscess, as are the opportunistic pathogens *Mycobacterium avium* complex, *Leishmania* spp., *Rhodococcus equi,* and *Pneumocystis jirovecii*. Sickle cell anemia has classically been associated with *Salmonella* infections of the spleen, but more recent series have noted a predominance of staphylococcal infection associated with this condition.[7] Many other organisms have been described as causative agents of splenic abscess at the case report level, including *Bartonella henselae*,[11] *Streptobacillus moniliformis*, and *Nocardia* spp.[4] In a series from Thailand, the agent of melioidosis, *Burkholderia pseudomallei*, was the cause of splenic abscess in 24 of 41 cases from which a pathogen was isolated.[12] Overall, blood cultures were positive in 24% to 60% of cases.[8,13]

CLINICAL PRESENTATION

Fever may be the only manifestation of splenic abscess, and fever is present in up to 95% of cases. Another frequent finding is abdominal pain, which is either generalized or localized to the left upper quadrant and may radiate to the left chest or shoulder. Nausea, vomiting, anorexia, and weakness are often present. Abdominal tenderness is present in only half of the cases, most often in the left upper quadrant. Splenomegaly can be detected in a similar number of cases. Chest findings, including dullness, rales, or both at the left base, have been detected in many patients. Other findings, less frequently present, include splenic friction rubs, hepatomegaly, tenderness at the costovertebral angle, and ascites. The only laboratory abnormality that is frequently present is leukocytosis, which is seen in 60% to 80% of cases.

DIAGNOSIS

Because the symptoms and findings of splenic abscess are most frequently nonspecific, diagnosis depends on appropriate imaging studies. Plain radiographs are surprisingly sensitive, with abnormalities detected in 50% to 80% of chest films and 25% of abdominal films (e.g., basilar infiltrates, pleural effusion, elevated hemidiaphragm, shift of viscera, presence of gas)[13]; however, the findings are most often nonspecific. The use of radionuclide scans as described in earlier literature, primarily technetium 99m sulfur-colloid liver-spleen scans, has been largely supplanted by ultrasonography, computed tomography (CT), and magnetic resonance imaging (MRI).

Ultrasonography. The advantages of ultrasonography in the evaluation of splenic abscess include low cost, portability, and relatively high sensitivity, reportedly ranging from 75% to 93%.[7,9,13,14] It is therefore appropriate in the initial assessment of most suspected splenic abscesses. Ultrasound typically demonstrates an area of decreased or absent echogenicity, sometimes with irregular areas of echodensity (debris) or a gas pattern within the lesion.[15] Splenomegaly can frequently be demonstrated. High-resolution (7.5 Mhz) ultrasonography can detect microabscesses in HIV-infected patients that are missed with conventional ultrasonography.[1]

Computed Tomography. CT appears to be the single most sensitive modality for the detection of splenic abscess, particularly if enhancement by intravenous contrast is used.[14] A sensitivity of greater than 90% has been seen in most series.[9] The abscess is seen as an area of low-density fluid or necrotic tissue within the relatively homogeneous spleen. Enhancement of the rim of the abscess cavity is seen in a minority of cases.

Magnetic Resonance Imaging. There is far less experience with MRI for the detection of splenic abscesses, and its role in the management is not yet established. MRI is sensitive for the detection of other abdominal abscesses, and its sensitivity in the discovery of splenic abscesses is probably similar. Nonetheless, although MRI has been successfully coupled with drainage procedures, it would appear to be more cumbersome and to offer fewer advantages than ultrasonography or CT.[16]

In the setting in which drainage may not be necessary—for example, in immunocompromised patients, in whom pathogens other than pyogenic bacteria are more common, or if a noninfectious diagnosis such as malignancy or cyst is likely—fine-needle aspiration under the guidance of diagnostic imaging may be useful.[17,18] The sensitivity of this method is variable, and its role remains the subject of investigation.

THERAPY

Untreated splenic abscess has a high mortality rate.[7] Splenectomy has been the traditional modality for treatment and remains the gold standard against which other therapies must be assessed. Antibiotics play an important role in the treatment of associated endocarditis and sepsis, in stabilization of the patient for splenectomy or a drainage procedure, and in treatment of selected pathogens (e.g., mycobacteria, fungi), but they are rarely curative alone for splenic abscess caused by pyogenic bacteria. Broad-spectrum empirical antibiotic therapy should be initiated as soon as splenic abscess is suspected, pending surgical or percutaneous drainage. Antibiotics should include agents active against streptococci, staphylococci, and aerobic gram-negative rods. Vancomycin or oxacillin plus an aminoglycoside, a third- or fourth-generation cephalosporin, or a fluoroquinolone would be reasonable empiric therapy. After blood or abscess culture results are obtained, antibiotic coverage can be narrowed accordingly. If splenectomy is a possibility, it is advisable to administer vaccinations for encapsulated bacterial pathogens as early as possible.

A limited experience of CT- and ultrasound-guided percutaneous aspiration of splenic abscesses has accumulated in recent decades. This procedure has the advantage of lower initial morbidity and mortality than splenectomy, and it allows for preservation of the spleen. Rates of success have ranged from 50% to 90% in several series.[7,9,19,20] In general, smaller (<3 cm), solitary, or unilocular abscesses have a higher rate of successful percutaneous drainage. In contrast, microabscesses, as well as complex, phlegmonous, or multilocular processes and those with thick fluid, tend to fare more poorly with this approach. Percutaneous drainage may be useful, at least initially, in those patients who are unstable or who present an unacceptably high surgical risk. Failure to achieve effective drainage or failure of the patient's condition to improve is an indication for definitive surgery. Aspirated abscess fluid should be sent for Gram staining; bacterial, fungal, and mycobacterial culture; and other studies as clinically indicated.

The optimal duration of antibiotic therapy for splenic abscess has not been established in any clinical trial. For some patients, such as those with bacterial endocarditis, the duration is dictated by the underlying condition. If splenectomy is performed and the focus of infection is eradicated, briefer durations may be possible. With percutaneous drainage, duration of therapy needs to be tailored to the clinical course, including resolution of the abscess as assessed by diagnostic imaging.

REFERENCES

1. Bernabeu-Wittel M, Villanueva JL, Pachon J, et al. Etiology, clinical features and outcome of splenic microabscesses in HIV-infected patients with prolonged fever. Eur J Clin Microbiol Infect Dis. 1999;18:324-329.
2. Altemeier WA, Culbertson WR, Fullen WD, Shook CD. Intra-abdominal abscesses. Am J Surg. 1973;125:70-79.
3. Sarr MG, Zuidema GD. Splenic abscess: Presentation, diagnosis, and treatment. Surgery. 1982;92:480-485.
4. Chulay JD, Lankerani MR. Splenic abscess: Report of 10 cases and review of the literature. Am J Med. 1976;61:513-522.
5. Alonso Cohen MA, Galera MJ, Ruiz M, et al. Splenic abscess. World J Surg. 1990;14:513-516; discussion, 516-517.
6. Paris S, Weiss SM, Ayers WH Jr, Clarke LE: Splenic abscess. Am Surg. 1994;60:358-361.
7. Nelken N, Ignatius J, Skinner M, Christensen N. Changing clinical spectrum of splenic abscess: A multicenter study and review of the literature. Am J Surg. 1987;154:27-34.
8. Chun CH, Raff MJ, Contreras L, et al. Splenic abscess. Medicine (Baltimore). 1980;59:50-65.
9. Ooi LL, Leong SS. Splenic abscesses from 1987 to 1995. Am J Surg. 1997;174:87-93.
10. Green BT. Splenic abscess: Report of six cases and review of the literature. Am Surg. 2001;67:80-85.
11. Rolain JM, Chanet V, Laurichesse H, et al. Cat scratch disease with lymphadenitis, vertebral osteomyelitis, and spleen abscesses. Ann N Y Acad Sci. 2003;990:397-403.
12. Sangchan A, Mootsikapun P, Mairiang P. Splenic abscess: Clinical features, microbiologic finding, treatment and outcome. J Med Assoc Thai. 2003;86:436-441.
13. Chiang IS, Lin TJ, Chiang IC, Tsai MS. Splenic abscesses: Review of 29 cases. Kaohsiung J Med Sci. 2003;19:510-515.
14. Johnson JD, Raff MJ, Drasin GF, Daffner RH. Radiology in the diagnosis of splenic abscess. Rev Infect Dis. 1985;7:10-20.
15. Changchien C-S, Tsai T-L, Hu T-H, et al. Sonographic patterns of splenic abscess: An analysis of 34 proven cases. Abdom Imaging. 2002;27:739-745.
16. Buecker A, Neuerburg JM, Adam GB, et al. MR-guided percutaneous drainage of abdominal fluid collections in combination with X-ray fluoroscopy: Initial clinical experience. Eur Radiol 2001;11:670-674.
17. Venkataramu NK, Gupta S, Sood BP, et al. Ultrasound guided fine needle aspiration biopsy of splenic lesions. Br J Radiol. 1999;72:953-956.
18. Tarantino L, Giorgio A, de Stefano G, et al. Disseminated mycobacterial infection in AIDS patients: Abdominal US features and value of fine-needle aspiration biopsy of lymph nodes and spleen. Abdom Imaging. 2003;28:602-608.
19. Gerzof SG, Robbins AH, Johnson WC, et al. Percutaneous catheter drainage of abdominal abscesses: A five-year experience. N Engl J Med. 1981;305:653-657.
20. Liu KY, Shyr YM, Su CH, et al. Splenic abscess: A changing trend in treatment. S Afr J Surg. 2000;38:55-57.

CHAPTER **72**

Appendicitis

COSTI D. SIFRI

LAWRENCE C. MADOFF

In 1886, Reginald Heber Fitz first described the natural course of acute inflammation of the appendix. In his seminal report, he coined the term *appendicitis* and advocated early surgical intervention.[1] Today, appendectomy is among the most common surgical emergencies of the abdomen; at least 290,000 nonincidental appendectomies are performed annually in the United States, accounting for 1 million inpatient hospital days.[2,3] With improvements in clinical assessment, antibiotic therapy, and surgical management, the overall mortality rate of acute appendicitis is less than 1%, although rates increase to 5% or more in the elderly.[3-5]

EPIDEMIOLOGY

The lifetime risk for appendicitis is 8.6% in men and 6.7% in women.[3] Although appendicitis is rare in infants, its incidence steadily increases through childhood and reaches a peak at 15 to 25 years of age for both men and women.[3,5,6] The incidence of appendicitis declines through adulthood, and fewer than 25% of cases occur in those older than 45 years of age.[3] Men have slightly higher rates of appendicitis than women, and the overall male-to-female rate ratio is 1.4:1.[3]

PATHOGENESIS

The appendix is a tube-shaped structure, usually 5 to 10 cm long in adults, that arises 2 to 3 cm below the terminal part of the ileum along the medial posterior wall of the cecum.[7] Typically, the appendix lies in an ascending retrocecal position, but atypical positions such as descending pelvic, transverse retrocecal, and ascending postileal are not uncommon and can alter the typical clinical features of acute appendicitis.[7] The appendix produces about 3 mL of mucus per day. Obstruction of the appendiceal lumen, usually by fecaliths, is thought to be the primary pathogenic mechanism of acute appendicitis.[8] Obstruction may also be caused by foreign bodies, tumor, stricture, parasites (e.g. *Enterobius vermicularis*, *Ascaris lumbricoides*, *Strongyloides stercoralis*) or lymphoid hyperplasia.[9-12] Mucus accumulates within the obstructed appendiceal lumen and intraluminal pressure increases, leading to compression of lymphatic and vascular drainage and causing ischemic damage of the mucosa followed by microbial invasion. Continued inflammation and ischemia, if left untreated, lead to gangrene and eventual perforation. The pathologic hallmark of acute appendicitis is the presence of polymorphonuclear cells within the appendiceal wall, accompanied by other markers of inflammation such as edema and vascular congestion. Obstruction is not found in a significant number of cases,[13] which has led to the speculation of other possible causes and cofactors, including dietary fiber,[14] familial susceptibility,[15] and primary infectious agents.

MICROBIOLOGY

Cultures of inflamed or gangrenous appendices typically yield 10 to 14 different organisms, which generally reflect the colonic microflora. A mixture of colonic anaerobic and facultative bacteria is usually recovered, predominantly *Escherichia coli*, *Bacteroides fragilis* group, pigmented *Prevotella* spp., *Bilophila wadsworthia*, *Peptostreptococcus* spp., Enterobacteriaceae, and viridans streptococci (particularly *Streptococcus anginosus* group).[16-18]

Yersinia enterocolitica and *Yersinia pseudotuberculosis* are thought to have a causative role in some cases of acute appendicitis.[19-21] More commonly, however, nonplague *Yersinia* causes ileocecitis or mesenteric adenitis, which mimic acute appendicitis with fever, leukocytosis, and acute right lower quadrant pain.[22-24] *Campylobacter* and nontyphoidal *Salmonella* can also cause ileocecitis and mesenteric adenitis.[23,25] Appendiceal or ileocecal tuberculosis, actinomycosis, and histoplasmosis are more likely to cause subacute or recurrent disease rather than classic acute appendicitis. Viral causes of mesenteric adenitis and, rarely, appendicitis include measles, Epstein-Barr virus, cytomegalovirus, and adenovirus.[26-29] In many cases of mesenteric adenitis, an infectious cause is not identified but is probably present.[30] The disorder is usually discovered at the time of surgery for suspected appendicitis; mesenteric lymph nodes of the right iliac fossa are enlarged, the adjacent bowel is only mildly inflamed, and the appendix appears normal. Nevertheless, an appendectomy should be performed to avoid the need to differentiate a recurrent attack from true appendicitis in the future.

CLINICAL MANIFESTATIONS

The clinical manifestations of acute appendicitis are distinctive and, in many cases, diagnostic. Appendicitis classically starts as colicky, visceral periumbilical pain that evolves for the next 6 to 24 hours to localized, somatic right lower quadrant abdominal pain after inflammation extends to the parietal peritoneum. If the inflamed appendix lies in the anterior position, tenderness is often maximal at or near McBurney's point, which lies 2 to 3 fingerbreadths above the right anterior superior iliac spine on a line with the umbilicus. If the appendix lies in a position relatively hidden from the parietal peritoneum, pain may remain poorly localized and migration to the right lower quadrant may be delayed or absent.[31] Pelvic appendices can cause pelvic or left lower quadrant pain. Third-trimester pregnancy or intestinal malrotation may shift pain to the right upper quadrant. Pain is often accompanied by mild fever, anorexia, nausea, and vomiting. Guarding is usually seen on examination of the abdomen. Rebound tenderness in the right lower quadrant with palpation of the left lower quadrant, known as Rovsing's sign, may be elicited. Other maneuvers that support the diagnosis of appendicitis include pain with active extension of the right hip, known as the psoas sign, and pain with internal rotation of the right hip, termed the obturator sign. High fever or a sudden reduction in pain suggests perforation, whereas abdominal rigidity suggests diffuse peritonitis. A palpable right lower quadrant mass may be indicative of a phlegmon or walled-off periappendiceal abscess[4,32] or, alternatively, a cecal carcinoma.[33] Most instances of perforation occur as the result of delays in seeking medical care.[34]

DIAGNOSIS

The diagnosis of acute appendicitis primarily is suggested by the history and physical examination findings. Acute onset of abdominal pain migrating over several hours to the right lower quadrant, with guarding and tenderness over McBurney's point, is most predictive of acute appendicitis; a history of previous pain, long duration of symptoms, and lack of migration to the right lower quadrant argue against it.[4,35] The serum concentration of β-human chorionic gonadotropin should be measured in all women of reproductive age to rule out a uterine or ectopic pregnancy. Most patients have a mild leukocytosis and elevated C-reactive protein. If inflammation extends to the ureter or bladder, sterile pyuria may be noted on urinalysis. Acute salpingitis with a tuboovarian abscess or impaction of a stone in the right ureter can be confused with acute appendicitis.

The appendix is found to be normal in approximately 8% to 25% of patients who undergo emergency appendectomy.[3,5,36-38] This "negative appendectomy rate" is significantly higher in women of childbearing age, young children, and the elderly.[37,39,40] Conversely, 20% of all cases of appendicitis are initially missed on presentation.[41-43] In an effort to improve diagnostic accuracy, scoring systems based on clinical findings and laboratory data have been developed to assist in the diagnosis of acute appendicitis.[44] In practice, however, they lack sufficient power to reproducibly discriminate acute appendicitis from other causes of pain in the right lower quadrant (Box 72-1).[45]

Observation, laparoscopy, and imaging are additional methods used to improve the diagnostic accuracy of acute appendicitis. If the clinical presentation is ambiguous, observation and reassessment can distinguish cases of evolving appendicitis from other causes of abdominal pain without increasing the risk of perforation.[46] Diagnostic laparoscopy is particularly effective in women of child-bearing age, in whom gynecologic causes of abdominal pain are common.[47,48] Diagnostic imaging, by ultrasonography or computed tomography (CT), has been shown to be very effective in the diagnosis of acute appendicitis. Ultrasonography is rapid and noninvasive, requires no contrast material, uses no ionizing radiation, and is excellent at visualizing gynecologic abnormalities. As such, it has proved to be particularly useful in the evaluation of young women, pregnant women, and children with suspected appendicitis.[49-51] Ultrasonography fails to visualize the appendix in 10% of cases[52] and is not as accurate as CT in diagnosing an abscess or phlegmon.[51]

CT, particularly focused helical appendiceal CT, has a reported sensitivity of 98% to 100%, a specificity of 95% to 98%, and an overall diagnostic rate of greater than 95% in patients with suspected appendicitis.[53,54] Appendiceal CT employs water-soluble contrast of the

Causes of Right Lower Quadrant Pain

Gastrointestinal
Appendicitis
Crohn's ileitis/cecitis
Cecal diverticulitis
Meckel's diverticulitis
Mesenteric lymphadenitis
Bacterial (*Yersinia, Campylobacter, Salmonella*) ileocolitis
Amebic colitis
Tuberculous colitis
Biliary colic
Epiploic appendagitis

Urinary Tract
Pyelonephritis
Renal colic

Neoplastic
Cecal adenocarcinoma
Carcinoid
Lymphoma
Metastasis

Gynecologic
Ovarian cyst
Ectopic pregnancy
Endometriosis
Cervicitis
Uterine leiomyoma
Tuboovarian abscess

Nonspecific Abdominal Pain

colon administered by enema and requires 15 minutes of scanner time (Fig. 72-1). CT imaging has the ability to avoid delays before necessary appendectomy, diagnose other pathologic conditions such as right-sided diverticulitis, reduce negative appendectomy rates, and prevent unnecessary hospital admissions.[53,55] However, more recent studies of the use of CT in the evaluation of suspected appendicitis have had inconsistent results.[56,57]

THERAPY

The primary treatment of appendicitis is surgery. Preoperative treatment includes fluid resuscitation and parenteral antibiotics. In cases of uncomplicated appendicitis, one or two doses of a second-generation cephalosporin (e.g., cefotetan) are effective.[58,59] In cases of ruptured appendicitis and secondary appendicitis, an antibiotic regimen that provides broad coverage for aerobic and anaerobic colonic flora should be used (see Chapter 68). Acute appendicitis, either without rupture or with perforation and secondary peritonitis, requires prompt surgical intervention. There is no clear consensus as to the optimal operative approach (open versus laparoscopic) in patients with suspected appendicitis. Laparoscopic appendectomy offers the advantage of allowing for further diagnostic evaluation if a normal appendix is found.[48] In addition, a meta-analysis of more than 40 studies suggested that patients have fewer wound infections, less postoperative pain, shorter hospital stays, and quicker returns to normal activity after laparoscopic appendectomy than after open appendectomy. However, laparoscopic appendectomies were associated with more frequent intra-abdominal abscesses, longer operative times, and higher total hospital costs.[60]

There is even less consensus on the optimal postoperative treatment of perforated appendicitis, including the duration of antibiotic therapy, use of parenteral versus oral agents, and duration of hospitalization.[61,62] In general, patients are treated with intravenous antibiotics for 5 to 10 days until fever resolves, the white blood cell count normalizes, and bowel function returns. Institutional clinical practice guidelines have been shown to reduce infectious complications and the cost of care.[63,64]

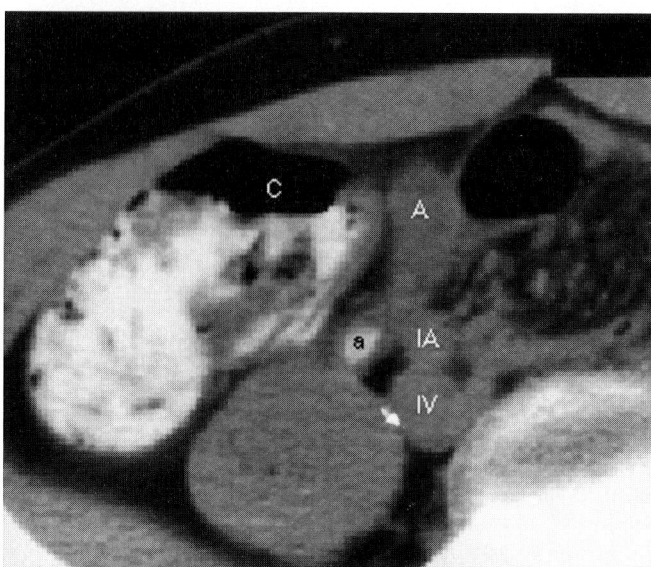

A

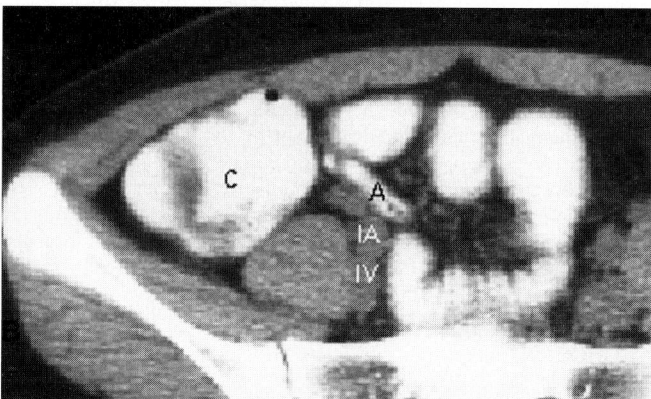

B

FIGURE 72-1. A, Computed tomographic scan of a 17-year-old boy with suspected appendicitis. The axial image shows an inflamed, unopacified appendix, 15 mm in diameter (A), with proximal appendolith (a). Also shown are the cecum (C) and the common iliac artery (IA) and vein (IV). **B,** Computed tomographic scan of a 21-year-old woman with suspected appendicitis. The axial image shows a tubular, opacified normal appendix. A, appendix; C, cecum; IA, common iliac artery; IV, common iliac vein. *(From Rao PM, Rhea JT, Novelline RA, et al. Effect of computed tomography of the appendix on treatment of patients and use of hospital resources. N Engl J Med. 1998;338:141-146. Copyright © 1998 Massachusetts Medical Society. All rights reserved.)*

In cases of appendicitis complicated by a contained perforation, antibiotic therapy and percutaneous drainage of the periappendiceal abscess, with ultrasound or CT guidance, can be initiated. If these maneuvers produce a response, interval appendectomy can be performed 6 to 8 weeks later, after inflammation subsides.[65-68] Historically, untreated appendicitis was a major cause of portal vein thrombophlebitis (pylephlebitis) and pyogenic liver abscess (see Chapter 69), but these complications are rare in the antibiotic era.[69]

REFERENCES

1. Fitz RH. Perforating inflammation of the vermiform appendix with special reference to its early diagnosis and treatment. Am J Med Sci. 1886;92:321-346.
2. Popovic JR, Hall MJ. 1999 National Hospital Discharge Survey: Advance data from vital and health statistics. Hyattsville, Md: National Center for Health Statistics; 2001.
3. Addiss DG, Shaffer N, Fowler BS, Tauxe RV. The epidemiology of appendicitis and appendectomy in the United States. Am J Epidemiol. 1990;132:910-925.

4. Wagner JM, McKinney WP, Carpenter JL. Does this patient have appendicitis? JAMA. 1996;276:1589-1594.

5. Hale DA, Molloy M, Pearl RH, et al. Appendectomy: A contemporary appraisal. Ann Surg. 1997;225:252-261.

6. Andersson RE, Olaison G, Tysk C, Ekbom A. Appendectomy and protection against ulcerative colitis. N Engl J Med. 2001;344:808-814.

7. Schumpelick V, Dreuw B, Ophoff K, Prescher A. Appendix and cecum: Embryology, anatomy, and surgical applications. Surg Clin North Am. 2000;80:295-318.

8. Wangensteen OH, Dennis C. Experimental proof of obstructive origin of appendicitis in man. Ann Surg. 1939;110:629-647.

9. Dorfman S, Talbot IC, Torres R, et al. Parasitic infestation in acute appendicitis. Ann Trop Med Parasitol. 1995;89:99-101.

10. Klingler PJ, Seelig MH, DeVault KR, et al. Ingested foreign bodies within the appendix: A 100-year review of the literature. Dig Dis. 1998;16:308-314.

11. Arnbjornsson E. Acute appendicitis as a sign of a colorectal carcinoma. J Surg Oncol. 1982;20:17-20.

12. Dymock RB. Pathological changes in the appendix: A review of 1000 cases. Pathology. 1977;9:331-339.

13. Arnbjornsson E, Bengmark S. Role of obstruction in the pathogenesis of acute appendicitis. Am J Surg. 1984;147:390-392.

14. Burkitt DP. The aetiology of appendicitis. Br J Surg. 1971;58:695-699.

15. Gauderer MW, Crane MM, Green JA, et al. Acute appendicitis in children: The importance of family history. J Pediatr Surg. 2001;36:1214-1217.

16. Bennion RS, Baron EJ, Thompson JE Jr, et al. The bacteriology of gangrenous and perforated appendicitis—Revisited. Ann Surg. 1990;211:165-171.

17. Rautio M, Saxen H, Siitonen A, et al. Bacteriology of histopathologically defined appendicitis in children. Pediatr Infect Dis J. 2000;19:1078-1083.

18. Bennion RS, Thompson JE, Baron EJ, Finegold SM. Gangrenous and perforated appendicitis with peritonitis: Treatment and bacteriology. Clin Ther. 1990;12(Suppl C): 31-44.

19. Attwood SE, Mealy K, Cafferkey MT, et al. *Yersinia* infection and acute abdominal pain. Lancet. 1987;1:529-533.

20. Bennion RS, Thompson JE Jr, Gil J, Schmit PJ. The role of *Yersinia enterocolitica* in appendicitis in the southwestern United States. Am Surg. 1991;57:766-768.

21. Lamps LW, Madhusudhan KT, Greenson JK, et al. The role of *Yersinia enterocolitica* and *Yersinia pseudotuberculosis* in granulomatous appendicitis: A histologic and molecular study. Am J Surg Pathol. 2001;25:508-515.

22. Weber J, Finlayson NB, Mark JB: Mesenteric lymphadenitis and terminal ileitis due to *Yersinia pseudotuberculosis*. N Engl J Med. 1970;283:172-174.

23. Van Noyen R, Selderslaghs R, Bekaert J, et al. Causative role of *Yersinia* and other enteric pathogens in the appendicular syndrome. Eur J Clin Microbiol Infect Dis. 1991;10:735-741.

24. Puylaert JB, Vermeijden RJ, van der Werf SD, et al. Incidence and sonographic diagnosis of bacterial ileocaecitis masquerading as appendicitis. Lancet. 1989;2:84-86.

25. Garcia-Corbeira P, Ramos JM, Aguado JM, Soriano F. Six cases in which mesenteric lymphadenitis due to non-typhi *Salmonella* caused an appendicitis-like syndrome. Clin Infect Dis. 1995;21:231-232.

26. Searle A, Owen WJ. Measles appendicitis. Br J Clin Pract. 1990;44:749.

27. Lopez-Navidad A, Domingo P, Cadafalch J, et al. Acute appendicitis complicating infectious mononucleosis: Case report and review. Rev Infect Dis. 1990;12:297-302.

28. Reif RM: Viral appendicitis. Hum Pathol. 1981;12:193-196.

29. Dieterich DT, Kim MH, McMeeding A, Rotterdam H. Cytomegalovirus appendicitis in a patient with acquired immune deficiency syndrome. Am J Gastroenterol. 1991;86:904-906.

30. Blattner RJ. Acute mesenteric lymphadenitis. J Pediatr. 1969;74:479-481.

31. Guidry SP, Poole GV. The anatomy of appendicitis. Am Surg. 1994;60:68-71.

32. Paulson EK, Kalady MF, Pappas TN. Clinical practice: Suspected appendicitis. N Engl J Med. 2003;348:236-242.

33. Peck JJ. Management of carcinoma discovered unexpectedly at operation for acute appendicitis. Am J Surg. 1988;155:683-685.

34. Temple CL, Huchcroft SA, Temple WJ. The natural history of appendicitis in adults: A prospective study. Ann Surg. 1995;221:278-281.

35. John H, Neff U, Kelemen M. Appendicitis diagnosis today: Clinical and ultrasonic deductions. World J Surg. 1993;17:243-249.

36. Blomqvist P, Ljung H, Nyren O, Ekbom A. Appendectomy in Sweden 1989-1993 assessed by the Inpatient Registry. J Clin Epidemiol. 1998;51:859-865.

37. Flum DR, Morris A, Koepsell T, Dellinger EP. Has misdiagnosis of appendicitis decreased over time? A population-based analysis. JAMA. 2001;286:1748-1753.

38. Smink DS, Finkelstein JA, Kleinman K, Fishman SJ. The effect of hospital volume of pediatric appendectomies on the misdiagnosis of appendicitis in children. Pediatrics. 2004;113:18-23.

39. Jess P, Bjerregaard B, Brynitz S, et al. Acute appendicitis: Prospective trial concerning diagnostic accuracy and complications. Am J Surg. 1981;141:232-234.

40. Andersson RE, Hugander A, Thulin AJ. Diagnostic accuracy and perforation rate in appendicitis: Association with age and sex of the patient and with appendicectomy rate. Eur J Surg. 1992;158:37-41.

41. Reynolds SL. Missed appendicitis in a pediatric emergency department. Pediatr Emerg Care. 1993;9:1-3.

42. Rothrock SG, Green SM, Dobson M, et al. Misdiagnosis of appendicitis in nonpregnant women of childbearing age. J Emerg Med. 1995;13:1-8.

43. McCallion J, Canning GP, Knight PV, McCallion JS. Acute appendicitis in the elderly: A 5-year retrospective study. Age Ageing. 1987;16:256-260.

44. Alvarado A. A practical score for the early diagnosis of acute appendicitis. Ann Emerg Med. 1986;15:557-564.

45. Ohmann C, Yang Q, Franke C. Diagnostic scores for acute appendicitis: Abdominal Pain Study Group. Eur J Surg. 1995;161:273-281.

46. Jones PF. Suspected acute appendicitis: Trends in management over 30 years. Br J Surg. 2001;88:1570-1577.

47. Sugarbaker PH, Sanders JH, Bloom BS, Wilson RE. Preoperative laparoscopy in diagnosis of acute abdominal pain. Lancet. 1975;1:442-445.

48. Thorell A, Grondal S, Schedvins K, Wallin G. Value of diagnostic laparoscopy in fertile women with suspected appendicitis. Eur J Surg. 1999;165:751-754.

49. Dilley A, Wesson D, Munden M, et al. The impact of ultrasound examinations on the management of children with suspected appendicitis: A 3-year analysis. J Pediatr Surg. 2001;36:303-308.

50. Cappell MS, Friedel D. Abdominal pain during pregnancy. Gastroenterol Clin North Am. 2003;32:1-58.

51. Birnbaum BA, Wilson SR. Appendicitis at the millennium. Radiology. 2000;215: 337-348.

52. Rettenbacher T, Hollerweger A, Gritzmann N, et al. Appendicitis: Should diagnostic imaging be performed if the clinical presentation is highly suggestive of the disease? Gastroenterology. 2002;123:992-998.

53. Rao PM, Rhea JT, Novelline RA, et al. Effect of computed tomography of the appendix on treatment of patients and use of hospital resources. N Engl J Med. 1998;338:141-146.

54. Rao PM, Rhea JT, Novelline RA, et al. Helical CT technique for the diagnosis of appendicitis: Prospective evaluation of a focused appendix CT examination. Radiology. 1997;202:139-144.

55. Rao PM, Rhea JT, Rattner DW, et al. Introduction of appendiceal CT: Impact on negative appendectomy and appendiceal perforation rates. Ann Surg. 1999;229:344-349.

56. Perez J, Barone JE, Wilbanks TO, et al. Liberal use of computed tomography scanning does not improve diagnostic accuracy in appendicitis. Am J Surg. 2003;185:194-197.

57. DeArmond GM, Dent DL, Myers JG, et al. Appendicitis: Selective use of abdominal CT reduces negative appendectomy rate. Surg Infect (Larchmt). 2003;4:213-218.

58. Andersen BR, Kallehave FL, Andersen HK. Antibiotics versus placebo for prevention of postoperative infection after appendicectomy. Cochrane Database Syst Rev 2003(2): D001439.

59. Liberman MA, Greason KL, Frame S, Ragland JJ. Single-dose cefotetan or cefoxitin versus multiple-dose cefoxitin as prophylaxis in patients undergoing appendectomy for acute nonperforated appendicitis. J Am Coll Surg. 1995;180:77-80.

60. Sauerland S, Lefering R, Neugebauer EA. Laparoscopic versus open surgery for suspected appendicitis. Cochrane Database Syst Rev 2002(1):CD001546.

61. Chen C, Botelho C, Cooper A, et al. Current practice patterns in the treatment of perforated appendicitis in children. J Am Coll Surg. 2003;196:212-221.

62. Newman K, Ponsky T, Kittle K, et al. Appendicitis 2000: Variability in practice, outcomes, and resource utilization at thirty pediatric hospitals. J Pediatr Surg. 2003;38:372-379; discussion, 372-379.

63. Helmer KS, Robinson EK, Lally KP, et al. Standardized patient care guidelines reduce infectious morbidity in appendectomy patients. Am J Surg. 2002;183:608-613.

64. Fishman SJ, Pelosi L, Klavon SL, O'Rourke EJ. Perforated appendicitis: Prospective outcome analysis for 150 children. J Pediatr Surg. 2000;35:923-926.

65. Weber TR, Keller MA, Bower RJ, et al. Is delayed operative treatment worth the trouble with perforated appendicitis in children? Am J Surg. 2003;186:685-689.

66. Nguyen DB, Silen W, Hodin RA. Interval appendectomy in the laparoscopic era. J Gastrointest Surg. 1999;3:189-193.

67. Vargas HI, Averbook A, Stamos MJ. Appendiceal mass: Conservative therapy followed by interval laparoscopic appendectomy. Am Surg. 1994;60:753-758.

68. Oliak D, Yamini D, Udani VM, et al. Initial nonoperative management for periappendiceal abscess. Dis Colon Rectum. 2001;44:936-941.

69. Johannsen EC, Sifri CD, Madoff LC. Pyogenic liver abscesses. Infect Dis Clin North Am. 2000;14:547-563, vii.

CHAPTER **73**

Diverticulitis and Typhlitis

COSTI D. SIFRI

LAWRENCE C. MADOFF

DIVERTICULITIS

Most colonic diverticula are pseudodiverticula that occur when the mucosa and submucosa herniate through the muscularis propria. These saccular herniations develop in areas of relative structural weakness of the colonic wall where small nutrient arteries supplying the colonic mucosa, the *vasa recta*, penetrate the circular muscle layer. In the West, the sigmoid and descending colons are most commonly affected. In Asia, colonic diverticula are predominantly right-sided. *Diverticulitis,* defined as inflammation and infection of the bowel wall associated with diverticula, is the most frequent complication of this disorder.

Epidemiology

Only 10% to 25% of patients with diverticulosis manifest clinical disease, making its true prevalence difficult to measure.[1] Although the disorder occurs worldwide, diverticulosis is particularly prominent in Western society, where the prevalence has been estimated to be 30% to 40%. In contrast, the prevalence of diverticulosis in rural Asia and Africa is estimated to be much less than 1%.[2] Increased prevalence is observed in populations that become westernized, presumably because of dietary changes or other environmental factors.[3-5] The prevalence of diverticulosis increases with age in the West, affecting 50% of those older than 70 years of age and up to 80% of those older than 85 years.[1,6] The complications of diverticulosis, including diverticulitis, also increase with age,[7] although some studies have suggested that diverticulitis may be more malignant in patients who are younger than 40 years of age.[8-10]

The most extensively studied risk factor for the development of diverticular disease is low dietary fiber intake. Diets with reduced dietary fiber are associated with more colonic diverticulosis[2] and with symptomatic diverticular disease.[11] Other risk factors for the development of diverticulitis are less well understood. Use of corticosteroids, nonsteroidal anti-inflammatory drugs, or opiates may be positively associated with diverticulitis, perforation, or both.[12-14] Lack of physical activity also may be an independent risk factor for symptomatic disease.[15] Tobacco, alcohol, and caffeine consumption do not appear to influence diverticular disease.[16,17]

Pathogenesis

The formation of diverticula is thought to be caused by a combination of increased intraluminal pressure and weakening of the bowel wall.[18] High dietary fiber increases stool volume and reduces bowel transit time, leading to decreased intracolonic pressures. The pathogenesis of diverticulitis is thought to be very similar to that of acute appendicitis: a fecalith obstructs the neck of the diverticulum,[19] causing mucus accumulation, bacterial overgrowth, perforation, and inflammation of the bowel wall and adjacent tissues. Microperforation may remain well localized, leading to limited colonic wall inflammation and the formation of a small peridiverticular phlegmon or abscess. Macroperforation results in larger abscesses; if not confined, its complications include distant abscesses, extension to other organs, spreading peritonitis, large inflammatory masses, and fistula formation.[6,18] Less commonly, gross fecal contamination can occur with free rupture of an unobstructed and uninflamed diverticulum into the peritoneal cavity. Rupture of a localized peridiverticular abscess into the peritoneal cavity does not result in gross fecal contamination, presumably because the diverticular neck is obstructed by a fecalith.[18]

Microbiology

Like most other cases of secondary peritonitis, acute diverticulitis is a polymicrobial infection caused by a variety of endogenous anaerobes and facultative bacteria. Commonly isolated organisms include *Bacteroides* spp., *Peptostreptococcus* spp., Enterobacteriaceae, viridans streptococci, and enterococci.[20,21]

Clinical Manifestations

The clinical manifestations of uncomplicated diverticulitis resemble those of appendicitis, but with findings typically on the left side of the abdomen. Diverticulitis often starts with visceral hypogastric pain that evolves to somatic pain which is localized, in the case of sigmoid disease, to the left lower quadrant. In contrast to acute appendicitis, the pain is often recurrent and is present for several days before presentation.[22] Fever, nausea and vomiting, changes in bowel habits, and urinary symptoms often accompany the pain. Leukocytosis is common but not invariably present (69% to 93% of cases).[23] Urinalysis may reveal sterile pyuria if inflammation extends

to the urinary tract system. Trace blood may be present in the stool, but hematochezia is uncommon and should raise suspicion for an alternative diagnosis. Low-grade fever is common in uncomplicated disease, and the physical examination typically reveals abdominal tenderness, guarding, and rebound tenderness in the left lower quadrant, the suprapubic area, or both; bowel sounds may be hypoactive or normal. A palpable abdominal mass may be caused by an inflammatory process but may also be indicative of cancer. High fever and abdominal rigidity suggest generalized peritonitis after perforation. Hyperactive bowel sounds suggest obstruction. Fistulization of the bladder or ureter with the colon may lead to pneumaturia and fecaluria[24]; passage of feces and flatus through the vagina occurs with fistula formation with the vagina or uterus.[25] Recurrent diverticulitis can lead to stricture and obstruction. Pyogenic liver abscess and pylephlebitis are rare complications.[25a]

Diagnosis

Although the diagnosis of acute diverticulitis can be made on the basis of the clinical evaluation,[23,26] more than half of patients with clinically suspected diverticulitis are found to have alternative conditions.[27] For this reason, diagnostic studies are performed in most cases of suspected diverticulitis,[28] and they are particularly important in the patient with an atypical presentation, a suspected complication, severe illness, or clinical deterioration.[26] Imaging modalities include computed tomography (CT) and ultrasonography. If complications such as macroperforation and generalized peritonitis are suspected, water-soluble contrast should be used. Double-contrast studies should be avoided, because insufflation of air could dislodge an obstructing fecalith and cause perforation.[18]

CT is now considered to be the diagnostic procedure of choice for patients with suspected acute diverticulitis.[18,26,31] Tomographic evidence of diverticulitis includes pericolic fat stranding (98%), diverticula (84%), bowel wall thickening (70%), and phlegmon or abscess formation (35%).[32] CT also offers the opportunity for therapeutic intervention: CT-guided percutaneous drainage can be temporizing in acutely ill patients with large abscesses (>5 cm in diameter), permitting curative surgery on an elective basis.[33,34] Immediate surgery is indicated, however, if the abscess cavity contains gross fecal material. Abdominal CT for suspected diverticulitis has traditionally employed oral, rectal, and, if not contraindicated, intravenous contrast. More recently, helical CT using colonic contrast alone has been shown to be highly effective in the evaluation of patients with left lower quadrant pain. Similar to appendiceal CT, "diverticular CT" has been shown to have high sensitivity (97%), specificity (100%), and overall diagnostic accuracy (99%) in the prospective evaluation of suspected diverticulitis.[27]

Acute diverticulitis can also be confirmed by ultrasonography, which is capable of delineating inflamed colonic segments, phlegmons, and abscesses.[35] In practice, however, ultrasonography is used much less frequently than CT or contrast enema for the evaluation of left lower quadrant pain, in contrast to right abdominal pain. The most useful role for ultrasound may be in the exclusion of gynecologic pathology in women of child-bearing age who present with left-sided abdominal pain.[26] Given the risk of perforation, endoscopy is avoided in the initial evaluation of patients with suspected acute diverticulitis. Occasionally, limited sigmoidoscopy with minimal air insufflation is performed in ambiguous cases to exclude other diagnoses, such as inflammatory bowel disease, carcinoma, or ischemic colitis.[18,26] A complete colonic evaluation should be performed 6 to 8 weeks after resolution of an episode of acute diverticulitis to rule out coexisting lesions, including colon cancer.

Therapy

A trial of outpatient therapy is indicated for acute, uncomplicated diverticulitis or for a well-localized, small (≤5 cm in diameter) peridiverticular abscess, provided the patient can tolerate oral hydration and 7 to 10 days of oral broad-spectrum antimicrobial therapy. Drugs must have an antimicrobial spectrum that includes aerobic and anaerobic colonic flora (e.g., quinolone/metronidazole, trimethoprim-sulfamethoxazole/metronidazole, amoxicillin/clavulanic acid).[36] If the patient is unable to tolerate oral hydration, requires narcotic analgesics, or fails to improve despite appropriate outpatient therapy, admission to the hospital for bowel rest, nasogastric tube placement, and parenteral antibiotics is indicated. Elderly patients and those with compromised immune systems or other comorbidities also should be hospitalized. Antibiotic recommendations are similar to those discussed for secondary peritonitis (see Chapter 68). Failure to respond to medical therapy within 48 to 72 hours should prompt repeat investigation for complications, consideration of alternative diagnoses, and surgical evaluation.[26]

Conservative medical therapy is successful in 70% to 80% of patients hospitalized with acute diverticulitis.[18,23] Indications for emergency colonic resection include uncontrolled sepsis, generalized peritonitis, acute clinical deterioration, persistent obstruction, and failure to respond to medical therapy. Under these circumstances, a two-stage operation, such as the Hartmann procedure, is usually performed.[23,37] The Hartmann procedure entails resection of the diseased colon, end colostomy, and closure of the distal loop or creation of a mucous fistula; colonic continuity can be restored several months later by elective anastomosis.[37] An alternative two-stage operation is primary resection of the diseased segment of colon with immediate anastomosis after intraoperative colonic lavage and proximal fecal diversion, followed later by elective stoma closure.[38]

Elective colonic resection is usually performed in cases of fistula formation or recurrent attacks of diverticulitis, or for complicated diverticulitis brought under control with conservative therapy.[23,26] In these cases, a one-stage procedure with primary resection and anastomosis can be performed, with lower morbidity and mortality and a shorter hospital length of stay than a two-stage procedure.[18,23] Elective surgery should also be considered for patients at high risk for complications of recurrent diverticulitis, including those with immunosuppressive conditions (e.g., organ transplantation, chronic corticosteroid therapy, renal failure)[39-43] and perhaps those younger than 40 years of age,[8] although this latter point is controversial.[44,45] Laparoscopic sigmoidectomy is an alternative to laparotomy in cases of mild-to-moderate disease.[46] Retrospective studies have reported that a one-stage procedure, combined with intraoperative colonic lavage but no protective diverting colostomy, may be feasible even in the moderate- to high-risk patient with colonic perforation.[47,48] Further studies, ideally prospective randomized trials, are needed to determine whether this approach is as safe and efficacious as the Hartmann procedure.

The classic three-stage procedure, consisting of drainage and proximal diverting colostomy, interval resection of diseased bowel with primary anastomosis, and stoma closure, has largely been abandoned, because failure to eliminate the source of peritoneal infection resulted in higher mortality rates compared with the two-stage procedure.[37]

TYPHLITIS (NEUTROPENIC ENTEROCOLITIS)

Typhlitis, also known as neutropenic enterocolitis, is a life-threatening complication of myelosuppressive chemotherapy administered for the treatment of hematologic and solid tissue malignancies.[49-51] It is also rarely seen in individuals with human immunodeficiency virus (HIV) infection[52] and in those with neutropenia caused by aplastic anemia, cyclic neutropenia, or acute leukemia before the initiation of chemotherapy.[50,53,54]

Pathogenesis

The pathologic characteristic of typhlitis is marked thickening and edema of the bowel wall, almost invariably involving the cecum and often extending to the ascending colon or terminal ileum or both.[53] Examination of the bowel wall reveals discrete or coalesced mucosal ulceration, intramural thrombocytopenic hemorrhage, and degeneration of the muscularis mucosa. Histologic specimens demonstrate mononuclear infiltrates and a variety of invading bacteria and fungi.

The pathogenesis is multifactorial and incompletely understood. A combination of neutropenia, mucosal injury (due to cytotoxic chemotherapy, radiotherapy, leukemic infiltrates, or some combination of these factors), and possibly ischemia due to cecal distention allows gut flora to opportunistically invade the bowel wall. In the setting of impaired host immunity, these organisms proliferate and cause local destruction by elaboration of exotoxins.[55]

Clinical Manifestations

Clinical manifestations are variable and depend on the extent of disease. Patients typically present with fever, nausea, vomiting, abdominal pain and tenderness, and diarrhea that is often bloody. Given the prominence of cecal involvement, typhlitis can mimic acute appendicitis with localization of abdominal pain and tenderness to the right lower quadrant.[56] Right lower abdominal pain is absent in 40% to 55% of cases, however,[57,58] and corticosteroid therapy may mask the symptoms of abdominal pain altogether.[53] Severe stomatitis and pharyngitis may be present and are markers of diffuse mucosal injury. Rapid progression to the development of an acute abdomen is not uncommon. Symptoms typically develop after 7 to 14 days of neutropenia (absolute neutrophil count, <500/mm³). Alternative diagnoses, in addition to acute appendicitis, include chemotherapy-induced mucositis, pseudomembranous colitis, chronic mucormycosis or aspergillosis, intussusception, ischemic colitis, bowel obstruction, Ogilvie's syndrome (colonic pseudoobstruction), ileus, acute cholecystitis, acute pancreatitis, cytomegalovirus enterocolitis, and herpes zoster.[59]

Diagnosis

Ultrasonography and computed tomography have largely supplanted plain radiography of the abdomen in the evaluation of suspected typhlitis.[51,59] The degree of bowel wall thickening, as measured by ultrasound, correlates with severity of disease: patients with bowel wall thickness greater than 10 mm had a 60% mortality rate, compared for 4% for those with a thickness of less than 10 mm.[60]

Cytotoxicity assays or other diagnostic tests for *Clostridium difficile* should be performed, and blood and stool cultures should be obtained. Bacteremia or fungemia occurs in 14% to 44% of patients, most commonly with *Pseudomonas aeruginosa*, Enterobacteriaceae, *Bacteroides fragilis*, viridans streptococci, enterococci, and *Candida* spp.[50,51,58,61,62] Patients with *Clostridium septicum* bacteremia may have a more fulminant, lethal course,[54,63] and this infection may represent a different syndrome.[64]

Therapy

The management of typhlitis is controversial. Although a number of early studies reported mortality rates greater than 50% and advocated early surgical intervention,[65,66] more recent studies have reported mortality rates of less than 20% with conservative medical therapy.[50,51,58,61,62] Management includes bowel rest, decompression, intravenous fluids, nutritional support, and broad-spectrum parenteral antibiotics. The antimicrobial regimen should cover enteric aerobic and anaerobic flora, *P. aeruginosa*, and perhaps yeast. Examples are imipenem or piperacillin/tazobactam, or cefepime and metronidazole, all with the possible addition of fluconazole. The regimen should also effectively treat *C. difficile*, if it has not been excluded as a possible cause. The indications for immediate surgical intervention include persistent gastrointestinal bleeding despite resolution of hematologic and clotting abnormalities, free intraperitoneal perforation, and clinical deterioration suggesting uncontrolled sepsis.[62]

REFERENCES

1. Parks TG. Natural history of diverticular disease of the colon. Clin Gastroenterol. 1975;4:53-69.
2. Painter NS, Burkitt DP. Diverticular disease of the colon: A deficiency disease of Western civilization. Br Med J. 1971;2:450-454.

3. Miura S, Kodaira S, Shatari T, et al. Recent trends in diverticulosis of the right colon in Japan: Retrospective review in a regional hospital. Dis Colon Rectum. 2000;43:1383-1389.

4. Levy N, Stermer E, Simon J. The changing epidemiology of diverticular disease in Israel. Dis Colon Rectum. 1985;28:416-418.

5. Lee YS. Diverticular disease of the large bowel in Singapore: An autopsy survey. Dis Colon Rectum. 1986;29:330-335.

6. Rodkey GV, Welch CE. Diverticulitis of the colon: Evolution in concept and therapy. Surg Clin North Am. 1965;45:1231-1243.

7. Mendeloff AI, Everhart JE. Diverticular disease of the colon. In: Everhart JE, ed. Digestive Diseases in the United States: Epidemiology and Impact. Washington, DC: National Institutes of Health, National Institute of Diabetes and Digestive and Kidney Diseases; 1994:551.

8. Cunningham MA, Davis JW, Kaups KL. Medical versus surgical management of diverticulitis in patients under age 40. Am J Surg. 1997;174:733-735; discussion, 735-736.

9. Schauer PR, Ramos R, Ghiatas AA, Sirinek KR. Virulent diverticular disease in young obese men. Am J Surg. 1992;164:443-446; discussion, 446-448.

10. Freischlag J, Bennion RS, Thompson JE Jr. Complications of diverticular disease of the colon in young people. Dis Colon Rectum. 1986;29:639-643.

11. Aldoori WH, Giovannucci EL, Rimm EB, et al. A prospective study of diet and the risk of symptomatic diverticular disease in men. Am J Clin Nutr. 1994;60:757-764.

12. Morris CR, Harvey IM, Stebbings WS, et al. Anti-inflammatory drugs, analgesics and the risk of perforated colonic diverticular disease. Br J Surg. 2003;90:1267-1272.

13. Goh H, Bourne R. Non-steroidal anti-inflammatory drugs and perforated diverticular disease: A case-control study. Ann R Coll Surg Engl. 2002;84:93-96.

14. Morris CR, Harvey IM, Stebbings WS, et al. Epidemiology of perforated colonic diverticular disease. Postgrad Med J. 2002;78:654-658.

15. Aldoori WH, Giovannucci EL, Rimm EB, et al. Prospective study of physical activity and the risk of symptomatic diverticular disease in men. Gut. 1995;36:276-282.

16. Aldoori WH, Giovannucci EL, Rimm EB, et al. A prospective study of alcohol, smoking, caffeine, and the risk of symptomatic diverticular disease in men. Ann Epidemiol. 1995;5:221-228.

17. Lin OS, Soon MS, Wu SS, et al. Dietary habits and right-sided colonic diverticulosis. Dis Colon Rectum. 2000;43:1412-1418.

18. Ferzoco LB, Raptopoulos V, Silen W. Acute diverticulitis. N Engl J Med. 1998;338:1521-1526.

19. Beer E. Some pathological and clinical aspects of acquired (false) diverticula of the intestine. Am J Med Sci. 1904;128:135-145.

20. Brook I, Frazier EH. Aerobic and anaerobic microbiology in intra-abdominal infections associated with diverticulitis. J Med Microbiol. 2000;49:827-830.

21. Walker AP, Krepel CJ, Gohr CM, Edmiston CE. Microflora of abdominal sepsis by locus of infection. J Clin Microbiol. 1994;32:557-558.

22. Rodkey GV, Welch CE. Changing patterns in the surgical treatment of diverticular disease. Ann Surg. 1984;200:466-478.

23. Wong WD, Wexner SD, Lowry A, et al. Practice parameters for the treatment of sigmoid diverticulitis: Supporting documentation. The Standards Task Force. The American Society of Colon and Rectal Surgeons. Dis Colon Rectum. 2000;43:290-297.

24. Krompier A, Howard R, Macewen A, et al. Vesicocolonic fistulas in diverticulitis. J Urol. 1976;115:664-666.

25. Grissom R, Snyder TE. Colovaginal fistula secondary to diverticular disease. Dis Colon Rectum. 1991;34:1043-1049.

25a. Johansen EC, Madoff LC. Pyogenic liver abscesses. Infect Dis Clin North Am. 2000;14:547-563.

26. Stollman NH, Raskin JB. Diagnosis and management of diverticular disease of the colon in adults. Ad Hoc Practice Parameters Committee of the American College of Gastroenterology. Am J Gastroenterol. 1999;94:3110-3121.

27. Rao PM, Rhea JT, Novelline RA, et al. Helical CT with only colonic contrast material for diagnosing diverticulitis: Prospective evaluation of 150 patients. AJR Am J Roentgenol. 1998;170:1445-1449.

28. Bahadursingh AM, Virgo KS, Kaminski DL, Longo WE. Spectrum of disease and outcome of complicated diverticular disease. Am J Surg. 2003;186:696-701.

29. Hiltunen KM, Kolehmainen H, Vuorinen T, Matikainen M. Early water-soluble contrast enema in the diagnosis of acute colonic diverticulitis. Int J Colorectal Dis. 1991;6:190-192.

30. Nicholas GG, Miller WT, Fitts WT, Tondreau RL. Diagnosis of diverticulitis of the colon: Role of the barium enema in defining pericolic inflammation. Ann Surg. 1972;176:205-209.

31. Ambrosetti P, Jenny A, Becker C, et al. Acute left colonic diverticulitis—compared performance of computed tomography and water-soluble contrast enema: Prospective evaluation of 420 patients. Dis Colon Rectum. 2000;43:1363-1367.

32. Hulnick DH, Megibow AJ, Balthazar EJ, et al. Computed tomography in the evaluation of diverticulitis. Radiology. 1984;152:491-495.

33. Neff CC, vanSonnenberg E, Casola G, et al. Diverticular abscesses: Percutaneous drainage. Radiology. 1987;163:15-18.

34. Gazelle GS, Mueller PR. Abdominal abscess: Imaging and intervention. Radiol Clin North Am. 1994;32:913-932.

35. Yacoe ME, Jeffrey RB Jr. Sonography of appendicitis and diverticulitis. Radiol Clin North Am. 1994;32:899-912.

36. Bohnen JM, Solomkin JS, Dellinger EP, et al. Guidelines for clinical care: Anti-infective agents for intra-abdominal infection. A Surgical Infection Society policy statement. Arch Surg. 1992;127:83-89; discussion, 89.

37. Nagorney DM, Adson MA, Pemberton JH. Sigmoid diverticulitis with perforation and generalized peritonitis. Dis Colon Rectum. 1985;28:71-75.

38. Deen KI, Madoff RD, Goldberg SM, Rothenberger DA. Surgical management of left colon obstruction: The University of Minnesota experience. J Am Coll Surg. 1998;187:573-576.

39. Lederman ED, Conti DJ, Lempert N, et al. Complicated diverticulitis following renal transplantation. Dis Colon Rectum. 1998;41:613-618.

40. Warshaw AL, Welch JP, Ottinger LW. Acute perforation of the colon associated with chronic corticosteroid therapy. Am J Surg 1976;131:442-446.

41. Tyau ES, Prystowsky JB, Joehl RJ, Nahrwold DL. Acute diverticulitis: A complicated problem in the immunocompromised patient. Arch Surg. 1991;126:855-858; discussion, 858-859.

42. Perkins JD, Shield CF 3rd, Chang FC, Farha GJ. Acute diverticulitis: Comparison of treatment in immunocompromised and nonimmunocompromised patients. Am J Surg. 1984;148:745-748.

43. Starnes HF Jr, Lazarus JM, Vineyard G. Surgery for diverticulitis in renal failure. Dis Colon Rectum. 1985;28:827-831.

44. West SD, Robinson EK, Delu AN, et al. Diverticulitis in the younger patient. Am J Surg. 2003;186:743-746.

45. Spivak H, Weinrauch S, Harvey JC, et al. Acute colonic diverticulitis in the young. Dis Colon Rectum. 1997;40:570-574.

46. Kohler L, Sauerland S, Neugebauer E. Diagnosis and treatment of diverticular disease: Results of a consensus development conference. The Scientific Committee of the European Association for Endoscopic Surgery. Surg Endosc. 1999;13:430-436.

47. Nespoli A, Ravizzini C, Trivella M, Segala M. The choice of surgical procedure for peritonitis due to colonic perforation. Arch Surg. 1993;128:814-818.

48. Schilling MK, Maurer CA, Kollmar O, Buchler MW. Primary vs. secondary anastomosis after sigmoid colon resection for perforated diverticulitis (Hinchey Stage III and IV): A prospective outcome and cost analysis. Dis Colon Rectum. 2001;44:699-703; discussion, 703-705.

49. Wagner ML, Rosenberg HS, Fernbach DJ, Singleton EB. Typhlitis: A complication of leukemia in childhood. Am J Roentgenol Radium Ther Nucl Med. 1970;109:341-350.

50. Sloas MM, Flynn PM, Kaste SC, Patrick CC. Typhlitis in children with cancer: A 30-year experience. Clin Infect Dis. 1993;17:484-490.

51. Song HK, Kreisel D, Canter R, et al. Changing presentation and management of neutropenic enterocolitis. Arch Surg. 1998;133:979-982.

52. Till M, Lee N, Soper WD, Murphy RL. Typhlitis in patients with HIV-1 infection. Ann Intern Med. 1992;116:998-1000.

53. Katz JA, Wagner ML, Gresik MV, et al. Typhlitis: An 18-year experience and post-mortem review. Cancer. 1990;65:1041-1047.

54. Hopkins DG, Kushner JP. Clostridial species in the pathogenesis of necrotizing enterocolitis in patients with neutropenia. Am J Hematol. 1983;14:289-295.

55. Prolla JC, Kirsner JB. The gastrointestinal lesions and complications of the leukemias. Ann Intern Med. 1964;61:1084-1103.

56. Wallace J, Schwaitzberg S, Miller K. Sometimes it really is appendicitis: Case of a CML patient with acute appendicitis. Ann Hematol. 1998;77:61-64.

57. Dosik GM, Luna M, Valdivieso M, et al. Necrotizing colitis in patients with cancer. Am J Med. 1979;67:646-656.

58. Gomez L, Martino R, Rolston KV. Neutropenic enterocolitis: Spectrum of the disease and comparison of definite and possible cases. Clin Infect Dis. 1998;27:695-699.

59. de Brito D, Barton E, Spears KL, et al. Acute right lower quadrant pain in a patient with leukemia. Ann Emerg Med. 1998;32:98-101.

60. Cartoni C, Dragoni F, Micozzi A, et al. Neutropenic enterocolitis in patients with acute leukemia: Prognostic significance of bowel wall thickening detected by ultrasonography. J Clin Oncol. 2001;19:756-761.

61. Schlatter M, Snyder K, Freyer D. Successful nonoperative management of typhlitis in pediatric oncology patients. J Pediatr Surg. 2002;37:1151-1155.

62. Shamberger RC, Weinstein HJ, Delorey MJ, Levey RH. The medical and surgical management of typhlitis in children with acute nonlymphocytic (myelogenous) leukemia. Cancer. 1986;57:603-609.

63. Anonymous. *Clostridium septicum* and neutropenic enterocolitis. Lancet. 1987;2:608.

64. Gorbach SL. Neutropenic enterocolitis. Clin Infect Dis. 1998;27:700-701.

65. Kunkel JM, Rosenthal D. Management of the ileocecal syndrome: Neutropenic enterocolitis. Dis Colon Rectum. 1986;29:196-199.

66. Wade DS, Nava HR, Douglass HO Jr. Neutropenic enterocolitis: Clinical diagnosis and treatment. Cancer. 1992;69:17-23.

SECTION G

CARDIOVASCULAR

INFECTIONS

CHAPTER **74**

Endocarditis and Intravascular Infections

VANCE G. FOWLER, Jr.
W. MICHAEL SCHELD
ARNOLD S. BAYER

INFECTIVE ENDOCARDITIS

The term *infective endocarditis* (IE) denotes infection of the endocardial surface of the heart and implies the physical presence of microorganisms in the lesion. Although the heart valves are affected most commonly, the disease also may occur within septal defects or on the mural endocardium. Infections of arteriovenous shunts and of arterioarterial shunts (patent ductus arteriosus) and infections related to coarctation of the aorta are included in the following discussion because the clinical manifestations are similar. The term *infective endocarditis,* first used by Thayer and later popularized by Lerner and Weinstein,[1] is preferable to the old term *bacterial endocarditis* because chlamydiae, rickettsiae, mycoplasmas, fungi, and perhaps even viruses may be responsible for the syndrome.

In the past, IE was classified as *acute* or *subacute.* This distinction was based on the usual progression of the untreated disease and is mainly of historical interest. The acute form follows a fulminant course, usually with high fever, systemic toxicity, and leukocytosis; death occurs in several days to less than 6 weeks. It classically is associated with infection caused by *Staphylococcus aureus, Streptococcus pyogenes, Streptococcus pneumoniae,* or *Neisseria gonorrhoeae.* The subacute (death occurring in 6 weeks to 3 months) and *chronic* (death occurring later than 3 months) forms usually are considered together. They commonly occur in the setting of prior valvular disease and are characterized by a slow, indolent course with low-grade fever, night sweats, weight loss, and vague systemic complaints. These two forms of IE classically are caused by the viridans streptococci. Although useful conceptually, this classification ignores the nonbacterial forms of IE and the frequent overlap in manifestations of infection by specific organisms, such as the enterococci. A classification based on the etiologic agent responsible is preferable because it has implications for the course usually followed, the likelihood of preexisting heart disease, and the appropriate antimicrobial agents to employ.

Although relatively uncommon, IE has received considerable attention by clinicians and scientists for the past century. The clinical manifestations of IE are so varied that they may be encountered in any of the medical subspecialties. Successful management depends on the close cooperation of medical and surgical disciplines. Endocarditis services have been created at several tertiary care centers in the United States. This collaboration has improved markedly the outcome of a disease that was universally fatal in the preantibiotic era. IE has attracted considerable investigative interest. Although the factors that influence its development now are identified more clearly, many questions remain about the unique aspects of this infection, in particular:

1. Why do organisms lodge specifically on the cardiac valves rather than elsewhere in the vascular tree?

2. What enables the microorganisms to survive on the valve surface after colonization?
3. What are the primary host defenses against induction and progression of the infection?
4. Why do only a relatively few strains of bacteria produce most cases of IE, whereas many others produce only bacteremia?
5. What factors are responsible for the marked variation in the manifestations of IE?
6. Why is the infection so difficult to eradicate with antibiotics even though the infecting organisms often are exquisitely sensitive to the drugs in vitro?

These questions are discussed in detail in the following sections.

Epidemiology

The incidence of IE is difficult to determine because the criteria for diagnosis and the methods of reporting vary with different series.[2,3] An analysis based on strict case definitions often reveals that only a small proportion ($\cong$20%) of clinically diagnosed cases are categorized as definite. Nevertheless, IE accounted for approximately 1 case per 1000 hospital admissions (range 0.16 to 5.4 cases per 1000 admissions) in a review of 10 large surveys.[2,4] This incidence has not changed since the 1970s.[5] The mean annual incidence was 3.8 per 100,000 person-years in Olmsted County, Minnesota, from 1950 to 1981, with no significant change during this interval.[6] A similar figure of 1.7 per 100,000 person-years was reported from a prospective survey in Louisiana[7] and is analogous to results from the United Kingdom[8] and France,[9,10] but this figure is less than incidence reports from the Delaware River Valley region (11.6/100,000 population).[11] A series of 210 episodes of IE seen at a large community hospital in Youngstown, Ohio, from 1980 through 1990 documented annual rates of 0.32 to 1.3 (mean 0.75) episodes per 1000 admissions per year.[12] In an autopsy study,[13] there was no change in the yearly number of cases of IE in the United Kingdom from 1939 to 1967. The proportion of acute cases has increased from approximately 20% in the preantibiotic era to 33%.[4,5] Despite these changes in the disease spectrum, IE remains a prevalent disease with a significant mortality in the antibiotic era.[12,14,15] Estimates from the American Heart Association (AHA) place the annual incidence of IE in the United States at 10,000 to 20,000 new cases.

The mean age of patients with IE has increased gradually in the antibiotic era. In 1926, the median age was younger than 30 years[16]; this had increased to 39 years by 1943; currently, greater than 50% of patients are older than 50 years.[5,12,17,18] Among approximately 2200 patients from seven centers in five countries with definite IE by the Duke criteria, the median age was 58 years.[19] The mean age of patients with IE caused by group D streptococci is older: 61 to 67 years.[20] The disease is uncommon in children, in whom it is associated primarily with (1) underlying structural congenital heart disease, particularly septal defects or complex lesions involving septal defects; (2) surgical repair of these defects; or (3) nosocomial catheter-related bacteremia, especially in infants.[21,22] The mean age for men is 6 to 7 years older than that for women, and men are affected more commonly (54% to 69% of the cases; the mean male-to-female ratio is 1.7:1, with a range of 1 to 3:1 in 18 large series).[4] In patients younger than age 35 years, more cases occur in women. Many factors may be related to this shift in age distribution. First, there has been a change in the nature of the underlying heart disease owing to a decline in the incidence of acute rheumatic fever and rheumatic heart disease countered by the increasing importance of degenerative heart disease in elderly patients. Second, the age of the population has been increasing steadily, and people with rheumatic or congenital heart disease are surviving longer. In addition, such patients increasingly are being subjected to prosthetic valve surgery, an important etiologic factor in the pathogenesis of IE. A new form of the disease—health care–associated IE—secondary to new therapeutic modalities (e.g., intravenous catheters, hyperalimentation lines, pacemakers, dialysis shunts) has emerged.[2,23-26] Of 125 cases of IE reviewed in Seattle, 35 were nosocomial in origin (28%).[27] Although nosocomial IE accounted for only 14.3% of cases in another study,

64% of patients were older than 60 years of age, and mortality was high.[28] The emerging importance of health care–associated IE in industrialized nations also may influence the microbiology of IE, with an increasing prevalence of *S. aureus* IE and decreasing prevalence of viridans streptococci among some U.S. tertiary care centers.[23]

The heart valve involved by the infection varies considerably with the proportion of acute cases reported in each series. The distribution ranges from 28% to 45% of cases for the mitral valve alone, 5% to 36% for the aortic valve alone, and 0% to 35% for the aortic and mitral valves combined. The tricuspid valve rarely is involved (0% to 6% of the cases), and the pulmonary valve is involved even less often (<1%).[17,20,27,29] Right-sided and left-sided disease are present in 0% to 4%. Involvement of the aortic valve alone is increasing in frequency and correlates with the increase in acute cases; the incidence was 5% in 1938 and increased to 39% by 1978.[17] The aortic valve is involved in 61% of cases in men but in only 31% of cases in women.[27]

Almost any type of structural heart disease may predispose to IE, especially when the defect results in turbulence of blood flow. Rheumatic heart disease has been the underlying lesion in 37% to 76% of infections in the past, and the mitral valve is involved in more than 85% of these cases.[4] If the mitral valve alone is involved, women outnumber men by 2 to 1. The aortic valve is affected in approximately 50% of these cases; if it alone is involved, men outnumber women by 4 to 1. Right-sided endocarditis is rare (except in intravenous drug users and patients with indwelling transvenous pacemakers) and accounts for less than 10% of all cases occurring in patients with rheumatic heart disease. In developed countries, the proportion of cases related to rheumatic heart disease has continued to decline to 25% or less in the past 2 decades,[30] whereas in developing countries, rheumatic heart disease remains the most common predisposing cardiac condition.[31,32] Congenital heart disease (especially patent ductus arteriosus, ventricular septal defect, coarctation of the aorta, bicuspid aortic valve, tetralogy of Fallot, and, rarely, pulmonic stenosis) is responsible in 6% to 24% of the cases.[4] IE is uncommon in the secundum atrial septal defects, probably because this lesion results in a low-pressure shunt with little turbulence. The congenitally bicuspid aortic valve, erroneously attributed to rheumatic carditis in the past,[33] now is recognized as an important condition in elderly patients (especially men), is the underlying lesion in more than 20% of the cases occurring past the age of 60, and is associated with a poor prognosis despite rapid valve replacement.[34] Marfan syndrome, when associated with aortic insufficiency, also has been associated with IE. Surgical closure of a ventricular septal defect lowers the risk of IE.[35]

The degenerative cardiac lesions (e.g., calcified mitral annulus, calcific nodular lesions secondary to arteriosclerotic cardiovascular disease, post–myocardial infarction thrombus) assume the greatest importance in the 30% to 40% of patients without any demonstrable underlying valvular disease. The actual contribution made by these lesions is unknown, but they occur with an increased incidence in the elderly. In one series, degenerative lesions were present in 50% of patients older than 60 years of age with native valve IE.[36] The contribution of these degenerative cardiac lesions to the development of IE is apparent in an analysis of 148 patients receiving treatment in London since 1970.[37,38] The underlying structural cardiac defects were as follows: rheumatic heart disease, present in 39 of the patients; congenital defects, in 13; and normal or degenerate valves, in 65. Similarly, only 31% of patients with IE in another series[39] had known cardiac disease. Although a calcified mitral annulus is fairly common in elderly women, this lesion rarely is complicated by IE (only 3 of 80 in one report).[40] When acute cases of IE are considered separately, more than 50% have no recognized underlying cardiac disease.[12]

Many other conditions, such as bicuspid aortic valve,[41] luetic heart disease, arterioarterial fistulas, hemodialysis shunts or fistulas, intracardiac pacemaker wires, and intracardiac prostheses, may predispose to IE. Prosthetic valve endocarditis is increasing in incidence in proportion to other forms of endocarditis and is discussed in Chapter 75. Intravascular infections involving cardiac devices (e.g., permanent cardiac pacemakers, defibrillators) also have increased signifi-

cantly since the 1990s.[42] IE also occurs more frequently in seriously ill hospitalized patients, who are compromised hosts and who are subjected to invasive intravascular access procedures (e.g., intravenous catheters, including central venous pressure monitoring lines; hyperalimentation lines; intracardiac pacemaker wires).[17] As noted previously, another group with an increased risk of IE comprises intravenous ("mainlining") drug users. (This group is considered in detail in a later section.) In this population, there is the added problem of a rapidly rising prevalence of IE in persons with human immunodeficiency virus (HIV) infection. In addition, intravenous drug users are the group at greatest risk for recurrent and polymicrobial IE.[4,43] Although the contribution of invasive procedures (e.g., sigmoidoscopy, colonoscopy) has been debated, native valve IE seems to be more common in patients with active inflammatory bowel disease (6 of 213 patients in one report[44]).

Although idiopathic hypertrophic subaortic stenosis or asymmetric hypertrophy of the interventricular septum classically has not been recognized as a condition leading to bacterial endocarditis, by 1982, 32 such cases had been reported in the literature.[45-47] In seven cases examined histologically, the infection was found on the aortic valve in three cases, mitral valve in two cases, both valves in one case, and the subaortic endocardium in one case. This distribution probably is related to the associated mitral regurgitation due to the displacement of the anterior leaflet by the abnormal ventricular architecture and by the turbulence of the jet stream affecting the aortic valve distal to the intraventricular obstruction. The age of patients developing IE ranged from 20 to 66 years, and in most cases (70%), the disease was produced by viridans streptococci. Approximately 5% of patients with idiopathic hypertrophic subaortic stenosis develop IE.[47] IE is more common in the subset of patients with idiopathic hypertrophic subaortic stenosis who have hemodynamically severe forms of the disease manifested by a higher peak systolic pressure gradient and a high prevalence of symptoms. New murmurs develop in 36% of patients with idiopathic hypertrophic subaortic stenosis complicated by IE, and this new physical finding correlates with a higher mortality rate.[47]

The association of the mitral prolapse syndrome and IE also has been recognized. Of 87 consecutive cases of IE reported from Stanford University, 10 (11%) occurred in patients with well-documented mitral valve prolapse.[48] These 10 cases represented more than one third of the 28 cases in which isolated mitral regurgitation was the predisposing condition. Four additional cases occurred in patients who were not studied by echocardiography or angiography but who had clinical evidence of the mitral prolapse syndrome. Of the cases of IE associated with isolated insufficient mitral valves, 40% to 50% probably occurred in patients with the mitral prolapse syndrome. In one series[29] of 63 cases of native valve endocarditis diagnosed in Memphis from 1980 to 1984, mitral valve prolapse was the most common underlying lesion (29%). In another study,[49] 5 of 58 patients with mitral valve prolapse followed prospectively for 9 to 22 years developed IE. This syndrome should be suspected in patients with midsystolic clicks with or without a late systolic murmur. The condition is common and has been recognized in 0.5% to 20% of otherwise healthy people, especially young women. It has become apparent that mitral valve prolapse is only one component of a developmental syndrome. This lesion often is associated with a distinct habitus in women,[50] von Willebrand's disease, or ophthalmoplegia. Some of these characteristics may be useful in identifying patients at high risk for IE. All 25 patients who developed IE on a prolapsing mitral valve had a holosystolic murmur, and none had the isolated click without a murmur.[48] The risk of IE seems to be increased in the subset of patients with mitral valve prolapse who exhibit thickened leaflets with valvular redundancy.[36] In addition, men older than 45 years who have mitral valve prolapse are at increased risk for IE.[51] Nevertheless, the risk of IE is higher in patients with mitral valve prolapse. In a careful retrospective, epidemiologic, matched case-control analysis, the calculated odds ratio (8.2; 95% confidence interval 2.4 to 28.4) indicated a substantially higher risk for the development of IE in these patients than in controls.[52] It seems that when IE develops in people with mitral valve prolapse, the symptoms and signs are more subtle and the mortality rate is less than in left-sided IE of other types.[53]

Pathogenesis and Pathophysiology

In vitro observations and studies in experimental animals have shown that the development of IE probably requires the simultaneous occurrence of several independent events, each of which may be influenced by a host of separate factors. The valve surface first must be altered to produce a suitable site for bacterial attachment and colonization. Surface changes may be produced by various local and systemic stresses, including blood turbulence. These alterations result in the deposition of platelets and fibrin and in the formation of so-called sterile vegetation—the lesions of nonbacterial thrombotic endocarditis (NBTE). Bacteria then must reach this site and adhere to the involved tissue to produce colonization. Certain strains seem to have a selective advantage in adhering to platelets or fibrin or both and produce the disease with a lower inoculum. After colonization, the surface is covered rapidly with a protective sheath of fibrin and platelets to produce an environment conducive to further bacterial multiplication and vegetative growth. The interaction of these events is depicted in Figure 74-1. In the following sections, these factors are considered independently (see elsewhere for in-depth discussions[54-57]).

Nonbacterial Thrombotic Endocarditis

Luschka, in 1852, first suggested that IE resulted when septic coronary emboli lodged in the vessels of the cardiac valve.[58] This hypothesis was discarded because cardiac valves are poorly vascularized.[56,59,60] It now is clear that the initial colonization occurs on the endothelial surface of the valve. In experimental animals, it is nearly impossible to produce IE with intravenous injections of bacteria, unless the valvular surface first is damaged or otherwise altered. When a polyethylene catheter is passed across the aortic valve of a rabbit, IE is produced with intravenously injected bacteria or fungi.[61,62] Microscopic examination of this early lesion shows the organisms intimately adherent to fibrin-platelet deposits overlying interstitial edema and mild cellular distortion that have formed in areas of valvular trauma.[63] Scanning electron micrographs of the damaged valvular surface confirm the adhesion

of microorganisms to these areas of fibrin-platelet deposition early in the disease course.[64] The organisms are covered rapidly by fibrin.[65] Opossums and pigs are the only animals known to develop IE readily without experimentally induced valvular alteration.[57,66] The stress of captivity is apparently sufficient in these animals to produce subtle valvular changes that lead to spontaneous endocarditis and a markedly increased susceptibility to the disease after the intravenous injection of bacteria. In other animals and probably in humans, alteration of the valve surface is a prerequisite for bacterial colonization. Angrist and Oka[59] first recognized the importance of these deposits as the crucial factor in allowing bacterial colonization of valve surfaces and suggested the term *nonbacterial thrombotic endocarditis*. Many forms of exogenous stress produce these lesions experimentally, including infection, hypersensitivity states, cold exposure, simulated high altitude, high cardiac output states, cardiac lymphatic obstruction, and hormonal manipulations.[57] These procedures all increase the susceptibility of the animals to IE.

NBTE has been found in patients with malignancy (particularly pancreatic, gastric, and lung carcinoma) and other chronic wasting diseases, rheumatic and congenital heart disease,[59] uremia, and connective tissue diseases such as systemic lupus erythematosus; after the placement of intracardiac catheters (e.g., Swan-Ganz); and after a self-limited acute illness. NBTE generally reflects one of two pathogenic mechanisms: hypercoagulability or endothelial damage. In a careful analysis performed in Japan, NBTE was found in 2.4% of 3404 autopsies, especially in elderly people with chronic wasting disease.[67] Among patients at high risk for NBTE, the rate may be greater. Cardiac valvular vegetations were found in 19% of 200 nonselected ambulatory patients with solid tumors undergoing prospective echocardiographic screening.[68] Valvular lesions were most common among patients with carcinoma of the pancreas and lung and lymphoma. NBTE is most common on the low-pressure side of the cardiac valves along the line of closure, precisely the site most often involved in IE. Whether this lesion is always essential for the development of IE in humans is unknown.

Hemodynamic Factors

IE characteristically occurs on the atrial surface of the mitral valve and the ventricular surface of the aortic valve when associated with valvular insufficiency. Rodbard[69] showed that this localization is related to a decrease in lateral pressure (presumably with decreased perfusion of the intima) immediately "downstream" from the regurgitant flow. Lesions with high degrees of turbulence (small ventricular septal defect with a jet lesion, valvular stenosis resulting from insufficient valves) readily create conditions that lead to bacterial colonization, whereas defects with a large surface area (large ventricular septal defect), low flow (ostium secundum atrial septal defect), or attenuation of turbulence (chronic congestive heart failure [CHF] with atrial fibrillation) rarely are implicated in IE. Cures of IE achieved with ligation alone of an arteriovenous fistula or patent ductus arteriosus also highlight the importance of hemodynamic factors. A hyperdynamic circulation itself, such as that developing after experimentally induced arteriovenous fistulas in dogs or after creation of fistulas and shunts in hemodialysis patients, indirectly may lead to IE by producing NBTE.[56,57]

The degree of mechanical stress exerted on the valve also affects the location of the IE.[70] In 1024 autopsy cases of IE reviewed through 1952, the incidence of valvular lesions was as follows: mitral, 86%; aortic, 55%; tricuspid, 19.6%; and pulmonic, 1.1%. This incidence correlates with the pressure resting on the closed valve: 116 mm Hg, 72 mm Hg, 24 mm Hg, and 5 mm Hg.

Transient Bacteremia

In the setting of preexistent NBTE, transient bacteremia may result in the colonization of these lesions and may lead to the development of IE.[71] Transient bacteremia occurs whenever a mucosal surface heavily colonized with bacteria is traumatized, such as with dental extractions and other dental procedures and gastrointestinal, urologic, and gynecologic procedures (Table 74-1).[71,72] The degree of bacteremia is pro-

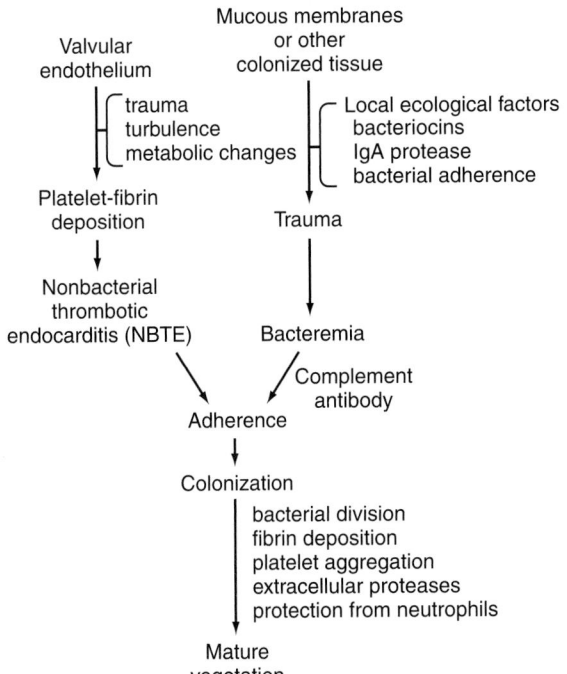

FIGURE 74-1. Proposed scheme for the pathogenesis of infective endocarditis.

portional to the trauma produced by the procedure and to the number of organisms inhabiting the surface, and the organisms isolated reflect the resident microbial flora. The bacteremia usually is low grade—with 10 or fewer colony-forming units (CFU)/mL—and transient; the blood stream usually is sterile in less than 15 to 30 minutes. In two studies in which blood cultures were drawn from patients with severe gingival disease before the dental procedure, spontaneous bacteremia was identified in 9% to 11%. Other studies have shown an even higher frequency of spontaneous bacteremia. Of the blood cultured from healthy people, 60% to 80% of specimens are positive when filters and anaerobic techniques were used.[73] The degree of bacteremia is low, however, with only 2 to 10 CFU/5 mL of blood isolated. "Nonpathogenic" organisms, such as *Propionibacterium acnes, Actinomyces viscosus, Staphylococcus epidermidis,* and other *Actinomyces* or streptococcal species, were responsible. Frequent episodes of silent bacteremia also are suggested by the identification of circulating humoral antibodies to the resident oral flora and by the noted increase in sensitized peripheral T cells to the flora of dental plaque.

Another crucial factor during the transient bacteremia stage is susceptibility of the potential pathogen to complement-mediated bactericidal activity. Only "serum-resistant," gram-negative aerobic bacilli (e.g., *Escherichia coli, Pseudomonas aeruginosa, Serratia marcescens*) reliably produce experimental IE in rabbits,[74,75] and this property is found in all isolates from human cases of IE. Although experimental IE can be induced in rats with "serum-sensitive" *E. coli,* the organisms are eliminated rapidly on catheter removal.[75]

Microorganism–Nonbacterial Thrombotic Endocarditis Interaction

The ability of certain organisms to adhere to NBTE lesions is a crucial early step in the development of IE. Gould and associates[76] showed that organisms commonly associated with IE (enterococci, viridans streptococci, *S. aureus, S. epidermidis, P. aeruginosa*) adhered more avidly to normal canine aortic leaflets in vitro than did organisms uncommon in IE (*Klebsiella pneumoniae, E. coli*). In addition, *S. aureus* and the viridans streptococci produce IE more readily than does *E. coli*

in the rabbit model of IE.[77] This observation correlates with the relative frequency with which these organisms produce the disease in humans. The rarity of IE due to gram-negative aerobic bacilli also may be related to their serum sensitivity, as noted previously.

Differences in the propensity to cause IE are apparent even within a single species. Eleven capsular serotypes of *S. aureus* have been described to date; highly mucoid strains (e.g., serotypes 1 and 2) rarely are recovered from clinical isolates, whereas types 5 and 8 account for approximately 75% of isolates. Nevertheless, mutant strains devoid of microencapsulation had significantly lower median infective dose (ID_{50}) values in a rat (catheter-induced NBTE) IE model[78] than wild-type parent strains. Microcapsule expression may attenuate *S. aureus* IE production by blocking bacterial cell surface adhesins, but this hypothesis requires confirmation. In addition, an increasing number of reports suggest that other specific pathogen characteristics in *S. aureus* are associated with the severity of infection caused by these strains in humans.[79-82]

Other studies using an elegant experimental model of IE after dental extraction in rats with periodontitis, which closely resembles the presumed pathogenetic sequence in humans, also suggest an important role for bacterial adhesion to NBTE in the early events. Although viridans streptococci were isolated much more commonly than were group G streptococci in blood cultures obtained 1 minute after extraction, the latter strains caused 83% of the IE episodes in this rat model.[83,84] This propensity to cause IE was associated with an increased adhesion of group G streptococci to fibrin-platelet matrices in vitro.[84]

The adherence of oral streptococci to NBTE may depend on the production of a complex extracellular polysaccharide, dextran. This polymer plays an essential role in the pathogenesis of dental caries by *Streptococcus mutans*.[85] Dextran allows the organism to adhere tightly to the surface of dental enamel. The enhanced ability to adhere to inert surfaces also may be important in IE. In an analysis of 719 cases of streptococcal infections in the United Kingdom, 317 cases of IE were found.[86] The most common etiologic agents were *Streptococcus sanguis* (16.4% of the cases), previously called *Streptococcus subacute bacterial endocarditis,* and *S. mutans* (14.2%). When a ratio denoting endocarditis to nonendocarditis bacteremia was derived (Table 74-2), the relative propensity for a particular organism to cause IE could be predicted. The ratios range from 14.2:1 for *S. mutans* to a reversed ratio of 1:32 for *S. pyogenes*. Only the first four organisms listed in Table 74-2 (all with ratios >3:1) produce extracellular dextran. This finding suggests that dextran production also may be a virulence factor in the pathogenesis of IE.

The role of dextran in the adherence of oral streptococci to NBTE also has been studied in vitro by using artificial fibrin-platelet matrices (simulating NBTE). The amount of dextran produced by the organism in broth correlated with adherence and was increased by incubating the organism in sucrose (which stimulates dextran production) and was decreased by the addition of dextranase (which removes the dextran from

---

TABLE 74-1 Incidence of Bacteremia after Various Procedures

Procedure/Manipulation	Percentage of Positive Blood Cultures
Dental	
Dental extraction	18-85
Periodontal surgery	32-88
Chewing candy or paraffin	17-51
Tooth brushing	0-26
Oral irrigation device	27-50
Upper Airway	
Bronchoscopy (rigid scope)	15
Tonsillectomy	28-38
Nasotracheal suctioning/intubation	16
Gastrointestinal	
Upper gastrointestinal endoscopy	8-12
Sigmoidoscopy/colonoscopy	0-9.5
Barium enema	11
Percutaneous needle biopsy of liver	3-13
Urologic	
Urethral dilation	18-33
Urethral catheterization	8
Cystoscopy	0-17
Transurethral prostatic resection	12-46
Obstetric/gynecologic	
Normal vaginal delivery	0-11
Punch biopsy of the cervix	0
Removal/insertion of IUD	0

IUD, intrauterine (contraceptive) device.
From Everett ED, Hirschmann JV. Transient bacteremia and endocarditis prophylaxis: A review. Medicine (Baltimore). 1977;56:61.

TABLE 74-2 Ratio of Infective Endocarditis Cases to Nonendocarditis Bacteremia Cases for Various Streptococci and Enterococci

Organism	Endocarditis:Nonendocarditis
Streptococcus mutans	14.2:1
Streptococcus bovis I	5.9:1
Dextran-positive *Streptococcus mitior*	3.3:1
Streptococcus sanguis	3:1
S. mitior	1.8:1
Unclassified viridans streptococci	1.4:1
Enterococcus faecalis	1:1.2
Miscellaneous streptococci	1:1.3
S. bovis II	1:1.7
Streptococcus anginosus	1:2.6
Group G streptococci	1:2.9
Group B streptococci	1:7.4
Group A streptococci	1:32

Modified from Parker MT, Ball LC. Streptococci and aerococci associated with systemic infection in man. J Med Microbiol. 1976;9:275.

the cell surface). The addition of exogenous dextran to *S. sanguis* grown in sucrose-free media increased adherence. Dextran production also correlated directly with the ability of these organisms to produce IE in vivo in the rabbit model.[87] The strain of *S. sanguis* produced IE less readily when incubated in dextranase than did control strains, and a strain that produced large quantities of dextran produced endocarditis more easily than did a strain that produced relatively small quantities of dextran. Dextran production also increases the adherence of *S. mutans* to traumatized canine aortic valves in vitro,[88] an effect dependent on polymers of higher molecular weight.[89] Dextran formation (or, more properly, exopolysaccharide or glycocalyx production) by oral streptococci may be a virulence factor for the production of IE by these organisms.[90] Continued in vivo synthesis of exopolysaccharide during experimental IE correlates with vegetation size and resistance to antimicrobial therapy.[91,92] Measurement of cell-adherent glycocalyx by a quantitative spectrophotometric tryptophan assay among viridans streptococci isolated from blood cultures has potential value as an independent predictor of the likelihood of IE.[93] Non–dextran-producing streptococci may produce IE in humans and adhere to artificial fibrin-platelet surfaces in vitro,[94] which suggests that other microbial surface characteristics are instrumental for this early event. Whatever the role of the extracellular glycocalyx in microbial adhesion, its presence may retard antimicrobial therapy for streptococcal endocarditis (see later).[91,92,95]

FimA is a surface adhesin expressed by viridans streptococci that serves as an important colonization factor in IE.[96] This 36-kD protein is located at the tips of the fimbriae and has been shown to mediate the attachment of such organisms to platelet-fibrin matrices in vitro and to experimental NBTE lesions in the animal model of IE.[97] Homologues of the *fimA* gene have been found widely distributed among clinical strains of viridans streptococci and enterococci, suggesting its importance in IE.[98] Several lines of experimental evidence have confirmed further the key role of FimA in the pathogenesis of IE. Inactivation of the *fimA* gene has yielded viridans streptococcal mutants exhibiting a significant decrease in virulence in experimental IE compared with the parental strain having intact FimA expression.[97] In addition, animals either passively immunized with anti-FimA antibody or actively immunized with a FimA vaccine were significantly less susceptible to experimental IE than nonimmunized controls.[98]

A similar important role of adhesion to NBTE in the pathogenesis of IE has been shown for yeasts. *Candida albicans* adheres to NBTE in vitro and produces IE in rabbits more readily than does *Candida krusei*, a nonadherent yeast rarely implicated in IE in humans.[99] Although microbial adhesion is a crucial early event in the pathogenesis of IE, the precise intracardiac loci are unknown and may differ among organisms. Most organisms probably adhere initially to a constituent of NBTE; some evidence implicates fibronectin as the host receptor within NBTE.[100] More recent studies[101,102] support this concept. Low-fibronectin-binding mutants of *S. aureus* and *S. sanguis* had decreased ability to produce IE in rats compared with high-fibronectin-binding parent strains. Other normal constituents of damaged endothelium or NBTE (e.g., fibrinogen, laminin, type 4 collagen[103]) also may serve to bind circulating bacteria. *Streptococcus defectivus*—the major species isolated in cases of IE due to nutritionally variant streptococci (NVS) (discussed subsequently)—bound the extracellular matrix of fibroblasts and endothelial cells in a saturable-specific manner, whereas *Streptococcus adjacens* and serotype III NVS strains did not bind.[104] A study also documented binding of *S. mutans*, *Streptococcus mitis*, *S. sanguis*, and *Enterococcus faecalis* to this extracellular matrix. Laminin-binding proteins (e.g., a 145-kD protein found in *Streptococcus gordonii* [formerly *S. sanguis* I]) have been found on the cell walls of organisms recovered from patients with IE,[105] and the level of protein expression seemed to be regulated by the presence of extracellular matrix proteins. Other organisms may bind directly to, or become ingested by, endothelial cells as the initial event[106-109]; this sequence appears important in the initiation of IE by *S. aureus* on "normal" cardiac valves. Many studies in experimental IE, using *S. aureus* as the study organism, have shed additional light on the importance of

microbial binding to specific matrix proteins found within the NBTE lesion on the development of IE. It seems that the key adhesin possessed by the organism for induction of IE is one or more of its several fibrinogen-binding proteins (e.g., clumping factor, coagulase[110,111]). Adhesins for other matrix molecules (e.g., fibronectin, collagen, thrombospondin[112-114]) are not involved pivotally in initial attachment of the organism to damaged endothelium but are crucial in the persistence of the microbe at this site. Additional virulence factors produced by this organism ((-toxin[115]) have been identified in the experimental IE model as important for the persistence and proliferation of the organism within maturing vegetations in the post–valvular colonization stage of infection. The fibronectin-binding adhesins of *S. aureus* seem to be crucial in the ability of the organism to invade cardiac endothelium and induce endothelial apoptosis.[116-118] Although the specific microbial surface–host receptor ligand relationship remains incompletely defined for all the major IE pathogens, this is an active area of investigation because inhibition of these events may provide novel prophylactic strategies.

The importance of adherence characteristics in the development of endocarditis also has been examined by using preincubation of organisms with antibiotics. Many classes of drugs, after incubation even at subinhibitory concentrations, decrease the adhesion of streptococcal species to fibrin-platelet matrices and damaged canine valves in vitro.[119] Several elegant studies in animal models have verified the significance of this in vitro observation because preincubation of the organism in subinhibitory antibiotic concentrations prevents the development of IE in vivo[120,121]; this has direct relevance to the chemoprophylactic prevention of IE (see Chapter 76). In one study, subinhibitory concentrations of penicillin were found to result in a loss of streptococcal lipoteichoic acid with reduced adhesion to NBTE-involved tissue and an impaired ability to produce IE in vivo.[122] Antibiotics may prevent IE by at least two mechanisms: (1) bacterial killing and (2) inhibition of adhesion to NBTE-involved tissue.[123]

Because platelets are (with fibrin) the major constituents of NBTE, the role of the platelet in the pathogenesis of IE also has been studied. Some strains of bacteria have been found to be potent stimulators of platelet aggregation and the release reaction.[124] In general, IE-producing strains of staphylococci and streptococci more actively aggregate platelets than do other bacteria that less frequently produce IE. Bacterial-platelet aggregates have been found in the peripheral blood in patients with bacteremia. The importance of these bacterial-platelet aggregates in the formation of the vegetation or, conversely, in the effect of the aggregation on the rate of removal of organisms from the circulation is unknown. In one study, even small numbers of platelets greatly increased the adherence of oral streptococci to fibrin in vitro.[86] Other studies[125] have shown that *S. sanguis*, an important cause of IE, aggregates platelets and adheres to these blood components by protease-sensitive components, not dextrans. A platelet receptor for ligands on certain strains of *S. sanguis* was suggested. This platelet aggregation by viridans streptococci requires, however, direct platelet binding and plasma components.[126] Other experiments implicate IgG in this specific streptococcal-platelet interaction and suggest that platelet activation is mediated through the platelet surface Fc receptor, with a molecular weight of 40,000.[127]

When the colonization of the valve occurs and a critical mass of adherent bacteria develops, the vegetation enlarges by further platelet-fibrin deposition and continued bacterial proliferation. There is a complex interplay among factors responsible for bacterial-platelet adhesion and aggregation. The ability of *S. sanguis* to induce platelet aggregation in vitro is conferred by two bacterial cell surface antigens: (1) class I antigen, which promotes adhesion of *S. sanguis* to platelets (adh+), and (2) coexpression of class II antigen, which promotes platelet adhesion or platelet aggregation (agg+). At least nine adh/agg phenotypes have been identified among naturally occurring variants, reflecting a range of platelet interactivity. Intravenous inoculation of agg+ *S. sanguis* strains into rabbits with catheter-induced aortic valve trauma leads to larger vegetations, a more severe clinical course, more gross lesions in major organs, and greater mortality than inoculation with an agg⁻ strain or the agg⁺ strains pretreated with Fab fragments specific for the platelet interactivity phenotype.[128] Platelet aggregation induced by *S. sanguis* in vivo seems to be an important virulence determinant of vegetation development and disease progression. Streptococcal exopolysaccharide production inversely correlates with platelet adhesion, while inhibiting aggregation,[129] indicating that these surface molecules may enhance endocarditis at some pathogenic steps but not others.

The manner in which *S. aureus* interacts with platelets in the pathogenesis of IE differs substantially from the viridans streptococci. This interaction does not require the presence of specific antistaphylococcal antibody and is not amplified by the platelet Fc receptor.[130] Platelet–*S. aureus* interactions for executing aggregation require fibrinogen as a bridging molecule but are independent of the primary platelet fibrinogen-binding site, the glycoprotein IIb/IIIa integrin receptor. In addition, it seems that *S. aureus* can bind to platelets via platelet-derived von Willebrand factor or directly to the von Willebrand factor receptor, at the von Willebrand factor–binding domain.[131-133] In experimental IE, transposon inactivation of the putative *S. aureus* platelet-binding adhesin gene results in mutants with diminished capacity to adhere to platelets in vitro in either suspension or surface-bound monolayers.[134] In experimental IE due to such low-platelet-binding mutants, the induction rates of IE were equivalent to the induction rates of the parental strain, presumably because of the microbe's ability to attach to damaged endothelium by multiple adhesive mechanisms. The capacity of the mutant to persist and proliferate within experimental vegetations and to disseminate hematogenously to the kidneys was impaired markedly, however, in the mutant strain.[134] This transposon defect was found to reside within the staphylococcal fibrinogen adhesin gene, clumping factor A (*clfA*).[135]

Platelets also may play a role in host defense within the cardiac vegetation during IE.[136] After specific exposure to thrombin, release of α-granule–derived platelet microbicidal proteins (PMPs), or thrombocidins, with bactericidal activity against most gram-positive cocci that cause IE has been shown.[137] Although the ability of *S. aureus* to adhere to and aggregate platelets is a related property, the resistance to PMPs is an independent phenotypic characteristic and a potential virulence factor.[138] PMPs are low-molecular-weight (approximately 8 to 10 kD) cationic proteins and may act primarily on the bacterial cell membrane or cell wall synergistically with antibiotics to kill bacteria. PMPs also may show fungicidal activity against some yeasts in vitro.[139] Microbial resistance to the cidal activity of PMPs may contribute to the pathogenesis of IE. This hypothesis is supported by a reduction in vegetation weight and bacterial concentration in rabbits with experimental aortic valve *S. aureus* endocarditis after treatment with aspirin.[140] In addition, three studies in experimental IE have confirmed the importance of the relationship of PMP resistance and the pathogenesis of IE. In experimental viridans streptococcal IE and *S. aureus* IE, PMP-resistant strains exhibit an enhanced capacity to persist at sites of valvular damage.[141,142] In addition, *S. aureus* strains exhibiting the PMP resistance phenotype in vitro are able to proliferate within the vegetation and hematogenously seeded extracardiac foci (kidneys, spleen) to a significantly greater extent than their isogenic counterparts that are PMP susceptible in vitro.[143,144] Several clinical studies also emphasize the important association between PMP resistance and the pathogenesis of intravascular infections. Blood-stream isolates of viridans streptococci and *S. aureus* from patients with IE tended to be substantially more resistant to PMPs in vitro.[142] *S. aureus* blood-stream isolates arising from an intravascular source (catheter or IE) were significantly more resistant than blood-stream isolates arising from a deep tissue source.[145] Finally, PMP-resistant *S. aureus* blood-stream isolates from patients with IE were significantly more likely to have arisen from an intravascular catheter source.[146]

The bacterial colonies are found beneath the surface of the vegetation (at variable depth, depending on the intracardiac location[147]), and infiltration by phagocyte cells is minimal; the vegetation creates an environment of impaired host resistance. These conditions allow for relatively unbridled bacterial growth, resulting in extremely high colony counts of 10⁹ to 10¹¹ bacteria per 1 g of tissue. Bacteria deep within the fibrin matrix have been shown by autoradiography to reach a state of reduced metabolic activity.[148] Studies by Yersin and Meddens and colleagues suggest that impairment of host defenses (e.g., neutropenia, corticosteroids) potentiates progression of the disease when the tricuspid, but not the aortic, valve is involved[149,150] but is largely dependent on the intracardiac location of the vegetation.[151] The role of granulocytes within the vegetation is unknown. When vegetation formation is retarded with anticoagulants in experimental animals with IE, the organisms seem to divide on the surface, total bacterial titers are lower, and the clinical disease is more explosive.[152,153] In addition, it has been suggested that phagocytosis of microorganisms by monocytes on or within the vegetation generates tissue thromboplastin formation; thromboplastin then acts as a stimulant to fibrin deposition and growth of the vegetation.[154] The best evidence suggests, however, that coagulation activation initiated by tissue factor,[155] with subsequent local thrombus formation, is responsible for the initiation of vegetation growth and persistence on the cardiac valve. It seems that some organisms (e.g., *S. aureus*) induce tissue factor production by endothelium without the necessity for host cytokines.[156]

Many important studies have elucidated the interaction between the invading microbe, the endothelium, the monocyte, and the pathogenesis of IE. After internalization by endothelial cells in vitro, microbes such as *S. aureus* evoke a potent proinflammatory chemokine response (e.g., increase in expression of interleukin-6 or interleukin-8 or of monocyte chemotactic peptide).[157,158] This event also is associated with increased expression on the endothelial cell surface of several key adhesion molecules, especially intercellular adhesion molecule 1 and vascular cell adhesion molecule 1.[109,157,158] Among other cells, monocytes are drawn into this endothelial cell microenvironment; via their appropriate counterreceptors, monocytes can bind avidly to such microbe-activated endothelial cells.[158] Extracellular bacteria circulating in the vascular system then bind directly to the monocyte surface, inducing the release of tissue thromboplastin (tissue factor).[159,160] This latter molecule participates in the catalytic conversion of prothrombin to thrombin, amplifying the procoagulant cascade at the site of endothelial cell colonization and leading to progressive evolution of the vegetative lesion in IE.

Immunopathologic Factors

IE causes the stimulation of humoral and cellular immunity as manifested by hypergammaglobulinemia, splenomegaly, and the presence of macrophages in the peripheral blood. The possibility that preformed antibody can increase the likelihood of the development of IE was suggested by the spontaneous occurrence of IE in horses receiving repeated immunizations with live pneumococci.[161] It was suggested that these antibodies produced bacterial agglutination in vivo, which increased the chances of valvular colonization. Studies in animals have suggested a protective role for circulating antibody. Rabbits preimmunized with heat-killed streptococci plus Freund's adjuvant had a significantly higher ID₅₀ than that noted for nonimmunized controls after aortic valve trauma.[162] Other studies have yielded similar results with *S. sanguis, S. mutans,* and *S. pneumoniae*.[163,164] In other experiments, antibody directed against cell surface components (including mannan) reduced the adhesion of *C. albicans* to fibrin and platelets in vitro and IE production in vivo.[165] This effect may depend on the infecting organism, however, because antibody to *S. epidermidis* and *S. aureus* does not prevent the development of IE in immunized animals or result in reduced bacterial concentrations in infected vegetations or kidneys,[166] perhaps because of the inability of immune sera to enhance opsonophagocytosis of staphylococci. The role of preformed antibody in the pathogenesis of IE is unclear. Intravascular agglutination of bacteria may decrease the frequency of IE by reducing the actual number of circulating organisms, but cross-protection is not achieved by passive transfer of high-titer immune globulin from *S. defectivus*–immunized rabbits to control animals.[164] Nitrogen mustard–treated immunized rabbits lose their ability to clear *S. defectivus* efficiently from the circulation, a process partially restored by neutrophil transfusion.[167]

The role of the glycocalyx of *S. aureus* and of antibodies directed against this exopolysaccharide in the pathogenesis of IE is controversial. Most experimental studies suggest that microencapsulation of strains by the common capsular types (5 and 8) may mitigate virulence of the organism in IE by obscuring key surface-expressed adhesins involved in colonization or persistence at endovascular damage sites.[168] Several more recent studies have suggested a salutary effect of active or passive immunization strategies against this glycocalyx in diminishing the induction, progression, or metastatic infection phases of experimental IE.[169,170]

Rheumatoid factor (anti-IgG IgM antibody) develops in about 50% of patients with IE of greater than 6 weeks' duration.[171] Rheumatoid factors have been found at the time of admission in 24% of patients with acute staphylococcal IE (<6 weeks' duration), and the frequency increased to 40% if fever persisted for 2 weeks after the initiation of antibiotic therapy.[172] More than two thirds of the patients became seronegative after 6 weeks of therapy, and two patients with a second episode of acute IE promptly redeveloped positive rheumatoid factors. The titers correlate with the level of hypergammaglobulinemia and decrease with therapy. Rheumatoid factor may play a role in the disease process by blocking IgG opsonic activity (by reacting with the Fc fragment), stimulating phagocytosis, or accelerating microvascular damage. Rheumatoid factor (IgM) has not been eluted from the immune complex glomerulonephritis associated with IE.[173] Antinuclear antibodies also occur in IE and may contribute to the musculoskeletal manifestations, low-grade fever, or pleuritic pain.[174]

IE, similar to malaria, schistosomiasis, syphilis, kala-azar, and leprosy, is associated with a constant intravascular antigenic challenge; the development of several classes of circulating antibody is not unexpected. Opsonic (IgG), agglutinating (IgG, IgM), and complement-fixing (IgG, IgM) antibodies and cryoglobulins (IgG, IgM, IgA, C3, fibrinogen); various antibodies to bacterial heat-shock proteins; and macroglobulins all have been described in IE.[175-177] Circulating immune complexes have been found in high titers in virtually all patients with IE.[178] Circulating immune complexes are found with increased frequency in connection with a long duration of illness, extravalvular manifestations, hypocomplementemia, and right-sided IE. Levels decrease and become undetectable with successful therapy. Patients with IE and circulating immune complexes may develop a diffuse glomerulonephritis that is analogous to the nephritis seen with infected ventriculoatrial shunts.[179] Corticosteroids have been used in a few patients with glomerulonephritis associated with IE.[180] Immune complexes plus complement are deposited subepithelially along the glomerular basement membrane to form a "lumpy-bumpy" pattern. Immune globulin eluted from these lesions has been shown to cross react with bacterial antigens.[181] In addition, bacterial antigens have been shown within circulating immune complexes.[182] Some of the peripheral manifestations of IE, such as Osler nodes, also may result from a deposition of circulating immune complexes. Pathologically, these lesions resemble an acute Arthus reaction. The finding of positive culture aspirates in Osler nodes[183] suggests, however, that they may be due to septic emboli rather than immune complex deposition. In some diffuse purpuric lesions in IE, immune complex deposits (IgG, IgM, and complement) have been shown in the dermal blood vessels by immunofluorescence.[184] Quantitative determinations of serum immune complex concentrations are useful in gauging the response to therapy. Effective treatment leads to a prompt decrease, with eventual disappearance of circulating immune complexes.[185] Conversely, therapeutic failures or relapses are characterized by rising titers or a reappearance of circulating immune complexes.[186]

Pathologic Changes

Heart

The classic vegetation of IE usually is located along the line of closure of a valve leaflet on the atrial surface for atrioventricular valves or the ventricular surface for semilunar valves. Vegetations may be single or multiple; are a few millimeters to several centimeters in size; and vary in color, consistency, and gross appearance. Microscopically the lesion consists primarily of fibrin, platelet aggregates, and bacterial masses; neutrophils and red blood cells are rare. Killed bacteria detectable by Gram stain within these vegetations sometimes may persist for months after therapy.[187] Destruction of the underlying valve may coexist. With treatment, healing occurs by fibrosis and occasionally calcification. The vegetation in acute cases is larger, softer, and more friable and may be associated with suppuration, more necrosis, and less healing than in subacute cases.[58,188] This infection may lead to perforation of the valve leaflet or rupture of the chordae tendineae, interventricular septum, or papillary muscle. Staphylococcal IE frequently results in valve ring abscesses[189] with fistula formation into areas of the myocardium or pericardial sac. Aneurysms of the valve leaflet or sinus of Valsalva also are common. Valvular stenosis may result from large vegetations. Myocarditis, myocardial infarction, and pericarditis[188,189] are found frequently at autopsy. Myocardial abscesses are found in 20% of the autopsy cases and are associated primarily with acute staphylococcal IE with hectic fever, a rapid onset of CHF, and conduction disturbances. Myocardial infarcts are found in 40% to 60% of the autopsied cases, often without diagnostic changes in the electrocardiogram. Pericarditis is much more common in acute IE.

Although echocardiographic abnormalities are common in patients with acquired immunodeficiency syndrome (AIDS), pericardial disease (pericarditis, effusions), myocardial disease leading to heart failure or arrhythmias, NBTE, and Kaposi's sarcoma all are more frequent than IE.[190] AIDS patients with IE usually are intravenous drug users with right-sided involvement, with an increase in the prevalence of cases due to *S. aureus* or fungi.[190,191] The clinical course in AIDS patients often is more fulminant than IE in intravenous drug users without AIDS; pneumonia and sepsis are common. IE also has been described in the transplanted heart.[192]

Embolic phenomena are common in IE. In the preantibiotic era, 70% to 95% of patients had clinically demonstrable embolic events, but this has decreased to 15% to 35% today. Pathologic evidence of embolization still is detected in 45% to 65% of autopsies, most frequently involving the renal, splenic, coronary, or cerebral circulation. Emboli and immune complex deposition contribute to the extracardiac manifestations of IE and may involve virtually any organ system. When large emboli occlude major vessels, fungal endocarditis, marantic endocarditis, or an intracardiac myxoma should be suspected.

Kidney

Three pathologic processes may be found in the kidney in IE: abscess, infarction, or glomerulonephritis. Abscesses are uncommon, but infarctions have been seen in 56% of the autopsy cases.[1] The kidney usually is normal in size but may be slightly swollen, and petechiae may be found in the capsule. When renal biopsy specimens are obtained during active IE, the renal architecture is abnormal in *all* cases,[193] even in the absence of clinical or biochemical evidence of renal disease. "Focal" glomerulonephritis is found in 48% to 88% of the cases but is rare in acute IE. It is a focal, local, and segmental process characterized by endothelial and mesangial proliferation, hemorrhage, neutrophilic infiltration, fibrinoid necrosis, crescent formation, and healing by fibrosis. Diffuse glomerulonephritis is found in 17% to 80% of the cases and consists of generalized cellular hyperplasia in all glomerular tufts. A less common condition called *membranoproliferative glomerulonephritis* is associated with IE due to *S. epidermidis* and is characterized by marked mesangial proliferation and by splitting of the glomerular basement membrane. Renal interstitial cellular infiltration is common.[193]

Of patients with IE, 10% to 15% exhibit an immune complex glomerulonephritis similar to that seen in lupus erythematosus.[179,181,185,186] The evidence for immune complex deposition rather than recurrent embolic phenomenon as the primary pathogenic mechanism includes the following:

1. Bacteria are rarely, if ever, seen in the lesions.
2. Glomerulonephritis can occur with right-sided IE.
3. Glomerulonephritis is rare in acute IE, even though large, friable vegetations result in widespread metastatic abscess formation.

4. Immunofluorescent staining with anti-immunoglobulin antibody reveals the typical lumpy-bumpy distribution seen in other forms of immune complex nephritis.

5. In diffuse glomerulonephritis, subepithelial electron-dense deposits are seen by electron microscopy, with IgG, IgM, IgA, or complement shown in these deposits by immunofluorescence.

6. Specific antibacterial antibody can be eluted from the lesions.[181]

7. Anti–glomerular basement membrane antibody has been found in a single case of IE with nephritis.

8. The glomerulonephritis often is accompanied by hypocomplementemia, with a positive result on serum assay for rheumatoid factor.

9. All these abnormalities usually resolve with successful antimicrobial therapy as the concentration of circulating immune complexes declines.

Mycotic Aneurysms

Mycotic aneurysms usually develop during active IE, but occasionally are detected months or years after successful treatment. They are more common with viridans streptococcal infections and are found in 10% to 15% of autopsied cases. They may arise by any of the following mechanisms: (1) direct bacterial invasion of the arterial wall with subsequent abscess formation or rupture, (2) septic or bland embolic occlusion of the vasa vasorum, or (3) immune complex deposition with resultant injury to the arterial wall. The aneurysms tend to occur at bifurcation points. They are found most commonly in the cerebral vessels (primarily the peripheral branches of the middle cerebral artery), but they also occur in the abdominal aorta; sinus of Valsalva; a ligated patent ductus arteriosus; and the splenic, coronary, pulmonary, and superior mesenteric arteries. Mycotic aneurysms usually are clinically silent until rupture occurs; consequently, their true incidence in active IE is unknown.[194]

Central Nervous System

Cerebral emboli are the most common neurologic manifestation of IE and occur in approximately 20% of all cases.[195,196] A multinational, prospective cohort investigation of 1024 cases of definite IE showed a cerebral embolization rate of 16.7%.[197] The middle cerebral artery and its branches are involved most commonly.[58] Three percent of the cerebral emboli from all causes are secondary to IE. Cerebral infarction, arteritis, abscesses, mycotic aneurysms, intracerebral or subarachnoid hemorrhage, encephalomalacia, cerebritis, and meningitis all have been reported.[198] Hemorrhagic transformation of an ischemic infarct due to septic emboli is the most common mechanism leading to fatal intracerebral hemorrhage during IE.[199] True acute purulent meningitis is rare except in pneumococcal endocarditis, but multiple microabscesses (cerebritis) due to *S. aureus* are relatively common in acute staphylococcal IE.

Spleen

Splenic infarctions have been reported in 44% of autopsy cases but often are clinically silent.[58] Splenic abscesses are an uncommon complication of IE and typically manifest with fever, left upper quadrant abdominal pain, and leukocytosis. Diagnosis is established by computed tomography (CT) or ultrasound.[200,201] Although splenectomy is a standard therapy for splenic abscess, percutaneous drainage may be an alternative in selected patients.[202] Splenic enlargement is common, and virtually all cases are associated with hyperplasia of the lymphoid follicles, an increase in secondary follicles, proliferation of reticuloendothelial cells, and scattered focal necrosis.[188] Occasional cases of spontaneous rupture of the spleen have been observed.

Lung

When right-sided IE is present, pulmonary embolism with or without infarction, acute pneumonia, pleural effusion, or empyema is common. The emboli may be septic or bland in type.[203]

Skin

Petechiae are found in 20% to 40% of cases (Fig. 74-2) (see later). Osler nodes consist microscopically of arteriolar intimal proliferation with extension to venules and capillaries and may be accompanied by

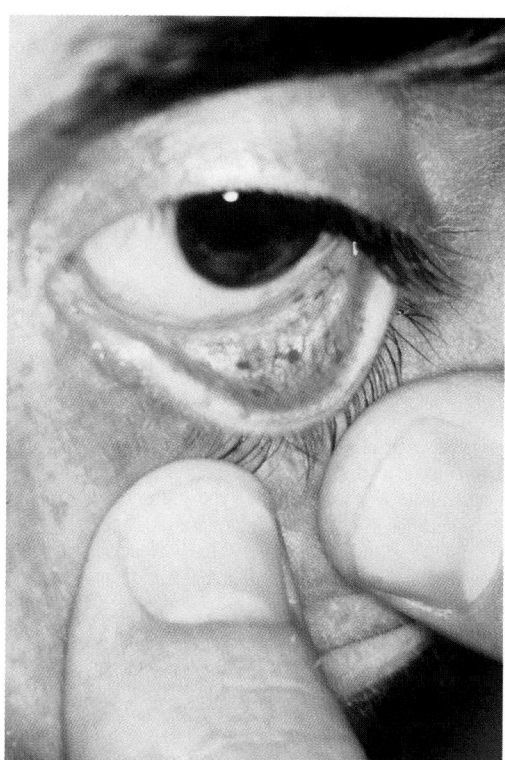

FIGURE 74-2. Conjunctival petechiae in a patient with bacterial endocarditis.

thrombosis and necrosis. A diffuse perivascular infiltrate consisting of neutrophils and monocytes surrounds the dermal vessels. Immune complexes have been shown in the dermal vessels. Janeway lesions consist of bacteria, neutrophilic infiltration, necrosis, and subcutaneous hemorrhage (Fig. 74-3). Janeway lesions are due to septic emboli and reveal subcutaneous abscesses on histologic examination.[204]

Eye

Roth spots consist microscopically of lymphocytes surrounded by edema and hemorrhage in the nerve fiber layer of the retina (Fig. 74-4).[205]

Clinical Manifestations

The interval between an event likely to produce high-grade bacteremia (e.g., dental extraction) and the onset of symptoms of IE, contrary to older estimates, is quite short. The so-called incubation period in 84% of 76 cases of streptococcal IE was less than 2 weeks.[206] The time from the onset of symptoms to diagnosis in the subacute form of IE is quite long, however, with a median interval of approximately 5 weeks. Symptom duration of cases managed in community hospitals is often shorter than in patients referred to a tertiary care center, reflecting "referral bias."[3]

The symptoms and signs (Table 74-3) are protean, and essentially any organ system may be involved. Four processes contribute to the clinical picture[58]: (1) the infectious process on the valve, including the local intracardiac complications; (2) bland or septic embolization to virtually any organ; (3) constant bacteremia, often with metastatic foci of infection; and (4) circulating immune complexes and other immunopathologic factors.[54-58,207,208] As a result, the clinical presentation of patients with IE is highly variable, and the differential diagnosis often is broad.[209] Because of its sometimes protean manifestations, the diagnosis of IE may be delayed or occasionally not clinically suspected and identified only on postmortem examination. In three different studies, 55% of 119 Danish patients with *S. aureus* IE identified from 1976 to 1981,[210] 32% of 260 Danish patients with *S. aureus* IE

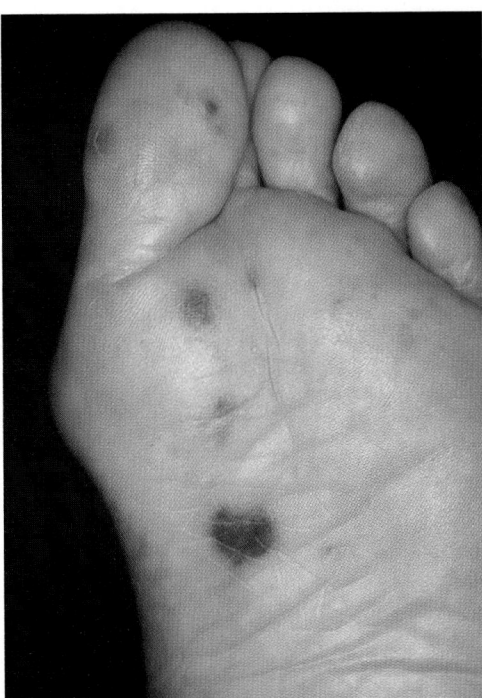

FIGURE 74-3. Janeway lesions in a patient with *Staphylococcus aureus* endocarditis. *(From Sande MA, Strausbaugh LJ. Infective endocarditis. In: Hook EW, Mandell GL, Gwaltney JM Jr, et al, eds. Current Concepts of Infectious Diseases. New York: Wiley Press; 1977. Copyright © 1977 Wiley Press. This material is used by permission of John Wiley & Sons, Inc.)*

identified from 1982 to 1991,[211] and 18% of 172 Brazilian IE patients[212] were not clinically suspected and were diagnosed with IE only at postmortem examination.

Fever is common but may be absent (5% of the cases), especially in the setting of CHF, renal failure, a terminal disease, old age,[213,214] or previous antibiotic therapy. The fever pattern is usually remittent, and the patient's temperature rarely exceeds 40° C (104° F) except in acute IE.[207] Persistent fever during antimicrobial therapy of IE is relatively uncommon but may be an ominous sign. In a review[215] of 123 patients

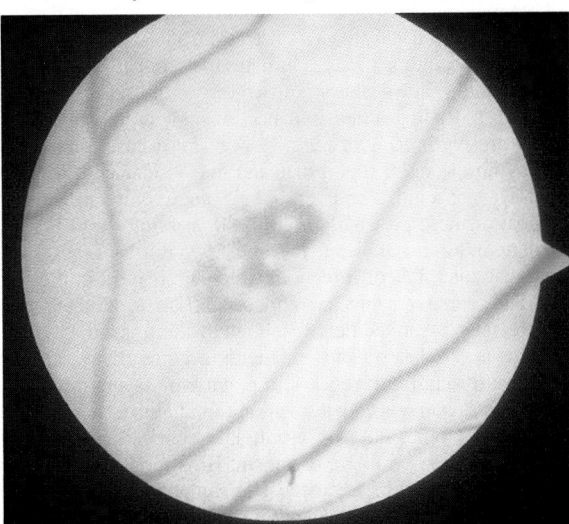

FIGURE 74-4. Retina from a patient with viridans streptococcal endocarditis showing Roth spots. *(From Sande MA, Strausbaugh LJ. Infective endocarditis. In: Hook EW, Mandell GL, Gwaltney JM Jr, et al, eds. Current Concepts of Infectious Diseases. New York: Wiley Press; 1977. Copyright © 1977 Wiley Press. This material is used by permission of John Wiley & Sons, Inc.)*

TABLE 74-3 Clinical Manifestations of Infective Endocarditis Myalgia/Arthralgia

Symptoms	Patients Affected (%)	Signs	Patients (%)
Fever	80	Fever	90
Chills	40	Heart murmur	85
Weakness	40	Changing murmur	5-10
Dyspnea	40	New murmur	3-5
Sweats	25	Embolic phenomenon	>50
Anorexia	25	Skin manifestations	18-50
Weight loss	25	Osler nodes	10-23
Malaise	25	Splinter hemorrhages	15
Cough	25	Petechiae	20-40
Skin lesions	20	Janeway lesion	<10
Stroke	20	Splenomegaly	20-57
Nausea/vomiting	20	Septic complications (e.g., pneumonia, meningitis)	20
Headache	20	Mycotic aneurysms	20
Myalgia/arthralgia	15	Clubbing	12-52
Edema	15	Retinal lesion	2-10
Chest pain	15	Signs of renal failure	10-25
Abdominal pain and delirium/coma	15		
Delirium/coma	10-15		
Hemoptysis	10		
Back pain	10		

Data from references 1, 27, 39 and 207.

with IE managed in Cleveland from 1972 to 1984, approximately half became afebrile within 3 days of the initiation of antibiotics; approximately 75% and approximately 90% had defervesced after 1 and 2 weeks of treatment. Prolonged fever ((2 weeks' duration) is associated with specific etiologic agents (i.e., *S. aureus,* gram-negative bacilli, fungi, culture-negative IE) and, perhaps more important, microvascular phenomena, embolization of major vessels, intracardiac (e.g., myocardial abscess) or peripheral complications, tissue infarction, a need for cardiac surgery, and a higher mortality rate.[215,216] Pulmonary emboli (bland), drug reactions, and nosocomial infection unrelated to IE also are causes of prolonged fever in this patient population.

Nonspecific symptoms, such as anorexia, weight loss, malaise, fatigue, chills, weakness, nausea, vomiting, and night sweats, are common, especially in subacute cases.[27] These nonspecific symptoms often result in an incorrect diagnosis of malignancy, collagen vascular disease, tuberculosis, or other chronic diseases.

Audible heart murmurs occur in greater than 85% of cases but may be absent with right-sided or mural infection. The classic "changing murmur" and the development of a new regurgitant murmur (usually aortic insufficiency) are uncommon and occur in 5% to 10% and in 3% to 5% of cases. When present, these are diagnostically useful signs and usually complicate acute staphylococcal disease. New or changing murmurs are less common in elderly patients and often lead to diagnostic confusion.[213,217] Greater than 90% of patients who show a new regurgitant murmur develop CHF. The incidence of CHF seems to be increasing (approximately 25% in 1966 and 67% in 1972),[27] and CHF now is the leading cause of death in IE. Pericarditis is rare but, when present, usually is accompanied by myocardial abscess formation as a complication of staphylococcal infection. Although valvular regurgitation is the most important hemodynamic complication of IE, hemodynamically significant valvular obstruction requiring surgery may occur rarely, even without a prior history of valvular stenosis.[218]

Although the classic peripheral manifestations previously were found in half of cases, the prevalence has decreased in recent years. Clubbing is present in 10% to 20%, especially if the disease is of long duration, and may recede with therapy. The complete syndrome of hypertrophic osteoarthropathy is rare. Splinter hemorrhages are linear red-to-brown streaks in the fingernails or toenails and are found commonly in IE. They are a nonspecific finding and are seen often in elderly patients or in patients with occupation-related trauma. These lesions are most suggestive of IE when located proximally in the nailbed. Petechiae are found in 20% to 40% of cases, particularly after a prolonged course, and usually appear in crops on the conjunctivae (see Fig. 74-2), buccal mucosa, palate, and extremities. These lesions initially are red and nonblanching but become brown and barely visible in 2 to 3 days. Petechiae may result from either local vasculitis or emboli. Osler nodes are small, painful, nodular lesions usually found in the pads of fingers or toes and occasionally in the thenar eminence. They are 2 to 15 mm in size and frequently are multiple and evanescent, disappearing in hours to days. Osler nodes are rare in acute cases of IE but occur in 10% to 25% of all cases. They are not specific for IE because they may be seen in systemic lupus erythematosus, marantic endocarditis, hemolytic anemia, and gonococcal infections and in extremities with cannulated radial arteries. Janeway lesions (see Fig. 74-3) are hemorrhagic, macular, painless plaques with a predilection for the palms or soles. They persist for several days and are thought to be embolic in origin and occur with greater frequency in staphylococcal IE. Roth spots (see Fig. 74-4) are oval, pale, retinal lesions surrounded by hemorrhage and usually are located near the optic disk. They occur in less than 5% of cases of IE; they also may be found in anemia, leukemia, and connective tissue disorders such as systemic lupus erythematosus.

Splenomegaly has been reported in 25% to 60% of all cases and is more common in patients with IE of prolonged duration. The incidence of splenomegaly seems to be decreasing progressively since the advent of antibiotics. Splenic septic emboli are common during IE, but localized signs and symptoms may be absent in approximately 90% of patients with this complication.[219] Abdominal CT is highly sensitive and should be employed in cases with prolonged fever or sepsis. Serial CT studies usually can distinguish between bland septic emboli and splenic abscess.[220]

Musculoskeletal manifestations are common in IE. In a review of 192 cases,[221] 44% of patients had musculoskeletal symptoms. These symptoms usually occurred early in the disease and were the only initial complaint in 15% of cases. They included proximal oligoarticular or monoarticular arthralgias (38%), lower extremity monoarticular or oligoarticular arthritis (31%), low back pain (23%), and diffuse myalgias (19%). The back pain may be severe, limiting movement, and may be the initial complaint in 5% to 10% of cases.[12] These findings may mimic findings in rheumatic disease, resulting in a diagnostic delay.

Major embolic episodes, as a group, are second only to CHF as a complication of IE and occur in at least one third of cases. Splenic artery emboli (as noted previously) with infarction may result in left upper quadrant abdominal pain with radiation to the left shoulder, a splenic or pleural rub, or a left pleural effusion. Renal infarctions may be associated with microscopic or gross hematuria, but renal failure, hypertension, and edema are uncommon. Retinal artery emboli are rare (occurring in <2% of the cases) and may be manifested by a sudden complete loss of vision. A panophthalmitis has been reported with pneumococcal IE. Pulmonary emboli secondary to right-sided IE constitute a common feature in narcotic addicts (see later). Coronary artery emboli usually arise from the aortic valve and may cause myocarditis with arrhythmias or myocardial infarction. This finding may be overlooked, especially given the time constraints of interventions such as thrombolytic therapy or angioplasty during acute myocardial infarction, resulting in serious complications in patients with IE presenting with an acute myocardial infarction.[222] Major vessel emboli (affecting the femoral, brachial, popliteal, or radial artery) are more common in fungal endocarditis.

Neurologic manifestations occur in 20% to 40% of cases and may dominate the clinical picture, especially in staphylococcal IE. Of patients with neurologic complications, 50% present with these signs and symptoms as the heralding features of their illness.[223,224] In a Finnish survey of 218 episodes of definite or possible IE, neurologic complications were identified in 55 episodes (25%), with an embolic event as the most common manifestation (23/55 [42%]). In most (76%) episodes, the neurologic manifestation was evident before antimicrobial treatment was started, being the first sign of IE in 47% of episodes.[195] The development of clinical neurologic deterioration during IE is

associated with a twofold to fourfold increase in mortality for the implicated etiologic microbe.[185] Mycotic aneurysms of the cerebral circulation occur in 2% to 10% of cases. They usually are single, small, and peripheral and may lead to devastating subarachnoid hemorrhage. Other features include seizures, severe headache, visual changes (particularly homonymous hemianopsias), choreoathetoid movements, mononeuropathy, and cranial nerve palsies. Toxic encephalopathy with symptoms ranging from a mild change in personality to frank psychosis may occur, especially in elderly patients.

Patients with IE may have symptoms of uremia. In the preantibiotic era, renal failure developed in 25% to 35% of the patients, but presently fewer than 10% are affected. When uremia does develop, diffuse glomerulonephritis with hypocomplementemia usually is found, but focal glomerulonephritis also has been implicated. Renal failure is more common with long-standing disease but usually is reversible with appropriate antimicrobial treatment alone. IE may be confused with thrombotic thrombocytopenic purpura when neurologic signs, fever, renal failure, anemia, and thrombocytopenia are present.[225]

Infective Endocarditis in Drug Addicts

Acute infection accounts for approximately 60% of hospital admissions among intravenous drug users; IE is implicated in 5% to 15% of these episodes.[226] It has proved difficult to predict accurately the presence of IE in a febrile drug addict,[227] especially from history and physical examination findings alone,[228] although cocaine use by an intravenous drug user should heighten the suspicion of IE.[229] Cocaine was associated strongly with the presence of IE in 102 intravenous drug users in San Francisco when findings were analyzed by logistic regression analysis, but no such correlation was found among febrile addicts who did not use cocaine. The most reliable predictors of IE in febrile parenteral drug users are visualization of vegetations by echocardiography and the presence of embolic phenomena.[228] Although many of the aforementioned clinical manifestations are seen in addicts with IE, several distinctions are noteworthy. In this group of patients, two thirds have no clinical evidence of underlying heart disease, and there is a predilection for the infection to affect the tricuspid valve. Only 35% of addicts ultimately proved to have IE show heart murmurs on admission.[226] The frequency of valvular involvement is as follows: tricuspid alone or in combination with others, 52.2%; aortic alone, 18.5%; mitral alone, 10.8%; and aortic plus mitral, 12.5%. Left-sided involvement has been more common in some series, however.[230] Data from Italy have suggested an increasing frequency of left-sided IE in the population.[231]

Of patients with tricuspid valve infection, 30% have pleuritic chest pain; pulmonary findings may dominate the clinical picture, and the chest radiograph shows abnormalities (e.g., infiltrates, effusion) in 75% to 85%.[232] Radiographic evidence of septic pulmonary emboli is eventually present in 87% of cases.[233] Signs of tricuspid insufficiency (gallop rhythm, systolic regurgitant murmur louder with inspiration, large V waves, or a pulsatile liver) are present in only one third of the cases. Most of these patients are 20 to 40 years old (80%), and men predominate in a ratio of 4 to 6:1. Almost two thirds of these patients have extravalvular sites of infection, which are helpful in the diagnosis.[232-234] The course of acute staphylococcal IE in an addict tends to be less severe than in nonaddicts,[232] although this may not be true in AIDS patients. HIV-seropositive patients acquire IE by one of two mechanisms: through intravenous drug abuse or as a complication of long-term central venous catheterization for administration of medications (e.g., for cytomegalovirus retinitis). In either situation, *S. aureus* is the most common etiologic organism. IE is more common among injection drug users with advanced HIV immunosuppression (CD4+ <200 cells/mm³) even after accounting for injection drug use behaviors.[234a] Conversely, among HIV-infected persons who do not practice injection drug use, IE is rare despite the increasing number of HIV-infected patients worldwide.[203] In the absence of intravenous drug abuse, HIV-seropositive patients develop left-sided and right-sided IE with equal frequencies.[235] In contrast, in the setting of intravenous drug abuse, HIV-seropositive patients develop predominantly right-sided IE.

The IE-related morbidity and mortality rates in HIV-seropositive patients who do not have an AIDS-defining illness or criteria are similar to rates in HIV-seronegative counterparts.[235]

Laboratory Findings

Hematologic parameters often are abnormal in IE, but none is diagnostic. Anemia is nearly always present (70% to 90% of cases), especially in subacute cases, and has the characteristics of the anemia of chronic disease, with normochromic, normocytic indices, a low serum iron concentration, and a low iron-binding capacity. The anemia tends to worsen with the duration of the illness. Thrombocytopenia occurs in 5% to 15% of cases but is common in neonatal IE. Leukocytosis is present in 20% to 30% of cases but is rare in the subacute variety, whereas counts of 15,000/mm³ to 25,000/mm³ are common in acute IE. The differential count usually is normal, but there may be a slight shift to the left. Leukopenia is uncommon (5% to 15%) and, when present, usually is associated with splenomegaly. Large mononuclear cells (histiocytes) can be detected in the peripheral blood in approximately 25% of patients, but the yield is higher in blood obtained by earlobe puncture. This finding is nonspecific because similar cells have been found in malaria, typhus, typhoid fever, and tuberculosis.

The erythrocyte sedimentation rate is nearly always (in 90% to 100% of cases) elevated, with a mean value of 57 mm/hr found in one large series.[27] In the absence of renal failure, CHF, or disseminated intravascular coagulation, a normal erythrocyte sedimentation rate is evidence against a diagnosis of IE. Hypergammaglobulinemia is detected in 20% to 30% of the cases and may be accompanied by a plasmacytosis in the bone marrow aspirate. A positive result on assay for rheumatoid factor is found in 40% to 50% of cases, especially when the duration of the illness is greater than 6 weeks.[171] Hypocomplementemia (seen in 5% to 15% of cases) parallels the incidence of abnormal renal function test results (elevated creatinine level in 5% to 15%). A false-positive result on Venereal Disease Research Laboratory testing is uncommon (0.2%). Lyme serologic tests may be positive in patients with IE living in areas endemic for Lyme disease, which may lead to diagnostic confusion and delay.[236]

The urinalysis frequently is abnormal; proteinuria occurs in 50% to 65% of cases, and microscopic hematuria occurs in 30 to 60%. Red blood cell casts may be seen in 12% of cases.[27] Gross hematuria, pyuria, white blood cell casts, and bacteriuria also may be found.

Circulating immune complexes can be detected in most cases of IE but also are found in 32% of patients with septicemia but without endocarditis, in 10% of healthy persons, and in 40% of noninfected narcotic addicts.[171] Levels of aggregated human immune globulin equivalent to or greater than 100 μg/mL were found only in IE (35% of the cases), however. Detection of high levels of immune complexes may be useful in the diagnosis of right-sided IE in narcotic addicts or in culture-negative cases. In addition, because the levels decline with appropriate treatment, serial measurement of immune complexes may assist in management of the disease.[185,186] Mixed-type cryoglobulins are detectable in 84% to 95% of patients with IE, but also constitute a nonspecific finding. Serial determination of the serum C-reactive protein concentration, although nonspecific and virtually always elevated in IE, may be useful to monitor therapy and detect intercurrent complications or infections.[237]

The detection of vegetations by gallium 67 myocardial imaging initially seemed to be a useful diagnostic tool. Of 11 patients in one study,[238] 7 had infected vegetations localized by scans, including one culture-negative case that was confirmed at autopsy. Further studies are needed to determine the potential value of noninvasive imaging of cardiac vegetations by using a radiolabeled compound, such as technetium 99m–labeled antibacterial antibody[239] and indium 111 (¹¹¹In)–labeled platelets[240]; both compounds have shown promise in experimental IE. At present, these techniques must be considered investigational. Radiographic techniques occasionally are useful in the diagnosis or in decisions regarding surgical intervention. CT of the abdomen detected splenic infarcts in 6 of 25 (24%) consecutive patients with IE in one series[241]; 2 of these 6 patients were asymptomatic.

The blood culture is the most important laboratory test performed in a diagnostic workup for IE. The bacteremia is usually continuous and low grade (80% of the cases have <100 CFU/mL of blood).[242] In approximately two thirds of cases, all the blood specimens drawn yield positive results on culture.[27] When bacteremia is present, the first two blood cultures yield the etiologic agent more than 90% of the time. In a review of 206 cases of IE seen over a 15-year period at The New York Hospital,[243] 95% of the blood cultures were positive. In streptococcal endocarditis, the first blood culture was positive in 96% of cases, and one of the first two cultures was positive in 98%. When antibiotics had been administered in the previous 2 weeks, the rate of positive cultures declined from 97% to 91% ($P < .02$). The influence of outpatient antibiotic administration on blood culture positivity was more significant in another retrospective analysis[244]; 64% of 88 cultures were positive in 17 patients receiving antibiotics before hospitalization versus 100% in 15 patients without antibiotic exposure. In nonstreptococcal IE, the first blood culture was positive in 86% of the cases, and when two cultures were taken, the first culture was positive in 100%. Most blood cultures contained only a few organisms; greater than 50% of the cultures contained 1 to 30 bacteria/mL. Only 17% of the cultures yielded more than 100 bacteria/mL. The bacteremia also was constant, with little variation in quantitative culture determinations in any individual patient. The sensitivity of blood cultures for the detection of streptococci is particularly susceptible to prior antibiotic therapy and is affected by the media employed.[245] Continuous monitoring blood culture systems (e.g., BACTEC, BacT/ALERT) are significantly more sensitive than conventional methods.

On the basis of these studies, the following procedures for culturing blood are recommended. At least three blood culture sets (no more than two bottles per venipuncture) should be obtained in the first 24 hours. More specimens may be necessary if the patient has received antibiotics in the preceding 2 weeks. At least 10 mL of blood (when feasible) should be injected into trypticase soy (or brain-heart infusion) and thioglycolate broth.[246,247] Supplementation with 15% sucrose (in an attempt to isolate cell wall–deficient forms) or the use of pre-reduced anaerobic media is unrewarding.[248] The newer commercial media also are effective, but comparative data are few. In general, culture of arterial blood offers no advantage over use of venous blood. Inspection for macroscopic growth should be performed daily, and routine subcultures should be done on days 1 and 3. The cultures should be held for at least 3 weeks. When gram-positive cocci grow on the initial isolation but fail to grow on subculture, nutritionally variant (thiol-dependent) streptococci (including *Granulicatella* spp.) should be suspected.[249] In this event, subculture inoculation should be onto media supplemented with either 0.05% to 0.1% L-cysteine or 0.001% pyridoxal phosphate.

Intraleukocytic bacteria have been visualized in peripheral blood in approximately 50% of cases[250] by a simple "monolayer" technique. This technique may be helpful in culture-negative cases or when patients have been receiving antibiotics.[251]

Ribitol teichoic acids are major constituents of the cell wall of staphylococci. Gel diffusion and counterimmunoelectrophoresis techniques have been used to detect teichoic acid antibodies in the serum of patients suspected of having *S. aureus* IE. Because of problems with false-positive and false-negative results, this test rarely is used now.

Special Diagnostic Tests

Special diagnostic tests are not used routinely (with the exception of echocardiography) in all cases of IE but may be useful in two situations: (1) in the diagnostic approach to culture-negative IE and (2) in decisions about surgical intervention during active infection. The incidence of so-called blood culture–negative endocarditis has ranged from 2.5% to 31% in published series.[252,253] If the patient has not received previous antibiotic therapy and the blood cultures are obtained as outlined, these cases should represent fewer than 5% of the total.[2] Some of the aforementioned tests (assays for rheumatoid factor and teichoic acid antibodies, examination of earlobe blood specimens for histiocytes, monolayer technique for detection of intraleukocytic bacteria) may be helpful in identifying such cases, but other procedures often are necessary. If the patient has received antibiotics, blood cultures in hypertonic media may allow detection of cell wall–defective organisms. Supplementation of media with vitamin B_6 or with cysteine may assist in the recovery of NVS. The lysis-centrifugation blood culture technique assists in the detection of staphylocci[254] and fungi, but NVS (now classified as *Abiotrophia* spp.) do not survive this procedure, and yields of pneumococci and anaerobes are decreased.[255] Routine use of this technique is not indicated, but it may be helpful in suspected culture-negative cases of IE. Because some anaerobes, *Brucella* spp., and members of the HACEK group (see "Unusual Gram-Negative Bacteria") are slow-growing organisms, holding cultures for 4 weeks may increase the recovery rate. Special efforts to neutralize or inactivate antimicrobial agents present in blood, such as the addition of penicillinase or of antibiotic-removal resins, do not enhance substantially the yield of positive blood cultures in IE and increase the incidence of laboratory contamination of the blood culture. These maneuvers are not recommended routinely.[256,257] Most automated blood culture detection systems use blood collection vials with antibiotic-binding resins. Cultures of bone marrow or urine rarely may be positive when blood cultures are negative. Serologic studies are necessary for the diagnosis of Q fever or murine typhus.[258] Psittacosis endocarditis usually is diagnosed with serologic methods, but one more recent case[259] yielded positive blood and pharyngeal cultures. Special culture techniques (e.g., for *Legionella* spp.[260]) are indicated in patients with suspected prosthetic valve IE when initial cultures are "negative." *Bartonella*, recognized as an important cause of apparent blood culture–negative IE (especially in homeless alcoholic patients), also can be isolated by prolonged incubation and subculture of the aerobic broth media.[261-265] Subculture on endothelial cell tissue may isolate *Bartonella* in certain cases.[261] Serologic strategies also may assist in the diagnosis of *Bartonella* IE.[262] In addition to blood culture and serodiagnostic strategies, as outlined previously, culture of valvular tissue or vegetations that have embolized to peripheral arteries and that have been removed surgically may yield the causative organism. Microscopy of these tissues, including direct fluorescence antibody techniques and electron microscopy, may assist in making the etiologic diagnosis, particularly in cases caused by fastidious or intracellular pathogens, such as *Tropheryma whippelii*,[266] *Chlamydia, Coxiella burnetii*,[267] and *Legionella*.[268] Molecular techniques to recover specific DNA or 16S ribosomal RNA from tissue samples have been useful diagnostically in selected cases,[269] and polymerase chain reaction studies performed on blood or serum may be useful for the diagnosis of IE caused by difficult-to-grow pathogens, such as *Bartonella*.[270] In an investigation comparing broad-range polymerase chain reaction results on resected endocardial specimens from 49 patients with suspected IE with results of culture and Gram staining of resected specimens and Duke criteria, bacterial DNA was shown within cardiac tissue in 18% of patients with sterile blood cultures.[271] Other tests to exclude collagen vascular diseases usually are necessary in patients undergoing evaluation for culture-negative native valve IE.[272]

Blood cultures are negative in more than 50% of cases of fungal IE.[273] The lysis-centrifugation method of blood culture also is useful in detecting fungi. This form of the disease is increasing in frequency and usually affects narcotic addicts, patients with prosthetic valves, or hospitalized patients receiving antibiotics or hyperalimentation or both.[274] Low-birth-weight neonates seem particularly prone to *Candida* IE, predominantly on the tricuspid valve or right atrial mural endocardium.[275] The rate of prosthetic valve endocarditis among fungemic patients with prosthetic heart valves was approximately 25% in one retrospective series.[276] The Castaneda principle (a culture of blood in a bottle containing agar and liquid broth) has been shown to increase the yield of fungal cultures.[248] Blastospores and pseudohyphae have been found in Wright-stained peripheral blood in at least one case of *Candida*-induced endocarditis.[277] Various serologic procedures have been used in an attempt to substantiate a diagnosis of fungal IE. Tests

for the determination of anti-*Candida* antibody are poorly standardized, variably sensitive, often nonspecific, and difficult to interpret.[278] In a rabbit model of *Candida*-induced endocarditis, precipitating and agglutinating antibodies were detected after 12 days of active infection, and titers rose progressively until death of the animals.[279] In contrast, animals without IE developed only a transient rise in antibody titers after a single intravenous injection of viable *C. albicans*. Tests for mannan antigenemia (a constituent of the cell wall of *Candida*) or enolase by hemagglutination inhibition and by enzyme-linked immunosorbent assay[280,281] have been reported as helpful in the diagnosis of disseminated candidiasis. In addition, a reliable radioimmunoassay for the detection of *Aspergillus* antigenemia currently is under investigation. When embolism to major vessels occurs, an embolectomy should be performed, and the material should be examined by special fungal stains and culture. Identification of the fungus by either technique is diagnostic of fungal IE even when blood cultures are sterile.

The use of echocardiography in the diagnosis of IE first was reported in 1973.[282] Echocardiograms have identified vegetations correctly on all valves. Most reports have focused on left-sided disease. The sensitivity and the specificity of this technique are uncertain; however, two studies correctly identified 33 of 52 vegetations documented surgically or at autopsy with transthoracic methods.[283,284] The characteristic finding is a shaggy, dense band of irregular echoes in a nonuniform distribution on one or more leaflets, with full unrestricted motion of the valve. The smallest vegetation detected was approximately 2 mm, but the acoustic impedance of the mass relative to the surrounding structures is a more important factor than size in identifying the vegetation. The use of two-dimensional, cross-sectional, real-time techniques improves the diagnostic accuracy over M-mode methods.[285] If the vegetation is calcified (which may occur early and independent of the healing process), the sensitivity of echocardiography may be increased. Echocardiography has localized vegetations correctly in culture-negative cases. Echocardiography may be of special value in the detection of the large friable vegetations characteristic of fungal IE. Use of M-mode or two-dimensional transthoracic techniques with prosthetic heart valves has been disappointing, however, because of the difficulty in resolution around the prosthetic device.

Many reports[286] have evaluated the role of transthoracic echocardiography (TTE) in the diagnosis and management of suspected IE and have been summarized in cogent analyses.[287,288] It seems from most analyses that TTE should be performed in all patients in whom IE seems to be a reasonable diagnosis. In contrast, TTE is not an appropriate screening test in the evaluation of febrile patients in whom IE is unlikely on clinical grounds or in bacteremic patients with organisms that rarely cause IE (e.g., *E. coli*), particularly if there is another obvious focus to explain the clinical syndrome; TTE may be overused in such low-risk situations.[289] TTE may be technically inadequate in 20% of adult patients owing to obesity, chronic obstructive pulmonary disease, or chest wall deformities. These studies also suggest the following: (1) TTE has variable sensitivity for the detection of vegetations (<50% to >90% positive), indicating that a negative study does not exclude IE; (2) the sensitivity of TTE for detecting vegetations is highest in right-sided IE because the tricuspid and pulmonic valves lie relatively close to the chest wall; (3) false-positive results are extremely rare; (4) only technically adequate studies are of value, a characteristic dependent on the experience of the person performing the examination; (5) echocardiography is extremely valuable in assessing local complications of IE, especially surrounding the aortic valve (however, the sensitivity for detecting these complications is relatively low for TTE [see later]); and (6) patients with a "vegetation" identified by echocardiography are at an increased risk for subsequent systemic emboli, CHF, the need for emergency surgery, and death, especially with aortic valve involvement. This apparent influence on prognosis has hastened earlier surgery in some cases,[290] but this point is controversial.[288,291]

Positive findings on the echocardiogram in a patient with IE should serve as adjunctive evidence, together with clinical parameters, in indicating surgical intervention. In one analysis from the Mayo Clinic,[292] emboli were not statistically more common in patients with left-sided native valve IE and echocardiographically documented vegetations within 72 hours of beginning antimicrobial therapy compared with patients without vegetations visualized by transthoracic techniques. The occurrence of emboli was correlated positively with the infecting microorganism, being more common in IE due to viridans streptococci than in IE due to *S. aureus*. Most studies suggest that mitral valve vegetations (particularly vegetations attached to the anterior leaflet), regardless of size, are associated with higher rates of embolization (25%) than are noted with aortic valve vegetations (10%). This association implicates the mechanical effects of abrupt mitral valve leaflet excursions, occurring twice per heart beat, in enhancing the embolic potential of vegetations.[293] Visualization of vegetations by echocardiography is not sufficient to prompt early surgery.[288,294] Serial echocardiograms often reveal the persistence of vegetations after successful therapy, but sequential studies may be useful in the timing of surgical intervention. Although still controversial, larger vegetation size has been associated with an increased risk of cerebral emboli. One large meta-analysis incorporating data from 10 studies on 738 patients showed that large vegetation size (>1 cm) was associated independently with increased risk for stroke.[295] Short-term changes in vegetation size during therapy do not correlate well with clinical outcome.[296]

A new technique, digital image processing of two-dimensional echocardiograms, may differentiate active from healed lesions.[297] If substantiated, this method may be useful in culture-negative cases (particularly with suspected recurrent IE) or when the response to therapy is suboptimal or inconclusive. One study suggested that an increase in vegetation size as seen by echocardiography during therapy of IE may identify a subset of patients with a higher rate of complications, independent of the presence of persistent bacteremia or overt clinical stigmata of IE.[298,299] Some studies have suggested that highly mobile vegetations constitute an independent increase in risk for complications in IE.[300] In other studies, vegetation mobility on echocardiography has not been an important independent risk factor for embolic events in IE because it is correlated strongly with vegetation size.[259,290]

One problem in considering the significance of these echocardiographic characteristics is the high degree of interobserver variability in interpreting the echocardiography images.[301] In one investigation involving four readers independently interpreting TTE studies from 41 cases of IE, investigators agreed on vegetation mobility in 57%, vegetation shape in 36%, and vegetation attachment in 40% of cases.[302] Transesophageal echocardiography (TEE) has altered the diagnostic approach to some patients with suspected IE.[303-308] TEE uses a 5-mHz phased array transducer with Doppler and color flow encoding capabilities mounted on the tip of a flexible endoscope. Biplane (horizontal and longitudinal) or omniplane imaging is preferred over TTE imaging because of (1) better spatial resolution with a higher frequency transducer; (2) lack of acoustic interference from the lungs, chest wall, and so forth; and (3) proximity to posterior structures (e.g., mitral valve, left atrium, interatrial septum, descending aorta).[305] TEE has proved useful in a wide variety of clinical situations, including detection of possible sources of emboli, diagnosis of thoracic aortic dissection, detection of prosthetic valve dysfunction, and evaluation of IE.[288,303-305] Intraoperative TEE imaging has become a valuable new tool, often providing real-time feedback to the surgical team during the procedure.

TEE is more sensitive than conventional TTE in the detection of intracardiac vegetations (approximately 95% and 60% to 65%), particularly in the setting of prosthetic valves (see Chapter 75). In one report of 96 patients with IE,[306] the sensitivity of TEE was 100% versus 63% for TTE, with identical specificity values (98%). The advantage of TEE was particularly evident for vegetations less than 10 mm in diameter. In another study,[307] vegetations were detected by TEE in 82% versus 69% for TTE. Although negative results on TEE do not exclude IE,[303-305,308] the procedure should be considered in patients with suspected IE and negative results on TTE. Potential sources of false-negative TEE studies include small vegetations and previous embolization of vegetations. When the clinical suspicion of IE is high and results of an initial TEE examination are negative, another TEE study is warranted within 7 to 10 days.[241] TEE also has become the procedure of choice for the detection of perivalvular extension of infection in patients with IE.[309,310] Daniel and colleagues[310] reported diagnostic sensitivity and specificity of 87% and 95% for TEE for detection of IE-related abscess versus 28% and 99% for TTE. Other investigations have shown TEE to be superior in the diagnosis of valvular perforation,[311] pacemaker IE,[312] eustachian valve IE,[313] IE in the elderly,[314] and other presentations. TEE should be performed (unless contraindicated, e.g., by significant esophageal disease) in all IE patients with a complicated course when perivalvular extension is suspected. Magnetic resonance imaging (MRI) also seems promising for the detection of these complications,[309] but clinical experience is limited.

TEE is not a screening or noninvasive procedure but is generally safe[315] in experienced hands, and it may alter management in selected patients with proved or suspected IE. Two cost-effectiveness analyses favor the increased use of TEE.[316,317] Using outcomes among a cohort of consecutive patients with intravascular catheter–associated *S. aureus* bacteremia, Rosen and colleagues[317] found that TEE was a cost-effective method of defining the duration of antibiotic therapy (2 weeks versus 4 weeks) compared with empirical courses of either 2 weeks or 4 weeks. Similarly a decision analysis by Heidenreich and co-workers[316] found TEE to be more cost-effective than TTE among patients with a high pretest probability of endocarditis (defined as 4% to 60%).

In conjunction with the physical examination, phonocardiography, and electrocardiography, the echocardiogram may play an important role in assessing the severity of acute aortic insufficiency in cases of active IE.[318] In this setting, classic signs, such as a wide pulse pressure and bounding pulses, often are absent; however, there is usually a reduction in intensity of the first heart sound, and Austin Flint murmurs may be audible. Findings on the chest roentgenogram and electrocardiogram may be normal. The degree of mitral valve preclosure (as determined by echocardiography) correlates with the acute elevation in left ventricular end-diastolic pressure. If this event occurs before the Q wave on the electrocardiogram, urgent surgical intervention is recommended.

Cardiac catheterization with quantitative blood cultures obtained proximal and distal to suspected sites of infection has been useful in selected cases in the localization of vegetations in right-sided and left-sided IE.[319] Multiple specimens from identical sites are necessary because minor fluctuations in bacteremia do occur. Cardiac catheterization provides valuable hemodynamic and anatomic information in patients with IE when surgical intervention is being considered.[234] Properly performed, the procedure is safe, as shown by the lack of postcatheterization emboli or hemodynamic deterioration in 35 consecutive patients in one series.[320]

Previous diagnostic criteria for IE were published in 1982 by von Reyn and colleagues[2] (Beth Israel criteria), but these criteria did not use echocardiographic findings in the case definitions, despite major improvements in echocardiographic technology (see previous discussion). In addition, the isolation of a "typical" IE pathogen from blood cultures was not considered in the Beth Israel definitions. Many presumptive cases of IE were classified as not *definite* but *probable*. With improved methodology *and* recognition of the central role of echocardiography in the evaluation of suspected IE, new case definitions and diagnostic criteria (the Duke criteria), proposed in 1994, now are used widely and have been accepted by most clinicians (Tables 74-4 and 74-5).[321] The new definitions retain, in slightly modified form, the pathologic parameters of the Beth Israel criteria[2] (see Table 74-4). The Duke criteria (modeled after the Jones criteria for diagnosing rheumatic fever[322]) build on the Beth Israel criteria by including echocardiographic demonstration of vegetations or paravalvular complications of IE and the isolation of typical IE pathogens from blood cultures as "major criteria" for the clinically definite categorization of IE. In addition, the presence of recent injection drug abuse is included in the Duke criteria as a "minor criterion" for diagnosing IE, recognizing the increased risk of IE in this patient population (see Table 74-5). Direct comparisons of the Duke and Beth Israel criteria have been done in 11 major studies, including nearly 1400 patients. Patient populations

TABLE 74-4 Proposed Criteria for Diagnosis of Infective Endocarditis

Definite infective endocarditis
  Pathologic criteria
    Microorganisms: shown by culture *or* histology in a vegetation, or in a vegetation that has embolized, or in an intracardiac abscess, *or*
    Pathologic lesions: vegetation or intracardiac abscess present, confirmed by histology showing active endocarditis
  Clinical criteria (using specific definitions for these terms [see Table 74-5])
    2 major criteria, *or*
    1 major and 3 minor criteria, *or*
    5 minor criteria
Possible infective endocarditis: findings consistent with infective endocarditis that fall short of *Definite*, but not *Rejected*
Rejected
  Firm alternate diagnosis explaining evidence of infective endocarditis, *or*
  Resolution of endocarditis syndrome, with antibiotic therapy for ≤4 days, *or*
  No pathologic evidence of infective endocarditis at surgery or autopsy, after antibiotic therapy for ≤4 days

Adapted from Durack DT, Lukes AS, Bright DK, et al. New criteria for diagnosis of infective endocarditis. Am J Med. 1994;96:200-209. With permission from Excerpta Medica, Inc.

from diverse geographic areas with presumed IE that have been studied include young, middle-aged, and elderly adults; pediatric patients; patients with native or prosthetic valve involvement; and injection drug abuse and non–injection drug abuse patients. These studies confirmed the increased sensitivity of the Duke criteria in clinically diagnosing IE and the diagnostic utility of echocardiography in identifying clinically definite cases (reviewed in detail by Bayer and associates[323]). Modifications of the Duke criteria, to provide a "floor" for diagnosis of putative cases as "possible IE," have yielded more specificity to the schema.[324]

TABLE 74-5 Terminology Used in the Proposed Criteria for Infective Endocarditis

Major Criteria
Positive blood culture for infective endocarditis
  Typical microorganism for infective endocarditis from 2 separate blood cultures
    Viridans streptococci, *Streptococcus bovis*, HACEK group*, *or*
    Community-acquired *Staphylococcus aureus* or enterococci, in the absence of a primary focus, *or*
  Persistently positive blood cultures for any microorganism (i.e., from blood cultures drawn >12 hours apart), *or*
  All of 3 or most of ≥4 separate blood cultures, with first and last specimens drawn at least 1 hour apart
Evidence of endocardial involvement
  Findings on echocardiogram positive for infective endocarditis
    Oscillating intracardiac mass on valve or supporting structures or in the path of regurgitant jets, or on iatrogenic devices, in the absence of an alternative anatomic explanation, *or*
    Abscess, *or*
    New partial dehiscence of prosthetic valve, *or*
  New valvular regurgitation (increase or change in preexisting murmur *not* sufficient)

Minor Criteria
Predisposition: predisposing heart condition *or* intravenous drug use
Fever: ≥38° C (≥100.4° F)
Vascular phenomena: arterial embolism, septic pulmonary infarcts, mycotic aneurysm, intracranial hemorrhage, Janeway lesions
Immunologic phenomena: glomerulonephritis, Osler nodes, Roth spots, rheumatoid factor
Echocardiogram: findings consistent with infective endocarditis but not meeting major criteria above
Microbiologic evidence: positive blood culture but not meeting major criteria above, *or* serologic evidence of active infection with organism consistent with infective endocarditis

*As discussed in the text later on, the HACEK organisms are *Haemophilus, Actinobacillus, Cardiobacterium, Eikenella,* and *Kingella.*
Adapted from Durack DT, Lukes AS, Bright DK, et al. New criteria for diagnosis of infective endocarditis. Am J Med. 1994;96:200-209.

Etiologic Agents

Streptococci

A plethora of microorganisms have been implicated in IE, but streptococci and staphylococci account for 80% to 90% of the cases in which identification is made. The most common etiologic agents are outlined in Table 74-6. The streptococci traditionally have been the most common cause of IE,[39] and many community hospitals still report viridans streptococci as the most common isolates among patients with IE.[325,236] Staphylococci have assumed increasing importance, however, among isolates in community hospitals in recent years (see later).[12,326] Viridans streptococci remain the major cause of IE in children. The disease usually runs a subacute course with multiple nonspecific symptoms (see Table 74-3). Greater than 80% of these patients have underlying heart disease. IE in young women with isolated mitral valve involvement almost universally is caused by viridans streptococci. Approximately 20% of cases are seen because of embolic phenomena. With modern medical and surgical management, the cure rate should exceed 90% in nonenterococcal streptococcal IE, although complications may ensue in more than 30% of cases.[325]

The nomenclature of the streptococci is confusing, and various authors differ in terminology used. As detailed in Chapter 192, current names for the α-hemolytic streptococci other than *S. pneumoniae* (i.e., viridans streptococci) causing IE are *S. mitis, S. sanguis, S. mutans, Streptococcus salivarius,* NVS (now classified as *Abiotrophia* spp.), and some isolates of the *Streptococcus intermedius* group (*S. intermedius* and *Streptococcus anginosus*). *Streptococcus morbillorum* now is classified as *Gemella morbillorum*; *Streptococcus mitior* now is considered to be a "genospecies" of *S. mitis.* The name *S. mitior* is embedded so deeply in the endocarditis literature, however, that it is retained in the discussion that follows. Group D streptococci are sometimes α-hemolytic, depending on the conditions and the isolate, but are not included among the viridans streptococci. Streptococci of the viridans group (not a true species) are α-hemolytic and usually nontypable by the Lancefield system.

The most common streptococci isolated from cases of IE are *S. sanguis, Streptococcus bovis, S. mutans,* and *S. mitior.*[86] In a series of 317 cases of streptococcal IE, the breakdown was as follows: α-hemolytic, 45%; nonhemolytic, non–group D, 21%; group D, 25%; pyogenic (groups A, B, C, G), 5%; miscellaneous, 3%; and aerococci, 1.3%. The α-hemolytic strains included *S. sanguis* (16.4% of all cases of IE), non–dextran-producing *S. mitior* (13.2%), dextran-positive *S. mitior* (7.3%), and an unclassified group (7.9%). Some isolates of *S. sanguis,* formerly called *Streptococcus SBE,* are in Lancefield group H; however, most are nontypable. *S. mutans* (14.2%), *S. anginosus* (5.4%), and *S. salivarius* (1.3%) composed the nonhemolytic, non–group D strains. Group D organisms included the enterococci (8%) and *S. bovis* (17%). In another analysis,[327] viridans streptococci caused 58% of cases of IE at The New York Hospital from 1970 to 1978. The various responsible species were as follows: *S. mitior,* 31%; *S. bovis,* 27%; *S. sanguis,* 24%; *S. mutans,* 7%; vitamin B$_6$–dependent *S. mitior,* 5%; *S. anginosus,* 4%; and others, 2%—all of which are

TABLE 74-6 Etiologic Agents in Infective Endocarditis

Agent	Cases (%)
Streptococci	60-80
Viridans streptococci	30-40
Enterococci	5-18
Other streptococci	15-25
Staphylococci	20-35
Coagulase-positive	10-27
Coagulase-negative	1-3
Gram-negative aerobic bacilli	1.5-13
Fungi	2-4
Miscellaneous bacteria	<5
Mixed infections	1-2
Culture-negative	<5-24

slightly different from the species reported from the United Kingdom. A similar species distribution was observed in 48 patients (with 51 episodes of IE) reported from Washington, DC.[328] By contrast, group D streptococci constituted 25% of all cases of IE within 6 regions of France representing 16 million inhabitants.[10] There seems to be no correlation, however, between the clinical outcome and the species involved,[238,325] with the exception of nutritionally deficient strains (see later). Viridans streptococci are the most commonly isolated pathogens in IE cases associated with mitral valve prolapse.[329] The relative role of each species overall is problematic, however, because species designations of identical strains among laboratories often are disparate,[325] and most blood and cerebrospinal fluid isolates of viridans or nonhemolytic streptococci are not from patients with IE.[330]

S. mutans, the etiologic agent in 14.2% of the cases in the review by Parker and Ball,[86] is microaerophilic, pleomorphic, and fastidious. Two thirds of strains hydrolyze bile-esculin,[331] a test used to identify group D organisms, and may be confused with enterococci. Other characteristics of *S. mutans* include the absence of group D antigen (some strains are positive for group E), production of acid from mannitol, a failure to hydrolyze hippurate, and the formation of gelatinous deposits (dextran) in media containing 5% sucrose. This organism may be difficult to isolate and to identify. It often requires more than 3 days for primary isolation, grows best on horse blood agar in 5% to 10% carbon dioxide on subculture, and is pleomorphic, resulting in confusion with diphtheroids. *S. mutans* first was isolated in 1924 by Clark from dental caries lesions of humans and first was reported in 1928 to cause IE. The central importance of this organism in dental caries has been amply documented.

S. bovis is a normal inhabitant of the gastrointestinal tract of humans and many animal species. The genetic diversity among organisms historically classified as *S. bovis* has been clarified to include biotypes I and II, *S. salivarius,* and *Streptococcus macedonicus.*[332] In addition, *S. bovis* has been subdivided further into *Streptococcus gallolyticus* and *Streptococcus infantarius.* It is important to separate this organism from the other members of group D (the enterococci) because the respective therapeutic approaches to infection by these organisms are different (see later). Group D organisms are identified presumptively by bile-esculin hydrolysis.[333,334] Only the enterococci (*E. faecalis* and its varieties *Enterococcus zymogenes* and *Enterococcus liquifaciens, Enterococcus faecium,* and *Enterococcus durans*) grow in 6.5% sodium chloride, whereas *S. bovis* and *Streptococcus equinus* (a rare cause of IE) are salt sensitive. Seventy-five percent of strains of *S. bovis* are heat tolerant, and they may grow and produce acid in *E. faecalis* broth; these methods are unreliable for separation.[335] Arginine hydrolysis by enterococci and starch hydrolysis by *S. bovis* are other means for reliable separation. The association of bacteremia due to *S. bovis* with carcinoma of the colon and other lesions of the gastrointestinal tract suggests that colonoscopy be performed when this organism is isolated from blood cultures.[336,337]

Enterococci are normal inhabitants of the gastrointestinal tract and occasionally the anterior urethra. All enterococci are in Lancefield group D; are catalase-negative and nonmotile; and may exhibit α-, β-, or γ-hemolysis on blood agar. They grow well in sodium azide (SF broth), 40% bile, 6.5% sodium chloride, and 0.1% methylene blue and can survive at 56° C for 30 minutes or at a pH of 9.6.[338] They should be separated from *S. bovis.* The *Enterococcus* group is responsible for 5% to 18% of the cases of IE, and the incidence seems to be increasing.[326,339,340] The disease usually runs a subacute course and affects older (mean age 59 years) men after genitourinary manipulation or younger (mean age 37 years) women after obstetric procedures. The mean duration of nonspecific symptoms, such as malaise, fatigue, anorexia, and weight loss, was 140 days in one review. Greater than 40% of the patients have no underlying heart disease, although more than 95% develop a heart murmur during the course of the illness. Classic peripheral manifestations are uncommon (<25% of the cases). Bacteriuria with enterococci is a helpful diagnostic clue and was found in 4 of 15 patients[338] in one study. Cure is difficult because of intrinsic resistance to many antibiotics, and a high mortality persists in this disease.

With the increasing usage of third-generation cephalosporins, which are relatively inactive against enterococci in vitro, and other contributing factors (e.g., indwelling urinary catheters), some reports[340-342] emphasized an alarming increase in enterococcal bacteremias during the past 2 decades. Most enterococcal bacteremias are nosocomial in origin, often polymicrobial (42% in one large series[343]), and are associated with serious underlying disorders. Factors that suggest IE in patients with enterococcal bacteremia include (1) community acquisition, (2) preexistent valvular heart disease, (3) cryptogenic source, and (4) absence of polymicrobial bacteremia.[343] Antibiotic usage patterns, the aging of the population, and more invasive procedures in hospitalized adults all portend a continued increase in serious enterococcal infections, including IE, in the future.

Before 1945, *S. pneumoniae* was responsible for approximately 10% of the cases of IE, but this has decreased to approximately 1% to 3% currently.[344] The course usually is fulminant and is often (in approximately one third of cases) associated with perivalvular abscess formation or pericarditis or both. Left-sided involvement is the rule, and there is a predilection for the aortic valve (approximately 70% of cases). Many patients with pneumococcal IE are alcoholics (approximately 40%), and concurrent meningitis is present in about 70% of cases.[344-346] The overall mortality rate is approximately 50% (approximately 60% to 65% in children[347]), with death usually due to rapid valvular destruction and hemodynamic compromise,[348] although indolent presentations of pneumococcal IE with a favorable outcome have been described.[349]

NVS may cause difficulties in isolation and were implicated in 5.4% of the cases of streptococcal IE at The New York Hospital.[350] The organisms do not grow on subculture unless L-cysteine or pyridoxal vitamin B_6 is provided. IE due to nutritionally deficient streptococci virtually always is indolent in onset and associated with preexisting heart disease.[351] Therapy is difficult because systemic embolization, relapse, and death are common (occurring in 17% to 27% of cases). A closely related species, *S. mitis,* although not nutritionally deficient, also causes serious infections, including IE, in adults[352] and has emerged as an important causative agent of IE among drug addicts in some areas (e.g., New York City[353]). Group B streptococci (*Streptococcus agalactiae*) are normal inhabitants of the mouth, vagina, and anterior urethra in 5% to 12% of the general population. In 149 patients with group B streptococcal infections, the serotypes isolated were Ia in 46%, II in 22%, and III in 11%.[354] Although long recognized as a cause of bacteremia and meningitis in neonates, serious *S. agalactiae* infections in adults also have been emphasized.[355,356] Risk factors for group B streptococcal sepsis and IE in adults include diabetes mellitus, carcinoma, alcoholism, hepatic failure, elective abortion, and intravenous drug use.[356-358] As with *S. bovis,* occasional cases occur in association with villous adenomas of the colon.[359] More than 90 cases of group B streptococcal IE have been reported.[357-361] Underlying heart disease is common, the male-to-female ratio is 1.4:1, the mean age is approximately 54 years, and left-sided involvement predominates. The overall mortality rate is nearly 50%. The organism does not produce fibrinolysin, which may be responsible for the large, friable vegetations and frequent major systemic emboli. A similar clinical picture with a destructive process, left-sided predominance, frequent complications, and high mortality (approximately 40%) has been observed in the 47 cases of group G streptococcal IE reported in the literature.[362,363] Most human infections with *Streptococcus suis* have presented as meningitis (with a striking predilection to cause deafness as a sequela) and sepsis with accompanying arthritis or endophthalmitis, but two cases of IE due to serotype 2 have been described.[364] A history of pig or raw pork contact was a feature in both patients. Group A streptococci remain a rare cause of IE associated with a high complication rate in adults and children.[365] *S. anginosus* is a rare cause of IE ($\cong$ 6% to 7% of cases) but is unusual among these streptococci in that it has a predilection to cause suppurative complications, including brain, liver, perinephric, and other abscesses and cholangitis, peritonitis, and empyema.[366-368] Some of these complications occur during IE due to this organism and may require surgical attention. Approximately 50% of *S. anginosus* strains carry the group F antigen.[367] IE caused by *S. anginosus* may result in "virulent" intracardiac complications (e.g., myocardial abscess, purulent pericarditis) more typical of *S. aureus* infections.[369]

IE due to *Gemella haemolysans* also has been reported.[370] This organism now is placed in genus V of the family Streptococcaceae. *Gemella* should be suspected if blood cultures reveal a variable morphology (with some organisms resembling diphtheroids) and an indeterminate Gram stain. The antimicrobial susceptibility of *Gemella* spp. is similar to that of the viridans streptococci. Although misidentification in the microbiology laboratory is presumably common, six cases of IE due to *G. haemolysans* have been reported since 1982.[371]

Staphylococci

Staphylococci cause at least 20% to 30% of the cases of IE, and 80% to 90% of these are due to coagulase-positive *S. aureus*. This species is the causative agent in most cases of acute IE, but only a few patients with *S. aureus* bacteremia have IE.[372,373] The organism may attack "normal" (defined as no clinically detectable cardiac disease) heart valves in approximately one third of the patients. The course frequently is fulminant when it involves the mitral or aortic valve, with widespread metastatic infection, and results in death in approximately 40% of patients.[374-377] As noted, the proportion of cases of IE due to *S. aureus* seems to be increasing at community and university hospitals.[12,325,326,378] It had been found previously that among cases of *S. aureus* IE, most were community acquired.[379] More recent experience from Duke University with 59 cases of definite *S. aureus* IE prospectively identified has suggested a demographic shift among patients with this infection.[380] In nearly half of cases, the IE was acquired nosocomially, frequently was caused by methicillin-resistant *S. aureus* (MRSA) strains, and often was associated with intravascular device–related *S. aureus* infection. These observations have been confirmed in a multinational cohort of 922 patients with definite IE. *S. aureus* was the most common cause of IE, accounting for 35.7% of all cases. Among *S. aureus* cases, 46% were presumed to be health care associated.[381] It seems that health care–associated *S. aureus* bacteremia should prompt a complete evaluation for underlying IE.

Myocardial abscesses (with conduction disturbances), purulent pericarditis, and valve ring abscesses are more common in staphylococcal endocarditis than in other forms of IE. Peripheral foci of suppuration (e.g., lung, brain, spleen, kidney) are common and affect more than 40% of these patients.[374,377,378] These extravascular sites of involvement may offer clues to an early diagnosis, especially in narcotic addicts.[232,233] This disease often is unsuspected and not clinically recognized in older patients, and mortality rates often are greater than 50% in patients older than 50 years of age, especially when the infection is nosocomially acquired.[378,382] The rare entity of neonatal IE also often is caused by *S. aureus*[383]; survival is unusual.

IE in narcotic addicts usually is due to *S. aureus*, but the disease tends to be less severe, with mortality rates of 2% to 6%.[232,233] The lower mortality is related directly to the preponderance of cases affecting the tricuspid valve, a syndrome that usually responds to antimicrobial therapy in most cases.[379] The emergence of MRSA in addicts with staphylococcal IE, first documented in the Detroit area, is disturbing.[226,384] Among 180 bacteremic addicts admitted to the Detroit Medical Center in 1 year, 24% grew MRSA, and 41% of the patients overall had IE. Previous hospitalizations, long-term addiction (particularly in men), and nonprescribed antibiotic use were predictive of MRSA acquisition (odds ratio 8.6:1).[384]

S. epidermidis is an important agent in prosthetic valve IE (see Chapter 75) and in infants with IE related to umbilical venous catheters in neonatal intensive care units.[385] Although such cases still are uncommon, some reports[386-388] have emphasized the importance of coagulase-negative staphylococci in native valve IE, particularly in patients with mitral valve prolapse.[386] Approximately two thirds of affected patients have preexistent valvular disease. Although the disease was indolent in onset, complications of IE were common; despite this, medical or surgical therapy or both usually was successful. Men predominate

among the 85 patients reported, and the incidence of emboli, skin manifestations, and CHF is low.[389] Separation of IE from uncomplicated bacteremias due to *S. epidermidis* (implicated in approximately 50% of cases of native valve coagulase-negative staphylococcal IE) may be difficult, but a solid-phase radioimmunoassay for the detection of IgG antibodies is promising.[390] In addition, IgG antibodies to a novel 30-kD cloned protein, termed *staphylococcal secretory antigen,* have been shown in patients with *S. epidermidis* IE but not in patients with uncomplicated *S. epidermidis* bacteremia or IE due to other pathogens.[391] Extensive laboratory evaluation[392] reveals that most *S. epidermidis* IE isolates are distinct and do not represent common-source outbreaks despite the frequent shift to a small-colony variant by many strains in vivo[393] and the description of polyclonal *S. epidermidis* IE.[394] Rare cases of IE due to other coagulase-negative staphylococci (e.g., *Staphylococcus saprophyticus, Staphylococcus capitis*) have been reported.[395,396] A growing number of reports of IE caused by a coagulase-negative staphylococcus called *Staphylococcus lugdunensis* have been published.[397-400] This organism tends to cause a substantially more virulent form of IE than that due to other coagulase-negative staphylococci, with high morbidity rates despite nearly uniform in vitro susceptibilities to most antibiotics, including penicillins and cephalosporins.[397-400] These strains frequently are misidentified as *S. aureus* because they often are yellow pigmented and yield complete hemolysis on blood agars. Their in vitro hemolytic capacities relate to the production of synergistic hemolysin. The differentiation of *S. lugdunensis* from *S. aureus* in the microbiology laboratory depends on the tube coagulase test and the ability of the former strains to cause ornithine decarboxylation. Distinguishing *S. lugdunensis* from other coagulase-negative staphylococci may be difficult using commercial identification schemata (e.g., API StaphIdent System[401]).

Gram-Negative Bacilli

Gram-negative aerobic bacilli have been reported to cause 1.3% to 4.8% of cases of IE, but in two reports[402,403] they accounted for more than 10% of cases. In the latter reports, approximately two thirds of the cases coexisted with or followed serious gram-positive infections. Despite an increasing incidence of gram-negative bacillary septicemia, IE due to these organisms remains uncommon, but the incidence is increasing. Only 1.7% of 452 valvular infections reported in the 1960s were caused by gram-negative organisms versus 7% to 15% in more recent series.[325,404] From 1958 to 1975, 56 cases of IE due to gram-negative bacteria were seen at the Mayo Clinic; 35 cases were seen from 1970 to 1975 alone.[405] Most cases were due to "fastidious" nonenteric organisms (see later); this group caused 10% of the IE cases seen at this institution. Narcotic addicts, prosthetic valve recipients, and patients with cirrhosis[406] seem to be at an increased risk for the development of gram-negative bacillary IE. The duration of illness is usually less than 6 weeks, most patients are 40 to 50 years old, and men and women are affected equally.[407] In gram-negative septicemia, the blood stream usually is cleared with appropriate antimicrobial agents. In contrast, in gram-negative bacillary IE, persistent bacteremia is common, even with high levels of antimicrobial activity. CHF is common, and the prognosis is poor. Most series report a mortality rate approaching 75% to 83%,[27,407] but more recent experience indicates a better prognosis,[405] with a cure rate of 62% in 21 patients infected with aerobic enteric bacilli. A heart murmur noted during an episode of gram-negative sepsis with unexplained anemia or the persistence of positive blood cultures despite adequate antibiotics may indicate IE. In the early postoperative period after prosthetic valve replacement, sustained gram-negative bacillary bacteremia does not imply IE,[408] and other foci of infection (e.g., sternal wound, pneumonia, urinary tract, intravenous catheters) should be sought carefully.

Among members of Enterobacteriaceae, *Salmonella* spp. were most common in early reports. These organisms have an affinity for abnormal cardiac valves, usually on the left side of the heart.[407,409] Although many serotypes have been implicated, most cases are due to *Salmonella choleraesuis, Salmonella typhimurium,* and *Salmonella enteritidis.* Valvular perforation or destruction, atrial thrombi, myocarditis, and pericarditis are common, and the outlook is grave. Salmonellae also may produce endarteritis in aneurysms of major vessels (see later).

In a review of 44 cases of Enterobacteriaceae IE due to species other than *Salmonella* spp.,[407] the following organisms were identified: *E. coli*, 17 cases; *Citrobacter* spp., 1 case; *Klebsiella-Enterobacter* spp., 9 cases; *S. marcescens*, 13 cases; *Proteus* spp. 2 cases; and *Providencia* spp., 2 cases. There were 19 additional cases of IE due to *S. marcescens* reported from San Francisco[410]; 17 occurred in narcotic addicts. Two thirds of these patients had previously normal heart valves, and most of the infections occurred on the aortic and mitral valves. The cases are characterized by large vegetations with near-total occlusion of the valve orifice in the absence of significant underlying valvular destruction. The overall mortality rate ranges from 68% to 73% because a cure of left-sided IE due to a member of Enterobacteriaceae is uncommon with medical therapy alone. Since 1974, 17 more cases of IE due to *S. marcescens* have been observed in the San Francisco area; 15 occurred in intravenous drug abusers. Only 3 of 10 patients with left-sided involvement survived despite antimicrobial combination therapy and high serum bactericidal activity. Valve replacement after approximately 7 to 10 days of antibiotics was recommended for these difficult infections.[411] Approximately 12 cases of IE due to *Campylobacter fetus* have been reported since the first case in 1955.[412]

The first case of *Pseudomonas*-induced IE was recognized in 1899; more than 200 cases subsequently have been reported.[226,384,406,413-416] Most (95%) of the patients have abused intravenous drugs.[384,413-416] The male-to-female ratio is 2.5:1, and the mean age is 30 years. The organism affects normal valves in most cases. Major embolic phenomena, inability to sterilize valves, neurologic complications (53%), ring and annular abscesses, splenic abscesses, bacteremic relapses, and rapidly progressive CHF are common. Ecthyma gangrenosum, the necrotizing cutaneous lesion characteristic of *Pseudomonas* bacteremia, occasionally has been noted, especially in cases of IE due to *Pseudomonas (Burkholderia) cepacia*.[417] The disease carries the highest mortality in patients older than age 30 (73% versus 33% in younger patients), when the duration of illness is less than 5 days (which raises the rate from 41% to 76%), and when there is left-sided cardiac involvement.[414,416,418] Owing to the poor prognosis and frequent complications,[226] early surgery is recommended by many authorities for left-sided *Pseudomonas* IE.[415,416] In contrast, high-dose regimens of antipseudomonal penicillins combined with aminoglycosides have had a salutary effect in most patients with isolated right-sided pseudomonal IE (see section on "Antimicrobial Therapy"). Nearly all addicts with *P. aeruginosa* IE in more recent reports[74,384,415,416] have abused tripelennamine and pentazocine ("T's and blues").

Unusual Gram-Negative Bacteria

IE produced by several other gram-negative species has received more recent attention. *N. gonorrhoeae* was responsible for at least 5% to 10% of the cases of IE before the introduction of penicillin but now is implicated rarely. In the older series, half of the patients with gonococcal IE had involvement of the right side of the heart and exhibited the characteristic double quotidian fever pattern. Of the cases of gonococcal IE reported since 1949,[419-421] most occurred in young men. Skin manifestations consistent with the gonococcal arthritis-dermatitis syndrome or IE are documented in only 20% of cases. Most of the cases of gonococcal IE now follow an indolent course, in contrast to the often fulminant progression in the preantibiotic era. Aortic valve involvement, large vegetations seen on TTE, associated valve ring abscesses, CHF, and nephritis are common.[421] A high frequency of late complement component deficiencies has been noted in patients with gonococcal IE. Sudden hemodynamic deterioration despite appropriate therapy may occur,[419-421] and the mortality rate is approximately 20%. "Nonpathogenic" *Neisseria* spp. (*Neisseria perflava*, *Neisseria flava*, *Neisseria pharyngis*, *Neisseria mucosa*, *Neisseria sicca*, *Neisseria flavescens*, and especially *Moraxella [Neisseria] catarrhalis* and *Neisseria elongata* subsp. *nitroreducens* [Centers for Disease

Control and Prevention group M-6]) now are isolated more frequently in IE than are gonococci, but they usually produce infection on abnormal or prosthetic heart valves.[422-424]

Haemophilus spp., predominantly *Haemophilus paraphrophilus*, *Haemophilus parainfluenzae*, and *Haemophilus aphrophilus*, account for 0.8% to 1.3% of all cases of IE.[425-428] This disease usually runs a subacute course and occurs in the setting of preexisting valvular disease. Emboli to major peripheral arteries were found in six of seven cases of *H. parainfluenzae* IE.[425] Major central nervous system complications are relatively common.[428] *H. aphrophilus* produced a similar clinical pattern and has been transmitted from dogs to humans. Single cases of IE due to *Haemophilus seguis* and *Haemophilus aegyptius* have been reported from Denmark and Israel.[429,430] A closely related organism, *Actinobacillus actinomycetemcomitans*, is a rare cause of subacute IE (with approximately 35 cases reported), with a mortality of 34%.[431,432] IE due to *Cardiobacterium hominis*[433] resembles the disease caused by *Haemophilus* spp.; 26 cases of IE due to this organism were reported by 1983. Only one extravascular infection due to *C. hominis* has been documented (meningitis during IE).

At least 28 cases of *Kingella* endocarditis (*Kingella kingae*, 25; *Kingella denitrificans*, 2; *Kingella indologenes*, 1) have been reported.[434] Approximately 50% of patients develop complications, including acute stroke in approximately 25%. A dozen cases of IE due to *Eikenella corrodens* have been reported; intravenous drug use (especially amphetamines) was implicated in five patients.[435,436] Dental infection or a history of dental procedures may be a feature, and drug users often have "cleaned" the injection site with saliva; *E. corrodens* is a usual habitant of the oropharynx. The disease generally has an indolent course but may present acutely.[436]

All of the aforementioned organisms—the HACEK group (*Haemophilus, Actinobacillus, Cardiobacterium, Eikenella, Kingella*)—are fastidious and may require 2 to 3 weeks for primary isolation. Routine subculturing onto supplemented chocolate agar or incubation in atmospheres of 5% to 10% carbon dioxide is necessary for the isolation of these organisms and should be performed in all culture-negative cases of IE. Granular growth in broth is characteristic and should suggest their presence. In addition, the clinical syndrome produced by this group is virtually identical with that in subacute IE: large friable vegetations, frequent emboli, and development of CHF and often the eventual need for valve replacement.[437]

Gram-Positive Bacilli

IE due to various species of corynebacteria (diphtheroids) is uncommon and usually occurs on damaged or prosthetic valves,[438] although native valve infections (e.g., *Arcanobacterium [Corynebacterium] haemolyticum* in a drug addict) are reported rarely. About 19 cases of IE due to *Corynebacterium pseudodiphtheriticum* (previously *Corynebacterium hofmannii*) have been reported; native valves were involved in approximately 50% of these cases.[439] *Corynebacterium xerosis* is a very rare cause of native valve IE. Nontoxigenic *Corynebacterium diphtheriae* IE has been reported in more than 40 patients. A cluster of seven cases in 1 year from New South Wales, Australia,[440] emphasized the aggressive nature of the infection, including major vascular complications, the frequent occurrence of septic arthritis (in four of seven patients), and involvement of native valves. Intravenous drug use also is a predisposing factor. *Listeria monocytogenes* has been isolated in 44 cases of IE.[441,442] Most cases of IE due to *Listeria* spp. have occurred in patients without any underlying defect in host defenses, although preexistent heart disease is present in approximately 50%. The mean age in the reported series was 51 years, and the overall mortality was 48%.[442] Lactobacilli also have been reported to cause a subacute form of IE, but these cases are rare (only 41 reported).[443,444] Despite an initial response to therapy, relapse of this infection is not unusual (approximately 60% of cases). Most cases occur on structurally abnormal native valves after dental manipulation.[444]

Therapy with single agents is often unsatisfactory because lactobacilli, similar to enterococci, are tolerant to penicillins. Medical cure has been difficult to achieve in the past. These organisms also may take several weeks for isolation on blood culture. Greater than 90% of 49 serious infections caused by *Erysipelothrix rhusiopathiae* were characterized as IE.[445] Occupational or vocational animal or fish exposure is a major risk factor, and approximately one third of patients are alcoholic. Most patients are men. A characteristic erysipeloid skin lesion is present in approximately 40% of cases, and the organism exhibits significant aortic valve tropism (involved in 70% of patients).[445] The overall mortality rate is 38%. Most cases of *Bacillus* IE involve the tricuspid valve in narcotic addicts, but nonaddicts and prosthetic valve recipients also have been affected.[446] *Rothia dentocariosa* is a rare cause of IE (six cases reported) but has led to significant central nervous system complications.[447,448]

Anaerobic Bacteria

Nonstreptococcal anaerobic bacteria were responsible for 1.3% of all the cases of IE in 1970.[449] *Bacteroides fragilis* was the predominant pathogen in a review of 67 cases from the literature.[450] The following organisms were isolated: *B. fragilis*, 35.8%; *Bacteroides oralis*, 3%; *Prevotella melaninogenica* (*Bacteroides melaninogenicus*), 3%; *Fusobacterium necrophorum*, 13.4%; *Fusobacterium nucleatum*, 9%; *Clostridium* spp., 13.4%; *P. acnes*, 7.5%; *Dialister granuliformans*, 1.5%; and unidentified, 16.4%. More than one third of the unidentified cases also were thought by the authors to represent *B. fragilis*. Approximately 25% of these cases were polymicrobial, usually mixed with anaerobic or microaerophilic streptococci. The portal of entry for *B. fragilis* was probably the gastrointestinal tract, whereas *B. oralis*, *P. melaninogenica* (*B. melaninogenicus*), or fusobacteria originated from the mouth or upper respiratory tract. Two thirds of the patients were older than age 40 and had preexisting heart disease. The course usually is subacute except for that with infection due to *F. necrophorum*, which characteristically produces a more fulminant disease. These organisms usually cause extensive valve destruction, CHF, and major systemic emboli (in 60% to 70% of the cases). Thromboembolic episodes are especially common in infections caused by *B. fragilis*, a phenomenon that may be related to the heparinase produced by this organism. The mortality rate in cases of anaerobic IE has ranged from 21% to 46%.[450] One series from California noted no deaths in seven patients with anaerobic or microaerophilic IE[451]; these cases constituted 10.6% of the IE cases seen. This is similar to a 7.7% incidence reported by other investigators[2] and suggests that anaerobic IE may be more prevalent now than it was in 1970.[452] Isolation of these organisms may be improved by the newer anaerobic culture techniques currently in use.

Other Bacteria

Many other bacteria have been described in cases of IE; however, consideration of these organisms separately is beyond the scope of this chapter. These include *Acinetobacter* (approximately 20 reported cases; a maculopapular rash on the palms and soles may be present),[453] *Actinomyces*,[454] *Alcaligenes*, *Bordetella*, *Flavobacterium*, *Micrococcus*, *Moraxella*, *Paracolon*, *Stomatococcus mucilaginosus* (four cases of IE),[455] *Streptobacillus moniliformis* (16 cases; usually damaged native valves are involved),[456] *Vibrio*, and *Yersinia*. *Brucella* spp. continue as important etiologic agents in Spain and in Saudi Arabia, where these organisms are responsible for approximately 10% of IE cases.[457] Aggressive medical therapy with valve replacement usually is necessary for a cure of *Brucella* IE.[458]

Etiology of Infective Endocarditis in Narcotic Addicts

The organisms responsible for IE in narcotic addicts require separate consideration because the distribution differs from that in other patients with IE. The frequencies of the etiologic agents isolated before 1977 in seven major series were as follows: *S. aureus*, 38%; *P. aeruginosa*, 14.2%; *Candida* spp., 13.8%; enterococci, 8.2%; viridans streptococci, 6%; *S. epidermidis*, 1.7%; gram-negative aerobic bacilli, 1.7% to 15%; other bacteria, 2.2%; mixed infections, 1.3%; and culture-negative, 12.9%. In addition, there seems to be an unexplained geographic variation in the causal agents of narcotic-associated IE. *S. aureus* predominated in

New York City, Washington, DC, Chicago, and Cincinnati; *P. aeruginosa* was isolated commonly in Detroit, but MRSA now predominates. A more recent compilation from Detroit indicates the distribution of causative agents in addicts with IE (*n* = 74) as follows: *S. aureus*, 60.8%; streptococci, 16.2%; *P. aeruginosa*, 13.5%; polymicrobial, 8.1%; and *Corynebacterium* JK, 1.4%. Polymicrobial IE (eight different pathogens have been recovered from blood cultures of an individual patient) is fairly common among drug addicts. Some authors have speculated that HIV infection predisposes intravenous drug users to IE due to unusual bacteria, including *Corynebacterium* or *Neisseria* spp.[459] Although *S. aureus* IE in this population usually was tricuspid, streptococci infected left-sided valves significantly more often than the other pathogens. Biventricular and multiple-valve infections occurred most commonly in *Pseudomonas* endocarditis; all of these patients abused T's and blues. Left-sided IE due to *P. aeruginosa* is a devastating disease and usually presents as an acute illness refractory to seemingly optimal antimicrobial regimens. Complications, including ring and annular abscesses, neurologic sequelae, CHF, and splenic abscesses, are common; surgery is often necessary for cure.[460] The overall mortality rate still approaches 60%, however. There is an increased incidence of enterococcal IE in Cleveland. *S. marcescens* previously was an important pathogen in San Francisco,[411] but at present *S. aureus* is the most common ((85%) etiologic agent (HF Chambers, personal communication). These differences do not correlate with contamination of "street" heroin.[461] The high incidence of staphylococcal endocarditis may be explained partially by an increase in nasal and oral carriage of this organism.[462] Heroin usage in the previous week was associated with an *S. aureus* isolation rate of 35% from skin, nose, or throat cultures; this rate declined to 11% (not significantly different from that in controls) if heroin had not been injected in the preceding 2 weeks. This suggests an endogenous source for the infecting organism because *S. aureus* is infrequently (in <5% of cases) isolated from street heroin or injection paraphernalia.

The exact incidence of IE in narcotic addicts is unknown. A conservative estimate is 1.5 to 2 cases of IE per 1000 addicts at risk per year.[463] Intravenous drug use is the most common risk factor for the development of recurrent native valve IE; 43% of 281 patients surveyed from 1975 to 1986 with this syndrome were addicts[464] (see earlier). A nested case-control study from Johns Hopkins University found that IE incidence was more common among injection drug users with advanced immunosuppression even after accounting for injection drug use behaviors. Analyses have shown that although *S. aureus* remains the most common cause of right-sided IE in injection drug users, cases of left-sided IE in the population are equally due to viridans group streptococci and *S. aureus*.[231]

Fungi

Most patients who have fungal IE can be grouped into three categories: (1) narcotic addicts, (2) patients who have undergone reconstructive cardiovascular surgery, and (3) patients who have received prolonged intravenous antibiotic therapy. In a review of 24 patients with fungal IE seen at the New York University Medical Center from 1968 to 1973,[273] 11 were heroin addicts, 9 had undergone cardiac surgery, and 5 had other serious illnesses requiring antibiotics or hyperalimentation. Underlying heart disease and a tendency for major systemic embolization were noted in two thirds of these patients. *Candida parapsilosis* and *Candida tropicalis* predominated in the addicts, whereas *C. albicans* and *Aspergillus* spp. caused most cases in nonaddicts. Evidence suggests a shift in the epidemiology of fungal IE toward patients receiving intensive medical care. The incidence of fungal sepsis increased 270% from 1980 to 2000.[465] Much of this increasing incidence in fungal sepsis likely was related to intensive health care contact. In a literature review of 152 cases of fungal IE published between 1995 and 2000, injection drug use was an identified risk factor in only 4.1% of cases, whereas other predisposing factors, such as cardiac abnormalities (47.3%), prosthetic valves (44.6%), and central venous catheters (30.4%), were more common.[274] In a review of 23 addicts, *C. parapsilosis* was responsible in 12 patients

(52%), and other *Candida* spp. (*Candida guilliermondii, Candida stellatoidea, C. krusei, C. tropicalis*) caused most of the remaining cases. *C. albicans* was isolated in only 1 of the 23 addicts. In contrast, in 82 patients who developed fungal IE after cardiac surgery, the reported distribution of causative organisms was different. *C. albicans* and *Aspergillus* spp. each accounted for approximately one third of the isolates. *C. parapsilosis* was found in fewer than 10%. Fungal IE was documented in 29 patients after prolonged intravenous therapy, and in 17 it developed during the treatment of bacterial IE. Half of these patients were infected with *C. albicans*.

The overall cure rate in cases of fungal IE is poor (14.5% in cases treated since 1968). The poor prognosis may be due to (1) large bulky vegetations, (2) tendency for fungal invasion of the myocardium, (3) widespread systemic septic emboli, (4) poor penetration of antifungal agents into the vegetation,[466] (5) low toxic-to-therapeutic ratio of the available antifungal agents, and (6) usual lack of fungicidal activity with these compounds. A cure is virtually impossible without surgical intervention (see later).[467] The role of promising antifungal agents, including caspofungin[468] and voriconazole,[469] in the management of fungal IE remains to be defined. Fatal IE due to *Candida* spp. also has followed Swan-Ganz catheterization.

In a review of 25 cases of *Aspergillus*-induced IE in which cultures were made,[470] the organisms isolated were as follows: *Aspergillus fumigatus*, 14; *Aspergillus flavus*, 4; *Aspergillus niger*, 3; and *Aspergillus ustus, Aspergillus sydowi, Aspergillus terreus,* and *Aspergillus glaucus*, 1 each. Only 5 of 34 patients in this series had positive blood cultures, and only 1 patient survived. A few cases, usually fatal, of *Aspergillus* IE after coronary artery bypass surgery have been described. *Aspergillus clavatus* was isolated in one case. Other fungi that have caused IE include *Histoplasma, Blastomyces, Coccidioides, Cryptococcus, Hansenula, Fonsecaea* (*Hormodendrum*), *Scedosporium prolificans, Mucor, Paecilomyces,* and *Phialophora*. *Histoplasma capsulatum* IE has been diagnosed rapidly using direct application of AccuProbe on an excised cardiac valve.[471] Of the eight reported cases of IE due to *Trichosporon beigelii*, six occurred on prosthetic valves; only two patients have survived a combined medical-surgical approach.[472] *Pseudallescheria boydii* has caused IE in approximately five reported patients; all were immunosuppressed (e.g., liver transplant, AIDS) or previous recipients of prosthetic heart valves.[473]

Fungal IE was unknown before 1945, and the incidence is increasing. At present, 1.2% to 2.6% of all cases of IE are due to fungi. IE also has been caused by higher bacteria, such as *Actinomyces, Nocardia,* and *Mycobacterium* spp.

Other Microorganisms

Five cases of IE due to *Spirillum minus,* a spirochete, have been reported.[474] This organism is distributed widely in nature, especially in fresh or salt water with organic debris. *S. minus* is the etiologic agent of rat-bite fever (sodoku), but rodent transmission was not documented in the cases of IE. Preexistent heart disease or severe underlying disease (e.g., aplastic anemia) is usually present, although one case occurred in an otherwise healthy person.

IE due to *C. burnetii* (the cause of Q fever) is well documented in the United Kingdom, the United States, Canada, France, the Middle East, and Australia.[475-477] Ten cases of Q fever IE were recognized in four Dublin teaching hospitals in only 3 years.[476] Q fever usually is a self-limited respiratory illness due to the inhalation of infected aerosols.[478] The first IE cases were reported in 1959. Men outnumber women by 6 to 1, and 90% of patients have preexisting heart disease. Most cases of IE are chronic, with a history of an influenza-like illness occurring 6 to 12 months previously. Risk factors may include exposure to parturient cats or rabbits and previous valvulopathy and pregnancy.[477] The aortic valve is involved in greater than 80% of the cases. Hematuria is uncommon, although it is observed frequently in acute Q fever. Hepatosplenomegaly and hepatitis, common features in other types of Q fever, are usual in IE caused by this organism. Other important clues are thrombocytopenia (seen in 90% of cases) and hypergammaglobulinemia. Immune complex–mediated glomerulonephritis

develops in approximately 25% of cases.[475,476,479] Histologically, Q fever IE is characterized by significant fibrosis and calcifications, slight inflammation and vascularization, and small or absent vegetations.[267] The rickettsiae were shown histologically in the valve tissue in 62% of the cases, and the organism was isolated in 83%, although this poses a significant laboratory hazard.[475] The diagnosis is best made serologically; a positive titer of antibody to the phase I antigen as measured by complement fixation or enzyme-linked immunosorbent assay indicates chronic infection, whereas a fourfold rise in titer of antibody to the phase II antigen is associated with active current infection. A phase I antibody titer (generally IgG or IgA or both) greater than 1:200 is considered virtually diagnostic of Q fever IE and may be useful to follow the response to therapy.[475,480] Isolation of *C. burnetii* by inoculation of valve suspensions into a human fetal diploid fibroblast cell line seems to be a promising technique.[481] DNA probes are under development. The prognosis with medical therapy alone is poor, and valve replacement often is necessary for a cure (see later). This agent also may cause endarteritis. A single case of IE due to the causative agent of murine typhus has been reported.[258]

Chlamydophila psittaci, the agent of psittacosis, has been implicated in at least 10 well-documented cases of IE.[482] This organism also may cause myocarditis or pericarditis. Most cases have been associated with psittacine bird exposure; in one case, chlamydiae were found in the liver of the suspected budgerigar. Transmission from pet cats also has been proposed. The course is subacute, and the diagnosis often is made retrospectively. Most patients had preexisting heart disease, with a striking propensity for aortic valve involvement, and rapid valvular destruction leading to surgical intervention or death. A diagnosis can be established with the demonstration of complement-fixing antibodies. Cure usually requires valve replacement and prolonged antibiotic therapy. The mortality rate in this small group was 40%. Two well-documented cases of IE due to *Chlamydia trachomatis* have been reported.[483] Microimmunofluorescence tests are necessary for a diagnosis. Several cases of probable *Chlamydia pneumoniae* IE have been reported.[484] IE due to *Mycoplasma pneumoniae* was proposed in one case report, but cultural confirmation was lacking.[485]

T. whippelii, the causative agent of Whipple's disease, is an occasional cause of IE and has been cultivated from human valvular tissue.[486] In a review of 35 reported cases of Whipple's IE, CHF, fever, and preceding valvular abnormalities all were less common in patients with Whipple's IE than in patients with IE due to other pathogens.[266]

The role of viruses in IE is unknown. Experimentally, coxsackie B virus has been shown to produce valvular and mural endocarditis in mice and cynomolgus monkeys.[487] In these studies, the viral antigen was shown in the valvular tissue by immunofluorescence techniques. Although the enteroviruses commonly are implicated in cases of myocarditis or pericarditis in humans, there is no proof that viral infections produce IE in humans. Adenoviruses also are capable of producing IE in mice. Persand[488] described a case of "cytomegalovirus endocarditis," but bacteria also were cultured from a mural lesion.

Culture-Negative Endocarditis

As discussed earlier, sterile blood cultures have been noted in 2.5% to 31% of cases of IE.[489,490] Blood cultures are negative, however, in only approximately 5% of patients with IE confirmed by strict diagnostic criteria.[491,492] Sterile blood cultures may be due to several factors: (1) subacute right-sided IE; (2) cultures taken toward the end of a chronic course (>3 months); (3) uremia supervening in a chronic course; (4) mural IE as in ventricular septal defects, post–myocardial infarction thrombi, or infection related to pacemaker wires; (5) slow growth of fastidious organisms, such as anaerobes, *Haemophilus* spp., *Actinobacillus* spp., *Cardiobacterium* spp., NVS, or *Brucella* spp; (6) prior administration of antibiotics[489,490]; (7) fungal IE; (8) IE caused by obligate intracellular parasites, such as rickettsiae, chlamydiae, *T. whippelii*,[266] and perhaps viruses; or (9) noninfective endocarditis or an incorrect diagnosis. Attention to the proper collection of blood culture specimens, care in the performance of serologic tests, and use of newer diagnostic techniques may reduce the proportion of culture-negative cases.

Polymicrobial Endocarditis

The proportion of IE cases due to more than one pathogen may be increasing. In a literature review spanning the 1980s,[493] 101 cases of polymicrobial IE were found. The mean age was 36.5 years, the male-to-female ratio was nearly 2:1, and 71 of the patients used intravenous drugs (as expected, tricuspid valve involvement with septic pulmonary emboli was common). Left-sided involvement, two organisms (versus three or more), and older age were associated with a higher mortality rate.

THERAPY FOR INFECTIVE ENDOCARDITIS

The response to antimicrobial therapy for IE is unique among bacterial infections. Although the organisms may exhibit exquisite susceptibility in vitro to the antibiotics used, complete eradication takes weeks to achieve, and relapse is not unusual. There are two possible explanations for these phenomena: (1) The infection exists in an area of impaired host defense and is encased tightly in a fibrin meshwork in which the bacterial colonies divide relatively free from interference from phagocytic cells, and (2) the bacteria in these vegetations reach tremendous population densities (often 10^9 to 10^{10} CFU/g). At these high populations, the organisms may exist in a state of reduced metabolic activity and cell division, as was suggested by Durack and Beeson[148] in studies of L-alanine incorporation into bacterial cell walls. A similar finding is observed in broth in vitro after 18 hours of incubation. In both situations, the bacteria are less susceptible to the bactericidal action of penicillin or other drugs that require cell wall synthesis and division for maximal activity. The relative importance of antimicrobial penetration into vegetations and the response to therapy is unresolved. Although multiple studies have examined antibiotic concentrations in human cardiac valve tissue obtained during surgery,[494] usually in close agreement with concurrent serum concentrations, the relevance of these data to therapy for IE is unknown so that current recommendations remain unaltered.

Information on antimicrobial concentration in vegetations, either in experimental models or in humans with IE, is sparse. Experiments after a single dose of radiolabeled antimicrobial agents with autoradiographic analysis of drug dispersion within vegetations of animals with experimental IE revealed three patterns[495]: (1) concentration at the periphery of the vegetation without diffusion into the core (e.g., teicoplanin); (2) progressive diffusion, but with a high gradient from periphery to core (e.g., ceftriaxone); or (3) homogeneous diffusion throughout the vegetation (e.g., several fluoroquinolones). The predictive value of these observations on therapeutic efficacy is unknown. The suboptimal clinical efficacy of teicoplanin in several clinical trials treating intravascular *S. aureus* infections may relate to the maldistribution of this agent within vegetations.[496] Analysis of pharmacodynamic variables (e.g., concentration-dependent bactericidal activity, postantibiotic effect) also may assist in the rational selection of regimens for the therapy of IE.[495] Studies in animals have confirmed that when vegetation formation is inhibited with anticoagulants, the organisms are eradicated more rapidly with penicillin treatment than in control animals with larger vegetations.[152] Enzymatic modification of the glycocalyx in the vegetations of experimental streptococcal IE by in vivo dextranase administration facilitates the bactericidal activity of penicillin by more rapid sterilization of the lesion.[497] In contrast, tissue-type plasminogen activator produced a concentration-dependent lysis of fibrin clots or vegetations infected with *S. epidermidis* or *S. sanguis* but did not enhance antimicrobial activity in in vitro models.[498,499] Several studies in experimental IE have confirmed the utility of aspirin in reducing the size of vegetations and the microbial densities within aortic vegetations.[500,501] In addition, one clinical study in patients with established IE suggested that aspirin could mitigate the growth of vegetative lesions (as monitored echocardiographically) and prevent cerebral emboli.[502]

Certain general principles have been accepted that provide the framework for the current recommendations for treatment of IE. Parenteral antibiotics are recommended over oral drugs in most circumstances because of the importance of sustained antibacterial activity.

Erratic absorption with many classes of agents makes oral drugs less desirable. Short-term therapy has been associated with relapse, and most current recommendations emphasize extended drug administration. Early studies by the British Medical Research Council[503] first emphasized the necessity for prolonged treatment. Bacteriostatic antibiotics are generally ineffective in the treatment of bacterial IE. Their use has been associated with frequent relapses, a failure to control the infection, or both. A symptomatic response to agents such as tetracycline, erythromycin, or, in some cases, clindamycin should not be accepted as indicative of successful treatment because when treatment with these agents is discontinued, relapse is common. Likewise, antibiotic combinations should produce a rapid bactericidal effect. This is seen with synergistic combinations, such as penicillin plus an aminoglycoside effective against most viridans streptococci or enterococci. In experimental animals, it has been shown that the rate of bactericidal action expressed by a drug or combination of drugs in broth is predictive of the relative rate at which the organisms would be eradicated from the cardiac vegetations in vivo. Antagonistic combinations, such as penicillin plus chloramphenicol, which are less rapidly bactericidal, are less effective in experimental IE than is the single bactericidal drug (penicillin) alone.[504] General guidelines for the evaluation of new antimicrobial agents for the therapy of IE were published in 1992.[505] Guidelines for outpatient parenteral antibiotic therapy for IE have been published. These guidelines outline a conservative approach (inpatient or daily outpatient follow-up) during the critical phase (weeks 0 to 2 of treatment) when complications are most likely, followed by outpatient parenteral antibiotic therapy for the continuation phase of antibiotic therapy.[506]

Patients with IE may have an associated myocarditis complicated by cardiac arrhythmias and CHF. These patients (with IE plus CHF) require close observation in an intensive care unit with electrocardiographic monitoring. As discussed subsequently, the selection of antibiotics should be based on antimicrobial susceptibility tests, and the treatment should be monitored clinically and with determination of antimicrobial blood levels when indicated. Blood cultures should be obtained during the early phase of therapy to ensure eradication of the bacteremia and in patients with persistent or recurrent fever during therapy. The use of anticoagulants during therapy for native valve IE has been associated with fatal subarachnoid hemorrhage and other bleeding complications. Most authorities agree that anticoagulant administration in this setting is contraindicated, but this area is controversial. In cases of IE localized to mechanical prosthetic valves, many clinicians maintain anticoagulation within therapeutic range, provided that the patient has no evidence of major vascular emboli (e.g., central nervous system signs or symptoms). One study concluded that oral anticoagulation should be discontinued among patients with *S. aureus* prosthetic valve IE until the septic phase of the disease is resolved (approximately first 10 days after beginning antimicrobial therapy).[507]

Patients with left-sided IE should be managed at least initially in facilities with access to cardiothoracic surgery. Although persistent or recurrent fever despite appropriate antimicrobial therapy may be due to pulmonary or systemic emboli or drug hypersensitivity, the most common cause is extensive valve ring or adjacent structure infection or metastatic infection.[508] Approximately one third of patients with left-sided IE require surgery during the acute stages of infection for either valve replacement or metastatic infection.[321] Close monitoring and early surgical consultation of patients with IE, particularly patients with signs of heart failure or persistent fever, are essential.

Tests Useful for Antimicrobial Treatment Monitoring

Management of IE demands careful consideration of the choice, dose, and duration of antimicrobial therapy. The following laboratory tests can help the physician to monitor treatment and can aid in rational therapeutic decisions. In every case of bacterial IE, the etiologic agent must be isolated in pure culture, and the minimal inhibitory concentration (MIC) and the minimal bactericidal concentration (MBC) must be determined for the usual antibiotics used (see later). Standard disk sensitivity testing is unreliable in the context of treating IE, and results may be misleading without the quantitative information provided by determining the MIC and MBC. During therapy, the serum can be monitored for bactericidal activity against the offending organism as originally described by Schlicter and MacIlean.[509] Performance method for this test varies greatly, and consequently there are disagreements in interpretation. The inoculum size, composition of the broth, timing of samples (peak versus trough), methods of dilution and subculture, and criteria for determination of the bactericidal end point are among the important variables. Perhaps because of these problems and the frequent adverse events unrelated to bactericidal effects, the serum bactericidal titer (SBT) often correlates poorly with the clinical outcome in patients with IE. There still is intense disagreement regarding the value of this test in monitoring therapy for IE. A retrospective review[510] of 17 reports published between 1948 and 1980 failed to confirm any correlation between an SBT of 1:8 or greater and therapeutic success.[511]

Controversy regarding the usefulness of peak versus trough SBT abounds.[512] When all of these variables are standardized,[513,514] the SBT test may be useful in selected patients with IE. One prospective multicenter study[515] evaluated a standardized SBT method in 129 patients with bacterial IE. Peak and trough SBT ratios of 1:64 or greater and 1:32 predicted bacteriologic cure in all patients, but specific levels could *not* be used to predict bacteriologic failure or clinical outcome accurately. Although there are problems with this study,[511] other data[515] support a role for the SBT when standardized and performed in the presence of 50% human serum: All patients with a peak SBT of 1:32 or greater were cured, whereas 7 of 21 (33%) with an SBT of 1:16 or less failed treatment.[516] Unless precluded by drug toxicity, it seems reasonable to attempt to achieve this level (1:8 to 1:16) of activity in patients, although this goal may be unattainable in some forms (e.g., gram-negative bacillary, enterococcal) of IE. Performance of the SBT test usually is unnecessary in patients with viridans streptococcal IE and other antibiotic-susceptible forms of IE, but the SBT may be useful when (1) the organism is inherently resistant or tolerant to one of the drugs administered or (2) the response to therapy is suboptimal.

In some forms of IE, combinations of antibiotics are used routinely.[517] These regimens are based on synergy studies performed in vitro and on results obtained in experimental animal models of IE. In difficult cases with a slow therapeutic response or in cases due to unusual organisms, a determination of synergistic combinations of antibiotics may be helpful. In these cases, tests for bactericidal synergism may be undertaken by standard techniques, such as broth dilution, microtiter "checkerboards," or time-kill curves in broth. Proper attention to standardized techniques, especially inoculum size, is crucial for a meaningful interpretation of the results.

When aminoglycosides are used in therapy, the concentration of antibiotic in the serum should be determined periodically. These agents have a low toxic-to-therapeutic ratio, especially in elderly patients or in patients with renal disease. Peak and trough concentrations should be measured, and the dose should be altered accordingly. This method is superior to reliance solely on nomograms for dosage changes. When synergy with another agent is demonstrable, serum concentrations of the aminoglycosides lower than those generally considered "therapeutic" may be adequate, lessening the potential for toxicity.

Antimicrobial Therapy

Wilson and colleagues[518] and the AHA Committee on Endocarditis reviewed the treatment of streptococcal, enterococcal, staphylococcal, and HACEK IE in detail. The role of aminoglycosides and other agents in combination therapy for IE also has been reviewed.[519]

Penicillin-Sensitive Streptococcal Endocarditis

Most strains of viridans streptococci, "other" streptococci (including *S. pyogenes*), and nonenterococcal group D streptococci (primarily *S. bovis*) are exquisitely sensitive to penicillins, with an MIC of less than 0.2 μg/mL. Of viridans streptococci, 15% to 20% are "resistant" to this arbitrary concentration of penicillin.[327,350] In addition, approximately

15% of the strains of *S. mutans* show a low MIC for penicillin (<0.1 μg/mL), but the MBC is considerably higher (1.25 to 50 μg/mL).[331] These organisms probably should be considered penicillin tolerant and should be treated accordingly. Although results depend on the in vitro methodology employed, studies suggest that tolerance to penicillin among viridans streptococci is more prevalent than previous reports suggested.[520] Of viridans streptococci cultured from gingiva and blood after dental procedures, 19% were tolerant,[521] especially among *S. mutans* (27%) and *S. mitior* (20%) isolates. Almost identical figures were reported among blood culture isolates of viridans streptococci,[522] with tolerance defined as a penicillin MBC-to-MIC ratio exceeding 10:1. Nearly all strains of nutritionally dependent streptococci are tolerant to penicillin.[523,524] The influence of the tolerance phenomenon on the response to penicillin therapy in experimental IE is not known; two studies yielded conflicting results.[525,526] Data on human infections with tolerant strains and the therapeutic results are unavailable. Except for NVS, we do not believe that the demonstration of tolerance by an isolate of viridans streptococci influences therapeutic decisions.

By broth dilution susceptibility tests, the usual MBC determinations for these so-called penicillin-sensitive streptococci are as follows: penicillin, 0.1 to 1 μg/mL; cephalothin, 0.15 to 1.25 μg/mL; vancomycin, 0.15 to 0.4 μg/mL; streptomycin, 6.25 to 50 μg/mL; and gentamicin, 1.56 to 3.12 μg/mL.[527,528] *S. bovis* is 10 to 5000 times more susceptible to penicillin than are the other group D species (enterococci). They also are relatively susceptible to oxacillin, methicillin, and lincomycin, whereas the enterococci are resistant.[334] Most streptococci in this group show synergism in vitro between penicillin or vancomycin and streptomycin, gentamicin, or kanamycin (see later).[529,530] The first strains of viridans streptococci with high-level streptomycin resistance (MIC ≥1000 μg/mL) were reported in 1982 from Paris. Although these strains are rare (2% to 8% of isolates in some locales),[531] the documentation of aminoglycoside-modifying enzymes and the lack of penicillin-streptomycin synergy in vitro and in experimental animal models[531,532] are alarming. These penicillin-susceptible strains are killed synergistically by penicillin-gentamicin combinations. Significant antibiotic antagonism has been shown with the combination of clindamycin and gentamicin for *S. mutans* IE. The in vitro synergism between penicillin and aminoglycosides has been found to correlate with a more rapid rate of eradication of bacteria from cardiac vegetations in vivo in the rabbit endocarditis model[533,534] for the common viridans streptococci. All of these studies have been summarized in reviews.[535-537] Low-level penicillin resistance (MIC 0.2 to 2 μg/mL) was found in 31% of viridans streptococci in Madrid in 1988 and 1989, and an additional 17% of strains showed high-level resistance.[538] Perhaps most important, streptomycin and cefotaxime resistance also was "common."[537] These authors suggested a vancomycin-gentamicin regimen for IE due to viridans streptococci in Spain.

The combination of penicillin and streptomycin has been used in more than 200 cases at The New York Hospital–Cornell Medical Center since 1959 without a documented relapse.[529] This clinical experience has been confirmed elsewhere, but the overall reported relapse rate is 1.4%.[536] This regimen is as follows: aqueous penicillin G, 10 million to 20 million U intravenously daily, or procaine penicillin G, 1.2 million units intramuscularly every 6 hours, for 4 weeks, combined with streptomycin, 0.5 g intramuscularly every 12 hours for the first 2 weeks. Studies by Wilson and colleagues at the Mayo Clinic[539,540] showed that a 2-week course of intramuscular procaine penicillin (1.2 million U every 6 hours) and streptomycin (0.5 g every 12 hours) cured at least 99% of patients with penicillin-sensitive streptococcal IE. These results are similar to results obtained with therapy consisting of β-lactams alone for a total of 4 weeks,[541,542] but significantly better than results obtained with penicillin alone for 2 weeks. The latter regimen was associated with a 50% relapse rate when low doses of penicillin were used and improved to 17% with higher penicillin dosages. The 2-week penicillin-streptomycin regimen is the most cost-effective and had been preferred therapy among the three regimens in uncomplicated penicillin-sensitive (MIC ≥ 0.1 μg/mL) streptococcal IE in young patients. With the advent of ceftriaxone-based regimens (featuring 2 weeks of ceftriaxone plus an aminoglycoside), many clinicians have opted for this approach[543,544] (see later). Four weeks of penicillin (or ceftriaxone; see later) alone is recommended in patients with impaired renal function or patients particularly susceptible to the low risk of streptomycin-induced ototoxicity (the elderly). The Cornell regimen of 4 weeks of penicillin with an initial 2 weeks of streptomycin has been recommended in patients with a complicated course, a history of disease exceeding 3 months' duration, or prosthetic valve IE due to these sensitive strains or when susceptibility testing reveals the rare penicillin-resistant streptococci.[545] The preferred regimen for IE due to penicillin-tolerant streptococci is not established.

Most of the published clinical data with β-lactam–aminoglycoside regimens for the therapy of viridans streptococcal IE involve the use of penicillin or ampicillin plus streptomycin. On the basis of extensive in vitro and animal data and a variety of other reasons, however, the AHA has deemed gentamicin as preferable to streptomycin in this context.[518] First, gentamicin currently is more widely available and used more often clinically than streptomycin in viridans streptococcal IE. Second, gentamicin (but not streptomycin) serum level determinations are performed routinely in most hospital laboratories. Third, gentamicin can be administered intravenously or intramuscularly, whereas streptomycin can be administered only intramuscularly. Because in vitro synergy against most viridans streptococci with penicillin or ampicillin in combination with gentamicin occurs at low gentamicin concentrations (1 to 3 μg/mL), most authorities recommend using gentamicin at a total daily dose of no more than 3 mg/day (intramuscularly or intravenously), split into either a twice-daily (every 12 hours) or thrice-daily (every 8 hours) dose regimen. A study using ceftriaxone plus gentamicin given as a once-daily dose had excellent efficacy in the therapy of penicillin-susceptible streptococcal IE, however, with no increases in aminoglycoside-associated nephrotoxicity.[544] Despite the apparent safety of once-daily aminoglycoside dosing in this latter IE study and in clinical trials involving patients with other infectious disorders,[546] the total number of patients receiving such regimens for 2 weeks or more is relatively limited. As with any patients receiving aminoglycosides, appropriate clinical and blood level monitoring to mitigate ototoxicity and nephrotoxicity should be employed. Nomograms for prudent monitoring and adjustments of aminoglycoside dosages when once-daily regimens are employed have been published.[545]

We believe that gentamicin, at a total daily dosage of 3 mg/kg, should be substituted for streptomycin in the aforementioned regimens when combination therapy is deemed advisable. In addition, a penicillin-gentamicin regimen is indicated for viridans streptococcal IE if high-level streptomycin resistance is present[531,532] or for strains with a penicillin MIC more than 0.2 μg/mL and less than 0.5 μg/mL.[518] Infections due to strains with a penicillin MIC more than 0.5 μg/mL should be treated as for enterococcal IE (see later). Owing to the enhanced rate of bacterial killing in animal models[547,548] and the high relapse rate of about 17%,[549] we also believe that the Cornell regimen (using gentamicin as the preferred aminoglycoside) should be employed for all patients with IE due to NVS. Although temafloxacin plus tobramycin was as effective as penicillin plus tobramycin in the therapy of experimental IE due to S. adjacens (an NVS species) in rabbits,[550] quinolones are best avoided for IE due to streptococci pending further data. In a penicillin-allergic patient when a cephalosporin is deemed safe, several regimens are acceptable for IE caused by penicillin-susceptible viridans streptococci: cefazolin, 1 to 2 g intramuscularly or intravenously every 8 hours for 4 weeks, combined with streptomycin, 0.5 g intramuscularly every 12 hours, or gentamicin (at the preceding dose regimens) for the initial 2 weeks or ceftriaxone, 2 g intravenously or intramuscularly daily alone for 4 weeks. The latter regimen has proven efficacy for the therapy of penicillin-sensitive streptococcal IE.[551,552] In one uncontrolled trial in Europe, 55 of 59 patients completed treatment with 4 months to 5 years of follow-up. Treatment was completely uneventful in 71% of patients, whereas valve replacement eventually was required in 10 patients. Ceftriaxone administered once daily may permit outpatient therapy in most stable patients with this disease. In addition,

ceftriaxone plus an aminoglycoside shows in vivo synergy in experimental viridans streptococcal IE.[553] Combination regimens of 2 weeks of once-daily ceftriaxone plus an aminoglycoside (netilmicin or gentamicin), which allows for shortened, predominantly outpatient regimens, have been studied in penicillin-susceptible viridans streptococcal IE.[543,544] These trials performed in Europe and North and South America documented efficacy in this form of IE comparable to other 2-week and 4-week regimens.[543,544] When treatment with β-lactams is contraindicated, the regimen of choice is vancomycin, 1 g intravenously every 12 hours for 4 weeks. A 4-week regimen of high-dose teicoplanin has been efficacious in a few patients with streptococcal IE,[554] but the occurrence of drug fever and infection with teicoplanin-tolerant S. bovis is cause for concern.

Penicillin-Resistant Streptococcal and Enterococcal Endocarditis (Minimal Inhibitory Concentration for Penicillin >1 μg/mL)[518]

IE due to enterococci is the third most common form of the disease and is the most resistant to therapy. The mortality rate still approximates 20%,[553] and relapses are common. By broth dilution susceptibility tests, the MIC determinations for many enterococci are as follows: penicillin, 0.4 to 12.5 μg/mL; ampicillin, less than 0.4 to 3.1 μg/mL; cephalothin, 12.5 to 25 μg/mL; vancomycin, 0.78 to 3.1 μg/mL; streptomycin, 3.1 to greater than 50 μg/mL; and gentamicin, 6.25 to 25 μg/mL. Ampicillin is approximately twice as active as penicillin by weight. In contrast, the usual MBC determinations are as follows: penicillin, greater than 6.25 μg/mL (in 80% of cases, >100 μg/mL); cephalothin, greater than 100 μg/mL; streptomycin, greater than 25 μg/mL; vancomycin, greater than 100 μg/mL; and gentamicin, 25 μg/mL or less.[555] E. faecium strains are more resistant to β-lactams than are E. faecalis strains.[556] In general these agents are bacteriostatic against the enterococci and should not be administered alone in this disease. This bacteriostatic action of agents known to inhibit cell wall synthesis is due to a defective bacterial autolytic enzyme system.[557,558] As stated before, all β-lactams, including imipenem, are bacteriostatic against enterococci in vitro, and combination regimens always are employed in treating IE.[559]

A new mechanism of penicillin resistance among E. faecalis strains was described in 1983: plasmid-mediated β-lactamase production. These strains remain relatively rare[560,561]; E. faecalis predominates, but β-lactamase production was documented in E. faecium.[562] Ampicillin-sulbactam overcomes the β-lactamase production and appears equivalent to vancomycin[563,564] (or teicoplanin[565]) in experimental IE due to these organisms and superior to therapy with ticarcillin-clavulanate.[564] Most β-lactamase–producing organisms also display high-level aminoglycoside resistance, further compromising and complicating the choice of available regimens (see later). Still other enterococci, particularly E. faecium or Enterococcus raffinosus, may display high-level penicillin resistance in the absence of β-lactamase production related to perturbations in various penicillin-binding proteins; experimental IE due to these organisms responds to therapy with daptomycin or vancomycin.[566] To date, the number of reported cases of enterococcal IE caused by β-lactamase–producing strains or cases with high-level penicillin resistance on a nonenzymatic basis is low. The traditional view of β-lactam tolerance among enterococci has been challenged[567] in that some strains show "paradoxical" tolerance (i.e., there is a higher percentage of survivors at higher antibiotic concentrations). This phenomenon is shown more easily in vitro at high bacterial densities in stationary growth phase, a situation presumably reflecting the in vivo conditions in the vegetation, and may be important in bacterial persistence or relapse during or after therapy of enterococcal IE.

Cell wall–active antibiotics plus an aminoglycoside are synergistic and produce a bactericidal effect in vitro against most enterococcal strains. Although successful treatment of enterococcal IE requires such combinations, aminoglycoside-associated nephrotoxicity and ototoxicity confer significant risk to patients whose antibiotic regimen includes an aminoglycoside. Studies in experimental models[568] suggest that "low-dose" streptomycin (peak serum concentrations of

9.1 μg/mL) in combination with penicillin is sufficient to treat streptomycin-susceptible enterococcal IE. "High-level" streptomycin resistance (MIC > 2000 μg/mL) is demonstrable in at least 60% of current enterococcal strains. This resistance correlates with an inability to show in vitro synergism between penicillin and streptomycin.[569] These highly resistant strains show synergism between a penicillin and gentamicin in vitro[570,571] at clinically achievable serum concentrations. Enhanced activity with the penicillin and gentamicin combination was seen in vivo for streptomycin-resistant and streptomycin-sensitive enterococci in the rabbit model of IE. No differences in results were seen when penicillin was combined with low-dose versus high-dose gentamicin (peak serum levels of 3.06 and 8.05 μg/mL) in the treatment of experimental streptomycin-resistant enterococcal IE.[572] Early reports[573,574] revealed high-level gentamicin resistance among enterococci in 14% of isolates beginning in 1979. This phenomenon has become increasingly prevalent in many areas[575-577] beginning with *E. faecalis*, but now includes *E. faecium* as well.[577-579] High-level gentamicin resistance (MIC ≥ 2000 μg/mL) now accounts for at least 35% of enterococcal blood isolates in many hospitals. The resistance is plasmid mediated via the production of aminoglycoside-modifying enzymes and can be transferred among strains. A clonal dissemination is not the cause of the increased frequency of these resistant strains because gentamicin resistance appears in a wide variety of different conjugative and nonconjugative plasmids among enterococci.[577] Although these strains seldom cause IE, they present major problems in nosocomial infections[510] and, because resistance to multiple aminoglycosides is common, represent a formidable therapeutic challenge.[580] In addition, penicillin-aminoglycoside or vancomycin-aminoglycoside synergy is not apparent against these organisms in vitro.

The optimal therapy for IE due to these highly resistant strains has not been established. None of the currently recommended regimens is bactericidal against these isolates, and valve replacement[581] may be necessary for a cure. When these isolates are encountered, all available aminoglycosides must be tested separately because the organism may be susceptible to one but resistant to others. Some isolates are sensitive to quinolones or daptomycin, but these agents have received scant attention in human infections. At this time, we favor long-term therapy (8 to 12 weeks) with high dosages of penicillin (20 to 40 million U intravenously daily in divided doses) or ampicillin (2 to 3 g intravenously every 4 hours or by continuous infusion) for IE due to these multiply aminoglycoside-resistant enterococci, pending further data. Although results vary among experimental animal models of IE due to these strains,[580,582] continuous infusion of high-dose ampicillin throughout the 24-hour period may be more effective than a divided-dose regimen and merits a trial in recalcitrant cases. Even higher dose aminoglycosides and trimethoprim-sulfamethoxazole were ineffective in animal models[583,584] and cannot be recommended. In vitro and experimental data have suggested the potential efficacy of double β-lactam combinations of third-generation cephalosporins and ampicillin in enterococcal IE.[585]

Vancomycin also is bacteriostatic against enterococci and exhibits synergy with the aminoglycosides in vitro. The vancomycin-streptomycin combination synergistically kills 40% to 80% of enterococcal strains, whereas the vancomycin-gentamicin combination shows synergy against 93% to 98%.[586] In one study, vancomycin therapy alone was ineffective in eradicating enterococci from cardiac vegetations in the rabbit model of IE, but the combination of vancomycin plus gentamicin rapidly achieved a bactericidal effect.[572] Vancomycin combined with rifampin has an indifferent effect against enterococci (43/48 strains) in vitro; antagonism is observed rarely.[587] Of some concern, outbreaks of infection due to vancomycin-resistant enterococci have been described.[588] Glycopeptide-resistant strains of enterococci first were isolated in France in 1986. These strains have emerged rapidly in recent years in many geographic areas worldwide (e.g., New York City[589]) as an important cause of nosocomial infections. The genetics of vancomycin resistance[590] is described elsewhere (see Chapter 189) and has been reviewed,[591] but multiple phenotypes exist that may confer cross-resistance to related agents (e.g., teicoplanin, daptomycin). Molecular

analyses suggest that a highly mobile genetic element (i.e., a transposon) is responsible for the rapid spread of vancomycin-resistant enterococci.[589] The molecular basis for some forms of this resistance (substitutions of D-alanine-D-lactate for D-alanine-D-alanine in the terminal pentapeptide chain) has been defined. IE due to vancomycin-resistant enterococci is unusual,[592] but has been reported in a variety of clinical settings,[593,594] including transplanted hearts.[595]

The therapy of vancomycin-resistant enterococcal IE is not established. All suspected strains should be tested quantitatively (e.g., by determination of MIC or MBC) in vitro for susceptibility to glycopeptides, penicillins, and aminoglycosides. Teicoplanin—or, potentially, daptomycin[596-598]—may be useful, in combination with gentamicin, against some isolates with low-level vancomycin resistance that do not exhibit cross-resistance. Anecdotal cases have been reported of cures after therapy with linezolid,[593] a combination of quinupristin-dalfopristin plus ampicillin and gentamicin in addition to aortic root replacement,[599] and chloramphenicol plus minocycline.[594] Ramoplanin, a cyclic lipoglycopeptide, is active against more than 90% of strains of highly vancomycin-resistant enterococci in vitro,[600] but clinical experience with IE is virtually nonexistent. A triple combination of high-dose penicillin plus vancomycin plus gentamicin seems promising in animal models of IE induced by such resistant enterococci[601,602] and should be employed if in vitro susceptibility test results suggest multiply-resistant isolates. The cephalosporins are relatively inactive against enterococci, even in combination with an aminoglycoside, and should not be used in this disease. The older generation quinolones (e.g., ciprofloxacin) do not seem promising for the treatment of enterococcal IE.[603] One study showed, however, that a newer quinolone agent with good in vitro spectrum against gram-positive cocci, trovafloxacin, had good in vivo activity against resistant enterococci in the experimental IE model.[604] This in vivo efficacy was noted for several resistant enterococcal strains, including a β-lactamase producer, and for strains exhibiting *vanA*-mediated and *vanB*-mediated resistance (especially when trovafloxacin was combined with ampicillin-sulbactam). In addition, there are limited human treatment data supporting the efficacy of the fixed streptogramin combination of quinupristin-dalfopristin in the therapy of serious vancomycin-resistant enterococcal infections.[605] Among 115 patients with bacteremia due to such strains, including 5 who had IE, the overall frequency of clearance of bacteremia and clinical efficacy approached 70%.[606]

Although controlled trials are lacking, clinical experience would dictate that enterococcal IE caused by strains with typical antibiotic susceptibility profiles be treated with combination antimicrobial therapy for at least 4 to 6 weeks.[535] The recommended regimen is as follows: aqueous penicillin G, 20 million U intravenously daily in divided doses (or ampicillin at doses as recommended for viridans streptococcal IE), combined with streptomycin, 0.5 g intramuscularly every 12 hours, or gentamicin, at the same regimen as that recommended for viridans streptococcal IE, for 4 to 6 weeks. Gentamicin should be given not once daily, but at least twice daily for enterococcal IE. Experimental studies in enterococcal IE models show a greater reduction in vegetation bacterial densities when the aminoglycoside is administered in multidosing rather than once-daily regimens.[607,608] If toxicity (vestibular, aural, or renal) occurs, the streptomycin dose is divided into an every-6-hour regimen. If the streptomycin MIC determined for the infecting strain is 2000 μg/mL or greater, gentamicin should be substituted for streptomycin, although relapses or therapeutic failures are unusual with penicillin plus streptomycin. We recommend penicillin plus gentamicin as the initial therapy. If the peak serum bactericidal titer is less than 1:8, the penicillin dose may be increased, or the aminoglycoside drug may be changed in accordance with in vitro test results.

Olaison and colleagues[609] conducted a 5-year nationwide prospective study in Sweden in which 93 episodes of enterococcal IE were identified. Although current AHA guidelines for the therapy of enterococcal IE recommend combined treatment with penicillin or ampicillin plus an aminoglycoside for 4 to 6 weeks, these investigators evaluated the clinical outcomes when the total duration of aminoglycoside therapy was reduced. Patients in this observational study had a median of 15 days of combined penicillin-ampicillin plus aminoglycoside. The overall cure rate of 81% (75/93) compares favorably with most historical control studies of enterococcal IE.[610,611] Olaison and colleagues[609] concluded that reducing the aminoglycoside duration to approximately 2 weeks would maintain clinical efficacy, while reducing potential toxicities in this high-risk patient population with enterococcal IE. Gavalda and co-workers[612] showed the efficacy of double β-lactam therapy for enterococcal IE, including many aminoglycoside-resistant strains. This approach takes advantage of the ability of agents such as ceftriaxone and ampicillin to saturate at least four of the five major penicillin-binding proteins of enterococci.

Wilson and associates[613] analyzed the experience at the Mayo Clinic with 56 patients who received treatment for 4 weeks with aqueous penicillin G (20 million U intravenously daily) combined with either streptomycin, 0.5 g intramuscularly every 12 hours, for enterococcal IE due to streptomycin-sensitive strains or gentamicin, 1 mg/kg intramuscularly every 8 hours, for IE due to streptomycin-resistant strains. Relapse rates were high (12.5%) for both regimens; however, all patients who relapsed had had symptoms suggestive of IE for longer than 3 months. Relapses also occurred only in patients with mitral valve involvement. All patients who received more than 3 mg/kg daily of gentamicin developed reversible nephrotoxicity (defined as a twofold increase in serum creatinine concentration), and 19% of patients receiving streptomycin for 4 weeks developed irreversible vestibular toxicity. Although this was not a prospective randomized trial, we believe that in selected cases, enterococcal IE may be treated with 4 weeks of combination therapy. Exceptions include mitral valve involvement, duration of symptomatic illness exceeding 3 months, enterococcal prosthetic valve endocarditis, and relapses of enterococcal IE.

A penicillin-allergic patient presents the clinician with a difficult therapeutic dilemma. Vancomycin as a single drug in a dose of 1 g intravenously every 12 hours has been used in the treatment of enterococcal IE. Experience is limited, however, and because of its lack of bactericidal activity in vitro and poor performance in experimental IE, vancomycin should be combined with gentamicin or streptomycin. This combination is potentially more nephrotoxic, and clinical proof of the superiority of such regimens over vancomycin alone is not available. The other therapeutic option in the allergic patient is "penicillin desensitization" followed by the administration of penicillin and an aminoglycoside. The therapy of enterococcal IE due to highly aminoglycoside-resistant or glycopeptide-resistant strains was discussed earlier.

Staphylococcal Endocarditis

The mortality rate in acute staphylococcal IE still approximates 40%, and the preferred antibiotic regimen is controversial. Mortality is highest for men, patients older than 50 years of age, and patients with left-sided involvement or central nervous system manifestations. In addition, narcotic addicts seem to have a lower mortality than do nonaddicts. Most *S. aureus* isolates, whether community or hospital acquired, are now resistant to penicillin G (MIC > 0.2 μg/mL). The current recommended regimen includes a penicillinase-resistant penicillin (nafcillin or oxacillin, 1.5 to 2 g intravenously every 4 hours) or a cephalosporin (cephalothin, 2 g intravenously every 4 hours, or cefazolin, 1 to 2 g intravenously or intramuscularly every 8 hours) given for 4 to 6 weeks.[518,614] The addition of gentamicin produces a synergistic effect against *S. aureus* in vitro and in experimental staphylococcal IE in rabbits.[615] The combination did not improve the survival rate (60%), however, over that observed with a penicillin derivative alone in a small group of patients.[377] Combination therapy did not improve the results of therapy for staphylococcal IE in addicts,[616] but the mortality rate is low in this subgroup of patients (2% to 8%) with this disease. Combination therapy may permit a shorter duration of therapy in addicts with *S. aureus* IE. Two weeks of nafcillin plus tobramycin (1 mg/kg intravenously every 8 hours) cured 47 of 50 (94%) intravenous drug users with right-sided IE[617] without evidence of renal failure, extrapulmonary metastatic infectious complications, aortic or mitral involvement, meningitis, or infection by MRSA.

Since this original experience with "short-course" parenteral therapy for right-sided *S. aureus* IE in addicts,[617] there have been three recent randomized, prospective trials of short-course regimens in this disease, comprising 121 patients (summarized by DiNubile).[618,619] The combination regimens employed included intravenous cloxacillin with either gentamicin or amikacin.[620-622] The overall clinical and microbiologic cure rates exceeded 90% in these studies. In patients with HIV seropositivity (most having CD4+ counts >300 × 10^6 cells) and in patients who had large tricuspid vegetations (≥10 mm in diameter), such regimens had excellent efficacy.[622] In this latter study, Ribera and co-workers[622] showed an efficacy of intravenous cloxacillin equivalent to that of the cloxacillin-plus-gentamicin regimen. It seems that for most addicted patients with uncomplicated right-sided *S. aureus* IE, short-course parenteral regimens of an antistaphylococcal semisynthetic penicillin plus an aminoglycoside are interchangeable with longer term (4 to 6 weeks) parenteral regimens. An investigation confirmed the relative ineffectiveness of a glycopeptide (teicoplanin or vancomycin) plus gentamicin–based, short-course regimen for right-sided *S. aureus* IE.[623] In addition, two studies have evaluated the use of predominantly oral 4-week antibiotic regimens (ciprofloxacin plus rifampin) for the therapy of uncomplicated right-sided *S. aureus* IE in addicts.[624,625] In each study, including one in which more than 70% of patients were HIV-seropositive,[625] cure rates exceeded 90%.

Anecdotal case reports in nonaddicts with staphylococcal IE suggest that the addition of gentamicin may be beneficial in patients failing to respond to nafcillin therapy.[626] This issue was addressed in a multicenter prospective trial comparing nafcillin alone with nafcillin plus gentamicin (for the initial 2 weeks) in the treatment of IE due to *S. aureus*.[627] Most of the patients in this study were nonaddicts who had left-sided IE. Although the combination resulted in a more rapid rate of eradication of the bacteremia, the incidence of nephrotoxicity was increased, and no improvement in mortality was achieved. Despite these results, many authorities still use combination therapy for short periods (e.g., 3 to 5 days) for left-sided *S. aureus* IE, especially in fulminant cases. For right-sided and left-sided *S. aureus* IE, there is little compelling evidence that adjunctive gentamicin therapy beyond 3 to 5 days adds any benefit to clinical outcomes in standard cases.[519] If the organism is susceptible to penicillin (MIC <0.1 (g/mL), this agent in a dose of 20 million U intravenously daily should be used. The response to treatment may be slow, often with fever and positive blood cultures lasting 1 week.[374]

The therapy of staphylococcal IE in penicillin-allergic patients, or when the isolate is methicillin-resistant (MRSA), is problematic. A decision analysis concluded that patients with a questionable history of immediate-type hypersensitivity to penicillin and methicillin-sensitive *S. aureus* IE should be skin tested before starting antibiotic therapy.[628] First-generation cephalosporins (as noted previously) generally are recommended in patients with non–life-threatening penicillin allergy, but nafcillin is more active in experimental methicillin-susceptible *S. aureus* endocarditis[629] and is preferred if results of skin tests for penicillin allergy are negative. With the exception of ceftazidime, the in vivo efficacy of cephalosporins in experimental *S. aureus* IE has a positive correlation with in vitro activity (MIC) and the time (percentage) during the dosing interval in which the drug serum level exceeds the MIC.[629] Vancomycin still is recommended for the therapy of *S. aureus* IE in patients with life-threatening penicillin allergy (e.g., anaphylaxis) or anaphylactoid reactions (e.g., giant urticaria) or when MRSA strains are involved; however, more recent experience suggests caution because suboptimal outcomes have been associated with the use of this agent in MRSA IE. Vancomycin is less rapidly bactericidal than nafcillin in vitro against *S. aureus,* especially at high inocula (approximately 10^7 CFU), mimicking intravegetation densities. Vancomycin therapy for complicated *S. aureus* bacteremia also has been associated with relapses as confirmed by pulsed-field gel electrophoresis.[630] Failure rates of approximately 40% have been documented in patients with *S. aureus* IE treated with vancomycin[631] despite right-sided involvement. In another study[632] using vancomycin-based regimens (with or without rifampin), blood cultures still were positive after

7 days of therapy in approximately 50% of patients, despite right-sided involvement and negative results in many echocardiographic studies. Daptomycin and teicoplanin appeared unlikely to be acceptable substitutes in early experiences, owing to unfavorable or unpredictable pharmacokinetics[633] or the development of resistance[634,635] during therapy. For methicillin-susceptible *S. aureus* IE in patients with anaphylactoid-type β-lactam allergy and suboptimal responses to vancomycin, the need for β-lactam desensitization should be considered.[636,637]

Clindamycin has been used to treat more than 60 cases of staphylococcal IE, but it is associated with an unacceptable relapse rate, and its use is not recommended.[638] The optimal therapy for IE due to "tolerant" strains of *S. aureus* is controversial.[639,640] One retrospective study[641] suggested that patients with IE due to these tolerant strains had a more complicated course; however, combination therapy did not seem to be beneficial. Tolerance does seem to influence the response to therapy in some experimental animal models of *S. aureus* IE,[642] and the use of combination regimens seems prudent when these strains are recovered from patients, but this is not universally accepted. Another controversial area is the adjunctive role of rifampin, the most active antibiotic currently available against *S. aureus* in vitro in therapy for IE. Owing to the emergence of resistant strains, this drug is ineffective alone. Results of in vitro studies on rifampin combinations with either β-lactam agents or vancomycin frequently are contradictory, and clinical outcomes with experimental IE induced by *S. aureus* depend on which drug in the combination exerts the greatest bactericidal activity in vivo.[643] At present, rifampin should be reserved for patients showing poor serum bactericidal activity during therapy with a β-lactam or vancomycin or in patients with suppurative complications (e.g., valve-ring abscesses, hematogenous osteomyelitis, meningitis). Resistance to clindamycin and rifampin has emerged during therapy of this condition, however.[644]

The therapy for IE due to *S. aureus* displaying borderline susceptibility to antistaphylococcal penicillins, first described by McDougal and Thornsberry in 1986,[645] is also a matter of debate. Experimental models of IE induced with these isolates suggest, however, that nafcillin (or oxacillin) or ampicillin-sulbactam should be effective.[646,647] Several newer agents, including teicoplanin, fosfomycin, and fluoroquinolones, are active against MRSA in vitro and are as rapidly bactericidal as vancomycin in experimental animal models of IE due to MRSA,[648-650] although resistance to the quinolones has emerged during therapy, and frank failures have been recorded.[637,651,652] For patients with MRSA IE not responding to vancomycin, several choices are available, including the addition of rifampin or gentamicin (or both) or other regimens including daptomycin, linezolid, quinupristin-dalfopristin, minocycline, trimethoprim-sulfamethoxazole, and ciprofloxacin-rifampin. Experience with these drugs in humans with *S. aureus* IE is limited.[653] According to some authors,[654] when *S. aureus* bacteremia occurs in a patient with a removable focus of infection, the risk of concurrent IE is low, and treatment schedules may be shortened to 2 to 3 weeks. This approach avoids the high costs and risks of superinfection or antibiotic reactions associated with prolonged therapy. In one study, 8 of 21 patients with an infected intravenous catheter as the suspected source of *S. aureus* bacteremia developed IE.[655]

Bayer and associates[637,656] identified four parameters predictive of the presence of IE in 72 patients with *S. aureus* bacteremia in a prospective study: (1) the absence of a primary site of infection, (2) community acquisition of infection, (3) metastatic sequelae, and (4) valvular vegetations detected by echocardiography. In another study of 724 prospectively identified patients with *S. aureus* bacteremia, clinical identifiers of complicated bacteremia included (1) community acquisition, (2) persistent fever at 72 hours, (3) skin examination suggesting the presence of acute systemic infection, and (4) positive blood culture 48 to 96 hours after the initial positive blood culture.[381] Although these clinical identifiers are useful methods to assist in the identification of clinically unsuspected IE, the role of echocardiography increasingly is being recognized.

Two decision analyses have shown the role of TEE in identifying the presence of IE and in helping to define duration of antibiotic therapy.

Heidenreich and colleagues[316] found that for patients whose prior probability of IE is 4% to 60%, initial use of TEE provided the greatest quality-adjusted survival at a cost within the range for commonly accepted health interventions. Rosen and colleagues[317] found that the use of TEE to determine the duration of therapy (2 weeks versus 4 weeks) for patients with intravascular catheter–associated *S. aureus* bacteremia was cost-effective and provided better outcomes than empirical 2-week or 4-week treatment strategies. While awaiting definitive trials, short-term therapy should be used only if IE can be excluded reasonably by methods previously discussed. Although some studies have suggested that occult IE in patients with nosocomial *S. aureus* bacteremia is uncommon,[636] a growing number of investigations have identified the increasing importance of health care–associated *S. aureus* IE.[23-26,657,658] Fowler and colleagues[657] documented an apparent increase in the proportion of cases of IE complicating nosocomially acquired *S. aureus* bacteremia (mainly from infected intravascular catheters). In this group of 27 patients, classic manifestations of IE were uncommon, and TEE was useful in diagnosis of IE. IE due to glycopeptide-intermediate *S. aureus* has been reported,[659,660] and soft tissue infections due to vancomycin-resistant *S. aureus*[661,662] have been reported and are cause for concern.

S. epidermidis is the most common etiologic agent in cases of prosthetic valve IE. Most of these strains (87%) are methicillin resistant when isolated within 1 year of valve implantation. One study[663] suggested that the optimal antimicrobial regimen for these infections is vancomycin plus rifampin, usually with the addition of an aminoglycoside. The emergence of vancomycin resistance among coagulase-negative staphylococci[664] is cause for concern. These concepts are discussed further in Chapter 75.

Endocarditis Due to Members of Enterobacteriaceae or *Pseudomonas* Species

Of 125 cases of IE reported from Seattle, 4.8% were due to gram-negative aerobic bacilli.[27] The mortality rate was 83%, and none of the patients in whom treatment did not include surgery survived. The prognosis is especially poor with left-sided cardiac involvement. Determinations of tube dilution MBC are necessary to guide therapy. Certain combinations of penicillins or cephalosporins and aminoglycosides have been shown to be synergistic against many of these strains and usually are recommended. For IE due to most strains of *E. coli* or *Proteus mirabilis,* a combination of a penicillin, either ampicillin (2 g intravenously every 4 hours) or penicillin (20 million U intravenously daily), and an aminoglycoside, usually gentamicin (1.7 mg/kg every 8 hours) or a broad-spectrum cephalosporin, is suggested. Third-generation cephalosporins are extremely active against *E. coli* in vitro, and some (e.g., ceftriaxone) have proved effective in experimental animal models of *E. coli* IE,[665] even when long dosing intervals were used. This group of agents merits further evaluation in humans for IE due to susceptible gram-negative bacilli. A combination of a third-generation cephalosporin and an aminoglycoside (either gentamicin or amikacin) is recommended for *Klebsiella* IE. Certain β-lactam/β-lactamase inhibitor combinations (e.g., piperacillin-tazobactam,[666] but not ceftriaxone-sulbactam[667]) are active in vivo in experimental models of *Klebsiella* IE in animals induced by TEM-3-producing isolates and merit further evaluation in combination with an aminoglycoside in humans with this disease. The specific aminoglycoside employed is a crucial variable and cannot be predicted totally from MIC data alone because pharmacodynamic characteristics differ markedly in animal models of IE due to gram-negative aerobic bacilli.[668,669] Endovascular *Salmonella* infections, including IE, also may respond to third-generation cephalosporins (see later).[670] Left-sided IE due to *S. marcescens* is refractory to medical therapy alone; valve replacement invariably is required to effect a cure.[411]

P. aeruginosa remains an important pathogen in drug addicts with IE. Medical therapy may be successful in *P. aeruginosa* IE involving the right side of the heart in 50% to 75% of cases. If the disease is refractory to antibiotics, tricuspid valvulectomy or "vegetectomy"[671] without valve replacement is indicated.[672] Although valve replacement often is necessary for a cure of left-sided IE due to *P. aeruginosa,*[673] results in a series of 10 patients (7 with left-sided involvement alone or in combination with tricuspid disease)[226] suggest that medical therapy alone occasionally is curative. Studies in animals with experimental *Pseudomonas* IE[674] offer a partial explanation for these disparate results: The penetration into vegetations and the time during which antibiotic concentrations exceeded the MBC were significantly greater with tricuspid than with aortic vegetations for ceftazidime and tobramycin.

Problems have emerged with all potential regimens in animal models of this disease: (1) Therapy with β-lactams (e.g., ceftazidime) has failed, owing to the selection of clones within valve vegetations that exhibit constitutive hyperproduction of type Id β-lactamase[675]; (2) isolates showing aminoglycoside resistance due to permeability defects emerge during therapy[676]; (3) no postantibiotic effect of β-lactams against *P. aeruginosa* is evident in vivo,[677] necessitating frequent (or continuous) drug administration; and (4) the alginate exopolysaccharide inhibits clearance of mucoid strains from the vegetation via cellular or antimicrobial mechanisms. This inhibition can be reversed partially by the coadministration of alginase in animal models of *Pseudomonas* IE.[678]

Treatment failures of *Pseudomonas* IE in humans also have been due to the selection of isolates with an enhanced production of type Id β-lactamase.[679] Based on clinical experience,[384,413,414] however, the preferred regimen for IE due to *P. aeruginosa* is high-dose tobramycin (8 mg/kg/day intravenously or intramuscularly in divided doses every 8 hours) with maintenance of peak and trough concentrations of 15 to 20 μg/mL and 2 μg/mL or less in combination with either an extended-spectrum penicillin (e.g., ticarcillin, piperacillin, azlocillin) or ceftazidime or cefepime in full doses. The toxicity associated with this regimen is low; combination treatment should be given for a minimum of 6 weeks. The use of quinolones (in combination with an aminoglycoside) seems promising for the treatment of *Pseudomonas* IE on the basis of favorable results in animal models[675] and in humans,[680] but the development of stepwise resistance during therapy may limit the efficacy of this class of drugs in the future. Based on limited experimental data,[681] ceftazidime-tobramycin is preferred over aztreonam-tobramycin for this disease. Approximately seven cases of *P. aeruginosa* IE have been treated successfully with imipenem plus an aminoglycoside,[682] but the potential for the development of resistance exists with any of these regimens.

In one study, IE due to *Haemophilus* spp. (and other members of the HACEK group) usually was responsive to ampicillin alone[405] administered for 3 weeks. β-lactamase–producing strains have been well documented, however. Because of difficulty in cultivating HACEK organisms in the laboratory, particularly for newer, automated susceptibility testing systems, such strains should be considered as ampicillin resistant. Ceftriaxone and cefotaxime have excellent in vitro activity against HACEK organisms and provide the potential for the avoidance of aminoglycoside-induced toxicity. Although clinical data are limited, the third-generation cephalosporins should be regarded as the drugs of choice for treatment of HACEK IE.[681] The place for quinolones (if any) in the therapy of these infections is not known.[683] Duration of treatment for HACEK IE should be 3 to 4 weeks for native valve infections and 6 weeks for prosthetic valve infections.[518,684] The foregoing recommendations offer only a rough guide for initial treatment. It is imperative that each isolate be subjected to quantitative sensitivity testing in vitro to ensure the optimal selection of antibiotics.

Endocarditis Due to Anaerobic Bacilli

Although IE caused by anaerobic bacilli is uncommon, the mortality is high. *B. fragilis* is isolated in many of these cases and is responsible for most fatalities. Most strains of anaerobic bacilli, with the exception of *B. fragilis,* are sensitive to penicillin in vitro, and use of this agent, in a dose of 20 million U intravenously daily, is the recommended therapy.[449,450] In addition, 33% of the strains of *B. fragilis* show an MIC for penicillin that is less than 0.25 μg/mL. Penicillin is only bacteriostatic

against these strains (MBC is invariably >100 μg/mL), however, and relapse is common. Although clindamycin and chloramphenicol readily inhibit most strains of *B. fragilis,* they lack bactericidal activity, and they are poor therapeutic choices, although several patients have been cured with high-dose penicillin, chloramphenicol (1 g intravenously every 6 hours), or clindamycin (600 mg intravenously every 6 hours). Owing to excellent bactericidal activity in vitro and the serum concentrations attained, metronidazole, ticarcillin plus clavulanic acid, piperacillin plus tazobactam, imipenem, and meropenem are reasonable choices for therapy for anaerobic IE.[451]

Pneumococcal, Gonococcal, and Meningococcal Endocarditis

IE caused by pneumococci, gonococci, or meningococci is now very rare. Pneumococcal IE must be considered in any patient with pneumococcal bacteremia, especially if meningitis is present. This form of IE is most common in alcoholics; the organism generally attacks the aortic valve and results in valvular insufficiency, often with perivalvular abscess formation or pericarditis. Type 12 pneumococci cause greater than 20% of the cases of pneumococcal IE, but are a rare (5% of cases) cause of pneumococcal pneumonia. Penicillin, 20 million U intravenously daily, or a third-generation cephalosporin for 4 weeks is recommended to treat pneumococcal IE. Although the impact of penicillin resistance on the outcome of pneumococcal IE is unresolved, one series of 63 patients with pneumococcal IE found that left-sided heart failure, but not penicillin resistance, was associated independently with a higher risk of death.[685] In the rare circumstance of IE due to strains either moderately resistant or highly resistant to penicillin G, a third-generation cephalosporin or vancomycin would be the preferred choice.

The gonococci that cause systemic infection usually are susceptible to penicillin.[686] IE due to these organisms and the meningococci can be treated effectively with the same penicillin regimen recommended for pneumococcal IE. Although IE due to penicillin-resistant gonococci (on either a β-lactamase production basis or due to chromosomally mediated mechanisms) has not been reported, ceftriaxone has been used successfully to treat gonococcal IE.[687]

Fungal Endocarditis

Since the 1990s, the incidence of fungal sepsis[465] and fungal IE has undergone a striking increase. Fungal IE occurs principally in a setting of narcotic addiction, after cardiac surgery, after the prolonged intravenous administration of drugs (especially broad-spectrum antibiotics), and in the compromised host (including preterm neonates). Although the survival rate in patients treated before 1974 was less than 20%,[273] survival in the current era has increased to approximately 40%, coincident with improved diagnostic techniques.[688] The preferred mode of therapy has not been determined. The use of antifungal agents alone has been almost universally unsuccessful in achieving a cure of this disease. The addition of surgical measures to antifungal therapy may result in an improvement in prognosis, but to date there is insufficient clinical experience. When fungal IE is diagnosed, a combined medical-surgical approach is recommended.[467,689]

The mainstay of antifungal drug therapy is amphotericin B. This agent is toxic and produces multiple side effects, including fever, chills, phlebitis, headache, anorexia, anemia, hypokalemia, renal tubular acidosis, nephrotoxicity, nausea, and vomiting. Drug toxicity is common and often necessitates alterations in the regimen. Dosages and the technique of administration are given in Chapter 36.

After 1 to 2 weeks of amphotericin B therapy at full dosages, surgery probably should be performed. If isolated tricuspid IE is present, as in a narcotic addict, total tricuspid valvulectomy usually can be performed. Rarely, removal of the vegetation alone is curative. Most patients tolerate the valvulectomy without the development of significant right-sided heart failure for at least 3 to 5 years. Valve replacement is necessary for left-sided fungal IE. The duration of antifungal therapy after surgery is empirical, but 6 to 8 weeks usually is recommended.

It is possible that combination antifungal therapy may improve the poor survival with fungal IE. Some strains of *Candida* spp. and *Cryptococcus neoformans* are inhibited in vitro by concentrations of 5-fluorocytosine achieved with the oral administration of 150 mg/kg/day in six divided doses. Synergism between 5-fluorocytosine and amphotericin B has been documented for these yeasts in vitro and in the treatment of cryptococcal meningitis. This combination was fungicidal and perhaps instrumental in the cure of one case of *Aspergillus* IE. In the rabbit model of IE due to *C. albicans,*[279] however, the addition of 5-fluorocytosine did not improve the rate of eradication of fungal organisms from the vegetation over that observed with amphotericin B alone. Potentiation of amphotericin B activity by rifampin has been noted for virtually all strains of *Candida* spp. tested and for a few isolates of *H. capsulatum.* The therapeutic advantage of the addition of 5-fluorocytosine or rifampin to amphotericin for fungal IE requires further investigation, but initial results in animal models of disseminated candidiasis are not encouraging.[690] On the basis of animal model data,[691] high-dose itraconazole may be of value in the treatment of *Aspergillus* IE, but valve replacement probably will remain imperative for a cure.[692] Amphotericin B is more effective than fluconazole for the prophylaxis and treatment of experimental *Candida* IE[693] and remains the agent of choice. The use of fluconazole apparently has led to long-term cures of *Candida* IE, however, in a limited number of patients[467,694-696] when valve replacement was considered to be contraindicated. This agent should be tried after an initial course of amphotericin B in this setting or used for long-term suppressive therapy. The role of amphotericin–lipid and liposomal complexes, voriconazole, and caspofungin in the treatment of fungal IE is unknown.

Q Fever Endocarditis

More than 1300 well-documented cases of Q fever have been reported[697]; the mortality exceeds 65%.[475,476,478-480] Prolonged therapy (≥4 years) with doxycycline and either trimethoprim-sulfamethoxazole or rifampin is considered to be the regimen of choice[475,698-700] (see Chapter 184). A fluoroquinolone may be a useful addition to doxycycline.[475,700] The acidic conditions of the phagolysosome, where the organism resides, may inhibit antibiotic activity.[700] Cure of the IE after treatment with a combination of doxycycline and hydroxychloroquine to alkalinize the phagolysosome for 1 year was reported in 20 patients.[475] Valve replacement often is required, and long-term prognosis is guarded. Careful follow-up to detect recrudescence of infection is essential. Most authorities recommend at least 3 to 4 years of therapy to eradicate valvular and extravalvular Q fever (usually in the liver). A combination regimen of doxycycline plus hydroxychloroquine for at least 18 months allowed shortening the duration of therapy and resulted in the reduction in the number of relapses.[697]

Infective Endocarditis Due to Chlamydiae

Albeit based on limited experience, a combination of valve replacement and prolonged (.3 months) tetracycline therapy seems justified in IE due to chlamydiae. Rifampin has cured at least one case of chlamydial IE after therapy with tetracyclines had failed, but exposure to this agent rapidly induces the emergence of drug resistance in *C. trachomatis* in tissue culture.[701] The role of combination regimens (e.g., rifampin plus erythromycin or tetracycline) merits further study.

Culture-Negative Endocarditis

The therapy for culture-negative IE in non–drug addicts is controversial, but the regimen usually used "covers" enterococci, the HACEK group, and NVS. This regimen consists of a combination of penicillin, 20 million U intravenously daily in divided doses, or ampicillin, 2 g intravenously every 4 hours, plus streptomycin, 0.5 g intramuscularly every 12 hours, or gentamicin, 1.7 mg/kg intramuscularly or intravenously every 8 hours, plus ceftriaxone, 2 g intravenously once daily. When staphylococcal IE is likely (as in narcotic addicts), a penicillinase-resistant penicillin or a cephalosporin in full dosage should be substituted in the aforementioned regimen. If clinical improvement occurs, some authorities recommend discontinuation of treatment with the aminoglycoside after 2 weeks. The other agents should be continued for a full 6 weeks of treatment. Continued surveillance for the causative agent and careful follow-up are mandatory. An analysis of any correlation between the response to empirical antimicrobial therapy and survival was performed in 52 patients with culture-negative IE[488]: 92% of the patients who became afebrile within the first week of therapy survived versus only 50% if fever persisted longer than 7 days. Most deaths were caused by major systemic emboli or uncontrollable CHF due to valvular insufficiency.

Surgical Therapy

Valve replacement has become an important adjunct to medical therapy in the management of IE and now is used in at least 25% of the cases. The generally accepted indications for surgical intervention during active IE are as follows: (1) refractory CHF; (2) more than one serious systemic embolic episode; (3) uncontrolled infection; (4) physiologically significant valve dysfunction as shown by echocardiography; (5) ineffective antimicrobial therapy (e.g., as in fungal IE); (6) resection of mycotic aneurysms; (7) most cases of prosthetic valve IE caused by more antibiotic-resistant pathogens (e.g., staphylococci, enteric gram-negative bacilli); and (8) local suppurative complications, including perivalvular or myocardial abscesses. The major indications in the past have been persistent infection and CHF[702-704] in adults and children.[705] CHF during active IE was the indication for surgery in 86% of 108 patients undergoing valve replacement at Stanford from 1963 to 1984.[704] The important role of valve replacement surgery has been emphasized for patients with *S. aureus* prosthetic valve IE.[706] Despite the widespread use of TTE and TEE at present in patients with IE, the indications for surgical intervention based on echocardiographic features remain controversial. The AHA Committee on IE, working from data reported in the recent literature, has identified the following echocardiographic features in IE as associated with a potential increased need for surgical intervention: (1) persistent vegetations after a major systemic embolic episode, (2) large (>1 cm in diameter) anterior mitral valve vegetations, (3) increase in vegetation size after 4 weeks of antibiotic therapy, (4) acute mitral insufficiency, (5) valve perforation or rupture, and (6) periannular extension of infection. (These data are reviewed in the article by Bayer and associates.[323]) Preliminary data from a tertiary cardiac surgical center in Europe have emphasized early mitral valve repair in IE where feasible to circumvent the eventual need for prosthetic valve placement in the decade after the episode of IE.[707] The most common causes of death in IE, in approximate order, are neurologic and septic complications,[708] CHF, embolic phenomena, rupture of a mycotic aneurysm, complications of cardiac surgery, lack of response to antimicrobial therapy, and prosthetic valve IE.[2,5-8,13,14,16-18,20,27]

A retrospective cohort study stratified adults with complicated left-sided native valve IE using baseline features into four groups of prognostic severity.[709] When acute aortic regurgitation complicated by CHF supervenes in IE, the mortality still exceeds 50%. The classic physical findings associated with chronic aortic regurgitation often are absent in these patients.[318] The current trend is to perform early surgery in this group of patients because nothing is gained by delay. The merits of early valve replacement surgery were confirmed in 1972.[710] In a series of 28 patients from Birmingham, Alabama, with acute aortic regurgitation, 4 had no CHF and were managed medically, and all survived. In contrast, 7 of 11 patients with mild CHF and 7 of 8 patients with moderate-to-severe CHF died during medical therapy, often suddenly and with pathologic evidence of coronary emboli and myocardial infarction. Four of five patients with moderately severe CHF who underwent surgery survived. These data suggest that early surgical intervention may improve survival in this setting. Valvular regurgitation on Doppler echocardiography is not predictive of death in the absence of CHF.[711]

The hemodynamic status of the patient, not the activity of the infection, is the crucial determining factor in the timing of cardiac valve replacement (i.e., development of CHF in the setting of IE generally dictates valvular surgery regardless of the acuity of infection or the amount of antibiotics already received by the patient).[712] The hemodynamic severity of the acute aortic regurgitation may be assessed by determining the degree of mitral valve preclosure by echocardiography. If premature closure of the mitral valve occurs before the Q wave of the electrocardiogram, the left ventricular end-diastolic pressure is very high, and surgical intervention is required urgently. Nothing is gained by temporizing, even if only a few hours of antibiotics can be administered. When CHF persists despite digoxin, diuretics, and other therapeutic modalities (e.g., left ventricular afterload reduction), surgery also is indicated. In 80 patients subjected to aortic valve replacement for IE, the surgical cure rate was 72%. There were no instances of subsequent infection of the prosthesis, but 16% developed paravalvular regurgitation. This latter complication usually was controlled easily medically. Organisms visible on Gram stain, positive cultures, or annular abscesses at the time of surgery are associated with late complications.[708] Although not systematically studied, most authorities suggest that if there is evidence of active IE at the time of valve replacement surgery, antibiotic therapy should be continued postoperatively for at least several weeks. This evidence includes vegetations that remain culture positive and vegetations with significant polymorphonuclear inflammation. An investigation by Morris and colleagues[187] found that dead bacteria may persist for months in sterile vegetations and concluded that only valve cultures should be considered when determining the duration of antibiotic therapy after valve replacement for IE. By contrast, routine valve cultures in patients undergoing native valve replacement for indications other than clinically suspected IE do not seem warranted.[713]

In contrast to left-sided IE, in which CHF is the usual indication for surgical intervention, persistent infection is the indication for surgery in greater than 70% of patients with right-sided IE. Most patients are narcotic addicts, with IE caused by organisms that are difficult to eradicate with antimicrobial therapy alone (e.g., fungi, gram-negative aerobic bacilli). Tricuspid valvulectomy or vegetectomy with valvuloplasty is now the procedure of choice for refractory right-sided IE.[714,715] Valve replacement at a second operation is advised only when medical management fails to control the hemodynamic manifestations and the patient has ceased using illicit drugs. Combination antimicrobial therapy should be continued for 4 to 6 weeks postoperatively. These patients may develop mild-to-moderate right-sided heart failure, but this is tolerated easily, and the success rate with this approach is greater than 70%. Eventual tricuspid valve replacement usually is required, however, for progressive right heart failure. Persistent fever, recurrent pulmonary emboli, or vegetations demonstrable by echocardiography usually do not necessitate tricuspid valvulectomy in this setting.[716] In addition, many surgeons contend that a return to the use of illicit drugs and reinfection of the valve after initial cure are contraindications to reoperation.[717]

Outstanding reviews on the indications for surgery during therapy for IE are available.[703,718-721] The rationale for surgical intervention, including major and minor criteria for valve replacement, is discussed in detail. A point system weighting multiple factors has been devised by Alsip and colleagues[718] to assist in decision making concerning surgery in patients with active IE. The value of this system remains to be defined. It has become apparent that most patients with prosthetic valve IE (except patients with late disease caused by penicillin-sensitive viridans streptococci) require valve replacement for consistent cures (see Chapter 66). Valve replacement also is necessary in a significant proportion of patients with IE on native valves after a medical cure; aortic involvement is a predictor of the need for surgery.[722]

SUPPURATIVE THROMBOPHLEBITIS

Suppurative thrombophlebitis is an inflammation of the vein wall due to the presence of microorganisms and frequently is associated with thrombosis and bacteremia. In the following discussion, suppurative thrombophlebitis is differentiated from catheter-related sepsis. Suppuration of the vein wall usually is absent in intravenous

catheter–related sepsis and bacteremia secondary to contaminated intravenous fluid but does occur. Suppurative thrombophlebitis may be classified into four forms: superficial, central (including pelvic), cavernous sinus, and infection of the portal vein (pyelophlebitis). The last two conditions have become rare since the introduction of antibiotics. Cavernous sinus thrombosis and thrombosis of the intracranial dural sinuses are discussed in Chapters 71 and 95. In contrast, superficial suppurative thrombophlebitis has been increasing steadily in incidence since the introduction of the plastic intravenous cannula. Superficial suppurative thrombophlebitis secondary to intravenous fluid therapy first was described in 1947,[723] when 93 cases were reported, 43 of which were amenable to surgical therapy.

Epidemiology

In 1973, approximately one of every four hospitalized patients received intravenous therapy, for a total of more than 10 million patients annually in the United States.[724] It is estimated that more than half of the 40 million patients admitted to U.S. hospitals each year undergo intravascular catheterization.[725] Suppurative thrombophlebitis is a particular problem in burned patients, for whom it represents a common cause of death due to infection. In several large series of burned patients,[726-729] suppurative thrombophlebitis developed in 4% to 8% and increased in frequency if cutdowns were performed. Suppurative thrombophlebitis also is found in other hospitalized patients (especially patients with cancer or patients receiving steroid therapy).[730,731] Seven cases were recognized in an 18-month period in Charleston, South Carolina, and 35 cases were identified in 7 years in Louisville, Kentucky.[732] Eight cases were encountered during an 8-month period in Johannesburg; suppurative thrombophlebitis was estimated to represent a minimum incidence of 0.12% of all admissions.[733] In a study using strict diagnostic criteria, 29 episodes of suppurative thrombophlebitis in 27 patients were identified in a large Air Force hospital within 4 years.[734] Using data from the National Nosocomial Infection Study, Rhame and associates[735] estimated the overall incidence of suppurative thrombophlebitis as 88 per 100,000 discharges, but this disease is underreported. Suppurative thrombophlebitis also is common in drug addicts, particularly when injections are made in large, central veins (e.g., jugular or subclavian veins).[736] This condition is unusual during childhood,[737] but may occur as a complication related to intravenous therapy.

Catheter-related sepsis without suppurative thrombophlebitis is much more common and affects at least 50,000 to 100,000 patients per year in the United States.[738,739] The risk of this complication is approximately 40 times higher with plastic cannulas (8%) than with steel or "scalp vein" cannulas (0.2%). Irritation to the vein wall with the subsequent development of suppurative thrombophlebitis is more common with polyethylene catheters than with catheters constructed of Teflon or Silastic material. Central venous catheterization has been employed for more than 35 years for hemodynamic monitoring, total parenteral nutrition, and infusion of drugs. The exact incidence of suppurative thrombophlebitis of the central veins commonly cannulated (i.e., jugulars, subclavian, venae cavae) is unknown. Catheter-induced thrombosis is relatively common. Autopsy series have revealed central venous thrombosis in 37% of catheterized subjects, but this diagnosis rarely is recognized because most patients are asymptomatic. When examined by phlebography at the time of catheter withdrawal, 42% of catheters have sleeve thrombi, and another 8% reveal veno-occlusive thrombi.[740] In addition, sepsis has been reported in approximately 7% of patients receiving total parenteral nutrition and other medications by the central route. When thrombosis and bacterial or fungal contamination or sepsis coexist, suppurative thrombophlebitis may intervene.[741] The role of hypercoagulability due to gene polymorphisms in catheter-associated infection and thrombosis has been evaluated[742] but is unresolved. At least 50 cases of suppurative thrombophlebitis of the great thoracic veins have been reported in the literature,[743-745] but this is almost certainly a gross underestimate of the problem. Eight cases in 8 years due to *Candida* spp. alone were observed at the University of Wisconsin.[746] As another example, 53 cancer patients with catheter-related *S. aureus* bacteremia were identified from 1986 to 1989 at the M.D. Anderson Cancer Center; septic thrombosis was diagnosed in 12 (23%) and suspected in another 3 (6%) patients. Five of these 12 patients developed deep-seated complications, including septic pulmonary emboli and endocarditis, versus 2 of 38 without septic thrombosis (P < .01). Persistent fever despite appropriate antistaphylococcal agents was an early clue to the diagnosis.[747] Septic atrial thrombosis, occasionally with a coexistent Budd-Chiari syndrome, has complicated Broviac catheter insertion in infants.[748]

Superficial suppurative thrombophlebitis is a complication of either dermal infection or use of an indwelling intravenous catheter. Pelvic suppurative thrombophlebitis is associated with parturition, abortion, gynecologic surgery, or a pelvic abscess. This is a disease of women of childbearing age, with most cases occurring between the ages of 15 and 40 years (mean 20 years). In 123 cases in two reports,[749,750] the predisposing conditions were as follows: vaginal delivery, 39 cases; cesarean section, 19 cases; abortion, 33 cases; and major gynecologic surgery, 32 cases. During a 9-year period in Atlanta, 27 cases of postpartum septic pelvic thrombophlebitis were identified in more than 54,000 deliveries.[750] The relative risks for this condition were as follows: parturition, 1/2000 (highest in the inner-city population); septic abortion, 1/200; and major gynecologic surgery, 1/800. The incidence of suppurative thrombophlebitis increases proportionally with the degree of trauma to the pelvic tissues.

Pathogenesis

The pathogenesis of suppurative thrombophlebitis (discussed in detail by Tornos and colleagues[722]) is poorly understood. A thrombus may act as a nidus for local entrapment and colonization of bacteria that gain access to the site from another focus. This is analogous to the proposed role of NBTE in the pathogenesis of IE. When superficial suppurative thrombophlebitis is associated with intravascular cannulas, the route of infection may be (1) migration from the skin between the catheter wall and perivascular tissue, (2) contamination of intravenous fluid, (3) contamination of the hub, or (4) hematogenous dissemination from an infected focus elsewhere. The relative contributions of these four routes are unknown, although most investigators believe that migration of organisms down the external surface of the catheter is the most important route of invasion.[725] The predominant organism in burn wounds, *P. aeruginosa,* is a rare cause of suppurative thrombophlebitis, however, and suppurative thrombophlebitis usually develops days to weeks after the cutdown incision is healed,[727,728] arguing against a local cutaneous source in burn patients.

The venous system draining the pelvis includes the intervertebral venous plexus, the lumbar venous plexus, the superficial and deep veins of the abdominal wall, and the hemorrhoidal plexus. Any component of this system may be affected in pelvic suppurative thrombophlebitis, but the veins draining the uterus, including the ovarian veins and the inferior vena cava, are involved most often.[751] Thrombus formation may result from stasis of blood flow due to the gravid uterus or from the hypercoagulable state of parturition. Normal residents of the vaginal or perineal bacterial flora gain access to the thrombus via the blood stream or regional lymphatics. There often is an associated endometritis or parametritis. Septic pulmonary emboli and metastatic abscess formation are common. Septic thrombosis of the portal vein often is associated with hepatic abscess (occurring in five of seven patients in one series[752]); an obvious extrahepatic source of intra-abdominal infection is usually absent.

Pathologic Changes

Regardless of the vein involved, the pathologic changes are similar. The vein is enlarged, tortuous, and thickened. There may be associated perivascular suppuration or hemorrhage or both, and the vein lumen usually contains pus and thrombus. Microscopically, endothelial damage, fibrinoid necrosis, and thickening of the vein wall are evident. Microabscesses may be present in the vein wall or in the surrounding tissue.[732,753] Gross periphlebitic abscesses are not unusual and may be evident on physical examination. Thrombi frequently extend beyond

the area of suppuration. In an autopsy series of peripheral suppurative thrombophlebitis in burned patients, extension of the clot into the great central veins was found in 18% of the cases.[727,729] Metastatic abscess formation and septic pulmonary emboli with infarction are found in more than 50% of the fatal cases. This may result from bacterial liquefaction and fragmentation of affected thrombi within the vein because clot liquefaction is noted commonly in autopsy series.

Clinical Manifestations

Superficial suppurative thrombophlebitis often is difficult to identify because local findings of inflammation may be absent. The disease occurs more frequently when plastic catheters are inserted in the lower extremities, a common practice in burned patients. In 132 cases of superficial suppurative thrombophlebitis reported from the burn center at Fort Sam Houston, Texas, the distribution of affected vessels was as follows: lower extremity (predominantly saphenous system), 100; upper extremity (predominantly antecubital fossa), 32; jugular vein, 7; and iliac vein, 4. The mean duration of preceding venous cannulation was 4.81 days, and the latent interval from removal of the catheter to the development of symptoms ranged from 2 to 10 days.[726,728] Fever was present in greater than 70% of the cases, but rigors were rare. Local findings, such as warmth, erythema, tenderness, swelling, or lymphangitis, were present in only 32% of the patients; however, bacteremia with signs of systemic sepsis was found in 84%. Septic pulmonary emboli with secondary pneumonia—often the first diagnostic clue—occurred in 44%. Pneumonia, sepsis, or metastatic abscess formation was the only manifestation of this disease in two thirds of the cases. The late onset of pneumonia or sepsis in a burned patient demands the careful inspection of all previously cannulated veins because untreated suppurative thrombophlebitis is associated with a high mortality. In another report, a dramatic increase in the overall insulin daily requirement heralded the onset of suppurative thrombophlebitis.[754] In these series, fewer than 50% of the cases were diagnosed antemortem.[727]

In contrast to the experience with suppurative thrombophlebitis in burned patients, most medical and postoperative patients develop the disorder in the upper extremities, and signs of local inflammation are present more commonly (94% in one series).[736] In a retrospective series of 21 children with superficial suppurative thrombophlebitis, 48% involved an upper extremity.[755] Many of these patients are elderly (20/35 >50 years old) with debilitating diseases and often are receiving antibiotics when superficial suppurative thrombophlebitis supervenes. As noted, the duration of intravenous catheterization is an important risk factor; 68% of implicated cannulas had been left in place for at least 5 days.[735,736] The frequency of catheter manipulations also has been linked to catheter infections.[756]

Subperiosteal abscesses of adjacent long bones may complicate superficial suppurative thrombophlebitis in children.[757] The local findings in this condition, including bone tenderness, erythema, warmth, and limitation of motion with occasional extension into the joint space, may overshadow the suppurative thrombophlebitis itself. Septic deep vein thrombosis of the femoral vessels with swollen, tender, and inflamed inguinal areas has been described in intravenous users of heroin and cocaine. Contiguous pelvic bone osteomyelitis is unusual.

Suppurative thrombophlebitis of the thoracic central veins occurs in critically ill patients with central catheters in place; in patients receiving total parenteral nutrition; or in patients after long-term cannulation with Broviac, Hickman, and other devices. The systemic findings associated with sepsis overshadow any local findings in venous occlusion (e.g., superior vena cava syndrome), which are rare in this setting. This syndrome should be suspected in any septic patient when bacteremia or fungemia fails to resolve on removal of the central catheter and institution of appropriate antimicrobial therapy.

Pelvic suppurative thrombophlebitis usually develops 1 to 2 weeks postpartum or postoperatively and is associated with high fever, chills, anorexia, nausea, vomiting, abdominal pain, and a protracted course.[750] Flank pain may result from ureteral obstruction by enlarged veins. Abdominal tenderness, usually in the right lower quadrant, may be mild to severe. Approximately 80% of cases are unilateral on the right side, 14% are bilateral, and only 6% are unilateral and left-sided. This distribution is thought to result from compression of the right ovarian vein at the pelvic brim by the enlarged uterus with retrograde flow on the left and protection from ascending infection. The physical examination may be normal, however. A tender vein can be palpated in 30% of the cases on pelvic or abdominal examination.[749,751] The uterus usually is freely movable. Spread of the process to the femoral vein with edema and tenderness of the lower extremity is unusual. Many of these patients are extremely ill, with an acute or chronic course characterized by little or no response to antibiotics and the development of multiple small septic pulmonary emboli. Because many of the manifestations are nonspecific, the differential diagnostic listing is broad and includes acute appendicitis, ureteral obstruction, torsion of an ovarian cyst, pyelonephritis, broad ligament hematoma, parametritis, endometritis, perinephric abscess, pelvic abscess, small bowel volvulus, pelvic inflammatory disease, sickle cell crisis, and ectopic pregnancy.

Laboratory Findings

Bacteremia occurs in 80% to 90% of the cases of superficial suppurative thrombophlebitis. Gross pus within the vein lumen is found in about half of cases, and this finding establishes a diagnosis of suppurative phlebitis. When infection of a venous catheter is suspected, the catheter should be removed and cultured. The results may be misleading, however, because even though bacteria are isolated in 60% of the cases, a positive culture does not correlate with inflammation.[758] The following semiquantitative culture technique has been developed in an attempt to differentiate catheter-related sepsis from suppurative thrombophlebitis. After preparing the skin with alcohol, the catheter is removed with sterile forceps (avoiding skin contact) and is placed in a sterile tube for transport. The catheter then is cut aseptically into 5.7-cm pieces, and each section is rolled across the surface of a 5% sheep blood agar plate. The growth of more than 15 colonies on the plate correlates well[758] with the presence of venous infection. In the few cases of suppurative thrombophlebitis studied by this technique, all catheters have yielded confluent growth. Because the standard 5.7-cm catheter retains approximately 0.7 to 1.5 mg of moisture on its surface and the plate growth has exceeded 1000 colonies in every case of suppurative thrombophlebitis, bacterial counts must exceed 10^6 organisms/g in the catheter wound. These titers are similar to titers found with other types of infected wounds. This technique is simple, rapid, and inexpensive and may prove useful in establishing the need for exploratory venotomy. Simple needle aspiration of the suspected vein also may be diagnostic. ^{111}In-labeled leukocyte imaging studies have detected superficial suppurative thrombophlebitis, but experience is limited.

Other laboratory findings in patients with superficial suppurative thrombophlebitis (e.g., leukocytosis) are nonspecific. The chest radiograph may reveal multiple peripheral densities or a pleural effusion consistent with pulmonary emboli, infarction, abscess, or empyema. The diagnosis of an associated subperiosteal abscess is difficult: Bone and gallium scans usually reveal hyperperfusion without definite osteomyelitis, routine radiographs virtually always show no abnormalities, and CT scans often show only soft tissue swelling with obliteration of tissue planes. The use of high-resolution CT scans may improve these results.[757] The diagnosis of deep central vein suppurative thrombophlebitis in the thorax is established by venography, with the demonstration of thrombi in a patient with positive blood cultures, but CT with contrast enhancement is probably as sensitive and is noninvasive. CT scans are useful in the diagnosis of suppurative phlebitis of the great central veins[759,760] and the portal vein[738]; gas may be detected in the venular lumen, which is diagnostic of this condition. Experience with MRI[761] and ^{111}In-labeled leukocytes is meager.

In most cases of pelvic suppurative thrombophlebitis, there is a peripheral blood leukocytosis, and the urinalysis is usually normal. The chest radiograph may reveal multiple septic pulmonary emboli. Intravenous pyelography can be useful in disclosing ureteral obstruction. Real-time ultrasonography is helpful in delineating the location

and extent of the thrombus, but the ileus that often is associated with this infection may render interpretation difficult. Ultrasonography also may show the presence of a periuterine, adnexal, or tubo-ovarian mass. CT reveals low attenuation with contrast enhancement in suppurative venous thrombosis and is sensitive in the diagnosis of pelvic suppurative thrombophlebitis.[762,763] MRI may be even more sensitive and can differentiate fresh thrombus ($\leq$1 week old) from organizing or subacute thrombus.[764] These sensitive and noninvasive techniques may lead to an increased recognition of pelvic suppurative thrombophlebitis, earlier diagnosis, and improved outcome. The role of newer diagnostic techniques, such as pelvic venography, transuterine phlebography, ^{111}In-labeled leukocyte scanning, and laparoscopy, still is undefined. Because bacteremia is shown in only 20% to 30%[749,750,765] of cases of pelvic suppurative thrombophlebitis, negative blood cultures do not exclude the diagnosis.

Etiologic Agents

S. aureus was the causative agent in 65% to 78% of the cases of superficial suppurative thrombophlebitis reported before 1968. Most cases now are due to a member of Enterobacteriaceae, especially *Klebsiella-Enterobacter* spp.[730,736] These agents are acquired nosocomially and often are resistant to multiple antibiotics. Nearly all patients with superficial suppurative thrombophlebitis due to gram-negative aerobic bacilli or fungi are receiving broad-spectrum antibiotics at the time the disease manifests. In a review of 86 cases compiled from the literature reported since 1970, the organisms isolated were as follows: *Klebsiella-Enterobacter* spp., in 34 cases; *Providencia* spp., in 5; *Proteus* spp., in 5; *Serratia* spp., in 3; *E. coli*, in 6; *P. aeruginosa*, in 3; *S. aureus*, in 15; *C. albicans*, in 9; *S. epidermidis*, in 4; and enterococci, in 2.[735,736] Suppurative thrombophlebitis due to gram-negative pathogens and *E. faecalis* is more common (than *S. aureus*) in patients with significant intra-abdominal pathology.[734] *S. aureus*, other gram-positive cocci, and *Candida* spp. were more common when this risk factor was absent. Multiple organisms are isolated in 14% of cases. Anaerobic isolates are extremely rare but have been described in pediatric patients.[766] An increase in the incidence of superficial suppurative thrombophlebitis due to *Candida* spp. has been reported[767,768]; all patients were receiving antibiotics without hyperalimentation. None were neutropenic or receiving corticosteroids. In one series of seven patients observed in a 15-month interval,[768] all had concomitant or preceding bacterial infections and had received multiple antibiotics (mean five antibiotics) for at least 2 weeks. Preceding candidal colonization at other sites (e.g., sputum, urine) often was present.[768] *Malassezia furfur* also is seen as an opportunistic pathogen of deep vein catheters, especially in premature infants[769] and other pediatric patients receiving lipid emulsions, but this risk factor is not present in all patients. Septic thrombosis, endocarditis, and other metastatic complications are common in this setting of disseminated *Malassezia* infection.[769] Although not documented by culture, histopathologic evidence suggests that cytomegalovirus may cause suppurative thrombophlebitis in patients with AIDS despite therapy with ganciclovir.[770]

The responsible agents in pelvic suppurative thrombophlebitis are poorly defined because blood cultures often are negative, and most investigators did not use adequate anaerobic techniques. The organisms isolated in approximate order of frequency are *Bacteroides* spp., microaerophilic or anaerobic streptococci, *E. coli* and other coliforms, and β-hemolytic streptococci. The predominance of *Bacteroides* may be related to the heparinase produced by this organism. A prolonged latent period (3 weeks) may occur before blood cultures become positive. The more extensive use of anaerobic isolation techniques and routine culturing of surgical specimens may serve to clarify the role of anaerobic bacteria in this entity.

Presumptive Therapy

Superficial suppurative thrombophlebitis is a lethal iatrogenic disease, and surgery often is necessary for cure. The first reported successful cure of suppurative thrombophlebitis followed surgical ligation of the vein by Hunter in 1784.[771] All authorities strongly endorse surgical excision as an integral part of treatment. In a review of 24 patients,[727] 14 were managed medically alone, and all died either directly from suppurative thrombophlebitis with persistent bacteremia or secondary to metastatic complications. Of 10 patients who underwent surgical exploration, 7 survived, and only 1 of the 3 deaths was attributable to suppurative thrombophlebitis. Antibiotics also should be used in the treatment of this disease; initial empirical treatment with a semisynthetic penicillin (e.g., nafcillin, 2 g intravenously every 4 to 6 hours) plus either an aminoglycoside (e.g., gentamicin, 1 to 1.7 mg/kg intravenously or intramuscularly every 8 hours) or a third-generation cephalosporin (e.g., cefotaxime) or a quinolone (e.g., ciprofloxacin) is recommended because members of Enterobacteriaceae or staphylococci are the usual etiologic agents. The optimal duration of therapy is unknown and largely empirical. The role of antifungal therapy for superficial suppurative thrombophlebitis due to *C. albicans* is controversial.[767,768] Most of these infections can be cured by vein excision. Because of the propensity of this pathogen to disseminate hematogenously to visceral organs (e.g., kidneys), however, a short course of amphotericin B (approximately 200 mg) or fluconazole (400 mg/day for 10 to 14 days) is advised postoperatively, pending further data. Antifungal therapy is mandatory in immunosuppressed patients or if signs of metastatic complications (e.g., endophthalmitis) develop.

When superficial suppurative thrombophlebitis is a likely diagnosis, an exploratory venotomy may be necessary. This procedure should be performed proximal to the suspected site; the vein should be ligated, then "milked" in an attempt to express purulent material for inspection by Gram stain and culture. If no pus is apparent, further surgical exploration is necessary to establish the diagnosis. In older literature, simple ligation was thought to be sufficient, but the rate of relapse with ongoing sepsis was high. The segment of vein and all its involved tributaries should be totally excised. Radical surgery from the ankle to the groin may be required in some burn patients. Nevertheless, local or regional anesthesia alone often is sufficient (approximately 90% of cases) for vein excision. Backbleeding, indicative of a patent lumen, should be evident at the point of vein transection. Vein excision usually is followed by prompt ($\leq$24 hours) defervescence. If systemic symptoms, bacteremia, or marked local manifestations persist after vein excision, reexploration is necessary, with careful attention to total removal of all involved veins and drainage of contiguous (e.g., periphlebitic, subperiosteal) abscesses. The role of less radical surgery in therapy for superficial suppurative thrombophlebitis has not been addressed adequately. Although the literature supports vein excision, this experience stems largely from burn centers. Despite infection with gram-negative bacilli or *Candida* spp., six of eight children with superficial suppurative thrombophlebitis were cured by local incision and drainage of the involved site plus parenteral antimicrobials.[734] Radical surgery with extensive excision perhaps can be reserved for patients in whom these measures fail. Delayed closure is preferred over primary wound closure. If osteomyelitis is documented in the adjacent long bones, antimicrobial therapy should be continued for at least 6 weeks. Resection of the involved vasculature in most patients with suppurative thrombophlebitis of the great central veins is technically impossible. Medical therapy is usually sufficient.[743,746,772] The recommended approach is catheter removal, full-dose anticoagulation with heparin,[772,773] and parenteral antibiotics. Although tissue plasminogen activator therapy has been used successfully in this setting,[774] experience is limited, and its use must be considered experimental. Septic thrombosis of the portal vein usually responds to systemic antimicrobial therapy directed at bowel flora with or without percutaneous drainage of any associated hepatic abscesses.[752]

The duration of therapy for septic phlebitis of deeper veins is unsettled; 2 to 3 weeks after catheter removal is suggested, with at least 4 weeks for *S. aureus* disease.[747] Experience with more potent agents (e.g., third-generation cephalosporins) for suppurative thrombophlebitis due to gram-negative bacilli is scant, but trials are indicated. Because heparin may precipitate vancomycin with a partial loss of antibacterial activity at concentrations present in intravenous lines,[773] these drugs should not be administered simultaneously by the same intravenous access line. In contrast to *Candida* IE, suppurative thrombophlebitis of the great central veins due to *Candida* spp. is curable medically, but antifungal regimens must be continued longer than is usually adequate for superficial suppurative thrombophlebitis. Based on limited data,[746] amphotericin B at a daily dose of 0.7 mg/kg, to a total dosage of at least 22 mg/kg, plus 5-fluorocytosine (100 to 150 mg/kg/day in four divided doses, if tolerable) is recommended after catheter removal. Fluconazole (400 mg/day) for 4 to 6 weeks is an alternative in patients not able to tolerate amphotericin B. Surgery may be essential, however, in patients with suppurative thrombophlebitis of the thoracic or neck veins when perivascular collections are present.

The optimal therapy for pelvic suppurative thrombophlebitis still is controversial. Because anaerobic streptococci and *Bacteroides* spp. predominate, the initial antibiotics of choice are aqueous penicillin G, 20 million U intravenously daily, plus either clindamycin, 450 to 600 mg intravenously every 6 hours, or metronidazole, 500 to 750 mg intravenously every 8 hours. The use of heparin is debated. The addition of heparin after several days of unsuccessful treatment with antibiotics itself may produce an antipyretic effect.[765] In one series of 46 patients with pelvic suppurative thrombophlebitis,[750] including 7 with massive ovarian vein involvement and 15 with septic pulmonary emboli, 42 patients become afebrile within 7 days (mean 2.5 days) while receiving penicillin, chloramphenicol, and heparin. Four patients required exploratory laparotomy, and pelvic abscesses were found in three. These results argue strongly that medical therapy alone often is effective, but no controlled studies on the use of heparin have been done. When medical therapy is unsatisfactory, surgery with drainage of abscesses and usually ligation of the implicated venous system must be performed. Some authorities[751] believe that ligation of the inferior vena cava or ovarian vein or both should be performed in all these cases, but the evidence for this approach is inconclusive.

Prevention

The incidence of superficial suppurative thrombophlebitis can be reduced by the same preventive procedures that are used for intravenous cannulas in general. These include the use of "scalp vein" cannulas whenever possible; the avoidance of lower extremity cannulations; insertion under aseptic conditions; secure anchoring of the cannula; and frequent replacement (at least every 48 to 72 hours) of intravenous fluid bottles, cannulas, and connecting tubing. Although neomycin–polymyxin B–bacitracin ointment is effective in reducing the incidence of cutdown infections,[775] use of this combination agent has not shown consistent benefit with intravenous cannulas.[776]

A detailed discussion of prevention strategies for vascular catheters has been published by the Centers for Disease Control and Prevention.[777] When clinical signs of bacteremia occur in a patient receiving intravenous fluids, the following steps should be taken: (1) Blood culture specimens should be obtained, (2) intravenous administration should be discontinued and all cannulas removed, (3) the intravenous fluid itself should be cultured, (4) the cannula should be cultured semiquantitatively on blood agar as described by Maki and associates,[758] and (5) appropriate antibiotic therapy should be instituted. If clinical signs of sepsis and bacteremia persist despite appropriate antibiotic therapy, an intravascular focus (e.g., suppurative thrombophlebitis at a previously cannulated vein) should be sought as discussed previously.

INFECTIVE ENDARTERITIS AND MYCOTIC ANEURYSMS

The term *mycotic aneurysm* was coined by Osler in 1885 to describe a mushroom-shaped aneurysm that developed in a patient with subacute bacterial endocarditis. At that time, the term *mycotic* was used to refer to all microorganisms. At present, the use of *mycotic* has been restricted specifically to fungal infections, but *mycotic aneurysm* still is used for all extracardiac (or intracardiac) aneurysms of infectious etiology except for syphilitic aortitis. This term also has been used to describe preexisting aneurysms secondarily infected from contiguous or distant foci or pseudoaneurysms arising from trauma or iatrogenic causes. *Endarteritis* refers to inflammation of the arterial wall, which may occur with or without coexistent aneurysmal dilation. Unless an aneurysm or coarctation of the aorta is present, infective endarteritis is usually a postmortem diagnosis. Because infected aneurysms differ in their pathogenesis, the various classifications (Table 74-7) are examined separately in the following discussion.[778] Infections of arterial prosthetic devices are discussed in detail in Chapter 66 and are not considered here.

Epidemiology

Although incidence figures are unavailable, a localized suppurative process of the arterial wall is rare. Estimates derived from autopsy series of aortic aneurysms are available but ignore infections at other locations in the arterial tree. In a review of more than 22,000 autopsies performed at the Boston City Hospital from 1902 to 1951,[779] aortic aneurysms were found in 1.5%. Mycotic aneurysms constituted only 2.6% of these lesions, however. In another review of 178 aneurysms found among more than 20,000 autopsies at the Mayo Clinic from 1925 to 1954,[780] only 6 were believed to be of infectious origin. Similarly, in a review[781] of 77 pure iliac artery aneurysms in 48 patients from a 21-year period, only 2 aneurysms (4.2%) were mycotic in origin. In the preantibiotic era, infected aneurysms were confined predominantly to patients with IE; in a series of 217 cases reported in 1923,[782] 86% were associated with IE. With the advent of antibiotics, mycotic aneurysms in IE have become less prevalent, and hematogenous seeding of a previously damaged arteriosclerotic vessel constitutes the most common mechanism. In one retrospective review of all emergency department cases seen at one city public hospital from 1994 to 1999, the annual prevalence of arterial mycotic aneurysms among injection drug users was 0.03%.[783]

Because most of these lesions arise in areas of severe atherosclerosis, men predominate over women by 3 to 1, and the average age has been 65 years. The mean age for mycotic aneurysms that occur with IE is younger (approximately 40 years), and men and women are affected approximately equally. Estimates of the incidence of mycotic aneurysms in patients with IE range up to 15%.[784-787] Approximately 2% to 4% of IE patients develop intracranial mycotic aneurysms,[787,788] although a neurologic presentation is common in patients with IE (noted in approximately 16% to 23% of cases), and at least 30% of the patients develop neurologic manifestations.[789,790] As discussed previously, the presence of such manifestations during IE has an adverse effect on the ultimate mortality rate. These lesions remain a significant cause of morbidity and mortality due to intracerebral and subarachnoid hemorrhage, especially in young people in developing countries, where acute rheumatic fever, rheumatic heart disease, and resultant IE still are prevalent.[791] Nine intracranial mycotic aneurysms associated with IE were treated in one neurosurgical unit in South Africa in an 18-month period, with five deaths.[791] In addition, aortic root complications, including abscess or mycotic aneurysm, are associated with a poor outcome from IE. In one review,[792] aortic root complications were documented in 23 of 50 cases of aortic valve IE (46%) over a 6-year period; prosthetic valve involvement was common, and the

surgical mortality rate and the incidence of postoperative aortic regurgitation were higher in the group with root complications.

Mycotic aneurysms are extremely rare in childhood[793] and, when present, are usually associated with IE, cardiovascular malformations, or connective tissue disorders. A specific disease entity first described in 1970 is aneurysm associated with umbilical artery catheterization in newborn infants.[794] These lesions are usually of staphylococcal etiology, and 34 cases had been reported in 1992, with the following distribution[794]: descending thoracic aorta, 14 cases; abdominal aorta, 10; iliac arteries, 6; and multiple sites, 4.

Pathogenesis

Four different mechanisms have been postulated to produce infection of the arterial wall: (1) formation of mycotic aneurysms secondary to septic microemboli to the vasa vasorum ("embolomycotic aneurysms"), (2) extension from a contiguous infected focus, (3) hematogenous seeding of the intima during bacteremia originating from a distant infection, and (4) trauma to the arterial wall with direct contamination.[795] Embolomycotic aneurysms usually occur in patients with active IE, and the incidence of this type has declined in the antibiotic era. The source of infection is the cardiac vegetation, with production of arterial emboli that lodge in the vasa vasorum, often at points of bifurcation of the affected artery. Contiguous foci of infection (e.g., a caseous tuberculous lymph node or pyogenic vertebral osteomyelitis) may extend directly to major vessels, with subsequent aneurysm formation. The normal arterial intima is very resistant to infection. When this lining is altered by congenital malformations (e.g., coarctation of the aorta) or acquired disease (especially atherosclerotic plaques or ulcers), however, resistance to infection is lowered, and the surface may become colonized by blood-borne organisms. This hypothesis is analogous to the central role of NBTE in the pathogenesis of IE. An intraluminal thrombus associated with an atherosclerotic vessel also may serve as a nidus for colonization. Atherosclerosis accounts for greater than 74% of secondarily infected aneurysms. Luetic arteritis and cystic medial necrosis also have been associated with secondary infection.[784] Trauma to the arterial wall with subsequent infection has been documented in narcotic addicts, in whom it is due to needle trauma,[796] and has been associated with gunshot wounds, vascular surgery, cardiac catheterization, percutaneous transluminal coronary angioplasty,[797,798] intravascular stent placement,[799] radial artery catheterization,[800] implantable ports for intra-arterial chemotherapy,[801] and puncture of a femoral artery for analysis of arterial blood gases.[778] These events, if associated with contamination, usually lead to pseudoaneurysm formation in a peripheral artery and a contiguous abscess in extravasated blood.

Pathologic Changes

Infection of the arterial tree has been recognized by pathologists for more than a century. Virchow first showed local dilation of the arterial wall at the site of a septic embolus in 1847. Infection superimposed on an atherosclerotic aorta first was reported by Koch in 1851. Stengel and Wolfroth[782] collected 217 cases of mycotic aneurysms in 1923. Because these lesions probably are underreported, pathologic material has been scant in recent years.

Most mycotic aneurysms that develop during the course of IE are situated in the sinus of Valsalva or in the supravalvular proximal thoracic aorta (>70% develop proximal to the aortic arch). Aneurysms are more common in the right or posterior sinus and may be complicated by acquired shunts (rupture into the right ventricle is the most common), tamponade, coronary artery occlusion, or an atrioventricular conduction block.[802] Less commonly, major visceral, intracranial, and peripheral arteries are involved. Intracranial mycotic aneurysms characteristically develop in the distribution of the middle cerebral artery at peripheral bifurcation points[789,790] versus a more proximal location for most congenital aneurysms. Multiple intracranial lesions may be present. Mycotic aneurysm of the extracranial carotid arteries is rare (26 case reports[803]), but most develop in association with IE, usually due to *S. aureus.* Less than 10% are found in

TABLE 74-7 Classification of Mycotic Aneurysms	
Preexistent Arterial Status	*Source of Infection*
Normal	Intravascular
Atherosclerotic	Embolism
Aneurysm	Bacteremia with seeding
Arterial prosthesis	Extension from adjacent endocardial focus on erosion
	Extravascular
	Contiguous site of infection
	Iatrogenic

the upper extremities, but these arteries usually are not examined adequately by pathologic or radiologic techniques. Infrafemoral aneurysms during IE or after its treatment[804] also are unusual. Multiple lesions are identified in many IE patients with mycotic aneurysms.[805] Saccular forms seem to be more common than fusiform ones.[779] The aneurysms vary in size from 1 mm to greater than 10 cm. As mentioned before, many of these aneurysms arise from emboli to the vasa vasorum, and occasionally the embolus can be shown grossly and microscopically. Acute and chronic inflammation is found diffusely through the arterial wall; necrosis, hemorrhage, abscess, and bacterial colonies all may be present in the sections. The elastica and muscularis layers usually are obliterated, but the intima often is intact. Rupture with surrounding hemorrhage and infection may be present.

Secondary infection of a preexisting aneurysm is found most commonly in the abdominal aorta (accounting for 70% of the cases) because this is the area most frequently and severely damaged by atherosclerosis. Ascending and descending aortic aneurysms each account for about 15% of the cases. The primary bacteremia most commonly originates from distal infections in soft tissue, lung, bone, or joint. The arterial infection usually begins in the distal abdominal aorta or iliac arteries as a focus of inflammation on an ulcerated atheromatous plaque. The wall of the aneurysm is thinned, and there is focal acute and chronic inflammation that may lead to arterial rupture. Even so-called bland aortic aneurysms commonly have some mild inflammation (characterized by a predominance of lymphocytes and mononuclear cells) in the wall; however, infected atherosclerotic aneurysms are characterized by acute inflammation with a predominance of polymorphonuclear leukocytes, necrosis, abscess formation, hemorrhage, and visible bacterial colonies. This lesion probably is underreported because the focal suppuration may be limited in extent and overlooked unless routine culture and histologic sections are examined on every aortic aneurysm specimen. Erosion and rupture may be present without aneurysmal dilation. Lumbar or thoracic osteomyelitis is present in one third of the cases[784] and may precede the aneurysm or develop secondary to contiguous spread from the vascular infection.

When contamination accompanies arterial injury, an infected pseudoaneurysm may result. These lesions are located in the extremities in greater than 80% of the cases and are characterized by more extensive local tissue inflammation than is seen with the two types mentioned previously. Infection as a cause of pseudoaneurysm formation is increasing; 17 of 57 (30%) lesions seen in the 1980s[806] were infected. When endarteritis develops after angioplasty, it usually follows a second procedure or repuncture, and this scenario should suggest the diagnosis; all cases have been due to *S. aureus*.[794,798] Distal emboli, pseudoaneurysm, and coexistent osteomyelitis are present in more than 50% of the cases. Infective aortic root aneurysm also has followed coronary artery bypass graft surgery, with disastrous results.[805,807,808] Subclavian artery aneurysms may be present, with systemic findings plus unilateral upper extremity rash or splinter hemorrhages.[809] Nineteen cases of intracavernous carotid artery aneurysms have been reported,[810] usually occurring with meningitis with or without IE.

Of special interest are mycotic aneurysms in renal transplant patients. In 640 renal transplants performed at the University of Minnesota over 8 years, perinephric infections developed in 28 patients, and 8 of these patients developed mycotic aneurysms.[811] These lesions were evident clinically 1.5 to 4 months after transplant. Six were located in the external iliac artery, with one each in the internal iliac artery and aorta. All these lesions were secondary to contiguous foci of infection in the deep tissues of the transplant wound.[812,813]

Clinical Manifestations

When mycotic aneurysms occur during the course of IE, manifestations of the underlying disease may be evident. Peripheral middle cerebral artery aneurysms constitute 2.5% to 6.2% of all intracranial aneurysms[787-791,813] and usually are secondary to infection. Intracranial mycotic aneurysms are usually clinically silent. When hemorrhage occurs, severe headache of sudden onset with rapid deterioration in the

level of consciousness is noted. The time interval from the diagnosis of IE to the onset of hemorrhage is variable (0 to 35 days), with a mean of 18 days.[788] Some lesions produce premonitory or herald neurologic signs, including focal deficits and seizures. These findings are relatively common in patients with IE without intracranial aneurysms, and the differential diagnosis and decisions regarding arteriography are difficult.[814] A sudden focal deficit consistent with embolism is seen in approximately 23% of patients and should prompt arteriography.[814] A high proportion of patients with intracranial mycotic aneurysm with severe, unremitting localized headache, often in association with homonymous hemianopsia (as a herald sign), has been reported in one series.[815] As noted, stroke syndromes may be seen and are manifested as focal neurologic deficits, headache, confusion, meningismus, seizures, or coma.[789,790] Contrary to popular belief, most intracranial hemorrhages associated with IE are due not to ruptured mycotic aneurysms but to septic necrotic arteritis.[789] Symptomatic intracranial hemorrhage was associated with a mortality rate of 60% to 90% in this study. Patients also may present with bilateral cortical blindness. Unusual location or etiology of an intracranial mycotic aneurysm suggests a diagnosis other than IE.[816] Mycotic aneurysms tend to occur more commonly in women of a younger age than does IE in general. They must be differentiated from aneurysms secondary to tumor emboli (especially choriocarcinoma or atrial myxoma), trauma, arteritis, moyamoya disease, and congenital aneurysms. Visceral artery aneurysms are uncommon but, when present, almost uniformly are due to infection[795] or polyarteritis nodosa. The most common location is in the superior mesenteric artery. Although superior mesenteric artery aneurysms account for only 8% of visceral artery aneurysms overall, most are of infectious etiology.[817] Symptoms include colicky abdominal pain of acute onset, but the presentation is variable. Hepatic artery aneurysms may produce colicky right upper quadrant pain, fever, jaundice, and gastrointestinal hemorrhage[818] or hemobilia.[819] More than 190 cases of this entity have been reported in the literature; 75% were extrahepatic and 25% were intrahepatic. Ruptured mycotic aneurysm of the celiac artery may present as hemoptysis or hemothorax.[820] When the external iliac artery is involved, a triad of clinical signs may be present: (1) pain in the lower extremity (especially the anterior aspect of the thigh) with quadriceps muscle wasting and a depressed knee jerk; (2) arterial insufficiency of the extremity with coolness, pallor, and depressed pulses; and (3) bacteremia.[821] Distal aneurysms (e.g., affecting the femoral artery) occasionally have unusual presenting manifestations, including arthritis and purpura in the affected limb.

When more peripheral arteries are involved (usually with a pseudoaneurysm), a tender, diffusely indurated mass is present in 92% of cases. The mass is pulsatile, with an associated bruit, in 50% to 60% of patients, and approximately 20% to 30% have decreased peripheral pulses, skin changes, or even frank gangrene.[796] Local suppuration, petechiae, and purpura are often present, and the lesion may be confused with localized cellulitis or an abscess without consideration of vascular involvement. In users of illicit drugs, the brachial, radial, or carotid arteries or arteries of the lower extremity may be involved.[783] Only 50% of these patients are febrile on admission.[783] A superimposed septic arthritis also may be present.[822]

Although most infected aortic atherosclerotic aneurysms occur in elderly men, no pathognomonic findings exist to separate these patients from patients with bland uninfected aneurysms. Fever is a helpful differentiating sign (present in .70% of patients) because it is uncommon in patients with bland aneurysms. Back pain or abdominal pain occurs in about a third of cases. A draining cutaneous sinus may be present. Separation of an infected aneurysm from the entity of inflammatory abdominal aortic aneurysm may be difficult. Inflammatory abdominal aortic aneurysms first were described in 1935 and account for 5% to 10% of abdominal aortic aneurysms; the lesions are usually infrarenal and often lead to ureteral obstruction, owing to the densely adherent fibrotic mass surrounding the vessel.[823] In a large series of 2816 patients undergoing repair of abdominal aortic aneurysms, 127 (4.5%) had inflammatory abdominal aortic aneurysms.[824] Most patients

(123/127) were men and heavy smokers. Inflammatory aortic aneurysms are associated with an elevated erythrocyte sedimentation rate (73% of cases), weight loss, symptoms (back or abdominal pain in 30% to 50%), and a high operative mortality. Continuing bacteremia despite "appropriate" antimicrobial therapy in an elderly (especially diabetic) patient with no signs of IE suggests an infected intravascular site. The aneurysm is palpable in 50% to 60% of the cases.[785,795] In most cases, the onset is insidious, and a low-grade fever may be present for several months before diagnosis. The nonspecificity of the clinical manifestations is reflected by the 75% preoperative rupture rate for this entity. Rupture may occur into the retroperitoneal space or peritoneal cavity (56%), pleural cavity (9%), duodenum (12%), esophagus (6%), mediastinum (3%), or pericardium (3%). The most common site of aortoenteric fistula is between the aorta and the third portion of the duodenum. Short periods of herald bleeding are common warning signs before exsanguinating hemorrhage occurs.[825] Severe pain and the rapid onset of shock usually accompany rupture of the aneurysm.

Laboratory Findings

There are no characteristic laboratory abnormalities in this group of diseases. When mycotic aneurysms occur with IE, alterations suggesting the underlying disease may be present. CT is useful in patients with neurologic manifestations of IE, especially for the demonstration of intracranial hemorrhage. CT is not sufficiently sensitive for the detection of intracranial mycotic aneurysms[789,790]; however, these lesions are not likely when the appearance on CT scan is completely normal. Diagnosis of intracranial mycotic aneurysm can be established by four-vessel cerebral arteriography, although two-dimensional and three-dimensional helical CT angiography,[826] magnetic resonance angiography,[790] and the less dangerous and invasive procedure of intravenous digital subtraction angiography[827] are promising. Magnetic resonance angiography may detect aneurysms only 2 to 3 mm in diameter, but false-negative results occur (in 8% to 10% of such studies); this modality cannot substitute for selective angiography.[828]

Patients with infected aortic aneurysms usually have a leukocytosis (65% to 83%), but this is nonspecific and may be present when the aneurysm is bland. Bacteremia is found in 53% to greater than 90% of the cases, is continuous, and usually does not clear with antibiotic therapy alone. Evidence for a primary source of bacteremia (e.g., pneumonia, osteomyelitis) may be present but is absent in 46% of the cases.[784] The abdominal aorta is noted to be calcified on abdominal radiographs in 47%,[786] and anterior vertebral body erosion has been shown in 18%. A lack of calcification suggests infection because 70% to 80% of bland aneurysms show calcification on abdominal radiographs. Certain procedures (e.g., intravenous pyelography, sonography, CT[829]) may reveal the presence of an aneurysm but often are not satisfactory for preoperative detail. The absence of intimal calcification, an associated perianeurysmal fluid collection or osteomyelitis (usually shown by CT), and the sudden appearance of an aneurysm in a septic patient all are features suggesting an infected abdominal aortic aneurysm.[830,831] Gas in the aortic wall is diagnostic, but rare. Although the sensitivity is unknown, gallium-67 and ^{111}In leukocyte imaging have been used to localize intra-arterial infections.[832] Occult infected aneurysms have been identified in patients with fever of unknown origin, and negative results on CT or MRI studies with gallium[833] or leukocyte scintigraphy[834] and may separate seroma or hematoma from adjacent infection. Leukocyte imaging with technetium-99m–labeled cells also seems promising, but false-positive results have been noted.[835] Nevertheless, preoperative angiography often is preferred to delineate precisely the extent of aneurysmal involvement.[836] This information may alter the operative approach and may minimize complications. Two-dimensional echocardiography (TTE or TEE) is a useful noninvasive technique for documenting mycotic aneurysms in the vicinity of the aortic valve (e.g., sinus of Valsalva, supravalvular, subvalvular), and this technique is adjunctive to aortic root angiography preoperatively.[837] Infective endarteritis or mycotic aneurysm in the vicinity of a patent ductus arteriosus also has been visualized successfully with two-dimensional and Doppler echocardiography.[838,839] Intraoperative epicardial echocardiography has been used to facilitate the surgical approach. When a hepatic aneurysm is suspected, liver scanning and ultrasonography performed before angiography may be helpful.[818]

Etiologic Agents

Before the antibiotic era, mycotic aneurysms associated with IE usually were due to the more "virulent" organisms, such as the β-hemolytic group A streptococci, pneumococci, or *H. influenzae*. With the decline of these organisms as causal agents in IE, most of these lesions now are due to streptococci or staphylococci (≥60% of cases) and follow the incidence patterns outlined in Table 74-4 for the underlying disease.

When bacteria "seed" a preexisting atherosclerotic vessel, the etiologic agents are markedly different from those found in mycotic aneurysms associated with IE. Gram-positive organisms cause approximately 60% of these lesions, but gram-negative bacilli (chiefly salmonellae) are isolated in 35%. Staphylococci are implicated in 40% of the cases overall,[786] and more than two thirds of these are *S. aureus*. The risk of vascular infection in adult patients with non-*typhi* Salmonella bacteremia has been reviewed.[840] Salmonellae cause 20% of the cases and involve, in order of frequency, the aorta and femoral and iliac arteries. Only 1 of 24 of such cases reported before 1974 was above the renal arteries.[841] Lumbar osteomyelitis due to *Salmonella* was present in one third of cases. The presumed portal of entry is the gastrointestinal tract.[842] *S. enteritidis* strains are isolated in 40% of cases, which is proportional to their overall rate of isolation in the United States. *S. choleraesuis*, an uncommon clinical isolate, seems to be particularly pathogenic in this condition because this species was isolated in 32% of the cases.[843] *Salmonella typhi* rarely is implicated in this disorder. *Salmonella* infections of aortic aneurysms first were reported in 1948. The predilection for involvement by this organism is not understood, but salmonellae tend to seed abnormal tissues during bacteremia (e.g., hematomas, malignant tumors, cysts, gallstones, bone infarcts, altered endothelium, aortic aneurysms). It has been estimated that 25% of patients older than age 50 with *Salmonella* bacteremia have an intravascular focus of infection.[844,845] *Arizona* spp. (especially *Arizona hinshawii*) are closely related to *Salmonella* spp., cause similar clinical syndromes, and infect aortic aneurysms in elderly diabetic men.[846] The following organisms also produce infection in atherosclerotic aneurysms: *E. coli, P. aeruginosa,*[847] *Proteus* spp., *Citrobacter freundii, Klebsiella-Enterobacter* spp., *Brucella* spp.,[848] *S. marcescens, C. fetus,*[849] *Listeria monocytogenes* (17 reported cases[850,851]), *B. fragilis,* gonococci, group B streptococci,[852] corynebacteria, *C. burnetii,*[853] *Clostridium septicum,*[854] enterococci, and pneumococci.[855] *Mycobacterium tuberculosis* is a rare cause of aortic mycotic aneurysms. Of the 41 cases reported in the literature since 1945, 75% seemed to result from erosion of the aortic wall by a contiguous focus, and 25% seemed to result from direct seeding of the aortic intima or via the vasa vasorum.[856]

Fungal mycotic aneurysms are rare in the intracranial compartment, with only 13 definite cases reported by 1981.[857] The most common etiologic agents are *Aspergillus* spp., agents of mucormycoses, and *Candida* spp. The first two agents may involve intracranial arteries by direct extension from foci of sinusitis. One case of multiple intracranial aneurysms due to *Coccidioides immitis* that occurred during therapy for basilar meningitis has been described. Fungal mycotic aneurysms tend to involve larger, more proximal vessels at the base of the brain (11/18 [61%] carotid or basilar) than those involved in bacterial cases of IE[858] and may complicate intracranial surgery. *Aspergillus* mycotic aneurysms have followed transsphenoidal resections. Fungi also may cause endarteritis in the aorta or on aortic grafts, including cases due to *Aspergillus* or *Bipolaris* spp.[859,860] Mycotic aneurysms with subarachnoid bleeding may complicate the course of neurobrucellosis.[861] Tuberculous aneurysms are now uncommon and when present are due to contiguous foci of infection.

Pseudoaneurysms resulting from intra-arterial or perivascular injection of illicit street drugs, often in addicts with sclerosed veins due to repeated intravenous inoculation, are associated with contiguous abscesses. The causative agents are *S. aureus* (in 76% of cases), *P. aeruginosa* (in 18%), and many others.[796]

Therapy

No uniformly acceptable approach has been devised for the treatment of mycotic aneurysms in IE. The treatment of intracranial mycotic aneurysms is particularly controversial. Some of these lesions seem to resolve with antimicrobial therapy alone. In a review of 56 aneurysms occurring in 45 patients,[862] 3 of 20 patients died when treatment was limited to antibiotics alone. Mild-to-moderate neurologic deficits were observed in 8 of the 17 survivors. Likewise, 6 of 25 patients in whom treatment included antibiotics and surgery died, and 9 of 19 survivors were left with mild-to-moderate neurologic deficits. In other studies, the investigators reported a different experience, with a higher mortality in the nonsurgical group,[788] but patients were selected only after subarachnoid hemorrhage had occurred. In a review of 13 intracranial mycotic aneurysms,[788] 6 of 8 patients who received treatment with antibiotics alone died; no deaths were observed in the surgical treatment group. In a review of 85 cases treated between 1954 and 1978, 20 of 38 patients managed solely with antibiotics died versus 8 of 30 patients operated on.[787] Endovascular stent-grafts combined with antibiotic therapy have been employed in a few patients with mycotic aneurysms of the descending thoracic aorta.[863] The distal location of most intracranial mycotic aneurysms associated with IE may permit ligation and excision with fewer complications compared with surgery for berry aneurysms in the circle of Willis. The mortality rate was low in patients with multiple aneurysms (4/15) who received treatment with antibiotics alone. In one series, the mortality rate was 29% after rupture of an intracranial mycotic aneurysm.

Serial angiographic studies may be useful in following these patients because the aneurysms may change in size, or new lesions may develop. In 21 patients studied by angiography, the mycotic aneurysm increased in size in 5 patients, did not change in 1 patient, became smaller in 6 patients, and completely resolved in 11 patients; new aneurysms developed in 2 patients. More than 50% of these peripheral intracranial aneurysms resolved with antibiotic therapy alone during the treatment of IE.[862] Surgery is indicated for aneurysms increasing in size on serial angiographic studies,[864-866] but may be deferred for 4 to 6 weeks for aneurysms remaining the same size (if the patient is an acceptable medical risk). The definitive treatment for aneurysms decreasing in size on subsequent serial angiographic studies repeated every 2 weeks is unclear. CT is not helpful in localizing the aneurysm but provides important information if hematomas, infarcts, or abscesses develop. The choice of antibiotics is governed by the etiologic agent of the IE, but therapy for intracranial mycotic aneurysms, especially multiple lesions, must be individualized[789,790] (see earlier discussion). The AHA has reviewed this topic.[323] It generally was concluded that a single intracranial mycotic aneurysm distal to the first bifurcation of a major artery (e.g., middle cerebral artery) should be followed with frequent serial angiograms and promptly excised if the aneurysm enlarges or bleeds. Multiple aneurysms similarly should be monitored, and any enlarging aneurysm should be managed surgically. Aneurysms proximal to the first bifurcation are less amenable to surgical therapy because they arise from major vessels, and their ligation may result in severe neurologic deficits. These latter lesions also should be assessed serially, and surgery should be pursued if enlargement or leakage occurs.

Peripheral vessels usually are involved when arterial trauma (narcotic addict, gunshot wound, iatrogenic) results in pseudoaneurysm formation with infection. Therapy with antibiotics, proximal ligation of the vessel, resection of the pseudoaneurysm, and appropriate drainage results in cures in 75% of the cases. Vascular reconstruction through uninfected tissue planes with autogenous grafts is necessary when limb viability depends on the affected vessel. This situation is encountered more frequently in the lower extremity. Severe ischemia developed in 9 of 28 patients after excision of mycotic aneurysms of the common femoral artery[796] in one series of 52 cases. Amputation was required in only 11% of a large series of 54 aneurysms among drug addicts seen at the Henry Ford Hospital; there were no deaths.[867]

The mortality rate in patients with infected atherosclerotic aneurysms often exceeds 90%; approximately 40 long-term survivors have been reported since 1962.[868-871] A high index of suspicion is necessary to allow surgical intervention before rupture occurs because this complication is uniformly fatal and occurs in about 80% of the cases. When gram-negative bacilli are the cause of the infection, "early" (e.g., within 2 weeks after the first positive blood culture) rupture occurs much more frequently (84%) than if gram-positive bacteria are isolated (10%). Survival after surgery also is more common (75%) for patients with aneurysms infected with gram-positive cocci than for patients with gram-negative bacilli (25%). Antibiotics should be used in this disease, however, even if the lesion is sterilized (reported in only three cases). The aneurysm still may continue to enlarge and rupture, and surgery is required.

At surgery, the aneurysm and any intraluminal thrombus must be sectioned and Gram stain performed, and specimens must be submitted for culture. If infection is present, all aneurysmal tissue and surrounding areas of inflammation must be resected before grafting. Basic principles of grafting in this situation include the use of autogenous rather than synthetic grafts and insertion only in clean, noninfected tissue planes. If the graft is placed in the infected area, continued infection, leakage, thrombus formation, abscess formation, or rupture usually results. Although some authorities have achieved a successful result by restoration of vascular continuity in situ after radical débridement,[868,870] this approach is not recommended in most cases. Nevertheless, the type of reconstruction must be individualized because results of in situ repair seem to be better when the aortic aneurysm is suprarenal[872-875] than when it is more distal in location if reconstruction is combined with prolonged courses of intravenous antimicrobial agents. Radical resection of intra-abdominal aortic aneurysms without prosthetic material also has been used in a few cases.[876] In a review of 24 patients with abdominal aortic aneurysms infected with salmonellae, 10 died after rupture without surgery, and another 7 patients survived grafting only to die because of continued leakage from the anastomosis (only 5 patients were long-term survivors). If a graft is inserted in situ and persistent fever with bacteremia or embolism in the lower extremities ensues, reoperation with extra-anatomic grafting is mandatory. Because the resected area is contaminated, special bypass techniques—especially thoracoiliac, transpubic, and axillofemoral—usually are required. When an axillofemoral approach is used, a single graft should be inserted for both lower extremities because patency is prolonged under these circumstances.[869,871] Bactericidal antibiotics should be continued for 6 to 8 weeks postoperatively. The choice of agents depends on the isolated organism (or the morphologic characteristics of the organisms in the surgical specimen) and on the results of in vitro susceptibility testing. Implantation of antibiotic-releasing carriers with in situ reconstruction has been used[877] but only in a few patients without controlled trials; use of such carriers remains of unproved benefit in therapy for mycotic aneurysm.

REFERENCES

1. Lerner PI, Weinstein L. Infective endocarditis in the antibiotic era. N Engl J Med. 1966;274:199.
2. von Reyn CF, Levy BS, Arbeit RD, et al. Infective endocarditis: An analysis based on strict case definitions. Ann Intern Med. 1982;94:505.
3. Steckelberg JM, Melton LJ III, Ilstrup DM, et al. Influence of referral bias on the apparent clinical spectrum of infective endocarditis. Am J Med. 1990;88:582.
4. Harris SL. Definitions and demographic characteristics. In: Kaye D, ed. Infective Endocarditis. New York: Raven Press; 1992:1.
5. Durack DT, Petersdorf RG. Changes in the epidemiology of endocarditis. In: Kaplan EL, Taranta AV, eds. Infective Endocarditis: An American Heart Association Symposium. Dallas: American Heart Association; 1977:3.
6. Griffin MR, Wilson WR, Edwards WD, et al. Infective endocarditis: Olmsted County, Minnesota, 1950 through 1981. JAMA. 1985;254:1199-1202.

7. King JW, Nguyen VQ, Conrad SA. Results of a prospective statewide reporting system for infective endocarditis. Am J Med Sci. 1988;295:517-527.

8. Shulman ST. Infective endocarditis—1986. Pediatr Infect Dis. 1986;5:691-694.

9. Delahaye F, Goulet V, Lacassin F, et al. Characteristics of infective endocarditis in France in 1991: A 1-year survey. Eur Heart J. 1995;16:394-401.

10. Hoen B, Alla F, Selton-Suty C, et al, and Association pour l'Etude et la Prevention de l'Endocardite Infectieuse (AEPEI) Study Group. Changing profile of infective endocarditis: Results of a 1-year survey in France. JAMA. 2002;288:75-81.

11. Berlin JA, Abrutyn E, Strom BL, et al. Incidence of infective endocarditis in the Delaware Valley, 1988-1990. Am J Cardiol. 1995;76:933-936.

12. Watanakunakorn C, Burkert T. Infective endocarditis at a large community teaching hospital, 1980-1990. Medicine. 1993;72:90.

13. Hayward GW. Infective endocarditis: A changing disease. BMJ. 1973;2:706.

14. Infective endocarditis (Editorial). BMJ. 1981;1:677.

15. Gold MJ. Cure rates and long term prognosis. In: Kaye D, ed. Infective Endocarditis. New York: Raven Press; 1992:455.

16. Thayer WS. Studies on bacterial (infective) endocarditis. Johns Hopkins Hosp Rep. 1926;22:1.

17. Garvey GJ, Neu HC. Infective endocarditis: An evolving disease. Medicine (Baltimore). 1978;57:105.

18. Lien EA, Solberg CO, Kalager T. Infective endocarditis 1973-1984 at the Bergen University Hospital: Clinical features, treatment and prognosis. Scand J Infect Dis. 1988;20:239-246.

19. Cabell CH, Abrutyn E. Progress toward a global understanding of infective endocarditis: Early lessons from the International Collaboration on Endocarditis investigation. Infect Dis Clin North Am. 2002;16:255-272.

20. Come PC. Infective endocarditis: Current perspectives. Compr Ther. 1982;8:57.

21. Kaplan EL. Infective endocarditis in the pediatric age group: An overview. In: Kaplan EL, Taranta AV, eds. Infective Endocarditis: An American Heart Association Symposium. Dallas: American Heart Association; 1977:51.

22. Baltimore RS. Infective endocarditis in children. Pediatr Infect Dis J. 1992;11:907.

23. Cabell CH, Jollis JG, Peterson GE, et al. Changing patient characteristics and the effect on mortality in endocarditis. Arch Intern Med. 2002;162:90-94.

24. Fernandez-Guerrero ML, Verdejo C, Azofra J, et al. Hospital-acquired infectious endocarditis not associated with cardiac surgery: An emerging problem. Clin Infect Dis. 1995;20:16-23.

25. Gouello JP, Asfar P, Brenet O, et al. Nosocomial endocarditis in the intensive care unit: An analysis of 22 cases. Crit Care Med. 2000;28:377-382.

26. Watanakunakorn C, Burkert T. Infective endocarditis at a large community teaching hospital, 1980-1990: A review of 210 episodes. Medicine. 1993;72:90-102.

27. Pelletier LL, Petersdorf RG. Infective endocarditis: A review of 125 cases from the University of Washington Hospitals, 1963-72. Medicine (Baltimore). 1977;56:287.

28. Terpenning MS, Buggy BP, Kaufmann CA. Hospital-acquired infective endocarditis. Arch Intern Med. 1988;148:1601-1603.

29. Roberts WC, Buchbinder NA. Right-sided valvular infective endocarditis: A clinicopathologic study of 12 necropsy patients. Am J Med. 1972;53:7.

30. Kaye D. Changing pattern of infective endocarditis. Am J Med. 1985;78(Suppl 6B):157-162.

31. Kanafani ZA, Mahfouz TH, Kanj SS. Infective endocarditis at a tertiary care centre in Lebanon: Predominance of streptococcal infection. J Infect. 2002;45:152-159.

32. Koegelenberg CF, Doubell AF, Orth H, et al. Infective endocarditis in the Western Cape Province of South Africa: A three-year prospective study. QJM. 2003;96:217-225.

33. Roberts WC, Perloff JK, Constantin T. Severe valvular aortic stenosis in patients over 65 years of age. Am J Cardiol. 1971;27:497.

34. Delahaye JP, Loire R, Milon H, et al. Infective endocarditis on stenotic aortic valves. Eur Heart J. 1988;9(Suppl E):S43-S49.

35. Gersony WM, Hayes CJ, Driscoll DJ, et al. Bacterial endocarditis in patients with aortic stenosis, pulmonary stenosis, or ventricular septal defect. Circulation. 1993;87(Suppl I):I-121.

36. McKinsey DS, Ratts TE, Bisno AL. Underlying cardiac lesions in adults with infective endocarditis: The changing spectrum. Am J Med. 1987;82:681-688.

37. Lowes JA, Hamer J, Williams G, et al. Ten years of infective endocarditis at St. Bartholomew's hospital: Analysis of clinical features and treatment in relation to prognosis and mortality. Lancet. 1980;1:133.

38. Moulsdale MT, Eykyn SJ, Phillips I. Infective endocarditis, 1970-1979: A study of culture-positive cases in St. Thomas' Hospital. QJM. 1980;49:315.

39. Venezio FR, Westenfelder GO, Cook FV, et al. Infective endocarditis in a community hospital. Arch Intern Med. 1982;142:789.

40. Fulkerson PK, Beaver BM, Aveson JC, et al. Calcification of the mitral annulus: Etiology, clinical associations, complications and therapy. Am J Med. 1979;66:967.

41. Lamas CC, Eykyn SJ. Bicuspid aortic valve—a silent danger: Analysis of 50 cases of infective endocarditis. Clin Infect Dis. 2000;30:336-341.

42. Cabell CH, Heidenreich PA, Chu VH, et al. Increasing rates of cardiac device infections among Medicare beneficiaries: 1990-1999. Am Heart J. 2004;147:582-586.

43. Welton DE, Young JB, Gentry LO, et al. Recurrent infective endocarditis: Analysis of predisposing factors and clinical features. Am J Med. 1979;66:932.

44. Kreuzpaintner G, Horstkotte D, Heyll A, et al. Increased risk of bacterial endocarditis in inflammatory bowel disease. Am J Med. 1992;92:391.

45. Cardelia JV, Befeler B, Hildner FJ, et al. Hypertrophic subaortic stenosis complicated by aortic insufficiency and subacute bacterial endocarditis. Am Heart J. 1971;81:543.

46. Wang K, Gobel FL, Gleason DF. Bacterial endocarditis in idiopathic hypertrophic subaortic stenosis. Am Heart J. 1975;89:359.

47. Chagnac A, Rudniki C, Loebel H, et al. Infectious endocarditis in idiopathic hypertrophic subaortic stenosis: Report of three cases and review of the literature. Chest. 1982;81:346.

48. Corrigan D, Bolen J, Hancock EW, et al. Mitral valve prolapse and infective endocarditis. Am J Med. 1977;63:215.

49. Jeresaty RM. Mitral valve prolapse-click syndrome. Prog Cardiovasc Dis. 1973;15:623.

50. Schutte JE, Gaffney FA, Blend L, et al. Distinctive anthropometric characteristics of women with mitral valve prolapse. Am J Med. 1981;71:533.

51. Devereux RB, Kramer-Fox R, Kligfield P. Mitral valve prolapse: Causes, clinical manifestations, and management. Ann Intern Med. 1989;111:305-317.

52. Clemens JD, Horwitz RI, Jaffe CC, et al. A controlled evaluation of the risk of bacterial endocarditis in persons with mitral-valve prolapse. N Engl J Med. 1982;307:776.

53. Nolan CM, Kane JJ, Grunow WA. Infective endocarditis and mitral prolapse: A comparison with other types of endocarditis. Arch Intern Med. 1981;141:447.

54. Scheld WM. Pathogenesis and pathophysiology of infective endocarditis. In: Sande MA, Kaye D, Root RK, eds. Endocarditis, v. 1. Contemporary Issues in Infectious Diseases. London: Churchill Livingstone; 1984:1-32.

55. Freedman LR. The pathogenesis of infective endocarditis. J Antimicrob Chemother. 1987;20(Suppl A):1-6.

56. Livornese LL Jr, Korzeniowski OM. Pathogenesis of infective endocarditis. In: Kaye D, ed. Infective Endocarditis. New York: Raven Press; 1992:19.

57. Tunkel AR, Scheld WM. Experimental models of endocarditis. In: Kaye D, ed. Infective Endocarditis. New York: Raven Press; 1992:37.

58. Weinstein L, Schlesinger JJ. Pathoanatomic, pathophysiologic, and clinical correlations in endocarditis (first of two parts). N Engl J Med. 1974;291:832.

59. Angrist AA, Oka M. Pathogenesis of bacterial endocarditis. JAMA. 1963;183:249.

60. Durack DT, Beeson PB. Pathogenesis of infective endocarditis. In: Rahimtoola SH, ed. Infective Endocarditis. New York: Grune & Stratton; 1978:1.

61. Durack DT, Beeson PB. Experimental bacterial endocarditis: I. Colonization of a sterile vegetation. Br J Exp Pathol. 1972;53:44.

62. Durack DT, Beeson PB, Petersdorf RG. Experimental endocarditis: III. Production and progress of the disease in rabbits. Br J Exp Pathol. 1973;54:142.

63. Durack DT. Experimental bacterial endocarditis: IV. Structure and function of very early lesions. J Pathol. 1975;115:81.

64. McGowan DA, Gillett R. Scanning electron microscopic observations of the surface of the initial lesion in experimental streptococcal endocarditis in the rabbit. Br J Exp Pathol. 1980;61:91.

65. Ferguson DJP, McColm AA, Ryan DM, et al. Experimental staphylococcal endocarditis and aortitis: Morphology of the initial colonization. Virchows Arch [A]. 1986;410:43-48.

66. Sherwood BF, Rowlands DT, Vakilzadeh J, et al. Experimental bacterial endocarditis in the opossum (Didelphis virginiana). Am J Pathol. 1971;64:513.

67. Chino F, Kodama A, Otake M, et al. Nonbacterial thrombotic endocarditis in a Japanese autopsy sample: A review of 80 cases. Am Heart J. 1975;90:190.

68. Edoute Y, Haim N, Rinkevich D, et al. Cardiac valvular vegetations in cancer patients: A prospective echocardiographic study of 200 patients. Am J Med. 1997;102:252-258.

69. Rodbard S. Blood velocity and endocarditis. Circulation. 1963;27:18.

70. Lepeschkin E. On the relation between the site of valvular involvement in endocarditis and the blood pressure resting on the valve. Am J Med Sci. 1952;224:318.

71. Okell CC, Elliott SD. Bacteraemia and oral sepsis: With special reference to the aetiology of subacute endocarditis. Lancet. 1935;2:869.

72. Everett ED, Hirschmann JV. Transient bacteremia and endocarditis prophylaxis: A review. Medicine (Baltimore). 1977;56:61.

73. Loesche WJ. Indigenous human flora and bacteremia. In: Kaplan EL, Taranta AV, eds. Infective Endocarditis: An American Heart Association Symposium. Dallas: American Heart Association; 1977:40.

74. Durack DT, Beeson PB. Protective role of complement in experimental Escherichia coli endocarditis. Infect Immun. 1977;16:213.

75. Yersin B, Glauser M-P, Guze L, et al. Experimental Escherichia coli endocarditis in rats: Roles of serum bactericidal activity and duration of catheter placement. Infect Immun. 1988;56:1273-1280.

76. Gould K, Ramirez-Ronda CH, Holmes RK, et al. Adherence of bacteria to heart valves in vitro. J Clin Invest. 1975;56:1364.

77. Freedman LR, Valone J Jr. Experimental infective endocarditis. Prog Cardiovasc Dis. 1979;22:169.

78. Baddour LM, Lowrance C, Albus A, et al. Staphylococcus aureus microcapsule expression attenuates bacterial virulence in a rat model of experimental endocarditis. J Infect Dis. 1992;165:749.

79. Baba T, Takeuchi F, Kuroda M, et al. Genome and virulence determinants of high virulence community-acquired MRSA. Lancet. 2002;359:1819-1827.

80. Gillet Y, Issartel B, Vanhems P, et al. Association between Staphylococcus aureus strains carrying gene for Panton-Valentine leukocidin and highly lethal necrotising pneumonia in young immunocompetent patients. Lancet. 2002;359:753-759.

81. Jarraud S, Mougel C, Thioulouse J, et al. Relationships between Staphylococcus aureus genetic background, virulence factors, agr groups (alleles), and human disease. Infect Immun. 2002;70:631-641.

82. Peacock SJ, Moore CE, Justice A, et al. Virulent combinations of adhesin and toxin genes in natural populations of Staphylococcus aureus. Infect Immun. 2002;70:4987-4996.

83. Overholser CD, Moreillon P, Glauser MP. Experimental bacterial endocarditis after dental extractions in rats with periodontitis. J Infect Dis. 1987;155:107-112.

84. Moreillon P, Overholser CD, Malinverni R, et al. Predictors of endocarditis in isolates from cultures of blood following dental extractions in rats with periodontal disease. J Infect Dis. 1988;157:990-995.

85. Gibbons RJ, Nygaard M. Synthesis of insoluble dextran and its significance in the formation of gelatinous deposits by plaque-forming streptococci. Arch Oral Biol. 1968;13:1249.

86. Parker MT, Ball LC. Streptococci and aerococci associated with systemic infection in man. J Med Microbiol. 1976;9:275.
87. Scheld WM, Valone JA, Sande MA. Bacterial adherence in the pathogenesis of endocarditis: Interaction of bacterial dextran, platelets, and fibrin. J Clin Invest. 1978;61:1394.
88. Ramirez-Ronda CH. Adherence of glucan-positive and glucan-negative streptococcal strains to normal and damaged heart valves. J Clin Invest. 1978;62:805.
89. Ramirez-Ronda CH. Effects of molecular weight of dextran on the adherence of *Streptococcus sanguis* to damaged heart valves. Infect Immun. 1980;29:1.
90. Pelletier LL Jr, Coyle M, Petersdorf R. Dextran production as a possible virulence factor in streptococcal endocarditis. Proc Soc Exp Biol Med. 1978;158:415.
91. Pulliam L, Dall L, Inokuchi S, et al. Enzymatic modification of the glycocalyx in experimental endocarditis due to viridans streptococci. J Infect Dis. 1987;156:736.
92. Dall L, Barnes WG, Lane JW, et al. Enzymatic modification of glycocalyx in the treatment of experimental endocarditis due to viridans streptococci. J Infect Dis. 1987;156:736-740.
93. Dall LH, Herndon BL. Association of cell adherent glycocalyx and endocarditis production by viridans group streptococci. J Clin Microbiol. 1990;28:1698.
94. Crawford I, Russell C. Comparative adhesion of seven species of streptococci isolated from the blood of patients with subacute bacterial endocarditis to fibrin-platelet clots in vitro. J Appl Bacteriol. 1986;60:127-133.
95. Dall L, Keihofner M, Herndon B, et al. Clindamycin effect on glycocalyx production in experimental viridans streptococcal endocarditis. J Infect Dis. 1990;161:1221.
96. Fenno JC, LeBlanc DJ, Fives-Taylor P. Nucleotide sequence analysis of a type 1 fimbrial gene of *Streptococcus sanguis* FW213. Infect Immun. 1989;57:3527-3533.
97. Burnette-Curley D, Wells V, Viscount H, et al: FimA, a major virulence determinant associated with *Streptococus parasanguis* endocarditis. Infect Immun. 1995;63:4669-4674.
98. Viscount HB, Munro CL, Burnette-Curley D, et al. Immunization with FimA protects against *Streptococcus parasanguis* endocarditis in rats. Infect Immun. 1997;65:994-1002.
99. Scheld WM, Calderone RA, Alliegro GM, et al. Yeast adherence in the pathogenesis of *Candida* endocarditis. Proc Soc Exp Biol Med. 1981;168:208.
100. Scheld WM, Strunk RW, Balian G, et al. Microbial adhesion to fibronectin in vitro correlates with production of endocarditis in rabbits. Proc Soc Exp Biol Med. 1985;180:474-482.
101. Kuypers JM, Proctor RA. Reduced adherence to traumatized rat heart valves by a low-fibronectin-binding mutant of *Staphylococcus aureus*. Infect Immun. 1989;57:2306.
102. Lowrance JH, Baddour LM, Simpson WA. The role of fibronectin binding in the rat model of experimental endocarditis caused by *Streptococcus sanguis*. J Clin Invest. 1990;86:7.
103. Becker RC, DiBello PM, Lucas FV. Bacterial tissue tropism: An in vitro model for infective endocarditis. Cardiovasc Res. 1987;21:813-820.
104. Tart RC, van de Rijn I. Analysis of adherence of *Streptococcus defectivus* and endocarditis-associated streptococci to extracellular matrix. Infect Immun. 1991;59:857.
105. Sommer P, Gleyzal C, Guerret S, et al. Induction of a putative laminin-binding protein of *Streptococcus gordonii* in human infective endocarditis. Infect Immun. 1992;60:360.
106. Vercellotti G, Lussenhop D, Peterson PK, et al. Bacterial adherence to fibronectin and endothelial cells: A possible mechanism for bacterial tissue tropism. J Lab Clin Med. 1984;103:34-43.
107. Ogawa SK, Yurberg ER, Hather VB, et al. Bacterial adherence to human endothelial cells in vitro. Infect Immun. 1985;50:218-224.
108. Hamill RJ, Vann JM, Proctor RA. Phagocytosis of *Staphylococcus aureus* by cultured bovine aortic-endothelial cells: Model for post adherence events in endovascular infections. Infect Immun. 1986;54:833-836.
109. Yao L, Benjualid V, Lowy FB, et al. Internalization of *Staphylococcus aureus* by endothelial cells induces cytokine gene expression. Infect Immun. 1995;63:1835-1839.
110. Devitt D, Francois P, Vaudaux P, et al. Molecular characterization of the clumping factor (fibrinogen receptor) of *Staphylococcus aureus*. Mol Microbiol. 1994;11:237-248.
111. Moreillon P, Entenza JM, Francioli P, et al. Role of *Staphylococcus aureus* coagulase and clumping factor in pathogenesis of experimental endocarditis. Infect Immun. 1995;63:4738-4743.
112. Flock J-I, Hienz SA, Heimdahl A, et al. Reconsideration of the role of fibronectin binding in endocarditis caused by *Staphylococcus aureus*. Infect Immun. 1996;64:1876-1878.
113. Heinz SA, Schennings T, Heimdahl A, et al. Collagen binding of *Staphylococcus aureus* is a virulence factor in experimental endocarditis. J Infect Dis. 1996;174:83-88.
114. Herrmann M, Suchard SJ, Boxer LA, et al. Thrombospondin binds to *Staphylococcus aureus* and promotes staphylococcal adherence to surfaces. Infect Immun. 1991;59:279-288.
115. Bayer AS, Ramos MD, Menzies BE, et al. Hyperproduction of α-toxin by *Staphylococcus aureus* results in paradoxically reduced virulence in experimental endocarditis-host defense role for platelet microbicidal proteins. Infect Immun. 1997;65:4652-4660.
116. Moreillon P, Que YA, Bayer AS. Pathogenesis of streptococcal and staphylococcal endocarditis. Infect Dis Clin North Am. 2002;16:297-318.
117. Piroth L, Que YA, Piu S, et al. Cooperation between the fibrinogen and fibronectin binding domains of *Staphylococcus aureus* FNBPA for infection in experimental endocarditis. Abstract 4. Abstracts of the Seventh International Symposium on Modern Concepts in Endocarditis and Cardiovascular Infections, Chamonix, France, June 26-28, 2003.
118. Que YA, Francois P, Haefliger JA, et al. Reassessing the role of *Staphylococcus aureus* clumping factor and fibronectin-binding protein by expression in *Lactococcus lactis*. Infect Immun. 2001;69:6296-6302.
119. Scheld WM, Zak O, Vosbeck K, et al. Bacterial adhesion in the pathogenesis of endocarditis: Effect of subinhibitory antibiotic concentrations on streptococcal adhesion in vitro and the development of endocarditis in rabbits. J Clin Invest. 1981;68:1381.
120. Bernard J-P, Francioli P, Glauser MP, et al. Vancomycin prophylaxis of experimental *Streptococcus sanguis* endocarditis: Inhibition of bacterial adherence rather than bacterial killing. J Clin Invest. 1981;68:1113.
121. Glauser MP, Francioli P. Successful prophylaxis against experimental streptococcal endocarditis with bacteriostatic antibiotics. J Infect Dis. 1982;146:806.
122. Lowry FD, Chang DS, Neuhaus EG, et al. Effect of penicillin on the adherence of *Streptococcus sanguis* in vitro and in the rabbit model of endocarditis. J Clin Invest. 1983;71:668.
123. Glauser MP, Bernard JP, Moreillon P, et al. Successful single-dose amoxicillin prophylaxis against experimental streptococcal endocarditis: Evidence for two mechanisms of protection. J Infect Dis. 1983;147:568.
124. Clawson CC, Rao Gunda HR, White JG. Platelet interaction with bacteria: IV. Stimulation of the release reaction. Am J Pathol. 1975;81:411.
125. Herzberg MC, Brintzenhofe KL, Clawson CC. Aggregation of human platelets and adhesion of *Streptococcus sanguis*. Infect Immun. 1983;39:1457.
126. Sullam PM, Valone FH, Mills J. Mechanisms of platelet aggregation by viridans group streptococci. Infect Immun. 1987;55:1743-1750.
127. Sullam PM, Jarvis GA, Valone FH. Role of immunoglobulin G in platelet aggregation by viridans group streptococci. Infect Immun. 1988;56:2907-2911.
128. Herzberg MC, MacFarlane GD, Gong K, et al. The platelet interactivity phenotype of *Streptococcus sanguis* influences the course of experimental endocarditis. Infect Immun. 1992;60:4809.
129. Sullam PM, Costerton JW, Yamasaki R, et al. Inhibition of platelet binding and aggregation by streptococcal exopolysaccharide. J Infect Dis. 1993;167:1123.
130. Bayer AS, Sullam PM, Ramos M, et al. *Staphylococcus aureus*–induced platelet aggregation—a fibrinogen-dependent mechanism that is integrin/RGD sequence-independent. Infect Immun. 1995;63:3634-3641.
131. Herrmann M, Hartleib J, Kehrel B, et al. Interaction of von Willebrand factor with *Staphylococcus aureus*. J Infect Dis. 1997;7:984-991.
132. Shenkman B, Varon D, Marinovitz U, et al. Mechanisms of *Staphylococcus aureus*–induced platelet aggregation: Involvement of glycoprotein Ib and glycoprotein IIb-IIIa. Abstract 50. Presented at the Annual Meeting of the Infectious Disease Society of America, San Francisco, Calif, September 1995.
133. Hartleib J, Kohler N, Dickinson RB, et al. Protein A is the von Willebrand factor binding protein on *Staphylococcus aureus*. Blood. 2000;96:2149-2156.
134. Sullam PM, Bayer AS, Foss W, et al. Reduced platelet binding capacity of *Staphylococcus aureus* in vitro diminishes induction frequency and metastatic complications of experimental endocarditis. Infect Immun. 1996;64:4915-4921.
135. Siboo IR, Cheung AL, Bayer AS, et al. Clumping factor A mediates binding of *Staphylococcus aureus* to human platelets. Infect Immun. 2001;69:3120-3127.
136. Kupferwasser LI, Yeaman MR, Shapiro SM, et al. Beneficial effects of thrombin-induced platelet microbicidal peptide in experimental *Staphylococcus aureus* endocarditis. Circulation. 1999;100:I-149.
137. Yeaman MR, Puentes SM, Norman DC, et al. Partial characterization and staphylocidal activity of thrombin-induced platelet microbicidal protein. Infect Immun. 1992;60:1202.
138. Yeaman MR, Norman DC, Bayer AS. *Staphylococcus aureus* susceptibility to thrombin-induced platelet microbicidal protein is independent of platelet adherence and aggregation in vitro. Infect Immun. 1992;60:2368.
139. Yeaman MR, Ibrahim AS, Edwards JE Jr, et al. Thrombin-induced rabbit platelet microbicidal protein is fungicidal in vitro. Antimicrob Agents Chemother. 1993;37:546.
140. Nicolau DP, Freeman CD, Nightingale CH, et al. Reduction of bacterial titers by low-dose aspirin in experimental aortic valve endocarditis. Infect Immun. 1993;61:1593.
141. Dankert J, van der Werff J, Saat SAJ, et al. Involvement of bactericidal factors from thrombin-stimulated platelets in clearance of adherent viridans streptococci in experimental infective endocarditis. Infect Immun. 1995;63:633-671.
142. Wu T, Yeaman MR, Bayer AS. Resistance to platelet microbicidal protein in vitro among bacteremic staphylococcal and viridans streptococcal isolates correlates with an endocarditis source. Antimicrob Agents Chemother. 1994;38:729-732.
143. Dhawan V, Yeaman MR, Kim E, et al. Phenotypic resistance to thrombin-induced platelet microbicidal protein in vitro correlates with enhanced virulence in experimental endocarditis due to *Staphylococcus aureus*. Infect Immun. 1997;65:3293-3299.
144. Dhawan VK, Bayer AS, Yeaman MR. Influence of in vitro susceptibility to thrombin-induced platelet microbicidal protein on the progression of experimental *Staphylococcus aureus* endocarditis. Infect Immun. 1998;66:3476-3479.
145. Bayer AS, Cheng D, Yeaman MR, et al. In vitro resistance to thrombin-induced platelet microbicidal protein among clinical bacteremic isolates of *Staphylococcus aureus* correlates with an endovascular infectious source. Antimicrob Agents Chemother. 1998;42:3169-3172.
146. Fowler VG Jr, McIntyre LM, Yeaman MR, et al. In vitro resistance to thrombin-induced platelet microbicidal protein in isolates of *Staphylococcus aureus* from endocarditis patients correlates with an intravascular device source. J Infect Dis. 2000;182:1251-1254.
147. Ferguson DJP, McColm AA, Ryan DM, et al. A morphological study of experimental staphylococcal endocarditis and aortitis: II. Inter-relationship of bacteria, vegetation and cardiovasculature in established infections. Br J Exp Pathol. 1986;67:679-686.
148. Durack DT, Beeson PB. Experimental bacterial endocarditis: II. Survival of bacteria in endocardial vegetations. Br J Exp Pathol. 1972;53:50.
149. Yersin BR, Glauser MP, Freedman LR. Effect of nitrogen mustard on natural history of right-sided streptococcal endocarditis: Role of cellular host defenses. Infect Immun. 1982;35:320.

150. Meddens MJM, Thompson J, Eulderink F, et al. Role of granulocytes in experimental *Streptococcus sanguis* endocarditis. Infect Immun. 1982;36:325.

151. Meddens MJM, Thompson J, Mattie H, et al. Role of granulocytes in the prevention and therapy of experimental *Streptococcus sanguis* endocarditis in rabbits. Antimicrob Agents Chemother. 1984;25:263-267.

152. Hook EW III, Sande MA. Role of the vegetation in experimental *Streptococcus viridans* endocarditis. Infect Immun. 1974;10:1433.

153. Thorig L, Thompson J, Eulderink F, et al. Effects of monocytopenia and anticoagulation in experimental *Streptococcus sanguis* endocarditis. Br J Exp Pathol. 1980;61:108.

154. van Ginkel CJW, Thorig L, Thompson J, et al. Enhancement of generation of monocyte tissue thromboplastin by bacterial phagocytosis: Possible pathway for fibrin formation on infected vegetations in bacterial endocarditis. Infect Immun. 1979;25:388.

155. Drake TA, Rodgers GM, Sande MA. Tissue factor is a major stimulus for vegetation formation in enterococcal endocarditis in rabbits. J Clin Invest. 1984;73:1750-1753.

156. Drake TA, Pang M. *Staphylococcus aureus* induces tissue factor expression in cultured human cardiac valve endothelium. J Infect Dis. 1988;157:749-756.

157. Yao L, Berman JW, Factor SM, et al. Correlation of histopathologic and bacteriologic changes with cytokine gene expression in an experimental murine model of bacteremic *Staphylococcus aureus* infection. Infect Immun. 1997;65:3889-3995.

158. Beekhuizen H, van de Gevel JS, Veltrop MHAM, et al. Bacterial colonization of vascular endothelium in the pathogenesis of endocarditis. Abstract 145. Presented at the Fourth International Symposium on Modern Concepts in Endocarditis and Cardiovascular Infections, Yverdon, Switzerland, May 24-26, 1997.

159. Veltrop MHAM, Beekhuizen H, Thompson J. Procoagulant properties of endothelial cells after infection with bacteria. Abstract 148. Presented at the Fourth International Symposium on Modern Concepts in Endocarditis and Cardiovascular Infections, Yverdon, Switzerland, May 1997.

160. Bansci MJLFM, Veltrop MHAM, Bertina RM, et al. Influence of monocytes and antibiotic treatment on tissue factor activity of endocardial vegetations in rabbits infected with *Streptococcus sanguis*. Infect Immun. 1996;64:448-451.

161. Mair W. Pneumococcal endocarditis in rabbits. J Pathol Bacteriol. 1923;26:426.

162. Scheld WM, Thomas JH, Sande MA. Influence of preformed antibody on experimental *Streptococcus sanguis* endocarditis. Infect Immun. 1979;25:781.

163. Durack DT, Gilliland BC, Petersdorf RG. Effect of immunization on susceptibility to experimental *Streptococcus mutans* and *Streptococcus sanguis* endocarditis. Infect Immun. 1978;22:52.

164. van de Rijn I. Analysis of cross-protection between serotypes and passively transferred immune globulin in experimental nutritionally variant streptococcal endocarditis. Infect Immun. 1988;56:117.

165. Scheld WM, Calderone RA, Brodeur JP, et al. Influence of preformed antibody on the pathogenesis of experimental *Candida albicans* endocarditis. Infect Immun. 1983;40:950.

166. Greenberg DP, Ward JI, Bayer AS. Influence of *Staphylococcus aureus* antibody on experimental endocarditis in rabbits. Infect Immun. 1987;55:3030-3034.

167. Sieling PJ, van de Rijn I. Evaluation of the immune response in protection against experimental *Streptococcus defectivus* endocarditis. J Lab Clin Med. 1991;117:402.

168. Albus A, Arbeit RD, Lee JC. Virulence of *Staphylococcus aureus* mutants altered in type 5 capsule production. Infect Immun. 1991;59:1008-1014.

169. Lee JC, Park J-S, Shepherd SE, Fattom A. Protective efficacy of antibodies to the *Staphylococcus aureus* type 5 capsular polysaccharide in a rat model of endocarditis. Infect Immun. 1997;65:4146-4151.

170. Bayer AS, Ing M, Kim E, et al. Role of anticapsular IgG in modifying the course of experimental *Staphylococcus aureus* endocarditis. Presented at the Thirty-sixth Interscience Conference on Antimicrobial Agents and Chemotherapy, Washington, DC, 1996.

171. Williams RC, Kunkel HG. Rheumatoid factors and their disappearance following therapy in patients with SBE. Arthritis Rheum. 1962;5:126.

172. Sheagren JN, Tuazon CV, Griffin C, et al. Rheumatoid factor in acute bacterial endocarditis. Arthritis Rheum. 1976;19:887.

173. Phair JP, Clarke J. Immunology of infective endocarditis. Prog Cardiovasc Dis. 1979;22:137.

174. Bacon PA, Davidson C, Smith B. Antibodies to *Candida* and autoantibodies in subacute bacterial endocarditis. QJM. 1974;43:537.

175. Laxdal T, Messner RP, Williams RC. Opsonic, agglutinating, and complement-fixing antibodies in patients with subacute bacterial endocarditis. J Lab Clin Med. 1968;71:638.

176. Horwitz D, Quismorio FP, Friou GJ. Cryoglobulinemia in patients with infectious endocarditis. Clin Exp Immunol. 1975;19:131.

177. Qoronfleh MW, Weraarchakul W, Wilkinson BJ. Antibodies to a range of *Staphylococcus aureus* and *Escherichia coli* heat shock proteins in sera from patients with *S. aureus* endocarditis. Infect Immun. 1993;61:1567.

178. Bayer AS, Theofilopoulos AN, Eisenberg R, et al. Circulating immune complexes in infective endocarditis. N Engl J Med. 1976;295:1500.

179. Gutman RA, Striker GE, Gilliland BC, et al. The immune complex glomerulonephritis of bacterial endocarditis. Medicine (Baltimore). 1972;51:1.

180. Le MV, Lacassin F, Delahousse M, et al. Use of corticosteroids in glomerulonephritis related to infective endocarditis: Three cases and review. Clin Infect Dis. 1999;28:1057-1061.

181. Levy RL, Hong R. The immune nature of subacute bacterial endocarditis (SBE) nephritis. Am J Med. 1973;54:645.

182. Inman RD, Redecha PB, Knechtle SJ, et al. Identification of bacterial antigens in circulating immune complexes of infective endocarditis. J Clin Invest. 1982;70:271.

183. Alpert JS, Krous HF, Dalen JE, et al. Pathogenesis of Osler's nodes. Ann Intern Med. 1976;85:471.

184. Lowenstein MB, Urman JD, Abeles M, et al. Skin immunofluorescence in infective endocarditis. JAMA. 1977;238:1163.

185. Cabane J, Godeau P, Herreman G, et al. Fate of circulating immune complexes in infective endocarditis. Am J Med. 1979;66:277.

186. Kauffman RH, Thompson J, Valentijn RM, et al. The clinical implications and the pathogenetic significance of circulating immune complexes in infective endocarditis. Am J Med. 1981;71:17.

187. Morris AJ, Drinkovic D, Pottumarthy S, et al. Gram stain, culture, and histopathological examination findings for heart valves removed because of infective endocarditis. Clin Infect Dis. 2003;36:697-704.

188. McFarland MM. Pathology of infective endocarditis. In: Kaye D, ed. Infective Endocarditis. New York: Raven Press; 1992:57.

189. Roberts WC. Characteristics and consequences of infective endocarditis (active or healed or both) learned from morphologic studies. In: Rahimtoola SH, ed. Infective Endocarditis. New York: Grune & Stratton; 1978:55.

190. Coplan NL, Bruno MS. Acquired immunodeficiency syndrome and heart disease: The present and future. Am Heart J. 1989;117:1175.

191. Francis CK. Cardiac involvement in AIDS. Curr Prob Cardiol. 1990;15:571.

192. Paterson DL, Dominguez EA, Chang FY, et al. Infective endocarditis in solid organ transplant recipients. Clin Infect Dis. 1998;26:689-694.

193. Morel-Maroger L, Sraer JD, Herreman G, et al. Kidney in subacute endocarditis: Pathological and immunofluorescence findings. Arch Pathol. 1913;94:205.

194. Anderson CB, Butcher HR, Ballinger WF. Mycotic aneurysms. Arch Surg. 1974;109:712.

195. Heiro M, Nikoskelainen J, Engblom E, et al. Neurologic manifestations of infective endocarditis: A 17-year experience in a teaching hospital in Finland. Arch Intern Med. 2000;160:2781-2787.

196. Mylonakis E, Calderwood SB. Infective endocarditis in adults. N Engl J Med. 2001;345:1318-1330.

197. Cabell CH, Barsic B, Bayer AS, et al. Clinical findings, complications, and outcomes in a large prospective study of definite endocarditis: The International Collaboration on Endocarditis—prospective cohort study. Abstract 22. Abstracts of the Seventh International Symposium on Modern Concepts in Endocarditis and Cardiovascular Infections, Chamonix, France, June 26-28, 2003.

198. Greenlee JE, Mandell GL. Neurological manifestations of infective endocarditis: A review. Stroke. 1973;4:958.

199. Masuda J, Yutani C, Waki R, et al. Histopathologic analysis of the mechanisms of intracranial hemorrhage complicating infective endocarditis. Stroke. 1992;23:843.

200. Changchien CS, Tsai TL, Hu TH, et al. Sonographic patterns of splenic abscess: An analysis of 34 proven cases. Abdom Imaging. 2002;27:739-745.

201. Ng KK, Lee TY, Wan YL, et al. Splenic abscess: Diagnosis and management. Hepatogastroenterology. 2002;49:567-571.

202. Thanos L, Dailiana T, Papaioannou G, et al. Percutaneous CT-guided drainage of splenic abscess. AJR Am J Roentgenol. 2002;179:629-632.

203. Miro JM, del Rio A, Mestres CA. Infective endocarditis in intravenous drug abusers and HIV-1 infected patients. Infect Dis Clin North Am. 2002;16:273-295.

204. Kerr A Jr, Tan JS. Biopsies of the Janeway lesion of infective endocarditis. J Cutan Pathol. 1979;6:124.

205. Silverberg HH. Roth spots. Mt Sinai J Med. 1970;37:77.

206. Starkebaum M, Durack D, Beeson P. The "incubation period" of subacute bacterial endocarditis. Yale J Biol Med. 1977;50:49.

207. Weinstein L, Rubin RH. Infective endocarditis—1973. Prog Cardiovasc Dis. 1973;16:239.

208. Freedman LR. Infective endocarditis and other intravascular infections. In: Braude AI, David CE, Fierer J, eds. Medical Microbiology and Infectious Diseases. Philadelphia: WB Saunders; 1981:1511.

209. Hermans PE. The clinical manifestations of infective endocarditis. Mayo Clin Proc. 1982;57:15.

210. Espersen F, Frimodt-Moller N. *Staphylococcus aureus* endocarditis: Review of 119 cases. Arch Intern Med. 1986;146:1118-1121.

211. Roder BL, Wandall DA, Frimodt-Moller N, et al. Clinical features of *Staphylococcus aureus* endocarditis: A 10-year experience in Denmark. Arch Intern Med. 1999;159:462-469.

212. Figueiredo LT, Ruiz-Junior E, Schirmbeck T. Infective endocarditis (IE) first diagnosed at autopsy: analysis of 31 cases in Ribeirao Preto, Brazil. Rev Inst Med Trop Sao Paulo. 2001;43:213-216.

213. Terpenning MS, Buggy BP, Kauffman CA. Infective endocarditis: Clinical features in young and elderly patients. Am J Med. 1987;83:626-634.

214. Bradley SF. *Staphylococcus aureus* infections and antibiotic resistance in older adults. Clin Infect Dis. 2002;34:211-216.

215. Lederman MM, Sprague L, Wallis RS, et al. Duration of fever during treatment of infective endocarditis. Medicine (Baltimore). 1992;71:52.

216. Blumberg EA, Robbins N, Adimora A, et al. Persistent fever in association with infective endocarditis. Clin Infect Dis. 1992;15:983.

217. Espersen F, Frimodt-Moller N. *Staphylococcus aureus* endocarditis: A review of 119 cases. Arch Intern Med. 1986;146:1118-1121.

218. Charney R, Keltz TN, Attai L, et al. Acute vavular obstruction from streptococcal endocarditis. Am Heart J. 1993;125:544.

219. Ting W, Silverman NA, Arzaman DA, et al. Splenic septic emboli in endocarditis. Circulation. 1990;82(Suppl IV):IV-105.

220. Mansur AJ, Grinberg M, DaLuz PL, et al. The complications of infective endocarditis—a reappraisal in the 1980s. Arch Intern Med. 1992;152:2428-2432.

221. Churchill MA, Geraci JE, Hunder GG. Musculoskeletal manifestations of bacterial endocarditis. Ann Intern Med. 1977;87:754.

222. Herzog CA, Henry TD, Zimmer SD. Bacterial endocarditis presenting as acute myocardial infarction: A cautionary note for the era of reperfusion. Am J Med. 1991;90:392.

223. Tunkel AR, Kaye D. Neurologic complications of infective endocarditis. Neurol Clin. 1993;11:419.

224. Selky AK, Roos KL. Neurologic complications of infective endocarditis. Semin Neurol. 1995;12:225.

225. Bayer AS, Theofilopulos AN, Eisenberg R, et al. Thrombotic thrombocytopenic purpura-like syndrome associated with infective endocarditis: A possible immune complex disorder. JAMA. 1977;238:408.

226. Levine DP, Crane LR, Zervos MJ. Bacteremia in narcotic addicts at the Detroit Medical Center: II. Infectious endocarditis: A prospective comparative study. Rev Infect Dis. 1986;8:374-396.

227. Marantz PR, Linzer M, Feiner CJ, et al. Inability to predict diagnosis in febrile intravenous drug abusers. Ann Intern Med. 1987;106:823-828.

228. Weisse AB, Heller DR, Schimenti RJ, et al. The febrile parenteral drug user: A prospective study in 121 patients. Am J Med. 1993;94:274.

229. Chambers HF, Morris DL, Tauber MG, et al. Cocaine use and the risk for endocarditis in intravenous drug users. Ann Intern Med. 1987;106:833-836.

230. Graves MK, Soto L. Left-sided endocarditis in parenteral drug abusers: Recent experience at a large community hospital. South Med J. 1992;85:387.

231. Carozza A, Romano G, De Feo M, et al. Infective endocarditis in intravenous drug users: Prevalence of left heart involvement and changing microbiologic profile. Abstract 53. Abstracts of the Seventh International Symposium on Modern Concepts in Endocarditis and Cardiovascular Infections, Chamonix, France, June 26-28, 2003.

232. Chambers HF, Korzeniowski OM, Sande MA, et al. *Staphylococcus aureus* endocarditis: Clinical manifestations in addicts and nonaddicts. Medicine (Baltimore). 1983;62:170.

233. Sklaver AR, Hoffman TA, Greenman RL. Staphylococcal endocarditis in addicts. South Med J. 1978;71:638.

234. Thadepalli H, Francis CK. Diagnostic clues in metastatic lesions of endocarditis in addicts. West J Med. 1978;128:1.

234a. Wilson LE, Thomas DL, Astemborski J, et al. Prospective study of infective endocarditis among injection drug users. J Infect Dis. 2002;185:1761-1766.

235. Nahass RG, Weinstein MP, Bartels J, et al. Infectious endocarditis in intravenous drug users: A comparison of human immunodeficiency virus type-1-negative and -positive patients. J Infect Dis. 1990;162:967-970.

236. Kaell AT, Volkman DJ, Gorevic PD, et al. Positive Lyme serology in subacute bacterial endocarditis. JAMA. 1990;264:2916.

237. McCartney AC, Orange GV, Pringle SD, et al. Serum C reactive protein in infective endocarditis. J Clin Pathol. 1988;41:44-48.

238. Wiseman J, Rouleau J, Rigo P, et al. Gallium-67 myocardial imaging for the detection of bacterial endocarditis. Radiology. 1976;120:135.

239. Wong DW, Dhawan VK, Tanaka T, et al. Imaging endocarditis with technetium 99m-labeled antibody—an experimental study: Concise communication. J Nucl Med. 1982;23:229.

240. Riba AL, Thakur ML, Gottschalk A, et al. Imaging experimental infective endocarditis with indium-111-labeled blood cellular components. Circulation. 1979;59:336.

241. Haft JI, Altieri J, Smight LG, et al. Computed tomography of the abdomen in the diagnosis of splenic emboli. Arch Intern Med. 1988;148:193-197.

242. Beeson PB, Brannon ES, Warren JV. Observations on the sites of removal of bacteria from the blood of patients with bacterial endocarditis. J Exp Med. 1945;81:9-23.

243. Werner AS, Cobbs CG, Kaye D, et al. Studies on the bacteremia of bacterial endocarditis. JAMA. 1967;202:199.

244. Pazin GJ, Saul S, Thompson ME. Blood culture positivity: Suppression by outpatient antibiotic therapy in patients with bacterial endocarditis. Arch Intern Med. 1982;142:263.

245. McKenzie R, Reimer LG. Effect of antimicrobials on blood cultures in endocarditis. Diagn Microbiol Infect Dis. 1987;8:165-172.

246. Aronson MD, Bos DH. Blood cultures. Ann Intern Med. 1987;106:246-253.

247. Washington JA II, Ilstrup DM. Blood cultures: Issues and controversies. Rev Infect Dis. 1986;8:792-802.

248. Washington JA II. The role of the microbiology laboratory in the diagnosis and antimicrobial treatment of infective endocarditis. Mayo Clin Proc. 1982;57:22.

249. Carey RB, Gross KC, Roberts RB. Vitamin-B₆-dependent *Streptococcus mitior (mitis)* isolated from patients with systemic infections. J Infect Dis. 1975;131:722.

250. Powers DL, Mandell GL. Intraleucocytic bacteria in endocarditis patients. JAMA. 1974;227:313.

251. Whitcomb DC. Bugs in the blood: Acute staphylococcal septicemia and endocarditis diagnosed by staining the buffy coat. NC Med J. 1986;47:293-295.

252. Cannady PB, Sanford JP. Negative blood cultures in infective endocarditis: A review. South Med J. 1976;69:1420.

253. Tunkel AR, Kaye D. Endocarditis with negative blood cultures. N Engl J Med. 1992;326:1215.

254. Walker RC, Henry NK, Washington JA II, et al. Lysis-centrifugation blood culture technique: Clinical impact in *Staphylococcus aureus* bacteremia. Arch Intern Med. 1986;146:2341-2343.

255. Washington JA II. The microbiological diagnosis of infective endocarditis. J Antimicrob Chemother. 1987;20(Suppl A):29-36.

256. Washington JA. The microbiologic diagnosis of infective endocarditis. J Antimicrob Chemother. 1987;20(Suppl A):29-36.

257. Tunkel AR, Kaye D. Endocarditis with negative blood cultures. N Engl J Med. 1992;326:1215-1217.

258. Austin SM, Smith SM, Co B, et al. Case report: Serologic evidence of acute murine typhus infection in a patient with culture-negative endocarditis. Am J Med Sci. 1987;293:320-323.

259. Shapiro DS, Kenney SC, Johnson M, et al. *Chlamydia psittaci* endocarditis diagnosed by blood culture. N Engl J Med. 1992;326:1192.

260. Tompkins LS, Roessler BJ, Redd SC, et al. *Legionella* prosthetic-valve endocarditis. N Engl J Med. 1988;318:530-535.

261. Spach DH, Kanter AS, Daniels NA, et al. *Bartonella (Rochalimaea)* species as a cause of apparent "culture-negative" endocarditis. Clin Infect Dis. 1995;20:1044-1047.

262. Larson AM, Cougherty MJ, Nowowiejski DJ, et al. Detection of *Bartonella (Rochalimaea)* by routine acridine orange staining of broth blood cultures. J Clin Microbiol. 1994;32:1492-1496.

263. Spach DH, Kanter AS, Dougherty MJ, et al. *Bartonella (Rochalimaea) quintana* bacteremia in inner-city patients with chronic alcoholism. N Engl J Med. 1995;332:419-423.

264. Drancourt M, Mainardi JL, Brouqui P, et al. *Bartonella (Rochalimaea) quintana* endocarditis in three homeless men. N Engl J Med. 1995;332:424-428.

265. Raoult D, Fournier PE, Drancourt M, et al. Diagnosis of 22 new cases of *Bartonella* endocarditis. Ann Intern Med. 1996;125:646-652.

266. Fenollar F, Lepidi H, Raoult D. Whipple's endocarditis: Review of the literature and comparisons with Q fever, *Bartonella* infection, and blood culture-positive endocarditis. Clin Infect Dis. 2001;33:1309-1316.

267. Lepidi H, Houpikian P, Liang Z, et al. Cardiac valves in patients with Q fever endocarditis: Microbiological, molecular, and histologic studies. J Infect Dis. 2003;187:1097-1106.

268. Brouqui P, Dumler JS, Raoult D. Immunohistologic demonstration of *Coxiella burnetii* in the valves of patients with Q fever endocarditis. Am J Med. 1994;97:451-458.

269. Hamed KA, Dormitzer PR, Su CK, et al. *Haemophilus parainfluenzae* endocarditis: Application of molecular approach for identification of pathogenetic bacterial species. Clin Infect Dis. 1994;19:677-683.

270. Zeaiter Z, Fournier PE, Greub G, et al. Diagnosis of *Bartonella* endocarditis by a real-time nested PCR assay using serum. J Clin Microbiol. 2003;41:919-925.

271. Bosshard PP, Kronenberg A, Zbinden R, et al. Etiologic diagnosis of infective endocarditis by broad-range polymerase chain reaction: A 3 year experience. Clin Infect Dis 2003;37:167-172.

272. Walterspiel JN, Kaplan SL. Incidence and clinical characteristics of "culture-negative" infective endocarditis in a pediatric population. Pediatr Infect Dis. 1986;5:328-332.

273. Rubenstein E, Noriega ER, Simberkoff MS, et al. Fungal endocarditis: Analysis of 24 cases and review of the literature. Medicine (Baltimore). 1975;54:331.

274. Pierrotti LC, Baddour LM. Fungal endocarditis, 1995-2000. Chest. 2002;122:302-310.

275. Mayayo E, Moralejo J, Camps J, et al. Fungal endocarditis in premature infants: Case report and review. Clin Infect Dis. 1996;22:366-368.

276. Nasser RM, Melgar GR, Longworth DL, et al. Incidence and risk of developing fungal prosthetic valve endocarditis after nosocomial candidemia. Am J Med. 1997;103:25-32.

277. Kobza K, Steenblock U. Demonstration of candida in blood smears. BMJ. 1977;1:1640.

278. Merz WG, Evans GL, Shadomy S, et al. Laboratory evaluation of serological tests for systemic candidiasis: A cooperative study. J Clin Microbiol. 1977;5:596.

279. Sande MA, Bowman CR, Calderone RA. Experimental *Candida albicans* endocarditis: Characterization of the disease and response to therapy. Infect Immun. 1977;17:140.

280. Warren RC, Bartlett A, Bidwell DE, et al. Diagnosis of invasive candidosis by enzyme immunoassay of serum antigen. BMJ. 1977;1:1183.

281. Scheld WM, Brown RS Jr, Harding SA, et al. Detection of circulating antigen in experimental *Candida albicans* endocarditis by an enzyme-linked immunosorbent assay. J Clin Microbiol. 1980;12:679.

282. Dillan JC, Feigenbaum H, Konecke LL, et al. Echocardiographic manifestations of valvular vegetations. Am Heart J. 1973;86:698.

283. Boucher CA, Fallion JT, Myers GS, et al. The value and limitations of echocardiography in recording mitral valve vegetations. Am Heart J. 1977;94:37.

284. Thomson KR, Nanda NC, Gramiak R. The reliability of echocardiography in the diagnosis of infective endocarditis. Radiology. 1977;125:473.

285. Melvin ET, Berger M, Lutzker LG, et al. Noninvasive methods for detection of valve vegetations in infective endocarditis. Am J Cardiol. 1981;47:271.

286. Mintz GS, Kotler MN. Clinical value and limitations of echocardiography: Its use in the study of patients with infectious endocarditis. Arch Intern Med. 1980;140:1022.

287. Popp RL. Echocardiography and infectious endocarditis. In: Remington JS, Swartz MN, eds. Current Clinical Topics in Infectious Diseases, v. 4. New York: McGraw-Hill; 1983:98.

288. Popp RL. Echocardiography. N Engl J Med. 1990;323:165.

289. Kuruppu JC, Corretti M, Mackowiak P, et al. Overuse of transthoracic echocardiography in the diagnosis of native valve endocarditis. Arch Intern Med. 2002;162:1715-1720.

290. Davis RS, Strom JA, Frishman W, et al. The demonstration of vegetations by echocardiography in bacterial endocarditis: An indication for early surgical intervention. Am J Med. 1980;57:69.

291. Martin RP, Mettzer RS, Chia EL, et al. Clinical utility of two-dimensional echocardiography in infective endocarditis. Am J Cardiol. 1980;46:379.

292. Steckelberg JM, Murphy JG, Ballard D, et al. Emboli in infective endocarditis: The prognostic value of echocardiography. Ann Intern Med. 1991;114:635.

293. Rohmann S, Erbel R, Gorge G, et al. Clinical relevance of vegetation localization by transesophageal echocardiography in infective endocarditis. Eur Heart J. 1992;13:446-452.

294. Bayer AS, Blomquist IK, Bello E, et al. Tricuspid valve endocarditis due to *Staphylococcus aureus:* Correlation of two-dimensional echocardiography with clinical outcome. Chest. 1988;93:247-253.

295. Tischler MD, Vaitkus PT. The ability of vegetation size on echocardiography to predict clinical complications: A meta-analysis. J Am Soc Echocardiogr. 1997;10:562-568.

296. Manolis AS, Melita H. Echocardiographic and clinical correlates in drug addicts with infective endocarditis: Implication of vegetation size. Arch Intern Med. 1988;148:2461-2465.

297. Tak T, Rahimtoola SH, Kumar A, et al. Value of digital image processing of two-dimensional echocardiograms in differentiating active from chronic vegetations of infective endocarditis. Circulation. 1988;78:116-123.

298. Rohmann S, Erbel R, Darius H, et al. Prediction of rapid versus prolonged healing of infective endocarditis by monitoring vegetation size. J Am Soc Echocardiogr. 1991;4:465-474.

299. Di Salvo G, Habib G, Pergola V, et al. Echocardiography predicts embolic events in infective endocarditis. J Am Coll Cardiol. 2001;37:1069-1076.

300. SanFilippo AJ, Picard MH, Newell JB, et al. Echocardiographic assessment of patients with infective endocarditis. J Am Coll Cardiol. 1991;18:1191-1199.

301. Sachdev M, Peterson GE, Jollis JG. Imaging techniques for diagnosis of infective endocarditis. Infect Dis Clin North Am. 2002;16:319-337.

302. Heinle S, Wilderman N, Harrison JK, et al. Value of transthoracic echocardiography in predicting embolic events in active infective endocarditis: Duke Endocarditis Service. Am J Cardiol. 1994;74:799-801.

303. Shapiro SM, Bayer AS. Transesophageal and Doppler echocardiography in the diagnosis and management of infective endocarditis. Chest. 1991;100:1125-1130.

304. Pearlman AS. Transesophageal echocardiography—sound diagnostic technique or two-edged sword? N Engl J Med. 1991;324:841.

305. Chamis AL, Gesty-Palmer D, Fowler VG, et al. Echocardiography for the diagnosis of Staphylococcus aureus infective endocarditis. Curr Infect Dis Rep. 1999;1:129-135.

306. Erbel R, Rohmann S, Drexler M, et al. Improved diagnostic value of echocardiography in patients with infective endocarditis by transesophageal approach: A prospective study. Eur Heart J. 1988;9:43.

307. Mügge A, Daniel WG, Frank G, et al. Echocardiography in infective endocarditis: Reassessment of prognostic implications of vegetation size determined by the transthoracic and transesophageal approach. J Am Coll Cardiol. 1989;14:631.

308. Sochowski RA, Chan K-L. Implication of negative results on a monoplane transesophageal echocardiographic study in patients with suspected infective endocarditis. J Am Coll Cardiol. 1993;21:216.

309. Carpenter JL. Perivalvular extension of infection in patients with infectious endocarditis. Rev Infect Dis. 1991;13:127.

310. Daniel WG, Mügge A, Martin RP, et al. Improvement in the diagnosis of abscesses associated with endocarditis by transesophageal echocardiography. N Engl J Med. 1991;324:795.

311. De Castro S, Cartoni D, d'Amati G, et al. Diagnostic accuracy of transthoracic and multiplane transesophageal echocardiography for valvular perforation in acute infective endocarditis: Correlation with anatomic findings. Clin Infect Dis. 2000;30:825-826.

312. Rallidis LS, Komninos KA, Papasteriadis EG. Pacemaker-related endocarditis: The value of transoesophageal echocardiography in diagnosis and treatment. Acta Cardiol. 2003;58:31-34.

313. Sawhney N, Palakodeti V, Raisinghani A, et al. Eustachian valve endocarditis: A case series and analysis of the literature. J Am Soc Echocardiogr. 2001;14:1139-1142.

314. Werner GS, Schulz R, Fuchs JB, et al. Infective endocarditis in the elderly in the era of transesophageal echocardiography: Clinical features and prognosis compared with younger patients. Am J Med. 1996;100:90-97.

315. Daniel WG, Erbel R, Kasper W, et al. Safety of transesophageal echocardiography: A multicenter survey of 10419 examinations. Circulation. 1991;83:817.

316. Heidenreich PA, Masoudi FA, Maini B, et al. Echocardiography in patients with suspected endocarditis: A cost-effectiveness analysis. Am J Med. 1999;107:198-208.

317. Rosen AB, Fowler VGJ, Corey GR, et al. Cost-effectiveness of transesophageal echocardiography to determine the duration of therapy for intravascular catheter-associated Staphylococcus aureus bacteremia. Ann Intern Med. 1999;130:810-820.

318. Mann T, McLaurin L, Grossman W, et al. Assessing the hemodynamic severity of acute aortic regurgitation due to infective endocarditis. N Engl J Med. 1975;293:108.

319. Mills J, Abbott J, Utley JR, et al. Role of cardiac catheterization in infective endocarditis. Chest. 1977;72:576.

320. Welton DE, Young JB, Raizner AE, et al. Value and safety of cardiac catheterization during active infective endocarditis. Am J Cardiol. 1979;44:1306.

321. Durack DT, Lukes AS, Bright DK, et al. New criteria for diagnosis of infective endocarditis. Am J Med. 1994;96:200-209.

322. Dajani AS, Ayoub E, Bierman FZ, et al. Guidelines for the diagnosis of rheumatic fever: Jones criteria, 1992 update. JAMA. 1992;69:203-208.

323. Bayer AS, Bolger AF, Taubert KA, et al. Diagnosis and management of infective endocarditis and its complications. Circulation. 1998;25:2936-2948.

324. Li JS, Sexton DJ, Mick N, et al. Proposed modifications to the Duke criteria for the diagnosis of infective endocarditis. Clin Infect Dis. 2000;30:633-638.

325. Kim EL, Ching DL, Pien FD. Bacterial endocarditis at a small community hospital. Am J Med Sci. 1990;299:87-93.

326. Kazanjian PH. Infective endocarditis: Review of 60 cases treated in community hospitals. Infect Dis Clin Pract. 1993;2:41.

327. Roberts RB, Krieger AG, Schiller NL, et al. Viridans streptococcal endocarditis: The role of various species, including pyridoxal-dependent streptococci. Rev Infect Dis. 1979;1:955.

328. Tuazon CV, Gill V, Gill F. Streptococcal endocarditis: Single vs. combination antibiotic therapy and the role of various species. Rev Infect Dis. 1986;8:54-60.

329. Baddour LM, Bisno AL. Infective endocarditis complicating mitral valve prolapse: Epidemiologic, clinical, and microbiologic aspects. Rev Infect Dis. 1986;8:117-137.

330. Hamoudi AC, Hribar MM, Marcon MJ, et al. Clinical relevance of viridans and non-hemolytic streptococci isolated from blood and cerebrospinal fluid in a pediatric population. Am J Clin Pathol. 1990;93:270.

331. Harder EJ, Wilkowske CJ, Washington JA, et al. Streptococcus mutans endocarditis. Ann Intern Med. 1974;80:364.

332. Facklam R. What happened to the streptococci: Overview of taxonomic and nomenclature changes. Clin Microbiol Rev. 2002;15:613-630.

333. Watanakunakorn C. Streptococcus bovis endocarditis. Am J Med. 1974;56:256.

334. Moellering RC, Watson BK, Kunz LJ. Endocarditis due to group D streptococci: Comparison of disease caused by Streptococcus bovis with that produced by the enterococci. Am J Med. 1974;57:239.

335. Hoppes WL, Lerner PI. Nonenterococcal group D streptococcal endocarditis caused by Streptococcus bovis. Ann Intern Med. 1974;81:588.

336. Klein RS, Reuco RA, Catalano MT, et al. Association of Streptococcus bovis with carcinoma of the colon. N Engl J Med. 1977;297:800.

337. Steinberg D, Naggar CZ. Streptococcus bovis endocarditis with carcinoma of the colon. N Engl J Med. 1977;297:1354.

338. Mandell GL, Kaye D, Levison ME, et al. Enterococcal endocarditis: An analysis of 38 patients observed at the New York Hospital-Cornell Medical Center. Arch Intern Med. 1970;125:258.

339. Serra P, Brandimarte C, Martino P, et al. Synergistic treatment of enterococcal endocarditis. Arch Intern Med. 1977;137:1562.

340. Mergran DW. Enterococcal endocarditis. Clin Infect Dis. 1992;15:63.

341. Malone DA, Wagner RA, Myers JP, et al. Enterococcal bacteremia in two large community teaching hospitals. Am J Med. 1986;81:601-606.

342. Hoffmann SA, Moellering RC Jr. The enterococcus: "Putting the bug in our ears." Ann Intern Med. 1987;106:757-561.

343. Maki DG, Agger WA. Enterococcal bacteremia: Clinical features, the risk of endocarditis, and management. Medicine (Baltimore). 1988;67:248-269.

344. Ugolini V, Pacifico A, Smitherman TC, et al. Pneumococcal endocarditis update: Analysis of 10 cases diagnosed between 1974 and 1984. Am Heart J. 1986;112:813-819.

345. Powderly WG, Stanley SL Jr, Medoff G. Pneumococcal endocarditis: Report of a series and review of the literature. Rev Infect Dis. 1986;8:786-791.

346. Bruyn GAW, Thompson J, van der Meer JWM. Pneumococcal endocarditis in adult patients: A report of five cases and review of the literature. QJM. 1990;74:33.

347. Elward K, Hruby N, Christy C. Pneumococcal endocarditis in infants and children: Report of a case and review of the literature. Pediatr Infect Dis J. 1990;9:652.

348. Lefort A, Mainardi JL, Selton-Suty C, et al. Streptococcus pneumoniae endocarditis in adults: A multicenter study in France in the era of penicillin resistance (1991-1998). The Pneumococcal Endocarditis Study Group. Medicine. 2000;79:327-337.

349. Gelfand MS, Threlkeld MG. Subacute bacterial endocarditis secondary to Streptococcus pneumoniae. Am J Med. 1992;93:91.

350. Carey RB, Brause BD, Roberts RB. Antimicrobial therapy of vitamin B₆-dependent streptococcal endocarditis. Ann Intern Med. 1977;87:150.

351. Stein DS, Nelson KE. Endocarditis due to nutritionally deficient streptococci: Therapeutic dilemma. Rev Infect Dis. 1987;9:908-916.

352. Catto BA, Jacobs MR, Shlaes DM. Streptococcus mitis: A cause of serious infection in adults. Arch Intern Med. 1987;147:885-888.

353. Rapeport KB, Giron JA, Rosner F. Streptococcus mitis endocarditis: Report of 17 cases. Arch Intern Med. 1986;146:2361-2363.

354. Hager WD, Speck EL, Mathew PK, et al. Endocarditis with myocardial abscesses and pericarditis in an adult: Group B streptococcus as a cause. Arch Intern Med. 1977;137:1725.

355. Sambola A, Miro JM, Tornos MP, et al. Streptococcus agalactiae infective endocarditis: Analysis of 30 cases and review of the literature, 1962-1998. Clin Infect Dis. 2002;34:1576-1584.

356. Opal SM, Cross A, Palmer M, et al. Group B streptococcal sepsis in adults and infants: Contrasts and comparisons. Arch Intern Med. 1988;148:641-645.

357. Gallagher PG, Watanakunakorn C. Group B streptococcal endocarditis: Report of seven cases and review of the literature, 1962-1985. Rev Infect Dis. 1986;8:175-188.

358. Scully BE, Spriggs D, Neu HC. Streptococcus agalactiae (group B) endocarditis—a description of twelve cases and review of the literature. Infection. 1987;15:169-176.

359. Wiseman A, Rene P, Crelinsten GL. Streptococcus agalactiae endocarditis: An association with villous adenomas of the large intestine. Ann Intern Med. 1985;103:893-894.

360. Vartrian CV, Septimus EJ. Tricuspid valve group B streptococcal endocarditis following elective abortion. Rev Infect Dis. 1991;13:997.

361. Baddour LM. Infective endocarditis caused by β-hemolytic streptococci. Clin Infect Dis. 1998;26:66-71.

362. Venezio FR, Gullberg RM, Westenfelder GO, et al. Group G streptococcal endocarditis and bacteremia. Am J Med. 1986;81:29-34.

363. Smyth EG, Pallett AP, Davidson RN. Group G streptococcal endocarditis: Two case reports, a review of the literature and recommendations for treatment. J Infect. 1988;16:169-176.

364. Ho AKC, Woo KS, Tse KK, et al. Infective endocarditis caused by Streptococcus suis serotype 2. J Infect. 1990;21:209.

365. Baddour LM. Infective endocarditis caused by beta-hemolytic streptococci: The Infectious Diseases Society of America's Emerging Infections Network. Clin Infect Dis. 1998;26:66-71.

366. Murray HW, Gross KC, Masur H, et al. Serious infections caused by Streptococcus milleri. Am J Med. 1978;64:759.

367. Shlaes DM, Lerner PI, Wolinsky E, et al. Infections due to Lancefield group F and related streptococci (S. milleri, S. anginosus). Medicine (Baltimore). 1981;60:197.

368. Gossling J. Occurrence and pathogenicity of the Streptococcus milleri group. Rev Infect Dis. 1988;10:257-285.

369. Hosea SW. Virulent Streptococcus viridans bacterial endocarditis. Am Heart J. 1981;101:174.

370. Buu-Joi A, Sapoetra A, Branger C, et al. Antimicrobial susceptibility of Gemella haemolysans isolated from patients with subacute endocarditis. Eur J Clin Microbiol. 1982;1:102.

371. Frésard A, Michel VP, Rueda X, et al. Gemella haemolysans endocarditis. Clin Infect Dis. 1993;16:586.

372. Mylotte JM, McDermott C, Spooner JA. Prospective study of 114 consecutive episodes of *Staphylococcus aureus* bacteremia. Rev Infect Dis. 1987;9:891-908.

373. Eykyn SJ. Staphylococcal sepsis: The changing pattern of disease and therapy. Lancet. 1988;1:100-104.

374. Watanakunakorn C, Tan JS, Phair JP. Some salient features of *Staphylococcus aureus* endocarditis. Am J Med. 1973;54:473.

375. Musher DM, McKenzie SO. Infection due to *Staphylococcus aureus*. Medicine (Baltimore). 1977;56:383.

376. Bayer AS. Staphylococcal bacteremia and endocarditis: State of the art. Arch Intern Med. 1982;142:1169.

377. Thompson RL. Staphylococcal infective endocarditis. Mayo Clin Proc. 1982;57:106.

378. Sanabria TJ, Alpert JS, Goldberg R, et al. Increasing frequency of staphylococcal infective endocarditis: Experience at a university hospital, 1981 through 1988. Arch Intern Med. 1990;150:1305.

379. Ing MB, Baddour LM, Bayer AS. Bacteremia and infective endocarditis: Pathogenesis, diagnosis and complications. In: Crossley KB, Archer GL, eds. The Staphylococci in Human Disease. New York: Churchill Livingstone; 1997:331-354.

380. Fowler VG, Sanders LL, Kong L, et al. *Staphylococcus aureus* endocarditis: 59 prospectively identified cases with followup. Clin Infect Dis. 1999;28:106-114.

381. Fowler VG Jr, Miro JM, Spelman D, et al. *Staphylococcus aureus* endocarditis throughout the world: A product of medical progress. Report from the ICE investigators. Abstracts of the 7th International Symposium on Modern Concepts in Endocarditis and Cardiovascular Infections. Chamonix, France, June 26-28, 2003.

382. Julander I. Unfavourable prognostic factors in *Staphylococcus aureus* septicemia and endocarditis. Scand J Infect Dis. 1985;17:179-187.

383. O'Callaghan C, McDougall P. Infective endocarditis in neonates. Arch Dis Child. 1988;63:53-57.

384. Crane LR, Levine DP, Zervos MJ, et al. Bacteremia in narcotic addicts at the Detroit Medical Center: I. Microbiology, epidemiology, risk factors, and empiric therapy. Rev Infect Dis. 1986;8:364-373.

385. Noel GJ, O'Loughlin JE, Edelson PJ. Neonatal *Staphylococcus epidermidis* right-sided endocarditis: Description of five catheterized infants. Pediatrics. 1988;82:234-239.

386. Baddour LM, Phillips TN, Bisno AL. Coagulase-negative staphylococcal endocarditis: Occurrence in patients with mitral valve prolapse. Arch Intern Med. 1986;146:119-121.

387. Harris LF, O'Shields H. Coagulase-negative staphylococcal endocarditis: A view from the community hospital. South Med J. 1986;79:1379-1386.

388. Caputo GM, Archer GL, Calderwood SB, et al. Native valve endocarditis due to coagulase-negative staphylococci: Clinical and microbiologic features. Am J Med. 1987;83:619-625.

389. Arber N, Militano A, Ben-Yehuda A, et al. Native valve *Staphylococcus epidermidis* endocarditis: Report of seven cases and review of the literature. Am J Med. 1991;90:758.

390. Espersen F, Wheat LJ, Bemis AT, et al. Solid-phase radio-immunoassay for IgG antibodies to *Staphylococcus epidermidis:* Use in serious coagulase-negative staphylococcal infections. Arch Intern Med. 1987;147:689-693.

391. Lang S, Livesley MA, Lambert PA, et al. Identification of a novel antigen from *Staphylococcus epidermidis.* FEMS Immun Med Microbiol. 2000;29:213-220.

392. Etienne J, Brun Y, El Solh N, et al. Characterization of clinically significant isolates of *Staphylococcus epidermidis* from patients with endocarditis. J Clin Microbiol. 1988;26:613-617.

393. Baddour LM, Simpson WA, Weems JJ Jr, et al. Phenotypic selection of small-colony variant forms of *Staphylococcus epidermidis* in a rat model of endocarditis. J Infect Dis. 1988;157:757-763.

394. Van Eldere J, Peetermans WE, Struelens M, et al. Polyclonal staphylococcal endocarditis caused by genetic variability. Clin Infect Dis. 2000;31:24-30.

395. Singh VR, Radd I. Fatal *Staphylococcus saprophyticus* native valve endocarditis in an intravenous drug addict. J Infect Dis. 1990;162:783.

396. Lina B, Celard M, Vandenesch F, et al. Infective endocarditis due to *Staphylococcus capitis.* Clin Infect Dis. 1992;15:173.

397. DeHondt G, Leven M, Vandermersch C, et al. Destructive endocarditis caused by *Staphylococcus lugdunensis*—case report and review of the literature. Acta Clin Belg. 1997;52:27-30.

398. Vandenesch F, Etienne J, Reverdy ME, et al. Endocarditis due to *Staphylococcus lugdunensis:* Report of 11 cases and review. Clin Infect Dis. 1993;17:871-876.

399. Celard M, Lelievre H, Obadia JF, et al. Long-standing bacteremia and endocarditis caused by *Staphylococcus lugdunensis* in a patient with an implantable cardioverter defibrillator. Clin Microbiol Infect. 1997;3:387-388.

400. Lessing MPA, Crook DWM, Bowler ICJ, et al. Native valve endocarditis caused by *Staphylococcus lugdunensis.* QJM. 1996;89:855-858.

401. Etienne J, Brun Y, Fleurette J. *Staphylococcus lugdunensis* endocarditis. J Clin Pathol. 1989;42:892-893.

402. Finland M, Barnes MW. Changing etiology of bacterial endocarditis in the antibacterial era: Experiences at Boston City Hospital 1933-1965. Ann Intern Med. 1970;72:341.

403. Pedersen FK, Petersen EA. Bacterial endocarditis of Blegdamshospitalet in Copenhagen 1944-1973. Scand J Infect Dis. 1976;8:99.

404. Cohen PS, Maguire JH, Weinstein L. Infective endocarditis caused by gram-negative bacteria: A review of the literature, 1945-1977. Prog Cardiovasc Dis. 1980;22:205.

405. Geraci JE, Wilson WR. Endocarditis due to gram-negative bacteria: Report of 56 cases. Mayo Clin Proc. 1982;57:145.

406. Snyder N, Atterbury CE, Correia JP, et al. Increased occurrence of cirrhosis and bacterial endocarditis. Gastroenterology. 1977;73:1107.

407. Carruthers M. Endocarditis due to enteric bacilli other than salmonellae: Case reports and literature review. Am J Med Sci. 1977;273:203.

408. Sande MA, Johnson WD, Hook EW, et al. Sustained bacteremia in patients with prosthetic cardiac valves. N Engl J Med. 1972;286:1067.

409. Schneider PJ, Nernoff J, Gold JA. Acute salmonella endocarditis: Report of a case and review. Arch Intern Med. 1967;120:478.

410. Mills J, Drew D. *Serratia marcescens* endocarditis. Ann Intern Med. 1976;85:397.

411. Cooper R, Mills J. Serratia endocarditis: A follow-up report. Arch Intern Med. 1980;140:199.

412. Caramelli B, Mansur AJ, Grinberg M, et al. *Campylobacter fetus* endocarditis on a prosthetic heart valve. South Med J. 1988;81:802-803.

413. Reyes MP, Brown WJ, Lerner AM. Treatment of patients with *Pseudomonas* endocarditis with high dose aminoglycoside and carbenicillin therapy. Medicine (Baltimore). 1978;57:57.

414. Reyes MP, Lerner AM. Current problems in the treatment of infective endocarditis due to *Pseudomonas aeruginosa.* Rev Infect Dis. 1983;5:314.

415. Wieland M, Lederman MM, Kline-King C, et al. Left-sided endocarditis due to *Pseudomonas aeruginosa:* A report of 10 cases and review of the literature. Medicine (Baltimore). 1986;65:180-189.

416. Komshian SV, Tablan OC, Palutke W, et al. Characteristics of left-sided endocarditis due to *Pseudomonas aeruginosa* in the Detroit Medical Center. Rev Infect Dis. 1990;12:693.

417. Noriega ER, Rubinstein E, Simberkoff M, et al. Subacute and acute endocarditis due to *Pseudomonas cepacia* in heroin addicts. Am J Med. 1975;59:29.

418. Reyes MP, Palutke WA, Wylin RF, et al. Pseudomonas endocarditis in the Detroit Medical Center 1969-1972. Medicine (Baltimore). 1973;52:173.

419. Jurica JV, Bomzer CA, England AC III. Gonococcal endocarditis: A case report and review of the literature. Sex Transm Dis. 1987;14:231-233.

420. Wall TC, Peyton RB, Corey GR. Gonococcal endocarditis: A new look at an old disease. Medicine. 1989;68:375.

421. Jackman JD Jr, Glamann DB. Gonococcal endocarditis: Twenty-five year experience. Am J Med Sci. 1991;301:221.

422. Wong JD, Janda JM. Association of an important *Neisseria* species, *Neisseria elongata* subsp. *nitroreducens,* with bacteremia, endocarditis, and osteomyelitis. J Clin Microbiol. 1992;30:719.

423. Ingram RJH, Cornere B, Ellis-Pegler RB. Endocarditis due to *Neisseria mucosa:* Two case reports and review. Clin Infect Dis. 1992;15:321.

424. Heiddal S, Sverrisson JT, Yngvason FE, et al. Native-valve endocarditis due to *Neisseria sicca:* Case report and review. Clin Infect Dis. 1993;16:667.

425. Chunn CJ, Jones SR, McCutchan JA, et al. *Haemophilus parainfluenzae* infective endocarditis. Medicine (Baltimore). 1977;56:99.

426. Lynn DJ, Kane JG, Parker RH. *Haemophilus parainfluenzae* and influenzae endocarditis: A review of forty cases. Medicine (Baltimore). 1977;56:115.

427. Geraci JE, Wilkowske CJ, Wilson WR, et al. Haemophilus endocarditis: Report of 14 cases. Mayo Clin Proc. 1977;52:209.

428. Parker SW, Apicella MA, Fuller CM. *Haemophilus* endocarditis: Two patients with complications. Arch Intern Med. 1983;143:48.

429. Bangsborg JM, Tuede M, Skinhoj P. *Haemophilus seguis* endocarditis. J Infect. 1988;16:81-85.

430. Porath A, Wanderman K, Simu A, et al. Case report: Endocarditis caused by *Haemophilus aegyptius.* Am J Med Sci. 1986;292:110-111.

431. Vandepitte J, DeGeest H, Jousten P. Subacute bacterial endocarditis due to *Actinobacillus actinomycetemcomitans:* Report of a case with a review of the literature. J Clin Pathol. 1977;30:842.

432. AhFat LNC, Patel BR, Pickens S. *Actinobacillus actinomycetemcomitans* endocarditis in hypertrophic obstructive cardiomyopathy. J Infect Dis. 1983;6:81.

433. Lane T, MacGregor RR, Wright D, et al. *Cardiobacterium hominis:* An elusive cause of endocarditis. J Infect. 1983;6:75.

434. Jenny DB, Letendre PW, Iverson G. Endocarditis due to *Kingella* species. Rev Infect Dis. 1988;10:1065-1066.

435. Decker MD, Graham BS, Hunter EB, et al. Endocarditis and infections of intravascular devices due to *Eikenella corrodens.* Am J Med Sci. 1986;292:209-212.

436. Patrick WD, Brown WD, Bowmer MI, et al. Infective endocarditis due to *Eikenella corrodens:* Case report and review of the literature. Can J Infect Dis. 1990;1:139.

437. Ellner JJ, Rosenthal MS, Lerner PI, et al. Infective endocarditis caused by slow-growing, fastidious, gram-negative bacteria. Medicine (Baltimore). 1979;58:145.

438. Gerry JL, Greenough WB. Diphtheroid endocarditis: Report of nine cases and review of the literature. Johns Hopkins Med J. 1976;139:61.

439. Morris A, Guild I. Endocarditis due to *Corynebacterium pseudodiphthericum:* Five case reports, review, and antibiotic susceptibilities of nine strains. Rev Infect Dis. 1991;13:887.

440. Tiley SM, Kociuba KR, Heron LG, et al. Infective endocarditis due to nontoxigenic *Corynebacterium diphtheriae:* Report of seven cases and review. Clin Infect Dis. 1993;16:271.

441. Bayer AS, Chow AW, Guze LB. *Listeria monocytogenes* endocarditis: Report of a case and review of the literature. Am J Med Sci. 1977;273:319.

442. Carvajal A, Frederiksen W. Fatal endocarditis due to *Listeria monocytogenes.* Rev Infect Dis. 1988;10:616-623.

443. Sussman JI, Baron EJ, Goldberg SM, et al. Clinical manifestations and therapy of *Lactobacillus* endocarditis: Report of a case and review of the literature. Rev Infect Dis. 1986;8:771-776.

444. Griffiths JK, Daly JS, Dodge RA. Two cases of endocarditis due to *Lactobacillus* species: Antimicrobial susceptibility, review, and discussion of therapy. Clin Infect Dis. 1992;15:250.

445. Gorby GL, Peacock JE Jr. *Erysipelothrix rhusiopathiae* endocarditis: Microbiologic, epidemiologic, and clinical features of an occupational disease. Rev Infect Dis. 1988;10:317-325.

446. Steen MK, Bruno-Murtha LA, Chaux G, et al. *Bacillus cereus* endocarditis: Report of a case and review. Clin Infect Dis. 1992;14:945.

447. Shands JW Jr. *Rothia dentocariosa* endocarditis. Am J Med. 1988;85:280-281.

448. Sudduth EJ, Rozich JD, Farrar WE. *Rothia dentocariosa* endocarditis complicated by perivalvular abscess. Clin Infect Dis. 1993;17:772.

449. Felner JM, Dowell UR. Anaerobic bacterial endocarditis. N Engl J Med. 1970;283:1188.

450. Nastro LJ, Finegold SM. Endocarditis due to anaerobic gram-negative bacilli. Am J Med. 1973;54:482.

451. Nastro FL, Sarma RJ. Infective endocarditis due to anaerobic and microaerophilic bacteria. West J Med. 1982;137:18.

452. Jackson RT, Dopp AC. *Bacteroides fragilis* endocarditis. South Med J. 1988;81:781-782.

453. Gradon JD, Chapnick EK, Lutwick LI. Infective endocarditis of a native valve due to *Acinetobacter*: Case report and review. Clin Infect Dis. 1992;14:1145.

454. Lam S, Samraj J, Rahman S, et al. Primary actinomycotic endocarditis: Case report and review. Clin Infect Dis. 1993;16:481.

455. Ascher DP, Zbick C, White C, et al. Infections due to *Stomatococcus mucilaginosus*: 10 cases and review. Rev Infect Dis. 1991;13:1048.

456. Rupp ME. *Streptobacillus moniliformis* endocarditis: Case report and review. Clin Infect Dis. 1992;14:769.

457. Al-Kasab S, Fagih MR, Al-Yousef S, et al. *Brucella* infective endocarditis: Successful combined medical and surgical therapy. J Thorac Cardiovasc Surg. 1988;95:862-867.

458. Jacobs F, Abramowicz D, Vereerstrater P, et al. *Brucella* endocarditis: The role of combined medical and surgical treatment. Rev Infect Dis. 1990;12:740-743.

459. Szabo S, Lieberman JP, Lue YA. Unusual pathogens in narcotic-associated endocarditis. Rev Infect Dis. 1990;12:412.

460. Komshian SV, Tablan OC, Palutke W, et al. Characteristics of left sided endocarditis due to *Pseudomonas aeruginosa* in the Detroit Medical Center. Rev Infect Dis. 1990;12:693.

461. Tuazon CW, Hill R, Sheagren JW. Microbiologic study of street heroin and injection paraphernalia. J Infect Dis. 1974;129:327.

462. Tuazon CW, Sheagren JW. Increased rate of carriage of *Staphylococcus aureus* among narcotic addicts. J Infect Dis. 1974;129:725.

463. Reisberg BE. Infective endocarditis in the narcotic addict. Prog Cardiovasc Dis. 1979;22:193.

464. Baddour LM. Twelve-year review of recurrent native-valve infective endocarditis: A disease of the modern antibiotic era. Rev Infect Dis. 1988;10:1163-1170.

465. Martin GS, Mannino DM, Eaton S, et al. The epidemiology of sepsis in the United States from 1979 through 2000. N Engl J Med. 2003;348:1546-1554.

466. Rubenstein E, Noriega ER, Simberkoff MS, et al. Tissue penetration of amphotericin B in *Candida* endocarditis. Chest. 1974;66:376.

467. Moyer D, Edwards JE. Fungal endocarditis. In: Kaye D, ed. Infective Endocarditis. New York: Raven Press; 1992:299-312.

468. Mora-Duarte J, Betts R, Rotstein C, et al, and Caspofungin Invasive Candidiasis Study Group. Comparison of caspofungin and amphotericin B for invasive candidiasis. N Engl J Med. 2002;347:2020-2029.

469. Herbrecht R, Denning DW, Patterson TF, et al, and Invasive Fungal Infections Group of the European Organisation for Research and Treatment of Cancer and the Global Aspergillus Study Group. Voriconazole versus amphotericin B for primary therapy of invasive aspergillosis. N Engl J Med. 2002;347:408-415.

470. Carrizosa J, Levison ME, Lawrence T, et al. Cure of *Aspergillus ustus* endocarditis of prosthetic valve. Arch Intern Med. 1974;133:486.

471. Chemaly RF, Tomford JW, Hall GS, et al. Rapid diagnosis of *Histoplasma capsulatum* endocarditis using the AccuProbe on an excised valve. J Clin Microbiol. 2001;39:2640-2641.

472. Keay S, Denning DW, Stevens DA. Endocarditis due to *Trichosporon beigelii*: In vitro susceptibility of isolates and review. Rev Infect Dis. 1991;13:383.

473. Welty FK, McLeod GX, Ezratty C, et al. *Pseudallescheria boydii* endocarditis of the pulmonic valve in a liver transplant recipient. Clin Infect Dis. 1992;15:858.

474. McIntosh CS, Nickers PJ, Isaqacs AJ. *Spirillum* endocarditis. Postgrad Med J. 1975;51:645.

475. Marrie T, Raoult D. Q fever. Clin Infect Dis. 1995;20:489-495.

476. Applefield MM, Billingsley LJ, Tucker HJ, et al. Q fever endocarditis—a case occurring in the United States. Am Heart J. 1977;93:669.

477. Raoult D, Tissot-Dupont H, Foucault C, et al. Q fever 1985-1998: Clinical and epidemiologic features of 1,383 infections. Medicine. 2000;79:109-123.

478. Maurin M, Raoult D. Q fever. Clin Microbiol Rev. 1999;12:518-553.

479. Tobin MJ, Cahill N, Gearty G, et al. Q fever endocarditis. Am J Med. 1982;72:396.

480. Peter O, Flepp M, Bestetti G, et al. Q fever endocarditis: Diagnostic approaches and monitoring of therapeutic effects. Clin Invest. 1992;70:932.

481. Fernandez-Guerrero ML, Muelas JM, Aquado JM. Q fever endocarditis on porcine bioprosthetic valves. Ann Intern Med. 1988;108:209-213.

482. Jones RB, Priest JB, Kuo C-C. Subacute chlamydial endocarditis. JAMA. 1982;247:655.

483. Brearley BF, Hutchinson DN. Endocarditis associated with *Chlamydia trachomatis* infection. Br Heart J. 1981;46:220.

484. Marrie TJ, Harczy M, Mann OE, et al. Culture-negative endocarditis probably due to *Chlamydia pneumoniae*. J Infect Dis. 1990;161:127.

485. Popat K, Barnardo D, Webb-Peploe M. *Mycoplasma pneumoniae* endocarditis. Br Heart J. 1980;44:111.

486. Raoult D, Birg ML, La Scola B, et al. Cultivation of the bacillus of Whipple's disease [erratum appears in N Engl J Med. 2000 May 18;342(20):1538]. N Engl J Med. 2000;342:620-625.

487. Burch GE, Tsui CY. Evolution of coxsackie viral valvular and mural endocarditis in mice. Br J Exp Pathol. 1971;52:360.

488. Persand V. Two unusual cases of mural endocarditis with a review of the literature. Am J Clin Pathol. 1970;53:832.

489. Van Scoy RE. Culture-negative endocarditis. Mayo Clin Proc. 1982;57:149.

490. Pesanti EL, Smith IM. Infective endocarditis with negative blood cultures: An analysis of 52 cases. Am J Med. 1979;66:43.

491. Hoen B, Selton-Suty C, Lacassin F, et al. Infective endocarditis in patients with negative blood cultures—analysis of 88 cases from a one-year nationwide survey in France. Clin Infect Dis. 1995;20:501-506.

492. Tunkel BR, Kaye D. Endocarditis with negative blood cultures. N Engl J Med. 1992;326:1215-1217.

493. Baddour LM, Meyer J, Henry B. Polymicrobial infective endocarditis in the 1980s. Rev Infect Dis. 1991;13:963.

494. Daschner FD, Frank V. Antimicrobial drugs in human cardiac valves and endocarditis lesions. J Antimicrob Chemother. 1988;12:776-782.

495. Cremieux A-C, Carbon C. Pharmacokinetic and pharmacodynamic requirements for antibiotic therapy of experimental endocarditis. Antimicrob Agents Chemother. 1992;36:2069.

496. Gilbert DN, Wood CA, Kimbrough RC, et al. Failure of treatment with teicoplanin at 6 milligrams/kg/day in patients with *Staphylococcus aureus* intravascular infections. Chemotherapy. 1991;115:674-680.

497. Dall L, Barnes WG, Lane JW, et al. Enzymatic modification of glycocalyx in the treatment of experimental endocarditis due to viridans streptococci. J Infect Dis. 1987;156:736-740.

498. Buiting AGM, Thompson J, Emeis JJ, et al. Effects of tissue-type plasminogen activator on *Staphylococcus epidermidis*–infected plasma clots as a model of infected endocardial vegetations. J Antimicrob Chemother. 1987;19:771-780.

499. Buiting AG, Thompson J, Emeis JJ, et al. Effects of tissue-type plasminogen activator (t-PA) on *Streptococcus sanguis*–infected endocardial vegetations in vitro. J Antimicrob Chemother. 1988;21:609-620.

500. Nicolau DP, Marangos MN, Nightingale CH, et al. Influence of aspirin on development and treatment of experimental *Staphylococcus aureus* endocarditis. Antimicrob Agents Chemother. 1995;39:1748-1751.

501. Kupferwasser LI, Yeaman MR, Shapiro SM, et al. Beneficial effects of aspirin in experimental *Staphylococcus aureus* endocarditis: Microbiologic, echocardiographic and histopathologic analyses. Presented at the Ninety-eighth General Meeting of the American Society for Microbiology, Atlanta, Ga, May 17-21, 1998.

502. Taha TH, Durrant SS, Mazeika PK, et al. Aspirin to prevent growth of vegetations and cerebral emboli in infective endocarditis. J Intern Med. 1992;231:543-546.

503. Cates JE, Christie RV. Subacute bacterial endocarditis. QJM. 1951;20:93.

504. Carrizosa J, Kobasa WD, Kaye D. Antagonism between chloramphenicol and penicillin in streptococcal endocarditis in rabbits. J Lab Clin Med. 1975;85:307.

505. Wilson WR, Gilbert DN, Bisno AL, et al. Evaluation of new anti-infective drugs for the treatment of infective endocarditis. Clin Infect Dis. 1992;15(Suppl 1):S89.

506. Andrews MM, von Reyn CF. Patient selection criteria and management guidelines for outpatient parenteral antibiotic therapy for native valve infective endocarditis. Clin Infect Dis. 2001;33:203-209.

507. Tornos P, Almirante B, Mirabet S, et al. Infective endocarditis due to *Staphylococcus aureus*: Deleterious effect of anticoagulant therapy. Arch Intern Med. 1999;159:473-475.

508. Douglas A, Moore-Gillon J, Eykyn S. Fever during treatment of infective endocarditis. Lancet. 1986;1:1341-1343.

509. Schlicter JG, MacIlean H. A method of determining the effective therapeutic level in the treatment of subacute bacterial endocarditis with penicillin. Am Heart J. 1947;34:209.

510. Coleman DL, Horwitz RI, Andriole VT. Association between serum inhibitory and bactericidal concentrations and therapeutic outcome in bacterial endocarditis. Am J Med. 1982;73:260.

511. Mellors JW, Coleman DL, Andriole VT. Value of serum bactericidal test in management of patients with bacterial endocarditis. Eur J Clin Microbiol. 1986;5:67-70.

512. Rahal JJ, Chan Y-K, Johnson G. Relationship of staphylococcal tolerance, teichoic acid antibody, and serum bactericidal activity to therapeutic outcome in *Staphylococcus aureus* bacteremia. Am J Med. 1986;81:43-52.

513. Wolfson JS, Swartz MN. Serum bactericidal activity as a monitor of antibiotic therapy. N Engl J Med. 1985;312:968-975.

514. Reller LB. The serum bactericidal test. Rev Infect Dis. 1986;8:803-808.

515. Weinstein MP, Stratton CW, Ackley A, et al. Multicenter collaborative evaluation of a standardized serum bactericidal test as a prognostic indicator in infective endocarditis. Am J Med. 1985;78:262-269.

516. Stratton CW. The role of the microbiology laboratory in the treatment of infective endocarditis. J Antimicrob Chemother. 1987;20(Suppl A):S41-S49.

517. Sande MA, Scheld WM. Combination antibiotic therapy of bacterial endocarditis. Ann Intern Med. 1980;92:390.

518. Wilson WR, Karchmer AW, Dajani AS, et al. Antibiotic treatment of adults with infective endocarditis due to streptococci, enterococci, staphylococci and HACEK microorganisms. JAMA. 1995;274:1706-1713.

519. Le T, Bayer AS. Combination antibiotic therapy for infective endocarditis. Clin Infect Dis. 2003;36:615-621.

520. Meylan PR, Francioloi P, Glauser MP. Discrepancies between MBC and actual killing by viridans group streptococci by cell-wall-active antibiotics. Antimicrob Agents Chemother. 1986;29:418-423.

521. Holloway Y, Pankert J, Hess J. Penicillin tolerance and bacterial endocarditis. Lancet. 1980;1:589.

522. Pulliam L, Inokuchi S, Hadley WK, et al. Penicillin tolerance in experimental streptococcal endocarditis. Lancet. 1979;2:957.

523. Gephart JF, Washington JA II. Antimicrobial susceptibilities of nutritionally variant streptococci. J Infect Dis. 1982;146:536.
524. Holloway Y, Dankert J. Penicillin tolerance in nutritionally variant streptococci. Antimicrob Agents Chemother. 1982;22:1073.
525. Lowry FD, Neuhas EG, Chang DS, et al. Penicillin therapy of experimental endocarditis caused by tolerant *Streptococcus sanguis* and nontolerant *Streptococcus mitis*. Antimicrob Agents Chemother. 1983;23:67.
526. Brennan RO, Durack DT. Therapeutic significance of penicillin tolerance in experimental streptococcal endocarditis. Antimicrob Agents Chemother. 1983;23:273.
527. Baker CW, Thornsberry C. Antimicrobial susceptibility of *Streptococcus mutans* isolated from patients with endocarditis. Antimicrob Agents Chemother. 1974;5:268.
528. Thornsberry C, Baker CN, Facklam RR. Antibiotic susceptibility of *Streptococcus bovis* and other group D streptococci causing endocarditis. Antimicrob Agents Chemother. 1974;5:228.
529. Wolfe JC, Johnson WD. Penicillin-sensitive steptococcal endocarditis: In vitro and clinical observations on penicillin-streptomycin therapy. Ann Intern Med. 1974;81:178.
530. Watanakunakorn C, Glotzbecker C. Synergism with aminoglycosides of penicillin, ampicillin, and vancomycin against nonenterococcal group D streptococci and viridans streptococci. J Med Microbiol. 1977;10:133.
531. Enzler MJ, Rouse MS, Henry NK, et al. In vitro and in vivo studies of streptomycin-resistant, penicillin-susceptible streptococci from patients with infective endocarditis. J Infect Dis. 1987;155:954-958.
532. Farber BF, Yee Y. High-level aminoglycoside resistance mediated by aminoglycoside-modifying enzymes among viridans streptococci: Implications for the therapy of endocarditis. J Infect Dis. 1987;155:948-953.
533. Sande MA, Irvin RG. Penicillin-aminoglycoside synergy in experimental *Streptococcus viridans* endocarditis. J Infect Dis. 1974;129:572.
534. Durack DT, Pelletier LL, Petersdorf RG. Chemotherapy of experimental streptococcal endocarditis: II. Synergism between penicillin and streptomycin against penicillin-sensitive streptococci. J Clin Invest. 1974;53:929.
535. Drake TA, Sande MA. Studies of the chemotherapy of endocarditis: Correlation of in vitro, animal model, and clinical studies. Rev Infect Dis. 1983;5(Suppl):S345.
536. Wilson WR, Geraci JE. Treatment of streptococcal infective endocarditis. Am J Med. 1985;78(Suppl 6B):S128-S137.
537. Scheld WM. Therapy of streptococcal endocarditis: Correlation of animal model and clinical studies. J Antimicrob Chemother. 1987;20(Suppl A):S71-S85.
538. Baquero F, Loza E. Penicillin resistance in Spain. Infect Dis Clin Pract. 1992;1:147.
539. Wilson WR, Geraci JE, Wilkowske CJ, et al. Short-term intramuscular therapy with procaine penicillin plus streptomycin for infective endocarditis due to viridans streptococci. Circulation. 1978;57:1158.
540. Wilson WR, Thompson RL, Wilkowske CJ, et al. Short-term therapy for streptococcal infective endocarditis: Combined intramuscular administration of penicillin and streptomycin. JAMA. 1981;245:360.
541. Karchmer AW, Mollering RC Jr, Maki DG, et al. Single antibiotic therapy for streptococcal endocarditis. JAMA. 1979;241:1801.
542. Malacoff RF, Frank E, Andriole VT. Streptococcal endocarditis (nonenterococcal, non-group A): Single vs. combination therapy. JAMA. 1979;241:1807.
543. Francioli P, Ruch W, Stamboulian D. Treatment of streptococcal endocarditis with a single daily dose of ceftriaxone and netilmicin for 14 days. Clin Infect Dis. 1995;21:1406-1410.
544. Sexton DJ, Tenenbaum MJ, Wilson WR, et al. Ceftriaxone once daily for 4 weeks compared to ceftriaxone plus gentamicin once daily for 2 weeks for treatment of penicillin-susceptible streptococcal endocarditis. Clin Infect Dis. 1998;27:1470-1474.
545. Parillo JE, Borst GC, Mazur MH, et al. Endocarditis due to resistant viridans streptococci during oral penicillin chemoprophylaxis. N Engl J Med. 1979;300:296.
546. Nicolau DP, Freeman CD, Belliveau PP, et al. Experience with once-daily aminoglycoside program administered to 2,184 adult patients. Antimicrob Agents Chemother. 1995;39:650-655.
547. Bouvet A, Cremieux AC, Contrepois A, et al. Comparison of penicillin and vancomycin, individually and in combination with gentamicin and amikacin, in the treatment of experimental endocarditis induced by nutritionally variant streptococci. Antimicrob Agents Chemother. 1985;28:607-611.
548. Henry NK, Wilson WR, Roberts RB, et al. Antimicrobial therapy of experimental endocarditis caused by nutritionally variant viridans group streptococci. Antimicrob Agents Chemother. 1986;30:465-467.
549. Stein DS, Nelson KE. Endocarditis due to nutritionally deficient streptococci: Therapeutic dilemma. Rev Infect Dis. 1987;9:908-916.
550. Cremieux A-C, Saleh-Mghir A, Vallois J-M, et al. Efficacy of temafloxacin in experimental *Streptococcus adjacens* endocarditis and autoradiographic diffusion pattern of [^{14}C] temafloxacin in cardiac vegetations. Antimicrob Agents Chemother. 1992;36:2216.
551. Stramboulian D, Bonvehi P, Arevalo C, et al. Antibiotic management of outpatients with endocarditis due to penicillin-susceptible streptococci. Rev Infect Dis. 1991;13(Suppl 2):S160.
552. Francioli P, Etienne J, Hoigué R, et al. Treatment of streptococcal endocarditis with a single daily dose of ceftriaxone sodium for 4 weeks: Efficacy and outpatient treatment feasibility. JAMA. 1992;267:264.
553. Francioli PB, Glauser MP. Synergistic activity of ceftriaxone combined with netilmicin administered once daily for treatment of experimental streptococcal endocarditis. Antimicrob Agents Chemother. 1993;37:207.
554. Yenditti M, Gelfusa V, Serra P, et al. 4-week treatment of streptococcal native valve endocarditis with high-dose teicoplanin. Antimicrob Agents Chemother. 1992;36:723.
555. Watanakunakorn C. Penicillin combined with gentamicin or streptomycin: Synergism against enterococci. J Infect Dis. 1971;124:581.
556. Moellering RC Jr, Korzeniowski OM, Sande MA, et al. Species-specific resistance to antimicrobial synergism in *Streptococcus faecium* and *Streptococcus faecalis*. J Infect Dis. 1979;140:203.
557. Krogstad DJ, Parquette AR. Defective killing of enterococci: A common property of antimicrobial agents acting on the cell wall. Antimicrob Agents Chemother. 1980;17:965.
558. Storch GA, Krogstad DA, Parquette AR. Antibiotic-induced lysis of enterococci. J Clin Invest. 1981;68:639.
559. Megran DW. Enterococcal endocarditis. Clin Infect Dis. 1992;15:63.
560. Murray BE, Church DA, Wanger A, et al. Comparison of two β-lactamase-producing strains of *Streptococcus faecalis*. Antimicrob Agents Chemother. 1986;30:861-864.
561. Ingerman M, Pitsakis PG, Rosenberg A, et al. β-Lactamase production in experimental endocarditis due to aminoglycoside-resistant *Streptococcus faecalis*. J Infect Dis. 1987;155:1226-1232.
562. Coudron PE, Markowitz SM, Wong ES. Isolation of a β-lactamase-producing, highly-gentamicin-resistant isolate of *Enterococcus faecalis*. Antimicrob Agents Chemother. 1992;36:1225.
563. Lavoie SR, Wong ES, Coudron PE, et al. Comparison of ampicillin-sulbactam with vancomycin for treatment of experimental endocarditis due to a β-lactamase-producing, highly-gentamicin-resistant isolate of *Enterococcus faecalis*. Antimicrob Agents Chemother. 1993;37:1447.
564. Thal LA, Vazquez J, Perri MB, et al. Activity of ampicillin plus sulbactam against β-lactamase-producing enterococci in experimental endocarditis. J Antimicrob Chemother. 1993;31:182.
565. Yao JDC, Thauvin-Eliopoulos C, Eliopoulos GM, et al. Efficacy of teicoplanin in two dosage regimens for experimental endocarditis caused by a β-lactamase-producing strain of *Enterococcus faecalis* with high level resistance to gentamicin. Antimicrob Agents Chemother. 1990;34:827.
566. Ramos MC, Grayson ML, Eliopoulos GM, et al. Comparison of daptomycin, vancomycin, and ampicillin-gentamicin for treatment of experimental endocarditis caused by penicillin-resistant enterococci. Antimicrob Agents Chemother. 1992;36:1864.
567. Fontana R, Grossato A, Ligozzi M, et al. In vitro response to bactericidal activity of cell wall-active antibiotics does not support the general opinion that enterococci are naturally tolerant to these antibiotics. Antimicrob Agents Chemother. 1990;34:1518.
568. Henry NK, Wilson WR, Geraci JE. Treatment of streptomycin-susceptible enterococcal experimental endocarditis with combinations of penicillin and low- or high-dose streptomycin. Antimicrob Agents Chemother. 1986;30:725-728.
569. Harwick HJ, Kalmanson GM, Guze LB. In vitro activity of ampicillin or vancomycin combined with gentamicin or streptomycin against enterococci. Antimicrob Agents Chemother. 1973;4:383.
570. Weinstein AJ, Moellering RC. Penicillin and gentamicin therapy for enterococcal infections. JAMA. 1973;223:1030.
571. Moellering RC, Wennersten C, Weinberg AW. Synergy of penicillin and gentamicin against enterococci. J Infect Dis. 1971;124(Suppl):S207.
572. Hook EW III, Roberts RB, Sande MA. Antimicrobial therapy of experimental enterococcal endocarditis. Antimicrob Agents Chemother. 1975;8:564.
573. Wright AJ, Wilson WR, Matsumoto JY, et al. Influence of gentamicin dose size on the efficacies of combinations of gentamicin and penicillin in experimental streptomycin-resistant enterococcal endocarditis. Antimicrob Agents Chemother. 1982;22:972.
574. Murray BE, Tsao J, Panida J. Enterococci from Bangkok, Thailand, with high-level resistance to currently available aminoglycosides. Antimicrob Agents Chemother. 1983;23:799.
575. Mederski-Samoraj BD, Murray BE. High-level resistance to gentamicin in clinical isolates of enterococci. J Infect Dis. 1983;147:751.
576. Zervos MJ, Dembinski S, Mikesell T, et al. High-level resistance to gentamicin in *Streptococcus faecalis*: Risk factors and evidence for exogenous acquisition of infection. J Infect Dis. 1986;153:1075-1083.
577. Patterson JE, Zervos MJ. High-level gentamicin resistance in *Enterococcus*: Microbiology, genetic basis, and epidemiology. Rev Infect Dis. 1990;12:644.
578. Zervos MJ, Terpenning MS, Schaberg DR, et al. High-level aminoglycoside-resistant enterococci. Arch Intern Med. 1987;147:1591-1594.
579. Eliopoulos GM, Wennersten C, Zighelboim-Daum S, et al. High-level resistance to gentamicin in clinical isolates of *Streptococcus (Enterococcus) faecium*. Antimicrob Agents Chemother. 1988;32:1528-1532.
580. Eliopoulos GM, Thauvin-Eliopoulos C, Moellering RC Jr. Contribution of animal models in the search for effective therapy for endocarditis due to enterococci with high-level resistance to gentamicin. Clin Infect Dis. 1992;15:58.
581. Fernandez-Guerrero ML, Barros C, Rodriguez Tudela JL, et al. Aortic endocarditis caused by gentamicin-resistant *Enterococcus faecalis*. Eur J Clin Microbiol. 1988;7:525-527.
582. Hellinger WC, Rouse MS, Robadan PM, et al. Continuous intravenous versus intermittent antimicrobial therapy of experimental endocarditis caused by aminoglycoside-resistant enterococci. Antimicrob Agents Chemother. 1992;36:1272.
583. Fantin B, Carbon C. Importance of the aminoglycoside dosing regimen in the penicillin-netilmicin combination for treatment of *Enterococcus faecalis*-induced experimental endocarditis. Antimicrob Agents Chemother. 1990;34:2387.
584. Grayson ML, Thauvin-Eliopoulos C, Eliopoulos GM, et al. Failure of trimethoprim-sulfamethoxazole therapy in experimental enterococcal endocarditis. Antimicrob Agents Chemother. 1990;34:1792.
585. Mainardi JL, Gutmann L, Acar JF, et al. Synergistic effect of amoxicillin and cefotaxime against *Enterococcus faecalis* [erratum appears in Antimicrob Agents Chemother. 1995 Dec;39(12):2835]. Antimicrob Agents Chemother. 1995;39:1984-1987.

586. Watanakunakorn C, Bakie C. Synergism of vancomycin-gentamicin and vancomycin-streptomycin against enterococci. Antimicrob Agents Chemother. 1973;4:120.

587. Watanakunakorn C, Tisone JC. Effects of a vancomycin-rifampin combination on enterococci. Antimicrob Agents Chemother. 1982;22:915.

588. Uttley AH, Collins CH, Naidoo J, et al. Vancomycin-resistant enterococci. Lancet. 1988;1:57-58.

589. Frieden TR, Munsiff SS, Low DE, et al. Emergence of vancomycin-resistant enterococci in New York City. Lancet. 1993;342:76.

590. Courvalin P. Resistance of enterococci to glycopeptides. Antimicrob Agents Chemother. 1990;34:2291.

591. Murray BE. Vancomycin-resistant enterococcal infections. N Engl J Med. 2000;342:710-721.

592. Murray BE. The life and times of the *Enterococcus*. Clin Microbiol Rev. 1990;3:46.

593. Babcock HM, Ritchie DJ, Christiansen E, et al. Successful treatment of vancomycin-resistant *Enterococcus* endocarditis with oral linezolid. Clin Infect Dis. 2001;32:1373-1375.

594. Safdar A, Bryan CS, Stinson S, et al. Prosthetic valve endocarditis due to vancomycin-resistant *Enterococcus faecium:* Treatment with chloramphenicol plus minocycline. Clin Infect Dis. 2002;34:E61-E63.

595. Venditti M, Biavasco F, Varaldo PE, et al. Catheter-related endocarditis due to glycopeptide-resistant *Enterococcus faecalis* in a transplanted heart. Clin Infect Dis. 1993;17:524.

596. Leclercq R, Derlot E, Dural J, et al. Plasmid-mediated resistance to vancomycin and teicoplanin in *Enterococcus faecium*. N Engl J Med. 1988;319:157-161.

597. Fantin B, Leclercq R, Arthur M, et al. Influence of low-level resistance to vancomycin on efficacy of teicoplanin and vancomycin for treatment of experimental endocarditis due to *Enterococcus faecium*. Antimicrob Agents Chemother. 1991;35:1570.

598. Caron F, Kitzis M-D, Gutmann L, et al. Daptomycin or teicoplanin in combination with gentamicin for treatment of experimental endocarditis due to a highly glycopeptide-resistant isolate of *Enterococcus faecium*. Antimicrob Agents Chemother. 1992;36:261.

599. Konstantinov IE, Zehr KJ. Aortic root replacement in a patient with vancomycin-resistant *Enterococcus faecium* endocarditis and leukemia. Chest. 2001;120:1744-1746.

600. Collins LA, Eliopoulos GM, Wennersten CB, et al. In vitro activity of ramoplanin against vancomycin-resistant gram-positive organisms. Antimicrob Agents Chemother. 1993;37:1364.

601. Caron F, Carbon C, Gutmann L. Triple-combination penicillin-vancomycin-gentamicin for experimental endocarditis caused by a moderately penicillin- and highly glycopeptide-resistant isolate of *Enterococcus faecium*. J Infect Dis. 1991;164:888.

602. Caron F, Lemeland J-F, Humbert G, et al. Triple combination penicillin-vancomycin-gentamicin for experimental endocarditis caused by a highly penicillin- and glycopeptide-resistant isolate of *Enterococcus faecium*. J Infect Dis. 1993;168:681.

603. Fernandez-Guerrero M, Rouse MS, Henry NK, et al. In vitro and in vivo activity of ciprofloxacin against enterococci isolated from patients with infective endocarditis. Antimicrob Agents Chemother. 1987;31:430-433.

604. Bayer AS, Li C, Kim E, et al. Efficacy of trovafloxacin (CP99219) in the therapy of experimental endocarditis due to drug-resistant enterococci. Abstract B257. Presented at the Thirty-sixth Interscience Conference on Antimicrobial Agents and Chemotherapy, New Orleans, September 1996.

605. Rubinstein E, Bompart F. Activity of quinupristin/dalfopristin against gram-positive bacteria: Clinical applications and therapeutic potential. J Antimicrob Ther. 1997;39(Suppl):S139-S143.

606. Moellering RC Jr. Early clinical results of RP59500 in bacteremia. Presented at the Third International Conference on the Macrolides, Azalides and Streptogramins, Lisbon, Portugal, 1996.

607. Fantin B, Carbon C. Importance of aminoglycoside dosing regimen in the penicillin-netilmicin combination for treatment of *Enterococcus faecalis*-induced experimental endocarditis. Antimicrob Agents Chemother. 1990;34:2387-2391.

608. Marangos MN, Nicolau DP, Nightingale CH, et al. Influence of gentamicin dosing interval on the efficacy of penicillin-containing regimens in experimental *Enterococcus faecalis* endocarditis. Presented at the Thirty-sixth Interscience Conference on Antimicrobial Agents and Chemotherapy, New Orleans, September 15-18, 1996.

609. Olaison L, Schadewitz K, and Swedish Society of Infectious Diseases Quality Assurance Study Group for Endocarditis. Enterococcal endocarditis in Sweden, 1995-1999: Can shorter therapy with aminoglycosides be used? Clin Infect Dis. 2002;34:159-166.

610. Mandell GL, Kaye D, Levison ME, et al. Enterococcal endocarditis: An analysis of 38 patients observed at the New York Hospital-Cornell Medical Center. Arch Intern Med. 1970;125:258-264.

611. Moellering RC Jr, Watson BK, Kunz LJ. Endocarditis due to group D streptococci: Comparison of disease caused by *Streptococcus bovis* with that produced by the enterococci. Am J Med 1974;57:239-250.

612. Gavalda J, Miro J, Torres C, et al. Efficacy of ampicillin plus ceftriaxone or cefotaxime in treatment of endocarditis due to *Enterococcus faecalis*. Abstract L1342. Abstracts of the Forty-first Interscience Conference on Antimicrobial Agents and Chemotherapy, Chicago, 2001.

613. Wilson WR, Wilkowski CJ, Wright AJ, et al. Treatment of streptomycin-susceptible and streptomycin-resistant enterococcal endocarditis. Ann Intern Med. 1984;100:816-823.

614. Karchmer AW. Staphylococcal endocarditis: Laboratory and clinical basis for antibiotic therapy. Am J Med. 1985;78(Suppl B):S116-S127.

615. Sande MA, Courtney KB. Nafcillin-gentamicin synergism in experimental staphylococcal endocarditis. J Lab Clin Med. 1976;88:118.

616. Abrams B, Sklaver A, Hoffman T, et al. Single or combination therapy of staphylococcal endocarditis in intravenous drug abusers. Ann Intern Med. 1979;90:789.

617. Chambers HF, Miller RT, Newman MD. Right-sided *Staphylococcus aureus* endocarditis in intravenous drug abusers: Two week combination therapy. Ann Intern Med. 1988;109:619-624.

618. DiNubile MJ. Abbreviated therapy for right sided *Staphylococcus aureus* endocarditis in injecting drug users: The time has come? Eur J Clin Microbiol Infect Dis. 1994;13:533-534.

619. DiNubile MJ. Short-course antibiotic therapy for right sided *Staphylococcus aureus* endocarditis in injection drug users. Ann Intern Med. 1994;121:873-876.

620. Torres-Tortosa M, de Cueto M, Vergara A, et al. Prospective evaluation of a two-week course of intravenous antibiotics in intravenous drug addicts with infective endocarditis. Eur J Clin Microbiol Infect Dis. 1994;13:559-564.

621. Espinosa FJ, Valdes M, Martin-Luengo M, et al. Right sided endocarditis caused by *Staphylococcus aureus* in parenteral drug addicts: Evaluation of a combined therapeutic scheme for 2 weeks versus conventional treatment. Enferm Infecc Microbiol Clin. 1993;11:235-240.

622. Ribera E, Gomez-Jimenez J, Cortes E, et al. Effectiveness of cloxacillin with and without gentamicin in short-term therapy for right-sided *Staphylococcus aureus* endocarditis: A randomized, controlled trial. Ann Intern Med. 1996;125:969-974.

623. Fortun J, Navas E, Martinez-Beltran J, et al. Short-course therapy for right-side endocarditis due to *Staphylococcus aureus* in drug abusers: cloxacillin versus glycopeptides in combination with gentamicin. Clin Infect Dis. 2001;33:120-125.

624. Dworkin RJ, Lee BL, Sande MA, Chambers HF. Treatment of right-sided *Staphylococcus aureus* endocarditis in intravenous drug users with ciprofloxacin and rifampicin. Lancet. 1989;2:1071-1073.

625. Heldman AW, Hartert TV, Ray SC, et al. Oral antibiotic treatment of right-sided staphylococcal endocarditis in injection drug users: Prospective randomized comparison with parenteral therapy. Am J Med. 1996;101:68-76.

626. Murray HW, Wigley FM, Mann JJ, et al. Combination antibiotic therapy in staphylococcal endocarditis: The use of methicillin sodium-gentamicin sulfate therapy. Arch Intern Med. 1976;136:480.

627. Korzeniowski OM, Sande MA, and The National Collaborative Endocarditis Study Group. Combination antimicrobial therapy for *Staphylococcus aureus* endocarditis in patients addicted to parenteral drugs and in nonaddicts: A prospective study. Ann Intern Med. 1982;97:496.

628. Dodek P, Phillips P. Questionable history of immediate-type hypersensitivity to penicillin in staphylococcal endocarditis: Treatment based on skin-test results versus empirical alternative treatment—a decision analysis. Clin Infect Dis. 1999;29:1251-1256.

629. Steckelberg JM, Rouse MS, Tallan BM, et al. Relative efficacies of broad-spectrum cephalosporins for treatment of methicillin-susceptible *Staphylococcus aureus* experimental infective endocarditis. Antimicrob Agents Chemother. 1993;37:554.

630. Fowler VGJ, Kong LK, Corey GR, et al. Recurrent *Staphylococcus aureus* bacteremia: Pulsed-field gel electrophoresis findings in 29 patients. J Infect Dis. 1999;179:1157-1161.

631. Small PM, Chambers HF. Vancomycin for *Staphylococcus aureus* endocarditis in intravenous drug users. Antimicrob Agents Chemother. 1990;34:1227.

632. Levine DP, Fromm BS, Reddy BR. Slow response to vancomycin or vancomycin plus rifampin in methicillin-resistant *Staphylococcus aureus* endocarditis. Ann Intern Med. 1991;115:674.

633. Rybak MJ, Bailey EM, Lamp KC, et al. Pharmacokinetics and bactericidal rates of daptomycin and vancomycin in intravenous drug abusers being treated for gram-positive endocarditis and bacteremia. Antimicrob Agents Chemother. 1992;36:1109.

634. Kaatz GW, Seo SM, Reddy VN, et al. Daptomycin compared with teicoplanin and vancomycin for therapy of experimental *Staphylococcus aureus* endocarditis. Antimicrob Agents Chemother. 1990;34:2081.

635. Kaatz GW, Seo SM, Dorman NJ, et al. Emergence of teicoplanin resistance during therapy of *Staphylococcus aureus* endocarditis. J Infect Dis. 1990;162:103.

636. Mortara LA, Bayer AS. *Staphylococcus aureus* bacteremia and endocarditis: New diagnostic and therapeutic concepts. Infect Dis Clin North Am. 1993;7:53.

637. Bayer AS. Infective endocarditis. Clin Infect Dis. 1993;17:313.

638. Watanakunakorn C. Clindamycin therapy of *Staphylococcus aureus* endocarditis: Clinical relapse and development of resistance to clindamycin, lincomycin, and erythromycin. Am J Med. 1976;60:419.

639. Kaye D. The clinical significance of tolerance of *Staphylococcus aureus*. Ann Intern Med. 1980;93:924.

640. Jackson MA, Hicks RA. Vancomycin failure in staphylococcal endocarditis. Pediatr Infect Dis J. 1987;6:750-752.

641. Rajashekaraiah KR, Rice T, Rao VS, et al. Clinical significance of tolerant strains of *Staphylococcus aureus* in patients with endocarditis. Ann Intern Med. 1980;93:796.

642. Voorn GP, Thompson J, Goessens WHF, et al. Role of tolerance in cloxacillin treatment of experimental *Staphylococcus aureus* endocarditis. J Infect Dis. 1991;163:640.

643. Zak O, Scheld WM, Sande MA. Rifampin in experimental endocarditis due to *Staphylococcus aureus* in rabbits. Rev Infect Dis. 1983;5(Suppl):481.

644. Tebas P, Martinez Ruiz R, Roman F, et al. Early resistance to rifampin and ciprofloxacin in the treatment of right-sided *Staphylococcus aureus* endocarditis. J Infect Dis. 1991;163:204.

645. McDougal LK, Thornsberry C: The role of β-lactamase in staphylococcal resistance to penicillinase-resistant penicillins and cephalosporins. J Clin Microbiol. 1986;23:832-839.

646. Hirano L, Bayer AS. β-Lactam-β-lactamase inhibitor combinations are active in experimental endocarditis caused by β-lactamase-producing oxacillin-resistant staphylococci. Antimicrob Agents Chemother. 1991;35:685.

647. Pefanis A, Thauvin-Eliopoulos C, Eliopoulos GM, et al. Activity of ampicillin-sulbactam and oxacillin in experimental endocarditis caused by β-lactamase-hyperproducing *Staphylococcus aureus*. Antimicrob Agents Chemother. 1993;37:507.

648. Fernandez-Guerrero M, Rouse M, Henry N, et al. Ciprofloxacin therapy of experimental endocarditis caused by methicillin-susceptible or methicillin-resistant *Staphylococcus aureus*. Antimicrob Agents Chemother. 1988;32:747-751.

649. Kaatz GW, Seo SM, Lamp KC, et al. CI-960, a new fluoroquinolone, for therapy of experimental ciprofloxacin-susceptible and -resistant *Staphylococcus aureus* endocarditis. Antimicrob Agents Chemother. 1992;36:1192.

650. Bayer AS, Li C, Ing M. Efficacy of trovafloxacin, a new quinolone antibiotic, in experimental staphylococcal endocarditis due to oxacillin-resistant strains. Antimicrob Agents Cheomother. 1998;42:1837-1841.

651. Kaatz GW, Seo SM, Barriere SL, et al. Development of resistance to fleroxacin during therapy of experimental methicillin-susceptible *Staphylococcus aureus* endocarditis. Antimicrob Agents Chemother. 1991;35:1547.

652. Munoz P, Berenguer J, Rodriguez-Creixems M, et al. Ciprofloxacin and infective endocarditis. Infect Dis Clin Pract. 1993;2:119.

653. Markowitz N, Quinn EL, Saravolatz LD. Trimethoprim-sulfamethoxazole compared with vancomycin for treatment of *Staphylococcus aureus* infection. Ann Intern Med. 1992;117:390-398.

654. Iannini PB, Crossley K. Therapy of *Staphylococcus aureus* bacteremia associated with a removable focus of infection. Ann Intern Med. 1976;84:558.

655. Watanakunakorn C, Baird IM. *Staphylococcus aureus* bacteremia and endocarditis associated with a removable infected intravenous device. Am J Med. 1977;63:253.

656. Bayer AS, Lam K, Ginzton L. *Staphylococcus aureus* bacteremia: Clinical, serologic, and echocardiographic findings in patients with and without endocarditis. Arch Intern Med. 1987;147:757-762.

657. Fowler VGJ, Sanders LL, Kong LK, et al. Infective endocarditis due to *Staphylococcus aureus:* 59 prospectively identified cases with follow-up. Clin Infect Dis. 1999;28:106-114.

658. Watanakunakorn C. *Staphylococcus aureus* endocarditis at a community teaching hospital, 1980 to 1991: An analysis of 106 cases. Arch Intern Med. 1994;154:2330-2335.

659. Andrade-Baiocchi S, Tognim MC, Baiocchi OC, et al. Endocarditis due to glycopeptide-intermediate *Staphylococcus aureus:* Case report and strain characterization. Diagn Microbiol Infect Dis. 2003;45:149-152.

660. Fridkin SK, Hageman J, McDougal LK, et al, and Vancomycin-Intermediate *Staphylococcus aureus* Epidemiology Study Group. Epidemiological and microbiological characterization of infections caused by *Staphylococcus aureus* with reduced susceptibility to vancomycin, United States, 1997-2001. Clin Infect Dis. 2003;36:429-439.

661. Vancomycin-resistant *Staphylococcus aureus*—Pennsylvania, 2002. MMWR Morbid Mortal Wkly Rep. 2002;51:902.

662. Chang S, Sievert DM, Hageman JC, et al, and Vancomycin-Resistant *Staphylococcus aureus* Investigative Team. Infection with vancomycin-resistant *Staphylococcus aureus* containing the vanA resistance gene. N Engl J Med. 2003;348:1342-1347.

663. Karchmer AW, Archer GL, Dismukes WE. *Staphylococcus epidermidis* causing prosthetic valve endocarditis: Microbiologic and clinical observations as guides to therapy. Ann Intern Med. 1983;98:447.

664. Schwalbe RS, Stapleton JT, Gilligan PH. Emergence of vancomycin resistance in coagulase-negative staphylococci. N Engl J Med. 1987;316:927-931.

665. Joly V, Parigon B, Vallois J-M, et al. Value of antibiotic levels in serum and cardiac vegetations for predicting antibacterial effect of ceftriaxone in experimental *Escherichia coli* endocarditis. Antimicrob Agents Chemother. 1987;31:1632-1639.

666. Caron F, Gutmann L, Bure A, et al. Ceftriaxone-sulbactam combination in rabbit endocarditis caused by a strain of *Klebsiella pneumoniae* producing extended-broad-spectrum TEM-3 β-lactamase. Antimicrob Agents Chemother. 1990;34:2070.

667. Mentec H, Vallois J-M, Bure A, et al. Piperacillin, tazobactam, and gentamicin alone or combined in an endocarditis model of infection by a TEM-3-producing strain of *Klebsiella pneumoniae* or its susceptible variant. Antimicrob Agents Chemother. 1992;36:1883.

668. Potel G, Caillon J, Fantin B, et al. Impact of dosage schedule on the efficacy of gentamicin, tobramycin, or amikacin in an experimental model of *Serratia marcescens* endocarditis: In vitro-in vivo correlation. Antimicrob Agents Chemother. 1991;35:111.

669. Potel G, Caillon J, LeGallou F, et al. Identification of factors affecting in vivo aminoglycoside activity in an experimental model of gram-negative endocarditis. Antimicrob Agents Chemother. 1992;36:774.

670. Rodriguez C, Olcoz MT, Izquierdo G, et al. Endocarditis due to ampicillin-resistant nontyphoid *Salmonella:* Cure with a third-generation cephalosporin. Rev Infect Dis. 1990;12:817.

671. Hughes CF, Noble N. Vegetectomy: An alternative surgical treatment for infective endocarditis of the atrioventricular valves in drug addicts. J Thorac Cardiovasc Surg. 1988;95:857-861.

672. Arbulu A, Thomas NW, Chiscano A, et al. Total tricuspid valvulectomy without replacement in the treatment of *Pseudomonas* endocarditis. Surg Forum. 1971;22:162.

673. Mammana RB, Levitsky S, Sernaque D, et al. Valve replacement for left-sided endocarditis in drug addicts. Ann Thorac Surg. 1983;35:436.

674. Bayer AS, Crowell DJ, Yih J, et al. Comparative pharmacokinetics and pharmacodynamics of amikacin and ceftazidime in tricuspid and aortic vegetations in experimental *Pseudomonas* endocarditis. J Infect Dis. 1988;158:355-359.

675. Bayer AS, Hirano L, Yih J. Development of β-lactam resistance and increased quinolone MIC's during therapy of experimental *Pseudomonas aeruginosa* endocarditis. Antimicrob Agents Chemother. 1988;32:231-235.

676. Parr TR Jr, Bayer AS. Mechanisms of aminoglycoside resistance in variants of *Pseudomonas aeruginosa* isolated during treatment of experimental endocarditis in rabbits. J Infect Dis. 1988;158:1003-1010.

677. Hessen MT, Pitsakis PG, Levison ME. Absence of a post-antibiotic effect in experimental *Pseudomonas* endocarditis treated with imipenem, with or without gentamicin. J Infect Dis. 1988;158:542-548.

678. Bayer AS, Park S, Ramos MC, et al. Effects of alginase on the natural history and antibiotic therapy of experimental endocarditis caused by mucoid *Pseudomonas aeruginosa*. Infect Immun. 1992;60:3979-3985.

679. Jimenez-Lucho VE, Saravolatz LD, Medeiros AA, et al. Failure of therapy in *Pseudomonas* endocarditis: Selection of resistant mutants. J Infect Dis. 1986;154:64-68.

680. Daikos GL, Kathopalia SB, Lolans VT, et al. Long-term oral ciprofloxacin: Experience in the treatment of incurable infective endocarditis. Am J Med. 1988;84:786-790.

681. Pefanis A, Giamarellou H, Karayiannakos P, et al. Efficacy of ceftazidime and aztreonam alone or in combination with amikacin in experimental left-sided *Pseudomonas aeruginosa* endocarditis. Antimicrob Agents Chemother. 1993;37:308.

682. Fichtenbaum CH, Smith MJ. Treatment of endocarditis due to *Pseudomonas aeruginosa* with imipenem. Clin Infect Dis. 1992;14:353.

683. Pavicic MJAMP, van Winkelhoff AJ, de Graaff J. In vitro susceptibilities of *Actinobacillus actinomycetemcomitans* to a number of antimicrobial combinations. Antimicrob Agents Chemother. 1992;36:2634.

684. Francioli PB. Ceftriaxone and outpatient treatment of infective endocarditis. Infect Dis Clin North Am. 1993;17:313-322.

685. Martinez E, Miro JM, Almirante B, et al, and Spanish Pneumococcal Endocarditis Study Group. Effect of penicillin resistance of *Streptococcus pneumoniae* on the presentation, prognosis, and treatment of pneumococcal endocarditis in adults. Clin Infect Dis. 2002;35:130-139.

686. Weisner PJ, Handsfield HH, Holmes KK. Low antibiotic resistance of gonococci causing disseminated infection. N Engl J Med. 1973;288:1221.

687. Black JR, Brint JM, Reichart CA. Successful treatment of gonococcal endocarditis with ceftriaxone. J Infect Dis. 1988;157:1281-1282.

688. Ellis ME, Al Abdely H, Sandridge A, et al. Fungal endocarditis: Evidence in the world literature, 1965-1995. Clin Infect Dis. 2001;32:50-62.

689. Melgar GR, Nasser RM, Gordon RM, et al. Fungal prosthetic valve endocarditis: An 11-year experience in a tertiary hospital. Medicine (Baltimore). 1997;76:94-103.

690. Ernst JD, Rusmak M, Sande MA. Combination antifungal chemotherapy for experimental disseminated candidiasis: Lack of correlation between in vitro and in vivo observations with amphotericin B and rifampin. Rev Infect Dis. 1983;5(Suppl):626.

691. Longman LP, Martin MV. A comparison of the efficacy of itraconazole, amphotericin B and 5-fluorocytosine in the treatment of *Aspergillus fumigatus* endocarditis in the rabbit. J Antimicrob Chemother. 1987;20:719-724.

692. Gumbo T, Taege AJ, Mawhorter S, et al. *Aspergillus* valve endocarditis in patients without prior cardiac surgery. Medicine. 2000;79:261-268.

693. Witt MD, Bayer AS. Comparison of fluconazole and amphotericin B for prevention and treatment of experimental *Candida* endocarditis. Antimicrob Agents Chemother. 1991;35:2481.

694. Venditti M, De Bernardis F, Micozzi A, et al. Fluconazole treatment of catheter-related right-sided endocarditis caused by *Candida albicans* and associated with endophthalmitis and folliculitis. Clin Infect Dis. 1992;14:422.

695. Czwerwiec FS, Bilsker MS, Kamerman ML, et al. Long-term survival after fluconazole therapy of candidal prosthetic valve endocarditis. Am J Med. 1993;94:545.

696. Nguyen MH, Nguyen ML, Yu VL, et al. *Candida* prosthetic valve endocarditis: Prospective study of six cases and review of the literature. Clin Infect Dis. 1996;22:262-267.

697. Raoult D, Houpikian P, Tissot DH, et al. Treatment of Q fever endocarditis: Comparison of 2 regimens containing doxycycline and ofloxacin or hydroxychloroquine. Arch Intern Med. 1999;159:167-173.

698. Haldane EV, Marrie TJ, Faulkner RS, et al. Endocarditis due to Q fever in Nova Scotia: Experience with five patients in 1981-1982. J Infect Dis. 1983;148:978-985.

699. Street AC, Durack DT. Experience with trimethoprim-sulfamethoxazole in treatment of infective endocarditis. Rev Infect Dis. 1988;10:915-922.

700. Levy PY, Drancourt M, Etienne J, et al. Comparison of different antibiotic regimens for therapy of 32 cases of Q fever endocarditis. Antimicrob Agents Chemother. 1991;35:533.

701. Jones JB, Ridgeway GL, Boulding S, et al. In vitro activity of rifamycins alone and in combination with other antibiotics against *Chlamydia trachomatis*. Rev Infect Dis. 1983;5(Suppl):556.

702. McAnulty JH, Rahimtoola SH. Surgery for infective endocarditis. JAMA. 1979;242:77.

703. Dinubile MJ. Surgery in active endocarditis. Ann Intern Med. 1980;96:650.

704. D'Agostino RS, Miller DC, Stinson EB, et al. Valve replacement in patients with native valve endocarditis: What really determines operative outcome? Ann Thorac Surg. 1985;40:429-438.

705. Tolan RW Jr, Kleiman MB, Frank M, et al. Operative intervention in active endocarditis in children: Report of a series of cases and review. Clin Infect Dis. 1992;14:852.

706. John MD, Hibberd PL, Karchmer AW, et al. *Staphylococcus aureus* prosthetic valve endocarditis: Optimal management and risk factors for death. Clin Infect Dis. 1998;26:1302-1309.

707. Dion R. Whom to operate and when/new techniques: Mitral valve. Abstract 25. Abstracts of the Seventh International Symposium on Modern Concepts in Endocarditis and Cardiovascular Infections, Chamonix, France, June 26-28, 2003.

708. Mansur AJ, Grinberg M, Lemosdaluz P, et al. The complications of infective endocarditis. Arch Intern Med. 1992;152:2428.

709. Hasbun R, Vikram HR, Barakat LA, et al. Complicated left-sided native valve endocarditis in adults: Risk classification for mortality. JAMA. 2003;289:1933-1940.
710. Griffin FM, Jones G, Cobb CG. Aortic insufficiency in bacterial endocarditis. Ann Intern Med. 1972;76:23-28.
711. Karalis DG, Blumberg AE, Vilaro JF, et al. Prognostic significance of valvular regurgitation in patients with infective endocarditis. Am J Med. 1991;90:193.
712. Wilson WR, Danielson GK, Giuliani ER, et al. Valve replacement in patients with active infective endocarditis. Circulation. 1978;58:585.
713. Chuard C, Antley CM, Reller LB. Clinical utility of cardiac valve Gram stain and culture in patients undergoing native valve replacement. Arch Pathol Lab Med. 1998;122:412-415.
714. Arbulu A, Asfaw I. Tricuspid valvulectomy without prosthetic replacement: Ten years of clinical experience. J Thorac Cardiovasc Surg. 1981;82:684.
715. Straumann E, Stulz P, Jenzer HR. Tricuspid valve endocarditis in the drug addict: A reconstructive approach ("vegetectomy"). Thorac Cardiovasc Surg. 1990;38:291.
716. DiNubile M. Surgery for addiction-related tricuspid valve endocarditis: Caveat emptor. Am J Med. 1987;82:811-813.
717. Arbulu A, Asfaw I. Management of infective endocarditis: Seventeen years' experience. Ann Thorac Surg. 1987;43:144-149.
718. Alsip SG, Blackstone EH, Kirklin JW, et al. Indications for cardiac surgery in patients with active infective endocarditis. Am J Med. 1985;78(Suppl 6B):S38-S48.
719. Blumberg EA, Karalis DA, Chandrase Karan K, et al. Endocarditis-associated paravalvular abscesses: Do clinical parameters predict the presence of abscess? Chest. 1995;107:898-903.
720. De Castro S, Magni G, Beni S, et al. Role of transthoracic echocardiography in predicting embolic events in patients with active endocarditis involving native cardiac valves. Am J Cardiol. 1997;57:339-343.
721. Moon MR, Stinson EB, Miller DC. Surgical treatment of endocarditis. Prog Cardiovasc Dis. 1997;40:239-264.
722. Tornos M-P, Permanyer-Miralda G, Olona M, et al. Long-term complications of native valve infective endocarditis in non-addicts: A 15-year follow-up study. Ann Intern Med. 1992;117:567.
723. Neuhof H, Seley GP. Acute suppurative phlebitis complicated by septicemia. Surgery. 1947;21:831.
724. Goldman DA, Maki DG, Rhame FS, et al. Guidelines for infection control in intravenous therapy. Ann Intern Med. 1973;79:848.
725. Rupp ME. Infections of intravascular catheters and vascular devices. In: Crossley KB, Archer GL, eds. The Staphylococci in Human Disease. New York: Churchill Livingstone; 1997:379-399.
726. O'Neill JA, Pruitt BA, Foley FD, et al. Suppurative thrombophlebitis—a lethal complication of intravenous therapy. J Trauma. 1968;8:256.
727. Stein JM, Pruitt BA. Suppurative thrombophlebitis: A lethal iatrogenic disease. N Engl J Med. 1970;282:1452.
728. Pruitt BA, Stein JM, Foley FD, et al. Intravenous therapy in burn patients: Suppurative thrombophlebitis and other life-threatening complications. Arch Surg. 1970;100:399.
729. Pruitt BA, McManus WF, Kim SH, et al. Diagnosis and treatment of cannula-related intravenous sepsis in burn patients. Ann Surg. 1980;191:546.
730. Garrison RN, Richardson JD, Fry DE. Catheter-associated septic thrombophlebitis. South Med J. 1982;75:917.
731. Sacks-Berg A, Strampfer MJ, Cunha BA. Suppurative thrombophlebitis caused by intravenous line sepsis. Heart Lung. 1987;16:318-320.
732. Munster AM. Septic thrombophlebitis: A surgical disorder. JAMA. 1974;230:1010.
733. Berkowitz FE, Argent AC, Baise T. Suppurative thrombophlebitis: A serious nosocomial infection. Pediatr Infect Dis J. 1987;6:64-67.
734. Johnson RA, Zajac RA, Evans ME. Suppurative thrombophlebitis: Correlation between pathogen and underlying disease. Infect Control. 1986;7:582-585.
735. Rhame FS, Maki DG, Bennett JV. Intravenous cannula-associated infections. In: Bennett JV, Brachman PS, eds. Hospital Infections. Boston: Little, Brown; 1979:433-442.
736. Baker CC, Peterson SR, Sheldon GF. Septic phlebitis: A neglected disease. Am J Surg. 1979;138:97.
737. Sears N, Grosfeld JL, Weber TR, et al. Suppurative thrombophlebitis in childhood. Pediatrics. 1981;68:630.
738. Zinner MJ, Zuidema GD, Lowery BD. Septic nonsuppurative thrombophlebitis. Arch Surg. 1976;111:122.
739. Maki DG. Infections due to infusion therapy. In: Bennett JV, Brachman PS, eds. Hospital Infections. Boston: Little, Brown; 1992:849.
740. Brismar B, Hardstedt C, Jacobson S. Diagnosis of thrombosis by catheter phlebography after prolonged central venous catheterization. Ann Surg. 1981;194:779-783.
741. Tagalakis V, Kahn SR, Libman M, et al. The epidemiology of peripheral vein infusion thrombophlebitis: A critical review. Am J Med. 2002;113:146-151.
742. Musher D, Goldsmith E, Dunbar S, et al. Association of hypercoagulable states and increased platelet adhesion and aggregation with bacterial colonization of intravenous catheters. J Infect Dis. 2002;186:769-773.
743. Slagle DC, Gates RH Jr. Unusual case of central vein thrombosis and sepsis. Am J Med. 1986;81:351-354.
744. Kaufman J, Demas C, Stark K, et al. Catheter-related septic central venous thrombosis—current therapeutic options. West J Med. 1986;145:200-203.
745. Veghese A, Widrich WC, Arbeit RD. Central venous septic thrombophlebitis—the role of medical therapy. Medicine (Baltimore). 1985;64:394-400.
746. Strinden WD, Helgerson RB, Maki DG. Candida septic thrombosis of the great central veins associated with central catheters: Clinical features and management. Ann Surg. 1985;202:653-658.
747. Raad I, Narro J, Khan A, et al. Serious complications of vascular catheter-related Staphylococcus aureus bacteremia in cancer patients. Eur J Clin Microbiol Infect Dis. 1992;11:675.
748. Haddad W, Idowu J, Georgeson K, et al. Septic atrial thrombosis: A potentially lethal complication of Broviac catheters in infants. Am J Dis Child. 1986;140:778-780.
749. Collins CG, MacCallum EA, Nelson EW, et al. Suppurative pelvic thrombophlebitis: I. Incidence, pathology, and etiology. Surgery. 1951;30:298.
750. Josey WE, Staggers SR. Heparin therapy in septic pelvic thrombophlebitis: A study of 46 cases. Am J Obstet Gynecol. 1974;120:228.
751. Collins CG. Suppurative pelvic thrombophlebitis: A study of 202 cases in which the disease was treated by ligation of the vena cava and ovarian vein. Am J Obstet Gynecol. 1970;108:681.
752. Lim GM, Jeffrey RB Jr, Ralls PW, et al. Septic thrombosis of the portal vein: CT and clinical observations. J Comput Assist Tomogr. 1989;13:656.
753. Barenholtz L, Kaminsky NI, Palmer DL. Venous intramural microabscesses: A cause of protracted sepsis with intravenous cannulas. Am J Med Sci. 1973;265:335.
754. Gillespie P, Siddiqui H, Clarke J. Cannula related suppurative thrombophlebitis in the burned patient. Burns. 2000;26:200-204.
755. Khan EA, Correa AG, Baker CJ. Suppurative thrombophlebitis in children: A ten-year experience. Pediatr Infect Dis J. 1997;16:63-67.
756. Syndman DR, Murray SA, Kornfeld SJ, et al. Total parenteral nutrition-related infections: Prospective epidemiologic study using semiquantitative methods. Am J Med. 1982;73:695.
757. Jupiter JB, Ehrlich MG, Novelline RA, et al. The association of septic thrombophlebitis with subperiosteal abscesses in children. J Pediatr. 1982;101:690.
758. Maki DG, Weise CE, Sarafin HW. A semiquantitative culture method for identifying intravenous-catheter-related infection. N Engl J Med. 1977;296:1305.
759. Ashkenazi S, Pickering LK, Robinson LH. Diagnosis and management of septic thrombosis of the inferior vena cava caused by Candida tropicalis. Pediatr Infect Dis J. 1990;9:446.
760. Mori H, Fukuda T, Isomoto I, et al. CT diagnosis of catheter-induced septic thrombosis of vena cava. J Comput Assist Tomogr. 1990;14:236.
761. Auber AE, Mancuso PA. Lemierre syndrome: magnetic resonance imaging and computed tomographic appearance. Milit Med. 2000;165:638-640.
762. Angel JL, Knuppel RA. Computed tomography in diagnosis of puerperal ovarian vein thrombosis. Obstet Gynecol. 1984;63:61-64.
763. Isada NB, Landy HJ, Larson JW Jr. Postabortal septic pelvic thrombophlebitis diagnosed with computed tomography. J Reprod Med. 1987;32:866-868.
764. Martin B, Molopulos GP, Bryan PJ. MRI of puerperal ovarian vein thrombosis. AJR Am J Roentgenol. 1986;147:291-292.
765. Josey WE, Cook CC. Septic pelvic thrombophlebitis: Report of 17 patients treated with heparin. Obstet Gynecol. 1970;35:891.
766. Brook I. Superficial suppurative thrombophlebitis in children, caused by anaerobic bacteria. J Pediatr Surg. 1998;33:1279-1282.
767. Torres-Rojas JR, Stratton CW, Sanders CV, et al. Candidal suppurative peripheral thrombophlebitis. Ann Intern Med. 1982;96:431.
768. Walsh TJ, Bustamante CI, Valhov D, et al. Candidal suppurative peripheral thrombophlebitis: Recognition, prevention, and management. Infect Control. 1986;7:16-22.
769. Shek YH, Tucker MC, Viciana AL, et al. Malassezia furfur—disseminated infection in premature infants. Am J Clin Pathol. 1989;92:595.
770. Peterson P, Stahl-Bayliss CM. Cytomegalovirus thrombophlebitis after successful DHPG therapy. Ann Intern Med. 1987;106:632-633.
771. Miller CJ. Ligation and excision of pelvic veins in treatment of puerperal pyaemia. Surg Gynecol Obstet. 1917;25:431.
772. Topiel MS, Bryan RT, Kessler CM, et al. Treatment of Silastic catheter-induced central vein septic thrombophlebitis. Am J Med Sci. 1986;291:425-428.
773. Barg NL, Supena RB, Fekety R. Persistent staphylococcal bacteremia in an intravenous drug abuser. Antimicrob Agents Chemother. 1986;29:209-211.
774. Schranz D, Haugwitz D, Zimmer B, et al. Successful lysis of a septic thrombosis of the superior vena cava using recombinant tissue-plasminogen activator. Klin Padiatr. 1991;203:363.
775. Moran JM, Atwood RP, Rowe MI. A clinical and bacteriologic study of infections associated with venous cutdowns. N Engl J Med. 1965;272:554.
776. Norden CW. Application of antibiotic ointment to the site of venous catheterization—a controlled trial. J Infect Dis. 1969;120:611.
777. Centers for Disease Control and Prevention. Part 1. Intravascular device–related infection: An overview. Part 2. Recommendations for prevention of intravascular device–related infections. Fed Reg. 1995;60:49978.
778. Patel S, Johnston KW. Classification and management of mycotic aneurysms. Surg Gynecol Obstet. 1977;144:691.
779. Parkhurst GF, Decker JP. Bacterial aortitis and mycotic aneurysms of the aorta: A report of 12 cases. Am J Pathol. 1955;31:821.
780. Sommerville RL, Allen EV, Edwards JE. Bland and infected arteriosclerotic abdominal aortic aneurysms: A clinicopathologic study. Medicine (Baltimore). 1959;38:207.
781. Sekkal S, Cornu E, Cristides C, et al. Isolated iliac aneurysms: Seventy-seven cases in forty-eight patients. J Mal Vasc. 1993;18:13.
782. Stengel A, Wolfroth CC. Mycotic (bacterial) aneurysms of intravascular origin. Arch Intern Med. 1923;31:527.
783. Tsao JW, Marder SR, Goldstone J, et al. Presentation, diagnosis, and management of arterial mycotic pseudoaneurysms in injection drug users. Ann Vasc Surg. 2002;16:652-662.
784. Bennett DE, Cherry JK. Bacterial infection of aortic aneurysms: A clinicopathologic study. Am J Surg. 1967;113:321.
785. Cliff MM, Soulen RL, Firestone AJ. Mycotic aneurysms: A challenge and a clue. Arch Intern Med. 1970;126:977.

786. Jarrett F, Darling C, Mundth ED, et al. Experience with infected aneurysms of the abdominal aorta. Arch Surg. 1975;110:1281.

787. Bohmfalk GL, Story JL, Wissenger JP, et al. Bacterial intracranial aneurysm. J Neurosurg. 1978;48:369.

788. Frazee JG, Cahan LD, Winter J. Bacterial intracranial aneurysms. J Neurosurg. 1980;53:633.

789. Selky AK, Roos KL. Neurologic complications of infective endocarditis. Semin Neurol. 1992;12:225.

790. Tunkel AR, Kaye D. Neurologic complications of infective endocarditis. Neurol Clin. 1993;11:419.

791. Bullock R, Van Dellen JR, Van den Heever CM. Intracranial mycotic aneurysms: A review of 9 cases. S Afr Med J. 1981;60:970.

792. John RM, Pugsley W, Treasure T, et al. Aortic root complications of infective endocarditis—influence on surgical outcome. Eur Heart J. 1991;12:241.

793. Hollingworth J, Palmer KS, Simms MH. Ruptured mycotic aneurysm of the abdominal aorta in childhood. Eur J Vasc Surg. 1992;6:665.

794. Cribari C, Meadors FA, Crawford ES, et al. Thoraco-abdominal aortic aneurysm associated with umbilical artery catheterization: Case report and review of the literature. J Vasc Surg. 1992;16:75.

795. Jarrett F, Darling RC, Mundth ED, et al. The management of infected arterial aneurysms. J Cardiovasc Surg. 1977;18:361.

796. Johnson JR, Ledgerwood AM, Lucas CE. Mycotic aneurysm: New concepts in therapy. Arch Surg. 1983;118:577.

797. Brummitt CF, Kravitz GR, Granrud GA, et al. Femoral endarteritis due to *Staphylococcus aureus* complicating percutaneous transluminal coronary angioplasty. Am J Med. 1989;86:822.

798. Frazee BW, Flaherty JP. Septic endarteritis of the femoral artery following angioplasty. Rev Infect Dis. 1991;13:620.

799. Pruitt A, Dodson TF, Najibi S, et al. Distal septic emboli and fatal brachiocephalic artery mycotic pseudoaneurysm as a complication of stenting. J Vasc Surg. 2002;36:625-628.

800. Tsao JW, Neymark E, Gooding GA. Radial artery mycotic pseudoaneurysm: An unusual complication of catheterization. J Clin Ultrasound. 2000;28:414-416.

801. Shindo S, Arai H, Kubota K, et al. Rupture of infected pseudoaneurysms in patients with implantable ports for intra-arterial infusion chemotherapy. J Cardiovasc Surg. 2000;41:95-98.

802. Feigl D, Feigl A, Edwards JE. Mycotic aneurysms of the aortic root: A pathologic study of 20 cases. Chest. 1986;90:553-557.

803. Jebara VA, Dervanian P, Acar C, et al. Mycotic aneurysm of the carotid artery secondary to acute bacterial endocarditis. Arch Mal Coeur Vaiss. 1992;85:1615.

804. Akers DL Jr, Fowl RJ, Kempczinski RF, et al. Mycotic aneurysm of the tibioperoneal trunk: Case report and review of the literature. J Vasc Surg. 1992;16:71.

805. Dean RH, Mecham PW, Weaver FA, et al. Mycotic embolism and embolomycotic aneurysms: Neglected lessons of the past. Ann Surg. 1986;204:300-307.

806. Sedwitz MM, Hye RJ, Stabile BE. The changing epidemiology of pseudoaneurysm: Therapeutic implications. Arch Surg. 1988;123:473-476.

807. Morgan MB, Cintron G, Balis JV. Infective "mycotic" aortic root aneurysm following coronary artery bypass grafting. Am J Med. 1993;94:550.

808. Prech M, Grajek S, CieSlinski A, et al. Mycotic aneurysm of the ascending aorta following CABG. Heart (British Cardiac Society). 2000;83:E3.

809. Vyas SK, Law NW, Loehry CA. Mycotic aneurysm of the left subclavian artery. Br Heart J. 1993;69:455.

810. Hurst RW, Choi IS, Persky M, et al. Mycotic aneurysms of the intracavernous carotid artery: A case report and review of the literature. Surg Neurol. 1992;37:142.

811. Kyriakides GK, Simmons RL, Najarian JS. Mycotic aneurysms in transplant patients. Arch Surg. 1976;111:472.

812. Smith EJ, Milligan SL, Filo RS. *Salmonella* mycotic aneurysms after renal transplantation. South Med J. 1981;74:1399.

813. Olmsted WW, McGee TP. The pathogenesis of peripheral aneurysms of the central nervous system: A subject review from the AFIP. Radiology. 1977;123:661.

814. Salgado AV, Furlan AJ, Keys TF. Mycotic aneurysm, subarachnoid hemorrhage, and indications for cerebral angiography in infective endocarditis. Stroke. 1987;18: 1057-1060.

815. Wilson WR, Lie JT, Houser OW, et al. The management of patients with mycotic aneurysm. Curr Clin Top Infect Dis. 1981;2:151.

816. Barrow DL, Prats AR. Infectious intracranial aneurysms: Comparison of groups with and without endocarditis. Neurosurgery. 1990;27:562.

817. Friedman SG, Pogo GJ, Moccio CG. Mycotic aneurysm of the superior mesenteric artery. J Vasc Surg. 1987;6:87-90.

818. Sukerkar AN, Dulay CC, Anandappa E, et al. Mycotic aneurysm of the hepatic artery. Radiology. 1977;124:444.

819. Khoda J, Lantsberg L, Sebbag G. Hepatic artery mycotic aneurysm as a cause of hemobilia. J Hepatol. 1993;17:131.

820. Carrel D, Cohle SD, Chapman AJ. Fatal hemothorax from mycotic celiac artery aneurysm. Am J Med Pathol. 1992;13:233.

821. Feinsod FM, Norfleet RG, Hoehn JL. Mycotic aneurysm of the external iliac artery: A triad of clinical signs facilitating early diagnosis. JAMA. 1977;238:245.

822. Merry M, Dunn J, Weissmann R, et al. Popliteal mycotic aneurysm presenting as septic arthritis and purpura. JAMA. 1972;221:58.

823. Plate G, Forsley N, Stigsson L, et al. Management of inflammatory abdominal aortic aneurysm. Acta Chir Scand. 1988;154:19-24.

824. Pennell RC, Hollier LH, Lie JT, et al. Inflammatory abdominal aortic aneurysms: A thirty year review. J Vasc Surg. 1985;2:859-869.

825. Morrow C, Safi H, Beall AC Jr. Primary aortoduodenal fistula caused by *Salmonella* aortitis. J Vasc Surg. 1987;6:415-418.

826. Villablanca JP, Jahan R, Hooshi P, et al. Detection and characterization of very small cerebral aneurysms by using 2D and 3D helical CT angiography. AJNR Am J Neuroradiol. 2002;23:1187-1198.

827. Kimura I, Okumura R, Yamashita K, et al. Mycotic aneurysm. Radiat Med. 1989;7:121.

828. Atlas SW. Magnetic resonance imaging of intracranial aneurysms. Neuroimaging Clin North Am. 1997;7:709-720.

829. Nguyen BT. Computed tomography diagnosis of thoracic aortic aneurysms. Semin Roentgenol. 2001;36:309-324.

830. Vogelzang RL, Sohaey R. Infected aortic aneurysms: CT appearance. J Comput Assist Tomogr. 1988;12:109-112.

831. Blair RH, Resnik MD, Polga JP. CT appearance of mycotic abdominal aortic aneurysms. J Comput Assist Tomogr. 1989;13:101.

832. Rivera JV, Blanco G, Perez M, et al. Gallium-67 localization in a mycotic aneurysm of the thoracic aorta. Clin Nucl Med. 1985;10:814-816.

833. Zwas ST, Lorberboyin M, Schechter M. Occult aortic arch mycotic aneurysm diagnosed by radio gallium scintigraphy. Clin Nucl Med. 1992;17:797.

834. Ben-Haim S, Seabold JE, Hawes DR, et al. Leukocyte scintigraphy in the diagnosis of mycotic aneurysm. J Nucl Med. 1992;33:1486.

835. Ramo OJ, Vorne M, Lantto E, et al. Postoperative graft incorporation after aortic reconstruction—comparison between computerized tomography and Tc-99m-HMPAO labelled leukocyte imaging. Eur J Vasc Surg. 1993;7:122.

836. Brewster DC, Retana A, Waltman AC, et al. Angiography in the management of aneurysms of the abdominal aorta. N Engl J Med. 1972;292:822.

837. Griffiths BE, Petch MC, English TAH. Echocardiographic detection of subvalvular aortic root aneurysm extending to mitral valve annulus as complication of aortic valve endocarditis. Br Heart J. 1982;47:392.

838. Ozkutlu S, Ozbarlas N, Bilgi CA, et al. Mycotic aneurysm of the descending aorta diagnosed by echocardiography. Int J Cardiol. 1992;37:112.

839. Vargas-Barron J, Avila-Rosales L, Romero-Cardenas A, et al. Echocardiographic diagnosis of a mycotic aneurysm of the main pulmonary artery and patent ductus arteriosus. Am Heart J. 1992;123:1707.

840. Benenson S, Raveh D, Schlesinger Y, et al. The risk of vascular infection in adult patients with nontyphi *Salmonella* bacteremia. Am J Med. 2001;110:60-63.

841. Kanwar YS, Malhotra U, Anderson BR, et al. Salmonellosis associated with abdominal aortic aneurysm. Arch Intern Med. 1974;134:1095.

842. Soravia-Dunand VA, Loo VG, Salit IE. Aortitis due to *Salmonella:* Report of 10 cases and comprehensive review of the literature. Clin Infect Dis. 1999;29:862-868.

843. Cohen JI, Bartlett JA, Corey GR. Extra-intestinal manifestations of *Salmonella* infections. Medicine (Baltimore). 1987;66:349-388.

844. Cohen OS, O'Brien TF, Schoenbaum SC, et al. The risk of endothelial infection in adults with *Salmonella* bacteremia. Ann Intern Med. 1978;89:931.

845. Flamand F, Harris KA, DeRose G, et al. Arteritis due to *Salmonella* with aneurysm formation: Two cases. Can J Surg. 1992;35:248.

846. McIntyre KE Jr, Malone JM, Richards E. Mycotic aortic pseudoaneurysm with aortoenteric fistula caused by *Arizona hinshawii.* Surgery. 1982;91:173.

847. Feltis BA, Lee DA, Beilman GJ. Mycotic aneurysm of the descending thoracic aorta caused by *Pseudomonas aeruginosa* in a solid organ transplant recipient: Case report and review. Surg Infect. 2002;3:29-33.

848. Kumar N, Prabhakar G, Kandeel M, et al. *Brucella* mycotic aneurysm of ascending aorta complicating discrete subaortic stenosis. Am Heart J. 1993;125:1780.

849. Anolik JR, Mildvan D, Winter JW, et al. Mycotic aortic aneurysm: A complication of *Campylobacter fetus* septicemia. Arch Intern Med. 1983;143:609.

850. Garto AR, Cone LA, Woodard DR, et al. Arterial infections due to *Listeria monocytogenes:* Report of four cases and review of world literature. Clin Infect Dis. 1992;14:23.

851. Clouse WD, DeWitt CC, Hagino RT, et al. Rapidly enlarging iliac aneurysm secondary to *Listeria monocytogenes* infection: A case report. Vasc Endovasc Surg. 2003;37:145-149.

852. Andreasen DA, Dimcecski G, Nielsen H. Mycotic aneurysm of the aorta caused by group B streptococcus. Scand J Infect Dis. 2002;34:208-209.

853. Fournier PE, Casalta JP, Piquet P, et al. *Coxiella burnetii* infection of aneurysms or vascular grafts: Report of seven cases and review. Clin Infect Dis. 1998;26:116-121.

854. Hurley L, Howe K. Mycotic aortic aneurysm infected by *Clostridium septicum*—a case history. Angiology. 1991;42:585.

855. Steig TA, Johannesen N, Schonheyder HC. Propensity of *Streptococcus pneumoniae* for the aorta: Report of 3 cases. Scand J Infect Dis. 2001;33:772-774.

856. Long R, Guzman R, Greenberg H, et al. Tuberculous mycotic aneurysm of the aorta: Review of published medical and surgical experience. Chest. 1999;115:522-531.

857. Mielke B, Weir B, Oldring D, et al. Fungal aneurysm: Case report and review of the literature. Neurosurgery. 1981;9:578.

858. Hadley MN, Martin NA, Spetzler RF, et al. Multiple intracranial aneurysms due to *Coccidioides immitis* infection. J Neurosurg. 1987;66:453-456.

859. Ogden PE, Hurley DL, Cain PT. Fatal fungal endarteritis caused by *Bipolaris spicifera* following replacement of the aortic valve. Clin Infect Dis. 1992;14:596.

860. Aguado JM, Valle R, Arjona R, et al. Aortic bypass graft infection due to *Aspergillus:* Report of a case and review. Clin Infect Dis. 1992;14:916.

861. McLean DR, Russell N, Khan MY. Neurobrucellosis: Clinical and therapeutic features. Clin Infect Dis. 1992;15:582.

862. Bingham WF. Treatment of mycotic intracranial aneurysms. J Neurosurg. 1977;46:428.

863. Semba CP, Sakai T, Slonim SM, et al. Mycotic aneurysms of the thoracic aorta: Repair with use of endovascular stent-grafts. J Vasc Interv Radiol. 1998;9:33-40.

864. Leipzig MJ, Brown FD. Treatment of mycotic aneurysms. Surg Neurol. 1985;23: 403-407.

865. Rodesch G, Noterman J, Thys JP, et al. Treatment of intracranial mycotic aneurysm: Surgery or not? Acta Neurochir. 1987;85:63-68.
866. Phuong LK, Link M, Wijdicks E. Management of intracranial infectious aneurysms: A series of 16 cases. Neurosurgery. 2002;51:1145-1151.
867. Reddy DJ, Smith RF, Elliott JP Jr, et al. Infected femoral artery false aneurysms in drug addicts: Evolution of selective vascular reconstruction. J Vasc Surg. 1986;3:718-724.
868. Johansen K, Devin J. Mycotic aortic aneurysms: A reappraisal. Arch Surg. 1983;118:583.
869. Parsons R, Gregory J, Palmer DL. *Salmonella* infections of the abdominal aorta. Rev Infect Dis. 1983;5:227.
870. Bitseff EJ, Edwards WH, Mulherin JL Jr, et al. Infected abdominal aortic aneurysms. South Med J. 1987;80:309-312.
871. Taylor LM Jr, Deitz DM, McConnell DB, et al. Treatment of infected abdominal aneurysms by extra anatomic bypass, aneurysm excision, and drainage. Am J Surg. 1988;155:655-658.
872. Pasic M, Carrel T, von Segesser L, et al. In situ repair of mycotic aneurysm of the ascending aorta. J Thorac Cardiovasc Surg. 1993;105:321.
873. Cull DL, Winter RP, Wheeler JR, et al. Mycotic aneurysm of the suprarenal abdominal aorta. J Thorac Cardiovasc Surg. 1992;33:181.
874. Robinson JA, Johansen K. Aortic sepsis: Is there a role for in situ graft reconstruction? J Vasc Surg. 1991;13:677.
875. Pasic M, Carrel T, Vogt M, et al. Treatment of mycotic aneurysm of the aorta and its branches: The location determines the operative technique. Eur J Vasc Surg. 1992;6:419.
876. Viglione G, Younes GA, Coste P, et al. Mycotic aneurysm of the celiac trunk: Radical resection and reconstruction without prosthetic material. J Cardiovasc Surg. 1993;34:73.
877. Pasic M, von Segesser L, Turina M. Implantation of antibiotic-releasing carriers and in situ reconstruction for treatment of mycotic aneurysm. Arch Surg. 1992;127:745.

TABLE 75-1 Nonvalvular Cardiovascular Device-Related Infections

Type of Device	Incidence of Infection (%)
Intracardiac	
Pacemakers (temporary and permanent)	0.13-19.9
Defibrillators	0-3.2
Left ventricular assist devices	25-70
Total artificial hearts	To be determined
Ventriculoatrial shunts	2.4-9.4
Pledgets (cardiac suture line)	Rare
Patent ductus arteriosus occlusion devices	Rare
Atrial septal defect closure devices	Rare
Conduits	Rare
Patches	Rare
Arterial	
Peripheral vascular stents	Rare
Vascular grafts, including hemodialysis	1-6
Intra-aortic balloon pumps	≤5-26
Angioplasty/angiography-related bacteremias	<1*
Coronary artery stents	Rare
Patches	1.8
Venous	
Vena caval filters	Rare

*Closure device use ≤1.9%.

CHAPTER 75

Infections of Prosthetic Valves and Other Cardiovascular Devices

LARRY M. BADDOUR
WALTER R. WILSON

Technologic advances in medicine since the 1950s have included the development of numerous implantable devices that improve or sustain life. Probably the two areas of medicine that have felt the most impact by these devices are cardiovascular and orthopedic medicine. During this period, we have witnessed not only the creation and use of these devices, but also the continuous improvement of them as newer generations of products are created.

Several cardiovascular devices (Table 75-1) are now in clinical use, and infection has complicated the use of each device. The infection risk has been wide ranging among the different devices (see Table 75-1). Infection of vena caval filters seems to be an extremely rare event, whereas infection complicating left ventricular assist device (LVAD) use is commonplace.

This chapter addresses infections related to cardiac valvular and nonvalvular cardiovascular devices. Intravascular catheter–related infections are reviewed in Chapter 300. The first part of this chapter reviews areas of commonality among the different devices. Subsequent sections discuss each device and characterize the unique features of each.

AREAS OF COMMONALITY

Epidemiology

Infections of cardiovascular devices can occur by one of three ways. First, microbial contamination of the device occurs at the time of device placement. If the device is implanted surgically, device infection can serve as an example of surgical site infection. The presence of foreign material in a surgical site can reduce greatly the infective dose of a contaminating strain, and the indwelling cardiovascular device is considered representative of this phenomenon. Second, cardiovascular devices can become infected as a result of hematogenous dissemination. Third, contiguous infection can spread and infect an indwelling cardiovascular device secondarily.

Pathogenesis

Microbial adherence (see Chapter 2) is the crucial first step in the establishment of infection. This step applies to native tissue and medical device–related infections. Because staphylococci account for most cardiovascular device–related infections, a limited overview of staphylococcal adherence is included. More detailed discussion can be found in Chapter 192.[1-3]

Investigative efforts have identified two mechanisms of staphylococcal adherence. In one paradigm, staphylococci attach to extracellular matrix proteins to initiate infection. These proteins coat the surface of the indwelling medical device. Extracellular matrix proteins also are exposed on the device surface after neointima formation and disruption of the endothelial cell layer by various factors, including stress forces caused by the presence of a medical device in the cardiovascular system. *Staphylococcus aureus* has a variety of virulence determinants, and some are adhesions, so-called MSCRAMMs (*m*icrobial *s*urface *c*omponents that are *r*esponsible for *a*ttachment to *m*olecular *m*olecules), that mediate attachment to medical devices via extracellular matrix proteins. Advances in molecular biology techniques have allowed investigations to define the role of *S. aureus* binding to fibrin(ogen), fibronectin, and collagen. Global gene regulators, accessory gene regulator (*agr*), and staphylococcal accessory regulator (*sar*) have been identified and coordinate the expression of adhesions (MSCRAMMs) that specifically bind to extracellular matrix proteins.[1,3] More recent work using a genetic transfer system[3] and a nonpathogenic organism (*Lactobacillus lactis*) has clarified further the important role of extracellular matrix protein binding of *S. aureus* in infection pathogenesis.

In the second paradigm, staphylococci attach to the surface of the cardiovascular device and form a biofilm. A *biofilm* is defined as "an assemblage of surface-associated microbial cells that is enclosed in an extracellular polymeric substance matrix."[2] Although much of the work has been directed toward coagulase-negative staphylococci and biofilm formation, *S. aureus* also is capable of producing biofilm on the surface of cardiovascular devices.[2] Biofilm-associated microorganisms are attached irreversibly to the surface of the foreign body, and device removal frequently is required for cure of infection in combination with antimicrobial therapy. The host immune response is not capable of clearing biofilm-associated staphylococci, and because of alterations in the metabolic state of bacteria in the biofilm, susceptibility to certain antibiotics may be reduced.

Microbiology

Bacteria and fungi are causes of cardiovascular device–related infections. Staphylococci are the most common pathogens among the bacterial group. *S. aureus* and coagulase-negative staphylococci are common causes of infection. Because device contamination occurs in the nosocomial setting at the time of device placement in many cases, multidrug resistance, including resistance to methicillin, characterizes these isolates. Coagulase-negative staphylococci harbor the highest rates of methicillin resistance, and among these strains, resistance to macrolides, aminoglycosides, and fluoroquinolones is typical. Other types of skin flora also cause device-related infection. *Corynebacterium* spp. are another group of bacteria that cause infection, and isolates often are multidrug resistant. *Propionibacterium acnes* can cause device infection and can be difficult to recover in cultures of clinical specimens, unless anaerobic cultures are obtained and held for extended periods.

A variety of streptococci cause cardiovascular device–related infection. Viridans group streptococci account for most of these infections. Although multidrug resistance has been described in numerous studies of bacteremic viridans group streptococcal isolates from patients with hematologic malignancies, to date, multidrug resistance has not characterized device-related infection strains. Varying degrees of penicillin resistance are well described, however, among device-related isolates. In addition, *Abiotrophia defectiva* and *Granulicatella* species, formally referred to as *nutritionally variant streptococci*, display fastidious growth, which makes in vitro susceptibility testing difficult. Because of this and higher relapse rates with monotherapy using penicillin G, treatment regimens that include aminoglycosides that are used for enterococci should be selected.

Enterococci produce device-related infections, and when nosocomially acquired, resistance to vancomycin increasingly is being reported. In addition, resistance to aminoglycosides in synergy testing with penicillin G is seen among vancomycin-susceptible and vancomycin-resistant enterococci.

Infections due to the HACEK (*Haemophilus parainfluenzae, Haemophilus aphrophilus, Actinobacillus actinomycetemcomitans, Cardiobacterium hominis, Eikenella corrodens,* and *Kingella kingae*) group of bacteria generally do not cause nosocomially acquired device-related infection but can produce late infections. An array of aerobic gram-negative bacilli causes cardiovascular device–related infections. Nosocomial acquisition is commonplace for these organisms, and multidrug resistance is common. Among this group, *Pseudomonas, Serratia, Acinetobacter,* and *Stenotrophomonas* spp. predominate. Anaerobic flora that normally inhabit the gastrointestinal tract are unusual causes of device-related infection. An exception includes aortic graft erosion into bowel lumen. Other unusual bacterial causes of cardiovascular device–related infection include *Legionella* spp., *Bartonella* spp., *Coxiella burnetii,* and nontuberculosis *Mycobacterium* spp.

Fungal infection of medical devices via nosocomial exposure has been seen more commonly in recent years. *Candida* spp. cause most of these infections, and *Candida albicans* is identified most often. *Candida parapsilosis* was the next most frequently isolated species, which supports the impression that *C. parapsilosis* has a proclivity to cause medical device–related infections; almost half of the cases involved prosthetic valves. Other non-*albicans* species of *Candida* also are recovered frequently and can be resistant (*C. glabrata, C. krusei*) to azoles. *Aspergillus* spp. cause a few infections and can be difficult to identify as causative pathogens because blood cultures usually are negative. Uncommon causes of fungal device-related infections include *Cryptococcus neoformans, Histoplasma capsulatum,* and an array of different molds.

Clinical Manifestations

Clinical signs and symptoms of cardiovascular device–related infection depend in part on the location of the infected portion of the device and the virulence of the infecting organism. For some pathogens with limited virulence, clinical presentations of infection are indolent and are ongoing for weeks to months before the correct diagnosis is considered. Bacteria, including coagulase-negative staphylococci, *P. acnes, Corynebacterium* spp., viridans group streptococci, and the HACEK group of organisms, usually cause more subtle infections, which are characterized by low-grade fever, weight loss, malaise, and myalgias. Blood cultures often return unexpectedly positive due to the lack of toxicity seen in many of these patients.

Blood-stream infection due to other organisms, including *S. aureus,* β-hemolytic streptococci, *Pseudomonas aeruginosa,* and *Candida* spp., is usually acute in presentation and associated with findings of sepsis, including high fever or hypothermia, tachypnea, tachycardia, and intermittent rigors. Complications of sepsis with shock, organ dysfunction, and coagulopathy also can occur.

Embolic events precipitating a stroke, pulmonary ischemia, myocardial infarction, bowel infarction, or loss of limb perfusion can complicate acute and subacute-to-chronic presentations. Vegetations are the source of emboli and form in a variety of cardiovascular device–related infections and are not limited to prosthetic cardiac valves.

Local signs of device infection at subcutaneous or percutaneous sites typically include erythema of the overlying or surrounding skin. Drainage with varying degrees of purulence, depending on the infecting organism, also may be seen.

Diagnosis

Fever with or without other symptoms is a usual complaint in patients with cardiovascular device–related infection. Fever without other findings may not prompt the attending clinician to consider the possibility of device infection. Empirical antibiotics may be administered without a bacterial process identified, which delays the diagnosis further due to resolution of fever or a diminution in specimen culture sensitivity if specimens are obtained after initiation of antibiotics.

Blood cultures are the best tool to show blood-stream infection. Blood cultures should be positive if there is infection of an intracardiac or intravascular portion of the device. Routine culture methods usually are sufficient for blood cultures. If fastidious or unusual organisms are considered as pathogens, additional methodologies are required.

Computed tomography (CT), ultrasonography, and magnetic resonance imaging (MRI) are useful in showing fluid collection around a device, which can indicate infection. Percutaneous aspirate of the fluid with ultrasound or CT guidance commonly is employed to confirm the diagnosis of device infection.

Echocardiography is sentinel in vegetation detection. Transesophageal echocardiography (TEE) frequently is required due to its increased sensitivity of visualization of vegetation in the proximity of foreign (medical device) material.

Treatment

There are two principles of treatment of cardiovascular device–related infections. The first is the provision of pathogen-specific antimicrobial therapy. Every effort should be made to obtain pertinent specimens for culture before initiation of antimicrobials. Without a pathogen identified, empirical therapy may not provide the most efficacious regimen and may include unnecessary agents that can result in toxicity without benefit; this is particularly true when therapy is extended for several weeks or longer. The ideal duration of antimicrobial treatment and route of drug administration currently are undefined for most device infections. Most experts believe, however, that a minimum of 4 weeks of parenteral therapy should be administered for device infection causing blood-stream infection. If infection is due to *S. aureus* or involves a cardiac prosthesis or vascular graft, more prolonged (6 to ≥8 weeks) courses of antimicrobials are used.

The second principle is device removal. In general, acceptable cure rates are achieved only with a combined treatment approach that includes medical therapy and device removal. Because many of the cardiovascular devices are life-sustaining, device replacement is required. For some patients, additional surgical procedures for device removal and new device placement are not a treatment option due to an unacceptably high risk of surgical mortality. In that case, initial control of infection by medical therapy is attempted. If control is achieved and the patient's cardiovascular status is stable, long-term (lifelong) oral suppressive antimicrobial therapy is administered. If initial control of infection is not achieved or if the patient has infection relapse despite long-term suppressive treatment, device removal should be reconsidered despite the increased operative risks.

Prevention

Several unique features of cardiovascular device–related infection should be reviewed when considering the use of peri-implantation prophylactic antimicrobials. First, the risk of infection due to the presence of a foreign body is enhanced markedly at an operative or implantation site. Second, device removal often is necessary to achieve cure of infection (with the administration of systemic antimicrobials). For a device that is life-sustaining, there can be a treatment conundrum if a patient, for any of variety of reasons, is deemed a nonsurgical candidate, and surgical intervention is required for device exchange and attempted infection cure. Third, infection due to multidrug-resistant staphylococci is seen frequently, and few antibiotic treatment options exist. Fourth, limited data are available that show the efficacy of perioperative prophylactic antimicrobials. As emphasized in a review,[4] the large number of patients required in a prophylaxis efficacy trial in the prevention of surgical implant infections is prohibitive. The estimated size of an adequately powered clinical trial to show a 25% reduction in the infection rate of prosthetic cardiac valves by the administration of perioperative antibiotic prophylaxis is more than 22,000 patients enrolled. Fifth, antimicrobial prophylaxis can be harmful.

Perhaps the most striking more recent example involved the application of "local" antimicrobial prophylaxis to prevent infection. A silver-coated sewing ring of a mechanical prosthetic cardiac valve (Silzone; St. Jude Medical Inc, Minneapolis, MN) was approved by the Food and Drug Administration (FDA) in the United States in March 1998. An interim analysis of data from an ongoing postmarketing trial (*Artificial Valve Endocarditis Reduction Trial* [AVERT])[5] that began patient enrollment in July 1998 indicated that early prosthetic paravalvular leak leading to valve replacement was more prevalent among the Silzone study arm. The manufacturer voluntarily withdrew the product in January 2000. The exact mechanisms responsible for the development of the paravalvular leak are yet to be defined. Culture-negative endocarditis involving the sewing ring, although initially thought to be operative, was not responsible. Explanted valves exhibited poor tissue ingrowth and loosening of sutures. This finding led some to speculate that the Silzone coating inhibited normal fibroblast response and incorporation of the sewing ring fabric into the surrounding cardiac tissue.[5] Continued clinical follow-up of 36,000 patients worldwide who received the Silzone prosthesis is ongoing and may improve understanding of the pathogenesis of poor tissue incorporation linked to local silver exposure.

PROSTHETIC VALVE ENDOCARDITIS

Incidence

Prosthetic valve endocarditis (PVE) is a life-threatening infectious complication that is seen frequently in medical centers that routinely care for patients with artificial cardiac valves. In more recently published large case series,[6-9] the prevalence of prosthetic valve infections among all cases of infective endocarditis ranged from 16% to 32%. Two population-based studies provide estimates of the overall incidence rate of PVE. One was conducted in the Netherlands as a nationwide, prospective investigation that included cases between 1986 and 1998.[10] The incidence of PVE in the Netherlands, 0.6 cases per 100,000 person-years, was similar to the incidence of PVE noted in

residents of the Delaware Valley in the United States between 1988 and 1990, 0.94 cases per 100,000 person-years.[11]

The incidence of PVE among prosthetic valve recipients is variable and depends on duration of follow-up. The risk of infection is highest within 1 year after valve placement,[12] with an incidence of 3.1% reported.[13] For intermediate (5 to 7 years) and long-term (15 years) follow-up, the incidence ranges from 3.8% to 6.4%[14,15] and 17%.[16]

An analysis of claims files from the Health Care Finance Administration for Medicare beneficiaries from 1990 through 1999 suggests that the incidences of prosthetic valve placement and infection are increasing.[17] The rate of prosthetic valve placement increased by 31% over the 10-year study period from 0.83 to 1.09 valve operations/1000 Medicare beneficiaries. The rate increase in valve infection was 50% for the same period, from 0.26 to 0.38 cases/1000 Medicare beneficiaries.

Epidemiology

The frequency of PVE ranges from 1% to 3% within the first year postoperatively; these rates have remained stable since the 1970s.[13,18-22] The risk of development of PVE is highest within the first 3 months postoperatively. After 6 months, the rate of PVE is low and remains at a relatively constant rate of approximately 0.4% annually.[22-24]

Many studies have evaluated the relative risk of PVE according to the type and location of valvular prosthesis. Studies suggest that there is no difference in the rate of PVE at the aortic compared with the mitral position.[13,20,24,25] There seems to be no difference in the overall risk of PVE associated with a mechanical prosthesis compared with a bioprosthetic device.[24-27] Although the overall risk of PVE is similar with a mechanical valve compared with a bioprosthetic valve, the risk of PVE was greater with a mechanical valve than with a bioprosthetic valve during the first 6 months postoperatively.[20] There was no significant difference in the frequency of PVE during the first 5 years postoperatively with mechanical valves (5%) compared with bioprosthetic valves (6.3%).[13] The risk of PVE 5 years or more postoperatively was greater for bioprostheses than for mechanical valves, presumably as a result of degenerative changes in the bioprosthetic leaflets that occur over time.[21,25] The risk of recurrent PVE after surgery to replace an infected valvular prosthesis is lower after use of a cryopreserved allograft than the risk associated with use of a mechanical prosthesis.[28]

Pathogenesis

The role and importance of microbial adherence in intravascular device infections were discussed previously. After cardiac valve prosthesis implantation, fibrin and platelet thrombi occur at the site of the sewing ring and anulus and serve as targets for adherence of microorganisms. As endothelialization occurs, this area becomes less susceptible to infection. *Staphylococcus epidermidis* or other coagulase-negative staphylococci, *S. aureus,* diphtheroids, and fungi most often cause early-onset PVE.[19] This spectrum of microorganisms suggests intraoperative contamination.[29] These microorganisms were recovered from cultures of intraoperative myocardial tissue, valvular prostheses, areas over the operative site, bypass pumps, and other surgical equipment.[29-34] Bacteremia occurring during the early postoperative period also may cause early-onset PVE. Contaminated intravenous catheters and bacteremia resulting from a wound infection were the most common factors associated with PVE secondary to early postoperative bacteremia.[22,35-39] Bacteremia caused by staphylococci is more likely to cause early-onset PVE than is bacteremia caused by gram-negative bacilli.[40,41]

Late-onset PVE most often results from the same pathophysiologic events that cause native valve endocarditis (NVE). With the passage of time postoperatively, bioprosthetic valve leaflets age and become sclerotic, resulting in blood flow turbulence and the deposition of nonbacterial fibrin platelet microthrombi. Despite the annular reepithelialization that occurs over time after mechanical valve implantation, blood flow turbulence occurs, and fibrin platelet deposition develops. These fibrin platelet matrices are targets for adherence of microorganisms in the blood during physiologic bacteremia or during bacteremia resulting from dental or other invasive procedures. Accordingly the microbiologic spectrum of late-onset PVE is similar to that of NVE except that endocarditis caused by coagulase-negative staphylococci is more common in PVE than in NVE.[19]

Pathology

Mechanical valve PVE usually is associated with perivalvular extension of infection with the formation of valve ring, aortic root, or myocardial abscesses, which result in partial or complete valve dehiscence.[42-46] Extension of infection into the septum may result in myocardial conduction defects.[43-45] Perivalvular extension of infection with valvular dehiscence was reported in 82% of patients with PVE at surgery or autopsy.[38] Vegetations may extend into the valvular aperture, causing obstruction, or they may prevent valvular closure, resulting in valvular incompetence.

PVE involving a bioprosthesis results in leaflet destruction or perforation. Perivalvular extension of infection also may occur and was reported in 36% to 54% of patients.[47-50] In mechanical and bioprosthetic valve PVE, perivalvular extension occurred more commonly and more extensively when PVE developed within the first year postoperatively, especially when caused by staphylococci, than when PVE occurred later than 1 year postoperatively.[48,51]

Microbiology

The microbiologic cause of PVE depends on whether the infection occurs early ($\leq$ 2 months) after cardiac valve replacement, after an intermediate period (2 to 12 months), or later ($\geq$ 12 months postoperatively). Approximately 40% to 60% of early-onset PVE is caused by staphylococci; *S. epidermidis* or other coagulase-negative staphylococci account for 30% to 35% of cases, and *S. aureus* accounts for 20% to 25%.[18,23,47,52-56] The remaining cases of early-onset infection are caused most often by gram-negative bacilli, diphtheroids, or fungi.[18,23,47,52-56] From 2 to 12 months, the distribution of microorganisms is similar to early-onset PVE except that the portion of infections caused by enteric gram-negative bacilli and diphtheroids is reduced greatly, and the frequency of streptococcal and enterococcal PVE is increased. PVE that occurs after 1 year postoperatively is caused by the same spectrum of microorganisms that causes community-acquired NVE except that coagulase-negative staphylococcal infection occurs more commonly (approximately 10% to 12% of cases) in PVE than in NVE.[13,39,57]

Most studies of coagulase-negative staphylococcal PVE have not reported the specific species. Cases occurring within 1 year postoperatively most often are caused by *S. epidermidis,* and 84% to 87% of these cases are methicillin resistant.[13,57] In contrast, at least 50% of coagulase-negative staphylococci that cause PVE more than 1 year postoperatively are a species other than *S. epidermidis,* and the frequency of methicillin resistance ranges from 22% to 30%.[13,57]

The microbial spectrum and susceptibility in vitro suggest that most cases of PVE that develop within 2 months postoperatively are nosocomially acquired, whereas cases that occur from 2 to 12 months are a mix of nosocomial and community-acquired infections, and cases that occur more than 1 year postoperatively are primarily community-acquired infections.

Diagnosis

The diagnosis of PVE depends on the clinical features of PVE, the laboratory findings, and the results of TEE. In the absence of operative or postmortem findings of PVE, there is no one specific test that is diagnostic of PVE.

Clinical Features

At least 95% of patients with PVE or NVE have fever. Otherwise, the signs and symptoms of PVE may differ from those of patients with NVE. In cases of early-onset PVE, especially when caused by staphylococci, the clinical findings often are related to the effects of sepsis and periannular extension of infection, such as shock, heart failure, myocardial conduction abnormalities, and peripheral emboli, particularly

those to the central nervous system (CNS).[18,54,55] Patients with late-onset PVE may present with a subacute or chronic course and may show classic peripheral stigmata of endocarditis, such as Osler nodes, Janeway lesions, and Roth spots. Late-onset PVE caused by *S. aureus* may resemble early-onset PVE with sepsis, shock, heart failure, and complications of perivalvular extension of infection. Early-onset or late-onset *S. aureus* PVE usually is a severe acute infection; stroke, hemorrhagic cerebritis, peripheral abscess formation, and intracardiac complications occur in at least 40% of patients.[55,58-60] Peripheral embolic events occur commonly in patients with PVE regardless of the microbiologic cause.[43-45] The overall frequency of clinically detectable emboli is approximately 40%, and CNS emboli occur in 20% to 40% of patients.[52,53,58,60,61]

In 1994, Durack and colleagues[62] proposed the Duke criteria for the diagnosis of patients with NVE. These criteria use echocardiographic findings together with a combination of major and minor criteria for the diagnosis. These criteria also may be used for the diagnosis of PVE.[63,64] *S. aureus* PVE may present with shock and heart failure without other typical manifestations of infectious endocarditis.[65] In these patients, TEE may be especially useful in the diagnosis of *S. aureus* PVE.[58,66,67] In patients suspected of having PVE who do not meet the Duke criteria for diagnosis, it is important to follow these patients carefully and use the Duke criteria and echocardiography during the period of observation.

Laboratory Diagnosis

Nonspecific laboratory findings, such as anemia, leukocytosis, elevated erythrocyte sedimentation rate, and elevated C-reactive protein, are often present in patients with PVE. In a patient with suspected PVE, a positive blood culture is essential to establish the accurate microbiologic diagnosis. In patients who have not received antimicrobial therapy, blood cultures are positive in at least 90% of patients. Similar to NVE, bacteremia usually is continuous in patients with PVE. Patients with a prosthetic cardiac valve who have *S. aureus* bacteremia in the early postoperative period or bacteremia that is community acquired always should be suspected of having PVE even in the absence of clinical findings suggesting PVE. In patients with a prosthetic cardiac valve, the recovery of microorganisms from blood cultures must be interpreted in the context of the clinical status of the patient. In the early postoperative period, gram-negative bacillary bacteremia may occur as the result of wound infection, urinary tract infection, presence of a urinary catheter, or other sources, but such bacteremia uncommonly causes PVE.[41] In these patients, if bacteremia or other signs of infection disappear promptly with antibiotic therapy, PVE is unlikely. If bacteremia persists or relapses after completion of a course of effective antimicrobial therapy, however, and no other source is identified, PVE is likely.

In the early postoperative period, patients may have a single or sporadic blood culture positive for microorganisms that are common blood culture contaminants, such as coagulase-negative staphylococci or diphtheroids. These organisms, especially coagulase-negative staphylococci, are common causes of early-onset or late-onset PVE. The diagnosis of PVE may become clear only later. In these patients, it is especially important to repeat blood cultures off antibiotic therapy, if possible, and to perform TEE. *S. epidermidis* PVE usually results from a single clone of microorganisms. Molecular evaluation of sporadically positive blood cultures that shows a single clone obtained from different blood cultures is unlikely to be a blood culture contaminant and is more likely PVE.[68]

The recovery of *A. defectiva* or *Granulicatella* species (nutritionally variant viridans streptococci) or a HACEK group microorganism from blood cultures is so suggestive of endocarditis, including late-onset PVE, that the mere appearance of these microorganisms in multiple blood cultures strongly suggests PVE.[66] These microorganisms are rarely contaminants of blood cultures. Similarly, community-acquired sustained viridans group streptococci or enterococcal bacteremia strongly suggest PVE. Viridans group streptococci in a single blood culture may be a contaminant, but contamination of blood cultures by enterococci is uncommon.

Culture-Negative Prosthetic Valve Endocarditis

Culture-negative PVE is more likely to be encountered in late-onset than early-onset PVE. True culture-negative PVE occurs in less than 5% of cases.[69-73] The most common cause of culture-negative PVE is the administration of antibiotics before obtaining blood cultures, which reduces the recovery rate of bacteria from blood by 35% to 40%.[69-73] The antimicrobial susceptibility of the organism and duration and nature of prior antimicrobial therapy affect the length of time blood cultures remain negative. In patients who have received partial or ineffective antimicrobial therapy and who are stable hemodynamically, it is preferable to delay the onset of antimicrobial therapy, observe the patient carefully, and repeat blood cultures.

Consultation with the microbiology laboratory should be done in all patients with suspected PVE whose blood cultures are negative. Some microorganisms, such as *A. defectiva, Granulicatella* species or the HACEK group, may be difficult to recover from routine blood culture systems. An extended period of incubation may be required. Special culture techniques enhance recovery of *Brucella* spp., *Bartonella* spp., and *Legionella* spp. Polymerase chain reaction performed on blood samples should be requested for *Tropheryma whippelii* and *Bartonella* spp. As experience with polymerase chain reaction on blood samples grows, this technique is likely to be helpful in the microbiologic diagnosis of PVE caused by other microorganisms.[74] Serologic testing for *Bartonella, Coxiella burnetii, Mycoplasma* spp., and *Chlamydia* spp. may be helpful in cases of culture-negative PVE.[75,76]

Cultures, histologic examination, and polymerase chain reaction performed on valvular tissue obtained at surgery or vegetations that have embolized to peripheral arteries may be useful in the microbiologic diagnosis of PVE. Standard blood cultures are negative in patients with *Aspergillus* PVE, and the diagnosis often is made by examination of a peripheral embolus.

Role of Echocardiography in the Diagnosis of Prosthetic Valve Endocarditis

TEE should be performed promptly in all patients with suspected PVE. Compared with transthoracic echocardiography, the TEE transducer is positioned in the esophagus, where it is in close physical proximity to the aortic root and septum, where most complications of perivalvular extension of infection of PVE occur. In patients with PVE, the detection of valvular vegetations and complications is substantially greater with TEE than with transthoracic echocardiography.[77-81] The sensitivity of detection of vegetations by TEE in patients with PVE was 86% to 94%, and specificity was 88% to 100%.[80,82-84] The preoperative presence of valvular dehiscence, abscess, or fistula

was detected in 87% of patients with TEE compared with 31% by transthoracic echocardiography.[83] The negative predictive value of TEE for PVE was 86% to 95%.[81,85-87] Patients with PVE and heart failure are considered candidates for urgent surgery. TEE is useful to identify whether the cause of heart failure is due to ventricular dysfunction rather than perivalvular extension of infection. The absence of perivalvular extension of infection detected by TEE identifies a subset of patients with PVE and heart failure who may respond favorably to medical therapy alone without surgical intervention. When the clinical suspicion of PVE is high, and the initial TEE does not show findings suggesting PVE, the TEE should be repeated within 1 week, and patients should be monitored by serial TEE and other laboratory tests to help establish the diagnosis.[66,77-89]

Antimicrobial Therapy

General Considerations

The management of patients with PVE depends on many factors. The most important of these are the microbiologic diagnosis and the functional hemodynamic status. TEE is used to assess the hemodynamic status, to identify complicating factors of PVE, and to monitor the patient for development of complications of PVE during antimicrobial therapy. This information determines whether patients may be treated successfully with medical therapy alone or with surgery combined with medical therapy.

All patients with PVE should be hospitalized initially. In patients who are stable hemodynamically, antimicrobial therapy should be withheld pending the results of blood cultures. In patients who have received suboptimal therapy and who are stable hemodynamically, it is preferable to delay the onset of antimicrobial therapy until a specific microbiologic diagnosis is identified. In patients with acute-onset PVE or in patients who are hemodynamically unstable, empirical antimicrobial therapy should be initiated immediately after obtaining three sets of blood cultures.

The choice of specific antimicrobial therapy for PVE is based on the specific etiologic microorganism and the results of in vitro susceptibility testing. Whenever possible, bactericidal therapy should be administered. The regimen should be administered for a minimum of 6 weeks. The suggested regimens for the treatment of PVE are shown in Tables 75-2 through 75-8.

Staphylococcal Prosthetic Valve Endocarditis. The therapy for staphylococcal PVE differs from that for staphylococcal NVE. In vitro studies, animal models of experimental infection, and clinical trials showed that regimens including rifampin are important for the treatment of staphylococcal foreign body infections.[48,57,90-93] Combinations includ-

TABLE 75-2 Therapy for Prosthetic Valve Endocarditis Caused by Staphylococci*

Regimen	Dosage and Route	Duration (wk)	Comments
Methicillin-Resistant Strains			
Vancomycin *plus*	15 mg/kg q12h in 2 equally divided doses	≥6	Initiate rifampin therapy on day 3 of therapy with vancomycin and gentamicin if susceptible to vancomycin and gentamicin, or on day 4-6 if resistant to gentamicin. Adjust vancomycin dosage to achieve 1-hour concentration in serum of 30-40 μg/mL and trough concentration of <12 μg/mL. See text for alternatives to gentamicin
Rifampin *plus*	300 mg PO or IV q8h	≥6	
Gentamicin[†]	3 mg/kg IM or IV single daily dose	2	
Methicillin-Susceptible Strains			
Nafcillin or oxacillin *plus*	2 g IV q4h	≥6	A first-generation cephalosporin may be substituted for nafcillin or oxacillin. Rifampin therapy should be initiated as above. Penicillin G, 24 million U/24 hr, may be used in place of nafcillin or oxacillin if strain is penicillin-susceptible (MIC ≤0.1 μg/mL) and does not produce β-lactamase
Rifampin *plus*	300 mg PO or IV q8h	≥6	
Gentamicin[†]	3 mg/kg IM or IV single daily dose	2	

*Dosages recommended are for patients with normal renal function.
[†]Gentamicin should be administered in close proximity to vancomycin, nafcillin, or oxacillin dose.
MIC, minimal inhibitory concentration.

TABLE 75-3 Therapy for Prosthetic Valve Endocarditis Caused by Viridans Streptococci, *Gemella* species, *Streptococcus agalactiae*, *Streptococcus pneumoniae*, *Streptococcus bovis*, *Abiotrophia defectiva*, or *Granulicatella* species*

Regimen	Dosage and Route	Duration (wk)	Comments
Penicillin-Susceptible Strain (MIC ≤ 0.1 µg/mL) of Viridans Streptococci, S. pneumoniae, S. bovis			
Either aqueous penicillin G *or*	12-18 million U/24 hr IV either continuously or in 6 divided doses	6	Penicillin or ceftriaxone together with gentamicin has not shown superior care rates compared with monotherapy with penicillin or ceftriaxone for patients with a highly susceptible strain. This regimen is preferred in most patients >65 years old or with impairment of eighth cranial nerve function. Gentamicin therapy should not be administered to patients with creatinine clearance 30 mL/min
Ceftriaxone	2 g once daily IV or IM	6	
With or without gentamicin[†]	3 mg/kg IM or IV single daily dose	2	
Vancomycin[‡]	15 mg/kg IV q12h in 2 equally divided doses	6	Vancomycin therapy is recommended only for patients unable to tolerate penicillin or ceftriaxone
Relatively or Fully Penicillin-Resistant Strain (MIC > 0.1 µg/mL) or **Gemella** species, **S. agalactiae**, **Abiotrophia defectiva**, **Granulicatella** species			
Either aqueous penicillin *or*	24 million U/24 hr IV either continuously or in 6 divided doses	6	
Ceftriaxone	2 g once daily IV or IM	6	
Plus gentamicin[†]	3 mg/kg IM or IV single daily dose	6	
Vancomycin[‡]	15 mg/kg q12h in 2 equally divided doses	6	Vancomycin therapy is recommended only for patients unable to tolerate penicillin or ceftriaxone

*Dosages recommended are for patients with normal renal function.
[†]Gentamicin should be administered in close proximity to the penicillin dose when penicillin therapy is administered in divided doses.
[‡]See Table 75-2 for appropriate dosing of vancomycin.
MIC, minimal inhibitory concentration.

ing rifampin are essential for the optimal treatment of staphylococcal PVE. Rifampin-resistant subpopulations of staphylococci may be encountered when there is a high density of microorganisms, such as occurs in PVE. Rifampin-resistant strains may be selected by the administration of ineffective rifampin-containing regimens.[48,92] We believe that rifampin therapy should not be initiated until therapy with two other antimicrobials known to be effective against the specific staphylococcus recovered from the patient with PVE has been administered for 2 days. If the staphylococcus is not susceptible to at least two other antimicrobials, therapy with a single effective agent should be administered for 3 to 5 days before initiation of rifampin therapy to reduce the staphylococcal population and the risk of selection of a rifampin-resistant subpopulation.

The antimicrobial therapy for staphylococcal PVE is based on in vitro susceptibility tests and not on the production of coagulase. The antimicrobial therapy for *S. aureus* PVE and coagulase-negative staphylococcal PVE is identical (Table 75-2). For methicillin-resistant staphylococcal PVE, therapy is initiated with vancomycin together with gentamicin, and rifampin is added to this regimen 2 days later if the isolate is susceptible to vancomycin and gentamicin. This triple-drug regimen is administered for the first 2 weeks of therapy. At the end of 2 weeks, gentamicin therapy is discontinued, and vancomycin together with rifampin is continued to complete at least a 6-week course of therapy. If the strain of staphylococcus is resistant to gentamicin and is susceptible to a fluoroquinolone and rifampin, a fluoroquinolone, such as moxifloxacin or gatifloxacin, may be administered in place of the aminoglycoside.[19,92-94] If the staphylococcus is susceptible to methicillin, nafcillin or a first-generation cephalosporin should be substituted for vancomycin in the combination regimen.

Streptococcal Prosthetic Valve Endocarditis. The regimens recommended[66,95] for treatment of viridans group streptococcal, *Streptococcus bovis, Streptococcus pneumoniae,* or other penicillin-susceptible streptococci are presented in Tables 75-3 and 75-4. In patients who can tolerate an aminoglycoside, gentamicin may be administered in a single daily dose for the first 2 weeks of therapy. If gentamicin therapy is relatively contraindicated, therapy should be administered for at least 6 weeks with penicillin, ceftriaxone, or vancomycin alone. For patients with PVE caused by a relatively or highly penicillin-resistant strain of streptococcus or by *Gemella* species, *Streptococcus agalactiae,* or *A. defectiva* or *Granulicatella* species, therapy should be administered with either penicillin or ceftriaxone combined with gentamicin for a minimum of 6 weeks (see Table 75-4). In patients who are unable to tolerate β-lactam therapy, monotherapy with vancomycin administered for at least 6 weeks is suggested. Short-course (2-week) therapy with a β-lactam combined with an aminoglycoside should not be administered to patients with streptococcal PVE.

Enterococcal Prosthetic Valve Endocarditis. Suggested regimens[19,95,96] for the treatment of enterococcal PVE are presented in Tables 75-5 through 75-7. A combination of penicillin, ampicillin, or vancomycin with an aminoglycoside is synergistic in vitro and in vivo against susceptible strains of enterococci. For patients with PVE caused by enterococci susceptible to penicillin and gentamicin, a combination

TABLE 75-4 Therapy for Prosthetic Valve Enterococcal Endocarditis Caused by Penicillin-Susceptible, Gentamicin-Resistant, Streptomycin-Susceptible, Vancomycin-Susceptible Strains*

Regimen	Dosage and Route	Duration (wk)	Comments
Either ampicillin *or*	2 g IV q4h	6	
Aqueous penicillin G* *plus*	18-30 million U/24 hr IV continuously or in 6 equally divided doses	6	
Streptomycin[†]	7.5 mg/kg IV or IM q12h	6	
Vancomycin[‡] *plus*	15 mg/kg IV q12h in 2 equally divided doses	6	
Streptomycin[†]	7.5 mg/kg IV or IM q12h	6	Vancomycin therapy recommended only for patients unable to tolerate penicillin or ampicillin

*Dosages suggested are for patients with normal renal function.
[†]See text for appropriate dosing of streptomycin.
[‡]See Table 75-2 for appropriate dosing of vancomycin.

TABLE 75-5 Therapy for Prosthetic Valve Enterococcal Endocarditis Caused by Penicillin-, Aminoglycoside-, Vancomycin-Susceptible Strains*

Regimen	Dosage and Route	Duration (wk)	Comments
Either ampicillin *or*	2 g IV q4h	6	
Aqueous penicillin G *plus*	18-30 million U/24 hr IV either continuously or in 6 divided doses	6	
Gentamicin[†]	1 mg/kg IV or IM q8h	6	
Vancomycin[‡] *plus*	15 mg/kg q12h IV in 2 equally divided doses	6	
Gentamicin[†]	1 mg/kg IV or IM q8h	6	Vancomycin therapy recommended only for patients unable to tolerate penicillin or ampicillin

*Dosages suggested for patients with normal renal function.
[†]The dosage of gentamicin should be adjusted to achieve a peak concentration in serum of approximately 3 μg/mL and a trough concentration of ≤1 mg/mL (see text). Dosage should be administered in close proximity to penicillin, ampicillin, or vancomycin dose.
[‡]See Table 75-2 for appropriate dosing of vancomycin.

of penicillin or ampicillin with gentamicin should be administered for 6 weeks (Table 75-5). Patients who are unable to tolerate β-lactams should be treated with vancomycin with gentamicin for 6 weeks. In contrast to patients with penicillin-susceptible streptococcal infection, gentamicin should not be administered in a single daily dose. For enterococcal PVE, gentamicin therapy should be administered every 8 hours in patients with normal renal function.[95,96] Concentrations of gentamicin in serum should be adjusted to achieve a 1-hour concentration of approximately 3 μg/mL and a trough concentration of less than 1 μg/mL.[96] Increasing the dose of gentamicin in these patients does not result in enhanced killing of enterococci and may result in an increased risk of nephrotoxicity.[96]

Multidrug-resistant strains of enterococci are increasing in frequency, and these strains may cause PVE. Tables 75-6 and 75-7 present suggested regimens for patients with PVE caused by antimicrobial-resistant enterococci. Approximately one third of high-level gentamicin-resistant (≥500 μg of gentamicin/mL) strains are susceptible in vitro to high levels of streptomycin (<2000 μg of streptomycin/mL),[96,97] and susceptibility at this level predicts synergism. All strains of enterococci recovered from patients with enterococcal PVE should be screened for susceptibility to gentamicin and streptomycin. If the strain is gentamicin resistant but streptomycin susceptible, streptomycin therapy may be combined with penicillin, ampicillin, or vancomycin for at least 6 weeks (see Table 75-6). The dosage of streptomycin should be adjusted to obtain a 1-hour concentration in serum of 20 to 30 μg/mL and a trough concentration less than 10 μg/mL.[96] Table 75-6 presents recommended regimens for the treatment of enterococcal PVE caused by penicillin-resistant, aminoglycoside-susceptible, and vancomycin-susceptible strains. Table 75-7 presents therapy suggested for multidrug-resistant enterococcal PVE. Patients with PVE caused by multidrug-resistant enterococci should be managed in consultation with an infectious diseases specialist and with the microbiology laboratory. A few reported cases of

multidrug-resistant enterococcal endocarditis were treated successfully with linezolid, quinupristin/dalfopristin, or a combination of imipenem/cilastatin and ampicillin.[98-100] Treatment failures also have been reported.[98-101] Patients with multidrug-resistant enterococcal PVE should undergo cardiac valve replacement combined with a long (at least 8 weeks) course of postoperative antimicrobial therapy.

HACEK Prosthetic Valve Endocarditis. HACEK PVE may be treated with the regimens presented in Table 75-8. Patients who are stable hemodynamically and with no evidence of valvular dysfunction may be treated successfully with antimicrobial therapy alone.[66]

Diphtheroid Prosthetic Valve Endocarditis. Diphtheroids may cause early-onset or late-onset PVE. β-Lactam–susceptible, gentamicin-susceptible strains of diphtheroids should be treated with a combination of penicillin or ampicillin with gentamicin for at least 6 weeks. The gentamicin dosage is the same as the dosage for patients with enterococcal PVE. In patients with penicillin-resistant or gentamicin-resistant diphtheroids or in patients who are unable to tolerate a β-lactam, monotherapy with vancomycin administered for at least 6 weeks is suggested.

Enteric Gram-Negative Bacillary Prosthetic Valve Endocarditis. The treatment of PVE caused by gram-negative bacilli is determined by the results of in vitro susceptibility testing. A combination of effective agents, such as a β-lactam with a fluoroquinolone, should be administered for at least 6 weeks. Patients with PVE caused by a multidrug-resistant gram-negative bacillus or by *Pseudomonas* spp. should be treated surgically with valve excision together with antimicrobial therapy.

Fungal Prosthetic Valve Endocarditis. Fungal PVE usually is caused by *Candida* spp. or *Aspergillus* spp. Medical therapy alone does not result in cure of fungal PVE. Patients with fungal PVE should undergo surgery followed by a long postoperative course of antifungal therapy. Historically, amphotericin B was considered to be the drug of choice for most cases of fungal PVE. In recent years, however, many

TABLE 75-6 Therapy for Prosthetic Valve Enterococcal Endocarditis Caused by Penicillin-Resistant, Aminoglycoside-Susceptible, Vancomycin-Susceptible Strains*

Regimen	Dosage and Route	Duration (wk)	Comments
β-Lactamase–Producing Strain			
Ampicillin-sulbactam *plus*	3 g IV q6h	6	
Gentamicin[†]	1 mg/kg IV or IM q8h	6	
Vancomycin[‡] *plus*	15 mg/kg IV q12h in 2 equally divided doses	6	Vancomycin therapy is recommended only for patients unable to tolerate ampicillin-sulbactam
Gentamicin[†]	1 mg/kg IV or IM q8h	6	
Intrinsic Penicillin Resistance			
Vancomycin[‡] *plus*	15 mg/kg IV q12h in 2 equally divided doses	6	
Gentamicin[†]	1 mg/kg IM or IV q8h	6	

*Dosages suggested are for patients with normal renal function.
[†]See text and Table 75-3 for appropriate dosing of gentamicin.
[‡]See Table 75-2 for appropriate dosing of vancomycin.

TABLE 75-7 Therapy for Prosthetic Valve Enterococcal Endocarditis Caused by Penicillin-, Aminoglycoside-, Vancomycin-Resistant Strains*

Regimen	Dosage and Route	Duration (wk)	Comments
β-Lactamase–Producing Strain			
Linezolid *or*	600 mg q12h PO or IV	≥ 8	Patients with endocarditis caused by these strains should be treated with infectious diseases and microbiology consultation. Cardiac valve replacement is necessary for bacteriologic cure. Severe, usually reversible thrombocytopenia may occur with linezolid therapy, especially after 2 weeks of therapy. Synercid is effective only against *Enterococcus faecium* and may be associated with severe myalgias, which may require discontinuation of therapy. There are only a few patients reported treated with imipenem/cilastatin-ampicillin.
Quinupristin-dalfopristin (Synercid) *or*	7.5 mg/kg IV q8h	≥8	
Imipenem/cilastatin *plus*	500 mg IV q6h	≥8	
Ampicillin sodium	2 g IV q4h	≥8	

*Dosages suggested are for patients with normal renal function.

antifungal compounds have been introduced that are at least as or more effective than amphotericin B and are associated with less toxicity. Lipid-containing preparations of amphotericin B, such as AmBisome and Abelcet, usually are better than amphotericin B in these patients. Other agents may be used, but clinical experience is limited. The choice of an individual agent depends on the species recovered and in vitro susceptibility tests. *Candida* spp. usually are susceptible to amphotericin B, fluconazole, caspofungin, or voriconazole, whereas *Aspergillus* spp. often are susceptible to amphotericin, caspofungin, or voriconazole. After cardiac valve replacement, a long course of postoperative therapy should be administered. Because of the tendency for fungal PVE to relapse despite appropriate therapy, some authorities suggest oral suppressive therapy with an antifungal agent, such as fluconazole or voriconazole, administered for an indefinite period, possibly lifelong. In patients with fungal PVE who are not considered surgical candidates, long-term suppressive therapy with an orally administered antifungal agent, such as fluconazole, has been suggested.[102-105]

Empirical Therapy

It may be necessary to begin empirical therapy for PVE in patients with acute-onset infection or with persistent culture-negative PVE. If the onset of PVE in these patients is less than 12 months from the time of surgery, therapy should be initiated with vancomycin, gentamicin, and rifampin. Gentamicin therapy may be discontinued after the first 2 weeks of therapy. If the onset of PVE is more than 12 months from the time of surgery, infection usually is caused by streptococci, enterococci, coagulase-negative staphylococci, or a HACEK group microorganism. In these patients, ceftriaxone therapy should be added to vancomycin, gentamicin, and rifampin. Because of the possibility of enterococcal or penicillin-resistant streptococcal PVE, gentamicin should be continued throughout the entire 6 weeks of treatment.

Surgical Treatment

General Considerations

Historically the mortality rate of patients with PVE was high—10% to 70%—despite administration of effective antimicrobial therapy, improved surgical techniques, and technologic advances in the management of critically ill patients.[18,19,39,106-109] More recent studies report lower mortality from PVE—4% to 20%.[28,66,110-115] Onset of infection within 1 year from the time of cardiac valve replacement, staphylococcal PVE, aortic position, patients with heart failure, and patients who are treated medically as opposed to with combined medical and surgical therapy have associated high mortality rates.[108,116-119] There is considerable debate about the selection of patients for medical compared with surgical therapy. Some authorities recommend surgical therapy for all patients with mechanical valve PVE.[120] Some studies report higher survival rates in surgically treated patients compared with patients treated with antibiotics alone.[108,120] Other studies report, however, that carefully selected patients may be treated medically with survival rates similar to patients treated surgically.[120-122] The decision to treat patients with PVE medically or surgically is individualized for each patient. In general, patients with complicated PVE should be treated surgically.

Complicated Prosthetic Valve Endocarditis

Perivalvular Extension of Infection. Most of the common serious complications of PVE result from extension of infection into the perivalvular or adjacent myocardial tissue. Perivalvular extension is considered more likely to occur in the aortic position than in the mitral position.[44,123-126] Perivalvular infection involving a mechanical prosthesis often results in valvular dehiscence with resultant valvular regurgitation and heart failure. Myocardial abscess may develop. Most patients with myocardial abscess require surgical intervention.[19,28,42,109,120] Some patients with myocardial abscess remain stable

TABLE 75-8 Therapy for Prosthetic Valve Endocarditis Due to HACEK* Microorganisms†

Regimen	Dosage and Route	Duration (wk)	Comments
Ceftriaxone *or*	2 g once daily IV or IM	6	Cefotaxime or other third-generation or fourth-generation cephalosporin may be substituted
Ampicillin-sulbactam	3 g IV q6h	6	
Ciprofloxacin‡	750 mg PO or 400 mg IV q12h	6	Recommended only for patients unable to tolerate cephalosporin or ampicillin therapy. Levofloxacin, gatifloxacin, or moxifloxacin in equivalent dosages may be substituted

Haemophilus parainfluenzae, Haemophilus aphrophilus, Actinobacillus actinomycetemcomitans, Cardiobacterium hominis, Eikenella corrodens, and *Kingella kingae.*
†Dosages suggested for patients with normal renal function.
‡Fluoroquinolones are highly active in vitro against HACEK microorganisms. There are minimal published data on the use of fluoroquinolone therapy for endocarditis caused by HACEK.

clinically and hemodynamically, however, and respond to medical therapy alone.[19,28,42,88,109,120] These patients should be monitored closely with serial TEE.[88,109] Perivalvular extension of infection also may result in prolonged fever and intermittently or consistently positive blood cultures despite administration of appropriate antibiotic therapy.

Heart Failure. Heart failure is the most common life-threatening complication of PVE and usually results from perivalvular extension and valvular dehiscence.[19,28,39,42,107,109,120] Patients with minimal or mild heart failure may respond to medical therapy alone. Patients with severe heart failure and patients with mild or moderate heart failure not responsive promptly to medical therapy should be considered candidates for urgent surgical intervention. Delay in surgery in an attempt to stabilize heart failure or to prolong a preoperative course of antibiotic therapy increases mortality and does not reduce the rate of postoperative infection.[19,127] Patients with moderate-to-severe heart failure due to valvular dehiscence rarely survive more than a few months unless they undergo surgery.[46,117,128]

Valvular Obstruction or Leaflet Destruction. PVE involving mechanical valves affects the perivalvular area. In some cases of mechanical valve PVE, large vegetations develop in the perivalvular area and may extend downward into the outflow tract of the prosthesis, resulting in mechanical obstruction or impairment of valve closure, resulting in valvular insufficiency. Bioprosthetic PVE begins on the surface of the cusp, resulting in vegetation formation and damage or perforation to the leaflets. Patients with obstruction, insufficiency, or valvular perforation should be treated surgically.[19,42,44]

Conduction Abnormalities. Newly developed conduction abnormalities result from perivalvular extension of infection, which involves the myocardial conduction system and is an indication for surgery. Preoperatively, insertion of a temporary pacemaker may be necessary. It is preferable to sterilize the blood before insertion of the temporary pacemaker to reduce the likelihood of pacemaker infection, which may cause infection of the newly inserted prosthesis. In patients with PVE who require urgent surgery, however, this may not be possible. If the pacemaker is inserted before control of sepsis or sterilization of the blood, the pacemaker should be removed, if technically possible, after surgery for PVE and preferably not reinserted until after 24 to 48 hours of antimicrobial therapy. After completion of antimicrobial therapy in surgically treated patients who require a pacemaker, follow-up blood cultures and TEE should be performed at 1- and 2-month intervals or earlier if necessary to ensure that neither the pacemaker nor the valvular prosthesis is infected.

Multiple Emboli. In NVE, multiple emboli that occur despite the administration of effective antimicrobial therapy are considered an indication for cardiac valve replacement.[66,109,129] The rate of embolization from NVE diminishes during antimicrobial therapy, especially during the first 2 weeks of therapy.[129] Such studies on the effect of antimicrobial therapy on the rate of embolization in PVE have not been published. Similar to patients with NVE, patients with PVE who have recurrent systemic embolization despite appropriate antibiotic therapy should be considered candidates for prompt surgical intervention.[66,109]

Microbiology. PVE that develops during the first year after surgery most often is caused by coagulase-negative staphylococci, especially *S. epidermidis* or *S. aureus*. The mortality resulting from staphylococcal PVE treated with medical therapy alone is 42% to 100%.[47,53,55,109,119,130,131] Most authorities believe that *S. aureus* or *Staphylococcus lugdunensis* PVE and early-onset, coagulase-negative staphylococcal PVE are by themselves indications for surgical therapy.[19,42,58,108,109,132]

Rarely, in our experience, patients with *S. aureus* or *S. lugdunensis* PVE or early-onset, coagulase-negative staphylococcal PVE may not develop significant perivalvular extension of infection or valvular dehiscence and may respond to antimicrobial therapy alone. These patients should be monitored closely with serial TEE and require close follow-up after completion of antimicrobial therapy for signs of relapse of infection or valvular dehiscence.

Most patients with early-onset PVE caused by enteric gram-negative bacilli, especially if due to *P. aeruginosa*, should be treated surgically. Medical therapy alone may be successful for patients with infection caused by a highly susceptible gram-negative bacillus, such as members of the HACEK group, and for patients who are stable clinically and echocardiographically. Similar to patients with staphylococcal PVE, these patients should be followed closely after completion of antimicrobial therapy. Patients with PVE caused by multiple antibiotic–resistant, gram-negative bacilli; vancomycin-resistant or aminoglycoside-resistant enterococci; or other multidrug-resistant organisms should be treated surgically.

PVE caused by fungi, most often *Candida* spp. or *Aspergillus* spp., is considered an indication for surgery.[19,106] Cure of fungal PVE does not seem to be possible without surgical removal of the infected prosthesis and thorough surgical débridement. Q fever and *Brucella* PVE also are considered indications for surgery.

Late-onset PVE most often is community acquired and is caused by the same spectrum of microorganisms that cause NVE in non–injection drug users, such as viridans group streptococci, other streptococci, enterococci, coagulase-negative staphylococci, and HACEK group microorganisms. Perivalvular extension of infection occurs less often in association with late-onset PVE caused by these microorganisms, and patients without complications respond satisfactorily to medical therapy alone.[19,42,66,88,107,109,120]

Persistent Sepsis. Patients with persistently positive blood cultures after 5 or more days of appropriate antibiotic therapy or patients with other signs of persistent sepsis should undergo surgery promptly. Persistent sepsis suggests the presence of extensive perivalvular infection, myocardial abscess, or infection caused by a highly resistant microorganism, such as *P. aeruginosa*, or a microorganism slowly responsive to antimicrobial therapy. Prolongation of antimicrobial therapy preoperatively in these patients does not result in control of infection, complicates the surgical procedure, limits surgical options, and increases mortality.[19,28,42,107,109] In patients with culture-negative PVE, persistent signs of infection, such as prolonged fever or hemodynamic instability, despite antimicrobial therapy are an indication for surgery. Cultures of vegetations or abscess material obtained during surgery may identify the causative microorganism and enhance the likelihood that specific, effective antimicrobial therapy may be administered postoperatively to these patients.

Relapse of Prosthetic Valve Endocarditis. Relapse of PVE, especially if caused by staphylococci or enteric gram-negative bacilli, should be considered an indication for surgery. Even in cases of nonstaphylococcal PVE that have relapsed after a course of appropriate antimicrobial therapy, it is unlikely that a repeat course of antibiotics would eradicate infection successfully without surgery.[19,42,66,109]

Transesophageal Echocardiography

TEE is an essential component in the management of patients with PVE. TEE is a sensitive method to identify patients who require surgery, such as patients with heart failure, perivalvular extension of infection, myocardial abscess, valvular dehiscence, obstruction, or perforation.[66,88,109] Alternatively, TEE findings may identify selected patients without complications who may respond to medical therapy alone.[66,88,109] In patients with heart failure, TEE is useful to determine whether heart failure is caused by ventricular dysfunction or valvular dehiscence. Patients with heart failure due to ventricular dysfunction may respond to medical therapy, whereas patients with heart failure caused by valvular dehiscence require surgery. In patients who are candidates for medical therapy alone, TEE should be performed weekly to detect the early development of complications. In surgically treated patients, serial TEE is performed postoperatively for early detection of complications, such as the development of heart failure or valvular dehiscence. TEE should be performed at 1- and 2-month intervals after completion of treatment for PVE to assess valvular and cardiac function.

Indications for and Timing of Surgery

Based on the aforementioned complicating factors, Table 75-9 lists criteria for surgery in patients with PVE. In general, patients with any

TABLE 75-9 Indications for Surgery in Patients with Prosthetic Valve Endocarditis

Severe heart failure; mild-to-moderate heart failure not responsive to medical therapy
Valvular dehiscence, obstruction, or leaflet perforation
Large myocardial abscess or myocardial abscess that increases in size during therapy
Newly developed conduction defects
Specific microorganisms
    Staphylococcus aureus
    Staphylococcus lugdunensis
    Coagulase-negative staphylococci—early onset (≤1 year from surgery)
    Fungi
    Multidrug-resistant gram-negative bacilli, gram-positive microorganisms, or enterococci
    Pseudomonas aeruginosa or other *Pseudomonas* spp.
    Coxiella burnetii, *Brucella* spp.
Relapse of infection after adequate therapy
Uncontrolled infection—intermittent or persistent positive blood cultures after ≥5 days of appropriate antimicrobial therapy
Culture-negative prosthetic valve endocarditis unresponsive to antimicrobial therapy
Multiple (>1) systemic emboli despite appropriate antimicrobial therapy

TABLE 75-11 Timing of Surgery for Prosthetic Valve Endocarditis

Urgent— ≤24 hours	1-7 days	>7 days
Severe heart failure	Moderate heart failure	Late development of heart failure caused by valvular dysfunction
	Mild heart failure unresponsive to medical therapy	
Acute valvular dysfunction	Subacute valvular dysfunction	Multiple (>1) systemic emboli. See text for CNS emboli
Unstable hemo-dynamically	Heart block Microorganism requiring surgery (see Table 75-9) Multiple (>1) systemic emboli. See text for CNS emboli	

CNS, central nervous system

one or a combination of these complications should undergo prompt surgical intervention combined with antimicrobial therapy. These indications for surgery are relative rather than absolute, and the decision for surgical intervention should be individualized for each patient. Table 75-10 lists patients who may respond satisfactorily to medical therapy alone. Patients treated medically without surgical intervention should be monitored carefully, however, for the development of complications during therapy, such as heart failure and valvular dehiscence. If complications occur, these patients should undergo surgery promptly.

Table 75-11 provides guidelines for the timing of surgery in patients with PVE. The hemodynamic status of the patient is the most important factor in determining the timing of surgery. The operative mortality is proportional to the degree of preoperative heart failure, hemodynamic instability, and renal or other organ dysfunction.[49,107,108,116,133] Prolonging antibiotic therapy in these patients does not reduce the risk of postoperative PVE or improve survival.[49,107-109,134] Patients with severe heart failure, patients who are unstable hemodynamically, and patients with severe acute valvular dysfunction should undergo urgent surgery regardless of the duration of preoperative antimicrobial therapy. The risk of postoperative PVE in these patients is surprisingly low even in patients with positive blood cultures on the day of surgery.[127] Among patients with indications for surgery who do not require urgent intervention, it is preferable to stabilize other acute comorbid conditions preoperatively that independently may increase surgical mortality, such as uncontrolled diabetes mellitus, nonvalvular cardiac conditions, or acute renal or respiratory failure. Surgery for PVE should be performed as soon as possible after these conditions are stabilized. If comorbid conditions do not respond promptly

to therapy, however, surgery should not be delayed because delay does not improve outcome and is associated with a higher surgical mortality.[49,107-109,116] Other patients with indications for surgery (see Table 75-9) who respond satisfactorily to medical therapy and remain stable hemodynamically require surgery later. In these patients, it is desirable to administer 1 week or more of antimicrobial therapy preoperatively to treat possible metastatic infections, which, if undiagnosed and untreated, may result in reinfection of the newly implanted prosthetic valvular prosthesis.

Type of Surgery for Prosthetic Valve Endocarditis

The decision to perform surgery in patients with PVE is complex and multifactorial. The surgery itself is highly complex, is technically demanding, and requires exceptional skill and experience from the surgical team. An extensive, thorough surgical débridement of all infected material and drainage of abscess are imperative before reconstruction and valvular reimplantation to reduce the risk of postoperative infection of the newly implanted prosthesis. Complex, elaborate reconstruction of the aortic valvular root, mitral valve, and supporting structures may be required depending on the extent of infection. Many different surgical options have been described,[28,120,135-138] including patch closure of annular or aortic leaflets and suture of the mechanical valve prosthesis to the patch,[139] supracoronary artery placement of the prosthetic valve with closure of the coronary ostia and bypass grafting,[140] composite prosthetic valve conduit replacement and reimplantation of the coronary ostia,[141] the Ross procedure,[142,143] and aortic root replacement with cryopreserved allograft.[28,114,136-138] Studies have shown that the use of cryopreserved allografts for surgical treatment of PVE in the aortic position has advantages over other surgical techniques.[28,137,138] The allograft is a biologic material that may be more resistant to infection than mechanical prostheses or procedures that require Dacron fabric grafting.[28,137] Because of the contiguous aortic wall and the anterior mitral valve leaflet contained in aortic allografts, complex annular defects are reconstructed more easily after trimming the allograft to conform to the residual defect.[28,137] The use of cryopreserved aortic allografts may have some disadvantages. The durability of aortic valve allografts reportedly is less than that of a mechanical prosthesis and similar to that of a xenograft valve prosthesis.[28,137,144] The development of significant aortic valve regurgitation after 5 years following allograft insertion has been reported.[28,137] Other authors have reported longer durability of allografts.[145-147] Heart block requiring a permanent pacemaker was reported in approximately one third of patients with aortic valve PVE treated with cryopreserved allograft.[28] This complication of allograft surgery resulted from the need for radical surgical débridement to remove perivalvular extension of infection.

TABLE 75-10 Patients with Prosthetic Valve Endocarditis Who Are Candidates for Medical Therapy without Surgical Intervention

Mild heart failure responsive to medical therapy
Stable hemodynamically and echocardiographically with no evidence of valvular dysfunction
Susceptible microorganisms
Viridans group streptococci or other streptococci
Enterococci
HACEK* group
Coagulase-negative staphylococci—late onset (>1 year after surgery)

Haemophilus parainfluenzae, Haemophilus aphrophilus, Actinobacillus actinomycetemcomitans, Cardiobacterium hominis, Eikenella corrodens, and *Kingella kingae.*

In desperate situations in which all other therapeutic options to treat PVE have failed, heart transplantation should be considered only as a last resort. Active bacterial infection is considered to be a contraindication to heart transplantation because of the risk of severe uncontrolled infection resulting from immunosuppressive therapy required in heart transplantation. Two cases of successful heart transplantation in patients with intractable PVE caused by microorganisms with relatively low virulence (viridans group streptococci and *Mycoplasma pneumoniae*) were reported.[148,149]

Outcome of Patients Treated Surgically for Prosthetic Valve Endocarditis

Mortality associated with surgical treatment using a mechanical or xenograft valve reportedly ranges from 10% to 50%—figures remarkably low considering a virtual 100% mortality in complicated PVE treated medically.[49,51,112,113,139,150-154] More recent studies have shown improved survival rates with the use of cryopreserved aortic allografts. Sabik and co-workers[28] reported a hospital mortality of only 4%. These authors reported an almost identical survival rate among patients who underwent aortic valve replacement for noninfectious indications.[28] The long-term risk of recurrence of PVE seems to be lower with the use of cryopreserved aortic allograft—5% at 10 years—compared with the risk after the use of mechanical or xenograft valves—15% to 18%.[113,136-138] After mechanical valve implantation, approximately 18% to 26% of patients require reoperation because of sterile prosthesis dehiscence.[49,51,112] The need for reoperation because of valvular deterioration in cryopreserved allografts was discussed previously.

Other Considerations Related to Surgery

Hemorrhagic CNS emboli complicate the surgical management of PVE. Patients who undergo cardiac valve replacement are placed on cardiopulmonary bypass and anticoagulation therapy. In patients with a recent CNS embolus, cardiopulmonary bypass and anticoagulation therapy may result in extension of an intracranial hemorrhage, which is associated with significant morbidity and mortality.[121] If cardiac hemodynamics permit, surgery for PVE in these patients may be done safely 4 weeks after cerebral infarction. If surgery is performed within 1 week after infarction, the frequency of neurologic deterioration is 40% compared with 10% if surgery is performed 15 to 21 days after cerebral infarction.[121] The use of a bioprosthesis that does not require long-term anticoagulant therapy is preferable to a mechanical valve in these patients.

Duration of Antimicrobial Therapy Postoperatively

The regimens and duration of therapy for patients with PVE are presented in Tables 75-2 through 75-8. The duration of postoperative antimicrobial therapy is based on the following: (1) operative findings, including pathology and the results of surgical cultures; (2) extracardiac infection (e.g., CNS or disk space infection); and (3) duration of preoperative antimicrobial therapy. Patients who undergo urgent surgery or patients with histopathologic indicators of acute infection or positive cultures of vegetations or abscess should receive a full course of antibiotics postoperatively. Patients with nonemergency surgery with no evidence of acute infection histopathologically and with negative operative cultures or patients with extracardiac infection should receive a course of antimicrobial therapy that when combined with the duration of preoperative therapy equals or exceeds the usual total duration of antibiotic therapy shown in Tables 75-2 through 75-8. Patients who have completed a full course of therapy preoperatively and have no evidence of active infection at surgery and no evidence of extracardiac infection should receive a short course of antimicrobial therapy postoperatively. Patients with fungal PVE who undergo surgery probably should receive lifelong, orally administered suppressive antifungal therapy.

Anticoagulation Therapy

Patients with most types of mechanical valvular prostheses require anticoagulation for the prevention of thromboemboli. Anticoagulation therapy should be continued in patients with PVE involving a mechanical prosthesis. This therapy reduced the frequency of stroke or hemorrhagic events in patients with PVE.[155,156] When anticoagulant therapy was discontinued, the frequency of CNS complications was nine times higher than in patients who continued to receive anticoagulation.[156] Patients with a bioprosthetic valvular prosthesis usually do not require anticoagulation. Similar to patients with NVE, anticoagulants should not be initiated in patients with bioprosthetic valve PVE, unless there are other independent medical conditions, such as a deep venous thrombosis, that require anticoagulation. Anticoagulant therapy per se does not have a therapeutic benefit in patients with endocarditis.[157,158]

If CNS emboli occur in patients with PVE, a bland infarct may develop into a hemorrhagic infarct, which may extend in size if anticoagulant therapy is continued. In these patients, anticoagulation should be reversed until the patient stabilizes and there is no further extension of hemorrhage, at which time anticoagulation should be resumed cautiously with heparin or a drug that interferes with platelet function.[19,66,158] Warfarin (Coumadin) therapy may be resumed cautiously later during the course of treatment of PVE, provided that there are no further thromboembolic events and no evidence of extension of CNS hemorrhage.

Prognosis

The prognosis of patients with PVE has improved since the 1990s. This improved outcome is related to many factors, including the use of TEE for early identification of perivalvular extension of infection and other complications, such as heart failure and myocardial abscess; improved surgical techniques; early surgical intervention in patients with complicated PVE, especially that caused by *S. aureus*; the use of cryopreserved aortic allografts; more effective antimicrobial therapy, including the recognition of the need for multidrug therapy, especially in patients with staphylococcal PVE; and improvements in the management of critically ill patients hospitalized in intensive care units.

Mortality is higher in early-onset PVE than in late-onset infection.[25,47,53,55,119] The mortality of late-onset PVE caused by susceptible microorganisms, such as viridans group streptococci and HACEK microorganisms, is less than 20%.[18,19,39,66,107] Calderwood and associates[107] reported an overall survival rate of 77% in patients with PVE. In this report, mortality was associated significantly with the extension of perivalvular infection rather than the time of onset of PVE postoperatively. Other more recent studies[28,137] reported a mortality rate of less than 4%.

Improved survival has noted been especially in patients with *S. aureus* PVE. Without surgery, the mortality approaches 100%. With early surgical intervention, mortality rates of less than 10% to 30% have been reported.[25,28,51,150-152] The impact of early surgery on reduced mortality in patients with complicated PVE strongly suggests that patients with PVE are managed best in facilities with medical and surgical experience in the treatment of this infection.

Prevention

Administration of prophylactic antibiotics is recommended perioperatively in patients who undergo cardiac valve replacement surgery. The administration of a first-generation cephalosporin, such as cefazolin, is recommended. Vancomycin may be used in patients unable to tolerate cefazolin therapy. Additionally, in facilities where methicillin-resistant *S. aureus* is a common cause of postoperative wound infection, vancomycin prophylaxis should be considered either as monotherapy or in combination with cefazolin.

Patients with prosthetic cardiac valves are considered to be at high risk for the development of PVE as defined by the American Heart Association.[159] Patients with a cardiac valvular prosthesis should be given the American Heart Association card on prevention of endocarditis. They should be informed about the importance of maintaining good oral hygiene to reduce the risk of late-onset PVE caused by oral cavity microflora, such as viridans group streptococci and HACEK group microorganisms.

ELECTROPHYSIOLOGIC CARDIAC DEVICES

Cardiac pacemakers and implantable cardioverter defibrillators are two of the more commonly used nonvalvular cardiovascular devices. Pacemakers have been in use for more than 4 decades and implantable cardioverter defibrillators for approximately 2 decades. More recently, combination devices that include pacing and cardioverter defibrillator capabilities have been available for selected patients. In contrast to years ago, when sternotomy or thoracotomy was required for epicardial lead placement, transvenous lead placement is used in almost all patients who require these devices. This change has led to a marked reduction in insertion-related morbidity and avoidance of potentially life-threatening infectious complications of major cardiothoracic surgical interventions. Nevertheless, surgery still is required to implant the pacemaker generator or the defibrillator into the subcutaneous tissues of the chest or upper abdominal wall and can be complicated by local or "pocket site" infection.

Pacemaker-related and cardioverter defibrillator–related infections have been classified temporarily according to symptom onset and date of device implantation. The studies have varied, however, in their respective designations of infection, which have included early, intermediate, late, and delayed types of labeling. Device-related infection also has been divided into anatomic area of infection, generator or defibrillator pocket site, along the subcutaneous endovascular or intracardiac locations of the leads, or both with the currently used transvenous system.

The incidence of device-related infection has been wide ranging. Current surveys indicate that less than 6% of implanted pacemakers and cardioverter defibrillators become infected, and many of these series report an infection rate of less than 2%.

No case-control investigations that include multivariate analyses have been conducted to identify statistically risk factors associated with pacemaker or defibrillator infections. Risk factors have been linked to electrophysiologic cardiac device infection, however, and include host-related and implantation-related factors. Host-related factors include factors that can cause abnormalities in the immunologic or coagulation systems, such as the administration of immunosuppressive agents including corticosteroids, cancer, malnutrition, underlying chronic skin conditions, and diabetes mellitus. Several of these factors predispose to bacteremia or fungemia, which can contaminate the indwelling device secondarily. Anticoagulation use predisposes to infection and probably does so by supporting hematoma formation at the pocket site that houses the pacemaker generator or the cardioverter defibrillator. Recurrent surgical manipulation of the pocket site is probably the most important surgery-related risk factor for pocket site infection. This manipulation often is due to the need to replace the generator's battery. Prolonged operative time and a two-staged implantation procedure also have been linked to infection. Temporary transvenous pacing is another potential risk factor for infection. The number of leads placed has not been identified as a risk factor for infection.

Staphylococci account for most electrophysiologic cardiac device infections, regardless of the timing of onset of infection after device placement. The most common staphylococcal pathogen in case series has varied. In some reports, *S. aureus* is more prevalent; in other surveys, coagulase-negative staphylococci are predominant.

In vitro drug resistance to multiple classes of antibiotics, including β-lactamase–resistant penicillins (i.e., methicillin), has characterized many of the staphylococcal isolates. Other normal skin flora can produce device infection and include *Propionibacterium acnes* and *Micrococcus* spp. These latter organisms and coagulase-negative staphylococci frequently are identified as pathogens in the setting of late pocket site infection and generator or defibrillator mechanical erosion through the chest wall skin. Less commonly, aerobic gram-negative bacilli are identified as pathogens. *Candida* spp. can produce electrophysiologic device infection, although other fungi have been recovered infrequently.

There are three important clinical presentations of pacemaker-related or cardioverter defibrillator–related infection. The most common presentation is that of pocket site infection. Dermal and subcutaneous inflammatory changes develop locally over the pocket site and may be associated with systemic manifestations in a few patients. The second presentation is that of occult bacteremia or fungemia and no local changes at the pocket sites. Some of these patients may manifest little systemic toxicity. The third presentation is that of right-sided infective endocarditis. Patients usually are bacteremic or fungemic and have pleuritic chest pain and multiple focal pulmonary infiltrates or abscesses on chest radiographs.

Diagnosis of pacemaker or defibrillator infection is apparent when pocket site inflammatory changes are manifest. For some patients, the diagnosis is more difficult to confirm, however. Occult bacteremia or fungemia with no other evidence of infection should raise serious concerns of device infection. The diagnosis of device infection becomes more difficult when there is evidence of infection at an ectopic site (e.g., vertebral diskitis or osteomyelitis). The question is whether the ectopic site is the source of blood-stream infection or whether the ectopic infection site is the result of hematogenous seeding from an infected electrophysiologic device.

In addition to blood cultures, other tools can be used to establish a diagnosis of device infection. Ultrasound is helpful in showing fluid collection at the pocket site. Although some fluid can be present early after surgical implantation of the generator or defibrillator, fluid accumulation months to years after device placement would be uncommon. Ultrasound-directed percutaneous aspiration should be considered when the diagnosis of infection is suspected. Indium-tagged leukocyte or gallium scanning may be helpful in differentiating an inflammatory fluid collection versus a noninfected pocket site fluid collection.

Echocardiography has been pivotal in securing a diagnosis of device-related infective endocarditis. Infected vegetations on leads are visualized by echocardiography. The vegetations are not restricted to the tricuspid valve but can develop anywhere along the intracardiac course of the lead. The diagnostic superiority of TEE over transthoracic echocardiography has been substantiated in multiple studies. Chest radiographs and CT scans may provide indirect evidence of lead infection if radiologic evidence of septic pulmonary emboli is found. Occasionally the diagnosis of lead infection is considered initially only after these studies are obtained to evaluate pulmonary complaints.

The primary focus of treatment should be complete removal of the pacemaker or cardioverter defibrillator system. Although no prospective, randomized trials have been conducted to evaluate the role of medical (antimicrobial) therapy alone versus combined medical-surgical treatment with device removal, data from several retrospective analyses show a clear and clinically important advantage of complete device removal. Infection relapse rates and mortality have been reduced by device removal.

When considering device removal, three factors must be addressed. First, removal of a lead that is embedded in the cardiac tissue can be difficult and potentially dangerous. Complications include tamponade due to tearing or perforation of the myocardial wall, laceration of the superior vena cava, and life-threatening arrhythmias. Newer techniques, including the use of a locking stylet, photoablation of fibrous attachments with a laser sheath, and minimally invasive video-assisted thoracoscopic techniques, are less invasive, safer methods of device removal.

Second, in cases in which larger ($\geq$10 mm in diameter) vegetations are attached to infected leads, embolic showering of the pulmonary vasculature with lead extraction is a concern. Data from two more recent studies[160,161] indicate that although there is a risk of embolization, death due to this complication did not occur, and only 1 of 14 patients developed symptoms due to pulmonary embolism.

Third, ongoing electrophysiologic support is required in most patients. Timing of removal of the infected device and reimplantation of a new device is controversial. In most cases, a temporary system is used for several days so that antimicrobial agents can be given and blood-stream infection cleared before implantation of the new device.

Use of a percutaneous, transverse temporary system, at least with pacemakers, has been associated with increased risk of permanent pacemaker infection. Some now advocate single-staged exchange with infected device removal and implantation of a new device at the same setting.[162] If this is done, a new pocket site is mandatory.

There is a clinically important subgroup of patients who either do not require continued use of the electrophysiologic device after the infected pacemaker or defibrillator is removed or refuse placement of a new system. The percentage of patients who do not require the replacement of a pacemaker has ranged from 13% to 52%.[163-165] Infection is an important event that leads to patient refusal of new cardioverter defibrillator implantation. In one survey[166] of causes and consequences of discontinuation of defibrillator therapy, 5 of 10 patients refused further defibrillator therapy after device removal due to infection. Three of the five patients had sudden cardiovascular events after device removal that included sudden death, recurrent ventricular tachycardia, and stroke.

The choice of antimicrobial therapy is dictated by identification of pathogen and its respective in vitro drug susceptibility profile. Intravenous administration of antimicrobials is recommended. Although no studies have been conducted that provide an evidence-based approach to duration of treatment, most authors believe that a minimum of 4 weeks of antimicrobial administration is appropriate for patients who have had complete removal of the infected device. For patients with complicating osteomyelitis or left-sided endocarditis, a 6-week parenteral treatment course is used widely.

Defining a prescribed duration of antimicrobial therapy for patients who harbor retained, infected hardware and are deemed ineligible for surgical intervention to remove an embedded lead has been more difficult. One approach is to provide initial "induction" parenteral antimicrobial therapy for a minimum of 4 weeks, then switch to an active orally administered regimen as long-term (i.e., lifelong) treatment.[167]

LEFT VENTRICULAR ASSIST DEVICES

The FDA first approved an LVAD for use in patients with end-stage heart failure in 1994.[168] The early model was pneumatically driven and was to be used as a "bridge to transplantation." An improved version that was self-contained, vented, and electric was approved as a temporary use device in 1998. For selected patients, the improvement in hemodynamic parameters results in marked clinical improvement with substantial increases in exercise tolerance and a reversal of metabolic and cellular abnormalities that characterize the heart failure syndrome.[169]

Three different devices are approved for use currently and include the HeartMate (Thoratec, Pleasanton, CA), Novacor (Baxter Healthcare, Oakland, CA), and Thoratec (Thoratec) systems. The Thoratec system includes a pneumatic pump that is paracorporeal. The HeartMate and Novacor systems include an electrically driven pump that is implanted surgically within the thoracic or abdominal cavity. Because each system has either cannulas (Thoratec) or drive lines (HeartMate and Novacor) that run percutaneously, risk of infection is substantial. This risk was highlighted in the rematch study.[168] This investigation examined the role of long-term LVAD use in patients who were deemed ineligible for cardiac transplantation and had symptoms of New York Heart Association class IV heart failure. Although patients who received the LVAD (HeartMate) had a longer survival and an improved quality of life compared with patients who were randomized to receive optimal medical therapy and no LVAD placement, it came at a cost. Patients in the LVAD group were more than twice as likely to have a serious adverse event compared with patients in the optimal medical therapy group. Infection and device failure were predominant factors that led to a limited 2-year survival rate of 23%. Within 3 months of LVAD placement, LVAD infection complicated 28% of cases. LVAD-related infections more commonly were limited to the driveline tract and pocket. Fatal sepsis also was seen and was twice as likely to occur in the LVAD-recipient group.

Development of a totally implanted system either as a left ventricular or as a biventricular pump (or artificial heart) is ongoing. In view of the extreme shortage of donor hearts that are available for a growing number of worthy recipients, it is pertinent that improvements in these devices continue and result in a reduced risk of device-related infection.

Three points should be emphasized when addressing the frequency of LVAD-related infections. First, most patients who need LVAD support are chronically ill, have prolonged stays in critical care areas, and require numerous modes of invasive monitoring and support, all of which predispose to nosocomial infection. Second, the incidence of LVAD-associated infections has been calculated in the past but has included all types of infections that occur during use of the LVAD and has not been limited to infections that involve only the device. Third, the risk of device infection is time dependent[170]; higher rates of device infection occur with more prolonged use of the device.

A cohort study[171] provides perhaps the most useful data in defining the incidence of device-related infection. The HeartMate was the LVAD used in this study. A total of 36 LVADs were implanted in 35 patients, and device use ranged from 2 days to 262 days (mean 73 days). Sixteen patients developed surgical site infections. The overall rate of surgical site infection was 44 per 100 LVAD implantations, or 6.2 infections per 1000 device days. Seven of these patients had superficial infection that involved the driveline incision (19.4 infections per 100 LVAD implantations). Three patients had sternal infections (8.2 infections per 100 LVAD implantations), and six had organ/space infections that involved either the LVAD or the preperitoneal pocket that contained the pump (16.7 infections per 100 LVAD implantations); two of these patients also developed mediastinitis.

Estimates of risk of device-related bacteremia have been calculated[172] in patients with LVAD placement. An LVAD-related bloodstream infection was defined as one in which the same pathogen was cultured from the device and the blood and no other source of bacteremia was identified. Overall, 140 nosocomial blood-stream infections occurred in 104 (49%) of 214 patients (7.9 blood-stream infections per 1000 LVAD days); 53 (38%) episodes were device related.

The impact of the LVAD on the immune system is speculated to be one factor that predisposes device recipients to infectious complications.[173,174] LVAD implantation is thought to predispose to infection through its effect of increasing the susceptibility of circulating CD4 T cells to activation-induced apoptosis; this leads to a progressive decline in CD4 T cells and cellular immunity. It is speculated that LVAD recipients are prone to opportunistic infections because of a defective cellular immune system. In one clinical survey,[174] LVAD recipients were at increased risk of developing candidal infections compared with controls (28% versus 3%; $P = .003$).

The most common clinical manifestations of LVAD infection are due to infection of the driveline. Erythema at the percutaneous exit sites that is more prominent than usually is seen is characteristic. Purulent drainage also can be seen. Surgical site infection is another localized form of device infection and involves the soft tissue pocket site where the device is placed. The pocket site can vary in location, and the superficial skin and soft tissues overlying the pocket site may or may not be involved in inflammatory changes.

Infection of the valves or other blood-contacting surfaces of the LVAD occurs less often. The clinical manifestations of this form of "endocardial" infection mirror the manifestations of NVE or PVE. Fever and other signs of sepsis may develop. Systemic or pulmonary (for LVADs that assist the right ventricle) embolic phenomena can be seen. Complications of sepsis or emboli can result in death. Mechanical dysfunction of the LVAD can occur if an obstructing pannus of infection develops within the internal lumen of the inflow or outflow cannulas that are anastomosed into the apex of the left ventricle and ascending aorta. Clinical worsening of cardiac function may develop despite initial improvement with LVAD placement.

LVAD removal is required in some patients to control infection. In others, suppressive antimicrobial therapy is effective in preventing the recurrence of clinical findings of infection until LVAD removal and cardiac transplantation is performed. LVAD infection is not a contraindication to cardiac transplantation. For some patients, cardiac transplantation is needed not only for cardiac dysfunction, but also for allowing removal of the infected device to achieve control of ongoing infection.

Prevention of LVAD infection is a worthy goal. The elimination of percutaneous drivelines with future generations of LVADs should reduce device infection considerably. Preliminary evaluation with the Jarvik-2000 LVAD (Jarvik Heart Inc., New York, NY) technically approaches this goal, and expectations are that the device would be useful long-term and could be transplantation saving.[175]

Until the Jarvik-2000 and similar models of ventricular assist pumps are approved for use by the FDA, other preventive measures currently are in use, including broad-spectrum antimicrobial administration (five agents in some centers) around the time of LVAD placement, limiting the use of central venous catheters and other types of temporary vascular devices, providing meticulous dressing change protocols at the driveline exit site, lengthening the driveline subcutaneous tunnel, immobilizing the driveline at the skin exit site, and impregnating the driveline with antimicrobials.

TOTAL ARTIFICIAL HEARTS

The remarkable evolution of the total artificial heart (TAH) continues. The thrombotic and infectious complications that plagued the use of the Jarvik-7 artificial heart in the 1980s served notice that major technical advances were needed before such a device could be employed for permanent use. Also, improvements in the design of ventricular assist devices have directed some of the focus away from development of the TAH.

The Cardiowest TAH (C-70 TAH; CardioWest Technologies, Inc, Tucson, AZ) is one newer generation version of the device that underwent study in the 1990s in the United States. It is pneumatically driven and is used as a bridge to cardiac transplantation. The infectious complications that occur in the Cardiowest C-70 TAH have been outlined.[176] Among 27 recipients of the device, 64 infections were described; 3 of the 27 patients experienced no infectious complications. Duration of implantation of the device may have been important. The 3 infection-free patients had the device an average of 32.3 days compared with the 24 patients with infection who used the TAH for an average of 57.3 days.

Most of the 45 systemic infections were of the respiratory tract (n = 24). Genitourinary (n = 9) and blood-borne (n = 7) infections also were common. Seven of the 19 local infections were of the driveline that had a percutaneous route. Nine infections occurred in one patient. Gram-positive cocci accounted for 66% and 80% of the blood-borne and local infections. Two patients had mediastinitis.

Two (7.4%) of the 27 patients died before undergoing heart transplantation. One death was due to disseminated infection caused by *Serratia marcescens*. Twenty-five patients were bridged to transplantation successfully. Based on the findings of this survey,[176] patients were less likely to die from infectious complications compared with patients who were implanted with the earlier Jarvik-7 artificial heart.

Further technical advances in TAH development have led to the first fully implantable device, the AbioCor Implantable Replacement Heart (Abiomed, Danvers, MA). As of March 2003, there have been 10 recipients of the AbioCor heart and the first heart was implanted on July 2, 2001. Data are available for the first seven patients who received the device, and none have experienced device infection.[177] Because recipients of the AbioCor heart have not been candidates for cardiac transplantation, the devices are expected to be used long-term.

The risk of device-related infection should remain lower than earlier versions of TAH that have drivelines that run percutaneously and predispose to local and systemic infections due to the duration of the skin barrier. Thrombotic events and the relatively large size of the AbioCor heart dictate that additional improvements in the device are in order.[178]

CENTRAL NERVOUS SYSTEM SHUNTS

CNS shunts have been used for 5 decades in the treatment of hydrocephalus. Shunting of cerebrospinal fluid is achieved by a variety of devices and implantation techniques (see Chapter 81). For the purposes of this chapter, the ventriculoatrial (VA) shunt and its infectious complications are reviewed. Today, the VA shunt is used much less commonly than the ventriculoperitoneal (VP) shunt, in part because of the more serious infectious complications of the VA device. Nevertheless, the VA shunt is an important alternative to VP shunting in patients whose peritoneum may not be an appropriate site for distal cerebrospinal fluid absorption because of prior abdominal surgery, peritonitis, or shunt infection.

The incidence of VA shunt infection in recent years has averaged less than 10% and is less than that seen decades ago when rates of 29% were recorded.[179] The incidence of infectious complications for VA and VP shunts seems equal. Most VA infections occur within 6 months of placement.

Staphylococci are the most commonly isolated pathogens. Coagulase-negative staphylococci outnumber *S. aureus* in most case series of VA shunt infection. Other skin flora, including *Corynebacterium jeikeium* and *P. acnes* and an array of other bacteria and yeasts, have been identified as causes of VA shunt infections.

The clinical manifestations of VA shunt infection are variable and depend on many factors, including site of shunt infection, whether proximal or distal, whether intraluminal or extraluminal, virulence of infecting pathogens, and presence or absence of shunt malfunction. Shunt malfunction can produce increased intracranial pressure and cause headache, nausea, vomiting, and mental status changes. Similar findings can occur with proximal site infection causing ventriculitis. Overt signs of meningitis are unusual because infected cerebrospinal fluid from the ventricles does not communicate with that in the subarachnoid space. Intraluminal infection can result in bacteremia and sepsis. Severe sepsis and septic shock are unusual. Right-sided infective endocarditis and septic pulmonary emboli have been described. In cases in which more subtle clinical features characterize the syndrome and lead to delays in treatment, immunologic sequelae, including nephritis, dermatologic abnormalities, and musculoskeletal findings, may develop. Infection of the external lumen of the VA shunt can occur as a complication of surgical site infection and lead to local findings of inflammation. Cutaneous tunnel is a classic manifestation of extraluminal shunt infection. In cases of infection due to pyogenic organisms, purulent drainage may be seen.

Blood cultures usually are positive when intraluminal infection is present and are important in securing a diagnosis of VA shunt infection. Blood cultures are not positive with extraluminal infection, and local inflammatory changes at the catheter tunnel site or surgical site can be helpful in diagnosis of extraluminal infection. In other cases in which clinical features of ventriculitis exist, sampling of the ventricular cerebrospinal fluid is required to establish a diagnosis. In one study,[180] the findings of fever and greater than 10% polymorphonuclear leukocytes in ventricular cerebrospinal fluid had a 99% specificity and a 93% positive predictive value for VA shunt infection. The absence of these two features had a 95% negative predictive value for shunt infection.

As with other types of cardiovascular device–related infections, foreign body removal coupled with antimicrobial therapy is the best treatment option. A published decision analysis[179] supports this approach. A two-staged exchange of the VA shunt and antimicrobial administration is employed. Temporary external ventricular drainage or serial ventricular taps are done to remove cerebrospinal fluid to relieve intraventricular pressure and to examine for sterility and instillation of antimicrobials. When sterility is achieved, a new VA shunt is placed.

CARDIAC SUTURE LINE INFECTIONS

Left ventriculotomy is performed for several reasons, including resection of aneurysms or scars, antiarrhythmic surgery, and placement of ventricular assist devices. A variety of devices are used to buttress sutures at the line of incision, including autologous or resorbable strips, but in many centers, Teflon pledgets or patches are employed. Despite the frequency of left ventriculotomy with suture line device support placement, infection of these devices has been described rarely. Two reports[181,182] in the same year described 29 patients with cardiac suture line infection. Because of the rarity of infection, the often prolonged (months to years) interval between ventriculotomy and onset of infection stigmata, and the syndrome similarities to other, more common clinical infection entities, the correct diagnosis frequently is delayed or not considered until surgical intervention or postmortem examination. As a result of a decline in performing autopsies in the United States, some cases of cardiac suture line infection likely go undiagnosed.[181]

Three clinical presentations have been appreciated: (1) chest wall or epigastric soft tissue infection, (2) bronchopulmonary infection, and (3) endocardial infection with bacteremia or fungemia. Chest wall or epigastric involvement is seen most commonly and presents as a chronic draining sinus, a subcutaneous mass, or local pain. A syndrome of endocardial infection is the next most common presentation, and bacteremia, often with sepsis, is seen. If the underlying diagnosis is not appreciated, relapsing bacteremia or fungemia can occur after discontinuation of antimicrobial treatment. In other cases, refractory blood-stream infection and sepsis are seen, and control of infection is not achieved until débridement is performed. Bronchopulmonary presentations are seen least often. Patients present with recurrent hemoptysis, purulent sputum production and bronchiectasis, and pneumonia with or without empyema. Some patients may present with a combination of clinical signs and symptoms that reflects more than one syndrome presentation.

Although staphylococci account for many of the cardiac suture line infections, a variety of other organisms cause these infections. Regardless of the cause of infection, treatment should include early surgical débridement of infected native and foreign tissues with pathogen-specific antimicrobial administration. Left ventricular false aneurysms commonly develop.[181,182] Evaluation in suspect cases should include echocardiography, CT, and coronary and left ventricular angiography. Of 29 patients in the two case series, 23 (79.3%) survived with combined débridement surgery and antimicrobial therapy. In four of the six patients who died, no débridement of the infected ventricular suture line was done.[181]

CLOSURE DEVICE TREATMENT OF PATENT DUCTUS ARTERIOSUS, ATRIAL SEPTAL DEFECT, AND VENTRICULAR SEPTAL DEFECT

Therapeutic cardiac catheterization with placement of closure devices for a variety of congenital defects is being used increasingly with good success and avoidance of surgery. Several different devices are in use and under investigation. Overall, complications related to device placement are seen infrequently. Infectious sequelae have been rare, and only two cases of infective endocarditis[183,184] have been described. Two different occlusion devices were used in the two cases. The epidemiology of infection was complicated in both cases, which was eventful in the period around device deployment; because of this, it is difficult to determine the interval between device placement and onset of occlusion device–related infection. Nevertheless, both infections occurred less than 3 months after device placement. Pathogens were identified in both cases and included *S. aureus* in one[184] and *Bacillus pumilus*[183] in the other. In both cases, device-related vegetations were shown by transthoracic echocardiography. After surgical excision of the devices, vegetations, and local infected tissues and parenteral antibiotic administration over 6 weeks, cure was achieved in both cases.

PERIPHERAL VASCULAR STENTS

Peripheral vascular stents are used commonly today in conjunction with percutaneous angioplasty procedures to treat complications of atherosclerosis nonsurgically. It has been estimated that more than 400,000 patients each year in the United States receive stents to optimize angioplasty results and prevent vessel restenosis.[185] Well-recognized compli-

cations of endovascular stent placement can occur and include vascular injury, thromboembolism, local delivery site/stent deployment irregularities, and hemorrhage.[186] In contrast, infection related to these devices rarely occurs. One estimate of infection risk has been calculated to be less than 1 in 10,000 cases.[185] Impressive case series from individual medical centers that characterize peripheral vascular stent infections are nonexistent. Perhaps the largest experience published to date was a detailed literature review[187]; 18 cases, excluding 3 cases of coronary artery stent infections, were analyzed and permit a description of the syndrome of peripheral vascular stent infection. A variety of different types of stents have been infected. No analysis of infection risk factors has been done, and owing to the rarity of the syndrome, risk factors are not likely to be confirmed statistically. Nevertheless, potential risk factors[187] include the prolonged use of an indwelling vascular catheter or sheath and reuse of the same sheath after 24 hours, usually in the patient who is undergoing thrombolytic therapy; recurrent use of the same femoral artery for vascular access within 1 week; local hematoma formation; prolonged stent insertion time; and multiple interventions on the same or adjacent tissues. The iliac artery stent site is involved most commonly and accounted for 9 of 18 infections.[187] Most (15 of 18 [83.3%]) patients in this series had clinical manifestations of stent infection appear within 28 days of stent placement. This finding supports the tenet that microbial stent site contamination occurs at the time of stent placement. Fever and sepsis are seen universally. Patients can present with local complaints, including pain in the area of stent placement. *S. aureus* has been the premiere pathogen in this syndrome and was isolated from blood or operative (stent excision) specimen cultures in 15 (83.3%) cases in the literature review. Initial and serial CT is a useful diagnostic tool. More than 90% of patients who have had CT performed have had radiologic findings suggesting infection. These findings have included pseudoaneurysm formation, mass formation, increased fat attenuation, abscess formation, perivascular fluid accumulation, and persistent inflammation.

Two treatment options for peripheral vascular stent infections have been used. Currently a combined medical-surgical approach is favored. Stent and vessel excision and extra-anatomic revascularization are the desired goals. To achieve these goals, several different surgical techniques have been employed. A second approach, which has been used in a smaller number of patients,[185,187] is antibiotic based and includes no surgery and no removal of the infected stent. CT scan and angiographic findings in these few patients support the correct diagnosis of stent infection. Patients are administered antibiotics either for a finite time or for the life of the patient and cure, or at least successful long-term suppression of infection, has been achieved. The latter approach is less favored and might be an option after careful consideration in patients deemed nonsurgical candidates because of host factors (patient age, severity of underlying medical conditions, limited expected life span) or technical surgery-related problems.

Morbidity and mortality are seen in patients with peripheral vascular stent infections. Some conditions, such as multiorgan dysfunction syndrome, adult respiratory distress, and disseminated intravascular coagulation, can complicate the syndrome and precipitate death. Limb or digit amputation may be required and can be due to embolic stents, prolonged hypotension due to sepsis or vessel rupture, thrombosis, or surgical disruption that leads to peripheral tissue death.

PROSTHETIC VASCULAR GRAFTS

The technical advances in nonvalvular cardiovascular devices have been most evident in the ongoing development of newer generations of prosthetic vascular grafts. Complications associated with the use of these grafts have declined due to graft design improvements. In addition, native tissue vascular grafts continue to be used in some clinical circumstances and are less likely to be complicated by infection compared with prosthetic vascular grafts. Despite these factors, devastating complications, including prosthetic vascular graft infection, occur in a few graft recipients and can lead to limb amputation or death.

Prosthetic vascular graft infection is defined by three different parameters: (1) perigraft infection or abscess formation, (2) exposed graft due to disruption of the more superficial soft tissue layers overlying the prosthesis, and (3) graft erosion or fistula formation involving a mucosal surface. The three are not mutually exclusive.

The incidence of prosthetic vascular graft infection is variable and depends on the anatomic location of the device. For aortic grafts limited to the abdomen, graft-related infections occur in 1% or less of recipients. The incidence of infection is higher (1.5% to 2%) for aortic grafts that extend to the femoral location. Infrainguinal vascular grafts that originate in the groin are at the highest (6%) risk of complicating infection.

Several distinct routes of microbial contamination are recognized as harbingers of vascular graft infection. Microbial seeding of the graft at the time of implantation or in the immediate postoperative period accounts for most graft infections. Vascular graft contamination can occur if there is adjacent infection. Colonization of thrombus in aneurysm sacs and in the atherosclerotic plaques in arterial walls is thought to be operative as one example of adjacent sites of infection. Superficial surgical site infection can result in graft infection. Subsequent manipulation of an implanted graft by either surgical or percutaneous procedures can predispose to graft infection. Finally, an anatomically remote site of infection can contribute indirectly to vascular prosthetic graft infection via seeding of the blood stream and secondary graft contamination.

The general expectation is that because intraoperative or immediate postoperative vascular graft contamination is the mechanism accounting for infection in most cases, clinical evidence of infection should be evident within 1 to 2 months after graft implantation. Although this is generally true for infrainguinal grafts that originate in the groin, the average delay in clinical onset of graft infection involving a graft restricted to the abdomen is measured in years. These tenets regarding onset of clinical symptoms depend to some degree on the virulence of the infecting pathogen. Currently, many less virulent bacteria that are part of the normal skin flora account for an increasing portion of vascular graft infections, including coagulase-negative staphylococci, *Corynebacterium* spp., and *P. acnes*. Graft infections caused by these organisms tend to be delayed in onset. In contrast, *S. aureus*–related graft infections occur early after graft implantation. In contrast to decades ago, when *S. aureus* was identified as the pathogen in most cases of graft infection, the administration of appropriate perioperative antibiotic prophylaxis coupled with improved operative techniques has resulted in sizable reductions in the prevalence of *S. aureus* graft infections. Enterococcal species and anaerobic bacteria, often as part of polymicrobial infection, have been identified as pathogens of vascular graft infections. *Candida* spp. have been isolated in cases of graft-related infections and have become important pathogens in a variety of cardiovascular device–related infections.

The clinical presentation of vascular graft infection is highly variable and can have a different compilation of signs and symptoms. Perhaps the best approach in categorizing the clinical features of infection is to divide the presentations into the early and late postoperative periods. In the former category, which extends to 3 months after graft implantation, local inflammatory findings indicating surgical site infection are present. Even when these findings are thought to be limited to superficial soft tissue structures that overlay the graft, graft infection is nevertheless a consideration. Abscess formation may occur locally. Other local manifestations include sinus tract formation, hemorrhage, graft occlusion, pseudoaneurysm, graft exposure, and poor tissue incorporation. Septic emboli and distal tissue ischemia also may be seen. Systemic signs of sepsis can accompany the local findings, particularly when more aggressive pathogens, including *S. aureus*, are present. Fever, chills, leukocytosis, and bacteremia or fungemia frequently are documented.

Late graft infection is characterized less often by systemic toxicity. The local stigmata of graft healing complications prevail. Cutaneous sinus tracts, lack of graft incorporation by surrounding tissue, anastomotic aneurysm, and graft-enteric erosions or fistula develop.[188] The formation of cutaneous sinus tracts is an obvious clue that underlying graft infection is present. Poor graft incorporation may not be apparent until intraoperative inspection of the implanted device is done. The clinical presentation of pseudoaneurysms is wide ranging. For some patients, little to no inflammatory response is manifested either systemically or locally even at intraoperative inspection of the graft. Culture of explanted graft material is positive, however. Other patients develop local pain with or without a palpable mass. Hemorrhage can occur and can be life-threatening. Distal ischemia with pain due to graft thrombosis or embolization also is seen. For one third of patients,[188] the clinical presentation of anastomotic pseudoaneurysm is emergent in regard to threat of life or limb.

Clinical symptoms due to prosthetic vascular graft–related enteric erosions and fistula usually are seen years after graft placement. Patients with graft-enteric erosions can present with systemic (sepsis) and local (abdominal pain) complaints. The aortic graft most often erodes the third or fourth portion of the duodenum. A prompt diagnosis of this condition is lifesaving because mortality is universal if the complication is left untreated.

Graft-enteric fistula complicating graft infection typically is seen years after graft placement. It is diagnosed in less than 5% of patients who undergo aortic graft placement, and similar to graft enteric erosions, the duodenum is the portion of bowel most often involved. Gastrointestinal tract bleeding, which ranges from subtle to massive, can present as hematemesis, hematochezia, or melena. Abdominal pain may be seen, and some patients develop systemic evidence of sepsis. Polymicrobial infection consisting of enteric flora usually is confirmed with blood and graft and perigraft tissue cultures.

Even when specific findings from a patient's history and physical examination strongly suggest graft infection, diagnostic procedures usually are performed to support the diagnosis further and to define extent of infection. CT is the best tool in the diagnostic evaluation of a patient with possible graft infection. Sensitivity and specificity of CT have been reported to be approximately 100%. Findings on CT that support a complicating infection include the presence of perigraft fluid not attributable to recent (≤3 months) graft implantation, increasing perigraft fluid in the early post–graft implantation setting, perigraft fluid with fat stranding of gas bubbles, lack of fat plane between graft and bowel, and anastomotic aneurysms.[189] These findings depend on an appropriate inflammatory response to infection. For less virulent pathogens, particularly coagulase-negative staphylococci, the inflammatory response may be limited, and the perigraft findings displayed on CT may be minimal to nonexistent. The sensitivity of CT is reduced considerably in patients with more indolent infections. In cases in which pseudoaneurysm is not detected on CT, an image-guided percutaneous aspiration of perigraft fluid should be considered at the time of the initial CT scan. Fluid should be sent for cytologic and microbiologic analysis.

Some of the same previously mentioned CT-related findings of infection are seen in the early postoperative state normally. Perigraft fluid can persist for 3 months after graft implantation. Perigraft air related to graft placement usually is absorbed within 1 week of surgery, although it can persist for 7 weeks.[190]

Experience with MRI is less extensive. Sensitivity and specificity of MRI have been cited as 85% and 100%.[191,192] MRI may be most beneficial in patients who have undergone CT with negative or unclear results due to infection with an indolent organism and little to no perigraft inflammatory response. MRI may be able better to show subtler perigraft inflammatory changes than CT.

Indium-labeled white cell scanning also has been used in the detection of graft-related infections. False-positive results, particularly seen soon after graft implantation, have an impact on test specificity. Prior antimicrobial therapy may reduce test sensitivity. This nuclear medicine scan is considered a second-tier diagnostic tool.

Additional evaluation techniques warrant comment. Ultrasonography's role is limited to detection of pseudoaneurysms. Sinography probably is used less often today than in years before the availability of CT. This situation has led to some centers having personnel with limited expertise in obtaining sinograms and can result in introducing potential pathogens into the perigraft location when high-pressure instillation of contrast material occurs. Endoscopic examination of the gastrointestinal tract is used to determine whether a graft enteric erosion or fistula is the cause of gastrointestinal bleeding. Angiography is not used diagnostically to detect vascular graft infection.

The overall health of the typical patient with prosthetic vascular graft infection is compromised. Often the consequences of accelerated atherogenesis due to decades of uncontrolled risk factor exposure have led to widespread cardiovascular complications. In addition, pulmonary disease and cancer have been diagnosed previously among patients who are long-term smokers. It is conceivable that limb-threatening and life-threatening complications are well recognized in patients with graft infections.

Management of graft infection is difficult, and a team of physicians from a variety of medical and surgical subspecialties is involved in the inpatient care of these patients. The length of stay that frequently is required to treat infected patients adequately often is weeks, not days. Preoperative and postoperative complications, including non–graft-related nosocomial infections, account for the prolonged hospitalization.

Four general principles are followed in the treatment of prosthetic vascular graft infections.[193] First, the infected graft must be excised. It is a foreign body that can allow infection to persist despite antimicrobial treatment and an intact immunologic response to infection. Also, infection involvement of the graft suture line mandates graft removal so that subsequent rupture at the anastomosis with hemorrhage does not occur. Second, complete débridement of all infected tissues, not limited to graft, is necessary. Residual infection must be resected so that graft stump healing is achieved. If perigraft tissue infection is not eliminated by combined aggressive débridement and antimicrobial therapy, stump blowout with hemorrhage may occur. Third, every effort should be made to identify the infecting pathogens so that directed parenteral antimicrobial therapy can be administered over an approximate 6-week course. Finally, the distal tissues that were dependent on blood flow via the graft prosthesis before infection dictate that revascularization be achieved. The best approach may be revascularization followed in 1 to 2 days by graft excision.[194] Autogenous vein or endarterectomy-treated artery is prepared over prosthetic conduits for use in revascularization with reconstruction through uninfected tissue planes.

All four principles—graft excision, local débridement, prolonged culture-directed antimicrobial coverage, and revascularization—are considered in all cases of prosthetic vascular graft infection. Treatment of graft infection must be individualized for each patient. Unique clinical features in each case, including urgency of the operation, mode of infection presentation, current vascular anatomy, patient comorbidities, pathogen virulence, and timing and type of infection, dictate an individualized treatment approach.[189] The vascular surgeon must be skilled in many graft techniques so that the most appropriate procedures are applied in each case.

Excision of the infected graft is performed in each case for at least two reasons. First, it is done to gain control of an infective process at a vascular site. If control is not achieved, particularly when infection is due to more aggressive pathogens, such as *S. aureus,* potentially life-threatening complications, including sepsis and catastrophic hemorrhage from an anastomotic site, can occur. Second, it is difficult to eradicate device-related infections with antimicrobial therapy alone. Even if control of infection is achieved without graft removal and infection is suppressed successfully with antimicrobial treatment, when antimicrobial therapy is discontinued, infection relapse occurs. There are cases in which additional surgical procedures are not a treatment option because of severe underlying comorbidities. In these cases in which infection has been controlled successfully by acute (induction) antimicrobial therapy, long-term (lifelong) antimicrobial suppressive therapy is administered, usually with oral agents on a daily basis.[167]

The temporal order of the surgical procedures varies. In medical centers where extra-anatomic bypass is preferred as the method of revascularization, the extra-anatomic bypass is done first and is followed by infected graft excision and local débridement. The latter procedures are done as either staged or sequenced interventions. The staged procedure of graft excision and local débridement is performed a few days after the extra-anatomic revascularization surgery. The sequenced procedure is done immediately after the revascularization and during the same anesthesia. The benefit of the staged operations is limiting the degree of physiologic stress that otherwise would accompany a single prolonged operation. The benefit of sequential operations, at least in the case of aortic graft infections, is a lower amputation rate. The concern of a theoretical increased risk of new graft seeding by the indwelling, infected old graft has not been realized. New graft infection rates after staged or sequenced operations may be less than rates seen with the traditional procedure of conducting the graft excision and débridement first. Two shortcomings of the extra-anatomic bypass revascularization method with graft excision and débridement for infected aortic grafts have been low limb salvage rates and aortic stump blowout, which is uniformly fatal with rare exceptions. The rates of these complications are approximately 20% to 30% for limb amputation and 20% for stump blowout. The reinfection rate has been estimated to be 20%.[189]

In situ bypass is another method of revascularization. Three types of grafts are available for use and include antibiotic-bonded prosthetic grafts, arterial allografts, and autogenous vein grafts. Rifampin has been studied most extensively for use in antibiotic-bonded prosthetic grafts. Fresh and cryopreserved arterial allografts are treatment options. One advantage of the allografts and autogenous vein grafts is the reduced likelihood of new graft infection because native tissue is placed in situ rather than prosthetic material. Having said this, relatively low "reinfection" rates are characteristic of the rifampin-bonded prosthetic grafts.

Additional advantages of in situ bypass over extra-anatomic bypass as a method of revascularization in aortic graft infection include reduced rates of lower extremity amputation, elimination of a need for a second operation for a staged extra-anatomic bypass, avoidance of creating an aortic stump that subsequently could blow out, and lack of anatomic limitations to placement. Other advantages depend on the type of in situ bypass. Rifampin-bonded prosthetic grafts are beneficial for patients who are poor surgical candidates and would benefit from the shortest operative time. Arterial allografts offer this same benefit, but the collective experience with these grafts is less, and they are more expensive and may be associated with graft failure.[189] The long-term patency of the autogenous vein graft is a major advantage of this type of in situ graft; the disadvantage is the prolongation of the operative time required for venectomy, which is not tolerated by many patients. In addition, early complications of deep vein harvest are seen in some patients.

Autogenous tissue coverage of the in situ graft is crucial in reducing the risk of graft reinfection. Vascularized tissue, which usually involves an omentum flap or, less often, a sartorius or rectus femoris muscle transposition or Gerota's fascia with perinephric fat, is used to surround the in situ graft completely. Vascular-rich tissue can absorb wound secretions and improve circulation, which should enhance the local immunologic response.[195]

Infection is a common malady among hemodialysis patients, and *S. aureus* is a commonly identified pathogen. Because of the frequent administration of antibiotics to this at-risk population, multidrug resistance has characterized strains of *S. aureus* and enterococci isolated from long-term hemodialysis patients. Most infections due to *S. aureus* that are intermediately resistant to vancomycin have been recovered from long-term hemodialysis patients. The single *S. aureus* isolate that is fully resistant to vancomycin that has been recovered to date produced infection in a hemodialysis patient. Because infection now is recognized as the second leading cause of death among patients with end-stage renal disease,[196] the Centers for Disease Control and Prevention[197] and the National Kidney Foundation[196] have established guidelines for infection prevention and national surveillance for hemodialysis-associated infections.

Vascular access site infections are a large part of the infection-related morbidity and mortality in long-term hemodialysis patients.

The infection-related morbidity and mortality are due in part to the widespread use of the prosthetic arteriovascular graft composed of polytetrafluoroethylene (PTFE), which is at increased risk of infection compared with the native arteriovenous fistula. In a national survey[197] conducted in 1995, the Centers for Disease Control and Prevention found that only 22% of long-term hemodialysis patients were dialyzed through a native arteriovenous fistula. The PTFE graft was prescribed in cases in which surgical formation of a native arteriovenous fistula was not anatomically feasible. The risk of infection with either funneled or temporary hemodialysis catheters is even higher. In one prospective survey,[196] the risks of infection (per 1000 dialysis sessions) in patients with arteriovenous grafts (2), funneled catheters (12.2), or temporary catheters (29.2) were much higher than the risks associated with the use of arteriovenous fistulas (0.9). It was estimated that if arteriovenous fistula use were increased from the current 16% of all vascular access use to 40%, the infection rate would decrease by 22%.

Risk factors for infection of PTFE grafts have been defined. Inherent to the use of the implanted device, the need for repetitive percutaneous cannulation is a risk. Additional risk factors include difficulty in cannulation, perigraft hematoma formation, prolonged postdialysis bleeding from the graft, breaks in sterile technique during cannulation, surgical manipulation of the graft, human immunodeficiency virus coinfection, poor patient hygiene, lower extremity (thigh) graft, and bacteremia or fungemia caused by an ectopic site of infection.[198]

As with other types of vascular graft infections, local findings of infection are seen commonly. Occult bacteremia or fungemia without local graft inflammatory changes also can be a manifestation of graft infection. This occult presentation has been highlighted[199] as a manifestation of old, nonfunctioning, thrombosed graft. Indium white blood cell scanning has been useful in detecting silent graft infection. In one investigation[200] of occult infection involving old, thrombosed grafts, the indium scan showed a sensitivity of 100% and a specificity of 75% in detecting graft infection.

Management decisions of PTFE graft infections often are affected by the need to preserve the vascular access site because other potential venous access sites have been exhausted. Parenteral antimicrobial therapy is curative in some cases of early graft infection, and graft removal is not required. The presence of purulence or abscess in the immediate graft area or aneurysmal graft formation mandates graft removal. Old, thrombosed, nonfunctioning grafts also should be removed when infection at this nidus is diagnosed.

There has been an upsurge in interest in preventing PTFE graft infections in hemodialysis patients. In addition to patient morbidity and mortality caused by arteriovenous graft infections, the financial burden on health care is substantial. A sizable portion of the total annual cost of vascular access morbidity in the United States is thought to be due to infection. The total annual cost of this morbidity has been projected to be more than $1 billion.[201]

Several interventions should be considered in an effort to reduce PTFE graft–related infections. Placement of an arteriovenous fistula instead of PTFE grafting always should be favored when anatomically feasible.

More aggressive use of intranasal mupirocin to eradicate *S. aureus* colonization among identified carriers has been advocated by some authors[202] to reduce *S. aureus* bacteremia rates. Antibiotics should be administered preoperatively at the time of graft placement and if subsequent operative graft manipulation is done. Proper infection control and graft cannulation techniques are mandatory. Cryopreserved vein allografts are gaining use in many centers and obviate the need for prosthetic graft placement in some scenarios.[203] The cryopreserved human femoral vein allograft has a reduced risk of infection and is being investigated actively as a long-term alternative dialysis conduit that may limit the future need for PTFE grafts. Perhaps the most exciting technical development of a tool used to prevent infection is a capsular polysaccharide-based vaccine used to prevent *S. aureus* infections. Active and passive immunization protocols are under investigation. The initial phase III trial of the active vaccine included only long-term hemodialysis patients and was shown to provide temporary protection against the development of *S. aureus* bacteremia.[203] Work to examine this vaccine and other *S. aureus*–derived immunogens further continues.

INTRA-AORTIC BALLOON COUNTERPULSATION

The intra-aortic balloon pump has been used since the 1970s to increase coronary perfusion by diastolic augmentation and to enhance cardiac performance by systolic unloading. The pump is used in a variety of clinical settings, including refractory cardiogenic shock, severely low cardiac output states, difficulty weaning from cardiopulmonary bypass, refractory myocardial ischemia, prevention of extension of a myocardial infarction in the preinfarction period, preoperative support in the presence of severe left ventricular dysfunction, and prophylactic insertion for catheterization or for operation in patients with severe left main coronary artery or triple-vessel disease.[204]

Two changes in balloon pump insertion have affected the risk of infection. First, an alternative percutaneous approach for placement of the pump into the common femoral artery was introduced in the 1980s and has reduced local infection risk. Before this time, surgical insertion of the pump was used. This procedure included placement of a woven Dacron graft that was anastomosed to the common femoral artery in end-to-side technique; the pump was inserted through this graft and into the artery. Second, the employment of a balloon catheter with a smaller diameter is complicated less often by infection.

Duration of placement of the balloon pump ranges from study to study and is important in its influence on the risk of infection. For surveys[205] in which the duration of balloon pump counterpulsation is measured in hours, infection rates are low. In other investigations[206] in which the duration of device use extends to 46 days, infection risks are higher. In the latter study, in which the mean insertion duration was 11.3 days, 13 (27%) of 49 patients developed infection. Seven had definite pump infection, four had probable pump infection, and two had local insertion site infection.

An analysis of complications of intra-aortic balloon pumping during the first 15 years of its use, which included insertion by surgical and percutaneous methods, suggests that there may be additional risk factors for infection.[207] A total of 733 patients with a range of balloon pump use up to 76 days were examined, and vascular and infectious complications were determined. Local infection, fever, and bacteremia were associated with device insertion under emergent conditions and in settings other than the operating room.

INVASIVE NONSURGICAL CARDIOLOGIC PROCEDURES

The array of invasive nonsurgical cardiologic procedures continues to expand. Three of the more common procedures include percutaneous transluminal coronary angioplasty (PTCA), diagnostic cardiac catheterization, and electrophysiologic studies. It is estimated that approximately 900,000 PTCA procedures are done annually worldwide. Most PTCA procedures involve stent placement. Although coronary stent infection is exceedingly rare (see later in this section), bacteremia complicating the procedure has been the topic of numerous reports. Local (groin) and metastatic infectious complications have been highlighted in other citations.

Bacteremia after invasive nonsurgical cardiologic procedures is the most common infectious complication. It can be a manifestation of local vascular or soft tissue infection or a cause of metastatic infection that can result in a variety of syndromes, including infective endocarditis, septic arthritis, and epidural abscess formation.

The incidence of bacteremia among patients who undergo invasive nonsurgical cardiologic procedures is low and was remarkably similar in two large retrospective surveys[208,209] and in one smaller prospective analysis[210] despite variable enrollment periods for procedure-related bacteremias that ranged from 36 hours to 7 weeks. In the two large retrospective analyses that were performed as part of case-control studies to determine infection risk factors, 22,006[208] and 4717[209] procedures were reviewed. In the much smaller prospective work,[210] 166

PTCA procedures were included. In one retrospective study,[208] which included cases of PTCA, diagnostic cardiac catheterization, and electrophysiologic studies, the incidence during the first 72 hours postprocedure was 0.11%. For PTCA, the bacteremia incidence was 0.24%.

In the second retrospective survey,[209] which was limited to PTCA procedures, the incidence of bacteremia was 0.64% and included bacteremia diagnosed 7 weeks after PTCA. Although the more prolonged enrollment period in the latter work likely contributed to increased incidence of bacteremia compared with the former study, most (93%) episodes of bacteremia occurred within the first week after PTCA. In the investigation by Munoz and colleagues,[208] bacteremia was detected a median 1.7 days after the procedure. The incidence of early (≤36 hours postprocedure) bacteremia in the prospective investigation[210] for patients who underwent PTCA was 0.61%.

Fever is the predominant symptom of complicating infection. Chills also are common, and local findings of infection in the femoral area are present among patients with femoral artery endarteritis, soft tissue infection, or pseudoaneurysm formation. Septic shock also can occur. Leukocytosis or bandemia (≥5% band forms) was seen in approximately three quarters of patients in one study.[209]

S. aureus has been the major pathogen in most case series and characteristically causes the most serious infections. Coagulase-negative staphylococci and enterococci are seen less commonly than gram-positive coccal pathogens. In only one case series,[208] gram-negative bacilli outnumbered gram-positive isolates as the cause of complicating bacteremia.

The designation of risk factors for the development of bacteremia after invasive nonsurgical cardiologic procedures has been the subject of several case series descriptions. These experiences have been anecdotal and based on relatively small numbers of cases. The two case-control studies that previously were cited[208,209] statistically evaluated purported risk factors. Multivariate analysis was used to identify independent risk factors. In the initial investigation,[209] five independent risk factors for PTCA-related bacteremia were described: duration of the procedure (odds ratio [OR] 2.9; $P = .04$), number of catheterizations at the same site (OR 4.0; $P = .015$), difficult vascular access (OR 14.9; $P = .007$), arterial sheath in place for more than 1 day (OR 6.8; $P = .025$), and congestive heart failure (OR 43.2; $P = .002$).

Data from the more recent case-control study[208] also identified congestive heart failure (OR 21; 95% confidence interval 6.8 to 66) as an independent risk factor for blood-stream infection. Age older than 60 years (OR 1.9; 95% CI 1.9 to 6.3) was the other independent risk factor determined by multivariate analysis. In this survey, the median length of hospital stay was 21 days and 6 days for patients with and without complicating bacteremia. This difference was significant statistically ($P = .001$). The overall mortality rate increased by almost 100-fold (8%) among patients who underwent the invasive cardiologic procedures and subsequently developed bacteremia compared with the mortality rate (0.009%) of patients who did not have blood-stream infection.

VASCULAR CLOSURE DEVICES

Since the 1990s, percutaneous arterial closure devices have been used for hemostasis of the femoral artery puncture site after catheterization. The advantages of their use, compared with the traditional methods of securing hemostasis by manual or mechanical compression, are that they decrease time to hemostasis and to ambulation. As a result, patients are more comfortable and have less pain after the procedure, and time to ambulation is abbreviated so that observation time (during which the patient is immobile and supine) and hospital length of stay are reduced.

The FDA has approved five devices for use to date, and newer and improved generations of vascular closure devices are being developed. The devices currently available have some commonality in that they involve the placement of foreign material in or at close proximity to the artery puncture site. Although the early experience with these devices showed little risk of infection, more recent surveys indicate that the risk of infection with use of these devices is higher than that seen with use of manual or mechanical compression. The infectious complications associated with the vascular closure devices are more severe and often require multiple surgical procedures as part of treatment. Limb amputation and death due to uncontrolled infection have been described. One retrospective analysis[211] that included 2003 cardiac catheterizations in 1 year is a representative example. Compared with a manual compression group, which had no infectious complications, the group that underwent femoral artery closure with a suture-based vascular closure device had five (1.6%, $P = .0003$) patients develop local infectious complications. Mycotic aneurysm (n = 3) and groin abscess (n = 2) were described. In four of the five cases, pathogens were recovered from infected tissue, and in three cases, *S. aureus* was identified. In two of three cases, *S. aureus* strains were methicillin resistant. In the remaining culture-positive case, *P. aeruginosa* was isolated. All five patients required operative intervention. Two patients died, one due to uncontrolled sepsis directly attributable to the femoral artery site infection caused by methicillin-resistant *S. aureus*. One patient underwent limb amputation before dying.

CORONARY ARTERY STENTS

Coronary artery stenting has been used since the 1980s. Stenting to prevent coronary artery abrupt closure and restenosis after PTCA now is used in greater than 60% of the more than 700,000 patients in the United States who undergo PTCA annually.[212] It is not surprising that the development of new types of stents has been described as a "booming business."[212]

Despite the prevalence of use of coronary artery stenting and the demonstrated risk of bacteremia associated with angioplasty,[213] infection of these stents has been reported rarely. No cases have been described to date in the United States. Five cases[214] have been reported from Western Europe. Reflective of the gender predilection for complications of atherosclerosis, four of the patients were men. The interval between coronary artery stent placement and onset of infectious symptoms ranged from 4 days to 4 weeks with four of the five patients developing symptoms within 1 week of stent placement. The acute onset of infection could be explained by the nature of the pathogens recovered in each case; *S. aureus* and *P. aeruginosa* were recovered in three cases and two cases. Pathogens were recovered from blood cultures in each case, and patients had infection syndromes that were consistent with that of infective endocarditis.

Complications were prevalent.[214] Three patients developed myocardial abscesses (cases 1, 4, and 5), two patients had pericardial empyemas (cases 1 and 3), and two patients had either true aneurysms (case 2) or pseudoaneurysms (case 3) of the coronary artery. Three of the five patients died as a result of infection and despite surgical excision of the stent and débridement of the involved coronary artery in two of the cases.

DACRON CAROTID PATCHES

Autologous saphenous vein patches increase the safety and durability of carotid endarterectomy compared with primary arteriotomy closure.[215] The risks of stroke, internal carotid thrombosis, and recurrent stenosis as a complication of carotid endarterectomy are less with saphenous vein patching. Synthetic carotid patches consisting of either Dacron or PTFE seem to have benefits similar to those of vein patches but are more convenient to use and avoid the lack of predictability of diameter size that characterizes vein grafts.

Synthetic carotid patch infection has been reported rarely but did occur in 1.8% (8 of 340) of synthetic patches applied in one 4-year institutional experience.[215] During this time, no patient who received either vein patch angioplasty (n = 843) or primary arteriotomy closure (n = 74) developed local infection.

Among the six patients who had medical records available for review, all six had received either perioperative cefuroxime or vancomycin (used in penicillin-allergic patients) at the time of Dacron patch placement. Dacron patch infections among the eight patients[215] clinically became apparent over a wide-ranging period—13 to 1060 days. Five of the eight patients were within 2 months of surgery, however, when local (carotid) infectious symptoms were noted. These local findings included abscess formation, draining sinus, pain, patch disruption with hemorrhage, and expanding pseudoaneurysm. Fever was described in only one of eight cases. Pathogens were cultured from operative specimens taken at the time of Dacron patch excision and débridement of surrounding inflammatory tissue in seven patients; operative cultures were negative in the remaining case. Recovered organisms included *S. aureus* (two cases), coagulase-negative staphylococci (two cases), and streptococci (three cases, two due to *Streptococcus milleri* and one due to *Streptococcus mitis*). Complications directly or indirectly related to Dacron graft excision were seen in four patients and included vocal cord paralysis, epidural abscess, myocardial infarction, stroke, and hypoglossal nerve injury. Vein patch replacement was used in the five patients with acute-onset Dacron graft infection. Vein grafts were employed in the three patients with late-onset infection. No infection relapse or infection-related deaths were observed during a mean follow-up of 17 months.

Sternbergh[216] reported his personal experience with Dacron patch closure. Two (1.2%) of 161 patients developed patch-related infection. Both infections were due to α-hemolytic streptococci, and local clinical findings of infection occurred 12 days and 17 days after Dacron carotid patch placement. All five infections in the two series[215,216] that were due to α-hemolytic streptococci were diagnosed early (mean 20.6 days) after Dacron patch placement. This early diagnosis is unanticipated, recognizing the relative indolence of infection caused by this group of organisms in immunocompetent hosts. In addition, no mention was made of invasive dental procedures being performed during this early postoperative period, which theoretically could cause seeding of the vascular patch. The more likely scenario was that patch site contamination occurred because of the anatomic proximity of the upper respiratory tract to the carotid incision.

VENA CAVA FILTERS

Inferior vena cava filters have been in use since the early 1970s, when the Greenfield filter was introduced.[217] Since that time, several hundred thousand patients with thromboembolic disease and a contraindication or prior complication to anticoagulation have received the device for protection from massive pulmonary embolism. There now are three versions of the Greenfield filter and three other types of filters available for use in the United States. Despite the widespread use of these devices, vena caval filter infection seems to be extremely rare. Five cases of infection have been described in the literature to date,[167,218-220] and in only three[218,219] was filter infection documented by culture of the explanted device. Blood cultures were positive in four of the five cases, and staphylococcal species were recovered in all five cases. In four of the five cases in which information was available, clinical onset of infection occurred 4 days, 5 days, 7 days, and 10 days after device placement. Two cases were complicated by lumbar spondylodiskitis.[219] One[220] of the five patients died as a result of sepsis related to vena caval filter infection. Three others[218,219] survived after filter removal. The remaining patient with presumed filter infection[167] was maintained on long-term antibiotic suppressive therapy, and the device was not removed.

REFERENCES

1. Baddour LM, Sullam PM, Bayer AS. Pathogenesis of infective endocarditis. In: Sussman M, ed. Molecular Medical Microbiology. London: Academic Press; 2002:999-1020.
2. Donlan RM. Biofilm formation: A clinically relevant microbiological process. Clin Infect Dis. 2001;33:1387-1392.
3. Moreillon P, Que YA, Bayer AS. Pathogenesis of streptococcal and staphylococcal endocarditis. Infect Dis Clin North Am. 2002;16:297-318.
4. Darouiche RO. Antimicrobial approaches for preventing infections associated with surgical implants. Clin Infect Dis. 2003;36:1284-1289.
5. Schaff HV, Carrel TP, Jamieson WRE, et al. Paravalvular leak and other events in Silzone-coated mechanical heart valves: A report from AVERT. Ann Thorac Surg. 2002;73:785-792.
6. Cabell CH, Jollis JG, Peterson GE, et al. Changing patient characteristics and the effect on mortality in endocarditis. Arch Intern Med. 2002;162:90-94.
7. Hoen B, Alla F, Selton-Suty C, et al. Changing profile of infective endocarditis: Results of a 1-year survey in France. JAMA. 2002;288:75-81.
8. Fefer P, Raveh D, Rudensky B, et al. Changing epidemiology of infective endocarditis: A retrospective survey of 108 cases, 1990-1999. Eur J Clin Microbiol Infect Dis. 2002;21:432-437.
9. Wallace SM, Walton BI, Kharbanda RK, et al. Mortality from infective endocarditis: Clinical predictors of outcome. Heart. 2002;88:53-60.
10. van der Meer JTM, Thompson J, Valkenburg HA, et al. Epidemiology of bacterial endocarditis in the Netherlands: 1. Patient characteristics. Arch Intern Med. 1992;152:1863-1868.
11. Berlin JA, Abrutyn E, Strom BL, et al. Incidence of infective endocarditis in the Delaware Valley, 1988-1990. Am J Cardiol. 1995;76:933-936.
12. Karchmer AW, Longworth DL. Infections of intracardiac devices. Infect Dis Clin North Am. 2002;16:477-505.
13. Calderwood SB, Swinski LA, Waternaux CM, et al. Risk factors for the development of prosthetic valve endocarditis. Circulation. 1985;72:31-37.
14. Grover FL, Cohen DJ, Oprian C, et al. Determinants of the occurrence of and survival from prosthetic valve endocarditis: Experience of the Veterans Affairs cooperative study on valvular heart disease. J Thorac Cardiovasc Surg. 1994;108:207-214.
15. Blackstone EH, Kirklin JW. Death and other time-related events after valve replacement. Circulation. 1985;72:753-767.
16. Hammermeister KE, Sethi G, Henderson WG, et al. Outcomes 15 years after valve replacement with a mechanical versus a bioprosthetic valve: Final report of the Veteran Affairs randomized trial. J Am Coll Cardiol. 2002;36:1152-1158.
17. Cabell CH, Heidenreich PA, Chu VH, et al. Increasing rate of cardiac device infections among Medicare beneficiaries: 1990-1999. Am Heart J. 2004;147:582-586.
18. Wilson WR, Jaumin PM, Danielson GK, et al. Prosthetic valve endocarditis. Ann Intern Med. 1975;82:751-756.
19. Karchmer AW. Infections of prosthetic valves and other intravascular devices. In: Mandell GL, Bennett JE, Dolin R, eds. Principles and Practice of Infectious Diseases. 5th ed. Philadelphia: Churchill Livingstone; 2000:903-917.
20. Ivert TSA, Dismukes WE, Cobbs CG, et al. Prosthetic valve endocarditis. Circulation. 1984;69:223-232.
21. Arvay A, Lengyel M. Incidence and risk factors of prosthetic valve endocarditis. Eur J Cardiothorac Surg. 1988;2:340-346.
22. Agnihotri AK, McGiffin DC, Galbraith AJ, et al. The prevalence of infective endocarditis after aortic valve replacement. J Thorac Cardiovasc Surg. 1995;110:1708-1724.
23. Horskotte D, Piper C, Niehues R, et al. Late prosthetic valve endocarditis. Eur Heart J. 1995;16(Suppl B):39-47.
24. Rutledge R, Kim J, Applebaum RE. Actuarial analysis of the risk of prosthetic valve endocarditis in 1598 patients with mechanical and bioprosthetic valves. Arch Surg. 1985;120:469-472.
25. Grover FL, Cohen DJ, Oprian C, et al. Determinants of the occurrence of and survival from prosthetic valve endocarditis. J Thorac Cardiovasc Surg. 1994;108:207-214.
26. Hammermeister KE, Sethi GK, Henderson WG. A comparison of outcomes eleven years after heart valve replacement with a mechanical valve or prosthesis. N Engl J Med. 1993;328:1289-1296.
27. Bloomfield P, Wheatley DJ, Prescott RJ. Twelve-year comparison of a Björk-Shiley mechanical heart valve with procine bioprostheses. N Engl J Med. 1991;324:573-579.
28. Sabik JF, Lytle BW, Blackstone EH, et al. Aortic root replacement with cryopreserved allograft for prosthetic valve endocarditis. Ann Thorac Surg. 2002;74:650-659.
29. Kluge RM, Calia FM, McLauglin JS, et al. Sources of contamination in open heart surgery. JAMA. 1974;230:1415-1418.
30. Blakemore WS, McGarrity GJ, Thurer RJ, et al. Infection by air-borne bacteria with cardiopulmonary bypass. Surgery. 1971;70:830-838.
31. Archer GL, Vishnaivsky N, Stiver HG. Plasmid pattern analysis of *Staphylococcus epidermidis* isolates from patients with prosthetic valve endocarditis. Infect Immun. 1982;35:627-632.
32. Boyce JM, Potter-Bynoe G, Opal SM, et al. A common-source outbreak of *Staphylococcus epidermidis* infections among patients undergoing cardiac surgery. J Infect Dis. 1990;161:493-499.
33. Mickelsen PA, Plorde JJ, Gordon KP, et al. Instability of antibiotic resistance in a strain of *Staphylococcus epidermidis* isolated from an outbreak of prosthetic valve endocarditis. J Infect Dis. 1985;152:50-58.
34. van den Broek PJ, Lampe AS, Berbee GAM, et al. Epidemic of prosthetic valve endocarditis caused by *Staphylococcus epidermidis*. BMJ. 1985;291:949-950.
35. Freeman R, King D. Analysis of results of catheter tip cultures in open heart surgery patients. Thorax. 1975;30:26-30.
36. Stiles GM, Singh L, Imazaki G, Stiles QR. Thermodilution cardiac output studies as a cause of prosthetic valve bacterial endocarditis. J Thorac Cardiovasc Surg. 1984;88:1035-1037.
37. Dismukes WE, Karchmer AW, Buckley MJ, et al. Prosthetic valve endocarditis: Analysis of 38 cases. Circulation. 1973;48:365-377.
38. Ismail MB, Hannachi N, Abid F, et al. Prosthetic valve endocarditis: A survey. Br Heart J. 1987;58:72-77.
39. Wilson WR. Prosthetic valve endocarditis: Incidence, anatomic location, cause, morbidity, and mortality. In: Duma RJ, ed. Infections of Prosthetic Heart Valves and Vascular Grafts: Prevention, Diagnosis, and Treatment. Baltimore: University Park Press; 1977:3-16.

40. Fang G, Keys TF, Gentry LO, et al. Prosthetic valve endocarditis resulting from nosocomial bacteremia: A prospective, multicenter study. Ann Intern Med. 1993;119:560-567.
41. Sande MA, Johnson WD, Hook EW, et al. Sustained bacteremia in patients with prosthetic cardiac valves. N Engl J Med. 1972;86:1067-1070.
42. San Román JA, Vilacosta I, Sarriá C, et al. Cinical course, microbiologic profile, and diagnosis of periannular complications in prosthetic valve endocarditis. Am J Cardiol. 1999;83:1075-1079.
43. Anderson DJ, Bulkley BH, Hutchins GM. A clinicopathologic study of prosthetic valve endocarditis in 22 patients: Morphologic basis for diagnosis and therapy. Am Heart J. 1977;94:325-332.
44. Arnett EN, Roberts WC. Prosthetic valve endocarditis: Clinicopathologic analysis of 22 necropsy patients with comparison of observations in 74 necropsy patients with active infective endocarditis involving natural left-sided cardiac valves. Am J Cardiol. 1976;38:281-291.
45. Rose AG. Prosthetic valve endocarditis: A clinicopathological study of 31 cases. S Afr Med J. 1986;69:441-445.
46. Richardson JV, Karp RB, Kirlin JW, et al. Treatment of infective endocarditis: A 10-year comparative analysis. Circulation. 1978;58:589-597.
47. Sett SS, Hudon MPJ, Jamieson WRE, et al. Prosthetic valve endocarditis: Experience with porcine bioprostheses. J Thorac Cardiovasc Surg. 1993;105:428-434.
48. Karchmer AW, Gibbons GW. Infections of prosthetic heart valves and vascular grafts. In: Bisno AL, Waldvogel FA, eds. Infections Associated with Indwelling Devices. 2nd ed. Washington, DC: American Society for Microbiology; 1994:213-249.
49. Baumgartner WA, Miller DC, Reitz BA, et al. Surgical treatment of prosthetic valve endocarditis. Ann Thorac Surg. 1983;35:87-102.
50. Fernicola DJ, Roberts WC. Frequency of ring abscess and cuspal infection in active infective endocarditis involving bioprosthetic valves. Am J Cardiol. 1993;72:314-323.
51. Lytle BW, Priest BP, Taylor PC, et al. Surgery for acquired heart disease: Surgical treatment of prosthetic valve endocarditis. J Thorac Cardiovasc Surg. 1996;111:198-210.
52. Chen SC, Sorrell TC, Dwyer DE, et al. Endocarditis associated with prosthetic cardiac valves. Med J Aust. 1990;152:458-463.
53. Tornos P, Sanz E, Permanyer-Miralda G, et al. Late prosthetic valve endocarditis: Immediate and long-term prognosis. Chest. 1992;101:37-41.
54. Keys TF. Early-onset prosthetic valve endocarditis. Cleve Clin J Med. 1993;60:455-459.
55. Wolff M, Witchitz S, Chastang C, et al. Prosthetic valve endocarditis in the ICU: Prognosis factors of overall survival in a series of 122 cases and consequences for treatment decision. Chest. 1995;108:688-694.
56. Piper C, Körfer R, Horstkotte D. Valve disease: Prosthetic valve endocarditis. Heart. 2001;85:590-593.
57. Karchmer AW, Archer GL, Dismukes WE. Staphylococcus epidermidis causing prosthetic valve endocarditis: Microbiologic and clinical observations as guides to therapy. Ann Intern Med. 1983;98:447-455.
58. John MVD, Hibberd PL, Karchmer AW, et al. Staphylococcus aureus prosthetic valve endocarditis: Optimal management and risk factors for death. Clin Infect Dis. 1998;26:1302-1309.
59. Ting W, Silverman NA, Arzouman DA. Splenic septic emboli in endocarditis. Circulation. 1990;82(Suppl IV):105-109.
60. Keyser DL, Biller J, Coffman TT, et al. Neurologic complications of late prosthetic valve endocarditis. Stroke. 1990;21:472-475.
61. Masur H, Johnson WD Jr. Prosthetic valve endocarditis. J Thorac Cardiovasc Surg. 1980;80:31-37.
62. Durack DT, Lukes AS, Bright DK. New criteria for diagnosis of infective endocarditis: Utilization of specific echocardiographic findings. Am J Med. 1994;96:200-209.
63. Nettles RE, McCarty DE, Corey RG, et al. An evaluation of the Duke criteria in 25 pathologically confirmed cases of prosthetic valve endocarditis. Clin Infect Dis. 1997;25:1401-1403.
64. Pérez-Vázquez A, Fariñas C, Garcia-Palomo D, et al. Evaluation of the Duke criteria in 93 episodes of prosthetic valve endocarditis. Arch Intern Med. 2000;160:1185-1191.
65. Røder BL, Wandall DA, Frimodt-Møller N, et al. Clinical features of Staphylococcus aureus endocarditis. Arch Intern Med. 1999;159:462-469.
66. Bayer AS, Bolger AF, Taubert KA, et al. Diagnosis and management of infective endocarditis and its complications. Circulation. 1998;98:2936-2948.
67. Rosen AB, Fowler VG Jr, Corey GR, et al. Cost-effectiveness of transesophageal echocardiography to determine the duration of therapy for intravascular catheter-associated Staphylococcus aureus bacteremia. Ann Intern Med. 1999;130:810-820.
68. Archer GL, Karchmer AW, Vishnaivsky N, et al. Plasmid-pattern analysis for the differentiation of infecting from non-infecting Staphylococcus epidermidis. J Infect Dis. 1984;149:913-920.
69. Washington JA. The microbiologic diagnosis of infective endocarditis. J Antimicrob Chemother. 1987;20(Suppl A):29-36.
70. Werner AS, Cobbs CG, Kaye D, et al. Studies on the bacteremia of bacterial endocarditis. JAMA. 1967;202:199-203.
71. Hoen B, Selton-Suty C, Lacassin F, et al. Infective endocarditis in patients with negative blood cultures: Analysis of 88 cases from a one-year nationwide survey in France. Clin Infect Dis. 1995;20:501-506.
72. Cannady PB Jr, Sanford JP. Negative blood cultures in infective endocarditis: A review. South Med J. 1976;69:1420-1424.
73. Pazin GJ, Saul S, Thompson ME. Blood culture positivity: Suppression by outpatient antibiotic therapy in patients with bacterial endocarditis. Arch Intern Med. 1982;142:263-268.
74. Bosshard PP, Kronenberg A, Zbinden R, et al. Etiologic diagnosis of infective endocarditis by broad-range polymerase chain reaction: A 3-year experience. Clin Infect Dis. 2003;37:167-172.
75. Raoult D, Fournier PE, Drancourt M, et al. Diagnosis of 22 new cases of Bartonella endocarditis. Ann Intern Med. 1996;125:646-652.
76. Shapiro DS, Kenney SC, Johnson M, et al. Brief report: Chlamydia psittaci endocarditis diagnosed by blood culture. N Engl J Med. 1992;326:1192-1195.
77. Khandheria BK. Transesophageal echocardiography in the evaluation of prosthetic valves. Am J Cardiac Imaging. 1995;9:106-114.
78. Stewart WJ, Shan K. The diagnosis of prosthetic valve endocarditis by echocardiography. Semin Thorac Cardiovasc Surg. 1995;16(Suppl B):63-67.
79. Bered Z, Mossinson D, Peleg E, et al. Echocardiographic assessment of prosthetic valve endocarditis. Eur Heart J. 1995;16(Suppl B):63-67.
80. Daniel WG, Mugge A, Grote J, et al. Comparison of transthoracic and transesophageal echocardiography for detection of abnormalities of prosthetic and bioprosthetic valves in the mitral and aortic positions. Am J Cardiol. 1993;71:210-215.
81. Morguet AJ, Werner GS, Andreas S, et al. Diagnostic value of transesophageal compared with transthoracic echocardiograhy in suspected prosthetic valve endocarditis. Herz. 1995;20:390-398.
82. Karalis DG, Bansal RC, Hauck AJ, et al. Transesophageal echocardiographic recognition of subaortic complications in aortic valve endocarditis: Clinical and surgical implications. Circulation. 1992;86:353-362.
83. Daniel WG, Mugge A, Martin RP, et al. Improvement in the diagnosis of abscesses associated with endocarditis by transesophageal echocardiography. N Engl J Med. 1991;324:795-800.
84. Birmingham GD, Rahko PS, Ballantyne F III. Improved detection of infective endocarditis with transesophageal echocardiography. Am Heart J. 1992;123:774-781.
85. Bayer AS. Infective endocarditis. Clin Infect Dis. 1993;17:313-320.
86. Ali AS, Trivedi V, Lesch M. Culture-negative endocarditis: A historical review and 1990s update. Prog Cardiovasc Dis. 1994;37:149-160.
87. Sochowski RA, Chan KL. Implication of negative results on a monoplane transesophageal echocardiographic study in patients with suspected infective endocarditis. J Am Coll Cardiol. 1993;21:216-221.
88. Bruss J, Jacobs LE, Kotler MN, et al. Utility of transesophageal echocardiography in the conservative management of prosthetic valve endocarditis. Chest. 1992;102:1886-1888.
89. Jacob S, Tong AT. Role of echocardiography in the diagnosis and management of infective endocarditis. Curr Opin Cardiol. 2002;17:478-485.
90. Archer GL, Johnston JL, Vazquez GJ, et al. Efficacy of antibiotic combinations including rifampin against methicillin-resistant Staphylococcus epidermidis: In vitro and in vivo studies. Rev Infect Dis. 1983;3(Suppl 3):S583-S542.
91. Kobasa WD, Kaye KL, Shapiro T, et al. Therapy for experimental endocarditis due to Staphylococcus epidermidis. Rev Infect Dis. 1983;5(Suppl 3):S533-537.
92. Chuard C, Hermann M, Vaudaux P, et al. Successful therapy of experimental chronic foreign-body infection due to methicillin-resistant Staphylococcus aureus by antimicrobial combinations. Antimicrob Agents Chemother. 1991;35:2611-2616.
93. Lucet JC, Hermann M, Rohner P, et al. Treatment of experimental foreign body infection caused by methicillin-resistant Staphylococcus aureus. Antimicrob Agents Chemother. 1990;34:2312-2317.
94. Rouse MS, Wilcox RM, Henry NK, et al. Ciprofloxacin therapy of experimental endocarditis caused by methicillin-resistant Staphylococcus epidermidis. Antimicrob Agents Chemother. 1990;34:273-276.
95. Wilson WR, Karchmer AW, Dajani AS, et al. Antibiotic treatment of adults with infective endocarditis due to streptococci, enterococci, staphylococci, and HACEK microorganisms. JAMA. 1995;274:1706-1713.
96. Wilson WR, Wilkowske CJ, Wright AJ, et al. Treatment of streptomycin-susceptible and streptomycin-resistant enterococcal endocarditis. Ann Intern Med. 1984;100:816-823.
97. Johnson, AP, Warner M, Woodford N, et al. Antibiotic resistance among enterococci causing endocarditis in the UK: Analysis of isolates referred to a reference laboratory. BMJ. 1998;317:629-630.
98. Birmingham MC, Rayner CR, Meagher AK, et al. Linezolid for the treatment of multidrug-resistant, gram-positive infections: Experience from a compassionate-use program. Clin Infect Dis. 2003;36:159-168.
99. Eliopoulos GM. Quinupristin-dalfopristin and linezolid: Evidence and opinion. Clin Infect Dis. 2003;36:473-481.
100. Rao N, White GJ. Successful treatment of Enterococcus faecalis prosthetic valve endocarditis with linezolid. Clin Infect Dis. 2002;35:902-904.
101. Ruiz ME, Guerrero IC, Tuazon CU. Endocarditis caused by methicillin-resistant Staphylococcus aureus: Treatment failure with linezolid. Clin Infect Dis. 2002;35:1018-1020.
102. Melgar GR, Nasser RM, Gordon SM, et al. Fungal prosthetic valve endocarditis in 16 patients: An 11 year experience in a tertiary care hospital. Medicine. 1997;76:94-103.
103. Gilbert HM, Peters ED, Lang SJ, et al. Successful treatment of fungal prosthetic valve endocarditis: Case report and review. Clin Infect Dis. 1996;22:348-354.
104. Nguyen MH, Nguyen ML, Yu VL, et al. Candida prosthetic valve endocarditis: Prospective study of six cases and review of the literature. Clin Infect Dis. 1996;22:262-267.
105. Pierrotti LC, Baddour LM. Fungal endocarditis, 1995-2000. Chest. 2002;122:302-310.
106. Wilson WR, Danielson GK, Giuliani ER, et al. Prosthetic valve endocarditis. Mayo Clin Proc. 1982;57:155-161.
107. Calderwood SB, Swinski LA, Karcherm AW. Prosthetic valve endocarditis: Analysis of factors affecting outcome of therapy. J Thorac Cardiovasc Surg. 1986;92:776-783.
108. Truninger K, Attenhofer Jost CH, Seifert B, et al. Long term follow-up of prosthetic valve endocarditis: What characteristics identify patients who were treated successfully with antibiotics alone? Heart. 1999;82:714-720.
109. Binder T, Maumgartner H, Maurer G. Diagnosis and management of prosthetic valve dysfunction. Curr Opin Cardiol. 1996;11:131-138.

110. Camacho MT, Cosgrove DM. Homografts in the treatment of prosthetic valve endocarditis. Semin Thorac Cardiovasc Surg. 1995;7:32-37.

111. Jault F, Gandjbakhch I, Chastre JC, et al. Prosthetic valve endocarditis with ring abscesses: Surgical management and long-term results. J Thorac Cardiovasc Surg. 1993;105:1106-1113.

112. Larbalestier RI, Kinchla NM, Aranki SF, et al. Acute bacterial endocarditis: Optimizing surgical results. Circulation. 1992;86(Suppl 2):68-74.

113. Dossche KM, Defau JJ, Ernst SM, et al. Allograft aortic root replacement in prosthetic aortic valve endocarditis: A review of 32 patients. Ann Thorac Surg. 1997;63:1644-1649.

114. Petrou M, Wong K, Albertucci M, et al. Evaluation of unstented aortic homografts for the treatment of prosthetic aortic valve endocarditis. Circulation. 1994;90(Suppl 2):198-204.

115. Aranki SF, Santini F, Adams DH, et al. Aortic valve endocarditis: Determinants of early survival and late morbidity. Circulation. 1994;90(Suppl 2):175-182.

116. Karchmer AW, Dismukes WE, Buckley MJ, et al. Late prosthetic valve endocarditis: Clinical features influencing therapy. Am J Med. 1978;64:199-206.

117. Saffle JR, Gardner P, Schoenbaum SC, et al. Prosthetic valve endocarditis: The case for prompt valve replacement. J Thorac Cardiovasc Surg. 1977;73:416-420.

118. Yu VL, Fang GD, Keys TF, et al. Prosthetic valve endocarditis: Superiority of surgical valve replacement versus medical therapy only. Ann Thorac Surg. 1994;58:1073-1077.

119. Akowuah EF, Davies W, Oliver S, et al. Prosthetic valve endocarditis: Early and late outcome following medical or surgical treatment. Heart. 2003;89:269-272.

120. David TE. The surgical treatment of patients with prosthetic valve endocarditis. Semin Thorac Cardiovasc Surg. 1995;7:47-53.

121. Yu VL, Fang GD, Keys TF, et al. Prosthetic valve endocarditis: Superiority of surgical valve replacement versus medical therapy only. Ann Thorac Surg. 1994;58:1073-1077.

122. Rocchiccioli C, Chastre J, Lecompte Y, et al. Prosthetic valve endocarditis: The case for prompt surgical management. J Thorac Cardiovasc Surg. 1985;92:784-789.

123. Omari B, Shapiro S, Giazton L, et al. Predictive risk factors for periannular extension of native valve endocarditis: Clinical and echocardiographic analyses. Chest. 1989;96:1273-1279.

124. Ellis SG, Goldstein J, Popp RL. Detection of endocarditis-associated abscesses by two dimensional echocardiography. J Am Coll Cardiol. 1985;5:647-653.

125. Seward JB, Khandheria BD, Edwards WD, et al. Biplanar transesophageal echocardiography: Anatomic correlations, image orientation, and clinical applications. Mayo Clin Proc. 1990;65:1193-1213.

126. Rohmann S, Seifert T, Erbel R, et al. Identification of abscess formation in native-valve infective endocarditis using transesophageal echocardiography: Implications for surgical treatment. J Thorac Cardiovasc Surg. 1991;39:273-280.

127. Wilson WR, Danielson GK, Giuliani ER, et al. Valve replacement in patients with active infective endocarditis. Circulation. 1978;58:585-588.

128. Horstkotte D, Bircks W, Loogen F. Infective endocarditis of native and prosthetic valves—the case for prompt surgical intervention? A retrospective analysis of factors affecting survival. Z Kardiol. 1986;75(Suppl 2):168-192.

129. Steckelberg JM, Murphy JG, Ballard D, et al. Emboli in infective endocarditis—the prognostic value of echocardiography. Ann Intern Med. 1991;114:635-640.

130. Roder BL, Wandall DA, Espersen F, et al. A study of 47 bacteremic *Staphylococcus aureus* endocarditis cases: 23 with native valves treated surgically and 24 with prosthetic valves. Scand Cardiovasc J. 1997;31:305-309.

131. Aragam JR, Weyman AE. Echocardiographic findings in infective endocarditis. In: Weyman AE, ed. Principles and Practice of Echocardiography. 2nd ed. Philadelphia: Lea & Febiger; 1994:1178-1197.

132. Jones RM, Jackson MA, Ong C, et al. Endocarditis caused by *Staphylococcus lugdunensis*. Pediatr Infect Dis J. 2002;21:265-268.

133. Reinhartz O, Hermann M, Redling F, et al. Timing of surgery in patients with acute infective endocarditis. J Cardiovasc Surg. 1996;37:397-400.

134. Boyd AD, Spencer FC, Isom OW, et al. Infective endocarditis: An analysis of 54 surgically treated patients. J Thorac Cardiovasc Surg. 1977;73:23-30.

135. Alexiou C, Langley SM, Stafford H, et al. Surgical treatment of infective mitral valve endocarditis: Predictors of early and late outcome. J Heart Valve Dis. 2000;9:327-334.

136. Cortina JM, Martinell J, Artiz V, et al. Surgical treatment of active prosthetic valve endocarditis: Results in 66 patients. Thorac Cardiovasc Surg. 1987;35:209-214.

137. Dearani JA, Orszulak TA, Schaff HV, et al. Surgery for acquired heart disease: Results of allograft aortic valve replacement for complex endocarditis. J Thorac Cardiovasc Surg. 1997;113:285-291.

138. Mestres CA, Ginel A, Cartana R, et al. Cryopreserved homografts in aortic and mitral prosthetic endocarditis: Expanding the use of biological tissues in complex cardiac infections. J Heart Valve Dis. 1993;2:679-683.

139. Symbas PN, Vlasis SE, Zacharopoulos L, et al. Acute endocarditis: Surgical treatment of aortic regurgitation and aortico-left ventricular discontinuity. J Thorac Cardiovasc Surg. 1982;84:291-296.

140. Reitz BA, Stinson EB, Watson DC, et al. Translocation of the aortic valve for prosthetic valve endocarditis. J Thorac Cardiovasc Surg. 1981;81:212-218.

141. Frantz PT, Murray GF, Wilcox BR. Surgical management of left ventricular-aortic discontinuity complicating bacterial endocarditis. Ann Thorac Surg. 1980;29:1-7.

142. Joyce F, Tingleff J, Pettersson G. The Ross operation in the treatment of prosthetic aortic valve endocarditis. Semin Thorac Cardiovasc Surg. 1995;7:38-46.

143. Ross DN. Homograft replacement of the aortic valve. Lancet. 1961;2:487-496.

144. Dearani JA, Orszulak TA, Daly RC, et al. Comparison of techniques for implantation of aortic valve allografts: Influence on subsequent aortic regurgitation. Ann Thorac Surg. 1996;62:1069-1075.

145. O'Brien MF, Stafford EG, Gardner MAH, et al. Allograft aortic valve replacement: Long-term follow-up. Ann Thorac Surg. 1995;60:565-570.

146. Miller DC, Shumway NE. "Fresh" aortic allografts: Long-term results with freehand aortic valve replacement. J Card Surg. 1978;2(Suppl):185-191.

147. Rubay JE, Raphael D, Sluysmans T, et al. Aortic valve replacement with allograft/autograft: Subcoronary versus intraluminal cylinder or root. Ann Thorac Surg. 1995;60:S78-82.

148. Park SJ, Sullivan HJ, Lonchyna V, et al. Heart transplantation for complicated and recurrent early prosthetic valve endocarditis. J Heart Lung Transplant. 1993;12:802-803.

149. DiSesa VJ, Sloss LJ, Cohn LH. Heart transplantation for intractable prosthetic valve endocarditis. J Heart Transplant. 1990;9:142-143.

150. Glazier JJ, Verwilghen J, Donaldson RM, et al. Treatment of complicated prosthetic aortic valve endocarditis with annular abscess formation by homograft aortic root replacement. J Am Coll Cardiol. 1991;17:1177-1182.

151. Olaison L, Petterson G. Current best practices and guidelines: Indications for surgical intervention in infective endocarditis. Infect Dis Clin North Am. 2002;16:453-475.

152. d'Udekem Y, David TE, Feindel CM, et al. Long-term results of operation for paravalvular abscess. Ann Thorac Surg. 1996;62:48-53.

153. David TE, Bos J, Christakis GT, et al. Heart valve operations in patients with active infective endocarditis. Ann Thorac Surg. 1990;49:701-705.

154. Mullany CJ, Chua YL, Schaff HV, et al. Early and late survival after surgical treatment of culture-positive endocarditis. Mayo Clin Proc. 1994;70:517-525.

155. Davenport J, Hart RG. Prosthetic valve endocarditis 1976-1987: Antibiotics, anticoagulation, and stroke. Stroke. 1990;21:993-999.

156. Wilson WR, Geraci JE, Danielson GK, et al. Anticoagulant therapy and central nervous system complications in patients with prosthetic valve endocarditis. Circulation. 1978;57:1004-1007.

157. Tornos P, Almirante B, Mirabet S, et al. Infective endocarditis due to *Staphylococcus aureus*: Deleterious effect of anticoagulant therapy. Arch Intern Med. 1999;159:473-475.

158. Delahaye JP, Poncet P, Malquarti V, et al. Cerebrovascular accidents in infective endocarditis: Role of anticoagulation. Eur Heart J. 1990;11:1074-1078.

159. Dajani AS, Taubert KA, Wilson WR, et al. Prevention of bacterial endocarditis: Recommendations by the American Heart Association, from the Committee on Rheumatic Fever, Endocarditis, and Kawasaki Disease, Council on Cardiovascular Diseases in the Young. JAMA. 1997;277:1794-1801.

160. Klug D, Lacroix D, Savoye C, et al. Systemic infection related to endocarditis on pacemaker leads: Clinical presentation and management. Circulation. 1997;95:2098-2107.

161. Victor F, De Place C, Camus C, et al. Pacemaker lead infection: Echocardiographic features, management and outcome. Heart. 1999;81:82-87.

162. Eggimann P, Waldrogel F. Pacemaker and defibrillator infections. In: Waldvogel FA, Bisno AL, eds. Infections Associated with Indwelling Medical Devices. Washington, DC: ASM Press; 2000:247-264.

163. Chua JD, Wilkoff BL, Lee I, et al. Diagnosis and management of infections involving implantable electrophysiologic cardiac devices. Ann Intern Med. 2000;133:604-608.

164. Cacoub P, Leprince P, Nataf P, et al. Pacemaker infective endocarditis. Am J Cardiol. 1998;82:480-484.

165. Bracke FA, Meijer A, van Gelder LM. Pacemaker lead complications: When is extraction appropriate and what can we learn from published data. Heart. 2001;85:254-259.

166. Li H, Natale A, Zhu W, et al. Causes and consequences of discontinuation of the implantable cardioverter-defibrillator therapy in non-terminally ill patients. Am J Cardiol. 1998;81:1203-1205.

167. Baddour LM, and the Infectious Diseases Society of America's Emerging Infectious Network. Long-term suppressive antimicrobial therapy for intravascular device-related infections. Am J Med Sci. 2001;322:209-212.

168. Rose EA, Gelijns AC, Moskowitz AJ, et al. Long-term use of a left ventricular assist device for end-stage heart failure. N Engl J Med. 2001;345:1435-1443.

169. Jessup M. Mechanical cardiac-support devices—dreams and devilish details. N Engl J Med. 2001;345:1490-1493.

170. Mekontso-Dessap A, Kirsch M, Vermes E, et al. Nosocomial infections occurring during receipt of circulatory support with the paracorporeal ventricular assist system. Clin Infect Dis. 2002;35:1308-1315.

171. Malani PN, Dyke DBS, Pagani FD, et al. Nosocomial infections in left ventricular assist device recipients. Clin Infect Dis. 2002;34:1295-1300.

172. Gordon SM, Schmitt SK, Jacobs M, et al. Nosocomial bloodstream infections in patients with implantable left ventricular assist devices. Am Thorac Surg. 2001;72:725-730.

173. Itescu S, Ankersmith J-H, Kocher AA, et al. Immunobiology of left ventricular assist devices. Prog Cardiovasc Dis. 2000;43:67-80.

174. Ankersmit H-J, Edwards NM, Schuster M, et al. Quantitative changes in T-cell populations after left ventricular assist device implantation: Relationship to T-cell apoptosis and soluble CD95. Circulation. 1999;100(Suppl II):211-215.

175. Westaby S, Frazier OH, Beyersdorf F, et al. The Jarvik 2000 Heart: Clinical validation of the intra-ventricular position. Eur J Cardiothorac Surg. 2002;22:228-232.

176. Arabia FA. Update on the total artificial heart. J Card Surg. 2001;16:222-227.

177. Ditlea S. The trials of an artificial heart. Sci Am. 2002;287:60-69.

178. Zareba KM. The artificial heart—past, present, and future. Med Sci Monit. 2002;8:RA72-77.

179. Schreffler RT, Schreffler AJ, Wittler RR. Treatment of cerebrospinal fluid shunt infections: A decision analysis. Pediatr Infect Dis J. 2002;21:632-636.

180. McClinton D, Carraccio C, Englander R. Predictors of ventriculoperitoneal shunt pathology. Pediatr Infect Dis J. 2001;20:593-598.

181. McHenry MC, Longworth DL, Rehm SJ, et al. Infections of the cardiac suture line after left ventricular surgery. Am J Med. 1988;85:292-300.

182. Wellens F, Vanermen H. Treatment of the infected cardiac suture line. J Card Surg. 1998;3:109-118.

183. Goldstein JA, Beardslee MA, Xu H, et al. Infective endocarditis resulting from CardioSEAL closure of a patent foramen ovale. Cathet Cardiovasc Intervent. 2002;55:217-220.

184. Bullock AM, Menahem S, Wilkinson JL. Infective endocarditis on an occluder closing an atrial septal defect. Cardiol Young. 1999;9:65-67.

185. Myles O, Thomas WJ, Daniels JT, et al. Infected endovascular stents managed with medical therapy alone. Cathet Cardiovasc Intervent. 2000;51:471-476.

186. Gordon GI, Vogelzang RL, Curry RH, et al. Endovascular infection after renal artery stent placement. J Vasc Intervent Radiol. 1996;7:669-672.

187. Dosluoglu HH, Curl GR, Doerr RJ, et al. Stent-related iliac artery and iliac vein infections: Two unreported presentations and review of the literature. J Endovasc Ther. 2001;8:202-209.

188. Pitsch RJ, Lawrence PF. Natural history of graft infections. In: Bunt TJ, ed. Vascular Graft Infections. Armonk, NY: Futura, 1994:31-42.

189. Oderich GS, Panneton JM. Aortic graft infection: What have we learned during the last decades? Acta Chir Belg. 2002;102:7-13.

190. Orton DF, LeVeen FR, Saigh JA, et al. Aortic prosthetic graft infections: Radiologic manifestations and implications for management. Radiographics. 2000;20:977-993.

191. Valentine RJ. Diagnosis and management of aortic graft infections. Semin Vasc Surg. 2001;14:292-301.

192. Yeager RA, Porter JM. Arterial and prosthetic graft infection. Ann Vasc Surg. 1992;6:485-491.

193. Bunt TJ. Vascular graft infections: An update. Cardiovasc Surg. 2001;9:225-233.

194. Angle N, Freischlag JA. Prosthetic graft infections. In: Moore WS, ed. Vascular Surgery: A Comprehensive Review. 6th ed. Philadelphia: WB Saunders 2002:741-750.

195. Chiesa R, Astore D, Frigerio S, et al. Vascular prosthetic graft infection: Epidemiology, bacteriology, pathogenesis, and treatment. Acta Clin Belg. 2002;102:238-247.

196. Stevenson KB, Hannah EL, Lowder CA, et al. Epidemiology of hemodialysis vascular access infections from longitudinal infection surveillance data: Predicting the impact of NKF-DOQI clinical practice guidelines for vascular access. Am J Kidney Dis. 2002;39:549-555.

197. Tokars JI, Miller ER, Stein G. New national surveillance system for hemodialysis-associated infections: Initial results. Am J Infect Control. 2002;20:288-295.

198. Nassar GM, Ayus JC. Infectious complications of the hemodialysis access. Kidney Int. 2001;60:1-13.

199. Nassar GM, Ayus JC. Infectious complications of old nonfunctioning arteriovenous grafts in renal transplant recipients: A case series. Am J Kidney Dis. 2002;40:832-836.

200. Ayus JC, Sheikh-Hammad D. Silent infection in clotted hemodialysis access grafts. J Am Soc Nephrol. 1998;9:1314-1317.

201. Feldman HI, Held PJ, Hutchinson JT, et al. Hemodialysis vascular access morbidity in the United States. Kidney Int. 1993;43:1091-1096.

202. Boelaert JR, van Landuyt HW, Gordts BZ, et al. Nasal and cutaneous carriage of Staphylococcus aureus in hemodialysis patients: The effects of nasal mupirocin. Infect Control Hosp Epidemiol. 1996;17:809-811.

203. Shinefield H, Black S, Fattom A, et al. Use of a Staphylococcus aureus conjugate vaccine in patients receiving hemodialysis. N Engl J Med. 2002;346:491-496.

204. Collier PE, Liebler GA, Park SB, et al. Is percutaneous insertion of the intraaortic balloon pump through the femoral artery the safest technique? J Vasc Surg. 1986;3:629-634.

205. Eltchaninoff H, Dimas AP, Whitlow PL. Complications associated with percutaneous placement and use of intra-aortic ballon counterpulsation. Am J Cardiol. 1993;71:328-332.

206. Lazar JM, Ziady GM, Dummer SJ. Outcome and complications of prolonged intra-aortic balloon counterpulsation in cardiac patients. Am J Cardiol. 1992;69:955-958.

207. Kantrowitz A, Tbonneland S, Freed PS, et al. Initial clinical experience with intraaortic balloon pumping in cardiogenic shock. JAMA. 1968;203:113-118.

208. Munoz P, Blanco R, Rodriquez-Creixems M, et al. Bloodstream infections after invasive nonsurgical cardiologic procedures. Arch Intern Med. 2001;161:2110-2115.

209. Samore MH, Wessolossky MA, Lewis SM, et al. Frequency, risk factors, and outcome for bacteremia after percutaneous transluminal coronary angioplasty. Am J Cardiol. 1997;79:873-877.

210. Shea KW, Schwartz RK, Gambino AT, et al. Bacteremia associated with percutaneous transluminal coronary angioplasty. Cathet Cardiovasc Diagn. 1995;36:5-9.

211. Smith TP, Cruz CP, Moursi MM, et al. Infectious complications resulting from use of hemostatic puncture closure devices. Am Thorac Surg. 2001;182:658-662.

212. Marso SP, Ellis SG, Russell R. Intracoronary stenting: An overview for the clinician. Cleve Clin J Med. 1999;66:434-442.

213. James E, Broadhurst P, Simpson A, et al. Bacteremia complicating coronary artery stenting. J Hosp Infect. 1998;38:154-155.

214. Gray NA, Baddour LM. Nonvalvular intravascular device-related infections. Curr Infect Dis Rep. 2002;4:293-298.

215. Rizzo RJ, Hertzer NR, O'Hara PJ, et al. Dacron carotid patch infection: A report of eight cases. J Vasc Surg. 2000;32:602-606.

216. Sternbergh WC III. Regarding "Dacron carotid patch infection: A report of eight cases." J Vasc Surg. 2001;33:663-664.

217. Greenfield LJ, Proctor MC. Filter complications and their management. Semin Vasc Surg. 2000;13:213-216.

218. Lin M, Soo TB, Horn LC. Successful retrieval of infected Günther Tulip IVC filter. J Vasc Intervent Radiol. 2000;11:1341-1343.

219. Herbiere P, Courouble Y, Bourgeois P, et al. Lumbar spondylodiscitis after insertion of a Mobin-Uddin caval "umbrella" filter. Nouv Presse Med. 1981;10:3715-3716.

220. Millward SF, Peterson RA, Mohr D, et al. LGM (vena tech) vena caval filter: Experience at a single institution. J Vasc Intervent Radiol. 1994;5:351-356.

Prophylaxis of Infective Endocarditis

DAVID T. DURACK

Prevention of infective endocarditis (IE) is important because this disease continues to cause serious morbidity and mortality. Despite advances in diagnosis and treatment, which have improved outcomes in some subgroups, the overall mortality of IE remains in the range of 20% to 30%, not significantly better than 50 years ago.[1] The etiologic organisms usually can be eradicated by antibiotics, but microbiologic cure often does not prevent permanent cardiac valvular damage and other early or late sequelae. Fewer than 20% of patients die during the active phase of endocardial infection,[2] but survival rates at 1, 5, and 10 years are notably lower. Many patients who have been "cured" of the infection suffer later complications, including recurrent IE, resulting in shortened life spans.[3-5] Furthermore, the increasing prevalence of antibiotic resistance among the common gram-positive cocci that cause most cases of endocarditis may further exacerbate the risks of IE and its complications.[6] Measures to prevent IE are clearly indicated,[7-11] but the determination of which potential interventions are effective, and cost-effective, remains an unanswered challenge.[8]

POTENTIAL INTERVENTIONS TO PREVENT ENDOCARDITIS

A variety of preventive measures potentially could interrupt the pathogenetic sequence that leads to endocarditis. These include treatment of predisposing cardiac conditions, elimination of portals of entry for organisms, immunization against bacteria that cause endocarditis, inhibition of bacterial adherence to the endocardium, topical application of antiseptics or antibiotics, and administration of systemic antibiotics. Administration of systemic antibiotics has received the most attention.

Elimination or Alleviation of Predisposing Conditions

Some abnormalities that predispose to endocarditis can be corrected. For example, surgical repair of a ventricular septal defect, patent ductus arteriosus, or coarctation of the aorta reduces or eliminates the significant risk for IE associated with these conditions. In the past, the lifetime risk for IE due to patent ductus arteriosus was 25% or more, high enough to indicate surgical repair for this reason alone. In recent years, the lifetime risk has fallen to less than 5%, probably too low to justify surgery unless it is required for other indications.[12]

Elimination of Portals of Entry for Organisms

Most cases of IE are caused by gram-positive cocci that originate from the mouth or the skin. Measures that reduce the frequency and intensity of bacteremias due to such organisms should be effective in preventing some cases of IE. It is therefore desirable to maintain optimal oral health, especially healthy gums. Periodontal probing can cause bacteremias,[13] and periodontitis may be an exacerbating factor.[14,15] Prevention and treatment of periodontal disease, and of other conditions associated with bacteremias (e.g., dental abscess), are strongly indicated in patients with cardiac conditions that predispose to IE. Likewise, prevention and prompt treatment of dermatologic infections such as furuncles or cellulitis caused by staphylococci and streptococci should reduce the risk posed by associated bacteremias, which can cause endocarditis in predisposed patients. Catheter-related bloodstream infections caused by gram-positive cocci and yeasts pose significant risk for development of nosocomial IE, especially if the pathogen is Staphylococcus aureus.[16] Nosocomial bacteremias due to S. aureus are common, and are increasing in frequency[6,16,17]; at least 5% of them are complicated by IE. Therefore, interventions to prevent or promptly detect and treat catheter-related blood-stream infections will prevent some cases of IE.

Immunization against Bacteria That Cause Endocarditis

Preexisting antibodies to bacteria that enter the blood potentially could either promote[18] or prevent[19-26] development of endocarditis. Under defined conditions, prior immunization can prevent streptococcal IE in rabbits.[22,23,26] A vaccine against FimA, a surface-associated protein found in about 80% of streptococci and enterococci that promotes adherence to fibrin, prevents experimental streptococcal endocarditis in rats.[19] Vaccines against various components of staphylococci that mediate adherence can prevent endocarditis,[24,25,27] catheter infection,[28] or septic death[29] in animal models, indicating that vaccines potentially could be developed to prevent staphylococcal bacteremias and therefore some cases of IE. However, assuming it were effective, vaccination would be difficult to validate as a preventive strategy against IE, and to this date no vaccine has been tested for this purpose in humans.

Inhibition of Bacterial Adherence to Endocardium

Adherence of bacteria to the endocardium and local deposition of platelets and fibrin are essential early events in development of IE. Inhibitors of these processes theoretically could prevent endocarditis. Anticoagulants have been tested in experimental animals but did not prevent infection.[30] As knowledge of the determinants of bacterial adherence progresses, new drugs that prevent attachment may be developed. A drug that prevented adherence of circulating bacteria might have advantages over antibiotics for prevention of endocarditis because it would not be limited by antibiotic resistance. No such drug is currently available.

Topical Application of Antiseptics or Antibiotics

The number of bacteria in the mouth and gingival crevices can be temporarily reduced by local irrigation with an antiseptic solution such as iodinated glycerol.[31] This might result in fewer or lower-density bacteremias after dental procedures. However, topical chlorhexidine was not effective.[32] Some dental experts have recommended application of this potentially useful degerming measure before dental extractions in patients at risk for IE, but it is not widely used in current practice. Topical application of antibiotics to the gums before dental procedures could theoretically reduce bacteremias, but topical amoxicillin proved ineffective in a human trial.[33] This approach could promote antibiotic resistance in oral flora, and therefore is not recommended.

Administration of Systemic Antibiotics

Administration of systemic antibiotics is a logical intervention, because many of the bacteria that cause endocarditis are killed or inhibited by commonly available antibiotics. However, development of recommendations for optimal use of antibiotics to prevent IE has been hampered by a serious lack of reliable data from human studies. There are no evidence-based answers to many basic questions. For example, what is the risk of developing IE after various procedures that cause bacteremia? Is antibiotic prophylaxis effective? If so, which procedures and operations should be covered by antibiotics? Which prophylactic antibiotic regimens are most effective? Several case-control studies have been performed, but it is unlikely that sufficient epidemiologic data can be accumulated to answer these questions definitively.

Random, low-grade bacteremias with organisms originating from the mouth, the gut, or the skin occur commonly, probably daily.[34,35] Therefore, patients with underlying heart conditions that predispose to bacterial colonization are continually at some risk of developing IE. In humans, it is usually impossible to determine with certainty which type of bacteremia—naturally occurring, or induced by a medical or dental procedure—was responsible for an episode of subacute IE. (Acute endocarditis that occurs after a nosocomial bacteremia caused by the same species is an exception to this general statement.)

Attempts to prevent endocarditis with antibiotics have usually been directed at the very brief bacteremias caused by dental, medical, and surgical interventions, but this approach may be misdirected. It has been argued that the continuing, cumulative risk posed by low-grade

daily bacteremias may be far higher than any risk attributable to highly episodic dental or medical bacteremias.[36] Clinical studies on the prophylactic efficacy of antibiotics are also unlikely to provide the answers because an excessively large number of patients would be required to reach a significant conclusion. To illustrate, let us assume that the risk of acquiring bacterial endocarditis after dental extraction is approximately 1 in 500,[37,38] that approval for a randomized trial of antibiotic versus a placebo could be obtained from an ethics review committee, and that an antibiotic regimen is available that is 100% effective in preventing endocarditis. An imaginary clinical trial under these admittedly arbitrary conditions might yield the following figures:

Treatment Group	No. Patients	No. Cases
Placebo	3000	6
Antibiotic	3000	0
Total	6000 ($\chi^2 = 4.2$, P $<$ .05)	

In this model, at least 6000 patients, *all with preexisting heart disease,* would have to be studied during dental procedures for the results to reach statistical significance. It is unlikely that such a large study could be successfully performed. However, it might be possible to demonstrate the efficacy of prophylaxis by selecting subgroups of patients at highest risk for endocarditis. Among patients with prosthetic heart valves who are undergoing various surgical procedures, no cases of endocarditis occurred after 287 procedures for which antibiotic prophylaxis was given, whereas 6 cases occurred after 390 procedures for which it was omitted.[38] This result just reaches statistical significance, but it has not been confirmed by any prospective randomized study.

Attempted prevention of bacterial infections with antibiotics is most likely to be effective and cost-effective when a single antimicrobial drug is directed against a single pathogen and when the disease occurs with fairly high frequency in the absence of prophylaxis.[39] In the past, prevention of recurrent rheumatic fever in young patients met these conditions, and several studies proved antimicrobial prophylaxis to be effective. Prevention of IE does not meet these ideals, because a variety of antibiotics are used against a variety of organisms and because the disease occurs rarely even if prophylactic antibiotics are not given. Furthermore, only a small proportion (perhaps 1% to 5%, or 15% at the most) of all cases of IE can be attributed to bacteremias caused by previous medical, surgical, or dental procedures.[34,40-42] It follows that the proportion of potentially preventable cases is also small.

Because definitive data are lacking, prevention of IE remains an empirical practice, characterized by uncertainty and controversy.[41,43-45] Nevertheless, most authorities agree that prophylaxis should be offered to susceptible patients during certain procedures known to be associated with bacteremia.[7,8,34,45-47] Controversy continues regarding the extent to which prophylaxis should be used and the specific risk factors and clinical situations that should be covered.

ESTIMATES OF RISK FOR INFECTIVE ENDOCARDITIS

To determine whether antibiotic prophylaxis should be given to an individual patient, it is necessary to estimate the patient's relative risk of developing endocarditis. This can be done by means of a matrix that relates the risk of bacteremia posed by the procedure to the risks posed by the underlying cardiac condition.

Procedures Causing Bacteremia

The incidence of transient bacteremia after various manipulations has been extensively studied.[32-35,48-63] Much of the literature on IE after dental procedures has emphasized tooth extraction, but bacteremias may occur after almost any form of dental manipulation.[34,35] It should be noted that the reported incidence of bacteremia varies quite widely between studies. Also, the presence in the blood of certain bacterial species associated with endocarditis, especially the viridans streptococci, may be more important than the overall frequency of bacteremia.[32] Some representative figures from selected studies are presented in Table 76-1.

TABLE 76-1 Representative Rates for Frequency of Bacteremia after Various Dental, Diagnostic, and Therapeutic Procedures

Procedure (%)	Bacteremia (%)	Range
None	0	0-3
Oral Cavity		
Extraction of teeth	60	18-85
Periodontal surgery	88	60-90
Brushing of teeth or irrigation	40	7-50
Tonsillectomy	35	33-38
Respiratory Tract		
Tracheal intubation	<10	0-16
Nasotracheal suctioning	16	NA
Bronchoscopy (rigid bronchoscope)	15	NA
Bronchoscopy (flexible bronchoscope)	0	NA
Genitourinary Tract		
Catheter insertion and removal	13	0-26
Prostatectomy (sterile urine)	12	11-13
Prostatectomy (infected urine)	60	58-82
Dilation of strictures	28	19-86
Normal delivery	3	1-5
Cesarean section	NA	NA
Intrauterine device insertion or removal	0	NA
Gastrointestinal Tract		
Upper gastrointestinal endoscopy	4	0-8
Transesophageal echocardiography	1	0-17
Endoscopic retrograde cholangiopancreatography	5	0-6
Barium enema	10	5-11
Colonoscopy	5	0-5
Sigmoidoscopy (rigid sigmoidoscope)	5	NA
Sigmoidoscopy (flexible sigmoidoscope)	0	NA
Proctoscopy	2	NA
Hemorrhoidectomy	8	NA
Esophageal dilation	45	NA
Echoendoscope-guided fine-needle aspiration	6	NA
Vascular System		
Cardiac catheterization	2	0-5
Other		
Insertion and removal of tympanostomy tubes	NA	NA

NA, not available, or insufficient data.
Data from multiple studies reviewed in references 8, 34, 54, 64.

BOX 76-1

Ranking of Risk for Infective Endocarditis After Dental, Diagnostic, and Therapeutic Procedures Related to Preexisting Cardiac Disorders

Higher Risk
Prosthetic heart valves
Previous infective endocarditis
Cyanotic congenital heart disease
Surgically constructed systemic-pulmonary shunts and conduits

Lower Risk
Mitral valve prolapse with regurgitation
Mitral regurgitation; stenosis; stenosis with regurgitation
Aortic regurgitation; stenosis; stenosis with regurgitation*
Tricuspid valve disease
Pulmonary stenosis
Ventricular septal defect
Patent ductus arteriosus
Coarctation of the aorta
Asymmetric septal hypertrophy
Calcific aortic sclerosis
Degenerative valvular disease in elderly patients
Surgically repaired intracardiac lesions with residual hemodynamic abnormality

Negligible Risk
Mitral valve prolapse without regurgitation
Minor valvular regurgitation by echocardiography without major structural abnormality
Isolated atrial septal defect
Arteriosclerotic plaques and coronary artery disease
Cardiac pacemakers
Surgically repaired intracardiac lesions with minimal or no hemodynamic abnormality

*Includes tricuspid, bicuspid, and unicuspid valves.
Adapted from Durack DT. Infective endocarditis. In: Alexander RW, Schlant RC, Fusterr V, O'Rourke RA, et al., eds. Hurst's The Heart, Arteries and Veins. New York: McGraw-Hill; 1998:2205-2239.

Several hundred cases of endocarditis that were attributed to prior dental procedures have been recorded in the literature.[34,65,66] In many of these, the first symptoms of endocarditis appeared less than 2 weeks after the procedure.[66] Although the incubation period of endocarditis is not known precisely, the onset of symptoms soon after dental operations in these cases makes a causal relationship likely. Similarly, more than 100 case reports provide reasonably good evidence that bacteremias originating from the genitourinary tract can cause endocarditis, especially when urologic or gynecologic operations are carried out in the presence of bacterial infections of the urinary or genital systems.[50] These uncontrolled case reports provide the basis for the belief that dental procedures often cause endocarditis—a belief that is widely but not universally accepted.[41,42,67-69]

The risk of developing IE from a dental procedure is certainly low, because such procedures are extremely common and often cause bacteremias, yet endocarditis is a relatively rare disease. It has been variously estimated that the risk for a predisposed patient is 1 in 533,[37] 1 in 115,500,[70] or even zero.[69] The risk may be as high as 1.5 in 100 for patients with prosthetic valves.[71] Most authorities would agree that dental operations do indeed pose some risk to susceptible patients, but it appears that the overall risk of acquiring IE is *less than 1%* for each procedure, even if no antibiotic prophylaxis is given.

Evidence that other medical and surgical procedures cause IE is sketchy. For example, only a few cases after miscellaneous operations such as drainage of soft tissue infections, abdominal surgery, diagnostic cardiac catheterization, and the use of oral irrigation devices have

been recorded.[34,72] The frequency of bacteremia during normal delivery is very low,[11,73,74] and few cases of endocarditis have been recorded in this setting.[74] Four cases occurring after skin biopsies have been reported, two of which were due to *S. aureus*.[75] Although bacteremias may occur during the performance of common diagnostic procedures such as endoscopies, barium enemas, and liver biopsies, very few cases of endocarditis attributable to these common procedures have been reported.[54,60,64,76-80] Estimates of the risks related to procedures that can cause bacteremias are offered in Box 76-1.

Underlying Cardiac Conditions

An assessment of risk in relation to the patient's underlying cardiac condition must also be made (Box 76-2). These estimates are based on the frequency with which various preexisting cardiac defects are found in patients with IE. Certain conditions clearly predispose to endocardial infection, including prosthetic valves, one or more previous episodes of IE, cyanotic congenital heart disease, congenital or acquired aortic valve disease, interventricular septal defects, and mitral stenosis or incompetence.[42,83] In a case-control study, the odds ratio was 75 for patients with a prosthetic valve, 37 for patients with a previous history of IE, and 17 for patients reporting any history of a cardiac valvular abnormality.[42] At the other end of the spectrum, uncomplicated secundum-type atrial septal defects carry such a low risk for IE[83] that prophylaxis is not recommended for these patients.[84]

Mitral valve prolapse presents a special problem because it is common in the general population (4% or more, according to the definition

BOX 76-2

Ranking of Risk for Infective Endocarditis Posed by Various Procedures That Might Cause Bacteremia

Higher-Risk Procedures
Dental procedures that involve the gingival crevice
Surgical procedures (including biopsies) inside the oral cavity
Genitourinary tract procedures when bacterial infection is present
Surgical procedures (including incision and drainage) when bacterial infection is present at the site

Lower-Risk Procedures
Injection of local anesthetic
Genitourinary tract procedures in absence of active bacterial infection
Surgery involving gastrointestinal or respiratory mucosa in absence of active bacterial infection
Skin biopsies and dermatologic procedures using standard antisepsis
Brochoscopy with or without biopsy
Gastrointestinal endoscopy, with or without biopsy
Cardiac catheterization
Transesophageal echocardiography
Esophageal dilatation and sclerotherapy of esophageal varices
Endotracheal tube insertion
Tympanostomy tube insertion
In the absence of active bacterial infection: urethral catheterization, laparoscopy, sterilization procedures, vaginal delivery, vaginal hysterectomy, cesarian section, therapeutic abortion, dilation and curettage, insertion or removal of intrauterine devices

Adapted from references 10, 45, 81, 82.

used).[85,86] Mitral valve prolapse increases a person's risk for endocarditis by fivefold to eightfold[83,85-87] and underlies 15% to 25% of cases of subacute bacterial endocarditis.[88-90] The risk appears to be greater for those patients with a systolic murmur[87,89] and for those with thickening and redundancy of the mitral leaflets on echocardiography.[86] Nevertheless, IE is an uncommon disease, so mitral valve prolapse cannot be regarded as a high-risk lesion,[85] even if a murmur is present. Many authorities currently recommend prophylaxis for patients with prolapse and regurgitation.[10] A study of benefits versus costs by decision analysis indicated that prophylaxis for mitral valve prolapse could prevent some cases of IE but probably would not be cost-effective.[91] Furthermore, because the incidence of endocarditis when a patient with prolapse undergoes a dental procedure without prophylaxis is very low, the years of life lost from anaphylaxis due to parenteral penicillin could exceed the years of life saved by prevention of endocarditis.[91]

The American Heart Association (AHA) guidelines[10] recommend that patients with mitral valve prolapse and regurgitation or thickening and redundancy of the leaflets by echocardiography should receive oral antibiotics before dental procedures, because the costs and risks of taking one oral dose of amoxicillin are small, and a serious disease may occasionally be prevented. However, the use of antibiotics could be considered optional rather than mandatory in this setting.[45] Parenteral prophylaxis should be avoided if possible.

INDIRECT EVIDENCE OF EFFICACY OF PROPHYLAXIS

In the absence of definitive data, recommendations for the prophylaxis of IE must be based on secondary sources of information. These include anecdotal clinical experience, in vitro studies of the organisms that cause bacteremia and endocarditis, and evaluation of the prevention of IE in experimental animals.

Uncontrolled Clinical Observations

Case reports describing patients who developed endocarditis after a procedure known to cause bacteremia despite the administration of

antibiotics provide anecdotal evidence that attempts to prevent endocarditis are not uniformly successful.[90,92] From 1979 to 1982, an AHA committee collected and recorded examples of apparent prevention failures.[90] Among 52 such cases, mitral valve prolapse was the single most common underlying cardiac lesion (33%), followed by various congenital abnormalities (29%), and rheumatic heart disease (21%). Nineteen percent had prosthetic valve endocarditis. Forty-eight cases (92%) occurred after a dental procedure, and 75% were caused by viridans streptococci. Symptoms began fairly soon after the procedure suspected to have caused endocarditis: 50% within 2 weeks and 79% within 5 weeks. Most patients received oral penicillin as prophylaxis. Sixty percent of organisms for which antimicrobial susceptibility was known were sensitive to the antibiotics used for prophylaxis. This experience, although anecdotal, indicates that failures of endocarditis prophylaxis may not be rare and may occur even if the infecting organism is susceptible to the antibiotics used. It confirms that mitral valve prolapse is a common underlying lesion in patients with streptococcal endocarditis.

Case-Control Studies and Decision Analysis

Several case-control studies have been performed. One indicated that prophylaxis appeared to be effective,[93] but only eight cases were analyzed, two of which were culture-negative. Two other large case-control studies concluded that attempted prevention with antibiotics in dental patients was of marginal or no value.[42,67] Decision analysis led the authors of one study to doubt that prophylaxis would be cost-effective, except in the highest-risk situations.[91] A cost-benefit analysis indicated that penicillin prophylaxis for dental patients would offer no net reduction in deaths.[94] These studies raise the possibility that the current practice of antibiotic prophylaxis for endocarditis is largely (or even entirely) ineffective.[45] It could even be counterproductive, by promoting antibiotic resistance and by diverting attention and resources from potentially more valuable interventions such as prevention of nosocomial bacteremias, patient education, and meticulous follow-up of patients at risk.

In Vitro Studies

A variety of organisms may be found in the blood stream after dental, surgical, and diagnostic procedures, including anaerobes and contaminants from the skin flora.[34,37,49,95] However, only gram-positive cocci such as viridans streptococci, enterococci, and staphylococci commonly cause IE in this setting. It is therefore appropriate to focus on the antibiotic susceptibilities of these organisms in attempting to formulate rational prophylactic programs. In the past, most of the bacteria in the oral flora that are likely to cause endocarditis were sensitive to penicillin G,[96] but some strains were partially resistant, with minimal bactericidal concentrations (MBCs) for penicillin G of 0.1 to 1.0 μg/mL or more.[97,98] Ampicillin and amoxicillin possess good in vitro activity against many strains of streptococci associated with endocarditis[96] and provide good serum concentrations.[99] However, penicillin resistance is increasing; a 1996 study in the United States found 43% intermediate and 13% high-level resistance among viridans streptococci.[100] Almost all strains of viridans streptococci, regardless of their MBCs, are killed more rapidly and more completely by a combination of a penicillin and an aminoglycoside than by a penicillin alone.[97,101] Many strains of enterococci, although more likely to be resistant to both penicillins and aminoglycosides, are killed synergistically by these drugs in combination, in vitro and in vivo.[98,102] However, many strains of enterococci have now developed high-level resistance to penicillins, aminoglycosides, or glycopeptides, posing new problems for prophylaxis and treatment.[103]

Experimental Infective Endocarditis

Study of the prevention of experimental IE in animal models has provided an important secondary source of information. In 1970, Garrison and Freedman[104] reported that placement of a polyethylene catheter in the rabbit heart led to the development of small, sterile vegetations at points of contact between the catheter and the endocardium.

If staphylococci were placed in the lumen of the catheter, staphylococcal endocarditis resulted. Modification of this model by injecting organisms intravenously[105] provided a suitable in vivo system for examining the efficacy of various antibiotic regimens for the prophylaxis of endocarditis.[102,106-109] A similar model in rats has also been used to investigate antibiotic prophylaxis.[15,110-114] Under experimental conditions, the time of onset of IE is known exactly. Another important advantage is that the incidence of infection in untreated animals can be adjusted easily by altering the size of the inoculum; therefore, the problem of very low infection rates in patients can be overcome by choosing an inoculum of the organism under investigation that is large enough to infect most of the animals. Significant differences among antibiotic regimens can then be demonstrated using manageable numbers of animals in each group.[15,102,106,108-113,115,116]

Early experiments comparing the success of various antibiotic regimens against viridans streptococci in these model systems showed that bacteriostatic antibiotics were usually ineffective, that penicillin in low doses or in high doses of brief duration was often ineffective, that high penicillin concentrations in serum for 12 hours or longer were more effective, that the combination of a penicillin plus an aminoglycoside was synergistic against viridans streptococci as well as enterococci, and that vancomycin provided an excellent alternative to regimens using penicillins.[102,106,107,109,115] Other antibiotics that have proved effective under controlled experimental conditions are ampicillin, amoxicillin,[108,112,113] ampicillin-sulbactam,[117] erythromycin,[113] clindamycin,[116] rifampin,[111] and azithromycin or clarithromycin.[118]

Further experiments have modified the view that bactericidal antibiotic activity is essential for prophylaxis. Streptomycin proved surprisingly effective in the prevention of experimental infection by some strains of enterococci, even though the serum concentrations of streptomycin were far too low to kill them.[102] Subinhibitory concentrations of certain antibiotics, especially vancomycin, can inhibit the adherence of streptococci to fibrin surfaces in vitro.[119] Other experiments have demonstrated successful prophylaxis for various streptococci with sublethal doses of vancomycin, clindamycin, erythromycin, and even a tetracycline.[113,115,116] Penicillin was much less effective in the prevention of experimental streptococcal endocarditis if the strain was tolerant to penicillin.[120] However, penicillin exhibited some prophylactic activity even if the strain was so tolerant that bactericidal concentrations of penicillin could not be achieved in serum.[120] All these findings suggest that prevention can sometimes be achieved by antibiotic effects that fall short of total bacterial killing, perhaps by an alteration of surface structures that mediate adherence to fibrin or by other unknown mechanisms. Bactericidal action may be sufficient but not necessary for prevention of endocarditis. The observation that successful prophylaxis with amoxicillin can be reversed by administration of penicillinase shortly *after* colonization of the vegetation shows that killing of organisms in the blood stream or prevention of their adherence to the endocardium is not essential for antibiotic prophylaxis in every situation.[110] The implications of these experimental findings for humans are uncertain. At present, it still seems prudent to choose bactericidal drugs for the prophylaxis of IE whenever possible.

To place these extensive experimental data into perspective, it should be emphasized that direct extrapolation of findings in animals to humans may not be meaningful. Although in vivo models provide a closer simulation of human endocarditis than any in vitro system could, there are at least two important differences. First, a foreign body was present throughout many of these experiments, because the intracardiac catheter often was left in place. The presence of a foreign body in tissue lowers the inoculum required to initiate infection and then makes infection harder to eradicate. Therefore, the animal models probably simulate patients with prosthetic valves more closely than they do patients with congenital or rheumatic valvular disease. Second, in many of the experiments a high inoculum was chosen deliberately, to make statistical comparisons possible with a relatively small number of animals. Because both the presence of a foreign body and the use of high inocula tend to make prevention harder to achieve, it is entirely possible that an antibiotic regimen that failed in animals might succeed in humans. Conversely, any regimen that proved effective under these rigorous experimental conditions would be likely to provide a wide margin of safety in clinical use.

With these reservations in mind, what has been the real contribution of experimental studies of prevention? Animal models provide a convenient in vivo method for ranking prophylactic antibiotic regimens in order of efficacy, but they cannot be used to prove whether any particular antibiotic regimen will or will not prevent endocarditis in patients. For example, experimental findings do not exclude the possibility that tetracycline or other bacteriostatic drugs may prevent endocarditis in some patients. They do support the conclusion that one of the optimal bactericidal regimens such as vancomycin, or penicillin plus an aminoglycoside, should provide a much wider margin of safety than does a lower-ranking regimen such as erythromycin or tetracycline.[109]

CARDIAC SURGERY

Most cardiovascular surgeons believe that the use of prophylactic antibiotics has reduced the incidence of postcardiotomy endocarditis. Although this is probably true, it should be noted that numerous technical improvements, introduced during the period when the incidence of postoperative endocarditis was falling, also may have contributed significantly. In fact, the efficacy of antibiotics for the prevention of postcardiotomy endocarditis has not yet been proved in any definitive controlled trial. However, the proven ability of antibiotics to prevent some other postoperative infections makes it difficult or impossible to obtain ethical approval for a placebo-controlled trial to address the question of efficacy for IE.

Early-onset postcardiotomy endocarditis is caused by a variety of organisms, including staphylococci, gram-negative bacteria, and, rarely, fungi. No single antibiotic regimen is effective against all of these organisms, and the use of broad-spectrum antibiotics may itself predispose to superinfection with resistant organisms. Therefore, attempts to prevent endocarditis with antibiotics during cardiac surgery should probably be limited to a short course of an antistaphylococcal agent such as a cephalosporin or vancomycin.[84] Some authorities recommend adding one concurrent dose of an aminoglycoside in the hope of taking advantage of possible synergism.

Diagnostic cardiac catheterizations (including Swan-Ganz catheters), insertion of pacemakers, coronary artery surgery, pericardial surgery, and the use of an intra-aortic balloon pump all appear to present little risk, and the administration of antibiotics specifically for the prevention of IE is not usually recommended during these operations. Pulmonary artery catheters have been reported to predispose to both nonbacterial and bacterial endocarditis in patients with severe burns, who often develop bacteremias, but because these catheters are often left in place for long periods, attempted antibiotic prophylaxis specifically for endocarditis is not indicated.[121]

Prosthetic Heart Valves

Extensive clinical experience has established that patients with prosthetic heart valves are at a relatively high risk for IE.[42,83,122-124] The high mortality and morbidity associated with prosthetic valve endocarditis and re-replacement of valves make its prevention a priority. Although the incidence of endocarditis after cardiac surgery has fallen steadily since these operations first became commonplace, the risk of early-onset endocarditis within 60 days after valve replacement remains in the region of 0.3% to 0.5%, and thereafter approximates 0.5% to 1% per year.[124] For comparison, the incidence of endocarditis is approximately 0.4% per year in patients with rheumatic heart disease.[125] It is important to recognize this risk and to take all possible steps to minimize it. Before elective valve replacement, the dental health of every patient should be evaluated and any necessary dental work completed under close observation and with appropriate antibiotic coverage. Healthy teeth should not be extracted, but if advanced dental or periodontal disease is present, extraction of all teeth should be considered. Thereafter, the patient should maintain good oral hygiene. Consultation between the patient's dentist and physician is important to ensure optimal antibiotic coverage during routine dental procedures.

Late-onset prosthetic valve endocarditis (60 days or more after the operation) is most likely to be caused by organisms originating in the oral cavity and reaching the valve via the blood stream, just as for native valve endocarditis. Attempted prophylaxis for endocarditis in the setting of a dental procedure should be directed primarily against streptococci, not staphylococci or gram-negative bacilli, just as for patients without prosthetic valves.

Many cardiac patients receive anticoagulant therapy, which may alter the choice of prophylactic antibiotics. Intramuscular injections are contraindicated in patients receiving heparin and should be avoided if possible in patients receiving Coumadin. Usually an oral dose is used, but if a parenteral antibiotic is given, the intravenous route should be used.

Timing of Prophylaxis

Antibiotics should be administered so as to provide the highest serum levels at the time when the procedure that might cause bacteremia is performed. There is no rationale to support the common practice of beginning antibiotic therapy earlier than is necessary to meet this criterion. Indeed, if antibiotics are given more than a few hours before the procedure, penicillin-sensitive oral flora may be replaced by penicillin-resistant organisms, and endocarditis, should it occur, may involve resistant organisms.[92] For most regimens, the administration of antibiotics 30 to 60 minutes before the procedure is appropriate. If the operation is delayed for longer than 1 or 2 hours, the dose should be repeated.

Duration of Prophylaxis

A single dose of antibiotic should suffice, based on the success of single-dose regimens in animal models.[105-107,109,112] Many practitioners continue prophylaxis for longer than is necessary.[90,126] This wastes antibiotic, may lead to the emergence of resistant organisms, and places the patient at an additional risk of adverse reactions. Moreover, a patient who is feeling perfectly well is unlikely to adhere to an unnecessarily prolonged regimen.

Prevention of Rheumatic Fever versus Prevention of Infective Endocarditis

Administration of low-dose penicillin orally or by monthly injection effectively prevents rheumatic fever but is *inadequate* to prevent IE. The incidence of IE in children who are receiving penicillin as prophylaxis for rheumatic fever is no less than in those with rheumatic heart disease who are not receiving prophylaxis.[125] Because patients taking low-dose oral penicillin for the prevention of rheumatic fever often carry moderately penicillin-resistant streptococci in the mouth, attempted prevention of IE with an oral penicillin regimen in these patients is not advisable. They should receive clindamycin as an alternative (Table 76-2).

Prophylaxis for Children

Because bacteremia during dental procedures appears to be somewhat less common in children than in adults, it has been suggested that antibiotic prophylaxis for IE is unnecessary in children.[128] However, careful studies indicate that bacteremia does indeed occur in a significant proportion of children after dental procedures,[129] and cases of endocarditis occurring soon after dental extraction have been reported.[129] The present consensus is that children should receive antibiotic prophylaxis for IE, with appropriate adjustment of dosages.

Compliance with Guidelines

Multiple studies and surveys have shown that most practitioners are aware of current recommendations, regarding them as authoritative. Nevertheless, they often do not follow them in practice,[130-132] for reasons that are unclear. Compliance may be improving gradually over time,[127] but it remains less than ideal.

THE MALPRACTICE DILEMMA

The issue of professional liability in the prophylaxis of endocarditis often has led to allegations of negligence and malpractice suits.[133] Clearly, the lack of basic factual information, referred to earlier, makes evaluation of such cases difficult. For example, it is hard to establish that any single procedure known to cause bacteremia was the "proximate cause" in a case of endocarditis. It is even harder to prove that the failure of a physician or dentist to administer antibiotics was the direct cause of a patient's acquiring endocarditis. If strict demonstration of proximate cause were always required, it is doubtful that any claim based on the failure to administer prophylaxis could succeed, but juries are sometimes capricious in deciding liability in malpractice cases. Another common problem for the defense in claims based on failure to administer prophylaxis is the lack of data on the upper limit of the incubation period of IE. Damages have been claimed in cases in which the first symptoms of endocarditis did not appear for months after tooth extractions without antibiotic cover. The likelihood of proximate cause here is remote, because review of case reports indicates that the incubation period is 2 weeks or less in most cases.[66]

A reasonable standard of care requires that health care professionals dealing with this question be aware of the factors that may increase the risk of IE. They should question the patient about underlying conditions that can predispose to endocarditis and should inform susceptible patients of the small risk that they may develop the disease. For the subgroup of patients judged to be at relatively high risk, an antibiotic regimen should be administered before selected dental, surgical, and genitourinary tract manipulations that might cause bacteremia.[10,45] Indications for prophylaxis outside these areas are less firmly established at present. A failure to use any recognized antibiotic regimen in preference to another should not be construed as negligence, because many different regimens have been recommended over the past 40 years. Although some authorities recognize evidence that certain antibiotic regimens probably provide a wider margin of efficacy than do others,[10,134] this evidence is not yet firm enough to make the choice of any particular regimen mandatory.

TABLE 76-2 Recommendations for Antibiotic Prophylaxis of Infective Endocarditis, Based on a Matrix Relating Underlying Cardiac Risk Factors (Box 76-1) and Risks Posed by Various Procedures (Box 76-2)*

	Underlying Cardiac Risk Factors (Box 76-1)		
Procedures (Box 76-2)	*Higher Risk*	*Lower Risk*	*Negligible Risk*
Higher-risk procedures	Prophylaxis recommended	Prophylaxis not recommended, but optional—clinical judgment needed	Prophylaxis not recommended
Lower-risk procedures	Prophylaxis not recommended, but optional—clinical judgment needed	Prophylaxis not recommended	Prophylaxis not recommended

*Note that antibiotics often may be given in these settings for prevention of infections other than endocarditis, or for other indications.

TABLE 76-3 Recommended Regimens for Prophylaxis of Endocarditis*

Indication	Regimen
Standard Regimen	
For dental procedures; oral or upper respiratory tract surgery; minor gastrointestinal (GI) or genitourinary (GU) tract procedures	Amoxicillin, 2.0 g PO 1 hr before procedure†
Special Regimens	
Oral regimens for penicillin-allergic patients (oral and respiratory tract only)	Clindamycin, 600 mg PO 1 hr before procedure *OR* Clarithromycin, 0.5 g PO 1 hr before procedure
Parenteral regimen for high-risk patients; also for GI or GU tract procedures	Ampicillin, 2.0 g IM or IV, 0.5 hr before procedure
Parenteral regimen for penicillin-allergic patients	Vancomycin, 1.0 g IV slowly over 1 hr starting 1 hr before procedure
Cardiac surgery including implantation of prosthetic valves	Cefazolin, 2.0 g IV at induction of anesthesia, repeated 8 and 16 hr later *OR* Vancomycin, 1.0 g IV slowly over 1 hr starting at induction of anesthesia, then 0.5 g IV 12 hr later

*Note: No regimen has been proved effective for the prevention of endocarditis, and prevention failures may occur with any regimen. These guidelines are not intended as the standard of care and are not intended to cover all clinical situations; the practitioner should use his or her own judgment on safety and cost-benefit issues in each individual case. One or two additional doses may be given if the period of risk for bacteremia is prolonged.

†Pediatric dosages: ampicillin, 50 mg/kg; cefazolin, 30 mg/kg; clindamycin, one-half of adult dose for child <60 lb (heavier child, same as adult dose); amoxicillin, one-half of adult dose for child <60 lb (heavier child, same as adult dose); amoxicillin, one-half of adult dose for child <60 lb (heavier child, same as adult dose); vancomycin, 20 mg/kg.

Adapted from references 9-11, 134.

The risks of toxicity from any prophylactic regimen must be considered carefully. Allergic reactions can occur after even low doses of penicillin; this risk is common to all regimens using penicillins as drugs of choice. However, the risk of anaphylaxis to penicillin is higher for parenteral than for oral administration. Other side effects are unlikely to occur with the very short courses (1 day or less) now used for the prophylaxis of IE.

CURRENT RECOMMENDATIONS

An AHA Committee[10] and various other authorities[9,11] have published guidelines for the prophylaxis of IE in the United States. Many groups in other countries have produced similar recommendations.[134] In view of continuing uncertainty and increasing skepticism[42,45,63,135] regarding the effectiveness and cost-effectiveness of systemic antibiotic prophylaxis for endocarditis, there is a trend toward limiting antibiotic prophylaxis to only the highest-risk situations, while giving more attention to patient education, follow-up, and surveillance. The author's current recommendations are listed in Tables 76-2 and 76-3.

REFERENCES

1. Durack DT. Evaluating and optimizing the results of surgery for infective endocarditis. JAMA. 2003;290:3250-3251.
2. Fonager K, Lindberg J. Incidence and short-term prognosis of infective endocarditis in Denmark, 1980-1997. Scand J Infect Dis. 2003;35:27-30.
3. Hasbun R, Vikram HR, Barakat LA, et al. Complicated left-sided native valve endocarditis in adults: Risk classification for mortality. JAMA. 2003;289:1933-1940.
4. Tornos M-P, Permanyer-Miralda G, Olona M, et al. Long-term complications of native valve infective endocarditis in non-addicts: A 15-year follow-up study. Ann Intern Med. 1992;117:567-572.
5. Ormiston JA, Neutze JM, Agnew TM, et al. Infective endocarditis: A lethal disease. Aust N Z J Med. 1981;11:620-629.
6. Chang FY, MacDonald BB, Peacock JE Jr, et al. A prospective multicenter study of Staphylococcus aureus bacteremia: Incidence of endocarditis, risk factors for mortality, and clinical impact of methicillin resistance. Medicine (Baltimore). 2003;82:322-332.
7. McGowan DA. A dental view of controversies in the prophylaxis of infective endocarditis. J Antimicrob Chemother. 1987;20(Suppl A):105-109.
8. Durack DT. Prevention of infective endocarditis. N Engl J Med. 1995;332:38-44.
9. American Society for Gastrointestinal Endoscopy. Antibiotic prophylaxis for gastrointestinal endoscopy. Gastrointest Endosc. 1995;42,630-635.
10. Dajani AS, Taubert KA, Wilson W, et al. Prevention of bacterial endocarditis: Recommendations by the American Heart Association. Circulation 1997;96:358-366.
11. American College of Obstetricians and Gynecologists. Prophylactic Antibiotics in Labor and Delivery. ACOG Practice Bulletin Number 47, October 2003. Obstet Gynecol. 2003;102;875-882.
12. Thilen U, Astrom-Olsson K. Does the risk of infective endarteritis justify routine patent ductus arteriosus closure? Eur Heart J. 1997;18:503-506.
13. Daly C, Mitchell D, Grossberg D, et al. Bacteraemia caused by periodontal probing. Aust Dent J. 1997;42:77-80.
14. Moreillon P, Overholser CD, Malinverni R, et al. Predictors of endocarditis in isolates from cultures of blood following dental extractions in rats with periodontal disease. J Infect Dis. 1988;157:990.
15. Overholser CD, Moreillon P, Glauser MP. Experimental bacterial endocarditis after dental extractions in rats with periodontitis. J Infect Dis. 1987;155:107-112.
16. Gottlieb GS, Fowler VG Jr, Kong LK, et al. Staphylococcus aureus bacteremia in the surgical patient: A prospective analysis of 73 postoperative patients who developed Staphylococcus aureus bacteremia at a tertiary care facility. J Am Coll Surg. 2000;190:50-57.
17. Lentino JR, Baddour LM, Wray M, et al. Staphylococcus aureus and other bacteremias in hemodialysis patients: Antibiotic therapy and surgical removal of access site. Infection. 2000;28:355-360.
18. Weinstein L, Schlesinger JJ. Pathoanatomic, pathophysiologic and clinical correlations in endocarditis (First of two parts). N Engl J Med. 1974;291:832-837.
19. Viscount HB, Munro CL, Burnette-Curley D, et al. Immunization with FimA protects against Streptococcus parasanguis endocarditis in rats. Infect Immun. 1997;65:994-1002.
20. Adler SW, Selinger DS, Reed WP. Effect of immunization on the genesis of pneumococcal endocarditis in rabbits. Infect Immun 1981;34:55-61.
21. Archer GL, Johnston JL. Effect of type-specific active immunization on the development and progression of experimental Pseudomonas aeruginosa endocarditis. Infect Immun. 1979;24:167-173.
22. Durack DT, Gilliland BC, Petersdorf RG. Effect of immunization on susceptibility to experimental Streptococcus mutans and Streptococcus sanguis endocarditis. Infect Immun. 1978;22:52-56.
23. Scheld WM, Thomas JH, Sande MA. Influence of preformed antibody on experimental Streptococcus sanguis endocarditis. Infect Immun. 1979;25:781-785.
24. Schennings T, Heimdahl A, Coster K, Flock JI. Immunization with fibronectin binding protein from Staphylococcus aureus protects against experimental endocarditis in rats. Microb Pathog. 1993;15:227-236.
25. Takeda S, Pier GB, Kojima Y, et al. Protection against endocarditis due to Staphylococcus epidermidis by immunization with capsular polysaccharide/adhesin. Circulation 1991;84:2539-2546.
26. van de Rijn I. Role of culture conditions and immunization in experimental nutritionally variant streptococcal endocarditis. Infect Immun. 1985;50:641-646.
27. Lee JC, Park JS, Shepherd SE, et al. Protective efficacy of antibodies to the Staphylococcus aureus type 5 capsular polysaccharide in a modified model of endocarditis in rats. Infect Immun. 1997;65:4146-4151.
28. Kojima Y, Tojo M, Goldmann DA, et al. Antibody to the capsular polysaccharide/adhesin protects rabbits against catheter-related bacteremia due to coagulase-negative staphylococci. J Infect Dis. 1990;162:435-441.
29. Nilsson IM, Patti JM, Bremell T, et al. Vaccination with a recombinant fragment of collagen adhesin provides protection against Staphylococcus aureus–mediated septic death. J Clin Invest. 1998;101:2640-2649.

30. Hook EW, Sande MA. Role of the vegetation in experimental *Streptococcus viridans* endocarditis. Infect Immun. 1974;10:1433-1438.

31. Bender IB, Naidorf IJ, Garvey GJ. Bacterial endocarditis: A consideration for physician and dentist. J Am Dent Assoc. 1984;109:415-450.

32. Lockhart PB. An analysis of bacteremias during dental extractions: A double-blind, placebo-controlled study of chlorhexidine. Arch Intern Med. 1996;156:513-520.

33. Vergis EN, Demas PN, Vaccarello SJ, Yu VL. Topical antibiotic prophylaxis for bacteremia after dental extractions. Oral Surg Oral Med Oral Pathol Oral Radiol Endod. 2001;91:162-165.

34. Everett ED, Hirschmann JV. Transient bacteremia and endocarditis prophylaxis: A review. Medicine (Baltimore). 1977;56:61-77.

35. Cobe HM. Oral medicine: Transitory bacteremia. Oral Surg Oral Med Oral Pathol 1954;7:609-615.

36. Roberts GJ. Dentists are innocent! "Everyday" bacteremia is the real culprit: A review and assessment of the evidence that dental surgical procedures are a principal cause of bacterial endocarditis in children. Pediatr Cardiol. 1999;20:317-325.

37. Kelson SR, White PD. Notes on 250 cases of subacute bacterial (streptococcal) endocarditis studied and treated between 1927 and 1939. Ann Intern Med. 1945;22: 40-60.

38. Horstkotte D, Friedrichs W, Pippert H, et al. Nutzen der endokarditisprophylaxe bei patienten mit prothetischen herzklappen. Z Kardiol. 1986;75:8-11.

39. Sanford JP. Prophylactic use of antibiotics: Basic considerations. South Med J. 1977;70(Suppl 1):2-3.

40. Freedman LR. Prophylaxis of intravascular infection. In: Freedman LR. Infective Endocarditis and Other Intravascular Infections. New York: Plenum; 1982.

41. Guntheroth WG. How important are dental procedures as a cause of infective endocarditis? Am J Cardiol. 1984;54:797-801.

42. Strom BL, Abrutyn E, Berlin JA, et al. Dental and cardiac risk factors for infective endocarditis: A population-based case-control study. Ann Intern Med. 1998;129: 761-769.

43. Kaplan EL. Bacterial endocarditis prophylaxis: Tradition or necessity? Am J Cardiol. 1986;57:478-479.

44. Chemoprophylaxis for infective endocarditis: Faith, hope, and charity challenged (Editorial). Lancet. 1992;339:525-526.

45. Durack DT. Antibiotics for prevention of endocarditis during dentistry: Time to scale back? Ann Intern Med. 1998;129:829-831.

46. Bisno AL. Antimicrobial prophylaxis for infective endocarditis. Hosp Pract. 1989:163-180.

47. Kaye D. Prevention of bacterial endocarditis: 1991. Ann Intern Med. 1991;114: 803-804.

48. Elliott SD. Bacteraemia and oral sepsis. Proc R Soc Med 1939;32:747-754.

49. Rogosa M, Hampp EG, Nevin TA, et al. Blood sampling and cultural studies in the detection of postoperative bacteremias. J Am Dent Assoc 1960;60:171-180.

50. Slade N. Bacteriaemia and septicaemia after urological operations. Proc R Soc Med 1958;51:331-334.

51. LeFrock JL, Ellis CA, Turchik JB, Weinstein L. Transient bacteremia associated with sigmoidoscopy. N Engl J Med 1973;289:467-469.

52. Le Frock J, Ellis CA, Klainer AS, Weinstein L. Transient bacteremia associated with barium enema. Arch Intern Med 1975;135:835-837.

53. Hoffman BI, Kobasa W, Kaye D. Bacteremia after rectal examination. Ann Intern Med 1978;88:658-659.

54. Shorvon PJ, Eykyn SJ, Cotton PB. Gastrointestinal instrumentation, bacteraemia, and endocarditis. Gut 1983;24:1078-1093.

55. Baltch AL, Pressman HL, Schaffer C, et al. Bacteremia in patients undergoing oral procedures: Study following parenteral antimicrobial prophylaxis as recommended by the American Heart Association, 1977. Arch Intern Med. 1988;148:1084-1088.

56. Lamich R, Alonso C, Guma JR, et al. Prospective study of bacteremia during transesophageal echocardiography. Am Heart J. 1993;125:1454-1455.

57. Botoman VA, Surawicz CM. Bacteremia with gastrointestinal endoscopic procedures. Gastrointest Endosc. 1986;32:342-346.

58. Low DE, Shoenut JP, Kennedy JK, et al. Risk of bacteremia with endoscopic sphincterotomy. Can J Surg. 1987;30:421-423.

59. Ho H, Zuckerman MJ, Wassem C. A prospective controlled study of the risk of bacteremia in emergency sclerotherapy of esophageal varices. Gastroenterology. 1991;101:1642-1648.

60. Rodriguez W, Levine JS. Enterococcal endocarditis following flexible sigmoidoscopy. West J Med. 1984;140:951-953.

61. Low DE, Shoenut JP, Kennedy JK, et al. Prospective assessment of risk of bacteremia with colonoscopy and polypectomy. Dig Dis Sci. 1987;32:1239-1243.

62. Wolf D, Fleischer D, Sivak MV Jr. Incidence of bacteremia with elective upper gastrointestinal endoscopic laser therapy. Gastrointest Endosc. 1985;31:247-250.

63. Lockhart PB, Durack DT. Oral microflora as a cause of endocarditis and other distant site infections. Infect Dis Clin North Am. 1999;13:833-850.

64. Levy MJ, Norton ID, Wiersema MJ, et al. Prospective risk assessment of bacteremia and other infectious complications in patients undergoing EUS-guided FNA. Gastrointest Endosc. 2003;57:672-678.

65. Sale L. Some tragic results following extraction of teeth: II. J Am Dent Assoc. 1939;26:1647-1651.

66. Starkebaum MK, Durack DT, Beeson PB. The "incubation period" of subacute bacterial endocarditis. Yale J Biol Med. 1977;50:49-58.

67. van der Meer JTM, Van Wijk W, Thompson J, et al. Efficacy of antibiotic prophylaxis for prevention of native-valve endocarditis. Lancet. 1992;339:135-140.

68. van der Meer JTM, Thompson J, Valkenburg HA, Michel MF. Epidemiology of bacterial endocarditis in the Netherlands: II. Antecedent procedures and use of prophylaxis. Arch Intern Med. 1992;152:1869-1873.

69. Schwartz SP, Salman I. The effects of oral surgery on the course of patients with diseases of the heart. Am J Orthod. 1942;28:331-345.

70. Pogrel MA, Welsby PD. The dentist and prevention of infective endocarditis. Br Dent J. 1975;139:12-16.

71. Horstkotte D, Rosin H, Friedrichs W, Loogen F. Contribution for choosing the optimal prophylaxis of bacterial endocarditis. Eur Heart J. 1987;8:379-381.

72. Drapkin MS. Endocarditis after the use of an oral irrigation device. Ann Intern Med. 1977;87:455.

73. Sugrue D, Blake S, Troy P, MacDonald D. Antibiotic prophylaxis against infective endocarditis after normal delivery: Is it necessary? Br Heart J. 1980;44:499-502.

74. Seaworth BJ, Durack DT. Infective endocarditis in obstetric and gynecologic practice. Am J Obstet Gynecol. 1986;154:180-188.

75. Spelman DW, Weinmann A, Spicer WJ. Endocarditis following skin procedures. J Infect. 1993;26:185-189.

76. Logan RF, Hastings JGM. Bacterial endocarditis: A complication of gastroscopy. BMJ. 1988;296:1107.

77. Pritchard TM, Foust RT, Cantey JR, Leman RB. Prosthetic valve endocarditis due to *Cardiobacterium hominis* occurring after upper gastrointestinal endoscopy. Am J Med. 1991;90:516-518.

78. Rigilino J, Mahapatra R, Barnhill J, Gutierrez J. Enterococcal endocarditis following sigmoidoscopy and mitral valve prolapse. Arch Intern Med. 1984;144:850-851.

79. Norfleet RG. Infectious endocarditis after fiberoptic sigmoidoscopy with a literature review. J Clin Gastroenterol. 1991;13:448-451.

80. Niv Y. Bacterial endocarditis after Hurst bougienage in a patient with a benign esophageal stricture and mitral valve prolapse. Gastrointest Endosc. 1985;31: 265-267.

81. Durack DT. Infective endocarditis. In: Alexander RW, Schlant RC, Fuster V, et al., eds. Hurst's The Heart, Arteries and Veins. New York: McGraw-Hill; 1998:2205-2239.

82. Babcock MD, Grekin RC. Antibiotic use in dermatologic surgery. Dermatol Clin. 2003;21:337-348.

83. Steckelberg JM, Wilson WR. Risk factors for infective endocarditis. Infect Dis Clin North Am. 1993;7:9-19.

84. Dajani AS, Bisno AL, Chung KJ, et al. Prevention of bacterial endocarditis: Recommendations by the American Heart Association. J Am Med Assoc. 1990; 264:2919-2922.

85. Clemens JD, Horwitz RI, Jaffe CC, et al. A controlled evaluation of the risk of bacterial endocarditis in persons with mitral-valve prolapse. N Engl J Med. 1982;307:776-781.

86. Marks AR, Choong CY, Sanfilippo AJ, Weyman AE. Identification of high-risk and low-risk subgroups of patients with mitral-valve prolapse. N Engl J Med. 1989; 320:1031-1036.

87. Danchin N, Voiriot P, Briancon S, et al. Mitral valve prolapse as a risk factor for infective endocarditis. Lancet. 1989;1:743-745.

88. Nolan CM, Kane JJ, Grunow WA. Infective endocarditis and mitral prolapse: A comparison with other types of endocarditis. Arch Intern Med. 1981;141:447-450.

89. MacMahon SW, Hickey AJ, Wilcken DEL, et al. Risk of infective endocarditis in mitral valve prolapse with and without precordial systolic murmurs. Am J Cardiol. 1986;58:105-108.

90. Durack DT, Kaplan EL, Bisno AL. Apparent failures of endocarditis prophylaxis: Analysis of 52 cases submitted to a national registry. J Am Med Assoc. 1983; 250:2318-2322.

91. Clemens JD, Ransohoff DF. A quantitative assessment of pre-dental antibiotic prophylaxis for patients with mitral-valve prolapse. J Chron Dis 1984;37:531-544.

92. Garrod LP, Waterworth PM. The risks of dental extraction during penicillin treatment. Br Heart J. 1962;24:39-46.

93. Imperiale TF, Horwitz RI. Does prophylaxis prevent postdental infective endocarditis? A controlled evaluation of protective efficacy. Am J Med. 1990;88:131-136.

94. Bor DH, Himmelstein DU. Endocarditis prophylaxis for patients with mitral valve prolapse: A quantitative analysis. Am J Med. 1984;76:711-717.

95. Nikutta P, Mantey-Stiers F, Becht I, et al. Risk of bacteremia induced by transesophageal echocardiography: Analysis of 100 consecutive procedures. J Am Soc Echocardiogr. 1992;5:168-172.

96. Basker MJ, Sutherland R. Activity of amoxicillin, alone, and in combination with aminoglycoside antibiotics against streptococci associated with bacterial endocarditis. J Antimicrob Chemother. 1977;3:273-282.

97. Blount JG. Bacterial endocarditis. Am J Med. 1965; 38:909-922.

98. Wilson WR, Geraci JE, Wilkowske CJ, Washington JA. Short-term intramuscular therapy with procaine penicillin plus streptomycin for infective endocarditis due to viridans streptococci. Circulation. 1978;57:1158-1161.

99. Shanson DC. The prophylaxis of infective endocarditis. J Antimicrob Chemother. 1978;4:2-4.

100. Doern GV, Ferraro MJ, Brueggmann AB, Ruoff KL. Emergence of high rates of antimicrobial resistance among viridans group streptococci in the United States. Antimicrob Agents Chemother. 1996;40:891-894.

101. Wolfe JC, Johnson WD. Penicillin-sensitive streptococcal endocarditis: In-vitro and clinical observations on penicillin-streptomycin therapy. Ann Intern Med. 1974;81:178-181.

102. Durack DT, Starkebaum MK, Petersdorf RG. Chemotherapy of experimental strepto-coccal endocarditis: VI. Prevention of enterococcal endocarditis. J Lab Clin Med. 1977;90:171-179.
103. Hoen B. Special issues in the management of infective endocarditis caused by gram-positive cocci. Infect Dis Clin North Am. 2002;16:437-452.
104. Garrison PK, Freedman LR. Experimental endocarditis: I. Staphylococcal endocardi-tis in rabbits resulting from placement of a polyethylene catheter in the right side of the heart. Yale J Biol Med. 1970;42:394-410.
105. Durack DT, Beeson PB, Petersdorf RG. Experimental bacterial endocarditis: III. Production and progress of the disease in rabbits. Br J Exp Pathol. 1973;54:142-151.
106. Durack DT, Petersdorf RG. Chemotherapy of experimental streptococcal endocardi-tis: I. Comparison of commonly recommended prophylactic regimens. J Clin Invest. 1973;52:592-598.
107. Pelletier LL Jr, Durack DT. Chemotherapy of experimental streptococcal endocardi-tis. J Clin Invest. 1975;56:319-330.
108. McGowan DA, Nair S, MacFarlane TW, MacKenzie D. Prophylaxis of experimental en-docarditis in rabbits using one or two doses of amoxicillin. Br Dent J. 1983;155:88-90.
109. Durack DT. Experience with prevention of experimental endocarditis. In: Kaplan EL, Taranta AV, eds. Infective Endocarditis: An American Heart Association Symposium. American Heart Association Monograph Number 52. Dallas: American Heart Association; 1977:28-32.
110. Moreillon P, Francioli P, Overholser D, et al. Mechanisms of successful amoxicillin prophylaxis of experimental endocarditis due to Streptococcus intermedius. J Infect Dis. 1986;154:801-807.
111. Malinverni R, Bille J, Glauser MP. Single-dose rifampin prophylaxis for experimen-tal endocarditis induced by high bacterial inocula of Viridans streptococci. J Infect Dis. 1987;156:151-157.
112. Malinverni R, Francioli PB, Glauser MP. Comparison of single and multiple doses of prophylactic antibiotics in experimental streptococcal endocarditis. Circulation. 1987;76:376-382.
113. Malinverni R, Overholser CD, Bille J, Glauser MP. Antibiotic prophylaxis of experi-mental endocarditis after dental extractions. Lab Invest. 1988;77:182-187.
114. Berney P, Francioli P. Successful prophylaxis of experimental streptococcal endo-carditis with single-dose amoxicillin administered after bacterial challenge. J Infect Dis. 1990;161:281-285.
115. Bernard J, Francioli P, Glauser MP. Vancomycin prophylaxis of experimental Streptococcus sanguis: Inhibition of bacterial adherence rather than bacterial killing. J Clin Invest. 1981;68:1113-1116.
116. Glauser MP, Francioli P. Successful prophylaxis against experimental streptococcal endocarditis with bacteriostatic antibiotics. J Infect Dis. 1982;146:806-810.
117. Ramos MC, Ing M, Kim E, et al. Ampicillin-sulbactam is effective in prevention and therapy of experimental endocarditis caused by beta-lactamase-producing coagulase-negative staphylococci. Antimicrob Agents Chemother. 1996;40:97-101.
118. Rouse MS, Steckelberg JM, Brandt CM, et al. Efficacy of azithromycin or clar-ithromycin for prophylaxis of viridans group streptococcus experimental endocardi-tis. Antimicrob Agents Chemother. 1997;41:1673-1676.
119. Scheld WM, Zak O, Vosbeck K, Sande MS. Bacterial adhesion in the pathogenesis of infective endocarditis: Effect of subinhibitory antibiotic concentrations on strepto-coccal adhesion in vitro and the development of endocarditis in rabbits. J Clin Invest. 1981;68:1381-1384.
120. Hess J, Dankert J, Durack DT. Significance of penicillin tolerance in endocarditis. Antimicrob Agents Chemother. 1983;11:555-564.
121. Ehrie M, Morgan AP, Moore FD, O'Connor NE. Endocarditis with the indwelling balloon-tipped pulmonary artery catheter in burn patients. J Trauma. 1978;18:665-666.
122. Horstkotte D, Friedrichs W, Pippert H, et al. Benefits of endocarditis prevention in pa-tients with prosthetic heart valves [German]. Z Kardiol. 1986;75:8-11.
123. Braimbridge MV, Eykyn SJ. Prosthetic valve endocarditis. J Antimicrob Chemother. 1987;20:173-180.
124. Eliopoulos GM. Enterococcal endocarditis. In: Kaye D, ed. Infective Endocarditis. New York: Raven Press; 1992:209-229.
125. Doyle EF, Spagnuolo M, Taranta A, et al. The risk of bacterial endocarditis during an-tirheumatic prophylaxis. J Am Med Assoc. 1967;201:129-134.
126. Brooks SL. Survey of compliance with American Heart Association guidelines for prevention of bacterial endocarditis. J Am Dent Assoc. 1980;101:41-43.
127. Brooks RG, Notario G, McCabe RE. Hospital survey of antimicrobial prophylaxis to prevent endocarditis in patients with prosthetic heart valves. Am J Med. 1988;84:617-621.
128. Hurwitz GA, Speck WT, Keller GB. Absence of bacteremia in children after prophy-laxis. Oral Surg Oral Med Oral Pathol. 1971;32:891-894.
129. Johnson DH, Rosenthal A, Nadas AS. A forty-year review of bacterial endocarditis in infancy and childhood. Circulation. 1975;51:581-588.
130. Kunzel C, Sadowsky D. Knowledge acquisition processes: Dissemination of expert recommendations to general practice dentists. J Health Soc Behav. 1989;30:330-343.
131. Sadowsky D, Kunzel C. Recommendations for prevention of bacterial endocarditis: Compliance by dental general practitioners. Circulation. 1988;77:1316-1318.
132. van der Meer JTM, Van Wijk W, Thompson J, et al. Awareness of need and actual use of prophylaxis: Lack of patient compliance in the prevention of bacterial endocardi-tis. J Antimicrob Chemother. 1992;29:187-194.
133. Martin MV, Butterworth ML, Longman LP. Infective endocarditis and the dental practitioner: A review of 53 cases involving litigation. Br Dent J. 1997;182:465-468.
134. Simmons NA. Recommendations for endocarditis prophylaxis. J Antimicrob Chemother. 1993;31:437-453.
135. van der Meer JT. Prophylaxis of endocarditis. Neth J Med 2002;60:423-427.

Myocarditis and Pericarditis

MARIA C. SAVOIA

MICHAEL N. OXMAN

Inflammatory processes affecting the heart frequently involve both the myocardium (myocarditis) and the pericardium (pericarditis). However, involvement of one or the other usually predominates, and the syndromes of myocarditis and pericarditis are sufficiently distinct in clinical presentation, etiology, and pathophysiology to warrant sep-arate consideration.

MYOCARDITIS

Myocarditis, literally "inflammation of the myocardium," is a protean disease with a wide variety of infectious and noninfectious causes. Postmortem examinations reveal evidence of previously unsuspected myocarditis in 1% to 4% of unselected cases,[1-3] with a higher inci-dence in young persons who have died suddenly.[4-7] The diagnosis of infectious myocarditis usually is considered when unexplained heart failure or arrhythmias occur in the setting of a systemic febrile illness or after symptoms of an upper respiratory tract infection. In some cases, however, the antecedent systemic illness is mild or long forgot-ten. In addition, myocarditis has been found histologically in 10% to 20% of cases of idiopathic dilated cardiomyopathy (DCM).[8-10] In myocarditis, the inflammatory process may affect myocytes, vascular elements, the conducting system, autonomic nerves, or the intersti-tium. One or more of at least four mechanisms appear to be involved: (1) direct damage to cells by an infectious agent; (2) cytotoxicity caused by a circulating toxin; (3) cytotoxicity caused by infection-induced immune reactions; and (4) nonspecific damage to myocytes as a result of an adjacent inflammatory process. Damage to the vascular endothelium may also result in indirect myocardial injury. A number of recent discoveries have revealed the complexities of the mecha-nisms involved in cardiac myocyte injury, especially injury caused by enteroviruses, and have also suggested targets for intervention.[11]

ETIOLOGIC AGENTS

In most cases of myocarditis, no definite cause is ever established. Almost every infectious agent is capable of causing myocarditis (Table 77-1), but viruses are the most important infectious cause of myocardi-tis in the United States and western Europe, and many cases of idio-pathic myocarditis are assumed to be viral in origin. Long before the era of modern virology, pericardial and myocardial involvement was recognized during outbreaks of mumps,[12] influenza,[13] measles,[14-16] po-liomyelitis,[17] and enterovirus-associated pleurodynia.[18] In modern times, enteroviruses[19,20] and especially group B coxsackieviruses,[21-25] have been the major agents implicated. These small, nonenveloped, sin-gle-stranded RNA viruses belonging to the Picornavirus family attach to specific receptors on myocardial cells.[19] When sensitive techniques such as in situ hybridization or the polymerase chain reaction (PCR) are used, enterovirus genomes, most of which are presumably group B coxsackievirus genomes, have been found in cardiac tissue from ap-proximately 25% of patients with myocarditis and in 10% to 30% of samples of patients with DCM.[23-27] A recent study using PCR to detect viral genomes in myocardial tissue from 624 patients with acute my-ocarditis and 149 patients with DCM identified adenoviruses in 23% of the patients with acute myocarditis and 12% of the patients with DCM.[28] Enterovirus genomes were detected in 14% of the patients with acute myocarditis and in 8% of the patients with DCM. Cytomegalovirus, parvovirus B19, influenza A virus, Epstein-Barr virus, herpes simplex virus, and respiratory syncytial virus were each identified in a small number of patients with acute myocarditis, but these agents were not detected in patients with DCM. Myocarditis has long been recognized in children with adenovirus pneumonia,[29-31] and other studies of myocarditis and DCM have also identified adenoviruses, especially in children.[24,28,32] Interestingly, enteroviruses were associated with a greater degree of myocardial inflammation than adenoviruses in patients with acute myocarditis and DCM.

There is considerable temporal and geographic variation in the prevalence of infections caused by various adenoviruses and enteroviruses, as well as marked seasonal variation in the prevalence of infections caused by other viruses associated with myocarditis, including parvovirus B19 and influenza A and B viruses. Moreover, the prevalence of infections caused by some viruses, for example, adenoviruses and parvovirus B19, is greater in children than in adults.[24,28,32,33] Consequently, the relative frequency with which different viruses are identified in acute myocarditis and DCM can be expected to vary from study to study.

The relatively high prevalence of human adenoviruses and group B coxsackieviruses, members of two very different virus families, as causes of viral myocarditis may be explained, at least in part, by the recent discovery that adenoviruses and group B coxsackieviruses both bind to a common receptor, the coxsackievirus-adenovirus receptor (CAR), that is expressed on the surface of cardiac myocytes.[11,34-37]

Symptomatic myocarditis or myopericarditis has also been reported in persons infected with many other viruses; additional viruses reported to cause myocarditis are listed in Table 77-1.

Myocardial involvement is the most common cause of death in diphtheria[147-149]; the toxin produced by *Corynebacterium diphtheriae* severely damages the myocardium and conduction system. The cardiac damage seen in patients with *Clostridium perfringens* may be the result of toxin, metastatic abscess formation, or both.[150,151] The immunologically mediated carditis associated with acute rheumatic fever[152] is discussed in Chapter 196.

Invasion of the blood stream by any bacterial pathogen may result in metastatic foci in the myocardium,[153] and myocarditis has been recognized in the course of meningococcemia,[154-156] salmonellosis,[157-159] *Campylobacter* infection,[161-163] brucellosis,[164-165] and bacteremias caused by streptococci,[166,167] staphylococci,[168-169] and *Listeria monocytogenes.*[170-172] More commonly, bacteria invade the myocardium as a complication of endocarditis by contiguous spread from valvular tissue or via septic embolization of the coronary arteries.[153,168,169]

Myocarditis is a rare complication during *Legionella* infection.[176] Myocarditis has also been observed in the course of *Mycoplasma pneumoniae,*[177-181] *Chlamydophila psittaci,*[182,183] and *Chlamydophila pneumoniae*[182,184,185] infections and is commonly seen in rickettsial infections,[153,186-189] especially scrub typhus.[153,188,189] Approximately 10% of patients with Lyme disease develop cardiac abnormalities, most commonly conduction system disturbances; full recovery is the norm.[192-199] In South America, the principal agent responsible for myocarditis is *Trypanosoma cruzi*, the protozoan that causes Chagas' disease. The initial infection is often asymptomatic, but it sometimes results in an acute illness complicated by myocarditis.[214,215] Myocarditis is the principal manifestation of chronic Chagas' disease, which occurs in approximately 30% of infected individuals. These patients typically have cardiomegaly, congestive heart failure (often predominantly right-sided), and conduction disturbances.[202,214,216-219] *Trypanosoma gambiense* and *Trypanosoma rhodesiense*, the agents of African trypanosomiasis, may also affect the heart with similar results, but central nervous system findings usually predominate.[220] Myocarditis is also observed in trichinosis[221-223] and is responsible for the occasional deaths that occur in severe infections.

In immunocompromised patients, myocarditis occurs as a consequence of a number of disseminated infections. Overt myocarditis is common in disseminated toxoplasmosis,[224-230] and systemic aspergillosis and candidiasis may also involve the heart.[201-208] Cryptococcal, *Toxoplasma*, and *Aspergillus* myocarditis have been reported in patients with the acquired immunodeficiency syndrome (AIDS).[206,211,212,226-228] Cardiac abnormalities in AIDS are common but are usually clinically silent.[133,145,146,233-235] A review of published autopsy series of AIDS cases by Kaul and associates suggested that the incidence of myocarditis in AIDS patients may be as high as 46%, although a strict definition of myocarditis requiring both myocardial inflammation and necrosis was not uniformly applied.[134] In a prospective study, DeCastro and colleagues[135] reported the presence of echocardiographic abnormalities in 47 of 72 AIDS patients (65.2%), with symptomatic cardiac involvement usually occurring late in the disease. Cardiac dysfunction is appreciated clinically in approximately 20% of AIDS patients and frequently takes the form of DCM, which is associated with a poor prognosis.[136] In a 1994 report, median survival time of patients at a similar stage of disease was reduced from 492 days to 101 days in those with cardiomyopathy.[137] A prospective study of 952 persons with human immunodeficiency virus (HIV) infection who did not use illicit drugs and had ratings of American Heart Association functional class I and US Centers for Disease Control and Prevention stage II showed that DCM developed in 76 (8%) during 5 years of follow-up.[138] A histologic diagnosis of myocarditis was made in 63 patients. HIV nucleic acid sequences were detected by in situ hybridization in biopsy samples of 36 (57%) of the patients with myocarditis. However, cultures were also positive for a group B coxsackievirus in four, and for Epstein-Barr virus in an additional four of the patients with myocarditis, and co-infection with HIV and another virus was documented in nine.[138] In this study, as in others,[135,139] cardiac dysfunction was highest in those with the most advanced disease. Although HIV has been cultured from endomyocardial biopsy samples[140,141,236] and identified by Southern blot analysis[237] or in situ hybridization,[137,138,141] in most AIDS patients with cardiac pathology HIV is found only rarely in myocytes,[137,142] and, when it is, there is often no correlation with histopathologic or clinical evidence of heart muscle disease.[141,145] The isolation of known cardiotropic viruses from AIDS patients is not infrequently reported,[100,136,137,236] and a causal relation

TABLE 77-1   Infectious Causes of Myocarditis

Viruses	Bacteria and rickettsiae
Coxsackie A[10,11,19-21,25-27,38-41]	*Corynebacterium*
Coxsackie B[10,11,19-27,38-50]	*diphtheriae*[147-149]
Echoviruses[10,11,26,51-53]	*Clostridium perfringens*[150,151]
Polio[17,54,55]	*Neisseria meningitidis*[154-156]
Nonpolio entero-	*Salmonella*[157-159]
viruses[10,11,19,25-28,41,56-63]	*Shigella*[160]
Adenovirus[11,26-32,63-65]	*Campylobacter*[161-163]
Mumps[12,66-68]	*Brucella*[164,165]
Rubeola[14-16,69]	*Streptococcus pyogenes*[166,167]
Influenza A and B[13,70-73]	*Staphylococcus aureus*[168,169]
Rabies[74]	*Listeria monocytogenes*[170,172]
Rubella[75,76]	*Vibrio cholerae*[173]
Dengue[77,78]	*Mycobacterium*
Chikungunya[78]	*tuberculosis*[174,175]
Yellow fever[79]	*Legionella pneumophila*[176]
Argentinian hemorrhagic fever[80]	*Mycoplasma pneumoniae*[177-181]
Bolivian hemorrhagic fever[80]	*Chlamydia psittaci*[182,183]
Lymphocytic choriomeningitis[81]	*Chlamydia pneumoniae*[182,184,185]
Lassa fever[82-84]	*Rickettsia rickettsii*[153,186]
Varicella-zoster[85-93]	*Rickettsia prowazekii*[153,187]
Cytomegalovirus[28,94-101]	*Rickettsia (Orientia)*
Epstein-Barr[28,102-109]	*tsutsugamushi*[153,188,189]
Herpes simplex[28,110-112]	*Coxiella burnetii*[190]
Variola[113]	*Ehrlichia*[191]
Vaccinia[114-119]	*Borrelia burgdorferi*[192-199]
Hepatitis B[120-122]	*Tropheryma whippelii*[200]
Hepatitis C[123-125]	**Fungi**
Respiratory syncytial virus[28,126,127]	*Aspergillus*[201-206]
Parvovirus B19[28,33,128-132]	*Candida* species[201-203,207,208]
Human immunodeficiency virus	*Blastomyces*[209]
(HIV)[100,133-146]	*Coccidioides immitis*[202,210]
	Cryptococcus
	neoformans[202,203,211,212]
	Histoplasma capsulatum[213]
	Parasites
	Trypanosoma cruzi[214-219]
	Trypanosoma gambiense[220]
	Trypanosoma rhodesiense[220]
	Trichinella spiralis[221-223]
	Toxoplasma gondii[224-230]
	Toxocara canis[231,232]

between HIV and myocarditis has yet to be firmly established. Malnutrition may also be a factor contributing to cardiac dysfunction in AIDS, and malnutrition and wasting are important independent predictors of cardiac morbidity and mortality.[143,144] Antimyosin and anti-cardiac mitochondrial adenine nucleotide translocator antibodies have been identified in some AIDS patients with cardiac dysfunction.[238]

PATHOLOGY AND PATHOGENESIS

Myocardial pathology depends on the infecting agent, the pathogenic mechanism involved, and the duration of the process. The hallmarks of myocarditis are an inflammatory infiltrate and injury to adjacent myocardial cells. Pathologic changes may be acute or chronic and vary markedly in severity, depending on the nature of the disease and the point in its course at which tissue is obtained. Some agents, such as the coxsackie B viruses, infect the myocytes themselves, whereas agents such as varicella-zoster virus, cytomegalovirus, and hepatitis B and C viruses appear to injure vascular endothelial cells. Although routine histology may help in the differential diagnosis, it rarely provides definitive information regarding an etiologic agent. Early in many viral infections, scattered hypereosinophilic myofibers, widespread edema, and only a few inflammatory cells may be present. Later, there is loss of striation, nuclear degeneration, and fragmentation of myofibers. The degenerating or partially necrotic myofibers are usually surrounded by lymphocytes, plasma cells, and macrophages.[21] The types of lymphocytes and macrophages that are present vary depending on the etiologic agent and the stage of infection.[142,239-241] Polymorphonuclear cells are occasionally seen[4] (Fig. 77-1). Return to normal cardiac function usually precedes resolution of the histologic abnormalities.[242] The acute process may resolve completely; healing and chronicity are reflected by the development of interstitial fibrosis and loss of myofibers.[243]

The pathogenesis of human viral myocarditis is incompletely understood. Mouse models of myocarditis induced by infection with either coxsackievirus B3 or encephalomyocarditis virus have revealed several possible pathogenetic mechanisms. Susceptibility to coxsackievirus B–induced myocarditis is age dependent and genetically determined.[244-248] Mechanisms of injury vary in different mouse strains.[244-248] In susceptible animals, acute myocarditis results from direct infection and cytolysis of myocytes.[3,4,8,249,250] In surviving animals, neutralizing antibody, perhaps in conjunction with macrophages[251,252] and natural killer cells,[253] appears to terminate virus replication by 7 to 9 days after infection.[19,254,255] Exercise[4,19,256] and corticosteroids[257] markedly enhance mortality during the early stages of infection. Studies in mice also demonstrated increased virulence of coxsackievirus B3 in selenium-deficient mice, suggesting that "oxidative stress" may contribute to myocardial damage.[258] The identification of coxsackie B viruses in the myocardium in patients with Keshan syndrome,[50] a form of myocarditis prevalent in a selenium-deficient region of China,[50] indicates that this murine model may have direct relevance to myocarditis in humans.

Nonsteroidal anti-inflammatory agents may also have deleterious effects,[259] perhaps through inhibition of interferon production.[260] Mice surviving the acute replicative phase of the virus infection may go on to develop severe myocarditis in the absence of recoverable virus.[8] This second phase of virus-induced myocardial destruction depends on the presence of cytolytic T cells,[21,261] which appear as productive virus replication ceases. Some of these cytolytic T cells recognize and lyse both infected and uninfected myocytes,[262] and their presence correlates with myocardial damage.[263,264] The severity of myocardial damage caused by this immune mechanism is greatest in male mice and pregnant female mice.[265] In some strains of mice that are less prone to myocarditis, the cytolytic T-cell response appears to be inhibited by suppressor cells.[266] Variants of coxsackievirus B3 that do not evoke cytolytic T cells directed against both infected and uninfected myocytes fail to cause myocarditis, even though they are indistinguishable from myocarditic strains in their ability to replicate and stimulate neutralizing antibodies.[267] The genetic loci responsible for the cardiovirulence of coxsackievirus B3 have been localized to two regions of the genome, the 5'-nontranslated region (NTR) and the capsid protein—encoding region.[268-270] Using two strains of coxsackievirus B3 that differ in their ability to produce autoimmunity, Weller and colleagues[271] demonstrated that the viruses used different re-

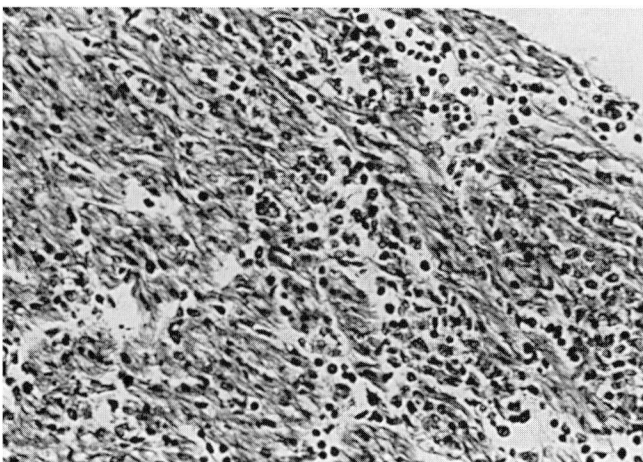

FIGURE 77-1. Coxsackievirus myocarditis with extensive infiltration of mononuclear cells, plasma cells, lymphocytes, and some eosinophils in the interstitial tissue (original magnification, ×250). *(From Bloor CM. Pericarditis and myocarditis. In: Cardiac Pathology. Philadelphia: JB Lippincott; 1978:265-295.)*

ceptors for cell entry, indicating that the receptor used by a virus may be important in triggering autosensitization. Interleukin (IL)-1, tumor necrosis factor (TNF), and bacterial lipopolysaccharide all enhance autoimmune injury and cause resistant mice to become susceptible.[272] Data demonstrating enhanced expression of intracellular adhesion molecule (ICAM)-1 in murine myocytes and both type I and type II major histocompatibility complex (MHC) antigens in human myocarditis also support the theory that autoimmunity plays a major role in the development of viral myocarditis.[273-276]

In situ hybridization studies suggest that the enterovirus genome can be found in all stages of acute and chronic infection and that virus persistence in the heart is characterized by restricted viral RNA and capsid protein synthesis. In one study, acute and chronic myocardial lesions were found consistently to be associated with infected myocardial cells, and mouse strains that cleared the virus after acute infection did not develop chronic disease.[277] Others have demonstrated the persistence of viral genome by PCR in mice after both culture and in situ hybridization techniques are negative.[278]

Mice and humans infected with coxsackievirus B3 also develop heart-reactive antibodies,[279-281] which may contribute to myocyte destruction.[246,282-286] Zhang and colleagues[287] demonstrated that a live attenuated variant of coxsackievirus B3 was able to protect mice against infection with the cardiovirulent wild-type strain. The attenuated virus was able to induce neutralizing antibodies, but, in contrast to wild-type virus, the attenuated virus failed to induce significant levels of antibody against cardiac myosin. In mice, susceptibility to damage from antimyosin antibodies is strain specific and appears to involve a genetically determined difference in target-organ sensitivity.[288] The role played by autoantibodies against structures such as the β-adrenoreceptors, myosin heavy chains, cardiac mitochondrial adenosine diphosphate/triphosphate carrier proteins, and aminin has not been clearly elucidated, but, for example, some antisarcolemmal antibodies that cross-react with enteroviral epitopes lyse myocytes.[282,284] Of note, Huber and associates[289] described three monoclonal antibodies to group A *Streptococcus* that also bind to various heart antigens and neutralize a myocarditic strain of coxsackievirus B3.

In human enteroviral infection, direct injury to myocytes appears to play a major role in neonatal myocarditis and in some cases of fulminant acute myocarditis in adults.[3,8,274,290] In situ hybridization studies have documented the presence of enterovirus genomes in 20% to 30% of cases of acute myocarditis and in many cases of DCM.[3,8,9,23-27] Patients with myocarditis also have been found to possess both cytotoxic lymphocytes that react with normal myocytes and high titers of antimyocyte antibodies.[3,8,246,274,290-292]

Recent observations have delineated potential mechanisms by which enteroviruses might cause acute myocarditis and DCM.[11,293-299] These observations suggest that the dystrophin-glycoprotein complex, a component of the extrasarcomeric cytoskeleton of cardiac myocytes that connects the internal F-actin cytoskeleton to laminin-2 in the extracellular matrix, may play a central role in the pathogenesis of myocarditis and DCM caused by enteroviruses.[11,293-299] The dystrophin-glycoprotein complex, which consists of dystrophin, a subsarcolemmal rod-shaped protein; four dystrophin-associated glycoproteins, α-, β-, γ-, and δ-dystroglycan; and sarcospan, a 25-kDa transmembrane protein, appear to transmit mechanical force from the sarcomere to the extracellular matrix and stabilize the sarcolemma.[11,293,294,300,301] Genetic defects in dystrophin cause Duchenne's and Becker's muscular dystrophy, both of which are associated with a high incidence of DCM, as well as X-linked cardiomyopathy, and genetic defects in the dystrophin-associated dystroglycans cause other forms of human muscular dystrophy and DCM.[11,293-295,300-302]

The demonstration by Badorff and colleagues[293,298,299] that enteroviral protease 2A, an essential viral gene product that cleaves the enteroviral polyprotein and inactivates eukaryotic initiation factor 4G (eIF4G), also cleaves dystrophin in the hinge 3 region provides a link between the mechanisms involved in viral and hereditary cardiomyopathy. Studies in mice and cell culture have shown that dystrophin deficiency markedly increases enterovirus replication and virus-induced disruption of the sarcolemmal membrane with the release of troponin I, whereas expression of wild-type dystrophin or a cleavage-resistant mutant dystrophin stabilizes the sarcolemmal membrane, reduces virus production, and protects cardiac myocytes from virus-induced cytopathic effects.[295] The capacity of enteroviral genomes to induce the cleavage of dystrophin and cause DCM in mice in the absence of virus replication[296] reveals a mechanism that could explain the induction of DCM by enteroviral genomes that have been found to persist in the heart following acute myocarditis in humans.

The innate immune system, equipped with pattern recognition receptors that recognize pathogen-associated molecular patterns, provides the first line of defense against invading microorganisms.[11,303] Recognition of pathogen-associated molecular patterns activates intracellular signaling pathways that lead to the expression of effector molecules such as cytokines, chemokines, and adhesion molecules involved in inflammation. Cardiac myocytes express mediators and effectors of the innate immune response, including proinflammatory cytokines (TNF-α, IL-1-β) and nitric oxide, in response to such pathogen-associated molecules as LPS and viral double-stranded RNA. Although these innate immune responses may have deleterious effects on cardiac function, they are also capable of inhibiting virus replication and dystrophin proteolysis by coxsackievirus protease 2A, thus protecting against enteroviral cardiomyopathy.[11,304] In this regard, it is noteworthy that patients who present with fulminant myocarditis, thought more severely ill, appear more likely to recover than do those with less severe acute myocarditis.[305]

Another mechanism that may explain the myocardial dysfunction and myocyte necrosis observed in viral myocarditis is damage to coronary vasculature with luminal narrowing, spasm, and obstruction leading to myocyte ischemia. This has been demonstrated in murine coxsackievirus B3 myocarditis,[306] and a similar mechanism appears to underlie the development of DCM in some humans after viral or idiopathic myocarditis.

In mouse models of cytomegalovirus myocarditis, genes linked to the H-2 complex influence susceptibility.[307] Cardiac lesions develop in and around the small penetrating blood vessels of the heart. When infected mice are depleted of CD4[+] T lymphocytes, myocardial lesions fail to develop even though viral titers may be increased.[308] Cytomegalovirus also induces antibodies that cross-react with cardiac myosin.[309] In contrast, in reovirus-induced murine myocarditis, myocarditis results from direct virus injury to myocytes; humoral immunity and cellular immunity protect against cardiac damage.[310]

In acute Chagas' disease, pathologic examination often reveals parasites within cardiac myocytes. When rupture of the cysts occurs, there is a marked inflammatory infiltrate consisting of lymphocytes,

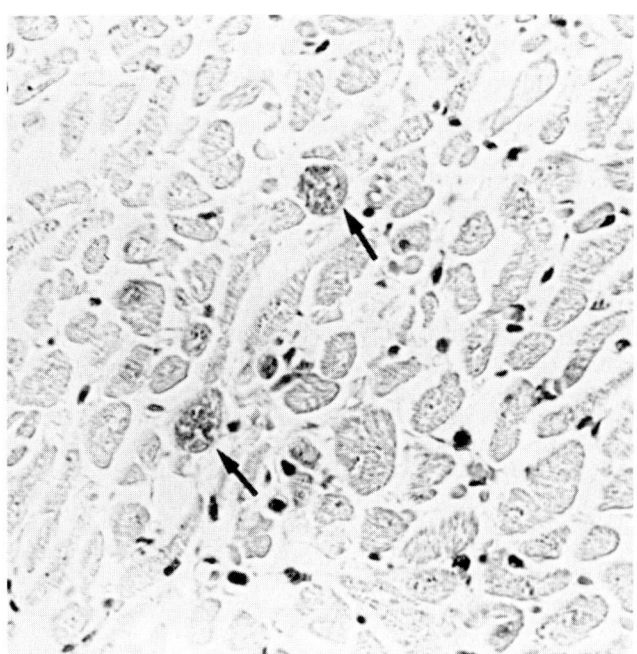

FIGURE 77-2. Cysts of *Toxoplasma gondii* (arrows) are easily visible in the heart of this immunosuppressed patient who died with disseminated toxoplasmosis.

plasma cells, macrophages, and some eosinophils.[202,214] In chronic Chagas' disease, the heart is often enlarged and flabby. Aneurysm formation may be present at the apex. The conduction system is often involved, and this is reflected by a high frequency of rhythm disturbances. Microscopic examination reveals focal mononuclear cell infiltrates and fibrosis.[202,214,217,218] In this stage, parasites can be identified only in 25% of patients.[218] Epitopes shared by *T. cruzi* and cardiac myocytes and recognized by cytotoxic T cells may play an important role in the progression of myocarditis late in the disease.[311]

The heart, as well as the central nervous system, is often prominently involved in disseminated toxoplasmosis. *Toxoplasma* pseudocysts containing numerous organisms may be readily identified in cardiac tissue, and there is a striking absence of cellular response around them (Fig. 77-2). Rupture of parasitized fibers is followed by infiltration of neutrophils and eosinophils.[202]

Myocardial microabscesses, affecting both myocytes and the conducting system, may occur in the course of systemic bacterial infections with organisms such as *Staphylococcus aureus*, but heart failure is rarely a direct consequence of such lesions.[168,169] In experimental animals, *Borrelia burgdorferi* has a predilection for connective tissue in the heart base, and disease severity correlates with the number of spirochetes found.[312] Mouse models suggest that infection with *B. burgdorferi* has a different pathogenesis than enterovirus myocarditis, because injury is independent of class II MHC:T-cell interactions and results from the response of macrophages to the spirochetes.[313]

Rickettsia and most fungi produce vasculitic lesions with surrounding inflammation. Damage to myocytes may be caused by the adjacent inflammatory process or may reflect anoxia caused by occlusion of small blood vessels.

Diphtheria toxin inhibits cellular protein synthesis. This results in hyaline degeneration and necrosis of myocardial fibers, with a secondary inflammatory response.[4,148]

CLINICAL MANIFESTATIONS

Patients with myocarditis may be asymptomatic, or they may have a rapidly progressive fatal disease. The diagnosis of infectious myocarditis usually is considered when a young person develops unexplained heart failure or arrhythmias, or when cardiac abnormalities occur in the course of a recognized systemic infection. Fever, malaise, arthralgias, upper respiratory tract symptoms, and chest pain may precede or accompany coxsackievirus myocarditis,[290,314,315] but these symptoms are not specific. Supraventricular tachycardia and ventricular extrasystoles are common.[316] Arrhythmias provide early evidence of involvement of the conduction system and are responsible for the occurrence of sudden death in patients with myocarditis. Myocarditis may mimic acute myocardial infarction,[317-321] but care should be taken not to mistake myocardial infarction occurring in a patient with infection for myocarditis.[42] In acute myocarditis, cardiac enzymes may be elevated and remain so for several days.[322,323] Symptomatic pericarditis may or may not be present.

DIAGNOSIS

Diagnosis of myocarditis requires a high index of suspicion. In infants, myocarditis is often just one manifestation of a widespread fulminant systemic infection. Involvement of the lungs, liver, and central nervous system; disseminated intravascular coagulation; and circulatory collapse may obscure the clinical signs of cardiac disease.[31,43,64,112] Recognition of myocarditis can also present difficulties in older children and adults when it occurs as part of an overwhelming systemic infection. When sought, however, signs of cardiac dysfunction usually are apparent. Even when cardiac signs and symptoms predominate, establishing a firm diagnosis may be difficult.

Nonspecific ST-segment and T-wave abnormalities on electrocardiography are frequently cited as presumptive evidence of myocarditis. Classically in myocarditis, there are sequential ST-segment elevations and T-wave inversions, which usually resolve in a month or two without the development of Q waves or R-wave depression.[314-316,324,382] The degree of ST-segment elevation and the extent and duration of later T-wave inversion have been reported to correlate with myocardial enzyme release and therefore with the amount of cell necrosis.[314-316,324,325] However, similar ST-segment and T-wave changes may also be seen with fever, hypoxia, tachycardia, and electrolyte disturbances, and they frequently occur during uncomplicated childhood viral infections.[326] Failure to reverse such ST-segment and T-wave changes with β-blockade is thought by some to be indicative of myocarditis,[327,328] but physicians should approach a diagnosis of myocarditis based solely on the presence of nonspecific ST-segment and T-wave abnormalities with skepticism.

Tachycardia out of proportion to the height of the fever, ventricular and supraventricular arrhythmias, and atrioventricular or intraventricular conduction disturbances may also be indicative of myocarditis. In a study of 45 patients with active myocarditis, the presence of Q waves in addition to ST-segment elevation frequently heralded a fulminant course, and abnormal QRS complexes and left bundle branch block were indicative of an increased risk of sudden cardiac death.[328]

The MB fraction of creatine kinase (CK-MB) is often elevated in the serum of patients with acute myocarditis and significant ST-segment elevation.[27,324] Elevated serum levels of troponin T and troponin I, components of the myocyte contractile apparatus, may persist in the serum for up to 14 days after myocyte injury.[27,324] Although elevations of cardiac troponins occur more frequently than do elevations of CK-MB, in one study only 34% (18 of 53) of those with biopsy-proved myocarditis had increased serum troponin levels, as did 11% (4 of 35) of patients without myocarditis.[322] An increased serum troponin level reflects cardiac injury, but it is neither sensitive nor specific for the diagnosis of myocarditis. A variety of heart-reactive antibodies have been detected in patients with myocarditis, and their persistence at high titer appears to be a poor prognostic sign. However, the clinical utility of these assays remains to be demonstrated.

Echocardiography is useful in detecting and quantifying impaired systolic function. Inflammation and edema may cause local thickening of the myocardium, and regional wall motion abnormalities are often observed.[329-332] Repeated echocardiographic examinations may be used to monitor the resolution or progression of myocarditis. Persistent wall motion abnormalities and ventricular dilation suggest the development of chronic myocarditis or DCM.

Indium 111–labeled antimyosin antibody imaging detects myocardial necrosis rather than inflammation, but it appears to be more sensitive for diagnosing myocarditis than endomyocardial biopsy.[27,198,199,333-337]

Increased myocardial uptake is observed in almost all patients with myocarditis who have positive endomyocardial biopsies, but it is also observed in many comparable patients with negative biopsies.[189,333-335] A negative ^{111}In-antimyosin antibody scan is highly predictive of a negative endomyocardial biopsy.[335] However, scans may continue to be positive long after the active phase of myocarditis, and this may account for at least some of the positive scans observed in biopsy-negative patients. In one study, 15 of 21 patients with DCM had positive scans before cardiac transplantation, but careful examination of their explanted hearts revealed histologic evidence of active myocarditis in only 7.[336] Indium 111 scanning has also been useful in distinguishing patients with acute myocarditis from those with acute myocardial infarction.[337]

Magnetic resonance imaging (MRI), which can detect small increases in the water content of tissues, has proved to be reliable in the diagnosis of cardiac allograft rejection.[338,339] Limited experience indicates that MRI also provides a sensitive means of detecting acute viral or idiopathic myocarditis.[340] In one study, MRI detected focal myocardial edema in two patients that corresponded anatomically to segmental wall-motion abnormalities detected by echocardiography and that normalized after the acute phase.[341] In another study, abnormal myocardial signal intensities indicative of edema were detected in six of six children with acute myocarditis proved by endomyocardial biopsy, but in none of the five biopsy-negative controls.[340] Both MRI and ^{111}In-antimyosin antibody scans were reported to be positive in a patient with endomyocardial biopsy–proved Lyme myocarditis.[199] Friedrich and co-workers[342] serially studied 19 patients who presented with symptoms of acute myocarditis using contrast medium–enhanced MRI and concluded that acute myocarditis evolves from a focal to a disseminated process during the first 2 weeks after the onset of symptoms.

The gold standard for the premortem diagnosis of myocarditis has traditionally been endomyocardial biopsy,[343-346] although some studies have questioned its value.[32,347,348] Biopsy confirmation of the clinical diagnosis of myocarditis is highly variable, ranging from 10% to 100% in different series.[346-354] Results of endomyocardial biopsy have also been highly variable in patients with unexplained congestive heart failure, with evidence of active myocarditis being found in 2% to 80% of these patients.[324,343,355-359] Several factors contribute to this variability and make interpretation of the literature difficult. These include lack of uniform clinical and histopathologic criteria for the diagnosis of myocarditis, a high degree of interobserver variability, sampling error, and marked variation in the timing of biopsies with respect to the onset of disease.[243,324-344,360-362] Agreement among pathologists on histopathologic criteria for the diagnosis of myocarditis (the *Dallas criteria*) has been a helpful development, but problems remain.[363] Scattered small collections of inflammatory cells with focal necrosis of myocytes may occur in response to stress or the administration of vasopressors,[327,346,363] and their presence in patients with heart failure may not be indicative of myocarditis. Conversely, a single small focus of myocarditis in the conducting system may be responsible for a fatal arrhythmia in someone without significant myocarditis elsewhere, and multiple endomyocardial biopsies are often necessary to establish the diagnosis.[347,348] Timing of biopsy is also critical. Early in enteroviral myocarditis there is necrosis of myocytes but not the lymphocytic infiltration demanded by the Dallas criteria.[44,53] Persistence of myocarditis is also highly variable; in some patients with acute enteroviral or idiopathic myocarditis, histopathologic abnormalities may resolve within a month or two after onset.[344-347,354,361]

DCM may represent, at least in some cases, the end stage of viral myocarditis.[3,8,9,324,364,365] This concept is supported by data from mouse models, by serial biopsies demonstrating progression to DCM in some patients with acute myocarditis, by evidence of active myocarditis in many patients with idiopathic DCM who undergo biopsy soon after the onset of their symptoms, and by the detection of enterovirus RNA in biopsies and explanted hearts.[3,8-11,21,23-28,57,58,246,343,344,349,355,364-367]

Proof of causation requires isolation of virus from the myocardium or demonstration of viral proteins or nucleic acids in the myocardium. Except in neonatal myocarditis and myocarditis occurring in immunocompromised patients, virus has rarely been isolated from cardiac tissue.[11,21,26,28,59] Detection of viral proteins has been difficult, primarily because lack of specificity has led to false-positive results, but the use of antiserum to purified coxsackievirus capsid proteins produced by recombinant DNA technology may overcome this difficulty.[368] To date, diagnosis of viral myocarditis has generally been based on the isolation of virus from another site (e.g., stool), the demonstration of a fourfold or greater rise in antibody titer from acute to convalescent sera, or the demonstration of a high titer of virus-specific immunoglobulin M antibody in serum.[11-22,290] At best, such data provide only circumstantial evidence of causation of myocarditis and must be interpreted with caution because of the prevalence of asymptomatic infections by the same agents that cause myocarditis. In a typical prospective study, 26% of patients without myocarditis had serologic evidence of infection with agents known to cause myocarditis.[316] These traditional methods have failed to provide a specific diagnosis in most patients with myocarditis of presumed viral origin.

The use of newer techniques for the detection and amplification of viral nucleic acids and their application to cardiac tissue obtained by endomyocardial biopsy is now providing interesting, but somewhat confusing, data on the viral etiology of myocarditis and DCM.[3,10,11,23-28,32,38,57-59,369-376] Cloned DNA fragments complementary to different regions of the enterovirus genome have served either as type-specific or as broadly cross-reactive hybridization probes, and PCR primers capable of detecting or amplifying nucleic acid sequences of a specific virus (e.g., coxsackievirus B3) or most enteroviruses or adenoviruses permit the detection of viral genomes with unprecedented sensitivity. In situ hybridization, although somewhat less sensitive than PCR, has the advantage of identifying the specific cells that are infected, whereas PCR can increase the sensitivity of the assay to between 1 and 10 viral genomes per milligram of tissue. Overall, enteroviral RNA has been detected by these techniques in approximately 25% of specimens from patients with myocarditis and in about 15% of specimens from patients with DCM. Similar figures have been reported for adenovirus DNA.

Results from individual studies have varied markedly, however. A large proportion of cases in which coxsackieviruses were implicated serologically did not give positive results by in situ hybridization.[38,374] Furthermore, the cells that contained enteroviral RNA were often not in areas of myocarditis,[38] and in some studies enteroviral RNA was also detected by PCR in cardiac tissue from control patients with a variety of other conditions, but not from noncardiac control tissues.[58] These results raise a number of difficult questions, including the specificity of the assays, the sensitivity and validity of the histopathologic assessments, and the pathogenetic significance of enteroviral RNA in the absence of inflammation or necrosis. The interpretation of such results is even more problematic when the viruses in question are members of the Herpesvirus family, which regularly persist in normal persons and which may even be present in the blood.[97] However, the recent demonstration by Wessely and co-workers[296] that the presence of coxsackie B virus genomes within cardiac myocytes can induce DCM in the absence of both virus replication and immune activation suggests that the mere presence of enterovirus RNA in the heart may have pathogenetic significance. In some studies the presence of enteroviral RNA in patients with myocarditis or DCM has been associated with a favorable prognosis,[60] but in other studies patients with demonstrated enteroviral RNA have had a poor outcome.[375,376]

The criteria for endomyocardial biopsy have evolved over time. At this time, myocardial biopsy is clearly indicated only in the monitoring of cardiac allograft rejection and anthracycline cardiotoxicity.[27,324,382] Many experts believe that endomyocardial biopsy is not warranted in most cases of myocarditis or DCM.[27,324,354,359,377,380,382] However, the availability of PCR and in situ hybridization techniques, and the development of antiviral drugs capable of inhibiting virus replication, may eventually justify endomyocardial biopsy during the acute phase of presumed infectious or idiopathic myocarditis in patients with positive ^{111}In-antimyosin antibody scans. Complications from right ventricular endomyocardial biopsy occur in approximately 6% of cases; serious adverse consequences (i.e., death, tamponade, perforation) occur in less than 1% if the operator is experienced.[359,381,382]

TABLE 77-2 Noninfectious Causes of Myocarditis

Collagen vascular disease[382-384]	Drug-induced (hypersensitivity)[383,400]
Systemic lupus erythematosus[385]	Methyldopa
Systemic sclerosis[386-388]	Sulfonamides
Rheumatoid arthritis[389,390]	Tetracycline
Dermatomyositis/	Scorpion, wasp, and spider stings[383,401]
polymyosisis[391,392]	Agents not yet identified
Still's disease[393]	Kawasaki disease[402]
Thyrotoxicosis[382,383]	Giant cell myocarditis[403]
Thrombotic thrombocytopenic	Sarcoid[404,405]
purpura[394]	
Pheochromocytoma[383]	
Peripartum[395]	
Radiation-induced[396-398]	
Drug-induced (direct toxic)[382,383,399]	
Cocaine	
Alcohol	
Emetine	
Catecholamines	
Arsenic	
Lead	
Cyclophosphamide	
Daunorubicin	
Adriamycin	

A wide variety of noninfectious diseases and agents may mimic infectious myocarditis and produce identical clinical syndromes (Table 77-2).

TREATMENT

Treatment of myocarditis should be directed at the specific etiologic agent involved whenever possible. Exercise has been shown to increase mortality in murine models of coxsackievirus B3 myocarditis and to worsen wall motion abnormalities in humans with myocarditis.[19,290,406,407] Thus, bed rest remains a very important part of therapy. Usual adjunctive care includes ensuring adequate oxygenation, avoiding and treating fluid overload if it develops, and monitoring for the development of ventricular arrhythmias. Some of the medications prescribed in the routine management of congestive heart failure may in the future play a more specific role in the treatment of myocarditis. In mice infected with either coxsackievirus B3 or encephalomyocarditis virus, treatment with captopril, an angiotensin-converting enzyme inhibitor used in the treatment of heart failure from a variety of causes, reduced inflammation and enhanced survival. Enalapril, however, did not reduce cardiac injury in a murine model of encephalomyocarditis virus-induced myocarditis,[408] suggesting that captopril's oxygen radical scavenging properties may be responsible for its beneficial effect.[409] Captopril has also been shown to ameliorate myocarditis in a mouse model of Chagas' disease.[410] Although verapamil and diltiazem are not useful agents in the treatment of human heart failure caused by ischemic disease,[411] experimental data in animals suggest that they may be useful in the treatment of some forms of infectious myocarditis.[412,413] Amlodipine, a novel dihydropyridine calcium channel blocker, both reduced myocardial injury in a murine myocarditis model (perhaps through an inhibition of nitric oxide)[414] and improved mortality in a double-blind, placebo-controlled study of patients with nonischemic DCM.[415]

Patients with rapidly progressive heart failure and cardiogenic shock are likely to benefit from circulatory support with a ventricular assist device, which can serve as a bridge to cardiac transplant or provide circulatory support until recovery from the acute phase of myocarditis.[416] Patients with fulminant myocarditis generally have a favorable long-term prognosis and should be given sufficient time to demonstrate recovery before being considered for cardiac transplantation.[305,372,416,417] In cases of severe myocarditis with progressive or fulminant heart failure, transplantation may be required if improvement does not occur with circulatory support by a ventricular assist device.

Most patients with viral myocarditis recover completely,[39,417,418] and the factors that predispose certain patients to a poor outcome are not clear. Early in experimental coxsackievirus B3 infection in mouse models, indomethacin, salicylates, and ibuprofen all increase viral replication and mortality.[259,409,419-421] No controlled data regarding their use in patients with myocarditis are available. Administration of glucocorticoids during the acute phase of viral myocarditis has been associated with rapid clinical deterioration, and the deleterious effects of these drugs have been clearly demonstrated in the acute phase of coxsackievirus infection in mice.[257,422] In some uncontrolled trials, patients with myocarditis proved by endomyocardial biopsy or with positive gallium scans who were given immunosuppressive agents showed improvement,[423-426] but controlled trials, with the exception of a methodolically flawed trial in children,[427] have failed to show benefit from treatment with prednisone alone or in combination with cyclosporine.[354,376-379] The largest controlled trial to date, which compared conventional therapy of congestive heart failure with conventional therapy plus prednisone and cyclosporine, failed to show benefit from immunosuppression.[354] An analysis of immunologic data from this study suggests that an early immune response may improve outcome, whereas an inadequate early immune response may predispose to viral persistence and chronic immunologic damage.[354] As knowledge of the pathogenesis of viral myocarditis increases and our ability to rapidly identify the etiologic agents improves, subgroups that might benefit from immunosuppressive therapy may emerge.

Data from mice and uncontrolled studies in humans suggest a beneficial role for immunoglobulins in the treatment of viral myocarditis and DCM. In mouse models of myocarditis induced by coxsackievirus B3 and encephalomyocarditis virus, immunoglobulin administration suppressed myocardial damage and increased survival, in association with a reduction in levels of proinflammatory cytokines and adhesion molecules, including TNF, interferon (IFN)-γ, IL-6, and ICAM-1.[428,429] Marsch and colleagues[430] demonstrated improvement of hemodynamic function and the eradication of virus after hyperimmunoglobulin treatment of patients with cytomegalovirus myocarditis. Immunoglobulin administration also led to significantly improved ejection fractions in 10 patients with new-onset DCM or myocarditis who had New York Heart Association class III/IV heart failure before therapy.[431] However, a follow-up study comparing intravenous immune globulin with placebo in adults with acute-onset DCM failed to demonstrate any benefit of treatment with intravenous immune globulin.[432]

The role for IFN in the treatment of acute myocarditis also remains to be elucidated. Studies in mice[433] and anecdotal reports[434-436] suggest potential benefit, although a small, single-center, matched-cohort trial demonstrated no significant difference in results between patients receiving IFN and controls.[437]

Studies in mouse models of viral myocarditis demonstrate a complex interplay between the virus and innate and adaptive host immune responses that inhibit virus replication and myocardial damage on the one hand and account for significant myocardial injury on the other.[3,8,9,11,27,240-243,268,273-277,288-304,419] The insights gained from these models are likely to be translated into new approaches to the treatment of myocarditis in humans. Cytokines and cytokine inhibitors are obvious candidates, as are inhibitors of signaling pathways involved in innate and adaptive immune responses, and inhibitors of the enteroviral protease 2A.[304,437]

Ganciclovir has been used successfully in the treatment of severe cytomegalovirus infection, including myocarditis.[438] No antiviral drugs with efficacy against the enteroviruses are commercially available at this time. Pleconaril, an experimental agent active against most members of the Picornavirus family including enteroviruses, has shown some benefit in clinical trials (see Chapter 38) but it is no longer available for compassionate use.[439-441] Pleconaril integrates into the picornavirus capsid and prevents the virus from attaching to cellular receptors and uncoating to release its RNA into the cell cytoplasm. WIN54954, an earlier compound in the same family, had potent antiviral effects in mouse models of coxsackievirus B3 myocarditis,[442-445] but adverse effects limited its development.

Prevention

The most effective means of preventing myocarditis is to eliminate its causes. To the extent that they have eliminated the diseases, vaccines against diphtheria, poliomyelitis, variola, measles, mumps, rubella, varicella, hepatitis virus A and B, influenza A and B, *Haemophilus influenza* type B, *Streptococcus pneumoniae,* and *Neisseria meningitidis* have eliminated myocarditis caused by the corresponding infectious agents. The fact that most cases of myocarditis and DCM in North America and Europe are caused by a limited group of viral pathogens, namely coxsackie B viruses, adenoviruses, and, perhaps, parvovirus B19, should make it possible to markedly reduce the incidence of myocarditis and DCM in these regions. A safe and effective vaccine against the coxsackie B viruses could be easily produced with the same technique currently used to produce inactivated polio vaccine. A safe and effective live attenuated oral adenovirus vaccine is currently administered to U.S. military recruits, and a multivalent adenovirus vaccine capable of markedly reducing the incidence of myocarditis and DCM caused by adenoviruses is feasible. Although no vaccine is currently available for parvovirus B19, vaccines have been produced against animal parvoviruses and the technology is readily available. The major impediments are cost and public acceptance. However, DCM occurs with an estimated annual incidence of 2 to 8 cases per 100,000, causes significant morbidity and mortality, and is the major reason for cardiac transplantation in the United States and Europe, and this should provide sufficient rationale for considering vaccine development.

PERICARDITIS

Pericarditis (inflammation of the pericardium) may be caused by any of a wide variety of infectious and noninfectious processes. It may be clinically silent or may result in severe hemodynamic compromise and death. In 1892, Sir William Osler called attention to the frequency with which pericarditis was overlooked by the practitioner,[446] and series indicate that this is still true today.[447-458] Advances in medicine, including antibiotic therapy, cardiac surgery, hemodialysis, cancer chemotherapy, and organ transplantation, as well as the current epidemic of HIV infection and AIDS, have altered the etiologic spectrum of pericarditis over the course of the 20th century. Idiopathic and viral pericarditis now predominate and usually result in a benign, self-limited disease. Purulent bacterial pericarditis and tuberculous pericarditis are now less common, but they still cause significant morbidity and mortality, and present a formidable diagnostic challenge.

ETIOLOGIC AGENTS

Because of the difficulty in establishing a specific diagnosis, the cause of acute, self-limited pericarditis in most cases is never determined and the disease is classified as idiopathic. In some series, idiopathic pericarditis accounted for 40% to 86% of patients hospitalized with acute pericarditis.[450-456] There are no clinical or epidemiologic features that distinguish idiopathic pericarditis from acute pericarditis of proven viral origin. Therefore, it is likely that viral infections are responsible for many, if not most, cases of acute pericarditis presently classified as idiopathic.

Most viruses infecting the heart affect both the myocardium and the pericardium (see previous discussion). Of the many viruses associated with heart disease, the enteroviruses, especially the coxsackieviruses, are most frequently implicated in pericarditis.[22,40,45,46,455] The association of myopericarditis with coxsackieviruses was first demonstrated in neonates with overwhelming, fatal systemic infections.[47] Pericarditis has also been recognized in the setting of epidemic coxsackievirus infection.[48,49] A century ago, cases of acute benign pericarditis were recognized during epidemics of Bornholm disease (epidemic pleurodynia), and it was postulated that the etiologic agent of the two diseases was the same.[18,48] Subsequently, the group B coxsackieviruses were shown to be the principal cause of epidemic pleurodynia, and their etiologic role in the associated cases of pericarditis was well established.[48,49]

Coxsackieviruses have only rarely been isolated from pericardial fluid[40,457,458] and, as with myocarditis, most diagnoses have been based on the isolation of virus from other body sites (e.g., stool) or the demonstration of a fourfold or greater rise in antibody titer after the acute illness, or both.[40,49,457-462] A number of other viruses have also been shown to cause pericarditis, but symptomatic involvement of the pericardium is uncommon. When it occurs, it is often a manifestation

TABLE 77-3 Infectious Causes of Pericarditis

Viruses
Coxsackie A[20,39,40,62,456,459-462]
Coxsackie B[20,22,24,40,43-49,62,456-462]
Echovirus[51-53,61,62,546,459,460]
Adenovirus[29,64,65,455,463,464]
Mumps[12,66,455,465]
Influenza A and B[13,70-73,466]
Lymphocytic
  choriomeningitis[81]
Lassa fever[82-84]
Varicella-zoster[467]
Cytomegalovirus[468-472]
Epstein-Barr[102,108,473,474]
Herpes simplex[475,476]
Variola[113]
Vaccinia[114-117]
Hepatitis B[121,477]
Human immunodeficiency virus
  (HIV)[133,135,136,139,143,146,233-235,478-481]

Fungi
Aspergillus[201-203,552-555]
Candida species[201-203,556-560]
Blastomyces[209]
Coccidioides immitis[210,561-564]
Cryptococcus
  neoformans[202,203,565]
Histoplasma capsulatum[213,566-568]

Protozoa
Entamoeba histolytica[569-573]
Toxoplasma gondii[224-226,574,575]
Toxocara canis[576]
Schistosoma[577]

Bacteria and Rickettsia
Streptococcus pneumoniae[482-485]
Other streptococcal species[166,486-491]
Staphylococcus
  aureus[168,169,447,482,483,492,493]
Neisseria meningitidis[155,156,494-496]
Neisseria gonorrhoeae[497,498]
Haemophilus influenzae[499-502]
Salmonella[157-159,503,504]
Yersinia[505]
Francisella tularensis[506-508]
Pseudomonas[509]
Campylobacter[510-511]
Brucella[512]
Listeria monocytogenes[172,513]
Nocardia[514]
Actinomyces[515,516]

Other anaerobic bacteria[517-520]
Mycobacterium tuberculosis[174,521-531]
Nontuberculous mycobacteria[532-536]
Legionella pneumophila[537-542]
Mycoplasma pneumoniae[180,181,543-546]
Coxiella burnetii[547]
Chlamydia[182]
Borrelia burgdorferi[192,193,196,199,548]

of severe disseminated infection. Viruses known to cause pericarditis are listed in Table 77-3.

A wide variety of bacteria can cause pericarditis. In the preantibiotic era, purulent pericarditis occurred primarily as a complication of pneumonia in previously healthy children and adults.[447,449-451,482,483] Of the 425 cases of purulent pericarditis reported in 1961 by Boyle and colleagues,[482] 43% were associated with pleuropulmonary infections. *S. pneumoniae* and *S. aureus* accounted for more than half of the cases. With the advent of antibiotics, the incidence of purulent pericarditis decreased markedly. Although staphylococci and streptococci are still etiologic in a substantial number of cases,[484-487,489-493] the incidence of pneumococcal pericarditis has declined substantially, and gram-negative bacilli have assumed a much more important role.[447-449,483,503-512] Patients with purulent pericarditis are now often older and have an underlying predisposing condition.[447-451,483] Recent reports emphasized the importance of anaerobic bacteria such as *Actinomyces, Prevotella, Fusobacteria, Peptostreptococcus,* and *Propionibacterium* in pericarditis complicating esophageal perforation and mediastinitis from head and neck infections,[515-520] but anaerobes can also seed the pericardium via the blood stream.[517-519] Purulent pericarditis may occur as a complication of meningococcal meningitis or fulminant meningococcemia, but *N. meningitidis*, especially serogroup C, also causes primary pericarditis.[494-496] A reactive, culture-negative pericarditis, presumably of immune origin, may also occur after successful treatment of meningococcal infection at another site.[494,495] *Neisseria gonorrhoeae* may also cause pericarditis, which may be either purulent or reactive.[497,498] *Mycoplasma pneumoniae* can cause pericarditis; although it is uncommon, this manifestation has been observed in almost 1% of patients hospitalized with *M. pneumoniae* infection.[180,181,543,546] *Legionella pneumophila* has been isolated from pericardial fluid,[537-539] and pericarditis has occurred in association with pneumonia[537-541] and endocarditis.[542] Pericarditis has been observed in children and adults with Lyme disease, but myocarditis is a more common manifestation of *B. burgdorferi* infection.[193,548] Bacterial infections account for proportionately more pericarditis in children; *S. aureus, Haemophilus influenzae,* and *N. meningitidis* are the most common etiologic agents.[499-502] Childhood immunization with *H. influenzae* type B conjugate vaccine has markedly reduced the frequency of *H. influenzae* type B infection in children, and this should result in a comparable reduction in the incidence of *H. influenzae* type B pericarditis.

Acute or chronic pericarditis is reported to occur in approximately 1% of patients with pulmonary tuberculosis.[523] Before the AIDS epidemic, because of the declining incidence of primary tuberculosis and the use of effective chemotherapy, *Mycobacterium tuberculosis* accounted for fewer than 5% of cases of acute pericarditis in Europe and North America.[521-525] In contrast, tuberculous pericarditis is a major cause of heart disease in Africa[526-528] and in patients with AIDS.[35,478,480,529] Diagnosis is difficult and mortality remains high.[521,522] *M. tuberculosis* continues to be an important treatable cause of chronic pericardial effusion and constrictive pericarditis[524,526-528,530,531,549-551] (see Chapter 248).

Primary pathogenic fungi are infrequently recognized as a cause of pericarditis. However, in large outbreaks, pericarditis occurred in 6% of patients with acute symptomatic histoplasmosis.[213,566] In most, it appeared to represent a sterile inflammatory response to infection in adjacent mediastinal lymph nodes and resolved spontaneously without specific therapy. In disseminated histoplasmosis the pericardium itself may be infected with *Histoplasma capsulatum*.[213,566] Pericarditis is rarely recognized in acute coccidioidomycosis. Spontaneously resolving cases resembling those seen in acute histoplasmosis have been described,[561] but most reported cases have occurred in the setting of disseminated coccidioidomycosis and represent *Coccidioides immitis* infection of the heart.[210,562-564] Fungal pericarditis (resulting from direct inoculation or extension of mediastinal infection) is seen with increasing frequency as a complication of cardiothoracic surgery.[483] Pericarditis caused by *Candida* spp., *Aspergillus* spp., *Cryptococcus neoformans*, and other fungi occurs as a consequence of disseminated infection, by direct extension, or following surgery, primarily in severely debilitated and immunocompromised patients, especially those with prolonged neutropenia who are receiving multiple courses of antibiotics.[201-203,209,552,556-560,565,578-580]

Pericardial effusions, most of which are asymptomatic, occur in 10% to 50% of patients with HIV infection and AIDS.[133-135,480] Although most are idiopathic, two thirds of the cases with tamponade are caused by infection or neoplasm; *M. tuberculosis* and nontuberculous mycobacteria, particularly *Mycobacterium avium-intracellulare* (MAI) and *Mycobacterium kansasii*, are responsible for 30% to 50%, and a wide variety of viral, bacterial, and fungal agents have also been isolated from the pericardial fluid.[133-135,479,480,532-535,581-583] Malignant effusions have also been observed, primarily Epstein-Barr virus–associated lymphomas and Kaposi's sarcoma.[133-135,479,480,581,583] As with myocarditis, pericardial effusions in HIV-infected patients are associated with advanced stages of infection.[479,480,581,583] The rare parasitic causes of pericarditis are referenced in Table 77-3.

PATHOLOGY, PATHOGENESIS, AND PATHOPHYSIOLOGY

The pericardium has two opposing mesothelial surfaces. The parietal pericardium forms a flask-shaped sac that encloses the heart and the origins of the great vessels. It consists of a 1-mm-thick layer of dense collagen lined by a single layer of mesothelial cells, which are covered by microvilli. The mesothelial cell layer is reflected onto the epicardial surface of the heart to form the visceral pericardium. The parietal pericardium has firm attachments to the sternum, the diaphragm, and the adventitia of the great vessels. The function of the normal pericardium has been a matter of considerable investigation and speculation.[584] It normally contains 15 to 50 mL of clear fluid, which may act as a lubricant. The pericardium reacts to acute injury by exuding fluid, fibrin, and cells in various combinations.[549,581,584,585] Acute pericarditis may resolve completely or progress to fibrous thickening, with or without constriction.

Cardiotropic viruses usually spread to the myocardium and pericardium hematogenously. Inflammation occurs in both visceral and parietal portions; effusion may develop and may be serous, serofibrinous, or serosanguineous. Concomitant myocarditis may or may not be evident. Although most patients with viral pericarditis recover completely, some have repeated disabling recurrences.[451,585-588] The pathophysiology of these recurrences has not been established, but it probably involves immunologic mechanisms and not recurrent or persistent virus replication. Rarely, viral pericarditis leads to constriction as a late complication.[462]

Bacterial pericarditis results from (1) spread from a contiguous focus of infection within the chest, either de novo or after surgery or trauma; (2) spread from a focus of infection within the heart, most commonly from endocarditis; (3) hematogenous infection; or (4) direct inoculation as a result of penetrating injury or cardiothoracic surgery. The incidence of purulent pericarditis arising from a contiguous pneumonia has steadily decreased and now usually occurs only when there has been significant delay in antibiotic therapy.[447,449,483,484] Pericarditis after cardiothoracic or esophageal surgery often occurs in patients with sternal wound infections or mediastinitis[447,483] and may be overlooked. Mortality is high. Pericarditis not infrequently accompanies fatal endocarditis,[168,169,589,590] especially that caused by *S. aureus*.[168] It often results from extension of a perivalvular abscess into the pericardium.[168,169,589,590] However, pericardial effusions in endocarditis may also be hemorrhagic[589] or sympathetic and sterile.[590] The presence of preexisting nonbacterial pericardial effusion may predispose to the development of purulent pericarditis in bacteremic patients. Although the pericardial fluid may initially be clear,[482,483] it is usually grossly purulent and may be loculated by the time the disease is clinically apparent. Subsequent organization with adhesions, obliteration of the pericardial space, and calcification may occur and result in constrictive pericarditis.

Tuberculous pericarditis may develop from a hematogenous focus present from the time of primary infection; as a result of lymphatic spread from peritracheal, peribronchial, or mediastinal lymph nodes; or by contiguous spread from a focus of infection in lung or pleura. Four pathologic stages in tuberculous pericarditis have been described.[522,525,531,549] In the first stage, there is diffuse fibrin deposition, and granulomas with viable mycobacteria are present (Fig. 77-3). A serous or serosanguineous pericardial effusion then develops, usually quite slowly and often without symptoms. Lymphocytes, monocytes, and plasma cells replace the polymorphonuclear cells that are present early in infection. In the third stage, the effusion is absorbed, the pericardium thickens, granulomas proliferate, and a thick coat of fibrin is deposited on the parietal pericardium. Acid-fast bacilli become difficult to find as dense fibrous tissue and collagen are deposited. In stage 4, which is associated with constriction, the pericardial space is obliterated by dense adhesions, the parietal pericardium is markedly thickened, and many granulomas are replaced by fibrous tissue. This is often followed by the accumulation of cholesterol crystals and calcification. Constrictive pericarditis may develop in up to 50% of patients with tuberculous pericarditis despite the use of antituberculous chemotherapy.[521,522,524,526,528,530,531,549,551,591] Although the incidence of tuberculosis has declined, it remains an important cause of constrictive pericarditis, especially in underdeveloped countries.[526-528,549]

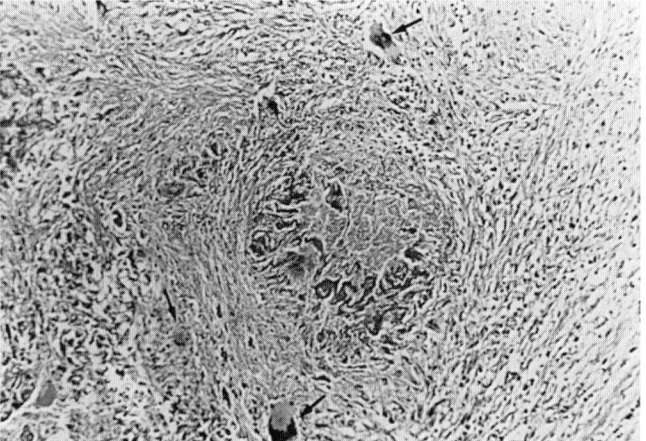

FIGURE 77-3. Tuberculous pericarditis, with a typical granuloma in the pericardium. There is central necrosis with aggregates of epithelioid cells at the periphery. Several multinucleated giant cells (arrows) are present (original magnification, × 40). *(From Bloor CM. Pericarditis and myocarditis. In: Cardiac Pathology. Philadelphia: JB Lippincott; 1978:265-295.)*

Regardless of the cause, if fluid accumulates rapidly in the pericardium and intrapericardial pressure rises, cardiac tamponade may result. Tamponade implies a progressive limitation of ventricular diastolic filling, with resultant reduction in stroke volume and cardiac output. In a series of medical patients with early cardiac tamponade, the cause was infectious in 12.5%, noninfectious in 74%, and undetermined in the remainder.[592] However, the proportion of cases that are idiopathic, associated with infection, or associated with other causes (e.g, cardiac surgery) will depend on the population studied.[448,452,459,478,480]

CLINICAL MANIFESTATIONS

The presentation of acute pericarditis varies depending on the cause. In viral or idiopathic pericarditis, chest pain is an important feature. This pain is often retrosternal, radiating to the shoulder and neck, and typically is aggravated by breathing, swallowing, and lying supine. In Smith's review of coxsackievirus B heart disease in adults,[46] 67% of patients had chest pain. Fever was present in 59%. A concurrent or prodromal flu-like illness with malaise, arthralgias, myalgias, and occasionally cough with sputum was present in 36%.

Bacterial pericarditis usually develops during the course of a severe systemic infection.[447-449,483] The patient is usually acutely ill; fever is almost always present, and dyspnea is common. However, chest pain is reported by only one third of patients with purulent pericarditis, and a pericardial friction rub, pathognomonic of pericarditis, is likewise present in only about one third.[447-449] The symptoms and signs of pericarditis that are present (i.e., fever, dyspnea, and tachycardia) are often attributed to the underlying disease. Consequently, purulent pericarditis is recognized in many patients only at necropsy or after severe hemodynamic compromise has developed.[447-449,581]

Tuberculous pericarditis most often has an insidious onset. Chest pain is present in 39% to 76%,[522,530,549,551] but it may be vague in nature. Weight loss, night sweats, cough, and dyspnea are common. Pericardial effusions in HIV-infected patients are usually asymptomatic or they may be overlooked in those with severe intercurrent illness.[479,480,583]

The classic physical finding in acute pericarditis is the three-component pericardial friction rub, which reflects cardiac motion during atrial systole, ventricular systole, and rapid ventricular filling in early diastole. This three-component rub was present in 50% of patients with acute pericarditis reported by Spodick.[593] The ventricular systolic component is often the loudest and most frequently appreciated. Rubs are often evanescent and may vary in quality; they are characteristically high-pitched, scratching, or grating. In the presence of significant pericardial effusion, there may be jugular venous distention—the most common physical finding in acute cardiac tamponade. Enlargement of the cardiac silhouette usually does not occur until at least 250 mL of fluid has accumulated in the pericardial space[581]; if fluid accumulates rapidly, tamponade may occur without detectable cardiomegaly. A pulsus paradoxus of more than 10 mm Hg and a prominent x descent with loss of the y descent in the jugular venous pressure may be present. Dyspnea is common, but signs of left-sided heart failure are usually absent in cardiac tamponade, and clear lung fields may help to differentiate tamponade from cardiogenic shock.

Constrictive pericarditis, with or without pericardial effusion, is observed in 10% to 20% of patients who present with clinical tamponade.[452] In recent series,[452,594] half of the cases of constrictive pericarditis were idiopathic, and most of the others were associated with previous cardiac surgery, thoracic radiation, neoplasms, or tuberculosis. In a series of 26 patients with surgically proved constrictive pericarditis, 18% were found to have no increase in pericardial thickness.[594]

Although the pericardium produces no electrical activity, the electrocardiogram is abnormal in 90% of patients with acute pericarditis,[581,584,585,595] reflecting diffuse subepicardial inflammation. Characteristic electrocardiographic changes are seen in approximately 50% of patients.[585,595] Early in pericarditis, ST-segment elevation without change in QRS morphology typically occurs in multiple leads. Several days later, the ST segment returns to baseline, and there is T-wave flattening. During these early stages, there may also be depression of the PR segment. In contrast to myocardial infarction, the T-wave inversions in pericarditis usually do not occur until after the ST segment has returned to baseline. These T-wave inversions may last for weeks or months. Large pericardial effusions may be associated with reduced QRS voltage and electrical alternans. Sinus tachycardia is common, but the presence of other arrhythmias suggests preexisting underlying heart disease or significant myocardial involvement.[596]

Echocardiography has proved to be an extremely useful tool for diagnosis of pericardial effusion and should be performed if the situation is not immediately life threatening. The size of the effusion can be roughly quantitated, and early hemodynamic compromise can often be detected.[581] Computed tomography has been useful in demonstrating pericardial thickening and, in some cases, in differentiating an uncomplicated transudate from a high-density exudates.[597,598] In addition, MRI techniques can easily detect pericardial fluid, pericardial thickening, and abnormal ventricular septal motion,[452,594,597-600] but they have no particular advantage over echocardiography.

DIAGNOSIS

A wide variety of agents and diseases can cause pericarditis and pericardial effusion (Tables 77-3 and 77-4). Low-grade fever is common to many. A careful history, knowledge of the clinical setting in which the pericarditis occurs, and a search for clues outside the cardiovascular system are helpful in establishing a diagnosis. In a young person without underlying illness who presents with acute pericardial pain, the most likely diagnosis is viral or idiopathic pericarditis. However, establishing a specific viral diagnosis is difficult, costly, and often possible only in retrospect. Virus isolation can be attempted from throat and stool, and acute and convalescent sera can be tested for antibodies to potential pathogens (e.g., the coxsackie B viruses and any other enteroviruses prevalent locally at the time), but these approaches frequently fail to yield a specific diagnosis. Viruses are rarely isolated from pericardial fluid, even in patients in whom the diagnosis of viral myocarditis is highly probable. The application of PCR technology using pathogen-specific primers and probes[32,369-371,374] to the detection of the genomes of pathogens in pericardial fluid, pericardial biopsy specimens, and, perhaps, peripheral blood should markedly increase the proportion of patients with pericarditis in whom an etiologic diagnosis is established.

If the clinical suspicion of viral or idiopathic pericarditis is strong in an otherwise healthy patient with uncomplicated pericarditis, pericardiocentesis or other invasive procedures add little diagnostically[525] and carry a small but definite risk.[601] After excluding patients with postpericardiotomy syndrome, myocardial infarction, renal failure, known neoplastic disease, trauma, and irradiation, Soler-Soler and colleagues[454]

prospectively evaluated 256 immunocompetent patients with primary acute pericardial disease. After thorough diagnostic evaluation, 221 (86%) were thought to have acute idiopathic pericarditis. Unsuspected neoplastic pericarditis was found in 12 (5%), tuberculosis in 11 (4%), and collagen vascular disease in 4 patients. Purulent pericarditis and viral pericarditis were each found in 3 patients, and *T. gondii* infection was found in 4. The diagnostic yield was substantial when pericardiocentesis or pericardiectomy with biopsy was done to relieve cardiac tamponade (28% and 54%, respectively) but led to a specific etiology in only 5% and 4%, respectively, when these procedures were done solely for the purpose of diagnosis. The authors concluded that the presence of a pericardial effusion per se is not an indication for an invasive procedure; in patients with pericardial effusion that has persisted for longer than 3 weeks, an invasive procedure may be indicated. In a similar study of patients with large (>20-mm echo-free space in diastole) pericardial effusions without tamponade physiology or suspected purulent pericarditis, the diagnostic yield for pericardiocentesis or surgery was only 7%.[602] Among those observed expectantly without a drainage procedure, no patient developed tamponade or died as a result of pericardial disease; moderate or large effusions persisted in only 2 of 45 patients.[602] Similarly, small, asymptomatic pericardial effusions in patients with HIV infection do not routinely require diagnostic evaluation.[480] In a study of 13 patients with AIDS who underwent surgical pericardial drainage, Kaposi's sarcoma was found in 3 (all with preexisting extracardiac lesions), but no other specific causes were identified.[603] However, in patients who are symptomatic, about two thirds of cases are caused by potentially treatable infections or neoplasms.[480]

When an invasive procedure is necessary, pericardiotomy with biopsy and drainage is preferable to pericardiocentesis because of greater diagnostic yield and fewer complications.[581] Pericardiocentesis alone establishes a specific etiologic diagnosis in 20% to 25% of cases; the availability of both fluid and tissue improves this yield to 54%.[525,551,604] The technique of percutaneous pericardial biopsy is an alternative to surgery for obtaining tissue, and it appears to be safe and effective in patients with a thickened pericardium.[605-607] Noninfectious diseases predominate as causes of significant pericardial effusion and cardiac tamponade,[452,525,581,583,594,604] but bacterial and tuberculous effusions are more likely to have serious hemodynamic consequences.[447,448,480,601] Untreated purulent pericarditis usually is rapidly fatal.[447-449,482,483,549] In acutely ill patients in whom purulent pericarditis is suspected, the diagnosis should be pursued quickly and aggressively.

TREATMENT

Bed rest, symptomatic therapy for pain, and careful monitoring for the development of hemodynamic compromise are the mainstays of treatment for presumed viral or idiopathic pericarditis. Nonsteroidal anti-inflammatory agents are often successful in relieving symptoms in acute pericardeitis,[608] but they should be avoided in patients with myocarditis, based on data from animal models.[259,260,421] Because myocarditis often accompanies viral pericarditis and steroids enhance myocardial injury during active virus replication, we believe that steroids should be avoided during the acute illness. Viral or idiopathic pericarditis is generally benign and self-limited, but recurrences[586-588] and late constriction[462] do occur. Although prospective, double-blind clinical trials are lacking, several studies have suggested that colchicine (1 mg/day) may be useful in limiting recurrences and may also be effective in the initial treatment of idiopathic pericarditis.[609-611] Steroids and other immunosuppressive agents have also been used to treat debilitating recurrences of idiopathic pericarditis, but controlled trials are lacking here also, and serious adverse effects with these regimens are more common.[612,613]

Surgical drainage of the pericardium, in addition to appropriate antibiotic therapy, is essential in almost all patients with purulent pericarditis.[482-484,500,518,614] Initial pericardiocentesis may be lifesaving, but fluid often reaccumulates, and constriction can develop rapidly.[500,524-527,614] There is little rationale for irrigating the pericardium with antibiotics, because penetration of antibiotics from serum is excellent.[607] With early diagnosis and aggressive therapy, *H. influenzae* pericarditis in young patients has a good prognosis.[500] However, overall mortality in bacte-

TABLE 77-4 Major Noninfectious Causes of Acute Pericarditis

Acute myocardial infarction[581,622-624]
Cardiac injury[581]
    Trauma (penetrating or blunt)[625]
    Myocardial infarction (Dressler's) syndrome[626]
    Postpericardiotomy[627]
Uremia[628,629]
Neoplasia[581]
    Primary
    Metastatic
Irradiation[396-398,581]
Dissecting aortic aneurysm[630]
Sarcoid[405,581]
Collagen vascular diseases[392,581]
    Systemic lupus erythematosus[385]
    Systemic sclerosis/scleroderma[387,388]
    Rheumatoid arthritis[389,390,631]
    Rheumatic fever[581]
Inflammatory bowel disease[632]
Myxedema[633]
Drug induced[581]
    Procainamide
    Hydralazine
    Other

rial pericarditis remains high (30%), especially when it develops after surgery or occurs in the course of endocarditis.[168,169,482-484,589,590]

Antituberculous therapy has reduced the mortality of tuberculous pericarditis substantially.[612] However, constrictive pericarditis may develop in 20% to 50% of patients despite appropriate treatment,[521-524,526-528,530,531,591] and patients with the clinical features of tamponade at presentation are at increased risk.[614] The addition of steroids to reduce inflammation and possibly avoid late constriction is favored by many, including the authors.[521,528,550,551,615,616] The use of corticosteroids, in addition to antituberculous therapy, is supported by the results of two large, controlled trials in Transkei reported by Strang and associates.[528,550] In patients with tuberculous pericardial effusions, the addition of prednisone to a four-drug antituberculosis regimen reduced the risk of death, the need for repeat pericardiocentesis, and the need for open surgical drainage because of rapid reaccumulation of pericardial fluid; constrictive pericarditis developed in 8% of steroid recipients and 12% of controls.[550] Prednisone was given in a dose of 60 mg daily for 4 weeks, followed by 30 mg daily for 4 weeks, 15 mg daily for 2 weeks, and 5 mg daily for 1 week. In a similar trial in patients with active tuberculous constrictive pericarditis, the addition of prednisone increased the rate of clinical improvement.[528] In 10 patients treated initially with 120 mg of prednisone daily, dramatic improvement occurred over a 1-week period, and the author suggested that higher initial doses might allow for a shorter duration of treatment. Early surgical intervention is advocated in patients with hemodynamic compromise from recurrent effusion or progressive pericardial thickening.[551,591,613,615-617]

In a retrospective study of children with tuberculous pericarditis reported from Africa, 5 (40%) of 12 patients with evidence of constriction at presentation required pericardiectomy.[618] These authors recommended observation for a period of 6 weeks to 3 months after the initiation of treatment, with pericardiectomy reserved for those who fail to improve or deteriorate. This procedure frequently results in striking hemodynamic improvement, but if diagnosis and therapy have been delayed, myocardial function may be affected, leading to less satisfactory results.[619,620] In some patients, resolution of venous congestion requires several months.[618] Patients with calcific tuberculous pericarditis have a poorer prognosis than those who undergo operation earlier in the course of their disease.[618,620] Early pericardial drainage and intrapericardial fibrinolysis by means of the instillation of streptokinase have been advocated to facilitate drainage, prevent loculation, and reduce the risk of constrictive pericarditis.[621] However, this approach has not yet been evaluated with appropriate clinical trials.

REFERENCES

1. Saphir O. Myocarditis: A general review with an analysis of two hundred and forty cases. Arch Pathol. 1941;32:1000-1051, and 1942;33:88-137.
2. Gravanis MG, Sterby NH. Incidence of myocarditis. Arch Pathol Lab Med. 1991;115:390-392.
3. Pisani B, Taylor DO, Mason JW. Inflammatory myocardial diseases and cardiomyopathies. Am J Med. 1997;102:459-469.
4. Bloor CM. Pericarditis and myocarditis. In: Cardiac Pathology. Philadelphia: JB Lippincott; 1978:265-295.
5. Bandt CM, Staley NA, Noren GR. Acute viral myocarditis: Clinical and histological changes. Minn Med. 1979;62:234-237.
6. Drory Y, Turetz Y, Hiss Y, et al. Sudden unexpected death in persons less than 40 years of age. Am J Cardiol. 1991;68:1388-1392.
7. Maron BJ. Medical progress: Sudden death in young athletes. N Engl J Med. 2003;349:1064-1075.
8. Mason JW. Myocarditis and dilated cardiomyopathy: An inflammatory link. Cardiovasc Res. 2003;60:5-10.
9. Kawai C. From myocarditis to cardiomyopathy: Mechanisms of inflammation and cell death: Learning from the past for the future. Circulation. 1999;99:1091-1100.
10. Baboonian C, Treasure T. Meta-analysis of the association of enteroviruses with human heart disease. Heart. 1997;78:539-543.
11. Bowles NE, Vallejo J. Viral causes of cardiac inflammation. Curr Opin Cardiol. 2003;18:182-188.
12. Bengtsson E, Orndahl G. Complications of mumps with special reference to the incidence of myocarditis. Acta Med Scand. 1954;149:381-388.
13. Lucke B, Wight T, Kime E. Pathologic anatomy and bacteriology of influenza: Epidemic of autumn 1918. Arch Intern Med. 1919;24:154-237.
14. Degen JA Jr. Visceral pathology in measles; clinicopathologic study of 100 fatal cases. Am J Med Sci. 1937;194:104-111.
15. Lucke B. Postmortem findings in measles bronchopneumonia and other acute infections. JAMA. 1918;70:2006-2011.
16. Frustaci A, Abdulla AK, Caldarulo M, et al. Fatal measles myocarditis. Cardiologia. 1990;35:347-349.
17. Saphir O, Wile SA. Myocarditis in poliomyelitis. Am J Med Sci. 1942;203:781-788.
18. Sylvest E. Epidemic myalgia: Bornholm disease. London: Oxford University Press; 1934.
19. Reyes MP, Lerner AM. Coxsackievirus myocarditis—with special reference to acute and chronic effects. Prog Cardiovasc Dis. 1985;27:373-394.
20. Hirschman SZ, Hammer GS. Coxsackie virus in myopericarditis. A microbiological and clinical review. Am J Cardiol. 1974;34:224-232.
21. Woodruff JF. Viral myocarditis. Am J Pathol. 1980;101:427-478.
22. Grist NR, Bell EJ. A six-year study of coxsackievirus B infections in heart disease. J Hyg (Lond.). 1974;71:165-172.
23. Kim KS, Hufnagel G, Chapman NM, Tracy S. The group B coxsackieviruses and myocarditis. Rev Med Virol. 2001;11:355-368.
24. Baboonian C, Davies MJ, Booth JC, McKenna W. Coxsackie B viruses and human heart disease. Curr Top Microbiol Immunol. 1997;223:31-52.
25. Martino TA, Liu P, Martin P, Sole MJ. Enteroviral myocarditis and dilated cardiomyopathy: A review of clinical and experimental studies. In: Rotbart HA, ed. Human Enterovirus Infections. Washington, DC: American Society for Microbiology; 1995:291-351.
26. Hyypia T. Etiologic diagnosis of viral heart disease. Scand J Infect Dis. 1993;88(Suppl):25-31.
27. Feldman AM, McNamara D. Myocarditis. N Engl J Med. 2000;343:1388-1398.
28. Bowles NE, Ni J, Kearney DL, et al. Detection of viruses in myocardial tissues by polymerase chain reaction: Evidence of adenovirus as a common cause of myocarditis in children and adults. J Am Coll Cardiol. 2003;42:466-472.
29. Chany C, Lepine P, Lelong M, et al. Severe and fatal pneumonia in infants and young children associated with adenovirus infections. Am J Hyg. 1958;67:367-378.
30. Berkovich S, Rodriguez-Torres R, Lin J-S. Virologic studies in children with acute myocarditis. Am J Dis Child. 1968;115:207-212.
31. Henson D, Mufson MA. Myocarditis and pneumonitis with type 21 adenovirus infection: Association with fatal myocarditis and pneumonitis. Am J Dis Child. 1971;121:334-336.
32. Martin AB, Webber S, Fricker FJ, et al. Acute myocarditis. Rapid diagnosis by PCR in children. Circulation. 1994;90:330-339.
33. Young NS, Brown KE. Mechanisms of disease: Parvovirus B19. N Engl J Med. 2004;350:586-597.
34. Bergelson JM, Cunningham JA, Droguett G, et al. Isolation of a common receptor for coxsackie B viruses and adenoviruses 2 and 5. Science. 1997;275:1320-1323.
35. Bergelson JM, Krithivas A, Celi L, et al. The murine CAR homolog is a receptor for coxsackie B viruses and adenoviruses. J Virol. 1998;72:415-419.
36. Roelvink PW, Lizonova A, Lee JG, et al. The coxsackievirus-adenovirus receptor protein can function as a cellular attachment protein for adenovirus serotypes from subgroups A, C, D, E and F. J Virol. 1998;72:7909-7915.
37. Noutsias M, Fechner H, de Jonge H, et al. Human coxsackie-adenovirus receptor is colocalized with integrins alpha(v)beta(3) and alpha(v)beta(5) on the cardiomyocyte sarcolemma and upregulated in dilated cardiomyopathy: Implications for cardiotropic viral infections. Circulation. 2001;104:265-280.
38. Easton AJ, Eglin RP. The detection of coxsackievirus RNA in cardiac tissue by in situ hybridization. J Gen Virol. 1988;69:285-291.
39. Remes J, Helin M, Vaino P, et al. Clinical outcome and left ventricular function 23 years after acute coxsackie virus myopericarditis. Eur Heart J. 1990;11:182-188.
40. Grist NR, Bell EJ. Coxsackie viruses and the heart. Am Heart J. 1969;77:295-300.
41. Karjalainen J, Heikkila J, Nieminen MS, et al. Etiology of mild acute infectious myocarditis. Relation to clinical features. Acta Med Scand. 1983;213:65-73.
42. Griffiths PD, Hannington G, Booth JC. Coxsackie B virus infections and myocardial infarction. Results from a prospective, epidemiologically controlled study. Lancet. 1980;1:1387-1389.
43. Kaplan MH, Kelin SW, McPhee J, et al. Group B coxsackievirus infection in infants younger than three months of age: A serious childhood illness. Rev Infect Dis. 1983;5:1019-1032.
44. Morita H, Kitaura Y, Deguchi H, et al. Coxsackie B5 myopericarditis in a young adult. Clinical course and endomyocardial biopsy findings. Jpn Circ J. 1983;47:1077-1083.
45. Koontz CH, Ray CG. The role of coxsackie group B virus infections in sporadic myopericarditis. Am Heart J. 1971;82:750-758.
46. Smith WG. Coxsackie B myopericarditis in adults. Am Heart J. 1970;80:34-46.
47. Montgomery J, Gear JHS, Prinslou FR, et al. Myocarditis of the newborn. An outbreak in a maternity home in Southern Rhodesia associated with coxsackie group-B virus infection. S Afr Med J. 1955;29:608-612.
48. Bain HW, McLean DM, Walker SJ. Epidemic pleurodynia (Bornholm disease) due to coxsackie B5 virus. Pediatrics. 1961;27:889-902.
49. Helin M, Savola J, Lapinleimu K. Cardiac manifestations during a coxsackie B5 epidemic. BMJ. 1968;2:97-99.
50. Bendig J, Franklin O, Hebden A, et al. Coxsackievirus B3 sequences in the blood of a neonate with congenital myocarditis, plus serological evidence of maternal infection. J Med Virol. 2003;70:606-609.
51. Russell SJM, Bell EJ. Echoviruses and carditis. Lancet. 1970;1:784-785.
52. Bell EJ, Grist NR. ECHO viruses, carditis and acute pleurodynia. Am Heart J. 1971;82:133-138.
53. Fukuhara T, Konoshita M, Bito K, et al. Myopericarditis associated with echovirus type 3 infection. A case report. Jpn Circ J. 1983;47:1274-1280.
54. Jungeblut CW, Edwards JE. Isolation of poliomyelitis virus from the heart in fatal cases. Am J Clin Pathol. 1951;21:601-623.
55. Weinstein L, Shelokov A. Cardiovascular manifestations in acute poliomyelitis. N Engl J Med. 1951;244:281-285.
56. Peng TLY, Yang Y, Niu C, et al. Characterization of enterovirus isolates from patients with heart muscle disease in a selenium-deficient area of China. J Clin Microbiol. 2000;38:3538-3543.
57. Weiss LM, Liu XF, Chang KL, et al. Detection of enteroviral RNA in idiopathic dilated cardiomyopathy and other human cardiac tissues. J Clin Invest. 1992;90:156-159.

58. Keeling PJ, Tracy S. Link between enteroviruses and dilated cardiomyopathy: Serological and molecular data. Br Heart J. 1994;72(Suppl):25-29.

59. Weinstein C, Fenoglio JJ. Myocarditis. Hum Pathol. 1987;18:613-618.

60. Figulla HR, Stille-Siegener M, Mall G, et al. Myocardial enterovirus infection with left ventricular dysfunction: A benign disease compared with idiopathic dilated cardiomyopathy. J Am Coll Cardiol. 1995;25:1170-1175.

61. Celers J, Celers P, Bertocchi A. Non-polio enterovirus in France from 1974 to 1985. Pathol Biol. 1988;36:1221-1226.

62. Grist NR, Bell EJ, Assaad F. Enteroviruses in human disease. Prog Med Virol. 1978;24:114-157.

63. Bowles NE, Ni J, Marcus F, et al. The detection of cardiotropic viruses in the myocardium of patients with arrhythmogenic right ventricular dysplasia/cardiomyopathy. J Am Coll Cardiol. 2002;39:892-895.

64. Nahmias AJ, Griffith D, Snitzer J. Fatal pneumonia associated with adenovirus type 7. Am J Dis Child. 1967;114:36-41.

65. Odio C, McCracken GH Jr, Nelson JD. Disseminated adenovirus infection: A case report and review of the literature. Pediatr Infect Dis. 1984;3:46-49.

66. Roberts WC, Fox SM III. Mumps of the heart: Clinical and pathological features. Circulation. 1965;32:342-345.

67. Chaudary S, Jaski BE. Fulminant mumps myocarditis. Ann Intern Med. 1989;110:569-570.

68. Kabakus N, Aydinoglue H, Yekeler H, Arslan IN. Fatal mumps nephritis and myocarditis. J Trop Pediatr. 1999;45:358-360.

69. Degen JA. Visceral pathology in measles. Am J Med Sci. 1937;194 (Suppl I):104-111.

70. Hamburger WW. The heart in influenza. Med Clin North Am. 1938;22:111-121.

71. Verel D, Warrack AJN, Potter CW, et al. Observations on the A2 England influenza epidemic. A clinicopathological study. Am Heart J. 1976;92:290-296.

72. Proby CM, Hacket D, Gupta S, et al. Acute myopericarditis in influenza A infection. QJM. 1986;60:887-892.

73. Adams CW. Postviral myopericarditis associated with the influenza virus: Report of 8 cases. Am J Cardiol. 1959;4:56-67.

74. Ross E, Armentrout SA. Myocarditis associated with rabies. Report of a case. N Engl J Med. 1962;266:1087-1089.

75. Ainger LE, Lawyer NG, Fitch CW. Neonatal rubella myocarditis. Br Heart J. 1966;28:691-697.

76. Kriseman T. Rubella myocarditis in a 9 year old patient. Clin Pediatr. 1984;23:240-241.

77. Chuah SK. Transient ventricular arrhythmia as a cardiac manifestation in dengue haemorrhagic fever—a case report. Singapore Med J. 1987;28:569-572.

78. Obeyesekere I, Hermon Y. Myocarditis and cardiomyopathy after arbovirus infections (dengue and chikungunya fever). Br Heart J. 1972;34:821-827.

79. Cannell DE. Myocardial degenerations in yellow fever. Am J Pathol. 1928;4:431-443.

80. Milei J, Bolomo NJ. Myocardial damage in viral hemorrhagic fevers. Am Heart J. 1982;104:1385-1391.

81. Thiede WH. Cardiac involvement in lymphocytic choriomeningitis. Arch Intern Med. 1962;109:50-54.

82. Cummins D, Bennett D, Fisher-Hoch SP, et al. Lassa fever encephalopathy: Clinical and laboratory findings. J Trop Med Hyg. 1992;95:197-201.

83. Cummins D, Bennett D, Fisher-Hoch SP, et al. Electrocardiographic abnormalities in patients with Lassa fever. J Trop Med Hyg. 1989;92:350-355.

84. Yanase O, Motomiya T, Watanabe K, et al. Lassa fever associated with effusive constrictive pericarditis and bilateral atrioventricular annular constriction: A case report. J Cardiol. 1989;19:1147-1156.

85. Waagner DC, Murphy TV. Varicella myocarditis. Pediatr Infect Dis J. 1990;9:360-363.

86. Alter P, Grimm W, Maisch B. Varicella myocarditis in an adult. Heart 2001;85:E2.

87. Woolf PK, Chung T-S, Stewart J, et al. Life-threatening dysrhythmias in varicella myocarditis. Clin Pediatr. 1987;26:480-482.

88. Coppack SW, Doshi R, Ghose AR. Fatal varicella in a healthy young adult. Postgrad Med J. 1985;61:529-531.

89. Tsintsof A, Delprado WJ, Keogh AM. Varicella zoster myocarditis progressing to cardiomyopathy and cardiac transplantation. Br Heart J. 1993;70:93-95.

90. Fiddler GI, Campbell RW, Pottage A, et al. Varicella myocarditis presenting with unusual ventricular arrhythmias. Br Heart J 1977;39:1150-1153.

91. Noren GR, Tobin JD Jr, Staley NA, et al. Association of varicella, myocarditis, and congestive cardiomyopathy. Pediatr Cardiol. 1982;3:53-57.

92. Lorber A, Zonis Z, Maisuls E, et al. The scale of myocardial involvement in varicella myocarditis. Int J Cardiol. 1988;20:257-262.

93. Kundu AK. Herpes zoster-induced myocarditis in a patient with diabetes mellitus. J Assoc Physicians India. 2001;49:286-7.

94. Tiula E, Leinikki P. Fatal cytomegalovirus infection in a previously healthy boy with myocarditis and consumption coagulopathy as presenting signs. Scand J Infect Dis. 1972;4:57-60.

95. Maisch B, Schonian U, Crombach M, et al. Cytomegalovirus-associated inflammatory heart muscle disease. Scand J Infect Dis. 1993;88:135-148.

96. Millett R, Tomita T, Marshall HE, et al. Cytomegalovirus endomyocarditis in a transplanted heart. A case report with in situ hybridization. Arch Pathol Lab Med. 1991;115:511-515.

97. Schonian U, Crombach M, Maisch B. Assessment of cytomegalovirus DNA and protein expression in patients with myocarditis. Clin Immunol Immunopathol. 1993;68:229-233.

98. Ando H, Shiramizu T, Hisanou R. Dilated cardiomyopathy caused by cytomegalovirus infection in a renal transplant recipient. Jpn Heart J. 1992;33:409-412.

99. Arbustini E, Grasso M, Diegoli M, et al. Histopathologic and molecular profile of human cytomegalovirus infections in patients with heart transplants. Am J Clin Pathol. 1992;98:205-213.

100. Wu TC, Pizzorno MC, Hayward GS, et al. In situ detection of human cytomegalovirus immediate-early gene transcripts within cardiac myocytes of patients with HIV-associated cardiomyopathy. AIDS 1992;6:777-785.

101. Powell KF, Bellamy AR, Catton MG. Cytomegalovirus myocarditis in a heart transplant recipient: Sensitive monitoring of viral DNA by the polymerase chain reaction. J Heart Transplant. 1989;8:465-470.

102. Webster BH. Cardiac complications of infectious mononucleosis: A review of the literature and report of five cases. Am J Med Sci. 1957;234:62-70.

103. Fraisse A, Paut O, Zandotti C, et al. Epstein-Barr virus. An unusual cause of acute myocarditis in children. Arch Pediatr. 2000;7:752-755.

104. Tyson AA Jr, Hackshaw BT, Kutcher MA. Acute Epstein-Barr virus myocarditis simulating myocardial infarction with cardiogenic shock. South Med J. 1989;82:1184-1187.

105. Hebert MM, Yu C, Towbin JA, Rogers BB. Fatal Epstein-Barr virus myocarditis in a child with repetitive myocarditis. Pediatr Pathol Lab Med. 1995;15:805-812.

106. Baykurt C, Caglar K, Ceviz N, et al. Successful treatment of Epstein-Barr virus infection associated with myocarditis. Pediatr Int. 1999;41:389-391.

107. Frishman W, Kraus ME, Zabkar J, et al. Infectious mononucleosis and fatal myocarditis. Chest. 1977;41:535-540.

108. Cheng TC. Severe chest pain due to infectious mononucleosis. Postgrad Med. 1983;73:149-152.

109. Tyson AA Jr, Hackshaw BT, Kutcher MA. Acute Epstein-Barr virus myocarditis simulating myocardial infarction with cardiogenic shock. S Med J. 1989;82:1184-1187.

110. Whorton CM, Thomas DM, Denham SW. Fatal systemic herpes simplex virus type 2 infection in a healthy young woman. South Med J. 1983;76:81-83.

111. Young EJ, Chafizadeh E, Oliveira VL, Genta RM. Disseminated herpesvirus infection during pregnancy. Clin Infect Dis. 1996;22:51-58.

112. Whitley RJ, Corey L, Arvin A, et al. Changing presentation of herpes simplex virus infection in neonates. J Infect Dis. 1988;158:109-116.

113. Anderson T, Foulis MA, Grist NR, et al. Clinical and laboratory observations in a smallpox outbreak. Lancet. 1951;1:1248-1252.

114. Macadam DB, Whitaker W. Cardiac complication after vaccination for smallpox. BMJ. 1962;5312:1099-1100.

115. Matthews AW, Griffiths ID. Post-vaccinal pericarditis and myocarditis. Br Heart J. 1974;36:1043-1045.

116. Halsell JS, Riddle JR, Atwood JE, et al. Myopericarditis following smallpox vaccination among vaccinia-naïve US military personnel. JAMA. 2003;289:3283-3289.

117. Centers for Disease Control and Prevention. Update: Cardiac-related events during the civilian smallpox vaccination program—United States, 2003. MMWR. 2003;52(21):492-496.

118. Saurina G, Shirazi S, Lane JM, et al. Myocarditis after smallpox vaccination: A case report. Clin Infect Dis. 2003;37:145-146.

119. Cono J, Casey C, Bell D. Smallpox vaccination and adverse reactions. MMWR. 2003;52(RR04):1-28.

120. Mahapatra RK, Ellis GH. Myocarditis and hepatitis B virus. Angiology. 1985;36:116-119.

121. Bell H. Cardiac manifestations of viral hepatitis. JAMA. 1971;218:387-391.

122. Ursell PC, Habib A, Sharma P, et al. Hepatitis B virus and myocarditis. Hum Pathol. 1984;15:481-484.

123. Matsumori A, Yutani C, Ikeda Y, et al. Hepatitis C virus from the hearts of patients with myocarditis and cardiomyopathy. Lab Invest. 2000;80:1137-1142.

124. Okabe M, Fukuda K, Arakawa K, et al. Chronic variant of myocarditis associated with hepatitis C virus infection. Circulation. 1997;96:22-24.

125. Matsumori A, Maloba Y, Sasayama S. Dilated cardiomyopathy associated with hepatitis C virus infection. Circulation. 1995;92:2519-2525.

126. Thomas JA, Raroque S, Scott WA, et al. Successful treatment of severe dysrhythmias in infants with respiratory syncytial virus infections: Two cases and a literature review. Crit Care Med. 1997;25:880-886.

127. Checchia PA, Appel HJ, Kahn S, et al. Myocardial injury in children with respiratory syncytial virus infection. Pediatr Crit Care Med. 2000;1:146-150.

128. Enders G, Deotsch J, Bauer J, et al. Life-threatening parvovirus B19–associated myocarditis and cardiac transplantation as possible therapy: Two case reports. Clin Infect Dis. 1998;26:355-358.

129. Schowengerdt KO, Ni J, Denfield SW, et al. Association of parvovirus B19 genome in children with myocarditis and cardiac allograft rejection: Diagnosis using the polymerase chain reaction. Circulation. 1997;96:3549-3554.

130. Munro K, Croxson MC, Thomas S, Wilson NJ. Three cases of myocarditis in childhood associated with parvovirus (B19 virus). Pediatr Cardiol. 2003;24:473-475.

131. Kuhl U, Pauschinger M, Bock T, et al. Parvovirus B19 infection mimicking acute myocardial infarction. Circulation. 2003;108:945-950.

132. Lamparter S, Schoppet M, Pankuweit S, Maisch B. Acute parvovirus B19 infection associated with myocarditis in an immunocompetent adult. Hum Pathol. 2003;34:725-728.

133. Yunis NA, Stone VE. Cardiac manifestations of HIV/AIDS: A review of disease spectrum and clinical management. J Acquir Immune Defic Syndr. 1998;18:145-154.

134. Kaul S, Fishbein MC, Siegel RJ. Cardiac manifestations of acquired immune deficiency syndrome: A 1991 update. Am Heart J. 1991;122:537-544.

135. De Castro S, Migliau G, Silvestri A, et al. Heart involvement in AIDS: A prospective study during various stages of the disease. Eur Heart J. 1992;13:1452-1459.

136. Cotter BR. Epidemiology of HIV cardiac disease. Prog Cardiovasc Dis. 2003;45:319-326.

137. Currie PF, Jacob AJ, Foreman AR, et al. Heart muscle disease related to HIV infection: Prognostic implications. BMJ. 1994;309:1605-1607.

138. Barbaro G, Di Lorenzo G, Grisorio B, et al. Incidence of dilated cardiomyopathy and detection of HIV in myocardial cells of HIV-positive patients. N Engl J Med. 1998;339:1093-1099.

139. Boller A-M, Al-Attar I, Orav EJ, Lipshultz SE. Cardiovascular morbidity and mortality in pediatric HIV infection. In: Lipshultz SE, ed. Cardiology in AIDS. New York: Chapman & Hall; 1998:77-94.

140. Calabrese LH, Proffitt MR, Yen-Lieberman B, et al. Congestive cardiomyopathy and illness related to the acquired immunodeficiency syndrome (AIDS) associated with isolation of retrovirus from myocardium. Ann Intern Med. 1987;107:691-692.

141. Grody W, Cheng L, Pang M, et al. Direct infection of the heart by human immunodeficiency virus (HIV). Circulation. 1989;80(Suppl II):665.

142. Beschorner WE, Baughman K, Turnicky RP, et al. HIV-associated myocarditis: Pathology and immunopathology. Am J Pathol. 1990;137:1365-1371.

143. Luginbuhl LM, Orav EJ, McIntosh K, Lipshultz SE. Cardiac morbidity and related mortality in children with HIV infection. JAMA. 1993;269:2869-2875.

144. Lipshultz SE. Dilated cardiomyopathy in HIV infected patients. N Engl J Med. 1998;339:1153-1154.
145. Baroldi G, Carallo S, Moroni M, et al. Focal lymphocytic myocarditis in acquired immunodeficiency syndrome (AIDS): A correlative morphologic and clinical study in 26 consecutive fatal cases. J Am Coll Cardiol. 1988;12:463-469.
146. Cammarosano C, Lewis W. Cardiac lesions in acquired immune deficiency syndrome (AIDS). J Am Coll Cardiol. 1985;5:703-706.
147. Hoyne A, Welford N. Diphtheritic myocarditis: A review of 496 cases. J Pediatr. 1934;5:642-653.
148. Gore I. Myocardial changes in fatal diphtheria; summary of observations in 221 cases. Am J Med Sci. 1948;215:257-266.
149. Havaldar PV, Sankpal MN, Doddannavar RP. Diphtheritic myocarditis: Clinical and laboratory parameters of prognosis and fatal outcome. Ann Trop Paediatr. 2000;20:209-215.
150. Roberts WC, Berard CW. Gas gangrene of the heart in clostridial septicemia. Am Heart J. 1967;74:482-488.
151. Guneratne F. Gas gangrene (abscess) of heart. N Y State J Med. 1975;75:1766-1769.
152. Stollerman GH. Rheumatic fever in the 21st century. Clin Infect Dis. 2001;33:806-814.
153. Gore I, Saphir O. Myocarditis. A classification of 1402 cases. Am Heart J. 1947;34: 827-830.
154. Garcia NS, Castelo JS, Ramos V, et al. Frequency of myocarditis in cases of fatal meningococcal infection in children: Observations on 31 cases studied at autopsy. Rev Soc Brasil Med Trop. 1999;32:517-522.
155. Brasier AR, Macklis JD, Vaughan D, et al. Myopericarditis as an initial presentation of meningococcemia. Unusual manifestation of infection with serotype W135. Am J Med. 1987;82:641-644.
156. Ejlersten T, Vesterlund T, Schmidt EB. Myopericarditis with cardiac tamponade caused by *Neisseria meningitidis* serogroup W135. Eur J Clin Microbiol Infect Dis. 1988;7: 403-404.
157. Cohen JI, Bartlett JA, Corey GR. Extra-intestinal manifestations of *Salmonella* infections. Medicine. 1987;66:349-388.
158. Wamder GS, Khurana SB, Puri S. *Salmonella* myopericarditis presenting with acute pulmonary oedema. Indian Heart J. 1992;44:55-56.
159. Baysal K, Sancak R, Ozturk F, et al. Cardiac involvement due to *Salmonella typhi* infections in children. Ann Trop Paediatr. 1998;188:23-25.
160. Rubenstein JS, Noah ZL, Zales VR, Shulman ST. Acute myocarditis associated with *Shigella sonnei* gastroenteritis. J Pediatr 1993;122:82-84.
161. Westling K, Evengard B. Myocarditis associated with *Campylobacter* infection. Scand J Infect Dis. 2001;33:877-878.
162. Cox ID, Fluck DS, Joy MD. *Campylobacter* myocarditis; loose bowels and a baggy heart. Eur J Heart Fail. 2001;3:105-107.
163. Cunningham C, Lee C. Myocarditis related to *Campylobacter jejuni* infection: A case report. BMC Infect Dis. 2003;3:16-20.
164. Jubber AS, Gunawardana DR, Lulu AR. Acute pulmonary edema in *Brucella* myocarditis and interstitial pneumonitis. Chest. 1990;97:1008-1009.
165. Lubani M, Sharda D, Helin I. Cardiac manifestations in brucellosis. Arch Dis Child. 1986;61:569-572.
166. Karjalainen J. Streptococcal tonsillitis and acute nonrheumatic myopericarditis. Chest. 1989;95:359-363.
167. Mattoo TK, al-Mutair A, al-Khatib, et al. Group A beta-hemolytic streptococcal infection and Henoch-Schonlein purpura with cardiac, renal and neurological complications. Ann Trop Paediatr. 1997;17:381-386.
168. Watanakunakorn C, Tan JS, Phair JP. Some salient features of *Staphylococcus aureus* endocarditis. Am J Med. 1973;54:473-481.
169. Buchbinder NA, Roberts WC. Left-sided valvular active infective endocarditis. A study of 45 necropsy patients. Am J Med. 1972;53:20-35.
170. McCue MJ, Moore EE. Myocarditis with microabscess formation caused by *Listeria monocytogenes* associated with myocardial infarct. Hum Pathol. 1979;10:469-472.
171. Stamm AM, Smith SH, Kirklin JK, et al. Listerial myocarditis in cardiac transplantation. Rev Infect Dis. 1990;12:820-823.
172. Tice AD, Nelson JS, Visconti EB. *Listeria monocytogenes* pericarditis and myocardial abscess. R I Med J. 1979;62:135-138.
173. Leon F, Badui E, Campos A, et al. Cholera and myocarditis: A case report. Angiology. 1997;48:545-549.
174. Dada MA, Lazarus NG, Kharsany ABM, Sturm AW. Sudden death caused by myocardial tuberculosis: Case report and review of the literature. Am J Forensic Med Pathol. 2000;21:385-388.
175. Diaz-Peromingo JA, Marino-Callejo AI, Gonzalez-Gonzalez C, et al. Tuberculous myocarditis presenting as long QT syndrome. Eur J Intern Med. 2000;11:340-342.
176. Armengol S, Domingo C, Mesalles E. Myocarditis: A rare complication during *Legionella* infection. Int J Cardiol. 1992;27:418-420.
177. Chen S-C, Tsai CC, Nouri S. Carditis associated with *Mycoplasma pneumoniae* infection. Am J Dis Child. 1986;140:471-472.
178. Lind K. Manifestation and complications of *Mycoplasma pneumoniae* disease: A review. Yale J Biol Med. 1983;56:461-468.
179. Karjalainen J. A loud third heart sound and asymptomatic myocarditis during *Mycoplasma pneumoniae* infection. Eur Heart J. 1990;11:960-963.
180. Linz DH, Tolle SW, Elliott DL. *Mycoplasma pneumoniae* pneumonia. Experience at a referral center. West J Med. 1984;140:895-900.
181. Ponka A. The occurrence and clinical picture of serologically verified *Mycoplasma pneumoniae* infections with emphases on central nervous system, cardiac and joint manifestations. Ann Clin Res. 1979;24:1-60.
182. Odeh M, Oliven A. Chlamydial infections of the heart. Eur J Clin Microbiol Infect Dis. 1992;11:885-893.
183. Dymock IW, Lawson JM, MacLennan WJ, et al. Myocarditis associated with psittacosis. Br J Clin Pract. 1971;25:240-242.
184. Gran JT, Hjetland R, Andreassen AH. Pneumonia, myocarditis and reactive arthritis due to *Chlamydia pneumoniae.* Scand J Rheumatol. 1993;22:43-44.
185. Wesslen LP, Pahlson C, Friman G, et al. Myocarditis caused by *Chlamydia pneumoniae* (TWAR) and sudden unexpected death in a Swedish elite orienteer (Letter). Lancet. 1992;340:427-428.
186. Marin-Garcia J, Mirvis DM. Myocardial disease in Rocky Mountain spotted fever: Clinical, functional, and pathologic findings. Pediatr Cardiol. 1984;5:149-154.
187. Diab SM, Araj GF, Fenech FF. Cardiovascular and pulmonary complications of epidemic typhus. Trop Geog Med. 1989;41:76-79.
188. Brown GW, Shirai A, Jegathesan M, et al. Febrile illness in Malaysia—an analysis of 1629 hospitalized patients. Am J Trop Med Hyg. 1984;33:311-315.
189. Ognibene AJ, O'Leary DS, Czarnecki SW, et al. Myocarditis and disseminated intravascular coagulation in scrub typhus. Am J Med Sci. 1971;262:233-239.
190. Fournier PE, Etienne J, Harle JR, et al. Myocarditis, a rare but severe manifestation of Q fever: a report of 8 cases and review of the literature. Clin Infect Dis. 2001;32:1440-1447.
191. Williams JD, Snow RM, Arciniegas JG. Myocardial involvement in a patient with human ehrlichiosis. Am J Med. 1995;98:414-415.
192. Segal LH. Early disseminated Lyme disease: Cardiac manifestations. Am J Med. 1995;98(Suppl 4A):258-285.
193. Horowitz HW, Belkin RN. Acute myopericarditis resulting from Lyme disease. Am Heart J. 1995;130:176-178.
194. Steere AC, Batsford WP, Weinberg M, et al. Lyme carditis: Cardiac abnormalities of Lyme disease. Ann Intern Med. 1980;93:8-16.
195. McAlister HF, Klementowicz PT, Andrews C, et al. Lyme carditis: An important cause of reversible heart block. Ann Intern Med. 1989;110:339-345.
196. van der Linde MR. Lyme carditis: Clinical characteristics of 105 cases. Scand J Infect Dis. 1991;77:81-84.
197. Midttun M, Lebech AM, Hansen K, et al. Lyme carditis: A clinical presentation and long time follow-up. Scand J Infect Dis. 1997;29:153-157.
198. Casans I, Villar A, Almenar V, et al. Lyme myocarditis diagnosed by indium-111 antimyosin scintigraphy. Eur J Nucl Med. 1989;15:330-331.
199. Bergler-Klein J, Sochor H, Stanek G, et al. Indium 111-monoclonal antimyosin antibody and magnetic resonance imaging in the diagnosis of acute Lyme myopericarditis. Arch Intern Med. 1993;153:2696-2700.
200. Silvestry FE, Kim B, Pollack BJ, et al. Cardiac Whipple disease: Identification of Whipple bacillus by electron microscopy of a patient before death. Ann Intern Med. 1997;126:214-216.
201. Atkinson JB, Connor DH, Robinowitz M, et al. Cardiac fungal infections: Review of autopsy findings in 60 patients. Hum Pathol. 1984;15:935-942.
202. Bloor CM. Protozoal, helminthic and fungal heart disease. In: Cardiac Pathology. Philadelphia: JB Lippincott; 1978:335-366.
203. Atkinson JB, Robinowitz M, McAllister HA Jr, et al. Cardiac infections in the immunosuppressed host. Cardiol Clin. 1984;2:671-686.
204. Williams AH. *Aspergillus* myocarditis. Am J Clin Pathol. 1974;61:247-256.
205. Rogers JG, Windle JR, McManus BM, et al. *Aspergillus* myocarditis presenting as myocardial infarction with complete heart block. Am Heart J. 1990;120:430-432.
206. Cox JN, Di Dio F, Pizzolato G-P, et al. *Aspergillus* endocarditis and myocarditis in a patient with the acquired immunodeficiency syndrome (AIDS): A review of the literature. Virchows Arch. 1990;417:255-259.
207. Franklin WG, Simon AB, Sodeman TM. *Candida* myocarditis without valvulitis. Am J Cardiol. 1976;38:924-928.
208. Einarsdottir HM, Danielsen R, Gottfredsson M. Successful treatment of *Candida glabrata* myocarditis with voriconazole. Scand J Infect Dis. 2002;34:778-780.
209. Witorsch P, Utz JP. North American blastomycosis: A study of 40 patients. Medicine. 1968;47:169-200.
210. Chapman MG, Kaplan L. Cardiac involvement in coccidioidomycosis. Am J Med. 1957;23:87-98.
211. Lewis W, Lipsick J, Cammarosano C. Cryptococcal myocarditis in acquired immune deficiency syndrome. Am J Cardiol. 1985;9:1240.
212. Lafont A, Wolff M, Marche C, et al. Overwhelming myocarditis due to *Cryptococcus neoformans* in an AIDS patient. Lancet. 1987;2:1145-1146.
213. Wheat J. Histoplasmosis. Experience during outbreaks in Indianapolis and review of the literature. Medicine. 1997;76:339-354.
214. Rosenbaum MB. Chagasic myocardiopathy. Prog Cardiovasc Dis. 1964;7:199-255.
215. Fuenmayor AJ, Fuenmayor AM, Carrasco H, et al. Results of electrophysiologic studies in patients with acute chagasic myocarditis. Clin Cardiol. 1997;20:1021-1024.
216. Mendoza I, Camardo J, Moleiro F, et al. Sustained ventricular tachycardia in chronic Chagasic myocarditis. Am J Cardiol. 1986;57:423-427.
217. Higuchi M de L. Chronic chagasic cardiopathy: The product of a turbulent host-parasite relationship. Rev Inst Med Trop Sao Paulo. 1997;39:53-60.
218. Mott KE, Hagstrom JWC. The pathologic lesions of the cardiac autonomic nervous system in chronic Chagas' myocarditis. Circulation. 1965;31:273-286.
219. de Carvalho VB, Sousa EF, Vila JH, et al. Heart transplantation in Chagas' disease. 10 years after the initial experience. Circulation. 1996;94:1815-1817.
220. Poltera AA, Owor R, Cox JN. Pathological aspects of human African trypanosomiasis in Uganda. Virchows Arch. 1977;373:249-265.
221. Barr R. Human trichinosis: Report of 4 cases with emphasis on central nervous system involvement and a survey of 500 consecutive autopsies at the Ottawa Civic Hospital. CMAJ. 1966;95:912-917.
222. Grey DF, Morse BS, Phillips WF. Trichinosis with neurologic and cardiac involvement. Review of the literature and report of three cases. Ann Intern Med. 1962;57:230-244.
223. Compton SJ, Celum CL, Lee C, et al. Trichinosis with ventilatory failure and persistent myocarditis. Clin Infect Dis. 1993;16:500-504.
224. Theologides A, Kennedy BJ. Toxoplasmic myocarditis and pericarditis. Am J Med. 1969;47:169-174.
225. Yermakov V, Rashid RK, Vuletin JC, et al. Disseminated toxoplasmosis. Case report and review of the literature. Arch Pathol Lab Med. 1982;106:524-528.
226. Matturri L, Quattrone P, Varesi C, et al. Cardiac toxoplasmosis in pathology of acquired immunodeficiency syndrome. Panminerva Med. 1990;32:194-196.
227. Hofman P, Drici MD, Gibelin P, et al. Prevalence of *Toxoplasma* myocarditis in patients with the acquired immunodeficiency syndrome. Br Heart J. 1993;70:376-381.
228. Montoya JG, Jordan R, Lingamneni S, et al. Toxoplasmic myocarditis and polymyositis in patients with acute acquired toxoplasmosis diagnosed during life. Clin Infect Dis. 1997;24:676-683.
229. Israelski DM, Remington JS. Toxoplasmosis in the non-AIDS immunocompromised host. Cur Clin Topics Infect Dis. 1993;13:322-356.
230. Duffield JS, Jacob AJ, Miller HC. Recurrent, life-threatening atrioventricular dissociation associated with toxoplasma myocarditis. Heart. 1996;76:453-454.
231. Dao AH, Virmani R. Visceral larval migrans involving the myocardium: Report of two cases and review of the literature. Pediatr Pathol. 1986:6:449-456.

232. Abe K, Shimokawa H, Kubota T, et al. Myocarditis associated with visceral larva migrans due to *Toxocara canis*. Ann Intern Med. 2002;41:7006-7008.
233. Welch K, Finkbeiner W, Alpers CE, et al. Autopsy findings in the acquired immune deficiency syndrome. JAMA. 1984;252:1152-1159.
234. Fink L, Reichek N, St. John Sutton MG. Cardiac abnormalities in acquired immune deficiency syndrome. Am J Cardiol. 1984;54:1161-1163.
235. Milei J, Grana D, Fernández Alonso G, et al. Cardiac involvement in acquired immunodeficiency syndrome—a review to push action. The Committee for the Study of Cardiac Involvement in AIDS. Clin Cardiol. 1998;21:465-472.
236. Dittrich H, Chow L, Denaro F, et al. Human immunodeficiency virus, coxsackievirus, and cardiomyopathy. Ann Intern Med. 1988;108:308-309.
237. Factor S, Flomenbaum M, Vdem S, et al. Proliferative membranopathy and human immunodeficiency virus in AIDS hearts. Circulation. 1989;80(Suppl II):535.
238. Herskowitz A, Ansori A, Neumann D, et al. Cardiomyopathy in acquired immunodeficiency syndrome: Evidence for autoimmunity. Circulation. 1989;80(Suppl II):322.
239. Parravicini C, Baroldi G, Gaiera G, et al. Phenotype of intramyocardial leukocytic infiltrates in acquired immunodeficiency syndrome (AIDS): A postmortem immunohistochemical study in 34 consecutive cases. Mod Pathol. 1991;4:559-565.
240. Mues B, Brisse E, Zwadlo G, et al. Phenotyping of macrophages with monoclonal antibodies in endomyocardial biopsies as a new approach to diagnosis of myocarditis. Eur Heart J. 1990;11:619-627.
241. Chow LH, Ye Y, Linder J, et al. Phenotypic analysis of infiltrating cells in human myocarditis. An immunohistological study in paraffin-embedded tissue. Arch Pathol Lab Med. 1989;113:1357-1362.
242. Keogh AM, Billingham ME, Schroeder JS. Rapid histological changes in endomyocardial biopsy specimens after myocarditis. Br Heart J. 1990;64:406-408.
243. Edwards WD. Myocarditis and endomyocardial biopsy. Cardiol Clin. 1984;2:647-656.
244. Lyden D, Olszewski J, Huber S. Variation in susceptibility of BALB/c mice to coxsackievirus group B type 3-induced myocarditis with age. Cell Immunol. 1987;105:332-339.
245. Herskowitz A, Wolfgram LJ, Rose NR, et al. Coxsackievirus B3, murine myocarditis: A pathologic spectrum of myocarditis in genetically defined inbred strains. J Am Coll Cardiol. 1987;9:1311-1319.
246. Huber SA, Lodge PA. Coxsackievirus B-3 myocarditis. Identification of different pathogenic mechanisms in DBA/2 and BALB/c mice. Am J Pathol. 1986;122:284-291.
247. Wolfgram LJ, Beisel KW, Herskowitz A, et al. Variations in the susceptibility to coxsackievirus B3-induced myocarditis among different strains of mice. J Immunol. 1986;136:1846-1852.
248. Khatib R, Probert A, Reyes MP, et al. Mouse strain-related variation as a factor in the pathogenesis of coxsackievirus B3 murine myocarditis. J Gen Virol. 1987;68:2981-2988.
249. Chow LH, Beisel KW, McManus BM. Enteroviral infection of mice with severe combined immunodeficiency. Evidence for direct viral pathogenesis of myocardial injury. Lab Invest. 1992;66:24-31.
250. McManus BM, Chow LH, Wilson JE, et al. Direct myocardial injury by enterovirus: A central role in the evolution of murine myocarditis. Clin Immunol Immunopathol. 1993;68:159-169.
251. Rager-Zisman B, Allison AC. The role of antibody and host cells in the resistance of mice against infection by coxsackie B-3 virus. J Gen Virol. 1973;19:329-338.
252. Woodruff JF. Lack of correlation between neutralizing antibody production and suppression of coxsackievirus B-3 replication in target organs: Evidence for involvement of mononuclear inflammatory cells in host defense. J Immunol. 1979;123:31-36.
253. Godeny EK, Gaunt CJ. In situ immune autoradiographic identification of cells in heart tissue of mice with coxsackievirus B3-induced myocarditis. Am J Pathol. 1987;129:267-276.
254. Godeny EK, Gaunt CJ. Murine natural killer cells limit coxsackievirus B3 replication. J Immunol. 1987;139:913-918.
255. Godeny EK, Gaunt CJ. Involvement of natural killer cells in coxsackievirus B3-induced murine myocarditis. J Immunol. 1986;137:1695-1702.
256. Keil RJ, Smith FE, Chason J, et al. Coxsackievirus B3 myocarditis in C3H/Hej mice: Description of an inbred model and the effect of exercise on virulence. Eur J Epidemiol. 1989;5:348-350.
257. Kilbourne ED, Wilson CB, Perrier D. The induction of gross myocardial lesions by a coxsackie (pleurodynia) virus and cortisone. J Clin Invest. 1956;35:362-370.
258. Beck MA, Kolbeck PC, Rohr LH, et al. Benign human enterovirus becomes virulent in selenium-deficient mice. J Med Virol. 1994;43:166-170.
259. Rezkalla S, Khatib G, Khatib R. Coxsackievirus B3 murine myocarditis: Deleterious effects of nonsteroidal anti-inflammatory agents. J Lab Clin Med. 1986;107:393-395.
260. Khatib R, Reyes MP, Smith F, et al. Enhancement of coxsackievirus B4 virulence by indomethacin. J Lab Clin Med. 1990;116:116-120.
261. Kishimoto C, Abekmann WH. In vivo significance of T cells in the development of coxsackievirus B3 myocarditis in mice. Immature but antigen-specific T cells aggravate cardiac injury. Circ Res. 1990;67:589-598.
262. Huber SA, Lodge PA. Coxsackievirus B-3 myocarditis in BALB/c mice. Evidence for autoimmunity to myocyte antigens. Am J Pathol. 1984;116:21-29.
263. Guthrie M, Lodge PA, Huber SA. Cardiac injury in myocarditis induced by coxsackievirus group B, type 3 in BALB/c mice is mediated by Lyt 2^+ cytolytic lymphocytes. Cell Immunol. 1984;88:558-567.
264. Kishimoto C, Kuribayashi K, Masuda T, et al. Immunologic behavior of lymphocytes in experimental viral myocarditis: Significance of T lymphocytes in the severity of myocarditis and silent myocarditis in BALB/c-nu/nu mice. Circulation. 1985;71:1247-1254.
265. Lyden DC, Huber SA. Aggravation of coxsackievirus, group B, type 3-induced myocarditis and increase in cellular immunity to myocyte antigens in pregnant BALB/c mice and animals treated with progesterone. Cell Immunol. 1984;87:462-472.
266. Job LP, Lyden DC, Huber SA. Demonstration of suppressor cells in coxsackievirus group B, type 3 infected female BALB/c mice which prevent myocarditis. Cell Immunol. 1986;98:104-113.
267. Huber SA, Job LP. Differences in cytolytic T cell response of BALB/c mice infected with myocarditic and non-myocarditic strains of coxsackievirus group B, type 3. Infect Immun. 1983;39:1419-1427.
268. Lee C, Maull E, Chapman N. Genomic regions of coxsackievirus B3-associated with cardiovirulence. J Med Virol. 1997;62:341-347.
269. Dunn JJ, Bradrick SS, Chapman NM, et al. The stem loop II within the 5′ nontranslated region of clinical coxsackievirus B3 genomes determines cardiovirulence phenotype in a murine model. J Infect Dis. 2003;187:1552-1561.
270. Huber SA, Sartini D, Exley M. Role of CD1d in coxsackievirus B3- induced myocarditis. J Immunol. 2003;170:3147-3153.
271. Weller AH, Simpson K, Herzum M, et al. Coxsackievirus B3-induced myocarditis: Virus receptor antibodies modulate myocarditis. J Immunol. 1989;143:1843-1850.
272. Lane JR, Neumann DA, Lafond-Walker A, et al. Role of IL-1 and tumor necrosis factor in coxsackievirus-induced autoimmune myocarditis. J Immunol. 1993;151:1682-1690.
273. Huber SA. Autoimmunity in myocarditis: Relevance of animal models. Clin Immunol Immunopathol. 1997;83:93-102.
274. Knowlton K, Badorff C. The immune system in viral myocarditis: Maintaining the balance. Circ Res. 1999;85:559-561.
275. Seko Y, Matsuda H, Kato K, et al. Expression of intercellular adhesion molecule-1 in murine hearts with acute myocarditis caused by coxsackievirus B3. J Clin Invest. 1993;91:1327-1336.
276. Herskowitz A, Admed-Ansari A, Neumann DA, et al. Induction of major histocompatibility complex antigens within the myocardium of patients with active myocarditis: A nonhistologic marker of myocarditis. J Am Coll Cardiol. 1990;15:624-632.
277. Kandolf R, Klingel K, Zell R, et al. Molecular pathogenesis of enterovirus-induced myocarditis: Virus persistence and chronic inflammation. Intervirology. 1993;35:140-151.
278. Rabausch-Starz A, Schwaiger K, Grunewald H-K, et al. Persistence of virus and viral genome in myocardium after coxsackievirus B3–induced murine myocarditis. Clin Exp Immunol. 1994; 96:69-74.
279. Wolfgram LJ, Beisel KW, Rose NR. Heart-specific autoantibodies following murine coxsackievirus B3 myocarditis. J Exp Med. 1985;161:1112-1121.
280. Neu N, Beisel KW, Traystman MD, et al. Autoantibodies specific for the cardiac myosin isoform are found in mice susceptible to coxsackievirus B3–induced myocarditis. J Immunol. 1987;138:2488-2492.
281. Gauntt C, Higdon A, Bowers D, et al. What lessons can be learned from animal model studies in viral heart disease? Scand J Infect Dis. 1993;88(Suppl):49-65.
282. Maisch B, Trostel-Soeder R, Stechemesser E, et al. Diagnostic relevance of humoral and cell-mediated immune reactions in patients with acute viral myocarditis. Clin Exp Immunol. 1982;48:533-545.
283. Shulze K, Becker B, Schauer R, Schultheib HP. Antibodies to the ADP-ATP carrier—an autoantigen in myocarditis and dilated cardiomyopathy—impair cardiac function. Circulation. 1990;81:959-969.
284. Maisch B, Deeg P, Liebau G, et al. Diagnostic relevance of humoral and cytotoxic immune reactions in primary and secondary dilated cardiomyopathy. Am J Cardiol. 1983;52:1072-1078.
285. Schultheib HP. The significance of autoantibodies against the ADP/ATP carrier for the pathogenesis of myocarditis and dilated cardiomyopathy—clinical and experimental data. Semin Immunopathol. 1993;68:229-233.
286. Neu N, Rose NR, Beisel KW, et al. Cardiac myosin induces myocarditis in genetically predisposed mice. J Immunol. 1987;139:3630-3636.
287. Zhang H, Morgan-Capner P, Latif N, et al. Coxsackievirus B3–induced myocarditis. Characterization of stable attenuated variants that protect against infection with the cardiovirulent wild-type strain. Am J Pathol. 1997;150:2197-2207.
288. Liao L, Sindhwani R, Rojkind M, et al. Antibody-mediated autoimmune myocarditis depends on genetically determined target organ sensitivity. J Exp Med. 1995;181:1123-1131.
289. Huber S, Polgar J, Moraska A, et al. T-lymphocyte responses in CVR3-induced murine myocarditis. Scand J Infect Dis. 1993;88(Suppl):67-78.
290. See DM, Tilles JG. Viral myocarditis. Rev Infect Dis. 1991;13:951-956.
291. Maisch B, Bauer E, Cirsi M, et al. Cytolytic cross-reactive antibodies directed against the cardiac membrane and viral proteins in coxsackievirus B3 and B4 myocarditis. Characterization and pathogenetic relevance. Circulation. 1993;87(Suppl 5):IV49-65.
292. Herzum M, Maisch B. Humoral and cellular immune reactions to the myocardium in myocarditis. Herz. 1992;17:91-96.
293. Badorff C, Lee GH, Lamphear BJ, et al. Enteroviral protease 2A cleaves dystrophin: evidence of cytoskeletal disruption in an acquired cardiomyopathy. Nat Med. 1999;5:320-326.
294. Lee GH, Badorff C, Knowlton KU. Dissociation of sarcoglycans and the dystrophin carboxyl terminus from the sarcolemma in enteroviral cardiomyopathy. Circulation Res. 2000;87:489-495.
295. Xiong DD, Lee GH, Badorff C. Dorner A, et al. Dystrophin deficiency markedly increases enterovirus-induced cardiomyopathy: A genetic predisposition to viral heart disease. J Nature Med. 2002;8:872-877.
296. Wessely R, Klingel K, Santana LF, et al. Transgenic expression of replication-restricted enteroviral genomes in heart muscle induces defective excitation-contraction coupling and dilated cardiomyopathy. J Clin Invest. 1998;102:1444-1453.
297. Wessely R, Lamphear BJ, Palakodeti R, et al. Coxsackieviral protease 2A is sufficient to induce a myocytopathic effect that can be rescued by expression of a mutant elF4G. Circulation. 1997;96:570-571.
298. Badorff C, Berkely N, Mehrotra S, et al. Enteroviral protease 2A directly cleaves dystrophin and is inhibited by a dystrophin-based substrate analogue. J Biol Chem. 2000;15:11191-11197.
299. Badorff C, Knowlton KU. Dystrophin disruption in enterovirus-induced myocarditis and dilated cardiomyopathy: from bench to bedside. Med Microbiol Immunol. 2004;193:121-126.
300. Straub V, Campbell KP. Muscular dystrophies and the dystrophin-glycoprotein complex. Curr Opin Neurol. 1997;10:168-175.
301. Towbin JA. The role of cytoskeletal proteins in cardiomyopathies. Curr Opin Cell Biol. 1998;10:131-139.
302. Towbin JA, Bowles KR, Bowles NE. Etiologies of cardiomyopathy and heart failure. Nat Med. 1999;5:266-267.
303. Medzhitov R, Janeway CA Jr. Innate immunity. N Engl J Med. 2000;343:338-344.
304. Badorff C, Fichtlscherer B, Rhoads RE, et al. Nitric oxide inhibits dystrophin proteolysis by coxsackieviral protease 2A through S-nitrosylation: A protective mechanism against enteroviral cardiomyopathy. Circulation. 2000;102:2276-2281.
305. McCarthy RE, Boehmer JP, Hruban RH, et al. Long-term outcome of fulminant myocarditis as compared with acute (nonfulminant) myocarditis. N Engl J Med. 2000;342:690-695.

306. Silver MA, Kowalczyk BS. Coronary microvascular narrowing in acute murine coxsackie B3 myocarditis. Am Heart J. 1989;118:173-174.

307. Lawson CM, O'Donoghue H, Bartholomaeus WN, et al. Genetic control of mouse cytomegalovirus-induced myocarditis. Immunology. 1990;69:20-26.

308. Craighead JE, Martin WB, Huber SA. Role of CD4+ (helper) T cells in the pathogenesis of murine cytomegalovirus myocarditis. Lab Invest. 1992;66:755-761.

309. Lawson CM, O'Donoghue HL, Reed WD. Mouse cytomegalovirus infection induces antibodies which cross-react with virus and cardiac myosin: A model for the study of molecular mimicry in the pathogenesis of viral myocarditis. Immunology. 1992;75:513-519.

310. Sherry B, Li XY, Tyler KL, et al. Lymphocytes protect against and are not required for reovirus-induced myocarditis. J Virol. 1993;67:6119-6124.

311. Felix JC, von Kreuter BF, Santos-Buch CA. Mimicry of heart cell surface epitopes in primary anti-*Trypanosoma cruzi* lyt 2+ T lymphocytes. Clin Immunol Immunopathol. 1993;68:141-146.

312. Armstrong AL, Barthold SW, Persing DH, et al. Carditis in Lyme disease: Susceptible and resistant strains of laboratory mice infected with *Borrelia burgdorferi*. Am J Trop Med Hyg. 1992;47:249-258.

313. Ruderman RM, Kerr JS, Telford SR III, et al. Early murine Lyme carditis has a macrophage predominance and is independent of major histocompatibility complex class II-CD4+ T cell interactions. J Infect Dis. 1995;171:362-370.

314. Mason JW. Myocarditis. Adv Int Med. 1999;44:293-310.

315. Kearney MT, Cotton JM, Richardson PJ, Shah AM. Viral myocarditis and dilated cardiomyopathy: mechanisms, manifestations, and management. Postgrad Med. J 2001;77:4-10.

316. Vikerfors T, Stjerna A, Olcen P, et al. Acute myocarditis. Serologic diagnosis, clinical findings and follow-up. Acta Med Scand. 1988;223:45-52.

317. Stratmann HG. Acute myocarditis versus myocardial infarction: Evaluation and management of the young patient with prolonged chest pain—case reports. Angiology. 1988;39:253-258.

318. Miklozek CL, Crumpacker CS, Royal HD, et al. Myocarditis presenting as acute myocardial infarction. Am Heart J. 1988; 115:768-776.

319. Spodick DH. Infection and infarction. Acute viral (and other) infection in the onset, pathogenesis, and mimicry of acute myocardial infarction. Am J Med. 1986;81:661-668.

320. Beaufils P, Slama R. Myocarditis confirmed by biopsy presenting as acute myocardial infarction. Br Heart J. 1986;4:420.

321. Dec GW Jr, Waldman H, Southern J, et al. Viral myocarditis mimicking acute myocardial infarction . J Am Coll Cardiol. 1992;20:85-89.

322. Smith SC, Landenson JH, Mason JW, et al. Elevations of cardiac troponin I associated with myocarditis. Experimental and clinical correlates. Circulation. 1997;95:163-168.

323. Heikkila J, Karjalainen J. Evaluation of mild acute infectious myocarditis. Br Heart J. 1982;47:381-391.

324. Karjalainen J. Clinical diagnosis of myocarditis and dilated cardiomyopathy. Scand J Infect Dis. 1993;88(Suppl):33-43.

325. Karjalainen J, Heikkila J. Acute pericarditis: Myocardial enzyme release as evidence for myocarditis. Am Heart J. 1986;111:546.

326. Scott LP III, Gutelius MF, Parrott RH. Children with acute respiratory tract infections. An electrocardiographic survey. Am J Dis Child. 1970;119:111-113.

327. Karjalainen J. Functional and myocarditis-induced T-wave abnormalities: Effect of orthostasis, beta blockade, and epinephrine. Chest. 1983;83:868-872.

328. Morgera T, Di Lenarda A, Dreas L, et al. Electrocardiography of myocarditis revisited: Clinical and prognostic significance of electrocardiographic changes. Am Heart J. 1992;124:455-467.

329. Weinhouse E, Wanderman KL, Sofer S, et al. Viral myocarditis simulating dilated cardiomyopathy in early childhood: Evaluation by serial echocardiography. Br Heart J. 1986;56:94-97.

330. Nieminen MS, Heikkila J, Karjalainen J. Echocardiography in acute infectious myocarditis: Relation to clinical and electrocardiographic findings. Am J Cardiol. 1984;53:1331-1337.

331. Kondo M, Takahashi M, Shimono Y, et al. Reversible asymmetric septal hypertrophy in acute myocarditis. Serial findings of two-dimensional echocardiogram and thallium-201 scintigram. Jpn Circ J. 1985;49:589-593.

332. Pinamonti B, Alberti E, Cigalotto A, et al. Echocardiographic findings in myocarditis. Am J Cardiol. 1988;62:285-291.

333. Yasuda T, Palacios IF, Dec W, et al. Indium-111 monoclonal antimyosin antibody imaging in the diagnosis of acute myocarditis. Circulation. 1987;76:306-311.

334. Carrio I, Berna L, Ballester M, et al. Indium-111 antimyosin scintigraphy to assess myocardial damage in patients with suspected myocarditis and cardiac rejection. J Nucl Med. 1988;29:1893-1900.

335. Dec W, Palacios I, Yasuda T, et al. Antimyosin antibody cardiac imaging: Its role in the diagnosis of myocarditis. J Am Coll Cardiol. 1990;16:97-104.

336. Obrador D, Ballester M, Carrio I, et al. Active myocardial damage without attending inflammatory response in dilated cardiomyopathy. J Am Coll Cardiol. 1993;21:1667-1671.

337. Narula J, Khaw BA, Dec GW Jr, et al. Brief report: Recognition of acute myocarditis masquerading as acute myocardial infarction. N Engl J Med. 1993;328:100-104.

338. Aherne T, Tscholakoff D, Finkbeiner W, et al. Magnetic resonance imaging of cardiac transplants: The evaluation of rejection of cardiac allografts with and without immunosuppression. Circulation. 1986;74:145-156.

339. Sasaki H, Sada M, Nishimura T, et al. The expanded scope of effectiveness of nuclear magnetic resonance imaging to determine cardiac allograft rejection. Transplant Proc. 1987;19:1062-1064.

340. Gagliardi MG, Bevilacqua M, Di Renzi P, et al. Usefulness of magnetic resonance imaging for diagnosis of acute myocarditis in infants and children, and comparison with endomyocardial biopsy. Am J Cardiol. 1991;68:1089-1091.

341. Chandraratna AN, Nimalasuriya A, Reid CL, et al. Left ventricular asynergy in acute myocarditis. Simulation of acute myocardial infarction. JAMA. 1983;250:1428-1430.

342. Friedrich MG, Strohm O, Schulz-Menger J, et al. Contrast media-enhanced magnetic resonance imaging visualizes myocardial changes in the course of viral myocarditis. Circulation. 1998;97:1802-1809.

343. O'Connell JB, Mason JW. Diagnosing and treating active myocarditis. West J Med. 1989;150:431-435.

344. Peters NS, Poole-Wilson PA. Myocarditis—continuing clinical and pathologic confusion. Am Heart J. 1991;121:942-947.

345. Billingham ME. The safety and utility of endomyocardial biopsy in infants, children and adolescents. J Am Coll Cardiol. 1990;15:443-445.

346. Fowles RE, Mason JW. Endomyocardial biopsy. Ann Intern Med. 1982;97:885-894.

347. Hauch AJ, Kearney DL, Edwards WD. Evaluation of postmortem endomyocardial biopsy specimens from 38 patients with lymphocytic myocarditis: Implications for the role of sampling error. Mayo Clin Proc. 1989;64:1235-1245.

348. Chow LH, Radio SJ, Sears TD, et al. Insensitivity of right ventricular endomyocardial biopsy in the diagnosis of myocarditis. J Am Coll Cardiol. 1989;14:915-920.

349. Nippoldt TB, Edwards WD, Holmes DR, et al. Right ventricular endomyocardial biopsy. Clinicopathologic correlates in 100 consecutive patients. Mayo Clin Proc. 1982;57:407-418.

350. Parrillo JE, Aretz HT, Palacios I, et al. The results of transvenous endomyocardial biopsy can frequently be used to diagnose myocardial diseases in patients with idiopathic heart failure. Endomyocardial biopsies in 100 consecutive patients revealed a substantial incidence of myocarditis. Circulation. 1984;69:93-101.

351. Takahashi O, Kamiya T, Echigo S, et al. Myocarditis in children—clinical findings and myocardial biopsy findings. Jpn Circ J. 1983;47:1298-1303.

352. Vasiljevic JD, Kanjuh V, Seferovic P, et al. The incidence of myocarditis in endomyocardial biopsy samples from patients with congestive heart failure. Am Heart J. 1990;120:1370-1377.

353. Herskowitz A, Campbell S, Deckers J. Demographic features and prevalence of idiopathic myocarditis in patients undergoing endomyocardial biopsy. Am J Cardiol. 1993;71:982-986.

354. Mason JW, O'Connell JB, Herskowitz A, et al. A clinical trial of immunosuppressive therapy for myocarditis. N Engl J Med. 1995;333:269-275.

355. Dec GW, Palacios IF, Fallon JT, et al. Active myocarditis in the spectrum of acute dilated cardiomyopathies. Clinical features, histologic correlates, and clinical outcome. N Engl J Med. 1985;312:885-890.

356. Zee-Cheng C-S, Tsai CC, Palmer DC, et al. High incidence of myocarditis by endomyocardial biopsy in patients with idiopathic congestive cardiomyopathy. J Am Coll Cardiol. 1984;3:63-70.

357. Fenoglio JJ, Ursell PC, Kellogg CF, et al. Diagnosis and classification of myocarditis by endomyocardial biopsy. N Engl J Med. 1983;308:12-18.

358. Mason JW, Billingham ME, Ricci DR. Treatment of acute inflammatory myocarditis assisted by endomyocardial biopsy. Am J Cardiol. 1980;45:1037-1044.

359. Chow LC, Dittrich HC, Shabetai R. Endomyocardial biopsy in patients with unexplained congestive heart failure. Ann Intern Med. 1988;109:535-539.

360. Shanes JG, Ghali J, Billingham ME, et al. Interobserver variability in the pathologic interpretation of endomyocardial biopsy results. Circulation. 1987;75:401-405.

361. Billingham M. Acute myocarditis: A diagnostic dilemma. Br Heart J. 1987;58:6-8.

362. Kereiakes DJ, Parmley WW. Myocarditis and cardiomyopathy. Am Heart J. 1984;108:1318-1326.

363. Aretz HT, Billingham ME, Edwards WD, et al. Myocarditis, a histopathologic definition and classification. Am J Cardiovasc Pathol. 1987;1:3-14.

364. Friman G, Fohlman J. The epidemiology of viral heart disease. Scand J Infect Dis. 1993;88(Suppl):7-10.

365. Kawai C, Matsumori A, Fujiwara H. Myocarditis and dilated cardiomyopathy. Annu Rev Med. 1987;38:221-239.

366. Kopecky SL, Gersh BJ. Dilated cardiomyopathy and myocarditis: Natural history, etiology, clinical manifestations, and management. In: O'Rourke RA, Crawford MH, eds. Current Problems in Cardiology. Chicago: Year Book Medical Publishers; 1987:569-647.

367. Lowry BS. Viruses and heart disease: A problem in pathogenesis. Ann Clin Lab Sci. 1986;16:358-364.

368. Zhang H, Li Y, McClean DR, et al. Detection of enterovirus capsid protein VP1 in myocardium from cases of myocarditis or dilated cardiomyopathy by immunohistochemistry: Further evidence of enterovirus persistence in myocytes. Med Microbiol Immunol. 2004;193:109-114.

369. Rotbart HA, Eastman PS, Ruth JL, et al. Nonisotopic oligomeric probes for the human enteroviruses. J Clin Microbiol. 1988;26:2669-2671.

370. Erlich HA, Gelfand DH, Saiki RK. Specific DNA amplification. Nature. 1988;331:461-462.

371. Schwaiger A, Umlauft F, Weyrer K, et al. Detection of enteroviral ribonucleic acid in myocardial biopsies from patients with idiopathic dilated cardiomyopathy by polymerase chain reaction. Am Heart J. 1993;126:406-410.

372. Wheeler DS, Kooy NW. A formidable challenge: The diagnosis and treatment of viral myocarditis in children. Crit Care Clin. 2003;19:365-391.

373. Caforio AL, Baboonian C, McKenna WJ. Postviral autoimmune heart disease—fact or fiction? Eur Heart J. 1997;18:1051-1055.

374. Tracy S, Wiegand V, McManus B, et al. Molecular approaches to enteroviral diagnosis in idiopathic cardiomyopathy and myocarditis. J Am Coll Cardiol. 1990;15:1688-1694.

375. Martino T, Liu P, Sole MJ. Viral infection and the pathogenesis of dilated cardiomyopathy. Circ Res. 1994;74:182-188.

376. Why HJ, Meany BT, Richardson PJ, et al. Clinical and prognostic significance of detection of enteroviral RNA in the myocardium of patients with myocarditis or dilated cardiomyopathy. Circulation. 1994;89:2582-2589.

377. McKenna WJ, Davies MJ. Immunosuppression for myocarditis. N Engl J Med. 1995;333:312-313.

378. Garg A, Shiau J, Guyatt G. The ineffectiveness of immunosuppressive therapy in lymphocytic myocarditis: An overview. Ann Intern Med. 1998;128:317-322.

379. Frustaci A, Chimenti C, Calabrese F, et al. Immunosuppressive therapy for active lymphocytic myocarditis: Virological and immunologic profile of responders versus nonresponders. Circulation 2003;107:857-863.

380. Grogan M, Redfield MM, Bailey KR, et al. Long-term outcomes of patients with biopsy-proven myocarditis: Comparison with idiopathic dilated cardiomyopathy. J Am Coll Cardiol. 1995;25:80-84.

381. Deckers JW, Hare JM, Baughman KL. Complications of transvenous right ventricular endomyocardial biopsy in adult patients with cardiomyopathy: A seven year survey of 516 consecutive diagnostic procedures in a tertiary referral center. J Am Coll Cardiol. 1992;19:43-47.
382. Wynne J, Braunwald E. The cardiomyopathies and myocarditides. In: Braunwald E, Zipes DP, Libby P. eds. Heart Disease, a Textbook of Cardiovascular Medicine. 6th ed. Philadelphia: WB Saunders; 2001:1751-1806.
383. Fowler NO. The secondary cardiomyopathies. In: Fowler NO. Myocardial Disease. New York: Grune & Stratton; 1973:337-359.
384. Vintila M, Tanaseanu S, Luca R, et al. Is cardiac involvement in collagen diseases important? A clinical study in 917 patients. Med Int. 1990;28:219-227.
385. Ansari A, Larson PH, Bates HD. Cardiovascular manifestations of systemic lupus erythematosus: Current perspective. Prog Cardiovasc Dis. 1985;27:421-434.
386. Clemson BS, Miller WR, Luck JC, et al. Acute myocarditis in fulminant systemic sclerosis. Chest. 1992;101:872-874.
387. McWhorter JE, LeRoy RC. Pericardial disease in scleroderma (systemic sclerosis). Am J Med. 1974;57:566-575.
388. Janosik DL, Osborn TG, Moore TL, et al. Heart disease in systemic sclerosis. Semin Arthritis Rheum. 1989;19:191.
389. Lebowitz WB. The heart in rheumatoid arthritis (rheumatoid disease). A clinical and pathological study of sixty-two cases. Ann Intern Med. 1963;58:102-123.
390. Goldenberg J, Ferraz MB, Pessoa AP, et al. Symptomatic cardiac involvement in juvenile rheumatoid arthritis. Int J Cardiol. 1992;34:57-62.
391. Askari AD, Huettner TL. Cardiac abnormalities in polymyositis/dermatomyositis. Semin Arthritis Rheum. 1982;12:208-219.
392. Tami LF, Bhasin S. Polymorphism of the cardiac manifestations in dermatomyositis. Clin Cardiol. 1993;16:260-264.
393. Bank I, Marboe CC, Redberg RF, et al. Myocarditis in adult Still's disease. Arthritis Rheum. 1985;28:452-454.
394. Webb JG, Butany J, Langer G, et al. Myocarditis and myocardial hemorrhage associated with thrombotic thrombocytopenic purpura. Arch Intern Med. 1990;150:1535-1537.
395. Midei MG, DeMent SH, Feldman AM, et al. Peripartum myocarditis and cardiomyopathy. Circulation. 1990;81:922-928.
396. Ikaheimo MJ, Niemela KO, Linnaluoto MM, et al. Early cardiac changes related to radiation therapy. Am J Cardiol. 1988;56:943-946.
397. Brosius FC, Waller BF, Roberts WC. Radiation heart disease. Am J Med. 1981;70: 519-530.
398. Stewart JR, Fajardo LF. Radiation-induced heart disease: An update. Prog Cardiovasc Dis. 1984;27:173.
399. Isner JM, Chokshi SK. Cardiac complications of cocaine abuse. Ann Rev Med. 1991;42: 133-138.
400. Taliercio CP, Olney BA, Lie JT. Myocarditis related to drug hypersensitivity. Mayo Clin Proc. 1985;60:463-468.
401. Brand A, Keren A, Kerem E, et al. Myocardial damage after a scorpion sting: Long-term echocardiographic follow-up. Pediatr Cardiol. 1988;9:59-61.
402. Matsuura H, Ishikita T, Yamamoto S, et al. Gallium-67 myocardial imaging for the detection of myocarditis in the acute phase of Kawasaki disease (mucocutaneous lymph node syndrome): The usefulness of single photon emission computed tomography. Br Heart J. 1987;58:385-392.
403. Humbert P, Faivre R, Fellman D, et al. Giant cell myocarditis: An autoimmune disease? Am Heart J. 1988;115:485-487.
404. Temple-Camp CR. Sarcoid myocarditis: A report of three cases. N Z Med J. 1989;102: 501-502.
405. Silverman KJ, Hutchins GM, Bulkley BH. Cardiac sarcoid: A clinicopathologic study of 84 unselected cases with systemic sarcoidosis. Circulation. 1978;58:1204-1211.
406. Tilles JG, Elson SH, Shaka JA, et al. Effects of exercise on coxsackie A9 myocarditis in adult mice. Proc Soc Exp Biol Med 1964;117:777-782.
407. Damm S, Andersson LG, Hendriksen E, et al. Wall motion abnormalities in male elite orienteers are aggravated by exercise. Clin Physiol 1999;19:121-126.
408. Suzuki H, Matsumori A, Kawai CH. Effects of angiotensin converting enzyme inhibitors on myocardial injury and congestive heart failure due to myocarditis in mice: Comparison with captopril and enalapril. Circulation. 1991;84(Suppl III):634.
409. Rezkalla SH, Raikar S, Kloner RA. Treatment of viral myocarditis with focus on captopril. Am J Cardiol. 1996;77:634-637.
410. Leon JS, Wang K, Engman DM. Captopril ameliorates myocarditis in acute experimental Chagas' disease. Circulation 2003;107:2264-2269.
411. Goldstein RE, Boccuzzi SJ, Cruess D, Nattel S. Diltiazem increases last-onset congestive heart failure in postinfarction patients with early reduction in ejection fraction. Circulation. 1991;83:52-60.
412. Factor SM, Minase T, Cho S, et al. Microvascular spasm in the cardiomyopathic Syrian hamster: A preventable cause of focal myocardial necroses. Circulation. 1982;66: 342-354.
413. Morris SA, Weiss LM, Factor S, et al. Verapamil ameliorates clinical, pathologic and biochemical manifestations of experimental chagasic cardiomyopathy in mice. J Am Coll Cardiol. 1989;14:782-789.
414. Wang WZ, Matsumori A, Yamada T, et al. Beneficial effects of amlodipine in a murine model of congestive heart failure induced by viral myocarditis. Circulation. 1997;95: 245-251.
415. Packer M, O'Connor CM, Ghali JK, et al. For the PRAISE study group. Effect of amlodipine on morbidity and mortality in severe chronic heart failure. N Engl J Med. 1996;335:1107-1114.
416. Maybaum S, Stockwell P, Naka Y, et al. Assessment of myocardial recovery in a patient with acute myocarditis supported with a left ventricular assist device. J Heart Lung Transplant. 2003;22:202-209.
417. Lee KJ, McCringle BW, Bohn DJ. Clinical outcome of acute myocarditis in children. Heart. 1999;82:226-233.
418. Hayakawa M, Inoh T, Yokota Y, et al. A long-term follow-up study of acute viral and idiopathic myocarditis. Jpn Circ J. 1983;47:1304-1309.
419. Vallejo J, Mann DL. Antiinflammatory therapy in myocarditis. Curr Opin Cardiol. 2003;18:189-193.
420. Khatib R, Reyes MP, Smith F, et al. Enhancement of coxsackie B3 virulence by indomethacin. J Lab Clin Med. 1990;116:116-120.
421. Costanzo-Norden MR, Reap EA, O'Connell JB, et al. A nonsteroid anti-inflammatory drug exacerbates coxsackie B3 murine myocarditis. J Am Coll Cardiol. 1985;6: 1078-1082.
422. Tomioka N, Kishimoto C, Matsumori A, et al. Effects of prednisolone on acute viral myocarditis in mice. J Am Coll Cardiol. 1986;7:868-872.
423. Ettinger J, Feucht H, Gartner R, et al. Cyclosporine A (CyA) for successful treatment of myocarditis (Letter). Eur Heart J. 1986;7:452.
424. Chan KY, Iwahara M, Benson LM, et al. Immunosuppressive therapy in the management of acute myocarditis in children: A clinical trial. J Am Coll Cardiol. 1991;17:458-460.
425. O'Connell JB, Robinson JA, Henkin RE, et al. Immunosuppressive therapy in patients with congestive cardiomyopathy and myocardial uptake of gallium-67. Circulation. 1981;64:780-786.
426. Anandasabapathy S, Frishman WH. Innovative drug treatments for viral and autoimmune myocarditis. J Clin Pharm. 1998;35:295-308.
427. Camargo PR, Snitcowsky R, da Luz PL, et al. Favorable effects of immunosuppressive therapy in children with dilated cardiomyopathy and active myocarditis. Pediatr Cardiol. 1995;16:61-68.
428. Takada H, Kishimoto C, Hiraoka Y. Therapy with immunoglobulin suppresses myocarditis in a murine coxsackie B3 model. Antiviral and antiinflammatory effects. Circulation. 1995;92:1604-1611.
429. Kishimoto C, Takada H, Kawamata H, et al. Immunoglobulin treatment prevents congestive heart failure in murine encephalomyocarditis viral myocarditis associated with reduction of inflammatory cytokines. J Pharmacol Exp Ther. 2001;299:645-651.
430. Maisch B, Herzum M, Hufnagel G, Schonean U. Immunosuppressive and immunomodulatory treatment for myocarditis. Curr Opin Cardiol. 1996;11:310-324.
431. McNamara DM, Rosemblum WD, Janosko KM, et al. Intravenous immune globulin in the therapy of myocarditis and acute cardiomyopathy. Circulation. 1997;95:2476-2478.
432. McNamara D, Holubkov R, Starling R, et al. Controlled trial of intravenous immune globulin in recent onset dilated cardiomyopathy. Circulation. 2001;103:2254-2259.
433. Kishimoto C, Crumpacker CS, Abelmann WH. Prevention of murine coxsackie B3 viral myocarditis and associated lymphoid organ atrophy with recombinant human leukocyte interferon alpha A/D. Cardiovasc Res. 1988;22:732-738.
434. Kuhl U, Pauschinger M, Schwimmbeck PL, et al. Interferon-beta treatment eliminates cardiotropic viruses and improves left ventricular function in patients with myocardial persistence of viral genomes and left ventricular dysfunction. Circulation. 2003;107:2793-2798.
435. Daliento L, Calabrese F, Tona F, Caforio AL, et al. Successful treatment of enterovirus-induced myocarditis with interferon-α. J Heart Lung Transplant. 2003;22:214-217.
436. Miric M, Vasilijevic J, Bojic M, et al. Long-term follow up of patients with dilated heart muscle disease treated with human leukocytic interferon alpha or thymic hormones. Initial results. Heart. 1996;75:596-601.
437. Matsumori A. The use of cytokine inhibitors: A new therapeutic insight into heart failure. Int J Cardiol. 1997;62:S3-S12.
438. McCormack JG, Bowler SD, Donnelly JE, Steadman C. Successful treatments of severe cytomegalovirus infection with ganciclovir in an immunocompetent host. Clin Infect Dis. 1998;26:1007-1008.
439. Rotbart HA, O'Connell JF, McKinlay MA. Treatment of human enterovirus infections. Antiviral Res. 1998;38:1-14.
440. Rotbart HA, Webster AD. Treatment of potentially life-threatening enterovirus infections with pleconaril. Clin Infect Dis. 2001;32:228-235.
441. Schiff GM, McKinlay MA, Sherwood JR. Oral efficacy of VP63843 in coxsackie A21–infected volunteers. Abstracts of the 36th Interscience Conference and Antimicrobial Agents and Chemotherapy, New Orleans, LA; 1996:171.
442. Woods MG, Diana GD, Rogge MC, et al. In vitro and in vivo activities of WIN 54954, a new broad-spectrum antipicornavirus drug. Antimicrob Agents Chemother. 1989;33:2069-2074.
443. Pauksen K, Ilback NG, Friman G, et al. Therapy of coxsackievirus B3–induced myocarditis with WIN 54954 in different formulations. Scand J Infect Dis. 1993;88 (Suppl):125-130.
444. See DM, Tilles JG. Treatment of coxsackievirus A9 myocarditis in mice with WIN 54954. Antimicrob Agents Chemother. 1993;36:425-428.
445. Fohlman J, Pauksen K, Hyypia T, et al. Antiviral treatment with WIN 54954 reduces mortality in murine coxsackie B2 myocarditis. Circulation. 1996;94:2254-2259.
446. Osler W. The Principles and Practice of Medicine. New York: D Appleton; 1892.
447. Klacsmann PG, Bulkley BH, Hutchins GM. The changed spectrum of purulent pericarditis: An 86-year autopsy experience in 200 patients. Am J Med. 1977;63:666-673.
448. Sagrista-Sauleda J, Barrabes JA, Permanyer-Miralda G, et al. Purulent pericarditis: Review of a 20 year experience in a general hospital. J Am Coll Cardiol. 1993;22: 1661-1665.
449. Park S, Bayer AS. Purulent pericarditis. Curr Clin Topics Infect Dis. 1992;12:56-82.
450. Gould K, Barnett JA, Sanford JP. Purulent pericarditis in the antibiotic era. Arch Intern Med. 1974;134:923-927.
451. Ilan Y, Oren R, Ben-Chetrit E. Acute pericarditis: Etiology, treatment and prognosis. Jpn Heart J. 1991;32:315-321.
452. Sagrista-Sauleda J, Angel J, Sanchez A, et al. Effusive-constrictive pericarditis. N Engl J Med. 2004;350:469-475.
453. Levy, P-Y, Corey R, Berger P, et al. Etiologic diagnosis of 204 pericardial effusions. Medicine. 2003;82:385-391.
454. Soler-Soler J, Permanyer-Miralda G, Sagrista-Sauleda J. A systematic diagnostic approach to primary acute pericardial disease. The Barcelona experience. Cardiol Clin. 1990;8: 609-620.
455. Maisch B, Ristic AD. The classification of pericardial disease in the age of modern medicine. Curr Cardiol Rep. 2002;4:13-21.
456. Johnson RT, Portnoy B, Rogers NG, et al. Acute benign pericarditis: Virologic study of 34 patients. Arch Intern Med. 1961;108:823.
457. Kagan H, Bernkopf H. Pericarditis caused by coxsackie virus B. Ann Pediatr. 1957;189: 44-50.
458. Brodie HR, Marchessault V. Acute benign pericarditis caused by coxsackie virus group B. N Engl J Med. 1960;262:1278-1280.

459. Van Reken D, Strauss A, Henandez A, et al. Infectious pericarditis in children. J Pediatr. 1974;85:165-169
460. Roberts R. Viral pericarditis. Med Serv J Can. 1961;17:588.
461. Movitt ER, Lenette EH, Mangum JF, et al. Acute benign pericarditis: Report of 2 cases associated with group A and group B coxsackie viruses. N Engl J Med. 1958;158: 1082-1086.
462. Matthews JD, Cameron SJ, George M. Constrictive pericarditis following coxsackie virus infection. Thorax. 1970;25:624-626.
463. Canas JA, Balsam D, Leggiadro RJ. Adenovirus pericarditis. N Y State J Med. 1986;86: 269-270.
464. Odie C, McCracken GH Jr, Nelson JD. Disseminated adenovirus infection: A case report and review of the literature. Pediatr Infect Dis. 1984;3:46-49.
465. Kleinfeld M, Milles S, Lidsky M. Mumps pericarditis: Review of the literature and report of a case. Am Heart J. 1958;55:153-156.
466. Hildenbrandt HM, Maassab HF, Willis PW III. Influenza virus pericarditis: Report of a case with isolation of Asian influenza virus from the pericardial fluid. Am J Dis Child. 1962;104:579.
467. Williams AJ, Freemont AJ, Barnett DB. Pericarditis and arthritis complicating chickenpox. Br J Clin Pract. 1983;37:226-227.
468. Kassab A, Demoulin JC, Vanlancker MA, et al. Cytomegalovirus hemopericarditis. Report of 1 case with histologic confirmation. Acta Cardiol. 1987;42:69-72.
469. Martin V, Miranda ML, Stiefel P, et al. Acute pericarditis caused by cytomegalovirus in a normal host (Letter). Enferm Infecc Microbiol Clin. 1989;7:515.
470. Nathan PE, Arsura EL, Zappi M. Pericarditis with tamponade due to cytomegalovirus in the acquired immunodeficiency syndrome. Chest. 1991;99:765-766.
471. Scott PJ, Conway SP, Da Costa P. Cardiac tamponade complicating cytomegalovirus pericarditis in a patient with AIDS. J Infect. 1990;20:92.
472. Campbell PT, Li JS, Wall TC, et al. Cytomegalovirus pericarditis: A case series and review of the literature. Am J Med Sci. 1995;309:229-234.
473. Shugoll GI. Pericarditis associated with infectious mononucleosis. Arch Intern Med. 1957;100:630-634.
474. Satoh T, Kojima M, Ohshima K. Demonstration of the Epstein-Barr genome by the polymerase chain reaction and in situ hybridization in a patient with viral pericarditis. Br Heart J. 1993;69:563-564.
475. Freedberg RS, Gindea AJ, Dieterich DT, et al. Herpes simplex pericarditis in AIDS. N Y State J Med. 1987;87:304-306.
476. Toma E, Poisson M, Claessens MR, et al. Herpes simplex type 2 pericarditis and bilateral facial palsy in a patient with AIDS. J Infect Dis. 1989;160:553-554.
477. Adler R, Takahashi M, Wright HT Jr. Acute pericarditis associated with hepatitis B infection. Pediatrics. 1978;61:716-719.
478. Kwan T, Karve MM, Emerole O. Cardiac tamponade in patients infected with HIV. Chest. 1993;104:1059-1062.
479. Moreno R, Villacastin J, Bueno H, et al. Clinical and echocardiographic findings in HIV patients with pericardial effusion. Cardiology. 1997;88:397-400.
480. Estok L, Wallach F. Cardiac tamponade in a patient with AIDS: A review of pericardial disease in patients with HIV infection. Mount Sinai J Med. 1998;65:33-39.
481. Chen Y, Brennessel D, Walters J, et al. Human immunodeficiency virus–associated pericardial effusion: Report of 40 cases and review of the literature. Am Heart J. 1999;137: 516-521.
482. Boyle JD, Pearce ML, Guze LB. Purulent pericarditis: Review of literature and report of eleven cases. Medicine. 1961;40:119-144.
483. Rubin RH, Moellering RC. Clinical, microbiologic and therapeutic aspects of purulent pericarditis. Am J Med. 1975;59:68-78.
484. Kauffman CA, Watanakunakorn C, Phair JP. Purulent pneumococcal pericarditis. A continuing problem in the antibiotic era. Am J Med. 1973;54:743-750.
485. Saenz RE, Sanders CV, Aldridge KE, et al. Purulent pericarditis with associated cardiac tamponade caused by a *Streptococcus pneumoniae* strain highly resistant to penicillin, cefotaxime, and ceftriaxone. Clin Infect Dis. 1998;26:762-763.
486. Pruitt JL. Group A streptococcal pericarditis in a previously well child. Pediatr Infect Dis J. 1989;8:338.
487. Karikm MA, Bach RG, Dressler F, et al. Purulent pericarditis caused by group B streptococcus with pericardial tamponade. Am Heart J. 1993;126:727-730.
488. Bateman AC, Richards M, Pallett AP. Fatal myocarditis associated with a Lancefield group B streptococcus. J Infect. 1998;36:354-355.
489. Kim NH, Park JP, Jeon SH, et al. Purulent pericarditis caused by group G streptococcus as an initial presentation of colon cancer. J Korean Med Sci. 2002;17:571-573.
490. Kumar VV, Herzog C. Purulent pericarditis caused by Group G streptococcus. JAMA. 1990;264:34-35.
491. Hirata K, Asato H, Maeshiro M. A case of effusive constrictive pericarditis caused by *Streptococcus milleri*. Jpn Circ J. 1991;55:154-158.
492. Kopec JS, Grifka RG, Karpawich PP. Isolated staphylococcal pericarditis following varicella in an adolescent: An unusual age-associated complication. Pediatr Emerg Care. 1990;6:38-39.
493. Demey HE, Eycken M, Vandermast M. Purulent pericarditis due to methicillin-resistant *Staphylococcus aureus*. A case report. Acta Cardiol. 1991;46:485-491.
494. Blaser MJ, Reingold AL, Alsever RN, et al. Primary meningococcal pericarditis: A disease of adults associated with serogroup C *Neisseria meningitidis*. Rev Infect Dis. 1984;6:625-632.
495. Finkelstein Y, Adler Y, Nussinovitch M, et al. A new classification for pericarditis associated with meningococcal infection. Eur J Pediatr. 1997;156:585-588.
496. Morgan DR, Spence M, Crowe M, O'Keeffe DB. Primary (isolated) meningococcal pericarditis. Clin Cardiol. 2002;25:305-307.
497. Coe MD, Hamer DH, Levy CS, et al. Gonococcal pericarditis with tamponade in a patient with systemic lupus erythematosus. Arthritis Rheum. 1990;33:1438-1441.
498. Wilson J, Zaman AG, Simmons AV. Gonococcal arthritis complicated by acute pericarditis and pericardial effusion. Br Heart J. 1990;63:134-135.
499. Dupuis C, Gronnier P, Kachaner J, et al. Bacterial pericarditis in infancy and childhood. Am J Cardiol. 1994;74:807-809.
500. Fyfe DA, Hagler DJ, Puga FJ, et al. Clinical and therapeutic aspects of *Haemophilus influenzae* pericarditis in pediatric patients. Mayo Clin Proc. 1984;59:415-422.
501. Schwartz KV, Guercio CA, Katz A. *Haemophilus influenza* pericarditis. Conn Med. 1987;51:423-424.
502. Welikovitch L, Knight JL, Burggraf GW, et al. Cardiac tamponade secondary to *Haemophilus* pericarditis: A case report. Can J Cardiol. 1992;8:303-305.
503. Yoshioka H, Shigemitsu K, Takeuchi M, et al. *Salmonella* pericarditis in a patient with primary idiopathic chylopericardium. Jpn J Thorac Cardiovasc Surg. 2003;51:16-17.
504. Sanchez-Guerrero J, Alarcon-Segovia D. *Salmonella* pericarditis with tamponade in systemic lupus erythematosus. Br J Rheumatol. 1990;29:69-71.
505. Lecomte F, Eustache M, Lemeland JF, et al. Purulent pericarditis due to *Yersinia enterocolitica*. J Infect Dis. 1989;159:363.
506. Marshall BW, Zimmerman SL. Tularemic pericarditis. AMA Arch Int Med. 1957;100: 300-304.
507. Adams CW. Tularemic pericarditis; report of two cases and review of the literature. Dis Chest. 1958;34:632-639.
508. Evans ME, Gregory DW, Schaffner W, McGee ZA. Tularemia: A 30-year experience with 88 cases. Medicine. 1985;64:251-269.
509. El Hassan N, Dbaibo G, Diab K, et al. *Pseudomonas* pericarditis in an immunocompetent newborn: Unusual presentation with review of the literature. J Infect. 2002;44:49-51.
510. Morrison VA, Lloyd BK, Chia JK, et al. Cardiovascular and bacteremic manifestations of *Campylobacter fetus* infection: Case report and review. Rev Infect Dis. 1990;12:387-392.
511. Kanj SS, Araj GF, Taher A, Reller LB. *Campylobacter fetus* pericarditis in a patient with beta-thalassemia: Case report and review of the literature. Clin Microbiol Infect. 2001;7:510-513.
512. Ugartemendia MC, Curos-Abadal A, Pujol-Rakosnik M, et al. *Brucella melitensis* pericarditis. Am Heart J. 1985;109:1108.
513. Ferguson R, Yee S, Finkle H, et al. *Listeria*-associated pericarditis in an AIDS patient. J Natl Med Assoc. 1991;85:225-228.
514. Poland GA, Jorgensen CR, Sarosi GA. *Nocardia asteroides* pericarditis: Report of a case and review of the literature. Mayo Clin Proc. 1990;65:819-824.
515. Ramsdale DR, Gautam PC, Perera B, et al. Cardiac tamponade due to actinomycosis. Thorax. 1984;39:473-474.
516. O'Sullivan RA, Armstrong JG, Rivers JT, et al. Pulmonary actinomycosis complicated by effusive constrictive pericarditis. Aust N Z J Med. 1991;21:879-880.
517. Skiest DJ, Steiner D, Werner M, et al. Anaerobic pericarditis: Case report and review. Clin Infect Dis. 1994;19:435-440.
518. Brook I. Pericarditis due to anaerobic bacteria. Cardiology. 2002;97:55-58.
519. Lam S, Greenberg R, Bank S. An unusual presentation of colon cancer: Purulent pericarditis and cardiac tamponade due to *Bacteroides fragilis*. Am J Gastroenterol. 1995;90: 1518-1520.
520. Touati GD, Carmi D, Nzomvuama A, Marticho P. Purulent pericarditis caused by malignant oesophago-pericardial fistula. Eur J Cardio Thorac Surg. 2003;24:847-849.
521. Rooney JJ, Crocco JA, Lyons HA. Tuberculous pericarditis. Ann Intern Med. 1970;72: 73-78.
522. Fowler NO. Tuberculous pericarditis. JAMA. 1991;266:99-103.
523. Larrieu AJ, Tyers GFO, Williams EH, et al. Recent experience with tuberculous pericarditis. Ann Thorac Surg. 1980; 29:464-468.
524. Sagrista-Sauleda J, Permanyer-Miralda G, Soler-Soler J. Tuberculous pericarditis: Ten year experience with a prospective protocol for diagnosis and treatment. J Am Coll Cardiol. 1988;11:724-728.
525. Permanyer-Miralda G, Sagrista-Sauleda J, Soler-Soler J. Primary acute pericardial disease: A prospective series of 231 consecutive patients. Am J Cardiol. 1985;56:623-630.
526. Desai HN. Tuberculous pericarditis. A review of 100 cases. S Afr Med J. 1979;55: 877-880.
527. Strang JIG. Tuberculous pericarditis in Transkei. Clin Cardiol. 1984;5:667.
528. Strang JI, Kakaza HH, Gibson DG, et al. Controlled clinical trial of complete open surgical drainage and of prednisone in treatment of tuberculous pericardial effusion in Transkei. Lancet. 1988;2:759-764.
529. D'Cruz IA, Sengupta EE, Abrahams C, et al. Cardiac involvement, including tuberculous pericardial effusion, complicating acquired immune deficiency syndrome. Am Heart J. 1986;5:1100.
530. Ortbals DW, Avioli LV. Tuberculous pericarditis. Arch Intern Med. 1979;139:231-234.
531. Peel AAF. Tuberculous pericarditis. Br Heart J. 1948;10:195-207.
532. Woods GL, Goldsmith JC. Fatal pericarditis due to *Mycobacterium avium-intracellulare* in acquired immunodeficiency syndrome. Chest. 1989;95:1355-1357.
533. Moreno F, Sharkey-Mathis PK, Mokulis E, et al. *Mycobacterium kansasii* pericarditis in patients with AIDS. Clin Infect Dis. 1994;19:967-969.
534. Campo RE, Campo CE. *Mycobacterium kansasii* disease in patients infected with human immunodeficiency virus. Clin Infect Dis. 1997;24:1233-1238.
535. Pintado V, Fortun J, Casado JL, Gomez-Mampaso E. *Mycobacterium kansasii* pericarditis as a presentation of AIDS. Infection. 2001;29:48-50.
536. Blaas SH, Bohm S, Martin G, et al. Pericarditis as primary manifestation of *Mycobacterium bovis* ssp. Caprae infection. Diag Microbiol Infect Dis. 2003;47:431-433.
537. Maycock R, Skale B, Kohler RB. *Legionella pneumophila* pericarditis proved by culture of pericardial fluid. Am J Med. 1983;75:534-536.
538. Reyes RR, Noble RC. Legionnaires' pericarditis. J Ky Med Assoc. 1983;81:757-758.
539. Luck PC, Helbig JH, Wunderlich E, et al. Isolation of *Legionella pneumophila* serogroup 3 from pericardial fluid in a case of pericarditis. Infection. 1989;17:388-390.
540. Svendsen JH, Jonsson V, Niebuhr U. Combined pericarditis and pneumonia caused by *Legionella* infection. Br Heart J. 1987;58:663-664.
541. Puleo J, Matar FA, McKeown PP, et al. *Legionella* pericarditis diagnosed by direct fluorescent antibody staining. Ann Thoracic Surg. 1995;60:444-446.
542. Friedland L, Snydman DR, Weingarden AS, et al. Ocular and pericardial involvement in Legionnaires' disease. Am J Med 1984;77:1105-1107.
543. Farraj RS, McCully RB, Ho JK, Smith TS. *Mycoplasma*-associated pericarditis. Mayo Clin Proc. 1997;72:33-36.

544. Balaguer A, Boronat M, Carrascosa A. Successful treatment of pericarditis associated with *Mycoplasma pneumoniae* infection. Pediatr Infect Dis J. 1990;9:141-143.
545. Kenny RT, Li JS, Clyde WA, et al. Mycoplasmal pericarditis: Evidence of invasive disease. Clin Infect Dis. 1993;1:S58-S62.
546. Sands MJ, Satz JE, Turner WE Jr, et al. Pericarditis and perimyocarditis associated with active *Mycoplasma pneumoniae* infection. Ann Intern Med. 1977;86:544-548.
547. Valero F, de Groote P, Millaire A, et al. Pericardial effusion as the initial feature of Q fever. Am Heart J 1995;130:1308-1309.
548. Bruyn GW, DeKoning J, Reijsoo FJ, et al. Lyme pericarditis leading to tamponade. Br J Rheumatol. 1994;33:862-866.
549. Roberts WC, Spray TL. Clinical and morphologic spectrum of pericardial heart disease. Curr Probl Cardiol. 1977;2:1-71.
550. Strang JI, Kakaza HH, Gibson DG, et al. Controlled trial of prednisolone as adjuvant in the treatment of tuberculous constrictive pericarditis in Transkei. Lancet. 1987;2:1418.
551. Traunter BW, Darouiche RO. Tuberculous pericarditis: Optimal diagnosis and management. Clin Infect Dis 2001;33:954-961.
552. Walsh TJ, Bulkley BH. *Aspergillus* pericarditis: Clinical and pathologic features in the immunocompromised patient. Cancer. 1982;49:48-54.
553. Cooper JAD, Weinbaum DL, Aldrich TK, et al. Invasive aspergillosis of the lung and pericardium in a nonimmunocompromised 33 year old man. Am J Med. 1981;71:903-907.
554. Ross EM, Macher AM, Roberts WC. *Aspergillus fumigatus* thrombi causing total occlusion of both coronary arterial ostia, all four major coronary arteries and coronary sinus and associated with purulent pericarditis. Am J Cardiol. 1985;56:499.
555. Le Moing V, Lortholary O, Timsit JF, et al. *Aspergillus* pericarditis with tamponade: Report of a successfully treated case and review. Clin Infect Dis. 1998;26:451-460.
556. Schrank JH, Dooley DP. Purulent pericarditis caused by *Candida* species: Case report and review. Clin Infect Dis. 1995;21:182-187.
557. Kraus WE, Valenstein PN, Corey GR. Purulent pericarditis caused by *Candida:* Report of three cases and identification of high-risk populations as an aid to early diagnosis. Rev Infect Dis. 1988;10:34-41.
558. Eng RHK, Sen P, Browne K, et al. *Candida* pericarditis. Am J Med. 1981:70:867-869.
559. Kaufman LD, Seifert FC, Eilbott DJ, et al. *Candida* pericarditis and tamponade in a patient with systemic lupus erythematosus. Arch Intern Med. 1988;148:715-717.
560. Neughebauer B, Alvarez V, Harb T, Keefer M. Constrictive pericarditis caused by *Candida glabrata* in an immunocompetent patient: Case report and review of the literature. Scand J Infect Dis. 2002;34:615-619.
561. Larson R, Scherb RI. Coccidioidal pericarditis. Circulation. 1953;7:211-217.
562. Schwartz EL, Waldmann EB, Payne RM, et al. Coccidioidal pericarditis. Chest. 1976;70: 670-672.
563. Amundson DE. Perplexing pericarditis caused by coccidioidomycosis. So Med J. 1993;86:694-696.
564. Oudiz R, Mahaisavariya P, Peng SK, et al. Disseminated coccidioidomycosis with rapid progression to effusive-constrictive pericarditis. J Am Soc Echocardiogr. 1995;8: 947-952.
565. Duvall CP, Carbone PP. *Cryptococcus neoformans* pericarditis associated with Hodgkin's disease. Ann Intern Med. 1966;64:850-856.
566. Wheat LJ, Stein L, Corya BC, et al. Pericarditis as a manifestation of histoplasmosis during two large urban outbreaks. Medicine. 1983;62:110-119.
567. Young EJ, Vainrub B, Musher DM. Pericarditis due to histoplasmosis. JAMA. 1978;240:1750.
568. Kilburn CD, McKinsey DS. Recurrent massive pleural effusion due to pleural, pericardial, and epicardial fibrosis in histoplasmosis. Chest. 1991;100:1715-1717.
569. Rab SW, Alam N, Hoda AN, et al. Amoebic liver abscess. Some unique presentations. Am J Med. 1967;43:811-816.
570. Baid CS, Varma AR, Lakhotia M. A case of subacute effusive constrictive pericarditis with a probable amoebic aetiology. Br Heart J. 1987;58:296-298.
571. Strang JIG. Two-dimensional echocardiography in the diagnosis of amoebic pericarditis. A case report. S Afr Med J. 1987;71:328-329.
572. Chao TH, Li YH, Tsai LM, et al. Amoebic liver abscess complicated with cardiac tamponade and mediastinal abscess. J Formosan Med Assoc. 1998;97:214-216.
573. Ibarra-Perez C, Green LS, Calvello-Juarez M, et al. Diagnosis and treatment of rupture of amebic abscess of the liver into the pericardium. J Thorac Cardiovasc Surg. 1972;64: 11-17.
574. Sagrista-Sauleda J, Permanyer-Miralda G, Juste-Sanchez C, et al. Huge chronic pericardial effusion caused by *Toxoplasma gondii.* Circulation. 1982;66:895-897.
575. Lyngberg KK, Vennervald BJ, Bygbjerg IC, et al. *Toxoplasma* pericarditis mimicking systemic lupus erythematosus. Diagnostic and treatment difficulties in one patient. Ann Med. 1992;24:337-340.
576. Herry I, Philippe B, Hennequin C. Acute life-threatening toxocaral tamponade. Chest. 1997;112:1692-1693.
577. Van der Horst R. Schistosomiasis of the pericardium. J R Soc Trop Med Hyg. 1979;73: 243-244.
578. Brusch JL. Cardiac infections in the immunosuppressed patient. Infect Dis Clin North Am. 2001;15:613-638.
579. Carrel TP, Schaffner A, Schmid ER, et al. Fatal fungal pericarditis after cardiac surgery and immunosuppression. J Thorac Cardiovasc Sur. 1991;101:161-164.
580. Canver CC, Patel AK, Kosolcharoen P, Voytovich MC. Fungal purulent constrictive pericarditis in a heart transplant patient. Ann Thorac Surg. 1998;65:1792-1794.
581. Spodick DH. Pericardial diseases. In: Braunwald E, Zipes DP, Libby P. eds. Heart Disease, a Textbook of Cardiovascular Medicine. 6th ed. Philadelphia: WB Saunders; 2001: 1823-1876.
582. Dalli E, Quesada A, Juan G, et al. Tuberculous pericarditis as the first manifestation of acquired immunodeficiency syndrome. Am Heart J. 1987;114:905-906.
583. Heidenreich PA, Eisenberg MJ, Kee LL, et al. Pericardial effusion in AIDS. Incidence and survival. Circulation. 1995;92:3229-3234.
584. Shabetai R. Function of the pericardium. In: Fowler NO, ed. The Pericardium in Health and Disease. Mount Kisco, NY: Futura; 1985:19-50.
585. Shabetai R. Acute pericarditis. Cardiol Clin. 1990;8:639-644.
586. Fowler NO. Recurrent pericarditis. Cardiol Clin. 1990;8:621-626.
587. Fowler NO, Harbin AD. Recurrent acute pericarditis: Follow-up study of 31 patients. J Am Coll Cardiol. 1986;7:300-305.
588. Raatikka M, Pelkonen PM, Karjalainen J, Jokinen ER. Recurrent pericarditis in children and adolescents. J Am Coll Cardiol. 2003;42:759-764.
589. Utley JR, Mills J. Annular erosion and pericarditis. Complications of endocarditis of the aortic root. J Thorac Cardiovasc Surg. 1972; 64:76-81.
590. Ribeiro P, Shapiro L, Nihoyannopoulos P, et al. Pericarditis in infective endocarditis. Eur Heart J. 1985;6:975-978.
591. Carson TJ, Murray GF, Wilcox BR, et al. The role of surgery in tuberculous pericarditis. Ann Thorac Surg. 1974;17:163-167.
592. Guberman BA, Fowler NO, Engel PJ, et al. Cardiac tamponade in medical patients. Circulation. 1981;64:633-640.
593. Spodick DH. Pericardial rub: Prospective multiple observer investigation of pericardial friction rub in 100 patients. Am J Cardiol. 1975;35:357-362.
594. Talreja DR, Edwards WD, Danielson GK, et al. Constrictive pericarditis in 26 patients with histologically normal pericardial thickness. Circulation. 2003;108:1852-1857.
595. Spodick DH. Electrocardiogram in acute pericarditis. Distributions of morphologic and axial changes by stages. Am J Cardiol. 1974;33:470-447.
596. Spodick DH. Frequency of arrhythmias in acute pericarditis determined by Holter monitoring. Am J Cardiol. 1984;53:842-845.
597. Isner JM, Carter BL, Bankoff MS, et al. Computed tomography in the diagnosis of pericardial heart disease. Ann Intern Med. 1982;97:473-479.
598. Tomoda H, Hoshiai M, Furuya H, et al. Evaluation of pericardial effusion with computed tomography. Am Heart J. 1980;99:701-706.
599. Sechtem U, Tscholakoff D, Higgins CB. MRI of the abnormal pericardium. AJR. 1986;147:245-252.
600. Giorgi B, Mollet NRA, Dymarkowski S, et al. Clinically suspected constrictive pericarditis: MR imaging assessment of ventricular septal motion and configuration in patients and healthy subjects. Radiology. 2003;228:417-424.
601. Krikorian JG, Hancock EW. Pericardiocentesis. Am J Med. 1978;65:808-814.
602. Mercé J, Sagristá-Sauleda J, Permanyer-Miralda G, et al. Should pericardial drainage be performed routinely in patients who have a large pericardial effusion without tamponade? Am J Med. 1998;105:106-109.
603. Gouny P, Lancelin C, Girard PM, et al. Pericardial effusion and AIDS: Benefits of surgical drainage. Eur J Cardiothorac Surg. 1998;13:165-169.
604. Corey GR, Campbell PT, Van Trigt P, et al. Etiology of large pericardial effusions. Am J Med. 1993;95:209-213.
605. Uthaman B, Endrys J, Abushaban L, et al. Percutaneous pericardial biopsy: Technique, efficacy, safety, and value in the management of pericardial effusion in children and adolescents. Pediatr Cardiol. 1997;18:414-418.
606. Selig MB. Percutaneous pericardial biopsy under echocardiographic guidance. Am Heart J. 1991;122:879-882.
607. Tan JS, Holmes JC, Fowler NO, et al. Antibiotic levels in pericardial fluid. J Clin Invest. 1974;53:7-12.
608. Schifferdecker B, Spodick DH. Nonsteroidal Anti-inflammatory Drugs in the Treatment of Pericarditis: Clinical Review. Cardiol Rev. 2003;11:211-217.
609. Adler Y, Finkelstein Y, Guindo J, et al. Colchicine treatment for recurrent pericarditis. A decade of experience. Circulation. 1998;97:2183-2185.
610. Guindo J, Adler Y, Spodick DH, et al. Colchicine for recurrent pericarditis: 51 patients followed up for 10 years. Circulation. 1997;96(Suppl I):1-29.
611. Millaire A, deGroote P, Docoulx E, et al. Treatment of recurrent pericarditis with colchicine. Eur Heart J. 1994;15:120-121.
612. Quale JM, Lipschik GY, Heurich AE. Management of tuberculous pericarditis. Ann Thorac Surg. 1987;43:653-655.
613. Marcolongo R, Russo R, Laveder F, et al. Immunosuppressive therapy prevents recurrent pericarditis. J Am Coll Cardiol. 1995;26:1276-1279.
614. Suwan PK, Potjalongslip S. Predictors of constructive pericarditis after tuberculous pericarditis. Br Heart J. 1995;73:187-189.
615. Dooley DP, Carpenter JL. Adjunctive corticosteroid therapy for tuberculosis: A critical reappraisal of the literature. Clin Infect Dis. 1997;25:872-887.
616. Alzeer AH, FitzGerald JM. Corticosteroids and tuberculosis: Risks and use as adjunct therapy. Tuber Lung Dis. 1993;74:6-11.
617. Wojnicz R, Nowalany-Kozielska E, Wokciechowska C, et al. Randomized, placebo-controlled study for immunosuppressive treatment of inflammatory dilated cardiomyopathy: Two year follow up results. Circulation. 2001;104:39-45.
618. Fennell WM. Surgical treatment of constrictive tuberculous carditis. S Afr Med J. 1982;62:353.
619. Arsan S, Mercan S, Sarigül A, et al. Long-term experience with pericardiectomy: Analysis of 105 consecutive patients. Thorac Cardiovasc Surg. 1994;42:340-344.
620. Bozbuga N, Erentug V, Eren E, et al. Pericardiectomy for chronic constrictive tuberculous pericarditis: Risks and predictors of survival. Tex Heart Inst J. 2003;30:180-185.
621. Ustunsoy H, Celkan MA, Sivrikoz MC, et al. Intrapericardial fibrinolytic therapy in purulent pericarditis. Eur J Cardio Thorac Surg. 2002;22:373-376.
622. Galve E, Garcia-del-Castillo H, Evangelista A, et al. Pericardial effusion in the course of myocardial infarction: Incidence, natural history, and clinical relevance. Circulation. 1986;73:294.
623. Gregoratos G. Pericardial involvement in acute myocardial infarction. Cardiol Clin. 1990;8:601-608.
624. Krainin FM, Flessas AP, Spodick DH. Infarction associated pericarditis. Rarity of diagnostic electrocardiogram. N Engl J Med. 1984;311:1211-1214.
625. Khan AH. The postcardiac injury syndromes. Clin Cardiol. 1992;15:67-72.
626. Dressler W. Post-myocardial infarction syndrome. JAMA. 1956;160:1379-1383.
627. Engle MA, Gay WA Jr, Zabriskie JB, et al. The post pericardiotomy syndrome: 25 years experience. J Cardiovasc Med. 1984;4:321-332.
628. Renfrew R, Buselmeier TJ, Kjeilstrand CM. Pericarditis and renal failure. Annu Rev Med. 1980;31:345-360.
629. Rutsky EA, Rostand SG. Treatment of uremic pericarditis and pericardial effusion. Am J Kidney Dis. 1987;10:2.

630. Saner HE, Gobel FL, Nicoloff DM, et al. Aortic dissection presenting as pericarditis. Chest. 1987;91:71.
631. Kelly CA, Bourke JP, Malcolm A, et al. Chronic pericardial disease in patients with rheumatoid arthritis: A longitudinal study. Q J Med. 1990;75:461-470.
632. Abid MA, Gitlin N. Pericarditis—an extraintestinal complication of inflammatory bowel disease. West J Med. 1990;153:314-315.
633. Zimmerman J, Yahalom J, Bar-On H. Clinical spectrum of pericardial effusion as the presenting feature of hypothyroidism. Am Heart J. 1983;106:770-771.

CHAPTER **78**

Mediastinitis

MARK E. RUPP

Acute mediastinitis is an uncommon, but potentially devastating, infection involving the structures of the mediastinum. Before the development of sophisticated techniques in cardiovascular and thoracic surgery, most cases resulted from esophageal perforation or contiguous spread from oropharyngeal foci. Mediastinitis now occurs most frequently as a postoperative infection after median sternotomy. Regardless of the pathogenesis of acute mediastinitis, a high index of clinical suspicion must be maintained for this serious infection in order to diagnose mediastinitis promptly and institute potentially life-saving medical and surgical therapy. Sclerosing mediastinitis, also known as fibrosing or granulomatous mediastinitis, often caused by *Histoplasma capsulatum,* is also discussed.

ANATOMIC CONSIDERATIONS

The mediastinum is the region within the thorax between the pleural sacs (Fig. 78-1). It extends from the diaphragm to the superior aperture of the thorax. The sternum and costal cartilages make up the anterior boundary, and the 12 thoracic vertebral bodies border the mediastinum posteriorly. The mediastinum is arbitrarily divided into four subdivisions: superior, posterior, anterior, and middle. Structures within the mediastinum include the heart and great vessels; the distal portion of the trachea and mainstem bronchi; the esophagus; the vagus nerves; the phrenic nerves; the remains of the thymus; and the thoracic duct. These structures are surrounded by adipose tissue, loose connective tissue, and lymph nodes. The mediastinum communicates with the structures of the head and neck via several fascial planes and potential spaces (see Chapter 57). Detailed descriptions of mediastinal anatomy are available,[1-4] and the major points are reviewed in the following sections. The three major routes by which infection spreads from the head and neck to the mediastinum are (1) the pretracheal space, (2) the long fascial planes of the posterior neck, and (3) the viscerovascular or lateral pharyngeal space. The long fascial planes of the posterior neck extend from the base of the skull to the diaphragm and are made up of the retropharyngeal or retrovisceral space, the prevertebral space, and the danger space. Pearse[1] attempted to delineate the relative importance of each route in the pathogenesis of mediastinitis and found the retropharyngeal space to be involved in 71% of cases, followed by the lateral pharyngeal space in 21% and the pretracheal space in 8%.

ACUTE MEDIASTINITIS

Epidemiology and Pathogenesis

Primary infection of the mediastinum is a rare event. Essentially all cases of mediastinitis occur because of the spread of infection from other sites or because of direct inoculation due to trauma. The causes of mediastinitis are summarized in Box 78-1 and can be grouped into the following four categories: esophageal perforation,[5-17] head and neck infection,[1,4,18-28] infection originating at another site,[2,29-33] and cardiothoracic surgery.[34-86] The pathogenesis, clinical manifestations, and treatment vary according to the underlying cause of mediastinitis.

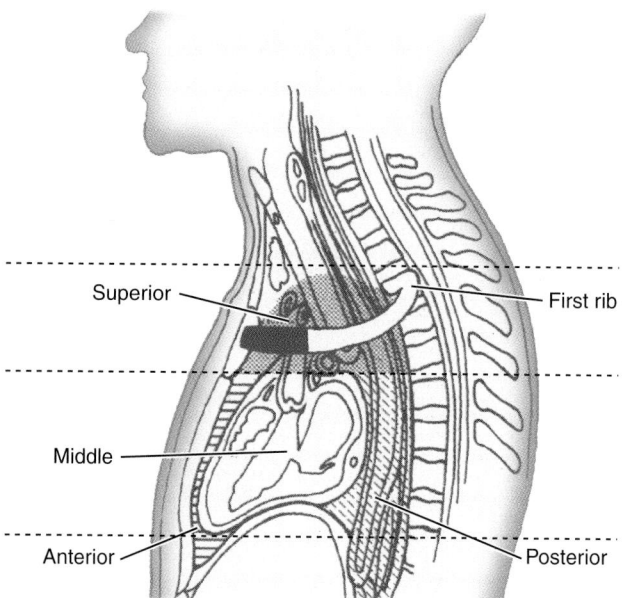

FIGURE 78-1. Anatomic boundaries and divisions of the mediastinum.

Mediastinitis Secondary to Infections of the Head and Neck and Other Contiguous Structures

Before the development of cardiac surgery, perforation of the esophagus was the leading cause of mediastinitis, followed by suppurative infections of the oropharynx.[1] In 1724, Herman Boerhaave described the first case of mediastinitis due to spontaneous rupture of the esophagus, in a Dutch admiral who self-induced emesis.[87,88] Subsequently, this entity, which is known as *Boerhaave syndrome,* continued to account for approximately 30% of cases of esophageal perforation.[89] Currently, esophageal perforation is most frequently caused by iatrogenic events.[6] Flexible fiberoptic endoscopy of the upper gastrointestinal tract is complicated by esophageal perforation in 0.074% to 0.4% of procedures.[4,12,90] This occurs more frequently during sclerotherapy or dilatation procedures.[6] Swallowed foreign bodies, esophageal carcinoma, and nonsurgical trauma may also result in perforation of the esophagus and mediastinitis.

Depending on where the esophageal perforation occurs, mediastinitis may result from direct spillage of esophageal contents into the posterior mediastinum or from migration of contents into the mediastinum via the fascial planes of the neck. A necrotizing chemical mediastinitis ensues that is followed by an aerobic and anaerobic bacterial mediastinitis. Often a synergistic necrotizing form of mediastinitis is observed.[18] Spread of infection from the neck into the mediastinum is influenced by respiratory dynamics, in which the negative intrathoracic pressure generated during respiration tends to force the infection into the mediastinum.[14]

Before antibiotics were widely available, odontogenic and pharyngeal infections accounted for 10% to 31% of cases of mediastinitis.[1,2,91] They are rare causes of mediastinitis today. The prototypic odontogenic infection leading to mediastinitis is Ludwig's angina. This typically arises from an infection of the second or third mandibular molar to involve the sublingual and submandibular spaces. From there, the infection can spread via the lateral pharyngeal space to involve the retropharyngeal space or carotid sheath and thus track into the mediastinum. During the antibiotic era, approximately 3.5% of cases of Ludwig's angina have been complicated by mediastinitis.[23] Mediastinitis resulting from infections involving the lateral pharyngeal space may originate from a number of sources, including the teeth, parotid glands, and tonsils, or, rarely, from otitis or mastoiditis. Lemierre's syndrome begins in the lateral pharyngeal space and extends into the mediastinum,

Causes of Acute Mediastinitis

Esophageal Perforation
Iatrogenic
  Esophagogastroduodenoscopy, esophageal dilation, esophageal variceal
    sclerotherapy, nasogastric tube, Sengstaken-Blakemore tube, endotracheal
    intubation, esophageal surgery, paraesophageal surgery, transesophageal
    echocardiography, anterior stabilization of cervical vertebral bodies
Swallowed foreign bodies
  Bones, coins, can pull-tabs, drug-filled condoms, swords, ball point pens
Trauma
  Penetrating
    Gunshot wound, knife wound
  Blunt
    Steering wheel injury, seatbelt injury, cardiopulmonary resuscitation,
      whiplash injury, barotrauma
  Spontaneous or other
    Emesis, cricoid pressure during anesthesia induction, heavy lifting, defecation,
      parturition, carcinoma

Head and Neck Infections
Odontogenic, Ludwig's angina, pharyngitis, tonsillitis, parotitis, epiglottitis,
  Lemierre's syndrome

Infection Originating at Another Site
Pneumonia; pleural space infection or empyema; subphrenic abscess;
  pancreatitis; cellulitis or soft tissue infection of the chest wall; osteomyelitis of
  sternum, clavicle, ribs, or vertebrae; hematogenous spread from distant foci
Lymph nodes: necrosis and hemorrhage (anthrax) or caseous necrosis
  (tuberculosis)

Cardiothoracic Surgery (Median Sternotomy)
Coronary artery bypass grafting, cardiac valve replacement, repair of congenital
  heart defect, heart transplantation, heart-lung transplantation, cardiac assist
  devices, other types of cardiothoracic surgery

accompanied by suppurative phlebitis of the jugular vein. Retropharyngeal space infections usually arise from perforation of the esophagus or by extension from pharyngitis, epiglottitis, or tonsillitis. From the long fascial planes of the neck, these infections easily spread into the superior mediastinum, or, if the danger space is involved, into the posterior mediastinum.[18,19] The pretracheal space descends into the anterior mediastinum and most often is involved in mediastinitis complicating surgery of the thyroid or trachea.[1]

Mediastinitis Secondary to Cardiothoracic Surgery

Since the refinement of cardiothoracic surgery in the 1960s and 1970s, mediastinitis has become largely a postsurgical infection. Numerous studies have documented the incidence of mediastinitis after cardiothoracic surgery and the risk factors for development of this serious complication. In 1984, Sar and colleagues[56] reviewed the available literature and found the incidence of mediastinitis to be 0.4% to 5% among patients undergoing median sternotomy. Since that time, studies documenting the experience of more than 150,000 patients have been published, with incidence rates ranging from 0.4% to 2.4%.[34,38-53,57,58,60,63,68,69] The incidence of mediastinitis during outbreaks has been as high as 5% to 23.7%.[92-96] Patients undergoing heart transplantation are at higher risk for development of mediastinitis, with incidences of 2.5% to 7.5%.[77-79,84] This increased risk of mediastinitis is even greater if a mechanical device, such as a left ventricular assist device or a total artificial heart, is used to support a patient who is awaiting a suitable donor heart. Incidences of mediastinitis in this situation range from 7.5% to 35.7%.[80-85] A sharp increase in the rate of mediastinitis after heart transplantation (up to 50%) was linked to changes in organ allocation that resulted in an increased pretransplantation hospital stay.[97] Rarely, donor-to-recipient transmission of bacteria has been observed to result in mediastinitis.[98]

A number of factors have been suggested to increase the risk of mediastinitis. The studies examining these risk factors are primarily retrospective case-control studies and therefore are limited by the problems inherent in retrospective surveys. Risk factors can be divided into the following groups: preoperative, intraoperative, and postoperative. Risk factors that can be identified preoperatively include diabetes mellitus, obesity, previous sternotomy, chronic obstructive pulmonary disease, peripheral vascular disease, a history of endocarditis, cigarette smoking, low cardiac output states, remote infection, hair removal with razor versus removal with electric clippers, and prolonged preoperative hospitalization.[34,37,39,40,42,44-47,49,51-56,59,63,99]

Intraoperative and surgical factors include the complexity of surgery, the type of bone saw used, the type of sternal closure, the use of internal mammary arteries in coronary artery bypass grafting, the use of bone wax, prolonged operative time, prolonged time on cardiopulmonary bypass, blood transfusions, the indiscriminate use of electrocautery, tearing of the aortic or femoral artery, prolonged aortic cross-clamp time, and antibiotic prophylaxis.[34-40,44-52,56,59,68,71-74,100,101] Postoperatively, patients at greater risk for mediastinitis have been found to have had reexploration to control bleeding, a prolonged length of stay in the intensive care unit, mechanical ventilation for longer than 24 to 48 hours, tracheostomy, cardiopulmonary resuscitation, temporary pacing wires, concurrent leg wound infection at the saphenous vein harvest site, and low cardiac-output states.[34,39,40,42,44-49,51,52,54,56,59-63,71,73,75]

There is not universal agreement regarding any of these factors. For instance, despite more than 3 decades of surgical experience, it is unclear whether the use of internal mammary artery grafts in coronary artery bypass surgery predisposes patients to mediastinitis. In 1972, Arnold[102] suggested that, based on anatomic studies of sternal blood supply, the use of the internal mammary artery in coronary artery bypass procedures might lead to significant sternal ischemia and thereby predispose patients to sternal osteomyelitis and mediastinitis. This hypothesis has been supported by several laboratory and clinical studies.[35,42,49,63,71,103] However, other investigators have observed no significant increase in sternal wound infections in patients undergoing coronary artery bypass grafting when the internal mammary artery was used.[34,35,37,48,55,104-107] Grover and colleagues[38] reviewed the data obtained from more than 14,000 patients in the Department of Veterans Affairs Cardiac Surgery Database. Although operative mortality was significantly decreased in patients who received internal mammary artery grafts, there was an increased risk of mediastinitis, particularly if multiple internal mammary artery grafts were used. Likewise, Walkes and associates[108] observed a higher incidence of mediastinitis in patients undergoing coronary artery bypass grafting when multiple internal mammary artery grafts were employed (4.4%), compared with single grafts (2.2%).

It is generally believed that the pathogenesis of mediastinitis after cardiac surgery is related to the inoculation of organisms from the patient's endogenous bacterial flora or from the surgical field into the operative wound. Bacteria are able to propagate in the relatively protected avascular area of the surgical wound and cause infection. Therefore, factors such as the length of time of surgery, the complexity of surgery, and the need for reexploration might be expected to increase the risk of mediastinitis. Outbreaks of mediastinitis that have been epidemiologically linked to sources such as bacteria from a surgeon's hands or nares lend support to this concept.[96,100,102-106,109] Ferrazzi and associates[67] observed a significant decrease in the incidence of gram-negative mediastinitis but no significant change in gram-positive infections with changes in the operating room environment, supporting the belief that many of these infections arise from a reservoir of gram-positive organisms resident on the patient's skin. Gummert and colleagues[42] observed a lower rate of wound infection and mediastinitis in 1070 patients undergoing cardiac surgery with minimally invasive techniques, compared with more than 9000 patients undergoing standard sternotomy procedures. Archer and Amstrong[110] demonstrated that patients are colonized by small numbers of antibiotic-resistant coagulase-negative staphylococci, which become the predominant species when subjected to the selective pressure of prophylactic antibiotics. In addition, various postulated immunosuppressive effects of cardiopulmonary bypass may contribute to the pathogenesis of mediastinitis after cardiac surgery.[111,112] However, no difference in infectious complications, including mediastinitis, was observed between 1741 patients undergoing coronary artery bypass grafting without the use of a cardiopulmonary bypass pump and 6126 patients undergoing traditional coronary artery bypass surgery.[43] Outbreaks of mediastinitis linked to environmental sources and poor hand-washing techniques have indicated the importance of postoperative factors.[92-95,113-115] Controlled prospective studies are needed to define better the factors that influence postcardiac surgery mediastinitis.[116]

Bacteriology

The bacteriology of mediastinitis related to cardiovascular surgery and that of mediastinitis that occurs secondary to odontogenic or other head and neck infections is strikingly different, as summarized in Box 78-2. Mediastinitis secondary to cardiothoracic surgery is primarily caused by gram-positive cocci, with lesser contributions by gram-negative bacilli. *Candida* appears to be responsible for a growing number of cases of mediastinitis after cardiothoracic surgery.[117-119] The bacteriology of mediastinitis secondary to extension from head and neck sources is largely polymicrobic. Often a synergistic infection made up of a number of oral anaerobes and gram-negative bacilli is present. The most frequently isolated organisms include viridans streptococci, peptococci, peptostreptococci, *Bacteroides* spp., and

Fusobacterium. The relative frequency with which these organisms are isolated is uncertain.[120,121]

Clinical Manifestations and Diagnosis

The clinical manifestations of mediastinitis also differ according to the underlying cause of disease. Patients with mediastinitis from extension of odontogenic or pharyngeal infections usually have obvious primary infections with significant pain, fever, and swelling at the affected site. Esophageal perforation may be clinically obvious or inapparent. Early in the course of mediastinitis, the signs and symptoms may be subtle, but as the condition progresses, patients note increasing chest pain, respiratory distress, and dysphagia. Chest pain, often the most prominent symptom, may localize depending on which portion of the mediastinum is involved. In anterior mediastinitis, pain is often located in the cervical or substernal region. Pain due to posterior mediastinitis may localize to the epigastric area with radiation to the interscapular region.[12,14,30,91] Pleuritic chest pain may also be experienced as a result of the relatively common complication of pleural effusion. Retroperitoneal extension may be accompanied by acute abdominal signs and may prompt unnecessary exploratory laparotomy.[18] Examination may reveal fever, tachycardia, crepitus, and edema of the chest or neck. Hamman's sign, a crunching, rasping sound heard over the precordium synchronous with the cardiac rhythm, caused by emphysema of the mediastinum, may be present in up to 50% of patients with pneumomediastinum.[122,123] Crepitus may appear in the supraclavicular area. The heart sounds may appear distant and dull. In the later stages of disease, signs of bacteremia and sepsis may predominate.

The early diagnosis of mediastinitis in the infant or neonate is particularly challenging. A peculiar, interrupted, staccato type of inspiration has been described in a number of cases.[124] The signs and symptoms of mediastinitis in older children are similar to those observed in adults.[125] Laboratory tests usually reveal a leukocytosis, with a leftward shift evident on the differential. Radiographically, plain films of the chest may reveal mediastinal widening, air-fluid levels, and subcutaneous or mediastinal emphysema (Fig. 78-2).[8,9,12,19,21,126] The lateral chest radiograph may be useful in demonstrating superior mediastinal gas not evident on upright films. Approximately 50% of cases of pneumomediastinum are not evident without lateral views.[127] Complications of mediastinitis, such as pleural effusion or pneumoperitoneum, may also be evident on the chest radiograph.

Esophageal perforation is best demonstrated by contrast esophagography, which reveals extravasation of dye in 59% to 100% of cases.[9,12,128,129] It is recommended that a water-soluble contrast agent be used initially to avoid the inflammation and granuloma formation evoked by extravasated barium.[130] If extravasation is not observed,

---

BOX 78-2

Microbiology of Mediastinitis

Organisms Frequently Recovered in Mediastinitis Secondary to Infection of the Head and Neck or Esophageal Perforation

Anaerobic
Gram-positive cocci: *Peptostreptococcus* spp.
Gram-positive bacilli: *Actinomyces, Eubacterium, Lactobacillus*
Gram-negative cocci: *Veillonella*
Gram-negative bacilli: *Bacteroides* spp., *Fusobacterium* spp., *Prevotella* spp., *Porphyromonas* spp.

Aerobic or Facultative
Gram-positive cocci: *Streptococcus* spp., *Staphylococcus* spp.
Gram-positive bacilli: *Corynebacterium*
Gram-negative cocci: *Branhamella*
Gram-negative bacilli: Enterobacteriaceae, *Pseudomonas* spp., *Eikenella corrodens*
Fungi: *Candida albicans*

Representative Organisms Recovered in Mediastinitis Secondary to Cardiothoracic Surgery, with Representative Rate (%) and Range
Gram-positive cocci
    Staphylococcus aureus, 25 (7.1-66.7)
    Staphylococcus epidermidis, 30 (6-45.5)
    Enterococcus spp., 10 (8-18.8)
    Streptococcus spp., 2 (0-18.2)
Gram-negative bacilli
    Escherichia coli, 5 (0-12.5)
    Enterobacter spp., 10 (4-21.4)
    Klebsiella spp., 3 (0-21.1)
    Proteus spp., 2 (0-7.1)
    Other Enterobacteriaceae, 2 (0-20)
    Pseudomonas spp., 2 (0-54)
Fungi
    C. albicans, <2 (0-14.3)
Polymicrobial, 10 (0-40)
Others occasionally reported: *Acinetobacter, Salmonella* spp., *Legionella* spp., *Bacteroides fragilis, Corynebacterium* spp., *Mycoplasma hominis, Candida tropicalis, Aspergillus* spp., *Nocardia* spp., *Kluyvera, Gordona sputi, Mycobacterium fortuitum, Mycobacterium chelonei, Rhodococcus bronchialis*

Other Unusual Causes of Mediastinitis
Anthrax, brucellosis, actinomycosis, paragonimiasis, *Streptococcus pneumoniae*

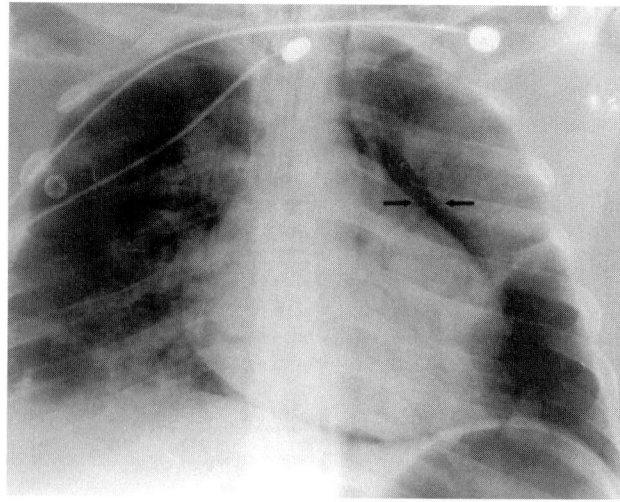

FIGURE 78-2. Chest radiograph demonstrating large pneumomediastinum and pneumopericardium *(arrows)* in a patient with mediastinitis.

barium should be used to detect subtle defects, because it provides a better definition of the anatomy.[130] Computed tomography (CT) is often helpful in cases in which the diagnosis is not evident clinically or on plain films (Fig. 78-3).[131,132] Transesophageal endosonography has been used to guide needle aspiration of the posterior mediastinum, particularly in cases in which the CT scan is inconclusive.[133] Technetium-labeled white blood cell scans have been reported to be helpful in the diagnosis of mediastinitis in specialized circumstances when CT scanning was not readily available.[134] Magnetic resonance imaging is very helpful in mediastinitis caused by esophageal perforation and may show air bubbles in the mediastinum adjacent to an esophageal perforation. Erosion of the anterior face of vertebral bodies from a periesophageal abscess or localized collections of pus may also be seen.

Recently, because of the intentional release of *Bacillus anthracis* via the United States Postal Service, great interest has been demonstrated in recognition, management, and prevention of inhalational anthrax, which typically manifests as hemorrhagic mediastinitis.[135-138] After inhalation, the 1- to 5-μm spores of *B. anthracis* are ingested by macrophages and transported to the mediastinal lymph nodes. Surviving spores travel from the lung to hilar and mediastinal nodes, germinate, propagate, and release toxins that lead to hemorrhage, edema, and necrosis. Approximately 90% of the recent patients with inhalational anthrax exhibited mediastinal adenopathy or widening on radiographic studies.[136,138] The finding of mediastinal adenopathy or widening in a febrile patient should trigger a strong suspicion for inhalational anthrax and institution of appropriate diagnostic and therapeutic measures (see Chapter 324).

Postcardiothoracic surgery mediastinitis usually manifests within the first 2 weeks after surgery.[44-47,53,56-59] However, rare cases have been described occurring up to 416 days postoperatively.[54] Infections caused by gram-negative organisms usually manifest earlier. One study found that all cases of mediastinitis occurring later than 2 weeks after surgery were caused by gram-positive organisms.[54] Usually, *Staphylococcus aureus* mediastinitis is readily diagnosed on clinical grounds, whereas the less virulent coagulase-negative staphylococci often cause more subtle cases that may be initially misdiagnosed as uninfected in up to 30% of cases.[139] El Oakley and Wright[140] proposed a classification system in which patients with postcardiothoracic surgery are divided into seven groups depending on time to presentation, underlying risk factors, and prior therapeutic efforts.

Mediastinitis may manifest fulminantly or subtly. Some patients have fever without localizing signs.[56] Patients may experience greater-than-normal postoperative pain, which may be pleuritic in nature.

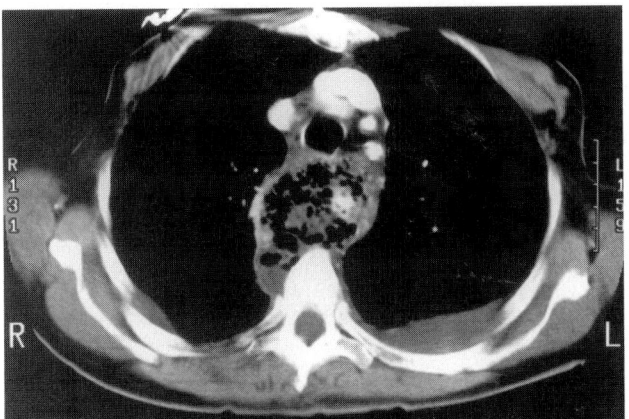

FIGURE 78-3. Computed tomograph of the chest at the level of the sixth thoracic vertebra, demonstrating a large abscess within the posterior mediastinum and a left-sided pleural effusion. The patient had experienced perforation of the esophagus due to a swallowed foreign body. *(From Rupp ME. Mediastinitis. In: Fishman AP, Elias JA, Fishman JA, et al, eds. Fishman's Pulmonary Diseases and Disorders, 3rd ed. New York: McGraw-Hill; 2036-2043.)*

Dysphagia is a rare complaint. Fever and an abnormal appearance of the surgical wound, characterized by erythema, cellulitis, or purulent discharge, are the most common signs of mediastinitis.[35,44-47,54,56,58,59,69,71] Sternal instability, dehiscence, and the observation of bubbles emanating from the sternal wound are less common findings. Occasionally, chest wall emphysema is observed. Poststernotomy mediastinitis manifesting as a deep neck abscess without abnormal findings on chest examination has been reported.[141] Laboratory tests usually show a moderate leukocytosis with a leftward shift on the white blood cell differential. Radiographically, mediastinal widening is a rare finding on plain chest films, and routine radiographs usually are of very little use in the diagnosis of mediastinitis after cardiothoracic surgery.[54,56,132] CT scanning has proved helpful in many cases of postoperative mediastinitis, particularly in differentiating superficial wound infections from deeper retrosternal processes.[131,132,142,143] Characteristic findings include soft tissue swelling, pleural effusion, subcutaneous fluid collection, and sternal erosion.[131,132,142,143] However, normal postoperative collections of fluid and gas are at times difficult to differentiate from early signs of mediastinitis.[131,144,145] Dressler's syndrome can be difficult to distinguish from mediastinitis after cardiac surgery. The diagnostic value of nuclear scans has been espoused by several investigators.[146-148]

Browdie and colleagues[149] studied the relative value of CT, indium 111–labeled leukocyte scanning, and epicardial pacer wire cultures in 24 patients being evaluated for possible mediastinitis. They found that CT had a sensitivity of 67% and a specificity of 71%. The ^{111}In-labeled leukocyte scan was 83% sensitive and 100% specific, and epicardial pacer wire cultures were reported to be 100% sensitive and 92% specific. On the other hand, Robicsek[150] found epicardial pacer wire cultures to be associated with an unacceptably high rate of false-positive findings, and Maroto and associates,[151] in a study of 565 patients, found epicardial wire cultures to be only 75% sensitive and 83.4% specific and to have positive and negative predictive values of 11.6% and 99.1%, respectively. The role of magnetic resonance imaging is not well delineated, and it is contraindicated in instances in which ferromagnetic metals are used in sternal wires, artificial heart valves, cardiac pacemakers, or vascular clips. Several investigators have found mediastinal needle aspiration to be useful in the diagnosis of mediastinitis.[48,49,56,69,152] This method, which has been reported to be successful in up to 100% of patients, appears to be particularly useful in diagnosing mediastinitis before it becomes more clinically obvious and has been associated with improved outcomes compared with diagnosis on the basis of delayed clinical signs.[48,49,152,153]

Treatment

Therapy that includes both medical and surgical techniques should be promptly initiated once the diagnosis of mediastinitis is made. Barrett[154] is credited with documenting the first successful treatment of mediastinitis caused by esophageal perforation. Since then, most authorities have recommended aggressive surgical drainage, débridement, and repair in cases of mediastinitis secondary to esophageal perforation.[7-9,12,128,155-157] However, based on experience with eight patients, Cameron and colleagues[158] identified a subset of mediastinitis that could be treated without surgical intervention: patients in this group have a well-contained disruption of the esophagus; the abscess drains back into the esophagus; minimal symptoms are present; and there is minimal evidence of clinical toxicity. Shaffer and coworkers[159] expanded on these recommendations based on the recognition of patients with esophageal perforation due to instrumentation before major mediastinal contamination occurred. Santos and Frator[160] recommended transesophageal irrigation for patients in whom primary repair of the esophagus is not possible because of advanced local infection with extensive tissue necrosis. CT-guided aspiration for culture is important for patients who do not undergo surgery, because the flora can be quite diverse.

Like cases of mediastinitis caused by esophageal perforation, cases secondary to descending odontogenic or pharyngeal infection require prompt surgical intervention. Several authors have warned that a transthoracic approach is necessary and that transcervical drainage is often inadequate.[18,19] Roberts and associates[161] reported the successful management of descending necrotizing mediastinitis by thoracoscopic drainage.

Although the importance of supportive therapy and surgical intervention cannot be overemphasized, the administration of appropriate antibiotics is an essential component of therapy. Empirical regimens are based on the underlying cause and should cover the major pathogens listed in Box 78-2. Penicillin G has traditionally been the antibiotic of choice in the treatment of anaerobic infections arising above the diaphragm and continues to exhibit excellent activity against most oral anaerobic bacteria. However, oral anaerobes such as *Prevotella* and *Porphyromonas* spp. (formerly *Bacteroides* spp.) are often resistant to penicillin G. If infection with those organisms is suspected, treatment with drugs that have activity against penicillin-resistant anaerobes as well as other oropharyngeal anaerobes, such as metronidazole, clindamycin, broad-spectrum β-lactam/β-lactamase combinations, imipenem, or meropenem, may be indicated.[120] In addition, gram-negative enteric bacilli are often implicated in mediastinitis and should be covered in initial empirical therapy. Antibiotic therapy should be more specifically tailored to the infecting organisms after definitive culture results are available, but therapy directed against anaerobic oropharyngeal organisms should probably be continued because of the difficulty in obtaining reliable anaerobic cultures.[120] The duration of therapy, which may range from weeks to months, is determined by the virulence of the bacteria, host factors, and the response to therapy.

The treatment of mediastinitis secondary to cardiac surgery requires aggressive surgical drainage and débridement. A small number of cases have been successfully treated by percutaneous catheter drainage.[162] Two approaches have been used in the surgical management of mediastinitis after cardiac surgery: an open technique and a closed technique. The open technique involves débridement of infected tissue and open packing of the wound with delayed closure.[34,48,49,56,68,71,163] Disadvantages of this technique include respiratory insufficiency resulting from a lack of mechanical support for the thorax, delayed healing and closure of the surgical wound, and hemorrhage from exposed vessels.[38,56,69,71] The closed method involves débridement of affected tissues, closure of the sternum, and postoperative irrigation through drainage tubes within the mediastinum.[34,48,49,56,68,71,163,164] Recently, vacuum-assisted closure therapy has been used successfully as a primary closure technique or to bridge between débridement and definitive flap closure.[165,166]

Irrigants have included a variety of antimicrobial and antiseptic solutions, such as an iodophor or Dakin's solution. They have been associated with a variety of complications, including the emergence of resistant organisms, pericardial and tissue toxicity, and systemic absorption and toxicity.[70,167-169] The most commonly employed irrigant is povidone-iodine. The use of povidone-iodine has been associated with iodine toxicity, renal failure, metabolic acidosis, and seizures.[170-172] Therefore, this agent must be used with caution, and it has been recommended that the serum iodide concentration be measured to ensure that toxic levels are not reached.[170-172] In cases of iodine toxicity and renal failure, iodine can be effectively cleared by hemodialysis.[173] A closed technique, employing Redon drainage devices, has been successfully used.[174,175] A number of investigators have reported the use of pectoralis muscle flaps and omental grafts, often at the time of initial débridement, to close mediastinal wounds with or without postoperative irrigation.[48,71,76,163,164,176-182]

The use of parenteral antibiotics has remained a cornerstone of therapy, although they are not sufficient alone. Empirical therapy should be directed at staphylococci and gram-negative aerobic bacilli until definitive culture results are available. As with mediastinitis secondary to infection of the head and neck, the duration of therapy is determined by a number of factors and can be prolonged. Treatment failure is more common in patients with mediastinitis caused by methicillin-resistant staphylococci than in those with infections caused by susceptible strains of *S. aureus*.[183] Also, there is some interest in the adjunctive use of intravenous immunoglobulin in the treatment of mediastinitis, but data from prospective, randomized trials are lacking.[184] In several cases of mediastinitis recalcitrant to more traditional therapy, packing of the wound with granulated sugar or honey has been used successfully to eradicate infection.[185-189] De Feo and colleagues[189] found in a group of 25 patients with recurrent staphylococcal mediastinitis that treatment with a granulated sugar dressing was significantly more effective than a traditional surgical regimen. It appears that the sugar lowers the water content of the tissue substrate to a level at which bacterial growth is inhibited.[186]

Antibiotic Prophylaxis

Although cardiothoracic surgical procedures are classified as clean procedures and the risk of infection is low, the consequences of infection can be devastating. Therefore, despite the lack of placebo-controlled studies documenting its efficacy in most cardiac procedures, antibiotic prophylaxis has become commonplace (see Chapter 316). A meta-analysis of seven randomized, placebo-controlled studies of antimicrobial prophylaxis for pacemaker placement showed a statistically significant reduction in the incidence of wound infection.[190] Cefazolin and cefuroxime have generally been regarded as the drugs of choice for prophylaxis.[191] In a comparison among vancomycin, cefazolin, and cefamandole, Maki and associates[192] demonstrated a significant reduction in postoperative wound infection in patients receiving vancomycin prophylaxis. Vancomycin should be considered for prophylaxis in medical centers in which there is a high prevalence of infections due to methicillin-resistant staphylococci. However, the use of vancomycin for surgical prophylaxis must be tempered by the risk of development of vancomycin resistance in enterococci and staphylococci.

Complications and Prognosis

Complications of mediastinitis include extension of the infection into a number of contiguous structures and spaces, including the pericardial space, resulting in pericardial effusion and tamponade; the pleural space; costochondral cartilages; and the peritoneum, resulting in peritonitis.[14,18] A major complication of mediastinitis after cardiac surgery is sternal osteomyelitis. Before the development of modern surgery and antibiotics, mediastinitis, caused primarily by esophageal perforation, was regarded as uniformly fatal. Since the time of Barrett's first successful surgical repair of the esophagus in 1946,[88] morbidity and mortality have remained high, with many studies recording mortality rates of 30% to 50%.[9,18,22,34,46,54] However, more recent studies have reported mortality rates of less than 10% to 15%.[39,44,45,140,163,164] In examining the economic ramifications of mediastinitis, Loop and coworkers[34] found that the hospital charges of patients undergoing coronary artery bypass surgery who experienced mediastinitis were 280% greater than those of patients with uncomplicated bypass surgery, and the median length of stay ranged from 38 to 51 days. Mossad and associates[47] found that patients with deep sternal wound infections caused by coagulase-negative staphylococci required an excess hospital stay of 21.5 days, at a cost of $20,000 per patient, compared with patients without infection. The most important factor in determining outcome has been the length of time to diagnosis and initiation of definitive therapy.[9,22,30,48,49,128] Other prognostic indicators have included the blood urea nitrogen level, white blood cell count, culture positivity, type of surgical repair, and cytomegalovirus shedding.[48,193,194]

SCLEROSING MEDIASTINITIS

The terms *sclerosing, fibrosing,* or *granulomatous mediastinitis* refer to a chronic form of mediastinitis characterized by an invasive and compressive inflammatory infiltrate. The first report of this entity, which can cause up 10% of all primary mediastinal masses,[195] was a description by Ulmont in 1855.[196] Although the causes of up to 83% of cases of sclerosing mediastinitis remain obscure,[195] many authorities believe that most cases are secondary to infection with *H. capsulatum*.[197-201]

Gryboski and associates[199] and Peabody and coworkers[200] found that up to 73% of cases previously characterized as nonspecific granulomatous mediastinitis could be reclassified as secondary to *H. capsulatum* infection by restaining of the tissue with fungal stains and a thorough review of the pathologic sections. Other reported infectious causes of this condition include tuberculosis[202,203] and, rarely, actinomycosis,[204,205] nocardiosis,[206] blastomycosis,[207] coccidioidomycosis,[208] aspergillosis,[208] *Rhizopus* spp. infection,[209] and *Wucheria bancrofti* infection.[210] Other conditions that closely mimic this entity include sarcoidosis,[195,211] silicosis,[195] lymphoma,[211] mesothelioma,[212] and mediastinal fibrosis associated with idiopathic retroperitoneal fibrosis, Riedel's struma, or sclerosing cholangitis.

Approximately 40% of patients with sclerosing mediastinitis are asymptomatic and come to medical attention when a chest roentgenogram incidentally reveals a mediastinal mass.[198] Symptomatic patients usually note symptoms related to invasion or obstruction of structures within or adjacent to the mediastinum (Box 78-3). Sclerosing mediastinitis is the most common nonmalignant cause of superior vena cava syndrome, responsible for up to 23% of cases.[213] These patients typically present with plethora and edema of the face, neck, and upper torso; neck vein distention; headache; and visual disturbances. Patients presenting with obstruction of the pulmonary arteries often note cough, dyspnea, and symptoms consistent with right-sided heart failure. Pulmonary infarction, although rare, has been reported to occur in patients with fibrosing mediastinitis.[214] Pulmonary venous obstruction causes patients to experience exertional dyspnea, easy fatigability, and sometimes hemoptysis. Patients with bronchial obstruction caused by sclerosing mediastinitis usually present with dry cough and recurrent episodes of bacterial bronchitis or pneumonia. Patients complaining of dysphagia may have esophageal obstruction due to posterior extension of the mediastinitis.

Radiographically, patients with fibrosing mediastinitis are often observed to have a mediastinal mass, most frequently located in the superior mediastinum at the level of the bifurcation of the trachea. Kerley B lines may be present.[215] CT sometimes reveals calcification in lymph nodes. Magnetic resonance angiography or pulmonary arteriography is helpful in the assessment of the vascular integrity.[216] Ventilation-perfusion lung scans often reveal large perfusion deficits caused by obstruction of the pulmonary vessels.

The diagnosis of fibrosing mediastinitis is often not confirmed by biopsy because of the hazard of uncontrolled venous bleeding or accidental ligation of collateral veins. There is a continuum of disease ranging from a predominantly granulomatous entity to an almost completely fibrosing process. Lesions described include caseating granuloma, dense hyalinized collagenous tissue, and infiltrations of lymphocytes, plasma cells, and giant cells. Specific stains for fungi often reveal organisms consistent with *Histoplasma*, if several areas with caseous necrosis are included in the section, but cultures are usually negative.[195,207]

The pathologic features of this disease suggest a marked inflammatory reaction. Several different mechanisms have been proposed to explain the pathology of fibrosing mediastinitis. Some investigators believe that a caseous lymph node from primary infection with *Histoplasma* ruptures into the mediastinum, invoking an intense inflammatory reaction.[195,207] However, the yeast is rarely found outside of a caseous lymph node. A second hypothesis is the development of a delayed hypersensitivity reaction caused by the spread of soluble *Histoplasma* antigens into the mediastinum.[217] An alternative explanation proposes that fibrosing mediastinitis represents an abnormality of collagen production and organization similar to that of idiopathic retroperitoneal fibrosis or Riedel's struma.[217] Noguchi and coworkers[218] incriminated the eosinophil in the pathogenesis of fibrosing mediastinitis by demonstrating eosinophils or major basic protein in tissue specimens from five of seven patients with this condition.

No controlled trials of medical or surgical therapy in the treatment of fibrosing mediastinitis have been conducted. Although there is some anecdotal evidence of a beneficial effect of antifungal agents,[219] most authorities believe that at the time of presentation there is little evidence of an active infection and antifungal agents are not indicated.[197,207,215] Because the natural history of this disease is variable, with some patients progressing to compression of vital structures and others seeming to have self-limited disease,[207] it is difficult to make recommendations regarding the timing or utility of surgical intervention. It has been suggested that early surgical intervention and removal of granulomatous tissue may prevent the development of subsequent end-stage fibrosis and involvement of vital structures.[220] Clearly, patients experiencing obstruction or invasion of mediastinal structures may require surgical exploration. Such surgery is hazardous and requires an experienced surgeon who is familiar with the disease.[207] Therapy with corticosteroids does not appear to have a role in the treatment of fibrosing mediastinitis.[221]

REFERENCES

1. Pearse HE Jr. Mediastinitis following cervical suppuration. Ann Surg. 1938;108: 588-611.
2. Neuhof H, Jemerin EE. Acute Infections of the Mediastinum. Baltimore: Williams & Wilkins; 1943.
3. De Marie S, Tjon A, Tham RTO, et al. Clinical infections and nonsurgical treatment of parapharyngeal infections complicating throat infection. Rev Infect Dis. 1989;11:975-982.
4. Chow AW. Life-threatening infections of the head and neck. Clin Infect Dis. 1992;14:991-1004.
5. Silvis SE, Nebel O, Rogers G, et al. Endoscopic complications: Results of the 1974 American gastrointestinal endoscopy survey. JAMA. 1976;235:928-930.
6. Michael L, Grillo HC, Malt RA. Esophageal perforation. Ann Thorac Surg. 1982;33:203-210.
7. Goldstein LA, Thompson WR. Esophageal perforations: A 15 year experience. Am J Surg. 1982;143:495-503.
8. Sarr MG, Pemberton JH, Payne WS. Management of instrumental perforations of the esophagus. J Thorac Cardiovasc Surg. 1982;84:211-218.
9. Moghissi K, Pender D. Instrumental perforations of the oesophagus and their management. Thorax. 1988;43:642-646.
10. Edling JE, Bacon BR. Pleuropulmonary complications of endoscopic variceal sclerotherapy. Chest. 1991;99:1252-1257.
11. Baydur A, Korula J. Cardiorespiratory effects of endoscopic esophageal variceal sclerotherapy. Am J Med. 1990;89:477-482.
12. Wychulis AR, Fontana RS, Payne WS. Noninstrumental perforations of the esophagus. Dis Chest. 1969;55:190-196.
13. Miller RH, Duplechain JK. Penetrating wounds of the neck. Otolaryngol Clin North Am. 1991;24:15-29.
14. Payne WS, Larson RH. Acute mediastinitis. Surg Clin North Am. 1969;49:999-1009.
15. Bennett DJ, Deveridge RJ, Wright JS. Spontaneous rupture of the esophagus: A review with reports of six cases. Surgery. 1970;68:766-770.
16. Derbes VJ, Mitchell RE Jr. Rupture of the esophagus. Surgery. 1956;39:688-709, 865-888.
17. Kimose HH, Lund O, Hasenkam JM, et al. Independent predictors of operative mortality and postoperative complications in surgically treated carcinomas of the oesophagus and cardia: Is the aggressive surgical approach worthwhile? Acta Chir Scand. 1990;156:373-382.
18. Estrera AS, Landay MJ, Grishom JM, et al. Descending necrotizing mediastinitis. Surg Gynecol Obstet. 1983;157:545-552.
19. Levine TM, Wurster CF, Krespi YP. Mediastinitis occurring as a complication of odontogenic infections. Laryngoscope. 1986;96:747-750.

BOX 78-3

Complications and Manifestations of Sclerosing Mediastinitis

Pulmonary venous or arterial obstruction
Superior vena cava obstruction
Inferior vena cava obstruction
Esophageal obstruction
Esophagobronchial obstruction
Tracheobronchial obstruction
Pulmonary venous or arterial obstruction
Pulmonary hypertension
Pulmonary infarction
Cor pulmonale
Thoracic duct obstruction
Constructive pericarditis
Coronary artery stenosis
Mediastinal nerve entrapment
Recurrent laryngeal nerve palsy

20. Moncada R, Warpeha R, Pickleman J, et al. Mediastinitis from odontogenic and deep cervical infection. Chest. 1978;73:497-500.
21. Rubin MM, Cozzi GM. Fatal necrotizing mediastinitis as a complication of an odontogenic infection. J Oral Maxillofac Surg. 1987;45:529-533.
22. Wheatley MJ, Stirling MC, Kirsh MM, et al. Descending necrotizing mediastinitis: Transcervical drainage is not enough. Ann Thorac Surg. 1990;49:780-484.
23. Moreland LW, Corey J, McKenzie R. Ludwig's angina: Report of a case and review of the literature. Arch Intern Med. 1988;148:461-466.
24. Van der Brempt X, Derue G, Severin F, et al. Ludwig's angina and mediastinitis due to *Streptococcus milleri*: Usefulness of computed tomography. Eur Respir J. 1990;3:728-731.
25. Baker AR, Moir AA, Donnelly PK. Life-threatening peripharyngeal sepsis with mediastinitis. Br J Clin Pract. 1990;44:640-641.
26. Zaltman C, Kallenbach J, Hockman M, et al. Fatal intrathoracic sepsis associated with neck space infection. Thorax. 1983;38:143-145.
27. Guardia SN, Cameron R, Phillips A. Fatal necrotizing mediastinitis secondary to acute suppurative parotitis. J Otolaryngol. 1991;20:54-56.
28. Chong WH, Woodhead MA, Millard FJC. Mediastinitis and bilateral thoracic empyemas complicating adult epiglottitis. Thorax. 1990;45:491-492.
29. Pane GA, Hamilton GC, Call E. Nontraumatic suppurative mediastinitis presenting as acute mediastinal widening. Ann Emerg Med. 1983;12:777-779.
30. Freidman BC, Pickul DC. Acute mediastinitis: What to do when the cause is nonsurgical. Postgrad Med. 1990;87:273-285.
31. Hardy CC, Raza SN, Isalska B, Barber PV. Atraumatic suppurative mediastinitis and purulent pericarditis due to *Eikenella corrodens*. Thorax. 1988;43:494-495.
32. Antreasian B. Mediastinal abscess: Two case reports. Indiana Med. 1988;81:528-532.
33. Smith A, Sinzobahamvya N. Anterior mediastinal abscess complicating septic arthritis. J Pediatr Surg. 1992;27:101-102.
34. Loop FD, Lytle BW, Cosgrove DM, et al. Sternal wound complications after isolated coronary artery bypass grafting: Early and late mortality, morbidity, and cost of care. Ann Thorac Surg. 1990;49:179-187.
35. Grossi EA, Esposito R, Harris LJ, et al. Sternal wound infections and use of internal mammary artery grafts. J Thorac Cardiovasc Surg. 1991;102:342-347.
36. Sethi GK, Copeland JG, Moritz T, et al. Comparison of postoperative complications between saphenous vein and IMA grafts to left anterior descending coronary artery. Ann Thorac Surg. 1991;51:733-738.
37. Sutherland RD, Martinez HE, Guynes WA, Miller L. Postoperative chest wound infections in patients requiring coronary bypass. J Thorac Cardiovasc Surg. 1977;73:944-947.
38. Grover FL, Johnson RR, Marshall G, Hammermeister KE. Impact of mammary grafts on coronary bypass operative mortality and morbidity. Ann Thorac Surg. 1994;57:559-569.
39. El Oakley R, Paul E, Wong PS, et al. Mediastinitis in patients undergoing cardiopulmonary bypass: Risk analysis and midterm results. J Cardiovasc Surg. 1997;38:595-600.
40. Milano CA, Kesler K, Archibald N, et al. Mediastinitis after coronary artery bypass graft surgery. Circulation. 1995;92:2245-2251.
41. Braxton JH, Marrin CAS, McGrath PD, et al. Mediastinitis and long-term survival after coronary artery bypass graft surgery. Ann Thorac Surg. 2000;70:2004-2007.
42. Gummert JF, Barten MJ, Hans C, et al. Mediastinitis and cardiac surgery: An updated risk factor analysis in 10,373 consecutive patients. Thorac Cardiovasc Surg. 2002;50:87-91.
43. Hernandez F, Cohn WE, Baribeau YR, et al. In-hospital outcomes of off-pump versus on-pump coronary artery bypass procedures: a multicenter experience. Ann Thorac Surg. 2001;72:1528-1534.
44. Munuz P, Menasalvas A, Bernaldo de Quiros JCL, et al. Postsurgical mediastinitis: A case-control study. Clin Infect Dis. 1997;25:1060-1064.
45. Bitkover CY, Garlund B. Mediastinitis after cardiovascular operations: A case-control study of risk factors. Ann Thorac Surg. 1998;65:36-40.
46. Farinas MC, Paralta FG, Bernal JM, et al. Suppurative mediastinitis after open-heart surgery: A case-control study covering a seven-year period in Santander, Spain. Clin Infect Dis. 1995;20:272-279.
47. Mossad SB, Serkey JM, Longworth DL, et al. Coagulase-negative staphylococcal sternal wound infections after open heart operations. Ann Thorac Surg. 1997;63:395-401.
48. Grossi EU, Culliford AT, Kriegu KH, et al. A survey of 77 major infectious complications of median sternotomy: A review of 7949 consecutive operative procedures. Ann Thorac Surg. 1985;40:214-223.
49. Culliford AT, Cunningham JN, Zeff RH, et al. Sternal and costochondral infections following open-heart surgery. J Thorac Cardiovasc Surg. 1976;72:714-726.
50. Hammermeister KE, Burchfiel C, Johnson R, Grover FL. Identification of patients at greatest risk for developing major complications at cardiac surgery. Circulation. 1990;82(Suppl 4):380-389.
51. Ottino G, De Paulis R, Pansini S, et al. Major sternal wound infection after open-heart surgery: A multivariate analysis of risk factors in 2579 consecutive operative procedures. Ann Thorac Surg 1987;44:173-179.
52. Newman LS, Szczukowski LC, Bain RP, Perlino CA. Suppurative mediastinitis after open heart surgery. Chest. 1988;94:546-553.
53. Nagachinta T, Stephens M, Reitz B, Polk BF. Risk factors for surgical-wound infection following cardiac surgery. J Infect Dis. 1987;156:967-973.
54. Bor DH, Rose RM, Modlin JF, et al. Mediastinitis after cardiovascular surgery. Rev Infect Dis. 1983;5:885-897.
55. Engleman RM, Williams CD, Gouge TH, et al. Mediastinitis following open-heart surgery. Arch Surg. 1973;107:772-778.
56. Sarr MG, Gott VL, Townsend TR. Mediastinal infection after cardiac surgery. Ann Thorac Surg. 1984;38:415-423.
57. Verkkala K, Jarvinen A. Mediastinal infection following open-heart surgery. Scand J Thor Cardiovasc Surg. 1986;20:203-207.
58. Kutsal A, Ibrisim E, Catav Z, et al. Mediastinitis after open heart surgery. J Cardiovasc Surg. 1991;32:38-41.
59. Farrington M, Webster M, Fenn A, Phillips I. Study of cardiothoracic wound infection at St. Thomas's hospital. Br J Surg. 1985;72:759-762.
60. Miholic J, Hudec M, Domanig E, et al. Risk factors for severe bacterial infections after valve replacement and aortocoronary bypass operations: Analysis of 246 cases by logistic regression. Ann Thorac Surg. 1985;40:224-228.
61. Serry C, Bleck PC, Javid H, et al. Sternal wound complications. J Thorac Cardiovasc Surg. 1980;80:861-867.
62. Sanfelippo PM, Danielson GK. Complications associated with median sternotomy. J Thorac Cardiovasc Surg. 1972;63:419-423.
63. Kouchoukos NT, Wareing TH, Murphy SF, et al. Risks of bilateral internal mammary artery bypass grafting. Ann Thorac Surg. 1990;49:210-219.
64. Nishida H, Grooters RK, Soltanzadeh H, et al. Discriminate use of electrocautery on the median sternotomy incision. J Thorac Cardiovasc Surg. 1991;101:488-494.
65. Doebbeling BN, Pfaller MA, Kuhns KR, et al. Cardiovascular surgery prophylaxis. J Thorac Cardiovasc Surg. 1990;99:981-989.
66. Ko W, Lazenby D, Zelano JA, et al. Effects of shaving methods and intraoperative irrigation on suppurative mediastinitis after bypass operations. Ann Thorac Surg. 1992;53:301-305.
67. Ferrazzi P, Allen R, Crupi G, et al. Reduction of infection after cardiac surgery. Ann Thorac Surg. 1986;42:321-325.
68. Cheung EH, Craver JM, Jones EL, et al. Mediastinitis after cardiac valve operations. J Thorac Cardiovasc Surg. 1985;90:517-522.
69. Jimenez-Martinez M, Arguero-Sanchez R, Perez-Alvarez JJ, Mina-Casteneda P. Anterior mediastinitis as a complication of median sternotomy incisions. Surgery. 1970;67:929-934.
70. Thurur RJ, Bognolo D, Vargas A, et al. The management of mediastinal infection following cardiac surgery. J Thorac Cardiovasc Surg. 1974;68:962-968.
71. Grmoljez PF, Barner HK, Willman VL, Kaiser GC. Major complications of median sternotomy. Am J Surg. 1975;130:679-681.
72. Firor WB. Infection following open-heart surgery, with special reference to the role of prophylactic antibiotics. J Thorac Cardiovasc Surg. 1967;53:371-378.
73. Brown AH, Baimbridge MV, Panagopoulos P, Sabar EF. The complications of median sternotomy. J Thorac Cardiovasc Surg. 1969;58:189-197.
74. Ochsner JL, Mills NL, Woolverton WC. Disruption and infection of the median sternotomy incision. J Cardiovasc Surg. 1972;13:394-399.
75. Rutledge R, Applbaum RE, Kim BJ. Mediastinal infection after open heart surgery. Surgery. 1985;97:88-92.
76. Stiegel RM, Beasley ME, Sink JD, et al. Management of postoperative mediastinitis in infants and children by muscle flap rotation. Ann Thorac Surg. 1988;46:45-46.
77. Miller R, Rudler J, Karwande SV, Burton NA. Treatment of mediastinitis after heart transplantation. J Heart Transplant. 1986;5:477-479.
78. Trento A, Dummer GS, Hardesty RL, et al. Mediastinitis following heart transplantation: Incidence, treatment, results. J Heart Transplant. 1984;3:336-340.
79. Baldwin RT, Radovancevic B, Sweeny MS, et al. Bacterial mediastinitis after heart transplantation. J Heart Lung Transplant. 1992;11:545-549.
80. Griffith BP, Kormos RK, Hardesty RL, et al. The artificial heart: Infection-related morbidity and its effect on transplantation. Ann Thorac Surg. 1988;45:409-414.
81. Pennington DG, McBride LR, Kanter KR, et al. Bridging to heart transplantation with circulatory support devices. J Heart Transplant. 1989;8:116-123.
82. Rooks JR, Burton NA, Lefrak EA, Macmanus Q. Mediastinitis complicating successful mechanical bridge to heart transplantation. J Heart Lung Transplant. 1992;11:261-264.
83. Phillips WS, Burton NA, Macmanus Q, Lefrak EA. Surgical complications in bridging to transplantation: The thermo-cardiosystems LVAD. Ann Thorac Surg. 1992;53:482-486.
84. Abid Q, Nkere UU, Hasan A, et al. Mediastinitis in heart and lung transplantation: 15 years experience. Ann Thorac Surg. 2003;75:1565-1571.
85. Didsheim P, Olsen DB, Farrar DJ, et al. Infections and thromboembolism with implantable cardiovascular devices. Trans Am Soc Artif Intern Organs. 1989;35:54-70.
86. Hazelrigg SR, Auer JE, Seifert PE. Experience in 100 transthoracic balloon pumps. Ann Thorac Surg. 1992;54:528-532.
87. Boerhaave H. Artocis, nec descripti prius Morbi Historia. Secundem Artis Leges Conscripta. Lugdunis Batavorum Bouresteniana; 1724.
88. Barrett NR. Spontaneous perforation of the oesophagus. Thorax. 1946;1:48-70.
89. Maier A, Pinter H, Anegg U, et al. Boerhaave's syndrome: A continuing challenge in thoracic surgery. Hepatogastroenterology. 2001;48:1368-1371.
90. Katz R. Morbidity and mortality in standard and flexible gastrointestinal endoscopy. Gastrointest Endosc. 1969;15:134-141.
91. Keefer CS. Acute and chronic mediastinitis. Arch Intern Med. 1938;62:109-136.
92. DeSilva MI, Rissing JP. Postoperative wound infections following cardiac surgery: Significance of contaminated cases performed in the preceding 48 hours. Infect Control. 1984;5:371-377.
93. Dandalides PC, Rutala WA, Sarubbi FA Jr. Postoperative infections following cardiac surgery: Association with an environmental reservoir in a cardiothoracic intensive care unit. Infect Control. 1984;5:378-384.
94. Palmer DL, Kuritsky JN, Lapham SC, et al. *Enterobacter* mediastinitis following cardiac surgery. Infect Control. 1985;6:115-119.
95. Ehrenkranz NJ, Pfaff SJ. Mediastinitis complicating cardiac operations: Evidence of postoperative causation. Rev Infect Dis. 1991;13:803-814.

96. Boyce JM, Bynoe GP, Opal SM, et al. A common-source outbreak of *Staphylococcus epidermidis* infections among patients undergoing cardiac surgery. J Infect Dis. 1990;161:493-499.

97. Samuel R, Axelrod P, St John K, et al. An outbreak of mediastinitis among heart transplant recipients apparently related to a change in the United Network for Organ Sharing guidelines. Infect Control Hosp Epidemiol. 2002;23:377-381.

98. Burket JS, Chenoweth CE, Meyer TL, Barg NL. Donor-to recipient transmission of bacteria as an unusual cause of mediastinitis. Infect Control Hosp Epidemiol. 1999;20:132-133.

99. Guvener M, Pasaoglu I, Demircin M, Oc M. Perioperative hyperglycemia is a strong correlate of postoperative infection in type II diabetic patients after coronary artery bypass grafting. Endocr J. 2002;49:531-537.

100. Nelson DR, Buxton TB, Luu QN, Rissing JP. The promotional effect of bone wax on experimental *Staphylococcus aureus* osteomyelitis. J Thorac Cardiovasc Surg. 1990; 99:977-980.

101. Chughtai T, Chen LQ, Salasidis G, et al. Clips versus suture technique: Is there a difference? Can J Cardiol. 2000;16:1403-1407.

102. Arnold M. The surgical anatomy of sternal blood supply. J Thorac Cardiovasc Surg. 1972;64:596-610.

103. Lust RM, Sun YS, Chitwood WR Jr. Internal mammary artery use: Sternal revascularization and experimental infection patterns. Circulation. 1991;84(Suppl 3):285-289.

104. Kay EB, Naraghipour H, Beg RA, et al. Internal mammary artery bypass graft: Long-term patency rate and follow-up. Ann Thorac Surg. 1974;18:269-279.

105. Green GE. Internal mammary artery to coronary artery anastomosis: Three-year experience with 165 patients. Ann Thorac Surg. 1972;14:260-265.

106. Tector AJ, Davis L, Gabiel R, et al. Experience with internal artery grafts in 298 patients. Ann Thorac Surg. 1976;22:515-519.

107. Danzer D, Christenson JT, Kalangos A, et al. Impact of double internal thoracic artery grafts on long-term outcomes in coronary artery bypass grafting. Tex Heart Inst J. 2001;28:89-95.

108. Walkes JC, Earle N, Reardon MJ, et al. Outcomes in single versus bilateral internal thoracic artery grafting in coronary artery bypass surgery. Curr Opin Cardiol. 2002;17:598-601.

109. Gaynes R, Marosok R, Hanley JM, et al. Mediastinitis following coronary artery bypass surgery: A 3-year review. J Infect Dis. 1991;163:117-121.

110. Archer GL, Armstrong BC. Alteration of staphylococcal flora in cardiac surgery patients receiving antibiotic prophylaxis. J Infect Dis. 1983;147:642-649.

111. Chenoweth DE, Cooper SW, Hugli TE, et al. Complement activation during cardiopulmonary bypass. N Engl J Med. 1981;304:497-503.

112. Kirklin JK, Westaby S, Blackstone EH, et al. Complement and the damaging effects of cardiopulmonary bypass. J Thorac Cardiovasc Surg. 1983;86:845-857.

113. Weinstein RA, Jones EL, Schwarzmann SW, Hatcher CR Jr. Sternal osteomyelitis and mediastinitis after open-heart operation: Pathogenesis and prevention. Ann Thorac Surg. 1976;21:442-444.

114. Rosendorf LL, Daicoff G, Baer H. Sources of gram-negative infection after open heart surgery. J Thorac Cardiovasc Surg. 1974;67:195-201.

115. Andersen BM, Sorlie D, Hotvedt R, et al. Multiply beta-lactam resistant *Enterobacter cloacae* infections linked to the environmental flora in a unit for cardiothoracic and vascular surgery. Scand J Infect Dis. 1989;21:181-191.

116. Kaiser AB. Risk factors for infection in cardiac surgery: Will the real culprit please stand up? Infect Control. 1984;5:369-370.

117. Glower DD, Douglas JM, Gaynor JW, et al. *Candida* mediastinitis after a cardiac operation. Ann Thorac Surg. 1990;49:157-163.

118. Clancy CJ, Nguyen MH, Morris AJ. Candidal mediastinitis: An emerging clinical entity. Clin Infect Dis. 1997;25:608-613.

119. Malani PN, McNeil SA, Bradley SF, Kauffman CA. *Candida albicans* sternal wound infections: A chronic and recurrent complication of median sternotomy. Clin Infect Dis. 2002;35:1316-1320.

120. Murray M, Finegold SM. Anaerobic mediastinitis. Rev Infect Dis. 1984;6:S123-S127.

121. Howell HS, Prinz RA, Pickleman JR. Anaerobic mediastinitis. Surg Gynecol Obstet. 1976;143:353-359.

122. Hamman L. Spontaneous mediastinal emphysema. Bull Johns Hopkins Hosp. 1939;64:1-21.

123. Aragon SB, Dolwick F, Buckley S. Pneumomediastinum and subcutaneous cervical emphysema during third molar extraction under general anesthesia. J Oral Maxillofac Surg. 1986;44:141-144.

124. Feldman R, Gromisch DS. Acute suppurative mediastinitis. Am J Dis Child. 1971; 121:79-81.

125. Meade RH. Laryngeal obstruction in children. Pediatr Clin North Am. 1962; 9:233-262.

126. Rossiter JL, Hendrix RA. Iatrogenic subcutaneous cervicofacial and mediastinal emphysema. J Otolaryngol. 1991;20:315-319.

127. Kirshner JA. Cervical mediastinal emphysema. Arch Otolaryngol. 1980;106:368-375.

128. Burnett CM, Rosemurgy AS, Pfeiffer EA. Life-threatening acute posterior mediastinitis due to esophageal perforation. Ann Thorac Surg. 1990;49:979-983.

129. Berry BE, Ochsner JL. Perforation of the esophagus: A 30 year review. J Thorac Cardiovasc Surg. 1973;65:1-7.

130. Vessal K, Mantali RJ, Larson SM, et al. Evaluation of barium and Gastrografin as contrast media for the diagnosis of esophageal ruptures or perforations. AJR Am J Roentgenol. 1975;123:307-319.

131. Carrol CL, Jeffrey B Jr, Federle MP, Vernacchia FS. CT evaluation of mediastinal infections. J Comput Assist Tomogr. 1987;11:449-454.

132. Breatnach E, Nath PH, Delany DJ. The role of computed tomography in acute and subacute mediastinitis. Clin Radiol. 1986;37:139-145.

133. Fritscher-Ravens A, Schirrow L, Pothmann W, et al. Critical care transesophageal endosonography and guided fine-needle aspiration for diagnosis and management of posterior mediastinitis. Crit Care Med. 2003;31:126-132.

134. Kao CH, Wang SJ. Spread of infectious complications of odontogenic abscess detected by technetium-99m-HMPAO-labeled WBC scan of occult sepsis in the intensive care unit. J Nucl Med. 1992;33:254-255.

135. Swartz MN. Recognition and management of anthrax: An update. N Engl J Med. 2001;345:1621-1626.

136. Jernigan JA, Stephens DS, Ashford DA, et al. Bioterrorism-related inhalational anthrax: The first 10 cases reported in the United States. Emerg Infect Dis. 2001;7:933-944.

137. Mina B, Dym JP, Kuepper F, et al. Fatal inhalational anthrax with unknown source of exposure in a 61-year-old woman in New York City. JAMA. 2002;287:858-862.

138. Inglesby TV, O'Toole T, Henderson DA, et al. Anthrax as a biological weapon, 2002. JAMA. 2002;287:2236-2252.

139. Tammelin A, Hambraeus A, Stahle E. Mediastinitis after cardiac surgery: Improvement of bacteriological diagnosis by use of multiple tissue samples and strain typing. J Clin Microbiol. 2002;40:2936-2941.

140. El Oakley RM, Wright JE. Postoperative mediastinitis: Classification and management. Ann Thorac Surg. 1996;61:1030-1036.

141. Simpson LC, Peters GE. Poststernotomy infections presenting as deep neck abscess. Arch Otolaryngol Head Neck Surg. 1988;114:909-912.

142. Kay HR, Goodman LR, Teplick SK, Mundth ED. Use of computed tomography to assess mediastinal complications after median sternotomy. Ann Thorac Surg. 1983; 36:706-714.

143. Misawa Y, Fuse K, Hasegwa T. Infectious mediastinitis after cardiac operations: Computed tomographic findings. Ann Thorac Surg. 1998;65:622-624.

144. Yamaguchi H, Yamauchi H, Yamada T, et al. Diagnostic validity of computed tomography for mediastinitis after cardiac surgery. Ann Thorac Cardiovasc Surg. 2001; 7:94-98.

145. Bitkover CY, Cederlund K, Aberg B, Vaage J. Computed tomography of the sternum and mediastinum after median sternotomy. Ann Thorac Surg. 1999;68:858-863.

146. Quirce R, Serano J, Arnal C, et al. Detection of mediastinitis after heart transplantation by gallium-67 scintigraphy. J Nucl Med. 1991;32:860-861.

147. Bahar RH, Shuhaiber HJ, Dayem HMA. The value of gallium-67 scintigraphy in localizing infection following cardiac surgery. Int J Cardiol. 1986;11:125-127.

148. Bitkover CY, Garlund B, Larsson SA, et al. Diagnosing sternal wound infections with 99mTc-labeled monoclonal granulocyte antibody scintigraphy. Ann Thorac Surg. 1996; 62:1412-1417.

149. Browdie DA, Bernstein RW, Agnew R, et al. Diagnosis of poststernotomy infection: Comparison of three means of assessment. Ann Thorac Surg 1991;51:290-292.

150. Robicsek F. Posternotomy infections. Ann Thorac Surg. 1991;52:896-900.

151. Maroto LC, Aguado JM, Carrascal Y, et al. Fulminant mediastinitis due to *Streptococcus pneumoniae* following cardiac surgery; report of a case. Clin Infect Dis. 1996;22:594-595.

152. Sarr MG, Watkins L Jr, Stewart JR. Mediastinal tap as useful method for the early diagnosis of mediastinal infection. Surg Gynecol Obstet. 1984;159:79-82.

153. Benlolo S, Mateo J, Raskine L, et al. Sternal puncture allows an early diagnosis of poststernotomy mediastinitis. J Thorac Cardiovasc Surg. 2003;125:611-617.

154. Barrett NR. Report of a case of spontaneous perforation of the oesophagus successfully treated by operation. Br J Surg. 1947;35:216-218.

155. Finley RJ, Pearson FG, Weisel RD, et al. The management of nonmalignant intrathoracic esophageal perforations. Ann Thorac Surg. 1980;30:575-583.

156. Trastek VF. Esophageal perforation: A reassessment of the criteria for choosing medical or surgical therapy. Arch Intern Med. 1992;152:693.

157. Kiernan PD, Conte JV Jr, Petri R, et al. Thoracic esophageal perforations at a Virginia hospital 1979-1990. Va Med Q. 1992;119:102-104.

158. Cameron JL, Kieffer RF, Hendrix TR, et al. Selective nonoperative management of contained intrathoracic esophageal disruptions. Ann Thorac Surg. 1979;27:404-408.

159. Shaffer HA, Valenzuela G, Mittal RK. Esophageal perforation. Arch Intern Med. 152:757-761.

160. Santos GH, Frater WM. Transesophageal irrigation for the treatment of mediastinitis produced by esophageal rupture. J Thorac Cardiovasc Surg. 1986;91:57-62.

161. Roberts JR, Smythe R, Weber RW, et al. Thoracoscopic management of descending necrotizing mediastinitis. Chest. 1997;112:850-854.

162. Gobien RP, Stanley JH, Gobien BS, et al. Percutaneous catheter aspiration and drainage of suspected mediastinal abscesses. Radiology. 1984;151:69-71.

163. Jones G, Jurkiewicz MJ, Bostwick J, et al. Management of the infected median sternotomy wound with muscle flaps. Ann Surg. 1997;225:766-778.

164. El Gamel A, Yonan NA, Hassan R, et al. Treatment of mediastinitis: Early modified Robicsek closure and pectoralis major advancement flaps. Ann Thorac Surg. 1998; 65:41-47.

165. Song DH, Wu LC, Lohman RF, et al. Vacuum assisted closure for the treatment of sternal wounds: The bridge between debridement and definitive closure. Plast Reconstr Surg. 2003;3:92-97.

166. Luckraz H, Murphy F, Bryant S, et al. Vacuum-assisted closure as a treatment modality for infections after cardiac surgery. J Thorac Cardiovasc Surg. 2003;125:301-305.

167. Gruhl VR. Renal failure, deafness, and brain lesions following irrigation of the mediastinum with neomycin. Ann Thorac Surg. 1971;11:376-379.

168. Kopel ME, Riemersma L, Finlayson DC, et al. Gentamicin solution for mediastinal irrigation: Systemic absorption, bactericidal activity, and toxicity. Ann Thorac Surg. 1989;48:228-231.

169. Kratz JM, Metcalf JS, Sade RM. Pericardial injury by antibacterial irrigants. J Thorac Cardiovasc Surg. 1983;86:785-787.

170. Zec N, Donovan JW, Kincaid RL, Demers LM. Seizures in a patient treated with continuous povidone-iodine mediastinal irrigation. N Engl J Med. 1992;326:1784.

171. Glick PL, Guglielmo BJ, Tranbaugh RF, Turley K. Iodine toxicity in a patient treated by continuous povidone-iodine mediastinal irrigation. Ann Thorac Surg. 1985;39:478-480.

172. Campistol JM, Abad C, Nogue S, Bertran A. Acute renal failure in a patient treated by continuous povidone-iodine mediastinal irrigation. J Cardiovasc Surg. 1988;29:410-412.

173. Kanakiriya S, DeChazal I, Nath KA, et al. Iodine toxicity treated with hemodialysis and continuous venovenous hemodiafiltration. Am J Kidney Dis. 2003;41:702-708.

174. Durandy Y, Batisse A, Bourel P, et al. Mediastinal infection after cardiac operation: A simple closed technique. J Thorac Cardiovasc Surg. 1989;97:282-285.

175. Kirsch M, Mekontso-Dessap A, Houel R, et al. Closed drainage using Redon catheters for poststernotomy mediastinitis: Results and risk factors for adverse outcome. Ann Thorac Surg. 2001;71:1580-1586.

176. Nahai F, Rand RP, Hester TR, et al. Primary treatment of the infected sternotomy wound with muscle flaps: A review of 211 consecutive cases. Plast Reconstr Surg. 1989;84:434-441.

177. Scully HE, Leclerc Y, Martin RD, et al. Comparison between antibiotic irrigation and mobilization of pectoral muscle flaps in treatment of deep sternal infections. J Thorac Cardiovasc Surg. 1985;90:523-231.

178. Majure JA, Albin RE, O'Donnell RS, Arganese TJ. Reconstruction of the infected median sternotomy wound. Ann Thorac Surg. 1986;42:9-12.

179. Miller JI, Nahai F. Repair of the dehisced median sternotomy incision. Surg Clin North Am. 1989;69:1091-1102.

180. Heath BJ, Bagnato VJ. Poststernotomy mediastinitis treated by omental transfer without postoperative irrigation or drainage. J Thorac Cardiovasc Surg. 1987;94:355-360.

181. Castello JR, Centella T, Garro L, et al. Muscle flap reconstruction for the treatment of major sternal wound infections after cardiac surgery: A 10-year analysis. Scand J Plast Reconstr Surg Hand Surg. 1999;33:17-24.

182. Schroeyers P, Wellens F, Degrieck I, et al. Aggressive primary treatment for poststernotomy acute mediastinitis: Our experience with omental- and muscle flaps surgery. Eur J Cardiothorac Surg. 2001;20:743-746.

183. Mekontso-Dessap A, Kirsch M, Brun-Buisson C, Loisance D. Poststernotomy mediastinitis due to *Staphylococcus aureus:* Comparison of methicillin-resistant and methicillin-susceptible cases. Clin Infect Dis. 2001;32:877-883.

184. Marggraf G, Neugebauer EA. A multicentre randomised placebo-controlled double-blind study on adjuvant treatment of mediastinitis with immunoglobulins (Pentaglobin) after cardiac surgery (ATMI): Outline and preliminary study protocol for discussion. Eur J Surg Suppl. 1999;584:26-32.

185. Szerafin T, Vaszily M, Peterffy A. Granulated sugar treatment of severe mediastinitis after open-heart surgery. Scand J Thorac Cardiovasc Surg. 1991;25:77-80.

186. Chirfe J, Scarmato G, Herszage L. Scientific basis for use of granulated sugar in treatment of infected wounds. Lancet. 1982;1:560-561.

187. Efem SEE. Clinical observations on the wound healing properties of honey. Br J Surg. 1988;75:679-681.

188. Trouillet JL, Chastre J, Fagon JY, et al. Use of granulated sugar in treatment of open mediastinitis after cardiac surgery. Lancet. 1985;2:180-184.

189. DeFeo M, De Santo LS, Romano G, et al. Treatment of recurrent staphylococcal mediastinitis: Still a controversial issue. Ann Thorac Surg. 2003;75:538-542.

190. Da Costa A, Kirkorian G, Cucherat M, et al. Antibiotic prophylaxis for permanent pacemaker implantation. Circulation. 1998;97:1796-1801.

191. Abramowicz M, ed. Antimicrobial prophylaxis in surgery. Med Lett. 2001;43:92-98.

192. Maki DG, Bohn MJ, Stolz SM, et al. Comparative study of cefazolin, cefamandole, and vancomycin for surgical prophylaxis in cardiac and vascular operations. J Thorac Cardiovasc Surg. 1992;104:1423-1434.

193. Hoen B, Gerard A, Berne C. Prognostic factors for mediastinitis following cardiac surgery. Abstract 1258. In: Abstracts of the 32nd Interscience Conference on Antimicrobial Agents and Chemotherapy. Washington, DC: American Society for Microbiology; 1992;320.

194. Domart Y, Trouillet JL, Fagon JY, et al. Incidence and morbidity of cytomegaloviral infection in patients with mediastinitis following cardiac surgery. Chest. 1990;97:18-22.

195. Schowengerdt CG, Suyemoto R, Main FB. Granulomatous and fibrous mediastinitis. J Thorac Cardiovasc Surg. 1969;57:365-379.

196. Hache L, Woolner LB, Bernatz PE. Idiopathic fibrous mediastinitis. Dis Chest. 1962;41:9-25.

197. Strimlan CV, Dines DE, Payne WS. Mediastinal granuloma. Mayo Clin Proc. 1975;50:702-705.

198. Dines DE, Payne WS, Bernatz PE, Pairolero PC. Mediastinal granuloma and fibrosing mediastinitis. Chest. 1979;75:320-324.

199. Gryboski WA, Crutcher RR, Holloway JB, et al. Surgical aspects of histoplasmosis. Arch Surg. 1963;87:590-599.

200. Peabody JW, Brown RB, Sullivan MB, Cannon A. Mediastinal granulomas. J Thorac Surg. 1958;35:384-396.

201. Goodwin RA, Loyd JE, Des Prez RM. Histoplasmosis in normal hosts. Medicine (Baltimore). 1981;60:231-266.

202. Ramakantan R, Shah P. Dysphagia due to mediastinal fibrosis in advanced pulmonary tuberculosis. AJR Am J Roentgenol. 1990;154:61-63.

203. Shah P, Ramakantan R. Hoarseness of the voice due to left recurrent laryngeal nerve palsy in tuberculous mediastinitis. Arch Otolaryngol Head Neck Surg. 1990;116:108.

204. Weese WC, Smith IM. A study of 57 cases of actinomycosis over a 36-year period. Arch Intern Med. 1975;135:1562-1568.

205. Bennhoff DF. Actinomycosis: Diagnostic and therapeutic considerations and a review of 32 cases. Laryngoscope. 1984;94:1198-1217.

206. Poland GA, Jorgensen CR, Sarosi GA. *Nocardia asteroides* pericarditis: Report of a case and review of the literature. Mayo Clin Proc. 1990;65:819-824.

207. Dunn EJ, Ulicny KS Jr, Wright CB, Gottesman L. Surgical implications of sclerosing mediastinitis. Chest. 1990;97:338-346.

208. Ahmad M, Weinstein AJ, Hughes JA, Cosgrove DE. Granulomatous mediastinitis due to *Aspergillus flavus* in a nonimmunocompromised patient. Am J Med. 1981;70:887-890.

209. Leong ASY. Granulomatous mediastinitis due to *Rhizopus* species. Am J Clin Pathol. 1978;70:103-107.

210. Gilbert HM, Hartman BJ. Short report: A case of fibrosing mediastinitis caused by *Wuchereria bancrofti.* Am J Trop Med Hyg. 1996;54:596-599.

211. Case records of the Massachusetts General Hospital (case 6-1989). N Engl J Med. 1989;320:380-389.

212. Grotty TB, Colby TV, Gay PC, Pisani RJ. Desmoplastic malignant mesothelioma masquerading as sclerosing mediastinitis. Hum Pathol. 1992;23:79-82.

213. Loeb JM, Lombard CM. Idiopathic mediastinitis with superior vena cava obstruction, cardiac tamponade, and cutaneous vasculitis. West J Med. 1991;155:296-299.

214. Williamson WA, Tronic BS, Levitan N, et al. Pulmonary venous infarction. Chest. 1992;102:937-940.

215. Berry DF, Buccigrossi BS, Peabody J, et al. Pulmonary vascular occlusion and fibrosing mediastinitis. Chest. 1986;89:296-301.

216. Rholl KS, Levitt RG, Glaser HS. Magnetic resonance imaging of fibrosing mediastinitis. AJR Am J Roentgenol. 1985;145:255-259.

217. Feigin DS, Eggleston JC, Siegelman SS. The multiple roentgen manifestations of sclerosing mediastinitis. Johns Hopkins Med J. 1979;144:1-8.

218. Noguchi H, Kephart GM, Colby TV, Gleich GJ. Tissue eosinophilia and eosinophil degranulation in syndromes associated with fibrosis. Am J Pathol. 1992;140:521-528.

219. Urschel HC Jr, Razzuk MA, Netto GJ, et al. Sclerosing mediastinitis: Improved management with histoplasmosis titer and ketoconazole. Ann Thorac Surg. 1990;50:215-221.

220. Zajtchuk R, Strevey TE, Heydorn WH, Treasure RL. Mediastinal histoplasmosis: Surgical considerations. J Thorac Cardiovasc Surg. 1973;66:300-304.

221. Cardasco EM Jr, Ahmad N, Mehta A, Rubio F. The effects of steroid therapy on pulmonary hypertension secondary to fibrosing mediastinitis. Cleve Clin J Med. 1990;57:647-652.

CHAPTER **79**

Approach to the Patient with Central Nervous System Infection

ALLAN R. TUNKEL

The central nervous system (CNS) may be infected by a variety of agents, including viruses, bacteria, fungi, protozoa, and other parasites. In addition, a number of noninfectious etiologies may account for syndromes that mimic CNS infections. These include neoplastic diseases, intracranial tumors and cysts, medications, collagen vascular disorders, and other systemic illnesses, and following various procedures that invade the CNS. The clinical presentation of a CNS infection may be acute, subacute, or chronic, and depends upon the virulence of the infecting agent and the location of the infection. Because CNS infections occur within the confines of the cranium or spinal column, they may be associated with significant morbidity and mortality, often necessitating emergent interventions to improve outcome. Here, I review the general approach to infections of the CNS, which are discussed in further detail in the following chapters of this section.

CLINICAL MANIFESTATIONS

The clinical presentation of a specific CNS infection depends upon the pathogenesis of spread of the infection to the CNS, the virulence of the etiologic agent, and the area of CNS involvement. Most patients with CNS infections present with the clinical features of fever, headache, altered mental status, or focal neurologic deficits. However, these findings are nonspecific and not all patients with CNS infections develop all of these clinical manifestations. In fact, the likelihood of any specific clinical finding is dependent upon the CNS syndrome caused by the infectious agent. These are reviewed subsequently.

Meningitis

Patients with acute meningitis most often present with fever, headache, meningismus, and altered mental status (see Chapter 80).[1] The typical adult patient with acute bacterial meningitis usually seeks medical attention within a few hours to several days after the onset of illness. The presentation may vary, however, depending upon the age of the patient and the presence of varying underlying conditions (e.g., head trauma, recent neurosurgery, the presence of a cerebrospinal fluid shunt [see Chapter 81], and the immunocompromised state). The presentation may also vary depending upon the microorganism causing meningitis. The common etiologic agents of acute meningitis are viruses (most often the enteroviruses, but also human immunodeficiency virus, mumps virus, and herpes simplex viruses) and bacteria (e.g., *Streptococcus pneumoniae, Neisseria meningitidis,* and *Listeria monocytogenes*). Less commonly, protozoa (e.g., *Naegleria fowleri*) and other parasites (e.g., *Angiostrongylus cantonensis)* may also cause acute meningitis.

In contrast, patients with subacute or chronic meningitis present over weeks to months, or even years (see Chapter 82). These patients may also have fever, headache, meningismus, and altered sensorium (as in patients with acute meningitis), but the onset is more gradual, fever is lower, and there may be associated lethargy and disability. These syndromes may be caused by mycobacteria (especially *Mycobacterium tuberculosis*), spirochetes (e.g., *Treponema pallidum* and *Borrelia burgdorferi),* and fungi (e.g., *Cryptococcus neoformans* and *Coccidioides* spp.).[1] Patients who develop meningitis caused by some of these agents are often immunocompromised, and the clinical presentation may vary from those who have intact immune systems. For example, the clinical presentation of cryptococcal meningitis is different in patients with and without the acquired immunodeficiency syndrome (AIDS). In non-AIDS patients, cryptococcal meningitis is typically a subacute process, in which patients have days to weeks of symptoms characterized by headache, fever, meningismus, and personality changes. In AIDS patients, the presentation is more subtle, with minimal, if any, symptoms; these patients may only present with headache and lethargy, with meningeal findings seen in only a minority of cases.

Encephalitis

The syndrome of acute encephalitis shares many features with acute meningitis (see Chapter 83).[2,3] Patients with both syndromes often present with the triad of fever, headache, and altered mental status. However, because the cerebral cortex is diffusely involved in patients with encephalitis, mental status changes early in the disease course, prior to the onset of obtundation or coma, are more common in patients with encephalitis. Other findings in patients with encephalitis include behavioral and speech disturbances, and focal or diffuse neurologic signs (e.g., seizures and hemiparesis). The syndrome may also coexist in the form of meningoencephalitis. A number of viruses have been shown to cause encephalitis and may be associated with specific manifestations that suggest their diagnosis. For example, herpes simplex virus affects the CNS focally (most often involving the temporal lobe), leading to clinical manifestations characterized by personality changes, altered mentation, a decreasing level of consciousness, seizures, and focal neurologic findings (e.g., dysphasia, weakness, and paresthesias). Other viral causes of acute encephalitis include the other herpesviruses (e.g., varicella-zoster virus, cytomegalovirus [CMV], and Epstein-Barr virus), arboviruses (e.g., West Nile, eastern equine, western equine, St. Louis, California, and Japanese encephalitis viruses), human immunodeficiency virus, rabies virus, and the enteroviruses. Although there may be overlapping clinical features with the viruses that cause encephalitis, the season of the year may offer a clue as to the specific etiologic agent. For example, arboviruses (e.g., eastern equine, western equine, St. Louis, and West Nile viruses) cause disease in summer or fall, whereas encephalitis caused by herpes simplex viruses and human immunodeficiency virus occurs sporadically throughout the year. Nonviral causes of encephalitis include *L. monocytogenes, Rickettsia* spp., *Bartonella* spp., and *Toxoplasma gondii* (more often seen in transplant patients with *Toxoplasma* encephalitis).

The clinical features in patients with chronic encephalitis may be similar to those seen in individuals with acute encephalitis, although the onset is more gradual. However, patients with chronic encephalitis may also progress to disability and death.

Focal Central Nervous System Syndromes

The clinical presentation in patients with focal CNS lesions (e.g., brain abscess, subdural empyema, and epidural abscess) depends upon the route of spread of the infection to the CNS, location of the lesion, and the severity of increased intracranial pressure (see Chapters 84 and 85). Patients develop brain abscesses via contiguous spread (e.g., from sinusitis, otitis media, or mastoiditis), hematogenous dissemination, or trauma. Initial clinical manifestations include headache, nausea, vomiting, and focal neurologic findings. Although patients may be brought to medical attention after development of a seizure or alteration in consciousness; fever is seen in less than 50% of patients. In patients with fungal brain abscess caused by *Aspergillus* spp. or the Mucorales, the clinical presentation may be that of a stroke syndrome because of the propensity of these organisms to invade blood vessels. In patients with focal infections that compress the spinal cord, the sequence of back pain, radiculopathy, and motor and sensory findings may eventually progress to complete paralysis, a clinical manifestation that is irreversible unless there is emergency intervention (see Chapter 85).

LUMBAR PUNCTURE

Lumbar puncture, with removal and analysis of cerebrospinal fluid (CSF), is an essential procedure in the diagnosis of many CNS infections,[1,4] most often in those with the clinical presentation of meningitis or encephalitis. In the performance of a lumbar puncture, the patient and the needle should be properly positioned to obtain adequate amounts of CSF; the patient is placed in either the lateral recumbent position on a firm surface with the back at the edge of the table and perpendicular to the table surface, or sitting with the back curved. Once the patient is properly positioned, the spinal needle (preferably 20 gauge or smaller) is inserted in the midline usually between the third and fourth lumbar vertebrae and perpendicular to the back. After needle insertion, frequent removal of the stylet can determine whether the subarachnoid space has been entered.

A number of complications have been associated with performance of the lumbar puncture.[1,4,5] These range from mild discomfort with insertion of the spinal needle to those that are life threatening. The most common complication following lumbar puncture is headache, which is observed in 10% to 25% of patients; the headache is characteristically absent when the patient is recumbent and appears rapidly when the patient stands. The headache is believed to be secondary to low CSF pressure as a result of continued leakage of CSF at the site of the lumbar puncture. The risk of headache may be reduced by using smaller-gauge needles (20 gauge or smaller); it has also been suggested that headache may be reduced by placing the patient in the prone position for several hours after the procedure, although it is not clear whether this maneuver is effective in reducing the likelihood of headache after lumbar puncture. The headache will usually resolve within hours to days after the procedure. Persistent headache can be treated by use of a "blood patch" in which some of the patient's own venous blood is injected outside the meninges at the site of the lumbar puncture; this procedure seals the site of CSF leakage.

Infection may occur after lumbar puncture, but the incidence of infection is low even in patients with concomitant bacteremia.[1] Although there have been conflicting studies on the risk of subsequent meningitis in patients who are bacteremic at the time of lumbar puncture, the importance of performing a diagnostic lumbar puncture in the appropriate clinical setting greatly outweighs any minor risk that the procedure itself might induce meningitis in a bacteremic patient. Lumbar puncture should not be performed in patients with established local infection in the lumbar space (e.g., spinal epidural abscess, spinal subdural empyema, or superficial or deep paraspinal infection); in these cases, CSF analysis should be obtained under fluoroscopic guidance via high cervical or cisternal puncture.

Local bleeding is a more common complication after lumbar puncture[1,4,5]; up to 20% of patients have a so-called traumatic tap.[6] Bleeding may occur from inadvertent puncture of the venous plexuses located dorsally and ventrally to the spinal dura or secondary to injury to vessels that accompany the cauda equina. This local bleeding rarely does harm to the patient, although patients with coagulation disturbances or who are receiving anticoagulants may develop continued bleeding with the development of spinal subdural or epidural hematomas that may compress the cauda equina and produce permanent neurologic injury.

Despite the complications listed above, the most feared complication following lumbar puncture is brain herniation, which may occur in the patient with an elevation of intracranial pressure.[1,4,5] In patients who undergo lumbar puncture, there is normally a mild, transient lowering of lumbar CSF pressure that is rapidly communicated throughout the

subarachnoid space. In patients with bacterial meningitis and suspected severe intracranial hypertension or impending herniation, a 22- or 25-gauge spinal needle should be used, with careful observation for several hours after removal of CSF; monitoring and treatment of increased intracranial pressure may need to be considered (see later). In patients who have an intracranial space-occupying lesion, particularly one located in the posterior fossa, there is already a relative pressure gradient (with downward displacement of the cerebrum and brain stem) that can be increased by lumbar puncture and precipitate brain herniation. Certain patients should therefore undergo neuroimaging studies (i.e., computed tomography [CT] or magnetic resonance imaging [MRI]) prior to lumbar puncture, if there is a suspicion that their neurologic presentation may be secondary to an intracranial mass lesion with accompanying mass effect. These include patients with the following characteristics: age older than 60 years, immunocompromised state, new-onset seizure, altered consciousness, papilledema, and/or focal neurologic deficit.[1,7]

Opening Pressure and Appearance

In the evaluation of CNS infections via lumbar puncture, a number of parameters should be assessed.[1,5,8] CSF opening pressure is measured with an air-water manometer; in adults placed in the lateral decubitus position, the normal CSF opening pressure ranges from 50 to 195 mm H_2O. Variation of pressure with deep respiration provides assurance that fluid flow into the manometer is unobstructed. Once obtained, CSF should be sent to the laboratory for analysis (Table 79-1). The CSF is normally clear and colorless, but may appear cloudy or turbid in patients with increased concentrations of white blood cells ($>200/mm^3$), red blood cells ($>400/mm^3$), bacteria ($>10^5$ colony-forming units [CFU]/mL), or protein. In patients with a traumatic tap, an initially bloody CSF (present when there are at least 6000 red blood cells/mm^3) should clear as flow of CSF continues. Xanthochromia, a yellow or yellow-orange supernatant of centrifuged CSF, is usually a result of red blood cell lysis and the presence of oxyhemoglobin, methemoglobin, and bilirubin; it characteristically appears 2 to 4 hours after red blood cells have entered the subarachnoid space, although has occasionally been seen for as long as 12 hours. The presence of xanthochromia distinguishes CSF that is bloody secondary to

---

TABLE 79-1 Tests of Cerebrospinal Fluid in Patients with Suspected Central Nervous System Infection

Routine Tests
White blood cell count with differential
Red blood cell count*
Glucose concentration[†]
Protein concentration
Gram stain
Bacterial culture

Selected Specific Tests Based on Clinical Suspicion
Viral culture[‡]
Smears and culture for acid-fast bacilli
Venereal Disease Research Laboratory (VDRL)
India ink prep
Cryptococcal polysaccharide antigen
Fungal culture
Antibody tests (IgM and/or IgG)[§]
Polymerase chain reaction[‖]
Cytology and flow cytometry[¶]

*Should be checked in the first and last tubes; in patients with a traumatic tap there should be a decrease in the number of red blood cells with continued flow of CSF. See text for formula for determining whether the numbers of CSF red blood cells and white blood cells are consistent with a traumatic tap.
[†]Compare to serum glucose drawn just before lumbar puncture.
[‡]Yield of viral culture may be low (see Chapters 80 and 83).
[§]May be useful for specific etiologies of meningitis and encephalitis (see Chapters 80, 82, and 83).
[‖]Most useful for specific viral etiologies of encephalitis and causes of chronic meningitis; see text and Chapters 82 and 83 for details.
[¶]In patients with suspected malignancy.

subarachnoid hemorrhage from CSF that is bloody secondary to a traumatic lumbar puncture, in which the centrifuged supernatant is clear. Xanthochromia has also been observed with elevated CSF protein concentrations of more than 150 mg/dL (Froin's syndrome) or as a consequence of systemic hyperbilirubinemia (>10-15 mg/dL). CSF with very high protein concentrations may clot, impairing the chemical, smear, and cytologic analyses.

In patients with meningitis, specific CSF results may vary depending upon the infectious agent (Table 79-2). For additional information on CSF results for specific etiologic agents of meningitis and encephalitis, please refer to the subsequent chapters in this section. Details of some CSF parameters are reviewed subsequently.

Cell Count

The normal CSF white blood cell count in children and adults is 0 to 5/mm^3. CSF white blood cell counts in term neonates may be up to 32/mm^3 (mean of 8-9/mm^3), although by 1 month of age normal CSF has fewer than 10 white blood cells/mm^3. Elevated CSF concentrations of white blood cells are seen in patients with meningitis, encephalitis, and parameningeal foci of infection (e.g., space-occupying lesions).[1,5] False-positive elevations of CSF white blood cell counts can be found after traumatic lumbar puncture, or in patients with intracerebral or subarachnoid hemorrhage in which both red blood cells and white blood cells are introduced into the subarachnoid space. In these instances, the following formula should be used as a correction factor for the true white blood cell (WBC) count in the presence of CSF red blood cells (RBC)[1]:

$$\text{True WBC in CSF} = \text{actual WBC in CSF} - \frac{\text{WBC in blood} \times \text{RBC in CSF}}{\text{RBC in blood}}$$

In the above equation the amount being subtracted is the predicted CSF WBC that would arise if all the CSF WBC were the result of blood contamination.[8]

Generalized seizures may also induce a transient CSF pleocytosis that is primarily neutrophilic, although the total WBC count should not exceed 80/mm^3. However, pleocytosis should not be ascribed to seizure activity alone unless the fluid is clear and colorless, the opening pressure and CSF glucose are normal, the CSF Gram stain is negative, and the patient has no clinical evidence of CNS infection.[1] In patients with CSF pleocytosis, differential counts should be performed; a neutrophilic, mononuclear, or eosinophilic predominance may be suggestive of certain etiologies in the right clinical setting (see Table 79-2 and Chapters 80 and 82).

Glucose and Protein

A CSF hypoglycorrhachia is seen in a number of CNS infections. The pathogenesis of CSF hypoglycorrhachia is multifactorial and may include an increased rate of macrovesicular glucose transport across arachnoid villi, increased glycolysis by leukocytes and bacteria, increased metabolic rate of the brain and spinal cord, and/or inhibition of glucose entry into the subarachnoid space caused by alterations in the membrane carrier system responsible for glucose transfer from

blood to CSF.[8] In addition, some infections of the CNS may result in cerebral vasculitis or a decrease in cerebral blood flow (as a result of increased intracranial pressure), or both, resulting in less delivery of glucose to the brain and glucose utilization by anaerobic glycolysis.[1] The actual CSF glucose concentration may be falsely low in the presence of hypoglycemia or may be incorrectly interpreted as normal when the patient is hyperglycemic (e.g., in diabetic patients). Therefore, the CSF glucose should always be compared with a simultaneous serum glucose that is drawn prior to lumbar puncture; the normal CSF:serum glucose ratio is approximately 0.6, and ratios less than 0.5 should be considered abnormal.[5]

The CSF protein concentration is also elevated in a number of CNS infections, presumably due to disruption of the blood-brain barrier, manifested morphologically by separation of intercellular tight junctions and increased numbers of pinocytotic vesicles in microvascular endothelial cells.[1] Lumbar CSF protein concentrations greater than 50 mg/dL and ventricular CSF concentrations greater than 15 mg/dL are considered abnormal. However, elevated CSF protein concentrations are among the most common and the least specific of all CSF parameters, and may be observed in a variety of infectious and noninfectious disorders of the CNS. In patients with a traumatic lumbar puncture, the true CSF protein concentration is determined by subtracting 1 mg/dL of protein for every 1000 RBC/mm^3, although these determinations must be made in the same CSF tube.[5]

Other Cerebrospinal Fluid Tests

Additional studies of CSF may be useful in determining a specific etiologic diagnosis in patients with meningitis and encephalitis.[1] Cultures are clearly important in attempts to identify a specific etiologic agent, but depending upon the pathogen, larger CSF volumes may be needed to increase the yield of a positive culture (e.g., for *M. tuberculosis* or fungi), CSF cultures may require prolonged incubation and special techniques for isolation of specific pathogens (see Chapters 80, 82, and 83). In some cases, simple stains of CSF specimens may establish the etiologic diagnosis. In patients with suspected bacterial meningitis, CSF Gram stain may provide a clue as to the etiologic diagnosis (see Chapter 80). The CSF Gram stain is positive in 60% to 90% of patients with acute bacterial meningitis, although this sensitivity varies depending upon the concentration of microorganisms in the CSF and the specific causative bacterium. However, not all specialized stains of CSF to identify specific microorganisms are as sensitive as the Gram stain. In patients with tuberculous meningitis, less than 15% to 25% of specimens are smear-positive by acid-fast stain, and up to 20% of patients with tuberculous meningitis have persistently negative CSF cultures. In patients with spirochetal meningitis (i.e., caused by *T. pallidum* or *B. burgdorferi*) and *Toxoplasma* encephalitis, there are no effective specialized stains that identify these organisms in CSF; in these cases, serum or CSF antibody studies are most often utilized to aid in the diagnosis (see Chapters 80 and 84). CSF India ink examination is positive in 50% to 75% of patients with cryptococcal meningitis, and the yield increases to 88% in patients with AIDS. However, the most important CSF test in the diagnosis of cryptococcal meningitis is the CSF latex agglutination

TABLE 79-2 Typical Cerebrospinal Fluid Findings in Patients with Selected Infectious Causes of Meningitis

Cause of Meningitis	White Blood Cell Count (cells/mm³)	Primary Cell Type	Glucose (mg/dL)	Protein (mg/dL)
Viral	50-1000	Mononuclear*	>45	<200
Bacterial	1000-5000[†]	Neutrophilic[‡]	<40[§]	100-500
Tuberculous	50-300	Mononuclear[‖]	<45	50-300
Cryptococcal	20-500[¶]	Mononuclear	<40	>45

*May be neutrophilic early in presentation (see Chapter 80).
[†]Range from fewer than 100 to more than 10,000 cells/mm³.
[‡]About 10% of patients have a CSF lymphocyte predominance.
[§]Should always be compared to a simultaneous serum glucose; ratio of CSF:serum glucose is equal to or less than 0.4 in the majority of cases (see Chapter 80).
[‖]May see a "therapeutic paradox" in which a mononuclear predominance becomes neutrophilic during antituberculous therapy.
[¶]More than 75% of patients with acquired immunodeficiency syndrome have fewer than 20 cells/mm³.

test for detection of cryptococcal polysaccharide antigen; a presumptive diagnosis is established by a CSF titer of at least 1:8.

Polymerase chain reaction (PCR) of CSF is a highly sensitive and specific test for the diagnosis of many CNS infections, and may be useful in providing a rapid diagnosis.[1] In patients with herpes simplex encephalitis, CSF PCR is 91% sensitive and 92% specific in patients with biopsy-proven disease,[9] although the specificity would have approached 100% in this study except that some tissue specimens were fixed in formalin, which killed infectious virus; the presence of RBCs in CSF may also inhibit the PCR reaction, giving a false-negative result. Diagnosis of CMV encephalitis by PCR has a high sensitivity and specificity for the diagnosis of CNS involvement[10]; the absence of CMV DNA by PCR has a high negative predictive value. Nucleic acid amplification with RT-PCR has also been found to be highly sensitive (86%-100%) and specific (92%-100%) for the diagnosis of enteroviral infections of the CNS.[11] The clinical utility of PCR in patients with bacterial meningitis has been investigated with use of a broad range of bacterial primers (i.e., broad-based PCR). In one study[12] the sensitivity of broad-based PCR was 100%, specificity 98.2%, and negative predictive value 100%, indicating that this test would be useful in excluding the diagnosis of bacterial meningitis and influencing decisions to initiate or discontinue antimicrobial therapy. Use of PCR to detect the fragments of mycobacterial DNA in CSF appears to be the most promising technique for the rapid diagnosis of tuberculous meningitis.[13] More information on the use of specialized CSF tests to establish an etiologic diagnosis, and use of other adjunctive tests, in patients with meningitis and encephalitis can be found in Chapters 80, 82, and 83.

NEUROIMAGING STUDIES

The use of neuroimaging studies, specifically CT and MRI, have been invaluable in localizing infectious processes within the CNS and in assessing response to therapy.[14] With CT scanning, areas of bone and blood appear as areas of high signal intensity, compared with brain and CSF, which appear as areas of low signal intensity. Following the intravenous administration of an iodinated contrast agent, increased intensity (i.e., contrast enhancement) is seen in areas of blood-brain barrier breakdown, thereby increasing the sensitivity for the diagnosis of certain abnormalities (e.g., brain abscesses). MRI directly generates images in all three planes (axial, coronal, and sagittal) to optimally evaluate brain morphology and pathology; MRI can also provide information about blood flow within arteries and veins, and demonstrates enhancement of specific lesions following intravenous administration of gadolinium diethylenetriaminepentaacetic acid (DTPA). Given the higher sensitivity of MRI compared with CT, MRI has become the preferred neuroimaging modality in the evaluation of many patients with suspected CNS infection. These modalities are reviewed in further detail, based on specific clinical syndrome, in the subsequent chapters of this section, but some examples are given here.

The most important and specific neuroimaging technique in patients with herpes simplex virus encephalitis is MRI with contrast enhancement, which demonstrates lesions earlier than CT[15]; MRI may also be useful in other causes of viral encephalitis (see Chapter 83). Neuroimaging studies are less important in the diagnosis of patients with bacterial meningitis, but may be useful in those who are not responding as expected—that is, have persistent or prolonged fever, clinical evidence of increased intracranial pressure, focal neurologic findings, new or recurrent seizures, enlarging head circumference (in neonates), persistent neurologic dysfunction, or persistently abnormal CSF parameters or cultures.[1] MRI is more sensitive than CT in the detection of focal CNS infections and has the advantages of early detection of cerebritis, cerebral edema with greater contrast between edema and adjacent brain, more conspicuous spread of inflammation into the ventricles and subarachnoid space, and earlier detection of satellite lesions (see Chapter 84). Contrast enhancement with gadolinium provides the added advantage of clear differentiation of the central abscess, surrounding enhancing rim, and cerebral edema surrounding the abscess. On T_2-weighted images, the zone of edema that surrounds the abscess is one of high signal intensity. In AIDS patients with positive immunoglobulin G (IgG) antibody titers to *T. gondii*, the detection of multiple ring–enhancing lesions by CT with contrast or MRI is enough evidence to initiate a trial of anti-*Toxoplasma* chemotherapy (see Chapter 84); CT or MRI is then repeated in 10 to 14 days to document a clinical response. Advancements in neuroimaging technology may further refine the approach to patients with CNS infections.

MANAGEMENT

Many infections of the CNS require emergent therapy to decrease the likelihood of serious morbidity and mortality. This involves use of empirical antimicrobial therapy to cover the likely pathogens based on the pathogenesis of spread of infection to the CNS, surgical therapy (e.g., abscess drainage) to establish the etiologic diagnosis and limit further neurologic dysfunction and damage, and adjunctive therapies, which may improve outcome and treat elevations in intracranial pressure.

Antimicrobial Therapy

Many factors influence the choice of a specific antimicrobial agent in the therapy of CNS infections. These factors have been best studied in experimental animal models of infections to evaluate use of antibacterial agents in the treatment of bacterial meningitis.[1,16] One important factor is the penetration of the antimicrobial agent into the CSF, in order to attain adequate drug concentrations to rapidly and effectively kill the meningeal pathogen. Drug penetration into CSF is dependent upon the status of the blood-brain barrier, which is disrupted in the presence of meningeal inflammation. Some agents (e.g., corticosteroids) may reduce meningeal inflammation and reduce blood-brain barrier penetration of antimicrobial agents. Entry of antimicrobial agents into CSF is also enhanced by drugs that have a low molecular weight, a low degree of ionization at physiologic pH, high lipid solubility, and a low degree of protein binding.

Once the antimicrobial agent penetrates the CSF, it must exhibit rapid bactericidal activity against the infecting pathogen because bacterial meningitis is an infection in an area of impaired host resistance. A final factor that contributes to response to antimicrobial therapy is pharmacodynamics, which is concerned with the time course of antimicrobial activity at the site of infection; these factors and whether the specific agent kills by concentration- or time-dependent killing are important to determine the dosing regimen for optimal effectiveness. These principles are reviewed in further detail in Chapter 80.

Many of the principles for the treatment of bacterial meningitis may also apply to treatment of other nonbacterial etiologies of meningitis and encephalitis. In addition, there are experimental and clinical studies that have examined the penetration of specific antimicrobial agents into brain abscesses, which may be important in the antimicrobial therapy of these infections. However, in the therapy of focal intracranial infections, clinicians often rely on agents that are known to have efficacy in experimental animal models (which includes extrapolating data from animal models of meningitis) and based on anecdotal case series or case reports. This approach is reasonable because these infections are not common, and randomized trials of specific agents are not likely to be performed.

Surgical Therapy

Many patients with focal CNS infections require surgical therapy for optimal management (see Chapters 84 and 85). Drainage of brain abscesses, subdural empyema, and epidural abscess is critical to establish a microbiologic diagnosis and to ensure a good outcome by relieving the increased intracranial pressure that is associated with these disorders. Aspiration can be performed via guidance by neuroimaging modalities (i.e., CT or MRI), which allows the surgeon rapid, accurate, and safe access to virtually any intracranial or parameningeal focus. Open craniotomy may be required for extensive intracranial infections that cannot be adequately drained via burr hole aspiration (e.g., in patients with cranial subdural empyema).

Although some patients with focal CNS infections can be treated with antimicrobial therapy alone, these patients must be carefully selected and followed to be certain that there is not development or progression of neurologic dysfunction.

Adjunctive Therapy

The morbidity and mortality in patients with infections of the CNS remain unacceptably high. Because CNS infections can be complicated by cerebral edema and increased intracranial pressure (with the potential for brain herniation), various adjunctive strategies have been examined for their efficacy in CNS infections. Among the best-studied agents are corticosteroids. For example, adjunctive dexamethasone (given concomitant with or just before the first antimicrobial dose) improves outcome in infants and children with *Haemophilus influenzae* type b and pneumococcal meningitis, and in adults with pneumococcal meningitis (see Chapter 80).[1,17,18] Corticosteroids may also be of benefit in patients with focal intracranial infections and cerebral edema associated with significant mass effect. Steroids may be beneficial in reduction of edema, leading to improvement of symptoms and signs of neurologic dysfunction until more definitive interventions can be performed.

Other adjunctive modalities in treatment of CNS infections are directed toward reduction of increased intracranial pressure, a complication that has been associated with cerebral ischemia and infarction.[1,19,20] Direct intracranial pressure monitoring is indicated in patients in whom there is clinical suspicion of increased intracranial pressure. Available methods include use of an intraventricular catheter, subarachnoid bolt, epidural fiber-optic catheter, or lumbar drain. Several simple methods are available to lower intracranial pressure: elevation of the head of the patient's bed to 30 degrees to maximize venous drainage with minimal compromise of cerebral perfusion; avoidance of turning the head to the side and hyperextending the neck, because these maneuvers may increase jugular venous pressure and block efflux of CSF through the foramen magnum; and avoidance of intratracheal suctioning or endotracheal intubation. Hyperventilation (to maintain the $PaCO_2$ between 27 and 30 mm Hg), which causes vasoconstriction and reduction in intracerebral volume, may also be employed to reduce intracranial pressure, although this maneuver may not be indicated in all patients with bacterial meningitis and elevated intracranial pressure (see Chapter 80). Hyperosmolar agents (e.g., mannitol) decrease intracranial pressure by making the intravascular space hyperosmolar relative to the brain, permitting movement of water from the brain tissue to the intravascular compartment. In patients who continue to have elevated intracranial pressure despite the above interventions, high-dose barbiturate therapy, which decreases cerebral metabolic demands and cerebral blood flow, may be indicated. Barbiturates can also cause vasoconstriction in normal tissue, thereby shunting blood to ischemic tissue and protecting the brain from ischemic insult; appropriate intracranial, electroencephalographic, and hemodynamic monitoring is necessary when barbiturates are utilized to reduce intracranial pressure.

Seizures may occur in patients with CNS infections, and must be managed quickly and aggressively to avoid permanent anoxic ischemic changes.[1,19,20] Status epilepticus that is continuous for 90 minutes or more can lead to permanent neurologic injury. Short-acting anticonvulsants with a rapid onset of action (e.g., lorazepam or diazepam) should be given, followed by a long-acting agent such as phenytoin. If these maneuvers fail to terminate the seizure, the patient should be intubated, mechanically ventilated, and treated with phenobarbital.

Fluid management is critical in patients with CNS infections.[1,20] Some patients may be volume depleted as a result of decreased oral intake, vomiting, and diarrhea. In these patients intravenous fluids are required to maintain systemic and cerebral perfusion. Hyponatremia (serum sodium < 135 mEq/L) may occur in patients with CNS infections, attributed to the syndrome of inappropriate secretion of antidiuretic hormone (SIADH). In these patients, restriction of fluids is important to correct the hyponatremia, although it is critical to maintain the patient in a euvolemic state.

Aggressive treatment of these complications in the critical care setting has improved the neurologic outcome of patients with CNS infections. The definitive treatment of specific infectious syndromes and the etiologic agents that cause them are reviewed in detail in the following chapters of this section.

REFERENCES

1. Tunkel AR. Bacterial meningitis. Philadelphia: Lippincott Williams & Wilkins; 2001.
2. Whitley RJ, Gnann JW. Viral encephalitis: Familiar infections and emerging pathogens. Lancet. 2002;359:507-513.
3. Cepelowicz J, Tunkel AR. Viral encephalitis. Curr Treat Op Infect Dis. 2003;5:11-19.
4. Marton KI, Gean AD. The spinal tap: A new look at an old test. Ann Intern Med. 1986;104:840-848.
5. Greenlee JE, Carroll KC. Cerebrospinal fluid in CNS Infections. In: Scheld WM, Whitley RJ, Durack DT, eds. Infections of the Central Nervous System. 2nd ed. Philadelphia: Lippincott-Raven Publishers; 1997:899-922.
6. Bonadio WA, Smith D, Goddard S, et al. Distinguishing cerebrospinal fluid abnormalities in children with bacterial meningitis and traumatic lumbar puncture. J Infect Dis. 1990;162:251-254.
7. Hasbun R, Abrahams J, Jekel J, Quagliarello VJ. Computed tomography of the head before lumbar puncture in adults with suspected meningitis. N Engl J Med. 2001;345:1727-1733.
8. Bonadio WA. The cerebrospinal fluid: Physiologic aspects and alterations associated with bacterial meningitis. Pediatr Infect Dis J. 1992;11:423-432.
9. Lakeman FD, Whitley RJ, and the Cooperative Antiviral Study Group. Diagnosis of herpes simplex encephalitis: Application of polymerase chain reaction to cerebrospinal fluid from brain-biopsied patients and correlation with disease. J Infect Dis. 1995;171:857-863.
10. Wildemann B, Haas J, Lynen N, et al. Diagnosis of cytomegalovirus central nervous system disease in AIDS patients by quantitation of cytomegalovirus genomes in cells of cerebrospinal fluid. Neurology. 1998;50:693-697.
11. Romero JR. Diagnosis and management of enteroviral infections of the central nervous system. Curr Infect Dis Rep. 2002;4:309-316.
12. Saravolatz LD, Manzor O, VanderVelde N, et al. Broad-range bacterial polymerase chain reaction for early detection of bacterial meningitis. Clin Infect Dis. 2003;36:40-45.
13. Sinner SW, Tunkel AR. Approach to the diagnosis and management of tuberculous meningitis. Curr Infect Dis Rep. 2002;4:324-331.
14. Zimmerman RA, Girard NJ. Imaging of intracranial infections. In: Scheld WM, Whitley RJ, Durack DT, eds. Infections of the Central Nervous System. 2nd ed. Philadelphia: Lippincott-Raven Publishers; 1997:923-944.
15. Johnson RT. Acute encephalitis. Clin Infect Dis. 1996;23:219-226.
16. Sinner SW, Tunkel AR. Antimicrobial agents in the treatment of acute bacterial meningitis. Infect Dis Clin North Am. 2004. In press.
17. McIntyre PB, Berkey CS, King SM, et al. Dexamethasone as adjunctive therapy in bacterial meningitis: A meta-analysis of randomized clinical trials since 1988. JAMA. 1997;278:925-931.
18. Tunkel AR, Scheld WM. Corticosteroids for everyone with meningitis? N Engl J Med. 2002;347:1613-1625.
19. Ling GSF, Hanley DF. Neurocritical care of CNS infections. In: Scheld WM, Whitley RJ, Durack DT, eds. Infections of the Central Nervous System. 2nd ed. Philadelphia: Lippincott-Raven Publishers; 1997:973-979.
20. Roos KL, Tunkel AR, Scheld WM. Acute bacterial meningitis. In: Scheld WM, Whitley RJ, Marra CM, eds. Infections of the Central Nervous System. 3rd ed. New York: Lippincott Williams & Wilkins; 2004. In press.

CHAPTER **80**

Acute Meningitis

ALLAN R. TUNKEL

W. MICHAEL SCHELD

Meningitis, or inflammation of the meninges, is identified by an abnormal number of white blood cells in cerebrospinal fluid (CSF). Acute meningitis is clinically defined as a syndrome characterized by the onset of meningeal symptoms over the course of hours to up to several days. Headache is a prominent early symptom, often followed later by confusion, stupor, or coma. Examination reveals few focal findings early during infection, although signs of meningeal irritation are common. The acute meningitis syndrome blurs imperceptibly into the syndromes of chronic meningitis (see Chapter 82) and encephalitis (see Chapter 83). Chronic meningitis has an onset measured in weeks to months (but is generally defined when symptoms, signs, and the CSF remain abnormal for at least 4 weeks), whereas encephalitis is distinguished by the presence of decreased mentation (i.e., confusion or stupor, with or without seizures) early in the course of disease with minimal meningeal signs. The distinction between these syndromes is clinically useful in guiding management but is clearly artificial in terms of etiology and pathology. For example, tuberculous meningitis may have a subacute or a chronic onset.

The acute meningitis syndrome may be caused by a wide variety of infectious agents and may also be a manifestation of noninfectious diseases (Table 80-1). Diseases in which meningeal symptoms occur but are not predominant (e.g., measles) are excluded from the table. Many of the causes of chronic meningitis, which can be manifested acutely, have been omitted but are listed in Chapter 82. Here, we review the common infectious causes of acute meningitis, with particular emphasis on epidemiology and etiology, pathogenesis and pathophysiology, clinical features, diagnosis, treatment, and prevention.

EPIDEMIOLOGY AND ETIOLOGY

Viral Meningitis

Viruses are the major cause of the *aseptic meningitis syndrome,* a term used to define any meningitis (infectious or noninfectious), particularly one with a lymphocytic pleocytosis, for which a cause is not apparent after initial evaluation and routine stains and cultures of CSF.[1,2] Common viral etiologic agents that cause the acute aseptic meningitis syndrome are discussed in the following paragraphs.

Enteroviruses

Enteroviruses, currently the leading recognizable cause of aseptic meningitis syndrome, account for 85% to 95% of all cases in which a pathogen is identified.[1,2] Estimates from the Centers for Disease Control and Prevention (CDC) indicate that 10 to 15 million symptomatic enteroviral infections occur annually in the United States, which includes 30,000 to 75,000 cases of meningitis.[3] However, these figures are most likely an underestimation of the true incidence because of underreporting of enteroviral cases from state laboratories to the CDC. Enteroviruses are worldwide in distribution. In temperate climates, they appear with a marked summer/fall seasonality, although in tropical and

---

TABLE 80-1 Differential Diagnosis of Acute Meningitis

Major infectious etiologies
  Viruses
    Nonpolio enteroviruses*
    Arboviruses†
    Herpesviruses‡
    Lymphocytic choriomeningitis virus
    Human immunodeficiency virus
    Adenovirus
    Parainfluenza virus type 3
    Influenza virus
    Measles virus
  Rickettsiae
    Rickettsia rickettsii
    Rickettsia conorii
    Rickettsia prowazekii
    Rickettsia typhi
    Orientia tsutsugamushi
    Ehrlichia and *Anaplasma* spp.
  Bacteria
    Haemophilus influenzae
    Neisseria meningitidis
    Streptococcus pneumoniae
    Listeria monocytogenes
    Escherichia coli
    Streptococcus agalactiae
    Propionibacterium acnes
    Staphylococcus aureus
    Staphylococcus epidermidis
    Enterococcus spp.
    Klebsiella pneumoniae
    Pseudomonas aeruginosa
    Salmonella spp.
    Acinetobacter spp.
    Viridans streptococci
    Streptococcus bovis
    Fusobacterium necrophorum
    Stenotrophomonas maltophilia
    Streptococcus pyogenes
    Pasteurella multocida
    Bacillus anthracis
    Capnocytophaga canimorsus
    Nocardia spp.
    Mycobacterium tuberculosis

Spirochetes
    Treponema pallidum (syphilis)
    Borrelia burgdorferi (Lyme disease)
    Leptospira spp.
Protozoa and helminths
    Naegleria fowleri
    Angiostrongylus cantonensis
    Baylisascaris procyonis
    Strongyloides stercoralis (hyperinfection syndrome)
Other infectious syndromes
    Parameningeal foci of infection§
    Infective endocarditis
    Viral postinfectious syndromes
    Postvaccination‖
Noninfectious etiologies and diseases of unknown etiology
  Intracranial tumors and cysts
    Craniopharyngioma
    Dermoid/epidermoid cyst
    Teratoma
  Medications
    Antimicrobial agents¶
    Nonsteroidal anti-inflammatory agents**
    Muromonab-CD3 (OKT3)
    Azathioprine
    Cytosine arabinoside (high dose)
    Carbamazepine††
    Immune globulin
    Ranitidine
    Phenazopyridine
  Systemic illnesses
    Systemic lupus erythematosus
    Vogt-Koyanagi-Harada syndrome
  Procedure-related
    Postneurosurgery
    Spinal anesthesia
    Intrathecal injections‡‡
    Chymopapain injection
  Miscellaneous
    Seizures
    Migraine or migraine-like syndromes
    Mollaret's meningitis

*Primarily echoviruses and coxsackieviruses.
†In the United States, the major etiologic agents are the mosquito-borne California, St. Louis, Eastern equine, Western equine, Venezuelan equine encephalitis, and West Nile viruses; and the tick-borne Colorado tick fever.
‡Primarily herpes simplex virus type 2, but also herpes simplex virus type 1, varicella-zoster virus, cytomegalovirus, Epstein-Barr virus, and human herpesvirus-6.
§Brain abscess, sinusitis, otitis, mastoiditis, subdural empyema, epidural abscess, venous sinus thrombophlebitis, pituitary abscess, cranial osteomyelitis.
‖Mumps, measles, polio, pertussis, rabies, vaccinia.
¶Trimethoprim, sulfamethoxazole, trimethoprim-sulfamethoxazole, ciprofloxacin, penicillin, isoniazid, metronidazole, cephalosporins, pyrazinamide.
**Ibuprofen, sulindac, naproxen, tolmetin, diclofenac, ketoprofen.
††In patients with connective tissue diseases.
‡‡Air, isotopes, antimicrobial agents, antineoplastic agents, steroids, radiographic contrast media.

subtropical areas, a high year-round incidence is observed. Periods of warm weather and wearing sparse clothing may facilitate the fecal-oral spread of these organisms; enteroviruses may also be recovered from houseflies, wastewater, and sewage.[2] In the United States, the 14 most commonly occurring enteroviral serotypes account for more than 80% of isolates.[3,4] Data from the CDC's National Enterovirus Surveillance System indicated that the predominant enteroviruses isolated from patients during the years 1997 through 1999 were (in decreasing order) echoviruses 30, 11, 9, 6, and 7; coxsackieviruses B2 and A9; echoviruses 18 and 16; coxsackieviruses B1 and B3; enterovirus 71; coxsackievirus B4; and echovirus 25. In addition, the newly numbered enteroviruses 70 and 71 have been reported to commonly cause central nervous system (CNS) disease.[5-7]

Infants and young children are the primary victims of enteroviral meningitis because they are the most susceptible host population (i.e., they are without previous exposure and immunity) within the community. In one large cohort study from Finland,[8] children younger than 1 year had an annual incidence of viral meningitis of 219 cases per 100,000 population, compared with an incidence of 19 cases per 100,000 population in children between the ages of 1 and 4 years; the incidence dropped even further with advancing age. The vast majority of these viral pathogens were enteroviruses. More than one episode of enteroviral meningitis may develop, although the same enteroviral serotype has not been implicated more than once in any immunocompetent patient.[2] Enteroviruses are also the most common causes of aseptic meningitis in adults.[9] Immunodeficiency (specifically congenital or acquired impaired humoral immunity) and possibly physical exercise may predispose to enteroviral meningitis.[2,4] Cases of enteroviral meningoencephalitis have also been seen in patients treated with the chimeric anti-CD20 monoclonal antibody rituximab.[10]

Arboviruses

The most common arthropod-transmitted cause of aseptic meningitis in the United States, until 2002, was St. Louis encephalitis virus, a flavivirus.[2] Aseptic meningitis accounts for about 15% of all symptomatic cases of St. Louis encephalitis and may be as high as 35% to 60% in children. Patients older than 60 years rarely present with aseptic meningitis if infected with St. Louis encephalitis virus; encephalitis is the more common finding. These infections are more frequent in warmer months, when contact with the insect vector is more likely. Vector exposure is more likely to occur indoors than outside because poorly sealed residences appear to be a risk factor. Other arboviruses reported to cause aseptic meningitis include the California encephalitis group of viruses (e.g., La Crosse, Jamestown Canyon, and snowshoe hare viruses, which are bunyaviruses) and the agent of Colorado tick fever, a coltivirus seen in the mountainous and western regions of the United States and Canada. Although encephalitis is the most common manifestation, West Nile virus may also cause aseptic meningitis or asymmetrical flaccid paralysis, indistinguishable from poliomyelitis (see Chapter 149).[114]

Mumps Virus

In an unimmunized population, mumps is one of the most common causes of aseptic meningitis and encephalitis; symptomatic meningitis is estimated to occur in 10% to 30% of mumps patients overall.[12] CNS disease caused by mumps virus can occur in patients without evidence of parotitis,[2,12] and 40% to 50% of patients with mumps meningitis have no evidence of salivary gland enlargement. Meningitis is the most common neurologic manifestation of infection with mumps virus[2,12] and is usually a benign and self-limited process. Males are affected two to five times more often than females, and the peak incidence is in children aged 5 to 9 years. Cases of vaccine-associated mumps meningitis have also been reported.

Lymphocytic Choriomeningitis Virus

Lymphocytic choriomeningitis virus was one of the earliest and seemingly most significant viruses to be associated with human aseptic meningitis[1,2]; this virus is now rarely reported as an etiologic agent.

Lymphocytic choriomeningitis virus is transmitted to humans by contact with rodents (e.g., hamsters, rats, mice) or their excreta; the greatest risk of infection is in laboratory workers, pet owners, and persons living in impoverished and nonhygienic situations. One outbreak was described in laboratory workers who were caring for nude mice that had been injected with lymphocytic choriomeningitis virus–infected tumor cell lines.[13] Presumed routes of transmission are ingestion of food contaminated with animal urine and exposure of open wounds to dirt. No evidence of human-to-human transmission has been reported.

Herpesviruses

Herpesviruses are DNA viruses and include herpes simplex virus types 1 and 2, varicella-zoster virus, cytomegalovirus, Epstein-Barr virus, and human herpesviruses 6, 7, and 8. Although neurologic complications are known to occur with some of these viruses,[14-16] complications associated with herpes simplex viruses are of the most significance. Overall, herpes simplex viruses account for approximately 0.5% to 3% of all cases of aseptic meningitis.[17] In patients beyond the neonatal period, it is critical to differentiate between herpes simplex encephalitis, a potentially fatal form of encephalitis, and herpes simplex meningitis, a self-limited syndrome. The syndrome of herpes simplex virus aseptic meningitis is most commonly associated with primary genital infection with herpes simplex virus type 2[14]; in one study, an aseptic meningitis syndrome developed in 36% of women and 13% of men concomitant with primary infection.[14] Meningitis is less likely with recurrences of genital herpes.[18] Primary genital infection with herpes simplex virus type 1 and nonprimary genital infection with herpes simplex virus of either type rarely result in meningitis.[14] Acute aseptic meningitis has also been associated with herpes zoster in patients with or without typical skin lesions,[15] the latter known as *zoster sine herpete*. DNA of herpes simplex virus (HSV) has been detected in the CSF of 50 published cases of Mollaret's recurrent meningitis, almost all being HSV-2, although a few cases associated with HSV-1 and Epstein-Barr virus have been reported.[19-22] Human herpesvirus 6 has also been associated with meningitis[23] in conjunction with roseola infantum; however, this virus can exhibit persistence in the CNS and has been demonstrated in the CSF of asymptomatic persons.[24] Cytomegalovirus and Epstein-Barr virus may cause aseptic meningitis in association with a mononucleosis syndrome,[25] particularly in an immunocompromised host.

Human Immunodeficiency Virus

Human immunodeficiency virus (HIV) can cross the meninges early and persist in the CNS after initial infection.[26] Meningitis associated with HIV may occur as part of the primary infection or may occur in an already infected patient[27]; HIV has been isolated from the CSF in some of these cases. However, acute meningitis does not occur in every individual who becomes infected, and it can be silent. Retrospective studies have noted that an acute meningoencephalitis is observed in 5% to 10% of HIV-infected patients during or after the mononucleosis-like syndrome that heralds the initial infection.[26,28]

Bacterial Meningitis

Bacterial meningitis remains a very important disease worldwide. Data defining the frequency of isolation of specific meningeal pathogens in cases of bacterial meningitis in the United States are shown in Table 80-2.[29-31] The overall annual attack rate for bacterial meningitis, as defined by a surveillance study of 27 states in the United States from 1978 through 1981, was approximately 3.0 cases per 100,000 population, although variability based on age, race, and sex was noted.[29] Unfortunately, there was significant underreporting in this study because no active effort was undertaken to detect cases. The three most common meningeal pathogens, *Haemophilus influenzae*, *Neisseria meningitidis*, and *Streptococcus pneumoniae*, accounted for more than 80% of cases. In a surveillance study conducted during 1995 in laboratories serving all the acute care hospitals in 22 counties of four states (>10 million population), the incidence of bacterial meningitis decreased dramatically.[31] This decrease, which was a result of a vaccine-related decline in meningitis caused by *H. influenzae* type B

TABLE 80-2 Etiology of Bacterial Meningitis in the United States

Organism	Percentage of Total Cases		
	1978-1981[29]	*1986*[30]	*1995*[31]
Haemophilus influenzae	48	45	7
Neisseria meningitidis	20	14	25
Streptococcus pneumoniae	13	18	47
Streptococcus agalactiae	3	6	12
Listeria monocytogenes	2	3	8
Other	8	14	—
Unknown	6	—	—

TABLE 80-4 Etiology of Bacterial Meningitis in Selected Series outside the United States

Organism	Percentage of Total Cases		
	United Kingdom (1980-1984)[36]	*Dakar, Senegal (1970-1979)*[37]	*Salvador, Brazil (1973-1982)*[38]
Haemophilus influenzae	29	20	23
Neisseria meningitidis	25	11	22
Streptococcus pneumoniae	20	29	17
Streptococcus agalactiae	7	4	—
Listeria monocytogenes	2	<0.5	—
Other	16	9	20
Unknown	—	26	18

(from 2.9 cases per 100,000 population in 1986 to 0.2 cases per 100,000 population in 1995),[30,31] means that in the United States, bacterial meningitis is now a disease predominantly of adults rather than of infants and children.

In patients 16 years old or older, the relative frequency of isolation of meningeal pathogens in patients with community-acquired bacterial meningitis is somewhat different (Table 80-3),[32-35] with most cases caused by *S. pneumoniae*, *N. meningitidis*, and *Listeria monocytogenes*. Case-fatality rates for single episodes of community-acquired meningitis were 25% in one study.[33] Risk factors for death among patients with community-acquired meningitis included age 60 years or older, obtunded mental status on admission, and seizures within the first 24 hours.

Bacterial meningitis is also a significant problem in hospitalized patients. In one review of 493 episodes of bacterial meningitis in adults 16 years old or older at the Massachusetts General Hospital from 1962 through 1988, 40% of episodes were nosocomial in origin, with most cases (38%) caused by gram-negative bacilli.[33] The overall case-fatality rate for patients with single episodes of nosocomial meningitis was 35% and did not vary significantly over the 27 years of the study.

In addition, bacterial meningitis is a major problem in other areas of the world (Table 80-4).[36-38] The largest review, of approximately 4100 cases of bacterial meningitis at Hospital Couta Maia in Salvador, Brazil, from 1973 through 1982, revealed an attack rate of 45.8 cases per 100,000 population.[38] The overall case-fatality rate was 33%, with 50% of deaths occurring within 48 hours of hospitalization. *H. influenzae*, *N. meningitidis*, and *S. pneumoniae* accounted for 62% of the cases and 70% of the deaths. The case-fatality rates for meningitis caused by Enterobacteriaceae was 86%; more than half of the cases in children younger than 24 months were caused by *Salmonella*, an unusual meningeal pathogen in industrialized nations.

The likely etiologic agents of bacterial meningitis vary according to the age and underlying disease status of the patient (Table 80-5). The following paragraphs review the epidemiology and etiology of specific meningeal pathogens.

Haemophilus influenzae

H. influenzae was previously isolated in 45% to 48% of all cases of bacterial meningitis in the United States[29,30]; this organism is now isolated in only 7% of cases.[31] The overall mortality rate is 3% to 6%.[29-31] Most episodes of meningitis previously occurred in infants and children younger than 6 years (peak incidence of 6 to 12 months), with 90% of cases caused by capsular type B strains. Isolation of this organism in older children and adults should suggest the presence of certain underlying conditions, including sinusitis, otitis media, epiglottitis, pneumonia, diabetes mellitus, alcoholism, splenectomy or asplenic states, head trauma with CSF leak, and immune deficiency (e.g., hypogammaglobulinemia).[39-41] A profound reduction has been seen in the incidence of invasive infections (including bacterial meningitis) caused by *H. influenzae* type B in the United States and Western Europe.[42] This decrease in infection is attributed, in part, to the widespread use of conjugate vaccines against *H. influenzae* type B that have been licensed for routine use in all children beginning at 2 months of age. The number of cases of *H. influenzae* type B meningitis since the introduction of vaccination has decreased more than

TABLE 80-3 Etiology of Bacterial Meningitis in Patients 16 Years of Age and Older

Organism	Percentage of Total Cases			
	United States (1962-1988)[33]	*Iceland (1975-1994)*[32]	*Canada (1985-1995)*[34]	*United States (1970-1998)*[35]
Haemophilus influenzae	4	5	8	4
Neisseria meningitidis	14	56	2	14
Streptococcus pneumoniae	38	20	53	48
Listeria monocytogenes	11	6	25	7
Other*	20	—	12	27
Unknown	13	8	—	—

*Includes gram-negative bacilli, streptococci, enterococci, *Staphylococcus aureus*, anaerobes, and diphtheroids.

TABLE 80-5 Relationship between Common Bacterial Pathogens and Factors Predisposing to Meningitis

Predisposing Factor	Bacterial Pathogens
Age	
<1 mo	*Streptococcus agalactiae, Escherichia coli, Listeria monocytogenes, Klebsiella pneumoniae*
1-23 mo	*S. agalactiae, E. coli, Haemophilus influenzae, Streptococcus pneumoniae, Neisseria meningitidis*
2-50 yr	*S. pneumoniae, N. meningitidis*
>50 yr	*S. pneumoniae, N. meningitidis, L. monocytogenes,* aerobic gram-negative bacilli
Immunocompromised state	*S. pneumoniae, N. meningitidis, L. monocytogenes,* aerobic gram-negative bacilli (including *Pseudomonas aeruginosa*)
Basilar skull fracture	*S. pneumoniae, H. influenzae,* group A β-hemolytic streptococci
Head trauma; postneurosurgery	*Staphylococcus aureus, Staphylococcus epidermidis,* aerobic gram-negative bacilli (including *P. aeruginosa*)

90%.[43-47] However, in developing countries, because of vaccine expense, the results are not as dramatic.

Neisseria meningitidis

N. meningitidis most commonly causes meningitis in children and young adults and is associated with an overall mortality rate of 3% to 13%.[29-31] Meningococci of serogroups B, C, and Y account for most of the endemic disease in the United States. During an active and ongoing, laboratory-based, population-based surveillance for meningococcal disease in the United States from 1992 to 1996, serogroup C caused 35%, serogroup B caused 32%, and serogroup Y caused 26% of cases.[48] In contrast, serogroup B accounted for 75% of isolates in Italy in a recent study.[49] Disease caused by serogroups A and C may occur in epidemics; group Y strains may be associated with pneumonia. Several outbreaks of disease caused by serogroup C meningococci have been reported in the United States, Canada, and Europe, with most caused by one strain of electrophoretic type 37 (ET-37) termed ET-15.[50-52] Isolates of the ET-37 complex were also responsible for most cases of sporadic serogroup C meningococcal disease in another study.[53] During the outbreak of meningococcal disease coinciding with the Hajj pilgrimage in March 2000, the attack rate of W135 disease was 25 cases per 100,000 pilgrims[54]; all outbreak-associated isolates of serogroup W135 were members of a single clone of the hypervirulent ET-37 complex, which occurred as the result of expansion of a clone that had been in circulation since 1970.[55] Respiratory tract infections, with viruses such as influenza virus, may play a role in the pathogenesis of invasive meningococcal disease.[56] Nasopharyngeal carriage of *N. meningitidis* is an important factor that leads to the development of invasive disease.[57] Patients with deficiencies in the terminal complement components (C5, C6, C7, C8, and perhaps C9), the so-called membrane attack complex, have a markedly increased incidence of neisserial infection,[58-60] including that caused by *N. meningitidis*, although mortality rates in patients with meningococcal disease are lower than those in patients with an intact complement system (3% versus 19% in the general population). An increased risk of invasive meningococcal disease has also been described in a Dutch family with dysfunctional properdin,[61] which suggests a potential role for the alternative pathway in complement-mediated resistance against meningococci. Because meningococcal meningitis occurs in approximately 39% of persons with late complement component deficiencies and 6% of those with properdin deficiencies, it has been suggested that a screening test for complement function (i.e., CH_{50}) should be performed for all patients who have invasive meningococcal infections, with consideration of direct assessment of terminal complement components and properdin proteins.[62]

Streptococcus pneumoniae

S. pneumoniae, the most frequently observed etiologic agent of bacterial meningitis in the United States, now accounts for 47% of the total cases[31]; the mortality rate ranges from 19% to 26%.[29-31] Of the more than 90 known pneumococcal serotypes, 18 are responsible for 82% of the cases of bacteremic pneumococcal pneumonia, with a close correlation between bacteremic subtypes and those implicated in meningitis. Patients often have contiguous or distant foci of pneumococcal infection such as pneumonia, otitis media, mastoiditis, sinusitis, and endocarditis. Serious infection may be observed in patients with various underlying conditions (e.g., splenectomy or asplenic states, multiple myeloma, hypogammaglobulinemia, alcoholism, malnutrition, chronic liver or renal disease, malignancy, and diabetes mellitus).[63-66] In children who develop second episodes of pneumococcal meningitis, screening for congenital immunoglobulin deficiencies should be performed.[62] The pneumococcus is the most common etiologic agent of meningitis in patients who have suffered basilar skull fracture with CSF leak.[67]

Listeria monocytogenes

L. monocytogenes causes 8% of cases of bacterial meningitis in the United States and carries a mortality rate of 15% to 29%.[29-31]

Serotypes 1/2b and 4b have been implicated in up to 80% of meningitis cases caused by this organism. *Listeria* has been isolated from dust, soil, water, sewage, and decaying vegetable matter (including animal feed and silage). Listerial infection is most common in infants younger than 1 month (up to 10% of cases), adults older than 60 years, alcoholics, cancer patients, those receiving corticosteroid therapy, and immunosuppressed adults (e.g., renal transplant recipients).[68-71] Other predisposing conditions include diabetes mellitus, liver disease, chronic renal disease, collagen-vascular diseases, and conditions associated with iron overload. Recently, *Listeria* meningitis has been reported in a patient with Crohn's disease after treatment with infliximab.[72] Although colonization rates are low, pregnant women (who account for 25% of all cases of listeriosis) may harbor the organism asymptomatically in their genital tract and rectum and transmit the infection to their infants. *Listeria* meningitis is found infrequently in patients with HIV infection[73,74] despite its increased incidence in patients with deficiencies in cell-mediated immunity. Adults less than 50 years of age who present with *Listeria* meningitis should be screened for HIV infection.[62] Meningitis can also occur in previously healthy adults.[75] Outbreaks of *Listeria* infection have been associated with the consumption of contaminated coleslaw, raw vegetables, milk, and cheese, with sporadic cases traced to contaminated cheese, turkey franks, alfalfa tablets, and processed meats, thus pointing to the intestinal tract as the usual portal of entry.[68-70]

Streptococcus agalactiae

Group B streptococcus is a common cause of meningitis in neonates,[76] with 52% of all cases in the United States reported during the first month of life.[31] In the United States, the overall mortality rate ranges from 7% to 27%.[29-31] Group B streptococcus has been isolated from the vaginal or rectal cultures of 15% to 35% of asymptomatic pregnant women[77]; colonization rates do not vary during pregnancy, and carriage may be chronic (40%), transient, or intermittent. The risk of transmission from mother to infant is increased when the inoculum of organisms and the number of sites of maternal colonization are increased; the route of delivery does not influence transmission. Horizontal transmission has also been documented from the hands of nursery personnel to the infant. Most cases of neonatal meningitis are caused by subtype III organisms and occur after the first week of life. Group B streptococcus can also cause meningitis in adults.[78-81] Risk factors in adults include age greater than 60 years, diabetes mellitus, pregnancy or the postpartum state, cardiac disease, collagen-vascular diseases, malignancy, alcoholism, hepatic failure, renal failure, previous stroke, neurogenic bladder, decubitus ulcers, and corticosteroid therapy; in one review of group B streptococcal meningitis in adults, no underlying illnesses were found in 43% of patients.[79]

Aerobic Gram-Negative Bacilli

Aerobic gram-negative bacilli (e.g., *Klebsiella* species, *Escherichia coli*, *Serratia marcescens*, *Pseudomonas aeruginosa*, *Salmonella* species) have become increasingly important as etiologic agents in patients with bacterial meningitis.[82-85] These agents may be isolated from the CSF of patients after head trauma or neurosurgical procedures[86-89] and may also be found in neonates, older adults, immunosuppressed patients, and patients with gram-negative septicemia. Some cases have been associated with disseminated strongyloidiasis in the hyperinfection syndrome, a condition in which meningitis caused by enteric bacteria occurs secondary to seeding of the meninges during persistent or recurrent bacteremias associated with the migration of infective larvae.[90] Alternatively, the larvae may carry enteric organisms on their surfaces or within their own gastrointestinal tracts as they exit the intestine and subsequently invade the meninges. In patients with *E. coli* meningitis, 75% of cases are caused by strains possessing the K1 antigen.[76] Almost half of pregnant women have this organism isolated on rectal culture, and as many as 75% of their infants will be colonized during the first days of life; horizontal transmission from nursery staff members or other infants has also been reported.

Staphylococci

Meningitis caused by *Staphylococcus aureus* is usually found in early postneurosurgical or post-trauma patients and in those with CSF shunts; other underlying conditions include diabetes mellitus, alcoholism, chronic renal failure requiring hemodialysis, injection drug use, and malignancies.[91-94] Thirty-five percent of cases are observed in the setting of head trauma or after neurosurgery, and an additional 20% of patients have underlying infective endocarditis or paraspinal infection. Other sources of community-acquired *S. aureus* meningitis include patients with sinusitis, osteomyelitis, and pneumonia. Mortality rates have ranged from 14% to 77% in various series. *Staphylococcus epidermidis* is the most common cause of meningitis in patients with CSF shunts (see Chapter 81).[95]

Other Bacteria

A review of 28 cases of nocardial meningitis revealed predisposing conditions in approximately 75% of patients,[96] including immunosuppressive drug therapy, malignancy, head trauma, CNS procedures, chronic granulomatous disease, and sarcoidosis. Anaerobic meningitis is unusual and is generally associated with contiguous foci of infection (e.g., otitis, sinusitis, pharyngitis, brain abscess, head and neck malignancy, recent head and neck surgery or wound infection, and CNS trauma and neurosurgery[97-100]); in many cases, more than one organism may be recovered. Enterococci are unusual etiologic agents of bacterial meningitis; most adult patients have underlying illnesses, and disease is often associated with immunosuppressive therapy, CNS trauma or surgery, or an enterococcal infection outside the CNS.[101] Despite the frequency with which the viridans streptococci cause bacteremia, they are unusual causes of meningitis (0.3% to 5% of culture-proven cases) (see Chapter 200).[102] Group A streptococcal meningitis is also unusual, generally seen in association with pharyngitis, otitis media, and sinusitis.[103] Diphtheroids, particularly *Propionibacterium acnes,* have become important etiologic agents of meningitis in patients with CNS shunt infections (see Chapter 203).[95] With continued increases in numbers of immunocompromised patients and use of invasive diagnostic or therapeutic devices within the CNS, other (more unusual) bacterial pathogens may be reported as etiologic agents of acute meningitis.

Spirochetal Meningitis

Treponema pallidum

T. pallidum disseminates to the CNS during early infection.[104] The organism can be isolated from the CSF of patients with primary syphilis, and CSF laboratory abnormalities are detected in 5% to 9% of patients with seronegative primary syphilis. The actual rate of invasion of the CNS during these early stages is likely to be considerably higher, however. Clinical neurosyphilis can be divided into four distinct syndromes[104]: syphilitic meningitis, meningovascular syphilis, parenchymatous neurosyphilis, and gummatous neurosyphilis. Some overlap may be seen in the clinical and laboratory findings of these syndromes. The incidence of syphilitic meningitis is greatest in the first 2 years after infection and is estimated to occur in only 0.3% to 2.4% of untreated syphilis cases. In contrast, meningovascular syphilis is found in 10% to 12% of individuals with CNS involvement[104,105] and occurs months to years after syphilis acquisition (peak incidence, approximately 7 years). Parenchymatous neurosyphilis has two variants, general paresis and tabes dorsalis. Both are relatively rare today and do not become apparent until 10 to 20 years after the acquisition of infection. Gummas are late manifestations of tertiary syphilis and may occur anywhere[104]; gummatous neurosyphilis is rare.

The overall incidence of neurosyphilis has increased, with many of the cases reported seen in patients with HIV infection.[106-108] In one report,[109] 44% of all patients with neurosyphilis had acquired immunodeficiency syndrome (AIDS); the remaining patients, who may have had HIV infection without AIDS, were not addressed in this report. The study also showed that 1.5% of patients with AIDS were found to have neurosyphilis at some point during the course of their disease. In a more recent review of neurosyphilis cases during the HIV era in San Francisco from 1985 to 1992, neurosyphilis was identified in young patients most often with HIV coinfection.[110]

Borrelia burgdorferi

The nervous system is eventually involved clinically in at least 10% to 15% of patients with Lyme disease, either while erythema migrans is still present or 1 to 6 months later.[111-113] A 1992 study used polymerase chain reaction (PCR) to detect spirochetal DNA in CSF samples from 8 of 12 patients with acute (<2 weeks) disseminated Lyme borreliosis,[114] which indicates that *B. burgdorferi* usually invades the CNS early in infection.

Protozoal and Helminthic Meningitis

Amebas

Despite the hundreds of species of free-living amebas that are known, only a few have been reported to infect humans.[115,116] The most important are in the genera *Naegleria* and *Acanthamoeba. Naegleria fowleri,* the main protozoan causing primary amebic meningoencephalitis in humans, has been recovered from lakes, puddles, pools, ponds, rivers, sewage sludge, tap water, air conditioner drains, and soil. Sporadic cases of primary amebic meningoencephalitis occur when persons, usually children and young adults, swim or play in water containing the amebas, or when swimming pools or water supplies have become contaminated, often through failure of chlorination. Asymptomatic carriage by humans can also occur. The incidence of infection is unknown, although a study of Florida lakes reported only seven documented cases of primary amebic meningoencephalitis in over 1 billion swimming episodes.[117] Several cases have been reported in HIV-infected patients, all with advanced HIV disease at the time of amebic infection.[118-120]

Angiostrongylus cantonensis

Infection of humans by larvae of the nematode *A. cantonensis* can lead to the development of an eosinophilic meningitis.[90,121,122] Humans become infected by eating infected intermediate (i.e., mollusks, such as snails and slugs) or paratenic (i.e., freshwater prawns, crabs, frogs, and planaria) hosts, or by eating food such as leafy green vegetables contaminated by these hosts.[123] The larvae invade the brain either directly from the blood stream or after migrating through other organs before reaching the spinal cord and brain. Once in the CNS, the larvae mature into adult worms that migrate through the brain. *A. cantonensis* is widespread and human infection is fairly common and reported from many parts of the world (Thailand, India, Malaysia, Vietnam, Indonesia, Papua New Guinea, Taiwan, and the Pacific Islands, including Hawaii).[90,121,123,124] The parasites may spread to many countries by rats moving freely from port to port on ships[121]; the rat infection rate in urban Bangkok has reached about 40%. More recently, cases have been reported in areas not previously considered risk regions. A large outbreak of *A. cantonensis* meningitis was recently described in North America in travelers who had visited the Caribbean[125]; in this outbreak, the lettuce in a Caesar salad shared by the case patients was the most likely mode of transmission. After this outbreak, parasitologic surveys documented *A. cantonensis* in the Jamaican rat and land snail populations.[126] Therefore, tourists and visitors to endemic areas are at risk of becoming infected with *A. cantonensis.*

Baylisascaris procyonis, a roundworm infection of raccoons, is emerging as an important helminthic zoonosis, principally affecting young children.[127] The parasite is widely distributed in raccoons in North America, and infected raccoons shed millions of *B. procyonis* eggs daily in their feces. This larval infection can invade the CNS, resulting in an eosinophilic meningoencephalitis. This parasite is discussed in more detail in Chapter 289.

PATHOGENESIS AND PATHOPHYSIOLOGY

Viral Meningitis

Initiation of Infection

After the colonization of selected mucosal surfaces in the body by various viruses, the host possesses numerous barriers to prevent viral entry.[128] For example, the respiratory tract contains a thin film of mucus and a mucociliary elevator that moves viral particles away from the lower respiratory tract; even if this barrier is crossed, alveolar macrophages are actively phagocytic for viral particles. Gastric acidity inactivates most swallowed viruses, and gastrointestinal enzymes and bile also disrupt viral envelopes, capsid proteins, and lipoprotein membranes; however, some nonenveloped, acid-resistant viruses (e.g., enteroviruses, adenoviruses, reoviruses, parvoviruses) are adapted for replication in the gastrointestinal tract. When the host has had previous contact with the viral agent, the mucosa of the gastrointestinal and respiratory tracts may be coated with secretory immunoglobulin A (IgA), which neutralizes the virus and prevents attachment and subsequent cell penetration. If certain viruses are able to escape initial host defense mechanisms, they may replicate and disseminate with the potential for CNS invasion.

Viremia and Central Nervous System Invasion

After hematogenous dissemination of the virus, CNS infection may occur. Most neurotropic viruses first multiply at extraneural sites (initially at the portal of entry), establish viremia, and then cross the blood-brain barrier (BBB) to invade the CNS.[129,130] For example, enteroviruses initially multiply in the peritonsillar lymphatics, Peyer's patches, the lamina propria of the intestine, and vascular and endothelial cells, depending on the particular agent. M cells may mediate virus penetration from the gut lumen to lymphoid cells. From this initial site, the virus then disseminates to vascular tissue (e.g., liver, spleen, and muscle), where further multiplication augments the viremia.[131] After viremia, viral particles are normally cleared by the reticuloendothelial system, with the speed of removal directly related to virus size (i.e., large viruses are cleared more promptly from the blood stream). Viruses may also elude host clearance by associating with certain cells. Some viruses (e.g., measles, herpes, mumps) grow in human leukocytes, which protects them from phagocytosis by the reticuloendothelial system, neutralization by circulating antibody, and inactivation by nonspecific serum inhibitors.

CNS invasion by viruses may occur via several mechanisms. Most viruses invade directly across cerebral capillary endothelial cells, the major site of the BBB. Some viruses directly infect cerebral microvascular endothelial cells before infection of adjacent glia and neurons,[131] whereas others initially infect glia without evidence of endothelial cell infection. Still other viruses may be carried between cerebral endothelial cells in infected leukocytes after BBB disruption. Another site of virus entry is the choroid plexus epithelium. Studies of mumps virus in hamsters have shown a sequence of infection from the choroid plexus to the ependyma to parenchymal cells; viral nucleocapsids have been found in the choroid plexus and ependymal cells of humans with mumps meningitis.

Viruses may reach the CNS by spread along olfactory nerves.[128,129,131,132] In an experimental hamster model,[128] intranasal inoculation of herpes simplex virus and togaviruses led to early infection of the olfactory bulb, which could be inhibited by cutting the olfactory tracts or chemical treatment of the olfactory mucosa. Peripheral nerve spread by viruses may also lead to CNS invasion. One study used a transgenic mouse model to demonstrate that after intramuscular inoculation of poliovirus in the limb, infectious poliovirus was first detected in the inferior segment of the spinal cord and then in the superior segment and the brain,[133] thus suggesting that poliovirus initially spreads to the CNS through peripheral nerve pathways.

Virus Spread within the Central Nervous System

Regardless of the mechanism of CNS invasion, the production of disease requires viral attachment to and penetration of susceptible cells, spread within the nervous system, and induction of cellular changes. Viral entry into the subarachnoid space via the choroid plexus leads to dispersion of virus within CSF in contact with meningeal and ependymal cells[128]; sequential spread of virus may then occur in a contiguous fashion to glia and neurons. Other viruses spread through extracellular gaps between cells and CNS processes (e.g., dendrites, axons, or glia), or they transit along the extensive axonal and dendritic ramifications of neurons by way of the glia, or they are carried by mobile leukocytes in the inflammatory response. Experimental evidence supports each mode of transit, and all may be involved to various degrees in different viral infections.

Once viral infection of the CNS occurs, inflammatory cells usually accumulate, although the mechanisms leading to recruitment of inflammatory cells and their role in viral CNS infections are only partially understood.[128,129] It appears that the initial inflammatory response is immunologically specific and consists of a population of lymphocytes sensitized by the virus. However, an inflammatory response may fail to develop in other viral CNS infections, and this may be dependent on host age rather than the virus itself. Sensitized lymphocytes probably respond to a virus-specific protein that diffuses or is transported to the luminal surface of the endothelium, with subsequent passage through endothelial cells and release of inflammatory cytokines. In an experimental mouse model of meningitis caused by lymphocytic choriomeningitis virus,[134] elevated CSF concentrations of interleukin (IL)-6 and interferon (IFN)-γ were demonstrated. CSF IL-6 concentrations began to rise 24 hours after intracerebral infection, followed by a rapid increase after day 4. IFN-γ was not detected in CSF until 5 to 6 days after infection, but then it markedly increased. CSF concentrations of these cytokines were only slightly and transiently elevated in athymic nude mice. In one review, IFN-γ was also detectable in the CSF in 75% of 16 patients with enteroviral meningitis,[135] with more consistent production and higher titers noted with coxsackievirus than with echovirus. Elevated CSF IL-6 concentrations were also detected in 12 of 15 samples from patients with acute aseptic meningitis.[134] More recently, CSF concentrations of IL-6 were found to be elevated during the initial stage (first 2 days) of enterovirus 71 CNS infection; cardiopulmonary failure or pulmonary edema also occurred during the early stage of enterovirus 71 CNS involvement.[136] Therefore, the systemic inflammatory response, coupled with CNS inflammation, may play an important role in the development of enterovirus 71–related pulmonary edema.

Other inflammatory cytokines have been measured in the CSF of patients with aseptic meningitis. In one study, CSF concentrations of tumor necrosis factor-α (TNF-α) and IL-1β were measured in 36 patients with aseptic meningitis, 13 of whom had culture-proven enteroviral meningitis, and in 14 controls.[137] None of the samples from the patients with aseptic meningitis or controls had detectable TNF-α activity, whereas 86% of patients with aseptic meningitis had detectable CSF IL-1β concentrations; only 2 of 14 control patients had elevated concentrations. The increased CSF IL-1β concentrations correlated with CSF white blood cell counts.

After development of a CSF inflammatory response, alterations in the BBB permit the traversal into CSF of serum proteins, including immunoglobulins. In addition, local CNS immunoglobulin synthesis occurs as B cells enter the CSF and differentiate into plasma cells. Intracerebral synthesis of immunoglobulins also occurs and is reflected by an increase in the CSF-to-serum ratios of specific immunoglobulins that persist for several weeks after infection.[128] The production of oligoclonal IgG proteins within the CNS has been demonstrated in patients with meningitis caused by mumps virus, varicella-zoster virus, and HIV.[12,15,138,139] Furthermore, elevated CSF concentrations of oligoclonal IgG may persist for up to 1 year in patients with mumps meningitis,[12] which suggests the possibility of viral persistence and ongoing antigenic stimulation.

An intact host immune response appears to be important for clearance of virus from the CNS[128,129]; T-cell responses appear to be more important than B-cell responses. Failure of an immune response to develop may be a result of immunologic tolerance, host immune defects, or the ability of the virus to escape immune surveillance. Chronic infections with varicella-zoster virus, cytomegalovirus, adenovirus, and measles virus have developed in patients with depressed cell-mediated immunity.

Bacterial Meningitis

Numerous investigations over the last 40 years have elucidated many of the pathogenic and pathophysiologic mechanisms operable in bacterial meningitis.[140-144] Figure 80-1 shows a simplistic hypothetical scheme of these mechanisms, which are discussed in greater detail in the following paragraphs.

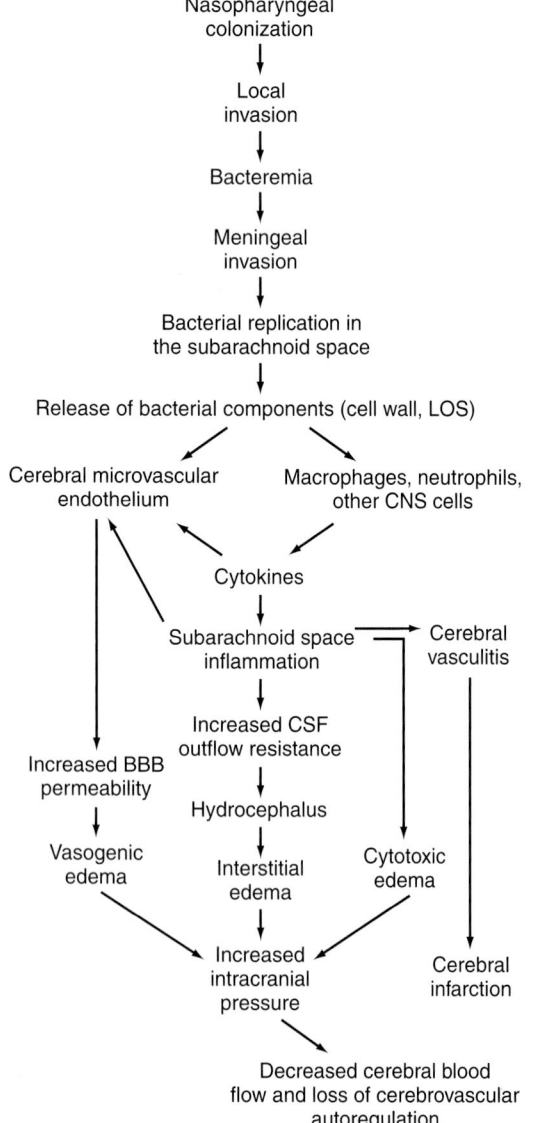

FIGURE 80-1. Pathogenesis and pathophysiology of bacterial meningitis. BBB, blood-brain barrier; IL-1, interleukin-1; LOS, lipo-oligosaccharide. *(From Tunkel AR, Scheld WM. Pathogenesis and pathophysiology of bacterial meningitis. Clin Microbiol Rev. 1993;6:118-136, with permission.)*

Mucosal Colonization and Systemic Invasion

The early pathogenic events that result in bacterial meningitis depend on an interplay between specific virulence factors and host defense mechanisms (Table 80-6). The initiation of infection with meningeal pathogens usually begins with host acquisition of a new organism by nasopharyngeal colonization.[145] Many of the major meningeal pathogens possess surface characteristics that enhance mucosal colonization. For example, the fimbriae (or pili) of *N. meningitidis* mediate adherence of this organism to nasopharyngeal epithelial cells; these fimbriated strains accounted for 80% of primary meningococcal isolates from nasopharyngeal carriers and from the CSF of patients with meningococcal meningitis,[142] although all fimbriae were lost on serial subculture in the laboratory. The fimbriae appear morphologically as aggregated bundles or single filaments. Aggregated bundles are found primarily among disease isolates exhibiting a low degree of adherence to human buccal epithelial cells, whereas the single filaments have medium to high adherence characteristics and are found predominantly among colonizing isolates. Once meningococci attach to nonciliated nasopharyngeal epithelial cells via a specific cell surface receptor (most likely CD46), they are transported across these cells within a phagocytic vacuole[145]; this process appears to be essential for the subsequent development of invasive meningococcal disease.

Fimbriae have also been implicated in the attachment of *H. influenzae* to upper respiratory tract epithelial cells,[142] although fimbriae have not been found on isolates from the CSF or blood of patients with invasive disease. This observation suggests that although fimbriae play an initial role in adherence of *H. influenzae* within the nasopharynx, their presence is not necessary for the development of invasive disease, including meningitis. Furthermore, the type of fimbriae expressed by *H. influenzae* type B strains may facilitate adherence to select nasopharyngeal sites: α-fimbriae enhance adherence in the anterior of the nasopharynx, whereas β-fimbriae facilitate the process more posteriorly. In addition, acquisition and colonization by *H. influenzae* type B may be promoted after respiratory tract infection by viral agents such as the influenza A/Victoria virus and respiratory syncytial virus, although the precise role of a preceding upper respiratory viral infection in the enhancement of nasopharyngeal colonization by *H. influenzae* type B is controversial. After nasopharyngeal colonization, invasion into the blood stream by *H. influenzae* appears to occur via a breakdown in the tight junctions between epithelial cells (in contrast to *N. meningitidis,* which invades via parasite-directed endocytosis), thereby leading to invasion by an intercellular mechanism.[145]

Surface encapsulation may also be an important virulence factor for nasopharyngeal colonization and systemic invasion of meningeal pathogens. Among the six encapsulated types of *H. influenzae* (A through F), type B strains constitute less than 5% of nasopharyngeal isolates but cause more than 95% of systemic and meningeal infections.[142,143] In an experimental infant rat model, it has been demonstrated that although all encapsulated strains of *H. influenzae* had the potential for systemic invasion after intraperitoneal inoculation, type B strains were the most virulent and were the only capsular types capable of systemic invasion after intranasal inoculation. Indeed, antibodies to type B capsule, which are almost uniformly detected in humans by the age of 4 years even in the absence of known exposure to *H. influenzae* type B, are protective against invasive disease. Polysaccharide capsule may also be an important virulence factor for the development of invasive disease by *S. pneumoniae*. In addition, in vivo capsular transformation events may equip pneumococcal strains with highly virulent blood-invasive phenotypes, thereby increasing the seriousness of pneumococcal infection, especially that caused by multidrug-resistant strains.[146]

Adherence of microorganisms to mucosal surfaces may be inhibited by natural antibodies found in mucosal secretions, such as IgA. However, it appears that the presence of high concentrations of circulating IgA antibodies to *N. meningitidis* may permit the development or progression of invasive disease by preferentially binding to the organism and blocking the beneficial effects of IgG and IgM antibodies.[142] In addition, species of many pathogenic bacteria (e.g., *Neisseria, Haemophilus, Streptococcus*) produce IgA$_1$ proteases that cleave IgA in the hinge region and facilitate the adherence of bacterial strains to mucosal surfaces through local destruction of IgA. However, the exact role of IgA protease production in this pathogenic sequence remains unclear. The presence of anticapsular polysaccharide antibodies may also be effective in decreasing nasopharyngeal carriage of meningeal pathogens. In an intralitter transmission model in which infant rats were intranasally inoculated with *S. pneumoniae* and placed in a cage with other infant rats, pretreatment of uninoculated rats with systemic IgG antibodies to pneumococcal polysaccharide reduced the intralitter transmission of *S. pneumoniae*,[147] which suggests that IgG antibodies to pneumococcal polysaccharide may be sufficient to reduce pneumococcal nasopharyngeal carriage in humans.

Intravascular Survival

Once bacteria cross the mucosal barrier and gain access to the blood stream, they must overcome additional host defense mechanisms to survive. The presence of bacterial capsule, by effectively inhibiting neutrophil phagocytosis and resisting classic complement–mediated bactericidal activity, may enhance blood-stream survival of the organism, thereby facilitating intravascular replication.[142] The most common meningeal pathogens *(H. influenzae, N. meningitidis, S. pneumoniae, E. coli, S. agalactiae)* are all encapsulated. In addition, certain capsular types are disproportionately associated with the development of meningitis. For example, about 84% of cases of neonatal meningitis caused by *E. coli* are caused by strains bearing the K1 antigen; in the absence of specific host antibody to the K1 capsule, these organisms are profoundly resistant to phagocytosis. Presence of the K1 capsule and a high degree of bacteremia are key determinants in the development of *E. coli* meningitis.[148] Recently, it has been shown that *E. coli* strain C5, which causes neonatal meningitis, harbors a pathogenicity island designated PAI I$_{C5}$ that contributes to the pathogenicity of *E. coli* meningitis by causing a high-grade bacteremia,[149] although further studies are needed to determine the importance of this factor in the development of *E. coli* meningitis.

The host possesses several defense mechanisms to counteract the antiphagocytic effects of bacterial capsule.[142] For example, activation of the alternative complement pathway by the capsular polysaccharide of *S. pneumoniae* results in the cleavage of C3 with attachment of C3 to the bacterial surface. This series of events facilitates opsonization, phagocytosis, and intravascular clearance of the organism. Impairment of the alternative complement pathway (e.g., in patients with sickle cell anemia and those who have undergone splenectomy) predisposes to the development of pneumococcal meningitis. *H. influenzae* type B also activates the complement cascade. Experimental studies in a rat model have shown that after intravenous or intraperitoneal challenge with *H. influenzae* of varying serotypes (A, B, C, or D), a greater incidence and magnitude of bacteremia developed in rats depleted of C3. Although the incidence of bacteremia caused by type B organisms increased from 63% to 95% in complement-depleted rats, the incidence and severity of meningitis were unaffected by complement depletion.

Complement system activation is also an essential host defense mechanism against invasive disease caused by *N. meningitidis*. Patients with deficiencies in the membrane attack complex are particularly prone to neisserial infections, although usually with a more favorable

outcome when appropriate therapy is instituted.[58] The reasons for the worse outcome in patients with an intact complement system are unclear, although a qualitative relationship can be shown between the concentration of circulating meningococcal lipo-oligosaccharide, a fatal outcome, and the degree of complement activation.[142]

Meningeal Invasion

The mechanisms by which meningeal pathogens gain access to the CNS remain unknown. The development of a sustained, high-grade bacteremia has been suggested as one important factor.[142,143] In one study, culture-positive meningitis was produced in an experimental infant rat model only after an intense bacteremia had been present for at least 6 hours. However, sustained bacteremia cannot be the sole factor responsible for meningeal invasion, because many other organisms (e.g., viridans streptococci) that produce high-grade bacteremia during infective endocarditis rarely produce meningitis.

The site of CNS invasion by meningeal pathogens is also unclear. Early studies suggested that invasion from the blood stream was via the dural venous sinus system, whereas other experiments suggested that the site of invasion was above the cribriform plate or via the choroid plexus (because of their exceptionally high rate of blood flow of approximately 200 mL/g/min).[142,143] Experimental studies, however, have demonstrated that receptors for some meningeal pathogens are present on cells of the choroid plexus and cerebral capillaries. In cryostat sections of infant rat brain cortical slices, *E. coli* strains possessing S fimbriae have been shown to bind specifically to the luminal surfaces of the vascular endothelium and the epithelium lining the choroid plexus and brain ventricles. Phase variation to the nonfimbriated form may then be necessary for these bacteria to invade the CNS. To understand the cellular mechanisms important for meningeal invasion, the invasion of *E. coli* into endothelial and epithelial cell cultures was studied. It appeared that microtubule-dependent and/or microfilament-dependent pathways, which rearrange the cell cytoskeleton, may be important for bacterial uptake and crossing of the BBB.[150] *N. meningitidis* was also shown to adhere in vivo to the endothelium of both the choroid plexus and the meninges in a fatal case of meningococcemia[151]; isolates obtained from the CSF expressed significantly more PilC protein than did the blood isolates, which suggests that PilC plays an important role for this organism to cross the BBB. Despite these studies, the importance of adherence of meningeal pathogens to sites within the CNS requires further investigation.

To further assess the molecular mechanisms important in meningeal invasion, the ability of strains of *E. coli* to invade endothelial cells was determined. A gene (termed *ibe10*) has been cloned and found to encode an 8.2-kilodalton protein that permits *E. coli* to invade brain microvascular endothelial cells both in vitro and in vivo.[152] The prevalence of *ibe10* was also increased in *E. coli* isolates from CSF compared with those from feces or blood,[153] although further studies are needed to assess the role of this virulence determinant in meningeal invasion. In addition, the *aslA* gene product of *E. coli* K12 has been shown to have homology to the DNA adjacent to the Tn*phoA* insertion site, which potentially contributes to the invasion process of meningitic *E. coli* into the BBB.[154]

Another determinant that has been identified to contribute to invasion of *E. coli* across brain microvascular endothelial cells is outer membrane protein A (OmpA). Both *OmpA* and *ibe10* deletion mutants

TABLE 80-6 Factors Involved in the Pathogenesis of Bacterial Meningitis

Pathogenic Event	*Bacterial Factors*	*Host Factors*
Mucosal colonization	Fimbriae, polysaccharide capsule, IgA protease production, bacteriocins	Mucosal epithelium, secretory IgA, ciliary activity, anticapsular antibodies
Intravascular survival	Polysaccharide capsule	Complement activation, organism-specific antibodies
Meningeal invasion	Fimbriae, association with monocytes, ibe10, OmpA, platelet-activating factor receptor, pneumococcal choline binding protein A	Blood-brain barrier
Survival in the subarachnoid space	Polysaccharide capsule	Poor opsonic activity

of *E. coli* were less invasive in vivo and in vitro, indicating the importance of each of these factors in the ability of *E. coli* to cross the BBB, although their contributions were not additive.[155] OmpA appears to be the most important factor for *E. coli* invasion and has been shown to bind to a 95-kD human brain microvascular endothelial cell receptor, Ecgp[156]; the N-terminal sequence of Ecgp is identical to gp96, a cell-surface glycoprotein related to heat shock protein. This receptor is present on endothelial cells from brain, but not on endothelial cells from other organs. OmpA of *E. coli* was also shown to interact with a gp96-like molecule on human brain microvascular endothelial cells, an interaction necessary for invasion.[157] In addition, cytotoxic necrotizing factor (CNF)-1, a dermonecrotic protein toxin produced by human and animal isolates of *E. coli,* was found to contribute to invasion of *E. coli* K1 across brain microvascular endothelial cells in vitro and to traversal of *E. coli* across the BBB in an experimental hematogenous animal model[158]; this effect was dependent on RhoA activation, indicating the CNF-1 may also contribute to *E. coli* invasion of brain microvascular endothelial cells. Despite the results summarized here, none of these determinants is sufficient by itself to account for the virulence properties of *E. coli* strains causing neonatal meningitis,[159] indicating that further studies are needed to elucidate the factors responsible for CNS invasion of *E. coli* and other meningeal pathogens.

Another pathogenic mechanism postulated to promote CNS invasion by meningeal pathogens is association of the organism with circulating monocytes. Histologic and scanning microscopic techniques were used to examine the neuraxes of pigs inoculated with a strain of *Streptococcus suis* type 2,[142,143] and the only pathologic lesions detected were associated with the choroid plexus and were manifested as brush-border disruption, decrease in the number of Kolmer cells, and exudation of fibrin and inflammatory cells into the ventricles. Intracellular bacteria were demonstrated in the parenchyma of the choroid plexus, in ventricular monocytes, and within circulating peripheral blood monocytes, thus suggesting that bacteria may gain access to the CSF in association with monocytes migrating along normal pathways.

Transcytosis through microvascular endothelial cells has been investigated as another possible mechanism of meningeal invasion during bacterial meningitis. In an in vitro model using rat and human brain microvascular endothelial cells,[160] the transparent phase variants of pneumococci that gained access to an intracellular vesicle from the apical side of the microvascular endothelial cell monolayer were able to transcytose to the basal surface of these cells in a manner dependent on the platelet-activating factor (PAF) receptor and the presence of pneumococcal choline-binding protein A; the remaining transparent bacteria entering the cell underwent a previously unrecognized recycling to the apical surface. These data suggest that interaction of pneumococci with the PAF receptor results in sorting so that bacteria can be transcytosed across the cell, whereas non-PAF receptor entry shunts bacteria for exit and reentry on the apical surface. This bidirectional trafficking of pneumococci represents an important potential bioprobe to investigate transport across mammalian cells. Direct uptake by endothelial cells of circulating bacteria is another mechanism by which *L. monocytogenes* may cross the BBB.[161] In an electron micrographic study of human brain-stem tissue, bacteria have been observed within endothelial cells or adhering to the luminal surface of the microvascular endothelium, consistent with in vitro data showing the ability of *L. monocytogenes* to invade cultured human brain microvascular endothelial cells. The listerial surface protein InlB (of the internalin family) is required for this invasion, indicating that specific bacterial molecules are actively involved with BBB interaction.

Bacterial Survival within the Subarachnoid Space

Once meningeal pathogens enter the subarachnoid space, host defense mechanisms are generally inadequate to control the infection.[142] CSF concentrations of complement components are absent or minimal; meningeal inflammation leads to increased, but low, CSF complement concentrations. This relative complement deficiency may be of critical importance because specific antibody or complement, or both,

are essential for opsonization of encapsulated meningeal pathogens and efficient phagocytosis. Observations in experimental animal models and in patients with meningitis have revealed absent or barely detectable opsonic and bactericidal activity. The explanation for this low level of complement components during bacterial meningitis is unclear. It has been suggested that degradation of complement components crossing the BBB by leukocyte proteases may result in inefficient opsonic activity at the site of infection. Indeed, in an experimental rabbit model of pneumococcal meningitis, the intracisternal inoculation of a nonspecific protease inhibitor (phenylmethylsulfonyl fluoride) led to a decline in pneumococcal concentrations in CSF when compared with saline-inoculated controls.

Immunoglobulin concentrations are also low in normal CSF (blood-to-CSF ratio of IgG of about 800:1), and although concentrations increase during bacterial meningitis, they remain low in comparison to simultaneous serum concentrations.[142] In an experimental rabbit model, the intravenous administration of a bactericidal monoclonal antibody against the polyribosylribitol phosphate of *H. influenzae* type B produced high serum antibody concentrations, but BBB permeability was poor (5.5% or less), even in the presence of meningeal inflammation, which suggests that systemic administration of type-specific antibodies alone is likely to be suboptimal in therapy for bacterial meningitis.

Bacterial meningitis is characterized by the development of a neutrophilic pleocytosis within the CSF, although the precise mechanism of leukocyte traversal across the BBB is undefined.[142] The complement component C5a has been suggested to be one chemotactic component, with chemotactic activity appearing 2 to 4 hours before neutrophil influx into CSF. In an experimental rabbit model, the intracisternal inoculation of C5a led to an influx of leukocytes into CSF 1 hour after inoculation, a response that was attenuated by co-administration of prostaglandin E_2 (PGE_2) in a dose- and time-dependent manner, which suggests a direct anti-inflammatory action of PGE_2 on C5a-induced CSF pleocytosis during bacterial meningitis. Elevated CSF concentrations of two alternative-pathway complement activation proteins, C3 and factor B, have also been found in mice and in patients with bacterial meningitis.[162,163] In the mouse model of *Listeria* meningitis,[162] intrathecal synthesis of C3 and factor B occurred during the course of the disease.

Studies have examined other chemotactic factors and their role in mediating CSF chemotactic activity. In an experimental mouse model of *Listeria* meningoencephalitis, the macrophage inflammatory proteins MIP-1α and MIP-2 were important in the recruitment of leukocytes into the CSF.[164] Elevated CSF concentrations of MIP-1α and MIP-1β, as well as other chemokines (IL-8, growth-related gene product-α, and monocyte chemotactic protein 1), have also been found to be increased in patients with bacterial meningitis.[165,166] However, no significant correlation was found between CSF leukocyte counts and chemokine concentrations or chemotactic activity mediated by CSF, suggesting that other factors influence the extent of CSF pleocytosis in vivo. In another study, the significant correlation of elevated CSF concentrations of IL-8 and growth-related gene product-α with the number of granulocytes that immigrated into the CSF of patients with bacterial meningitis[167] suggested the importance of these chemokines in the recruitment of leukocytes into the subarachnoid space.

Despite this early influx of leukocytes in bacterial meningitis, host defense in CSF remains suboptimal because of the lack of functional opsonic and bactericidal activity. With inefficient phagocytosis, bacteria can multiply to huge concentrations in the CSF during meningitis.

The precise pathway of leukocyte traversal into the CSF is unknown, although adherence to vascular endothelial cells is a likely prerequisite. Pretreatment of noncerebral endothelial cells in culture with lipo-oligosaccharide or cytokines (IL-1 or TNF) has been shown to induce the formation of specific adhesion molecules such as endothelial leukocyte adhesion molecule 1 and intercellular adhesion molecule 1 (ICAM-1).[141] It is unclear whether similar adhesion mechanisms exist between neutrophils and cerebral vascular endothelium. In an infant mouse model of hematogenous bacterial meningitis,[168] mice genetically deficient in the gene coding for ICAM-1 production had a higher incidence of *H. influenzae* type B bacteremia than did wild-type mice, and more ICAM-1–deficient mice had positive CSF cultures for *H. influenzae* type B. In contrast, the incidence of *S. pneumoniae* bacteremia was equivalent in both groups of mice, and all were CSF culture positive, although mortality was higher for ICAM-1–deficient mice at 24 hours. These results suggested that ICAM-1 deficiency may be protective early in *H. influenzae* type B infection but detrimental in *S. pneumoniae* infection. In an experimental rat model, a monoclonal antibody (CD54) directed against ICAM-1 significantly reduced the accumulation of leukocytes in CSF during the early phase of bacterial meningitis,[169] which makes this adhesion molecule a promising target in the development of adjunctive strategies to treat bacterial meningitis.

Other families of leukocyte receptors have also been studied to determine their role in leukocyte-mediated damage in bacterial meningitis. In an experimental rabbit model, the intravenous inoculation of a monoclonal antibody (IB4) directed against the CD18 family of receptors on leukocytes (leukocyte integrins) blocked the accumulation of leukocytes in CSF despite the intracisternal inoculation of *H. influenzae* type B, *N. meningitidis*, pneumococcal cell wall, or lipo-oligosaccharide[170]; increased protein concentrations in CSF were also attenuated by IB4. In addition, the monoclonal antibody prevented the development of cerebral edema and death in animals challenged with lethal doses of *S. pneumoniae*. CSF penetration of antibiotics, CSF bactericidal concentrations, and the bactericidal response to ampicillin therapy were not affected by administration of the monoclonal antibody, although the onset of bacteremia was delayed and the CSF inflammatory response was attenuated after ampicillin-induced bacterial killing.

Selectins also play an important role in promoting the margination and reversible rolling of leukocytes at sites of tissue inflammation. After intravenous administration of prokaryotic peptides that mimic selectins (the S2 and S3 subunits of pertussis toxin) and competitively inhibit adherence of neutrophils to endothelial cells in vitro, recruitment of leukocytes into the CSF of rabbits with pneumococcal meningitis was disrupted, thus suggesting that these peptides have therapeutic anti-inflammatory potential.[171] An anti-CD11b monoclonal antibody (IB6) was studied in an infant rat model of *H. influenzae* sepsis and meningitis[172]; IB6 played a role in inhibiting neutrophil emigration to sites of inflammation within the CNS but was not beneficial in decreasing mortality in this model. Furthermore, in an experimental cytokine-induced model of meningitis, mice deficient in P- and E-selectins displayed nearly complete inhibition in CSF leukocyte accumulation and BBB permeability versus only partial inhibition in P-selectin–deficient mice.[173] In additional studies, after intravenous treatment with the polysaccharide fucoidin, a homopolymer of sulfated L-fucose known to block the function of the leukocyte "rolling receptor" L-selectin,[174] leukocyte rolling was rapidly and profoundly reduced (confirmed by intravital microscopy in muscle), and the accumulation of both leukocytes and plasma proteins in the CSF of rabbits challenged intrathecally with pneumococcal antigen was profoundly reduced. These findings suggest that inhibition of selectin-mediated leukocyte rolling may be an effective therapeutic approach to the attenuation of leukocyte-mediated damage during bacterial meningitis.[175]

The dynamic aspects of these leukocyte–endothelial cell interactions were also examined in a meningitis model by means of confocal laser scanning microscopy, a new microscopic technique with much improved depth-discrimination properties. In an experimental model of pneumococcal meningitis, the behavior of rhodamine 6G–labeled leukocytes in pial vessels was determined.[176] When compared with controls, the number of adherent leukocytes significantly increased within 1 hour after intracisternal challenge with *S. pneumoniae*, with further increases noted up to 6 hours after infection. Pretreatment with dexamethasone significantly attenuated the adherence and transendothelial passage of leukocytes. In another study using this technique, heparin was found to significantly attenuate leukocyte rolling, as well as leukocyte sticking, after the induction of pneumococcal meningitis.[177] Therefore, this technique has potential usefulness

in investigation of the efficacy of anti-inflammatory agents that may interfere with leukocyte adherence.

Meningeal and perivascular macrophages may have an important role in the influx of leukocytes across the BBB. In an experimental rat meningitis model, a single intraventricular injection of mannosylated clodronate liposomes, which deplete meningeal and perivascular macrophages, resulted in increased illness after pneumococcal challenge[178]; the illness correlated with higher bacterial counts in blood and CSF, associated with a decreased influx of leukocytes into CSF. Therefore, meningeal and perivascular macrophages may play a protective role during bacterial meningitis secondary to their supportive role on the traversal of leukocytes across the BBB. Further studies are needed to define the importance of macrophages in this process.

Induction of Subarachnoid Space Inflammation

The induction of a marked subarachnoid space inflammatory response by meningeal pathogens contributes to many of the pathophysiologic consequences of bacterial meningitis and therefore to significant morbidity and mortality from this disorder. Recent experimental studies have focused on the virulence factors of meningeal pathogens and the specific inflammatory mediators that they induce (Table 80-7) to learn more about the mechanisms responsible for subarachnoid space inflammation.

Despite the importance of the bacterial polysaccharide capsule to the survival of meningeal pathogens in the intravascular and subarachnoid space, capsular polysaccharides are remarkably noninflammatory even when inoculated in purified form into the CSF of animals. In contrast, the cell walls of *S. pneumoniae* are potent inducers of CSF inflammation,[142,143] and even independent intracisternal inoculation of the major components of the pneumococcal cell wall, teichoic acid and peptidoglycan, induces CSF inflammation. These findings lend support to the concept that release of pneumococcal cell wall lytic products during antibiotic-induced autolysis in the treatment of bacterial meningitis contributes to an accentuated host inflammatory response in the subarachnoid space. Pneumolysin, an intracellular polypeptide toxin of *S. pneumoniae* that is released after bacterial cell lysis, does not appear to play a role in postantibiotic enhancement of meningeal inflammation. Subarachnoid space inflammation is also induced by the intracisternal inoculation of purified *H. influenzae* type B lipo-oligosaccharide, a response blocked by pretreatment of lipo-oligosaccharide with polymyxin B or neutrophil acyloxyacyl hydrolase, thus supporting the importance of the lipid A region of the lipo-oligosaccharide molecule in the induction of inflammation.

Recently, however, experimental evidence has supported the concept that pneumococcal cell wall or lipo-oligosaccharide does not induce subarachnoid space inflammation directly but does so through the local CNS release of inflammatory mediators such as IL-1, TNF, and prostaglandins.[142,143] In an experimental rat model, the intracisternal

TABLE 80-7 Potential Factors Contributing to Subarachnoid Space Inflammation

Bacterial factors
    Cell wall components
    Lipo-oligosaccharide
    Outer membrane vesicles
    Peptidoglycan
Host factors
    Prostaglandins (PGE$_2$, prostacyclin)
    Interleukins (IL-1β, IL-6, IL-8, IL-12, IL-16)
    Interferon-γ
    Growth-related gene product-α
    Tumor necrosis factor-α
    Platelet-activating factor
    Macrophage inflammatory proteins 1 and 2
    Leukocyte integrins (CD18)
    Leukocyte selectins
    Endothelial leukocyte adhesion molecule 1
    Intercellular adhesion molecule 1 (ICAM-1)
    Reactive nitrogen intermediates
    Peroxynitrite

inoculation of purified *H. influenzae* type B lipo-oligosaccharide led to elevated CSF concentrations of IL-1 and TNF within 30 to 120 minutes; elevated CSF concentrations of TNF have also been found in an experimental rabbit model, with peak activity at 2 hours and persistence for about 5 hours. Similar results were observed after intracisternal challenge with live *H. influenzae* type B, although TNF activity persisted longer (about 14 hours). The TNF was produced principally within the CNS (i.e., no TNF activity was detected in serum samples) in this experimental animal model system, a finding that has also been observed in patients with bacterial meningitis. In addition, the finding of increased CSF concentrations of TNF-α may be specific for bacterial meningitis. The presence of TNF-α in CSF appears to be indicative of a bacterial etiology, although the absence of TNF-α does not exclude the diagnosis of bacterial meningitis. Furthermore, elevated CSF concentrations of PGE$_2$, prostacyclin, IL-1β, and TNF have been found in most infants and children with bacterial meningitis.

Direct intracisternal inoculation of these inflammatory mediators can also induce CSF inflammation.[142,143] In an experimental rabbit model, injection of purified rabbit TNF-α or human recombinant IL-1β produced significant CSF inflammation. This effect was synergistic when lower doses of each cytokine were administered simultaneously, with more rapid and significantly increased leukocyte influx than when each cytokine was administered alone. In contrast, in an experimental rabbit model of pneumococcal meningitis, the parameters of CSF leukocytosis, BBB permeability, and brain edema were induced by intracisternal inoculation of human recombinant TNF-α, MIP-1 and MIP-2, and IL-α, but not by IL-1β. Leukocytosis and brain edema were inhibited by antibodies homologous to each mediator, as well as in rabbits treated with a monoclonal antibody to CD18 to render neutrophil–endothelial cell interactions dysfunctional. PAF is also inflammatory in the CNS and causes significant BBB permeability and cerebral edema; at higher doses, these effects are accompanied by CSF leukocytosis, which can be inhibited by the administration of antibody to the CD18 family of leukocyte adhesion molecules. In an experimental rabbit model, treatment with a PAF receptor antagonist decreased CSF cytochemical values induced by intracisternal challenge with pneumococci but not with *H. influenzae*, thus suggesting a specific role for PAF in pneumococcal disease. In addition, another study using an experimental rat model found that PAF augmented the meningeal inflammation and BBB permeability elicited by *H. influenzae* type B lipo-oligosaccharide. It would appear that these inflammatory mediators have multiple complex and interrelated activities in the CNS that contribute to inflammation and tissue damage during bacterial meningitis.

These findings have importance with regard to outcome in patients with bacterial meningitis.[142,143] Outcome after gram-negative bacillary meningitis has been correlated with the persistence of organisms and higher concentrations of endotoxin (as measured by the *Limulus* lysate assay) in CSF. In children with *H. influenzae* type B meningitis, CSF concentrations of free lipo-oligosaccharide correlated with the Herson-Todd severity score and the number of febrile hospital days. In an experimental rabbit model of *E. coli* meningitis, a single intravenous dose of an antimicrobial agent (cefotaxime, cefpirome, meropenem, chloramphenicol, or gentamicin) caused a 2- to 10-fold increase in free CSF lipopolysaccharide concentrations within 2 hours, although free lipopolysaccharide concentrations increased almost 100-fold in untreated animals 4 hours later as bacteria continued to multiply. The degree of elevated CSF concentrations of IL-1β also correlated with outcome after neonatal gram-negative bacillary meningitis. Furthermore, among infants and children with predominantly *H. influenzae* type B meningitis, those with CSF concentrations of IL-1β of 500 pg/mL or more were more likely to have neurologic sequelae; elevated CSF concentrations of TNF were not associated with outcome. Elevated CSF concentrations of PAF have been demonstrated in children with *H. influenzae* meningitis and correlate with bacterial density and with CSF concentrations of lipo-oligosaccharide and TNF-α; these increased concentrations of TNF-α and PAF were associated with severity of disease. This association

was confirmed in more recent studies that demonstrated that elevated CSF concentrations of TNF-α and soluble TNF receptor, the natural homeostatic regulator of the actions of TNF-α, were important for predicting neurologic sequelae in bacterial meningitis. In an experimental rabbit model, intracisternal inoculation of rabbit recombinant IL-1β and TNF-α combined with IL-1 receptor antagonist and soluble TNF receptor produced less inflammation in rabbits than after inoculation of these cytokines alone.[179] However, IL-1 receptor antagonist and soluble TNF receptor did not reduce the meningeal inflammatory response associated with intracisternal inoculation of *H. influenzae* type B lipo-oligosaccharide, thus indicating that these cytokine inhibitors may not be effective in modulating inflammation induced by a broad inflammatory stimulus such as gram-negative bacteria or their products.

More recently, the role of other cytokines in the subarachnoid space inflammatory response in bacterial meningitis has been studied. Elevated CSF concentrations of IL-6 have been observed in the CSF of patients with bacterial meningitis[142,143,180]; these increased concentrations occurred after the release of TNF-α and before neutrophilic infiltration into CSF. IL-8, a cytokine with potent chemoattractant and activating effects on neutrophils, has been detected in the CSF of patients with bacterial meningitis[181-183]; IL-8 may also have a role as a neutrophil chemotactic factor in nonbacterial meningitis. In a rabbit model of pneumococcal meningitis, intravenous, but not intracisternal, administration of anti-IL-8 attenuated CSF pleocytosis,[184] suggesting that the functional activity of IL-8 appears to be at the blood-stream side of the microvascular endothelium. IL-10, an anti-inflammatory protein formed by T lymphocytes and monocytes, inhibits the production of proinflammatory cytokines such as TNF-α and has been detected in the CSF of animals and humans with bacterial meningitis.[185-188] In an experimental rabbit model, IL-10 modulated CSF TNF-α concentrations in experimental meningitis caused by *H. influenzae* type B lipo-oligosaccharide, *H. influenzae* type B, or *L. monocytogenes*, an effect that was maximal when IL-10 was combined with dexamethasone.[189] In IL-10–deficient mice challenged with *S. pneumoniae,* the absence of IL-10 was associated with higher cytokine and chemokine concentrations and a more pronounced infiltrate, but it had no influence on antibacterial defense or animal survival,[190] suggesting that IL-10 does not play an essential role in host defense during murine pneumococcal meningitis. Production of IFN-γ was induced by IL-12 (which is produced by phagocytic cells in response to infection and stimulates adaptive immunity), with TNF-α as a costimulator, and was inhibited by IL-10[191]; this IFN-γ production may contribute to the natural immunity against microorganisms in CSF during the acute phase of bacterial meningitis. Concentrations of IL-16, an immunomodulatory cytokine characterized by chemotactic activity and stimulation of proinflammatory cytokine expression in monocytic cells, have been shown to rise transiently in the CSF during the initial stage of meningitis (both bacterial and viral) in children[192]; these results suggest that IL-16 may promote an inflammatory response during meningitis in concert with other proinflammatory cytokines. Therefore, it appears that release of inflammatory mediators in the CNS is responsible for induction of a marked subarachnoid space inflammatory response and may correlate with morbidity and mortality in patients with bacterial meningitis.

Toll-like receptor (TLR)-2, which plays a crucial role in the detection of microbial infection and activation of the inflammatory response, may also have an important role in subarachnoid space inflammation during bacterial meningitis. In an experimental murine model of pneumococcal meningitis, TLR-2 participated in the sensing and activation of the initial immune response to intracisternal challenge with *S. pneumoniae*.[193] Deficiency of TLR-2 was associated with higher cerebellar bacterial titers, supporting the concept that the subarachnoid space is a localized area of host immunodeficiency that allows the unrestrained proliferation of pneumococci, which, if untreated, overwhelms the host until death. Mice deficient in TLR-2 are highly susceptible to *S. pneumoniae* meningitis secondary to reduced bacterial clearing (with early death) and enhanced inflammation.[194]

Alterations of the Blood-Brain Barrier

Bacterial meningitis has been shown to increase permeability across the BBB, which is composed of the arachnoid membrane, choroid plexus epithelium, and cerebral microvascular endothelium; the cerebral microvascular endothelium has been the site of intensive study in bacterial meningitis.[141-143] An adult experimental rat model was used to examine the propensity for meningeal pathogens to induce functional and morphologic alterations of the BBB. After intracisternal inoculation of either *E. coli, S. pneumoniae,* or *H. influenzae* type B, alterations of the BBB were found with all three pathogens and were manifested morphologically by an early and sustained increase in pinocytotic vesicle formation and progressive separation of intercellular tight junctions; these morphologic changes correlated with the functional penetration of albumin, a molecule normally excluded by an intact BBB, into the CSF. Intracisternal inoculation of an unencapsulated strain of *H. influenzae* caused an increase in pinocytotic vesicle formation without separation of intercellular tight junctions, which suggests that encapsulation of *H. influenzae* was not essential for BBB injury but facilitated its progression by avoidance of host defense mechanisms. The increased BBB permeability was observed in both normal and leukopenic animals, although permeability was augmented by the presence of leukocytes. The site of BBB injury was subsequently examined by in situ tracer perfusion and immunolabeling procedures to identify the topography and microvascular exit pathways of bovine serum albumin (BSA). Exit of both perfused colloidal gold–BSA and immunodetectable BSA was through open intercellular junctions of venules in the pia-arachnoid, thus specifically and topographically localizing the BBB injury in bacterial meningitis to the meningeal venules.

Because surface encapsulation was not an essential virulence factor for the production of BBB injury, BBB permeability was examined after the intracisternal inoculation of purified *H. influenzae* type B lipo-oligosaccharide.[142,143] Purified lipo-oligosaccharide was shown to increase BBB permeability in an experimental rat model in a manner that was both dose and time dependent (maximum change at a dose of 20 ng 4 hours after intracisternal inoculation), with a close correlation between permeability and CSF pleocytosis 4 hours after intracisternal inoculation. Increased BBB permeability was also observed after the intracisternal inoculation of *H. influenzae* type B outer-membrane vesicles, an effect that was blocked by preincubation with polymyxin B but not by a monoclonal antibody directed against the oligosaccharide side chain of the lipo-oligosaccharide; no change in permeability was observed in leukopenic animals. *H. influenzae* type B peptidoglycan has also been shown to induce meningeal inflammation and BBB permeability in an infant rat model.

Further experiments demonstrated that lipo-oligosaccharide did not directly mediate the increased BBB permeability but did so by inducing the production of various inflammatory cytokines (e.g., IL-1 and TNF) within the CNS; intracisternal inoculation of purified lipo-oligosaccharide led to increased CSF concentrations of both IL-1 and TNF within 30 to 120 minutes.[142,143] Furthermore, the intracisternal inoculation of human recombinant IL-1β into rats led to a peak increase in BBB permeability about 3 hours after inoculation, earlier than the peak response obtained after inoculation with lipo-oligosaccharide (4 hours). No permeability changes were induced after the intracisternal inoculation of human recombinant TNF-α, although all available evidence suggests that these cytokines act synergistically inasmuch as inoculation with submaximal doses of IL-1β plus TNF-α, at concentrations that produced no changes individually, enhanced BBB permeability. In contrast, in a study of patients with bacterial meningitis, CSF concentrations of TNF-α, but not of IL-1β, correlated with BBB disruption (assessed by CSF protein concentrations); synergy between IL-1β and TNF-α was also noted in this study.

The effects of lipo-oligosaccharide on BBB permeability in the experimental rat model have also been examined in an in vitro model by growing purified preparations of cerebral microvascular endothelium on a semipermeable support.[142,143] Several investigators have demonstrated increased permeability across this monolayer after exposure to *H. influenzae* type B or purified lipo-oligosaccharide. The mechanism for this increased permeability is unclear, however. It may be related to a direct cytotoxic effect of lipo-oligosaccharide, for instance, through effects of serum components such as lipo-oligosaccharide–binding protein on the cerebral microvascular endothelium, or it could be related to lipo-oligosaccharide–induced formation of various second messengers (e.g., cyclic adenosine or guanosine monophosphate) by endothelial cells.

Matrix metalloproteinases (MMPs), a family of zinc-dependent endopeptidases that degrade the components of the extracellular matrix, may also be involved in BBB alterations during bacterial meningitis. In a rat model of meningococcal meningitis, increased CSF concentrations of MMP-9 were seen 6 hours after meningococcal challenge[143]; batimastat, an MMP inhibitor, significantly reduced BBB disruption and intracranial pressure but failed to significantly reduce CSF white blood cell counts. MMP-9 appears to be activated by a reactive oxygen species–dependent pathway.[195] Treatment with the MMP inhibitor GM6001 reduced CSF concentrations of MMP-9 and significantly attenuated brain damage in an experimental rat model of pneumococcal meningitis.[196] MMPs may alter BBB permeability by degrading components of the extracellular matrix that contribute to BBB integrity. Furthermore, MMPs and TNF-α–converting enzyme (TACE), which proteolytically releases several cell-surface proteins including TNF-α and its receptor, appear to act synergistically; treatment with BB-1101, a hydroxaminic acid–based inhibitor of MMP and TACE, downregulated the CSF concentrations of TNF-α and decreased the incidence of seizures and mortality in an infant rat model of pneumococcal meningitis.[197] Therapy with BB-1101, when combined with antimicrobial therapy, attenuated neuronal necrosis in the cortex and hippocampus, suggesting that inhibition of MMP and TACE offers a novel therapeutic strategy to prevent brain injury and neurologic sequelae in bacterial meningitis.

Increased Intracranial Pressure

Cerebral edema is the major element contributing to increased intracranial pressure during bacterial meningitis and may result in life-threatening cerebral herniation and other complications.[142,143] The origin of the cerebral edema may be vasogenic, cytotoxic, or interstitial, or any combination of the three; all three elements probably contribute to cerebral edema during bacterial meningitis. Vasogenic cerebral edema is primarily a consequence of increased BBB permeability; cytotoxic cerebral edema results from swelling of the cellular elements of the brain, most likely through release of toxic factors from neutrophils, bacteria, or both; and interstitial cerebral edema reflects obstruction of the flow of normal CSF as in hydrocephalus. The last factor has been examined in an experimental rabbit model of pneumococcal or *E. coli* meningitis in which the CSF outflow resistance (defined as factors that inhibit the flow of CSF from the subarachnoid space to the major dural sinuses) was markedly elevated and remained elevated for as long as 2 weeks despite rapid CSF sterilization with penicillin therapy.

These concepts have been examined in greater detail in an experimental animal model of pneumococcal meningitis by measuring brain water content (indicative of cerebral edema if elevated), CSF lactate concentrations, and CSF pressure.[142,143] All three parameters were elevated in infected animals. Although treatment with ampicillin rapidly sterilized the CSF and normalized the brain water content and CSF pressure, the CSF lactate concentration remained elevated. The bacterial virulence factor responsible for the production of brain edema was subsequently examined in an experimental animal model of *E. coli* meningitis in which therapy with cefotaxime, but not chloramphenicol, induced a marked rise in CSF endotoxin concentrations that was associated with increased brain water content. The peptidoglycan of the *H. influenzae* cell wall also induced cerebral edema without perturbing the other parameters of inflammation (e.g., increased BBB permeability), which suggests that peptidoglycan induces cytotoxic rather than vasogenic cerebral edema. Neutrophils appeared to contribute to the development of cerebral edema if adequately stimulated, although the parameters of increased intracranial pressure and increased CSF concentrations of lactate and protein were unrelated to the presence of neutrophils. However, this area remains controversial because neutrophils are required for the increased BBB permeability seen in response to the intracisternal inoculation of bacterial virulence factors and inflammatory mediators.

Variability among bacterial strains may also be an important determinant in production of the subarachnoid space inflammatory response and brain edema in bacterial meningitis. Intracisternal inoculation of three different pneumococcal isolates resulted in pronounced differences in the pathophysiologic profiles 24 hours after challenge.[143] When pneumococcal cell wall fragments were inoculated intracisternally, the chemical composition of the fragments, specifically the degree of teichoication, influenced the induction of brain edema. In a subsequent study in an experimental rabbit model, serotype-specific characteristics of pneumococci were found to play a major role in the subarachnoid space inflammatory process, although significant differences in brain water content were observed only with one of the serotypes tested.[198] It is unclear, however, whether these differences affect the clinical expression of disease in patients with bacterial meningitis.

The infusion of hypertonic mannitol to treat increased intracranial pressure has been evaluated in a rabbit model of *H. influenzae* type B meningitis.[142] In all animals, mannitol consistently reduced intracisternal pressure, although the magnitude of reduction was greater in infected animals, and brain water content was no different in mannitol-treated animals than in untreated ones. In contrast, in an experimental rat model of pneumococcal meningitis, mannitol modulated changes in cerebral blood flow, intracranial pressure, and brain water content,[199] perhaps by a mechanism of scavenging hydroxyl radicals, which have been shown to be involved in the pathogenesis and pathophysiology of cerebral ischemia and neuronal injury in bacterial meningitis (see later).

Other modalities have been recently examined to determine their effectiveness in reduction of increased intracranial pressure in bacterial meningitis. In an experimental rat model of pneumococcal meningitis, nimodipine (an L-type calcium channel blocker) attenuated CSF pleocytosis and decreased intracranial pressure, possibly by mechanisms including reduction of reactive oxygen species and IL-6 production.[200] Triptans, which inhibit the release of proinflammatory neuropeptides from perivascular nerve fibers, reduced the influx of leukocytes into CSF, attenuated the increase in regional cerebral blood flow, and reduced elevated intracranial pressure and brain water content in an experimental rat model.[201] These modalities may offer new options as adjunctive agents in bacterial meningitis and require further study.

Alterations in Cerebral Blood Flow

Bacterial meningitis exerts profound effects on blood vessels that course through the subarachnoid space,[142,143] and the resulting vasculitis leads to narrowing or thrombosis of cerebral blood vessels and the propensity for ischemia and/or infarction of underlying brain. In combination with increased intracranial pressure, these changes may result in altered cerebral blood flow in patients with bacterial meningitis. An infant rhesus monkey model of *H. influenzae* meningitis demonstrated that cerebral cortical hypoperfusion occurs during meningitis and causes relative cerebral anoxia. Cerebrovascular autoregulation, in which cerebral blood flow is unchanged despite alterations of blood pressure over a wide range, is also lost during experimental bacterial meningitis. Furthermore, studies in an experimental rabbit model of pneumococcal meningitis have demonstrated that animals given a lower intravenous fluid regimen (50 mL/kg/24 hours) of normal saline had a lower mean arterial pressure, lower cerebral blood flow, and a higher concentration of CSF lactate than did animals that received a higher fluid regimen (150 mL/kg/24 hours). In the first 4 to 6 hours of antibiotic administration, rabbits receiving lower fluid regimens had a significant decrease in mean arterial pressure and cerebral blood flow and a significant increase in CSF lactate concentrations when compared with rabbits receiving higher fluid regimens. These results, in combination with other experimental studies that have noted an increase in

cerebral blood flow within the first few hours of intracisternal inoculation of either live pneumococci or pneumococcal cell wall fragments, have suggested that maintenance of adequate intravascular volume and minimization of stimuli that increase systemic blood pressure may be important in the treatment of bacterial meningitis. These findings may also be of potential clinical relevance inasmuch as inadvertent increases in mean arterial pressure directly increase cerebral blood flow and intracranial pressure and depletion of intravascular volume with decreases in mean arterial pressure can cause parallel decreases in cerebral blood flow and a reduction in substrate delivery to the brain. Therefore, the brain is at risk from either hypoperfusion or hyperperfusion. As demonstrated by near-infrared spectroscopy in conjunction with measurement of cerebral blood flow in an experimental rabbit model of pneumococcal meningitis, infected animals had a relative increase in the deoxygenated hemoglobin fraction and a decrease in the oxygenated hemoglobin fraction, thus supporting the possibility of cerebral venous engorgement in bacterial meningitis, which may contribute to intracranial hypertension in this disorder.

Additional studies have examined the importance of the subarachnoid space inflammatory response in alterations of cerebral blood flow during bacterial meningitis. In an experimental rabbit model of *H. influenzae* type B meningitis, CSF leukocytes were found to be not responsible for the hyperemic response,[202] which suggests that cerebral hyperemia in bacterial meningitis is induced directly by bacterial components or indirectly by components of the inflammatory cascade. More recently, endothelin (which has been found to regulate vascular tone and integrity and to act as a mediator of inflammation) has been investigated as a possible mediator of cerebrovascular complications in bacterial meningitis. In an experimental rat model of pneumococcal meningitis, endothelin contributed to the increased cerebral blood flow (as measured by laser Doppler flowmetry), intracranial pressure, brain water content, and CSF pleocytosis.[203] Elevated CSF concentrations of endothelin have also been found in patients during the acute stage of bacterial meningitis,[204] which suggests a potential role for endothelin in mediation of meningitis-induced cerebral hypoperfusion and brain infarction. In an infant rat model of pneumococcal meningitis, intraperitoneal treatment with bosentan, an endothelin antagonist, restored cerebral blood flow to control levels,[205] indicating that endothelin contributes to neuronal injury by causing cerebral ischemia.

Cerebral blood flow has been measured in patients with bacterial meningitis. In an early study,[142,143] measurement of cerebral blood flow (by the xenon 133 intra-arterial injection method) revealed a 30% to 40% reduction in average total blood flow in five patients with pneumococcal meningitis (mean age, 54 years), but not in five patients with meningococcal meningitis (mean age, 20 years). An inverse relationship between cerebral blood flow and intracranial pressure has been observed in infants with bacterial meningitis; among eight patients, alterations were noted only in the four older infants (age range, 3 to 10 months) and not in the four neonates (age range, 5 to 30 days) in whom no changes in cerebral blood flow velocity were detected. In another study of 17 children (aged 8 days to 6 years) with bacterial meningitis, transcranial Doppler ultrasound monitoring demonstrated an improvement in cerebral blood flow velocity with resolution of meningitis. This observation suggests that in the early phase of bacterial meningitis, increased cerebrovascular resistance may contribute to a relative impairment in cerebral perfusion; transcranial Doppler ultrasound may be a useful technique for the early detection of deterioration in cerebral hemodynamics.

In a subsequent study in 20 children seriously ill with bacterial meningitis, total and regional cerebral blood flow measured by stable xenon computed tomography (CT) revealed a global decrease in flow and even more regional variability.[142,143] Although autoregulation of cerebral blood flow was preserved in the patients studied, hyperventilation reduced flow below the ischemic threshold, which raises important concerns about the routine use of hyperventilation in the management of increased intracranial pressure in patients with bacterial meningitis. In contrast, in another study of nine patients with bacterial meningitis, eight of whom had impaired cerebral blood flow autoregulation, autoregulation was partially or completely restored in six of eight patients by short-term hyperventilation[206]; this recovery may protect the brain from fluctuations in perfusion pressure. Further studies are needed before recommendations are made regarding the implementation of therapies that reduce cerebral blood flow in patients with bacterial meningitis. In another study of 86 adult patients with bacterial meningitis, cerebral angiography was performed on 27 patients who had focal deficits (either clinically, on cranial CT, or both) and who had persistent coma without an explained cause despite 3 days of antimicrobial therapy.[207] Thirteen of the patients who underwent angiography had alterations in their blood vessel system; the prognosis in these patients was poor. However, definitive changes in cerebral blood flow during bacterial meningitis are controversial and may vary with the stage of disease. These blood flow alterations may lead to regional hypoxia, increased lactate concentrations in the brain secondary to utilization of glucose by anaerobic glycolysis, and CSF acidosis, which may be a precursor to encephalopathy.[208]

Neuronal Injury

Data have suggested that oxygen radicals may contribute to the increased brain water content, intracranial pressure, and changes in regional blood flow in bacterial meningitis. In an experimental rat model of pneumococcal meningitis after intracisternal inoculation of live pneumococci or pneumococcal cell wall components,[209] the increases in brain water content and intracranial pressure were prevented, and the increase in regional blood flow was significantly attenuated by conjugated superoxide dismutase and deferoxamine. Catalase, which eliminates hydrogen peroxide, also significantly attenuated the increase in regional blood flow and brain water content, although only a trend toward a reduction in intracranial pressure was observed.[210] Furthermore, in a neonatal rat model of group B streptococcal meningitis, generation of reactive oxygen intermediates (localized to cells constituting the subarachnoid and ventricular inflammation and to the cerebral vasculature) was a major contributor to cerebral ischemia and necrotic and apoptotic neuronal injury[211]; the free radical scavenger α-phenyl-tert-butyl nitrone inhibited the biologic effect of the reactive oxygen intermediates, thereby improving cerebral cortical perfusion and reducing the extent of both necrotic and apoptotic neuronal injury. It also appeared that TNF-α plays a critical role in neuronal apoptosis in the hippocampus in rats with group B streptococcal meningitis,[212] although it was not essential for the development of inflammation and cortical injury in this model. A number of other agents that interfere with reactive oxygen intermediates have also been examined for their efficacy in experimental animal models of bacterial meningitis. Rifampin was shown to reduce the release of reactive oxygen intermediates and decrease secondary brain injury in an experimental model of pneumococcal meningitis.[213] In another study utilizing an experimental pneumococcal meningitis model, three clinically used antioxidants (*N*-acetylcysteine, deferoxamine, and tirilazad mesylate) all reduced cortical, but not hippocampal, injury[214]; an ideal agent should act at both the cortex and the hippocampus.

Additional studies have attempted to clarify the mechanisms responsible for apoptosis in bacterial meningitis. In an in vitro model, exposure of microglia or neurons to live pneumococci led to rapid apoptosis[215]; this was attributed to mitochondrial damage and was followed by mitochondrial release of apoptosis-inducing factor (AIF). The apoptosis was markedly impaired by intracytoplasmic microinjection of AIF-specific antiserum, indicating the AIF may play a central role in brain cell apoptosis during bacterial meningitis. In an experimental model of pneumococcal meningitis, the pneumococcal toxin pneumolysin colocalized with apoptotic neurons of the hippocampus[216]; infection with pneumococci unable to produce pneumolysin and hydrogen peroxide significantly reduced damage. Apoptosis was induced by translocation of AIF, suggesting potentially

new protective strategies for pneumococcal meningitis. Another study assessed the role of poly(adenosine diphosphate-ribose) polymerase (PARP) activation in experimental pneumococcal meningitis.[217] Mice with a targeted disruption of the PARP 1 gene were protected against meningitis-associated CNS complications and by PARP inhibition using 3-aminobenzamide, indicating that PARP activation seems to play a crucial role in development of CNS complications and pneumococcus-induced endothelial injury. The activity of caspase-3, an enzyme required for the morphologic changes associated with apoptosis, was significantly increased in the hippocampal tissue of rats with pneumococcal meningitis and was localized to the immature cells of the dentate gyrus[218]; intracisternal administration of a caspase-3–specific inhibitor, Ac-DEVD-CHO, reduced apoptosis but did not affect inflammation (as assessed by TNF-α and IL-1β concentrations in CSF). Therefore, caspase-3 is a key effector of neuronal apoptosis in pneumococcal meningitis.

Evidence has suggested that reactive nitrogen intermediates may also play a role in the inflammatory process and other pathophysiologic events during bacterial meningitis.[144,219,220] In an experimental rat model of pneumococcal meningitis utilizing treatment with the nitric oxide synthase inhibitor *N*-nitro-L-arginine, it was determined that nitric oxide accounted for the regional cerebral blood flow changes and pial arteriolar vasodilation in the early phase of meningitis and was involved as a mediator of brain edema and meningeal inflammation[221]; stimulation of cerebral endothelial cells with pneumococci released nitric oxide, presumably via inducible nitric oxide synthase. In addition, inhibition of the neuronal nitric oxide synthase pathway with 7-nitroindazole also prevented pneumococci-induced pial arteriolar vasodilation.[222] Similarly, in another rat model of meningitis, CSF concentrations of nitrite (a major metabolic product of nitric oxide in vivo) rose after challenge with live *H. influenzae* type B or *H. influenzae* type B lipo-oligosaccharide, in direct correlation with increased permeability of the BBB.[223] This result was confirmed by another study in an experimental rat model in which excessive nitric oxide production contributed to BBB disruption[224]; administration of aminoguanidine, an inhibitor of inducible nitric oxide synthase, during meningeal inflammation significantly diminished meningeal nitric oxide production, attenuated white blood cell migration into the CSF, and maintained normal BBB permeability. A subsequent study also demonstrated that inhibition of nitric oxide production with aminoguanidine increased cortical hypoperfusion and ischemic neuronal injury,[225] which suggests that nitric oxide attenuates the development of cortical ischemia and neuronal injury in bacterial meningitis. A nonselective nitric oxide synthase (NOS) inhibitor L-NAME (N[omega]-nitro-L-arginine methyl ester) has been shown to attenuate the acute inflammatory response and brain injury in neonatal *E. coli* meningitis.[226] Because both nitric oxide and prostaglandins are inflammatory mediators produced during bacterial meningitis, the in vivo relationships between PGE$_2$ and nitric oxide during bacterial meningitis were assessed, as well as whether pharmacologic inhibition of cyclooxygenase-2 (COX-2) and inducible NOS (iNOS) would affect BBB permeability.[227] After the intracisternal inoculation of lipopolysaccharide in an experimental rat model, inhibition of prostaglandin synthesis via COX-2 did not prevent or reduce BBB disruption, although nimesulide inhibition of COX-2 elicited significantly higher concentrations of meningeal nitric oxide. These data suggest that the presence of prostaglandin, or some component of COX-2 activity, may contribute to an inhibitory feedback loop for iNOS activity under inflammatory conditions, leading to promotion of nitric oxide toxicity through enhanced nitric oxide synthesis during neuroinflammation. Endothelial NOS (eNOS) may also have a role in bacterial meningitis. In an experimental model of pneumococcal meningitis, the accumulation of CSF leukocytes, BBB disruption, and increased intracranial pressure were more pronounced in eNOS-deficient mice, indicating that eNOS deficiency is detrimental in bacterial meningitis.[228] Both iNOS and eNOS are upregulated in the acute phase of experimental bacterial meningitis, and iNOS-derived nitric oxide contributes to peroxynitrite formation (see later) and breaching of the BBB. Reactive nitrogen species were also involved in the breeching of the blood-labyrinth barrier during meningogenic pneumococcal labyrinthitis,[229] indicating that the nitric oxide produced by eNOS and iNOS may contribute to oxidative cochlear damage and sensorineural damage in bacterial meningitis.

The role of nitric oxide has also been examined in patients with bacterial meningitis. It has been suggested that nitric oxide may contribute to anaerobic glycolysis and neurologic damage in children with bacterial meningitis.[230] The induction of nitric oxide synthase, and consequently the production of nitric oxide, may be induced by TNF in CSF,[231] which in turn mediates the increased BBB permeability in bacterial meningitis.

Current interest is focusing on the role of peroxynitrite, a powerful oxidative agent, in the pathogenesis of neuronal injury in bacterial meningitis.[232] In an adult rat model of pneumococcal meningitis, treatment of infected rats with uric acid, a scavenger of peroxynitrite, significantly attenuated intracranial pressure, CSF white blood cell count, and BBB leakage.[233] Similarly, the elevation of serum uric acid concentrations, to those found in humans, led to a reduction of CSF pleocytosis and intracranial pressure in a dose-dependent manner.[234] In advanced bacterial meningitis, markedly increased concentrations of uric acid are found in CSF and cerebral cortex,[235] suggesting that its production may be a protective brain response. Peroxynitrite has also been involved in the pathophysiology of bacterial meningitis in humans. In brain specimens obtained at autopsy, a strong increase in tyrosine nitration was detected by immunohistochemical staining that was most evident in the inflammatory cells and blood vessels in the subarachnoid space[236]; increased CSF nitrotyrosine was accompanied by depletion of the antioxidant ascorbic acid and an increased oxidation of the natural peroxynitrite scavenger uric acid to allantoin. Treatment with scavengers of peroxynitrite have marked anti-inflammatory effects and have been shown to reduce intracranial hypertension in an experimental rat model of pneumococcal meningitis without accelerating bacterial growth or delaying the sterilization of CSF.[237] Therefore, these agents hold promise in the adjunctive therapy of bacterial meningitis.

A potential role for excitatory amino acids in the pathogenesis of brain injury in bacterial meningitis has been proposed. In an experimental rabbit model, intracisternal inoculation of S. pneumoniae led to significant increases in CSF concentrations of glutamate, aspartate, glycine, taurine, and alanine[238]; elevated glutamate concentrations were also found in the brain extracellular space, which suggests that excitotoxic neuronal injury may play a role in bacterial meningitis. In an experimental rat model of group B streptococcal meningitis, administration of kynurenic acid attenuated the toxic effects of glutamate by inhibition of neuronal excitatory amino acid receptors, and treated animals showed significantly less neuronal injury in the cortex and hippocampus than did untreated controls,[239] thus demonstrating the important contribution of glutamate to neurotoxicity in bacterial meningitis. Excess CSF concentrations of glutamate have also been detected in patients with bacterial meningitis[240,241]; a prolonged increase in CSF glutamate concentrations may predict a poor outcome in patients with bacterial meningitis, possibly because of the sustained neurotoxic effects of this excitatory neurotransmitter.

Finally, tissue plasminogen activator (tPA), which converts plasminogen to plasmin, has been shown to increase neuronal cell death during excitotoxicity and cerebral ischemia, leading to degradation of the extracellular matrix, MMP activation, and processing of growth factors and cytokines. Both serum and CSF tPA concentrations are increased in patients with bacterial meningitis,[242] which may promote BBB disruption, proinflammatory signaling, and neuronal damage. Specifically, urokinase plasminogen activator has been shown to be involved in leukocyte recruitment and breeching of the BBB[243]; CSF concentrations of urokinase plasminogen activator exceeded those in serum, suggesting production of this factor in the CNS. Further studies on the pathogenesis of neuronal injury in bacterial meningitis may lead to the development of adjunctive strategies to prevent or modify this devastating consequence of bacterial meningitis.

CLINICAL FEATURES

Viral Meningitis

Enteroviruses

The clinical manifestations of enteroviral meningitis depend on host age and immune status.[2,4] In neonates (2 weeks of age or younger) with proven enteroviral meningitis, fever is a ubiquitous finding and is usually accompanied by any combination of vomiting, anorexia, rash, and upper respiratory symptoms and signs. Neurologic involvement may be associated with nuchal rigidity and a bulging anterior fontanelle, although infants younger than 1 year are less likely to demonstrate meningeal signs. Mental status may be altered, but focal neurologic signs are uncommon. A more severe form of meningoencephalitis may be seen in neonates, who appear to be at greatest risk for morbidity and mortality (rates as high as 74% and 10%, respectively), particularly when symptoms and signs develop during the first day of life (after presumed transplacental transmission of the virus). With disease progression, a sepsis-like syndrome characterized by multiorgan involvement (e.g., hepatic necrosis, myocarditis, and necrotizing enterocolitis), disseminated intravascular coagulation, and cardiovascular collapse may develop. Findings in the CNS are of an encephalitis associated with seizures and focal neurologic signs. Lack of humoral antibody may contribute to the severity of neonatal infection.

The findings in neonates contrast with the clinical findings of enteroviral meningitis beyond the neonatal period (older than 2 weeks), in which severe disease and poor outcome are rare.[2,4] In this patient population, the onset of illness is usually sudden, with fever present in 76% to 100% of patients; the fever may be biphasic, initially appearing with nonspecific constitutional symptoms, disappearing, and then reappearing with the onset of meningeal signs. More than half of patients have nuchal rigidity, which is more frequently present in older toddlers, children, adolescents, and adults. Headache (often severe and frontal in location) is nearly always present in adults; photophobia is also common in older patients. Nonspecific symptoms and signs include vomiting, anorexia, rash, diarrhea, cough, upper respiratory findings (especially pharyngitis), and myalgias. Other clues to the presence of enteroviral disease, in addition to the time of year and known epidemic disease in the community, include the presence of exanthems, myopericarditis, conjunctivitis, and specifically recognizable enteroviral syndromes such as pleurodynia, herpangina, and hand-foot-and-mouth disease.[1] In addition, specific clinical stigmata may be associated with certain enteroviral serotypes.[2] For example, echovirus 9 is associated with scattered maculopapular rashes. Herpangina, in particular the finding of painful vesicles on the posterior oropharynx, is associated with coxsackievirus A; the presence of pericarditis or pleurisy may identify coxsackievirus B. The duration of illness in enteroviral meningitis is usually less than 1 week, with many patients reporting improvement after lumbar puncture, presumably as a result of a reduction in intracranial pressure. In contrast, during an outbreak of enterovirus 71 infection in Taiwan in patients 3 months to 8.2 years of age, the chief neurologic complaint was rhombencephalitis (seen in 90% of children), which carried a case-fatality rate of 14%.[6] In another outbreak in young children with enterovirus 71 infection in Perth, Western Australia,[7] neurologic syndromes included aseptic meningitis, Guillain-Barré syndrome, acute transverse myelitis, acute cerebellar ataxia, opsomyoclonus syndrome, benign intracranial hypertension, and febrile convulsions; this contrasts to previous epidemics, in which damage to gray matter was the most frequent cause of neurologic disease.

A unique clinical situation is seen in children and adults with absent or deficient humoral immunity that impairs clearance of enteroviruses. In persons who are agammaglobulinemic, a chronic enteroviral meningitis or meningoencephalitis may develop and last several years, often with a fatal outcome[2,4]; this syndrome has been designated chronic enteroviral meningoencephalitis in agammaglobulinemia (CEMA). CEMA is a constellation of neurologic symptoms

TABLE 80-8 Presenting Symptoms and Signs in Patients with Central Nervous System Mumps

Symptom or Sign	Relative Frequency (%)
Fever	88-100
Vomiting	68-94
Headache	47-88
Salivary gland swelling	47-62
Meningismus	43-93
Lethargy	28-69
Abdominal pain	14-23
Seizures	14-18

Adapted from Gnann JW Jr. Meningitis and encephalitis caused by mumps virus. In: Scheld WM, Whitley RJ, Durack DT, eds. Infections of the Central Nervous System. 2nd ed. Philadelphia: Lippincott-Raven; 1997:169-180, with permission.

that includes headache, seizures, hearing loss, lethargy/coma, weakness, ataxia, paresthesias, and loss of cognitive skills. In about half of these patients, a rheumatologic syndrome, usually dermatomyositis, also develops, probably as a direct result of enteroviral invasion of affected tissues.

Mumps Virus

In patients with mumps, CNS symptoms usually follow the onset of parotitis, when present, by about 5 days. The most frequent clinical manifestation of mumps CNS infection is the triad of fever, vomiting, and headache (Table 80-8).[12] The fever is usually high and lasts for 72 to 96 hours. Salivary gland enlargement is present in only about 50% of patients. Other findings include neck stiffness, lethargy or somnolence, and abdominal pain. Most patients have signs of meningitis but no evidence of cortical dysfunction. Defervescence is usually accompanied by clinical recovery, and in uncomplicated cases, the total duration of illness is 7 to 10 days. Rarely, mumps may cause encephalitis, seizures, polyradiculitis, polyneuritis, cranial nerve palsies, myelitis, Guillain-Barré syndrome, and fatality.[12]

Lymphocytic Choriomeningitis Virus

Lymphocytic choriomeningitis virus infection begins with nonspecific viral symptoms. After a brief period of improvement, severe headache, photophobia, lightheadedness, lumbar myalgias, and pharyngitis develop in approximately 15% of patients.[1] Occasionally, orchitis, arthritis, myopericarditis, and alopecia are also seen, usually as late manifestations.

Herpesviruses

Meningitis associated with herpes simplex virus type 2 infection is usually characterized by stiff neck, headache, and fever.[14] In one review of 27 patients with herpes simplex virus type 2 meningitis,[18] neurologic complications were found in 37% of cases and consisted of urinary retention, dysesthesias, paresthesias, neuralgia, motor weakness, paraparesis, concentration difficulties of about 3 months' duration, and impaired hearing. All complications, however, subsided within 6 months in all patients. Recurrent meningitis was documented in five patients. Pharyngitis, lymphadenopathy, and splenomegaly should suggest Epstein-Barr virus infection. A diffuse vesiculopustular rash may be seen in meningitis caused by varicella-zoster virus.

Human Immunodeficiency Virus

HIV-infected patients may present with a typical aseptic meningitis syndrome associated with acute infection (i.e., the mononucleosis-like syndrome).[26-28] In addition, some patients may present with an atypical aseptic meningitis that is often chronic, tends to recur, and often includes cranial neuropathies (usually cranial nerves V, VII, and VIII) or long-tract findings.[244] The most common features are headache, fever, and meningeal signs. The illness is self-limited or recurrent rather than progressive.

TABLE 80-9 Presenting Symptoms and Signs in Patients with Bacterial Meningitis

Symptom or Sign	Relative Frequency (%)
Headache	≥90
Fever	≥90
Meningismus	≥85
Altered sensorium	>80
Vomiting	~35
Seizures	~30
Focal neurologic findings	10-20
Papilledema	<5

Bacterial Meningitis

Patients with bacterial meningitis classically present with fever, headache, meningismus, and signs of cerebral dysfunction (i.e., confusion, delirium, or a declining level of consciousness ranging from lethargy to coma) (Table 80-9).[63,143] In a review of 493 cases of acute bacterial meningitis in adults,[33] the classic triad of fever, nuchal rigidity, and change in mental status was found in only two thirds of patients, but all had at least one of these findings. The meningismus may be subtle, marked, or accompanied by Kernig's or Brudzinski's sign, or both.[245] Kernig's sign is elicited with the patient in the supine position, with the thigh flexed on the abdomen and the knee flexed. The leg is then passively extended, and in the presence of meningeal inflammation, the patient resists leg extension; this technique differs somewhat from the maneuver as first described by Kernig, in which the patient was initially placed in the seated position. Several signs were described by Brudzinski, although the best known is the nape-of-the-neck sign, in which passive flexion of the neck results in flexion of the hips and knees. However, in a recent prospective study that examined the diagnostic accuracy of meningeal signs in adults with suspected meningitis, the sensitivity of these findings was 5% for Kernig's sign, 5% for Brudzinski's sign, and 30% for nuchal rigidity,[246] indicating that they did not accurately distinguish patients with meningitis from those without meningitis. Therefore, the absence of these findings does not rule out the diagnosis of bacterial meningitis. Cranial nerve palsies (especially those involving cranial nerves III, IV, VI, and VII) and focal cerebral signs are seen in 10% to 20% of cases. Cranial nerve palsies probably develop as the nerve becomes enveloped by exudate in the arachnoid sheath surrounding the nerve, or they may be a sign of increased intracranial pressure. Seizures occur in about 30% of patients. Focal neurologic deficits and seizures arise from cortical and subcortical ischemia, which results from inflammation and thrombosis of blood vessels, often within the subarachnoid space. Hemiparesis may also result from the presence of a large subdural effusion and arises when infection in the adjacent subarachnoid space leads to increased permeability of the thin-walled capillaries and veins of the inner layer of the dura; this condition is usually self-limited, although an enlarging effusion can lead to a mass effect with resultant hemiparesis. Papilledema is seen in less than 5% of cases early in infection, and its presence should suggest an alternative diagnosis. With disease progression, signs of increased intracranial pressure may develop, including coma, hypertension, bradycardia, and palsy of cranial nerve III.

To further characterize the accuracy and precision of the clinical examination in adult patients with acute meningitis, patient data from 845 episodes of acute meningitis (confirmed by lumbar puncture or autopsy) in patients aged 16 to 95 years were reviewed[247]; the majority of patients in this review had acute bacterial meningitis, although 62 had tuberculous or "aseptic" meningitis. The results demonstrated that individual items of the clinical history (i.e., headache, nausea, and vomiting) had a low accuracy for the diagnosis of acute meningitis in adults. However, on review of the accuracy of physical examination findings, the absence of fever, neck stiffness, and altered mental status effectively eliminated the likelihood of acute meningitis; the sensitivity was 99% to 100% for the presence of one of these findings in the diagnosis of acute meningitis.

Despite these findings, however, physicians should have a low threshold for lumbar puncture in patients at high risk for bacterial meningitis, given the serious nature of this disease.

A specific etiologic diagnosis in patients with bacterial meningitis may be suggested by certain symptoms or signs.[143] About 50% of patients with meningococcemia, with or without meningitis, present with a prominent rash located principally on the extremities. Early in the course of illness, the rash is typically erythematous and macular, but it quickly evolves into a petechial phase with further coalescence into a purpuric form. The rash often matures rapidly, with new petechial lesions appearing during the physical examination. In one review of the clinical features of 255 patients with acute meningococcal meningitis,[248] a petechial rash was observed in three quarters of the patients; the rash was more commonly seen in children and adults younger than 30 years (81%) than in patients 30 years and older (62%). A similar rash may also be seen in splenectomized patients with rapidly overwhelming sepsis caused by *S. pneumoniae* or *H. influenzae* type B. In patients who have suffered a basilar skull fracture in which a dural fistula is produced between the subarachnoid space and the nasal cavity, paranasal sinuses, or middle ear, a common finding is rhinorrhea or otorrhea secondary to a CSF leak[67]; in these patients, meningitis may be recurrent and is most commonly caused by *S. pneumoniae*. Patients with *L. monocytogenes* meningitis have an increased tendency to have seizures and focal deficits early in the course of infection, and some patients may present with ataxia, cranial nerve palsies, or nystagmus secondary to rhombencephalitis[68-70]; however, patients with *Listeria* meningitis may not present with any focal signs. In a large review (367 episodes) of CNS infections caused by *L. monocytogenes*,[71] the most frequent findings were fever (92%) and altered sensorium (65%); only about 50% of patients had headache.

Some categories of patients may not manifest many of the classic symptoms and signs of bacterial meningitis.[143] For example, neonates with bacterial meningitis usually do not have meningismus.[76,249] Clinical clues to the presence of meningitis in neonates are temperature instability (hypothermia or hyperthermia), listlessness, high-pitched crying, fretfulness, lethargy, refusal to feed, weak suck, irritability, jaundice, vomiting, diarrhea, or respiratory distress. A change in the child's affect or state of alertness is one of the most important signs of meningitis. A bulging fontanelle (seen in one third of cases) usually occurs late during the course of illness; seizures are observed in 40% of neonates with bacterial meningitis. In children 1 to 4 years of age, fever (94%), vomiting (82%), and nuchal rigidity (77%) are the most common initial symptoms.[250] Older adult patients, especially those with underlying conditions (e.g., diabetes mellitus or cardiopulmonary disease), may present insidiously with lethargy or obtundation, no fever, and variable signs of meningeal inflammation.[251] In one review,[252] confusion was very common in older adult patients on initial examination and occurred in 92% and 78% of those with pneumococcal and gram-negative bacillary meningitis, respectively. Older adult patients may also present with an antecedent or concurrent bronchitis, pneumonia, or paranasal sinusitis. The diagnosis of bacterial meningitis in neutropenic patients requires a high index of suspicion, because symptoms and signs may initially be subtle because of the impaired ability of the patient to mount a subarachnoid space inflammatory response.[253] In patients with head trauma, the symptoms and signs of meningitis may be present as a result of the underlying injury and not meningitis.[67] In all of these subgroups of patients, altered or changed mental status should not be ascribed to other causes until bacterial meningitis has been excluded by CSF examination.

Spirochetal Meningitis

Treponema pallidum

The clinical features of neurosyphilis that have been described are based on studies compiled before the availability of penicillin, and it is not known whether the clinical findings of symptomatic neurosyphilis have been modified in the antibiotic era or by associated HIV infection.[104] Although the clinical features of neurosyphilis are numerous, only patients with acute meningitis and meningovascular syphilis are discussed here.

Patients with syphilitic meningitis usually present in a manner similar to that of patients with other forms of aseptic meningitis: they have complaints of headache, nausea, and vomiting. In one series, these complaints were present in 91% of patients.[254] Meningismus occurred in 59% and fever in less than half of the patients with syphilitic meningitis. Seizures occurred in 17% of patients, whereas cranial nerve palsies were found in 45% of cases (most commonly cranial nerves VII and VIII, followed by II, III, VI, and V). Focal abnormalities such as hemiplegia, aphasia, and mental status changes were seen less commonly. Syphilitic meningitis rarely affects the spinal cord.

Meningovascular syphilis is clinically distinguished from syphilitic meningitis temporally and on the basis of focal neurologic findings as a result of focal syphilitic arteritis, which almost always occurs in association with meningeal inflammation.[104,105,255] Most patients experience weeks to months of episodic prodromal symptoms and signs, including headache or vertiginous episodes, personality changes (e.g., apathy or inattention), behavioral changes (e.g., irritability or memory impairment), insomnia, or seizures. Focal deficits, which reflect episodes of ischemia in regions of the brain by involved blood vessels (usually in the distribution of the middle cerebral artery), may also occur; if untreated, these deficits may progress to a stroke syndrome with attendant irreversible neurologic deficits.

Coinfection with HIV may modify the clinical spectrum of syphilis. Case reports and small series have suggested that patients with HIV infection are more likely to progress to neurosyphilis and have accelerated disease courses.[106-109,256] However, few clinical data currently support these hypotheses. In one study of HIV-infected and HIV-uninfected patients with syphilis at sexually transmitted disease clinics in Baltimore,[257] no significant differences were observed in clinical stage or in disease progression.

Borrelia burgdorferi

Meningitis is the most important neurologic abnormality of acute disseminated Lyme disease, usually following erythema migrans by 2 to 10 weeks[111]; however, only about 40% (range, 10% to 90%) of cases of Lyme meningitis are preceded by this characteristic rash.[113,258] Headache is the single most common symptom (30% to 90% of patients) in Lyme meningitis, whereas neck stiffness is seen in only 10% to 20% of cases.[111] Photophobia, nausea, and vomiting are intermediate in frequency between headache and neck stiffness. About two thirds of patients have accompanying systemic symptoms, including malaise, fatigue, myalgias, fever, arthralgias, and involuntary weight loss. In untreated cases, the duration of symptoms ranges from 1 to 9 months. Patients typically experience recurrent attacks of meningeal symptoms lasting several weeks and alternating with similar periods of milder symptoms.[111-113,258]

About half of patients with Lyme meningitis have mild cerebral symptoms consisting most commonly of somnolence, emotional lability, depression, impaired memory and concentration, and behavioral symptoms.[111-113,258] These symptoms may fluctuate in severity in untreated patients before resolution. Transverse myelitis, spastic paraparesis or quadriparesis, disturbances of micturition, and Babinski's sign are also reported during this stage. Approximately 50% of patients also have cranial neuropathies. Facial nerve palsy is the most common (80% to 90%) of the cranial nerve palsies overall and occurs with rapid onset (often in 1 to 2 days), frequently accompanied by slight ipsilateral facial numbness or tingling or ipsilateral ear or jaw pain. The facial palsy is bilateral in 30% to 70% of cases, although the two sides are affected asynchronously in most cases. Other cranial nerves affected less commonly are cranial nerves II, III, the sensory portion of V, VI, and the acoustic portion of VIII. Recovery usually takes place within 2 months.

Protozoal and Helminthic Meningitis

Amebas

Primary amebic meningoencephalitis occurs in two forms.[115,116] The acute form (incubation period, 3 to 8 days) is characterized by the sudden onset of high fever, photophobia, headache, and progression to stupor or coma and is usually indistinguishable from acute bacterial meningitis, although focal signs and seizures are more common in amebic meningoencephalitis. Because of early involvement of the olfactory area, early symptoms of abnormal smell or taste may be reported. Confusion, irritability, and restlessness progress to delirium, stupor, and finally, coma. Death in untreated patients generally occurs within 2 to 3 days from the onset of symptoms.

In contrast, the subacute or chronic form of primary amebic meningoencephalitis is manifested more insidiously by low-grade fever, headache, and focal signs (e.g., hemiparesis, aphasia, cranial nerve palsies, visual field disturbances, diplopia, ataxia, seizures)[115,116]; the olfactory bulbs are usually spared. Deterioration occurs over a period of 2 to 4 weeks until death. However, longer durations of illness have also been reported (range, 5 to 18 months).

Angiostrongylus cantonensis

Symptoms of meningitis begin 6 to 30 days (typically 1 to 2 weeks) after the ingestion of raw mollusks or other sources of the parasite.[90,123,259] Findings include severe headache (90%), stiff neck (56%), paresthesias (54%), and vomiting (56%). Moderate fever is present in about half of the cases. In a recent outbreak in 12 people with a common foodborne exposure in Jamaica, the mean incubation period was 11 days (range, 6 to 31 days).[125] Headache was the most frequent symptom. Visual disturbances or photophobia were seen in 92% of patients, and nuchal rigidity or neck pain and fatigue in 80% of cases. Hyperesthesias or paresthesias were present in 75% of patients, and were present in a patchy distribution of the extremities or trunk and did not correspond to any dermatomal pattern.

DIAGNOSIS

Viral Meningitis

Cerebrospinal Fluid Examination

CSF pleocytosis is almost always present in patients with enteroviral meningitis, although some enteroviruses have been isolated from young infants with clinical evidence of meningitis but no CSF white blood cells.[1,2] The cell count is usually 100 to 1000/mm³, although counts in the several thousands have also been reported; higher CSF white blood cell counts have been associated with a greater likelihood of isolating the causative enterovirus.[260] Early in infection, neutrophils may dominate the CSF profile, although this situation quickly gives way to a lymphocytic predominance over the first 6 to 48 hours. However, in a recent retrospective chart review of 158 cases of meningitis (138 aseptic and 20 bacterial), 51% of the 53 patients with aseptic meningitis and duration of symptoms of more than 24 hours had a neutrophil predominance in CSF,[261] suggesting that a CSF neutrophil predominance is not useful as a sole criterion in distinguishing between aseptic and bacterial meningitis. Elevated CSF protein and decreased CSF glucose concentrations, if present, are usually mild, although extreme degrees of both have been reported. A specific virologic diagnosis of enteroviral meningitis depends on isolation of the virus from the CSF in tissue culture,[262] although the sensitivity for enteroviral serotypes is only 65% to 75%, largely a result of the inability to grow many coxsackievirus A serotypes, which require suckling mouse inoculations.[2] The difficulty in isolation of enteroviruses from CSF may also relate to the low titers of enterovirus in CSF (as low as a median tissue culture infective dose of 10^1 to 10^3 per milliliter of CSF), and that no single cell line is optimal for the detection of all members of the genus.[4] Furthermore, the time required for identifying an enterovirus from CSF using cell cultures is too long to be of clinical

utility in establishing the diagnosis; the mean time for CSF enteroviruses to grow is 3.7 to 8.2 days. Although isolation of a nonpolio enterovirus from the throat or rectum of a patient with aseptic meningitis is suggestive of an etiologic diagnosis, the mean shedding periods from those sites after infection are 1 week and several weeks, respectively. In addition, viral shedding can occur in 7.5% of healthy controls during enterovirus epidemics.[1] Therefore, shedding from a past infection cannot be ruled out. Furthermore, a study found that non-CSF viral cultures were not helpful in predicting enteroviral CNS infection inasmuch as enteroviruses were isolated at the same frequency from non-CSF sites in infants in whom enteroviruses were cultured from CSF as in hospitalized infants with an acute illness whose CSF was negative.[263] Follow-up acute and convalescent serologic testing for the specific isolated strain may confirm the etiologic diagnosis.[1] Magnetic resonance imaging (MRI) of patients with rhombencephalitis has demonstrated high-intensity lesions in the brain stem, most commonly located in the tegmentum.[4]

Rapid diagnosis of enterovirus infection by immunoassay techniques has been hampered by the lack of a common antigen among the various serotypes and the low concentrations of virus in body fluids.[1,2] PCR is the most promising alternative to viral culture for the diagnosis of enteroviral meningitis. All the primers are directed at highly conserved regions of the 5′-noncoding region of the viral genome and designed for reverse transcription combined with PCR. Enteroviral reverse transcription PCR (RT-PCR) has been tested in clinical settings by numerous investigators and found to be more sensitive than culture for the detection of the enterovirus; the sensitivity has ranged from 86% to 100% and specificity from 92% to 100% for the diagnosis of enteroviral meningitis.[2,4,264-266] In addition, the time to identification of the enterovirus using RT-PCR is significantly reduced (hours to a day) compared with cell culture, which may lead to shortened patient hospitalization, less use of antimicrobial agents for treatment of presumptive bacterial meningitis, and reduction of the need for ancillary diagnostic tests.[267]

Patients with mumps meningitis almost always have CSF pleocytosis (usually less than 500/mm³), primarily mononuclear cells (greater than 80% lymphocytes in 80% to 90% of patients); the pleocytosis may persist for weeks. CSF protein levels are reported in one series to be normal in more than half of patients with mumps meningitis.[12] The CSF glucose content is normal in most patients, but it may be depressed in up to 25% of cases. Complement fixation and hemagglutination inhibition on serum specimens are the most reliable serologic tests for the diagnosis of mumps. Testing of paired acute and convalescent sera should demonstrate a diagnostic fourfold rise in mumps antibody titer. Mumps virus can be grown from CSF in tissue culture for at least 1 week after the onset of disease, but the sensitivity of this technique is highly variable (30% to 50% if collected from CSF early during the course of mumps CNS infection).[12] Application of molecular diagnostic techniques such as PCR may make the diagnosis of mumps faster and more reliable in the future.

The CSF of patients with meningitis caused by lymphocytic choriomeningitis virus typically shows a lymphocytic pleocytosis (usually less than 750/mm³, although counts up to several thousand may be seen).[1] Hypoglycorrhachia is seen in up to 25% of cases. No rapid detection method is available. The virus may be cultured from blood and CSF early in infection and later from urine. The diagnosis is usually made by a fourfold rise between acute and convalescent sera.

Patients with herpes simplex virus type 2 meningitis also have a lymphocytic meningitis (less than 500/mm³) and a normal glucose content.[1] The virus has been cultured from the CSF and buffy coat of some patients. PCR appears promising for the diagnosis of CNS infections caused by herpes simplex virus. With PCR, herpes simplex virus type 2 has been strongly associated with typical cases of Mollaret's meningitis in patients without symptoms or signs of genital infection.[20,21] PCR has also been used to confirm the presence of varicella-zoster viral DNA in the CSF of patients with herpes zoster meningitis.[268,269] The CSF in HIV-infected patients during the acute retroviral syndrome typically shows a mild lymphocytic pleocytosis ($< 200/mm^3$), mildly elevated protein concentrations, and a normal or slightly decreased glucose content[28,244]; these CSF parameters improve and sometimes resolve within 2 weeks. HIV has been isolated from the CSF of some patients with neurologic disease,[28,270] although it can be isolated from HIV-infected patients without neurologic symptoms or signs.[270,271] HIV RNA has also been detected in the CSF of patients with meningitic disease.[272,273] A few mononuclear cells and elevated protein concentrations in CSF are commonly documented in HIV-positive patients throughout the course of infection. The CSF findings in patients with arboviral meningitis are similar to those caused by enteroviruses.[1,2] Virus has been cultured from blood and CSF, but the diagnosis is usually made by comparison of acute and convalescent sera.

Bacterial Meningitis

Cerebrospinal Fluid Examination

The diagnosis of bacterial meningitis rests on CSF examination by lumbar puncture[143,249,274,275]; typical CSF findings in acute bacterial meningitis are shown in Table 80-10. In virtually all cases, the opening pressure is elevated, with values over 600 mm H_2O suggesting the presence of cerebral edema, intracranial suppurative foci, or communicating hydrocephalus. The white blood cell count is elevated in untreated bacterial meningitis, usually 1000 to $5000/mm^3$ (range of less than 100 to more than $10,000/mm^3$). Neutrophils usually predominate, although approximately 10% of patients with acute bacterial meningitis present with a predominance of lymphocytes in spinal fluid; such predominance is more common in neonatal gram-negative bacillary meningitis and meningitis caused by *L. monocytogenes* (about 30% of cases). Patients with very low CSF white cell counts (0 to $20/mm^3$) despite high CSF bacterial concentrations tend to have a poor prognosis. The absence of a CSF pleocytosis can characterize up to 4% of cases of bacterial meningitis overall,[276] most commonly in premature neonates (up to 15% of cases) and infants younger than 4 weeks (17% of cases). In addition, normal CSF white blood cell counts have been seen in patients with meningococcal meningitis[277,278] and accounted for almost 10% of all cases of meningococcal meningitis in one study.[277] Therefore, a Gram stain and culture should be performed on all spinal fluid specimens even if the white blood cell count is normal. A CSF glucose concentration decreased to less than 40 mg/dL is found in about 60% of patients and a CSF-to-serum glucose ratio less than 0.31 in about 70% of patients. CSF protein concentrations are elevated in virtually all patients, presumably because of disruption of the BBB. However, a normal CSF white blood cell count and protein concentration may be seen in specimens obtained at the onset of meningitis, in some cases of neonatal meningitis, and in severely immunocompromised patients. A CSF glucose concentration less than 34 mg/dL, a CSF-to-blood glucose ratio less than 0.23, a CSF protein concentration greater than 220 mg/dL, more than 2000 leukocytes per cubic millimeter of CSF, and more than 1180 neutrophils per cubic millimeter of CSF were found to be individual predictors of bacterial rather than viral meningitis, with 99% certainty or better.[279] This model was validated in one retrospective review of patients with meningitis,[280]

TABLE 80-10 Typical Cerebrospinal Fluid Findings in Patients with Bacterial Meningitis

Cerebrospinal Fluid Parameter	Typical Finding
Opening pressure	200-500 mm H_2O
White blood cell count	1000-5000/mm³ (range, <100 to >10,000)
Percentage of neutrophils	≥ 80%
Protein	100-500 mg/dL
Glucose	≤40 mg/dL
CSF-to-serum glucose ratio	≤0.4
Gram stain	Positive in 60%-90%
Culture	Positive in 70%-85%
Polymerase chain reaction	Promising*

*See text for details.

although proof of the utility of this model will require a prospective application. Elevated CSF lactate concentrations (especially above 35 mg/dL) may also be useful in differentiating bacterial from nonbacterial meningitis in patients who have not received prior antimicrobial therapy[281]; despite the high sensitivity of the CSF lactate concentration in the diagnosis of acute bacterial meningitis, the results are generally nonspecific and provide little additional diagnostic information.

Gram stain examination of CSF permits rapid, accurate identification of the causative microorganism in 60% to 90% of patients with bacterial meningitis and has a specificity of nearly 100%.[143,249] The likelihood of detecting the organism by Gram stain correlates with the concentration of bacteria in CSF; concentrations of 10^3 or fewer colony-forming units per milliliter are associated with positive Gram stains about 25% of the time, whereas CSF concentrations of bacteria of 10^5 or greater lead to positive microscopy results in up to 97% of cases. The clinical utility of the Gram stain also depends on the bacterial pathogen[282,283]: bacteria have been observed in 90% of cases of meningitis caused by *S. pneumoniae*, 86% of cases caused by *H. influenzae*, 75% of cases caused by *N. meningitidis*, and 50% of cases caused by gram-negative bacilli; the CSF Gram stain is positive in less than 50% of patients with *L. monocytogenes* meningitis. In addition, the probability of identifying the organism may decrease in patients who have received prior antimicrobial therapy (40% to 60% and less than 50% positivity on Gram stain and culture, respectively). In studies of infants and children with bacterial meningitis, initially positive CSF cultures became sterile in 90% to 100% of patients within 24 to 36 hours of administration of "appropriate" antimicrobial therapy.[276] More recently, it has been suggested that CSF sterilization may occur more rapidly after initiation of parenteral antimicrobial therapy than previously suggested, with complete sterilization of CSF containing meningococcus within 2 hours and the beginning of sterilization of pneumococcus by 4 hours into therapy.[284] However, in most infants and children with bacterial meningitis who have received prior antimicrobial therapy, no significant differences in the CSF indices occur, although two studies revealed significantly lower CSF protein concentrations and rates of Gram stain positivity.[143]

Several rapid diagnostic tests have been developed to aid in the diagnosis of bacterial meningitis.[143,283] Latex agglutination techniques detect the antigens of *H. influenzae* type B, *S. pneumoniae*, *N. meningitidis*, *E. coli* K1, and the group B streptococci. However, many of the test kits do not include tests for group B meningococci, and other kits are probably poor because of the limited immunogenicity of group B meningococcal polysaccharide. Performance of one of these rapid diagnostic tests may be considered on CSF specimens from patients with presumed bacterial meningitis and a negative CSF Gram stain, although it must be emphasized that a negative test does not rule out infection caused by a specific meningeal pathogen. Recently, the routine use of CSF bacterial antigen tests for the etiologic diagnosis of bacterial meningitis has been questioned. In one study of 901 CSF bacterial antigen tests performed over a 37-month period, no modification of therapy occurred in 22 of 26 patients with positive results.[143] False-positive results have occasionally resulted in unnecessary treatment and prolonged hospitalization. Another study of 344 CSF specimens submitted for bacterial antigen assays found that 10 specimens represented true infections (by culture criteria), for a sensitivity and specificity of 70% and 99.4%, respectively[285]; a positive CSF antigen test did not affect clinical therapy or hospital course. Furthermore, in patients with culture-negative meningitis, CSF latex agglutination had a sensitivity of only 7% in one study.[286]

PCR has been used to amplify DNA from patients with meningitis caused by several meningeal pathogens.[143,249] In one study of CSF samples from patients with meningococcal meningitis,[287] the sensitivity and specificity of PCR were both 91%. More recently, the clinical utility of PCR for the diagnosis of meningitis was assessed with the use of a broad range of bacterial primers. The test characteristics for broad-based bacterial PCR demonstrated a sensitivity of 100%, a specificity of 98.2%, a positive predictive value of 98.2%, and a negative predictive value of 100%.[288] Therefore, broad-based bacterial

PCR may be useful for excluding the diagnosis of meningitis, with the potential of influencing decisions to initiate or discontinue antimicrobial therapy. PCR may be particularly useful in patients with bacterial meningitis who have received prior antimicrobial therapy and are more likely to have negative CSF cultures.[289] Problems with false-positive results arise when using PCR, although further refinements in this technique may lead to its usefulness in the diagnosis of bacterial meningitis, particularly when CSF Gram stain and cultures are negative. Another potential application of PCR is rapid detection of the in vitro susceptibility of meningeal pathogens to specific antimicrobial agents. In a recent report, a novel real-time PCR-hybridization assay was developed for the rapid detection of penicillin susceptibility in *S. pneumoniae;* when applied to 24 pneumococcal DNA–positive CSF extracts, penicillin-sensitive *S. pneumoniae* was detected in all instances.[290] Further studies may establish the usefulness of this rapid technique in allowing clinicians to decide on the use of specific antimicrobial therapy in patients with bacterial meningitis (see later).

C-Reactive Protein and Procalcitonin

Several proteins have been examined for their usefulness in the diagnosis of acute bacterial meningitis. Specifically, C-reactive protein (CRP), detected either in serum or CSF, and serum procalcitonin concentrations have been elevated in patients with acute bacterial meningitis and may be useful in discriminating between bacterial and viral meningitis. In one study, serum CRP was capable of distinguishing Gram stain–negative bacterial meningitis from viral meningitis on admission with a sensitivity of 96%, a specificity of 93%, and a negative predictive value of 99%.[291] In another study, a serum procalcitonin concentration of more than 0.2 ng/mL had a sensitivity and specificity of up to 100% in the diagnosis of bacterial meningitis,[292] although false-negative results have been reported.[293] In patients with meningitis in whom the CSF Gram stain is negative and analysis of other parameters is inconclusive, serum concentrations of CRP or procalcitonin that are normal or below the limit of detection have a high negative predictive value in the diagnosis of bacterial meningitis, so that these patients (i.e., with a presumptive diagnosis of viral meningitis) can be carefully observed without initiation of antimicrobial therapy.[294]

Radiography

Cranial computed tomography (CT) or MRI does not aid in the diagnosis of acute bacterial meningitis. However, one of these modalities should be considered during the course of illness in patients who have persistent or prolonged fever, clinical evidence of increased intracranial pressure, focal neurologic findings or seizures, enlarging head circumference (in neonates), persistent neurologic dysfunction, or persistently abnormal CSF parameters or cultures (Fig. 80-2).[76,143,274] However, cranial CT may underestimate the possibility of increased intracranial pressure in patients with pneumococcal meningitis,[295] so intracranial pressure monitoring should be considered in patients with prolonged coma. Cranial CT or MRI has been recommended at the end of antimicrobial therapy in newborn infants to be certain that no intracranial complications have occurred.[76] In one review of 107 children with bacterial meningitis who underwent CT scanning,[296] one or more abnormalities were found in 52% of cases, although most findings did not require specific intervention. However, children with fever and subdural collections detected by CT may require a drainage procedure.

Radiographic studies may be useful in the subset of patients with meningitis as a result of a basilar skull fracture with CSF leak.[67,95] CT scanning may detect air-fluid levels, opacification of the paranasal sinuses, or intracranial air; CT scanning with sagittal reconstruction can also be used to document or localize fracture sites. Radioisotope cisternography with cottonoid pledgets placed at the outlet of the sinuses within the nasal passage can be used to document a CSF leak, although high-resolution CT scanning with water-soluble contrast enhancement of the CSF (metrizamide cisternography) is the best test for defining the site of leakage.

Spirochetal Meningitis

Treponema pallidum

For the diagnosis of CNS involvement in patients with syphilis, no single routine laboratory test is definitive. CSF cellular and protein abnormalities have been reported to occur in 10% to 20% of patients with primary syphilis, 30% to 70% of patients with secondary syphilis, and 10% to 30% of patients with latent syphilis.[108] CSF abnormalities are

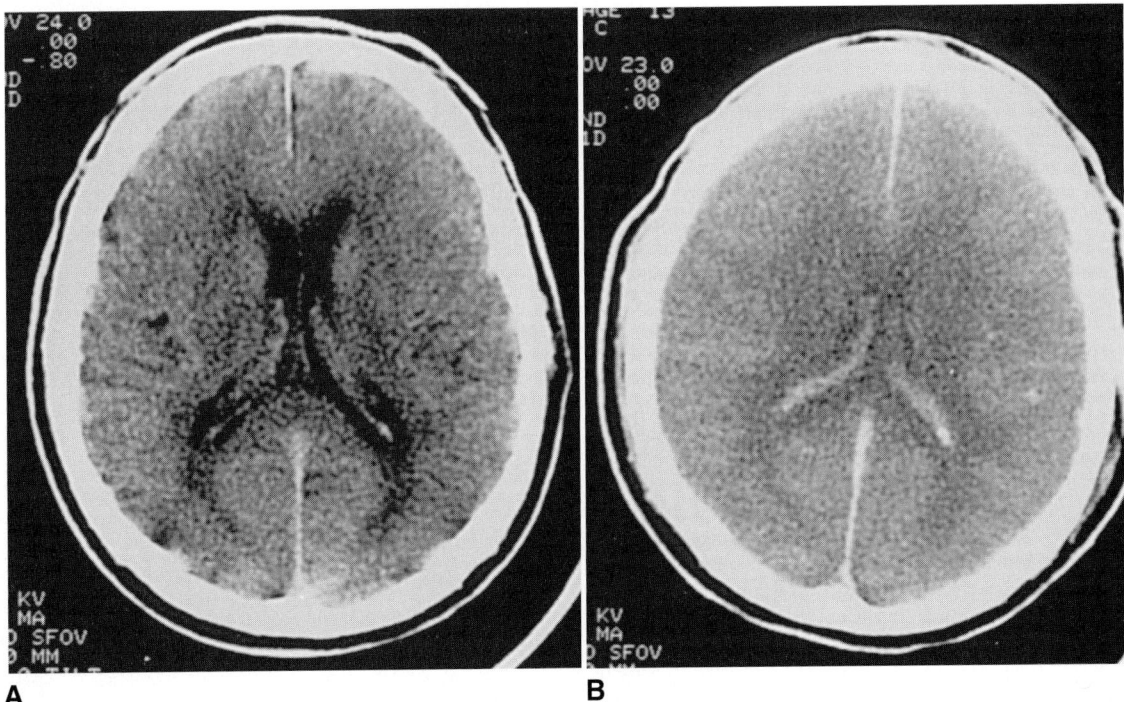

A   **B**

FIGURE 80-2. Computed tomography (CT) scans of the head in a patient with pneumococcal meningitis. **A,** CT scan on presentation reveals moderate cortical atrophy. **B,** CT scan 3 days later reveals diffuse swelling of the cerebral hemispheres bilaterally, with effacement of the ventricular system.

common in patients with syphilitic meningitis, but they are nonspecific. Findings include a mononuclear pleocytosis (more than 10 cells/mm³ in most patients), elevated CSF protein concentrations (78% of patients), and mild decreases in CSF glucose concentrations (less than 50 mg/dL in 55% of patients).[254] Oligoclonal bands and intrathecally produced antitreponemal antibodies are frequently present. Recovery of *T. pallidum* from CSF specimens is difficult, expensive, time consuming, and not routinely performed.[108]

Given the difficulties in the diagnosis of neurosyphilis, other CSF laboratory tests, particularly serologic testing (i.e., Venereal Disease Research Laboratory [VDRL] and fluorescent treponemal antibody tests) have been used.[108,254,297] However, serologic testing of CSF in patients with syphilis is problematic. For example, CSF collected by lumbar puncture is subject to blood contamination in about 10% of patients, which may lead to contamination of CSF and, therefore, a false-positive serologic test result[104]; the likelihood of a false-positive test depends on the relative amount of contamination, the antibody titer in blood, and the sensitivity of the test. For patients with a serum VDRL value of 1:256 or less, sufficient blood contamination to be visible to the naked eye is required to cause false-positive CSF VDRL results. Although the specificity of the CSF VDRL test for the diagnosis of neurosyphilis is high, the sensitivity is low (reactive tests in only 30% to 70% of patients).[297] Therefore, a reactive CSF VDRL test in the absence of blood contamination is sufficient to diagnose neurosyphilis; a nonreactive result does not exclude the diagnosis. The CSF fluorescent treponemal antibody absorption (FTA-ABS) test has also been examined as a possible diagnostic test for neurosyphilis.[104,297,298] A nonreactive test effectively rules out the likelihood of neurosyphilis, but the specificity of the test is much less than the CSF VDRL test because of the possibility of leakage of small amounts of antibody from the serum into CSF. Furthermore, no compelling data confirm the significance of a reactive CSF FTA-ABS as being useful for the diagnosis of neurosyphilis.[104] PCR has been used to detect *T. pallidum* DNA in CSF samples in patients with acute symptomatic neurosyphilis.[299] Further large-scale studies are needed to determine the sensitivity and specificity of this technique. Because of the low sensitivity of the CSF VDRL test, and until further studies demonstrate the usefulness of rapid diagnostic techniques, the diagnosis of neurosyphilis is based on elevated CSF concentrations of white blood cells, protein, or both in the appropriate clinical and serologic setting.

Borrelia burgdorferi

Typical CSF changes in patients with Lyme meningitis are a pleocytosis (usually fewer than 500 cells/mm³, but up to 3500 cells/mm³), with more than 90% lymphocytes in 75% of cases[111]; plasma cells may also be present. CSF protein concentrations are usually elevated (up to 620 mg/dL) and the CSF glucose concentration is usually normal, although glucose can be low in patients with illness of long duration. Oligoclonal banding may be present, with the bands reactive to *B. burgdorferi* antigens.

The best currently available laboratory test for the diagnosis of Lyme disease is demonstration of specific serum antibody to *B. burgdorferi*, and this positive test in a patient with a compatible neurologic abnormality is strong evidence for the diagnosis.[111,300] However, these tests are not standardized, and marked variability is seen between laboratories.[301] Most laboratories now use an enzyme-linked immunosorbent assay (ELISA) with sonicated *B. burgdorferi* as the antigen, although others still use the immunofluorescence technique. By the time that subacute disseminated (i.e., stage II) disease develops in most patients, they have elevated serum concentrations of IgG antibody to *B. burgdorferi*. False-positive reactions have been reported in patients with rheumatoid arthritis, Rocky Mountain spotted fever, infectious mononucleosis, tuberculous meningitis, leptospirosis, yaws, syphilis, and relapsing fever,[111] although high titers of cross-reacting IgG antibodies have been detected only in patients with syphilis or relapsing fever. False-negative results may be obtained from an unreliable assay, early infection, or early antibiotic use, which may blunt the normal humoral immune response. It is currently recommended

that when the pretest probability of Lyme disease is 0.20 to 0.80, sequential testing with ELISA and Western blot is the most accurate method for ruling in or out the possibility of Lyme disease.[302,303] Specific antibody against *B. burgdorferi* also appears in the CSF, and calculation of a specific antibody-IgG index for serum and CSF may indicate intrathecal antibody synthesis,[111] although demonstration of the usefulness of CSF antibody must await prospective studies with adequate sample size.[302] The technique of PCR on CSF samples has also been successfully used to identify *B. burgdorferi* DNA in patients with Lyme neuroborreliosis[304,305] (see Chapter 239), although PCR must still be considered experimental in the diagnosis of CNS Lyme disease.

Radiologic studies may also be useful in patients with CNS manifestations of Lyme disease. CT has shown both enhancing and nonenhancing low-density lesions, mass effect, and cerebral demyelination. MRI may reveal punctate hyperresonant areas without mass effect within the cerebral white matter (Fig. 80-3).

Protozoal and Helminthic Meningitis

Amebas

The CSF formula in patients with the acute form of primary amebic meningoencephalitis reveals a neutrophilic pleocytosis, low glucose concentration, an elevated protein concentration, and red blood cells.[115,116] Gram stain is always negative. However, examination of fresh, warm specimens of CSF can reveal the ameboid movements of motile trophozoites.[306] After their death, trophozoites can be demonstrated by light or electron microscopy of brain tissue.

Patients with the subacute or chronic form of the illness have a less florid CSF inflammatory response with a predominant mononuclear leukocytosis. The CSF protein concentration is elevated, and the glucose content is often normal or slightly reduced. Because amebas are not found in CSF, the diagnosis usually requires examination of a biopsy or necropsy specimen revealing the characteristic cysts. The

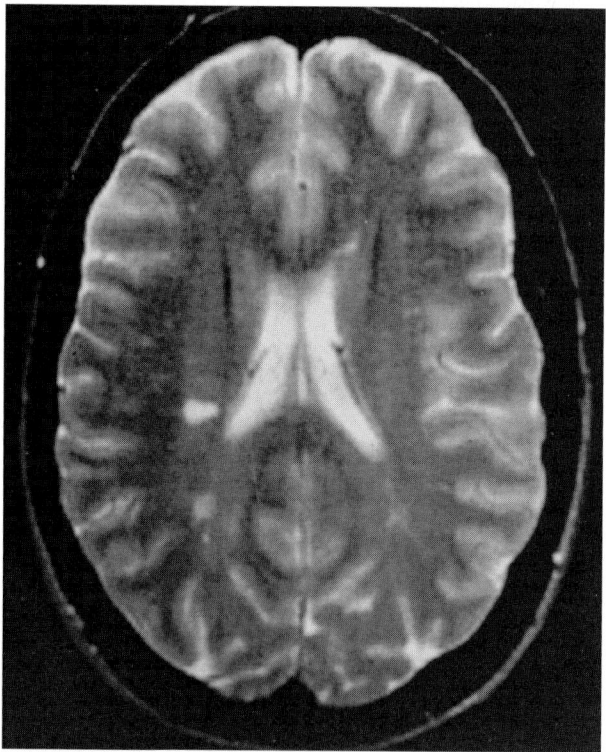

FIGURE 80-3 T₂-weighted magnetic resonance imaging scan in a patient with Lyme disease reveals areas of increased signal intensity in the cerebral white matter.

value of serologic tests is variable.[115] Serum immunofluorescence, amebic immobilization titers, and complement-fixing antibodies support the diagnosis, although demonstration of rising titers is necessary to establish the diagnosis because some healthy persons have circulating antibodies.

Angiostrongylus cantonensis

The combination of a history of ingestion of suspected food, moderate to high peripheral eosinophilia, and CSF eosinophilia leads to the suspicion of angiostrongyloidiasis.[115] The CSF leukocytosis is moderate, with 16% to 72% eosinophils and an increased protein concentration, but the glucose is normal. However, eosinophilia is not always present in the peripheral blood or in CSF on initial evaluation.[123] In the Jamaican outbreak, eosinophilia was not present in nearly half of the patients at the time of hospital admission, initially present in 56% and 44% of CSF and peripheral blood specimens, respectively.[125] Larvae are occasionally found on microscopy of CSF and are seen more often in pediatric patients than in adults. Serologic studies for *A. cantonensis* are not widely available and are not available in a timely manner for making clinical decisions.[123]

INITIAL MANAGEMENT OF PATIENTS WITH ACUTE MENINGITIS

The initial management of a patient with presumed bacterial meningitis includes performance of a lumbar puncture to determine whether the CSF formula is consistent with that diagnosis (Fig. 80-4).[143,307] If purulent meningitis is present, institution of antimicrobial therapy should be based on the results of Gram staining (Table 80-11). However, if no etiologic agent can be identified by this means or if performance of the lumbar puncture is delayed, institution of empirical antimicrobial therapy should be based on the patient's age and underlying disease status (Table 80-12). Although no prospective data are available on the timing of administration of antimicrobial therapy in patients with bacterial meningitis, a retrospective cohort study in patients with community-acquired bacterial meningitis demonstrated that a delay in initiation of antimicrobial therapy after patient arrival in the emergency department was associated with an adverse clinical

outcome when the patient's condition advanced to a high stage of prognostic severity,[308] thus supporting the assumption that treatment of bacterial meningitis before it advances to a high level of clinical severity improves clinical outcome. This concept has also been supported by two recent retrospective studies: one demonstrated a reduction in mortality with early administration of antimicrobial therapy,[309] and the other showed a benefit in terms of neurologic outcome and survival in patients who received antimicrobial therapy before the patient's level of consciousness deteriorated to a Glasgow Coma Scale lower than 10.[310] In patients who present with focal neurologic findings, or who have papilledema and suspected bacterial meningitis, a CT scan of the head should be performed before lumbar puncture to rule out the presence of an intracranial mass lesion because of the potential risk of herniation[143]; the true incidence of this problem is unclear but has been suggested to be less than 1.2% in patients with papilledema and about 12% in patients without papilledema but with elevated intracranial pressure. However, the time involved in waiting for a CT scan significantly delays the initiation of antimicrobial therapy, with the potential for increased morbidity and mortality in patients with bacterial meningitis. Therefore, emergency empirical antimicrobial therapy, after obtaining blood cultures, should be initiated before sending the patient to the CT scanner. Although CSF cultures may be sterile after the initiation of antimicrobial therapy, pretreatment blood

TABLE 80-11 Recommended Antimicrobial Therapy for Acute Bacterial Meningitis

Microorganism*	Antimicrobial Therapy
Haemophilus influenzae type B	Third-generation cephalosporin[†]
Neisseria meningitidis	Penicillin G or ampicillin[‡]
Streptococcus pneumoniae	Vancomycin plus a third-generation cephalosporin[†]
Listeria monocytogenes	Ampicillin or penicillin G[§]
Streptococcus agalactiae	Ampicillin or penicillin G[§]
Escherichia coli	Third-generation cephalosporin[†]

*Pathogen presumptively identified by positive Gram stain or bacterial antigen test.

[†]Cefotaxime or ceftriaxone; the fourth-generation cephalosporin cefepime may also be used.

[‡]Some authorities would prefer a third-generation cephalosporin if a resistant organism is suspected; the superiority of a third-generation cephalosporin over penicillin for these organisms has not been proved.

[§]Addition of an aminoglycoside should be considered.

From Tunkel AR, Scheld WM. Acute bacterial meningitis. Lancet. 1995;346:1675-1680. Reprinted with permission from Elsevier.

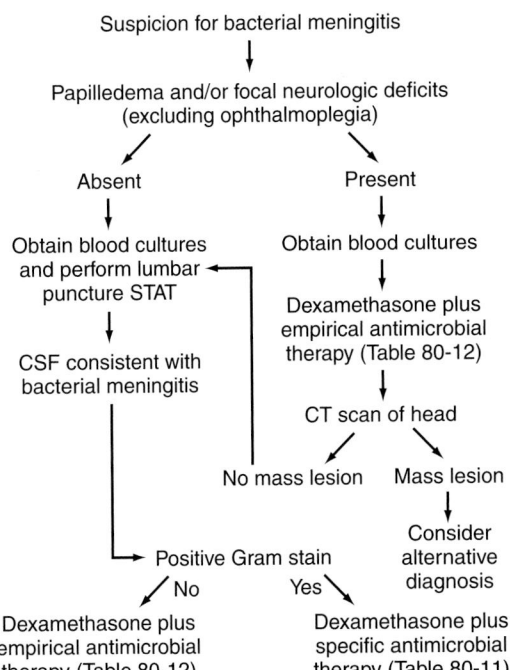

FIGURE 80-4. Algorithm for the initial management of the patient with meningitis. See text for recommendations for dexamethasone use.

TABLE 80-12 Empirical Therapy for Purulent Meningitis

Predisposing Factor	Antimicrobial Therapy
Age	
<1 mo	Ampicillin plus cefotaxime; or ampicillin plus an aminoglycoside
1-23 mo	Vancomycin plus a third-generation cephalosporin*; or vancomycin plus ampicillin plus chloramphenicol
2-50 yr	Vancomycin plus a third-generation cephalosporin*,[†]
>50 yr	Vancomycin plus ampicillin plus a third-generation cephalosporin*
Immunocompromised state	Vancomycin plus ampicillin plus either ceftazidime or cefepime
Basilar skull fracture	Vancomycin plus a third-generation cephalosporin*
Head trauma; postneurosurgery	Vancomycin plus ceftazidime or cefepime

*Cefotaxime or ceftriaxone; the fourth-generation cephalosporin cefepime may also be used.

[†]Add ampicillin if meningitis caused by *Listeria monocytogenes* is suspected.

cultures and the CSF formula or Gram stain will provide evidence for or against a diagnosis of bacterial meningitis. In one retrospective review of 177 patients (39 of whom had received prior antimicrobial therapy) with CSF culture–proven bacterial meningitis,[311] the combination of blood culture and CSF Gram strain, with or without latex agglutination, identified the causative bacterium in 92% of patients. Although some clinicians routinely order CT scans of the head before performance of a lumbar puncture in adults with suspected bacterial meningitis, this is not necessary in most patients. In a recent study of 301 patients with bacterial meningitis,[312] the clinical features at baseline that were associated with an abnormal finding on CT scan of the head were an age of at least 60 years, immunocompromised status, a history of CNS disease, a history of seizure within 1 week before presentation, and the following neurologic abnormalities: an abnormal level of consciousness, an inability to answer two consecutive questions correctly or to follow two consecutive commands, gaze palsy, abnormal visual fields, facial palsy, arm drift, leg drift, and abnormal language. The decision to perform a CT prior to lumbar puncture must be individualized, although these guidelines are useful in determining the patient groups that are more likely to have abnormal findings on neuroimaging studies.

Once the infecting meningeal pathogen is isolated and susceptibility testing known, antimicrobial therapy can be modified for optimal treatment (Table 80-13).[143] Recommended dosages of antimicrobial agents for adults with infections of the CNS are shown in Table 80-14, and those for neonates, infants, and children are presented in Table 80-15.

In addition, certain patients should receive adjunctive dexamethasone therapy when presenting with suspected or proven bacterial meningitis.[143,249,307] As stated earlier (see "Pathogenesis and Pathophysiology"), generation of pneumococcal cell wall components in an experimental animal model of pneumococcal meningitis

after treatment with bacteriolytic antibiotics may contribute to the inflammatory response in the subarachnoid space. The inflammatory response induced by either live pneumococci or pneumococcal cell wall was reduced by agents (e.g., methylprednisolone, oxindanac) that inhibit the cyclooxygenase pathway of arachidonic acid metabolism, and a correlation was noted between CSF concentrations of the arachidonic acid metabolite PGE_2 and CSF leukocytes. In another study, administration of the anti-inflammatory agent indomethacin decreased both brain water content and CSF concentrations of PGE_2 during experimental pneumococcal meningitis, although intracranial pressure was not reduced. In addition, the administration of either dexamethasone or oxindanac lessened the massive influx of serum albumin and other proteins of high and low molecular weight into the CSF during the early stages of experimental pneumococcal meningitis. Several corticosteroid agents have also been examined in experimental animal models of meningitis. Early studies revealed that methylprednisolone administration led to a significant reduction in the mass of leukocytes within the meninges of rabbits with pneumococcal meningitis. Another study demonstrated that CSF outflow resistance was reduced by methylprednisolone therapy and to a greater extent than in untreated or penicillin-treated rabbits with pneumococcal meningitis. In further studies that examined the effects of corticosteroids (methylprednisolone or dexamethasone) on brain water content, CSF pressure, and CSF lactate in rabbits with pneumococcal meningitis, it was found that both agents completely reversed the development of brain edema, but that only dexamethasone led to a reduction in CSF pressure and lactate; however, neither agent was superior to therapy with ampicillin alone in reducing cerebral edema or intracranial pressure, and no comparison was made between ampicillin alone and the combination of ampicillin plus corticosteroids, a comparison that would have been relevant to the potential clinical usefulness

TABLE 80-13   Specific Antimicrobial Therapy for Acute Meningitis

Microorganism	Standard Therapy	Alternative Therapies
Bacteria		
Haemophilus influenzae		
β-Lactamase negative	Ampicillin	Third-generation cephalosporin*; cefepime; chloramphenicol; aztreonam
β-Lactamase positive	Third-generation cephalosporin*	Cefepime; chloramphenicol; aztreonam; fluoroquinolone
Neisseria meningitidis		
Penicillin MIC < 0.1 μg/mL	Penicillin G or ampicillin	Third-generation cephalosporin*; chloramphenicol
Penicillin MIC 0.1-1.0 μg/mL	Third-generation cephalosporin*,†	Chloramphenicol; fluoroquinolone
Streptococcus pneumoniae		
Penicillin MIC < 0.1 μg/mL	Penicillin G or ampicillin	Third-generation cephalosporin*; vancomycin
Penicillin MIC 0.1-1.0 μg/mL	Third-generation cephalosporin*	Meropenem; vancomycin‡
Penicillin MIC ≥ 2.0 μg/mL	Vancomycin plus a third-generation cephalosporin*,‡	Third-generation cephalosporin plus a fluoroquinolone§
Enterobacteriaceae	Third-generation cephalosporin*	Aztreonam; fluoroquinolone; trimethoprim-sulfamethoxazole; meropenem
Pseudomonas aeruginosa	Ceftazidime‖ or cefepime‖	Aztreonam‖; fluoroquinolone‖; meropenem‖
Listeria monocytogenes	Ampicillin or penicillin G‖	Trimethoprim-sulfamethoxazole
Streptococcus agalactiae	Ampicillin or penicillin G‖	Third-generation cephalosporin*; vancomycin
Staphylococcus aureus		
Methicillin-sensitive	Nafcillin or oxacillin	Vancomycin
Methicillin-resistant	Vancomycin	—
Staphylococcus epidermidis	Vancomycin‡	—
Spirochetes		
Treponema pallidum	Penicillin G	Ceftriaxone¶
Borrelia burgdorferi	Third-generation cephalosporin*	Penicillin G; doxycycline
Protozoa/helminths		
Naegleria fowleri	Amphotericin B** plus rifampin plus doxycycline	—

*Cefotaxime or ceftriaxone; the fourth-generation cephalosporin cefepime may also be used.
†Superiority of a third-generation cephalosporin over penicillin has not been established.
‡Addition of rifampin may be considered; see text for indications.
§No clinical data available on the use of this combination; fluoroquinolones with in vitro activity against *S. pneumoniae* should be used (see text for details).
‖Addition of an aminoglycoside should be considered.
¶Value of these antimicrobial agents has not been established.
**Intravenous and intraventricular administration.
MIC, minimum inhibitory concentration.

TABLE 80-14 Recommended Dosages of Antimicrobial Agents for Meningitis in Adults with Normal Renal and Hepatic Function

Antimicrobial Agent*	Total Daily Dose	Dosing Interval (Hours)
Amikacin[†]	15 mg/kg	8
Ampicillin	12 g	4
Aztreonam	6-8 g	6-8
Cefepime	6 g	8
Cefotaxime	8-12 g	4-6
Ceftazidime	6 g	8
Ceftriaxone	4 g	12-24
Chloramphenicol[‡]	4-6 g	6
Ciprofloxacin	800-1200 mg	8-12
Doxycycline	200-400 mg	12
Gentamicin[†]	5 mg/kg	8
Meropenem	6 g	8
Nafcillin	9-12 g	4
Oxacillin	9-12 g	4
Penicillin G	24 million units	4
Rifampin[§]	600 mg	24
Tobramycin[†]	5 mg/kg	8
Trimethoprim-sulfamethoxazole[‖]	10-20 mg/kg	6-12
Vancomycin[†,¶]	30-40 mg/kg	8-12

*Unless indicated, therapy is administered intravenously.
[†]Need to monitor peak and trough serum concentrations.
[‡]Higher dose recommended for pneumococcal meningitis.
[§]Oral administration.
[‖]Dosage based on trimethoprim component.
[¶]May need to monitor cerebrospinal fluid concentrations in severely ill patients.

of adjunctive corticosteroid therapy in bacterial meningitis. A subsequent study did examine treatment with ceftriaxone versus ceftriaxone plus dexamethasone in an experimental rabbit model of *H. influenzae* meningitis. Although combination therapy consistently reduced the brain water content, CSF pressure, and CSF lactate to a greater degree than ceftriaxone alone did, the differences were not statistically significant. The authors suggested, however, that adjunctive dexamethasone might be more beneficial if administered early or even before antibiotic-induced bacterial lysis and release of microbial products. In a subsequent analysis using the experimental rabbit model of *H. influenzae* type B meningitis, ceftriaxone administration led to a significant increase in CSF endotoxin concentrations 2 hours after administration, which was followed by a rise in CSF TNF con-

centrations. Simultaneous administration of dexamethasone and ceftriaxone did not affect the release of endotoxin into CSF, but it markedly attenuated CSF concentrations of TNF measured 8 hours later. Adjunctive dexamethasone therapy also resulted in a significant decrease in CSF leukocytosis and a trend toward earlier improvement in CSF concentrations of glucose, lactate, and protein. These parameters improved without any apparent decrease in the rate of bacterial killing within the CSF in vivo.

On the basis of these observations, numerous clinical trials were undertaken to determine the effects of adjunctive dexamethasone on outcome in patients with bacterial meningitis (Table 80-16).[313-331] One meta-analysis of these clinical studies confirms the benefit of adjunctive dexamethasone (0.15 mg/kg every 6 hours for 2 to 4 days) for *H. influenzae* type B meningitis and, if commenced with or before parenteral antimicrobial therapy, suggests benefit for pneumococcal meningitis in childhood.[332] Evidence of clinical benefit was strongest for hearing outcomes. In contrast, a retrospective, nonrandomized study of children with pneumococcal meningitis published after the meta-analysis demonstrated that the use of adjunctive dexamethasone was not associated with a beneficial effect,[325] although the dexamethasone was administered before or within 1 hour of the first dose of antibiotic and the children in the dexamethasone group had a higher severity of illness. In addition, in a recently published double-blind, placebo-controlled trial of adjunctive dexamethasone in Malawi,[330] the overall number of deaths in the two treatment groups was similar, as was the frequency of neurologic sequelae (see Table 80-16). The factors that may have accounted for these results include the fact that Malawian children had severe disease associated with undernutrition and HIV infection, and the fact that they presented for medical attention after a delay, which resulted in very high case-fatality rates and significant long-term morbidity.[333] Corticosteroids do not reverse CNS damage that has already resulted from the pathophysiologic consequences of bacterial meningitis (e.g., cerebral edema and increased intracranial pressure). However, even in children with bacterial meningitis in the developing world, adjunctive dexamethasone should be used, because no adverse effects were attributable to its administration in this trial and its use may benefit some of the children with this devastating disorder.

In adult patients with bacterial meningitis, the routine use of adjunctive dexamethasone was controversial, until recently. In a prospective, randomized, double-blind trial in 301 adults with bacterial meningitis,[331] adjunctive dexamethasone was associated with a reduction in

TABLE 80-15 Recommended Dosages of Antimicrobial Agents for Meningitis in Neonates, Infants, and Children with Normal Renal and Hepatic Function

Antimicrobial Agent*	Total Daily Dose (Dosing Interval in Hours)		
	Neonates (0-7 Days Old)[†]	Neonates (8-28 Days Old)[†]	Infants and Children
Amikacin[‡]	15-20 mg/kg (12)	30 mg/kg (8)	20-30 mg/kg (8)
Ampicillin	150 mg/kg (8)	200 mg/kg (6-8)	300 mg/kg (6)
Cefepime	—	—	150 mg/kg (8)
Cefotaxime	100-150 mg/kg (8-12)	150-200 mg/kg (6-8)	225-300 mg/kg (6-8)
Ceftazidime	100-150 mg/kg (8-12)	150 mg/kg (8)	150 mg/kg (8)
Ceftriaxone	—	—	80-100 mg/kg (12-24)
Chloramphenicol	25 mg/kg (24)	50 mg/kg (12-24)	75-100 mg/kg (6)
Gentamicin[‡]	5 mg/kg (12)	7.5 mg/kg (8)	7.5 mg/kg (8)
Meropenem	—	—	120 mg/kg (8)
Nafcillin	75 mg/kg (8-12)	100-150 mg/kg (6-8)	200 mg/kg (6)
Penicillin G	0.15 mU/kg (8-12)	0.2 mU/kg (6-8)	0.3 mU/kg (4-6)
Rifampin[§,‖]	—	—	10-20 mg/kg (12-24)
Tobramycin[‡]	5 mg/kg (12)	7.5 mg/kg (8)	7.5 mg/kg (8)
Trimethoprim-sulfamethoxazole[¶]	—	—	10-20 mg/kg (6-12)
Vancomycin[‡]	20-30 mg/kg (8-12)	30-45 mg/kg (6-8)	60 mg/kg (6)

*Unless indicated, therapy is administered intravenously.
[†]Smaller dosages and longer intervals of administration may be advisable for very low birth weight neonates (<2000 g).
[‡]Need to monitor peak and trough serum concentrations.
[§]Oral administration.
[‖]Maximum daily dosage of 600 mg.
[¶]Dosage based on trimethoprim component.

TABLE 80-16 Outcome in Patients Receiving Adjunctive Dexamethasone Therapy for Bacterial Meningitis in Clinical Trials (1988-1998)

Study	Design	Antimicrobial Regimen	Results	Concerns
Lebel et al.[313]	Randomized, placebo-controlled; 200 infants and children 2 mo to 16 yr old; 77% of cases caused by *Haemophilus influenzae* type B	Cefuroxime or ceftriaxone	More rapid normalization of CSF parameters (glucose, protein, lactate) and temperature; lower incidence of moderate to severe bilateral sensorineural hearing loss (15.5% vs 3.3%, $p < .01$)	Audiologic sequelae significantly reduced only in patients receiving cefuroxime; four patients receiving dexamethasone developed gastrointestinal hemorrhage
Lebel et al[314]	Randomized, placebo-controlled; 60 infants and children 3 mo to 16 yr old; 75% of cases caused by *H. influenzae* type B	Cefuroxime	No significant differences in audiologic or neurologic sequelae	Small study size
Girgis et al[315]	Randomized, not placebo-controlled; 429 children and adults 3 mo to 60 yr old; 62% of cases caused by *Neisseria meningitidis*; 25% by *Streptococcus pneumoniae*; 13% by *H. influenzae* type B	Ampicillin plus chloramphenicol	Lower mortality rate in patients with pneumococcal meningitis (13.5% vs 40.7%, $p < .01$); lower incidence of sensorineural hearing loss in patients with pneumococcal meningitis (0% vs 12.5%, $p < .05$)	No differences in normalization of CSF parameters; no documentation of possible adverse effects; high percentage (>60%) of patients presented in a comatose state; most patients (370 of 429) received inadequate therapy for 3-5 days before hospitalization; antibiotics administered intramuscularly; no differences in outcome in patients with meningitis caused by *N. meningitidis* or *H. influenzae* type B
Odio et al[316]	Randomized, placebo-controlled; 101 infants and children 6 wk to 13 yr old; dexamethasone given 15-20 min before antibiotic; 78% of cases caused by *H. influenzae* type B	Cefotaxime	Significantly better clinical condition and mean prognostic score at 24 hr ($p \leq .001$); by 12 hr all indices of CSF inflammation improved with dexamethasone associated with a decrease in TNF-α and PAF; decreased incidence of one or more neurologic sequelae in patients followed a mean of 15 mo (10% vs 31%, $p = .008$); trend in reduction of audiologic sequelae in patients followed a mean of 15 mo (6% vs 16%, $p = .18$)	—
Kennedy et al[317]	Retrospective; 97 infants and children 2 mo to 15 yr old; 100% of cases caused by *S. pneumoniae*	Cefotaxime, ceftriaxone, cefuroxime, ampicillin, or penicillin	Significant reduction in total long-term neurologic outcome (11% vs 33%, $p = .033$); trend to reduction in neurologic (6% vs 16%, $p = .18$) and audiologic outcome (9% vs 21%, $p = .14$)	Retrospective review; no data on differences with regard to specific antibiotic used
Schaad et al[318]	Randomized, placebo-controlled; 115 infants and children 3 mo to 16 yr old; dexamethasone given 10 min before antibiotic; 58% of cases caused by *H. influenzae* type B, 24% by *N. meningitidis*	Ceftriaxone	Reduction in one or more neurologic or audiologic sequelae 15 mo after discharge (5% vs 16%, $p = .066$); relative risk of sequelae of 3.27 in patients receiving placebo	Dexamethasone given every 12 hr for 2 days
King et al[319]	Randomized, placebo-controlled; 101 children 1 mo to 18 yr old; 55% of cases caused by *H. influenzae* type B, 18% by *N. meningitidis*, 13% by *S. pneumoniae*	Ceftriaxone	No significant reduction in audiologic sequelae (10.4% vs 11.1% in placebo recipients); no significant reduction in neurologic sequelae (10.9% vs 8.6% in placebo recipients)	Dexamethasone given within 24 hr of antibiotic (median of 11 hr); only 8 of 50 patients received dexamethasone within 4 hr; study stopped prematurely because standard of care became early administration of dexamethasone
Wald et al[320]	Randomized, placebo-controlled; 143 infants and children 8 wk to 12 yr old; 53% of cases caused by *H. influenzae* type B, 23% by *S. pneumoniae*, 16% by *N. meningitidis*	Ceftriaxone	No significant differences in neurologic sequelae or developmental outcome; no significant differences in unilateral (10.3% vs 13.5% in placebo recipients) or bilateral (4.4% vs 9.4% in placebo recipients; $p = .33$) deafness; of 22 children who were deaf at entry, there were no significant differences in resolution of hearing impairment	Dexamethasone given within 4 hr of first dose of antibiotic; lack of follow-up for 13% of study population and incomplete follow-up for an additional 18%

CSF, cerebrospinal fluid; HIV, human immunodeficiency virus; PAF, platelet-activating factor; TNF, tumor necrosis factor; WBC, white blood cell count.

TABLE 80-16 Outcome in Patients Receiving Adjunctive Dexamethasone Therapy for Bacterial Meningitis in Clinical Trials (1988-1998)—cont'd

Study	Design	Antimicrobial Regimen	Results	Concerns
Kanra et al[321]	Randomized, placebo-controlled; 56 children 2 to 16 yr old; 100% of cases caused by *S. pneumoniae*	Ampicillin-sulbactam	No significant differences in moderate or severe unilateral or bilateral sensorineural hearing loss or neurologic sequelae at 6 wk (7.4% vs 23% in the placebo group; $p = .11$) or 1 yr (7.4% vs 26.9% in the placebo group; $p = .062$); significant reduction in hearing impairment at 3 mo (3.7% vs 23%, $p = .044$)	Did not use standard antibiotic therapy for bacterial meningitis; no data on antimicrobial resistance of pneumococcal isolates; Glasgow Coma Scale significantly lower in the dexamethasone group ($p = .004$)
Kilpi et al[322]	Randomized, not placebo-controlled; 122 infants and children 3 mo to 15 yr old; 53% of cases caused by *H. influenzae* type B, 33% by *N. meningitidis*, 10% by *S. pneumoniae*	Ceftriaxone	Dexamethasone recipients showed only a tendency to less severe hearing impairment	Some patients in each group also received therapy with oral glycerol; small sample size
Macaluso et al[323]	Retrospective; 179 children 1 mo to 16 yr old; 37% of cases caused by *H. influenzae* type B, 22% by *N. meningitidis*, 9% by *S. pneumoniae*	Benzyl penicillin plus chloramphenicol	Rate of discharge without sequelae was higher in the dexamethasone group (70% vs 56%, $p = .07$); in children aged 6-59 mo, those treated with dexamethasone had a significantly lower case-fatality rate (11% vs 25%, $p = .05$) and a better rate of discharge without sequelae (73% vs 52%, $p = .02$)	Retrospective; benefits observed only for children aged 6-59 mo; no causative organism identified in 27% of cases; no follow-up to assess the incidence of permanent neurologic sequelae
Qazi et al[324]	Randomized, placebo-controlled; 89 children 2 mo to 12 yr old; 20% of cases caused by *H. influenzae* type B, 9% by *N. meningitidis*, 7% by *S. pneumoniae*	Ampicillin plus chloramphenicol	Higher mortality rate in patients treated with adjunctive dexamethasone (25% vs 12%); in the survivors who received dexamethasone, the frequency of neurologic sequelae was 26.5% (vs 24% in the placebo recipients) and the frequency of hearing impairment was 42.3% (vs 30% in the placebo recipients)	No causative organism identified in 55% of cases; differences in mortality were not statistically significant due to small sample size; no correlation of severity of illness with outcome; not all patients may have received appropriate intensive care
Arditi et al[325]	Retrospective; children 3 days to 16.5 yr old; 100% of cases caused by *S. pneumoniae*	Variable	In the dexamethasone group, there was a higher incidence of any moderate or severe hearing loss (46% vs 23%, $p = .016$) or of any neurologic deficits (55% vs 33%, $p = .02$); no significant differences in deafness ($p = .06$) or neurologic sequelae ($p = .10$) when data controlled for severity of disease	Retrospective; children in the dexamethasone group more frequently required intubation and mechanical ventilation, and had a lower initial CSF glucose concentration; no data on use of specific antimicrobial agents in each group; no long-term follow-up of patients with hearing loss or neurologic deficits
Daoud et al[326]	Randomized, but not placebo-controlled; 52 full-term infants	Cefotaxime plus ampicillin	Mortality was 22% in the treated group vs 28% in the control group ($p = .87$); at follow-up examination up to age of 2 yr, 30% of dexamethasone recipients and 39% of control group had neurologic sequelae	Small study size
Thomas et al[327]	Randomized, placebo-controlled; 60 patients 18-79 yr old; 52% of cases caused by *S. pneumoniae* and 30% caused by *N. meningitidis*	Amoxicillin	No significant differences in the rate of cured patients without any neurologic sequelae (74.2% in the dexamethasone group vs 51.7% in the placebo group; $p = .07$)	Study stopped prematurely because of a new recommendation to use vancomycin plus a third-generation cephalosporin in meningitis; amoxicillin may have been inadequate for meningitis caused by resistant pneumococci; dexamethasone given within 3 hr of first antibiotic dose; patients in the dexamethasone group were significantly younger and less ill
Gijwani et al[328]	Prospective, placebo-controlled; 40 patients >10 yr old	Ceftriaxone	Clinical improvement of signs of meningeal irritation more rapid in dexamethasone group, but no differences in regard to resolution of fever, headache, and vomiting; neurologic complications and hearing loss were more common and severe in placebo group ($p < .05$)	Small sample size; secondary fever, gastrointestinal tract bleeding, and psychiatric manifestations were more common in the dexamethasone group

Continued

TABLE 80-16 Outcome in Patients Receiving Adjunctive Dexamethasone Therapy for Bacterial Meningitis in Clinical Trials (1988-1998)—cont'd

Study	Design	Antimicrobial Regimen	Results	Concerns
Ahsan et al[329]	Systematic sampling open-cohort study; not placebo-controlled; 68 patients 12-85 yr old	Benzyl penicillin plus chloramphenicol	Early resolution of fever, headache, and altered consciousness in the dexamethasone group; CSF inflammatory parameters (WBC count, glucose, protein) resolved earlier in the dexamethasone group by day 5; no difference in occurrence of other focal neurologic deficits; mortality lower in the dexamethasone group, but not statistically significant	Not placebo-controlled
Molyneux et al[330]	Double-blind, placebo-controlled; 598 children 2 mo to 13 yr old; 40% of cases caused by *S. pneumoniae*, 28% of cases caused by *H. influenzae* type B, 11% of cases caused by *N. meningitidis*, and 5% caused by *Salmonella* spp; 13% of patients had no growth on culture	Benzyl penicillin plus chloramphenicol; ceftriaxone could be added as second-line antibiotic	The overall numbers of deaths in the two treatment groups were similar (31% vs 31%, $p = .93$), with no significant differences based on isolated microorganism; at final outcome, sequelae were identified in 28% of children who received dexamethasone and 28% of those who received placebo ($p = .97$)	Patients had severe disease associated with undernutrition and HIV infection; patients presented for medical attention after a significant delay that resulted in high case-fatality rates and significant long-term morbidity; over one third of children received antimicrobial therapy prior to admission; 30% of children were placed on second-line antimicrobial therapy because of inadequate microbiologic or clinical response
de Gans and van de Beek[331]	Prospective, randomized, placebo-controlled, double-blind trial; 301 adults ≥ 17 yr old; 36% of cases caused by *S. pneumoniae*, 33% caused by *N. meningitidis*; 22% of patients had negative bacterial cultures	Amoxicillin	At 8 wk, the percentage of patients with an unfavorable outcome was significantly smaller in the dexamethasone group (15% vs 25%, $p = .03$) and the number of patients who died was significantly smaller in the dexamethasone group (7% vs 15%, $p = .04$); benefits were most striking in the subset of patients with pneumococcal meningitis, with the dexamethasone group having a lower percentage of patients with unfavorable outcome (26% vs 52%, $p = .006$) and death (14% vs 34%, $p = .02$); dexamethasone was most beneficial in patients with moderate to severe disease on the Glasgow Coma Scale	Higher percentage of patients in the dexamethasone group had seizures (10% vs 5%); only 72% of pneumococcal isolates were submitted for in vitro susceptibility testing and all were susceptible to penicillin; no data on effects of adjunctive dexamethasone in patients with pneumococcal meningitis caused by penicillin- or cephalosporin-resistant strains

CSF, cerebrospinal fluid; HIV, human immunodeficiency virus; PAF, platelet-activating factor; TNF, tumor necrosis factor; WBC, white blood cell count.

the proportion of patients who had unfavorable outcomes and in the proportion of patients who died (see Table 80-16). The benefits were most striking in the subgroup of patients with pneumococcal meningitis and in those with moderate-to-severe disease as assessed by the admission Glasgow Coma Scale. On the basis of these data and the apparent absence of serious adverse outcomes in the patients who received dexamethasone, the routine use of adjunctive dexamethasone (given concomitant with or just prior to the first dose of an antimicrobial agent for maximal attenuation of the subarachnoid space inflammatory response) is warranted in most adults with pneumococcal meningitis.[334] Adjunctive dexamethasone should not be used in patients who have already received antimicrobial therapy; if the meningitis is subsequently found not to be caused by *S. pneumoniae*, dexamethasone should be discontinued. The use of adjunctive dexamethasone is of particular concern in patients with pneumococcal meningitis caused by highly penicillin- and cephalosporin-resistant strains, in which case patients may require antimicrobial therapy with vancomycin. A diminished CSF inflammatory response after dexamethasone administration might significantly reduce vancomycin penetration into CSF and delay CSF sterilization, as shown in an experimental rabbit model of penicillin- and cephalosporin-resistant pneumococcal meningitis.[335] This result was confirmed in another rabbit model of pneumococcal meningitis in which significantly lower CSF vancomycin concentrations and differences in bacterial killing were found in the dexamethasone-treated rabbits.[336] However, CSF vancomycin penetration was not reduced by dexamethasone in a study in children.[337] CSF concentrations of ceftriaxone are not significantly altered in animals or patients treated with adjunctive dexamethasone.[335,338,339] In contrast, in an experimental rabbit model of cephalosporin-resistant pneumococcal meningitis,[340] concomitant use of dexamethasone with ceftriaxone resulted in higher CSF bacterial counts and a higher number of therapeutic failures. For any patient receiving adjunctive dexamethasone who is not improving as expected or who has a pneumococcal isolate for which the cefotaxime or ceftriaxone minimal inhibitory concentration (MIC) is 2.0 µg/mL or greater, a repeat lumbar puncture 36 to 48 hours after initiation of antimicrobial therapy is recommended to document the sterility of CSF.[341,342] In the study cited earlier, only 78 (72%) of 108 CSF cultures that were positive for *S. pneumoniae* were submitted for in vitro susceptibility testing and all were susceptible to penicillin,[331] a finding that is unusual in many areas of the world. In patients with pneumococcal meningitis caused by strains that are highly resistant to penicillin or cephalosporins, careful observation and follow-up are critical to determine whether use of adjunctive dexamethasone is associated with adverse clinical outcome in these patients.[334]

ANTIMICROBIAL THERAPY

Viral Meningitis

Specific antiviral chemotherapy for the enteroviruses is not currently available; treatment is supportive. However, this may change in the future. Pleconaril is an agent that is being evaluated in serious enteroviral infections.[4] Pleconaril is a novel compound that integrates into the hydrophobic pocket of picornaviruses (including enteroviruses) and prevents viral replication by inhibiting viral uncoating and blocking viral attachment to host cell receptors. It is orally bioavailable in all age groups, and CNS concentrations are four times higher than those in serum. In a preliminary report on the outcome of potentially life-threatening enterovirus infections in patients treated with pleconaril by compassionate-use protocol,[343] the drug had beneficial effects on the clinical, virologic, laboratory, and radiologic parameters in patients with enterovirus infections. Of the 16 patients with chronic enteroviral meningoencephalitis in agammaglobulinemia (CEMA), 12 improved on pleconaril and four were unchanged and stable. In placebo-controlled clinical studies of pleconaril treatment of adults and children with non–life-threatening enteroviral meningitis, clinical (i.e., faster resolution of headache and return to work or school) and virologic benefits, and a favorable safety profile, were documented.[4] In a double-blind, placebo-controlled trial in infants (<12 months of age) with enteroviral meningitis, efficacy of pleconaril was not demonstrated, which may have been due to the low yield of serial viral cultures, relatively short and benign clinical courses, and the small number of subjects enrolled.[344] Further data are needed to determine the efficacy of pleconaril in more serious enteroviral infections (e.g., neonatal enteroviral sepsis), and careful surveillance for adverse events is necessary, particularly in infants who are treated with this agent.

No specific antiviral therapy exists for the arboviruses, mumps virus, or lymphocytic choriomeningitis virus. Antiretroviral therapy for HIV-infected patients is discussed in Chapter 124. Recovery of patients with herpes simplex virus type 2 meningitis is usually complete without neurologic sequelae. It is not clear whether antiviral treatment alters the course of mild meningitis. However, treatment with acyclovir is generally indicated for primary genital herpes infection (see Chapter 132).[17] Intravenous acyclovir is used if meningitis is associated with genital herpes simplex infection.

Bacterial Meningitis

Principles of Therapy

Many factors influence the choice of an antimicrobial agent in the treatment of bacterial meningitis. Utilization of animal models of infection has permitted quantification of the relative penetration of drug into CSF, the effects of meningitis on this entry parameter, and the relative bactericidal efficacy (defined as the rate of bacterial eradication) within purulent CSF.[143]

The first factor relates to penetration of the antimicrobial agent into CSF, which depends, to a great extent, on the status of the BBB.[140,143] For example, β-lactam antibiotics such as penicillin penetrate into CSF poorly (about 0.5% to 2.0% of peak serum concentrations) when the BBB is normal. In the presence of meningeal inflammation, CSF penetration of the antibiotic is enhanced because of increased permeability across the BBB, perhaps as a result of separation of intercellular light junctions and increased numbers of pinocytotic vesicles in

cerebral microvascular endothelial cells. Antimicrobial entry decreases as inflammation subsides, indicating that maximal parenteral doses of antimicrobial agents should be continued throughout the course of therapy to maintain adequate CSF concentrations. Antibiotic entry into CSF is also enhanced by drugs with a high lipid solubility, low molecular weight, low degree of protein binding in serum, and low degree of ionization at physiologic pH.

The second factor is the bactericidal activity of the antimicrobial agent within purulent CSF.[140,143] Because of the accumulation of lactate in CSF during bacterial meningitis, the pH of CSF is decreased, thereby inhibiting the bactericidal activity of the aminoglycosides; this is likely to have contributed to the poor response observed with the aminoglycosides in the therapy of meningitis in experimental animal models and in patients. Elevated CSF protein concentrations may decrease the efficacy of antimicrobial agents that are highly protein bound because free drug is needed for the antibacterial effect. Drug that penetrates the CSF may be removed by an active transport system that exists in the choroid plexus (as for the penicillins and cephalosporins), or it may be converted to an inactive metabolite. In addition, other drugs may influence antibiotic activity within purulent CSF. In experimental animal models of meningitis, antagonism has been shown when a bactericidal agent is co-administered with a bacteriostatic antibiotic (e.g., chloramphenicol plus gentamicin). However, in other instances the combination of antibiotics may be synergistic, as in the combination of penicillin or ampicillin with gentamicin in *L. monocytogenes* meningitis, and ampicillin plus gentamicin against *S. agalactiae*.

A third factor concerns the importance of bactericidal activity in CSF for optimal therapy inasmuch as bacterial meningitis represents an infection in an area of impaired host defense. Multiple studies in experimental animal models have shown that rapid bacterial killing is observed in vivo only when CSF concentrations of β-lactams or aminoglycosides exceed the minimal bactericidal concentration (MBC) by about 10- to 20-fold.[143] The importance of rapid bacterial killing has also been examined in patients with bacterial meningitis. One study that compared outcomes in infants and children with bacterial meningitis who had negative or positive CSF cultures 18 to 36 hours after the initiation of antimicrobial therapy revealed an increased rate of neurologic complications (i.e., ataxia, hemiparesis, developmental delay, moderate to severe hearing impairment) in the group in whom the causative organism could still be recovered after this interval.[345]

A final factor that may contribute to response to antimicrobial therapy in bacterial meningitis is pharmacodynamics,[143,346,347] which is concerned with the time course of antimicrobial therapy at the site of infection and is important to determine a dosing regimen for optimal effectiveness. In time-dependent antimicrobial activity, as observed with β-lactam agents, the bactericidal activity of an antimicrobial agent depends on the time that its concentration exceeds the MIC as a proportion of the dosing interval. As stated earlier, CSF concentrations of β-lactams need to exceed the MBC by at least 10- to 20-fold to obtain the maximal bactericidal effect, although peak CSF antimicrobial concentrations and the time that the antimicrobial concentrations exceed the MBC (T > MBC) are interrelated, and T-greater-than-MBC increased in parallel with peak CSF concentrations. This explains why the bactericidal effect did not improve with larger antimicrobial doses. The second pattern of antimicrobial activity is concentration dependent, and it is characterized by killing over a wide range of antimicrobial concentrations and a prolonged recovery period (i.e., postantibiotic effect) after drug concentrations fall below the MIC; this is seen with the aminoglycosides and fluoroquinolones. Although single-dose gentamicin therapy was as effective as divided-dosage regimens in an experimental animal model despite different times that CSF gentamicin concentrations exceeded the MBC, the applicability of these findings to humans needs to be established. The pharmacodynamic characteristics of the fluoroquinolones are very similar to those of the aminoglycosides, although features of both time dependency and concentration dependency have been demonstrated with the fluoroquinolones in animal models of meningitis.

Specific Antimicrobial Therapy

Haemophilus influenzae. Therapy for meningitis caused by *H. influenzae* type B has been markedly altered by the emergence of β-lactamase–producing strains.[143] These strains accounted for approximately 24% of all CSF isolates in the United States based on a surveillance study of 27 states from 1978 through 1981.[29] A subsequent surveillance study of five states and Los Angeles County in 1986 found the incidence of these β-lactamase-producing strains to be 32%.[30] Resistance of *H. influenzae* to chloramphenicol has also been described, although more commonly from areas such as Spain (more than 50% of isolates) than the United States (less than 1% of isolates). In Brazil, the prevalence of β-lactamase–producing strains of *H. influenzae* was 18.4% (range, 6.6% to 57.7%), with almost 17% of strains also resistant to chloramphenicol.[348] Chloramphenicol resistance is of particular concern in developing countries of the world, where it is used as first-line treatment for suspected bacterial meningitis. In an observational study with a retrospective control group conducted in Papua New Guinea, where chloramphenicol was used as empiric treatment followed by ceftriaxone when in vitro resistance to chloramphenicol was found in *H. influenzae,* there was invariably a very poor outcome (i.e., death or severe neurologic sequelae) in patients with chloramphenicol-resistant disease (71% versus 9% when chloramphenicol was used as first-line therapy).[349] Even in patients with chloramphenicol-sensitive isolates, a prospective study found chloramphenicol to be bacteriologically and clinically inferior to ampicillin, ceftriaxone, or cefotaxime in the treatment of childhood bacterial meningitis caused predominantly by *H. influenzae* type B.[350] Furthermore, the use of chloramphenicol can be problematic because of its unpredictable metabolism in young infants and its pharmacologic interactions with other concomitantly administered drugs such as phenobarbital, rifampin, phenytoin, and acetaminophen, which increase the likelihood of toxicity.[249]

Several studies have documented the efficacy of third-generation cephalosporins (particularly cefotaxime or ceftriaxone) to be similar to that of the combination of ampicillin plus chloramphenicol for bacterial meningitis.[143] Based on these findings, the American Academy of Pediatrics has recommended the use of a third-generation cephalosporin as empirical antimicrobial therapy for children with bacterial meningitis. The second-generation cephalosporins should not be used for therapy of bacterial meningitis. A prospective randomized study comparing ceftriaxone with cefuroxime for the treatment of childhood bacterial meningitis documented more rapid CSF sterilization (2% versus 12% of CSF cultures positive at 18 to 36 hours, $p = .11$) and a lower incidence of hearing impairment (4% versus 17%, $p = .05$) in the patients receiving ceftriaxone.[351] Cefepime has been studied in the treatment of bacterial meningitis.[352] Cefepime has in vitro activity and cure rates similar to those of cefotaxime and ceftriaxone in patients with meningitis caused by *H. influenzae, N. meningitidis,* and *S. pneumoniae;* it also has greater in vitro activity against *Enterobacter* species and *P. aeruginosa.* In a prospective randomized comparison of cefepime and cefotaxime for the treatment of bacterial meningitis in infants and children,[353] cefepime was found to be safe and therapeutically equivalent to cefotaxime and can be considered a suitable therapeutic alternative for the treatment of patients with this disease.

Neisseria meningitidis. Penicillin G and ampicillin are the antimicrobial agents of choice for meningitis caused by *N. meningitidis.*[143] However, these recommendations may need to be modified in the future because of trends in the antimicrobial susceptibility of meningococci. Meningococcal strains that are relatively resistant to penicillin G and have an MIC range of 0.1 to 1.0 μg/mL have recently been reported from several areas (particularly Spain). For example, of 3264 strains of *N. meningitidis* isolated from blood and CSF in Spain during 1978 to 1985,[354] only one resistant isolate was observed, whereas 9 (5%) of 168 invasive isolates relatively resistant to penicillin G were found in the first 6 months of 1986; this figure reached 20% in 1989. This resistance was reported to be mediated by a reduced affinity of the antibiotic for penicillin-binding proteins 2 and 3. Decreased

meningococcal susceptibility to penicillin has also been reported from Greece, Switzerland, Romania, France, Belgium, the United Kingdom, Malawi, South Africa, Canada, Croatia, and Turkey.[143,355-357] High-level penicillin resistance resulting from β-lactamase production has also been reported, and the MICs for these strains may be as high as 256 μg/mL.[358] Furthermore, high-level chloramphenicol resistance (MIC ≥ 64 μg/mL) has been described as resulting from the presence of the *catP* gene on a truncated transposon that has lost mobility because of internal deletions[359]; transmission of genetic material between strains of *N. meningitidis* probably played an important role in dissemination of the gene.

In the United States, meningococcal strains relatively resistant to penicillin have also been described.[360-362] In a population-based surveillance study of invasive meningococcal disease in selected areas of the United States, 3 of 100 isolates had penicillin MICs of 0.125 μg/mL.[360] In another active, population-based surveillance in seven geographically dispersed areas of the United States during 1997,[363] 3 of 90 isolates were intermediately resistant to penicillin (MIC, 0.12 μg/mL), whereas 49 of the remaining 87 isolates had MICs of 0.06 μg/mL. These data indicate the importance of continued surveillance for these resistant strains.

The clinical significance of these isolates is unclear at present because many patients with meningitis caused by relatively penicillin-resistant meningococci have recovered with standard penicillin therapy. However, isolated reports of treatment failure have been described.[364,365] Furthermore, in a study from Spain, reduced susceptibility of *N. meningitidis* to penicillin was seen in 34% of 213 children with meningococcal meningitis[366]; in this report, reduced penicillin susceptibility was more frequent in strains responsible for death or sequelae (60% versus 32%, $p = .04$). On the basis of these data, some authorities would treat patients who had meningococcal meningitis with a third-generation cephalosporin (either cefotaxime or ceftriaxone), and these agents are likely to emerge as first-line treatment in the future. Susceptibility testing of the isolate should be performed for patients who fail to respond appropriately. Trovafloxacin was found to be equivalent to ceftriaxone in children with meningococcal meningitis in one report,[367] although this study has been published only in abstract form. Further studies are needed before any fluoroquinolone can be recommended as first-line treatment of patients with meningococcal meningitis.

Streptococcus pneumoniae. Therapy for meningitis caused by the pneumococcus has recently been modified according to current pneumococcal susceptibility patterns.[143,307,341,342,368] In the past, pneumococci were uniformly susceptible to penicillin, with MICs of 0.06 μg/mL or less. Numerous reports from throughout the world have now documented strains of pneumococci that are relatively resistant to penicillin (MIC range, 0.1 to 1.0 μg/mL), as well as strains that are highly resistant to penicillin (MIC, 2.0 μg/mL or higher). The mechanism of this resistance is an alteration in the structure and molecular size of penicillin-binding proteins. Resistance has been reported in several different pneumococcal serotypes, although the overwhelming majority of resistant strains are serotypes 6, 14, 19, and 23; most of the multiresistant strains isolated in the United States disseminated from a multiresistant serotype 23F clone of *S. pneumoniae* that was isolated in Spain as early as 1978. Results of recent surveillance studies in the United States show that the prevalence of penicillin-nonsusceptible *S. pneumoniae* ranges from 25% to more than 50%[369]; rates are as high as 60% in some parts of Latin America and as high as 80% in some countries in Asia. Factors reported to predispose to resistance include the patient's age (younger than 10 or older than 50 years), immunosuppression, prolonged hospital stay, children in daycare settings, infection by serotypes 14 and 23, and frequent, prolonged, or prophylactic use of antimicrobial therapy.

Several alternative agents for the treatment of meningitis caused by penicillin-resistant pneumococci have been evaluated by in vitro susceptibility testing, in animal models, and in patients.[143,307,368] Here, we will restrict our discussion to agents that have been examined in clinical trials, unless animal model data have influenced treatment recommendations.

Chloramphenicol is one agent that has been studied for the treatment of pneumococcal meningitis. However, clinical failures with chloramphenicol have been reported in patients with penicillin-resistant isolates, probably because of the poor bactericidal activity of chloramphenicol against these strains; 20 of 25 children had an unsatisfactory outcome (i.e., death, serious neurologic deficit, poor clinical response) in one study.[370] Despite susceptibility on disk testing, chloramphenicol MBCs of the penicillin-resistant pneumococcal isolates were significantly higher than those for the penicillin-sensitive isolates, with subsequent subtherapeutic bactericidal activity and treatment failure.

Third-generation cephalosporins have been considered the treatment of choice in relatively penicillin-resistant pneumococcal meningitis.[143,307,368] Cefotaxime and ceftriaxone are the third-generation agents of choice; ceftizoxime is not recommended because its MIC to resistant pneumococci tends to be higher than that of either cefotaxime or ceftriaxone. However, some reports of meningitis treatment failure with the third-generation cephalosporins have appeared, and pneumococcal strains have emerged that are resistant to these agents (MIC ≥ 2 μg/mL). When the MIC to the third-generation cephalosporin is 1 μg/mL or less, some patients have been treated successfully with either high-dose cefotaxime or ceftriaxone alone, although one study found that high-dose cefotaxime did not have reliably sufficient CSF bactericidal activity against cephalosporin-resistant pneumococci.

Vancomycin has been evaluated in 11 adult patients with meningitis caused by relatively penicillin-resistant pneumococcal strains.[371] This therapy was associated with clinical failure in four patients; no failures occurred in 14 subsequent patients treated with ceftriaxone. In two of the failures, CSF vancomycin concentrations were undetectable at 48 hours, and in a third patient, symptoms recurred on the 8th day of antimicrobial therapy. The concomitant administration of dexamethasone and the subsequent decreased inflammation and poor entry of vancomycin into CSF may have contributed to this negative outcome; this explanation has been supported in an experimental rabbit model of pneumococcal meningitis.[335] These data support the concept that vancomycin should not be used alone for the treatment of pneumococcal meningitis. Of additional concern is the recent description of *S. pneumoniae* strains that are tolerant to vancomycin.[372,373] A vancomycin- and cephalosporin-tolerant strain of *S. pneumoniae* was isolated from the CSF of a patient with meningitis who then developed recrudescence of meningitis despite therapy with vancomycin plus a third-generation cephalosporin.[374] Because tolerance is a precursor phenotype to the development of resistance, these data have important implications in the use of vancomycin for pneumococcal meningitis.

In view of the aforementioned data, penicillin can never be recommended as empirical therapy in patients with suspected pneumococcal meningitis. As an empirical regimen, the combination of vancomycin plus a third-generation cephalosporin (either cefotaxime or ceftriaxone) is recommended.[143,307,368] This combination was synergistic in a rabbit model of penicillin-resistant pneumococcal meningitis and was synergistic, or at least additive, in the CSF of children with meningitis. The addition of rifampin to vancomycin with or without a third-generation cephalosporin has been recommended by some authorities, although clinical data are lacking; rifampin should be added only if the organism is demonstrated to be susceptible, the expected clinical or bacteriologic response is delayed, or the pneumococcal isolate has a cefotaxime/ceftriaxone MIC greater than 4.0 μg/mL.[341,342] Any patient who is not improving as expected or has a pneumococcal isolate for which the cefotaxime/ceftriaxone MIC is greater than 2.0 μg/mL should undergo a repeat lumbar puncture to document sterility of CSF after 36 to 48 hours of therapy; this may be especially important for patients who are receiving adjunctive dexamethasone therapy. In patients not responding, intrathecal or intraventricular vancomycin also remains a reasonable option.[375] Once susceptibility studies of the isolated pneumococcus are performed, antimicrobial therapy can be modified for optimal treatment (see Table 80-13).

With continued emergence of penicillin- and cephalosporin-resistant strains of *S. pneumoniae*, other antimicrobial agents have been evaluated for their efficacy in pneumococcal meningitis.[143,368] Meropenem, a carbapenem with a broad spectrum of in vitro activity, including activity against penicillin-resistant pneumococci, has been approved by the U.S. Food and Drug Administration for the treatment of bacterial meningitis in children 3 months old and older. Meropenem has been studied for the treatment of meningitis in both adults and children in several clinical trials,[376] with microbiologic and clinical outcomes similar to those with either cefotaxime or ceftriaxone. Meropenem was also used successfully in one patient with multiply resistant pneumococcal meningitis.[377] In one prospective study of 258 children with bacterial meningitis, patients were randomly assigned to receive either meropenem or cefotaxime; there were no significant differences in outcome, with clinical cure (with or without sequelae) in 97% and 96% of patients treated with meropenem and cefotaxime, respectively.[378] Further studies are needed to determine the efficacy of meropenem in pneumococcal meningitis caused by penicillin- and cephalosporin-resistant strains, although isolated case reports have shown efficacy.

The fluoroquinolones have generally lacked sufficient in vitro activity against *S. pneumoniae* to warrant their investigation in the treatment of CNS infections. However, newer agents (moxifloxacin, gemifloxacin, gatifloxacin, garenoxacin) have shown excellent in vitro activity and have been evaluated in experimental animal models of infection.[379] Trovafloxacin has been compared with ceftriaxone with or without vancomycin in a multicenter, randomized, comparative trial enrolling 311 children from 11 countries; *S. pneumoniae* was isolated in 27% of cases.[380] The overall efficacy of both treatment groups was comparable in terms of CSF sterilization (94% in the trovafloxacin group and 96% in the comparator) and clinical success at the end of treatment (75% in the trovafloxacin group and 82% for the comparator). Although trovafloxacin is no longer utilized because of concerns about liver toxicity, these data suggest the potential usefulness of the newer fluoroquinolones in the treatment of bacterial meningitis.[379,381] However, further clinical trials are needed before these agents can be recommended. Of concern are the reports of decreased pneumococcal susceptibility to the fluoroquinolones,[382] the development of fluoroquinolone-resistant *S. pneumoniae* associated with levofloxacin therapy,[383] and the report of a case of fatal meningitis caused by a levofloxacin-resistant strain of *S. pneumoniae*[384]; these data highlight the need to monitor the in vitro susceptibility of pneumococci to these agents. Nevertheless, a combination regimen of a third-generation cephalosporin plus a newer-generation fluoroquinolone may emerge as the treatment option of choice for pneumococcal meningitis in the future.

Listeria monocytogenes. Despite their broad range of in vitro activity, third-generation cephalosporins are inactive in meningitis caused by *L. monocytogenes*. For patients with *Listeria* meningitis, therapy should consist of ampicillin or penicillin G[68-71,143]; the addition of an aminoglycoside should be considered in proven infection because of in vitro synergy and enhanced killing in vivo, as documented in a variety of animal models of *Listeria* infection. Nevertheless, it is important to emphasize that a controlled clinical trial comparing ampicillin alone with ampicillin plus gentamicin has never been performed in humans with listeriosis. An alternative agent in a penicillin-allergic patient is trimethoprim-sulfamethoxazole, which is bactericidal against *Listeria* in vitro. Although chloramphenicol has varying activity against *Listeria* in vitro, its use has been associated with an unacceptably high failure rate in patients with *Listeria* meningitis. Vancomycin is also unsatisfactory for *Listeria* meningitis despite favorable in vitro susceptibility results. However, intraventricular administration of vancomycin was successful in one case of recurrent *L. monocytogenes* meningitis. Rifampin is bacteriostatic against *L. monocytogenes* in vitro and was no better than penicillin alone when evaluated in the experimental rabbit model of meningitis. Meropenem is active in vitro and in experimental animal models of *L. monocytogenes* meningitis and may be a useful alternative if found to be clinically efficacious.

Streptococcus agalactiae. Standard therapy for neonatal meningitis caused by the group B streptococcus is the combination of ampicillin plus an aminoglycoside,[76,249] which is also recommended for adult patients with meningitis caused by this organism[79]; this combination is recommended because of documented in vitro synergy and recent reports detailing the presence of penicillin-tolerant strains. Alternative agents are the third-generation cephalosporins; vancomycin is reserved for patients who are allergic to penicillin.

Aerobic Gram-Negative Bacilli. Treatment of bacterial meningitis caused by enteric gram-negative bacilli has been revolutionized by the availability of third-generation cephalosporins.[143] Previous mortality rates with standard regimens (usually an aminoglycoside with or without chloramphenicol) ranged from 40% to 90% versus cure rates of 78% to 94% with the third-generation cephalosporins. Cefotaxime is preferred over ceftriaxone as the third-generation cephalosporin for use in neonates because it has been used more extensively and is not excreted in bile, which may have an inhibitory effect on the bacterial flora of the intestinal tract[274]; ceftriaxone also has increased protein binding. One particular third-generation cephalosporin, ceftazidime, has enhanced in vitro activity against *P. aeruginosa* and resulted in the cure of 19 of 24 patients in one study of *P. aeruginosa* meningitis when administered alone or in combination with an aminoglycoside.[385] In another study of 10 pediatric patients with *Pseudomonas* meningitis, seven patients were cured clinically and nine were cured bacteriologically when treated with ceftazidime-containing regimens.[386]

Concomitant intrathecal or intraventricular aminoglycoside therapy should be considered in patients with gram-negative meningitis who are not responding to conventional parenteral therapy. However, this mode of administration is rarely needed at present and was associated with a higher mortality rate than was systemic therapy alone in infants with gram-negative meningitis and ventriculitis.

Several other antimicrobial agents have been used in patients with meningitis caused by aerobic gram-negative bacilli.[143,368] Aztreonam attains excellent CSF concentrations and has been shown to be efficacious in the treatment of gram-negative meningitis. Imipenem was found to be efficacious in one case of *Acinetobacter* meningitis and in eradication of bacteria from CSF in a recent study of 21 children with bacterial meningitis (most cases caused by *H. influenzae* type B and *N. meningitidis*), although a high rate of seizure activity (33%) limits its usefulness in the treatment of bacterial meningitis. High-dose meropenem (2 g every 8 hours) given for 18 weeks was successful in a lymphoma patient with *P. aeruginosa* meningitis who had failed therapy with ceftazidime plus gentamicin, as well as in a patient with post-traumatic meningitis caused by *P. aeruginosa*. Cefepime was successful in a patient with postoperative meningitis caused by *Enterobacter aerogenes*.[387] Intravenous colistin (5 mg/kg/day) was successfully used to treat a patient with meningitis caused by a multidrug-resistant *Acinetobacter baumannii*[388]; intrathecal colistin was also efficacious in another case of meningitis caused by this same multidrug-resistant organism.[389] The fluoroquinolones (e.g., ciprofloxacin, pefloxacin) have been used successfully in some patients with gram-negative meningitis.[379,381] In one case series of 12 neonates and infants with nosocomial meningitis (in which 6 cases were attributed to gram-negative bacilli), 10 patients were cured, and in 7 children, no neurologic sequelae appeared after a 2- to 4-year follow-up.[390] Another patient who developed *P. aeruginosa* meningitis after a laminectomy was cured by the addition of high-dose ciprofloxacin (400 mg intravenously every 8 hours) to the previous regimen of ceftazidime and gentamicin,[391] and a preterm infant with *Stenotrophomonas maltophilia* meningitis was successfully treated with ciprofloxacin.[392] The limited published literature on use of the fluoroquinolones suggests that the primary area of usefulness of these agents is for the treatment of multidrug-resistant gram-negative organisms (e.g., *P. aeruginosa*) or when the response to conventional β-lactam therapy is slow (e.g., meningitis caused by *Salmonella* species). Data are currently insufficient to recommend any fluoroquinolone for empirical therapy in any patient with community-acquired bacterial meningitis.

Staphylococci. *S. aureus* should be treated with nafcillin or oxacillin,[92] and vancomycin should be reserved for patients allergic to penicillin or when methicillin-resistant organisms are suspected or isolated. However, given the likelihood of methicillin-resistant *S. aureus* in patients with *S. aureus* meningitis, vancomycin should be utilized as empirical therapy pending results of in vitro susceptibility testing.[393] The addition of rifampin should be considered in patients not responding to therapy. Meningitis caused by coagulase-negative staphylococci, the most commonly encountered organisms in CSF shunt infections, should be treated with vancomycin; rifampin should be added if the patient fails to improve.[95] Removal of the shunt is often necessary to optimize therapy (see Chapter 81).

Other Bacteria. *Salmonella* meningitis should be treated with a third-generation cephalosporin, with or without a fluoroquinolone, because use of conventional antimicrobial agents (e.g., chloramphenicol, ampicillin, cotrimoxazole) have an unacceptable cure rate (about 41%), relapse rate (about 12%), and high associated mortality (about 45%)[394]; the fluoroquinolones have a cure rate of approximately 89% and the third-generation cephalosporins a cure rate of about 85%. Ampicillin plus gentamicin should be used for enterococcal meningitis caused by susceptible strains; vancomycin, or ampicillin-sulbactam, is substituted for ampicillin for β-lactamase–producing strains. In patients with meningitis caused by vancomycin-resistant *E. faecium*, several case reports have shown successful treatment with intravenous linezolid[395-398]; given the failures associated with other alternative agents, use of linezolid is reasonable in meningitis caused by this multidrug-resistant organism.

Duration of Therapy

The duration of therapy for bacterial meningitis has been based more on tradition than on scientific evidence.[143,399] The duration of antimicrobial therapy in patients with bacterial meningitis has been 10 to 14 days for cases of nonmeningococcal meningitis. Several studies comparing 7 with 10 days of treatment in infants and children with *H. influenzae* type B meningitis, however, have documented that 7 days of therapy is safe and effective, although therapy must be individualized and some patients may require longer courses. Meningococcal meningitis can be treated for 7 days with intravenous penicillin, and some authors have also suggested that 4 days of therapy is adequate; this study requires confirmation because only 50 patients were studied and no control group was included. A single dose, or even two to three doses, of long-acting penicillin or chloramphenicol has been used successfully in developing countries to treat meningococcal meningitis, although this therapy is not considered standard. In one randomized trial of 4 versus 7 days of ceftriaxone therapy in children with bacterial meningitis who had an initial rapid recovery,[400] no significant differences in outcome were observed in the two groups at completion of therapy or at a follow-up of 1 to 3 months after discharge. In another trial, the clinical outcome of patients treated with 7 days' ceftriaxone therapy was similar to 10 days' therapy for acute bacterial meningitis in children in developing countries[401] and was associated with a lower incidence of nosocomial infection and earlier hospital discharge. In adults with meningitis caused by enteric gram-negative bacilli, treatment regimens should be continued for 3 weeks because of the high rate of relapse in patients treated with shorter courses of therapy. Ten to 14 days is recommended for the treatment of meningitis caused by *S. pneumoniae* and 14 to 21 days for group B streptococci. *L. monocytogenes* meningitis should be treated for at least 21 days.[70,71]

Outpatient antimicrobial therapy may also be appropriate for certain patients with bacterial meningitis. The following criteria have been suggested to guide outpatient antimicrobial therapy[402]: inpatient therapy for at least 6 days; no fever for at least 24 to 48 hours before initiation of outpatient therapy; no significant neurologic dysfunction, focal findings, or seizure activity; clinically stable or improving condition; intake of all fluids by mouth; first dose of outpatient antimicrobial therapy given under medical supervision and without reaction;

access to home health nursing for antimicrobial administration; reliable intravenous line and infusion device, if needed; daily examination by a physician, and an established plan for physician visits, nurse visits, laboratory monitoring, and emergencies; patient and/or family compliance with the program; and a safe environment with access to a telephone, utilities, food, and a refrigerator. In addition, completion of antimicrobial therapy in a skilled nursing facility may be appropriate for selected patients who need continued care but do not require acute hospitalization.

Spirochetal Meningitis

Treponema pallidum

In syphilis patients with CSF abnormalities but without clinically apparent disease, the goals of therapy are to prevent progression to symptomatic disease and ameliorate the laboratory abnormalities thought to indicate disease activity.[104] For patients with clinical neurosyphilis syndromes, the goal may be to reverse clinical symptoms and signs or to arrest disease progression. In patients with syphilitic meningitis whose clinical picture is that of meningeal inflammation as a result of the acute inflammatory response, clinical findings other than cranial nerve abnormalities usually resolve without therapy. In patients with meningovascular syphilis, the prognosis after therapy is quite good, except perhaps in patients with larger, clinically apparent neurologic deficits before therapy; therapy in this situation may halt progression and prevent further ischemic events caused by neurosyphilis.

The drug of choice for the treatment of neurosyphilis is penicillin G (see Table 80-14), although considerable controversy remains regarding the most appropriate total dose and the formulation and duration of therapy.[104,108] Therapy with benzathine penicillin (2.4 million units intramuscularly) does not reliably produce CSF penicillin concentrations above 0.018 μg/mL and should not be used for the treatment of neurosyphilis. Furthermore, a small but poorly defined proportion of patients with syphilis treated with benzathine penicillin fails therapy, defined as persistent CSF abnormalities with clinically apparent neurosyphilis. However, many patients treated with benzathine penicillin resolve their CSF abnormalities and do not progress, which suggests that factors other than CSF concentrations of penicillin play a role in response to therapy.

The preferred antimicrobial regimen for the treatment of CNS syphilis is intravenous aqueous crystalline penicillin G at a dose of 12 to 24 million units daily in divided doses every 4 hours for 10 to 14 days.[104] Alternatively, procaine penicillin, 2.4 million units intramuscularly daily, plus probenecid, 500 mg orally four times daily, both for 10 to 14 days, can be used. Some experts also recommend follow-up therapy with one injection of benzathine penicillin G (2.4 million units intramuscularly), although no data support this recommendation. No large studies have been performed to evaluate alternative antimicrobial agents for neurosyphilis. On the basis of case reports, clinical experience, and extrapolations from experimental animal studies, the tetracyclines, chloramphenicol, and ceftriaxone have all been described to be of potential clinical utility in penicillin-allergic patients. One experimental study, however, suggested that ceftriaxone may not be adequate therapy for neurosyphilis.[403] Furthermore, a study of 43 HIV-infected patients with latent syphilis or neurosyphilis treated with ceftriaxone (1 or 2 g daily for 10 to 14 days) had a 23% failure rate,[404] similar to that seen in 13 HIV-infected patients with latent syphilis or neurosyphilis treated with benzathine penicillin (30%). Erythromycin is not recommended because of treatment failures in erythromycin-treated patients. In HIV-infected patients with neurosyphilis, careful monitoring for response to therapy is needed.[107,405] Follow-up lumbar puncture should be performed every 6 months in all patients until the CSF changes have normalized. Several reports of failures in HIV-infected patients receiving standard therapy for neurosyphilis have appeared; these failures probably occurred because the patient's immunologic response

has an important role in controlling the infection even in the presence of "adequate" antimicrobial therapy.

Borrelia burgdorferi

Parenteral antimicrobial therapy is usually needed to treat the neurologic manifestations of Lyme disease, including meningitis (see Table 80-14).[111,300,406] Initial studies used high-dose (15 to 20 million units daily) intravenous penicillin G for 10 to 14 days, although one author found the benefits limited to patients treated within 5 weeks of the onset of neurologic symptoms. The meningeal and systemic reactions tend to improve within days, whereas radicular pain and motor deficits improve over many weeks. CNS abnormalities are arrested by treatment and may slowly improve, but some residual deficit is common. Some patients have also responded to treatment with oral or intravenous doxycycline, which has been found to be as efficacious as penicillin in several studies.[407,408] Patients who have failed to respond to intravenous penicillin have responded to therapy with intravenous cefotaxime, ceftriaxone, or chloramphenicol.[111] In one prospective randomized trial,[409] ceftriaxone was superior to penicillin in therapy for late Lyme borreliosis. The current recommendation is to treat most patients with Lyme meningitis with intravenous ceftriaxone at a dosage of 2 g daily for 2 to 4 weeks[30,111,406]; the literature contains no agreement on the duration of therapy or on the minimal adequate dose of the antimicrobial. No evidence supports treatment durations longer than 4 weeks. However, no regimen has proved to be universally effective. Although one report has indicated that high-dose oral doxycycline may produce inhibitory concentrations against B. burgdorferi in CSF,[410] parenteral regimens are generally necessary for CNS infection.

Protozoal and Helminthic Meningitis

Amebas

Many antimicrobial agents, including amphotericin B, the tetracyclines, the imidazoles, artemisin compounds, and rifampin, have in vitro activity against free-living amebas[136]; phenothiazines are amebicidal only at high concentrations (100 μm). Amphotericin B is rapidly amebicidal against N. fowleri in vitro, but it is much less active against Acanthamoeba. Fewer than 10 patients reported in the literature have survived after therapy for primary amebic meningoencephalitis.[115,411-413] All received amphotericin B along with various other antimicrobial agents. One documented survivor received amphotericin B and miconazole intravenously and intrathecally, rifampin, sulfisoxazole, and dexamethasone. Another received amphotericin B, rifampicin, and ornidazole.[413] However, no effective regimen has been established. Therapy with parenteral and intracisternal amphotericin B combined with rifampin and tetracycline has been suggested[116]; the addition of experimental therapies such as one of the phenothiazines or artemisin compounds, may also be justified in view of the extremely poor outcome in patients with primary amebic meningoencephalitis. Therapy is continued for 2 to 3 weeks if the clinical response is good and no complications occur.

Angiostrongylus cantonensis

Treatment of symptoms such as headache, nausea, and vomiting with analgesics and rehydration is indicated for eosinophilic meningitis caused by A. cantonensis.[115,123] Most patients recover within 1 to 2 weeks. Treatment with specific anthelminthic agents is controversial; exacerbation of neurologic symptoms after larval death is a theoretical complication of anthelminthic therapy. The benzimidazoles have been tried in humans without definite benefit; thiabendazole cleared A. cantonensis from rats in one study.[121] Thiabendazole has been used in the early stages of migration of the larvae of A. cantonensis, but the drug fails as soon as the worm reaches the CNS. Clinicians in Taiwan routinely treat eosinophilic meningitis with anthelminthics[123]; agents utilized have included mebendazole, levamisole, and albendazole. However, no randomized study of use of anthelminthic agents for eosinophilic meningitis has been reported and there are insufficient data to recommend their use.

ADJUNCTIVE THERAPY

Viral Meningitis

Adjunctive measures have been used in seriously ill patients with enteroviral meningitis. Because enteroviral clearance from the host is antibody mediated, exogenously administered antibody has been examined.[2,4] Administration of immune globulin by multiple routes (including directly into the CNS) has led to stabilization or improvement of agammaglobulinemic patients with chronic enteroviral meningitis or meningoencephalitis, but results have varied. Neonates with overwhelming enteroviral sepsis and meningitis have received intravenous immune globulin, maternal plasma, and exchange transfusions with occasional success. In a single randomized trial of intravenous immune globulin plus standard therapy versus standard therapy alone in neonates suspected of having enteroviral infection during the first 2 weeks of life, intravenous immune globulin failed to reduce viremia or lead to significant outcome differences, although the study enrolled too few patients for a definitive conclusion[414]; 75% of these patients had clinical or laboratory evidence of meningitis.

Specific hyperimmune globulin has been shown to reduce the incidence of orchitis in a single prospective controlled trial in patients with mumps,[2] but no benefit in neurologic syndromes has been proved. Anecdotal reports have appeared on the use of corticosteroids in patients with mumps encephalitis,[12] but no benefits have been documented.

Bacterial Meningitis

Anti-inflammatory Agents

Despite the availability of effective bactericidal antimicrobial agents in the treatment of bacterial meningitis, morbidity and mortality from this disorder remain unacceptably high. Because the subarachnoid space inflammatory response is a major factor contributing to morbidity and mortality, investigators have examined whether attenuation of this response would improve outcome in bacterial meningitis. Adjunctive dexamethasone has been the agent most extensively studied in experimental animal models and in patients, and it should now be utilized in the initial approach to most patients with acute bacterial meningitis (see "Initial Management of Patients with Meningitis," earlier, for a description of experimental studies and clinical trials of adjunctive dexamethasone in bacterial meningitis).

Other agents that reduce subarachnoid space inflammation have also been examined as possible adjuncts in the treatment of bacterial meningitis. Pentoxifylline, a phosphodiesterase inhibitor that decreases endotoxin-induced TNF-α production, attenuates the inflammatory action of IL-1 and TNF on leukocyte function, and blocks the lipo-oligosaccharide–induced release of TNF and IL-1 from microglial cell cultures, has been examined in an experimental rabbit model of *H. influenzae* type B meningitis.[415] Administration of pentoxifylline 20 minutes before intracisternal challenge with *H. influenzae* type B lipo-oligosaccharide significantly reduced CSF concentrations of leukocytes, protein, and lactate. However, dexamethasone was superior to pentoxifylline in modulation of these CSF inflammatory changes, and no appreciable synergism was observed when both agents were administered. Thalidomide, which also inhibits TNF-α production, was studied in an experimental rabbit model of meningitis. Thalidomide reduced TNF-α production after intracisternal challenge with either *H. influenzae* type B or *S. pneumoniae,* although it had a relatively greater effect on the inflammatory response to *S. pneumoniae.*[416]

Other studies have examined the effects of a monoclonal antibody (IB4) directed against the CD18 family of receptors on leukocytes to reduce CSF inflammation. Intravenous inoculation of IB4 blocked the accumulation of leukocytes in CSF despite intracisternal challenge with *H. influenzae* type B, *N. meningitidis,* pneumococcal cell wall, or lipo-oligosaccharide.[170] Furthermore, the monoclonal antibody was effective

in preventing the development of cerebral edema and death in animals challenged with lethal doses of *S. pneumoniae*. In a second study using an experimental rabbit model of *H. influenzae* type B meningitis,[417] the concomitant administration of dexamethasone and IB4 led to a marked attenuation of all indices of meningeal inflammation and a reduction in brain water content when compared with the results obtained in untreated animals or when each agent was used alone. Clinical trials with this agent, perhaps in conjunction with dexamethasone, will be needed to determine whether outcome (i.e., morbidity or mortality) can be improved by the administration of IB4 in patients with bacterial meningitis.

Bactericidal/permeability-increasing protein, which is present in the azurophilic granules of neutrophils and binds to and neutralizes the biologic activity of the lipid A portion of lipo-oligosaccharide, has also been studied for its effects on CSF inflammation in bacterial meningitis. In an experimental rabbit model, the intracisternal inoculation of recombinant bactericidal/permeability-increasing protein significantly reduced CSF inflammation in response to meningococcal endotoxin[418]; this effect was not seen after systemic administration, probably because of failure of this protein to cross the BBB.

Although experimental results with these agents have shown a benefit in reduction of CSF inflammation in animals with bacterial meningitis, none has been studied in clinical trials. Therefore, their use in patients cannot be recommended at present.

Reduction of Intracranial Pressure

Patients with bacterial meningitis who have signs of increased intracranial pressure (e.g., altered level of consciousness; dilated, poorly reactive, or nonreactive pupils; ocular movement disorders) and who are stuporous or comatose may benefit from the insertion of an intracranial pressure–monitoring device.[143,419] Intracranial pressures exceeding 20 mm Hg are abnormal and should be treated. Furthermore, there is rationale for treating smaller pressure elevations (i.e., above 15 mm Hg) to avoid larger elevations, so-called plateau waves, that can lead to cerebral herniation and irreversible brain-stem injury.

Several methods are available to reduce intracranial pressure,[143,419] including elevation of the head of the bed to 30 degrees to maximize venous drainage with minimal compromise of cerebral perfusion; hyperventilation to maintain the Paco$_2$ between 27 and 30 mm Hg, which causes cerebral vasoconstriction and a reduction in cerebral blood volume; use of hyperosmolar agents (e.g., mannitol) to make the intravascular space hyperosmolar to the brain and permit movement of water from brain tissue into the intravascular compartment; and corticosteroids. However, some experts have questioned the routine use of hyperventilation to reduce intracranial pressure in patients with bacterial meningitis.[420] In infants and children with bacterial meningitis who have initially normal CT scans of the head, hyperventilation can safely reduce elevated intracranial pressure because it is unlikely that cerebral blood flow would be reduced to ischemic thresholds. However, in children with cerebral edema evident on head CT, cerebral blood flow is more likely to be normal or reduced. Although hyperventilation might decrease intracranial pressure, it would do so at the cost of a significant reduction in cerebral blood flow, possibly approaching ischemic thresholds. These patients may benefit more from the early use of diuretics, osmotically dehydrating agents (provided that intravascular volume is protected), and corticosteroids; however, controlled trials exploring these issues have yet to be performed.

Glycerol, an osmotic dehydrating agent that can be given orally, has been evaluated in a trial of 122 infants and children with bacterial meningitis.[322] Patients in this study were randomized to receive adjunctive intravenous dexamethasone, oral glycerol, dexamethasone plus glycerol, or neither. Seven percent of the glycerol-treated patients and 19% of those not given glycerol had audiologic or neurologic sequelae ($p = .052$). However, further placebo-controlled, blinded studies are required before glycerol can be routinely recommended in patients with bacterial meningitis.

Patients who continue to have elevated intracranial pressures despite the aforementioned measures may be treated with high-dose barbiturate therapy,[143,419] which decreases cerebral metabolic demands and cerebral blood flow. Barbiturates can also cause vasoconstriction in normal tissue, thereby shunting blood to ischemic tissue and protecting the brain from ischemic insult. During the administration of pentobarbital, the patient is monitored to measure decreases in intracranial pressure, or the dose can be titrated to the development of a burst suppression pattern on the electroencephalogram. Cardiac parameters also need to be monitored (by placement of a Swan-Ganz catheter) because of the risk of cardiac toxicity (e.g., decreased cardiac output, decreased contractile force, arrhythmias) with high-dose barbiturate therapy. This mode of treatment for meningitis and elevated intracranial pressure is of unproven benefit, however, and must be considered experimental.

Surgery

Surgical intervention may be required in some patients with bacterial meningitis. Patients who have suffered a basilar skull fracture with CSF leak may have persistent dural defects that can lead to recurrent episodes of bacterial meningitis.[67] Many leaks will cease spontaneously, but surgery is indicated for leaks that persist for several weeks or in patients who present with delayed or recurrent infection. Surgery is not indicated in the acute phase (before 7 days) of leakage; no difference in outcome is seen when patients with acutely repaired leaks are compared with those whose leaks stop spontaneously within 7 days. Surgical intervention may also be required in patients in whom recurrent meningitis develops from congenital or acquired cranial defects and dermal sinuses.[95]

Helminthic Meningitis

In seriously ill patients with *A. cantonensis* meningitis, the major treatment objective is control of intracranial pressure; repeated lumbar punctures can produce dramatic, though transient, clinical improvement.[123] Anecdotal case series have shown benefits of corticosteroids, although one large observational study in Thailand concluded that prednisone was not effective. However, in a recent placebo-controlled study from Thailand, a 2-week course of prednisolone (60 mg/day) was effective and safe in patients with eosinophilic meningitis (most cases presumptively caused by *A. cantonensis*).[421] Those patients who received corticosteroids demonstrated improved rates of headache resolution, a more rapid improvement in symptoms, and less need for repeat lumbar punctures. In another report, three patients with severe headaches underwent repeated lumbar punctures and received corticosteroids[125]; two of these patients had marked improvement in symptoms and all three had a decrease in opening CSF pressure.

PREVENTION

Viral Meningitis: Immunoprophylaxis

The cornerstone of prevention of mumps is active immunization with the live-attenuated mumps vaccine. Administration is in the second year of life, and protective serum antibody concentrations are seen in more than 97% of patients.[12] Widespread use of the mumps vaccine has greatly reduced the incidence of mumps and mumps meningoencephalitis. By the mid-1980s, mumps was the seventh most common cause of viral encephalitis in the United States (approximately 0.5% of cases), whereas it was the leading cause of viral encephalitis through the mid-1960s.[12] Mumps meningitis has been reported in children 11 days to 2 months after vaccine administration, although it is not clear whether these cases represented vaccine failure or meningitis from the vaccine strain of mumps virus.

Bacterial Meningitis

Haemophilus influenzae

Chemoprophylaxis. It has become clear that the spread of several types of bacterial meningitis can be prevented by prophylaxis of contacts of cases with antimicrobial agents. Several studies have documented the transmission of *H. influenzae* type B from patients with meningitis to household contacts.[143] The risk is markedly age dependent, highest for children younger than 2 years. Most secondary cases (75%) occur within 6 days of onset of the index case, although untreated household contacts remain at increased risk for *H. influenzae* type B disease for at least 1 month after onset in the index case. Daycare outside the home is considered another risk factor for transmission[29]; secondary disease is more likely to develop in children younger than 2 years. Controversy regarding the magnitude of the risk to children in daycare settings, however, has led to disagreement concerning the recommendation for chemoprophylaxis of children in these facilities.

The rationale for the use of chemoprophylaxis for prevention of secondary disease is eradication of nasopharyngeal colonization of *H. influenzae* type B, thereby preventing transmission to young, susceptible contacts and the development of invasive disease in those already colonized. The recommended chemoprophylactic agent of choice is rifampin (20 mg/kg daily for 4 days) for all individuals, including adults, in households with at least one unvaccinated or incompletely vaccinated child younger than 48 months (see Chapter 222).[143] One study suggested that 2 days of rifampin therapy was as efficacious as 4 days' treatment, although further study is required before a recommendation to shorten the duration of prophylaxis can be made. The index patient may also need to receive rifampin prophylaxis. Ampicillin and chloramphenicol, unlike ceftriaxone and cefotaxime, do not effectively eliminate nasopharyngeal colonization. Rifampin is not recommended for pregnant women who are contacts of infected infants because the risk of rifampin to the fetus has not been established. Chemoprophylaxis is not currently recommended for daycare contacts 2 years old or older unless two or more cases occur in the daycare center within a 60-day period. For children younger than 2 years, the CDC recommends prophylaxis for daycare contacts, whereas the American Academy of Pediatrics does not in most cases. The question of whether to administer prophylaxis in this setting needs to be individualized and should be considered more strongly in daycare centers that resemble households, where children have prolonged contact.

Neisseria meningitidis

Chemoprophylaxis. Chemoprophylaxis is also necessary for close contacts of patients with invasive meningococcal disease[143]; up to 10% of meningococcal meningitis cases have had contact with another known case. The estimated prevalence of meningococcal carriage in the United States is 5% to 10% under nonepidemic conditions. In closed populations such as military recruits, carriage rates can reach levels of 40% to 90%. Carriage may last for a long time (at least months) in about 25% of carriers, is intermittent in one third, and is transient or infrequent in the remaining 40%.[57] Household contacts exposed to a case of meningococcal disease have a 500- to 800-fold to 3000- to 4000-fold increased risk of invasive disease.[143] Secondary systemic meningococcal disease often develops within 5 days of recognition of the index case, with 70% to 80% of secondary cases occurring within 14 days of the primary case; in one report, 9 of 17 (53%) secondary cases occurred 5 to 39 weeks after the primary case. Transmission of *N. meningitidis* has also been documented in a campus bar, a dance club, and a sports club.[422-424]

Chemoprophylaxis is recommended for close contacts of the index case, defined as household contacts, daycare center members, and anyone directly exposed to the patient's oral secretions (e.g., through kissing, mouth-to-mouth resuscitation, endotracheal intubation, or endotracheal tube management).[425] Chemoprophylaxis is not recommended for school, work, or transportation contacts. Chemoprophylaxis may also need to be administered to the index case before hospital discharge because certain antimicrobial agents (e.g., high-dose penicillin or chloramphenicol) do not reliably eradicate meningococci from the nasopharynx of colonized patients. Chemoprophylaxis should be administered as soon as possible (ideally within 24 hours) after the case is identified; administration 14 or more days after the onset of illness in the index patient is probably of limited value.

The optimal chemoprophylactic agent to prevent invasive meningococcal disease is controversial.[143] The CDC currently recommends the administration of rifampin at 12-hour intervals for 2 days in the following dosages: adults, 600 mg; children 1 month or older, 10 mg/kg; and infants younger than 1 month, 5 mg/kg.[425] However, rifampin has several shortcomings, including nasopharyngeal eradication rates of only about 80%, adverse events, necessity for multiple doses over a 2-day period, and emergence of resistant organisms (up to 10% to 27% of isolates), which may then cause invasive disease. In the search for alternative agents, ceftriaxone (intramuscular administration of 250 mg in adults and 125 mg in children) eliminated the serogroup A carrier state in 97% of patients in one study for up to 2 weeks,[426] although parenteral administration is required. Additional studies have demonstrated a single dose of oral ciprofloxacin (500 mg in adults) to be very effective in elimination of the nasopharyngeal carriage of *N. meningitidis*.[381] Ciprofloxacin concentrations in nasal secretions have been shown to exceed the MIC_{90} for meningococci. Ciprofloxacin may well supplant rifampin for chemoprophylaxis in adults. Ciprofloxacin is not recommended for use in children because of concern regarding cartilage damage. In pregnant patients, ceftriaxone is probably the safest alternative agent for chemoprophylaxis. Azithromycin (500 mg orally once) was also shown to be as effective as a four-dose regimen of rifampin in the eradication of meningococci from the nasopharynx.[427] Widespread chemoprophylaxis to low-risk contacts should be discouraged because of the concern over emergence of resistant organisms and possible future limitations on this approach.

Streptococcus pneumoniae

Chemoprophylaxis. The risk of secondary pneumococcal disease in contacts of infected patients has not been defined, although outbreaks have been described in closed populations such as gold miners, military recruits, and jail inmates.[143] In one outbreak in a daycare center,[428] treatment of 97% of the daycare center children and staff with rifampin (10 mg/kg twice daily for 2 days) resulted in a 70% reduction (i.e., only partial eradication) of positive nasopharyngeal cultures for *S. pneumoniae* but did not prevent new acquisition of this organism by three children and one family member. Further studies are needed before chemoprophylaxis is recommended for contacts of patients with pneumococcal meningitis. Some authors do recommend prophylaxis with oral penicillin in patients with sickle cell disease; therapy in such patients has been shown to reduce the incidence of pneumococcal bacteremia by 84%.[143] The CDC has recommended daily penicillin prophylaxis for children with sickle cell hemoglobinopathy beginning before 4 months of age,[429] although consensus has not been reached regarding the age when prophylaxis should be discontinued.

Streptococcus agalactiae

Chemoprophylaxis. Administration of ampicillin during labor to mothers with prenatal vaginal or rectal group B streptococcal colonization and obstetric risk factors (e.g., premature labor, prolonged rupture of membranes, or intrapartum fever) has been associated with reduced rates of colonization and early-onset streptococcal sepsis in the neonate.[430] The CDC has established guidelines for the prevention of group B streptococcal infection by chemoprophylaxis.[431,432] All pregnant women should be screened at 35 to 37 weeks' gestation for anogenital colonization with group B streptococci. Maternal group B streptococcal carriers, identified either antepartum or intrapartum, should receive chemoprophylaxis if one or more of the following risk factors are present: preterm labor at less than 37 weeks' gestation, fever (temperature of 38° C or higher) during labor, or membrane rupture 18 or more hours previously. Furthermore, previous delivery of a sibling with invasive group B streptococcal disease warrants intrapartum maternal chemoprophylaxis in each subsequent pregnancy. Chemoprophylaxis should consist of intrapartum intravenous ampicillin (2 g initially, and then 1 to 2 g every 4 hours) or penicillin G (5 million units initially, and then 2.5 million units every 4 hours) until delivery; intravenous clindamycin or erythromycin should be used in penicillin-allergic patients.

Basilar Skull Fracture. A number of studies have used prophylactic antibiotics in patients with basilar skull fractures and CSF leak on the premise that in patients with a dural defect, the CSF is exposed to pathogenic organisms from the nasopharynx, nasal or mastoid sinuses, or external auditory canal.[67,95] Interpretation and comparison of the various studies examining this question are confounded by multiple variables, including patient selection, choice of antimicrobial agents, and definition of infection. No prospective controlled trials have examined the efficacy of prophylactic antimicrobial agents in these patients, although a meta-analysis suggested that antibiotic prophylaxis did not prevent meningitis in patients with basilar skull fracture.[433] Antibiotic use does not appear to change the incidence of posttraumatic bacterial meningitis and may result in the selection and growth of resistant organisms.

Haemophilus influenzae

Immunoprophylaxis. Vaccination to prevent infection with specific meningeal pathogens is a very useful measure for decreasing the incidence of bacterial meningitis. For *H. influenzae* type B, the availability of conjugate vaccines has decreased the number of cases of *H. influenzae* type B meningitis more than 90% in recent years.[31,43-46] Three *H. influenzae* type B conjugate vaccines are now licensed for infant immunization. The American Academy of Pediatrics has recommended vaccine doses at 2, 4, and 6 months of age[434]; if PRP-OMP (PedvaxHIB) is administered at 2 and 4 months, a dose at 6 months is not required. A booster dose of vaccine is also administered at 12 to 15 months of age no matter which vaccine was administered for the primary series. In addition to preventing invasive disease caused by *H. influenzae* type B, conjugate vaccines are effective in reducing nasopharyngeal colonization and therefore may confer protection to populations not targeted for immunization through herd immunity. However, this reduction may open ecologic niches for non–type B strains of *H. influenzae*. In a surveillance study recently conducted in Brazil before and after the introduction of *H. influenzae* type B conjugate vaccine immunization, the incidence of *H. influenzae* type B meningitis decreased by 69%, but the incidence of *H. influenzae* type A meningitis increased eightfold,[435] highlighting the importance of maintaining surveillance to monitor potential increases in disease due to serotype replacement. Of additional concern is the recent report of cases of invasive *H. influenzae* type B disease in children previously vaccinated against this disease in Nottingham, United Kingdom.[436] There are several possible reasons for this increase, most notably that the vaccination schedule used in the United Kingdom is to vaccinate at 2, 3, and 4 months of age; the absence of a booster dose may have led to this increase in invasive disease.[437]

Neisseria meningitidis

Immunoprophylaxis. Monovalent vaccines using purified serogroup capsular polysaccharide antigens of *N. meningitidis* have been shown to be immunogenic in humans,[438,439] although the serogroup C component is poorly immunogenic in recipients younger than 2 years of age. Serogroup A and C vaccines have demonstrated clinical efficacies of approximately 85% to 100% in older children and adults and are useful in controlling epidemics. The duration of efficacy, however, decreases markedly during the first 3 years after a single dose of vaccine, a decrease that occurs more rapidly in infants and children than in adults. Bactericidal antibody responses are also elicited in adults with the licensed quadrivalent vaccine (activity against serogroups A, C, Y, and W135). Vaccination with the quadrivalent meningococcal vaccine is currently recommended for patients in certain high-risk groups, including those with terminal complement component or properdin deficiency or dysfunction, patients with anatomic or functional asplenia, those who travel to areas with hyperendemic or epidemic meningococcal disease (e.g., the African meningitis belt during the dry season from December to June), military recruits, and those who are close contacts of the primary case, as an adjunct to chemoprophylaxis, although this use is controversial and of unproven efficacy.[143,439,440] Since introduction of routine immunization of military recruits in 1971, meningococcal disease rates decreased by about 94% from 1964 to 1998 in the military.[441] Research, industrial, and clinical laboratory personnel who are routinely exposed to *N. meningitidis* in solutions that may be aerosolized should also be considered for vaccination. The vaccine is not recommended for routine use in the United States because of the overall low risk of infection, the inability to protect against serogroup B disease, and the inability to provide lasting immunity to young children. However, because of the recent increase in invasive meningococcal disease in adolescents and young adults of high school and college age in the United States, the Advisory Committee on Immunization Practices has recommended that college freshman dormitory residents and their parents be provided information about meningococcal infection and the benefits of vaccination, and that other undergraduate students wishing to reduce their risk of meningococcal disease can also choose to be vaccinated.[442,443]

On the basis of the success of conjugate *H. influenzae* type B conjugate vaccines (see earlier), conjugate vaccines for use against disease caused by serogroups A and C meningococci have been developed. The United Kingdom became the world's first country to implement vaccination with a monovalent serogroup C conjugate meningococcal vaccine, in which children are vaccinated at 2, 3, and 4 months of age.[143] The efficacy of the meningococcal serogroup C conjugate vaccine in adolescents and toddlers was evaluated after the first 9 months after vaccine introduction in a catch-up program in which toddlers and adolescents received a single dose of CRM_{197}-meningococcal C vaccine.[444] The short-term vaccine efficacies in toddlers and adolescents were 92% and 97%, respectively. In an update of the epidemiologic effect of the first 18 months of the U.K. meningococcal C conjugate vaccine program, the overall reduction of cases of serogroup C disease from 1998-99 to 2000-01 was 81%,[445] with some variability based on age group. In another case-control study in teenagers in the United Kingdom to assess vaccine efficacy, the protective effectiveness of the vaccine was 93%.[446] Furthermore, carriage of meningococci was reduced by 66% in students aged 15 to 17 years,[447] demonstrating that meningococcal C conjugate vaccines protect against carriage of meningococci that express serogroup C polysaccharide capsules. On the basis of these data, licensure of the vaccine is likely to be considered in other countries; the National Advisory Committee on Immunization in Canada has recently recommended the use of meningococcal vaccine for infants, children, adolescents, and young adults.[439] However, one significant obstacle to control of invasive meningococcal disease worldwide is the lack of a suitable vaccine against serogroup B.[438]

Streptococcus pneumoniae

Immunoprophylaxis. Use of the current 23-valent pneumococcal vaccine is currently recommended for prevention of bacteremic pneumococcal disease in certain high-risk groups[429]: persons 65 years and older; persons aged 2 to 64 years with chronic cardiovascular disease, chronic pulmonary disease, diabetes mellitus, alcoholism, chronic liver disease, CSF leaks, or functional or anatomic asplenia; and those living in special environments or social settings (including Alaskan natives and certain Native American populations). Immunocompromised persons 2 years or older with HIV infection, hematologic or generalized malignancies, chronic renal failure, or nephrotic syndrome; those receiving immunosuppressive chemotherapy (including corticosteroids); and those who have received an organ or bone marrow transplant should also be vaccinated. Efficacy of the vaccine in prevention of pneumococcal meningitis has never been proved, although it may be assumed that the overall efficacy of the vaccine is about 50% against pneumococcal meningitis (with a wide 95% confidence interval); in addition, no data have proved efficacy in infants and very young chil-

dren.[143] One recent study examined the efficacy of a heptavalent conjugate pneumococcal vaccine (administered in four doses at 2, 4, 6, and 12 to 15 months of age) in 37,868 infants and children and demonstrated an efficacy of 97.4% in the prevention of invasive pneumococcal disease in fully vaccinated children.[448] In a cost-effectiveness analysis of pneumococcal conjugate vaccination of healthy infants and children in a hypothetical United States birth cohort of 3.8 million infants, it was estimated that vaccination would prevent more than 12,000 cases of meningitis and bacteremia, and 112 deaths caused by pneumococcal infection for each United States birth cohort.[449] On the basis of the preceding information, the American Academy of Pediatrics Committee on Infectious Diseases has recommended vaccination of all infants less than 2 years of age with the currently licensed heptavalent pneumococcal conjugate vaccine (Prevnar)[450]; the vaccine is administered in four doses at 2, 4, 6, and 12 to 15 months of age. In a study conducted in Israel, administration of a nine-valent pneumococcal conjugate vaccine to toddlers attending daycare centers led to a reduction in nasopharyngeal carriage of *S. pneumoniae*,[451] suggesting that widespread vaccination may result in marked herd immunity. In a study of population-based data from the Active Bacterial Core Surveillance of the CDC on trends in the rate of invasive pneumococcal disease after licensure of the heptavalent pneumococcal vaccine, there was a decline in the rate of invasive pneumococcal disease, with the largest decline (69%) in children under 2 years of age.[452] Disease also fell in adults (32% lower for those 20 to 39 years of age, 8% lower for those 40 to 64 years of age, and 18% lower for those 65 years of age and older), and in persons with invasive disease caused by pneumococcal strains that were not susceptible to penicillin (35% reduction). Continued surveillance of pneumococcal serotypes causing invasive disease is critical and may have implications for the serotype formulation of future conjugate vaccines.[453-455]

REFERENCES

1. Connolly KJ, Hammer SM. The acute aseptic meningitis syndrome. Infect Dis Clin North Am. 1990;4:599-622.
2. Rotbart HA. Viral meningitis and the aseptic meningitis syndrome. In: Scheld WM, Whitley RJ, Durack DT, eds. Infections of the Central Nervous System. 2nd ed. Philadelphia: Lippincott-Raven; 1997:23-46.
3. Centers for Disease Control and Prevention. Enterovirus surveillance—United States, 1997-1999. MMWR Morb Mortal Wkly Rep. 2000;49:913.
4. Romero JR. Diagnosis and management of enteroviral infections of the central nervous system. Curr Infect Dis Rep. 2002;4:309-316.
5. Ho M, Chen ER, Parker RA. An epidemic of enterovirus 71 infection in Taiwan. N Engl J Med. 1999;341:929-935.
6. Huang CC, Liu CC, Chang UC, et al. Neurologic complications in children with enterovirus 71 infection. N Engl J Med. 1999;341:936-942.
7. McMinn P, Stratov I, Nagarajan L, Davis S. Neurological manifestations of enterovirus 71 infection in children during an outbreak of hand, foot, and mouth disease in western Australia. Clin Infect Dis. 2001;32:236-242.
8. Rantakallio P, Leskinen M, von Wendt L. Incidence and prognosis of central nervous system infections in a birth cohort of 12,000 children. Scand J Infect Dis. 1986; 18:287-294.
9. Rotbart HA, Brennan PJ, Fife KH, et al. Enterovirus meningitis in adults. Clin Infect Dis. 1998;27:896-898.
10. Quartier P, Tournilhac O, Archimbaud C, et al. Enteroviral meningoencephalitis after anti-CD20 (rituximab) treatment. Clin Infect Dis. 2003;36:e47-49.
11. Nash D, Mostashari F, Fine A, et al. The outbreak of West Nile virus infection in the New York City area in 1999. N Engl J Med. 2001;344:1807-1814.
12. Gnann JW Jr. Meningitis and encephalitis caused by mumps virus. In: Scheld WM, Whitley RJ, Durack DT, eds. Infections of the Central Nervous System. 2nd ed. Philadelphia: Lippincott-Raven; 1997:169-180.
13. Dykewicz CA, Dato VM, Fisher-Hoch SP, et al. Lymphocytic choriomeningitis outbreak associated with nude mice in a research institute. JAMA. 1992;267:1349-1353.
14. Corey L, Adams HG, Brown ZA, et al. Genital herpes simplex virus infection: Clinical manifestations, course, and complications. Ann Intern Med. 1983;98: 958-972.
15. Echevarria JM, Martinez-Martin P, Tellaz A, et al. Aseptic meningitis due to varicella-zoster virus: Serum antibody levels and local synthesis of specific IgG, IgM, and IgA. J Infect Dis. 1987;155:959-967.
16. Barnes DW, Whitley RJ. CNS diseases associated with varicella zoster virus and herpes simplex virus infection: Pathogenesis and current therapy. Neurol Clin. 1986;4:265-283.
17. Corey L, Spear PG. Infections with herpes simplex viruses (2). N Engl J Med. 1986;314:749-757.

18. Bergström T, Vahlne A, Alestig K, et al. Primary and recurrent herpes simplex virus type 2-induced meningitis. J Infect Dis. 1990;162:322-330.

19. Yamamoto LJ, Tedder DG, Ashley R, et al. Herpes simplex virus type 1 DNA in cerebrospinal fluid of a patient with Mollaret's meningitis. N Engl J Med. 1991;325:1082-1085.

20. Tedder DG, Ashley R, Tyler KL, Levin MJ. Herpes simplex virus infection as a cause of benign recurrent lymphocytic meningitis. Ann Intern Med. 1994;121:334-338.

21. Kojima Y, Hashiguchi H, Hashimoto T, et al. Recurrent herpes simplex virus type 2 meningitis: A case report of Mollaret's meningitis. Jpn J Infect Dis. 2002;55:85-88.

22. Graman PS. Mollaret's meningitis associated with acute Epstein-Barr virus mononucleosis. Arch Neurol. 1987;44:1204-1205.

23. Huang LM, Lee CY, Lee PI, et al. Meningitis caused by human herpesvirus-6. Arch Dis Child. 1991;66:1443-1444.

24. Caserta MT, Hall CB, Schnabel K, et al. Neuroinvasion and persistence of human herpesvirus 6 in children. J Infect Dis. 1994;170:1586-1589.

25. Silverstein A, Steinberg G, Nathanson M. Nervous system involvement in infectious mononucleosis. Arch Neurol. 1972;26:353-358.

26. Berger JR, Simpson DM. Neurological complications of AIDS. In: Scheld WM, Whitley RJ, Durack DT, eds. Infections of the Central Nervous System. 2nd ed. Philadelphia: Lippincott-Raven; 1997:255-271.

27. McArthur JC. Neurologic manifestations of AIDS. Medicine (Baltimore). 1987;66:407-437.

28. Hollander H, Stringari S. Human immunodeficiency virus-associated meningitis: Clinical course and correlations. Am J Med. 1987;83:813-816.

29. Schlech WF III, Ward JI, Band JD, et al. Bacterial meningitis in the United States, 1978 through 1981. The National Bacterial Meningitis Surveillance Study. JAMA. 1985;253:1749-1754.

30. Wenger JD, Hightower AW, Facklam RR, et al. Bacterial meningitis in the United States, 1986: Report of a multistate surveillance study. J Infect Dis. 1990;162:1316-1323.

31. Schuchat A, Robinson K, Wenger JD, et al. Bacterial meningitis in the United States in 1995. N Engl J Med. 1997;337:970-976.

32. Sigurdardottir B, Bjornsson OM, Jonsdottir KE, et al. Acute bacterial meningitis in adults: A 20-year overview. Arch Intern Med. 1997;157:425-430.

33. Durand ML, Calderwood SB, Weber DJ, et al. Acute bacterial meningitis in adults: A review of 493 episodes. N Engl J Med. 1993;328:21-28.

34. Hussein AS, Shafran SD. Acute bacterial meningitis in adults: A 12-year review. Medicine (Baltimore). 2000;79:360-368.

35. McMillan DA, Lin CY, Aronin SI, Quagliarello VJ. Community-acquired bacterial meningitis in adults: Categorization of causes and timing of death. Clin Infect Dis. 2001;33:969-975.

36. Noah ND. Epidemiology of bacterial meningitis: UK and USA. In: Williams JD, Burnie J, eds. Bacterial Meningitis. London: Academic; 1987:93-115.

37. Greenwood BM. The epidemiology of acute bacterial meningitis in tropical Africa. In: Williams JD, Burnie J, eds. Bacterial Meningitis. London: Academic; 1987:61-91.

38. Bryan JP, de Silva HR, Tavares A, et al. Etiology and mortality of bacterial meningitis in northeastern Brazil. Rev Infect Dis. 1990;12:128-135.

39. Spagnuolo PJ, Ellner JJ, Lerner PI, et al. *Haemophilus influenzae* meningitis: The spectrum of disease in adults. Medicine (Baltimore). 1982;61:74-85.

40. Takala AK, Eskola J, van Alphen L. Spectrum of invasive *Haemophilus influenzae* type b disease in adults. Arch Intern Med. 1990;150:2573-2576.

41. Farley MM, Stephens DS, Brachman PS, et al. Invasive *Haemophilus influenzae* disease in adults: A prospective, population-based surveillance. Ann Intern Med. 1992;116:806-812.

42. Robbins JB, Schneerson R, Anderson P, Smith DH. Prevention of systemic infections, especially meningitis, caused by *Haemophilus influenzae* type b. JAMA. 1996;276:1181-1185.

43. Garpenholt O, Silverdal SA, Hugosson S, et al. The impact of *Haemophilus influenzae* type b vaccination in Sweden. Scand J Infect Dis. 1996;28:165-169.

44. Van Alphen L, Spanjaard L, Van der Ende A, et al. Effect of nationwide vaccination of 3-month-old infants in The Netherlands with conjugate *Haemophilus influenzae* type b vaccine: High efficacy and lack of herd immunity. J Pediatr. 1997;131:869-873.

45. Mulholland K, Hilton S, Adegbola R, et al. Randomised trial of *Haemophilus influenzae* type-b tetanus protein conjugate for prevention of pneumonia and meningitis in Gambian infants. Lancet. 1997;349:1191-1197.

46. Steinhoff MC. *Haemophilus influenzae* type b infections are preventable everywhere. Lancet. 1997;349:1186-1187.

47. Kyaw MH, Christie P, Jones IG, Campbell H. The changing epidemiology of bacterial meningitis and invasive non-meningitic bacterial disease in Scotland during the period 1983-99. Scand J Infect Dis. 2002;34:289-298.

48. Rosenstein NE, Perkins BA, Stephens DS, et al. The changing epidemiology of meningococcal disease in the United States, 1992-1996. J Infect Dis. 1999;180:1894-1901.

49. Mastrantonio P, Stefanelli P, Fazio C, et al. Serotype distribution, antibiotic susceptibility, and genetic relatedness of *Neisseria meningitidis* strains recently isolated in Italy. Clin Infect Dis. 2003;36:422-428.

50. Jackson LA, Schuchat A, Reeves MW, Wenger JD. Serogroup C meningococcal outbreaks in the United States: An emerging threat. JAMA. 1995;273:383-389.

51. Whalen CM, Hockin JC, Ryan A, Ashton R. The changing epidemiology of invasive meningococcal disease in Canada, 1985 through 1992: Emergence of a virulent clone of *Neisseria meningitidis*. JAMA. 1995;273:390-394.

52. Berron S, La Fuente LD, Martin E, et al. Increasing incidence of meningococcal disease in Spain associated with variant of serogroup C. Eur J Clin Microbiol Infect Dis. 1998;17:85-89.

53. Raymond NJ, Reeves M, Ajello G, et al. Molecular epidemiology of sporadic (endemic) serogroup C meningococcal disease. J Infect Dis. 1997;176:1277-1284.

54. Wilder-Smith A, Goh KT, Barkham T, Paton NI. Hajj-associated outbreak of *Neisseria meningitidis* serogroup W135: Estimates of the attack rate in a defined population and the risk of invasive disease developing in carriers. Clin Infect Dis. 2003;36:679-683.

55. Mayer LW, Reeves MW, Al-Hamdan N, et al. Outbreak of W135 meningococcal disease in 2000: Not emergence of a new W135 strain but clonal expansion with the electrophoretic type-37 complex. J Infect Dis. 2002;185:1596-1605.

56. Makras P, Alexiou-Daniel S, Antoniadis A, Hatzigeorgiou D. Outbreak of meningococcal disease after an influenza B epidemic at a Hellenic Air Force recruit training center. Clin Infect Dis. 2001;33:e48-50.

57. Stephens DS. Uncloaking the meningococcus: Dynamics of carriage and disease. Lancet. 1999;353:941-942.

58. Ross SC, Densen P. Complement deficiency states and infection: Epidemiology, pathogenesis and consequences of neisserial and other infections in an immune deficiency. Medicine (Baltimore). 1984;64:243-273.

59. Zoppi M, Weiss M, Nydegger UE, et al. Recurrent meningitis in a patient with congenital deficiency of the C9 component of complement: First case of C9 deficiency in Europe. Arch Intern Med. 1990;150:2395-2399.

60. Fijen CAP, Kuijper EJ, Tjia HG, et al. Complement deficiency predisposes for meningitis due to nongroupable meningococci and *Neisseria*-related bacteria. Clin Infect Dis. 1994;18:780-784.

61. Sjöholm AG, Kuijper EJ, Tijssen CC, et al. Dysfunctional properdin in a Dutch family with meningococcal disease. N Engl J Med. 1988;319:33-37.

62. Overturf GD. Indications for the immunological evaluation of patients with meningitis. Clin Infect Dis. 2003;36:189-194.

63. Geiseler PJ, Nelson KE, Levin S, et al. Community-acquired purulent meningitis: A review of 1,316 cases during the antibiotic era, 1954-1976. Rev Infect Dis. 1980;2:725-745.

64. Burman LA, Norrby R, Trollfors B. Invasive pneumococcal infections: Incidence, predisposing factors, and prognosis. Rev Infect Dis. 1985;7:133-142.

65. Musher DM. Infections caused by *Streptococcus pneumoniae*: Clinical spectrum, pathogenesis, immunity, and treatment. Clin Infect Dis. 1992;14:801-809.

66. Kragsbjerg P, Kallman J, Olcen P. Pneumococcal meningitis in adults. Scand J Infect Dis. 1994;26:659-666.

67. Tunkel AR, Scheld WM. Acute infectious complications of head trauma. In: Braakman R, ed. Handbook of Clinical Neurology, Head Injury. Amsterdam: Elsevier; 1990:317-326.

68. Gellin BG, Broome CV. Listeriosis. JAMA. 1989;261:1313-1320.

69. Cherubin CE, Appleman MD, Heseltine PNR, et al. Epidemiological spectrum and current treatment of listeriosis. Rev Infect Dis. 1991;13:1108-1114.

70. Lorber B. Listeriosis. Clin Infect Dis. 1997;24:1-11.

71. Mylonakis E, Hohmann EL, Calderwood SB. Central nervous system infection with *Listeria monocytogenes*. 33 years' experience at a general hospital and review of 776 episodes from the literature. Medicine (Baltimore). 1998;77:313-336.

72. Kamath BM, Mamula P, Baldassano RN, Markowitz JE. *Listeria* meningitis after treatment with infliximab. J Pediatr Gastroenterol Nutr. 2002;34:410-412.

73. Decker CF, Simon GL, DiGioia RA, et al. *Listeria monocytogenes* infections in patients with AIDS: Report of five cases and review. Rev Infect Dis. 1991;13:413-417.

74. Berenguer J, Solera J, Diaz MD, et al. Listeriosis in patients infected with human immunodeficiency virus. Rev Infect Dis. 1991;13:115-119.

75. Zuniga M, Aguado JM, Vada J. *Listeria monocytogenes* meningitis in previously healthy adults: Long-term follow-up. Q J Med. 1992;85:911-915.

76. Saez-Llorens X, McCracken GH Jr. Bacterial meningitis in neonates and children. Infect Dis Clin North Am. 1990;4:623-644.

77. Schuchat A. Epidemiology of group B streptococcal disease in the United States: Shifting paradigms. Clin Microbiol Rev. 1998;11:497-513.

78. Farley MM, Harvey RC, Stull T, et al. A population-based assessment of invasive disease due to group B streptococci in nonpregnant adults. N Engl J Med. 1993;328:1807-1811.

79. Dunne DW, Quagliarello V. Group B streptococcal meningitis in adults. Medicine (Baltimore). 1993;72:1-10.

80. Jackson LA, Hilsdon R, Farley MM, et al. Risk factors for group B streptococcal disease in adults. Ann Intern Med. 1995;123:415-420.

81. Domingo P, Barquet N, Alvarez M, et al. Group B streptococcal meningitis in adults: Report of twelve cases and review. Clin Infect Dis. 1997;25:1180-1187.

82. Mangi RJ, Quintiliani R, Andriole VT. Gram-negative bacillary meningitis. Am J Med. 1975;59:829-836.

83. Cherubin CE, Marr JS, Sierra MF, et al. *Listeria* and gram-negative bacillary meningitis in New York City, 1972-1979. Am J Med. 1981;71:199-209.

84. Unhanand M, Mustafa MM, McCracken GH Jr, et al. Gram-negative enteric bacillary meningitis: A twenty-one-year experience. J Pediatr. 1993;122:15-21.

85. Leonard MK, Murrow JR, Jurado R, Gaynes R. *Salmonella* meningitis in adults infected with HIV: Case report and review of the literature. Am J Med Sci. 2002;323:266-268.

86. Tang LM, Chen ST. *Klebsiella oxytoca* meningitis: Frequent association with neurosurgical procedures. Infection. 1995;23:163-167.

87. Papadakis KA, Vartivarian SE, Vassilaki ME, Anaissie EJ. *Stenotrophomonas maltophilia* meningitis: Report of two cases and review of the literature. J Neurosurg. 1997;87:106-108.

88. Chang WN, Tsai YC, Chien CC, et al. Frequent association with neurosurgical conditions in adult *Proteus mirabilis* meningitis: Report of five cases. Clin Neurol Neurosurg. 2002;104:121-124.

89. Reichert MCF, Medeiros EAS, Ferraz FAP. Hospital-acquired meningitis in patients undergoing craniotomy: Incidence, evolution, and risk factors. Am J Infect Control. 2002;30:158-164.

90. Cameron ML, Durack DT. Helminthic infections of the central nervous system. In: Scheld WM, Whitley RJ, Durack DT, eds. Infections of the Central Nervous System. 2nd ed. Philadelphia: Lippincott-Raven; 1997:845-878.

91. Gordon JJ, Harter DH, Phair JP. Meningitis due to Staphylococcus aureus. Am J Med. 1985;78:965-970.

92. Schlesinger LS, Ross SC, Schaberg DR. Staphylococcus aureus meningitis: A broad-based epidemiologic study. Medicine (Baltimore). 1987;66:148-156.

93. Jensen AG, Espersen F, Skinhoj P, et al. Staphylococcus aureus meningitis: A review of 104 nationwide, consecutive cases. Arch Intern Med. 1993;153:1902-1908.

94. Lerche A, Rasmussen N, Wandall JH, Bohr VA. Staphylococcus aureus meningitis: A review of 28 consecutive community-acquired cases. Scand J Infect Dis. 1995;27:560-573.

95. Kaufman BA, Tunkel AR, Pryor JC, et al. Meningitis in the neurosurgical patient. Infect Dis Clin North Am. 1990;4:677-701.

96. Bross JE, Gordon G. Nocardial meningitis: Case reports and review. Rev Infect Dis. 1991;13:160-165.

97. Heerema MS, Ein ME, Musher DM, et al. Anaerobic bacterial meningitis. Am J Med. 1979;67:219-227.

98. Feder HM Jr. Bacteroides fragilis meningitis. Rev Infect Dis. 1987;9:783-786.

99. Law DA, Aronoff SC. Anaerobic meningitis in children: Case report and review of the literature. Pediatr Infect Dis J. 1992;11:968-971.

100. Korman TM, Athan E, Spelman DW. Anaerobic meningitis due to Peptostreptococcus species: Case report and review. Clin Infect Dis. 1997;25:1462-1464.

101. Stevenson KB, Murray EW, Sarubbi FA. Enterococcal meningitis: Report of four cases and review. Clin Infect Dis. 1994;18:233-239.

102. Lu CH, Chang WN, Chang HW. Adults with meningitis caused by viridans streptococci. Infection. 2001;29:305-309.

103. van de Beek D, de Gans J, Spanjaard L, et al. Group A streptococcal meningitis in adults: Report of 41 cases and a review of the literature. Clin Infect Dis. 2002;34: e32-36.

104. Hook EW III. Central nervous system syphilis. In: Scheld WM, Whitley RJ, Durack DT, eds. Infections of the Central Nervous System. 2nd ed. Philadelphia: Lippincott-Raven; 1997:669-684.

105. Simon RP. Neurosyphilis. Arch Neurol. 1985;42:606-613.

106. Hook EW III. Syphilis and HIV infection. J Infect Dis. 1989;160:530-534.

107. Musher DM, Hamill RJ, Baughn RE. Effect of human immunodeficiency virus (HIV) infection on the course of syphilis and on the response to treatment. Ann Intern Med. 1990;113:872-881.

108. Hook EW III, Marra CM. Acquired syphilis in adults. N Engl J Med. 1992;326: 1060-1069.

109. Katz DA, Berger JR. Neurosyphilis in acquired immunodeficiency syndrome. Arch Neurol. 1989;46:895-898.

110. Flood JM, Weinstock HS, Guroy ME, et al. Neurosyphilis during the AIDS epidemic, San Francisco, 1985-1992. J Infect Dis. 1998;177:931-940.

111. Reik L Jr. Lyme disease. In: Scheld WM, Whitley RJ, Durack DT, eds. Infections of the Central Nervous System. 2nd ed. Philadelphia: Lippincott-Raven; 1997:685-718.

112. Reik L, Steere AC, Bartenhagen NH, et al. Neurologic abnormalities of Lyme disease. Medicine (Baltimore). 1979;58:281-294.

113. Pachner AR, Steere AC. The triad of neurologic manifestations of Lyme disease: Meningitis, cranial neuritis and radiculoneuritis. Neurology. 1985;35:47-53.

114. Luft BJ, Steinman CR, Neimark HC, et al. Invasion of the central nervous system by Borrelia burgdorferi in acute disseminated infection. JAMA. 1992;267:1364-1367.

115. Niu MT, Duma RJ. Meningitis due to protozoa and helminths. Infect Dis Clin North Am. 1990;4:809-841.

116. Durack DT. Amebic infections. In: Scheld WM, Whitley RJ, Durack DT, eds. Infections of the Central Nervous System. 2nd ed. Philadelphia: Lippincott-Raven; 1997:831-844.

117. Wellings FM, Amuso PT, Chang SL, et al. Isolation and identification of pathogenic Naegleria from Florida lakes. Appl Environ Microbiol. 1977;34:661-667.

118. Gardner HAR, Martinez AJ, Visvesvara GS, et al. Granulomatous amebic encephalitis in an AIDS patient. Neurology. 1991;41:1993-1995.

119. Di Gregorio C, Rivasi R, Mongiardo N, et al. Acanthamoeba meningoencephalitis in a patient with acquired immunodeficiency syndrome. Arch Pathol Lab Med. 1992;116:1363-1365.

120. Gordon SM, Steinberg JP, DuPuis MH, et al. Culture isolation of Acanthamoeba species and leptomyxid amebas from patients with amebic meningoencephalitis, including two patients with AIDS. Clin Infect Dis. 1992;15:1024-1030.

121. Koo J, Pien F, Kliks MM. Angiostrongylus (Parastrongylus) eosinophilic meningitis. Rev Infect Dis. 1988;10:1155-1162.

122. Re V, Gluckman SJ. Eosinophilic meningitis. Am J Med. 2003;114:217-223.

123. Slom T, Johnson S. Eosinophilic meningitis. Curr Infect Dis Rep. 2003;5:322-328.

124. Tsai HC, Liu YC, Kunin CM, et al. Eosinophilic meningitis caused by Angiostrongylus cantonensis: Report of 17 cases. Am J Med. 2001;111:109-114.

125. Slom TJ, Cortese MM, Gerber SI, et al. An outbreak of eosinophilic meningitis caused by Angiostrongylus cantonensis in travelers returning from the Caribbean. N Engl J Med. 2002;346:668-675.

126. Lindo JF, Waugh C, Hall J, et al. Enzootic Angiostrongylus cantonensis in rats and snails after an outbreak of human eosinophilic meningitis, Jamaica. Emerg Infect Dis. 2002;8:324-326.

127. Sorvillo F, Ash LR, Berlin OG, Morse SA. Baylisascaris procyonis: An emerging helminthic zoonosis. Emerg Infect Dis. 2002;8:355-359.

128. Johnson RT. Pathogenesis of CNS infections. In: Viral Infections of the Central Nervous System. New York: Raven; 1982:37-60.

129. Tunkel AR, Wispelwey B, Scheld WM. Pathogenesis and pathophysiology of meningitis. Infect Dis Clin North Am. 1990;4:555-581.

130. Cassady KA, Whitley RJ. Pathogenesis and pathophysiology of viral infections of the central nervous system. In: Scheld WM, Whitley RJ, Durack DT, eds. Infections of the Central Nervous System. 2nd ed. Philadelphia: Lippincott-Raven; 1997:7-22.

131. Johnson RT, Mims CA. Pathogenesis of viral infections of the nervous system. N Engl J Med. 1968;278:23-30, 84-92.

132. Kristensson K, Ghetti B, Wisniewski HM. Study on the propagation of herpes simplex virus (type 2) into brain after intraocular injection. Brain Res. 1974;69:189-201.

133. Ren R, Racaniello VR. Poliovirus spreads from muscle to the central nervous system by neural pathways. J Infect Dis. 1992;166:747-752.

134. Frei K, Leist TP, Meager A, et al. Production of B cell stimulatory factor-2 and interferon-γ in the central nervous system during viral meningitis and encephalitis: Evaluation in a murine model infection and in patients. J Exp Med. 1988;168: 449-453.

135. Chonmaitree T, Baron S. Bacteria and viruses induce production of interferon in the cerebrospinal fluid of children with acute meningitis: A study of 57 cases and review. Rev Infect Dis. 1991;13:1061-1065.

136. Lin TY, Hsia SH, Huang YC, et al. Proinflammatory cytokine reactions in enterovirus 71 infections of the central nervous system. Clin Infect Dis. 2003;269-274.

137. Ramilo O, Mustafa MM, Porter J, et al. Detection of interleukin 1β but not tumor necrosis factor-α in cerebrospinal fluid of children with aseptic meningitis. Am J Dis Child. 1990;144:349-352.

138. Resnick L, diMarzo-Veronese F, Schüpbach J, et al. Intra-blood-brain-barrier synthesis of HTLV-III-specific IgG in patients with neurologic symptoms associated with AIDS or AIDS-related complex. N Engl J Med. 1985;313:1498-1504.

139. Gnann JW Jr, Whitley RJ. Neurologic manifestations of varicella and herpes zoster. In: Scheld WM, Whitley RJ, Durack DT, eds. Infections of the Central Nervous System. 2nd ed. Philadelphia: Lippincott-Raven; 1997:91-105.

140. Tunkel AR, Wispelwey B, Scheld WM. Bacterial meningitis: Recent advances in pathophysiology and treatment. Ann Intern Med. 1990;112:610-623.

141. Quagliarello V, Scheld WM. Bacterial meningitis: Pathogenesis, pathophysiology, and progress. N Engl J Med. 1992;327:864-872.

142. Tunkel AR, Scheld WM. Pathogenesis and pathophysiology of bacterial meningitis. Clin Microbiol Rev. 1993;6:118-136.

143. Tunkel AR. Bacterial Meningitis. Philadelphia: Lippincott, Williams & Wilkins; 2001.

144. Scheld WM, Koedel U, Nathan B, Pfister HW. Pathophysiology of bacterial meningitis: Mechanisms of neuronal injury. J Infect Dis. 2002;186:S225-S233.

145. Stephens DS, Farley MM. Pathogenic events during infection of the human nasopharynx with Neisseria meningitidis and Haemophilus influenzae. Rev Infect Dis. 1991;13:22-33.

146. Nesin M, Ramirez M, Tomasz A. Capsular transformation of a multidrug-resistant Streptococcus pneumoniae in vitro. J Infect Dis. 1998;177:707-713.

147. Malley R, Stack AM, Ferretti ML, et al. Anticapsular polysaccharide antibodies and nasopharyngeal colonization with Streptococcus pneumoniae in infant rats. J Infect Dis. 1998;178:878-882.

148. Kim KS, Itabashi H, Genski P, et al. The K1 capsule is the critical determinant in the development of Escherichia coli meningitis in the rat. J Clin Invest. 1992;90:897-905.

149. Houdouin V, Bonacorsi S, Brahimi N, et al. A uropathogenicity island contributes to the pathogenicity of Escherichia coli strains that cause neonatal meningitis. Infect Immun. 2002;70:5865-5869.

150. Meier C, Oelschlaeger TA, Merkert H, et al. Ability of Escherichia coli isolates that cause meningitis in newborns to invade epithelial and endothelial cells. Infect Immun. 1996;64:2391-2399.

151. Pron B, Taha MK, Rambaud C, et al. Interaction of Neisseria meningitidis with the components of the blood-brain barrier correlates with an increased expression of PilC. J Infect Dis. 1997;176:1285-1292.

152. Huang SH, Wass C, Fu Q, et al. Escherichia coli invasion of brain microvascular endothelial cells in vitro and in vivo: Molecular cloning and characterization of invasion gene ibe10. Infect Immun. 1995;63:4470-4475.

153. Bingen E, Bonacorsi S, Brahimi N, et al. Virulence patterns of Escherichia coli K1 strains associated with neonatal meningitis. J Clin Microbiol. 1997;35:2981-2982.

154. Huang SH, Wan ZS, Chen YH, et al. Further characterization of Escherichia coli brain microvascular endothelial cell invasion gene ibe10 by deletion, complementation, and protein expression. J Infect Dis. 2001;183:1071-1078.

155. Wang Y, Kim KW. Role of OmpA and ibe10 in Escherichia coli K1 invasion of brain microvascular endothelial cells in vitro and in vivo. Pediatr Res. 2002;511:559-563.

156. Prasadarao NV. Identification of Escherichia coli outer membrane protein A receptor on human brain microvascular endothelial cells. Infect Immun. 2002;70:4556-4563.

157. Prasadarao NV, Srivastava PK, Rudrabhatia RS, et al. Cloning and expression of the Escherichia coli K1 outer membrane A receptor, a gp96 homologue. Infect Immun. 2003;71:1680-1688.

158. Khan NA, Wang Y, Kim KJ, et al. Cytotoxic necrotizing factor-1 contributes to Escherichia coli invasion of the central nervous system. J Biol Chem. 2002;277:15607-15612.

159. Kim KS. Strategy of Escherichia coli for crossing the blood-brain barrier. J Infect Dis. 2002;186:S220-S224.

160. Ring A, Weiser JN, Tuomanen EI. Pneumococcal trafficking across the blood-brain barrier: Molecular analysis of a novel bidirectional pathway. J Clin Invest. 1998;102:347-360.

161. Vazquez-Boland JA, Kuhn M, Berche P, et al. Listeria pathogenesis and molecular virulence determinants. Clin Microbiol Rev. 2001;14:584-640.

162. Stahel PF, Frei K, Fontana A, et al. Evidence for intrathecal synthesis of alternative pathway complement activation proteins in experimental meningitis. Am J Pathol. 1997;151:897-904.

163. Stahel PF, Nadal D, Pfister HW, et al. Complement C3 and factor B cerebrospinal fluid concentrations in bacterial and aseptic meningitis. Lancet. 1997;349:1886-1887.

164. Seebach J, Bartholdi D, Frei K, et al. Experimental *Listeria* meningoencephalitis: Macrophage inflammatory protein-1α and -2 are produced intrathecally and mediate chemotactic activity in cerebrospinal fluid of infected mice. J Immunol. 1995;155:4367-4375.

165. Inaba Y, Ishiguro A, Shimbo T. The production of macrophage inflammatory protein-1α in the cerebrospinal fluid at the initial stage of meningitis in children. Pediatr Res. 1997;42:788-793.

166. Spanaus KS, Nadal D, Pfister HW, et al. C-X-C and C-C chemokines are expressed in the cerebrospinal fluid in bacterial meningitis and mediate chemotactic activity on peripheral blood-derived polymorphonuclear and mononuclear cells in vitro. J Immunol. 1997;158:1956-1964.

167. Sprenger H, Rosler A, Tonn P, et al. Chemokines in the cerebrospinal fluid of patients with meningitis. Clin Immunol Immunopathol. 1996;80:155-161.

168. Tan TQ, Smith W, Hawkins EP, et al. Hematogenous bacterial meningitis in an intercellular adhesion molecule-1-deficient infant mouse model. J Infect Dis. 1995;171:342-349.

169. Weber JR, Angstwurm K, Burger W, et al. Anti ICAM (CD 54) monoclonal antibody reduces inflammatory changes in experimental bacterial meningitis. J Neuroimmunol. 1995;63:63-68.

170. Tuomanen EI, Saukkonen K, Sande S, et al. Reduction of inflammation, tissue damage, and mortality in bacterial meningitis in rabbits treated with monoclonal antibodies against adhesion-promoting receptors of leukocytes. J Exp Med. 1989;170:959-968.

171. Rozdzinski E, Jones T, Burnette WN, et al. Antiinflammatory effects in experimental meningitis of prokaryotic peptides that mimic selectins. J Infect Dis. 1993;168:1422-1428.

172. Tan TQ, Smith W, Hawkins EP, Kaplan SL. Anti-CD11b monoclonal antibody in an infant rat model of *Haemophilus influenzae* type b sepsis and meningitis. J Antimicrob Chemother. 1997;39:209-216.

173. Tang T, Frenette PS, Hynes RO, et al. Cytokine-induced meningitis is dramatically attenuated in mice deficient in endothelial selectins. J Clin Invest. 1996;97:2485-2490.

174. Granert C, Raud J, Xie I, et al. Inhibition of leukocyte rolling with polysaccharide fucoidin prevents pleocytosis in experimental meningitis in the rabbit. J Clin Invest. 1994;93:929-936.

175. Tuomanen E. A spoonful of sugar to control inflammation? J Clin Invest. 1994;93:917-918.

176. Lorenzl S, Loedel U, Dirnagl U, et al. Imaging of leukocyte-endothelium interaction using in vivo confocal laser scanning microscopy during the early phase of experimental pneumococcal meningitis. J Infect Dis. 1993;168:927-933.

177. Weber JR, Angstwurm K, Rosenkranz T, et al. Heparin inhibits leukocyte rolling in pial vessels and attenuates inflammatory changes in a rat model of experimental bacterial meningitis. J Cereb Blood Flow Metab. 1997;17:1221-1229.

178. Polfliet MMJ, Zwijnenburg PJG, van Furth AM, et al. Meningeal and perivascular macrophages of the central nervous system play a protective role during bacterial meningitis. J Immunol. 2001;167:4644-4650.

179. Paris MM, Friedland IR, Ehrett S, et al. Effect of interleukin-1 receptor antagonist and soluble tumor necrosis factor receptor in animal models of infection. J Infect Dis. 1995;171:161-169.

180. Azuma H, Tsuda N, Sasaki K, Okuno A. Clinical significance of cytokine measurements for detection of meningitis. J Pediatr. 1997;131:463-465.

181. Halstensen A, Ceska M, Brandtzaeg P, et al. Interleukin-8 in serum and cerebrospinal fluid from patients with meningococcal disease. J Infect Dis. 1993;167:471-475.

182. Lopez-Cortes LF, Cruz-Ruiz M, Gomez-Mateos J, et al. Interleukin-8 in cerebrospinal fluid from patients with meningitis of different etiologies: Its possible role as neutrophil chemotactic factor. J Infect Dis. 1995;172:581-584.

183. Ostergaard C, Benfield TL, Sellebjerg F, et al. Interleukin-8 in cerebrospinal fluid from patients with septic and aseptic meningitis. Eur J Clin Microbiol Infect Dis. 1996;15:166-169.

184. Ostergaard C, Yieng-Kow RV, Larson CG, et al. Treatment with a monoclonal antibody to IL-8 attenuates the pleocytosis in experimental pneumococcal meningitis in rabbits when given intravenously, but not intracisternally. Clin Exp Immunol. 2000;122:207-211.

185. Frei K, Nadal D, Pfister HW, Fontana A. *Listeria* meningitis: Identification of a cerebrospinal fluid inhibitor of macrophage listericidal function as interleukin-10. J Exp Med. 1993;178:1255-1261.

186. van Furth AM, Seijmonsbergen EM, Langermans JAM, et al. High levels of interleukin-10 and tumor necrosis factor in cerebrospinal fluid during the onset of bacterial meningitis. Clin Infect Dis. 1996;21:220-222.

187. Diab A, Zhu J, Lindquist L, et al. Cytokine mRNA profiles during the course of experimental *Haemophilus influenzae* bacterial meningitis. Clin Immunol Immunopathol. 1997;85:236-245.

188. Kornelisse RF, Savelkoul HFJ, Mulder PHG, et al. Interleukin-10 and soluble tumor necrosis factor receptors in cerebrospinal fluid of children with bacterial meningitis. J Infect Dis. 1996;173:1498-1502.

189. Paris MM, Hickey SM, Trujillo M, et al. The effect of interleukin-10 on meningeal inflammation in experimental bacterial meningitis. J Infect Dis. 1997;176:1239-1246.

190. Zwijnenburg PJG, van der Poll T, Florquin S, et al. Interleukin-10 negatively regulates local cytokine and chemokine production but does not influence antibacterial host defense during murine pneumococcal meningitis. Infect Immun. 2003;71:2276-2279.

191. Kornelisse RF, Hack CE, Savelkoul HFJ, et al. Intrathecal production of interleukin-12 and gamma interferon in patients with bacterial meningitis. Infect Immun. 1997;65:877-881.

192. Suzuki T, Ishiguro A, Shimbo T. Transient elevation of interleukin-16 levels at the initial stage of meningitis in children. Clin Exp Immunol. 2003;131:484-489.

193. Koedel U, Angele B, Rupprecht T, et al. Toll-like receptor-2 participates in mediation of immune response in experimental pneumococcal meningitis. J Immunol. 2003;170:438-444.

194. Echchannaoui H, Frei K, Schnell C, et al. Toll-like receptor 2-deficient mice are highly susceptible to *Streptococcus pneumoniae* meningitis because of reduced bacterial clearing and enhanced inflammation. J Infect Dis. 2002;186:798-806.

195. Meli DN, Christian JM, Leib SL. Matrix metalloproteinase-9 in pneumococcal meningitis: Activation via an oxidative pathway. J Infect Dis. 2003;187:1411-1415.

196. Leib SL, Leppert D, Clements J, Täuber MG. Matrix metalloproteinases contribute to brain damage in experimental pneumococcal meningitis. Infect Immun. 2000;68:615-620.

197. Leib SL, Clements JM, Lindberg RLP, et al. Inhibition of matrix metalloproteinases and tumor necrosis factor converting enzyme α as adjuvant therapy in pneumococcal meningitis. Brain. 2001;124:1734-1742.

198. Engelhard D, Pomeranz S, Gallily R, et al. Serotype-related differences in inflammatory response to *Streptococcus pneumoniae* in experimental meningitis. J Infect Dis. 1997;175:979-982.

199. Lorenzl S, Koedel U, Pfister HW. Mannitol, but not allopurinol, modulates changes in cerebral blood flow, intracranial pressure, and brain water content during pneumococcal meningitis in the rat. Crit Care Med. 1996;24:1874-1880.

200. Paul R, Koedel U, Pfister HW. Reduction of intracranial pressure by nimodipine in experimental pneumococcal meningitis. Crit Care Med. 2000;28:2552-2556.

201. Hoffmann O, Keilwerth N, Bille MB, et al. Triptans reduce the inflammatory response in bacterial meningitis. J Cereb Blood Flow Metab. 2002;22:988-996.

202. Slater AJ, Berkowitz ID, Wilson DA, Traystman RJ. Role of leukocytes in cerebral autoregulation and hyperemia in bacterial meningitis in rabbits. Am J Physiol. 1997;42:H380-H386.

203. Koedel U, Lorenzl S, Gorriz C, et al. Endothelin B receptor-mediated increase of cerebral blood flow in experimental pneumococcal meningitis. J Cereb Blood Flow Metab. 1998;18:67-74.

204. Koedel U, Gorriz C, Lorenzl S, Pfister HW. Increased endothelin levels in cerebrospinal fluid samples from adults with bacterial meningitis. Clin Infect Dis. 1997;25:329-330.

205. Pfister LA, Tureen JH, Shaw S, et al. Endothelin inhibition improves cerebral blood flow and is neuroprotective in pneumococcal meningitis. Ann Neurol. 2000;47:329-335.

206. Moller K, Skinhoj P, Knudsen GM, et al. Effect of short-term hyperventilation on cerebral blood flow autoregulation in patients with acute bacterial meningitis. Stroke. 2000;31:1116-1122.

207. Pfister HW, Borasio GD, Dirnagl U, et al. Cerebrovascular complications of bacterial meningitis in adults. Neurology. 1992;42:1497-1504.

208. Guerra-Romero L, Täuber MG, Fournier MA, et al. Lactate and glucose concentrations in brain interstitial fluid, cerebrospinal fluid, and serum during experimental pneumococcal meningitis. J Infect Dis. 1992;166:546-550.

209. Pfister HW, Koedel U, Lorenzl S, et al. Antioxidants attenuate microvascular changes in the early phase of experimental pneumococcal meningitis in rats. Stroke. 1992;23:1798-1804.

210. Pfister HW, Ködel U, Dirnagl U, et al. Effect of catalase on regional cerebral blood flow and brain edema during the early phase of experimental pneumococcal meningitis. J Infect Dis. 1992;166:1442-1445.

211. Leib SL, Kim YS, Chow LL, et al. Reactive oxygen intermediates contribute to necrotic and apoptotic neuronal injury in an infant rat model of bacterial meningitis due to group B streptococci. J Clin Invest. 1996;98:2632-2639.

212. Bogdan I, Leib SL, Bergeron M, et al. Tumor necrosis factor-α contributes to apoptosis in hippocampal neurons during experimental group B streptococcal meningitis. J Infect Dis. 1997;176:693-697.

213. Bottcher T, Gerber J, Wellmer A, et al. Rifampin reduces production of reactive oxygen species of cerebrospinal fluid phagocytes and hippocampal neuronal apoptosis in experimental *Streptococcus pneumoniae* meningitis. J Infect Dis. 2000;181:2095-2098.

214. Auer M, Pfister LA, Leppert D, et al. Effects of clinically used antioxidants in experimental pneumococcal meningitis. J Infect Dis. 2000;182:347-350.

215. Braun JS, Novack R, Murray PJ, et al. Apoptosis-induced factor mediates microglial and neuronal apoptosis caused by pneumococcus. J Infect Dis. 2001;184:1300-1309.

216. Braun JS, Sublett JE, Freyer D, et al. Pneumococcal pneumolysin and H_2O_2 mediate brain cell apoptosis during meningitis. J Clin Invest. 2002;109:19-27.

217. Koedel U, Winkler F, Angele B, et al. Meningitis-associated central nervous system complications are mediated by the activation of poly(ADP-ribose) polymerase. J Cereb Blood Flow Metab. 2002;22:39-49.

218. Gianinazzi C, Grandgirard D, Imboden H, et al. Caspase-3 mediates hippocampal apoptosis in pneumococcal meningitis. Acta Neuropathol. 2003;105:499-507.

219. Shenep JL, Tuomanen E. Perspective: Targeting nitric oxide in the adjuvant therapy of sepsis and meningitis. J Infect Dis. 1998;177:766-769.

220. Kortytko PJ, Boje KMK. Pharmacological characterization of nitric oxide production in a rat model of meningitis. Neuropharmacology. 1996;35:231-237.

221. Koedel U, Bernatowicz A, Paul R, et al. Experimental pneumococcal meningitis: Cerebrovascular alterations, brain edema, and meningeal inflammation are linked to the production of nitric oxide. Ann Neurol. 1995;37:313-323.

222. Paul R, Koedel U, Pfister HW. 7-Nitroindazole inhibits pial vasodilation in a rat model of pneumococcal meningitis. J Cereb Blood Flow Metab. 1997;17:985-991.

223. Buster BL, Weintrob AC, Townsend GC, Scheld WM. Potential role of nitric oxide in the pathophysiology of experimental bacterial meningitis in the rat. Infect Immun. 1995;63:3835-3839.
224. Boje KMK. Inhibition of nitric oxide synthase attenuates blood-brain barrier disruption during experimental meningitis. Brain Res. 1996;720:75-83.
225. Leib SL, Kim YS, Black SM, et al. Inducible nitric oxide synthase and the effect of aminoguanidine in experimental neonatal meningitis. J Infect Dis. 1998;177:692-700.
226. Park WS, Chang YS, Lee M. N(Omega)-nitro-L-arginine methyl ester (L-NAME) attenuates the acute inflammatory responses and brain injury during the early phase of experimental Escherichia coli meningitis in the newborn piglet. Neurol Res. 2001;23:862-868.
227. Boje KMK, Jaworowicz D Jr, Raybon JJ. Neuroinflammatory role of prostaglandins during experimental meningitis: Evidence suggestive of an in vivo relationship between nitric oxide and prostaglandins. Pharmacology. 2003;304:319-325.
228. Koedel U, Paul R, Winkler F, et al. Lack of endothelial nitric oxide synthase aggravates murine pneumococcal meningitis. J Neuropathol Exp Neurol. 2001;60:1041-1050.
229. Kastenbauer S, Klein M, Koedel U, Pfister HW. Reactive oxygen species contribute to blood-labyrinth barrier disruption in suppurative labyrinthitis complicating experimental pneumococcal meningitis in the rat. Brain Res. 2001;904:208-217.
230. Kornelisse RF, Hoekman K, Visser JJ, et al. The role of nitric oxide in bacterial meningitis in children. J Infect Dis. 1996;174:120-126.
231. van Furth AM, Seijmonsbergen EM, Groeneveld PHP, et al. Levels of nitric oxide correlate with high levels of tumor necrosis factor α in cerebrospinal fluid samples from children with bacterial meningitis. Clin Infect Dis. 1996;22:876-878.
232. Leib SL, Täuber MG. Pathogenesis of bacterial meningitis. Infect Dis Clin North Am. 1999;13:527-548.
233. Kastenbauer S, Koedel U, Pfister HW. Role of peroxynitrite as a mediator of pathophysiological alterations in experimental pneumococcal meningitis. J Infect Dis. 1999;180:1164-1170.
234. Kastenbauer S, Koedel U, Becker BF, Pfister HW. Experimental meningitis in the rat: Protection by uric acid at human physiologic blood concentrations. Eur J Pharmacol. 2001;425:149-152.
235. Christen S, Bifrare YD, Siegenthaler C, et al. Marked elevation in cortical urate and xanthine oxidoreductase activity in experimental bacterial meningitis. Brain Res. 2001;900:244-251.
236. Kastenbauer S, Koedel U, Becker BF, Pfister HW. Oxidative stress in bacterial meningitis in humans. Neurology. 2002;58:186-191.
237. Kastenbauer S, Koedel U, Becker BF, Pfister HW. Pneumococcal meningitis in the rat: Evaluation of peroxynitrite scavengers for adjunctive therapy. Eur J Pharmacol. 2002;449:177-181.
238. Guerra-Romero L, Tureen JH, Fournier MA, et al. Amino acids in cerebrospinal and brain interstitial fluid in experimental pneumococcal meningitis. Pediatr Res. 1993;33:510-513.
239. Leib SL, Kim YS, Ferriero DM, Täuber MG. Neuroprotective effect of excitatory amino acid antagonist kynurenic acid in experimental bacterial meningitis. J Infect Dis. 1996;173:166-171.
240. Spranger M, Krempien S, Schwab S, et al. Excess glutamate in the cerebrospinal fluid in bacterial meningitis. J Neurol Sci. 1996;143:126-131.
241. Spranger M, Schwab S, Krempien S, et al. Excess glutamate levels in the cerebrospinal fluid predict clinical outcome of bacterial meningitis. Arch Neurol. 1996;53:992-996.
242. Winkler F, Kastenbauer S, Koedel U, Pfister HW. Increased serum concentrations of tissue plasminogen activator correlate with an adverse clinical outcome in patients with bacterial meningitis. J Neurol Neurosurg Psychiatry 2002;73:456.
243. Winkler F, Kastenbauer S, Koedel U, Pfister HW. Role of urokinase plasminogen activator system in patients with bacterial meningitis. Neurology. 2002;59:1350-1355.
244. Gaduzda DH, Hirsch MS. Neurologic manifestations of infection with human immunodeficiency virus: Clinical features and pathogenesis. Ann Intern Med. 1987;107:383-391.
245. Verghese A, Gallemore G. Kernig's and Brudzinski's signs revisited. Rev Infect Dis. 1987;9:1187-1192.
246. Thomas KE, Hasbun R, Jekel J, Quagliarello VJ. The diagnostic accuracy of Kernig's sign, Brudzinski's sign, and nuchal rigidity in adults with suspected meningitis. Clin Infect Dis. 2002;35:46-52.
247. Attia J, Hatala R, Cook DJ, et al. Does this patient have acute meningitis? JAMA. 1999;282:175-181.
248. Anderson J, Backer V, Voldsgaard P, et al. Acute meningococcal meningitis: Analysis of features of the disease according to the age of 255 patients. J Infect. 1997;34:227-235.
249. Saez-Llorens X, McCracken GH Jr. Bacterial meningitis in children. Lancet. 2003;361:2139-2148.
250. Ashwal S, Perkin RM, Thompson JR, et al. Bacterial meningitis in children: Current concepts of neurologic management. Curr Probl Pediatr. 1994;24:267-284.
251. Choi C. Bacterial meningitis in aging adults. Clin Infect Dis. 2001;33:1380-1385.
252. Gorse GJ, Thrupp LD, Nudleman KL, et al. Bacterial meningitis in the elderly. Arch Intern Med. 1989;149:1603-1606.
253. Tunkel AR, Scheld WM. Central nervous system infection in the compromised host. In: Rubin RH, Young LS, eds. Clinical Approach to Infection in the Compromised Host. 4th ed. New York: Kluwer Academic/Plenum; 2002:163-214.
254. Merritt HH, Moore M. Acute syphilitic meningitis. Medicine (Baltimore). 1935;14:119-183.
255. Holmes MD, Zawadzki B, Simon RP. Clinical features of meningovascular syphilis. Neurology. 1984;34:553-555.
256. Johns DR, Tierney M, Felsenstein D. Alteration in the natural history of neurosyphilis by concurrent infection with the human immunodeficiency virus. N Engl J Med. 1987;316:1569-1572.
257. Hutchinson CM, Rompalo AM, Reichart CA, et al. Characteristics of patients with syphilis attending Baltimore STD clinics: Multiple, high-risk subgroups and interactions with human immunodeficiency virus infection. Arch Intern Med. 1991;151:511-516.
258. Reik L, Burgdorfer W, Donaldson JO. Neurologic abnormalities in Lyme disease without erythema chronicum migrans. Am J Med. 1986;81:73-78.
259. Kuberski T, Wallace GD. Clinical manifestations of eosinophilic meningitis due to Angiostrongylus cantonensis. Neurology. 1979;29:1566-1570.
260. Dagan R, Henista JA, Menegus MA. Association of clinical presentation, laboratory findings, and virus serotypes with the presence of meningitis in hospitalized infants with enterovirus infection. J Pediatr. 1988;113:975-978.
261. Negrini B, Kelleher KJ, Wald ER. Cerebrospinal fluid findings in aseptic versus bacterial meningitis. Pediatrics. 2000;105:316-319.
262. Chonmaitree T, Baldwin CD, Lucia HL. Role of the virology laboratory in diagnosis and management of patients with central nervous system disease. Clin Microbiol Rev. 1989;2:1-14.
263. Johnson GM, McAbee GA, Seaton ED, et al. Suspect value of non-CSF viral cultures in the diagnosis of enteroviral CNS infections in young infants. Dev Med Child Neurol. 1992;34:876-884.
264. Rotbart HA. Diagnosis of enteroviral meningitis with the polymerase chain reaction. J Pediatr. 1990;117:85-89.
265. Sawyer MH, Holland D, Aintablian N. Diagnosis of enteroviral central nervous system infection by polymerase chain reaction during a large community outbreak. Pediatr Infect Dis J. 1994;13:177-182.
266. Ahmed A, Brito F, Goto C, et al. Clinical utility of polymerase chain reaction for diagnosis of enteroviral meningitis in infancy. J Pediatr. 1997;131:393-397.
267. Ramers C, Billman G, Hartin M, et al. Impact of a diagnostic cerebrospinal fluid enterovirus polymerase chain reaction test on patient management. JAMA. 2000;283:2680-2685.
268. Echevarria JM, Cases I, Tenorio A, et al. Detection of varicella-zoster virus-specific DNA sequences in cerebrospinal fluid from patients with acute aseptic meningitis and no cutaneous lesions. J Med Virol. 1994;43:331-335.
269. Shoji H, Honda Y, Murai I, et al. Detection of varicella-zoster virus DNA by polymerase chain reaction in cerebrospinal fluid of patients with herpes zoster meningitis. J Neurol. 1992;239:69-70.
270. Hollander H, Levy JA. Neurologic abnormalities and recovery of human immunodeficiency virus from cerebrospinal fluid. Ann Intern Med. 1987;106:692-695.
271. Chalmers AC, Aprill BS, Shephard H. Cerebrospinal fluid and human immunodeficiency virus: Findings in healthy, asymptomatic, seropositive men. Arch Intern Med. 1990;150:1538-1540.
272. Pratt RD, Nichols S, McKinney N, et al. Virologic markers of human immunodeficiency virus type 1 in cerebrospinal fluid of infected children. J Infect Dis. 1996;174:288-293.
273. Conrad AJ, Schmid P, Syndulko K, et al. Quantifying HIV-1 RNA using the polymerase chain reaction on cerebrospinal fluid and serum of seropositive individuals with and without neurologic abnormalities. J Acquir Immune Defic Syndr. 1995;10:425-435.
274. Feigin RD, McCracken GH Jr, Klein JO. Diagnosis and management of meningitis. Pediatr Infect Dis J. 1992;11:785-814.
275. Kaplan SL. Clinical presentation, diagnosis, and prognostic factors of bacterial meningitis. Infect Dis Clin North Am. 1999;13:579-594.
276. Bonadio WA. The cerebrospinal fluid: Physiologic aspects and alterations associated with bacterial meningitis. Pediatr Infect Dis J. 1992;11:423-432.
277. Coll MT, Uriz MS, Pineda V, et al. Meningococcal meningitis with "normal" cerebrospinal fluid. J Infect. 1994;29:289-294.
278. Sivakmaran M. Meningococcal meningitis revisited: Normocellular CSF. Clin Pediatr (Phila). 1997;36:351-355.
279. Spanos A, Harrell FE Jr, Durack DT. Differential diagnosis of acute meningitis: An analysis of the predictive value of initial observation. JAMA. 1989;262:2700-2707.
280. McKinney WP, Heudebert GR, Harper SA, et al. Validation of a clinical prediction rule for the differential diagnosis of acute meningitis. J Gen Intern Med. 1994;9:8-12.
281. Genton B, Berger JP. Cerebrospinal fluid lactate in 78 cases of adult meningitis. Intensive Care Med. 1990;16:196-200.
282. Greenlee JE. Approach to diagnosis of meningitis: Cerebrospinal fluid evaluation. Infect Dis Clin North Am. 1990;4:583-597.
283. Gray LD, Fedorko DP. Laboratory diagnosis of bacterial meningitis. Clin Microbiol Rev. 1992;5:130-145.
284. Kanegaye JT, Soliemanzadeh P, Bradley JS. Lumbar puncture in pediatric bacterial meningitis: Defining the time interval for recovery of cerebrospinal fluid pathogens after parenteral antibiotic pretreatment. Pediatrics. 2001;108:1169-1174.
285. Hayden RT, Frenkel LD. More laboratory testing: Greater cost but not necessarily better. Pediatr Infect Dis J. 2000;19:290-292.
286. Tarafdar K, Rao S, Recco RA, Zaman MM. Lack of sensitivity of the latex agglutination test to detect bacterial antigen in the cerebrospinal fluid of patients with culture-negative meningitis. Clin Infect Dis. 2001;33:406-408.
287. Ni H, Knight AI, Cartwright K, et al. Polymerase chain reaction for diagnosis of meningococcal meningitis. Lancet. 1992;340:1432-1434.
288. Saravolatz LD, Manzor O, VanderVelde N, et al. Broad-range bacterial polymerase chain reaction for early detection of bacterial meningitis. Clin Infect Dis. 2003;36:40-45.

289. Singhi SC, Mohankumar D, Singhi PD, et al. Evaluation of polymerase chain reaction (PCR) for diagnosing *Haemophilus influenzae* b meningitis. Ann Trop Pediatr. 2002;22:347-353.

290. Kearns AM, Graham C, Burdess D, et al. Rapid real-time PCR for determination of penicillin susceptibility in pneumococcal meningitis, including culture-negative cases. J Clin Microbiol. 2002;40:682-684.

291. Sormunen P, Kallio MJT, Kilpi T, Peltola H. C-reactive protein is useful in distinguishing Gram stain-negative bacterial meningitis from viral meningitis in children. J Pediatr. 1999;134:725-729.

292. Viallon A, Zeni F, Lambert C, et al. High sensitivity and specificity of serum procalcitonin levels in adults with bacterial meningitis. Clin Infect Dis. 1999;28:1313-1316.

293. Schwarz S, Bertram M, Schwab S, et al. Serum procalcitonin levels in bacterial and abacterial meningitis. Crit Care Med. 2000;28:1828-1832.

294. Nathan BR, Scheld WM. The potential roles of C-reactive protein and procalcitonin concentrations in the serum and cerebrospinal fluid in the diagnosis of bacterial meningitis. Curr Clin Top Infect Dis. 2002;22:155-165.

295. Winkler F, Kastenbauer S, Yousry TA, et al. Discrepancies between brain CT imaging and severely raised intracranial pressure proven by ventriculostomy in adults with pneumococcal meningitis. J Neurol. 2002;249:1292-1297.

296. Friedland IR, Paris MM, Rinderknecht S, et al. Cranial computed tomographic scans have little impact on management of bacterial meningitis. Am J Dis Child. 1992;146:1484-1487.

297. Hart G. Syphilis tests in diagnostic and therapeutic decision making. Ann Intern Med. 1986;104:368-376.

298. Davis LE, Schmitt JW. Clinical significance of cerebrospinal fluid tests for neurosyphilis. Ann Neurol. 1989;25:50-55.

299. Noordhoek GT, Wolters EC, de Jonge MEJ, van Embden JDA. Detection by polymerase chain reaction of *Treponema pallidum* DNA in cerebrospinal fluid from neurosyphilis patients before and after antibiotic treatment. J Clin Microbiol. 1991;29:1976-1984.

300. Steere AC. Lyme disease. N Engl J Med. 1989;321:586-596.

301. Corpuz M, Hilton E, Lardis MP, et al. Problems in the use of serologic tests for the diagnosis of Lyme disease. Arch Intern Med. 1991;151:1837-1840.

302. American College of Physicians. Guidelines for laboratory evaluation in the diagnosis of Lyme disease. Ann Intern Med. 1997;127:1106-1108.

303. Tugwell P, Dennis DT, Weinstein A, et al. Laboratory evaluation in the diagnosis of Lyme disease. Ann Intern Med. 1997;127:1109-1123.

304. Keller TL, Halperin JJ, Whitman M. PCR detection of *Borrelia burgdorferi* DNA in cerebrospinal fluid of Lyme neuroborreliosis patients. Neurology. 1992;42:32-42.

305. Lebech AM, Hansen K. Detection of *Borrelia burgdorferi* DNA in urine samples and cerebrospinal fluid samples from patients with early and late Lyme neuroborreliosis by polymerase chain reaction. J Clin Microbiol. 1992;30:1646-1653.

306. Martinez AJ, Visvesvara GS. Laboratory diagnosis of pathogenic free-living amoebas: *Naegleria, Acanthamoeba* and *Leptomyxid*. Clin Lab Med. 1991;11:861-872.

307. Tunkel AR, Scheld WM. Acute bacterial meningitis. Lancet. 1995;346:1675-1680.

308. Aronin SI, Peduzzi P, Quagliarello VJ. Community-acquired bacterial meningitis: Risk stratification for adverse clinical outcome and effect of antibiotic timing. Ann Intern Med. 1998;129:862-869.

309. Miner JR, Heegaard W, Mapes A, Biros M. Presentation, time to antibiotics, and mortality of patients with bacterial meningitis at an urban county medical center. J Emerg Med. 2001;21:387-392.

310. Lu CH, Huang CR, Chang WN, et al. Community-acquired bacterial meningitis in adults: The epidemiology, timing of appropriate antimicrobial therapy, and prognostic factors. Clin Neurol Neurosurg. 2002;104:352-358.

311. Coant PN, Kornberg AE, Duffy LC, et al. Blood culture results as determinants in the organism identification of bacterial meningitis. Pediatr Emerg Care. 1992;8:200-205.

312. Hasbun R, Abrahams J, Jekel J, Quagliarello VJ. Computed tomography of the head before lumbar puncture in adults with suspected meningitis. N Engl J Med. 2001;345:1727-1733.

313. Lebel MH, Freij BJ, Syrogiannopoulos GA, et al. Dexamethasone therapy for bacterial meningitis: Results of two double-blind, placebo-controlled trials. N Engl J Med. 1988;319:964-971.

314. Lebel MH, Hoyt MJ, Waagner DC, et al. Magnetic resonance imaging and dexamethasone therapy for bacterial meningitis. Am J Dis Child. 1989;143:301-306.

315. Girgis NI, Farid Z, Mikhail IA, et al. Dexamethasone treatment for bacterial meningitis in children and adults. Pediatr Infect Dis J. 1989;8:848-851.

316. Odio CM, Faingezicht I, Paris M, et al. The beneficial effects of early dexamethasone administration in infants and children with bacterial meningitis. N Engl J Med. 1991;324:1525-1531.

317. Kennedy WA, Hoyt MJ, McCracken GH Jr. The role of corticosteroid therapy in children with pneumococcal meningitis. Am J Dis Child. 1991;145:1374-1378.

318. Schaad UB, Lips U, Gnehm HE, et al. Dexamethasone therapy for bacterial meningitis in children. Lancet. 1993;342:457-461.

319. King SM, Law B, Langley JM, Heurter H. Dexamethasone therapy for bacterial meningitis: Better never than late? Can J Infect Dis. 1994;5:1-7.

320. Wald ER, Kaplan SL, Mason EO Jr, et al. Dexamethasone therapy for children with bacterial meningitis. Pediatrics. 1995;95:21-28.

321. Kanra GY, Ozen H, Secmeer G, et al. The beneficial effects of dexamethasone in children with pneumococcal meningitis. Pediatr Infect Dis J. 1995;14:490-494.

322. Kilpi T, Peltola H, Jauhiainen T, et al. Oral glycerol and intravenous dexamethasone in preventing neurologic and audiologic sequelae of childhood bacterial meningitis. Pediatr Infect Dis J. 1995;14:270-278.

323. Macaluso A, Pivetta S, Maggi RS, et al. Dexamethasone adjunctive therapy for bacterial meningitis in children: A retrospective study in Brazil. Ann Trop Paediatr. 1996;16:193-198.

324. Qazi SA, Khan MA, Mughal N, et al. Dexamethasone and bacterial meningitis in Pakistan. Arch Dis Child. 1996;75:482-488.

325. Arditi M, Mason EO Jr, Bradley JS, et al. Three-year multicenter surveillance of pneumococcal meningitis in children: Clinical characteristics, and outcome related to penicillin susceptibility and dexamethasone use. Pediatrics. 1998;102:1087-1097.

326. Daoud AS, Batieha A, Al-Sheyyab M, et al. Lack of effectiveness of dexamethasone in neonatal bacterial meningitis. Eur J Pediatr. 1999;158:230-233.

327. Thomas R, Le Tulzo Y, Bouget J, et al. Trial of dexamethasone treatment for severe bacterial meningitis in adults. Intensive Care Med. 1999;25:475-480.

328. Gijwani D, Kumhar MR, Singh VB, et al. Dexamethasone therapy for bacterial meningitis in adults: A double blind placebo control study. Neurol India. 2002;50:63-67.

329. Ahsan T, Shahid M, Mahmood T, et al. Role of dexamethasone in acute bacterial meningitis in adults. J Pak Med Assoc. 2002;52:233-239.

330. Molyneux EM, Walsh AL, Forsyth H, et al. Dexamethasone treatment in childhood bacterial meningitis in Malawi: A randomized controlled trial. Lancet. 2002;360:211-218.

331. de Gans J, van de Beek D. Dexamethasone in adults with bacterial meningitis. N Engl J Med. 2002;347:1549-1556.

332. McIntyre PB, Berkey CS, King SM, et al. Dexamethasone as adjunctive therapy in bacterial meningitis: A meta-analysis of randomized clinical trials since 1988. JAMA. 1997;278:925-931.

333. McCracken GH Jr. Rich nations, poor nations, and bacterial meningitis. Lancet. 2002;360:183.

334. Tunkel AR, Scheld WM. Corticosteroids for everyone with meningitis? N Engl J Med. 2002;347:1613-1615.

335. Paris MM, Hickey SM, Uscher MI, et al. Effect of dexamethasone on therapy of experimental penicillin- and cephalosporin-resistant pneumococcal meningitis. Antimicrob Agents Chemother. 1994;38:1320-1324.

336. Cabellos C, Martinez-Lacasa J, Martox A, et al. Influence of dexamethasone on efficacy of ceftriaxone and vancomycin therapy in experimental pneumococcal meningitis. Antimicrob Agents Chemother. 1995;39:2158-2160.

337. Klugman KP, Friedland IR, Bradley JS. Bactericidal activity against cephalosporin-resistant *Streptococcus pneumoniae* in cerebrospinal fluid of children with acute bacterial meningitis. Antimicrob Agents Chemother. 1995;39:1988-1992.

338. Gaillard JL, Abadie V, Cheron G, et al. Concentrations of ceftriaxone in cerebrospinal fluid of children with meningitis receiving adjunctive dexamethasone therapy. Antimicrob Agents Chemother. 1994;38:1209-1210.

339. Buke AC, Cavusoglu C, Karasulu E, Karakartal G. Does dexamethasone affect ceftriaxone penetration into cerebrospinal fluid in adult bacterial meningitis? Int J Antimicrob Agents. 2003;21:452-456.

340. Cabellos C, Martinez-Lacasa J, Tubau F, et al. Evaluation of combined ceftriaxone and dexamethasone therapy in experimental cephalosporin-resistant pneumococcal meningitis. J Antimicrob Chemother. 2000;45:315-320.

341. Kaplan SL, Mason EO Jr. Management of infections due to antibiotic-resistant *Streptococcus pneumoniae*. Clin Microbiol Rev. 1998;11:628-644.

342. Kaplan SL. Management of pneumococcal meningitis. Pediatr Infect Dis J. 2002;21:589-591.

343. Rotbart HA, Webster AD. Treatment of potentially life-threatening enterovirus infections with pleconaril. Clin Infect Dis. 2001;32:228-235.

344. Abzug MJ, Cloud G, Bradley J, et al. Double blind placebo-controlled trial of pleconaril in infants with enterovirus meningitis. Pediatr Infect Dis J. 2003;22:335-340.

345. Lebel MH, McCracken GH Jr. Delayed cerebrospinal fluid sterilization and adverse outcome of bacterial meningitis in infants and children. Pediatrics. 1989;83:161-167.

346. Lustar I, McCracken GH Jr. Antibiotic pharmacodynamics in cerebrospinal fluid. Clin Infect Dis. 1998;27:1117-1129.

347. Andes DR, Craig WA. Pharmacokinetics and pharmacodynamics of antibiotics in meningitis. Infect Dis Clin North Am. 1999;13:595-618.

348. Casagrande ST, Landgraf IM, Kobata AM, et al. Antimicrobial resistance among invasive *Haemophilus influenzae* strains: Results of a Brazilian study carried out from 1996 through 2000. Braz J Med Biol Res. 2002;35:1293-1300.

349. Duke T, Michael A, Mokela D, et al. Chloramphenicol or ceftriaxone, or both, as treatment for meningitis in developing countries? Arch Dis Child. 2003;88:536-539.

350. Peltola J, Anttila M, Renkonen OV, The Finnish Study Group. Randomised comparison of chloramphenicol, ampicillin, cefotaxime, and ceftriaxone for childhood bacterial meningitis. Lancet. 1989;1:1281-1287.

351. Schaad UB, Suter S, Gianella-Borradori A, et al. A comparison of ceftriaxone and cefuroxime for the treatment of bacterial meningitis in children. N Engl J Med. 1990;322:141-147.

352. Saez-Llorens X, O'Ryan M. Cefepime in the empiric treatment of meningitis in children. Pediatr Infect Dis J. 2001;20:356-361.

353. Saez-Llorens X, Castano E, Garcia R, et al. Prospective randomized comparison of cefepime and cefotaxime for treatment of bacterial meningitis in infants and children. Antimicrob Agents Chemother. 1995;39:937-940.

354. Saez-Nieto JA, Lujan R, Berron S, et al. Epidemiology and molecular basis of penicillin-resistant *Neisseria meningitidis* in Spain: A 5-year history (1985-1989). Clin Infect Dis. 1992;14:394-402.

355. van Deuren M, Brandtzaeg P, van der Meer JWM. Update on meningococcal disease with emphasis on pathogenesis and clinical management. Clin Microbiol Rev. 2000;13:144-166.

356. Boras A, Bozinovic D, Tenover FC, Popovic T. First report of *Neisseria meningitidis* intermediately resistant to penicillin in Croatia. J Clin Microbiol. 2001;39:823.

357. Punar M, Eraksoy H, Cagatay AA, et al. *Neisseria meningitidis* with decreased susceptibility to penicillin in Istanbul, Turkey. Scand J Infect Dis. 2002;34:11-13.

358. Oppenheim BA. Antibiotic resistance in *Neisseria meningitidis*. Clin Infect Dis. 1997;24(Suppl 1):S98-S101.
359. Galimand M, Gerbaud G, Guibourdenche M, et al. High-level chloramphenicol resistance in *Neisseria meningitidis*. N Engl J Med. 1998;339:868-874.
360. Jackson LA, Tenover FC, Baker C, et al. Prevalence of *Neisseria meningitidis* relatively resistant to penicillin in the United States, 1991. J Infect Dis. 1994;169:438-441.
361. Buck GE, Adams M. *Meningococcus* with reduced susceptibility to penicillin isolated in the United States. Pediatr Infect Dis J. 1994;13:156-157.
362. Woods CR, Smith AL, Wasilauskas BL, et al. Invasive disease caused by *Neisseria meningitidis* relatively resistant to penicillin in North Carolina. J Infect Dis. 1994;170:453-456.
363. Rosenstein NE, Stocker SA, Popovic T, et al. Antimicrobial resistance of *Neisseria meningitidis* in the United States, 1997. Clin Infect Dis. 2000;30:212-213.
364. Casado-Flores J, Osona B, Comingo P, Barquet N. Meningococcal meningitis during penicillin therapy for meningococcemia. Clin Infect Dis. 1997;25:1479.
365. Goldani LZ. Inducement of *Neisseria meningitidis* resistance to ampicillin and penicillin in a patient with meningococcemia treated with high doses of ampicillin. Clin Infect Dis. 1998;26:772.
366. Cubells CL, Garcia JJG, Martinez JR, Otin CL. Clinical data in children with meningococcal meningitis in a Spanish hospital. Acta Paediatr. 1997;86:26-29.
367. Hopkins S, Williams D, Dunne M, et al. A randomized, controlled trial of oral or IV trovafloxacin vs. ceftriaxone in the treatment of epidemic meningococcal meningitis. In: Program and Abstracts of the 36th Interscience Conference on Antimicrobial Agents and Chemotherapy. Washington, DC: American Society for Microbiology; 1996.
368. Tunkel AR, Scheld WM. Treatment of bacterial meningitis. Curr Infect Dis Rep. 2002;4:7-16.
369. Appelbaum PC. Resistance among *Streptococcus pneumoniae:* Implications for drug selection. Clin Infect Dis. 2002;34:1613-1620.
370. Friedland IR, Klugman KP. Failure of chloramphenicol therapy in penicillin-resistant pneumococcal meningitis. Lancet. 1992;339:405-408.
371. Viladrich PF, Gudiol F, Linares J, et al. Evaluation of vancomycin for therapy of adult pneumococcal meningitis. Antimicrob Agents Chemother. 1991;35:2467-2472.
372. Novak R, Henriques B, Charpentier E, et al. Emergence of vancomycin tolerance in *Streptococcus pneumoniae*. Nature. 1999;399:590-593.
373. Gilmore MS, Hoch JA. A vancomycin surprise. Nature. 1999;399:524-527.
374. McCullers JA, English BK, Novak R. Isolation and characterization of vancomycin-tolerant *Streptococcus pneumoniae* from the cerebrospinal fluid of a patient who developed recrudescent meningitis. J Infect Dis. 2000;181:369-373.
375. Ahmed A. A critical evaluation of vancomycin for treatment of bacterial meningitis. Pediatr Infect Dis J. 1997;16:895-903.
376. Bradley JS, Scheld WM. The challenge of penicillin-resistant *Streptococcus pneumoniae* meningitis: Current antibiotic therapy in the 1990s. Clin Infect Dis. 1997;24 (Suppl 2):S213-S221.
377. John CC, Aouad G, Berman B, Schreiber JR. Successful meropenem treatment of multiply resistant pneumococcal meningitis. Pediatr Infect Dis J. 1997;16:1009-1011.
378. Odio CM, Puig JR, Feris JM, et al. Prospective, randomized, investigator-blinded study of the efficacy and safety of meropenem vs. cefotaxime therapy in bacterial meningitis in children. Pediatr Infect Dis J. 1999;18:581-590.
379. Cottagnoud P, Tuber MG. Fluoroquinolones in the treatment of meningitis. Curr Infect Dis Rep. 2003;5:329-336.
380. Saez-Llorens X, McCoig C, Feris JM, et al. Quinolone treatment for pediatric bacterial meningitis: A comparative study of trovafloxacin and ceftriaxone with or without vancomycin. Pediatr Infect Dis J. 2002;21:14-22.
381. Tunkel AR, Scheld WM. Treatment of meningitis and other central nervous system infections. In: Hooper DC, Rubinstein E, eds. Quinolone Antimicrobial Agents. 3rd ed. Washington, DC: American Society for Microbiology; 2003.
382. Chen DK, McGeer A, de Azavedo JC, et al. Decreased susceptibility of *Streptococcus pneumoniae* to fluoroquinolones in Canada. N Engl J Med. 1999;341:233-239.
383. Urban C, Rahman N, Zhao X, et al. Fluoroquinolone-resistant *Streptococcus pneumoniae* associated with levofloxacin therapy. Clin Infect Dis. 2001;184:794-798.
384. Wortmann GW, Bennett SP. Fatal meningitis due to levofloxacin-resistant *Streptococcus pneumoniae*. Clin Infect Dis. 1999;29:1599-1600.
385. Fong IW, Tomkins KB. Review of *Pseudomonas aeruginosa* meningitis with special emphasis on treatment with ceftazidime. Rev Infect Dis. 1985;7:604-612.
386. Rodriguez WJ, Khan WN, Cocchetto DM, et al. Treatment of *Pseudomonas* meningitis with ceftazidime with or without concurrent therapy. Pediatr Infect Dis J. 1990;9:83-87.
387. Rousseau JM, Soullie B, Villevielle T, Koeck JT. Efficacy of cefepime in postoperative meningitis attributable to *Enterobacter aerogenes*. J Trauma. 2001;50:971.
388. Jimenez-Mejias ME, Pichardo-Guerrero C, Marquez-Rivas FJ, et al. Cerebrospinal fluid penetration and pharmacokinetic/pharmacodynamic parameters of intravenously administered colistin in a case of multidrug-resistant *Acinetobacter baumannii* meningitis. Eur J Clin Microbiol Infect Dis. 2002;21:212-214.
389. Vasan N, Desmery P, Ilutovich S, et al. Intrathecal use of colistin. J Clin Microbiol. 2000;38:3523.
390. Kremery V Jr, Filka J, Uher J, et al. Ciprofloxacin in treatment of nosocomial meningitis in neonates and in infants: Report of 12 cases and review. Diagn Microbiol Infect Dis. 1999;35:75-80.
391. Lipman J, Allworth A, Walis SC. Cerebrospinal penetration of high doses of intravenous ciprofloxacin in meningitis. Clin Infect Dis. 2000;31:1131-1133.
392. Lo WT, Wang CC, Lee CM, Chu ML. Successful treatment of multi-resistant *Stenotrophomonas maltophilia* meningitis with ciprofloxacin in a pre-term infant. Eur J Pediatr. 2002;161:680-682.
393. Chang WN, Lu CH, Wu JJ, et al. *Staphylococcus aureus* meningitis in adults: A clinical comparison of infections caused by methicillin-resistant and methicillin-sensitive strains. Infection. 2001;29:245-250.
394. Owusu-Ofori A, Scheld WM. Treatment of *Salmonella* meningitis: Two case reports and review of the literature. Int J Infect Dis. 2003;7:53-57.
395. Zeana C, Kubin CJ, Della-Latta P, Hammer SM. Vancomycin-resistant *Enterococcus faecium* meningitis successfully managed with linezolid: Case report and review of the literature. Clin Infect Dis. 2001;33:477-482.
396. Shaikj ZHA, Peloquin CA, Ericsson CD. Successful treatment of vancomycin-resistant *Enterococcus faecium* meningitis with linezolid: Case report and literature review. Scand J Infect Dis. 2001;33:375-379.
397. Hachem R, Afif C, Gokaslan Z, Raad I. Successful treatment of vancomycin-resistant *Enterococcus* meningitis with linezolid. Eur J Clin Microbiol Infect Dis. 2001;20:432-434.
398. Steinmetz MP, Vogelbaum MA, De Georgia MA, et al. Successful treatment of vancomycin-resistant *Enterococcus* meningitis with linezolid: Case report and review of the literature. Crit Care Med. 2001;29:2383-2385.
399. Radetsky M. Duration of treatment in bacterial meningitis: A historical inquiry. Pediatr Infect Dis J. 1990;9:2-9.
400. Roine I, Ledermann W, Foncea ML, et al. Randomized trial of four vs. seven days of ceftriaxone treatment for bacterial meningitis in children with rapid initial recovery. Pediatr Infect Dis J. 2000;19:219-222.
401. Singhi P, Kaushal M, Singhi S, Ray P. Seven days vs. 10 days ceftriaxone therapy in bacterial meningitis. J Trop Pediatr. 2002;48:273-279.
402. Tice AC, Strait K, Ramey R, et al. Outpatient parenteral antimicrobial therapy for central nervous system infections. Clin Infect Dis. 1999;29:1394-1399.
403. Marra CM, Slatter V, Tartaglione TA, et al. Evaluation of aqueous penicillin G and ceftriaxone for experimental neurosyphilis. J Infect Dis. 1991;165:396-397.
404. Dowell ME, Ross PG, Musher DM, et al. Response of latent syphilis or neurosyphilis to ceftriaxone therapy in persons infected with human immunodeficiency virus. Am J Med. 1992;93:481-488.
405. Hook EW III. Management of syphilis in human immunodeficiency virus-infected patients. Am J Med. 1992;93:477-479.
406. Wormser GP, Nadelman RB, Dattwyler RJ, et al. Practice guidelines for the treatment of Lyme disease. Clin Infect Dis. 2000;13:S1-14.
407. Kohlhepp W, Oschmann P, Mertens HG. Treatment of Lyme borreliosis: Randomized comparison of doxycycline and penicillin G. J Neurol. 1989;236:464-469.
408. Karlsson M, Hammers-Berggren S, Lindquist L, et al. Comparison of intravenous penicillin G and oral doxycycline for treatment of Lyme neuroborreliosis. Neurology. 1994;44:1203-1207.
409. Dattwyler RJ, Halperin JJ, Volkman DJ, et al. Treatment of late Lyme borreliosis: Randomised comparison of ceftriaxone and penicillin. Lancet. 1988;1:1191-1194.
410. Dotevall L, Hagberg L. Penetration of doxycycline into cerebrospinal fluid in patients treated for suspected Lyme neuroborreliosis. Antimicrob Agents Chemother. 1989;33:1078-1080.
411. Sischel JS, Harmatz P, Visvesvara GS, et al. Successful treatment of primary amebic meningoencephalitis. N Engl J Med. 1982;306:346-348.
412. Brown RL. Successful treatment of primary amebic meningoencephalitis. Arch Intern Med. 1991;151:1201-1202.
413. Jain R, Prabhakar S, Modi M, et al. *Naegleria* meningitis: A rare survival. Neurol India. 2002;50:470-472.
414. Abzug MJ, Keyserling HL, Lee ML, et al. Neonatal enterovirus infection: Virology, serology, and effects of intravenous immune globulin. Clin Infect Dis. 1995;20:1201-1206.
415. Saez-Llorens X, Ramilo O, Mustafa MM, et al. Pentoxifylline modulates meningeal inflammation in experimental bacterial meningitis. Antimicrob Agents Chemother. 1990;34:837-843.
416. Burroughs MH, Tsenova-Berkova L, Sokol K, et al. Effect of thalidomide on the inflammatory response in cerebrospinal fluid in experimental bacterial meningitis. Microb Pathog. 1995;19:245-255.
417. Saez-Llorens X, Jafari HS, Severien C, et al. Enhanced attenuation of meningeal inflammation and brain edema by concomitant administration of anti-CD18 monoclonal antibodies and dexamethasone in experimental *Haemophilus* meningitis. J Clin Invest. 1991;88:2003-2011.
418. Kartalija M, Kim Y, White ML, et al. Effect of recombinant N-terminal fragment of bactericidal/permeability-increasing protein (rBPI$_{23}$) on cerebrospinal fluid inflammation induced by endotoxin. J Infect Dis. 1995;171:948-953.
419. Lyons MK, Meyer FB. Cerebrospinal fluid physiology and the management of increased intracranial pressure. Mayo Clin Proc. 1990;65:684-707.
420. Ashwal S, Stringer W, Tomasi L, et al. Cerebral blood flow and carbon dioxide reactivity in children with bacterial meningitis. J Pediatr. 1990;117:523-530.
421. Chotmongkol V, Sawanyawisuth K, Thavornpitak Y. Corticosteroid treatment of eosinophilic meningitis. Clin Infect Dis. 2000;31:660-662.
422. Imrey PB, Jackson LA, Ludwinski PH, et al. Meningococcal carriage, alcohol consumption, and campus bar patronage in a serogroup C meningococcal disease outbreak. Antimicrob Agents Chemother. 1995;33:3133-3137.
423. Cookson ST, Corrales JL, Lotero JO, et al. Disco fever: Epidemic meningococcal disease in northeastern Argentina associated with disco patronage. J Infect Dis. 1998;178:266-269.
424. Koh YM, Barnes GH, Kaczmarski E, Stuart JM. Outbreak of meningococcal disease linked to a sports club. Lancet. 1998;352:706-707.

425. Centers for Disease Control and Prevention. Control and prevention of meningococcal disease and control and prevention of serogroup C meningococcal disease: Evaluation and management of suspected outbreaks. MMWR Morb Mortal Wkly Rep. 1997;46(RR-5):1-11.

426. Schwartz B, Al-Tobaiqi A, Al-Ruwais A, et al. Comparative efficacy of ceftriaxone and rifampicin in eradicating pharyngeal carriage of group A *Neisseria meningitidis.* Lancet. 1988;1:1239-1242.

427. Girgis N, Sultan Y, Frenck RW Jr, et al. Azithromycin compared with rifampin for eradication of nasopharyngeal colonization by *Neisseria meningitidis.* Pediatr Infect Dis J. 1998;17:816-819.

428. Rauch AM, O'Ryan M, Van R, et al. Invasive disease due to multiply resistant *Streptococcus pneumoniae* in a Houston, Tex, day-care center. Am J Dis Child. 1990;144:923-927.

429. Centers for Disease Control and Prevention. Prevention of pneumococcal disease: Recommendations of the Advisory Committee on Immunization Practices (ACIP). MMWR Morb Mortal Wkly Rep. 1997;46(RR-8):1-23.

430. Zangwill KM, Schuchat A, Wenger JD, Group B Streptococcal Disease Study Group. Group B streptococcal disease in the United States, 1990: Report from a multistate active surveillance system. MMWR Morb Mortal Wkly Rep. 1992;41:25-32.

431. Centers for Disease Control and Prevention. Prevention of perinatal group B streptococcal disease: A public health perspective. MMWR Morb Mortal Wkly Rep. 1996;45(RR-7):1-24.

432. Schuchat A. Group B streptococcus. Lancet. 1999;353:51-56.

433. Villalobos T, Arango C, Kubilis P, Rathore M. Antibiotic prophylaxis after basilar skull fracture. Clin Infect Dis. 1998;27:364-369.

434. American Academy of Pediatrics, Committee on Infectious Diseases. Recommended childhood immunization schedule—United States, January-December 2002. Pediatrics. 2002;109:162.

435. Ribeiro GS, Reis JN, Cordeiro SM, et al. Prevention of *Haemophilus influenzae* type B (Hib) meningitis and emergence of serotype replacement with type A strains after introduction of Hib immunization in Brazil. J Infect Dis. 2003;187:109-116.

436. Garner J, Weston V. Effectiveness of vaccination for *Haemophilus influenzae* type B. Lancet. 2003;361:395-437.

437. Steinhoff M, Goldblatt D. Conjugate Hib vaccines. Lancet. 2003;361:360-361.

438. Jodar L, Feavers IM, Salisbury D, Granoff DM. Development of vaccines against meningococcal disease. Lancet. 2002;359:1499-1508.

439. Wildes SS, Tunkel AR. Meningococcal vaccines: A progress report. Biodrugs. 2002;16:321-329.

440. Memish ZA. Meningococcal disease and travel. Clin Infect Dis. 2002;34:84-90.

441. Brundage JF, Ryan MAK, Feighner BH, Erdtmann FJ. Meningococcal disease among United States military service members in relation to routine use of vaccines with different serogroup-specific components, 1964-1998. Clin Infect Dis. 2002;35:1376-1381.

442. Harrison LH. Preventing meningococcal infection in college students. Clin Infect Dis. 2000;30:648-651.

443. American Academy of Pediatrics, Committee on Infectious Diseases. Meningococcal disease prevention and control strategies for practice-based physicians (addendum: recommendations for college students). Pediatrics. 2000;106:1500-1504.

444. Ramsay MA, Andrews N, Kaczmarski EB, et al. Efficacy of meningococcal serogroup C conjugate vaccine in teenagers and toddlers in England. Lancet. 2001;357:195-196.

445. Miller E, Salisbury D, Ramsay M. Planning, registration, and implementation of an immunization campaign against meningococcal serogroup C disease in the UK: A success story. Vaccine. 2001;20:S58-67.

446. Bose A, Coen P, Tully J, et al. Effectiveness of meningococcal C conjugate vaccine in teenagers in England. Lancet. 2003;361:675-676.

447. Maiden MCJ, Stuart JM. Carriage of serogroup C meningococci 1 year after meningococcal C conjugate polysaccharide vaccination. Lancet. 2002;359:1829-1830.

448. Black S, Shinefield H, Fireman B, et al. Efficacy, safety and immunogenicity of heptavalent pneumococcal conjugate vaccine in children. Pediatr Infect Dis J. 2000;19:187-195.

449. Lieu TA, Ray GT, Black SB, et al. Projected cost-effectiveness of pneumococcal conjugate vaccination of healthy infants and young children. JAMA. 2000;283:1460-1468.

450. American Academy of Pediatrics, Committee on Infectious Diseases. Policy statement: Recommendations for the prevention of pneumococcal infections, including use of pneumococcal conjugate vaccine (Prevnar), pneumococcal polysaccharide vaccine, and antibiotic prophylaxis. Pediatrics. 2000;106:362-366.

451. Dagan R, Givon-Lavi N, Zamir O, et al. Reduction of nasopharyngeal carriage of *Streptococcus pneumoniae* after administration of a 9-valent pneumococcal conjugate vaccine to toddlers attending day care centers. J Infect Dis. 2002;185:927-936.

452. Whitney CG, Farley MM, Hadler J, et al. Decline in invasive pneumococcal disease after the introduction of protein-polysaccharide conjugate vaccine. N Engl J Med. 2003;348:1737-1746.

453. Hausdorff WP, Bryant J, Paradiso PR, et al. Which pneumococcal serogroups cause the most invasive disease: Implication for conjugate vaccine formulation and use, part I. Clin Infect Dis. 2000;30:100-121.

454. Hausdorff WP, Bryant J, Kloek C, et al. The contribution of specific pneumococcal serogroups to different disease manifestations: Implications for conjugate vaccine formulation and use, part II. Clin Infect Dis. 2000;30:122-140.

455. Brandileone MCC, de Andrade ALSG, Di Fabio JL, et al. Appropriateness of a pneumococcal conjugate vaccine in Brazil: Potential impact of age and clinical diagnosis, with emphasis on meningitis. J Infect Dis. 2003;187:1206-1212.

CHAPTER 81

Cerebrospinal Fluid Shunt Infections

ALLAN R. TUNKEL

BRUCE A. KAUFMAN

In the United States hydrocephalus accounts for approximately 70,000 annual hospital admissions.[1] In patients with hydrocephalus, effective treatment includes the diversion of cerebrospinal fluid (CSF) to another part of the body for absorption, a process known as shunting.[2,3] The typical CSF shunt has a proximal portion that enters the CSF space, and a distal portion that is internalized and terminates in either the peritoneal, pleural, or vascular space; or one that is externalized from the patient (for temporary use). The proximal portion of the system usually consists of a catheter inserted into one of the cerebral ventricles, an intracranial cyst, or into the lumbar subarachnoid space. Most neurosurgeons prefer the peritoneal cavity as the shunt terminus (that is, a ventriculoperitoneal [VP] shunt) over shunts that terminate in the vascular space (ventriculoatrial [VA] shunt) because VP shunts require fewer revisions, are easier to place and revise, and have fewer serious complications.[4] Part of the system (as a separate component) is a pressure-regulating valve that is usually placed just outside the skull or as an integral part of the distal tubing. Reservoirs for intermittent percutaneous access can also be added to the system or incorporated into the valve assembly. Additional hardware includes antisiphon valves and various connectors, allowing interconnection of more than one catheter or device.

Externalized devices are most commonly used to treat infected CSF shunts (see later), for intracranial pressure (ICP) monitoring, or for temporary diversion of the CSF from an obstructed ventricular system (an external ventriculostomy).[4,5] Temporary intraventricular catheters are particularly useful for the management of patients with elevated ICP secondary to acute hydrocephalus caused by subarachnoid hemorrhage, intracranial hemorrhage, intraventricular hemorrhage, and neoplasms obstructing the CSF circulation.

The placement of internalized and externalized devices for drainage of CSF may be associated with an increased risk of infection, leading to a permanent adverse outcome. In the following sections we review the epidemiology and etiology, clinical features, and management approach to CSF shunt infections.

EPIDEMIOLOGY AND ETIOLOGY

The case incidence of CSF shunt infection (i.e., the occurrence of infection in any given patient) has ranged from 5% to 41% in various series,[4] although the incidence is usually in the range of 5% to 15%.[6-11] The operative incidence (i.e., the occurrence of infection per procedure) has ranged from 2.8% to 14%,[4] although more recent series have reported operative infection rates of less than 4%.[12-14] A number of factors have been reported to be associated with an increased risk of CSF shunt infection (Table 81-1). A higher case incidence rate may be related to the infection rate with succeeding shunt revisions[15]; infection may be especially high in those undergoing three or more revisions,[16] although that has not been observed in all studies.[9] In patients undergoing revision after treatment for an infected CSF shunt, the operative incidence of infection is considerably higher (12%-20%)[4]; the same microorganism has been cultured at least 50% of the time, suggesting that the initial infection was not adequately treated. Premature birth, previous shunt infection, and intraoperative use of the neuroendoscope were identified as independent risk factors in a recent study of patients with VP shunt infections.[17]

TABLE 81-1 Factors Associated with an Increased Risk of Cerebrospinal Fluid Shunt (CSF) Infection*

Premature birth
Previous shunt infection
Experience of the neurosurgeon
Number of people traversing the operating theater
Intraoperative use of the neuroendoscope
Length of the shunt procedure
Insertion of catheter below T7 in ventriculoatrial shunting†
Patient skin preparation
Shaving of skin
Exposure of large areas of patient's skin during the procedure
Shunt revision‡

*Not all studies have found all of these factors to be associated with an increased risk of CSF shunt infection.
†Presence of foreign-body irritation on the tricuspid valve, with thrombus formation and subsequent infection during bacteremia.
‡The risk may be especially high in patients undergoing three or more revisions.

In patients with externalized devices, infectious complications have ranged from zero to 22%, although most are in the range of 5% to 10%.[4,5] Factors associated with an increased risk of infection are intraventricular hemorrhage, subarachnoid hemorrhage, cranial fracture with CSF leak, catheter irrigation, craniotomy, and duration of catheterization. Although there is controversy regarding the relationship between the duration of catheterization and risk of infection, most studies consider extended catheter duration to be an important risk factor for subsequent infection.[5]

The etiologic agents identified in CSF shunt infections are shown in Table 81-2.[4] Staphylococcal species account for more than two thirds of CSF shunt infections, with *Staphylococcus epidermidis* most frequently isolated (47%-64% of infections), followed by *Staphylococcus aureus* (12%-29% of infections). The most common isolated gram-negative species are *Escherichia coli*, *Klebsiella*, *Proteus*, and *Pseudomonas*; cases of nosocomial *Acinetobacter* meningitis have also been reported in patients with VP shunts.[18-20] The usual etiologic agents of community-acquired bacterial meningitis (i.e., *Haemophilus influenze*, *Streptococcus pneumoniae*, and *Neisseria meningitidis*) are only isolated in about 5% of CSF shunt infections. In 10% to 15% of cases, more than one microorganism is isolated, usually including a staphylococcus or *E. coli*. In recent years an increasing prevalence of diphtheroids (including *Propionibacterium acnes*) have been found in CSF shunt infections, isolated in up to 50% of cases in one series.[21] However, it may be that the incidence is not increasing, but rather that the diagnosis was not made because isolation of these organisms was not considered to be significant, or inadequate culture techniques were utilized.[22] Fungal shunt infections are rare, although the frequency of *Candida* shunt infections has increased in recent years (range of 6%-17% in one review).[23] Fungal shunt infections may be seen in patients receiving broad-spectrum antimicrobial therapy, corticosteroids, hyperalimentation, and in those with indwelling intravascular catheters or who are immunocompromised. A previous ventricular shunt may also increase the risk of subsequent *Candida* meningitis.[24]

TABLE 81-2 Bacterial Etiologic Agents in Cerebrospinal Fluid Shunt Infections.

Etiologic Agent	Incidence (%)
Staphylococci*	65-85
Gram-negative bacteria	6-20
Streptococci	8-10
Corynebacteria	1-14
Anaerobes	6
Mixed cultures	10-15

*The majority are caused by coagulase-negative staphylococci.

Different microorganisms may be isolated depending on the type of shunt. Shunts terminating in the peritoneal cavity may have a greater risk of infection with gram-negative organisms[15,25]; mixed infections may be seen when the catheter has perforated a hollow viscus.[26-28] Although some investigators have found an increased prevalence of gram-negative shunt infections in patients with a peritoneal termination,[29] others have found no difference in the bacterial spectrum in those with VP or VA shunts.[30] Lumboperitoneal shunts have similar distributions of infecting organisms to those originating in the ventricles.[29,30] Gram-positive cocci account for the majority of cases of meningitis associated with external drains, but infections caused by gram-negative bacilli, gram-positive bacilli, fungi, and antimicrobial-resistant bacteria have also been described.[5]

PATHOGENESIS AND PATHOPHYSIOLOGY

There are four mechanisms by which CSF shunts may become infected.[4] The first mechanism is retrograde infection from the distal end of the shunt. This mode is found frequently in patients with ureteral shunts,[30,31] with gram-negative organisms accounting for 35% of infections. Bowel perforation can also lead to distal catheter contamination. Retrograde infection is the most likely mechanism of infection of externalized devices[32]; microorganisms may enter the device by tracking from the exit site alongside the device, gaining access into the fluid column that drains CSF, or may be introduced from injection through the tubing to maintain tubular function.

The second mechanism is wound or skin breakdown overlying the shunt, which allows direct access of microorganisms to the shunt.[4] The infection may be surgically acquired (i.e., when the incision fails to heal), or because the patient scratches the open wound (often seen in infants and small children). In debilitated or immobile patients, a decubitus ulcer may develop over the shunt. Infection of tissues near the shunt site may also lead to direct inoculation of microorganisms. Accessing the shunt by needle puncture may inoculate skin microorganisms into the shunt.

A third mechanism is hematogenous seeding. Patients with venous shunts who have a foreign body in the vascular system are at continued risk of infection from bacteremia (with a retrograde infection). However, the susceptibility of nonvascular shunts to an infection that is spread hematogenously is less clear.

The final, and most frequent, mechanism is colonization of the shunt at the time of surgery.[4] This mechanism is suggested by the timing of most shunt infections (usually within several weeks of operation) and by the microorganisms that are isolated. At the time of implantation, direct exposure and handling of the shunt can allow bacterial contamination. However, in multiple studies utilizing surveillance culture techniques, less than 50% of the microorganisms cultured from the wound or infected shunt could be traced directly to the patient,[4,26,33] suggesting that there are other factors that affect colonization and subsequent CSF shunt infection.

There are no animal models that have specifically examined the role of CSF shunts in the initiation or propagation of central nervous system (CNS) infection. Characteristically, foreign body infections require a low-infecting organism inoculum to establish disease, evolve over a protracted course, do not spread beyond the vicinity of the foreign body, and require removal of the device for optimal management of the condition. A guinea pig model has been developed to study prosthetic device infections, which involves the subcutaneous implantation of a perforated polymer cylinder.[34] This tissue-cage model permits analysis of the natural history and pathogenicity of various microorganisms in foreign-body infections, testing of different prosthetic materials, study of bacterial adherence to foreign bodies, and elucidation of the local host defense mechanisms in the area of the foreign body. Although this model is somewhat artificial (because it does not perform any mechanical function), it is inexpensive, reproducible, and permits serial evaluation of the biologic characteristics of an individual infection. The following sections review the bacterial virulence factors and host defense mechanisms that are likely operable in CSF shunt infections.

Bacterial Virulence Factors

The vast majority of CSF shunt infections are caused by staphylococci that colonize the wound at the time of shunt placement.[30] These organisms can adhere directly to prosthetic material and produce substances that protect them from phagocytosis and the actions of antimicrobial agents.[35,36] Adherence is an important step in the pathogenesis of foreign-body infections, although the exact mechanism of invasion remains undefined. *S. epidermidis* strains may excavate into some polymer surfaces,[37] hydrolyzing the plastic as a food source. In addition, host proteins such as fibronectin and collagen may enhance staphylococcal adherence to foreign surfaces,[38,39] although strains of *S. epidermidis* adhere quite avidly even in the absence of these plasma proteins. Further study is needed to define the precise role of host-derived molecules in the pathogenesis of foreign-body infections.

Another mechanism of attachment may involve the production of an extracellular slime substance by these microorganisms. Slime is water soluble and contains 40% sugar and 27% protein, although this percentage may vary in different organisms.[36] Slime production by coagulase-negative staphylococci may be important in the pathogenesis of foreign-body infections,[40,41] and has been specifically examined in coagulase-negative staphylococci from patients with CSF shunt infections.[42,43] In one study[42] it was determined that 88% of CSF shunt isolates were adherent to plastic tissue-culture plates and that antimicrobial therapy was ineffective in patients with these adherent strains unless the colonized shunt was removed. Although all slime-producing strains were adherent, not all of the adherent strains produced slime. Slime production by other microorganisms (e.g., *Pseudomonas aeruginosa* and *Corynebacterium* spp.) may also contribute to virulence in foreign-body infections.[44,45] However, other factors undoubtedly play an important role in the pathogenesis of CSF shunt infections.

Host Defense Mechanisms

The persistence of CSF shunt infections probably relates not only to specific virulence factors but also to the inadequacy of host defense mechanisms in the CNS; the foreign body itself may also interfere with host defenses. In the tissue-cage model of foreign-body infections,[34] complement concentrations and opsonic titers are decreased relative to those in serum, with presumed impairment of efficient phagocytosis within the infected site. Granulocytes harvested from the tissue cage showed diminished phagocytic activity against *S. aureus* (strain Wood 46), manifested by a decreased ingestion rate, granular enzyme activity, and oxidative metabolism.[34,46] The explanation for this finding is unclear, although there is evidence that contact between neutrophils and foreign bodies can lead to increased release of lysosomal enzymes and oxygen free radicals that, in turn, cause leukocyte damage and inefficient phagocytosis and killing.[47] This resistance to phagocytosis may be related to the adherence of the organism to the foreign body,[48] or the shunt catheter itself may interfere with phagocytosis; neutrophils adhered poorly to the catheters, leading to inefficient ingestion of the bacteria despite qualitatively normal phagocytosis.[49]

Slime from coagulase-negative staphylococci may also protect organisms from host defenses by altering neutrophil function and interfering with the cellular immune system,[48,50,51] thereby impairing the inflammatory response and leading to persistence of disease. All of these findings support removal of an infected CSF shunt as an important adjunctive measure for optimal therapy in the eradication of this infection (see later).

CLINICAL FEATURES

The clinical features of CSF shunt infection can be quite variable and depend on the pathogenesis of infection, organism virulence, and type of shunt.[4,16,29,30,52] The most frequent symptoms are headache, nausea, lethargy, and change in mental status (seen in up to 65% of infected patients); these symptoms occur as a result of shunt malfunction secondary to the infection. Fever is reported in as little as 14% to as much as 92% of cases, so the absence of fever cannot exclude the possibility

of infection. Pain, often related to infection at the peritoneal or pleural endings of the shunt, may be absent in up to 60% of infections.

Symptoms and signs of a CSF shunt infection may be referable to either the proximal or distal portions of the shunt. Infection beginning in the proximal portion of the shunt (i.e., the catheter within the CSF space) results in meningitis or ventriculitis in about 30% of cases, and may cause shunt obstruction or decreased function.[4,15,30,52] However, meningeal symptoms should not be expected with infected ventricular shunts because communication between the infected ventricles and the CSF in contact with the meninges is usually absent; this may be because of the original reason for the shunting, or secondary to an aqueductal stenosis acquired after ventricular shunting in patients with communicating hydrocephalus. Rarely, intracranial empyemas and abscesses may occur secondary to a poorly treated infection, in the presence of retained hardware, or in patients with externalized monitors.

Symptoms of infection referable to the distal portion of the shunt are more specific to terminus location.[4,15] Infected vascular shunts lead to bacteremia, which may occur secondary to infected CSF directly entering the blood stream, from an infected thrombus at the end of the vascular catheter, or from true bacterial endocarditis. However, the clinical presentation of an infected vascular shunt is usually nonspecific, with fever and lethargy often seen. One unique complication of a chronic vascular shunt is shunt nephritis,[4,10,30,53,54] which is observed in 4% to 14% of patients. The majority of isolated bacteria in patients with shunt nephritis are usually coagulase-negative staphylococci, although diphtheroids and other pathogens have been isolated. The pathogenesis of shunt nephritis is similar to that of subacute bacterial endocarditis, with deposition of immunoglobulin M (IgM) and IgG antigen-antibody complexes in the renal glomeruli. The complement system is activated, with subsequent depletion of circulating complement factors C3 and C4. Failure to detect this condition can lead to permanent renal failure. Treatment usually, but not always, leads to resolution of the renal dysfunction.

Infected shunts that terminate in the pleural or peritoneal space may lead to an inflammatory response in the absorbing tissue (i.e., pleuritis or peritonitis).[4] In patients with infected VP shunts, symptoms of peritonitis appear as the peritoneal inflammation becomes more severe, in which patients develop fever, anorexia, and other signs and symptoms of an acute abdomen.[55,56] In the peritoneal cavity, host defense mechanisms attempt to limit the infection, often resulting in the encystment of the shunt catheter, fluid buildup within the cyst, and loculation of pockets of fluid within the abdomen. These fluid collections can grow quite large, because deposited CSF is not absorbed by the peritoneal cavity.

Some shunt infections, however, are insidious and cause few or no symptoms, perhaps only an intermittent low-grade fever or general malaise. The presentation may be that of an unexplained occlusion of an open-ended peritoneal catheter or failure of peritoneal CSF absorption. Therefore the clinician must consider the possibility of CSF shunt infection in these patients and institute an appropriate diagnostic workup (see later).

Patients with external devices can have infection of the wounds or infection of the proximal end, manifested as ventriculitis, meningitis, or (rarely) an abscess.[4,57,58] Wound infections are more frequent with external devices than CSF shunts. The change in mental status that occurs in patients who develop meningitis or ventriculitis, however, may be difficult to distinguish from the impaired level of consciousness that is a manifestation of the patient's underlying disease. Fever that occurs in these patients may also be from other sources of infection. It is important to carefully observe wounds and frequently culture CSF to diagnose the infections in patients with external CSF drainage devices.

DIAGNOSIS

The diagnosis of CSF shunt infections is established by direct culture of the shunt, or of fluid within or around the shunt.[4,21,30,31,52] To obtain fluid from a ventricular shunt, there must be a reservoir that can be tapped. These reservoirs are typically located in an easily accessible subcutaneous location. Following sterile preparation, the reservoir is percutaneously punctured. Introduction of infection is a possible risk of this procedure, and was reported to be as high as 12% in patients undergoing frequent, repeated aspirations.[59] In patients with infected ventricular shunts, sampling of the lumbar CSF may not reflect the state of the ventricular fluid or may not reveal the presence of an infection because the lumbar fluid is not in direct connection with the proximal portion of the shunt.

Once obtained, CSF should be sent for cell count with differential, chemistries (glucose and protein), Gram stain, and culture. High white blood cell (WBC) counts correlate with the presence of infection, but infection may be present even in patients with normal CSF WBC counts. CSF eosinophilia (>8% of differential count) has been associated with an indolent infection.[60] The cell count may be obscured by recent surgery that may have spilled blood into CSF, or the surgery may have caused an inflammatory reaction, so-called chemical meningitis. A negative CSF Gram stain does not exclude the likelihood of infection. CSF culture from the shunt is the most important test to establish the diagnosis of shunt infection; the culture will usually be positive in patients with an infected shunt even when there is no pleocytosis or alterations in CSF chemistries. CSF cultures may require several days to weeks of incubation before they can be called negative, or the results may be confounded in patients who have received prior antimicrobial therapy. Occasionally, shunts may be tapped for evaluation of function in patients with no clinical evidence of infection and may be found to be culture positive. In this situation, contamination may be responsible for the positive culture, but true infection must be strongly considered. The shunt should be retapped, and a positive culture with the same microorganism is usually indicative of true infection.

In patients with external ventricular drains (ventriculostomies), definite infection is defined as a positive CSF culture (obtained from the ventricular catheter or after lumbar puncture) associated with CSF pleocytosis and a paucity of clinical symptoms other than fever[5,57,61]; this progresses to ventriculitis when accompanied by high-grade fever and clinical signs of meningitis. A progressively declining CSF glucose and increasing CSF protein accompanied by advancing CSF pleocytosis, in the absence of positive CSF cultures or Gram stain, characterizes a suspected infection. A contaminating microorganism is defined as an isolated positive CSF culture and/or Gram stain with an expected CSF cell count, CSF glucose, and CSF protein; ventriculostomy colonization has a similar definition except that there are multiple positive CSF cultures and/or Gram stains and a lack of clinical symptoms (other than fever).

In patients with VA shunts, blood cultures should also be performed because bacteremia is invariably present in patients with infected VA shunts (positive blood cultures in more than 90% of cases).[4] This contrasts with infections in other types of CSF shunts, in which the incidence of negative blood cultures approaches 80%.[30,52]

The diagnosis of CSF shunt infection may be more difficult to establish when the distal portion of the VP shunt is infected.[4] The shunt tap may be normal with negative cultures if the patient has not yet developed a retrograde infection. VP shunts with distal occlusion, but no symptoms or signs of infection, should be investigated for possible infection at the time of revision, including Gram stain and culture of the distal tubing. Computed tomography (CT) scanning or ultrasound of the abdomen may identify CSF loculations at the shunt terminus. Although some free fluid in the pleural or peritoneal cavities is normal, it should not be confused with the larger volumes and cysts seen with infection at the shunt terminus.

Neuroimaging studies are not useful in identifying CSF shunt infection, but may show evidence of shunt malfunction. Rarely, a subdural empyema or brain abscess may be the first indication of a shunt infection.

TREATMENT

Numerous methods of treating CSF shunt infections have been reported, but no randomized, prospective studies have been performed.[4] The therapeutic approach to an infected CSF shunt must take into account the need for a functioning device during or after treatment. For example, in patients with noncommunicating hydrocephalus and persistent infection, an endoscopic third ventriculostomy may permit removal of the shunt and clearing of the infection.[62] Factors to be considered in the therapy of an infected CSF shunt include selection of antimicrobial therapy, timing of hardware removal, timing of shunt replacement, and duration of antimicrobial therapy; these therapeutic approaches, however, have not been standardized in published studies.

Antimicrobial Therapy

The principles of antimicrobial therapy for CSF shunt infections are generally the same as for acute bacterial meningitis (see Chapter 80)—the agent selected must penetrate the CNS and have bactericidal activity against the infecting pathogen. If CSF pleocytosis is present, antimicrobial therapy should be initiated before culture results are available. The most likely microorganisms associated with CSF shunt infection are coagulase-negative staphylococci (*S. epidermidis*), *S. aureus*, diphtheroids (including *P. acnes*), and gram-negative bacilli (including *P. aeruginosa*). Empirical therapy with vancomycin plus either cefepime, ceftazidime, or meropenem is appropriate, pending culture results and in vitro susceptibility testing of the isolated pathogen. The empirical choice to treat a presumptive gram-negative pathogen should be based on the local antimicrobial resistance patterns of these pathogens. If staphylococci are isolated and the organism is methicillin susceptible, therapy should be changed to either nafcillin or oxacillin; the addition of rifampin to an antistaphylococcal agent may augment treatment.[63] One patient with a *S. epidermidis* VP shunt infection was cured with shunt removal and intravenous linezolid,[64] although linezolid cannot be considered as first-line therapy for this infection. Recommended antimicrobial agents (based on isolated pathogen) and dosages of these agents for use in CNS infections in neonates, children, and adults are found in Chapter 80. Intravenous amphotericin B, often combined with 5-flucytosine, or fluconazole is recommended for *Candida* shunt infection.

Direct instillation of antimicrobial agents into the ventricles (i.e., through an external ventriculostomy or shunt reservoir) is occasionally necessary in patients with shunt infections that are difficult to eradicate or when the patient is unable to undergo the surgical components of therapy (see later),[4,65] although the indications for intraventricular administration are not well defined. No antimicrobial agent has been approved by the U.S Food and Drug Administration (FDA) for intraventricular use. The dosages of antimicrobial agents for intraventricular use have been determined empirically (Table 81-3), with adjustments of dose and dosing interval based on the ability of the agent to achieve adequate CSF concentrations.[66-69] Efficacy and tolerability of intraventricular drug are affected by continued drainage of the ventri-

TABLE 81-3 Antimicrobial Agents Administered by the Intraventricular Route*

Antimicrobial Agent	Daily Intraventricular Dose
Vancomycin	5-20 mg[†]
Gentamicin	1-8 mg
Tobramycin	5-20 mg
Amikacin	5-50 mg[‡]
Polymyxin B	5 mg[§]
Colistin	10 mg[‖]
Teicoplanin	5-40 mg[¶]
Quinupristin/dalfopristin	2-5 mg
Amphotericin B	0.1-0.5 mg[**]

*There are no specific data that define the exact dose of intraventricular antimicrobial agents that should be used in cerebrospinal fluid shunt infections; see text for details of specific studies.
[†]Most studies have used a 10- or 20-mg dose.
[‡]30 mg daily is the usual intraventricular dose.
[§]Dosage of 2 mg daily in children.
[‖]In one published trial,[75] patient received 5 mg on day 1 followed by 10 mg daily to complete a 21-day course of therapy.
[¶]5 to 10 mg/kg every 48 to 72 hours used in one study.
[**]Dosage for *Candida* shunt infection.

cle, which allows the drug to pass rapidly out of the ventricle into the shunt or ventriculostomy. Very little drug may enter the rest of the ventricular system. Vancomycin has been directly instilled into the ventricles to overcome the relatively meager CSF penetration of this agent after intravenous administration; daily dosages have ranged from 5 to 20 mg. In one report, 20 shunt infections were successfully treated with 20 mg of intraventricular vancomycin in adults and 10 mg in children administered from 5 to 19 days.[70] The British Society for Antimicrobial Chemotherapy Working Party on Infection in Neurosurgery has recommended that after shunt removal and establishment of external ventricular drainage (see later), intraventricular vancomycin be administered at a dosage of 20 mg daily combined with intravenous or oral rifampicin.[71] In another study in three patients with CSF shunt infections treated with intraventricular vancomycin,[72] peak and trough CSF vancomycin concentrations were 292.9 μg/mL and 7.6 μg/mL, respectively. Gentamicin (1 to 2 mg daily for infants and children and 4 to 8 mg daily for adults) has been administered, but always in combination with a parenteral agent (e.g., a β-lactam), for infections caused by susceptible gram-negative organisms. To determine additional intraventricular dosages of these agents, a sample of CSF is withdrawn immediately prior to instillation of the agent to obtain a "trough" CSF concentration. The trough CSF concentration divided by the minimal inhibitory concentration (MIC) of the agent for the isolated bacterial pathogen is termed the "inhibitory quotient," which should exceed 10 to 20 for consistent CSF sterilization.[4] Although not standardized, this approach is reasonable to ensure that adequate CSF concentrations of these agents are obtained.

Intravenous and intraventricular quinupristin/dalfopristin has been used successfully to treat a patient with ventriculostomy-related meningitis caused by vancomycin-resistant *Enterococcus faecium*.[73] Teicoplanin, a glycopeptide antimicrobial agent not currently licensed in the United States, was also found to be successful after intraventricular administration in seven patients with staphylococcal neurosurgical shunt infections.[74] Intraventricular polymyxin B[65] and intrathecal colistin[75] have been utilized in the treatment of gram-negative meningitis, but these agents should be reserved for patients with meningitis caused by multidrug-resistant gram-negative bacteria. Intraventricular amphotericin B may be required for *Candida* shunt infections that fail to respond to parenteral therapy and shunt removal. Penicillins and cephalosporins should not be given by the intrathecal route because they have been associated with significant neurotoxicity, especially seizures.[65,75,76]

Shunt Removal

The approaches to the therapy of CSF shunt infections in the published literature have included antimicrobial therapy with or without shunt removal.[4,15,29,30,52,75,77-83] In early attempts to treat CSF shunt infections, intravenous antimicrobial agents were used exclusively to avoid additional operations and to maintain CSF diversion during treatment; success with this approach, however, was low (about 24%) and carried a high mortality rate. The instillation of antimicrobial agents into CSF, in conjunction with parenteral therapy, increased the success rate to approximately 40%, but often required a lengthy hospitalization, and the frequency of an adverse outcome was unacceptably high; the ability of many of these organisms to adhere to prostheses and survive antimicrobial therapy likely precluded optimal treatment in situ. Combining the removal of shunt hardware with immediate shunt replacement and intravenous antimicrobial therapy cures roughly 75% of patients with shunt infections, although the failure and reinfection rates still remained quite significant with this approach. The other option is shunt removal with delayed replacement (in order to treat the infection with antimicrobial therapy in the absence of any foreign devices), although this approach leaves untreated the reason for the initial shunt placement.[84]

Antimicrobial use with removal of all components of the infected shunt along with use of some component of external drainage appears to be the most effective treatment for CSF shunt infections; the ventriculitis of shunt infections appears to clear more quickly with external

drainage. The presence of a drainage catheter also allows for monitoring of CSF parameters and continued treatment of the underlying hydrocephalus, and avoids the complications associated with only shunt removal. With this approach, treatment success is usually greater than 90%. The most important risk of the external ventricular drain is that of secondary infection[4,5,85-87]; longer duration of the ventriculostomy placement appears to increase the risk, although prophylactic catheter exchange performed every 5 days does not significantly reduce the likelihood of CSF infection.[88,89] In one randomized controlled trial in 103 patients who required external ventricular drains for more than 5 days,[89] the CSF infection rate was 7.8% for the group that underwent catheter exchange every 5 days and 3.8% for the no-change group ($P = 0.5$), suggesting that a single external ventricular catheter can be employed for as long as clinically indicated unless a change is necessary because of CSF infection or catheter malfunction. Attention to maintaining a sterile, closed system with avoidance of injections into the system and surveillance of the draining CSF will usually keep this risk to less than 5%. In the treatment of infection caused by an external ventricular device, removal of the device is an important adjunctive measure.

Duration of Antimicrobial Therapy and Shunt Reimplantation

The duration of antimicrobial therapy for CSF shunt infections is not completely defined and is dependent on the isolated microorganism, the extent of infection as defined by cultures obtained after externalization, and occasionally on CSF findings.[4] In patients with shunt infection caused by coagulase-negative staphylococci and with normal CSF findings, the presence of negative CSF cultures for 48 hours after externalization generally confirms that removal of the hardware effected a cure and the patient can be reshunted on the third day after removal. If the coagulase-negative staphylococcus was isolated in association with CSF abnormalities (i.e., CSF pleocytosis, abnormal chemistries), a true infection was likely present. If repeat cultures are negative, 7 days of antimicrobial therapy are recommended prior to reshunting, but if repeat cultures are positive, antimicrobial treatment is continued until CSF cultures remain negative for 10 consecutive days before a new CSF shunt is placed. For shunt infections caused by *S. aureus*, 10 days of antimicrobial therapy with negative cultures are recommended prior to reshunting. When gram-negative bacilli are isolated, a 21-day course of antimicrobial therapy should be utilized, although some experts have recommended shorter durations (i.e., 14 days) in shunt infections caused by these microorganisms.[90] Some experts also suggest that consideration be given to a 3-day period off antimicrobial therapy to verify clearing of the infection prior to shunt reimplantation, although this observation period is optional and may not be necessary in all patients.[4] It is important to note, however, that these recommendations have not been rigorously studied and some patients may require a longer duration of antimicrobial therapy before a new CSF shunt is placed. Careful follow-up after reimplantation is also critical to ensure that the patient has been cured.

REFERENCES

1. Bondurant CP, Jimenez DF. Epidemiology of cerebrospinal fluid shunting. Pediatr Neurosurg. 1995;23:254-258.
2. Aronyk KE. The history and classification of hydrocephalus. Neurosurg Clin North Am. 1993;4:599-609.
3. Hirsch JF. Surgery of hydrocephalus: Past, present, and future. Acta Neurochir (Wien). 1992;116:155-160.
4. Kaufman BA. Infections of cerebrospinal fluid shunts. In: Scheld WM, Whitley RJ, Durack DT, eds. Infections of the Central Nervous System. 2nd ed. Philadelphia: Lippincott-Raven; 1997:555-577.
5. Lozier AP, Sciacca RRE, Romagnoli MF, Connolly ES Jr. Ventriculostomy-related infections: A critical review of the literature. Neurosurgery. 2002;51:170-182.
6. Piatt JH Jr, Carlson CV. A search for determinants of cerebrospinal fluid shunt survival: Retrospective analysis of a 14-year institutional experience. Pediatr Neurosurg. 1993;19:233-241.
7. McGirt MJ, Leveque JC, Wellons JC Jr, et al. Cerebrospinal fluid shunt survival and etiology of failures: A seven-year institutional experience. Pediatr Neurosurg. 2002;36:248-255.
8. Quigley MR, Reigel DH, Kortyna R. Cerebrospinal fluid shunt infections: Report of 41 cases and a critical review of the literature. Pediatr Neurosci. 1989;15:111-120.

9. Renier D, Lacombe J, Pierre-Kahn A, et al. Factors causing acute shunt infection: Computer analysis of 1174 operations. J Neurosurg. 1984;61:1072-1078.
10. Kontny U, Hofling B, Gutjahr P, et al. CSF shunt infections in children. Infection. 1993;21:89-92.
11. Younger JJ, Simmons JC, Barrett FF. Operative related infection rates for ventriculoperitoneal shunt procedures in a children's hospital. Infect Control. 1987;8:67-70.
12. Choux M, Genitori L, Lang D, Lena G. Shunt implantation: Reducing the incidence of shunt infection. J Neurosurg. 1992;77:875-880.
13. Winston KR. Hair and neurosurgery. Neurosurgery. 1992;31:320-329.
14. Morissette I, Gourdeau M, Francoeur J. CSF shunt infections: A fifteen-year experience with emphasis on management and outcome. Can J Neurol Sci. 1993;20:118-122.
15. Odio C, McCracken GH Jr, Nelson JD. CSF shunt infections in pediatrics. Am J Dis Child. 1984;138:1103-1108.
16. George R, Leibrock L, Epstein M. Long-term analysis of cerebrospinal fluid shunt infections: A 25-year experience. J Neurosurg. 1979;51:804-811.
17. McGirt MJ, Zaas A, Fuchs HE, et al. Risk factors for pediatric ventriculoperitoneal shunt infection and predictors of infectious pathogens. Clin Infect Dis. 2003;36:858-862.
18. Seifert H, Richter W, Pulverer G. Clinical and bacteriological features of relapsing shunt-associated meningitis due to *Acinetobacter baumannii*. Eur J Clin Microbiol Infect Dis. 1995;14:130-134.
19. Kralinsky K, Krcmeryova T, Tuharsky J, Krcmery V. Nosocomial *Acinetobacter* meningitis. Pediatr Infect Dis J. 2000;19:270.
20. Filka J, Huttova M, Schwartzova D, et al. Nosocomial meningitis due to *Acinetobacter calcoaceticus* in 10 children after ventriculoperitoneal shunt insertion. J Hosp Infect. 2000;44:76-77.
21. Rekate HL, Ruch T, Nulsen FE. Diphtheroid infections of cerebrospinal fluid shunts. J Neurosurg. 1980;25:553-556.
22. Brook I. Meningitis and shunt infection caused by anaerobic bacteria in children. Pediatr Neurol. 2002;26:99-105.
23. Montero A, Romero J, Vargas JA, et al. *Candida* infection of cerebrospinal fluid shunt devices: Report of two cases and review of the literature. Acta Neurochir. 2000;142:67-74.
24. Chen TL, Tsai CA, Fung CP, et al. Clinical significance of *Candida* species isolated from cerebrospinal fluid. J Microbiol Immunol Infect. 2002;35:249-254.
25. Yogev R. Cerebrospinal fluid shunt infections: A personal view. Pediatr Infect Dis J. 1985;4:113-118.
26. Shapiro S, Boaz J, Kleiman M, et al. Origin of organisms infecting ventricular shunts. Neurosurgery. 1988;22:868-872.
27. Ho KJ. Recurrent meningitis associated with intragastric migration of a ventriculoperitoneal shunt catheter in a patient with normal-pressure hydrocephalus. South Med J. 1992;85:1145-1148.
28. Ibrahim AW. *E. coli* meningitis as an indicator of intestinal perforation by V-P shunt tube. Neurosurg Rev. 1998;21:194-197.
29. Walters BC, Hoffman HJ, Mendrick EB, Humphreys RP. Cerebrospinal fluid shunt infection—Influences on initial management and subsequent outcome. J Neurosurg. 1984;60:1014-1021.
30. Schoenbaum SC, Gardner P, Shillito J. Infections of cerebrospinal fluid shunts: Epidemiology, clinical manifestations, and therapy. J Infect Dis. 1975;131:543-552.
31. Gardner P, Leipzig T, Phillips P. Infections of central nervous system shunts. Med Clin North Am. 1985;69:297-314.
32. Paramore CG, Turner DA. Relative risks of ventriculostomy infection and morbidity. Acta Neurochir (Wien). 1994;127:79-84.
33. Pople IK, Bayston R, Hayward RD. Infection of cerebrospinal fluid shunts in infants: A study of etiological factors. J Neurosurg. 1992;77:29-36.
34. Zimmerli W, Waldvogel FA, Vaudaux P, Nydegger UE. Pathogenesis of foreign body infection: Description and characteristics of an animal model. J Infect Dis. 1982;146:487-497.
35. Quie PG, Belani KK. Coagulase-negative staphylococcal adherence and persistence. J Infect Dis. 1987;156:543-547.
36. Dougherty SH. Pathobiology of infection in prosthetic devices. Rev Infect Dis. 1988;10:1102-1117.
37. Peters G, Locci R, Pulverer G. Adherence and growth of coagulase-negative staphylococci on surfaces of intravenous catheters. J Infect Dis. 1982;146:479-482.
38. Vaudaux P, Suzuki R, Waldvogel FA, et al. Foreign body infection: Role of fibronectin as a ligand for the adherence of *Staphylococcus aureus*. J Infect Dis. 1984;150:546-553.
39. Maxe I, Ryden C, Wadstrom T, Rubin K. Specific attachment of *Staphylococcus aureus* to immobilized fibronectin. Infect Immun. 1986;54:768-774.
40. Bayston R, Penny SR. Excessive production of mucoid substance in *Staphylococcus* SIIA: A possible factor in colonization of Holter shunts. Dev Med Child Neurol (Suppl). 1972;27:25-28.
41. Christensen GD, Simpson WA, Bisno AL, Beachey EH. Adherence of slime-producing strains of *Staphylococcus epidermidis* to smooth surfaces. Infect Immun. 1982;37:318-326.
42. Younger JJ, Christensen GD, Bartley DL, et al. Coagulase-negative staphylococci isolated from cerebrospinal fluid shunts: Importance of slime production, species identification, and shunt removal to clinical outcome. J Infect Dis. 1987;156:548-554.
43. Diaz-Mitoma F, Harding GKM, Hoban DJ, et al. Clinical significance of a test for slime production in ventriculoperitoneal shunt infections caused by coagulase-negative staphylococci. J Infect Dis. 1987;156:555-560.
44. Pollack M. The virulence of *Pseudomonas aeruginosa*. Rev Infect Dis. 1984;6:S617-S626.
45. Bayston R, Comton C, Richards K. Production of extracellular slime by coryneforms colonizing hydrocephalus shunts. J Clin Microbiol. 1994;32:1705-1709.
46. Zimmerli W, Lew PD, Waldvogel FA. Pathogenesis of foreign body infection: Evidence for a local granulocyte defect. J Clin Invest. 1984;73:1191-1200.
47. Dougherty SH, Simmons RL. Endogenous factors contributing to prosthetic device infections. Infect Dis Clin North Am. 1989;3:199-209.
48. Vaudaux PE, Zulian G, Huggler E, Waldvogel FA. Attachment of *Staphylococcus aureus* to polymethylmethacrylate increases its resistance of phagocytosis in foreign body infections. Infect Immun. 1985;50:472-477.
49. Borges LF. Cerebrospinal fluid shunts interfere with host defenses. Neurosurgery. 1982;10:55-60.
50. Johnson GM, Lee DA, Regelmann WE, et al. Interference with granulocyte function by *Staphylococcus epidermidis* slime. Infect Immun. 1986;54:13-20.
51. Gray ED, Peters G, Verstegen M, Regelmann WE. Effect of extracellular slime substance from *Staphylococcus epidermidis* on the human cellular immune response. Lancet. 1984;1:365-367.
52. Forward KR, Fewer HD, Stiver HG. Cerebrospinal fluid shunt infections—A review of 35 infections in 32 patients. J Neurosurg. 1983;59:389-394.
53. Arze RS, Rashid H, Morley R, et al. Shunt nephritis: Report of two cases and review of the literature. Clin Nephrol. 1983;19:48-53.
54. Samtleben W, Bauriedel G, Bosch T, et al. Renal complications of infected ventriculoatrial shunts. Artif Organs. 1993;17:695-701.
55. Reynolds M, Sherman JO, McLone DG. Ventriculoperitoneal shunt infection masquerading as an acute surgical abdomen. J Pediatr Surg. 1983;18:951-954.
56. Rekate HL, Yonas H, White RJ, Nulsen PE. The acute abdomen in patients with ventriculoperitoneal shunts. Surg Neurol. 1979;11:442-445.
57. Mayhall CG, Archer NH, Lamb VA, et al. Ventriculostomy related infections—A prospective epidemiologic study. N Engl J Med. 1984;310:553-559.
58. Gerner-Smidt P, Stenager E, Kock-Jensen C. Treatment of ventriculostomy-related infections. Acta Neurochir (Wien). 1988;91:47-49.
59. Siegel T, Pfeffer R, Steiner I. Antibiotic therapy for infected Ommaya reservoir systems. Neurosurgery. 1988;22:97-100.
60. Tung H, Raffel C, McComb JG. Ventricular cerebrospinal fluid eosinophilia in children with ventriculoperitoneal shunts. J Neurosurg. 1991;75:541-544.
61. Sundbarg G, Nordstrom CH, Soderstrom S. Complications due to prolonged ventricular fluid pressure recording. Br J Neurosurg. 1988;2:485-495.
62. Jones RF, Stening WA, Kwok BC, Sands TM. Third ventriculostomy for shunt infections in children. Neurosurgery. 1993;32:855-859.
63. Gombert ME, Landesman SH, Corrado ML, et al. Vancomycin and rifampin therapy for *Staphylococcus epidermidis* meningitis associated with CSF shunts. J Neurosurg. 1981;55:633-636.
64. Gill CJ, Murphy MA, Hamer DH. Treatment of *Staphylococcus epidermidis* ventriculo-peritoneal shunt infection with linezolid. J Infect. 2002;45:129-132.
65. Wen DY, Bottini AG, Hall WA, Haines SJ. The intraventricular use of antibiotics. Neurosurg Clin North Am. 1992;3:343-354.
66. James HE, Wilson HD, Connor JD, Walsh JW. Intraventricular cerebrospinal fluid antibiotic concentrations in patients with intraventricular infections. Neurosurgery. 1982;10:50-54.
67. Ressor C, Chow AW, Kureishi A, Jewesson PJ. Kinetics of intraventricular vancomycin in infections of cerebrospinal fluid shunts. J Infect Dis. 1988;158:1142-1143.
68. Wilson HD, Bean JR, James HE, Pendley MM. Cerebrospinal fluid antibiotic concentrations in ventricular shunt infections. Child's Brain. 1978;4:74-82.
69. Bayston R, Hart CA, Barnicot M. Intraventricular vancomycin in the treatment of ventriculitis associated with cerebrospinal fluid shunting and drainage. J Neurol Neurosurg Psychiatry 1987;50:1419-1423.
70. Swayne R, Rampling A, Newsome SWB. Intraventricular vancomycin for treatment of shunt associated ventriculitis. J Antimicrob Chemother. 1987;19:249-253.
71. Bayston R. Epidemiology, diagnosis, treatment, and prevention of cerebrospinal fluid shunt infections. Neurosurg Clin North Am. 2001;36:703-708.
72. Pfausler B, Haring HP, Kampfl A, et al. Cerebrospinal fluid (CSF) pharmacokinetics of intraventricular vancomycin in patients with staphylococcal ventriculitis associated with external CSF drainage. Clin Infect Dis. 1997;25:733-735.
73. Williamson JC, Glazier SS, Peacock JE Jr. Successful treatment of ventriculostomy-related meningitis caused by vancomycin-resistant *Enterococcus* with intravenous and intraventricular quinupristin/dalfopristin. Clin Neurol Neurosurg. 2002;104:54-56.
74. Cruciani M, Navarra A, Di Perri G, et al. Evaluation of intraventricular teicoplanin for the treatment of neurosurgical shunt infections. Clin Infect Dis. 1992;15:285-289.
75. Vasen W, Desmery P, Ilutovich S, et al. Intrathecal use of colistin. J Clin Microbiol. 2000;38:3523.
76. Manzella JP, Paul RL, Butler IL. CNS toxicity associated with intraventricular injection of cefazolin. J Neurosurg. 1988;68:970-971.
77. Nelson JD. Cerebrospinal fluid shunt infections. Pediatr Infect Dis J. 1984;3:30-32.
78. James HE, Walsh JW, Wilson HD, et al. Prospective randomized study of therapy in cerebrospinal fluid shunt infection. Neurosurgery. 1980;7:459-463.
79. James HE, Walsh JW, Wilson HD, Connor JD. The management of cerebrospinal fluid shunt infections—A clinical experience. Acta Neurochir (Wien). 1981;59:157-166.
80. Shurtleff DB, Foltz EL, Weeks RD, Loeser J. Therapy of *Staphylococcus epidermidis*: Infections associated with cerebrospinal fluid shunts. Pediatrics. 1974;53:55-62.
81. Mates S, Glaser J, Shapiro K. Treatment of cerebrospinal fluid shunt infections with medical therapy alone. Neurosurgery. 1982;11:781-783.
82. Frame PT, McLaurin RL. Treatment of CSF shunt infections with intrashunt plus oral antibiotic therapy. J Neurosurg. 1984;60:354-360.
83. Salmon JH. Adult hydrocephalus: Evaluation of shunt therapy in 80 patients. J Neurosurg. 1972;37:423-428.

84. Walters BC. Cerebrospinal fluid shunt infection. Neurosurg Clin North Am. 1992;3:387-401.
85. Sayers MP. Shunt complications. Clin Neurosurg. 1976;23:393-400.
86. Smith RW, Alksne JF. Infections complicating the use of external ventriculostomy. J Neurosurg. 1976;44:567-570.
87. Lyke KE, Obasanjo OO, Williams MA, et al. Ventriculitis complicating use of intraventricular catheters in adult neurosurgical patients. Clin Infect Dis. 2001;33:2028-2033.
88. Holloway KL, Barnes T, Choi S, et al. Ventriculostomy infections: The effect of monitoring duration and catheter exchange in 584 patients. J Neurosurg. 1996;85:419-424.
89. Wong GKC, Poon WS, Wai S, et al. Failure of regular external ventricular drain exchange to reduce cerebrospinal fluid infection: Result of a randomized controlled trial. J Neurol Neurosurg Psychiatry 2002;73:759-761.
90. Chapman PH, Borges LF. Shunt infections: Prevention and treatment. Clin Neurosurg. 1985;32:652-664.

CHAPTER **82**

Chronic Meningitis

IRMGARD BEHLAU

JERROLD J. ELLNER

A large number of infectious and noninfectious diseases can cause the clinical syndrome of chronic meningitis (Tables 82-1 and 82-2). The onset of symptoms in such cases typically is subacute to chronic with signs of meningoencephalitis such as fever, headache, lethargy, confusion, nausea, vomiting, and stiff neck. Cerebrospinal fluid (CSF) is abnormal with elevated protein concentrations, a pleocytosis that usually is predominantly lymphocytic, and sometimes a low glucose level. The major difficulty during initial evaluation is in distinguishing the rare patient with chronic meningitis from those patients with the more common syndromes of acute meningitis and encephalitis. If the neurologic symptoms and signs either persist or progress clinically and the CSF remains abnormal for at least 4 weeks, the diagnosis of chronic meningitis is appropriate.[1-9] The diagnosis of chronic meningitis has important implications that relate to etiology, management, and prognosis. This duration of symptoms helps distinguish between patients with chronic progressive disease and those with self-limited processes. Because patients may be seen within 1 to 4 weeks after the onset of symptoms, prompt diagnosis and appropriate treatment may abort the neurologic process before the criteria for chronic meningitis are fulfilled.

Central nervous system (CNS) involvement by most diseases causing chronic meningitis has a high morbidity and mortality when unrecognized. Successful intervention requires the early administration of specific, often potentially toxic forms of therapy. Furthermore,

TABLE 82-2 Noninfectious Causes of Chronic Meningitis

Behçet's disease
Chronic benign lymphocytic meningitis
Chronic meningitis of unknown cause
Connective tissue disease (SLE, polyarteritis nodosa, Sjögren's syndrome, Wegener's granulomatosis)
Granulomatous angiitis
Neoplastic meningitis
Sarcoidosis
Uveomeningoencephalitis

SLE, systemic lupus erythematosus.

drugs appropriate for treating one cause of chronic meningitis may be contraindicated in others. Therefore, a precise etiologic diagnosis is critical in modifying the course of this syndrome, and broad empirical therapeutic regimens are a poor and sometimes hazardous substitute. Because up to one third of patients with chronic meningitis are undiagnosed, certain aspects of the presentation may be helpful in determining causality or at least limiting the differential diagnosis.

HISTORY

The exposure history (Table 82-3) may be important in suggesting certain infectious diseases such as tuberculosis, coccidioidomycosis, histoplasmosis, brucellosis, cysticercosis, syphilis, Lyme disease, and, especially, acquired immunodeficiency syndrome (AIDS) with its distinctive spectrum of opportunistic pathogens. The exposure history should direct the evaluation to include specific serologic studies and other diagnostic tests. Because the presence of human immunodeficiency virus (HIV) infection significantly alters the differential diagnosis, HIV testing should be done on all patients with chronic meningitis. This chapter discusses chronic meningitis in the HIV-seronegative patient, except where specifically noted.

The history also is of importance in distinguishing chronic meningitis from two superficially similar syndromes, acute meningitis (or encephalitis) with a protracted recovery period and recurrent meningitis. In chronic meningitis, onset is insidious and symptoms are chronic, although they may wax and wane. Episodes of acute neurologic deterioration sometimes punctuate the clinical course and may be caused by cerebral edema, hydrocephalus, cerebrovascular occlusions, or seizures. Even when symptoms temporarily regress, CSF abnormalities persist and reflect continued disease activity. In the protracted recovery period that sometimes follows pyogenic or aseptic meningitis and viral encephalitis, actual progression of disease is confined to the acute stages of the illness; clearing of the signs, symptoms, and CSF abnormalities, although gradual, may occur during observation. The second syndrome that must be differentiated from chronic meningitis is recurrent meningitis.[10] Patients with recurrent meningitis usually have repeated episodes of acute disease followed by periods during which signs and symptoms are absent and the CSF is normal (Table 82-4).

TABLE 82-1 Infectious Diseases That May Manifest as Chronic Meningitis: Usual Presentation in the Central Nervous System

Meningitis	*Focal Lesions*	*Encephalitis*
Acanthamoeba infection	Actinomycosis	African trypanosomiasis
Angiostrongylus cantonensis infection	Blastomycosis	Cytomegalovirus infection
Brucellosis	Coenurosis	Enterovirus (patients with agammaglobulinemia)
Candidiasis	Cysticercosis	Measles (subacute sclerosing panencephalitis)
Coccidioidomycosis	Molds: aspergillosis, phaeohyphomycosis, pseudallescheriasis	Rabies
Cryptococcosis	Nocardiosis	Viral encephalitis (see Chapter 83)
Histoplasmosis	Schistosomiasis	
Lyme disease	Toxoplasmosis	
Sporotrichosis		
Syphilis		
Tuberculosis		

TABLE 82-3 Evaluation of Patients with Chronic Meningitis

Initial Evaluation of All Patients
History: travel to southwestern United States, developing countries, or tropical Africa; new sexual partner, high-risk activity for HIV, household member with tuberculosis; brucellosis exposure such as unpasteurized milk or meat packing, intravenous drug abuse, history of a skin lesion resembling erythema migrans, childhood measles

Physical examination: complete examination, including search for skin lesions or subcutaneous nodules; ocular examination for retinal lesions, papilledema, uveitis, or iritis; lymphadenopathy; hepatosplenomegaly; neurologic examination

Laboratory tests: complete blood count with differential analysis and sedimentation rate; liver and renal function; PPD; chest radiograph; MRI with gadolinium enhancement or CT (with special attention for parameningeal foci in paranasal sinus or mastoids, intracerebral lesions, epidermoid cysts, and hydrocephalus); blood culture for fungi and mycobacteria by lysis centrifugation; urine culture for fungi and mycobacteria; serology for HIV, syphilis, cryptococcal antigen, and antinuclear antibody; lumbar puncture for opening pressure, leukocytes, protein, glucose (simultaneous blood glucose), cytospin cytology, VDRL, cryptococcal antigen, India ink, acid-fast stain, *Mycobacterium tuberculosis* PCR and large-volume (3-5 mL) cultures each for fungus, mycobacteria

Radiographic tests: MRI with gadolinium of head and spine to evaluate for parameningeal and parenchymal lesions; CT scan with contrast if MRI unavailable

Tests Indicated by Appropriate Exposure History
Serum serology for antibody to *Histoplasma, Coccidioides, Brucella,* and *Borrelia burgdorferi* (Lyme disease agent)

Cerebrospinal fluid antibody to *Histoplasma, Coccidioides, Blastomyces, Taenia solium* (cysticercosis), *Brucella,* and measles virus; *Histoplasma* antigen; stain CSF leukocytes for eosinophils; *Brucella* culture; blood smear for trypanosomes

Enigmatic Cases
Repeat PPD in 2 to 4 weeks; serum immunoglobulins and angiotensin-converting enzyme; CSF for antibody to *Sporothrix;* enteroviral culture and PCR (if low serum immunoglobulin G), repeat cytology and PCR for lymphocyte gene rearrangement. Biopsy of extraneural sites such as lymph nodes, bone marrow, liver, skin, or muscle. Consider brain biopsy for diffuse carcinomatosis or gliomatosis, *Acanthamoeba,* mold infections, granulomatous angiitis, or in patients who are rapidly deteriorating despite treatment.

CSF, cerebrospinal fluid; CT, computed tomography; HIV, human immunodeficiency virus; MRI, magnetic resonance imaging; PCR, polymerase chain reaction; PPD, purified protein derivative of tuberculin; VDRL, Venereal Disease Research Laboratory test for syphilis.

The history also is important in defining the cause of meningitis in those instances in which CNS extension occurs as a late manifestation of a previously diagnosed systemic disease. These conditions include acute leukemia, lymphoma, blastomycosis, and Behçet's disease.

PHYSICAL EXAMINATION

Diagnostic physical findings are rare. However, physical examination (see Table 82-3) may delineate signs of an associated systemic disease that provide a potential source of rapid diagnosis. Skin lesions, although infrequent, are particularly important for their diagnostic value. Even benign-appearing superficial lesions, subcutaneous nodules and abscesses, or draining sinuses should be cultured and biopsy

TABLE 82-4 Differential Diagnosis of Recurrent Meningitis

Drug-induced (with rechallenge)[11-13]
Parameningeal focus
   Infection (sinusitis, mastoiditis, osteomyelitis, brain abscess)
   Tumor (epidermoid cyst, craniopharyngioma)[14-15]
Post-traumatic (bacterial)
Mollaret's meningitis[16-19]
Systemic lupus erythematosus[20-21]
Herpes simplex virus

specimens obtained. Among the causes of chronic meningitis that are notable for manifesting with skin lesions are cryptococcosis (Fig. 82-1), sarcoidosis, *Acanthamoeba* infection, coccidioidomycosis, blastomycosis, and secondary syphilis; in addition, the subcutaneous nodules of cysticercosis and metastatic carcinoma (e.g., breast, melanoma) are important signs. The eye examination may be helpful if such lesions as choroidal tubercles, sarcoid granulomas, or uveitis are demonstrable. The finding of papilledema also is of significance because it alters the course of the neurologic workup and contraindicates lumbar puncture. Hepatomegaly may reflect systemic disease involving the liver and increases the potential diagnostic yield of a liver biopsy.

Neurologic examination is of obvious importance in delineating the extent of CNS involvement. However, it is of limited use in differentiating among specific causes because mental status changes, meningismus, oculomotor palsies, and, less frequently, focal findings, evidence of increased intracranial pressure, and spinal cord signs can be caused by most processes associated with chronic meningitis. Focal signs, however, often reflect a parenchymal mass such as an abscess or granuloma that would dictate specific diagnostic and therapeutic maneuvers. Involvement of multiple levels of the neuraxis is suggestive of meningeal carcinomatosis. Hydrocephalus may complicate chronic meningitis, and appropriate neuroradiographic evaluation should be initiated when the constellation of headache, nausea, vomiting, mental changes, ataxia, incontinence, and papilledema is present. The finding of hydrocephalus, particularly with associated cranial neuropathies, is suggestive of an infectious cause with basilar leptomeningitis, although

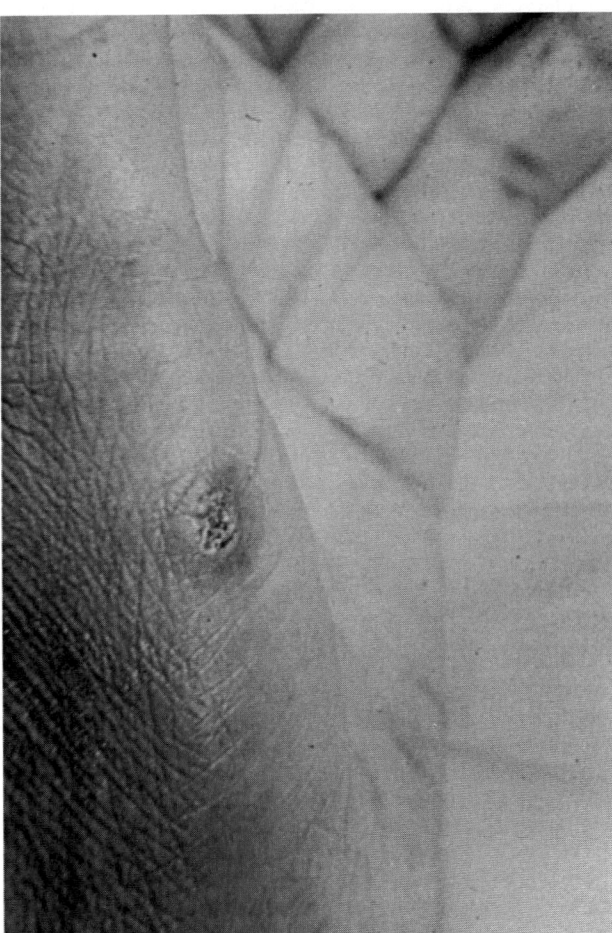

FIGURE 82-1. Skin lesion of a woman with chronic lymphocytic leukemia treated with corticosteroids and cytotoxic drugs, admitted with chronic meningitis. Material expressed from the lesion was positive on India ink preparation and culture for *Cryptococcus neoformans.*

hydrocephalus also may complicate sarcoidosis, cysticercosis, and CNS tumor. Peripheral neuropathy is noted uncommonly in chronic meningitis and is suggestive of sarcoidosis or Lyme disease. In patients infected with HIV-1, radiculomyelitis should suggest cytomegalovirus infection.

LABORATORY EVALUATION

The cause of chronic meningitis ultimately must be established in the laboratory (see Table 82-3).

The CSF formula is never itself diagnostic; however, certain abnormalities and patterns are more characteristic of a restricted group of causes of chronic meningitis (Table 82-5). Lumbar puncture must be repeated periodically both for culture and cytology, and to follow the course of meningeal inflammation. Among the infectious diseases, tuberculosis meningitis clearly is the most common etiology and far outranks all others in the immunologically intact host. Likewise, in the immunocompromised host, and in the AIDS era, cryptococcal meningitis is most likely. Both cultures and India ink preparations should be made from the sediment of 3 to 5 mL of CSF. The India ink preparation is more likely to be positive in patients with relatively acute presentations and in immunosuppressed patients with lymphoma or AIDS. In the latter setting, yeast organisms often far outnumber leukocytes in the CSF. Due to the combined high sensitivity of CSF and serum serology for cryptococcal antigen, serology has essentially supplanted the India ink smear.

Cultures are mandatory even when a specific diagnosis is suggested by serology or other studies. CSF should be cultured at least three times for bacteria, acid-fast bacilli, and fungi, and more numerous samples should be obtained and cultured in their entirety when the cause of the meningitis remains uncertain after the initial diagnostic evaluation is complete. The low density of mycobacteria and fungi in the CSF and the difficulty in culturing certain organisms may delay the diagnosis of these infections. In mycotic infections the yield can be improved by inoculating Sabouraud's agar layered on the bottom of Erlenmeyer flasks with large volumes of CSF. The finding of even a single colony of an organism capable of causing chronic meningitis such as *Sporothrix schenckii* should never be disregarded as a contaminant (Fig. 82-2).[24] In fact, it may be useful to continue to examine fungal cultures for at least 4 to 6 weeks because the growth of such organisms can be exceedingly slow. Dependent on the organism, obtaining both lumbar and ventricular CSF needs to be considered.[25] Urine, sputum, and blood cultures should be obtained and processed routinely for mycobacteria and fungi even in the absence of clinical evidence of extraneural infection. These ancillary cultures frequently are positive in cases of cryptococcosis, tuberculosis, histoplasmosis, and blastomycosis. Special culture techniques such as anaerobiasis or increased carbon dioxide tension also are appropriate in the search for certain pathogens such as *Actinomyces* spp. and *Brucella abortus,*

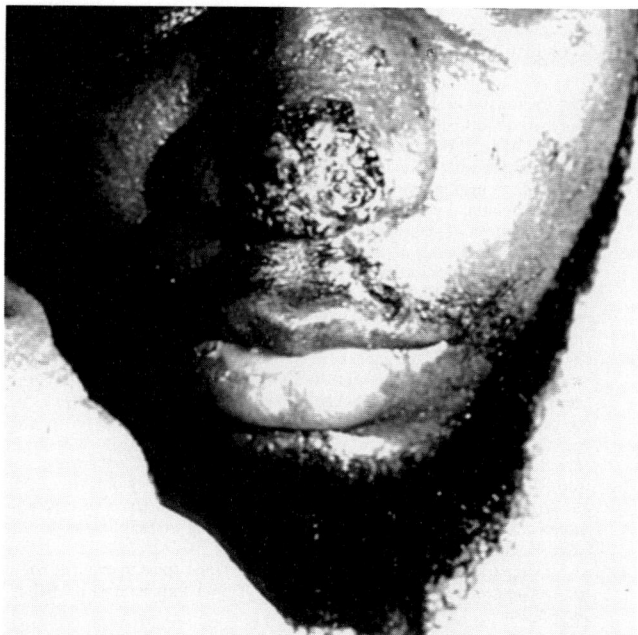

FIGURE 82-2. Skin lesions developed in this patient with enigmatic chronic meningitis after ventriculojugular shunting for hydrocephalus. A discarded cerebrospinal fluid culture from an earlier admission was found overgrown with mold, subsequently identified as *Sporothrix schenckii.*

respectively. Consultation with a clinical microbiologist may be helpful in difficult cases.

CSF cytologic studies are indicated in all patients with chronic meningitis. Multiple specimens may be necessary and negative cytologic studies do not preclude this possibility. Demonstration of a clonal origin of CSF lymphocytes with the use of B- and T-cell immunologic markers also is helpful in the diagnosis of lymphomatous meningitis,[26] as is polymerase chain reaction (PCR) detection of clonal immunoglobulin or T-cell receptor rearrangement.[27]

Serologic studies of serum and CSF are extremely important in evaluating the patient for coccidioidomycosis, cryptococcosis, and syphilis and should be performed routinely. In the case of cryptococcal meningitis, testing for cryptococcal polysaccharide antigen is helpful; testing for antibody is not useful. Serum antibodies to *Brucella* and *Toxoplasma* also may suggest these infections when they are present in high or increasing titers. Serum antibodies to *Histoplasma* are found in 60% of patients with *Histoplasma* meningitis.[28] Complement-

TABLE 82-5 Cerebrospinal Fluid Characteristics of Various Causes of Chronic Meningitis			
Pleocytosis <50 Cells/μL	*Neutrophilic Pleocytosis*[22]	*Eosinophilic Pleocytosis*[23]	*Low Glucose*
Behçet's disease	Bacteria	Chemical	Bacteria
Benign lymphocytic meningitis	*Actinomyces*	*Coccidioides*	*Actinomyces*
Carcinoma	*Nocardia*	Lymphoma	*Nocardia*
Cryptococcus in HIV-infected patients	Chemical	Parasites	Carcinoma
Sarcoidosis	CMV in HIV-infected patients	*Angiostrongylus*	*Cysticercus*
Vasculitis	Early *Mycobacterium tuberculosis* infection	*Cysticercus*	Fungi (all)
	Fungi	*Schistosoma*	*M. tuberculosis*
	Aspergillus		Postsubarachnoid hemorrhage
	Candida		Sarcoidosis
	Systemic lupus erythematosus		Syphilis
			Toxoplasma
			Viral
			Chronic enterovirus
			CMV in HIV-infected patients

CMV, cytomegalovirus; HIV, human immunodeficiency virus.

fixing antibodies to *Histoplasma* are found in the CSF of most patients with CNS histoplasmosis, although they may also be detected in coccidioidal and cryptococcal infection.[29] More specific is the detection of *Histoplasma capsulatum* antigen in serum, urine, or CSF by enzyme-linked immunosorbent assay (ELISA); however, this assay is less sensitive, with only 25% of patients with meningitis caused by this organism having detectable antigen in the CSF.[30] The antigen test is more likely to be positive in HIV-infected persons with *Histoplasma* meningitis.[28] The ELISA for antibody to *S. schenckii* in CSF has also been useful, although the disease rarely causes meningitis.[31] Identification of *Mycobacterium tuberculosis* DNA in CSF by PCR is more sensitive than culture, detecting 27% to 85% of cases of presumed tuberculous meningitis that responded to therapy.[32-36]

Skin testing should be limited to tuberculin purified protein derivative (PPD). Anergy testing is no longer recommended. Repeated skin testing may be helpful when tuberculosis is a possibility. Fungal skin test antigens should not be used.

Biopsy of specific tissues should be directed by abnormal findings on physical examination. Skin, lymph node, and liver biopsy specimens may demonstrate granulomas, sometimes with caseation and occasionally with an organism demonstrable on special staining. Caseation is suggestive of tuberculosis, histoplasmosis, or coccidioidomycosis. Focal necrosis may be found in brucellosis. All biopsy specimens should be cultured for bacteria, fungi, and mycobacteria. Bone marrow biopsy and culture are particularly useful in tuberculosis and histoplasmosis. Liver biopsy is indicated when miliary tuberculosis is suspected, and it has a greater yield when liver function tests suggest an infiltrative process (increased alkaline phosphatase and glutamyltranspeptidase).

Brain and meningeal biopsy should be considered in undiagnosed cases with a deteriorating course, recognizing that the yield of treatable causative organisms is low. In series reported from referral centers, the yield of a definitive diagnosis from leptomeningeal brain biopsy in chronic meningitis was 20% to 39%,[7,8] and the most common diagnosis at biopsy was sarcoidosis (31%) and carcinomatous meningitis (25%). However, if the biopsy was in a site of gadolinium-enhanced meninges on a magnetic resonance imaging (MRI) study, the diagnostic yield increased to 80%.[7] Despite the low yield, patients with hypoglycorrhachia and CSF pleocytosis greater than 50 cells/μL progressing on empirical antituberculosis therapy should be considered for biopsy. Earlier biopsy may be indicated, especially if the PPD skin test result is negative and the clinical course is deteriorating without a diagnosis.

RADIOGRAPHIC TECHNIQUES

Abnormalities on chest radiographs or chest computed tomography (CT) may reflect systemic involvement by the underlying infectious process, carcinoma, or sarcoidosis. These findings should be pursued in an attempt to define the cause of the meningitis. In more enigmatic cases, biopsy of lung lesions may be indicated; this is associated with less morbidity and greater yield than is a brain biopsy.

The decision of whether to do brain MRI or head CT or both depends on the clinical situation. MRI is becoming the preferred choice; in general, it is more sensitive. It is clearly the procedure of choice in herpes simplex virus (HSV) encephalitis, spinal and epidural abscesses, and identification of cerebritis adjacent to parameningeal infections. MRI provides greater specificity in distinguishing gray from white matter disease. It is also able to identify necrosis, inflammation, hemorrhage, demyelination, fluid collections, infection of the paranasal sinuses and mastoids, and small focal lesions that may be amenable to stereotactic biopsy. The T_2-weighted image is very sensitive for edema. The T_1-weighted image with gadolinium provides additional specificity and shows enhancement in areas of breakdown of the blood-brain barrier. Gadolinium diethylenetriaminepentaacetic acid (Gd-DTPA) MRI is able to distinguish between leptomeningitis, which correlates with infectious etiologies, and pachymeningitis, which may be more typical of carcinomas.[37,38] The disadvantage of MRI is its expense and limited availability. The use of newer techniques such as technetium-99m hexamethylpropyleneamine oxime (99m Tc HMPAO) single photon emission CT (SPECT) and proton spectroscopy may someday prove to make the early detection of certain diseases possible[39]; their more immediate role may be monitoring the response to certain therapies.

Ancillary procedures such as mammography and gastrointestinal radiographic series may be appropriate in the search for a primary carcinoma when meningeal carcinomatosis is suspected.

THERAPEUTIC TRIALS

Therapeutic trials are indicated when the specific cause remains uncertain despite comprehensive evaluation. However, further attempts at establishing a diagnosis should be continued actively during such trials. Interpretation of the response to empirically administered drugs may be difficult because clinical improvement is often slow, even when the agent selected is appropriate. When the patient is stable, sequential trials are indicated.

Tuberculous meningitis is the most common cause of chronic meningitis[4] where tuberculosis is endemic; therefore, an empirical trial of antituberculosis drugs clearly is appropriate when the presentation and CSF formula are consistent with tuberculosis and there is evidence of active or prior tuberculous infection. Studies suggest that initial tuberculin skin test results are negative in up to two thirds of patients with tuberculous meningitis.[40-42] Therefore empirical antituberculosis therapy is indicated in many cases of undiagnosed chronic meningitis. Adequate cultures of CSF, urine, sputum, or gastric aspirates must be obtained before therapy is begun, and biopsy specimens of liver and bone marrow should be included if miliary disease is suspected. Repeat intermediate-strength PPD skin testing after 2 to 4 weeks should be done if the initial studies are negative.[42] Positive cultures or a clinical response to antituberculosis treatment despite negative cultures would be an indication to complete a full course of therapy.

Fluconazole is potentially useful as empirical therapy for chronic meningitis caused by *Cryptococcus neoformans, Coccidioides* spp., and *Candida albicans*. No clinical trials have been published to guide empirical use. The diagnostic value of empirical fluconazole is limited by the slow response known to occur in documented cases. Improvement may not be obvious for several months, during which time meningitis resulting from other causes may irreversibly deteriorate. If such a trial is attempted, a dose of 400 mg/day is indicated, and repeated CSF examinations should be obtained to monitor the results of therapy. Should the patient respond but the condition remain undiagnosed, a minimum course would probably be at least 6 months.

Traditionally, empirical trials of corticosteroids have been avoided because of the potential catastrophic adverse effects in patients with unrecognized tuberculosis or fungal meningitis. However, chronic meningitis in areas where tuberculosis is not endemic usually is not infectious, sarcoidosis accounting for 31%.[6,7] Of 49 patients with chronic idiopathic meningitis at the Mayo Clinic from 1978 through 1990, 85% had a prolonged but benign course, with 50% responding promptly to empirical corticosteroids. No patient responded to empirical tuberculosis therapy.[6] In selected patients in whom an infectious cause has been fairly excluded, serious consideration should be given to an empirical trial of corticosteroid therapy. Negative tests on serum and CSF should include cryptococcal antigen, *Histoplasma* antigen and antibody, and, depending on endemic area, *Coccidioides* and Lyme disease antibody. Normal chest radiograph and negative PPD skin test results, no history of exposure to tuberculosis, and CSF cell count less than 20 leukocytes/mm³ would also support this consideration.

DIFFERENTIAL DIAGNOSIS

A number of conditions can cause syndromes resembling chronic meningitis superficially but are usually distinguishable from it on clinical grounds at presentation or during evaluation and observation of the patient (Table 82-6). In addition, a careful history is important to differentiate

TABLE 82-6 Diseases That Sometimes Resemble Chronic Meningitis

Infectious diseases
  Aseptic meningitis
  Infective endocarditis
  Parameningeal infections
  Partially treated bacterial meningitis
  Viral and nonviral encephalitis
Noninfectious diseases
  Brain tumor
  Giant cell arteritis
  Metabolic and other encephalopathies
  Multiple sclerosis
  Postinfectious encephalitis
  Sarcoidosis
  Subarachnoid hemorrhage
  Subdural hematoma
  Systemic lupus erythematosus
  Thrombotic thrombocytopenic purpura

between recurrent and chronic meningitis, because the former syndrome connotes a different spectrum of diseases (see Table 82-4).

Those infections causing the syndrome of chronic meningitis (see Table 82-1) are discussed in detail in other chapters. Features that are important in establishing the cause of the chronic meningitis are reviewed here.

Tuberculous Meningitis

Tuberculous meningitis[40-51] results from rupture of a superficial infective focus into the subarachnoid space. In younger patients this event typically is associated with active, progressive systemic disease. Stigmata of miliary tuberculosis may be present on physical examination and on chest radiographs. Tuberculin skin test results frequently are negative initially but convert on repeated testing. The diagnosis of tuberculosis usually is confirmed by smear, biopsy, and cultures obtained from extraneural specimens as well as CSF culture. In contrast, tuberculous meningitis in the adult more frequently results from the discharge of an old tuberculous focus into the subarachnoid space. As a result, physical examination, chest radiographs, and extraneural cultures often are not helpful; despite presumably long-standing tuberculous infection, series indicate that the initial tuberculin skin test result is negative in 50% to 65% of patients.[40-42] The diagnosis rests on the outcome of CSF cultures. As a result of the frequent early use of antituberculous therapy empirically, more cases now are "unproved" microbiologically but with the diagnosis of tuberculosis suggested by an apparent response to treatment.

It is often difficult to distinguish the clinical syndrome of tuberculous meningitis from other causes of chronic meningitis. Diagnostic criteria as proposed by Thwaites and colleagues[43] looked at five features (age, length of history, white blood cell [WBC] count, total CSF WBC count, and CSF neutrophil percentage) and found fairly high sensitivity (86%-97%) and fair specificity (70%-91%) for tuberculous meningitis. Yet caution must be exercised if the study population to which these criteria are applied to does not mirror the high prevalence of tuberculosis and relatively lower prevalence of HIV coinfection of their Vietnamese study population. About 50% of patients with tuberculous meningitis have had symptoms for longer than 2 weeks. Ocular palsies, particularly those caused by involvement of cranial nerve VI, are found in 30% to 70% of the cases.[51] The typical CSF findings consist of a lymphocytic pleocytosis (usually of 100 to 500 cells/mm³), increased protein concentration, and depressed glucose levels in two thirds of the patients on the initial lumbar puncture. This formula also is not specific for tuberculous meningitis. However, in unclear cases, progressive decrease in CSF glucose in the absence of specific treatment may be useful in distinguishing tuberculosis from aseptic meningitis and viral encephalitis. Cytologic examination of CSF often shows activated monocytoid cells and rarely Langerhans cells.[46] It should be noted that neutrophils may predominate, particularly during the first 10 days of symptoms.[40] CSF smears contain acid-fast bacilli in 10% to

22% of cases.[40,41,50] Proteinaceous spinal fluid contains fibrinogen and forms a clot or pellicle on standing; staining of the pellicle may increase the yield of the direct smear.[47] CSF cultures are positive in 38% to 88% of the cases, and sputum in about 14% to 50%.

CSF tests evaluated for the presumptive diagnosis of tuberculous meningitis have included various antibody and antigen detection assays[52]; currently, detection of mycobacterial DNA by PCR has become standard and is routinely performed, often being the first confirmatory test.[53-55] Sensitivity of PCR ranges from 27% to 85% in series, with specificity of 95% to 100%. The low amount of mycobacterial DNA in the CSF limits the sensitivity, but in most studies it is significantly greater than that of culture.[32-36] The Gen-Probe MTD and Roche Amplicor tests are only approved for detection of mycobacterial nucleic acid in respiratory specimens but can also be used with nonrespiratory specimens including CSF (see Chapter 15). Adenosine deaminase is released by T lymphocytes, and increased CSF levels are found in tuberculous meningitis but not in viral or bacterial meningitides.[53,56-58] Specificity is not perfect, because elevations are seen also in lymphomatous meningitis, neurosarcoidosis, and brucellosis. Prognostic factors associated with increased mortality include high lactate levels, low WBCs, especially neutrophils, and low CSF glucose levels.[59]

Cryptococcal Meningitis

Cryptococcal meningitis[40,60-67] manifests in several different fashions, but the most characteristic, that of a subacute to chronic meningoencephalitis, is not at all distinctive among the causes of chronic meningitis. Exposure history is of little value clinically because the yeastlike fungus *C. neoformans* var. *neoformans* is a widespread saprophyte with a worldwide distribution. However, *C. neoformans* var. *gattii* is most often found in the tropical and subtropical areas of Australia, Southeast Asia, Africa, and South America. More patients infected with the latter variety were previously normal, more have indolent onset, and they more often have focal CNS lesions on MRI than those infected with *C. neoformans* var. *neoformans*.[68,69] Although half of patients in the pre-AIDS era lacked clinically apparent immunologic deficits, an underlying cellular immune dysfunction was known to predispose to this infection. The development of chronic meningitis in patients with Hodgkin's disease or lymphosarcoma, in persons receiving high-dose daily corticosteroid therapy, or in persons at risk for AIDS suggests cryptococcal meningitis.

In the previously healthy person, cryptococcal meningitis may cause an extremely indolent illness with gradual progression of dementia. The India ink preparation frequently is negative in such cases. More commonly the onset of disease is subacute, at times mimicking a brain tumor, particularly when signs of increased intracranial pressure are present. In patients with hematologic malignancies or AIDS, the initial manifestation of cryptococcosis may be unexplained fever. However, CNS involvement often proceeds rapidly. CSF abnormalities include a lymphocytic pleocytosis (usually with 40 to 400 cells/mm³) and a depressed glucose level in 55% of cases. In patients with AIDS the CSF often shows little evidence of an inflammatory response, but in contrast with the HIV-negative patient, this has not been a risk factor for poor outcome.[63,64,66] Overall, the India ink preparation suggests the diagnosis of cryptococcal meningitis in more than 50% of cases. The yield is highest in patients with an acute syndrome. More than 85% of patients have cryptococcal polysaccharide antigen in the CSF. However, serum also should be processed for this antigen; the overlap between significant antigen titers in the serum and in the CSF allows a presumptive diagnosis of cryptococcosis in 94% of cases. The use of serum cryptococcal antigen to monitor response to therapy appears less reliable and should not be depended upon.[70]

Negative serology findings do not exclude a diagnosis of cryptococcal meningitis,[71] and false-positive tests are not rare. Cultural confirmation of the diagnosis is mandatory. The initial CSF culture is positive in three quarters of patients; additional CSF cultures increase this yield and are indicated. Cultures of urine, sputum, and blood also should be obtained. They have both diagnostic and prognostic value and frequently are positive in the absence of overt signs of extraneural infection. CSF cultures and serologies also are indicated in all patients with extraneural cryptococcal infection because they may have subclinical CNS disease; this is particularly likely in the immunocompromised host. Experimental PCR-based assays appear comparable to positive CSF cultures,[72-74] but are still not in widespread use for diagnosis and monitoring of treatment.

Coccidioidal Meningitis

Exposure history is important in the diagnosis of coccidioidal meningitis, because this infection is endemic in certain arid and semiarid areas of the Western Hemisphere.[75-83] CNS infection may be a part of generalized coccidioidomycosis, or it may represent the sole extrapulmonary site of active clinical disease. One third of patients with extrapulmonary coccidioidomycosis have meningeal involvement. Meningitis usually occurs within 6 months after the primary pulmonary infection; however, it has developed as long as 12 years after the initial infection.[79] Headache is the most prominent finding in patients with coccidioidal meningitis; the clinical syndrome is, however, in no way distinctive from the other causes of chronic meningitis. Skin tests with Spherulin are positive in 33% to 50% of patients with meningitis, though neither this antigen nor the earlier antigen, coccidioidin, is now commercially available.[78,79] Complement-fixing antibody to the causative organism is found in the CSF of 55% to 95% of such patients. One study suggests that detection of CSF antibodies to a 33-kD antigen from the spherule by ELISA is more sensitive than detection of complement fixation antibodies.[82] Eosinophils are commonly seen in the CSF of patients with coccidioidal meningitis, with 30% of patients having more than 10 eosinophils/mm^3.[80] A presumptive diagnosis is possible when chronic meningitis occurs in the presence of demonstrated systemic coccidioidomycosis or a serum complement fixation titer to *Coccidioides* spp. of at least 1:16. CSF findings resemble those of cryptococcal meningitis; CSF cultures are positive in one third to 50% of cases, and spherules of *Coccidioides* spp. are sometimes present on a smear. MRI findings typically show signs of meningitis with focal enhancement in the basal cisterns, sylvian fissures, or pericallosal region. Communicating hydrocephalus and deep infarcts are associated findings.[83]

Histoplasma Meningitis

Histoplasma meningitis[28-30,84-86] is a rare complication of infection with *H. capsulatum.* However, in one fourth of cases of *Histoplasma* meningitis, disease is limited to the CNS. Clinical presentation is not differentiable from that seen with other causes of chronic meningitis; fever is almost universally present.[28] Symptoms may have been present for weeks or many months. Oral mucosal lesions, although found in only 16% of patients with *Histoplasma* meningitis, can be diagnostic if present and are more common than skin lesions. CSF cultures are positive in only 27% to 65% of cases, making diagnosis problematic. Blood cultures should always be done; use of isolator tubes significantly increased the yield of blood cultures in a study of AIDS patients.[86] As discussed, detection of serum and CSF antibodies to the fungus is the most sensitive test for histoplasmosis; however, it is not specific because the antibodies may cross react with other fungi. Persons with positive *Histoplasma* serology should have their cryptococcal antigen level checked; if the patient is from an endemic area, coccidioidal serology should also be done to detect a false-positive test result. The serum antibody tests are negative in 10% to 40% of proven cases of *Histoplasma* meningitis. *Histoplasma* polysaccharide antigen may be detected in urine, blood, or CSF in 61% of patients with *Histoplasma* meningitis[28]; yields are even higher in HIV-infected persons.[86] The outcome of CNS histoplasmosis is often unfavorable. Some reports have concluded that amphotericin B–fluconazole combination therapy is antagonistic and should not be used in *Histoplasma* meningitis.[87,88] Treatment is discussed in Chapter 262.

Lyme Disease

Infection with the spirochete *Borrelia burgdorferi* frequently involves the CNS.[89-93] The spirochete is introduced into its human host by an often unrecognized bite of the small deer tick, *Ixodes scapularis (dammini).* Early infection is characterized by a flulike syndrome and the pathognomonic rash of erythema chronicum migrans. Neurologic symptoms follow the rash by a median of 4 weeks; headache and lymphocytic pleocytosis are seen in almost all patients with neuroborreliosis. Cranial nerve palsies (especially facial nerve) and peripheral neuropathies may be prominent and help to differentiate Lyme disease from the other chronic meningitides except sarcoidosis, which can manifest similarly. Exposure history is key in guiding appropriate serologic testing; in the absence of exposure, a positive serology result is more likely to represent a false-positive test than to be diagnostic for Lyme disease.[94] False-positive tests have been associated with infectious mononucleosis, rheumatoid arthritis, systemic lupus erythematosus, other spirochetal disease such as syphilis and periodontal disease, and malignancy. However, in endemic areas, up to 25% of healthy people are seropositive, so antibody detection in serum alone is not diagnostic. Persons in an endemic area who have an appropriate clinical presentation and positive serology results should be treated as having neuroborreliosis. Almost all persons with CNS Lyme disease have positive serologic evidence of Lyme disease and CSF pleocytosis.[94] The most specific test is the detection of synthesis of intrathecal antibody to *B. burgdorferi* in the CNS.[94,95] PCR detection of *Borrelia* DNA in the CSF is specific but has limited sensitivity for neuroborreliosis (38% in acute cases and 25% in chronic cases).[96,97]

Cysticercosis

Cysticercosis[98-106] is the most common parasitic disease of the CNS. Highly endemic areas include Mexico, central and upper South America, China, India, sub-Saharan Africa, and the Caribbean. In the United States, immigrants from Mexico are the largest infected population and can present with symptoms up to 25 years after leaving Mexico. The infection is acquired by eating food contaminated with stool containing the eggs of the tapeworm *Taenia solium;* these hatch in the small intestine, with the larvae invading the blood stream and infecting muscle, eye, and brain. In these sites the larvae mature into cysts and remain asymptomatic for an average of 4 to 5 years. The person develops symptoms as the larvae begin to die, inciting an increased inflammatory response. Symptoms vary depending on the part of the brain infected; intraparenchymal neurocysticercosis (the most common manifestation) results in seizures and focal neurologic deficits. Cysts in the subarachnoid space can collect in the basilar cisterns and induce a chronic basilar meningitis with hydrocephalus. CSF shows a lymphocytic pleocytosis, and hypoglycorrhachia occurs in up to 25% of patients. Cysts can also occur in the ventricles, causing ventriculitis or internal hydrocephalus.

Diagnosis is suggested by characteristic multiple cystic or calcified lesions detected by head CT scan or MRI in a person who has been in an endemic area; early in infection the calcium may not be present. CT is able to better define calcified lesions, but MRI is the modality of choice for the evaluation of intraventricular cysticercosis, brain-stem cysts, and small cysts located over the convexity of the cerebral hemispheres. Its high-contrast resolution allows MRI to recognize many forms of cysticercosis not visualized on CT.[100] Accurately defining the number, location, and viability of the parasites in the nervous system is important to individualize therapeutic decisions, including whether to use antiparasitic drugs, and follow response to therapy.[101] Subcutaneous cysts may be present in 25% of patients with neurocysticercosis; biopsy is diagnostic for the larval tapeworm. Skeletal muscle calcification on plain film is also suggestive of cysticercosis; however, the yield was low (< 10%) in a series from the United States.[102] Serologic studies of serum and particularly of CSF are helpful, but negative serology studies do not rule out neurocysticercosis, because serum antibodies are negative in up to 50% of cases. The yield in CSF is high (up to 84% positive serology findings) in patients with meningitis or hydrocephalus. The introduction of new CSF ELISA for detection of cysticercal antigens (sensitivity 86%)[103] not only provides a diagnostic tool for viable metacestodes but also may guide drug treatment. Diagnostic criteria for neurocysticercosis have been proposed based on histology, neuroimaging findings, immunologic data, response to treatment, and epidemiologic data.[104]

Other Infectious Causes

Candida meningitis[5,107-111] is rare and often associated with widely disseminated disease. Risk factors for meningitis are similar to those for candidemia, including prolonged antimicrobial therapy, indwelling venous catheters, hyperalimentation, corticosteroid use, recent intraabdominal surgery, and intravenous drug abuse. CSF shunts and ventricular catheters have also been associated specifically with meningitis. Neonates, and especially premature infants, seem to be at increased risk for candidal meningitis and *Candida* meningitis is associated with a poor outcome.[108-110] Presentation ranges from subacute to indolent, with the interval from onset of symptoms to diagnosis ranging from days to months. Most commonly the disease manifests acutely as a complication of disseminated *Candida* infection; the clinical presentation and CSF findings can mimic those of bacterial meningitis. However, *Candida* meningitis can manifest as chronic meningitis progressing over months, similar to the endemic fungi.[111] CSF shows pleocytosis with a predominance of neutrophils in 50% of cases and hypoglycorrhachia in 60%. Gram staining reveals yeast in 33% of smears, and CSF culture is usually diagnostic. However, culture of large volumes of CSF and filtering of CSF with culture of the filter contents may be necessary.[111]

Syphilitic meningitis[112-118] is a rare but easily diagnosed and treated form of secondary syphilis. The disease is usually subacute, with the symptoms persisting for longer than 1 month in about 25% of cases. Meningitis is the first overt sign of syphilis in 25% of meningitic patients. When extraneural manifestations occur, they generally precede CNS involvement by less than 2 years. Any patient with eye findings consistent with syphilis should undergo examination of the CSF.[117] The clinical presentation and CSF abnormalities resemble those of the other causes of chronic meningitis; however, cranial nerve palsies are seen in almost 50% of cases, with a special predilection for nerves VII and VIII. Hypoglycorrhachia is present in 55% of cases. The diagnosis of syphilitic meningitis is suggested by positive CSF and serum serology results for syphilis. Detection of *Treponema pallidum* DNA by PCR has been reported in neurosyphilis, but this test is not as sensitive as CSF–Venereal Disease Research Laboratory (VDRL) with conventional CSF analysis.[116] Transient dramatic deterioration of patients with meningitis after the initiation of penicillin therapy should suggest a Jarisch-Herxheimer reaction and the possibility of syphilis. MRI findings are nonspecific, but may manifest as vascular occlusive disease such as cerebral infarction or arteritis, nonspecific white matter lesions, and enhancing cortical lesions with or without adjacent meningeal enhancement.[118]

A meningoencephalomyelitis may follow the initial manifestations of brucellosis by 2 months to 2 years in less than 5% of cases.[119-123] Exposure to unpasteurized milk products or contact with cows, goats, sheep, swine, or their carcasses suggests the diagnosis. The patient also may have current or past symptoms and signs of systemic brucellosis, such as night sweats, unexplained fever, orchitis, and hepatosplenomegaly. The clinical manifestations of the meningitis and CSF abnormalities usually are nonspecific, with a lymphocytic pleocytosis in all and hypoglycorrhachia in 50% of cases. However, transient episodes of hemianesthesia or paresthesia can be prominent in neurobrucellosis. In chronic cases, calcified foci may be noted in the liver and spleen on abdominal x-ray films. Cultures should be maintained in an increased carbon dioxide atmosphere for 3 weeks. CSF cultures are positive for *Brucella* in less than 50% of cases. Blood cultures occasionally are positive. The diagnosis is made by detection of *Brucella* antibodies in the serum and CSF.

S. schenckii has been described as a cause of chronic meningitis,[24,31,124] and the CSF may demonstrate *Sporothrix* antibody before the fungus is recovered by culture.[31] *Angiostrongylus cantonensis* is a nematode endemic to Southeast Asia and the Pacific Islands and is the most common cause worldwide of eosinophilic meningitis.[125,126] Symptoms develop approximately 1 week after ingestion of raw fish or snails and persist for 2 to 4 weeks, usually resolving spontaneously. Rarely, the living larvae may be found in the CSF or eye; however, the diagnosis is usually made clinically (eosinophilic meningitis with the correct exposure

history). Hyperintense basal ganglia lesions on T_1-weighted MRI scans have been associated with *A. cantonensis* meningitis.[127]

CNS involvement in a large number of infections commonly is expressed as brain abscesses or other focal lesions occurring by hematogenous seeding or direct extension from clinically apparent extraneural sites. Rarely, the syndrome of chronic meningitis may be caused by these agents, sometimes without other stigmata of infection. Infectious diseases belonging in this category include North American blastomycosis,[128-130] paracoccidioidomycosis,[131] cerebral phaeohyphomycosis,[132] actinomycosis,[133] nocardiosis,[134-136] and toxoplasmosis.[137-141] Several infectious agents have been documented to cause chronic meningitis in unique epidemiologic circumstances (*Coenurus cerebralis, Toxocara canis*)[1,142,143] or in isolated case reports (*Leptospira icterohaemorrhagiae,* mucormycosis)[1,144] and are not discussed here. Other infections in which CNS involvement is a late manifestation with few related symptoms, or leptomeningitis is noted pathologically but not clinically, also are not reviewed.

Mollaret's Meningitis

Mollaret's meningitis[145] is not a chronic meningitis; rather, it is a rare syndrome in which recurrent episodes of aseptic meningitis are characterized by acute onset of fever, headache, photophobia, and nuchal rigidity.[10,145] The symptoms resolve spontaneously within 2 to 5 days, and the patient returns to normal, only to undergo recurrent attacks weeks to months later.

This disease is most commonly seen in young adults, although the age range of reported cases is 5 to 57 years. There is no predisposition by sex. Lumbar puncture reveals a mixed lymphocytic and polymorphonuclear pleocytosis, with leukocytes ranging from hundreds to thousands per cubic millimeter. The protein concentration is only mildly elevated, usually being less than 100 mg/mL, and the glucose concentration is usually normal. Early in an attack, large, fragile mononuclear cells are seen. Mollaret called these "endothelial" cells.[145] However, electron microscopy and monoclonal antibody techniques have demonstrated that these cells are monocytes.[146,147] After 24 hours the CSF pleocytosis has greatly decreased and is mainly lymphocytic; Mollaret's "endothelial" cells and neutrophils have disappeared. By 1 week, the CSF has completely normalized. Rarely, focal neurologic deficits have been associated with acute episodes, but they are self-limited and resolve during the episode without sequelae.

Studies have shown a probable link between HSV and some cases of Mollaret's meningitis.[16-19,148-152] HSV-2 (and less commonly HSV-1) DNA has been detected in the CSF by PCR in patients with benign recurrent aseptic meningitis. In a few reports, the classic Mollaret cells were seen in the same CSF samples that contained the HSV DNA.[17,149] CSF from patients between episodes or from control patients without a recurrent meningitis syndrome did not have the viral DNA. This association with HSV has potential therapeutic importance because acyclovir therapy might prevent further recurrences.

Neoplastic Meningitis

The noninfectious diseases causing chronic meningitis may be difficult to diagnose and distinguish from occult infections (see Table 82-2). The frequency of neoplastic meningitis (4%-7% of patients with extraneural cancer) is increasing due to longer survival in patients with extraneural cancer and improved neuroimaging techniques.[153] Primary and metastatic, hematologic, and solid tumors all may involve the meninges diffusely to cause a similar clinical syndrome. In the case of acute leukemia and lymphoma,[154-156] CNS involvement usually occurs in the setting of known underlying malignancy. The major diagnostic problem is to distinguish CNS involvement by the tumor from superimposed CNS infection and the uncommon paraneoplastic syndromes. Primary brain tumors, including gliomas, pinealomas, ependymomas, and choroid plexus tumors, may involve the meninges diffusely,[157] sometimes without gross parenchymal involvement. A diagnosis can be difficult in such cases. In metastatic "meningeal carcinomatosis,"[158-162] the nature of the meningeal process also may be difficult to ascertain. In one large series, the primary tumor had not been diagnosed by the time of onset of neurologic symptoms in 75% of the patients.[159] Typically the onset of symptoms is subacute, with intractable headache a prominent complaint along with mental changes. Cranial neuropathy occurs in 50% of cases, and meningismus in about 20%. Fever usually is absent, or when it occurs is associated with an intercurrent infection. Characteristically, neurologic signs far exceed symptoms and indicate widespread neurologic dysfunction; cerebral, cranial nerve, and spinal involvement are noted in 50% of patients on initial physical examination.

The CSF is abnormal; 72% of patients have a pleocytosis, often minimal, although some patients have a marked cellular response. The glucose content is depressed in 38% of patients initially and in 72% during serial examinations. The finding of marked hypoglycorrhachia in the presence of minimal pleocytosis should suggest this diagnosis. In one series, CSF cytology results were diagnostic in 42% of patients in the first study and in 74% when multiple specimens were processed.[162] Of the ancillary neurodiagnostic tests, the myelogram was particularly helpful diagnostically and revealed multiple nodular deposits on nerve roots in 39% of the cases. MRI of the brain with gadolinium reveals enhancement and thickening in the meninges with better sensitivity than CT scan.[163,164] In contrast to the observation that leptomeningeal involvement is fairly specific for infectious etiologies, demonstration of pachymeningitis appears less specific for cancer.[37,38] The finding of markedly elevated CSF levels of β-glucuronidase is suggestive of meningeal carcinomatosis.[165,166] The most common primary sites of malignancy causing this syndrome are the breast, lung, stomach, pancreas, and skin (melanoma). Although neurologic signs may fluctuate and even partly regress, the course of meningeal carcinomatosis usually is rapidly progressive with involvement of all parts of the neuraxis. Because the primary tumor may be occult and extraneural metastatic sites lacking, cytologic examination of multiple CSF specimens is appropriate in all patients with undiagnosed chronic meningitis.

Sarcoid Meningitis

Neurologic involvement is seen in 5% of patients with sarcoidosis[167-173]; however, among these patients, almost 33% present with neurologic signs as their initial indication of sarcoidosis and 17% have neurologic signs as the sole manifestation of the disease.[171] The clinical syndrome of sarcoid meningitis often includes cranial nerve palsies, long-tract and cerebellar abnormalities, and changes in mentation. Peripheral seventh cranial nerve paralysis is the most common manifestation of neurosarcoidosis.[174] The predilection for the basilar meninges with extension to the hypothalamus results in diabetes insipidus in 14% to 30% of cases; this is of diagnostic significance because it rarely occurs in other forms of chronic meningitis. In addition, peripheral neuropathies accompany CNS sarcoidosis in 14% of patients but generally are unusual in chronic meningitis except for Lyme disease. Seizures occur in 15% of patients and are associated with an acute, severe, progressive, and relapsing course.[175]

Characteristic CSF abnormalities consist of a minimal lymphocytic pleocytosis in 60% of patients and hypoglycorrhachia in 10% to 18%. The diagnosis of CNS sarcoidosis in patients with classic systemic manifestations of the disease is complicated by the necessity of excluding superimposed tuberculosis or cryptococcosis, both of which occur with increased frequency in patients with sarcoidosis and in patients receiving corticosteroid therapy. The diagnosis is more difficult when disease is limited to the CNS. Even the demonstration of granulomas in meningeal biopsy specimens is not specific. Serum and CSF concentrations of angiotensin-converting enzyme may be elevated in neurosarcoidosis,[176-178] although increased concentrations also are seen in malignant and bacterial meningitis.[177] More than two thirds of patients with neurosarcoidosis have evidence of thoracic disease; chest radiography and gallium scanning may be helpful in locating a site for diagnostic biopsy.[171,172] Prolonged corticosteroid therapy is recommended for the treatment of CNS sarcoidosis; cytotoxic drug therapy may be required in some cases.[174,179] Cyclosporine also has been used in refractory cases.[180]

Low-dose irradiation of the CNS has been used with apparent advantage in several patients.[171,181] Overall prognosis is good.[171]

Other Noninfectious Causes

Granulomatous angiitis is a necrotizing vasculitis of small leptomeningeal and perforating arteries and veins usually isolated to the CNS.[182-187] The process usually manifests as headache, confusion, focal neurologic findings, and CSF pleocytosis. Mean age of onset is the mid-40s. CSF findings include a lymphocytic pleocytosis and increased protein levels. Cerebral angiograms show a "string of beads" appearance in 27% to 65% of patients with primary angiitis of the CNS; however, a normal angiogram is seen in 13% to 44% of reported cases.[184] MRI findings are highly variable from normal to diffusely abnormal; high signal on T_2-weighted images may be seen, both focal or diffuse, and mainly in deep and subcortical white matter.[188] Biopsy is the gold standard for diagnosis; because of the focal nature of the disease, the sensitivity is only 71%.[189] Untreated, this disease is thought to be uniformly fatal. Successful long-term outcomes have been reported with a combination of corticosteroid and cytotoxic immunosuppressive therapy.[183] On clinical and pathologic grounds, this syndrome is distinct from sarcoidosis, giant cell arteritis, and Wegener's granulomatosis. An ipsilateral granulomatous angiitis of the middle cerebral artery may follow ophthalmic zoster; in some instances, varicella-zoster virus has been cultured from involved cerebral blood vessels.

A subacute meningoencephalitis usually occurs early in the course of the Vogt-Koyanagi-Harada syndrome (uveomeningoencephalitis).[190-194] The clinical diagnosis is established by the development of severe, protracted, granulomatous uveitis; depigmentary skin changes such as poliosis (whitening of the eyebrows and eyelashes) and vitiligo; and dysacusis and tinnitus 3 months or more into the illness. The CSF shows predominantly lymphocytic pleocytosis. The CNS disease gradually resolves spontaneously. This syndrome is considered to be an autoimmune disease directed against an antigenic component of the melanocytes, possibly tyrosinase or a tyrosinase-related protein. It has a predilection for races with greater pigmentation: Asians, Latinos, Native Americans, and Asian Indians. Corticosteroids have been reported to preserve visual acuity.[192-194]

Of the patients with Behçet's disease (recurrent oral and genital ulcerations and uveitis), CNS involvement develops in 10% to 25%.[195-201] The neurologic manifestations include aseptic meningitis, meningoencephalitis, seizures, cranial nerve palsies, and hemiparesis. Occasionally they precede other features of the syndrome. Neurologic involvement is caused by primary neural parenchymal disease or secondary to major vascular involvement. CSF abnormalities include an elevation of protein concentrations, normal glucose, and minimal pleocytosis (usually fewer than 60 cells/mm³ with both lymphocytes and polymorphonuclear cells reported). Poor prognostic signs are parenchymal involvement, brain-stem involvement, elevated protein and/or pleocytosis in the CSF, and relapse during steroid taper.[201]

Other connective tissue diseases that may mimic chronic meningitis include systemic lupus erythematosus (SLE), Sjögren's syndrome, polyarteritis nodosa, and Wegener's granulomatosis. SLE can manifest as acute aseptic meningitis (less than 5% of patients with SLE),[202] but most SLE patients presenting with meningitis have an infectious cause.[203,204] Polyarteritis nodosa involves the CNS in 23% to 53% of cases, but almost all have evidence of systemic disease also (e.g., abdominal pain, renal dysfunction).[205] Although CNS involvement in Wegener's granulomatosis occurs in 25% to 50% of cases, meningitis is a rare manifestation, causing headache, cranial neuropathies, and a mild lymphocytic pleocytosis.[206] Rarely, meningitis is the presenting sign.[207] Sjögren's syndrome has been associated with a chronic inflammatory meningoencephalitis mimicking Alzheimer's dementia; the CSF is remarkably normal, but perivascular inflammation is seen on brain biopsy. This complication of Sjögren's syndrome responds dramatically to glucocorticoid therapy.[208]

A syndrome of chronic benign lymphocytic meningitis was first reported in 1973 from the National Hospitals for Nervous Diseases in London.[209] Over a 6-year period, observers identified 12 cases of idiopathic chronic meningitis. Five patients had very low CSF glucose or severe neurologic deficit, which distinguished them from the seven other patients with chronic benign lymphocytic meningitis. The CSF of these patients had only mildly elevated protein, modest CSF pleocytosis (usually <50 cells/mm³), and normal glucose. Three patients were treated with glucocorticoids, and two improved on this therapy. Patients observed for 1 to 9 years had persistent pleocytosis but no significant clinical deterioration.

Three more studies have supported the existence of a benign or steroid-responsive chronic meningitis.[4,6,7] In a retrospective review of chronic meningitis in a New Zealand hospital, 28 of 83 patients had idiopathic meningitis.[4] Of these, 50% responded to empirical antituberculosis therapy, 33% responded to steroids, and 14% improved on no therapy. A distinguishing feature of the steroid-responsive group was a normal CSF glucose concentration. Two patients died after withdrawal of glucocorticoid therapy. In a series of 37 patients who underwent brain biopsy for chronic meningitis at the Mayo Clinic between 1989 and 1993,[7] 66% of patients ultimately were treated with glucocorticoids after the biopsy revealed chronic inflammation. Half of these patients improved, and none was reported to have deteriorated on corticosteroid therapy. Of note, 33% were sarcoid meningitis. A larger series from the Mayo Clinic reported on 49 patients with chronic idiopathic meningitis seen between 1978 and 1990.[6] Although only 10 of these patients ultimately had a definitive diagnosis, of whom 8 had neoplastic meningitis, the follow-up observations of the 39 idiopathic cases revealed that 85% had a good outcome despite a prolonged illness. Approximately half of the patients received glucocorticoid therapy, often with prompt resolution of symptoms. No patient responded to empirical antituberculosis therapy. Therefore, in their study population, the most useful empirical therapy was corticosteroids rather than antituberculosis medications.

In contrast to the patients with unexplained minimal, self-limited disease, an additional group of patients has an enigmatic chronic meningitis with significant neurologic involvement, a high CSF protein concentration, and sometimes a depressed glucose level.[1] The prognosis in this group is poor. Therapeutic trials may alter the course of the disease, the cultures, and the pathologic findings. A specific diagnosis may be apparent at autopsy, but this is not always the case. A temporal response to antifungal therapy in some cases has implicated an infectious cause; mycotic meningitis too often is associated with negative CSF cultures and only diagnosed after death. Therefore, a thorough diagnostic evaluation followed ultimately by meningeal and brain biopsy and, if appropriate, an empirical trial of amphotericin B or fluconazole with or without glucocorticoid therapy is indicated.

THE IMMUNOCOMPROMISED PATIENT

Chronic meningitis in the immunosuppressed patient with impaired cellular immunity requires special consideration because of the distinctive differential diagnosis. The distribution of pathogens is determined by the nature of the host defense defect.[210] Among renal transplant recipients and patients with lymphoma or leukemia, *C. neoformans* is the most common cause of chronic meningitis.[211] *M. tuberculosis*, *Toxoplasma gondii*, *Nocardia*, *Histoplasma*, and *Coccidioides* also cause chronic meningitis more often in such patients. Progressive multifocal leukoencephalopathy (caused by papovaviruses) may produce profound focal neurologic deficits with minimal or no abnormalities in the CSF. JC virus DNA can be detected in the CSF by PCR.[212] MRI demonstrates progressive lesions in the white matter and is preferred over CT. Hypogammaglobulinemic patients are susceptible to chronic meningoencephalitis secondary to enteroviral infections.[213] Symptoms include headache, seizures, lethargy, weakness, and ataxia; the CSF shows lymphocytic pleocytosis with hypoglycorrhachia.

HIV-1 is associated with multiple neurologic complications either due to the HIV-1 infection,[214-216] opportunistic infections,[217-227] or neoplasm.[221] The neurologic manifestations of HIV are further discussed in Chapter 120 and the management of opportunistic infections in patients with AIDS in Chapter 125 as well as in individual chapters dealing with the specific microbial pathogens. Following are some notable distinguishing characteristics due to HIV infection.

Aseptic meningitis with fever, headache, and meningismus is common in primary HIV infection[215]; symptoms resolve rapidly, but CSF pleocytosis can be found in 10% of asymptomatic HIV-infected patients.[214,216] A mild elevation in protein is also seen, but glucose remains normal. Of note, chronic inflammatory CSF changes can be ascribed to HIV infection only after exclusion of secondary pathogens and neoplasms.

Cryptococcus, the most common opportunistic pathogen to cause meningitis in patients with AIDS, occurs in about 1% to 2% of patients in the United States, the incidence having fallen since highly active antiretroviral therapy became available.[217] Tuberculous meningitis is a more common complication of tuberculosis in HIV-infected persons, occurring in 10% of tuberculosis patients with HIV disease and only 2% of tuberculosis patients without HIV infection in Spain.[218] Clinical presentation, CSF findings, and mortality in HIV-infected patients were similar to those in HIV-negative patients with tuberculous meningitis.[218,219] Risk factors for poor outcome were duration of symptoms greater than 2 weeks before admission and a CD4-positive T-lymphocyte count less than 200 cells/mm³.[218] Meningitis secondary to *Coccidioides*,[220] *Histoplasma*,[86] and *Blastomyces*[129] has also been reported with HIV. Reactivation of *T. gondii* is common in AIDS patients but usually causes ring-enhancing mass lesions rather than meningitis. CNS lymphoma similarly manifests more frequently as mass lesions; lymphocytic meningitis is much less common. PCR detection of Epstein-Barr viral DNA in the CSF suggests primary CNS lymphoma.[221] End-stage AIDS patients are at risk for cytomegalovirus ventriculoencephalitis[222,223]; presenting symptoms include cranial nerve palsies, nystagmus, and confusion, usually in patients with previously diagnosed cytomegalovirus end-organ disease (e.g., retinitis). MRI scans show ependymal enhancement; the CSF has a neutrophilic pleocytosis with hypoglycorrhachia. Cytomegalovirus DNA is detectable by PCR in the CSF.[221] An associated ascending radiculomyelitis with flaccid weakness and hyporeflexia is often seen. Prognosis is grim, with death occurring a median of 4 weeks after diagnosis despite antiviral chemotherapy. Progression of syphilis is accelerated in HIV-infected patients, with more syphilitic meningitis and uveitis seen[224]; usually routine serologic tests confirm the diagnosis.[115,225] Negative serology results in patients with frank syphilitic meningitis have been reported, but follow-up serologic studies were positive.[224,226] Thirty percent of patients with advanced HIV infection and a documented previous history of syphilis have a negative fluorescent treponemal antibody absorption (FTA-ABS) test, calling into question the interpretation of negative serologic findings in AIDS patients.[227] When clinical suspicion for syphilis is high, serologic studies should be repeated in follow-up, looking for delayed seroconversion.

REFERENCES

1. Ellner JJ, Bennett JE. Chronic meningitis. Medicine (Baltimore). 1976;55:341-369.
2. Wilhelm C, Ellner JJ. Chronic meningitis. Neurol Clin. 1986;4:115-141.
3. Swartz M. Chronic meningitis: Many causes to consider. N Engl J Med. 1987;317:957-959.
4. Anderson NE, Willoughby EW. Chronic meningitis without predisposing illness: A review of 83 cases. Q J Med. 1987;63:283-295.
5. Salaki JS, Louria DB, Chmel H. Fungal and yeast infections of the central nervous system: A clinical review. Medicine (Baltimore). 1984;63:108-132.
6. Smith JE, Asamit AJ. Outcome of chronic idiopathic meningitis. Mayo Clin Proc. 1994;69:548-556.
7. Cheng TM, O'Neill BP, Scheithauer BW, et al. Chronic meningitis: The role of meningeal or cortical biopsy. Neurosurgery. 1994;34:590-596.
8. Anderson NE, Willoughby EW, Synek BJL. Leptomeningeal and brain biopsy in chronic meningitis. Aust N Z J Med. 1995;25:703-706.
9. Gripshover BM, Ellner JJ. Chronic meningitis syndrome and meningitis of noninfective or uncertain etiology. In: Scheld WM, Whitley RJ, Durak DT: Infections of the Central Nervous System. Philadelphia: Lippincott Raven; 1997:881-896.
10. Hermans PE, Goldstein NP, Wellman WE. Mollaret's meningitis and differential diagnosis of recurrent meningitis. Am J Med. 1972;52:128-140.
11. Joffle AM, Farley JD, Linden D, et al. Trimethoprim-sulfamethoxazole-associated aseptic meningitis: Case reports and review of the literature. Am J Med. 1989;87:332-338.

12. Marinac JS. Drug- and chemical-induced aseptic meningitis: A review of the literature. Ann Pharmacother. 1992;26:813-821.

13. River Y, Averbuch-Heller L, Weinberger M, et al. Antibiotic induced meningitis. J Neurol Neurosurg Psychiatry. 1994;57:705-708.

14. Lunardi P, Missori P. Cranial and spinal tumors with meningitic onset. Ital J Neurol Sci. 1990;11:145-151.

15. Achard JM, Lallement PY, Veyssier P. Recurrent aseptic meningitis secondary to intracranial epidermoid cyst and Mollaret's meningitis: Two distinct entities or a single disease? A case report and a nosologic discussion. Am J Med. 1990;89:807-810.

16. Berger JR. Benign aseptic (Mollaret's) meningitis after genital herpes. Lancet. 1991;337:1360-1361.

17. Picard FJ, Dekaban GA, Silva J, et al. Mollaret's meningitis associated with herpes simplex type 2 infection. Neurology. 1993;43:1722-1727.

18. Tedder DG, Ashley R, Tyler KL, et al. Herpes simplex virus infection as a cause of benign recurrent lymphocytic meningitis. Ann Intern Med. 1994;121:334-338.

19. Monteyne P, Sindic CJM, Laterre EC. Recurrent meningitis and encephalitis associated with herpes simplex type 2: Demonstration by polymerase chain reaction. Eur Neurol. 1996;36:176-177.

20. Pasquale M, Finelli F, Yockey CC, et al. Recurrent aseptic meningitis in an elderly man: Unusual prodrome of systemic lupus erythematosus. JAMA. 1976;235:1142-1144.

21. Kanekura T, Mizumoto J, Setoyama M. A case of lupus meningitis treated successfully with methylprednisolone pulse therapy. J Dermatol. 1993;20:566-571.

22. Peacock JE Jr, McGinnis MR, Cohen MS. Persistent neutrophilic meningitis: Report of four cases and review of the literature. Medicine (Baltimore). 1984;63:379-395.

23. Weller PF. Eosinophilic meningitis. Am J Med. 1993;95:250-253.

24. Ewing GE, Bose GJ, Petersen PK. *Sporothrix schenckii* meningitis in a farmer with Hodgkin's disease. Am J Med. 1980;68:455-457.

25. Kravitz GR, Davies SF, Eckman MR, et al. Chronic blastomycotic meningitis. Am J Med. 1981;71:501.

26. Kranz BR, Thiel E, Thierfelde M. Immunocytochemical identification of meningeal leukemia and lymphoma: Poly-L-lysine-coated slides permit multimarker analysis even with minute cerebrospinal fluid cell specimens. Blood. 1989;73:1942-1950.

27. Rhodes CH, Glantz MJ, Glantz L, et al. A comparison of polymerase chain reaction examination of cerebral spinal fluid and conventional cytology in the diagnosis of lymphomatous meningitis. Cancer. 1996;77:543-548.

28. Wheat LJ, Batteiger BE, Sathapatayarongs B. *Histoplasma capsulatum* infections of the central nervous system: A clinical review. Medicine (Baltimore). 1990;69:244-260.

29. Wheat J, French M, Batteiger B, et al. Cerebrospinal fluid *Histoplasma* antibodies in central nervous system histoplasmosis. Arch Intern Med. 1985;145:1237-1240.

30. Wheat LJ, Kohler RB, Tewari RP, et al. Significance of *Histoplasma* antigen in the cerebrospinal fluid of patients with meningitis. Arch Intern Med. 1989;149:302-304.

31. Scott EN, Kaufman L, Brown AC, et al. Serologic studies in the diagnosis and management of meningitis due to *Sporothrix schenckii*. N Engl J Med. 1987;317:935-940.

32. Kox LFF, Kuijper S, Kolk AHJ. Early diagnosis of tuberculous meningitis by polymerase chain reaction. Neurology. 1995;45:2228-2232.

33. Lin JJ, Harn HJ, Hsu YD, et al. Rapid diagnosis of tuberculous meningitis by polymerase chain reaction assay of cerebrospinal fluid. J Neurol. 1995;242:147-152.

34. Miorner H, Sjobring U, Nayak P, et al. Diagnosis of tuberculous meningitis: A comparative analysis of 3 immunoassays, an immune complex assay and the polymerase chain reaction. Tuber Lung Dis. 1995;76:381-386.

35. Bonington A, Strang JIG, Klapper PE, et al. Use of Roche AMPLICOR *Mycobacterium tuberculosis* PCR in early diagnosis of tuberculous meningitis. J Clin Microbiol. 1998;36:1251-1254.

36. Rajo MC, Perez Del Molina ML, Lado Lado FL, et al. Rapid diagnosis of tuberculous meningitis by ligase chain reaction amplification. Scand J Infect Dis. 2002;34:14-16.

37. Kioumehr F, Dadsetan MR, Feldman N, et al. Postcontrast MRI of cranial meninges: Leptomeningitis versus pachymeningitis. J Comput Assist Tomogr 1995;19:713-720.

38. Phillips ME, Ryals TJ, Kambhu SA, Yuh WT. Neoplastic vs inflammatory meningeal enhancement with Gd-DPTA. J Comput Assist Tomogr 1990;14:536-541.

39. Takahashi M. Infection of the central nervous system. Curr Opin Neurol Neurosurg. 1992;5:849-853.

40. Stocksill MT, Kauffman CA. Comparison of cryptococcal and tuberculous meningitis. Arch Neurol. 1983;40:81-85.

41. Klein NC, Damsker B, Hirschman SZ. Mycobacterial meningitis: Retrospective analysis from 1970-1983. Am J Med. 1985;79:29-34.

42. Kent SJ, Crowe SM, Yung A, et al. Tuberculous meningitis: A thirty year review. Clin Infect Dis. 1993;17:987-994.

43. Thwaites GE, Chau TTH, Stepniewska K, et al. Diagnosis of adult tuberculous meningitis by use of clinical and laboratory features. Lancet. 2002;360:1287-1292.

44. Rich AR, McCordock HA. The pathogenesis of tuberculous meningitis. Bull Johns Hopkins Hosp. 1933;52:5-38.

45. Merritt HH, Fremont-Smith F. Cerebrospinal fluid in tuberculous meningitis. Arch Neurol Psychol. 1935;33:516-536.

46. Jeren T, Beus I. Characteristics of cerebrospinal fluid in tuberculous meningitis. Acta Cytol. 1982;26:678.

47. Johnson JL, Ellner JJ. Tuberculous meningitis. In: Evans RW, Baskin DS, Vatsu FM, eds. Prognosis in Neurological Disease. New York: Oxford University Press; 1991:209-225.

48. Yechoor VK, Shandera WX, Rodriguez P, et al. Tuberculous meningitis among adults with and without HIV infection. Arch Intern Med. 1996;156:1710-1716.

49. Girgis NI, Sultan Y, Farid Z, et al. Tuberculosis meningitis, Abbassia Fever Hospital Naval Medical Research Unit No. 3-Cairo, Egypt, from 1976 to 1996. Am J Trop Med Hyg. 1998;58:28-34.

50. Verdon R, Chevret S, Laissy JP, et al. Tuberculous meningitis in adults: A review of 48 cases. Clin Infect Dis. 1996;22:982-988.

51. Kent SJ, Crowe SM, Yung A, et al. Tuberculous meningitis: A 30-year review. Clin Infect Dis. 1993;17:987-994.

52. Daniel TM. New approaches to the rapid diagnosis of tuberculous meningitis. J Infect Dis. 1987;155:599-602.

53. Thomson RB Jr, Bertram H. Laboratory diagnosis of central nervous system infections. Infect Dis Clin North Am. 2001;15:1047-1071.

54. Mak W, Cheung RT, Ho SL, et al. Tuberculosis meningitis in Hong Kong: Experience in a regional hospital. Int J Tuberc Lung Dis. 1998;2:1040-1043.

55. Correa MF, Armas E, Diaz D, et al. Diagnosis of tuberculosis meningitis by detection of adenosine deaminase activity and amplification of nucleotide sequences with PCR. Acta Cient Venez. 2001;52(Suppl 1):52-54 (Spanish).

56. Ribera E, Martinez-Vazquez JM, Ocana I, et al. Activity of adenosine deaminase in cerebrospinal fluid for the diagnosis and follow up of tuberculous meningitis in adults. J Infect Dis. 1987;155:603-607.

57. Petterson T, Klockars M, Weber TH, et al. Diagnostic value of cerebrospinal fluid adenosine deaminase determination. Scand J Infect Dis. 1991;23:97-100.

58. Lopez-Cortez LF, Cruz-Ruiz M, Gomez-Mateous J, et al. Adenosine deaminase activity in the CSF of patients with aseptic meningitis: Utility in the diagnosis of tuberculous meningitis or neurobrucellosis. Clin Infect Dis. 1995;20:525-530.

59. Thwaites GE, Simmons CP, Than Ha Quyen N, et al. Pathophysiology and prognosis in Vietnamese adults with tuberculous meningitis. J Infect Dis. 2003;188:1105-1115.

60. Butler WT, Alling DW, Spickard A, et al. Diagnostic and prognostic value of clinical and laboratory findings in cryptococcal meningitis: A follow-up study of forty patients. N Engl J Med. 1964;270:59-66.

61. Littman ML, Walter JE. Cryptococcosis: Current status. Am J Med. 1968;45:922-932.

62. Diamond RD, Bennett JE. Prognostic factors in cryptococcal meningitis: A study of 111 cases. Ann Intern Med. 1974;80:176-181.

63. Chuck SZ, Sande MA. Infections with *Cryptococcus neoformans* in the acquired immunodeficiency syndrome. N Engl J Med. 1989;321:794-799.

64. Clark RA, Greer D, Atkinson W, et al. Spectrum of *Cryptococcus neoformans* infection in 68 patients infected with human immunodeficiency virus. Rev Infect Dis. 1990;12:768-777.

65. Saag MS, Powderly WG, Cloud GA, et al. Comparison of amphotericin B with fluconazole in the treatment of acute AIDS-associated cryptococcal meningitis. N Engl J Med. 1992;326:83-89.

66. Darras-Joly C, Chevret S, Wolff M, et al. *Cryptococcus neoformans* infection in France: Epidemiologic features of and early prognostic parameters for 76 patients who were infected with human immunodeficiency virus. Clin Infect Dis. 1996;23:369-376.

67. Van der Horst CM, Saag MS, Cloud GA, et al. Treatment of cryptococcal meningitis associated with the acquired immunodeficiency syndrome. N Engl J Med. 1997;337:15-21.

68. Mitchell DH, Sorrell TC, Allworth AM, et al. Cryptococcal disease of the CNS in immunocompetent hosts: Influence of cryptococcal variety on clinical manifestations and outcome. Clin Infect Dis. 1995;20:611-616.

69. Speed B, Dunt D. Clinical and host differences between infections with the two varieties of *Cryptococcus neoformans*. Clin Infect Dis. 1995;21:28-34.

70. Aberg JA, Watson J, Segal M, Chang LW. Clinical utility of monitoring serum cryptococcal antigen (sCRAG) titers in patients with AIDS-related cryptococcal disease. HIV Clin Trials. 2000;1:1-6.

71. Currie BP, Freundlich LF, Soto MA, et al. False-negative cerebrospinal fluid cryptococcal latex agglutination tests for patients with culture-positive cryptococcal meningitis. J Clin Microbiol. 1993;31:2519-2522.

72. Iyer RS, Banker DD. Cryptococcal meningitis in AIDS. Indian J Med Sci. 2002;56:593-597.

73. Rappelli P, Are R, Casu G, et al. Development of a nested PCR for detection of *Cryptococcus neoformans* in cerebrospinal fluid. J Clin Microbiol. 1998;36:3438-3440.

74. Bialek R, Weiss M, Bekure-Nemariam K, et al. Detection of *Cryptococcus neoformans* DNA in tissue samples by nested and real-time PCR assays. Clin Diagn Lab Immunol. 2002;9:461-469.

75. Smith CE, Saito MT, Simons SA. Pattern of 39,500 serologic tests in coccidioidomycosis. JAMA. 1956;160:546.

76. Winn WA. Coccidioidal meningitis: A follow-up report. In: Ajello L, ed. Coccidioidomycosis. Tucson: University of Arizona Press; 1967:55.

77. Deresinski SC, Stevens DA. Coccidioidomycosis in compromised hosts. Medicine (Baltimore). 1974;54:377.

78. Bouza E, Dreyer JS, Hewitt WL, et al. Coccidioidal meningitis: An analysis of 31 cases and review of the literature. Medicine (Baltimore). 1981;60:139-171.

79. Vincent T, Galgiani JN, Huppert M, et al. The natural history of coccidioidal meningitis: VA-Armed Forces cooperative studies 1955-1958. Clin Infect Dis. 1993;16:247-254.

80. Ragland S, Arsura E, Ismail Y, et al. Eosinophilic pleocytosis in coccidioidal meningitis: Frequency and significance. Am J Med. 1993;95:254-257.

81. Tucker RM, Denning DW, Dupont B, et al. Itraconazole therapy for chronic coccidioidal meningitis. Ann Intern Med. 1990;112:108-112.

82. Galgiani JN, Peng T, Lewis ML, et al. Cerebrospinal fluid antibodies detected by ELISA against a 33-kDa antigen from spherules of *Coccidioides immitis* in patients with coccidioidal meningitis. J Infect Dis. 1996;173:499-502.

83. Erly WK, Bellon RJ, Seeger JF, Carmody RF. MR imaging of acute coccidioidal meningitis. Am J Neuroradiol. 1999;20(3):509-514.

84. Tynes BS, Crutcher JC, Utz JP. *Histoplasma* meningitis. Ann Intern Med. 1963;59:615-621.

85. Gelfand JA, Bennett JE. Active *Histoplasma* meningitis of 22 years duration. JAMA. 1975;233:1294-1295.
86. Wheat LJ, Connolly-Stringfield PA, Baker RJ, et al. Disseminated histoplasmosis in the acquired immunodeficiency syndrome: Review of the literature. Medicine (Baltimore). 1990;69:361-374.
87. LeMonte AM, Washum KE, Smedema ML, et al. Amphotericin B combined with itraconazole or fluconazole for treatment of histoplasmosis. J Infect Dis 2000;182: 545-550.
88. Haynes RR, Connolly PA, Durkin MM, et al. Antifungal therapy for central nervous system histoplasmosis, using newly developed intracranial model of infection. J Infect Dis. 2002;185:1830-1832.
89. Pachner AR, Steere AC. The triad of neurologic manifestations of Lyme disease: Meningitis, cranial neuritis, and radiculoneuritis. Neurology (NY). 1985;35:47-53.
90. Pachner AR. Neurologic manifestations of Lyme disease, the new "Great Imitator." Rev Infect Dis. 1989;11:S1482-S1486.
91. Halperin JJ, Volkeman DJ, Wu P. Central nervous system abnormalities in Lyme neuroborreliosis. Neurology. 1991;41:1571-1582.
92. Shapiro Ed, Gerber MA. Lyme disease. Clin Infect Dis. 2000;31:533-542.
93. Pachner AR. Early disseminated Lyme disease: Lyme meningitis. Am J Med. 1995;98:4A30S-4A43S.
94. Tugwell P, Dennis DT, Weinstein A, et al. Laboratory evaluation in the diagnosis of Lyme disease. Ann Intern Med. 1997;127:1109-1123.
95. Steere AC, Berrardi VP, Weeks KE, et al. Evaluation of the intrathecal antibody response to *Borrelia burgdorferi* as a diagnostic test for Lyme neuroborreliosis. J Infect Dis. 1990;761:1203-1209.
96. Nocton JJ, Bloom BJ, Rutledge BJ, et al. Detection of *Borrelia burgdorferi* DNA by polymerase chain reaction in cerebrospinal fluid in Lyme neuroborreliosis. J Infect Dis. 1996;174:623-627.
97. Schwaiger M, Peter O, Cassinotti P. Routine diagnosis of *Borrelia burgdorferi* (sensu lato) infections using a real-time PCR assay. Clin Microbiol Infect. 2001;7:461-469.
98. Denti JH. Cysticercosis cerebri-cestode infestation of the human brain. JAMA. 1957;164:401.
99. Garcia HH, Gonzalez AE, Evans CA, et al; Cysticercosis Working Group in Peru. *Taenia solium* cysticercosis. Lancet. 2003;362:547-556.
100. Garcia HH, Del Brutto OH. Imaging findings in neurocysticercosis. Acta Trop. 2003;87:71-78.
101. Garcia HH, Evans CA, Nash TE, et al. Current consensus guidelines for treatment of neurocysticercosis. Clin Microbiol Rev. 2002;15:747-756.
102. Earnest MP, Reller LD, Filley CM, et al. Neurocysticercosis in the United States: 35 cases and a review. Rev Infect Dis. 1987;9:961-979.
103. Garcia HH, Harrison LJ, Parkhouse RM, et al. A specific antigen-detection ELISA for the diagnosis of human neurocysticercosis. The Cysticercosis Working Group in Peru. Trans R Soc Trop Med Hyg. 1998;92:411-414.
104. DelBrutto OH, Rajshekhar V, White AC Jr, et al. Proposed diagnostic criteria for neurocysticercosis. Neurology. 2001;57:177-183.
105. Garcia HH, Gonzalez AE, Giman RH. Cysticercosis Working Group in Peru. Diagnosis, treatment, and control of *Taenia solium* cysticercosis. Curr Opin Infect Dis. 2003;16:411-419.
106. Shandera WX, White AC, Chen JC, et al. Neurocysticercosis in Houston, Texas: A report of 112 cases. Medicine (Baltimore). 1994;73:37-52.
107. Bayer AS, Edwards JE Jr, Seidel JS, et al. *Candida* meningitis. Medicine (Baltimore). 1976;55:477-486.
108. Fernandiz M, Moylett EH, Noyola DE, Baker CJ. Candidal meningitis in neonates: A 10-year review. Clin Infect Dis. 2000;31:458-463.
109. Moylett EH. Neonatal *Candida* meningitis. Semin Pediatr Infect Dis. 2003;14:115-122.
110. Doctor BA, Newman N, Minich NM, et al. Clinical outcomes of neonatal meningitis in very-low-birth-weight infants. Clin Pediatr (Phila). 2001;40(9):473-480.
111. Voice RA, Bradley SF, Sangeorzan JA, et al. Chronic candidal meningitis: An uncommon manifestation of candidiasis. Clin Infect Dis. 1994;19:60-66.
112. Merritt HH, Adams RD, Solomon HC. Neurosyphilis. New York: Oxford University Press; 1946:24.
113. Hooshmand H, Escobar MR, Kopf SW. Neurosyphilis: A study of 241 patients. JAMA. 1972;219:726-729.
114. Katz DA, Berger JR, Duncan RC. Neurosyphilis: A comparative study of the effects of infection with human immunodeficiency virus. Arch Neurol. 1993;50:243-249.
115. Flood J, Weinstock HS, Guroy M, et al. Neurosyphilis during the AIDS epidemic, San Francisco, 1985-1992. J Infect Dis. 1998;177:931-940.
116. Marra CM, Gary DW, Kuypers J, et al. Diagnosis of neurosyphilis in patients infected with human immunodeficiency virus type 1. J Infect Dis. 1996;174:219-221.
117. Ormerod LD, Puklin JE, Sobel JD. Syphilitic posterior uveitis: Correlative findings and significance. Clin Infect Dis. 2001;32(12):1661-1673.
118. Brightbill TC, Ihmeidan IH, Post MJ, et al. Neurosyphilis in HIV-positive and HIV-negative patients: Neuroimaging findings. Am J Neuroradiol. 1995;16(4):703-711.
119. Nichols E. Meningoencephalitis due to brucellosis. Ann Intern Med. 1951;35:673.
120. Bouza E, Garcia de la Torre M, Parras F, et al. *Brucella* meningitis. Rev Infect Dis. 1987;9:810-822.
121. McLean DR, Russell N, Khan MY. Neurobrucellosis: Clinical and therapeutic features. Clin Infect Dis. 1992;15:582-590.
122. Akdeniz H, Irmak H, Anlar O, et al. Central nervous system brucellosis: Presentation, diagnosis and treatment. J Infect. 1998;36:297-301.
123. Bodur H, Erbay A, Akinci E, et al. Neurobrucellosis in an endemic area of brucellosis. Scand J Infect Dis. 2003;35:94-97.
124. Kaufman CA, Hajjeh R, Chapman SW. Practice guidelines for the management of patients with sporotrichosis. For the Mycoses Study Group. Infectious Diseases Society of America. Clin Infect Dis. 2000;30:684-687.
125. Koo J, Pien F, Kliks MM. *Angiostrongylus (Parastrongylus)* eosinophilic meningitis. Rev Infect Dis. 1988;10:1155-1162.
126. Slom T, Johnson S. Eosinophilic meningitis. Curr Infect Dis Rep. 2003;5:322-328.
127. Tsai HC, Liu YC, Kunin CM, et al. Eosinophilic meningitis caused by *Angiostrongylus cantonensis* associated with eating raw snails: Correlation of brain magnetic resonance imaging scans with clinical findings. Am J Trop Med Hyg. 2003;68:281-285.
128. Wilhelmj CM. The primary meningeal form of systemic blastomycosis. Am J Med Sci. 1925;169:172.
129. Pappas PG, Pottage JC, Powderly WF, et al. Blastomycosis in patients with the acquired immunodeficiency syndrome. Ann Intern Med. 1992;116:847-853.
130. Friedman JA, Wijdicks EF, Fulgham JR, Wright AJ. Meningoencephalitis due to *Blastomyces dermatitidis:* Case report and literature review. Mayo Clin Proc. 2000;75:403-408.
131. Pereira WC, Raphael A, Tehuto RA, et al. Localizacao encefalica da blastomicose sulAmericana: Consideracoes a proposito de 9 casos. Arq Neuropsiquiatr. 1965; 23:113.
132. Bennett JE, Bonner H, Jennings AE, et al. Chronic meningitis caused by *Cladosporium trichoides*. Am J Clin Pathol. 1973;59:398-407.
133. Smego RA Jr. Actinomycosis of the central nervous system. Rev Infect Dis. 1987;9:855-865.
134. Richter RW, Silva M, Neu HC, et al. The neurological aspects of *Nocardia asteroides* infection. Infect Nerv Sys. 1968;44:424.
135. Bross JE, Gordon G. Nocardial meningitis: Case reports and review. Rev Infect Dis. 1991;13:160-165.
136. Mok CC, Lau CS, Poon SP. Primary nocardial meningitis in systemic lupus erythematosus. Br J Rheumatol. 1995;34:178-181.
137. Townsend JJ, Wolinsky JS, Baringer JR, et al. Acquired toxoplasmosis: A neglected cause of treatable nervous system disease. Arch Neurol. 1975;32:335-343.
138. Grines C, Plouffe JF, Baird IM, et al. *Toxoplasma* meningoencephalitis with hypoglycorrhachia. Arch Intern Med. 1981;141:935.
139. Cohen BA. Neurologic manifestations of toxoplasmosis in AIDS. Semin Neurol. 1999;19:201-211.
140. Montoya JG. Laboratory diagnosis of *Toxoplasma gondii* infection and toxoplasmosis. J Infect Dis. 2002;185(Suppl 1):S73-S82.
141. Miller RF, Hall-Craggs MA, Costa DC, et al. Magnetic resonance imaging, thallium-210 SPECT scanning, and laboratory analyses for discrimination of cerebral lymphoma and toxoplasmosis in AIDS. Sex Transm Infect. 1998;74:258-264.
142. Vidal JE, Sztajnbok J, Seguro AC. Eosinophilic meningoencephalitis due to *Toxocara canis*: Case report and review of the literature. Am J Trop Med Hyg. 2003;69; 341-343.
143. Xinou E, Lefkopoulos A, Gelagoti M, et al. CT and MR imaging findings in cerebral toxocaral disease. Am J Neuroradiol. 2003;24;714-718.
144. Jones PG, Gilman RM, Medeiros AA, et al. Focal intracranial mucormycosis presenting as chronic meningitis. JAMA. 1981;24:2063.
145. Mollaret MP. La meningite endothelio-leucotaire multirecurrent benigne: Syndrome nouveau ou maladie nouvelle? Rev Neurol. 1981;9:81-84.
146. Lowe E. Mollaret's meningitis: A case report. Acta Cytol. 1982;26:338-340.
147. Stoppe G, Stark E, Patzold U. Mollaret's meningitis: CSF immunohistological examinations. J Neurol. 1987;234:103-106.
148. Yamamoto LJ, Tedder DG, Ashley R, et al. Herpes simplex virus type 1 DNA in the cerebrospinal fluid of a patient with Mollaret's meningitis. N Engl J Med. 1991;325:1082-1085.
149. Picard FJ, Dekaban GA, Silva J, et al. Mollaret's meningitis associated with herpes simplex type 2 infection. Neurology. 1993;43:1722-1727.
150. Chan TY, Parwani AV, Levi AW, et al. Mollaret's meningitis: Cytopathologic analysis of 14 cases. Diagn Cytopathol. 2003;28:227-231.
151. Kojima Y, Hashiguchi H, Hashimoto T, et al. Recurrent herpes simplex virus type 2: A case report of Mollaret's meningitis. Jpn J Infect Dis. 2002;55; 85-88.
152. Tang YW, Cleavinger PJ, Li H, et al. Analysis of candidate host immunogenetic determinants in HSV-associated Mollaret's meningitis. Clin Infect Dis. 2000;30: 176-178.
153. Kim L, Glantz MJ. Neoplastic meningitis. Curr Treat Options Oncol. 2001;2:517-527.
154. Moore EW, Thomas LB, Shaw RK, et al. The central nervous system in acute leukemia. Arch Intern Med. 1960;105:451.
155. Griffin JW, Thompson RW, Mitchinson MJ, et al. Lymphomatous leptomeningitis. Am J Med. 1971;51:200-208.
156. Hoffman MA, Valderrama E, Fuchs A, et al. Leukemic meningitis in B-cell prolymphocytic leukemia. Cancer. 1995;75:1100-1103.
157. Berg L. Hypoglycorrhachia of noninfectious origin: Diffuse meningeal neoplasia. Neurology (Minn). 1953;3:811-824.
158. Fischer-Williams M, Bosanquet FD, Daniel P. Carcinomatosis of the meninges. Brain. 1955;78:42-58.
159. Vital C, Bruno-Martin F, Henry P, et al. La carcinomatose méningée. Bordeaux Med. 1970;12:2927-2944.
160. Wasserstrom WR, Glass P, Posner JB. Diagnosis and treatment of leptomeningeal metastases from solid tumors. Cancer. 1982;49:759-772.
161. Rosen ST, Aisner J, Makuch RW. Carcinomatous leptomeningitis in small cell lung cancer. Medicine (Baltimore). 1982;61:45-53.
162. Olson ME, Chernik NL, Posner JH. Infiltration of the leptomeninges by systemic cancer: A clinical and pathologic study. Arch Neurol. 1974;30:122-137.

163. Sze G, Soletsky S, Bronen R, et al. MR imaging of the cranial meninges with emphasis on contrast enhancement and meningeal carcinomatosis. AJNR Am J Neuroradiol. 1989;10:965-975.
164. Phillips ME, Ryals TJ, Kambhu SA, et al. Neoplastic vs. inflammatory meningeal enhancement with Gd-DTPA. J Comput Assist Tomogr. 1990;14:536-541.
165. Shuttleworth E, Allen N. CSF β-glucuronidase assay in the diagnosis of neoplastic meningitis. Arch Neurol. 1980;37:684-687.
166. Tallman RD, Kimbrough SM, O'Brien JF, et al. Assay for β-glucuronidase in cerebrospinal fluid: Usefulness for the detection of neoplastic meningitis. Mayo Clin Proc. 1985;60:293-298.
167. Wiederholt WC, Siekert RB. Neurological manifestations of sarcoidosis. Neurology (Minn). 1965;15:1147-1154.
168. Gaines JD, Eckman PB, Remington JS. Low CSF glucose level in sarcoidosis involving the central nervous system. Arch Intern Med. 1970;125:333-336.
169. Delaney P. Neurological manifestations in sarcoidosis. Ann Intern Med. 1977;87:336-345.
170. Stern BJ, Krumholz A, Scott P, et al. Sarcoidosis and its neurological manifestations. Arch Neurol. 1985;42:909-917.
171. Chapelon C, Ziza JM, Piette JC, et al. Neurosarcoidosis: Signs, course and treatment in 35 confirmed cases. Medicine (Baltimore). 1990;69:261-276.
172. Sharma OP. Neurosarcoidosis: A personal perspective based on the study of 37 patients. Chest. 1997;112:220-228.
173. Nowak DA, Widenka DC. Neurosarcoidosis: A review of its intracranial manifestation. J Neurol. 2001;248:363-372.
174. Lower EE, Broderick JP, Brott TG, et al. Diagnosis and management of neurological sarcoidosis. Arch Intern Med. 1997;157:1864-1868.
175. Krumholz A, Stern BJ, Stern EG. Clinical implications of seizures in neurosarcoidosis. Arch Neurol. 1991;48:842-844.
176. Chan Seu CP, Norfolk G, Spokes EG. CSF angiotensin-converting enzyme in neurosarcoidosis. Lancet. 1985;1:456-457.
177. Jones DB, Mitchell D, Horn DB, et al. Cerebrospinal fluid angiotensin converting enzyme levels in the diagnosis of neurosarcoidosis. Scott Med J. 1991;36:144-145.
178. Agobogu BN, Stern BJ, Sewell C, et al. Therapeutic considerations in patients with refractory neurosarcoidosis. Arch Neurol. 1995;52:875-879.
180. Stern BJ, Schonfield SA, Sewell C, et al. The treatment of neurosarcoidosis with cyclosporine. Arch Neurol. 1992;49:1065-1072.
181. Menninger MD, Amdur RJ, Marcus RB Jr. Role of radiotherapy in the treatment of neurosarcoidosis. Am J Clin Oncol. 2003;26:E115-E118.
182. Kolodny EM, Rebeiz JJ, Caviness VS, et al. Granulomatous angiitis of the central nervous system. Arch Neurol. 1968;19:510-524.
183. Cupps TR, Moore PM, Fauci AS. Isolated angiitis of the central nervous system: Prospective diagnostic and therapeutic experience. Am J Med. 1983;74:97-105.
184. Stein RL, Martino CR, Weinert DM, et al. Cerebral angiography as a guide for therapy in isolated central nervous system vasculitis. JAMA. 1987;257:2193-2196.
185. Calabrese LH, Mallek JA. Primary angiitis of the central nervous system: Report of 8 new cases, review of the literature and proposal for new diagnostic criteria. Medicine (Baltimore). 1987;67:20-39.
186. Lie JT. Primary (granulomatous) angiitis of the central nervous system: A clinicopathologic analysis of 15 new cases and a review of the literature. Hum Pathol. 1992;23:164-171.
187. Vollmer TL, Guarnaccia J, Harrington W, et al. Idiopathic granulomatous angiitis of the central nervous system. Arch Neurol. 1993;50:925-930.
188. Campi A, Benndorf G, Filippi M, et al. Primary angiitis of the central nervous system: Serial MRI of the brain and spinal cord. Neuroradiology 2001;43:599-607.
189. Parisi JE, Moore PM. The role of biopsy in vasculitis of the central nervous system. Semin Neurol. 1994;14:341-348.
190. Cowper AR. Harada's disease and Vogt-Koyanagi syndrome. Arch Ophthalmol. 1951;45:367.
191. Pattison EM. Uveomeningoencephalitis syndrome. Arch Neurol. 1965;12:197-205.
192. Moorthy RS, Inomata H, Rao NA. Vogt-Koyanagi-Harada syndrome. Surv Ophthalmol. 1995;39:265-292.
193. Read RW, Rao NA, Cunningham ET. Vogt-Koyanagi-Harada disease. Curr Opin Ophthalmol. 2000;11:437-442.
194. Read RW, Rechodouni A, Butani N, et al. Complications and prognostic factors in Vogt-Koyanagi-Harada disease. 2001;131:599-606.
195. Schotland DL, Wolf SM, White HH, et al. Neurologic aspects of Behçet's disease. Am J Med. 1963;34:544-552.
196. Wolf SM. Involvement of nervous system in Behçet's syndrome. Arch Neurol. 1965;12:315-325.
197. Chajek T, Fainaru M. Behçet's disease: Report of 41 cases and a review of the literature. Medicine (Baltimore). 1975;54:179-196.
198. Serdaroglu P. Behçet's disease and the nervous system. J Neurol. 1998;245:197-205.
199. Kocer N, Islak C, Siva A, et al. CNS involvement in neuro-Behçet syndrome: An MR study. Am J Neuroradiol. 1999;20:1015-1024.
200. Al-Araji A, Sharquie K, Al-Rawi Z. Prevalence and patterns of neurological involvement in Behçet's disease: A prospective study from Iraq. J Neurol Neurosurg Psychiatry. 2003;74:608-613.
201. Akman-Demir G, Serdaroglu P, Tasci B. Clinical patterns of neurological involvement in Behçet's disease: Evaluation of 200 patients. The Neuro-Behçet Study Group. Brain. 1999;122(Pt 11):2171-2182.
202. Sergent JS, Lockshin MD, Klempner MS, et al. Central nervous system disease in systemic lupus erythematosus: Therapy and prognosis. Am J Med. 1975;58:644-654.
203. Wong KL, Woo EK, Yu YL, et al. Neurological manifestations of systemic lupus erythematosus: A prospective study. Q J Med. 1991;81:857-870.

204. Paton NI. Infections in systemic erythematosus patients. Ann Acad Med Singapore. 1997;26:694-700.
205. Sigal LH. The neurological presentation of vasculitic and rheumatologic syndromes. Medicine (Baltimore). 1987;66:157-179.
206. Jinnah HA, Dixon A, Brat DJ, et al. Chronic meningitis with cranial neuropathies in Wegener's granulomatosis. Arthritis Rheum. 1997;40:573-577.
207. Yasuhara T, Fukuhara T, Nakagawa M, et al. Wegener granulomatosis manifesting as meningitis. Case Report. J Neurosurg. 2002;97;1229-1232.
208. Casselli RJ, Scheithauer BW, O'Duffy JD, et al. Chronic inflammatory meningoencephalitis should not be mistaken for Alzheimer's disease. Mayo Clin Proc. 1993;68:846-853.
209. Hopkins AP, Harvey PKP. Chronic benign lymphocytic meningitis. J Neurol Sci. 1973;18:443-453.
210. Cunha BA. Central nervous system infections in the compromised host: A diagnostic approach. Infect Dis Clin North Am. 2001;15:567-590.
211. Hooper DC, Pruitt AA, Rubin RH. Central nervous system infection in the chronically immunosuppressed. Medicine (Baltimore). 1982;61:166-188.
212. Fong IW, Britton CB, Luinstra KE, et al. Diagnostic value of detecting JC virus DNA in cerebrospinal fluid of patients with progressive multifocal leukoencephalopathy. J Clin Microbiol. 1995;33:484-486.
213. McKinney RE, Katz SL, Wilfert CM. Chronic enteroviral meningoencephalitis in agammaglobulinemic patients. Rev Infect Dis. 1987;9:334-356.
214. Mamidi A, DeSimone JA, Pomerantz RJ. Central nervous system infections in individuals with HIV-1 infection. J. Neurovirol. 2002;8:158-167.
215. Schacker T, Collier AC, Hughes J, et al. Clinical and epidemiologic features of primary HIV infection. Ann Intern Med. 1996;125:257-264.
216. Appleman ME, Marshall DW, Porey RL, et al. Cerebrospinal fluid abnormalities in patients without AIDS who are seropositive for the human immunodeficiency virus. J Infect Dis. 1988;158:193-199.
217. Collazos J. Opportunistic infections of the CNS in patients with AIDS: Diagnosis and management. CNS Drugs. 2003;17(12):869-887.
218. Berenguera J, Moreno S, Laguna F, et al. Tuberculous meningitis in patients infected with the human immunodeficiency virus. N Engl J Med. 1992;326:668-672.
219. Sanchez-Portocarrero J, Perez-Cecila E, Jimenez-Escrig A, et al. Tuberculous meningitis: Clinical characteristics and comparison with cryptococcal meningitis in patients with human immunodeficiency virus infection. Arch Neurol. 1996;53:671-676.
220. Fish DG, Ampel NM, Galgiani JN, et al. Coccidioidomycosis during human immunodeficiency virus infection: A review of 77 patients. Medicine (Baltimore).1990;69: 384-391.
221. Cinque P, Scarpellini P, Vago L, et al. Diagnosis of central nervous system complications in HIV-infected patients: Cerebrospinal fluid analysis by the polymerase chain reaction. AIDS. 1997;11:1-17.
222. Kalayjian RC, Cohen MC, Bonomo RA, et al. Cytomegalovirus ventriculoencephalitis in AIDS: A syndrome with distinct clinical and pathological features. Medicine (Baltimore). 1993;72:67-77.
223. McCutchan JA. Cytomegalovirus infections of the nervous system in patients with AIDS. Clin Infect Dis. 1995;20:747-754.
224. Feraru ER, Aronow HA, Lipton RB. Neurosyphilis in AIDS patients: Initial CSF VDRL may be negative. Neurology. 1990;40:541-543.
225. Matlow AG, Rachlis AR. Syphilis serology in human immunodeficiency virus-infected patients with symptomatic neurosyphilis: Case report and review. Rev Infect Dis. 1990;12:703-707.
226. Hicks CB, Benson PM, Lupton GP, et al. Seronegative secondary syphilis in a patient infected with the human immunodeficiency virus (HIV) with Kaposi's sarcoma. Ann Intern Med. 1987;107:492-495.
227. Haas JS, Bolan G, Larse SA, et al. Sensitivity of treponemal tests for detecting prior treated syphilis during human immunodeficiency virus infection. J Infect Dis. 1990;162:862-866.

CHAPTER **83**

Encephalitis, Myelitis, and Neuritis

DIANE E. GRIFFIN

The terms *encephalitis*, *myelitis*, and *neuritis* refer to inflammations of brain, spinal cord, and peripheral nerves, respectively. If sensory or motor spinal roots are specifically involved, the term *radiculitis* may be used. Because meningeal inflammation often accompanies these inflammatory processes, compounded terms such as *meningoencephalitis* and *meningoencephalomyelitis* are sometimes used. None of these terms, however, differentiates between the inflammatory diseases caused by direct invasion of agents and the postinfectious or parainfectious processes that may involve the brain, spinal cord, or peripheral nerves. Because of the diversity of clinical symptoms and signs that can occur with these inflammatory diseases, infectious or parainfectious causes must be entertained in the differential diagnosis of a great variety of neurologic diseases. As with all neurologic diseases, the differential diagnosis is determined by the temporal evolution of signs and symptoms and by the localization of the disease process to one or more anatomic sites by physical findings. Systemic involvement (skin, lung, salivary glands, liver, gastrointestinal tract) or fever may suggest an infectious cause, but these signs may also be absent.

ENCEPHALITIS AND MYELITIS

This section deals with infectious and postinfectious encephalitis and myelitis together because they are often considered in the same differential diagnosis and have considerable overlap in manifestation and causation. Peripheral neuropathies caused by infectious agents are considered, along with tetanus and botulism, in a separate section.

Pathogenesis and Pathologic Characteristics

Infectious agents can produce clinical symptoms and signs within the central nervous system (CNS) by either direct or indirect involvement of neural tissue. Infectious agents can invade the CNS by several pathways. The most common is through the blood. This is best documented for viral infections but is probably also important in rickettsial, bacterial, and fungal infections.[1-3] The initial site of entry of a pathogen and the primary site of replication may be the respiratory tract (e.g., measles, mumps, varicella-zoster, Nipah viruses, *Mycobacterium tuberculosis*, *Cryptococcus neoformans*), the gastrointestinal tract (e.g., poliovirus, echovirus, *Listeria monocytogenes*), the genital tract (e.g., herpes simplex virus), or subcutaneous tissue (e.g., arthropod-borne viruses, *Rickettsia rickettsii*, *Rickettsia typhi*, trypanosomes). Involvement of the CNS is, for the most part, an infrequent consequence of common infections.

In certain viral infections, entry into the CNS occurs by way of the peripheral nerves. Transport systems within motor and sensory axons carry substances from the cell body to the periphery (anterograde transport) and from the periphery to the cell body (retrograde transport). The neural route of entry is important in viral infections such as rabies[4] and poliomyelitis.[5] Retrograde transport from the skin or mucous membranes moves herpes simplex and varicella-zoster viruses into sensory ganglia at the time of primary infection, and anterograde transport carries reactivated virus from the ganglia to the periphery during reactivation.[6] On occasion, reactivated virus may also be carried retrograde to the CNS.

Entry of infectious agents into the CNS by way of the exposed olfactory nerves in the nasal mucosa has been demonstrated in experimental animals[7,8] but is of proven clinical importance only for free-living amebas, which enter the olfactory and frontal lobes of the brain through the nasal mucosa and across the cribriform plate.[9]

When the infective agent is within the CNS, only certain cells may be infected. This gives rise to variations in clinical manifestations. Neuronal infection may cause seizure activity, which, depending on the areas involved, may be focal or generalized. Infection of oligodendroglia may cause demyelination alone. Cortical infection or reactive parenchymal swelling may give rise to changes in the state of consciousness,[10] and infection of specific brain-stem neurons can cause coma or respiratory failure.[11] Infection of microglia and macrophages may lead to neurologic dysfunction through indirect effects on neuronal function.[12,13]

In fatal viral encephalitis, an inflammatory reaction is usually prominent in the meninges and in a perivascular distribution within the brain. Although the perivascular inflammatory reaction is composed predominantly of mononuclear cells, polymorphonuclear cells may be evident. Neural cells may show degenerative changes, and apparent phagocytosis of neurons by macrophages or microglial cells (neuronophagia) is often found. Multinucleated giant cells containing viral antigen are found in the brains of patients with encephalitis induced by

human immunodeficiency virus (HIV).[14] CNS lesions in HIV infections may also include myelin pallor, vacuolar myelopathy, and gracile tract degeneration.[14,15] Whether these pathologic changes are direct or indirect consequences of viral infection is not yet clear. Intranuclear inclusion bodies are seen in herpesvirus,[6] adenovirus,[16] and subacute and chronic forms of measles virus infections.[17] Cytomegalovirus infections produce characteristic pathologic changes with the induction of cytomegalic cells containing inclusion bodies.[18] Negri bodies are found in rabies virus encephalitis.[19]

Rickettsiae tend to invade and to multiply in vascular endothelial cells, resulting in widespread vasculitis of capillaries, arterioles, and small arteries,[20] including the retina.

Infectious agents can give rise to signs or symptoms suggesting encephalitis or myelitis without actually invading CNS parenchyma. One mechanism is the development of adhesive meningitis and vasculitis during the course of subacute or chronic leptomeningeal infection. In chronic tuberculous, fungal, or syphilitic meningitis or untreated or partially treated bacterial meningitis, the chronic meningeal reaction may cause obstruction of cerebrospinal fluid (CSF) flow, resulting in hydrocephalus, cranial nerve palsies, or gliosis in the underlying cerebral cortex. In addition, vasculitis involving large vessels may lead to infarctions of brain and focal neurologic deficits. This sequence of events is frequently observed in tuberculosis,[21] aspergillosis,[22] and meningovascular neurosyphilis[23] and occasionally in coccidioidomycosis[24] and herpes zoster.[25] Syphilis of the meningovascular type appears relatively early in the course of this disease, and, in contrast to the parenchymatous manifestations (tabes dorsalis and paresis) that appear later, it is inflammatory and often reversible. *Cryptococcus* produces a chronic meningitis with little inflammatory reaction even in the immunologically healthy host.[26] In chronic bacterial or fungal meningitis, organization of a subarachnoid exudate at the base of the brain may lead to communicating hydrocephalus and cranial nerve palsies.[3,27]

When acute demyelinating disease complicates viral exanthems or respiratory or gastrointestinal infections, it is not known whether invasion of the virus into the CNS is a prerequisite to disease. The pathogenesis of this syndrome is thought to be related to induction of an immune response to CNS myelin.[28] This mechanism is analogous to that of neurologic complications of neural tissue–derived rabies vaccines.[29]

The pathologic changes of postinfectious and postvaccinal encephalomyelitis are characterized by perivascular infiltration of mononuclear inflammatory cells and perivenous demyelination. Acute hemorrhagic leukoencephalitis, characterized by fibrinoid necrosis of arterioles and hemorrhage in addition to the perivenular demyelination, represents a more severe form of postinfectious encephalomyelitis.[30]

On the other hand, Reye's syndrome is a distinct acute encephalopathy associated with mitochondrial dysfunction that usually follows a viral infection. This syndrome affects children and is characterized by acute fatty liver and noninflammatory cerebral edema. Reye's syndrome has been most commonly associated with varicella and influenza virus infections and has been epidemiologically related to administration of salicylates during infection.[31]

Neurotoxins produced by bacteria infecting gastrointestinal and respiratory sites have been postulated to cause the acute CNS diseases seen occasionally with shigellosis[32] and melioidosis.[33] The role of the organism in the encephalopathy associated with *Bartonella henselae* infection (cat-scratch disease) is unknown.[34]

Clinical Findings

Infections limited to the leptomeninges manifest with signs and symptoms of meningeal irritation: headache, stiff neck, and pleocytosis. If the meningeal process is chronic, as in tuberculosis, manifesting symptoms and signs may be those of a communicating hydrocephalus (headache, nausea and vomiting, mental deterioration, or spastic paraparesis), a localized infarction secondary to vasculitis, or both.[35] The chronic form of cryptococcal meningitis may manifest as progressive mental deterioration rather than with headache, fever, and meningismus, as is seen in the more acute form.[27,36]

Patients with viral encephalitis usually have signs and symptoms of meningeal inflammation, but, in addition to headache, fever, and nuchal rigidity, their encephalitis is characterized by alterations of consciousness: mild lethargy may progress to confusion, stupor, and coma. Focal neurologic signs usually develop, and seizures are common. Motor weakness, with or without accentuated deep tendon reflexes, and extensor plantar responses may be observed. Abnormal movements are seen in some cases of encephalitis, and, rarely, a tremor characteristic of Parkinson's disease may develop. The hypothalamic-pituitary axis may be involved, causing severe hyperthermia or poikilothermia, diabetes insipidus, and inappropriate antidiuretic hormone secretion. Involvement of the spinal cord can lead to flaccid paralysis, depression of tendon reflexes, and paralysis of bowel and bladder. Increased intracranial pressure can cause papilledema and third and sixth cranial nerve palsies.

In herpes simplex encephalitis, signs often include personality change, hallucinations, and aphasia, suggesting the temporal lobe localization typical of that infection.[6,37] Rabies may begin with local paresthesia at the site of the bite.[38] A parkinsonian syndrome is common in Japanese encephalitis virus infection.[39] Acute contralateral hemiparesis may occur after herpes zoster ophthalmicus infection related to a localized cerebral angiitis, causing frontal lobe infarction.[25] With Lyme neuroborreliosis, both peripheral nervous system and CNS complications occur, ranging from severe meningoencephalitis to isolated cranial nerve palsies.[40,41]

Myelitis can occur, with or without encephalitis. Transverse myelitis simulates acute transection of the cord, with rostral limb weakness, sensory level, and loss of bowel and bladder control. Ascending myelitis leads to an ascending flaccid paralysis and rising sensory deficit and is characterized by early bowel and bladder involvement. Poliomyelitis, in which anterior horn cells are involved primarily, typically causes asymmetrical flaccid paralysis and muscular pain without sensory loss or bladder dysfunction. This syndrome is seen in infections caused by flaviviruses such as Japanese encephalitis, West Nile, and tick-borne encephalitis viruses[42,43] as well as enteroviruses such as poliovirus and enterovirus 71.[44]

In postinfectious encephalomyelitis, the time lapse between manifestations of the primary infection and onset of symptoms referable to the nervous system ranges between 2 and 12 days. The onset is often abrupt, with depression of consciousness or seizure.[28,30]

Systemic findings of particular importance are the rashes of Lyme disease, Rocky Mountain spotted fever (palms and soles), typhus, varicella, herpes B virus, and herpes zoster. An exanthem is also occasionally seen with *Mycoplasma*, coxsackievirus, and echovirus infections. A history of tick bite is often obtained in Rocky Mountain spotted fever, Lyme disease, ehrlichiosis, tick-borne encephalitis, and Colorado tick fever. A history of animal or bat bite may be obtained in rabies, although most patients in the United States never give such a history.[45]

Mycobacterial and fungal infections often manifest as chronic and, on occasion, fluctuating disease, but in certain cases (including mucormycosis) they may progress very rapidly.

Bacterial infections usually manifest with an acute onset, but certain infections such as neurosyphilis, Lyme disease, relapsing fever, brain abscess, brucellosis, and Whipple's disease can have an insidious onset and an indolent, chronic, or even fluctuating course. The neurologic features of *Tropheryma whippelii* infection (Whipple's disease) may occur without significant manifestations of malabsorption and can include dementia, supranuclear ophthalmoplegia, myoclonus, spastic paresis, ataxia, and papilledema.[46] The rickettsial diseases are usually acute in onset, causing fever, headache, and myalgias. Rocky Mountain spotted fever and typhus are associated with a rash before or after neurologic disease,[47,48] whereas a rash is rarely present in ehrlichiosis.[49]

Viral infections may also be acute, subacute, or chronic. Encephalitis caused by adenovirus and enteroviruses has occurred both as acute disease in immunologically healthy persons and as subacute disease in immunologically compromised persons.[1,16] A number of CNS infections such as Creutzfeldt-Jakob disease, subacute sclerosing panencephalitis, rubella panencephalitis, HIV encephalopathy

and myelopathy, tropical spastic paraparesis, and progressive multifocal leukoencephalopathy are slowly progressive diseases with an insidious onset and absence of fever.[1,50-52]

Laboratory Findings

Peripheral blood counts are rarely helpful in this group of diseases because they may be normal or may show a moderate leukocytosis or leukopenia. Peripheral blood smears may show atypical lymphocytes in Epstein-Barr virus infections, the diagnostic gametocytes of *Plasmodium falciparum* in malaria, the morulae of *Ehrlichia* and *Anaplasma*, the borreliae in relapsing fever, or the trypanosomes in trypanosomiasis. The serum amylase concentration may be elevated in mumps virus infection. Pulmonary infiltrates may accompany lymphocytic choriomeningitis virus, typhus, *Legionella*, *Chlamydia*, and *Mycoplasma* infections.

CSF examination is essential. The pleocytosis of viral encephalomyelitis is variable (10 to 2000 cells/mm³), and mononuclear cells usually predominate; however, early in any of these diseases there may be no cells, or polymorphonuclear cells may be present in considerable numbers. Repeated examination of the CSF in 24 hours is often useful.[53] Significant numbers of red blood cells may be found in herpes simplex encephalitis,[54] acute necrotizing hemorrhagic leukoencephalitis,[30] and *Naegleria* encephalitis.[9] In the chronic fungal and bacterial meningitides, a moderate mononuclear pleocytosis is usually found.[27] Meningoencephalitis caused by *Naegleria*, *Nocardia*, *Actinomyces*, *Candida*, or *Aspergillus* elicits a polymorphonuclear response.[55,56] Helminth infections and coccidioidomycosis meningitis elicit eosinophils.[57]

The CSF protein level is usually increased in encephalomyelitis, and in chronic infections an increased proportion of this protein is immunoglobulin G (IgG) (normal is less than 12%). Under normal conditions, CSF IgG is derived primarily from the serum, and antibodies are present in the CSF at a ratio of about 1:200 with the serum concentration.[58] During acute inflammatory reactions a transudate of protein occurs, including serum immunoglobulins. Increased IgM is typical of African trypanosomiasis[59] and virus-specific IgM may be diagnostic.[60,61] During convalescence, plasma cells may produce pathogen-specific IgG within the CNS, as is seen after Japanese encephalitis,[62] herpes simplex,[54] and varicella-zoster virus[63] encephalitides. In chronic infection, examination of the CSF for specific IgG can be diagnostic in syphilis,[64] Lyme disease,[65] tropical spastic paraparesis,[50] subacute sclerosing panencephalitis,[66] progressive multifocal leukoencephalopathy,[67] and rubella panencephalitis[68] and may be more useful than serum determinations in the viral, rickettsial, fungal, and bacterial encephalitides for which antibody tests are available. If antibody to a particular pathogen is present at a comparable or higher amount in CSF than in serum and the CSF protein is only moderately elevated, it is indicative of CNS infection with the agent.

For diagnosis by serum antibodies, it is important to obtain serum early in the course (acute phase) for comparison with serum taken after 1 to 3 weeks of illness to demonstrate a significant antibody increase.[69] Tests for specific IgM in serum and CSF often allow earlier and more specific diagnoses.[60,61,70] This diagnosis is often of more than academic interest because presumptive therapy begun early may be discontinued if a diagnosis is established. Tests for cold agglutinins and heterophile antibody may yield false-negative results in the diagnosis of *Mycoplasma* and Epstein-Barr virus infections, respectively; therefore, organism-specific antibody tests are preferred.

The CSF glucose level is usually within the normal range during viral or rickettsial infections of the CNS, although a mild depression may be seen. The glucose level is usually low in tuberculous,[71] fungal,[27] bacterial, or amebic[55] infections.

Direct examination of the CSF by Gram stain for bacteria, by acid-fast stain for mycobacteria, and by India ink for *Cryptococcus* should be performed and may be diagnostic. Wet preparation of CSF may reveal free-living amebas, and Giemsa stain identifies trypanosomes. Bacteria, mycobacteria, fungi, amebas, and viruses may also be recovered from the CSF by appropriate culture techniques. Microbial antigen detection methods have proved particularly useful in cryptococcal disease.[36] Detection of nucleic acid in CSF by polymerase chain reaction (PCR) is useful for a number of viral infections, particularly herpesviruses, enteroviruses, and polyomavirus.[37,72] PCR performed early in disease may be negative and should be repeated after 48 to 72 hours.[73]

The electroencephalogram is often abnormal in acute and chronic forms of herpes simplex encephalitis and may provide early localizing information in herpesvirus encephalitis. The computed tomographic scan is useful for ruling out space-occupying lesions but is often unrevealing in encephalitis and myelitis. Magnetic resonance imaging allows better visualization of the spinal cord, is a sensitive indicator of demyelination, and can detect the edematous changes that are often an early feature of encephalitis.

TABLE 83-1 Viral Causes of Acute Encephalomyelitis	
Direct Infection	*Postinfection*
Togaviridae	
Alphaviruses	
Eastern equine	
Western equine	
Venezuelan equine	Togaviridae
Flaviviridae	Rubivirus
St. Louis	Rubella
Murray Valley	Orthomyxoviridae
West Nile	Influenza
Japanese	Paramyxoviridae
Dengue	Rubulavirus
Tick-borne complex	Mumps
Bunyaviridae	Morbillivirus
La Crosse	Measles
Rift Valley	Poxviridae
Toscana	Orthopoxvirus
Paramyxoviridae	Vaccinia
Paramyxovirus	Herpesviridae
Mumps	Herpesvirus
Morbillivirus	Varicella-zoster virus
Measles	Epstein-Barr virus
Henipavirus	
Hendra	
Nipah (Hendra-like)	
Arenaviridae	
Arenavirus	
Lymphocytic choriomeningitis	
Machupo	
Lassa	
Junin	
Picornaviridae	
Enterovirus	
Poliovirus	
Coxsackievirus	
Echovirus	
Hepatitis A	
Reoviridae	
Colorado tick fever	
Rhabdoviridae	
Lyssavirus	
Rabies	
Filoviridae	
Ebola	
Marburg	
Retroviridae	
Lentivirus	
Human immunodeficiency virus	
Herpesviridae	
Alphaherpesvirus	
Herpes simplex virus types 1 and 2	
Varicella-zoster virus	
Herpes B virus	
Betaherpesvirus	
Cytomegalovirus	
Human herpesvirus 6	
Human herpesvirus 7	
Gammaherpesvirus	
Epstein-Barr virus	
Adenoviridae	
Adenovirus	

Etiology of Encephalomyelitis

Table 83-1 lists the viruses known to cause acute encephalitis or myelitis and those associated with postinfectious encephalomyelitis. This list is undoubtedly incomplete, and most cases of encephalitis do not have an identified etiology.[74-76] Many of the infections known to cause encephalomyelitis have distinct seasonal variations that are helpful in narrowing the differential diagnosis (Fig. 83-1). The alphavirus, flavivirus, and bunyavirus encephalitides are arthropod borne and therefore occur when their insect vectors are biting. The mosquito-borne encephalitides peak in late summer in temperate regions.[77] The tick-borne diseases occur most often in spring and early summer.[78,79] Enteroviruses are the most common cause of viral encephalitis and occur primarily in late summer and fall. In contrast, the herpesvirus encephalitides occur throughout the year. Lymphocytic choriomeningitis virus is most common in the winter, when rodents come indoors, and leptospirosis is more common in the warm months, when rodents and people are in contact with ponds and streams.[69]

In addition to the season, geographic and travel histories may be helpful in the diagnosis of vector-borne encephalitides. For instance, eastern equine encephalitis is most common in the Great Lakes region and along the Atlantic and Gulf coasts, whereas La Crosse and St. Louis virus encephalitides are widespread in the United States.[1,80] West Nile virus encephalitis is widespread in North America and in eastern Europe and the Middle East.[81] *Borrelia* is endemic in the northeast and upper midwestern United States and in Europe.[82] Japanese encephalitis is found in most of Asia and the Indian subcontinent,[83] and tick-borne encephalitis occurs over a wide area of eastern Europe and northern Asia.[84]

Exposure to infected animals can transmit viral agents of encephalitis, even when the animals do not appear ill. Herpes B virus encephalitis may occur in monkey handlers who have been bitten or scratched by infected monkeys. Hendra virus has caused encephalitis in a few Australian horse handlers, and Nipah virus caused a large outbreak of encephalitis in Malaysia in persons in contact with swine.[85,86] The natural reservoirs for both Hendra and Nipah viruses are pteropid bats.[87]

Encephalitis occurs most commonly in young children and adults older than 65 years.[74] However, infection with eastern equine encephalitis virus produces clinically evident encephalitis with high frequency in all age groups.[88] For other causes of viral encephalitis, a large majority of the infections are subclinical. Encephalomyelitis with St. Louis and West Nile viruses occurs in about 1% of infections,[80,89] and California or La Crosse virus produces encephalitis predominantly in

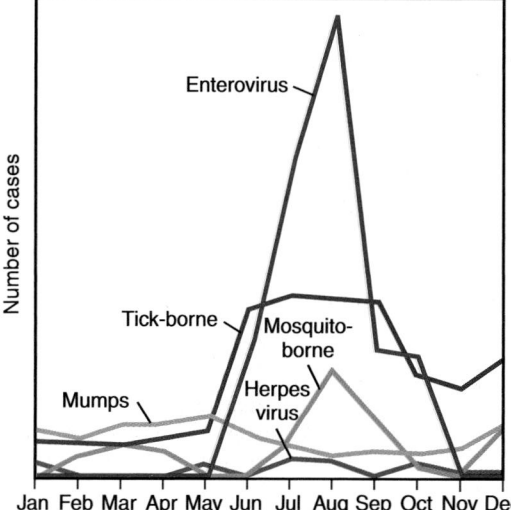

FIGURE 83-1 Seasonal variation in temperate zones of the Northern Hemisphere for the encephalitides caused by mosquito-borne viruses, enteroviruses, mumps virus, herpesvirus, and tick-borne diseases.

children.[90] Venezuelan equine encephalitis virus primarily causes an influenza-like illness in humans but can produce encephalitis in any age group.[91]

Nonviral causes of encephalomyelitis are listed in Table 83-2. Some of these diseases are of known and others of unknown cause, and the clinical presentations are often indistinguishable from those of viral encephalitis.[75,76,92,93] They include drug reactions such as the neuroleptic malignant syndrome[94] and chemotherapy-induced leukoencephalopathy,[95] which may be confused with infection. Many are treatable. One of the most important concerns in evaluating a patient with encephalomyelitis is consideration of treatable entities.

The cause of encephalitis is frequently different in immunodeficient patients. Patients with hypogammaglobulinemia may have chronic encephalitis with enterovirus.[96] Patients with defects in cell-mediated immunity have unusual forms of encephalitis or myelitis with herpesviruses,[18,25,97] a subacute inclusion body encephalitis with measles,[3,17] meningoencephalitis with adenovirus,[16] and *Acanthamoeba*.[98] In acquired immunodeficiency syndrome (AIDS) a number of unusual agents, principally *Toxoplasma, Pneumocystis, Cryptococcus, Histoplasma*, cytomegalovirus, and papovavirus (progressive multifocal leukoencephalopathy), may cause CNS disease, either singly or in combination.[18,36,98-101]

Transverse myelitis caused by a vasculitis of the anterior spinal artery has been seen in varicella-zoster virus infections, tuberculosis, syphilis, and schistosomiasis.[3,102,103] Postinfectious transverse myelitis has been associated with vaccinia, measles, rubella, mumps, and upper respiratory tract diseases.[104,105] Direct infection of the spinal cord with varicella-zoster virus or *Borrelia* may also produce a transverse myelitis.[3,25] Infection with human T-lymphotropic virus type I causes disease primarily in the thoracic cord, leading to progressive spastic paraparesis.[50] Infection with HIV causes myelopathy manifested by spastic paraparesis and sensory ataxia.[106,107] An ascending myelitis may also occur in rabies.[108] The lower motor neuron variety of myelitis causing flaccid paralysis (poliomyelitis) may be produced by a number of enteroviruses, particularly poliovirus and enterovirus 71,[3,44,109] as well as arboviruses[42,43] and rabies virus.[110]

Presumptive Treatment

Specific therapy is available for most of the diseases listed in Table 83-2 and should be instituted as soon as possible if a presumptive diagnosis can be made. In addition, effective therapy is available with acyclovir for herpes simplex, varicella-zoster, and herpes B[111-114] virus encephalitis. Cytomegalovirus encephalitis and radiculomyelitis can be treated with ganciclovir or foscarnet.[18,115] HIV-associated neurologic disease is delayed or prevented and, in previously untreated individuals, may improve with antiretroviral treatment.[106,116,117] None of these treatments eliminates the latent state of these viruses in the nervous system.

TABLE 83-2 Nonviral Causes of Encephalomyelitis

Subacute bacterial endocarditis	Actinomycosis
Rocky Mountain spotted fever	Tuberculosis
Typhus	*Cryptococcus*
Ehrlichia	*Histoplasma*
Q fever	*Naegleria*
Chlamydia	*Acanthamoeba*
Mycoplasma	*Ballamuthia mandrillaris*
Legionella	*Toxoplasma*
Brucellosis	*Plasmodium falciparum*
Subacute bacterial endocarditis	Trypanosomiasis
Listeria	Behçet's disease
Whipple's disease	Vasculitis
Cat-scratch disease	Carcinoma
Syphilis (meningovascular)	Drug reactions
Relapsing fever	
Lyme disease	
Leptospirosis	
Nocardia	

Patients in coma caused by encephalitis or postinfectious encephalomyelitis may make remarkable recoveries even after prolonged periods of unconsciousness. For this reason vigorous supportive treatment is indicated, and the complications of ventilator therapy, catheters, intravenous lines, and so forth should be avoided if possible and should be treated vigorously if they occur. Blood glucose levels and electrolytes should be monitored closely because the hypothalamic area may be involved in the encephalitic process. Seizures should be controlled, if they occur. Some fever may be beneficial, but extreme hyperthermia may exacerbate seizures, as may hypoxia. Cerebral edema can be damaging in itself and should be controlled with drugs as necessary.

NEURITIS

Neuritis is an inflammatory disease involving the peripheral nerves. Leprosy, trypanosomes, microsporidia, and cytomegalovirus cause a direct infection of nerves leading to clinical signs of peripheral neuropathy.[115,118-120] Neuroborreliosis frequently causes radiculoneuritis and cranial neuritis associated pathologically with inflammation.[3,121] Herpes simplex virus and varicella-zoster virus infect sensory ganglia, and reactivation may be associated with radicular pain. Herpes zoster may also be complicated by a postherpetic pain syndrome in the distribution of nerves supplied by the affected ganglia. Three bacterial toxins affect peripheral nerves either directly (diphtheria) or indirectly (tetanus, botulism), each causing distinct syndromes. The Guillain-Barré syndrome is a postinfectious inflammatory process of peripheral nerves that can involve destruction of axons or myelin.[122,123]

Pathologic Characteristics and Pathogenesis

In lepromatous leprosy the immunologic response does not effectively control the infection. There is a widespread distribution of *Mycobacterium leprae*. Nerves in the skin may exhibit only minor changes, but larger peripheral nerves contain many leprosy bacilli in Schwann cells.[124] The organisms grow best in the cooler parts of the body, and nerves close to skin surface and distal nerves are affected preferentially.[125] In late stages of the disease, extensive axonal degeneration may occur.

Tuberculoid leprosy is characterized by a marked granulomatous reaction to the infection and few demonstrable bacilli.[124] Cutaneous nerves beneath the skin macules are destroyed, producing anesthesia. The peripheral nerves are nodular and thickened, with destruction of the normal architecture. Segmental demyelination and axonal degeneration result in nerve destruction and severe fibrosis.[125]

Trypanosoma cruzi, Trypanosoma gambiense, and *Trypanosoma rhodesiense* can invade and replicate in tissue of the peripheral nervous system as well as the CNS. *T. cruzi* preferentially damages cells of the autonomic nervous system by replicating in the supporting Schwann cells, satellite cells, and capsular fibroblasts rather than in the neurons. In Africa, trypanosomiasis patients dying with encephalomyelitis often have evidence of neuritis. The microsporidia *Nosema connori* can invade the nerve fibers of Auerbach's plexus, causing nerve dysfunction.

Tetanus toxin, produced by *Clostridium tetani* under anaerobic conditions, is transported up the axon and binds to the presynaptic endings on motor neurons in the anterior horns of the spinal cord, where it cleaves synaptic vesicle components, blocking inhibitory input.[3,126] This action results in uncontrolled motor input to skeletal muscle and the spasms typical of this disease. Because of this transport mechanism for entry into the CNS, patients may have only localized disease in the area of the wound.

Botulinum toxin is produced during anaerobic metabolism of *Clostridium botulinum* and may be either ingested as preformed toxin (food botulism) or produced by organisms that are in the intestine (infant botulism) or are introduced into a wound (wound botulism). Botulinum toxin binds to the presynaptic axon terminal of the neuromuscular junction and cleaves components of exocytic synaptic vesicles, preventing release of acetylcholine and leading to flaccid paralysis.[3,126] Little, if any, histologic abnormality is seen in either tetanus or botulism.

Diphtheria toxin is produced by *Corynebacterium diphtheriae* lysogenized by a phage coding for this toxin. The toxin is a protein with two subunits; subunit A inhibits protein synthesis by adenosine diphosphate ribosylation of elongation factor 2, and subunit B binds to cell membranes and enables the active subunit A to enter the cell.[127-129] The effect of this toxin on peripheral nerves is to cause a noninflammatory demyelination. Both cranial and peripheral nerves may be demyelinated, although cranial nerves are more frequently affected.[130]

The Guillain-Barré syndrome usually follows within 4 weeks after a respiratory or gastrointestinal infection, immunization, trauma, or metabolic insult. Infections with *Campylobacter jejuni*, herpesviruses, *Mycoplasma pneumoniae*, and a few other organisms have been associated with this syndrome.[123,131] Two types of nerve pathology are recognized: mononuclear inflammation with demyelination and axonal degeneration.[123,132] *C. jejuni* is the most common preceding infection, particularly in patients with axonal degeneration and in children, and infection with specific strains may be involved.[122,133,134] Induction of antibodies that react with gangliosides in the nervous system (molecular mimicry) appears to mediate many forms of this disease.[122,133]

Clinical Findings

Leprosy has two distinctive manifestations, depending on the cellular immune response, which determines whether the disease is of the tuberculoid or the lepromatous type. Tuberculoid leprosy produces a mononeuropathy beneath sharply demarcated skin patches. Peripheral nerves may be palpably and visibly enlarged, and the neurologic involvement is a prominent part of the disease. In lepromatous leprosy, a distal hypesthesia with selective loss of pain and temperature is most common, although a mononeuropathy may be present. Cooler areas of the body are more strikingly affected, and the loss of pain sensation results in mutilation and eventual loss of digits.[135]

Tetanus usually manifests with rigidity of muscles, which may be painful. The initial manifestation may be "local tetanus," in which the rigidity affects only the limb or area of the body in which the *Clostridium*-containing wound is located. Stiffness of the jaw muscles causes trismus, and stiffness of the facial muscles may cause a change of expression. This mild picture can progress to generalized rigidity with reflex spasms and dysphagia. The disease is most common in elderly individuals and usually follows a recognized injury.[136] The wound may have seemed insignificant at the time of the injury and may appear well healed at the time of the neurologic disease.[3,137]

Botulism characteristically manifests 12 to 36 hours after ingestion of the toxin with weakness, dizziness, and dryness of the mouth. More severe neurologic symptoms follow within 12 to 72 hours with blurred vision, diplopia, dysphonia, dysphagia, and muscle weakness. Infants may present with constipation and poor feeding.[138] On examination, sensation is preserved, the tendon reflexes are depressed or absent, and the paralysis is flaccid.[3] The same picture can develop more gradually in a patient with wound botulism. The original wound is usually of a rather severe traumatic nature and may appear to be healing well at the time of neurologic disease.[3,139,140]

The earliest sign of pharyngeal diphtheria (5 to 12 days) is paralysis of the palate, which produces a nasal quality of the voice and an increasing tendency to regurgitate fluids through the nose. Other cranial nerves (particularly III, VI, VII, IX, and X) may become involved, with blurring of vision and inability to accommodate as early symptoms. Later in the course of the disease, often after the previous symptoms have subsided (2 to 6 weeks), a predominantly motor polyneuropathy involving bulbar dysfunction and symmetrical weakness of distal extremities occurs and may appear similar to Guillain-Barré syndrome.[130] There is a flaccid paralysis with loss of deep tendon reflexes that may be accompanied by the signs and symptoms of a diphtheritic myocarditis.

Neuropathies associated with HIV infection include acute and chronic inflammatory demyelinating polyneuropathies, sensory ganglioneuritis, and polyradiculopathy early in infection and a distal, symmetrical, primarily sensory neuropathy later, after AIDS has developed.[120]

In approximately 60% to 70% of cases, Guillain-Barré syndrome follows an infection or immunization.[123,131] Clinically it manifests with subjective paresthesias or weakness, or both, which may continue to progress for up to 4 weeks.[141,142] Examination typically reveals a flaccid paralysis with loss of deep tendon reflexes. Involvement of the autonomic nervous system resulting in lability of blood pressure, inappropriate antidiuretic hormone secretion, and inability to compensate for volume changes occurs in approximately 20% of the cases.[143] These problems frequently necessitate the management of patients in an intensive care unit even though they may not require ventilatory assistance. The condition of an individual patient can change rapidly either during progression or during recovery. Improvement is often slow, however, and may continue for up to 12 months.[123,130,141,142,144]

Laboratory Findings

Routine blood chemistry analyses are not helpful in this group of diseases. If botulism is suspected, serum for mouse inoculation should be procured and CSF should also be obtained. In Guillain-Barré syndrome or diphtheritic polyneuritis, an increased protein level, with few cells (albuminocytologic dissociation) in the CSF, is the characteristic finding; however, some patients have a normal protein level, particularly early in the disease. Others, especially those with HIV infection, also have a moderate pleocytosis. The CSF findings are normal in tetanus, botulism, and leprosy. Neurometric tests that aid in localization of the pathologic changes and therefore the diagnosis are (1) measurement of nerve conduction times, to look for the slowed conduction found in the peripheral nerve lesions of Guillain-Barré syndrome and diphtheria (F-wave measurements may allow identification of abnormalities if lesions are very proximal), and (2) recording from muscle during repetitive nerve stimulation, to look for the incremental response characteristic of botulism and not found in Guillain-Barré syndrome.[139,145] Nerve biopsies or aspirations may be useful in identifying the granulomas or acid-fast bacilli, or both, of leprosy.[124]

Presumptive Treatment

In this group of clinically distinctive diseases, it is important to recognize the disease and to treat it appropriately. Current treatment for leprosy involves a combination of rifampicin, clofazimine, and dapsone.[135] In toxin-mediated diseases, antitoxin should be used. Most patients with Guillain-Barré syndrome benefit from plasmapheresis or intravenous immunoglobulin therapy, especially early in the disease.[146] Patients must be closely monitored for vital capacity, electrolytes, blood pressure, temperature, and heart rate, and those with respiratory failure should be ventilated mechanically. Patients with autonomic nervous system dysfunction should be treated with short-acting drugs because autonomic function in these patients can be very labile. A patient who is hypertensive in the morning may be distressingly hypotensive in the evening and vice versa. Patients may not adjust to abrupt changes in intravascular volume, and intravenous fluids should be carefully controlled.

REFERENCES

1. Johnson RT. Viral Infections of the Nervous System. 2nd ed. Philadelphia: Lippincott-Raven; 1998.
2. Mims CA. The Pathogenesis of Infectious Disease. 4th ed. New York: Academic Press; 1995.
3. Scheld WM, Whitley RJ, Durack DT. Infections of the Central Nervous System. 2nd ed. Philadelphia: Lippincott-Raven; 1997.
4. Tsiang H, Ceccaldi PE, Lycke E. Rabies virus infection and transport in human sensory dorsal root ganglia neurons. J Gen Virol. 1991;72:1191-1194.
5. Wyatt HV. Incubation of poliomyelitis as calculated from the time of entry into the central nervous system via the peripheral nerve pathways. Rev Infect Dis. 1990;12:547-556.
6. Whitley RJ, Kimberlin DW, Roizman B. Herpes simplex viruses. Clin Infect Dis. 1998;26:541-553.
7. Monath TP, Cropp CP, Harrison AK. Mode of entry of a neurotropic arbovirus into the central nervous system. Reinvestigation of an old controversy. Lab Invest. 1983;48:399-410.

8. Charles PC, Walters E, Margolis F, et al. Mechanism of neuroinvasion of Venezuelan equine encephalitis virus in the mouse. Virology. 1995;208:662-671.

9. Ma P, Visvesvara GS, Martinez AJ, et al. *Naegleria* and *Acanthamoeba* infections: Review. Rev Infect Dis. 1990;12:490-513.

10. Johnson RT. Selective vulnerability of neural cells to viral infections. Brain. 1980;103:447-472.

11. Johnson RT, Burke DS, Elwell M, et al. Japanese encephalitis: Immunocytochemical studies of viral antigen and inflammatory cells in fatal cases. Ann Neurol. 1985;18:567-573.

12. Kaul M, Garden GA, Lipton SA. Pathways to neuronal injury and apoptosis in HIV-associated dementia. Nature. 2001;410:988-994.

13. Power C, Johnson RT. Neuroimmune and neurovirological aspects of human immunodeficiency virus infection. Adv Virus Res. 2001;56:389-433.

14. Budka H. Neuropathology of human immunodeficiency virus infection. Brain Pathol. 1991;1:163-175.

15. Rance NE, McArthur JC, Cornblath DR, et al. Gracile tract degeneration in patients with sensory neuropathy and AIDS. Neurology. 1988;38:265-271.

16. Carrigan DR. Adenovirus infections in immunocompromised patients. Am J Med. 1997;102:71-74.

17. Roos RP, Graves MC, Wollmann RL, et al. Immunologic and virologic studies of measles inclusion body encephalitis in an immunosuppressed host: The relationship to subacute sclerosing panencephalitis. Neurology. 1981;31:1263-1270.

18. McCutchan JA. Cytomegalovirus infections of the nervous system in patients with AIDS. Clin Infect Dis. 1995;20:747-754.

19. Dupont JR, Earle KM. Human rabies encephalitis. A study of forty nine fatal cases with a review of the literature. Neurology. 1965;15:1023-1034.

20. Miller JQ, Price TR. The nervous system in Rocky Mountain spotted fever. Neurology. 1972;22:561-566.

21. Dastur DK, Lalitha VS, Udani PM, Parekh U. The brain and meninges in tuberculous meningitis—Gross pathology in 100 cases and pathogenesis. Neurol India. 1970;18:86-100.

22. Walsh TJ, Hier DB, Caplan LR. Aspergillosis of the central nervous system: Clinicopathological analysis of 17 patients. Ann Neurol. 1985;18:574-582.

23. Greenfield JG. Infectious diseases of the central nervous system: Neurosyphilis. In: Blackwood W, McMenemey WH, Meyer A, eds. Greenfields' Neuropathology. Baltimore: Williams & Wilkins; 1963:164.

24. Mischel PS, Vinters HV. Coccidioidomycosis of the central nervous system: Neuropathological and vasculopathic manifestations and clinical correlates. Clin Infect Dis. 1995;20:400-405.

25. Gray F, Belec L, Lescs MC, et al. Varicella-zoster virus infection of the central nervous system in the acquired immune deficiency syndrome. Brain. 1994;117:987-999.

26. Baker RD, Haugen RK. Tissue changes and tissue diagnosis in cryptococcosis: A study of 26 cases. J Clin Pathol. 1955;25:14-24.

27. Ellner JJ, Bennett JE. Chronic meningitis. Medicine (Baltimore). 1976;55:341-369.

28. Johnson RT, Griffin DE, Hirsch RL, et al. Measles encephalomyelitis—Clinical and immunologic studies. N Engl J Med. 1984;310:137-141.

29. Hemachudha T, Griffin DE, Giffels JJ, et al. Myelin basic protein as an encephalitogen in encephalomyelitis and polyneuritis following rabies vaccination. N Engl J Med. 1987;316:369-374.

30. Dangond F, Lacomis D, Schwartz RB, et al. Acute disseminated encephalomyelitis progressing to hemorrhagic encephalitis. Neurology. 1991;41:1697-1698.

31. Hardie RM, Newton LH, Bruce JC, et al. The changing clinical pattern of Reye's syndrome 1982-1990. Arch Dis Child. 1996;74:400-405.

32. Goren A, Freier S, Passwell JH. Lethal toxic encephalopathy due to childhood shigellosis in a developed country. Pediatrics. 1992;89:1189-1193.

33. Woods ML II, Currie BJ, Howard DM, et al. Neurological melioidosis: Seven cases from the Northern Territory of Australia. Clin Infect Dis. 1992;15:163-169.

34. Marra CM. Neurologic complications of *Bartonella henselae* infection. Curr Opin Neurol. 1995;8:164-169.

35. Osuntokun BO, Adeuja AOG, Familusi JB. Tuberculous meningitis in Nigerians: A study of 1974 patients. Trop Geogr Med. 1971;23:225-231.

36. Moosa MY, Coovadia YM. Cryptococcal meningitis in Durban, South Africa: A comparison of clinical features, laboratory findings, and outcome for human immunodeficiency virus (HIV)-positive and HIV-negative patients. Clin Infect Dis. 1997;24:131-134.

37. Domingues RB, Tsanaclis AM, Pannuti CS, et al. Evaluation of the range of clinical presentations of herpes simplex encephalitis by using polymerase chain reaction assay of cerebrospinal fluid samples. Clin Infect Dis. 1997;25:86-91.

38. Hattwick MAW. Human rabies. Public Health Rep. 1981;96:580-584.

39. Misra UK, Kalita J. Movement disorders in Japanese encephalitis. J Neurol. 1997;244:299-303.

40. Halperin JJ, Volkman DJ, Wu P. Central nervous system abnormalities in Lyme neuroborreliosis. Neurology. 1991;41:1571-1582.

41. Coyle PK, Schutzer SE. Neurologic aspects of Lyme disease. Med Clin North Am. 2002;86:261-284.

42. Li J, Loeb JA, Shy ME, et al. Asymmetric flaccid paralysis: A neuromuscular presentation of West Nile virus infection. Ann Neurol. 2003;53:703-710.

43. Solomon T, Kneen R, Dung NM, et al. Poliomyelitis-like illness due to Japanese encephalitis virus. Lancet. 1998;351:1094-1097.

44. Hayward JC, Gillespie SM, Kaplan KM, et al. Outbreak of poliomyelitis-like paralysis associated with enterovirus 71. Pediatr Infect Dis J. 1989;8:611-616.

45. Messenger SL, Smith JS, Rupprecht CE. Emerging epidemiology of bat-associated cryptic cases of rabies in humans in the United States. Clin Infect Dis. 2002;35:738-747.

46. Gerard A, Sarrot-Reynauld F, Liozon E, et al. Neurologic presentation of Whipple disease: Report of 12 cases and review of the literature. Medicine (Baltimore). 2002;81:443-457.

47. Kirk JL. Rocky Mountain spotted fever: A clinical review based on 48 confirmed cases, 1943-1986. Medicine (Baltimore). 1990;69:35-45.

48. Pai H, Sohn S, Seong Y, et al. Central nervous system involvement in patients with scrub typhus. Clin Infect Dis. 1997;24:436-440.

49. Ratnasamy N, Everett ED, Roland WE, et al. Central nervous system manifestations of human ehrlichiosis. Clin Infect Dis. 1996;23:314-319.

50. Levin MC, Jacobson S. HTLV-I associated myelopathy/tropical spastic paraparesis (HAM/TSP): A chronic progressive neurologic disease associated with immunologically mediated damage to the central nervous system. J Neurovirol. 1997;3:126-140.

51. Spencer MD, Knight RS, Will RG. First hundred cases of variant Creutzfeldt-Jakob disease: Retrospective case note review of early psychiatric and neurological features. BMJ. 2002;324:1479-1482.

52. McArthur JC, Haughey N, Gartner S, et al. Human immunodeficiency virus-associated dementia: An evolving disease. J Neurovirol. 2003;9:205-221.

53. Feigin RD, Shackelford PG. Value of repeat lumbar puncture in the differential diagnosis of meningitis. N Engl J Med. 1973;289:571-574.

54. Koskiniemi M, Vaheri A, Taskinen E. Cerebrospinal fluid alterations in herpes simplex virus encephalitis. Rev Infect Dis. 1984;6:608-618.

55. Carter RF. Primary amoebic meningoencephalitis: An appraisal of present knowledge. Trans R Soc Trop Med Hyg. 1972;66:193-213.

56. Peacock JE Jr, McGinnis MR, Cohen MS. Persistent neutrophilic meningitis: Report of four cases and review of the literature. Medicine (Baltimore). 1984;63:379-395.

57. Kuberski T. Eosinophils in the cerebrospinal fluid. Ann Intern Med. 1979;91:70-75.

58. Sindic CJ, Van Antwerpen MP, Goffette S. The intrathecal humoral immune response: Laboratory analysis and clinical relevance. Clin Chem Lab Med. 2001;39:333-340.

59. Lejon V, Reiber H, Legros D, et al. Intrathecal immune response pattern for improved diagnosis of central nervous system involvement in trypanosomiasis. J Infect Dis. 2003;187:1475-1483.

60. Solomon T, Thao LT, Dung NM, et al. Rapid diagnosis of Japanese encephalitis by using an immunoglobulin M dot enzyme immunoassay. J Clin Microbiol. 1998;36:2030-2034.

61. Martin DA, Biggerstaff BJ, Allen B, et al. Use of immunoglobulin M cross-reactions in differential diagnosis of human flaviviral encephalitis infections in the United States. Clin Diagn Lab Immunol. 2002;9:544-549.

62. Burke DS, Nisalak A, Ussery MA, et al. Kinetics of Japanese encephalitis virus immunoglobulin M and G antibodies in human serum and cerebrospinal fluid. J Infect Dis. 1985;151:1093-1099.

63. Vartdal F, Vandvik B, Norrby E. Intrathecal synthesis of virus specific oligoclonal IgG, IgA and IgM antibodies in a case of varicella zoster meningoencephalitis. J Neurol Sci. 1982;57:121-132.

64. Vartdal F, Vandvik B, Michaelsen TE, et al. Neurosyphilis: Intrathecal synthesis of oligoclonal antibodies to *Treponema pallidum*. Ann Neurol. 1982;11:35-40.

65. Steere AC, Berardi VP, Weeks KE, et al. Evaluation of the intrathecal antibody response to *Borrelia burgdorferi* as a diagnostic test for Lyme neuroborreliosis. J Infect Dis. 1990;161:1203-1209.

66. Salmi AA, Norrby E, Panelius M. Identification of different measles virus-specific antibodies in the serum and cerebrospinal fluid from patients with subacute sclerosing panencephalitis and multiple sclerosis. Infect Immun. 1972;6:248-254.

67. Weber T, Weber F, Petry H, et al. Immune response in progressive multifocal leukoencephalopathy: An overview. J Neurovirol. 2001;7:311-317.

68. Townsend JJ, Baringer JR, Wolinsky JS, et al. Progressive rubella panencephalitis: Late onset after congenital rubella. N Engl J Med. 1975;292:990-993.

69. Meyer HM, Johnson RT, Crawford IP. Central nervous system syndromes of "viral" etiology: A study of 713 cases. Am J Med. 1960;29:334-347.

70. Calisher CH, Berardi VP, Muth DJ, et al. Specificity of immunoglobulin M and G antibody responses in humans infected with eastern and western equine encephalitis viruses: Application to rapid serodiagnosis. J Clin Microbiol. 1986;23:369-372.

71. Ogawa SK, Smith MA, Brennessel DJ, et al. Tuberculous meningitis in an urban medical center. Medicine (Baltimore). 1987;66:317-326.

72. Hukkanen V, Vuorinen T. Herpesviruses and enteroviruses in infections of the central nervous system: A study using time-resolved fluorometry PCR. J Clin Virol. 2002;25 (Suppl 1):S87-S94.

73. De Tiaga X, Heron B, Lebon P, et al. Limits of early diagnosis of herpes simplex encephalitis in children: A retrospective study of 38 cases. Clin Infect Dis. 2003;36:1335-1339.

74. Khetsuriani N, Holman RC, Anderson LJ. Burden of encephalitis-associated hospitalizations in the United States, 1988-1997. Clin Infect Dis. 2002;35:175-182.

75. Glaser CA, Gilliam S, Schnurr D, et al. In search of encephalitis etiologies: Diagnostic challenges in the California Encephalitis Project, 1998-2000. Clin Infect Dis. 2003;36:731-742.

76. Kolski H, Ford-Jones EL, Richardson S, et al. Etiology of acute childhood encephalitis at The Hospital for Sick Children, Toronto, 1994-1995. Clin Infect Dis. 1998;26:398-409.

77. Petersen LR, Marfin AA. West Nile virus: A primer for the clinician. Ann Intern Med. 2002;137:173-179.

78. Wilfert CM, MacCormack JN, Kleeman K, et al. Epidemiology of Rocky Mountain spotted fever as determined by active surveillance. J Infect Dis. 1984;150:469-479.

79. Ciesielski CA, Hightower AW, Horsley R, et al. The geographic distribution of Lyme disease in the United States. Ann NY Acad Sci. 1990;539:283-288.

80. Calisher CH. Medically important arboviruses of the United States and Canada. Clin Microbiol Rev. 1994;7:89-116.

81. Petersen LR, Roehrig JT. West Nile virus: A reemerging global pathogen. Emerg Infect Dis. 2001;7:611-614.
82. Schmid GP. The global distribution of Lyme disease. Rev Infect Dis. 1985;7:41-50.
83. Solomon T, Ni H, Beasley DW, et al. Origin and evolution of Japanese encephalitis virus in southeast Asia. J Virol. 2003;77:3091-3098.
84. Zanotto PM, Gao GF, Gritsun T, et al. An arbovirus cline across the northern hemisphere. Virology. 1995;210:152-159.
85. Lam SK, Chua KB. Nipah virus encephalitis outbreak in Malaysia. Clin Infect Dis. 2002;34(Suppl 2):S48-S51.
86. O'Sullivan JD, Allworth AM, Paterson DL, et al. Fatal encephalitis due to novel paramyxovirus transmitted from horses. Lancet. 1997;349:93-95.
87. Field H, Young P, Yob JM, et al. The natural history of Hendra and Nipah viruses. Microbes Infect. 2001;3:307-314.
88. Przelomiski MM, O'Rourke E, Grady GF, et al. Eastern equine encephalitis in Massachusetts: A report of 16 cases, 1970-1984. Neurology. 1988;38:736-739.
89. Meehan PJ, Wells DL, Paul W, et al. Epidemiological features of and public health response to a St. Louis encephalitis epidemic in Florida, 1990-1. Epidemiol Infect. 2000;125:181-188.
90. Woodruff BA, Baron RC, Tsai TF. Symptomatic La Crosse virus infections of the central nervous system: A study of risk factors in an endemic area. Am J Epidemiol. 1992;136:320-327.
91. Rivas F, Diaz LA, Cardenas VM, et al. Epidemic Venezuelan equine encephalitis in La Guajira, Colombia, 1995. J Infect Dis. 1997;175:828-832.
92. Johnson JD, Raff MJ, Van Arsdall JA. Neurologic manifestations of Legionnaires' disease. Medicine (Baltimore). 1984;63:303-310.
93. Korman TM, Turnidge JD, Grayson ML. Neurological complications of chlamydial infections: Case report and review. Clin Infect Dis. 1997;25:847-851.
94. Bristow MF, Kohen D. Neuroleptic malignant syndrome. Br J Hosp Med. 1996; 55:517-520.
95. Glass JP, Lee YY, Bruner J, et al. Treatment-related leukoencephalopathy. A study of three cases and literature review. Medicine (Baltimore). 1986;65:154-162.
96. McKinney RE Jr, Katz SL, Wilfert CM. Chronic enteroviral meningoencephalitis in agammaglobulinemic patients. Rev Infect Dis. 1987;9:334-356.
97. Chretien F, Belec L, Hilton DA, et al. Herpes simplex virus type 1 encephalitis in acquired immunodeficiency syndrome. Neuropathol Appl Neurobiol. 1996; 22:394-404.
98. Gordon SM, Steinberg JP, DuPuis MH, et al. Culture isolation of Acanthamoeba species and leptomyxid amebas from patients with amebic meningoencephalitis, including two patients with AIDS. Clin Infect Dis. 1992;15:1024-1030.
99. Mamidi A, DeSimone JA, Pomerantz RJ. Central nervous system infections in individuals with HIV-1 infection. J Neurovirol. 2002;8:158-167.
100. Skiest DJ. Focal neurological disease in patients with acquired immunodeficiency syndrome. Clin Infect Dis. 2002;34:103-115.
101. Fong IW, Toma E. The natural history of progressive multifocal leukoencephalopathy in patients with AIDS. Canadian PML Study Group. Clin Infect Dis. 1995;20:1305-1310.
102. Kenyon LC, Dulaney E, Montone KT, et al. Varicella-zoster ventriculo-encephalitis and spinal cord infarction in a patient with AIDS. Acta Neuropathol (Berl). 1996; 92:202-205.
103. Pittella JE. Neuroschistosomiasis. Brain Pathol. 1997;7:649-662.
104. Kerr DA, Ayetey H. Immunopathogenesis of acute transverse myelitis. Curr Opin Neurol. 2002;15:339-347.
105. Christensen PB, Wermuth L, Hinge HH, et al. Clinical course and long-term prognosis of acute transverse myelopathy. Acta Neurol Scand. 1990;81:431-435.
106. Eggers C. HIV-1 associated encephalopathy and myelopathy. J Neurol. 2002; 249:1132-1136.
107. Berger JR, Sabet A. Infectious myelopathies. Semin Neurol. 2002;22:133-142.
108. Chopra JS, Banerjee AK, Murthy JM, et al. Paralytic rabies: A clinico-pathological study. Brain. 1980;103:789-802.
109. Melnick JL. Enterovirus type 71 infections: A varied clinical pattern sometimes mimicking paralytic poliomyelitis. Rev Infect Dis. 1984;6:S387-S390.
110. Hemachudha T, Laothamatas J, Rupprecht CE. Human rabies: A disease of complex neuropathogenetic mechanisms and diagnostic challenges. Lancet Neurol. 2002;1:101-109.
111. Whitley RJ, Roizman B. Herpes simplex virus infections. Lancet. 2001;357:1513-1518.
112. Whitley RJ, Bnann JW, Hinthorn D, et al. Disseminated herpes zoster in the immunocompromised host: A comparative trial of acyclovir and vidarabine. J Infect Dis. 1992;165:450-455.
113. Cohen JI, Davenport DS, Stewart JA, et al. Recommendations for prevention of and therapy for exposure to B virus (cercopithecine herpesvirus 1). Clin Infect Dis. 2002;35:1191-1203.
114. Raschilas F, Wolff M, Delatour F, et al. Outcome of and prognostic factors for herpes simplex encephalitis in adult patients: Results of a multicenter study. Clin Infect Dis. 2002;35:254-260.
115. Cinque P, Cleator GM, Weber T, et al. Diagnosis and clinical management of neurological disorders caused by cytomegalovirus in AIDS patients. European Union Concerted Action on Virus Meningitis and Encephalitis. J Neurovirol. 1998;4: 120-132.
116. von Giesen HJ, Arendt G. Drug treatment for HIV-1-associated dementia. Curr Opin Investig Drugs. 2002;3:1643-1646.
117. Langford TD, Letendre SL, Larrea GJ, et al. Changing patterns in the neuropathogenesis of HIV during the HAART era. Brain Pathol. 2003;13:195-210.
118. Sasaki S, Takeshita F, Okuda K, et al. Mycobacterium leprae and leprosy: A compendium. Microbiol Immunol. 2001;45:729-736.
119. Scollard DM. Endothelial cells and the pathogenesis of lepromatous neuritis: Insights from the armadillo model. Microbes Infect. 2000;2:1835-1843.
120. Simpson DM. Selected peripheral neuropathies associated with human immunodeficiency virus infection and antiretroviral therapy. J Neurovirol. 2002;8(Suppl 2):33-41.
121. Cadavid D, Barbour AG. Neuroborreliosis during relapsing fever: Review of the clinical manifestations, pathology, and treatment of infections in humans and experimental animals. Clin Infect Dis. 1998;26:151-164.
122. Yuki N. Infectious origins of, and molecular mimicry in, Guillain-Barré and Fisher syndromes. Lancet Infect Dis. 2001;1:29-37.
123. Govoni V, Granieri E. Epidemiology of the Guillain-Barré syndrome. Curr Opin Neurol. 2001;14:605-613.
124. Singh N, Malik A, Arora VK, et al. Fine needle aspiration cytology of leprous neuritis. Acta Cytol. 2003;47:368-372.
125. Nations SP, Katz JS, Lyde CB, et al. Leprous neuropathy: An American perspective. Semin Neurol. 1998;18:113-124.
126. Turton K, Chaddock JA, Acharya KR. Botulinum and tetanus neurotoxins: Structure, function and therapeutic utility. Trends Biochem Sci. 2002;27:552-558.
127. Holmes RK. Biology and molecular epidemiology of diphtheria toxin and the tox gene. J Infect Dis. 2000;181(Suppl 1):S156-S167.
128. Falnes PO, Sandvig K. Penetration of protein toxins into cells. Curr Opin Cell Biol. 2000;12:407-413.
129. Collier RJ. Understanding the mode of action of diphtheria toxin: A perspective on progress during the 20th century. Toxicon. 2001;39:1793-1803.
130. Logina I, Donaghy M. Diphtheritic polyneuropathy: A clinical study and comparison with Guillain-Barré syndrome. J Neurol Neurosurg Psychiatry. 1999;67:433-438.
131. Hadden RD, Karch H, Hartung HP, et al. Preceding infections, immune factors, and outcome in Guillain-Barré syndrome. Neurology. 2001;56:758-765.
132. Lu JL, Sheikh KA, Wu HS, et al. Physiologic-pathologic correlation in Guillain-Barré syndrome in children. Neurology. 2000;54:33-39.
133. Willison HJ, Yuki N. Peripheral neuropathies and anti-glycolipid antibodies. Brain. 2002;125:2591-2625.
134. Tsang RS. The relationship of Campylobacter jejuni infection and the development of Guillain-Barré syndrome. Curr Opin Infect Dis. 2002;15:221-228.
135. Ramos-e-Silva M, Rebello PF. Leprosy. Recognition and treatment. Am J Clin Dermatol. 2001;2:203-211.
136. Izurieta HS, Sutter RW, Strebel PM, et al. Tetanus surveillance—United States, 1991-1994. MMWR CDC Surveill Summ. 1997;46:15-25.
137. Weinstein L. Tetanus. N Engl J Med. 1973;289:1293-1296.
138. Cox N, Hinkle R. Infant botulism. Am Fam Physician. 2002;65:1388-1392.
139. Cherington M. Clinical spectrum of botulism. Muscle Nerve. 1998;21:701-710.
140. Weber JT, Goodpasture HC, Alexander H, et al. Wound botulism in a patient with a tooth abscess: Case report and review. Clin Infect Dis. 1993;16:635-639.
141. Barohn RJ, Saperstein DS. Guillain-Barré syndrome and chronic inflammatory demyelinating polyneuropathy. Semin Neurol. 1998;18:49-61.
142. Hughes RA, Rees JH. Clinical and epidemiologic features of Guillain-Barré syndrome. J Infect Dis. 1997;176(Suppl 2):S92-S98.
143. Lichtenfeld P. Autonomic dysfunction in the Guillain-Barré syndrome. Am J Med. 1971;50:772-780.
144. Ho TW, Li CY, Cornblath DR, et al. Patterns of recovery in the Guillain-Barré syndromes. Neurology. 1997;48:695-700.
145. Hadden RD, Cornblath DR, Hughes RA, et al. Electrophysiological classification of Guillain-Barré syndrome: Clinical associations and outcome. Plasma Exchange/Sandoglobulin Guillain-Barré Syndrome Trial Group. Ann Neurol. 1998;44:780-788.
146. Kieseier BC, Hartung HP. Therapeutic strategies in the Guillain-Barré syndrome. Semin Neurol. 2003;23:159-168.

CHAPTER **84**

Brain Abscess

ALLAN R. TUNKEL

Brain abscess is a focal, intracerebral infection that begins as a localized area of cerebritis and develops into a collection of pus surrounded by a well-vascularized capsule.[1] Brain abscess was an almost uniformly fatal disease before the late 1800s, when surgical techniques (i.e., drainage) led to cure in selected patients.[2] Further advances in the management of brain abscess were made after the introduction of antimicrobial therapy and stereotactic brain biopsy and aspiration techniques. Here we review the common bacterial, fungal, and protozoal causes of brain abscess, highlighting the clinical presentation, diagnosis, and approach to management.

EPIDEMIOLOGY AND ETIOLOGY

Brain abscess is one of the most serious complications of head and neck infections. Before the advent of human immunodeficiency virus (HIV) infection, brain abscess accounted for about 1 in 10,000 general hospital admissions, with 1500 to 2500 cases treated in the United States each year.[3] In most pediatric and adult series, a male predominance exists with a median age between 30 and 40 years, although the age distribution varies depending on the predisposing condition leading to the formation of brain abscess. When the abscess is related to a focus in the paranasal sinuses, most patients are 10 to 30 years of age; when the abscess is from an otitic focus, patients are younger than 20 or older than 40 years.[3,4] Overall, about 25% of brain abscess cases occur in children, most in the 4- to 7-year age group, and usually they originate from an otitic focus or in patients with cyanotic congenital heart disease. Brain abscess is extremely rare in patients younger than 2 years.

Case-fatality rates in patients with brain abscess, even in the antibiotic era, have ranged from 30% to 60% (similar to the rates in the pre-antibiotic era) until the period since the late 1970s, when the overall mortality rate has ranged from 0% to 24%.[3-5] This improvement has been attributed to the availability of more effective antimicrobial regimens (e.g., the addition of metronidazole), new surgical techniques, and, most importantly, the availability of computed tomography (CT) scanning. Data from the University of California in San Francisco demonstrated a decrease in the overall mortality rate from 44% during the 3 years before CT scanning to zero for the 3 years following the introduction of CT scanning in 1977.[6] This lower mortality rate was principally related to early diagnosis and an accurate method of postoperative follow-up with CT. The incidence of neurologic sequelae in patients who survive a brain abscess has ranged from 20% to 70%. In one study of factors influencing the outcome in 39 cases of bacterial brain abscess, the prognosis was primarily determined by the rapidity of progression of the disease before hospitalization and the patient's mental status on admission.[7] Therefore, early recognition of predisposing conditions is important for improving the outcome in this disorder.

When the microorganisms likely to be responsible for causing brain abscesses are evaluated, the isolation frequency depends on the predisposing condition (Table 84-1).[3] Improved microbiologic culture techniques, particularly for anaerobes, have had a significant impact on the awareness of microorganisms that are found in brain abscesses. The following paragraphs review the common bacteria, fungi, protozoa, and helminths that can produce brain abscess.

TABLE 84-1 Predisposing Conditions and Microbiology of Brain Abscess

Predisposing Condition	Usual Microbial Isolates
Otitis media or mastoiditis	Streptococci (anaerobic or aerobic), *Bacteroides* and *Prevotella* spp., Enterobacteriaceae
Sinusitis (frontoethmoid or sphenoid)	Streptococci, *Bacteroides* spp., Enterobacteriaceae, *Staphylococcus aureus, Haemophilus* spp.
Dental sepsis	Mixed *Fusobacterium, Prevotella* and *Bacteroides* spp., streptococci
Penetrating trauma or postneurosurgical	*S. aureus,* streptococci, Enterobacteriaceae, *Clostridium* spp.
Lung abscess, empyema, bronchiectasis	*Fusobacterium, Actinomyces, Bacteroides* and *Prevotella* spp., streptococci, *Nocardia* spp.
Bacterial endocarditis	*S. aureus,* streptococci
Congenital heart disease	Streptococci, *Haemophilus* spp.
Neutropenia	Aerobic gram-negative bacilli, *Aspergillus* spp., Mucorales, *Candida* spp.
Transplantation	*Aspergillus* spp., *Candida* spp., Mucorales, Enterobacteriaceae, *Nocardia* spp., *Toxoplasma gondii*
Human immunodeficiency virus infection	*T. gondii, Nocardia* spp., *Mycobacterium* spp., *Listeria monocytogenes, Cryptococcus neoformans*

Bacterial Brain Abscess

Streptococci (aerobic, anaerobic, and microaerophilic) are the bacteria most commonly (up to 70% of cases) cultured from patients with bacterial brain abscess, and they are frequently isolated in mixed infections (30% to 60% of cases).[3] These bacteria, especially the *Streptococcus anginosus (milleri)* group (*Streptococcus anginosus, Streptococcus constellatus,* and *Streptococcus intermedius*), normally reside in the oral cavity, appendix, and female genital tract, and they have a proclivity for abscess formation (see Chapter 201). Although streptococcal brain abscesses are seen most often in patients with otopharyngeal infections or infective endocarditis, they are also isolated after neurosurgical or other medical procedures.[8] *Staphylococcus aureus* accounts for 10% to 15% of isolates, usually in patients with cranial trauma or infective endocarditis, and it is often isolated in pure culture. The attention to proper culture techniques has increased the isolation of anaerobes from brain abscesses (40% to 100% of cases) with *Bacteroides* and *Prevotella* species isolated in 20% to 40% of patients, often in mixed culture.[9,10] Enteric gram-negative bacilli (e.g., *Proteus* species, *Escherichia coli, Klebsiella* species, and *Pseudomonas* species) are isolated in 23% to 33% of patients, often in those with otitic foci of infection, those with septicemia, those who have had neurosurgical procedures, or those who are immunocompromised. At one center, *Klebsiella* was the most prevalent pathogen (usually associated with hematogenous dissemination or postneurosurgical states),[11,12] followed by *Proteus* and *Enterobacter* species.[13] In one review of 41 patients with otogenic brain abscess, *Proteus* was isolated in 41% of cases.[14] The incidence of negative cultures has ranged from 0% to 43% in selected series,[3,9,14-16] with the frequency often correlating with prior use of antimicrobial therapy.

Other bacterial pathogens may be isolated from brain abscesses in selected patients or from those who are immunocompromised. Although *Haemophilus influenzae, Streptococcus pneumoniae,* and *Listeria monocytogenes* are common etiologic agents of bacterial meningitis, they are rarely isolated from patients with pyogenic brain abscesses (<1% of cases).[17-20] Brain abscess accounts for about 10% of central nervous system (CNS) infections caused by *L. monocytogenes.*[19] *Listeria* brain abscess is usually seen in immunocompromised patients. In a review of 39 cases of *Listeria* brain abscess, 85% of the patients had significant underlying conditions (including leukemia, lymphoma, HIV infection, and various conditions requiring corticosteroids or other immunosuppression), and disease was often associated with concomitant meningitis (38% of cases) and bacteremia (86% of cases).[20] In contrast, although meningitis caused by other facultative gram-negative organisms (e.g., *Citrobacter diversus, Proteus* species, *Serratia marcescens,* or *Enterobacter* species) is infrequent, it is associated with concomitant brain abscess in more than 75% of cases[1,21-23]; children with bacteremia or meningitis caused by these organisms should be evaluated for the possibility of brain abscess. Cerebral abscesses may also be a complication of neurologic infection with *Burkholderia pseudomallei.*[24] Actinomycosis of the CNS may present as brain abscess, usually secondary to hematogenous spread from a primary infection in the lung, abdomen, or pelvis, although contiguous spread from foci of infection in the ears, paranasal sinuses, or cervicofacial regions may occur.[25] Nocardial brain abscess may occur as an isolated CNS lesion or as part of a disseminated infection in association with pulmonary or cutaneous disease.[1] This organism is most often isolated in patients with defects in cell-mediated immunity (secondary to corticosteroid therapy, in organ transplant recipients, in patients infected with HIV, and in patients with neoplastic disease),[26-29] although up to 50% of patients with nocardiosis have no underlying conditions. Cases of nocardial brain abscess have also been seen in pregnant patients.[30] *Mycobacterium tuberculosis* and nontuberculous mycobacteria have been increasingly observed to cause focal CNS lesions,[1,3,31] with several cases reported in patients with HIV infection.[32-34]

Fungal Brain Abscess

The incidence of fungal brain abscess has increased as a result of the prevalent administration of immunosuppressive agents, broad-spectrum antimicrobial therapy, and corticosteroids.[35-39] Unfortunately, the diagnosis of fungal brain abscess is often unexpected, and many cases are not discovered until autopsy. In autopsy studies, *Candida* species have emerged as the most prevalent etiologic agents[40,41]; neuropathologic lesions include microabscesses, macroabscesses, noncaseating granulomas, and diffuse glial nodules. Risk factors for invasive *Candida* infection include the use of corticosteroids, broad-spectrum antimicrobial therapy, and hyperalimentation; disease is also seen in premature infants; in patients with malignancy, neutropenia, chronic granulomatous disease, diabetes mellitus, or thermal injuries; and in those with a central venous catheter in place.[36,39,42] However, several other pathogenic fungi should be considered in the differential diagnosis of fungal brain abscess, particularly in the immunosuppressed patient.

Cases of intracranial infection caused by *Aspergillus* species have been reported worldwide, with most cases occurring in adults. Cerebral aspergillosis is reported in 10% to 20% of all cases of invasive aspergillosis, and only rarely is the brain the only site of infection.[43] The lungs are the usual site of primary infection, and intracranial seeding occurs during dissemination of the organism or by direct extension from an area anatomically adjacent to the brain (e.g., the paranasal sinuses).[39] Most cases of invasive aspergillosis are found in neutropenic patients who have an underlying hematologic malignancy. Other risk groups include patients with hepatic disease, Cushing's syndrome, diabetes mellitus, chronic granulomatous disease, or HIV infection; injection drug abusers; postcraniotomy patients; organ transplant recipients; and patients receiving chronic corticosteroid therapy.[35,43-46]

Mucormycosis (zygomycosis, phycomycosis) is one of the most acute, fulminant fungal infections known. Many predisposing conditions to mucormycosis have been described including diabetes mellitus (70% of cases), usually in association with acidosis, acidemia from profound systemic illnesses (e.g., sepsis, severe dehydration, severe diarrhea, chronic renal failure), hematologic neoplasms, renal transplantation, injection drug use, and the use of deferoxamine.[39,47-51] Less than 5% of cases involve normal hosts. CNS disease may result from direct extension of the rhinocerebral form of mucormycosis, by open head trauma, or by hematogenous dissemination. The order Mucorales includes many species that have caused brain lesions (see Chapter 257), with *Rhizopus arrhizus (oryzae)* being one of the most common.[52]

Pseudallescheria boydii is a common mold readily isolated from soil that may cause CNS disease in both normal and immunocompromised hosts (e.g., those with neutropenia or cellular immunodeficiency).[39,53-56] This organism is being increasingly referred to as *Scedosporium apiospermum*, the asexual form of *P. boydii*. *P. boydii* may enter the CNS by direct trauma, by hematogenous dissemination from a pulmonary route, by way of an intravenous catheter, or by direct extension from infected sinuses. Brain abscess is the usual CNS manifestation, although meningitis and ventriculitis have also been reported. There is an association between near-drowning and subsequent illness, resulting from the pathogen's presence in contaminated water and manure.

Many of the etiologic agents of fungal meningitis may also cause brain abscess (e.g., *Cryptococcus neoformans, Coccidioides* spp., *Histoplasma capsulatum,* and *Blastomyces dermatitidis*); the epidemiologic and etiologic characteristics of these organisms are described in other chapters of this book. In addition, many of the dematiaceous and other fungi have also been reported to cause brain abscess; these include, in particular, *Cladophialophora bantiana, Bipolaris hawaiiensis, Bipolaris spicifera, Exophiala (Wangiella) dermatitidis, Ochroconis gallopava (Dactylaria constricta* var. *gallopava), Ramichloridium mackenziei, Curvularia pallescens,* and *Acrophialophora fusispora.*

Protozoal and Helminthic Brain Abscess

Several protozoa and helminths have been reported to produce brain abscess.[1,3,57] These include *Trypanosoma cruzi, Entamoeba histolytica, Schistosoma* species, and *Paragonimus* species.[57-60] Neurocysticercosis, caused by the larval form of *Taenia solium,* is a major cause of brain lesions in the developing world.[61] The epidemiologic features and approach to diagnosis and management of these organisms are discussed in other chapters of this book.

Disease caused by *Toxoplasma gondii* is the most common protozoal cause of brain abscess. The incidence of human infection caused by *T. gondii* depends on dietary habits (especially the amount of meat consumed and whether eaten rare, raw, or well done), the number of stray cats living in close proximity to humans, climatic conditions (moderate temperatures and high humidity favor oocyst survival in soil), and the overall level of sanitation and hygiene.[62] *T. gondii* infection of the CNS appears in a variety of syndromes but is usually associated with the development of intracerebral mass lesions or encephalitis in immunocompromised hosts. In the past, most cases of CNS toxoplasmosis occurred from reactivation of disease in patients with reticuloendothelial malignancies (either due to the malignancy itself or associated immunosuppressive or cytotoxic therapy), or in patients receiving immunosuppressive therapy after organ or bone marrow transplantation or for treatment of collagen vascular disorders.[63-68] Disease in organ transplant recipients not only occurs secondary to reactivation but may occur after the transfer of infected cysts in the allograft, most commonly in heart transplant recipients.

The number of cases of CNS toxoplasmosis has increased dramatically since 1981, specifically in patients with HIV infection.[69-72] Studies prior to the advent of highly active antiretroviral therapy (HAART) estimated that 5% to 47% of patients latently infected with *T. gondii* would develop CNS disease.[73] The use of trimethoprim-sulfamethoxazole prophylaxis of *Pneumocystis jirovecii* pneumonia and HAART has now decreased the incidence of *Toxoplasma* encephalitis substantially.[74,75]

PATHOGENESIS AND PATHOPHYSIOLOGY

Pathogenesis

Microorganisms can reach the brain by several different mechanisms (see Table 84-1).[1,3-5,15,17] The most common pathogenic mechanism of brain abscess formation is spread from a contiguous focus of infection, most often in the middle ear, mastoid cells, or paranasal sinuses. Brain abscess occurring secondary to otitis media is usually localized to the temporal lobe or the cerebellum; in one review of 41 cases of brain abscess from an otogenic source, 54% were in the temporal lobe, 44% in the cerebellum, and 2% in both locations.[14] Early studies reported that 40% of brain abscesses were associated with otitis media, but this number has been decreasing. However, if antimicrobial therapy of otitis is neglected, there is an increased risk of intracranial complications.[14] Paranasal sinusitis continues to be an important condition predisposing to brain abscess. The frontal lobe is the predominant abscess site, although when brain abscess complicates sphenoid sinusitis, the temporal lobe or sella turcica is usually involved. Dental infections are a less common cause of brain abscess[76]; infections of molar teeth seem most often to be the inciting factor. The frontal lobe is the usual site of the abscess after dental infection, but temporal lobe extension has also been reported.

A second mechanism of brain abscess formation is hematogenous dissemination to the brain from a distant focus of infection. These abscesses are usually multiple and multiloculated, and they have a higher mortality rate than abscesses that arise secondary to contiguous foci of infection.[3,4] The most common sources of initial infection in adults are chronic pyogenic lung diseases, especially lung abscess, bronchiectasis, empyema, and cystic fibrosis. Brain abscess may also occur hematogenously from wound and skin infections, osteomyelitis, pelvic infection, cholecystitis, and other intra-abdominal infections. Another predisposing factor leading to hematogenously acquired brain abscess is cyanotic congenital heart disease,[77-79] which accounts for about 5% to 15% of all brain abscess cases, with higher percentages in some pediatric series. These are most commonly seen in patients with tetralogy of Fallot or transposition of the great vessels. Brain abscess is rare after bacterial endocarditis (less than 5% of cases in most series),[80-82] despite the presence of continuous bacteremia. Hereditary hemorrhagic telangiectasia is a predisposing factor for brain abscess (occurring in about 1% of patients) and is almost always observed in patients with coexisting pulmonary arteriovenous malformations, perhaps by allowing septic emboli to cross the pulmonary circulation without capillary filtration or by bacterial seeding of an ischemic portion of the brain after paradoxical sterile emboli.[83-87] Brain abscesses have also developed after esophageal dilation and after sclerosing therapy for esophageal varices.[88,89]

Trauma is a third pathogenic mechanism in the development of brain abscess when it occurs secondary to an open cranial fracture with dural breach, or as a result of neurosurgery or a foreign body injury.[90] Four cases of brain abscess were recently reported in patients with malignant gliomas after craniotomy. These patients were treated with Gliadel wafers,[91] which are placed locally in the tumor bed and release carmustine after they undergo hydrolysis. The wafers may serve as a nidus for subsequent infection. The incidence of brain abscess formation after head trauma ranges from 3% to 17% in military populations, where it is usually secondary to retained bone fragments or contamination of initially "sterile" missile sites with bacteria from skin, clothes, and the environment.[92] However, in a recent study of 160 war missile penetrating craniocerebral injuries in Croatia in which 21 skull base injuries were treated surgically,[93] the authors did not attempt to remove all retained metallic or bone fragments but only the accessible ones. Retained foreign bodies did not seem to increase the infection rate, except in cases with an in-driven cluster of bone fragments or cerebrospinal fluid (CSF) leak; three cases of brain abscess were seen, for which repeat surgery was required. These findings were confirmed in another retrospective study from Croatia in 88 patients with missile brain wounds in which only accessible bone/metallic fragments were removed during intracranial débridement[94]; there were nine cases of brain abscess, and retained fragments were not responsible for an increased rate of infection. In another study of 43 patients who survived low-velocity missile injuries of the brain during military conflicts and who had retained intracranial fragments,[95] suppurative sequelae were seen in six patients, and two of these progressed to brain abscess. Traumatic predisposing conditions to brain abscess formation in the civilian population include compound depressed skull fractures, dog bites, rooster pecking, tongue piercing, and, especially in children, injury from lawn darts and pencil tips.[96-98]

Brain abscess is cryptogenic in about 20% of patients. Patent foramen ovale has been suggested as a possible predisposing condition in patients with cryptogenic brain abscess,[99] although this report of two patients does not establish patent foramen ovale as a definitive risk factor.

Initiation of Infection

Few studies have focused on the identification of the specific virulence factors of microorganisms that produce brain abscess. Contrary to common views, the brain may be more susceptible to infection than many other tissues. For example, compared with skin, the brain is significantly more susceptible to appropriate bacterial challenge. This was studied in a rat model of experimental brain abscess in which injections of 10^4 colony-forming units (CFU) of *S. aureus* or 10^6 CFU of *E. coli* failed to cause infection in the skin, whereas brain tissue was susceptible to as few as 10^2 CFU of either organism, with resultant abscess formation.[100] The brain may also have different susceptibilities to infection by different organisms. In a rat model of experimental brain abscess, strains of *E. coli* were more virulent (i.e., leading to abscess formation at lower inocula) than either *Pseudomonas aeruginosa, S. aureus,* or *Streptococcus pyogenes.*[101] Furthermore, *E. coli* strains possessing the K1 antigen were more infective than K1-negative strains, indicating that certain encapsulated strains may be more virulent in the production of brain abscess. However, the role of capsule among other bacterial species in the pathogenesis of brain abscess has not been evaluated. The inoculation of *Bacteroides fragilis* or microaerophilic organisms such as *S. intermedius* into rat brain failed to produce infection and abscess formation, although these organisms account for a high percentage of isolates from brain abscess patients (see earlier).

This discrepancy may be explained because brain abscess is often a result of contiguous spread of chronic otitic or sinus infections, and the synergistic infectivity of mixed populations of anaerobes plus a facultative organism may be necessary to establish the disease.[102,103] In an experimental dog model of brain abscess formation, the inoculation of *B. fragilis* in mixed culture with *Staphylococcus epidermidis* caused a virulent reaction,[104] but each organism was not tested separately.

The role of other bacterial virulence factors in brain abscess formation has not been evaluated. Despite extensive evidence implicating bacterial lipopolysaccharide in the pathogenesis of bacterial meningitis (see Chapter 80), similar studies on the effect, if any, of lipopolysaccharide on brain abscess formation and evolution are unavailable. *B. fragilis,* a major pathogen producing brain abscess, has a lipopolysaccharide that is chemically distinct from the lipopolysaccharide of aerobic gram-negative bacilli, but the biologic function of *B. fragilis* lipopolysaccharide is poorly defined and is unknown in the CNS.

An additional concern is the formation of brain abscesses in patients with bacterial meningitis. Brain abscess is a rare complication of bacterial meningitis, with the exception of the high prevalence of abscess formation in neonates with *C. diversus* meningitis.[22,23] In this disease, there is a propensity for contiguous inflammation in the cerebral white matter, which may reflect the effects of endotoxin on the small penetrating vessels in this area. This was examined in an infant rat model, in which infection was initiated with a high-grade bacteremia, followed by infiltration of the leptomeninges and the development of ventriculitis.[105] Brain abscesses in these animals were found exclusively in the periventricular white matter, apparently from disruption of the ventricular ependymal lining and direct extension of the infection into the parenchyma. The virulence factors responsible for the propensity of this organism to cause brain abscess are undefined, although a minor outer-membrane protein (32 kilodaltons) may be a marker for strains more likely to produce ventriculitis and brain abscess[106]; strains that lack the 32-kD outer-membrane protein cause more bacteremia, meningitis, and death. Other factors, such as fimbriation, biotype, and hemolysis, did not correlate with CNS invasion.

Natural History of Infection

Several animal models have been used to examine the pathophysiologic consequences and temporal course of brain abscesses after the initiation of infection. A canine model was utilized to define the pathologic stages of brain abscess formation after the inoculation of α-hemolytic streptococci.[107] On the basis of detailed histologic evaluation, four stages of brain abscess evolution were defined: early cerebritis (days 1 to 3), late cerebritis (days 4 to 9), early capsule formation (days 10 to 13), and late capsule formation (day 14 and later after initial inoculation). Although these stages are somewhat arbitrary, they are useful in classification and in comparing organisms with regard to their virulence in the production of brain abscess. The early cerebritis stage is characterized by an acute inflammatory infiltrate with visible bacteria on Gram stain and marked edema surrounding the lesion. The center of the lesion becomes necrotic during the late cerebritis stage, and macrophages and fibroblasts begin to invade the periphery. With early capsule formation, the necrotic center begins to decrease in size with simultaneous development of a collagenous capsule that is less prominent on the ventricular side of the lesion; cerebral edema also starts to regress during this stage. In this canine model, the collagen capsule was complete circumferentially by the end of the second week and then increased in density and thickness. Similar neuropathologic findings have been observed in a model of experimental anaerobic brain abscess,[104] although capsule formation could not be divided into early and late stages because of delayed encapsulation. A subsequent study revealed that *S. aureus* was more virulent than the α-hemolytic streptococci in brain abscess formation[108]; the amount of necrosis, the total area of involvement after staphylococcal challenge, the course of infection as it progressed toward resolution, the time for the abscess to reach a stable size, and the time to contain the necrotic region with a collagenous capsule were all longer after inoculation of *S. aureus*. Capsule formation was less prominent on the ventricular than on the cortical surface in these studies,[104,107,108] perhaps because differences in vascularity between cortical gray and white matter allowed greater fibroblast proliferation on the cortical side of the abscess. This may explain the tendency for brain abscesses to rupture into the ventricular system rather than into the subarachnoid space. An alternative hypothesis was supported in an experimental rat model after inoculation of *E. coli*.[109] It was suggested in this study that brain abscesses tended to rupture intraventricularly because the infectious process is directed along the major white matter tracts (areas of low tissue resistance) rather than as a result of asymmetrical collagen deposition. The importance of virulence factor production in brain abscess development was demonstrated by the inability of heat-inactivated *S. aureus* to induce proinflammatory cytokine or chemokine expression in an experimental murine model[110]; alpha-toxin was identified as a key virulence factor for survival of *S. aureus* in the brain and the subsequent development of brain abscess.

Host Defense Mechanisms

The brain is usually protected from infection by an intact blood-brain barrier. However, once brain infection is established, immune defenses are inadequate to control the infection. Because local opsonization is deficient, encapsulated bacteria such as *E. coli* and *B. fragilis* may escape efficient phagocytosis within the brain parenchyma. Several studies have shown that phagocytosis of *Bacteroides* species requires heat-labile serum factors (e.g., complement, lysozyme),[111,112] and these factors are likely to be absent, or at very low concentrations, even in the presence of CNS inflammation early in disease. In addition, an outer-membrane component of *Bacteroides* species may be important in the inhibition of neutrophil chemotaxis, thus reducing the host response to brain abscess associated with this organism.[113]

The host inflammatory response after the initiation of infection has been evaluated by serial pathologic analysis in several animal models of brain abscess formation.[104,107,108] During the early cerebritis stage, a border around the initial area of inoculation, composed of acute inflammatory cells, is observed, and this is accompanied by the rapid development of a perivascular infiltration consisting of neutrophils, plasma cells, and mononuclear cells. In an experimental rat model of *S. aureus* brain abscess,[114] production of the proinflammatory cytokines interleukin (IL)-1α, IL-1β, IL-6, and tumor necrosis factor (TNF)-α occurred as early as 1 to 6 hours after *S. aureus* exposure. This was followed by enhanced concentrations of the CXC chemokine KC, 24 hours after bacterial exposure, which correlated with the appearance of neutrophils in the abscess. To address the importance of neutrophils in the early containment of *S. aureus* infection in the brain, mice transiently depleted of neutrophils prior to implantation of bacteria-laden beads had higher CNS bacterial burdens than control animals.[115] Both macrophage inflammatory protein (MIP)-2 and KC/CXCL1, two neutrophil-attracting CXC chemokines, were significantly elevated in the brain after *S. aureus* exposure, indicating the importance of the CXCR2 ligands MIP-2 and KC, and neutrophils, in the acute host response to *S. aureus* in the brain. With progression to the late cerebritis stage, the acute inflammatory cells become mixed with macrophages and fibroblasts, and reticulin formation surrounds the necrotic center. As the capsule begins to form, increased numbers of fibroblasts and macrophages infiltrate the periphery, and mature collagen is deposited to form a capsule. With further encapsulation, the necrotic center continues to decrease in size while marked gliosis develops outside the capsule.

The importance of this host inflammatory response in containment of the brain abscess has been examined in immunosuppressed animals. Initial studies in the dog model of experimental brain abscess with *S. aureus* or *Proteus mirabilis* demonstrated that the administration of dexamethasone slowed, but did not fully impair, capsule formation.[116] In contrast, in another study no evidence of encapsulation was found when dexamethasone was given to rabbits at the same time as inoculation of either *S. pyogenes* or *S. aureus*.[117] In an experimental rat model of *E. coli* brain abscess, dexamethasone administration led to a

reduction in the macrophage and glial response, collagen deposition, and host survival, with an increased number of viable bacteria in the brain abscess.[109] Co-administration of dexamethasone also impaired the lymphocytic and fibroblastic response in a rat model of experimental *S. aureus* brain abscess[118] but did not entirely halt the encapsulation or reduce the associated cerebral edema. Another study utilized dogs that were immunosuppressed with azathioprine and prednisone 7 days before the intracerebral inoculation of α-hemolytic streptococci.[119] The immunosuppressed animals manifested a decreased inflammatory response characterized by a reduction in neutrophils and macrophages in the lesion, a decrease and delay in collagen deposition, and persistence of viable organisms into the late capsule stage. Neutrophils, plasma cells, lymphocytes, and macrophages were markedly reduced in the areas surrounding the necrotic center of the abscess, and cerebritis was also decreased outside the developing capsule. Gliosis, however, was markedly increased in the area surrounding the collagen capsule in these immunosuppressed dogs. Although this decreased inflammatory response and edema formation resulted in less mass effect initially, the eventual size and area of the abscess may have become larger as a result of the diminished host response.

CLINICAL PRESENTATION

The clinical course of brain abscess may range from indolent to fulminant.[1,3,5,7,15,17,120] Most of the clinical manifestations (Table 84-2) are not due to the systemic signs of infection but rather to the size and location of a space-occupying lesion within the brain and the virulence of the infecting microorganism. Headache is the most common presenting symptom and is observed in approximately 70% of patients. The headache may be moderate to severe and hemicranial or generalized in location, but it is without particularly distinguishing features, accounting for frequent delays in diagnosis. Sudden worsening of the headache, accompanied by a new onset of meningismus, may signify rupture of the abscess into the ventricular space[121]; this complication is often associated with a high mortality rate (up to 80% in some series). In a recent study of 33 consecutive patients with intraventricular rupture of brain abscess, severe headaches and signs of meningeal irritation were prominent before rupture, with a rapidly deteriorating clinical condition developing within 10 days after the signs of meningeal irritation[122]; CT scanning prior to rupture demonstrated localized enhancement of the ventricular wall adjacent to the abscess, most likely because capsule formation was more complete on the cortical side than on the ventricular side of the abscess. Less than 50% of patients with brain abscess present with the classic triad of fever, headache, and focal neurologic deficit. In addition, the clinical presentation of brain abscess in the immunocompromised patient may be masked by the diminished inflammatory response.[35,37] In a recent study of 123 patients with brain abscess, the most common manifestations were fever, headache, altered consciousness, and hemiparesis, occurring in 58%, 55%, 50%, and 44% of patients, respectively.[12]

The location in the brain abscess defines the clinical presentation.[3,5,15,17] Patients with a frontal lobe abscess often present with headache, drowsiness, inattention, deterioration of mental status, hemiparesis with unilateral motor signs, and a motor speech disorder.

TABLE 84-2 Common Symptoms and Signs in Brain Abscess

Symptom or Sign	Frequency (%)
Headache	~70
Mental status changes	≤70
Focal neurologic deficits	>60
Fever	45-50
Triad of headache, fever, and focal deficit	<50
Seizures	25-35
Nausea and vomiting	25-50
Nuchal rigidity	~25
Papilledema	~25

The clinical presentation of cerebellar abscesses includes ataxia, nystagmus, vomiting, and dysmetria. Temporal lobe abscesses may cause ipsilateral headache and aphasia if the lesion is in the dominant hemisphere; a visual field defect (e.g., an upper homonymous quadrantanopsia) may be the only presenting sign of a temporal lobe abscess. Abscesses of the brain stem usually manifest with facial weakness, fever, headache, hemiparesis, dysphagia, and vomiting.[123,124] The classic findings of a well-defined brain-stem syndrome is frequently lacking in patients with brain-stem abscesses because the abscess is likely to extend longitudinally along fiber tracts rather than expanding transversely.[1]

Certain pathogens may lead to the development of specific clinical characteristics after CNS infection. In patients with nocardial brain abscess, the presentation is generally nonspecific with fever, headache, and focal deficits determined by the site and size of the lesion.[26-30,125] The clinical suspicion of nocardial brain abscess may be increased by the presence of pulmonary, skin, or muscle lesions, which are present concurrently in many, but not all, cases. All patients with pulmonary nocardiosis should undergo evaluation to exclude CNS disease.

Patients with *Aspergillus* brain abscess most commonly manifest signs of a stroke syndrome (secondary to ischemia or intracerebral hemorrhage, or both) referable to the involved area of brain.[39] Headache, encephalopathy, and seizures may also occur. Fever is not a consistent feature, and signs of meningeal irritation are rare. Patients who are severely immunocompromised usually present with nonspecific findings (i.e., alteration in mental status, or seizures, or both) shortly before death, whereas those patients less immunocompromised are more likely to have headache and focal neurologic deficits.[43] Patients with *Aspergillus* brain abscess commonly have evidence of aspergillosis involving other organ systems.[45,126]

Rhinocerebral mucormycosis initially manifests with complaints referable to the eyes or sinuses including headache (often unilateral), facial pain, diplopia, lacrimation, and nasal stuffiness or epistaxis[39,43,48,127]; fever is usual. As the infection spreads to contiguous structures, necrotic lesions appear in the turbinates, nose, paranasal skin, or hard palate. Chemosis, proptosis, and external ophthalmoplegia may occur. Cranial nerve abnormalities are common (including cranial nerves II through VII, IX, and X), and blindness may occur as a result of invasion of the cavernous sinus, ophthalmic artery, and orbit. Thrombosis is a striking feature of this disease because the organism has a proclivity for blood vessel invasion. Focal neurologic deficits such as hemiparesis, seizures, or monocular blindness suggest far-advanced disease. With further progression, invasion of the internal carotid artery in the cavernous sinus can occur, accompanied by metastatic lesions in the frontoparietal cortex and deepening coma.[128] In patients with nonrhinocerebral brain abscess caused by the Mucorales, fever, headache, or focal neurologic deficits were present in more than half the patients. In one review of 22 cases,[49] 50% of the patients were injection drug users and the basal ganglia were the most commonly involved CNS site (83% of patients).

Brain abscess due to *P. boydii* tends to occur in immunocompromised patients or in patients 15 to 30 days after an episode of near-drowning.[54,55] Brain abscesses can be located in the cerebrum, cerebellum, or brain stem; clinical presentations include seizures, altered consciousness, headache, meningeal irritation, focal neurologic deficits, abnormal behavior, and aphasia. The clinical manifestations of CNS disease caused by *Cryptococcus, Histoplasma, Coccidioides, Candida,* and other fungal pathogens depend on the intracranial location of the abscess. In one review, nearly one third of bone marrow transplant recipients with brain abscess caused by *Candida* species had no signs or symptoms[37]; these infections were commonly diagnosed postmortem.

The clinical manifestations of CNS toxoplasmosis in the immunocompromised patient are variable, ranging from an insidious process evolving over several weeks to acute onset with a confusional state; the initial symptoms and signs may be focal or nonfocal, or both.[62] *T. gondii* has a predilection to localize in the basal ganglia and brain stem, producing extrapyramidal symptoms resembling those of Parkinson's disease. Generally, patients who present with nonfocal abnormalities develop signs of focal neurologic disease as the infection progresses, although some patients develop a diffuse, rapidly fatal encephalopathic process. Nonfocal evidence of neurologic dysfunction may predominate and includes generalized weakness, headache, confusion, lethargy, alteration of mental status, personality changes, and coma. CNS toxoplasmosis may also present differently depending on the risk group. Infection in transplant recipients is often diffuse, disseminated disease.[64,67] Localizing neurologic signs tend to occur late in the course of infection in transplant recipients or not at all. In patients with underlying malignancies (e.g., Hodgkin's disease), the presentation of toxoplasmic encephalitis is evenly distributed between focal and nonfocal manifestations of encephalitis.[63-65]

Patients with acquired immunodeficiency syndrome (AIDS) often present subacutely with nonspecific symptoms such as neuropsychiatric complaints, headache, disorientation, confusion, and lethargy progressing over 2 to 8 weeks; associated fever and weight loss are also common.[62,69-71,73] Patients then develop clinical evidence of focal CNS mass lesions with ataxia, aphasia, hemiparesis, visual field loss, and vomiting, or a more generalized encephalitis with increasing confusion, dementia, and stupor; seizures are common and may be the presenting clinical manifestation of CNS toxoplasmosis in patients with AIDS.

DIAGNOSIS

CT has revolutionized the diagnosis of brain abscess. Before the advent of CT, delays in diagnosis contributed significantly to the high morbidity and mortality in patients with brain abscess. CT has rendered diagnostic tests such as angiography, ventriculography, pneumoencephalography, and radionuclide brain scanning virtually obsolete[129]; therefore, these modalities will not be discussed here. CT is not only an excellent means of examination of the brain parenchyma but is superior to these standard radiographic procedures for examination of the paranasal sinuses, mastoids, and middle ear.[130,131] The characteristic CT appearance of brain abscess is that of a hypodense center with a peripheral uniform ring enhancement following the injection of contrast material; this is surrounded by a variable hypodense area of brain edema (Fig. 84-1). Other CT findings include nodular enhancement and areas of low attenuation without enhancement, the latter of which is observed during the early cerebritis stage before abscess formation; as the abscess progresses, contrast enhancement is observed. Once the abscess becomes encapsulated in the later stages, contrast material no longer differentiates the lucent center and the CT appearance is similar to that of the early cerebritis stage. CT scanning is also useful for following the course of brain abscess, although after aspiration, improvement in the CT appearance may not be seen for up to 5 weeks or longer.

Magnetic resonance imaging (MRI) has been extensively evaluated in the diagnosis of brain abscess and is the first imaging choice in the evaluation of a patient suspected of having this disorder. MRI is more sensitive than CT and therefore offers significant advantages in the early detection of cerebritis, including greater contrast between cerebral edema and adjacent brain, more conspicuous spread of inflammation into the ventricles and subarachnoid space, and earlier detection of satellite lesions (Fig. 84-2).[132] On T_1-weighted images, the abscess capsule often appears as a discrete rim that is isointense to mildly hyperintense. Contrast enhancement with the paramagnetic agent gadolinium diethylenetriaminepentaacetic acid provides the added advantage of clearly differentiating the central abscess, the surrounding enhancing rim, and the cerebral edema surrounding the abscess.

On T_1-weighted images, enhancement of the abscess capsule occurs. On T_2-weighted images, the zone of edema that surrounds the abscess is one of marked high signal intensity; the capsule now appears as a well-defined hypointense rim at the margin of the abscess. It is important to note that therapy with corticosteroids can decrease enhancement seen with both CT and MRI. Magnetic resonance spectroscopy, in combination with MRI, was useful in diagnosing two

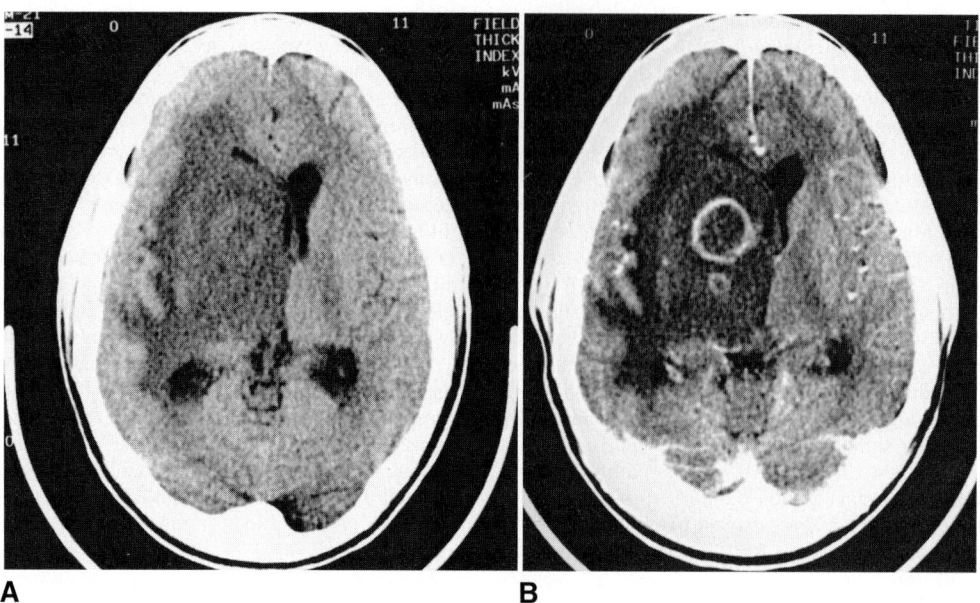

FIGURE 84-1. Computed tomography scan of the head reveals a large rounded area of low attenuation in the right lentiform nucleus, with compression of the right horn of the right lateral ventricle and a shift to the left with vasogenic edema. **A,** Unenhanced scan reveals increased signal within the center of the area of low attenuation. **B,** After the administration of intravenous contrast, there is ring enhancement of the abscess and evidence of a smaller satellite lesion.

cases of bacterial brain abscess,[133] although further studies are needed to verify the diagnostic utility of this technique.

CT and MRI are also quite sensitive in defining the lesions in patients with fungal brain abscess; these modalities, however, are not specific, although some exceptions do exist. The finding of a cerebral infarct in a patient with risk factors for invasive aspergillosis should suggest that diagnosis.[39] The areas of infarction typically develop into either single or multiple abscesses involving the cerebrum (usually frontal or temporal lobes) or cerebellum. In patients with rhinocerebral mucormycosis, CT and MRI may show characteristic changes, including sinus opacification, erosion of bone, and obliteration of

deep fascial planes.[134,135] Frontal lobe involvement in mucormycosis may show little or no ring enhancement; the lack of contrast enhancement is a poor prognostic sign as it indicates failure of host defense mechanisms to isolate or encapsulate the offending organism. Cavernous sinus involvement may be seen on MRI.

CT and MRI are both extremely useful in the diagnosis of CNS toxoplasmosis.[62,70] The characteristic CT appearance (seen in 90% of patients) is that of rounded isodense or hypodense lesions with ring enhancement after the administration of contrast material; however, homogeneous enhancement or no enhancement can also be seen. There are multiple lesions in 70% to 80% of cases, often involving the

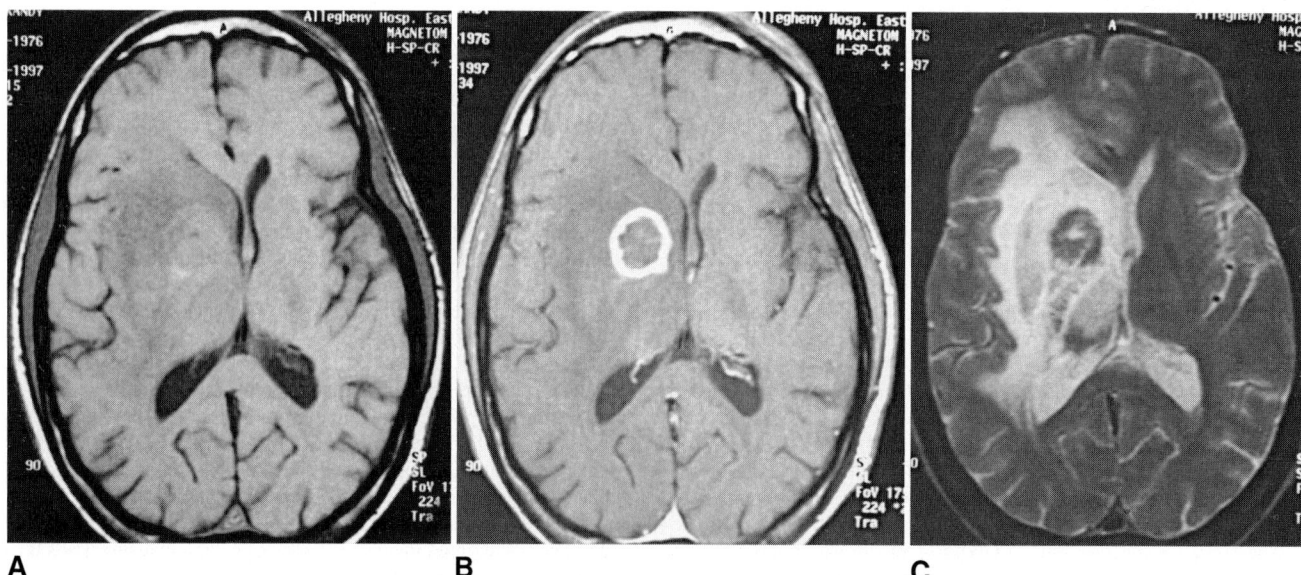

FIGURE 84-2. Magnetic resonance imaging of the brain (same patient as shown in Fig. 84-1) reveals a 2-cm, round, ring-enhancing lesion in the right lentiform nucleus with associated vasogenic edema and midline shift to the left. **A,** T_1-weighted image reveals an ill-defined area of low attenuation. **B,** T_1-weighted image after administration of gadolinium, which reveals ring enhancement of the abscess. **C,** T_2-weighted image demonstrates hypointensity of the rim of the abscess with a large area of high signal intensity consistent with cerebral edema.

corticomedullary junction and the basal ganglia, although any part of the CNS may be involved. Marked edema and a mass effect are also frequently observed. A double-dose delayed-contrast study may be a more sensitive method for delineating the true extent of disease. Unfortunately, CT usually underestimates the number of lesions documented pathologically at autopsy.[69] MRI has a greater sensitivity than CT and has detected lesions in patients with active toxoplasmic encephalitis whose CT scans were normal. Therefore, MRI should be performed in patients with AIDS and neurologic symptoms in whom CT shows no abnormality (or only cerebral atrophy). CT and MRI may also be useful in following the response to therapy, as most patients demonstrate radiographic evidence of improvement within 10 to 14 days of initiation of anti-*Toxoplasma* therapy.[72,136]

In the immunosuppressed host with presumed toxoplasmic encephalitis, serologic testing is of value to aid in the diagnosis. For example, in patients with AIDS, toxoplasmic encephalitis occurs as a result of a recrudescence of a latent infection.[69-71] In this situation, the presence of anti-*Toxoplasma* immunoglobulin G (IgG) antibody can almost uniformly be demonstrated before the development of the encephalitis. More than 97% of patients with AIDS and toxoplasmic encephalitis have serum IgG antibody titers against *T. gondii* ranging from 1:8 to more than 1:1024[62]; the predictive value of a positive serologic result in patients with characteristic abnormalities on radiographic studies may be as high as 80% in the United States.[70,137] In contrast, in a retrospective review of 115 patients with AIDS and CNS toxoplasmosis at San Francisco General Hospital between 1981 and 1990, 4 of 18 patients with pathologically confirmed disease had undetectable anti-*Toxoplasma* IgG antibody by an indirect immunofluorescence assay.[72] Despite these conflicting data, many physicians in the United States initiate a therapeutic trial of anti-*Toxoplasma* chemotherapy in a patient with AIDS who is seropositive for *T. gondii* and has characteristic neuroradiographic abnormalities.[138] This is generally a valid approach in patients with AIDS and presumed CNS toxoplasmosis (see Chapter 276).

CSF polymerase chain reaction (PCR) has also been utilized as a diagnostic test for toxoplasmic encephalitis; CSF PCR has a specificity of 96% to 100%, but a sensitivity of only about 50% in the diagnosis of CNS toxoplasmosis.[73] In contrast, in a study of 12 HIV-infected patients with suspected cerebral toxoplasmosis who neither met the diagnostic criteria from the Centers for Disease Control and Prevention nor had positive mouse inoculation tests,[139] 11 patients with confirmed toxoplasmosis had positive PCR results in either blood or CSF, suggesting a high sensitivity, specificity, and clinical utility of this test in the diagnosis of toxoplasmic encephalitis. However, further studies are needed to determine the utility of CSF PCR in the diagnosis of toxoplasmic encephalitis.

A major advance in the use of CT scanning in patients with suspected brain abscess is the ability to perform stereotactic CT-guided aspiration to facilitate microbiologic diagnosis and guide antimicrobial therapy. Ultrasound-guided aspiration, via transdural insonation, has also been performed through a single bur hole and showed excellent abscess visualization in 10 patients in one study,[140] although aspiration by CT guidance is generally the preferred method. Aspiration during the cerebritis stage, however, may be complicated by hemorrhage.

At the time of aspiration, specimens should be sent for Gram stain, routine aerobic and anaerobic cultures, and cultures for mycobacteria and fungi. In addition, other special stains such as acid-fast stains for mycobacteria, modified acid-fast stains for *Nocardia,* and special stains (e.g., mucicarmine, methenamine silver) for fungi should be used to aid in making an etiologic diagnosis. For example, *Aspergillus* species manifest as septate hyphae in tissue sections with acute-angle, dichotomous branching. Biopsy of cerebral lesions in mucormycosis usually demonstrates irregular hyphae, right-angle branching, and a lack of septa. *P. boydii, Scedosporium prolificans,* and *Fusarium* hyphae cannot be distinguished reliably from *Aspergillus* species.[54] Hyphae of dematiaceous fungi in the brain may be brownish on hematoxylin and eosin stain and tend to have swollen and constricted areas in the hyphae, but they are not reliably distinguished from other molds. In pa-

tients with CNS toxoplasmosis,[62] diagnosis may require specialized immunohistochemical techniques (peroxidase-antiperoxidase) to detect the organisms or its antigens. Pseudocysts and tachyzoites, which are easily identifiable by histopathologic stains, may not be found in the center of the necrotic lesion and are best identified at the periphery of the lesion or within normal brain tissue. A sensitive test for rapid diagnosis is the immunofluorescence technique, using monoclonal anti-*Toxoplasma* antibodies on brain touch preparations.

INITIAL MANAGEMENT OF THE PATIENT WITH BRAIN ABSCESS

The initial approach to the patient with a suspected brain abscess is a multidisciplinary one and should include a neuroradiologist, a neurosurgeon, and an infectious diseases specialist. The following steps are a recommended approach to the patient with a suspected brain abscess[139]:

1. Contrast CT or MRI should be performed to verify the suspicion of brain abscess.
2. If single or multiple ring-enhancing lesions are found, the patient should be taken urgently to surgery. All lesions greater than 2.5 cm in diameter should be excised or stereotactically aspirated and specimens sent to the microbiology and pathology laboratories (see earlier paragraphs). For abscesses in the early cerebritis stage or when the abscesses are 2.5 cm in diameter or less, the largest lesion should be aspirated for diagnosis and organism identification.
3. Once abscess material has been obtained for microbiologic and histopathologic studies, empirical antimicrobial therapy should be initiated on the basis of the patient's predisposing conditions and the presumed pathogenesis of abscess formation (Table 84-3). If a primary source of infection outside the CNS is recognized as potentially having led to formation of the brain abscess, empirical antimicrobial therapy can be begun on the basis of microbiologic studies from the other source (e.g., positive blood cultures in a patient with infective endocarditis).
4. Therapy with corticosteroids should be initiated in patients with significant edema and an associated mass effect that is causing increased intracranial pressure or a predisposition to transtentorial herniation. Phenytoin should be considered to prevent seizures during early stages of therapy.

The empirical approach to antimicrobial therapy for bacterial brain abscess should take into account the frequency of isolation of certain organisms.[3] Because of the high rate of isolation of streptococci (particularly the *S. anginosus [milleri]* group) from brain abscesses of various causes, high-dose intravenous penicillin G or another drug (e.g., a third-generation cephalosporin, either cefotaxime or ceftriaxone) active against this organism should be included in the initial therapeutic regimen. Penicillin G is also active against most anaerobic species with the notable exception of *B. fragilis,* which may be isolated in a high percentage of brain abscess cases; metronidazole should be included in the initial regimen when this organism is suspected. Metronidazole has bactericidal activity against *B. fragilis* and *Prevotella melaninogenica* and attains high concentrations in brain abscess pus, and its entry into cerebral abscesses is not affected by concomitant corticosteroid therapy.[140-142] When *S. aureus* is considered a likely pathogen (e.g., after cranial trauma or after neurosurgery), nafcillin should be used, with vancomycin reserved for patients allergic to penicillin or when methicillin-resistant organisms are suspected or isolated.[143] Because an increase in community-acquired methicillin-resistant *S. aureus* has been observed in recent years, vancomycin should be used empirically when *S. aureus* brain abscess is suspected or proven,[144] until in vitro susceptibility testing is performed. If *P. aeruginosa* is a likely infecting pathogen, ceftazidime or cefepime is the agent of choice. In patients with a bacterial brain abscess of unclear pathogenesis, empirical therapy with vancomycin, metronidazole, and a third- or fourth-generation cephalosporin (cefotaxime or ceftriaxone, or ceftazidime or cefepime if *P. aeruginosa* is suspected) is recommended pending culture results.

TABLE 84-3 Empirical Antimicrobial Therapy for Bacterial Brain Abscess

Predisposing Condition	Antimicrobial Regimen
Otitis media or mastoiditis	Metronidazole + a third-generation cephalosporin*
Sinusitis (frontoethmoid or sphenoid)	Metronidazole + a third-generation cephalosporin*,†
Dental sepsis	Penicillin + metronidazole
Penetrating trauma or postneurosurgical	Vancomycin + a third-generation cephalosporin*,‡
Lung abscess, empyema, bronchiectasis	Penicillin + metronidazole + a sulfonamide§
Bacterial endocarditis	Vancomycin + gentamicin *or* nafcillin + ampicillin + gentamicin
Congenital heart disease	Third-generation cephalosporin*
Unknown	Vancomycin + metronidazole + a third-generation cephalosporin*,‡

*Cefotaxime, ceftriaxone, or cefepime.
†Add vancomycin when infection caused by methicillin-resistant *Staphylococcus aureus* is suspected.
‡Use ceftazidime or cefepime as the third-generation cephalosporin if *Pseudomonas aeruginosa* is suspected.
§Trimethoprim-sulfamethoxazole; include if a *Nocardia* species is suspected.

In HIV-infected patients with CNS mass lesions, the initial approach to management is somewhat different because of the high likelihood of the diagnosis of toxoplasmic encephalitis.[70,145] For patients with large lesions demonstrating a mass effect and threatening impending herniation, open biopsy with decompression is the standard. In HIV-infected patients with multiple ring-enhancing lesions on contrast CT or MRI and positive anti-*Toxoplasma* IgG serologic tests, empirical therapy for toxoplasmic encephalitis should be initiated (Table 84-4); clinical and radiographic improvement should be observed within 10 to 14 days in 95% of patients with toxoplasmic encephalitis.[73,136] For patients with positive anti-*Toxoplasma* IgG serologic tests and a single lesion identified by MRI, consideration should be given to thallium 201 single photon emission computed tomography (^{201}Tl-SPECT) scanning. Although ^{201}Tl-SPECT scans are not sensitive, positive scans are highly specific for the diagnosis of primary CNS lymphoma and would warrant stereotactic brain biopsy.[146-148] A compilation of published studies revealed a mean sensitivity and specificity of 92% and 89%, respectively, for ^{201}Tl-SPECT in distinguishing cerebral lymphoma from toxoplasmic encephalitis in patients with AIDS.[73] However, ^{201}Tl-SPECT was positive in one patient with chronic lymphocytic leukemia and a *Nocardia* brain abscess.[149] In addition, a recent prospective study of 14 HIV-infected patients (12 diagnosed by biopsy and 2 by clinical course and response to therapy) suggested limited accuracy of ^{201}Tl-SPECT in differentiating lymphoma from non-neoplastic disease, in which a low uptake ratio did not exclude lymphoma and a high uptake ratio did not exclude an infectious cause.[150] The accuracy of ^{201}Tl-SPECT can be affected by the size of the lesion, grade of the malignancy, presence of necrotic areas in the tumor, and location of the lesion. Similar results have been obtained with positron-emission tomography (PET) scanning

TABLE 84-4 Antimicrobial Therapy for Brain Abscess

Organism	Standard Therapy	Alternative Therapies
Bacteria*		
Actinomyces spp.	Penicillin G	Clindamycin
Bacteroides fragilis	Metronidazole	Clindamycin
Enterobacteriaceae	Third-generation cephalosporin†	Aztreonam, trimethoprim-sulfamethoxazole, fluoroquinolone, meropenem
Fusobacterium spp.	Penicillin G	Metronidazole
Haemophilus spp.	Third-generation cephalosporin†	Aztreonam, trimethoprim-sulfamethoxazole
Listeria monocytogenes	Ampicillin or penicillin G‡	Trimethoprim-sulfamethoxazole
Mycobacterium tuberculosis	Isoniazid + rifampin + pyrazinamide ± ethambutol	—
Nocardia spp.	Trimethoprim-sulfamethoxazole or sulfadiazine	Minocycline, imipenem, meropenem, a third-generation cephalosporin,† amikacin
Prevotella melaninogenica	Metronidazole	Clindamycin, cefotaxime
Pseudomonas aeruginosa	Ceftazidime‡ or cefepime‡	Aztreonam,‡ fluoroquinolone,‡ meropenem‡
Staphylococcus aureus		
Methicillin-sensitive	Nafcillin or oxacillin	Vancomycin
Methicillin-resistant	Vancomycin	—
Streptococcus anginosus (*milleri*) group, other streptococci	Penicillin G	Third-generation cephalosporin,† vancomycin
Fungi		
Aspergillus spp.	Voriconazole	Amphotericin B lipid complex, liposomal amphotericin B
Candida spp.	Amphotericin B§	Fluconazole, liposomal amphotericin B,‖ amphotericin B lipid complex‖
Cryptococcus neoformans	Amphotericin B§	Fluconazole, liposomal amphotericin B,‖ amphotericin B lipid complex‖
Mucorales	Amphotericin B	Liposomal amphotericin B,‖ amphotericin B lipid complex‖
Pseudallescheria boydii	Voriconazole	Itraconazole,‖ posaconazole¶
Protozoa		
Toxoplasma gondii	Pyrimethamine + sulfadiazine	Pyrimethamine + clindamycin; pyrimethamine + azithromycin, clarithromycin, atovaquone, or dapsone

*Depending on the pathogenesis of bacterial brain abscess (see text), these bacteria may be isolated as part of a mixed infection.
†Cefotaxime, ceftriaxone, or cefepime.
‡Addition of an aminoglycoside should be considered.
§Addition of flucytosine should be considered.
‖Efficacy not yet proved in brain abscess caused by this organism.
¶Not yet licensed for clinical use.

employing ^{18}F-fluorodeoxyglucose (^{18}FDG-PET),[151,152] although this technology is not yet widely available.[73] In patients with mass lesions and negative anti-*Toxoplasma* IgG serologic tests, the diagnosis of toxoplasmic encephalitis is possible, but unlikely; scanning with ^{201}Tl-SPECT or ^{18}FDG-PET may be helpful in this setting, although each test has limitations and should not be relied on in isolation because specific expertise is required for interpretation, the tests are costly, and rigid diagnostic criteria have not yet been determined.[73] Brain biopsy is optimal, although some experts have recommended an empirical trial of therapy for toxoplasmic encephalitis in patients with multiple ring-enhancing lesions even if the anti-*Toxoplasma* IgG serologic test is negative.[145] However, brain biopsy should be performed in patients who fail to respond. Patients with single lesions on MRI and negative serologic tests should undergo a stereotactic brain biopsy. A strategy for the management of suspected *Toxoplasma* CNS lesions in HIV-infected patients can be found in Chapter 276.

THERAPY

Once the infecting pathogen is isolated, antimicrobial agents can be modified for optimal therapy. My recommendations for standard therapy, with alternative agents, are shown in Table 84-4. Doses of these agents used for CNS infections are in Table 84-5. The following paragraphs review the principles of antimicrobial use and surgical therapy for bacterial and fungal brain abscesses. The therapeutic approach to toxoplasmic encephalitis is discussed in Chapter 276.

Bacterial Brain Abscess

Antimicrobial Therapy

The antimicrobial agents used to treat bacterial brain abscess should be able to penetrate into the abscess cavity and should have in vitro activity against the pathogens isolated.[1,3-5,153,154] The few studies that have addressed the penetration of antimicrobials into brain abscess fluid have included limited numbers of patients. Concentrations of penicillin G have been measured in brain abscess pus but were detected consistently only if the daily dosage in adults exceeded 24 million units; in some cases, penicillin G may be inactivated in pus, with the result that bacteria can still be cultured despite adequate penicillin concentrations.[155] Limited data are available on the penetration of the semisynthetic penicillins (e.g., nafcillin, oxacillin) into brain abscesses, although some studies suggest that concentrations of these drugs in brain abscess fluid are variable.[9] Metronidazole has excellent in vitro activity against strict anaerobes, making it an important agent for the therapy of patients with brain abscess.[142] Its excellent pharmacokinetic profile (i.e., good oral absorption and penetration into brain abscess cavities) has made metronidazole a more attractive antianaerobic agent than chloramphenicol for therapy of brain abscess. However, metronidazole must always be used in combination with an antimicrobial agent effective against streptococci, because polymicrobial infections are common in patients with brain abscesses. Vancomycin has also been shown to demonstrate excellent concentrations in brain abscess fluid (90% of serum concentrations) after prolonged therapy.[143]

The role of newer antimicrobial agents in the therapy of brain abscess is evolving. The third-generation cephalosporins are attractive agents for the therapy of brain abscess, given their good CNS penetration and excellent in vitro activity against many of the pathogens isolated from bacterial brain abscesses. When cefotaxime is given in high doses (3 g every 8 hours), brain abscess concentrations of cefotaxime and its active metabolite, desacetylcefotaxime, were above the minimal inhibitory concentrations of the majority of gram-positive and gram-negative organisms against which cefotaxime is used systemically. When combined with metronidazole and used in conjunction with surgical excision, high doses of cefotaxime have also been effective clinically in the treatment of brain abscess.[156] Ceftriaxone, ceftizoxime, and ceftazidime have all been used in the treatment of brain abscess,[157,158] although only a small number of patients have been studied.

TABLE 84-5 Recommended Dosages of Antimicrobial Agents for Central Nervous System Infections in Adults[*]

Antimicrobial Agent	Total Daily Dosage	Dosing Interval (hr)
Amikacin[†]	15 mg/kg	8
Amphotericin B	0.6-1.0 mg/kg[‡]	24
Amphotericin B lipid formulation	5 mg/kg	24
Ampicillin	12 g	4
Atovaquone	3000 mg	6
Azithromycin	1200-1500 mg	24
Aztreonam	6-8 g	6-8
Cefepime	4-6 g	8-12
Cefotaxime	8-12 g	4-6
Ceftazidime	6 g	8
Ceftriaxone	4 g	12
Chloramphenicol	4-6 g	6
Ciprofloxacin	800-1200 mg	8-12
Clindamycin	2400-4800 mg[§]	6
Dapsone[‖]	100 mg	24
Ethambutol[‖]	15 mg/kg	24
Fluconazole	400-800 mg	24
Flucytosine[‖]	100 mg/kg	6
Gentamicin[†]	3-5 mg/kg	8
Isoniazid[‖]	300 mg	24
Itraconazole	400 mg	12
Liposomal amphotericin B (AmBisome)	5 mg/kg	24
Meropenem	6 g	8
Metronidazole	30 mg/kg	6
Nafcillin	9-12 g	4
Oxacillin	9-12 g	4
Penicillin	24 million units	4
Pyrazinamide[‖]	15-30 mg/kg	24
Pyrimethamine[‖]	25-75 mg[§]	24
Rifampin[‖]	600 mg	24
Sulfadiazine[‖]	4-6 g	6
Tobramycin[‖]	3-5 mg/kg	8
Trimethoprim-sulfamethoxazole	10-20 mg/kg[¶]	6-12
Vancomycin[†]	2-3 g	8-12
Voriconazole[**]	8 mg/kg	12

[*]Patients with normal renal and hepatic function. Unless indicated, the intravenous mode of administration is used.
[†]Need to monitor peak and trough serum concentrations.
[‡]Dosages up to 1.5 mg/kg/day may be used for aspergillosis or mucormycosis.
[§]Higher dosages utilized in acquired immunodeficiency syndrome patients with toxoplasmic encephalitis; load with 100 to 200 mg.
[‖]Dosage for oral administration.
[¶]Dosage based on trimethoprim component; higher dose utilized for *Nocardia* brain abscess.
[**]Load with 6 mg/kg IV every 12 hours for two doses.

Ampicillin-sulbactam has also demonstrated therapeutic success in patients with brain abscesses[159]; intracavitary concentrations were variable, but adequate, in most cases.

Imipenem has been used successfully for the treatment of pyogenic and nocardial brain abscesses,[160,161] although the use of imipenem has been associated with an increased risk of seizures, limiting its usefulness in patients with CNS mass lesions. Meropenem, a carbapenem antimicrobial agent similar to imipenem, was successful in one case of an *Enterobacter cloacae* brain abscess,[162] suggesting that this agent may be useful in brain abscess cases, especially when caused by resistant pathogens. The fluoroquinolones have good CNS penetration and have been used anecdotally in the treatment of brain abscess patients,[163] although further data are needed to determine the efficacy of the fluoroquinolones for the therapy of brain abscess.

Antimicrobial therapy with high-dose intravenous antibiotics has traditionally been administered for 6 to 8 weeks in patients with bacterial brain abscesses.[1] This is often followed by oral antibiotic therapy for 2 to 6 months if an appropriate agent or agents are available, although the efficacy and necessity of this approach has not been established. Shorter courses (3 to 4 weeks) of antimicrobial therapy may be adequate for patients who have undergone surgical excision of the abscess. Surgical therapy (i.e., excision or aspiration) is often required for the optimal management of brain abscess (see later), although certain subsets of patients may be treated with antimicrobial therapy alone.[124,164-166] These are patients with medical conditions that increase the risk of surgery, multiple abscesses, abscesses in a deep or dominant location, concomitant meningitis or ependymitis, early abscess reduction with clinical improvement after antimicrobial therapy, and abscess size under 3 cm. However, in one series, no abscess larger than 2.5 cm resolved without surgical therapy.[164] Furthermore, patients treated with antimicrobial therapy alone may require prolonged (up to 12 weeks) courses of parenteral treatment, and must receive careful clinical and radiographic follow-up. In one small series, eight selected patients with abscess size less than 3 cm were successfully treated with short-course intravenous antimicrobial therapy (6 to 12 days), followed by prolonged oral antimicrobial therapy (15 to 19 weeks),[167] although this approach cannot be considered standard therapy in most patients with bacterial brain abscess.

When a brain abscess due to *Nocardia* is suspected or proved, the sulfonamides, with or without trimethoprim, are recommended as first-line therapy,[168,169] although treatment failures have been reported.[170] Alternative agents include minocycline, amikacin, imipenem, the third-generation cephalosporins, and linezolid, which are among the most active agents against *Nocardia* in vitro.[171-173] However, in vitro activity may not always correlate with clinical efficacy. Combination therapies have been studied,[174-178] and combination regimens containing the third-generation cephalosporins or imipenem along with a sulfonamide or amikacin should be considered for immunocompromised patients or those in whom therapy fails.[1,179] Linezolid was also recently shown to be efficacious in two patients with multiple *Nocardia* brain abscesses,[180] although therapy was changed in one patient as a result of an adverse effect from linezolid. The duration of antimicrobial therapy for nocardial brain abscess has ranged from 3 to 12 months.[27,181] However, therapy in immunosuppressed patients should probably be continued for up to 1 year,[125] with careful follow-up to monitor for relapse.

Surgical Therapy

Most patients with bacterial brain abscess require surgical management for optimal therapy. The two procedures available are aspiration of the abscess after bur hole placement and complete excision after craniotomy.[16,17,182] No prospective trial comparing the two procedures has ever been performed. Therefore, the choice of procedure must be individualized for each patient. Aspiration may be performed by a stereotactic procedure utilizing CT or MRI guidance, which affords the surgeon rapid, accurate, and safe access to virtually any intracranial point, including those areas located in deep critical regions of the CNS (e.g., brain stem, cerebellum, or diencephalic structures adjacent to the ventricles)[158,183-188]; aspiration can also be used for swift relief of increased intracranial pressure. In one series of patients with brain abscess from an initially otitic focus, immediate radical mastoidectomy was utilized followed by evacuation of the abscess through the mastoidectomy cavity.[14]

Complete excision by craniotomy is now infrequently performed because of the development of the aspiration and closed drainage techniques described previously, but it may be required in patients with multiloculated abscesses (for whom aspiration techniques have failed) or for abscesses that fail to resolve. Craniotomy with total excision is difficult in cases of nocardial brain abscess, because these abscesses are usually multiloculated.[125] In one review of 11 patients with nocardial brain abscess,[189] aspiration alone (which was repeated as clinically indicated) was a safe, efficacious treatment for 9 patients. In another series of three patients with nocardial brain abscess, cure was achieved only after neurosurgical enucleation,[190] suggesting that an aggressive approach should be utilized. In patients with intraventricular rupture of a purulent brain abscess who have dilated ventricles and ventriculitis, ventricular drainage combined with the administration of appropriate intravenous or intrathecal antimicrobial agents, or both, is recommended.[122]

Fungal Brain Abscess

The optimal therapy for fungal brain abscesses usually requires a combined medical and surgical approach; surgery includes either excision or drainage of the abscess. However, therapy of fungal brain abscess in immunocompromised patients carries a high mortality rate despite surgery and antifungal therapy. Nevertheless, early recognition of this infection can lead to a successful outcome, especially if leukocyte counts return to normal or if the dosages of immunosuppressive agents can be reduced.[1] The mainstay of medical therapy for candidal brain abscess is amphotericin B plus 5-flucytosine.[41] The efficacy of fluconazole in the therapy of *Candida* brain abscess has not been evaluated, although one case report in a premature infant with *Candida albicans* brain abscess demonstrated a decrease in abscess size after the addition of fluconazole to amphotericin B plus 5-flucytosine.[191]

The antifungal therapy of choice for *Aspergillus* brain abscess has been amphotericin B deoxycholate (0.8 to 1.25 mg/kg/day); doses up to 1.5 mg/kg/day have been used, depending on the clinical response.[192] However, few instances of survival have been recorded in CNS aspergillosis despite the administration of this agent. Most patients have required a total of more than 3 g of amphotericin B for eradication of CNS disease. Itraconazole has in vitro activity against *Aspergillus,* and high-dose therapy (800 mg daily for 5 months, followed by 400 mg daily for 4.5 months) resulted in complete resolution of cerebral abscesses caused by *Aspergillus fumigatus* in an older asthmatic patient who was treated with corticosteroids.[193] Despite this and a few other case reports of the successful use of high-dose itraconazole, the unreliable absorption and very modest reported experience in *Aspergillus* brain abscess makes itraconazole more promising as an extension of successful therapy than as primary therapy. One patient with chronic granulomatous disease and an *Aspergillus* brain abscess was successfully treated with amphotericin B, itraconazole, and interferon-γ, with the amphotericin B discontinued after the first 3 weeks of therapy.[194] Amphotericin B has also been applied to the abscess cavity in patients with aspergillosis though the drug is neurotoxic on injection into the brain.[195]

Voriconazole appears to be the drug of choice in patients with *Aspergillus* brain abscess.[196] In one review of voriconazole in the treatment of invasive aspergillosis that included 19 patients with cerebral disease, 3 (16%) patients had a partial response to treatment.[197] Excisional surgery or drainage was a key factor in the successful management of several cases of CNS aspergillosis.[44,198-200]

Mucormycosis should also be treated with amphotericin B, along with correction of underlying metabolic derangements and aggressive surgical débridement.[39,47,48,201,202] The role of surgery in the treatment of cerebral mucormycosis cannot be overemphasized. Because of their propensity for invading blood vessels, the Mucorales cause extensive tissue infarction, thereby impairing the delivery of antifungal agents to the site of infection. This often leaves surgery as the only modality that may effectively eliminate the invading microorganisms. Amphotericin B has also been applied topically in the orbital cavities in patients with rhinocerebral mucormycosis,[202] although it is not clear if this is beneficial. Hyperbaric oxygen therapy has been reported to be a useful adjunct in cerebral mucormycosis,[203,204] although no prospective, controlled trials have been performed to adequately assess its efficacy.

For *P. boydii* brain abscess, surgical drainage is the cornerstone of effective therapy.[54] The organism demonstrates in vitro resistance to amphotericin B. Previously, the antifungal treatment of choice was intravenous miconazole,[54,55,205,206] although failures and relapses are common and few hospitals stock the drug.[39] Despite the report of partial response to fluconazole (600 to 800 mg/day), activity of this azole against molds has been modest or nonexistent.[207] Itraconazole has been used successfully to treat pulmonary infection,[208] but its efficacy in CNS disease is unknown. One patient was successfully treated with surgical drainage and systemic voriconazole.[209] Another patient with acute lymphoblastic lymphoma and multiple *P. boydii* (*S. apiospermum*) brain abscesses who did not respond to neurosurgical drainage and treatment with itraconazole, amphotericin B, and ketoconazole, had complete resolution of the abscesses after treatment with posaconazole[210]; posaconazole, however, is not yet licensed by the

U.S. Food and Drug Administration (FDA), and no parenteral formulation is available. Based on clinical experience and the absence of good alternative agents,[196] voriconazole is now the antifungal agent of choice for treatment of *P. boydii* brain abscess.

The addition of granulocyte or macrophage colony-stimulating factors, which enhanced neutrophil-mediated killing of fungi in vitro,[211,212] may deserve study in fungal brain abscess. Administration of these agents may be considered in patients who fail conventional therapy.

REFERENCES

1. Mathisen GE, Johnson JP. Brain abscess. Clin Infect Dis. 1997;25:763-781.
2. Canale DJ. William Macewen and the treatment of brain abscesses: Revisited after one hundred years. J Neurosurg. 1996;84:133-142.
3. Wispelwey B, Dacey RG Jr, Scheld WM. Brain abscess. In: Scheld WM, Whitley RJ, Durack DT, eds. Infections of the Central Nervous System. 2nd ed. Philadelphia: Lippincott-Raven; 1997:463-493.
4. Heilpern KL, Lorber B. Focal intracranial infections. Infect Dis Clin North Am. 1996;10:879-898.
5. Kaplan K. Brain abscess. Med Clin North Am. 1985;69:345-360.
6. Rosenblum ML, Joff JT, Norman D, et al. Decreased mortality from brain abscesses since advent of computerized tomography. J Neurosurg. 1978;49:658-668.
7. Seydoux C, Francioli P. Bacterial brain abscess: Factors influencing mortality and sequelae. Clin Infect Dis. 1992;15:394-401.
8. Su TM, Lin YC, Lu CH, et al. Streptococcal brain abscess: Analysis of clinical features in 20 patients. Surg Neurol. 2001;56:189-194.
9. De Louvois J, Gortvai P, Hurley R. Bacteriology of abscesses of the central nervous system: A multicentre prospective study. Br Med J. 1977;2:981-984.
10. De Louvois J. The bacteriology and chemotherapy of brain abscess. J Antimicrob Chemother. 1978;4:395-413.
11. Liliang PC, Lin YC, Su TM, et al. Klebsiella brain abscess in adults. Infection. 2001;29:81-86.
12. Lu CH, Chang WN, Lin YC, et al. Bacterial brain abscess: Microbiological features, epidemiological trends and therapeutic outcomes. Q J Med. 2002;95:501-509.
13. Rau CS, Chang WN, Lin YC, et al. Brain abscess caused by aerobic gram-negative bacilli: Clinical features and therapeutic outcomes. Clin Neurol Neurosurg. 2002;105:60-65.
14. Sennaroglu L, Sozeri B. Otogenic brain abscess: Review of 41 cases. Otolaryngol Head Neck Surg. 2000;123:751-755.
15. Yang SY. Brain abscess: A review of 400 cases. J Neurosurg. 1981;55:794-799.
16. Mampalam TJ, Rosenblum ML. Trends in the management of bacterial brain abscesses: A review of 102 cases over 17 years. Neurosurgery. 1988;23:451-458.
17. Chun CH, Johnson JD, Hofstetter M, et al. Brain abscess: A study of 45 consecutive cases. Medicine. 1986;65:415-431.
18. Grigoriadis E, Gold WL. Pyogenic brain abscess caused by Streptococcus pneumoniae: Case report and review. Clin Infect Dis. 1997;25:1108-1112.
19. Lorber B. Listeriosis. Clin Infect Dis. 1997;24:1-11.
20. Eckburg PB, Montoya JG, Vosti KL. Brain abscess due to Listeria monocytogenes: Five cases and a review of the literature. Medicine (Baltimore). 2001;80:223-235.
21. Renier D, Flandin C, Hirsch E, Hirsch JF. Brain abscesses in neonates: A study of 30 cases. J Neurosurg. 1988;69:877-882.
22. Kline MW. Citrobacter meningitis and brain abscess in infancy: Epidemiology, pathogenesis, and treatment. J Pediatr. 1988;113:430-434.
23. Morgan MG, Stuart C, Leonard AT, et al. Citrobacter diversus brain abscess: Case reports and molecular epidemiology. J Med Microbiol. 1992;36:273-278.
24. Chadwick DR, Ang B, Sitoh YY, Lee CC. Cerebral melioidosis in Singapore: A review of five cases. Trans R Soc Trop Med Hyg. 2002;96:72-76.
25. Smego RA Jr, Foglia G. Actinomycosis. Clin Infect Dis. 1998;26:1255-1263.
26. Wilson JP, Turner HR, Kirchner KA, et al. Nocardial infections in renal transplant recipients. Medicine. 1989;68:38-57.
27. Berkey P, Bodey GP. Nocardial infection in patients with neoplastic disease. Rev Infect Dis. 1989;11:407-412.
28. Kim J, Minamoto GY, Grieco MH. Nocardial infection as a complication of AIDS: Report of six cases and review. Rev Infect Dis. 1991;13:624-629.
29. Lerner PI. Nocardiosis. Clin Infect Dis. 1996;22:891-905.
30. Braun TI, Kerson LA, Eisenberg FP. Nocardial brain abscesses in a pregnant woman. Rev Infect Dis. 1991;13:630-632.
31. Kumar R, Pandey CK, Bose N, Sahay S. Tuberculous brain abscess: Clinical presentation, pathophysiology and treatment (in children). Childs Nerv Syst. 2002;18:118-123.
32. Farrar DJ, Flanigan TP, Gordon NM, et al. Tuberculous brain abscess in a patient with HIV infection: Case report and review. Am J Med. 1997;102:297-301.
33. Gordon SM, Blumberg HM. Mycobacterium kansasii brain abscess in a patient with AIDS. Clin Infect Dis. 1992;14:789-790.
34. Monno L, Carbonara S, Costa D, et al. Cerebral lesions in two patients with AIDS: The possible role of Mycobacterium kansasii. Clin Infect Dis. 1996;22:1130-1131.
35. Salaki JS, Louria DB, Chmel H. Fungal and yeast infections of the central nervous system: A clinical review. Medicine. 1984;63:108-132.
36. Burgert SJ, Classen DC, Burke JP, Blatter DD. Candidal brain abscess associated with vascular invasion: A devastating complication of vascular catheter-related candidemia. Clin Infect Dis. 1995;21:202-205.
37. Hagensee ME, Bauwens JE, Kjos B, Bowden RA. Brain abscess following marrow transplantation: Experience at the Fred Hutchinson Cancer Center, 1984-1992. Clin Infect Dis. 1994;19:402-408.
38. Selby R, Ramirez CB, Singh R, et al. Brain abscess in solid organ transplant recipients receiving cyclosporine-based immunosuppression. Arch Surg. 1997;132:304-310.
39. Sepkowitz K, Armstrong D. Space-occupying fungal lesions. In: Scheld WM, Whitley RJ, Durack DT, eds. Infections of the Central Nervous System. 2nd ed. Philadelphia: Lippincott-Raven; 1997:741-762.
40. Lipton SA, Hickey WF, Morris JH, et al. Candidal infection in the central nervous system. Am J Med. 1984;76:101-108.
41. Sanchez-Portocarrero J, Perez-Cecilia E, Corral O, et al. The central nervous system and infection by Candida species. Diagn Microbiol Infect Dis. 2000;37:169-179.
42. Walsh TJ, Hier DB, Caplan LP. Fungal infections of the central nervous system: Comparative analysis of risk factors and clinical signs in 57 patients. Neurology. 1985;35:1654-1657.
43. Denning DW. Invasive aspergillosis. Clin Infect Dis. 1998;26:781-805.
44. Green M, Wald ER, Tzakis A, et al. Aspergillosis of the CNS in a pediatric liver transplant recipient: Case report and review. Rev Infect Dis. 1991;13:653-657.
45. Beal MF, O'Carroll P, Kleinman GM, et al. Aspergillosis of the nervous system. Neurology. 1982;32:473-479.
46. Minamoto GY, Barlam TF, Vander Els NJ. Invasive aspergillosis in patients with AIDS. Clin Infect Dis. 1992;14:66-74.
47. Parfrey NZ. Improved diagnosis and prognosis of mucormycosis. Medicine. 1986;65:113-123.
48. Morduchowicz G, Shmueli D, Shapira Z, et al. Rhinocerebral mucormycosis in renal transplant recipients. Rev Infect Dis. 1986;8:441-446.
49. Stave GM, Heimberger T, Kerkering TM. Zygomycosis of the basal ganglia in intravenous drug users. Am J Med. 1989;86:115-117.
50. Daly AL, Velazquez LA, Bradley SF, et al. Mucormycosis: Association with deferoxamine therapy. Am J Med. 1989;87:468-471.
51. Sugar AM. Mucormycosis. Clin Infect Dis. 1992;14:S126-S129.
52. Rinaldi MG. Zygomycosis. Infect Dis Clin North Am. 1989;3:19-41.
53. Travis LB, Roberts GD, Wilson WR. Clinical significance of Pseudallescheria boydii: A review of ten years' experience. Mayo Clin Proc. 1985;60:531-537.
54. Berenguer J, Diaz-Mediavilla J, Urra D, et al. Central nervous system infection caused by Pseudallescheria boydii. Rev Infect Dis. 1989;11:890-896.
55. Dworzack DL, Clark RB, Borkowski WJ, et al. Pseudallescheria boydii brain abscess: Association with near-drowning and efficacy of high-dose, prolonged miconazole therapy in patients with multiple abscesses. Medicine. 1989;68:218-224.
56. Kershaw P, Freeman R, Templeton D, et al. Pseudallescheria boydii infection of the central nervous system. Arch Neurol. 1990;47:468-472.
57. Bia FJ, Barry M. Parasitic infections of the central nervous system. Neurol Clin. 1986;4:171-206.
58. Solari A, Saavefra H, Sepulveda G, et al. Successful treatment of Trypanosoma cruzi encephalitis in a patient with hemophilia and AIDS. Clin Infect Dis. 1993;16:255-259.
59. Ohnishi K, Murata M, Kojima H, et al. Brain abscess due to infection with Entamoeba histolytica. Am J Trop Med Hyg. 1994;51:180-182.
60. Campbell S. Amebic brain abscess and meningoencephalitis. Semin Neurol. 1993;13:153-160.
61. White AC Jr. Neurocysticercosis: A major cause of neurological disease worldwide. Clin Infect Dis. 1997;24:101-115.
62. Dukes CS, Luft BJ, Durack DT. Toxoplasmosis of the central nervous system. In: Scheld WM, Whitley RJ, Durack DT, eds. Infections of the Central Nervous System. 2nd ed. Philadelphia: Lippincott-Raven; 1997:785-806.
63. Carey RM, Kimball AC, Armstrong D, et al. Toxoplasmosis. Clinical experiences in a cancer hospital. Am J Med. 1973;54:30-38.
64. Ruskin J, Remington JS. Toxoplasmosis in the compromised host. Ann Intern Med. 1976;84:193-199.
65. Hakes TB, Armstrong D. Toxoplasmosis. Problems in diagnosis and treatment. Cancer. 1983;52:1535-1540.
66. Deleze M, Mintz G, Carmen Majia MD. Toxoplasma gondii encephalitis in systemic lupus erythematosus, a neglected cause of treatable nervous system infection. J Rheumatol. 1985;12:994-996.
67. Luft BJ, Naot Y, Araujo FG, et al. Primary and reactivated Toxoplasma infection in patients with cardiac transplants. Ann Intern Med. 1983;99:27-31.
68. Mele A, Paterson PJ, Prentice HG, et al. Toxoplasmosis in bone marrow transplantation: A report of two cases and systematic review of the literature. Bone Marrow Transplant. 2002;29:691-698.
69. Navia BA, Petito CK, Gold JWM, et al. Cerebral toxoplasmosis complicating the acquired immune deficiency syndrome: Clinical and neuropathological findings in 27 patients. Ann Neurol. 1986;19:224-238.
70. Luft BJ, Remington JS. Toxoplasmic encephalitis in AIDS. Clin Infect Dis. 1992;15:211-222.
71. Renold C, Sugar A, Chave JP, et al. Toxoplasma encephalitis in patients with acquired immunodeficiency syndrome. Medicine. 1992;71:224-239.
72. Porter SB, Sande MA. Toxoplasmosis of the central nervous system in the acquired immunodeficiency syndrome. N Engl J Med. 1992;327:1643-1648.
73. Skiest DJ. Focal neurological disease in patients with acquired immunodeficiency syndrome. Clin Infect Dis. 2002;34:103-115.
74. Sacktor N, Lyles RH, Skolasky R, et al. HIV-associated neurologic disease incidence changes: Multicenter AIDS Cohort Study, 1990-1998. Neurology. 2001;56:257-260.

75. Abgrall S, Rabaud C, Costagliola D, et al. Incidence and risk factors for toxoplasmic encephalitis in human immunodeficiency virus-infected patients before and during the highly active antiretroviral therapy era. Clin Infect Dis. 2001;33:1747-1755.

76. Corson MA, Postlethwaite KP, Seymour RA. Are dental infections a cause of brain abscess? Case report and review of the literature. Oral Dis. 2001;7:61-65.

77. Yang SY. Brain abscess associated with congenital heart disease. Surg Neurol. 1989;31:129-132.

78. Park SC, Neeches WH. The neurologic complications of congenital heart disease. Neurol Clin. 1993;11:441-462.

79. Takeshita M, Kagawa M, Yato S, et al. Current treatment of brain abscess in patients with congenital cyanotic heart disease. Neurosurgery. 1997;41:1270-1279.

80. Pruitt AA, Rubin RHJ, Karchmer AW, Duncan GW. Neurologic complications of bacterial endocarditis. Medicine. 1978;57:329-343.

81. Tunkel AR, Kaye D. Neurologic complications of infective endocarditis. Neurol Clin. 1993;11:419-440.

82. Tunkel AR, Pradhan SK. Central nervous system infections in injection drug users. Infect Dis Clin North Am. 2002;16:589-605.

83. Press OW, Ramsey PG. Central nervous system infections associated with hereditary hemorrhagic telangiectasia. Am J Med. 1984;77:86-92.

84. Gelfand MS, Stephens DS, Howell EI, et al. Brain abscess: Association with pulmonary arteriovenous fistula and hereditary hemorrhagic telangiectasia—Report of three cases. Am J Med. 1988;85:718-720.

85. Walder LA, Anastasia LF, Spodick DH. Pulmonary arteriovenous malformations with brain abscess. Am Heart J. 1994;127:227-232.

86. Thurnheer R, Vernazza PL, Galeazzi RL. Recurrent brain abscesses in an HIV-positive patient with hereditary hemorrhagic telangiectasia and arteriovenous malformation of the lung. Eur J Clin Microbiol Infect Dis. 1996;15:407-410.

87. Dong SL, Reynolds SF, Steiner IP. Brain abscess in patients with hereditary hemorrhagic telangiectasia: Case report and literature review. J Emerg Med. 2001;20:247-251.

88. Kuman P, Mehta SK, Deri BI, et al. Pyogenic meningitis and cerebral abscesses after endoscopic injection sclerotherapy. Am J Gastroenterol. 1991;86:1672-1674.

89. Algood L, Boon P, DeVos M, et al. Brain abscess after esophageal dilatation for stenosis. Clin Neurol Neurosurg. 1992;94:169-172.

90. Tunkel AR, Scheld WM. Acute infectious complications of head injury. In: Braakant R, ed. Handbook of Clinical Neurology, vol. 57: Head Injury. Amsterdam: Elsevier Science; 1990:317-326.

91. McGovern PC, Lautenbach E, Brennan PJ, et al. Risk factors for postcraniotomy surgical site infection after 1,3-bis (2-chloroethyl)-1-nitrosourea (Gliadel) wafer placement. Clin Infect Dis. 2003;36:759-765.

92. Rish BL, Careness WF, Dillon JD, et al. Analysis of brain abscess after penetrating craniocerebral injuries in Vietnam. Neurosurgery. 1981;9:535-541.

93. Splavski B, Sisljagic V, Peric LJ, et al. Intracranial infection as a common complication following war missile skull base injury. Injury. 2000;31:233-237.

94. Hecimovic I, Dmitrovic B, Kurbel S, et al. Intracranial infection after missile brain wound: 15 war cases. Zentralblatt Neurochir. 2000;61:95-102.

95. Bhatoe HS. Retained intracranial splinters: A follow up study in survivors of low intensity military conflicts. Neurol India. 2001;49:29-32.

96. Foy P, Schair M. Cerebral abscesses in children after pencil tip injuries. Lancet. 1980;2:662-663.

97. Tay JS, Garland JS. Serious head injuries from lawn darts. Pediatrics. 1987;79:260-263.

98. Martinello RA, Cooney EL. Cerebellar brain abscess associated with tongue piercing. Clin Infect Dis. 2003;36:e32-34.

99. Kawamata T, Takeshita M, Ishizuka N, Hori T. Patent foramen ovale as a possible risk factor for cryptogenic brain abscess: Report of two cases. Neurosurgery. 2001;49:204-207.

100. Mendes M, Moore P, Wheeler CB, et al. Susceptibility of brain and skin to bacterial challenge. J Neurosurg. 1980;52:772-775.

101. Costello GT, Heppe R, Winn HR, et al. Susceptibility of brain to aerobic, anaerobic, and fungal organisms. Neurosurgery. 1983;41:535-539.

102. Onderonk AB, Kasper DL, Cisneros RL, Bartlett JG. The capsular polysaccharide of Bacteroides fragilis as a virulence factor: Comparison of the pathogenic potential of encapsulated and unencapsulated strains. J Infect Dis. 1977;136:82-89.

103. Onderonk AB, Kasper DL, Mansheim BJ, et al. Experimental animal models for anaerobic infections. Rev Infect Dis. 1979;1:291-301.

104. Britt RH, Enzmann DR, Placone RC Jr, et al. Experimental anaerobic brain abscess: Computerized tomographic and neuropathological correlations. J Neurosurg. 1984;60:1148-1159.

105. Kline MW, Kaplan SL, Hawkins EP, Mason EO Jr. Pathogenesis of brain abscess formation in an infant rat model of Citrobacter diversus bacteremia and meningitis. J Infect Dis. 1988;157:106-112.

106. Kline MW, Mason EO Jr, Kaplan SL. Characterization of Citrobacter diversus strains causing neonatal meningitis. J Infect Dis. 1988;157:101-105.

107. Britt RH, Enzmann DR, Yeager AS. Neuropathological and computerized tomographic findings in experimental brain abscess. J Neurosurg. 1981;55:590-603.

108. Enzmann DR, Britt RR, Obana WG, et al. Experimental Staphylococcus aureus brain abscess. Am J Neuroradiol. 1986;7:395-402.

109. Neuwelt EA, Lawrence MS, Blank NK. Effect of gentamicin and dexamethasone on the natural history of the rat Escherichia coli brain abscess model with histopathological correlation. Neurosurgery. 1984;15:475-483.

110. Kielian T, Cheung A, Hickey WF. Diminished virulence of an alpha-toxin mutant of Staphylococcus aureus in experimental brain abscess. Infect Immun. 2001;69:6902-6911.

111. Casciato DA, Rosenblatt JE, Goldberg LS, Bluestone R. In vitro interaction of Bacteroides fragilis with polymorphonuclear leukocytes and serum factors. Infect Immun. 1975;11:337-342.

112. Ingham HR, Sisson PR, Middleton RL, et al. Phagocytosis and killing of bacteria in aerobic and anaerobic conditions. Med Microbiol. 1981;14:391-399.

113. Adamu SA, Sperry JF. Polymorphonuclear neutrophil chemotaxis induced and inhibited by Bacteroides spp. Infect Immun. 1981;33:806-810.

114. Kielian T, Hickey WF. Proinflammatory cytokine, chemokine, and cellular adhesion molecule expression during the acute phase of experimental brain abscess development. Am J Pathol. 2000;157:647-658.

115. Kielian T, Barry B, Hickey WF. CXC chemokine receptor-2 ligands are required for neutrophil-mediated host defense in experimental brain abscesses. J Immunol. 2001;166:4634-4643.

116. Long WD, Meacham WF. Experimental method for producing brain abscess in dogs with evaluation of the effect of dexamethasone and antibiotic therapy on the pathogenesis of intracerebral abscesses. Surg Forum. 1968;19:437-438.

117. Quartey GRC, Johnston JA, Rozdilsky B. Decadron in the treatment of cerebral abscess: An experimental study. J Neurosurg. 1976;45:301-310.

118. Yildizhan A, Pasaoglu A, Kandemir B. Effect of dexamethasone on various stages of experimental brain abscess. Acta Neurochir. 1989;96:141-148.

119. Obana WG, Britt RH, Placone RC, et al. Experimental brain abscess development in the chronically immunosuppressed host: Computerized tomographic and neuropathologic correlations. J Neurosurg. 1986;65:382-391.

120. Brewer NS, MacCarty CS, Wellman WE. Brain abscess: A review of recent experience. Ann Intern Med. 1985;82:571-576.

121. Zeidman SM, Geisler FH, Olivi A. Intraventricular rupture of a purulent brain abscess: Case report. Neurosurgery. 1995;36:189-193.

122. Takeshita M, Kawamata T, Izawa M, Hori T. Prodromal signs and clinical factors influencing outcome in patients with intraventricular rupture of purulent brain abscess. Neurosurgery. 2001;48:310-317.

123. Dake MD, McMurdo SK, Rosenblum ML, et al. Pyogenic abscess of the medulla oblongata. Neurosurgery. 1986;18:370-372.

124. Carpenter JL. Brain stem abscesses: Cure with medical therapy, case report, and review. Clin Infect Dis. 1994;18:219-226.

125. Mamelak AN, Obana WG, Flaherty JF, Rosenblum ML. Nocardial brain abscess: Treatment strategies and factors influencing outcome. Neurosurgery. 1994;35:622-631.

126. Walsh TJ, Hier DB, Caplan LR. Aspergillosis of the central nervous system: Clinicopathological analysis of 17 patients. Ann Neurol. 1985;18:574-582.

127. Rangel-Guerra R, Martinez HR, Saenz C. Mucormycosis: Report of 11 cases. Arch Neurol. 1985;42:578-581.

128. Anaissie EJ, Shikhani AH. Rhinocerebral mucormycosis with internal carotid occlusion: Report of two cases and review of the literature. Laryngoscope. 1985;95:1107-1113.

129. Osenbach RK, Loftus CM. Diagnosis and management of brain abscess. Neurosurg Clin North Am. 1992;3:403-420.

130. Miller ES, Psrilal SD, Uttley D. CT scanning in the management of intracranial abscess: A review of 100 cases. Br J Neurosurg. 1988;2:439-446.

131. Zimmerman RD, Weingarten K. Neuroimaging of cerebral abscesses. Neuroimaging Clin North Am. 1991;1:1-16.

132. Zimmerman RA, Girard NJ. Imaging of intracranial infections. In: Scheld WM, Whitley RJ, Durack DT, eds. Infections of the Central Nervous System. 2nd ed. Philadelphia: Lippincott-Raven; 1997:923-944.

133. Martinez-Perez I, Moreno A, Alonso J, et al. Diagnosis of brain abscess by magnetic resonance spectroscopy: Report of two cases. J Neurosurg. 1997;86:708-713.

134. Anderson D, Matick H, Naheedy MH, et al. Rhinocerebral mucormycosis with CT scan findings. Comput Radiol. 1984;8:113-117.

135. Press GA, Weindling SM, Hesselink JR, et al. Rhinocerebral mucormycosis: MR manifestations. J Comput Assist Tomogr. 1988;12:744-749.

136. Luft BJ, Hafner R, Korzun AH, et al. Toxoplasmic encephalitis in patients with the acquired immunodeficiency syndrome. N Engl J Med. 1993;329:995-1000.

137. Cohn JA, McMeeking A, Cohen W, et al. Evaluation of the policy of empiric treatment of suspected Toxoplasma encephalitis in patients with the acquired immunodeficiency syndrome. Am J Med. 1989;86:521-527.

138. Cimino C, Lipton RB, Williams A, et al. The evaluation of patients with human immunodeficiency virus-related disorders and brain mass lesions. Arch Intern Med. 1991;151:1381-1384.

139. Joseph P, Calderon MM, Gilman RH, et al. Optimization and evaluation of a PCR assay for detecting toxoplasmic encephalitis in patients with AIDS. J Clin Microbiol. 2002;40:4499-4503.

140. Strowitzki M, Schwerdtfeger K, Steudel WI. Ultrasound-guided aspiration of brain abscess through a single burr hole. Minim Invasive Neurosurg. 2001;44:135-140.

141. Mamelak AN, Mampalam TJ, Obana WG, Rosenblum ML. Improved management of multiple brain abscesses: A combined surgical and medical approach. Neurosurgery. 1995;36:76-86.

142. Alderson D, Strong AJ, Ingham MR, et al. Fifteen year review of the mortality of brain abscess. Neurosurgery. 1981;8:1-6.

143. Levy RM, Gutin PH, Baskin DS, et al. Vancomycin penetration of a brain abscess: Case report and review of the literature. Neurosurgery. 1986;18:633-636.

144. Khan MA, Greig JR, Jayamohan J. Community-acquired methicillin-resistant Staphylococcus aureus brain abscess in an immunocompetent individual. Scand J Infect Dis. 2000;32:423-424.

145. Quality Standards Subcommittee of the American Academy of Neurology. Evaluation and management of intracranial mass lesions in AIDS. Neurology. 1998;50:21-26.

146. Ruiz A, Ganz WI, Post MJD, et al. Use of thallium-201 brain SPECT to differentiate cerebral lymphoma from *Toxoplasma* encephalitis in AIDS patients. AJNR Am J Neuroradiol. 1994;15:1885-1894.

147. Berry I, Gaillard JF, Guo Z, et al. Cerebral lesions in AIDS: What can be expected from scintigraphy? Cerebral tomographic scintigraphy using thallium-201: A contribution to the differential diagnosis of lymphomas and infectious lesions. J Neuroradiol. 1995;22:218-228.

148. O'Malley JP, Ziessman HA, Kumar PN, et al. Diagnosis of intracranial lymphoma in patients with AIDS: Value of 201 Tl single-photon emission computed tomography. AJR Am J Roentgenol. 1994;163:417-421.

149. Garcia-Morales F, Chengazi VU, O'Mara RE. *Nocardia* brain abscess identification with Tl-201 SPECT. Clin Nucl Med. 2001;26:981-982.

150. Licho R, Litofsky NS, Senitko M, George M. Inaccuracy of Tl-201 SPECT in distinguishing cerebral infections from lymphoma in patient with AIDS. Clin Nucl Med. 2002;27:81-86.

151. Hoffman JM, Waskin HA, Schifter T, et al. FDG-PET in differentiating lymphoma from nonmalignant central nervous system lesions in patients with AIDS. J Nucl Med. 1993;34:567-575.

152. Pierce MA, Johnson MD, Maciunas RJ, et al. Evaluating contrast-enhancing brain lesions in patients with AIDS by using positron emission tomography. Ann Intern Med. 1995;123:594-598.

153. De Louvois J. Antimicrobial chemotherapy in the treatment of brain abscess. J Antimicrob Chemother. 1983;11:205-207.

154. Black P, Graybill JR, Charache P. Penetration of brain abscess by systemically administered antibiotics. J Neurosurg. 1973;38:705-709.

155. De Louvois J, Gortvai P, Hurley R. Antibiotic treatment of abscesses of the central nervous system. Br Med J. 1977;2:985-987.

156. Sjolin J, Lilja A, Eriksson N, et al. Treatment of brain abscess with cefotaxime and metronidazole: Prospective study on 15 consecutive patients. Clin Infect Dis. 1993;17:857-863.

157. Green HT, O'Donoghue MAT, Shaw MDM, Dowling C. Penetration of ceftazidime into intracranial abscesses. J Antimicrob Chemother. 1989;24:431-436.

158. Skrap M, Melatini A, Vassallo A, Sidoti C. Stereotactic aspiration and drainage of brain abscesses: Experience with 9 cases. Minim Invasive Neurosurg. 1996;39:108-112.

159. Adova M, Akalin HE, Korten V, et al. Treatment of intracranial abscesses: Experience with sulbactam/ampicillin. J Chemother. 1993;5:181-185.

160. Aseni V, Carton JA, Maradona JA, et al. Imipenem therapy of brain abscesses. Eur J Clin Microbiol Infect Dis. 1996;15:653-657.

161. Aseni V, Carton JA, Maradona JA, et al. Therapy of brain abscess with imipenem— A safe therapeutic choice? J Antimicrob Chemother. 1996;37:200-203.

162. Meis JFGM, Groot-Loonen J, Hoogkamp-Korstanje JAA. A brain abscess due to multiply-resistant *Enterobacter cloacae* successfully treated with meropenem. Clin Infect Dis. 1995;20:1567.

163. Wessalowksi R, Thomas L, Kivit J, Voit T. Multiple brain abscesses caused by *Salmonella enteritidis* in a neonate: Successful treatment with ciprofloxacin. Pediatr Infect Dis J. 1993;12:683-688.

164. Rosenblum ML, Hoff JT, Norman D, et al. Nonoperative treatment of brain abscesses in selected high-risk patients. J Neurosurg. 1980;52:217-225.

165. Boom WH, Tuazon CU. Successful treatment of multiple brain abscesses with antibiotics alone. Rev Infect Dis. 1985;7:189-199.

166. Fulgham JR, Wijdicks EFM, Wright AJ. Cure of a solitary brainstem abscess with antibiotic therapy: Case report. Neurology. 1996;46:1451-1454.

167. Skoutelis AT, Gogos CA, Maraziotis TE, Bassaris HP. Management of brain abscesses with sequential intravenous/oral antibiotic therapy. Eur J Clin Microbiol Infect Dis. 2000;19:332-335.

168. Wallace RJ Jr, Septimus EJ, Williams TW Jr, et al. Use of trimethoprim-sulfamethoxazole for treatment of infections due to *Nocardia*. Rev Infect Dis. 1982;4:315-325.

169. Smego RA Jr, Moeller MB, Gallis HA. Trimethoprim-sulfamethoxazole therapy for *Nocardia* infections. Arch Intern Med. 1983;143:711-718.

170. Overkamp D, Waldmann B, Lins T, et al. Successful treatment of brain abscess caused by *Nocardia* in an immunocompromised patient after failure of co-trimoxazole. Infection. 1992;20:365-366.

171. Wallace RJ Jr, Steele LC, Sumter G, et al. Antimicrobial susceptibility patterns of *Nocardia asteroides*. Antimicrob Agents Chemother. 1988;32:1776-1779.

172. Berkey P, Moore D, Rolston K. In vitro susceptibilities of *Nocardia* species to newer antimicrobial agents. Antimicrob Agents Chemother. 1988;32:1078-1079.

173. Brown-Elliott BA, Warad SC, Crist CJ, et al. In vitro activities of linezolid against multiple *Nocardia* species. Antimicrob Agents Chemother. 2001;45:1295-1297.

174. Krone A, Schaal KP, Brawanski A, Schuknecht B. Nocardial cerebral abscess cured with imipenem/amikacin and enucleation. Neurosurg Rev. 1989;12:333-340.

175. Kim J, Minamoto GY, Hoy CD, et al. Presumptive cerebral *Nocardia asteroides* infection in AIDS: Treatment with ceftriaxone and minocycline. Am J Med. 1991;90:656-658.

176. Garlando F, Bodmer T, Lee C, et al. Successful treatment of disseminated nocardiosis complicated by cerebral abscess with ceftriaxone and amikacin: Case report. Clin Infect Dis. 1992;15:1039-1040.

177. Jansen C, Frenay HM, Vandertop WP, Visser MR. Intracerebral *Nocardia asteroides* abscess treated by neurosurgical aspiration and combined therapy with sulfadiazine and cefotaxime. Clin Neurol Neurosurg. 1991;93:253-255.

178. Gombert ME, du Bouchet L, Aulicino TM, Berkowitz LB. Antimicrobial synergism in the therapy of experimental cerebral nocardiosis. J Antimicrob Chemother. 1989;24:39-43.

179. Fleetwood IG, Embil JM, Ross IB. *Nocardia asteroides* cerebral abscess in immunocompetent hosts: Report of three cases and review of surgical recommendations. Surg Neurol. 2000;53:605-610.

180. Moylett EH, Pacheco SE, Brown-Elliott BA, et al. Clinical experience with linezolid for the treatment of *Nocardia* infection. Clin Infect Dis. 2003;36:313-318.

181. Filice GA, Simpson GL. Management of *Nocardia* infections. In: Remington JS, Swartz MN, eds. Current Clinical Topics in Infectious Diseases. New York: McGraw-Hill; 1984:49-64.

182. Stephanov S. Surgical treatment of brain abscess. Neurosurgery. 1988;22:724-730.

183. Dyste GN, Hitchon PW, Menezes AH, et al. Stereotaxic surgery in the treatment of multiple brain abscesses. J Neurosurg. 1988;69:188-194.

184. Rossitch E, Alexander E, Schiff SJ, et al. The use of computed tomography-guided stereotactic techniques in the treatment of brain stem abscesses. Clin Neurol Neurosurg. 1988;90:365-368.

185. Itakura T, Yokote H, Ozaki F, et al. Stereotactic operation for brain abscess. Surg Neurol. 1987;28:196-200.

186. Lunsford LD. Stereotactic drainage of brain abscesses. Neurol Res. 1987;9:270-274.

187. Shahzadi S, Lozano AM, Bernstein M, et al. Stereotactic management of bacterial brain abscesses. Can J Neurol Sci. 1996;23:34-39.

188. Laborde G, Klimek L, Harders A, Gilsbach J. Frameless stereotactic drainage of intracranial abscesses. Surg Neurol. 1993;40:16-21.

189. Lee GYF, Daniel RT, Brophy BP, Reilly PL. Surgical treatment of nocardial brain abscesses. Neurosurgery. 2002;51:668-672.

190. Valarezo J, Cohen JE, Valarezo L, et al. Nocardial cerebral abscess: Report of three cases and review of the current neurosurgical management. Neurol Res. 2003;25:27-30.

191. Kamitsuka MD, Nugent NA, Conrad PD, Swanson TN. *Candida albicans* brain abscesses in a premature infant treated with amphotericin B, flucytosine and fluconazole. Pediatr Infect Dis J. 1995;14:329-331.

192. Denning DW, Stevens DA. Antifungal and surgical treatment of invasive aspergillosis: Review of 2,121 published cases. Rev Infect Dis. 1990;12:1147-1201.

193. Sanchez C, Mauri E, Dalmau D, et al. Treatment of cerebral aspergillosis with itraconazole: Do high doses improve the prognosis? Clin Infect Dis. 1995;21:1485-1487.

194. Saulsbury FT. Successful treatment of *Aspergillus* brain abscess with itraconazole and interferon-gamma in a patient with chronic granulomatous disease. Clin Infect Dis. 2001;32:e137-139.

195. Erdogan E, Beyzadeoglu M, Arpaci F, Celasun B. Cerebellar aspergillosis: Case report and literature review. Neurosurgery. 2002;50:874-876.

196. Johnson LB. Kauffman CA. Voriconazole: A new triazole antifungal agent. Clin Infect Dis. 2003;36:630-637.

197. Denning DW, Ribaud P, Milpied N, et al. Efficacy and safety of voriconazole in the treatment of acute invasive aspergillosis. Clin Infect Dis. 2002;34:563-571.

198. Goodman ML, Coffey RJ. Stereotactic drainage of *Aspergillus* brain abscess with long-term survival: Case report and review. Neurosurgery. 1989;24:96-99.

199. Venugopal PV, Venugopal TV, Thiruneelakantan K, et al. Cerebral aspergillosis: Report of two cases. Sabouraudia. 1977;15:225-230.

200. Klein HJ, Richter HP, Schachenmayr W. Intracerebral *Aspergillus* abscess: Case report. Neurosurgery. 1983;13:306-309.

201. Ochi JW, Harris JP, Feldman JI, et al. Rhinocerebral mucormycosis: Results of aggressive surgical debridement and amphotericin B. Laryngoscope. 1988;98:1339-1342.

202. Talmi YP, Goldschmied-Reouven A, Bakon M, et al. Rhino-orbital and rhino-orbital-cerebral mucormycosis. Otolaryngol Head Neck Surg. 2002;127:22-31.

203. Couch L, Theilen F, Mader JT. Rhinocerebral mucormycosis with cerebral extension successfully treated with adjunctive hyperbaric oxygen therapy. Arch Otolaryngol Head Neck Surg. 1988;114:791-794.

204. Ferguson BJ, Mitchell TG, Moon R, et al. Adjunctive hyperbaric oxygen for treatment of rhinocerebral mucormycosis. Rev Infect Dis. 1988;10:551-559.

205. Fisher JF, Shadomy S, Teabeaut JR, et al. Near-drowning complicated by brain abscess due to *Petriellidium boydii*. Arch Neurol. 1982;39:511-513.

206. Perez RE, Smith M, McClendon J, et al. *Pseudallescheria boydii* brain abscess: Complication of an intravenous catheter. Am J Med. 1988;84:359-362.

207. Bailey T, Graham MB, Powderly W. Disseminated *Pseudallescheria boydii* infection treated with fluconazole (Abstract 71). In: Sixth International Symposium on Infections in the Immunocompromised Host, Peebles, Scotland, 1990.

208. Nomdedeu J, Brunet S, Martino R, et al. Successful treatment of pneumonia due to *Scedosporium apiospermum* with itraconazole: Case report. Clin Infect Dis. 1993;16:731-733.

209. Nesky MA, McDougal EC, Peacock JE Jr. *Pseudallescheria boydii* brain abscess successfully treated with voriconazole and surgical drainage: Case report and literature review of central nervous system pseudallescheriasis. Clin Infect Dis. 2000;31:673-677.

210. Mellinghoff IK, Winston DJ, Mukwaya G, Schiller GJ. Treatment of *Scedosporium apiospermum* brain abscess with posaconazole. Clin Infect Dis. 2002;34:1648-1650.

211. Roilides E, Sein T, Holmes A, et al. Effects of macrophage colony-stimulating factor on antifungal activity of mononuclear phagocytes against *Aspergillus fumigatus*. J Infect Dis. 1995;172:1028-1034.

212. Dale DW, Liles C, Summer WR, Nelson S. Granulocyte colony-stimulating factor—:Role and relationships in infectious diseases. J Infect Dis. 1995;172:1061-1075.

Subdural Empyema, Epidural Abscess, and Suppurative Intracranial Thrombophlebitis

ALLAN R. TUNKEL

SUBDURAL EMPYEMA

Epidemiology and Etiology

Subdural empyema refers to a collection of pus in the space between the dura and arachnoid. It accounts for 15% to 20% of all localized intracranial infections. Before the advent of antimicrobial therapy, the disease was essentially fatal (almost 100% mortality), but with current methods of diagnosis and treatment, mortality rates are approximately 10% to 20%.[1-5] The most common predisposing conditions to cranial subdural empyema are otorhinologic infections, especially of the paranasal sinuses, which are affected in 50% to 80% of cases[1,2,4-6]; this percentage may even be higher in children.[7,8] The pathogenesis involves spread of the infection to the subdural space via valveless emissary veins in association with thrombophlebitis, or via extension of an osteomyelitis of the skull with accompanying epidural abscess. Once the infection reaches the subdural space, it can spread without interruption over the convexities of the brain. The mastoid and middle ear are the source in 10% to 20% of patients, especially in geographic areas where cases of otitis media are not treated promptly with antimicrobial therapy. Other predisposing conditions in patients with subdural empyema include skull trauma, neurosurgical procedures, and infection of a preexisting subdural hematoma.[4,5,9-13] The infection is metastatic in about 5% of cases, principally from a pulmonary source. Rare predisposing factors include cranial traction devices, nasal surgery, ethmoidectomy, and polypectomy.[4] In infants with subdural empyema, meningitis is an important predisposing condition.[14] Subdural empyema occurs in about 2% to 10% of infants with bacterial meningitis,[5,15] presumably secondary to infection of an initially sterile subdural effusion. However, *Haemophilus influenzae* type b immunization has decreased the incidence of bacterial meningitis in infants and children (see Chapter 80), and cranial subdural empyema is now more commonly seen in teens and young adults.[16]

A number of bacterial species have been isolated in patients with cranial subdural empyema,[3-6,17] including aerobic streptococci (25% to 45% of cases), staphylococci (10% to 15% of cases), aerobic gram-negative bacilli (3% to 10% of cases), and anaerobic streptococci and other anaerobes (33% to as much as 100% in some small series in which careful culturing was performed).[4,18] Polymicrobial infections are common. These organisms make up the microbial flora that is frequently isolated from patients with chronic sinusitis or cranial abscess. Postoperative and post-traumatic infections are more commonly caused by staphylococci and aerobic gram-negative bacilli. Unusual pathogens include *Salmonella* species[19,20] and *Propionibacterium acnes*,[21,22] the latter microorganism isolated after trauma or neurosurgical procedures. In two series, 17%[5] and 21%[4] of samples taken from patients with cranial subdural empyema were sterile. Cranial subdural empyema caused by *Mycobacterium tuberculosis*[23] and *Candida* species[24] have also been reported.

Spinal subdural empyema is a rare condition that usually occurs secondary to metastatic infection from a distant site.[25,26] The most frequent microbial isolate is *Staphylococcus aureus*, with streptococci, coagulase-negative staphylococci, and gram-negative bacilli found less frequently.[27]

Clinical Features

The clinical presentation of cranial subdural empyema can be rapidly progressive, with symptoms and signs secondary to the presence of increased intracranial pressure, meningeal irritation, or focal cortical inflammation.[1-5,27] This acute presentation of subdural empyema is seen most often in patients with contiguous spread of infection. Fever greater than 39° C is present in most cases. Headache, which may be localized to the infected sinus or ear, is a prominent complaint and becomes generalized as the infection progresses. Vomiting is common as intracranial pressure increases. Altered mental status (i.e., drowsiness and disorientation), which progresses to obtundation or coma if the infection is not treated, is seen in more than two thirds of cases. Focal neurologic signs appear in 24 to 48 hours and progress rapidly, with eventual involvement of the entire cerebral hemisphere. The most common focal signs are hemiparesis and hemiplegia; ocular palsies, dysphasia, homonymous hemianopsia, dilated pupils, and cerebellar signs have all been reported. However, in one study, no focal signs were observed in 41% of 699 patients with cranial subdural empyema.[5] One third of patients in this series also presented with subgaleal abscesses. Seizures (either focal or generalized) are seen in up to 50% of cases. Signs of meningeal irritation are present in about 80% of patients, although fewer have either Kernig's or Brudzinski's sign. In untreated patients, there is rapid neurologic deterioration with signs of increased intracranial pressure and cerebral herniation, although papilledema develops in fewer than 50% of cases. This fulminant presentation, however, may not be seen in patients who have subdural empyema after cranial surgery or trauma, in those who have received prior antimicrobial therapy, in those with infected subdural hematomas, or in those with infections metastatic to the subdural space. In one review of 55 patients with traumatic cranial subdural empyema,[13] headache (84% of cases), fever (69% of cases), and neck stiffness (65% of cases) were the most common clinical features, and the mean time from initial trauma to presentation was 19 days (range, 4 to 60 days). In subdural empyema of infancy (which results in patients with bacterial meningitis), persistent fever, declining neurologic status, seizures, or some combination of these are most frequently observed.[16]

The clinical presentation of spinal subdural empyema is usually one of radicular pain and symptoms of spinal cord compression, which may occur at multiple levels.[25,27] The clinical presentation is difficult to distinguish from that of spinal epidural abscess (see later discussion).

Diagnosis

The diagnosis of cranial subdural empyema should be considered for any patient who presents with meningeal signs and a focal neurologic deficit.[1-5] A lumbar puncture with cerebrospinal fluid (CSF) analysis is contraindicated because of the risk of cerebral herniation. In one large series,[5] 280 patients with cranial subdural empyema underwent lumbar puncture; 33 patients were thought to have experienced neurologic deterioration as a direct result of this procedure, with 3 unnecessary deaths. In patients in whom a lumbar puncture has been done, CSF findings have been nonspecific and have included an elevated opening pressure, neutrophilic pleocytosis (although in up to 40% of cases there may be a mononuclear pleocytosis), and an increased CSF protein concentration[26]; CSF Gram stain and cultures are negative, unless the course is complicated by the presence of bacterial meningitis. Skull radiographs may show evidence of concurrent sinusitis or osteomyelitis, but they are not useful in establishing the diagnosis of subdural empyema.

Diagnostic procedures for cranial subdural empyema are either computed tomography (CT) with contrast or magnetic resonance imaging (MRI).[1,26,27] The typical CT appearance is that of a crescentic or elliptical area of hypodensity below the cranial vault or adjacent to the falx cerebri; loculations may also be seen. Depending on the extent of disease, there may be an associated mass effect with displacement of midline structures. After the administration of intravenous contrast, a fine, intense line of enhancement can be visualized between the subdural collection and the cerebral cortex. MRI provides better clarity of morphologic detail and may detect the presence of a subdural empyema not seen on CT; it is particularly helpful in detecting subdural empyemas located at the base of the brain, along the falx cerebri, or in the posterior fossa. MRI can also differentiate extra-axial empyemas from most sterile effusions and subdural hematomas. Based on these differences, MRI is now considered the diagnostic procedure of choice for cranial subdural empyema (Fig. 85-1). Both CT and MRI are also useful for demonstrating sinusitis and otitis. MRI is the diagnostic procedure of choice for spinal subdural empyema,[26,28] because it is better than CT in defining the extent of the lesion.

Management and Outcome

Subdural empyema is a medical emergency, and its treatment optimally requires a combined medical and surgical approach. Surgery (i.e., drainage) is needed, because antimicrobial agents alone do not reliably sterilize the empyema. Cultures (aerobic and anaerobic) of purulent material are needed to guide use of specific antimicrobial agents, and surgical decompression is useful for controlling increased intracranial pressure. Once purulent material has been aspirated via craniotomy or bur hole placement, antimicrobial therapy should be initiated based on results of the Gram stain and on the likely predisposing factor that led to the development of the subdural empyema. If *S. aureus* is a suspected pathogen, vancomycin should be used empirically but changed to nafcillin if the organism is found to be methicillin susceptible and the patient is not allergic to penicillin. Metronidazole is recommended if anaerobes are suspected. For infection likely caused by aerobic gram-negative bacilli, empirical therapy with cefepime, ceftazidime, or meropenem is appropriate, pending microorganism identification and in vitro susceptibility testing. Dosing for these agents can be found in Chapter 84. Depending on the clinical response, parenteral antimicrobial therapy should be continued for 3 to 4 weeks after drainage, although there are no firm data to support a specific duration of antimicrobial therapy in patients with subdural empyema; longer periods of intravenous, and perhaps oral, therapy may be required if the patient has accompanying osteomyelitis. There have been anecdotal cases in which cranial subdural empyema was treated with antimicrobial therapy alone. This approach may be appropriate in patients with minimal or no impairment of consciousness, no major neurologic deficit, limited extension of the empyema without midline shift, and early improvement with antimicrobial therapy alone.[4,16] However, these selected patients need careful clinical and radiographic monitoring, and probably longer courses of antimicrobial therapy.

The goals of surgical therapy in cranial subdural empyema are to achieve adequate decompression of the brain and to completely evacuate the empyema. The optimal surgical approach in patients with cranial subdural empyema (drainage via craniotomy or bur holes) is controversial.[1,16,27] Some studies have demonstrated a lower mortality rate in patients who have undergone craniotomy, although it may be that a larger number of patients treated with bur hole drainage were more ill and had a greater surgical risk. Use of bur holes with irrigation may be more efficacious for drainage in the early stages of subdural empyema, when the pus is liquid,[29,30] allowing easier aspiration. If drainage is accomplished via bur holes, multiple bur holes may be needed to allow for extensive irrigation. When the pus becomes thickened and loculated as the disease progresses, these patients should undergo craniotomy. However, craniotomy may be essential for posterior fossa subdural empyema or if drainage is inadequate after bur holes.

If craniotomy is performed, wide exposure is needed to allow adequate exploration of all areas where the empyema is suspected. The neurosurgeon may also elect to leave drains or catheters in the subdural space, although this may increase the subsequent risk of nosocomial infections. In one report,[31] the efficacy of craniotomy versus CT-guided bur hole or craniectomy drainage was analyzed during the periods 1983-1987 (189 patients) and 1988-1997 (509 patients). At operation, the empyema collections were sometimes found to be more loculated, tenacious, and extensive than indicated by neuroimaging studies; based on this experience, craniotomy became the preferred method of drainage for these authors beginning in 1988. A significant improvement in outcome was demonstrated between the 1983-1987 study period (good outcome in 71.4% of patients) and the 1988-1997 period (good outcome in 86.1%; $P = .001$). Analysis of the entire database (1983 through 1997) revealed that the mortality rates were higher for patients treated only with drainage via bur holes (23.3%), compared with those who underwent craniectomies (11.5%) or craniotomies (8.4%). Patients with multiple bur holes or craniectomy drainage not only required more frequent operations to drain recurrent or remaining pus but also exhibited higher mortality rates and poorer outcomes. The authors recommended limited procedures (i.e., bur hole drainage or craniectomy) only for patients with septic shock, patients with localized parafalcine collections, and children with subdural empyemas secondary to meningitis (because there is usually no brain swelling and the pus is thin). Regardless of the initial surgical approach, several studies have shown that a number of patients require reoperation; in one study, reoperation was required in half of those patients treated with bur hole drainage and one fifth of those initially treated with craniotomy.[32] Surgical correction of the antecedent otorhinologic infection may also be required.

In the modern era, survival rates among patients with cranial subdural empyema are greater than 90% for those who are awake and alert at presentation but less than 50% for those who present unresponsive to pain.[27] Furthermore, 10% to 44% of patients may experience permanent neurologic deficits.[4,5,16] Cranial subdural empyemas may also be complicated by septic venous thrombosis, localized cerebritis, and cerebral abscesses.

In patients with spinal subdural empyema, empirical antimicrobial therapy should be directed against staphylococci, streptococci, and aerobic gram-negative bacilli,[27] with adjustments based on culture results. Laminectomy is also necessary for drainage of the infection.

EPIDURAL ABSCESS

Epidemiology and Etiology

Epidural abscess refers to a localized collection of pus between the dura mater and the overlying skull or vertebral column. Because cranial epidural abscess can cross the cranial dura along emissary veins, an accompanying subdural empyema is often present.[1] Therefore, the bacterial etiology and pathogenesis of cranial epidural abscess are usually identical to those described earlier for cranial subdural empyema, with the initial focus usually in the paranasal sinuses, middle ear, or mastoid cells. Cranial epidural abscess may also occur after trauma, fetal scalp monitoring, halo pin penetration, or craniotomy.[12,16,33,34]

Spinal epidural abscess usually occurs secondary to hematogenous dissemination from foci elsewhere in the body to the epidural space, or by extension from vertebral osteomyelitis.[35-43] Bacteremia may be an important predisposing factor, because the incidence of spinal epidural abscess is increased in patients who use injection drugs[44,45] and in those who have intravenous catheters or infective endocarditis. Diabetes mellitus also appears to be an important risk factor; it has been identified in up to 50% of patients.[38,40,42,43,46] Hematogenous spread occurs in 25% to 50% of cases, secondary to infections of the skin (e.g., furuncles, cellulitis, infected acne), urinary tract infections, periodontal abscesses, pharyngitis, pneumonia, or mastoiditis. Mild blunt spinal trauma (a history elicited from 15% to 35% of patients) may provide a devitalized site that is susceptible to transient bacteremia, although it is unclear whether this represents a true risk factor for the subsequent development of spinal epidural abscess. A primary source of infection is not identified in 20% to 40% of patients.[35-38] Infection of the epidural space has also been reported after penetrating injuries, extension of decubitus ulcers or paraspinal abscesses, back surgery, lumbar puncture, CT-guided needle biopsies, and administration of epidural anesthesia or analgesia.[47-51]

The infecting microorganism in most (50% to 90%) of the patients with spinal epidural abscess is *S. aureus*.[35-43,46,52,53] Other isolates include aerobic and anaerobic streptococci (8% to 17% of cases) and aerobic gram-negative bacilli (12% to 17% of cases), especially

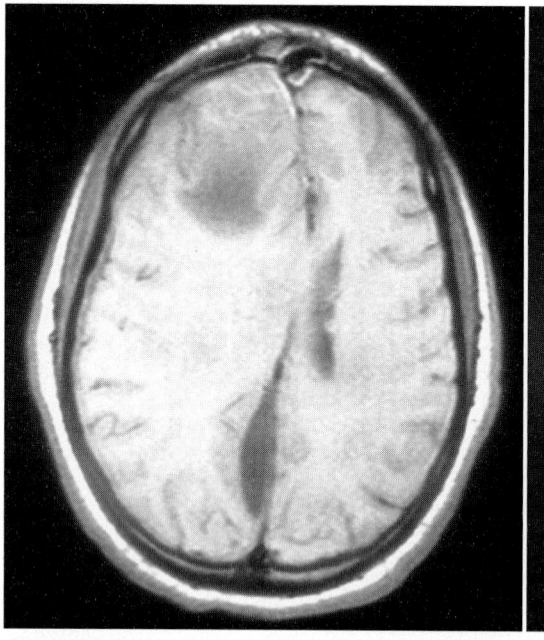

A

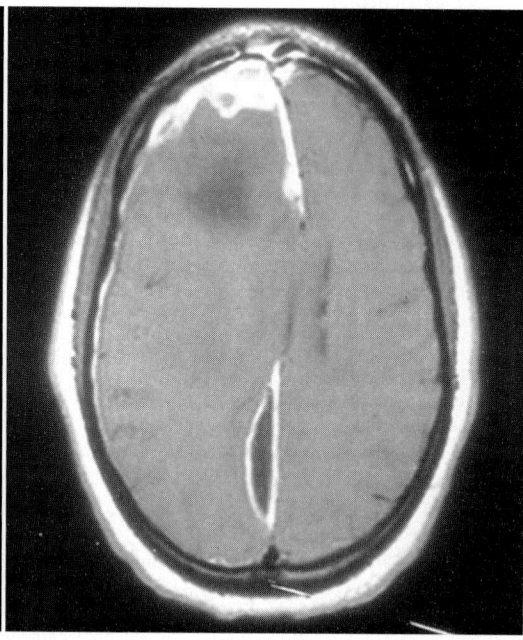

B

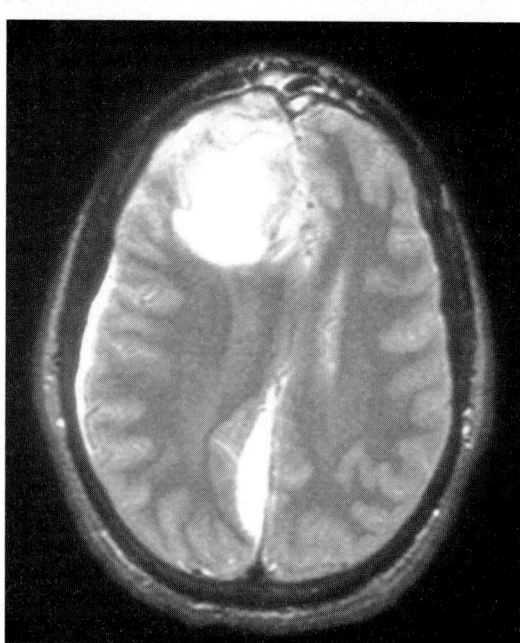

C

FIGURE 85-1. A, T_1-weighted axial magnetic resonance image of the brain showing a hypodense mass in the right frontal region with marked meningeal thickening, midline shift, and effacement of the right lateral ventricle. **B,** T_1-weighted axial magnetic resonance image of the brain in the same patient with gadolinium enhancement, showing abnormal enhancement. Posteriorly, there is an elliptically shaped density in the interhemispheric fissure. *(From Tunkel AR, Scheld WM. Focal central nervous system infections. In: Root RK, ed. Clinical Infectious Diseases: A Practical Approach. New York: Oxford University Press; 1999:723-731, with permission.)* **C,** T_2-weighted axial magnetic resonance image of the brain in the same patient, showing high signal intensity in the right frontal region and interhemispheric fissure.

Escherichia coli and *Pseudomonas aeruginosa*; recent case series have noted an increased incidence of aerobic gram-negative bacilli, streptococci, and anaerobes. More than one microorganism is isolated in about 5% to 10% of cases.[35,38,39,45] In addition to numerous case reports of patients with spinal epidural abscess caused by other bacteria, epidural infection can also be caused by *Nocardia* species,[54] *M. tuberculosis*,[55,56] and fungi.[39,57-59]

Clinical Features

The clinical presentation in patients with cranial epidural abscess may be insidious and overshadowed by the primary focus of infection (i.e., sinusitis or otitis media).[1,16,39] Headache is a usual complaint, but the patient may otherwise feel well (leading to a delay in diagnosis) unless the clinical course is complicated (e.g., by development of subdural empyema, brain abscess, or meningitis). This insidious presentation occurs because the dura is closely opposed to the inner surface of the cranium, so that the abscess usually enlarges too slowly to produce the sudden onset of major neurologic deficits (in contrast to the presentation in patients with cranial subdural empyema) unless there is deeper intracranial extension. Eventually, focal neurologic signs and seizures (either focal or generalized) may develop. In the untreated patient, papilledema and other signs of increased intracranial pressure develop as the abscess enlarges. A cranial epidural abscess near the petrous bone may result in Gradenigo's syndrome, which is characterized by involvement of cranial nerves V and VI, with unilateral facial pain and weakness of the lateral rectus muscle.

The clinical findings in patients with spinal epidural abscess may develop within hours to days (usually after hematogenous seeding), or the course may be more chronic, over weeks to months (usually in association with vertebral osteomyelitis or another contiguous focus of infection).[35-43,46,60] The presentation in most patients with spinal epidural abscesses progresses through the following four clinical stages: (1) backache and focal vertebral pain, with tenderness on examination; (2) nerve root pain, manifested by radiculopathy or paresthesias, or both; (3) spinal cord dysfunction, characterized by defects of motor, sensory, or sphincter function; and (4) complete paralysis. Pain is the most consistent symptom (70% to 90% of cases) and is usually accompanied by local tenderness at the affected level. Fever is reported in 60% to 70% of patients, although it was noted in only 32% of patients in one study.[40] The specific neurologic signs depend on the level of spinal cord involvement; the most common locations are the thoracic and lumbar epidural spaces. Because the neurologic manifestations are usually reversible before complete paralysis occurs, emergency imaging studies and intervention are necessary if the diagnosis is being considered (see later discussion).

Diagnosis

MRI (with gadolinium enhancement) is the diagnostic procedure of choice for cranial epidural abscess. It demonstrates a superficial, circumscribed area of diminished intensity with pachymeningeal enhancement; the possibility of adjacent subdural empyema or other intracranial infection can also be assessed.[1,39] CT scanning may be used to image bone or if MRI is not available. MRI is superior to CT in the identification and delineation of the collections, and it has the ability to differentiate epidural abscesses from sterile effusions and hematomas that may occur in patients after trauma or cranial surgery.

MRI is also the diagnostic procedure of choice in cases of suspected spinal epidural abscess (Fig. 85-2).[39-41,43,52] MRI is recommended over CT because it can better visualize the spinal cord and epidural space in both sagittal and transverse sections and can also identify accompanying osteomyelitis, intramedullary spinal cord lesions, and diskitis. The epidural mass may be isointense or hypointense on T_1-weighted images and hyperintense on T_2-weighted

images. Gadolinium enhancement typically demonstrates linear enhancement surrounding nonenhancing purulent or necrotic matter. MRI can also readily assess the response to therapy (see later discussion). CT myelography may be performed if MRI is unavailable or contraindicated.[40,43]

Management and Outcome

The management of cranial epidural abscess requires a combined medical and surgical approach. Empirical antimicrobial therapy for cranial epidural abscess is similar to that for cranial subdural empyema (see earlier discussion); therapy is usually continued for 3 to 6 weeks after surgical drainage, or longer (6 to 8 weeks) if osteomyelitis is present.[16] Surgical drainage is also required; craniotomy or craniectomy is generally preferred over bur hole placement or aspiration of purulent material through the scalp.[1,12,16,33]

The principles of therapy for spinal epidural abscess are prompt surgical decompression, drainage of the abscess, and long-term antimicrobial therapy. Empirical antimicrobial therapy for spinal epidural abscess must include a first-line antistaphylococcal agent (i.e., vancomycin pending organism identification and in vitro susceptibility testing) plus coverage for aerobic gram-negative bacilli (e.g., cefepime, ceftazidime, meropenem), especially for any patient with a history of spinal procedure or injection drug use.[36,39] Once the infecting pathogen is identified, antimicrobial therapy can be modified based on in vitro susceptibility testing. One study suggested that relapse was less likely in patients who received at least 8 weeks of antimicrobial therapy.[61]

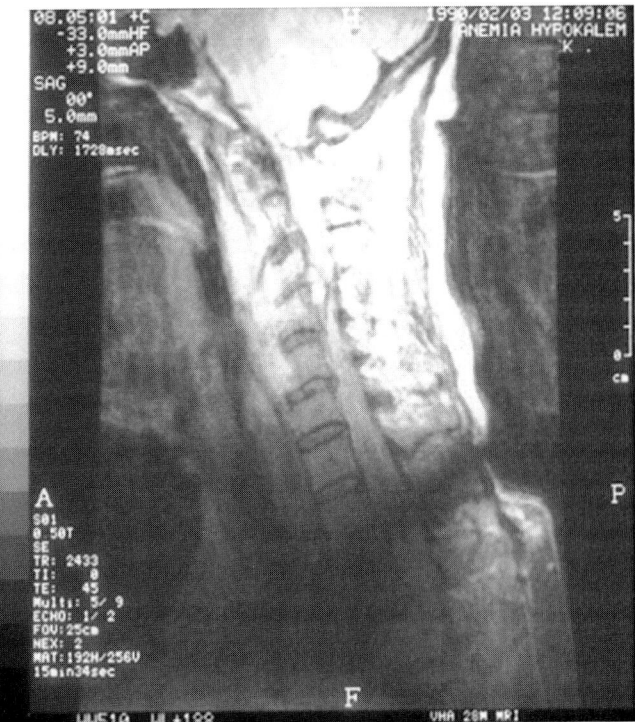

FIGURE 85-2. Proton-weighted sagittal magnetic resonance image of the cervical spine showing an epidural collection at the C3-C4 level that is compressing the spinal cord. *(From Tunkel AR, Scheld WM. Focal central nervous system infections. In: Root RK, Waldvogel F, Corey L, Stamm WE, eds. Clinical Infectious Diseases: A Practical Approach. New York: Oxford University Press; 1999:723-731. Copyright 1999 by Oxford University Press, Inc. Used by permission of Oxford University Press, Inc.)*

Patients with spinal epidural abscess and neurologic dysfunction require laminectomy with decompression and drainage performed as a surgical emergency to minimize the likelihood of permanent neurologic sequelae.[35-43] CT-guided aspiration may be used in place of laminectomy in selected patients,[62] although there are no data to indicate that this approach reduces the need for surgical intervention. There have been no randomized, prospective trials that have compared the efficacy of antimicrobial therapy plus surgery with that of antimicrobial therapy alone in patients with spinal epidural abscess. However, in one literature review of 38 patients with spinal epidural abscess treated with antimicrobial therapy alone,[63] 23 patients recovered, 2 died, 1 worsened, and the rest remained the same or improved. Antimicrobial therapy alone can be considered in patients who have localized pain or radicular symptoms without long-tract findings. However, these patients require frequent neurologic examinations and serial MRI studies to demonstrate resolution of the abscess. Emergency surgical decompression should be performed for any patient with increasing neurologic deficit, persistent severe pain, or increasing fever or peripheral white blood cell count.[64] Surgery is not likely to be a viable therapeutic option in patients who have experienced complete paralysis for longer than 24 hours,[38] although some authors would perform surgical therapy in patients if complete paralysis has lasted less than 72 hours.[42]

Mortality rates for spinal epidural abscess ranged from 5% to 23% in recent series.[37,38,40,41,43,45] The final neurologic outcome in patients with spinal epidural abscess is related to the severity of neurologic impairment before initiation of appropriate therapy.[38-41,46,56] Complete recovery with return of full neurologic function is most likely if neurologic signs are present for less than 24 hours before initiation of therapy; complete recovery is less likely if symptoms persist for longer than 36 to 48 hours. Worse outcome has been observed in patients with multiple medical problems, increasing age, prior spinal surgery, cervical or thoracic abscess location, leukocytosis ($>$14,000/mm^3 at admission), thrombocytopenia ($<$100,000/mm^3), elevated serum C-reactive protein concentrations during the second postoperative week, isolation of methicillin-resistant staphylococci, and degree of thecal sac compression ($>$50% spinal canal involvement).[40,43,46]

SUPPURATIVE INTRACRANIAL THROMBOPHLEBITIS

Epidemiology and Etiology

Suppurative intracranial thrombophlebitis includes both venous thrombosis and suppuration. It may begin within veins or venous sinuses, or it may occur after infection of the paranasal sinuses, middle ear, mastoid, face, or oropharynx.[65-67] Additional vessels may be involved by propagation or discontinuous spread. Suppurative thrombophlebitis also occurs in association with epidural abscess, subdural empyema, or bacterial meningitis. Occasionally, there is metastatic spread from a distant site of infection. Conditions that increase blood viscosity or coagulability (e.g., dehydration, polycythemia, pregnancy, oral contraceptive use, sickle cell disease, malignancy, trauma, Behçet's disease, antiphospholipid antibodies, systemic lupus erythematosus, and deficiencies in protein C, protein S, or antithrombin III) have been associated with an increase in the likelihood of thrombosis.[65,68,69]

The development of septic intracranial venous sinus thrombosis depends on the close proximity of various structures to the dural venous sinuses. The usual predisposing condition for septic cavernous sinus thrombosis is paranasal sinusitis (especially of the frontal, ethmoid, or sphenoid sinuses)[65,66,70,71]; infections of the face and mouth are less commonly the primary sources of infection in the antimicrobial era. Otitis media and mastoiditis are infections that are associated with lateral sinus thrombosis[65,72-74] and infection of the superior and inferior petrosal sinuses. Infections of the face, scalp, subdural space, epidural space, and meninges are associated with septic thrombophlebitis of the superior sagittal sinus. In all of these infections, the likely microorganisms depend on the associated primary condition. The most important

infecting microorganism in septic cavernous sinus thrombosis is *S. aureus*, which is isolated in 60% to 70% of patients.[65,70,71] However, the likely infecting bacterial pathogens depends on the pathogenesis of infection: staphylococci, streptococci, gram-negative bacilli, and anaerobes if the antecedent condition is sinusitis; and predominantly *S. aureus* in the case of facial infections. *S. aureus*, streptococci, and *E. coli* are commonly reported as pathogens in patients with lateral sinus thrombosis,[65,73] although in one study *Fusobacterium necrophorum* was the microorganism isolated in four of six children with lateral sinus thrombosis.[74] In another study of patients with lateral sinus thrombosis secondary to chronic ear infection,[73] all patients had mixed infections and *Bacteroides fragilis* was isolated in five of six cases. Venous sinus thrombosis may also be seen in patients with rhinocerebral mucormycosis[75] or invasive aspergillosis.[76]

Clinical Features

The clinical findings in patients with suppurative intracranial thrombophlebitis depend on the sinus involved.[65,66] The two cavernous sinuses are positioned on either side of the sella turcica; they are connected by anterior and posterior intercavernous sinuses that encircle the pituitary gland.[70,71] The horizontal segment of the internal carotid artery and cranial nerve VI run through the lumen, and cranial nerves III, IV, and the ophthalmic and maxillary branches of cranial nerve V run through the outside layers of the lateral walls of the cavernous sinuses. The clinical manifestations may relate to damage to the nerves that traverse the cavernous sinuses. The most common complaints in patients with septic cavernous sinus thrombosis are periorbital swelling (73% of cases) and headache (52% of cases)[65]; headache is more common if the antecedent condition is sinusitis rather than a facial infection. Other symptoms include drowsiness, diplopia, eye tearing, photophobia, and ptosis. Signs include fever (present in more than 90% of patients), proptosis, chemosis, periorbital edema, and weakness of the extraocular muscles (secondary to involvement of cranial nerves III, IV, and VI)[65,66,70,71]; because cranial nerve VI is the only cranial nerve traversing the interior of the cavernous sinus, a lateral gaze palsy may be an early neurologic finding. Papilledema or venous engorgement is observed in 65% of patients, and a change in mental status in 55%. Meningismus is present in as many as 40% of patients, usually secondary to retrograde spread of the thrombophlebitis. Fewer than 50% of patients have dilated or sluggishly reactive pupils, decreased visual acuity (which may progress to blindness), and dysfunction of cranial nerve V. As infection spreads to the opposite cavernous sinus through the intercavernous sinuses, findings are duplicated in the opposite eye, usually within 24 to 48 hours after the initial unilateral periorbital edema. Cortical vein thrombophlebitis is a particularly serious complication of septic cavernous sinus thrombosis because it carries the risk of cerebral hemorrhagic infarction.[65,71]

Persons with septic cavernous sinus thrombosis may present with either acute or chronic illness.[65,66] In the acute presentation (usually secondary to facial infection), the time between primary infection and cavernous sinus thrombosis is short (usually less than 1 week), and the patient presents in a significantly toxic state, with rapid development of the signs and symptoms described earlier; there is also rapid progression to bilateral eye signs. In contrast, in the more indolent form of cavernous sinus thrombosis, which usually occurs secondary to dental infection, otitis media, or paranasal sinusitis, the orbital manifestations are often unimpressive and involvement of the contralateral eye is a late and inconsistent finding.

Patients with septic lateral sinus thrombosis complain predominantly of headache (more than 80% of cases); photophobia, earache, vomiting, and vertigo may also occur, because otitis media is a common predisposing condition.[65,73,74] Fever and abnormal ear findings are observed in most patients (79% and 98%, respectively), and palsy of cranial nerve VII, facial pain and altered facial sensation, papilledema, mastoid tenderness, and nuchal rigidity may also be present.

Thrombosis of the superior sagittal sinus produces an abnormal mental status, motor deficits, nuchal rigidity, and papilledema.[65]

Seizures occur in more than half of these patients. Patients with sinusitis as a predisposing condition tend to have a subacute onset of symptoms. Involvement of the inferior petrosal sinus may produce ipsilateral facial pain and lateral rectus muscle involvement (Gradenigo's syndrome).

Diagnosis

Laboratory studies are usually nonspecific in suppurative intracranial thrombophlebitis.[65,66] Lumbar puncture demonstrates a mild pleocytosis (either mononuclear, neutrophilic, or mixed) and an elevated CSF protein concentration (consistent with a parameningeal focus of infection), although there may be findings of frank meningitis in patients with septic thrombosis of the superior sagittal sinus, and the causative microorganism may be isolated on culture of CSF. Blood cultures may be positive, especially in patients with a rapidly progressive course. Chest radiographs may reveal evidence of septic pulmonary emboli after propagation of the thrombus into the inferior petrosal sinus and jugular vein. Sinus radiographs may document involvement of the paranasal sinuses, although conventional radiographs are inferior to CT or MRI in the detection of sphenoid sinusitis.

The noninvasive diagnostic procedure of choice for suppurative intracranial thrombophlebitis is MRI (Fig. 85-3).[67,77,78] Cross-sectional MRI demonstrates areas of cerebral edema and, potentially, regions of abnormal blood-brain barrier breakdown with associated contrast enhancement. Magnetic resonance angiography and venography can directly visualize the cerebral vasculature, differentiating thrombus from normal blood flow. It can also reveal the evolution and resolution of the entire veno-occlusive process. As an alternative, high-resolution CT (with and without intravenous contrast) with a slice thickness of 3 mm or less permits diagnosis of venous sinus thrombosis,[79] although it is considerably less sensitive and less reliable than MRI. In patients with septic cavernous sinus thrombosis, CT usually reveals unilateral or bilateral multiple irregular filling defects in the enhancing cavernous sinus, with or without orbital inflammatory change, or enlargement or expansion of the cavernous sinus with lateral wall flattening or convexity rather than the normal concavity. An additional benefit of both MRI and CT is the ability to fully evaluate the paranasal sinuses and to provide information concerning subdural and epidural infection, cerebral infarction, cerebritis, hemorrhage, and cerebral edema.

Management and Outcome

Before the availability of antimicrobial therapy, suppurative intracranial thrombophlebitis carried a mortality rate of 80% to 100%. Since 1940, mortality rates have ranged from 0% to 16% in patients with septic lateral sinus thrombosis[73] and from 13% to 30% in patients with septic cavernous sinus thrombosis,[65,70] although in one series of 14 pediatric patients with septic cavernous sinus thrombosis, 79% died despite parenteral antimicrobial therapy.[80] Selection of appropriate antimicrobial therapy for suppurative intracranial thrombophlebitis depends on the antecedent clinical condition; the likely microorganisms are similar to those observed in cranial subdural empyema and cranial epidural abscess (see earlier discussions). If the antecedent clinical condition is paranasal sinusitis, empirical antimicrobial therapy should be directed toward staphylococci, streptococci, aerobic gram-negative bacilli, and anaerobes. In septic cavernous sinus thrombosis, an antistaphylococcal agent should always be included because of the high likelihood of isolation of *S. aureus*; vancomycin is recommended empirically, pending results of in vitro susceptibility testing. An appropriate empirical regimen is vancomycin, metronidazole, and a third- or fourth-generation cephalosporin, pending culture results and in vitro susceptibility testing. Intravenous antimicrobial therapy is usually continued for at least 3 to 4 weeks, but the duration needs to be individualized depending on the clinical response.

Surgery may also be needed for optimal treatment of septic intracranial thrombophlebitis.[65,66,70,71] Surgical therapy for infected sinuses is necessary if antimicrobial therapy alone is ineffective; this is especially important in patients with cavernous sinus thrombosis secondary to sphenoid sinusitis. In fact, some authors have recommended operative intervention for patients who develop cavernous sinus thrombosis as a complication of sinusitis. Internal jugular vein ligation has been used for lateral sinus vein thrombosis, and thrombectomy has also been used in some situations,[73] but the efficacy of these proce-

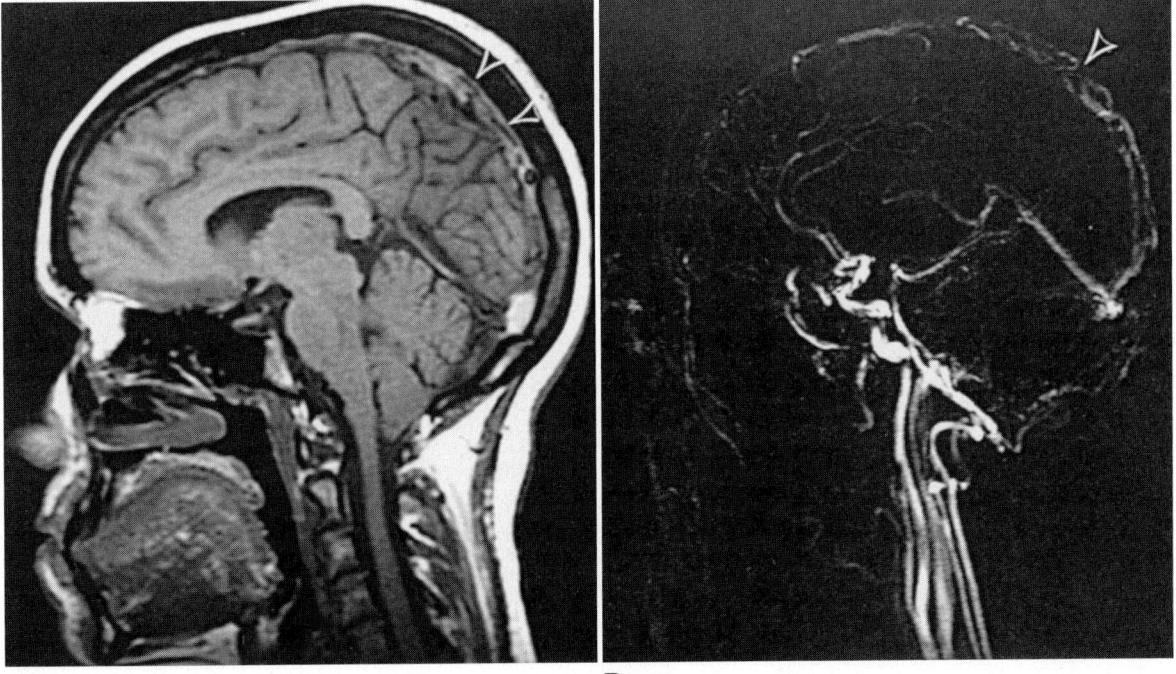

A   **B**

FIGURE 85-3. A, Magnetic resonance image of superior sagittal sinus thrombosis. There is increased signal within the vessel on the T$_2$-weighted image *(arrows)*, indicating the presence of thrombus. **B,** Magnetic resonance angiogram in the same patient, showing nonfilling of the superior sagittal sinus. The sinus is surrounded by tortuous collateral vessels *(arrow)*. *(Courtesy of Dr. Wayne Davis, University of Utah.)*

dures is poorly defined. Some authors have recommended ligation of the internal jugular vein for patients who develop septic embolization despite antimicrobial therapy and surgical drainage.[74,81] Surgical therapy may also be required for other infections (e.g., dental abscesses, mastoiditis, complicating brain abscess, or subdural empyema).

The use of anticoagulation in suppurative intracranial thrombophlebitis is controversial. There is support in the literature for the use of anticoagulation (i.e., heparin) to prevent spread of the thrombus from the cavernous sinus to other dural venous sinuses and cerebral veins.[65,66,70,71] Retrospective evidence indicates that anticoagulation, in combination with antimicrobial therapy, reduces mortality and is most beneficial if given early (within 7 days after hospitalization) in the treatment of cavernous sinus thrombosis.[65,82] However, it must be recognized that anticoagulation carries the risk of intracranial hemorrhage from sites of cortical venous infarction or from sites on the intracavernous walls of the carotid artery. Some authors have not recommended anticoagulation in patients with septic lateral sinus or superior sagittal sinus thrombosis because of the high number of venous hemorrhagic infarcts observed postmortem.[65] In the absence of prospective data, anticoagulation should be used in the treatment of septic cavernous sinus thrombosis unless there are contraindications or documented hemorrhagic intracranial complications on neuroimaging studies; however, some practitioners use anticoagulation only as an adjunct to antimicrobial therapy in patients with a deteriorating clinical condition.[71] The duration of anticoagulation has varied from 2 weeks to several months; some have continued anticoagulation until complete thrombus resolution has been documented on neuroimaging studies.

Among patients who survive their episode of septic cavernous sinus thrombosis, up to 50% are left with long-term cranial nerve deficits,[65,71] although they may continue to improve for several months after completion of therapy. Partial or complete visual loss is seen in 7% to 22% of cases. Patients should be observed for several months after completion of antimicrobial therapy, because isolated relapses have been documented within 6 weeks after apparent clinical resolution, and intracranial abscesses have been demonstrated up to 8 months later.[71]

REFERENCES

1. Silverberg AL, DiNubile MJ. Subdural empyema and cranial epidural abscess. Med Clin North Am. 1985;69:361-374.
2. Coonrad JD, Dans PE. Subdural empyema. Am J Med. 1972;53:85-91.
3. Kaufman DM, Miller MH, Steigbigel NH. Subdural empyema: Analysis of 17 recent cases and review of the literature. Medicine (Baltimore). 1975;54:485-498.
4. Dill SR, Cobbs CG, McDonald CK. Subdural empyema: Analysis of 32 cases and review. Clin Infect Dis. 1995;20:372-386.
5. Nathoo N, Nadvi SS, van Dellen JR, Gouws E. Intracranial subdural empyemas in the era of computed tomography: A review of 699 cases. Neurosurgery. 1999;44:529-535.
6. Kaufman DM, Litman N, Miller MH. Sinusitis-induced subdural empyema. Neurology. 1983;33:123-132.
7. Giannoni C, Sulek M, Friedman EM. Intracranial complications of sinusitis: A pediatric series. Am J Rhinol. 1998;12:173-178.
8. Ong YK, Tan HKK. Suppurative intracranial complications of sinusitis in children. Int J Pediatr Otorhinolaryngol. 2002;66:49-54.
9. Dee KE, Newell DW, Cohen WA. Subdural empyema after depressed frontal sinus fracture. AJR Am J Roentgenol. 1998;170:790.
10. Levy I, Sood S. Staphylococcus aureus dissemination to a preexisting subdural hematoma. Pediatr Infect Dis J. 1996;15:1139-1140.
11. Bakker S, Kluytmans J, den Hollander JC, Lie ST. Subdural empyema caused by Escherichia coli: Hematogenous dissemination to a preexisting chronic subdural hematoma. Clin Infect Dis. 1995;21:458-459.
12. Hlavin ML, Kaminski HJ, Fenstermaker RA, White RJ. Intracranial suppuration: A modern decade of postoperative subdural empyema and epidural abscess. Neurosurgery. 1994;34:974-980.
13. Nathoo N, Nadvi SS, van Dellen JR. Traumatic cranial empyemas: A review of 55 patients. Br J Neurosurg. 2000;14:326-330.
14. Chang YC, Huang CC, Wang ST, Chio CC. Risk factor of complications requiring neurosurgical intervention in infants with bacterial meningitis. Pediatr Neurol. 1997;17:144-149.
15. Jacobson PL, Farmer TW. Subdural empyema complicating meningitis in infants: Improved prognosis. Neurology. 1981;31:190-193.
16. Bockova J, Rigamonti D. Intracranial empyema. Pediatr Infect Dis J. 2000;19:735-737.
17. Yoshikawa TT, Chow AW, Guze LB. Role of anaerobic bacteria in subdural empyema: Report of four cases and review of 327 cases from the English literature. Am J Med. 1975;58:99-104.
18. Brook I. Aerobic and anaerobic bacteriology of intracranial abscesses. Pediatr Neurol. 1992;8:210-214.
19. Aliaga L, Mediavilla JD, Lopez de la Osa A, et al. Nontyphoidal Salmonella intracranial infections in HIV-infected patients. Clin Infect Dis. 1997;25:1118-1120.
20. Mahapatra AK, Pawar SJ, Sharma RR. Intracranial Salmonella infections: Meningitis, subdural collections and brain abscess. A series of six surgically managed cases with follow-up results. Pediatr Neurosurg. 2002;36:8-13.
21. Jallo GI, Koslow M, Hanna BA, Carson LA. Propionibacterium as a cause of postneurosurgical infection in patients with dural allografts: Report of three cases. Neurosurgery. 1999;44:1138-1141.
22. Chu RM, Tummala RP, Hall WA. Focal intracranial infections due to Propionibacterium acnes: Report of three cases. Neurosurgery. 2001;49:717-720.
23. van Dellen A, Nadvi SS, Nathoo N, Ramdial PK. Intracranial tuberculous subdural empyema: Case report. Neurosurgery. 1998;43:370-373.
24. Duffner F, Brandner S, Opitz H, et al. Primary Candida albicans empyema associated with epidural hematomas in craniocervical junction. Clin Neuropathol. 1997;16:143-146.
25. Dacey RG, Winn HR, Jane JA, Butler AB. Spinal subdural empyema: Report of two cases. Neurosurgery. 1978;3:400-403.
26. Levy ML, Wieder BH, Schneider J, et al. Subdural empyema of the cervical spine: Clinicopathologic correlates and magnetic resonance imaging. J Neurosurg. 1993;79:929-935.
27. Helfgott DC, Weingarten K, Hartman BJ. Subdural empyema. In: Scheld WM, Whitley RJ, Durack DT, eds. Infections of the Central Nervous System. 2nd ed. Philadelphia: Lippincott-Raven; 1997:495-505.
28. Weingarten K, Zimmerman RD, Becker RD, et al. Subdural and epidural empyemas: MR imaging. AJR Am J Roentgenol. 1989;152:615-621.
29. De Falco R, Scarano E, Cigliano A, et al. Surgical treatment of subdural empyema: A critical review. J Neurosurg Sci. 1996;40:53-58.
30. Ak HE, Ozkan U, Devecioglu C, Kemaloglu MS. Treatment of subdural empyema by burr hole. Isr J Med Sci. 1996;32:542-544.
31. Nathoo N, Nadvi SS, Gouws E, van Dellen JR. Craniotomy improves outcomes for cranial subdural empyemas: Computed tomography-era experience with 699 patients. Neurosurgery. 2001;49:872-878.
32. Mauser HW, van Houwelingen HC, Tulleken CA. Factors affecting the outcome of subdural empyema. J Neurol Neurosurg Psychiatry 1987;50:1136-1141.
33. Harris LF, Haws FP, Triplett JN Jr. Subdural empyema and epidural abscess: Recent experience in a community hospital. South Med J. 1987;80:1254-1258.
34. Papagelopoulos PJ, Sapkas GS, Kateros KT, et al. Halo pin intracranial penetration and epidural abscess in a patient with a previous cranioplasty: Case report and review of the literature. Spine. 2001;26:E463-E467.
35. Baker AS, Ojemann RG, Swartz MN, Richardson EP Jr. Spinal epidural abscess. N Engl J Med. 1975;293:463-468.
36. Danner RL, Hartman BJ. Update on spinal epidural abscess: 35 cases and review of the literature. Rev Infect Dis. 1987;9:265-274.
37. Hlavin ML, Kaminski HJ, Ross JS, Ganz E. Spinal epidural abscess: A ten-year perspective. Neurosurgery. 1990;27:177-184.
38. Dar* Dariouiche RO, Hamill RJ, Greenberg SB, et al. Bacterial spinal epidural abscess: Review of 43 cases and literature survey. Medicine (Baltimore). 1992;71:369-385.
39. Gellin BG, Weingarten K, Gamache FW Jr, Hartman BJ. Epidural abscess. In: Scheld WM, Whitley RJ, Durack DT, eds. Infections of the Central Nervous System. 2nd ed. Philadelphia: Lippincott-Raven; 1997:507-522.
40. Rigamonti D, Liem L, Sampath P, et al. Spinal epidural abscess: Contemporary trends in etiology, evaluation, and management. Surg Neurol. 1999;52:189-197.
41. Reihsaus E, Waldbaur H, Seeling W. Spinal epidural abscess: A meta-analysis of 915 patients. Neurosurg Rev. 2000;23:175-204.
42. Tang HJ, Lin HJ, Liu YC, Li CM. Spinal epidural abscess: Experience with 46 patients and evaluation of prognostic factors. J Infect. 2002;45:76-81.
43. Soehle M, Wallenfang T. Spinal epidural abscess: Clinical manifestations, prognostic factors, and outcomes. Neurosurgery. 2002;51:79-87.
44. Koppel BS, Tuchman AJ, Mangiardi JR, et al. Epidural spinal infection in intravenous drug abusers. Arch Neurol. 1988;45:1331-1337.
45. Nussbaum ES, Rigamonti D, Standiford H, et al. Spinal epidural abscess: A report of 40 cases and review. Surg Neurol. 1992;38:225-231.
46. Khanna RK, Malik GM, Rock JP, Rosenblum ML. Spinal epidural abscess: Evaluation of factors influencing outcome. Neurosurgery. 1996;39:958-964.
47. Shintani S, Tanaka H, Irifune A, et al. Iatrogenic acute spinal epidural abscess with septic meningitis: MR findings. Clin Neurol Neurosurg. 1992;94:253-255.
48. Smitt PS, Tsafka A, Ten-van de Zande F, et al. Outcome and complications of epidural anesthesia in patients with chronic cancer pain. Cancer. 1998;83:2015-2022.
49. Knight JW, Cordingley JJ, Palazzo MG. Epidural abscess following epidural steroid and local anaesthetic injection. Anaesthesia. 1997;52:576-578.
50. Koka VK, Potti A. Spinal epidural abscess after corticosteroid injections. South Med J. 2002;95:772-774.

51. Phillips JMG, Stedeford JC, Hartsilver E, Roberts C. Epidural abscess complicating insertion of epidural catheters. Br J Anaesth. 2002;89:778-782.
52. Auletta JJ, John CC. Spinal epidural abscesses in children: A 15-year experience and review of the literature. Clin Infect Dis. 2001;32:9-16.
53. Khan SH, Hussain MS, Griebel RW, Hattingh S. Comparison of primary and secondary spinal epidural abscesses: A retrospective analysis of 29 cases. Surg Neurol. 2003;59:28-33.
54. Siao P, McCabe P, Yagnick P. Nocardial spinal epidural abscess. Neurology. 1989;39:996.
55. Kaufman DM, Kaplan JG, Litman N. Infectious agents in spinal epidural abscesses. Neurology. 1980;30:844-850.
56. Lu CH, Chang WN, Lui CC, et al. Adult spinal epidural abscess: Clinical features and prognostic factors. Clin Neurol Neurosurg. 2002;104:306-310.
57. Bonomo RA, Strauss M, Glinkhorn R, Salata RA. *Torulopsis (Candida) glabrata*: A new pathogen found in spinal epidural abscess. Clin Infect Dis. 1996;22:588-589.
58. Liang JD, Tang CT, Chen YC, et al. *Candida albicans* spinal epidural abscess secondary to prosthetic valve endocarditis. Diagn Microbiol Infect Dis. 2001;40:121-123.
59. Gupta PK, Mahapatra AK, Gaind R, et al. *Aspergillus* spinal epidural abscess. Pediatr Neurosurg. 2001;35:18-23.
60. Lasker BR, Harter DH. Cervical epidural abscess. Neurology. 1987;37:1747-1753.
61. Mackenzie AR, Laing RB, Smith CC, et al. Spinal epidural abscess: The importance of early diagnosis and treatment. J Neurol Neurosurg Psychiatry. 1998;65:209-212.
62. Lyu RK, Chen CJ, Tang LM, Chen ST. Spinal epidural abscess successfully treated with percutaneous, computed tomography-guided, needle aspiration and parenteral antibiotic therapy: Case report and review of the literature. Neurosurgery. 2002;51:509-512.
63. Wheeler D, Keiser P, Rigamonti D, Keay S. Medical management of spinal epidural abscess: Case report and review. Clin Infect Dis. 1992;15:22-27.
64. Baker AS, Ojemann RG, Baker RA. To decompress or not to decompress: Spinal epidural abscess. Clin Infect Dis. 1992;15:28-29.
65. Southwick FS, Richardson EP Jr, Swartz MN. Septic thrombosis of the dural venous sinuses. Medicine (Baltimore). 1985;65:82-106.
66. DiNubile MJ. Septic thrombosis of the cavernous sinuses. Arch Neurol. 1988;45:567-572.
67. Gallagher RM, Gross CW, Phillips CD. Suppurative intracranial complications of sinusitis. Laryngoscope. 1998;108:1635-1642.
68. Wechsler B, Vidailhet M, Piette JC, et al. Cerebral venous thrombosis in Behçet's disease: Clinical study and long term follow up of 25 cases. Neurology. 1992;42:614-618.
69. Daif A, Adnan A, Al-Rajeh S, et al. Cerebral venous thrombosis in adults: A study of 40 cases from Saudi Arabia. Stroke. 1995;26:1193-1195.
70. Ebright JR, Pace MT, Niazi AF. Septic thrombosis of the cavernous sinuses. Arch Intern Med. 2001;161:2671-2676.
71. Bhatia K, Jones NS. Septic cavernous sinus thrombosis secondary to sinusitis: Are anticoagulants indicated? A review of the literature. J Laryngol Otol. 2002;116:667-676.
72. Samuel J, Fernandes CMC. Lateral sinus thrombosis (a review of 45 cases). J Laryngol Otol. 1987;101:1227-1229.
73. Syms MJ, Tsai PD, Holtel MR. Management of lateral sinus thrombosis. Laryngoscope. 1999;109:1616-1620.
74. Holzmann D, Huisman T, Linder TE. Lateral dural sinus thrombosis in childhood. Laryngoscope. 1999;109:645-651.
75. Estrem SA, Tully R, Davis WE. Rhinocerebral mucormycosis: Computed tomographic imaging of cavernous sinus thrombosis. Ann Otol Rhinol Laryngol. 1990;99:160-161.
76. Sekhar LN. Carotid-cavernous sinus thrombosis caused by *Aspergillus fumigatus*. J Neurosurg. 1980;67:219-222.
77. Medlock MD, Olivero WC, Hanigan WC, et al. Children with cerebral venous thrombosis diagnosed with magnetic resonance imaging and magnetic resonance angiography. Neurosurgery. 1992;31:870-876.
78. Igarashi H, Igarashi S, Fujio N, et al. Magnetic resonance imaging in the early diagnosis of cavernous sinus thrombosis. Ophthalmologica. 1995;209:292-296.
79. Schuknecht B, Simmen D, Yuksel C, Valavania A. Tributary venosinus occlusion and septic cavernous sinus thrombosis: CT and MR findings. Am J Neuroradiol. 1998;19:617-626.
80. Ali SM, Ahmed SH. Cavernous sinus thrombosis in children. J Trop Pediatr. 1992;38:194-195.
81. Singh B. The management of lateral sinus thrombosis. J Laryngol Otol. 1993;107:803-808.
82. Levine SR, Twyman RE, Gilman S. The role of anticoagulation in cavernous sinus thrombosis. Neurology. 1988;38:517-522.
83. Tunkel AR, Scheld WM. Focal central nervous system infections. In: Root RK, ed. Clinical Infectious Diseases: A Practical Approach. New York: Oxford University Press; 1999:723-731.

CHAPTER **86**

Cellulitis and Subcutaneous Tissue Infections

MORTON N. SWARTZ

MARK S. PASTERNACK

CELLULITIS AND SUPERFICIAL INFECTIONS

Major attention should be directed to determination of the specific microbial cause of any infection involving the skin. This chapter considers bacterial and mycotic infections, exclusive of those caused by the common dermatophytes. Classification of cutaneous infections on morphologic and clinical grounds can be very helpful in providing initial clues regarding the most likely responsible infectious agents (Table 86-1).

Primary Pyodermas

Impetigo

Impetigo is an initially vesicular, later crusted, superficial infection of the skin. Most cases occur in children. Previously, group A streptococcus was considered the principal cause of impetigo and was isolated from about 80% of cases, either alone or mixed with *Staphylococcus aureus.*[1] In the past 15 years, group A streptococcus has been found less commonly (20% to 30%) in impetigo and appears to have been supplanted by *S. aureus* in frequency.[2-4] However, studies occasionally implicate group A streptococci as a major cause of impetigo.[5] These differences may well reflect geographic shifts in streptococcal hyperendemicity over time. As a cautionary note, the role of staphylococci may be overestimated inasmuch as these organisms are common secondary invaders, and some strains appear to produce bacteriocins that may make it more difficult to isolate group A streptococci in their presence.[6]

Pathologic Characteristics and Pathogenesis. Histopathologically, impetigo consists of a superficial, intraepidermal, unilocular vesicopustule. In epidemiologic studies, group A streptococcal acquisition on normal skin antedates the appearance of impetigo by about 10 days.[1] During that time, minor trauma (e.g., insect bite, abrasion) predisposes to the development of infected lesions. Impetigo is most common during hot, humid summer weather. Two to 3 weeks after skin acquisition of streptococci, pharyngeal colonization by the same organism occurs in about 30% of children with skin lesions. (The sporadic cases of facial impetigo occurring in cooler climates probably result from contiguous spread from an initial nasopharyngeal infection, and the serotypes involved are those commonly causing pharyngeal disease.) In contrast, in the cases of staphylococcal impetigo (in which *S. aureus* is the only pathogen), nasal colonization precedes that of the normal skin; skin lesions then occur after such colonization.[7,8]

Evidence suggests that nonbullous impetigo caused by group A streptococcus (*Streptococcus pyogenes*) begins when the corneal layer of the epidermis is disrupted and the bacteria gain access to highly differentiated subcorneal keratinocytes. Adherence of impetigo strains, but not pharyngeal strains, of *S. pyogenes* is furthered by keratinocyte differentiation.[9] M protein of *S. pyogenes* mediates binding of the bacteria to keratinocytes.[10] A second streptococcal surface protein, protein F, or fibronectin-binding protein, mediates adherence to antigen-presenting Langerhans' cells located along the basal layer of the epidermis.

Impetigo is a highly communicable infection. Spread in families (particularly among preschool children) is facilitated by crowding and poor hygiene.

Clinical Findings. Streptococcal impetigo begins as small vesicles, sometimes with narrow inflammatory halos, that rapidly pustulate and readily rupture. The purulent discharge dries and forms the characteristic thick, golden-yellow, "stuck-on" crusts. Exposed areas are the most common sites for lesions. Pruritus is common, and scratching of lesions can spread infection. Occasionally, large crusts are produced by coalescence of smaller pustules. The lesions remain superficial and do not ulcerate or infiltrate the dermis, and mild regional lymphadenopathy is common. Healing occurs without scarring. The lesions are painless, and constitutional manifestations are minimal.

Laboratory Findings. Gram-stained smears of vesicles show gram-positive cocci. Culture of exudate beneath an unroofed crust reveals *S. aureus*, group A streptococci, or a mixture of streptococci and *S. aureus.* The anti–streptolysin O titer after streptococcal impetigo is scant, probably related to inhibition of streptolysin O by skin lipids at the infection site. In contrast, the anti-DNase B response readily occurs (elevated titers in 90% of patients with nephritis complicating streptococcal skin infections).[11]

Etiologic Agents. The group A streptococci responsible for impetigo usually belong to different M serotypes (e.g., 2, 49, 52, 55, 57, 59, 60, 61) from those of strains that produce pharyngitis (e.g., 1, 2, 4, 6, 25).

M surface proteins, many of which are key virulence factors, are encoded in emm genes. Five major emm chromosomal patterns (groups A through E) have been described based on the number and arrangement of specific nucleotide sequences encoding part of the peptidoglycan-spanning M-protein domain.[12] Almost all group A streptococcal impetigo isolates belong to emm chromosomal patterns D and, to a lesser extent, E, whereas most isolates from patients with either uncomplicated pharyngitis or acute rheumatic fever belong to emm chromosomal pattern groups A, B, or C. Consistent with these epidemiologic findings, pattern D strains had a higher gross pathology score than did pattern A, B, or C strains in a humanized in vivo model (human skin–severe combined immunodeficiency [SCID] mouse chimera) for streptococcal impetigo.[13] Further, a plasminogen-binding domain genotype (designated plasminogen-binding group A streptococcal M protein, or PAM) is widely distributed among emm pattern D isolates, in contrast to patterns A, B, C and E organisms, in which the PAM genotype is uncommon.[14]

Group C and group G streptococci may rarely cause impetigo; group B streptococci have been associated with impetigo in newborns.

Differential Diagnosis. Although the initial vesicular lesions may resemble early varicella, the crusts of the latter are darker brown and harder. The central clearing of a confluent cluster of lesions of impetigo may suggest tinea circinata but can be distinguished by the thick crusts, which are not formed in the fungus infection. When the vesicles of herpes simplex become turbid, they may look like impetigo. Acute palmoplantar pustulosis, a sterile, idiopathic, self-limited pustular eruption on the palms and soles that sometimes occurs after pharyngitis, may initially resemble impetigo.[15] Localized acute pustular psoriasis may also be mistaken for impetigo. Primary cutaneous listeriosis, an occupational disease of veterinarians and farmers involved in calving, is characterized by papulovesicular and pustular lesions on the forearms that may resemble those of impetigo.[16]

Presumptive Therapy. Penicillin was the drug of choice in the past for the treatment of ordinary impetigo, because of the predominant role of group A streptococci and the possible occurrence of acute glomerulonephritis as a sequela of such infections. Because of delay in seeking medical attention for such a mild infection, it remains

TABLE 86-1 Classification of Bacterial and Mycotic Infections of the Skin

Type of Lesion	Etiologic Agents
Primary Pyodermas	
Impetigo	*Staphylococcus aureus*, group A streptococci
Folliculitis	*S. aureus, Candida, Pseudomonas aeruginosa, Pityrosporum ovale*
Furuncles and carbuncles	*S. aureus*
Paronychia	*S. aureus*, group A streptococci, *Candida, P. aeruginosa*
Ecthyma	Group A streptococci
Erysipelas	Group A streptococci
Chancriform lesions	*Treponema pallidum, Haemophilus ducreyi, Sporothrix, Bacillus anthracis, Francisella tularensis, Mycobacterium ulcerans, Mycobacterium marinum*
Membranous ulcers	*Corynebacterium diphtheriae*
Cellulitis	Group A streptococci, *S. aureus*; rarely, various other organisms
Infectious Gangrene and Gangrenous Cellulitis	
Streptococcal gangrene and necrotizing fasciitis	Group A streptococci, mixed infections with Enterobacteriaceae and anaerobes
Progressive bacterial synergistic gangrene	Anaerobic streptococci plus a second organism (*S. aureus, Proteus*)
Gangrenous balanitis and perineal phlegmon	Group A streptococci, mixed infections with enteric bacteria (e.g., *Escherichia coli, Klebsiella*) and anaerobes
Gas gangrene, crepitant cellulitis	*Clostridium perfringens* and other clostridial species; *Bacteroides*, peptostreptococci, *Klebsiella, E. coli*
Gangrenous cellulitis in immunosuppressed patients	*Pseudomonas, Aspergillus*, agents of mucormycosis
Erythrasma	*Corynebacterium minutissimum*
Nodular Lesions	*Candida, Sporothrix, S. aureus* (botryomycosis), *M. marinum, Nocardia brasiliensis, Leishmania brasiliensis*
Hyperplastic (Pseudoepitheliomatous) and Proliferative Lesions (e.g., Mycetomas)	*Nocardia, Pseudallescheria boydii, Blastomyces dermatitidis, Paracoccidioides brasiliensis, Phialophora, Cladosporium*
Vascular Papules/Nodules (Bacillary Angiomatosis, Epithelioid Angiomatosis)	*Bartonella henselae, Bartonella quintana*
Annular Erythema (Erythema Chronicum Migrans)	*Borrelia burgdorferi*
Secondary Bacterial Infections Complicating Preexisting Skin Lesions	
Burns	*P. aeruginosa, Enterobacter*, various other gram-negative bacilli, various streptococci, *S. aureus, Candida, Aspergillus*
Eczematous dermatitis and exfoliative erythrodermas	*S. aureus*, group A streptococci
Chronic ulcers (varicose, decubitus)	Coliform bacteria, *P. aeruginosa*, peptostreptococci, enterococci, *Bacteroides, C. perfringens*
Dermatophytosis	*S. aureus*, group A streptococci
Traumatic lesions (e.g., abrasions, animal bites, insect bites)	*Pasturella multocida, C. diphtheriae, S. aureus*, group A streptococci
Vesicular or bullous eruptions (varicella, pemphigus)	*S. aureus*, group A streptococci
Acne conglabata	*Propionibacterium acnes*
Hidradenitis suppurativa	*S. aureus, Proteus* and other coliforms, streptococci, peptostreptococci, *Bacteroides*
Intertrigo	*S. aureus*, coliforms, *Candida*
Pilonidal and sebaceous cysts	Peptostreptococci, *Bacteroides*, coliforms
Pyoderma gangrenosa	*S. aureus*, peptostreptococci, *Proteus* and other coliforms, *P. aeruginosa*
Cutaneous Involvement in Systemic Bacterial and Mycotic Infections	
Bacteremias	*S. aureus*, group A streptococci (also other groups such as D), *Neisseria meningitidis, Neisseria gonorrhoeae, P. aeruginosa, Salmonella typhi; Haemophilus influenzae*
Endocarditis	Viridans streptococci, *S. aureus*, group D streptococci, and others
Fungemias	*Candida, Cryptococcus, Blastomyces dermatitidis, Fusarium*
Listeriosis	*Listeria monocytogenes*
Leptospirosis (Weil's disease and pretibial fever)	*Leptospira interrogans* serotypes
Rat-bite fever	*Streptobacillus moniliformis, Spirillum minus*
Melioidosis	*Burkholderia pseudomallei*
Glanders	*Burkholderia mallei*
Carrión's disease (verruga peruana)	*Bartonella bacilliformis*
Scarlet fever syndromes	
Scarlet fever	Group A streptococci, rarely *S. aureus*
Scalded skin syndrome	*S. aureus* (phage group II)
Toxic shock syndrome	*S. aureus* (pyrogenic toxin–producing strains)
Parainfectious and postinfectious nonsuppurative complications	
Purpura fulminans (manifestation of disseminated intravascular coagulation)	Group A streptococci, *S. aureus*, pneumococcus
Erythema nodosum	Group A streptococci, *Mycobacterium tuberculosis, Mycobacterium leprae, Coccicidioides immitis, Leptospira autumnalis, Yersinia enterocolitica, Legionella pneumophila*
Erythema multiforme–like lesions (rarely), guttate psoriasis	Group A streptococci

unclear whether penicillin therapy is effective in reducing the incidence of streptococcal pyoderma-associated nephritis. Penicillin is administered either as a single intramuscular injection of benzathine penicillin (child, 300,000 to 600,000 units; adult, 1,200,000 units), as oral penicillin V (10-50 mg/kg/day in divided doses every 6 to 8 hours for 10 days), or as amoxicillin (500 mg orally q8h for adults).

Erythromycin (child, 30 to 50 mg/kg/day in divided doses every 6 hours for 10 days; adult, 250 to 500 mg orally every 6 hours) is an alternative for penicillin-allergic patients. The efficacy of erythromycin may be reduced in areas where erythromycin-resistant streptococci (and staphylococci) are prevalent. Local care (removal of crusts by soaking with soap and water) is helpful.

Mixed streptococcal-staphylococcal impetigo has the same crusted lesions and clinical course as streptococcal impetigo and may respond to treatment with penicillin G.[17] However, because S. aureus, either alone or in concert with S. pyogenes as the cause of impetigo, commonly produces penicillinase, treatment with penicillin alone often fails. Penicillinase-resistant oral penicillins (e.g., dicloxacillin) or cephalosporins (e.g., cephalexin, cefadroxil) are very effective[2,18] (see later discussion).

A topical antibiotic, mupirocin ointment in a polyethylene glycol base, was shown to be as effective as oral erythromycin in the treatment of impetigo,[3] and more effective when erythromycin-resistant S. aureus strains were involved.[4] Another topical antimicrobial agent, fusidic acid cream, is available in Europe and was shown to be much more effective than a placebo cream in treatment of childhood impetigo caused, in most of the cases, by S. aureus.[19] Gentle application of topical agents is important to minimize tissue maceration and spread of infection. Systemic therapy is preferred for the treatment of widespread impetigo. With the increased frequency of isolation of S. aureus from the lesions of patients with impetigo, some physicians favor alternative (but more expensive) initial approaches, such as the use of cephalexin (child, 25 to 50 mg/kg orally per day in two divided doses), cefadroxil (child, 30 mg/kg orally per day in two divided doses), or dicloxacillin (child, 12.5 mg/kg orally per day in four divided doses).[18] For most patients with nonbullous impetigo, erythromycin (or penicillin) or topical mupirocin is appropriate therapy unless problems in the community with erythromycin-resistant organisms are suspected.

Mupirocin has also been used topically to eradicate methicillin-resistant S. aureus (MRSA) from secondarily infected skin lesions and from colonized patients. However, because resistance in S. aureus strains has emerged sooner than anticipated after the introduction of mupirocin, particularly when long-term therapy was used, prolonged administration should probably be avoided.

Bullous Impetigo

Clinical Findings. The bullous form of impetigo is caused by S. aureus of phage group II (usually type 71); it occurs principally in newborns and young children and accounts for about 10% of all cases of impetigo. The lesions begin as vesicles that turn into flaccid bullae initially containing clear yellow fluid. No erythematous areola is noted, and the Nikolsky sign is absent. The bullae quickly rupture, leave a moist red surface, and then form thin, "varnish-like," light brown crusts. Bullous impetigo, like the staphylococcal scalded skin syndrome (SSSS) and the staphylococcal scarlatiniform syndrome, represents a form of cutaneous response to the two extracellular exfoliative toxins produced by S. aureus of phage group II. The gene for one of the toxins (ETA) is chromosomal in origin, and that of the other (ETB) is located on a plasmid[20]; ETA appears to have an amino acid sequence similar to that of an S. aureus serine protease. The toxin acts extracellularly locally at the site of cutaneus infection in bullous impetigo and systemically in causing generalized blistering from toxin produced at a site of S. aureus infection in the skin or elsewhere. It causes subcorneal separation of cells of the epidermis by cleaving desmoglein 1, a transmembrane glycoprotein of desmosomes.[20,21] Staphylococci are regularly isolated from the skin lesions of bullous impetigo. Streptococcal superinfection rarely complicates bullous impetigo, probably because type 71 strains of S. aureus produce a bacteriocin that inhibits streptococci. Fever and constitutional symptoms are uncommon, and healing occurs without scarring.

Presumptive Therapy. Extensive bullous impetigo responds to treatment with a penicillinase-resistant penicillin (e.g., dicloxacillin, 25 to 50 mg/kg daily in divided doses orally every 6 hours for a child), a cephalosporin (e.g., cephalexin, 25 to 50 mg/kg daily in divided doses orally every 8 to 12 hours for a child) or erythromycin in a penicillin-allergic patient.

Staphylococcal Scalded Skin Syndrome

SSSS is the most severe manifestation of infection with S. aureus strains producing an exfoliative exotoxin; it is characterized by widespread bullae and exfoliation.[22-24] Pemphigus neonatorum (Ritter's disease) is SSSS in the newborn. The more general term *toxic epidermal necrolysis* is often used to encompass both SSSS and a morphologically identical syndrome of various causes (drug reactions, viral illnesses) (see Chapter 192).

Clinical Findings. SSSS usually occurs in younger children, but it can rarely develop in adults. Epidemics have occurred in neonatal nurseries.[25] SSSS begins abruptly (sometimes a few days after a recognized staphylococcal infection) with fever, skin tenderness, and a scarlatiniform rash. The Nikolsky sign can be demonstrated. Large, flaccid, clear bullae form, promptly rupture, and result in the separation of sheets of skin. New bullae appear over a period of 2 to 3 days. Exfoliation exposes large areas of bright red skin surface (Fig. 86-1). With appropriate fluid replacement and antimicrobial therapy, the skin lesions heal within 2 weeks, in contrast to drug-induced toxic epidermal necrolysis, in which recovery is more prolonged because the entire epidermis must be replaced and scarring is more frequent. The mortality rate from SSSS in children is less than 3%, but in adults it can be up to 60%.[20,21]

Presumptive Therapy. Intravenous use of a penicillinase-resistant penicillin (e.g., nafcillin, 100 mg/kg/day for newborns, 100 to 200 mg/kg/day for older children) is indicated in the initial treatment of SSSS, because of the presence of active staphylococcal infection and rapid progression of the skin lesions. Topical treatment consists of cool saline compresses. Systemic corticosteroids alone should not be used in the treatment of SSSS, although they may be indicated in therapy for drug-induced toxic epidermal necrolysis.

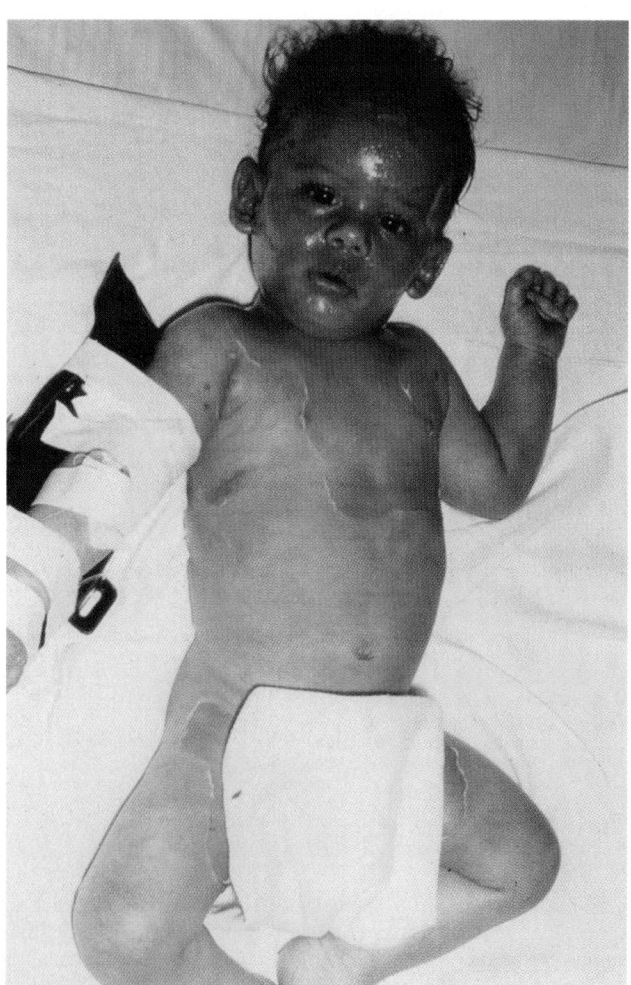

FIGURE 86-1. Staphylococcal scalded skin syndrome in a young infant. Exfoliation has occurred on the face, chest, and groin, exposing areas of bright red skin surface.

Staphylococcal Scarlet Fever

Staphylococcal scarlet fever is fundamentally a forme fruste of SSSS that does not progress beyond the initial stage of a generalized erythematous eruption. However, *S. aureus* enterotoxins (A through D) and toxic shock syndrome toxin 1 are more frequently associated with staphylococcal scarlet fever than are ETA and ETB.[26] The rash is indistinguishable from that of scarlet fever, and Pastia's lines can develop. However, pharyngitis is not usually present, and an enanthem does not develop. Desquamation, beginning on the face and involving most of the body, occurs 2 to 5 days after onset of the scarlatiniform rash. Antibiotic treatment with penicillinase-resistant penicillins is indicated.

Toxic Shock Syndrome

Toxic shock syndrome is another acute febrile illness with a generalized scarlatiniform eruption associated with *S. aureus* infection. Other elements of the syndrome include (1) hypotension (shock), (2) functional abnormalities of three or more organ systems, and (3) desquamation in the evolution of the skin lesions[27-29] (see Chapter 192).

Folliculitis

Folliculitis is a pyoderma located within hair follicles and the apocrine regions. The lesions consist of small (2 to 5 mm), erythematous, sometimes pruritic papules often topped by a central pustule. Sycosis barbae is a distinctive form of deep folliculitis, often chronic, that occurs on bearded areas. *S. aureus* is the usual cause of folliculitis. *Pseudomonas aeruginosa* (most often serotype O-11) has been responsible for folliculitis acquired from swimming pools and whirlpools contaminated with large numbers of these organisms.[30] This type of skin infection produces pruritic, sometimes tender papulourticarial lesions (appearing within 48 hours after exposure) that eventuate in pustule formation. Lesions in different stages of development (macules, papules, papulopustules) are present simultaneously. Preferred sites include the buttocks, hips, and axillae; the palms and soles are spared. Otitis externa is also a common manifestation. Healing occurs spontaneously within 5 days, either by drainage or by regression. Scarring develops rarely, when an occasional pustule has progressed to furuncle formation. If folliculitis is acquired in a whirlpool, the lesions are sharply limited to the trunk below the upper part of the chest or neck. Inadequate chlorine levels in whirlpools, hot tubs, and swimming pools have been responsible for many of the outbreaks reported. *P. aeruginosa* can also cause superinfection in acne and rosacea after prolonged broad-spectrum antibiotic therapy. In granulocytopenic and immunosuppressed hospitalized patients, *P. aeruginosa* O-11 from tap water used for washing was implicated in folliculitis that rapidly progressed to ecthyma gangrenosum.[31] *Pseudomonas* folliculitis developed in a toddler who was exposed to a contaminated wash cloth and bath mat.[32]

Folliculitis, often perioral and perinasal, caused by Enterobacteriaceae, can occur as a complication in patients with acne and rosacea, usually during prolonged courses of oral antibiotic therapy.[33,34]

Candida is sometimes the cause of folliculitis. It produces pruritic satellite lesions surrounding areas of intertriginous candidiasis, particularly in patients receiving prolonged antibiotic or corticosteroid therapy. *Malassezia furfur,* a common skin saprophyte, may also produce a folliculitis with pruritic erythematous papules and papulopustules on the trunk, upper extremities, and face, particularly in the setting of diabetes mellitus, corticosteroid administration, or granulocytopenia.[35-37] These lesions, particularly the early papular nodular ones, may suggest those of systemic candidiasis, a diagnosis that may seem to be supported by the presence of budding yeast forms on Gram-stained material from unroofed lesions. Unlike *Candida, M. furfur* requires lipid-supplemented media for primary isolation. Eosinophilic pustular folliculitis, a rare pruritic dermatosis characterized by recurrent crops of follicular papules and pustules with eosinophilic infiltration of perifollicular dermis, occurs particularly in the setting of acquired immunodeficiency syndrome (AIDS). It resembles bacterial or mycotic folliculitis but is a sterile process.[38]

Local measures (saline compresses and topical antibacterials or antifungals such as clotrimazole) are usually sufficient to control the infection.

Furuncles and Carbuncles

Definition and Pathologic Characteristics. A furuncle is a deep inflammatory nodule that usually develops from preceding folliculitis. A carbuncle is a more extensive process that extends into the subcutaneous fat in areas covered by thick, inelastic skin. In the latter, multiple abscesses separated by connective tissue septa develop and drain to the surface along hair follicles. *S. aureus* is almost invariably the etiologic agent (see also Chapter 192).

Clinical Findings. Furuncles occur in skin areas that are subject to friction and perspiration and contain hair follicles (neck, face, axillae, buttocks). Predisposing factors include obesity, blood dyscrasias, treatment with corticosteroids, defects in neutrophil function, and probably diabetes mellitus. A furuncle begins as a firm, tender, red nodule that soon becomes painful and fluctuant. Spontaneous drainage of pus commonly occurs, and the lesion subsides. A carbuncle is a larger, deeper, indurated, more serious lesion, usually located at the nape of the neck, on the back, or on the thighs. Fever and malaise are frequently present, and some patients are acutely ill. As the lesion progresses, drainage occurs externally along the course of multiple hair follicles. A leukocytosis occurs, particularly if the lesion contains a large amount of undrained pus or if a complicating cellulitis or bacteremia is present.

Blood stream invasion can occur unpredictably (but is sometimes precipitated by manipulation of the lesions) and can result in osteomyelitis, endocarditis, or other metastatic foci. Lesions about the upper lip and nose present the special problem of spread of infection via the facial and angular emissary veins to the cavernous sinus.

Presumptive Therapy. Most furuncles are satisfactorily treated by the application of moist heat, which promotes localization and drainage of the process. A carbuncle, a furuncle with surrounding cellulitis or fever, or a furuncle located about the midface should be treated with an antistaphylococcal antibiotic (e.g., dicloxacillin, 0.25 g orally every 6 hours for an adult). In a penicillin-allergic adult, clindamycin (150 to 300 mg orally every 6 hours) or erythromycin (0.25 to 0.5 g orally every 6 hours) is an alternative. If the lesions are large and fluctuant, surgical drainage is indicated. Antibiotic treatment should be continued until evidence of acute inflammation has subsided. If the patient has been recently hospitalized, methicillin-resistant staphylococcal infection should be considered. These infections are best treated with vancomycin or linezolid or daptomycin (see Chapter 192).

Management of recurrent furunculosis presents a troublesome problem. This disease does not appear to be caused by specific staphylococcal strains with special biologic properties, and most patients do not have definable underlying defects in host defenses. Prophylaxis of recurrent episodes involves several measures:

1. *Antibiotic treatment.* Systemic antibiotic treatment, as described earlier, should be administered for the most recent episode. Prolonged treatment (2 months) is no more effective than a 10- to 14-day course in preventing recurrences.[39]
2. *General skin care.* Soap and water should be used to reduce the number of *S. aureus* organisms on the body surface, and careful hand washing should be performed after contact with lesions. A separate towel and washcloth (carefully washed in hot water before reuse) should be reserved for the patient. Chlorhexidine solution (4%), an antimicrobial skin cleanser, or hexachlorophene may be used to further decrease staphylococcal skin colonization. Hexachlorophene is contraindicated for use in newborns and infants because of potential neurotoxicity.
3. *Care of clothing.* Sheets and underclothing should be laundered at high temperatures and changed daily for problem patients.
4. *Care of dressings.* Draining lesions should be covered at all times with sterile dressings to prevent autoinoculation, and the dressings should be wrapped and promptly disposed of after removal.

Further measures aimed at elimination of nasal carriage and subsequent shedding of *S. aureus* (methicillin-susceptible or methicillin-resistant strains) onto the skin may be warranted in the management of refractory cases. Intranasal application of a 2% mupirocin calcium ointment in a white, soft paraffin base for 5 days can eliminate *S. aureus* carriage in healthy persons for up to 90 days[40] (bacitracin and neomycin ointments were previously used for the same purpose). Similarly, prophylaxis with antibiotic ointment (fusidic acid) in the nares twice daily every fourth week (along with a peroral antistaphylococcal antimicrobial agent for 10 to 14 days) has been used with some success in patients and family members who are nasal carriers.[39] Oral antibiotics such as rifampin (600 mg daily for 10 days) have been effective in eradicating coagulase-positive staphylococci from most nasal carriers for periods up to 3 months.[41] Such use of rifampin to eliminate nasal carriage of *S. aureus* and interrupt a continuing cycle of recurrent furunculosis might be considered in patients for whom other measures have failed. However, such therapy can lead to rapid selection of rifampin-resistant strains. The addition of a second drug (dicloxacillin if the *S. aureus* is methicillin susceptible; trimethoprim-sulfamethoxazole, ciprofloxacin, or minocycline if the strain is methicillin resistant) has been used to reduce the emergence of rifampin resistance.[42] In one very limited study, prophylaxis with oral clindamycin alone (150 mg daily for 3 months), without an accompanying intranasal antimicrobial agent, reduced the frequency of recurrent staphylococcal skin infection.[43] Various staphylococcal vaccines have not proved effective in preventing recurrent furunculosis.

Ecthyma

Clinical Findings. The lesions of ecthyma begin in a fashion similar to those of impetigo but penetrate through the epidermis. Group A streptococci either produce the lesions de novo or secondarily infect preexisting superficial lesions (e.g., insect bites, excoriations), with both mechanisms resulting in the same clinical picture.[44] Ecthyma lesions most frequently occur on the lower extremities, particularly in children and the elderly. They consist of "punched-out" ulcers covered by greenish yellow crusts that extend deeply into the dermis and are surrounded by raised violaceous margins. Treatment is the same as for impetigo. Very extensive involvement with complicating bacteremia was reported in a patient with AIDS.[45]

Chancriform Lesions: Anthrax

A variety of infections, often with systemic consequences, are characterized by an initial chancriform lesion (see Table 86-1). Of the nonvenereal infections, anthrax has one of the most prominent chancriform lesions. (See Chapter 205 for a detailed discussion of anthrax.)

Pathogenesis. In the 20 years before 2001, naturally acquired anthrax infections, occurring in persons working with raw imported wool and other animal products contaminated with highly resistant spores of *Bacillus anthracis,* were rare (less than 1 case per year) in the United States. Routine safety measures for employees in wool plants and similar situations have virtually eliminated anthrax from this group; sporadic cases still occur in transient workers in factories (e.g., ventilation repairmen) and in persons directly importing wool for their own weaving. Most infections occur on the face, neck, or arms in an area with a minor abrasion. Rarely, pulmonary infection occurs after inhalation of *B. anthracis,* or intestinal anthrax results from ingestion of the organism.

A bioterrorism-associated anthrax outbreak occurred suddenly in the United States in the autumn of 2001, when *B. anthracis* spores were sent through the mail in letters to addresses in Washington, D.C., New York City, and Florida.[46] Twenty-two cases of anthrax ensued, 11 of the cutaneous form and 11 of the inhalation form (see Chapter 324).

Clinical Findings. After an incubation period of 1 to 8 days, a painless, sometimes pruritic, papule develops on an exposed area. The lesion enlarges, vesiculates ("malignant pustule"), and becomes surrounded by a wide zone of brawny, erythematous, gelatinous, nonpitting edema.[47–49] The edema may become massive, in young infants and in individuals with lesions on the face or neck, and may suggest the diagnosis of

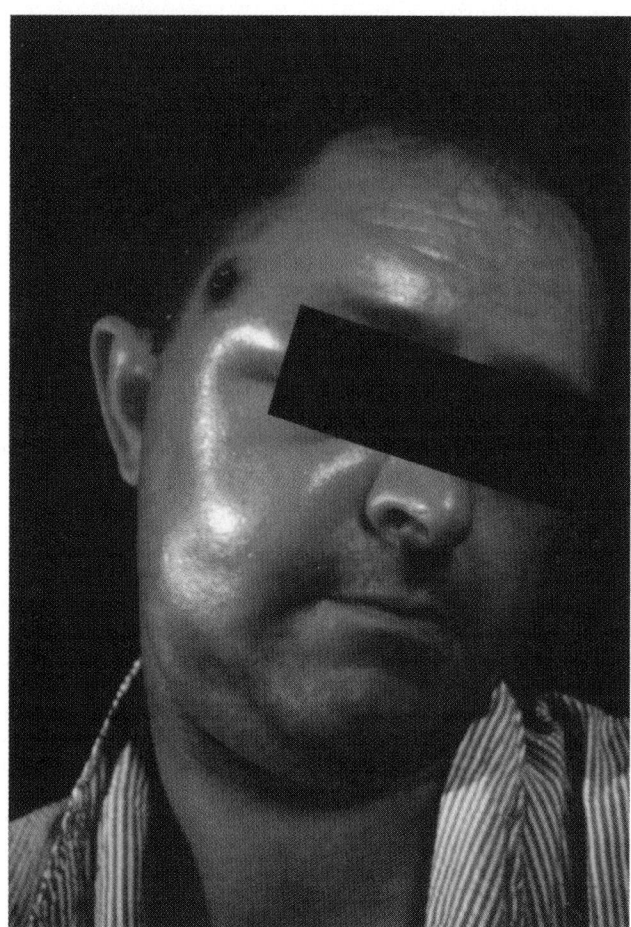

FIGURE 86-2. Chancriform lesion of anthrax on the forehead. There is a prominent surrounding zone of gelatinous edema that is most evident on the eyelids. *(Courtesy of Dr. Louis Weinstein, Boston, Mass.)*

cellulitis. Malaise and low-grade fever are present. As the lesion evolves, the initial vesicle enlarges and becomes hemorrhagic, necrotic, and covered by an eschar of variable dimensions (Fig. 86-2). Frequently, regional lymphadenopathy is present. Uncommonly, lymphangitis occurs from the initial process or from secondary infection. At all stages, the lesion remains painless. If untreated, bacteremic dissemination of infection from a skin site may occur, accompanied by high fever and hypotension. Meningitis may complicate such a bacteremic infection or primary pulmonary anthrax.

The epidemiologic background and the striking appearance of extensive gelatinous edema serve to distinguish anthrax from other types of chancriform lesions. A staphylococcal pustule or carbuncle with a necrotic eschar may be mistaken for early anthrax. However, the former is very painful and tender, and the etiologic agent can usually be demonstrated on a Gram-stained smear of material from the lesion. Other lesions mimicking the eschar of anthrax include ecthyma (usually lacking edema), ecthyma gangrenosum (usually in neutropenic patients with *P. aeruginosa* bacteremia), brown recluse spider bite (in rural areas, painful during incipient necrosis), orf (exposure to sheep, scab but without large eschar or gelatinous edema), and other infection-associated eschars at sites of tick or mite bites (tularemia, rickettsial spotted fevers, scrub typhus).

Presumptive Treatment. Incision and débridement should be avoided because they may increase the likelihood of bacteremia, but skin punch biopsy after initiation of antimicrobial therapy may be necessary to establish the diagnosis by culture, immunohistochemical staining, or polymerase chain reaction testing for *B. anthracis*. Almost

TABLE 86-2 Initial Oral Antimicrobial Therapy for Cutaneous Anthrax Where Risk of Bioterrrorism Exists

Drug	Dosage	Duration
Adults		
Ciprofloxacin	500 mg q12h	60 days[*†]
OR		
Doxycycline	100 mg q12h	
Children		
Ciprofloxacin	10-15 mg/kg q12h (not to exceed 1 g/day)	60 days[*†]
OR		
Doxycycline[‡]		
>8 yr and >45 kg	100 mg q12h	
>8 yr and ≤45 kg	2.2 mg/kg q12h	
≤8 yr	2.2 mg/kg q12h	

[*]Previously, treatment recommended for cutaneous anthrax was for 7-10 days; this was increased to 60 days in the setting of bioterrorism risks because of the likelihood of concomitant aerosol exposure.

[†]Amoxicillin, 500 mg orally q8h for an adult (or 80 mg/kg/day, divided q8h for a child), is an option for completion of treatment after clinical improvement.

[‡]Use of tetracyclines is warranted in children because of the seriousness of the infection.

Modified from Centers for Disease Control and Prevention. Update: Investigation of bioterrorism-related anthrax and interim guidelines for exposure management and antimicrobial therapy, October 2001. MMWR Morb Mortal Wkly Rep. 2001;50:909. (See also Chapter 324.)

all naturally occurring strains are susceptible to penicillin, and it has been the drug of choice for decades. With the concern that strains used in bioterrorist attacks might have been deliberately modified to be resistant to penicillins (and other commonly used antimicrobial agents), initial treatment of cutaneous anthrax with oral ciprofloxacin or doxycycline has been recommended (Table 86-2)[50] (see Chapter 324). Susceptibility studies of *B. anthracis* strains (both naturally occurring strains and those from the recent bioterrorism attack) indicate them to be susceptible to ciprofloxacin, various tetracyclines, clindamycin, imipenem, rifampin, chloramphenicol, aminoglycosides, cefazolin, vancomycin, macrolides, and linezolid.

Erysipelas

Erysipelas is a distinctive type of superficial cellulitis of the skin with prominent lymphatic involvement. It is almost always caused by group A streptococci (uncommonly, by group C or G streptococci). Group B streptococci have produced erysipelas in newborns. Evidence of streptococcal infection (groups A, G, and C) was found in 26 of 27 patients with clinical erysipelas by the combination of direct immunofluorescence and cultures of punch biopsy specimens along with serologic titers.[51] Very rarely, a similar skin lesion is caused by *S. aureus*.

Clinical Findings. Erysipelas is more common in infants, young children, and older adults. Formerly, the face was most commonly involved, and an antecedent streptococcal respiratory tract infection preceded cutaneous involvement in about one third of patients, even though streptococci might not be found on culture at the time that the skin lesion became evident. Now, the distribution of erysipelas has changed: 70% to 80% of the lesions are on the lower extremities, and 5% to 20% are on the face.[52] Portals of entry may be skin ulcers, local trauma or abrasions, psoriatic or eczematous lesions, or fungal infections, but often the skin of the involved area is intact. In the neonate, erysipelas may develop from an infection of the umbilical stump. Predisposing factors include venous stasis, paraparesis, diabetes mellitus, and alcohol abuse. Patients with the nephrotic syndrome are particularly susceptible. Erysipelas tends to occur in areas of preexisting lymphatic obstruction or edema (e.g., after a radical mastectomy). Also, because erysipelas itself produces lymphatic obstruction, it tends to recur in an area of earlier infection. Over a 3-year period, the recurrence rate is about 30%,[52] predominantly in individuals with venous insufficiency or lymphedema. Asymptomatic anal colonization

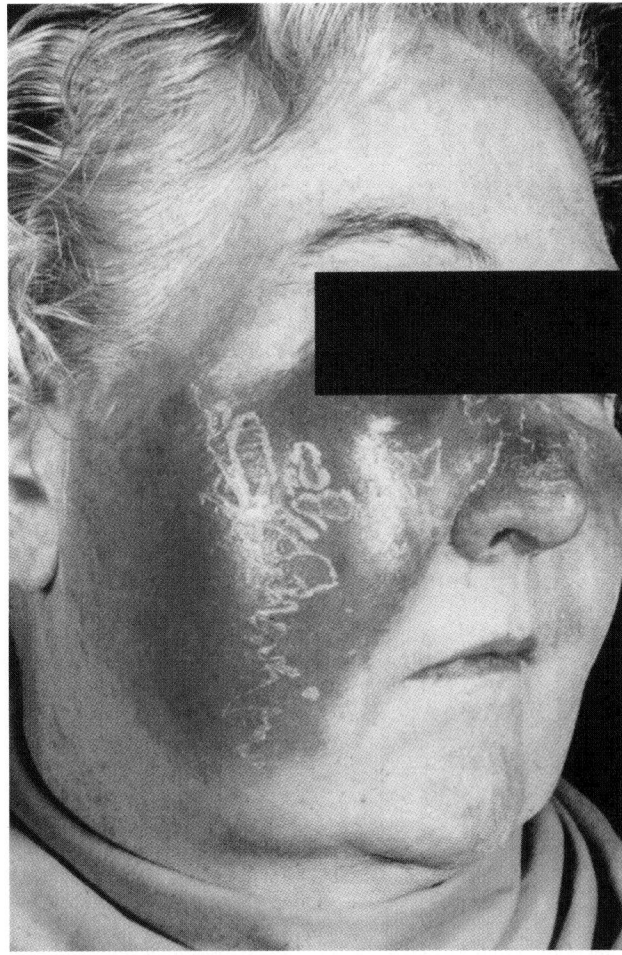

FIGURE 86-3. Facial erysipelas involving both cheeks and the bridge of the nose. The sharp demarcation between the bright red area of erythema and the normal surrounding skin is evident. *(From Fitzpatrick TB, Eisen AZ, Wolff K, et al, eds. Dermatology in General Medicine. New York: McGraw-Hill; 1971.)*

with group A or G streptococci may serve as a reservoir in such individuals with relapsing erysipelas (or cellulitis).[53]

Streptococcal bacteremia occurs in about 5% of patients with erysipelas; group A, C, or G streptococci can be isolated on throat culture in about 20% of the cases.[52]

Erysipelas is a painful lesion with a bright red, edematous, indurated ("peau d'orange") appearance and an advancing, raised border that is sharply demarcated from the adjacent normal skin (Fig. 86-3). Fever is a feature. A common form of erysipelas involves the bridge of the nose and the cheeks. Uncomplicated erysipelas remains confined primarily to the lymphatics and the dermis. Bullous erysipelas is a complication of severe disease observed in about 5% of cases of erysipelas. The bullae are flaccid and intraepidermal, and cultures of blister fluid are sterile before erosion occurs.[55] Occasionally, the infection extends more deeply and produces cellulitis, subcutaneous abscess, and necrotizing fasciitis.

Leukocytosis is common with erysipelas. Group A streptococci usually cannot be cultured from the surface of the skin lesion, and only rarely can they be isolated from tissue fluid aspirated from the advancing edge of the lesion. In cases of erysipelas complicating infected ulcers, group A streptococci have been isolated from the ulcerated area in 30% of patients.

Differential Diagnosis. The diagnosis is made on the basis of the appearance of the lesion and the clinical setting. Early herpes zoster involving the second division of the fifth cranial nerve may resemble unilateral facial erysipelas but can be distinguished by the pain and hyperesthesia preceding the skin lesions. Occasionally, contact dermatitis or giant urticaria may look like erysipelas but can be distinguished by the absence of fever and the presence of pruritus. Lesions closely resembling erysipelas, but apparently not caused by streptococcal infection, may occur repeatedly in patients with familial Mediterranean fever. Diffuse inflammatory carcinoma of the breast may mimic low-grade erysipelas. Erythema chronicum migrans, the cutaneous lesion of Lyme disease, resembles erysipelas but is not painful and progresses much more slowly, and the associated fever is less marked. An erysipelas-like skin lesion was reported in several patients with hypogammaglobulinemia and *Campylobacter jejuni* bacteremia.[56]

Presumptive Therapy. Mild early cases of erysipelas in an adult may be treated with intramuscular procaine penicillin (600,000 units once or twice daily) or oral penicillin V (250 to 500 mg every 6 hours). Erythromycin (250 to 500 mg orally every 6 hours) is a suitable alternative. For more extensive erysipelas, patients should be hospitalized and should receive parenteral aqueous penicillin G (2,000,000 units every 6 hours). Treatment with oral pristinamycin (a streptogramin antibiotic used in Europe but not approved in the United States) was shown to be comparable to intravenous, followed by oral, penicillin therapy in hospitalized patients with nonsevere erysipelas.[57] Although typical erysipelas can be readily distinguished from cellulitis (which can be of staphylococcal or streptococcal origin), the differentiation occasionally may not be clearcut. Under such conditions, particularly in an acutely ill patient, intravenous administration of a penicillinase-resistant penicillin (nafcillin or oxacillin) or a first-generation cephalosporin is warranted.

Cellulitis

Cellulitis is an acute, spreading infection of the skin that extends deeper than erysipelas and involves the subcutaneous tissues. Group A streptococcus or *S. aureus* is the most common etiologic agent.

Clinical Findings. Previous trauma (laceration, puncture wound) or an underlying skin lesion (furuncle, ulcer) predisposes to the development of cellulitis. Occasionally, cellulitis results from blood-borne spread of infection to the skin and subcutaneous tissues; rarely, it is caused by direct spread from subjacent infections (subcutaneous abscesses, fistulas from osteomyelitis). Within several days after the inciting trauma, local tenderness, pain, and erythema develop and rapidly intensify. Malaise, fever, and chills develop. The involved area is often extensive and the lesion is very red, hot, and swollen. In contrast to erysipelas, the borders of an area of cellulitis are not elevated and sharply demarcated; patchy involvement with skip areas may occur. Regional lymphadenopathy is common, and bacteremia can occur. Local abscesses may develop, and small patches of overlying skin may subsequently undergo necrosis. Superinfection with gram-negative bacilli may supervene.

Cellulitis caused by group A streptococci may occur as a postoperative wound infection. Although it is uncommon today, it is particularly noteworthy because of the rapidity with which it can spread and invade the blood stream. Such infection may be manifested within 6 to 48 hours after surgery (comparable to the short incubation period of postoperative clostridial myonecrosis), earlier than the usual postoperative staphylococcal infection, which is not evident for at least several days after surgery. Hypotension, often caused by bacteremia, may be the initial sign of infection, before significant erythema is evident about the incision. A thin, serous discharge may be expressed on compression of the wound margins, and streptococci can be identified on a Gram-stained smear.

Cellulitis is a serious disease because of the propensity of infection to spread via the lymphatics and blood stream. Cellulitis of the lower extremities in older patients may be complicated by thrombophlebitis. In patients with chronic dependent edema, cellulitis may spread extremely rapidly.

A form of cellulitis that is distinctive by virtue of the clinical setting occurs in the lower extremities of patients whose saphenous veins have been removed for coronary artery bypass surgery.[58] Occasionally, an associated lymphangitis is present. In some patients, episodes of cellulitis are recurrent. Systemic manifestations such as chills, high fever, and toxicity are prominent. The area of cellulitis extends along the course of the saphenous venectomy. Edema, erythema, and tenderness are marked. Occasionally, the involved areas are somewhat similar to those observed in erysipelas ("pseudoerysipelas"). Although a bacterial cause has not been defined in most cases, isolates available from involved skin or blood implicate non–group A β-hemolytic streptococci (groups C, G, and B) as major causes.[59] The portal of entry of the infection is often an associated area of tinea pedis. The combination of compromised lymphatic drainage and minor venous insufficiency secondary to saphenous venectomy may result in lower leg edema, a favorable setting for cellulitis. The inflammation from an initial episode of cellulitis, erysipelas, or lymphangitis obstructs lymphatic drainage, enhancing the predisposition to further episodes of infection. Other specific anatomic variants of or predispositions to cellulitis have been described (Table 86-3).[60]

Recurrent episodes of cellulitis or pseudoerysipelas caused by group B and G streptococci have occurred in patients with lower-extremity lymphedema secondary to radical pelvic surgery, radiation therapy, or neoplastic involvement of pelvic lymph nodes.[60] Typically, the cellulitis involves the vulva, inguinal areas, and both lower extremities. In this setting, recurrent episodes have occurred in association with recent coitus.[64]

Before routine immunization of infants with the conjugated protein-polysaccharide *Haemophilus influenzae* type B vaccine, buccal cellulitis, originating in the upper respiratory tract and caused by *H. influenzae* type B, accounted for up to 25% of cases of facial cellulitis in infants in the 3- to 24-month age group.[61] Complicating bacteremia

---

TABLE 86-3 Anatomic Variants of or Predispositions to Cellulitis

Anatomic Variant/Predisposition	Location	Likely Bacterial Cause
Periorbital cellulitis	Periorbital	*Staphylococcus aureus, Streptococcus pneumoniae,* group A streptococci
Buccal cellulitis	Cheek	*Haemophilus influenzae*
Cellulitis complicating body piercing	Ear, nose, umbilicus	*S. aureus,* group A streptococci
After mastectomy (with axillary node dissection)[63]	Ipsilateral upper extremity	Non–group A β-hemolytic streptococci
After lumpectomy (with limited axillary node dissection, breast radiotherapy[64])	Ipsilateral breast	Non–group A β-hemolytic streptococci
After saphenous vein harvest for coronary artery bypass	Ipsilateral leg	Group A or non–group A β-hemolytic streptococci
After radical pelvic surgery, radiation therapy	Vulva, inguinal areas, legs	Group B and group G streptococci
After liposuction	Thigh, abdominal wall	Group A streptococci, peptostreptococci
Postoperative (very early) wound infection	Abdomen, chest, hip	Group A streptococci
Injection drug use ("skin popping")	Extremities, neck	*S. aureus,* streptococci (groups A, C, F, G)*
Perianal cellulitis	Perineum	Group A streptococcus

*Other bacteria to consider based on isolation from skin or abscesses in this setting include *Enterococcus faecalis,* viridans group streptococci, coagulase-negative staphylococci, anaerobes (including *Bacteroides* and *Clostridium* spp.), and Enterobacteriaceae.

Modified with permission from Swartz, MN. Clinical Practice. Cellulitis. N Engl J Med. 2004;350:904-912. Copyright © 2004 Massachusetts Medical Society. All rights reserved.

was frequently present. The cellulitis can have a bluish ("blue dome") appearance, but usually it appears similar to streptococcal cellulitis.

An uncommon but distinctive form of cellulitis, perianal streptococcal (group A) cellulitis, occurs principally in children.[65] The clinical features consist of perianal pruritus, purulent secretions, intense perianal erythema, pain on defecation, blood-streaked stools from anal fissures, and chronicity (months) if not treated with penicillin. Relapse is common despite appropriate systemic oral therapy.

A rare but particularly troublesome, chronic, and progressive form of cellulitis, known as dissecting cellulitis of the scalp or perifolliculitis capitis, is probably similar to hydradenitis suppurativa and acne conglobata in pathogenesis. The clinical features consist of recurrent painful, fluctuant dermal and subcutaneous nodules, purulent drainage from burrowing interconnecting abscesses, scarring, and alopecia. *S. aureus* is most commonly isolated. Effective treatment has involved wide excision and skin grafting.

Lymphatic cutaneous metastases from neoplasms, particularly adenocarcinoma, may produce a localized, edematous, erythematous lesion resembling cellulitis. Inflammatory carcinoma of the breast, or carcinoma erysipeloides, involves the skin overlying the site of the primary tumor. Very rarely, lymphomatous involvement of subpectoral or retromammary nodes may produce an erythematous lymphedema of the breast, suggesting subacute cellulitis or inflammatory carcinoma of the breast.

A polymorphonuclear leukocytosis is usually present regardless of the bacterial etiology. Although culture of needle aspirates from areas of cellulitis is not indicated ordinarily, data from studies employing this methodology have provided the best information on the most likely pathogens.[66-71] A pathogen was identified in 30% of 284 patients. Gram-positive bacteria (mainly *S. aureus*, group A streptococci, group B streptococci, viridans streptococci, and *Enterococcus faecalis*) represented 79%; the remainder were gram-negative bacilli (Enterobacteriaceae, *H. influenzae, Pasteurella multocida, P. aeruginosa,* and *Acinetobacter* spp). Cultures of ulcers and abrasions contiguous with areas of cellulitis have shown similar likely gram-positive pathogens (*S. aureus* or group A streptococci or both). In view of the overall limited yield of pathogens with aspiration of areas of cellulitis, it is reasonable to use this procedure only if unusual pathogens are suspected (e.g., in immunocompromised patients), fluctuant areas are detected, or initial antimicrobial therapy has been unsuccessful.

A broader spectrum of pathogens has been isolated from deep wounds or débrided tissue in diabetic patients with limb-threatening infections (including cellulitis).[72] These comprised gram-positive aerobes in 56% of patients (*S. aureus, Enterococcus* spp., and various streptococcal species); gram-negative aerobes in 22% (Enterobacteriaceae, *Acinetobacter, P. aeruginosa*); and anaerobes in 22% (*Bacteroides, Peptococcus*). In cellulitis complicating decubitus ulcers, this broad range of microorganisms also should be considered as potential pathogens. If this complication develops in a hospitalized patient, resistant nosocomial pathogens should be considered when deciding on empirical antibiotic coverage.

Blood cultures are positive in only 2% to 4% of patients with community-acquired cellulitis.[66,67,69-71,73] About two thirds of isolates are group A or G streptococci or *S. aureus*, and the remainder are *H. influenzae, P. multocida,* or *Vibrio vulnificus*. Blood cultures appear to be positive more frequently with cellulitis superimposed on lymphedema.[74]

Erysipelothrix rhusiopathiae is the etiologic agent of erysipeloid, a somewhat indolent cellulitis occurring principally in persons who handle saltwater fish, shellfish, poultry, meat, and hides (see Chapter 207). The infection, which usually occurs in the summer, is introduced through an abrasion on the hands. A painful violaceous area appears within 1 week after the injury. As the process spreads peripherally with distinct raised borders, the central portion of the lesion clears. Ulceration is not a feature. Occasionally, an adjacent joint is involved; rarely, bacteremia and endocarditis may follow. The causative organism is not usually observed in Gram-stained drainage from the lesion but may be isolated on culture of a biopsy specimen

taken from the advancing margin of the lesion. The development of a typical lesion in a person handling fish or meat products suggests the diagnosis. Other forms of bacterial cellulitis or erysipelas may resemble erysipeloid, particularly if the lesion is on the hand. A somewhat similar lesion of unknown origin, called "seal finger," occurs in aquarium workers and veterinarians secondary to seal bites or trauma sustained in caring for these animals. Whereas penicillin is the antibiotic of choice in the treatment of erysipeloid, it appears that seal finger responds to tetracycline.[75]

Rare cases of pneumococcal cellulitis acquired through the bacteremic route have been reported.[76] Soft tissue infections by the pneumococcus can bear a striking resemblance to streptococcal erysipelas. A variety of bacteria (*Serratia, Proteus,* other Enterobacteriaceae, and *Helicobacter cinaedi*) and fungi (*Cryptococcus neoformans, Fusarium* spp.) that are not the cause of cellulitis in healthy individuals may produce blood-borne cellulitis in an immunocompromised or granulocytopenic patient.[77,78] *Legionella* spp. have very rarely produced cellulitis—*Legionella pneumophila* in association with pneumonia[79] and *Legionella micdadei* in a renal transplant recipient.[80] Spontaneous *Escherichia coli* cellulitis occurs in children with the nephrotic syndrome in relapse.[81]

An environmental gram-negative bacillus found particularly in lakes, rivers, and soil, *Aeromonas hydrophila* may produce an acute cellulitis after introduction of the organism through a laceration acquired during swimming in fresh water.[82]

Cellulitis, bullous lesions, or necrotic ulcers may complicate infection of a traumatic wound sustained in salt water (or brackish inland waters) or from exposure to drippings from raw seafood. Such infections, caused by *Vibrio* spp. (primarily *V. vulnificus* but also occasionally *Vibrio alginolyticus,* non–serogroup 01 *Vibrio cholerae,* and *Vibrio parahaemolyticus*), can result in bacteremia and progress to necrosis, which requires extensive surgical débridement.[83,84] A rapidly progressive primary septicemia caused by *V. vulnificus* may occur after entry of the organism through the gastrointestinal tract (e.g., consumption of raw oysters) rather than through abraded skin. Cellulitis with hemorrhagic skin bullae often occurs rapidly after the bacteremia. Particularly at risk for the septicemic form of disease are patients with alcoholic cirrhosis, hemochromatosis, or thalassemia—presumably as a result of enhanced growth of *V. vulnificus* mediated by these processes with enhanced iron storage.[85] These vibrios are generally susceptible in vitro to tetracyclines, chloramphenicol, the aminoglycosides, and third-generation cephalosporins. Tetracyclines have been considered the treatment of *V. vulnificus* infections, with cefotaxime and ciprofloxacin as alternatives.

A variety of processes that resemble cellulitis in appearance should be distinguished from it. These include infections as well as inflammatory and neoplastic entities (Box 86-1).

Envenomation after puncture wounds by the spines of a stonefish (indigenous to shallow waters of the South Pacific) produces local edema and erythema that may suggest acute bacterial cellulitis acquired in seawater.[86] This reaction may be accompanied by serious systemic toxicity, including acute pulmonary edema.

Familial Mediterranean fever is seen in Sephardic Jews and in individuals from the Middle East. Patients have a history of previous bouts of fever, sometimes accompanied by cellulitis-like, noninfectious episodes of localized erythema, and by often crises of abdominal pain.[87]

Sweet's syndrome consists of the acute development of tender erythematous pseudovesiculated plaques, fever, and neutrophilic leucocytosis, often associated with malignancy. If lesions occur on the face, they may suggest erysipelas or periorbital cellulitis.[88]

Kawasaki disease occurs in infancy or childhood and is characterized by fever, conjunctivitis, acute cervical lymphadenopathy, and a macular eruption. The facial appearance with conjunctivitis may suggest periorbital cellulitis.[89] Polymorphic rashes on the trunk and especially the perineum of children with Kawasaki disease can be seen. Although cellulitis may be considered, the constellation of findings typically supports the diagnosis of Kawasaki disease.

Processes to Be Distinguished from Cellulitis

Infections
Necrotizing fasciitis types I and II
Anaerobic myonecrosis (gas gangrene)
Cutaneous anthrax with prominent surrounding gelatinous edema
Prominent response to vaccination with vaccinia
Erythema chronicum migrans lesion of Lyme disease

Inflammatory and Neoplastic Processes
Insect bite (hypersensitivity response)
Fixed drug reaction
Envenomation from spines of stonefish
Acute gout
Deep venous thrombophlebitis of lower extremity
Familial Mediterranean fever–associated cellulitis-like erythema
Pyoderma gangrenosa (particularly lesions starting in subcutaneous fat as acute panniculitis)
Sweet's syndrome (acute febrile neutrophilic dermatosis)
Kawasaki disease
Wells' syndrome (eosinophilic cellulitis/fasciitis)
Carcinoma erysipeloides

Modified from Swartz MN. Cellulitis. N Engl J Med. 2004;350:904.

The appearance and clinical features of Wells' syndrome (eosinophilic cellulitis) consist of urticaria-like, moderately erythematous and edematous lesions that develop rapidly and are often accompanied by fever. It can be distinguished from the usual bacterial cellulitis by its minimal tenderness, lack of local heat, and failure to respond to antibiotics. Biopsy of the early lesion shows marked infiltration of the dermis with eosinophils. The lesions resolve in several weeks but frequently recur.[90]

Carcinoma erysipeloides is a form of metastatic carcinoma with prominent lymphatic involvement. It can occur close to the site of the primary tumor (e.g., on the anterior chest wall with cancer of the breast) or at sites of distant metastases. Progression is slower than that of cellulitis, and fever is not a feature.[91,92]

Presumptive Therapy. β-Lactam antibiotics active against penicillinase-producing *S. aureus* are the usual drugs of choice for initial treatment of cellulitis in view of the fact that the great majority of cases are caused by streptococci or *S. aureus*. Administration should be by the intravenous route in hospital if the lesion is rapidly spreading, if the systemic response is prominent, or if there are significant comorbidities (asplenia, neutropenia, immunocompromise, cirrhosis, cardiac or renal failure, or preexisting edema). Cefazolin (1.0 g intravenously every 6 to 8 hours) or nafcillin (1.0 to 1.5 g intravenously every 4 hours) is a reasonable choice for an adult. If MRSA is the suspected cause (nosocomial infection or infection with community-acquired MRSA in areas of prevalence of such strains[93]) and in penicillin-allergic individuals, vancomycin (1.0 g intravenously every 12 hours) or linezolid[94] (0.6 g intravenously every 12 hours) is indicated. Once-daily intravenous daptomycin is an option for treatment of methicillin-resistant staphylococcal soft tissue infections. A switch to oral therapy (dicloxacillin, 0.5 g every 6 hours) may be made after fever abates and skin lesions begin to resolve. Alternative oral therapy might consist of cephradine or cephalexin in the same dosage, or cefadroxil at a dosage of 0.5 to 1.0 g orally every 12 to 24 hours. Follow-up oral therapy in the case of MRSA requires linezolid 0.6 g every 12 hours. If the cellulitis is very early and mild and no significant comorbidities are present, initial therapy with the above-noted oral follow-up antimicrobial agents may be employed initially.

Cellulitis in the setting of a diabetic foot infection may involve a much wider spectrum of potential pathogens and warrants broader antimicrobial coverage, such as ampicillin/sulbactam (3.0 g intravenously every 6 hours in adults), imipenem/cilastatin or meropenem, or other antimicrobial combinations targeting anaerobes as well as gram-positive and gram-negative aerobes.[72]

Specially tailored initial antimicrobial therapy is warranted if additional bacterial species are likely to be involved in cellulitis after unusual exposures. These include human or animal bites, for which initial therapy might involve ampicillin/sulbactam intravenously or amoxicillin/clavulanate (500 mg orally every 8 hours in an adult). In the setting of cellulitis after an abrasion or laceration occurring with salt water exposure, where *V. vulnificus* might be the pathogen, treatment with doxycycline (200 mg intravenously per day in two divided doses) along with an antimicrobial targeted to the common pathogens is appropriate. Similarly, in the setting of cellulitis after an abrasion or laceration occurring with fresh water exposure, where *A. hydrophila* might be involved, treatment with ciprofloxacin (400 mg intravenously every 12 hours) along with an antimicrobial targeted to the common pathogens is indicated; alternatively, a combination of ceftazidime plus gentamicin may be used.

Initial local care of cellulitis includes immobilization and elevation of the involved limb to reduce swelling and application of a cool, sterile saline dressing to remove purulent exudate from any associated ulcer or infected abrasion and decrease local pain.

Patients who have cellulitis at the saphenous site after coronary bypass surgery and fungal infection in the interdigital spaces should be treated topically for the latter with miconazole, clotrimazole, or terbinafine. The initial antibiotic (e.g., cefazolin) should be given by the intravenous route for 3 to 5 days until fever abates and skin findings begin to resolve, to ensure prompt resolution before switching to other routes of therapy. Attention to the problem of tinea pedis before bypass surgery can prevent this form of cellulitis. Similar prompt attention to pedal epidermophytosis in patients who have had one such episode of cellulitis can obviate subsequent episodes.

Recurrent episodes of cellulitis usually occur in patients with peripheral edema. The use of support stockings and good skin hygiene can reduce its frequency or eliminate recurrences. In the occasional patient who continues to have frequent episodes of cellulitis or erysipelas despite such measures, prophylactic penicillin V (250 to 500 mg orally twice daily), or erythromycin (250 mg orally once or twice daily) for the penicillin-allergic patient, may be indicated.[95]

Membranous Ulcers

Infected ulcers of varied or mixed bacterial origin may be covered at their base by a layer of necrotic debris resembling a membrane. The latter is not usually strongly adherent and can be removed without much difficulty. In addition, such a lesion has abundant purulent drainage, attributable to infection with pyogenic bacteria. Membrane-covered lesions (both superficial and deep ulcers) are also produced by cutaneous infection with *Corynebacterium diphtheriae*.

Cutaneous Diphtheria

Cutaneous diphtheria (see Chapter 202) is uncommon in developed countries; most cases occur among unimmunized persons in overcrowded, underdeveloped parts of the world, particularly in tropical areas, and are associated with skin trauma and poor hygiene. Recent increases in cutaneous diphtheria in the United States have been noted in the Pacific Northwest and the South.

Clinical Findings. Three types of cutaneous lesions have been described in cutaneous diphtheria: (1) wound diphtheria—secondary *C. diphtheriae* infection of a preexisting wound, which becomes partially covered by a membrane and encircled by a zone of erythema; (2) primary cutaneous diphtheria—a disease of the tropics that begins as a single or as several pustules, usually on a lower extremity, and progresses to form a punched-out ulcer covered by a gray-brown membrane; and (3) superinfection of eczematized skin lesions—a superficial membranous infection. *C. diphtheriae* has also been isolated from lesions resembling impetigo, ecthyma, and infected insect bites, where they may represent true infections or merely a cutaneous carrier state.[96] Chronic, nonhealing skin ulcers in intravenous drug users that are caused by trauma and are infected with *S. aureus* or various types of streptococci have been found on occasion to be superinfected with nontoxigenic strains of *C. diphtheriae*.[97] Cutaneous diphtheria may be as contagious as the respiratory form of the disease among schoolchildren.

Occasionally, membranous pharyngitis accompanies cutaneous diphtheria. However, 20% to 40% of patients with cutaneous diphtheria carry *C. diphtheriae* in their upper respiratory tract.[96,98] Myocarditis is extremely rare as a complication of cutaneous diphtheria, but cranial nerve palsies and Guillain-Barré syndrome occur in 3% to 5% of patients with membranous diphtheritic skin ulcers.

Laboratory Findings. Characteristic beaded, metachromatically staining bacilli can be found in methylene blue–stained smears of the edge of the membrane. However, the diagnosis can be established only by isolation of *C. diphtheriae* from a suggestive skin lesion. Selective media (cysteine-tellurite blood agar or fresh Tinsdale's medium) are necessary for isolation to inhibit other bacteria in skin ulcers. In addition to isolation of the organism, toxigenicity should be demonstrated by an Elek plate (agar diffusion precipitin reaction) or by guinea pig inoculation (dermonecrosis).

Differential Diagnosis. Pyogenic infection of ulcerated traumatic lesions is usually purulent, and the lesions are not covered by a membrane. Cutaneous fungal infections have more proliferative and irregular margins. The early stages of primary cutaneous diphtheria and secondary infection of insect bites and abrasions with *C. diphtheriae* may closely resemble impetigo.

Presumptive Therapy. If a presumptive diagnosis of ulcerative cutaneous diphtheria is made on clinical grounds and on the basis of preliminary bacteriologic findings, antitoxin (20,000 to 40,000 units intramuscularly or intravenously) is administered after testing for sensitivity to horse serum. Antibiotic administration (erythromycin 2.0 g/day orally or procaine penicillin 1.2 to 2.4 million units/day intramuscularly for 7 to 10 days in an adult) also assists in elimination of the convalescent carrier state. Removal of necrotic debris aids in healing of the lesions.

Infectious Gangrene (Gangrenous Cellulitis)

Infectious gangrene is a cellulitis that has rapidly progressed, with extensive necrosis of subcutaneous tissues and the overlying skin. Several different clinically distinguishable pictures may be produced, depending to varying extents on the specific causative organism, the anatomic location of the infection, and the predisposing conditions. Such clinical entities include (1) necrotizing fasciitis (type I, or polymicrobial, often including Enterobacteriaceae and anaerobes; type II, or streptococcal gangrene caused by *S. pyogenes*); (2) gas gangrene (clostridial myonecrosis) and anaerobic cellulitis; (3) progressive bacterial synergistic gangrene; (4) synergistic necrotizing cellulitis, perineal phlegmon, and gangrenous balanitis; (5) gangrenous cellulitis in an immunosuppressed patient; and (6) very localized areas of skin necrosis complicating conventional cellulitis.

Pathologic Characteristics and Pathogenesis. The pathologic changes of gangrenous cellulitis are those of necrosis and some hemorrhage in the skin and subcutaneous tissues. In most types of gangrenous cellulitis an abundant polymorphonuclear leukocytic exudate is present, but in clostridial myonecrosis the exudate is thin and consists of fluid, fibrin, and gas but few leukocytes. In most types of gangrenous cellulitis (particularly streptococcal gangrene), fibrin thrombi are present in small arteries and veins of the dermis and subcutaneous fat.[99] In most instances, gangrenous cellulitis has developed secondary to introduction of the infecting organism at the infected site. It may also result from extension of infection from a deeper site to involve the subcutaneous tissues and skin, as in clostridial myonecrosis after intestinal surgery or in perineal phlegmon after dissection of infection from a perirectal abscess. Occasionally, gangrenous cellulitis begins at a site of metastatic infection in the course of a bacteremia (clostridial myonecrosis caused by *Clostridium septicum* at a peripheral site secondary to spread from an associated colonic neoplasm; *Pseudomonas* gangrenous cellulitis).

Clinical Findings

Streptococcal Gangrene. Streptococcal gangrene is a rare form of gangrene caused by group A (or C or G) streptococci that usually develops at a site of trauma on an extremity but may occur in the absence of an obvious portal of entry (see later discussion of necrotizing fasciitis, type II). The lesion begins as a local, exquisitely painful area of erythema and edema. The extent of this aggressive process initially is often underestimated, because it spreads widely in deep fascial planes with relative sparing of overlying skin.[100] The streptococcal toxic shock syndrome may evolve rapidly and be the most prominent feature.[101] Over the next 1 to 3 days, the skin becomes dusky. Bullae containing yellowish to red-black fluid develop and rupture.[102] The lesion evolves into a sharply demarcated area covered by necrotic eschar and surrounded by a border of erythema. The process at this point resembles a third-degree burn, for which it could be mistaken if a history were not available. Lymphangitis is rarely evident. Extensive necrotic sloughing can result because of deep penetration of the infection along fascial planes. Bacteremia, metastatic abscesses, and death may result from this life-threatening illness if appropriate combined antibiotic therapy and surgical exploration are not initiated promptly. Secondary thrombophlebitis may be a complication if the lower extremities are involved. Streptococci can usually be cultured from the early bullous lesions and frequently from blood.

Progressive Bacterial Synergistic Gangrene. This distinctive lesion usually occurs after infection at an abdominal operative wound site (frequently when wire sutures have been used), about an ileostomy or colostomy, at the exit of a fistulous tract, or in proximity to chronic ulceration on an extremity.[103,104] It begins as a local, tender area of swelling and erythema that subsequently ulcerates. The painful, shaggy ulcer gradually enlarges and is characteristically encircled by a margin of gangrenous skin (Fig. 86-4). Surrounding the latter is a violaceous

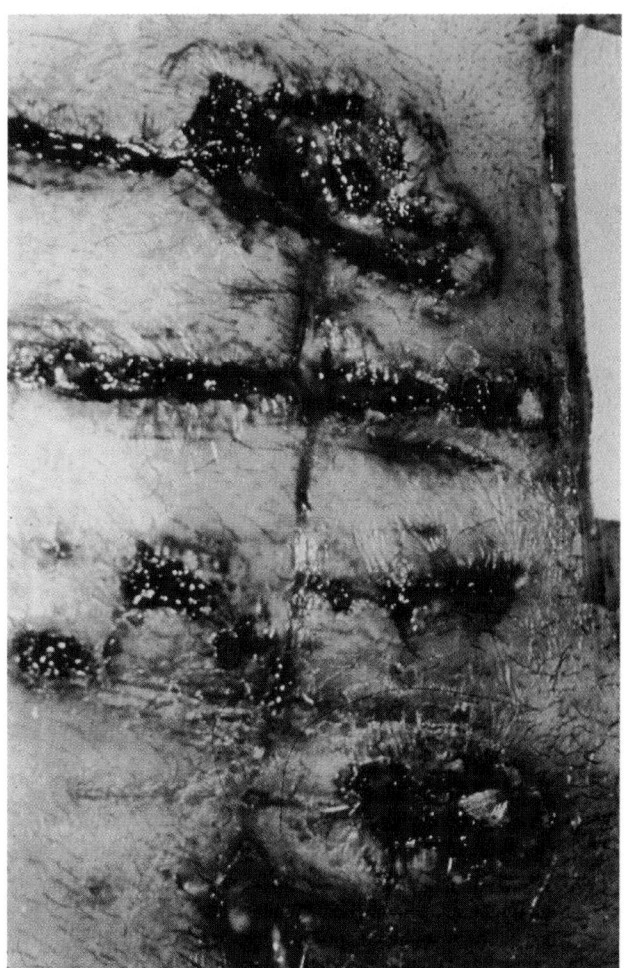

FIGURE 86-4. Progressive bacterial synergistic gangrene of the abdominal wall. Ulcerated areas had developed about wire stay sutures that have since been removed. *(From Bornstein DL, Weinberg AN, Swartz MN, et al. Anaerobic infections. Review of current experience. Medicine [Baltimore]. 1964;43:207.)*

zone that fades into an outer, pink, edematous border area. If untreated, the process extends slowly but relentlessly, ultimately producing an enormous ulceration.

Microaerophilic or anaerobic streptococci can be recovered from aspirates of the advancing margin of the lesion, and *S. aureus* (or occasionally *Proteus* or other gram-negative bacilli) are present in the ulcerated area. Meleney reproduced the same type of lesions by experimentally injecting both microaerophilic streptococci and *S. aureus* (but not either alone) into the skin of animals. The similarity of appearance between Meleney's progressive bacterial synergistic gangrene and amebic *(Entamoeba histolytica)* skin gangrene, as well as the usual occurrence of both processes at abdominal or thoracic operative wound sites, led to the suggestion that *E. histolytica* is the principal cause.[106] However, development of the latter infection after gynecologic surgery and its occurrence in countries where amebic infections are rare argue against this concept of pathogenesis. Nonetheless, the capacity of amebic infection to involve the skin of the abdominal wall in a gangrenous process after abdominal surgery should not be overlooked,[107] and appropriate measures (stool examination for amebas, serologic tests, periodic acid–Schiff stain of scrapings, or biopsy of the lesion) should be undertaken to exclude this diagnosis.

Gas Gangrene, Anaerobic Cellulitis, and Other Forms of Crepitant Cellulitis. See Chapters 87 and 244 and "Subcutaneous Tissue Infections and Abscesses" in this chapter.

Gangrenous Cellulitis in a Predisposed Host. The etiologic considerations for cellulitis occurring in a compromised host include agents that produce such infections in healthy persons as well as a variety of other organisms not ordinarily regarded as causes of cellulitis. Mucormycotic gangrenous cellulitis may be engrafted on an extensive burn wound, or it may rarely develop in patients with diabetes mellitus or in those who are receiving immunosuppressive therapy. Local factors (open fracture sites, ileostomy stomas, fistulous tracts) also play a predisposing role in this type of infection. Spores of *Rhizopus* spp. (members of the Mucoraceae) contaminating Elastoplast tape used for occlusive dressings have resulted in progressive local and disseminated infection in immunosuppressed patients.[108] The infection may exhibit an indolent course with minimal fever and a slowly enlarging black ulcer, or it may follow a rapidly progressive febrile course. The characteristic lesion consists of a central anesthetic, black, necrotic area with a surrounding raised zone of violaceous cellulitis and edema.[109] Superficial vesicles and blistering may occur in the gangrenous area. Hematogenous dissemination is not ordinarily demonstrable, and the skin infection usually does not result from an initial pulmonary or rhinocerebral focus. Cultures of the necrotic skin or aspirates from the advancing margin usually do not reveal the fungus. Identification of the cause is best obtained from biopsy specimens: fungal wet mount on a crushed tissue preparation, tissue sections stained with hematoxylin and eosin (showing tissue and vascular invasion by characteristic broad hyphae), and culture. Necrotizing angioinvasive cellulitis caused by the zygomycete *Apophysomyces elegans* has occurred in a small number of nonimmunocompromised patients after traumatic injury potentially contaminated with soil.[110]

Pseudomonas bacteremia may also produce a gangrenous cellulitis (see "Cutaneous Involvement in Systemic Bacterial and Mycotic Infections") in immunocompromised hosts, patients with thermal burns, and others. In similar settings, gangrenous skin lesions may occur with disseminated aspergillosis.

Prominent necrosis of skin and subcutaneous fat occurs rarely in patients who have chronic renal failure (with secondary hyperparathyroidism), in those receiving chronic dialysis therapy, in patients with extensive calcification of the small arteries of subcutaneous tissue, and in those in whom the calcium-phosphate product is markedly elevated.[111] The process that results in acute local calcification has been termed calciphylaxis.[112] Precipitating factors for the development of calciphylaxis are poorly defined but include local trauma and systemic infection. The skin lesions begin as dark red, irregular areas resembling livido reticularis. They become plaquelike or nodular, are painful, and rapidly increase in size but remain well demarcated. They

progress to gangrenous necrosis with eschar formation. Secondary infection of necrotic areas may follow. Histologically, involved areas show extensive vascular calcification, calcinosis cutis, and ischemic skin necrosis. Bacteremia originating elsewhere may contribute to the local ischemic process through further lesional thromboses mediated by disseminated intravascular coagulopathy. These necrotic skin ulcers in patients with chronic renal failure resemble those of infective gangrenous cellulitis, particularly if they become secondarily infected.

Differential Diagnosis. See Table 86-4. The bite of the brown recluse house spider can produce a necrotizing skin lesion that resembles infectious gangrenous cellulitis. The occurrence of fever and chills 24 to 48 hours after the bite enhances the mimicry.

Presumptive Therapy. Treatment of streptococcal gangrene consists of immediate surgical exploration with longitudinal incisions extending through the deep fascia and beyond the involved gangrenous and undermined areas.[102] Initial resuscitation measures with intravenous fluids are essential in the presence of hypotension caused by accompanying streptococcal bacteremia or the streptococcal toxic shock–like syndrome.[113] Areas of cutaneous necrosis are excised, and nonviable fascia is débrided. Reexploration is commonly performed within 24 hours. Antibiotic therapy consists of high-dose intravenous aqueous penicillin G (3 to 4 million units every 4 hours). In the treatment of streptococcal gangrene and streptococcal toxic shock, the addition of clindamycin to penicillin is reasonable, because it has been shown to reduce the early in vitro release of streptococcal pyrogenic exotoxin A.[114]

If there is any question regarding the etiologic agent (e.g., possibly *S. aureus* rather than group A streptococcus), nafcillin (1.5 to 2.0 g intravenously every 4 to 6 hours) should be used. Necrotizing fasciitis resulting from mixed anaerobes and facultative organisms (synergistic necrotizing cellulitis) can usually be suspected at the outset from the foul odor and the appearance of the exudate on a Gram-stained smear. After surgery, the wound is treated with elevation and moist dressings. Skin grafting is usually required later.

Progressive bacterial synergistic gangrene is very difficult to treat. Local irrigation with bacitracin and systemic therapy with parenteral penicillin (12 to 18 million units/day intravenously) and a second drug (based on antibiotic susceptibility testing of bacteria other than microaerophilic streptococci isolated from the lesion) are sometimes helpful. The initial use of a β-lactam/β-lactamase combination such as piperacillin/tazobactam or a carbapenem agent such as meropenem may be a reasonable empirical strategy until microbiologic data can be used to refine therapy. However, wide excision of all necrotic tissue (extending well into normal tissue), combined with antibiotic treatment, is usually required.

Erythrasma

Clinical Findings. Erythrasma is a common superficial bacterial infection of the skin characterized by slowly spreading, pruritic, reddish-brown macular patches, usually located in the genitocrural area.[115] The lesions are finely scaled and finely wrinkled, and they are more common in men and in obese individuals with diabetes mellitus. The disease may be asymptomatic or may undergo periodic exacerbations. The cause appears to be bacterial: *Corynebacterium minutissimum,* a species that can be grown aerobically. Gram-stained imprints of the skin surface show large numbers of small gram-positive bacilli. Examination of the lesions under Wood's lamp reveals a distinctive coral-red fluorescence.

The principal superficial skin infections to be considered in the differential diagnosis are tinea versicolor lesions on the trunk and tinea cruris (a deeper, more inflammatory, and more rapidly progressive process).

Treatment with oral erythromycin (1.0 g/day for 5 to 7 days) is usually efficacious and clears the lesions within several weeks. Topical treatment with an aqueous solution of 2% clindamycin hydrochloride can also be effective.[116]

C. minutissimum is also the causative agent of pitted keratolysis, a superficial process consisting of crateriform pits up to 7 mm in width occurring on the pressure-bearing areas of the sole and on the

TABLE 86-4 Differential Diagnosis of Infectious Gangrene and Gangrenous Cellulitis

Factor	Progressive Bacterial Synergistic Gangrene	Synergistic Necrotizing Cellulitis*	Streptococcal Gangrene†	Clostridial Myonecrosis (Gas Gangrene)	Necrotizing Cutaneous Mucormycosis	Bacteremic Pseudomonas Gangrenous Cellulitis	Pyoderma Gangrenosum
Predisposing conditions	Surgery, draining sinus	Diabetes common	Occasionally diabetes or myxedema, after abdominal surgery	Local trauma	Diabetes, corticosteroid therapy	Burns, immunosuppression	Ulcerative colitis, rheumatoid arthritis
Pain	Prominent	Prominent	Prominent	Prominent	Minimal	Mild	Moderate
Systemic toxicity	Minimal	Marked	Marked	Very marked	Variable	Marked	Minimal
Course	Slow	Rapid	Very rapid	Extremely rapid	Rapid	Rapid	Slow
Fever	Minimal or absent	Moderate	High	Moderate or high	Low grade	High	Low grade
Anesthesia of lesion	−	−	±	−	+	±	−
Crepitus	−	Often present	−	+	−	−	−
Appearance of the involved area	Central shaggy, necrotic ulcer surrounded by dusky margin and erythematous periphery	Crepitant cellulitis; thick, copious, foul-smelling "dishwater" drainage from scattered areas of skin necrosis	Necrosis of subcutaneous tissue and fascia with black, necrotic, "burned" appearance of overlying skin	Marked swelling, yellow-bronze discoloration of skin, brown bullae, green-black patches of necrosis, serosanguineous discharge	Usually a central black, necrotic area with a purple raised margin; may also appear as just a black ulcer	A sharply demarcated, necrotic area with black eschar and surrounding erythema resembling a decubitus ulcer; may evolve from initial hemorrhagic bulla	Begin as bullae, pustules, or erythematous nodules that ulcerate deeply; often multiple, large, and coalescing; usually on lower extremities or abdomen
Etiology	Microaerophilic streptococci plus *Staphylococcus aureus* (or *Proteus* sometimes)	Usually a mixture of organisms (e.g., *Bacteroides*, peptostreptococci, *Escherichia coli*)	Primarily group A streptococci; if secondary to abdominal surgery, enteric bacteria also involved	*Clostridium perfringens* (occasionally other clostridia)	*Rhizopus, Mucor, Absidia*	*Pseudomonas aeruginosa*	Not an infection primarily; may be confused with such resulting from secondary colonization by Enterobacteriaceae, microaerophilic streptococci, *P. aeruginosa, S. aureus*

−, absent; +, present; ±, occasionally present.
*Similar to necrotizing fasciitis type I.
†Necrotizing fasciitis type II.
Modified with permission from Swartz MN. Clinical practice. Cellulitis. N Engl J Med. 2004;350:904-912. Copyright © 2004 Massachusetts Medical Society. All rights reserved.

ventral aspect of the toes.[117] The lesions are malodorous and are associated with hyperhidrosis.

Secondary Bacterial Infections Complicating Preexisting Skin Lesions

A variety of skin lesions (e.g., burns, eczematous dermatitides, traumatic lesions) may become secondarily infected (see Table 86-1). Such infected lesions usually do not exhibit distinctive morphologic characteristics based on the infecting organism. Rather, the appearance of the lesions is determined to a large measure by the nature of the preexisting injury or dermatosis, such as dermatophytosis and acne conglobata, which are often treated primarily by dermatologists. Several of the other secondarily infected dermatoses have some distinctive clinical and bacteriologic features and merit brief consideration.

Diabetic Foot and Other Chronic Superficial Skin Ulcers

A variety of aerobic and facultative organisms (e.g., *Pseudomonas, Proteus,* enterococci) colonize and secondarily infect decubitus ulcers. Only in recent years has the prominent role of anaerobic bacteria in such infections been recognized. The character of the ulcers (extensive undermining and necrosis of tissue) and their location, frequently in proximity to the anus, provide the opportunity for invasion by anaerobes. *Bacteroides fragilis,* other Bacteroidaceae, and *Clostridium perfringens* have commonly been isolated from infected decubitus ulcers. Such lesions have been the source of symptomatic bacteremias caused by *B. fragilis, Peptostreptococcus* spp., *S. aureus, Enterococcus,* various streptococci, and a variety of facultative gram-negative bacilli.[118]

Chronic foot infections in patients with diabetes mellitus are common and difficult problems. They usually begin after minor trauma in patients with peripheral neuropathy, neuropathic ulcers, and arterial vascular insufficiency and take the form of cellulitis, soft tissue necrosis, or osteomyelitis with a draining sinus. For convenience, foot infections in diabetic patients are classified into two categories[119]: (1) non–limb-threatening infections, which are superficial, lack systemic toxicity, have minimal cellulitis extending less than 2 cm from the portal of entry, have ulceration (if present) not fully extending through the skin, and lack significant ischemia, and (2) limb-threatening infections, which exhibit more extensive cellulitis, lymphangitis, ulcers penetrating through the skin into subcutaneous tissue, and prominent ischemia. In the former group, *S. aureus* is the major pathogen, facultative streptococci are isolated in about one third of patients, and facultative gram-negative bacilli and anaerobes are uncommonly isolated. In the limb-threatening category, in contrast, infection is commonly polymicrobial.[119-121] *S. aureus,* group B streptococci, *Enterococcus,* and facultative gram-negative bacilli are major pathogens in this situation, along with anaerobic gram-positive cocci and *Bacteroides* species.

Deep tissue cultures provide the most reliable bacteriologic information in diabetic foot infections. If they are not available, cultures and Gram-stained smears of material obtained from curettage of the base of the ulcer or from a purulent exudate may provide the information needed to guide antimicrobial therapy. Gas present in surrounding tissues on radiologic examination may represent air introduced through the ulcer or gas generated in soft tissues by the infecting anaerobic or coliform organisms.

Antibiotic treatment of infected diabetic foot ulcers is based on meaningful bacteriologic data, if available. Initial antimicrobial treatment in a previously untreated patient with a non–limb-threatening infection is focused primarily on staphylococci and streptococci. For mild infections that can be treated at home, oral clindamycin or cephalexin for 2 weeks has been satisfactory.[119] Similarly, dicloxacillin may be effective. If superficial ulcers are complicated by cellulitis warranting parenteral antibiotics, intravenous cefazolin is effective.[119] Initial antimicrobial treatment of limb-threatening infections involves the use of broad-spectrum antibiotics aimed at its polymicrobial nature (group B streptococci, other streptococci, Enterobacteriaceae, anaerobic gram-positive cocci, and *Bacteroides* spp., including *B. fragilis*). In the past, the combination of clindamycin and an aminoglycoside has often been administered. In addition, cefoxitin or ceftizoxime has been used. Although ciprofloxacin has been successful as monotherapy, potential problems are presented by the possible role of *Bacteroides* spp. in these infections and by the emerging resistance to this drug among *S. aureus* strains. Currently, a variety of regimens are advocated for initial empirical therapy for limb-threatening infections[119]: ampicillin-sulbactam or imipenem,[72] clindamycin plus a third-generation cephalosporin, ticarcillin-clavulanate, and clindamycin plus ciprofloxacin. Aminoglycoside therapy is less attractive in this setting because of the advanced age of patients and frequent associated diabetic nephropathy.

Initial surgical management includes unroofing of encrusted areas and probing the wound to determine the extent of tissue destruction and possible bone involvement. Edema should be reduced by bed rest, elevation, and diuretic therapy as indicated. Control of diabetes is of considerable importance. Open ulcers should be gently packed three times daily with sterile gauze moistened with normal saline or one-quarter strength povidone-iodine (Betadine). Surgical débridement and drainage should be carried out promptly in patients with deep ulcers extending to subcutaneous tissue or if deep tissue necrosis or suppuration is present.[119]

Occupationally related contaminated traumatic wounds often involve loss of skin and subcutaneous tissue, with ensuing cellulitis and deeper infections. Comparison of the bacteriology of initial wounds sustained in factories with those sustained on farms (associated with corn-harvesting machinery) indicates that gram-negative bacilli (particularly *Enterobacter* spp. and *Stenotrophomonas maltophilia*) are 10 times more common in the latter.[122]

A newly described, often occupationally related (fish farmers, fish cutters, cooks) form of cellulitis caused by *Streptococcus iniae* has occurred in individuals exposed to aquacultured fish, primarily tilapia.[123] *S. iniae* is a fish pathogen that has caused outbreaks of invasive disease with high mortality among tilapia in aquaculture farms or merely colonization of the surface of fish. Human infection occurs after a puncture wound of the hand by a fish bone or knife while handling or preparing fish. Cellulitis develops rapidly (within 6 to 24 hours after the injury). Fever, lymphangitis originating from the site of injury, and bacteremia are frequently observed. Metastatic infections such as septic arthritis, meningitis, and endocarditis may occur. Bulla formation and skin necrosis are not features. Penicillin G is the treatment of choice, but *S. iniae* is also susceptible in vitro to cefazolin and ceftriaxone.

Sport fishing in fresh water may result in puncture wounds or lacerations incurred from the venomous spines of catfish.[124] Such wounds may rapidly become secondarily infected, particularly by gram-negative bacilli found in ponds and lakes (e.g., *A. hydrophila, Klebsiella, E. coli*).

Post-traumatic Opportunistic Skin Infections in Immunocompromised Patients

A variety of unusual pathogens may invade the skin of immunocompromised patients after local, often minor laceration or abrasion. Such pathogens include fungi (*Paecilomyces, Penicillium, Trichosporon, Fusarium, Alternaria*), mycobacteria (*Mycobacterium marinum*), and even algae (*Prototheca wickerhamii*).[108] The lesions are usually ulcerative or nodular,[125] but, in the case of *M. marinum,* they may take the form of a nodular lymphangitis extending from the original focus. Cutaneous protothecosis (*P. wickerhamii*) occurs occasionally in patients with AIDS or other immunosuppressed states.[126] Protothecosis occurs rarely in nonimmunosuppressed patients who have been exposed to trauma, water, or local corticosteroid injections.[127] Excision therapy or the use of amphotericin B has been successful. A typical dermatophyte, *Trichophyton rubrum,* which ordinarily produces only superficial skin infections, may invade the deeper subcutaneous tissues of immunosuppressed hosts and produce multiple nodular or fluctuant masses.[128] Primary cutaneous *Bacillus cereus* infection can occur in neutropenic patients[129] and has been reported in a patient with severe combined immunodeficiency disease.[130] The lesions are vesicular or pustular and usually occur on the hand or on an extremity during warm weather. Bacteremia is not a feature. Intravenous vancomycin is the preferred treatment.[129]

Rarely, scattered papular and nodular lesions in patients with AIDS show on biopsy an abscess containing a granule consisting of basophilic-staining cocci surrounded by eosinophilic material (Splendore-Hoeppli phenomenon). This particle superficially resembles a "sulfur granule" of actinomycosis or a mycetoma, but it is the lesion of botryomycosis and is caused by *S. aureus*.[131] Botryomycosis also occurs in immunocompetent patients; a foreign body may play a role in initiating or perpetuating the lesion, which has the gross appearance of a small infected sebaceous cyst or may resemble prurigo nodulans. Several cases of botryomycosis have occurred in patients with the hyperimmunoglobulin E syndrome associated with recurrent staphylococcal infections.

Bacillary Angiomatosis in Patients with Acquired Immunodeficiency Syndrome

Bacillary angiomatosis (epithelioid angiomatosis) is an infection that involves primarily the skin but also visceral organs in patients with AIDS, occasionally in patients with other forms of immunosuppression (e.g., with renal transplantation[132]), and rarely even in an immunocompetent individual (e.g., at the site of healing second-degree burns[133]) (see Chapter 232). The lesions begin as tiny red papules that enlarge to become exophytic or pedunculated nodules, occasionally reaching several centimeters in diameter.[134] They are often dome-shaped, vascular lesions with a collarette of scale.[135] Deeper nodules that may occur in the dermis or subcutaneous tissue are flesh colored, with a somewhat rubbery to firm consistency; they may be movable or fixed to underlying structures. The lesions bleed readily if incised. Only a few may be present, or they may number in the hundreds and cover the body. Oral, nasal, conjunctival, genital, and anal mucosal lesions occur. Visceral involvement takes the form of bacillary peliosis hepatis, with hypodense lesions of the liver and spleen demonstrable on abdominal computed tomographic scans.

The lesions of bacillary angiomatosis grossly resemble those of Kaposi's sarcoma, pyogenic granuloma, hemangioma, subcutaneous tumors, or verruga peruana (eruptive phase of bartonellosis in Peru and Ecuador). Histologically, bacillary angiomatosis consists of a circumscribed, lobular proliferation of capillaries lined with prominent large endothelial cells, an inflammatory infiltrate with neutrophils, and, characteristically, aggregates of bacillary bodies that are demonstrable on Warthin-Starry silver stain.

The initially uncultivatable etiologic agent of bacillary angiomatosis was first defined in tissue samples as a rickettsia-like organism closely related to *Bartonella quintana* by techniques used to analyze phylogenetic relatedness of eubacterial 16S ribosomal gene fragments.[136] A more recently described species of *Bartonella, Bartonella henselae,* a fastidious gram-negative organism, was then isolated in blood cultures of immunocompromised and nonimmunocompromised patients with an abrupt febrile illness and from cutaneous and osseous lesions of patients with bacillary angiomatosis.[135] *B. quintana* was cultured from other patients with bacillary angiomatosis.

Based on results of an immunofluorescence assay for antibody to *B. henselae* and on isolation of this organism from the lymph nodes of several nonimmunosuppressed patients with clinical cat-scratch disease, *B. henselae* (or a closely related organism) appears to be the causative agent in most cases of cat-scratch disease. Many patients with bacillary angiomatosis have a history of cat contact or cat scratches.

The diagnosis of bacillary angiomatosis is made by the clinical appearance of the lesions in a patient with human immunodeficiency virus (HIV) infection and confirmed on biopsy (Warthin-Starry silver stain). Because the skin lesions are often extensive and systemic manifestations (fever, peliosis hepatis) can be features, antimicrobial treatment is indicated. Erythromycin (0.5 g orally four times daily for 2 to 8 weeks) or another macrolide is the drug of choice. Some patients have responded to doxycycline, and azithromycin (1.0 g orally once daily) was used successfully in a patient with skin lesions, fever, and bacillary peliosis hepatis.

Hidradenitis Suppurativa

Hidradenitis suppurativa is an extremely troublesome, chronic, suppurative, cicatricial disease of apocrine glands in the axillary, genital, and perianal areas. The primary lesion appears to be an unexplained keratinous plugging of the ducts of the apocrine glands that results in dilatation and eventually rupture of the gland and surrounding tissue inflammation. The initial lesions are reddish-purple nodules that slowly become fluctuant and drain. Irregular sinus tracts are formed with repeated crops of lesions; reparative processes are only partially successful. Ultimately, the involved areas show a mixture of burrowing, draining tracts and cicatricial scarring. In some patients, hidradenitis suppurativa is associated with acne conglobata or dissecting cellulitis of the scalp. In such patients, a distinctive spondyloarthropathy may occur.[137] Squamous cell carcinoma is a rare complication of the lesions of hidradenitis suppurativa.[138]

Although not initially infected, the lesions frequently become infected secondarily.[139] Staphylococci, nonhemolytic streptococci, *Streptococcus anginosus* group, *E. coli, Proteus,* and *Pseudomonas* are often isolated from draining lesions. Anaerobic organisms (*Bacteroides,* anaerobic gram-positive cocci) have also been reported from such lesions. The foul odor of the discharge from such lesions suggests the presence of anaerobes.

Treatment of hidradenitis suppurativa is difficult, particularly when the process is chronic and extensive, because of the multiple deep-seated sites of secondary infection that are inaccessible to antibiotics. Antimicrobial therapy (based on Gram-stained smears and culture results) and local moist heat to establish drainage are helpful in treatment of the initial phases of infection. Surgical drainage is required in the management of large abscesses. In severe, resistant cases exhibiting chronicity and scarring, unroofing of sinus tracts and marsupialization or radical excision of most of the involved area, followed by skin grafting, may become necessary.[138]

Infected Epidermal Cysts

Epidermal cysts are closed sacs lined with proliferating epidermal cells located about the head, trunk, extremities, and vulvovaginal and scrotal areas. Lacking communication with the skin surface, they can become infected and result in abscess formation. *S. aureus* (frequently present as the sole aerobic organism) and various streptococci are the principal aerobic/facultative isolates from these abscesses. *Peptostreptococcus* and *Bacteroides* spp., the primary anaerobic isolates, are often present in polymicrobial mixtures in cyst abscesses about the head, perineum, and vulvovaginal area.[140] Treatment consists principally of surgical drainage, and initial antimicrobial therapy (clindamycin, cefoxitin, or amoxicillin-clavulanate), if needed, is aimed at *S. aureus* and the probable anaerobes pending results of Gram-stained smears and cultures.

Self-Induced Skin Infections

Rarely, persisting unexplained skin ulcers are self-induced. Their colonization with a variety of gram-negative and gram-positive bacteria is inevitable. However, the continuing ulceration is the result of repeated, self-induced trauma rather than bacterial infection per se. Very rarely, unexplained continuing or recurrent polymicrobial (oral or intestinal flora) cellulitis or a subcutaneous abscess is the result of injection of foreign material containing saliva or contaminated fluids into subcutaneous tissue. Examination of biopsy specimens from the involved area by polarizing microscopy may reveal the presence of birefringent foreign bodies, which suggest the true diagnosis.

Cutaneous Involvement in Systemic Bacterial and Mycotic Infections

Cutaneous manifestations may be a feature of a variety of bacteremias, fungemias, and systemic bacterial infections[141] (see Table 86-1). In leptospirosis, rat-bite fever, and listeriosis, cutaneous manifestations are a small part of the total clinical picture; these conditions are considered in the chapters dealing with the responsible organisms. In some systemic infections, cutaneous manifestations are noninfectious complications of the illness (erythema nodosum, purpura fulminans).

Bacteremias

Staphylococcus aureus. The occurrence of skin lesions (pustules, subcutaneous abscesses, purulent purpura) in the course of bacteremia or endocarditis secondary to *S. aureus* can provide a clue to the nature of the infecting organism. The most distinctive of these lesions is purulent purpura, a small area of purpura with a white, purulent center. Aspiration of the contents of the central portion reveals staphylococci and polymorphonuclear leukocytes. Rarely, scattered tender subcutaneous nodules may develop during *S. aureus* bacteremia.

Pseudomonas aeruginosa. Five types of skin lesion have been described in the course of *Pseudomonas* septicemia:

1. *Vesicles and bullae.* These lesions occur as isolated bullae or occasionally in small clusters anywhere on the skin surface. They rapidly become hemorrhagic and have a narrow encircling zone of dusky erythema. Occasionally, in infants, the lesions are surrounded by large, erythematous halos resembling insect bites or erythema multiforme.
2. *Ecthyma gangrenosum.* This lesion is a round, indurated, ulcerated, painless area with a central gray-black eschar and a surrounding narrow zone of erythema. These lesions may develop de novo, or they may evolve from an initial bullous lesion.
3. *Subcutaneous nodules.* Solitary or multiple, minimally fluctuant, subcutaneous nodules are uncommon features of *Pseudomonas* bacteremia, primarily in immunocompromised hosts.[142] Similar nodules in immunocompromised patients may have other infectious etiologies: *S. aureus* and botryomycosis, mycobacterial infections, candidiasis and other deep mycoses, protothecosis, *Acanthamoeba* infection, and bacillary angiomatosis.
4. *Gangrenous cellulitis.* Gangrenous cellulitis is either a superficial, sharply demarcated necrotic area that may resemble a decubitus ulcer or an area of cellulitis with edema and some necrosis of the overlying skin.
5. *Macular or maculopapular lesions.* These lesions are small, oval, erythematous macules located predominantly over the trunk that resemble the "rose spots" of typhoid fever. Such lesions have been reported, particularly in the tropics, in association with fever and diarrhea in the syndrome described as Shanghai fever.

The foregoing types of metastatic lesions contain numerous gram-negative bacilli but relatively few polymorphonuclear leukocytes. The development of such lesions in a febrile patient with leukemia who is undergoing induction chemotherapy or on uninvolved skin areas of a patient with extensive thermal burns should strongly suggest the presence of *Pseudomonas* bacteremia. Presumptive antibiotic management should be aimed at *P. aeruginosa* and includes a combination of ceftazidime or ticarcillin with tobramycin or a fluoroquinolone. Rarely, ecthyma gangrenosum occurs in the course of bacteremia caused by other gram-negative bacilli or in disseminated candidiasis, or it may occur in the absence of bacteremia as progression of *Pseudomonas* folliculitis in an immunocompromised patient.[143]

Neisseria meningitidis. The skin lesions of acute meningococcemia consist of erythematous macules (initially), petechiae, purpura, and ecchymoses located on the extremities and trunk. Extensive gun-metal gray, hemorrhagic, necrotic patches can develop by confluence of petechial and purpuric lesions in fulminant meningococcemia. Symmetric peripheral gangrene and purpura fulminans occur with prominent disseminated intravascular coagulation. Occasionally, gram-negative diplococci can be observed on smears of serum obtained from the skin lesions of patients with acute meningococcemia.

Skin lesions are an important feature of the unusual syndrome of chronic meningococcemia, which is characterized by recurrent cycles of fever, arthralgia, and rash over a period of 2 to 3 months.[144] The rash appears in crops, each consisting of a small number of individual lesions during febrile episodes. The lesions are generally located on the extremities, particularly about joints. They may consist of erythematous maculopapules, petechiae, petechiae with vesiculopustular centers, petechiae with small areolas of pale erythema, suggillations, or

tender erythema nodosum–like nodules. Biopsy specimens of the lesions reveal the histologic picture of leukocytoclastic angiitis, a finding that may erroneously direct attention toward the diagnosis of a small vessel hypersensitivity vasculitis and away from that of vasculitis secondary to systemic infection.

Neisseria gonorrhoeae. The skin lesions of gonococcemia consist of a mixture of pustules surrounded by a thin zone of purpura, macules, papules, purpuric vesicles and bullae, and purpuric infarcts. The lesions are few, scattered over the distal ends of extremities in particular, and frequently painful. They are part of the gonococcemic dermatitis-arthritis syndrome.[145] *Neisseria gonorrhoeae* is isolated from fewer than 5% of skin lesions, but in one study gonococcal antigens were identified by immunofluorescent staining procedures in most lesions. In addition to arthralgias and frank arthritis, tenosynovitis may be a conspicuous feature.

Salmonella typhi. "Rose spots" frequently appear 7 to 10 days into the febrile course of untreated typhoid fever. The lesions are slightly raised, small (1 to 3 mm), pink papules that tend to occur in crops of 10 to 20 lesions. They are found most commonly on the upper part of the abdomen, the lower part of the chest, and the back. Rose spots are less frequently found in enteric fever caused by *Salmonella* spp. other than *Salmonella typhi.* Early treatment with ciprofloxacin or chloramphenicol prevents the appearance of these skin lesions. *S. typhi* can sometimes be found on Gram-stained preparations from the papules and isolated on culture.

Haemophilus influenzae. Cellulitis involving the face, neck, or upper extremities occasionally occurs with bacteremic *H. influenzae* type B infection in children, particularly those younger than 3 years of age. Although commonly described as having a peculiar purple-red or blue-red hue, the lesion most often is erythematous, indurated, and indistinguishable from cellulitis caused by streptococci or staphylococci. The site of primary infection is the pharynx, the middle ear, or elsewhere in the upper respiratory tract. Direct invasion across traumatized buccal mucous membranes by *H. influenzae* type B colonizing the respiratory tract has been suggested as the pathogenesis of most cases of buccal cellulitis in children.[146] This infection is life-threatening and acute, and bacteremia (sometimes complicated by meningitis) occurs in about 80% of the cases.[147] A few cases have been reported in adults with epiglottitis or other forms of upper respiratory disease caused by *H. influenzae.*[148] *H. influenzae* type B cellulitis in children has almost disappeared in developed countries since widespread immunization with conjugate vaccines was introduced more than a decade ago. Although almost all cases of *H. influenzae* cellulitis in adults have involved cervical or thoracic areas, one case of bacteremic *H. influenzae* type B cellulitis occurred on the foot of an otherwise healthy octogenarian.[149] In view of the increased incidence of ampicillin resistance in clinical strains of *H. influenzae* type B, provisional antibiotic therapy should use a third-generation cephalosporin or chloramphenicol (either alone or in combination with ampicillin) until the isolate can be tested for β-lactamase activity.

Helicobacter cinaedi. A syndrome of *Helicobacter cinaedi* febrile, indolent bacteremia with resultant recurrent multifocal cellulitis has been described.[77] Although *H. cinaedi* was originally described in homosexual men with gastroenteritis, gastroenteritis has not been a feature of patients with the bacteremia-cellulitis syndrome. The patients have been immunocompromised to a large extent, often with HIV infection. In the latter group, the infection may be sexually transmitted. The cellulitis in some patients is described as having an atypical appearance: red-brown or copper-colored and lacking the expected local heat. *H. cinaedi* is susceptible to tetracyclines, aminoglycosides, rifampin, and often ciprofloxacin. Prolonged therapy (2 to 6 weeks) is usually required to ensure resolution of symptoms and prevent recurrence.[150]

Infective Endocarditis

The cutaneous lesions of subacute bacterial endocarditis consist of petechiae, subungual "splinter" hemorrhages, Osler's nodes, and Janeway lesions (see figures in Chapter 74). Petechiae tend to occur in small crops, particularly in the conjunctivae, on the palate, and on the upper part of the chest and extremities, and they are the most common skin lesions of endocarditis. Rarely, petechiae are extremely numerous, particularly on the lower extremities, and suggest a primary vasculitis. Osler's nodes are split pea–sized, erythematous, tender nodules located principally on the pads of the fingers and toes. They are few at any given time and occur in about 15% of patients with subacute bacterial endocarditis. The lesions are usually transient and clear in 1 to 2 days. Similar lesions may also occur in acute endocarditis (e.g., secondary to *S. aureus*). Histologic examination of such lesions in several cases of acute endocarditis has suggested septic embolization in their pathogenesis.[151] The genesis of Osler's nodes in subacute bacterial endocarditis may have a different basis, perhaps sterile embolization or an allergic vasculitis. Janeway lesions are painless, small, erythematous macules or minimally nodular hemorrhages in the palms or soles that occur in either acute or subacute endocarditis—more commonly in the former, particularly if *S. aureus* is the cause, in which case it occurs in 6% of patients.[152] Histologic findings in a case of *S. aureus* endocarditis indicate that Janeway lesions are caused by septic microembolization.[153]

Fungemias: *Candida albicans*

Systemic candidiasis developing in the setting of leukemia, immunosuppression, extensive antibiotic therapy, hyperalimentation, heroin addiction, cardiac surgery, and so on may be difficult to diagnose clinically until the organism is isolated from routine blood cultures. The portal for disseminated candidiasis (or aspergillosis) may be an area of skin injured in the course of intravenous therapy (or trauma induced by adhesive tape or extravasation of intravenous fluid).[108] Examination of the optic fundi (for evidence of candidal ophthalmitis) and a search for *Candida* pseudohyphae and yeast forms on a smear of buffy coat of venous blood are sometimes helpful in making an early diagnosis of candidal fungemia while awaiting isolation of the organism from blood cultures. In neutropenic patients, the appearance of multiple, discrete (2 to 5 mm), pink maculopapules (sometimes with pale centers) on the trunk or extremities can suggest the diagnosis.[154] In some of these patients, severe diffuse muscle tenderness is present, and muscle biopsy specimens have shown necrosis with yeast and pseudohyphal forms.[155] Occasionally, subcutaneous abscesses caused by *Candida* may develop in the course of fungemia. Aspiration of such abscesses reveals the cause on stained smear. Punch biopsy specimens of the maculopapular lesions provide a more accurate diagnosis than simple culture does, because histologic sections can reveal yeast cells in blood vessels and pseudohyphae in adjacent soft tissue. Isolation of *Candida* from an unroofed lesion may represent only surface colonization or may be consistent with *Candida* folliculitis rather than disseminated candidiasis. *M. furfur* folliculitis can be mistaken for hematogenous *Candida* lesions on appearance and histopathology.

SUBCUTANEOUS TISSUE INFECTIONS AND ABSCESSES

Exact categorization of some bacterial infections of the soft tissues (skin, subcutaneous tissue, fascia, and skeletal muscle) may be difficult. Although differences between a superficial pyoderma and a necrotizing myositis[105] such as gas gangrene are readily apparent, distinctions between many other types of soft tissue infection are sometimes blurred. Classification is usually based on features such as the anatomic structure involved, the infecting organisms, and the clinical picture. Some infections may involve several components of the soft tissue, and multiple bacterial species may produce infections with the same clinical appearance.

To further compound the problem of classification, a variety of designations have been given to closely related or virtually identical processes. For example, streptococcal gangrene has also been referred to as necrotizing fasciitis. After the initial descriptions of this condition, it became apparent that it was sometimes caused by bacteria other than group A streptococci.[156] Therefore, streptococcal gangrene can be considered the major subset of necrotizing fasciitis. For conve-

nience, because a major feature of its manifestation is cutaneous gangrene, streptococcal gangrene was considered in the preceding section with cellulitis and infectious cutaneous gangrene. Necrotizing fasciitis is reconsidered in this section on subcutaneous tissue infections, particularly in relation to its nonstreptococcal causes. Another example of the problems in nomenclature is that presented by infections that involve multiple soft tissue strata and can be caused by a variety of bacterial species. For example, the condition known as synergistic necrotizing cellulitis has also been described as gram-negative anaerobic cutaneous gangrene and as synergistic nonclostridial anaerobic myonecrosis.[157,158] Because of the prominence of subcutaneous tissue involvement in this condition, it is considered primarily in this part of the chapter, although it could be considered almost as readily in the first part ("Cellulitis and Superficial Infections") or in the chapter on myositis (see Chapter 87).

Clostridial Anaerobic Cellulitis

Clostridial anaerobic cellulitis is a necrotizing clostridial infection of devitalized subcutaneous tissue. Deep fascia is not appreciably involved, and, ordinarily, no associated myositis is present. Gas formation is common and often extensive. Anaerobic cellulitis is several times more common than gas gangrene in war wounds.

Pathogenesis and Pathologic Characteristics. Clostridial species, usually *C. perfringens,* are introduced into subcutaneous tissue through a dirty or inadequately débrided traumatic wound, through contamination at surgery, or from a preexisting localized infection. The last is frequently located in the perineum, abdominal wall, buttocks, or lower extremities, areas that are readily contaminated with fecal flora. The presence of foreign debris and necrotic tissue in the depths of a wound provides a suitable anaerobic milieu for clostridial proliferation. Very rarely, clostridial anaerobic cellulitis develops not after primary cutaneous injury, but rather as a consequence of *C. septicum* bacteremia in the setting of leukemia and granulocytopenia.[159] Intestinal erosions are the presumed initial portals of entry. This type of *C. septicum* cellulitis should be distinguished from the even more life-threatening bacteremic *C. septicum* myonecrosis, which is often associated with a cryptic underlying colonic neoplasm (see Chapter 87).

Clinical Findings. The incubation period is several days, longer than the 1 to 2 days for clostridial myonecrosis. The onset is gradual, but the process may subsequently spread rapidly.[160] Local pain, tissue swelling, and systemic toxicity are not prominent features, and the relative mildness of the process helps distinguish it from true gas gangrene. The dark blebs and bronzing of the skin seen in gas gangrene are not usually features of clostridial cellulitis. Thin, dark, sometimes foul-smelling drainage from the wound (often containing fat globules) is characteristic, as is extensive tissue gas formation, more prominent than that observed in clostridial myonecrosis. Frank crepitus is present in the involved area and may extend very widely, even beyond the limits of the active infection. *C. perfringens* cellulitis has been recurrent in the setting of retained foreign bodies.[161]

Gram-stained smears of drainage material show numerous bluntended, thick, gram-positive bacilli and variable numbers of polymorphonuclear leukocytes. Soft tissue roentgenograms show abundant gas, but not usually in the feathery linear pattern in muscles that is observed in clostridial myonecrosis.

Etiologic Agents. *C. perfringens* is the most common clostridial species responsible for this infection, but *C. septicum* and other species have been isolated. Sometimes, clostridia are present in mixed culture with facultative organisms.

Differential Diagnosis. If crepitus is observed with a wound, a variety of possibilities must be considered in the differential diagnosis (Table 86-5). The first is clostridial myonecrosis (gas gangrene), because of the fulminant nature of the infection and the requirement for emergency surgery. At the same time, distinguishing between clostridial gas gangrene and anaerobic cellulitis is essential to avoid performing unnecessarily extensive surgery. Ultimately, the two processes are differentiated in the operating room, when the wound is

TABLE 86-5 Differential Diagnosis of Crepitant Soft Tissue Wounds*

Factor	Clostridial Cellulitis	Nonclostridial Anaerobic Cellulitis	Clostridial Myonecrosis (Gas Gangrene)	Anaerobic Streptococcal Myositis	Necrotizing Fasciitis (Type I)†	Infected Vascular Gangrene	Synergistic Necrotizing Cellulitis‡	Noninfectious Causes of Gas in Tissues
Predisposing conditions	Local trauma or surgery	Diabetes mellitus, preexisting localized infection	Local trauma or surgery	Local trauma	Diabetes mellitus, abdominal surgery, perineal infection	Peripheral arterial insufficiency	Diabetes mellitus, cardiorenal disease, obesity, perirectal infection	Mechanical effects of penetrating trauma, injuries involving the use of compressed air, entrapment of air under loosely sutured wounds or under ulcers, irrigation of wounds with hydrogen peroxide, intravenous catheter placement, dissection of air from tracheostomy or spontaneous mediastinal emphysema
Incubation period	Usually >3 days	Several days	1-2 days	3-4 days	1-4 days	>5 days	3-14 days	Less than 1 hour
Onset	Gradual	Gradual or rapid	Acute	Not as rapid as gas gangrene	Acute	Gradual	Acute	Usually present immediately after trauma or manipulation; may not be recognized until examination several hours later
Pain	Mild	Mild	Marked	Occurs late, marked	Moderate or severe	Variable	Severe	Mild
Swelling	Moderate	Moderate	Marked	Moderate	Marked	Moderate or marked	Moderate or marked	Slight or absent
Skin appearance	Minimal discoloration	Minimal discoloration	Yellow-bronze, dark bullae, green-black patches of necrosis	Erythema	Erythematous cellulitis, areas of skin necrosis	Discolored or black	Scattered areas of skin necrosis	Only those resulting from the initiating trauma
Exudate	Thin, dark	Dark pus	Serosanguineous	Abundant, seropurulent	Seropurulent	None	"Dishwater" pus	None
Gas	++++	++++	++	±	++	+++	++	Variable but present; does not extend
Odor	Sometimes foul	Foul	Variable, slightly foul or peculiarly sweet	Slight; "sour"	Foul	Foul	Foul	None
Systemic toxicity	Minimal	Moderate	Marked	Only late in course	Moderate or marked	Minimal	Marked	None
Muscle involvement	None	None	++++	+++	None	Dead	++	None

±, rarely present; ++, present to mild extent; +++, present to moderate extent; ++++, extensive.
*In addition to the causes of crepitant infections listed in this table, *Aeromonas hydrophila* myositis may be associated with gas in soft tissues.
†The term necrotizing fasciitis is used here to designate other forms of this syndrome other than streptococcal gangrene.
‡Synergistic necrotizing cellulitis is essentially the same process as type I necrotizing fasciitis. Because the former occasionally tends to involve muscle, it is given a separate designation here; however, the two processes are clinically indistinguishable in most instances.
Modified from Finegold SM. Anaerobic Bacteria in Human Disease. New York: Academic Press; 1977.

laid open and the viability and appearance of the muscle are observed. The muscle is normal (pink) in clostridial cellulitis but distinctly abnormal in clostridial myonecrosis: it is discolored, fails to contract on stimulation, and does not bleed from a cut surface (see Chapter 87).

Presumptive Therapy. Surgical exploration is essential to determine the presence of any muscle involvement. If no myonecrosis is found, treatment should be limited to débridement of necrotic tissue and drainage of pus after the wound is opened widely. Initial antimicrobial management of clostridial cellulitis requires the use of several antibiotics, because until surgical exploration has been carried out to distinguish between clostridial myonecrosis and anaerobic cellulitis and until Gram-stained smears of material from the lesion have been evaluated, gas gangrene or a potentially polymicrobial infection is an important consideration. Intravenous penicillin (2 million units every 3 hours or 3 to 4 million units every 4 hours) or ampicillin (1.5 to 2 g every 4 hours), plus intravenous clindamycin (0.6 g every 6 to 8 hours) or metronidazole (1 g loading dose followed by 0.5 g every 6 hours), provides a two-drug combination for treatment of the anaerobic organisms likely to be involved. Use of an additional antimicrobial agent (an aminoglycoside, ciprofloxacin, or third-generation cephalosporin) aimed at aerobic gram-negative bacilli is based on evaluation of Gram-stained smears of exudate and tissue. Definitive selection of antimicrobial agents is subsequently based on results of cultures and antimicrobial-susceptibility tests.

Nonclostridial Anaerobic Cellulitis

A clinical picture very similar to that of clostridial anaerobic cellulitis can be produced by infection with a variety of non–spore-forming anaerobic bacteria (various *Bacteroides* species, peptostreptococci, and peptococci, either alone or as mixed infections).[158] The anaerobic bacteria may be present along with facultative species (coliform bacilli, various streptococci, staphylococci) in a mixed infection. Gas-forming soft tissue infections have been produced by *E. coli, Klebsiella, Aeromonas,* and perhaps other facultative bacteria.[105,163]

Because the clinical features and setting are very similar to those of clostridial anaerobic cellulitis, the same initial antimicrobial therapy (see earlier description) is appropriate to cover the mixed bacterial nature of the infection. In the past, the combination of penicillin or ampicillin (aimed at *Peptostreptococcus, Peptococcus, Clostridium,* and various streptococcal species) plus chloramphenicol (directed at *Bacteroides* spp. and facultative gram-negative bacilli) has been used as preliminary therapy and is still favored by some. Ampicillin-sulbactam may also be used as initial therapy. Evaluation of Gram-stained smears of exudate aspirated from the lesion supplies a more focused basis for initial antimicrobial therapy. Subsequent results of cultures and susceptibility testing of aspirates or tissue removed at surgical exploration provide the information needed for narrowing (or extending) antimicrobial therapy. The surgical approach used is the same as in the treatment of clostridial anaerobic cellulitis.

Necrotizing Fasciitis

The term *necrotizing fasciitis* encompasses two bacteriologic entities.[164] In *type I,* at least one anaerobic species (most commonly *Bacteroides* or *Peptostreptococcus*) is isolated in combination with one or more facultative anaerobic species such as streptococci (other than group A) and members of the Enterobacteriaceae (e.g., *E. coli, Enterobacter, Klebsiella, Proteus*). An obligate aerobe such as *P. aeruginosa* is only rarely a component of such a mixed infection. Cases in which only anaerobes are present appear to be rare.

In *type II* (corresponding to the entity also known as hemolytic streptococcal gangrene), group A streptococci are isolated either alone or in combination with other species, most commonly *S. aureus.* Streptococcal gangrene was considered in the first part of this chapter as a form of gangrenous cellulitis. In this section, specific comments about streptococcal gangrene are limited to the expanded setting in which the disease can appear, as well as the changes in clinical features noted with the recent apparent increase in bacteremic and severe invasive group A streptococcal infections and their association with the streptococcal toxic shock–like syndrome.[2,100,165]

Hemolytic streptococcal gangrene occurs after minor trauma, stab wounds, or surgery, particularly in the context of diabetes and peripheral vascular disease, but cirrhosis and corticosteroid therapy have also been predisposing factors.[100] In outbreaks of streptococcal toxic shock–like syndrome, chills, fever (or profound hypothermia and shock), confusion, vomiting, diarrhea, tachycardia, hypotension, and multiorgan failure are prominent features. Necrotizing fasciitis is present in about half of cases of streptococcal toxic shock–like syndrome.[2] Streptococcal strains of M protein types 1, 3, 12, and 28 are most commonly involved, and, in the United States, they usually elaborate pyrogenic exotoxin A. The use of nonsteroidal anti-inflammatory agents may mask and delay the diagnosis by reducing the inflammatory features. Leukocytosis, thrombocytopenia, azotemia, and increased serum levels of creatine phosphokinase are commonly present. Rising creatine phosphokinase levels may serve as an indication of progression of streptococcal cellulitis to necrotizing fasciitis and myositis. Unlike many earlier cases of hemolytic streptococcal gangrene, which affected older individuals with underlying diseases, a more recent outbreak of streptococcal toxic shock–like syndrome occurred primarily in young, previously healthy adults after minor trauma. In 70% of the patients, soft tissue findings progressed to hemolytic streptococcal gangrene with the development of vesicles, violaceous bullae, and necrosis of subcutaneous tissues typical of necrotizing fasciitis (or myositis) and requiring surgical débridement.[101] The mortality rate was about 30%. In young children, the skin lesions of varicella can be superinfected with group A streptococci and become a risk factor for group A streptococcal necrotizing fasciitis.[166,167]

In a study in Ontario, Canada, in the late 1980s, a primary site of infection could be defined in 38 (76%) of 50 cases of severe, invasive group A streptococcal infection. Skin and soft tissue infections were present in 26 (68%) of these cases, and necrotizing fasciitis in 15 (57%). The most common group A streptococci in several outbreaks have been M1/T1 or M12/T12 types containing pyrogenic exotoxin A (spe A) or C (spe C) genes[168] and M1 or M3 types producing pyrogenic exotoxins A or B.[165] Examination of type M1 and M3 isolates from cases of streptococcal toxic shock–like syndrome suggests their possible clonal origin.[169] The finding of a characteristic restriction enzyme fragment profile of streptococcal DNA (hybridized with an spe A probe) from patients with serious streptococcal disease (mainly toxic shock–like syndrome) of several different serotypes further suggests that the invasive strains are not serotype specific but, rather, that a strain of a given serotype can acquire a new gene (toxin gene) and, with it, enhanced virulence.[170] The more general features of necrotizing fasciitis are now considered.

Clinical Findings. Necrotizing fasciitis is an uncommon severe infection involving the subcutaneous soft tissues, particularly the superficial (and often the deep) fascia. It is usually an acute process but rarely may follow a subacute progressive course. Necrotizing fasciitis can affect any part of the body but is most common on the extremities, particularly the legs. Other sites of predilection are the abdominal wall, perianal and groin areas, and postoperative wounds.[171] The portal of entry is usually a site of trauma (laceration, abrasion, burn, insect bite), a laparotomy performed in the presence of peritoneal soiling (penetrating abdominal trauma or perforated viscus) or another surgical procedure (e.g., hemorrhoidectomy, vasectomy), perirectal abscess, decubitus ulcer, or an intestinal perforation. The last may be secondary to occult diverticulitis,[172,173] rectosigmoid neoplasm, or a foreign body such as a chicken bone or toothpick. Necrotizing fasciitis from such intestinal sources may occur in the lower extremity (extension along the psoas muscle), as well as in the groin or abdominal wall (via a colocutaneous fistula). Particular clinical settings in which necrotizing fasciitis may develop include diabetes mellitus, alcoholism, and parenteral drug abuse.[174]

In the newborn, necrotizing fasciitis can be a serious complication of omphalitis. Initial swelling and erythema about the umbilicus can progress over several hours to several days and result in purplish discoloration and periumbilical necrosis.[175] Involvement of the anterior abdominal wall frequently extends to the flanks and even onto the chest wall.

The affected area is initially erythematous, swollen, without sharp margins, hot, shiny, exquisitely tender, and painful.[176] Lymphangitis and lymphadenitis are infrequent. The process progresses rapidly over several days, with sequential skin color changes from red-purple to patches of blue-gray. Within 3 to 5 days after onset, skin breakdown with bullae (containing thick pink or purple fluid) and frank cutaneous gangrene (resembling a thermal burn) can be seen. By this time, the involved area is no longer tender but has become anesthetic secondary to thrombosis of small blood vessels and destruction of superficial nerves located in the necrotic, undermined subcutaneous tissue. The development of anesthesia may antedate the appearance of skin necrosis and provide a clue that the process is necrotizing fasciitis and not a simple cellulitis. Marked swelling and edema may produce a compartment syndrome with complicating extensive myonecrosis requiring prompt fasciotomy. Measurement of compartment pressure may aid the evaluation in early situations in which marked pain and swelling are present without concomitant skin changes that would indicate the diagnosis.[2] Subcutaneous gas is often present in the polymicrobial form of necrotizing fasciitis, particularly in patients with diabetes mellitus. Systemic toxicity is prominent, and the temperature is elevated in the range of 38.9° C to 40.5° C (102° F to 105° F). On probing of the lesion with a hemostat through a limited incision, the instrument easily passes along a plane just superficial to the deep fascia. Such easy passage would not occur with ordinary cellulitis.

Leukocytosis is commonly present. Gram-stained smears of exudate usually reveal a mixture of organisms or, in the case of streptococcal gangrene, chains of gram-positive cocci. In one instance, we observed numerous long gram-positive bacilli with subterminal spores (along with gram-negative bacilli) in the foul-smelling, purulent exudate of a patient with crepitant necrotizing fasciitis after a lower leg amputation for peripheral vascular disease. The presence of numerous spores in the wound exudate indicated that the gram-positive bacilli were unlikely to be *C. perfringens.* Before surgery the patient had *Clostridium difficile* enterocolitis, and *C. difficile* was isolated along with several members of the Enterobacteriaceae from the wound drainage material.

Blood cultures are frequently positive. Hypocalcemia (without tetany) may occur if necrosis of subcutaneous fat is extensive.

Fournier's Gangrene. A form of necrotizing fasciitis occurring about the male genitals is known as Fournier's gangrene[158,164] (idiopathic gangrene of the scrotum, streptococcal scrotal gangrene, perineal phlegmon). It may be confined to the scrotum, or it may extend to involve the perineum, penis, and abdominal wall. Predisposing factors include diabetes mellitus, local trauma, paraphimosis, periurethral extravasation of urine, perirectal or perianal infection,[177] and surgery in the area (circumcision, herniorrhaphy). In cases originating in the genitalia, the infecting bacteria probably pass through Buck's fascia of the penis and spread along the dartos fascia of the scrotum and penis, Colles' fascia of the perineum, and Scarpa's fascia of the anterior abdominal wall. In view of the typical foul odor associated with this form of necrotizing fasciitis, a major role for anaerobic bacteria is likely. Mixed cultures containing facultative organisms (*E. coli, Klebsiella,* enterococci), along with anaerobes (*Bacteroides, Fusobacterium, Clostridium,* anaerobic or microaerophilic streptococci), have been obtained from the lesions in the limited number of cases studied. Rarely, group A streptococcal gangrene evolving from streptococcal balanitis can also involve the male genital area.

The infection commonly starts as cellulitis adjacent to the portal of entry. Early in the course of Fournier's gangrene, the involved area is swollen, erythematous, and tender as the infection begins to involve the deep fascia. Pain is prominent; fever and systemic toxicity are marked.[178] Swelling and crepitus of the scrotum quickly increase, and dark purple areas develop and progress to extensive scrotal gangrene. If the abdominal wall becomes involved in an obese patient with diabetes, the process can spread extremely rapidly.

Other Special Anatomic Forms of Necrotizing Fasciitis. Necrotizing fasciitis of the face and eyelids,[179] the neck,[180] and the lip[181] is an uncommon but life-threatening form of this disease. It is most often caused by group A streptococci, alone or with *S. aureus,* and represents streptococcal gangrene; occasionally, it represents mixed infections of group A streptococcus with Enterobacteriaceae or oral *Bacteroides* spp. Although necrotizing fasciitis of the head and neck is often considered a single entity, in fact it represents two conditions etiologically.[182] Craniofacial necrotizing fasciitis is commonly caused by group A streptococci, whereas cervical necrotizing fasciitis often represents a polymicrobial process (e.g., group A streptococci, various other streptococcal species, *Bacteroides* spp., *Peptostreptococcus* spp.). In mixed infections, crepitus may be a feature, as may necrosis of the epidermis and superficial fascia. Trauma is the usual precipitating cause of necrotizing fasciitis of the periorbital areas and face; dental, oral, and pharyngeal infections predispose to cervical necrotizing fasciitis. Differentiation of the latter from cervical soft tissue infection of odontogenic origin can be difficult, but rapid spread of infection to other areas of the neck, severe pain, and systemic symptoms along with subcutaneous crepitus suggest the diagnosis of necrotizing fasciitis. If crepitus is not palpable, soft tissue radiographs may help in the diagnosis by demonstrating subcutaneous gas. The mortality associated with cervical necrotizing fasciitis is about four times as high as that from craniofacial necrotizing fasciitis.[182]

Other Microbial Etiologies of Necrotizing Fasciitis. Necrotizing fasciitis in neutropenic children receiving cancer chemotherapy may be caused by *P. aeruginosa* or Enterobacteriaceae.[183] The acute cellulitis caused by *V. vulnificus* and other *Vibrio* species (described earlier) may extend to the superficial and deep fascia and produce necrotizing fasciitis. Very rare causes of necrotizing fasciitis include environmental species such as *Flavobacterium odoratum,*[184] *Serratia marcescens,*[185] and *Ochrobactrum anthropi.*[186]

Differential Diagnosis. See Table 86-5 for the differential diagnosis of necrotizing fasciitis.

Presumptive Therapy. Prompt diagnosis is of paramount importance because of the rapidity with which the process can progress. The mortality rate of necrotizing fasciitis ranges from 20% to 47% overall (13% and 22% for Fournier's gangrene).[177,178] Among patients with either type I or type II necrotizing fasciitis in whom the diagnosis is made within 4 days after appearance of the initial symptoms, the mortality rate is reduced to 12%.[187] Early clinical differentiation of necrotizing fasciitis from cellulitis can be difficult because the initial signs—including pain, edema, and erythema—are not distinctive. However, the presence of marked systemic toxicity out of proportion to the local findings should alert the physician. Computed tomography and magnetic resonance imaging can demonstrate subcutaneous and fascial edema, as well as tissue gas, in patients with necrotizing fasciitis and distinguish this process from cellulitis.[188,189] However, in patients in whom the diagnosis is clearly suspected, the most expeditious route to diagnosis is through surgical exploration or biopsy without introducing delay for imaging studies. Imaging studies can be most useful early in the process, when pain and swelling are evident but cutaneous changes are absent and the diagnosis is uncertain. Imaging studies may also be helpful in monitoring clinical progress after surgical débridement, when further surgery may need to be considered. Additionally, imaging studies are useful in the diagnosis and management of necrotizing fasciitis in areas of the body where the process is more inaccessible (e.g., retroperitoneal involvement) or may readily spread to other tissue compartments (e.g., cervical fasciitis spreading to the mediastinum, pleura, and pericardium). Frozen-section examination of biopsy specimens (including dermis, infected subcutaneous tissue, fascia, and underlying muscle) has been found to be helpful for early diagnosis.[187]

Once the diagnosis is made, immediate surgical débridement is essential. In patients in whom the diagnosis is clearly suspected on clinical grounds (deep pain with patchy areas of surface hypoesthesia, crepitation, or bullae and skin necrosis), direct operative intervention is indicated. Extensive incisions should be made through the skin and subcutaneous tissues and should go beyond the area of involvement until normal fascia is found. Necrotic fat and fascia should be excised, and the wound should be left open. A second-look procedure is frequently necessary 24 hours later to ensure adequacy of the initial débridement.[176] In the case of Fournier's gangrene, orchiectomy is almost never required because the testes have their own blood supply, independent of the compromised fascial and cutaneous circulation of the scrotum. Initial antimicrobial therapy is based on the evidence for prominent roles of anaerobic bacteria, Enterobacteriaceae, and various streptococci in this process and on the specific findings on Gram-stained smears. Antibiotics used before bacteriologic data area are obtained include combinations of ampicillin, gentamicin, and clindamycin; ampicillin, gentamicin, and metronidazole; ampicillin-sulbactam and gentamicin; and imipenem or meropenem. For group A streptococcal necrotizing fasciitis, penicillin or ampicillin plus clindamycin is recommended (see Chapter 195).

Several ancillary therapies, neither a substitute for prompt surgical débridement nor of proven efficacy, have been described. One is the use of intravenous immune globulin to treat the streptococcal toxic shock–like syndrome accompanying the treatment of group A streptococcal necrotizing fasciitis.[2] The other is the use of hyperbaric oxygen in the treatment of polymicrobial necrotizing fasciitis, particularly of the trunk.[164]

Synergistic Necrotizing Cellulitis

Clinical Findings. Synergistic necrotizing cellulitis (gram-negative anaerobic cutaneous gangrene, necrotizing cutaneous myositis, synergistic nonclostridial anaerobic myonecrosis) is a variant of necrotizing fasciitis, with prominent involvement of skin and muscle, as well as subcutaneous tissue and fascia. Some cases of Fournier's gangrene extending onto the abdominal wall are examples of this condition. Predisposing factors include diabetes mellitus, obesity, advanced age, and cardiorenal disease. Most infections are located on the lower extremities or near the perineum (e.g., originating in a perirectal abscess).[157]

The lesion may first be manifested as small skin ulcers draining foul-smelling, reddish-brown ("dishwater") pus. Circumscribed areas of blue-gray gangrene surround these draining sites, but the intervening skin appears normal despite necrosis of underlying subcutaneous tissue, fascia, and muscle. Local pain and tenderness are marked. Tissue gas is noted in about one fourth of patients. Systemic toxicity is a feature; about half of the patients have bacteremia.

Etiologic Agents. Cultures consistently show mixtures of anaerobic bacteria (anaerobic streptococci, *Bacteroides,* or both) and facultative bacteria *(Klebsiella-Enterobacter, E. coli, Proteus).*[157] *Bacteroides* has been reported as the major pathogen on occasion.[190]

Presumptive Therapy. Initial surgery involves incision and drainage, but radical débridement is often necessary because of extensive involvement of deep fascia and muscle.[157,190] Amputation may be required. Antibiotic management is initially based on the results of Gram-stained smears of wound exudates, but it should include an antimicrobial agent effective against *Bacteroides* (see earlier discussion of presumptive therapy for type I necrotizing fasciitis).

Miscellaneous Infections Secondary to Trauma

Bite Infections. Infections secondary to bites are discussed in Chapter 318.[191]

Burn Infections. Infections secondary to burns are discussed in Chapter 317.

Injection Site Abscesses. Subcutaneous and intramuscular abscesses infrequently occur after therapeutic injections. *S. aureus,* facultative gram-negative bacilli, and anaerobic bacteria are usually implicated. Hematomas may represent sites of delayed infection. Gas gangrene has occurred after various injections, particularly epinephrine in oil.[105] Subcutaneous and intramuscular abscesses caused by a variety of oral anaerobes and streptococci have occurred after "skin popping" or attempted intravenous injections by narcotic addicts.[158] In the case of subcutaneous abscesses secondary to intravenous drug abuse, appropriate débridement and drainage should include excision of involved veins, which often contain pus or an infected thrombus.[192]

Factitial Disease (Self-Induced Abscesses). Occasionally, subcutaneous abscesses and cellulitis are produced when a patient deliberately injects or inserts contaminated substances into the skin.[193,194] Such abscesses are often recurrent and may be of monomicrobial or polymicrobial origin (often consisting of oral or fecal flora). Sterile abscesses may be induced by the introduction of foreign material without bacterial contamination. Such foreign material may be identified by examination of biopsy specimens with polarizing microscopy.

Subcutaneous Infections Originating in Contiguous Foci

Osteomyelitis. Occasionally, most commonly in a child, acute hematogenous osteomyelitis is manifested as subcutaneous abscess. Under these circumstances, a subperiosteal abscess has ruptured through intervening tissue into the subcutaneous tissue. *S. aureus* is the most common etiologic agent in such infections. It is important to recognize the nature of the process because of the different therapeutic programs required for osteomyelitis and for a subcutaneous abscess of cutaneous origin. Involvement of subcutaneous tissue as a consequence of osteomyelitis may also occur in the form of a draining sinus associated with chronic osteomyelitis and sequestrum formation. Multiple draining sinuses may occur as a result of multiple foci of osteomyelitis in disseminated blastomycosis.

Actinomycosis. Subcutaneous abscesses frequently develop in the course of cervical, thoracic, or sometimes abdominal actinomycosis. Draining sinuses ultimately result (see Chapter 253).

Primary Pyodermas. On occasion, more superficial skin infections beginning as folliculitis, furunculosis, or cellulitis may progress into the deeper subcutaneous tissue and form a subcutaneous (sometimes "cold") abscess. *S. aureus* is commonly the cause. Such progression occurring repeatedly might suggest certain underlying phagocytic cell defects, such as chronic granulomatous disease of childhood or hyperimmunoglobulin E syndrome (Job's syndrome).[195,196]

In a cataloging of the bacteriology of a large number of cutaneous abscesses (with unspecified individual predisposing causes), *S. aureus* was the single most common aerobic/facultative isolate, followed in frequency by streptococci, both groupable (A, B, C, D) and nongroupable.[197] Among anaerobic isolates, *Bacteroides* spp. (most commonly *B. fragilis* group) were most frequent, followed by *Peptostreptococcus* spp. and *Clostridium* spp. These abscesses are commonly polymicrobial (mixed aerobic-anaerobic). As might be predicted, *S. aureus* is the principal isolate in infections (both abscesses and wounds) of the extremities and trunk, whereas anaerobes are more numerous than aerobic/facultative species in such infections in the genital, perirectal, inguinal, and head and neck areas.

Subcutaneous Abscesses in the Course of Bacteremic Infections

Metastatic pyogenic infections can occur during the course of bacteremias or endocarditis caused by various common invasive organisms (e.g., *S. aureus*) in subcutaneous tissue, as well as a variety of other organs and tissues. These abscesses are tender and fluctuant. Rarely, multiple, firm, nodular, subcutaneous lesions clinically resembling those of Weber-Christian disease occur in the course of a staphylococcal bacteremia. If promptly identified and treated, the process may be aborted before frank abscess formation occurs.

Less common bacterial pathogens, infrequently responsible for bacteremia (e.g., *Nocardia* spp.,[198] *Corynebacterium jeikeium*[199]) may also occasionally produce metastatic cutaneous abscesses in immunocompromised or debilitated individuals.

Mycetoma

See Chapter 260.

REFERENCES

1. Ferrieri P, Dajani AS, Wannamaker LW, et al. Natural history of impetigo: I. Site sequence of acquisition and familial patterns of spread of cutaneous streptococci. J Clin Invest. 1972;51:2851.
2. Bisno AL, Stevens DL. Streptococcal infections of skin and soft tissues. N Engl J Med. 1996;334:240.

3. Britton JW, Fajardo JE, Krafte-Jacobs B. Comparison of mupirocin and erythromycin in the treatment of impetigo. J Pediatr. 1990;117:827.

4. Dagan R, Bar-David Y. Double-blind study comparing erythromycin and mupirocin for treatment of impetigo in children: Implications of a high prevalence of erythromycin-resistant Staphylococcus aureus strains. Antimicrob Agents Chemother. 1992;36:287.

5. Esterly NB, Nelson DB, Dunne WM Jr. Impetigo. Am J Dis Child. 1991;145:125.

6. Dajani AS, Wannamaker LW. Experimental infection of the skin in the hamster simulating human impetigo: III. Interaction between staphylococci and group A streptococci. J Exp Med. 1971;134:588.

7. Dajani AS, Ferrieri P, Wannamaker LW. Natural history of impetigo: II. Etiologic agents and bacterial interactions. J Clin Invest. 1972;51:2863.

8. Dillon HC. Impetigo contagiosa: Suppurative and non-suppurative complications. I: Clinical, bacteriologic, and epidemiologic characteristics of impetigo. Am J Dis Child. 1968;115:530.

9. Darmstadt GL, Fleckman P, Jonas M, et al. Differentiation of cultured keratinocytes promotes the adherence of Streptococcus pyogenes. J Clin Invest. 1998;101:128.

10. Okada N, Pentland AP, Falk P, et al. M protein and protein F act as important determinations of cell-specific tropism of Streptococcus pyogenes in skin tissue. J Clin Invest. 1994;94:965.

11. Dillon HC. Post-streptococcal glomerulonephritis following pyoderma. Rev Infect Dis. 1979;1:935.

12. Bessen DE, Sotir CM, Readdy TL, et al. Genetic correlates of throat and skin isolates of group A streptococci. J Infect Dis. 1996;173:896.

13. Scaramuzzino DA, McNiff JM, Bessen DE. Humanized in vivo model for streptococcal impetigo. Infect Immun. 2000;68:2880

14. Svensson MD, Sjöbring U, Bessen DE. Selective distribution of a high affinity plasminogen-binding site among group A streptococcus associated with impetigo. Infect Immun. 1999;67:3915.

15. Burge SM, Ryan TJ. Acute palmoplantar pustulosis. Br J Dermatol. 1985;113:77.

16. McLaughlin J, Low JC. Primary cutaneous listeriosis in adults: An ocupational disease of veterinarians and farmers. Vet Rec. 1994;135:615.

17. Baltimore RS. Treatment of impetigo: A review. Pediatr Infect Dis. 1985;4:597.

18. Feder HM Jr, Abrahamian LM, Grant-Kels JM. Is penicillin still the drug of choice for non-bullous impetigo? Lancet. 1991;2:803.

19. Konig S, van Suylekom-Smit LWA, Nouen JL, et al. Fusidic acid cream in the treatment of impetigo in general practice: Double blind randomized placebo controlled trial. BMJ. 2002;324:203.

20. Gemmell CG. Staphylococcal scalded skin syndrome. J Med Microbiol. 1995;43:318.

21. Hanakawa Y, Schechter NM, Lin C, et al. Molecular mechanisms of blister formation in bullous impetigo and staphylococcal scalded skin syndrome. J Clin Invest. 2002;110:53.

22. Dajani AS. The scalded-skin syndrome: Relation to phage group II staphylococci. J Infect Dis. 1972;125:548.

23. Melish ME, Glascow LA, Turner MD, et al. The staphylococcal epidermolytic toxin: Its isolation, characterization, and site of action. Ann N Y Acad Sci. 1974;236:317.

24. Elias PM, Fritsch P, Epstein EH Jr. Staphylococcal scalded skin syndrome: Clinical features, pathogenesis, and recent microbiological and biochemical developments. Arch Dermatol. 1977;113:207.

25. Curran JP, Al-Salihi FL. Neonatal staphylococcal scalded skin syndrome: Massive outbreak due to an unusual phage type. Pediatrics. 1980;66:285.

26. Lina G, Gillet Y, Vandenesch F, et al. Toxin involvement in staphylococcal scalded skin syndrome. Clin Infect Dis. 1997;25:1369.

27. Shands KN, Schmid GP, Dan BB, et al. Toxic-shock syndrome in menstruating women: Its association with tampon use and Staphylococcus aureus and the clinical features in 52 cases. N Engl J Med. 1980;303:1436.

28. Institute of Medicine, National Academy of Science. Conference on the Toxic Shock Syndrome. Ann Intern Med. 1978;96:835.

29. Todd JT, Fishaut M, Kapral F, et al. Toxic shock syndrome associated with phage-group-I staphylococci. Lancet. 1978;2:1116.

30. Gustafson LT, Band JD, Hutcheson RH, et al. Pseudomonas folliculitis: An outbreak and review. Rev Infect Dis. 1983;5:1.

31. El Baze P, Thyss A, Caldini C, et al. Pseudomonas aeruginosa 0-11 folliculitis: Development into ecthyma gangrenosum in immunosuppressed patients. Arch Dermatol. 1985;121:873.

32. Stähelin-Massik J, Gnehm HE, Itin PH. Pseudomonas folliculitis in a young child. Pediatr Infect Dis J. 2000;19:362.

33. Noble WC. Gram-negative bacterial skin infections. Semin Dermatol. 1993;12:336.

34. Neubert U, Jansen H, Plewig G. Bacteriologic and immunologic aspects of gram-negative folliculitis: A study of 46 patients. Int J Dermatol. 1999;38:270.

35. Klotz SA, Drutz DJ, Huppert M, et al. Pityrosporum folliculitis: Its potential for confusion with skin lesions of systemic candidiasis. Arch Intern Med. 1982;142:2126.

36. Bufill JA, Lum LG, Caya JG, et al. Pityrosporum folliculitis after bone marrow transplantation. Ann Intern Med. 1988;108:560.

37. Archer-Dubon C, Icaza-Chivez ME, Orozco-Topete R. An epidemic outbreak of Malassezia folliculitis in three adult patients in an intensive care unit: A previously unrecognized nosocomial infection. Int J Dermatol. 1999;38:453.

38. Buchness MR, Lim HW, Hatcher VA, et al. Eosinophilic pustular folliculitis in the acquired immunodeficiency syndrome. N Engl J Med. 1988;318:1183.

39. Hedstrom SA. Treatment and prevention of recurrent staphylococcal furunculosis: Clinical and bacteriologic follow-up. Scand J Infect Dis. 1985;17:55.

40. Reagan DR, Doebbeling BN, Pfaller AM, et al. Elimination of coincident Staphylococcus aureus nasal and hand carriage with intranasal application of mupirocin calcium ointment. Ann Intern Med. 1991;114:101.

41. Wheat LJ, Kohler RB, Luft FC, et al. Long-term studies of the effect of rifampin on nasal carriage of coagulase-positive staphylococci. Rev Infect Dis. 1983;5 (Suppl):S459.

42. Darouiche R, Wright C, Hammill R, et al. Eradication of colonization by methicillin-resistant Staphylococcus aureus using oral minocycline-rifampin and topical mupirocin. Antimicrob Agents Chemother. 1991;35:1612.

43. Klempner MS, Styrt B. Prevention of recurrent staphylococcal skin infections with low-dose oral clindamycin therapy. JAMA. 1988;260:2682.

44. Allen AM, Taplin D, Twigg L. Cutaneous streptococcal infections in Vietnam. Arch Dermatol. 1971;104:271.

45. Hewitt WD, Farrar WE. Case report: Bacteremia and ecthyma caused by Streptococcus pyogenes in a patient with acquired immunodeficiency syndrome. Am J Med Sci. 1988;295:52.

46. Inglesby TV, O'Toole T, Henderson DA, et al. Anthrax as a biological weapon 2002: Updated recommendations for management. JAMA. 2002;287:2236.

47. Smego RA, Gebrain B, Desmangels G. Cutaneous manifestations of anthrax in rural Haiti. Clin Infect Dis. 1998;26:97.

48. Aksaray N, Cinaz P, Coskum U, et al. Cutaneous anthrax. Trop Geogr Med. 1990;42:168.

49. Swartz MN. Recognition and treatment of anthrax: An update. N Engl J Med. 2001;345:1621.

50. Centers for Disease Control and Prevention. Update: Investigation of bioterrorism-related anthrax and interim guidelines for exposure management and antimicrobial therapy, October 2001. MMWR Morb Mortal Wkly Rep. 2001;50:909.

51. Bernard P, Bedame C, Mounier M, et al. Streptococcal cause of erysipelas and cellulitis in adults. Arch Dermatol. 1989;125:779.

52. Jorup-Ronstrom C. Epidemiological, bacteriological and complicating features of erysipelas. Scand J Infect Dis. 1986;18:519.

53. Eriksson BKG. Anal colonization of group G β-hemolytic streptococci in relapsing erysipelas of the lower extremity. Clin Infect Dis. 1999;29:1319.

54. Fitzpatrick TB, Eisen AZ, Wolff K, et al, eds. Dermatology in General Medicine. New York: McGraw-Hill; 1971.

55. Guberman D, Gilead LT, Zlotogorski A, et al. Bullous erysipelas: A retrospective study of 26 patients. J Am Acad Dermatol. 1999;41:733.

56. Kerstens PJ, Endtz HP, Meis JF, et al. Erysipelas-like lesions associated with Campylobacter jejuni septicemia in patients with hypogammaglobulinemia. Eur J Clin Microbiol Infect Dis. 1992;11:842.

57. Bernard P, Chosidow O, Vaillant L, et al.. Oral pristinamycin versus standard penicillin regimen to treat erysipelas in adults: Randomized, non-inferiority open trial. BMJ. 2002;325:864.

58. Baddour LM, Bisno AL. Recurrent cellulitis after saphenous venectomy for coronary bypass surgery. Ann Intern Med. 1982;97:493.

59. Baddour LM, Bisno AL. Non-group A beta-hemolytic streptococcal cellulitis: Association with venous and lymphatic compromise. Am J Med. 1985;79:155.

60. Chmel H, Hamdy M. Recurrent streptococcal cellulitis complicating radical hysterectomy and radiation therapy. Obstet Gynecol. 1984;63:862.

61. Swartz MN. Cellulitis. N Engl J Med. 2004;350:904.

62. Simon MS, Cody RL. Cellulitis after axillary lymph node dissection for carcinoma of the breast. Am J Med. 1992;93:543.

63. Mertz KR, Baddour LM, Bell JL, et al. Breast cellulitis following breast conservation therapy: A novel complication of medical progress. Clin Infect Dis. 1998;26:481.

64. Ellison RT III, McGregor JA. Recurrent postcoital lower extremity streptococcal erythroderma in women: Streptococcal-sex syndrome. JAMA. 1987;257:3260.

65. Barzilae A, Choen HA. Isolation of group A streptococci from children with perianal cellulitis and from their siblings. Pediatr Infect Dis J. 1998;17:358.

66. Kielhofer MA, Brown B, Dall L. Influence of underlying disease process on the utility of cellulitis needle aspirates. Arch Intern Med. 1988;148:2451.

67. Sachs MK. The optimum use of needle aspiration in the bacteriologic diagnosis of cellulitis in adults. Arch Intern Med. 1980;150:1907.

68. Durvanel T, Auckenthaler R, Rohner P, et al. Quantitative cultures of biopsy specimens from cutaneous cellulitis. Arch Intern Med. 1989;149:293.

69. Sigurdsson AF, Gudmundsson S. The etiology of bacterial cellulitis as determined by fine-needle aspiration. Scand J Infect Dis. 1989;21:537.

70. Hook EW III, Hooton TM, Horton CA, et al. Microbiologic evaluation of cutaneous cellulitis in adults. Arch Intern Med. 1986;146:295.

71. Howe PM, Fajardo JE, Orcutt MA. Etiologic diagnosis of cellulitis: Comparison of aspirates obtained from the leading edge and the point of maximal inflammation. Pediatr Infect Dis J. 1987;6:685.

72. Grayson ML, Gibbons GW, Habershaw GM, et al. Use of ampicillin/sulbactam versus imipenem/cilastatin in the treatment of limb-threatening foot infections in diabetic patients. Clin Infect Dis. 1994;18:683.

73. Perl B, Gottehrer NP, Ravek D, et al. Cost effectiveness of blood cultures for adult patients with cellulitis. Clin Infect Dis. 1999;29:1483.

74. Woo PGY, Lum PML, Wong SSY, et al. Cellulitis complicating lymphedema. Eur J Clin Microbiol Infect Dis. 2000;19:294.

75. Markham RB, Polk BF. Seal finger. Rev Infect Dis. 1979;1:567.

76. Patel M, Ahrens JC, Moyer DV, et al. Pneumococcal soft-tissue infections: A problem deserving more recognition. Clin Infect Dis. 1994;19:149.

77. Kielbauch JA, Tauxe RV, Baker CN, et al. Helicobacter cinaedi associated bacteremia and cellulitis in immunocompromised patients. Ann Intern Med. 1994;121:90.

78. Horrevorts AM, Huysmans FTM, Koopman RJJ, et al. Cellulitis as first clinical presentation of disseminated cryptococcosis in renal transplant recipients. Scand J Infect Dis. 1994;26:623.

79. Waldor MK, Wilson B, Swartz M. Cellulitis caused by Legionella pneumophila. Clin Infect Dis. 1993;16:51.

80. Kilborn JA, Manz LA, O'Brien M, et al. Necrotizing cellulitis caused by *Legionella micdadei*. Am J Med. 1992;92:104.
81. Asmar BI, Bashour BN, Fleischmann LE. *Escherichia coli* cellulitis in children with idiopathic nephrotic syndrome. Clin Pediatr (Phila). 1987;26:592.
82. Gold WL, Salit IE. *Aeromonas hydrophila* infections of skin and soft tissue: Report of 11 cases and review. Clin Infect Dis. 1993;16:69.
83. Bonner JR, Coker AS, Berryman CR, et al. Spectrum of *Vibrio* infections in a Gulf Coast community. Ann Intern Med. 1983;99:464.
84. Chuang Y-C, Yuan C-Y, Liu C-Y, et al. *Vibrio vulnificus* infection in Taiwan: Report of 28 cases and review of clinical manifestations and treatment. Clin Infect Dis. 1992;15:271.
85. Arnold M, Woo M-L, French GL. *Vibrio vulnificus* septicemia presenting as spontaneous necrotizing cellulitis in a woman with hepatic cirrhosis. Scand J Infect Dis. 1989;21:727.
86. Lehman DF, Hardy JC. Stonefish envenomation. N Engl J Med. 1993;329:510.
87. Majeed HA, Quabazard Z, Hijasi Z, et al. The cutaneous manifestations in children with familial Mediterranean fever (recurrent hereditary polyserositis): A six-year study. QJM. 1990;75;607.
88. Morgan KW, Callen JP. Sweet's syndrome in acute myelogenous leukemia presenting as periorbital cellulitis with an infiltrate of leukemic cells. J Am Acad Dermatol. 2001;45:590.
89. Sheard RM, Pandey KR, Barnes ND, et al. Kawasaki disease presenting as orbital cellulitis. J Pediatr Ophthal Strabis. 2000;37:123.
90. Saulsbury FT, Cooper PH, Bracikowski A, et al. Eosinophilic cellulitis in a child. J Pediatr. 1983;102:266.
91. Taylor GW, Metzger A. Inflammatory carcinoma of the breast. Am J Cancer. 1938;33:33.
92. Faber K. Schroeder L, Thill M-P, et al. Carcinoma erysipeloides of the neck. Lancet. 2002;359:1025.
93. Groom AV, Wolsey DH, Naimi TS, et al. Community-acquired methicillin resistant *Staphylococcus aureus* in a rural American Indian Community. JAMA. 2001; 286:1201.
94. Stevens DL, Herr D, Lamperkis H, et al. Linezolid versus vancomycin for the treatment of methicillin-resistant *Staphylococcus aureus* infections. Clin Infect Dis. 2002;34:1481.
95. Kremer M, Zuckerman R, Avraham Z, et al. Long-term antimicrobial therapy in the prevention of recurrent soft-tissue infections. J Infect. 1991;22:37.
96. Belsey MA, Sinclair M, Roder MR, et al. *Corynebacterium diphtheriae* skin infections in Alabama and Louisiana: A factor in the epidemiology of diphtheria. N Engl J Med. 1969;280:135.
97. Gruner E, Opravil M, Altwegg M, et al. Nontoxigenic *Corynebacterium diphtheriae* isolated from intravenous drug users. Clin Infect Dis. 1994;18:94.
98. Koopman JS, Campbell J. The role of cutaneous diphtheria infections in a diphtheria epidemic. J Infect Dis. 1975;131:239.
99. Barker FG, Leppard BJ, Seal DV. Streptococcal necrotizing fasciitis: Comparison between histological and clinical features. J Clin Pathol. 1987;40:335.
100. Aitken DR, MaCkett MC, Smith LL. The changing pattern of hemolytic streptococcal gangrene. Ann Surg. 1982;117:561.
101. Stevens DL, Tanner MH, Winship J, et al. Severe group A streptococcal infections associated with a toxic shock-like syndrome and a scarlet fever toxin A. N Engl J Med. 1989;321:1.
102. Strasberg SM, Silver MS. Hemolytic streptococcus gangrene: An uncommon but frequently fatal infection in the antibiotic era. Am J Surg. 1968;115:763.
103. Meleney FL. Bacterial synergism in disease processes with a confirmation of the synergistic bacterial etiology of a certain type of progressive gangrene of the abdominal wall. Ann Surg. 1931;94:961.
104. Husseinzadeh N, Nahas WA, Manders EK, et al. Spontaneous occurrence of synergistic bacterial gangrene following external pelvic irradiation. Obstet Gynecol. 1984;63:859.
105. Bornstein DL, Weinberg AN, Swartz MN, et al. Anaerobic infections: Review of current experience. Medicine (Baltimore). 1964;43:207.
106. Davson J, Jones DM, Turner L. Diagnosis of Meleney's synergistic gangrene. Br J Surg. 1988;75:267.
107. Turner L, Jones DM, Davson J. Cutaneous amoebiasis: Case report. BMJ. 1985; 291:635.
108. Wolfson JS, Sober AJ, Rubin RH. Dermatologic manifestations in the compromised host. Annu Rev Med. 1983;14:205.
109. Wilson CB, Siber GR, O'Brein TF, et al. Phycomycotic gangrenous cellulitis. Arch Surg. 1976;111:531.
110. Weinberg WG, Wade BH, Cierny G III, et al. Invasive infection due to *Apophysomyces elegans* in immunocompetent hosts. Clin Infect Dis. 1993;17:881.
111. Case Records of the Massachusetts General Hospital: Case 31-2001: A 70-year old woman with end-stage renal disease and cutaneous ulcers. N Engl J Med. 2001; 345:1119.
112. Khalif RA, DeLima C, Silverberg A, et al. Calciphylaxis and systemic calcinosis. Arch Intern Med. 1990;150:956.
113. Cone LA, Woodward DA, Schlievert PM, et al. Clinical and bacteriologic observations of a toxic-shock-like syndrome due to *Streptococcus pyogenes*. N Engl J Med. 1987;317:146.
114. Coyle EA, Cha R, Ryback MJ. Influences of linezolid, penicillin, and clindamycin alone and in combination, on streptococcal pyrogenic exotoxin A release. Antimicrob Agents Chemother. 2003;47:1752.
115. Sarkany I, Taplin D, Blank H. The etiology and treatment of erythrasma. J Invest Dermatol. 1961;37:283.
116. Sindhuphak W, MacDonald E, Smith EB. Erythrasma: Overlooked or misdiagnosed. Int J Dermatol. 1985;24:95.
117. Takama H, Tamada Y, Yano K, et al. Pitted keratolysis: Clinical manifestations in 53 cases. Br J Dermatol. 1997;137:282.
118. Allman RM. Pressure ulcers among the elderly. N Engl J Med. 1989;320:850.
119. Karchmer AW, Gibbons GW. Foot infections in diabetes: Evaluation and management. In: Remington JS, Swartz MN, eds. Current Clinical Topics in Infectious Diseases, v. 14. Boston: Blackwell; 1994:7-10.
120. Gerding DM. Foot infections in diabetic patients: Role of anaerobes. Clin Infect Dis. 1995;20:5283.
121. Wheat LJ, Allen SD, Henry M, et al. Diabetic foot infections: Bacteriologic analysis. Arch Intern Med. 1986;146:1935.
122. Agger WA, Cogbill TH, Busch H Jr, et al. Wounds caused by corn-harvesting machines: An unusual source of infection due to gram-negative bacilli. Rev Infect Dis. 1986;8:927.
123. Weinstein MR, Litt M, Kertess DA, et al. Invasive infections due to a fish pathogen. N Engl J Med. 1997;337:589.
124. Baack BR, Kucan JO, Zook EG, et al. Hand infections secondary to catfish spines: Case reports and literature review. J Trauma. 1991;31:1432.
125. Benedict LM, Kusne S, Torre-Cisneros J, et al. Primary cutaneous fungal infection after solid-organ transplantation: Report of five cases and review. Clin Infect Dis. 1992;15:17.
126. Carey WP, Kaykova Y, Bandres JC, et al. Cutaneous protothecosis in a patient with AIDS and a severe functional neutrophil defect: Successful therapy with amphotericin B. Clin Infect Dis. 1997;25:1265.
127. Walsh SV, Johnson RA, Tahan SR. Protothecosis: An unusual cause of chronic subcutaneous and soft tissue infection. Am J Dermatopathol. 1998;20:379.
128. Novick NL, Tapia L, Bottone EJ. Invasive *Trichophyton rubrum* infection in an immunocompromised host. Am J Med. 1987;82:321.
129. Henrickson KJ, Flynn PM, Shenep JL, et al. Primary cutaneous *Bacillus cereus* infection in neutropenic children. Lancet. 1989;1:601.
130. Machado LS, Sleasman JW, Ford MJ. *Bacillus* species infection of the skin as a presentation of severe combined immunodeficiency disease. J Am Acad Dermatol. 1998;39:285.
131. Patterson JW, Kitces EN, Neafie RC. Cutaneous botryomycosis in a patient with acquired immunodeficiency syndrome. J Am Acad Dermatol. 1987;16:238.
132. Cline MS, Cummings OW, Goldman M, et al. Bacillary angiomatosis in a renal transplant recipient. Transplantation. 1999;67:296.
133. Karakas M, Aksungur VL, Homan S, et al. Bacillary angiomatosis on a region of burned skin in an immunocompetent patient. Br J Dermatol. 2000;143:609.
134. Cockerell CJ, LeBoit PE. Bacillary angiomatosis: A newly characterized, pseudoneoplastic, infectious, cutaneous vascular disorder. J Am Acad Dermatol. 1990;22:501.
135. Schwartzman WA. Infections due to *Rochalimaea:* The expanding clinical spectrum. Clin Infect Dis. 1992;15:893.
136. Relman DA, Loutit JS, Schmidt TM, et al. The agent of bacillary angiomatosis: An approach to the identification of uncultured pathogens. N Engl J Med. 1990;323:1573.
137. Olafsson S, Khan MA. Musculoskeletal features of acne, hidradenitis suppurativa, and dissecting cellulitis of the scalp. Rheum Dis Clin North Am. 1992;18:215.
138. Mitchell KM, Beck DF. Hidradenitis suppurativa. Surg Clin North Am. 2002;82:1187.
139. Jemec GBE, Faber M, Gutschik E, et al. The bacteriology of hidradenitis suppurativa. Dermatology. 1996;193:203.
140. Brook I. Microbiology of infected epidermal cysts. Arch Dermatol. 1989;125:1658.
141. Kingston ME, Mackey D. Skin clues in the diagnosis of life-threatening infections. Rev Infect Dis. 1986;8:1.
142. Bourelly PE, Grossman ME. Subcutaneous nodule as a manifestation of *Pseudomonas* sepsis in an immunocompromised host. Clin Infect Dis. 1998;26:188.
143. Huminer D, Siegman-Igra Y, Morduchowicz G, et al. Ecthyma gangrenosum without bacteremia: Report of six cases and review of the literature. Arch Intern Med. 1987;147:299.
144. Benoit FL. Chronic meningococcemia. Am J Med. 1963;35:103.
145. O'Brien JP, Goldenberg DL, Rice PA. Disseminated gonococcal infection: A prospective analysis of 49 patients and a review of pathophysiology and immune mechanisms. Medicine (Baltimore). 1983;62:395.
146. Chartrand SA, Harrison CJ. Buccal cellulitis reevaluated. Am J Dis Child. 1986; 140:891.
147. Walker JS, Corcoran KJ. Buccal cellulitis. Am J Emerg Med. 1990;8:542.
148. Drapkin MS, Wilson ME, Shrager SM, et al. Bacteremic *Hemophilus influenzae* type B cellulitis in the adult. Am J Med. 1977;63:449.
149. Bernard P, Mounier M, Acouturier P, et al. *Haemophilus influenzae* type B cellulitis of the lower extremity in a non-immunosuppressed elderly patient. Acta Dermatol Venereol (Stockh). 1990;70:359.
150. Burman WJ, Cohn DL, Reves RR, et al. Multifocal cellulitis and monarticular arthritis as manifestations of *Helicobacter cinaedi* bacteremia. Clin Infect Dis. 1995;20:564.
151. Alpert JS, Krous HF, Dalen JE. Pathogenesis of Osler's nodes. Ann Intern Med. 1976;85:471.
152. Roder BL, Wandall DA, Frimodt-Moller N, et al. Clinical features of *Staphylococcus aureus* endocarditis: A 10-year experience in Denmark. Arch Intern Med. 1999;159:462.
153. Cardullo AC, Silvers DN, Grossman ME. Janeway lesions and Osler's nodes: A review of histopathologic findings. J Am Acad Dermatol. 1990;22:1088.

154. Balandral L, Rothschild H, Pugh N, et al. A cutaneous manifestation of systemic candidiasis. Ann Intern Med. 1973;78:400.

155. Jarowski CI, Fialk MA, Murray HW, et al. Fever, rash, and muscle tenderness: A distinctive clinical presentation of disseminated candidiasis. Arch Intern Med. 1978;138:544.

156. Wilson HD, Haltalin KC. Acute necrotizing fasciitis in childhood. Am J Dis Child. 1973;125:591.

157. Stone HH, Martin JJ Jr. Synergistic necrotizing cellulitis. Ann Surg. 1972;175:702.

158. George WL. Other infections of skin, soft tissue, and muscle. In: Finegold SM, George WL, eds. Anaerobic Infections in Humans. New York: Academic; 1989; 492-504.

159. Moses AE, Hardan I, Simhon A, et al. *Clostridium septicum* bacteremia and diffuse spreading cellulitis of the head and neck in a leukemic patient. Rev Infect Dis. 1991;15:525.

160. MacLennan JD. The histotoxic clostridial infections of man. Bacteriol Rev. 1962; 26:177.

161. Bryant P, Carapetis J, Matussek J, et al. Recurrent crepitant cellulitis caused by *Clostridium perfringens*. Pediatr Infect. Dis J. 2002;21:1173.

162. Finegold SM. Anaerobic Bacteria in Human Disease. New York: Academic Press; 1977.

163. Bessman AN, Wagner W. Nonclostridial gas gangrene. JAMA. 1975;233:958.

164. Green RJ, Dafoe DC, Raffin TA. Necrotizing fasciitis. Chest. 1996;110:219.

165. Stevens SL. Invasive group A streptococcus infections. Clin Infect Dis. 1992;14:2.

166. Brogan TV, Nizet V, Waldhausen JHT, et al. Group A streptococcal necrotizing fasciitis complicating varicella: A series of fourteen patients. Pediatr Infect Dis J. 1995;14:588.

167. Wilson GJ, Talkington DF, Guber W, et al. Group A streptococcal necrotizing fasciitis following varicella in children: Case reports and review. Clin Infect Dis. 1995;20:1333.

168. Demers B, Simor AE, Vellend H, et al. Severe invasive group A streptococcal infections in Ontario, Canada: 1987-1991. Clin Infect Dis. 1993;16:792.

169. Musser JM, Hauser AR, Kim MH, et al. *Streptococcus pyogenes* causing toxic-shock-syndrome and other invasive diseases: Clonal diversity and pyrogenic exotoxin expression. Proc Natl Acad Sci U S A. 1991;88:2668.

170. Cleary PP, Kaplan EL, Handley JP, et al. Clonal basis for resurgence of serious *Streptococcus pyogenes* disease in the 1980s. Lancet. 1992;339:518.

171. Casali RE, Tucker WE, Petrino RA, et al. Postoperative necrotizing fasciitis of the abdominal wall. Am J Surg. 1980;140:787.

172. Galbut DL, Gerber DL, Belgraier AH. Spontaneous necrotizing fasciitis: Occurrence secondary to occult diverticulitis. JAMA. 1977;238:2302.

173. Barza MJ, Proppe KH. Case records of the Massachusetts General Hospital. N Engl J Med. 1979;301.370.

174. Schecter W, Meyer A, Schecter G, et al. Necrotizing fasciitis of the upper extremity. J Hand Surg. 1982;7:15.

175. Lally KP, Atkinson JB, Woolley MM, et al. Necrotizing fasciitis: A serious sequela of omphalitis in the newborn. Ann Surg. 1984;199;101.

176. Sudarsky LA, Laschinger JC, Coppa GF, et al. Improved results from a standardized approach in treating patients with necrotizing fasciitis. Ann Surg. 1987;206:661.

177. Iorianni P, Oliver GC. Synergistic soft tissue infections of the perineum. Dis Colon Rectum. 1992;35:640.

178. Nickel JC, Morales A. Necrotizing fasciitis of the male genitalia (Fournier's gangrene). Can Med Assoc J. 1983;129:445.

179. Kronish JW, McLeish WM. Eyelid necrosis and periorbital necrotizing fasciitis: Report of a case and review of the literature. Ophthalmology. 1991;98:92.

180. Rapoport Y, Himelfarb MZ, Zikk D, et al. Cervical necrotizing fasciitis of odontogenic origin. Oral Surg Oral Med Oral Pathol. 1991;72:15.

181. Margolis RD, Cohen KR, Loftus MJ, et al. Nonodontogenic β-hemolytic necrotizing fasciitis of the face. J Oral Maxillofac Surg. 1989;47:1098.

182. Banerjee AR, Murty GE, Moir AA, et al. Cervical necrotizing fasciitis: A distinct clinocopathological entity? J Laryngol Otol. 1996;110:81.

183. Murphy JJ, Granger R, Blair GK, et al. Necrotizing fasciitis in childhood. J Pediatr Surg. 1995;30:1131.

184. Hsueh P-R, Wu J-J, Hsiue T-R, et al. Bacteremic necrotizing fasciitis due to *Flavobacterium odoratum*. Clin Infect Dis. 1995;21:1337.

185. Zipper RP, Bustamente MA, Khatib R. *Serratia marcescens:* A single pathogen in necrotizing fasciitis. Clin Infect Dis. 1996;23:648.

186. Brivet F, Guibert M, Kiredjian M, et al. Necrotizing fasciitis, bacteremia, and multiorgan failure caused by *Ochrobactrum anthropi*. Clin Infect Dis. 1993;17:516.

187. Stamenkovic I, Lew PD. Early recognition of potentially fatal necrotizing fasciitis: Use of frozen-section biopsy. N Engl J Med. 1984;310:1689.

188. Walshaw CF, Deans H. CT findings in necrotizing fasciitis—a report of four cases. Clin Radiol. 1996;51:429.

189. Schmid MR, Kossman T, Duewell S. Differentiation of necrotizing fasciitis and cellulitis using MR imaging. AJR Am J Roentgenol. 1998;170:615.

190. Baxter CR. Surgical management of soft tissue infections. Surg Clin North Am. 1972;52:1483.

191. Talan DA, Citron DM, Abrahamian FM, et al. Bacteriologic analysis of infected dog and cat bites. N Engl J Med. 1999;340:85.

192. Biderman P, Hiatt JR. Management of soft-tissue infections of the upper extremity in parenteral drug abusers. Am J Surg. 1987;154:526.

193. Aduan RP, Fauci AS, Dale DC, et al. Factitious fever and self-induced infection: A report of 32 cases and review of the literature. Ann Intern Med. 1979;90:230.

194. Reich P, Gottfried LA. Factitious disorders in a teaching hospital. Ann Intern Med. 1983;99:240.

195. Dreskin SC, Gallin JI. Evolution of the hyperimmunoglobulin E and recurrent infection (HIE, Job's) syndrome in a young girl. J Allergy Clin Immunol. 1987;80:746.

196. Curnutte JT, Boxer LA. Clinically significant phagocytic cell defects. In: Remington JS, Swartz MN, eds. Current Clinical Topics in Infectious Diseases, v. 6. New York: McGraw-Hill; 1985:103-156.

197. Brook I, Frazier EH. Aerobic and anaerobic bacteriology of wounds and cutaneous abscesses. Arch Surg. 1990;125:1990.

198. Curley RK, Hayward T, Holden CA. Cutaneous abscesses due to systemic nocardiosis. Clin Exp Dermatol. 1990;15:459.

199. Dan M, Somer I, Knobel B, et al. Cutaneous manifestations of infection with *Corynebacterium* group JK. Rev Infect Dis. 1988;10:1204.

CHAPTER **87**

Myositis

MARK S. PASTERNACK
MORTON N. SWARTZ

Infection of skeletal muscle (infectious myositis) is uncommon. When it occurs, a wide range of organisms may be responsible: bacteria, mycobacteria, fungi, viruses, and parasitic agents. Bacteria invade muscle either from contiguous sites of infection (skin and subcutaneous abscesses, penetrating wounds, decubitus ulcers, osteomyelitis) or by hematogenous spread from a distant focus. It is helpful to categorize infectious myositis on the basis of clinical manifestations. These may be very distinctive, as in clostridial gas gangrene, and suggest the specific etiologic agent; or they may be very nonspecific, as in the myalgias of viral infections and infective endocarditis (Table 87-1). In certain instances (e.g., psoas abscess), it is the anatomic location rather than the morphologic characteristics of the lesion or the nature of the infecting agent that distinguishes the particular type of muscle infection.

PYOMYOSITIS

Pyomyositis is an acute bacterial infection of skeletal muscle that usually is caused by *Staphylococcus aureus.* The accumulation of pus is always intramuscular initially and is not secondary to infection of adjacent skin, soft tissue, or bone. Clinically, it is characterized by fever, localized muscle pain and stiffness, swelling, and tenderness.

Pathogenesis and Pathologic Characteristics

Bacterial infections of muscle usually occur after a penetrating wound, prolonged vascular insufficiency in an extremity, or a contiguous infection. Bacteremic spread of infection to skeletal muscle is extremely uncommon. Among fatal cases of staphylococcal septicemia, abscesses in skeletal muscle are found in fewer than 1%.[1] Pyomyositis (primary muscle abscess) is a bacterial infection of muscle that occurs in the absence of a predisposing site of infection. *S. aureus* is the most common cause.[2,3] Blood cultures are positive in 5% to 35% of the cases at the time of clinical manifestation; metastatic infections in tissue other than muscle are rare.

Most cases of pyomyositis occur in the tropics; hence, the term *tropical pyomyositis.* It accounts for 1% to 4% of hospital admissions in some tropical areas.[2,4] In the United States, pyomyositis is very uncommon (only about 100 cases reported between 1970 and 1990 in North America); it occurs both in persons who have recently immigrated from the tropics and in those who have always resided in a temperate climate.[5,6] It occurs at all ages—in the tropics more frequently among children, but in North America more often in adults and the elderly.[5] As yet, no convincing evidence relating pyomyositis causally to predisposing circumstances peculiar to the tropics (e.g., malaria, filariasis, arbovirus infection) has been developed. However, an association between *Toxocara canis* infection (visceral larva migrans) and staphylococcal pyomyositis has been proposed.[7] Migration of the guinea worm, *Dracunculus medinensis,* in the deep connective tissues

TABLE 87-1 Classification of Infectious Myositis

Type of Process	Clinical Pattern	Principal Specific Causes

Pyogenic and predominantly localized (spreading by contiguity)	Pyomyositis	*Staphylococcus aureus*
		Group A streptococcus (occasionally)
		Other gram-positive cocci (rarely):
		    Group B, C, or G streptococci
		    Streptococcus pneumoniae
		Gram-negative bacilli (rarely)
		Anaerobic bacteria (rarely):
		    Fusobacterium necrophorum
		    Clostridia
		Mycobacteria (rarely):
		    Mycobacterium tuberculosis
		    Mycobacterium avium-intracellulare
		Fungi (rarely):
		    Cryptococcus neoformans

	Gas gangrene	*Clostridium perfringens*; occasionally other histotoxic clostridial species

	Nonclostridial (crepitant) myositis
	    Anaerobic streptococcal gangrene
	    Group A streptococcal necrotizing myositis
	    Synergistic nonclostridial anaerobic myonecrosis
		
		Peptostreptococcus (plus group A streptococci or *S. aureus*)
		Group A streptococcus
		Mixed infections: *Bacteroides* and other anaerobic non–spore-forming gram-negative bacilli; *Peptostreptococcus* and various streptococci; *Escherichia coli; Klebsiella; Enterobacter*

	Infected vascular gangrene *Aeromonas hydrophila* myonecrosis Psoas abscess	Same as for synergistic nonclostridial anaerobic myonecrosis *A. hydrophila* Gram-negative bacilli; *S. aureus;* mixed infections; *M. tuberculosis*
Nonpyogenic and predominantly generalized	Myalgias	Viral infections (e.g., influenza, dengue); infective endocarditis; bacteremias (e.g., meningococcemia); rickettsioses (e.g., Rocky Mountain spotted fever): toxoplasmosis
	Pleurodynia Myalgias with eosinophilia Trichinosis Cysticercosis (also subcutaneous nodules) Muscle degeneration and destruction associated with infections elsewhere	Coxsackievirus B *Trichinella spiralis* *Taenia solium*
	Acute rhabdomyolysis	Influenza, echovirus, coxsackie and Epstein-Barr viruses, *Legionella*

of the lower extremities may be complicated by staphylococcal abscesses. However, these are located between muscle groups and are not the intramuscular abscesses typical of pyomyositis. About 40% of cases in temperate climates lack any relevant underlying disease, but the remainder have possible predisposing conditions: diabetes mellitus; alcoholic liver disease; corticosteroid therapy; immunosuppressive illnesses such as leukemia, lymphoma, or other hematologic processes (Felty's syndrome, myelodysplasia, sickle cell disease, cyclic neutropenia) and their cytotoxic therapies; and human immunodeficiency virus (HIV) infection.[5,6]

Pyomyositis has been reported in more than 50 patients with HIV infection, with or without acquired immunodeficiency syndrome (AIDS) (including one neonate); in the majority of these patients, it was caused by *S. aureus*.[5,8-13] The predisposition to pyomyositis in patients with AIDS probably stems from the combination of defective bactericidal activity of neutrophils,[14,15] the underlying cell-mediated immunodeficiency, and the potential for muscle injury (HIV myopathy, zidovudine-associated mitochondrial myopathy, myositis from parasitic disease, *Mycobacterium avium* complex infection) associated with this disease. Although *S. aureus* is the etiologic agent in the majority of HIV-associated cases, *Salmonella* accounts for 10% and streptococci 5% of pyomyositis episodes in this population.[13] Pyomyositis has been reported in 12 intravenous drug abusers; it was caused by *S. aureus* in half of these patients and by either gram-negative bacilli or multiple organisms (including anaerobes) in the remainder.[16] AIDS was a contributing factor in five patients. Although pyomyositis is a rare complication of bacterial endocarditis, it was observed in an intravenous drug abuser who had left-sided *S. aureus* endocarditis.[17]

The presumed pathogenesis of pyomyositis involves a prior bacteremia, commonly asymptomatic and transient. Because traumatizing of muscle (locus minoris resistentiae) is necessary to produce pyomyositis in experimental animals after intravenous injection of *S. aureus*,[18] a role for local mechanical injury has been hypothesized.

Clinical Findings

In 20% to 50% of cases, there has been recent blunt trauma to or vigorous exercise of the involved area. The clinical picture often involves three stages. In the first or invasive stage, the onset is subacute with variable fever, local swelling with or without erythema, mild pain, and minimal tenderness. The area is indurated or has a wooden consistency. This stage is often overlooked. Because the initial swelling is firm and pain is not striking, attention is directed away from an infectious cause. Aspiration, if attempted, yields no pus. The second or suppurative stage occurs 10 to 21 or more days later, and this is the time when most patients are seen and diagnosed. Distinct muscle tenderness and swelling (tending to conform to the shape of the involved muscle) are present, and the patient is febrile. The overlying skin is intact and warm, and erythema is commonly absent. At this point, pus can be aspirated from the involved muscle. In the third stage, systemic manifestations of sepsis and local findings of erythema, exquisite tenderness, and fluctuance are striking. If untreated, the infection can progress to metastatic abscesses, shock, and renal failure. The progression of pyomyositis from the initial invasive stage, associated with muscle inflammation and swelling, to the suppurative stage with focal abscess formation, was documented by serial imaging in a patient whose infection was initially managed with antibiotic therapy.[19]

Occasionally, the onset is acute rather than subacute, with malaise, chills, and high fever. Rarely, the clinical picture is combined with that of toxic shock syndrome.[20,21] This is a particular risk of myositis caused by group A β-hemolytic streptococci (see later discussion). Because the muscle abscesses are contained by the overlying fascia, local erythema and heat may be minimal until the process extends through to the subcutaneous tissues some days to weeks later. Regional lymphadenitis is not a feature. Usually only a single muscle group is involved, but multiple muscle abscesses occur in up to 40% of the patients. The most frequent sites of involvement are the large muscles of the lower extremities (e.g., quadriceps femoris, gluteus

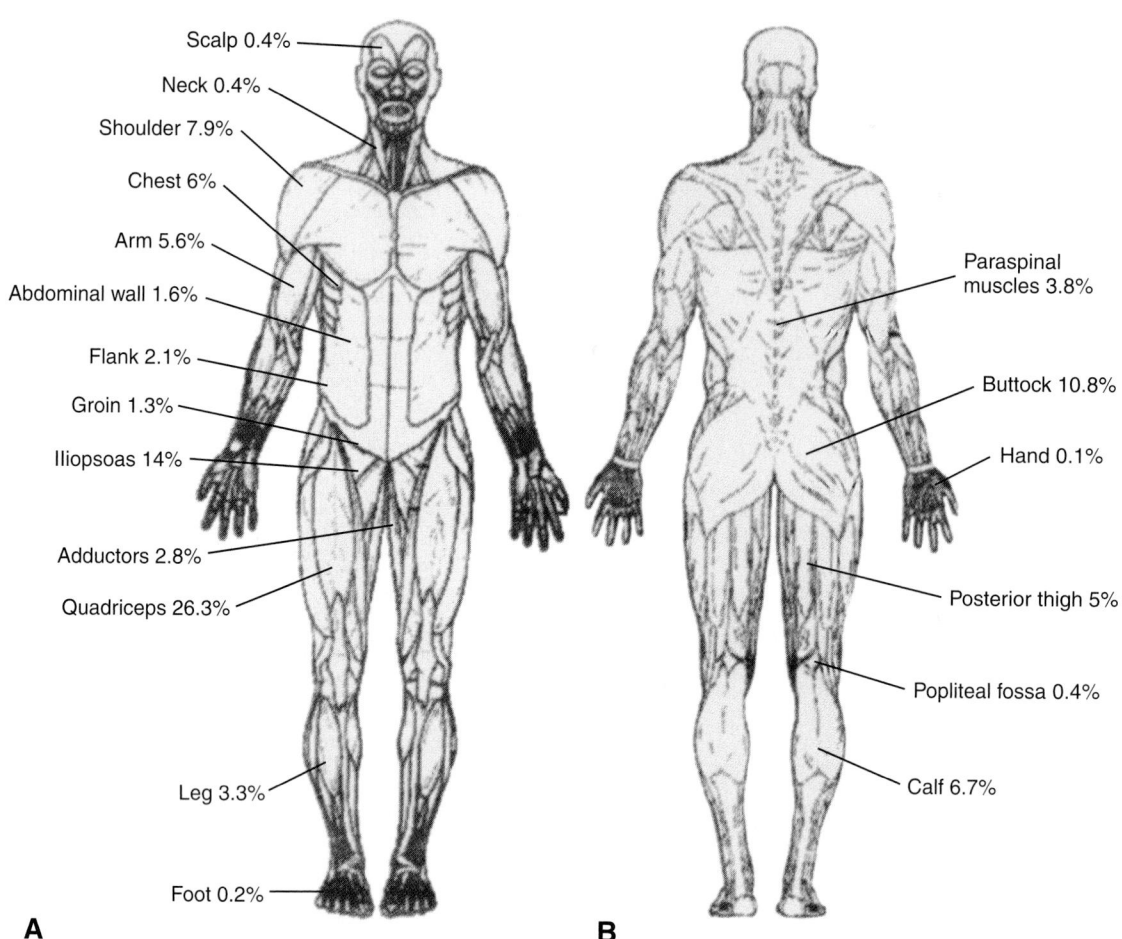

FIGURE 87-1. A and **B,** Distribution of sites of pyomyositis. *(Adapted from Bickels J, Ben-Sira L, Kessler A, Wientroub S. Primary pyomyositis. J Bone Joint Surg Am. 2002;84:2277-2286. Copyright © 2002. The Journal of Bone and Joint Surgery, Inc.)*

group) and the trunk muscles, but a variety of other muscles can be involved (Fig. 87-1). Involvement of the abdominal muscles is uncommon but noteworthy, because it may mimic an acute abdomen.[16,22]

A leukocytosis occurs. Eosinophilia is common in patients with tropical pyomyositis (even in the presence of a prominent leukocytosis) and appears to reflect the prevalence of parasitic infestation. Serum muscle enzyme levels may be elevated, particularly with severe streptococcal disease, but they frequently are normal despite gross muscle destruction. However, marked rhabdomyolysis with myoglobinuria and acute renal failure was reported in a patient with pyomyositis.[23]

Etiologic Agents

S. aureus is responsible for 95% of the cases in tropical areas. In North America, *S. aureus* is the cause of 66% to 70% of cases.[5,6] Group A streptococci account for 1% to 5% of the cases. Other gram-positive organisms uncommonly implicated in pyomyositis include various streptococci (groups B, C, and G), *Streptococcus pneumoniae,*[24] and *Streptococcus anginosus.* Other very rare causes include Enterobacteriaceae *(Escherichia coli, Klebsiella oxytoca, Klebsiella pneumoniae, Serratia marcescens, Morganella morganii,*[11] *Citrobacter freundii, Salmonella* spp.[25]*), Yersinia enterocolitica, Neisseria gonorrhoeae, Haemophilus influenzae,* and *Aeromonas hydrophila.*[3,5,6] Anaerobes *(Fusobacterium nucleatum, Fusobacterium necrophorum,*[26] *Veillonella* spp.,[27] oral anaerobic streptococci,[28] and *Clostridium septicum)* have been the cause in several cases. *Burkholderia mallei* and *Burkholderia pseudomallei* in the past have very rarely caused abscesses in muscle in the septicemic or chronic suppurative forms of the diseases they produce (glanders and melioidosis, respectively).

Aspergillus fumigatus has caused a localized muscle abscess in rare patients with myelodysplasia or AIDS and in patients who have received corticosteroids. Pathogenic yeasts can cause myositis on rare occasion. Pyomyositis due to *Cryptococcus neoformans* was reported in an immunocompromised host.[29] Hematogenously disseminated candidiasis in neutropenic patients can manifest with fever and muscle pain. The scattered *Candida* abscesses in the muscle are too small to localize by symptoms and physical examination, but myositis in these patients is often accompanied by small, tender, erythematous skin lesions. Punch biopsy of a skin lesion shows numerous *Candida* organisms in the dermis. Tuberculous pyomyositis occurred in a patient with disseminated tuberculosis,[30,31] and necrotizing pyomyositis due to *M. avium* complex occurred in a patient with AIDS.[12] Extrapulmonary *Pneumocystis jirovecii* infection is relatively uncommon in patients with AIDS, but in one patient it manifested as an intramuscular, localized, painful thigh swelling with typical granulomatous histopathology.[32]

Differential Diagnosis

Early in the course of pyomyositis, other diagnoses may be suspected, particularly in nontropical areas: fever of obscure origin (in the early phase, when localizing findings may be minimal or absent), osteomyelitis, septic arthritis, appendicitis or diverticulitis, muscle strain, contusion or hematoma, muscle rupture, and thrombophlebitis. Iliopsoas myositis has mimicked appendicitis[33]; iliacus pyomyositis has mimicked septic arthritis of the hip[34]; and pyriformis muscle pyomyositis has simulated an epidural abscess because of severe back and radiating (sciatic) leg pain.[35] Muscle infarction is an uncommon condition that occurs most frequently in the quadriceps in poorly controlled diabetics with nephropathy, neuropathy, and hypertension. It may suggest pyomyositis because of the acute onset of pain and presence of tender local swelling, but, in contrast to pyomyositis, fever is absent.[36] In the patient with multiple sites of muscle involvement and eosinophilia (from incidental parasitic infestation), the picture may suggest trichinosis. This resemblance ends after localized swellings become prominent and markedly tender. Rupture of the muscle abscess through the fascia into subcutaneous tissues may suggest the diagnosis of cellulitis. The presence of a slowly enlarging, painful mass in an extremity of a patient with only low-grade fever may suggest the diagnosis of sarcoma. Pyomyositis of the pectoral muscle can pose a particular problem in diagnosis because it must be distinguished not only from muscle rupture, hematoma, and sarcoma but also from cryptic abscessed subpectoral nodes developing via lymphatic extension of an initiating infection on the thumb or index finger of the ipsilateral hand. Streptococcal necrotizing fasciitis, like gangrenous streptococcal myositis, manifests initially with local pain disproportionate to any physical findings. Localized swelling, tenderness, and erythema ensue, but only in advanced stages are the characteristic violaceous skin changes, bullae, and frank skin necrosis seen overlying areas of fascial necrosis. Rapid frozen-section biopsy or surgical exploration may be needed to distinguish among these processes.

Diagnosis

Prompt imaging is essential in the evaluation of patients with focal soft tissue pain and fever. Plain films can demonstrate focal soft tissue swelling, the presence of gas in the soft tissues, and the presence of any primary skeletal abnormalities (e.g., osteomyelitis, osteosarcoma). Ultrasonography is readily accessible and can demonstrate muscle enlargement in the initial stage of pyomyositis; it can also show the presence of focal abscess formation in the suppurative stage of disease, through the presence of hypoechoic areas with internal echoes,[37] especially if symptoms are localized in an extremity. Ultrasound assessment of the hip can detect the presence of a joint effusion, but it may be less sensitive in assessing the deep pelvic musculature. Ultrasonography is almost always followed by cross-sectional imaging to gain greater anatomic detail and should not delay definitive imaging studies in acutely ill patients.

Magnetic resonance imaging (MRI) has proved invaluable in the assessment of patients with pyomyositis because it identifies focal muscle edema and localizes the presence of focal abscess formation with great precision. MRI scanning can demonstrate enlargement of involved muscles and a slight increase in signal intensity on T_1-weighted images in the involved area, with a hypointense central area and a surrounding gadolinium-enhanced rim; it also shows a diffuse increase in signal intensity on T_2-weighted images, with a central high-signal-intensity fluid collection surrounded by a low-intensity rim.[38] Computed tomographic (CT) scanning is an alternative cross-sectional modality that provides less anatomic detail at the inflammatory stage of myositis but is helpful when used to guide percutaneous drainage of an established muscle abscess. CT can reveal low-density areas with loss of muscle planes, a central fluid collection, and a surrounding rim of contrast enhancement characteristic of pyomyositis.[38] Enlargement of the involved muscle is usually evident. A superimposed cellulitis may sometimes be evident on CT, namely, skin thickening, stranding of subcutaneous fat with blurring of fat and fascial planes, and subcutaneous venous distention. Radionuclide (gallium 67) scanning shows diffuse uptake in the involved area but does not differentiate an intramuscular abscess from necrotizing myositis or necrotizing fasciitis. It may be helpful on occasion when several areas of pyomyositis are present, or in patients with diffuse myalgias in the early phase of the disease. The need for delayed imaging limits its utility in the routine management of myositis.

Presumptive Therapy

Surgical (open, ultrasound- or CT-guided percutaneous) drainage of all abscesses is essential. Initial antibiotic therapy should consist of intravenous administration of a β-lactamase–resistant penicillin because of the preponderance of penicillin-resistant *S. aureus* isolates from such abscesses. In a chronically ill and often-hospitalized patient, the possibility of primary methicillin-resistant *S. aureus* (MRSA) infection should lead to the consideration of initial empiric vancomycin therapy. If a group A streptococcus is isolated, treatment should be changed to high-dose penicillin G and clindamycin (see later discussion). Early modification of initial antimicrobial therapy is based on interpretation of a Gram-stained smear of pus and subsequent results of cultures and susceptibility testing. Continued fever after surgical or percutaneous needle drainage of a muscle abscess while the patient is receiving appropriate antimicrobial therapy should suggest the presence of other undrained suppurative foci. Pyomyositis may be complicated by a compartment syndrome, particularly if it occurs in the anterior tibial compartment, and may require additional surgical drainage, fasciotomies, and débridement beyond simple percutaneous drainage.[39]

The prognosis after definitive treatment for pyomyositis is excellent, unless staphylococcal or streptococcal infection is complicated by the presence of the toxic shock syndrome.[20,21] The multiorgan failure associated with established toxic shock carries a disturbingly high mortality rate. In the absence of toxic shock, definitive drainage accompanied by prolonged effective antibiotic therapy usually leads to complete resolution of infection with little or no long-term morbidity, even in immunocompromised individuals. Delays in diagnosis and definitive drainage (when drainage is necessary) have led to muscle fibrosis and/or the need for widespread excision and subsequent functional disability.

GROUP A STREPTOCOCCAL NECROTIZING MYOSITIS

In addition to producing an occasional case of typical pyomyositis with abscess formation, on rare occasions group A streptococci cause a fulminant form of myositis (peracute streptococcal pyomyositis, streptococcal necrotizing myositis, streptococcal myonecrosis or spontaneous streptococcal gangrenous myositis).[40-42] Reports such as that of 1 case of myositis and 3 cases of myositis with necrotizing fasciitis, among 20 patients in an outbreak of invasive group A streptococcal infections associated with a toxic shock–like syndrome, suggest that this form of infection may be more frequent now than in the past.[42,43] The entire clinical course may be telescoped to 2 to 3 days. The clinical features are usually intense pain, boardlike swelling of the affected muscle, and fever. The overlying skin may be uninvolved, or it may become erythematous or violaceous and contain petechiae and bullae.[44] Most cases involve the extremities and appear to develop spontaneously without antecedent pharyngitis or tonsillitis. Bacteremia and toxemia are prominent features and contribute to the very high mortality rate (80% to 100%).[43] The rapid spread of infection in a closed compartment of muscles can markedly raise intramuscular pressure, resulting in further necrosis of muscle.[44,45] However, both processes can be simultaneously present in the same area. The compartment syndrome with group A streptococcal myositis (e.g., a tibial compartment syndrome) may develop in the absence of fascial and muscle necrosis but be associated with muscle bulging secondary to edema and serosanguineous exudate.[46] Compartment pressures are elevated. The clinical features of such a syndrome include weakness of the compartment muscles, which are swollen and tender; severe pain on movement of the lower leg; and overlying cutaneous hyperesthesia.

Streptococcal necrotizing fasciitis may resemble streptococcal myositis clinically, although the presence of tense bullae and areas of skin necrosis are more suggestive of the former. Sometimes both conditions are present together. MRI may disclose the predominantly involved structure, but urgent surgical exploration, always necessary in the setting of suspected toxic shock associated with focal pain and swelling, should provide a clear answer. A rare case of acute streptococcal myositis with the toxic shock syndrome caused by group G streptococcus has been reported.[47]

Laboratory findings include a leukocytosis and an elevated serum creatine phosphokinase level. This is in marked distinction to non-streptococcal forms of pyomyositis, in which little if any elevation of the creatine phosphokinase concentration is seen. This disease is a medical emergency requiring prompt clinical diagnosis with verification at surgery. Distinguishing group A streptococcal necrotizing myositis from streptococcal necrotizing fasciitis and spontaneous clostridial myonecrosis may be difficult clinically, but gas in the tissue suggests spontaneous clostridial myonecrosis. In any case, all three diseases require prompt surgical exploration. Sonography, CT, or MRI scanning usually reveals muscle swelling and fluid collection in muscle compartments. If prolonged delays are encountered in the pursuit of imaging studies, proceeding directly to surgical exploration with an initial limited surgical approach for diagnostic purposes is justified. Early, aggressive surgical intervention with fasciotomy and débridement of necrotic tissue is indicated; in some instances, amputation is required. If the operative Gram stain suggests streptococcal infection, antibiotic therapy should consist of high doses of penicillin G (3 million units intravenously every 3 hours, or 4 million units every 4 hours, or adjusted appropriately for renal insufficiency) along with clindamycin (600 mg intravenously every 6 to 8 hours).[48] Clinical experience suggests that clindamycin has greater efficacy against group A streptococci in this life-threatening infection ("Eagle effect"), because of its greater activity against large bacterial populations in stationary phase growth, its more sustained postantibiotic effect, and its suppression of the production of toxin and other virulence factors by virtue of its inhibition of bacterial protein synthesis.[42] The use of intravenous immunoglobulin G as an adjunct in the treatment of streptococcal toxic shock, to neutralize streptococcal exotoxins and perhaps to modulate the host immune response, has gained popularity on the basis of retrospective studies and one small prospective randomized trial,[49] but conclusive evidence supporting its use remains limited.[50]

GAS GANGRENE (CLOSTRIDIAL MYONECROSIS)

Gas gangrene is a rapidly progressive, life-threatening, toxemic infection of skeletal muscle caused by clostridia (principally *Clostridium perfringens*). It usually occurs after muscle injury and contamination, as in a dirty traumatic wound, or sometimes after surgery. Nontraumatic gas gangrene, usually caused by *Clostridium septicum,* is a complication of bacteremia, which often is the result of an occult gastrointestinal mucosal lesion such as an adenocarcinoma or a complication of neutropenic colitis.

Pathogenesis and Pathologic Characteristics

Gas gangrene occurs in settings that have in common muscle injury and contamination with soil or other foreign material containing spores of *C. perfringens* or other histotoxic clostridial species. These include (1) accidental traumatic civilian injuries such as compound fracture[51]; (2) penetrating war wounds[52]; (3) surgical wounds, particularly after bowel or biliary tract surgery[53] or septic abortion; and (4) arterial insufficiency in an extremity.[53] Rare cases of gas gangrene have occurred after parenteral injection of medication, particularly epinephrine in oil; subcutaneous insulin administration[54]; and parenteral injection of methamphetamine or heroin.[55] A fulminant case was described as beginning at the site of a simple venipuncture in a granulocytopenic patient.[53] *C. perfringens* organisms usually are present in large numbers as normal flora in human feces and therefore can endogenously contaminate skin surfaces. Despite a high frequency (up to 88%) of clostridial contamination of major traumatic, open wounds, the incidence of gas gangrene in this setting is only 1% to 2%,[56] emphasizing the importance of devitalized tissue and the presence of foreign bodies in the pathogenesis of gas gangrene. The minimal dose of *C. perfringens* needed to produce fatal gas gangrene in experimental animals is reduced by a factor of 10^6 if the organism is injected into devitalized muscle contaminated with sterile dirt rather than into normal muscle. The policy of prompt, thorough débridement and of leaving

wounds open has decreased the incidence of gas gangrene in wartime injuries; only 22 cases among 139,000 combat casualties in Vietnam were reported.[57]

Gas gangrene may occasionally develop in the absence of an obvious external wound. This form of clostridial myonecrosis is designated spontaneous, nontraumatic gas gangrene. Its principal cause is *C. septicum,* a relatively aerotolerant species, which is spread by the bacteremic route and is apparently more capable of establishing infection without significant antecedent tissue injury than are other clostridia. Intestinal tract abnormalities (colon cancer, diverticulitis, bowel infarction, necrotizing enterocolitis, volvulus) are the major predisposing conditions.[58] Colon cancer, often cryptic, is the most common of these, occurring in up to 88% of patients with *C. septicum* bacteremia. Other predisposing disorders include leukemia, other causes of neutropenia, and diabetes mellitus. The primary source of the organism is probably mucosal ulceration or perforation of the intestinal tract. The spread by the bacteremic route probably accounts for the bilateral (but separated) involvement observed in a few patients with spontaneous gas gangrene. However, it may manifest in the buttocks or flanks as the consequence of an intra-abdominal catastrophe, with rapid extension of infection along the iliopsoas or other deep muscle groups. The progression of *C. septicum* spontaneous gas gangrene may be even more fulminant than that of traumatic *C. perfringens* gas gangrene; the mortality rate of the former is 67% to 100%, with most patients dying within 24 hours after onset.[58]

The involved muscle undergoes rapid disintegration. Initially, it may exhibit only pallor, edema, and loss of elasticity. When examined in the operating room, it fails to contract on stimulation and does not bleed from a cut surface. Later it becomes discolored (reddish-purple, then greenish-purple and gangrenous) and friable. Histologically, the muscle fibers show coagulation necrosis, cavities caused by gas production, and a loss of supporting connective tissue; numerous gram-positive bacilli are present. Few if any inflammatory cells are present. Evidence suggests that the α and θ toxins of *C. perfringens* are major virulence factors that play important roles in myonecrosis and reduction of the inflammatory response at the site of infection.[59] Intravascular thrombosis due to the local effects of α toxin on platelets and granulocytes appears to be responsible for the severe herald pain (which may be ischemic in nature) and extensive myonecrosis.[60] In addition to these local effects, the α toxin provokes systemic hypotension by directly suppressing myocardial contractility and triggering the release of endogenous inflammatory mediators.[61]

Clinical Findings

The usual incubation period between injury and the development of clostridial myonecrosis is 2 to 3 days, but it may be as short as 6 hours. The onset is acute. Pain is the earliest and most important symptom, although on occasion a sense of heaviness may be the only initial symptom. Pain rapidly increases in intensity, is more severe than what would generally be associated with the preceding injury or surgical procedure, and may become excruciating. The patient soon appears severely ill, pale, and sweaty. The pulse is rapid, the blood pressure falls, and shock and renal failure follow. The patient may be apathetic or may be apprehensive and restless but mentally clear. Delirium, stupor, and unconsciousness may supervene. Fever is frequently present, but often with a temperature of less than 38.3 °C (101° F). Hypothermia is a poor prognostic sign and is usually associated with shock. Jaundice may become evident. The process may rapidly progress over a period of hours, with a fatal outcome if not properly treated.

Very early, tense edema and local tenderness may be the only findings of local lesions. If an open wound is present, swollen muscle may herniate through. A serosanguineous, dirty-appearing discharge, containing numerous organisms but few leukocytes, escapes from the wound. The wound has a peculiar foul odor. Gas bubbles may be visible in the discharge. Crepitus usually is present but not prominent; sometimes it is completely obscured by very marked edema. The skin adjacent to the wound is initially swollen and white but rapidly takes

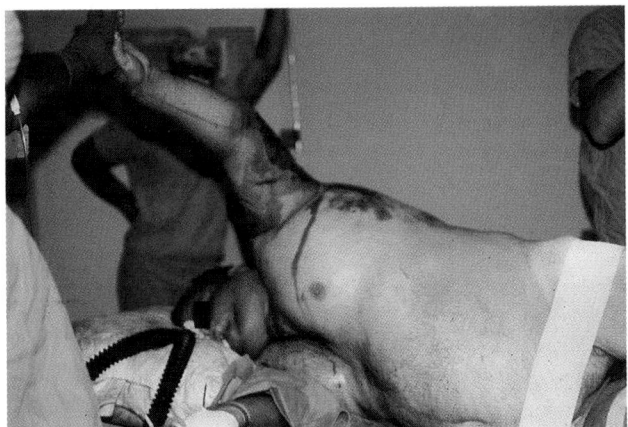

FIGURE 87-2. Clostridial gas gangrene of the left upper extremity. There is prominent characteristic bronze discoloration of the skin extending over the shoulder. Crepitus could be palpated beyond the area of discoloration onto the back.

on a yellowish or bronze discoloration (Fig. 87-2). Tense blebs containing thin, serosanguineous or dark fluid develop in the overlying skin, and areas of green-black cutaneous necrosis appear. In fulminant cases, progression of the changes occurs over 2 to 4 hours, as indicated by the advance of the area of edema and crepitation.

Laboratory Findings

The hematocrit level is usually reduced, despite progressive local edema and expected hemoconcentration, because of the lysolecithinase activity of clostridial α toxin and acute hemolysis. *C. perfringens* bacteremia occurs in about 15% of patients with gas gangrene.[62] Intense bacteremia (with associated intravascular hemolysis) is more likely to occur as a complication of uterine infection.[63] An initial leukocytosis is common.

A Gram-stained smear of the wound exudate or of an aspirate from one of the blebs reveals many large, gram-positive bacilli with blunt ends but few polymorphonuclear leukocytes (see Chapter 244). In almost all cases, spores are not evident. The presence of spores (subterminal) might suggest *C. septicum*.[64] Not infrequently, scattered gram-negative bacilli are also present, particularly in grossly contaminated wounds. The growth of *C. perfringens* in culture can be extraordinarily rapid (generation time, as little as 8 minutes), paralleling the rapidity of advance of the infection in devitalized tissue. Examination of liquid anaerobic cultures for gas production ("stormy fermentation") and subsequent Gram-stain examination as little as 6 hours after inoculation may provide an early presumptive diagnosis of the infecting species. Radiographic films of the involved areas show extensive and progressive gaseous dissection of muscle and fascial planes.

Etiologic Agents

C. perfringens is most commonly isolated from the lesions of gas gangrene (80% to 95% of the cases).[51,57] *Clostridium novyi* is involved in 10% to 40% of the cases, and *C. septicum* in 5% to 20%. Other clostridial species (*Clostridium bifermentans, Clostridium histolyticum, Clostridium fallax, Clostridium ramosum, Clostridium sordellii*) have been implicated on rare occasions. In addition to clostridia, other organisms (e.g., *E. coli, Enterobacter* spp., enterococci) are sometimes isolated from the lesions of gas gangrene, reflecting the contaminated character of the initiating trauma or lesion.[62]

Differential Diagnosis

The major considerations in differential diagnosis are gas-forming infections of the soft tissues (clostridial anaerobic cellulitis, nonclostridial crepitant myositis, nonclostridial crepitant cellulitis). Clostridial anaerobic cellulitis (see Chapter 86) is more gradual in onset and progression, and the systemic manifestations of illness are much milder than in gas gangrene. Local pain is relatively mild, and the skin lesions of gas gangrene (bronzing, dark blebs) do not develop. Gas formation is often much more extensive in clostridial cellulitis than in gas gangrene. Clinically, it is often difficult to distinguish between early clostridial cellulitis and myonecrosis. Definitive evaluation requires examination in the operating room for the characteristic changes of myonecrosis described earlier. The clinical picture of nonclostridial crepitant cellulitis is very similar to that of clostridial cellulitis. Although contamination of an operative or traumatic wound may be the source of infection in both types of cellulitis, nonclostridial crepitant cellulitis frequently develops in the setting of vascular insufficiency or perirectal infection. Bacteria isolated from nonclostridial crepitant cellulitis include facultative species (*E. coli, Klebsiella,* various streptococci) and anaerobic bacteria (*Bacteroides, Peptostreptococcus*). Commonly, these are present in mixed culture and can be seen on the Gram-stained smear of a wound aspirate.

Presumptive Therapy

Treatment includes emergency surgical exploration, both to define the nature of the process (gas gangrene versus crepitant cellulitis) by direct examination of muscles at the site of infection and to carry out appropriate débridement. Prompt and extensive surgery is the principal element in the treatment of gas gangrene. This includes excision of involved muscles (or amputation if necessary) and fasciotomies to decompress and drain the swollen fascial compartments. Antibiotic therapy is an important adjunct to surgical management. Penicillin G, the antibiotic of choice in the past, is administered intravenously in a dosage of 2 million units every 2 to 3 hours (or adjusted for acute renal insufficiency) for an adult. Currently, the combination of penicillin with clindamycin (600 mg intravenously every 6 to 8 hours) is widely used in treatment. The addition of clindamycin is based on results of experimental studies of fulminant clostridial myonecrosis in mice, in which clindamycin, metronidazole, and tetracycline were each more effective than penicillin.[65] In vitro, the addition of penicillin to metronidazole antagonizes the activity of the latter; in contrast, the combination of penicillin with clindamycin provides slightly greater efficacy than clindamycin alone but significantly enhanced efficacy over that of penicillin alone.[66]

An additional antimicrobial agent (e.g., ciprofloxacin, a third-generation cephalosporin, chloramphenicol) may be employed initially if Gram-stained smears of the wound exudate show gram-negative bacilli as well as the predominant gram-positive bacilli. In addition to clindamycin, chloramphenicol is a good alternative drug in the highly penicillin-allergic patient; it is preferable to tetracycline in view of the resistance of some clostridia to the latter. Although the majority of *C. perfringens* isolates are susceptible in vitro to first-, second-, and third-generation cephalosporins, the minimum inhibitory concentrations for at least 10% of isolates are greater than levels readily achievable in vivo.[57] The demonstration that plasmids mediate transferable drug resistance (tetracycline and chloramphenicol; perhaps erythromycin and clindamycin) in *C. perfringens*[67] suggests the need for periodic monitoring of antibiotic susceptibilities of clinical isolates. Some strains of this organism may be showing somewhat less susceptibility in vitro to penicillin than was formerly the case.[68] *C. perfringens* is susceptible in vitro to metronidazole, but experience with the clinical use of this drug alone in clostridial myonecrosis is lacking.

The role of hyperbaric oxygen therapy is still under debate (see Chapter 40).[69,70] The rarity of clostridial myonecrosis and the limited availability of hyperbaric oxygen facilities has made prospective controlled clinical trials impractical. Its use should never delay immediate surgical débridement if possible. Its most appropriate role at present would appear to be in the management of extensive involvement of the trunk, for which complete surgical excision would be impossible (paraspinal sites) or mutilating.[71] In a murine model of *C. perfringens* myonecrosis initiated with a high inoculum, clindamycin therapy was more effective than hyperbaric oxygen, and the addition of the latter provided no further efficacy to use of clindamycin alone.[72] Initial hyperbaric oxygen therapy may reduce the extent of débridement that is necessary under these circumstances. The efficacy of intravenously administered polyvalent gas gangrene antitoxin has never been established clinically, and it is no longer available. Ancillary therapy is essential in the management of gas gangrene. This includes attention to fluid and electrolyte replacement and maintenance of adequate hematocrit levels by means of transfusions.

NONCLOSTRIDIAL (CREPITANT) MYOSITIS

Nonclostridial (crepitant) myositis includes four relatively distinct entities that differ from gas gangrene in their clinical picture and bacteriologic characteristics: (1) anaerobic streptococcal myonecrosis, (2) synergistic nonclostridial anaerobic myonecrosis, (3) infected vascular gangrene, and (4) *A. hydrophila* myonecrosis.

Anaerobic Streptococcal Myonecrosis

Anaerobic streptococcal myonecrosis is an acute interstitial myositis that clinically resembles subacute clostridial gas gangrene. The initial manifestations are swelling and a copious, seropurulent exudate occurring 3 to 4 days after an injury. Pain develops later, unlike the early occurrence of pain in gas gangrene. Tissue gas is present in muscle and fascial planes but is not extensive. The wound has an unpleasant, sour odor. The involved muscles are discolored but do react to stimulation. In contrast to gas gangrene, early cutaneous erythema is prominent. If it is not adequately treated, the infection progresses, with the development of toxemia, frank gangrene, and shock.

Numerous streptococci and polymorphonuclear leukocytes are present in the exudate. The infection is usually mixed (anaerobic streptococci with group A streptococci or *S. aureus*). A mixed infection of muscle with both peptostreptococci and *Bacillus subtilis* has been observed on several occasions in the setting of vascular injury. The clinical picture, along with the appearance of the Gram-stained smear, initially might suggest the diagnosis of clostridial myonecrosis.[73] Treatment involves the use of large doses of penicillin (and an antistaphylococcal agent, if indicated) and surgical débridement.

Synergistic Nonclostridial Anaerobic Myonecrosis

Synergistic nonclostridial anaerobic myonecrosis, a severe infection seen particularly in diabetics and in neutropenic individuals, is also known as synergistic necrotizing cellulitis (see Chapter 86). It involves skin, subcutaneous tissue, fascia, and muscle. The most extensive involvement is in the subcutaneous tissues and fascia; changes in overlying skin and underlying muscle are usually secondary. Although a mixture of anaerobic and facultative organisms is commonly recovered at surgical exploration, on rare occasions crepitant myonecrosis may be caused by *K. pneumoniae*[74] or *Enterobacter cloacae*,[75] unaccompanied by other organisms (aerobic or anaerobic), in high-risk patients. The clinical course is rapidly progressive, often leading to a fatal outcome despite emergency surgical exploration and débridement of necrotic tissue.

Infected Vascular Gangrene

Infected vascular gangrene is a mixed infection that develops in a group of muscles or in a limb that is devitalized as a result of arterial insufficiency, particularly in patients with diabetes mellitus. *Proteus* spp., *Bacteroides* spp., and anaerobic streptococci are among the bacteria found in such lesions. Gas formation and foul-smelling pus are prominent. The infection does not extend beyond the area of vascular gangrene to involve healthy muscle. *Bacillus cereus* infection has been associated with myonecrosis with slight crepitus after thrombosis of arterial grafts.[76]

Aeromonas hydrophila Myonecrosis

Rapidly progressive myonecrosis caused by *A. hydrophila,* a facultatively anaerobic, gram-negative bacillus, may occur after penetrating trauma in a freshwater environment or in association with fish or other aquatic animals.[77,78] Although *Aeromonas* was associated with pyomyositis and a compartment syndrome in one neutropenic pa-

tient,[79] spontaneous (nontraumatic) myonecrosis due to *Aeromonas* has not been reported. In a few instances, myonecrosis has been accompanied by gas spreading extensively in soft tissue planes. The rapid onset (24 to 48 hours) and rapid progression after trauma resemble those of clostridial gas gangrene. The prominence of pain, marked edema, serosanguineous bullae, and toxicity, in addition to the presence of gas in fascial planes, adds to the similarity of these conditions. Bacteremia is frequently present. Treatment consists of extensive surgical débridement and prompt initiation of antimicrobial therapy. Most isolates of *Aeromonas* are susceptible in vitro to gentamicin, tobramycin, trimethoprim-sulfamethoxazole, chloramphenicol, and ciprofloxacin.[80] Third-generation cephalosporins, carbapenems, and aztreonam also appear to be active, although individual strains may express β-lactamases that selectively hydrolyze cephalosporins or carbapenems.

PSOAS ABSCESS

Infection of the psoas muscle takes the form of either an abscess or a phlegmon. Unlike primary pyomyositis of other muscle groups, psoas infections are usually the consequence of spread of infection from an adjacent structure. Rarely, primary psoas abscesses develop by the hematogenous route[81]; in children particularly, there may be no prior inciting event such as trauma or preceding infection, and *S. aureus* is the most common cause in this setting.[82] In adult women, hematogenous psoas abscesses have been observed as a complication of spontaneous vaginal delivery.[83] Psoas abscess usually is confined within the psoas fascia, but occasionally, because of anatomic relations, infection extends to the buttock, hip, or upper thigh. Psoas abscess may complicate pyogenic or tuberculous or blastomycotic vertebral osteomyelitis. Tuberculosis was formerly the principal cause of psoas abscesses; now they most commonly result from direct extension of intra-abdominal infections (e.g., diverticulitis, appendicitis, Crohn's disease).[84] Occasionally, a psoas abscess results from extension of a perinephric abscess or from secondary infection of a retroperitoneal hematoma. The organisms involved in spread of infection from an intestinal site are usually members of the aerobic and anaerobic bowel flora. *S. aureus* is the most common cause of psoas abscess secondary to vertebral osteomyelitis.

The iliacus muscle, applied to the ilium in the iliac fossa, forms a conjoined tendon with the lower portion of the psoas muscle. Osteomyelitis of the ilium or septic arthritis of the sacroiliac joint can penetrate the sheaths of either or both muscles in this location, producing an iliacus or psoas abscess.[85]

Clinical manifestations of a psoas abscess include fever, lower abdominal or back pain, or pain referred to the hip or knee. A limp may be evident, and flexion deformity of the hip may develop from reflex spasm, suggesting septic arthritis of the hip. The psoas sign is evident. Often a tender mass can be palpated in the groin.

Roentgenograms may show a bulge produced by a psoas muscle abscess or the presence of gas within the psoas sheath. Calcification in a psoas abscess strongly suggests a tuberculous cause. Of the five noninvasive techniques currently available for visualization of the psoas and iliacus muscles, CT scanning is the most rapid and sensitive. Ultrasound is less reliable for detecting small lesions or a phlegmon. Gallium scanning does not provide as sharp a localization and takes up to 72 hours; indium-labeled leukocyte scanning may be preferable. CT scanning may show diffuse enlargement of the psoas (phlegmon) or a sharply circumscribed, low-density fluid collections (abscess) within the muscle, or it may demonstrate the presence of gas within the muscle (indicative of abscess).[86] MRI scanning of the pelvis can show enlarged psoas and iliacus muscles displaying grossly abnormal signal intensities.

Pyogenic psoas abscesses are treated by surgical drainage and provisional initial antibiotic therapy based on knowledge of the origin of the infection. CT scanning may be of considerable value for guidance of direct needle aspiration of an abscess for culture or for drainage if the direct surgical approach is not preferable or warranted. Although culture-negative psoas abscesses can be seen when drainage procedures follow an initial course of empiric antibiotic therapy, pseudo-psoas abscesses associated with erosive discitis due to calcium pyrophosphate deposition have been reported.[87] If the process appears to be a phlegmon, repeated CT scanning during the course of antibiotic therapy can confirm resolution of the anatomic changes.

OTHER SPECIFIC SITES OF MUSCLE ABSCESSES

Infective myositis or pyomyositis may occasionally occur in unusual anatomic areas for these processes and mimic other, more common infections. Iliacus pyomyositis[34] and pyomyositis of the adductor muscles or the obturator internus[88] may mimic septic arthritis of the hip; pyriformis pyomyositis may suggest a spinal epidural abscess[35] or pelvic osteomyelitis[89]; iliopsoas myositis[33] may mimic appendicitis.

MYALGIAS

Myalgias are prominent features of a variety of infections such as dengue, influenza, and Rocky Mountain spotted fever. Little information is available on the presence of specific histologic findings indicative of myositis. In addition to the focal myositis syndromes discussed earlier, a variety of pathogens are associated with acute diffuse muscle injury (culminating in rhabdomyolysis) or with chronic diffuse muscle injury mimicking autoimmune polymyositis (see Table 87-1).[90] The histopathologic similarities observed between autoimmune muscle injury and the polymyositis associated with certain infectious processes, as well as the antigen specificities of infiltrating lymphocytes, suggest that infection in at least some instances may trigger an autoimmune attack on myocytes.[91]

Influenza

Muscle aches are common early in the course of influenza. Occasionally, severe bilateral muscle pains in the lower limbs may develop in the recovery phase of influenza A or influenza B, particularly in young children[92,93]; this has been termed "acute benign myositis."[94,95] Muscle tenderness is demonstrable, principally in the gastrocnemius and soleus muscles, and calf swelling may be present. Deep tendon reflexes and muscle strength are normal, but there is considerable difficulty in walking. The leg pains and muscle tenderness subside in less than 1 week. Mild elevations of serum concentrations of aldolase and creatine phosphokinase occur. The few biopsies performed have shown either nonspecific degenerative changes or muscle necrosis with polymorphonuclear leukocytic infiltration. Whether this "myositis" is caused by direct viral invasion or by some immunologic or other response is unknown. However, influenza A virus was isolated from the muscle biopsy specimen of an adult with generalized muscle weakness occurring during an influenza A outbreak.[96] Life-threatening rhabdomyolysis with extreme elevations of creatine kinase and myoglobin-induced acute renal failure are rarely seen after influenza A infection; the prognosis is favorable but may require short-term dialysis.[97] Isolated influenza myocarditis, sometimes quite severe, can occur in the absence of generalized rhabdomyolysis (see Chapter 162).[98]

Infective Endocarditis

Prominent myalgias occur in about 15% of patients with infective endocarditis.[99] They may be either diffuse or localized. The pathogenesis is not known, but in one instance muscle biopsy specimens showed a small focus of muscle fiber destruction and leukocytic infiltration consistent with embolization to a small artery.[99] On rare occasions, infective endocarditis may lead to frank pyomyositis.[17]

Toxoplasmosis

The major features of acute acquired disseminated toxoplasmosis are those of meningoencephalitis, myocarditis, pneumonitis, skin rash, and occasionally hepatitis (see Chapter 276). In rare instances, particularly in immunocompromised hosts (e.g., HIV infection, chronic immunosuppressive therapy after organ transplantation, CD4 lymphopenia[100]), polymyositis may be a prominent clinical manifestation resembling autoimmune polymyositis. Marked myalgias, muscle weakness and swelling, and fasciculations occur in such patients. Muscle biopsy specimens show interstitial myositis with destruction of muscle fibers, and pseudocysts of *Toxoplasma gondii* can be found in areas that are of muscle free of inflammatory reaction. In several cases, these organisms have been isolated by animal inoculation.[101,102]

Other Causes

Occasionally, the only clinical manifestations of initial infection with HIV-1 are those of polymyositis (myalgias, muscle weakness, and increased serum levels of muscle enzymes). HIV-1 viral antigens can be found in CD4+ T lymphocytes in areas of muscle fiber inflammation and necrosis.[103] During the subsequent course of HIV-1 infection, various forms of muscular involvement may develop, including generalized or localized myalgias, HIV myopathy (polymyositis),[104] muscle atrophy secondary to the anorexia and cachexia of the "wasting syndrome" of AIDS,[105] and the mitochondrial myopathy related to prolonged zidovudine therapy.[106] The clinical presentation of HIV-1 myopathy (inflammatory polymyositis) is that of progressive proximal muscle weakness. Elevated serum creatine phosphokinase and electromyographic changes assist in diagnosis. Muscle biopsy material consists of either of two histologic patterns alone or both in combination: (1) an inflammatory myopathy with lymphocytic infiltration and muscle fiber necrosis, and (2) abundant nemaline rod bodies and muscle fiber necrosis. In patients receiving prolonged zidovudine therapy in whom myopathy develops, muscle biopsy material shows a combination of endomysial inflammatory infiltrate (CD8+ T cells and macrophages) and a mitochondrial myopathy characterized by proliferation of large numbers of abnormal mitochondria ("ragged-red fibers") in the subsarcolemmal spaces.[107] The mitochondrial changes appear to represent toxic changes associated with zidovudine therapy, and clinical improvement in some patients may occur after discontinuance of the drug. The inflammatory myopathy may represent primarily an HIV-associated autoimmune process and may respond clinically to prednisone.

Inflammatory myositis with a lymphoplasmacytic cellular response has been documented in patients with human T-cell lymphotropic virus-1 (HTLV-1)–associated polymyositis, and muscle-infiltrating lymphocytes specific for viral and class I major histocompatability determinants were demonstrated.[91] Inflammatory myositis was the major feature in a case of Lyme disease.[108] Spirochetes morphologically similar to *Borrelia burgdorferi* were present on Dieterle silver stain of biopsied muscle. Rarely, infection by *Sarcocystis* (an intracellular sporozoan parasite) has been observed in histologic sections of muscle of individuals with muscle pain or weakness, mainly outside the United States.[109] Microsporidia myositis was reported in a patient with AIDS.[110]

PLEURODYNIA SYNDROMES

Epidemic pleurodynia is an acute, febrile disease caused by group B coxsackieviruses that is characterized by the sudden onset of sharp chest pain over the lower ribs or sternum (see Chapter 169). Paroxysms of knifelike pain are precipitated by voluntary or respiratory movements. Muscle tenderness may be present. Abdominal pain may also be present in some patients; in others, abdominal pain may be the sole manifestation, simulating intraperitoneal processes.

Group B coxsackieviruses produce visceral lesions and also some focal myositis in experimental animals. Myositis has not been demonstrated as a feature pathologically, either in fatal cases of severe neonatal coxsackievirus B infection or in the few biopsy specimens obtained from affected muscles of patients with epidemic pleurodynia,[111,112] but it has been associated with rhabdomyolysis complicating mild exercise in the recovery phase of illness.[113]

MYALGIAS WITH EOSINOPHILIA (PARASITIC MYOSITIS)

Trichinosis

Trichinosis is acquired by ingestion of insufficiently cooked pork or, less commonly, bear meat, wild boar, or walrus. The prominent clinical manifestations of trichinosis include fever, myositis, periorbital edema, and eosinophilia. An initial intestinal phase (nausea, vomiting, nonbloody diarrhea) during the first week is followed during the second week by larval invasion of skeletal muscle (see Chapter 286). Serious complications in the form of myocarditis, meningoencephalitis, and pneumonitis can occur.[114] Myalgias, frequently accompanied by muscle swelling and weakness and occasionally associated with fasciculations, are present in most patients with the disease. Muscles commonly involved include the extraocular muscles, flexor muscles of the extremities, back muscles, and the muscles used in chewing and swallowing. Periorbital edema, chemosis, and conjunctival hemorrhages are related to larval invasion of extraocular muscles. The inflammatory response in muscle produces increased serum levels of muscle enzymes.

Muscle biopsy specimens reveal encysted larval trichinae in necrotic muscle fibers, surrounded by inflammatory cells (predominantly eosinophils and neutrophils, but also lymphocytes). Severe skeletal muscle involvement was reported in a case of trichinosis in an immunosuppressed patient.[115] Although granulomatous reactions have been observed in the heart and lungs in fatal cases, larval encystment does not take place in organs other than skeletal muscle.

Trichinella spiralis is the most common cause of human trichinosis, but other species can infect humans. *Trichinella pseudospiralis* caused a large outbreak of trichinosis in Thailand.[116] Because this species, unlike *T. spiralis,* does not undergo encystment in skeletal muscle, prolonged larval migration and clinical symptoms ensue.

Diagnosis of trichinosis is made on the basis of the clinical picture, eosinophilia, serology (enzyme-linked immunosorbent assay, bentonite flocculation), and, if needed, muscle biopsy.

Benzimidazole compounds (thiabendazole, mebendazole, albendazole) are the most effective therapies early in the illness. Albendazole may have the advantage of being better tolerated.[116]

Trichinosis should be distinguished from the eosinophilia-myalgia syndrome, which results from the ingestion of certain tryptophan products and is characterized by prominent myalgias, fatigue, and eosinophilia, followed, in some instances, by development of neurologic and scleroderma-like skin changes.[117]

Cysticercosis (Cysticercus Cellulosal Myositis)

Human cysticercosis is rare in the United States but common in Latin America and Asia. It results from the ingestion and subsequent hatching of viable eggs of *Taenia solium* into the larval form (cysticercus) of the parasite (formerly known as *Cysticercus cellulosae*) (see Chapter 288). Eggs reach the upper intestinal tract in food contaminated by feces from a person parasitized by the adult worm. Autoinfection can occur through the fecal-oral route and possibly by reverse peristalsis, with introduction of egg-laden proglottids back into the duodenum or stomach, where they hatch. From the stomach, they are distributed widely (skeletal muscle, subcutaneous tissues, heart, eye, central nervous system).

Symptomatic involvement of muscle is uncommon. Occasionally, the stage of invasion is characterized by fever, muscle tenderness, and eosinophilia. More characteristically, asymptomatic calcified cysts ("puffed rice" appearance) are detected in muscles on soft tissue radiographic films of patients with neurologic manifestations.

MUSCLE DEGENERATION ASSOCIATED WITH INFECTIONS AT OTHER SITES

Acute Rhabdomyolysis

Myoglobinuria occasionally occurs after an acute illness with symptoms suggesting an upper respiratory tract infection. Scattered cases have been shown to follow documented influenza A virus infections in children and adults,[118] legionnaires' disease, *Mycoplasma pneumoniae,*[119] leptospirosis (Weil's disease),[120] pneumococcal sepsis,[121] meningococcal sepsis,[122] echovirus infection,[123] and infections caused by coxsackievirus, Epstein-Barr virus, and adenovirus.[124] Diffuse muscle pains (especially in the extremities), weakness, swelling, and tenderness are prominent features, along with myoglobinuria. Rhabdomyolysis has occurred in patients with no previous episodes and no family history of this condition. Like the myositis that occurs after influenza in children, it develops when respiratory symptoms are resolving.

Muscle Proteolysis and Mediators of Fever in Patients with Sepsis

Muscle involvement, in the form of myalgias and weakness, is common in the course of systemic infections. Accelerated catabolism of skeletal muscle contributes to the marked weakness and muscle wasting that can be observed in systemic infections. This appears to be part of a protective "acute phase" host response to sepsis and trauma. Important roles are played by interleukin-1 (IL-1), tumor necrosis factor, interferon-α, and IL-6. The intracellular events accompanying muscle catabolism involve direct cleavage of actomyosin by caspase 3[125] and subsequent degradation by proteasomes; additional mechanisms also help regulate the process of muscle cachexia.[126] A polypeptide (possibly a breakdown product of IL-1) that produces a rapid increase in protein degradation in rat or human muscle preparations[127] has been observed in the plasma of patients with sepsis. Similar changes are produced by IL-1 itself.[128] This accelerated proteolysis is effected through increased synthesis in muscle of prostaglandin E_2, which in turn activates proteases in muscle-cell lysosomes. This catabolic activity is accompanied by IL-1–stimulated hepatic protein synthesis (using the newly generated source of amino acids) and other elements of the acute phase response and by fever (also generated by IL-1 and mediated by prostaglandin E_2). The important role of prostaglandin E_2 in the generation of the muscle aches and fever of infection is consistent with the amelioration of these symptoms produced by inhibitors of prostaglandin synthesis (e.g., aspirin).

REFERENCES

1. Smith IM, Vickers AB. Natural history of 338 treated and untreated patients with staphylococcal septicaemia. Lancet. 1960;1:1318-1322.
2. Levin MJ, Gardner P, Waldvogel FA. "Tropical" pyomyositis: An unusual infection due to *Staphylococcus aureus*. N Engl J Med. 1971;284:196-198.
3. Bickels J, Ben-Sira L, Kessler A, Wientroub S. Primary pyomyositis. J Bone Joint Surg Am. 2002;84:2277-2286.
4. Horn CV, Master S. Pyomyositis tropicans in Uganda. E Afr Med J. 1968;45:463-471.
5. Christin L, Sarosi GA. Pyomyositis in North America: Case reports and review. Clin Infect Dis. 1992;15:668-677.
6. Harbarth SJ, Lew DP. Pyomyositis as a nontropical disease. In: Remington J, Swartz MN, eds. Current Clinical Topics in Infectious Diseases, v. 17. Malden, Mass.: Blackwell Science Publishers; 1997:37-50.
7. Rayes AA, Nobre V, Teixeira DM, et al. Tropical pyomyositis and human toxocariasis: A clinical and experimental study. Am J Med. 2000;109:422-425.
8. Gardiner JS, Zauk AM, Minnefor AB, et al. Pyomyositis in an HIV-positive premature infant: Case report and review of the literature. J Pediatr Orthop. 1990;10:791-793.
9. Rodgers WB, Yodlowski ML, Mintzer CM. Pyomyositis in patients who have the human immunodeficiency virus: Case report and review of the literature. J Bone Joint Surg Am. 1993;75:588-592.
10. Medina F, Fuentes M, Jara LJ, et al. Salmonella pyomyositis in patients with the human immunodeficiency virus. J Rheumatol. 1995;34:568-571.
11. Arranz-Caso JA, Cuadrado-Gomez LM, Romanik-Cabrera J, et al. Pyomyositis caused by *Morganella morganii* in a patient with AIDS. Clin Infect Dis. 1996;22:372-373.
12. Miralles GD, Bregman Z. Necrotizing pyomyositis caused by *Mycobacterium avium* complex in a patient with AIDS. Clin Infect Dis. 1994;18:833-834.
13. Vassilopoulos D, Chalasani P, Jurado RL, et al. Musculoskeletal infections in patients with human immunodeficiency virus infection. Medicine (Baltimore). 1997;76:284-294.
14. Mylonakis E, Rich JD, Flanigan T, et al. Muscle abscess due to *Aspergillus fumigatus* in a patient with AIDS. Clin Infect Dis. 1996;23:1323-1324.
15. Murphy PM, Lane HC, Fauci AS, et al. Impairment of neutrophil bactericidal capacity in patients with AIDS. J Infect Dis. 1988;158:627-630.

16. Hsueh P-R, Hsiue TR, Hsieh W-C. Pyomyositis in intravenous drug abusers: Report of a unique case and review of the literature. Clin Infect Dis. 1996;22:858-860.

17. Lo TS, Mooers MG, Wright LJ. Pyomyositis complicating acute bacterial endocarditis in an intravenous drug user. N Engl J Med. 2000;342:1614-1615.

18. Miyake H. Beitrag zur Kenntniss des sogenannten Myositis infectiosa. Mitt Grenzgeb Med Chir. 1904;13:155.

19. Flier S, Dolgin SE, Saphir RL, et al. A case confirming the progressive stages of pyomyositis. J Pediatr Surg. 2003;38:1551-1553.

20. Immerman RP, Greenman RL. Toxic shock syndrome associated with pyomyositis caused by a strain of *Staphylococcus aureus* that does not produce toxic-shock-syndrome toxin-1. Infect Dis. 1987;156:505-507.

21. Wolfe MW, Bennett JT. Pyomyositis with toxic shock syndrome presenting as back pain and fever: A case report and literature review. Am J Orthop. 1997;26:135-137.

22. Kennedy CA, Mathisen G, Goetz MB. Tropical pyomyositis of the abdominal wall musculature mimicking acute abdomen. West J Med. 1990;152:296-298.

23. Armstrong JH. Tropical pyomyositis and myoglobinuria. Arch Intern Med. 1978;138:1145-1446.

24. Collazos J, Fernandez A, Martinez E, et al. Pneumococcal pyomyositis: Case report, review of the literature, and comparison with classic pyomyositis caused by other bacteria. Arch Intern Med. 1996;156:1470-1474.

25. Collazos J, Mayo J, Martinez E, Blanco MS. Muscle infections caused by *Salmonella* species: Case report and review. Clin Infect Dis. 1999; 29: 673-677.

26. Liu AC, Argent JD. Necrobacillosis: A resurgence? Clin Radiol. 2002;57:332-338.

27. Beumont MG, Duncan J, Mitchell SD, et al. Veillonella myositis in an immunocompromised patient. Clin Infect Dis. 1995;21:678-679.

28. Brook I. Pyomyositis in children, caused by anaerobic bacteria. J Pediatr Surg. 1996;31:394-396.

29. Flagg SD, Chang YJ, Masuell CP, et al. Myositis resulting from disseminated cryptococcosis in a patient with hepatitis C cirrhosis. Clin Infect Dis. 2001;32:1104-1107.

30. Bonomo RA, Graham R, Makley JT, et al. Tuberculous pyomyositis: An unusual presentation of disseminated *Mycobacterium tuberculosis* infection. Clin Infect Dis. 1995;20:1576-1577.

31. Ahmed J, Homans J. Tuberculosis pyomyositis of the soleus muscle in a fifteen-year-old boy. Pediatr Infect Dis J. 2002;21:1169-1171.

32. Pearl GS, Sieger B. Granulomatous *Pneumocystis carinii* myositis presenting as an intramuscular mass. Clin Infect Dis. 1996;22:577-578.

33. Wysoki MG, Angeid-Backman E, Izes BA. Iliopsoas myositis mimicking appendicitis: MRI diagnosis. Skeletal Radiol. 1997;26:316-318.

34. Chen W-S, Wan Y-L. Iliacus pyomyositis mimicking septic arthritis of the hip joint. Arch Orthop Trauma Surg. 1996;115:233-235.

35. Chusid MJ, Hill WC, Bevan JA, et al. Proteus pyomyositis of the pyriformis muscle in a swimmer. Clin Infect Dis. 1998;26:194-195.

36. Case Records of the Massachusetts General Hospital. Skeletal muscle infarction associated with diabetes mellitus. N Engl J Med. 1997;337:839-845.

37. Quillin SP, McAlister WH. Rapidly progressive pyomyositis: Diagnosis by repeat sonography. J Ultrasound Med. 1991;10:181-184.

38. Gordon BA, Martinez S, Collins AJ. Pyomyositis: Characteristics at CT and MRI imaging. Radiology. 1995;197:279-286.

39. Cone LA, Lamb RB, Graff-Radford A, et al. Pyomyositis of the anterior tibial compartment. Clin Infect Dis; 1997:25:146-148.

40. Svane S. Peracute spontaneous streptococcal myositis. Acta Chir Scand. 1971;137:155-163.

41. Moore DL, Delage G, Labelle H, et al. Peracute streptococcal pyomyositis: Report of two cases and review of the literature. J Pediatr Orthop. 1986;6:232-235.

42. Stevens DL. Streptococcal toxic shock syndrome associated with necrotizing fasciitis. Annu Rev Med. 2000;51:271-288.

43. Stevens DL, Tanner MH, Winship J, et al. Severe group A streptococcal infections associated with a toxic shock-like syndrome and scarlet fever toxin A. N Engl J Med. 1989;321:1-7.

44. Jahnson L, Berggren L, Björsell-Östling E, et al. Streptococcal myositis. Scand J Infect Dis. 1992;24:661-665.

45. Yoder EL, Mendez J, Khatib R. Spontaneous gangrenous myositis induced by *Streptococcus pyogenes:* Case report and review of the literature. Rev Infect Dis. 1987;9:382-385.

46. Case Records of the Massachusetts General Hospital. Group A beta-hemolytic streptococcus infection, with the compartment and toxic shock syndrome. N Engl J Med. 1995;333:113-119.

47. Wagner JG, Schlievert PM, Assimacopoulos AP, et al. Acute Group G streptococcal myositis associated with streptococcal toxic shock syndrome: Case report and review. Clin Infect Dis. 1996;23:1159-1161.

48. Stevens DL, Gibbons AE, Bergstrom R, et al. The Eagle effect revisited: Efficacy of clindamycin, erythromycin, and penicillin in the treatment of streptococcal myositis. J Infect Dis. 1988;158:23-28.

49. Darenberg J, Ihendyane N, Sjolin J, et al. Intravenous immunoglobulin G therapy in streptococcal toxic shock syndrome: A European randomized, double-blind, placebo-controlled trial. Clin Infect Dis. 2003;37:333-340.

50. Stevens DL. Dilemmas in the treatment of invasive *Streptococcus pyogenes* infections. Clin Infect Dis. 2003;37:341-343.

51. Altemeier WA, Fullen WD. Prevention and treatment of gas gangrene. JAMA. 1971;217:806-813.

52. MacLennan JD. The histotoxic clostridial infections of man. Bacteriol Rev. 1962;26:177-276.

53. Bornstein DL, Weinberg AN, Swartz MN, et al. Anaerobic infections: Review of current experience. Medicine (Baltimore). 1964;43:207-232.

54. Chin RL, Martinez R, Garmel G. Gas gangrene from subcutaneous insulin administration. Am J Emerg Med. 1993;11:622-625.

55. Bangsberg DR, Rosen JI, Aragon T, et al. Clostridial myonecrosis cluster among injection drug users: A molecular epidemiology investigation. Arch Intern Med. 2002;162:517-522.

56. Altemeier WA, Furste WL. Gas gangrene. Surg Gynecol Obstet. 1947;84:507-523.

57. Finegold SM. Anaerobic Bacteria in Human Disease. New York: Academic Press; 1977:424.

58. Stevens DL, Musher DM, Watson DA, et al. Spontaneous, nontraumatic gangrene due to *Clostridium septicum.* Rev Infect Dis. 1990;12:286-296.

59. Stevens DL, Tweten RK, Awad MM, et al. Clostridial gas gangrene: Evidence that α and θ toxins differentially modulate the immune response and induce acute tissue necrosis. J Infect Dis. 1997;176:189-195.

60. Bryant AE. Biology and pathogenesis of thrombosis and procoagulant activity in invasive infections caused by group A streptococci and *Clostridium perfringens.* Clin Microbiol Rev. 2003;16:451-462.

61. Stevens DL, Bryant AE. The role of clostridial toxins in the pathogenesis of gas gangrene. Clin Infect Dis. 2002;35:S93-S100.

62. Caplan ES, Kluge RM. Gas gangrene: Review of 34 cases. Arch Intern Med. 1976;136:788-791.

63. Dylewski J, Wiesenfeld H, Latour A. Postpartum uterine infection with *Clostridium perfringens.* Rev Infect Dis. 1989;11:470-473.

64. Case Records of the Massachusetts General Hospital: Weekly clinicopathological exercises. Case 5-1993: An 81-year-old man with pain and crepitus in the shoulder. N Engl J Med. 1993;328:340-346.

65. Stevens DL, Maier KA, Laine BM, et al. Comparison of clindamycin, rifampin, tetracycline, metronidazole, and penicillin for efficacy in prevention of experimental gas gangrene due to *Clostridium perfringens.* J Infect Dis. 1987;155:220-228.

66. Stevens DL, Laine BM, Mitten JE. Comparison of single and combination antimicrobial agents for prevention of experimental gas gangrene caused by *Clostridium perfringens.* Antimicrob Agents Chemother. 1987;31:312-316.

67. Brefort G, Magot M, Ionesco H, et al. Characterization and transferability of *Clostridium perfringens* plasmids. Plasmid. 1977;1:52-66.

68. Marrie TJ, Haldane EV, Swantee CA, et al. Susceptibility of anaerobic bacteria to nine antimicrobial agents and demonstration of decreased susceptibility of *Clostridium perfringens* to penicillin. Antimicrob Agents Chemother. 1981;19:51-55.

69. Stephens MB. Gas gangrene: Potential for hyperbaric oxygen therapy. Postgrad Med. 1996;99:217-220.

70. Wang C, Schwaitzberg S, Berliner E, et al. Hyperbaric oxygen for treating wounds: A systematic review of the literature. Arch Surg. 2003;138:272-279.

71. Shupak A, Halpern P, Ziser A, et al. Hyperbaric oxygen therapy for gas gangrene casualties in the Lebanon War, 1982. Isr J Med Sci. 1984;20:323-326.

72. Stevens DL, Bryant AE, Adams K, et al. Evaluation of therapy with hyperbaric oxygen for experimental infection with *Clostridium perfringens.* Clin Infect Dis. 1993;17:231-237.

73. Chambers CH, Bond GF, Morris JH. Synergistic necrotizing myositis complicating vascular injury. J Trauma. 1974;14:980-984.

74. Bruno-Murtha LA, Sedghivaziri MA, Arbeit RD. Crepitant myonecrosis caused by *Klebsiella pneumoniae* in an immunocompromised diabetic patient. J Infect Dis. 1990;162:1415-1416.

75. Fata F, Chittivelu S, Tessler S, Kupfer Y. Gas gangrene of the arm due to *Enterobacter cloacae* in a neutropenic patient. South Med J. 1996;89:1095-1096.

76. Johnson DA, Aulicino PL, Newby JG. *Bacillus cereus*-induced myonecrosis. J Trauma. 1984;24:267-270.

77. Davis WA, Kane JG, Garagusi VF. Human *Aeromonas* infections: A review of the literature and case report of endocarditis. Medicine (Baltimore). 1978;57:267-277.

78. Heckerling PS, Stine TM, Pottage JC, et al. *Aeromonas hydrophila* myonecrosis and gas gangrene in a nonimmunocompromised host. Arch Intern Med. 1983;143:2005-2007.

79. Cone LA, Lamb RB, Graff-Radford A, et al. Pyomyositis of the anterior tibial compartment. Clin Infect Dis. 1997;25:146-148.

80. San Joaquin VH, Scribner RK, Pickett DA, et al. Antimicrobial susceptibility of *Aeromonas* species isolated from patients with diarrhea. Antimicrob Agents Chemother. 1986;30:794-795.

81. Steiner JL, Septimus EJ, Vartian CV. Infection of the psoas muscle secondary to *Streptococcus pneumoniae* infection. Clin Infect Dis. 1992;15:1047-1048.

82. Desandre AR, Cottone FJ, Evers ML. Iliopsoas abscess: Etiology, diagnosis, and treatment. Am Surg. 1995;61:1087-1091.

83. Shahabi S, Klein JP, Rinaudo PF. Primary psoas abscess complicating a normal vaginal delivery. Obstet Gynecol. 2002;99:906-909.

84. Kyle J. Psoas abscess in Crohn's disease. Gastroenterology. 1971;61:149-155.

85. Simons GW, Sty JR, Starshak RJ, et al. Retroperitoneal and retrofascial abscesses. J Bone Joint Surg Am. 1983;65:1041-1058.

86. Gordin F, Stamler C, Mills J. Pyogenic psoas abscesses: Noninvasive diagnostic techniques and review of the literature. Rev Infect Dis. 1983;5:1003-1011.

87. Dudler J, Stucki RF, Gerster JC. Aseptic psoas pyomyositis and erosive discitis in a case of calcium pyrophosphate crystal deposition disease. Rheumatology. 2000;39:1290-1292.

88. Viani RM, Bromberg K, Bradley JS. Obturator internus muscle abscess in children: Report of seven cases and review. Clin Infect Dis. 1999;28:117-122.

89. Hernandez RJ, Strouse PJ, Craig CL, Farley FA. Focal pyomyositis of the perisciatic muscles in children. AJR Am J Roentgenol. 2002;179:1267-1271.

90. Ytterberg SR. The relationship of infectious agents to inflammatory myositis. Rheum Dis Clin North Am. 1994;20:995-1015.

91. Saito M, Higuchi I, Saito A, et al. Molecular analysis of T cell clonotypes in muscle-infiltrating lymphocytes from patients with human T lymphotropic virus type 1 polymyositis. J Infect Dis. 2002;186:1231-1241.
92. Middleton PJ, Alexander RM, Szymanski MT. Severe myositis during recovery from influenza. Lancet. 1970;2:533-535.
93. Mejlszenkier JD, Safran AP, Healy JJ, et al. The myositis of influenza. Arch Neurol. 1973;29:441-443.
94. McIntyre PG, Doherty C. Acute benign myositis during childhood: Report of five cases. Clin Infect Dis. 1995;20:722.
95. Karpathios T, Kostaki M, Drakonaki S, et al. An epidemic with influenza B virus causing benign acute myositis in ten boys and two girls. Eur J Pediatr. 1995;154:334-336.
96. Kessler HA, Trenholme GM, Harris AA, et al. Acute myopathy associated with influenza A/Texas/1/77 infection. JAMA. 1980;243:461-462.
97. Morton SE, Mathai M, Byrd RP Jr, et al. Influenza A pneumonia with rhabdomyolysis. South Med J. 2001;94:67-69.
98. Craver RD, Sorrells K, Gohd R. Myocarditis with influenza B infection. Pediatr Infect Dis J. 1997;16:629-630.
99. Churchill MA, Geraci JE, Hunder GG. Musculoskeletal manifestations of bacterial endocarditis. Ann Intern Med. 1977;87:754-759.
100. Plonquet A, Bassez G, Authier FJ, et al. Toxoplasmic myositis as a presenting manifestation of idiopathic CD4 lymphocytopenia. Muscle Nerve. 2003;27:761-765.
101. Greenlee JE, Johnson WD, Campa JF, et al. Adult toxoplasmosis presenting as polymyositis and cerebral ataxia. Ann Intern Med. 1975;82:367-371.
102. Kass EH, Andrus SB, Adams RD, et al. Toxoplasmosis in the human adult. Arch Intern Med. 1952;89:759-782.
103. Dalakas MC, Pezeshkpour GH, Gravell M, et al. Polymyositis associated with AIDS retrovirus. JAMA. 1986;256:2381-2383.
104. Simpson DM, Bender AN. Human immunodeficiency virus-associated myopathy: Analysis of 11 patients. Ann Neurol. 1988;24:79-84.
105. Grunfeld C, Feingold KR. Metabolic disturbances and wasting in the acquired immunodeficiency syndrome. N Engl J Med. 1992;327:329-337.
106. Till M, MacDonell KB. Myopathy with human immunodeficiency virus type 1 (HIV-1) infection: HIV-1 or zidovudine? Ann Intern Med. 1990;113:492-494.
107. Dalakas MC, Illa I, Pezeshkpour GH, et al. Mitochondrial myopathy caused by long-term zidovudine therapy. N Engl J Med. 1990;322:1098-1105.
108. Atlas E, Novak SN, Duray P, et al. Lyme myositis: Muscle invasion by *Borrelia burgdorferi.* Ann Intern Med. 1988;109:245-246.
109. Beaver PC, Gadgil RK, Morera P. Sarcocystis: A review and report of five cases. Am J Trop Med Hyg. 1979;28:819-844.
110. Ledford DK, Overman MD, Gonzalvo A, et al. Microsporidiosis myositis in a patient with the acquired immunodeficiency syndrome. Ann Intern Med. 1985;102:628-630.
111. Adams RD. Diseases of Muscle: A Study in Pathology. Hagerstown, Md.: Harper & Row; 1975:318.
112. Cherry JD. Enteroviruses. In: Remington JS, Klein JO, eds. Infectious Diseases of the Fetus and Newborn Infant. 5th ed. Philadelphia: WB Saunders; 2001:477.
113. Marinella MA. Exertional rhabdomyolysis after recent coxsackie B virus infection. South Med J. 1998;91:1057-1059.
114. Clausen MR, Meyer CN, Krantz T, et al. Trichinella infection and clinical disease. Q J Med. 1996;89:631-636.
115. Jacobson ES, Jacobson HG. Trichinosis in an immunosuppressed human host. Am J Clin Pathol. 1977;68:791-794.
116. Cabié A, Bouchard O, Houzés, et al. Albendazole versus thiabendazole as therapy for trichinosis: A retrospective study. Clin Infect Dis. 1996;22:1033-1035.
117. Culpepper RC, Williams RG, Mease PJ, et al. Natural history of the eosinophilia-myalgia syndrome. Ann Intern Med. 1991;115:437-442.
118. Minow RA, Gorbach S, Johnson BL, et al. Myoglobinuria associated with influenza A infection. Ann Intern Med. 1974;80:359-361.
119. Berger RP, Wadowksy RM. Rhabdomyolysis associated with infection by *Mycoplasma pneumoniae:* A case report. Pediatrics. 2000;105:433-436.
120. Solbrig MV, Sher JH, Kula RW. Rhabdomyolysis in leptospirosis (Weil's disease). J Infect Dis. 1987;156:692-693.
121. Naschitz JE, Yeshurun D, Shagrawi I. Rhabdomyolysis in pneumococcal sepsis. Am J Med. 1989;87:479-480.
122. Van Deuren M, Neeleman C, Assmann KJM, et al. Rhabdomyolysis during the subacute stage of meningococcal sepsis. Clin Infect Dis. 1998;26:214-215.
123. Josselson J, Pula T, Sadler JH. Acute rhabdomyolysis associated with an echovirus 9 infection. Arch Intern Med. 1980;140:1671-1672.
124. Meshkinpour H, Vaziri ND. Acute rhabdomyolysis associated with adenovirus infection. J Infect Dis. 1981;143:133.
125. Du J, Wang X, Miereles C. et al. Activation of caspase-3 is an initial step triggering accelerated muscle proteolysis in catabolic conditions J. Clin. Invest. 2004;113:115-123.
126. Hasselgren PO, Wray C, Mammen J. Molecular regulation of muscle cachexia: It may be more than the proteasome. Biochem Biophys Res Commun. 2002;290:1-10.
127. Clowes GHA Jr, George BC, Villee CA Jr, et al. Muscle proteolysis induced by a circulating peptide in patients with sepsis or trauma. N Engl J Med. 1983;308:545-552.
128. Baracos V, Rodemann HP, Dinarello CA, et al. Stimulation of muscle protein degradation and prostaglandin E_2 release by leukocytic pyrogen (interleukin-1): A mechanism for the increased degradation of muscle proteins during fever. N Engl J Med. 1983;308:553-558.

CHAPTER 88

Lymphadenitis and Lymphangitis

MARK S. PASTERNACK
MORTON N. SWARTZ

LYMPHADENITis

Lymphadenitis is an acute or chronic inflammation of lymph nodes. It may be restricted to a solitary node or to a localized group of nodes draining an anatomic area (regional lymphadenitis), or the involvement can be generalized during a systemic infection. The gross features may be those of nonsuppurative, suppurative, necrotizing, or caseous inflammation, depending on the nature of the infecting microorganism.

Pathogenesis and Pathologic Changes

Acute Lymphadenitis

Lymph nodes serve as filters, removing infectious agents from lymphatics, draining areas of acute inflammation. The initial histologic response consists of swelling and hyperplasia of sinusoidal lining cells and the infiltration of leukocytes. Depending on the nature of the infecting organism, host defenses, and antimicrobial therapy, the process may or may not progress to abscess formation. With some microorganisms, a more distinctive pathologic picture may be seen: caseation necrosis with infections due to *Mycobacterium tuberculosis, Histoplasma capsulatum, Coccidioides immitis*, and various atypical mycobacteria; stellate abscesses surrounded by palisading epithelioid cells ("granulomatous abscess")[1] with lymphogranuloma venereum, cat-scratch disease, tularemia, yersiniosis, fungal lymphadenitis, and chronic granulomatous disease; or reactive follicular hyperplasia with scattered clusters of epithelioid histiocytes, located in cortical and paracortical zones and characteristically blurring the margins of germinal centers, along with focal distention of subcapsular and trabecular sinuses by monocytoid cells (monocytoid B cells), in toxoplasmosis.[2] The necrotizing granulomatous lymphadenitis that occurs in tularemia can resemble that occurring in cat-scratch disease but often exhibits more granulomatous inflammation. *Yersinia (Yersinia pseudotuberculosis* or *Yersinia enterocolitica)* infection in mesenteric lymph nodes can also cause a necrotizing lymphadenitis. Necrotizing nongranulomatous lymphadenitis may be a feature of processes to which an infectious cause has not yet been ascribed: Kikuchi's necrotizing lymphadenitis, Kawasaki's syndrome, and systemic lupus erythematosus.[3] Necrotizing viral lymphadenitis has been documented due to herpes simplex virus, primarily in individuals with underlying hematologic disorders,[4,5] and due to parvovirus B19 in healthy individuals, as well as in patients with systemic lupus erythematosus.[6]

Chronic Lymphadenitis

Histologically the response is proliferative with hyperplasia of reticuloendothelial cells, prominent germinal centers, and dilated lymph sinuses filled with mononuclear cells. This picture is nonspecific, can be seen with a variety of infections, and may be observed initially on biopsy in a patient subsequently proven to have a lymphoproliferative disorder. Noncaseous granulomatous lymphadenitis is characteristic of sarcoidosis. More destructive granulomatous lymphadenitis with necrosis or caseation may occur in tuberculous or fungal lymphadenitis.

Dermatopathic lymphadenitis is a distinctive form of chronic lymphadenitis involving lymph nodes draining sites of chronic pruritic dermatitides. Histologically the enlarged nodes show hyperplasia of reticulum cells in the germinal follicles and of sinusoidal lining cells, as well as the accumulation of lipid and melanin in macrophages (released from the inflammatory process in the skin). The latter feature is the basis for the pathologic designation *lipomelanotic reticuloendotheliosis*. The hyperplastic appearance of such nodes may be so prominent as to suggest erroneously the diagnosis of a lymphoproliferative disorder.

Clinical Findings

Acute Regional Lymphadenitis Due to Pyogenic Bacteria

Palpable lymph nodes do not always indicate serious or ongoing disease. Some degree of inguinal lymphadenopathy is relatively common, reflecting prior episodes of infection in the lower extremities (e.g., interdigital web infections secondary to epidermophytosis); similarly, minor enlargement of cervical nodes may be the residual from previous pharyngeal or dental infections. Lymphadenopathy in certain anatomic areas (preauricular, posterior auricular, supraclavicular, deltoidopectoral, and pectoral) should be viewed with greater suspicion because these nodes are not frequently enlarged as a result of local subclinical infections or minor trauma. Enlargement of superficial lymph nodes along the external jugular vein, as well as of nodes that drain the earlobe and the floor of the external acoustic meatus, is very infrequent but may be associated with superficial infection accompanying recent initial earring insertion. Rarely, a firm mass in the tail or lateral aspect of the breast, suggestive of carcinoma, proves to be an enlarged lymph node in an unusual location due to toxoplasmosis.[2]

Acute suppurative lymphadenitis is far more common in children than in adults. In the past four decades, *Staphylococcus aureus* has superseded group A streptococci as the most frequent etiologic agent. The most common sites of involvement are, in descending order, submandibular (submaxillary), anterior and posterior cervical, inguinal, and axillary lymph nodes. The portal of entry for infection is frequently difficult to determine in children when cervical lymph nodes are involved. The recovery of a variety of anaerobic pathogens in cervical lymph node aspirates from some patients suggests that in addition to cutaneous foci, primary dental or pharyngeal infections may lead to suppurative lymphadenitis.[7,8]

On examination, the involved area is swollen, and the node(s) is usually at least 3 cm in diameter and tender. Fever is commonly present. The node(s) may be very firm or frankly fluctuant. The overlying skin is warm and often erythematous and edematous.

Syndromes Due to Suppurative Lymphadenitis at Specific Anatomic Sites

Cervical Lymphadenitis

Acute unilateral adenitis of pyogenic origin occurs most often in preschool-aged children. Fever (38° C-39° C) is common, and local swelling may have been present for some days before the patient is seen by a physician. In only a minority of the cases is there a history of sore throat. However, in the past, group A streptococci have been implicated in about 75% of the cases of untreated suppurative cervical lymphadenitis in children.[9,10] *S. aureus*, or a combination of *S. aureus* and group A streptococci, is often the etiologic agent of suppurative cervical lymphadenitis associated with pyodermas of the face and scalp. Improved anaerobic culture techniques have demonstrated a variety of oral anaerobes in percutaneous needle aspirates in up to 40% of patients, either as pure anaerobic infections or as mixed infections with conventional gram-positive aerobes.[7,8] Acute torticollis may result from cervical lymphadenitis, of either bacterial or viral (e.g., infectious mononucleosis) origin, and may be the initial symptom that brings the child to the physician.[11]

On examination, there is prominent swelling of the neck or face owing to the enlargement of a single node or a matted collection of adjacent lymph nodes, which may be walnut sized. The mass is exquis-

itely tender and firm but may be fluctuant at presentation, or may become fluctuant during the course of therapy. The swelling may be sufficiently marked to interfere with opening of the mouth. A leukocytosis with a white blood cell count of 12,000 to 25,000/mm³ is a common finding.

Acute bilateral cervical adenitis usually involves multiple nodes that are enlarged and somewhat tender in association with viral pharyngitis, infectious mononucleosis, streptococcal pharyngitis, or periodontal infection. Such lymphadenopathy does not ordinarily go on to suppuration unless the symptomatic streptococcal pharyngitis or periodontal infection is ignored.

Acute Axillary Lymphadenitis

This process, when due to *Staphylococcus pyogenes*, is characterized by an abrupt onset with chills, fever, marked axillary pain, and prominent edema of the shoulder, arm, axilla, supraclavicular fossa, and pectoral areas.[12] The site of initiating infection is usually a pustule or traumatic lesion on the hand or arm. The involved area, although edematous, does not have features of cellulitis, lymphangitis, or erysipelas. Ipsilateral pleural effusion may develop owing to blockage of lymphatic vessels draining the parietal pleura into involved lymph nodes at the junction of the internal jugular and subclavian veins. Thrombosis of the axillary and subclavian veins may be a complication.

Subpectoral Lymphadenitis

An unusual course may be taken occasionally by infection (usually streptococcal but sometimes staphylococcal) of the thumb or of the interdigital web between the thumb and index finger. Lymphatics from this area do not pass through the epitrochlear nodes but drain directly into the axillary nodes, which in turn communicate with the subpectoral nodes. If infection is not contained in the axillary nodes, subpectoral lymphadenitis develops.[13] Suppuration of these subpectoral nodes can follow. Infection in this area may dissect downward and manifest as cellulitis over the lower chest and upper abdomen, suggesting an intra-abdominal infection. Occasionally, large subpectoral abscesses may suggest a tumor because the overlying pectoralis major obscures the local warmth and erythema commonly associated with infection. Rarely, contraction of the pectoral muscle (as on elevating the arm) causes cephalic movement of the pectoral area swelling, suggesting avulsion of the inferior attachments of this muscle to the sternum, sixth costal cartilage, and the aponeurosis of the external abdominal oblique muscle. The suppurating nodes may drain onto the chest wall. A pleural effusion may develop on the involved side.

Acute Mediastinal Lymphadenitis

Acute suppurative mediastinal lymphadenitis is usually recognized in the course of managing bacterial mediastinitis, a fulminant process typically complicating progressive infections of the upper respiratory tract, or perforation of the esophagus or bronchial tree as the result of trauma or surgery. Rarely, odontogenic foci of infection may lead to progressive mediastinal lymphadenitis without apparent progressive infection of the head and neck. Suppurative mediastinal lymphadenitis is one of the benign causes of the superior vena cava (SVC) syndrome.[14] The superior vena cava syndrome has also been attributed to marked reactive lymphadenopathy in the setting of cystic fibrosis without frank mediastinal suppuration.[15] Prominent acute hemorrhagic thoracic lymphadenitis is a feature of inhalation anthrax, an aspect reemphasized in the 2001 bioterrorism-related anthrax outbreak.[16]

Acute Suppurative Epitrochlear Lymphadenitis

The epitrochlear nodes receive lymphatic drainage from the middle, ring, and little fingers and from the medial portion of the hand and the ulnar aspect of the forearm. Acute suppurative epitrochlear lymphadenitis is uncommon. The site of the initiating infection in most patients is a primary pyoderma or secondarily infected skin lesion. Unilateral tender swelling, erythema, and induration of the epitrochlear area develop and may subsequently spread along the medial aspect of the arm and forearm. Pain on movement of the elbow is evident. There is often a moderate fever and leukocytosis. The diagnosis is apparent when a discrete, tender nodular swelling can be palpated; but when the area is diffusely swollen and movement at the elbow is limited, the picture may suggest septic arthritis, osteomyelitis, or olecranon bursitis.[17] Group A streptococci and *S. aureus* are implicated most commonly.

Suppurative Iliac Lymphadenitis

The iliac lymph nodes are located along the external and common iliac arteries in the anterior retroperitoneal space. They receive deep lymphatic drainage from the lower abdominal wall and afferents from the superficial and deep inguinal nodes. Iliac lymphadenitis may develop secondary to infection of the lower extremities, lower abdominal wall, perineum, and so forth, or rarely, it may result from hematogenous infection. After infection develops, it appears to break through fascial compartments in the iliac fossa, and abscess formation ensues. Formerly, most cases occurred in children and young adults, but more recently there appears to be no age predilection. The suppurative lymphadenitis progresses to abscess formation in the space between the posterior peritoneum and the psoas and iliacus fascia.[18] An unexplained limp may be the initial symptom; an acute picture with fever may not occur for some days or weeks. Back and hip pain becomes prominent; extension of the thigh is very painful, but abduction and adduction of the hip evoke minimal discomfort. The symptomatology and clinical findings direct attention to the diagnostic possibilities of septic arthritis and osteomyelitis. Only after some days or weeks does lower abdominal pain develop, and the patient becomes acutely ill with high fever and marked leukocytosis. Examination at this point reveals a tightly flexed hip, rectus muscle spasm on the affected side, possibly a tender posterolateral pelvic mass, or a tender inguinal mass suggesting an incarcerated inguinal hernia. By this stage, the abscess may be sizable and may produce elevation and medial displacement of the sigmoid colon and medial displacement of the lower third of the ureter. When the symptoms are on the right side, the diagnosis of *retrocecal* appendicitis with abscess may be suggested, but the antecedent limp is an important clinical clue. Other diagnoses that may be suggested by the clinical manifestations include tuberculosis of the spine with psoas abscess formation, pelvic inflammatory disease, and tumor of the thigh.[19] Cross-sectional imaging via body computed tomography (CT) or magnetic resonance imaging (MRI) can be very helpful in defining an inflammatory collection abutting the psoas and iliacus muscles. *S. aureus* is the microorganism most commonly implicated, followed in frequency by streptococci.

Acute Regional Lymphadenitis Due to Infecting Agents Other Than Pyogenic Bacteria

A variety of organisms other than the common pyogens may produce localized lymphadenitis (in some cases, going on to abscess and sinus tract formation). These infections resemble pyogenic lymphadenitis but are distinguishable by a prolonged and indolent course, the atypical anatomic areas involved, the lack of prior pyogenic infection, and sometimes by clues in the history (e.g., scratch by a cat, previous tuberculosis, recent sexual exposure). Occasionally the nature of the clinical setting and host immunodeficiency broaden the spectrum of microorganisms to be considered as the cause of firm or fluctuant lymphadenitis. Mycotic (*Candida albicans, Aspergillus* spp.) cervical lymphadenitis has occurred after oral mucositis in neutropenic children with leukemia,[2] but a rare case of bilateral cervical lymphadenopathy due to *Aspergillus fumigatus* has been described in a young girl without underlying disease, neutropenia, or immunosuppression.[21] In patients with suppurative lymphadenitis complicating chronic granulomatous disease, the microbial etiology is usually a catalase-positive pathogen. In addition to the commonly involved *S. aureus*, these include members of the family Enterobacteriaceae (*Klebsiella, Serratia, Salmonella*), *Pseudomonas* (often *Pseudomonas cepacia*), *Aspergillus, Nocardia,* Calmette-Guérin bacillus (BCG), and *Chromobacterium violaceum.*[22-24]

A variety of opportunistic pathogens rarely may be responsible for peripheral lymphadenitis in patients with HIV infection. These include *H. capsulatum, Cryptococcus neoformans,*[25] *Pneumocystis jirovecii,*[26] and *Bartonella henselae*[27] (bacillary angiomatosis). In addition, unusual pathogens have been responsible for lymphadenitis on rare occasions in immunocompetent persons. Such microorganisms include *Rhodococcus equi*[28] and *Y. pseudotuberculosis.*[29]

Specific Types of Nonpyogenic Regional Lymphadenitis

Scrofula (Tuberculous Cervical Lymphadenitis)

Tuberculous cervical adenitis, formerly a common disease in children and young adults, has become infrequent. It is still occasionally seen in older adults who many years earlier had immigrated to this country from endemic areas (British Isles, Europe, and the Far East) or who lived in rural areas in this country. In this setting it represents breakdown of prior cervical node tuberculosis, acquired either by ingestion of infected milk (bovine tuberculosis) or by lymphohematogenous spread of infection from an initial pulmonary focus to this group of lymph nodes. *M. tuberculosis* is seen in this country as the etiologic agent of cervical adenitis also in adults of particular ethnic groups: Native Americans, Latinos, and recent immigrants from Haiti and Asia. In the United States, mycobacterial cervical lymphadenitis (scrofula) is four or five times more frequently due to atypical mycobacteria, commonly *Mycobacterium scrofulaceum* in children,[30] than to *M. tuberculosis.* In certain areas of the United States, *Mycobacterium avium-intracellulare* complex is the principal etiologic agent[31-32] in children and in adults. Recently, newly recognized, difficult-to-isolate, and uncommon mycobacterial species have been reported as occasionally causing childhood cervical lymphadenitis[31]: *Mycobacterium interjectum, Mycobacterium malmoense, Mycobacterium haemophilum, Mycobacterium xenopi,* and *Mycobacterium szulgai.* Two additional newly described slowly growing mycobacterial species have been described very recently: one, *Mycobacterium lentiflavum,*[33] is yellow pigmented, and the other, *Mycobacterium heidelbergense,*[34] is nonphotochromogenic. *M. tuberculosis* infections, including cervical lymphadenitis, are frequent in the human immunodeficiency virus (HIV)-infected population. *M. tuberculosis* lymphadenitis in the HIV-infected patient differs in several respects from the infection in HIV-negative patients: higher frequency of fever, often negative results on purified protein derivative (PPD) skin testing (anergy), and higher frequency of positive smears for acid-fast bacilli (and greater numbers of organisms) on fine-needle aspirates of involved lymph nodes.[35] In parts of the world where BCG vaccination of infants is commonly practiced, subcutaneous abscesses and regional lymphadenitis are not uncommon complications, occurring 2 to 8 weeks after vaccination, but these usually resolve spontaneously. Occasionally the regional (axillary, supraclavicular, or cervical) lymphadenitis progressively enlarges and goes on to caseating suppuration.[36] This has been reported to occur at a frequency of 0.1 to 4.3 cases per 100,000 doses administered to children younger than 2 years of age.[37]

The onset of scrofula is insidious, and fever and other systemic manifestations are generally absent. Several nodes are enlarged and matted together; the mass so formed may develop a swollen fluctuant area, and this brings the patient to medical attention. The process is usually painless. In most cases, clinical evidence of tuberculosis elsewhere is absent. Spontaneous drainage of caseous material onto the skin surface (scrofuloderma) may eventually occur.

Definition of the mycobacterial species involved is important. The atypical mycobacteria causing cervical lymphadenitis are frequently resistant to conventional antituberculous chemotherapy, and surgical excision of the involved fluctuant node or nodes is indicated.[38-40] Adjunctive therapy with rifampin and clarithromycin is sometimes considered when treating *M. avium-intracellulare* lymphadenitis, especially when imaging by ultrasound or computed tomography demonstrates extensive deep lymph node involvement or involvement of submandibular nodes abutting the facial nerve, which preclude total excision.[32,40] Antituberculous therapy is usually not needed for BCG nonsuppurative lymphadenitis, but if suppurative lymphadenitis develops, aspiration[41] or complete excision[37] and antituberculous chemotherapy are indicated.

Granulomatous Lymphadenitis Caused by Nondiphtheria *Corynebacteria*

Subacute or chronic relapsing lymphadenitis has been reported occasionally to be due to *Corynebacterium pseudotuberculosis (Corynebacterium ovis)*.[42] Most patients have lived in Australia[43] and have had extensive contact with animals, particularly sheep in which *C. pseudotuberculosis* is a common cause of caseous lymphadenitis. The histologic picture is that of a suppurative or necrotizing granulomatous process. Treatment consists of prolonged antibiotic (erythromycin or penicillin) therapy combined with surgical drainage or excision of the involved nodes.

Oculoglandular (Parinaud's) Syndrome

Preauricular lymphadenopathy can occur secondary to granulomatous nodular conjunctival infection caused by the introduction of certain pathogens onto the external eye. Oculoglandular syndromes occur occasionally in tularemia, cat-scratch disease,[44,45] listeriosis, sporotrichosis, adenovirus infection, and lymphogranuloma venereum. Epidemic keratoconjunctivitis due to adenoviruses is often associated with an enlarged preauricular lymph node as well.

Cat-Scratch Disease

Cat-scratch disease[44] is a slowly progressive and sometimes chronic form of regional lymphadenitis caused by *B. henselae* (see Chapter 232). Although cat-scratch disease is usually a benign and ultimately self-limited process, it may be complicated by acute encephalitis, hepatitis, osteolysis, neuroretinitis, arthritis, pleuritis, atypical pneumonia, hilar adenopathy, and thrombocytopenia.

B. henselae bacilli are slow growing, requiring 2 to 6 weeks' incubation in a moist environment (e.g., in a sealed gas-permeable plastic bag) under 5% CO_2 for growth on blood agar plates (human blood is preferable to sheep or horse blood).[46]

About 90% of patients with cat-scratch disease give a history of contact with cats (most often kittens), and most have been scratched. A primary lesion (small papule or vesicle resembling an insect bite) develops at the site of the scratch 7 to 14 days after contact with the animal. This primary lesion lasts for several weeks to months and may be helpful in diagnosis. Lymphadenopathy develops within 1 to 2 weeks of the appearance of the skin papule.[47] There is no lymphangitis. The lymphadenopathy progresses to suppuration in 10% to 50% of cases, but the course is slower than that of suppurative lymphadenitis due to pyogenic bacteria, and most patients are only mildly ill. Regional lymphadenitis is the sole manifestation of cat-scratch disease in half of the cases. Almost any peripheral lymph node may be involved, but the axillary nodes are most commonly affected. The nodes are tender, acutely so when there is frank suppuration. Fever is present in only about a third of patients and is low grade. About 10% to 15% of patients suffer features of a more systemic illness: anorexia, headache, weight loss, and hepatosplenomegaly. Unusual clinical presentations include Parinaud's oculoglandular syndrome (conjunctivitis from ocular inoculation associated with ipsilateral preauricular lymphadenopathy) in 4% of patients, neuroretinitis, and, rarely, acute encephalitis/encephalopathy, usually with a sudden seizure as the initial neurologic manifestation, occurring several weeks after the first symptoms of cat-scratch disease. In one patient with cervical lymphadenopathy and another patient with Parinaud's oculoglandular syndrome, *B. henselae* was isolated on blood culture after prolonged incubation (9 days in one case).[48] *B. henselae* infection has been confirmed by polymerase chain reaction (PCR) testing of biopsy tissue[49] within the first 6 weeks of lymphadenopathy, and from conjunctival scraping in the setting of Parinaud's oculoglandular syndrome.[45] *B. henselae* infections can be confirmed serologically at the Centers for Disease Control and Prevention.

Mediastinal Lymphadenopathy

In contrast to acute or subacute peripheral regional lymphadenitis where local signs and symptoms prompt medical attention, mediastinal lymphadenitis is sometimes detected only in the course of evaluation of nonlocalizing systemic complaints such as fever and weight loss, or primarily pulmonary symptoms such as cough and sputum production. Distinctive radiologic features may support particular diagnoses. Symmetric hilar adenopathy with clear lung fields or symmetric interstitial fibrosis is consistent with sarcoidosis, particularly when accompanied by any of a variety of extrathoracic manifestations. Asymmetric or unilateral hilar adenopathy, particularly when associated with ipsilateral chronic focal lung disease with calcification, fibrosis, and/or cavitation, suggests tuberculosis or fungal infection. The presence of mediastinal widening in association with subacute or chronic mediastinal lymphadenopathy strongly suggests histoplasmosis. *Cryptococcus* can cause suppurative mediastinitis in HIV patients as part of the acquired immunodeficiency syndrome. The underlying health, travel history, extrapulmonary signs and symptoms, and ancillary laboratory tests (gallium scanning, angiotensin-converting enzyme levels, anergy) all contribute to a presumptive diagnosis, but in most adults, lymph node biopsy or transbronchial lung biopsy is necessary for pathologic and microbiologic confirmation.

Inguinal Buboes of Sexually Transmitted Disease

Inguinal lymphadenopathy due to pyogenic infections or cat-scratch disease is usually unilateral. Prominent bilateral (or unilateral) adenopathy, particularly in men, is suggestive of several sexually transmitted diseases. The genital chancre of primary syphilis is usually accompanied by one or several discrete, firm, nonsuppurative, painless, enlarged nodes in one or both inguinal areas. Constitutional signs are lacking. The overlying skin is uninflamed. In secondary syphilis, the lymphadenopathy is generalized and painless and usually precedes the cutaneous eruption.

Lymphogranuloma venereum (LGV) infections arise following the sexual transmission of selected *Chlamydia trachomatis* serovars. The primary genital lesion (painless papule, vesicle, or erosion) is usually transient and asymptomatic. The initial manifestation of the disease is usually the characteristic inguinal bubo, occurring 10 to 30 days after sexual exposure and 1 to 2 weeks after the primary lesion. The adenopathy is more commonly unilateral. Initially the node is tender, discrete, hard, and movable, but subsequently the inflammatory process involves multiple nodes in the area. Chills, fever, and constitutional symptoms are common at this stage. As a result of periadenitis, the nodes become fixed and matted into an oval or lobulated mass. The mass is adherent to the overlying skin, which is purplish. Foci of suppuration develop, with multiple fistulous tracts. A central lengthwise linear depression (so-called groove sign of LGV) is produced by involvement of nodes above and below the inguinal ligament. Although characteristic of LGV, the groove sign may rarely be produced by suppurative bacterial lymphadenitis or by lymphomatous involvement of inguinal nodes.

Chancroid is usually accompanied by painful, tender inguinal adenopathy. The primary lesion is a papule or pustule that progresses to form an extremely painful and tender but nonindurated ulceration with undermined edges, quite in contrast to a syphilitic chancre. Autoinoculation is common with lesions on opposing or contiguous areas of the skin. The adenopathy of chancroid develops about 1 week after the primary lesion appears and, unlike in LGV, is present while the ulcer is still active. Systemic symptoms accompany chancroid only rarely. The chancroidal bubo is typically unilateral and made up of fused inguinal nodes and is more painful than that of LGV. Unilocular suppuration may develop. However, in most patients, the lymphadenitis subsides without suppuration.

Primary genital herpes simplex infection in men and women is often associated with tender inguinal adenopathy. Histologically, the nodes show paracortical hyperplasia (with a prominent admixture of immunoblasts, plasma cells, and macrophages), along with sinus histiocytosis, discrete foci of necrosis, and intranuclear inclusions within scattered mononuclear and giant cells. Similar, histologically proven, recurrent, localized as well as generalized herpetic lymphadenitis can occur in immunocompromised patients in the absence of overt mucocutaneous lesions.[50,51] The "pseudobuboes" of granuloma inguinale are produced by subcutaneous granulomatous infection rather than by suppurative lymphadenitis.

Suppurative inguinal lymphadenitis due to group A streptococci has been superimposed on chronic lymphadenopathy in homosexual men.[52]

Inguinal Buboes of Other Than Sexually Transmitted Disease Origin

Inguinal or femoral buboes occur in bubonic plague, because the flea bite initiating the infection is commonly on a lower extremity.[53] However, involvement of most other peripheral nodes can occur. The disease begins with fever, malaise, headache, and tender regional adenopathy after an incubation period of 2 to 6 days. Only rarely is a lesion (papule, pustule) at the site of the insect bite evident at the onset of clinical illness. A large, matted collection of lymph nodes with surrounding edema quickly develops and may go on to suppuration and spontaneous drainage. If not treated promptly the infection rapidly progresses to a septicemic phase. The diagnosis should be suspected in a febrile, acutely ill patient with a large cluster of extremely tender lymph nodes and a history of exposure to fleas, rodents, or rabbits in the western United States (see Chapter 226). (Tularemia may mimic the epidemiologic and clinical features of bubonic plague but is more likely to produce an *ulceroglandular syndrome* [Table 88-1], with a primary lesion at the site of inoculation.[54]) Cutaneous anthrax is another cause of ulceroglandular infection, but the marked local edema and eschar formation at the site of inoculation dominate the clinical picture.[16] Diagnostic procedures include blood cultures (which yield uniformly positive results in the septicemic phase of plague), as well as cultures and stained smears of carefully obtained bubo aspirates. Appropriate treatment (see later) should be instituted immediately, before results of cultures become available, if bubonic plague is suspected. Cat-scratch disease also may present as unilateral inguinal bubo.

Generalized Lymphadenitis Associated with Systemic Infections

Widespread lymphadenitis is a feature of a variety of infections disseminated by the blood stream. In most instances, suppuration of the involved nodes does not occur. Generalized lymphadenopathy is a feature, for example, of secondary syphilis, HIV infection, infectious mononucleosis, acute toxoplasmosis, leptospirosis, and miliary tuberculosis. Generalized lymphadenopathy associated with infections is commonly due to the presence of the invading microorganism in the nodes. Generalized lymph node enlargement is a feature of a variety of infectious diseases due to bacterial, rickettsial, chlamydial, spirochetal, viral, protozoal, and helminthic agents (see Table 88-1). In immunocompromised hosts, particularly following organ transplantation, Epstein-Barr virus infection may evolve into a lymphoproliferative disorder (post-transplantation lymphoproliferative disorder) that requires reduction in immunosuppressive therapy and antiviral therapy.[55]

Recurrent Lymphadenitis

Periodic Fever, Aphthous Ulcers, Pharyngitis, and Adenitis Syndrome (PFAPA)

There are several periodic fever syndromes that possess well-defined genetic defects or readily identifiable laboratory abnormalities in addition to distinctive patterns of illness. Lymph node involvement is generally not a prominent feature of these diseases. However, recurrent cervical lymphadenitis is a prominent feature of PFAPA (Marshall's) syndrome, a disease of unknown etiology.[56,57] This syndrome, which has its onset primarily, but not exclusively, in young children, is recognized by roughly monthly sudden bouts of high fever associated with oropharyngeal involvement (aphthous ulcers, pharyngitis) and cervical adenitis. Febrile episodes are accompanied by leukocytosis and elevation of the erythrocyte sedimentation rate. Patients become entirely well after 4 to 5 days of fever, and remain asymptomatic, with normal laboratory studies, until the next bout of fever. The syndrome persists for an average of 4 to 5 years. The acute febrile symptomatic episodes can be promptly aborted by single doses of prednisone (1-2 mg/kg).[58] Tonsillectomy has been reported to induce permanent remission of symptoms in some patient series,[58,59] and cimetidine has also been suggested to modulate clinical illness.[58,60]

Filarial Lymphangitis

Recurrent inguinal lymphadenitis, accompanied by lymphangitis, is a common problem in individuals with bancroftian filariasis. These acute inflammatory episodes (acute filarial lymphangitis) are thought to reflect the death of adult filariae with elicitation of a brisk host response, but at times may represent bacterial infection which complicates adult worm-induced lymphectasia (see later).[61]

Etiologic Agents and Differential Diagnosis

It is helpful for purposes of the differential diagnosis to consider infective lymphadenitis in several categories (see Table 88-1): (1) regional lymphadenopathy, (2) regional lymphadenopathy with breakdown of nodes, (3) inguinal bubo formation, (4) ulceroglandular syndrome, (5) oculoglandular syndrome, and (6) generalized lymphadenopathy.

In distinguishing among the causes of fluctuant cervical lymphadenitis, the history may suggest a streptococcal (preceding tonsillitis), staphylococcal (recent facial or neck infection), or tuberculous (prior exposure to tuberculosis) disease or cat-scratch disease (exposure to cat) as the causative disorder. In a study of suppurative cervical adenitis, *S. aureus* was the etiologic agent more frequently than group A streptococci (36% versus 26%), and in another 25% of the cases, a bacteriologic diagnosis could not be made.[62] A subacute clinical course with little fever and a normal leukocyte count would be more consistent with cat-scratch disease or mycobacterial involvement. Sinus tract formation suggests infection due to *M. tuberculosis* or an atypical mycobacterium. Gram-stained and Ziehl-Neelsen smears and culture (including cultures for mycobacteria) of material aspirated or drained from suppurating nodes provides a diagnosis in about two thirds of such cases of cervical lymphadenitis. Further information may be provided by skin tests (PPD), serologic tests (antistreptolysin O or anti-DNase B antibody titers), and histologic examination (e.g., caseation necrosis suggesting mycobacterial infection or bimorphic appearance suggesting cat-scratch disease) of an excised node when culture of aspirated material is unrevealing. Surgical exploration affords both diagnosis and therapy of suppurative lymphadenitis. Although simple incision and drainage are satisfactory for bacterial or *B. henselae* lymphadenitis, complete excisional biopsy is preferred when exploring mycobacterial adenitis to reduce the risk of poor wound healing and unsightly scar formation; thus the presenting clinical features must guide surgical strategy.

A variety of noninfectious processes may resemble unilateral cervical lymphadenitis. Lymphoma may be suggested by the indolent course of cat-scratch disease. Kawasaki disease, (acute febrile mucocutaneous lymph node syndrome), a disease of unknown etiology almost exclusively affecting infants and young children, is characterized by nonsuppurative cervical lymphadenopathy.[63,64] The age of the patient, febrile course, conjunctival injection, erythematous rash, and subsequent desquamation suggest the diagnosis. In some patients, unilateral lymphadenitis may precede mucocutaneous manifestations and make diagnosis more difficult by initially suggesting bacterial involvement.[65] A variety of additional clinical (uveitis, hydrops of the gallbladder) and laboratory findings (sterile pyuria, inflammatory synovitis, aseptic meningitis, thrombocytosis, elevated erythrocyte sedimentation rate and C-reactive protein) may also be present.

TABLE 88-1 Clinical Patterns and Microbial Agents of Infectious Lymphadenitis

Disease	Infecting Organism	Regional	Regional with Suppuration (or Caseation)	Inguinal Bubo Formation	Ulceroglandular	Oculoglandular	Generalized
Bacterial							
Pyogenic	Group A or B streptococci Staphylococcus aureus	+	+				
Scarlet fever	Group A streptococci	+	+				+
Diptheria	Corynebacterium diptheriae	+					
Fusospirochetal angina	Prevotella melaninogenica; peptostreptococci, etc.	+					
Scrofula	Mycobacterium tuberculosis	+	+				
	Mycobacterium scrofulaceum; Mycobacterium avium-intracellulare	+	+				
Miliary tuberculosis	M. tuberculosis						+
Brucellosis	Brucella						+
Leptospirosis	Leptospira						+
Syphilis	Treponema pallidum	+					
Chancroid	Haemophilus ducreyi			+			
Plague	Yersinia pestis	+	+	+			
Tularemia	Francisella tularensis		+		+	+	
Rat-bite fever	Streptobacillus moniliformis; Spirillum minus	+ +			+		
Anthrax	Bacillus anthracis	+			+		
Listeriosis	Listeria monocytogenes					+	
Melioidosis	Burkholderia pseudomallei	+	+				+
Glanders	Burkholderia mallei	+	+				+
Cat-scratch fever	Batonella henselae	+	+		±	+	
Typhoid fever	Salmonella typhi						+
Mycotic							
Histoplasmosis	Histoplasma capsulatum						+
	H. capsulatum var duboisii	+					
Coccidiodomycosis	Coccidioides immitis	+					
Paracoccidioidomycosis	Paracoccidioides brasiliensis	+					
Cryptococcosis	Cryptococcus neoformans	+					+
Rickettsial							
Boutonneuse fever, etc.	Rickettsia conorii				+		
Scrub typhus	Rickettsia tsutsugamushi	+					
Rickettsialpox	Rickettsia akari	+					+
Chlamydial							
Lymphogranuloma venereum	Chlamydia trachomatis			+		+	+
Viral							
Measles	Measles virus						+
Rubella	Rubella virus						+
Infectious mononucleosis	Epstein-Barr virus						+
Cytomegalovirus mononucleosis	Cytomegalovirus						+
Dengue fever	Dengue virus						+
West Nile fever	West Nile virus						+
Lassa fever	Lassa fever virus						+
Genital herpes infection	Herpes simplex virus type 2	+					
Pharyngoconjunctival fever	Adenovirus (types 3 and 7)	+				+	
Epidemic keratoconjunctivitis	Adenovirus (types 8 and 19)					+	
AIDS; AIDS-related complex	Human immunodeficiency virus						+
Protozoan							
Kala azar	Leishmania donovani						+
African trypanosomiasis	Trypanosoma brucei	+					+
Chagas' disease	Trypanosoma cruzi					+	+
Toxoplasmosis	Toxoplasma gondii						+
Helminthic							
Filariasis	Wuchereria bancrofti						+
	Brugia malayi						+
Loiasis	Loa loa			+			
Onchocerciasis	Onchocerca volvulus			+			

AIDS, acquired immunodeficiency syndrome; +, present.

A more recently described benign disorder of lymph nodes, histiocytic necrotizing lymphadenitis or Kikuchi's disease, was first recognized in Japan and now has been observed in the United States.[66] Clinical features consist of localized, sometimes tender cervical lymphadenopathy, often with an upper respiratory prodrome and associated in some patients with fever or rash.[67] Most cases occur in women, commonly younger than 40 years of age. The involved nodes are usually rubbery or firm, discrete, and rarely greater than 2 cm in diameter.[68] Occasional patients present with generalized lymphadenopathy, and rarely, hepatosplenomegaly occurs.[69] Less frequent symptoms include nausea, vomiting, weight loss, and night sweats, suggesting the diagnosis of lymphoma. Mild leukopenia and lymphocytosis may suggest infectious mononucleosis. The illness does not respond to antibiotics, but it usually resolves spontaneously within 1 or 2 months. Occasionally recurrences may be a feature. Histologically, surgical biopsy specimens may be erroneously interpreted as lymphoma, but the principal findings are those of focal or confluent nodules (made up of crescentic histiocytes, plasmacytoid monocytes, immunoblasts and karyorrhectic debris) combined with patchy areas of coagulative necrosis. Neutrophils are few or absent. Diagnosis has been made in some cases by fine-needle aspiration cytology.[70] Histologically, the lymph node appearance in systemic lupus erythematosus is very similar to that in Kikuchi's disease, but hematoxylin bodies are characteristic of the former. Serologic studies (e.g., antinuclear antibody or anti–deoxyribonucleic acid [DNA] antibody assays) are warranted to help distinguish between the two processes. Although a viral origin is suspected on the basis of the clinical features, serologic and ultrastructural studies have failed to identify a specific agent. A case of parvovirus B19–associated hemophagocytic syndrome causing cervical lymphadenopathy with histologic features resembling those of Kikuchi's disease was recently described.[71]

Bronchial cleft cysts and cystic hygromas may be mistaken for cervical lymphadenitis, particularly if infected; thyroglossal duct cysts may suggest infected submental nodes. Infections of these congenital structures must be considered, particularly if a patient presents with what appears to be recurrent bacterial cervical adenitis. Lymphoepithelial cysts, indolent lesions of the salivary glands (usually the parotid) occurring in HIV-infected patients, may mimic preauricular lymphadenopathy or suggest Sjögren's syndrome.[72] Submaxillary sialadenitis or salivary gland tumors may mimic submandibular lymphadenitis. Bimanual (intraoral and submandibular) palpation can be helpful in distinguishing between these processes.

Isolated inguinal lymphadenitis or bubo formation in the adult suggests venereal disease (syphilis, LGV, chancroid). Distinctive associated primary lesions are usually features of syphilis and chancroid but not of LGV, but in some individuals a syphilitic chancre may not be visible because of vaginal, cervical, or rectal inoculation. The inguinal adenopathy of primary syphilis consists of painless, firm, discrete, movable nodes without erythema of the overlying skin. The nodes do not suppurate, whereas spontaneous rupture of the buboes of LGV and chancroid may occur. The groove sign is suggestive of LGV. The buboes of chancroid are characteristically painful. Axillary, cervical, and inguinal buboes may occur with plague and tularemia. In plague an inguinal location is common. The geographic locale and a history of animal exposure are important clues to the diagnosis. Inguinal and femoral nodes can be involved in cat-scratch disease, although much less frequently than axillary or cervical nodes.

Generalized lymphadenopathy is frequently a manifestation of disseminated infection (see Table 88-1). Clues may be provided by the age of the patient and the presence of a characteristic rash (childhood exanthems, secondary syphilis); geographic factors (dengue, filariasis, localized *Leishmania* lymphadenitis,[73] histoplasmosis); occupation and dietary history (brucellosis, toxoplasmosis); exposure to animals and their excreta, e.g., standing water (leptospirosis); and the presence of atypical lymphocytes (infectious mononucleosis, cytomegalovirus infection). Diagnosis of toxoplasmic lymphadenitis in the immunocompetent patient is based primarily on serologic testing, although

sometimes a node biopsy is performed because of initial concern for lymphoma. A negative result on the Sabin-Feldman dye test or on a comparable test for *Toxoplasma* IgG antibody (indirect immunofluorescence [IIF], passive hemagglutination [PHA], or enzyme-linked immunosorbent assay [ELISA]) practically excludes the diagnosis. Between 3 and 6 months after clinical onset of *Toxoplasma* lymphadenitis, Sabin-Feldman dye titers are 1:1024 or greater.[74] With toxoplasmosis the ELISA is positive for IgM antibodies within the first 3 months of infection in most patients. In the occasional patient with negative, low-positive, or equivocal titers of IgM antibodies, diagnosis may be made by detection of IgA or IgE antibodies or an acute pattern in the differential agglutination test (comparing titers obtained with formalin-fixed tachyzoites with those obtained with acetone-fixed or methanol-fixed tachyzoites-essentially differentiating between avidity of IgG antibodies in acute and nonacute infections). In a study of serodiagnosis in 40 consecutive patients with biopsy-confirmed toxoplasmic lymphadenitis, a serologic profile (dye test; IgM, IgG, and IgE antibody titers; and differential agglutination test) had a sensitivity of 100% with use of the first serum specimen drawn after clinical onset of lymphadenitis.[74]

Laboratory diagnosis of acute toxoplasmic lymphadenitis can also be made by seroconversion from a negative to a positive result on IgG antibody testing or by demonstration of a fourfold rise in titer over 3 weeks. In endemic areas, generalized nonsuppurative (and, very rarely, suppurative) lymphadenopathy occurs in typhoid fever.[75]

Widespread suppurative infections of lymph nodes occur as a result of the microbicidal defect characteristic of neutrophils and monocytes of patients with chronic granulomatous disease. Recurrent infections (involving skin, bones, lungs, and liver, as well as lymph nodes) beginning in childhood and due to *S. aureus* and certain gram-negative bacilli (*Escherichia coli*, salmonellae, *Serratia marcescens*) suggest the diagnosis. Suppurative lymphadenitis can also be seen in patients lacking the early complement factor C3.[76]

Widespread lymphadenopathy may be a feature of many noninfectious diseases, particularly infiltrative processes such as lymphoma and reticuloendothelioses. Prominent peripheral lymphadenopathy may be a feature of rheumatoid arthritis. Lymphadenopathy may occur as an adverse effect of prolonged use of phenytoin. Widespread lymphadenopathy is a feature of the syndrome of immunoblastic lymphadenopathy, which is often accompanied by skin rash, polyclonal hypergammaglobulinemia, and immunosuppression. This disorder of immune regulation often eventuates in B-cell or T-cell lymphomas.[77]

Sinus histiocytosis with massive lymphadenopathy (Rosai-Dorfman disease) is another benign process that produces extensive, painless lymphadenopathy in the cervical areas in children and adolescents.[78] It is often accompanied by fever, neutrophilic leukocytosis, and polyclonal hypergammaglobulinemia. Histologically there is extensive proliferation of histiocyte-like cells within the sinuses of the involved lymph nodes.[79] The etiology is unknown, and the prognosis is favorable. A very rare form of regional lymphadenopathy, showing sinus histiocytosis (with the cells seen to contain metal granules) histologically, can be the result of wear-induced debris from an adjacent metallic prosthesis.[80,81] Similarly, enlarged regional lymph nodes (showing noncaseating granulomas containing silicone or histiocytic necrotizing lymphadenitis[82,83]) have been described draining areas in which a silicone mammary prosthesis or a Silastic joint prosthesis[84] had been inserted previously.

Generalized Lymphadenopathy with the Acquired Immunodeficiency Syndrome

Patients with acquired immunodeficiency syndrome (AIDS) or with the AIDS-related complex may have generalized lymphadenopathy in which involvement with opportunistic infection or neoplastic disease (particularly Kaposi's sarcoma) is evident on histologic examination. The infections have included those due to cytomegalovirus and *M. avium-intracellulare*.[85] Those caused by the latter usually show a few poorly formed or no granulomas and a prominent histiocytic reaction. Large clusters ("globi") of acid-fast bacilli are present within the cytoplasm of histiocytes. Kaposi's sarcoma in patients with AIDS may follow the pattern of generalized lymph node involvement and a fulminant course with mucosal and visceral lesions.[86] In AIDS, other neoplasms can involve lymph nodes. These are primarily of the B-cell type and include B-cell immunoblastic sarcomas, small noncleaved-cell Burkitt-type lymphoma, and plasmacytoid lymphocytic lymphoma.[87]

Lymphadenopathy occurs in 50% to 75% of patients at risk for AIDS who develop an acute illness approximately 3 to 6 weeks after initial exposure to HIV.[88,89] It often is one feature of a mononucleosis-like syndrome consisting of fever, malaise, myalgias, headaches, sore throat, diarrhea, leukopenia, thrombocytopenia, and a maculopapular rash. After the acute clinical illness subsides, lymphadenopathy may remain as persistent generalized lymphadenopathy, involving at least several extrainguinal sites, of at least 3 months' duration. This progressive lymphadenopathy early in the course of this infection may be the result of an active immune response against HIV in the affected lymph nodes (see Chapter 117).[90] The nodes are discrete and nontender; suppuration does not occur. HIV replication takes place in such lymph nodes, which histologically show follicular hyperplasia or mixed follicular and interfollicular hyperplasia.[91] Regression of the lymphadenopathy may occur after 8 to 19 months in some patients.

Presumptive Treatment

Initial treatment of infective lymphadenitis requires some narrowing of the diagnostic possibilities (see Table 88-1). Localized pyogenic lymphadenitis responds well to early antibiotic treatment. When cervical lymphadenitis has developed from a pharyngeal or periodontal portal, initial treatment with penicillin is appropriate (procaine penicillin G, 600,000 units intramuscularly every 12 to 24 hours initially to ensure receipt of the therapeutic agent when the patient may be nauseated; subsequently, 500 mg of penicillin V may be administered orally every 6 hours, or 500 mg of amoxicillin every 8 hours, for at least 20 days in older children and adults). In patients who are more acutely ill, larger doses of aqueous penicillin G administered parenterally are indicated. Erythromycin (20 to 40 mg/kg/day orally in divided doses every 6 hours) or clindamycin (600 mg intravenously followed by 300 mg orally three times daily or 30 mg/kg/day in three divided doses for children) are alternatives for patients allergic to penicillin.

Pyogenic lymphadenitis complicating skin infections may be of staphylococcal or streptococcal etiology, and a penicillinase-resistant penicillin is the drug of choice (e.g., dicloxacillin or cephalexin, 0.5 g orally every 6 hours for the older child or an adult). In the more acutely ill patient, intravenous administration of a semisynthetic penicillinase-resistant penicillin (e.g., nafcillin) or a first-generation cephalosporin should be employed. Failure to show improvement, or progression to suppuration, is an indication for imaging by ultrasound or computed tomography scanning and consideration for percutaneous needle aspiration (for bacteriologic diagnosis and treatment) or surgical drainage. Many patients who present with acute suppurative lymphadenitis lack a history of prior focal infection; in these individuals, antistaphylococcal therapy is appropriate. Surgical exploration prior to the evolution of frank suppuration is associated with difficult dissection and recovery of little if any purulent material. Hence exploration is usually reserved for clearcut suppurative adenitis manifested by palpable fluctuance or the demonstration of necrotic nodes by cross-sectional imaging in the setting of continued fever and toxicity. In some centers needle aspiration is performed rather than open surgical drainage.[92] The small but growing incidence of primary community-acquired methicillin-resistant *S. aureus* (MRSA) must be considered when there is a failure to respond to conventional antistaphylococcal medical therapy. Recovery of MRSA at the time of a drainage procedure is invaluable to guide appropriate postoperative antibiotic therapy.

For cat-scratch disease, usually a self-limited process resolving in 2 to 4 months, treatment is principally symptomatic. If the nodes become fluctuant, aspiration is appropriate both for relief of pain and for bacteriologic diagnosis. The few strains of *B. henselae* from

cases of cat-scratch disease that have been studied show in vitro susceptibility to a variety of antimicrobial agents, with the notable exception of first-generation cephalosporins.[46] In a retrospective review of antimicrobial treatment of several hundred patients with cat-scratch disease, clinical efficacy (58%-87%) was attributed to four drugs (in increasing order): trimethoprim-sulfamethoxazole, gentamicin, ciprofloxacin, and rifampin.[93] Azithromycin has also been used to treat *B. henselae* lymphadenitis[94,95]; the intracellular concentration of this agent may offer a therapeutic advantage over other macrolides but clinical trials comparing these agents are not available. Antimicrobial therapy may be reasonable in patients with more severe or extranodal cat-scratch disease. Oral corticosteroids have been used in individuals with *B. henselae* lymphadenitis[96] or hepatosplenic infection[97] refractory to antibiotic therapy. Bacillary angiomatosis and bacillary peliosis hepatitis, infections in patients with AIDS that are due to *B. henselae* or a closely related Bartonellaceae species, appear to respond to prolonged antimicrobial therapy with either erythromycin, doxycycline, or rifampin.[98]

If the diagnosis of bubonic plague is suspected, antibiotic treatment should be instituted promptly. Streptomycin (1 g intramuscularly every 12 hours in adults), alone or in combination with tetracycline (0.5 g orally every 6 hours in adults), are the preferred drugs, and treatment is continued for 10 days. If streptomycin is not readily available, intravenous gentamicin should be considered, although clinical experience is more limited.[99]

LYMPHANGITIS

Lymphangitis is an inflammation of lymphatic channels, usually in the subcutaneous tissues. It occurs either as an acute process of bacterial origin or as a chronic process of mycotic, mycobacterial, or filarial etiology.

Pathologic Changes and Pathogenesis

The visible red streaking in acute lymphangitis stems from the inflammatory process in the walls (and surrounding tissue spaces) of dilated lymphatic channels. Lymphatic obstruction often occurs on healing, resulting sometimes in persistent lymphedema. Cutaneous lymphatic sporotrichosis, a form of chronic lymphangitis, produces a combined suppurative and granulomatous response.

Clinical Findings

Acute Lymphangitis

Acute lymphangitis develops when an infection, commonly on an extremity, is not contained locally but spreads along lymphatic channels. Such infections are most often due to group A streptococci (and occasionally are due to streptococci of other groups and, very rarely, to *S. aureus* or *Pasteurella multocida* following a cat bite). Systemic manifestations may develop rapidly before evidence of infection becomes apparent at the site of inoculation of organisms, and they may be more prominent than might be anticipated on the basis of local pain and erythema. Red linear streaks, a few millimeters to several centimeters in width, extend from the initial site of infection toward the regional lymph nodes, which are enlarged and tender. Peripheral edema of the involved extremity often occurs. The time course of this type of infection can be accelerated from initial lesion to lymphangitis to complicating bacteremia in 24 to 48 hours. Occasionally recurrent episodes of lymphangitis occur, with the initial episode causing some degree of chronic lymphedema, in turn predisposing to another episode. Rarely, elephantiasis nostras, a temperate-zone (nonfilarial) form of progressive lymphatic obstruction of a lower limb, can follow recurrent episodes of streptococcal lymphangitis. With each episode, further localized edema occurs, eventuating in grotesque enlargement of the extremity due to permanent solid edema, fibrosis of dermis and subcutaneous tissues, and verrucous pachyderma.[100]

The peripheral white blood cell count is commonly elevated. The etiologic agent often can be identified on Gram-stained smears and cultures obtained from the initial lesion. Blood cultures also may reveal the causative organism.

Acute lymphangitis or lymphadenitis, usually involving the lower extremities, is a feature of filariasis due to *Wuchereria bancrofti* (and sometimes to *Brugia malayi*).[61,101] These mosquito-borne diseases are endemic to Africa, Southeast Asia and the Pacific, and tropical South America. The acute form of disease is characterized by recurrent episodes of headache, backache, lymphangitis, lymphadenitis, epididymitis, and orchitis. Bancroftian lymphangitis may involve the breast, with a clinical appearance suggesting carcinoma.[102] Fever is uncommon. The adult filariae reside in lymphatics and lymph nodes and discharge microfilariae into the blood stream. With prolonged exposure in an endemic area, chronic lymphatic obstruction can develop with elephantiasis of the skin and scrotum.[103] In this setting, recurrent episodes of lymphangitis (dermatolymphangioadenitis, DLA) may be the result of both the parasitic infestation and superimposed streptococcal infections (to which the chronic lymphedema predisposes).[61,104] Serologic tests for filariasis may be helpful in diagnosis if microfilariae are not found, but results of such tests are positive in many other filarial infections. Lymph node or lymphatic vessel biopsy may be necessary for diagnosis.

Chronic Granulomatous Lymphangitis

Unlike acute lymphangitis, chronic granulomatous lymphangitis is an indolent process associated with little pain or systemic evidence of infection. Sporotrichosis is most commonly the underlying disease.[105] This infection frequently is introduced by minor trauma (e.g., from a thorn of a barberry or rose bush) into the skin of a gardener. An erythematous subcutaneous nodule (often becoming fluctuant) or a chancriform ulcer subsequently develops at the site of inoculation of *Sporothrix schenckii* (present on some plants and in sphagnum moss used in gardening) on the hand or finger. The lesion does not respond to local treatment or to administration of the common antibacterial agents. Slowly, multiple subcutaneous nodules appear and extend proximally along the course of regional lymphatics, which become thickened. Other infections producing a sporotrichoid pattern are characterized as nodular lymphangitis.[106,107]

Cutaneous infection ("swimming pool granuloma") with *Mycobacterium marinum*—an atypical mycobacterium that grows optimally at 25° C to 32° C and is found in swimming pools and fish tanks—produces a chronic nodular, verrucous or ulcerative lesion at the site of an abrasion, usually about the knees or elbows. The lesion is usually solitary, but in an occasional patient new lesions develop proximally, as in sporotrichosis. Multiple sporotrichoid lesions have occurred in occasional infections due to *Nocardia brasiliensis*[107,108] and in rare infections due to *Mycobacterium kansasii*, *Mycobacterium chelonae*, and *Nocardia asteroides*. Even rarer causes of nodular lymphangitis include leishmaniasis,[107,109] staphylococcal lymphangitis,[110] botryomycosis, and tularemia (reported earlier this century but not in the past 40 years).[106]

A very rare but most troublesome process is localized granulomatous lymphangitis of the penile and scrotal skin with resulting chronic edema of the genital area. It may be associated with lymphogranuloma venereum, granuloma inguinale, Milroy's disease, self-inflicted trauma, Melkersson-Rosenthal syndrome, or Crohn's disease, or it may be idiopathic.[111] Penile edema either can be an initial manifestation of Crohn's disease or may develop as a late complication of well-established gastrointestinal disease.

Pseudolymphangitis

Exogenous liquid chemical agents that drain along the skin may produce localized linear inflammatory reactions and mimic superficial lymphangitis. When the provoking agent is directly toxic, the etiology of the rash is obvious. However, certain plant products can serve as photosensitizing agents, and the history of initial contact is not recalled by the patient. In particular, lime rinds and lime juice contain several coumarin moieties that can provoke phytophotodermatitis.[112]

TABLE 88-2 Causes of Lymphangitis

Clinical Form	Etiologic Agent	Relative Frequency as Cause of Lymphangitis
Acute	Group A streptococci	Common
	Staphylococcus aureus	Occasional
	Pasteurella multocida	Occasional
	Spirillum minus (rat-bite fever)	Rare
	Wuchereria bancrofti; *Brugia malayi* (filariasis)	Rare (only in immigrants from endemic areas)
Chronic	*Sporothrix schenckii* (sporotrichosis)	Occasional
	Mycobacterium marinum (swimming pool granuloma)	Occasional
	Mycobacterium kansasii	Rare
	Nocardia brasiliensis	Rare
	W. bancrofti; B. malayi	Rare (only in immigrants from endemic areas)
	Nocardia asteroides	Very rare
	Mycobacterium chelonae	Very rare
	S. aureus (botryomycosis)	Very rare
	Leishmania brasiliensis or *Leishmania mexicana*	Very rare
	Francisella tularensis	Very rare

Etiologic Agents

In the United States, acute lymphangitis is most commonly due to group A streptococci, and chronic lymphangitis is usually caused by *S. schenckii*. Other infectious agents occasionally produce lymphangitis (Table 88-2).

Differential Diagnosis

The combination of a peripheral infection or traumatic lesion and the acute onset of fever with proximal red linear streaks directed toward regional lymph nodes is diagnostic of acute lymphangitis. In the legs, thrombophlebitis may produce linear areas of tender erythema, but the absence of an initiating lesion and of tender regional adenopathy is helpful in distinguishing it from lymphangitis. It is important to note that on occasion severe lymphangitis may be complicated by the development of thrombophlebitis. A history of rat bite and the subsequent development of lymphangitis suggest *Spirillum minus* infection. Filariasis is a consideration when an appropriate geographic history is obtained. Sporotrichosis is considered when chronic ulcerative lymphangitis develops in a person working with plants, soil, or timbers. *M. marinum* is suggested as the etiologic agent when sporotrichoid lesions develop in a person who has been around swimming pools and fish tanks.

Presumptive Therapy

Penicillin therapy is the recommended initial treatment for acute lymphangitis. Prompt empiric therapy is crucial because disease progression may be quite rapid. Initially, procaine penicillin G, 600,000 units intramuscularly administered every 12 to 24 hours to ensure prompt and reliable drug delivery, may be considered; a single dose of ceftriaxone (1 g intramuscularly) may be administered if more readily available, followed by high-dose oral therapy with penicillin V or amoxicillin (500 mg every 6 hours) if the patient is not toxic and close monitoring is possible. Oral dicloxacillin or cephalexin (500 mg every 6 hours) may be given if there is concern regarding a possible staphylococcal etiology. More acutely ill patients, particularly those in whom bacteremia may have developed, should be hospitalized and given parenteral aqueous penicillin G (e.g., 2 million units every 4 to 6 hours). If a staphylococcal etiology is suspected, a penicillinase-resistant penicillin such as nafcillin (e.g., 2 g every 4-6 hours) is used.

Clindamycin may be considered for the patient with significant β-lactam allergy.

The initial treatment of presumptive lymphocutaneous sporotrichosis is itraconazole; saturated solution of potassium iodide is also effective (see Chapter 258).[106] If sporotrichoid *M. marinum* infection is suspected, the diagnosis should be confirmed by demonstration of acid-fast bacilli and by isolation of the organism at 30° C on appropriate media. Localized swimming pool granulomas are often treated by surgical excision. Chemotherapy is reserved for more extensive and sporotrichoid forms of infection. On the basis of limited data, the combination of choice would appear to be rifampin and ethambutol (see Chapter 251).[106,113] Prolonged tetracycline or minocycline therapy has also been reported as successful in a small number of cases,[106,114] but in vitro resistance to and treatment failure with doxycycline have been reported.[115] Trimethoprim-sulfamethoxazole has been reported as effective in several studies. However, in vitro activity requires drug concentrations greater than those usually achieved in serum and tissues.[116]

Chronic lymphedema, a complication of recurrent lymphangitis, has been treated primarily in the past with elevation and elastic hosiery. Newer and more successful methods to increase lymph drainage for problematic patients have recently been developed and include remedial exercises, manual massage, multilayered bandage wrapping, and intermittent pneumatic compression massage.[117] Individuals with frequent episodes of recurrent cellulitis occurring in the setting of chronic lymphedema may benefit from chronic suppressive therapy with oral penicillin (e.g., 250 mg orally twice daily).

REFERENCES

1. Case Records of the Massachusetts General Hospital. N Engl J Med. 1993;329:714.
2. McCabe RE, Brooks RG, Dorfman RF, et al. Clinical spectrum in 107 cases of toxoplasmic lymphadenopathy. Rev Infect Dis. 1987;9:754.
3. Strickler JG, Warnke RA, Weiss LM. Necrosis in lymph nodes. Pathol Annu. 1987;2:253-282.
4. Higgins JPT, Warnke RA. Herpes lymphadenitis in association with chronic lymphocytic leukemia. Cancer. 1999;86:1210-1215.
5. Witt MD, Torno MS, Sun N, Stein T. Herpes simplex virus lymphadenitis: Case report and review of the literature. Clin Infect Dis. 2002;34:1-6.
6. Johnson LB, Pasumarthy A, Saravolatz LD. Parvovirus B19 infection presenting with necrotizing lymphadenitis. Am J Med. 2003;114:340-341.
7. Brook I, Frazier EH. Microbiology of cervical lymphadenitis in adults. Acta Otolaryngol. 1998;118:443-446.
8. Brook I. Aerobic and anaerobic bacteriology of cervical adenitis in children. Clin Pediatr. 1980;19:693-696.
9. Scobie W. Acute suppurative adenitis in children. Scot Med J. 1969;14:352-354.
10. Dajani AS, Garcia RE, Wolinski E. Etiology of cervical lymphadenitis in children. N Engl J Med. 1963;268:1329-1333.
11. Bredenkamp JK, Maceri DR. Inflammatory torticollis in children. Arch Otolaryngol Head Neck Surg. 1990;116:310-313.
12. Boyce JM. Severe streptococcal lymphadenitis. N Engl J Med. 1990;323:655-658.
13. Amren DP. Unusual forms of streptococcal disease. In: Wannamaker LW, Matsen JM, eds. Streptococci and Streptococcal Disease. New York: Academic Press; 1972:545.
14. Roy D, Thompson KC, Price JP. Benign superior vena cava syndrome due to suppurative mediastinal lymphadenitis: Anterior mediastinoscopic management. Mayo Clin Proc. 1998;73:1185-1187.
15. Chow BJW, McKim DA, Shennib H, Dales RE. Superior vena cava obstruction secondary to mediastinal lymphadenopathy in a patient with cystic fibrosis. Chest. 1997;112:1438-1441.
16. Swartz MN. Recognition and management of anthrax—An update. N Engl J Med. 2001;345:1621-1626.
17. Currarino G. Acute epitrochlear lymphadenitis. Pediatr Radiol. 1977;6:160-163.
18. Maull KI, Sachatello CR. Retroperitoneal iliac fossa abscess. A complication of suppurative iliac lymphadenitis. Am J Surg. 1974;127:270-274.
19. Oliff M, Chuang VP. Retroperitoneal iliac fossa pyogenic abscess. Radiology. 1978;126:647-652.
20. Shenep JL, Kalwinsky DK, Feldman S, et al. Mycotic cervical lymphadenitis following oral mucositis in children with leukemia. J Pediatr. 1985;106:243-246.
21. Mazzoni A, Ferrarese M, Manfredi R, et al. Primary lymph node invasive aspergillosis. Infection. 1996;24:37-42.
22. Curnutte JT, Boxer LA. Clinically significant phagocytic cell defects. In: Remington JS, Swartz MN, eds. Current Clinical Topics in Infectious Diseases, v. 4. New York: McGraw-Hill; 1985;103-155.
23. Sorensen RU, Jacobs MR, Shurin SB. *Chromobacterium violaceum* adenitis acquired in the northern United States as a complication of chronic granulomatous disease. Pediatr Infect Dis. 1985;4:701-702.
24. Kobayashi Y, Komazawa Y, Kobayashi M, et al. Presumed BCG infection in a boy with chronic granulomatous disease. A report of a case and review of the literature. Clin Pediatr. 1984;23:586-589.
25. Alfonso F, Gallo L, Winkler B, et al. Fine needle aspiration cytology of peripheral lymph node cryptococcosis. Acta Cytol. 1994;38:459-462.
26. Ramponi A, Angeli G, Rizzo GM, et al. Laterocervical lymphadenitis caused by *Pneumocystis carinii* in a patient with AIDS. Histopathology. 1994;24:91-93.
27. Haught WH, Steinbach J, Zander DS, et al. Case report: Bacillary angiomatosis with massive visceral lymphadenopathy. Am J Med Sci. 1993;306:236-240.
28. Lee-Chiong T, Saigh M, Simms M, et al. Case reports: Pericarditis and lymphadenitis due to *Rhodococcus equi*. Am J Med Sci. 1995;310:31-33.
29. Pouchot J, Bortolotti V, Sterkers O, et al. Cervical suppurative lymphadenitis due to *Yersinia pseudotuberculosis*. Clin Infect Dis. 1995;21:1063-1064.
30. Lincoln EM, Gilbert LA. Disease in children due to mycobacteria other than *Mycobacterium tuberculosis*. Am Rev Respir Dis. 1972;105:683-714.
31. Wolinsky E. Mycobacterial lymphadenitis in children; a prospective study of 105 nontuberculous cases with long-term follow-up. Clin Infect Dis. 1995;20:954-963.
32. Hazra R, Robson CD, Perez-Atayde AR, Husson RN. Lymphadenitis due to nontuberculous mycobacteria in children: Presentation and response to therapy. Clin Infect Dis. 1999;28:123-129.
33. Haase G, Kentrup H, Skopnik H, et al. *Mycobacterium lentiflavum*: An etiologic agent of cervical lymphadenitis. Clin Infect Dis. 1997;25:1245-1246.
34. Haas WH, Butler WR, Kirschner P, et al. A new agent of mycobacterial lymphadenitis in children: *Mycobacterium heidelbergense* sp. Nov. J Clin Microbiol. 1997;35:3203-3209.
35. Shriner KA, Mathisen GE, Goetz MB. Comparison of mycobacterial lymphadenitis among persons infected with human immunodeficiency virus and seronegative controls. Clin Infect Dis. 1992;15:601-605.
36. Victoria MS, Shah BR. Bacillus Calmette-Guérin lymphadenitis: A case report and review of the literature. Pediatr Infect Dis. 1985;4:295-296.
37. Oguz F, Mujgan S, Alper G, et al. Treatment of bacillus Calmette-Guérin-associated lymphadenitis. Pediatr Infect Dis. J. 1992;11:887-888.
38. Mandell DL, Wald ER, Michaels MG, Dohar JE. Management of nontuberculous mycobacterial cervical lymphadenitis. Arch Otolaryngol Head Neck Surg. 2003;129:341-344.
39. Panesar J, Higgins K, Daya H, et al. Nontuberculous mycobacterial cervical adenitis: A ten-year retrospective review. Laryngoscope 2003;113:149-154.
40. Rahal A, Abela A, Arcand PH, et al. Nontuberculous mycobacterial adenitis of the head and neck in children: Experience from a tertiary care pediatric center. Laryngoscope. 2001;111:1791-1796.
41. Goraya JS, Virdi S. Bacille Calmette-Guerin lymphadenitis. Postgrad Med J. 2002;78:327-329.
42. Lipsky BA, Goldberger AC, Tompkins LS, et al. Infections caused by non-diphtheria corynebacteria. Rev Infect Dis. 1982;4:1220-1235.
43. Peel MM, Palmer GG, Stacpoole AM, et al. Human lymphadenitis due to *Corynebacterium pseudotuberculosis*: Report of ten cases from Australia and review. Clin Infect Dis. 1997;24:185-191.
44. Carithers HA, Carithers CM, Edwards RO Jr. Cat-scratch disease. Its natural history. JAMA. 1969;207:312-316.
45. Grando D, Sullivan LJ, Flexman JP, Watson MW, Andrew JH. *Bartonella henselae* associated with Parinaud's oculoglandular syndrome. Clin Infect Dis. 1999;28: 1156-1158.
46. Dolan MJ, Wong MT, Regnery RL, et al. Syndrome of *Rochalimaea henselae* adenitis suggesting cat scratch disease. Ann Intern Med. 1993;118:331-336.
47. Carithers HA. Cat-scratch disease. An overview based on a study of 1,200 patients. Am J Dis Child. 1985;139:1124-1133.
48. Wong MT, Dolan MJ, Lattuada CP, et al. Neuroretinitis, aseptic meningitis, and lymphadenitis associated with *Bartonella (Rochalimaea) henselae* infection in immunocompetent patients and patients infected with human immunodeficiency virus type 1. Clin Infect Dis. 1995;21:352-360.
49. Ridder GJ, Boedeker CC, Technau-Ihling K, et al. Role of cat-scratch disease in lymphadenopathy in the head and neck. Clin Infect Dis. 2002;35:643-649.
50. Epstein JI, Ambinder RF, Kuhajda FP, et al. Localized herpes simplex lymphadenitis. Am J Clin Pathol. 1986;86:444-448.
51. Miliauskas JR, Leong AS. Localized herpes simplex lymphadenitis: Report of three cases and review of the literature. Histopathology. 1991;19:355-360.
52. Ho DD, Murata GH. Streptococcal lymphadenitis in homosexual men with chronic lymphadenopathy. Am J Med. 1984;77:151-153.
53. Reed WP, Palmer DL, Williams RC, et al. Bubonic plague in southwestern United States. Medicine. Baltimore 1970;49:465-486.
54. Young LS, Bicknell DS, Archer BG, et al. Tularemia epidemic: Vermont 1968. Forty-seven cases linked to contact with muskrats. N Engl J Med. 1969;280:1253-1260.
55. Posey LA, Kerschner JE, Conley SF. Posttransplantation lymphoproliferative disease in children: otolaryngologic manifestations and management. South Med J. 1999;92:1079-1082.
56. Padeh S, Brezniak N, Zemer D, et al. Periodic fever, aphthous stomatitis, pharyngitis, and adenopathy syndrome: Clinical characteristics and outcome. J Pediatr. 1999;135:98-101.
57. Long SS. Syndrome of periodic fever, aphthous stomatitis, pharyngitis, and adenitis (PFAPA)—What it isn't. What is it? (editorial). J Pediatr. 1999;135:1-5.
58. Thomas KT, Feder HM, Lawton AR, Edwards KM. Periodic fever syndrome in children J Pediatr. 1999;135:15-21.
59. Berlucchi M, Meini A, Plebani A, et al. Update on treatment of Marshall's syndrome (PFAPA syndrome): Report of five cases with review of the literature. Ann Otol Rhinol Laryngol. 2003;112:365-369.

60. Lee WI, Yang MH, Lee KF, et al. PFAPA syndrome (periodic fever, aphthous stomatitis, pharyngitis, adenitis). Clin Rheumatol. 1999;18:27-213.

61. Dreyer G, Noroes J, Figueredo-Silva J, Piessens WF. Pathogenesis of lymphatic disease in Bancroftian filariasis: A clinical perspective. Parasitol Today. 2000;16:544-548.

62. Barton LL, Feigin RD. Childhood cervical lymphadenitis: A reappraisal. J Pediatr. 1974;84:846-852.

63. Feigin RD, Schleien CI. Kawasaki's disease. In: Remington J, Swartz MN, eds. Current Clinical Topics in Infectious Disease, v. 4. New York: McGraw-Hill; 1983;30.

64. Mason WH, Takahashi M. Kawasaki syndrome. Clin Infect Dis. 1999;28:169-185.

65. Waggoner-Fountain LA, Hayden GF, Hendley JO. Kawasaki syndrome masquerading as bacterial lymphadenitis. Clin Pediatr. 1995;34:185-189.

66. Unger PD, Rappaport KM, Strauchen JA. Necrotizing lymphadenitis (Kikuchi's disease). Arch Pathol Lab Med. 1987;111:1031-1034.

67. Spies J, Foucar K, Thompson CT, LeBoit PE. The histopathology of cutaneous lesions of Kikuchi's disease (necrotizing lymphadenitis): A report of five cases. Am J Surg Pathol. 1999;23:1040-1047.

68. Tsang WYW, Chan JKC, Ng CS. Kikuchi's lymphadenitis: A morphologic analysis of 75 cases with special reference to unusual features. Am J Surg Pathol. 1994;18:219-231.

69. Dorfman RF. Histiocytic necrotizing lymphadenitis of Kikuchi and Fujimoto. Arch Pathol Lab Med. 1987;111:1026-1029.

70. Tsang WYW, Chan JKC. Fine needle aspiration cytologic diagnosis of Kikuchi's lymphadenitis. A report of 27 cases. Am J Clin Pathol. 1994;102:454-458.

71. Yufu Y, Matsumoto M, Miyamura T, et al. Parvovirus B19-associated haemophagocytic syndrome with lymphadenopathy resembling histiocytic necrotizing lymphadenitis (Kikuchi's disease). Br J Haematol. 1997;96:868-871.

72. Maiorano E, Favia G, Viale G. Lymphoepithelial cysts of salivary glands: An immunohistochemical study of HIV-related and HIV-unrelated lesions. Hum Pathol. 1998;29:260-265.

73. Garcia-González R, Sanz I, Saus C, et al. Localized lymphadenitis due to Leishmania. Diagnosis by fine needle aspiration cytology. Postgrad Med J. 1990;66:326.

74. Montoya JG, Remington JS. Studies on the serodiagnosis of toxoplasmic lymphadenitis. Clin Infect Dis. 1995;20:781-789.

75. Naqvi SH, Thobani S, Moazam F, et al. Generalized suppurative lymphadenitis with typhoidal salmonellosis. Pediatr Infect Dis J. 1988;7:882-883.

76. Alper CA, Abramson N, Johnston RB, et al. Increased susceptibility to infection associated with abnormalities of complement mediated functions and of the third component of complement C3. New Engl J Med. 1970;282:349-354.

77. Abruzzo LV, Schmidt K, Weiss LM, et al. B-cell lymphoma after angioimmunoblastic lymphadenopathy: A case with oligoclonal gene rearrangements associated with Epstein-Barr virus. Blood. 1993;82:241-246.

78. Rosai J, Dorfman RF. Sinus histiocytosis with massive lymphadenopathy, a pseudolymphomatous benign disorder: Analysis of 34 cases. Cancer. 1972;30:1174-1188.

79. Paulli M, Locatelli F, Kindl S, et al. Sinus histiocytosis with massive lymphadenopathy (Rosai-Dorfman disease). Clinico-pathological analysis of a paediatric case. Eur J Pediatr. 1992;151:672-675.

80. Shinto Y, Uchida A, Yoshikawa H, et al. Inguinal lymphadenopathy due to metal release from a prosthesis. J Bone Joint Surg. 1993;75B:266-269.

81. O'Connell JX, Rosenberg AE. Histiocytic lymphadenitis associated with a large joint prosthesis. Am J Clin Pathol. 1993;99:314-316.

82. van Diest PJ, Beekman WH, Hage JJ. Pathology of silicone leakage from breast implants. J Clin Pathol. 1998;51:493-497.

83. Sever CE, Leith CP, Appenzaller J, Foucar K. Kikuchi's histiocytic necrotizing lymphadenitis associated with ruptured silicone breast implant. Arch Pathol Lab Med. 1996;120:380-385.

84. Rogers LA, Longtine JA, Garnick MB, et al. Silicone lymphadenopathy in a long distance runner: Complication of a Silastic prosthesis. Hum Pathol. 1988;19:1237-1239.

85. Fauci AS, Macher AM, Longo DL, et al. Acquired immunodeficiency syndrome: Epidemiologic, clinical, immunologic, and therapeutic considerations. Ann Intern Med. 1984;100:92-106.

86. Gottlieb MS, Groopman JE, Weinstein WM, et al. The acquired immunodeficiency syndrome. Ann Intern Med. 1983;99:208-220.

87. Levine AM, Meyer PR, Begandy MK, et al. Development of B-cell lymphoma in homosexual men: Clinical and immunological findings. Ann Intern Med. 1984;100:7-13.

88. Kinloch-de Loës S, deSaussure P, Saurat J-H, et al. Symptomatic primary infection due to human immunodeficiency virus type 1: Review of 31 cases. Clin Infect Dis. 1993;17:59-65.

89. Clark SJ, Saag MS, Decker WD, et al. High titers of cytopathic virus in plasma of patients with symptomatic primary HIV-1 infection. N Engl J Med. 1991;324:954-960.

90. Pantaleo G, Graziosi C, Fauci AS. New concepts in the immunopathogenesis of human immunodeficiency virus infection. N Engl J Med. 1993;328:327-335.

91. Baroni CD, Uccini S. The lymphadenopathy of HIV infection. Am J Clin Pathol. 1993;99:397-401.

92. Serour F, Gorenstein A, Somekh E. Needle aspiration for suppurative cervical lymphadenitis. Clin Pediatr (Phila). 2002;41:471-474.

93. Margileth AM. Antibiotic therapy for cat-scratch disease: Clinical study of therapeutic outcome in 268 patients and a review of the literature. Pediatr Infect Dis J. 1992;11:474-478.

94. Chia JK, Nakata MM, Lami JL, et al. Azithromycin for the treatment of cat-scratch disease. Clin Infect Dis. 1998;26:193-194.

95. Bass JW, Freitas BC, Freitas AD, et al. Prospective randomized double blind placebo-controlled evaluation of azithromycin for treatment of cat-scratch disease. Pediatr Infect Dis J. 1998;17:447-452.

96. Lerdluedeeporn P, Krogstad P, Roberts RL, Stiehm ER. Oral corticosteroids in cat-scratch disease. Clin Pediatr (Phila). 2003;42:71-73.

97. Bryant K, Marshall GS. Hepatosplenic cat scratch disease treated with corticosteroids. Arch Dis Child. 2003;88:345-346.

98. Koehler JE, Quinn FD, Berger TG. Isolation of Rochalimaea species from cutaneous and osseous lesions of bacillary angiomatosis. N Engl J Med. 1992;327:1625-1631.

99. Inglesby TV, Dennis DT, Henderson DA, et al, for the Working Group on Civilian Biodefense. Plague as a biological weapon: Medical and public health management. JAMA. 2000;283:2281-2290.

100. Sanders LJ, Slomsky JM, Burger-Caplan C. Elephantiasis nostras: An eight year observation of progressive nonfilarial elephantiasis of the lower extremity. Cutis. 1988;42:406-411.

101. Grove DI, Warren KS, Mahmoud AAF. Algorithms in the diagnosis and management of exotic diseases. VI. The filariases. J Infect Dis. 1975;132:340-352.

102. Jungmann P, Figueredo-Silva J, Dreyer G. Bancroftian lymphangitis in north-eastern Brazil: A histopathological study of 17 cases. J Trop Med Hyg. 1992;95:114-118.

103. Pani SP, Yuvaraj J, Vanamial P, et al. Episodic adenolymphangitis and lymphoedema in patients with bancroftian filariasis. Trans R Soc Trop Med Hyg. 1995;89:72-74.

104. Gyapong JO, Gyapong M, Adjel S. The epidemiology of acute adenolymphangitis due to lymphatic filariasis in northern Ghana. Am J Trop Med Hyg. 1996;54:591-595.

105. Orr ER, Riley HD Jr. Sporotrichosis in childhood: Report of ten cases. J Pediatr. 1971;78:951-957.

106. Heller HM, Swartz MN. Nodular lymphangitis: Clinical features, differential diagnosis and management. In: Remington JS, Swartz MN, eds. Current Clinical Topics in Infectious Diseases, v. 14. Boston: Blackwell Scientific; 1994:142-158.

107. Smego RA, Castiglia M, Asperilla MO. Lymphocutaneous syndrome: A review of non-Sporothrix causes. Medicine. 1999;78:38-63.

108. Sachs MK. Lymphocutaneous Nocardia brasiliensis infection acquired from a cat scratch: Case report and review. Clin Infect Dis. 1992;15:710.

109. Gaafar A, Ismail A, El Kadaro AY, et al. Necrotizing and suppurative lymphadenitis in Leishmania major infections. Trop Med Int Health. 1996;1:243-250.

110. Lieberman AA, Grossman ME, Bloomgarden D. Sporotrichoid lymphangitis due to Staphylococcus aureus in a diabetic patient. Clin Infect Dis. 1995;21:433-434.

111. Mors Y, Zaidi SZ, Rose DSC, et al. Granulomatous lymphangitis of the penile skin as a cause of penile swelling in children. J Urol. 1997;158:591-592.

112. Ahmed I, Charles-Holmes R. Phytophotodermatitis mimicking superficial lymphangitis. Br J Dermatol. 2000;142:1047-1069.

113. Van Dyke JJ, Lake KB. Chemotherapy for aquarium granuloma. JAMA. 1975;233:1380-1381.

114. Izumi AK, Hanke CW, Higaki M. Mycobacterium marinum infections treated with tetracycline. Arch Dermatol. 1977;1313:1067-1068.

115. Ljungberg B, Christensson B, Grubb R. Failure of doxycycline treatment in aquarium-associated Mycobacterium marinum infections. Scand J Infect Dis. 1987;19:539-543.

116. Sanders WJ, Wolinsky E. In vitro susceptibility of Mycobacterium marinum to eight antimicrobial agents. Antimicrob Agents Chemother. 1980;18:529-531.

117. Consensus Document of the International Society of Lymphology. The diagnosis and treatment of peripheral lymphedema. Lymphology. 2003;36:84-91.

CHAPTER **89**

Principles and Syndromes of Enteric Infection

RICHARD L. GUERRANT
THEODORE S. STEINER

Gastrointestinal infections encompass a wide variety of symptom complexes and recognized infectious agents. With the exception of *Helicobacter pylori* gastritis, the term *gastroenteritis* is applied to syndromes of diarrhea or vomiting that tend to involve noninflammatory infection in the upper small bowel or inflammatory infection in the colon. Other enteric infections and infestations cause predominantly systemic symptoms. Infections of the gastrointestinal tract, especially infectious diarrhea, are among the most common debilitating infectious diseases, afflicting people of all ages around the world. In many heavily populated areas, deaths from diarrheal illnesses exceed those from any other single cause.

In the absence of demonstrable causal forces, many descriptive terms have arisen through the years. Names such as Montezuma's revenge, Delhi belly, Aden gut, gyppi tummy, Aztec two-step, Greek gallop, Rome runs, Hong Kong dog, Turkey trots, la turista, Basra belly, and back door sprint illustrate the widespread occurrence of these infections. Although an etiologic agent is not found in many cases, the infectious nature of most acute diarrheal diseases is suggested by their epidemiologic behavior showing case clustering, spread in families and other groups, and occurrence among travelers. In the last three decades, much has been learned about bacterial, protozoal, and viral agents capable of causing acute gastrointestinal illnesses. These include *Escherichia coli* strains that produce enterotoxins (which cause fluid secretion), other *E. coli* strains capable of causing tissue destruction and inflammation, and pathogens such as *Vibrio, Salmonella, Yersinia, Campylobacter, Clostridium, Cryptosporidium, Cyclospora,* rotaviruses, and noroviruses. With the development of new tools for diagnosis, important information has been gained in our understanding of the causes, pathogenesis, epidemiology, and control of acute gastrointestinal infections.

OCCURRENCE AND SCOPE OF GASTROINTESTINAL INFECTIONS

On a global scale, diarrheal diseases are a leading cause of childhood death and are an even greater cause of lasting morbidity, especially with the longer-term impact of early childhood diarrhea on growth and development.[1,2] Estimates are that over 2 million children still die each year (>6000/day) in Asia, Africa, and Latin America,[3,4] and that more than 10,000 die from diarrhea each year in the United States.[1,2,5] Although the global mortality is decreasing (especially with oral rehydration therapy [ORT]),[6] in some areas diarrhea mortality is increasing[7] and prolonged diarrhea is emerging as a major cause of

death.[8] Even greater than the mortality is the serious morbidity from diarrheal diseases, especially in association with malabsorption and malnutrition in tropical and developing areas. In areas such as Bangladesh, India, Guatemala, and Brazil, the attack rates often reach six or more episodes per person per year among children younger than 2 years of age.[6,7,9-11] The attack rate is highest at the time of weaning.[7]

Children dying with diarrhea in developing areas often also have nutritional deficiencies as associated causes of death, and a vicious cycle of diarrhea and malnutrition has been documented.[8] Acute infectious diarrhea exacerbates nutritional deficiencies in several ways. As with any acute infection, caloric demands are increased, and often catabolic steroids, glucagon, and adrenergic amines cause increased breakdown of structural proteins. Through vicious cycles of transient malabsorption and anorexia, repeated bouts of acute diarrhea are major contributors to malnutrition.[8,12] The reverse is also true: undernutrition appears to reduce resistance to acute infectious diarrhea. Increased attack rates and increased mortality from acute infectious diarrheal illnesses occur with progressive severity of malnutrition. As a specific example, shigellae are shed longer and there is an increased relapse rate in children if they are malnourished.[13] In addition, malnutrition appears to predispose to more prolonged diarrheal illnesses.

More recent data suggest that there is also a complex interaction between poor nutritional status and persistent diarrheal illnesses, usually defined as diarrhea lasting longer than 14 days. These illnesses constituted a majority of total diarrheal burden in studies of several cohorts of children living in impoverished areas.[7,14] A bidirectional interaction exists between malnutrition and persistent diarrhea. Malnutrition (as measured by growth shortfalls) predisposes to subsequent persistent diarrheal illness, and each persistent diarrheal illness during the first 2 years of life may itself be associated with subsequent growth shortfalls.[6] Moreover, studies have demonstrated that carriage of the persistent diarrheal pathogens *Cryptosporidium parvum, Giardia lamblia,* and enteroaggregative *E. coli* is associated with poor growth even in the absence of diarrhea.[6,15-17] These findings taken with the long-term developmental impact of diarrhea suggest that the overall global impact of childhood diarrheal illnesses may be much greater than previously suspected.

Military history indicates that acute diarrheal illnesses have played decisive roles in numerous campaigns. Diarrheal diseases and enteric infections were the major nontraumatic cause of hospitalization among U.S. troops in Vietnam and in Saudi Arabia, their number approaching the number of hospitalizations resulting from injuries due to hostile action.[18] Overall rates of gastrointestinal illness in the United States ranged from 1.5 to 5 illnesses per person per year in studies done in communities and in daycare centers, respectively.[5,19] Rates are highest in young children but may sometimes increase during young adulthood (as with *Campylobacter jejuni* in the "second weaning") or in older adults (as with *Clostridium difficile* and *Salmonella*).[5,20] Acute "gastroenteritis" is second only to respiratory diseases in community-based studies and often leads to physician visits and symptomatic or other medications.[5]

EPIDEMIOLOGIC AND ENVIRONMENTAL FACTORS

The frequency, type, and severity of enteric infections are determined by *who* you are, *where* you are, and *when* you are there.

Who is at risk of acquiring a gastrointestinal infection varies greatly with age, living conditions, personal and cultural habits, and group exposures. Although the infant who is being breastfed is relatively protected from contaminated food and water and probably to some degree by maternal colostral antibodies and lactoferrin, at weaning there is a great increase in the risk of diarrheal illness. Adults, particularly if they live for many years in the same environment, may become asymptomatic reservoirs of microorganisms that cause diarrhea in the immunologically untutored child or visitor. Living conditions often reflect socioeconomic conditions, and type of housing, population density, sanitation facilities, and water sources are major determinants of environmental exposure to enteric pathogens. The impact of water quality and quantity cannot be overemphasized. As shown in

TABLE 89-1	Types of Water-Related Diseases
Waterborne	Diseases transmitted by ingestion of contaminated drinking water. Examples: cholera, typhoid fever, cryptosporidiosis.
Water-carried	Diseases acquired by accidental ingestion of, or exposure to, contaminated recreational water. Examples: cryptosporidiosis, giardiasis, *Pseudomonas* dermatitis.
Water-washed	Diseases transmitted person-to-person as a result of poor sanitation due to inadequate quantities of water for washing hands, utensils, and so on. Examples: shigellosis, hepatitis A, cryptosporidiosis.
Water-based	Diseases caused by pathogens with an obligatory life-cycle phase occurring in the water. Examples: schistosomiasis, dracunculiasis.
Water-vectored	Diseases transmitted by insects that breed or bite in or near water. Examples: malaria, yellow fever, dengue, African trypanosomiasis.

Adapted from data published in Steiner TS, Theilman NM, Guerrant RL. Protozoal agents: What are the dangers for the public water supply? Annu Rev Med. 1997;48:329-340.

Table 89-1, there are five basic ways in which a shortage of clean water can lead to transmission of enteric infections.[21] Personal hygiene habits determine how many organisms are ingested. Although the infectious dose varies with the organism, relatively small inocula of certain organisms may result in disease. Shigellae are acquired with an unusually low infectious dose and are often spread by direct contact among children in daycare centers. On the other hand, *C. difficile* colitis occurs with increasing frequency with age. The majority of nonspecific diarrheal illnesses acquired in communities occur in family clusters, often with small children having the first illness. Of great importance whenever a patient has an enteric illness is a careful history of other illnesses in the family or community. Multiple illnesses and common exposure may be clues to a foodborne outbreak or to the causative agent.

The second epidemiologic determinant of risk for enteric infection is *where* you are. The pattern of illnesses and the etiologic agents vary greatly with climate. For example, enterotoxigenic, enteropathogenic, and enteroaggregative *E. coli* cause disease primarily in the tropics, where the heaviest burden of parasites also occurs. In contrast, enterohemorrhagic *E. coli* has been found largely in developed areas such as Japan, North America, and Europe. Viral causes of common enteric illnesses have been found among young children in temperate and tropical climates. Despite their clustering, however, many community cases of diarrhea remain unexplained.

Finally, the third determinant of risk is *when* you are there. The majority of enteric illnesses in temperate climates occur during winter months. The opposite is true in tropical countries, where distinct summer peaks of illnesses are common. The role of rainfall is uncertain, and some adjacent areas with similar monsoon climates have opposite seasons of major diarrheal illnesses, as illustrated by the peak seasons for cholera in different parts of Bengal. In Dhaka, endemic cholera occurs during the winter dry months; less than 200 miles away, the peak cholera season in Calcutta occurs during the summer monsoon.

HOST FACTORS

Considering the ubiquity of potential enteric pathogens, it is surprising that enteric infections are not even more common. After exposure to infectious agents, several host factors determine who becomes ill. Several enteric host defenses provide substantial protection against many intestinal pathogens (Table 89-2).

Host Species, Genotype, and Age

Host species, genotype, and age are complex but major determinants of susceptibility to colonization and disease with enteric pathogens. Although a broad spectrum of animal hosts can be infected with pathogens such as *Salmonella enteritidis* and *C. jejuni,* only primates

TABLE 89-2	Enteric Host Defenses

Host species, genotype, and age factors
Personal hygiene
Gastric acidity and other physical barriers
Intestinal motility
Enteric microflora
Immunity
    Phagocytic
    Humoral
    Cell-mediated
Nonspecific protective factors in human milk
Intestinal receptors

and humans are characteristically infected with *Salmonella typhi* or *Shigella* species. In addition, attachment traits of enteropathogenic and some enterotoxigenic *E. coli* are largely species specific. Interspecies variation and host genotype are also important. Persons with blood group O appear to be more susceptible to cholera, and possibly those with type A to giardiasis.[22] Such species or even genotype specificities play important roles in determining host susceptibility and the epidemiology of these infections. Genotypic differences in susceptibility to enteric infections may have far-reaching implications. For example, it has been suggested that the high prevalence of mutations in the cystic fibrosis transmembrane regulatory protein in whites may have been maintained by a selective heterozygote advantage in susceptibility to *S. typhi.*[23]

The role of age in determining host susceptibility is complex. In animals, a narrow age-window of susceptibility to specific enteric infections is well recognized. In humans, the tendency of rotaviral and enteropathogenic *E. coli* (EPEC) infections to affect young children is impressive. The explanations probably reside in age-related changes in gut mucus, cell surface factors, microbial flora, environmental exposure, and specific immune factors. In addition, specific receptors for microbial adhesins or toxins may be developmentally regulated, such as those for *Shigella,* Shiga-like, cholera, *E. coli,* and *C. difficile* enterotoxins.[24,25] This may explain in part the predisposition to hemolytic-uremic syndrome in children. Moreover, like certain strains of rotavirus, toxigenic strains of *C. difficile* are carried frequently by healthy young infants, in whom they seldom cause disease.

Specific receptor components or antagonists (e.g., monosaccharides such as *N*-acetylneuraminic acid) can be added exogenously and compete with intestinal binding sites for *E. coli.*[26] Furthermore, lectin-like substances that bind to the intestinal cell receptors may compete with the bacterial attachment factors. Positive chemotaxis of *Vibrio cholerae, E. coli,* and *Salmonella typhimurium* has been shown toward rabbit ileal mucosa, and a role of negative chemotactic factors as a new type of host defense has been postulated.[27]

Personal Hygiene

Whether a person acquires an enteric infection depends first on the number of pathogens ingested. Almost all agents of concern are acquired by the oral route. The majority of identified enteric pathogens have come from other mammalian intestinal tracts; often, a human fecal-oral route can be traced. A plentiful, conveniently located supply of uncontaminated water, in conjunction with improved sanitary facilities, is critically important in reducing this mode of spread. Studies of presumptive viral agents that have not yet been defined strongly implicate the human fecal-oral route of infection.[28] Usually in bacterial infections, a large number of organisms (100,000 to 100 million) must be ingested to overcome host defenses and cause disease (Table 89-3). Such numbers may result from growth in food that is allowed to stand unrefrigerated for several hours after the initial contaminating inoculum. Exceptions to the large number of organisms usually required for an infecting dose are *Shigella* and cysts of certain parasites, which can be reproducibly transmitted with only 10 to 100 organisms. A mathematical model based on a large waterborne outbreak of cryptosporidiosis in Milwaukee, Wisconsin, in 1993 suggested that some people may have been infected after ingesting a single oocyst.[29] This

TABLE 89-3 Infectious Doses of Enteric Pathogens	
Shigella	10 to 10^2
Campylobacter jejuni	10^2 to 10^6
Salmonella	10^5
Escherichia coli	10^8
Vibrio cholerae	10^8
Giardia lamblia	10 to 10^2 cysts
Entamoeba histolytica	10 to 10^2 cysts
Cryptosporidium parvum	1 to 10^3 oocysts

small inoculum can readily be transmitted directly by person-to-person contact (as in daycare centers). This is an unusual route of spread for other bacterial enteric pathogens except in hosts with impaired defenses and newborn infants. However, secondary spread of enterohemorrhagic *E. coli* (EHEC) in some outbreaks and the possible transmission by houseflies suggests that some strains of this organism might infect with a relatively low inoculum and, hence, have the potential for person-to-person transmission.[30-33]

Gastric Acidity and Other Physical Barriers

Most bacterial pathogens that are ingested never reach the intestinal tract because of the normal gastric acid barrier. When this barrier is neutralized with antacids, both the susceptibility and the severity of several enteric bacterial and parasitic infections are increased. At normal gastric pH (<4), more than 99.9% of ingested coliform bacteria are killed within 30 minutes. In contrast, there is no reduction of an experimental bacterial inoculum in achlorhydric stomachs after 1 hour. Not surprisingly, then, the gastric coliform flora in fasting subjects (normally fewer than 10 organisms per milliliter) exceeds 10,000/mL in the majority of achlorhydric patients.[34] Excessive numbers of normal bacterial flora in the upper small bowel may contribute to malabsorption and diarrheal syndromes.

The inoculum of *V. cholerae* required to cause disease can be reduced 10,000-fold (from 10^8 to 10^4 organisms) by neutralization of gastric acid with 2 g of sodium bicarbonate. In an outbreak of cholera in Israel, 25% of the patients had had previous gastric resection, whereas none of a comparable control group had had gastric surgery. A similar association of previous gastric surgery or achlorhydria with increased frequency and severity of *Salmonella* infections has also been noted. Likewise, the frequency of enteric multiplication of a vaccine strain of *Shigella flexneri* increases threefold with sodium bicarbonate neutralization of gastric acid. With *C. jejuni*, a substantial range in infectious doses has been documented with different strains. Although gastric acidity may enhance the process of excystation and infection by some parasites after ingestion of the ova, it may provide protection against other parasites. The fragile trophozoite of *G. lamblia* (requiring a pH of 6.4 to 7.1) causes more severe symptoms in association with hypochlorhydria or achlorhydria, perhaps because of increased survival of trophozoites refluxed to the stomach and proximal duodenum. The association of achlorhydria and hypochlorhydria with symptomatic strongyloidiasis has also been noted. Some have suggested that vitamin B_{12} deficiency occurs more often in association with fish tapeworm (*Diphyllobothrium latum*) in patients who are achlorhydric and who have high jejunal infestations. Finally, certain parasitic, viral, or bacterial processes such as *H. pylori* infections may in themselves alter gastric acidity and thereby increase host susceptibility to other enteric pathogens.[35] The further importance of gastric acidity in preventing gastric, pharyngeal, and tracheal colonization by gram-negative bacilli and even nosocomial pneumonia has been shown by the increased risk of patients taking antacids or histamine (H_2) blockers compared with sucralfate, which preserves gastric acidity.[36]

Other physical barriers such as mucus and mucosal tissue integrity are important resistance factors in healthy hosts and work in concert with gastric acidity and intestinal motility to clear many bacteria from the upper small bowel. Continuous removal and renewal of gastrointestinal mucus may bind organisms and toxins and further aid in protecting the intact mucosa from enzymatic and microbial attack.[37]

Intestinal Motility

Intestinal motility plays several important roles in normal intestinal physiology: (1) in the fluid absorptive process, (2) in maintaining the appropriate distribution of indigenous enteric microflora, and (3) in ridding the host of pathogenic microorganisms. Motility also helps to maintain normal distribution and flow of microflora. The risk of bowel stasis is evident in the bacterial overgrowth syndromes in the small bowel and in the added risk of "toxic megacolon" in inflammatory bowel disease after antimotility drugs are administered.

In addition, intestinal motility appears to play a role in providing protection from enteric pathogens. Experimental animals are much more easily infected with enteric pathogens after inhibition of gut motility with opiates. *Salmonella* bacteremia may develop in patients after opiates are taken for relatively mild gastroenteritis.[38] A controlled study of adults with shigellosis treated with diphenoxylate hydrochloride with atropine (Lomotil) revealed that the antimotility drug abolished antibiotic effectiveness in reducing diarrhea and positive cultures and was associated with prolonged fever and shedding of the *Shigella* organisms.[39] Moreover, case reports suggest that complications of *Campylobacter* and *C. difficile* enteritis are more common in patients who have received antimotility agents. These drugs also predispose patients to hemolytic-uremic syndrome after infection with EHEC.[40] Gut motility and diarrhea, which help rid the host of offending pathogens, may therefore be analogous to the cough in pulmonary infections as a mechanism to expel pathogens.

Normal Enteric Microflora

It is recognized that 99.9% of the normal enteric bacterial flora are anaerobes (approximately 10^{11} organisms per gram of normal feces). These organisms (*Bacteroides, Clostridium*, peptostreptococci, peptococci, and others) far exceed the number of aerobes. *E. coli* number 10^8 per gram; *Klebsiella, Proteus*, enterococci, and other species number approximately 10^5 to 10^7 per gram. The role of normal flora as an extremely important and often overlooked host defense is beginning to be appreciated. In several situations, the normal bacterial flora can be shown to be highly effective in resisting colonization by potentially pathogenic invaders. The loss of normal flora or a shift in the balance of these organisms caused by use of antibiotics often leads to their replacement by organisms such as *Pseudomonas, Klebsiella, Clostridium*, and *Candida*. When these organisms take up residence, they may cause serious systemic infections, especially in a nosocomial setting. There are numerous examples of increased susceptibility to infection in patients with reduced bacterial flora.[41] Several enteric infections, such as infant botulism, nosocomial salmonellosis, and EPEC infection, occur with increased frequency in newborn infants who have not yet acquired a normal enteric flora. Diarrhea associated with the use of antibiotics is common and in many cases is probably related to an alteration in the balance of normal enteric microflora.

The basis for the resistance provided by normal bacterial flora in the intestinal tract was elucidated in an elegant series of studies.[42] In experimental mice, the researchers showed that the protective effect of normal flora is eradicated by a single injection of streptomycin. The infecting dose of *S. typhimurium* was reduced more than 100,000-fold by the administration of a single dose of streptomycin. This reduced resistance correlated with the reduction in the normal colonic flora and their toxic acidic products. Resistance was restored with the return of enteric flora (especially *Bacteroides*), either by inoculation or naturally.

Indigenous microbes such as *Lactobacillus, Bacteroides*, and *Clostridium* species attach to the intestinal epithelial surface and act synergistically with the host immunity to interfere with experimental *S. typhimurium* challenge. The protective role of normal enteric bacterial flora in humans was documented by the increased frequency of *Salmonella* infections among Swedish tourists who took a prophylactic antibiotic compared with those who took no antimicrobial agent.[41] In a huge outbreak of antimicrobial-resistant *S. typhimurium* enteritis involving almost 200,000 people in Illinois in the spring of 1985, there was a significant association of illness with a history of having taken antimicrobial drugs the month before the illness. There was a fivefold difference (6% versus 30%) between well controls and ill persons in the percentage who took antibiotics to which the outbreak strain was resistant.[43] Others have reported an increased risk of infection with antimicrobial-sensitive *Salmonella* after antimicrobial exposure.[44] Some have even used normal colonic or other competing bacterial flora to treat refractory *C. difficile* colitis. In addition, cytotoxic chemotherapy with agents such as methotrexate, cyclophosphamide, or fluorouracil may also suppress normal flora and predispose to *C. difficile* colitis.[45] The protective benefits of normal intestinal flora have led to a large interest in the field of probiotics, or ingestion of "healthy" bacteria, to prevent or treat diarrheal disease. Clinical trials of probiotics have been promising in certain settings, including reducing the incidence of antibiotic-associated diarrhea (but not *C. difficile* colitis)[46] and improving symptom duration in rotavirus diarrhea in children.[47-49] Smaller studies have suggested a benefit of probiotic treatments with the yeast *Saccharomyces boulardii* or with various mixtures of lactobacilli, bifidobacteria, and other nonpathogenic bacteria in specific diseases such as recurrent *C. difficile* colitis and ulcerative pouchitis.[50-53]

Intestinal Immunity

The human immune system is commonly divided into two complementary armies: innate and adaptive immunity. Innate immunity, the more primitive system, shares elements with invertebrates and plants. In mammals, innate immunity consists of the physical barriers discussed earlier, as well as a system of cells that perform active surveillance and killing of pathogens and abnormal host tissue. In the gut, these cells include intestinal epithelial cells, phagocytes, natural killer lymphocytes, and dendritic cells. Another important element of innate immunity is the elaboration of host factors with direct effects on microorganisms. These factors include small molecules (such as nitric oxide and hydrogen peroxide) that cause physical damage by generating reactive oxygen species, as well as large molecules such as complement components and antimicrobial peptides. Emerging evidence suggests that expression of antimicrobial peptides is a major task of the Paneth cells that line intestinal crypts.[54,55] The common feature of innate immune mediators is that they appear to target broad classes of organisms rather than specific species or groups. This is accomplished in part through the actions of pattern recognition receptors, host proteins that recognize "molecular signatures" unique to certain classes of microorganisms. For example, intestinal epithelial cells recognize and respond to bacterial components such as lipopolysaccharide, unmethylated CpG DNA, peptidoglycan, and flagellin via different members of the Toll-like receptor family. In contrast, adaptive immune responses, whether humoral or cell mediated, are directed toward specific protein, lipid, or carbohydrate epitopes regardless of their origin. The resulting antibodies and T-cell immunity provide specific anamnestic protection against individual pathogens.

Each component of immunity makes specific contributions to host resistance to enteric infections as demonstrated by the consequences of various inborn or acquired immune defects. The importance of intact innate immunity becomes evident when neutrophils are absent in hosts, who then become particularly susceptible to gram-negative rod infections that often originate in the gastrointestinal tract. In addition, neutropenic patients may develop stomatitis or necrotizing typhlitis (with fever, abdominal pain, cecal necrosis and edema, and sometimes bloody diarrhea).[56] Patients with chronic granulomatous disease, who have an impaired neutrophil oxidative burst, are particularly susceptible to *Salmonella* bacteremia in addition to many extraintestinal infections.[57] The importance of innate immunity is also demonstrated by the potentially severe adenoviral, rotaviral, enteroviral, and *C. difficile* infections in patients undergoing bone marrow transplantation, who suffer defects in cell population numbers as well as loss of intestinal integrity as a result of conditioning chemotherapy and graft-versus-host disease. More subtle defects in innate immunity may explain some of

the heterogeneity of responses to enteric pathogens. For example, people with a particular polymorphism leading to increased expression of the neutrophil chemokine interleukin (IL)-8 appear to have increased susceptibility to enteroaggregative *E. coli* (EAEC) infection.[58]

The importance of adaptive immunity is most profoundly demonstrated in patients with the acquired immunodeficiency syndrome (AIDS), which selectively depletes the lymphocyte armies required for adaptive immune responses. Patients with AIDS who are unable to receive highly active antiretroviral therapy are at risk for devastating diarrheal infections. Most such infections have a documentable cause, such as cytomegalovirus, *Entamoeba histolytica*, *Cryptosporidium*, microsporidia, *Salmonella*, *Giardia*, *C. jejuni*, *Shigella*, *Mycobacterium*, *Cyclospora*, EAEC, or herpes simplex virus. In Haiti and Africa, up to 95% of patients with AIDS initially present with diarrhea; up to 50% have *Cryptosporidium* infections, and 15% have *Isospora belli*.[59-62]

Humoral intestinal immunity (coproantibody) arises either from a leakage of serum immunoglobulin (predominantly IgG or IgM) or from the formation of IgA by plasma cells located predominantly in the lamina propria. Secretory IgA (an 11S dimer [molecular weight, M_r, 390,000] with a secretory piece [M_r 60,000] from the mucosal epithelial cells) is found in the lumen.[63] Selective deficiency of secretory component has been associated with intestinal candidiasis.[64] Certain mucosal pathogens produce an IgA protease or degrade IgA.[65] Both serum and secretory antibody responses have been demonstrated in response to parenteral and intraluminal challenge with cholera toxoid. Secretory IgA is resistant to intraluminal degradation by enzymatic proteolysis and sulfhydryl reduction. Passively acquired IgA probably accounts for part of the protection against enteric infections in infants who are breastfed. Colostral antibody against rotaviruses and the enterotoxins of *V. cholerae* and *E. coli* have been demonstrated in breast milk. Interestingly, however, patients with antibody deficiency (including common variable immunodeficiency and IgA deficiency) do not appear to be at significantly increased risk of enteric infections, with the exception of giardiasis.[66,67]

Other Protective Factors in Human Milk and Serum

The protection afforded by breast-feeding probably relates to several passively transmitted factors and to reduced exposure to a contaminated environment.[67,68] In addition to antibody, these factors include lactoferrin, lysozyme, phagocytes, high lactose, low protein, low phosphate, low pH (in part from bifidobacteria), and oligosaccharide fractions.[69-71] The role of lactoferrin in human milk is suggested by the abolition of milk's bacteriostatic properties against *V. cholerae* and EPEC by saturation with iron. In addition, patients with chronic iron excess from hemolytic processes such as malaria, sickle cell anemia, and Oroya fever are at increased risk of infection with organisms such as *Salmonella*, and patients receiving the iron-chelating drug desferrioxamine may be at increased risk for infection with *Yersinia enterocolitica*.[71] Some bacteriostatic properties of normal serum are abolished when iron-binding proteins are saturated with iron.

MICROBIAL FACTORS

A number of bacterial virulence traits determine the pathogenic mechanisms responsible for diarrhea. Many of these traits are demonstrated by the various pathotypes of diarrheogenic *E. coli*, as summarized in Table 89-4. This versatile species may form the predominant normal aerobic colonic flora or may be a urinary, bacteremic, or enteric pathogen. Depending largely on virulence traits encoded on plasmids, chromosomal pathogenicity islands, or phage, *E. coli* may produce one of several families of enterotoxins, may be invasive (enteroinvasive *E. coli* [EIEC]), may cause hemorrhagic colitis (EHEC), or may exhibit adherence to epithelial cells leading to direct or indirect tissue damage (EPEC, EAEC, or diffusely adherent *E. coli* [DAEC]). Study of *E. coli* with these varied pathogenic traits has greatly helped to unravel the mechanisms by which enteric pathogens alter normal intestinal absorptive function to cause diarrheal diseases.[72,73]

TABLE 89-4 Pathogenic Mechanisms of *Escherichia coli* Diarrhea*

Type	Mechanism	Model	Gene Code	Predominant Serogroups
I. Enterotoxigenic *E. coli* (ETEC)	Adherence via CFA-I through CFA-IV	Mannose-resistant hemagglutination (for most)	Plasmid	—
LT *E. coli*	Adenylate cyclase–like cholera toxin	Rabbit ileal loops (18 hr), CHO, Y1 cell immunoassay	LT-I plasmid, LT-II chromosome	LT + ST: O groups 11, 15, 20, 25, 27, 60, 63, 75, 80, 85, 88, 89, 99, 101, 109, 114, 139, 153
STa *E. coli*	Guanylate cyclase	Suckling mice	Plasmid	ST: O groups 12, 78, 115, 148, 149, 153, 159, 166, 167
STb *E. coli*	Cyclic nucleotide–independent bicarbonate secretion	Piglet ileal loops	Plasmid	—
II. Enterohemorrhagic *E. coli* (EHEC)	Attaching/effacing (analogous to EPEC), Shiga-like (Vero) toxin 1 or 2 inhibits protein synthesis	HeLa cell cytotoxicity Fluorescent actin staining	Chromosome (pathogenicity island), phage	Predominantly O157:H7; O26:H11, O103:H2, O111:H⁻, O113:H21⁺, and some 50 others
III. Enteroinvasive *E. coli* (EIEC)	Local mucosal invasion, EIET	Sereny test, rabbit ileal loops, Ussing chambers	Plasmid, chromosome	O groups 11, 28ac, 29, 112ac, 115, 124, 136, 143, 144, 147, 152, 164, 167, 173
IV. Enteropathogenic *E. coli* (EPEC)				
Locally adherent attaching and effacing *E. coli*	Adhere focally via bundle-forming pili Attach to and efface brush border epithelium via injection and phosphorylation of Tir and subsequent intimin binding	Localized HEp-2 cell adherence Fluorescent actin staining	Plasmid (60 MDa, pMAR2, with EAF and bfpA) Chromosome locus of enterocyte effacement (LEE)	O18:H⁻, 7, 14; O26:H⁻, 11; O44:H18, 44; O55:H⁻, 6, 7; O86:H34; O88; O111:H⁻, 2, 12, 21; O114:H2; O119:H⁻, 27; O127:H⁻†; O128ab: H2, 7; O142:H6; O145; O157:H8; 158:H23
V. Enteroaggregative *E. coli* (EaggEC)	Aggregative adherence to Hep-2 cells	Aggregative pattern of HEp-2 cell adherence	Plasmid	O3:H2; O44; O78:H33; O15:H11; O77:H18; O51:H11
EAST-1	Guanylate cyclase	Ussing chamber	Plasmid	O?:H10, among others (O78, 86, 91, 92)
PET	Secretion, cytotoxicity	Ussing chamber	Plasmid	—
VI. Diffusely adherent *E. coli* (DAEC)	Diffuse adherence	Diffuse adherence to HEp-2 cells	Chromosomal	(Strain F1845, 189, 57-1)
Normal enteric flora	?Adherence traits	—	—	O groups 1, 2, 4, 6, 7, 25, 45, 75, 81
Genitourinary, blood stream, or meningeal pathogens	?Capsular polysaccharide ± adherence pili, CNF-I and CNF-II; adenosine diphosphate-ribosylate Rho proteins	Several animals (mice, rabbits), cytotoxicity	Plasmid (CNF-II)	O groups 1, 2, 4, 6, 7, 11, 18, 22, 25, 45, 62, 75, 81 (K antigens 1, 2, 3, 5, 13)

*In addition, nontoxigenic *E. coli* with recognized or new colonization factor fimbriae can cause diarrhea, as documented in experimental animals and in human volunteers; several reviews comment on O and H serotypes.

†O127:H6 is the focally HEp-2 cell adherent strain (E2348) from which the plasmid pMAR-2 was isolated.

CFA, colonization factor antigen; CHO, Chinese hamster ovary; CNF, colony necrotizing factor; EAF, enteroadherence factor; EAST, enteroaggregative STa-like toxin; EIEC, enteroinvasive *E. coli;* LT, heat-labile; ST, heat-stable; PET, plasmid-encoded toxin.

Toxins

Toxic microbial components or products are implicated in the disease-producing capacity of several enteric pathogens. Culture filtrates of toxigenic microorganisms are capable of altering gastrointestinal structure or function in the absence of the organisms themselves. Toxins produced by enteric pathogens can be classified as *neurotoxins, enterotoxins,* or *cytotoxins* (Table 89-5), although certain toxins fit into more than one category.

Neurotoxins

Neurotoxins are usually ingested as preformed toxins that often cause enteric symptoms. These include staphylococcal, *Bacillus cereus,* and botulinum toxins. Although staphylococcal food poisoning is an abrupt upper gastrointestinal syndrome attributed to staphylococcal enterotoxin, the effect appears to be caused by the action of this superantigen toxin on the central autonomic nervous system rather than by destruction or fluid secretion in the intestine per se.[74,75] An exotoxin related to enterotoxin A may cause fluid accumulation in rabbit ileal loops directly. A different staphylococcal α-toxin elicits hyperperistalsis. Certain strains of *B. cereus* isolated from patients with acute food poisoning also produce a highly heat-stable emetic toxin (especially when cultured with rice) that is a small (M_r <5000), nonantigenic polypeptide capable of causing vomiting in monkeys, much like staphylococcal enterotoxin.[76] Botulinum toxin has a primary effect on

the neuromuscular junction to prevent the release of acetylcholine from the presynaptic vesicle.[74] Finally, several neurotoxins are found in seafood and can cause severe disease when ingested. These include tetrodotoxin and the agents of paralytic shellfish poisoning and ciguatera. Although diarrhea may occur after ingestion of these toxins, the predominant effects result from systemic neurotoxicity.

Enterotoxins

True enterotoxins are defined as those having a direct effect on the intestinal mucosa to elicit net fluid secretion. The classic enterotoxin, cholera toxin, has been extensively studied and causes fluid secretion after the ganglioside-binding B subunit releases the A2 toxin subunit, which activates basolateral epithelial adenylate cyclase via adenosine diphosphate-ribosylation of Gsα to increase concentrations of intestinal cyclic adenosine monophosphate (cAMP).[77] In addition, prostaglandins, platelet-activating factor, and possibly neurohumoral mediators such as serotonin may be involved in the secretory or tissue culture responses to cholera toxin.[78] Antigenically and mechanistically similar toxins have been described for other closely related vibrios[79] and *E. coli.*[80]

Because there are no reliable markers such as serotype or biotype for enterotoxigenicity, demonstration of the toxin itself or the genes encoding it is necessary to identify which *E. coli* strains are enterotoxigenic. The genetic codes for enterotoxigenicity reside on transmissible

TABLE 89-5 Enteric Bacterial Toxins

Neurotoxin group
  Clostridium botulinum
  Staphylococcus aureus (enterotoxin b)
  Bacillus cereus (emetic toxin)
Secretory enterotoxin group
  Vibrio cholerae (cAMP)
Noncholera vibrios
  Escherichia coli, LT (cAMP)
  E. coli, STa (cGMP)
  E. coli, STb
  Salmonella
  Klebsiella
  Clostridium perfringens (A)
  Shigella dysenteriae
  B. cereus
Possible enterotoxins
  E. coli: EIET, EAST, EALT, PET
  V. cholerae: Ace, Zot
  Bacteroides fragilis
Cytotoxin group
  Shigella
  C. perfringens (A)
  Vibrio parahaemolyticus
  S. aureus
  Clostridium difficile (A and B)
  E. coli (EHEC) (certain O groups: 26, 39, 128, 157)
  Campylobacter jejuni
  Helicobacter pylori

cAMP, cyclic adenosine monophosphate; cGMP, cyclic guanosine monophosphate; EALT, enteroaggregative *E. coli* heat-labile toxin; EAST, enteroaggregative STa-like toxin; EHEC, enterohemorrhagic *E. coli*; EIEC, enteroinvasive *E. coli*; LT, heat-labile; PET, plasmid-encoded toxin; ST, heat-stable.

plasmids that can be lost or transferred to other *E. coli* strains by conjugation or by phage transduction.[81] Prior to the development of molecular diagnostics, enterotoxins could be identified only by bioassays of culture filtrates of the organisms in question. At one time, this required inoculation into a ligated rabbit ileal segment or into rabbit skin to test for a toxin-associated permeability factor. The ability of the heat-labile enterotoxin of *E. coli* (LT) to activate adenylate cyclase has been used in the development of tissue culture bioassays.[82,83] Its similar antigenicity to cholera toxin provided immunoassay techniques as well. Oligonucleotide gene probes for LT and the heat-stable enterotoxin (STa) are now available with nonradioactive enzyme markers and provide a simple, sensitive, and highly specific detection method for these enterotoxins.[84] More recently, polymerase chain reaction (PCR)-based diagnostic methods have been shown to be highly sensitive and specific, and when incorporated into a multiplex assay, have the capability of identifying a number of *E. coli* virulence traits, including toxins and adherence factors.[85-87]

The LT-producing *E. coli* are associated with watery diarrhea among adults in Asia, travelers to Central America, and children in a number of areas.[88-93] In addition, *Klebsiella, Citrobacter, Salmonella,* and *C. jejuni* produce cholera-like heat-labile toxins that also activate adenylate cyclase, bind to ganglioside, and share some immunogenicity with *E. coli* LT.[94,95]

The ST-producing *E. coli,* first described as a cause of diarrhea in piglets and calves, are capable of causing diarrhea in human volunteers as well.[96] STa from enterotoxigenic *E. coli* (ETEC) appears to be significantly associated with diarrhea among tourists to Central America, in occasional newborn nursery outbreaks in this country, and among adults with noninflammatory diarrhea on a Navajo reservation and in Brazil.[97,98] The mechanism of action of STa involves the specific activation of intestinal guanylate cyclase.[99-101] Like cAMP, cyclic guanosine monophosphate (cGMP) analogues (e.g., 8Br-GMP) can mimic the secretory effect of the enterotoxin. STa and its homologues in *Yersinia*, non-O1 *V. cholerae,* and *Citrobacter freundii* consist of 17 to 19 amino acids with conservation of six cysteines (with three disulfide bonds) and a central Asp-Pro-Ala region that is required for binding to and activation of enterocyte guanylate cyclase. Another *E. coli* guanylate cyclase–activating peptide toxin, known as EAST-1, is found in a majority of EHEC and EAEC isolates and in some atypical EPEC and *Salmonella* isolates as well.[102-105] These toxins may mimic endogenous ST-like compounds such as guanylin that have been isolated from mammalian cells and may play key roles in normal intestinal and renal physiology.[106,107]

Several other bacterial products induce intestinal secretion via electrogenic ion secretion. These include a chromosomally mediated 68- to 80-kDa secretory toxin produced in iron-deprived conditions by EIEC called EIET,[108,109] and the thermostable direct hemolysin of *Vibrio parahaemolyticus.* A protein neuroenterotoxin isolated from *Shigella dysenteriae* 1 (which may be responsible for the headache, meningismus, and seizures) also causes fluid secretion in rabbit ileal loops. Although experimental findings have been contradictory, the activation of adenylate cyclase by this *Shigella* enterotoxin has been demonstrated in rabbit ileal loops.[110] Certain strains of *B. cereus* have also been reported to produce a heat-labile, adenylate cyclase–activating, rabbit ileal loop–positive, dermonecrotic, and intestinonecrotic enterotoxin.[76] Other enteric organisms with enterotoxin-like activity include *Salmonella, Klebsiella, Citrobacter, Aeromonas,* and *Enterobacter* species.[93,111-115] Both heat-labile and heat-stable toxins have been reported. Although these enterotoxigenic organisms appear to be infrequent, much needs to be learned about the occurrence and the mechanism of action of enterotoxins from these organisms other than *E. coli.*

Cytotoxins and Mixed Toxins

Cytotoxic products of several enteric pathogens are responsible for the mucosal destruction that often results in inflammatory colitis. One prototype intestinal cytotoxin is the Shiga toxin from *S. dysenteriae* type 1. This cytotoxin may play a role in the colonic mucosal destructive process of shigellosis, leading to bacillary dysentery.[116] A role for Shiga-like toxins is more pronounced in EHEC that cause hemorrhagic colitis or the hemolytic-uremic syndrome (O groups 26, 39, 111, 113, 121, 128, and 157).[117-119] These toxins, known as SLT-1 and SLT-2, are associated with bacteriophage in *E. coli* O157:H7.[120] Following the multistate outbreak of hemorrhagic colitis with *E. coli* O157:H7 in 1982,[119] it was found that SLT-1 is nearly identical to the Shiga toxin from *S. dysenteriae* 1. Since that time, EHEC has caused numerous outbreaks and sporadic cases of hemorrhagic colitis or childhood hemolytic-uremic syndrome in schools, daycare centers, nursing homes, and communities, including more than 500 documented cases and four deaths in four western states associated with a single hamburger chain in 1993.[119,121-125] A massive outbreak in 1996 involving more than 10,000 Japanese schoolchildren was presumptively traced to contaminated radish sprouts; there was a relatively low incidence of hemolytic-uremic syndrome in this outbreak.[126,127]

Like Shiga toxin, *E. coli* SLT-1 has binding and active subunits, is neutralized by anti-Shiga toxin antibody, and binds to globotriaosylceramide (Gb3) via its B subunit. After this, the enzymatic A subunit (analogous to that of the plant toxin, ricin) cleaves the *N*-glycoside bond of adenine at position 4324 in the 28 srRNA of the 60S ribosomal subunit to prevent elongation factor 1–dependent aminoacyl transfer RNA binding to the ribosome, thereby halting protein synthesis.[128] Subtle differences in the B-subunit specificities for Gb4 or Gb5 (globotetraosyl or globopentaosyl ceramide, respectively) and for Gb3 may help explain differences in cell culture effects and in the disease manifestations of SLT-1 and SLT-2, SLT-2vh, and SLT-2vp (to cause bloody diarrhea or hemolytic-uremic syndrome in patients or edema diseases in swine).[129]

Clostridium perfringens enterotoxin also produces cytotoxicity similar to that of *S. dysenteriae* toxin in HeLa cells and in animal models.[130] Vero cells have been used to detect a cytotoxicity in fecal filtrates that is neutralized by specific antiserum or toxin fragments.[131,132] These methods have enabled studies that implicate enterocytotoxigenic *C. perfringens* in geriatric institutions and in cases of antibiotic-associated diarrhea.[133] *C. perfringens* type C produces a trypsin-sensitive β-toxin.[134] Another enteric pathogen that releases a cytotoxin is *V. parahaemolyticus,* an important cause of seafood-borne diarrheal illness outbreaks. There is a strong association between clinical disease and the presence of the gene for thermostable direct hemolysin,[135,136] a toxin with both cytotoxic (believed to be a result of pore-forming ability)[137] and enterotoxic (via mobilization of intracellular calcium in rabbit loops) activities.[138] Others have noted the tendency of *V. parahaemolyticus* to penetrate and cause bacteremia in animal models[139] or an invasive colitis in patients.[140] *V. parahaemolyticus* typically causes explosive watery diarrhea in foodborne outbreaks in coastal areas of the United States.[141]

Another mechanism of several bacterial toxins is cytoskeletal disruption, which can lead to loss of tight junctions and perturbations in absorptive and barrier function of the intestinal epithelium. For example, the Bft toxin identified from *Bacteroides fragilis* isolates from children and adults with diarrhea in Montana and Arizona disrupts tight junctions by proteolytically cleaving E-cadherin in intestinal epithelial cells.[116,142] The toxins of *C. difficile* disrupt epithelial integrity by performing an enzymatic monoglucosylation of the Thr-37 residue of small GTP-binding proteins of the Rho family, leading to their inactivation.[143,144] The zonula occludens toxin of *V. cholerae,* which causes paracellular leak, may contribute to the diarrhea of cholera.[145] The plasmid-encoded cytotoxin (Pet) from EAEC isolated from children with diarrhea in Mexico City causes both fluid secretion and unique ultrastructural changes in the intestinal epithelium. Pet is a member of the serine protease autotransporter family of bacterial toxins, and cleaves the cytoskeletal proteins spectrin and fodrin, although the full spectrum of its activity is not yet known.[146]

In addition to direct effects on mucosal integrity, disruption of tight junctions and other cytoskeletal elements can trigger a cascade of inflammation in the gut epithelium, contributing to symptoms of infection. For example, the role of inflammatory mediators in *C. difficile* diarrhea is suggested by the prevention of hemorrhagic fluid accumulation in experimental animals by anti-inflammatory compounds, including receptor antagonists for platelet-activating factor or substance P, blocking antibodies against leukocyte adhesion molecules, ketotifen (which inhibits mast-cell activation), and indomethacin.[147-151]

A number of other cytotoxic enteric pathogens have been identified. *Staphylococcus aureus* produces a nonantigenic Δ-toxin that impairs water absorption and causes cytotoxic disruption of intestinal mucosa or cells in tissue culture.[152] In addition, a 110-kDa heat- and trypsin-labile cytotoxin that is distinct from Shiga toxin has been implicated in patients with seizures or encephalopathy with shigellosis.[153] Cytolethal distending toxin, a family of related proteins found in some *E. coli* and *Campylobacter* isolates, causes a cell cycle arrest leading to cell death.[154-156] A novel cytotoxic enterotoxin, Act, has been found in many diarrheogenic *Aeromonas* strains.[157] Genomic analysis of EPEC and EHEC led to the identification of a lymphostatin, a large protein with homology to *C. difficile* toxins that inhibits lymphocyte proliferation in vitro.[158] Finally, the pathogenesis of *C. jejuni* and *H. pylori* may involve cytotoxins that have been described.[159-162] As the genomes of more diarrheal pathogens are sequenced, additional protein toxins will undoubtedly be discovered.

Attachment

The ability of many enteric pathogens to cause disease depends not only on the organism's ability to penetrate the mucosa or to produce enterotoxin or cytotoxin but also on its ability to adhere to and colonize the mucosa. This adherence capacity has been well described with ETEC, which, to cause disease, must first adhere to and colonize the upper small bowel of humans or animals. This adherence capacity for *E. coli* is variously called K88, K99, or CFA for strains affecting piglets, calves, and humans, respectively. As with enterotoxigenicity, the production of these adherence antigens appears to be genetically encoded by transmissible plasmids. These fimbriate bacterial surface adhesins are distinct from type 1 pili and from recognized urinary tract adhesins[163-165] and usually cause hemagglutination that is mannose re-

sistant.[166,167] Although these adhesins hold great promise for immunization against colonization, there are now at least five different types of CFAs among human ETEC: CFA-I, CFA-II, E8775, 260-1, and O159:H4.[162,168-170]

Like ETEC adhesins, fimbriate or fibrillar adhesins may also aid in the initial colonization of EHEC, EPEC, and EAEC. The Shiga-like toxin–producing EHEC O26 has been shown to adhere to the mucosa of human fetal small intestinal tissue in vitro in a mannose-resistant fashion, a trait that is transmissible by a colicinogenic conjugative plasmid.[171] In addition, EHEC strain O157:H7 has been shown to have a 60-MDa plasmid that encodes a new type of fimbria that appear to mediate attachment to Henle 407 cells in tissue culture.[172]

The complexity of bacterial adherence is demonstrated in EPEC, which uses plasmid- and chromosomally encoded traits to produce its characteristic attaching and effacing phenotype. The 50- to 60-MDa plasmid in EPEC encodes inducible, bundle-forming pili that share amino-terminal sequence homology with the toxin-coregulated pili in *V. cholerae* and are responsible for efficient adherence to human laryngeal tumor cells (HEp-2) in "localized" colonies.[173-175] This is followed by injection of a 90-kDa protein known as Tir (translocated intimin receptor) directly into the host cytosol via a type III secretion system (TTSS). Tir then acts as a receptor for the 94-kDa bacterial chromosomally encoded protein intimin, which leads to intimate attachment to intestinal epithelial cells. Subsequent actin accumulation and microvillus effacement requires tyrosine phosphorylation of Tir within the cell to create the characteristic "pedestal" on which the bacterium sits.[176-179] Other mediators injected or secreted by the TTSS have profound effects on cell physiology, although the contribution of these mediators to EPEC disease is still being determined. EHEC O157:H7 and several animal pathogens (rabbit diarrheogenic *E. coli* [RDEC] and *Citrobacter rodentium*)[180-182] produce similar attaching and effacing lesions via a TTSS, although there are significant differences between them. For example, the EHEC pedestal has a qualitatively different appearance from the EPEC pedestal, and unlike EPEC, EHEC Tir does not require tyrosine phosphorylation to produce pedestals.[183-185]

Distinct from the localized adherence of EPEC to HEp-2 cells are the "aggregative" and "diffuse" adherence patterns (AA and DA, respectively), for which gene probes have been developed that detect some, but not all, *E. coli* with these phenotypes.[186-190] EAEC have been associated with persistent diarrhea in children in a number of developing areas, in adults with AIDS, in a large outbreak in Japanese schoolchildren, and, increasingly, in travelers to developing areas.[191-197] Unlike EPEC and EHEC, EAEC does not appear to intimately attach to cells but instead resides within a dense "slime" layer on the epithelial surface, utilizing one of several families of aggregative adherence fimbriae. Coordinated regulation of dispersin, an anti-aggregative factor,[198] and Pic, a mucinase,[199] allows the bacteria to approach the epithelial surface, create a niche within the mucus layer, and adhere to each other and to the epithelium in a manner resembling biofilm.

DAEC represent several serotypes as identified by gene probes for strain 1845[200] and for a 100-kilobase plasmid–encoded 100-kDa protein adhesin (AIDA-I) from strain 2787 (O126:H27).[201] Because DAEC have been variably seen in association with diarrhea and controls, a pathogenic role has not yet been established.[202,203] However, a unique ultrastructural phenotype of DAEC adherence to epithelial cells has been observed. The bacteria adhere within the forest of microvilli, and in some cases elongated microvilli appear to embrace and surround the bacteria. This phenotype is associated with binding and clustering of decay-accelerating factor in regions of the apical membrane.[204]

Bacterial adherence itself can produce diarrhea in some settings. Enteric bacterial pathogens engineered to express the colonization traits mentioned previously, but lacking enterotoxin production, can still cause diarrhea. An engineered, colonizing, multiply toxin-deleted *V. cholerae* vaccine strain (lacking proteins ctxA, zot, ace, and hly) caused diarrhea in animals[205-207] and in human volunteers. This diarrhea was associated with modest elevations in fecal lactoferrin, implying an inflammatory component.[208] Whether naturally occurring colonizing bacteria are responsible, alone or in part, for cases of acute or prolonged diarrhea remains to be determined.

Invasiveness

The capacity of organisms such as *Shigella* and certain invasive strains of *E. coli* to invade and destroy epithelial cells is responsible for the inflammatory or dysenteric diarrhea they cause. This capacity is demonstrated in the laboratory by the guinea pig conjunctivitis (Sereny) test.[209] There is cell destruction and superficial inflammatory invasion of the cornea similar to that noted in colonic mucosa. Modifications in the specific components of the O side chain of the cell wall lipopolysaccharide alter this invasive property in *Shigella*.[210] There is also evidence that the invasiveness of certain *E. coli* may be reflected in their O antigens or serotype.[211,212] Invasiveness is also associated with large, 120- to 140-MDa plasmids in *Shigella sonnei*,[213] *S. flexneri*,[214] and invasive *E. coli*.[215] HeLa cell, rabbit loop, and Sereny's test invasiveness can be genetically constructed by the sequential transfer of defined chromosomal and plasmid genes for *S. flexneri* to *E. coli* K12.[216]

Cell invasion, unlike superficial colonization, may involve attachment to transmembrane glycoproteins (instead of carbohydrates and glycolipids) such as integrin bound by *Yersinia* invasin.[217] The expression of "invasiveness" is complex. In *Shigella* and EIEC, it appears to involve a series of plasmid-encoded invasion and adhesin proteins (ipaA through ipaD) that are regulated by key chromosomal codons (e.g., kcpA).[216-218] Once *Shigella* enters the host cell, a complex array of proteins induces condensation of host actin in a polar fashion by the protein IcsA, which allows the bacterium to propel itself through the cytoplasm to enhance its invasive properties.[219] In *Salmonella*, adherence and invasion appear to be closely linked and may require bacterial proteins that are induced by trypsin- and neuraminidase-sensitive structures present on the epithelial cell surface.[220] Adherence and invasion phenotypes of *Salmonella* require the SPI-1 chromosomal pathogenicity island, whereas subsequent survival within intracellular vacuoles requires genes in a second pathogenicity island, termed SPI-2.[221-223] The capacity of *E. histolytica* to adhere and "invade" relates, at least in part, to a GalNAc-inhibitable amebic lectin that leads to contact-dependent cytolysis of host cells, particularly attracted neutrophils.[224-226] As discussed previously, cytotoxic exotoxins may well play roles in the invasive and destructive properties of certain shigellae, *V. parahaemolyticus*, staphylococci, and clostridia.

Finally, many enteric pathogens include a vigorous host response that in and of itself can lead to diarrhea. For example, invasion by *Shigella* or *Salmonella* and adherence by *E. histolytica* lead to release of a wide array of proinflammatory cytokines from intestinal epithelial cells.[227] In addition, secreted or otherwise released culture products of several bacteria (including EAEC, *H. pylori*, and *C. difficile*) have been shown to cause release of IL-8 from intestinal epithelial cells.[17,228,229] This leads to accumulation of neutrophils within the lamina propria. These neutrophils can damage host tissue directly, or they can migrate through tight junctions into the lumen (under the influence of host or pathogen chemotactic factors), where they release 5'-AMP, which is cleaved to adenosine by an apical 5'-nucleotidase, causing electrogenic chloride secretion.[230] *S. typhimurium* infection of polarized epithelial cells in vitro is associated with translocation of flagellin to the basolateral surface, where it acts through Toll-like receptor 5 to trigger IL-8 release and, possibly, other inflammatory responses.[231,232] Even noninvasive, nontoxigenic organisms may induce fluid secretion by causing subepithelial cells to secrete prostaglandins or other secretory mediators. In the case of *C. parvum*, this host response is vigorous enough to create a secretory effect of stool from infected patients in the absence of any identifiable enterotoxin.[233] Whether induction of host inflammation is of itself a pathogenic feature of these organisms remains to be determined.

Other Virulence Factors

In addition to enterotoxin production and adherence, an orchestrated set of additional virulence traits appears to be critical to the ability of pathogens such as *V. cholerae* to succeed in colonizing the intestinal mucosa. These include motility,[234,235] chemotaxis,[27,236] and mucinase production,[237,238] any one of which can be missing and lead to reduced virulence. The virulence of certain enteric pathogens such as *S. typhi* appears to be related to the Vi antigen[236] and to the polysaccharide composition of the O side chain of its lipopolysaccharide cell wall content,[239,240] both of which have been used in vaccine production.[240-243] Finally, several enteric pathogens (EPEC, EHEC, *Salmonella*, *Yersinia*) express type III secretion systems, which enable export and delivery of toxic proteins directly into the host cytoplasm. The list of organisms expressing such secretion systems and the effectors they produce is rapidly expanding.

Still another way that organisms can cause diarrhea involves the selective destruction of absorptive cells (villus tip cells) in the mucosa, leaving secretory cells (crypt cells) intact.[244-247] Both the rotaviruses and the noroviruses (Norwalk-like viruses), which selectively infect and disrupt the villus tip cells, alter the normal absorptive fluid balance, and reduce the brush-border digestive enzymes present during active infection.[246,247] Such an imbalanced disruption of the specialized absorptive surface may also be involved in other small bowel infections that are often associated with villus tip flattening or microvillus destruction, including bacterial overgrowth syndromes, EPEC infections, giardiasis, strongyloidiasis, and cryptosporidiosis.

MAJOR SYNDROMES OF DERANGED GASTROINTESTINAL PHYSIOLOGY

The elements of net fluid balance in the healthy adult intestinal tract are shown diagrammatically in Figure 89-1. With a daily oral intake of 1.5 L, salivary, gastric, biliary, and pancreatic secretions contribute a total of approximately 8.5 L of fluid that enters the upper gastrointestinal tract each day. However, daily fecal fluid excretion is normally less than 150 mL, indicating a net absorption of more than 8 L each day by the intestinal tract. More than 90% of this net absorption occurs in the small bowel, where there is a massive bidirectional flux that probably exceeds 50 L/day. A relatively slight shift in the bidirectional flux can result in substantial overload of the colonic absorptive capacity, which rarely exceeds 2 to 3 L/day. As in the kidney, there are hormonal,

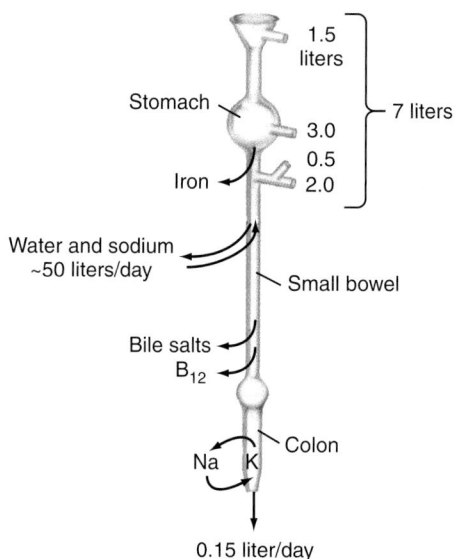

FIGURE 89-1. Diagram of fluid balance in the gastrointestinal tract of a healthy adult.

physical, and osmotic factors active in the intestinal tract. Aldosterone, for example, enhances intestinal sodium absorption at the expense of potassium.[248,249] Excessive fluid volume results in a "third factor" effect that may elicit or prolong diarrhea,[250] and osmotic laxatives are as familiar as osmotic diuretics.

Enteric disease can be produced by microbe-host interactions that alter normal intestinal physiology in one of three fundamental ways: (1) by a shift in the delicate balance of bidirectional water and electrolyte fluxes in the upper small bowel by intraluminal toxins or minimally invasive organisms (e.g., *Giardia, Cryptosporidium*), (2) by inflammatory or cytotoxic destruction of the ileal or colonic mucosa, or (3) by penetration through an intact mucosa to the reticuloendothelial system. These three types of enteric infections are outlined in Table 89-6. They can often be distinguished by a quick, simple examination. Mucus from a fresh stool specimen is mixed with a drop of methylene blue on a slide and examined for the presence of fecal leukocytes.[251,252] In most cases, no leukocytes are noted. This suggests a noninflammatory process in which diarrhea usually arises from the upper small bowel by the action of a true enterotoxin or agents such as *Giardia* or viruses. The secretory effects of certain enterotoxins share similar mechanisms with noninfectious endocrine causes of diarrhea such as non–β-cell islet tumors, medullary carcinoma of the thyroid, carcinoid tumors, and other benign or malignant neoplasms that are associated with increased serum prostaglandins, vasoactive intestinal polypeptide, or changes in cyclic nucleotide concentrations. Impaired small bowel absorption is important in tropical sprue, enzyme deficiencies, and solute loads. Enhanced colonic secretion without an inflammatory response characteristic of microbial or ulcerative colitis may result from excessive bile salts or fatty acids or from neoplasms such as villous adenomas.

The presence of numerous polymorphonuclear leukocytes documents an inflammatory or invasive process that usually arises from the colon or distal small bowel. Amebic colitis can often be distinguished from bacterial dysenteries by microscopic fecal examination. In addition to the amebic trophozoites or cysts, fecal neutrophils are usually pyknotic or absent with amebiasis, probably because of the cytopathic effect of virulent amebae on mammalian cells, including neutrophils.[253] Impaired colonic absorption may contribute to the diarrhea in inflammatory colitis caused by shigellosis, pseudomembranous enterocolitis, amebic colitis, or idiopathic ulcerative colitis. In addition, evidence suggests that the products of the lipoxygenase and other pathways in neutrophils may also contribute to a secretory process.[254,255] Agents that cause an inflammatory colitis may require specific antimicrobial intervention as well as supportive fluid therapy.[252]

The third type of enteric infection is caused by organisms that penetrate the intact intestinal mucosa, often in the distal small bowel, to multiply in the lymphatic or reticuloendothelial cells. This usually results in a febrile systemic illness with or without diarrhea. The classic example of this type of enteric pathogen is *S. typhi*. If diarrhea is present, mononuclear leukocytes may be found in the stools of these patients.[251] Cultural documentation of the pathogen is important, because a bacteremia that necessitates specific antimicrobial therapy may result in this setting.

The tripartite distinction among enteric infections is by no means absolute. For example, *C. difficile* colitis is pathophysiologically an inflammatory diarrhea, although there are often no visible fecal leukocytes. In addition, certain pathogens considered noninflammatory (e.g., *Cryptosporidium*, EPEC, EAEC) are actually associated with varying degrees of villus destruction and inflammation, as measured both by histopathology and by more sensitive assays for fecal inflammatory markers such as lactoferrin, IL-1, and IL-8.[17,254] Even cholera, the prototype secretory diarrhea, can be associated with intestinal inflammation, as evidenced by volunteer studies using toxin-negative vaccine candidates.[208] Finally, EHEC infection, although characterized by colonic tissue damage, may present with the absence of fecal leukocytes or low levels of fecal lactoferrin.[255] As more of the pathophysiology of enteric infections is understood, these categories may require further revision.

DIAGNOSTIC APPROACH TO ENTERIC INFECTIONS

The appropriate diagnostic approach to diarrheal illness is determined by the patient's age, the severity of illness, the duration of illness, the type of illness, and the available facilities. Of greatest importance in patients with diarrhea are evaluation and treatment of dehydration and a careful history, physical examination, and, if in doubt about whether an inflammatory process is present, examination of a specimen for fecal lactoferrin or leukocytes. A history of recent antibiotic use, weight loss, underlying diseases, other illnesses in the family or in other contacts, or travel outside the United States, to the seacoast, or to rural mountainous areas should elicit a more careful investigation of specific etiologic agents. A prompt evaluation of physical signs of fever, toxicity, or severe dehydration may result in lifesaving supportive fluid therapy. Particularly worrisome signs of severe dehydration, especially in children, include lethargy, postural hypotension and tachycardia,

TABLE 89-6 Comparison of the Three Types of Enteric Infection

	Type I	Type II	Type III
Mechanism	Noninflammatory (enterotoxin or adherence/superficial invasion)	Inflammatory (invasion, cytotoxin)	Penetrating
Location	Proximal small bowel	Colon	Distal small bowel
Illness	Watery diarrhea	Dysentery	Enteric fever
Stool examination	No fecal leukocytes	Fecal polymorphonuclear leukocytes	Fecal mononuclear leukocytes
	Mild or no ↑ lactoferrin	↑↑Lactoferrin	—
Examples	*Vibrio cholerae*	*Shigella*	*Salmonella typhi*
	Escherichia coli (ETEC, LT, ST)	*E. coli* (EIEC, EHEC)	*Yersinia enterocolitica*
	Clostridium perfringens	*Salmonella enteritidis*	?*Campylobacter fetus*
	Bacillus cereus	*Vibrio parahaemolyticus*	
	Staphylococcus aureus	*Clostridium difficile*	
	Also[†]:	*Campylobacter jejuni*	
	Giardia lamblia	*Entamoeba histolytica*[*]	
	Rotavirus		
	Norwalk-like viruses		
	Cryptosporidium parvum		
	E. coli (EPEC, EAEC)		
	Microsporidia		
	Cyclospora cayetanensis		

[*]Although amebic dysentery involves tissue inflammation, the leukocytes are characteristically pyknotic or absent, having been destroyed by the virulent amebae.
[†]Although not typically enterotoxic, these pathogens alter bowel physiology via adherence, superficial cell entry, cytokine induction, or toxins that inhibit cell function.
EAEC, enteroaggregative *E. coli;* EHEC, enterohemorrhagic *E. coli;* EIEC, enteroinvasive *E. coli;* EPEC, enteropathogenic *E. coli;* ETEC, enterotoxigenic *E. coli;* LT, heat-labile; ST, heat-stable.

sunken fontanelles, and dry skin (with decreased turgor), dry eyes, or dry mucous membranes.[256]

As noted in Figure 89-2, selective fecal testing is indicated for severe, bloody, febrile, dysenteric, nosocomial, or persistent diarrheal illnesses.[5] Indeed, Infectious Diseases Society of America guidelines suggest that the approach shown in Figure 89-2 should replace traditional orders for stool cultures or for ova and parasite exams.[5] Examination of a fresh stool specimen, preferably collected in a cup, is particularly valuable. First, it provides the physician with an objective determination of the patient's subjective complaints. Second, a gross description of the stool as watery, mucoid, or bloody provides important clues about its cause and appropriate management. Third, testing for fecal lactoferrin or a microscopic examination for fecal leukocytes may reveal heavy parasites or maldigested fat or meat fibers suggesting pancreatic insufficiency, or lipid droplets suggesting malabsorption with steatorrhea. If fever or fecal lactoferrin or neutrophils are present, the physician should selectively take a culture for the most commonly recognized invasive pathogens—*C. jejuni, Salmonella,* and *Shigella.*[252] Swab or diaper specimens appear to be less sensitive than cup specimens for fecal leukocytes.[257] A newer and simpler test for fecal lactoferrin provides a rapid, sensitive marker for fecal leukocytes that is effective even with swab or refrigerated samples.[258]

Any grossly bloody stool specimen should also be examined for *E. coli* O157 by growth on sorbitol–MacConkey's agar and for other SLT-producing *E. coli* by a specific SLT assay. In the United States, EHEC is the most common cause of bloody diarrhea and should be suspected particularly if fever is absent.[40] Any patient with a history of recent antibiotic or antineoplastic drug use should have a stool assay for *C. difficile* toxins, regardless of the results of the microscopic stool examination. A history of recent antibiotic use, weight loss, and chronic diarrhea (>10 days); seacoast or other exposures; or immunocompromised states should prompt the physician to consider other agents as noted.

Other diagnostic studies that can be made on fecal specimens include special stains for fat or muscle and determinations of pH and reducing substances. A Sudan stain may reveal many large (10 to 75 μm), orange-stained globules of fat, suggesting malabsorption, or smaller (1 to 4 μm) globules or needle-like crystals of fatty acid that may be normal. Numerous undigested muscle fibers may be seen with an aqueous 2% eosin stain and suggest pancreatic insufficiency and maldigestion.

An acidic stool pH can be helpful in the identification of lactose intolerance, especially in children with diarrhea. Although breastfed infants have a fecal pH ranging from 4.7 to 5.1, stool pH usually exceeds 7.0 if the infant is on a regular milk-containing diet. On a regular diet, a fecal pH less than 5.0 suggests the presence of lactic acid from the action of colonic bacterial flora on unabsorbed lactose. Stool-reducing substances may also be helpful in the detection of carbohydrate malabsorption. A simple test uses copper sulfate (Clinitest) tablets. Mix 1 mL stool with 2 mL water, add 15 drops of this mixture to a test tube, and then add one copper sulfate tablet. A reduction positive for "sugar" indicates reducing substances. Positive tests for blood may suggest an invasive process such as amebiasis or shigellosis. Although this is usually evident from a gross examination of the stool, tests for occult blood are much more sensitive but less specific. Tests for hemoglobin peroxidase use orthotoluidine, benzidine, or guaiac reagents, in descending order of sensitivity. Some are so sensitive that they may be positive with ingested meat myoglobin. Twenty-four-hour determinations for fecal fat (normal, <7.2 g/day fecal fat or <150 to 200 g/day total stool weight) may also be of value.

For culture of enteric pathogens, the specimen should be inoculated onto culture plates as promptly as possible. The media used are selective and often contain indicator substances that aid in initial identification. Routine techniques must include selective culture for *C. jejuni,* in a selective atmosphere of reduced oxygen (4% to 6%) and increased carbon dioxide (6% to 10%) at 42° C. Routine stool culture also includes a medium, such as MacConkey's or eosin methylene blue (EMB) agar, that inhibits gram-positive organisms and selects predominantly for aerobic gram-negative rods. In addition, more se-

lective media (e.g., xylose-lysine-deoxycholate, *Salmonella-Shigella* agar) and enrichment broths (e.g., gram-negative, selenite, and tetrathionate broths) that inhibit most organisms except *Salmonella* and *Shigella* should be used. However, because highly selective media are also more inhibitory, the less selective MacConkey's and EMB agar should also be examined for non–lactose-fermenting (colorless) colonies that may be salmonellae or shigellae. Even the best techniques with fresh specimens may miss fragile organisms such as shigellae. Fecal cultures failed to yield shigellae in 40% of volunteers with inflammatory diarrhea from experimental *Shigella* infection.[251] When immediate culture is impossible, specimens may be transported to a laboratory in a non-nutrient holding medium, such as Cary-Blair soft agar, that prevents drying and overgrowth of normal flora.

Culture of vibrios (*V. cholerae, V. parahaemolyticus,* and others), which should be suspected after any exposure to coastal areas or seafood, requires the highly selective thiosulfate citrate bile salt sucrose agar. Culture of *Y. enterocolitica* may require the selective process of cold enrichment on sheep blood agar or phosphate-buffered saline for 2 to 3 weeks and should be considered particularly for patients receiving desferrioxamine or with a history of raw pork consumption.

E. coli that grow readily as dry, lactose-fermenting (purple) colonies on EMB or MacConkey's agar are major aerobic constituents of normal fecal flora but should also be considered potential pathogens. However, routine analysis of *E. coli* in sporadic cases is of limited value and should be considered a special tool for investigating epidemic diarrhea in settings such as newborn nurseries or unexplained dysentery. Commonly used tests for diarrheogenic *E. coli* include gene probes or PCR to detect toxin genes, and the HEp-2 adherence assay to identify EPEC, EAEC, and DAEC. Special tests for secretory enterotoxins include the rabbit ileal loop, rabbit skin permeability, Chinese hamster ovary cell, Y1 adrenal cell, immunoassay, and suckling mouse assay. EIEC may be identified by inoculation into the conjunctival sac of guinea pigs (Sereny test).[209]

When diarrhea persists unexplained, especially with blood or weight loss, examinations for protozoa and *Strongyloides stercoralis* are indicated, using specific techniques for the pathogens suspected. An acid-fast stain detects *Cryptosporidium* and *Cyclospora;* more sensitive enzyme immunoassay or fluorescent-tagged antibody stains are now available for *Cryptosporidium* and *Giardia.* A modified trichrome stain for microsporidia should also be considered for patients with AIDS. If *E. histolytica* is suspected, specific immunoassays offer improved alternatives to microscopic examination.

Proctoscopic examination can be very helpful in the differential diagnosis, especially when inflammatory colitis is present. Although necrotic ulcers may be seen in acute shigellosis, discrete ulcers are more suggestive of amebiasis or Crohn's disease. Mucosal friability is more suggestive of inflammatory bowel disease (e.g., ulcerative colitis). The appearance of raised, plaquelike pseudomembranes is diagnostic of pseudomembranous colitis due to toxigenic *C. difficile.* Large amounts of mucus may be present in "mucous colitis" or with a villous adenoma; melanosis coli may suggest laxative abuse.

Rectal mucosal biopsy specimens, especially when ulcers are present, can be of great help for identification of the parasite *E. histolytica,* granulomata, amyloidosis (with Congo red stain), or Whipple's disease (with periodic acid–Schiff stain). Small bowel biopsy specimens may also be diagnostic in Whipple's disease, giardiasis, amyloidosis, a β-lipoproteinemia, lymphoma, cryptosporidiosis, giardiasis, microsporidiosis, or mast-cell disease. Characteristic but not necessarily diagnostic histopathologic changes may be seen in celiac disease, tropical sprue, eosinophilic gastroenteritis, dermatitis herpetiformis, and dysgammaglobulinemia. However, several conditions, including Crohn's disease, bacterial overgrowth syndrome, and pancreatic or bile salt insufficiency, may be associated with normal small bowel histologic findings or with nonspecific changes.

Radiologic studies of the intestinal tract may reveal toxic megacolon, pancreatic calcifications, or nodular adrenal calcifications suggestive of tuberculosis or histoplasmosis. Colonic mucosal edema

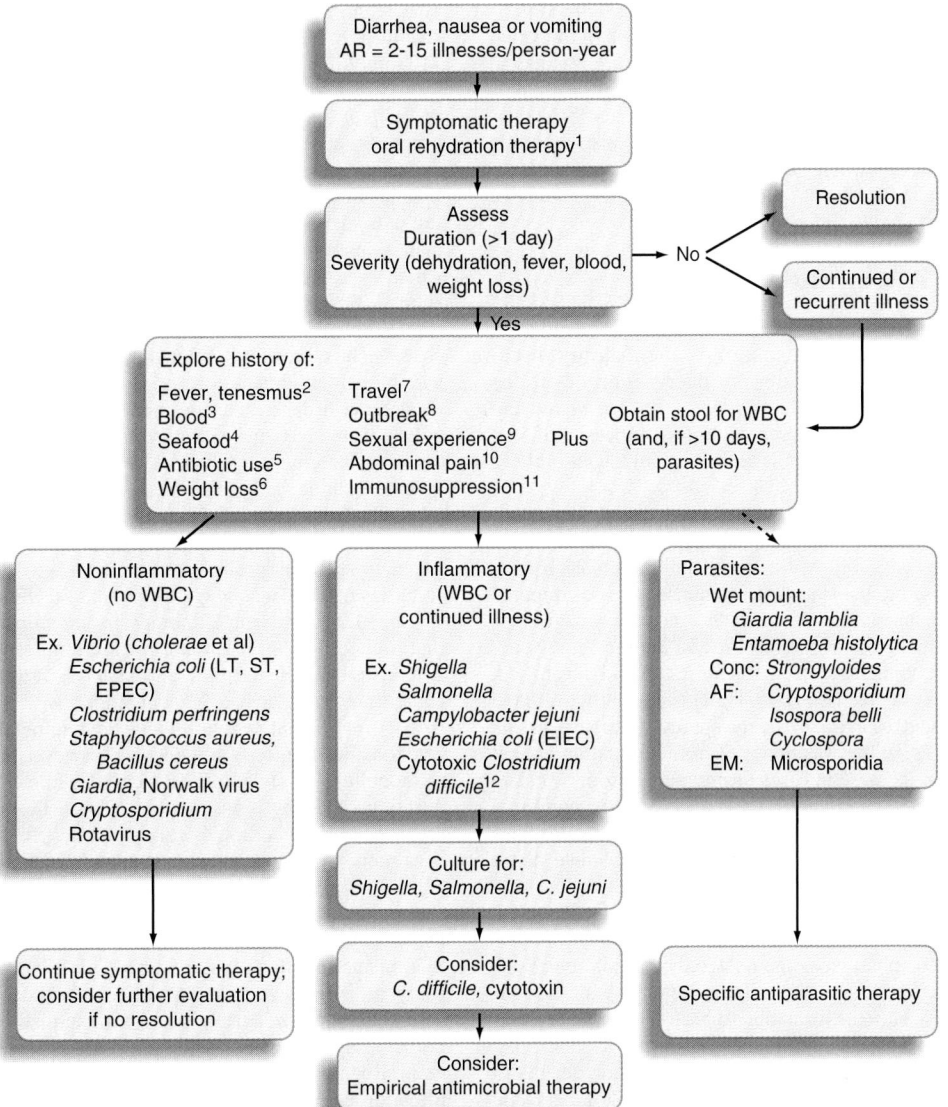

FIGURE 89-2. Approach to diagnosis and management of infectious diarrhea. Key to superscripts: *1.* Oral rehydration solution (ORS) can be prepared by adding 3.5 g NaCl, 2.5 g NaHCO$_3$ (or 2.9 g sodium citrate), 1.5 g KCl, and 20 g glucose or glucose polymer (e.g., 40 g sucrose; 4 tablespoons sugar; 50 to 60 g cereal flour such as rice, maize, sorghum, millet, wheat, or potato flour) to 1 L (1.05 quart) of clean water. This makes approximately Na 90, K 20, Cl 80, HCO$_3$ 30, and glucose 111 mmol/L. One level teaspoon table salt and 8 level teaspoons table sugar per liter makes about 86 mmol Na and 30 g sucrose/L, to which one could add 1 cup orange juice or two bananas for potassium. *2.* Fever or tenesmus suggests an inflammatory proctocolitis. *3.* Diarrhea with blood, especially without fecal leukocytes, suggests enterohemorrhagic (Shiga-like toxin–producing) *Escherichia coli* or amebiasis (in which leukocytes are destroyed by the parasite). *4.* Ingestion of inadequately cooked seafood should prompt consideration of infections with *Vibrio* or Norwalk-like viruses. *5.* Antibiotics should be stopped if possible and cytotoxigenic *Clostridium difficile* considered. Antibiotics may also predispose to other infections such as salmonellosis. *6.* Persistence (>10 days) with weight loss should prompt consideration of giardiasis, cyclosporiasis, cryptosporidiosis. *7.* Travel to tropical areas increases the chance of developing enterotoxigenic *E. coli* (ETEC) as well as viral (Norwalk-like or rotaviral), parasitic *(Giardia, Entamoeba, Strongyloides, Cryptosporidium),* and, if fecal leukocytes are present, invasive bacterial infections as noted in the algorithm. *8.* Outbreaks should prompt consideration of *Staphylococcus aureus, Bacillus cereus,* anisakiasis (incubation period <6 hours), *Clostridium perfringens, Cryptosporidium,* ETEC, *Vibrio, Salmonella, Campylobacter, Shigella,* or enteroinvasive *E. coli* (EIEC) infection. During spring and summer months, *Cyclospora* should also be considered. Consider saving *E. coli* for LT, ST, invasiveness, and adherence testing, and for serotyping; stool for rotavirus testing; and stool plus paired sera for Norwalk-like virus or toxin testing. *9.* Sigmoidoscopy in symptomatic homosexual men should distinguish proctitis in the distal 15 cm only (caused by herpesvirus, gonococcal, chlamydial, or syphilitic infection) from colitis (*Campylobacter, Shigella, C. difficile,* or chlamydial [LGV serotypes] infection) or noninflammatory diarrhea (giardiasis). *10.* If unexplained abdominal pain and fever persist or suggest an appendicitis-like syndrome, culture for *Yersinia enterocolitica* with cold enrichment. *11.* In immunocompromised hosts, a wide range of viral (cytomegalovirus, herpes simplex virus, coxsackievirus, rotavirus), bacterial (*Salmonella, Mycobacterium avium* complex), and parasitic (*Cryptosporidium, Isospora, Strongyloides, Entamoeba,* and *Giardia*) agents should be considered. *12.* If the fecal lactoferrin latex agglutination titer is 1:50 or higher, even if fecal leukocytes are absent, an inflammatory diarrhea should be considered, because some inflammatory colonic pathogens such as cytotoxigenic *C. difficile* or *Entamoeba histolytica* can destroy fecal leukocyte morphology. AF, *acid-fast;* EM, *electron microscopy;* EPEC, enteropathogenic *E. coli;* LT, heat-labile; ST, heat-stable; WBC, white blood cell. *(Adapted from Guerrant RL, Bobak DA. Bacterial and protozoal gastroenteritis. N Engl J Med. 1991;325:327-340, with permission.)*

with a "thumbprint" appearance has been reported on barium enema studies of patients with bloody diarrhea and *E. coli* O157 infection.[259] Although barium studies may reveal nonspecific changes in the small bowel (giardiasis) or colon (inflammatory colitis), they are less useful in diagnosing microbial diarrheas. Indeed, the barium contrast material renders a microscopic examination of stool virtually useless.

Bacterial overgrowth syndrome may result in deconjugation of bile salts that can be tested with a ^{14}C-glycocholic acid breath test. ^{14}C-carbon dioxide in the breath represents the degradation product of bacterial deconjugation of bile salts.

PREVENTION, CONTROL, AND THERAPY

The public health measures of improved water supply and sanitation facilities are most important for the control of the majority of enteric infections. Another important area for intervention lies in the quality control of commercial products such as bottled water and beverages. These may have been responsible for outbreaks of significant enteric infections such as cholera in Portugal[260] and typhoid fever in Mexico.[261]

Nonspecific host factors should be appreciated to minimize their violation. Examples include careful personal hygiene and limited, judicious use of antacids, antimotility drugs, and antimicrobial agents.

Vaccines may be used to boost specific immune processes directed against the bacteria themselves, or against adherence appendages, cytotoxins, or enterotoxins. Perhaps the most useful are the Vi polysaccharide capsule and conjugate vaccines against typhoid fever.[242] A live-attenuated cholera vaccine (CVD-103HgR) is currently available in Europe. A tetravalent rotavirus vaccine approved for use in the United States was effective but was removed from circulation after it was associated with an increase in cases of intussusception.[262-264] The most recent addition to the armamentarium is a vaccine to a combination of killed whole cell bacteria and LT-B subunit, which provides short-term protection against ETEC infection.[259,265,266] To date, there are no effective vaccines against a parasitic enteric infection, and much new work is required to improve the understanding of host defenses against enteric parasitic processes.

New possibilities for pharmacologic antagonists to microbial adherence or to toxin action are on the horizon. New types of "antibiotics" may work by blocking the formation of bacterial adherence factors, binding bacterial adherence appendages, or acting as lectin-like competitors for the host cell receptors that enable microorganisms to colonize the gastrointestinal tract. Pharmacologic reversal of the cyclic nucleotide–associated secretory process may also be possible. Such a mechanism has been suggested for bismuth subsalicylate (Pepto-Bismol). Finally, specific competitors for either the binding or the action of enterotoxins hold promise. For example, monosialoganglioside (G_{m1}) successfully binds cholera toxin or the heat-labile enterotoxin of *E. coli* in vitro and in animal experiments. Clinical trials of oligosaccharide competitors to receptors for Shiga-like toxins and *C. difficile* toxins are currently underway.

Of greatest importance in the treatment of microbial diarrhea, regardless of the cause or category, is ORT. The degree of volume depletion must first be assessed by examining the turgor of the skin and mucous membranes, by noting the amount of lacrimation, and by obtaining a history of urinary output. Postural lightheadedness with changes in pulse and blood pressure are helpful objective parameters of volume depletion. It has been documented that, despite the severest form of secretory derangement in cholera, glucose absorption and its coupled sodium and water absorption remain intact in the upper small bowel. Therefore, many patients can be completely rehydrated and maintained by a simple oral glucose-containing electrolyte solution. A controlled study of patients with cholera and other noninflammatory watery diarrheal diseases in Dacca, Bangladesh, documented the efficacy of both sucrose (table sugar) and glucose in the ORT solution.[267] Electrolyte losses in severe watery diarrhea are similar to the electrolyte composition of serum, and fluid replacement should contain approximately these concentrations of electrolytes.

A standard ORT regimen contains 3.5 g NaCl, 2.5 g NaHCO$_3$, 1.5 g KCl, and 20 g glucose per liter of boiled water. This corresponds to sodium 90, potassium 20, bicarbonate 30, chloride 80, and glucose 110 mmol/L.[268] A similar solution may be prepared with 3 level tablespoons of sugar, $\frac{3}{4}$ teaspoon salt, and $\frac{1}{2}$ teaspoon sodium bicarbonate in 1 cup of orange juice to make up 1 L (1.05 quart) in water. If there is concern about hypertonicity, particularly in children, the salt can be reduced in cases of milder diarrhea, and the solution should be given with ad libitum water. Still another alternative is 1 level teaspoon of salt and 8 level teaspoons of sugar per liter (or quart) of water, which makes approximately 86 mmol sodium and 30 g sucrose per liter, to which one could add 1 cup of orange juice or two bananas for potassium. A further improvement can be made by substituting 40 to 50 g cereal flour (rice, maize, sorghum, millet, wheat, or potato) for glucose.[269] The electrolyte contents of commonly available soft drinks are variable, although solutions of similar electrolyte composition to the ideal described here can be made in dilute solutions of bouillon or gelatin water. New developments in ORT include the use of rice powder or other glucose polymers, and the use of amino acids such as glycine, alanine, and glutamine, which enhance sodium absorption independently of glucose. Glutamine-containing ORT solutions are of particular interest because of the importance of glutamine as the major enterocyte energy source; current studies examining whether these solutions offer an advantage over standard ORT appear promising.

Specific antimicrobial therapy for infectious diarrhea is indicated in a limited number of situations. Randomized controlled trials have demonstrated a benefit of antibacterial drugs in the treatment of acute traveler's diarrhea,[270,271] in shigellosis,[272] and in campylobacteriosis.[5,273,274] Treatment is always recommended for typhoid fever and for bacteremic salmonellosis. However, antibiotic treatment of salmonellosis in uncomplicated cases, while effective in reducing the duration of illness, has been associated in some trials with an increased risk of clinical relapse and prolonged shedding.[275,276] Treatment is even more controversial for EHEC infections, as uncontrolled reports have suggested a greater risk of subsequent hemolytic-uremic syndrome in patients who received antibiotics.[277,278] One study in the mouse model found an increase in mortality and SLT phage transfer after treatment with ciprofloxacin but not fosfomycin.[279] However, a mouse infection model using levofloxacin,[280] a small randomized trial,[281] and a meta-analysis of human case reports[282] failed to demonstrate any harmful effect of antibiotic treatment. Regardless of antibiotic use, the principles of oral rehydration, infection control, and avoidance of antimotility agents in bloody or inflammatory diarrhea are nearly universally applicable.

REFERENCES

1. Kosek M, Bern C, Guerrant RL. The global burden of diarrheal disease, as estimated from studies published between 1992 and 2000. Bull World Health Organ. 2003;81:197-204.
2. Guerrant RL, Kosek M, Lima AAM, et al. Updating the DALYs for diarrheal disease. Trends Parasitol. 2002;18:191-193.
4. Yunes J. Evaluation of infant mortality and proportional infant mortality in Brazil. World Health Stats Q. 1981;34:200-219.
5. McAuliffe JF, Shields DS, de Souza MA, et al. Prolonged and recurring diarrhea in the northeast of Brazil: Examination of cases from a community-based study. J Pediatr Gastroenterol Nutr. 1986;5:902-906.
3. Guerrant RL, Van Gilder T, Steiner TS, et al. Practice guidelines for the management of infectious diarrhea. Clin Infect Dis. 2001;32:331-350.
6. Schorling JB, Wanke CA, Schorling SK, et al. A prospective study of persistent diarrhea among children in an urban Brazilian slum. Am J Epidemiol. 1990;132:144-156.
7. Bhatnager S, Dosajh U. Diarrhoeal disease morbidity in children below 5 years in urban slums of Delhi. Indian J Med Res. 1986;84:53-58.
8. Black RE, Brown KH, Becker S, et al. Longitudinal studies of infectious diseases and physical growth of children in rural Bangladesh. Am J Epidemiol. 1982;115:315-324.
9. Lima AAM, Moore SR, Barboza MS Jr, et al. Persistent diarrhea signals a critical period of increased diarrhea burdens and nutritional shortfalls: A prospective cohort study among children in northeastern Brazil. J Infect Dis. 2000;181:1643-1651.
10. Guerrant RL, Kirchhoff LV, Shields DS, et al. Prospective study of diarrheal illness in northeastern Brazil: Patterns of disease, nutritional impact, etiologies and risk factors. J Infect Dis. 1983;148:986.
11. Schorling JB, Guerrant RL. Diarrhea and catch-up growth. Lancet. 1990;335:599-600.

12. Guerrant RL, Schorling JB, McAuliffe JF, et al. Diarrhea as a cause and effect of malnutrition: Diarrhea prevents catch-up growth and malnutrition increases diarrhea frequency and duration. Am J Trop Med Hyg. 1992;47:28-35.

13. Gordon JE, Guzman MA, Ascoli W, et al. Acute diarrhoeal disease in less developed countries: 2. Patterns of epidemiological behaviour in rural Guatemalan villages. Bull World Health Organ. 1964;31:9.

14. Schorling JB, Wanke CA, Schorling SK, et al. A prospective study of persistent diarrhea among children in an urban Brazilian slum. Am J Epidemiol. 1990;132:144-156.

15. Checkley W, Gilman RH, Epstein LD, et al. Asymptomatic and symptomatic cryptosporidiosis: Their acute effect on weight gain in Peruvian children. Am J Epidemiol. 1997;145:156-163.

16. Agnew DG, Lima AAM, Newman RD, et al. Cryptosporidiosis in northeastern Brazilian children: Association with increased diarrheal morbidity. J Infect Dis. 1998;177:754-760.

17. Steiner T, Lima A, Nataro J, et al. Enteroaggregative Escherichia coli produce intestinal inflammation and growth impairment and cause interleukin-8 release from intestinal epithelial cells. J Infect Dis. 1998;177:88-96.

18. Hyams KC, Malone JD, Kapikian AZ, et al. Norwalk virus infection among Desert Storm troops. J Infect Dis. 1993;167:986-987.

19. Bartlett AV, Moore M, Gary GW, et al. Diarrheal illness among infants and toddlers in daycare centers: II. Comparison with daycare home and households. J Pediatr. 1985;107:503-509.

20. Tauxe RV, Deming MS, Blake PA. Campylobacter jejuni infections on college campuses: A national survey. Am J Public Health. 1985;75:659-660.

21. Steiner TS, Thielman NM, Guerrant RL. Protozoal agents: What are the dangers for the public water supply? Annu Rev Med. 1997;48:329-340.

22. Levine MM, Nalin DR, Rennels MB, et al. Genetic susceptibility to cholera. Ann Hum Biol. 1979;6:369-379.

23. Pier GB, Grout M, Zaidi T, et al. Salmonella typhi uses CFTR to enter intestinal epithelial cells. Nature. 1998;393:79-82.

24. Mobassaleh M, Koul O, Mishra K, et al. The developmental pattern of the regulatory enzymes involved in the synthesis and breakdown of the Shiga toxin receptor in rabbit small intestine. Gastroenterology. 1992;102:A567.

25. Chu SW, Walker WA. Bacterial toxin interaction with the developing intestine: A possible explanation for toxigenic diarrhea of infancy. Gastroenterology. 1993;104:916-925.

26. Bergman MJ, Evans DG, Sullivan JA, et al. Attachment of E. coli to human intestinal epithelial cells: A functional in vitro test for intestinal colonization factor. Trans Assoc Am Physicians. 1978;91:80.

27. Allweiss B, Dostal J, Carey KE, et al. The role of chemotaxis in the ecology of bacterial pathogens of mucosal surfaces. Nature. 1977;266:448.

28. Blackow NR, Greenberg HB. Viral gastroenteritis. N Engl J Med. 1991;325:252-264.

29. Haas CN, Rose JB. Reconciliation of microbial risk models and outbreak epidemiology: The case of the Milwaukee outbreak. Proc Am Water Works Assoc. 1994;517-523.

30. Kobayashi M, Sasaki T, Saito N, et al. Houseflies: Not simple mechanical vectors of enterohemorrhagic Escherichia coli O157:H7. Am J Trop Med Hyg 1999;61:625.

31. O'Donnell JM, Thornton L, McNamara EB, et al. Outbreak of Vero cytotoxin-producing Escherichia coli O157 in a child day care facility. Commun Dis Public Health. 2002;5:54.

32. Spika JS, Parsons JE, Nordenberg D, et al. Hemolytic uremic syndrome and diarrhea associated with Escherichia coli O157:H7 in a day care center. J Pediatr. 1986;109:287.

33. Carter AO, Borczyk AA, Carlson JA, et al. A severe outbreak of Escherichia coli O157:H7: Associated hemorrhagic colitis in a nursing home. N Engl J Med. 1987;317:1496.

34. Giannella RA, Broitman SA, Zamcheck N. Influence of gastric acidity on bacterial and parasitic enteric infections: A perspective. Ann Intern Med. 1973;78:271.

35. Nurko SS, Garcia-Aranda JA, Consuelo A, et al. Is Helicobacter pylori a significant risk factor for persistent diarrhea in Mexican children? (Abstract). Gastroenterology. 1993;104:A160.

36. Driks MR, Craven DE, Celli BR, et al. Nosocomial pneumonia in intubated patients given sucralfate as compared with antacids or histamine type 2 blockers: The role of gastric colonization. N Engl J Med. 1987;317:1376.

37. Schrager J. The chemical composition and function of gastrointestinal mucus. Gut. 1970;11:450.

38. Sprinz H. Pathogenesis of intestinal infections. Arch Pathol. 1969;87:556.

39. DuPont HL, Hornick RB. Adverse effect of Lomotil therapy in shigellosis. JAMA. 1973;226:1525.

40. Slutsker L, Ries AA, Greene KD, et al. Escherichia coli O157:H7 diarrhea in the United States: Clinical and epidemiologic features. Ann Intern Med. 1997;126:505-513.

41. Mentzing LO, Ringertz O. Salmonella infection in tourists: 2. Prophylaxis against salmonellosis. Acta Pathol Microbiol Scand. 1968;74:405.

42. Bohnhoff M, Miller CP, Martin WR. Resistance of the mouse's intestinal track to experimental Salmonella infections. J Exp Med. 1964;120:805.

43. Ryan CA, Nickels MK, Hargrett-Bean NT, et al. Massive outbreak of antimicrobial-resistant salmonellosis traced to pasteurized milk. JAMA. 1987;258:3269-3274.

44. Pavia AT, Shipman LD, Wells JG, et al. Epidemiologic evidence that prior antimicrobial exposure decreases resistance to infection by antimicrobial-sensitive Salmonella. J Infect Dis. 1990;161:255-260.

45. Cuzzolin L, Zambreri D, Donini M, et al. Influence of radiotherapy on intestinal microflora in cancer patients. J Chemother. 1992;4:176-179.

46. D'Souza AL, Rajkumar C, Cooke J, Bulpitt CJ. Probiotics in prevention of antibiotic associated diarrhoea: Meta-analysis. BMJ. 2002;324:1361.

47. Huang JS, Bousvaros A, Lee JW, et al. Efficacy of probiotic use in acute diarrhea in children: A meta-analysis. Dig Dis Sci. 2002;47:2625.

48. Rosenfeldt V, Michaelsen KF, Jakobsen M, et al. Effect of probiotic Lactobacillus strains on acute diarrhea in a cohort of nonhospitalized children attending day-care centers. Pediatr Infect Dis J. 2002;21:417.

49. Rosenfeldt V, Michaelsen KF, Jakobsen M, et al. Effect of probiotic Lactobacillus strains in young children hospitalized with acute diarrhea. Pediatr Infect Dis J. 2002;21:411.

50. Buts JP, Corthier G, Delmee M. Saccharomyces boulardii for Clostridium difficile-associated enteropathies in infants. J Pediatr Gastroenterol Nutr. 1993;16:419.

51. Kimmey MB, Elmer GW, Surawicz CM, McFarland LV. Prevention of further recurrences of Clostridium difficile colitis with Saccharomyces boulardii. Dig Dis Sci. 1990;35:897.

52. Gionchetti P, Rizzello F, Helwig U, et al. Prophylaxis of pouchitis onset with probiotic therapy: A double-blind, placebo-controlled trial. Gastroenterology. 2003;124:1202.

53. Gionchetti P, Rizzello F, Venturi A, et al. Oral bacteriotherapy as maintenance treatment in patients with chronic pouchitis: A double-blind, placebo-controlled trial. Gastroenterology. 2000;119:305.

54. Jones DE, Bevins CL. Paneth cells of the human small intestine express an antimicrobial peptide gene. J Biol Chem. 1992;267:23216.

55. Ouellette AJ. IV. Paneth cell antimicrobial peptides and the biology of the mucosal barrier. Am J Physiol. 1999;277:G257.

56. Bodey GD, Fainstein V, Guerrant RL. Infections of the gastrointestinal tract in the immunocompromised patient. Annu Rev Med. 1986;37:271-281.

57. Winkelstein JA, Marino MC, Johnston RB Jr, et al. Chronic granulomatous disease: Report on a national registry of 368 patients. Medicine (Baltimore). 2000;79:155.

58. Jiang Z, Okhuysen P, Gho D, et al. A single nucleotide polymorphism in the interleukin-8 (IL-8) promoter region is associated with diarrhea due to enteroaggregative Escherichia coli (EAEC). In: 40th Annual Meeting of the Infectious Diseases Society of America, Chicago, 2002.

59. Thielman NM, Guerrant RL. An algorithmic approach to the workup and management of HIV-related diarrhea. J Clin Outcomes Manag. 1997;4:36-47.

60. Wanke CA, Mayer H, Weber R, et al. Enteroaggregative Escherichia coli as a potential cause of diarrheal disease in adults infected with human immunodeficiency virus. J Infect Dis. 1998;178:185-190.

61. Sewankambo N, Mugerwa RD, Goodgame R, et al. Enteropathic AIDS in Uganda: An endoscopic, histological and microbiological study. AIDS. 1987;1:9-13.

62. Verdier RI, Fitzgerald DW, Johnson WD, Pape JW. Trimethoprim-sulfamethoxazole compared with ciprofloxacin for the treatment and prophylaxis of Isospora belli and Cyclospora cayetanensis infection in HIV-infected patients: A randomized, controlled trial. Ann Intern Med. 2000;132:885-888.

63. Bull DM, Tomasi TB. Deficiency of immunoglobulin A in intestinal disease. Gastroenterology. 1968;54:313.

64. Strober W, Krakauer R, Klaeveman HL, et al. Secretory component deficiency: A disorder of the IgA immune system. N Engl J Med. 1976;294:351-356.

65. Plaut AG. The IgAI proteases of pathogenic bacteria. Annu Rev Microbiol. 1983;37:603-622.

66. Zinneman HH, Kaplan AP. The association of giardiasis with reduced intestinal secretory immunoglobulin A. Am J Dig Dis. 1972;17:793-797.

67. Ament ME, Ochs HD, Davis SD. Structure and function of the gastrointestinal tract in primary immunodeficiency syndromes: A study of 39 patients. Medicine. 1973;52:227.

68. Welsh JK, May JT. Anti-infective properties of breast milk. J Pediatr. 1979;94:1.

69. McClelland DBL, McGrath J, Samson RR. Antimicrobial factors in human milk: Studies of concentration and transfer to the infant during the early stages of lactation. Acta Paediatr Scand. 1978;27(Suppl):1.

70. Cravioto A, Tello A, Villafán H, et al. Inhibition of localized adhesion of enteropathogenic Escherichia coli to HEp-2 cells by immunoglobulin and oligosaccharide fractions of human colostrum and breast milk. J Infect Dis. 1991;163:1247-1255.

71. Robins-Browne RM, Prpic JK. Effects of iron and desferrioxamine on infections with Yersinia enterocolitica. Infect Immun. 1985;47:774-779.

72. Levine MM. Escherichia coli that cause diarrhea: Enterotoxigenic enteropathogenic, enteroinvasive, enterohemorrhagic, and enteroadherent. J Infect Dis. 1987;155:377-388.

73. Schlager TA, Guerrant RL. Seven possible pathogenic mechanisms for Escherichia coli diarrhea. Infect Dis Clin North Am. 1988;2:1-18.

74. Bobak DA, Guerrant RL. New developments in enteric bacterial toxins. Adv Pharmacol. 1992;23:85-108.

75. Freer JH, Arbuthnott JP. Toxins of Staphylococcus aureus. In: Dorner F, Drews J, eds. Pharmacology of Bacterial Toxins. Oxford: Pergamon Press; 1986:581-633.

76. Turnbull PCB. Bacillus cereus toxins. In: Dorner F, Drews J, eds. Pharmacology of Bacterial Toxins. Oxford: Pergamon Press; 1986:397-448.

77. Guerrant RL, Chen LC, Sharp GWG. Intestinal adenyl-cyclase activity in canine cholera: Correlation with fluid accumulation. J Infect Dis. 1972;125:377.

78. Peterson JW, Ochoa G. Role of prostaglandins and cAMP in the secretory effects of cholera toxin. Science. 1989;245:857-859.

79. Blake PA, Weaver RE, Hollis DG. Diseases of humans (other than cholera) caused by vibrios. Annu Rev Microbiol. 1980;34:341.

80. Guerrant RL, Ganguly U, Casper AGT, et al. Effect of Escherichia coli on fluid transport across canine small bowel: Mechanism and time-course with enterotoxin and whole bacterial cell. J Clin Invest. 1973;52:1707.

81. Takeda Y, Murphy J. Bacteriophage conversion of heat-labile enterotoxin in Escherichia coli. J Bacteriol. 1978;133:172.

82. Guerrant RL, Brunton LL, Schnaitman TC, et al. Cyclic adenosine monophosphate and alteration of Chinese hamster ovary cell morphology: A rapid, sensitive in vitro assay for the enterotoxins of *Vibrio cholerae* and *Escherichia coli*. Infect Immun. 1974;10:320.

83. Donta ST, Moon HW, Whipp SC. Detection of heat-labile *Escherichia coli* enterotoxins with the use of adrenal cells in tissue culture. Science. 1974;183:334.

84. Sommerfelt H, Svennerholm AM, Kalland KH, et al. Comparative study of colony hybridizations with synthetic oligonucleotide probes and enzyme-linked immunosorbent assay for identification of *Escherichia coli*. J Clin Microbiol. 1988;26:530-534.

85. Caeiro JP, Estrada-Garcia MT, Jiang ZD, et al. Improved detection of enterotoxigenic *Escherichia coli* among patients with travelers' diarrhea, by use of the polymerase chain reaction technique. J Infect Dis. 1999;180:2053.

86. Osek J, Gallien P, Protz D, Truszczynski M. Rapid and specific differentiation of enterotoxin-producing *Escherichia coli* strains from other gram-negative enteric bacteria using multiplex PCR. Berl Munch Tierarztl Wochenschr. 2000;113:265.

87. Rappelli P, Maddau G, Mannu F, et al. Development of a set of multiplex PCR assays for the simultaneous identification of enterotoxigenic, enteropathogenic, enterohemorrhagic and enteroinvasive *Escherichia coli*. New Microbiol. 2001;24:77.

88. Gorbach SL, Banwell JG, Chatterjee BD, et al. Acute undifferentiated human diarrhea in the tropics: I. Alterations in intestinal microflora. J Clin Invest. 1971;50:881.

89. Guerrant RL, Rouse JD, Hughes JM. Turista among members of the Yale Glee Club in Latin America. Am J Trop Med Hyg. 1980;29:895.

90. Sack RB, Hirschhorn N, Brownlee I, et al. Enterotoxigenic *Escherichia coli*-associated diarrheal disease in Apache children. N Engl J Med. 1975;292:1041.

91. Guerrant RL, Moore RA, Kirschenfeld PM, et al. Role of toxigenic and invasive bacteria in acute diarrhea of childhood. N Engl J Med. 1975;293:567.

92. Guerrant RL, Dickens MD, Wenzel RP, et al. Toxigenic bacterial diarrhea: Nursery outbreak involving multiple bacterial strains. J Pediatr. 1976;89:885-891.

93. Wachsmuth K, Wells J, Shipley P. Heat-labile enterotoxin production in isolates from a shipboard outbreak of human diarrheal illness. Infect Immun. 1979;24:793-797.

94. Sandefur PD, Peterson JW. Neutralization of *Salmonella* toxin-induced elongation of Chinese hamster ovary cells by cholera antitoxin. Infect Immun. 1977;15:988-992.

95. Ruiz-Palacios GM, Torres J, Torres NI, et al. Cholera-like enterotoxin produced by *Campylobacter jejuni*: Characterization and clinical significance. Lancet. 1983;2:250-253.

96. Levine MM, Caplan ES, Waterman D, et al. Diarrhea caused by *Escherichia coli* that produce only heat-stable enterotoxins. Infect Immun. 1977;17:78-82.

97. Ryder RW, Wachsmuth IK, Buxton AE, et al. Infantile diarrhea produced by heat-stable enterotoxin *Escherichia coli*. N Engl J Med. 1976;295:849.

98. Hughes JM, Rouse JD, Barada FA, et al. Etiology of summer diarrhea among the Navajo. Am J Trop Med Hyg. 1980;29:613.

99. Hughes JM, Murad F, Chang B, et al. Role of cyclic GMP in the action of heat-stable enterotoxin of *Escherichia coli*. Nature. 1978;271:755.

100. Field M, Graf LH Jr, Laird WJ, et al. Heat stable enterotoxin of E. coli: In vitro effects on guanylate cyclase activity, cyclic GMP concentration, and ion transport in small intestine. Proc Natl Acad Sci U S A. 1978;75:2800.

101. Guerrant RL, Hughes JM, Chang B, et al. Activation of intestinal guanylate cyclase by heat-stable enterotoxin of E. coli: Studies of tissue specificity, potential receptors and intermediates. J Infect Dis. 1980;142:220.

102. Savarino S, Fasano A, Watson J, et al. Enteroaggregative *Escherichia coli* heat-stable enterotoxin 1 represents another subfamily of E. coli heat-stable toxin. Proc Natl Acad Sci U S A. 1993;90:3093.

103. Yamamoto T, Echeverria P. Detection of the enteroaggregative *Escherichia coli* heat-stable enterotoxin-1 gene sequences in enterotoxigenic E. coli strains pathogenic for humans. Infect Immun. 1996;64:1441.

104. Savarino S, Fasano A, Robertson D, Levine M. Enteroaggregative *Escherichia coli* elaborate a heat-stable enterotoxin demonstrable in an in vitro intestinal model. J Clin Invest. 1991;87:1450.

105. Savarino S, McVeigh A, Watson J, et al. Enteroaggregative *Escherichia coli* heat-stable enterotoxin is not restricted to enteroaggregative E. coli. J Infect Dis. 1996;173:1019.

106. Currie MG, Fok KF, Kato J, et al. Guanylin: An endogenous activator of intestinal guanylate cyclase. Proc Natl Acad Sci U S A. 1992;89:947-951.

107. Hamra FK, Forte LR, Eber SL, et al. Uroguanylin: Structure and activity of a second endogenous peptide that stimulates intestinal guanylate cyclase. Proc Natl Acad Sci U S A. 1993;90:10464.

108. Fasano A, Kay BA, Russell RG, et al. Enterotoxin and cytotoxin production by enteroinvasive *Escherichia coli*. Infect Immun. 1990;58:3717-3723.

109. Navarro-Garcia F, Eslava C, Villaseca JM, et al. In vitro effects of a high-molecular-weight heat-labile enterotoxin from enteroaggregative *Escherichia coli*. Infect Immun. 1998;66:3149-3154.

110. Keusch GT. Invasive bacterial diarrhea. In: LC Chen, Scrimshaw NS, eds. Diarrhea and Malnutrition. New York: Plenum Press; 1983:45.

111. Dubey RS, Sanyal SC. Characterisation and neutralisation of *Aeromonas hydrophila* enterotoxin in the rabbit ileal-loop model. J Med Microbiol. 1979;12:347.

112. Koupal LR, Deibel RH. Assay, characterization and localization of an enterotoxin produced by *Salmonella*. Infect Immun. 1975;11:14.

113. Klipstein FA, Holdeman LV, Corcino JJ. Enterotoxigenic intestinal bacteria in tropical sprue. Ann Intern Med. 1973;79:632.

114. Wasdstrom T, Aust-Kettis A, Habte D, et al. Enterotoxin-producing bacteria and parasites in stools of Ethiopian children with diarrhoeal disease. Arch Dis Child. 1976;51:865.

115. Ljungh A, Popoff M, Wadstrom T. *Aeromonas hydrophila* in acute diarrheal disease: Detection of enterotoxin and biotyping of strains. J Clin Microbiol. 1977;6:96.

116. Saidi RF, Jaeger K, Montrose MH, et al. *Bacteroides fragilis* toxin rearranges the actin cytoskeleton of HT29/C1 cells without direct proteolysis of actin or decrease in F-actin. Cell Motil Cytoskeleton. 1997;37:159-165.

117. Konowalchuk J, Speirs JI, Stavric S. Vero response to a cytotoxin of *Escherichia coli*. Infect Immun. 1977;18:775.

118. Scotland SM, Day NP, Willshaw GA, et al. Cytotoxic enteropathogenic *Escherichia coli*. Lancet. 1980;1:90.

119. Riley LW, Remia RS, Helgerson SD, et al. Outbreaks of hemorrhagic colitis associated with a rare *Escherichia coli* serotype. N Engl J Med. 1983;308:681.

120. Strockbine NA, Marques LRM, Newland JW, et al. Two toxin-converting phages from E. coli O157:H7 strains 933 encode antigenically distinct toxins with similar biologic activities. Infect Immun. 1986;53:135-140.

121. Karmali MA, Petric M, Lim C, et al. The association between idiopathic hemolytic uremic syndrome and infection by verotoxin producing E. coli. J Infect Dis. 1985;151:775-782.

122. Pai CH, Gordon R, Sims HU, et al. Sporadic cases of hemorrhagic colitis associated with E. coli O157:H7. Ann Intern Med. 1984;101:738-742.

123. Carter AO, Borczyk AA, Carlson AK, et al. A severe outbreak of E. coli O157:H7 associated hemorrhagic colitis in a nursing home. N Engl J Med. 1987;317:1496-1500.

124. Griffin PM, Tauxe RV. The epidemiology of infections caused by *Escherichia coli* O157:H7, other enterohemorrhagic E. coli, and the associated hemolytic uremic syndrome. Epidemiol Rev. 1991;13:60-98.

125. Centers for Disease Control and Prevention. Update: Multistate outbreak of *Escherichia coli* O157:H7 infections from hamburgers: Western United States, 1992-1993. MMWR Morb Mortal Wkly Rep. 1993;42:258-263.

126. Watanabe H, Wada A, Inagaki Y, et al. Outbreaks of enterohaemorrhagic *Escherichia coli* O157:H7 infection by two different genotype strains in Japan. Lancet. 1996;348:831-832.

127. Watanabe H, Guerrant RL. Summary: Nagasaki enterohemorrhagic *Escherichia coli* meeting and workshop. J Infect Dis. 1997;176:247-249.

128. O'Brien AD, Holmes RK. Shiga and Shiga-like toxins. Microbiol Rev. 1987;51:206-220.

129. Samuel JE, Perera LP, Ward S, et al. Comparison of the glycolipid receptor specificities of Shiga-like toxin type II and Shiga-like toxin type II variants. Infect Immun. 1990;58:611-618.

130. McDonel JL, Duncan CL. Histopathological effect of *Clostridium perfringens* enterotoxin in the rabbit ileum. Infect Immun. 1975;12:1214.

131. Bartholomew BA, Stringer MF. Observations on the purification of *Clostridium perfringens* type A enterotoxin and the production of a specific antiserum. FEMS Microbiol Lett. 1983;18:43-48.

132. Horiguchi Y, Akai T, Sakaguchi G. Isolation and function of a *Clostridium perfringens* enterotoxin fragment. Infect Immun. 1987;55:2912-2915.

133. Borriello SP, Barclay F, Welch AR, et al. Epidemiology of diarrhea caused by enterotoxigenic *Clostridium perfringens*. J Med Microbiol. 1985;20:363-372.

134. Lawrence GW, Lehmann D, Anian G, et al. Impact of active immunization against enteritis necroticans in Papua New Guinea. Lancet. 1990;336:1165-1167.

135. Sanyal SC, Sen PC. Human volunteer study on the pathogenicity of *Vibrio parahaemolyticus*. In: International Symposium on *Vibrio parahaemolyticus*. Tokyo, Japan, Sept. 17-18, 1973. Tokyo: Saikon; 227-230.

136. Shirai H, Ito H, Hirayama T, et al. Molecular epidemiologic evidence of association of thermostable direct hemolysin (TDH) and TDH-related hemolysin of *Vibrio parahaemolyticus*. Infect Immun. 1990;58:3568-3573.

137. Huntley JS, Hall AC. Nature of the cation leak induced in erythrocyte membranes by Kanagawa hemolysin of *Vibrio parahaemolyticus*. Biochem Biophys Acta. 1996;1281:220-226.

138. Raimondi F, Kao JP, Kaper JB, et al. Calcium-dependent intestinal chloride secretion by *Vibrio parahaemolyticus* thermostable direct hemolysin in a rabbit model. Gastroenterology. 1995;109:381-386.

139. Calia FM, Johnson DE. Bacteremia in suckling rabbits after oral challenge with *Vibrio parahaemolyticus*. Infect Immun. 1975;11:1222.

140. Bolen JL, Zamiska SA, Grennough WB III. Clinical features in enteritis due to *Vibrio parahaemolyticus*. Am J Med. 1974;57:638.

141. Barker WH, MacKowiak PA, Fishbein M, et al. *Vibrio parahaemolyticus* gastroenteritis outbreak in Covington, Louisiana, in August 1972. Am J Epidemiol. 1974;100:316.

142. Wu S, Lim KC, Huang J, et al. *Bacteroides fragilis* enterotoxin cleaves the zonula adherens protein, E-cadherin. Proc Natl Acad Sci U S A. 1998;95:14979.

143. Just I, Wilm M, Selzer J, et al. The enterotoxin from *Clostridium difficile* (ToxA) monoglucosylates the Rho proteins. J Biol Chem. 1995;270:13932-13936.

144. Just I, Wilm M, Selzer J, et al. Glucosylation of Rho proteins by *Clostridium difficile* toxin B. Nature. 1995;375:500-503.

145. Fasano A, Uzzau S, Fiore C, et al. The enterotoxic effect of zonula occludens toxin on rabbit small intestine involves the paracellular pathway. Gastroenterology. 1997;112:839-846.

146. Villaseca JM, Navarro-Garcia F, Mendoza-Hernandez G, et al. Pet toxin from enteroaggregative *Escherichia coli* produces cellular damage associated with fodrin disruption. Infect Immun. 2000;68:5920.

147. Kelly CP, Becker S, Linevsky JK, et al. Neutrophil recruitment in *Clostridium difficile* toxin A enteritis in the rabbit. J Clin Invest. 1994;93:1257-1265.

148. Pothoulakis C, Casagiuolo I, LaMont JT, et al. CP-96,345, a substance P antagonist, inhibits rat intestinal responses to *Clostridium difficile* toxin A but not cholera toxin. Proc Natl Acad Sci U S A. 1994;91:947-951.

149. Fang GD, Lima AAM, Thielman NM, et al. Role of phospholipase A2 in the histologic, epithelial, and secretory responses to *Clostridium difficile* toxin A. Biomed J. 1994;1:71-76.

150. Fonteles M, Fang G, Thielman NM, et al. Role of platelet activating factor in the inflammatory and secretory effects of *Clostridium difficile* toxin A. J Lipid Mediat Cell Signal. 1995;11:133-143.

151. Pothoulakis C, Karmeli F, Kelly CP, et al. Ketotifen inhibits *Clostridium difficile* toxin A-induced enteritis in rat ileum. Gastroenterology. 1993;105:701-707.

152. Kapral FA, O'Brien AD, Ruff PD, et al. Inhibition of water absorption in the intestine by *Staphylococcus aureus* delta toxin. Infect Immun. 1976;13:140.

153. Ashkenazi A, Cleary KR, Pickering LK, et al. The association of Shiga toxin and other cytotoxins with the neurologic manifestations of shigellosis. J Infect Dis. 1990;161:961-965.

154. Bouzari S, Varghese A. Cytolethal distending toxin (CLDT) production by enteropathogenic *Escherichia coli* (EPEC). FEMS Microbiol Lett. 1990;59:193.

155. Johnson WM, Lior H. A new heat-labile cytolethal distending toxin (CLDT) produced by *Campylobacter* spp. Microb Pathog. 1988;4:115.

156. Johnson WM, Lior H. A new heat-labile cytolethal distending toxin (CLDT) produced by *Escherichia coli* isolates from clinical material. Microb Pathog. 1988;4:103.

157. Ferguson MR, Xu XJ, Houston CW, et al. Hyperproduction, purification, and mechanism of action of the cytotoxic enterotoxin produced by *Aeromonas hydrophila*. Infect Immun 1997;65:4299.

158. Klapproth JM, Scaletsky IC, McNamara BP, et al. A large toxin from pathogenic *Escherichia coli* strains that inhibits lymphocyte activation. Infect Immun. 2000;68:2148.

159. Perez-Perez GL, Cohn DL, Guerrant RL, et al. Clinical and immunologic significance of cholera-like toxin and cytotoxin production by *Campylobacter* species in patients with acute inflammatory diarrhea in the USA. J Infect Dis. 1989;160:460-467.

160. Leunk RD, Johnson PT, David BC, et al. Cytotoxic activity in broth-culture filtrates of *Campylobacter pylori*. J Med Microbiol. 1988;26:93-99.

161. Leunk RD, Ferguson MA, Morgan DR, et al. Antibody to cytotoxin in infection by *Helicobacter pylori*. J Clin Microbiol. 1990;28:1181-1184.

162. Guerrant RL, Lingwood CA. Glycoconjugate receptors for adhesins and toxins. In: Marshall BJ, McCallum RW, Guerrant RL, eds. *Helicobacter pylori* in Peptic Ulceration and Gastritis. Boston: Blackwell Scientific; 1991:66-80.

163. Salit IE, Gostchlich EC. Type I *Escherichia coli* pili: Characterization of binding to monkey kidney cells. J Exp Med. 1977;146:1182.

164. Silverblatt FJ. Host parasitic in the rat renal pelvis: A possible role for pili in the pathogenesis of pyelonephritis. J Exp Med. 1974;140:1696.

165. Eden CS, Hausson S, Jodal U, et al. Host-parasite interaction in the urinary tract. J Infect Dis. 1988;157:421-426.

166. Evans DG, Satterwhite TK, Evans DJ Jr, et al. Differences in serological responses and excretion patterns of volunteers challenged with enterotoxigenic *Escherichia coli* with and without the colonization factor antigen. Infect Immun. 1978;19:883.

167. Bergman MJ, Updike WS, Wood SJ, et al. Attachment factors among enterotoxigenic *Escherichia coli* from patients with acute diarrhea from diverse geographic areas. Infect Immun. 1981;32:881.

168. Thomas LV, Cravioto A, Scotland SM, et al. New fimbrial antigenic type E8775 that may represent a colonization factor in enterotoxigenic *E. coli* in humans. Infect Immun. 1982;35:1119-1124.

169. Honda T, Arita M, Miwatani T: Characterization of new hydrophobic pili of human enterotoxigenic *Escherichia coli*: A possible new colonization factor. Infect Immun. 1984;43:959-965.

170. Tacket CO, Maneval DR, Levine MM. Purification, morphology, and genetics of a new fimbrial putative colonization factor of enterotoxigenic *Escherichia coli* O159:H4. Infect Immun. 1987;55:1063-1069.

171. Williams PH, Sedgwick MI, Evans N, et al. Adherence of an enteropathogenic strain of *Escherichia coli* is mediated by a colicinogenic conjugative plasmid. Infect Immun. 1978;22:393.

172. Karch H, Heesemann J, Laufs R, et al. A plasmid of enterohemorrhagic *Escherichia coli* O157:H7 is required for expression of a new fimbrial antigen and for adhesion to epithelial cells. Infect Immun. 1987;55:455-461.

173. Francis CL, Jerse AE, Kaper JB, et al. Characterization of interactions of enteropathogenic *Escherichia coli* O127:H6 with mammalian cells in vitro. J Infect Dis. 1991;164:693-703.

174. Vuopio-Varkila J, Schoolnik GK. Localized adherence by enteropathogenic *Escherichia coli* is an inducible phenotype associated with the expression of new outer membrane proteins. J Exp Med. 1991;174:1167-1177.

175. Girón JA, Ho ASY, Schoolnik GK. An inducible bundle-forming pilus of enteropathogenic *Escherichia coli*. Science. 1992;254:710.

176. Kenny B, DeVinney R, Stein M, et al. Enteropathogenic *E. coli* (EPEC) transfers its receptor for intimate adherence into mammalian cells. Cell. 1997;91:511-520.

177. Rosenshine I, Ruschkowski S, Stein M, et al. A pathogenic bacterium triggers epithelial signals to form a functional bacterial receptor that mediates actin pseudopod formation. EMBO J. 1996;15:2613-2624.

178. Goosney DL, DeVinney R, Finlay BB. Recruitment of cytoskeletal and signaling proteins to enteropathogenic and enterohemorrhagic *Escherichia coli* pedestals. Infect Immun. 2001;69:3315.

179. Gruenheid S, DeVinney R, Bladt F, et al. Enteropathogenic *E. coli* Tir binds Nck to initiate actin pedestal formation in host cells. Nat Cell Biol. 2001;3:856.

180. Deng W, Li Y, Vallance BA, Finlay BB. Locus of enterocyte effacement from *Citrobacter rodentium*: Sequence analysis and evidence for horizontal transfer among attaching and effacing pathogens. Infect Immun. 2001;69:6323.

181. Deng W, Vallance BA, Li Y, et al. *Citrobacter rodentium* translocated intimin receptor (Tir) is an essential virulence factor needed for actin condensation, intestinal colonization and colonic hyperplasia in mice. Mol Microbiol. 2003;48:95.

182. De Rycke J, Comtet E, Chalareng C, et al. Enteropathogenic *Escherichia coli* O103 from rabbit elicits actin stress fibers and focal adhesions in HeLa epithelial cells, cytopathic effects that are linked to an analog of the locus of enterocyte effacement. Infect Immun. 1997;65:2555.

183. DeVinney R, Puente JL, Gauthier A, et al. Enterohaemorrhagic and enteropathogenic *Escherichia coli* use a different Tir-based mechanism for pedestal formation. Mol Microbiol. 2001;41:1445.

184. DeVinney R, Stein M, Reinscheid D, et al. Enterohemorrhagic *Escherichia coli* O157:H7 produces Tir, which is translocated to the host cell membrane but is not tyrosine phosphorylated. Infect Immun. 1999;67:2389.

185. Yamamoto T. Distinct attaching and effacing phenomena observed with enterohemorrhagic *Escherichia coli* (EHEC) and enteropathogenic *E. coli* (EPEC). 33rd U.S.-Japan Cholera and Related Diarrheal Diseases Joint Panel Meeting. The United States-Japan Cooperative Medical Sciences Program: Clearwater Beach, Fla, Dec. 23-25, 1997:126-130.

186. Nataro JP, Kaper JB, Robins-Browne R, et al. Patterns of adherence of diarrheagenic *Escherichia coli* to HEp-2 cells. Pediatr Infect Dis J. 1987;6:829-831.

187. Mathewson JJ, Johnson PC, Dupont HL, et al. Pathogenicity of enteroadherent *Escherichia coli* in adult volunteers. J Infect Dis. 1986;154:524-527.

188. Scaletsky ICA, Silva MLM, Toledo MRF, et al. Correlation between adherence to HeLa cells and serogroups, serotypes, and bioserotypes of *Escherichia coli*. Infect Immun. 1985;49:528-532.

189. Mathewson JJ, Cravioto A. HEp-2 cell adherence as an assay for virulence among diarrheagenic *Escherichia coli*. J Infect Dis. 1989;159:1057-1060.

190. Baudry B, Savarino SJ, Vial P, et al. A sensitive and specific DNA probe to identify enteroaggregative *Escherichia coli*, a recently discovered diarrheal pathogen. J Infect Dis. 1990;161:1249-1251.

191. Bhan MK, Raj P, Levine MM, et al. Enteroaggregative *Escherichia coli* associated with persistent diarrhea in a cohort of rural children in India. J Infect Dis. 1989;159:1061-1064.

192. Bhan MK, Khoshoo V, Sommerfelt H, et al. Enteroaggregative *Escherichia coli* and *Salmonella* associated with nondysenteric persistent diarrhea. Pediatr Infect Dis J. 1989;8:499-502.

193. Wanke CA, Schorling JB, Barrett LJ, et al. Adherence traits of *Escherichia coli*, alone and in association with other stool pathogens: Potential role in pathogenesis of persistent diarrhea in an urban Brazilian slum. Pediatr J Infect Dis. 1991;10:746-751.

194. Itoh Y, Nagano I, Kunishima M, et al. Laboratory investigation of enteroaggregative *Escherichia coli* O untypable:H10 associated with a massive outbreak of gastrointestinal illness. J Clin Microbiol. 1997;35:2546-2550.

195. Adachi J, Glandt M, Jiang Z-D, et al. Enteroaggregative *Escherichia coli* as a major etiologic agent in travelers' diarrhea in three regions of the world. In: 37th Annual Meeting of the Infectious Diseases Society of America, Philadelphia, 1999.

196. Adachi JA, Jiang ZD, Mathewson JJ, et al. Enteroaggregative *Escherichia coli* as a major etiologic agent in traveler's diarrhea in 3 regions of the world. Clin Infect Dis. 2001;32:1706-1709.

197. Greenberg DE, Jiang ZD, Steffen R, et al. Markers of inflammation in bacterial diarrhea among travelers, with a focus on enteroaggregative *Escherichia coli* pathogenicity. J Infect Dis. 2002;185:944.

198. Sheikh J, Czeczulin JR, Harrington S, et al. A novel dispersin protein in enteroaggregative *Escherichia coli*. J Clin Invest. 2002;110:1329.

199. Henderson IR, Czeczulin J, Eslava C, et al. Characterization of pic, a secreted protease of *Shigella flexneri* and enteroaggregative *Escherichia coli*. Infect Immun. 1999;67:5587.

200. Bilge SS, Clausen CR, Lau W, et al. Molecular characterization of a fimbrial adhesin, F1845, mediating diffuse adherence of diarrhea-associated *Escherichia coli* to HEp-2 cells. J Bacteriol. 1989;171:4281-4289.

201. Benz I, Schmidt MA. Isolation and serologic characterization of AIDA-I, the adhesin mediating the diffuse adherence phenotype of the diarrhea-associated *Escherichia coli* strain 2787 (O126:H27). Infect Immun. 1992;60:13-18.

202. Girón JA, Fry J, Frankel G, et al. Diffuse-adhering *Escherichia coli* (DAEC) as a putative cause of diarrhea in Mayan children in Mexico. J Infect Dis. 1991;163:507-513.

203. Baqui AH, Sack RB, Black RE, et al. Enteropathogens associated with acute and persistent diarrhea in Bangladeshi children <5 years of age. J Infect Dis. 1992;166:792-796.

204. Bernet-Camard M, Coconnier M, Hudualt S, Servin A. Pathogenicity of the diffusely adhering strain *Escherichia coli* C1845/F1845 adhesin-decay accelerating factor interaction, brush border microvillus injury, and actin disassembly in cultured human intestinal epithelial cells. Infect Immun. 1996;64:1918.

205. Wanke C, Guerrant RL. Small-bowel colonization alone is a cause of diarrhea. Infect Immun. 1987;55:1924-1926.

206. Schlager TA, Wanke CA, Guerrant RL. Net fluid secretion and impaired villous function induced by colonization of the small intestine by nontoxigenic colonizing *Escherichia coli*. Infect Immun. 1990;58:1337-1343.

207. Tacket CO, Losonsky G, Nataro JP, et al. Safety, immunogenicity and transmissibility of live oral cholera vaccine candidate CVD110, a ΔCTXA ΔZOT Δace derivative of El Tor Ogawa *Vibrio cholerae*. J Infect Dis. 1993;168:1536-1540.

208. Silva TM, Schleupner MA, Tacket CO, et al. New evidence for an inflammatory component in diarrhea caused by selected new, live attenuated cholera vaccines and by El Tor and O139 *Vibrio cholerae*. Infect Immun. 1996;64:2362-2364.

209. Sereny B. Experimental *Shigella* keratoconjunctivitis: A preliminary report. Acta Microbiol Acad Sci Hung. 1955;2:293.

210. Gemski P Jr, Sheahan DG, Washington O, et al. Virulence of *Shigella flexneri* hybrids expressing *Escherichia coli* somatic antigens. Infect Immun. 1972;6:104.

211. Trabulsi LR, Fernandes MFR. *Escherichia coli* serogroup O115 isolated from patients with enteritis: Biochemical characteristics and experimental pathogenicity. Rev Inst Med Trop Sao Paulo. 1969;11:358.

212. DuPont HL, Formal SB, Hornick RB, et al. Pathogenesis of *Escherichia coli* diarrhea. N Engl J Med. 1971;285:1.

213. Charney AN, Gots RE, Formal SB, et al. Activation of intestinal mucosal adenylate cyclase by *Shigella dysenteriae* I enterotoxin. Gastroenterology. 1976;70:1085.

214. Sansonetti PJ, Kopecko DJ, Formal SB. Involvement of a plasmid in the invasive ability of *Shigella flexneri*. Infect Immun. 1982;35:852.

215. Harris JR, Wachsmuth IK, Davis BR, et al. High-molecular-weight plasmid correlates with *Escherichia coli* invasiveness. Infect Immun. 1982;37:1295.

216. Sansonetti PJ, Hale TL, Oaks EV. Genetics of virulence in enteroinvasive *Escherichia coli*. In: Microbiology: New Concepts in the Pathogenesis of *Escherichia coli* Diarrhea. Washington, DC: American Society for Microbiology; 1985:74-77.

217. Isberg RR. Discrimination between intracellular uptake and surface adhesion of bacterial pathogens. Science. 1991;252:934-938.

218. Maurelli AT, Sansonetti P. Identification of a chromosomal gene controlling temperature-regulated expression of *Shigella* virulence. Proc Natl Acad Sci U S A. 1988;85:2820-2824.

219. Bernardini ML, Mounier J, D'Hauteville H, et al. Identification of *icsA*, a plasmid locus that governs intra- and intercellular spread through interaction with F-actin. Proc Natl Acad Sci U S A. 1989;86:3867-3871.

220. Finlay BB, Heffron F, Falkow S. Epithelial cell surfaces induce *Salmonella* proteins required for bacterial adherence and invasion. Science. 1989;243:940-943.

221. Pfeifer CG, Marcus SL, Steele-Mortimer O, et al. *Salmonella typhimurium* virulence genes are induced upon bacterial invasion into phagocytic and nonphagocytic cells. Infect Immun. 1999;67:5690.

222. Hensel M, Shea JE, Waterman SR, et al. Genes encoding putative effector proteins of the type III secretion system of *Salmonella* pathogenicity island 2 are required for bacterial virulence and proliferation in macrophages. Mol Microbiol. 1998;30:163.

223. Steele-Mortimer O, Brumell JH, Knodler LA, et al. The invasion-associated type III secretion system of *Salmonella enterica* serovar *Typhimurium* is necessary for intracellular proliferation and vacuole biogenesis in epithelial cells. Cell Microbiol. 2002;4:43.

224. Ravdin JI, Guerrant RL. Role of adherence in cytopathogenic mechanisms of *Entamoeba histolytica*. J Clin Invest. 1981;68:1305-1313.

225. Guerrant RL, Brush JE, Ravdin JI, et al. Interaction between *Entamoeba histolytica* and human polymorphonuclear leukocytes. J Infect Dis. 1981;143:83-93.

226. Petri WA Jr, Chapman MD, Snodgrass T, et al. Subunit structure of the galactose and N-acetyl-D-galactosamine-inhibitable adherence lectin of *Entamoeba histolytica*. J Biol Chem. 1989;264:3007-3012.

227. Jung HC, Eckmann L, Yang SK, et al. A distinct array of proinflammatory cytokines is expressed in human colon epithelial cells in response to bacterial invasion. J Clin Invest. 1995;95:55-65.

228. Aihara M, Tsuchimoto D, Takizawa H, et al. Mechanisms involved in *Helicobacter pylori*-induced interleukin-8 production by a gastric cancer cell line, MKN45. Infect Immun. 1997;65:3218-3224.

229. Mahida YR, Makh S, Hyde S, et al. Effect of *Clostridium difficile* toxin A on human intestinal epithelial cells: Induction of interleukin-8 production and apoptosis after cell detachment. Gut. 1996;38:337-347.

230. Madara JL, Patapoff TW, Gillece-Castro B, et al. 5′-Adenosine monophosphate is the neutrophil-derived paracrine factor that elicits chloride secretion from T84 intestinal epithelial cells. J Clin Invest. 1993;91:2320-2325.

231. Gewirtz AT, Navas TA, Lyons S, et al. Cutting edge: Bacterial flagellin activates basolaterally expressed Tir5 to induce epithelial proinflammatory gene expression. J Immunol. 2001;167:1882.

232. Gewirtz AT, Simon P Jr, Schmitt CK, et al. *Salmonella typhimurium* translocates flagellin across intestinal epithelia, inducing a proinflammatory response. J Clin Invest. 2001;107:99.

233. Guarino A, Canani RB, Pozio E, et al. Enterotoxic effect of stool supernatant of *Cryptosporidium*-infected calves on human jejunum. Gastroenterology. 1994;106:28.

234. Guentzel MN, Berry LJ. Motility as a virulence factor for *Vibrio cholerae*. Infect Immun. 1975;2:890-897.

235. Freter R, Allweiss B, O'Brien PC, et al. Role of chemotaxis in the association of motile bacteria with intestinal mucosa: In vitro studies. Infect Immun. 1981;34:241-249.

236. Hornick RB, Greisman SE, Woodward TE, et al. Typhoid fever: Pathogenesis and immunologic control. N Engl J Med. 1970;283:686.

237. Schneider DR, Parker CD. Isolation and characterization of protease-deficient mutants of *Vibrio cholerae*. J Infect Dis. 1978;138:143-151.

238. Schneider DR, Parker CD. Purification and characterization of the mucinase of *Vibrio cholerae*. J Infect Dis. 1982;145:474-482.

239. Robbins PW, Uchida T. Determinants of specificity in *Salmonella*: Changes in antigenic structure mediated by bacteriophage. Immunochemistry. 1962;21:702.

240. Germanier R, Furer E. Isolation and characterization of Gal E mutant Ty 21a of *Salmonella typhi*: A candidate strain for a live, oral typhoid vaccine. J Infect Dis. 1975;131:533.

241. Levine MM, Kaper JB, Black RE, et al. New knowledge on pathogenesis of bacterial enteric infections as applied to vaccine development. Microbiol Rev. 1983;47:510-550.

242. Acharya IL, Lowe CU, Thapa R, et al. Prevention of typhoid fever in Nepal with the Vi capsular polysaccharide of *Salmonella typhi*. N Engl J Med. 1987;317:1102-1104.

243. Klugman KP, Koornhof H, Schneerson R, et al. Protective activity of Vi capsular polysaccharide vaccine against typhoid fever. Lancet. 1987;2:1165-1167.

244. Perez-Perez GI, Hopkins JA, Blaser MJ. Antigenic heterogeneity of lipopolysaccharides from *Campylobacter jejuni* and *Campylobacter fetus*. Infect Immun. 1985;48:528-533.

245. Field M. Cholera toxin, adenylate cyclase, and the process of active secretion in the small intestine: The pathogenesis of diarrhea in cholera. In: Andreoli TE, Hoffman JF, Fauestil DD, eds. Physiology of Membrane Disorder. New York: Plenum Press; 1978.

246. Davidson GP, Barnes GL. Structural and functional abnormalities of the small intestine in infants and young children with rotavirus enteritis. Acta Paediatr Scand. 1979;68:181.

247. Agus SG, Dolin R, Wyatt RG, et al. Acute infectious nonbacterial gastroenteritis: Intestinal histopathology, histologic and enzymatic alterations during illness produced by Norwalk agent in man. Ann Intern Med. 1973;79:18.

248. Levitan R, Ingelfinger FJ. Effect of D-aldosterone on salt and water absorption from the intact human colon. J Clin Invest. 1965;44:801.

249. Guerrant RL, Chen LC, Rohde JE. Effect of spironolactone on stool electrolyte losses during human cholera. Gut. 1972;13:197.

250. Guerrant RL, Carpenter CC. Diarrheagenic effect of volume expansion: Intestinal fluid secretion without mucosal adenyl cyclase stimulation. Johns Hopkins Med J. 1975;136:209-211.

251. Harris JC, DuPont HL, Hornick RB. Fecal leukocytes in diarrheal illness. Ann Intern Med. 1972;76:697.

252. Guerrant RL, Shields DS, Thorson SM, et al. Evaluation and diagnosis of acute infectious diarrhea. Am J Med. 1985;78:91-98.

253. Guerrant RL, Brush JE, Ravdin JI, et al. The interaction between *Entamoeba histolytica* and human polymorphonuclear leukocytes. J Infect Dis. 1981;143:83.

254. Seydel KB, Zhang T, Champion AB, et al. *Cryptosporidium parvum* infection of human intestinal xenografts in SCID mice induces production of human tumor necrosis factor and interleukin-8. Infect Immun. 1998;66:2379-2382.

255. Iida T, Naka A, Suthienkul O, et al. Measurement of fecal lactoferrin for rapid diagnosis of enterohemorrhagic *Escherichia coli* infection. Clin Infect Dis. 1997;25:167.

256. Thielman NM, Guerrant RL. Clinical practice: Acute infectious diarrhea. N Engl J Med. 2004;350:38-47.

257. Korzeniowski OM, Basada FA, Rouse JD, et al. Value of examination for fecal leukocytes in the early diagnosis of shigellosis. Am J Trop Med Hyg. 1979;28:1031-1035.

258. Guerrant RL, Araujo V, Soares E, et al. Measurement of fecal lactoferrin as a marker of fecal leukocytes. J Clin Microbiol. 1992;30:1238-1242.

259. Blake PA, Rosenberg ML, Florencia J, et al. Cholera in Portugal, 1974. Am J Epidemiol. 1977;105:344.

260. Lee JA, Kean BH. International Conference on the Diarrhea of Travelers. New Directions in Research: A summary. J Infect Dis. 1978;137:360.

261. Perez-Schael I, Guntinas MJ, Perez M, et al. Efficacy of the rhesus rotavirus-based quadrivalent vaccine in infants and young children in Venezuela. N Engl J Med. 1997;337:1181-1187.

262. Intussusception among recipients of rotavirus vaccine—United States, 1998-1999. MMWR Morb Mortal Wkly Rep. 1999;48:577.

263. Kramarz P, France EK, Destefano F, et al. Population-based study of rotavirus vaccination and intussusception. Pediatr Infect Dis J. 2001;20:410.

264. Cohen D, Orr N, Haim M, et al. Safety and immunogenicity of two different lots of the oral, killed enterotoxigenic *Escherichia coli*-cholera toxin B subunit vaccine in Israeli young adults. Infect Immun. 2000;68:4492.

265. Scerpella EG, Sanchez JL, Mathewson IJ, et al. Safety, immunogenicity, and protective efficacy of the whole-cell/recombinant B subunit (WC/rBS) oral cholera vaccine against travelers' diarrhea. J Travel Med. 1995;2:22.

266. Savarino SJ, Hall ER, Bassily S, et al. Oral, inactivated, whole cell enterotoxigenic *Escherichia coli* plus cholera toxin B subunit vaccine: Results of the initial evaluation in children. PRIDE Study Group. J Infect Dis. 1999;179:107.

267. Palmer DL, Koster FT, Islam AF, et al. Comparison of sucrose and glucose in oral electrolyte treatment of cholera and other severe diarrheas. N Engl J Med. 1977;297:1107-1110.

268. Oral glucose/electrolyte therapy for acute diarrhea (Editorial). Lancet. 1975;1:79.

269. Molla AM, Molla A, Nath SK, et al. Food-based oral rehydration salt solutions for acute childhood diarrhoea. Lancet. 1989;2:429-431.

270. DuPont HL, Reves RR, Galindo E, et al. Treatment of travelers' diarrhea with trimethoprim/sulfamethoxazole and with trimethoprim alone. N Engl J Med. 1982;307:841.

271. Adachi JA, Ostrosky-Zeichner L, DuPont HL, Ericsson CD. Empirical antimicrobial therapy for traveler's diarrhea. Clin Infect Dis. 2000;31:1079.

272. Mabadeje AF. A controlled clinical trial of trimethoprim-sulphamethoxazole in shigella dysentery. J Trop Med Hyg. 1974;77:50.

273. Anders BJ, Lauer BA, Paisley JW, Reller LB. Double-blind placebo controlled trial of erythromycin for treatment of *Campylobacter* enteritis. Lancet. 1982;1:131.

274. Salazar-Lindo E, Sack RB, Chea-Woo E, et al. Early treatment with erythromycin of *Campylobacter jejuni*-associated dysentery in children. J Pediatr. 1986;109:355.

275. Sanchez C, Garcia-Restoy E, Garau J, et al. Ciprofloxacin and trimethoprim-sulfamethoxazole versus placebo in acute uncomplicated *Salmonella* enteritis: A double-blind trial. J Infect Dis. 1993;168:1304.

276. Nelson JD, Kusmiesz H, Jackson LH, Woodman E. Treatment of *Salmonella* gastroenteritis with ampicillin, amoxicillin, or placebo. Pediatrics. 1980;65:1125.

277. Wong CS, Jelacic S, Habeeb RL, et al. The risk of the hemolytic-uremic syndrome after antibiotic treatment of *Escherichia coli* O157:H7 infections. N Engl J Med. 2000;342:1930.

278. Pavia AT, Nichols CR, Green DP, et al. Hemolytic-uremic syndrome during an outbreak of *Escherichia coli* O157:H7 infections in institutions for mentally retarded persons: Clinical and epidemiologic observations. J Pediatr. 1990;116:544.

279. Zhang X, McDaniel AD, Wolf LE, et al. Quinolone antibiotics induce Shiga toxin-encoding bacteriophages, toxin production, and death in mice. J Infect Dis. 2000;181:664.

280. Isogai E, Isogai H, Hayashi S, et al. Effect of antibiotics, levofloxacin and fosfomycin, on a mouse model with *Escherichia coli* O157 infection. Microbiol Immunol. 2000;44:89.

281. Proulx F, Turgeon JP, Delage G, et al. Randomized, controlled trial of antibiotic therapy for *Escherichia coli* O157:H7 enteritis. J Pediatr. 1992;121:299.

282. Safdar N, Said A, Gangnon RE, Maki DG. Risk of hemolytic uremic syndrome after antibiotic treatment of *Escherichia coli* O157:H7 enteritis: A meta-analysis. JAMA. 2002;288:996.

CHAPTER **90**

Esophagitis

PAUL S. GRAMAN

Esophagitis, or inflammation of the esophagus, is most often caused by noninfectious conditions, of which gastroesophageal reflux disease is the most common. Esophageal infection occurs predominantly in patients with impaired immunity resulting from cancer chemotherapy, transplantation, or human immunodeficiency virus (HIV) infection and occasionally in persons who are otherwise healthy. *Candida albicans*, cytomegalovirus (CMV), and herpes simplex virus (HSV) are the leading etiologic agents of esophageal infection. Among patients with HIV infection, aphthous ulceration of the esophagus is a well-recognized entity. Acute HIV infection may also be a direct cause of esophageal ulceration.[1] A variety of other fungal, viral, mycobacterial, and parasitic agents have been shown to cause esophagitis on rare occasion. Pill-induced esophagitis resulting from local mucosal injury has been attributed to almost 100 different drugs, particularly if they are ingested without water or in the supine position; antibiotics and antiviral agents are implicated in 50% of cases.[2,3] Infectious and noninfectious causes of esophagitis are listed in Table 90-1. Multiple concomitant causes of esophagitis are not uncommon in patients who are significantly immunosuppressed or critically ill.[11]

TABLE 90-1 **Etiology of Esophagitis**

Common	Rare
Infectious	
Candidiasis	*Mycobacterium tuberculosis*[4-8]
Cytomegalovirus	*Mycobacterium avium* complex[9,10]
Herpes simplex virus	*Cryptococcus neoformans*[11,12]
HIV infection, acute	*Histoplasma capsulatum*[13]
	Actinomyces[14,15]
	Saccharomyces cerevisiae[16]
	Cryptosporidium[17]
	Pneumocystis jirovecii[18]
	Varicella-zoster virus[19-21]
	Epstein-Barr virus[22]
Noninfectious	
Gastroesophageal reflux	Ingestion of corrosives (e.g., lye)
Mucositis from cancer chemotherapy	Local mucositis from tablets or capsules[2,3] (e.g., doxycycline, zidovudine,[23] ddC[24])
Mucositis from radiation therapy	
Aphthous ulcers	

ddC, dideoxycytidine (zalcitabine); HIV, human immunodeficiency virus.

CLINICAL MANIFESTATIONS

Most patients with esophagitis present with odynophagia (pain on swallowing) or dysphagia, described as difficulty swallowing or a sense of obstruction—either substernal, epigastric, or in the throat. Liquids are often better tolerated than solids such as meats, which may worsen both odynophagia and dysphagia. Pain may be exacerbated by the ingestion of acidic liquids and by eructation. Ulcerative esophagitis is characterized primarily by odynophagia, which can be severe, at times to the point of limiting oral intake and resulting in weight loss and dehydration. Spontaneous substernal pain or burning may also occur intermittently, unrelated to swallowing. Gastrointestinal bleeding is rarely the initial manifestation of esophagitis, but it does occur.[25] Among patients evaluated for nausea and vomiting or abdominal pain, endoscopically proven esophagitis may be present in the absence of specific esophageal symptoms. In one review, odynophagia or dysphagia was absent in 21% to 41% of patients with documented esophagitis caused by *Candida*, HSV, CMV, or, rarely, *Mycobacterium tuberculosis*.[26] Fever accompanied esophagitis in 20% of patients with CMV or mycobacterial infection but was less common among those with *Candida* or HSV. Nausea and vomiting were most common (42%) in patients with CMV esophagitis, possibly reflecting the fact that CMV infection is seldom confined to the esophagus. Oral lesions frequently provide clues to the diagnosis of esophagitis, particularly in patients with acquired immunodeficiency syndrome (AIDS). Oral thrush is seen in most patients with esophageal candidiasis and AIDS.[27] The finding of oropharyngeal candidiasis in a patient with esophageal symptoms and AIDS has a positive predictive value of 70% or greater for esophageal involvement.[9,11,28-30] Similarly, oropharyngeal vesicles or ulcerations may suggest, but do not prove, concomitant esophageal HSV or aphthous ulceration in a symptomatic patient.

SPECIFIC ETIOLOGIC AGENTS

Candida Esophagitis

C. albicans is the predominant pathogen of esophagitis. Non-*albicans* species of *Candida*, including *Candida tropicalis*, *Candida parapsilosis*, *Candida krusei*, and *Candida glabrata*, are implicated less often but may play a greater role as a result of selective pressure among patients who have received antifungal agents.[31,32] Small numbers of *C. albicans* are part of the normal oral flora; esophageal colonization may be present in up to 20% of the population,[33] particularly in patients treated with histamine type 2 blockers.[34] Colonization is the initial process whereby superficial adherence and proliferation of organisms remain confined to the superficial mucosa, without penetration or inflammation of the epithelium. Colonization progresses to infection if systemic and local defenses are inadequate to prevent invasion into deeper epithelial layers, with pseudohyphae seen at the advancing margin of tissue involvement. On endoscopic examination, the esophagus appears hyperemic with discrete, yellow-white mucosal plaques that are firmly adherent and, when removed, reveal an underlying rough and friable surface (Fig. 90-1). Lesions are most frequently located in the distal third of the esophagus. Disease may progress to involve large confluent plaques, ulceration, luminal narrowing, strictures, and necrosis.[2,35] Perforation of the esophagus is a rare complication of necrotizing esophagitis that may necessitate surgical intervention.[36]

Systemic host factors predisposing to esophageal candidiasis include acute[37] and advanced HIV infection, diabetes mellitus, leukemia and lymphoma, broad-spectrum antimicrobial therapy, antineoplastic therapy, corticosteroid therapy, and bone marrow or solid organ transplantation. In addition to immune dysfunction, contributing local factors are those that impair esophageal motility (e.g., systemic sclerosis, achalasia, esophageal webs or rings, obstructing esophageal cancer) and conditions that result in mucosal injury (e.g., reflux, HSV esophagitis). Esophageal symptoms occur in up to half of all patients with AIDS,[9,38] and *Candida* accounts for 50% or more of these

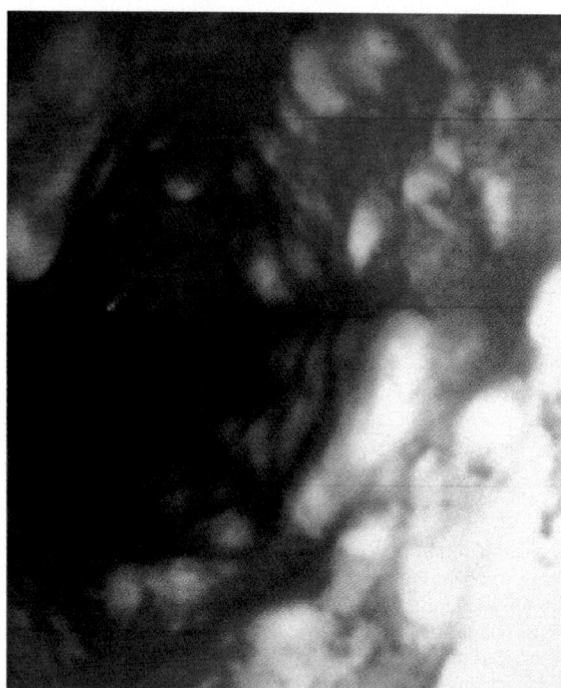

FIGURE 90-1. Endoscopic appearance of esophageal candidiasis, showing typical white plaques and nodules, in a patient with multiple myeloma. *(Courtesy of Dr. Arthur DeCross, Rochester, N.Y.)*

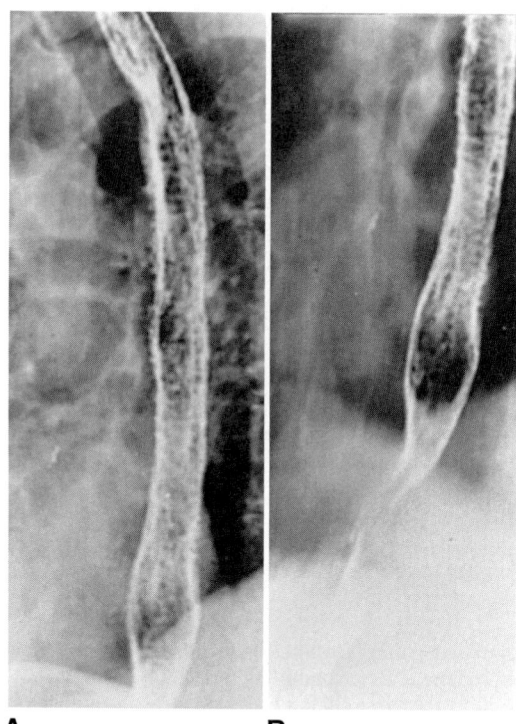

A **B**

FIGURE 90-2. A and **B,** Barium contrast esophagograms of *Candida* esophagitis showing a markedly irregular esophagus due to multiple plaques in a patient with acquired immunodeficiency syndrome and severe odynophagia. *(From Polis M. Esophagitis. In: Mandell GL, Bennett JE, Dolin R, eds. Principles and Practice of Infectious Diseases. 4th ed. New York: Churchill Livingstone; 1995:962-965.)*

cases.[11,30] Porro and colleagues[29] documented esophageal candidiasis in 48% of AIDS patients admitted to a hospital, although 40% of those infected reported no esophageal symptoms. Transplant recipients, many of whom receive routine antifungal prophylaxis, appear less susceptible to *Candida* esophagitis, which developed in 5 (2.2%) of 224 renal transplant recipients[39] and none of 304 cardiac transplant recipients.[40] Among symptomatic bone marrow transplant recipients, esophageal infection was diagnosed in 21 of 46 endoscopic examinations, but *Candida* accounted for only 5 of the 21 infections, the remainder being caused by CMV, HSV, or both.[41]

Accurate diagnosis of esophageal candidiasis is established by endoscopy with directed brushings and biopsies. The characteristic gross appearance of candidiasis is suggestive but occasionally misleading, inasmuch as white exudative lesions may also be visualized with HSV or CMV infection or pill esophagitis. Brushings of exudative lesions and ulcer craters are obtained with a sheathed cytology brush, smeared onto slides, and submitted for periodic acid–Schiff, silver, or Gram stain. Biopsies of lesions and the edges of ulcers are submitted for histopathologic examination and for viral culture to identify CMV and HSV. Masses of yeast and pseudohyphae seen in tissue or brushings are diagnostic of *Candida* infection. Fungal cultures are not generally helpful, except to identify the pathogen in cases of fungal esophagitis that are refractory to treatment. Blind brushing of the esophagus via a nasogastric tube has been advocated as an alternative to endoscopy in patients with HIV infection and suspected esophagitis; this technique was 96% sensitive and 87% specific for the diagnosis of candidiasis.[28]

Radiologic contrast studies are of limited diagnostic value and are seldom performed in patients with esophagitis. Although focal or confluent plaques or a diffuse, "shaggy" appearance is characteristic of candidiasis on the esophagogram (Fig. 90-2), the examination result may be normal in some patients, and visualized abnormalities such as plaques, ulcerations, fistulas, or masses are often nonspecific; concurrent infections are likely to be missed.[25,42] Radiographic studies may be useful if endoscopy is unavailable. Computed tomographic scanning may demonstrate thickening of the esophageal wall in patients with esophagitis, but this finding is neither sensitive nor specific for infection.[43]

Cytomegalovirus Esophagitis

CMV esophagitis occurs most often in patients with AIDS or severe immunosuppression. CMV was an esophageal pathogen or copathogen in 33 (30%) of 110 patients with HIV infection and esophageal symptoms[11] and in 7 (33%) of 21 symptomatic recipients of bone marrow transplants.[41] Rare cases in immunocompetent hosts have been reported.[44] Symptoms are indistinguishable from those associated with *Candida* or HSV esophagitis. The endoscopic appearance of CMV esophagitis is typified by large (>10 cm^2), shallow, "punched-out" ulcers, solitary or multiple in number, located in the middle to distal part of the esophagus.[45] The ulcer margins are distinct, and the intervening mucosa appears relatively normal. Isolation of CMV in culture is not diagnostic, because virus harbored in blood or saliva may contaminate esophageal specimens. Conversely, culture is not positive in all cases. Histopathologic examination is the most reliable diagnostic method when mucosal and submucosal biopsies are obtained from the ulcer edge and ulcer base; routine hematoxylin and eosin staining demonstrates enlarged endothelial cells or fibroblasts containing large, dense intranuclear inclusions.[45] Immunohistochemical and direct fluorescent staining techniques, highly specific for CMV and HSV, may also help establish these diagnoses. Coinfections of the esophagus are common in patients with CMV; concomitant candidiasis (73%) and HSV (12%) have been reported among these patients.[11]

Herpes Simplex Virus Esophagitis

Herpes simplex esophagitis is usually identified in patients with AIDS or other significant immunosuppressive conditions, although cases in healthy adults are also seen. Among 23 patients with HSV esophagitis reported by McBane and associates,[46] 7 (30%) had hematologic malignancies, 4 (17%) had received chemotherapy or irradiation for solid tumors, 8 (35%) had been treated with immunosuppressive agents for

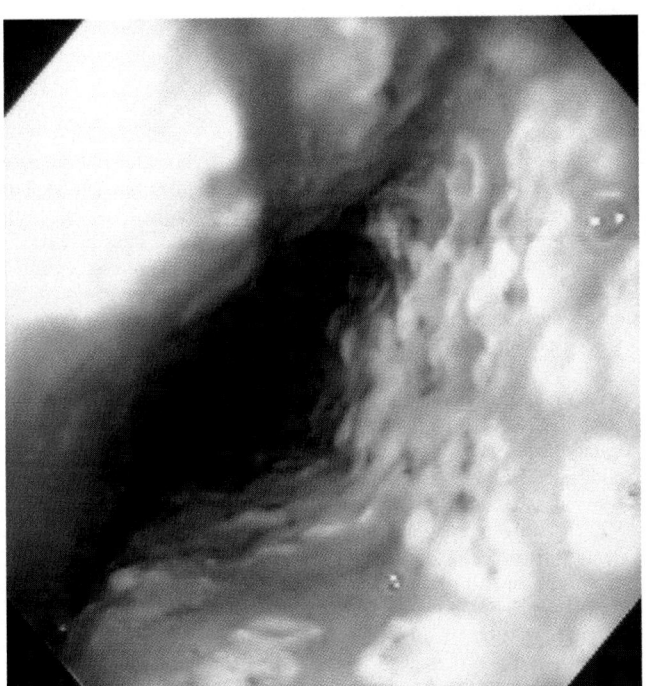

FIGURE 90-3. Herpes simplex esophagitis, characterized by numerous small ulcerations, in an immunocompetent adult with fever and odynophagia. *(Courtesy of Dr. Charles Michalko, Rochester, N.Y.)*

biopsies is the most sensitive diagnostic tool and is positive for HSV-1 in most (but not all) cases; HSV-2 has rarely been implicated.[50,51] Histologic examination may show characteristic ballooning degeneration, multinucleated giant cells, and prominent intranuclear Cowdry type A inclusion bodies in 55% to 70% of biopsy specimens. Superficial candidal invasion of HSV ulcers is often seen on biopsy.

Aphthous (Idiopathic) Ulceration of the Esophagus

Aphthous or idiopathic ulceration, an important variant of esophagitis in patients with advanced HIV infection, accounts for approximately 5% of AIDS patients with esophagitis.[9,11] No specific cause is evident in 40% of AIDS patients with esophageal ulceration,[52] and painful ulcers are often present in the oropharynx as well.[53] Esophageal ulceration has also been described in patients with acute HIV infection who present initially with odynophagia, and detection of HIV virions by electron microscopy in the margins of these ulcers has suggested to some a direct pathogenic role for HIV itself.[1] Others, having detected HIV nucleic acid by in situ hybridization or polymerase chain reaction in the esophageal mucosa of up to 80% of AIDS patients with idiopathic ulceration or with specific etiologic diagnoses (*Candida*, CMV, or HSV esophagitis), have concluded that HIV is not a primary pathogen in ulcerative disease.[30,54] Other, unrecognized infectious agents may contribute to the pathogenesis of these idiopathic ulcerations.

MANAGEMENT OF ESOPHAGEAL INFECTION

General Considerations in Therapy

Specific therapies for infectious causes of esophagitis are listed in Table 90-2. The approach to diagnosis and therapy in a particular patient often depends on the presence of underlying disease and the severity of immunosuppression (Table 90-3).

Patients receiving cancer chemotherapy may experience severe mucositis with odynophagia that is clinically indistinguishable from fungal or viral esophagitis. Oropharyngeal candidiasis is highly predictive of esophageal candidiasis in patients with cancer, particularly in patients with mucositis after chemotherapy.[60] Diagnostic endoscopy should be pursued whenever possible, but in practice the procedure is frequently deferred because of bleeding, severe pain, mucosal friability, or critical illness; empirical therapy for *Candida* and HSV is appropriate in the interim period, particularly if oral thrush or mucocutaneous HSV lesions are clinically evident or cultures are positive. Patients with fever and neutropenia (<100 neutrophils/mm³) are usually treated empirically with systemic antifungal agents (amphotericin B, lipid formulations of amphotericin, caspofungin, or voriconazole) in doses sufficient to treat either esophageal or disseminated candidiasis. Intravenous acyclovir is often administered in this acute setting if HSV stomatitis or labialis is present or if esophageal symptoms are severe.

nonmalignant conditions, and 1 was otherwise healthy. HSV esophagitis accounts for 6% to 16% of HIV-infected patients with esophageal symptoms.[38] In a series of 21 bone marrow transplant recipients with esophagitis, HSV was identified in 48%.[41] More than 40 cases of HSV esophagitis have been described in immunocompetent hosts, predominantly men, in whom the infection is typically self-limited.[47,48] Odynophagia, chest pain, fever, nausea, and vomiting are the most common initial symptoms; clinically significant gastrointestinal bleeding occurs in 15% to 25%.[46] Esophageal rupture is a rare complication.[49] Oral, labial, or cutaneous HSV is clinically evident in only 19% to 38% of cases.[47,50] Typical lesions appear endoscopically as multiple, small, superficial ulcers in the distal third of the esophagus; larger confluent ulcers, pseudomembranes, or diffusely denuded epithelium may be seen as the infection progresses (Fig. 90-3). "Volcano ulcers" may have raised margins around the central crater. Vesicles are rarely visualized. Double-contrast esophagography demonstrates ulcerative irregularities that are not specific or diagnostic. Viral culture of brushings or

TABLE 90-2 Treatment of Esophagitis		
Cause	*Usual Treatment (Adult Dose)*	*Alternative Drugs*
Candida	Fluconazole, 100-200 mg/day PO or IV for 14-21 days; maintenance suppressive therapy may be necessary in AIDS (fluconazole, 100-200 mg/day PO)	Itraconazole, 100-200 mg bid oral suspension PO Amphotericin B, 0.2-0.4 mg/kg/day IV for 7 days Caspofungin, 50 mg/day IV after 70-mg loading dose Voriconazole,[55] 200 mg bid PO*
Herpes simplex	Acyclovir, 5 mg/kg IV q8h for 7-14 days *or* 400 mg 5 times daily PO for 14-21 days, or valacyclovir, 1g PO tid for 14-21 days*; maintenance suppressive therapy may be necessary in AIDS	Famciclovir, 500 mg bid PO for 14-21 days (not for acyclovir-resistant infection) Foscarnet, 90 mg/kg q12h IV for 7-14 days (used for acyclovir-resistant infection)
Cytomegalovirus	Ganciclovir, 5 mg/kg IV q12h for 14-21 days; maintenance suppressive therapy usually is necessary in AIDS (ganciclovir, 5 mg/kg/day IV 7 days/wk *or* 6 mg/kg/day IV 5 days/wk)	Foscarnet, 90 mg/kg q12h IV for 14-21 days; suppression with foscarnet, 90–120 mg/kg/d IV Valganciclovir, 900 mg bid PO for treatment, and 900 mg qd for maintenance/suppression*
Aphthous (in AIDS)	Prednisone,[56] 40 mg/day PO for 14 days, then taper	Thalidomide,[57,58] 200 mg/day PO*

*Not approved by the U.S. Food and Drug Administration for this indication.
AIDS, acquired immunodeficiency syndrome.

TABLE 90-3 Causes of Esophagitis in Symptomatic Patients with Underlying Disease*

Cause	AIDS† (n = 183)	Bone Marrow Transplant‡ (n = 39)	Solid Organ Transplant§ (n = 88)
Candida alone	38	10	3
Candida + other	22	3	—
Cytomegalovirus	21	26	6
Herpes simplex virus	11	26	7
Aphthous ulceration	4	—	—
Kaposi's sarcoma	7	—	—

*Patients on whom upper endoscopy was performed to evaluate odynophagia, dysphagia, epigastric pain, nausea and vomiting, or gastrointestinal bleeding. Values represent percentages of patients.
†Data from refs. 9, 11, 30.
‡Data from ref. 41.
§Data from refs. 40, 59.

Allogeneic bone marrow transplant recipients who are neutropenic commonly receive antiviral prophylaxis until engraftment occurs. Esophageal infections in bone marrow transplantation patients usually begin more than 40 days after transplantation, and neutrophil counts are usually within the normal range at that time; CMV and HSV are at least as common as *Candida* in this group of patients, and treatment should be guided by the results of endoscopic diagnosis.[41] Similarly, treatment of esophagitis in solid organ transplant recipients or immunocompetent hosts should be guided by endoscopic appearance, culture data, and histopathology. Tacrolimus and cyclosporine levels may be elevated and should be monitored in transplantation patients who are receiving concomitant fluconazole or itraconazole.

Esophagitis in Patients with Acquired Immunodeficiency Syndrome

Esophageal symptoms occur in 40% to 50% of patients with AIDS at some point in the course of their disease and may have a significant impact on nutritional status and overall morbidity.[9,25,38] The frequencies of various causes are shown in Table 90-3, and treatment regimens are listed in Table 90-2. *Candida* esophagitis is the most common type; it is treated empirically with oral fluconazole or itraconazole solution[61] in the symptomatic patient, particularly if oropharyngeal candidiasis is also observed. Oral thrush is predictive of esophageal involvement in more than 70% of such cases.[9,11,28-30,62,63] Ketoconazole tablets and itraconazole capsules are erratically absorbed and are less effective.[64] Complete symptomatic response can be expected in more than 80% of patients treated empirically, usually within 1 week. If there is no response to empirical azole therapy within 7 days, endoscopy should be performed to establish a diagnosis.[65] Among patients for whom empirical azole therapy for esophageal symptoms has failed, endoscopy demonstrates ulceration of the esophagus in 62% to 77%, attributable most often to CMV (32% to 40%), aphthous disease (27% to 32%), or HSV (5% to 8%).[66,67] Early endoscopy is appropriate in patients with severe symptoms or gastrointestinal bleeding. The incidence of esophageal candidiasis has declined by 30% to 50% in the current era of highly active antiretroviral therapy.[68-70]

A viral cause is identified in approximately one third of cases, often in association with candidiasis. Empirical antiviral therapy for CMV or HSV is discouraged. Patients with CMV esophagitis confirmed by culture and histopathologic examination are treated with ganciclovir, 5 mg/kg intravenously every 12 hours. Cases refractory to ganciclovir may respond to foscarnet, 90 mg/kg intravenously every 12 hours. A partial or complete response to induction therapy is observed in 75% to 85% of patients treated with either ganciclovir or foscarnet,[71-73] but relapses are common with or without maintenance therapy. Documented HSV esophagitis is usually treated with intravenous acyclovir initially in severe cases; therapy may be continued with oral acyclovir, valacyclovir, or famciclovir. Complete resolution is reported in 70% of patients treated with acyclovir, but relapse occurs in 15% of

patients with HSV esophagitis within 4 months.[50] If acyclovir therapy has failed because of resistance, no response to ganciclovir is expected, and foscarnet should be given.

Patients with aphthous ulceration of the esophagus have improved with a regimen of prednisone, 40 mg daily for 2 weeks, in more than 90% of cases.[56] A placebo-controlled trial demonstrated complete healing of AIDS-associated oropharyngeal aphthous ulcers in 55% of 29 patients treated with thalidomide, 200 mg daily for 1 month, compared with only 7% of patients in the placebo group.[57] In a similar randomized study of 24 HIV-infected patients with biopsy-confirmed aphthous ulceration of the esophagus, the same regimen of thalidomide resulted in complete healing at 4 weeks in 73% of treated subjects, compared with 23% of placebo recipients (P = .033).[74] In a series of 12 patients with idiopathic esophageal ulceration, 92% experienced complete resolution of symptoms with this treatment regimen.[75] Use of these therapies should be considered for patients with esophageal ulcerations not attributable to specific pathogens. Thalidomide in lower doses of 100 mg three times per week was not effective in preventing recurrences of oral and esophageal aphthous ulcers in HIV-infected patients.[74] Zidovudine and zalcitabine (ddC) capsules may also cause esophageal ulceration; patients should be advised to take these and all oral medications in the upright position and with sufficient water.[23,24]

Approximately 5% of cases of endoscopically proven *Candida* esophagitis are refractory to fluconazole therapy because of either acquisition of a resistant strain or gradual emergence of resistance over time. Refractory candidiasis, most common in patients with advanced AIDS, a CD4 T-cell count lower than 50/mm³, and long-term exposure to azole antifungal agents, is an indicator of poor disease prognosis.[76] Patients unresponsive to fluconazole, 200 mg daily for 2 weeks, may respond to higher doses, at least transiently; 50% to 60% of such patients have responded to itraconazole oral solution, 200 to 400 mg daily.[76,77] Chronic prophylaxis with itraconazole is associated with reduced susceptibility to itraconazole and cross-resistance to fluconazole.[78] Oral voriconazole is as effective as fluconazole in treatment of esophageal candidiasis; its role in management of fluconazole-refractory cases remains to be studied.[55] Amphotericin B oral solution is no longer available in the United States but was reported to be an effective alternative in 43% of fluconazole-refractory patients.[79] Parenteral amphotericin has been reserved for patients who fail other therapies; doses of 15 to 20 mg daily are often sufficient. Caspofungin has proved at least as effective and better tolerated than amphotericin B; however, response rates to either drug are reduced in patients for whom fluconazole previously failed, probably because of more severe immunosuppression in this group.[80-82] Relapse rates are higher with refractory candidiasis, and maintenance therapy is almost always required. Highly active antiretroviral therapy is critical in such patients and must be optimized. To reduce the risk of refractory disease, continuous antifungal prophylaxis should be avoided in most AIDS patients with mucosal candidiasis unless recurrences are particularly frequent or severe.[76]

Various other pathogens have caused rare cases of esophagitis in patients with AIDS, including *Pneumocystis jirovecii*,[18] Epstein-Barr virus,[22] *Mycobacterium avium* complex,[9,10] *Histoplasma capsulatum*,[13] *Cryptococcus neoformans*,[11] *Cryptosporidium*,[17] *Actinomyces*,[14,15] *Trichomonas*,[83] and *Saccharomyces*.[16] Therapy is the same as for infections with these agents at other sites. Kaposi's sarcoma involving the esophagus has been documented in up to 7% of AIDS patients with esophageal symptoms.[9,11,30]

REFERENCES

1. Rabeneck L, Popovic M, Gartner S, et al. Acute HIV infection presenting with painful swallowing and esophageal ulcers. JAMA. 1990;263:2318-2322.
2. Baehr PH, McDonald GB. Esophageal disorders caused by infection, systemic illness, medications, radiation, and trauma. In: Feldman M, Scharschmidt BF, Sleisenger MH, eds. Gastrointestinal and Liver Disease. 6th ed. Philadelphia: WB Saunders; 1998:519-539.
3. Kikendall JW. Pill esophagitis. J Clin Gastroenterol. 1999;28:298-305.

4. Monig SP, Schmidt R, Wolters U, Krug B. Esophageal tuberculosis: A differential diagnostic challenge. Am J Gastroenterol. 1995;90:153-154.
5. Mokoena T, Shama DM, Ngakane H, Bryer JV. Oesophageal tuberculosis: A review of eleven cases. Postgrad Med J. 1992;68:110-115.
6. Rosario MT, Raso CL, Comer GM. Esophageal tuberculosis. Dig Dis Sci. 1989;34:1281-1284.
7. Garcia Sepulcre MF, Casellas Valde JA, Alonso Maillo G, et al. Esophageal tuberculosis with fistula to mediastinum. Am J Gastroenterol. 1995;90:2074-2075.
8. Griga T, Duchna HW, Orth M, et al. Tuberculous involvement of the oesophagus with oesophagobroncheal fistula. Dig Liver Dis. 2002;34:528-531.
9. Connolly GM, Hawkins D, Harcourt-Webster JN, et al. Oesophageal symptoms, their causes, treatment, and prognosis in patients with the acquired immunodeficiency syndrome. Gut. 1989;30:1033-1039.
10. El-Serag HB, Johnston DE. *Mycobacterium avium* complex esophagitis. Am J Gastroenterol. 1997;92:1561-1563.
11. Bonacini M, Young T, Laine L. The causes of esophageal symptoms in human immunodeficiency virus infection: A prospective study of 110 patients. Arch Intern Med. 1991;151:1567-1572.
12. Jacobs DH, Macher AM, Handler R, et al. Esophageal cryptococcosis in a patient with the hyperimmunoglobulin E-recurrent infection (Job's) syndrome. Gastroenterology. 1984;87:201-203.
13. Forsmark CE, Wilcox CM, Darragh TM, Cello JP. Disseminated histoplasmosis in AIDS: An unusual case of esophageal involvement and gastrointestinal bleeding. Gastrointest Endosc. 1990;36:604-605.
14. Poles MA, McMeeking AA, Scholes JV, Dieterich DT. *Actinomyces* infection of a cytomegalovirus esophageal ulcer in two patients with acquired immunodeficiency syndrome. Am J Gastroenterol. 1994;89:1569-1572.
15. Spencer GM, Roach D, Skucas J. Actinomycosis of the esophagus in a patient with AIDS: Findings on barium esophagograms. AJR Am J Roentgenol. 1993;161:795-796.
16. Konecny P, Drummond FM, Tish KN, Tapsall JW. *Saccharomyces cerevisiae* oesophagitis in an HIV-infected patient. Int J STD AIDS. 1999;10:821-822.
17. Kazlow PG, Shah K, Benkov KJ, et al. Esophageal cryptosporidiosis in a child with acquired immune deficiency syndrome. Gastroenterology. 1986;91:1301-1303.
18. Grimes MM, LaPook JD, Bar MH, et al. Disseminated *Pneumocystis carinii* infection in a patient with acquired immunodeficiency syndrome. Hum Pathol. 1987;18:307-308.
19. Sherman RA, Silva J Jr, Gandour-Edwards R. Fatal varicella in an adult: Case report and review of the gastrointestinal complications of chickenpox. Rev Infect Dis. 1991;13:424-427.
20. Gill RA, Gebhard RL, Dozeman RL, Sumner HW. Shingles esophagitis: Endoscopic diagnosis in two patients. Gastrointest Endosc. 1984;30:26-27.
21. Lawn SD, Venkatesan P. Chickenpox oesophagitis and haematemesis in an immunocompetent adult. J Infection. 2002;44:206.
22. Kitchen VS, Helbert M, Francis ND, et al. Epstein-Barr virus associated oesophageal ulcers in AIDS. Gut. 1990;31:1223-1225.
23. Edwards P, Turner J, Gold J, Cooper DA. Esophageal ulceration induced by zidovudine. Ann Intern Med. 1990;112:65-66.
24. Indorf AS, Pegram PS. Esophageal ulceration related to zalcitabine (ddC). Ann Intern Med. 1992;117:133-134.
25. Wilcox CM. Esophageal disease in the acquired immunodeficiency syndrome: Etiology, diagnosis, and management. Am J Med. 1992;92:412-421.
26. Baehr PH, McDonald GB. Esophageal infections: Risk factors, presentation, diagnosis, and treatment. Gastroenterology. 1994;106:509-532.
27. Tavitian A, Raufman JP, Rosenthal LE. Oral candidiasis as a marker for esophageal candidiasis in the acquired immunodeficiency syndrome. Ann Intern Med. 1986;104:54-55.
28. Bonacini M, Laine L, Gal AA, et al. Prospective evaluation of blind brushing of the esophagus for *Candida* esophagitis in patients with human immunodeficiency virus infection. Am J Gastroenterol. 1990;85:385-389.
29. Porro GB, Parente F, Cernuschi M. The diagnosis of esophageal candidiasis in patients with acquired immune deficiency syndrome: Is endoscopy always necessary? Am J Gastroenterol. 1989;84:143-146.
30. Smith PD, Eisner MS, Manischewitz JF, et al. Esophageal disease in AIDS is associated with pathologic processes rather than mucosal human immunodeficiency virus type 1. J Infect Dis. 1993;167:547-552.
31. Mukherjee S. Torulopsis glabrata esophagitis. Am J Gastroenterol. 2000;95:1106-1107.
32. Wingard JR, Merz WG, Rinaldi MG, et al. Increase in *Candida krusei* infection among patients with bone marrow transplantation and neutropenia treated prophylactically with fluconazole. N Engl J Med. 1991;325:1274-1277.
33. Andersen LI, Frederiksen HJ, Appleyard M. Prevalence of esophageal *Candida* colonization in a Danish population: Special reference to esophageal symptoms, benign esophageal disorders, and pulmonary disease. J Infect Dis. 1992;165:389-392.
34. Vermeersch B, Rysselaere M, Dekeyser K, et al. Fungal colonization of the esophagus. Am J Gastroenterol. 1989;84:1079-1083.
35. Wilcox CM. Esophageal strictures complicating ulcerative esophagitis in patients with AIDS. Am J Gastroenterol. 1999;94:339-343.
36. Gaissert HA, Roper CL, Patterson GA, Grillo HC. Infectious necrotizing esophagitis: Outcome after medical and surgical intervention. Ann Thoracic Surg. 2003;75:342-347.
37. Decker CF, Tiernan R, Paparello SF. Esophageal candidiasis associated with acute infection due to human immunodeficiency virus. Clin Infect Dis. 1992;14:791.
38. Laine L, Bonacini M. Esophageal disease in human immunodeficiency virus infection. Arch Intern Med. 1994;154:1577-1582.
39. Frick T, Fryd DS, Goodale RL, et al. Incidence and treatment of candida esophagitis in patients undergoing renal transplantation. Data from the Minnesota prospective randomized trial of cyclosporine versus antilymphocyte globulin-azathioprine. Am J Surg. 1988;155:311-313.
40. Johnson R, Peitzman AB, Webster MW, et al. Upper gastrointestinal endoscopy after cardiac transplantation. Surgery. 1988;103:300-304.
41. McDonald GB, Sharma P, Hackman RC, et al. Esophageal infections in immunosuppressed patients after marrow transplantation. Gastroenterology. 1985;88:1111-1117.
42. Levine MS, Macones AJ Jr, Laufer I. *Candida* esophagitis: Accuracy of radiographic diagnosis. Radiology. 1985;154:581-587.
43. Berkovich GY, Levine MS, Miller WT Jr. CT findings in patients with esophagitis. AJR Am J Roentgenol. 2000;175:1431-1434.
44. Altman C, Bedossa P, Dussaix E, Buffet C. Cytomegalovirus infection of esophagus in immunocompetent adult. Dig Dis Sci. 1995;40:606-608.
45. Wilcox CM, Diehl DL, Cello JP, et al. Cytomegalovirus esophagitis in patients with AIDS: A clinical, endoscopic, and pathologic correlation. Ann Intern Med. 1990;113:589-593.
46. McBane RD, Gross JB Jr. Herpes esophagitis: Clinical syndrome, endoscopic appearance, and diagnosis in 23 patients. Gastrointest Endosc. 1991;37:600-603.
47. Galbraith JC, Shafran SD. Herpes simplex esophagitis in the immunocompetent patient: Report of four cases and review. Clin Infect Dis. 1992;14:894-901.
48. Ramanathan J, Rammouni M, Baran J Jr, Khatib R. Herpes simplex virus esophagitis in the immunocompetent host: An overview. Am J Gastroenterol. 2000;95:2171-2176.
49. Dieckhaus KD, Hill DR. Boerhaave's syndrome due to herpes simplex virus type 1 esophagitis in a patient with AIDS. Clin Infect Dis. 1998;26:1244-1245.
50. Genereau T, Lortholary O, Bouchaud O, et al. Herpes simplex esophagitis in patients with AIDS: Report of 34 cases. The Cooperative Study Group on Herpetic Esophagitis in HIV Infection. Clin Infect Dis. 1996;22:926-931.
51. Wishingrad M. Sexually transmitted esophagitis: Primary herpes simplex virus type 2 infection in a healthy man. Gastrointest Endosc. 1999;50:845-846.
52. Wilcox CM, Schwartz DA, Clark WS. Esophageal ulceration in human immunodeficiency virus infection: Causes, response to therapy, and long-term outcome. Ann Intern Med. 1995;123:143-149.
53. Bach MC, Howell DA, Valenti AJ, et al. Aphthous ulceration of the gastrointestinal tract in patients with the acquired immunodeficiency syndrome (AIDS). Ann Intern Med. 1990;112:465-467.
54. Wilcox CM, Zaki SR, Coffield LM, et al. Evaluation of idiopathic esophageal ulceration for human immunodeficiency virus. Mod Pathol. 1995;8:568-572.
55. Ally R, Schurmann D, Kreisel W, et al. A randomized, double-blind, double-dummy, multicenter trial of voriconazole and fluconazole in the treatment of esophageal candidiasis in immunocompromised patients. Esophageal Candidiasis Study Group. Clin Infect Dis. 2001;33:1447-1454.
56. Wilcox CM, Schwartz DA. Comparison of two corticosteroid regimens for the treatment of HIV-associated idiopathic esophageal ulcer. Am J Gastroenterol. 1994;89:2163-2167.
57. Jacobson JM, Greenspan JS, Spritzler J, et al. Thalidomide for the treatment of oral aphthous ulcers in patients with human immunodeficiency virus infection. N Engl J Med. 1997;336:1487-1493.
58. Jacobson JM, Spritzler J, Fox L, et al. Thalidomide for the treatment of esophageal aphthous ulcers in patients with human immunodeficiency virus infection. J Infect Dis. 1999;180:61-67.
59. Alexander JA, Brouillette DE, Chien MC, et al. Infectious esophagitis following liver and renal transplantation. Dig Dis Sci. 1988;33:1121-1126.
60. Samonis G, Skordilis P, Maraki S, et al. Oropharyngeal candidiasis as a marker for esophageal candidiasis in patients with cancer. Clin Infect Dis. 1998;27:283-286.
61. Graybill JR, Vazquez J, Darouiche RO, et al. Randomized trial of itraconazole oral solution for oropharyngeal candidiasis in HIV/AIDS patients. Am J Med. 1998;104:33-39.
62. Darouiche RO. Oropharyngeal and esophageal candidiasis in immunocompromised patients: Treatment issues. Clin Infect Dis 1998;26:259-274.
63. Rex JH, Walsh TJ, Sobel JD, et al. Practice guidelines for the treatment of candidiasis. Infectious Disease Society of America (IDSA). Clin Infect Dis. 2000;30:662-678.
64. Barbaro G, Barbarini G, Calderon W, et al. Fluconazole versus itraconazole for candida esophagitis in acquired immunodeficiency syndrome. Gastroenterology. 1996;111:1169-1177.
65. Wilcox CM, Alexander LN, Clark WS, Thompson SE. Fluconazole compared with endoscopy for human immunodeficiency virus-infected patients with esophageal symptoms. Gastroenterology. 1996;110:1803-1809.
66. Wilcox CM, Straub RF, Alexander LN, Clark WS. Etiology of esophageal disease in human immunodeficiency virus-infected patients who fail antifungal therapy. Am J Med. 1996;101:599-604.
67. Bini EJ, Micale PL, Weinshel EH. Natural history of HIV-associated esophageal disease in the era of protease inhibitor therapy. Dig Dis Sci. 2000;45:1301-1307.
68. Detels R, Tarwater P, Phair JP, et al. Effectiveness of potent antiretroviral therapies on the incidence of opportunistic infections before and after AIDS diagnosis. Multicenter AIDS Cohort Study. AIDS. 2001;15:347-355.
69. Kaplan JE, Hanson D, Dworkin MS, et al. Epidemiology of human immunodeficiency virus-associated opportunistic infections in the United States in the era of highly active antiretroviral therapy. Clin Infect Dis. 2000;30(Suppl 1):S5-S14.
70. San-Andres FJ, Rubio R, Castilla J, et al. Incidence of acquired immunodeficiency syndrome-associated opportunistic diseases and the effect of treatment on a cohort of 1115 patients infected with human immunodeficiency virus, 1989-1997. Clin Infect Dis. 2003;36:1177-1185.

71. Wilcox CM, Straub RF, Schwartz DA. Cytomegalovirus esophagitis in AIDS: A prospective evaluation of clinical response to ganciclovir therapy, relapse rate, and long-term outcome. Am J Med. 1995;98:169-176.

72. Parente F, Bianchi Porro G. Treatment of cytomegalovirus esophagitis in patients with acquired immune deficiency syndrome: A randomized controlled study of foscarnet versus ganciclovir. Am J Gastroenterol. 1998;93:317-322.

73. Blanshard C, Benhamou Y, Dohin E, et al. Treatment of AIDS-associated gastrointestinal cytomegalovirus infection with foscarnet and ganciclovir: A randomized comparison. J Infect Dis. 1995;172:622-628.

74. Jacobson JM, Greenspan JS, Spritzler J, et al. Thalidomide in low intermittent doses does not prevent recurrence of human immunodeficiency virus-associated aphthous ulcers. J Infect Dis. 2001;183:343-346.

75. Alexander LN, Wilcox CM. A prospective trial of thalidomide for the treatment of HIV-associated idiopathic esophageal ulcers. AIDS Res Hum Retroviruses. 1997;13:301-304.

76. Fichtenbaum CJ, Koletar S, Yiannoutsos C, et al. Refractory mucosal candidiasis in advanced human immunodeficiency virus infection. Clin Infect Dis. 2000;30:749-756.

77. Wilcox CM, Darouiche RO, Laine L, et al. A randomized, double-blind comparison of itraconazole oral solution and fluconazole tablets in the treatment of esophageal candidiasis. J Infect Dis. 1997;176:227-232.

78. Goldman M, Cloud GA, Smedema M, et al. Does long-term itraconazole prophylaxis result in in vitro azole resistance in mucosal *Candida albicans* isolates from persons with advanced human immunodeficiency virus infection? Antimicrob Agents Chemother. 2000;44:1585-1587.

79. Fichtenbaum CJ, Zackin R, Rajicic N, et al. Amphotericin B oral suspension for fluconazole-refractory oral candidiasis in persons with HIV infection. AIDS. 2000;14:845-852.

80. Villanueva A, Arathoon EG, Gotuzzo E, et al. A randomized double-blind study of caspofungin versus amphotericin for the treatment of candidal esophagitis. Clin Infect Dis. 2001;33:1529-1535.

81. Arathoon EG, Gotuzzo E, Noriega LM, et al. Randomized, double-blind, multicenter study of caspofungin versus amphotericin B for treatment of oropharyngeal and esophageal candidiases. Antimicrob Agents Chemother. 2002;46:451-457.

82. Kartsonis N, DiNubile MJ, Bartizal K, et al. Efficacy of caspofungin in the treatment of esophageal candidiasis resistant to fluconazole. JAIDS J Acquir Immun Defic Syndr. 2002;31:183-187.

83. Borczuk AC, Hagan R, Chipty F, Brandt LJ. Cytologic detection of *Trichomonas* esophagitis in a patient with acquired immunodeficiency syndrome. Diagn Cytopathol. 1998;19:313-316.

CHAPTER **91**

Nausea, Vomiting, and Noninflammatory Diarrhea

RICHARD L. GUERRANT

DAVID A. BOBAK

The vast majority of acute gastrointestinal illnesses do not involve a recognizable inflammatory process.[1] Although there is considerable inflammatory enteritis during summer months in warm areas with poor sanitation, most cases of diarrhea in these areas are noninflammatory, which suggests an enterotoxic bacterial, viral, or noninvasive parasitic process.[2,3]

EPIDEMIC DIARRHEA IN NEWBORN NURSERIES

Epidemic infantile diarrhea has long been recognized as a potentially serious problem that occurs in newborn nurseries. The mortality rate in this disease has been as high as 24% to 50%.[4,5] Epidemic diarrhea among hospitalized newborns has been associated with certain enteropathogenic serotypes of *Escherichia coli* (EPEC). EPEC serotypes have been associated with diarrhea in hospitalized infants younger than 4 months.

The unusual susceptibility of newborns may be explained by their unique host status; they have not yet acquired a normal intestinal flora or specific immunity. In infants in special care nurseries, this situation is compounded by severe underlying conditions such as prematurity or congenital cardiac or pulmonary disease. The consequences of diarrhea in the newborn are unusually severe because of poorly developed homeostatic mechanisms and limited water and electrolyte reserves. Nosocomial transmission may occur because the newborn nurseries may be crowded with susceptible infants.[6] A nursery outbreak can go unrecognized because infants may develop diarrhea after being discharged.

The onset is insidious, with the development of listlessness, irritability, and poor feeding over a period of 3 to 6 days.[5,7,8] Vomiting and fever are infrequent, and the stools tend to be watery, yellow-green in color, and usually without mucus, pus, or blood. Early signs such as failure to gain weight or a slight weight loss and abdominal distention may be subtle. The disease may progress to more severe signs of dehydration and shock with depressed sensorium, drowsiness, coma, sunken eyes, circumoral cyanosis, and grayish discoloration of the skin. Shock without hyperpnea often occurs in this setting despite the development of severe acidosis. Poorly nourished infants with decreased protein and potassium reserves may have severe hypokalemia, hyponatremic dehydration, and paradoxical edema. The illness usually lasts 5 to 15 days but may persist or relapse over the course of several weeks. Complications may include intercurrent otitis media, pneumonia, bacteremia, peritonitis, and renal vein or cerebral sinus thrombosis. Dissemination of EPEC to the lungs has been demonstrated by immunofluorescence staining of tissue at autopsy.[9] Although the mortality may be quite high, as noted previously, South[10] and Kaslow and colleagues[11] have reported a milder illness with lower morbidity and mortality. However, in many areas such as South Africa and southern Brazil, EPEC organisms remain among the most common causes of diarrhea in infants and young children, especially during the summer months.[12-14] Endemic childhood diarrheal illness in areas such as England and Canada also remains associated with EPEC in 6% to 18% of cases.[12,13]

Several potentially life-threatening processes may mimic this infantile diarrhea syndrome. So-called parenteral diarrhea refers to the well-recognized but poorly understood tendency for systemic infections or localized infections elsewhere (such as otitis or meningitis) to be manifest clinically with diarrhea. Likewise, a strangulated hernia, intussusception, or torsion of an ovary or testis may be manifested by abdominal pain or diarrhea.

Appropriate antibiotic therapy must be tailored to the specific sensitivity pattern of the organism isolated.[10] If systemic infection is suspected, parenteral therapy should be started and should be tailored to the antibiotic sensitivity pattern of the organism isolated. Appropriate preventive measures include forming cohorts of nursery admissions, avoidance of overcrowding in nurseries, utilization of individual units and equipment, careful formula preparation, isolation of infants with diarrhea, and careful hand washing by hospital personnel.

The association of a certain strain of *E. coli* with infantile diarrhea was first demonstrated by slide agglutination by Bray and Beavan[15] in 1945 and reported in further details in 1948. They identified serologically homogeneous *E. coli* organisms in most infants with summer diarrhea (87.5% versus 4% of the control subjects); half of the cases were hospital acquired. Varela and associates[16] and Olarte and Varela[17] subsequently found this strain (called *E. coli*-gomez by Varela and associates) in cases of infantile diarrhea in Mexico. A second serotype, initially designated as β to distinguish it from the earlier serotype called α, was described by Giles and Sangster[18] as the cause of an outbreak of infantile gastroenteritis in Aberdeen.

E. coli strains are classified into a large number of serotypes on the basis of three major types of antigens: the O or heat-stable somatic antigen (lipopolysaccharide endotoxin), which forms the basis for 169 serogroups; an outer, heat-labile capsular antigen called K, which may inhibit O agglutination; and, for motile organisms, the H or flagellar antigen, which is also heat labile. Three different kinds of K antigens have been identified, L, A, and B, the latter (B) being of importance in the identification of EPEC serotypes. The original α and β serotypes of *E. coli* were subsequently associated with several outbreaks of infantile epidemic gastroenteritis and were classified as serotypes O111-B4 and O55-B5, respectively, by Kaufmann and Dupont.[19] As shown

TABLE 91-1 Enteropathogenic and Enterohemorrhagic *Escherichia coli* Serotypes Classically Recognized in Infantile Diarrhea Outbreaks*

Serotype	Difco Serogroup (References)
Class I (EAF-positive) EPEC	
055-K59(B5): H⁻/6/7	A (18-20)
0111ab-K58(B4):H⁻/5/12	A (15-17, 19, 20)
0127a-K63(B8):H6	A (20)
0119-K69(B14)	B (20)
0125ac-K70(B15):H21	B (20)
0126-K71(B10):H⁻/H2	B (20)
0128ab-K67(B12)	B (20)
0142	(6, 20, 21)
0158	(20, 22)
Class II (EAF-negative) EPEC	
044-K74	C (20)
0114	(4, 20, 23, 24)
086a-K61(B7)	B (20)
0157-H7	(25-27)
026-B6	A (20)

*See also Table 91-4.

EAF, enteroadherence factor probe for focal HEp-2 cell adherence plasmid pMAR2; EHEC, enterohemorrhagic *E. coli;* EPEC, enteropathogenic *E. coli.*

in Table 91-1, exclusive of certain invasive serotypes (see Table 93-2 in Chapter 93), there are 14 classically recognized EPEC *E. coli* serotypes, including O111-K58 (α), O55-K59 (β), O127-K63, O128-K67, O26-B6, O86-K61, O119-K69, O125-K70, O126-K71, O20-B7, and O44-K74. Additional serotypes recognized as causes of epidemic infantile diarrhea include O114,[4,23,24] O142,[6,21] and O158.[22] *E. coli* O157-H7 and other enterohemorrhagic *E. coli* strains that make a Shiga-like toxin have caused hemorrhagic diarrhea with minimal inflammation and hemolytic-uremic syndrome (HUS) in several outbreaks as well as sporadic cases.[25-29]

The mechanism by which most EPEC organisms cause disease involves a complex set of attachment and effacement traits, as detailed in Chapter 89. Although most are not invasive and do not produce conventionally recognized heat-labile or heat-stable enterotoxins, these organisms are capable of causing diarrheal disease in human volunteers, from whom the organism can be reisolated and in whom an antibody response can be documented.[7,30] EPEC diarrhea continues to occur in some areas, especially urban hospitals in subtropical areas.[31,32] Studies in adult human volunteers suggest that EPEC diarrhea may be more inflammatory than previously recognized.[33]

Epidemic infantile diarrhea may also be caused by enterotoxigenic organisms that are not limited to certain serotypes of *E. coli.* An outbreak has been described in which multiple serotypes of different organisms (*E. coli, Klebsiella,* and *Citrobacter*) that were demonstrated to be transiently enterotoxigenic were isolated,[34] which suggests the transmission of enterotoxigenicity among etiologic strains by plasmids[35] or by bacteriophages.[36] An investigation of a subsequent outbreak of diarrhea on a cruise ship also documented the association of enterotoxigenic *Klebsiella* and *Citrobacter* as well as *E. coli* with watery diarrhea.[37] Another report of sporadic diarrhea among infants and children in Africa has shown that enteric organisms other than *E. coli* may produce an enterotoxin.[38] Enterotoxigenicity is not limited to specific serotypes, and most EPEC serotypes do not produce recognizable enterotoxins.[38-41] However, a number of serotypes of *E. coli* are identified more often among enterotoxigenic isolates, as shown in Table 91-2.[20,42] Whether these organisms are better recipients for enterotoxin plasmids or are simply better adapted to maintaining these plasmids is not known.

A 9-month-long outbreak of diarrhea in the special care nurseries of a pediatric hospital has been reported in association with a multiple-drug–resistant *E. coli* O78 that produced only the heat-stable type of enterotoxin.[43] Another outbreak of diarrhea lasting 3 months in a newborn nursery in Scotland was related to heat-stable enterotoxin (ST)-producing *E. coli* O159.[44] Other bacterial causes of diarrhea, such as shigellosis[45] and epidemic salmonellosis,[46,47] may also spread readily in the newborn nursery setting. Potential viral causes of epidemic infantile diarrhea include echoviruses,[48] coxsackieviruses,[49] adenoviruses,[50] and rotaviruses.[51-56] Echovirus 18 was isolated from 10 of 12 infants who had watery noninflammatory diarrhea in a 21-patient premature nursery. The virus was also isolated from two nurses, one of whom was implicated in the spread of the agent to five other babies in another ward.[48] The role of enteroviruses as causes of acute gastroenteritis remains controversial. Hospital acquisition of rotaviruses may be common among newborns; some investigators suggest that mild diarrhea develops relatively infrequently.[57] However, rotaviruses have been clearly implicated in epidemic neonatal diarrhea[54-56] as well as in sporadic infantile diarrhea after the neonatal period.

WEANLING DIARRHEA

Weanling diarrhea usually occurs in the second year of life in areas where sanitation is poor. The greatest attack rate of diarrhea in the community occurs at the time of weaning, usually between 6 and 24 months of age.[5,6,58,59] As noted in Chapter 89, weanling diarrhea is a major cause of mortality around the world. The increased susceptibility of a recently weaned infant is related to several factors.[60] In areas with poor sanitation, the infant ingests large numbers of many new organisms at the time of weaning. In developing countries, weaning foods prepared under conditions of poor hygiene are frequently found to be contaminated with large numbers of potential pathogens.[61,62] A second contributing factor is the deteriorating nutritional status that may occur with weaning in many parts of the world.[63,64] Finally, cellular and humoral factors passively transferred in human breast milk convey resistance to agents that commonly cause diarrhea in this age group.[65-69] Weanling diarrhea is manifest clinically as an acute, sporadic, watery diarrheal illness that occurs with increased frequency, especially in the summer months, in areas with poor sanitation. In the well-nourished infant, the disease is usually short lived and resolves within 2 to 3 days with adequate hydration. A low-grade fever may be present, and vomiting is common.[39,59] Diarrhea in the malnourished child tends to persist or to recur and is often much more severe.

Weanling diarrhea is usually an acute, noninflammatory process. Acute diarrhea in children 6 to 24 months of age has been commonly associated with rotaviruses[39,70,71] and with enterotoxigenic *E. coli.*[38,40,72] Shigellosis may also occur in this setting. From 16% to 83% of acute diarrheal illnesses among infants and young children have been associated with enterotoxigenic *E. coli.*[38,40,72,73] Most of these reports involve studies of the summer peak of diarrhea in areas with poor sanitation. The presence of antibody to the heat-labile enterotoxin (LT) of *E. coli* in colostrum[65,66] may provide some protection against LT-producing *E. coli* diarrhea among breastfed infants exposed to unsanitary conditions. The demonstration of passive protection against experimental enterotoxigenic *E. coli* infections in human volunteers with immune bovine colostrum further documents the potential protective role of passive antibody in colostrum or milk.[74] The role of enterotoxigenic

TABLE 91-2 Serotypes of *Escherichia coli* That Appear with Increased Frequency among Enterotoxigenic Isolates

LT *E. coli*	ST *E. coli*
O6-K15:H16	078-H11, 078-H12
08-K40:H9, 08-K25:H9	0115-H40
LT + ST *E. coli*	0128-H7
011-H27	0148-H28
020-H⁻, 020:H11	0153
025-K7:H42	0159-H20
025-K98:H⁻	0166, 0167
027-H7	
063-H12	
080, 085, 0139	

LT, heat-labile; ST, heat-stable.

E. coli in causing infantile diarrhea in temperate climates is less clear. Enterotoxigenic *E. coli* serotypes were uncommon among children with diarrhea in studies from Massachusetts and Virginia.[75-77]

The ability of enteric organisms other than *E. coli* to produce enterotoxins has been suggested, but these organisms appear to be considerably less common than enterotoxigenic *E. coli*. Studies from Ethiopia suggested that young children with sporadic diarrhea may have *Klebsiella*, *Citrobacter*, *Aeromonas*, or *E. coli* that produce an LT-like toxin.[78] However, in Brazil, enterotoxigenic *Klebsiella* organisms were found in only 2 of 40 patients, both of whom also had enterotoxigenic *E. coli*.[72] Diarrhea produced by LT shares the adenylate cyclase–activating mechanism with cholera toxin,[79-83] whereas the heat-stable toxin (STa) activates intestinal guanylate cyclase.[84-86]

The major nonbacterial causes of weanling diarrhea are rotaviruses (see Chapter 146).[52,53,87,88] Worldwide, rotaviruses cause more than 100 million cases of gastroenteritis and up to 600,000 deaths each year in children younger than 5 years.[53,89] Of these deaths, more than 80% occur to children residing in the poorest areas of the world. Although most adults have demonstrable antibody to rotaviruses that may protect against symptomatic disease, children younger than 2 years throughout temperate and tropical climates appear to be highly susceptible to rotavirus diarrhea,[53] which occurs most frequently in the winter or cooler, dry months[39,70,75,90-96] and occasionally in the summer months.[97] Rotavirus diarrhea appears to be associated with low humidity and possibly indoor crowding to a greater extent than with low temperature or inadequate sanitation.[98-100] The illness is usually mild and without fever and is often associated with vomiting.[39,52,70,87,101] Rotaviruses have been associated with initial bouts of weanling diarrhea in Aboriginal communities,[102] and antirotavirus antibody has been demonstrated in human colostrum among patients in Costa Rica and Brazil.[66,68] There is a high frequency of rotavirus shedding or seroconversion among parents and other household contacts of cases of rotavirus-associated diarrhea.[39,103,104] Up to 40% of these infected adult contacts may experience mild abdominal cramps or diarrhea.[105]

The human rotaviruses demonstrate antigenic cross-reactivity with several animal strains, including the Nebraska calf diarrhea virus (NCDV), the agent of epizootic diarrhea of infant mice, simian rotavirus (SA-11), and the O agent of monkeys.[39,106] However, there are different antigenic types of rotaviruses,[107-110] and multiple attacks may occur.[111] Five major serotypes, A to E, have been described for rotavirus strains, with group A strains further subdivided into G (glycoprotein) types and P (protease) types.[87,112-114] Worldwide, five serotypes (G1 to G4 and G9) are the most prevalent.[87,112,115] Although rotavirus infection is classically described in young children, subclinical infections remain common in adults and symptomatic outbreaks have been reported as well. Three U.S. outbreaks of rotavirus gastroenteritis in adults were reported over a 2-year period, 1998 to 2000.[116] Two of these episodes were associated with nursing homes and one with a university. Each outbreak, although geographically distinct, was caused by the same rotavirus G2 strain, suggesting that natural immunity may be less efficacious for certain G2 strains. This same strain of rotavirus (G2 [P4] type) has been shown to cause a more severe form of infection in children than other more common serotypes.[117,118] This epidemiologic information is important to consider in the context of new attempts to develop an effective rotavirus vaccine for humans, as discussed later.

The laboratory diagnosis of rotavirus diarrhea may be made by examining the stool directly for viruses or by a variety of molecular assays designed to detect virus-specific antigens, antibodies, or nucleic acids.[119] Rotaviruses can be detected in fecal material by direct electron microscopy or by using immunologic techniques such as enzyme-linked immunosorbent assay (ELISA),[120] radioimmunoassay,[121] counterimmunoelectrophoresis,[122] or fluorescence antibody staining of stool or biopsy specimens.[123,124] Immunoassays for rotaviral antigen are available, with ELISA being the most sensitive. Simple rapid latex agglutination assays with 86% sensitivity and 95% specificity have been developed.[125] Detection of rotaviral genomic RNA in stools by means of dot hybridization using labeled RNA probes appears to be sensitive, specific, and convenient.[126] Methods for detecting serum antibody titers to rotaviruses use their cross-reactivity with NCDV, SA-11, or O agents of animals that can be cultivated in bovine embryonic kidney cells or in African green monkey kidney cells in tissue culture. Serum antibody has been measured by immune electron microscopy,[92,127] complement fixation,[39,92] and immunofluorescence[75] with one of the substitute antigens.

Much has been learned about the pathogenesis and the pathologic characteristics of intestinal rotavirus infections.[87,88] Biopsy specimens from confirmed cases have shown transient, patchy, irregular inflammatory responses in the lamina propria and immature, cuboidal epithelium with 70- to 90-nm rotavirus particles in the distended cisternae of the endoplasmic reticulum.[90] Normal columnar epithelium at the villus tips was replaced by irregular cuboidal cryptlike cells. As would be expected from the destruction of villus-type epithelial cells, a transient brush border disaccharidase deficiency in the duodenal and upper jejunal mucosa and, despite the efficacy of oral therapy with glucose-electrolyte solutions, increased fecal reducing substances have been noted in children with rotavirus diarrhea.[128-131] The degree of microvillus damage parallels the severity of diarrhea and dehydration.[132] As with transmissible gastroenteritis in piglets, studies of experimental rotaviral infections in animals confirm the shortened villi, reduced sucrase activity, increased thymidine kinase activity, lack of change in cyclic adenosine monophosphate (AMP) concentrations, and blunted glucose-induced sodium absorption.[133,134] As noted in Chapter 89, this loss of absorptive villus tip cells may be responsible for the fluid imbalance and nutritional impact of rotaviral infections. In certain in vitro and murine models of rotavirus infection, a virally encoded nonstructural protein (NSP4) has been shown to induce Ca^{2+}-dependent enterotoxigenic effects.[87,88,113,114] The primary effects of the putative rotavirus enterotoxin are independent of cyclic AMP and also do not stimulate any significant level of inflammatory response.[87,88]

No specific antiviral therapy is available for rotaviral infections and therapy should be supportive, directed first at the immediate restoration of fluid balance by intravenous or oral glucose-electrolyte therapy and then at restoration of the nutritional state to normal. Prevention is the key to controlling rotavirus epidemics. Reasonable preventive measures include the provision of improved sanitation facilities and safe water supplies as well as efforts to develop protective antibacterial, antitoxic, or antiviral immunity.[135] Because of the great global burden of childhood rotavirus gastroenteritis, there continues to be great interest in multinational efforts to develop an effective rotavirus vaccine.

On the basis of a number of effective clinical trials in infants worldwide,[136-141] the U.S. Food and Drug Administration approved the rhesus-human reassortant rotavirus tetravalent vaccine (RRV-TV) in August 1998 for use in infants. Less than 1 year later, case-control and cohort studies suggesting an association between administration of the vaccine and an increased risk of intussusception led the U.S. Advisory Committee on Immunization Practices to withdraw its recommendation for use of RRV-TV.[140-144] The etiology of this association remains unknown. Because certain viral forms of gastroenteritis, including rotavirus forms, appear themselves to be associated with a somewhat increased risk of intussusception, the significance of the apparent RRV-TV association with intussusception has been extensively reexamined but without a consensus opinion.[140,141] Vaccine development continues, with candidate vaccines entering or nearing clinical trials.[145-149] In addition, other ongoing studies, in anticipation of the new vaccine trials, are examining the relationship between natural rotavirus infection and the risk of intussusception in infants.[150]

ACUTE NAUSEA AND VOMITING (WINTER VOMITING DISEASE)

The syndrome of acute nausea and vomiting, "intestinal flu," or "viral gastroenteritis" commonly occurs in winter months in temperate climates. Although there is some overlap of this syndrome with rotavirus-associated infantile gastroenteritis, rotaviruses appear to be a relatively uncommon cause of winter vomiting disease in older children and adults. The Cleveland family studies of Dingle and co-workers[151] showed that enteritis was second only to upper respiratory infection as a cause of illness in homes. Gastrointestinal illnesses were most common between the ages of 1 and 10 years, when approximately two illnesses occurred per person per year. The peak season for these gastrointestinal illnesses was November through February, with June being the month of lowest frequency over this continuous study period. Most illnesses were of less than 1 to 3 days' duration; 20% occurred with respiratory symptoms, and 20% involved only diarrhea.

Illnesses tended to occur in one of two patterns: (1) mild afebrile illness with watery diarrhea or (2) a more severe febrile illness with vomiting, headache, and constitutional symptoms. Although etiologic agents were rarely identified, these two patterns of illness subsequently developed among volunteers who ingested filtrates prepared from the feces of ill patients.[152-154] Studies done in 1975 to 1977 in Charlottesville, Virginia, confirmed this pattern of winter illnesses, with clustering in families, highest attack rates in children, and the absence of identifiable etiologic agents in most cases despite the application of techniques for virologic and enterotoxin studies.[76,77]

Although there has been little consistent documentation of enteroviruses in association with febrile winter vomiting disease, echovirus type 11 has been demonstrated in association with a small laboratory outbreak of febrile vomiting disease.[155] Abdominal pain and vomiting have been described with influenza B infections in children between the ages of 4 and 10 years.[156]

Noroviruses are now recognized as major causes of acute gastroenteritis (see Chapter 172). Their individual names were derived originally from the sites of outbreaks where they have been implicated. These include the following viral agents: Norwalk,[157-159] Hawaii,[160] Snow Mountain,[161] Taunton, and W agent.[162] These viruses cause illness throughout the year, consisting of low-grade fever and various combinations of abdominal cramps, vomiting, and diarrhea. Person-to-person spread is common, and secondary attack rates can be high. Biopsy specimens of subjects with norovirus illness revealed an intact small intestinal mucosa but blunted villi, shortened microvilli, and dilation of the endoplasmic reticulum with intracellular multivesiculate bodies. Dilated mitochondria and intercellular spaces were observed.[163] There was a transient decrease in the activities of the brush border enzymes, alkaline phosphatase, sucrase, and trehalase. The colon is relatively spared, and fecal leukocytes are absent in this noninflammatory type of diarrhea.

The pathophysiologic features of winter vomiting disease caused by noroviruses may be parallel in some respects to the features mentioned in the previous section for rotaviruses. Both cause mucosal villus disruption and transient brush border enzyme deficiencies in the upper portion of the small bowel without any alteration in adenylate cyclase activity.[109,164,165] The roles of transient enzyme deficiency, malabsorption of xylose and lactose, and the slight increase in the number of bacteria present during the norovirus illness remain unclear.[164,166]

In addition to the preceding viruses, several other groups of viral pathogens have been identified in endemic and epidemic cases of gastroenteritis (Table 91-3)[52,119,167-169]: (1) caliciviruses with characteristic "chalice-like" surface hollows (including agents described in the United States, United Kingdom, Europe, and Japan); (2) astroviruses, with a five- or six-pointed star–like surface structure (including Marin County,[170] UK1-5, and Japan agents); and (3) other less well-defined viral agents. Because many of these agents have either not yet been cultivated in vitro or lack a convenient animal model, study of their role as enteric pathogens has been limited. Other viral agents, including enteroviruses (especially echovirus types 11, 14, and 18), enteric adenoviruses (said to cause up to 9% of pediatric inpatient diarrhea),[171] human coronaviruses (isolated from infants with gastroenteritis),[172,173] pestiviruses,[174] toroviruses,[175,176] and picobirnaviruses,[177] are becoming more well recognized as pathogens in children and adults; more detailed discussion of these agents may be found in Chapters 169, 172, and 173. More than one third of outbreaks of nonbacterial gastroenteritis in the United States have been associated with noroviruses.[178,179] Astroviruses have been found to be among the most common causes of viral gastroenteritis in the pediatric age group.[180-183] Infection with

TABLE 91-3   Viral Pathogens Causing Gastroenteritis

Established pathogens[*]	Likely and emerging pathogens[*]
Adenoviruses (enteric types)	Coronaviruses
Astroviruses	Enteroviruses (various)
Caliciviruses	Picobirnaviruses, picotrirnaviruses
Noroviruses	Pestiviruses
Rotoviruses groups A-C	Toroviruses
Cytomegalovirus	

[*]Data from references 52, 119, 168, 169.

astrovirus occasionally occurs in association with other enteric pathogens; in these cases, the illness is more severe and protracted.[182] In a review of electron microscopic findings from 10 centers in the United States and Canada over 6 years, a viral agent was seen in 16% of cases, including rotavirus, adenovirus, small round virus, astroviruses, and caliciviruses, the latter three being associated with nosocomial diarrhea.[183]

Identification of noroviruses requires immune electron microscopy[159] or radioimmunoassay for demonstration of a serologic response.[184] In vitro expression of the Norwalk virus capsid protein results in the production of capsid structures resembling clinical isolates of this agent.[185] These recombinant particles may facilitate generation of clinically useful diagnostic tests for noroviruses (see Chapter 172). It is clear that there are multiple antigenic types of these agents that are capable of causing similar disease and that resistance may be related to individual (genetic) differences rather than to lasting protective immunity after symptomatic infection.[185,186] Methods for detection of other viral causes of gastroenteritis include monoclonal antibody–based enzyme immunoassay,[174,187] tissue culture,[188] and gene probes.[189] Finally, additional viral agents are being recognized as potential causes of diarrhea in children in developing and developed areas.[175,176]

ACUTE NONINFLAMMATORY DIARRHEA IN ADULTS

In temperate climates, acute noninflammatory diarrhea in adults may be caused by rotaviruses[190,191] or by Norwalk-like viruses.[105,109,158,190] The association of rotaviruses as well as adenoviruses, coxsackieviruses, and toxigenic *Clostridium difficile* with diarrhea, abdominal cramps, and a higher mortality among adult bone marrow transplant recipients has also been noted.[192] In addition, several agents of food poisoning such as *Clostridium perfringens*, *Bacillus cereus*, and *Staphylococcus aureus* commonly cause noninflammatory diarrheal syndromes in adults (see Chapter 95).

In adults living in areas with poor sanitation, several other agents commonly cause sporadic noninflammatory diarrhea. In certain areas in South Asia, cholera is an endemic cause of severe watery diarrhea. With the increased infection-to-case ratio of El Tor cholera, the seventh pandemic has swept most of the continents of the Eastern Hemisphere, including Asia, Africa, and the Mediterranean portions of Europe.[193] Isolated cases have also occurred in the United States.[194,195] Outbreaks have been related to contaminated mineral water[196] and to undercooked shellfish.[197,198] Beginning in Madras, India, in late 1992 and rapidly spreading to Calcutta and Bangladesh in 1993, a new strain of non-O1 *Vibrio cholerae*—O139, called Bengal—is causing epidemic cholera gravis and may represent the beginning of an eighth pandemic.[199-203] Cholera should be suspected in any patient who has severe dehydration and watery diarrhea, especially if the patient has a history of recent travel to a cholera-endemic area. The disease can be so fulminant as to cause hypovolemic shock and death from the outpouring of fluid into the upper portion of the small bowel before the first diarrheal stool occurs.[204] As discussed in detail in Chapter 211, the entire dehydrating syndrome of cholera appears to be related to the activation of intestinal adenylate cyclase by the potent cholera enterotoxin.[79,80] To make the diagnosis of cholera bacteriologically, stool specimens should be cultured onto thiosulfate citrate bile salts–sucrose agar. Of prime importance in therapy is fluid replacement, accomplished either intravenously with isotonic fluids or orally with glucose-electrolyte solutions.

Patients from whom *V. cholerae* cannot be isolated may also have a cholera-like syndrome. In 1956, De and associates[205] demonstrated that *E. coli* isolated from adults and children with this syndrome caused fluid accumulation similar to that seen with *V. cholerae* in ligated rabbit ileal loops. In the early 1960s, Trabulsi,[206] working in São Paulo, reported similar findings with "toxigenic" *E. coli*. Subsequently, Taylor and colleagues[207,208] demonstrated that enterotoxigenicity correlated poorly with classical serotypes and that viable organisms were not required. Smith and Halls[209] identified several enterotoxigenic strains in association with animal diarrhea. Other workers showed that several adult cases of "acute undifferentiated diarrhea" in tropical Bengal were due to enterotoxigenic *E. coli* strains that were usually not of the classically recognized pathogenic serotypes.[210-213] These strains were transiently present during acute illness and elicited net jejunal fluid secretion. The toxic material present in the culture filtrate of these *E. coli* strains was demonstrated to be heat labile and nondialyzable and was precipitated in 40% ammonium sulfate. Subsequent studies have demonstrated that two types of enterotoxin are produced by *E. coli*: an LT and an ST.[214] Like cholera toxin, the *E. coli* LT activates mucosal adenylate cyclase.[64-66] LT is larger, inactivated by heating at 60° C for 30 minutes, and antigenically and mechanistically similar to cholera toxin, with a lag period before the activation of adenylate cyclase. LT is detected by several bioassay systems that use the adenylate cyclase–activating property of this toxin[215-217] or by immunoassay methods.[218] In contrast, STa activates guanylate cyclase,[84-86] has an earlier onset of action,[214] has greater tissue specificity,[86] and has a much lower molecular weight than LT.[219] It is assayed in suckling mice.[220] The role of yet a different type of enterotoxin, STb, that causes secretion in piglets without altering intestinal cyclic AMP or cyclic guanosine monophosphate remains unclear in humans at present.[221-223]

Methods for demonstrating enterotoxigenic *E. coli* are limited by the lack of a selective culture process (as routinely used, for example, to identify salmonellae or shigellae) and the necessity to pick a few random colonies of *E. coli* for enterotoxin testing. Data from a common-source outbreak of enterotoxigenic *E. coli* diarrhea in Crater Lake National Park in Oregon demonstrate the insensitivity of nonselective culture methods.[224] Fourteen patients in this outbreak had enterotoxigenic *E. coli* diarrhea by epidemiologic and clinical criteria, and each had multiple, random *E. coli* stool isolates tested for enterotoxin as well as paired sera examined for antitoxic immunity. Only 43% had enterotoxigenic *E. coli* identified, 36% had significant serum antitoxin antibody titer increases, and only 64% had either one or the other. Thirty-six percent of the cases could not be confirmed by current, nonselective methods. The lack of a serum antibody response in many patients with this intraluminal toxinosis is not surprising.

Other studies have shown that, in addition to the association with diarrhea in children, strains producing LT only, ST only, and LT plus ST are associated with adult diarrhea.[71] Adults living in areas of poor sanitation may often carry LT-producing *E. coli* asymptomatically.[225,226] In contrast, ST-producing *E. coli* strains are significantly associated with diarrheal disease and are less frequently present in asymptomatic control patients living in areas with poor sanitation. However, studies suggest that enterotoxigenic *E. coli* serotypes are uncommonly associated with diarrhea in the United States.[75,76]

A cause of acute, noninflammatory, self-limited diarrhea among persons exposed to infected animals, food, drinking or recreational water, or other infected patients is cryptosporidiosis.[227-230] The agent, a tiny coccidian protozoal parasite composed of more than 20 "named" species, causes more a severe, watery, prolonged diarrhea in immunocompromised hosts.[227,229-232] In addition to supportive care, described subsequently, several international studies in children have demonstrated efficacy of the antiparasitic agent nitazoxanide in patients with cryptosporidiosis.[230,233-236]

Treatment of diarrhea in adults consists primarily of rehydration.[237] If glucose or sucrose accompanies the isotonic fluid taken orally, the coupled absorption of sodium and water is often sufficient to replace fluid loss.[238] Bismuth subsalicylate (Pepto-Bismol) may reduce enterotoxin action,[239] and if there is no significant febrile or inflammatory process, low doses of antimotility agents may offer some relief with minimal risk if cramping is severe. Studies also suggest that novel analogues of glutamine may be beneficial in reducing the severity and extent of symptoms associated with certain forms of infectious diarrhea.[240] There has been considerable emerging interest in the use of probiotic compounds for the treatment of various forms of diarrhea. Few controlled studies have addressed the efficacy of probiotics as adjunct therapy for the management of infectious diarrhea, although these agents may be of some benefit in selected cases.[241-243]

DIARRHEA IN PATIENTS WITH ACQUIRED IMMUNODEFICIENCY SYNDROME

Patients with the acquired immunodeficiency syndrome (AIDS) often develop or present with diarrhea. Among patients with AIDS in the United States, 30% to 60% present with diarrhea,[223,224,227,244-248] a number that reaches 95% in tropical developing areas such as Africa or Haiti.[247] In many of these patients, diarrhea becomes prolonged and life threatening and may pose major difficulties in management. Although some investigators have reported an enteropathy without identifiable pathogens[249,250] or with primary human immunodeficiency virus (HIV) infection of enterochromaffin cells in the bowel mucosal crypts and lamina propria,[251] others report one or more enteric pathogens in 55% to 85% of patients with AIDS and diarrhea.[248,252,253] Sexually promiscuous homosexual males often become infected with *Giardia lamblia*, *Entamoeba histolytica*, *Campylobacter jejuni*, *Shigella*, *Chlamydia trachomatis*, or *C. difficile* or (with proctitis) *Neisseria gonorrhoeae*, herpes simplex virus, or *Treponema pallidum*.[254] As shown in Table 91-4, the leading agents found in patients with AIDS and diarrhea are cytomegalovirus, *Cryptosporidium*, microsporidia, *E. histolytica*, *G. lamblia*, *Salmonella*, *Campylobacter*, *Shigella*, *C. difficile*, *Vibrio parahaemolyticus*, and *Mycobacterium* spp.[252,253,255-257] *Cyclospora* and *Isospora belli* infections are also potentially treatable causes of persistent diarrhea in patients with AIDS, especially in tropical areas such as Haiti.[248,258-260] Even *Pneumocystis carinii* can occasionally involve the intestinal tract in this setting.[261]

TABLE 91-4 Possible Enteric Pathogens in Patients with Acquired Immunodeficiency Syndrome

Pathogen	Diarrhea (%) (n = 181)	No Diarrhea (%) (n = 28)
Cytomegalovirus	12-45	15
Cryptosporidium	14-30	0
Microsporidia	7.5-33	0
Entamoeba histolytica	0-15	0
Giardia lamblia	2-15	5
Salmonella spp.	0-15	0
Campylobacter spp.	2-11	8
Shigella spp.	5-10	0
Clostridium difficile toxin	6-7	0
Vibrio parahaemolyticus	4	0
Mycobacterium spp.	2-25	0
Isospora belli	2-6	0
Cyclospora	0-11	0
Blastocystis hominis	2-15	16
Candida albicans	6-53	24
Herpes simplex	5-18	40
Chlamydia trachomatis	11	13
Strongyloides	0-6	0
Intestinal spirochetes	11	11
One or more pathogens	55-86	39

Data from references 255, 256, 258, 259.

Although eradicative treatment may be difficult, most of these patients respond to specific antimicrobial or antiparasitic therapy, emphasizing the need to identify the etiologic agent in these infections whenever possible. The antiviral agent ganciclovir can transiently reverse intestinal cytomegalovirus infection,[262] and most bacterial and parasitic infections can be treated with the expectation of some improvement. *Cryptosporidium*, which infects 3% to 21% of patients with AIDS in the United States, can be found in as many as 50% of patients with AIDS and diarrhea in Africa and Haiti.[227-230,247] *Cryptosporidium* may also extend into the biliary tract in this setting. The same acid-fast stain that detects *Cryptosporidium* or *Mycobacterium* in fecal specimens may also reveal *I. belli* and *Cyclospora* in 2% to 15% of AIDS patients with diarrhea in the United States and Africa, respectively.[247,248,259,260,263] *Cryptosporidium* and microsporidial infections are associated with villus atrophy, crypt hyperplasia, increased intraepithelial lymphocytes, and D-xylose malabsorption.[255] An increased yield for pathogens may be found when there is a 5- to 10-kg weight loss or an abnormal result on the Schilling test.[256] Nontyphoidal *Salmonella* infections occur with an estimated 20-fold increase in frequency as well as with increased severity in patients with AIDS.[264-267] Enteric viruses have also emerged as significant potential pathogens seen with diarrhea in HIV-infected individuals. In one study, astrovirus, picobirnavirus, calicivirus, and adenovirus were found in 6% to 12% of HIV-positive patients with diarrhea.[268] Other common enteric infections include esophagitis or stomatitis with *Candida* or herpes simplex virus.

Several practical algorithmic approaches to the diagnosis and management of diarrhea in the HIV-infected patient have been published.[244,245,248] These strategies favor the use of early noninvasive stool studies and practical empirical treatment trials followed by more invasive tests (e.g., endoscopy with biopsy) for patients with refractory or more severe presentations. Highly active antiretroviral therapy (HAART) has decreased the incidence of several important opportunistic infections, including certain causes of gastroenteritis. Most notably, there has been a dramatic decline in the incidence of tissue-invasive infections caused by cytomegalovirus, including luminal gastrointestinal disease.[269,270] The influence of HAART on other opportunistic pathogens causing gastroenteritis is less well described but undoubtedly will come to light in the near future. The treatment regimens available for many agents causing infectious gastroenteritis in HIV-infected patients are less than satisfactory, but judicious adherence to safe food and water guidelines can help prevent serious enteric infections.[271]

DIARRHEA IN INSTITUTIONS

Institutions provide special host and environmental settings for the acquisition of certain enteric pathogens. As with diarrhea in patients with AIDS and traveler's diarrhea, most cases of institution-acquired diarrhea are still noninflammatory; however, an increased frequency of certain causes of inflammatory diarrhea should prompt a careful search for fecal leukocytes in sporadic or clustered cases in hospitals, chronic care facilities, or daycare centers.[272]

Hospitals

Nosocomial diarrhea is among the most common nosocomial outbreaks reported to the Centers for Disease Control and Prevention and accounted for 21% of all 223 nosocomial outbreaks reported from 1956 to 1979.[273] However, its frequency is often overlooked, and it has been suggested to be the most common nosocomial infection in some areas.[274] Furthermore, nosocomial diarrhea appears to be a significant factor predisposing to other nosocomial infections such as urinary tract infection.[275] Overall rates range from 2.3 to 4.1 illnesses per 100 admissions on pediatric wards[274,276] and from 7.7 per 100 admissions to 41% of adults hospitalized in intensive care units.[274,277]

C. difficile remains the most common and most costly infectious cause of nosocomial diarrhea in hospitalized patients.[278-280] In particular, *C. difficile*–associated diarrhea is an important emerging nosocomial infection worldwide, especially in elderly hospitalized patients as well as patients occupying beds in surgical wards or intensive care units.[280-283] Most sporadic and outbreak cases of *C. difficile*–associated disease appear to be caused by exposure to contaminated environmental surfaces rather than direct contact with an index case.[284-286] *Salmonella* is the most common cause in reported outbreaks of nosocomial gastroenteritis.[273] One study suggested that *Cryptosporidium* may be associated with cases of nosocomial diarrhea involving chronically ill, elderly patients in addition to HIV-positive patients.[287] In young children and in immunocompromised hosts, viral agents (rotaviruses, adenoviruses, coxsackieviruses, and others) are often found as well.[276,288] In addition, there has been a newfound appreciation for the roles of various viruses as causes of nosocomial diarrhea, especially in children and neonates and in intensive care unit settings.[289-291]

Long-Term Care Facilities

Diarrheal illnesses also constitute a significant problem in extended-care facilities for elderly persons. A conservative estimate based on passively reported illness rates is that one third of patients in long-term care facilities experience diarrhea each year.[292-294] *C. difficile* cytotoxin is present in about one fourth of these patients, one third of whom are symptomatic with diarrhea.[295,296] More than 20% have fecal cytotoxin on admission, and a comparable number acquire cytotoxigenic *C. difficile* in the institution.[296] When patients with diarrhea are studied, 18% to 53% have cytotoxin or *C. difficile*, respectively.[295,297] The frequency of potentially transmissible enteric pathogens emphasizes the importance of careful hand washing in situations in which hygiene is often difficult. Similar problems have long been recognized in mental institutions, where hepatitis, *Strongyloides* infection, and amebiasis are readily acquired.

Daycare Centers

Another special institutional setting in which hygiene is difficult and enteric infections are increasingly appreciated is daycare centers. Numerous outbreaks have been reported in association with viruses, bacteria, or parasites. Most common in infants and children younger than 2 years are rotaviruses, whereas older toddlers are more likely to acquire *G. lamblia*.[298] Newer diagnostic tests, based on immunoassays and reverse transcriptase–polymerase chain reaction (RT-PCR), have been used to detect a greater number of etiologic agents, such as astrovirus, in many diarrhea outbreaks in daycare centers.[299,300] A clinical syndrome of prolonged noninflammatory diarrhea may be associated with *Cryptosporidium* in daycare centers.[301-303] Outbreaks of inflammatory diarrhea in the daycare center setting include those related to *Shigella*, *C. jejuni*, and *C. difficile*.[304,305]

TRAVELER'S DIARRHEA (TURISTA)

Whether it "arouses one from bed with a start at 4 AM for a record-breaking race to the bathroom to begin a staccato ballet"[306] or produces the poetry of the psalmist, "I am poured out like water . . . my heart like wax is melted in the midst of my bowels,"[307] traveler's diarrhea has a major impact each year on the 300 million to 500 million international travelers and probably on the distribution of well over $100 billion in international tourism receipts.[308,309] Sixteen million people (8 million from the United States) travel from industrialized to developing countries. This type of diarrhea is by far the most common and among the most disconcerting illnesses that threaten the traveler.[310-312] Many studies have focused on North Americans and northern Europeans, who appear to be the groups at greatest risk when they travel to Latin America, southern Europe, Africa, or Asia.[313-316] Traveler's diarrhea, which may be severe and incapacitating (albeit rarely if ever fatal), is by far the most common health problem encountered with travel to developing countries.[317] The global nature of the problem and some suggested causal forces are illustrated by its more euphemistic names: "Delhi belly," "Gyppi tummy," "GIs," "Rome runs," "Greek gallop," "Turkey trots," "Montezuma's revenge," "Aztec two-step," "Aden gut," "San Franciscitis," "Basra belly," "la turista," "backdoor sprint," "summer complaint," "coeliac flux," "Canary disease," "passion," "Hong Kong dog," "Poona poohs," "Casablanca crud," "tourist trots," "Malta dog," and many more.

The onset in the vast majority of cases of traveler's diarrhea is usually between 5 and 15 days after arrival, with a range from 3 to 31 days in several reported series.[263,304,318-323] The illness is typically manifested by malaise, anorexia, and abdominal cramps, followed by the sudden onset of watery diarrhea. Nausea and vomiting may accompany 10% to 25% of the illnesses. The diarrhea is usually noninflammatory, without blood or pus. A low-grade fever may be present in approximately a third of the cases. The duration is usually 1 to 5 days, but a significant number of people (19% to 50%) have an illness that continues beyond 5 to 10 days.

The attack rate ranges from 7% after 2 weeks in Aden[319] to 54% after 8 days in Mexico[313] and was 4% to 51% over a 14-day period among 17,280 Swiss tourists, depending on where they went.[316] One report of British tourists noted an attack rate ranging from 26% in Africa to 7.7% in North America. In descending order of risk after Africa in this study were the Middle East, southern Europe, central Europe, Asia (including India and Pakistan), South America, Australia, and North America.[323,324] In general, it appears that the risk of acquiring turista during travel to a tropical country from a temperate climate for 2 weeks or more approaches 50%. The attack rate also appears to decrease with age after 25 years, an observation that may reflect different habits and exposures rather than inherent susceptibility.[306,316] Expatriate residents appear to be at persistent risk for diarrhea of infectious causes; one study showed an attack rate of 49% per month during the first 2 years of residence in Nepal.[325]

For many years, the etiology of turista was an enigma; only infrequently have parasites or bacteria such as amebas, *Giardia*, *Salmonella*, or *Shigella* been identified. Likewise, viral studies have failed to elucidate significant viral causes of traveler's diarrhea. The first suggestion that an infectious bacterial process was likely came from the effective reduction in the attack rate by the use of prophylactic antimicrobial agents.[223,318,323,326] Studies by Kean[306] suggested that *E. coli* of certain enteropathogenic serotypes might be involved in up to one third of the cases. The involvement of *E. coli* was further confirmed in an outbreak of traveler's diarrhea among British troops in Aden, where *E. coli* O148 was identified among 54% of the British troops with diarrhea.[319]

Subsequent studies have demonstrated enterotoxigenic *E. coli* in approximately 50% (range 20% to 75%) of cases of traveler's diarrhea in Latin America, Africa, and Asia (Table 91-5).[304,305] The attack rate ranged from 20% to 100% (median 52% to 54%) in 26 studies reviewed (see Table 91-5).[324,327] Enterotoxigenic *E. coli* organisms were almost never present before the travel; such organisms were acquired by only 14 of 111 (12.6%) fellow travelers who did not become ill.[263,321,322] The type of enterotoxin produced by *E. coli* associated with traveler's diarrhea may be the LT type, the ST type, or both LT and ST (Table 91-6). In contrast to adults who live in tropical areas and may often carry enterotoxigenic *E. coli* asymptomatically, the traveler appears to be susceptible to illness caused by enterotoxin-producing *E. coli*. Salmonellae, shigellae, or vibrios are present in only 1% to 16% of the patients with traveler's diarrhea. *Aeromonas* spp. have also been implicated in causing a small percentage of cases of traveler's diarrhea.[328,329] Rotavirus infections have been described in 0% to 36% of cases of traveler's diarrhea, often in association with bacterial or parasitic pathogens.[330] In a study of Panamanian tourists to Mexico, rotavirus or Norwalk virus was found in 41%, *Campylobacter* in 11%, and enterotoxigenic *E. coli* in only one case of diarrhea.[331] Noroviruses have been implicated in outbreaks of gastroenteritis on cruise ships.[332-334] In many respects, however, cruise ship–associated outbreaks of gastroenteritis share more epidemiologic characteristics with institution-associated gastroenteritis than with the classical form of traveler's diarrhea.

Intestinal protozoa are rare causes of acute cases of traveler's diarrhea, but agents such as *Cryptosporidium parvum*, *Cyclospora cayetanensis*, and various microsporidia (*Enterocytozoon* and *Encephalitozoon* spp.) are important causes of persistent, noninflam-

TABLE 91-5 Etiology of Traveler's Diarrhea

Characteristic	Latin America (15 Studies)	Africa (3 Studies)	Asia (8 Studies)
Duration of stay (days)	21 (2-42)*	28 (28-35)	(28-42)
Attack rate (%)	52 (21-100)	54 (36-62)	(39-57)
Percentage with			
Enerotoxigenic *Escherichia coli*	46 (28-72)	36 (31-75)	(20-34)
Shigella	0 (0-30)	0 (0-15)	(4-7)
Salmonella		0 (0-0)	(11-15)
Campylobacter jejuni	—	—	(2-15)
Vibrio parahaemolyticus	—	—	(1-13)
Rotavirus	23 (0-36)	0 (0-0)	—

*Medium (range) from 26 studies.[328,329]

matory diarrhea in returned international travelers.[335-337] Other protozoal parasites such as *I. belli* and *Blastocystis hominis* can be commonly identified in the stools of persons traveling to developing countries. However, it has been difficult to ascertain whether these organisms actually cause disease in this population or are merely a commensal.[338-340] Cholera is rarely a problem for U.S. travelers.[316,341] A subset of patients have persistent diarrhea for which no infectious agent can be implicated. Chronic idiopathic diarrhea, referred to as Brainerd diarrhea, has been reported to occur in outbreaks in the United States and in a group of North American travelers to the Galapagos Islands.[342-345]

In contrast to the frequent identification of potential etiologic agents among travelers to tropical areas who develop diarrhea, careful studies of a group of marines who developed diarrhea upon arrival in temperate South Korea (21% in 3 weeks) failed to reveal any evidence of bacterial, parasitic, or rotaviral pathogens.[346] Travelers to certain areas such as Russia and national parks in the United States may be especially susceptible to development of the more insidious watery diarrhea seen with giardiasis or cryptosporidiosis.[347-350] Strongyloidiasis may also be acquired in tropical areas and may cause noninflammatory diarrhea, abdominal pain, and eosinophilia.[351]

Several other potentially serious infections manifested initially by diarrhea or abdominal pain may be acquired by travelers. Malaria may be manifested initially as "gastroenteritis" with nausea, vomiting, diarrhea, or abdominal pain in 30% to 50% of the cases.[352] The physician caring for world travelers should also remember to consider typhoid fever and other infections that may be manifested with a "typhoidal pattern" including plague, melioidosis, typhus, and arboviral hemorrhagic fevers.[352,353]

The desire to control the bothersome problem of diarrhea in travelers has led to extreme and sometimes irrational attempts at management.[306] Some travelers persist in using iodochlorhydroxyquin (Entero-Vioform, clioquinol), which has been shown not only to be ineffective for traveler's diarrhea[313,354] but also to carry a risk of severe subacute myelo-optic atrophy.[355] Other commonly used remedies such as diphenoxylate-atropine (Lomotil) and kaolin-pectin suspension were of no value in treating children with acute diarrhea in Guatemala.[356] The former and other antimotility agents may actually worsen the illness with inflammatory processes such as shigellosis.[357] Bismuth subsalicylate (Pepto-Bismol) has been shown to inhibit enterotoxin activity in experimental animal models[289] and has been recommended for symptomatic therapy and, in doses as low as 1.05 g/day (two tablets twice a day), for prophylaxis.[357-359] The mainstay of therapy, as with any diarrheal illness, is adequate hydration with an oral glucose- or sucrose-electrolyte solution.

Prevention of traveler's diarrhea should be directed toward reducing the consumption of infectious agents in food and water. Salads, raw vegetables, and untreated water (or ice) are high-risk foods.[310-312,360] Bottled, noncarbonated water cannot be considered safe because outbreaks of cholera[196] and typhoid fever[361,362] have been traced to bottled

TABLE 91-6 Frequency of Enterotoxigenic *Escherichia coli* in Association with Traveler's Diarrhea in Latin America, Africa, and Asia

| | Reported Frequency | | | | |
Feature	Gastroenterologists in Mexico[174]	Peace Corps Volunteers in Kenya[175]	Yale Glee Club in Latin America[176]	Japanese Travelers Returning to Tokyo from India, Southeast Asia, Orient[329]	Total
Illness attack rate	49% in 16 days	69% in 5 wk	74% in 1 mo	—	
Type of enterotoxin					
LT only	16%	33%	25%	4.8%	21%
LT and ST	16%	15%	12.5%	11.8%	38%
ST only	9.8%	2%	19%	13.6%	41%
Total	21/51 cases	14/27 cases	9/16 cases	270/843 cases	
Percentage of illness with ETEC	41%	52%	56%	30.2%	32%

ETEC, enterotoxigenic *E. coli;* LT, heat-labile; ST, heat-stable.

water and beverages, respectively. It has been suggested that even brief, 10-minute heating to 50° C to 55° C (the temperature of some hot tap water, "too hot for the hand to tolerate") may kill many enteric bacterial and parasitic pathogens.[363] Care in eating and drinking may reduce one's risk even in highly endemic areas to less than 15%.[360,364]

The efficacy of prophylactic antimicrobial agents has been documented in several studies.[318,323,365] However, multiple-drug–resistant enterotoxigenic *E. coli* strains occur and have demonstrated cotransfer of enterotoxigenicity and drug resistance.[366,367] The increased risk of acquiring a more severe infection such as salmonellosis,[368] the risk of drug side effects (such as photosensitivity in the tropics), and the emergence of drug-resistant organisms should preclude the widespread use of antibiotic prophylaxis at this time. Because treatment regimens combining loperamide with antibiotic are rapidly effective in controlling traveler's diarrhea (<10 hours), most experts consider prophylactic therapy only in travelers with special considerations (e.g., high risk of infection, importance to remain disease-free during the trip).[369,370] Although, as discussed later, quinolone-resistant *Campylobacter* infections are common in South Asia, treatment of traveler's diarrhea elsewhere with a fluoroquinolone such as ciprofloxacin or levofloxacin for 1 to 3 days can significantly reduce the duration and severity of the disease.[310-312,329,371-373]

Travelers to developing countries should be generally be given a fluoroquinolone for empirical self-treatment if needed. Fluoroquinolone drugs are contraindicated in pregnant women (a nonabsorbable agent such as attapulgite can be tried)[310-312,370,372] and children younger than 16 years. Therapy with trimethoprim-sulfamethoxazole has traditionally been suggested for children, but because of resistance, most experts currently recommend the use of a macrolide, such as azithromycin.[310-312,374] The emergence of fluoroquinolone-resistant strains of *Campylobacter* spp. is of concern especially for travelers to many areas of the world, most notably to Thailand and other portions of Southeast Asia.[375-378] Consideration should be given to providing travelers to areas of the world where endemic enteric bacteria are known to have high levels of fluoroquinolone resistance with an agent such as azithromycin for empirical self-treatment of traveler's diarrhea.

DIFFERENTIAL DIAGNOSIS OF ACUTE NONINFLAMMATORY DIARRHEA

Acute noninflammatory diarrhea may also be a consequence of several noninfectious processes. As with agents that effect an osmotic diuresis, nonabsorbable agents such as sorbitol may cause diarrhea if consumed in excess. Ipecac fluid extract used by mistake instead of ipecac syrup may cause watery diarrhea instead of vomiting. Heavy metal poisoning (with As, Sn, Fe, Cd, Hg, or Pb) is often associated with diarrhea, probably as a result of toxic effects on the rapidly growing mucosal epithelium. Endocrine causes of diarrhea that may share the adenylate cyclase–activating mechanism with enterotoxins include non–β islet cell tumors, medullary carcinoma of the thyroid, carcinoid tumors, and others that are associated with increased serum prostaglandins or vasoactive intestinal polypeptide.[379] Patients with thyrotoxicosis and adrenal or parathyroid insufficiency may also have diarrhea. Congenital and acquired enzyme deficiencies include lactase deficiency and pancreatic or biliary insufficiency, in which inadequately degraded or absorbed nutrients may promote an osmotic diarrhea. A child with diarrhea as well as with edema, hypertension, or petechiae should be suspected of having hemolytic-uremic syndrome with or without enterohemorrhagic *E. coli* O157-H7. Patients with dermatitis herpetiformis may also have diarrhea that may respond to sulfone or sulfapyridine therapy or to a gluten-free diet.

CHRONIC NONINFLAMMATORY DIARRHEA

Syndromes of chronic noninflammatory diarrhea of infectious etiology include giardiasis, tropical spruelike syndromes, syndromes of bacterial "overgrowth," and *Cryptosporidium* or *I. belli* infection (especially in immunocompromised hosts).[247,251,273,380,381]

The patient with weight loss, malaise, and watery or fatty stools should be suspected of having giardiasis or some other cause of a malabsorption syndrome. This syndrome may also be associated with hypocalcemia, with iron or folate deficiency anemia, or with vitamin D, vitamin K, or protein deficiency.

Giardiasis may go undiagnosed for weeks. Although it is endemic throughout most of the United States and much of the world, giardiasis received attention when it was acquired in Rocky Mountain ski resorts and in Leningrad.[382,383] Effective management requires a high index of suspicion followed by a careful search by a competent experienced person for the trophozoite or cyst of *G. lamblia* in multiple stool specimens or in a small bowel aspirate or "string" (Enterotest; Hedeco, Palo Alto, California) sample. Recommended therapy is administration of metronidazole (Flagyl), 250 mg three times a day for 7 to 10 days, with a reported 70% cure rate.[381] Higher doses of metronidazole may be more effective. Furazolidone, which is available in liquid form for pediatric use, divided into three daily doses with meals (total, 8 mg/kg/day) for 10 days is often used in children.[384]

The diagnosis of *Cryptosporidium, Cyclospora,* or *I. belli* infection is best made by phase microscopic or modified Kinyoun acid–fast stain examination of fecal specimens with or without sugar flotation.[247,251,382] The diagnosis of *Cryptosporidium* and *Giardia* infections is also now facilitated by an enzyme immunoassay or fluorescence antibody test.

BACTERIAL OVERGROWTH SYNDROMES

Many syndromes have been described in which impaired absorption was attributed to abnormal bacterial colonization in the upper segment of the small bowel.[383] Whether these organisms are virulent pathogens or simply part of the normal colonic flora abnormally distributed is unclear at present.

Normally, the upper portion of the small bowel is relatively sparsely populated, with fewer than 10^5 organisms per milliliter; these are predominantly facultative gram-positive organisms (diphtheroids, streptococci, and lactobacilli).[385] The organisms most often incriminated in bacterial overgrowth syndromes in the small bowel are aerobic enteric coliforms (members of the family Enterobacteriaceae) and anaerobic gram-negative fecal flora (*Bacteroides* and other genera). Other organisms such as *Plesiomonas shigelloides* may occasionally be responsible.[386] Bacterial colonization in the upper part of the small bowel may be associated with malabsorption or chronic diarrhea in the absence of significant histopathologic changes. Small bowel overgrowth is usually associated with a predisposing bowel abnormality such as achlorhydria (from gastritis, pernicious anemia, or gastric surgery), blind-loop syndromes, cholangitis, impaired motility (scleroderma, diabetic neuropathy, vagotomy), surgery, strictures, diverticula, or radiation damage.[387,388] Malnutrition, especially with protein, folate, or vitamin B_{12} deficiency, may also render the bowel more susceptible to microbial colonization and injury.[385,389] An episode of acute infectious diarrhea may also provide the initiating event in the establishment of small bowel colonization and chronic diarrhea.[385,390,391] Lindenbaum and colleagues[392] described spruelike morphologic changes in the upper portion of the small bowel in association with increased numbers of bacteria and malabsorption among Peace Corps volunteers living in Pakistan.

The mechanism by which fecal flora in the small bowel causes malabsorption may involve bacterial binding or utilization of nutrients (such as vitamin B_{12} or carbohydrates, respectively), deconjugation of bile salts by bacteria such as enterococci and anaerobes,[393] or the toxic effects of bacterial products such as fatty acids or amines.[385] Indeed, *E. coli* organisms that lack other recognized virulence traits but that colonize the bowel have been shown to cause prolonged diarrhea in a rabbit model,[394] with an associated impairment in water and electrolyte absorption as well as disaccharidase activity.[395]

The approach to the patient suspected of having bacterial overgrowth as a cause of malabsorption or chronic diarrhea should include quantitative aerobic and anaerobic cultures of the upper small bowel contents obtained by intubation or string passage. Because the critical number of organisms appears to be approximately 10^5 organisms per milliliter, semiquantitative estimates from a Gram stain analogous to the urine Gram stain may also prove to be of value. Roberts and associates[390] have suggested that unexplained malnutrition in elderly persons may be due to clinically inapparent bacterial overgrowth that can be detected by the [^{14}C]glycocholic acid breath test for bacterial deconjugation of bile salts. Tests for urinary indican (from bacterial conversion of tryptophan) have proved to be insensitive and nonspecific for bacterial overgrowth syndromes.[396]

Patients with diarrhea or malabsorption and bacterial overgrowth are potential candidates for antibiotic therapy, especially if predisposing conditions such as achlorhydria, scleroderma, or diabetes are present. Depending on results of quantitative cultures of upper small bowel aspirates, therapy may need to be directed against anaerobes as well as aerobic coliform organisms.[385,390] Although small amounts of antibiotics have been used to improve the nutritional status of animals and poultry and even of malnourished children,[397] the potential risks of widespread antibiotic use[398] must be weighed against potential benefits.

Noninfectious causes of chronic noninflammatory diarrhea should also be considered in the differential diagnosis. These include congenital deficiency syndromes and food allergies, certain neoplastic and endocrine processes, and less well understood functional disorders. Causative disorders to be considered in the first two categories are milk allergies, disaccharidase deficiencies, gluten enteropathy, acrodermatitis enteropathica, β-lipoprotein deficiency, familial hyperchloremic alkalosis (congenital "chloridorrhea"), Leiner's disease, and Wiskott-Aldrich syndrome. Neoplastic and endocrine causes of diarrhea include carcinoid, Werner's syndrome (multiple endocrine adenomatosis), Zollinger-Ellison syndrome (gastrinoma), "pancreatic cholera" syndromes, medullary carcinoma of the thyroid, and thyrotoxicosis.

Patients with partial mechanical bowel obstruction or pellagra may also have chronic diarrhea. Finally, frequent small stools may suggest an irritable bowel syndrome of presumed functional etiology. However, a search for the infectious agents of treatable diarrheal illness reviewed in this chapter should always precede the latter diagnosis.

REFERENCES

1. Field M. Intestinal ion transport and the pathophysiology of diarrhea. J Clin Invest. 2003;111:931.
2. Guerrant RL, Kosek M, Moore S, et al. Magnitude and impact of diarrheal diseases. Arch Med Res. 2002;33:35.
3. Kosek M, Bern C, Guerrant RL. The global burden of diarrhoeal disease, as estimated from studies published between 1992 and 2000. Bull World Health Organ. 2003;81:197.
4. Jacobs SI, Holzel A, Wolman B, et al. Outbreak of infantile gastroenteritis caused by *Escherichia coli* O114. Arch Dis Child. 1970;45:656.
5. Neter E. Enteritis due to enteropathogenic *Escherichia coli*: Present-day status and unsolved problems. J Pediatr. 1959;55:223.
6. Hone R, Fitzpatrick S, Keane C, et al. Infantile enteritis in Dublin caused by *Escherichia coli* O142. Med Microbiol. 1973;6:505.
7. Levine MM, Nalin DR, Hornick RB, et al. *Escherichia coli* strains that cause diarrhea but do not produce heat-labile or heat-stable enterotoxins and are noninvasive. Lancet. 1978;1:1119.
8. Nelson JD, Haltalin KC. Accuracy of diagnosis of bacterial diarrheal disease by clinical features. J Pediatr. 1971;78:519.
9. Drucker MM, Polliack A, Yeivin R, et al. Immunofluorescent demonstration of enteropathogenic *Escherichia coli* in tissues of infants dying with enteritis. Pediatrics. 1970;46:855.
10. South MA: Enteropathogenic *Escherichia coli* disease: New developments and perspectives. J Pediatr. 1971;79:1.
11. Kaslow RA, Taylor A, Dweck HS, et al. Enteropathogenic *Escherichia coli* infection in a newborn nursery. Am J Dis Child. 1974;128:797.
12. Levine MM, Edelman R. Enteropathogenic *Escherichia coli* of classic serotypes associated with infant diarrhea: Epidemiology and pathogenesis. Epidemiol Rev. 1984;6:31-51.
13. Gurwith M, Hinde D, Gross R, et al. A prospective study of enteropathogenic *E. coli* in endemic diarrheal disease. J Infect Dis. 1978;137:292.
14. Toledo MRF, Alvariza MCB, Murahovschi J, et al. Enteropathogenic *Escherichia coli* serotypes and endemic diarrhea in infants. Infect Immun. 1983;39:586-589.
15. Bray J, Beavan TED. Slide agglutination of *Bacterium coli* var. *Neopolitanum* in summer diarrhea. J Pathol Bacteriol. 1948;60:395.
16. Varela G, Aguirre A, Grillo J. *Escherichia coli*-gomez, nueva especie aislada de un caso mortal de diarrea. Bol Med Hosp Infantil Mexico. 1946;3:3.
17. Olarte J, Varela G. A complete somatic antigen common to *Salmonella adelaide*, *Escherichia coli*-gomez and *Escherichia coli* O111:B4. J Lab Clin Med. 1952;40:252.
18. Giles C, Sangster G. An outbreak of infantile gastro-enteritis in Aberdeen. J Hyg (Camb). 1948;46:1.
19. Kaufmann F, Dupont A. *Escherichia* strains from infantile epidemic gastroenteritis. Acta Pathol Microbiol Scand. 1950;27:552.
20. rskov I, rskov F, Jann B, et al. Serology, chemistry and genetics of O and K antigens of *Escherichia coli*. Bacteriol Rev. 1977;41:667.
21. Rowe B, Gion RJ. *Escherichia coli* O142 and infantile enteritis in Scotland. Lancet. 1971;1:649.
22. Rowe B, Gross J, Lindop R, et al. A new *E. coli* O group O158 associated with an outbreak of infantile enteritis. J Clin Pathol. 1974;27:832.
23. Rogers KB, Cracknell VM. Epidemic infantile gastro-enteritis due to *Escherichia coli* type O114. J Pathol Bacteriol. 1956;72:27.
24. Charter RE. *Escherichia coli* type O114 isolated from infantile diarrhea and calf scours. J Pathol Bacteriol. 1956;72:33.
25. Riley LW, Remis RS, Helgerson SD, et al. Outbreaks of hemorrhagic colitis associated with a rare *Escherichia coli* serotype. N Engl J Med. 1983;308:681.
26. Johnson WM, Lior H, Bezanson GS. Cytotoxic *Escherichia coli* O157:H7 associated with hemorrhagic colitis in Canada. Lancet. 1983;1:76.
27. Outbreak of hemorrhagic colitis—Ottawa, Canada. MMWR Morb Mortal Wkly Rep. 1983;32:133.
28. Slutsker LM, Ries AA, Greene KD, et al. *Escherichia coli* O157:H7 diarrhea in the United States: Clinical and epidemiologic features. Ann Intern Med. 1994;126:505-513.
29. Iida T, Naka A, Suthienkul O, et al. Measurement of fecal lactoferrin for rapid diagnosis of enterohemorrhagic *Escherichia coli* infection. Clin Infect Dis. 1997;25:167.
30. Neter E, Shumway CN. *E. coli* serotype D433: Occurrence in intestinal and respiratory tracts, cultural characteristics, pathogenicity, sensitivity to antibiotics. Proc Soc Exp Biol Med. 1950;74:504.
31. Thielman NM, Guerrant RL. Enteric *Escherichia coli* infections. In: Guerrant RL, Walker DA, Weller PF, eds. Tropical Infectious Diseases: Principles, Pathogens, and Practice. Philadelphia: WB Saunders; 1999;261-276.
32. Donnenberg MS. Enteropathogenic *Escherichia coli*. In: Blaser MJ, Smith PD, Ravdin JR, et al, eds. Infections of the Gastrointestinal Tract. New York: Raven; 1995;709-726.
33. Miller JR, Barrett LJ, Kotloff K, Guerrant RL. A rapid test for infectious and inflammatory enteritis. Arch Intern Med. 1994;154:2660-2664.

34. Guerrant RL, Dickens MD, Wenzel RP, et al. Toxigenic bacterial diarrhea: Nursery outbreak involving multiple bacterial strains. J Pediatr. 1976;89:885.

35. Skerman FJ, Formal SB, Falkow S. Plasmid-associated enterotoxin production in a strain of Escherichia coli isolated from humans. Infect Immun. 1972;5:622.

36. Takeda Y, Murphy J. Bacteriophage conversion of heat labile enterotoxin in Escherichia coli. J Bacteriol. 1978;133:172.

37. Wachsmith K, Wells J, Shipley P, et al. Heat-labile enterotoxin production in isolates from a shipboard outbreak of human diarrheal illness. Infect Immun. 1979;24: 793-797.

38. Schorling JB, Wanke CA, Schorling SK, et al. A prospective study of persistent diarrhea among children in an urban Brazilian slum. Am J Epidemiol. 1990;132:144-156.

39. Ryder TW, Sack DA, Kapikian AZ, et al. Enterotoxigenic Escherichia coli and reovirus-like agent in rural Bangladesh. Lancet. 1976;1:659.

40. Sack RB, Hirschhorn N, Brownlee I, et al. Enterotoxigenic Escherichia coli–associated diarrheal disease in Apache children. N Engl J Med. 1975;292:1041.

41. Sack RB. Human diarrheal disease caused by enterotoxigenic Escherichia coli. Annu Rev Microbiol. 1975;29:333.

42. Merson MH, Black RE, Gross RJ, et al. Use of antisera for identification of enterotoxigenic E. coli. Lancet. 1980;2:222.

43. Ryder RW, Wachsmuth IK, Buxton AE, et al. Infantile diarrhea produced by heat-stable enterotoxigenic Escherichia coli. N Engl J Med. 1976;295:849.

44. Gross RJ, Rowe B, Henderson A, et al. A new Escherichia coli O-group, O159, associated with outbreaks of enteritis in infants. Scand J Infect Dis. 1976;8:195.

45. Haltalin KC. Neonatal shigellosis. Am J Dis Child. 1967;114:603.

46. Schroeder SA, Aserkoff B, Brachman PS. Epidemic salmonellosis in hospitals and institutions. N Engl J Med. 1968;279:674.

47. Rice PA, Craven PC, Wells JG. Salmonella heidelberg enteritis and bacteremia. An epidemic on two pediatric wards. Am J Med. 1976;60:509.

48. Eichenwald HF, Ababio A, Arky AM, et al. Epidemic diarrhea in premature and older infants caused by echo virus type 18. JAMA. 1958;166:1563.

49. Yow MD, Melnick JL, Blattner RJ, et al. The association of viruses and bacteria with infantile diarrhea. Am J Epidemiol. 1970;92:33.

50. Moffet HL, Shulenberger HK, Burkholder ER. Epidemiology and etiology of severe infantile diarrhea. J Pediatr. 1968;72:1.

51. Bishop RF, Barnes GC. Neonatal rotavirus infection. J Paediatr Child Health. 1997;33(1):80.

52. Goodgame RW. Viral causes of diarrhea. Gastroenterol Clin North Am. 2001;30:77.

53. Parashar UD, Hummelman EG, Bresee JS, et al. Global illness and deaths caused by rotavirus disease in children. Emerg Infect Dis. 2003;9:565.

54. Murphy AM, Albrey MB, Crew EB. Rotavirus infections of neonates. Lancet. 1977;2:1149.

55. Cameron DJS, Bishop RF, Davidson GP, et al. New virus associated with diarrhea in neonates. Med J Aust. 1976;1:85.

56. Bishop RF, Hewstone AS, Davidson GP, et al. An epidemic of diarrhea in human neonates involving a reoviruslike agent and "enteropathogenic" serotypes of Escherichia coli. J Clin Pathol. 1976;29:46.

57. Chrystie IL, Totterdell BM, Banatvala JE. Asymptomatic endemic rotavirus infections in the newborn. Lancet. 1978;1:1176.

58. Guerrant RL, Kirchoff LV, Shields DS, et al. Prospective study of diarrheal illnesses in northeastern Brazil: Patterns of disease, nutritional impact and risk factors. J Infect Dis. 1983;148:986.

59. Gordon JE, Chitkara ID, Wyon JB. Weanling diarrhea. Am J Med Sci. 1963;245:345.

60. Welsh JK, May JT. Anti-infective properties of breast milk. J Pediatr. 1979;94:1.

61. Motarjemi Y, Kaferstein F, Moy G, Quevedo F. Contaminated weaning food: A major risk factor for diarrhoea and associated malnutrition. Bull World Health Organ. 1993;71:79-92.

62. King J, Ashworth A. Contemporary feeding practices in infancy and early childhood in developing countries. In: King J, Ashworth A, eds. Infant and Child Nutrition, Worldwide Issues and Perspectives. Boca Raton, Fla: CRC Press; 1991:141-174.

63. Gordon JE, Guzman MA, Ascoli W, et al. Acute diarrhoeal disease in less developed countries. Bull World Health Organ. 1964;31:9.

64. Reddy V, Rashuramulu N, Bhaskaram C. Secretory IgA in protein-calorie malnutrition. Arch Dis Child. 1976;51:871.

65. Stollar OA, Kaniecki-Green E, Pelley RP, et al. Secretory IgA against enterotoxins in breast milk. Lancet. 1976;1:1258.

66. Brown SE III, Sauer KT, Nations MK, et al. Comparison of paired whole milk and dried filter paper samples for anti-enterotoxin and antirotavirus activities. J Clin Microbiol. 1982;16:103.

67. Bullen CL, Willis AT. Resistance of the breast-fed infant to gastroenteritis. BMJ. 1971;3:338.

68. Bullen JJ, Rogers HJ, Leigh L. Iron-binding proteins in milk and resistance to Escherichia coli infection in infants. BMJ. 1972;1:69.

69. Simhon A, Mata L. Anti-rotavirus antibody in human colostrum. Lancet. 1978;1:39.

70. Kapikian AZ, Kim H-W, Wyatt RG, et al. Human reovirus-like agent as the pathogen associated with "winter" gastroenteritis in hospitalized infants and young children. N Engl J Med. 1976;294:965.

71. Black RE, Merson MH, Huq I, et al. Incidence and severity of rotavirus and E. coli diarrhea in rural Bangladesh. Lancet. 1981;1:141.

72. Guerrant RL, Moore RA, Kirschenfeld PM, et al. Role of toxigenic and invasive bacteria in acute diarrhea of childhood. N Engl J Med. 1975;293:567.

73. Gorbach SL, Khurana CM. Toxigenic Escherichia coli: A cause of infantile diarrhea in Chicago. N Engl J Med. 1972;287:791.

74. Tacket CO, Losonsky G, Link H, et al. Protection by milk immunoglobulin concentrate against oral challenge with enterotoxigenic Escherichia coli. N Engl J Med. 1988;318:1240-1243.

75. Echeverria P, Blacklow NR, Smith DH. Role of heat-labile toxigenic Escherichia coli and reovirus-like agent in diarrhea in Boston children. Lancet. 1975;2:1113.

76. Hughes JM, Gwaltney JM, Hughes DH, et al. Acute gastrointestinal illness in Charlottesville: A prospective family study (Abstract). Clin Res. 1978;26:24.

77. Guerrant RL, Hughes JM, Lima NL, et al. Microbiology of diarrhea in developed and developing countries. Rev Infect Dis. 1990;12(Suppl):S41-S50.

78. Wadstrom T, Aust-Kettis A, Habte D, et al. Enterotoxin-producing bacteria and parasites in stool of Ethiopian children with diarrheal disease. Arch Dis Child. 1976;51:865.

79. Chen LC, Rohde JE, Sharp GWG. Intestinal adenyl-cyclase activity in human cholera. Lancet. 1971;1:939.

80. Guerrant RL, Chen LC, Sharp GWG. Intestinal adenyl-cyclase activity in canine cholera: Correlation with fluid accumulation. J Infect Dis. 1972;125:377.

81. Evans DJ Jr, Chen LC, Curlin GT, et al. Stimulation of adenyl cyclase by Escherichia coli enterotoxin. Nature. 1972;236:137.

82. Guerrant RL, Ganguly U, Casper AGT, et al. Effect of Escherichia coli on fluid transport across canine small bowel: Mechanism and time course-with enterotoxin and whole bacterial cells. J Clin Invest. 1973;52:1707.

83. Kantor HS, Tao P, Gorbach SL. Stimulation of intestinal adenyl cyclase by Escherichia coli enterotoxin: Comparison of strains from an infant and an adult with diarrhea. J Infect Dis. 1974;129:1.

84. Hughes JM, Murad F, Chang B, et al. Role of cyclic GMP in the action of heat stable enterotoxin of Escherichia coli. Nature. 1978;271:755.

85. Field M, Graf LH Jr, Laird WJ, et al. Heat-stable enterotoxin of Escherichia coli: In vitro effects on guanylate cyclase activity, cyclic GMP concentration, and ion transport in small intestine. Proc Natl Acad Sci U S A. 1978;75:2800.

86. Guerrant RL, Hughes JM, Chang B, et al. Activation of intestinal guanylate cyclase by heat stable enterotoxin of E. coli: Studies of tissue specificity, potential receptors, and intermediates. J Infect Dis. 1980;142:220.

87. Lundgren O, Svensson L. Pathogenesis of rotavirus diarrhea. Microbes Infect. 2001;3:1145.

88. Morris AP, Estes MK. Microbes and microbial toxins: Paradigms for microbial-mucosal interactions. VIII. Pathological consequences of rotavirus infection and its enterotoxin. Am J Physiol 2001;281:G303.

89. de Zoysa I, Feachem RG. Interventions for the control of diarrhoeal diseases among young children: Rotavirus and cholera immunization. Bull World Health Organ. 1985;63:569.

90. Bishop RF, Davidson GP, Holmes IH, et al. Virus particles in epithelial cells of duodenal mucosa from children with acute non-bacterial gastroenteritis. Lancet. 1973;2:1281.

91. Flewett TH, Bryden AS, Davies H. Virus particles in gastroenteritis. Lancet. 1973;2:1497.

92. Kapikian AZ, Kim HW, Wyatt RG, et al. Reoviruslike agent in stools: Association with infantile diarrhea and development of serologic tests. Science. 1974;185:1049.

93. Virus of infantile gastroenteritis (Editorial). BMJ. 1975;3:555.

94. Rotaviruses of man and animals (Editorial). Lancet. 1975;1:257.

95. Mata L, Simhon A, Padilla R, et al. Diarrhea associated with rotaviruses, enterotoxigenic E. coli, Campylobacter, and other agents in Costa Rican children, 1976-1981. Am J Trop Med Hyg. 1983;32:146.

96. Black RE, Merson MH, Rahman ASMM, et al. A two-year study of bacterial, viral, and parasitic agents associated with diarrhea in rural Bangladesh. J Infect Dis. 1980;142:660.

97. Echeverria P, Ho MT, Blacklow NR, et al. Relative importance of viruses and bacteria in the etiology of pediatric diarrhea in Taiwan. J Infect Dis. 1977;136:383.

98. Paul MO, Erinle EA. Influence of humidity on rotavirus prevalence among Nigerian infants and young children with gastroenteritis. J Clin Microbiol. 1982;15:212.

99. Brandt CD, Kim HW, Rodriguez WJ. Rotavirus gastroenteritis and weather. J Clin Microbiol. 1982;16:478.

100. Gurwith M, Wenman W, Gurwith D, et al. Diarrhea among infants and young children in Canada: A longitudinal study in three northern communities. J Infect Dis. 1983;147:685.

101. Shepherd RW, Truslow S, Walker-Smith JA. Infantile gastroenteritis: A clinical study of reovirus-like agent infection. Lancet. 1975;2:1082.

102. Sexton M, Davidson GP, Bishop RF, et al. Viruses in gastroenteritis. Lancet. 1974;2:355.

103. Tallett S, MacKenzie C, Middleton P, et al. Clinical, laboratory, and epidemiologic features of a viral gastroenteritis in infants and children. Pediatrics. 1977;60:217.

104. Kim HW, Brandt CD, Kapikian AZ, et al. Human reoviruslike agent infection. Occurrence in adult contacts of pediatric patients with gastroenteritis. JAMA. 1977;238:404.

105. Wenman WM, Hinde D, Feltham S, et al. Rotavirus infection in adults: Results of a prospective family study. N Engl J Med. 1979;301:303.

106. Kapikian AZ, Dienstag JL, Purcell RH. Immune electron microscopy as a method for the detection, identification, and characterization of agents not cultivable in an in vitro system. In: Rose NR, Friedman H, eds. Manual of Clinical Immunology. Washington, DC: American Society for Microbiology; 1976.

107. Zissis G, Lambert JP. Different serotypes of human rotaviruses. Lancet. 1978;1:38.

108. Beards GM, Pilford JN, Thouless ME, et al. Rotavirus serotypes by serum neutralization. J Med Virol. 1980;5:231.

109. Blacklow NR, Cukor G. Viral gastroenteritis. N Engl J Med. 1981;304:397.

110. Urasawa S, Urasawa T, Taniguchi K. Three human rotavirus serotypes demonstrated by plaque neutralization of isolated strains. Infect Immun. 1982;38:781.

111. Fonteyne J, Zissis G, Lambert JP. Recurrent rotavirus gastroenteritis. Lancet. 1978;1:983.

112. Desselberger U, Iturriza-Gomara M, Gray JJ. Rotavirus epidemiology and surveillance. Novartis Found Symp. 2001;238:125.

113. Estes MK. Rotaviruses and their replication. In: Fields BN, Knipe DM, Howley PM, eds. Fields Virology. 4th ed. Philadelphia: Lippincott-Raven; 2001:1747-1785.

114. Kapikan A, Channock RM. Rotaviruses. In: Fields BN, Knipe DM, Howley PM, eds. Fields Virology. 4th ed. Philadelphia: Lippincott-Raven; 2001:1787-1833.

115. Fischer TK, Page NA, Griffin DD, et al. Characterization of incompletely typed rotavirus strains from Guinea-Bissau: Identification of G8 and G9 types and a high frequency of mixed infections. Virology. 2003;311(1):125-133.

116. Griffin DD, Fletcher M, Levy ME, et al. Outbreaks of adult gastroenteritis traced to a single genotype of rotavirus. J Infect Dis. 2002;185:1502.

117. Bern C, Unicomb L, Gentsch JR, et al. Rotavirus diarrhea in Bangladeshi children: Correlation of disease severity with serotypes. J Clin Microbiol. 1992;30:3234.

118. Cascio A, Vizzi E, Alaimo C, Arista S. Rotavirus gastroenteritis in Italian children: Can severity of symptoms be related to the infecting virus? Clin Infect Dis. 2001;32:1126-1132.

119. Atmar RL, Estes MK. Diagnosis of noncultivatable gastroenteritis viruses, the human caliciviruses. Clin Microbiol Rev. 2001;14:15.

120. Yolken R, Kim HW, Clem T, et al. Enzyme immunoassay (ELISA) for the detection of human reovirus-like agent in human stools. Lancet. 1977;2:263.

121. Kalica AR, Purcell RH, Sereno NM, et al. Microtiter solid phase radioimmunoassay for detection of the human reovirus-like agent in stools. J Immunol. 1977;118:1275.

122. Middleton PJ, Petrie M, Hewitt CM, et al. Counter-immunoelectro-osmophoresis for the detection of infantile gastroenteritis virus (orbi group) antigen and antibody. J Clin Pathol. 1976;29:191.

123. Middleton PJ, Szymanski MT, Abbott GD, et al. Orbivirus acute gastroenteritis of infancy. Lancet. 1974;1:1241.

124. Davidson GP, Goller I, Bishop RF, et al. Immunofluorescence in duodenal mucosa of children with acute enteritis due to a new virus. J Clin Pathol. 1975;28:263.

125. Thomas EE, Puterman ML, Kawano E, et al. Evaluation of seven immunoassays for detection of rotavirus in pediatric stool samples. J Clin Microbiol. 1988;26: 1189-1193.

126. Flores J, Purcell RH, Perez I, et al. A dot hybridization assay for detection of rotavirus. Lancet. 1983;1:555.

127. Flewett TH, Bryden AS, Davies H, et al. Relation between viruses from acute gastroenteritis of children and newborn calves. Lancet. 1974;2:61.

128. Guerrant RL. Pathophysiology of the enterotoxic and viral diarrhea. In: Chen LC, Scrimshaw NS, eds. Diarrhea and Malnutrition: Interactions, Mechanisms and Interventions. New York: Plenum; 1983;23-43.

129. Middleton PJ, Szymanski MT, Abbott GD, et al. Orbivirus acute gastroenteritis of infancy. Lancet. 1974;1:1241.

130. Davidson GP, Goller I, Bishop RF, et al. Immunofluorescence in duodenal mucosa of children with acute enteritis due to a new virus. J Clin Pathol. 1974;28:263.

131. Sack DA, Chowdhury AMAK, Eusof A, et al. Oral hydration in rotavirus diarrhea: A double blind comparison of sucrose with glucose electrolyte solution. Lancet. 1978;2:280.

132. Davidson GP, Barnes GL. Structural and functional abnormalities of the small intestine in infants and young children with rotavirus enteritis. Acta Paediatr Scand. 1979;68:181.

133. Shepherd RW, Butler DG, Cutz E, et al. The mucosal lesion in viral enteritis: Extent and dynamics of the epithelial response to virus invasion in transmissible gastroenteritis of piglets. Gastroenterology. 1979;76:770.

134. Davidson GP, Gall DG, Petric M, et al. Human rotavirus enteritis induced in conventional piglets: Intestinal structure and transport. J Clin Invest. 1977;60:1402.

135. Glass RI, Kilgore PE, Holman RC, et al. The epidemiology of rotavirus diarrhea in the United States: Surveillance and estimates of disease burden. J Infect Dis. 1996;174(Suppl 1):S5-S11.

136. Perez-Schael I, Guntinas MJ, Perez M, et al. Efficacy of the rhesus rotavirus-based quadrivalent vaccine in infants and young children in Venezuela. N Engl J Med. 1997;337:1181-1187.

137. Bernstein DI, Glass RI, Rodgers G, et al. Evaluation of rhesus rotavirus monovalent and tetravalent reassortant vaccines in US children. US Rotavirus Vaccine Efficacy Group. JAMA. 1995;273:1191-1196.

138. Rennels MB, Glass RI, Dennehy PH, et al. Safety and efficacy of high-dose rhesushuman reassortant rotavirus vaccines—Report of the National Multicenter Trial. United States Rotavirus Vaccine Efficacy Group. Pediatrics. 1996;97:7-13.

139. Joensu J, Koskenniemi E, Pang XL, Vesikari T. Randomised placebo-controlled trial of rhesus-human reassortant rotavirus vaccine for prevention of severe rotavirus gastroenteritis. Lancet. 1997;350:1205-1209.

140. Murphy BR, Morens DM, Simonsen L, et al. Reappraisal of the association of intussusception with the licensed live rotavirus vaccine challenges initial conclusions. J Infect Dis. 2003;187:1301.

141. Murphy TV, Smith PJ, Gargiullo PM, Schwartz B. The first rotavirus vaccine and intussusception: Epidemiological studies and policy decisions. J Infect Dis. 2003;187:1309.

142. Murphy TV, Gargiullo PM, Massoudi MS, et al. Intussusception among infants given an oral rotavirus vaccine. N Engl J Med. 2001;344:564. Erratum in N Engl J Med 2001;344:1564.

143. Centers for Disease Control and Prevention. Intussusception among recipients of rotavirus vaccine—United States, 1998-1999. MMWR 1999;48:577-581.

144. Nakagomi T. Rotavirus infection and intussusception: A view from retrospect. Microbiol Immunol. 2000;44:619.

145. Barnes GL, Lund JS, Mitchell SV, et al. Early phase II trial of human rotavirus vaccine candidate RV3. Vaccine. 2002;20:2950.

146. Offit PA. The future of rotavirus vaccines. Semin Pediatr Infect Dis. 2002;13:19.

147. Hoshino Y, Jones RW, Chanock RM, Kapikian AZ. Generation and characterization of six single VP4 gene substitution reassortant rotavirus vaccine candidates: Each bears a single human rotavirus VP4 gene encoding P serotype 1A[8] or 1B[4] and the remaining 10 genes of rhesus monkey rotavirus MMU18006 or bovine rotavirus UK. Vaccine. 2002;20:3576.

148. Ward RL. Possible mechanisms of protection elicited by candidate rotavirus vaccines as determined with the adult mouse model. Viral Immunol. 2003;16:17.

149. Rotavirus vaccines, an update. Wkly Epidemiol Rec. 2003;78:2.

150. Perez-Schael I, Escalona M, Salinas B, et al. Intussusception-associated hospitalization among Venezuelan infants during 1998 through 2001: Anticipating rotavirus vaccines. Pediatr Infect Dis J. 2003;22:234.

151. Dingle JH, Badger GF, Jordan WS Jr. Illnesses in the Home: A Study of 25,000 Illnesses in a Group of Cleveland Families. Cleveland: Press of Western Reserve University; 1964.

152. Gordon I, Ingraham HS, Korns RF. Transmission of epidemic gastroenteritis to human volunteers by oral administration of fecal filtrates. J Exp Med. 1947;86:409.

153. Jordan WS, Gordon I, Dorrance WR. A study of illness in a group of Cleveland families. VII. Transmission of acute nonbacterial gastroenteritis to volunteers: Evidence for two different etiologic agents. J Exp Med. 1953;98:461.

154. Kojima S, Fukumi H, Kusama H, et al. Studies on the causative agent of the infectious diarrhea; records of the experiments on human volunteers. Jpn Med J. 1948;1:467.

155. Klein JO, Lerner AM, Finland M. Acute gastroenteritis associated with echo virus, type II. Am J Med Sci. 1950;240:749.

156. Kerr AA, McQuillin J, Downham MAPS, et al. Gastric "flu" influenza B causing abdominal symptoms in children. Lancet. 1975;1:291.

157. Adler JL, Zickl R. Winter vomiting disease. J Infect Dis. 1969;119:668.

158. Dolin R, Blacklow NR, DuPont H, et al. Transmission of acute infectious nonbacterial gastroenteritis to volunteers by oral administration of stool filtrates. J Infect Dis. 1971;123:307.

159. Kapikian AZ, Wyatt RG, Dolin R, et al. Visualization by immune electron microscopy of a 27-nm particle associated with acute infectious nonbacterial gastroenteritis. J Virol. 1972;10:1075.

160. Wyatt RG, Dolin R, Blacklow NR, et al. Comparison of three agents of acute infectious nonbacterial gastroenteritis by cross-challenge in volunteers. J Infect Dis. 1974;129:709.

161. Dolin R, Treanor JJ, Madore HP. Novel agents of viral enteritis in humans. J Infect Dis. 1987;155:365-376.

162. Clarke SKR, Cook GT, Egglestone SI, et al. A virus from epidemic vomiting disease. Br Med J. 1972;3:86.

163. Agus SG, Dolin R, Wyatt RG, et al. Acute infectious nonbacterial gastroenteritis. Intestinal histopathology. Ann Intern Med. 1973;79:18.

164. Schreiber DS, Trier JS, Blacklow NR. Recent advances in viral gastroenteritis. Gastroenterology. 1977;73:174.

165. Levy AG, Widerlite L, Schwartz CJ, et al. Jejunal adenylate cyclase activity in human subjects during viral gastroenteritis. Gastroenterology. 1976;70:321.

166. Blacklow NR, Dolin R, Fedson DS, et al. Acute infectious nonbacterial gastroenteritis: Etiology and pathogenesis. Ann Intern Med. 1972;76:993.

167. Glass RI, Noel J, Ando T, et al. The epidemiology of enteric caliciviruses from humans: A reassessment using new diagnostics. J Infect Dis. 2000;181(Suppl 2):S254.

168. Koopmans M, von Bonsdorff C-H, Vinje J, et al. Foodborne viruses. FEMS Microbiol Rev. 2002;26:187.

169. Wilhelmi I, Roman E, Sanchez-Fauquier A. Viruses causing gastroenteritis. Clin Microbiol Infect. 2003;9:247.

170. Oshiro LS, Haley CE, Roberto RR, et al. A 27-nm virus isolated during an outbreak of acute infectious nonbacterial gastroenteritis in a convalescent hospital: A possible new serotype. J Infect Dis. 1981;143:791.

171. Brandt CD, Kim HW, Rodriguez WJ, et al. Adenoviruses and pediatric gastroenteritis. J Infect Dis. 1985;151:437-443.

172. Gerna G, Passarani N, Battaglia M, et al. Human enteric coronaviruses: Antigenic relatedness to human coronavirus OC43 and possible etiologic role in viral gastroenteritis. J Infect Dis. 1985;151:796-802.

173. Battaglia M, Passarani N, DiMatteo A, et al. Human enteric coronaviruses: Further characterization and immunoblotting of viral proteins. J Infect Dis. 1987;144: 140-143.

174. Yolken R, Santosham M, Reid R, et al. Pestiviruses: Major etiological agents of gastroenteritis in human infants and children (Abstract). Clin Res. 1988;36:780.

175. Koopmans MG, Goosen ESM, Lima AAM, et al. Association of torovirus with acute and persistent diarrhea in children. Pediatr Infect Dis J. 1997;16:504-507.

176. Koopmans M, Petric M, Glass RI, Monroe SS. Enzyme-linked immunosorbent assay reactivity of torovirus-like particles in fecal specimens from humans with diarrhea. J Clin Microbiol. 1993;31:2738-2744.

177. Grohmann GS, Glass RI, Pereira HG, et al. Enteric viruses and diarrhea in HIV-infected patients. N Engl J Med. 1993;329:14-20.

178. Greenberg HB, Valdesuso J, Yolken RH, et al. Role of Norwalk virus in outbreaks of nonbacterial gastroenteritis. J Infect Dis. 1979;139:564.

179. Kaplan JE, Gary GW Jr, Baron RC, et al. Epidemiology of Norwalk gastroenteritis and the role of the Norwalk virus in outbreaks of nonbacterial gastroenteritis. Ann Intern Med. 1982;96:756.

180. Moe CL, Monroe SS, Gary HE Jr, et al. Detection of astrovirus in pediatric stool samples by immunoassay and RNA probe. J Clin Microbiol. 1991;29:2390-2396.

181. Lew JF, Moe CL, Monroe SS, et al. Astrovirus and adenovirus associated with diarrhea in children in day care settings. J Infect Dis. 1991;164:673-678.

182. Cruz JR, Bartlett AV, Herrmann JE, et al. Astrovirus-associated diarrhea among Guatemalan ambulatory, rural children. J Clin Microbiol. 1992;30:1140-1144.

183. Lew JF, Glass RI, Petric M, et al. Six-year retrospective surveillance of gastroenteritis virus identified at ten electron microscopy centers in the United States and Canada. Pediatr Infect Dis. 1990;9:709-714.

184. Greenberg HB, Wyatt RG, Valdesuso J, et al. Solid-phase microtiter radioimmunoassay for detection of the Norwalk strain of acute nonbacterial, epidemic gastroenteritis virus and its antibodies. J Med Virol. 1978;2:97.

185. Jiang X, Wang M, Graham DY, et al. Expression, self-assembly, and antigenicity of the Norwalk virus capsid protein. J Virol. 1992;66:6527-6232.

186. Parrino TA, Schreiber DS, Trier JS, et al. Clinical immunity in acute gastroenteritis caused by Norwalk agent. N Engl J Med. 1977;297:86-89.

187. Herrmann JE, Perron-Henry DM, Blacklow NR. Antigen detection with monoclonal antibodies for the diagnosis of adenovirus gastroenteritis. J Infect Dis. 1987;155:1167-1171.

188. Shinozaki T, Araki K, Ushijima H, et al. Use of Graham 293 cells in suspension for isolating enteric adenoviruses from the stools of patients with acute gastroenteritis. J Infect Dis. 1987;156:246.

189. Neil C, Gomes SA, Leite JPG, et al. Direct detection and differentiation of fastidious and nonfastidious adenoviruses in stools by using a specific nonradioactive probe. J Clin Microbiol. 1986;24:785-789.

190. von Bonsdorff CH, Hovi T, Makela P, et al. Rotavirus associated with acute gastroenteritis in adults. Lancet. 1976;2:423.

191. Wenman WM, Hinde D, Feltham S, et al. Rotavirus infection in adults. Results of a prospective study. N Engl J Med. 1979;301:306.

192. Yolken RH, Bishop CA, Townsend TR, et al. Infectious gastroenteritis in bone-marrow transplant recipients. N Engl J Med. 1982;306:1099.

193. Goodgame RW, Greenough WB III. Cholera in Africa: A message for the west. Ann Intern Med. 1975;82:101.

194. Weissman JB, DeWitt WE, Thompson J, et al. A case of cholera in Texas, 1973. Am J Epidemiol. 1975;100:487.

195. Blake PA, Allegra DT, Snyder JD, et al. Cholera: A possible endemic focus in the United States. N Engl J Med. 1980;302:305.

196. Blake PA, Rosenberg ML, Florencia J, et al. Cholera in Portugal, 1974. II. Transmission by bottled mineral water. Am J Epidemiol. 1977;105:344.

197. Baine WB, Mazzotti M, Greco D, et al. Epidemiology of cholera in Italy in 1973. Lancet. 1974;2:1370.

198. Gitelson S. Gastrectomy, achlorhydria and cholera. Isr J Med Sci. 1971;7:663.

199. Ramamurthy T, Garg S, Sharma R, et al. Emergence of novel strain of Vibrio cholerae with epidemic potential in southern and eastern India (Letter). Lancet. 1993;341:703-704.

200. Albert MJ, Siddique AK, Islam MS, et al. Large outbreak of clinical cholera due to Vibrio cholerae non-O1 in Bangladesh (Letter). Lancet. 1993;341:704.

201. Bhattacharya MK, Bhattacharya SK, Garg S, et al. Outbreak of Vibrio cholerae non-O1 in India and Bangladesh (Letter). Lancet. 1993;341:1346-1347.

202. Shimada T, Nair GB, Deb BC, et al. Outbreak of Vibrio cholerae non-O1 in India and Bangladesh (Letter). Lancet. 1993;341:1347.

203. Centers for Disease Control and Prevention. Emerging infectious diseases: Imported cholera associated with a newly described toxigenic Vibrio cholerae O139 strain-California, 1993. MMWR Morb Mortal Wkly Rep. 1993;42:501-503.

204. Snow J. On the Mode of Communication of Cholera. 2nd ed. London: Churchill; 1855.

205. De SN, Bhattacharya K, Sarkar JK. A study of the pathogenicity of strains of Bacterium coli from acute and chronic enteritis. J Pathol Bacteriol. 1956;71:201.

206. Trabulsi LR. Revelação de colibacilos associados as diarreias infantis pelo metodo da infecão experimental da alca ligade do intestino do coelho. Rev Inst Med Trop Sao Paulo. 1964;6:197.

207. Taylor J, Wilkins MP, Payne JM. Relation of rabbit gut reaction to enteropathogenic Escherichia coli. Br J Exp Pathol. 1961;42:43.

208. Taylor J, Bettleheim KA. The action of chloroform-killed suspensions of enteropathogenic Escherichia coli on ligated rabbit-gut segments. J Gen Microbiol. 1966; 42:309.

209. Smith HW, Halls S. Studies on Escherichia coli enterotoxin. J Pathol Bacteriol. 1967;93:531.

210. Gorbach SL, Banwell JG, Chatterjee BD, et al. Acute undifferentiated human diarrhea in the tropics. I. Alterations in intestinal microflora. J Clin Invest. 1971;50:881.

211. Banwell JG, Gorbach SL, Pierce NF, et al. Acute undifferentiated human diarrhea in the tropics. II. Alterations in intestinal fluid and electrolyte movements. J Clin Invest. 1971;50:890.

212. Sack RB, Gorbach SL, Banwell JG, et al. Enterotoxigenic Escherichia coli isolated from patients with severe cholera-like disease. J Infect Dis. 1971;123:378.

213. DuPont HL, Formal SB, Hornick RB, et al. Pathogenesis of Escherichia coli diarrhea. N Engl J Med. 1971;285:1.

214. Evans DG, Evans DJ Jr, Pierce NF. Differences in the response of rabbit small intestine to heat-labile and heat-stable enterotoxins of Escherichia coli. Infect Immun. 1973;7:873.

215. Guerrant RL, Brunton LL, Schnaitman TC, et al. Cyclic adenosine monophosphate and alteration of Chinese hamster ovary cell morphology: A rapid, sensitive in vitro assay for the enterotoxins of Vibrio cholerae and Escherichia coli. Infect Immun. 1974;10:320.

216. Donta ST, Moon HW, Whipp SC. Detection of heat-labile Escherichia coli enterotoxin with the use of adrenal cells in tissue culture. Science. 1974;183:334.

217. Guerrant RL, Brunton LL. Characterization of the Chinese hamster ovary cell assay for the enterotoxins of Vibrio cholerae and Escherichia coli and for antitoxin: Differential inhibition by gangliosides, specific antisera, and toxoid. J Infect Dis. 1977;135:720.

218. Honda T, Arita M, Takeda Y, et al. Further evaluation of the Biken test (modified Elek test) for detection of enterotoxigenic E. coli producing heat-labile enterotoxin and application of the test to sampling of heat-stable enterotoxin. J Clin Microbiol. 1982;16:60.

219. Alderete JF, Robertson DC. Purification and chemical characterization of the heat-stable enterotoxin produced by porcine strains of enterotoxigenic Escherichia coli. Infect Immun. 1978;19:1021.

220. Dean AG, Ching YC, Williams RG, et al. Test for Escherichia coli enterotoxin using infant mice: Application in a study of diarrhea in children in Honolulu. J Infect Dis. 1972;125:407.

221. Gyles CL. Limitation of the infant mouse test for E. coli heat-stable enterotoxin. Can J Comp Med. 1979;43:371-379.

222. Kennedy DJ, Greenberg RN, Dunn JA, et al. Effects of Escherichia coli heat stable enterotoxin STb on intestines of mice, rats, rabbits and piglets. Infect Immun. 1984;46:639-643.

223. Weikel CS, Mellans HN, Guerrant RL. In vivo and in vitro effects of a novel enterotoxin, STb, produced by Escherichia coli. J Infect Dis. 1986;153:893-901.

224. Rosenberg ML, Koplan JP, Wachsmuth IK, et al. Epidemic diarrhea at Crater Lake from enterotoxigenic Escherichia coli. A large, waterborne outbreak. Ann Intern Med. 1977;86:714.

225. Korzeniowski OM, Dantas W, Trabulsi LR, et al. A controlled study of endemic sporadic diarrhea among adult residents of southern Brazil. Trans R Soc Trop Med Hyg. 1984;78:363-369.

226. Hughes JM, Rouse JD, Barada FA, et al. Etiology of summer diarrhea among the Navajo. Am J Trop Med Hyg. 1980;29:613.

227. Katz DE, Taylor DN. Parasitic infections of the gastrointestinal tract. Gastroenterol Clin North Am. 2001;30:79.

228. Chappell CL, Okhuysen PC. Cryptosporidiosis. Curr Opin Infect Dis. 2002;15:523.

229. Dillingham RA, Lima AA, Guerrant RL. Cryptosporidiosis: Epidemiology and impact. Microbes Infect. 2002;4:105.

230. Leav BA, Mackay M, Ward HD. Cryptosporidium species: New insights and old challenges. Clin Infect Dis. 2003;36:903.

231. Tzipori S, Ward H. Cryptosporidiosis: Biology, pathogenesis and disease. Microbes Infect. 2002;4:1047.

232. Riggs MW. Recent advances in cryptosporidiosis: The immune response. Microbes Infect. 2002;4:1067-1080.

233. Amadi B, Mwiya M, Musuku J, et al. Effect of nitazoxanide on morbidity and mortality in Zambian children with cryptosporidiosis: A randomised controlled trial. Lancet. 2002;360:1375.

234. Cedillo-Rivera R, Chavez B, Gonzalez-Robles A, et al. In vitro effect of nitazoxanide against Entamoeba histolytica, Giardia intestinalis and Trichomonas vaginalis trophozoites. J Eukaryot Microbiol. 2002;49:20.

235. Gilles HM, Hoffman PS. Treatment of intestinal parasitic infections: A review of nitazoxanide. Trends Parasitol. 2002;18:95.

236. Diaz E, Mondragon J, Ramirez E, Bernal R. Epidemiology and control of intestinal parasites with nitazoxanide in children in Mexico. Am J Trop Med Hyg. 2003;68:384.

237. Guerrant RL, Van Gilder T, Steiner TS, et al. Practice guidelines for the management of infectious diarrhea. Clin Infect Dis. 2001;32:33.

238. Palmer DL, Koster FT, Islam AFMR, et al. A comparison of sucrose and glucose in oral electrolyte therapy of cholera and other severe diarrheas. N Engl J Med. 1977;297:1107.

239. Ericsson CD, Evans DG, DuPont HL, et al. Bismuth subsalicylate inhibits activity of crude toxins of Escherichia coli and Vibrio cholerae. J Infect Dis. 1977;136:693.

240. Carneiro-Filho BA, Bushen OY, Brito GA, et al. Glutamine analogues as adjunctive therapy for infectious diarrhea. Curr Infect Dis Rep. 2003;5:114.

241. Cremonini F, Di Caro S, Nista EC, et al. Meta-analysis: The effect of probiotic administration on antibiotic-associated diarrhoea. Aliment Pharmacol Ther. 2002;16:1461.

242. D'Souza AL, Rajkumar C, Cooke J, Bulpitt CJ. Probiotics in prevention of antibiotic associated diarrhoea: meta-analysis. BMJ. 2002;324:136.

243. Isolauri E. Probiotics for infectious diarrhoea. Gut. 2003;52:436.

244. Cohen J, West AB, Bini EJ. Infectious diarrhea in human immunodeficiency virus. Gastroenterol Clin North Am. 2001;30:637.

245. Oldfield EC 3rd. Evaluation of chronic diarrhea in patients with human immunodeficiency virus infection. Rev Gastroenterol Disord. 2002;2:176.

246. Gelb A, Miller S. AIDS and gastroenterology. Am J Gastroenterol. 1986;81:619-622.

247. Soave R, Johnson WD. Cryptosporidium and Isospora belli infections. J Infect Dis. 1988;157:225-229.

248. Guerrant RL, Thielman NM. Emerging enteric protozoa: Cryptosporidium, Cyclospora and microsporidia. In: Scheld WM, Armstrong D, Hughes JM, eds. Emerging Infections. Washington, DC: ASM Press; 1997:233-245.

249. Kotler DP, Goetz HP, Lange M, et al. Enteropathy associated with the acquired immunodeficiency syndrome. Ann Intern Med. 1984;101:421-428.

250. Gillin JS, Shike M, Alcock N, et al. Malabsorption and mucosal abnormalities of the small intestine in the acquired immunodeficiency syndrome. Ann Intern Med. 1985;102:619-622.

251. Current WL, Reese NC, Ernst JV, et al. Human cryptosporidiosis in immunocompetent and immunodeficient persons. N Engl J Med. 1983;308:1252.

252. Smith PD, Lance C, Gill VJ, et al. Intestinal infections in patients with the acquired immunodeficiency syndrome (AIDS). Ann Intern Med. 1988;108:328-333.

253. Laughon BE, Druckman DA, Vernon A, et al. Prevalence of enteric pathogens in homosexual men with and without acquired immunodeficiency syndrome. Gastroenterology. 1988;94:984.

254. Quinn TC, Stamm WE, Goodell SE, et al. The polymicrobial origin of intestinal infections in homosexual men. N Engl J Med. 1983;309:576-582.

255. Kotler DP, Francisco A, Clayton F, et al. Small intestinal injury and parasitic diseases in AIDS. Ann Intern Med. 1990;113:444-449.

256. Connolly GM, Forbes A, Gazzard BG. Investigation of seemingly pathogen-negative diarrhoea in patients infected with HIV1. Gut 1990;31:886-889.

257. Guerrant RL, Bobak DA. Bacterial and protozoal gastroenteritis. N Engl J Med. 1991;325:327-340.

258. DeHovitz JA, Pape JW, Boncy M, Johnson WD Jr. Clinical manifestations and therapy of *Isospora belli* infection in patients with the acquired immunodeficiency syndrome. N Engl J Med. 1986;315:87-90.

259. Pape JW, Verdier RI, Boncy M, et al. *Cyclospora* infection in adults infected with HIV. Clinical manifestations, treatment, and prophylaxis. Ann Intern Med. 1994;121:654-657.

260. Guerrant RL, Thielman NM. Emerging enteric protozoa: *Cryptosporidium, Cyclospora,* and Microsporidia. In: Scheld WM, Armstrong D, Hughes JM, eds. Emerging Infections. Washington, DC: ASM Press; 1998:233-245.

261. Carter TR, Cooper PH, Petri WA Jr, et al. *Pneumocystis carinii* infection of the small intestine in a patient with acquired immune deficiency syndrome. Am J Clin Pathol. 1988;89:679-683.

262. Chachoua A, Dieterich D, Krasinski K, et al. 9-(1,3-Dihydroxy-2-propoxy-methyl)guanine (ganciclovir) in the treatment of cytomegalovirus gastrointestinal disease with the acquired immunodeficiency syndrome. Ann Intern Med. 1987;107:133-137.

263. Merson MH, Morris GK, Sack DA, et al. Travelers' diarrhea in Mexico, a prospective study of physicians and family members attending a congress. N Engl J Med. 1976; 294:1299.

264. Celum CL, Chaisson RE, Rutherford GW, et al. Incidence of salmonellosis in patients with AIDS. J Infect Dis. 1987;156:998-1002.

265. Jacobs JL, Gold JWM, Murray HW, et al. *Salmonella* infections in patients with the acquired immunodeficiency syndrome. Ann Intern Med. 1985;102:186-188.

266. Glaser JB, Morton-Kute L, Berger SR, et al. Recurrent *Salmonella typhimurium* bacteremia associated with the acquired immunodeficiency syndrome. Ann Intern Med. 1985;102:189-193.

267. Sperber SJ, Schleupner CJ: Salmonellosis during infection with human immunodeficiency virus. Rev Infect Dis. 1987;9:925-934.

268. Grohman GS, Glass RI, Pereira HG, et al. Enteric viruses and diarrhea in HIV-infected patients. N Engl J Med. 1993;329:14-20.

269. Bobak DA. Gastrointestinal infections caused by cytomegalovirus. Curr Infect Dis Rep. 2003;5:10.

270. Drew WL. Cytomegalovirus disease in the highly active antiretroviral therapy era. Curr Infect Dis Rep. 2003;5:25.

271. Hayes C, Elliot E, Krales E, Downer G. Food and water safety for persons infected with human immunodeficiency virus. Clin Infect Dis. 2003;36(Suppl 2):S106.

272. Guerrant RL, Hughes JM, Lima NL, et al. Microbiology of diarrhea in developed and developing countries. Rev Infect Dis. 1990;12(Suppl):S41-S50.

273. Stamm WE, Weinstein RA, Dixon RE. Comparison of endemic and epidemic nosocomial infections. Am J Med. 1981;70:393-397.

274. Lima N, Searcy M, Guerrant R. Nosocomial diarrhea rates exceed those of other nosocomial infections on ICU and pediatric wards. Abstract 1050. Presented at the Twenty-Sixth Interscience Conference on Antimicrobial Agents and Chemotherapy, New Orleans, 1986.

275. Lima NL, Guerrant RL, Kaiser DL, et al. Nosocomial diarrhea: A possible risk factor for nosocomial infections (Abstract). Clin Res. 1988;36:580.

276. Welliver RC, McLaughlin S. Unique epidemiology of nosocomial infection in a children's hospital. Am J Dis Child. 1984;138:131-135.

277. Kelly WJ, Patrick MR, Hilman KM. Study of diarrhea in critically ill patients. Crit Care Med. 1983;1:7-9.

278. Ciesla WP, Bobak DA. Management and prevention of *Clostridium difficile*–associated diarrhea. Curr Infect Dis Rep. 2001;3:109.

279. Bartlett JG. *Clostridium difficile*–associated enteric disease. Curr Infect Dis Rep. 2002;4:477.

280. Kyne L, Hamel MB, Polavaram R, Kelly CP. Health care costs and mortality associated with nosocomial diarrhea due to *Clostridium difficile*. Clin Infect Dis. 2002;34:346.

281. Barbut F, Petit JC. Epidemiology of *Clostridium difficile*–associated infections. Clin Microbiol Infect. 2001;7:405.

282. Kent KC, Rubin MS, Wroblewski L, et al. The impact of *Clostridium difficile* on a surgical service: A prospective study of 374 patients. Ann Surg. 1998;227:296-301.

283. Brown E, Talbot GH, Axelrod P, et al. Risk factors for *Clostridium difficile* toxin–associated diarrhea. Infect Control Hosp Epidemiol. 1990;11:283-290.

284. Samore MH, Venkataraman L, DeGirolami PC, et al. Clinical and molecular epidemiology of sporadic and clustered cases of nosocomial *Clostridium difficile* diarrhea. Am J Med. 1996;100:32-40.

285. McFarland LV. Epidemiology, risk factors, and treatments for antibiotic-associated diarrhea. Dig Dis. 1998;16:292-307.

286. Samore MH, Bettin KM, DeGirolami PC, et al. Wide diversity of *Clostridium difficile* types at a tertiary referral hospital. J Infect Dis. 1994;170:615-621.

287. Neill MA, Rice SK, Ahmad NV, Flanigan TP. Cryptosporidiosis: An unrecognized cause of diarrhea in elderly hospitalized patients. Clin Infect Dis. 1996;22:168-170.

288. Yolken RJ, Bishop CA, Towsend R, et al. Infectious gastroenteritis in bone marrow transplant recipients. N Engl J Med. 1982;306:1009-1012.

289. Chadwick PR, Beards G, Brown D, et al. Management of hospital outbreaks of gastroenteritis due to small roundstructured viruses. J Hosp Infect. 2000;45:1.

290. Dennehy PH, Nelson SM, Spangenberger S, et al. A prospective case-control study of the role of astrovirus in acute diarrhea among hospitalized young children. J Infect Dis. 2001;184:10.

291. Gelber SE, Ratner AJ. Hospital-acquired viral pathogens in the neonatal intensive care unit. Semin Perinatol. 2002;26:346.

292. Farber BF, Brennen JC, Puntereri AJ, et al. A prospective study of nosocomial infections in a chronic care facility. J Am Geriatr Soc. 1984;32:499.

293. Nicolle LE, McIntyre M, Zacharias H, et al. Twelve-month surveillance of infections in institutionalized elderly men. J Am Geriatr Soc. 1984;32:513.

294. Sims RV, Hauser RJ, Adewale AO, et al. Acute gastroenteritis in three community-based nursing homes. J Gerontol [A] Biol Sci Med Sci. 1995;50:M252-M256.

295. Simor AE, Bradley SF, Strausbaugh LJ, et al. *Clostridium difficile* in long-term-care facilities for the elderly. Infect Control Hosp Epidemiol. 2002;23:696.

296. Bender BS, Laughon BE, Gaydos C, et al. Is *Clostridium difficile* endemic in chronic-care facilities? Lancet. 1986;2:1279.

297. Treolar AJ, Kalra L. Mortality and *Clostridium difficile* diarrhoea in the elderly. Lancet. 1987;2:1279.

298. Pickering LK, Evans DG, Dupont HL, et al. Diarrhea caused by *Shigella*, rotavirus and *Giardia* in day care centers: Prospective study. J Pediatr. 1981;99:51-56.

299. Mitchell DK, Monroe SS, Jiang X, et al. Virologic features of an astrovirus diarrhea outbreak in a day care center revealed by reverse transcriptase–polymerase chain reaction. J Infect Dis. 1995;172:1437-1444.

300. Mitchell DK, Van R, Morrow AL, et al. Outbreaks of astrovirus gastroenteritis in day care centers. J Pediatr. 1993;123:725-732.

301. Centers for Disease Control and Prevention. Cryptosporidiosis among children attending day-care centers: Georgia, Pennsylvania, Michigan, California, New Mexico. MMWR Morb Mortal Wkly Rep. 1984;33:599.

302. Alpert G, Bell LM, Kirkpatrick CE, et al. Cryptosporidiosis in a day-care center. N Engl J Med. 1984;311:860-861.

303. Taylor JP, Perdue JN, Dingley D, et al. Cryptosporidiosis outbreak in a day-care center. Am J Dis Child. 1985;139:1023-1025.

304. Bartlett AV, Moore M, Gary GW, et al. Diarrheal illness among infants and toddlers in daycare centers. I. Epidemiology and pathogens. J Pediatr. 1985;107:495-502.

305. Guerrant RL, Lohr JA, Williams EK. Acute infectious diarrhea. I. Epidemiology, etiology, and pathogenesis. Pediatr Infect Dis. 1986;5:353-359.

306. Kean BH. The diarrhea of travelers to Mexico. Summary of five-year study. Ann Intern Med. 1963;59:605.

307. Psalms 22:14.

308. Consensus development conference statement on travelers' diarrhea. Rev Infect Dis. 1986;8(Suppl):227-233.

309. Keystone JS, Kozarsky PE. Health advice for international travel. In: Guerrant RL, Walker DH, Weller PF, eds. Tropical Infectious Diseases: Principles, Pathogens and Practice. Philadelphia: WB Saunders; 1999:1345-1365.

310. Ramzan NN. Traveler's diarrhea. Gastroenterol Clin North Am. 2001;30:665.

311. Chen LH, Wilson ME. Recent advances and new challenges in travel medicine. Curr Infect Dis Rep. 2002;4:50

312. Cheng AC, Thielman NM. Update on traveler's diarrhea. Curr Infect Dis Rep. 2002;4:70.

313. Lowenstein MS, Balows A, Gangarosa EJ. Turista at an international congress in Mexico. Lancet. 1973;1:529.

314. The diarrhea of travelers: Turista (Editorial). JAMA. 1962;180:402.

315. Higgens AR. Observations on the health of United States personnel living in Cairo, Egypt. Am J Trop Med Hyg. 1955;4:970.

316. Steffen R. Epidemiologic studies of travelers' diarrhea, severe gastrointestinal infections, and cholera. Rev Infect Dis. 1986;8(Suppl 2):122-130.

317. Steffen R, Rickernbach M, Wilhelm U, et al. Health problems after travel to developing countries. J Infect Dis. 1987;156:84-91.

318. Kean BH, Schaffner W, Brennan RW. The diarrhea of travelers. V. Prophylaxis with phthalylsulfathiazole and neomycin sulphate. JAMA. 1962;180:367-371.

319. Rowe B, Taylor J, Bettelheim KA. An investigation of travelers' diarrhea. Lancet. 1970;1:1.

320. Gorbach SL, Kean BH, Evans DG, et al. Travelers' diarrhea and toxigenic *Escherichia coli*. N Engl J Med. 1975;292:933.

321. Sack DA, Kaminsky DC, Sack RB, et al. Enterotoxigenic *Escherichia coli* diarrhea of travelers: A prospective study of American Peace Corps volunteers. Johns Hopkins Med J. 1977;141:63.

322. Guerrant RL, Rouse JD, Hughes JM. Turista among members of the Yale Glee Club in Latin America. Am J Trop Med Hyg. 1980;29:895.

323. Turner AC. Travelers' diarrhoea: A survey of symptoms, occurrence, and possible prophylaxis. BMJ. 1967;4:453-454.

324. Black RE. Pathogens that cause travelers' diarrhea in Latin America and Africa. Rev Infect Dis. 1986;8(Suppl 2):131-135.

325. Hoge CW, Shlim DR, Echeverria P, et al. Epidemiology of diarrhea among expatriate residents living in a highly endemic environment. JAMA. 1996;275:533-538.

326. Wolfson JS, Richter JM, Waldron MA, et al. Cryptosporidiosis in immunocompetent patients. N Engl J Med. 1985;312:1278-1282.

327. Taylor DN, Echeverria P. Etiology and epidemiology of travelers' diarrhea in Asia. Rev Infect Dis. 1986;8(Suppl 2):136-141.

328. Castelli F, Carosi G. Epidemiology of traveler's diarrhea. Chemotherapy. 1995;41(Suppl):32.

329. Wolfe MS. Protection of travelers. Clin Infect Dis. 1997;25:177-184.

330. Bolivar R, Conklin RH, Vollet JJ, et al. Rotavirus in travelers' diarrhea: Study of an adult student population in Mexico. J Infect Dis. 1978;137:324.

331. Ryder RW, Oquist CA, Greenberg H, et al. Travelers' diarrhea in Panamanian tourists in Mexico. J Infect Dis. 1981;144:442.

332. Gunn RA, Terranova WA, Greenberg HB, et al. Norwalk virus gastroenteritis aboard a cruise ship: An outbreak for five consecutive cruises. Am J Epidemiol. 1980;112:820-827.

333. Cramer EH, Gu DX, Durbin RE, et al. Diarrheal disease on cruise ships, 1990-2000: The impact of environmental health programs. Am J Prev Med. 2003;24:227.

334. CDC. Outbreaks of gastroenteritis associated with noroviruses on cruise ships—United States, 2002. MMWR Morb Mortal Wkly Rep. 2002;51:1112.

335. Okhuysen PC. Traveler's diarrhea due to intestinal protozoa. Clin Infect Dis. 2001;33:110.

336. Goodgame R. Emerging causes of traveler's diarrhea: *Cryptosporidium, Cyclospora, Isospora,* and *Microsporidia*. Curr Infect Dis Rep. 2003;5:66.

337. Jelinek T, Lotze M, Eichenlaub S, et al. Prevalence of infection with *Cryptosporidium parvum* and *Cyclospora cayetanensis* among international travellers. Gut. 1997;41:801-804.
338. Shlim DR, Hoge CW, Rajah R, et al. Is *Blastocystis hominis* a cause of diarrhea in travelers? A prospective controlled study in Nepal. Clin Infect Dis. 1995;21:97-101.
339. Keystone JS. *Blastocystis hominis* and traveler's diarrhea (Editorial). Clin Infect Dis. 1995;21:102-103.
340. Jelinek T, Peyerl G, Loscher T, et al. The role of *Blastocystis hominis* as a possible intestinal pathogen in travellers. J Infect. 1997;35:63-66.
341. Snyder JD, Blake PA. Is cholera a problem for US travelers? JAMA. 1982;247:2268.
342. DuPont HL. Pathogenesis of traveler's diarrhea. Chemotherapy. 1995;41(Suppl):9.
343. Osterholm MT, MacDonald KL, White KE, et al. An outbreak of a newly recognized chronic diarrhea syndrome associated with raw milk consumption. JAMA. 1986;256:484-490.
344. Parsonnet J, Trock SC, Bopp CA, et al. Chronic diarrhea associated with drinking untreated water. Ann Intern Med. 1989;110:985-991.
345. Mintz ED, Weber JT, Guris D, et al. An outbreak of Brainerd diarrhea among travelers to the Galapagos Islands. J Infect Dis. 1998;177:1041-1045.
346. Echeverria P, Hodge FA, Blacklow NR, et al. Travelers' diarrhea among United States marines in South Korea. Am J Epidemiol. 1978;108:68.
347. Wolfe MS. Current concepts in parasitology. Giardiasis. N Engl J Med. 1978;298:319.
348. Brodsky RE, Spencer HC Jr, Schultz MG. Giardiasis in American travelers to the Soviet Union. J Infect Dis. 1974;130:319.
349. Soave R, Armstrong D. *Cryptosporidium* and cryptosporidiosis. Rev Infect Dis. 1986;8:1012-1023.
350. Jokipii L, Pohjola S, Jokipii AMM. *Cryptosporidium*: A frequent finding in patients with gastrointestinal symptoms. Lancet. 1983;2:358-360.
351. Kean BH, Reilly PC. Malaria—The mime. Recent lessons from a group of civilian travelers. Am J Med. 1976;61:159.
352. Pearson RD, Hewlett EL, Guerrant RL. Tropical diseases in North America. Dis Mon. 1984;30:1-68.
353. Hill DR, Pearson RD. Health advice for international travel. Ann Intern Med. 1988;108:839-852.
354. Kean BH, Waters SR. Diarrhea of travelers. III. Drug prophylaxis in Mexico. N Engl J Med. 1959;261:71.
355. Oakley GP. The neurotoxicity of the halogenated hydroxyquinolines. JAMA. 1973;225:395.
356. Portnoy BL, DuPont HL, Pruitt D, et al. Antidiarrheal agents in the treatment of acute diarrhea in children. JAMA. 1976;236:844.
357. DuPont HL, Hornick RB. Adverse effect of Lomotil therapy in shigellosis. JAMA. 1973;226:1525.
358. DuPont HL, Sullivan P, Pickering LK, et al. Symptomatic treatment of diarrhea with bismuth subsalicylate among students attending a Mexican university. Gastroenterology. 1977;73:715.
359. Steffen R, Heusser R, DuPont HL. Prevention of travelers' diarrhea by non-antibiotic drugs. Rev Infect Dis. 1986;8(Suppl 2):151-159.
360. Blaser MJ. Environmental interventions for the prevention of travelers' diarrhea. Rev Infect Dis. 1986;8(Suppl 2):142-150.
361. Gonzales-Cortez A, Gangarosa EJ, Parrilla C, et al. Bottled beverages and typhoid fever: The Mexican epidemic of 1972-3. Am J Public Health. 1982;72:844.
362. Harris JR. Are bottled beverages safe for travelers? Am J Public Health. 1982;72:787.
363. Neumann HH. Travellers' diarrhea. Lancet. 1970;1:420.
364. Tjoa W, DuPont HL, Sullivan P, et al. Location of food consumption and travelers' diarrhea. Am J Epidemiol. 1977;106:61.
365. Sack DA, Kaminsky DC, Sack RB, et al. Prophylactic doxycycline for travelers' diarrhea, results of a prospective double-blind study of Peace Corps volunteers in Kenya. N Engl J Med. 1978;298:758.
366. Echeverria P, Verhaert L, Ulyangco CV, et al. Antimicrobial resistance and enterotoxin production among isolates of *Escherichia coli* in the Far East. Lancet. 1978;2:589.
367. Murray BE. Resistance of *Shigella*, *Salmonella* and other selected enteric pathogens. Rev Infect Dis. 1986;8(Suppl 2):172-181.
368. Mentzing LO, Ringertz O. *Salmonella* infection in tourists. 2. Prophylaxis against salmonellosis. Acta Pathol Microbiol Scand. 1968;74:405.
369. Ericsson CD, DuPont HL, Matthewson JJ, et al. Treatment of travelers' diarrhea with sulfamethoxazole and trimethoprim and loperamide. JAMA. 1990;263:257-261.
370. DuPont HL, Ericsson CD. Prevention and treatment of travelers' diarrhea. N Engl J Med. 1993;328:1821-1826.
371. DuPont HL, Reves RR, Galindo E, et al. Treatment of travelers' diarrhea with trimethoprim/sulfamethoxazole and with trimethoprim alone. N Engl J Med. 1983;307:841-844.
372. Statement on travellers' diarrhea. Committee to Advise on Tropical Medicine and Travel. CMAJ. 1995;152:205-212.
373. Petruccelli BP, Murphy GS, Sanchez JL, et al. Treatment of traveler's diarrhea with ciprofloxacin and loperamide. J Infect Dis. 1992;165:557-560.
374. Stauffer WM, Konop RJ, Kamat D. Traveling with infants and young children. Part III: Travelers' diarrhea. J Travel Med. 2002;9:141.
375. Kariuki S, Hart CA. Global aspects of antimicrobial-resistant enteric bacteria. Curr Opin Infect Dis. 2001;14:579.
376. Sanders JW, Isenbarger DW, Walz SE, et al. An observational clinic-based study of diarrheal illness in deployed United States military personnel in Thailand: Presentation and outcome of *Campylobacter* infection. Am J Trop Med Hyg. 2002;67:533.
377. Hakanen A, Jousimies-Somer H, Siitonen A, et al. Fluoroquinolone resistance in *Campylobacter jejuni* isolates in travelers returning to Finland: Association of ciprofloxacin resistance to travel destination. Emerg Infect Dis. 2003;9:267.
378. Tjaniadi P, Lesmana M, Subekti D, et al. Antimicrobial resistance of bacterial pathogens associated with diarrheal patients in Indonesia. Am J Trop Med Hyg. 2003;68:666.
379. Said SI, Faloona GR. Elevated plasma and tissue levels of vasoactive intestinal polypeptide in the watery diarrhea syndrome due to pancreatic, bronchogenic, and other tumors. N Engl J Med. 1975;293:155.
380. Tzipori S. Cryptosporidiosis in animals and humans. Microbiol Rev. 1983;47:84.
381. Wolff MS. Giardiasis. JAMA. 1975;233:1362.
382. Ma P, Soave R. Three-step stool examination for cryptosporidiosis in 10 homosexual men with protracted watery diarrhea. J Infect Dis. 1983;147:824.
383. Donaldson RM Jr. Small bowel bacterial overgrowth. Adv Intern Med. 1970;16:191.
384. Murphy TV, Nelson JD. Five vs ten days' therapy with furazolidone for giardiasis. Am J Dis Child. 1983;137:267.
385. Gorbach SL. Intestinal microflora. Gastroenterology. 1971;60:1110.
386. Penn RG, Giger DK, Knoop FC, et al. *Plesiomonas shigelloides* overgrowth in the small intestine. J Clin Microbiol. 1982;15:869.
387. Scott AJ, Khan GA. Partial biliary obstruction with cholangitis producing a blind loop syndrome. Gut. 1968;9:187.
388. Vantrappen G, Janssens J, Hellemans J, et al. Interdigestive motor complex of normal subjects and patients with bacterial overgrowth of the small intestine. J Clin Invest. 1977;59:1158.
389. Heyworth B, Brown J. Jejunal microflora in malnourished Gambian children. Arch Dis Child. 1975;50:27.
390. Roberts SH, James O, Jarvis EH. Bacterial overgrowth syndrome without "blind loop": A cause for malnutrition in the elderly. Lancet. 1977;2:1193.
391. Ruiz-Palacios GM, DuPont HL. Bacterial overgrowth syndrome after acute nonspecific diarrhoea. Lancet. 1978;1:337.
392. Lindenbaum J, Kent TH, Sprinz H. Malabsorption and jejunitis in American Peace Corps volunteers in Pakistan. Ann Intern Med. 1955;65:1201.
393. Shimada K, Bricknell KS, Finegold SM. Deconjugation of bile acids by intestinal bacteria: Review of literature and additional studies. J Infect Dis. 1969;119:273.
394. Wanke CA, Guerrant RL. Small bowel colonization alone is a cause of diarrhea. Infect Immun. 1987;55:1924-1926.
395. Schlager TA, Wanke CA, Guerrant RL. Net fluid secretion and impaired villous function induced by small intestinal colonization by non-toxigenic, colonizing *E. coli*. Infect Immun. 1990;58:1337.
396. Hamilton JD, Dyer NH, Dawson AM, et al. Assessment and significance of bacterial overgrowth in the small bowel. Q J Med. 1970;39:265.
397. MacDougall LG. The effect of aureomycin on undernourished African children. J Trop Pediatr. 1957;3:74.
398. Levy SB, FitzGerald GB, Macone AB. Changes in intestinal flora of farm personnel after introduction of a tetracycline-supplemented feed on a farm. N Engl J Med. 1976;295:583.

CHAPTER **92**

Antibiotic-Associated Colitis

NATHAN M. THIELMAN
KENNETH H. WILSON

Diarrhea is one of the most common complications associated with antibiotic therapy, and colitis is one of the most serious. Attack rates vary depending on the antimicrobial agent used, the epidemiologic setting, and the host. Overall, attack rates for antibiotic-associated diarrhea in hospitals range from 3.2% to 29%.[1] Almost 15% of hospitalized patients receiving β-lactam antibiotics develop diarrhea, and rates for those receiving clindamycin range from 10% to 25%.[2] Predisposing host factors and circumstances affecting the frequency and severity of disease include advanced age, underlying illness, recent surgery, and recent administration of drugs that alter bowel motility.

Clostridium difficile is now recognized as a frequent cause of antibiotic-associated diarrhea and colitis, and the incidence of *C. difficile*–associated diarrhea appears to be increasing.[3] It is implicated in 20% to 30% of patients with antibiotic-associated diarrhea, in 50% to 75% of those with antibiotic-associated colitis, and in more than 90% of those with antibiotic-associated pseudomembranous colitis.[4] In a Swedish study, *C. difficile*–associated diarrhea was almost twice as prevalent as all other diagnosed domestic cases of reportable bacterial and protozoal diarrhea combined.[5]

The etiology of antibiotic-associated diarrhea and colitis that is *not* caused by *C. difficile* is poorly understood. *Staphylococcus aureus*, once implicated as the agent of antibiotic-associated colitis, is now rarely appreciated (see "Historical Overview"). Receiving more attention in the last decade has been a possible link with *Candida* spp., particularly among hospitalized elderly patients.[6] In most but not all patients, colitis is absent, and in almost all reported cases, therapy with oral nystatin leads to improvement. However, definitive data establishing the pathogenicity of *Candida* in diarrhea are lacking, and dense colonization has been observed in the absence of diarrhea. Enterotoxigenic *Clostridium perfringens* has also been cited as a possible cause of antibiotic-associated diarrhea, and 8% of patients with antibiotic-associated diarrhea were found to have *C. perfringens* enterotoxin present in stool in one study.[7] Recent antibiotic exposure has emerged as a distinct risk factor in both sporadic cases and outbreaks of salmonellosis.[8] A nosocomial outbreak of fluoroquinolone-resistant salmonellosis has been reported; treatment with a fluoroquinolone posed a significant risk for infection in a case-controlled analysis.[9] Changes in carbohydrate and short-chain fatty acid metabolism may also play a role in antibiotic-associated diarrhea not caused by infectious agents.[10]

Although the morbidity and economic burden of broadly characterized antibiotic-associated diarrhea are difficult to quantify, relevant data for *C. difficile*–associated diarrhea have been reported. A prospective case-control analysis conducted in a geriatric population documented significantly higher death rates and increased hospital costs—in excess of $5000 per case—among patients with *C. difficile*–associated diarrhea hospitalized in Britain.[11] In the United States, charges incurred when the admitting diagnosis was *C. difficile*–associated diarrhea averaged $5000 per case in 1991 in a community hospital, and charges for cases acquired in the hospital were almost $2000 per patient.[12] In a U.S.-based national referral study of recurrent *C. difficile*–associated disease, the mean lifetime cost of direct medical care approached $11,000.[13] It is not surprising that several studies have reported substantial increases in length of hospital stay associated with this disease.[11,14]

HISTORICAL OVERVIEW

Paradoxically, the major pathologic feature of antibiotic-associated colitis—pseudomembrane formation—was first described in the pre-antibiotic era. Finney[15] reported the case of a 22-year-old woman who developed hemorrhagic diarrhea 10 days after gastric surgery and eventually died; the autopsy report described "diphtheritic colitis." This historic description, published more than 40 years prior to the introduction of antibiotics, illustrates the importance of abdominal surgery, hospitalization, and impaired intestinal motility (after administration of opiates) in the pathogenesis of this process. As early as 1948, staphylococci were implicated in a case of fatal enteritis in an infant after administration of oral streptomycin.[16] Thereafter, Bennett and colleagues[17] at Johns Hopkins Hospital resectioned and reexamined the original pathologic specimens from Finney's case and found "myriads of gram-positive cocci." In the 1950s and 1960s, several reports of staphylococcal enterocolitis were based merely on culturing of staphylococci in diarrheal stools or pathology specimens[16,18]; in other reports, the organism was actually demonstrated within pseudomembranes or intestinal tissue sections (Fig. 92-1). Noting the absence of *S. aureus* in 11 of 18 patients with pseudomembranous enterocolitis, Dearing and associates[18] concluded that such findings "cast doubt on the concept that all cases of pseudomembranous enteritis are produced by *S. aureus* in the intestine." Since the late 1960s, and after the discovery of *C. difficile* as the major cause of antibiotic-associated colitis in 1977, antibiotic-associated staphylococcal diarrhea has virtually disappeared from the medical literature, with only a few pur-

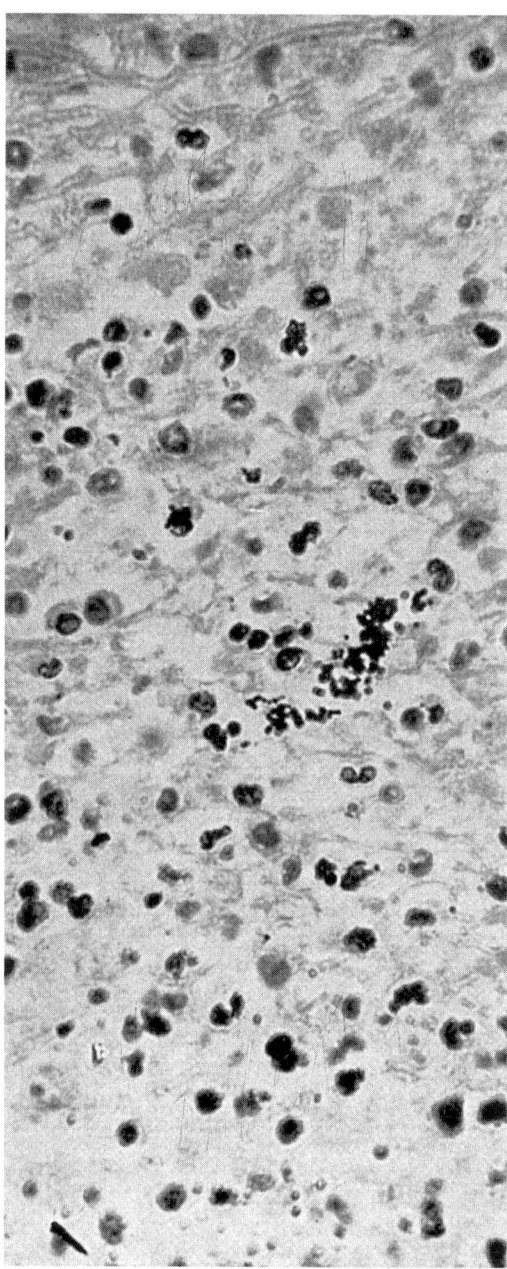

FIGURE 92-1. Section of pseudomembrane demonstrating inflammatory cells, fibrin, and gram-positive cocci, from a 1956 report of a fatal case of staphylococcal pseudomembranous enteritis. *(From Corridan M. Antibiotic-resistant staphylococcal pseudomembranous enteritis. J Clin Pathol. 1956;9:131-135.)*

ported cases in the United States and Japan.[19] There are at least three potential explanations for the dramatic decline in the number of reported cases of staphylococcal enterocolitis: (1) staphylococci were wrongly implicated and actually played no role in pseudomembranous enterocolitis[20]; (2) the actual incidence of the disease decreased dramatically after the introduction of β-lactamase–stable penicillins[21]; or (3) the entity still exists but is ignored because of the emphasis on *C. difficile* toxin testing and the use of empirical vancomycin for antibiotic-associated diarrhea.[19]

The literature from the mid-1970s emphasized the attack rates for diarrhea and pseudomembranous colitis associated with the use of individual antibiotics. Several studies reported rates of clindamycin (and lincomycin)–associated diarrhea ranging from 7% to 21%[22] and rates

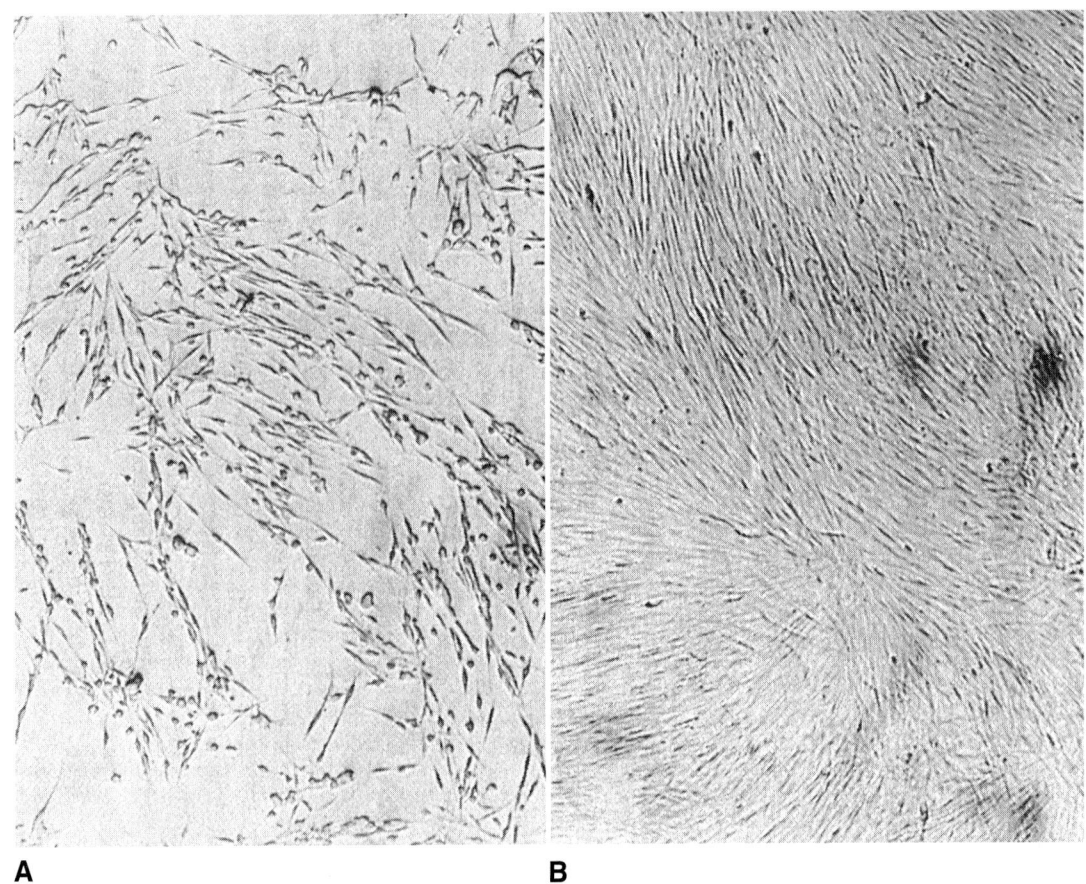

A   **B**

FIGURE 92-2. A, Toxic cytopathic effect of fecal suspension in human embryonic lung fibroblasts (MRC 5 cells) from 12-year-old girl with pseudomembranous colitis. **B,** Uninoculated tissue cultures. These figures accompanied one of the first reports to implicate a bacterial toxin in pseudomembranous colitis; 7 months later, the same investigators reported that this effect was neutralized by *Clostridium sordellii* antitoxin. *(From Larson HE, Perry JV, Price AB, et al. Undescribed toxin in pseudomembranous colitis. BMJ. 1977;1:1246-1248.)*

of ampicillin-associated diarrhea from 4% to 17%.[22-24] In a now classic prospective clinical investigation, Tedesco[24] found diarrhea in 21% of 200 patients receiving clindamycin and described "clindamycin colitis" in fully 10%. Although proctoscopic examination confirmed the presence of pseudomembranous colitis in the latter group, the investigators found little to suggest an underlying bacterial cause, and results of cultures of plaque-like lesions, mucosal smears, and stool for staphylococci were negative.[25] Prompted by these data and additional reports, in 1979 the Committee on Safety of Medicines in the United Kingdom recommended that clindamycin and lincomycin "should in general be reserved for severe or life-threatening conditions where other antibiotic therapy is ineffective or undesirable"; similar warnings had already been issued in the United States.[20,26,27]

In the late 1970s, a series of investigations established toxigenic *C. difficile* as the cause of pseudomembranous colitis. First, Larson and colleagues,[28] in attempts to isolate viruses from the feces of a 12-year-old girl with a prior history of penicillin exposure, diarrhea, negative results on stool cultures, and endoscopically proven pseudomembranous colitis, suggested a role for bacterial toxins in this process. Fecal suspensions from the patient (and subsequently those from four of five others with pseudomembranous colitis) demonstrated cytopathic effects on HeLa cells, Rhesus monkey kidney cells, and human embryonic lung fibroblast cells (Fig. 92-2).[28] Within a short period, several other reports shed light on this observation. Bartlett and co-workers,[29] using a Syrian hamster model of clindamycin-associated enterocolitis, found that intracecal material transferred the disease from affected hamsters to healthy ones, that broth cultures of *Clostridia* and their cell-free supernatants produced this disease, and that this activity was neutralized by gas gangrene antiserum. Rifkin and associates[30] re-

ported at about the same time that stool filtrates from humans with pseudomembranous colitis were lethal for hamsters; caused edema, hemorrhage, and increased vascular permeability in rabbit skin; and possessed cytotoxic activity that was neutralized by *Clostridium sordellii* antitoxin. Larson and colleagues' original observation was followed by identification of a toxin in stool neutralized by *C. sordellii* antitoxin in nine of nine patients with pseudomembranous colitis and two of two others with antibiotic-associated nonspecific colitis.[31] Other investigators soon implicated the species *C. difficile*, demonstrating the presence of toxigenic strains in the stool of patients with pseudomembranous colitis.[32]

MICROBIOLOGY

Forty-three years before *C. difficile* was established as a pathogen, Hall and O'Toole[33] isolated this organism during a study of intestinal biota of newborn infants. They described an obligately anaerobic, spore-producing, gram-positive rod that was toxigenic. Because of "the unusual difficulty which was encountered in its isolation and study," it was first named *Bacillus difficilis*[34]; 3 years later it was renamed *Clostridium difficile*. Ribosomal DNA sequence analysis indicates that *C. difficile* is closely related to *C. sordellii* but not to other toxigenic clostridia, such as *C. perfringens*, *Clostridium botulinum*, and *Clostridium tetani*. It is relatively large (2 to 17 μm in length) and fast-growing. Many strains are seen on electron microscopy to produce flagellae or fimbria-like structures.[35] Surface-layer proteins confer serologic specificity.[36] Production of toxin is controlled at the transcriptional level by a sigma factor (component of RNA polymerase) that is expressed optimally at body temperature.[37]

Cycloserine, cefoxitin, and fructose agar in an egg-yolk agar base are the constituents of CCFA medium, shown by George and colleagues[38] to be highly selective for *C. difficile*. Detecting as few as 2000 organisms in a total of 6×10^{10} bacteria per gram of wet feces,[39] the medium is relatively insensitive at detecting spores unless a primary bile salt is added.[40] This medium has demonstrated growth characteristics (in plates anaerobically reduced for 4 hours before use) that are superior to those for cycloserine-mannitol blood agar.[41] Once growth is sustained on CCFA, if colonial morphology and Gram staining do not presumptively identify the organism, commercial identification kits are typically used.

EPIDEMIOLOGY

Prevalence of Symptomatic Disease in Hospitals and Extended-Care Facilities and among Outpatients

The incidence of antibiotic-associated diarrhea and colitis varies greatly, depending on the offending antibiotic and its spectrum of activity and pharmacokinetic properties, as well as the epidemiologic setting. Toxigenic *C. difficile* remains the most common cause of nosocomial diarrhea and is implicated in 10% to 30% of such cases. Local nosocomial diarrhea prevalence rates may vary considerably depending on antibiotic prescribing patterns, endemic strains, and criteria used to define antibiotic-associated diarrhea.[42] The reported frequency of *C. difficile* colitis among acute care hospitalized patients ranges between 1 and 10 cases per 1000 discharges.[43] In a given hospital the rate may vary considerably over time, as evidenced in a 10-year prospective study at the Veterans Affairs Hospital in Minneapolis, where the annual rate of *C. difficile*–associated diarrhea ranged from 3.2 to 9.9 cases per 1000 discharges.[44] At a tertiary university hospital with about 29,000 admissions per year, the incidence of *C. difficile* colitis increased from 0.68% to 1.2% between 1989 and 2000, and the incidence of fulminant, life-threatening disease doubled to 3.2%.[3] Although colonization with toxigenic *C. difficile* is frequent among residents of some extended-care and rehabilitation facilities (see later discussion), only a minority of infected patients develop symptomatic disease.[45,46] Conversely, *C. difficile* infection was identified in 25% of patients undergoing diagnostic evaluation for diarrhea in two rehabilitation hospitals.[47] Among outpatients exposed to antibiotics, in contrast, clinically recognized *C. difficile*–associated diarrhea is uncommon. A retrospective cohort study of a 265,000-member health maintenance organization revealed an overall risk of less than 1 case per 10,000 antibiotic prescriptions.[48] The rate of hospitalization in this study was between 0.5 and 1 hospital admission per 100,000 person-years, a rate similar to that previously reported.

Inciting Agents

Although almost all antibiotic classes have been associated with the disease (Table 92-1), reports of large clinical series most commonly implicate clindamycin, penicillins, and cephalosporins.[23,42,49,50] Several noteworthy studies primarily implicated clindamycin and ampicillin in the 1970s,[22,24,25] and clindamycin-resistant strains of *C. difficile* were implicated in outbreaks of diarrhea strongly associated with clindamycin use between 1989 and 1992.[51] Other reports have emphasized an association with cephalosporins.[49,50,52]

Third-generation cephalosporins have been implicated in particular and appear to predispose to *C. difficile*–associated disease more commonly than the narrow-spectrum penicillins (i.e., penicillin V and penicillin G) or the β-lactamase–stable penicillins do.[52] Ticarcillin-clavulanate appears to be associated infrequently with the disease. In a 2-year retrospective study of 61,000 courses of ticarcillin-clavulanate therapy, no *C. difficile*–induced disease was identified.[52] However, other studies have reported an association.[53] Several case reports and a case-control study have implicated fluoroquinolones in *C. difficile* disease.[43,54] In the hamster model, the following drugs regularly produce lethal hemorrhagic cecitis due to *C. difficile*: ampicillin, carbenicillin, cefamandole, cefaclor, cefazolin, cefoxitin, cephalexin, cephaloridine, cephalothin, cephradine, clindamycin, oral gentamicin,

TABLE 92-1 Antimicrobial and Chemotherapeutic Agents Associated with *Clostridium difficile* Diarrhea or Colitis

More Frequently Associated Agents	Less Frequently Associated Agents
Cephalosporins (especially second- and third-generation agents)	Ticarcillin-clavulanate
Ampicillin and amoxicillin	Chloramphenicol
Clindamycin	Metronidazole
Other penicillins, including β-lactamase–stable penicillins	Amphotericin B
	Quinolones
Erythromycin and other macrolides	Rifampin
Tetracyclines	5-Fluorouracil
Trimethoprim-sulfamethoxazole	Methotrexate
	Doxorubicin
	Cyclophosphamide
	Aminoglycosides
	Sulfonamides

Data from Bartlett,[2] Kelly et al.,[4] and Thielman and Guerrant.[251]

imipenem, metronidazole, nafcillin, penicillin, ticarcillin, and vancomycin; only rarely do tetracyclines, chloramphenicol, sulfonamides, and trimethoprim-sulfamethoxazole produce disease.[2,55]

Changes in antibiotic restriction policies have been associated with varying *C. difficile*–associated diarrhea attack rates, and policies limiting the use of clindamycin[56] and cefotaxime[57] in different hospital outbreaks have reduced the number of new cases. Because the reduction in new cases seen in some outbreaks is greater than that predicted by the number of patients for whom the antimicrobial agent was avoided, a "herd immunity" model of *C. difficile*–associated diarrhea has been proposed.[58] This paradigm takes into account the risk of disease associated with the use of certain antimicrobials for an entire population rather than solely for individuals.

A number of antineoplastic agents, particularly those with modest antibacterial activity, have been associated with *C. difficile* diarrheal disease, including doxorubicin, cisplatin, cyclophosphamide, 5-fluorouracil, chlorambucil, and methotrexate.[59]

Rarely, the disease occurs without exposure to agents known to alter the microecology of the gut.[60]

Contributing Factors

In addition to the use of antimicrobials, certain host and environmental factors also predispose to *C. difficile*–associated disease. In a comprehensive prospective study of risk factors in hospitalized patients, McFarland and associates[49] identified advanced age and severity of underlying illness as factors associated with increased risk of *C. difficile* carriage and diarrhea and found that agents that alter normal intestinal motility—specifically enemas and gastrointestinal stimulants, as well as stool softeners—also contributed to the risk of *C. difficile*–associated diarrhea.[49] Given the tendency of this disease to affect ill, elderly patients who receive antibiotics, it is no surprise that patients with *C. difficile* disease are also at risk for colonization by vancomycin-resistant enterococci (VRE).[61-63] Other investigators have reported that critically ill burned patients,[64] uremic patients,[65] patients with hematologic malignancies,[66] and those undergoing gastrointestinal surgery[67] are at increased risk for *C. difficile* diarrhea and colitis. Emerging evidence suggests that immunologic susceptibility may play a critical role in *C. difficile*–associated infection. Host immunoglobulin G (IgG) responses have been shown to protect against symptomatic disease[68] and relapse.[69] Human immunodeficiency virus (HIV) infection per se does not appear to predispose to *C. difficile* colonization,[70] and specific risk factors for *C. difficile*–associated disease among HIV-infected patients appear to be similar to those in HIV-seronegative persons.[71] Patients with very low CD4+ T-lymphocyte counts ($<50/mm^3$) may be at increased risk by virtue of their increased exposure to antibiotics.[72] Although some reports[72,73] have suggested that *C. difficile* disease is more severe in HIV-infected patients, others have found that the disease behaves no differently in this group than in HIV-negative controls.[74]

Reservoirs

The source of *C. difficile* may be either endogenous or environmental. Since Hall and O'Toole's original description of the organism in healthy neonates,[33] studies have documented the prevalence of *C. difficile* (or one of its toxins) in 15% to 70% of stools of healthy neonates.[75-78] Despite the presence of toxin-producing organisms in this population, the prevalence of *C. difficile* colitis remains relatively low.[77] Enhanced chemotactic responses of granulocytes to toxin A in older persons[79] and the absence of high-affinity receptors for toxin A in neonates (in a rabbit model)[80] have been cited as possible reasons for this age-dependent susceptibility (see "Pathogenesis"). The ability of *C. difficile* to temporarily colonize newborn humans and hamsters[81] suggests that the gastrointestinal tracts of very young mammals may be a major reservoir.

In healthy adults, intestinal carriage rates of toxigenic *C. difficile* are typically 3% or less and not greater than 8%.[82] Asymptomatic intestinal carriage rates are higher (approximately 20%) among hospitalized adults, particularly those who have received antibiotics.[2] The prevalence of *C. difficile* colonization has been documented in particular patient populations, including 13% of patients on admission to an infectious diseases ward (70% of whom were seropositive for HIV), 2% to 8% of elderly nursing home residents, and 7% to 14% of elderly hospitalized patients.[70] It is important to note that although *C. difficile* carriage rates may be quite high in asymptomatic adults, rarely do these persons harbor significant quantities of toxin A or toxin B in stool (the basis for the clinical diagnosis in most cases).

The frequency of extraintestinal carriage of this organism is not clearly defined. Whereas *C. difficile* was isolated from the vast majority of urethral and vaginal cultures in men and women attending a sexually transmitted diseases clinic,[83] other studies reported vaginal carriage in fewer than 18% of pregnant women,[84] and still others were unable to detect urogenital colonization at all.[85]

Clearly, a preexisting endogenous reservoir of *C. difficile* is not a prerequisite for symptomatic infection, and the majority of disease-causing organisms appear to be acquired from exogenous sources. In a prospective cohort study of patients admitted to a Seattle teaching hospital, acquisition of the organism was documented in 21% of 399 patients who initially had negative culture results; of these patients, 37% developed diarrhea.[86] Arguing for the significance of environmental acquisition of *C. difficile* is the number of outbreaks that have been reported in hospitals,[87,88] chronic-care facilities,[46,89] and daycare centers.[90] Even the classic "clindamycin colitis" study[25] is now retrospectively recognized as a report of the first confirmed hospital epidemic—owing to the unusually high rates of *C. difficile* toxin in subsequent stool analysis. In such settings, *C. difficile* is readily cultured from multiple inanimate environmental sources and from the hands of hospital personnel.[86] Among hospital personnel caring for patients shedding *C. difficile*, 59% had positive results on culture for *C. difficile* from their hands in one report.[86]

In addition, *C. difficile* is found in many sources outside the hospital and has been cultured from soil, swimming pools, and beaches, as well as sea, river, and tap water, and from several animals. Carriage rates in household pets such as dogs and cats range from 20% to 40%, and some authorities propose that it may be zoonotically acquired.[91] Food-borne transmission has also been suggested, but neither food-borne nor zoonotic transmission has been definitively documented.

Epidemic Strains

There are ample approaches to type strains of *C. difficile*, although none is ideal. Because serologic reagents are less available than reagents for molecular typing, molecular methods are supplanting the former. Pulsed-field gel electrophoresis (PFGE), the gold standard for many bacterial species, is limited by production of nucleases in at least 10% of *C. difficile* strains.[92,93] Arbitrarily primed polymerase chain reaction (PCR) assays, as in other applications,

lack reproducibility. Ribotyping by PCR is highly reproducible but lacks discrimination compared with PFGE.[92] Analysis of amplified fragment length polymorphisms, the current method for typing the highly monomorphic *Bacillus anthracis*,[94] promises to be both discriminating and reproducible.[93]

Numerous strains with varying virulence potential may circulate simultaneously in a hospital.[95] As in the hamster model,[96,97] nontoxigenic strains appear to protect against the disease.[98] Numerous outbreaks featuring a predominant pathogenic strain or a closely related group of *C. difficile* strains have been reported,[56,71,88,99] possibly reflecting antimicrobial use patterns, increased virulence or resistance among particular strains, or breakdowns in infection control. Molecular typing analysis implicated either a single strain or a set of genetically closely related strains among multiple isolates in five of six outbreaks in different regions in North America. Similar methodology resolved a few distinct and genetically stable serogroup C strains associated with outbreaks in Belgium, France, and Benin spanning more than a decade.[99] More recently, a strain of clindamycin-resistant *C. difficile* was reported to cause four geographically dispersed epidemics in the United States.[51] With the exception of the macrolide-lincosamide resistance seen in several clindamycin-associated outbreaks, it is not known why a given strain sometimes becomes predominant and causes an epidemic. Despite the many clusters of infection attributed to specific strains, a high incidence of *C. difficile* diarrhea in a given facility does not necessarily suggest a clonal outbreak. Significant clonal diversity was recently documented at a New England hospital, with 55 distinct types isolated from 106 patients, including asymptomatic patients with culture-proven colonization and those with diarrhea.[100] Divergent strains predominated in a typing analysis of endemic *C. difficile* isolates from patients and the environment on an oncology ward[101] and among elderly residents in a long-term care facility.

CLINICAL MANIFESTATIONS

Infection with toxigenic *C. difficile* causes a spectrum of disease ranging from asymptomatic carriage (particularly in neonates) to a fulminant, relapsing, and occasionally fatal colitis. When *C. difficile* produces clinical disease, the onset of signs and symptoms typically occurs after 5 to 10 days of antibacterial treatment, but diarrhea may develop as early as the first day of therapy or as late as 10 weeks after cessation of therapy.[102] *C. difficile*–associated diarrhea may be brief and self-limited, or it may be cholera-like, resulting in more than 20 stools per day.[2] Accompanying findings often include fever (30% to 50% of patients),[42,103,104] leukocytosis (50% to 60%),[42,52,104] and abdominal pain or cramping (20% to 33%).[103-106] The mean peripheral leukocyte count of patients with *C. difficile*–associated diarrhea is typically 15,000 to 16,000/mm^3,[107,108] and in one series *C. difficile* infection was noted in 25% of patients with white blood cell counts of greater than 35,000/mm^3 who did not have hematologic malignancy.[109] Nausea, malaise, anorexia, hypoalbuminemia, occult colonic bleeding, and dehydration have also been reported.[2,4,110] Infrequently, *C. difficile* colitis manifests without diarrhea as an acute abdominal syndrome or toxic megacolon (Fig. 92-3).[111,112] In one report, 5 of 97 patients with *C. difficile* disease (only 1 of whom had profuse diarrhea) presented initially with marked leukocytosis (white blood cell count ≥25,000/mm^3) and right lower quadrant peritoneal signs mimicking those of acute peritonitis.[113] Toxic megacolon is suggested by acute dilatation of the colon to a diameter greater than 6 cm, associated systemic toxicity, and the absence of mechanical obstruction. It carries a high mortality rate (64% in one series of 11 patients).[114]

Other intra-abdominal complications include colonic perforation,[115] transverse volvulus,[116] protein-losing enteropathy,[117] and recurrent *C. difficile*–associated diarrhea, the last occurring in approximately 20% of patients.[118,119]

Extraintestinal manifestations occur more rarely and include bacteremia, often with concurrent isolation of other constituent organisms in the bowel flora,[53,120] splenic abscess,[121] and osteomyelitis.[122] In ad-

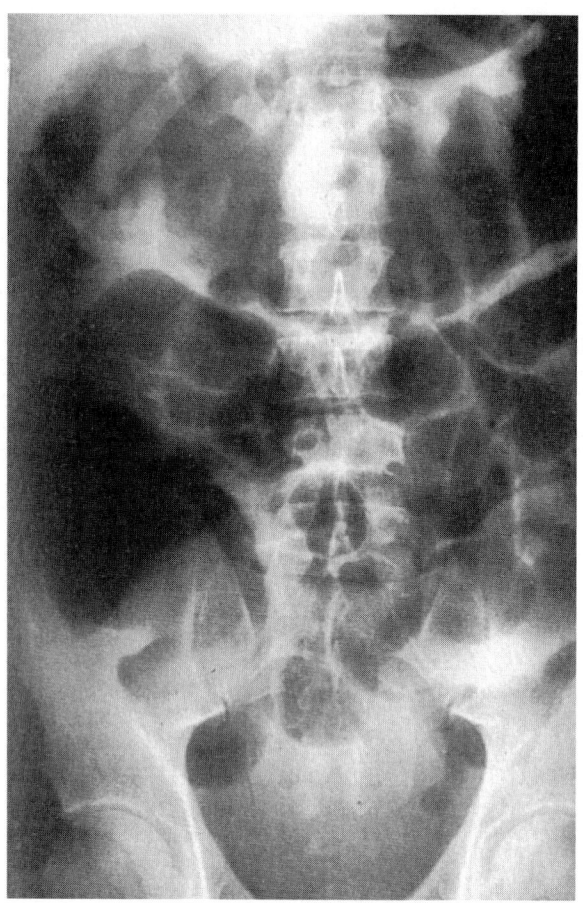

FIGURE 92-3. Abdominal radiograph demonstrating markedly dilated colon, wall edema, and loss of haustration in a patient with *Clostridium difficile*–associated pseudomembranous colitis complicated by toxic megacolon. *(From Agnifili A, Gola P, Manno M, et al. The role and timing of surgery in the treatment of pseudomembranous colitis: A case complicated by toxic megacolon. Hepatogastroenterology. 1994;41:394-396.)*

dition, multiple reports have described reactive arthritis or tenosynovitis or both,[123-126] some cases including features of Reiter's syndrome[124] and others occurring in patients with preexisting Reiter's syndrome.[127] As with other reactive arthritides after enteric infections, many of these patients are positive for the human leukocyte antigen HLA-B27.[123,124,126]

Considerations in the differential diagnosis of antibiotic-associated colitis include diarrhea caused by other enteric pathogens (especially *Salmonella*), adverse reactions to other medications, ischemic colitis, inflammatory bowel disease, and intra-abdominal sepsis.[110]

PATHOGENESIS

Key steps in the pathogenesis of *C. difficile*–mediated diarrhea and colitis include (1) disruption of normal colonic biota by antibiotics or antineoplastic agents with antibacterial activity, (2) colonization with toxigenic *C. difficile*, (3) elaboration of toxin A and/or toxin B, both of which mediate cytoskeletal derangement in target cells, and (4) mucosal injury and inflammation.

The indigenous microbiota of the gut constitutes a complex and poorly understood host defense system. This dense biomass, which typically contains 10^{11} to 10^{12} bacteria per gram of feces, is dominated by four phylogenetic groups of bacteria,[128-130] including two established genera (*Bacteroides* and *Bifidobacterium*) and two clusters of diversely named organisms related to *Clostridium coccoides* and

Clostridium leptum, respectively. Both classical and molecular studies indicate that hundreds of distinct organisms comprise this ecosystem.[131] Animal models demonstrate that these organisms *en masse* confer resistance to *C. difficile* colonization,[132] and that disruption of this microbial ecosystem with antibiotics is a prerequisite for establishing *C. difficile* disease.[55] Studies of a carefully documented in vitro continuous-flow culture model of mouse microbiota indicated that the normally present organisms efficiently deplete carbon sources required for growth of *C. difficile,* especially certain monosaccharide components of mucin.[133] Because they are known to metabolize mucin,[134] are related phylogenetically to *C. difficile,* and have been shown to suppress this pathogen in a continuous-flow culture model,[135] *C. coccoides* and relatives are likely candidates for exerting the key suppressive effect. *Clostridium cocleatum,* phylogenetically a member of the less related *Clostridium ramosum* assemblage, has shown a suppressive effect in gnotobiotic mice.[136]

Once antibiotics have rendered the gut more susceptible to *C. difficile* infection, colonization occurs by fecal-oral transmission. Whereas most vegetative cells are killed in the acidic environment of the stomach, acid-resistant spores pass through relatively undamaged and convert to vegetative forms in the small bowel after exposure to primary bile acid.[137,138] Colony counts of more than 10^8 colony-forming units (CFUs) per gram of feces are typical in patients with *C. difficile* disease, and it appears likely that the organism grows throughout the lumen of the colon, rather than attaching to specific colonocyte receptors.[139] Although some *C. difficile* strains possess various structures shown to mediate adhesion in vitro, the roles of these factors in colonization and virulence remain unclear.[140] As *C. difficile* becomes more genetically tractable, it may become possible to test the roles of these potential virulence determinants directly.

As pathogenic *C. difficile* organisms multiply at steady state in the colon, they release two potent toxins that ultimately mediate diarrhea and colitis. These large exotoxins—toxin A, a 308-kd enterotoxin, and toxin B, a 269-kd cytotoxin[141]—rank among the most lethal bacterial toxins studied[142] and have proved active against the more than 20 cell lines from different mammalian species and tissues tested to date.[34,143] These toxins, which exhibit an overall homology of greater than 45% at the amino acid level, contain a complex series of contiguous repeated units at the carboxyl terminus.[139] For toxin A, these repeating units appear to be responsible for carbohydrate receptor binding[144] and for antibody binding in the enzyme-linked immunosorbent assay (ELISA).[145,146] In humans and rodents, toxin A binds to specific carbohydrate receptors containing the carbohydrate moiety galactose-β-1,4-*N*-acetylglucosamine.[147] Three carbohydrate antigens bearing this structure—Lewis I, X, and Y, which exist on human intestinal epithelium—bind toxin A.[147,148] Because of its self-aggregative qualities, toxin B is more difficult to work with, and its receptors have not yet been identified.

Once they gain access to the cytoplasm, both toxin A and toxin B inactivate Rho proteins, a family of small guanosine triphosphate (GTP)–binding proteins that regulate actin cytoskeleton and various signal transduction processes.[149] Specifically, using uridine diphosphate (UDP)–glucose as cosubstrate, the toxins catalyze monoglucosylation of Rho at the threonine 37 position.[150] Ultimately, the toxin-induced dysregulation of Rho leads to cytoskeletal disruption, cell rounding and retraction, and apoptosis in cultured cell lines[151,152]; it also probably explains the profound effect of toxin A on intercellular tight junctions of epithelial cell monolayers and cytoskeletal derangements in neutrophils.[153,154]

In intact animal models, *C. difficile* toxin A causes intestinal fluid secretion, mucosal injury, and inflammation. If instilled in equimolar amounts into ligated loops of rabbit small intestine, toxin A stimulates fluid secretion as efficiently as cholera toxin, although the mechanisms of action for the two are completely different.[155] A sequential study[156] of early histopathologic changes in rabbit small intestine exposed to toxin A revealed an initial diffuse lymphocytic infiltrate in the lamina propria, followed by edema and bulging of the lamina propria in the apical portions of villi and, eventually, cytolysis and separation of the basal portions of the apical epithelial cells. An acute inflammatory response also occurs, with polymorphonuclear leukocyte and mononuclear cell infiltration into the lamina propria.[157]

Key mediators implicated in the inflammatory and secretory responses of toxin A include arachidonic acid metabolites (prostaglandins, leukotrienes, and platelet-activating factor),[158] substance P,[159] leptin,[160] and, potentially, monocyte-derived interleukins IL-8 and IL-6, tumor necrosis factor (TNF), and IL-1.[151,161-163]

Neutrophils, which are found within pseudomembranes and within the intestinal mucosal layer underneath pseudomembranes, play a pivotal role in the pathophysiology of this disease. Via a pertussis toxin–inhibitable G protein, toxin A directly activates human granulocytes in vitro, inducing a transient rise in unbound cytosolic calcium that is both rapid and dose dependent.[164] Toxin A has been shown to promote chemotaxis and chemokinesis in some conditions,[164] whereas in others it clearly impairs directed and nondirected migration and induces striking morphologic changes.[154] Monoclonal antibodies directed against the neutrophil adhesion molecule CD11/18 markedly inhibit both neutrophil infiltration and intestinal secretory responses in a rabbit model of *C. difficile* disease.[165] Mast cells also participate in these responses in mouse and rat models, in pathways that appear to involve substance P.[166]

Although toxin B has no demonstrable effect on permeability, fluid secretion, neutrophil migration, or changes in intestinal morphology in the rabbit model,[157] it also disrupts tight junctions in human epithelial cell monolayers,[167] and it is approximately 10 times more potent on a molar basis than toxin A in mediating damage to human colonic mucosa in the Ussing chamber model.[168] Strains lacking toxin A can show the full range of virulence in humans.[145] In a rat model of neutrophil migration, toxin B also stimulated intense neutrophil recruitment via macrophage-derived TNF-α and lipoxygenase.[169]

PATHOLOGY

A distinct macroscopic appearance characterizes pseudomembranous colitis at endoscopy (Fig. 92-4). The colonic mucosa is studded with adherent, raised, white and yellowish plaques. Initially, these lesions are small and discrete and are easily dislodged; the intervening mucosa may be inflamed and covered with mucus, but often it appears entirely normal.

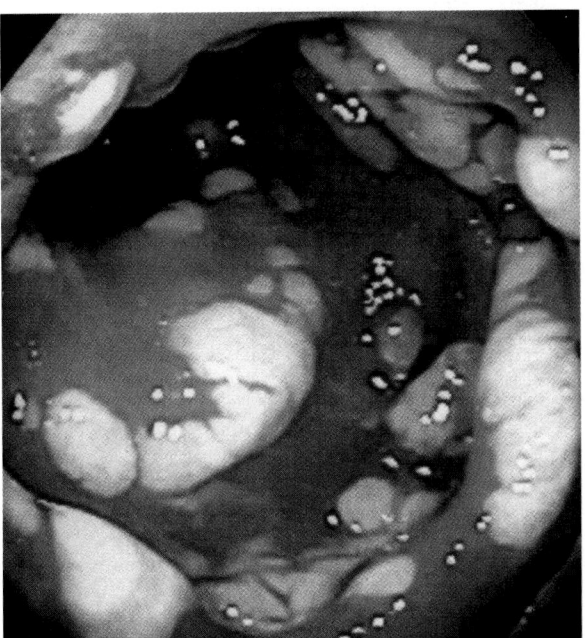

FIGURE 92-4. Endoscopic view of multiple scattered, yellowish plaques consistent with pseudomembranous colitis. *(From Iseman DT, Hamza SH, Eloubeidi MA. Pseudomembranous [Clostridium difficile] colitis. Gastrointest Endosc. 2002;56:907.)*

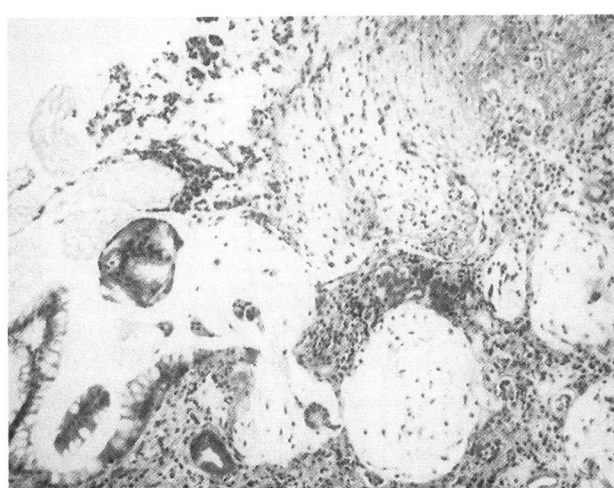

FIGURE 92-5. Biopsy specimen from pseudomembranous colitis showing denudation of superficial epithelium, neutrophilic infiltrate in the lamina propria, and mucopurulent exudates erupting to mucosal surface. *(From Iseman DT, Hamza SH, Eloubeidi MA. Pseudomembranous [Clostridium difficile] colitis. Gastrointest Endosc. 2002;56:907.)*

tirely normal. With progression of disease, pseudomembranous plaques may enlarge and coalesce. Pseudomembranes can exist throughout the entire colon, but they are usually most pronounced in the rectosigmoid colon; rarely does the disease progress proximal to the ileocecal valve.

Histologic criteria for pseudomembranous colitis and a method for grading lesions have been described. The principal features are inflamed mucosa with a neutrophilic predominance and mucin-distended glands. Attached pseudomembranes are composed of a loose network of mucin, neutrophils, fibrin, and nuclear debris (Fig. 92-5).

DIAGNOSIS

C. difficile–associated disease should be suspected in patients with diarrhea who have received antibiotics within the previous 2 months or whose diarrhea begins 72 hours after hospitalization.[110] In most instances, toxin testing or *C. difficile* culture of a single stool specimen effectively establishes the diagnosis; however, repeat testing or endoscopy, or both, may be necessary. Table 92-2 summarizes characteristics of the various tests used in the diagnosis of *C. difficile*–associated diarrhea.

Detection of *Clostridium difficile* Toxins

The most widely used means of diagnosing *C. difficile*–associated diarrhea and colitis clinically is detection of *C. difficile* toxins in stool specimens. The cytotoxicity assay has been considered the gold standard for diagnosis, but most clinical laboratories use various enzyme immunoassays (EIA), which perform reasonably well compared with cytotoxicity testing. As in the original descriptions of *C. difficile* cytotoxin assays,[28,30] stool filtrates are incubated with a mammalian tissue culture cell line with and without toxin-neutralizing antibody. If cytotoxic activity, usually manifested as rounding of cultured cells, is noted in the well with the stool filtrate but not in the well containing both stool filtrate and toxin-neutralizing antibody, the test result for the specimen is considered to be positive (see Fig. 92-2).[28] If used in the appropriate clinical setting, this test is both sensitive and specific; more than 90% of patients with pseudomembranous colitis have cytotoxic activity in their stools detected by this assay.[143] However, sensitivity may vary with the use of different cell lines and because of potential inactivation of toxin B during storage and handling of samples. Additional disadvantages

TABLE 92-2 **Sensitivity and Specificity of Tests for the Diagnosis of *Clostridium difficile*-Associated Disease**

Test	Sensitivity (%)*	Specificity (%)*	Utility of Test
Endoscopy	51	Approximately 100	Diagnostic of PMC
Culture for *C. difficile*	89-100	84-99	Highly sensitive; confirmation of organism toxicity optimal
Cell culture cytotoxin test	67-100	85-100	With clinical data, diagnostic of CDAD
EIA toxin test	63-99	75-100	With clinical data, diagnostic of CDAD
Latex test for *C. difficile* antigen	58-92	80-96	Less sensitive and specific than other tests; rapid results
PCR toxin gene detection	Undetermined	Undetermined	Research test

*Using both clinical and test-based criteria.
CDAD, *Clostridium difficile*-associated disease; EIA, enzyme immunoassay; PCR, polymerase chain reaction; PMC, pseudomembranous colitis.
Modified from Gerding DN, Johnson S, Peterson LR, et al. *Clostridium difficile*–associated diarrhea and colitis. Infect Control Hosp Epidemiol. 1995;16:459-477.

of the cytotoxicity assay include its expense, lack of standardization, slow turnaround time (up to 2 days), and, in most cases, the need for a tissue culture facility (commercial kits may not require this). Finally, although the cytotoxicity assay is widely considered the best single test for *C. difficile*–associated enteric disease, its sensitivity was cited as being as low as 67% when a combination of clinical and laboratory criteria was used to confirm the diagnosis.[169a]

At least eight commercial ELISA kits that detect toxin A or B or both are available, and their performance characteristics have been studied extensively.[170-172] In general, they are rapid, relatively inexpensive, and specific, but they lack the sensitivity of the technically more cumbersome cytotoxin assays. If measured against the strictest diagnostic criteria that include clinical diarrhea, along with positive cytotoxin assay and culture results, their sensitivity ranges from 63% to 94%, with a specificity of 75% to 100%.[173] Repeated testing can boost sensitivity. Assays targeting the detection of both toxins are preferred and have the advantage of detecting strains that are negative for toxin A but positive for toxin B, which are missed by toxin A assays.[145] As with many laboratory tests, those with greatest sensitivity often have poorer specificity, and some have a relatively broad indeterminate range, necessitating either repeat testing or use of a different method on the same sample.

Culture for *Clostridium difficile*

Anaerobic culture for *C. difficile*, the most sensitive test in many laboratories, remains essential for epidemiologic studies of outbreaks. However, cost and convenience issues have driven many hospital laboratories to replace routine cultures with the more rapid and less expensive ELISA-based assays, sometimes in combination with cytotoxin assays. Most clinical microbiology laboratories are not equipped to distinguish between toxigenic and nonpathogenic, nontoxigenic strains, and testing schemes that rely solely on *C. difficile* cultures yield a significant number of false-positive results. (In some hospitals, 20% to 25% of *C. difficile* isolates are nontoxigenic.[101]) Testing for stool toxin simultaneously or using in vitro toxin production assays may help to resolve this problem,[173] but at considerable additional expense. Furthermore, the diagnostic accuracy of testing isolates for toxin production is not established.

Additional Tests for *Clostridium difficile*

The latex agglutination test is rapid and simple but relatively insensitive and nonspecific. Originally thought to detect toxin A, this inexpensive test actually detects glutamate dehydrogenase, a protein that has no definable role in enteric disease,[174,175] and organisms other than *C. difficile* produce antigens that cross react with the antibody used in this assay.[176] Because of its overall poor performance and the availability of other rapid tests that are more sensitive and more specific, use of the latex agglutination test is not recommended.[173]

Oligonucleotide probes to identify *C. difficile* have been known for 15 years,[177] and it has been possible to amplify the pathogen's toxin genes for 10 years,[178] but there are as yet no commercially available molecular tests for *C. difficile* disease. Gene amplification has been shown repeatedly to compare favorably with testing for cytotoxin, widely considered to be the most accurate laboratory test

for the disease.[178-183] It therefore seems likely that, as the technology becomes more cost efficient, such tests will become useful in clinical practice.

Role of Endoscopy

Direct visualization of exudative plaques, or pseudomembranes, on colonic mucosa establishes the diagnosis of pseudomembranous colitis. The pathognomonic lesion is characteristically raised, yellowish, and usually 2 to 10 mm in diameter with "skip" areas of normal mucosa, but in severe disease, lesions may coalesce to form plaques.[110] At least 90% of patients with pseudomembranous colitis demonstrate either *C. difficile* or its toxin in stool samples.[103,181-183]

Flexible sigmoidoscopy alone fails to detect up to 10% of cases without colonoscopy.[184] If *C. difficile* colitis is not accompanied by pseudomembrane formation, endoscopic findings are relatively nonspecific, but biopsy may reveal changes typical of pseudomembranous colitis.

Because of its cost, risk to the patient, and the availability of other diagnostic tests, endoscopy is usually reserved for special situations. The American College of Gastroenterology Guidelines[110] recommend endoscopy for situations such as the following: (1) a rapid diagnosis is needed and test results are delayed or insensitive tests are used, (2) the patient has an ileus and stool is not available, or (3) other colonic diseases that can be diagnosed with endoscopy are being considered.

Testing Strategies

The proper use of the aforementioned tests necessitates an understanding of which patients should be tested. According to a clinical prediction rule derived and validated in a relatively narrow patient population, hospitalized patients without a history of antimicrobial use within the past 30 days *and* without either significant diarrhea (defined as three or more stools of decreased consistency within 24 hours) or abdominal pain would be expected to have a negative result on cytotoxin assay for *C. difficile*.[105,106] The clinical utility of this rule is its negative predictive value: 94% to 97% of such patients are cytotoxin-negative. Therefore, in such circumstances, cytotoxin testing usually is not required. Katz and associates[105,106] calculated that, with the use of this rule, 29% to 39% of cytotoxin tests ordered in such study populations could have been avoided or deferred. In addition, *C. difficile* testing is not recommended for patients with nondiarrheal stool specimens (unless ileus due to *C. difficile* is suspected); for infants younger than 1 year of age (in whom clinical illness does not correlate with presence of toxin in stools); or for "test of cure."[173]

No single best laboratory testing scheme for the diagnosis of *C. difficile*–associated diarrhea and colitis has been established. The Society for Healthcare Epidemiology Association (SHEA)[173] and other authorities[185] recommend combining tissue culture cytotoxin testing with stool culture for optimal diagnostic sensitivity (culture) and specificity (cytotoxin assay). However, many laboratories no longer culture *C. difficile*,[170,186] and stool cytotoxin testing is costly and time-consuming. Although toxin ELISAs sacrifice some sensitivity, because of their relatively good specificity, rapid turnaround time, convenience, and cost they are considered reasonable alternatives to cytotoxin assays and are widely used.[4,110,173] A combination of EIA testing and cytotoxin testing is used sequentially in some laboratories.[104,170,187] Manabe and co-workers[104] found that the addition of a tissue culture assay to EIA testing improved the diagnostic sensitivity of the first stool specimen from 72% to 81%. If initial stool studies are negative and the patient's diarrhea persists without any other obvious cause, repeating the studies may increase the rate of detection significantly[104] and has been recommended,[110] although not all authorities support this practice.[188]

Because stool toxin testing can take up to 2 to 3 days to perform (depending on the assay used), testing for the presence of fecal inflammatory markers may assist with clinical decision making in some instances. For *C. difficile*–associated disease, the sensitivity of the fecal lactoferrin assay ranges from 75% to 90%,[104,189] but the test is not very specific (46% in one study).[189] In comparison, microscopy for fecal leukocytes is less sensitive (28% to 40%) but more specific (92%).[189,190]

TREATMENT

General Considerations

Both the American College of Gastroenterology and the SHEA have prepared management recommendations for *C. difficile*–associated disease (Table 92-3).[173] Initial therapy for pseudomembranous colitis should include discontinuation of the offending antibiotic regimen, if possible, and replacement of fluid and electrolyte losses. In a prospective treatment trial, the diarrhea resolved before initiation of therapy in 23% of 149 patients,[191] but most patients require specific antibacterial therapy. If the offending antibiotic cannot be discontinued or cannot be safely replaced by another antibiotic that is less likely to predispose to *C. difficile*–associated disease (see Table 92-1), antibacterial therapy with oral metronidazole is preferred.

Oral Metronidazole

Although metronidazole and vancomycin are equally effective for treating *C. difficile*–associated disease,[191] metronidazole is now considered the drug of choice for most cases because of cost and concerns regarding the emergence of VRE.[4,110,173,192] Most *C. difficile* isolates are highly susceptible to metronidazole, with the minimal inhibitory concentration for 90% of the organisms (MIC$_{90}$) in most studies ranging from 0.25 to 1.0 μg/mL in several studies from different geographic regions.[193,194] However, resistance was reported to be 6% in one recent study.[195] In patients with *C. difficile*–associated diarrhea, bactericidal fecal levels are readily achievable; in one study, nine patients had bactericidal fecal concentrations of metronidazole (mean, 9.3 ± 7.5 μg/g of wet stool) and of its hydroxymetabolite during therapy for *C. difficile*–associated diarrhea.[196] As the patients' diarrhea abated, metronidazole and hydroxymetronidazole levels fell, with neither detectable after recovery. In other settings, after administration of oral metronidazole, patients with severe Crohn's disease had higher intraluminal levels than in those with more quiescent disease,[197] and fecal levels were either undetectable or minimally detectable in healthy volunteers[198] and in asymptomatic *C. difficile* carriers.[45] The decline in fecal levels of metronidazole during therapy parallels expected decreases in mucosal inflammation and may be explained by decreased exudation of metronidazole through less inflamed mucosa. It is also possible that, with clinical improvement, decreased intestinal motility increases metronidazole transit time, enabling more complete absorption.[196] This phenomenon has been invoked as a potential explanation for the relapses seen with metronidazole.

Despite these concerns, oral metronidazole is highly effective clinically, with cure rates of 94% to 95% and relapse rates of 5% to 16% in two prospective randomized trials.[191,199] The largest recorded experience with metronidazole comes from the Minneapolis Veterans Affairs Hospital, where oral metronidazole therapy was used in 632 patients with *C. difficile*–associated diarrhea between 1982 and 1991. Metronidazole was judged to be highly effective in this observational report, with intolerance, failure, and relapse rates of 1%, 2%, and 7%, respectively.[44]

TABLE 92-3 Recommendations for Treatment of *Clostridium difficile*-Associated Diarrhea and Colitis

If clinical situation allows, discontinue offending antibiotic and/or modify regimen to agent less commonly associated with *C. difficile* disease (see Table 92-1).

Replace fluid and electrolyte losses.

Avoid antiperistaltic agents.

If above conservative measures are not effective or not practical, institute specific therapy with oral metronidazole, 250 mg qid for 10 days.

Do not treat asymptomatic colonization.

Re-treat first-time recurrences with the same regimen used to treat the initial episode.

Avoid vancomycin use, if possible.*

*In general vancomycin should be reserved for patients who (1) fail or cannot take metronidazole (e.g., intolerance, coadministration of ethanol-containing solutions, pregnancy, child younger than 10 years of age); (2) have *C. difficile* disease associated with metronidazole-resistant strain, or, (3) are critically ill because of *C. difficile*–associated disease.

Adapted with permission from The American Gastroenterological Association, from the American College of Gastroenterology Practice Guidelines as reported by Fekety R. *Am J Gastroenterol*. 1997;92:739-750; and from the Society for Healthcare Epidemiology Association position paper presented by Gerding DN, Johnson S, Peterson LR, et al. *Clostridium difficile*–associated diarrhea and colitis. *Infect Control Hosp Epidemiol*. 1995;16:459-477.

Oral Vancomycin

Multiple randomized, comparative studies have documented the efficacy of oral vancomycin for *C. difficile*–associated diarrhea and colitis.[191,199-202] Despite concerns for cost and the emergence of VRE, it is cited as the preferred drug for severe disease.[110,192] However, there is little published evidence showing superiority to metronidazole with regard to clinical end points. Most *C. difficile* isolates are susceptible to an MIC of 1 μg/mL, and virtually all are susceptible to 16 μg/mL, levels that are orders of magnitude lower than the intraluminal levels achieved with oral vancomycin.[203] Oral vancomycin is rarely absorbed to any appreciable degree, and multiple studies report levels in stool in excess of 1000 to 3000 μg/mL,[200,204,205] which, unlike those of metronidazole, are maintained for the duration of antimicrobial therapy. Although higher doses may achieve greater fecal concentrations,[204,205] there is no evidence that higher dosing regimens (which are considerably more expensive) offer any clinical benefit. Doses of 125 mg four times daily for 10 days effected no fewer cures than did 500 mg four times daily in one study, but the trial lacked sufficient statistical power to prove the equivalence of the two regimens.[206] One case report documented enteral absorption of vancomycin leading to significant serum levels (up to 20 μg/mL) in a patient with pseudomembranous colitis and renal failure.[207]

Comparative prospective studies with various doses of vancomycin have documented clinical response rates of 86% to 100%, with relapses in 15% to 33%.[199-202,206] A retrospective review[207] of clinical outcome in 189 patients receiving oral vancomycin (at dosages ranging from 0.5 to 2.0 g/day, usually for 7 to 14 days) identified treatment failures in only 3%. Overall treatment response was judged to be good (i.e., prompt improvement and recovery without a change in the specific therapy) in 87%, with relapses occurring in 24%.[208]

Oral vancomycin therapy is a significant risk factor for colonization and infection with VRE,[209] and the Hospital Infection Control Practice Advisory Committee (HICPAC) recommends vancomycin for antibiotic-associated colitis only if metronidazole fails or if the disease is severe and potentially life-threatening.[192] It should be noted, however, that some of these same studies also identified metronidazole use as a risk factor for VRE colonization or infection.[209] The issue is clouded by the fact that *C. difficile* disease itself is associated with carriage of VRE.

Second-Line Agents

A number of other antibacterials and toxin-binding preparations have been evaluated for the treatment of primary *C. difficile* disease. The results of prospective randomized studies[200,201] using oral bacitracin are summarized in Table 92-4. Given the overall relatively poor efficacy of

TABLE 92-4 Efficacy and Cost of Oral Antibiotics for *Clostridium difficile*-Associated Diarrhea and Colitis

Drug (Range of Dosing Regimens Reported)	Response Rate (%)	Relapse Rate (%)	Mean Days to Improvement or Resolution
Metronidazole (250 mg qid to 500 mg tid × 10 days)	94-95	5-16	2.4-3.2
Vancomycin (125 mg qid × 7 days to 500 mg qid × 10 days)	86-100	15-33	2.6-4.2
Bacitracin (20,000 to 25,000 U qid × 7-10 days)	76-80	42	2.4-4.1
Teicoplanin* (100 to 400 mg bid × 10 days)	96-98	8	2.8-3.4
Fusidic acid* (500 mg tid × 10 days)	93	28	3.8

*Not available in the United States.

Data from prospective, randomized trials reported by Teasley,[191] Wenisch,[199] Young,[200] Dudley,[201] de Lalla,[202] and Fekety[206] and their respective co-workers.

this agent compared with oral vancomycin or metronidazole, its higher cost (which is increased by the need for compounding by a pharmacist), and its lack of palatability, oral bacitracin should be considered only in rare circumstances in which oral metronidazole or vancomycin cannot be used. Oral teicoplanin and fusidic acid, neither of which is available in the United States, had efficacy similar to that of oral vancomycin or metronidazole in two small but well-designed clinical studies. However, experience with these glycopeptides for *C. difficile* disease remains limited.

The anion-exchange resins cholestyramine and colestipol, which bind *C. difficile* cytotoxin,[210] have been proposed as potential nonantibiotic treatments for milder cases and for consolidation therapy, after the use of first-line agents, for relapses.[203] The following findings argue against their routine use: (1) only 5 of 14 patients with either toxin- or culture-positive diarrhea responded to colestipol in a prospective evaluation[211]; (2) unsatisfactory results were reported retrospectively in 37% of 19 patients receiving cholestyramine[208]; and (3) systemic absorption of cholestyramine has been documented.[212] In vivo studies have demonstrated the potential to inhibit toxin B at its intracellular site of action by exposing cells to inactive mutated toxin B,[213] suggesting a possibility for novel therapeutic agents. The potential of antibody therapy is discussed later (see "Recurrent Disease").

Therapy for Patients Who Lack Oral Access

No single regimen has demonstrated superiority in patients who are unable to take or tolerate oral metronidazole or vancomycin because of paralytic ileus, nasogastric suctioning, intestinal obstruction, or diversion. After intravenous administration of metronidazole, three patients with documented *C. difficile*–associated diarrhea responded clinically, and fecal concentrations of metronidazole and its hydroxymetabolite were documented at concentrations well in excess of the MIC for *C. difficile*.[196] Intravenous metronidazole was also used successfully in six patients with acute abdomen, antibiotic-associated colitis (pseudomembranous in five), and positive results on latex agglutination testing for *C. difficile* (three also received vancomycin via nasogastric tube).[111] Parenteral metronidazole failures have also been reported.[214]

Fewer clearcut treatment successes with intravenous vancomycin have been reported,[215] and failures have been clearly documented.[214,216] In one such failure, fecal levels of vancomycin could not be detected despite 5 days of parenteral therapy.[216] Anecdotal reports of adjunctive therapy with rectal vancomycin (coadministered with intravenous or nasogastric vancomycin or metronidazole) pepper the literature,[217,218] and the drug has been administered both as an enema and through a long catheter placed during colonoscopy.[217] However, the safety and efficacy of this practice have not been established, and systemic absorption after long-catheter colonic instillation of vancomycin has been reported.[218]

The absence of controlled, prospective trials of treatment in patients who lack oral access precludes definitive recommendations; however, intravenous metronidazole (500 mg every 6 to 8 hours),

or vancomycin retention enemas (500 mg every 4 to 8 hours) or vancomycin via colonic catheter should be considered.[215-219] Rarely, extremely ill patients with ileus may benefit from surgical decompression and direct instillation of vancomycin or metronidazole through the stoma. Alternatively, in toxic megacolon, colonoscopic decompression with vancomycin instillation has been used successfully.[220]

Antimotility Agents

Antiperistaltic agents, such as loperamide and diphenoxylate hydrochloride with atropine, should be avoided. There is little evidence that such agents lead to symptomatic improvement, and in one study predating the discovery of *C. difficile* as a pathogen,[221] diarrhea was actually more common among patients receiving diphenoxylate-atropine plus lincomycin than among those receiving placebo plus lincomycin. Several anecdotes and case series have associated the use of diphenoxylate, and of loperamide and other antiperistaltic agents, with the development of toxic megacolon in patients with *C. difficile* disease[113,114] or pseudomembranous colitis. Because these agents promote colonic stasis, there is a theoretical risk of further damage and inflammation with prolonged mucosal exposure to *C. difficile* toxins.

Surgery

Although rarely necessary, surgical intervention can be lifesaving, particularly in cases complicated by toxic megacolon or colonic perforation. Reported rates of surgery necessitated by *C. difficile* disease range from 0.39% of 3300 toxin-positive assays in a 6-year survey at Johns Hopkins Medical Institutions[222] to 3.6% of 138 such cases during a 6-month outbreak in Dublin.[223] The University of Pittsburgh Medical Center recorded colectomies in 1.9% of 2334 hospitalized patients with *C. difficile* colitis between 1989 and 2000.[3] Various surgical approaches for management of toxic megacolon have been described, including diversion of the fecal stream by ileostomy, cecostomy, or decompressive colostomy or by subtotal colectomy. The last-named has been advocated as the procedure of choice for serious disease, including fulminant toxic megacolon associated with pseudomembranous colitis.[224] Two patterns of perforation have been described: multiple perforations involving a large portion of the colon, associated with a higher mortality rate, and a single perforation, associated with relatively lower mortality. With localized perforation, limited segmental resection may be successful. The overall mortality rate in cases requiring surgery is between 30% and 35%,[222] although some series report mortality rates in excess of 50%.[114,223]

RECURRENT DISEASE

Despite initial adequate antimicrobial treatment, recurrent *C. difficile*–associated diarrhea has been reported in 5% to 50% of patients in several small studies[191,200,201]; in 24% of 189 patients who had received vancomycin therapy, as determined by retrospective analysis[208]; and in 7% of 754 patients in whom either metronidazole or vancomycin treatment was initially successful in the Minneapolis experience.[44] A multiple relapse pattern, characterized by five or more relapses after intervening treatments, has been described and may be seen in 5% to 8% of patients who receive specific drug therapy.[44] Risk factors for recurrent disease identified in prospective studies include increased age, recent abdominal surgery, increased number of *C. difficile* diarrheal episodes, and, oddly, onset of initial disease in spring.[119,120] Additional risk factors suggested by retrospective analysis include leukocytosis, chronic renal failure, initial presentation of community-acquired disease, infection with certain immunoblot types, and female gender.[118,119]

Relapse occurs as a result of several factors. Antibiotics do nothing to restore the gut biota's integrity, disturbance of which allowed *C. difficile* to colonize in the first place. Also, patients who recover from *C. difficile* disease typically have mounted an IgG response to one or both toxins.[225] In one recent study, patients having a poor antibody response to toxin A had a 48-fold risk of developing recurrent disease.[68] Finally, antibiotics do not damage bacterial spores, and *C. difficile* spores can survive even high intraluminal levels of vancomycin and remain cultivable from feces during and after therapy.[204] Alternatively, patients with recurrent disease may reacquire the original strain from exogenous environmental sources, or they may acquire a new strain altogether. Although one study found the same strain type in both first and second episodes in 7 of 8 cases,[118] larger studies using varied typing methods have demonstrated new strains in approximately 50% of recurrences.[226]

The treatment of relapsing *C. difficile* disease remains problematic. Patients who experience relapses usually respond to a repeated course of either metronidazole or vancomycin.[44] The only critical comparative trial for treatment of relapsing *C. difficile* disease evaluated the effectiveness of the yeast *Saccharomyces boulardii*. This multicenter, placebo-controlled trial demonstrated that 4 weeks of 3 × 10[10] *S. boulardii* ingested daily, in addition to standard antimicrobial therapy, yielded significantly fewer treatment failures in recurrent but not initial *C. difficile* disease.[227] A variety of other approaches have been reported anecdotally.[228] Tedesco and coinvestigators[229] successfully treated 22 patients with recurrent disease by administering a tapering and then intermittent low dose of oral vancomycin over 6 weeks (125 mg q6h for 1 week, 125 mg q12h for 1 week, 125 mg daily for 1 week, 125 mg every other day for 1 week, and finally 125 mg every 3 days for 2 weeks). Vancomycin (125 mg four times daily) combined with rifampin (600 mg twice daily) for 7 days was reported to be successful in 7 patients.[230] Administration of *C. sordellii* antitoxin prevented disease in the hamster model.[231] Intravenous immune globulin contains significant levels of antibodies to *C. difficile* toxins,[232,233] and there are more than 10 case reports of its successful use for treatment of relapsing disease.[233,234] Administration of fecal suspensions to reestablish the colonic biota has an excellent rationale, was shown to prevent disease in hamsters[228] and in mice,[132] and has been used in approximately 20 reported cases to resolve relapsing disease in humans.[235,236] However, the safety and esthetics of this approach remain a concern. Possibly safer and more palatable, a synthetic biota consisting of 10 bacterial strains including predominant anaerobes was reported to succeed in 6 patients.[237] An extended course of cholestyramine, which binds the cytotoxin,[238] has been successful in a handful of patients.[239-241] Lactobacillus GG ingestion was reported to have been successful in 9 patients with relapsing disease,[242] but, given what is known of the microecology of *C. difficile* and the numeric insignificance of lactobacilli in human biota, the rationale for its use is not clear. No animal studies or continuous-flow culture studies support this approach. Whole-bowel irrigation with a polyethylene glycol solution also has been suggested.[240] In most of these reports, the interventions were used after multiple failed attempts with traditional therapy or as adjunctive therapy. Some of these therapies are riskier than others, and insufficient scientific rigor precludes any specific recommendations.

PREVENTION

The prevention and control of *C. difficile*–associated diarrhea and colitis are thoroughly reviewed in the SHEA position paper.[173] Because in the hospital setting cases tend to cluster in time and space,[238,244] careful monitoring for cases can be rewarding. Simple infection control measures, such as scrupulous glove use during the handling of any body substance[245] and replacement of electronic thermometers with single-use disposable ones,[246] are of proven benefit for decreasing *C. difficile* transmission in health care settings. Good hand washing and environmental cleaning and disinfection are prudent for many reasons and may be effective in reducing the incidence of *C. difficile* disease.[86,247] Screening to identify asymptomatic carriers for specific drug therapy is neither practicable nor enduringly effective. In one study, although treatment with vancomycin was temporarily effective in eradicating asymptomatic *C. difficile* excretion in hospitalized patients, they began to excrete the organism again soon after cessation of therapy.[45]

Limiting the use of certain antimicrobials (particularly those associated with *C. difficile* disease in a given institution) has proved an effective means of control in some outbreaks.[56,248] In particular, restriction of clindamycin use in outbreaks caused by clindamycin-resistant strains resulted in fewer *C. difficile* infections[51,56] and was associated with a return of clindamycin susceptibility and overall cost savings.[56]

Because the population size of *C. difficile* is controlled by the normal biota, introduction of competing, nonpathogenic organisms into the intestinal tract should be useful to prevent antibiotic-associated diarrhea. However, the basic scientific underpinnings to support such an approach are not yet in place. Alternatively, several approaches to vaccination against *C. difficile* toxins have shown promise.[249,250] It seems probable that in the future this disease will be both preventable and reliably curable.

REFERENCES

1. McFarland LV, Surawicz CM, Greenberg RN, et al. Prevention of beta-lactam–associated diarrhea by *Saccharomyces boulardii* compared with placebo. Am J Gastroenterol. 1995;90:439-448.
2. Bartlett JG. Antibiotic-associated diarrhea. Clin Infect Dis. 1992;15:573-581.
3. Dallal RM, Harbrecht BG, Boujoukas AJ, et al. Fulminant *Clostridium difficile:* An underappreciated and increasing cause of death and complications. Ann Surg. 2002;235:363-372.
4. Kelly CP, Pothoulakis C, LaMont JT. *Clostridium difficile* colitis. N Engl J Med. 1994;330:257-262.
5. Karlstrom O, Fryklund B, Tullus K, Burman LG. A prospective nationwide study of *Clostridium difficile*–associated diarrhea in Sweden. The Swedish *C. difficile* Study Group. Clin Infect Dis. 1998;26:141-145.
6. Levine J, Dykoski RK, Janoff EN. *Candida*-associated diarrhea: A syndrome in search of credibility. Clin Infect Dis. 1995;21:881-886.
7. Asha NJ, Wilcox MH. Laboratory diagnosis of *Clostridium perfringens* antibiotic-associated diarrhoea. J Med Microbiol. 2002;51:891-894.
8. Neal KR, Briji SO, Slack RC, et al. Recent treatment with H₂ antagonists and antibiotics and gastric surgery as risk factors for *Salmonella* infection. BMJ. 1994;308:176.
9. Olsen, SJ, DeBess, EE, McGivern, TE, et al. A nosocomial outbreak of fluoroquinolone-resistant salmonella infection. N Engl J Med. 2001;344:1572-1579.
10. Hove H, Tvede M, Mortensen PB. Antibiotic-associated diarrhoea, *Clostridium difficile,* and short-chain fatty acids. Scand J Gastroenterol. 1996;31:688-693.
11. Wilcox MH, Cunniffe JG, Trundle C, Redpath C. Financial burden of hospital-acquired *Clostridium difficile* infection. J Hosp Infect. 1996;34:23-30.
12. Kofsky P, Rosen L, Reed J, et al. *Clostridium difficile:* A common and costly colitis. Dis Colon Rectum. 1991;34:244-248.
13. McFarland LV, Surawicz CM, Rubin M, et al. Recurrent *Clostridium difficile* disease: Epidemiology and clinical characteristics. Infect Control Hosp Epidemiol. 1999;20:43-50.
14. Macgowan AP, Brown I, Feeney R, et al. *Clostridium difficile*–associated diarrhoea and length of hospital stay. J Hosp Infect. 1995;31:241-244.
15. Finney J. Gastro-enterostomy for cicatrizing ulcer of the pylorus. Johns Hopkins Hosp Bull. 1893;4:53-55.
16. Kramer IRH. Fatal staphylococcal enteritis developing during streptomycin therapy by mouth. Lancet. 1948;1:646-647.
17. Bennett IL, Wood JS, Yardley HH. Staphylococcal pseudomembranous enterocolitis in chinchillas: A clinico-pathologic study. Trans Assoc Am Physician. 1956;69:116.
18. Dearing WH, Baggenstoss AH, Weed LA. Studies on the relationship of *Staphylococcus aureus* to pseudomembranous enteritis and to postantibiotic enteritis. Gastroenterology. 1960;38:441-451.

19. Fekety R. Staphylococcal diarrhea and enterocolitis. In: Crossley KB, Archer GL, eds. The Staphylococci in Human Disease. New York: Churchill Livingstone; 1997:545-563.

20. Bartlett JG, Gorbach SL. Pseudomembranous enterocolitis (antibiotic-related colitis). Adv Intern Med. 1977;22:455-476.

21. Willis TA. Historical aspects. In: Rolfe RD, Finegold SM, eds. Clostridium difficile: Its Role in Intestinal Disease. San Diego: Academic Press; 1988:15-28.

22. Lusk RH, Fekety FR Jr, Silva J Jr, et al. Gastrointestinal side effects of clindamycin and ampicillin therapy. J Infect Dis. 1977;135(Suppl):S111-S119.

23. Robertson MB, Breen KJ, Desmond PV, et al. Incidence of antibiotic-related diarrhoea and pseudomembranous colitis: A prospective study of lincomycin, clindamycin and ampicillin. Med J Aust. 1977;1:243-246.

24. Tedesco FJ. Ampicillin-associated diarrhea: A prospective study. Am J Dig Dis. 1975;20:295-297.

25. Tedesco FJ, Barton RW, Alpers DH. Clindamycin-associated colitis. Ann Intern Med. 1974;81:429-433.

26. Colitis associated with clindamycin. Med Lett Drugs Ther. 1974;16:73-74.

27. Warning on antibiotic-induced colitis. Lancet. 1979;1:1306.

28. Larson HE, Parry JV, Price AB, et al. Undescribed toxin in pseudomembranous colitis. BMJ. 1977;1:1246-1248.

29. Bartlett JG, Onderdonk AB, Cisneros RL, Kasper DL. Clindamycin-associated colitis due to a toxin-producing species of Clostridium in hamsters. J Infect Dis. 1977;136:701-705.

30. Rifkin GD, Fekety FR, Silva J Jr. Antibiotic-induced colitis: Implication of a toxin neutralised by Clostridium sordellii antitoxin. Lancet. 1977;2:1103-1106.

31. Larson HE, Price AB. Pseudomembranous colitis: Presence of clostridial toxin. Lancet. 1977;2:1312-1314.

32. Bartlett JG, Chang TW, Gurwith M, et al. Antibiotic-associated pseudomembranous colitis due to toxin-producing clostridia. N Engl J Med. 1978;298:531-534.

33. Hall IC, O'Toole E. Intestinal flora in new-born infants. Am J Dis Child. 1935;49:390-402.

34. Thielman NM, Guerrant RL. Clostridium difficile and its toxins. In: Moss J, Iglewski B, Vaughn M, Tue AT, eds. Bacterial Toxins and Virulence Factors in Disease. New York: Marcel Dekker; 1995:327-366.

35. Tasteyre A, Barc MC, Karjalainen T, et al. A Clostridium difficile gene encoding flagellin. Microbiology 2000;146:957-966.

36. Karjalainen T, Saumier N, Barc MC, et al. Clostridium difficile genotyping based on slpA variable region in S-layer gene sequence: An alternative to serotyping. J Clin Microbiol. 2002;40:2452-2458.

37. Mani N, Dupuy B. Regulation of toxin synthesis in Clostridium difficile by an alternative RNA polymerase sigma factor. Proc Nat Acad Sci U S A. 2001;98:5844-5849.

38. George WL, Sutter VL, Citron D, Finegold SM. Selective and differential medium for isolation of Clostridium difficile. J Clin Microbiol. 1979;9:214-219.

39. Lyerly DM, Allen SD. The clostridia. In: Emmerson AM, Hawkey PM, Gillespie SH, eds. Principles and Practice of Clinical Bacteriology. Chichester: John Wiley & Sons; 1997:599-623.

40. Wilson KH, Kennedy MJ, Fekety FR. Use of sodium taurocholate to enhance spore recovery on a medium selective for Clostridium difficile. J Clin Microbiol. 1982;15:443-446.

41. Mundy LS, Shanholtzer CJ, Willard KE, et al. Laboratory detection of Clostridium difficile. A comparison of media and incubation systems. Am J Clin Pathol. 1995;103:52-56.

42. Gerding DN, Olson MM, Peterson LR, et al. Clostridium difficile-associated diarrhea and colitis in adults: A prospective case-controlled epidemiologic study. Arch Intern Med. 1986;146:95-100.

43. Lai KK, Melvin ZS, Menard MJ, et al. Clostridium difficile-associated diarrhea: Epidemiology, risk factors, and infection control. Infect Control Hosp Epidemiol. 1997;18:628-632.

44. Olson MM, Shanholtzer CJ, Lee JT Jr, Gerding DN. Ten years of prospective Clostridium difficile-associated disease surveillance and treatment at the Minneapolis VA Medical Center, 1982-1991. Infect Control Hosp Epidemiol. 1994;15:371-381.

45. Johnson S, Homann SR, Bettin KM, et al. Treatment of asymptomatic Clostridium difficile carriers (fecal excretors) with vancomycin or metronidazole: A randomized, placebo-controlled trial. Ann Intern Med. 1992;117:297-302.

46. Bender BS, Bennett R, Laughon BE, et al. Is Clostridium difficile endemic in chronic-care facilities? Lancet. 1986;2:11-13.

47. Yablon SA, Krotenberg R, Fruhmann K. Clostridium difficile-related disease: Evaluation and prevalence among inpatients with diarrhea in two freestanding rehabilitation hospitals. Arch Phys Med Rehabil. 1993;74:9-13.

48. Hirschhorn LR, Trnka Y, Onderdonk A, et al. Epidemiology of community-acquired Clostridium difficile-associated diarrhea. J Infect Dis. 1994;169:127-133.

49. McFarland LV, Surawicz CM, Stamm WE. Risk factors for Clostridium difficile carriage and C. difficile-associated diarrhea in a cohort of hospitalized patients. J Infect Dis. 1990;162:678-684.

50. Wistrom J, Norrby SR, Myhre EB, et al. Frequency of antibiotic-associated diarrhoea in 2462 antibiotic-treated hospitalized patients: A prospective study. J Antimicrob Chemother. 2001;47:43-50.

51. Johnson S, Samore MH, Farrow KA, et al. Epidemics of diarrhea caused by a clindamycin-resistant strain of Clostridium difficile in four hospitals. N Engl J Med. 1999;341:1645-1651.

52. Anand A, Bashey B, Mir T, Glatt AE. Epidemiology, clinical manifestations, and outcome of Clostridium difficile-associated diarrhea. Am J Gastroenterol. 1994;89:519-523.

53. Feldman RJ, Kallich M, Weinstein MP. Bacteremia due to Clostridium difficile: Case report and review of extraintestinal C. difficile infections. Clin Infect Dis. 1995;20:1560-1562.

54. Bauwens JE, McFarland LV, Melcher SA. Recurrent Clostridium difficile disease following ciprofloxacin use. Ann Pharmacother. 1997;31:1090.

55. Small JD. Drugs used in hamsters with a review of antibiotic-associated colitis in the laboratory hamster. In: Van Hoosier GL, McPherson CW, eds. Laboratory Hamsters. Orlando: Academic Press; 1987:179-199.

56. Climo MW, Israel DS, Wong ES, et al. Hospital-wide restriction of clindamycin: Effect on the incidence of Clostridium difficile-associated diarrhea and cost. Ann Intern Med. 1998;128:989-995.

57. Impallomeni M, Galletly NP, Wort SJ, et al. Increased risk of diarrhoea caused by Clostridium difficile in elderly patients receiving cefotaxime. BMJ. 1995;311:1345-1346.

58. Starr JM, Rogers TR, Impallomeni M. Hospital-acquired Clostridium difficile diarrhoea and herd immunity. Lancet. 1997;349:426-428.

59. Anand A, Glatt AE. Clostridium difficile infection associated with antineoplastic chemotherapy: A review. Clin Infect Dis. 1993;17:109-113.

60. Moskovitz M, Bartlett JG. Recurrent pseudomembranous colitis unassociated with prior antibiotic therapy. Arch Intern Med. 1981;141:663-664.

61. Ray AJ, Donskey CJ. Clostridium difficile infection and concurrent vancomycin-resistant Enterococcus stool colonization in a health care worker: Cse report and review of the literature. Am J Infect Control. 2003;31:54-56.

62. Ray AJ, Hoyen CK, Das SM, et al. Undetected vancomycin-resistant Enterococcus stool colonization in a Veterans Affairs Hospital using a Clostridium difficile-focused surveillance strategy. Infect Control Hosp Epidemiol. 2002;23:474-477.

63. Leber AL, Hindler JF, Kato EO, et al. Laboratory-based surveillance for vancomycin-resistant enterococci: Utility of screening stool specimens submitted for Clostridium difficile toxin assay. Infect Control Hosp Epidemiol. 2001;22:160-164.

64. Grube BJ, Heimbach DM, Marvin JA. Clostridium difficile diarrhea in critically ill burned patients. Arch Surg. 1987;122:655-661.

65. Aronsson B, Barany P, Nord CE, et al. Clostridium difficile-associated diarrhoea in uremic patients. Eur J Clin Microbiol. 1987;6:352-356.

66. Heard SR, Wren B, Barnett MJ, et al. Clostridium difficile infection in patients with haematological malignant disease: Risk factors, faecal toxins and pathogenic strains. Epidemiol Infect. 1988;100:63-72.

67. Keighley MR, Burdon DW, Alexander-Williams J, et al. Diarrhoea and pseudomembranous colitis after gastrointestinal operations: A prospective study. Lancet. 1978;2:1165-1167.

68. Kyne L, Warny M, Qamar A, et al. Asymptomatic carriage of Clostridium difficile and serum levels of IgG antibody against toxin A. N Engl J Med. 2000;342:390-397.

69. Kyne L, Warny M, Qamar A, et al. Association between antibody response to toxin A and protection against recurrent Clostridium difficile diarrhoea. Lancet. 2001;357:189-193.

70. Hutin Y, Casin I, Lesprit P, et al. Prevalence of and risk factors for Clostridium difficile colonization at admission to an infectious diseases ward. Clin Infect Dis. 1997;24:920-924.

71. Hutin Y, Molina JM, Casin I, et al. Risk factors for Clostridium difficile-associated diarrhoea in HIV-infected patients. AIDS. 1993;7:1441-1447.

72. Tumbarello M, Tacconelli E, Leone F, et al. Clostridium difficile-associated diarrhoea in patients with human immunodeficiency virus infection: A case-control study. Eur J Gastroenterol Hepatol. 1995;7:259-263.

73. Cappell MS, Philogene C. Clostridium difficile infection is a treatable cause of diarrhea in patients with advanced human immunodeficiency virus infection: A study of seven consecutive patients admitted from 1986 to 1992 to a university teaching hospital. Am J Gastroenterol. 1993;88:891-897.

74. Lu SS, Schwartz JM, Simon DM, Brandt LJ. Clostridium difficile-associated diarrhea in patients with HIV positivity and AIDS: A prospective controlled study. Am J Gastroenterol. 1994;89:1226-1229.

75. Bolton RP, Tait SK, Dear PR, Losowsky MS. Asymptomatic neonatal colonisation by Clostridium difficile. Arch Dis Child. 1984;59:466-472.

76. Al-Jumaili I, Shibley M, Lishman AH, Record CO. Incidence and origin of Clostridium difficile in neonates. J Clin Microbiol. 1984;19:77-78.

77. el-Mohandes AE, Keiser JF, Refat M, Jackson BJ. Prevalence and toxigenicity of Clostridium difficile isolates in fecal microflora of preterm infants in the intensive care nursery. Biol Neonate. 1993;63:225-229.

78. Zedd AJ, Sell TL, Schaberg DR, et al. Nosocomial Clostridium difficile reservoir in a neonatal intensive care unit. Pediatr Infect Dis. 1984;3:429-432.

79. Triadafilopoulos G, Shah MH, Pothoulakis C. The chemotactic response of human granulocytes to Clostridium difficile toxin A is age dependent. Am J Gastroenterol. 1991;86:1461-1465.

80. Eglow R, Pothoulakis C, Itzkowitz S, et al. Diminished Clostridium difficile toxin A sensitivity in newborn rabbit ileum is associated with decreased toxin A receptor. J Clin Invest. 1992;90:822-829.

81. Rolfe R, Iaconis JP. Intestinal colonization of infant hamsters with Clostridium difficile. Infect Immun. 1983;42:480-486.

82. Nakamura S, Mikawa M, Nakashio S, et al. Isolation of Clostridium difficile from the feces and the antibody in sera of young and elderly adults. Microbiol Immunol. 1981;25:345-351.

83. Hafiz S, Morton R, McEntegart M, et al. Clostridium difficile in the urogenital tract of males and females. Lancet. 1975;1:420-421.

84. Tabaqchali S, O'Farrell S, Nash JQ, Wilks M. Vaginal carriage and neonatal acquisition of Clostridium difficile. J Med Microbiol. 1984;18:47-53.

85. Larson HE, Barclay FE, Honour P, Hill ID. Epidemiology of *Clostridium difficile* in infants. J Infect Dis. 1982;146:727-733.

86. McFarland LV, Mulligan ME, Kwok RY, Stamm WE. Nosocomial acquisition of *Clostridium difficile* infection. N Engl J Med. 1989;320:204-210.

87. Poxton IR, Aronsson B, Möllby R, et al. Immunochemical fingerprinting of *Clostridium difficile* strains isolated from an outbreak of antibiotic-associated colitis and diarrhoea. J Med Microbiol. 1984;17:317-324.

88. Nath SK, Thornley JH, Kelly M, et al. A sustained outbreak of *Clostridium difficile* in a general hospital: Persistence of a toxigenic clone in four units. Infect Control Hosp Epidemiol. 1994;15:382-389.

89. Bennett RG, Laughon BE, Mundy LM, et al. Evaluation of a latex agglutination test for *Clostridium difficile* in two nursing home outbreaks. J Clin Microbiol. 1989;27:889-893.

90. Kim K, DuPont HL, Pickering LK. Outbreaks of diarrhea associated with *Clostridium difficile* and its toxin in day-care centers: Evidence of person-to-person spread. J Pediatr. 1983;102:376-382.

91. Borriello SP, Honour P, Turner T, Barclay F. Household pets as a potential reservoir for *Clostridium difficile* infection. J Clin Pathol. 1983;36:84-87.

92. Bidet P, Lalande V, Salauze B, et al. Comparison of PCR-ribotyping, arbitrarily primed PCR, and pulsed-field gel electrophoresis for typing *Clostridium difficile*. J Clin Microbiol. 2000;38:2484-2487.

93. Klaassen CH, van Haren HA, Horrevorts AM. Molecular fingerprinting of *Clostridium difficile* isolates: Pulsed-field gel electrophoresis versus amplified fragment length polymorphism. J Clin Microbiol 2002;40:101-104.

94. Keim P, Price LB, Klevytska AM, et al. Multiple-locus variable-number tandem repeat analysis reveals genetic relationships within *Bacillus anthracis*. J Bacteriol. 2000;182:2928-2936.

95. Johnson S, Clabots CR, Linn FV, et al. Noscomial *Clostridium difficile* colonisation and disease. 1990;336:97-100.

96. Wilson KH, Sheagren JN. Antagonism of toxigenic *Clostridium difficile* by nontoxigenic C. difficile. J Infect Dis. 1983;147:733-736.

97. Borriello SP, Barclay FE. Protection of hamsters against *Clostridium difficile* ileocaecitis by prior colonisation with non-pathogenic strains. J Med Microbiol. 1985;19:339-350.

98. Seal D, Borriello SP, Barclay FE, et al. Treatment of relapsing *Clostridium difficile* diarrhea by administration of a nontoxigenic strain. Eur J Clin Microbiol. 1987;6:51-53.

99. van Dijck P, Avesani V, Delmee M. Genotyping of outbreak-related and sporadic isolates of *Clostridium difficile* belonging to serogroup C. J Clin Microbiol. 1996;34:3049-3055.

100. Samore MH, Bettin KM, DeGirolami PC, et al. Wide diversity of *Clostridium difficile* types at a tertiary referral hospital. J Infect Dis. 1994;170:615-621.

101. Cohen SH, Tang YJ, Muenzer J, et al. Isolation of various genotypes of *Clostridium difficile* from patients and the environment in an oncology ward. Clin Infect Dis. 1997;24:889-893.

102. Tedesco FJ. Pseudomembranous colitis. Med Clin North Am. 1982;66:655-664.

103. Gebhard RL, Gerding DN, Olson MM, et al. Clinical and endoscopic findings in patients early in the course of *Clostridium difficile*-associated pseudomembranous colitis. Am J Med. 1985;78:45-48.

104. Manabe YC, Vinetz JM, Moore RD, et al. *Clostridium difficile* colitis: An efficient clinical approach to diagnosis. Ann Intern Med. 1995;123:835-840.

105. Katz DA, Lynch ME, Littenberg B. Clinical prediction rules to optimize cytotoxin testing for *Clostridium difficile* in hospitalized patients with diarrhea. Am J Med. 1996;100:487-495.

106. Katz DA, Bates DW, Rittenberg E, et al. Predicting *Clostridium difficile* stool cytotoxin results in hospitalized patients with diarrhea. J Gen Intern Med. 1997;12:57-62.

107. Bulusu M, Narayan S, Shetler K, et al. Leukocytosis as a harbinger and surrogate marker of Clostridium difficile infection in hospitalized patients with diarrhea. Am J Gastroenterol. 2000;95:3137-3141.

108. Bartlett JG. Leukocytosis and *Clostridium difficile*–associated diarrhea. Am J Gastroenterol. 2000;95:3023-3024.

109. Wanahita A, Goldsmith EA, Musher DM. Conditions associated with leukocytosis in a tertiary care hospital, with particular attention to the role of infection caused by *Clostridium difficile*. Clin Infect Dis. 2002;34:1585-1592.

110. Fekety R. Guidelines for the diagnosis and management of *Clostridium difficile*–associated diarrhea and colitis. American College of Gastroenterology, Practice Parameters Committee. Am J Gastroenterol. 1997;92:739-750.

111. Triadafilopoulos G, Hallstone AE. Acute abdomen as the first presentation of pseudomembranous colitis. Gastroenterology. 1991;101:685-691.

112. Burke GW, Wilson ME, Mehrez IO. Absence of diarrhea in toxic megacolon complicating *Clostridium difficile* pseudomembranous colitis. Am J Gastroenterol. 1988;83:304-307.

113. Drapkin MS, Worthington MG, Chang TW, Razvi SA. *Clostridium difficile* mimicking acute peritonitis. Arch Surg. 1985;120:1321-1322.

114. Trudel JL, Deschenes M, Mayrand S, Barkun AN. Toxic megacolon complicating pseudomembranous enterocolitis. Dis Colon Rectum. 1995;38:1033-1038.

115. Snooks SJ, Hughes A, Horsburgh AG. Perforated colon complicating pseudomembranous colitis. Br J Surg. 1984;71:291-292.

116. Yaseen ZH, Watson RE, Dean HA, Wilson ME. Case report: Transverse colon volvulus in a patient with *Clostridium difficile* pseudomembranous colitis. Am J Med Sci. 1994;308:247-250.

117. Rybolt AH, Bennett RG, Laughon BE, et al. Protein-losing enteropathy associated with *Clostridium difficile* infection. Lancet. 1989;1:1353-1355.

118. Do AN, Fridkin SK, Yechouron A, et al. Risk factors for early recurrent *Clostridium difficile*–associated diarrhea. Clin Infect Dis. 1998;26:954-959.

119. Fekety R, McFarland LV, Surawicz CM, et al. Recurrent *Clostridium difficile* diarrhea: Characteristics of and risk factors for patients enrolled in a prospective, randomized, double-blinded trial. Clin Infect Dis. 1997;24:324-333.

120. Byl B, Jacobs F, Struelens MJ, Thys JP. Extraintestinal *Clostridium difficile* infections. Clin Infect Dis. 1996;22:712.

121. Saginur R, Fogel R, Begin L, et al. Splenic abscess due to *Clostridium difficile*. J Infect Dis. 1983;147:1105.

122. Pron B, Merckx J, Touzet P, et al. Chronic septic arthritis and osteomyelitis in a prosthetic knee joint due to *Clostridium difficile*. Eur J Clin Microbiol Infect Dis. 1995;14:599-601.

123. Atkinson MH, McLeod BD. Reactive arthritis associated with *Clostridium difficile* enteritis. J Rheumatol. 1988;15:520-522.

124. Hayward RS, Wensel RH, Kibsey P. Relapsing *Clostridium difficile* colitis and Reiter's syndrome. Am J Gastroenterol. 1990;85:752-756.

125. Putterman C, Rubinow A. Reactive arthritis associated with *Clostridium difficile* pseudomembranous colitis. Semin Arthritis Rheum. 1993;22:420-426.

126. Lofgren RP, Tadlock LM, Soltis RD. Acute oligoarthritis associated with *Clostridium difficile* pseudomembranous colitis. Arch Intern Med. 1984;144:617-619.

127. Case records of the Massachusetts General Hospital. Weekly clinicopathological exercises. Case 19-1998: A 70-year-old man with diarrhea, polyarthritis, and a history of Reiter's syndrome. N Engl J Med. 1998;338:1830-1836.

128. Wilson KH, Blitchington RB. Human colonic biota studied by ribosomal DNA sequence analysis. 1996;62:2273-2278.

129. Wilson KH, Ikeda JS, Blitchington RB. Phylogenetic placement of community members in human colonic biota. Clin Infect Dis. 1997;25:S114-S116.

130. Suau A, Bonnet R, Sutren M, et al. Direct analysis of genes encoding 16S rRNA from complex communities reveals many novel molecular species within the human gut. Appl Environ Microbiol. 1999;65:4799-4807.

131. Moore WEC, Holdeman LV. Human fecal flora: The normal flora of 20 Japanese-Hawaiians. Appl Microbiol. 1974;27:961-979.

132. Wilson KH, Freter R. Interactions of *Clostridium difficile* and *E. coli* with microfloras in continuous-flow cultures and gnotobiotic mice. Infect Immun. 1986;54:354-358.

133. Wilson KH, Perini F. Role of competition for nutrients in suppression of *Clostridium difficile* by the colonic microflora. Infect Immun. 1988;56:2610-2614.

134. Miller RS, Hoskins LC. Mucin degradation in human colonic ecosystems: Fecal population densities of mucin-degrading bacteria estimated by a "most probable number" method. Gastroenterology. 1981;81:759-765.

135. Wilson KH, Brown RS. Isolates belonging to the *Clostridium coccoides* group suppress *Clostridium difficile* in a continuous-flow culture model. Presented at the Annual Meeting of the American Society for Microbiology, Washington, DC, May 18-22, 2003.

136. Boureau H, Decre D, Carlier JP, et al. Identification of a *Clostridium cocleatum* strain involved in an anti–*Clostridium difficile* barrier effect and determination of its mucin-degrading enzymes. Res Microbiol. 1993;144:405-410.

137. Wilson KH. The microecology of *Clostridium difficile*. Clin Infect Dis. 1993;16(Suppl 4):S214-S218.

138. Wilson KH, Sheagren JN, Freter R. Population dynamics of ingested *Clostridium difficile* in the gastrointestinal tract of the Syrian hamster. J Infect Dis. 1985;151:355-361.

139. Lyerly DM, Wilkins TD. *Clostridium difficile*. In: Blaser MJ, Smith PD, Ravdin JI, et al., eds. Infections of the Gastrointestinal Tract. New York: Raven; 1995:867-891.

140. Borriello SP, Davies HA, Barclay FE. Detection of fimbriae amongst strains of *Clostridium difficile*. FEMS Microbiol Lett. 1988;49:65-67.

141. von Eichel-Streiber C, Laufenberg-Feldmann R, Sartingen S, et al. Comparative sequence analysis of the *Clostridium difficile* toxins A and B. Mol Gen Genet. 1992;233:260-268.

142. Gill DM. Bacterial toxins: A table of lethal amounts. Microbiol Rev. 1982;46:86-94.

143. Lyerly DM, Krivan HC, Wilkins TD. *Clostridium difficile*: Its disease and toxins. Clin Microbiol Rev. 1988;1:1-18.

144. Price SB, Phelps CJ, Wilkins TD, Johnson JL. Cloning of the carbohydrate-binding portion of the toxin A gene of *Clostridium difficile*. Curr Microbiol. 1987;16:55-60.

145. Alfa MJ, Kabani A, Lyerly D, et al. Characterization of a toxin A-negative, toxin B-positive strain of *Clostridium difficile* responsible for a nosocomial outbreak of *Clostridium difficile*–associated diarrhea. J Clin Microbiol. 2000;38:2706-2714.

146. Barbut F, Lalande V, Burghoffer B, et al. Prevalence and genetic characterization of toxin A variant strains of *Clostridium difficile* among adults and children with diarrhea in France. J Clin Microbiol 2002;40:2079-2083.

147. Tucker KD, Wilkins TD. Toxin A of *Clostridium difficile* binds to the human carbohydrate antigens I, X, and Y. Infect Immun. 1991;59:73-78.

148. Smith JA, Cooke DL, Hyde S, et al. *Clostridium difficile* toxin A binding to human intestinal epithelial cells. J Med Microbiol. 1997;46:953-958.

149. Hippenstiel S, Kratz T, Krull M, et al. Rho protein inhibition blocks protein kinase C translocation and activation. Biochem Biophys Res Commun. 1998;245:830-834.

150. Just I, Selzer J, Wilm M, et al. Glucosylation of Rho proteins by *Clostridium difficile* toxin B. Nature. 1995;375:500-503.

151. Mahida YR, Makh S, Hyde S, et al. Effect of *Clostridium difficile* toxin A on human intestinal epithelial cells: Induction of interleukin 8 production and apoptosis after cell detachment. Gut. 1996;38:337-347.

152. Brito GA, Fujii J, Carneiro-Filho BA, et al. Mechanism of *Clostridium difficile* toxin A–induced apoptosis in T84 cells. J Infect Dis. 2002;186:1438-1447.

153. Moore R, Pothoulakis C, LaMont JT, et al. C. difficile toxin A increases intestinal permeability and induces Cl- secretion. Am J Physiol. 1990;259:G165-G172.

154. Brito GA, Sullivan GW, Ciesla WP Jr, et al. *Clostridium difficile* toxin A alters in vitro–adherent neutrophil morphology and function. J Infect Dis. 2002;185:1297-1306.

155. Lima AA, Lyerly DM, Wilkins TD, et al. Effects of *Clostridium difficile* toxins A and B in rabbit small and large intestine in vivo and on cultured cells in vitro. Infect Immun. 1988;56:582-588.

156. Lima AA, Innes D Jr, Chadee K, et al. *Clostridium difficile* toxin A: Interactions with mucus and early sequential histopathologic effects in rabbit small intestine. Lab Invest. 1989;61:419-425.

157. Triadafilopoulos G, Pothoulakis C, O'Brien MJ, LaMont JT. Differential effects of *Clostridium difficile* toxins A and B on rabbit ileum. Gastroenterology. 1987;93: 273-279.

158. Fonteles M, Fang G, Thielman NM, et al. Role of platelet activating factor in the inflammatory and secretory effects of *Clostridium difficile* toxin A. J Lipid Mediat Cell Signal. 1995;11:133-143.

159. Castagliuolo I, Keates AC, Qiu B, et al. Increased substance P responses in dorsal root ganglia and intestinal macrophages during *Clostridium difficile* toxin A enteritis in rats. Proc Natl Acad Sci U S A. 1997;94:4788-4793.

160. Mykoniatis A, Anton PM, Wlk M, et al. Leptin mediates *Clostridium difficile* toxin A–induced enteritis in mice. Gastroenterology. 2003;124:683-691.

161. Steiner TS, Flores CA, Pizarro TT, Guerrant RL. Fecal lactoferrin, interleukin-1beta, and interleukin-8 are elevated in patients with severe *Clostridium difficile* colitis. Clin Diagn Lab Immunol. 1997;4:719-722.

162. Linevsky JK, Pothoulakis C, Keates S, et al. IL-8 release and neutrophil activation by *Clostridium difficile* toxin–exposed human monocytes. Am J Physiol. 1997;273(6 Pt 1):G1333-G1340.

163. Melo Filho AA, Souza MH, Lyerly DM, et al. Role of tumor necrosis factor and nitric oxide in the cytotoxic effects of *Clostridium difficile* toxin A and toxin B on macrophages. Toxicon. 1997;35:743-752.

164. Pothoulakis C, Sullivan R, Melnick DA, et al. *Clostridium difficile* toxin A stimulates intracellular calcium release and chemotactic response in human granulocytes. J Clin Invest. 1988;81:1741-1745.

165. Kelly CP, Becker S, Linevsky JK, et al. Neutrophil recruitment in *Clostridium difficile* toxin A enteritis in the rabbit. J Clin Invest. 1994;93:1257-1265.

166. Wershil BK, Castagliuolo I, Pothoulakis C. Direct evidence of mast cell involvement in *Clostridium difficile* toxin A–induced enteritis in mice. Gastroenterology. 1998;114:956-964.

167. Hecht G, Koutsouris A, Pothoulakis C, et al. *Clostridium difficile* toxin B disrupts the barrier function of T84 monolayers. Gastroenterology. 1992;102:416-423.

168. Riegler M, Sedivy R, Pothoulakis C, et al. *Clostridium difficile* toxin B is more potent than toxin A in damaging human colonic epithelium in vitro. J Clin Invest. 1995;95:2004-2011.

169. Souza MH, Melo-Filho AA, Rocha MF, et al. The involvement of macrophage-derived tumour necrosis factor and lipoxygenase products on the neutrophil recruitment induced by *Clostridium difficile* toxin B. Immunology. 1997;91:281-288.

169a. Peterson LR, Kelly PJ. The role of the clinical microbiology laboratory in the management of *Clostridium difficile*–associated diarrhea. Infect Dis Clin North Am. 1993;7:277-293.

170. Groschel DH. *Clostridium difficile* infection. Crit Rev Clin Lab Sci. 1996;33:203-245.

171. Altaie SS, Meyer P, Dryja D. Comparison of two commercially available enzyme immunoassays for detection of *Clostridium difficile* in stool specimens. J Clin Microbiol. 1994;32:51-53.

172. Turgeon DK, Novicki TJ, Quick J, et al. Six rapid tests for direct detection of *Clostridium difficile* and its toxins in fecal samples compared with the fibroblast cytotoxicity assay. J Clin Microbiol. 2003;41:667-670.

173. Gerding DN, Johnson S, Peterson LR, et al. *Clostridium difficile*–associated diarrhea and colitis. Infect Control Hosp Epidemiol. 1995;16:459-477.

174. Lyerly DM, Wilkins TD. Commercial latex test for *Clostridium difficile* toxin A does not detect toxin A. J Clin Microbiol. 1986;23:622-623.

175. Lyerly DM, Ball DW, Toth J, Wilkins TD. Characterization of cross-reactive proteins detected by Culturette Brand Rapid Latex Test for *Clostridium difficile*. J Clin Microbiol. 1988;26:397-400.

176. Wongwanich S, Kusum M, Phan-Urai R. Reactivity of the CD D-1 latex test with *Clostridium difficile* and other bacteria. Southeast Asian J Trop Med Public Health. 1994;25:321-323.

177. Wilson KH, Blitchington R, Hindenach B, Greene RC. Species-specific oligonucleotide probes for rRNA of *Clostridium difficile* and related species. J Clin Microbiol. 1988;26:2484-2488.

178. Gumerlock PH, Tang YJ, Weiss JB, Silva J Jr. Specific detection of toxigenic strains of *Clostridium difficile* in stool specimens. J Clin Microbiol. 1993;31:507-511.

179. Guilbault C, Labbe AC, Poirier L, et al. Development and evaluation of a PCR method for detection of the *Clostridium difficile* toxin B gene in stool specimens. J Clin Microbiol. 2002;40:2288-2290.

180. Belanger SD, Boissinot M, Clairoux N, et al. Rapid detection of *Clostridium difficile* in feces by real-time PCR. J Clin Microbiol. 2003;41:730-734.

181. Wolfhagen MJ, Fluit AC, Torensma R, et al. Rapid detection of toxigenic *Clostridium difficile* in fecal samples by magnetic immuno PCR assay. J Clin Microbiol. 1994;3:1629-1633.

182. Gumerlock PH, Tang YJ, Weiss JB, Silva J Jr. Specific detection of toxigenic strains of *Clostridium difficile* in stool specimens. J Clin Microbiol. 1993;31:507-511.

183. Tang YJ, Gumerlock PH, Weiss JB, Silva J Jr. Specific detection of *Clostridium difficile* toxin A gene sequences in clinical isolates. Mol Cell Probes. 1993;8:463-467.

184. Tedesco FJ, Corless JK, Brownstein RE. Rectal sparing in antibiotic-associated pseudomembranous colitis: A prospective study. Gastroenterology. 1982;83:1259-1260.

185. Fang FC, Gerding DN, Peterson LR. Diagnosis of *Clostridium difficile* colitis. Ann Intern Med. 1996;125:515; discussion 516.

186. Vinetz J, Manabe Y, Bartlett J. Diagnosis of *Clostridium difficile* colitis. Ann Intern Med. 1996;125:516.

187. Schleupner MA, Garner DC, Sosnowski KM, et al. Concurrence of *Clostridium difficile* toxin A enzyme-linked immunosorbent assay, fecal lactoferrin assay, and clinical criteria with *C. difficile* cytotoxin titer in two patient cohorts. J Clin Microbiol. 1995;33:1755-1759.

188. Renshaw AA, Stelling JM, Doolittle MH. The lack of value of repeated *Clostridium difficile* cytotoxicity assays. Arch Pathol Lab Med. 1996;120:49-52.

189. Yong WH, Mattia AR, Ferraro MJ. Comparison of fecal lactoferrin latex agglutination assay and methylene blue microscopy for detection of fecal leukocytes in *Clostridium difficile*–associated disease. J Clin Microbiol. 1994;32:1360-1361.

190. Marx CE, Morris A, Wilson ML, Reller LB. Fecal leukocytes in stool specimens submitted for *Clostridium difficile* toxin assay. Diagn Microbiol Infect Dis. 1993;16:313-315.

191. Teasley DG, Gerding DN, Olson MM, et al. Prospective randomised trial of metronidazole versus vancomycin for *Clostridium difficile*-associated diarrhoea and colitis. Lancet. 1983;2:1043-1046.

192. Recommendations for preventing the spread of vancomycin resistance. Recommendations of the Hospital Infection Control Practices Advisory Committee (HICPAC). MMWR Morb Mortal Wkly Rep. 1995;44(RR-12):1-13.

193. Chow AW, Cheng N, Bartlett KH. In vitro susceptibility of *Clostridium difficile* to new beta-lactam and quinolone antibiotics. Antimicrob Agents Chemother. 1985;28:842-844.

194. Bacon AE, McGrath S, Fekety R, Holloway WJ. In vitro synergy studies with *Clostridium difficile*. Antimicrob Agents Chemother. 1991;35:582-583.

195. Pelaez T, Alcala L, Alonso R, et al. Reassessment of *Clostridium difficile* susceptibility to metronidazole and vancomycin. Antimicrob Agents Chemother. 2002;46:1647-1650.

196. Bolton RP, Culshaw MA. Faecal metronidazole concentrations during oral and intravenous therapy for antibiotic-associated colitis due to *Clostridium difficile*. Gut. 1986;27:1169-1172.

197. Krook A, Lindstrom B, Kjellander J, et al. Relation between concentrations of metronidazole and *Bacteroides* spp in faeces of patients with Crohn's disease and healthy individuals. J Clin Pathol. 1981;34:645-650.

198. Arabi Y, Dimock F, Burdon DW, et al. Influence of neomycin and metronidazole on colonic microflora of volunteers. J Antimicrob Chemother. 1979;5:531-537.

199. Wenisch C, Parschalk B, Hasenhundl M, et al. Comparison of vancomycin, teicoplanin, metronidazole, and fusidic acid for the treatment of *Clostridium difficile*–associated diarrhea. Clin Infect Dis. 1996;22:813-818.

200. Young GP, Ward PB, Bayley N, et al. Antibiotic-associated colitis due to *Clostridium difficile*: Double-blind comparison of vancomycin with bacitracin. Gastroenterology. 1985;89:1038-1045.

201. Dudley MN, McLaughlin JC, Carrington G, et al. Oral bacitracin vs vancomycin therapy for *Clostridium difficile*–induced diarrhea: A randomized double-blind trial. Arch Intern Med. 1986;146:1101-1104.

202. de Lalla F, Nicolin R, Rinaldi E, et al. Prospective study of oral teicoplanin versus oral vancomycin for therapy of pseudomembranous colitis and *Clostridium difficile*–associated diarrhea. Antimicrob Agents Chemother. 1992;36:2192-2196.

203. Finegold SM, George WL. Therapy directed against *Clostridium difficile* and its toxins: Complications of therapy. In: Rolfe RD, Finegold SM, eds. *Clostridium difficile*: Its Role in Intestinal Disease. San Diego: Academic Press; 1988:341-366.

204. Baird DR. Comparison of two oral formulations of vancomycin for treatment of diarrhoea associated with *Clostridium difficile*. J Antimicrob Chemother. 1989;23:167-169.

205. Keighley MR, Burdon DW, Arabi Y, et al. Randomised controlled trial of vancomycin for pseudomembranous colitis and postoperative diarrhoea. BMJ. 1978;2:1667-1669.

206. Fekety R, Silva J, Kauffman C, et al. Treatment of antibiotic-associated *Clostridium difficile* colitis with oral vancomycin: Comparison of two dosage regimens. Am J Med. 1989;86:15-19.

207. Spitzer PG, Eliopoulos GM. Systemic absorption of enteral vancomycin in a patient with pseudomembranous colitis. Ann Intern Med. 1984;100:533-534.

208. Bartlett JG. Treatment of antibiotic-associated pseudomembranous colitis. Rev Infect Dis. 1984;6(Suppl 1):S235-S241.

209. Morris JG Jr, Shay DK, Hebden JN, et al. Enterococci resistant to multiple antimicrobial agents, including vancomycin: Establishment of endemicity in a university medical center. Ann Intern Med. 1995;123:250-259.

210. Taylor NS, Bartlett JG. Binding of *Clostridium difficile* cytotoxin and vancomycin by anion-exchange resins. J Infect Dis. 1980;141:92-97.

211. Keighley MRB. Antibiotic-associated colitis: Pathogenesis and management. Drugs. 1980;20:49-56.

212. McDonald GB, Vracko R. Systemic absorption of oral cholestyramine. Gastroenterology. 1984;87:213-215.

213. Spyres LM, Daniel J, Hensley A, et al. Mutational analysis of the enzymatic domain of *Clostridium difficile* toxin B reveals novel inhibitors of the wild-type toxin. Infect Immun. 2003;71:3294-3301.

214. Oliva SL, Guglielmo BJ, Jacobs R, Pons VG. Failure of intravenous vancomycin and intravenous metronidazole to prevent or treat antibiotic-associated pseudomembranous colitis. J Infect Dis. 1989;159:1154-1155.

215. Cohen H, Brocavich JM. Managing *Clostridium difficile* colitis in patients who lack oral access. Infect Med. 1996;13:101-109.

216. Tedesco F, Markham R, Gurwith M, et al. Oral vancomycin for antibiotic-associated pseudomembranous colitis. Lancet. 1978;2:226-228.

217. Pasic M, Jost R, Carrel T, et al. Intracolonic vancomycin for pseudomembranous colitis. N Engl J Med. 1993;329:583.

218. Pasic M, Carrel T, Opravil M, et al. Systemic absorption after local intracolonic vancomycin in pseudomembranous colitis. Lancet. 1993;342:443.

219. Apisarnthanarak A, Razavi B, Mundy LM. Adjunctive intracolonic vancomycin for severe *Clostridium difficile* colitis: Case series and review of the literature. Clin Infect Dis. 2002;35:690-696.

220. Shetler K, Nieuwenhuis R, Wren SM, Triadafilopoulos G. Decompressive colonoscopy with intracolonic vancomycin administration for the treatment of severe pseudomembranous colitis. Surg Endosc. 2001;15:653-659.

221. Novak E, Lee JG, Seckman CE, et al. Unfavorable effect of atropine-diphenoxylate (Lomotil) therapy in lincomycin-caused diarrhea. JAMA. 1976;235:1451-1454.

222. Lipsett PA, Samantaray DK, Tam ML, et al. Pseudomembranous colitis: A surgical disease? Surgery. 1994;116:491-496.

223. Synnott K, Mealy K, Merry C, et al. Timing of surgery for fulminating pseudomembranous colitis. Br J Surg. 1998;85:229-231.

224. Agnifili A, Gola P, Marino M, et al. The role and timing of surgery in the treatment of pseudomembranous colitis: A case complicated by toxic megacolon. Hepatogastroenterology. 1994;41:394-396.

225. Viscidi R, Laughon BE, Yolken R, et al. Serum antibody response to toxins A and B of *Clostridium difficile*. J Infect Dis. 1983;148:93-100.

226. O'Neill GL, Beaman MH, Riley TV. Relapse versus reinfection with *Clostridium difficile*. Epidemiol Infect. 1991;107:627-635.

227. McFarland LV, Surawicz CM, Greenberg RN, et al. A randomized placebo-controlled trial of *Saccharomyces boulardii* in combination with standard antibiotics for *Clostridium difficile* disease. JAMA. 1994;271:1913-1918.

228. Wilson KH, Silva J, Fekety FR. Suppression of *Clostridium difficile* by normal hamster flora and prevention of antibiotic-associated cecitis. Infect Immun. 1981;34:626-628.

229. Tedesco FJ, Gordon D, Fortson WC. Approach to patients with multiple relapses of antibiotic-associated pseudomembranous colitis. Am J Gastroenterol. 1985;80:867-868.

230. Buggy BP, Fekety R, Silva J Jr. Therapy of relapsing *Clostridium difficile*–associated diarrhea and colitis with the combination of vancomycin and rifampin. J Clin Gastroenterol. 1987;9:155-159.

231. Allo M, Silva J Jr, Fekety R, et al. Prevention of clindamycin-induced colitis in hamsters by *Clostridium sordellii* antitoxin. Gastroenterology. 1979;76:351-355.

232. Leung DY, Kelly CP, Boguniewicz M, et al. Treatment with intravenously administered gamma globulin of chronic relapsing colitis induced by *Clostridium difficile* toxin. J Pediatr. 1991;118:633-637.

233. Salcedo J, Keates S, Pothoulakis C, et al. Intravenous immunoglobulin therapy for severe *Clostridium difficile* colitis. Gut. 1997;41:366-370.

234. Beales IL. Intravenous immunoglobulin for recurrent *Clostridium difficile* diarrhoea. Gut. 2002;51:456.

235. Aas J, Gessert CE, Bakken JS. Recurrent *Clostridium difficile* colitis: Case series involving 18 patients treated with donor stool administered via a nasogastric tube. Clin Infect Dis. 2003;36:580-585.

236. Schwan A, Sjölin S, Trottestam U, Aronsson B. Relapsing *Clostridium difficile* enterocolitis cured by rectal infusion of normal faeces. Scand J Infect Dis. 1984;16:211-215.

237. Tvede M, Rask-Madsen J. Bacteriotherapy for chronic relapsing *Clostridium difficile* diarrhoea in six patients. Lancet. 1989;1:1156-1160.

238. Mody LR, Smith SM, Dever LL. *Clostridium difficile*–associated diarrhea in a VA medical center: Clustering of cases, association with antibiotic usage, and impact on HIV-infected patients. Infect Control Hosp Epidemiol. 2001;22:42-45.

239. Pruksananonda P, Powell KR. Multiple relapses of *Clostridium difficile*–associated diarrhea responding to an extended course of cholestyramine. Pediatr Infect Dis J. 1989;8:175-178.

240. Kunimoto D, Thomson AB. Recurrent *Clostridium difficile*–associated colitis responding to cholestyramine. Digestion. 1986;33:225-228.

241. Moncino MD, Falletta JM. Multiple relapses of *Clostridium difficile*–associated diarrhea in a cancer patient: Successful control with long-term cholestyramine therapy. Am J Pediatr Hematol Oncol. 1992;14:361-364.

242. Gorbach SL, Chang TW, Goldin B. Successful treatment of relapsing *Clostridium difficile* colitis with *Lactobacillus* GG. Lancet. 1987;2:1519.

243. Liacouras CA, Piccoli DA. Whole-bowel irrigation as an adjunct to the treatment of chronic, relapsing *Clostridium difficile* colitis. J Clin Gastroenterol. 1996;22:186-189.

244. Kroker PB, Bower M, Azadian B. *Clostridium difficile* infection, hospital geography and time-space clustering. QJM. 2001;94:223-225.

245. Johnson S, Gerding DN, Olson MM, et al. Prospective, controlled study of vinyl glove use to interrupt *Clostridium difficile* nosocomical transmission. Am J Med. 1990;88:137-140.

246. Brooks SE, Veal RO, Kramer M, et al. Reduction in the incidence of *Clostridium difficile*–associated diarrhea in an acute care hospital and a skilled nursing facility following replacement of electronic thermometers with single-use disposables. Infect Control Hosp Epidemiol. 1992;13:98-103.

247. Mayfield JL, Leet T, Miller J, Mundy LM. Environmental control to reduce transmission of *Clostridium difficile*. Clin Infect Dis. 2000;31:995-1000.

248. Brown E, Talbot GH, Axelrod P, et al. Risk factors for *Clostridium difficile* toxin–associated diarrhea. Infect Control Hosp Epidemiol. 1990;11:283-290.

249. Kotloff KL, Wasserman SS, Losonsky GA, et al. Safety and immunogenicity of increasing doses of a *Clostridium difficile* toxoid vaccine administered to healthy adults. Infect Immun. 2001;69:988-995.

250. Ward SJ, Douce G, Figueiredo D, et al. Immunogenicity of a *Salmonella typhimurium* aroA aroD vaccine expressing a nontoxic domain of *Clostridium difficile* toxin A. Infect Immun. 1999;67:2145-2152.

251. Thielman NM, Guerrant RL. *Clostridium difficile*. In: Burg FD, Ingelfinger JR, Wald ER, Polin RA, eds. Gellis and Kagan's Current Pediatric Therapy. 15th ed. Philadelphia: WB Saunders; 1995:584-586.

Inflammatory Enteritides

RICHARD L. GUERRANT

ALDO A. M. LIMA

The acute inflammatory enteritides include several specific distal small bowel and colonic infections such as campylobacteriosis, salmonellosis, shigellosis, and amebiasis, as well as the syndromes of necrotizing enteritis and antibiotic-associated pseudomembranous enterocolitis. Several other infectious agents cause chronic enteric inflammatory processes that may result in syndromes of abdominal pain, weight loss, diarrhea, or malabsorption. These include such processes as gastrointestinal mycoses, mycobacterioses, bacterial infections, and certain parasitic infections such as coccidiosis.

ACUTE DYSENTERY: HISTORY, EPIDEMIOLOGY, AND DIAGNOSIS

Syndromes of acute dysentery with fecal blood and pus have been well recognized since the days of Hippocrates. Dysentery is defined as frequent, small bowel movements accompanied by blood and mucus with tenesmus, or pain on defecation. This syndrome implies an inflammatory invasion of the colonic mucosa resulting from bacterial, cytotoxic, or parasitic destruction.

The pathologic changes of inflammatory colitis range from a superficial intense exudative inflammatory process involving the colonic mucosa, as seen in infection by shigellae or invasive *Escherichia coli* organisms, to deeper, penetrating, "flask-shaped" ulcers with undermined edges, as seen in amebic dysentery. The pathogenesis of the inflammatory colitides may involve cytotoxic products of shigellae,[1] certain *E. coli* strains,[2] clostridia, or other organisms.

The epidemiologic patterns of acute dysenteric syndromes are influenced by the unusually low inoculum required by organisms such as shigellae or amebae for infection. As few as 100 shigellae or as few as 10 cysts of enteric parasites such as *Entamoeba coli* or *Giardia lamblia* have been found to result in infection in adult volunteers.[3,4] Consequently, there is a substantial risk of person-to-person spread in daycare centers,[5] institutions, or other areas where nonhygienic conditions may allow direct fecal-oral spread. The cysts of parasites such as *Entamoeba histolytica* or *Balantidium coli* often resist chlorination and therefore may cause waterborne outbreaks of dysenteric illnesses. Saltwater or seafood exposure should lead to consideration of *Vibrio parahaemolyticus* as a cause of inflammatory colitis, and farm or domestic animal exposure might lead to consideration of nontyphoid *Salmonella* species, *Campylobacter jejuni*, or *Yersinia enterocolitica*. In addition, when typhoid fever is present with diarrhea in an endemic area, the diarrhea is often inflammatory, with many fecal polymorphonuclear or mononuclear leukocytes seen on microscopic examination.[6] A history of travel to areas of poor sanitation may implicate any of the aforementioned pathogens. Finally, venereal exposure, particularly among male homosexuals, may implicate gonococci, herpes simplex virus, *Chlamydia trachomatis*, or *Treponema pallidum* as a cause of proctitis, or *Campylobacter*, *Shigella*, *C. trachomatis* (lymphogranuloma venereum serotypes), *E. histolytica*, or *Clostridium difficile* as a cause of colitis.[7]

Examination for fecal leukocytes often reveals sheets of polymorphonuclear leukocytes in clumps of mucus even in the absence of gross blood in the stool specimen (Fig. 93-1).[8,9] Fewer pyknotic leukocytes are reported in amebic dysentery[10-12]; this may be attributable to the deeper, undermining ulcers characteristic of intestinal amebiasis or

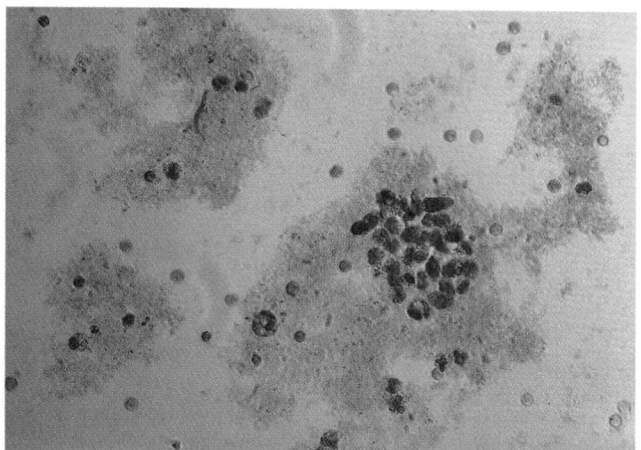

FIGURE 93-1. Methylene blue stain of fecal leukocytes from patient with colitis. This exudative response may be seen in shigellosis, salmonellosis, *Campylobacter* infection, and colitis due to invasive *Escherichia coli*.

TABLE 93-1 Differential Diagnosis of Acute Dysentery and Inflammatory Enterocolitis

Specific Infectious Processes
Bacillary dysentery (*Shigella dysenteriae, Shigella flexneri, Shigella sonnei, Shigella boydii;* invasive *Escherichia coli*)
Campylobacteriosis (*Campylobacter jejuni*)
Amebic dysentery (*Entamoeba histolytica*)
Ciliary dysentery (*Balantidium coli*)
Bilharzial dysentery (*Schistosoma japonicum, Schistosoma mansoni*)
Other parasitic infections (*Trichinella spiralis*)
Vibriosis (*Vibrio parahaemolyticus*)
Salmonellosis (*Salmonella typhimurium*)
Typhoid fever (*Salmonella typhi*)
Enteric fever (*Salmonella choleraesuis, Salmonella paratyphi*)
Yersiniosis (*Yersinia enterocolitica*)
Spirillar dysentery (*Spirillum* spp.)

Proctitis
Gonococcal (*Neisseria gonorrhoeae*)
Herpetic (herpes simplex virus)
Chlamydial (*Chlamydia trachomatis*)
Syphilitic (*Treponema pallidum*)

Other Syndromes
Necrotizing enterocolitis of the newborn
Enteritis necroticans
Pseudomembranous enterocolitis (*Clostridium difficile*)
Diverticulitis
Typhlitis

Chronic Inflammatory Processes
Enteropathogenic and enteroaggregative *E. coli*
Syphilis
Gastrointestinal tuberculosis
Gastrointestinal mycosis
Parasitic enteritis

Syndromes without Known Infectious Etiology
Idiopathic ulcerative colitis
Crohn's disease
Radiation enteritis
Ischemic colitis
Allergic enteritis

to a contact-dependent cytolytic effect of the ameba on leukocytes. The use of fresh specimens promptly plated onto appropriate enteric culture media is very important in the isolation of shigellae.[13] Specialized techniques are required to isolate *Vibrio* (thiosulfate citrate bile salts [TCBS] agar),[14] *Yersinia* (cold enrichment),[15] or *C. jejuni*.[16] The identification of toxigenic *C. difficile* is done by immunoassay or cell culture cytotoxicity assay for *C. difficile* toxin A or B, respectively.[17-19] Leukocytosis or even a leukemoid reaction has been described in colitis due to *C. difficile*.

Sigmoidoscopic examination, especially with biopsy, may be useful in the diagnosis of a pseudomembranous enterocolitis or in the identification of parasites such as *E. histolytica* (with special periodic acid–Schiff [PAS] stain) or *Balantidium coli*. Amebic colitis is associated with discrete small ulcerations with undermined edges amid relatively normal mucosa. Acute shigellosis causes more widespread, shallow, 3- to 7-mm ulcers with a more intense inflammatory exudate. Barium studies are unnecessary and are relatively contraindicated in toxic patients with acute colitis. Therapy consists of careful supportive fluid management with specific antimicrobial therapy directed at a specific pathogen if suspected on the basis of the epidemiologic setting or culture results.

The potential causes of acute dysentery are listed in Table 93-1.

Shigellosis and Enteroinvasive *Escherichia coli*

It is estimated that *Shigella* species (see Chapter 221) infect over 200 million people and cause 650,000 deaths each year worldwide.[20] The four *Shigella* species are classified in subgroups A to D: *Shigella dysenteriae, Shigella flexneri, Shigella sonnei,* and *Shigella boydii,* respectively. These *Shigella* species are capable of elaborating a potent toxin with enterotoxic, cytotoxic, and neurotoxic properties (Shiga toxin).[21] Shigellae are facultative intracellular pathogens and may cause acute bloody dysentery with high fever and systemic manifestations of malaise, headache, and abdominal pain. The incubation period ranges from 6 hours to 9 days but is usually less than 72 hours. *Shigella* species are the most common cause of bloody diarrhea in children, and the syndrome may be particularly severe in poorly nourished children.[22]

Despite the intense superficial destructive process in the colonic epithelium that typifies acute shigellosis, bacteremia and disseminated infection are relatively rare.[23] *S. flexneri* invades and causes inflammatory destruction of the human colonic epithelium. The cell and tissue invasion results from a type III secretion system that delivers effector protein into target eukaryotic cells.[24] Acute shigellosis by *S. dysenteriae* type I induces apoptotic cell death in rectal tissues that is associated with increased production of Fas/Fas ligand, perforin, caspase-1, and caspase-3 but reduced production of Bcl-2 and interleukin-2.[25] *Shigella* infection (especially with *S. dysenteriae* type 1) is associated with enteric protein loss that ceases after appropriate antimicrobial therapy.[26] This protein loss may contribute to increased susceptibility to secondary infections or growth stunting.[27,28] A complication of severe shigellosis in childhood is a hemolytic–uremic syndrome (HUS), which may be associated with a leukemoid reaction, pseudomembranous colitis (Fig. 93-2), circulating immune complexes, and circulating endotoxin, usually in the absence of demonstrable bacteremia.[29]

Intestinal obstruction, which occurs in about 3% of patients, is a poor prognostic sign, not infrequently associated with death or the development of HUS.[30] Other, more common extraintestinal manifestations of shigellosis are headache, meningismus, and even seizures, especially in children.[31] These findings may be attributable to a neurotoxin that has been demonstrated with *S. dysenteriae* type 1.[1,32] A serious arthritis similar to that seen in Reiter's syndrome has been described in up to 10% of patients 2 to 5 weeks after the dysenteric illness that characteristically occurs in patients with histocompatibility antigen HLA-B27.[33] Culture-positive conjunctivitis during acute shigellosis has also been described and may represent autoinoculation of the conjunctiva analogous to that induced in guinea pigs in the Sereny test.[34] Arthritis syndromes have also been described after inflammatory colitis with *Y. enterocolitica, Salmonella enteritidis,* or *C. difficile,* again in association with HLA-B27.[35] The diagnosis of shigellosis is made using bacterial cultures or polymerase chain reaction (PCR) for the invasiveness plasmid in organisms isolated from stool, rectal swab, or endoscopic biopsy specimens.[36]

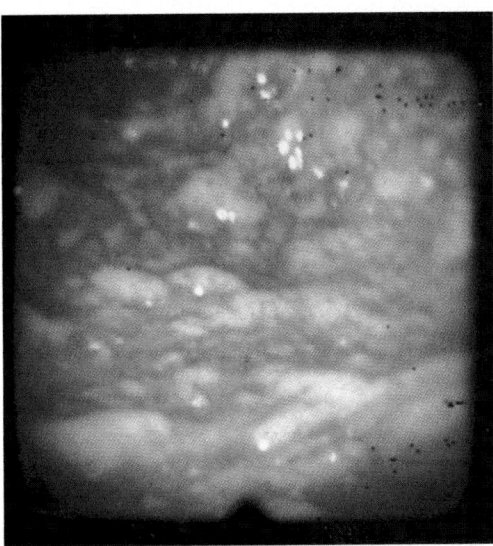

FIGURE 93-2. Proctoscopic view of pseudomembranous colitis in a patient who received clindamycin. Note the 4- to 8-mm raised, white plaques overlying an erythematous mucosa. *(From Tedesco FJ, Barton RW, Alpers DH: Clindamycin-associated colitis. Ann Intern Med 1974;81:429.)*

Certain *E. coli* strains may produce a syndrome identical to that seen with acute shigellosis. The incubation period is usually 2 to 3 days after ingestion. Although invasive *E. coli* organisms appear to be limited to certain serotypes (Table 93-2),[34,37,38] to confirm the presence of such organisms their invasive potential should be demonstrated with the guinea pig conjunctivitis (Sereny's) test[39] or in HeLa cells,[40] or the 120- to 140-MD plasmid that is associated with invasiveness in *Shigella* and invasive *E. coli* should be identified.[41] Invasive *E. coli* organisms were responsible for a single widespread outbreak of dysentery associated with imported French Camembert cheese.[38,42] Although they have been identified as occasional causes of diarrhea in Brazil,[34] invasive *E. coli* organisms do not appear to be frequent causes of sporadic diarrhea in the United States. Because they are often slow to ferment lactose in the laboratory, invasive *E. coli* organisms may be initially mistaken for shigellae,[34,38,40] to which they are closely related. Invasive *E. coli* organisms are also usually lysine negative, are often nonmotile,[43] and are antigenically related to *Shigella*.[44]

Early administration of empiric antibiotic treatment is justified in children hospitalized for clinical dysentery.[45] Short-course (3 days) oral ciprofloxacin for *S. dysenteriae* type 1 dysentery in children was effective.[46] Oral rehydration salts (ORS) solution (World Health Organization formula) is recommended for oral rehydration therapy.[47]

Enterohemorrhagic *Escherichia coli* Diarrhea

A significant cause of bloody diarrhea and potentially fatal HUS is now recognized to be enterohemorrhagic *E. coli* organisms (EHEC) (see Chapter 215), which produce Shiga-like toxin, although the frequency with which they cause inflammatory diarrhea is not clear.[2,48] These organisms have attracted particular attention because of widespread outbreaks in popular hamburger chain restaurants.[49] While they account for only 0.8% to 3.0% of all cases of diarrhea in the United States and Canada, EHEC (of serotype O157) are estimated to account for 15% to 36% of cases of bloody diarrhea.[2] The majority of recognized EHEC strains are of serotype O157; others include O26:K60:H11; O103:H2; O91:H2; O145:H-; O111:K58:H-; O38:H21; O6:H-; O5:H-; O128; O139; O113:K75; O121; and O172.[2,37,50] EHEC were the most commonly recognized cause of diarrhea (3%) among 5415 patients studied in Calgary in Alberta, Canada, where such cases showed a summer seasonal peak.[51] In addition to causing 15% to 36% of all cases of bloody diarrhea, including outbreaks of hemorrhagic colitis, EHEC are associated with 75% to 90% of cases of HUS in North America, a complication that develops in 8% of EHEC infections.[2]

The incubation period is usually 3 to 4 days after the ingestion of contaminated food or water. Cattle are the major reservoir of the organism. The consumption of inadequately cooked beef, raw milk, or other products contaminated by the intestinal contents of cattle, and occasionally of contaminated water, has been recognized as important sources of O157:H7 infection.[52] A waterborne outbreak of *E. coli* O157:H7 has been documented in upstate New York at a county fair.[53] The infection causes abdominal cramps and watery diarrhea that is followed by bloody diarrhea.[54] The HUS and thrombocytopenia may occur 2 to 4 days after the onset of diarrhea, especially in children under 5 years of age and in older adults. EHEC O157:H7 forms characteristic actin pedestals on infected mammalian cells.[55] EHEC secrete their own translocated intimin receptor (Tir) molecule (via a type II secretion system) into the plasma membranes of host cells.[56] The attachment of the organism via its Tir receptor is required to trigger the assembly of actin into focused pedestals beneath bound bacteria. EHEC produces Stx1 or Stx2—the latter is more associated with HUS.[57] Another EHEC virulence factor, H7 flagellin, is also associated with activation of proinflammatory signals in human colonic epithelial cells in response to this noninvasive pathogen.[56] The diagnosis of infection with EHEC depends on culturing stool on MacConkey's culture medium, where it yields sorbitol-negative colonies.[58] The isolated *E. coli* is serotyped for somatic (O) and flagellar (H) antigens. Rapid methods for detection of Shiga toxins in the stool samples are now in development.[59,60] Antibiotic therapy has not been shown to be effective for disease caused by EHEC or EIEC. Some EHEC strains may increase their phage-mediated production of Shiga-like toxins when exposed to antibiotic to which they are sensitive, such as ampicillin, tetracycline, and norfloxacin.[61]

Campylobacter Enteritis

Campylobacter jejuni (formerly *Campylobacter fetus* or "*Vibrio fetus*") systemic infections (see Chapter 213) have been recognized for many years. Although the majority of *Campylobacter* blood-stream infections in humans are with *C. fetus* (old subspecies, *intestinalis*),[62] *C. jejuni* commonly causes an enteric infection in all age groups. This organism was recognized many years ago as a cause of swine dysentery. Commercially available techniques of fecal culture have enabled the culture of *C. jejuni* on highly selective media at 42° C from fecal specimens of patients with diarrhea.[16] This organism causes a syndrome of severe abdominal pain, fever, and acute inflammatory enteritis that may range from watery diarrhea to severe dysentery with blood and pus in the stools.[63] This infection has also been associated with sequelae of reactive arthritis and Guillain-Barré syndrome.[64] Cross-reacting antibodies recognizing both *C. jejuni* lipopolysaccharide (LPS) and antigenic determinants of nerve gangliosides are speculated to contribute to the development of the nerve damage after *C. jejuni* infection. Reports from Belgium, England, and central Africa reveal that in 5% to 14% of unselected cases of diarrhea, *C. jejuni* is present,[63,65] and outbreaks of *Campylobacter* enteritis have been associated with ingestion of contaminated water, raw milk, and uncooked

TABLE 93-2	Enteroinvasive *Escherichia coli* Serotypes	
Serotype	*Difco Serogroup*	*References*
O28 ac	C	34, 166
O29	—	37
O112 a,c	C	166
O124	B	34, 38, 166
O136	C (Trabulsi's 193-T-64)	38, 166
O143	—	166
O144	—	38, 166
O152	(Trabulsi's 185-T-64)	38, 166

meat and poultry. The roles of toxins, adhesins, and LPSs in the pathogenesis of *Campylobacter* enteritis remain uncertain.[66]

Most patients with mild to moderate *C. jejuni* enterocolitis do not benefit from antibiotic treatment. Severely ill patients, especially debilitated or immunocompromised persons, appear to benefit from antibiotic therapy, and erythromycin or ciprofloxacin are the drugs of choice. Increased fluoroquinolone resistance in *Campylobacter* species from man and animals, the result of mutations in topoisomerase genes, has been documented.[67]

Amebic Dysentery

An estimated 40,000 to 100,000 people die yearly from amebiasis, making this disease the second leading cause of death from parasitic diseases (after malaria[68]). There are two morphologically identical *Entamoeba* species: *E. histolytica* and *Entamoeba dispar* (see Chapter 270).[69] The former is a pathogen and is responsible for invasive amebiasis, whereas the latter is a gut commensal. *E. histolytica* cysts are ingested, pass through the gastric acidity, and undergo digestion of the capsule in the small bowel. Trophozoites then invade the colonic mucosa and produce shallow, flask-shaped, undermining ulcers. The capacity of this parasite to invade tissue has been attributed to histolytic enzymes, but invasion probably also involves contact-dependent cytolysis of target cells, especially polymorphonuclear leukocytes, which then discharge their cytolytic contents.[70-72] After their invasion of the intestine, amebae may then seed the liver via the portal vein, from which extension may occur to the skin, diaphragm, lung, or pericardium. Although extraintestinal amebiasis occurs with less than one-tenth the frequency of symptomatic intestinal amebic dysentery, dissemination is reportedly more common in states of undernutrition, with cytotoxic or steroid medication, during late pregnancy, and with carcinoma or other overwhelming systemic diseases. Asymptomatic cyst carriage occurs in 1% to 5% of the population in the southern United States. The frequency of amebiasis is greater in rural and lower socioeconomic groups and in institutions where fecal-oral spread of this human parasite may occur. Fulminant amebic colitis is a rare disease but may be associated with diabetes mellitus and chronic alcoholism.[73]

To distinguish between *E. histolytica* and *E. dispar*, an enzyme-linked immunosorbent assay (ELISA) is available commercially that identifies *E. histolytica* antigens in stool.[74] The PCR techniques used in research could become another diagnostic method.[75] The diagnosis of amebic liver abscess relies on computed tomography (CT) scans of the liver and on amebic serology, which is highly sensitive (>94%) and highly specific (>95%).[74]

Amebic colitis is treated by a nitroimidazole derivative (metronidazole, tinidazole, or ornidazole), followed by a luminal agent (diloxanide furoate, paromomycin, or iodoquinol) to eradicate colonization.[67] The treatment of amebic liver abscess is a single course of metronidazole; surgical drainage should be avoided in uncomplicated amebic liver abscesses.

Ciliary Dysentery

Balantidium coli (see Chapter 281) is the only ciliated parasite that is pathogenic for humans. The most common reservoir is swine. Like *E. histolytica*, this parasite excysts in the small bowel, invades the terminal ileum and colon, and may cause appendicitis or a dysenteric syndrome with rectosigmoid ulceration (with heaped-up edges around 1.5- to 3-cm ulcers) and secondary bacteremia. However, there is no extraintestinal extension of *B. coli* infection, as may be seen with amebiasis. The diagnosis is made by scraping the margin of the ulcer and examining microscopically for the ciliate trophozoite. Mucosal invasion is usually limited to the rectal vault. Symptoms may last for 1 to 4 weeks and may recur several times a year if the infection goes untreated. Therapy with tetracycline is usually successful.

Bilharzial Dysentery

Schistosomiasis may involve acute bloody diarrhea, abdominal pain, and weight loss when the adult schistosomes (usually *Schistosoma japonicum* or *Schistosoma mansoni* [see Chapter 287]) migrate to the intestinal tract, where they begin egg deposition.[76] This occurs 3 to 8 weeks after initial skin exposure to the cercariae and may last for several weeks. Fecal examination reveals blood, pus, and numerous ova. Fever, leukocytosis, and increasing eosinophilia may be associated with this illness, and hepatosplenic disease may follow. *S. mansoni* may also cause chronic blood or protein loss via inflammatory "polyps."

The detection of schistosome eggs in feces or urine is diagnostic of schistosomiasis. The use of formalin-based techniques for sedimentation and concentration may increase the diagnostic yield.[77] Praziquantel is the drug of choice for treatment of schistosomiasis. This drug causes tetanic contractions and tegumental vacuoles in the worms, resulting in their death and detachment from the wall of the vein.

Trichinosis

Another potential parasitic cause of inflammatory enteritis is acute trichinosis (see Chapter 286). Approximately 24 hours after the ingestion of infested pork, the larvae excyst and invade the intestinal mucosa, often resulting in nausea, vomiting, diarrhea, and abdominal pain. This precedes the systemic manifestation of periorbital edema, fever, myositis, and eosinophilia by 1 to 2 weeks.

Vibriosis

In addition to classic and El Tor *Vibrio cholerae* O1, non-O1 *V. cholerae* and several halophilic *Vibrio* species (see Chapters 211 and 212) are now recognized to cause diarrhea and occasional wound or bloodstream infection.[78] The most common and best characterized is *V. parahaemolyticus*, which has been recognized since 1950 in Japan and was identified as a vibrio in 1963. *V. parahaemolyticus* is a cause of seafood poisoning, with onset of signs and symptoms 9 to 25 hours after the ingestion of inadequately cooked fish or shellfish. This has been reported throughout the coastal areas of the United States and on cruise ships and is the most common form of food poisoning in Japan, where raw seafood is commonly eaten.[79] Diarrhea may be explosive and watery or may be characterized by full-blown dysentery with blood and pus and superficial ulceration on proctoscopic examination.[80] The latter syndrome may be associated with cramps, nausea, vomiting, headache, and fever. The illness is usually self-limited, resolving within 3 to 4 days. The pathogenic Kanagawa-positive strains from patients produce β-hemolysis on special (Wagatsuma) medium—in contrast to environmental isolates—and are best isolated as blue-green colonies (alkaline) on TCBS agar.[14] A PCR method was recently developed as a species-specific probe for *V. parahaemolyticus*, *Vibrio alginolyticus*, *Vibrio anguillarum*, and a cluster of related species.[81] Antibiotic treatment with tetracycline or doxycycline can diminish the duration and severity of gastrointestinal symptoms. To prevent *V. parahaemolyticus* infections, consumption of raw or undercooked shellfish and exposure of wounds to seawater should be avoided.[82]

Other halophilic vibrios include *V. alginolyticus*, *Vibrio fluvialis*, *Vibrio hollisae*, *Vibrio damsela*, and *Vibrio vulnificus*, which have been associated with enteric, wound, or systemic infections in humans.[78] *V. vulnificus* has been associated with life-threatening septicemia occurring within 24 hours of ingesting raw oysters.[78,83]

Salmonellosis and Typhoid Fever

Salmonella enterocolitis is characterized by fever, cramping, abdominal pain, and diarrhea that begins 8 to 48 hours after ingestion of an infective dose, usually with food, and usually lasts 3 to 5 days (see Chapter 220). The diarrheal stools of patients with salmonellosis often contain a moderate number of polymorphonuclear leukocytes, usually fewer than is typical of shigellosis.

Although *Salmonella* enteritis involves predominantly the lamina propria in the small bowel, several reports have noted *Salmonella typhimurium* as a cause of colitis, with crypt abscesses and erosion and ulcerations of the colonic mucosa, which result in blood and pus in the stool.[84] Certain other strains of salmonella (*Salmonella choleraesuis* and *Salmonella paratyphi*), like *Salmonella typhi*, tend to elicit a mononuclear response and cause a bacteremia characteristic of enteric fever. Antibiotic therapy is not required, but patients who are severely ill or those with risk factors for developing extraintestinal spread of infection should be treated with fluoroquinolones or third-generation cephalosporins.

Typhoid fever may lead to an erosion of the blood vessels in Peyer's patches that without appropriate treatment may result in gross blood in the feces in 10% to 20% of the patients. Severe intestinal hemorrhage may complicate approximately 2% of the cases late in the course of untreated typhoid fever. Such intestinal bleeding may precede perforation, another complication of typhoid fever.[85]

Yersiniosis

Yersinia enterocolitica (see Chapter 226) is another increasingly recognized enteric pathogen that may be responsible for an enteric fever–like illness, mesenteric adenitis (which may mimic acute appendicitis), or an inflammatory ileitis or ulcerative colitis syndrome with fecal neutrophils and mononuclear cells.[86] *Y. enterocolitica* and *Yersinia pseudotuberculosis* may cause similar symptoms and signs. The virulence of *Yersinia* is associated with the direct injection of proteins, such as *Yersinia* protein kinase A (YpkA) and YopE, into eukaryotic cells.[87,88] *Yersinia* infection may also be associated with migratory polyarthritis, Reiter's syndrome, or erythema nodosum. A syndrome of acute diarrhea and vomiting is especially common in young children. The organism may cause disseminated abscesses in the liver and spleen[89] or an inflammatory colitis.[90] The causative agent, a gram-negative member of the family Enterobacteriaceae, is in the same genus as the plague bacillus *Yersinia pestis* and is sometimes mistaken for *Proteus* on initial culture plates.

Cultivation may require cold enrichment techniques.[15] PCR methods for detection of pathogenic *Y. enterocolitica* are more sensitive than culture methods.[91] *Yersinia* infection is usually self-limiting; however, patients with severe illness or systemic infection are usually treated with tetracycline, chloramphenicol, or ciprofloxacin.

Gonococcal Proctitis

Neisseria gonorrhoeae (see Chapter 209) may be the cause of ulcerative proctitis, usually acquired by anal intercourse.[7] The resultant purulent proctitis is accompanied by an erythematous, friable mucous membrane in the rectal vault and occasional abscess or fistula formation. Although copious purulent discharge, tenesmus, and burning rectal pain may be noted, two thirds of the culture-positive patients with anorectal gonococcal infection are asymptomatic.[92] Additional diagnostic possibilities in cases of venereally acquired proctitis are syphilitic, herpetic, and chlamydial proctitis.[93]

Unusual Causes of Dysentery

"Spirillar" or "spirochetal" dysentery has been reported to occur in southern France and has been attributed to *Spirillum* species. Although severe mucoid diarrhea or dysentery has been associated with intestinal spirochetes, their frequency and role in causing enteric disease is unclear. A DNA probe for the 16S recombinant RNA (rRNA) of the agent of swine dysentery, *Treponema hyodysenteriae*, has been developed and may open new approaches to the recognition of similar infections in humans.[94]

Other unusual causes of colitis include brucellosis[95] and adenovirus infections.[96,97]

APPROACH TO DIAGNOSIS AND TREATMENT OF ACUTE DYSENTERY

Any of the aforementioned microorganisms may cause an acute dysentery syndrome with blood and pus in the stool; examination for leukocytes or for fecal lactoferrin[98] may suggest intestinal inflammation even if blood is not present in the stool on gross examination. Other considerations in the differential diagnosis of inflammatory colitis are pseudomembranous enterocolitis, which may be associated with antibiotic use, and the potentially rapidly progres-

sive necrotizing enterocolitis syndromes, which are discussed in Chapters 92 and 93. These diagnoses are suggested by the setting, clinical course, history, and findings on radiologic and proctoscopic examinations. Noninfectious syndromes that may be manifested as acute inflammatory enterocolitis include idiopathic ulcerative colitis and Crohn's disease.

Presumptive therapy for the inflammatory colitides varies greatly with the different organisms and is influenced by the increasing resistance of enteric pathogens to antimicrobial therapy[99] (see Chapter 93). For example, an acute febrile dysenteric illness in a young child with daycare exposure or in an area where shigellosis is common should be treated with an antimicrobial agent such as one of the fluoroquinolones. If the *Shigella* organism is sensitive, prompt therapy can successfully stop the diarrhea, alleviate systemic symptoms, and reduce shedding of the organisms in the feces.[100-102] Because shigellae are increasingly resistant to multiple antibiotics,[103,104] the practitioner must be familiar with the local resistance pattern of shigellae to appropriately treat acute shigellosis when it is first suspected. Although at present the fluoroquinolones are not approved for use in children in the United States, the available data suggest that a short course of therapy is safe.[105] Although ciprofloxacin may shorten the clinical course of *Salmonella* infections, it does not eradicate the organism.[106] Recent studies show increasing resistance of *Campylobacter* and even *Salmonella* to quinolones.[107,108] Azithromycin may reduce the duration of symptoms.[109] Vitamin A has also been used to reduce both severity and mortality from shigellosis.[110]

Amebic dysentery is traditionally diagnosed by direct examination of wet mounts of fresh fecal or proctoscopic specimens, which reveal *E. histolytica* trophozoites or cysts characterized by four or fewer delicate nuclei with central karyosomes. Additional patients may be diagnosed by biopsy, which may reveal periodic acid–Schiff (PAS)-positive trophozoites or cysts in the undermining ulcer in the lamina propria, or by a fecal or serum *E. histolytica*–specific antigen test, which distinguishes virulent *E. histolytica* from avirulent *E. dispar* infections.[74]

Necrotizing Enterocolitis in the Newborn

The syndrome of diffuse fulminating necrotizing colitis has been recognized in infants since the 1960s. This syndrome probably represents the same entity described as "spontaneous" intestinal perforation and peritonitis as early as 1838.[111] Although milder forms of the syndrome doubtless exist, the syndrome of necrotizing enterocolitis (NEC) is defined by the presence of air in the wall of the intestine, portal venous system, or peritoneal cavity, or by necrosis of the bowel wall with mucosal sloughing. This fulminant syndrome often leads to intestinal perforation, peritonitis, and bacteremia. It is a major cause of mortality in low-birth-weight infants (<1500 g) after the first week of life.[112] The diffuse necrotic changes that characterize this syndrome most often occur in the terminal ileum but may be seen in the colon or in the proximal portion of the gastrointestinal tract.

The pathogenesis of NEC appears to involve mucosal injury that is most often of ischemic origin from hypoxemic or hypotensive episodes that may occur in premature infants or in the presence of complicating factors such as an umbilical vein exchange transfusion. Ischemia may also result from the effects of endotoxemia followed by the effects of epinephrine, to which the vessels supplying the terminal ileum may be especially sensitive. Other factors predisposing to mucosal ischemia include asphyxia in association with hyaline membrane disease in premature infants or cyanotic heart disease. Increased intraluminal pressures may contribute to ischemia and pneumatosis, a process that may also play a role in previously normal infants who develop necrotizing colitis after protracted periods of diarrhea. Some investigators have suggested a localized Shwartzman reaction to endotoxemia or gram-negative bacteria.[113] The absence of lysozyme (normally present in human breast milk) may allow overgrowth of gram-negative bacilli. "Enteropathogenic" *E. coli* serotype O111:B4 has also been associated with NEC.[114] Because of the association with use of umbilical vein polyvinylchloride catheters and feeding tubes, the toxic effect of plasticizers leached from the polyvinylchloride materials has also been suggested.[115] Reports of outbreaks of NEC in newborn intensive care units[116,117] have led to a careful search for infectious agents including viral, fungal, and bacterial pathogens.[118] Among bacteria, *Pseudomonas, Klebsiella,*[119] certain *E. coli* strains,[114,120] *Salmonella,*[121] and *Clostridium butyricum*[117] have been implicated. The roles of both ischemia and bacteria have been suggested by Barlow and colleagues with work in an experimental rat model of NEC, in which breast milk was shown to be protective.[122] On the basis of acidic intraluminal pH (<5.0) and organic acids in human neonates with NEC,[123] increased numbers of lactose-fermenting *Klebsiella* organisms have been postulated to play a role in the pathogenesis.[124] Other investigators have suggested a role for platelet-activating factor (PAF), and protection by superoxide dismutase or by endogenous nitric oxide.[125]

Clinical features of this serious condition in newborn infants include apneic spells, vomiting, abdominal distention, and occasionally bloody diarrhea. Most infants are less than 1 week of age, and there is an association with prematurity, maternal infections during delivery (such as amnionitis with prolonged post–ruptured membranes status), and exchange transfusion via the umbilical vein. There is no sex or seasonal predilection. The disease often progresses rapidly to intestinal perforation, shock, septicemia, and pneumatosis intestinalis. Air may also be evident in the portal venous system or biliary tract on plain roentgenograms. This syndrome is associated with a mortality rate that is often in excess of 70%.

The diagnosis of NEC should be considered in any premature infant with altered gastrointestinal function, abdominal distention, or apneic spells. Further investigation should include examination of the stool for occult blood and for the presence of reducing substances. Plain abdominal roentgenograms may reveal air in the bowel wall, peritoneal cavity, or portal venous system, and there may be bloody diarrhea late in the course of the disease. Management must be initiated early and aggressively for any infant suspected of having NEC. Umbilical catheters should be removed, oral feeding should be stopped, and nasogastric aspiration should be initiated. Intravenous fluid therapy is of paramount importance. Laparotomy and excision of the necrotic bowel are often necessary and should be done aggressively if there is any evidence of peritonitis or obstruction.[126]

Prevention of NEC includes avoidance of risk factors and careful infection control measures in newborn intensive care units. Hypertonic elemental formulas have been implicated and should be avoided in high-risk patients. NEC rarely occurs in breast-fed infants. Explanations for the advantage of human breast milk include the presence of lysozyme, antibodies, and cellular elements that may play a protective role against potential infectious agents. Although oral prophylactic nonabsorbable antibiotics have been suggested, serious questions remain about the use of prophylactic antibiotics, even in high-risk newborn infants weighing less than 1500 g.

Darmbrand, Pig-Bel, Necrotizing Enteritis in Adults (Enteritis Necroticans)

First described as *Darmbrand* (meaning "fire bowels") in epidemics of enteritis necroticans in northern Germany in the immediate postwar period in the mid-1940s, a severe necrotizing jejunitis has also been recognized in both epidemic and sporadic forms after pork feasting in the highlands of Papua New Guinea.[127] *Pig-bel* was the name given to the syndrome of abdominal discomfort that followed a large pork meal, commonly eaten after a large "pig kill," which takes place every 3 to 10 years among the highland Melanesians of Papua New Guinea. Sporadic cases have been reported from other parts of the world, including the United States.[128]

The pathologic findings are those of acute, patchy, necrotizing disease of the small bowel in previously healthy people that may proceed rapidly to segmental gangrene with small amounts of gas in the mucosa, mesentery, or nodes.

Several theories of pathogenesis have been suggested, most of which involve the toxic products of *Clostridium perfringens* type C, including α- and β-toxins. Sporadic cases of NEC have been noted in association with nutritional disorders, alcoholism, and malabsorption, and after pancreatic or gastric resection.[129] After gastric surgery, increased numbers of *C. perfringens* organisms and increased levels of α-toxin have been noted in the upper small bowel and stomach. Whether α- or β-toxins are capable of causing the necrotizing enteritis alone or whether they initiate the invasion of the mucosa by other organisms such as gram-negative rods is currently unclear. An attractive hypothesis has been suggested by Lawrence and Walker that could explain the association of necrotizing enteritis with poor nutrition and episodic dietetic overindulgence.[129] The low-protein diet of Papua New Guinea highlanders is associated with low levels of digestive proteases in the intestinal lumen, which can be shown to inactivate the β-toxin. The proteases can be further blocked by the oral intake of trypsin inhibitors, which are found in such dietary staples as sweet potatoes in this population. Proteases return with improved diet, as occurred in postwar Germany. This hypothesis has been confirmed in an animal model that required protease inhibitors for symptomatic infection.[130]

The clinical syndromes of necrotizing enteritis range from anorexia, vomiting, severe abdominal pain, and bloody diarrhea to fulminant toxemia and shock. Acute complications that necessitate emergency surgery include paralytic ileus, bowel strangulation, and bowel perforation with peritonitis. These complications are common in the first 2 weeks of illness. Later complications that may also necessitate surgery include scarring leading to stenosis, obstruction, malabsorption, and fistulas. Necrotizing enteritis occurs with greater frequency and greater severity in children under 10 years of age. In contrast to European controls who rarely have antibody, 70% of the healthy adults in Papua New Guinea have demonstrable antibody to clostridial β-toxin.[127,129]

The syndrome is defined by the pathologic findings but should be suspected in patients who develop severe abdominal pain, bloody diarrhea, ileus, and toxemia. The course is often too fulminant for radiographic detection of air in the bowel wall to be of any diagnostic value.

Etiologic agents held responsible for necrotizing enteritis include *C. perfringens* type C, once designated as type F in the older classification of *Clostridium welchii*. The majority of surgically resected bowel specimens from patients with necrotizing enteritis contain *C. perfringens*, over half of which are type C. Furthermore, 12 of 21 cases described had a significant change in serum β-antitoxin titer after illness with pig-bel in Papua New Guinea.[127] Although polyvalent gas gangrene antiserum was ineffective, administration of type C antiserum resulted in a 30% decrease in the need for surgery, and a mortality reduced from 43% to 19%.[127] Furthermore, active immunization against the β-toxin has also proved effective in preventing pig-bel.[131]

Some have suggested that type A *C. perfringens,* staphylococci, or even hepatitis virus may be responsible for necrotizing enteritis. The syndrome of "enteritis gravis" has been described in association with infectious hepatitis, although no viral etiology has been documented.

Considerations in the differential diagnosis of necrotizing enteritis include acute shigellosis, acute food poisoning syndromes, antibiotic-associated pseudomembranous colitis, and acute ulcerative colitis. The absence of colonic involvement, the epidemiologic setting, especially in poorly nourished patients, and the rapid progression to toxemia and shock are strongly suggestive of necrotizing enteritis.

Therapy for NEC includes careful supportive care and bowel decompression. Fluid requirements may be substantially greater than what is indicated by fecal output. Resection of the involved bowel must be considered if there is a persistence of paralytic ileus, a rapid increase in signs of toxemia, localized or diffuse signs of peritonitis, persistent pain, or a palpable mass lesion. If subacute obstruction or malabsorption is suspected on the basis of weight loss, elective surgery may be required up to 6 months after the acute illness. Raw peanut or soybean diets should be avoided because they contain trypsin inhibitors. *C. perfringens* type C antiserum containing β-antitoxin or the active β-toxin vaccine should be available for use in areas where necrotizing enteritis can be expected to occur.

Pseudomembranous enterocolitis and nosocomial *C. difficile* colitis are discussed in Chapter 92.

CHRONIC INFLAMMATORY PROCESSES

Chronic inflammatory enteritides are often indolent, slowly progressive infections. Often there is a history of weeks or months of fever, abdominal pain, weight loss, or other systemic manifestations. Recurring or relapsing symptoms may be seen with *C. jejuni* or *Salmonella* gastroenteritis. In addition, 16% of cases of shigellosis may become prolonged, lasting for 3 weeks or longer.[132] Any diarrheal illness that extends beyond 2 weeks is considered severe and is associated with a high risk of nutritional morbidity in children who live in tropical, developing areas.[133-135]

Enteropathogenic and Enteroaggregative *Escherichia coli*

Enteropathogenic *E. coli* organisms that cause acute diarrhea in infants may rarely be associated with an insidious persistent or relapsing illness.[136] *E. coli* organisms in O groups 1, 2, 4, 7, and 75 that produce hemolysin and necrotoxin have been isolated from patients with ulcerative colitis. These toxic organisms are not present in healthy people or in patients with acute diarrheal syndromes.[137] In addition, enteroaggregative *E. coli* organisms are recognized as a cause of persistent diarrhea in India, Brazil, and Mexico.[138-140] Enteroaggregative *E. coli* (EAEC) infections are an emerging problem, and enteropathogenic *E. coli* (EPEC) infections remain important in many parts of the world.[141,142] Enteroaggregative *E. coli* organisms have been associated with intestinal inflammation and malnutrition, even in the absence of diarrhea.[143] The effects of antibiotic treatment constitute a topic of current interest, and such therapy may be feasible.[144]

Syphilis

Syphilis (see Chapter 235) can also involve the gastrointestinal tract, usually in the upper part of the small bowel or stomach. An acute erosive and infiltrative gastritis with motile spirochetes and a positive specific response on treponemal immunofluorescence testing has been reported in late secondary syphilis.[145] The initial complaints are upper abdominal pain, vomiting, and weight loss. More classic are the late gastrointestinal manifestations of lues: pyloric obstruction, "hourglass" constriction, and linitis plastica of the stomach. Less commonly, gumma may be seen in the small bowel or colon.

Gastrointestinal Tuberculosis

Intestinal tuberculosis, once considered common, had become a relatively rare disease but is now reemerging in association with acquired immunodeficiency syndrome (AIDS) and with multidrug-resistant *Mycobacterium tuberculosis* (see Chapter 248).[146] Intestinal involvement with tuberculosis may be either *primary,* from ingestion of the organisms or *secondary,* usually from a pulmonary source.

Primary intestinal tuberculosis without pulmonary disease often results in hypertrophic mucosal changes. Nearly two thirds of cases of acute miliary tuberculosis may also have gastrointestinal involvement.[147] Patients with primary intestinal tuberculosis may present with abdominal pain, fever, and a tender, fixed palpable mass in the ileocecal area. Primary hypertrophic intestinal tuberculosis continues to occur in the Near East[148] and in India.[149] Intestinal involvement secondary to pulmonary tuberculosis may result from swallowing infected sputum or from biliary excretion of the organism from an infected liver. The frequency of secondary intestinal tuberculosis increases with far-advanced pulmonary disease. Hippocrates stated that "diarrhea attacking a person with phthisis is a mortal symptom."

Tuberculosis may involve any part of the gastrointestinal tract, but most ulcerative and hypertrophic types occur in the ileocecal region, where there is a predominance of submucosal lymphatic tissue. The most common features are fever and abdominal pain that is often relieved by defecation or vomiting. Weight loss is more common in secondary intestinal tuberculosis. Only one third of the patients with gastrointestinal tuberculosis have diarrhea. Diarrhea may be related to exacerbations of abdominal pain and occasionally occurs with extensive involvement of the small intestine, which may cause steatorrhea and a malabsorption syndrome. Although ulceration and mucous diarrhea are relatively common with secondary intestinal tuberculosis, hemorrhage and the presence of gross blood in the stool are distinctly uncommon, perhaps because of the associated obliterative endarteritis.

The diagnosis of gastrointestinal tuberculosis may be very difficult radiologically and even histologically. It must be distinguished from regional enteritis, sarcoidosis, actinomycosis, ameboma, carcinoma, and periappendiceal abscess. In contrast to Crohn's disease, gastrointestinal tuberculosis rarely causes anal lesions, fistulas, or perforation. It is often associated with miliary nodules on the serosa, it rarely causes strictures longer than 3 cm, and it may cause circumferential transverse ulcers. Tuberculosis may also cause fibrosis of the muscularis mucosa, pyloric metaplasia, and epithelial regeneration.[150] There may be minimal or no radiologic changes in the bowel mucosa. Small mucosal ulcerations may result in tiny calcified nodules in the mucosa in association with calcified mesenteric lymph nodes analogous to those seen in the pulmonary Ghon complex. The ileocecal region often reveals radiologic evidence of irritability and hypermotility, with hypersegmentation of the mucosal folds or poor filling of the ileocecal region detected by barium enema. Occasionally, frank ulcerations can be noted on contrast studies, and late in the course there is scarring. The diagnosis requires a careful examination of involved tissue for acid-fast bacilli by special stain and culture. Caseous necrosis is more frequently found in the mesenteric nodes than in intestinal tissue itself. Complications of intestinal tuberculosis include perforation, peritonitis, and obstruction from either hypertrophy, scarring, or tuberculoma.

Gastrointestinal Mycosis

Candida albicans (see Chapter 255) can cause ulcerations in any part of the gastrointestinal tract.[151] Although shallow invasion of gastric or duodenal ulcers may have no obvious clinical consequence in the nonimmunosuppressed patient, ulcerations anywhere from the distal third of the esophagus to the rectum may be deeply invaded and numerous in the neutropenic patient, constituting an important entry site for hematogenously disseminated candidiasis. Patients infected with human immunodeficiency virus type 1 (HIV-1) are prone to esophageal candidiasis.[152] Several reports have implicated *Candida* species as a cause of diarrhea.[153,154] Although *Candida* organisms may reach high concentrations in the stool of patients receiving antimicrobial agents, and some have suggested that it may cause diarrhea, *Candida* has no clearly established role in the etiology of diarrhea.

Whereas gastrointestinal involvement with the North American blastomycosis is quite rare, South American blastomycosis (due to *Paracoccidioides brasiliensis* [see Chapter 266) is often manifested as lesions of the skin, oral mucosa, or intestinal tract, where it causes granulomatous or ulcerative disease.[155] The most common intestinal sites of involvement are the appendix, cecum, and anorectal areas. There is often abscess formation and lymphatic spread to regional nodes and to the spleen, the liver, or even the lungs. The major symptoms are abdominal pain and ulcerative, granulomatous lesions, especially in the oropharynx. Palpable, tender abdominal masses in the ileocecal region may be noted on physical examination. Peritoneal signs are often absent. Diagnosis is made by biopsy, stain, and culture of the ulcerative lesion.

Other fungi usually involve the intestinal tract as only one feature of disseminated granulomatous disease; some of these pathogens may be acquired through a gastrointestinal portal of entry. Phycomycetes

(*Absidia*, *Rhizopus*, and *Mucor* species) may invade the predisposed host via the gastrointestinal tract,[156] or phycomycosis may involve the gastrointestinal tract by hematogenous spread and cause abdominal pain, diarrhea, gastrointestinal bleeding, and peritonitis.[157]

Histoplasmosis (see Chapter 262) may also involve the intestinal tract as a part of disseminated infection. In the gastrointestinal tract, histoplasmosis is manifested as ulceration, bleeding, obstruction, or, rarely, protein-losing enteropathy.[158,159] Lesions tend to be single and may be initially considered to be neoplastic.

Parasitic Enteritis

Parasitic enteritides that should be considered among causes of chronic inflammatory bowel processes include coccidiosis, chronic or recurrent amebiasis, and the rare invasive, inflammatory form of giardiasis.

Human coccidiosis is an upper small bowel inflammatory process caused by *Isospora belli* (see Chapter 281) that should be considered in patients (especially AIDS patients[160]) with chronic diarrhea of obscure origin and eosinophilia.[161] Weight loss, fever, headache, and colicky abdominal pain may also be present, with steatorrhea and malabsorption. The causative unicellular sporozoan parasite undergoes asexual schizogony in the intestinal epithelial cells, from which merozoites are released. Like malarial plasmodia, merozoites may then invade other cells and repeat the asexual schizogony cycle or may mature into sexual gametocytes and form zygotes and then sporulated oocysts that rupture to yield sporozoites that restart the enterocyte cycle. Sporulated oocysts are the infective form and have caused laboratory-acquired infections. The diagnosis is made by careful examination of multiple serial sections of intestinal biopsy specimens for any stage of the parasite, or by examining small bowel contents for oocysts. Stool oocysts may be seen after staining with a modified acid-fast stain as for *Cryptosporidium* or may be demonstrated, rarely and with some difficulty, by incubating a specimen at room temperature for 1 to 2 days to permit their maturation before examination, and then using a concentration technique such as zinc sulfate flotation. Sulfamethoxazole-trimethoprim is effective even in AIDS patients, in whom multiple courses or suppressive therapy may be required.[160]

The protozoan parasite *Cryptosporidium* (see Chapter 280) is a cause of severe chronic diarrhea in immunosuppressed persons. It is typically self-limited after 2 to 4 weeks in normal hosts. Unlike *Isospora* organisms, cryptosporidia usually infect only the surface of the mucosal epithelium, and the process is less inflammatory. The organism may be identified by sugar flotation or modified acid-fast stains of fecal specimens.[162]

Cyclospora (see Chapter 281) has also now been associated with persistent diarrhea in travelers, those living in tropical areas, health care workers, and AIDS patients.[163]

Invasive syndromes may occur over a long period of time or in a recurring pattern with intestinal amebiasis. This syndrome may even extend into an entity called ulcerative postdysenteric colitis, which may no longer respond to antiamebic therapy.[164]

Inflammatory small bowel disease may occur with unusually severe *G. lamblia* infection (see Chapter 277). This may result in severe villus atrophy, with dense plasma cell infiltration and acute inflammation in the lamina propria.[165]

Considerations in the differential diagnosis of chronic inflammatory diarrhea include several syndromes of noninfectious or unknown causes. Idiopathic inflammatory bowel disease including regional enteritis, granulomatous colitis, and ulcerative colitis may be difficult to distinguish from infectious enteritides. Other conditions that often require biopsy and culture to exclude infectious processes include intestinal involvement with sarcoidosis, lymphoma, and carcinoma. Radiation enterocolitis, ischemic colitis, and diverticulitis may also be manifested as chronic inflammatory diarrhea.

REFERENCES

1. Keusch GT, Jacewicz M. The pathogenesis of *Shigella* diarrhea: V. Relationship of Shiga enterotoxin, neurotoxin and cytotoxin. J Infect Dis. 1975;131(Suppl):33.
2. Edelman R, Karmali MA, Fleming PA. Summary of the International Symposium and Workshop on Infections Due to Verocytotoxin (Shiga-like Toxin)-Producing *Escherichia coli*. J Infect Dis. 1988;157:1102-1104.
3. Blacklow NR, Dolin R, Fedson DS, et al. Acute infectious nonbacterial gastroenteritis: Etiology and pathogenesis. Ann Intern Med. 1972;76:993.
4. Rendtorff RC. The experimental transmission of human intestinal protozoan parasites. Am J Hyg. 1954;59:196.
5. Weissman JB, Schmerler A, Gangarosa EJ, et al. Shigellosis in day-care centres. Lancet. 1975;1:88.
6. Roy SK, Speelman P, Butler T, et al. Diarrhea associated with typhoid fever. J Infect Dis. 1985;151:1138-1143.
7. Quinn TC, Stamm WE, Goodell SE, et al. The polymicrobial origin of intestinal infections in homosexual men. N Engl J Med. 1983;309:576.
8. Korzeniowski OM, Barada FA, Rouse JD, et al. Value of examination for fecal leukocytes in the early diagnosis of shigellosis. Am J Trop Med Hyg. 1979;28:1031.
9. Pickering LK, DuPont HL, Olarte J, et al. Fecal leukocytes in enteric infections. Am J Clin Pathol. 1977;68:562-565.
10. Haugwout FG. The microscopic diagnosis of the dysenteries at their onset. JAMA. 1924;83:1156.
11. Guerrant RL, Brush JE, Ravdin JI, et al. Interaction between *Entamoeba histolytica* and human polymorphonuclear neutrophils. J Infect Dis. 1981;143:83-93.
12. Speelman P, McGlaughlin R, Kabir I, et al. Differential clinical features and stool findings in shigellosis and amebic dysentery. Trans R Soc Trop Med Hyg. 1987;81:549-551.
13. Rahaman MM, Khan MM, Azi KMS, et al. An outbreak of dysentery caused by *Shigella dysenteriae* type I on a coral island in the Bay of Bengal. J Infect Dis. 1975;132:15.
14. Feeley JC, Balows A. *Vibrio*. In: Lennette EH, Spaulding EH, Truant JP, eds. Manual of Clinical Microbiology. Washington, DC: American Society for Microbiology; 1974:238-245.
15. Morris GK, Feeley JC, Martin WT, et al. Isolation and identification of *Yersinia enterocolitica*. Public Health Lab. 1977;35:217.
16. Skirrow MB. *Campylobacter* enteritis: A "new" disease. BMJ. 1972;2:9.
17. Lyerly DM, Krivan HC, Wilkins TD. *Clostridium difficile*: Its disease and toxins. J Clin Microbiol. 1988;1:1-18.
18. Doern GV, Coughlin RT, Wu L. Laboratory diagnosis of *Clostridium difficile*–associated gastrointestinal disease: Comparison of a monoclonal antibody enzyme immunoassay for toxins A and B with a monoclonal antibody enzyme immunoassay for toxin A only and two cytotoxicity assays. J Clin Microbiol. 1992;30:2042-2046.
19. Lima AAM, Lyerly DM, Wilkins TD, et al. Effects of *Clostridium difficile* toxins A and B in rabbit small and large intestine *in vitro* and on cultured cells *in vitro*. Infect Immun. 1988;56:582-588.
20. Lindberg AA, Pal T. Strategies for development of potential candidate *Shigella* vaccines. Vaccine. 1993;11:168-179.
21. Sandvig K. Shiga toxins. Toxicon. 2001;39:1629.
22. Townes JM, Quick R, Gonzales OY, et al. Etiology of bloody diarrhea in Bolivian children: Implications for empiric therapy. J Infect Dis. 1997;175:1527-1530.
23. Struelens MJ, Mondal G, Roberts M, et al. Role of bacterial and host factors in the pathogenesis of *Shigella* septicemia. Eur J Clin Microbiol Infect Dis. 1990;9:337-344.
24. D'Hauteville H, Khan S, Maskell DJ, et al. Two msbB genes encoding maximal acylation of lipid A are required for invasive *Shigella flexneri* to mediate inflammatory rupture and destruction of the intestinal epithelium. J Immunol. 2002;168:5240.
25. Raqib R, Ekberg C, Sharkar P, et al. Apoptosis in acute shigellosis is associated with increased production of Fas/Fas ligand, perforin, caspase-1, and caspase-3 but reduced production of Bcl-2 and interleukin-2. Infect Immun. 2002;70:3199.
26. Bennish ML, Salam MA, Wahed MA. Enteric protein loss during shigellosis. Am J Gastroenterol. 1993;88:53-57.
27. Black RE, Brown KH, Becker S. Effects of diarrhea associated with specific enteropathogens on the growth of children in rural Bangladesh. Pediatrics. 1984;73:799-805.
28. Henry FJ, Alam N, Aziz KM, Rahaman MM. Dysentery, not watery diarrhoea, is associated with stunting in Bangladeshi children. Hum Nutr Clin Nutr. 1987;41C:243-249.
29. Koster F, Levin J, Walker L, et al. Hemolytic uremic syndrome after shigellosis: Relation to endotoxemia and circulating immune complexes. N Engl J Med 1978;298:927.
30. Bennish ML, Azad AK, Yousefzadeh D. Intestinal obstruction during shigellosis: Incidence, clinical features, risk factors, and outcome. Gastroenterology. 1991;101:626-634.
31. Barrett-Connor E, Connor JD. Extraintestinal manifestations of shigellosis. Am J Gastroenterol. 1970;53:234.
32. Keusch GT, Grady GF, Mata LJ, et al. The pathogenesis of *Shigella* diarrhea: I. Enterotoxin production by *Shigella dysenteriae* 1. J Clin Invest. 1972;51:1212.
33. Aho K, Ahvonen P, Alkio P, et al. HLA-27 in reactive arthritis following infection. Ann Rheum Dis. 1975;34(Suppl):29.
34. Trabulsi LR, Fernandes MFR, Zuliani ME. Noval bacterias pathogenicas para o intestino do homn. Rev Inst Med Trop Sao Paulo. 1967;9:31.

35. Mermel LA, Osborn TG. *Clostridium difficile* associated reactive arthritis in an HLA-B27 positive female: Report and literature review. J Rheumatol. 1989;16:133-135.

36. Luo W, Wang S, Peng X. Identification of Shiga toxin–producing bacteria by a new immuno-capture toxin gene PCR. FEMS Microbiol Lett. 2002;216:39.

37. Levine MM. *Escherichia coli* that cause diarrhea: Enterotoxigenic, enteropathogenic, enteroinvasive, enterohemorrhagic, and enteroadherent. J Infect Dis. 1987;155:377-389.

38. Tulloch EF Jr, Ryan KJ, Formal SB, et al. Invasive enteropathic *Escherichia coli* dysentery: An outbreak in 28 adults. Ann Intern Med. 1973;79:13.

39. Sereny B. Experimental shigella keratoconjunctivitis: A preliminary report. Acta Microbiol Acad Sci Hung. 1955;2:293.

40. DuPont HL, Formal SB, Hornick R. Pathogenesis of *E. coli* diarrhea. N Engl J Med. 1971;285:1-9.

41. Harris JR, Wachsmuth IK, Davis BF, et al. High molecular weight plasmid correlates with *E. coli* enteroinvasiveness. Infect Immun. 1982;37:1295-1298.

42. Marier R, Wells JG, Swanson RC, et al. An outbreak of enteropathogenic *Escherichia coli* foodborne disease traced to imported French cheese. Lancet. 1973;2:1376.

43. Silva RM, Toledo MRF, Trabulsi LF. Biochemical and cultural characteristics of invasive *Escherichia coli*. J Clin Microbiol. 1980;11:441.

44. Pal T, Pasca S, Emody L, et al. Antigenic relationship among virulent enteroinvasive *E. coli, Shigella flexneri* and *Shigella sonnei* detected by ELISA. Lancet. 1983;2:102.

45. Finkelstein Y, Moran O, Avitzur Y, et al. Clinical dysentery in hospitalized children. Infection. 2002;30:132.

46. Zimbabwe, Bangladesh, South Africa (Zimbasa) Dysentery Study Group. Pediatr Infect Dis J. 2002;21:1136

47. Alam NH, Ashraf H. Treatment of infectious diarrhea in children. Paediatr Drugs. 2003;5:151.

48. O'Brien AD, Newland JW, Miller SF, et al. Shiga-like toxin-converting phages from *Escherichia coli* strains that cause hemorrhagic colitis or infantile diarrhea. Science. 1984;226:694-696.

49. Riley LW, Remis RS, Helgerson SD, et al. Outbreak of hemorrhagic colitis associated with a rare *E. coli* serotype. N Engl J Med. 1983;308:681-685.

50. Orskov I, Wachsmuth IK, Taylor DN, et al. Two new *Escherichia coli* O groups: O172 from "Shiga-like" toxin II–producing strains (EHEC) and O173 from enteroinvasive *E. coli* (EIEC). Acta Patho Microbiol Immunol Scand. 1991;99:30-32.

51. Pai CH, Ahmed N, Lior H, et al. Epidemiology of sporadic diarrhea due to verocytotoxin-producing *Escherichia coli:* A two-year prospective study. J Infect Dis. 1988;157:1054-1057.

52. Pruett WP, Biela T, Lattuada CP, et al. Incidence of *Escherichia coli* O157:H7 in frozen beef patties produced over an 8-hour shift. J Food Prot. 2002;65:1363-1370.

53. Bopp DJ, Sauders BD, Waring AL, et al. Detection, isolation, and molecular subtyping of *Escherichia coli* O157:H7 and *Campylobacter jejuni* associated with a large waterborne outbreak. J Clin Microbiol. 2003;41:174.

54. Ina K, Kusugam K, Ohta M. Bacterial hemorrhagic enterocolitis. J Gastroenterol. 2003;38:111.

55. Campellone KG, Leong JM. Tails of two tirs: Actin pedestal formation by enteropathogenic *E. coli* and enterohemorrhagic *E. coli* O157:H7. Curr Opin Microbiol. 2003;6:82.

56. Berin MC, Darfeuille-Michaud A, Egan LJ, et al. Role of EHEC O157:H7 virulence factors in the activation of intestinal epithelial cell NF-kappaB and MAP kinase pathways and the upregulation expression of interleukin 8. Cell Microbiol. 2002;4:635-648.

57. Lee JE, Kim JS, Choi IH, et al. Cytokine expression in the renal tubular epithelial cells stimulated by Shiga toxin 2 of *Escherichia coli* O157:H7. Ren Fail. 2002;24:567.

58. Fujisawa T, Sata S, Aikawa K, et al. Evaluation of sorbitol-salicin MacConkey medium containing cefixime and tellurite (CT-SSMAC medium) for isolation of *Escherichia coli* O157:H7 from raw vegetables. Int J Food Microbiol. 2002;74:161-163.

59. Paton JC, Paton AW. Methods for detection of STEC in humans: An overview. Methods Mol Med. 2003;73:9-26.

60. Park CH, Kim HJ, Hixon DL. Importance of testing stool specimens for Shiga toxins. J Clin Microbiol. 2002;40:3542-3543.

61. Wong CS, Brandt JR. Risk of hemolytic uremic syndrome from antibiotic treatment of *Escherichia coli* O157:H7 colitis. JAMA. 2002;288:996.

62. Guerrant RL, Lahita RG, Winn WC, et al. Campylobacteriosis in man: Pathogenic mechanisms and review of 91 bloodstream infections. Am J Med. 1978;65:584.

63. Blaser MJ, Reller LB. *Campylobacter* enteritis. N Engl J Med. 1981;305:1444.

64. Scott DA. Vaccines against *Campylobacter jejuni*. J Infect Dis. 1997;2:S183-S188.

65. DeMol P, Bosmans E. *Campylobacter* enteritis in Central Africa. Lancet. 1978;1:604.

66. Perez-Perez GL, Cohn DL, Guerrant RL, et al. Clinical and immunologic significance of choleralike toxin and cytotoxin production by *Campylobacter* species in patients with acute inflammatory diarrhea in the USA. J Infect Dis. 1989;160:460-467.

67. Piddock LJ, Ricci V, Pumbwe L, et al. Fluoroquinolone resistance in *Campylobacter* species from man and animals: detection of mutations in topoisomerase genes. J Antimicrob Chemother. 2003;51:19.

68. Stanley SL Jr. Amoebiasis. Lancet. 2003;361:1025-1034.

69. Jackson TF. *Entamoeba histolytica* and *Entamoeba dispar* are distinct species: Clinical, epidemiological and serological evidence. Int J Parasitol. 1998;1:181-186.

70. Ravdin JI, Croft BY, Guerrant RL. Cytopathologic mechanisms of *Entamoeba histolytica*. J Exp Med. 1980;152:377.

71. Ravdin JI, Guerrant RL. A review of the parasite cellular mechanisms involved in the pathogenesis of amebiasis. Rev Infect Dis. 1982;4:1185-1207.

72. Petri WA Jr, Chapman MD, Snodgrass T, et al. Subunit structure of the galactose and *N*-acetyl-D-galactosamine-inhibitable adherence lectin of *Entamoeba histolytica*. J Biol Chem. 1989;264:3007-3012.

73. Takahashi T, Gamboa-Dominguez A, Gomez-Mendez TJ, et al. Fulminant amebic colitis: Analysis of 55 cases. Dis Colon Rectum. 1997;40:1362-1367.

74. Haque R, Mollah NU, Ali IK, et al. Diagnosis of amebic liver abscess and intestinal infection with the TechLab *Entamoeba histolytica* II antigen detection and antibody tests. J Clin Microbiol. 2000;38:3235.

75. Ayeh-Kumi PF, Ali IM, Lockhart LA, et al. *Entamoeba histolytica:* Genetic diversity of clinical isolates from Bangladesh as demonstrated by polymorphisms in the serine-rich gene. Exp Parasitol. 2001;99:80.

76. Ross AGP, Bartley PB, Sleigh AC, et al. Schistosomiasis. N Engl J Med. 2002;346:1212.

77. Garcia LS, Shimizu RY, Palmer JC. Algorithms for detection and identification of parasites. In: Murray PR, ed. Manual of Clinical Microbiology. 7th ed. Washington, DC: American Society for Microbiology Press, 1999:1336.

78. Morris JG, Black RE. Cholera and other vibrioses in the United States. N Engl J Med. 1985;312:343.

79. Hughes JM, Boyce JM, Aleem AR, et al. *Vibrio parahemolyticus* enterocolitis in Bangladesh: Report of an outbreak. Am J Trop Med Hyg. 1978;27:106-112.

80. Bolen JL, Zamiska SA, Greenough WB III. Clinical features in enteritis due to *Vibrio parahemolyticus*. Am J Med. 1974;57:638.

81. Sparagano OA, Robertson PA, Purdom I, et al. PCR and molecular detection for differentiating *Vibrio* species. Ann N Y Acad Sci. 2002;969:60.

82. Daniels NA, MacKinnon L, Bishop R, et al. *Vibrio parahaemolyticus* infections in the United States, 1973-1998. J Infect Dis. 2000;181:1661.

83. Blake PA, Merson MH, Weaver RE, et al. Disease caused by a marine vibrio: Clinical characteristics and epidemiology. N Engl J Med. 1979;300:1.

84. Radsel-Medvescek A, Zargi R, Acko M, et al. Colonic involvement in salmonellosis. Lancet. 1977;1:601.

85. Rowland HAK. The complications of typhoid fever. J Trop Med Hyg. 1961;64:143.

86. Black RE, Jackson RJ, Tsai T, et al. Epidemic *Yersinia enterocolitica* infection due to contaminated chocolate milk. N Engl J Med. 1978;298:76.

87. Dukuzummuremyi JM, Rosqvist R, Hallberg B, et al. The *Yersinia* protein kinase A is a host-factor inducible RhoA/Rac-binding virulence factor. J Biol Chem. 2000;275:35281.

88. Tafazoli F, Holmstrom A, Forsberg A, et al. Apically exposed and YopE-mediated perturbation of epithelial barriers by wild-type *Yersinia* bacteria. Infect Immun. 2000;68:5335.

89. Rabson AR, Hallett AF, Koornhof HJ. Generalized *Yersinia enterocolitica* infection. J Infect Dis. 1975;131:447.

90. Bradford WD, Noce PS, Gutman LT. Pathologic features of enteric infection with *Yersinia enterocolitica*. Arch Pathol. 1974;98:7.

91. Fredriksson-Ahomaa M, Korkeala H. Low occurrence of pathogenic *Yersinia enterocolitica* in clinical, food, and environmental samples: A methodological problem. Clin Microbiol Rev. 2003;16:220.

92. Klein EJ, Fisher LS, Chow AW. Anorectal gonococcal infection. Ann Intern Med. 1977;86:340.

93. Quinn TC, Stamm WE, Gardell SE. The polymicrobial etiology of intestinal infections in homosexual men. N Engl J Med. 1983;309:576-582.

94. Jensen NS, Casey TA, Stanton TB. Detection and identification of *Treponema hyodysenteriae* by using oligodeoxynucleotide probes complementary to 16S rRNA. J Clin Microbiol. 1990;28:2717-2721.

95. Stermer E, Levy N, Potasman I, et al. Brucellosis as a cause of severe colitis. Am J Gastroenterol. 1991;86:917-919.

96. Krajden M. Brown M, Petrasek A, et al. Clinical features of adenovirus enteritis: A review of 127 cases. Pediatr Infect Dis J. 1990;9:636-641.

97. Janoff EN, Orenstein JM, Manischewitz JF, et al. Adenovirus colitis in the acquired immunodeficiency syndrome. Gastroenterology. 1991;100:976-979.

98. Guerrant RL, Araujo V, Cooper WH, et al. Measurement of fecal lactoferrin as a marker of fecal leukocytes and inflammatory enteritis. J Clin Microbiol. 1992;30:1238-1242.

99. Nataro JP. Treatment of bacterial enteritis. Pediatr Infect Dis. 1998;17:420-421.

100. Haltalin KC, Nelson JD, Ring R III, et al. Double-blind treatment study of shigellosis comparing ampicillin, sulfadiazine, and placebo. J Pediatr. 1967;70:970.

101. Tong MJ, Martin DG, Cunningham JJ, et al. Clinical and bacteriological elevation of antibiotic treatment in shigellosis. JAMA. 1970;214:1841.

102. Barada FA, Guerrant RL. Sulfamethoxazole-trimethoprim versus ampicillin in treatment of acute invasive diarrhea in adults. Antimicrob Agents Chemother. 1980;17:961.

103. Farrar WE Jr, Eidson M: Antibiotic resistance to *Shigella* mediated by R factors. J Infect Dis. 1971;123:477.

104. Ross S, Controni G, Khan W. Resistance of shigellae to ampicillin and other antibiotics: Its clinical and epidemiological implications. JAMA. 1972;221:45.

105. Salam MA, Dhar U, Khan WA, Bennish ML. Randomised comparison of ciprofloxacin suspension and pivmecillinam for childhood shigellosis. Lancet. 1998;352:522-527.

106. Neill MA, Opal SM, Heelan J, et al. Failure of ciprofloxacin to eradicate convalescent fecal excretion after acute salmonellosis: Experience during an outbreak in health care workers. Ann Intern Med. 1991;114:195-199.

107. Smith KE, Besser JM, Hedberg CW, et al. Quinolone-resistant *Campylobacter jejuni* infections in Minnesota, 1992-1998. N Engl J Med. 1999;340:1525-1532.
108. Molbak K, Bagessen DL, Aarestrup FM, et al. An outbreak of multidrug-resistant, quinolone-resistant *Salmonella enterica* serotype typhimurium DT104. N Engl J Med. 1999;341:1420-1425.
109. Kuschner RA, Trofa AF, Thomas RJ, et al. Use of azithromycin for the treatment of *Campylobacter* enteritis in travelers to Thailand, an area where ciprofloxacin resistance is prevalent. Clin Infect Dis. 1995;21:536-541.
110. Hossain S, Biswas R, Kabir I, et al. Single dose vitamin A treatment in acute shigellosis in Bangladesh children: Randomised double blind controlled trial. BMJ. 1998;316:422-426.
111. Simpson JY. Peritonitis in the fetus in uterus. Edinb Med Surg J. 1838;15:390.
112. Wilson R, Kanto WP, McCarthy BJ, et al. Epidemiologic characteristics of necrotizing enterocolitis: A population-based study. Am J Epidemiol. 1981;114:880.
113. Hermann RE. Perforation of the colon from necrotizing colitis in the newborn: Report of a survival and a new etiologic concept. Surgery. 1965;58:436-441.
114. McKay DG, Wahle GH. Epidemic gastroenteritis due to *Escherichia coli* O111B4. Arch Pathol. 1955;60:679.
115. Rogers AF, Dunn PM. Intestinal perforation, exchange transfusion and P.V.C. Lancet. 1969;2:1246.
116. Book LS, Overall JC, Herbst JJ, et al. Clustering of necrotizing enterocolitis: Interruption by infection-control measures. N Engl J Med. 1977;297:984.
117. Howard FM, Flynn DM, Bradley JM, et al. Outbreak of necrotizing enterocolitis caused by *Clostridium butyricum*. Lancet. 1977;2:1099.
118. Frantz ID, L'Heureux P, Engel RR, et al. Necrotizing enterocolitis. J Pediatr. 1975;86:259.
119. Olarte J, Ferguson WW, Henderson ND, Torregrosa L. *Klebsiella* strains isolated from diarrheal infants: Human volunteer studies. Am J Dis Child. 1961;101:763-770.
120. Speer ME, Taber LH, Yow MD, et al. Fulminant neonatal sepsis and necrotizing enterocolitis associated with a "nonenteropathogenic" strain of *Escherichia coli*. J Pediatr. 1976;89:91.
121. Stein H, Beck J, Solomon A, et al. Gastroenteritis with necrotizing enterocolitis in premature babies. Br Med J. 1972;2:616.
122. Barlow B, Santulli TV, Heird WC, et al. An experimental study of acute neonatal enterocolitis: The importance of breast milk. J Pediatr Surg. 1974;9:587.
123. Clark DA, Thompson JE, Weiner LB, et al. Necrotizing enterocolitis: Intraluminal biochemistry in human neonates and a rabbit model. Pediatr Res. 1985;19:919-921.
124. Carbonaro CA, Clark DA, Elseviers D. A bacterial pathogenicity determinant associated with necrotizing enterocolitis. Microb Pathogen. 1988;5:427-436.
125. MacKendrick W, Caplan M, Hsueh W. Endogenous nitric oxide protects against platelet-activating factor-induced bowel injury in the rat. Pediatr Res. 1993;34:222-228.
126. Stevenson JK, Oliver TK, Graham CB, et al. Aggressive treatment of neonatal necrotizing enterocolitis: Thirty-eight patients with 25 survivors. J Pediatr Surg. 1971;6:28.
127. Murrell TGC, Roth L, Egerton J, et al. Pig-bel: Enteritis necroticans. Lancet. 1966;1:217.
128. Patterson M, Rosenbaum HD. Enteritis necroticans. Gastroenterology. 1952;21:110.
129. Lawrence G, Walker PD. Pathogenesis of enteritis necroticans in Papua New Guinea. Lancet. 1976;1:125-126.
130. Lawrence G, Coake R. Experimental pigbel: The production and pathology of necrotizing enteritis due to *Clostridium welchii* type C in the guinea pig. Br J Exp Pathol. 1980;61:261-271.
131. Lawrence GW, Lehmann D, Anian G, et al. Impact of active immunization against enteritis necroticans in Papua New Guinea. Lancet. 1990;336:1165-1167.
132. Black RE, Merson MH, Rahaman SMM, et al. Prospective study of bacterial, viral, and parasitic agents associated with diarrhea in rural Bangladesh. J Infect Dis. 1980;142:660.
133. McAuliffe JF, Shields DS, de Souza MA, et al. Prolonged and recurring diarrhea in the northeast of Brazil: Examination of cases from a community-based study. J Pediatr Gastroenterol Nutr. 1986;5:902-906.
134. Schorling JB, Wanke CA, Schorling SK, et al. A prospective study of persistent diarrhea among children in an urban Brazilian slum. Am J Epidemiol. 1990;132:144-156.
135. Guerrant RL, Schorling JB, McAuliffe JF, et al. Diarrhea as a cause and effect of malnutrition: Diarrhea prevents catch-up growth and malnutrition increases diarrhea frequency and duration. Am J Trop Med Hyg. 1992;47:28-35.
136. Nelson JD, Haltalin KC. Accuracy of diagnosis of bacterial diarrheal disease by clinical features. J Pediatr. 1971;78:519.
137. Cooke EM. Properties of strains of *Escherichia coli* isolated from the feces of patients with ulcerative colitis, patients with acute diarrhea and normal persons. J Pathol Bacteriol. 1968;95:101.
138. Bhan MK, Raj P, Levine MM, et al. Enteroaggregative *Escherichia coli* associated with persistent diarrhea in a cohort of rural children in India. J Infect Dis. 1989;159:1061-1064.
139. Wanke CA, Schorling JB, Barrett LJ, et al. Adherence traits of *Escherichia coli*, alone and in association with other stool pathogens: Potential role in pathogenesis of persistent diarrhea in an urban Brazilian slum. Pediatr J Infect Dis. 1991;10:746-751.
140. Carvioto A, Tello A, Navarro A, et al. Association of *Escherichia coli* Hep-2 adherence patterns with type and duration of diarrhoea. Lancet. 1991;337:262-264.
141. Nataro JP, Kaper JB. Diarrheagenic *Escherichia coli*. Clin Microbiol Rev. 1998;11:142-201.
142. Lima AAM, Moore SR, Barboza Jr MS, et al. Persistent diarrhea signals a critical period of increased diarrhea burdens and nutritional shortfalls: A prospective cohort study among children in Northeastern Brazil. J Infect Dis. 2000;181:1643.
143. Steiner TS, Lima AA, Nataro JP, Guerrant RL. Enteroaggregative *Escherichia coli* produce intestinal inflammation and growth impairment and cause interleukin-8 release from intestinal epithelial cells. J Infect Dis. 1998;177:88-96.
144. Wanke CA, Mayer H, Weber R, et al. Enteroaggregative *Escherichia coli* as a potential cause of diarrheal disease in adults infected with human immunodeficiency virus. J Infect Dis. 1998;178:185-190.
145. Sachar DB, Klein RS, Swerdlow F. Erosive syphilitic gastritis: Dark-field and immunofluorescent diagnosis from biopsy specimen. Ann Intern Med. 1974;80:512.
146. Fischl MA, Daikos GL, Uttamchandani RB, et al. Clinical presentation and outcome of patients with HIV infection and tuberculosis caused by multiple-drug-resistant bacilli. Ann Intern Med. 1992;117:184-190.
147. Cullen JH. Intestinal tuberculosis: A clinicopathologic study. Q Bull Sea View Hosp. 1940;5:143.
148. Hamandi WJ, Thamer MA. Tuberculosis of the bowel in Iraq: A study of 86 cases. Dis Colon Rectum. 1965;8:158.
149. Anand SS. Hypertrophic ileo-cecal tuberculosis in India with a record of fifty hemicolectomies. Ann R Coll Surg Engl. 1956;19:205.
150. Tandon HD, Prakach A. Pathology of intestinal tuberculosis and its distinction from Crohn's disease. Gut. 1972;13:260.
151. Eras P, Goldstein MJ, Sherlock P. *Candida* infection of the gastrointestinal tract. Medicine (Baltimore). 1972;51:367.
152. Smith PD, Lane C, Gill VJ, et al. Intestinal infections in patients with the acquired immunodeficiency syndrome (AIDS): Etiology and response to therapy. Ann Intern Med. 1988;108:328-333.
153. Gupta TP, Ehrinpreis MN. *Candida* associated diarrhea in hospitalized patients. Gastroenterology. 1990;98:780-785.
154. Zaidi M, Ponce de Leon S, Ortiz RM, et al. Hospital-acquired diarrhea in adults: A prospective case-controlled study in Mexico. Infect Control Hosp Epidemiol. 1991;12:349-355.
155. Restrepo A, Robledo M, Gutierrey F, et al. Paracoccidioidomycosis (South American blastomycosis). Am J Trop Med Hyg. 1970;19:68.
156. Satir AA, Alla MD, Mahgoub S, et al. Systemic phycomycosis. Br Med J. 1971;1:440.
157. Smith JMB. Mycoses of the alimentary tract. Gut. 1969;10:1035.
158. Bank S, Trey C, Gans I, et al. Histoplasmosis of the small bowel with "giant" intestinal villi and secondary protein-losing enteropathy. Am J Med. 1965;39:492.
159. Shull HJ. Human histoplasmosis: Disease with protean manifestations, often with digestive system involvement. Gastroenterology. 1953;25:582.
160. Pape JW, Verdier R, Johnson WD. Treatment and prophylaxis of *Isospora belli* infection in patients with the acquired immunodeficiency syndrome. N Engl J Med. 1989;320:1044-1047.
161. Trier JS, Moxey PC, Schimmel EM, et al. Chronic intestinal coccidiosis in man: Intestinal morphology and response to treatment. Gastroenterology. 1974;66:923.
162. Alcantara CE, Yang C-H, Steiner TS, et al. Interleukin-8, tumor necrosis factor-α, and lactoferrin in immunocompetent hosts with experimental and Brazilian children with acquired cryptosporidiosis. Am J Trop Med Hyg. 2003;68:325-328.
163. Herwaldt BL. Cyclospora cayetanensis: A review, focusing on the outbreaks of cyclosporiasis in the 1990s. Clin Infect Dis. 2000;31:1040-1057.
164. Powell SJ, Wilmot AJ. Ulcerative post-dysenteric colitis. Gut. 1966;7:438.
165. Blenkinsopp WK, Gibson JA, Haffenden GP. Giardiasis and severe jejunal abnormality. Lancet. 1978;1:994.
166. Ørskov F. Virulence factors of the bacterial cell surface. J Infect Dis. 1978;137:630.

Enteric Fever and Other Causes of Abdominal Symptoms with Fever

NATHAN M. THIELMAN
RICHARD L. GUERRANT

Typhoid fever and several other enteric infections are characterized by abdominal pain and fever. The portal of entry of the responsible infectious agents is usually the gastrointestinal tract. After a systemic phase, these infections may subsequently involve intestinal tissue and then manifest as one of three clinical syndromes. (1) Enteric fever, characterized by sustained fever, headache, abdominal pain, splenomegaly, bacteremia, and occasionally skin rash, is the most serious of these syndromes and may result from infection by several bacteria. A number of systemic bacterial, rickettsial, viral, fungal, and parasitic infections, such as malaria, may mimic enteric fever, and a delay in diagnosis can be life threatening. They are discussed later in the chapter. (2) Mesenteric adenitis, a syndrome that may mimic acute appendicitis, can be caused by several bacteria. (3) Eosinophilia, associated with abdominal cramps or diarrhea often accompanied by fever, may be caused by a number of parasites, usually helminths, several diseases of unknown cause, and neoplasms.

We focus on the differential diagnosis of these syndromes. Important clinical and epidemiologic features, appropriate diagnostic approaches, and antimicrobial therapeutic considerations are discussed.

ENTERIC FEVER

The classic syndrome of enteric fever is an acute illness, the first typical manifestations of which are fever, headache, abdominal pain, relative bradycardia, splenomegaly, and leukopenia. The prototype of the syndrome is typhoid fever caused by *Salmonella enterica* serotype typhi (see Chapter 220). Fever is present in 75% to 100% of cases[1] and is often initially of the remittent type, rising in a stepwise fashion during the first week of illness, after which it becomes sustained.[2,3] Typhoid fever is a major problem for people living in developing areas with poor sanitation and fecal contamination of food and water. It is estimated that there are at least 16 million new cases of typhoid fever each year and 600,000 deaths.[4] In the United States, 2445 cases were reported to the Centers for Disease Control and Prevention between 1985 and 1994, 72% of which were imported, most frequently from Mexico or India.[5] In addition, 60 relatively small outbreaks have been reported in the United States from 1960 to 1999 and their average frequency per year appears to be decreasing.[6]

Pathogenesis

S. enterica serotype typhi and other bacteria that cause the enteric fever syndrome are ingested and survive exposure to gastric acid before gaining access to the small bowel, where they penetrate the intestinal epithelium possibly through microfold cells over Peyer's patches. During an incubation period of 7 to 14 days, they multiply in intestinal lymphoid tissue and then disseminate by the lymphatic or hematogenous route. *Salmonella* spp. grow intracellularly, primarily in reticuloendothelial cells in lymph nodes, spleen, liver, and bone

marrow. Animal models for this syndrome in which mice are infected orally with *Salmonella enteritidis* or *Yersinia enterocolitica* have been developed.[7]

Clinical Features

The organism classically responsible for the enteric fever syndrome is *S. enterica* serotype typhi (formerly *S. typhi*). Other salmonellae, especially *Salmonella paratyphi* A, *Salmonella schottmuelleri* (formerly *S. paratyphi* B), *Salmonella hirschfeldii* (formerly *S. paratyphi* C), and *Salmonella choleraesuis*, may cause a similar clinical syndrome (Table 94-1). Other diseases that may mimic enteric fever and that must be included in the differential diagnosis of enteric fever are also summarized in Table 94-1; important clinical and epidemiologic clues to these specific diagnoses are indicated.

Symptoms

Classic "typhoidal" fever begins with a remittent fever pattern that becomes sustained over the first few days of illness. The frequencies of reported symptoms from several series of patients infected by *S. typhi* and *S. paratyphi* A and *S. schottmuelleri* are summarized in Table 94-2. Most patients report fever and headache. Although reports from the preantibiotic era suggest that constipation occurred more frequently than diarrhea (79% versus 43%),[3] more recent reports suggest that these symptoms occur with approximately equal frequency or that diarrhea may be more common, particularly in young children and in adults with human immunodeficiency virus (HIV) infection.[8,9,11-13] Extraintestinal symptoms reported by patients include cough and conjunctivitis. Although enteric fever caused by salmonellae other than *S. typhi* is usually less severe and of shorter duration than typhoid fever, the syndromes are not sufficiently different to permit clinical separation of individual cases.

Physical Findings

In evaluating patients with possible enteric fever syndrome, the physical examination should focus on characteristics of the fever curve and accompanying pulse, skin, eyes, oral cavity and oropharynx, chest, abdomen, and lymph nodes. The frequencies of commonly reported physical findings are summarized in Table 94-2. Fever is present in most series in more than 90% of the cases. However, bacteriologic confirmation of typhoid fever has been obtained in patients who were afebrile when the culture was obtained. Classically, the fever is remittent during the first week, rising in a stepwise fashion in both naturally acquired infection and volunteer studies[2]; after the first week, the fever usually becomes sustained. Deviations from this classic pattern frequently occur, particularly in endemic areas. In studies from India, fever was remittent in 30% and 60% of the cases, sustained in 22% to 25%, and intermittent in 15% to 46%.[1] Relative bradycardia suggests the diagnosis of enteric fever. The presence of rose spots, blanching erythematous maculopapular lesions 2 to 4 mm in diameter, although not pathognomonic, is extremely helpful in confirming the impression of enteric fever; however, they are observed in less than half of the patients and are even less common in dark-skinned people.[3] Rose spots may be observed more frequently in infection caused by *S. typhi* than in other forms of enteric fever.[14,15] Conjunctivitis has been reported in up to 44% of the patients with enteric fever, but it is usually less common.[3] Pharyngitis is infrequent and usually not a prominent feature. Rales may be present on examination of the chest. Abdominal tenderness may be diffuse or localized, most often in the right lower quadrant. Splenomegaly is noted more frequently than hepatomegaly. Two physical findings, lymphadenopathy and herpes simplex labialis, are useful in suggesting alternative diagnoses because they rarely occur in patients with enteric fever.

Laboratory Findings

The definitive diagnosis of enteric fever is made by isolating *S. typhi* or another *Salmonella* sp. from blood, bone marrow, stool, or urine. Cultures of blood as well as stool and urine should be obtained before the initiation of antimicrobial therapy. If multiple blood cultures are

The authors thank Dr. Richard D. Pearson, who coauthored this chapter in previous editions, for his important input.

TABLE 94-1 Clinical, Epidemiologic, and Laboratory Clues to the Causes of Enteric Fever and Conditions That May Mimic Enteric Fever

Etiologic Agent or Disease	Clinical Clues in Addition to Fever	Epidemiologic Clues	Laboratory Clues
Causes of Enteric Fever			
Salmonella enterica serotype Typhi Salmonella paratyphi A Salmonella schottmuelleri Salmonella choleraesuis	Relative bradycardia, splenomegaly, rose spots, conjunctivitis	Young adults, travel, especially to India, Mexico, and other tropical areas,* exposure to known carrier	Cultures (B, BM, U, F), serology, leukopenia
Yersinia enterocolitica Yersinia pseudotuberculosis	Chronic liver or other underlying disease, arthritis, erythema nodosum	Older adults, ± pet exposure	Cultures (B, F, J), serology
Campylobacter fetus	Stigmata or chronic liver disease, phlebitis	Older adults, ± farm or small-animal contact	Cultures (B, F), serology
Brucellosis (Brucella spp.)	Paucity of physical findings	Occupation (abattoir employee, butcher), animal contact (goats, sheep, cattle), diet (unpasteurized cheese)	Cultures (B, BM), serology, leukopenia
Typhoidal tularemia (Francisella tularensis)	Severe prostration, splenomegaly	Animal contact (especially rabbits), vector exposure (ticks)	Serology
Conditions That May Mimic Enteric Fever			
Bacterial infections			
Septicemic plague (Yersinia pestis)	Severe prostration	Rodent contact, vector exposure (fleas), travel	Cultures (B), serology
Intestinal anthrax (Bacillus anthracis)	Severe prostration	Travel,* diet (undercooked meat)	Cultures (B, F)
Septicemia melioidosis (Burkholderia pseudomallei)	Severe prostration, pustular skin lesions	Travel,* especially Southeast Asia	Cultures (B), serology, chest radiograph
Acute bartonellosis (Bartonella bacilliformis)	Severe prostration, hemolysis, renal failure	Travel to Andean valleys in Peru, Ecuador, and Colombia,* vector exposure (sand fly)	Cultures (B), blood smear, acute hemolysis
Leptospirosis (Leptospira spp.)	Relative bradycardia, conjunctival suffusion	Occupation (farmers, abattoir and sewer workers, veterinarians), animal contact (especially cattle, dogs), swimming†	Cultures (B, CSF, U), serology, hepatorenal dysfunction
Relapsing fever (Borrelia spp.)	Fever pattern, conjunctival suffusion, splenomegaly, skin rash	Travel, especially to Southeast Asia, Far East, Ethiopia, and the western United States,* vector exposure (louse, tick)	Blood smear
Legionellosis (Legionella spp.)	Pneumonia, CNS symptoms	Normal or compromised host	Chest radiograph, purulent sputum, DFA of sputum, urine antigen
Intestinal tuberculosis (Mycobacterium tuberculosis, Mycobacterium avium-intracellulare)	Stigmata of tuberculosis or AIDS	Exposure to known case ± travel* ± diet (unpasteurized milk and milk products), malnourished children, HIV infection	Cultures (S, G, BM, L), radiograph (UGI, SBFT)
Abdominal actinomycosis (Actinomyces spp.)	Abdominal mass, fistula	Men	Culture (FD, A), radiograph (UGI, SBFT), CT with oral contrast medium
Intra-abdominal abscess	Spiking daily fever, reduced diaphragmatic excursion, intraabdominal or diaphragmatic pain	Previous surgery, bowel or biliary tract disease	Leukocytosis, CT, gallium scan, sonography, fluoroscopy
Rat bite fever			
Streptobacillus moniliformis	Headache, nausea, vomiting, rash, myalgia, polyarthritis	Rat bite or food-borne outbreak	Culture (B, J), serology
Spirillum minus	Headache, nausea, adenopathy, roseolar-urticarial rash	Rat bite	Serology
Mycoplasma pneumoniae	Cough, headache, bullous myringitis	Children and adolescents	Serology
Chlamydophila psittaci	Headache, nausea, vomiting, arthralgias, cough	Exposure to parrots, parakeets, related birds	Serology
Bacterial pneumonia (Streptococcus pneumoniae, Haemophilus influenzae spp.)	Cough, sputum, rales, headache, delirium, pulmonary infiltrates	Older adults, smoking, underlying diseases	Sputum Gram stain, culture (S, B), chest radiograph
Viral infections			
Hepatitis	Jaundice, arthritis (with hepatitis B)	Exposure to known case, drug abuse, travel*	Liver dysfunction, antibody and/or antigen detection
Dengue	Relative bradycardia, myalgia, conjunctival suffusion, rash	Travel,* vector exposure (mosquito)	Culture (B), serology, leukopenia, thrombocytopenia
Infectious mononucleosis	Pharyngitis, lymphadenopathy, splenomegaly, rash	Young adults	Serology, lymphocyte morphology

*Travel to endemic areas, either domestic or foreign.
†Swimming in contaminated surface water.

A, Abscess; AIDS, acquired immunodeficiency syndrome; ANA, antinuclear antibody; B, blood; BM, bone marrow; C′, complement; CNS, central nervous system; CSF, cerebrospinal fluid; CT, computed tomography; DFA, direct fluorescent antibody test; F, feces; FD, fistula drainage; G, gastric aspirate; HIV, human immunodeficiency virus; J, joint fluid; L, liver; LN, lymph node; MM, mucous membrane; N, nasal; O&P, ova and parasite; S, sputum; T, throat; U, urine; UGI, SBFT, upper gastrointestinal tract with small bowel follow-through.

TABLE 94-1   Clinical, Epidemiologic, and Laboratory Clues to the Causes of Enteric Fever and Conditions That May Mimic Enteric Fever—cont'd

Etiologic Agent or Disease	Clinical Clues in Addition to Fever	Epidemiologic Clues	Laboratory Clues
Rickettsial infections			
Rocky Mountain spotted fever	Rash, headache, myalgias	Travel,* vector exposure (tick)	Serology, skin biopsy
Epidemic typhus	Conjunctival suffusion, rash, severe prostration	Travel,* vector exposure (louse)	Serology
Brill-Zinsser disease	Rash	Older adults, remote travel* history	Serology
Endemic typhus	Conjunctival suffusion, rash, splenomegaly	Rat contact, vector exposure (flea)	Serology
Scrub typhus	Conjunctival suffusion, rash, lymphadenopathy	Travel,* vector exposure (mites)	Serology
Q fever	Pneumonia, hepatitis	Animal contact (especially livestock), ± travel, ± diet (especially unpasteurized milk)	Serology, chest radiograph, liver dysfunction
Ehrlichiosis	Headache, myalgia, rash (occasional)	Travel,* vector exposure (tick)	Serology, leukopenia, thrombocytopenia
Mycotic infections			
Disseminated histoplasmosis	Mucocutaneous lesions, adrenal insufficiency	Travel,* animal contact (chicken, birds, bats), hobby (cave exploration)	Culture (B, BM, L, MM), biopsy (BM, L, MM), chest radiograph, urine antigen
Penicillium marneffei	Umbilicated skin lesions, lymphadenopathy, cough, hepatomegaly	Travel,* concurrent AIDS	Culture (B, BM, LN), chest radiograph
Parasitic Infections			
Malaria	Fever pattern, splenomegaly	Travel,* vector exposure (mosquito)	Blood smear
Amebiasis	Colitis, liver abscess	Travel*	Stool examination, serology, liver scan, sonography, CT, colon biopsy
Babesiosis	Paucity of physical findings	Travel,* splenectomy, vector exposure (tick)	Blood smear, serology
Toxoplasmosis	Lymphadenopathy	Animal contact (cat); diet (undercooked pork)	Serology, biopsy (lymph node)
Trichinosis	Periorbital edema, muscle tenderness	Diet (undercooked pork or bear meat)	Serology, eosinophilia, biopsy (muscle)
Katayama fever (acute schistosomiasis)	Urticaria, lymphadenopathy	Travel,* swimming or other freshwater exposure	Eosinophilia, serology, stool O&P
Visceral larva migrans	Hepatosplenomegaly, rash, bronchospasm, ocular lesions	Young children with history of pica, animal contact (dog, cat)	Serology, biopsy (L), eosinophilia
Noninfectious causes			
Malignancy	Adenopathy, anergy, weight loss	Family history or prior malignancy	Sonography, CT, gallium scan, biopsy
Collagen vascular or granulomatous disease (e.g., sarcoidosis, granulomatous hepatitis, ulcerative colitis, Crohn's disease, Still's disease, vasculitis, etc.)	Skin lesions, arthritis, serositis, multiple organ involvement	Family history	Biopsy of involved tissue, serology (ANA, C'), exclusion of other causes

obtained, 73% to 97% of the cases are confirmed.[3] Patients with severe disease are the most likely to have positive cultures. Culture of the blood clot after the serum is removed and large volume (15 mL in adults) blood cultures improve culture sensitivity.[11] Bone marrow cultures may be positive when blood cultures are negative, even after antibiotics have been administered.[12,13] Stool cultures are positive in less than half the patients, and urine cultures are even less frequently positive.[3,12] If patients have received antimicrobial therapy, blood cultures are often negative. Cultures of biopsy specimens of rose spots have been reported to be positive in nearly two thirds of patients, including some who previously received antimicrobial therapy.[12]

The Widal test has been used to detect anti-*S. typhi* antibodies for more than 100 years, but its role in the diagnosis of typhoid fever is limited.[14] The minimal titers defined as positive for the O (surface polysaccharide) antigens and H (flagellar) antigens must be determined for individual geographic areas and are higher in developing regions than in the United States.[11] Cross-reactions occur with both non–*S. typhi* group D salmonellae and salmonellae from other groups. When paired acute and convalescent samples are studied, a fourfold or greater increase is considered positive.

The Widal test has been reported to be positive in 46% to 94% of patients with typhoid fever.[14,16] The test is most reliable in areas in which data on the titers in control groups without enteric fever are available; the sensitivity of the test can be improved when diseases such as rheumatoid arthritis, which are associated with false-positive reactions, are ruled out by other assays. Although the criteria vary, a single elevated titer for O equal to or greater than 1:320 or H equal to or greater than 1:640 is considered positive. A fourfold or greater titer rise demonstrated in paired serum specimens obtained 2 to 3 weeks apart is also diagnostic, but it is of no value in the acute setting. The potential for either false-positive or false-negative responses limits the value of the Widal test in the diagnosis of typhoid fever.[14,16] Finally, the Widal test is not helpful in the diagnosis of enteric fever caused by organisms other than *S. typhi*.

A number of other assays have been used to detect antibodies against other *S. typhi* antigens or circulating antigens themselves. They include rapid tests for antibodies to lipopolysaccharide or outer-membrane proteins.[17,18] Finally, polymerase chain reaction assays are now available in research settings but seem impractical in resource-poor regions most affected by the disease.[15,19]

TABLE 94-2 Frequency of Symptoms and Physical Findings in Patients with Enteric Fever

	Typhoid Fever* (%)	Paratyphoid A and B† (%)
Symptoms		
Fever	39-100	92-100
Headache	43-90	60-100
Nausea	23-36	33-58
Vomiting	24-35	22-45
Abdominal cramps	8-52	29-92
Diarrhea	30-57	17-68
Constipation	10-79	2-29
Cough	11-86	10-68
Physical findings		
Fever	98-100	100
Abdominal tenderness	33-84	6-29
Splenomegaly	23-65	0-74
Hepatomegaly	15-52	16-32
Relative bradycardia	17-50	11-100
Rose spots	2-46	0-3
Rales or rhonchi	4-84	2-87
Epistaxis	1-21	2-13
Meningismus	1-12	0-3

*Data from references 2, 3, 5, 10-13.
†Data from references 10, 14, 15.

Additional laboratory tests that may be of value include the white blood cell count and differential, liver function tests, urinalysis, and chest radiograph. Leukopenia is reported in 16% to 46% of the cases. In some series, two thirds of patients had no eosinophils on peripheral smear,[1] a finding that may be helpful in areas in which helminthic diseases are prevalent and eosinophilia is common. Liver function tests may reveal a mildly elevated bilirubin level and a slight to threefold elevation in alkaline phosphatase and transaminase levels in one third to two thirds of the patients; on occasion, hepatic manifestations may be prominent.[20] Urinalysis frequently reveals proteinuria, pyuria, and casts[3]; immune complex glomerulonephritis with red blood cell casts occasionally occurs.[21] Coagulation abnormalities compatible with mild disseminated intravascular coagulation are common, but the syndrome is rarely clinically apparent.[22] Chest radiographic films reveal infiltrates in 2% to 11% of the cases.[3] In patients with diarrhea, a methylene blue stain of a fresh stool specimen for fecal leukocytes may reveal mononuclear cells.[23]

Epidemiology

Certain epidemiologic data may be of value in the diagnosis of enteric fever. Typhoid fever is more common in children and young adults both in the United States[24] and abroad. In the United States, cases occur throughout the year. Because humans are the only reservoir for *S. typhi*, a history of being abroad in settings where sanitation is poor or with a known typhoid case or carrier is useful, but a specific contact is identified in a minority of cases.[5] The proportion of the cases in the United States that were acquired abroad has increased dramatically; during 1985 to 1994, 72% of the cases were acquired abroad.[5] Six countries accounted for 80% of the cases: Mexico (28%), India (25%), the Philippines (10%), Pakistan (8%), El Salvador (5%), and Haiti (4%). The percentage of cases associated with visiting Mexico decreased from 46% in 1985 to 23% in 1994, whereas the percentage of cases associated with visiting the Indian subcontinent increased from 25% in 1985 to 37% in 1994. The incidence among U.S. citizens traveling to the Indian subcontinent was at least 18 times higher than that in people traveling to any other geographic region.[5] Patients who acquire infection abroad are usually older than those who acquire disease in the United States.

The importance of the microbiology laboratory as a source of domestic *S. typhi* infection has also been recognized.[25,26] In most laboratory-acquired cases, *S. typhi* had been used for proficiency testing or research. Most patients with enteric fever caused by *S. paratyphi* A or *S. schottmuelleri* acquire their infection abroad; *S. schottmuel-*

leri is only occasionally and *S. paratyphi* A rarely isolated in the United States.

Differential Diagnosis

Enteric Fever–like Syndromes Caused by Other Bacteria

Y. enterocolitica, Yersinia pseudotuberculosis, and *Campylobacter fetus* can each produce an illness characterized by fever, headache, and abdominal pain that may be clinically indistinguishable from enteric fever caused by *S. typhi* or other salmonellae (see Table 94-1). However, certain features of these infections may differentiate them from true enteric fever. Acute diarrhea is often a prominent feature of enteric fever–like illnesses caused by *Y. enterocolitica*[27,28] and occasionally *Y. pseudotuberculosis.*[29,30] Diarrhea is less frequent in enteric fever–like illness caused by *C. fetus*; the acute gastrointestinal symptoms of nausea, vomiting, abdominal cramps, and diarrhea were present in only 27% of bacteremic illnesses caused by *C. fetus.*[31] A clue to the diagnosis of *Campylobacter* infection is associated phlebitis.[31,32]

The enteric fever–like syndromes caused by *Y. enterocolitica, Y. pseudotuberculosis,* and *C. fetus* tend to occur in patients with significant underlying disease. Of 31 patients with *Y. enterocolitica* bacteremia for whom information was available, 12 had cirrhosis of the liver, 4 others had thalassemia, and 1 had kwashiorkor.[27] Only five were known to be free of underlying disease. In another series, five of seven patients with the acute septicemic or typhoidal form of *Y. enterocolitica* infection had evidence of liver disease; in addition, all six patients with the subacute, localized form of the disease characterized by hepatic and splenic abscesses had cirrhosis of the liver.[27] Of 20 patients with the enteric fever–like syndrome caused by *Y. pseudotuberculosis,* 11 had evidence of significant underlying disease; the liver was involved in 10 of these patients.[29] In a series of patients with bacteremia *C. fetus* illness, 73% had a significant underlying disease, frequently involving the liver.[31]

Epidemiologic clues in differentiating true enteric fever from these enteric fever–like syndromes include the patient's age, residence, and recent travel history. Patients with *Salmonella*-induced enteric fever are most often younger than 30 years, whereas the vast majority of patients with non-*Salmonella* enteric fever–like syndromes are older than 40.[27-32] As with typhoid fever, men are more frequently affected than women. Patients with *Salmonella*-induced enteric fever frequently have a history of recent foreign travel, most often to developing countries. Diseases caused by *Y. enterocolitica* and *Y. pseudotuberculosis* appear to be common in Europe, particularly in Scandinavia,[33] and are not frequently reported from developing countries. Infections caused by both *Y. enterocolitica* and *Y. pseudotuberculosis* may be acquired in the United States as well.[34] Although bacteremic *C. fetus* infection is relatively rarely documented, the majority of cases have been reported from the United States, and foreign travel has not appeared to be a significant predisposing factor.[31]

A pulse-temperature deficit similar to that observed in typhoid fever has been reported in enteric fever–like illness caused by *Y. enterocolitica*[28,34,35] and *Y. pseudotuberculosis*[29] but not in that caused by *C. fetus.*[31] An additional clue may be provided by the fever pattern. In contrast to *Salmonella*-induced enteric fevers in which sustained fever is common, intermittent fever throughout the illness caused by *Y. enterocolitica* has been reported.[36] Because of the increased frequency of chronic liver disease in patients with these enteric fever–like syndromes, physical examination is more likely to reveal stigmata of chronic liver disease such as spider angiomas, gynecomastia, ascites, and testicular atrophy. In addition, hepatomegaly is frequent and may be more pronounced than in patients with typhoid fever.[28] Both erythema nodosum and polyarthritis may occur in patients with illnesses caused by *Y. enterocolitica* and *Y. pseudotuberculosis*; in one series, 55% of the patients with yersiniosis had arthritis, and 88% of those had multiple joint involvement.[33] Nonsuppurative arthritis is more common in infections caused by *Y. enterocolitica* (43%) than in those caused by *Y. pseudotuberculosis* (10%).[37] Patients with bacteremic infection caused by *Y. enterocolitica* and *C. fetus* may also have acute septic arthritis,[28,31,34,35] a condition that is infrequently found in patients with classic enteric fever. Erythema nodosum has been reported in 15% to 24% of patients with *Yersinia* and may be slightly more common with *Y. pseudotuberculosis* infection than with *Y. enterocolitica* infection.[33,37] Thrombophlebitis has been reported in patients with *C. fetus* bacteremia and may be an additional diagnostic clue.[31,32]

As in the *Salmonella*-induced enteric fevers, blood cultures are the key to the diagnosis. Each of the three organisms is more frequently isolated from blood than from other specimens.[27-31] The isolation rate from stool cultures is improved if cold-enrichment techniques are used for *Yersinia*[38] and if special selective media are used for *Campylobacter*. However, because of its sensitivity to cephalosporins, *C. fetus* cannot be cultured from stool on commonly used *Campylobacter jejuni*–selective agars if they contain cephalosporins. In addition, serologic tests are available for documenting infection with *Y. enterocolitica* and *Y. pseudotuberculosis* and appear to be more sensitive and more specific than those for *Salmonella* infection. Polymerase chain reaction–based assays for *Y. enterocolitica*, *Y. pseudotuberculosis*, and *C. fetus* appear promising, but they are available only in research settings.

Leukopenia is infrequent in patients with enteric fever–like syndromes; its presence suggests that salmonellae are responsible. Findings on abdominal computed tomography (CT) or ultrasonography suggestive of hepatic or splenic abscesses favor the diagnosis of yersiniosis.[27] Glomerulitis complicating both typhoid fever and *Y. enterocolitica* has been reported; therefore, the presence of protein, red blood cells, and red blood cell casts in the urine is compatible with either of these syndromes.[21,39]

Patients with typhoidal tularemia may be clinically indistinguishable from those with enteric fever. The epidemiologic history may be of value. A history of rabbit or tick exposure within 7 days before the onset of illness supports the diagnosis of tularemia.[40] Although potentially dangerous, *Francisella tularensis* may be isolated from blood if the appropriate medium is used. More often, serologic tests are used to confirm the diagnosis.

Acute brucellosis may manifest with fever, myalgias, and splenomegaly.[41] As in typhoid fever, white blood cell counts are frequently normal or low. Skin lesions are uncommon in brucellosis. Blood and bone marrow cultures and serologic testing permit separation of these entities.

Systemic Infections That May Mimic Enteric Fever

A number of other serious infections may be initially confused with enteric fever. These are particularly important because several are potentially fatal if not promptly recognized and treated. Among the most common serious febrile illnesses associated with travel to tropical areas is malaria, which should be considered even in individuals who claim to have been compliant in avoiding mosquitoes and taking malarial prophylaxis. It is characterized by fever, headache, myalgias, and, in some patients, gastrointestinal complaints. Intestinal and extraintestinal amebiases may arise as acute or subacute febrile illnesses. Dengue fever can begin up to 9 days after exposure in an endemic area. Other, less common infectious causes of fever and enteric symptoms are discussed later. Some are endemic in North America, whereas others are not. In addition, persons with pneumococcal, *Legionella*, or *Mycoplasma* pneumonia may have enteric symptoms along with respiratory complaints.

Septicemic plague can mimic enteric fever. The diagnosis of plague is suggested by a sudden onset and rapid progression of illness. The history may again provide a clue to the diagnosis; plague is present in wild rodents in the southwestern United States and in endemic areas abroad. A history of travel to those areas, particularly if there is exposure to rodents during the previous 2 weeks, supports the diagnosis of plague.[42] Blood cultures, methylene blue stains of peripheral blood,[43] and serologic testing aid in the diagnosis.

Intestinal anthrax may be characterized by fever and severe abdominal pain. It is typically acute in onset and rapid in progression. Patients usually die during the first few days of their illness. A history of in-

gesting raw or undercooked meat in an area where anthrax is endemic suggests the diagnosis.[44]

Acute septicemic melioidosis may be confused clinically with enteric fever; this disease is endemic in Southeast Asia. Physical findings that support the diagnosis of melioidosis include pustular skin lesions.[45] The chest radiograph may reveal nodular pulmonary densities. Blood cultures and serologic studies again permit differentiation from typhoid fever.

Acute bartonellosis (Oroya fever) may manifest with fever, headache, and abdominal pain. Because this disease occurs only in certain valleys in the Andes mountains of Peru, Ecuador, and Colombia, a lack of travel in the preceding month is helpful in excluding this possibility.[46] Evidence of acute hemolysis suggests the diagnosis. The causative organisms may be seen on a stained peripheral blood smear. Because Oroya fever predisposes to *Salmonella*-induced bacteremia, both infections may be encountered simultaneously.[47] A fever surveillance study in Egypt identified brucellosis as an important cause of prolonged fever that was frequently mistaken clinically as typhoid fever; 87% of patients with brucellosis were diagnosed with and treated for typhoid.[48]

Rat-bite fever caused by *Streptobacillus moniliformis* may mimic enteric fever when the rat puncture site is not clinically evident or when the infection is foodborne.[49] This illness may also mimic enteric fever–like syndromes. History of a recent rat bite suggests the diagnosis.[49] Cultures of blood and joint fluid may confirm the diagnosis; serologic tests may also be helpful. The other cause of rat-bite fever, *Spirillum minus*, causes subacute fever, headache, nausea, and vomiting, often with an urticarial rash (sodoku), 1 to 4 weeks after a rat bite. There is usually regional adenopathy.[50,51] Spirillary fever causes a false-positive serologic test for syphilis in the majority of cases. *S. minus* requires mouse inoculation for its isolation or demonstration of the 2- to 5-μm twisted gram-negative rod in tissue or blood for diagnosis. Like syphilis and relapsing fever, spirillary fever is often associated with a Herxheimer reaction when treatment with penicillin G is initiated.

Leptospirosis frequently manifests with fever and headache and is most prevalent in young adults. Abdominal pain occurs in approximately 30% of cases.[52] Diarrhea and constipation are less frequent. Muscle pain and tenderness occur in nearly 70% of the patients, more frequently than in enteric fever. Additional differentiating features are the fever curve and clinical course; leptospirosis is characteristically a biphasic illness.[53] Evidence of liver dysfunction is present in approximately 50% of the patients with leptospirosis.[52] Although conjunctival suffusion is characteristic of leptospirosis and is reported in one third of patients, conjunctivitis occurs in enteric fever as well. Two findings that would favor the diagnosis of leptospirosis are azotemia (26% of cases) and cerebrospinal fluid pleocytosis (47% of cases).[52] Serologic tests are of value in confirming the diagnosis of leptospirosis.

Relapsing fever caused by *Borrelia hermsii* may be confused with enteric fever. A history of travel during the previous 3 weeks to an area where louse-borne relapsing fever is endemic (Ethiopia, South America, Far East) raises the possibility of this diagnosis. Tick-borne relapsing fever can also be acquired in the western United States.[54] Conjunctivitis, rash, and hepatosplenomegaly are common. However, in contrast to patients with enteric fever, patients with tick-borne relapsing fever have a fever that resolves in a crisis during the first week only to recur later.[55] Giemsa or Wright stain of peripheral blood during a febrile episode may confirm the presence of spirochetes.

Patients with intestinal tuberculosis may have fever and findings referable to the gastrointestinal tract. The areas most commonly affected are jejunoileum and ileocecum. Radiologic studies of the terminal ileum may show evidence of a terminal ileitis that can be confused with the terminal ileitis of typhoid fever or *Y. enterocolitica* infection. Imaging features that suggest tuberculosis include cecal amputation, ileocecal thickening and inflammation, mesenteric adenopathy, and evidence of associated peritonitis.[56] Intestinal tuberculosis, once a rare disease in the United States, has become more common as a consequence of the acquired immunodeficiency syndrome (AIDS) epidemic, and it remains an important problem in developing areas.[57] Evidence of active pulmonary tuberculosis, which is present in approximately 20% of cases, and a positive purified protein derivative test support the diagnosis.

Abdominal actinomycosis may also mimic enteric fever. Physical examination may reveal an abdominal mass; the presence of a draining sinus tract strongly favors this diagnosis.[58] The diagnosis is confirmed by culture.

Intra-abdominal pyogenic abscesses can pose difficult diagnostic challenges and remain high on the list of undiagnosed causes of fever.[59] They should be suspected when fever persists or recurs and may be detected by sonography, CT, or magnetic resonance imaging.

Patients with *Mycoplasma pneumoniae* infection rarely have a course suggestive of enteric fever. Fever and headache may be prominent. The presence of tracheobronchitis with severe, nonproductive cough or pneumonia identified by physical examination or on the chest radiograph suggests this diagnosis, although infiltrates may also occur in patients with enteric fever caused by *S. typhi*. The presence of bullous myringitis suggests *M. pneumoniae* infection.[60] The appearance of upper or lower respiratory illness in friends or members of the patient's family also favors this diagnosis. Serologic studies can be used to confirm *M. pneumoniae* infection.

Patients with psittacosis frequently have an illness characterized by fever, headache, myalgia, abdominal pain, vomiting, and diarrhea. On physical examination a faint macular rash may be noted; splenomegaly occurs in some patients.[61] A history of exposure to birds suggests the diagnosis, and serologic testing is helpful in confirmation.

Several rickettsial infections, especially epidemic typhus, Brill-Zinsser disease, endemic typhus, Rocky Mountain spotted fever, and scrub typhus as well as Q fever, are characterized by fever, headache, myalgia, and, except in Q fever, skin rash. Of these, Rocky Mountain spotted fever is the most likely to be encountered in the United States.[62,63] The gastrointestinal manifestations of Rocky Mountain spotted fever include abdominal pain, diarrhea, vomiting, and upper gastrointestinal tract bleeding, and a diagnosis of appendicitis, cholecystitis, or gastroenteritis may initially be considered.[64-66] A history of recent tick exposure suggests the diagnosis. Although failure of the characteristic rash to develop may lead to a fatal delay in diagnosis and treatment, once the characteristic rash associated with these illnesses appears, the diagnostic confusion is lessened. Serologic testing provides documentation of rickettsial infections. In addition, fluorescent antibody techniques can be used to demonstrate *Rickettsia rickettsii* in biopsy specimens of involved skin.[67] Sporadic cases of epidemic typhus associated with flying squirrels have been reported in the United States since 1976.[68,69] The majority of these have occurred in southeastern states during the winter months. Q fever is associated with cattle and sheep exposure or the ingestion of unpasteurized milk.[70]

Monocytotropic and granulocytotropic ehrlichiosis, other tick-borne diseases, may also arise with typhoid-like symptoms including fever, myalgias, vomiting, diarrhea, headache, and, in some cases, rash, with elevated liver enzyme levels, leukopenia, and anemia.[71,72] A history of tick exposure in an endemic area is helpful. The diagnosis can be confirmed by serologic tests.

Legionella infections in normal or immunocompromised hosts may arise with gastrointestinal symptoms of abdominal pain, nausea, vomiting, or diarrhea that is usually watery and noninflammatory.[73] Patients with disseminated histoplasmosis may have fever, abdominal pain, nausea, vomiting, and diarrhea.[74] The diagnosis may be suggested by the presence of mucous membrane lesions or adrenal insufficiency. Biopsy specimens and cultures of liver, blood, urine, and bone marrow may be useful in confirming the diagnosis.

Several acute viral infections have gastrointestinal manifestations. Abdominal pain, nausea, and vomiting are frequent symptoms in patients with hepatitis. However, the severity of jaundice and the extent of elevation of transaminase levels are much greater than those observed in enteric fever. Influenza (particularly type B) may manifest with fever, headache, and abdominal pain. Serologic studies and, in the case of influenza, nasopharyngeal swabs are useful in distinguishing these illnesses. Infectious mononucleosis may mimic enteric fever, particu-

larly when acute pharyngitis is not prominent. Examination of the peripheral blood smear and studies for heterophil or Epstein-Barr virus–specific antibodies are helpful in differentiating this illness from enteric fever.

In dengue fever, an important mosquito-borne viral disease in the tropics, headache, severe myalgias, and leukopenia are common. The maculopapular skin rash that characteristically appears on the trunk on the third to fifth day of illness and subsequently spreads peripherally, the biphasic clinical course, and a history of recent travel (within the previous 9 days) to areas in which dengue is endemic suggest the diagnosis.

A number of protozoal and helminthic infections can also mimic typhoid fever. Malaria is endemic in many areas of the world in which typhoid fever is also relatively common. Both diseases may arise with fever, headache, abdominal pain, and other gastrointestinal symptoms. Two thirds of 25 cases of malaria in one series presented with prominent gastrointestinal symptoms (nausea, vomiting, abdominal pain, or diarrhea) that might have misled physicians from an early diagnosis of malaria.[75] When present, intermittent fever suggests the diagnosis of malaria, but it is not observed in the majority of nonimmune individuals with the disease. Peripheral blood smears confirm the diagnosis of malaria.

Fever, chills, and hemolytic anemia in a person with exposure to an area with *Ixodes scapularis* ticks and white-footed mice (*Peromyscus* spp.) or white-tailed deer (*Odocoileus virginianus*) may be due to infection with *Babesia microti*, especially in an asplenic patient.[76,77]

Either intestinal or hepatic amebiasis may mimic acute enteric fever. In patients with hepatic abscesses, documentation of a single abscess cavity favors the diagnosis of amebiasis.[78] The diagnosis may be confirmed by means of a positive indirect hemagglutination test. Patients with visceral leishmaniasis frequently present with fever, malaise, hepatosplenomegaly, weight loss, anemia, thrombocytopenia, and leukopenia. Massive splenomegaly suggests visceral leishmaniasis. The diagnosis is made by identifying leishmanial amastigotes within mononuclear phagocytes in aspirates of the spleen or bone marrow or by culturing leishmania from those specimens.

Several helminthic infections may cause an enteric fever–like syndrome, but they are usually associated with eosinophilia as discussed later. Patients with trichinosis typically present with fever, headache, myalgias, abdominal pain, diarrhea, periorbital edema, and rash. The presence of eosinophilia, rather than the eosinopenia frequently noted in enteric fever, helps in the differentiation. The history of recent ingestion of raw or undercooked pork suggests trichinosis. It can be confirmed by acute and convalescent serologic tests or biopsy, but the latter is seldom necessary.

Patients with visceral larva migrans may also have fever and hepatomegaly. In more severe infections, splenomegaly, rash, and pneumonitis may also occur. In contrast to enteric fever, visceral larva migrans is typically associated with pronounced eosinophilia. The diagnosis is suggested by a history of pica. Serologic tests may confirm the diagnosis of *Toxocara* spp. infection.

Patients with acute schistosomiasis (Katayama's fever) may also present with an enteric fever syndrome. Again, eosinophilia is helpful in separating these possibilities. The history of swimming in fresh water during the previous month in areas where schistosomiasis is endemic further suggests schistosomiasis. The diagnosis is suggested by serologic tests and confirmed by the eventual identification of ova in the stool.

Noninfectious causes of fever and abdominal pain such as eosinophilic gastroenteritis, hematologic and other malignancies involving abdominal lymph nodes or the intestine, vasculitides, and granulomatous diseases must also be considered. Diagnosis in such cases often requires radiographic studies, biopsy of involved tissues, and the exclusion of other processes as discussed later. See Chapter 48 for a discussion of the differential diagnosis of fever of unknown origin.

Therapy for Enteric Fever

In patients with the enteric fever syndrome, it is advisable to consider empirical antimicrobial therapy for typhoid fever before the diagnosis is confirmed by culture. Multiple-drug–resistant isolates of *S. typhi* unresponsive to ampicillin, trimethoprim-sulfamethoxazole, and chloramphenicol are increasingly prevalent around the world.[79-81] Fluoroquinolones, such as ciprofloxacin or ofloxacin,[82-84] are now widely used, but resistance to them has been reported in a number of areas.[85-87] The fluoroquinolones achieve high concentration in phagocytic cells and in bile. They are usually well tolerated and, provided the infecting strain is sensitive, result in faster defervescence than cephalosporins. Fluoroquinolones are not approved for use in children in the United States because of their potential to damage cartilage and tendons, but accumulating evidence of their safe use with children with typhoid, bacillary dysentery, and cystic fibrosis has led to their increased use in this population.[88-90] For uncomplicated quinolone-resistant typhoid, therapy with azithromycin is considered first-line therapy.[4] Third-generation cephalosporins, such as ceftriaxone,[91-93] and the monobactam aztreonam are also effective.[94] For sensitive *S. typhi*, ampicillin, trimethoprim-sulfamethoxazole, or chloramphenicol can be used. Strains may occasionally acquire resistance during therapy. A patient's recent travel and exposure history should be considered in selecting additional empirical antimicrobial drugs to cover other possible causes of the enteric syndrome, pending the results of cultures and other diagnostic tests.

MESENTERIC ADENITIS

Patients with mesenteric adenitis typically have a history of fever and abdominal pain, frequently with localization to the right lower quadrant. The illness is similar to acute appendicitis. Few data are available on the incidence of this syndrome, and it may vary with the geographic location. In one series of hospitalized patients, 50 of 651 (7.7%) admitted with a diagnosis of appendicitis had a discharge diagnosis of mesenteric adenitis.[95]

Etiologic Agents and Pathogenesis

The most frequently reported causes of the syndrome of mesenteric adenitis are *Y. enterocolitica* and *Y. pseudotuberculosis*. These organisms seem to be more prevalent in Europe than in the United States. Among 2861 consecutive patients undergoing appendectomy for suspected appendicitis in a Belgian hospital, *Y. enterocolitica* was isolated from the appendix or stool in 3.6%. Of those with histologically confirmed mesenteric adenitis or terminal ileitis without appendicitis, or both, *Y. enterocolitica* was cultured in 75%.[96] In another report, five of eight patients (63%) who had mesenteric adenitis confirmed at surgery also had serologic evidence of recent *Y. enterocolitica* infection.[97] Of 20 patients with mesenteric adenitis reported by Mair and associates, 17 were adequately studied; 3 (18%) had evidence of infection with *Y. pseudotuberculosis*.[98] In a school-related outbreak of *Y. pseudotuberculosis* among 34 children in Finland, 3 children went to surgery for suspected appendicitis and were found to have mesenteric lymphadenitis.[99] In a mouse model, after intragastric administration of *Y. enterocolitica*, polymorphonuclear leukocytes appeared in Peyer's patches within 24 hours. The infection then spread to the mesenteric lymph nodes, where abscesses developed.[100]

Mesenteric adenitis can theoretically occur with any pathogen that affects lymph nodes. It has also been associated with nontyphoidal *Salmonella* spp. infections,[101,102] *S. typhi* infections,[103] tuberculous mesenteric lymphadenitis, intestinal anthrax, and, in children with HIV infections in Southeast Asia, *Penicillium marneffei* infection.[104]

In the preantibiotic era, hemolytic streptococci were frequently reported as etiologic agents. In one study, 19 of 36 patients (53%) with mesenteric adenitis in whom cultures were obtained had hemolytic streptococci and 4 (11%) had *Escherichia coli*. Of interest is the fact that 37 of 39 patients (97%) had throat cultures positive for hemolytic streptococci, and 35 of these had a history of a recent sore throat.[105] Although now uncommon, hemolytic streptococci have been isolated in a few cases of mesenteric adenitis in the antibiotic era as well.[98,106,107] Asch and colleagues reported on one patient from whom β-hemolytic streptococci were isolated from an inflamed mesenteric node and in whom subsequent studies revealed an elevated anti–streptolysin O

titer.[106] *Staphylococcus aureus* alone or with β-hemolytic streptococci has also been isolated from inflamed mesenteric nodes in the absence of appendicitis.[107] In a report of two patients with mesenteric abscesses secondary to suppurative mesenteric adenitis, one had enterococci and an unidentified hemolytic bacillus isolated from an abscess, whereas the other had *Bacteroides* and *Clostridium* spp.; in both cases the appendix was normal.[108] Viruses have also been occasionally reported as causes of mesenteric adenitis.

Clinical Features of Mesenteric Lymphadenitis Caused by *Yersinia* Species

Symptoms

Y. enterocolitica produces a spectrum of disease, including acute enterocolitis, terminal ileitis, and mesenteric adenitis. *Y. pseudotuberculosis*, which commonly infects animals, is a less frequent cause of human disease. It typically produces mesenteric adenitis, especially in older children and adults.

Regardless of the cause, persons with mesenteric adenitis present with fever and right lower quadrant pain, making the syndrome indistinguishable from acute appendicitis.[109] The symptoms reported by persons in four common-source outbreaks of *Yersinia* infection are summarized in Table 94-3.[110-112] Fever, abdominal pain, vomiting, and diarrhea were frequent. In a series of 37 sporadic cases of *Yersinia*-induced enteritis reported from Belgium, 84% of the patients had abdominal pain, 78% had diarrhea, 43% had fever, and 22% reported anorexia; 13% had nausea and 8% vomiting.[113] Patients with mesenteric adenitis caused by *Yersinia* may have a history of biphasic illness.[114] Consumption of raw pork in the 2 weeks before illness has been associated with *Y. enterocolitica* infection in the most highly endemic country, Belgium, and consumption of chitterlings before the onset of illness has been reported in the United States.[115,116]

Physical Examination

The physical findings of mesenteric adenitis typically include fever, right lower quadrant tenderness, and often rebound tenderness. Rectal tenderness was present in nearly one third of people examined in one epidemic.[112] In contrast to the enteric fever syndromes, a pulse-temperature deficit is not found.

Laboratory Findings

Leukocytosis is usually present in patients with *Yersinia*-associated mesenteric adenitis[115-118]; white blood cell counts typically are between 10,000 and 15,000/mm³. Examination of feces may reveal polymorphonuclear leukocytes.[119] Blood cultures are rarely positive, but *Y. enterocolitica* or *Y. pseudotuberculosis* may be isolated from stool cultures. The frequency of isolation is improved by the use of cold-enrichment techniques.[120] Stool cultures were positive in 56% of hospitalized patients with the syndrome in one common-source outbreak[112]; the isolation of *Y. pseudotuberculosis* from feces seems to occur less frequently but has been reported.[121] Serologic testing may be

TABLE 94-3 Symptoms in Four Outbreaks of Mesenteric Adenitis Caused by *Yersinia enterocolitica*

Location	Japan (110)	Japan (111)	Japan (111)	United States (112)
Serotype	03	03	03	08
Number ill	198	188	544	38
Percentage with				
Abdominal pain	76	86	64	97
Fever	61	76	50	100
Diarrhea	36	60	32	47
Vomiting	12	4	11	—
Percentage undergoing appendectomy	2	—	—	42

helpful in the diagnosis, but agglutinins are rarely present during the first week of illness,[113] and cross-reactions can occur with *Brucella* spp., *Vibrio* spp., and some Enterobacteriaceae. Serologic confirmation was obtained in 84% of the hospitalized patients in one outbreak. The isolation of *Y. enterocolitica* from a stool culture should be considered significant; the organism is rarely isolated from control subjects.[122]

Sonographic, radiographic contrast studies, or CT examination may provide clues that are helpful in differentiating mesenteric lymphadenitis from appendicitis. Of 170 patients presenting with a clinical syndrome suggesting acute appendicitis or mesenteric lymphadenitis who underwent sonography using graded compression, 14 had only enlarged mesenteric nodes with mural thickening of the terminal ileum (without visualization of the appendix); none of the 14 had appendicitis; and 8 (of 9 cultured) had *Y. enterocolitica* in the stool.[123] In another study of 609 patients with suspected appendicitis, graded ultrasonography suggested a spectrum of other diseases in addition to appendicitis, but in 3 cases there were incorrect sonographic diagnoses with serious sequelae.[124] In a series of 37 adult patients who had documented *Y. enterocolitica* infection, 40% had symptoms compatible with appendicitis; 21 of the 24 patients studied with radiographic contrast material had abnormalities of the terminal ileum consisting of coarse mucosal folds in 67%, nodularity in 45%, and ulceration in 45%.[113] Although radiologic studies of the colon were normal in these patients, sigmoidoscopic or colonoscopic examination in 13 revealed evidence of colitis in 6 and aphthoid ulceration in 2, indicating that colonic involvement may occur. In another series of 25 patients with *Yersinia* infection who were given the clinical diagnosis of acute appendicitis and underwent appendectomy, acute terminal ileitis was confirmed at surgery. When these patients were examined within 1 week of surgery by a barium contrast study of the small bowel, abnormalities were confined to the distal 20 cm of the ileum. The lesions evolved from an initial nodular pattern to an edematous pattern before resolution within 10 weeks in all cases.[124]

Helical appendiceal CT can also be used to diagnose appendicitis. An enlarged appendix with periappendiceal fat stranding occurs in 93% of cases of appendicitis. Less common but specific changes are cecal apical changes and an appendolith or appendoliths.[125] In a series of 18 patients with a discharge diagnosis of mesenteric lymphadenitis, the CT scan showed three or more nodes measuring 5 mm in the shortest axis clustered in the right lower quadrant, with a normal appendix.[95] Eight patients had associated ileal or ileocecal wall thickening. As promising as sonography, radiography, and CT appear, they are still not sufficiently sensitive and specific to preclude surgery in most instances.

At surgery, patients with mesenteric adenitis may also have evidence of acute appendicitis, but the organ is rarely severely inflamed or ruptured. Patients may also have evidence of acute terminal ileitis.[97,109,118,124] Culture of the terminal ileum at surgery may yield the organism.[117] Histopathologic examination of resected mesenteric lymph nodes in cases of *Y. enterocolitica* infection frequently reveals histiocytic infiltration and the presence of large pyroninophilic cells; abscesses are typically absent.[126,127] In contrast, although reticulum cell hyperplasia is frequently seen in nodes infected with *Y. pseudotuberculosis*, granulomas, polymorphonuclear leukocyte infiltration, and abscess formation are more frequent.[98,117,126,128] In both infections, tissue Gram stain may reveal the bacteria. Two fatal cases occurred in a *Y. enterocolitica* outbreak among four families in North Carolina.[129] Postmortem examination revealed extensive ulceration and necrosis extending from the stomach or small bowel to the colon. Mesenteric lymph nodes were necrotic in one case, and the sinusoids were filled with leukocytes and mononuclear cells. In the second case, the lymph nodes were large, firm, and edematous. There was reticuloendothelial hyperplasia with abundant histiocytes and plasma cells within the sinusoids.[119]

Epidemiology

Mesenteric adenitis caused by *Y. enterocolitica* or *Y. pseudotuberculosis* is a syndrome of children and young adults, is most frequent in people between 5 and 14 years of age, is more common in boys, and is most often encountered during the winter and spring. This seasonal pattern is reported from both the preantibiotic[105] and antibiotic[130] eras.

The mode of transmission of *Y. enterocolitica* and *Y. pseudotuberculosis* has not been well defined; outbreaks involving several members of several families[129] or people from the same school have been reported. In these and other episodes of *Yersinia* infection, simultaneous documentation of infection in family pets has been obtained[131]; whether these animals were the source of the human infection or merely acquired the infection simultaneously is unknown. Person-to-person spread to family members does occur.[122] Large common-source outbreaks of mesenteric adenitis have also been reported[110-112,132,133]; in one of these, chocolate milk was the vehicle of transmission.[112] *Y. enterocolitica* has been isolated from drinking water,[103,134] but waterborne transmission of these organisms has not been well documented. Results of one study in Wisconsin suggested that *Y. enterocolitica* infection was more common in rural areas.[135]

Differential Diagnosis

The major consideration in the differential diagnosis of mesenteric adenitis is acute appendicitis. Other infectious diseases characteristically involving the terminal ileum or mesenteric lymph nodes, or both, such as tuberculosis, nontyphoidal *Salmonella* infections,[101,102] *S. enterica* serotype typhi infections,[102] actinomycosis, *Mycobacterium avium-intracellulare* infection in patients with AIDS,[136] or *P. marneffei* infections in children with HIV infection in Southeast Asia,[104] must be considered. Inflammatory reactions to latent mycobacterial infections after initiation of highly active antiretroviral therapy in patients with AIDS may also cause mesenteric lymphadenitis. Viruses have been occasionally implicated as causes of mesenteric lymphadenitis, including parvovirus B19 as a cause of pseudoappendicitis[137] and Epstein-Barr virus as a cause of mesenteric lymphadenopathy.[138] Adenovirus infection has been associated with mesenteric lymph node hypertrophy and intussusception.[139] *Angiostrongylus costaricensis* may produce an appendicitis-like syndrome but is usually associated with eosinophilia as described later.[140]

Therapy

Mesenteric adenitis is a self-limited illness in the vast majority of cases. Specific antimicrobial therapy is often not required. In patients who are severely ill or who have evidence of systemic disease, the selection of an antimicrobial agent should be based, if possible, on the results of antimicrobial sensitivity tests. When these data are not available, therapeutic agents to be considered for *Y. enterocolitica* include trimethoprim-sulfamethoxazole, second- and third-generation cephalosporins, ciprofloxacin and other fluoroquinolones, piperacillin, imipenem, tetracycline, and chloramphenicol.[141-143] *Y. enterocolitica* is often resistant to amoxicillin, cefazolin, and macrolides.[144-146] Although *Y. enterocolitica* isolates may be sensitive in vitro to aminoglycosides,[114] these drugs should not be the initial choice for treatment because of the reported failure of these agents to eradicate systemic infection.[27] *Y. pseudotuberculosis* is usually sensitive to tetracycline, cephalosporins, aminoglycosides, and chloramphenicol. The optimal management of focal mycobacterial lymphadenitis after initiation of highly active antiretroviral therapy has not been established.

SYNDROME OF ABDOMINAL PAIN OR DIARRHEA WITH EOSINOPHILIA

The differential diagnosis and etiologic considerations for the syndrome of abdominal pain, diarrhea, and eosinophilia as well as useful diagnostic tests are summarized in Table 94-4. Most cases are caused by helminths. Additional diagnostic considerations include eosinophilic gastroenteritis, dermatitis herpetiformis, polyarteritis nodosa, regional enteritis, and ulcerative colitis. In addition, lymphomas and some solid tumors may manifest with abdominal pain and eosinophilia. Epidemiologic data, particularly dietary and travel histories, may provide important clues to the diagnosis. Valuable laboratory tests in these patients include examination of stool and small bowel contents for ova and parasites, specific serologic tests, and, in some cases, radiologic studies or biopsy.

TABLE 94-4 Etiologic Agents and Useful Laboratory Studies in the Differential Diagnosis of Infectious Causes of the Syndrome of Abdominal Pain and/or Diarrhea with Eosinophilia

Etiologic Agents or Disease	Stool Examination	Small Bowel Fluid Examination or Biopsy	Tissue Biopsy	Serology	Radiologic and Other Studies
Nematodes					
Strongyloides stercoralis	+	+	−	+	−
Ascaris lumbricoides	+	±	−	−	± (small bowel)
Visceral larva migrans (*Toxocara canis, Toxocara cati*, and others)	−	−	+ (liver)	+	−
Trichinella spiralis	−	−	+ (muscle)	+	−
Anisakiasis (*Anisakis* spp. and other genera)	−	−	−	−	+ (endoscopy)
Capillaria philippinensis	+	+	−	−	−
Angiostrongylus costaricensis	−	−	+ (ileum, colon)	+	+ (UGI series; small bowel)
Trematodes					
Schistosoma spp.	+	−	+ (rectum)	+	−
Clonorchis sinensis (Chinese liver fluke)	+	−	−	−	± (biliary tract abnormalities)
Opisthorchis spp. (Southeast Asian liver fluke)	+	−	−	−	± (biliary tract abnormalities)
Metorchis conjunctus (North American liver fluke)	+	−	−	+	−
Fasciola hepatica (sheep liver fluke)	+	−	−	−	+ (ultrasound, liver CT scan)
Fasciolopsis buski (intestinal fluke)	+	−	−	−	−
Heterophyes heterophyes (intestinal fluke)	+	−	−	−	−
Metagonimus yokogawi (intestinal fluke)	+	−	−	−	−
Nanophyetus salmincola (intestinal fluke)	+	−	−	−	−
Cestodes					
Echinococcosis	−	−	−	+	+ (chest radiograph, abdominal ultrasound or CT scan)
Protozoa					
Isospora belli	+	+	−	−	−
Dientamoeba fragilis	+	−	−	−	−
Diseases of unknown cause					
Eosinophilic gastroenteritis	−	+	−	−	+ (UGI series; small bowel CT scan)
Polyarteritis nodosa and other forms of vasculitis	−	−	+ (skin, muscle, kidney)	−	+ (angiography)
Inflammatory bowel disease	−	−	+ (colon)	−	+ (small bowel, colonoscopy)
Malignancies	−	−	+ (lymph nodes, liver, bone marrow)	−	+ (UGI series, barium enema, CT scan, ultrasound)

+, Feature present; −, feature absent; CT, computed tomography; UGI, upper gastrointestinal.

Differential Diagnosis

Strongyloides stercoralis is unique among intestinal nematodes in its ability to persist for many years through autoinfection and to produce life-threatening hyperinfection in immunocompromised hosts.[147] It infects people in areas where sanitation is poor. Patients with strongyloidiasis frequently have abdominal pain, diarrhea, or a sense of bloating and eosinophilia. Pain is often epigastric, although some patients report pain in the right upper and right lower quadrants or in the periumbilical region. Ninety percent of those infected have eosinophilia. Cases of hyperinfection have occurred in persons who are immunosuppressed after organ transplantation and in association with malnutrition, lymphoma, cimetidine therapy, or HIV infection, although hyperinfection has been observed less commonly than expected with HIV infection.[147-150] *Strongyloides* hyperinfection can result in secondary bacteremia, meningitis, urinary tract infection, or pneumonia related to enteric bacteria on the surface of migrating larvae. On the other hand, infection with human T-cell lymphotropic virus type 1 (HTLV-1) is clearly associated with severe disseminated and recurrent strongyloidiasis. In contrast to HIV infection, HTLV-1 infection triggers immortalization of CD4 lymphocytes, increased interferon-γ and Th1 responses, and reduced Th2 responses, with reduced interleukin-4 (IL-4), IL-5, IL-13, and immunoglobulin E responses needed to protect against helminthic infections.[151,152]

In the United States, strongyloidiasis is most often diagnosed in immigrants, residents of the Southeast, or veterans who served in endemic areas abroad. Prolonged infections have been demonstrated in troops and former prisoners in World War II who served in Southeast Asia.[153] A prospective study in rural Tennessee documented *S. stercoralis* in 6.1% of patients at a Veterans Affairs hospital and in 2.6% of their household contacts.[154] The diagnosis of strongyloidiasis can be confirmed by demonstration of larvae in fresh stool specimens, but the sensitivity is low. The sensitivity can be enhanced by studying multiple specimens or by using the Baermann funnel gauze test[155,156] or the agar plate method, which is probably the diagnostic measure of choice.[157] Larvae can also be identified in some cases in duodenal contents[158-160] and in sputum in some patients with disseminated hyperinfection. Immunofluorescence assay or enzyme-linked immunosorbent assay (ELISA) can be used to detect anti-*Strongyloides* antibodies,[161-163] but both false-positive and false-negative results can occur. Eosinophilia is often absent in immunocompromised patients, particularly those taking corticosteroids.[148,149]

Most patients infected with *Ascaris lumbricoides* are asymptomatic. Although ascariasis is not usually associated with diarrhea, severe abdominal pain may occur when patients with heavy worm burdens develop intestinal obstruction or adult worms migrate into or occlude the biliary or pancreatic ducts.[164-166] These complications are most frequent in young children. It is estimated that acute intestinal obstruction caused by *Ascaris* may occur in as many as 1 in 1000 persons in endemic areas. Ascariasis is most common in areas where sanitation is poor. Eggs are ingested in contaminated food or water or, by children, in dirt. In the United States, *Ascaris* infection was once common in the southeastern states, but symptomatic infections are now rare. Eosinophilia may or may not be present. The diagnosis is made by the demonstration of ova in stool specimens. Because a single worm produces large numbers of eggs, concentration of feces is not necessary. In patients with intestinal or biliary tract obstruction, sonographic, radiologic, or CT studies may reveal the presence of an adult worm, and there may be elevations of liver or pancreatic enzyme levels.[166]

Patients with toxocariasis (visceral larva migrans) caused by animal nematodes such as *Toxocara canis* may present with abdominal pain and eosinophilia. In temperate climates, *T. canis* is the most important etiologic agent.[167] The abdominal pain may be associated with the presence of tender hepatomegaly. Clinical clues to the diagnosis include the simultaneous occurrence of splenomegaly or pneumonitis with bronchospasm.[168-170] Patients may have pruritic rashes on the trunk or lower extremities. The presence of a granuloma in the ocular fundus or other evidence of ocular inflammation, high titers of isoagglutinins, and hypergammaglobulinemia provide additional diagnostic clues. The total white blood cell count is often elevated, and eosinophils may exceed 50%. Patients are usually young children; additional epidemiologic clues are a history of pica or close contact with dogs. As many as 10% to 30% of the soil samples in public playgrounds and parks in the United States have been found to be contaminated with *Toxocara* eggs.[167] Serologic tests are available; ELISA seems to be the most sensitive and specific.[168-170] On rare occasions, larvae are identified in biopsies of the liver or other organs.

The onset of infection with *Trichinella spiralis* may be characterized initially by diarrhea, which occurs in approximately 40% of the cases; abdominal pain, which occurs in approximately 20%; or constipation.[171,172] The intestinal symptoms, which are attributed to the presence of adult worms or invading larvae in the intestinal tract, occur during the first week of illness and may precede the appearance of eosinophilia. Infection occurs by the ingestion of raw or undercooked pork or pork products such as sausage; bear, walrus, cougar, and horse meat; and occasionally by other vehicles such as ground beef contaminated during processing with pork.[172-175] Trichinellosis cases appear to be declining in the United States (probably because of decreased prevalence of *T. spiralis* in domestic swine, increased use of home freezers, and the practice of thoroughly cooking pork), but the proportion of cases attributable to ingestion of wild game meat has increased.[176] Myalgias, periorbital edema, muscle tenderness, splinter hemorrhages, and evidence of myocarditis or central nervous system involvement with eosinophilia further suggest the diagnosis. Prolonged diarrhea has been the dominant symptom among Inuit inhabitants of northern Canada who become reinfected with *Trichinella nativa* after eating contaminated, uncooked walrus meat. Myalgia and muscle weakness are less prominent complaints in that setting.[144,145] The diagnosis of trichinosis is usually made on clinical grounds and confirmed by serologic tests, but antibodies do not typically become positive until several weeks into infection.[146] A definitive diagnosis may be made by the demonstration of larvae in muscle, although biopsy is seldom necessary.

Patients with anisakiasis caused by nematodes of the family Anisakidae and related parasites of fish may have an acute illness characterized by epigastric pain, nausea, and vomiting or a chronic illness characterized by abdominal pain and fever. The disease is caused by larvae that migrate from the viscera to the muscle of fish after they are caught and penetrate the human gastrointestinal tract after fish is eaten raw or inadequately cooked. The stomach, small bowel, or colon may be involved. Necrotizing eosinophilic granulomatous inflammation with peripheral eosinophilia occur at the sites where larvae attempt to invade.[177-179] The pathologic and radiologic manifestations may resemble those of regional enteritis[180]; mass lesions resembling malignancies may also occur.[181] The disease is rarely reported in the United States; it is most common in the Netherlands and Japan. The infection is ac-

quired by the ingestion of raw or undercooked marine fish such as cod, salmon, and herring. In Japan, raw or pickled marine fish are common vehicles; in the Netherlands, raw or slightly salted herring is the most common source of infection.[177,178] Therefore, the travel or dietary history may suggest the diagnosis. Confirmation is obtained by identification of the larvae by endoscopy or in tissue specimens. Eustrongylidiasis is another helminthic infection associated with abdominal pain, diarrhea, and eosinophilia after the ingestion of contaminated uncooked fish or minnows.[182]

Capillaria philippinensis is a rare but important cause of intestinal disease in endemic regions of the Philippines. Sporadic cases have also been reported from Thailand, Egypt, and other areas of the world. Those infected typically give a history of vague abdominal pain and voluminous watery diarrhea.[183] The illness is characterized by a protein-losing enteropathy and malabsorption, which may be severe. Electrolyte abnormalities and hypoproteinemia are common. Weight loss, muscle wasting, weakness, hyporeflexia, and edema occur.[184] Worms are found in the small bowel, especially in the jejunum, and the adults are partially embedded in the mucosa. The intestinal villi are flattened in focal areas.[185] The life cycle involves birds and freshwater fish, which appear to be the vehicle of transmission when eaten raw or poorly cooked. The finding of eggs, adult worms, and larvae in small bowel contents suggests that autoinfection may occur. Travel and dietary histories may provide a clue to the diagnosis. The diagnosis is confirmed by identifying ova of *C. philippinensis* in fecal specimens.

Angiostrongylus costaricensis lives in the lumen of mesenteric arteries of the ileocecal region of rodents and occasionally involves the same site in humans.[186,187] Eggs form emboli to terminal branches of the mesenteric arteries. Disease, usually encountered in children, may arise as an acute abdominal infection with fever, nausea, vomiting, pain, and sometimes a right lower quadrant mass. Leukocytosis and eosinophilia (11% to 82%) are common. In some cases it may be impossible to distinguish infection with *A. costaricensis* from acute appendicitis on clinical grounds.[186] Humans become infected by ingesting material contaminated by infected slugs or land snails, which are intermediate hosts. *A. costaricensis* is endemic in areas of Central America and South America. Infection has also been acquired in the United States.[187] The diagnosis is suggested by the clinical syndrome and history of exposure. Antibodies can be detected by ELISA or latex agglutination tests.[186] The diagnosis is frequently made after surgical exploration and resection by identifying adult worms and eggs in tissue.

Patients with schistosomiasis and other trematode infections may present with gastrointestinal complaints and eosinophilia. Katayama's fever, a serum sickness–like syndrome characterized by fever, headache, diarrhea, hepatosplenomegaly, generalized lymphadenopathy, urticaria, and eosinophilia, can occur within 4 to 8 weeks after primary exposure to schistosomes. The syndrome is seen in persons with heavy infections. It occurs most frequently with *Schistosoma japonicum*, less frequently with *Schistosoma mansoni*, and rarely with *Schistosoma haematobium* infections.[188] The acute manifestations of schistosomiasis are usually self-limited, although death may occur. The diagnosis of Katayama's fever should be suspected in patients with a serum sickness–like illness accompanied by eosinophilia who have had exposure to schistosomes during the previous 4 to 8 weeks through swimming or bathing in fresh water in an endemic area.[157,189] Serologic tests provide suggestive evidence of disease. The diagnosis is confirmed by the demonstration of ova in feces[188] or in a rectal biopsy specimen.

Acute infections with the Chinese fluke, *Clonorchis sinensis*, the Southeast Asian liver fluke, *Opisthorchis viverrini*, or the North American liver fluke, *Metorchis conjunctus*, are acquired through the ingestion of raw or inadequately cooked freshwater fish.[190-192] Persons infected may present with fever, abdominal pain, diarrhea, hepatomegaly, and eosinophilia. Those with established *C. sinensis* and *O. viverrini* infections are usually free of abdominal discomfort and eosinophilia, but they are at increased risk for ascending cholangitis and cholangiocarcinoma. Acute infection with *Fasciola hepatica*, the sheep liver fluke, is endemic in many cattle- and sheep-raising areas of the world. It is characterized by fever and pain in the right upper quadrant, hepatomegaly, and often marked eosinophilia.[193] Human infections are acquired by the ingestion of metacercariae that encyst on aquatic plants such as wild watercress. Infections have been reported from South America, Africa, Europe, China, and Australia. The diagnosis is confirmed by the identification of characteristic ova in the feces or bile or ELISA. Concentration techniques increase the likelihood of finding ova.

Several trematodes that inhabit the gastrointestinal tract can produce abdominal pain, diarrhea, and eosinophilia. Infections with *Heterophyes heterophyes*, *Metagonimus yokogawai*, and *Nanophyetus salmincola* are acquired through the ingestion of raw or undercooked freshwater fish.[194-197] *Fasciolopsis buski* is acquired through the ingestion of water chestnuts or the peeling of other freshwater plants with the teeth before ingestion.[194] Infection with these flukes may be asymptomatic, but patients with heavy infections often develop both abdominal pain and diarrhea. The diagnosis is suggested by a history of exposure in an endemic area and the dietary history. The diagnosis is made by the demonstration of ova in feces and may require concentration techniques. *Echinostoma* spp. may cause a similar syndrome after ingestion of raw, infected snails, amphibians, or fish.[198]

Adult tapeworm infestations with *Taenia solium*, the pork tapeworm, *Taenia saginata*, the beef tapeworm, *Diphyllobothrium latum*, the fish tapeworm, and *Hymenolepis nana*, the dwarf tapeworm, are usually asymptomatic, but they can on occasion be associated with abdominal discomfort, diarrhea, or eosinophilia.[199] In patients with echinococcosis, eosinophilia may occur in conjunction with abdominal pain or occasionally anaphylaxis when cysts leak.[200] The diagnosis of echinococcosis should be suspected in patients who have lived or traveled in endemic areas. The diagnosis is usually made on the basis of sonographic or CT findings and serologic studies.[201]

Patients with enteric protozoal infections (e.g., *Entamoeba histolytica*) usually do not have eosinophilia. *Isospora belli* is an exception.[202] It can cause abdominal pain, watery diarrhea, and malabsorption in association with eosinophilia. Infection is usually encountered in the tropics where sanitation is poor. In healthy adults, *I. belli* produces a self-limited disease, but it is an important cause of severe, chronic diarrhea and weight loss in Haitians and others with AIDS.[203] The diagnosis is suggested by a history of potential exposure and confirmed by the demonstration of oocysts in feces; concentration techniques and acid-fast staining are helpful.[204,205] Examinations of duodenal contents or small bowel biopsy specimens are more sensitive diagnostic techniques. *Dientamoeba fragilis* is another protozoan that can cause diarrhea and abdominal discomfort. It has been associated with pinworm infection and eosinophilia.[206,207]

Eosinophilic gastroenteritis is a rare disease of uncertain cause characterized by eosinophilic infiltration of the gastrointestinal tract, peripheral eosinophilia in the majority of cases, and clinical manifestations that may include abdominal pain, diarrhea, protein-losing enteropathy, malabsorption, or gastric outlet obstruction in the absence of documented helminthic infestation.[208] The clinical manifestations depend both on the portion of bowel involved (stomach, duodenum, jejunum, or ileum) and on the layer involved (mucosa, muscular layer, or submucosa). The stomach and small intestine are the most common sites, but eosinophilic ileocolitis has also been reported.[209] Patients frequently have a history of allergic diathesis.[208,209] The sedimentation rate is usually normal or only mildly elevated, and Charcot-Leyden crystals may be seen in the stool. Radiologic studies may reveal polypoid gastric or duodenal mucosal folds and rigid dilated loops of jejunum with a sawtooth mucosal pattern. The diagnosis is usually made by endoscopic biopsy. Histologic examination of involved tissue reveals eosinophilia in the absence of granulomas, vasculitis, and helminths. Because the involvement may be patchy, multiple biopsy specimens should be taken. Biopsies may be negative if the disease involves only the muscular or subserosal layers. In the latter case, the presence of eosinophils in ascitic fluid is suggestive of the diagnosis. Eosinophilic gastroenteritis is chronic and occasionally fatal, but most patients respond to corticosteroid therapy.[208,209] As previously discussed, a number of intestinal helminths that infect humans, such as the dog hookworm

Ancylostoma caninum, which can produce eosinophilic enteritis in humans, and nematodes of fish that cause anisakiasis can produce eosinophilic enteritis or gastroenteritis and must be excluded before a diagnosis of idiopathic eosinophilic gastroenteritis is made.

Gastrointestinal involvement with eosinophilia can also occur as a manifestation of vasculitis.[210] Up to 25% of the patients with polyarteritis nodosa have involvement of the gastrointestinal tract. It is the initial manifestation of disease in 15% of patients. Abdominal pain is a prominent symptom, and eosinophilia is frequent. The clue to the diagnosis, which may be confirmed by biopsy or angiography, is provided by the systemic nature of the disease with frequent involvement of the kidneys, heart, and musculoskeletal and nervous systems. In allergic angiitis and granulomatosis of the Churg-Strauss syndrome type, lung involvement is pronounced, patients manifest prominent eosinophilia, and there is a strong allergic diathesis, often with asthma.[210] Some of the patients with this syndrome also have abdominal involvement and have been classified as having a polyangiitis overlap syndrome.[211]

Abdominal pain and diarrhea accompanied by eosinophilia may occur in patients with regional enteritis, Whipple's disease, or ulcerative colitis.[25,212] In one series, 32% of the patients with radiologically or surgically proven regional enteritis had eosinophilia on more than one occasion.[212] The average elevated eosinophil count was 6.2%; the range was from 4% to 22%.[212] On occasion, the extraintestinal manifestations of inflammatory bowel diseases provide clues to their diagnosis.

Patients with solid tumors and lymphomas may also have abdominal pain, diarrhea, and eosinophilia.[213] Eosinophilia is most commonly associated with solid tumors after metastasis has occurred. Among solid tumors, frequently implicated malignancies are gastric, colonic, lung, pancreatic, and uterine carcinomas. A history of weight loss and the presence of melena or guaiac-positive stools and anemia suggest the diagnosis of cancer in the gastrointestinal tract, which may be confirmed by appropriate radiographic or endoscopic studies. Both Hodgkin's disease and non-Hodgkin's lymphomas may also be associated with eosinophilia, diarrhea, and abdominal pain when the bowel or abdominal or retroperitoneal nodes are involved.

REFERENCES

1. Gulati PD, Saxena SN, Gupta PS, et al. Changing pattern of typhoid fever. Am J Med. 1968;45:544-548.
2. Hornick RB, Greisman SE, Woodward TE, et al. Typhoid fever: Pathogenesis and immunologic control. N Engl J Med. 1970;283:686-691.
3. Stuart BM, Pullen RL. Typhoid: Clinical analysis of three hundred and sixty cases. Arch Intern Med. 1946;78:629-661.
4. Parry CM, Hien TT, Dougan G, et al. Typhoid fever. N Engl J Med. 2002;347:1770-1782.
5. Mermin JH, Townes JM, Gerber M, et al. Typhoid fever in the United States, 1985-1994: Changing risks of international travel and increasing antibiotic resistance. Arch Intern Med. 1998;158:633-638.
6. Olsen SJ, Bleasdale SC, Magnano AR, et al. Outbreaks of typhoid fever in the United States, 1960-99. Epidemiol Infect. 2003;130:13-21.
7. Carter PB, Collins FM. The route of enteric infection in normal mice. J Exp Med. 1974;139:1189-1203.
8. Gotuzzo E, Frisancho O, Sanchez J, et al. Association between the acquired immunodeficiency syndrome and infection with *Salmonella typhi* or *Salmonella paratyphi* in an endemic typhoid area. Arch Intern Med. 1991;151:381-382.
9. Vinh H, Wain J, Vo TN, et al. Two or three days of ofloxacin treatment for uncomplicated multidrug-resistant typhoid fever in children. Antimicrob Agents Chemother. 1996;40:958-961.
10. Meals RA. Paratyphoid fever: A report of 62 cases with several unusual findings and a review of the literature. Arch Intern Med. 1976;136:1422-1428.
11. Watson KC. Laboratory and clinical investigation of recovery of *Salmonella typhi* from blood. J Clin Microbiol. 1978;7:122-126.
12. Gilman RH, Terminel M, Levine MM, et al. Relative efficacy of blood, urine, rectal swab, bone-marrow, and rose-spot cultures for recovery of *Salmonella typhi* in typhoid fever. Lancet. 1975;1:1211-1213.
13. Gasem MH, Dolmans WM, Isbandrio BB, et al. Culture of *Salmonella typhi* and *Salmonella paratyphi* from blood and bone marrow in suspected typhoid fever. Trop Geogr Med. 1995;47:164-167.
14. Shukla S, Patel B, Chitnis DS. 100 years of Widal test and its reappraisal in an endemic area. Indian J Med Res. 1997;105:53-57.
15. Cocolin L, Manzano M, Astori G, et al. A highly sensitive and fast non-radioactive method for the detection of polymerase chain reaction products from *Salmonella* serovars, such as *Salmonella typhi*, in blood specimens. FEMS Immunol Med Microbiol. 1998;22:233-239.

16. Levine MM, Grados O, Gilman RH, et al. Diagnostic value of the Widal test in areas endemic for typhoid fever. Am J Trop Med Hyg. 1978;27:795-800.
17. Lim PL, Tam FC, Cheong YM, Jegathesan M. One-step 2-minute test to detect typhoid-specific antibodies based on particle separation in tubes. J Clin Microbiol. 1998;36:2271-2278.
18. Bhutta ZA, Mansurali N. Rapid serologic diagnosis of pediatric typhoid fever in an endemic area: A prospective comparative evaluation of two dot-enzyme immunoassays and the Widal test. Am J Trop Med Hyg. 1999;61:654-657.
19. Chaudhry R, Laxmi BV, Nisar N, et al. Standardization of polymerase chain reaction for the detection of *Salmonella typhi* in typhoid fever. J Clin Pathol. 1997;50:437-439.
20. Ramachandran S, Godfrey JJ, Perera MVF. Typhoid hepatitis. JAMA. 1974;230:236-242.
21. Sitprija V, Pipatanagul V, Boonpucknavig V, et al. Glomerulitis in typhoid fever. Ann Intern Med. 1974;81:210-213.
22. Butler W, Bell WR, Levin J, et al. Typhoid fever: Studies of blood coagulation, bacteremia, and endotoxemia. Arch Intern Med. 1978;138:407-410.
23. Harris JC, DuPont HL, Hornick RB. Fecal leukocytes in diarrheal illness. Ann Intern Med. 1972;76:697-703.
24. Misra S, Diaz PS, Rowley AH. Characteristics of typhoid fever in children and adolescents in a major metropolitan area in the United States. Clin Infect Dis. 1997;24:998-1000.
25. Blaser MJ, Hickman FW, Farmer JJ III, et al. *Salmonella typhi*: The laboratory as a reservoir of infection. J Infect Dis. 1980;142:934-938.
26. Blaser MJ, Lofgren JP. Fatal salmonellosis originating in a clinical microbiology laboratory. J Clin Microbiol. 1981;13:855-858.
27. Rabson AR, Hallett AF, Koornhof JH. Generalized *Yersinia enterocolitica* infection. J Infect Dis. 1975;131:447-451.
28. Spira TJ, Kabins SA. *Yersinia enterocolitica* septicemia with septic arthritis. Arch Intern Med. 1976;136:1305-1308.
29. Marlon A, Gentry L, Merigan TC. Septicemia with *Pasteurella pseudotuberculosis* and liver disease. Arch Intern Med. 1971;127:947-949.
30. Ljungberg P, Valtonen M, Harjola VP, et al. Report of four cases of *Yersinia pseudotuberculosis* septicemia and a literature review. Eur J Clin Microbiol Infect Dis. 1995;14:804-810.
31. Guerrant RL, Lahita RG, Winn WC Jr, et al. Campylobacteriosis in man: Pathogenic mechanisms and review of 91 bloodstream infections. Am J Med. 1978;65:584-592.
32. Carbone KM, Heinrich MC, Quinn TC. Thrombophlebitis and cellulitis due to *Campylobacter fetus* spp *fetus*. Medicine (Baltimore). 1984;64:244-250.
33. Leino R, Kalliomaki JL. Yersiniosis as an internal disease. Ann Intern Med. 1974;81:458-461.
34. Keet EE. *Yersinia enterocolitica* septicemia: Source of infection and incubation period identified. NY State J Med. 1974;74:2226-2230.
35. Taykor BG, Zafarzai MZ, Humphreys DW, et al. Nodular pulmonary infiltrates and septic arthritis associated with *Yersinia enterocolitica* bacteremia. Am Rev Respir Dis. 1977;116:525-529.
36. Bliddal J, Kaliszan S. Prolonged monosymptomatic fever due to *Yersinia enterocolitica*. Acta Med Scand. 1977;201:387-389.
37. Ahvonen P. Human yersiniosis in Finland. II. Clinical features. Ann Clin Res. 1972;4:39-48.
38. Greenwood JR, Flanigan SW, Pickett MJ, et al. Clinical isolation of *Yersinia enterocolitica*: Cold temperature enrichment. J Clin Microbiol. 1975;2:559-560.
39. Forrsstrom J, Viander M, Lehtonen A, et al. Case report: *Yersinia enterocolitica* infection complicated by glomerulonephritis. Scand J Infect Dis. 1977;9:253-256.
40. Guerrant RL, Humphries MK Jr, Butler JE, et al. Tickborne oculoglandular tularemia. Arch Intern Med. 1976;136:811-813.
41. Buchanan TM, Faber LC, Feldman RA. Brucellosis in the United States, 1960-1972: An abattoir-associated disease. I. Clinical features and therapy. Medicine (Baltimore). 1974;53:403-413.
42. Reed WP, Palmer DL, Williams RC Jr, et al. Bubonic plague in the southwestern United States: A review of recent experience. Medicine (Baltimore). 1970;49:465-486.
43. Ferguson NE, Steele L, Crawford CY, et al. Bioterrorism web site resources for infectious disease clinicians and epidemiologists. Clin Infect Dis. 2003;36:1458-1473. Epub 2003 May 22.
44. Mansour-Ghanaei F, Zareh S, Salimi A. GI anthrax: Report of one case confirmed with autopsy. Med Sci Monit. 2002;8:CS73-CS76.
45. Brundage WG, Thuss CJ Jr, Walden DG. Four fatal cases of melioidosis in US soldiers in Vietnam: Bacteriologic and pathologic characteristics. Am J Trop Med Hyg. 1968;17:183-191.
46. Schwartzman W. *Bartonella* (*Rochalimaea*) infections: Beyond cat scratch. Annu Rev Med. 1996;47:355-364.
47. Cuadra M. Salmonellosis complication in human bartonellosis. Tex Rep Biol Med. 1956;14:97-113.
48. Crump JA, Youssef FG, Luby SP, et al. Estimating the incidence of typhoid fever and other febrile illnesses in developing countries. Emerg Infect Dis. 2003;9:539-544.
49. Cunningham BB, Paller AS, Katz BZ. Rat bite fever in a pet lover. J Am Acad Dermatol. 1998;38:330-332.
50. Kowal J. Spirillum fever: Report of a case and review of the literature. N Engl J Med. 1961;264:123-128.
51. Anderson LC, Leary SL, Manning PJ. Rat bite fever in animal research laboratory personnel. Lab Anim Sci. 1983;33:292-294.
52. Heath CW Jr, Alexander AD, Galton MM. Leptospirosis in the United States: Analysis of 483 cases in man, 1949-1961. N Engl J Med. 1965;273:857-864.
53. Edwards GA, Domm BM. Human leptospirosis. Medicine (Baltimore). 1960;39:117-156.
54. Trevejo RT, Schriefer ME, Gage KL, et al. An interstate outbreak of tick-borne relapsing fever among vacationers at a Rocky Mountain cabin. Am J Trop Med Hyg. 1998;58:743-747.
55. Dworkin MS, Anderson DE Jr, Schwan TG, et al. Tick-borne relapsing fever in the northeastern United States and southeastern Canada. Clin Infect Dis. 1998;26:122-131.
56. Jadvar H, Mindelzun RE, Olcott EW, et al. Still the great mimicker: Abdominal tuberculosis. AJR. 1997;168:1455-1460.
57. Horvath KD, Whelan RL. Intestinal tuberculosis: Return of an old disease. Am J Gastroenterol. 1998;93:692-696.
58. Smego RA Jr, Foglia G. Actinomycosis. Clin Infect Dis. 1998;26:1255-1261.
59. Larson EB, Featherstone HJ, Petersdorf RG. Fever of undetermined origin: Diagnosis and follow-up of 105 cases, 1970-1980. Medicine (Baltimore). 1982;61:269-292.
60. Murray HW, Masur H, Senterfit LB, et al. The protean manifestations of *Mycoplasma pneumoniae* infection in adults. Am J Med. 1975;58:229-242.
61. Gregory DW, Schaffner W. Psittacosis. Semin Respir Infect. 1997;12:7-11.
62. Walker DH. Rocky Mountain spotted fever: A seasonal alert. Clin Infect Dis. 1995;20:1111-1117.
63. Dalton MJ, Clarke MJ, Holman RC, et al. National surveillance for Rocky Mountain spotted fever, 1981-1992: Epidemiologic summary and evaluation of risk factors for fatal outcome. Am J Trop Med Hyg. 1995;52:405-413.
64. Walker DH. Gastroenterology of Rocky Mountain spotted fever. Pract Gastroenterol. 1986;10:25-39.
65. Jiminez J, Byrne WJ, Seibert JJ, et al. Gastrointestinal symptoms in Rocky Mountain spotted fever: Histopathologic finding of ulcerative enteritis with vasculitis. Clin Pediatr. 1982;21:581-584.
66. Middleton DB. Rocky Mountain spotted fever: Gastrointestinal and laboratory manifestations. South Med J. 1978;71:629-632.
67. Woodward TE, Pedersen CE Jr, Oster CN, et al. Prompt confirmation of Rocky Mountain spotted fever: Identification of rickettsiae in skin tissues. J Infect Dis. 1976;134:297-301.
68. Duma RJ, Sonenshine DE, Bozeman FM, et al. Epidemic typhus in the United States associated with flying squirrels. JAMA. 1981;245:2318-2323.
69. Centers for Disease Control. Epidemic typhus associated with flying squirrels: United States. MMWR Morb Mortal Wkly Rep. 1982;31:555-561.
70. Marrie TJ, Schlech WF III, Williams JC, et al. Q fever pneumonia associated with exposure to wild rabbits. Lancet. 1986;1:427-429.
71. Bakken JS, Krueth J, Wilson-Nordskog C, et al. Clinical and laboratory characteristics of human granulocytic ehrlichiosis. JAMA. 1996;275:199-205.
72. Jacobs RF, Schultz GE. Ehrlichiosis in children. J Pediatr. 1997;131:184-192.
73. Chow JW, Lu VL. New perspectives on *Legionella* pneumonia: Diagnosis, management and prevention. J Crit Illness. 1988;3:17-27.
74. Sturim HS, Kouchonkos NT, Ahlvin RC. Gastrointestinal manifestations of disseminated histoplasmosis. Am J Surg. 1965;110:435-440.
75. Gordon S, Brennessel DJ, Goldstein JA, et al. Malaria: A city hospital experience. Arch Intern Med. 1988;148:1569-1571.
76. Gorenflot A, Moubri K, Precigout E, et al. Human babesiosis. Ann Trop Med Parasitol. 1998;92:489-501.
77. Boustani MR, Gelfand JA. Babesiosis. Clin Infect Dis. 1996;22:611-615.
78. Lee KC, Yamazaki O, Hamba H, et al. Analysis of 69 patients with amebic liver abscess. J Gastroenterol. 1996;31:40-45.
79. Butler T, Arnold K, Linh NN, et al. Chloramphenicol-resistant typhoid fever in Vietnam associated with R factor. Lancet. 1973;2:983-991.
80. Brown JD, Mo DH, Rhoades ER. Chloramphenicol-resistant *Salmonella typhi* in Saigon. JAMA. 1975;231:162-166.
81. Bhutta ZA, Naqvi SH, Razzaq RA, et al. Multidrug-resistant typhoid in children. Presentation and clinical features. Rev Infect Dis. 1991;13:832-836.
82. Chew SK, Monteiro EH, Lim YS, et al. A 7-day course of ciprofloxacin for enteric fever. J Infect. 1992;25:267-271.
83. Uwaydah AK, al Soub H, Matar I. Randomized prospective study comparing two dosage regimens of ciprofloxacin for the treatment of typhoid fever. J Antimicrob Chemother. 1992;30:707-711.
84. Dutta P, Rasaily R, Saha MR, et al. Ciprofloxacin for treatment of severe typhoid fever in children. Antimicrob Agents Chemother. 1993;37:1197-1199.
85. Murdock DA, Banatvala NA, Bone A, et al. Epidemic ciprofloxacin-resistant *Salmonella typhi* in Tajikistan. Lancet. 1998;351:339.
86. Wain J, Hoa NT, Chinh NT, et al. Quinolone-resistant *Salmonella typhi* in Viet Nam: Molecular basis of resistance and clinical response to treatment. Clin Infect Dis. 1997;25:1401-1410.
87. Rowe B, Ward LR, Threlfall EJ. Multidrug-resistant *Salmonella typhi*: A worldwide epidemic. Clin Infect Dis. 1997;24(Suppl):S106-S109.
88. Schaad UB, abdus Salam M, Aujard Y, et al. Use of fluoroquinolones in pediatrics: Consensus report of an International Society of Chemotherapy commission. Pediatr Infect Dis J. 1995;14:1-9.
89. Doherty CP, Saha SK, Cutting WA. Typhoid fever, ciprofloxacin and growth in young children. Ann Trop Paediatr. 2000;20:297-303.
90. Bethell DB, Hien TT, Phi LT, et al. Effects on growth of single short courses of fluoroquinolones. Arch Dis Child. 1996;74:44-46.
91. Lasserre R, Sangalang RP, Santiago L. Three-day treatment of typhoid fever with two different doses of ceftriaxone, compared to 14-day therapy with chloramphenicol: A randomized trial. J Antimicrob Chemother. 1991;28:765-772.
92. Soe GB, Overturf GD. Treatment of typhoid fever and other systemic salmonellosis with cefotaxime, ceftriaxone, cefoperazone and other newer cephalosporins. Rev Infect Dis. 1987;9:719-736.
93. Memon IA, Billoo AG, Memon HI. Cefixime: An oral option for the treatment of multidrug-resistant enteric fever in children. South Med J. 1997;90:1204-1207.
94. Girgis NI, Sultan Y, Hammad O, et al. Comparison of the efficacy, safety and cost of cefixime, ceftriaxone and aztreonam in the treatment of multi-drug resistant *Salmonella typhi* septicemia in children. Pediatr Infect Dis J. 1995;14:603-605.

95. Rao PM, Rhea JT, Novelline RA. CT diagnosis of mesenteric adenitis. Radiology. 1997;202:145-149.
96. Van Noyen R, Selderslaghs R, Bekaert J, et al. Causative role of *Yersinia* and other enteric pathogens in the appendicular syndrome. Eur J Clin Microbiol Infect Dis. 1991;10:735-741.
97. Winblad S, Nilehn B, Sternby NJ. *Yersinia enterocolitica (Pasteurella X)* in human enteric infections. Br Med J. 1966;2:1363-1366.
98. Mair NS, Mair HJ, Stirk EM, et al. Three cases of acute mesenteric lymphadenitis due to *Pasteurella pseudotuberculosis.* J Clin Pathol. 1960;13:432-439.
99. Tertti R, Vuento R, Mikkola P, et al. Clinical manifestations of *Yersinia pseudotuberculosis* infection in children. Eur J Clin Microbiol Infect Dis. 1989;8:587-591.
100. Carter PB. Pathogenicity of *Yersinia enterocolitica* for mice. Infect Immun. 1975;11:164-170.
101. Garcia-Corbeira P, Ramos JM, Aguado JM, et al. Six cases in which mesenteric lymphadenitis due to non-typhi *Salmonella* caused an appendicitis-like syndrome. Clin Infect Dis. 1995;21:231-232.
102. Lee JH, Rhee PL, Lee JK, et al. The etiology and clinical characteristics of mesenteric adenitis in Korean adults. J Korean Med Sci. 1997;12:105-110.
103. Laasen J. *Yersinia enterocolitica* in drinking-water. Scand J Infect Dis. 1972;4:125-127.
104. Ukarapol N, Sirisanthana V, Wongsawasdi L. *Penicillium marneffei* mesenteric lymphadenitis in human immunodeficiency virus–infected children. J Med Assoc Thai. 1998;81:637-640.
105. Collins DC. Mesenteric lymphadenitis in adolescents simulating appendicitis. Can Med Assoc J. 1936;34:402-405.
106. Asch MJ, Amoury RA, Touloukian RJ, et al. Suppurative mesenteric lymphadenitis: A report of two cases and review of the literature. Am J Surg. 1968;115:570-573.
107. Constantinides CG, Davies MRQ, Cywes S. Suppurative mesenteric lymphadenitis in children: Case reports. S Afr Med J. 1981;60:629-631.
108. Dudley HAF, MacLaren IF. Primary mesenteric abscess. Lancet. 1956;2:1182-1184.
109. Jepsen OB, Korner B, Lauritsen KB, et al. *Yersinia enterocolitica* infection in patients with acute surgical abdominal disease: A prospective study. Scand J Infect Dis. 1976;8:189-194.
110. Zen-Yoji H, Maruyama T, Sakai S, et al. An outbreak of enteritis due to *Yersinia enterocolitica* occurring at a junior high school. Jpn J Microbiol. 1973;17:220-222.
111. Asakawa Y, Akahane S, Kagata N, et al. Two community outbreaks of human infection with *Yersinia enterocolitica.* J Hyg (Lond). 1973;71:715-723.
112. Black RE, Jackson RJ, Tsai T, et al. Epidemic *Yersinia enterocolitica* infection due to contaminated chocolate milk. N Engl J Med. 1978;298:76-79.
113. Vantrappen G, Agg HO, Ponette E, et al. *Yersinia* enteritis and enterocolitis: Gastroenterological aspects. Gastroenterology. 1977;72:220-227.
114. Hammerberg S, Sorger S, Marks MI. Antimicrobial susceptibilities of *Yersinia enterocolitica* biotype 4, serotype O:3. Antimicrob Agents Chemother. 1977;11:566-568.
115. Abdel-Haq NM, Asmar BI, Abuhammour WM, Brown WJ. *Yersinia enterocolitica* infection in children. Pediatr Infect Dis J. 2000;19:954-958.
116. Tauxe RV, Vandepitte J, Wauters G, et al. *Yersinia enterocolitica* infections and pork: The missing link. Lancet. 1987;1:1129-1132.
117. Weber J, Finlayson NB, Mark JBD. Mesenteric lymphadenitis and terminal ileitis due to *Yersinia pseudotuberculosis.* N Engl J Med. 1970;283:172-174.
118. Saari TN, Triplett DA. *Yersinia pseudotuberculosis* mesenteric adenitis. J Pediatr. 1974;85:656-659.
119. Bradford WD, Noce PS, Gutman LT. Pathologic features of enteric infection with *Yersinia enterocolitica.* Arch Pathol. 1974;98:17-22.
120. Weissfeld AS, Sonnenwirth AC. *Yersinia enterocolitica* in adults with gastrointestinal disturbances: Need for cold enrichment. J Clin Microbiol. 1980;11:196-197.
121. Daniels JJHM. Enteral infection with *Pasteurella pseudotuberculosis*: Isolation of the organism from human feces. Br Med J. 1961;2:997.
122. Marks MI, Pai CH, Lafleur L, et al. *Yersinia enterocolitica* gastroenteritis: A prospective study of clinical, bacteriologic, and epidemiologic features. J Pediatr. 1980;96:26-31.
123. Puylaert JB. Mesenteric adenitis and acute terminal ileitis: Ultrasound evaluation using graded compression. Radiology. 1986;161:691-695.
124. Ekberg O, Sjostrom B, Brahme F. Radiological findings in *Yersinia* ileitis. Radiology. 1977;123:15-19.
125. Rao PM, Rhea JT, Novelline RA. Sensitivity and specificity of the individual CT signs of appendicitis: Experience with 200 helical appendiceal CT examinations. J Comput Assist Tomogr. 1997;21:686-692.
126. Ahlqvist J, Ahvonen P, Rasanen JA, Wallgren GR. Enteric infection with *Yersinia enterocolitica*: Large pyroninophilic cell reproduction in mesenteric lymph nodes associated with early production of specific antibodies. Acta Pathol Microbiol Scand [A]. 1971;79:109-122.
127. Braunstein H, Tucker EB, Gibson BC. Mesenteric lymphadenitis due to *Yersinia enterocolitica*: Report of a case. Am J Clin Pathol. 1971;55:506-510.
128. El-Maraghi NRH, Mair NS. The histopathology of enteric infection with *Yersinia pseudotuberculosis.* Am J Clin Pathol. 1979;71:631-639.
129. Gutman LT, Ottesen EA, Quan TJ, et al. An inter-familial outbreak of *Yersinia enterocolitica* enteritis. N Engl J Med. 1973;288:1372-1377.
130. Arvastson B, Damgaard K, Winblad S. Clinical symptoms of infection with *Yersinia enterocolitica.* Scand J Infect Dis. 1971;3:37-40.
131. Wilson HD, McCormick JB, Feeley JC. *Yersinia enterocolitica* infection in a 4-month-old infant associated with infection in household dogs. J Pediatr. 1976;89:767-768.
132. Tacket CO, Narain JP, Sattin R, et al. A multistate outbreak of infections caused by *Yersinia enterocolitica* transmitted by pasteurized milk. JAMA. 1984;251:483-486.
133. Outbreak of *Yersinia enterocolitica*—Washington State. MMWR Morb Mortal Wkly Rep. 1982;31:562-564.
134. Highsmith AK, Feeley JC, Skaliy P, et al. Isolation of *Yersinia enterocolitica* from well water and growth in distilled water. Appl Environ Microbiol. 1977;34:745-750.
135. Snyder JD, Christenson E, Feldman RA. Human *Yersinia enterocolitica* infections in Wisconsin. Am J Med. 1982;72:768-774.
136. Berkowitz FE, Nesheim S. Chylous ascites caused by *Mycobacterium avium* complex and mesenteric lymphadenitis in a child with the acquired immunodeficiency syndrome. Pediatr Infect Dis J. 1993;12:99-101.
137. Morinet F, Monsuez JJ, Roger P, et al. Parvovirus B19 associated with pseudoappendicitis (Letter). Lancet. 1987;2:1466.
138. Chen CM, Chao K, Su IJ. Acute primary Epstein-Barr virus infection presenting as acute abdomen. Pediatr Infect Dis J. 1991;10:471-473.
139. Bhisitkul DM, Tod KM, Listernick R. Adenovirus infection and childhood intussusception. Am J Dis Child. 1992;146:1331-1341.
140. Loria-Cortes R, Lobo-Sanahuja JF. Clinical abdominal angiostrongylosis: A study of 116 children with intestinal eosinophilic granuloma caused by *Angiostrongylus costaricensis.* Am J Trop Med Hyg. 1980;29:538-544.
141. Gutman LT, Wilfert CM, Quan T. Susceptibility of *Yersinia enterocolitica* to trimethoprim-sulfamethoxazole. J Infect Dis. 1973;128(Suppl):S538.
142. Hornstein MJ, Jupeau AM, Scavizzi MR, et al. In vitro susceptibilities of 126 clinical isolates of *Yersinia enterocolitica* to 21 β-lactam antibiotics. Antimicrob Agents Chemother. 1985;27:806-811.
143. Stolk-Engelaar VM, Meis JF, Mulder JA, et al. In-vitro antimicrobial susceptibility of *Yersinia enterocolitica* isolates from stools in The Netherlands from 1982-1991. J Antimicrob Chemother. 1995;36:839-843.
144. Viallet J, MacLean JD, Goresky CA, et al. Arctic trichinosis presenting as prolonged diarrhea. Gastroenterology. 1986;91:938-946.
145. MacLean JD, Poirier L, Gyorkos TW, et al. Epidemiologic and serologic definition of primary and secondary trichinosis in the Arctic. J Infect Dis. 1992;165:908-912.
146. Kagan IG. Serodiagnosis of trichinosis. In: Cohen S, Sadun EH, eds. Immunology of Parasitic Infections. Oxford: Blackwell Scientific; 1976:143-151.
147. Mahmoud AAF. Strongyloidiasis. Clin Infect Dis. 1996;23:949-952.
148. Scowden EB, Schaffner W, Stone WJ. Overwhelming strongyloidiasis: An unappreciated opportunistic infection. Medicine (Baltimore). 1978;57:527-544.
149. Morgan JS, Schaffner W, Stone WJ. Opportunistic strongyloidiasis in renal transplant recipients. Transplantation. 1986;42:518-524.
150. Cadranel JF, Eugene C. Another example of *Strongyloides stercoralis* infection associated with cimetidine in an immunosuppressed patient. Gut. 1986;27:1229.
151. Brosset C, Hovette P, Raphenon G, et al. HTLV1 and coinfections. Med Trop (Mars). 1991;51:399-406.
152. Porto MA, Muniz A, Oliveira J Jr, Carvalho EM. Clinical and immunological consequences of the association between HTLV-1 and strongyloidiasis. Rev Soc Bras Med Trop. 2002;35:641-649. Epub 2003 February 26.
153. Pelletier LL Jr, Baker CB, Gam AA, et al. Diagnosis and evaluation of treatment of chronic strongyloidiasis in ex-prisoners of war. J Infect Dis. 1988;157:573-576.
154. Berk SL, Verghese A, Alvarez S, et al. Clinical and epidemiologic features of strongyloidiasis: A prospective study in rural Tennessee. Arch Intern Med. 1987;147:1257-1261.
155. Lima JP, Delgado PG. Diagnosis of strongyloidiasis: Importance of Baermann's method. Am J Diagn Dis. 1961;6:899-904.
156. De Kaminsky RG. Evaluation of three methods for laboratory diagnosis of *Strongyloides stercoralis* infection. J Parasitol. 1993;79:277-280.
157. Elliot DE. Schistosomiasis. Pathophysiology, diagnosis, and treatment. Gastroenterol Clin North Am. 1996;25:599-625.
158. Salazar SA, Gutierrez C, Berk SL. Value of the agar plate method for the diagnosis of intestinal strongyloides. Diagn Microbiol Infect Dis. 1995;23:141-145.
159. Jongwutiwes S, Charoenkorn M, Sitthichareonchai P, et al. Increased sensitivity of routine laboratory detection of *Strongyloides stercoralis* and hookworm by agar-plate culture. Trans R Soc Trop Med Hyg. 1999;93:398-400.
160. Beal CB, Viens P, Grant RGL, Hughes JM. A new technique for sampling duodenal contents: Demonstration of upper small-bowel pathogens. Am J Trop Med Hyg. 1970;19:349-352.
161. Genta RM. Predictive value of an enzyme-linked immunosorbent assay (ELISA) for the serodiagnosis of strongyloidiasis. Am J Clin Pathol. 1988;89:391-394.
162. Gyorkos TW, Genta RM, Viens P, MacLean JD. Seroepidemiology of *Strongyloides* infection in the Southeast Asian refugee population in Canada. Am J Epidemiol. 1990;132:257-264.
163. Gam AA, Neva FA, Krotoski WA. Comparative sensitivity and specificity of ELISA and IHA for serodiagnosis of strongyloidiasis with larval antigens. Am J Trop Med Hyg. 1987;37:157-161.
164. Blumenthal DS, Schultz MG. Incidence of intestinal obstruction in children infected with *Ascaris lumbricoides.* Am J Trop Med Hyg. 1975;24:801-805.
165. Akgun Y. Intestinal obstruction caused by *Ascaris lumbricoides.* Dis Colon Rectum. 1996;39:1159-1163.
166. Krige JEJ, Lewis G, Bornman PC. Recurrent pancreatitis caused by a calcified ascaris in the duct of Wirsung. Am J Gastroenterol. 1987;82:256-257.
167. Schantz PM, Glickman LT. Toxocaral visceral larva migrans. N Engl J Med. 1978;298:436-439.
168. Glickman LT, Magnaval JF. Zoonotic roundworm infections. Infect Dis Clin North Am. 1993;7:717-732.
169. Thompson DE, Bundy DAP, Cooper ES, et al. Epidemiological characteristics of *Toxocara canis* zoonotic infection of children in a Caribbean community. Bull World Health Organ. 1986;64:283-290.
170. Glickman LT, Magnaval J-F, Domanski LM, et al. Visceral larva migrans in French adults: A new disease syndrome. Am J Epidemiol. 1987;125:1019-1034.

171. Grove DI, Warren KS, Mahmoud AAF. Algorithms in the diagnosis and management of exotic diseases. VII. Trichinosis. J Infect Dis. 1975;132:485-488.

172. Campbell WC. Trichinella and Trichinosis. New York: Plenum; 1983.

173. Singal M, Schantz PM, Werner SB. Trichinosis acquired at sea: Report of an outbreak. Am J Trop Med Hyg. 1976;25:675-681.

174. Petri WA Jr, Holsinger JR, Pearson RD. Common-source outbreak of trichinosis associated with eating raw home-butchered pork. South Med J. 1988;81:1056-1058.

175. Trichinosis outbreaks associated with horsemeat. Parasitol Today. 1986;2:295.

176. Moorhead A, Grunenwald PE, Dietz VJ, Schantz PM. Trichinellosis in the United States, 1991-1996: Declining but not gone. Am J Trop Med Hyg. 1999;60:66-69.

177. Kwee HG, Sautter RL. Anisakiasis. Am Fam Physician. 1987;36:137-140.

178. Smith JW, Wooten R. Anisakis and anisakiasis. Adv Parasitol. 1978;16:93-163.

179. Pinkus GS, Coolidge C. Intestinal anisakiasis: First case report from North America. Am J Med. 1975;59:114-120.

180. Richman RH, Lewicki AM. Right ileocolitis secondary to anisakiasis. Am J Roentgenol Radium Ther Nucl Med. 1973;119:329-331.

181. Yokogawa M, Yoshimura H. Clinicopathologic studies on larval anisakiasis in Japan. Am J Trop Med Hyg. 1967;16:723-734.

182. Whittner M, Turner JW, Jacquette G, et al. Eustrongylidiasis—A parasitic infection acquired by eating sushi. N Engl J Med. 1989;320:1124-1126.

183. Cross JH. Intestinal capillariasis. Clin Microbiol Rev. 1992;5:120-129.

184. Dronda F, Chaves F, Sanz A, et al. Human intestinal capillariasis in an area of nonendemicity: Case report and review. Clin Infect Dis. 1993;17:909-912.

185. Fresh JW, Cross JH, Reyes V, et al. Necropsy findings in intestinal capillariasis. Am J Trop Med Hyg. 1972;21:169-173.

186. Morera P. Abdominal angiostrongyliasis. Clin Trop Med Commun Dis. 1987;2:747-754.

187. Hulbert TV, Larsen RA, Chandrasoma PT. Abdominal angiostrongyliasis mimicking acute appendicitis and Meckel's diverticulum: Report of a case in the United States and review. Clin Infect Dis. 1992;14:836-840.

188. Mahmoud AA. Schistosomiasis. N Engl J Med. 1977;297:1329-1331.

189. Farid Z, Trabolsi B, Hafez A. Acute schistosomiasis mansoni (Katayama syndrome). Ann Trop Med Parasitol. 1986;80:563-564.

190. Brockelman WY, Upatham ES, Viyanant V, et al. Measurement of incidence of the human liver fluke, Opisthorchis viverrini, in northeast Thailand. Trans R Soc Trop Med Hyg. 1987;81:327-335.

191. MacLean JD, Arthur JR, Ward BJ, et al. Common-source outbreak of acute infection due to the North American liver fluke Metorchis conjunctus. Lancet. 1996;347:154-158.

192. Liu LX, Harinasuta KT. Liver and intestinal flukes. Gastroenterol Clin North Am. 1996;25:627-636.

193. Arjona R, Riancho JA, Aguado JM, et al. Fascioliasis in developed countries: A review of class and aberrant forms of the disease. Medicine (Baltimore). 1995;74:13-23.

194. Warren KS, Mahmoud AAF. Algorithms in the diagnosis and management of exotic diseases. XXI. Liver, intestinal and lung flukes. J Infect Dis. 1977;135:692-696.

195. Adams KO, Jungkind DL, Bergquist EJ, et al. Intestinal fluke infection as a result of eating sushi. Am J Clin Pathol. 1986;86:688-689.

196. Goldsmith RS. Chronic diarrhea in returning travelers: Intestinal parasite infection with the fluke Metagonimus yokogawai. South Med J. 1978;71:1513-1515.

197. Harrell LW, Deardorff TL. Human nanophyetiasis: Transmission by handling naturally infected coho salmon (Oncorhynchus kisutch). J Infect Dis. 1990;161:146-148.

198. Huffman JE, Fried B. Echinostoma and echinostomiasis. Adv Parasitol. 1990;29:215-269.

199. Schantz PM. Tapeworms (cestodiasis). Gastroenterol Clin North Am. 1996;25:637-653.

200. Ammann RW, Eckert J. Cestodes. Echinococcus. Gastroenterol Clin North Am. 1996;25:655-689.

201. Craig PS, Rogan MT, Allan JC. Detection, screening and community epidemiology of taeniid cestode zoonoses: cystic echinococcosis, alveolar echinococcosis and neurocysticercosis. Adv Parasitol. 1996;38:169-250.

202. Ackers JP. Gut coccidia—Isospora, Cryptosporidium, Cyclospora and Sarcocystis. Semin Gastrointest Dis. 1997;8:33-44.

203. DeHovitz JA, Page JW, Boncy M, et al. Clinical manifestations and therapy of Isospora belli infection in patients with the acquired immunodeficiency syndrome. N Engl J Med. 1986;315:87-90.

204. Guerrant RL, Bobak DA. Bacterial and protozoal gastroenteritis. N Engl J Med. 1991;325:327-340.

205. Pape JW, Verdier R, Johnson WD. Treatment and prophylaxis of Isospora belli infection in patients with the acquired immunodeficiency syndrome. N Engl J Med. 1989;320:1044-1047.

206. Butler WP. Dientamoeba fragilis. An unusual intestinal pathogen. Dig Dis Sci. 1996;41:1811-1813.

207. Cuffari C, Oligny L, Seidman EG. Dientamoeba fragilis masquerading as allergic colitis. J Pediatr Gastroenterol Nutr. 1998;26:16-20.

208. Lee M, Hodges WG, Huggins TL, Lee EL. Eosinophilic gastroenteritis. South Med J. 1996;89:189-194.

209. Schoonbroodt D, Horsmans Y, Laka A, et al. Eosinophilic gastroenteritis presenting with colitis and cholangitis. Dig Dis Sci. 1995;40:308-314.

210. Cupps TR, Fauci AS. The Vasculitides. Philadelphia: WB Saunders; 1981.

211. Lhote F, Cohen P, Guillevin L. Polyarteritis nodosa, microscopic polyangiitis and Churg-Strauss syndrome. Lupus. 1998;7:238-258.

212. Haeberle MG, Griffen WO Jr. Eosinophilia and regional enteritis: A possible diagnostic aid. Am J Dig Dis. 1972;17:200-204.

213. Beeson P. Cancer and eosinophilia. N Engl J Med. 1983;309:792-793.

CHAPTER 95

Foodborne Disease

ALICIA M. FRY

CHRISTOPHER R. BRADEN

PATRICIA M. GRIFFIN

JAMES M. HUGHES

Foodborne diseases result from ingestion of a wide variety of foods contaminated with pathogenic microorganisms, microbial toxins, or chemicals. From 1993 to 1997, a mean of approximately 550 outbreaks of foodborne disease affecting over 17,000 persons in the United States were reported annually to the Centers for Disease Control and Prevention (CDC).[1] These figures certainly underestimate the magnitude of the problem. The actual incidence of foodborne disease is unknown, but it is estimated to be approximately 76 million cases, with 325,000 hospitalizations and 5000 deaths each year.[2] Trends in the incidence of a number of bacterial foodborne pathogens have been followed by CDC's Foodborne Diseases Active Surveillance Network (FoodNet). FoodNet has conducted surveillance for nine foodborne pathogens since 1996 in several states, with 13% of the U.S. population in active surveillance catchment areas in 2002. Analysis of surveillance data from 1996 through 2002 has shown a decrease in the incidence of illnesses due to a number of important pathogens: the incidence of *Campylobacter* isolates identified decreased by 24%, that of *Listeria* decreased 38%, and that of *Yersinia* decreased 43%, indicating important advances in food safety (Figure 95-1).[3] In contrast, the incidences of *Salmonella,* of *Escherichia coli* O157, and of *Shigella* isolates did not change significantly.[3] Certain serotypes of *Salmonella* had important increases, such as *Salmonella* Newport, which increased 87%. In addition, *Vibrio* isolates increased 126% from 1996 to 2002.[3] Table 95-1 shows the incidences of isolates identified for seven foodborne pathogens in 2002. Clearly, foodborne diseases are common and can be severe, and food safety programs need to be intensified.

Although a wide variety of microorganisms and toxins can cause foodborne disease, this discussion focuses mostly on foodborne disease syndromes that are acute and whose clinical features include gastrointestinal manifestations. The diseases to be discussed and the frequency with which outbreaks were reported to the CDC from 1973 to 2000 are indicated in Table 95-2.

The spectrum of foodborne diseases has expanded in recent years. New foodborne agents causing severe disease have emerged (e.g., *E. coli* O157-H7, *Cyclospora cayetanensis*)[4]; previously uncommon food vehicles such as fresh fruits and vegetables have become important sources of foodborne disease; and *Salmonella* and *Campylobacter* have become increasingly resistant to antimicrobial drugs. Important food sources have been defined for other established pathogens, such as *Vibrio cholerae* O1 and *Listeria monocytogenes*. Postinfectious syndromes have been recognized as important sequelae of foodborne infections, including hemolytic uremic syndrome after infections with *E. coli* O157-H7,[5] Reiter's syndrome after salmonellosis,[6] and Guillain-Barré syndrome after campylobacteriosis.[7] Centralization of the food supply increases the risk for nationwide outbreaks. Globalization of the food supply has facilitated exposure to foodborne pathogens from other parts of the world. The growing population of persons with immunosuppressive conditions or treatments and the increasing number of institutionalized older persons mean that more of the population is exquisitely susceptible to microbial contamination of food.

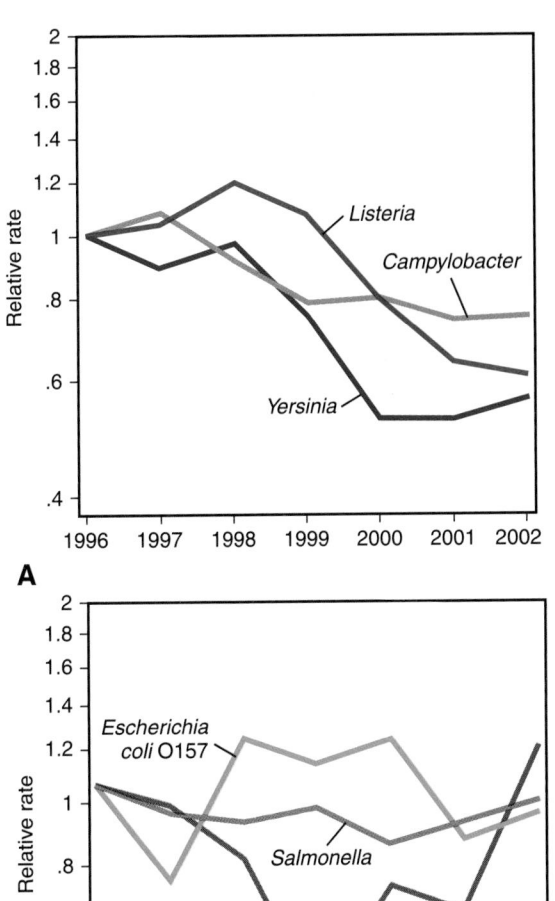

FIGURE 95-1. Foodborne Diseases Active Surveillance Network, United States, 1996-2002. **A,** Relative rates (compared with 1996) of laboratory-diagnosed cases of *Campylobacter, Listeria,* and *Yersinia,* by year. **B,** Relative rates (compared with 1996) of laboratory-diagnosed cases of *Escherichia coli* O157, *Salmonella,* and *Shigella,* by year.

TABLE 95-1 Annual Incidence of Diagnosed Infections Identified through Active Surveillance in the Foodborne Disease Active Surveillance Network—United States, 2002

Pathogen	Incidence per 100,000 Population
Campylobacter	13.17
Escherichia coli O157	1.73
Listeria	0.27
Salmonella	16.10
Shigella	10.34
Vibrio	0.27
Yersinia	0.44
Cryptosporidium	1.42
Cyclospora	0.11
Hemolytic uremic syndrome*	1.78

*Incidence per 100,000 children aged less than 5 years.

TABLE 95-2 Foodborne Disease Outbreak-Associated Cases of Known Cause Reported to the CDC, 1973-2000

Etiologic Agent	Outbreaks Number	Outbreaks %	Outbreak-Associated Cases Number	Outbreak-Associated Cases %
Bacterial				
Bacillus cereus	121	2.0	2787	1.2
Campylobacter	140	2.3	3696	1.5
Clostridium botulinum	316	5.2	713	0.3
Clostridium perfringens	364	5.9	22,885	9.5
Escherichia coli	202	3.3	7692	3.2
Listeria monocytogenes	13	0.2	466	0.2
Salmonella	2147	35.1	102,574	42.7
Shigella	216	3.5	24,631	10.2
Staphylococcus aureus	517	8.4	22,000	9.2
Streptococcus, group A	16	0.3	2178	0.9
Vibrio cholerae	13	0.2	960	0.4
Vibrio cholerae non-O1	3	0.0	13	0.0
Vibrio parahaemolyticus	51	0.8	1371	0.6
Yersinia enterocolitica	11	0.2	844	0.4
Other bacteria	27	0.4	1170	0.5
Chemical				
Ciguatoxin	376	6.1	1610	0.7
Heavy metals	58	0.9	826	0.3
Mushroom poisoning	75	1.2	239	0.1
Scombroid toxin	423	6.9	2309	1.0
Shellfish	37	0.6	283	0.1
Other chemical	161	2.6	1443	0.6
Parasitic				
Giardia	22	0.4	547	0.2
Trichinella spiralis	152	2.5	1113	0.5
Other parasites	29	0.5	2531	1.1
Viral				
Hepatitis A	219	3.6	7188	3.0
Norovirus	390	6.4	26,374	11.0
Other viruses	24	0.4	1985	0.8
Total	6123	100	240,428	100

CDC, Centers for Disease Control and Prevention.

PATHOGENESIS AND CLINICAL FEATURES

Foodborne disease can appear as an isolated sporadic case or, less frequently, as an outbreak of illnesses affecting a group of people after a common food exposure. The diagnosis of foodborne disease should be considered when an acute illness with gastrointestinal or neurologic manifestations affects two or more persons who have shared a meal during the previous week. Important clues to the etiologic agent are provided by both the symptoms and the incubation period.

Foodborne Disease Caused by Microbial Agents or Their Toxins

The toxic mechanisms of foodborne bacterial disease are summarized in Table 95-3.

Nausea and Vomiting within 1 to 6 Hours. The major etiologic considerations are *Staphylococcus aureus* and *Bacillus cereus.* The relatively short incubation period reflects the fact that these diseases are caused by a preformed enterotoxin. Staphylococcal food poisoning is characterized by vomiting (82% of cases) and diarrhea (68%); fever is relatively uncommon (16%).[8] Staphylococci responsible for episodes of food poisoning produce one or more enterotoxins; multiple serologically distinct enterotoxins have been and continue to be identified (currently, A through Q, excluding F) but not all are emetic.[9] The staphylococcal enterotoxins are grouped together with toxic shock syndrome toxin-1 (TSST-1) as pyrogenic toxin superantigens; enterotoxin B and C have been implicated in nonmenstrual toxic shock syndrome.[9] Although the mechanism of action of these enterotoxins in humans has not been clarified, studies in monkeys and cats suggest that the enterotoxin produces its emetic action after interaction with abdominal viscera,

TABLE 95-3 Pathogenic Mechanisms in Bacterial Foodborne Disease

Preformed Toxin	Toxin Production in Vivo	Tissue Invasion	Toxin Production and/or Tissue Invasion
Staphylococcus aureus Bacillus cereus (short incubation) Clostridium botulinum	Clostridium perfringens B. cereus (long incubation) C. botulinum (infant botulism) Enterotoxigenic Escherichia coli Vibrio cholerae O1 or O139 V. cholerae non-O1 Shiga toxin–producing E. coli	Campylobacter jejuni Salmonella Shigella Invasive E. coli	Vibrio parahaemolyticus Yersinia enterocolitica

and that the sensory stimulus is carried to the vomiting center in the brain by the vagus and sympathetic nerves.[9]

Enterotoxigenic staphylococci isolated from implicated foods in outbreaks are most often lysed by group III phages; less commonly, they are lysed by both group I and group III phages or by group I phages alone.[10] More than 99% of enterotoxigenic staphylococci associated with food poisoning are coagulase positive; occasionally, an outbreak caused by enterotoxigenic *Staphylococcus epidermidis* has been reported.[11] In the past, strains producing type A enterotoxin alone accounted for most of the reported outbreaks of staphylococcal food poisoning in the United States.[8]

B. cereus strains can cause two types of food poisoning syndromes, one characterized primarily by nausea and vomiting with an incubation period of 1 to 6 hours (short-incubation "emetic" syndrome) and a second manifested primarily by abdominal cramps and diarrhea with an incubation period of 8 to 16 hours (long-incubation "diarrhea" syndrome).[12] The short-incubation syndrome, characterized by vomiting (100% of cases), abdominal cramps (100%), and, less frequently, diarrhea (33%),[13] is caused by a toxin resistant to heat, pH, and proteolysis. Although its structure has long been a mystery, recent detection by the use of Hep-2 cells allowed its isolation and structure determination. It has been named cereulide and consists of a ring structure of three repeats of four amino acids with a molecular weight of 1.2 kilodaltons. The complete mechanism of action remains to be determined, but it has been shown to bind to the 5-hydroxytryptamine-3 (5-HT$_3$) receptor of the vagus afferent nerve.[12]

Another clue to the cause of both staphylococcal and short-incubation *B. cereus* outbreaks is provided by the fact that the illnesses are of short duration, usually lasting less than 12 hours.[8,13]

Abdominal Cramps and Diarrhea within 8 to 16 Hours. The major etiologic considerations for this syndrome, which is also enterotoxin mediated, are *Clostridium perfringens* and *B. cereus*. In contrast to staphylococcal food poisoning and the short-incubation *B. cereus* disease, which are caused by ingestion of preformed enterotoxins in food, *C. perfringens* and long-incubation *B. cereus* food poisoning are caused by toxins produced in vivo, accounting for the longer incubation period. In *C. perfringens* food poisoning, the most common symptoms are diarrhea and abdominal cramps. Although nausea may occur, vomiting and fever are uncommon, occurring in less than 10% of the patients.[14,15] Although five types of *C. perfringens* toxin have been described, type A is almost always the toxin causing this food poisoning syndrome.[15] *C. perfringens* enterotoxin is a heat-labile protein with a molecular weight of approximately 35,000 daltons[16] and synthesized by the vegetative cells of *C. perfringens* in the gastrointestinal tract; the enterotoxin is produced during sporulation.[17] Studies in rabbits and rats indicate that the enterotoxin is active throughout the small intestine, with greatest activity in the ileum, in which net secretion of sodium and fluid and inhibition of chloride and glucose absorption occur.[18,19] The enterotoxin damages brush borders of epithelial cells at villus tips.[19]

B. cereus strains, which cause a similar long-incubation syndrome that produces diarrhea (96%) and abdominal cramps (75%), sometimes vomiting (33%), and rarely fever,[13] elaborate two different three-component enterotoxins.[12] Some strains produce both of the three-component enterotoxins, whereas other strains contain genes for only one of them. One toxin has dermonecrotic and vascular permeability activity and causes fluid accumulation in rabbit ileal loops.[12]

Although nausea occurs in many patients with *C. perfringens* and long-incubation *B. cereus* food poisoning, vomiting occurs infrequently. In fact, occurrence of vomiting in more than one third of affected persons suggests that these organisms are not involved. Although these illnesses last longer than staphylococcal and short-incubation *B. cereus* food poisoning last, symptoms usually resolve within 24 hours.[13,20] However, in some long-incubation *B. cereus* outbreaks, the mean duration of illness can be more than 2 days, and occasionally illness may last several weeks.[21-23]

Fever, Abdominal Cramps, and Diarrhea within 16 to 48 Hours. The major etiologic considerations for this syndrome are *Salmonella*, *Shigella*, *Campylobacter jejuni*, *Vibrio parahaemolyticus*, and *E. coli*. Bloody diarrhea and vomiting occur in a varying proportion of patients infected with these pathogens. These illnesses usually resolve within 2 to 7 days.

C. jejuni is the most common foodborne bacterial pathogen.[2] In contrast to the illnesses caused by other organisms in this group, *C. jejuni* food poisoning is characterized by a longer incubation period of typically 3 to 4 days.[24] Nontyphoidal *Salmonella* is the second most common foodborne bacterial pathogen and the most common bacterial pathogen associated with foodborne outbreaks.[1,2] The median incubation period is 6 to 48 hours.[25] Like *C. jejuni* food poisoning, *E. coli* O157-H7 food poisoning has a median incubation period of 3 to 4 days.[26]

Infrequently, outbreaks of a febrile gastroenteritis caused by *L. monocytogenes* in previously healthy persons have been reported.[27-30] This syndrome is characterized by watery and frequent diarrhea, fever, abdominal cramps, headache, and myalgias, with a median incubation period of 20 to 31 hours.

The diarrhea experienced by patients with *V. cholerae* non-O1 infection is sometimes bloody, and fever may be present.[31,32]

Abdominal Cramps and Watery Diarrhea within 16 to 72 Hours. The major etiologic considerations in this syndrome are enterotoxigenic strains of *E. coli*, *V. parahaemolyticus*, *V. cholerae* non-O1, and, in endemic areas, *V. cholerae* O1 and O139; *C. jejuni*, *Salmonella*, and *Shigella* may also cause this syndrome. Enterotoxins synthesized in vivo are responsible for the syndrome caused by *V. cholerae* O1, *V. cholerae* non-O1,[33] and enterotoxigenic strains of *E. coli*[34]; enterotoxigenic or cytotoxic substances, or both, may also play a role in the pathogenesis of this syndrome when it is caused by *Salmonella*,[35,36] *Shigella*,[37-39] or *V. parahaemolyticus*.[40,41]

Severe cholera manifests as a profuse, watery diarrhea accompanied by muscular cramps. With the other infections, fever and vomiting occur in a minority of cases.[31] With the exception of cholera, which may last for 5 days, and disease caused by *V. cholerae* non-O1, which may last for 2 to 12 days, these illnesses usually resolve within 72 to 96 hours. However, in one documented enterotoxigenic *E. coli* outbreak, the median duration of illness was 7 days.[42]

Vomiting and Nonbloody Diarrhea within 24 to 48 Hours. Noroviruses (formerly Norwalk-like viruses) are the most common of known foodborne pathogens, causing an estimated 9.2 million illnesses per year, or two thirds of all foodborne illnesses caused by known pathogens.[2] Even more cases of acute gastroenteritis are caused by non-foodborne transmission of noroviruses, such as person-to-person or fomite contamination.[43] Vomiting and diarrhea are often the presenting symptoms, with onset 1 to 2 days after exposure. The syndrome progresses to include watery, nonbloody diarrhea, abdominal pain, and nausea. Vomiting is more common among children, whereas diarrhea is more likely to predominate among adults; however, both symptoms occur in most patients regardless of age.[43] Fever occurs in one third to one half of patients, is usually low grade, and lasts for less than 24 hours. Symptoms usually resolve in 1 to 3 days.[43] A group of related viruses in the *Caliciviridae* family, most notably the sapoviruses, may also cause similar foodborne illness, but such reports are few.

It is impossible to distinguish between norovirus and some bacterial causes of gastroenteritis, such as enterotoxigenic strains of *E. coli* (ETEC), for a single patient based on clinical course, but a few simple criteria have been used epidemiologically to assess whether norovirus was the likely cause of outbreaks. Criteria that suggest norovirus infection include (1) failure to detect a bacterial or parasitic pathogen in stool specimens, (2) the occurrence of vomiting in greater than 50% of patients, (3) a mean duration of illness of 12 to 60 hours, and (4) a mean incubation period of 24 to 48 hours.[43]

Fever and Abdominal Cramps within 16 to 48 Hours, without Diarrhea. *Yersinia enterocolitica* has been incriminated as a cause of foodborne outbreaks in the United States and is a more common cause of foodborne disease in Northern Europe and Canada.[44-47] In young children, febrile diarrhea is the most common presentation.[44] In older children and adults, the clinical illness may be prolonged, and one syndrome may closely resemble acute appendicitis; nausea and vomiting are relatively uncommon, occurring in less than 25% to 40% of the cases.[47-49] Duration of the illness ranges from 24 hours to 4 weeks.[45,49]

Bloody Diarrhea without Fever within 72 to 120 Hours. The distinctive syndrome of hemorrhagic colitis has been linked to Shiga toxin–producing strains of *E. coli*, most often serotype O157-H7.[50,51] These strains produce cytotoxins that affect Vero kidney cell cultures and are neutralized by antiserum to Shiga toxin; they have been called Shiga toxins or verotoxins.[52,53] The toxins are absorbed from the gut and damage vascular endothelial cells in target organs such as the gut and kidney.[54] The illness is characterized by severe abdominal cramping and diarrhea, which is initially watery but may later be grossly bloody.[51] Patients with uncomplicated infection usually remain afebrile. The mean incubation period in outbreaks is 3 to 8 days. The duration of uncomplicated illness ranges from 1 to 12 days. The development of fever and leukocytosis may herald hemolytic uremic syndrome, which has a 3% to 5% mortality rate in children.[55] Hemolytic uremic syndrome occurs in 8% of infections in children, with onset about 1 week after the beginning of the diarrheal illness.[56] The case-fatality rate in outbreaks has been 0% to 2%, but rates as high as 16% to 35% have been observed in nursing homes.[56] Other *E. coli* serogroups that produce Shiga toxins can also cause hemorrhagic colitis and hemolytic uremic syndrome, and two, O104 and O111, have caused outbreaks in the United States.[57-59]

Nausea, Vomiting, Diarrhea, and Paralysis within 18 to 36 Hours. The occurrence of acute gastrointestinal symptoms simultaneously with or just before the onset of descending weakness or paralysis strongly suggests the diagnosis of foodborne botulism. Constipation is common once the neurologic syndrome is well established, but nausea and vomiting occur at onset in 50% of the patients, and diarrhea occurs in approximately 20% to 25%.[60-62] The pathogenesis of the acute gastrointestinal symptoms is not understood; the botulinal toxins, which inhibit acetylcholine release from nerve endings,[63,64] do not appear to be responsible. The disease in humans is usually caused by one of three immunologically distinct, heat-labile protein neurotoxins, designated A, B, and E,[65] which are produced after germination of *Clostridium botulinum* spores in inadequately processed foods. The disease in older children and adults results from ingestion of preformed toxin. The syndrome of infant botulism results from ingestion of spores, with subsequent toxin production in vivo.[66-68] Both illnesses last from several weeks to several months. Clinical suspicion is critical if the disease is to be correctly diagnosed.[69]

Guillain-Barré syndrome has been associated with serologic evidence of recent infection with *C. jejuni*.[7] In a multicenter study of 118 patients in the United States with Guillain-Barré syndrome, 36% had serologic evidence of a preceding *C. jejuni* infection.[7] When preceding

diarrheal illness is reported, it typically occurs 1 to 3 weeks before the onset of neurologic symptoms.[7] In contrast to botulism, this syndrome is usually manifested by an ascending paralysis accompanied by sensory findings and abnormal nerve conduction velocity.

Systemic Illness. This discussion has focused on diseases often transmitted by foods and manifested primarily by gastrointestinal or neurologic symptoms and signs. However, some foodborne diseases manifest mainly as invasive infections in immunocompromised patients. Listeriosis typically affects pregnant women, fetuses, and persons with compromised cellular immunity, who present with fever, myalgias, and primary bacteremia or meningitis.[70] Identified sources are most often foods, including cold processed meats and dairy products.[70-72] The incubation period is prolonged, ranging from 2 to 6 weeks, and the case-fatality rate is 23%.[73] *Vibrio vulnificus* infections cause fulminant myonecrosis or primary bacteremia after ingestion of raw oysters. This severe syndrome is seen almost exclusively in patients with underlying liver disease, especially if associated with iron-overload states.[74]

Other infectious diseases with primary symptoms outside the gastrointestinal and neurologic systems that can be transmitted by foods include group A β-hemolytic streptococci (most commonly in potato and egg salads), typhoid fever (shellfish), brucellosis (goat's milk cheese), anthrax (meat), tuberculosis (milk), Q fever (milk), hepatitis A (shellfish, fresh produce), trichinosis (pork), toxoplasmosis (beef), anisakiasis (fish), and tapeworms (beef, pork, and fish).

Postinfection Syndromes. Reactive arthritis (Reiter's syndrome) may develop after infection with *Salmonella, Yersinia, Campylobacter,* or *Shigella*, as well as after nonfoodborne infections such nongonococcal urethritis and *Cyclospora* infection.[75,76] Reiter's syndrome consists of the classic triad of aseptic inflammatory polyarthritis, urethritis, and conjunctivitis, although not all components occur in all patients. Over two thirds of patients are HLA-B27 positive, suggesting an important component of genetic predisposition.[75] Among 217 patients in an outbreak caused by *Salmonella* serotype Enteritidis enterocolitis in Washington state, 32% had symptoms of reactive arthritis and 3% had Reiter's syndrome.[77] Increased severity and longer duration of diarrheal illness were associated with the development of reactive arthritis.

Foodborne Disease Caused by Nonbacterial Toxins

Nausea, Vomiting, and Abdominal Cramps within 1 Hour. The major etiologic considerations for this syndrome are heavy metals; copper, zinc, tin, and cadmium have caused foodborne outbreaks.[78-82] Incubation periods most often range from 5 to 15 minutes. Nausea, vomiting, and abdominal cramps result from irritation of the gastric mucosa and usually resolve within 2 to 3 hours after removal of the offending agent during emesis.

Paresthesias within 1 Hour. When patients have this symptom, fish poisoning, shellfish poisoning (Table 95-4), the so-called Chinese restaurant syndrome, and niacin poisoning are the major possibilities. Histamine fish poisoning (scombroid) is characterized by symptoms resembling those of a histamine reaction. Burning of the mouth and throat, flushing, headache, and dizziness are common; abdominal cramps, nausea, vomiting, and diarrhea also occur in most cases.[83] In severe cases, urticaria and bronchospasm may also occur. Symptoms are thought to result from histamine and inhibitors of histamine degradation produced in fish flesh by the enzymatic decarboxylation of histidine by certain marine bacteria.[84,85] In an outbreak traced to tuna sashimi, a strain of *Klebsiella pneumoniae* capable of producing large quantities of histamine was implicated.[86] Symptoms usually resolve in a few hours.

Three types of shellfish poisoning should be considered: paralytic (PSP), neurotoxic (NSP), and amnesic (ASP).[87,88] PSP is characterized by paresthesias of the mouth, lips, face, and extremities.[89-93] In severe cases, dyspnea, dysphagia, muscle weakness or frank paralysis, ataxia, and respiratory insufficiency may occur.[91,92] Respiratory failure may occur during the first 12 hours of the illness.[91] Some patients also have nausea, vomiting, and diarrhea.[87] The disease is caused by neurotoxic substances in dinoflagellates, one of which is known as *saxitoxin*.

TABLE 95-4 Fish and Shellfish Poisoning Syndromes

Syndrome	Incubation Period	Duration	Geographic Location*	Season
Histamine fish poisoning (scombroid)	5 min-1hr	Few hours	Primarily coastal areas (Hawaii, California)	Year-round
Ciguatera	1-6 hr	Few days to few months	35 degrees N to 35 degrees S latitude (Hawaii, Florida)	Feb.-Sept.
Paralytic shellfish poisoning	5 min-4 hr	Few hours to few days	Above 30 degrees N and below 30 degrees S latitude (New England, West Coast)	May-Nov.
Neurotoxic shellfish poisoning	5 min-4 hr	Few hours to few days	Gulf and Atlantic coasts of Florida (Florida)	Spring, Fall
Amnesic shellfish poisoning	15 min-6 hr	Few days to permanent	Coastal areas?	Uncertain

*Location of U.S. outbreaks in parentheses.

Bivalve mollusks feed on these dinoflagellates; the toxins are concentrated in their flesh but do not affect the mollusks.[89] Saxitoxin appears to be the only neurotoxin produced by *Gonyaulax catenella*, whereas *Gonyaulax tamarensis* produces saxitoxin and several additional neurotoxic substances.[94-96] The structure of saxitoxin has been determined[97]; it is heat stable and blocks the propagation of nerve and muscle action potentials by interfering with the increase in sodium permeability by acting at a metal cation-binding site in the sodium channels or nerve membranes.[98-100] The mechanisms of action of the other neurotoxins are unknown. Duration of the illness ranges from a few hours to a few days.[90]

Although many patients with PSP experience the onset of symptoms within 1 hour of ingestion, the incubation period is often inversely related to the amount of toxin ingested. A European outbreak involved 120 patients who ingested contaminated mussels; the median incubation period in this outbreak was 3.5 hours, with a range of 1 to 10 hours.[90]

The clinical features of NSP are similar to those of PSP, but paralysis does not occur.[87,89] Several poorly characterized neurotoxins responsible for this illness are found in *Gymnodinium breve,* the responsible dinoflagellate.[101,102] One of these neurotoxins stimulates postganglionic cholinergic nerve fibers.[103] Duration of the illness ranges from a few hours to a few days.[87]

The clinical features of ASP are initially nonspecific and include vomiting, abdominal cramping, and diarrhea. Confusion, amnesia, coma, and cardiovascular instability follow within hours in severe cases; these signs tend to occur in older persons and in persons with underlying renal disease. The hallmark of the disease is antegrade amnesia, which was reported in 25% of affected persons in a large Canadian outbreak.[88] The disease is caused by domoic acid, a toxin produced by the dinoflagellate *Nitzschia pungens* and concentrated in the flesh of mollusks. Amnesia is the result of bilateral destruction of the hippocampi by the toxin and can be permanent.[104]

The Chinese restaurant syndrome is characterized by a burning sensation in the neck, chest, abdomen, or arms and by a sensation of tightness over the face and chest.[105] Headache, flushing, diaphoresis, lacrimation, weakness, nausea, abdominal cramps, and thirst frequently occur.[105,106] Symptoms appear to be caused by excessive amounts of monosodium L-glutamate in foods, although other undefined substances may also play a role.[105,106] The illness usually resolves within several hours.

Niacin poisoning produces a burning facial erythema within 20 minutes of ingestion, which rapidly resolves.[107]

Paresthesias within 1 to 6 Hours. The major diagnostic considerations for this syndrome are PSP and ciguatera fish poisoning (see Table 95-4). Ciguatera is characterized by an onset of abdominal cramps, nausea, vomiting, and diarrhea, preceded or followed by numbness and paresthesias of the lips, tongue, and throat.[108-110] Malaise, headache, pruritus, dry mouth, metallic taste, myalgias, arthralgias, blurred vision, photophobia, and transient blindness have also been reported.[111-113] Sharp shooting pains in the legs and a sensation of looseness and pain in the teeth are characteristic.[110] In severe cases, reversal of hot and cold temperature sensations, sinus bradycardia, hypotension, cranial nerve palsies, and respiratory paralysis may occur.[110,111,114]

The illness is caused by ciguatoxin, a poorly characterized, lipid-soluble, relatively heat-stable compound[115] that is acquired by fish through the food chain.[116] The dinoflagellate *Gambierdiscus toxicus* and algae that grow on reefs have been identified as the source of the toxin in the food chain.[117] Ciguatoxin inhibits red blood cell cholinesterase activity,[118] increases membrane sodium permeability,[119] and changes the electrical potential of cells through its action on sodium channels.[120,121] Duration of the acute illness ranges from a few days to a few months; pain in the extremities has been reported to occur intermittently for years after an episode of ciguatera. Other natural marine toxins have been associated with similar syndromes, including scaritoxin, maitotoxin, and palytoxin.[117]

Miscellaneous Mushroom Poisoning Syndromes with Onset within 2 Hours. At least five clinical syndromes may occur within 2 hours of ingestion of toxic mushrooms (Table 95-5).[122-125] Species containing ibotenic acid and muscimol cause an illness that mimics acute alcoholic intoxication and is characterized by confusion, restlessness, and visual disturbances followed by lethargy; symptoms resolve within 24 hours. Species containing muscarine cause an illness characterized by evidence of parasympathetic hyperactivity (e.g., salivation, lacrimation, diaphoresis, blurred vision, abdominal cramps, diarrhea). Some patients experience miosis, bradycardia, and bronchospasm. Symptoms usually resolve within 24 hours. Species containing the toxic substances psilocybin and psilocin cause an acute psychotic reaction manifested by hallucinations and inappropriate behavior, which usually resolves within 12 hours. The mushroom *Coprinus atramentarius* contains a disulfiram-like substance that can result in headache, flushing, paresthesias, nausea, vomiting, and tachycardia if alcohol is consumed during the 48-hour period after ingestion. The fifth clinical syndrome is characterized by nausea, vomiting, abdominal cramps, and diarrhea after the ingestion of mushrooms containing gastrointestinal irritants that are not well characterized.

Abdominal Cramps and Diarrhea within 6 to 24 Hours, Followed by Hepatorenal Failure. Species of poisonous mushrooms containing amatoxins and phallotoxins are responsible for this syndrome (see Table 95-5).[122,123,125] The most common implicated species are *Amanita phalloides, Amanita virosa,* and *Amanita verna.*[126,127] The illness is typically biphasic; the abdominal cramps and diarrhea, which may be severe, usually resolve within 24 hours. The patient then remains well for 1 to 2 days before evidence of hepatic and renal failure supervenes. A mortality rate of 20% to 50% has been reported.[128-130]

A similar clinical syndrome occurs after ingestion of mushrooms of the *Gyromitra* genus, which contain the toxic substance gyromitrin. Hemolysis, seizures, and coma can occur, but this toxin does not cause acute renal failure.[131]

Persistent Diarrhea within 1 to 3 Weeks. Two distinctive persistent diarrheal syndromes can be foodborne: cyclosporiasis and Brainerd diarrhea. Cyclosporiasis emerged as a major foodborne infection in the United States in 1996, when it caused many outbreaks related to imported raspberries. In 1997 and 1999, outbreaks of cyclosporiasis were associated with fresh mesclun and fresh basil. The diarrhea is often intermittent and relapsing; is associated with anorexia, weight loss, nausea and profound fatigue; and begins after a median in-

TABLE 95-5 Mushroom Poisoning Syndromes

Syndrome	Mushroom Species	Toxins
Short Incubation		
Delirium	*Amanita muscaria, Amanita pantherina*	Ibotenic acid, muscimol
Parasympathetic hyperactivity	*Inocybe* spp.	Muscarine
	Clitocybe spp.	Muscarine
Hallucinations	*Psilocybe* spp.	Psilocybin, psilocin
	Panaeolus spp.	Psilocybin
Disulfiram reaction	*Coprinus atramentarius*	Disulfiram-like substance
Gastroenteritis	Many	?
Long Incubation		
Gastroenteritis, hepatorenal failure	*Amanita phalloides*	Amatoxins, phallotoxins
	Amanita virosa	Amatoxins
	Amanita verna	Amatoxins
	Galerina autumnalis	Amatoxins
	Galerina marginata	Amatoxins
	Galerina venenata	Amatoxins
Gastroenteritis, hepatic failure, hemolysis, seizures, coma	*Gyromitra* spp.	Gyromitrin

cubation period of 7 days.[132] A distinctive chronic watery diarrhea, known as Brainerd diarrhea, was first described in persons who had consumed raw milk.[133] After a mean incubation period of 15 days, affected persons developed acute, watery diarrhea with marked urgency and abdominal cramping. Diarrhea persisted for a mean of 2 years. No etiologic agent was identified. A restaurant-associated outbreak and a cruise ship–associated outbreak of a similar illness suggests that other vehicles may also be involved.[134,135]

Waterborne Disease

The evaluation of a suspected foodborne outbreak may reveal that water was the vehicle. Pathogens incriminated in waterborne outbreaks are different from those most often responsible for foodborne disease; the responsible etiologic agents for waterborne outbreaks reported to the CDC from 1972 through 2000 are shown in Table 95-6.[136-156] *Giardia lamblia* is the most frequently recognized pathogen in the United States and has been responsible for several large outbreaks traced to municipal water supplies.[151-153] This illness is characterized by abdominal pain, bloating, flatulence, and occasionally malabsorption. The incubation period is typically 1 to 4 weeks, and the duration of illness may be several weeks. Large waterborne outbreaks caused by *Cryptosporidium parvum*,[157] *E. coli* O157-H7,[158,159] shigellae,[160] hepati-

tis A,[161] *Salmonella* serotype Typhi,[162] nontyphoid salmonellae,[163] ETEC,[164] *C. jejuni*,[165,166] Brainerd diarrhea,[167] noroviruses,[168-170] and *Toxoplasma*[171] have been reported. The majority of waterborne outbreaks are of unknown cause.

EPIDEMIOLOGY

In addition to the clinical syndrome and incubation period, other clues to the cause of an outbreak of foodborne disease may be provided by the type of food responsible and the setting in which it is eaten (Table 95-7).

Foods

Outbreaks of staphylococcal food poisoning are associated with foods of high protein content, such as ham, poultry, potato and egg salads, and cream-filled pastries, which are thought to be contaminated during preparation by a food handler. In the classic staphylococcal foodborne outbreak, a food handler's hand has a purulent skin lesion, but this is true in only a minority of outbreaks. In contrast, outbreaks of *B. cereus* food poisoning of the short-incubation type are most often associated with fried rice that has been cooked and held warm for extended periods. The growth of *B. cereus* under similar experimental conditions in rice has been well documented.[172]

C. perfringens outbreaks usually occur after the ingestion of meat (especially beef and poultry) and gravies; organisms have been isolated from 16% to 85% of raw meat, poultry, and fish specimens.[173] Outbreaks are more likely to occur when these items are prepared in large quantities for banquets or in institutional settings, without adequate final reheating.[173] Long-incubation *B. cereus* food poisoning is frequently associated with meat or vegetable dishes. In addition to being a frequent contaminant of raw meats, vegetables, and milk products, *B. cereus* has been isolated from 25% of dried foods such as seasoning mixes, spices, and dried potatoes[174] and from more than 50% of dried beans and cereals.[175] A long-incubation *B. cereus* outbreak was traced to a meal delivery service operation in which food was held at and above room temperature for an extended period.[176]

E. coli O157-H7 outbreaks were initially recognized mostly after consumption of undercooked ground beef.[55] However, more recent *E. coli* O157 outbreaks have been traced to a broad range of foods, including lettuce, apple cider, alfalfa sprouts, venison, and salami. Healthy cattle commonly carry *E. coli* O157-H7 in their intestines and excrete it in manure. Produce may become contaminated with *E. coli* O157-H7 through use of manure as fertilizer or use of water in processing that has been contaminated with fecal matter. Outbreaks have also been caused by consumption of contaminated drinking and swimming water and by person-to-person transmission in daycare centers.[55,58]

Salmonella foodborne outbreaks most frequently occur after ingestion of poultry, beef, egg, dairy products, or produce. Internally contaminated

TABLE 95-6 Waterborne Disease Outbreaks of Known Cause, Associated with Drinking Water, Reported to the CDC, 1972-2000

	Outbreaks	
Etiologic Agent	Number	%
Giardia lamblia	119	35.8
Shigella spp.	38	11.4
Hepatitis A	21	6.3
Noroviruses	19	5.7
Campylobacter jejuni	15	4.5
Cryptosporidium	14	4.2
Salmonella, nontyphoidal	13	3.9
Escherichia coli O157-H7	8	2.4
Salmonella serotype Typhi	5	1.5
Vibrio cholerae	2	0.6
Enterotoxigenic *Escherichia coli*	1	0.3
Yersinia enterocolitica	1	0.3
Rotavirus	1	0.3
Entamoeba histolytica	1	0.3
Plesiomonas shigelloides	1	0.3
Small round virus	1	0.3
Miscellaneous chemicals	72	21.7
Total	332	100

CDC, Centers for Disease Control and Prevention.

TABLE 95-7 Etiology of Foodborne Disease Outbreaks by Food, Season, and Geographic Predilection

Etiology	Foods	Season	Geographic Predilection
Bacterial			
Salmonella	Beef, poultry, eggs, dairy products, produce	Summer, fall	None
Staphylococcus aureus	Ham, poultry, and egg salads, pastries	Summer	None
Campylobacter jejuni	Poultry, raw milk	Spring, summer	None
Clostridium botulinum	Vegetables, fruits, fish, often home-preserved honey (infants)	Summer, fall	None
Clostridium perfringens	Beef, poultry, gravy, Mexican food	Fall, winter, spring	None
Shigella	Egg salad, lettuce	Summer	None
Vibrio parahaemolyticus	Shellfish	Spring, summer, fall	Coastal states
Bacillus cereus	Fried rice, meats, vegetables	Year round	None
Yersinia enterocolitica	Milk, pork, chitterling	Winter	Unknown
Vibrio cholerae O1	Shellfish	Variable	Tropical, Gulf Coast, Latin America
Vibrio cholerae non-O1	Shellfish	Unknown	Tropical, Gulf Coast
Shiga toxin–producing Escherichia coli	Ground beef, raw milk, fresh produce	Summer, fall	Northern states
Viral			
Noroviruses	Shellfish, salads	Year round	None
Chemical			
Ciguatera	Barracuda, snapper, amberjack, grouper	Spring, summer (in Florida)	Tropical reefs
Histamine fish poisoning (scombroid)	Tuna, mackerel, bonito, skipjack, mahi-mahi	Year round	Coastal
Mushroom poisoning	Mushrooms	Spring, fall	Temperate
Heavy metals	Acidic beverages	Year round	None
Monosodium-L-glutamate	Chinese food	Year round	None
Paralytic shellfish poisoning	Shellfish	Summer, fall	Temperate coastal zones
Neurotoxic shellfish poisoning	Shellfish	Spring, fall	Subtropical

shell eggs cause many outbreaks of infections with *Salmonella* serotype Enteritidis.[177] Foods made with raw or undercooked shell eggs are a dominant source of outbreaks and sporadic cases of *S.* serotype Enteritidis infection in the United States.[178] Despite its risks, raw milk is still legally sold in many states and is sometimes given to school groups who visit dairy farms. During 1972 to 2000, a total of 58 raw milk–associated outbreaks were reported to CDC, of which 17 (29%) were caused by *Salmonella.*[179] Outbreaks also have been traced to fresh produce, including melons, tomatoes, unpasteurized orange juice, and alfalfa sprouts.[180-184] Large international outbreaks have been caused by contaminated chocolate candy, peanut snacks, and cereals.[185-187] *Shigella* outbreaks are most often associated with cool, moist foods, such as potato and egg salads, that require much handling after cooking. Outbreaks have been caused by fresh produce, including raw vegetables at a salad bar, parsley, scallions, and lettuce.[188-191] *C. jejuni* infection most often follows the ingestion of undercooked poultry, although outbreaks have also occurred from raw or contaminated milk and contaminated water sources.[192] *V. parahaemolyticus* outbreaks in the United States are associated with the ingestion of bivalve mollusks and crustaceans.[193]

V. cholerae O1 and non-O1 outbreaks have been traced to contaminated shellfish eaten raw or inadequately cooked.[194] Crabs, shrimp, and raw oysters were implicated as the vehicles of transmission of a unique strain of *V. cholerae* O1 in Louisiana.[195] Crabs brought in travelers' luggage from Latin America have caused cholera in the United States.[196] Sporadic cases of diarrhea associated with *V. cholerae* non-O1 strains in the United States have also been linked to shellfish ingestion.[31]

Foodborne infections with *Y. enterocolitica* have been caused by consumption of raw pork and contaminated milk and by cross-contamination from the preparation of pork chitterlings in the household.[44-49] Traveler's diarrhea caused by ETEC was associated with consumption of salads in Mexico,[197] and a foodborne outbreak of ETEC occurred after ingestion of imported cheese.[198] Traveler's diarrhea due to ETEC among cruise ship passengers has been linked to water bunkered in foreign ports.[199] In recent years, outbreaks of "traveler's diarrhea at home" related to consumption of fresh produce have become more common.[200,201]

Botulism outbreaks are most often associated with the ingestion of low-acid (pH ≥ 4.4) home-canned vegetables, fruits, and fish. Outbreaks of botulism have also occurred after ingestion of unusual vehicles, in-

cluding baked potatoes, sautéed onions, and chopped garlic.[69,202] Honey was the source of *C. botulinum* in some cases of infant botulism.[203]

In norovirus outbreaks, contamination of food by an ill food handler has been documented and very likely occurs frequently.[43] Less commonly, contaminations of shellfish, salads, imported frozen raspberries, and ice have been implicated.[43,204-207] In one large multistate outbreak, steamed shellfish from the Gulf Coast were implicated. These were probably contaminated by ill oystermen themselves, who, lacking toilet facilities on their oyster boats, defecated and vomited directly into the shallow oyster beds.[208] In 1996 and 1997, large outbreaks of *Cyclospora* infections were linked to consumption of raspberries imported from Central America.[131] Outbreaks have also been associated with mesclun mix lettuce and basil sauce.[209,210]

Outbreaks of heavy metal poisoning are most often associated with acidic beverages such as lemonade, fruit punch, and carbonated drinks that have been stored in corroded metallic containers such as punch bowls[79] or that have been in contact with metallic tubing (e.g., in vending machines)[211] for periods sufficient to leach the metallic ions from the container.

Histamine fish poisoning outbreaks are associated with scombroid fish, the most common of which are tuna, mackerel, bonito, and skipjack. In addition, the nonscombroid fish mahi-mahi has caused outbreaks of scombroid-like fish poisoning. Ciguatera fish poisoning has been associated with more than 400 species of fish. Barracuda, red snapper, amberjack, and grouper are most commonly implicated. The disease is more often associated with large fish; in one study, 69% of red snapper weighing 2.8 kg or more were toxic, compared with only 18% of smaller fish.[212] PSP, NSP, and ASP occur after ingestion of bivalve mollusks, most often oysters, clams, and mussels.

The possibility that foodborne illness could be the result of an intentional contamination should also be considered. An outbreak of salmonellosis in Oregon in 1984 involved 751 persons who ate or worked at 10 area restaurants. Epidemiologic investigation determined that illness was associated with eating from salad bars, but no single item was implicated. A subsequent criminal investigation revealed that members of a religious commune had deliberately contaminated the salad bars.[213] In 1996, an outbreak of *Shigella dysenteriae* type 2 affecting 12 laboratory workers was caused by consumption of deliberately contaminated muffins.[214] The use of botulinum toxin by terrorists has also become a concern.[60,215]

Changes in the Population

The increasing average age in many countries means that more of the population has a heightened susceptibility to severe foodborne infections. In the United States, a growing segment of the population has immune impairment as a consequence of infection with the human immunodeficiency virus (HIV) or underlying chronic disease. People with compromised immunity due to infection with HIV have higher reported rates of salmonellosis, campylobacteriosis, and listeriosis than do persons not infected with HIV.[216,217] *Salmonella* and possibly *Campylobacter* infections are more likely to be severe, recurrent, or persistent in such patients. Furthermore, extraintestinal disease caused by *Salmonella* and *L. monocytogenes* infection are more likely to be reported among HIV-infected persons than in the general population.[216,217]

Seasonality

The time of year may also provide a clue to the cause of a foodborne outbreak. Outbreaks caused by the bacterial pathogens *S. aureus*, *Salmonella*, and *Shigella* are most common during the summer months. *C. jejuni* outbreaks are more common during the spring and fall. *C. perfringens* outbreaks occur throughout the year but least often during the summer months, and botulism outbreaks are more common during the summer and fall. Shellfish-associated *Vibrio* infections are largely limited to late summer and early fall and are closely related to the temperature of the water in the oyster beds.[218] *Y. enterocolitica* is typically a winter infection, often occurring after winter holidays at which pork chitterlings are served.[44]

In general, chemical food poisoning occurs throughout the year. Exceptions are PSP, which often occurs in association with a red tide[219] and is most common in the summer and fall; ciguatera, which is most common in the spring and summer in Florida[220]; and mushroom poisoning, which is most common in the spring, late summer, and fall.

Geographic Location

The geographic setting may also provide a clue to the cause of foodborne disease. *E. coli* O157-H7 infections are more common in the northern tier of states bordering Canada, for unexplained reasons.[50] *Salmonella* serotype Enteritidis infections have been most common in the Northeast but are increasing in frequency in the rest of the country.[178] *V. parahaemolyticus* outbreaks are most frequently reported from coastal states.[221,222] An outbreak of cholera and sporadic cases of *V. cholerae* O1 and non-O1 infection have been reported from the Gulf Coast of the United States.[195] Type A botulism outbreaks are most common west of the Mississippi River, whereas type B outbreaks are most common in the East and type E outbreaks are most common in Alaska.[65]

Ciguatera outbreaks occur in tropical and subtropical regions between 35 degrees N and 35 degrees S latitudes. More than 90% of outbreaks in the United States have been reported from Florida or Hawaii.[86] Ciguatera is common in the Virgin Islands,[223] and travelers who return with the characteristic syndrome should be questioned regarding fish consumption. PSP and NSP outbreaks occur in coastal areas.

Epidemiologic Assessment

If an outbreak of foodborne disease is suspected, public health authorities should be contacted so that it can be investigated. Investigating the outbreak is important to identify and rapidly control the source and to prevent similar outbreaks from happening again. Once a common meal is identified through interviews with ill people, food-specific attack rates should be determined for all foods and beverages served at the meal (Table 95-8). People who were present at the same meal but did not become ill must also be interviewed. Food-specific attack rates may identify the responsible vehicle of transmission. To be adequately incriminated, a food must have a significantly higher attack rate for those who ate it than for those who did not, and most of those who became ill must have eaten the food. On occasion, more than one food item may be incriminated. On these occasions, a stratified analysis may indicate whether both items were contaminated by the etiologic agent or whether both were eaten by most people at the meal (e.g., meat and

TABLE 95-8 Example of Use of Food-Specific Attack Rates and Cross-Table Analysis to Identify Food Vehicle in a Foodborne Outbreak

	Food-Specific Attack Rates					
	No. of People Eating Food			No. of People Not Eating Food		
Food	Total	Ill	Percent Ill	Total	Ill	Percent Ill
Meatloaf	100	88	88*	10	2	20*
Gravy	80	80	100†	30	10	33†
Potatoes	95	78	82	15	12	80
Salad	90	74	82	20	16	80
Water	70	58	82	40	32	80

	Cross-Table Analysis					
	No. of People Eating Meatloaf			No. of People Not Eating Meatloaf		
	Total	Ill	Percent Ill	Total	Ill	Percent Ill
No. of people eating gravy	75	67	89†	5	1	20*
No. of people not eating gravy	25	21	84†	5	1	20*

*$p < .05$ (Fisher's exact test).
†$p < .05$ (chi-square analysis).

gravy) (see Table 95-8). For example, if meatloaf and gravy were both incriminated, subsequent analysis may indicate that attack rates were high for those who ate meatloaf regardless of whether they ate gravy, and were low for those who did not eat meatloaf regardless of whether they ate gravy, indicating that the meatloaf alone was responsible for the outbreak.

Once a food vehicle for the infections is identified, the investigation turns to the question of how contamination is likely to have occurred. Steps of food preparation are reviewed with the chef, and the safety of the various ingredients and the hygienic circumstances in the kitchen are assessed. In complex outbreaks, detailed epidemiologic investigation into the sources of food ingredients and replication of the cooking protocol may be needed to explain the event.

LABORATORY DIAGNOSIS

Appropriate specimens for laboratory confirmation vary with the etiologic agents but include feces, vomitus, serum, and blood (Table 95-9). In addition, cultures from the leftover food, the food preparation environment, and food handlers may be indicated. The laboratory should be alerted to suspected causes so that special techniques can be used for identification of *C. perfringens*, vibrios, *C. jejuni*, *E. coli* O157-H7, *Cyclospora*, and *Y. enterocolitica* and so that organisms considered part of the normal flora (other *E. coli*, *B. cereus*) are not overlooked.

Careful specimen collection and transport is critical to successful diagnosis.[224] Rectal or stool swabs for bacteriologic diagnosis should be collected from patients not already treated with antimicrobials and should be transported under refrigeration to the laboratory in Cary-Blair or another suitable transport medium. They should be frozen if they cannot be plated within 48 hours. For optimal viral diagnosis, liquid stools should be collected early in the illness and transported under refrigeration without freezing. Parasitic diagnosis depends on collection of a stool sample and its transport in specialized parasitic transport media. Additional information on the collection of specimens for diagnosis and investigation of foodborne outbreaks is available on the World Wide Web at http://www.cdc.gov/foodborneoutbreaks/guide_sc.htm.

To confirm the etiologic agent in outbreaks, specimens should be collected and tested from multiple ill people involved in the outbreak. Foods may also be collected and tested to confirm the etiology and food

TABLE 95-9 Appropriate Laboratory Specimens for Documenting the Cause of a Foodborne Outbreak

	Patient			Food Handler				Environment	
	Stools	Vomitus	Urine	Blood	Stools	Nose	Hands	Food	Food-Preparation Environment
Bacterial									
Salmonella	C	—	—	C	C	—	—	C	C
Staphylococcus aureus	C	C	—	—	—	C	C	C,T	—
Campylobacter jejuni	C	—	—	—	C	—	—	C	C
Clostridium botulinum	C,T	C,T	T	—	—	—	—	C,T	—
Clostridium perfringens	C,T	—	—	—	—	—	—	C	—
Shigella	C	—	—	—	C	—	—	C	—
Vibrio parahaemolyticus	C	—	—	—	—	—	—	C	C
Bacillus cereus	C	C	—	—	—	—	—	C	—
Yersinia enterocolitica	C	—	—	S	C	—	—	C	C
Vibrio cholerae O1 and non-O1	C	—	—	S	C	—	—	C	C
Shiga toxin–producing Escherichia coli	C,T	—	—	S	C	—	—	C	—
Viral									
Norwalk agent	I,P	—	—	S	I,P	—	—	P	—
Chemical									
Ciguatera	—	—	—	—	—	—	—	T	—
Histamine fish poisoning (scombroid)	—	—	—	—	—	—	—	T	—
Mushroom	T	T	T	T	—	—	—	T	—
Heavy metals	—	—	—	—	—	—	—	T	—
Monosodium-L-glutamate	—	—	—	—	—	—	—	T	—
Paralytic shellfish poisoning	—	—	—	—	—	—	—	T	—
Neurotoxic shellfish poisoning	—	—	—	—	—	—	—	T	—

C, culture; I, immune electron microscopy; P, polymerase chain reaction probe; S, serology; T, toxin testing.

vehicle for a foodborne outbreak. Many of the tests used for outbreak identification and confirmation are available only in specialized public health or food microbiology laboratories.

The identification, investigation, and confirmation of foodborne outbreaks of bacterial etiology has been aided greatly by the establishment of standardized pulsed field gel electrophoresis (PFGE) methods used by public health laboratories in the United States and Canada in a molecular subtyping network called PulseNet. Pathogens routinely subtyped by PFGE include *E. coli* O157-H7, *Salmonella, Shigella, Listeria,* and *Campylobacter.* Standard PFGE methods are being developed for other pathogens.[225] PulseNet is growing internationally, which will enable better identification of outbreaks of international scale. Additional information concerning PulseNet is available at http://www.cdc.gov/pulsenet.

Outbreaks of staphylococcal food poisoning may be confirmed by the isolation of *S. aureus* of the same phage type or PFGE pattern from vomitus or feces of two or more ill people. The detection of enterotoxin or the isolation of greater than 10^5 organisms per gram in epidemiologically implicated food may also be confirmatory. The demonstration of *S. aureus* enterotoxin may be accomplished by gel diffusion, by radioimmunoassay (RIA), or by enzyme-linked immunosorbent assay (ELISA).[226]

B. cereus outbreaks may be documented by the isolation of organisms from the feces of two or more ill people who shared the same meal or by the isolation of 10^5 or more *B. cereus* organisms per gram of incriminated food. Serotyping, if available, may be of value in confirming that isolates were derived from a common source, as 14% of healthy adults have been reported to have transient gastrointestinal colonization with *B. cereus.*[227] Plasmid analysis may also be useful.[228] Commercial immunoassays are available for the diarrheogenic toxin of *B. cereus.*[229]

The laboratory confirmation of *C. perfringens* outbreaks is more difficult. Because both heat-sensitive and heat-resistant strains of *C. perfringens* type A have been implicated as causes of food poisoning, selective isolation procedures involving heat treatment of food and fecal specimens should not be used. Because *C. perfringens* organisms are part of the normal flora in most healthy people, the number of organisms should be greater than 10^5 per gram of stool in two or more ill people to confirm *C. perfringens* as the etiologic agent in an outbreak. Confirmation may also be attained by the demonstration of the enterotoxin in the stool of two or more ill people or isolation of greater than

10^5 organisms per gram of epidemiologically implicated food.[230,231] Demonstration of *C. perfringens* enterotoxin in stools of ill people and not in those of control subjects is possible with ELISA or latex agglutination, although these tests are investigational.[232-234] *Salmonella, Shigella, C. jejuni, V. cholerae* O1 and O139, *V. parahaemolyticus,* and *Y. enterocolitica* outbreaks may be confirmed by isolation and serotyping of the organisms from the feces of ill people. In *Salmonella* outbreaks, PFGE, and for *S.* serotype Enteritidis, *S.* serotype Typhi, and *S.* serotype Typhimurium, phage type determination, may be helpful.[178,180] Strains of *V. parahaemolyticus* isolated from patients usually produce a thermostable direct hemolysin (TDH) on special blood agar medium (Kanagawa-positive strains). Isolation and serotyping of *Salmonella, Shigella, C. jejuni, Vibrio,* and *Y. enterocolitica* from the incriminated food may also be confirmatory. Molecular characterization of *V. cholerae* O1 with PFGE may help to define the geographic origins of the infecting organism.[235] Because *V. parahaemolyticus* in low numbers is a frequent contaminant of shellfish, a count of 10^5 or more organisms per gram of shellfish meat is required for confirmation; food isolates are usually TDH negative. Serologic testing of acute and convalescent sera may be helpful in confirming the diagnosis of patients in outbreaks of cholera, typhoid fever, and Shiga toxin–producing *E. coli,* but it currently plays no important role in the investigation of nontyphoid *Salmonella, Shigella, C. jejuni,* and *V. parahaemolyticus* outbreaks.

Infection with *E. coli* O157-H7 can be diagnosed by isolating sorbitol-negative *E. coli* from stools of ill persons on sorbitol-MacConkey medium and confirming the serotype. Infection with other Shiga toxin–producing *E. coli* can be diagnosed by demonstration of Shiga toxin in broth culture of a stool specimen, or by isolation of other Shiga toxin–producing strains from stools from ill persons.[55] Isolates of Shiga toxin–producing *E. coli* should be forwarded to the jurisdiction public health laboratory for full characterization and PFGE analysis for surveillance and outbreak detection purposes. In the outbreak setting, ETEC can be identified by detecting heat-stable and heat-labile toxins in stool using a commercial latex agglutination assay or ELISA.[236] Enterotoxigenic, enteroinvasive, and enteropathogenic *E. coli* may be identified in the stool of ill persons or foods by gene detection assays (gene probes or polymerase chain reaction [PCR] assays).[236] For outbreaks caused by diarrheogenic *E. coli* or for well-characterized outbreaks with no identifiable etiologic agent, arrangements can be made through state health departments to send *E. coli* isolates to the CDC for virulence testing and serotyping.

Botulism outbreaks may be confirmed by the demonstration of botulinum toxin in the serum or stool of ill people or in incriminated food by the mouse neutralization test, or by the isolation of *C. botulinum* from the feces of ill people or from the incriminated food.[237,238] Laboratory confirmation by testing of clinical specimens can be obtained in approximately 70% to 75% of the cases of botulism.[237,238] Outbreaks of norovirus or other human caliciviruses may be confirmed by the detection of viral genes in stools of ill persons by PCR.[43] Laboratory diagnosis of parasitic pathogens typically depends on visualization of characteristic forms in the feces. The enteric parasites *Cyclospora* and *Cryptosporidium* are identified after specialized concentration and staining methods.[239,240] Additional information concerning the diagnosis of *Cyclospora*, and other parasitic infections, can be found at http://www.dpd.cdc.gov/dpdx.

Outbreaks caused by heavy metals or chemicals, such as pesticides, may be documented by demonstration of the metallic ion or chemical in the incriminated food. Chemicals and their metabolic breakdown products may be detected in urine specimens from ill persons collected within 48 hours of exposure, as well as in the first vomitus after exposure. Histamine fish poisoning may be confirmed by demonstration of histamine in the fish; concentrations of 100 mg in 100 g of fish flesh correlate with toxicity. The diagnosis of ciguatera is usually based on the clinical picture. However, ciguatera outbreaks may be documented by demonstration of ciguatoxin in the incriminated fish using ELISA techniques.[241] Shellfish poisoning may be confirmed either by demonstration of the toxin in mollusks by the mouse bioassay technique or by finding elevated numbers of the responsible dinoflagellate in the water from which the mollusks were obtained. Outbreaks of Chinese restaurant syndrome may be confirmed by demonstration of elevated monosodium L-glutamate levels in the food. Mushroom poisoning may be confirmed either by the identification of the responsible toxin in gastric contents, blood, urine, or fecal specimens by thin-layer chromatography or RIA or by the identification of the mushroom by a mycologist.

More than 50% of the reported foodborne disease outbreaks in the United States are of unknown cause. In some cases, appropriate diagnostic procedures are not conducted. In others, diagnostic specimens are not collected or transported properly. In still others, no agent is identified despite testing, raising the possibility that other etiologic agents are responsible; possibilities include ETEC, *Plesiomonas shigelloides,* rotaviruses, and norovirus. Although enterococci and gram-negative rods (*Aeromonas hydrophila, Klebsiella, Enterobacter, Proteus, Citrobacter,* and *Pseudomonas*) have been reported as causes of foodborne outbreaks on rare occasions, their role has not been well documented, and they may be present in foods without causing illness. Because these organisms may be part of the normal fecal flora, documentation of their presence in ill people and their absence from well people is required to confirm their role in foodborne outbreaks.

THERAPY

Supportive measures are the mainstay of therapy in most cases of food poisoning. Most diarrheal diseases can be managed with oral rehydration.[242] Antiemetics and antiperistaltic agents offer symptomatic relief, although the latter are contraindicated in patients with high fever, bloody diarrhea, or fecal leukocytes indicative of an invasive infection. Fatalities can still occur (Table 95-10). The most lethal foodborne diseases are botulism, listeriosis (affecting neonates and immunocompromised persons), *V. vulnificus* infection (in those with impaired hepatic function), paralytic shellfish poisoning, and long-incubation mushroom poisoning. With other pathogens, fatalities may occur because the patient is extremely young, is extremely old, or has compromised host defenses; because the dose is overwhelming; or because the pathogen is resistant to treatment.

In any diarrheal illness, gastrointestinal fluid losses should be replaced either orally or parenterally. Antimicrobial agents may be used in the treatment of shigellosis and cholera and are lifesaving in invasive

TABLE 95-10 Estimated Frequency of Hospitalizations and Deaths for Known Foodborne Pathogens, United States, 1997

Disease or Agent	Percent Hospitalized	Percent Died
Bacterial		
Bacillus cereus	0.6	0.00
Botulism, foodborne	80.0	7.69
Brucella spp.	55.0	5.00
Campylobacter spp.	10.2	0.10
Clostridium perfringens	0.3	0.05
Escherichia coli O157-H7	29.5	0.83
E. coli, non-O157 STEC	29.5	0.83
E. coli, enterotoxigenic	0.5	0.01
E. coli, other diarrheogenic	0.5	0.01
Listeria monocytogenes	92.2	20.00
Salmonella serotype Typhi	75.0	0.40
Salmonella, nontyphoidal	22.1	0.78
Shigella spp.	13.9	0.16
Staphylococcus food poisoning	18.0	0.02
Streptococcus, foodborne	13.3	0.00
Vibrio cholerae, toxigenic	34.0	0.60
Vibrio vulnificus	91.0	39.00
Other vibrios	12.6	2.50
Yersinia enterocolitica	24.2	0.05
Parasitic		
Cryptosporidium parvum	15.0	0.50
Cyclospora cayetanensis	2.0	0.05
Giardia lamblia	n/a	n/a
Toxoplasma gondii	n/a	n/a
Trichinella spiralis	8.1	0.30
Viral		
Norwalk-like viruses	n/a	n/a
Rotavirus	n/a	n/a
Astrovirus	n/a	n/a
Hepatitis A virus	13.0	0.30

STEC, Shiga toxin–producing *E. coli.*
Modified from Mead PS, Slutsker L, Dietz V, et al. Food-related illness and death in the United States. Emerg Infect Dis. 1999;5:607-624.

salmonellosis and typhoid fever, but they should be avoided in uncomplicated gastrointestinal infection caused by nontyphoid salmonellae.[242] Tetracycline shortens both the duration of clinical cholera and the excretion of *V. cholerae* O1. Fluoroquinolone-resistant *Campylobacter* infections emerged after the approval of these agents for use in poultry; such infections may be worsened with fluoroquinolone treatment. Erythromycin eradicates carriage of susceptible *C. jejuni* and may shorten the duration of illness if given early in the disease. *Cyclospora* infection can be treated with high-dose trimethoprim-sulfamethoxazole.[242] The role of antimicrobial agents in the management of food poisoning caused by *V. parahaemolyticus;* by enterotoxigenic, Shiga toxin–producing, or invasive *E. coli;* or by *Y. enterocolitica* is unsettled but probably minimal.[242] Patients with *E. coli* O157-H7 infection should be hydrated well and evaluated expectantly for the development of hemolytic uremic syndrome, which often requires transfusion, renal dialysis, and prolonged intensive care.[243] Antimicrobial agents are of no value in the management of staphylococcal, *C. perfringens,* or *B. cereus* food poisoning.

A multiple-drug–resistant strain of *Salmonella* serotype Typhimurium definitive type 104 (DT 104) has emerged in Europe and the United States. By 1996, DT 104 was the second most common cause of human salmonellosis in England and Wales, and it accounted for 8% of all salmonellosis in the United States.[244,245] More than 90% of all DT 104 isolates were resistant to ampicillin, chloramphenicol, streptomycin, sulfonamides, and tetracycline (R-type ACSSuT), and 30% of strains also showed resistance to trimethoprim and ciprofloxacin.[244] Surveillance for DT 104 infections in the United Kingdom indicates high hospitalization and fatality rates compared with infections caused by other *Salmonella* serotypes. In one study, 41% of patients with multidrug-resistant DT 104 infection required hospitalization, and 3% died.[246] The appearance of this highly resistant strain can complicate treatment for any infection, because an inapparent subclinical DT 104 infection can be changed to severe salmonellosis by exposure to an antimicrobial agent to which DT 104 is resistant.[247] The emergence of this resistant strain is probably related to agricultural uses of antimicrobials. This highlights the interconnected pool of pathogens between animal reservoirs and people and underlines the need for prudent use of antimicrobials in both sectors.

A multiple-drug–resistant strain of *Salmonella* serotype Newport that is associated with eating raw or undercooked ground beef has recently been described in the United States.[248] This strain is resistant to amoxicillin/clavulanate, ampicillin, cefoxitin, cephalothin, chloramphenicol, streptomycin, sulfonamides, and tetracycline and exhibits decreased susceptibility to ceftriaxone. Isolates with this resistance pattern have plasmids that carry the *bla*$_{CMY}$ gene.

Patients with botulism present several additional therapeutic problems, which are discussed in Chapter 243. Medical care providers who suspect botulism in a patient should immediately call their state health department's emergency 24-hour telephone number. The state health department will contact the CDC to arrange for a clinical consultation by telephone and, if indicated, release of botulinum antitoxin. The CDC's 24-hour telephone number for state health departments to report suspected botulism cases, obtain clinical consultation on botulism cases, and request botulinum antitoxin release is 770-488-7100.

Patients with PSP and some patients with ciguatera may require ventilatory support, usually for only a few days. Reports suggest that intravenous mannitol may ameliorate the acute neurologic symptoms of severe ciguatera, and that tocainide may improve persistent dysesthesias.[249,250] Therapy is otherwise supportive; no antitoxins are available. If not contraindicated by the presence of ileus, enemas or cathartics may be administered in an effort to remove unabsorbed toxin from the intestinal tract. Because of the severe dysesthesias associated with ciguatera, analgesics may also be required. Symptoms of histamine fish poisoning may be relieved by antihistamines. In severe cases with bronchospasm, epinephrine or aminophylline may be required.

Therapy for short-incubation types of mushroom poisoning is primarily supportive.[251] Patients who have ingested species containing pharmacologically active amounts of muscarine and who manifest evidence of parasympathetic hyperactivity may be treated with atropine. Patients who are severely ill after ingestion of species containing ibotenic acid and muscimol may be treated with physostigmine. Therapy for the long-incubation illness includes cathartics and enemas to remove unabsorbed toxin, and a number of specific and supportive measures.[251] Because hypoglycemia often occurs, intravenous glucose may be required. Liver failure may ultimately require transplantation. α-Lipoic acid (thioctic acid) is an experimental drug that appears to be an effective antidote in these patients[126]; the drug may be obtained from Burton M. Berkson, M.D., Ph.D., in Las Cruces, New Mexico (505-524-3720 or 505-521-1609). Pyridoxine is indicated in the management of patients poisoned with *Gyromitra* species.

Therapy for acute heavy metal poisoning is supportive. Emesis should be induced if it does not occur spontaneously. Antiemetics are contraindicated, because retention of the toxic ions in the gut and subsequent systemic absorption may result. In severe cases with systemic manifestations of heavy metal toxicity, use of specific antidotes may be considered, but this is rarely necessary in these outbreaks.

SURVEILLANCE

Public health authorities monitor trends in specific diseases through reports of diagnosed cases provided by clinicians and microbiologists. State public health laws determine reportable conditions for each state and who is responsible for reporting. In turn, state public health officials voluntarily submit reports of nationally notifiable diseases to the CDC for the compilation of nationwide surveillance data. Disease conditions reportable by law may vary from one state to another; the information about reportable conditions is available through state and local health departments. Disease and case definitions for nationally notifiable infectious diseases are available at http://www.cdc.gov/epo/dphsi/phs/infdis.htm.

Reports from physicians, nurses, laboratorians, and other potential reporting groups are the starting point for public health activities that can prevent further cases from occurring— activities such as education, identification of potentially hazardous events, and epidemiologic investigation. Increasingly, public health notification occurs most rapidly through the clinical laboratory. For *Salmonella, Shigella,* Shiga toxin–producing *E. coli,* and *Listeria,* the bacterial isolate itself should be referred to a public health laboratory for serotyping and molecular subtyping. Although knowing the specific serotype is rarely of importance in the management of a single case, it is fundamental to the recognition of outbreaks and in monitoring the success of control efforts. This means that ordering the diagnostic tests needed to determine the nature of the illness is of benefit not only to the patient but to society as a whole. A single case of illness reported from a daycare center or family gathering not infrequently leads to discovery of an entire outbreak. Outbreaks can be apparent even though the specific diagnosis is not in hand, and investigation can succeed in identifying and controlling a source even without knowing the cause. This means that the astute clinician or microbiologist who calls the public health department epidemiologist to discuss a potential outbreak plays an important role in the control of foodborne and other diseases.

PREVENTION

Prevention of foodborne disease depends on careful handling of raw products and finished foods all the way from the farm to the table, and on technologies that reduce or eliminate contamination in food.[252] Raw animal products, including meat, milk, eggs, and shellfish, are common sources of contamination leading to foodborne diseases. Contamination of raw animal products can be reduced by better animal production and slaughter practices. Monitoring of the safety of industrial food processing is increasingly important as the nation's food supply becomes more centralized and preprocessed for the convenience of the consumer. One approach to risk reduction, called the Hazard Analysis Critical Control Point (HACCP) program, was originally developed to ensure the safety of foods used in the space program. This approach requires a food producer to identify points where the risk of contamination can be controlled and to use production systems that eliminate these hazards. HACCP programs focus on preventing food contamination rather than relying on a final inspection step to detect it after it has occurred. Milk pasteurization and commercial canning practices are early examples of technologies that make foods safe. Strategies being explored now include provision of microbiologically safe food and water to animals, environmental microbiologic testing on the farm or in the processing plant to identify and eliminate pathogens in the environment prior to food contamination, acid rinses and steam scalding of carcasses, and gamma and electron-beam irradiation of meats and produce.[253]

Renewed efforts are also being focused on identification of sites and sources of contamination of fresh produce harvested in the United States, Mexico, and Central America. There are many points where produce can become contaminated during growth and harvesting, processing and washing, transport, and final processing.[254] The surface of plants and fruits may be contaminated by soil, manure, or feces of animals or agricultural workers. Guidelines for produce growers and processors are available to minimize the microbial hazards associated with sources of contamination through the U.S. Food and Drug Administration (FDA) website at http://www.cfsan.fda.gov/~dms/prodguid.html. It is unknown whether contamination is more likely to occur when produce is grown outside the United States; however, water quality in the developing world is a particular concern. Unclean water supplies can lead to contamination because water is used to irrigate and wash produce and to make the ice that is used to keep produce cool during trucking. The extra handling required to prepare salads and salad bars, and the time delay between preparation and consumption associated with salad bars, may increase the potential for produce to cause illness.[255] Pasteurizing juice and implementing HACCP programs will help decrease the risk associated with consumption of produce.

Much foodborne disease can be prevented if food is selected, prepared, and stored properly. In large kitchens and in homes, careful cooking and storage are necessary to kill pathogens and to prevent their growth when food is recontaminated after cooking. Because they serve high-risk populations, the kitchens of hospitals and nursing homes must pay particular attention to food safety. For example, routine use of pasteurized eggs instead of shell eggs prevents many nosocomial outbreaks of foodborne salmonellosis. A common error is storage of food at inappropriate temperatures.[1] Bacterial pathogens grow in food at temperatures ranging from 40° F to 140° F; growth may be prevented if cold food is adequately refrigerated and hot food is held at temperatures higher than 140° F before serving.

The usual source of contamination for *Salmonella, Campylobacter, C. perfringens,* vibrios, *Y. enterocolitica,* and other zoonoses is raw food of animal origin, not infected food handlers. However, poor personal hygiene by food handlers frequently contributes to *Staphylococcus, Shigella,* hepatitis A, and norovirus outbreaks. Although thorough cooking of food just before consumption eliminates the risk of many illnesses, protection against staphylococcal food poisoning is not provided because the staphylococcal enterotoxins are heat stable, and moreover, many foods, such as fresh produce, are not cooked at all. Inadequate heat processing of home-canned foods can lead to botulism, and the use of contaminated equipment such as knives and meat slicers can result in *E. coli* O157-H7 infections and nontyphoid salmonellosis.[256,257] Particular care in handling and cooking of raw poultry, beef, pork, shellfish, and eggs is important to prevent many foodborne diseases. Avoiding consumption of raw milk is important to prevent *Salmonella* and *C. jejuni* infections.[179,192]

Food-handling errors resulting in chemical intoxication are different from those leading to bacterial outbreaks. Heavy metal poisoning occurs when acidic beverages are stored in defective metallic containers or when valves in vending machines malfunction. Ciguatera and shellfish poisoning occur when fish or shellfish are obtained from unsafe sources. Items contaminated with these toxins appear and taste normal; in addition, cooking of these items does not provide protection, because the toxins are heat stable.

The role of the clinician goes beyond that of diagnosis and treatment to prevention. This means warning high-risk patients (e.g., those infected with HIV, infants and older adults, and those with chronic medical conditions) of the hazards of raw oysters, raw eggs, and unpasteurized milk.[217,258] Although listeriosis is a rare disease, the infec-

tion is often deadly. Pregnant women, persons at the extremes of age, and immunocompromised individuals at risk for listeriosis should be informed about and may choose to abide by general precautions and avoidance of relatively high risk foods as outlined in Table 95-11.

Clinicians and microbiologists have an important role in the detection of outbreaks, in particular in obtaining appropriate diagnostic tests for foodborne pathogens and reporting them to public health authorities. Public health surveillance of foodborne infections and outbreaks is important for appreciating the magnitude and complexity of the problem and guiding targeted prevention efforts. Reporting is essential if investigations are to be conducted to identify the source of the outbreak so that it can be corrected. Prompt reporting may also lead to the prevention of additional cases; there are well-documented outbreaks of botulism,[67,259] salmonellosis,[260] and *E. coli* O157-H7[261] in which recognition and reporting of the initial illness could have prevented many subsequent cases. Diagnosing and reporting of illnesses with the potential for intrafamilial spread, or for spread within institutions such as child care centers (e.g., shigellosis, *E. coli* O157-H7 infection), can prevent secondary transmission. Reporting has been critical to stimulate concerted action to control major new hazards, such as *Salmonella* serotype Enteritidis in eggs, or *E. coli* O157-H7 in beef. As we embark on the 21st century, clinicians, laboratory workers, public health authorities, food safety officials, and members of industry can all play critical roles in decreasing the burden of foodborne illnesses.

REFERENCES

1. Olson SJ, MacKinon LC, Goulding JS, et al. Surveillance for foodborne disease outbreaks: United States, 1993-1997. MMWR Morb Mortal Wkly Rep. 2000;49(SS01):1-51.
2. Mead PS, Slutsker L, Dietz V, et al. Food-related illness and death in the United States. Emerg Infect Dis. 1999;5:607-624.
3. Centers for Disease Control. Preliminary FoodNet data on the incidence of foodborne illness: Selected sites, United States, 2002. MMWR Morb Mortal Wkly Rep. 2003;52:340-343.
4. Tauxe RV. Emerging foodborne diseases: An evolving public health challenge. Emerg Infect Dis. 1997;3:425-434.
5. Mead PS, Griffin PM. *Escherichia coli* O157:H7. Lancet. 1998;352:1207-1212.
6. Swerdlow DL, Lee LA, Tauxe RV, et al. Reactive arthropathy following a multistate outbreak of *Salmonella typhimurium* infections (Abstract 916). 30th Interscience Conference on Antimicrobial Agents and Chemotherapy. Atlanta, October 21-24, 1990.
7. Mishu B, Ilyas AA, Kosli CL, et al. Serologic evidence of previous *Campylobacter jejuni* infections in patients with the Guillain-Barré syndrome. Ann Intern Med. 1993;118:947-953.
8. Holmberg SD, Blake PA. Staphylococcal food poisoning in the United States: New facts and old misconceptions. JAMA. 1984;251:487.
9. Dinges MM, Orwin PM, Schlievert PM. Exotoxins of *Staphylococcus aureus*. Clin Microbiol Rev. 2000;13:16-34.
10. Gilbert RJ. Staphylococcal food poisoning and botulism. Postgrad Med J. 1974;50:603.
11. Breckinridge JC, Bergdoll MS. Outbreak of foodborne gastroenteritis due to a coagulase-negative enterotoxin-producing staphylococcus. N Engl J Med. 1971;284:541.
12. Granum PE, Lund T. Bacillus cereus and its food poisonings toxins. FEMS Microbiol Lett. 1997;157:223-228.
13. Terranova W, Blake PA. *Bacillus cereus* food poisoning. N Engl J Med. 1978;298:143.
14. Hobbs BC, Smith ME, Oakley CL, et al. *Clostridium welchii* food poisoning. J Hyg. 1953;51:75.
15. Shandera WX, Tacket CO, Blake PA. Food poisoning due to *Clostridium perfringens* in the United States. J Infect Dis. 1983;147:167.
16. Stark RL, Duncan CL. Purification and biochemical properties of *Clostridium perfringens* type A enterotoxin. Infect Immun. 1972;6:662.
17. Rood JI, Cole ST. Molecular genetics and pathogenesis of *Clostridium perfringens*. Microbiol Rev. 1990;55:621-648.
18. McDonel JL, Duncan CL. Regional localization of activity of *Clostridium perfringens* type A enterotoxin in the rabbit ileum, jejunum, and duodenum. J Infect Dis. 1977;136:661.
19. McDonel JL. The molecular mode of action of *Clostridium perfringens* enterotoxin. Am J Clin Nutr. 1979;32:210.
20. Loewenstein MS. Epidemiology of *Clostridium perfringens* food poisoning. N Engl J Med. 1972;286:1026.
21. Giannella RA, Brasile L: A hospital food-borne outbreak of diarrhea caused by *Bacillus cereus:* Clinical, epidemiologic, and microbiologic studies. J Infect Dis. 1979;139:366.
22. Granum PE. *Bacillus cereus* and food hygiene. Norsk Vet Tidskr. 1994;106:911-914.
23. Granum PE, Næstvold A, Gundersby KN. *Bacillus cereus* food poisoning during Norwegian Ski Championship for juniors. Norsk Vet Tidskr. 1995;107:945-948.

TABLE 95-11 Recommendations for the Prevention of Listeriosis from the Centers for Disease Control and Prevention

General Recommendations
- Thoroughly cook raw food from animal sources, such as beef, pork, or poultry.
- Wash raw vegetables thoroughly before eating.
- Keep uncooked meats separate from vegetables and from cooked foods and ready-to-eat foods.
- Avoid unpasteurized (raw) milk or foods made from unpasteurized milk.
- Wash hands, knives, and cutting boards after handling uncooked foods.

Recommendations for Persons at High Risk, Such as Pregnant Women and Persons with Weakened Immune Systems, in Addition to the Recommendations Listed Above:
- Do not eat hot dogs, luncheon meats, or deli meats, unless they are reheated until steaming hot.
- Avoid getting fluid from hot dog packages on other foods, utensils, and food preparation surfaces, and wash hands after handling hot dogs, luncheon meats, and deli meats.
- Do not eat soft cheeses such as feta, Brie, and Camembert, blue-veined cheeses, and Mexican-style cheeses such as queso blanco, queso fesco, and Panela, unless they have labels that clearly state they are made from pasteurized milk.
- Do not eat refrigerated pâtés or meat spreads. Canned or shelf-stable pâtés and meat spreads may be eaten.
- Do not eat refrigerated smoked seafood, unless it is contained in a cooked dish, such as a casserole. Refrigerated smoked seafood, such as salmon, trout, whitefish, cod, tuna, and mackerel, is most often labeled as "nova-style," "lox," "kippered," "smoked," or "jerky." The fish is found in the refrigerator section or sold at deli counters of grocery stores and delicatessens. Canned or shelf-stable smoked seafood may be eaten.

24. Blaser MJ, Wells JG, Feldman RA. *Campylobacter* enteritis in the United States: A multicenter study. Ann Intern Med. 1983;98:360.

25. Saphra I, Winter JW. Clinical manifestations of salmonellosis in man: An evaluation of 7779 human infections identified in New York *Salmonella* Center. N Engl J Med. 1957;256:1128.

26. Ostroff SM, Griffin PM, Tauxe RV, et al. A statewide outbreak of *E. coli* O157:H7 infections in Washington state. Am J Epidemiol. 1990;132:239-247.

27. Dalton CB, Austin CC, Sobel J, et al. An outbreak of gastroenteritis and fever due to *Listeria monocytogenes* in milk. N Engl J Med. 1997;336:100.

28. Frye DM, Zweig R, Sturgeon J, et al. An outbreak of febrile gastroenteritis associated with delicatessen meat contaminated with *Listeria monocytogenes*. Clin Infect Dis. 2002;35:943-949.

29. Miettinen MK, Siitonen A, Heiskanen P, et al. Molecular epidemiology of an outbreak of febrile gastroenteritis caused by *Listeria monocytogenes* in cold-smoked rainbow trout. J Clin Microbiol. 1999;37:2358-2360.

30. Aureli P, Fiorucci GC, Caroli D, et al. An outbreak of febrile gastroenteritis associated with corn contaminated with *Listeria monocytogenes*. N Engl J Med. 2000;343:1236-1241.

31. Morris JG Jr. Non-O1 group 1 *Vibrio cholerae* strains not associated with epidemic disease. In: Wachsmuth IK, Blake PA, Olsvik O, eds. *Vibrio cholerae* and Cholera: Molecular to Global Perspectives. Washington, DC: American Society for Microbiology; 1994:103-116.

32. Wilson R, Lieb S, Roberts A, et al. Non-O group 1 *Vibrio cholerae* gastroenteritis associated with eating raw oysters. Am J Epidemiol. 1981;114:293.

33. Reidl J, Klose KE. *Vibrio cholerae* and cholera: Out of the water and into the host. FEMS Microbiol Rev. 2002;26:125-139.

34. Sack RB. Human diarrheal disease caused by enterotoxigenic *Escherichia coli*. Annu Rev Microbiol. 1975;29:333.

35. Sandefur PD, Peterson JW. Neutralization of *Salmonella* toxin-induced elongation of Chinese hamster ovary cells by cholera antitoxin. Infect Immun. 1977;15:988.

36. Sedlock DM, Deibel RH. Detection of *Salmonella* enterotoxin using rabbit ileal loops. Can J Microbiol. 1978;24:268.

37. Keusch GT, Donta ST. Classification of enterotoxins on the basis of activity in cell culture. J Infect Dis. 1975;131:58.

38. Keusch GT, Jacewicz M. The pathogenesis of *Shigella* diarrhea: IV. Toxin and antitoxin in *Shigella flexneri* and *Shigella sonnei* infections in humans. J Infect Dis. 1977;135:552.

39. O'Brien AD, Gentry MK, Thompson MR, et al. Shigellosis and *Escherichia coli* diarrhea: Relative importance of invasive and toxigenic mechanisms. Am J Clin Nutr. 1979;32:229.

40. Honda T, Shimizu M, Takeda Y, et al. Isolation of a factor causing morphological changes of Chinese hamster ovary cells from the culture filtrate of *Vibrio parahaemolyticus*. Infect Immun. 1976;14:1028.

41. Carruthers MM. Cytotoxicity of *Vibrio parahaemolyticus* in HeLa cell culture. J Infect Dis. 1975;132:555.

42. Taylor WR, Schell WL, Wells JG, et al. A foodborne outbreak of enterotoxigenic *Escherichia coli* diarrhea. N Engl J Med. 1982;306:1093.

43. Bresee JS, Widdowson M, Monroe SS, et al. Foodborne viral gastroenteritis: Challenges and opportunities. Clin Infect Dis. 2002;35:748-753.

44. Lee LA, Gerber AR, Lonsway DR, et al. *Yersinia enterocolitica* O:3 infections in infants and children, associated with household preparation of chitterlings. N Engl J Med. 1990;322:984-987.

45. Ostroff SM, Kapperud G, Lassen J, et al. Clinical features of sporadic *Yersinia enterocolitica* infections in Norway. J Infect Dis. 1992;166:812-817.

46. Tauxe RV, Vandepitte J, Wauters G, et al. *Yersinia enterocolitica* infections and pork: The missing link. Lancet. 1987;1:1129-1132.

47. Black RE, Jackson RJ, Tsai T, et al. Epidemic *Yersinia enterocolitica* infection due to contaminated chocolate milk. N Engl J Med. 1978;298:76.

48. Ackers ML, Schoenfeld S, Markman J, et al. An outbreak of *Yersinia enterocolitica* O:8 infections associated with pasteurized milk. J Infect Dis. 2000;181:1834-1837.

49. Asakawa Y, Akahane S, Kagata N, et al. Two community outbreaks of human infection with *Yersinia enterocolitica*. J Hyg (Lond). 1973;71:715.

50. Slutsker L, Ries AA, Greene KD, et al. *Escherichia coli* O157:H7 diarrhea in the United States: Clinical and epidemiologic features. Ann Intern Med. 1997;126:505.

51. Griffin PM, Ostroff SM, Tauxe RV, et al. Illnesses associated with *Escherichia coli* O157:H7 infections: A broad clinical spectrum. Ann Intern Med. 1988;109:705-712.

52. Johnson WM, Lior H, Bezanson GS. Cytotoxic *Escherichia coli* O157:H7 associated with haemorrhagic colitis in Canada. Lancet. 1983;1:76.

53. O'Brien AD, Lively TA, Chen ME, et al. *Escherichia coli* O157:H7 strains associated with haemorrhagic colitis in the United States produce a *Shigella dysenteriae* 1 (Shiga) like cytotoxin. Lancet. 1983;1:702.

54. Lingwood CA, Mylvaganam M, Arab S, et al. Shiga toxin (verotoxin) binding to its receptor glycolipid. In: Kaper JB, O'Brien AD, eds. *Escherichia coli* O157:H7 and Other Shiga Toxin–Producing *E. coli* Strains. Washington, DC: American Society for Microbiology; 1998:129-139.

55. Griffin PM, Mead PS, Sivapalasingam S. *Escherichia coli* O157:H7 and Other enterohemorrhagic *E. coli*. In: Blaser MJ, Smith PD, Ravdin JI, eds. Infections of the Gastrointestinal Tract. 2nd ed. Philadelphia: Lippincott Williams and Wilkins; 2002:627-642.

56. Boyce TG, Swerdlow DL, Griffin PM. *Escherichia coli* O157:H7 and the hemolytic-uremic syndrome. N Engl J Med. 1995;333:364-367.

57. Centers for Disease Control and Prevention. Outbreak of acute gastroenteritis attributable to *Escherichia coli* serotype O104:H21-Montana. MMWR Morb Mortal Wkly Rep. 1995;44:501-504.

58. Banatvala N, Debeukelaer MM, Griffin PM, et al. Shiga-like toxin-producing *Escherichia coli* O111 and associated hemolytic uremic syndrome: A family outbreak. Pediatr Infect Dis J. 1996;15:1008-1011.

59. Centers for Disease Control and Prevention. *Escherichia coli* O111:H8 outbreak among teenage campers—Texas, 1999. MMWR Morb Mortal Wkly Rep. 2000;49:321-324.

60. Shapiro RL, Hatheway C, Swerdlow DL. Botulism in the United States: A clinical and epidemiological review. Ann Intern Med. 1998;129:221-228.

61. Woodruff BA, Griffin PM, McCroskey LM, et al. Clinical and laboratory comparison of botulism from toxin types A, B, and E in the United States, 1975-1988. J Infect Dis. 1992;166:1281-1286.

62. Hughes JM, Blumenthal JR, Merson MH, et al. Clinical features of types A and B food-borne botulism. Ann Intern Med. 1981;95:442.

63. Kao I, Drachman DB, Price DL. Botulinum toxin: Mechanism of presynaptic blockade. Science. 1976;193:1256.

64. Simpson LL. The origin, structure, and pharmacological activity of botulinum toxin. Pharmacol Rev. 1981;33:155.

65. Horwitz MA, Hughes JM, Merson MH, et al. Food-borne botulism in the United States, 1970-1975. J Infect Dis. 1977;136:153.

66. Midura TF, Arnon SS. Infant botulism: Identification of *Clostridium botulinum* and its toxins in feces. Lancet. 1976;2:934.

67. Arnon SS. Infant botulism. In: Feigen RD, Cherry JD, eds. Textbook of Pediatric Infectious Diseases. 4th ed. Philadelphia: WB Saunders; 1998:1570-1577.

68. Sugiyama H, Mills DC. Intraintestinal toxin in infant mice challenged intragastrically with *Clostridium botulinum* spores. Infect Immun. 1978;21:59.

69. St Louis ME, Shaun HS, Peck MB, et al. Botulism from chopped garlic: Delayed recognition of a major outbreak. Ann Intern Med. 1988;108:363-368.

70. Mead P, Slutsker L, Gellin B. Listeriosis. In: Ryser ET, Marth EH, eds. Listeria, Listeriosis, and Food Safety. 2nd ed. New York: Marcel Dekker; 1999:801-811.

71. Centers for Disease Control and Prevention. Outbreak of listeriosis: Northeastern United States, 2002. MMWR Morb Mortal Wkly Rep. 2002;51:950.

72. Centers for Disease Control and Prevention. Multistate outbreak of listeriosis—United States, 2000. MMWR Morb Mortal Wkly Rep. 2000;50:101.

73. Jackson LA, Wenger JD. Listeriosis: A foodborne disease. Infect Med. 1993;10:61-66.

74. Blake PA, Merson MH, Weaver RE, et al. Disease caused by a marine *Vibrio:* Clinical characteristics and epidemiology. N Engl J Med. 1979;300:1-5.

75. Barth WF, Segal K. Reactive arthritis (Reiter's syndrome). Am Fam Physician. 1999;60:499-507.

76. Conner BA, Johnson E, Soave R. Reiter's syndrome following protracted symptoms of *Cyclospora* infection. Emerg Inf Dis. 2001;7:453-454.

77. Dworkin MS, Shoemaker PC, Goldoft MJ, Kobayashi JM. Reactive arthritis and Reiter's syndrome following an outbreak of gastroenteritis caused by *Salmonella enteritidis*. Clin Infect Dis. 2001;33:1010-1014.

78. Semple AB, Parry WH, Phillips DE. Acute copper poisoning: An outbreak traced to contaminated water from a corroded geyser. Lancet. 1960;2:700.

79. Brown MA, Thom JV, Orth GL, et al. Food poisoning involving zinc contamination. Arch Environ Health. 1964;8:657.

80. Centers for Disease Control and Prevention. Illness associated with elevated levels of zinc in fruit punch: New Mexico. MMWR Morb Mortal Wkly Rep. 1983;32:257.

81. Barker WH Jr, Runte V. Tomato juice-associated gastroenteritis, Washington and Oregon, 1969. Am J Epidemiol. 1972;96:219.

82. Baker TD, Hafner WG. Cadmium poisoning from a refrigerator shelf used as an improvised barbecue grill. Public Health Rep. 1961;76:543.

83. Merson MH, Baine WB, Gangarosa EJ, et al. Scombroid fish poisoning: Outbreak traced to commercially canned tuna fish. JAMA. 1974;228:1268.

84. Taylor SL. Histamine food poisoning: Toxicology and clinical aspects. CRC Crit Rev Toxicol. 1986;17:91-128.

85. Lehane L, Olley J. Histamine food poisoning revisited. Int J Food Microbiol. 2000;58:1-37.

86. Taylor SL, Guthertz LS, Leatherwood M, et al. Histamine production by *Klebsiella pneumoniae* and an incident of scombroid fish poisoning. Appl Environ Microbiol. 1979;37:274.

87. Hughes JM, Merson MH. Fish and shellfish poisoning. N Engl J Med. 1976; 295:1117.

88. Perl TM, Bedard L, Kosatsky T, et al. An outbreak of toxic encephalopathy caused by eating mussels contaminated with domoic acid. New Engl J Med. 1990;322:1775-1780.

89. Halstead BW, Courville DA. Poisonous and Venomous Marine Animals of the World, v. 1. Invertebrates. Washington, DC: Government Printing Office; 1965:157.

90. Zwahlen A, Blanc MH, Robert M. Epidémie d'intoxication par les moules ("Paralytic shellfish poisoning"). Schweiz Med Wochenschr. 1977;107:226.

91. Acres J, Gray J. Paralytic shellfish poisoning. Can Med Assoc J. 1978;119: 1195-1197.

92. Rodriguez DC, Etzel RA, Hall S, et al. Lethal paralytic shellfish poisoning in Guatemala. Am J Trop Med Hyg. 1990;42:267-271.

93. Centers for Disease Control and Prevention. Neurologic illness associated with eating Florida pufferfish, 2002. MMWR Morb Mortal Wkly Rep. 2002;51:321-323.

94. Proctor NH, Chan SL, Trevor AJ. Production of saxitoxin by cultures of *Gonyaulax catenella*. Toxicon. 1975;13:1-9.

95. Ghazarossian VE, Schantz EJ, Schnoes HK, et al. Identification of a poison in toxic scallops from a *Gonyaulax tamarensis* red tide. Biochem Biophys Res Comm. 1974;59:1219.

96. Shimizu Y, Buckley LJ, Alam M, et al. Structures of gonyautoxin II and III from the East Coast toxic dinoflagellate *Gonyaulax tamarensis*. J Am Chem Soc. 1976;98:5414.

97. Schantz EJ, Ghazarossian VE, Schnoes HK, et al. The structure of saxitoxin. J Am Chem Soc. 1975;97:1238.

98. Henderson R, Ritchie JM, Strichartz GR. The binding of labelled saxitoxin to the sodium channels in nerve membranes. J Physiol. 1973;235:783.

99. Henderson R, Ritchie JM, Strichartz GR. Evidence that tetrodotoxin and saxitoxin act at a metal cation binding site in the sodium channels of nerve membrane. Proc Natl Acad Sci U S A. 1974;71:3936.

100. Catterall WA. Neurotoxins that act on voltage-sensitive sodium channels in excitable membranes. Annu Rev Pharmacol Toxicol. 1980;20:15.

101. Spiegelstein MY, Paster Z, Abbott BC. Purification and biological activity of Gymnodinium breve toxins. Toxicon. 1973;11:85.

102. Kim YS, Padilla GM. Purification of the ichthyotoxic component of Gymnodinium breve (red tide dinoflagellate) toxin by high pressure liquid chromatography. Toxicon. 1976;14:379.

103. Grunfeld Y, Spiegelstein MY. Effects of Gymnodinium breve toxin on the smooth muscle preparation of guinea-pig ileum. Br J Pharmacol. 1974;51:67.

104. Teitlebaum JS, Zatorre RJ, Carpenter S, et al. Neurologic sequelae of domoic acid intoxication due to the ingestion of contaminated mussels. N Engl J Med. 1990;322:1781-1787.

105. Schaumburg HH, Byck R, Gerstl R, et al. Monosodium L-glutamate: Its pharmacology and role in the Chinese restaurant syndrome. Science. 1969;163:826.

106. Reif-Lehrer L. A questionnaire study of the prevalence of Chinese restaurant syndrome. Fed Proc. 1977;36:1617.

107. Hudson PJ, Vogt RL. A foodborne outbreak traced to niacin overenrichment. J Food Protection. 1985;48:249-251.

108. Barkin RM. Ciguatera poisoning: A common source outbreak. South Med J. 1974;67:13.

109. Halstead BW. Fish poisoning: The diagnosis, pharmacology and treatment. Clin Pharmacol Ther. 1964;5:615.

110. Russell FE. Ciguatera poisoning: A report of 35 cases. Toxicon. 1975;13:383.

111. Halstead BW, Courville DA. Poisonous and Venomous Marine Animals of the World, v. 1. Vertebrates. Washington, DC: Government Printing Office; 1967:63.

112. Engleberg NC, Morris JG Jr, Lewis J, et al. Ciguatera fish poisoning: A major common-source outbreak in the U.S. Virgin Islands. Ann Intern Med. 1983;98:336.

113. Bagnis R, Kuberski T, Laugier S. Clinical observations on 3,009 cases of ciguatera (fish poisoning) in the South Pacific. Am J Trop Med Hyg. 1979;28:1067.

114. Morris JG Jr, Lewin P, Hargrett NT, et al. Clinical features of ciguatera fish poisoning: A study of the disease in the U.S. Virgin Islands. Arch Intern Med. 1982;142:1090.

115. Scheuer PJ, Takahashi W, Tsutsumi J, et al. Ciguatoxin: Isolation and chemical nature. Science. 1967;155:1267.

116. Helfrich P, Banner AH. Experimental induction of ciguatera: Toxicity in fish through diet. Nature. 1963;197:1025.

117. Morris JG Jr. Natural toxins associated with fish and shellfish. In: Blaser MJ, Smith PD, Ravdin JI, eds. Infections of the Gastrointestinal Tract. 2nd ed. Philadelphia: Lippincott Williams and Wilkins; 2002:215-221.

118. Li K-M. Ciguatera fish poison: A cholinesterase inhibitor. Science. 1965;147:1580.

119. Halstead BW. Current status of marine biotoxicology: An overview. Clin Toxicol. 1981;18:1.

120. Le Grand AM, Galonnier M, Bagnis R. Studies on the mode of action of ciguateric toxins. Toxicon. 1982;20:311-315.

121. Bidard JN, Vijverberg HPM, Frelin C, et al. Ciguatoxin is a novel type of Na⁺ channel toxin. J Biol Chem. 1984;259:8353-8357.

122. Lampe KF. Current concepts of therapy in mushroom intoxication. Clin Toxicol. 1974;7:115.

123. Becker CE, Tong TG, Boerner U, et al. Diagnosis and treatment of Amanita phalloides-type mushroom poisoning: Use of thioctic acid. West J Med. 1976;125:100.

124. Hall AH, Spoerke DG, Rumack BH. Mushroom poisoning: Identification, diagnosis, and treatment. Pediatr Rev. 1987;8:291-298.

125. Lampe KF. Toxic fungi. Annu Rev Pharmacol Toxicol. 1979;19:85.

126. Paaso B, Harrison DC. A new look at an old problem: Mushroom poisoning. Am J Med. 1975;58:505.

127. Hughes JM, Horwitz MA, Merson MH, et al. Foodborne disease outbreaks of chemical etiology in the United States, 1970-1974. Am J Epidemiol. 1977;105:233.

128. Editorial: Death-cap poisoning. Lancet. 1972;1:1320.

129. Centers for Disease Control and Prevention. Mushroom poisoning among Laotian refugees: 1981. MMWR Morb Mortal Wkly Rep. 1982;31:287.

130. Centers for Disease Control and Prevention. Amanita phalloides mushroom poisoning: Northern California, January 1997. MMWR Morb Mortal Wkly Rep. 1997;46:489-492.

131. Wieland T, Wieland O. The toxic peptides of Amanita species. In: Kadis S, Ciegler A, Aji SJ, eds. Microbiol Toxins, v. 8: Fungal Toxins. New York: Academic Press; 1972:249.

132. Herwaldt BL. Cyclospora cayetanensis: A review, focusing on the outbreaks of cyclosporiasis in the 1990s. Clin Infect Dis. 2000;31:1040-1057.

133. Osterholm MT, MacDonald KL, White KE, et al. An outbreak of a newly recognized chronic diarrhea syndrome associated with raw milk consumption. JAMA. 1986;256:484-490.

134. Martin DL, Hoberman LJ. A point source outbreak of chronic diarrhea in Texas: No known exposure to raw milk. JAMA. 1986;256:469.

135. Mintz ED, Weber JT, Guris D, et al. An outbreak of Brainerd diarrhea among travelers to the Galapagos Islands. J Infect Dis. 1998;177:1041.

136. Merson MH, Barker WH Jr, Craun GF, et al. Outbreaks of waterborne disease in the United States, 1971-1972. J Infect Dis. 1974;129:614.

137. Hughes JM, Merson MH, Craun GF, et al. Outbreaks of waterborne disease in the United States, 1973. J Infect Dis. 1975;132:336.

138. Horwitz MA, Hughes JM, Craun GF. Outbreaks of waterborne disease in the United States, 1974. J Infect Dis. 1976;133:588.

139. Black RE, Horwitz MA, Craun GF. Outbreaks of waterborne disease in the United States, 1975. J Infect Dis. 1978;137:370.

140. Centers for Disease Control and Prevention. Foodborne and Waterborne Disease Outbreaks Annual Summary 1976. October 1977.

141. Centers for Disease Control and Prevention. Foodborne and Waterborne Disease Surveillance Annual Summary 1977. August 1979.

142. Centers for Disease Control and Prevention. Water-Related Disease Outbreaks Surveillance Annual Summary 1978. May 1980.

143. Centers for Disease Control and Prevention. Water-Related Disease Outbreaks Surveillance Annual Summary 1979. September 1981.

144. Centers for Disease Control and Prevention. Water-Related Disease Outbreaks Surveillance Annual Summary 1980. February 1982.

145. Centers for Disease Control and Prevention. Water-Related Disease Outbreaks Surveillance Annual Summary 1981. September 1982.

146. Centers for Disease Control and Prevention. Water-Related Disease Outbreaks Surveillance Annual Summary 1982. Centers for Disease Control. 1983;1-15.

147. Centers for Disease Control and Prevention. Water-Related Disease Outbreaks Surveillance Annual Summary 1983. 1984;1-15.

148. Centers for Disease Control and Prevention. Water-Related Disease Outbreaks Surveillance Annual Summary 1984. 1985;1-15.

149. St Louis ME. Water-Related Disease Outbreaks, 1985. CDC surveillance summaries. MMWR Morb Mortal Wkly Rep. 1986;37(SS-2):15-24.

150. Levine WC, Stephenson WT, Craun GF. Waterborne disease outbreaks, 1986-1988. Centers for Disease Control Surveillance Summaries, March 1990. MMWR Morb Mortal Wkly Rep. 1990;39(SS-1):1-13.

151. Herwaldt BL, Craun GF, Stokes SL, et al. Waterborne disease outbreaks, 1989-1990. Centers for Disease Control Surveillance Summaries, December 1991. MMWR Morb Mortal Wkly Rep. 1991;40(SS-3):1-21.

152. Moore AC, Herwaldt BL, Craun GC, et al. Surveillance for waterborne disease outbreaks: United States, 1991-1992. MMWR Morb Mortal Wkly Rep. 1993;42(SS-5):1.

153. Kramer MH, Herwaldt BL, Craun GC, et al. Surveillance for waterborne disease outbreaks: United States, 1993-1994. MMWR Morb Mortal Wkly Rep. 1996;45(SS-1):1.

154. Levy DA, Bens MS, Craun GC, et al. Surveillance for waterborne disease outbreaks: United States, 1995-1996. MMWR Morb Mortal Wkly Rep. 1998;47(SS-5):1.

155. Barwick RS, Levy DA, Bens MS, Craun GC, et al. Surveillance for waterborne disease outbreaks: United States, 1997-1998. MMWR Morb Mortal Wkly Rep. 2000;49(SS-4):1.

156. Lee S, Levy DA, Craun GC, et al. Surveillance for waterborne disease outbreaks: United States, 1999-2000. MMWR Morb Mortal Wkly Rep. 2000;51(SS-8):1.

157. MacKenzie WR, Hoxie NJ, Proctor ME, et al. A massive outbreak in Milwaukee of Cryptosporidium infection transmitted through the public water supply. N Engl J Med. 1994;331:161.

158. Swerdlow DL, Woodruff BA, Brady RC, et al. A waterborne outbreak in Missouri of Escherichia coli O157:H7 associated with bloody diarrhea and death. Ann Intern Med. 1992;117:812-819.

159. Olsen SJ, Miller G, Breuer T, et al. Waterborne outbreak of Escherichia coli O157:H7 infections and hemolytic uremic syndrome: Implications for rural water systems. Emerg Infect Dis. 2002;8:370-375.

160. Weissman JB, Craun GF, Lawrence DN, et al. An epidemic of gastroenteritis traced to a contaminated public water supply. Am J Epidemiol. 1976;103:391.

161. Mosley JW. Water-borne infectious hepatitis. N Engl J Med. 1959;261:703.

162. Feldman RE, Baine WB, Nitzkin JL, et al. Epidemiology of Salmonella typhi infection in a migrant labor camp in Dade County, Florida. J Infect Dis. 1974;130:334.

163. A collaborative report. A waterborne epidemic of salmonellosis in Riverside, California, 1965: Epidemiologic aspects. Am J Epidemiol. 1971;93:33.

164. Rosenberg ML, Koplan JP, Wachsmuth IK, et al. Epidemic diarrhea at Crater Lake from enterotoxigenic Escherichia coli: A large waterborne outbreak. Ann Intern Med. 1977;86:714.

165. Vogt RL, Sours HE, Barrett T, et al. Campylobacter enteritis associated with contaminated water. Ann Intern Med. 1982;96:292.

166. Palmer SR, Gully PR, White JM, et al. Water-borne outbreak of Campylobacter gastroenteritis. Lancet. 1983;1:287.

167. Parsonnet J, Trock SC, Bopp CA, et al. Chronic diarrhea associated with drinking untreated water. Ann Intern Med. 1989;110:985-991.

168. Wilson R, Anderson LJ, Holman RC, et al. Waterborne gastroenteritis due to the Norwalk agent: Clinical and epidemiologic investigation. Am J Public Health. 1982;72:72.

169. Kaplan JE, Goodman RA, Schonberger LB, et al. Gastroenteritis due to Norwalk virus: An outbreak associated with a municipal water system. J Infect Dis. 1982;146:190.

170. Anderson AD, Heryford AG, Sarisky JP, et al. A waterborne outbreak of Norwalk-like virus among snowmobilers: Wyoming, 2001. J Infect Dis. 2003;187:303-306.

171. Bowie WR, King AS, Werker DH, et al. Outbreak of toxoplasmosis associated with municipal drinking water. The BC Toxoplasma Investigation Team. Lancet. 1997;350:173-177.

172. Gilbert RJ, Stringer MF, Peace TC. The survival and growth of Bacillus cereus in boiled and fried rice in relation to outbreaks of food poisoning. J Hyg (Lond). 1974;73:433.

173. McClane B. Clostridium perfringens. In: Doyle MP, Beuchat LR, Montville TJ, eds. Food Microbiology: Fundamentals and Frontiers. Washington, DC: American Society for Microbiology; 1997:305-326.

174. Kim HU, Goepfert JM. Enumeration and identification of *Bacillus cereus* in foods: I. 24-hour presumptive test medium. Appl Microbiol. 1971;22:581.

175. Blakey LJ, Priest FG. The occurrence of *Bacillus cereus* in some dried foods including pulses and cereals. J Appl Bacteriol. 1980;48:297.

176. Jephcott AE, Barton BW, Gilbert RJ, et al. An unusual outbreak of food-poisoning associated with meals-on-wheels. Lancet. 1977;2:129.

177. St. Louis ME, Morse DL, Potter ME, et al. The emergence of grade A eggs as a major source of *Salmonella enteritidis* infections. JAMA. 1988;259:2103-2107.

178. Centers for Disease Control and Prevention. Outbreaks of *Salmonella* serotype Enteritidis infections associated with eating shell eggs: United States, 1999-2001. MMWR Morb Mortal Wkly Rep. 2003;51:1149-1152.

179. Centers for Disease Control and Prevention. Multistate outbreak of *Salmonella* serotype Typhimurium infections associated with drinking unpasteurized milk: Illinois, Indiana, Ohio and Tennessee, 2002-2003. MMWR Morb Mortal Wkly Rep. 2003;52:613-615.

180. Centers for Disease Control and Prevention. Multistate outbreaks of *Salmonella* serotype Poona infections associated with eating cantaloupe from Mexico: United States and Canada, 2000-2002. MMWR Morb Mortal Wkly Rep. 2002;51:1044-1047.

181. Centers for Disease Control and Prevention. Outbreak of *Salmonella* serotype Javiana infections: Orlando, Florida, June 2002. MMWR Morb Mortal Wkly Rep. 2002;51:683-684.

182. Centers for Disease Control and Prevention. Outbreak of *Salmonella* serotype Muenchen infections associated with unpasteurized orange juice: United States and Canada, June 1999. MMWR Morb Mortal Wkly Rep. 1999;48:582-585.

183. Centers for Disease Control and Prevention. Outbreak of *Salmonella* serotype Kottbus infections associated with eating alfalfa sprouts: Arizona, California, Colorado, and New Mexico, February-April 2001. MMWR Morb Mortal Wkly Rep. 2002;51:7-9.

184. Mahon BE, Pönkä A, Hall WN, et al. An international outbreak of *Salmonella* infections caused by alfalfa sprouts grown from contaminated seeds. J Infect Dis. 1997;175:876-882.

185. Gill ON, Bartlett CLR, Sockett PN, et al. Outbreak of *Salmonella napoli* infection caused by contaminated chocolate bars. Lancet. 1983;1:574.

186. Killalea D, Ward LR, Roberts D, et al. International epidemiological and microbiological study of outbreak of *Salmonella agona* infection from a ready to eat savoury snack: I. England and Wales and the United States. BMJ. 1996;313:1105-1107.

187. Centers for Disease Control and Prevention. Multistate outbreak of *Salmonella* serotype Agona infections linked to toasted oats cereal: United States, April-May, 1998. MMWR Morb Mortal Wkly Rep. 1998;47:462-464.

188. Centers for Disease Control and Prevention. Outbreaks of *Shigella sonnei* infection associated with eating fresh parsley: United States and Canada, July-August 1998. MMWR Morb Mortal Wkly Rep. 1999;48:285-289.

189. Centers for Disease Control and Prevention. Hospital-associated outbreak of *Shigella dysenteriae* type 2: Maryland. MMWR Morb Mortal Wkly Rep. 1983;32:250.

190. Cook KA, Boyce T, Langkop C, et al. Scallions and shigellosis: A multistate outbreak traced to imported green onions (Abstract). Proceedings of the 44th Annual Conference of the Epidemic Intelligence Service. Atlanta, Ga: Centers for Disease Control and Prevention; 1995:36.

191. Frost JA, McEvoy MB, Bentley CA, et al. An outbreak of *Shigella sonnei* infection associated with consumption of iceberg lettuce. Emerg Infect Dis. 1995;1:6-9.

192. Friedman, CR, Neiman J, Wegener HC, Tauxe RV. Epidemiology of *Campylobacter jejuni* infections in the United States and other industrialized nations. In: Nachamkin I, Blaser ML, Tompkins L, eds. *Campylobacter jejuni:* Current Status and Future Trends. 2nd ed. Washington, DC: American Society of Microbiology; 2000:121-137.

193. Daniels NA, MacKinnon L, Bishop R, et al. *Vibrio parahaemolyticus* infections in the United States, 1973-1998. J Infect Dis. 2000;181:1661-1666.

194. Mintz ED, Popovic T, Blake PA. Transmission of *Vibrio cholerae* O1. In: Wachsmuth IK, Blake PA, Olsvik O, eds. *Vibrio cholerae* and Cholera: Molecular to Global Perspectives. Washington, DC: American Society for Microbiology; 1994:345-356.

195. Blake PA. Endemic cholera in Australia and the United States. In: Wachsmuth IK, Blake PA, Olsvik O, eds. *Vibrio cholerae* and Cholera: Molecular to Global Perspectives. Washington, DC: American Society for Microbiology; 1994:309-320.

196. Finelli L, Swerdlow D, Mertz K, et al. Outbreak of cholera associated with crab brought from an area with epidemic disease. J Infect Dis. 1992;166:1433-1435.

197. Merson MH, Morris GH, Sack DA, et al. Travelers' diarrhea in Mexico. N Engl J Med. 1976;294:1299.

198. MacDonald KL, Eidson M, Strohmeyer C, et al. A multistate outbreak of gastrointestinal illness caused by enterotoxigenic *Escherichia coli* in imported semisoft cheese. J Infect Dis. 1985;151:716-720.

199. Daniels NA, Neimann J, Karpati A, et al. Traveler's diarrhea at sea: Three outbreaks of waterborne enterotoxigenic *Escherichia coli* on cruise ships. J Infect Dis. 2000;181:1491-1495.

200. Dalton C, Mintz ED, Wells JG, et al. Outbreaks of enterotoxigenic *Escherichia coli* infection in American adults: A clinical and epidemiologic profile. Epidemiol Infect. 1999;123:9-16.

201. Centers for Disease Control and Prevention. Foodborne outbreaks of enterotoxigenic *Escherichia coli*—Rhode Island and New Hampshire, 1993. MMWR Morb Mortal Wkly Rep. 1994;43:87-88.

202. MacDonald KL, Cohen ML, Blake PA. The changing epidemiology of adult botulism in the United States. Am J Epidemiol. 1986;124:794-799.

203. Spika JS, Shaffer N, Hargrett-Bean N. Risk factors for infant botulism in the United States. Am J Dis Child. 1989;143:828-832.

204. Murphy AM, Grohmann GS, Christopher PJ, et al. An Australia-wide outbreak of gastroenteritis from oysters caused by Norwalk virus. Med J Aust. 1979;2:329.

205. Morse DL, Guzewich JJ, Hanrahan JP, et al. Widespread outbreaks of clam- and oyster-associated gastroenteritis: Role of Norwalk virus. N Engl J Med. 1986;314:678-681.

206. Gunn RA, Janowski HT, Lieb S, et al. Norwalk virus gastroenteritis following raw oyster consumption. Am J Epidemiol. 1982;115:348.

207. Griffin MR, Surowiec JJ, McCloskey DI, et al. Foodborne Norwalk virus. Am J Epidemiol. 1982;115:178.

208. Kohn MA, Farley TA, Ando T, et al. An outbreak of Norwalk virus gastroenteritis associated with eating raw oysters. JAMA. 1995;273:466-471.

209. Centers for Disease Control and Prevention. Update: Outbreaks of cyclosporiasis. MMWR Morb Mortal Wkly Rep. 1997;46:521-523.

210. Centers for Disease Control and Prevention. Outbreaks of cyclosporiasis-Northern Virginia/Washington, DC/Baltimore, Maryland Metropolitan Area, 1997. MMWR Morb Mortal Wkly Rep. 1997;46:689-691.

211. Hopper SH, Adams HS. Copper poisoning from vending machines. Public Health Rep. 1958;73:910.

212. Hesse IDW, Halstead BW, Peckham NH. Marine biotoxins. I. Ciguatera poison: Some biological and chemical aspects. Ann N Y Acad Sci. 1960;90:788-797.

213. Török TJ, Tauxe RV, Wise RP, et al. A large community outbreak of salmonellosis caused by intentional contamination of restaurant salad bars. JAMA. 1997;278:389-395.

214. Kolavic SA, Kimura A, Simons SL, et al. An outbreak of *Shigella dysenteriae* type 2 among laboratory workers due to intentional food contamination. JAMA. 1997;278:396-398.

215. Arnon SS, Schechter R, Inglesby TV, et al. Botulinum toxin as a biological weapon: Medical and public health management. JAMA. 2001;285:1059-1070.

216. Altekruse SF, Hyman FH, Klontz KC, et al. Foodborne bacterial infections in individuals with the human immunodeficiency virus. South Med J. 1994;87:169-173.

217. Angulo FJ, Swerdlow DL. Bacterial enteric infections in persons infected with human immunodeficiency virus. Clin Infect Dis. 1995;21(Suppl 1):S84-S93.

218. Shapiro RL, Altekruse S, Hutwagner L, et al. The role of Gulf Coast oysters harvested in warmer months in *Vibrio vulnificus* infections in the United States, 1988-1996. J Infect Dis. 1998;178:752-759.

219. Collins JC, Bicknell WJ. The red tide: A public-health emergency. N Engl J Med. 1974;288:1126.

220. Lawrence DN, Enriquez MB, Lumish RM, et al. Ciguatera fish poisoning in Miami. JAMA. 1980;244:254.

221. Barker WH Jr. *Vibrio parahaemolyticus* outbreaks in the United States. Lancet. 1974;1:551.

222. Centers for Disease Control and Prevention. Outbreak of *Vibrio parahaemolyticus* infections associated with eating raw oysters-Pacific Northwest, 1997. MMWR Morb Mortal Wkly Rep. 1998;47:457-462.

223. Morris JG Jr, Lewin P, Smith CW, et al. Ciguatera fish poisoning: Epidemiology of the disease on St. Thomas, U.S. Virgin Islands. Am J Trop Med Hyg. 1982;31:574.

224. Lew JF, LeBaron CW, Glass RI, et al. Recommendations for collection of laboratory specimens associated with outbreaks of gastroenteritis. MMWR Morb Mortal Wkly Rep. 1990;39(RR 14):1-13.

225. Swaminathan B, Barrett TJ, Hunter SB, Tauxe RV, CDC PulseNet Task Force. PulseNet: The molecular subtyping network for foodborne bacterial diseases surveillance, United States. Emerg Infect Dis. 2001;7:382-389.

226. Jablonski LM, Bohach GA. *Staphylococcus aureus*. In: Doyle MP, Beuchat LR, Montville TJ, eds. Food Microbiology: Fundamentals and Frontiers. Washington, DC: ASM Press; 1997:353-375.

227. Ghosh AC. Prevalence of *Bacillus cereus* in the faeces of healthy adults. J Hyg (Lond). 1978;80:233.

228. De Buono BA, Brondum J, Kramer JM, et al. Plasmid, serotypic, and enterotoxin analysis of *Bacillus cereus* in an outbreak setting. J Clin Microbiol. 1988;26:1571-1574.

229. Feng P. Detecting foodborne pathogens and their toxins: Conventional versus rapid and automated methods. In: Doyle MP, Beuchat LR, Montville TJ, eds. Food Microbiology: Fundamentals and Frontiers. 2nd ed. Washington, DC: ASM Press; 2001:775-796.

230. Hauschild AHW. Criteria and procedures for implicating *Clostridium perfringens* in food-borne outbreaks. Can J Public Health. 1975;66:388.

231. Schiemann DA. Laboratory confirmation of an outbreak of *Clostridium perfringens* food poisoning. Health Lab Sci. 1977;14:35-38.

232. Harmon SM, Kautter DA. Evaluation of a reversed passive latex agglutination test kit for *Clostridium perfringens* enterotoxin. J Food Protection. 1986;49:523-525.

233. McClane BA, Strouse RJ. Rapid detection of *Clostridium perfringens* type A enterotoxin by enzyme-linked immunosorbent assay. J Clin Microbiol. 1984;19:112-115.

234. Birkhead G, Vogt RL, Heun EM, et al. Characterization of an outbreak of *Clostridium perfringens* food poisoning by quantitative fecal culture and fecal enterotoxin measurement. J Clin Microbiol. 1988;26:471-474.

235. Wachsmuth IK, Evins GM, Fields PI, et al. The molecular epidemiology of cholera in Latin America. J Infect Dis. 1993;167:621-626.

236. Bopp CA, Brenner FW, Fields PI, et al. *Escherichia, Shigella,* and *Salmonella*. In: Murray PR, Baron EJ, Jorgensen JH, et al, eds. Manual of Clinical Microbiology. 8th ed. Washington, DC: American Society of Microbiologists. 2003:654-671.

237. Dowell VR Jr, McCroskey LM, Hatheway CL, et al. Coproexamination for botulinal toxin and *Clostridium botulinum*. JAMA. 1977;238:1829.

238. Mann JM, Hatheway CL, Gardiner TM. Laboratory diagnosis in a large outbreak of type A botulism. Am J Epidemiol. 1982;115:598.

239. Eberhard ML, Pieniazek NJ, Arrowood MJ. Laboratory diagnosis of *Cyclospora* infections. Arch Pathol Lab Med. 1997;121:792.

240. Garcia LS, Bruckner DA. Diagnostic medical parasitology. 3rd ed. Washington, DC: American Society for Microbiology; 1997:66-69.

241. Hokama Y, Abad MA, Kimura LH. A rapid enzyme-immunoassay for the detection of ciguatoxin in contaminated fish tissues. Toxicon. 1983;21:817-824.

242. Guerrant RL, Van Gilder T, Thielman NM, et al. Practice guidelines for the management of infectious diarrhea. Clin Infect Dis. 2001;32:331-350.

243. Meyers KEC, Schulman SL, Kaplan BS. Principles of the treatment of Shiga toxin-associated hemolytic uremic syndrome: Pay meticulous attention to detail and do no harm. In: Kaper JB, O'Brien AD, eds. *Escherichia coli* O157:H7 and Other Shiga Toxin-Producing *E. coli* Strains. Washington, DC: American Society for Microbiology; 1998:364.

244. Wall PG, Ross D, Van Somern P, et al. Features of the epidemiology of multidrug resistant *Salmonella typhimurium* DT 104 in England and Wales. Proceedings of *Salmonella* and Salmonellosis, 97. Ploufragan, France, 1997:565-567.

245. Glynn MK, Bopp C, DeWitt W, et al. Emergence of multidrug-resistant *Salmonella enterica* serotype Typhimurium DT 104 infections in the United States. N Engl J Med. 1998;338:1333-1338.

246. Wall PG, Morgan D, Lamden K, et al. A case control study of infection with an epidemic strain of multiresistant *Salmonella typhimurium* DT 104 in England and Wales. Commun Dis Rep. 1994;4:R130-R135.

247. Cohen ML, Tauxe RV. Drug-resistant *Salmonella* in the United States: An epidemiologic perspective. Science. 1986;234:964-969.

248. Centers for Disease Control and Prevention. Outbreak of multidrug-resistant *Salmonella* Newport: United States, January-April 2002. MMWR Morb Mortal Wkly Rep. 2002;51:545-548.

249. Swift AEB, Swift TR. Ciguatera. Clin Toxicol. 1993;31:1-29.

250. Lange WR, Kreider SD, Hatwick M, et al. Potential benefit of tocainide in the treatment of ciguatera: Report of three cases. Am J Med. 1988;84:1087-1088.

251. Mitchel DH. *Amanita* mushroom poisoning. Ann Rev Med. 1980;31:51.

252. Osterholm MT, Potter ME. Irradiation pasteurization of solid foods: Taking food safety to the next level. Emerg Infect Dis. 1997;3:575-577.

253. Steele JH, Engel RE. Radiation processing of foods. J Am Vet Med Assoc. 1992;201:1522-1529.

254. Tauxe RV, Kruse H, Hedberg C, et al. Microbial hazards and emerging issues associated with produce: A preliminary report to the National Advisory Committee on Microbiologic Criteria for Foods. J Food Protection. 1997;60:1400-1408.

255. Hedberg CW, MacDonald KL, Osterholm MT. Changing epidemiology of food-borne disease: A Minnesota perspective. Clin Infect Dis. 1994;18:671-682.

256. Jordan MC, Powell KE, Corothers TE, et al. Salmonellosis among restaurant patrons: The incisive role of a meat slicer. Am J Public Health. 1973;63:982.

257. Banatvala N, Magnano AR, Cartter ML, et al. Meat grinders and molecular epidemiology: Two supermarket outbreaks of *Escherichia coli* O157:H7 infections. J Infect Dis. 1996;173:480-483.

258. Tuttle J, Kellerman S, Tauxe RV. The risks of raw shellfish: What every transplant patient should know. J Transpl Coord. 1994;4:60-63.

259. Horwitz MA, Marr JS, Merson MH, et al. A continuing common-source outbreak of botulism in a family. Lancet. 1975;2:861.

260. Payne DJH, Scudamore JM. Outbreaks of salmonella food poisoning over a period of eight years from a common source. Lancet. 1977;1:1249.

261. Cieslak PR, Noble SJ, Maxson DJ, et al. Hamburger-associated *Escherichia coli* O157:H7 infection in Las Vegas: A hidden epidemic. Am J Public Health. 1997;87:176-180.

CHAPTER **96**

Tropical Sprue/Enteropathy

CHRISTINE A. WANKE

Tropical sprue, also called *postinfectious tropical malabsorption,* is a syndrome of enigmatic origin that is characterized by a prolonged diarrheal illness and malabsorption of two or more substances in persons in the tropics who have no other obvious reason for malabsorption. Tropical sprue has been recognized since the 2nd or 3rd century AD, when Aretaeus of Cappadocchia reported on "The Coeliac Affection." The first mention of sprue in the modern medical literature was in 1747, when Hillary emigrated from England to Barbados and published his observations on a prolonged tropical diarrheal disease in native islanders. The English term *sprue* is an adaptation from the Dutch *sprouw,* which originally was used to refer to persistent diarrheal disease in Holland (probably celiac disease). The term *sprue* first was used in 1880 by Manson for the persistent wasting diarrhea that occurred in tropical countries.[1] Knowledge about the cause or pathogenesis of sprue did not advance significantly until investigations were begun after recognized outbreaks during World War II. The distinction between celiac sprue and tropical sprue was not clear until the early 1970s.

EPIDEMIOLOGY

Although sprue is considered a disease of tropical locales, there are distinct geographic areas of risk within the tropics. Tropical sprue has been identified most readily in Asia and the Caribbean islands, and there are isolated areas of particular risk within both hemispheres. Sprue is relatively common among the indigenous populations of Puerto Rico, Haiti, the Dominican Republic, and Cuba, but it is not seen in the rest of the Caribbean islands and no longer is recognized in Barbados.[2,3] It is seen in northern South America, in Venezuela and Colombia, but rarely in Central America or Mexico. It is common on the Indian subcontinent, from the Himalayas to the south, and it has been recognized in Myanmar and the Philippines.[4-6] Little tropical sprue was documented in Africa until the 1970s; cases have been recognized in Rhodesia and South Africa, and tropical sprue has developed among expatriates living in Nigeria.[7] There may be endemic foci of tropical sprue in the Middle East as well, with a spruelike illness recognized in Turkey.

In contrast to other endemic diarrheal illnesses in the tropical world, tropical sprue is a disease mainly of adults. Children are thought to be relatively spared, although disease has been documented in all age groups. Very young children have not been found to have tropical sprue; this may represent a beneficial effect of breast-feeding. In studies of family outbreaks of tropical sprue in South India, even older children developed disease at a significantly lower rate than adults.[8] The reason for this is not clear. Persistent diarrhea develops in children more commonly in parts of the world where the environment is contaminated more heavily with potentially disease-causing microorganisms.[9] Tropical sprue may be one of the causes of prolonged diarrhea and wasting in this age group as well, but studies such as small bowel intubation and cultures or biopsy have shown conflicting results regarding the correlation of small bowel colonization with persistent diarrhea.[10-12]

Some patterns of disease expression are of particular interest in tropical sprue. There are clear epidemics of the disease, which have been documented best in families and villages in South India.[8] There have been descriptions of sprue houses, in which successive tenants have developed disease, and an outbreak was described in which more than half of the exposed persons in an isolated extended family developed tropical sprue within 3 months of onset of disease in the index case. Well-documented outbreaks of sprue affecting entire villages also have been reported, mostly from the Indian subcontinent. Such an epidemic pattern suggests an underlying infectious cause.

There has been seasonal variation in outbreaks of tropical sprue as well. An increased rate of mild tropical sprue in the setting of an increased rate of diarrheal disease was seen more often from March to July than at other times of the year for at least 4 years at an American military base in the Philippines.[6] In these outbreaks, sprue occurred among American military personnel and their dependents, who were eating a high-calorie, Western-style diet. A seasonal variation also has been documented in the rate of occurrence of tropical sprue in the indigenous population of Puerto Rico.[3] This seasonal variation also lends credence to the possibility of an underlying infectious cause.

As suggested by the outbreaks among American military personnel, tropical sprue occurs among expatriates living in endemic areas.[13] Tropical sprue originally was recognized among expatriates and British colonists in India in the early 19th century and subsequently among the Dutch in Java; the French in Indochina; and Americans in the Philippines, Vietnam, and Puerto Rico. Tropical sprue or malabsorption with jejunitis (*tropical enteropathy*) has been described among Peace Corps volunteers and has occurred sporadically among travelers.[14] Generally, tropical sprue develops in an expatriate who has lived for a prolonged time (6 months to 1 year) in an endemic area. Rare cases also have been described among short-term travelers.[15]

Tropical sprue also is recognized among immigrants who leave endemic areas, although they may not complain of gastrointestinal symptoms until they have been out of the endemic area for a prolonged period.[16,17] These exposure data also suggest an infectious origin for tropical sprue.

ETIOLOGY

There is a strong presumption that tropical sprue is caused by an enteric infection, perhaps in individuals predisposed by some nutritional deficiency. The facts lending support to this theory include the following: (1) Often the prolonged episode of tropical sprue is initiated by an episode of acute diarrheal disease; (2) there is an epidemic and seasonal nature to the epidemiology of the disease, as discussed previously; and (3) the disease responds most often to treatment with antibiotics with or without nutritional supplements. The precise nature of the infection that leads to development of tropical sprue is less clear.

Multiple studies in Asia and the Caribbean have shown small bowel bacterial overgrowth in patients with tropical sprue.[14,18,19] Although some bacteria normally live in the upper small bowel of healthy persons, the organisms isolated from this region of the gut in healthy asymptomatic individuals most often are gram-positive. Streptococci, staphylococci, and lactobacilli are among the common isolates, and these are present in small numbers. In the distal small bowel, the cecum, and the colon, anaerobes and facultative gram-negative organisms predominate in normal persons. Small bowel cultures from travelers with tropical sprue show increased numbers of gram-negative rods, including *Alcaligenes, Enterobacter aerogenes,* and *Hafnia* spp. In small bowel cultures from persons with tropical sprue who were native to India, Haiti, or Puerto Rico, *Klebsiella, Escherichia coli,* and *Enterobacter cloacae* were the most common organisms. Carefully done studies in South Africa and India documented similar organisms in similar concentrations in the small bowel of asymptomatic control patients and in patients with tropical sprue, suggesting that environmental contamination may predispose to increased small bowel flora.[14,18,19] In another series of patients from India, the number of organisms found in the small bowel of tropical sprue patients was the same as that found in the small bowel of healthy controls, but the type of organisms isolated varied.[18] Other organisms, especially *Enterobacter* and *Veillonella,* were isolated more frequently from the small bowel of patients with tropical sprue than from healthy controls.[20] Demonstration of organisms does not prove cause and effect, however.

Gram-negative organisms isolated from the small bowel of tropical sprue patients in Haiti were found to have a secretory effect, presumably by toxin production, in rabbit ileal loops and rat perfusion studies.[21,22] These supposedly enterotoxigenic organisms have not been studied for the presence of any of the recognized secretory toxins by currently available methods, such as DNA probes or enzyme-linked immunosorbent assay; these organisms have not been studied for the presence of colonizing factors, such as pili or the hydrophobic surface proteins that are found in many enteric pathogens. *E. coli* and *Klebsiella* isolated from Indian patients with tropical sprue were not found to produce heat-stabile or heat-labile enterotoxins when they were tested.[23] Some animal studies have suggested that small bowel overgrowth by colonizing nontoxigenic *E. coli* can produce a secretory diarrheal syndrome if the level of colonization reaches a high enough concentration within the small bowel.[24,25]

More recent data suggest further that enteroaggregative *E. coli* are associated with malnutrition, with or without persistent diarrhea, and with intestinal inflammation and cytokine production.[26-30] In addition to its association with persistent diarrhea among children in tropical developing areas, enteroaggregative *E. coli* in patients with acquired immunodeficiency syndrome is associated with persistent diarrhea that improves with antimicrobial therapy.[31,32] Strains of *E. coli* from patients with tropical sprue have not been examined for aggregative adherence. The presence of bacteria in the small bowel may potentiate the symptoms caused by the small bowel parasite *Giardia lamblia,* and the interaction of small bowel bacteria and parasites has been consid-

ered as a possible cause of tropical sprue.[33] Infection with hookworm or *Strongyloides stercoralis* also has been discussed as a possible cause for tropical sprue. Reports of tropical sprue occurring in the presence of orthomyxovirus or coronavirus particles in the stool also have appeared in the literature. Cases of tropical sprue have been reported after an intestinal infection with either fungus or the blue-green algae *Prototheca*.[34,35] Although the traditional definition of tropical sprue excludes patients with diarrhea on the basis of recognized pathogens, it is possible that improvements in diagnostic techniques would permit the identification of organisms that are or have been associated with tropical sprue but previously were not able to be isolated or identified. Sequence-based microbial identification is an example of a new technique that may be beneficial in elucidating further the infectious etiology of tropical sprue.[36] Better techniques to diagnose cyclosporiasis and microsporidiosis also may be revealing.[37,38]

That small bowel overgrowth, as it occurs spontaneously in a certain segment of the population in less developed countries or after an acute enteric infection, may precipitate a series of intestinal insults that proceed to full-blown tropical sprue in susceptible persons is at present the most likely etiologic explanation for tropical sprue. The predisposition for progression from intestinal insult to tropical sprue is less easy to explain. Malnutrition, whether generalized or presenting as specific micronutrient deficiencies, may be a predisposing factor, but it is neither necessary nor sufficient, as shown by the occurrence of tropical sprue among apparently well-nourished military personnel and their dependents. Small bowel overgrowth may alter intestinal transit time and promote further overgrowth and intestinal stasis, but it cannot explain the initial colonization that induces the episode.

In vitro data suggest that small bowel colonization by *E. coli* may be increased by low levels of cytokines, as might be expected in chronic parasitic infections in the developing world.[39] As noted previously, certain organisms, such as enteroaggregative *E. coli,* can alter the intestinal environment by the induction of intestinal proinflammatory cytokines and intestinal inflammation.[26] There has been no genetic predisposition noted for tropical sprue as there has been for celiac sprue, and the inflammatory cytokine profile in the lymphocytes of the small bowel in patients with tropical sprue has not been described.

The processes that control the normal colonization of the small bowel are not well understood; the forces that may disrupt these normal processes to permit abnormal colonization are even less well understood. Some of the factors that can affect the normal small bowel colonization process include gastric acidity, which controls the entry of viable organisms into the small bowel, and intestinal mucin glycoprotein, which contains receptors for and specifically binds a variety of bacteria within the small bowel lumen.[40] *Helicobacter pylori* may impair gastric acidity and predispose to small bowel colonization or persistent diarrhea.[41,42]

Bacterial binding to mucin is presumed to promote clearance of pathogenic organisms to protect the small bowel, but it may promote colonization by nonpathogenic organisms or promote small bowel colonization by pathogens when the mucin is damaged by malnutrition, an inflammatory process, or bacterial proteases or mucinases. Some loss of the protective mucin layer in tropical sprue is suggested by evidence that the bacteria visualized often are associated tightly within the mucosa rather than being free within the lumen of the gut.[1] Damage to the protective mucin layer also may permit epithelial cell damage by food or other small bowel antigens. The presence of free bile acids within the upper small bowel can alter intestinal bacterial growth rates and colonization, but bile acid concentrations have not been abnormal in patients with tropical sprue, and the bacterial organisms that have been cultured from patients with tropical sprue are not organisms that classically alter bile salt metabolism.[23]

Intestinal immunologic dysfunction has been suggested as a factor that might predispose to abnormal bacterial colonization in tropical sprue. Patients with deficiencies of secretory IgA are subject to more frequent and severe bouts of enteric infections. In addition to secretory IgA, lymphoid tissue is present throughout the small bowel focally in Peyer's patches and diffusely as mucosal lymphocytes. When small bowel lymphocytes were characterized in patients with tropical sprue and in control patients with irritable bowel syndrome in southern India, there was no difference in the number of IgA-producing, IgG-producing, or IgM-producing lymphocytes between the two groups.[43,44] Patients with sprue had increased numbers of lymphocytes in the crypt epithelium, with a higher percentage of immunoblasts and a higher mitotic index.[45] These data can be interpreted as evidence that lymphoid activation does occur in tropical sprue, but that it is probably secondary to whatever primary process institutes the disease, rather than being an inciting process itself.

It also has been postulated that dietary fat might play a role in tropical sprue. Similar to the permissive effect of protein ingestion in the pathogenesis of pig bel, the intake of long-chain fatty acids has been studied as a potential etiologic factor for tropical sprue.[46] The seasonal epidemic occurrence of tropical sprue in Puerto Rico immediately follows a traditional holiday feast of pork, which is rich in long-chain fatty acids.[47] There are several mechanisms by which these long-chain fatty acids might contribute to the production of clinical tropical sprue. Long-chain fatty acids can alter intestinal motility and delay intestinal transit time. Plasma levels of enteroglucagon and motilin are increased significantly in patients with tropical sprue; motilin slows gastric emptying, and enteroglucagon slows intestinal transit.[48] Intubation studies have shown that intestinal infusions of fat increase plasma enteroglucagon levels and decrease intestinal motor activity. Fat within the gut lumen also inhibits the mucosal sodium-potassium fluxes and the magnesium adenosine triphosphatases, which can contribute to malabsorption of water and electrolytes in the intestine and raise the pH of the mucosal microenvironment.[46,49] The elevated mucosal pH produced by intestinal fats also has been associated with increased growth of gram-negative bacteria in the lumen of the small bowel.[15,50]

The elevation of mucosal pH and the presence of fatty acids within the lumen of the gut also may impair the ability of the intestine to absorb folate; folate deficiency may potentiate the intestinal dysfunction that precedes it.[51] Folate deficiency leads to a decreased number of gut epithelial cells, as assessed by DNA concentrations, and to villus atrophy. Additional structural alterations are seen in the intestine with folate deficiency, including crypt hypertrophy, villus blunting, and megaloblastic changes in the epithelial cells. These changes are nonspecific and are similar to those seen with vitamin B_{12} deficiency or with tropical sprue. Functionally the folate-deficient gut is less efficient in absorbing water, electrolytes, and carbohydrates than the normal small bowel.[52] It is likely that whatever the initial insult to the gut may be in tropical sprue, the resulting folate malabsorption and deficiency contribute to the further pathogenesis of disease (Fig. 96-1).

Exocrine pancreatic insufficiency has been documented in patients with tropical sprue by the indirect pancriolauryl test. The pancriolauryl test was abnormally low in patients with tropical sprue and was correlated with damage seen on intestinal biopsy.[53] Pancreatic function improved with therapy in this study.

CLINICAL MANIFESTATIONS

The classic clinical features of tropical sprue are nonspecific and simply reflect the symptoms of malabsorption. Malabsorption is so frequent in the developing world that it is difficult to know where on the spectrum of malabsorption that tropical sprue begins. It has been suggested that the malabsorption seen with sprue is only the tip of the malabsorption iceberg.[54] Studies done in the Gambia suggest that abnormal intestinal permeability as determined by lactulose/mannitol absorption is a major factor in growth faltering in children younger than age 2 years. Although lactulose/mannitol permeability improves with increasing age in children, the abnormality may persist into adulthood.[55] Malabsorptive symptoms include prolonged diarrhea, abdominal cramping, and anorexia, with or without nausea and secondary weight loss. Other associated, but less common symptoms, also related to the malabsorption of nutrients and subsequent malnutrition, include peripheral edema, glossitis, stomatitis, and dermatitis.[15,16] Fever may occur at the onset of diarrhea (especially in Asia); although

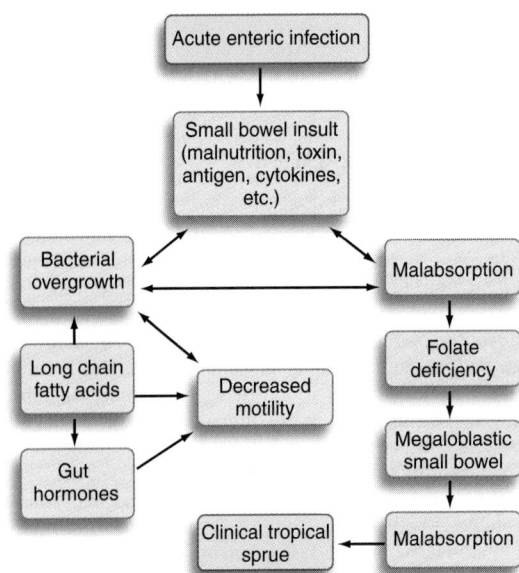

FIGURE 96-1. Proposed pathogenesis of tropical sprue. The complex vicious cycle of small bowel insult that results in bacterial overgrowth and malabsorption and further small bowel damage by luminal long-chain fatty acids and dysregulation of intestinal hormones may promote disease in susceptible persons after an acute enteric infection.

the presence of fever has been suggested as a means to distinguish Caribbean from Asian sprue, this distinction has not been observed consistently. Fever rarely persists for the course of disease, which may span months to years. Signs and symptoms related to anemia also may occur; pallor and weakness are most common early in disease. Later in the course of tropical sprue, peripheral neuropathy, confusion, and, if the anemia is severe enough, congestive symptoms reflecting high-output failure may occur.

Many patients can pinpoint the onset of disease; tropical sprue rarely has an insidious onset and far more often is associated with an obvious acute episode of diarrhea that then becomes prolonged. Patients with tropical sprue may recall other people with similar acute illnesses or being exposed to someone with an acute illness just before getting sick themselves. Because the operative definition of tropical sprue implies that the function of the gut was normal before the development of the disease, ideally the alteration of bowel habits from a normal pattern by the inciting episode of acute diarrheal disease should be notable. In practice, especially in the developing world, the distinction between normal and abnormal bowel habits may not be so clear.

Patients describe crampy abdominal pain, multiple soft or loose stools daily often with mucus, and exacerbation of symptoms with food consumption. Patients also may complain of nausea and bloating that lead to decreased appetite and decreased oral intake. The precise presentation of a patient with tropical sprue depends on the duration of illness and the extent of malabsorption.

Malabsorption of specific nutrients may lead to other symptoms and syndromes.[56] Lactose intolerance often develops early in the course of tropical sprue. The anemia of tropical sprue is most often macrocytic and related to vitamin B_{12} and folate malabsorption. Iron deficiency also may occur, related to malabsorption, and may turn a macrocytic anemia into a normocytic anemia. Impaired absorption of calcium, vitamin D, and magnesium may occur, with resulting osteopenia.[57] Patients with tropical sprue also have malabsorption of fats and, depending on the severity of fat malabsorption, may complain of bulky, floating, or foul-smelling stools.

Spontaneous recovery may occur, but this is not inevitable. Spontaneous recovery is more common in travelers to areas endemic for tropical sprue who return to their native environments. Patients who have emigrated from endemic areas and patients living in endemic areas often require medical therapy to alleviate symptoms. Because the clinical manifestations of tropical sprue are nonspecific, symptomatic response to specific therapy can be considered additional evidence that the patient had tropical sprue.

INTESTINAL ABNORMALITIES

Although the secretory and malabsorptive syndrome seen in tropical sprue suggests preferential damage to the small bowel, which has greater nutrient absorptive capabilities and a greater secretory capacity than the colon, functional abnormalities are seen in the small and the large bowel in tropical sprue. Functional changes in the small bowel mirror the morphologic changes seen and are most prominent in the ileum and jejunum. In tropical sprue, the jejunum is in a net secretory state, with active secretion of water, sodium, and chloride[58]; however, glucose-linked absorption remains intact, as it does for many other secretory infectious diarrheal syndromes.[59] In tropical sprue, there is malabsorption of bile acids and vitamin B_{12} in the ileum. Bile acid malabsorption leads to fat malabsorption and malabsorption of the fat-soluble vitamins D, A, K, and E. Brush-border enzymes are decreased functionally and are less efficient in digesting and absorbing disaccharides, such as lactose.[60,61] Xylose, glucose, and folate malabsorption occur, as does malabsorption of minerals, such as calcium and magnesium. Amino acid malabsorption occurs; protein metabolism is complicated further by loss of albumin in the lumen of the damaged small bowel.[62]

Most of the functional changes in tropical sprue may be related to small bowel mucosal damage represented by the morphologic changes seen, but the hormonal regulation of the gut also is dysfunctional in this disease.[63] Postprandial insulin and gastric inhibitory peptide are reduced in tropical sprue; enteroglucagon and motilin levels are increased. In chronic tropical sprue, gastric acid secretion and secretion of intrinsic factor also may be affected. Transit time through the small bowel is slowed, as measured by breath hydrogen testing.[64,65]

The colon normally serves as a storage and absorptive organ, absorbing 4 to 7 L of water and 100 to 160 mmol of carbohydrates per day. In the few studies of colonic function in tropical sprue that have been done, the ability of the colon to absorb water is decreased in patients compared with controls. There is speculation that the dysfunction of colonic cells may be related to damage by excess fatty acids in the gut lumen or bacterial toxins or infection. Although there is physiologic confirmation of the ability of fatty acids to disturb the absorptive function of colonocytes and small bowel enterocytes, data suggesting that colonic infections are important in the pathogenesis of tropical sprue are lacking.

MORPHOLOGY

Partial villus atrophy is the hallmark histologic change seen in the small bowel in tropical sprue, as opposed to the flattened mucosa that is characteristic of celiac sprue.[66] The villi in tropical sprue progressively shorten and thicken, forming fused leaves after about 4 months of illness. These histologic changes are seen in the jejunum and the ileum, where the changes in absorption also are localized. These histologic changes are not specific for tropical sprue but may be present in severe folate deficiency or with bacterial overgrowth.

Microscopically the mucosa is thin, with an infiltrate of chronic inflammatory cells consisting of plasma cells, histiocytes, lymphocytes, and eosinophils. As mentioned previously, these lymphocytes have been characterized, and IgA, IgG, and IgM lymphocytes are present in numbers equal to those of asymptomatic control patients.[43,44] An increased mitotic index can be seen in the crypt cells; the nuclei of the crypt cells also may appear megaloblastic.[62,67] An increased number of goblet cells may be present, and lipoid vacuoles have been seen within the basement membrane. To date, there is no convincing evidence that tropical sprue is an immunologically mediated disease.

DIAGNOSIS

Because the symptom complex of tropical sprue is nonspecific, the travel and exposure history of the patient is crucial in making the diagnosis. Tropical sprue should be considered in a patient who presents with chronic diarrhea, weight loss, and evidence of malabsorption. Attempts should be made to elicit the onset of the diarrheal illness; the duration of diarrheal illness; the degree of weight loss; the frequency and character of the stool; and any other systemic complaints, such as prolonged fever, jaundice, or itching, that might suggest alternative explanations for the diarrheal illness. Information regarding travel to, residence in, or emigration from the tropics should be requested; although there are sporadic case reports of mild spruelike illnesses occurring after diarrheal illnesses in temperate climates, this so-called temperate sprue is rare, and a history of exposure to an endemic area should be present to entertain the diagnosis of tropical sprue.[47]

Pertinent medical history also should be obtained, with particular emphasis on any surgical procedures that may have altered the anatomy of the bowel, predisposing to a blind loop syndrome, or any medications that may predispose to small bowel overgrowth. Social history, in addition to travel and exposures, should include questions relating to possible human immunodeficiency virus (HIV) exposures because HIV infection is a major risk factor for the development of chronic diarrhea.[68] History pertaining to symptoms of specific nutrient deficiencies, such as night blindness secondary to malabsorption of vitamin A, would be expected only in prolonged disease.

There are no diagnostic physical findings for tropical sprue. The physical examination should document presence or absence of fever, volume status by any orthostatic changes, body weight, evidence of weight loss such as temporal wasting, and presence or absence of significant lymphadenopathy or abdominal masses. Hyperactive bowel sounds may be the only pertinent abdominal finding. Signs of anemia, such as pallor, are notoriously nonspecific but can be looked for. Signs of specific nutrient deficiencies also may be present on physical examination: Cheilosis, stomatitis, glossitis, rashes, dermatitis, koilonychia, muscle pain or weakness, peripheral neuropathy, or edema can suggest deficiencies of iron, zinc, vitamin B_{12}, folate, vitamins D and E, or protein. Deficiencies of any of these nutrients could be present in tropical sprue because of malabsorption by the damaged small bowel.

Laboratory evaluation of a patient with suspected tropical sprue can be minimal or extensive, depending on the degree of suspicion and the urgency for diagnosis. A simple complete blood count showing a macrocytic anemia in a high-risk patient in the appropriate clinical setting could be sufficient to proceed with other, more confirmatory diagnostic tests, such as a small bowel biopsy. A more complete laboratory evaluation includes serum vitamin B_{12} level and red blood cell folate levels, serum carotene concentration, or, preferably, a 72-hour fecal fat determination. Stool examination to exclude *Giardia* is useful; stool culture looking for bacterial pathogens is less likely to be helpful in chronic diarrhea.

Ultimately a small bowel series with small bowel follow-through showing flattened mucosal folds, luminal dilation, or flocculation of the barium meal can suggest tropical sprue.[68] An upper endoscopy with duodenal aspirate for parasites, biopsy, and quantitative small bowel culture, if available, can be diagnostic of tropical sprue in the appropriate clinical setting. Documentation of abnormal transit time by small bowel follow-through or breath hydrogen testing, which also can imply bacterial overgrowth, suggests but is not diagnostic of tropical sprue. The differential diagnosis that must be considered in a patient with chronic diarrhea, weight loss, and malabsorption, even in a clinical setting consistent with tropical sprue, should include giardiasis, cryptosporidiosis, coccidiosis (*Isospora belli*), capillariasis, strongyloidiasis, celiac sprue (gluten enteropathy), lymphoma, intestinal tuberculosis, blind loop syndrome, pancreatic tumors, Whipple's disease, and microsporidia-associated HIV enteropathy.

TREATMENT

Treatment with folate alone improves the symptoms of tropical sprue but does not cure the diarrhea. Combination therapy with tetracycline and folate seems to be most effective in symptom resolution and cure of diarrhea with promotion of weight gain.[69,70] Treatment with 250 mg of tetracycline four times daily and 5 mg of folate daily for 1 month has been effective for travelers with tropical sprue, but therapy must be prolonged for 6 months or longer for residents of the tropics who have had long-term disease. Even with prolonged therapy, relapses have been seen in this population, although these may have been caused by reexposure to an infecting organism and represent recurrent rather than relapsing disease.[71] Reports have suggested that tropical sprue in the Caribbean is more amenable to therapy than sprue in India, but these studies are difficult to compare.[72] Poorly absorbed sulfa drugs are an acceptable alternative to tetracycline in children or pregnant women.[73] A favorable symptomatic response to therapy with folate and antibiotics can provide additional evidence that tropical sprue was the cause of chronic diarrhea and malabsorption in a patient; however, even this is not specific because bacterial overgrowth in a blind loop syndrome also would be expected to respond.

REFERENCES

1. Bartholomew C. William Hillary and sprue in the Caribbean: 230 years later. Gut Festschr. 1989;30:17-21.
2. Klipstein FA, Samloff IM, Smarth G, et al. Treatment of overt and subclinical malabsorption in Haiti. Gut. 1969;10:315-322.
3. Klipstein FA, Corcino JJ. Seasonal occurrence of overt and subclinical tropical malabsorption in Puerto Rico. Am J Trop Med Hyg. 1974;23:1189-1196.
4. Gorbach SL, Banwell JG, Jacobs B, et al. Tropical sprue and malnutrition in West Bengal. Am J Clin Nutr. 1970;23:1515-1558.
5. Mathan VI, Baker SJ. Epidemic tropical sprue and other epidemics of diarrhea in South Indian villages. Am J Clin Nutr. 1968;21:1077-1087.
6. Jones TC, Dean AG, Parker GW. Seasonal gastroenteritis and malabsorption at an American military base in the Philippines. Am J Epidemiol. 1973;95:128-139.
7. Thomas G, Clain DJ, Wicks CB. Tropical enteropathy in Rhodesia. Gut. 1976;17:888-894.
8. Mathan VI, Ignatius M, Baker SJ. A household epidemic of tropical sprue. Gut. 1966;7:490.
9. Schorling JB, Wanke CA, Schorling SK, et al. A prospective study of persistent diarrhea among children in an urban Brazilian slum. Am J Epidemiol. 1990;132:144-156.
10. Wanke CA, Guerrant RL. Pathogenesis of persistent diarrhea. In: Guerrant RL, de Souza MA, Nations MK, eds. At the Edge of Development: Health Crises in a Transitional Society. Durham, NC: Carolina Academic Press; 1996:177-201.
11. Lima AA, Fang G, Schorling JB, et al. Persistent diarrhea in northeast Brazil: Etiologies and interactions with malnutrition. Acta Paediatr Scand. 1992;381(Suppl):39-44.
12. Penny ME, Scotland SM, Smith HR, et al. Virulence properties of Enterobacteriaceae isolated from the small intestine of children with diarrhea. Pediatr Infect Dis J. 1992;11:623-630.
13. Klipstein FA. Tropical sprue in travelers and expatriates living abroad. Gastroenterology. 1981;80:590.
14. Lindenbaum J, Kent TH, Sprine H. Malabsorption and jejunitis in American Peace Corps volunteers in Pakistan. Ann Intern Med. 1966;65:1201.
15. Davis JS, Klipstein FA. Tropical sprue in visitor to Mexico. Lancet. 1985;1:454.
16. Klipstein FA, Falaiye JM. Tropical sprue in expatriates from the tropics living in the continental United States. Medicine (Baltimore). 1969;48:475.
17. Montgomery RD, Beale DJ, Sammons HG, et al. Postinfective malabsorption: A sprue syndrome. BMJ. 1973;2:265-268.
18. Appelbaum PC, Moshal MG, Hift W, et al. Intestinal bacteria in patients with tropical sprue. S Afr Med J. 1980;57:1081.
19. Bhat P, Shantakumari S, Rajan D, et al. Bacterial flora of the gastrointestinal tract in southern Indian control subjects and patients with tropical sprue. Gastroenterology. 1972;62:11.
20. Tomkins AM, Drasbar BS, James WPT. Bacterial colonisation of jejunal mucosa in acute tropical sprue. Lancet. 1975;1:59.
21. Klipstein FA, Engert RF, Short HB. Enterotoxigenicity of colonising coliform bacteria in tropical sprue and blind-loop syndrome. Lancet. 1978;342.
22. Klipstein FA, Holdeman LV, Corcino JJ. Enterotoxigenic intestinal bacteria in tropical sprue. Ann Intern Med. 1973;79:632-641.
23. Ramakrishna BS, Mathan VI. Role of bacterial toxins, bile acids, and free fatty acids in colonic water malabsorption in tropical sprue. Dig Dis Sci. 1987;32:500-505.
24. Wanke CA, Guerrant RL. Small-bowel colonization alone is a cause of diarrhea. Infect Immun. 1987;55:1924-1926.
25. Schlager TA, Wanke CA, Guerrant RL. Net fluid secretion and impaired villous function induced by colonization of the small intestine by non-toxigenic, colonizing E. coli. Infect Immun. 1990;58:1337-1343.
26. Steiner TS, Lima AM, Nataro JP, et al. Enteroaggregative Escherichia coli produce intestinal inflammation and growth impairment and cause interleukin-8 release from intestinal epithelial cells. J Infect Dis. 1998;177:88-96.
27. Nataro JP, Steiner TS, Guerrant RL. Enteroaggregative Escherichia coli (EAEC): An emerging cause of diarrhea and malnutrition. Emerg Infect Dis. 1998;4:251-261.
28. Bhan MK, Raj P, Levine MM, et al. Enteroaggregative Escherichia coli associated with persistent diarrhea in a cohort of rural children in India. J Infect Dis. 1989;159:1061-1064.
29. Cravioto A, Tello A, Navarro A, et al. Association of Escherichia coli HEp-2 adherence patterns with type and duration of diarrhoea. Lancet. 1991;337:262-264.
30. Wanke CA, Schorling JB, Barrett LJ, et al. Potential role of adherence traits of Escherichia coli in persistent diarrhea in an urban Brazilian slum. Pediatr Infect Dis J. 1991;10:746-751.
31. Wanke CA, Mayer H, Weber R, et al. Enteroaggregative Escherichia coli as a potential cause of diarrheal disease in adults infected with human immunodeficiency virus. J Infect Dis. 1998;178:185-190.
32. Wanke CA, Gerrior J, Blais V, et al. Successful treatment of diarrheal disease associated with enteroaggregative E. coli in adults infected with human immunodeficiency virus. J Infect Dis. 1998;178:1369-1372.
33. Tomkins AM, Wright SG, Drasbar BS, et al. Bacterial colonization of jejunal mucosa in giardiasis. Trans R Soc Trop Med Hyg. 1978;72:33.
34. Klipstein FA, Schneider R. Prototheca and sprue. Gastroenterology. 1975;69:1372.
35. Swanson VL, Haley LD, Wheby MS. Mycological study of jejunal biopsy specimens from patients with tropical sprue. Am J Trop Med Hyg. 1965;14:1066.
36. Fredricks DN, Relman DA. Infectious agents and etiology of chronic idiopathic diseases. Curr Clin Top Infect Dis. 1998;18:180-200.
37. Cook GC. Tropical sprue: Some early investigators favoured an infective cause, but was a coccidian protozoan involved? Gut. 1997;40:428-429.
38. Farthing MJ. Tropical malabsorption. Semin Gastrointest Dis. 2002;13:221-231.
39. Wanke CA, Cronan S, Bistrian B. Recombinant tumor necrosis factor and recombinant murine IL-1 alter binding of Escherichia coli to intestinal mucin and the HT29 intestinal cell line. Nutrition. 1997;13:959-964.
40. Wanke CA, Cronan S, Goss C, et al. Characterization of binding of Escherichia coli strains which are enteropathogens to small-bowel mucin. Infect Immun. 1990;58:794-800.
41. Graham D, Alpert L, Smith J, et al. Iatrogenic Campylobacter pylori infection is a cause of epidemic achlorhydria. Am J Gastroenterol. 1988;83:974.
42. Nurko SS, García-Aranda JA, Consuelo A, et al. Is Helicobacter pylori a significant risk factor for persistent diarrhea in Mexican children? Gastroenterology. 1993;104:A160.
43. Malik AK, Mehta SK, Chandrashekhar Y, et al. Quantitation of immunoglobin-containing cells in the jejunal lamina propria in tropical sprue. J Clin Gastroenterol. 1992;14:163-166.
44. Marsh MN. Functional and structural aspects of the epithelial lymphocyte, with implications for coeliac disease and tropical sprue. Scand J Gastroenterol. 1985;115:55-75.
45. Marsh MN, Mathan M, Mathan VI. Studies of intestinal lymphoid tissue: VII. The secondary nature of lymphoid cell "activation" in the jejunal lesion of tropical sprue. Am J Pathol. 1983;112:302-312.
46. Tiruppathi C, Balasubramanian KA, Hill PG, et al. Faecal free fatty acids in tropical sprue and their possible role in the production of diarrhoea by inhibition of ATPases. Gut. 1983;24:300-305.
47. Glynn J. Tropical sprue: Its aetiology and pathogenesis. J R Soc Med. 1986;79:599.
48. Cook GC. Aetiology and pathogenesis of postinfective tropical malabsorption (tropical sprue). Lancet. 1984;1:721.
49. Ramakrishna BS, Mathan VI. Absorption of water and sodium and activity of adenosine triphosphatases in the rectal mucosa in tropical sprue. Gut. 1988;29:665-668.
50. Lucas ML, Mathan VI. Jejunal surface pH measurements in tropical sprue. Trans R Soc Trop Med Hyg. 1989;83:138-142.
51. Kesavan V, Noronha JM. An ATPase dependent, radio sensitive, acidic microclimate essential for folate absorption. J Physiol. 1978;280:1-7.
52. Davidson GP, Townley RRW. Structural and functional abnormalities of the small bowel due to nutritional folate deficiency in infancy. J Pediatr. 1977;90:590-594.
53. Mittal SK, Rajeshwari K, Kalra KK, et al. Tropical sprue in north Indian children. Trop Gastroenterol. 2001;22:146-148.
54. Rosenberg IH. Tropical enteritis: Nutritional consequences and connections with the riddle of cholera. J Nutr. 2003;133:333S-335S.
55. Campbell DI, Lunn PG, Elia M. Age-related association of small intestinal mucosal enteropathy with nutritional status in rural Gambian children. Br J Nutr. 2002;88:499-505.
56. Chacko A, Begum A, Mathan VI. Absorption of nutrient energy in southern Indian control subjects and patients with tropical sprue. Am J Clin Nutr. 1984;40:771-775.
57. Haddock L, Vazquez MDC, Rivera R, et al. The kinetics of D3-3H metabolism in tropical sprue. P R Health Sci J. 1985;4:47.
58. Tompkins A. Tropical malabsorption: Recent concepts in pathogenesis and nutritional significance. Clin Sci. 1981;60:131-137.
59. Rolston DDK, Mathan VI. Jejunal and ileal glucose-stimulated water and sodium absorption in tropical enteropathy: Implications for oral rehydration therapy. Digestion. 1990;46:55-60.
60. Batt RM, Bush BM, Peters TJ. Subcellular biochemical studies of a naturally occurring enteropathy in the dog resembling chronic tropical sprue in human beings. Am J Vet Res. 1993;44:1492.
61. Cook GC, Menzies IS. Intestinal absorption and unmediated permeation of sugars in post-infective tropical malabsorption (tropical sprue). Digestion. 1986;33:109-116.
62. Westergaard H. Southwestern Internal Medicine Conference. The sprue syndromes. Am J Med Sci. 1985;290:249-262.

63. Besterman HS, Cook GC, Sarson DL, et al. Gut hormones in tropical malabsorption. BMJ. 1979;1252-1255.
64. Cook GC. Delayed small-intestinal transit in tropical malabsorption. BMJ. 1978;2:238-240.
65. Jayanthi V, Chacko A, Gani IK, et al. Intestinal transit in healthy southern Indian subjects and in patients with tropical sprue. Gut. 1989;30:35-38.
66. Tawil SC, Brandt LJ, Bernstein LH. Scalloping of the valvulae conniventes and mosaic mucosa in tropical sprue. Gastroenterology. 1991;37:365.
67. Mathan MM, Ponniah J, Mathan VI. Epithelial cell renewal and turnover and relationship to morphologic abnormalities in jejunal mucosa in tropical sprue. Dig Dis Sci. 1986;31:586-592.
68. Thielman NM, Guerrant RL. An algorithmic approach to the workup and management of HIV-related diarrhea. J Clin Outcomes Management. 1997;4:36-47.
69. Scully RE, Mark EJ, McNeely WF, et al. Weekly clinicopathologic exercises: Case 15-1990. N Engl J Med. 1990;322:1067-1075.
70. Guerra R, Wheby MS, Bayless TM. Long-term antibiotic therapy in tropical sprue. Ann Intern Med. 1965;63:619.
71. Rickles FR, Klipstein FA, Tomasini J, et al. Long-term follow-up of antibiotic-treated tropical sprue. Ann Intern Med. 1972;76:203-210.
72. Gerson CD, Kent TH, Saha JR, et al. Recovery of small-intestinal structure and function after residence in the tropics: II. Studies in Indians and Pakistanis living in New York City. Ann Intern Med. 1971;75:41-48.
73. Maldonado N, Horta E, Guerra R, Perez-Santiago H. Poorly absorbed sulfonamides in the treatment of tropical sprue. Gastroenterology. 1969;57:559.

CHAPTER **97**

Whipple's Disease

THOMAS MARTH

Whipple's disease is a rare systemic infectious disorder. This chronic disease, first described in 1907 by Whipple as intestinal lipodystrophy, affects preferentially middle-aged white men who may present with weight loss, arthralgia, diarrhea, and abdominal pain. A variety of other clinical patterns, such as involvement of the heart, lung, or central nervous system (CNS), are frequent. The diagnosis often is established by small bowel biopsy, which is characterized by periodic acid–Schiff (PAS)–positive inclusions representing the causative bacteria. These organisms have been classified phylogenetically as actinomycetes and can be detected by specific polymerase chain reaction (PCR). The causative bacteria have been cultured, and the official name of this species is *Tropheryma whipplei*. Other studies have shown that subtle defects of the cell-mediated immunity exist in active and inactive Whipple's disease that may predispose certain individuals to a clinical manifestation of *T. whipplei* infection. Most patients respond well to antibiotic treatment, but some patients with relapsing disease or CNS manifestation may have a poor prognosis. More recent findings may allow development of new strategies for diagnosis, treatment, and monitoring of patients with Whipple's disease.

ETIOLOGY

Whipple found rod-shaped structures with silver stain in his original case but noted: "Whether this is the active agent in this peculiar pathological complex cannot be determined from the study of this single case but its distribution in the glands is very suggestive."[1] In 1960, a characteristic, rod-shaped (0.25 × 1.5 to 2.5 μm in size) organism was observed by electron microscopy within cells in various stages of degradation and in the extracellular space (Fig. 97-1).[2] Morphologically the organism possesses uniformly a trilaminar plasma membrane and a surrounding homogeneous cell wall of 20-nm thickness with two inner layers and an outer trilaminar membrane–like stucture.[3] The bacillus can be found typically in macrophages of the lamina propria of the small intestine and its lymphatic drainage, but also has been observed in, among

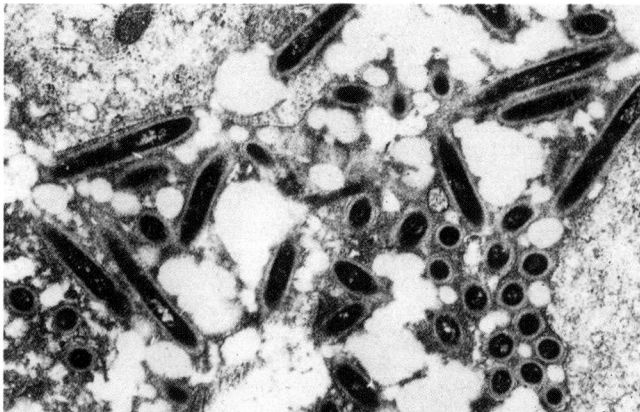

FIGURE 97-1. Electron microscopic view of the Whipple bacillus, designated *Tropheryma whipplei*. The characteristic, rod-shaped (0.25 × 1.5 to 2.5 μm in size) organism can be observed in the extracellular space in florid disease or within cells in various stages of degradation. The bacillus is found typically and in the highest frequency in macrophages of the lamina propria of the small intestine and its lymphatic drainage. *T. whipplei* is characterized by a trilaminar plasma membrane, a surrounding homogeneous cell wall of 20-nm thickness, and an outer trilaminar membrane–like structure usually seen in gram-negative bacteria. Other characteristics, including the central location of tubules and vesicles, are typical of gram-positive organisms. (×20,000.)

others, endothelial and epithelial cells, muscle cells, and various cells of the immune system, including polymorphonuclear leukocytes, plasma cells, mast cells, and intraepithelial lymphocytes.[3,4] The organisms disappear from the lamina propria on antibiotic-induced clinical improvement, which argued for their etiologic significance.[5] The unique nature of the Whipple's disease organism also was suggested by its distinct cross-reactivity with streptococcal (groups A, B, and G) and shigella (group B) antisera on fixed tissues.[6,7]

In 1991/1992, specific segments of bacterial 16S ribosomal RNA from duodenal lesions of diseased patients were amplified genomically using PCR[8,9] with the use of broad-range and specific primers. The sequence analysis enabled the classification of the causative organism phylogenetically as a new genus and species,[8,9] and the name *Tropheryma whippelii* (*trophe,* "nourishment," and *eryma,* "barrier") was proposed.[9]

After several unsuccessful attempts at culture, the Whipple's bacillus isolated from heart valve tissue tentatively had been propagated in peripheral blood mononuclear cells deactivated by interleukin (IL)-4 and IL-10.[10] In 1999, the growth of the organism was established in human fibroblast (HEL) cells (in minimal essential medium with 10% calf serum).[11] As the bacterial strains have been deposited in bacterial collections, the name of the Whipple's bacillus officially was corrected to *Tropheryma whipplei.*[12] Raoult and co-workers[11] showed that the bacterium is slowly growing with an estimated doubling time of 17 days. An animal model for Whipple's disease is not yet available. The site of multiplication of *T. whipplei* in vivo is controversial. It has been suggested that bacteria multiply in the digestive lumen, become phagocytized, and then degraded in macrophages.[4] In vitro, the bacteria do grow also in cell-free media. *T. whipplei* replicates within peripheral blood mononuclear cells (which release the bacteria) and within HeLa cells, where the bacillus actively multiplies in acidic vacuoles at pH 5.[13] Because high acidity may impair antibiotic activity, this may be a cause for the lack of efficacy of some antibiotics.[13] The genome of *T. whipplei* has been sequenced and deposited in Genbank.[14,14a] *T. whipplei* has a single circular chromosome and small genome size (925 kb)[14,14a] and seems to possess characteristics that suggest immune evasion and host interaction play an important role in its replication.[14,14a] In particular, *T. whipplei* seems to have a high degree of sequence variation and lacks several important biochemical pathways, including deficiencies in amino acid biosynthesis and carbohydrate metabolism, suggesting a host-dependent lifestyle.[14,14a]

The organism has been placed phylogenetically within the subdivision of gram-positive bacteria with high guanine and cytosine content, the actinomycetes, and is in close relationship to several actinobacteria, nocardioforms, and cellulomonads, including *Dermatophilus congolensis, Arthrobacter globiformis, Terrabacter tumescens, Cellulomonas cellulans, Corynebacterium aquaticus,* the human pathogenetic *Rothia dentocariosa,* and *Rhodococcus* spp.; *T. whipplei* is related more weakly to *Streptomyces* spp. and *Mycobacterium* spp.[8,9,13] The bacteria of the *T. whipplei* species show some degree of genetic heterogenicity as shown by sequencing of 16S-23S rDNA interspacer[15] and of the 23S rDNA. The genomic variants may be associated with the geographic residence of the patients. It has been suggested that some strains may be nonpathogenic; some may cause typical Whipple's disease; and some may cause atypical clinical forms, such as infectious endocarditis.[16] *T. whipplei* seems to occur, similar to some of its phylogenetic relatives, in the environment as it was found by PCR in sewage water[17] and in human feces.[13] It is speculated that it may contaminate people through drinking water. PCR-based studies have shown that *T. whipplei* could be amplified from saliva, gastric fluid, and duodenal biopsy specimens of people without Whipple's disease.[18] The prevalence of *T. whipplei* PCR-positive samples in asymptomatic subjects seems to depend on the geographic origin of subjects, which might explain why other authors did not find such results in other areas.

EPIDEMIOLOGY AND PATHOGENESIS

Because Whipple's disease is rare, no valid estimation on the incidence is available. The disorder has been described most frequently in whites. Only rare occurrence is reported in Hispanics, blacks, Indians, and Asians.[4] It has been presumed that the disease may occur in local clusters, that many patients stem from rural areas, and that farming often is found among the documented occupations.[4,13] Specific environmental factors or habits have not yet been associated with Whipple's disease, however.

Whipple's disease occurs usually late in life (i.e., primarily in middle-aged individuals with a mean age at diagnosis of about 50 years). The disease is approximately eight times more common in men than in women.[4,13] Although there are several case reports of familial clusters (brother pairs, father/daughter), most of the analyzed cases do not exhibit familial components. A genetic susceptibility is suggested by HLA-B27 positivity in approximately 26% of patients (three to four times higher than expected)[4,19]; however, this is not found in all populations (not in Italy and not in Argentina). The presumed immunologic defect in Whipple's disease is likely to be subtle and specific for the Whipple's disease organism because patients with the disease usually are not predisposed to infections with other organisms. This holds true for most patients, although some case reports have pointed out that Whipple's disease also may occur in immunodeficiency, in immunosuppression, or concomitant with other infections (e.g., in patients with acquired immunodeficiency syndrome [AIDS] or in patients with *Nocardia* or *Giardia* infections).[13,20] Newer data point to the possibility that intestinal manifestation of Whipple's disease is triggered by medical immunosuppression (which is given for the treatment of arthropathy) (unpublished data).

The immunohistologic features of the lamina propria in Whipple's disease is unique because the intestinal tissue shows a relative paucity of lymphocytic infiltration, including plasma cells, despite the massive influx of macrophages.[4,21] Although the lack of lymphocytic infiltrate and disturbed immunity in Whipple's disease could be attributed partially to an intestinal lymphangiectasia, many studies have found a more profound phenotypic and functional alteration of immunologic features in Whipple's disease patients. It has been shown that lamina propria and circulating T-cell populations in active Whipple's disease are characterized by a reduced CD4/CD8 T-cell ratio, a shift toward mature T-cell subpopulations (e.g., CD45RO expression increased, CD45RA expression decreased), and increased cell activation markers.[22] These changes

are accompanied by disturbed function of peripheral T cells (i.e., by reduced T-cell proliferative responses to a variety of stimuli [phytohemagglutinin, concanavalin A, and anti-CD2 antibodies]), and in several instances, as yet unidentified serum factors have been found that downregulate T cell–mediated responses.[13,22,23] In addition, impaired delayed-type hypersensitivity reaction to skin antigens (mostly recall antigens) can be detected in many cases.[22,23] Although the aforementioned alterations are present most clearly in acutely ill patients, they may be found even in patients with long-standing remission.

Studies have found reduced numbers of IgA-positive B cells but increased numbers of surface IgM-positive B cells in the lamina propria.[24] Secretory IgA levels determined from intestinal aspirates have been found normal.[4] Humoral immune responses to infectious agents in the periphery and total serum IgG levels usually are normal, whereas IgM often is decreased and IgA is increased in acute stages of the disease.[4,13] One study from our laboratory showed decreased IgG2 subclass levels in a small patient group.[25] IgG2 is a subclass of antibody that is produced in response to infection with encapsulated bacteria and that presumably is regulated by cell-mediated immune and interferon (IFN)-γ responses.

Studies on macrophages in Whipple's disease are sparse. Macrophages from Whipple's disease patients manifested decreased intracellular degradation of several organisms,[26] and intestinal macrophages showed some decrease of phagocytosis. In addition, we have shown that patients with active and inactive Whipple's disease have reduced numbers of circulating cells expressing CD11b, the α-chain of complement receptor 3, which serves as a facilitator of microbial phagocytosis, plays a role in antigen processing, and mediates IFN-γ-induced intracellular killing of ingested bacteria.[25]

As shown in one of our series, impaired functions of antigen-presenting cells in Whipple's disease may be related to reduced macrophage IL-12 production,[27] a cytokine that has important functions in regulating cell-mediated immune responses There is an increase in functional Th2 responses in peripheral T cells,[27] lending support to the observation that *T. whipplei* replicates in cytokine (IL-4 and IL-10)–deactivated macrophages.[10] As a further indication for the pathogenetic relevance of the impaired cellular immune responses, it was reported that in one patient with Whipple's disease refractory to antibiotic regimens and with reduced IFN-γ levels in vitro, treatment with antimicrobials and supplemental recombinant IFN-γ led to the clearance of the infection.[28]

Collectively, cellular immunity and the activation and interaction of macrophages and T cells seem to be disturbed in a subtle but persistent manner. This disturbance may be the cause for a disturbed phagocytosis and intracellular degradation of *T. whipplei* and may allow the invasion of the bacillus. The exact nature of these defects and possible genetic components in the etiology have to be clarified.

PATHOLOGY

On gross inspection, the duodenum and jejunum, which are the sites most frequently affected, often appear thickened and edematous.[4,29] The infiltration of the bowel wall is associated with a widening and flattening of the villi with dilated lacteals containing yellow lipid deposits, which are the result of a villous lymphatics blockade. Based on these and similar observations in the draining mesenteric lymph nodes, Whipple assumed a disorder of fat metabolism and suggested the name *intestinal lipodystrophy.*[1] Pathophysiologically the disturbance of the villous architecture is presumably the cause of the steatorrhea and the subsequent malabsorption syndrome that accompany the disease. In addition, the intestinal lymphangiectasia and protein-losing enteropathy seem to be mainly secondary to the lymphatic blockage.

Light microscopic examination of duodenal biopsy specimens in Whipple's disease reveals usually the pathognomonic infiltration of the lamina propria with large macrophages (also called *sickle-form particle-containing cells*) containing granular-foamy, purple-stained, PAS-positive inclusions that are diastase-resistant, silver-positive, and often gram-positive; they represent more or less intact remnants of ingested

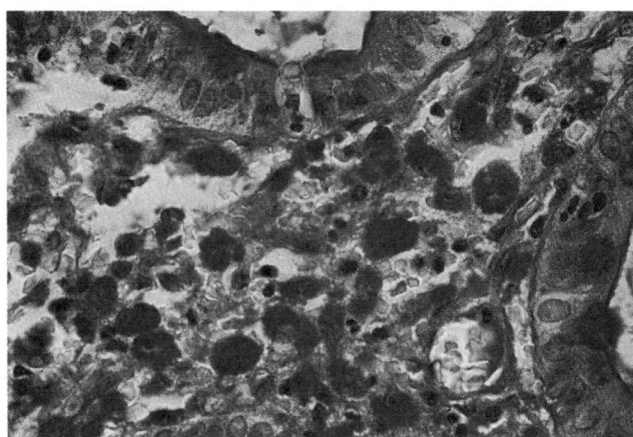

FIGURE 97-2. Periodic acid–Schiff stain of a duodenal biopsy specimen in a patient with Whipple's disease. Large numbers of purple-stained macrophages in the lamina propria can be seen. (×40.)

TABLE 97-1 Signs and Symptoms in Whipple's Disease

	Approximate Percentage of Incidence*
Major Clinical Features	
Weight loss	95 (85-100)
Arthropathy	85 (70-100)
Diarrhea	75 (70-85)
Abdominal pain	65 (50-90)
Frequent Signs and Symptoms	
Fever	50 (40-60)
Lymphadenopathy	50 (40-60)
Hyperpigmentation	45 (35-60)
Hypotension	40 (30-80)
Peripheral edema	35 (20-45)
Cardiac murmurs	35 (30-40)
Occult bleeding	25 (20-30)
Myalgia	25
Abdominal mass	20 (15-25)
Chronic cough	20
Splenomegaly	15 (5-20)
Hepatomegaly	15
Ascites	10
Other Clinical Features	
Pleuritis	
Pleural effusion	
Endocarditis	
Muscle wasting	
Glossitis	
Peripheral neuropathy	
Eye involvement (e.g., visual loss, uveitis, retinitis)	
CNS involvement (e.g., dementia, ophthalmoplegia, myoclonus, ataxia, nystagmus)	
Organ-Specific Involvement	
Gastrointestinal tract	100 (95-100)
Cardiac involvement	55
Pulmonary involvement	50
CNS	25 (20-30)
Ocular involvement	10

*Approximate frequencies reported in literature in parentheses.[4,31,34,44]
CNS, central nervous system.

bacteria (Fig. 97-2).[1,4,29] The PAS positivity is believed to be a reaction with bacterial capsular mucopolysaccharides located in the cell wall, as noted first in 1949.[30] In florid disease, undigested extracellular bacteria also are seen.[7,9] Although it seems reasonable to assume that the route of infection occurs through the intestinal lumen resulting in a secondary accumulation of *T. whipplei* in the cells of the lamina propria, another possibility is penetration of the bacillus through the intestinal lymphatics because the most viable organisms were seen at the base and not the apex of the epithelial cells.[4,13]

Because Whipple's disease is a systemic disease, PAS-positive macrophages and electron microscopically–detectable bacilli have been shown in many cell types, as noted earlier, and in almost all organs and in body fluids, including the heart, lung, CNS, cerebrospinal fluid (CSF), eye, vitreous humor, liver, spleen, ascites, lymph nodes, endocrine glands, joints, synovium, and bone marrow.[4,29] The involvement of heart valves, mostly the aortic and mitral valves, deserves special mention because it leads frequently to clinical symptoms and is present in more than one third of autopsy cases. Other frequent pathologic features include pericarditis or myocarditis, pleuritis, hepatosplenomegaly, ascites or polyserositis, uveitis and ependymitis, cortical atrophy, and demyelination of the CNS.[4]

CLINICAL FEATURES AND DIAGNOSIS

The leading symptoms of Whipple's disease are weight loss, diarrhea, and arthropathies, and in 75% of cases, these symptoms are found together by the time of diagnosis.[13,31] The clinical presentation of patients may vary to a great extent, however, owing to the differential organ involvement and the stage of the disease. Cardiac and CNS involvement may occur in the absence of gastrointestinal involvement.[32,33]

In many instances (63% in our large series),[31] the disease begins insidiously with arthropathy. This symptom, often associated with positivity for HLA-B27, may precede the diagnosis by a considerable length of time (mean 8 years in one series)[31] and consists usually of chronic migratory, nondestructive, and seronegative joint disease involving predominantly the peripheral joints; in addition, it often is accompanied by myalgias.[4,13,34] As new diagnostic tools enable detection of *T. whipplei* in the synovial fluid,[35] these patients may be diagnosed earlier in the future.

Weight loss is found nearly invariably in all patients at the time of diagnosis. We found that weight loss was present in two thirds of patients more than 4 years before diagnosis and was clinically relevant (often 20%) (unpublished data).[31]

Gastrointestinal symptoms, which usually begin later and ultimately often lead to diagnosis, consist of episodic and watery diarrhea or steatorrhea in many cases accompanied by colicky abdominal pain and, in 20% to 30% of patients, occult blood in the stool.[4,13,34] These

symptoms and concomitant anorexia may lead to the full picture of a malabsorption syndrome with severe weight loss, weakness, general cachexia, and associated secondary signs and symptoms (Table 97-1).

Systemic symptoms occur frequently (i.e., in about half of patients with Whipple's disease) (see Table 97-1). These symptoms consist of intermittent, mostly low-grade fever and night sweats. Frequent features of Whipple's disease also are peripheral and abdominal lymphadenopathy; mesenteric lymphadenopathy is found often in radiologic investigations but also may present as an abdominal mass. Skin hyperpigmentation, particularly affecting light-exposed areas and suggesting Addison's disease (which has not yet been reported in patients with Whipple's disease), has been observed in one third of patients in large series. Chronic, nonproductive cough or chest pain indicating lung involvement or pleuritis, polyserositis, ascites, hypotension, and edema are among other frequently found signs and symptoms. Hepatomegaly or splenomegaly may be present in some patients with this disorder (see Table 97-1). Less frequent involvement of the genitourinary system and the endocrine system has been reported.[4,13,32,34]

Cardiac involvement is frequent and has been reported increasingly to be of clinical relevance. It may present with cardiac murmurs, valve (aortic or mitral) insufficiency leading to valve replacement, or the clinical picture of blood culture–negative endocarditis; many of these cases were diagnosed histologically on cardiac valve examination. In these patients, endocarditis frequently is an isolated finding (i.e., no other evidence of clinical Whipple's disease is observed and duodenal biopsy may be negative).[32]

A major and frequently overlooked area of involvement in Whipple's disease is the CNS. This involvement manifests most often as memory disorders, personality changes, and dementia. Other frequent clinical signs may be ophthalmoplegia, nystagmus, or myoclonia. These may be found often in combination with a disturbed sleep pattern, ataxia, seizure, or symptoms of cerebral compression (due to hydrocephalus). A variety of cranial nerve symptoms, such as hearing loss and blurred vision, have been reported. In some patients, a specific, if not pathognomonic, oculomasticatory myorhythmia or myoclonus with ophthalmoplegia has been described. These CNS symptoms have a frequency of 15% and may occur with minimal or absent gastrointestinal involvement.[4,33,36]

The diagnosis of Whipple's disease usually is made by upper endoscopy. Endoscopically, Whipple's disease findings often are described as a pale yellow shaggy mucosa alternating with an erythematous, erosive, or mildly friable mucosa in the postbulbar region of the duodenum or the jejunum; alternatively, whitish yellow plaques may be seen.[37] Small bowel biopsy specimens should be taken from the proximal and the distal duodenum or the jejunum because involvement can be patchy. The diagnosis usually can be established if the characteristic PAS-positive material is present in the lesions. Endoscopy is an important part in patient follow-up. The duodenal mucosa recovers during the first weeks to months under antibiotic therapy, whereas the PAS-positive material in the macrophages may persist in single cases several years; a reincrease of PAS-positive material may be the first indicator of a relapse.[31,37] Based on clinical manifestations, other samples may be tested, such as CSF, cardiac valve tissue, lymph nodes, or synovial tissue.[13]

There are several histopathologic pitfalls in making a diagnosis of Whipple's disease. Involvement of the gastrointestinal tract or lymphatic tissue may be accompanied by noncaseating, epithelioid cells (sarcoid-like) granulomas. Infections with *Rhodococcus equii* and *Mycobacterium avium-intracellulare* complex in patients with AIDS, but also infection with fungi, *Histoplasma* spp., and others are histologically similar to Whipple's disease, some of which may be ruled out by a Ziehl-Neelsen stain. Lipid deposits and lymphangiectasia must be differentiated from other causes. Biopsy specimens taken from the colon or the rectum, sites that are only infrequently involved, can be misleading due to other conditions that are accompanied by PAS-positive cells (e.g., melanosis coli or histiocytosis); in these cases, the presence of *T. whipplei* should be shown by other techniques as well.[4,29,38]

Although the clinical picture together with a pathognomonic PAS-positive histology from the duodenum usually is sufficient to establish the diagnosis, a specific diagnostic test, such as PCR or electron microscopy, is recommended in every newly identified patient; it is mandatory in cases of doubt or if the diagnosis is based on extraduodenal tissue. This recommendation reflects the fact that PAS staining is of limited value in extraintestinal tissue and for monitoring the effect of therapy. Formerly, electron microscopic examination of the biopsy material often was and still may be helpful to confirm the diagnosis; however, its application is inconvenient.

In recent years, a considerable amount of experience has been gained with PCR-based detection of *T. whipplei* DNA. Several studies[8,9] showed that the original PCR primers could identify *T. whipplei* in a variety of tissues (fresh or embedded), and newer work has shown that many alternative primer pairs may be useful in diagnostic procedures as well.[16,39,40] There is currently controversy, however, regarding the reliability and sensitivity of PCR tests performed in patients without Whipple's disease. Positive PCR results were reported when testing gastric fluid small bowel biopsy specimens and saliva[18] of patients without disease, but these results could not be confirmed by other investigators. Several target gene sequences currently are available based on 16S rRNA (e.g., interspacer), 23S rRNA, or RpoB.[13,41] Sample specimens usable for PCR are duodenal biopsy, synovial fluid, lymph node, cardiac valve, vitreous humor, and CSF.[13,38,41] Blood has not been a good sample for this purpose.[42] The quantitative detection of *T. whipplei* by real-time PCR is promising and deserves to be evaluated against other PCR techniques. Before definitive diagnosis, and particularly when atypical cases are reported, the use of at least two PCR tests based on primers obtained from two different genes is recommended to avoid a false positivity caused by contamination.[13]

The detection of *T. whipplei* by immunohistochemistry using monoclonal antibodies has been shown on lymph node sections and in circulating monocytes of patients with active Whipple's disease.[7,43,44] The first antibody-based serology tests gave promising results[11] and deserve further development. Culture of *T. whipplei* is currently performed only in highly specialized laboratories on an experimental basis and to date is problematic because of the slow growth of the organism, the risk of contamination, and the preclusion of culture by prior antibiotic treatment.[13]

The clinician always has to interpret the histopathologic and laboratory findings—in diagnostic and monitoring situations—in the view of the clinical features of the patient (i.e., a positive PCR test without clinical correlation should not result in the initiation of a treatment). Specialists usually should be consulted.

Laboratory testing often reveals evidence of malabsorption and protein-losing enteropathy: reduced serum levels of beta carotene, various vitamins (B_{12}, D, K, and folic acid), albumin, cholesterol, and electrolytes; lymphocytopenia; elevated stool fat excretion; and reduced D-xylose absorption.[4,34] For unexplained reasons, some Whipple's disease patients have eosinophilia and abnormalities of serum immunoglobulins, such as low IgM or high IgA.[4,41,45] Finally, other, less specific, laboratory abnormalities in Whipple's disease include elevated erythrocyte sedimentation rate, elevated acute-phase proteins such as C-reactive protein, thrombocytosis, and hypochromic anemia.[4,34]

TREATMENT AND PROGNOSIS

Whipple's disease was considered to be a fatal disorder before empirical establishment of antibiotic therapy (the first case was treated with chloramphenicol) in the 1950s.[46] Many studies since have proved that antibiotic therapy leads to a rapid improvement of the clinical status in most patients with Whipple's disease and to a lasting remission. Diarrhea and fever may disappear within 1 week of therapy, whereas arthropathy and other symptoms often are improved after 2 to 4 weeks. The laboratory findings normalize often over several weeks. The clinical improvement usually is accompanied by a gradual reconstitution of the villous architecture of the small intestine and by a disappearance of the bacteria over several weeks.[4,5,31] Finally, immunologic parameters, such as increased IgA or shifts in T-cell subpopulations, return to normal within months. In contrast, the subtle defect in cell-mediated immunity persists for years, if not indefinitely.[22]

A variety of antibiotic regimens have proved beneficial in Whipple's disease patients. Until the 1980s, many patients were treated with a 2-week systemic course of penicillin plus streptomycin followed by oral tetracycline.[47] Because this treatment regimen may be associated with a higher frequency of relapses, including relapses involving the CNS,[31] and because of the high proportion of patients with a positive PCR for *T. whipplei* in the CSF at time of diagnosis,[39] trimethoprim-sulfamethoxazole, which readily crosses the blood-brain barrier, now usually is recommended for long-term oral therapy (160/800 mg twice daily for at least 1 year). This therapy also seems to be clinically superior to tetracycline for patients with and without CNS symptoms.[31] Although the cultivation of *T. whipplei* and the resulting susceptibility tests may soon allow one to define more adequately treatment regimens for Whipple's disease,[47a] there still are no results of prospective studies available on the choice or the duration of antibiotic therapy. We strongly encourage early contact with specialized centers for newly diagnosed and refractory patients. In Europe, different long-term therapies—possibly based on data of susceptibility testing—will be compared (for information, see European Project on Whipple's Disease at www.whipplesdisease.info) (Table 97-2).

Oral therapy should be preceded, especially in severely ill patients, by 2 weeks of parenteral therapy. The institution of ceftriaxone (i.e., a 2-week course of ceftriaxone, 2 g/day intravenously) is recommended and often has prompt clinical effects.[36,48] On the basis of case reports and personal experience, ceftriaxone probably is superior to the empirical regimen of systemic penicillin plus streptomycin, but it is not clear whether it is equivalent to intravenous meropenem, a hypothesis that

TABLE 97-2 Recommended Treatment in Whipple's Disease

Initial parenteral therapy (IV)
  2 weeks of ceftriaxone, 2 g daily
  Alternatively: meropenem or penicillin plus streptomycin
Long-term therapy (oral)
  At least 1 year of trimethoprim-sulfamethoxazole, 160/800 mg twice daily
  Alternatively: doxycycline or a cephalosporin

currently is being tested in the first prospective and randomized clinical trial (SIMW initiated by Feurle; for information, see www.whipplesdisease.info). In patients with endocarditis, prolonged intravenous therapy (4 to 8 weeks) has been suggested (see Table 97-2).

In the case of an intolerance to sulfonamides, doxycycline therapy can be instituted. Other antibiotics, such as cephalosporins and fluoroquinolones, have been used in individual cases.[45,47] Rarely a Jarisch-Herxheimer reaction has been described after the initiation of antibiotic therapy in Whipple's disease.[45]

The patient should be followed with duodenal biopsies and in case of cerebral involvement with CSF analysis at 6 months and 1 year after diagnosis. If PAS-positive material is absent after 1 year and no bacteria are detected by PCR or by electron microscopy, antibiotic treatment can be stopped. We recommend, even in successfully treated patients in whom therapy has been discontinued, performing follow-up biopsies at increasingly longer intervals 5 years after the establishment of diagnosis. If bacterial material persists after 1 year of treatment, therapy must be continued. Therapy probably can be stopped safely if the histology has been stationary for 2 years. Monitoring of therapy in the future may be improved with the use of serology, PCR, or immunohistology.

In severely ill patients, replacement therapy is indicated similar to other malabsorption syndromes. This therapy includes vitamin D and calcium supplementation in patients with steatorrhoea, fluid and electrolyte replacement in cachectic patients, iron in anemic patients, and a high calorie/protein/vitamin diet.

Relapses become evident mostly within a few years after diagnosis and usually are treated successfully with the reinstitution of the primary antibiotic regimen. CNS manifestations seem to be more frequent at relapses.[4,13,33,36,45,46] Some patients have an antibiotic-refractory disease course, and in some patients with primary or recurrent CNS manifestation, a beneficial treatment needs to be defined. A combination of antibiotic treatment and immunotherapy (e.g., with recombinant IFN-γ) may be beneficial.[28]

REFERENCES

1. Whipple GH. A hitherto undescribed disease characterized anatomically by deposits of fat and fatty acids in the intestinal and mesenteric lymphatic tissues. Johns Hopkins Hosp Bull. 1907;18:382-391.
2. Cohen AS, Schimmel EM, Holt PR, Isselbacher KJ. Ultrastructural abnormalities in Whipple's disease. Proc Soc Exp Biol Med. 1960;105:411-414.
3. Silva MT, Macedo PM, Nunes JFM. Ultrastructure of bacilli and bacillary origin of the macrophagic inclusions in Whipple's disease. J Gen Microbiol. 1985;131:1001-1013.
4. Dobbins WO III. Whipple's Disease. Springfield, IL: Charles C Thomas; 1987.
5. Trier JS, Phelps PC, Eidelmann S, Rubin CE. Whipple's disease: Light and electron microscope correlation of jejunal mucosal histology with antibiotic treatment and clinical status. Gastroenterology. 1965;48:684-707.
6. Keren DF. Whipple's disease: A review emphasizing immunology and microbiology. Crit Rev Clin Lab Sci. 1981;14:75-108.
7. Lepidi H, Costedoat N, Piette JC, et al. Immunohistological detection of Tropheryma whipplei (Whipple bacillus) in lymph nodes. Am J Med. 2002;113:334-336.
8. Wilson KH, Blitchington R, Frothingham R, Wilson JAP. Phylogeny of the Whipple's disease-associated bacterium. Lancet. 1991;338:474-475.
9. Relman DA, Schmidt TM, Macdermott RP, Falkow S. Identification of the uncultured bacillus of Whipple's disease. N Engl J Med. 1992;327:293-301.
10. Schoedon G, Goldenberger D, Forrer R, et al. Deactivation of macrophages with interleukin-4 is the key to the isolation of Tropheryma whippelii. J Infect Dis. 1997;176:672-677.
11. Raoult D, Birg ML, La Scola B, et al. Cultivation of the bacillus of Whipple's disease. N Engl J Med. 2000;342:620-625.
12. La Scola B, Fenollar F, Fournier PE, Altwegg M, et al. Description of Tropheryma whipplei gen.nov., sp.nov., the Whipple's disease bacillus. Int J Syst Evol Mic. 2001;51:1471-1479.
13. Marth T, Raoult D. Whipple's disease. Lancet. 2003;361:239-246.
14. Bentley S, Maiwald M, Murphy LD, et al. Sequencing and analysis of the genome of the Whipple's disease bacterium Tropheryma whipplei. Lancet. 2003;361:637-644.
14a. Raoult D, Ogata H, Audic S, et al. Tropheryma whipplei Twist: A human pathogenic Actinobacteria with a reduced genome. Genome Res. 2003;13:1800-1809.
15. Maiwald M, Ditton HJ, von Herbay A, et al. Reassessment of the phylogenetic position of the bacterium associated with Whipple's disease and determination of the 16S-23S ribosomal intergenic spacer sequence. Int J Syst Bacteriol. 1996;46:1078-1082.
16. Hinrikson HP, Dutly F, Nair S, Altwegg M. Detection of three different types of 'Tropheryma whippelii' directly from clinical specimens by sequencing, single-strand conformation polymorphism (SSCP) analysis and type-specific PCR of their 16S-23S ribosomal intergenic spacer region. Int J Syst Bacteriol. 1999;4:1701-1706.
17. Maiwald M, Schuhmacher F, Ditton, HJ, von Herbay A. Environmental occurrence of the Whipple's disease bacterium (Tropheryma whippelii). Appl Environment Microbiol. 1998;64:760-762.
18. Dutly F, Hinrikson HP, Seidel T, et al. Tropheryma whippelii DNA in saliva of patients without Whipple's disease. Infection. 2000;28:219-222.
19. Feurle GE, Dörken B, Schöpf E, Lenhard V. HLA-B27 and defects in the T-cell system in Whipple's disease. Eur J Clin Invest. 1979;9:385-389.
20. Meier-Willersen HJ, Maiwald M, von Herbay A. Whipple's disease associated with opportunistic infections. Dtsch Med Wochenschr. 1993;118:854-860.
21. Maxwell JD, Ferguson A, McCay AM, et al. Lymphocytes in Whipple's disease. Lancet. 1968;1:887-889.
22. Marth T, Roux M, von Herbay A, et al. Persistent reduction of complement receptor 3 alpha-chain expressing mononuclear blood cells and transient inhibitory serum factors in Whipple's disease. Clin Immunol Immunopathol. 1994;72:217-226.
23. Groll A, Valberg LS, Simon JB, et al. Immunological defect in Whipple's disease. Gastroenterology. 1972;63:943-950.
24. Eck M, Kreipe H, Harmsen D, Müller-Hermelink HK. Invasion and destruction of mucosal plasma cells by Tropheryma whippelii. Hum Pathol. 1997;28:1424-1428.
25. Marth T, Neurath M, Cuccherini BA, Strober W. Defects of monocyte interleukin-12 production and humoral immunity in Whipple's disease. Gastroenterology. 1997;113:442-448.
26. Bai JC, Sen L, Diez R, et al. Impaired monocyte function in patients successfully treated for Whipple's disease. Acta Gastroenterol Latinoam. 1996;26:85-89.
27. Marth T, Kleen N, Stallmach A, et al. Dysregulated peripheral and mucosal Th1/Th2 response in Whipple's disease. Gastroenterology. 2002;123:1468-1477.
28. Schneider T, Stallmach A, von Herbay A, et al. Treatment of refractory Whipple's disease with recombinant interferon-gamma. Ann Intern Med. 1998;129:875-877.
29. Enzinger FM, Helwig EB. Whipple's disease: A review of the literature and report of 15 patients. Virchows Arch. 1963;336:238-268.
30. Black-Schaffer B. Tinctorial demonstration of a glycoprotein in Whipple's disease. Proc Soc Exp Biol Med. 1949;72:225-227.
31. Feurle GE, Marth T. An evaluation of antimicrobial treatment for Whipple's disease—tetracycline versus trimethoprim-sulfamethoxazole. Dig Dis Sci. 1994;39:1642-1648.
32. Fenollar F, Lepidi H, Raoult D. Whipple's endocarditis: Review of the literature and comparisons with Q fever, Bartonella infection, and blood culture-positive endocarditis. Clin Infect Dis. 2001;33:1309-1316.
33. Feurle GE, Volk B, Waldherr R. Cerebral Whipple's disease with negative jejunal histology. N Engl J Med. 1979;300:907-908.
34. Fleming JL, Wiesner RH, Shorter RG. Whipple's disease: Clinical, biochemical and histopathological features and assessment of treatment in 29 patients. Mayo Clin Proc. 1988;63:539-551.
35. O'Duffy JD, Griffing WL, Li CY, et al. Whipple's arthritis: Direct detection of Tropheryma whippelii in synovial fluid and tissue. Arthritis Rheum. 1999;42:812-817.
36. Gerard A, Sarrot-Reynauld F, Liozon E, et al. Neurologic presentation of Whipple disease: Report of 12 cases and review of the literature. Medicine. 2002;81:443-457.
37. Geboes K, Ectors N, Heidbuchel H, et al. Whipple's disease: The value of upper gastrointestinal endoscopy for the diagnosis and follow-up. Acta Gastroenterol Belg. 1992;55:209-219.
38. Ectors N, Geboes K, De Vos R, et al. Whipple's disease: A histological, immunocytochemical and electronmicroscopic study of the immune response in the small intestinal mucosa. Histopathology. 1992;21:1-12.
39. von Herbay A, Ditton HJ, Schuhmacher F, Maiwald M. Whipple's disease: Staging and monitoring by cytology and polymerase chain reaction of cerebrospinal fluid. Gastroenterology. 1997;113:434-441.
40. Ramzan NN, Loftus E, Burgart LJ, et al. Diagnosis and monitoring of Whipple's disease by polymerase chain reaction. Ann Intern Med. 1997;126:520-527.
41. Fenollar F, Raoult D. Whipple's disease. Clin Diagn Lab Immunol. 2001;8:1-8.
42. Marth T, Fredericks D, Strober W, Relman DA. Limited role for PCR-based diagnosis of Whipple's disease from peripheral blood mononuclear cells. Lancet. 1996;348:66-67.
43. Raoult D, Lepidi H, Harle JR. Tropheryma whipplei circulating in blood monocytes. N Engl J Med. 2001;345:548.
44. Raoult D, La Scola B, Lecocq P, et al. Culture and immunological detection of Tropheryma whippleii from the duodenum of a patient with Whipple disease. JAMA. 2001;285:1039-1043.
45. Durand DV, Lecomte C, Cathébras P, et al. Whipple disease: Clinical review of 52 cases. Medicine. 1997;76:170-184.
46. Paulley JW. A case of Whipple's disease (intestinal lipodystrophy). Gastroenterology. 1952;22:128-133.
47. Keinath RD, Merrell DE, Vlietstra R, Dobbins WO III. Antibiotic treatment and relapse in Whipple's disease. Gastroenterology. 1985;88:1867-1873.
47a. Boulos A, Rolain JM, Raoult D. Antibiotic susceptibility of Tropheryma whipplei in MRC5 cells. Antimicrob Agents Chemother. 2004;48(3):747-752.
48. Adler CH, Galetta SL. Oculo-facial-skeletal myorhythmia in Whipple's disease: Treatment with ceftriaxone. Ann Intern Med. 1990;112:467-469.

CHAPTER **98**

Infectious Arthritis of Native Joints

CHRISTOPHER A. OHL

Infectious arthritis of single or multiple joints may be caused by any of a number of diverse microorganisms. Bacterial arthritis, also known as *suppurative*, *pyogenic*, or *septic arthritis*, is the most common, and arguably most important, joint infection and is considered a rheumatologic emergency because of its potential for rapid joint destruction with irreversible loss of function. Viral arthritis often involves multiple joints as a component of a systemic infection and generally does not lead to long-term morbidity. In contrast to the acute presentation of bacterial and viral arthritis, joint infection caused by mycobacteria and non-*Candida* fungi usually arises as chronic, slowly progressive monoarticular arthritis. In addition to the arthritis caused by direct joint infection by these microbes, a reactive or sterile arthritis is occasionally associated with systemic or local infection at a site remote from the joint. For patients with infectious arthritis, a prompt and thorough clinical evaluation and early institution of specific treatment are essential in order to limit long-term sequelae. This chapter primarily discusses infections of native joints. For a detailed discussion of infections involving prosthetic arthroplasty, see Chapter 100.

ACUTE BACTERIAL ARTHRITIS

The reported incidence of native joint septic arthritis in the general population is between 2 and 10 cases per 100,000 per year and may be increasing because of a larger number of at-risk patients and surgical joint procedures.[1-4] Estimates of the incidence in patients with rheumatoid arthritis are much higher, ranging from 28 to 38 per 100,000 per year. The published mortality rates of bacterial arthritis in adults vary between 10% and 30%, although it is difficult to determine the proportion that is directly attributable to acute joint infection and its sequelae versus that related to patients' comorbidity or underlying disease.[5-7] The morbidity of septic arthritis is considerable, with up to 50% of patients reporting decreased joint function or mobility after infection.[8,9] Despite improved antimicrobial agents, adjunct treatment measures, and hospital care, the morbidity and mortality of septic arthritis have not changed appreciably in the past two to three decades.[10]

Bacterial arthritis is usually hematogenously acquired. The extremely vascular synovial membrane of the joint lacks a limiting basement membrane and is particularly susceptible to the deposition of bacteria during occult or clinically apparent bacteremia.[3,8,11] Other routes of infection include direct inoculation of bacteria into the joint through surgery, trauma, percutaneous puncture (such as from a nail, needle, or thorn), or contiguous spread from adjacent infected soft tissue or bone.[3,4] Septic arthritis is an unusual complication of total knee arthroscopy, occurring in only 0.04% to 0.4% of procedures, although the use of perioperative, intra-articular corticosteroids appears to increase this risk.[12,13] Similarly, it is also rare for infection to follow a single joint aspiration or corticosteroid injection. In addition, bacterial arthritis has been reported as a complication of reconstructive surgery of the knee in which contaminated cadaveric bone or tendon allografts are inadvertently utilized.[14-16]

TABLE 98-1   **Predisposing Factors in Bacterial Arthritis**

Joint disease
    Rheumatoid arthritis
    Crystal-induced arthritis
    Osteoarthritis
    Charcot's arthropathy
Chronic systemic disease
    Diabetes mellitus
    Chronic renal failure
    Chronic liver disease
    Collagen vascular disease
    Malignancy
    Sickle cell disease
Immunosuppression
    Human immunodeficiency virus (HIV) infection
    Immunosuppressant therapy including systemic steroids
    Organ and bone marrow transplantation
    Hypogammaglobulinemia
Trauma
    Surgery (including arthroscopic)
    Penetrating injury
    Intra-articular injection (e.g., glucocorticoids)
Prosthetic joint
Intravenous drug use
Endocarditis

From references 2, 3, 5, 7, 8, 17.

Normal, diseased, and prosthetic joints are all susceptible to infection, although abnormal joint architecture in the latter cases greatly increases the risk. Additional predisposing host factors include immunosuppression, diabetes mellitus, malignancy, chronic renal failure, and intravenous drug abuse (Table 98-1). Patients with human immunodeficiency virus (HIV) infection are probably at higher risk for septic arthritis, although it is difficult to know how much of this risk is due to recreational intravenous drug use.[17] Skin disease or lesions, with or without concomitant infection, are an important source of hematogenously derived joint sepsis.[2,3] The clinical manifestations, severity, treatment, and prognosis of septic arthritis are dependent on the identity and virulence of the infecting bacterium, source of joint infection, and certain underlying host factors such as immune status, comorbid illness, and abnormal joint architecture resulting from disease or surgery.

Nongonococcal Arthritis

Pathophysiology

The pathophysiology of acute nongonococcal septic arthritis is complex and dependent on adherence of organisms to and colonization of the synovial membrane, bacterial proliferation in synovial fluid, and a resultant synovial infection with generation of a host inflammatory response. Much of our understanding of these pathophysiologic mechanisms comes from study of animal models of joint infection, particularly with *Staphylococcus aureus*. After hematogenous or direct entry into the joint, bacterial adherence is facilitated by the low-shear conditions of synovial fluid and in some cases by joint disease or injury (traumatic or surgical) that results in an increased amount or exposure of host-derived extracellular matrix proteins such as fibronectin, collagen, laminin, elastin, and hyaluronic acid that promote bacterial attachment.[11] Certain bacteria (e.g., *S. aureus*, *Streptococcus* spp., and *Neisseria gonorrhoeae*) display a tropism for synovial infection, at least in part because of adherence characteristics of the organism. For example, *S. aureus* has surface receptors such as fibronectin-binding protein and microbial surface components recognizing adhesive matrix molecules (MSCRAMMs) that recognize selected host proteins and mediate adherence to the joint extracellular matrix.[18,19] A number of *S. aureus* genes have been found encoding these surface receptors, and mutation in some of these genes strongly reduces the ability of staphylococci to produce joint infection in experimental animals.[20-22]

Although certain bacterial products or toxins, including bacterial DNA and staphylococcal α-hemolysin, may directly increase tissue damage in the infected joint,[11] it is the host inflammatory response to infection that is responsible for much of the joint injury.[23] In response to replicating bacteria and a number of bacterial products, an inflammatory cell response is rapidly noted within the joint synovial membrane, which then responds with a proliferative lining-cell hyperplasia.[24] An influx of acute and chronic inflammatory cells results in the characteristic purulent inflammation of the joint and its synovial fluid. Leukocyte-derived proteases and inflammatory cytokines including interleukin (IL)-1, IL-6, and tumor necrosis factor-α either directly or indirectly result in cartilage degradation, inhibition of cartilage synthesis, and subchondral bone loss.[11] Intra-articular cartilage destruction may be seen in as little as 3 days.[25] In addition, the inflammatory joint infusion increases intra-articular pressure, hampering capillary blood flow to the joint and resulting in cartilage and synovial ischemia and necrosis.[8] Over time, cartilage destruction leads to joint space narrowing and further erosive damage to the cartilage and underlying bone. If untreated, infection can spread from the joint to surrounding soft tissue, disrupting ligaments, tendons, and other periarticular structures and occasionally forming sinus tracts.[26,27]

Microbiology

Nongonococcal septic arthritis is caused by a multitude of pathogenic bacteria (Table 98-2). The most common etiologic agent in adults is *S. aureus*, which is responsible for 37% to 65% of cases depending on geographic location, incidence of comorbid rheumatic disease, and proportion of infections involving native joints.[3-5,7,28-30] For patients with rheumatoid arthritis, the proportion of septic arthritis caused by *S. aureus* has been reported to be higher (approximately 75%),[26,31] although a more recent study found it to be similar to that seen in the population at large.[6] Anecdotal reports suggest that methicillin-resistant *S. aureus* (MRSA) is increasingly isolated from joints in both nosocomial and community-acquired infectious arthritis and that previous colonization or infection of the patient by MRSA increases this risk.[32-36]

Streptococcus spp. are the bacteria next most frequently isolated from adults with native joint septic arthritis.[11,28,29] *Streptococcus pyogenes* and other β-hemolytic streptococci from Lancefield groups C, F, and G are important pathogens within this group. Group B streptococci have emerged as an important cause of bacterial arthritis in adults with diabetes, malignancy, and genitourinary structural abnormalities.[11,37] *Streptococcus pneumoniae*, traditionally thought of as a rare cause of hematogenous septic arthritis in the antibiotic era, was found to cause 6% of cases in a systematic review.[29] Enterococci are rare causes of bacterial arthritis in native joints.

Gram-negative bacilli are cultured from approximately 5% to 20% of patients with bacterial arthritis, particularly from neonates, elderly people, intravenous drug users, and immunocompromised hosts.[11] The coliform bacteria are most commonly isolated, particularly *Escherichia coli*.[3,29,30] *Pseudomonas aeruginosa*, an important pathogen in intravenous drug users, has a particular affinity for fibrocartilaginous articular structures such as the pubic symphysis and sternoclavicular, sternochondral, and sacroiliac joints.[38,39] *Haemophilus influenzae*, once an important pathogen in young children, now rarely causes septic arthritis in populations in which *H. influenzae* type b vaccine is widely employed.[40] For children younger than 2 years, *Kingella kingae*, a resident of the normal oral flora, has replaced *H. influenzae* as the principal gram-negative cause of hematogenous bacterial arthritis.[41]

Other nongonococcal bacteria identified in infected joints include anaerobes, corynebacteria, *Salmonella* spp., *Neisseria meningitidis*, *Brucella* spp., *Mycoplasma hominis*, and *Ureaplasma urealyticum*. Unusual bacterial pathogens causing contiguous septic arthritis after a dog or cat bite include *Pasteurella multocida* and *Capnocytophaga* spp. And, in the case of a human bite, *Eikenella corrodens* and *Fusobacterium nucleatum*.[42-44] *Streptobacillus moniliformis*, a causative agent of rat-bite fever, is occasionally isolated from the blood in patients with a polyarticular arthritis after a rat bite.[45] Table 98-3 lists selected clinical and epidemiologic associations with septic arthritis and the likely causative bacteria.

Cultures of synovial fluid or blood from patients diagnosed with septic arthritis remain negative in 10% to 20% of cases[30] and yield polymicrobial flora in up to 8% of cases.[29] Important causes of bacterial arthritis in which a pathogen is not isolated from blood or joint fluid using conventional culture techniques are *Borrelia burgdorferi* and *Tropheryma whipplei*, agents associated with Lyme and Whipple's disease, respectively.[46,47]

TABLE 98-2 Bacteria Isolated in 2302 Compiled Cases of Bacterial Septic Arthritis

Organism	Isolates No. (% of total)
Gram-Positive	
Staphylococcus aureus	1066 (46)
Staphylococci, coagulase negative	84 (4)
Streptococci	512 (22)
Streptococcus pyogenes	183 (8)
Streptococcus pneumoniae	156 (7)
Streptococcus agalactiae	69 (3)
Other streptococci	104 (5)
Gram-Negative	
Escherichia coli	91 (4)
Haemophilus influenzae	104 (5)
Neisseria gonorrhoeae	77 (3)
Neisseria meningitidis	28 (1)
Pseudomonas aeruginosa	36 (2)
Salmonella spp.	25 (1)
Other gram-negative rods	110 (5)
Miscellaneous (including anaerobes)	136 (6)
Polymicrobial	33 (1)

Adapted from Ross JJ, Saltzman CL, Carling P, Shapiro DS. Pneumococcal septic arthritis: Review of 190 cases. Clin Infect Dis. 2003;36:319-327.

TABLE 98-3 Clinical and Epidemiologic Features Associated with Selected Bacterial Causes of Septic Arthritis

Clinical or Epidemiologic Feature	Etiologic Agent
Rheumatoid arthritis	*Staphylococcus aureus*
Intravenous drug use	*S. aureus, Pseudomonas aeruginosa*
Diabetes, malignancy	*S. aureus*, group B streptococci
Immunocompromised hosts	*S. aureus*, streptococci, enteric gram-negative bacilli
Neonates, children younger than 2 years	Gram-negative bacilli, *Kingella kingae*
Young adults, menstruating females, associated skin lesions	*Neisseria gonorrhoeae*
Fibrocartilaginous joints (e.g., pubic symphysis)	*S. aureus, P. aeruginosa*
Cat or dog bite	*Pasteurella multocida, Capnocytophaga* sp., anaerobes
Human bite	*Eikenella corrodens*, anaerobes, other oral flora (e.g., viridans streptococci)
Rat bite	*Streptobacillus moniliformis*
Postpartum women	*Mycoplasma hominis*
Ingestion of unpasteurized dairy products, residents or travelers from endemic areas	*Brucella* sp.
Residents or travelers to Southeast Asia	*Burkholderia pseudomallei* (melioidosis)
Status after reconstructive surgery of the knee involving cadaveric bone or tendon graft	*Clostridium* sp.

Adapted from Smith JW, Hasan M. Infectious arthritis. In: Mandell G, Bennett J, Dolin R, eds. Principles and Practice of Infectious Diseases. Philadelphia: Churchill Livingstone; 2000:1175-1182.

Clinical Features

Nongonococcal septic arthritis is monarticular in 80% to 90% of cases, with the knee being the site of infection in approximately 50% of patients.[1,48-50] Other native joints that are frequently involved in adults include the shoulder, wrist, and ankle. In children, hip infections predominate and frequently affect a native joint, whereas in adults the majority of infections in this joint involve prosthetic or osteosynthetic material.[3] Infections of the peripheral joints of the hands are unusual except in the setting of trauma, particularly animal or human bites.[43] Septic arthritis of the small joints of the foot is most often secondary to contiguous spread from skin and soft tissue ulcerations or adjacent osteomyelitis and is mostly seen in diabetic patients.[51] Sternoclavicular or costochondral joint infections are uncommon except in intravenous drug users and occasionally as a complication of subclavian vein catheterization.[52,53] Risk factors for septic arthritis of the pubic symphysis include female urinary incontinence surgery, participation in athletics, pelvic malignancy, and intravenous drug use.[39] Nongonococcal polyarticular bacterial arthritis is observed in 10% to 20% of patients, especially in those with rheumatoid arthritis, immunosuppression, or prolonged or intense bacteremia, and is usually caused by *S. aureus*.[54]

Most patients with acute bacterial arthritis present with the cardinal symptoms of arthritis—pain and loss of function of one or more joints. In addition to intense pain and decreased range of motion, other symptoms of nongonococcal bacterial arthritis include swelling, redness, and increased warmth of the infected joint.[8] Joint pain is often the only focal symptom of deep or axial joint infection. In the case of sacroiliac or pubic symphysis septic arthritis, pain is intensely exacerbated by ambulation and often radiates to the back or groin, respectively, and to the hip and proximal leg in either case.[39,55] Although fever and malaise are commonly associated with bacterial arthritis in adults, high fevers with rigors and shaking chills are typically not apparent.[8,49]

Physical examination findings in infected peripheral joints include focal joint tenderness, inflammation, and effusion (Fig. 98-1). Active and passive range of motion of the joint is usually limited and results in considerable discomfort. Examination findings in patients with bacterial arthritis of the nonperipheral joints may be limited to focal tenderness over the affected area. Children with septic arthritis of the hip characteristically hold the hip in a flexed and externally rotated position and resist any range of motion. A source of infection distant from the afflicted joint may be discovered after careful clinical evaluation in 50% of patients.[49]

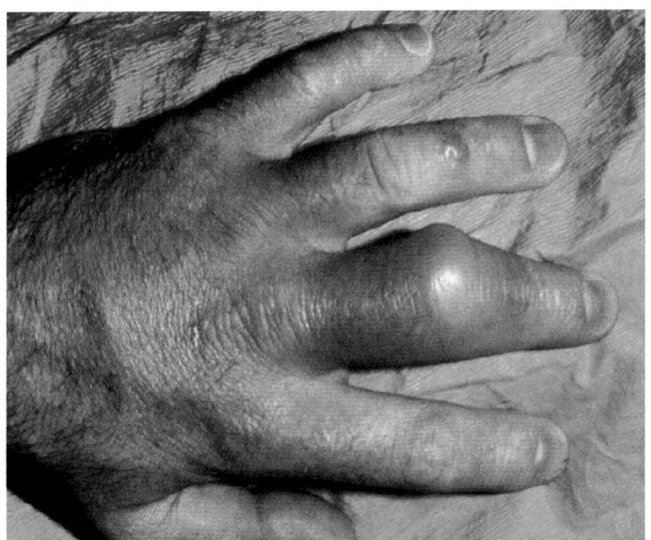

FIGURE 98-1. Bacterial arthritis of the third proximal interphalangeal joint demonstrating redness, swelling, and effusion.

Patients who are immunocompromised, have comorbid illnesses (including rheumatoid arthritis), or are at the extremes of age often present with significantly more subtle symptoms and signs of joint infection, frequently resulting in a delay in diagnosis.[1,5,56,57] For patients afflicted with rheumatoid arthritis or other chronic joint disease, particularly those receiving systemic or intra-articular steroids, manifestations of a complicating joint infection may be limited to a modest increase in the severity of chronic articular inflammation and loss of function and can be difficult to differentiate from an exacerbation of their underlying disease.[6,48]

Laboratory evaluation frequently shows an elevated erythrocyte sedimentation rate and C-reactive protein, although both tests are relatively nonspecific. The peripheral blood leukocyte count is usually increased in older children but may be normal in adults and neonates. Arthrocentesis of an affected joint reveals purulent, low-viscosity synovial fluid with a markedly elevated polymorphonuclear neutrophil count. Synovial fluid culture in nongonococcal infection yields bacterial growth up to 80% to 90% of the time; however, Gram staining is diagnostic in only 50% of these cases.[30] False-positive Gram stains of synovial fluid can occur because of artifacts from stain, mucin, and cellular debris. There is some evidence that direct inoculation of synovial fluid into pediatric or adult blood culture medium bottles improves the recovery of pathogens,[58,59] although one investigation comparing the BACTEC blood culture bottle with lysis centrifugation and conventional agar plate culture techniques found similar yields from all three methods.[60] Blood cultures are positive in 50% to 70% of patients with nongonococcal bacterial arthritis.[49] Synovial fluid and blood culture sensitivity declines in patients after antimicrobial therapy has been initiated.

Radiographic Features

Imaging studies of joints and periarticular structures affected by bacterial arthritis often yield additional information helpful for establishing the diagnosis or evaluating for complications of infection. Plain film roentgenography in early infection typically shows periarticular soft tissue swelling and fat pad edema but normal osseous structures.[61] In advanced infection, findings may include periarticular osteoporosis, joint space loss, periosteal reaction, marginal and central erosions, and destruction of subchondral bone. Plain films are useful for assessment of preexisting joint disease, metallic foreign bodies, and simultaneous osteomyelitis or as a baseline image in monitoring for sequelae of infection. Ultrasonography, another simple technique, is an extremely sensitive test to confirm the presence of an effusion and guide needle aspiration of certain joints.[62]

Scintigraphy, computed tomography (CT), and magnetic resonance imaging (MRI) are highly sensitive techniques for imaging early septic arthritis. Scintigraphy, including three- or four-phase bone scanning using technetium 99m methylene diphosphonate, is a sensitive indicator of increased blood flow adjacent to the joint and altered osteoblastic activity in periarticular bone, nonspecific indications of joint inflammation or infection.[61] CT is useful for the detection of erosive bone changes, subchondral cysts, joint effusions, and periarticular soft tissue extension of infection, particularly in deep articulations such as the hip, sacroiliac, and sternoclavicular joints and the pubic symphysis (Fig. 98-2).[39,55,61,63,64] Similarly to bone scanning and CT, MRI is an extremely sensitive procedure for the evaluation of bacterial arthritis but is more specific than these other modalities.[65] MRI is particularly valuable for the detection of joint inflammation, effusion, and articular cartilage destruction as well as for periarticular cellulitis, fistula, abscess, or osteomyelitis. However, MRI may have difficulty distinguishing septic arthritis from other sterile inflammatory arthropathies, cannot be used with certain metal joint implants, and has lower resolution for the bony cortex than CT.[11,65]

Gonococcal Arthritis

N. gonorrhoeae is an important cause of bacterial arthritis in sexually active adults and adolescents, with the majority of cases occurring in persons younger than 30 years.[66] Gonococcal arthritis is one of two

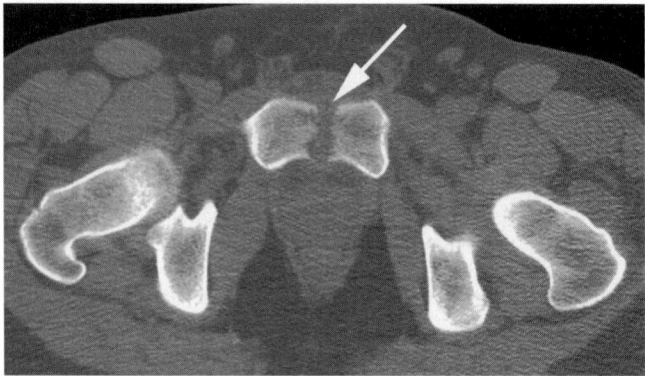

A

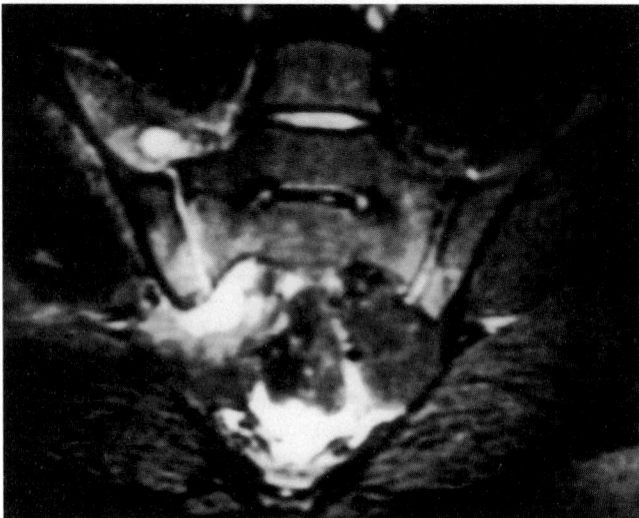

B

FIGURE 98-2. A, Septic arthritis of the symphysis pubis. Computed tomography of the pelvis reveals joint space widening with subchondral bone resorption and disruption of the articular cortical margins. **B,** Septic sacroiliac joint. Coronal T2-weighted magnetic resonance image demonstrates fluid within the right sacroiliac joint, spreading superiorly and inferiorly to form soft tissue abscesses. *(From Chew FS, Maldjian C, Leffler SG. Musculoskeletal Imaging: A Teaching File. Philadelphia: Lippincott Williams & Wilkins; 1999:267.)*

clinical presentations of disseminated gonococcal infection (DGI), the other being a syndrome of tenosynovitis, dermatitis, and polyarthralgia without purulent joint infection.[67] There is overlap between the two conditions, and in some patients disseminated infection may progress from a bacteremic tenosynovitis-dermatitis syndrome to localized joint infection. Septic mon- or oligoarticular arthritis occurs in 42% to 85% of patients with DGI.[68]

DGI is approximately four times more common in women than men and complicates 0.5% to 3% of cases of mucosal gonococcal infection.[66,69] Epidemiologic characteristics associated with DGI consist of lower socioeconomic status, nonwhite ethnicity, men having sex with men, multiple sexual partners, and illicit drug use.[67] The incidence is markedly less in Europe than in North America and is considerably higher in the developing world.[66] In the United States, although statistics are not kept for DGI, the incidence has probably declined as the rate of mucosal gonorrhea has decreased by approximately 75% between 1975 and 2002.[70]

Pathogenesis

Gonococcal arthritis and DGI occur as a result of occult bacteremia secondary to mucosal infection of the urethra, uterine cervix, rec-

tum, or oropharynx. Asymptomatic mucosal infection is much more likely to result in DGI than symptomatic infection and may have been sexually contracted days to months before dissemination. This, at least in part, accounts for the increased risk of disease in women, in whom endocervical gonorrhea may persist without symptoms for extended periods. In addition, for women with *N. gonorrhoeae* infection of the uterine cervix the risk of DGI increases substantially during menstruation, pregnancy, and the direct postpartum period. One third to one half of all women who present with DGI do so during these times,[68,71,72] probably as a result of alterations in vaginal pH, cervical mucus, genital flora, and increased endometrial exposure of submucosal vessels to the infecting organism.[67,69] Other host factors that increase the risk of DGI are complement deficiencies, particularly the terminal components C5 to C8,[73,74] and systemic lupus erythematosus.[75] Immune mechanisms, including circulating immune complexes, may also play a part in the pathogenesis of DGI and gonococcal arthritis.[76]

N. gonorrhoeae possesses several virulence factors, many of them cell surface proteins, which influence pathogenesis and the ability of the organism to disseminate widely from infected mucosa. Microbial attachment to mucosal and synovial epithelium is facilitated by long pili that also play a role in inhibiting host leukocyte phagocytosis.[77] Gonococcal strains with the ability to disseminate are serum resistant and almost always express protein 1A, a principal outer-membrane protein.[69,78,79] Other characteristics of strains with an increased propensity to disseminate include lack of outer-membrane protein II, also called opacity protein, and nutritional requirements for arginine, hypoxanthine, and uracil.[11,66] The lipooligosaccharide of *N. gonorrhoeae* contributes to synovial damage and also plays a role in the serum resistance exhibited by this organism.[80,81]

N. gonorrhoeae displays acquired resistance to several antimicrobials including penicillin, tetracycline, and rarely cephalosporins or spectinomycin.[70] Although still uncommon, fluoroquinolone resistance has emerged in *N. gonorrhoeae*, particularly in Asia and the Pacific Rim. In Hawaii and the U.S. West Coast in 2002, 11.3% of gonococci were resistant to fluoroquinolones.[70] Even though the vast majority of ciprofloxacin-resistant gonococcal isolates worldwide are from mucosal sites, treatment recommendations for DGI and gonococcal arthritis have been modified to reflect growing resistance to this class of antimicrobials.[82]

Clinical Features

Patients with DGI typically present with the classical triad of dermatitis, tenosynovitis, and migratory polyarthralgia or polyarthritis.[67,68,71,75,83] Joint symptoms may be quite severe and are often asymmetric. Moderate fevers, chills, and general malaise are usually present. Two thirds of patients develop tenosynovitis, usually in the fingers, hands and wrists, although the distal large and small joints of the lower limbs can also be involved.[68,84] The hip is rarely affected.[85] Less than one half of patients have a true septic arthritis with a purulent joint effusion. The lesions of dermatitis are seen in two thirds of DGI patients; they are painless and nonpruritic, few in number, and may not be noticed by the patient.[66,67,84] Macules, papules, and pustules on an erythematous base are most commonly seen and often develop central necrosis (Fig. 98-3). The rash characteristically appears simultaneously with tenosynovitis and is seen in various stages of development involving the limbs and hands (including the palms and soles), less often the torso, and rarely the face. Lesions resolve after 4 to 5 days even if untreated, and new lesions may materialize after antimicrobial therapy is initiated.[67]

Septic gonococcal arthritis arising without tenosynovitis or skin lesions is less common than the so-called bacteremic form described previously and is clinically indistinguishable from bacterial arthritis caused by other organisms. The knees, wrists, and ankles are most commonly affected and monoarthritis is more common than polyarthritis. Joints tend to be markedly inflamed with large effusions. A syndrome of tenosynovitis with skin lesions may have occurred before the patient sought medical care. Mucosal infection is usually present

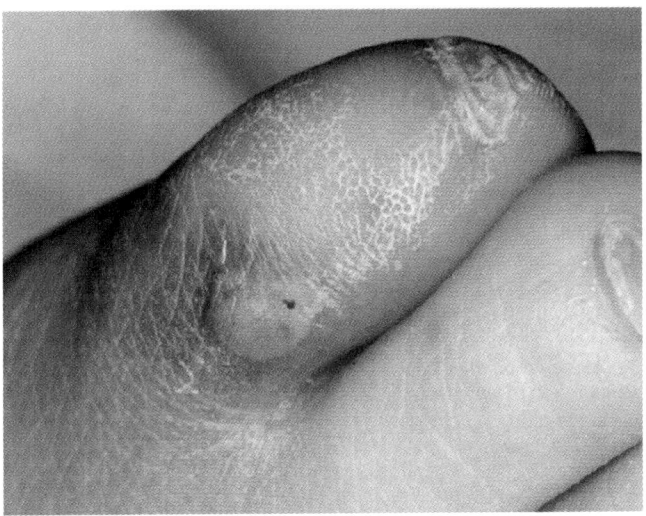

FIGURE 98-3. Pustular lesion overlying the fifth toe in a patient with disseminated gonococcal infection. *(Courtesy of the Graham International Dermatopathology Learning Center.)*

in patients with DGI and purulent gonococcal arthritis, although it is usually asymptomatic.

As with nongonococcal septic arthritis, the laboratory findings of gonococcal arthritis and DGI include mild leucocytosis and elevated erythrocyte sedimentation rate over 50 mm/hour in about 50% of patients.[67,68] Synovial fluid from joint effusions of patients afflicted with gonococcal arthritis frequently has 50,000 to 100,000 white blood cells/mm³, predominately neutrophils, whereas joint aspirates from patients with DGI without frank suppurative arthritis exhibit lower white blood cell counts.[67] *N. gonorrhoeae* is cultured from synovial fluid in approximately 50% of these cases and in 20% to 30% of patients with DGI.[66-68] This difference may be due in part to the fastidious growth properties of the organism or possibly to sub-threshold numbers of gonococci present in synovial fluid. Only 25% of Gram-stained joint aspirates from patients with suppurative gonococcal arthritis reveal intra- and extracellular gram-negative diplococci. Significantly higher proportions of patients with DGI are found to have *N. gonorrhoeae* identified in synovial fluid by polymerase chain reaction (PCR) testing than by conventional culture, with reported sensitivities of PCR estimated as 80%.[86-88] Positive blood cultures are exhibited by less than 30% of patients and are more common in those with dermatitis and tenosynovitis.[66,83,84,89] Gram staining and bacterial culture of skin lesions rarely yield organisms.

For patients with DGI and gonococcal arthritis, culture yield of *N. gonorrhoeae* is much higher from mucosal sites than from synovial fluid or blood. Cultures are positive for uterine cervical swabs in 80% to 90% of women and urethral swabs in 50% to 70% of men.[67,68,71] Culture yields from rectal and oropharyngeal swabs are lower but still occasionally give positive results. Although not studied in patients with DGI, nucleic acid amplification techniques performed on urethral or cervical swabs or freshly voided urine should give similar results.[90]

Management of Acute Bacterial Arthritis

Approach to the Patient

The diagnosis of bacterial arthritis should be suspected in any patient with acute mon- or polyarticular arthritis. Features of the patient's demographics, clinical history, physical examination, laboratory evaluation, and imaging studies may suggest an infecting pathogen; however, because of the diverse number of possible organisms and the need for prolonged courses of pathogen-specific antimicrobial therapy, a definitive etiologic diagnosis should always be sought. Antimicrobial therapy should be delayed until arthrocentesis and appropriate diagnostic

cultures are obtained unless the patient shows signs of sepsis. Bacterial cultures should be obtained from blood, any wound contiguous with the affected joint, and skin lesions, if present. If gonococcal arthritis is suspected, nucleic acid amplification tests for *N. gonorrhoeae* should be obtained using genitourinary sites or freshly voided urine, or both, in addition to cultures of genitourinary mucosa, rectum, and oropharynx.

The definitive diagnosis of bacterial arthritis requires identification of bacteria from synovial fluid obtained through arthrocentesis. This procedure should be performed in all patients with inflammatory arthritis in whom septic arthritis is within the differential diagnosis. Skin visibly involved with cellulitis should be avoided when entering the joint. For cases of polyarticular arthritis, multiple affected joints should be aspirated. For axial and deep joints difficult to aspirate at the bedside (e.g., sacroiliac or pubic symphysis) or in the event of a "dry tap" of a peripheral joint, fluoroscopic or CT-guided arthrocentesis is indicated. Synovial fluid examination should include cell count and leukocyte differential. Other tests that may be helpful include viscosity, total protein, lactate dehydrogenase, glucose, and crystal examination under polarized light. Gram stain, aerobic and anaerobic bacterial culture, and, in some cases, fungal and mycobacterial smears and cultures should be performed. Additional serologic testing for *B. burgdorferi* is indicated for patients in endemic areas with clinical features of Lyme arthritis, especially if they are at risk for tick bites. Serology may also be helpful in the diagnosis of the various viral arthritides, including parvovirus B19. Bacterial antigen testing of serum or synovial fluid is seldom diagnostic. Identification of bacterial or viral DNA in synovial fluid through PCR testing may be useful in some exceptional cases of acute arthritis but is not readily available for widespread clinical application.[91] CT or MRI is indicated to assess for septic arthritis in deep axial joints and if soft tissue or osteomyelitic extension is suspected.

Differential Diagnosis

The differential diagnosis of pyogenic arthritis includes several inflammatory joint diseases of noninfectious causes in addition to joint infections caused by nonbacterial pathogens. Acute attacks of the crystalline joint diseases, gout and pseudogout, are perhaps the greatest mimics of bacterial arthritis. For patients with a history of gouty attacks in stereotypical joints, acute joint inflammation is more likely to be due to crystalline than bacterial arthritis; however, in such attacks arthrocentesis is necessary to rule out concomitant bacterial infection.

Rheumatoid arthritis, systemic lupus erythematosus, spondyloarthropathy, Still's disease, rheumatic fever, and Kawasaki syndrome typically arise with subacute polyarticular arthritis associated with specific symptoms and signs of the respective diseases. Although these conditions may be confused with viral arthritides, especially parvoviral B19 arthritis, they are usually easily differentiated from bacterial arthritis. More important, however, are the recognition and diagnosis of bacterial arthritis in a patient with preexisting rheumatoid or other inflammatory arthritis. A sudden increase in inflammation of one or two joints in such patients should raise suspicion of complicating bacterial arthritis, even if it is not accompanied by fever or other systemic evidence of infection, and joint aspiration should be performed.

Reiter's syndrome and other reactive arthritides may occur spontaneously or after a recent gastrointestinal or genitourinary infection, particularly in men. The oligoarticular arthritis of Reiter's syndrome may be associated with tenosynovitis and urethritis, mimicking disseminated gonorrhea. Patients with Reiter's syndrome, however, do not display the characteristic rash of DGI and often have concomitant sacroiliitis, conjunctivitis, circinate balanitis, or keratoderma blennorrhagica—all conditions absent in DGI.

Arthralgias and myalgias are typical symptoms of subacute bacterial endocarditis, and sometimes an acute, sterile synovitis or tenosynovitis may be seen. Purulent joint or bone infection is not a common complication of endovascular infection.

Treatment

The management of acute bacterial arthritis requires prompt joint drainage in addition to antimicrobial therapy. One approach to drainage is through daily closed needle aspiration of affected joints until the amount and degree of purulence of synovial fluid are minimal. Another effective modality is arthroscopy, which allows better visualization and irrigation of the joint, lysis of adhesions, and removal of thick purulent material.[92] Arthroscopy is particularly effective for débridement of the knee, shoulder, and ankle. Open surgical drainage is recommended for septic arthritis of the hip and when repeated joint aspiration or arthroscopy is impractical or fails to control infection.[92] Prosthetic joint infections, particularly those arising more than 3 months after arthroplasty, usually necessitate prosthesis removal in conjunction with extensive joint débridement.[49] When joint infection is under control, early passive joint mobilization facilitates recovery and improves ultimate joint function.[92]

Initial antimicrobial therapy of native joint bacterial arthritis is dictated by synovial fluid Gram staining or likely infecting pathogens, or both, as determined by the clinical presentation (Table 98-4; see Table 98-2). Definitive treatment should be based on the identity and antimicrobial susceptibility of bacteria identified in synovial fluid, blood, or in some cases ancillary cultures (e.g., mucosal cultures for gonococcus). The penetration of inflamed joints is adequate for most intravenous and some oral antimicrobials, whereas in osteomyelitis an optimal bone concentration is difficult to achieve.[93] For septic arthritis related to animal or human bites, antimicrobials should be chosen that have activity against aerobic and anaerobic oral flora, for example, ampicillin-sulbactam or amoxicillin-clavulanate and, in the penicillin-allergic patient, clindamycin plus ciprofloxacin. For patients with native joint bacterial arthritis related to MRSA, intravenous vancomycin is recommended. Linezolid and daptomycin, two new drugs with activity against MRSA, may be an option for patients with joint infection with this organism who are allergic to, intolerant of, or not clinically responding after 3 to 5 days of vancomycin (neither drug is approved by the U.S. Food and Drug Administration for this indication).

TABLE 98-4 Recommended Empirical Therapy for Adult Native Joint Bacterial Arthritis

Gram Stain	Antimicrobial*
Gram-positive cocci	
No risk factors for MRSA[†]	Nafcillin/oxacillin 2 g q4h *or* Cefazolin 2 g q8h *or* PCN/CEPH allergic: clindamycin 900 mg q8h or vancomycin 1 g q12h
Risk factors for MRSA[†]	Vancomycin 1 g q12h
Gram-negative cocci	Ceftriaxone 1 g q24h
Gram-negative rods	Ceftazidime or cefepime 2 g q8h *or* piperacillin-tazobactam 4.5 g q6h *or* carbapenem (imipenem 500 mg q6h or meropenem 1 g q8h) PCN/CEPH allergic: aztreonam 2 g q8h *or* FQ (ciprofloxacin 400 mg IV q12h or levofloxacin 750 mg q24h)[‡]
Gram stain negative	Regimen for gram-positive cocci above *plus* Ceftazidime *or* fluoroquinolone (ciprofloxacin or levofloxacin)[‡] *or* aminoglycoside (tobramycin or gentamicin 5-7 mg/kg once daily or 5 mg/kg in three divided doses per day)

*All indicated dosages are intravenous for patients with normal renal function.
[†]Risk factors for MRSA include previous infection or colonization with MRSA, chronic renal failure or other debilitating illness, and frequent or prolonged hospitalization.
[‡]Can be given orally as ciprofloxacin 750 mg q12h or levofloxacin 750 mg q24h.
CEPH, cephalosporin; FQ, fluoroquinolone; MRSA, methicillin-resistant *Staphylococcus aureus*; PCN, penicillin.

Gonococcal arthritis is best treated initially with ceftriaxone, cefotaxime, or ceftizoxime; in regions without appreciable fluoroquinolone resistance, oral ciprofloxacin or levofloxacin may be substituted as the patient improves.[82]

Intravenous antimicrobials are usually continued for 2 to 4 weeks, although infections with *S. aureus*, including MRSA, and gram-negative bacilli generally require 4 weeks of treatment. For gram-negative septic arthritis in which the organism is susceptible to fluoroquinolones, oral ciprofloxacin or levofloxacin can be considered as an alternative to intravenous treatment during the latter half of a course of therapy. Gonococcal arthritis is typically treated with 2 weeks of antibiotics.

Adjuvant, short-course systemic corticosteroid treatment for children with hematogenous bacterial arthritis was shown in a randomized, double-blind, placebo-controlled study to reduce significantly the duration of symptoms and residual joint dysfunction.[94] Application of these findings to clinical practice is pending confirmatory studies in other populations of patients.

VIRAL ARTHRITIS

Arthritis or arthropathy caused by viral agents is often acute, occurs concurrently with signs and symptoms of febrile systemic illness, and resolves along with other manifestations of illness. Viruses may cause arthritis directly by infecting the synovium or indirectly through host immune-mediated responses, and much of the pathogenesis is poorly understood.[95]

Perhaps the most common form of viral arthritis in developed countries is caused by human parvovirus B19 (HPV-B19). In children, HPV-B19 infection arises with fever, rash, coryza, headache, and malaise.[96] The rash classically appears with bright red "slapped cheeks" and a lacy, reticular exanthem on the torso and extremities. Arthritis occurs in only a small percentage of afflicted children and tends to be asymmetric and pauciarticular.[97]

Adults who become infected with HPV-B19 do not display the classical facial erythema noted in children and present with a febrile, influenza-like illness with prominent polyarthralgia and joint inflammation.[98-100] Cases are usually seen in late winter and early spring, and regional outbreaks of disease have been reported.[101,102] An associated exanthem, if apparent, is a fleeting and difficult to appreciate rash on the torso and less often on the extremities that may show some of the reticular aspects exhibited by children (Fig. 98-4). Arthritis or prominent arthralgias are more common in women than men with HPV-B19 infection, affecting 60% and 30% of individuals, respectively.[99] Characteristically, an acute and moderately severe, symmetrical poly-

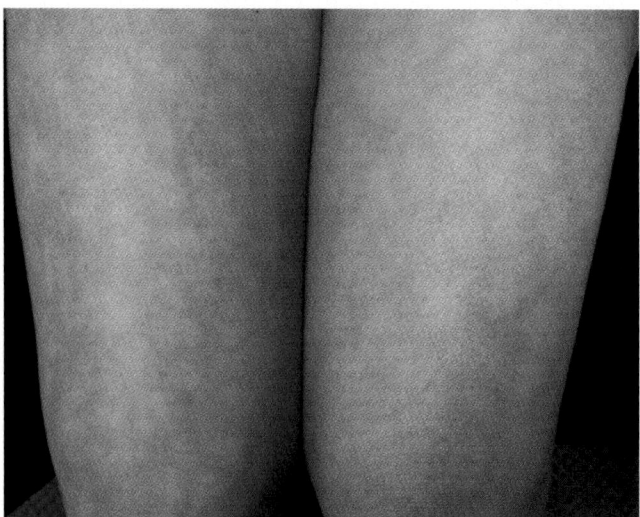

FIGURE 98-4. Faint, lacy reticular rash of the proximal lower extremities characteristic of adult human parvovirus B19 infection.

arthritis of the proximal interphalangeal and metacarpophalangeal joints is associated with morning stiffness and somewhat resembles rheumatoid arthritis.[96] Knees, wrists, and ankles may also be involved. In approximately one third of patients, particularly women, joint symptoms occur in episodic flares with symptom-free intervals.[96] Diagnosis is made clinically, and a positive serologic or peripheral blood PCR test supports the diagnosis, although false-positive and -negative results occur with both tests.[96]

Although joint symptoms usually resolve within 2 weeks, persistent polyarticular arthritis may follow acute HPV-B19 infection in up to 20% of female patients and in some individuals may last up to several months, occasionally longer.[96,100] In such patients, joint erosions and objective evidence of synovial inflammation do not develop[96] and follow-up studies do not demonstrate long-term joint swelling or restricted range of motion consistent with true chronic arthritis.[103]

Rubella is another important cause of viral arthritis in adults, particularly in the developing world where childhood vaccination is not widespread. Joint inflammation may follow natural infection or immunization with live-attenuated vaccine. Arthritis is thought to occur by direct infection of joint synovial tissue rather than through immune mechanisms.[104] As with HPV-B19, the polyarthritis that is associated with rubella affects predominantly women and most frequently involves the small joints of the hands, less commonly the knees, wrists, and ankles.[105] Joint symptoms occur simultaneously or within a few days of the rash in 52% of adult female subjects with infection by wild-type virus and within 2 to 3 weeks in 14% of adults receiving rubella vaccine.[105] A placebo-controlled, randomized trial showed that 30% of seronegative adult women receiving rubella vaccine developed acute arthropathy after vaccination, as opposed to 20% of those receiving placebo, a significant difference.[106] Arthritis after rubella vaccination or natural infection may persist for several weeks, but chronic or recurring arthritis is unusual.[104]

In acute hepatitis B infections, arthritis may be seen during the febrile prodrome before the onset of jaundice and is often seen together with urticaria.[107] A symmetrical, polyarticular arthritis typically involves the hands and resolves with the onset of jaundice. In chronic essential mixed cryoglobulinemia induced by hepatitis B or C, arthralgias and fibromyalgia are described as occurring in approximately one third of patients, although frank arthritis is not usually observed.[108-110]

Both HIV-1 and human T-cell lymphotropic virus type I (HTLV-I) are retroviruses with the ability to cause arthritis or arthropathy.[95] Articular manifestations of HIV-1 are uncommon and include nonspecific arthralgia and oligoarticular arthritis.[111] In addition, a "painful articular syndrome" with joint pain lasting less than 24 hours has rarely been reported.[112] Humans infected with HTLV-I have been described with a chronic joint infection termed HTLV-I–associated arthropathy that closely resembles rheumatoid arthritis.[95,113]

Several alphaviruses cause arthritis in Africa, Asia, and Australia but are usually not seen outside their endemic regions.[114] These include Chikungunya, O'nyong-nyong, Mayaro, Sindbis, and Ross River viruses. Other viruses rarely associated with arthritis or arthropathies include mumps,[115] herpes simplex virus type 1,[116] cytomegalovirus,[117] varicella-zoster virus,[118] variola major-minor (smallpox), lymphocytic choriomeningitis, and possibly the human retrovirus HRV-5.[119]

CHRONIC INFECTIOUS ARTHRITIS

Chronic infectious arthritis consists of a constellation of monarticular or less commonly oligoarticular joint infections that are characterized by an insidious onset and indolent course, a paucity of symptoms, and progressive joint destruction that may result in considerable loss of articular function. Many of these infections arise with few symptoms and signs of joint inflammation other than subacute or chronic joint swelling, with or without effusion, and pain and stiffness during active range of motion. Although this form of infectious arthritis remains relatively uncommon compared with acute septic arthritis, it is a significant component of the differential diagnosis of subacute or chronic

joint inflammation. An increasing number of anecdotal reports indicate that it is an emerging problem in immunocompromised or chronically ill hosts. Noteworthy aspects of this entity include its ability to mimic other inflammatory joint disorders such as rheumatoid arthritis and its ability to arouse little clinical suspicion, resulting in considerable delays in diagnosis. Moreover, establishing a pathogen-specific diagnosis is difficult, and the response to treatment is slow and often incomplete. Inappropriate treatment, for example, systemic or intra-articular steroids for a tentative diagnosis of rheumatoid arthritis, is not uncommon and can further delay diagnosis or lead to more rapid or severe joint destruction. Subacute or chronic infectious arthritis is usually caused by mycobacteria or fungi and occasionally by bacteria, such as *B. burgdorferi* (Lyme disease),[47] *T. whipplei* (Whipple's disease),[46] *Treponema pallidum* (tertiary syphilis),[120] and *Nocardia*[121] (Table 98-5). Chronic arthritis caused by parasitic infection is rarely described with various helminths and filariae despite the large number of persons infected with these parasites each year.[122]

Fungal Arthritis

Fungal arthritis may sometimes occur in healthy hosts; however, in immunocompromised or chronically ill persons a steadily increasing frequency of infection and diversity of infecting mycotic pathogens are apparent.[123] Although there is some overlap between the two groups, the most common fungal pathogens isolated from infectious arthritis in healthy hosts residing in endemic regions for the dimorphic fungi are *Blastomyces dermatitidis*, *Coccidioides* spp., *Paracoccidioides brasiliensis*, and *Sporothrix schenckii*, whereas in immunocompromised hosts *Candida* spp., *Cryptococcus*, and *Aspergillus*, are more often observed.[124] Joint infection in these cases usually results from hematogenous dissemination of the organism and, except for *Candida*, has as its source a symptomatic or subclinical pneumonitis. Fungal arthritis caused by *Fusarium* spp., *Curvularia* spp., *Trichosporon asahii*, *Scedosporium prolificans*, and *Pseudallescheria boydii* may be seen in either immunocompetent or immunocompromised patients. In the noncompromised host, infection is typically introduced into the joint by direct trauma or injury, sometimes associated with a penetrating foreign body.[123,125,126] In the immunocompromised host, either penetrating injury or hematogenous spread may infect the joint.

Candida arthritis afflicts both native and prosthetic joints and has been increasing in frequency over the past two decades paralleling the rising incidence of systemic and focal infections due to this organism in hospitalized and chronically ill patients.[127] Risk factors for candidal joint infection with this organism include loss of skin integrity, diabetes, malignancy, malnutrition, premature birth, intravenous drug use, immunosuppressive therapy including glucocorticoids; and the prolonged use of broad-spectrum antimicrobials, hyperalimentation fluid, and central intravenous catheters.[127] In most cases, articular infection occurs through the hematogenous route, with normal joints typically infected in a monarticular or pauciarticular pattern; but infection can occur by direct inoculation of the joint through surgery or corticosteroid injection, particularly in arthritic or surgically altered

TABLE 98-5 Infectious Causes of Chronic Monarticular or Oligoarticular Arthritis

Bacterial	Mycobacteria
Borrelia burgdorferi	M. tuberculosis
Tropheryma whipplei	M. kansasii
Treponema pallidum	M. marinum
Nocardia sp.	M. avium-intracellulare complex
Fungi	M. terrae
Candida sp.	M. fortuitum, M. chelonae, M. abscessus
Cryptococcus neoformans	M. haemophilum
Blastomyces dermatitidis	M. leprae
Coccidioides spp.	
Paracoccidioides brasiliensis	**Parasites**
Sporothrix schenckii	Helminths
Aspergillus sp.	Filariae
Pseudallescheria, Fusarium	

joints.[128] *Candida albicans* is the most commonly isolated species, followed by *Candida tropicalis*, *Candida parapsilosis*, *Candida guilliermondii*, and *Candida glabrata*.[127-130] As in bacterial arthritis, the knee is affected in the majority of cases.[127] In intravenous drug abusers, fibrocartilaginous joints including the sternoclavicular, sacroiliac, and costochondral joints may be involved. Prosthetic joint infections with *Candida* may occur immediately after surgery but are often delayed by months or years.[131]

Candida arthritis may arise acutely with complaints of marked joint inflammation and associated fever and constitutional symptoms, especially in cases in which it is accompanied by systemic candidiasis, or more insidiously with chronic, indolent joint pain and stiffness and minimal systemic manifestations.[128] Synovial fluid analysis characteristically shows polymorphonuclear leukocytosis with cell counts above 50,000 cells/mm³ and low measured glucose. Gram staining of synovial fluid is not usually diagnostic, although bacterial or fungal culture yields *Candida* spp. in most cases. In cases of hematogenous *Candida* arthritis, extra-articular cultures including urine, oropharynx, or sputum are often positive for *Candida* spp., suggesting widespread colonization of the patient.[128] Blood cultures are diagnostic in 50% or less of patients.

Cryptococcus neoformans causes skeletal infections in less than 10% of patients with disseminated infection with this organism.[132] Cryptococcal arthritis is considerably less common than cryptococcal osteomyelitis, and the latter is frequently the nidus of infection for the former with local contiguous spread.[133] The majority of patients with joint infection with this organism are immunocompromised because of various conditions, including the acquired immunodeficiency syndrome (AIDS).[134] The presentation of cryptococcal arthritis and associated osteomyelitis is that of a chronic joint infection. A serum cryptococcal antigen test may be positive.[133] Diagnosis requires joint aspiration or synovial biopsy with appropriate synovial fluid or tissue fungal cultures.

Acute infection with *Coccidioides immitis* occurs in the southwestern region of the United States, northern Mexico, and a few regions of Central America and South America, causing a symptomatic or subclinical primary pneumonitis. Migratory polyarthralgias and polyarticular arthritis occur in approximately one third of these patients, manifesting as a self-limited hypersensitivity syndrome termed "desert rheumatism" or "valley fever."[123] In about 1% of persons with coccidioidomycosis dissemination occurs, and although any host may be afflicted, it is more likely in men, pregnant females, blacks, Filipinos, and immunocompromised persons.[135] Skeletal involvement occurs in 10% to 50% of such cases and results in a chronic granulomatous infection of bones, joints, and periarticular tissues.[124] Joint infection may be primary or secondary to extension from contiguous osteomyelitis. Weight-bearing joints, particularly the knees, are most frequently affected, but any joint may be involved.[124,136] Presentation is that of subacute or chronic mon- or polyarticular arthritis with effusion.[137] Synovial fluid leukocyte counts are moderately elevated with a lymphocytic predominance. Coccidioidal arthritis should be considered in patients presenting with chronic progressive arthritis in endemic areas. Diagnosis is suggested by an elevated titer against coccidioidal antigens on serologic testing of serum and confirmed by fungal culture of synovial fluid or histopathologic examination and culture of synovial or periarticular tissues.

Like coccidioidomycosis, blastomycosis and histoplasmosis are primarily pulmonary infections that may later disseminate, potentially involving the bones and joints. Skeletal infection caused by *B. dermatitidis* occurs in about one fourth of patients with disseminated infection, and joint infection in most cases is associated with juxta-articular osteomyelitis.[138] Monoarticular arthritis of the knee is most common, followed by the ankle, elbow, wrist, and hand.[123] An acute arthritis with abrupt onset and a more chronic joint infection are both described.[139] Concomitant blastomycotic pneumonia and skin lesions are frequently evident on examination, and periarticular draining sinus tracts are occasionally seen.[123] Synovial fluid is purulent and organ-

isms are readily demonstrated on cytologic examination or microscopic examination of a wet mount (see Chapter 15).[140] Cultures of synovial fluid or other affected locations usually confirm the diagnosis. *Histoplasma capsulatum* is an extremely rare cause of fungal arthritis in endemic areas and is usually associated with immunosuppression. A chronic monarticular arthritis of native and prosthetic knee joints has been described.[141,142] In addition, a hypersensitivity syndrome may accompany *Histoplasma* primary infection that is similar to that in coccidioidomycosis.[143,144]

Sporotrichosis is a chronic infection caused by *S. schenckii* that primarily affects the skin and secondarily the lymphatics after percutaneous inoculation by a contaminated foreign body that is often composed of plant or soil material. In contrast to the other endemic mycoses, primary pulmonary infection is uncommon. Osteoarticular sporotrichosis rarely originates in the skin, but occasionally hematogenous spread to the skin occurs at the same time. The portal of entry is usually not apparent. Only 0.3% of patients develop arthritis as a complication of infection.[145] Immunocompromised patients (including those with AIDS), patients with diabetes, and alcoholic patients are at higher risk for disseminated infection and arthritis caused by *S. schenckii*,[146-148] and the typical patient is a male involved in gardening, farming, or an outdoor occupation.[149,150] Chronic monoarticular or polyarticular arthritis arises in the knees, hands, and wrists, and a tenosynovitis has also been reported.[150,151] Symptoms and signs are more prominent in the small joints of the wrist and ankle. Fever is uncommon, and there are usually no other focal symptoms or signs of infection, including pulmonary or cutaneous, before or during the course of sporotrichal arthritis.[148,150] Diagnosis is difficult as organisms are rarely found on histologic examination of joint fluid or tissue and fungal cultures of these specimens are often negative. Repeated aspiration and biopsy of affected joints are frequently necessary. As a result, extremely long diagnostic delays and permanent joint sequelae are common.[152]

Treatment

A combined approach to therapy for fungal arthritis utilizing medical and surgical modalities is necessary for optimal results. Open or arthroscopic débridement and drainage should be performed, at which time tissue and fluid specimens can be obtained for histopathologic and microbiologic testing if diagnostic uncertainty remains. Fungal prosthetic joint infections almost always require resection arthroplasty for eradication of infection.

In the past, most of the clinical experience with therapy for fungal arthritis was with amphotericin B, with or without the addition of flucytosine. Azole antifungals have expanded the therapeutic options available for selected fungal pathogens, and lipid preparations of amphotericin B have modestly reduced the toxicity of this drug, increasing the safety of long-term therapy. Treatment recommendations for native joint *Candida* arthritis are for amphotericin B deoxycholate (0.5 to 1 mg/kg/day) for 2 to 3 weeks followed by fluconazole to complete a total duration of therapy of 6 to 12 months.[153] Limited experience suggests that fluconazole as initial therapy (6 mg/kg/day) and continued for 6 to 12 months may also be effective for joint infections with susceptible *Candida* spp. Fluconazole, if used, may be given orally. Although not licensed for this indication, the echinocandin caspofungin may be an option for *Candida* spp. isolates that are resistant to azole drugs in patients who are intolerant of amphotericin B preparations. For cryptococcal arthritis, the choice of treatment depends on the extent of disseminated disease and the immune status of the patient. In general, initial therapy with an amphotericin B preparation followed by oral fluconazole is appropriate.[154] The preferred treatment of isolated joint infection without central nervous system involvement caused by the endemic mycoses, including *Coccidioides*, *Blastomyces*, *Histoplasma*, and *Sporothrix*, is with itraconazole (200 to 400 mg/day) for 12 months.[155-158] Available evidence suggests that for these pathogens therapy with itraconazole is equivalent to that with amphotericin B. The new azole antifungal voriconazole has not been studied in fungal musculoskeletal infections, and clinical experience with this drug for these infections is limited. Because of its enhanced activity against *Aspergillus*, *Pseudallescheria*, and *Fusarium*, voriconazole may have a future role in treatment of bone and joint infections with these pathogens.

Mycobacterial Arthritis

Worldwide, approximately 10% to 11% of extrapulmonary tuberculosis (TB) involves the bone and joints, accounting for 1% to 3% of all TB cases.[159] The incidence is higher in the developing world and is increasing because of the escalating prevalence of HIV disease. In endemic regions of the developing world, TB arthritis is mostly a disease of children and young adults, whereas in other regions older adults and immunocompromised hosts are predominately afflicted. Risk factors for TB arthritis include lower socioeconomic class, incarceration, alcohol abuse, debilitating illness, intravenous drug use, immunosuppressive drug therapy (including corticosteroids), HIV infection, and preexisting joint disease.[159] A study of patients with TB in the United States found women, non-Hispanic blacks, and HIV-infected individuals to be at higher risk for extrapulmonary disease.[160]

Mycobacterium tuberculosis causes a chronic granulomatous monoarthritis that is usually a result of the hematogenous dissemination associated with primary pulmonary TB.[160] Articular infection may remain latent for long periods before clinical presentation. It typically involves the knee, hip, and ankle but can involve any joint.[161] The clinical presentation is that of chronic arthritis, indistinguishable from that with other potential infectious or noninfectious causes. Long-standing cases may develop an articular-cutaneous fistula, whereas TB arthritis of the wrist may involve the periarticular tendon sheaths and arise with a carpal tunnel syndrome.[161,162] Coexisting pulmonary or other extra-articular infection may be evident, but in more than half of cases it is not.[161] Fever and other constitutional symptoms of TB are often absent. Tuberculin skin testing is positive in 90% of patients.[163]

In order to prevent unacceptable delays in diagnosis and further joint destruction, a high index of suspicion for TB arthritis must be maintained, particularly for patients with risk factors for TB or a remote or currently positive tuberculin skin test, or both. In the absence of known extra-articular TB, diagnosis requires synovial fluid analysis and in most cases synovial biopsy. Synovial fluid demonstrates inflammatory changes with leukocyte counts characteristically between 10,000 and 20,000 cells/mm³, although higher counts in the range seen with bacterial arthritis may be present.[161] Staining of synovial fluid demonstrates acid-fast bacilli in a minority of joint aspirates; however, mycobacterial culture yields *M. tuberculosis* 80% of the time. The most sensitive means of confirming the diagnosis is synovial biopsy, in which the characteristic histopathology of caseating or noncaseating granulomas can be correlated with tissue mycobacterial staining and culture, the latter being positive in about 90% of specimens.[161] Mycobacterial susceptibility tests should be performed on all culture isolates. Direct amplification testing of synovial fluid for *M. tuberculosis* by PCR is a potentially promising technique for the rapid diagnosis of tuberculous arthritis; however, the performance of currently available commercial tests for this purpose is still under investigation (see Chapter 15).[164]

Current recommendations from the Centers for Disease Control and Prevention for the treatment of skeletal TB in adults without pulmonary TB are identical to those for extrapulmonary TB (including patients with HIV or other immunosuppressive states): isoniazid, rifampin, ethambutol, and pyrazinamide for 8 weeks (ethambutol may be discontinued for isolates known to be without drug resistance), followed by isoniazid and rifampin to complete 6 months of therapy (see Chapter 248).[165] Directly observed therapy is advisable for most patients. If the condition is treated early, residual joint disease is uncommon and negligible. Adjuvant surgical therapy is required only for reconstruction of unstable joints or osseous structures or drainage of periarticular abscesses.

Nontuberculous mycobacterial arthritis, unlike that caused by *M. tuberculosis*, is usually due to direct percutaneous inoculation of these opportunistic mycobacteria into the skin, joint, or periarticular structures. Soil and water are the usual sources of these uncommon joint infections. *Mycobacterium avium-intracellulare*, *Mycobacterium kansasii*, *Mycobacterium marinum*, and *Mycobacterium terrae* are the most common causes, although virtually any atypical mycobacteria may be involved.[166] Skeletal infections with the so-called rapid growers *Mycobacterium chelonae*, *Mycobacterium fortuitum*, and *Mycobacterium abscessus* may follow trauma, surgery, or rarely joint injection.[166-169] Occasional atypical mycobacterial joint infection is acquired through the hematogenous route, usually in immunocompromised hosts, and has been reported with *M. avium-intracellulare*, *Mycobacterium haemophilum*, *M. kansasii*, and *M. chelonei* (see Chapters 250 and 251).[170]

Chronic monarticular arthritis and tenosynovitis of the hands caused by nontuberculous mycobacteria are well described.[166] *M. marinum* arthritis most often affects the small joints of the hand or wrist and their overlying tendon sheaths.[171] Infection is acquired from preexisting or concomitant skin trauma, often minor; contact with fresh, brackish, or salt water; or marine animals such as fish and crustaceans. Diagnosis of atypical mycobacterial joint or tendon infections usually requires biopsy of infected structures for histopathologic examination and culture. If *M. marinum* is suspected, cultures should be incubated at 30° C in addition to 37° C to facilitate growth of this organism. Treatment varies depending on the identity of the isolated mycobacteria. Susceptibility testing can be performed in reference laboratories and is useful in directing therapy for some of these organisms.

Mycobacterium leprae has also rarely been associated with an inflammatory arthritis that often arises in conjunction with erythema nodosa leprosum (type 2 lepra reaction) (see Chapter 249).[122] This systemic reaction is caused by circulating immune complexes and in its most severe form arises with diffuse soft tissue, eye, ear, and nerve swelling with acute polyarthritis, particularly of the hands, wrists, and ankles. In addition, advanced Hansen's disease may be associated with chronic neuropathic (Charcot) arthritis of the peripheral joints.

SEPTIC BURSITIS

Septic bursitis is common, usually affecting the subcutaneous olecranon or prepatellar bursae. Bacteria are most often introduced through trauma or accidental percutaneous punctures and rarely through intrabursal injection of corticosteroids.[172,173] Infection of deep bursae is rare and is usually secondary to contiguous spread from an adjacent joint infection. More than 80% of septic bursitis is due to *S. aureus*, with the remainder due to *Streptococcus* spp. and various gram-negative bacteria, mycobacteria, and fungi.[172] Olecranon septic bursitis caused by the algal agent *Prototheca* has been reported.[174] Patients with olecranon or prepatellar bacterial bursitis present with painful swelling, redness, and increased warmth of the affected bursae. Evidence of an overlying cutaneous injury or lesion is often present. In moderate or severe cases, pain may be extreme and the range of motion of the underlying joint reduced. Soft tissue edema and erythema may extend along the extremity and circumferentially about the joint. Associated systemic symptoms potentially include fever, chills, and malaise.

The diagnosis of septic bursitis is made by aspirating the affected bursae and analyzing the fluid for white blood cell count and crystals. Gram staining and culture should also be performed. The differential diagnosis includes gout, acute arthritis, and traumatic and rheumatic bursitis. To distinguish septic olecranon bursitis from acute arthritis of the elbow, it is helpful to evaluate whether pain is worsened by elbow extension or flexion. Bursal pressures are increased in the latter case. Thus, for patients with septic bursitis, elbow pain is increased with joint flexion, whereas for patients with septic arthritis, synovial pressures are increased during elbow joint extension and pain is greatest in this position.[172]

Treatment for septic bursitis includes antibiotics and daily aspiration of the bursae until sterile fluid is obtained. Oral antimicrobials with antistaphylococcal activity are initially indicated for mild cases afflicting healthy patients with good access to medical care. For more severe cases or patients with chronic illness or immunosuppression, intravenous antimicrobials should be selected that are active against organisms identified on bursal fluid Gram staining. In both cases, definitive antibiotic therapy should be selected on the basis of the identity and susceptibilities of cultured bacteria and continued to complete a 14- to 21-day course. The prognosis of prepatellar or olecranon septic bursitis is generally quite good, although recurrences are common and may require bursectomy when infection is quiescent.

REFERENCES

1. Cooper C, Cawley MI. Bacterial arthritis in an English health district: A 10 year review. Ann Rheum Dis. 1986;45:458-463.
2. Kaandorp CJ, van Schaardenburg D, Krijnen P, et al. Risk factors for septic arthritis in patients with joint disease. A prospective study. Arthritis Rheum. 1995;38:1819-1825.
3. Kaandorp CJ, Dinant HJ, van de Laar MA, et al. Incidence and sources of native and prosthetic joint infection: A community based prospective survey. Ann Rheum Dis. 1997;56:470-475.
4. Morgan DS, Fisher D, Merianos A, Currie BJ. An 18 year clinical review of septic arthritis from tropical Australia. Epidemiol Infect. 1996;117:423-428.
5. Gupta MN, Sturrock RD, Field M. A prospective 2-year study of 75 patients with adult-onset septic arthritis. Rheumatology (Oxford). 2001;40:24-30.
6. Nolla JM, Gomez-Vaquero C, Fiter J, et al. Pyarthrosis in patients with rheumatoid arthritis: A detailed analysis of 10 cases and literature review. Semin Arthritis Rheum. 2000;30:121-126.
7. Weston VC, Jones AC, Bradbury N, et al. Clinical features and outcome of septic arthritis in a single UK Health District 1982-1991. Ann Rheum Dis. 1999;58:214-219.
8. Goldenberg DL, Reed JI. Bacterial arthritis. N Engl J Med. 1985;312:764-771.
9. Kaandorp CJE, Krijnen P, Moens HJB, et al. The outcome of bacterial arthritis: A prospective community-based study. Arthritis Rheum. 1997;40:884-892.
10. Garcia-De La Torre I. Advances in the management of septic arthritis. Rheum Dis Clin North Am. 2003;29:61-75.
11. Shirtliff ME, Mader JT. Acute septic arthritis. Clin Microbiol Rev. 2002;15:527-544.
12. Armstrong RW, Bolding F. Septic arthritis after arthroscopy: The contributing roles of intraarticular steroids and environmental factors. Am J Infect Control. 1994;22:16-18.
13. Karchmer T, Song X, Perl T. Risk factors (RF) for developing septic arthritis following arthroscopic knee surgery. Presented at the Society for Health Care Epidemiology of America, Toronto, April 2, 2001.
14. Septic arthritis following anterior cruciate ligament reconstruction using tendon allografts-Florida and Louisiana, 2000. MMWR Morb Mortal Wkly Rep. 2001;50:1081-1083.
15. Update: allograft-associated bacterial infections—United States, 2002. MMWR Morb Mortal Wkly Rep. 2002;51:207-210.
16. Matava MJ, Evans TA, Wright RW, Shively RA. Septic arthritis of the knee following anterior cruciate ligament reconstruction: Results of a survey of sports medicine fellowship directors. Arthroscopy. 1998;14:717-725.
17. Vassilopoulos D, Chalasani P, Jurado RL, et al. Musculoskeletal infections in patients with human immunodeficiency virus infection. Medicine (Baltimore). 1997;76:284-294.
18. Fischer B, Vaudaux P, Magnin M, et al. Novel animal model for studying the molecular mechanisms of bacterial adhesion to bone-implanted metallic devices: Role of fibronectin in Staphylococcus aureus adhesion. J Orthop Res. 1996;14:914-920.
19. Ryden C, Tung HS, Nikolaev V, et al. Staphylococcus aureus causing osteomyelitis binds to a nonapeptide sequence in bone sialoprotein. Biochem J. 1997;327:825-829.
20. Jonsson K, Signas C, Muller HP, Lindberg M. Two different genes encode fibronectin binding proteins in Staphylococcus aureus. The complete nucleotide sequence and characterization of the second gene. Eur J Biochem. 1991;202:1041-1048.
21. Park PW, Rosenbloom J, Abrams WR, et al. Molecular cloning and expression of the gene for elastin-binding protein (ebpS) in Staphylococcus aureus. J Biol Chem. 1996;271:15803-15809.
22. Switalski LM, Patti JM, Butcher W, et al. A collagen receptor on Staphylococcus aureus strains isolated from patients with septic arthritis mediates adhesion to cartilage. Mol Microbiol. 1993;7:99-107.
23. Mader JT, Shirtliff M, Calhoun JH. The host and the skeletal infection: Classification and pathogenesis of acute bacterial bone and joint sepsis. Baillieres Best Pract Res Clin Rheumatol. 1999;13:1-20.
24. Goldenberg DL, Chisholm PL, Rice PA. Experimental models of bacterial arthritis: A microbiologic and histopathological characterization of the arthritis after the intraarticular injections of Neisseria gonorrhoeae, Staphylococcus aureus, group A streptococci, and Escherichia coli. J Rheumatol. 1983;10:5-11.
25. Roy S, Bhawan J. Ultrastructure of articular cartilage in pyogenic arthritis. Arch Pathol. 1975;99:44-47.
26. Gardner GC, Weisman MH. Pyarthrosis in patients with rheumatoid arthritis: A report of 13 cases and a review of the literature from the past 40 years. Am J Med. 1990;88:503-511.
27. Rosenthal J, Bole GG, Robinson WD. Acute nongonococcal infectious arthritis. Evaluation of risk factors, therapy, and outcome. Arthritis Rheum. 1980;23:889-897.
28. Dubost JJ, Soubrier M, De Champs C, et al. No changes in the distribution of organisms responsible for septic arthritis over a 20 year period. Ann Rheum Dis. 2002;61:267-269.
29. Ross JJ, Saltzman CL, Carling P, Shapiro DS. Pneumococcal septic arthritis: Review of 190 cases. Clin Infect Dis. 2003;36:319-327.
30. Ryan MJ, Kavanagh R, Wall PG, Hazleman BL. Bacterial joint infections in England and Wales: Analysis of bacterial isolates over a four year period. Br J Rheumatol. 1997;36:370-373.
31. Goldenberg DL. Infectious arthritis complicating rheumatoid arthritis and other chronic rheumatic disorders. Arthritis Rheum. 1989;32:496-502.
32. Ang-Fonte GZ, Rozboril MB, Thompson GR. Changes in nongonococcal septic arthritis: Drug abuse and methicillin-resistant Staphylococcus aureus. Arthritis Rheum. 1985;28:210-213.
33. Byrne PA, Hosein IK, Camilleri J. Methicillin-resistant Staphylococcus aureus septic arthritis: Urgent and emergent. Clin Rheumatol. 1998;17:407-408.
34. Huang SS, Platt R. Risk of methicillin-resistant Staphylococcus aureus infection after previous infection or colonization. Clin Infect Dis. 2003;36:281-285.
35. Kallarackal G, Lawson TM, Williams BD. Community-acquired septic arthritis due to methicillin-resistant Staphylococcus aureus. Rheumatology (Oxford). 2000;39:1304-1305.
36. Stott NS. Review article: Paediatric bone and joint infection. J Orthop Surg (Hong Kong). 2001;9:83-90.
37. Schattner A, Vosti KL. Bacterial arthritis due to beta-hemolytic streptococci of serogroups A, B, C, F, and G. Analysis of 23 cases and a review of the literature. Medicine (Baltimore). 1998;77:122-139.
38. Ohl C, Pollack M. Pseudomonas aeruginosa and related bacteria. In: Gorbach SL, Bartlett JG, Blacklow NR, eds. Infectious Diseases. Philadelphia: Lippincott Williams & Wilkins; 2004:1703-1707.
39. Ross JJ, Hu LT. Septic arthritis of the pubic symphysis: Review of 100 cases. Medicine (Baltimore). 2003;82:340-345.
40. Bowerman SG, Green NE, Mencio GA. Decline of bone and joint infections attributable to Haemophilus influenzae type b. Clin Orthop. 1997;August:128-133.
41. Yagupsky P, Dagan R. Kingella kingae: An emerging cause of invasive infections in young children. Clin Infect Dis. 1997;24:860-866.
42. Ewing R, Fainstein V, Musher DM, et al. Articular and skeletal infections caused by Pasteurella multocida. South Med J. 1980;73:1349-1352.
43. Murray PM. Septic arthritis of the hand and wrist. Hand Clin. 1998;14:579-587, viii.
44. Resnick D, Pineda CJ, Weisman MH, Kerr R. Osteomyelitis and septic arthritis of the hand following human bites. Skeletal Radiol. 1985;14:263-266.
45. Thong BY, Barkham TM. Suppurative polyarthritis following a rat bite. Ann Rheum Dis. 2003;62:805-806.
46. Puechal X. Whipple disease and arthritis. Curr Opin Rheumatol. 2001;13:74-79.
47. Steere AC. Diagnosis and treatment of Lyme arthritis. Med Clin North Am. 1997;81:179-194.
48. Dubost JJ, Soubrier M, Sauvezie B. Pyogenic arthritis in adults. Joint Bone Spine. 2000;67:11-21.
49. Goldenberg DL. Septic arthritis. Lancet. 1998;351:197-202.
50. Smith JW, Hasan M. Infectious arthritis. In: Mandell G, Bennett J, Dolin R, eds. Principles and Practice of Infectious Diseases. Philadelphia: Churchill Livingstone; 2000:1175-1182.
51. Ledermann HP, Morrison WB, Schweitzer ME. MR image analysis of pedal osteomyelitis: Distribution, patterns of spread, and frequency of associated ulceration and septic arthritis. Radiology. 2002;223:747-755.
52. Aglas F, Gretler J, Rainer F, Krejs GJ. Sternoclavicular septic arthritis: A rare but serious complication of subclavian venous catheterization. Clin Rheumatol. 1994;13:507-512.
53. Brancos MA, Peris P, Miro JM, et al. Septic arthritis in heroin addicts. Semin Arthritis Rheum. 1991;21:81-87.
54. Dubost JJ, Fis I, Denis P, et al. Polyarticular septic arthritis. Medicine (Baltimore). 1993;72:296-310.
55. Vyskocil JJ, McIlroy MA, Brennan TA, Wilson FM. Pyogenic infection of the sacroiliac joint. Case reports and review of the literature. Medicine (Baltimore). 1991;70:188-197.
56. Cooper C, Cawley MI. Bacterial arthritis in the elderly. Gerontology 1986;32:222-227.
57. Nade S. Septic arthritis. Best Pract Res Clin Rheumatol. 2003;17:183-200.
58. Hughes JG, Vetter EA, Patel R, et al. Culture with BACTEC Peds Plus/F bottle compared with conventional methods for detection of bacteria in synovial fluid. J Clin Microbiol. 2001;39:4468-4471.
59. von Essen R. Culture of joint specimens in bacterial arthritis. Impact of blood culture bottle utilization. Scand J Rheumatol. 1997;26:293-300.
60. Kortekangas P, Aro HT, Lehtonen OP. Synovial fluid culture and blood culture in acute arthritis. A multi-case report of 90 patients. Scand J Rheumatol. 1995;24:44-47.
61. Greenspan A, Tehranzadeh J. Imaging of infectious arthritis. Radiol Clin North Am. 2001;39:267-276.
62. Chhem RK, Kaplan PA, Dussault RG. Ultrasonography of the musculoskeletal system. Radiol Clin North Am. 1994;32:275-289.
63. Akkasilpa S, Osiri M, Ukritchon S, et al. Clinical features of septic arthritis of sternoclavicular joint. J Med Assoc Thai. 2001;84:63-68.
64. Coan MR, Demos TC, Lomasney L, Pangan A. Radiologic case study. Pyogenic left sacroiliac infection. Orthopedics. 2002;25:122, 197-200.
65. Learch TJ, Farooki S. Magnetic resonance imaging of septic arthritis. Clin Imaging. 2000;24:236-242.

66. Bardin T. Gonococcal arthritis. Best Pract Res Clin Rheumatol. 2003;17:201-208.
67. Cucurull E, Espinoza LR. Gonococcal arthritis. Rheum Dis Clin North Am. 1998;24:305-322.
68. O'Brien JP, Goldenberg DL, Rice PA. Disseminated gonococcal infection: A prospective analysis of 49 patients and a review of pathophysiology and immune mechanisms. Medicine (Baltimore). 1983;62:395-406.
69. Britigan BE, Cohen MS, Sparling PF. Gonococcal infection: A model of molecular pathogenesis. N Engl J Med. 1985;312:1683-1694.
70. Centers for Disease Control and Prevention. Sexually Transmitted Disease Surveillance, 2002. Atlanta: U.S. Department of Health and Human Services, Centers for Disease Control and Prevention; September 2003.
71. Masi AT, Eisenstein BI. Disseminated gonococcal infection (DGI) and gonococcal arthritis (GCA): II. Clinical manifestations, diagnosis, complications, treatment, and prevention. Semin Arthritis Rheum. 1981;10:173-197.
72. Zbella EA, Deppe G, Elrad H. Gonococcal arthritis in pregnancy. Obstet Gynecol Surv. 1984;39:8-12.
73. Joiner KA, Warren KA, Brown EJ, et al. Studies on the mechanism of bacterial resistance to complement-mediated killing. IV. C5b-9 forms high molecular weight complexes with bacterial outer membrane constituents on serum-resistant but not on serum-sensitive Neisseria gonorrhoeae. J Immunol. 1983;131:1443-1451.
74. Petersen BH, Lee TJ, Snyderman R, Brooks GF. Neisseria meningitidis and Neisseria gonorrhoeae bacteremia associated with C6, C7, or C8 deficiency. Ann Intern Med. 1979;90:917-920.
75. Wise CM, Morris CR, Wasilauskas BL, Salzer WL. Gonococcal arthritis in an era of increasing penicillin resistance. Presentations and outcomes in 41 recent cases (1985-1991). Arch Intern Med. 1994;154:2690-2695.
76. Goldenberg DL, Sexton DJ. Disseminated gonococcal infection. UpToDate. 2003. Available at www.uptodate.com.
77. Blake M, Swanson J. Studies on gonococcus infection. IX. In vitro decreased association of pilated gonococci with mouse peritoneal macrophages. Infect Immun. 1975;11:1402-1404.
78. Ram S, Mackinnon FG, Gulati S, et al. The contrasting mechanisms of serum resistance of Neisseria gonorrhoeae and group B Neisseria meningitidis. Mol Immunol. 1999;36:915-928.
79. Vogel U, Frosch M. Mechanisms of neisserial serum resistance. Mol Microbiol. 1999;32:1133-1139.
80. Goldenberg DL, Reed JI, Rice PA. Arthritis in rabbits induced by killed Neisseria gonorrhoeae and gonococcal lipopolysaccharide. J Rheumatol. 1984;11:3-8.
81. Wetzler LM, Barry K, Blake MS, Gotschlich EC. Gonococcal lipooligosaccharide sialylation prevents complement-dependent killing by immune sera. Infect Immun. 1992;60:39-43.
82. Centers for Disease Control and Prevention. Sexually transmitted diseases treatment guidelines 2002. MMWR Morb Mortal Wkly Rep. 2003;51:36-39.
83. Scopelitis E, Martinez-Osuna P. Gonococcal arthritis. Rheum Dis Clin North Am. 1993;19:363-377.
84. Brogadir SP, Schimmer BM, Myers AR. Spectrum of the gonococcal arthritis-dermatitis syndrome. Semin Arthritis Rheum. 1979;8:177-183.
85. Lee AH, Chin AE, Ramanujam T, et al. Gonococcal septic arthritis of the hip. J Rheumatol. 1991;18:1932-1933.
86. Li F, Bulbul R, Schumacher HR Jr, et al. Molecular detection of bacterial DNA in venereal-associated arthritis. Arthritis Rheum. 1996;39:950-958.
87. Muralidhar B, Rumore PM, Steinman CR. Use of the polymerase chain reaction to study arthritis due to Neisseria gonorrhoeae. Arthritis Rheum. 1994;37:710-717.
88. Liebling MR, Arkfeld DG, Michelini GA, et al. Identification of Neisseria gonorrhoeae in synovial fluid using the polymerase chain reaction. Arthritis Rheum. 1994;37:702-709.
89. Gelfand SG, Masi AT, Garcia-Kutzbach A. Spectrum of gonococcal arthritis: Evidence for sequential stages and clinical subgroups. J Rheumatol. 1975;2:83-90.
90. Van Der Pol B, Ferrero DV, Buck-Barrington L, et al. Multicenter evaluation of the BDProbeTec ET System for detection of Chlamydia trachomatis and Neisseria gonorrhoeae in urine specimens, female endocervical swabs, and male urethral swabs. J Clin Microbiol. 2001;39:1008-1016.
91. Louie JS, Liebling MR. The polymerase chain reaction in infectious and post-infectious arthritis. A review. Rheum Dis Clin North Am. 1998;24:227-236.
92. Donatto KC. Orthopedic management of septic arthritis. Rheum Dis Clin North Am. 1998;24:275-286.
93. Stengel D, Bauwens K, Sehouli J, et al. Systematic review and meta-analysis of antibiotic therapy for bone and joint infections. Lancet Infect Dis. 2001;1:175-188.
94. Odio CM, Ramirez T, Arias G, et al. Double blind, randomized, placebo-controlled study of dexamethasone therapy for hematogenous septic arthritis in children. Pediatr Infect Dis J. 2003;22:883-888.
95. Masuko-Hongo K, Kato T, Nishioka K. Virus-associated arthritis. Best Pract Res Clin Rheumatol. 2003;17:309-318.
96. Naides SJ. Rheumatic manifestations of parvovirus B19 infection. Rheum Dis Clin North Am. 1998;24:375-401.
97. Nocton JJ, Miller LC, Tucker LB, Schaller JG. Human parvovirus B19–associated arthritis in children. J Pediatr. 1993;122:186-190.
98. Anderson MJ, Higgins PG, Davis LR, et al. Experimental parvoviral infection in humans. J Infect Dis. 1985;152:257-265.
99. Torok TJ. Parvovirus B19 and human disease. Adv Intern Med. 1992;37:431-455.
100. Woolf AD, Campion GV, Chishick A, et al. Clinical manifestations of human parvovirus B19 in adults. Arch Intern Med. 1989;149:1153-1156.
101. Habib GS, Zisman D. Unusual cluster of parvovirus arthritis. Isr Med Assoc J. 2002;4:314.
102. Scroggie DA, Carpenter MT, Cooper RI, Higgs JB. Parvovirus arthropathy outbreak in southwestern United States. J Rheumatol. 2000;27:2444-2448.
103. Speyer I, Breedveld FC, Dijkmans BA. Human parvovirus B19 infection is not followed by inflammatory joint disease during long term follow-up. A retrospective study of 54 patients. Clin Exp Rheumatol. 1998;16:576-578.
104. Smith CA, Petty RE, Tingle AJ. Rubella virus and arthritis. Rheum Dis Clin North Am. 1987;13:265-274.
105. Tingle AJ, Allen M, Petty RE, et al. Rubella-associated arthritis. I. Comparative study of joint manifestations associated with natural rubella infection and RA 27/3 rubella immunisation. Ann Rheum Dis. 1986;45:110-114.
106. Tingle AJ, Mitchell LA, Grace M, et al. Randomised double-blind placebo-controlled study on adverse effects of rubella immunisation in seronegative women. Lancet. 1997;349:1277-1281.
107. Inman RD. Rheumatic manifestations of hepatitis B virus infection. Semin Arthritis Rheum. 1982;11:406-420.
108. Buskila D, Shnaider A, Neumann L, et al. Musculoskeletal manifestations and autoantibody profile in 90 hepatitis C virus infected Israeli patients. Semin Arthritis Rheum. 1998;28:107-113.
109. Cesur S, Akin K, Kurt H. The significance of cryoglobulinemia in patients with chronic hepatitis B and C virus infection. Hepatogastroenterology. 2003;50:1487-1489.
110. Vassilopoulos D, Calabrese LH. Rheumatic manifestations of hepatitis C infection. Curr Rheumatol Rep. 2003;5:200-204.
111. Mody GM, Parke FA, Reveille JD. Articular manifestations of human immunodeficiency virus infection. Best Pract Res Clin Rheumatol. 2003;17:265-287.
112. Pouchot J, Simonpoli AM, Bortolotti V, et al. Painful articular syndrome and human immunodeficiency virus infection. Arch Intern Med. 1992;152:646, 649.
113. Nishioka K, Nakajima T, Hasunuma T, Sato K. Rheumatic manifestation of human leukemia virus infection. Rheum Dis Clin North Am. 1993;19:489-503.
114. Smith JW, Piercy EA. Infectious arthritis. Clin Infect Dis. 1995;20:225-230.
115. Nussinovitch M, Volovitz B, Varsano I. Complications of mumps requiring hospitalization in children. Eur J Pediatr. 1995;154:732-734.
116. Brna JA, Hall RF Jr. Acute monoarticular herpetic arthritis. A case report. J Bone Joint Surg Am. 1984;66:623.
117. Burns LJ, Gingrich RD. Cytomegalovirus infection presenting as polyarticular arthritis following autologous BMT. Bone Marrow Transplant. 1993;11:77-79.
118. Evans E, Dawes PT, Mattey DL. An unusual case of adult varicella-associated arthritis. Rheumatology (Oxford). 2000;39:806-808.
119. Brand A, Griffiths DJ, Herve C, et al. Human retrovirus-5 in rheumatic diseases. J. Autoimmun. 1999;13:149-154.
120. Reginato AJ. Syphilitic arthritis and osteitis. Rheum Dis Clin North Am. 1993;19:379-398.
121. Koll BS, Brown AE, Kiehn TE, Armstrong D. Disseminated Nocardia brasiliensis infection with septic arthritis. Clin Infect Dis. 1992;15:469-472.
122. McGill PE. Geographically specific infections and arthritis, including rheumatic syndromes associated with certain fungi and parasites, Brucella species and Mycobacterium leprae. Best Pract Res Clin Rheumatol. 2003;17:289-307.
123. Cuellar ML, Silveira LH, Espinoza LR. Fungal arthritis. Ann Rheum Dis. 1992;51:690-697.
124. Cuellar ML, Silveira LH, Citera G, et al. Other fungal arthritides. Rheum Dis Clin North Am. 1993;19:439-455.
125. Hospenthal D, Bennett J. Miscellaneous fungi and prototheca. In: Mandell G, Bennett J, Dolin R, eds. Principles and Practice of Infectious Diseases. Philadelphia: Churchill Livingstone; 2000:2772-2780.
126. Dellestable F, Kures L, Mainard D, et al. Fungal arthritis due to Pseudallescheria boydii (Scedosporium apiospermum). J Rheumatol. 1994;21:766-768.
127. Silveira LH, Cuellar ML, Citera G, et al. Candida arthritis. Rheum Dis Clin North Am. 1993;19:427-437.
128. Cuende E, Barbadillo C, Mazzucchelli R, et al. Candida arthritis in adult patients who are not intravenous drug addicts: Report of three cases and review of the literature. Semin Arthritis Rheum. 1993;22:224-241.
129. Weems JJ Jr. Candida parapsilosis: Epidemiology, pathogenicity, clinical manifestations, and antimicrobial susceptibility. Clin Infect Dis. 1992;14:756-766.
130. Zmierczak H, Goemaere S, Mielants H, et al. Candida glabrata arthritis: Case report and review of the literature of Candida arthritis. Clin Rheumatol. 1999;18:406-409.
131. Lambertus M, Thordarson D, Goetz MB. Fungal prosthetic arthritis: Presentation of two cases and review of the literature. Rev Infect Dis. 1988;10:1038-1043.
132. Italiano A, Yen BC, Rosenthal SA, Rafii M. Cryptococcal osteomyelitis with septic arthritis. Orthopedics. 2001;24:59-60.
133. Stead KJ, Klugman KP, Painter ML, Koornhof HJ. Septic arthritis due to Cryptococcus neoformans. J Infect. 1988;17:139-145.
134. Behrman RE, Masci JR, Nicholas P. Cryptococcal skeletal infections: Case report and review. Rev Infect Dis. 1990;12:181-190.
135. Galgiani J. Coccidioides immitis. In: Mandell G, Bennett J, Dolin R, eds. Principles and Practice of Infectious Diseases. Philadelphia: Churchill Livingstone; 2000:2746-2757.
136. Kushwaha VP, Shaw BA, Gerardi JA, Oppenheim WL. Musculoskeletal coccidioidomycosis. A review of 25 cases. Clin Orthop. 1996;November:190-199.
137. Bayer AS, Guze LB. Fungal arthritis. II. Coccidioidal synovitis: Clinical, diagnostic, therapeutic, and prognostic considerations. Semin Arthritis Rheum. 1979;8:200-211.
138. MacDonald PB, Black GB, MacKenzie R. Orthopaedic manifestations of blastomycosis. J Bone Joint Surg Am. 1990;72:860-864.
139. Bayer AS, Scott VJ, Guze LB. Fungal arthritis. IV. Blastomycotic arthritis. Semin Arthritis Rheum. 1979;9:145-151.

140. George AL Jr, Hays JT, Graham BS. Blastomycosis presenting as monoarticular arthritis. The role of synovial fluid cytology. Arthritis Rheum. 1985;28:516-521.
141. Darouiche RO, Cadle RM, Zenon GJ, et al. Articular histoplasmosis. J Rheumatol. 1992;19:1991-1993.
142. Fowler VG Jr, Nacinovich FM, Alspaugh JA, Corey GR. Prosthetic joint infection due to *Histoplasma capsulatum*: Case report and review. Clin Infect Dis. 1998;26:1017.
143. Friedman SJ, Black JL, Duffy J. Histoplasmosis presenting as erythema multiforme and polyarthritis. Cutis. 1984;34:396-398.
144. Rosenthal J, Brandt KD, Wheat LJ, Slama TG. Rheumatologic manifestations of histoplasmosis in the recent Indianapolis epidemic. Arthritis Rheum. 1983;26:1065-1070.
145. Vismer HF, Hull PR. Prevalence, epidemiology and geographical distribution of *Sporothrix schenckii* infections in Gauteng, South Africa. Mycopathologia. 1997;137:137-143.
146. Gottlieb GS, Lesser CF, Holmes KK, Wald A. Disseminated sporotrichosis associated with treatment with immunosuppressants and tumor necrosis factor-alpha antagonists. Clin Infect Dis. 2003;37:838-840.
147. Heller HM, Fuhrer J. Disseminated sporotrichosis in patients with AIDS: Case report and review of the literature. AIDS. 1991;5:1243-1246.
148. Howell SJ, Toohey JS. Sporotrichal arthritis in south central Kansas. Clin Orthop. 1998;January:207-214.
149. Bayer AS, Scott VJ, Guze LB. Fungal arthritis. III. Sporotrichal arthritis. Semin Arthritis Rheum. 1979;9:66-74.
150. Chowdhary G, Weinstein A, Klein R, Mascarenhas BR. Sporotrichal arthritis. Ann Rheum Dis. 1991;50:112-114.
151. Jones N. Photo quiz: Osteoarticular sporotrichosis. Clin Infect Dis. 1999;29:59, 202-203.
152. Crout JE, Brewer NS, Tompkins RB. Sporotrichosis arthritis: Clinical features in seven patients. Ann Intern Med. 1977;86:294-297.
153. Pappas PG, Rex JH, Sobel JD, et al. Guidelines for treatment of candidiasis. Clin Infect Dis. 2004;38:161-189.
154. Saag MS, Graybill RJ, Larsen RA, et al. Practice guidelines for the management of cryptococcal disease. Infectious Diseases Society of America. Clin Infect Dis. 2000;30:710-718.
155. Chapman SW, Bradsher RW Jr, Campbell GD Jr, et al. Practice guidelines for the management of patients with blastomycosis. Infectious Diseases Society of America. Clin Infect Dis. 2000;30:679-683.
156. Galgiani JN, Ampel NM, Catanzaro A, et al. Practice guideline for the treatment of coccidioidomycosis. Infectious Diseases Society of America. Clin Infect Dis. 2000;30:658-661.
157. Kauffman CA, Hajjeh R, Chapman SW. Practice guidelines for the management of patients with sporotrichosis. For the Mycoses Study Group. Infectious Diseases Society of America. Clin Infect Dis. 2000;30:684-687.
158. Wheat J, Sarosi G, McKinsey D, et al. Practice guidelines for the management of patients with histoplasmosis. Infectious Diseases Society of America. Clin Infect Dis. 2000;30:688-695.
159. Malaviya AN, Kotwal PP. Arthritis associated with tuberculosis. Best Pract Res Clin Rheumatol. 2003;17:319-343.
160. Yang Z, Kong Y, Wilson F, et al. Identification of risk factors for extrapulmonary tuberculosis. Clin Infect Dis. 2004;38:199-205.
161. Garrido G, Gomez-Reino JJ, Fernandez-Dapica P, et al. A review of peripheral tuberculous arthritis. Semin Arthritis Rheum. 1988;18:142-149.
162. Klofkorn RW, Steigerwald JC. Carpal tunnel syndrome as the initial manifestation of tuberculosis. Am J Med. 1976;60:583-586.
163. Kramer N, Rosenstein ED. Rheumatologic manifestations of tuberculosis. Bull Rheum Dis. 1997;46:5-8.
164. Harrington JT. The evolving role of direct amplification tests in diagnosing osteoarticular infections caused by mycobacteria and fungi. Curr Opin Rheumatol. 1999;11:289-292.
165. Blumberg HM, Burman WJ, Chaisson RE, et al. American Thoracic Society/Centers for Disease Control and Prevention/Infectious Diseases Society of America: Treatment of tuberculosis. Am J Respir Crit Care Med. 2003;167:603-662.
166. Kozin SH, Bishop AT. Atypical *Mycobacterium* infections of the upper extremity. J Hand Surg [Am]. 1994;19:480-487.
167. Ip FK, Chow SP. *Mycobacterium fortuitum* infections of the hand. Report of five cases. J Hand Surg [Br]. 1992;17:675-677.
168. Wallace RJ Jr, Brown BA, Onyi GO. Skin, soft tissue, and bone infections due to *Mycobacterium chelonae chelonae*: Importance of prior corticosteroid therapy, frequency of disseminated infections, and resistance to oral antimicrobials other than clarithromycin. J Infect Dis. 1992;166:405-412.
169. Khermosh O, Weintroub S, Topilsky M, Baratz M. *Mycobacterium abscessus* (*M. chelonei*) infection of the knee joint: Report of two cases following intra-articular injection of corticosteroids. Clin Orthop. 1979;May:162-168.
170. Meier JL, Beekmann SE. Mycobacterial and fungal infections of bone and joints. Curr Opin Rheumatol. 1995;7:329-336.
171. Harth M, Ralph ED, Faraawi R. Septic arthritis due to *Mycobacterium marinum*. J Rheumatol. 1994;21:957-960.
172. Canoso JJ, Barza M. Soft tissue infections. Rheum Dis Clin North Am. 1993;19:293-309.
173. Weinstein PS, Canoso JJ, Wohlgethan JR. Long-term follow-up of corticosteroid injection for traumatic olecranon bursitis. Ann Rheum Dis. 1984;43:44-46.
174. de Montclos M, Chatte G, Perrin-Fayolle M, Flandrois JP. Olecranon bursitis due to *Prototheca wickerhamii*, an algal opportunistic pathogen. Eur J Clin Microbiol Infect Dis. 1995;14:561-562.

CHAPTER **99**

Osteomyelitis

ELIE F. BERBARI

JAMES M. STECKELBERG

DOUGLAS R. OSMON

CLASSIFICATION

Osteomyelitis is a heterogeneous disease in its pathophysiology, clinical presentation, and management. It is a disease of antiquity and is one of the most difficult to treat infectious diseases. Progressive destruction of the bone and the formation of sequestra are characteristics of this disease. Osteomyelitis can be due to contiguous spread from adjacent soft tissues and joints, hematogenous seeding, or direct inoculation of microorganism into the bone as a result of trauma or surgery. When established, bacteria produce a local inflammatory reaction that promotes bone necrosis and the formation of sequestra. *Staphylococcus aureus,* the most common microorganism recovered in osteomyelitis, preferentially causes this disease through the expression of receptors for fibronectin, laminin, collagen, or sialoglycoprotein present on the bone surface. The economic impact of osteomyelitis is tremendous. In a cohort study by Ramsey and colleagues[1] of 8905 patients with diabetes mellitus, 5.8% developed a foot ulcer during the study period, of which 15% developed osteomyelitis. In this study, the attributable cost for a man 40 to 65 years old with a new foot ulcer was $27,987 for the 2 years after diagnosis.

There are two major osteomyelitis classification schemes. Cierny and Mader classified osteomyelitis based on the affected portion of the bone, the physiologic status of the host, and the local environment (Table 99-1).[2] This classification lends itself to the treatment and prognosis of osteomyelitis. Stage 1 osteomyelitis typically can be treated with antimicrobial therapy alone, whereas stage 3 disease most often is managed with aggressive surgical débridement, antimicrobial therapy, and delayed orthopedic reconstruction. Lee and Waldvogel[3] classified osteomyelitis based on the duration of illness (acute versus chronic), the

TABLE 99-1 Staging System of Osteomyelitis

Anatomic Type
Stage 1: Medullary osteomyelitis
Stage 2: Superficial osteomyelitis
Stage 3: Localized osteomyelitis
Stage 4: Diffuse osteomyelitis

Physiologic Class
A Host: Normal host
B Host: Systemic compromise (Bs)
    Local compromise (Bi)
    Systemic and local compromise (Bis)
C Host: Treatment worse than the disease

Systemic or Local Factors That Affect Immune Surveillance, Metabolism, and Local Vascularity

Systemic (Bs)	Local (Bi)
Malnutrition	Chronic lymphedema
Renal, hepatic failure	Major vessel compromise
Diabetes mellitus	Small vessel disease
Chronic hypoxia	Vasculitis
Immune disease	Venous stasis
Malignancy	Extensive scarring
Extremes of age	Radiation fibrosis
Immunosuppression	Neuropathy
	Tobacco abuse

From Mader JT, Shirtliff M, Calhoun JH. Staging and staging application osteomyelitis. Clin Infect Dis. 1997;25:1303-1309.

TABLE 99-2 Microbiology of Osteomyelitis

Common (>50% of Cases)
Staphylococcus aureus
Coagulase-negative staphylococci

Occasionally Encountered (>25% of Cases)
Streptococci
Enterococci
Pseudomonas spp.
Enterobacter spp.
Proteus spp.
Escherichia coli
Serratia spp.
Anaerobes (*Peptostreptococcus* spp., *Clostridium* spp., *Bacteroides fragilis* group)

Rarely Encountered (<5% of Cases)
Mycobacterium tuberculosis
Mycobacterium avium complex
Rapidly growing mycobacteria
Dimorphic fungi
Candida spp.
Aspergillus spp.
Mycoplasma spp.
Tropheryma whipplei
Brucella spp.
Salmonella spp.
Actinomyces

mechanism of infection (hematogenous versus contiguous), and the presence of vascular insufficiency (Table 99-2). In contrast to the Cierny and Mader classification, the Waldvogel classification is an etiologic classification and does not implicate a specific therapeutic strategy.[4]

Because of differences in pathophysiology, diagnosis, and management, long bone osteomyelitis, osteomyelitis due to open fractures, vertebral osteomyelitis, osteomyelitis in patients with diabetes mellitus and peripheral vascular insufficiency, acute hematogenous osteomyelitis, and SAPHO syndrome are discussed separately. In addition, osteomyelitis in specific hosts (e.g., sickle cell disease), in unusual locations (e.g., clavicle), and secondary to unusual microorganisms are reviewed.

LESSONS FROM EXPERIMENTAL MODELS

Because of the lack of well-designed prospective clinical trials to guide the management of patients with osteomyelitis, recommendations about management of this disease have been primarily derived from experimental animal models, expert opinion, and retrospective cohort studies. Experimental models have been developed mainly to study the pathogenesis and treatment of osteomyelitis and offer a more controlled approach to a heterogeneous disease.[5]

In experimental models, normal bone is highly resistant to infection. Osteomyelitis in this setting can be created only after inoculation of large inocula, as a result of bone trauma, or due to the presence of foreign bodies.[3,5] When digested by osteoblasts, *S. aureus* can survive in a dormant and phenotypically altered state for a long time. This altered state renders *S. aureus* more resistant to the action of antimicrobials. This characteristic might explain in part the high relapse rate of osteomyelitis treated with a short course of antimicrobials and the long incubation period.[3,5] Muller and associates[6] studied leukocyte mobilization and phagocytosis in a guinea pig model of posttraumatic osteomyelitis. In this model, leukocyte locomotion was reduced after trauma and infection with *S. aureus* for 90 days.[6]

Norden and co-workers[7] analyzed the effect of the duration of antimicrobial therapy on the rate of bone sterilization in an experimental model of chronic *S. aureus* osteomyelitis that did not include surgical débridement as part of the experimental treatment. Of cultures, 78% and 16% yielded bacterial growth after 14 and 28 days of clindamycin therapy. These data support the need for a prolonged course of an-

timicrobial therapy in osteomyelitis. To our knowledge, the optimal duration of antimicrobial therapy after surgical débridement in an experimental model has not been studied.

Given the importance of biofilm production and the role of rifampin in killing microorganisms present in biofilms, several animal models of staphylococcal osteomyelitis have analyzed the efficacy of rifampin alone or in combination with β-lactams, vancomycin, macrolides, and quinolones. Combinations of rifampin with other antimicrobial agents generally were more effective in sterilizing the bone.[8-11]

The effect of fluoroquinolones on the healing process of bone fractures was assessed by Huddleston and colleagues.[12] In this study, 60 rats were divided equally into three groups, each group receiving ciprofloxacin, cefazolin, or no treatment for 3 weeks. Radiographs revealed significantly impaired healing of fractures in the ciprofloxacin-treated group compared with fractures in the cefazolin-treated group. Additional studies have shown this effect with other fluoroquinolones but not with vancomycin or gentamicin.[13,14] We have interpreted these data to mean that quinolones should be used cautiously and when other antimicrobials are not available in cases of osteomyelitis in which fracture healing needs to occur concomitantly with antimicrobial administration. Given the inherent difficulties of conducting large prospective clinical trials in humans, the management of osteomyelitis is likely to continue to be guided by lessons learned from experimental animal models.[5]

GENERAL PRINCIPLES

Osteomyelitis can be hematogenous or contiguous to a soft tissue infection. Acute hematogenous infectious osteomyelitis in children is discussed separately. Adults usually have vague symptoms with a subacute-to-chronic presentation. Nonspecific pain around the involved site with the absence of systemic signs and symptoms is normal. Fever, chills, local swelling, and erythema in the proximity of the involved bone are seldom seen. A draining sinus tract may be present over the involved bone. It usually evolves over several months and sometimes years.

The diagnosis of osteomyelitis is first suspected on clinical grounds. Confirmation usually entails a combination of radiologic, microbiologic, and pathologic tests. The erythrocyte sedimentation rate (ESR) and C-reactive protein are often elevated. The white blood cell count can be normal or elevated.

Although insensitive, a conventional radiograph is inexpensive and readily available. Abnormalities are usually seen 10 to 14 days after onset of the infection. Nuclear bone scans, although sensitive, are expensive and sometimes nonspecific. Technetium-99m methylene diphosphonate, gallium Ga 67 citrate, and indium-111-labeled white blood cells commonly are used as tracers (Fig. 99-1). Degenerative joint disease, bone tumors, and recent surgery can give false-positive results. Cross-sectional imaging modalities, such as computed tomography (CT) and magnetic resonance imaging (MRI), are now considered standard of care in the diagnosis of osteomyelitis. Although expensive, theses modalities are sensitive and specific. They provide excellent anatomic delineation of the infectious process and resolution of the surrounding soft tissue envelope. The presence of hardware may preclude the use of MRI and might create imaging artifacts with the use of CT. Nuclear imaging studies, such as bone scans and indium-labeled white blood cell scans, can be helpful in this situation and provide reasonable sensitivity and specificity.[15] The experience with positron emission tomography for the diagnosis of osteomyelitis is limited but seems promising.[16]

The identification of a causative microorganism is crucial. The type of organism and the associated in vitro susceptibility data help optimize medical therapy. Organism identification is best accomplished by surgical sampling or by needle aspiration under radiologic guidance to obtain tissues for histopathologic examination and bacterial and anaerobic culture.

Contrary to common belief, swab cultures from draining wounds and sinus tracts can be of diagnostic benefit for two main reasons. The

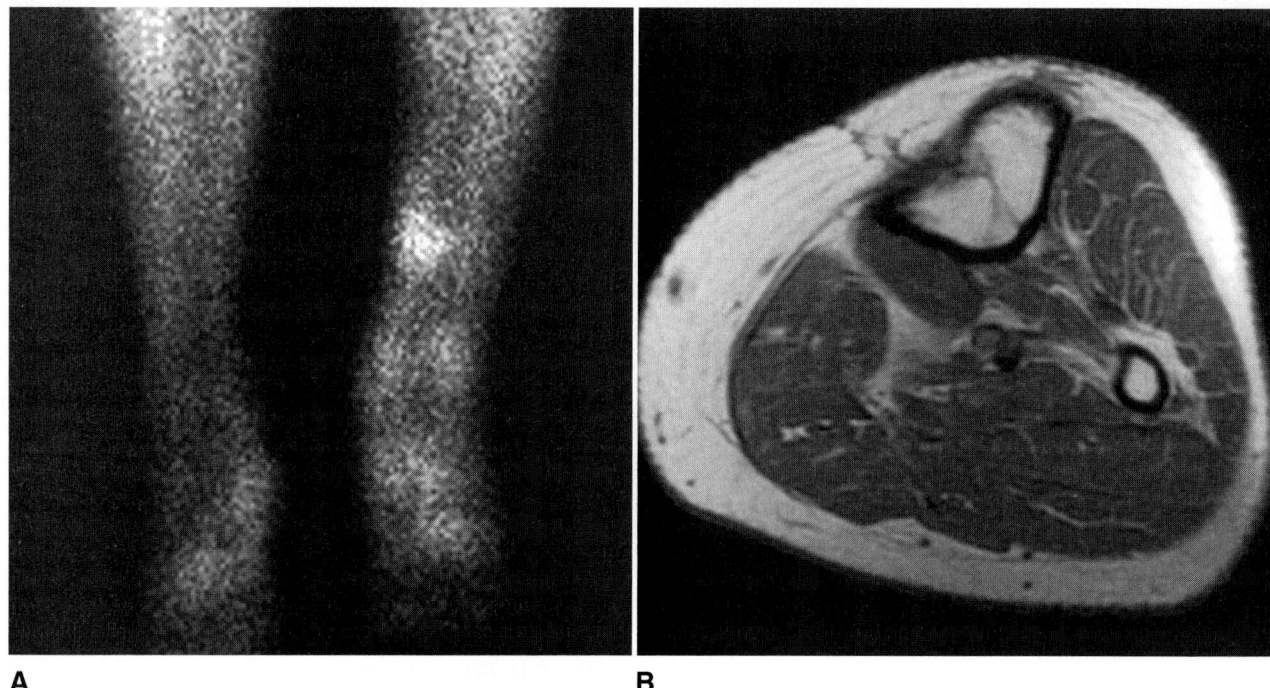

FIGURE 99-1. A, Indium scan showing increased uptake of the distal tibia in a patient with a history of open tibial fracture 40 years ago. **B,** Magnetic resonance imaging of the distal tibia with a sinus tract extending to the tibial cortex.

identification of certain resistant microorganisms (e.g., methicillin-resistant *S. aureus,* vancomycin-resistant enterococcus) indicates the need for infection control measures. Second, the isolation of *S. aureus* from superficial cultures has a high degree of correlation with deep cultures.[17] The recovery of other microorganisms correlates poorly with deep cultures.

In hematogenous long bone osteomyelitis, the infection is usually monobacterial, whereas in contiguous infection it is usually polymicrobial. *S. aureus,* coagulase-negative staphylococci, aerobic gram-negative bacteria, and *Peptostreptococcus* spp. are the most common organisms encountered (see Table 99-2).[15]

The goal of therapy of osteomyelitis is to eradicate the infection and to restore function. Most cases of osteomyelitis in adults require a

combination of medical and surgical therapy for successful eradication of the infection. It has long been recognized that antimicrobial therapy alone is not curative in most cases of osteomyelitis. In 1944, with the introduction of penicillin, Key[18] wrote: "continuous drug over a long period of time will lessen the amount of discharge, but it will not cure the disease because it cannot sterilize dead bone or cavities with necrotic content and rigid walls." All antimicrobials should be withheld if possible until percutaneous aspirate or surgical deep cultures have been obtained, unless there is concomitant soft tissue infection or sepsis syndrome. Antimicrobials are usually started (Table 99-3) immediately after surgical débridement (Table 99-4).

β-Lactams and vancomycin are the most commonly used antimicrobials in the medical management of osteomyelitis.[19] Cephalosporins

TABLE 99-3 Antimicrobial Therapy of Chronic Osteomyelitis in Adults for Selected Microorganisms

Microorganisms	First Choice*	Alternative Choice*
Staphylococci		
Oxacillin sensitive	Nafcillin sodium or oxacillin sodium, 1.5-2 g IV q 4 hr for 4-6 wk, *or* cefazolin, 1-2 g IV q 8 hr for 4-6 wk	Vancomycin, 15 mg/kg IV q 12 hr for 4-6 wk; some add rifampin, 600 mg PO qd, to nafcillin/oxacillin
Oxacillin resistant (MRSA)	Vancomycin†, 15 mg/kg IV q 12 hr for 4-6 wk	Linezolid, 600 mg PO/IV q 12 hr for 6 wk, *or* levofloxacin†, 500-750 mg PO/IV daily, plus rifampin, 600-900 mg/day PO for 6 wk if susceptible to both drugs
Penicillin-sensitive streptococci	Aqueous crystalline penicillin G, 20 × 10⁶ U/24 hr IV either continuously or in 6 equally divided daily doses for 4-6 wk, *or* ceftriaxone, 1-2 g IV or IM q 24 hr for 4-6 wk, *or* cefazolin, 1-2 g IV q 8 hr for 4-6 wk	Vancomycin, 15 mg/kg IV q 12 hr for 4-6 wk
Enterococci or streptococci with MIC ≥0.5 μg/mL, *Abiotrophia* and *Granulicatella* spp.	Aqueous crystalline penicillin G, 20 × 10⁶ U/24 hr IV either continuously or in 6 equally divided daily doses for 4-6 wk, *or* ampicillin sodium, 12 g/24 hr IV either continuously or in 6 equally divided daily doses; the addition of gentamicin sulfate, 1 mg/kg IV or IM q 8 hr for 1-2 wk is *optional*	Vancomycin†, 15 mg/kg IV q 12 hr for 4-6 wk; the addition of gentamicin sulfate, 1 mg/kg IV or IM q 8 hr for 1-2 wk is *optional*
Enterobacteriaceae	Ceftriaxone, 1-2 g IV q 24 hr for 4-6 wk	Ciprofloxacin†, 500-750 mg PO q 12 hr for 4-6 wk
Pseudomonas aeruginosa or *Enterobacter* spp.	Cefepime, 2 g IV q 12 hr for 4-6 weeks, *or* meropenem 1 g IV q 8 hr for 4-6 wk	Ciprofloxacin†, 750 mg PO q 12 hr for 4-6 wk, *or* ceftazidime, 2 g IV q 8 hr

*Antimicrobial selection should be based on in vitro sensitivity data.
†Should be avoided if possible in pediatric patients and in osteomyelitis associated with fractures.

TABLE 99-4 Surgical Principles in Osteomyelitis

Adequate drainage of all infected tissue
Extensive débridement of all infected tissue
Removal of all hardware
Management of dead space (flap)
Complete wound closure
Stability of infected fracture

and penicillinase-resistant penicillin are commonly used in patients with osteomyelitis because of their low toxicity profile and their spectrum of activity against staphylococci and other common bacterial pathogens that cause osteomyelitis. Cefazolin has excellent activity against methicillin-sensitive staphylococci, is safe, is inexpensive, and has been used extensively in the medical therapy of osteomyelitis.[19] Although ceftriaxone once daily is convenient for outpatient therapy, its use in methicillin-sensitive staphylococcal osteomyelitis is controversial.[20,21] We reserve the use of ceftriaxone for patients with penicillin-sensitive staphylococci, streptococci, or susceptible aerobic gram-negative bacilli other than *Pseudomonas aeruginosa* and *Enterobacter* spp.

Vancomycin is used commonly in the treatment of osteomyelitis due to methicillin-resistant staphylococci and ampicillin-resistant enterococci. Until more recently, it was the only available antimicrobial agent that was effective against these organisms despite its known lack of efficacy compared with β-lactams when treating susceptible organisms. In a large cohort study of 450 patients with osteomyelitis who were followed for 10 years, vancomycin was associated with a 2.5 relative risk of recurrence compared with a penicillinase-resistant penicillin in a univariate analysis.[19] Vancomycin infrequently can cause significant ototoxicity and renal toxicity, although this is controversial.

Linezolid is the first approved drug in the new oxazolidinone class of antimicrobials. It has excellent activity against staphylococci, streptococci, and vancomycin-resistant enterococci. Linezolid has excellent bioavailability when administered orally. For all these characteristics, linezolid has been used in patients with infections due to vancomycin-resistant enterococci or when β-lactams or vancomycin cannot be used.[22,23] Prolonged used of linezolid has been associated with significant pancytopenia and peripheral neuropathy.[24] Because of its toxicity profile, high cost, and experimental models showing a high failure rate, the use of linezolid in patients with osteomyelitis typically has been limited to patients with osteomyelitis due to vancomycin-resistant enterococci or patients who are intolerant of vancomycin.[25]

Daptomycin, a more recently approved cyclic lipopeptide antimicrobial agent, has bactericidal activity against aerobic and facultative gram-positive pathogens. The use of daptomycin in the therapy of experimental methicillin-resistant *S. aureus* osteomyelitis in rabbits yielded results similar to vancomycin.[26] Daptomycin's role in the therapy of patients with osteomyelitis in clinical practice has yet to be defined.

The optimal duration of antimicrobial therapy in osteomyelitis is unknown because of the lack of prospective randomized clinical trials assessing the length of antimicrobial therapy in patients with osteomyelitis and the heterogeneous nature of the disease. In experimental models, 4 weeks of therapy was more effective in sterilizing the bone than 2 weeks of therapy. Surgical débridement was not part of these models, however, and shorter courses of therapy may be as effective when extensive surgical débridement is accomplished.[7] Because it takes 6 weeks for the débrided bone to be covered by vascularized soft tissue, and because of anecdotal experiences suggesting a higher relapse rate with a short duration of therapy, many experts advocate a total duration of 4 to 6 weeks of parenteral antimicrobial therapy. When the surgical débridement of all infected bone is complete or the osteomyelitic bone has been resected, some experts advocate a short duration of antimicrobial therapy. When stable, patients can be dismissed from the hospital, and parenteral antimicrobial therapy can be continued on an outpatient basis. Using long-term intravenous catheters, such as peripherally inserted central catheters, can facilitate this task.[27]

Hyperbaric oxygen therapy has been used as an adjunctive measure for patients with chronic or refractory osteomyelitis.[28,29] It is hypothesized that an adequate oxygen tension is necessary for oxygen-dependent killing of organisms by the polymorphonuclear leukocytes and for fibroblast activity leading to angiogenesis and wound healing. In addition, hyperbaric oxygen has a direct bactericidal or bacteriostatic effect on anaerobic organisms. Randomized studies in animals showed that hyperbaric oxygen therapy was effective in reducing the number of bacterial colonies compared with antimicrobial therapy alone.[28,29] Anecdotal experience in humans includes patients with recurrent and refractory osteomyelitis (see Chapter 40). To our knowledge, there are no adequate randomized trials assessing the efficacy of hyperbaric oxygen therapy in humans with chronic or refractory osteomyelitis.

OSTEOMYELITIS AFTER A CONTAMINATED OPEN FRACTURE

Contaminated open fractures can lead to the development of osteomyelitis of the fractured bone typically at the fracture site in 3% to 25% of cases depending on the type of fracture, the level of contamination, the degree of soft tissue injury, and whether systemic and local antimicrobial therapy have been administered (Fig. 99-2).[30-37] Patients with open fractures are usually young men in their teens or 20s. The bones of the lower extremity are typically involved, most often the tibia or fibula. Early contamination after the open fracture of bone and soft tissue eventually can lead to the development of osteomyelitis at the fracture site. Untreated, infection ultimately may lead to nonunion of the infected site, chronic osteomyelitis, or amputation.

The microorganisms isolated late in this type of osteomyelitis correlate in 25% with the initial culture results at the time of débridement.[38] A variety of microorganisms have been implicated. Pathogens can include normal skin flora that contaminate the wound, organisms

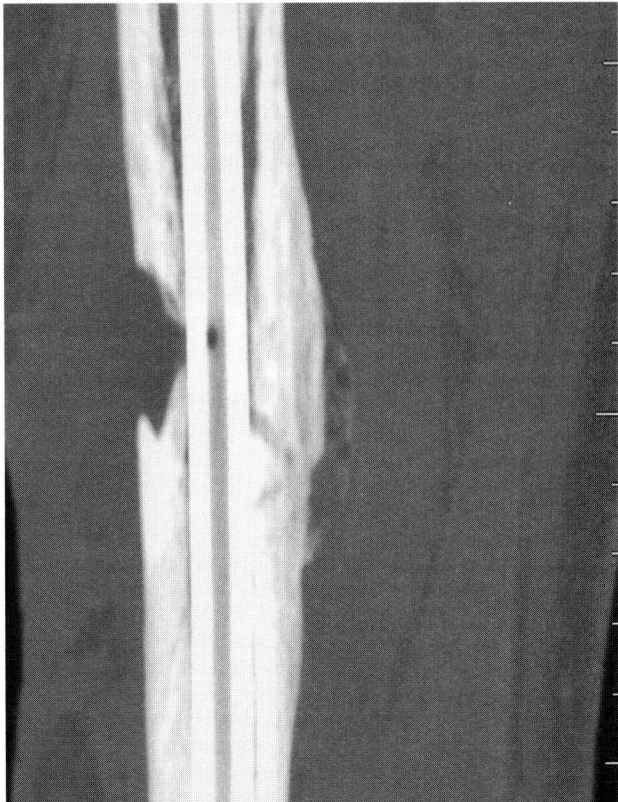

FIGURE 99-2. Computed tomography reconstruction images of a nonunited femur fracture 6 months after intramedullary nailing. Surgical cultures grew *Pseudomonas aeruginosa* and *Propionibacterium acnes*.

from contaminated soil, or nosocomial pathogens acquired because of the multiple operations that often are required to repair surgically the fracture and surrounding soft tissue envelope. Staphylococci and aerobic gram-negative bacilli are the two most common groups of microorganisms implicated in this type of osteomyelitis. Several other unusual microorganisms, such as enterococci, fungi, and atypical mycobacteria, also have been implicated.

Current management of open contaminated fractures entails early aggressive wound irrigation and débridement, administration of parenteral antimicrobials, fracture fixation, and soft tissue coverage. In one study, a delay of 5 hours in surgical débridement was associated with a higher incidence of infection.[38] Randomized clinical trials performed by Patzakis and colleagues[39] established the efficacy of a short duration of antimicrobial prophylaxis in the prevention of osteomyelitis in patients treated for open contaminated fractures. The use of prolonged antimicrobial therapy for prevention does not decrease the risk of infection and potentially can lead to the development of resistant microorganisms.[40] More recent cohort studies have shown the efficacy of antibiotic-impregnated polymethyl methacrylate beads temporarily placed in and around the fracture site in the prevention of osteomyelitis after a contaminated open fracture.[34-36] The choice between external versus intramedullary fracture fixation devices in contaminated open fractures is controversial and discussed in detail elsewhere.[41-44]

Signs and symptoms of infection typically appear several months after an open fracture. The hallmark of osteomyelitis after open fracture is nonunion of the fracture site or poor wound healing after wound closure or soft tissue coverage. Other symptoms, such as local erythema or fever and chills, are less common. MRI or radionuclide imaging studies are typically neither sensitive nor specific for the presence of infection because of the abnormalities created by the recent previous surgery and the presence of foreign bodies.

Management of established osteomyelitis or infected nonunion after an open fracture requires débridement of the surgical site, identification of the causative microorganisms, and pathogen-directed antimicrobial therapy (see Table 99-3). If foreign bodies are retained, long-term oral antimicrobial suppression may be helpful until fracture healing occurs, at which time oral antimicrobial suppression could be discontinued. The use of quinolone and rifampin combinations has been studied in staphylococcal fracture fixation device infection.[45,46] In sensitive staphylococcal hardware-associated osteomyelitis, a 3- to 6-month course of a quinolone and rifampin eradicated the infection in more than 80% of cases.[45,46] Given the good outcome of patients treated with other antimicrobials and the concerns of the effect of quinolones on bone healing, we have not universally adopted this strategy. If recurrence of the infection occurs after discontinuation of long-term oral antimicrobial suppression and fracture bone healing, definitive therapy with removal of the foreign bodies and pathogen-directed antimicrobial therapy usually can be undertaken without compromising limb function. This is in contrast to prosthetic joint infection treated with débridement and retention of components, in which removal of the prosthesis typically compromises limb function.

VERTEBRAL OSTEOMYELITIS, SPONDYLODISKITIS, AND EPIDURAL ABSCESS

Infection of the intervertebral disk and the adjacent vertebrae, variably referred to as *spondylodiskitis, disk space infection,* and *vertebral osteomyelitis,* all with or without associated epidural or psoas abscesses, is hematogenous in origin in most cases. It is believed that the hematogenous infection of the vertebrae occurs via the segmental artery supplying the vertebrae.[47] Potential sources of hematogenous infection are skin and soft tissue infection, genitourinary tract, infective endocarditis, infected intravenous sites, intravenous drug abuse, and respiratory tract infection.[48] Infection of the disk space and contiguous vertebra also can occur postoperatively.[49] Several studies have established the efficacy of antimicrobial prophylaxis before spinal surgery in reducing the risk of postoperative superficial or deep infection, including vertebral osteomyelitis. In one study by Schnoring and

Brock,[50] 0.2% of patients receiving antimicrobial prophylaxis developed a surgical site infection, whereas 2.8% of patients developed surgical site infection when antimicrobial prophylaxis was withheld.

The clinical presentation of vertebral osteomyelitis includes localized insidious pain and tenderness in the spine area in 90% of patients. Fever is present in less than 50% of cases. Motor and sensory deficits, owing to spinal cord or nerve root compression, are present in 15% of patients.[48,49,51-53]

S. aureus and coagulase-negative staphylococci are the most common microorganisms encountered in vertebral osteomyelitis. *Mycobacterium tuberculosis* and *Brucella* spondylodiskitis are common in endemic regions. Spine infections due to gram-negative aerobic bacteria and *Candida* spp. are seen more commonly in intravenous drug abusers, immunosuppressed patients, and postoperative patients.

The diagnosis of vertebral osteomyelitis requires a high index of suspicion in at-risk patients presenting with compatible signs and symptoms. The goal of the diagnostic evaluation is to identify the organism and to determine the extent of infection. Neurologic function and spinal stability always should be assessed carefully. An elevation of the ESR is present in more than 90% of cases, whereas the white blood cell count is elevated in less than 50% of patients. Blood cultures may be positive, and if they are, infective endocarditis may be present.[54,55]

Plain spinal radiographs are not sensitive in the diagnosis of disk space infection. In one study, 32% of radiographs obtained suggested diskitis.[54] MRI has proved to be an invaluable tool in detecting disk space infection and spinal cord compression (Fig. 99-3). Gallium citrate Ga 67 scanning seems to be a sensitive and specific method used to diagnose diskitis. In a study of 41 patients with suspected spondylodiskitis, gallium scanning proved to be 100% sensitive, specific, and accurate.[56] We use gallium scanning when MRI cannot be performed and in cases in which MRI is inconclusive.

CT-guided percutaneous biopsy and aspiration has a sensitivity of 50%.[57] If the results of the first aspirate are inconclusive, a repeat as-

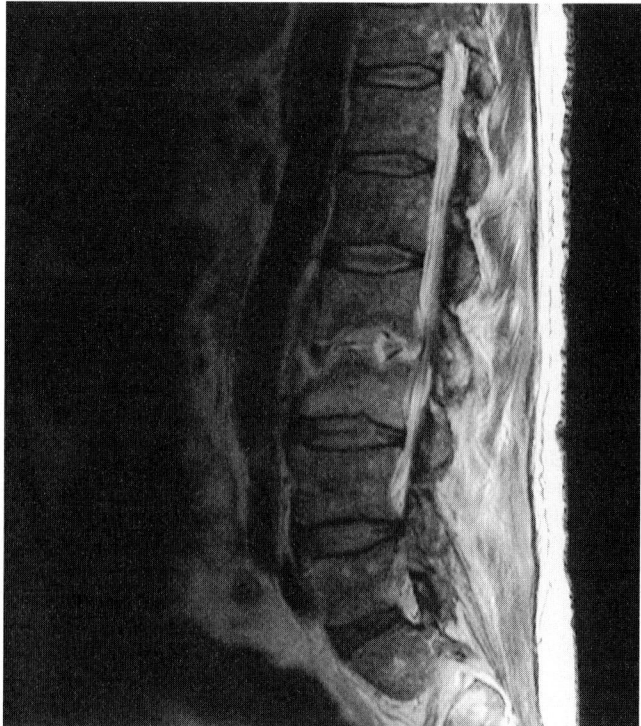

FIGURE 99-3. T1-weighted magnetic resonance images show an abnormal signal in the disk between L2 and L3 with associated vertebral osteomyelitis. A fluid collection is located in the posterior part of L2 and L3 resulting in the elevation of the posterior ligament. A computed tomography–guided aspirate grew *Staphylococcus aureus.*

pirate should be performed if possible so that a microbiologic diagnosis can be obtained and pathogen-specific antimicrobial therapy administered. An open biopsy should be reserved for patients with a nondiagnostic percutaneous biopsy or in patients not responding to empirical antimicrobial therapy administered in the situation in which the diagnosis of infection is made, a microbiologic diagnosis could not be obtained, and an open biopsy is not performed.[57]

The goals of therapy should include eradicating the infection, relieving pain, preserving or restoring neurologic function, and maintaining spinal stability. Complete bed rest is not often necessary. The spine could be externally stabilized using a corset or a body brace. The treatment of vertebral osteomyelitis requires an initial 4- to 6-week course of antimicrobial therapy (see Table 99-3). Parenteral antimicrobial treatment may be extended in difficult cases or in cases in which undrained abscesses are being treated and do not resolve after 4 to 6 weeks. Surgical therapy is not necessary in most cases. Surgical débridement should be considered in patients with large paravertebral or epidural abscesses associated with neurologic deficits, when the diagnosis is in doubt even after a CT-guided aspirate, when medical management fails, or when the spine is mechanically unstable. In selected cases, percutaneous transpedicular débridement and diskectomy, performed under fluoroscopic guidance, may prevent the progression of bone destruction and deformity in the early stages of vertebral osteomyelitis and spondylodiskitis.[58] The neurologic status of the patient must be monitored closely. With effective antimicrobial medical therapy, spontaneous bone fusion occurs in 12 to 24 months. Carragee and associates[59] examined the value of serial measurements of the ESR. In their study, a rapid decline of the ESR (>50% in the first month) after institution of effective antimicrobial therapy was rarely seen in treatment failure. Follow-up MRI may give the impression of clinical progression even though there is otherwise clinical improvement.[60]

Early postoperative hardware-associated spine infection is treated initially with surgical débridement and retention of the hardware. Removal of spinal hardware in this situation would compromise the stability of the spine and the spinal cord. In this setting, surgical débridement is followed by a course of parenteral antimicrobial therapy (see Table 99-3).[61] Although not recommended by all experts, parenteral antimicrobial therapy at our institution is typically followed by the use of long-term oral antimicrobial suppression in this situation. Long-term antimicrobial suppression should be continued until there is radiologic evidence of bone vertebral fusion. This modality is highly successful in our institution. Complete bone remodeling and fusion typically are complete after 2 years. At that time, long-term oral suppression may be discontinued, with a low risk of recurrence. If there is recurrence, the spinal hardware can be removed without compromising the stability of the spine.[60]

OSTEOMYELITIS IN PATIENTS WITH DIABETES MELLITUS OR VASCULAR INSUFFICIENCY

Osteomyelitis in patients with diabetes mellitus is typically found in the foot and less often in the hand.[62] The economic consequences of this type of osteomyelitis are enormous. Currently the cost of therapy for an episode of diabetic foot infection averages $17,000, and the hospitalization of a patient with a diabetic foot infection that leads to amputation averages $35,000. Fifteen percent of patients with diabetes mellitus develop foot ulcers during their lifetime, and 6% require hospitalization for foot ulcers.[63,64] Several factors can lead to the development of a diabetic foot infection. Neuropathy, vascular insufficiency, and hyperglycemia can lead to a variety of consequences that ultimately lead to the development of a skin ulcer and subsequently to contiguous osteomyelitis.

Early recognition and management of factors that can lead to the development of foot ulcers in patients with diabetes mellitus are key to the delay or even prevention of osteomyelitis. In assessing the risk of subsequent foot ulcer in patients with diabetes mellitus, the treating physician should pay special attention to several factors (Table 99-5). The lower extremity macrovascular and microvascular circulation supply can be assessed by physical examination of the pedal pulses, noninvasive vascular assessments, or measurement of transcutaneous oxygen pressures.[65] The severity of peripheral neuropathy can be assessed early by examining motor nerve conduction velocity in the lower extremities.[66] All patients with diabetes mellitus or vascular insufficiency should have an annual complete foot examination performed by a health care professional.[67,68] Strict glycemic control and smoking cessation can reduce the rate of progression of vascular diseases and neuropathy. Patients with evidence of increased local pressure should be offered well-cushioned walking shoes that redistribute the pressure in their feet.[69,70]

As discussed earlier, the diagnosis of osteomyelitis in patients with diabetes or vascular insufficiency often requires multiple modalities, including measurement of the ESR or C-reactive protein, nuclear imaging studies, and MRI. When osteomyelitis of the foot bones is being sought, an additional useful, inexpensive test is the "probe to bone test." This test, which involves palpation of bone through a contiguous ulcer with a metal probe, has a positive predictive value of 89% and a negative predictive value of 56%.[71]

As in other forms of osteomyelitis, combined surgical and medical therapy is most often warranted (see Tables 99-3 and 99-4). Treatment failure is often due to lack of adequate débridement or the lack of adequate oxygen tension in the bone and surrounding soft tissue.[72]

In patients with poor arterial vascular supply, revascularization should be done if possible to provide blood flow to the débrided area or to minimize the extent of any amputation that may be required. In this subset of patients, the infected and necrotic bone is usually exposed and surrounded by poorly vascularized soft tissue. Management of dead space and adequate surgical drainage of infected bone and soft tissue often are required. Antimicrobial therapy should be withheld until intraoperative deep cultures have been obtained. Antimicrobials should be administered before culture results, however, in patients with local or systemic signs of an infectious process (cellulitis, acute soft tissue infection, fever, and hemodynamic compromise).

Because most of these infections are polymicrobial, including multiple aerobic and anaerobic microorganisms, broad-spectrum antimicrobial therapy often is required. Multiple antimicrobial regimens have been used, including piperacillin-tazobactam, ampicillin-sulbactam, ticarcillin-clavulanic acid, and other β-lactams combined with metronidazole.[72] The use of a quinolone combined with metronidazole or clindamycin also is considered an acceptable alternative. Quinolones, clindamycin, and metronidazole also have excellent bioavailability when taken orally. First-generation quinolones, such as ciprofloxacin, have little activity against staphylococci, streptococci, and enterococci and no activity against anaerobes. Levofloxacin has good streptococcal and staphylococcal activity but variable and minimal anaerobic activity. The latest generation quinolones, such as gatifloxacin and moxifloxacin, are broad-spectrum antimicrobials with excellent activity against gram-negative and gram-positive organisms and improved anaerobic activity. Quinolones often are used in combination with metronidazole or clindamycin for the treatment of osteomyelitis in patients with diabetes and peripheral vascular disease.[72,73]

TABLE 99-5 Factors Associated with Increased Risk of Foot Ulcers in Patients with Diabetes Mellitus

Diabetes mellitus duration >10 yr
Poor glucose control
Cardiovascular disease
Renal or retinal complications
Peripheral neuropathy
Evidence of increased local pressure (callus, erythema)
Limited joint mobility
Peripheral vascular disease
Prior history of foot ulcer
Prior history of amputation

The long-term safety of quinolones, specifically levofloxacin, has been analyzed in patients with chronic osteomyelitis, chronic sinusitis, and multidrug-resistant tuberculosis. Patients with multidrug-resistant tuberculosis were treated with a 1000-mg daily dose for a median duration of 266 days. No significant toxicity was encountered. These data showed that levofloxacin at a dose of 1000 mg was safe and effective.[74-76] Fewer data are available on the long-term safety of gatifloxacin and moxifloxacin.

The efficacy of linezolid in the treatment of diabetic foot infection was evaluated in a large randomized clinical trial. In this study, linezolid with or without aztreonam was compared with an aminopenicillin/β-lactamase inhibitor. The linezolid arm was comparable to the aminopenicillin arm in terms of safety, clinical efficacy, and microbiologic efficacy.[77] Surgical therapy was performed as clinically indicated.

Whether patients with grade 2 contiguous osteomyelitis (minimal cortical osteomyelitis diagnosed on imaging studies) can be treated with prolonged antimicrobial therapy without surgical débridement is subject to debate.[73] Patients should be treated for at least 4 weeks.[72] Some experts argue that antimicrobial therapy should be extended until the soft tissue defect and the skin have completely healed.

ACUTE HEMATOGENOUS OSTEOMYELITIS

Hematogenous seeding of bones, albeit rare, potentially can affect any bone in the body. Acute hematogenous osteomyelitis of long bones occurs mainly in prepubertal children, elderly patients, intravenous drug abusers, and patients with indwelling central catheters.[15] Hematogenous seeding of an intervertebral disk space can occur in adults and was discussed in earlier. This section discusses mainly acute hematogenous osteomyelitis in prepubertal children.

Acute hematogenous osteomyelitis involves mostly the metaphyses of long bones (Cierny-Mader classification stage I). The tibia and femur are affected in most cases.[78] In neonates, the infection can spread to the adjacent joint space. The infection can involve multiple osseous sites. Because the infection is not confined to the metaphyses, approximately half of cases of neonatal osteomyelitis also have involvement of the adjacent joint with development of septic arthritis. The predilection of infection to the metaphyseal region is explained by its peculiar anatomy.[79] Capillary ends of the nutrient artery make sharp loops under the growth plate. This nonanastomosing capillary system feeds into large venous sinusoids, where the blood flow becomes slow and turbulent. An obstruction of these capillaries can lead to an area of avascular necrosis. Metaphyseal capillaries lack phagocytic lining cells.[80] Any minor trauma can lead to the development of a small hematoma, vascular obstruction, and subsequent bone necrosis. This area can be seeded from a transient bacteremia.[80] The acute infection initially produces an inflammatory infiltration, increased bone pressure, decreased pH, and decreased oxygen tension. These factors compromise the medullary circulation and enhance the spread of infection. In infants, the infection may proceed laterally through the bone cortex or through the epiphysis and joint surfaces through capillaries that cross the growth plate.

The most common microorganisms isolated in cases of hematogenous osteomyelitis are *S. aureus* and *Streptococcus pneumoniae*. *Haemophilus influenzae* type b, historically a common cause of long bone osteomyelitis, has become exceedingly rare since the development and widespread use of an effective vaccine in children.[78] Osteomyelitis in neonates results from hematogenous spread, especially in infants with indwelling central venous catheters. Common causative organisms in osteomyelitis of the neonate are organisms that frequently cause neonatal sepsis, such as group B *Streptococcus* spp. and *Escherichia coli*. *Candida* spp. and *P. aeruginosa* are more commonly encountered in intravenous drug abusers and patients with indwelling central catheters.

In children, the diagnosis often is made in a patient with compatible radiologic and clinical findings with positive blood cultures. In adults, a CT-guided aspirate or an open biopsy is often necessary to establish a definitive diagnosis.

Most cases of acute hematogenous osteomyelitis in children can be treated with antimicrobial therapy alone. Surgical débridement and intramedullary reaming are indicated if the diagnosis is in doubt, the patient has not responded clinically to antimicrobial therapy within 48 hours, infection extends into the joint, or an adequate course of antimicrobial therapy fails to cure the infection. After obtaining microbiologic specimens, empirical antimicrobial therapy is started to cover clinically suspected organisms. When an organism is identified, the antimicrobial therapy can be changed accordingly (see Table 99-3). Switching from parenteral therapy to oral antimicrobial therapy can be done when the patient is afebrile and able to tolerate oral antimicrobials. Oral antimicrobial therapy should be given to compliant patients with close follow-up. The typical duration of antimicrobial therapy in children is 3 weeks (see Table 99-3). Dosages of antimicrobials should be adapted to the pediatric population. Quinolones are contraindicated in pediatric patients. In adults, surgical therapy often is required followed by appropriate antimicrobial therapy based on culture and sensitivity data.

SAPHO SYNDROME

SAPHO, an acronym for *s*ynovitis, *a*cne, *p*lantar pustulosis, *h*yperostosis, and *o*steitis, is a disease of unknown cause. This syndrome was first described in 1972 by Giedion and co-workers.[81] The pathogenesis of this disease is unclear. Several postulated infectious, autoimmune, hereditary, and immunodeficiency mechanisms exist. Inflammatory-type pain is present in most cases. Local swelling and tenderness of affected bones is often present. Systemic symptoms of fever, weight loss, and generalized malaise are rare. Osteitis typically is multifocal and affects several bones, including the chest wall bones (63%), pelvis (40%), and spine (33%).[82]

Bones of the lower limbs are affected in only 6% of cases. The mean number of active lesions per patient is five. The disease is self-limited, with spontaneous intermittent periods of exacerbation and remission. The differential diagnosis includes infectious osteomyelitis, bone malignancy, and other inflammatory arthritides. Patients require bone biopsy and cultures for diagnosis to exclude infectious osteomyelitis.

There are no specific laboratory tests to diagnose SAPHO syndrome. The ESR is increased in 65% of cases. Bone radiographs may show lytic erosions similar to those of infectious osteomyelitis affecting the metaphysis. With time, a rime of reactive hyperostosis can develop. Histopathology typically is nonspecific with a combination of acute and chronic inflammatory cells. Cultures of biopsy material are negative for bacteria, fungi, and mycobacteria.[83] When used, antimicrobials seem to have no impact on the course of this illness. Several therapeutic modalities, including nonsteroidal anti-inflammatory drugs, pamidronate, glucocorticoids, sulfadiazine, methotrexate, and interferon-γ, have been used in case reports and small case series.[84,85]

Another closely related syndrome is chronic recurrent multifocal osteitis.[82] This syndrome mainly affects children and adolescents and typically affects bones of the lower extremities.

OTHER FORMS OF OSTEOMYELITIS: SPECIFIC HOSTS, UNUSUAL LOCATIONS, OR UNUSUAL ORGANISMS

Osteitis Pubis

Osteitis pubis is an infection of the symphysis pubis. It was recognized as a complication in the early era of gynecourologic surgery. Early reports postulated that this disease was not infectious because of the nonresponse to antimicrobials and the "nonvirulent organisms" recovered during cultures. The disease is encountered after a variety of urologic and gynecologic surgical procedures, including Marshall-Marchetti-Krantz urethropexy, prolonged catheterization, inguinal hernia repair, and vaginal delivery.[86-88] *S. aureus*, *Enterococcus* spp., *E. coli*, *Pseudomonas* spp., and *Proteus* spp. are the most commonly encountered organisms. Some patients might present with a sterile form of osteitis pubis. It is believed that this form is due to an aseptic inflammation that could be triggered by surgery or by bone infarction. Most patients present with suprapubic pain and difficulty and pain with ambulation. In one study, the time between surgery and the diagnosis ranged from 2 to 18 months.[87] Fever and leukocytosis rarely are present.[88] An elevated ESR (>20 mm/hr) is present in 67% of patients.[88] Plain radiographs may be normal early in the disease. Radiographs performed 6 months later can reveal pubic bone sclerosis, widening of the joint spaces, and rarefaction. CT and MRI are more sensitive than plain radiography and can define the soft tissue much better. Bone or indium-labeled white blood cell scan is sensitive. Fine-needle aspirate is sometimes helpful. The aseptic form of osteitis pubis could be managed with nonsteroidal anti-inflammatory drugs and corticosteroids. Antimicrobial therapy should be administered in all other cases. In one study, surgical débridement of infected bone was required in more than 70% of cases.[88]

Osteomyelitis of the Clavicle

Osteomyelitis of the clavicle represents less than 3% of osteomyelitis cases.[89-91] It may be hematogenous or related to subclavian vein catheterization and neck surgery. *S. aureus* is the most common organism. A variety of other microorganisms have been described, including gram-negative bacteria and *M. tuberculosis*. Given the nontraumatic nature, most cases of clavicular osteomyelitis present as a therapeutic challenge. The disease may present as acute local pain and swelling with positive blood cultures (i.e., *S. aureus*) or may be more chronic and indolent in nature (i.e., *M. tuberculosis*). In one study, the clinical duration of the symptoms ranged from 2 weeks to 1.5 years.[89] All patients typically present with clavicular site pain. Fever, localized swelling or a mass, and soft tissue abscesses are present in 60%, 30%, and 30% of cases.[89] Plain radiographs of the clavicle can show sclerotic or lytic changes. Acute cases secondary to *S. aureus* can be treated with parenteral antimicrobial therapy alone (see Table 99-3). Chronic cases should be treated with surgical débridement followed by antimicrobial therapy.

Sacroiliac Joint Infection

Sacroiliac joint infection is an uncommon metastatic infection of *S. aureus* bacteremia.[92] Nevertheless, sacroiliac infection is caused most often by *S. aureus*. Intravenous drug abusers and patients with indwelling catheters are at risk. Patients typically present with acute onset of sacral or pelvic pain and leukocytosis. Blood cultures are often positive. Patients should be evaluated for the presence of concomitant infective endocarditis. Brucellosis causes a chronic unilateral osteomyelitis of the sacroiliac joint that must be distinguished from similar lesions caused by inflammatory bowel disease and ankylosing spondylitis (see Chapter 223).

Osteomyelitis in Hemodialysis Patients

Patients undergoing long-term hemodialysis are at an increased risk for osteomyelitis. Hematogenous infections are common, usually affecting the disk space and resulting in vertebral osteomyelitis; this is the result of repetitive access of the arteriovenous fistula or the dialysis catheter. Because of a higher rate of *S. aureus* colonization in this patient population, most cases of hematogenous osteomyelitis are due to this microorganism. Oxacillin resistance is common among *S. aureus* isolates in these patients. Advanced diabetes mellitus and peripheral vascular disease are common among patients undergoing hemodialysis. These conditions put them at risk for contiguous osteomyelitis of the extremities (see earlier).[93]

Osteomyelitis in Patients with Sickle Cell Disease

Patients with sickle cell disease are at increased risk for osteoarticular infections. Acute and long bone osteomyelitis and septic arthritis are the most commonly encountered syndromes. In a large cohort study of 299 patients in France with homozygous sickle cell anemia, the prevalence of osteomyelitis was 12%.[94] It seemed that the HLA class II DRB1* 15 had a protective effect against infectious complications, including osteomyelitis, whereas patients with HLA class II DQB1* 03

were more susceptible to serious infections.[95] *Salmonella* spp. and *S. aureus* remain the most commonly encountered microorganisms in sickle cell anemia patients with osteomyelitis.[96,97] Most patients are children.[94,97] Although osteomyelitis could be multifocal in this setting, long bones are commonly affected.

The differentiation between bone infarction and osteomyelitis could be challenging because their clinical and radiologic presentation is similar. A history of bone pain and fever followed in 1 to 2 weeks by the onset of spiking fever, chills, and leukocytosis suggests osteomyelitis. Sequential radionuclide bone marrow and bone scans can aid in the differentiation process.[98] CT-guided aspirate or an open biopsy with cultures sometimes is needed for a more definitive diagnosis, but the procedure can infect previously sterile, infarcted bone. Surgical and medical therapy is similar to osteomyelitis in patients without sickle cell disease. Empirical antimicrobial therapy should be directed against *Salmonella* and *S. aureus*.

Osteomyelitis in Injection Drug Users

Osteoarticular infections occur more commonly in injection drug users (see Chapter 309).[99-101] Pathogens can reach the bones by hematogenous routes or by contiguous or direct inoculation. Multiple skeletal sites can be affected. Unusual sites of infection outside this setting are common in these patients, such as sternoclavicular, sternochondral joint, sacroiliac joint, and pubic symphysis. *S. aureus, Pseudomonas* spp., and *Candida* spp. are the most commonly encountered organisms in these patients. *M. tuberculosis* can cause vertebral osteomyelitis in these patients. *Eikenella corrodens,* a normal oral flora microorganism, can cause osteomyelitis in injection drug users who lick the needle tip or the skin before injection ("needle licker osteomyelitis").[102] Surgical and medical therapy of osteomyelitis in these patients is similar to therapy in other groups with osteomyelitis. Outpatient parenteral antimicrobial therapy and central venous access catheters should be used with caution in these patients.[27]

Skeletal Mycobacterial Infection

Extrapulmonary disease represents 20% of all tuberculosis (see Chapter 248). Infection of the musculoskeletal system represents 1% to 5% of all tuberculosis cases. Osteomyelitis due to *M. tuberculosis* often affects the spine or a para-articular focus. Most cases are the result of a hematogenous spread from a pulmonary source.[103-114]

The clinician should consider tuberculous osteomyelitis in patients with a past medical history of treated or untreated tuberculosis with new back pain, patients with a known positive tuberculin skin test, young patients, patients coming from endemic areas with chest-x-ray findings consistent with active tuberculosis or old healed tuberculosis, patients with a household member who had tuberculosis, patients with negative bacterial cultures, or patients whose biopsy specimen of infected bone shows granulomatous inflammation.[108] Clinical features of osteomyelitis due to *M. tuberculosis* are pain and swelling with abscess and sinus formation. Radiographs reveal irregular cavities and areas of bone destruction with little surrounding sclerosis. Because of the presence of a sinus tract, secondary bacterial infection does occur.[107,112]

Vertebral osteomyelitis due to *M. tuberculosis,* also called *Pott's disease,* is among the most common osteoarticular manifestations of tuberculosis. In this form of vertebral osteomyelitis, in contrast to bacterial vertebral osteomyelitis, systemic symptoms are often absent. Back pain or stiffness is commonly the only symptom, and a delay in the diagnosis is often the norm. In 50% of patients with spinal tuberculosis, MRI reveals paravertebral soft tissue abscesses in addition to the bone lesion. The infection has a predilection to the anterior superior or inferior angles of the vertebral bodies, especially in the early phases of the disease.[108,109,113]

Significant overlap in imaging appearances between tuberculous osteomyelitis and other forms of osteomyelitis exists. The diagnosis should rely on the presence of *M. tuberculosis* on stain or culture of a biopsy specimen. Chest radiographs show an abnormality in less than 50% of patients with musculoskeletal tuberculosis but should be obtained routinely because the existence of concomitant pulmonary tuberculosis has infection control ramifications and may provide for an alternative area from which to obtain culture specimens. The therapy of skeletal tuberculosis is discussed in Chapter 246.

Osteoarticular infections with nontuberculous mycobacteria also can occur. It is commonly seen in immunocompromised patients[114] or after contamination of a wound after trauma or surgery. *Mycobacterium marinum, Mycobacterium avium-intracellulare, Mycobacterium fortuitum, Mycobacterium chelonae, Mycobacterium ulcerans, Mycobacterium kansasii, Mycobacterium xenopi,* and *Mycobacterium haemophilum* all have been associated with infection.[114-117] Disseminated osteoarticular infection with *Mycobacterium bovis* after bacille Calmette-Guérin vaccination and intravesicular installation of bacille Calmette-Guérin also has been reported.[118]

Medical therapy alone is often curative, although in selected cases surgical débridement is required. Antimicrobial agents typically used in the treatment of osteoarticular infection due to atypical mycobacteria are the same as agents used to treat infection at other sites and are discussed in Chapter 249.

Fungal Osteomyelitis

Osteomyelitis due to fungi is uncommon. Several observational studies and case reports have been published.[119-131] Bone lesions are most common in blastomycosis, disseminated coccidioidomycosis, and extracutaneous sporotrichosis, but are seen occasionally in cryptococcosis, candidiasis, and aspergillosis. The typical epidemiologic risk factors and host characteristics that predispose to mycoses often provides clues as to the fungal etiology. Although most fungal osteomyelitis is hematogenous, trauma with contamination of a wound is a risk factor for fungal osteomyelitis due to molds, including *Pseudallescheria boydii, Scedosporium prolificans,* and *Fusarium* spp. Hematogenous fungal osteomyelitis usually presents clinically as a "cold abscess" and radiologically as a well-defined osteolytic lesion with adjacent soft tissue abscess. In contrast, extracutaneous sporotrichosis causes patchy bone loss and commonly extends to contiguous joints. Surgical débridement of contiguous soft tissue should be done in patients with large collections of pus, but the role of surgery is usually limited to biopsy for diagnosis. Therapy of specific mycoses is discussed in other chapters and in treatment guidelines.[125-131]

Brodie's Abscess

Brodie's abscess refers to a chronic localized bone abscess. Patient with subacute cases may present with fever, pain, and periosteal elevation, whereas patients with chronic Brodie's abscess are often afebrile and present with long-standing dull pain. The most common site of involvement is the distal part of the tibia. The lesion is typically single and located near the metaphysis. Of patients, 75% are younger than 25 years old. Surgical débridement and culture-directed antibiotics are often curative. Cultures may be negative.

Culture-Negative Osteomyelitis

Rarely, bone culture specimens are sterile despite clinical, radiologic, and pathologic evidence of osteomyelitis. Brodie's abscess and bone infarcts due to Gaucher's disease or sickle cell disease should be considered. At our institution, most of these cases are due to prior use of antimicrobial therapy. For indolent cases not responding to therapy, consideration should be given to stopping antibiotics and waiting for at least 1 month before repeating the culture.[132] Antimicrobial therapy may slow the growth of ordinarily hardy organisms.[133] When aerobic and anaerobic bacterial specimens are sterile, cultures should be obtained for fungi and mycobacteria. In selected cases, polymerase chain reaction analysis with use of 16S rRNA gene primers with a broad specificity for detecting bacterial DNA in bone and purulent material can be helpful.[134] If all cultures are negative, we believe that the antimicrobial regimen should be designed to cover the commonly encountered organisms that are clinically suspected, taking into account the history of prior use of antimicrobial agents.

SUMMARY

Despite important medical and surgical advances in management of patients, osteomyelitis remains extremely difficult to treat. The relapse rate can be 20%. The optimal management of osteomyelitis requires a multidisciplinary team of physicians, including an orthopedic surgeon, neurosurgeon, oral surgeon, plastic surgeon, vascular surgeon, invasive radiologist, and infectious disease specialist. The usual goal of therapy is the eradication of the infection and restoration of function. Treatment of chronic osteomyelitis usually requires aggressive surgical débridement and prolonged antimicrobial therapy.

REFERENCES

1. Ramsey SD, Newton K, Blough D, et al. Incidence, outcomes, and cost of foot ulcers in patients with diabetes. Diabetes Care. 1999;22:382-387.
2. Mader JT, Shirtliff M, Calhoun JH. Staging and staging application osteomyelitis. Clin Infect Dis. 1997;25:1303-1309.
3. Lew DP, Waldvogel FA. Osteomyelitis. N Engl J Med. 1997;336:999-1007.
4. Waldvogel FA, Medoff G, Swartz MN. Osteomyelitis. A review of clinical features, therapeutic considerations and unusual aspects. N Engl J Med. 1970;282:316-322.
5. Norden CW. Lessons learned from animal models of osteomyelitis. Rev Infect Dis. 1988;10:103-110.
6. Muller C, Zielinski CC, Passl R, et al. Divergent patterns of leucocyte locomotion in experimental post-traumatic osteomyelitis. Br J Exp Pathol.1984;65:299-303.
7. Norden CW, Shinners E, Niederriter K. Clindamycin treatment of experimental chronic osteomyelitis due to *Staphylococcus aureus*. J Infect Dis.1986;153:956-959.
8. Norden CW. Experimental chronic staphylococcal osteomyelitis in rabbits: Treatment with rifampin alone and in combination with other antimicrobial agents. Rev Infect Dis. 1983;5(Suppl 3):S491-S494.
9. Shirtliff ME, Mader JT, Calhoun J. Oral rifampin plus azithromycin or clarithromycin to treat osteomyelitis in rabbits. Clin Orthop.1999;359:229-236.
10. O'Reilly T, Kunz S, Sande E, et al. Relationship between antibiotic concentration in bone and efficacy of treatment of staphylococcal osteomyelitis in rats: Azithromycin compared with clindamycin and rifampin. Antimicrob Agents Chemother.1992;36:2693-2697.
11. Henry NK, Rouse MS, Whitesell AL, et al. Treatment of methicillin-resistant *Staphylococcus aureus* experimental osteomyelitis with ciprofloxacin or vancomycin alone or in combination with rifampin. Am J Med.1987;82:73-75.
12. Huddleston PM, Steckelberg JM, Hanssen AD, et al. Ciprofloxacin inhibition of experimental fracture-healing. J Bone Joint Surg Am. 2000;82:161-173.
13. Perry AC, Prpa B, Rouse MS, et al. Levofloxacin and trovafloxacin inhibition of experimental fracture-healing. Clin Orthop. 2003;414:95-100.
14. Haleem AA, Rouse MS, Lewallen DG, et al. Effect of gentamicin or vancomycin on experimental fracture healing. (Abstract). Musculoskeletal Infection Society, Aspen, CO, August 2003.
15. Berbari EF, Osmon DR. Osteomyelitis and septic arthritis. In Badour L, Gorbach SL, eds. Therapy of Infectious Diseases. Philadelphia: WB Saunders; 2003:331-342.
16. De Winter F, Vogelaers D, Gemmel F, et al. Promising role of 18-F-fluoro-D-deoxyglucose positron emission tomography in clinical infectious diseases. Eur J Clin Microbiol Infect Dis. 2002;21:247-257.
17. Mackowiak PA, Jones SR, Smith JW. Diagnostic value of sinus-tract cultures in chronic osteomyelitis. JAMA. 1978;239:2772-2775.
18. Key JA. Sulfonamides in the treatment of chronic osteomyelitis. J Bone Joint Surg. 1944;26:63.
19. Tice AD, Hoaglund PA, Shoultz DA. Outcomes of osteomyelitis among patients treated with outpatient parenteral antimicrobial therapy. Am J Med. 2003;114:723-728.
20. Tice AD. Ceftriaxone in treatment of serious infections: Osteomyelitis. Hosp Pract (Office Edition). 1991;26(Suppl 5):31-36.
21. Guglielmo BJ, Luber AD, Paletta D Jr, et al. Ceftriaxone therapy for staphylococcal osteomyelitis: A review. Clin Infect Dis. 2000;30:205-207.
22. Till M, Wixson RL, Pertel PE. Linezolid treatment for osteomyelitis due to vancomycin-resistant *Enterococcus faecium*. Clin Infect Dis. 2002;34:1412-1414.
23. Prokop A, Isenberg J, Seifert H, et al. Linezolid—a new antibiotic for treatment of methicillin resistant *Staphylococcus aureus* infections in trauma surgery? Report of 2 cases. Unfallchirurg. 2002;105:287-291.
24. Waldrep TW, Skiest DJ. Linezolid-induced anemia and thrombocytopenia. Pharmacotherapy. 2002;22:109-112.
25. Patel R, Piper KE, Rouse MS, Steckelberg JM. Linezolid therapy of *Staphylococcus aureus* experimental osteomyelitis. Antimicrob Agents Chemother. 2000;44:3438-3440.
26. Mader JT, Adams K. Comparative evaluation of daptomycin (LY146032) and vancomycin in the treatment of experimental methicillin-resistant *Staphylococcus aureus* osteomyelitis in rabbits. Antimicrob Agents Chemother.1989;33:689-692.
27. Williams DN, Rehm SJ, Tice AD, et al. Practice guidelines for community-based parenteral anti-infective therapy. Clin Infect Dis. 1997;25:787-801.
28. Mendel V, Reichert B, Simanowski HJ, et al. Therapy with hyperbaric oxygen and cefazolin for experimental osteomyelitis due to *Staphylococcus aureus* in rats. Undersea Hyperb Med. 1999;26:169-174.
29. Morrey BF, Dunn JM, Heimbach RD, et al. Hyperbaric oxygen and chronic osteomyelitis. Clin Orthop. 1979;144:121-127.
30. Merritt K. Factors increasing the risk of infection in patients with open fractures. J Trauma. 1988;28:823-827.

31. DeLong WG Jr, Born CT, Wei SY, et al. Aggressive treatment of 119 open fracture wounds. J Trauma. 1999;46:1049-1054.
32. Puno RM, Grossfeld SL, Henry SL, et al. Functional outcome of patients with salvageable limbs with grades III-B and III-C open fractures of the tibia. Microsurgery. 1996;17:167-173.
33. Sterett WI, Ertl JP, Chapman MW, et al. Open tibia fractures in the splenectomized trauma patient: Results of treatment with locking, intramedullary fixation. J Trauma. 1995;38:639-641.
34. Holcombe SJ, Schneider RK, Bramlage LR, et al. Use of antibiotic-impregnated polymethyl methacrylate in horses with open or infected fractures or joints: 19 cases (1987-1995). J Am Vet Med Assoc. 1997;211:889-893.
35. Ostermann PA, Seligson D, Henry SL. Local antibiotic therapy for severe open fractures: A review of 1085 consecutive cases. J Bone Joint Surg Br. 1995;77:93-97.
36. Henry SL, Ostermann PA, Seligson D. The prophylactic use of antibiotic impregnated beads in open fractures. J Trauma. 1990;30:1231-1238.
37. Worlock P, Slack R, Harvey L, et al. The prevention of infection in open fractures: An experimental study of the effect of antibiotic therapy. J Bone Joint Surg Am. 1988;70:1341-1347.
38. Kindsfater K, Jonassen EA. Osteomyelitis in grade II and III open tibia fractures with late debridement. J Orthop Trauma. 1995;9:121-127.
39. Patzakis MJ, Wilkins J, Moore TM. Use of antibiotics in open tibial fractures. Clin Orthop. 1983;178:31-35.
40. Dellinger EP, Caplan ES, Weaver LD, et al. Duration of preventive antibiotic administration for open extremity fractures. Arch Surg. 1988;123:333-339.
41. Clifford RP, Beauchamp CG, Kellam JF, et al. Plate fixation of open fractures of the tibia. J Bone Joint Surg Br. 1988;70:644-648.
42. Clifford RP, Lyons TJ, Webb JK. Complications of external fixation of open fractures of the tibia. Injury. 1987;18:174-176.
43. Chapman MW. The role of intramedullary fixation in open fractures. Clin Orthop. 1986;212:26-34.
44. Etter C, Burri C, Claes L, et al. Treatment by external fixation of open fractures associated with severe soft tissue damage of the leg: Biomechanical principles and clinical experience. Clin Orthop. 1983;178:80-88.
45. Zimmerli W, Widmer AF, Blatter M, et al. Role of rifampin for treatment of orthopedic implant-related staphylococcal infections: A randomized controlled trial. Foreign-Body Infection (FBI) Study Group. JAMA. 1998;279:1537-1541.
46. Drancourt M, Stein A, Argenson JN, et al. Oral rifampin plus ofloxacin for treatment of *Staphylococcus*-infected orthopedic implants. Antimicrob Agents Chemother. 1993;37:1214-1218.
47. Wiley AM, Trueta J. The vascular anatomy of the spine and its relationship to pyogenic vertebral osteomyelitis. J Bone Joint Surg Br. 1959;41:796-804.
48. Honan M, White GW, Eisenberg GM. Spontaneous infectious discitis in adults. Am J Med. 1996;100:85-89.
49. Song KS, Ogden JA, Ganey T, et al. Contiguous discitis and osteomyelitis in children. J Pediatr Orthop. 1997;17:470-477.
50. Schnoring M, Brock M. Prophylactic antibiotics in lumbar disc surgery: Analysis of 1,030 procedures. Z Neurochir. 2003;64:24-29.
51. Pertuiset E, Beaudreuil J, Liote F, et al. Spinal tuberculosis in adults: A study of 103 cases in a developed country, 1980-1994. Medicine. 1999;78:309-320.
52. Maiuri F, Iaconetta G, Gallicchio B, et al. Spondylodiscitis: Clinical and magnetic resonance diagnosis. Spine. 1997;22:1741-1746.
53. Skolnick AA. Interventional radiological treatments tested. JAMA. 1997;277:1424-1425.
54. Hopkinson N, Stevenson J, Benjamin S. A case ascertainment study of septic discitis: Clinical, microbiological and radiological features. QJM. 2001;94:465-470.
55. Vlahakis NE, Temesgen Z, Berbari EF, et al. Osteoarticular infection complicating enterococcal endocarditis. Mayo Clin Proc. 2003;78:623-628.
56. Hadjipavlou AG, Cesani-Vazquez F, Villaneuva-Meyer J, et al. The effectiveness of gallium citrate Ga 67 radionuclide imaging in vertebral osteomyelitis revisited. Am J Orthop. 1998;27:179-183.
57. Nolla JM, Ariza J, Gomez-Vaquero C, et al. Spontaneous pyogenic vertebral osteomyelitis in nondrug users. Semin Arthritis Rheum. 2002;31:271-278.
58. Hadjipavlou AG, Crow WN, Borowski A, et al. Percutaneous transpedicular discectomy and drainage in pyogenic spondylodiscitis. Am J Orthop. 1988;27:188-197.
59. Carragee EJ, Kim D, van der Vlugt T, et al. The clinical use of erythrocyte sedimentation rate in pyogenic vertebral osteomyelitis. Spine. 1997;22:2089-2093.
60. Carragee EJ. The clinical use of magnetic resonance imaging in pyogenic vertebral osteomyelitis. Spine. 1997;22:780-785.
61. Carragee EJ. Instrumentation of the infected and unstable spine: A review of 17 cases from the thoracic and lumbar spine with pyogenic infections. J Spinal Disord. 1997;10:317-324.
62. Barbieri RA, Freeland AE. Osteomyelitis of the hand. Hand Clin.1998;14:589-603.
63. Ramsey SD, Newton K, Blough D, et al. Incidence, outcomes, and cost of foot ulcers in patients with diabetes. Diabetes Care. 1999;22:382-387.
64. Devendra D, Farmer K, Bruce G, et al. Diagnosing osteomyelitis in patients with diabetic neuropathic osteoarthropathy. Diabetes Care. 2001;24:2154-2155.
65. Caputo GM, Cavanagh PR, Ulbrecht JS, et al. Assessment and management of foot disease in patients with diabetes. N Engl J Med. 1994;331:854-860.
66. Carrington AL, Shaw JE, Van Schie CH, et al. Can motor nerve conduction velocity predict foot problems in diabetic subjects over a 6-year outcome period? Diabetes Care. 2002;25:2010-2015.
67. Mason J, O'Keeffe C, Hutchinson A, et al. A systematic review of foot ulcer in patients with type 2 diabetes mellitus: II. Treatment. Diabetic Med.1999;16:889-909.
68. American Diabetes Association. Preventive foot care in people with diabetes. Diabetes Care. 1998;21:2178-2179.
69. Dargis V, Pantelejeva O, Jonushaite A, et al. Benefits of a multidisciplinary approach in the management of recurrent diabetic foot ulceration in Lithuania: A prospective study. Diabetes Care. 1999;22:1428-1431.
70. Faglia E, Favales F, Morabito A. New ulceration, new major amputation, and survival rates in diabetic subjects hospitalized for foot ulceration from 1990 to 1993: A 6.5-year follow-up. Diabetes Care. 2001;24:78-83.
71. Grayson ML, Gibbons GW, Balogh K, et al. Probing to bone in infected pedal ulcers: A clinical sign of underlying osteomyelitis in diabetic patients. JAMA. 1995;273:721-723.
72. Calhoun JH, Overgaard KA, Stevens CM, et al. Diabetic foot ulcers and infections: Current concepts. Adv Skin Wound Care. 2002;15:31-42.
73. Snyder RJ, Cohen MM, Sun C, et al. Osteomyelitis in the diabetic patient: Diagnosis and treatment: Part 2. Medical, surgical, and alternative treatments. Ostomy Wound Manage. 2001;47:24-30, 32-41.
74. Senneville E, Yazdanpanah Y, Cazaubiel M, et al. Rifampicin-ofloxacin oral regimen for the treatment of mild to moderate diabetic foot osteomyelitis. J Antimicrob Chemother. 2001;48:927-930.
75. Ortega M, Soriano A, Garcia S, et al. Tolerability and safety of Levofloxacin long-term treatment. Rev Esp Quimioterapia. 2000;13:263-266.
76. Castineiras AA, Perez-Pascual P, Zarranz JE, et al. Bacteriological conversion in twenty urinary tuberculosis patients treated with ofloxacin, rifampin and isoniazid: A 10-year follow-up study. Int Microbiol. 2002;5:139-144.
77. Lipsky BA, Armstrong D, Acin F, et al. Treating diabetic foot infection with linezolid vs. aminopenicillins: A randomized international multicenter trial (Abstract #189). Presented at Infectious Diseases Society of America meeting, San Francisco, 2002.
78. Vazquez M. Osteomyelitis in children. Curr Opin Pediatr.2002;14:112-115.
79. Trueta J, Morgan JD. The vascular contribution to osteogenesis: I. Studies by the injection method. J Bone Joint Surg Br. 1960;42:97-109.
80. Morrissy RT, Haynes DW. Acute hematogenous osteomyelitis: A model with trauma as an etiologic agent (Abstract). Kappa Delta Paper 2. Presented at American Academy of Orthopedic Surgeons Fifty-first Annual Meeting, Atlanta, GA, 1984.
81. Giedion A, Holthusen W, Masal LF, et al. Subacute and chronic "symmetrical" osteomyelitis. Ann Radiol. 1972;15:329-342.
82. Job-Deslandre C, Krebs S, Kahan A. Chronic recurrent multifocal osteomyelitis: Five-year outcomes in 14 pediatric cases. Joint Bone Spine Rev Rhumatisme. 2001;68:245-251.
83. Beretta-Piccoli BC, Sauvain MJ, Gal I, et al. Synovitis, acne, pustulosis, hyperostosis, osteitis (SAPHO) syndrome in childhood: A report of ten cases and review of the literature. Eur J Pediatr. 2000;159:594-601.
84. Guignard S, Job-Deslandre C, Sayag-Boukris V, et al. Pamidronate treatment in SAPHO syndrome. Joint Bone Spine Rev Rhumatisme. 2002;69:392-396.
85. Olivieri I, Padula A, Ciancio G, et al. Successful treatment of SAPHO syndrome with infliximab: Report of two cases. Ann Rheum Dis. 2002;61:375-376.
86. Mader R, Yeromenco E. Pseudomonas osteomyelitis of the symphysis pubis after inguinal hernia repair. Clin Rheumatol. 1999;18:167-169.
87. Graham CW, Dmochowski RR, Faerber GJ, et al. Pubic osteomyelitis following bladder neck surgery using bone anchors: A report of 9 cases. J Urol. 2002;168:2055-2057.
88. Kammerer-Doak DN, Cornella JL, Magrina JF, et al. Osteitis pubis after Marshall-Marchetti-Krantz urethropexy: A pubic osteomyelitis. Am J Obstet Gynecol. 1998;179(3 Pt 1):586-590.
89. Gerscovich EO, Greenspan A. Osteomyelitis of the clavicle: Clinical, radiologic, and bacteriologic findings in ten patients. Skeletal Radiol. 1994;23:205-210.
90. Alessi DM, Sercarz JA, Calcaterra TC. Osteomyelitis of the clavicle. Arch Otolaryngol Head Neck Surg. 1988;114:1000-1002.
91. Lowden CM, Walsh SJ. Acute staphylococcal osteomyelitis of the clavicle. J Pediatr Orthop. 1997;17:467-469.
92. Hodgson BF. Pyogenic sacroiliac joint infection. Clin Orthop. 1989;246:146-149.
93. Nicholls A, Edward N, Catto GR. Staphylococcal septicaemia, endocarditis, and osteomyelitis in dialysis and renal transplant patients. Postgrad Med J. 1980;56:642-648.
94. Neonato MG, Guilloud-Bataille M, Beauvais P, et al. Acute clinical events in 299 homozygous sickle cell patients living in France. French Study Group on Sickle Cell Disease. Eur J Haematol. 2000;65:155-164.
95. Tamouza R, Neonato MG, Busson M, et al. Infectious complications in sickle cell disease are influenced by HLA class II alleles. Hum Immunol. 2002;63:194-199.
96. Epps CH Jr, Bryant DD 3rd, Coles MJ, et al. Osteomyelitis in patients who have sickle-cell disease: Diagnosis and management. J Bone Joint Surg Am. 1991;73:1281-1294.
97. Chambers JB, Forsythe DA, Bertrand SL, et al. Retrospective review of osteoarticular infections in a pediatric sickle cell age group. J Pediatr Orthop. 2000;20:682-685.
98. Skaggs DL, Kim SK, Greene NW, et al. Differentiation between bone infarction and acute osteomyelitis in children with sickle-cell disease with use of sequential radionuclide bone-marrow and bone scans. J Bone Joint Surg Am. 2001;83:1810-1813.
99. Gifford DB, Patzakis M, Ivler D, et al. Septic arthritis due to *Pseudomonas* in heroin addicts. J Bone Joint Surg Am. 1975;57:631-635.
100. Roca RPP, Yoshikawa TT. Primary skeletal infections in heroin users: A clinical characterization, diagnosis, and therapy. Clin Orthop. 1979;144:238-248.
101. Chandrasekar PH, Narula AP. Bone and joint infections in intravenous drug abusers. Rev Infect Dis. 1986;8:904-911.
102. Kak V, Chandrasekar PH. Bone and joint infections in injection drug users. Infect Dis Clin North Am. 2002;16:681-695.
103. Wallace R, Cohen AS. Tuberculosis arthritis: A report of two cases with review of biopsy and synovial fluid findings. Am J Med. 1976;61:277-282.
104. Gorse GJ, Pais MJ, Kusske JA, et al. Tuberculosis spondylitis: A report of six cases and a review of the literature. Medicine. 1983;62:178-193.
105. Davidson PT, Horowitz I. Skeletal tuberculosis: A review with patient presentations and discussion. Am J Med. 1970;48:77-84.
106. Marchevsky A, Damsker B, Green S, et al. The clinicopathological spectrum of non-tuberculous mycobacterial osteoarticular infection. J Bone Joint Surg Am. 1985;67:925-929.

107. Watts HG, Lifeso RM. Tuberculosis of bones and joints. J Bone Joint Surg Am. 1996;78:288-298.
108. Ikem IC, Bamgboye EA, Olasinde AA. Spinal tuberculosis: A 15 year review at OAUTHC Ile-Ife. Nigerian Postgrad Med J. 2001;8:22-25.
109. Lo Re V 3rd, Barton T, Feiner S. A pain in the back. N Engl J Med. 2001;344:456-457.
110. Babhulkar SS, Pande SK. Unusual manifestations of osteoarticular tuberculosis. Clin Orthop. 2002;398:114-120.
111. Wallace R, Cohen AS. Tuberculosis arthritis: A report of two cases with review of biopsy and synovial fluid findings. Am J Med. 1976;61:277-282.
112. Falk A. Results of long-term chemotherapy in spinal tuberculosis: XVII. A follow-up study of 235 patients. Am Rev Respir Dis. 1967;95:1-5.
113. Gorse GJ, Pais MJ, Kusske JA, et al. Tuberculosis spondylitis: A report of six cases and a review of the literature. Medicine. 1983;62:178-193.
114. Sarria JC, Chutkan NB, Figueroa JE, Hull A. Atypical mycobacterial vertebral osteomyelitis: Case report and review. Clin Infect Dis. 1998;26:503-505.
115. Barbari EF, Hanssen AD, Duffy MG, et al. Prosthetic joint infection due to *Mycobacterium tuberculosis*. Am J Orthop. 1998;27:219-227.
116. Corrales IF, Cortes JA, Mesa ML, et al. Sternal osteomyelitis and scrofuloderma due to BCG vaccination. Biomedica. 2003;23:202-207.
117. Sampaio JL, Alves VA, Leao SC, et al. *Mycobacterium haemophilum*: Emerging or underdiagnosed in Brazil? Emerging Infect Dis. 2002;8:1359-1360.
118. Abu-Nader R, Terrell CL. *Mycobacterium bovis* vertebral osteomyelitis as a complication of intravesical BCG use. Mayo Clin Proc. 2002;77:393-397.
119. Chi CY, Fung CP, Liu CY. *Aspergillus flavus* epidural abscess and osteomyelitis in a diabetic patient. J Microbiol Immunol Infection. 2003;36:145-148.
120. Garbino J, Schnyder I, Lew D, et al. An unusual cause of vertebral osteomyelitis: *Candida* species. Scand J Infect Dis. 2003;35:288-291.
122. Dotis J, Panagopoulou P, Filioti J, et al. Femoral osteomyelitis due to *Aspergillus nidulans* in a patient with chronic granulomatous disease. Infection. 2003;31:121-124.
123. Kaneko J, Sugawara Y, Makuuchi M. Aspergillus osteomyelitis after liver transplantation. Liver Transplant. 2002;8:1073-1075.
124. Maliner LI. Successful treatment of cryptococcal osteomyelitis and paraspinous abscess. South Med J. 2002;95:945.
125. Rex JH, Walsh TJ, Sobel JD, et al. Practice guidelines for the treatment of candidiasis. Clin Infect Dis. 2000;30:662-678.
126. Galgiani JN, Ampel NM, Catanzaro A, et al. Practice guidelines for the treatment of coccidioidomycosis. Clin Infect Dis. 2000;38:656-661.
127. Stevens A, Williams PL. Practice guidelines for the treatment of coccidioidomycosis. Clin Infect Dis. 2000;30:658-661.
128. Chapman SW, Bradsher RW Jr, Campbell GD Jr, et al. Practice guidelines for the management of patients with blastomycosis. Clin Infect Dis. 2000;30:679-683.
129. Stevens DA, Kan VL, Judson MA, et al. Practice guidelines for diseases caused by *Aspergillus*. Clin Infect Dis. 2000;30:696-709.
130. Kauffman CA, Hajjeh R, Chapman SW. Practice guidelines for the management of patients with sporotrichosis. Clin Infect Dis. 2000;30:684-687.
131. Saag MS, Graybill RJ, Larsen RA, et al. Practice guidelines for the management of cryptococcal disease. Clin Infect Dis. 2000;30:710-718.
132. Trampuz A, Hanssen AD, Osmon DR, et al. The role of preoperative antimicrobial therapy on culture sensitivity of joint fluid, periprosthetic tissue, and explant sonicate in the diagnosis of prosthetic joint infection (Abstract). Musculoskeletal Infection Society, Aspen, CO, August 2003.
133. Von Eiff C, Bettin D, Proctor RA, et al. Recovery of small colony variants of *Staphylococcus aureus* following gentamicin bead placement for osteomyelitis. Clin Infect Dis. 1997;25:1250-1251.
134. La Scola B, Michel G, Raoult D. Use of amplification and sequencing of the 16S rRNA gene to diagnose *Mycoplasma pneumoniae* osteomyelitis in a patient with hypogammaglobulinemia. Clin Infect Dis. 1997;24:1161-1163.

CHAPTER **100**

Infections with Prostheses in Bones and Joints

BARRY D. BRAUSE

Prosthetic replacement surgery for hip, knee, shoulder, and elbow joints has become commonplace because of the magnificent success of these procedures in restoring function to persons disabled by arthritis. Patients receiving total joint replacements number in the hundreds of thousands each year worldwide, and millions of people have in-dwelling prosthetic articulations. Between 1% and 5% of indwelling prostheses become infected; this is a calamity for the patient, and it is associated with significant morbidity and occasionally with death. Prosthesis removal, which usually is necessary to treat these infections, produces large skeletal defects, shortening of the extremity, and severe functional impairment. The health care cost of treating a single septic prosthetic joint has been estimated conservatively at $50,000 to $60,000, with an extrapolated expenditure of more than $200 million to $250 million per year in the United States alone.[1] The patient faces protracted hospitalization, sizable financial expense, and potentially renewed disability.

PATHOGENESIS

Certain patient populations have been identified as being predisposed toward infection of their prosthetic joints. These include patients with prior surgery at the site of the prosthesis, rheumatoid arthritis, immunocompromised states, diabetes mellitus, poor nutritional status, obesity, psoriasis, or extremely advanced age.[2-4] Infection usually occurs in osseous tissue adjacent to the foreign body. Because most prostheses are cemented in place with polymethylmethacrylate, infection develops at the bone-cement interface. Sepsis involving cementless prostheses develops in the bone contiguous with the metallic alloy.

Prosthetic joints become infected by two different pathogenetic routes: locally introduced and hematogenous types of osteomyelitis. The locally introduced form of infection is the result of wound sepsis contiguous to the prosthesis or operative contamination. Any factor or event that delays wound healing increases the risk of infection. Ischemic necrosis, infected wound hematomas, wound infection (with or without identifiable cellulitis), and suture abscesses are common preceding events for joint replacement sepsis. During the early postimplantation period, when these superficial infections develop, the fascial layers have not yet healed and the deep, periprosthesis tissue is not protected by the usual physical barriers. These infections usually are caused by a single pathogen, but polymicrobial sepsis with as many as five different organisms is observed. Coagulase-negative staphylococci are the most common etiologic agents in this clinical setting. Infrequently, latent foci of chronic, quiescent osteomyelitis are reactivated by the disruption of tissue associated with implantation surgery. Although bone cultures at the time of the joint replacement operation may be sterile, old *Staphylococcus aureus* and *Mycobacterium tuberculosis* infections can recrudesce postoperatively.[3,5,6]

Any bacteremia can induce infection of a total joint replacement by the hematogenous route.[7-9] A recent prospective study documented a 34% incidence of prosthetic joint infection after *S. aureus* bacteremia.[10] Dentogingival infections and manipulations are known causes of viridans streptococcal and anaerobic *(Peptococcus, Peptostreptococcus)* infections in prostheses. Pyogenic skin processes can cause staphylococcal *(S. aureus, Staphylococcus epidermidis)* and streptococcal (groups A, B, C, and G streptococci) infections of joint replacements. Genitourinary and gastrointestinal tract procedures or infections are associated with gram-negative bacillary, enterococcal, and anaerobic infections of prostheses. Between 20% and 40% of prosthetic joint infections arise by the hematogenous route; the remainder are of the locally introduced type.

The frequency of the presence of specific etiologic microorganisms in prosthetic joint sepsis varies among the published studies, but a general view of the spectrum of this bacteriology and the prominence of certain microbial groups is given in Table 100-1. Staphylococci (coagulase-negative staphylococci and *S. aureus*) are the principal causative agents; aerobic streptococci and gram-negative bacilli are each responsible for 20% to 25%; and anaerobes represent 10% of these infections. The spectrum of microbial agents capable of causing prosthetic joint infection is unlimited and includes organisms ordinarily considered "contaminants" of cultures, such as corynebacteria, propionibacteria, and *Bacillus* spp. Although infections with fungi (particularly *Candida*) and mycobacteria (*M. tuberculosis*) are rare, these infections and proposed treatments have been described.[3,6,11,12]

TABLE 100-1 Bacteriology of Prosthetic Joint Infection

Pathogens	Frequency (%)
Coagulase-negative staphylococci	22
Staphylococcus aureus	22
α-Hemolytic streptococci	9
β-Hemolytic streptococci groups A, B, G	5
Enterococci	7
Gram-negative aerobic bacilli	25
Obligate anaerobes	10

TABLE 100-2 Presenting Symptoms of Prosthetic Joint Infection

Symptom	Frequency (%)
Joint pain	95
Fever	43
Periarticular swelling	38
Wound or cutaneous sinus drainage	32

As foreign bodies, the indwelling metallic prosthesis and the polymethylmethacrylate cement, which binds the metal alloy to adjacent bone, predispose both joint space and osseous tissue to septic processes. Foreign substances contribute to local sepsis experimentally by decreasing the quantity of bacteria necessary to establish infection and by permitting pathogens to persist on their avascular surface, sequestered from circulating immunologic defenses (leukocytes, antibodies, and complement) and from systemic antibiotics.[3,13] Polymethylmethacrylate cement appears to predispose toward infection to an extent beyond that of other inert foreign substances. The cement in unpolymerized form has been shown to inhibit phagocytic, lymphocytic, and complement function in vitro.[14,15] The polymerization process itself appears to enhance the risk of infection, possibly because of the substantial heat generated by this in vivo reaction.[14] In an effort to provide total joint replacement without polymethylmethacrylate, cementless prostheses have been designed. These devices have textured surfaces to provide for fixation by the growth of adjacent bone into the "porous" interface of the prosthesis. The current data on this form of arthroplasty reveal no apparent effect on the occurrence of infection.[16]

Host responses to methylmethacrylate also may play a role in the pathogenesis of infection. Fibronectin, a connective tissue and plasma glycoprotein, appears to enhance *S. aureus* adherence to polymethylmethacrylate in vivo and may contribute to the occurrence of sepsis.[17,18] Microbial products may assist the development and persistence of infection in association with foreign substances. In the presence of prosthetic devices, many bacteria elaborate a fibrous exopolysaccharide material called *glycocalyx*. Organisms can grow within this matrix and form thick biofilms that are protected at least in part from host defense mechanisms.[2,19] Bacteria adherent to biomaterials demonstrate decreased quantitative susceptibility to antibiotics both in vitro and in vivo.[20-22]

CLINICAL PRESENTATION

Prosthetic joint sepsis produces the cardinal symptoms of inflammation with a wide spectrum of severity. Most patients present with a long, indolent course characterized by a progressive increase in joint pain and occasionally by the formation of cutaneous draining sinuses, but not by fever, soft tissue swelling, or systemic toxicity. Others present with an acute, fulminant illness with high fever, severe joint pain, local swelling, and erythema. The frequencies of these presenting symptoms are listed in Table 100-2.[23]

The pattern of clinical presentation is determined largely by three factors: the virulence of the infecting pathogen, the nature of the host tissue in which the microorganism grows, and the route of infection. *S. aureus* is a particularly virulent pathogen in this setting and usually produces a fulminant infection (occasionally with septic shock). β-Hemolytic streptococci and aerobic gram-negative bacilli are also capable of causing this clinical picture. Alternatively, the relatively avirulent but tenacious coagulase-negative staphylococci are consistently associated with an indolent course.

Characteristics of the involved tissue can influence the type of presentation on the basis of their support of microbial growth. Wound hematomas (as well as seromas and hemarthroses), fresh operative wounds, ischemic wounds, and tissues in diabetic and steroid-treated patients all enhance the ability of bacteria to multiply rapidly in ex-

pansive tissue planes. These factors promote the development of a more fulminant infection if a large inoculum of bacteria is allowed access to deep tissue compartments during surgery or in a slowly healing wound postoperatively.

The hematogenous route of infection theoretically seeds the bone-cement interface with a relatively small number of organisms. When a bloodborne infection arises in a prosthetic joint several months or years after implantation surgery, the fully healed connective tissue often is capable of restricting the septic process to a relatively small but critical focus at the bone-cement interface. Joint pain is the principal symptom of deep tissue infection regardless of the mode of presentation. It suggests either acute inflammation of periarticular tissue or loosening of the prosthesis as a result of subacute erosion of bone at the bone-cement interface.

DIAGNOSIS

The clinical manifestations previously described (i.e., joint pain, swelling, erythema, and warmth) all reflect an underlying inflammatory process in the surrounding tissues but are not specific for infection. If a painful prosthesis is accompanied by a fever or purulent drainage from overlying cutaneous sinuses, infection may be presumed, pending further confirmatory tests. However, in most cases, infection must be differentiated from aseptic and mechanical problems (e.g., hemarthrosis, gout, bland loosening, dislocation, metallic debris-induced synovitis, osteolysis), which are more common causes of pain and inflammatory symptoms in these patients.

Constant joint pain is suggestive of infection, whereas mechanical loosening commonly causes pain only with motion and weight bearing.[2] Plain radiographs can reveal (1) abnormal lucencies greater than 2 mm in width at the bone-cement interface, (2) changes in the position of prosthetic components, (3) cement fractures, (4) periosteal reaction, or (5) motion of components on stress views. In addition, the intra-articular injection of dye (arthrography) may reveal abnormal communications between the joint space and multiple defects in the bone-cement interface. These radiologic abnormalities (Fig. 100-1) are found in 50% of septic prostheses. They are generally related to the duration of infection, because 3 to 6 months may be required before manifestation of such changes. If both distal and proximal components of a prosthetic joint demonstrate radiographic pathology, sepsis is more likely than is simple mechanical loosening. However, these changes seen on radiography are not specific for infection, because they are also seen frequently with aseptic processes.

Radioisotopic scans with technetium diphosphonate demonstrate increased uptake in areas of bone with enhanced blood supply or increased metabolic activity. Increased technetium uptake is seen routinely around normal prostheses for 6 months after arthroplasty. Positive scan findings after this period are abnormal and reflect inflammation and possible loosening but not specifically infection of the implant. Sequential technetium-gallium bone scanning is also nondiagnostic because of unacceptable sensitivity (66%) and specificity (81%).[24] Indium-labeled leukocyte scanning is inconsistently sensitive and provides only nonspecific results.[25,26] A normal or negative technetium scan can be considered evidence against the presence of infection, but a positive radioisotopic scan, of any type, is not definitive in establishing the diagnosis of arthroplasty infection. Elevated peripheral

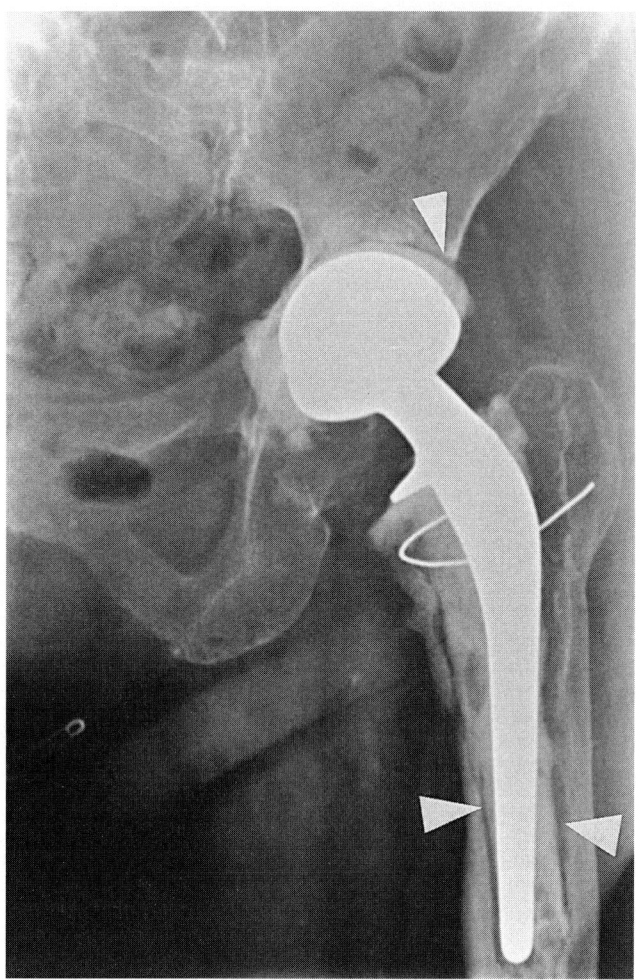

FIGURE 100-1. A plain radiograph of an infected total hip prosthesis demonstrates lucencies at the bone-cement interface of both femoral and acetabular components *(arrowheads).*

TABLE 100-3 Diagnostic Value of the Number of Positive Operative Cultures (for the Same Organism) When Three to Six Specimens Are Examined

Number Positive	Probability of Infection (%)
3	94.8
2	20.4
1	13.3
0	3.4

From Atkins BL, Athanasou N, Deeks JJ, et al. Prospective evaluation of criteria for microbiologic diagnosis of prosthetic-joint infection at revision arthroplasty. J Clin Microbiol. 1998;36:2932-2939.

ficulty is encountered in obtaining intra-articular fluid, irrigation with sterile normal saline solution (without antiseptic preservative additives) can be used to provide the necessary fluid for culture. If initial cultures reveal a relatively avirulent organism (*S. epidermidis,* corynebacteria, propionibacteria, or *Bacillus* spp.), a second aspirate should be considered to reconfirm the bacteriologic diagnosis and to eliminate the possibility that the isolate is artifactual.

Operative cultures are used to definitively diagnose prosthetic joint infection; therefore, the patient should not receive antimicrobial therapy for several weeks before surgery. Optimally several (five to seven) specimens of tissue and fluid should be submitted for culture. Atkins and colleagues[28] calculated the diagnostic value of the number of positive operative cultures (for the same organism). If three to six specimens are submitted to the microbiology laboratory, then a finding of no positive cultures represents a 3.4 % probability of infection; one positive culture represents a 13.3% probability, two positive cultures a 20.4% probability, and three positive cultures a 94.8% probability of prosthetic joint infection (Table 100-3). The results of these microbiologic techniques and analyses should confirm the presence and nature of the infection and allow for optimal treatment. In the uncommon circumstance in which the clinical suggestion of sepsis is strong but the cultures are sterile, fastidious organisms (particularly anaerobes) should be suspected. Mycobacteria and fungi should also be considered as possible etiologic pathogens in appropriate clinical circumstances. To design the most efficacious and least toxic antimicrobial therapy, the patient's infecting strain of bacteria must first be available for in vitro evaluation (described later).

THERAPY

Successful treatment of a total joint arthroplasty infection depends on extensive and meticulous surgical débridement and effective antimicrobial therapy. Simple surgical drainage (with retention of the prosthesis in situ) followed by antibiotic therapy has been successful in only 20% to 36% of cases.[29-31] The results of recent attempts to avoid removal of infected prostheses suggest that treatment without prosthesis removal is more likely to be successful if there has been a short duration of symptoms and signs or in cases of infection with certain specific pathogens.[30,31,32-35] Early postoperative infections (<1 month after implantation) and early hematogenous infections (<1 month of symptoms) treated without prosthesis removal have had reported success rates of approximately 71% in small numbers of patients receiving a single débridement followed by 4 to 6 weeks of antibiotic therapy.[32,33] Some of these cases may have had false-positive cultures in this setting, which could inflate the success rate; other studies have been far less successful.[30,31,34] In one group of patients with hip prostheses, débridement with retention of the implant was successful in only 23% of those who had had symptoms for less than 2 weeks; if symptoms had been present for longer than 2 weeks, no patients were successfully treated.[30] Another study reported only a 38% overall success rate with implant retention and noted that patients in whom treatment was successful had been symptomatic for an average of 5 days, whereas those for whom treatment failed had been symptomatic for a mean of 54 days.[34]

leukocyte counts, erythrocyte sedimentation rates, and C-reactive protein levels, although suggestive, also are inadequate to diagnose sepsis in this clinical setting.[26]

The specific diagnosis of joint replacement infection depends, in large part, on isolation of the pathogen by aspiration of joint fluid or by culture of tissue obtained at arthrotomy.[26,27] Analysis of joint fluid often reveals a high leukocyte count (mainly polymorphonuclear cells), a high protein content, and a low glucose concentration. However, these changes are only variably present and are neither prerequisites for making the diagnosis of joint replacement infection nor specific for this entity. Histopathologic examination of periprosthetic tissue frequently reveals an infiltration of polymorphonuclear leukocytes, indicative of an acute inflammatory reaction, but this parameter is only variably present (probably because of the sampling limitations of frozen-section histopathology) and also may not be sufficiently specific. Therefore, the single observation that delineates the presence of implant infection is isolation of the pathogen by arthrocentesis or surgical débridement.

Because fastidious microorganisms, including anaerobes, may be etiologic agents in prosthetic arthroplasty infections, multiple specimens should be obtained and rapidly cultured in appropriate media. Arthrocentesis demonstrated the pathogen with sensitivities of 86% to 92% and specificities of 82% to 97% in the larger studies.[26,27] Gram staining is positive in 32% of cases. Fluoroscopic guidance and arthrography are useful to document accurate needle placement. If dif-

Antibiotic therapy with prosthesis retention eradicated only 36% of *S. aureus* infections in another study.[31] The cumulative probability of failure of treatment within the first 2 years in these patients was 50% if symptoms were present for 2 days or less and 90% if symptoms were present for longer than 2 days. In contradistinction to these reports, 89.5% of patients whose prosthetic joints were infected with penicillin-susceptible streptococci, all of whom had been symptomatic for 10 days or less, were successfully treated without implant removal.[35]

Success with long courses (3 to 6 months) of antibiotic therapy using rifampin in combination with other antimicrobial agents was reported in selected patients with retained orthopedic implants.[36] However, most of these infected implants were fracture fixation devices and not septic total joint prostheses; infections of the latter appear to be more difficult to cure. Nonetheless, rifampin, as a zwitterion, has an enhanced capacity to penetrate membranes and biofilms and therefore may be a critically important antibiotic in the treatment of infected prosthetic articulations.

For more predictably effective treatment of prosthetic joint infection, complete removal of all foreign materials (metallic prosthesis, cement, and any accompanying biofilm) is essential. Prosthesis extraction and reimplantation can be accomplished in a single-stage (exchange) procedure or in a more efficacious two-stage approach.

The most successful protocol incorporates standardized antimicrobial therapy with a two-stage surgical procedure. Removal of the prosthesis and cement is followed by a 6-week course of bactericidal antibiotic therapy chosen on the basis of quantitative in vitro susceptibility studies. Reimplantation is performed at the conclusion of the 6-week antibiotic course. Use of methylmethacrylate cement impregnated with an antimicrobial agent (usually tobramycin or gentamicin with or without vancomycin) has not been subjected to controlled trials but is commonly practiced. The antimicrobial agents leach out from the hardened plastic (cement) to produce variable but high initial release and protracted diffusion of antibiotic into surrounding tissues at the bone-cement interface.[37-39] Antibiotic-loaded polymethylmethacrylate is also commonly used in cement spacers inserted after prosthesis removal to facilitate delayed reimplantation. With this protocol, a 90% to 96% success rate has been achieved in total hip replacement infections, and a 97% success rate in total knee replacement infections.[4,40-44] The success of this regimen relies on thorough débridement techniques and effective antimicrobial therapy. In this manner, both gram-positive bacteria (including multidrug-resistant staphylococci and enterococci) and gram-negative bacteria (including *Pseudomonas aeruginosa*) can be eliminated if the specific sensitivity of each isolate allows eradication.[45] The empirical selection of a 6-week duration of antibiotic therapy may be critical for efficacy. Others have employed a similar approach to therapy but with only a 2-week course of antibiotic treatment before reinsertion of the prosthesis.[46] With this protocol, the pathogen was eradicated in only 79% of the cases, and only 35% of the patients obtained good function with the new prosthesis.

The alternative method of treatment involves extraction of the metallic joint and cement with immediate reimplantation of a new prosthesis in a one-stage surgical procedure (exchange operation) accompanied by antimicrobial therapy. Antibiotic-loaded methylmethacrylate cement is used during reimplantation. The protocol is effective in 70% to 83% of cases.[4,47-50] If the exchange operation is repeated (in those for whom the first replacement failed) and antibiotic-laden cement is used, the success rate is increased to 90%.[48] It has been suggested that this mode of therapy is applicable only to infections with the less virulent microorganisms, because high failure rates are observed when the pathogen is *S. aureus* or a gram-negative bacillus.[51] Systemic antibiotics are administered rarely and without standardization in this regimen. Moreover, the customary selection of an aminoglycoside as a component in the recementing phase of these operations may not reflect the susceptibility of the pathogen being treated. Currently, surgeons have the additional option of including vancomycin with the aminoglycoside in loading the cement; this should increase the effectiveness of this local, depot administration of antibiotic therapy.[38,39] Although the two-stage removal-reimplantation approach is more effective, the one-stage procedure is often used for elderly or infirm patients who might not tolerate protracted bed rest and a second major operation.[52]

Present therapeutic interventions include the most efficacious parts of these two protocols, combining a 6-week antibiotic regimen and two-stage prosthesis removal-reimplantation surgery with the incorporation of antibiotic-impregnated cement during arthroplasty reinsertion.[43,44] In those clinical situations in which adequate antimicrobial potency cannot be achieved, arthrodesis or resection arthroplasty is recommended, rather than an attempt at prosthesis reimplantation. However, with the advent of antibiotic-impregnated cement incorporating new antimicrobial agents, even patients in these difficult cases may be candidates for another total joint arthroplasty.

SUPPRESSIVE ANTIBIOTIC THERAPY

Although removal of the implanted prosthesis is necessary to confidently eradicate deep infection associated with these devices, this therapeutic approach is not always available. Occasionally, surgical excision is contraindicated as a result of medical and surgical conditions or patient refusal. Because it is likely that the pathogen will be able to persist at the undébrided bone-cement interface despite high-dose, finite systemic antimicrobial therapy, lifelong oral antibiotic treatment may be considered to suppress the infection and retain the usefulness of the total joint replacement. In selected cases in which (1) prosthesis removal is not possible, (2) the pathogen is relatively avirulent, (3) the pathogen is exquisitely sensitive to an orally absorbed antibiotic, (4) the patient can tolerate an appropriate oral antibiotic, and (5) the prosthesis is not loose, suppressive oral antimicrobial therapy may be of value. Successful retention of a functioning hip arthroplasty was observed in 63% of patients when all five criteria were fulfilled.[53] However, when similar therapy was employed in total knee replacements infected with a variety of microorganisms (both virulent and relatively avirulent), successful joint function was only variably maintained in 26% to 82% of patients.[54,55] The suppressive approach is not without risk. Serial radiographs are needed over the course of treatment to monitor for progressive bone resorption at the bone-cement interface, which could reduce the success of any future revision surgery. Secondary resistance can emerge, and, despite continual antibiotic therapy, the localized septic process can extend into adjacent tissue compartments or become a systemic infection.[36,56] Moreover, the patient is subjected to the potential side effects of chronic antibiotic administration.

PREVENTION OF JOINT PROSTHESIS INFECTION

In view of the catastrophic effects of prosthetic arthroplasty infection, prevention of these septic processes is of prime importance. In anticipation of elective total joint replacement surgery, the patient should be evaluated for the presence of pyogenic dentogingival pathology, obstructive uropathy, and dermatologic conditions that might predispose to infection and bacteremia. Strong consideration should be given to reducing the risks represented by these factors (i.e., dental extraction, prostatic resection, control of dermatitis) before insertion of the prosthesis. Perioperative antibiotic prophylaxis has been shown to reduce deep wound infection effectively in total joint replacement surgery.[57] Oxacillin or cefazolin is commonly administered as an antistaphylococcal agent immediately before the operation and for 1 to 2 days thereafter. The use of aminoglycoside-impregnated cement during implantation may additionally decrease the incidence of infection.[58] Filtered laminar airflow systems in the operating room further reduce infection rates, especially if whole-body, exhaust-ventilated suits are worn by the operating team.[59,60] For patients with indwelling joint prostheses, early recognition and prompt therapy for infection in any location is critical to reduce the risk of seeding the joint implant hematogenously. Situations that are likely to cause bacteremia should be avoided. The use of prophylactic antibiotics in anticipation of bacteremic events (i.e., dental surgery, cystoscopy, colonoscopic biopsy, surgical procedures on infected or contaminated tissues) has been suggested on the same empirical basis on which endocarditis prophylaxis is recommended.[3,8] This approach to prevention is controversial, and no data are available with which to determine the adequacy or the cost-effectiveness of such measures. The American Dental Association and the American Academy of Orthopedic Surgeons have jointly advised that a single dose of prophylactic antibiotic be given to selected patients undergoing dental procedures associated with significant bleeding (including periodontal scaling).[61] The selected patient populations include patients with inflammatory arthropathies, immunosuppression, diabetes mellitus, malnutrition, hemophilia, or previous prosthetic joint infection, as well as all patients undergoing these procedures within 2 years after joint replacement. More recently, the American Urologic Association and the American Academy of Orthopedic Surgeons have jointly advised that prophylactic antibiotics be considered in similar selected patient populations undergoing urologic procedures with higher bacteremic risk.[62] Clinical decisions regarding prophylactic antibiotics for expected bacteremias in patients with prosthetic joints should be made on an individual basis.

REFERENCES

1. Sculco TP. The economic impact of infected joint arthroplasty. Orthopedics. 1995;18:871-873.
2. Gristina AG, Kolkin J. Total joint replacement and sepsis. J Bone Joint Surg Am. 1983;65:128-134.
3. Brause BD. Prosthetic joint infections. Curr Opin Rheumatol. 1989;1:194-198.
4. Hanssen AD, Rand JA. Evaluation and treatment of infection at the site of a total hip or knee arthroplasty. J Bone Joint Surg Am. 1998;80:910-922.
5. Kim Y-H, Oh S-H, Kim J-S. Total hip arthroplasty in adult patients who had childhood infection of the hip. J Bone Joint Surg Am. 2003;85:198-204.
6. Hugate R Jr, Pellegrini VD Jr. Reactivation of ancient tuberculous arthritis of the hip following total hip arthroplasty. J Bone Joint Surg Am. 2002;84:101-105.
7. Ahlberg A, Carlsson AS, Lindberg L. Hematogenous infection in total joint replacement. Clin Orthop. 1978;137:69-75.
8. Maderazo EG, Judson S, Pasternak H. Late infections of total joint prostheses: A review and recommendations for prevention. Clin Orthop. 1988;229:131-142.
9. Lindqvist C, Slatis P. Dental bacteremia: A neglected cause of arthroplasty infections? Acta Orthop Scand. 1985;56:506-508.
10. Murdoch DR, Roberts SA, Fowler VG Jr, et al. Infection of orthopedic prostheses after *Staphylococcus aureus* bacteremia. Clin Infect Dis. 2001;32:647-649.
11. Phelan DM, Osmon DR, Keatnig MR, Hanssen AD. Delayed reimplantation arthroplasty for candidal prosthetic joint infection: A report of 4 cases and review of the literature. Clin Infect Dis. 2002;34:930-938.
12. Simonian PT, Brause BD, Wickiewicz TL. *Candida* infection after total knee arthroplasty: Management without resection or amphotericin B. J Arthroplasty. 1997;12:825-829.
13. Petty W, Spanier S, Shuster JJ, et al. The influence of skeletal implants on incidence of infection. J Bone Joint Surg Am. 1985;67:1236-1244.
14. Petty W. The effect of methylmethacrylate on bacterial inhibiting properties of normal human serum. Clin Orthop. 1978;132:266-277.
15. Petty W. The effect of methylmethacrylate on bacterial phagocytosis and killing by human polymorphonuclear leukocytes. J Bone Joint Surg Am. 1978;60:752-757.
16. Nestor BJ, Hanssen AD, Ferrer-Gonzalez R, Fitzgerald RH. The use of porous prostheses in delayed reconstruction of total hip replacements that have failed because of infection. J Bone Joint Surg Am. 1994;76:349-359.
17. Vaudaux P, Suzuki R, Waldvogel FA, et al. Foreign-body infection: Role of fibronectin as a ligand for the adherence of *Staphylococcus aureus*. J Infect Dis. 1984;150:546-553.
18. Darouiche RO. Device-associated infections: A macroproblem that starts with microadherence. Clin Infect Dis. 2001;33:1567-1572.
19. Costerton JW, Irvin RT, Cheng K-J. The bacterial glycocalyx in nature and disease. Annu Rev Microbiol. 1981;35:299-324.
20. Gristina AG, Jennings RA, Naylor PT, et al. Comparative in vitro antibiotic resistance of surface-colonizing coagulase-negative staphylococci. Antimicrob Agents Chemother. 1989;33:813-816.
21. Widmer AF, Frei R, Rajacic Z, et al. Correlation between in vivo and in vitro efficacy of antimicrobial agents against foreign body infections. J Infect Dis. 1990;162: 96-102.
22. Donlon RM. Biofilm formation: A clinically relevant microbiologic process. Clin Infect Dis. 2001;33:1387-1392.
23. Inman JN, Gallegos KV, Brause BD, et al. Clinical and microbial features of prosthetic joint infection. Am J Med. 1984;77:47-53.
24. Merkel KD, Brown ML, Fitzgerald RH. Sequential technetium-99m HMDP-gallium-67 citrate imaging for the evaluation of infection in the painful prosthesis. J Nucl Med. 1986;27:1413-1417.
25. Lentino JR. Prosthetic joint infections: Bane of orthopedists, challenge for infectious disease specialists. Clin Infect Dis. 2003;36:1157-1161.
26. Spangehl MJ, Younger ASE, Masri BA, et al. Diagnosis of infection following total hip arthroplasty. J Bone Joint Surg Am. 1997;79:1578-1588.
27. Lachiewicz PF, Rogers GD, Thomason HG. Aspiration of the hip joint before revision total hip arthroplasty. J Bone Joint Surg Am. 1996;78:749-754.
28. Atkins BL, Athanasou N, Deeks JJ, et al. Prospective evaluation of criteria for microbiologic diagnosis of prosthetic-joint infection at revision arthroplasty. J Clin Microbiol. 1998;36:2932-2939.
29. Fitzgerald RH, Nolan DR, Ilstrup DM, et al. Deep wound sepsis following total hip arthroplasty. J Bone Joint Surg Am. 1977;59:847-855.
30. Crockarell JR, Hanssen AD, Osmon DR, Morrey BF. Treatment of infection with debridement and retention of the components following hip arthroplasty. J Bone Joint Surg Am. 1998;80:1306-1313.
31. Brandt CM, Sistrunk WW, Duffy MC, et al. *Staphylococcus aureus* prosthetic joint infection treated with debridement and prosthesis retention. Clin Infect Dis. 1997;24:914-919.
32. Tsukayama DT, Estrada R, Gustilo RB. Infection after total hip arthroplasty. J Bone Joint Surg Am. 1996;78:512-523.
33. Mont MA, Waldman B, Banerjee C, et al. Multiple irrigation, debridement, and retention of components in infected total knee arthroplasty. J Arthroplasty. 1997;12:426-433.
34. Tattevin P, Cremieux A-C, Pottier P, et al. Prosthetic joint infection: When can prosthesis salvage be considered? Clin Infect Dis. 1999;29:292-295.
35. Meehan AM, Osmon DR, Duffy MCT, et al. Outcome of penicillin-susceptible streptococcal prosthetic joint infection treated with debridement and retention of the prosthesis. Clin Infect Dis. 2003;36:845-849.
36. Zimmerli W, Widmer AF, Blatter M, et al. Role of rifampin for treatment of orthopedic implant-related staphylococcal infections. JAMA. 1998;279:1537-1541.
37. Wininger DA, Fass RJ. Antibiotic impregnated cement and beads for orthopedic infections. Antimicrob Agents Chemother. 1996;40:2675-2679.
38. Gonzales Della Valle A, Bostrom M, Brause B, et al. Effective bactericidal activity of tobramycin and vancomycin eluted from acrylic bone cement. Acta Orthop Scand. 2001;72:237-240.
39. Masri BA, Duncan CP, Beauchamp CP. Long-term elution of antibiotics from bonecement: An in vivo study using the prosthesis of antibiotic-loaded acrylic cement (PROSTALAC) system. J Arthroplasty.1998;13:331-338.
40. Callaghan JJ, Salvati EA, Brause BD, et al. Reimplantation for salvage of the infected hip. In: The Hip: Proceedings of the 14th Open Scientific Meeting of The Hip Society. St Louis: CV Mosby; 1986:65-94.
41. Windsor RE, Insall JN, Urs WK, et al. Two-stage reimplantation for the salvage of total knee arthroplasty complicated by infection. J Bone Joint Surg Am. 1990;72: 272-278.
42. Salvati EA, Chekofsky KM, Brause BD, et al. Reimplantation in infection. Clin Orthop. 1982;170:62-75.
43. Lieberman JR, Callaway GH, Salvati EA, et al. Treatment of the infected total hip arthroplasty with a two-stage reimplantation protocol. Clin Orthop. 1994;301: 205-212.
44. Garvin KL, Salvati EA, Brause BD. Role of gentamicin-impregnated cement in total joint arthroplasty. Orthop Clin North Am. 1988;19:605-610.
45. Kilgus DJ, Howe DJ, Strang A. Results of periprosthetic hip and knee infections caused by resistant bacteria. Clin Orthop. 2002;404:116-124.
46. Rand JA, Bryan RS. Reimplantation for the salvage of an infected total knee arthroplasty. J Bone Joint Surg Am. 1983;65:1081-1086.
47. Buchholz HW, Elson RA, Lodenkamper H. The infected joint implant. In: McKibbin B, ed. Recent Advances in Orthopedics. Edinburgh: Churchill Livingstone; 1979: 139-161.
48. Buchholz HW, Elson R, Engelbrecht E. Management of deep infection of total hip replacement. J Bone Joint Surg Br. 1981;63:342-353.
49. Carlsson AS, Josefsson G, Lindberg L. Revision with gentamicin-impregnated cement for deep infection in total hip arthroplasties. J Bone Joint Surg Am. 1978;60:1059-1064.
50. Jackson WO, Schmalzried TP. Limited role of direct exchange arthroplasty in the treatment of infected total hip replacements. Clin Orthop. 2000;381:101-105.
51. Fitzgerald RH, Jones DR. Hip implant infection. Am J Med. 1986;78(Suppl 6B): 225-228.
52. Garvin KL, Hanssen AD. Infection after total hip arthroplasty. J Bone Joint Surg Am. 1995;77:1576-1588.
53. Goulet JA, Pellicci PM, Brause BD, et al. Prolonged suppression of infection in total hip arthroplasty. J Arthroplasty. 1988;3:109-116.
54. Ayers DC, Dennis DA, Johanson NA. Common complications of total knee arthroplasty. J Bone Joint Surg Am. 1997;79:278-311.
55. Segreti J, Nelson JA, Trenholme GM. Prolonged suppressive antibiotic therapy for infected orthopedic prostheses. Clin Infect Dis. 1998;27:711-713.
56. Thornes B, Murray P, Bouchier-Hayes D. Development of resistant strains of *Staphylococcus epidermidis* on gentamicin-loaded bone cement in vivo. J Bone Joint Surg Br. 2002;84:758-760.
57. Norden C. A critical review of antibiotic prophylaxis in orthopedic surgery. Rev Infect Dis. 1983;5:928-932.
58. Espehaug B, Engesaeter LB, Vollset SE, et al. Antibiotic prophylaxis in total hip arthroplasty. J Bone Joint Surg Br. 1997;79:590-595.

59. Lidwell O, Lowbury E, Whyte E. Effect of ultraclean air in operating rooms on deep sepsis in the joint after total hip or total knee replacement. BMJ. 1982;285:10-14.

60. Salvati EA, Robinson RP, Zeno SM, et al. Infection rates after 3175 total hip and total knee replacements performed with and without a horizontal unidirectional filtered air-flow system. J Bone Joint Surg Am. 1982;64:525-535.

61. American Dental Association, American Academy of Orthopaedic Surgeons. Advisory statement: Antibiotic prophylaxis for dental patients with total joint replacements. J Am Dental Assoc. 1997;128:1004-1007.

62. American Urologic Association, American Academy of Orthopaedic Surgeons. Advisory statement: Antibiotic prophylaxis for urologic patients with total joint replacements. J Urol 2003;169:1796-1797.

CHAPTER **101**

Genital Skin and Mucous Membrane Lesions

MICHAEL H. AUGENBRAUN

Genital lesions are of uncertain historical pedigree. Ancient Chinese medical writings dating back perhaps to as early as 2500 BC appear to have alluded to a "corroding ulcer" of the genitals developing a few days after coitus.[1] There are references throughout the Old Testament to genital pathology that may have been infectious in nature. Ancient Greek, Roman, and Arabic medical texts also suggest a familiarity with acute genital infections, but the descriptions are difficult to associate with any specific clinical syndrome recognized today.[2,3]

Although genital lesions originate from a wide range of infectious processes, they most commonly result from sexually transmitted diseases or venereal infections (Box 101-1).[4-7] Other pathologic processes, including chemical and mechanical trauma, neoplasia, and immunologic phenomena, can also cause genital lesions (Box 101-2). The term "venereal" as it relates to disease dates to the 15th century. Its root comes from the Latin *venereus* or *venus,* meaning "from sexual love or desire." In the United States, the most common causes of sexually transmitted genital lesions are herpes simplex virus type 2 (HSV-2), *Treponema pallidum* (syphilis), *Haemophilus ducreyi* (chancroid), and human papillomavirus (HPV).[8]

BOX 101-1

Infectious Causes of Genital Lesions

Sexually Transmitted Infections
Syphilis
   Primary (chancre)
   Secondary (condyloma latum)
Herpes simplex virus types 1 and 2
Chancroid (*Haemophilus ducreyi*)
Lymphogranuloma venereum
Granuloma inguinale (donovanosis)
Human papillomavirus
Sarcoptes scabiei
Molluscum contagiosum

Nonsexually Transmitted Infections
Folliculitis
Tuberculosis
Tularemia
Histoplasmosis
Candida (balanitis or vaginitis)
Amebiasis

BOX 101-2

Nonvenereal Causes of Genital Lesions

Trauma
Malignancies (e.g., squamous cell carcinoma)
Behçet's syndrome
Fixed drug eruption
Eczema
Psoriasis
Inflammatory bowel disease
Contact dermatitis
Lichen planus
Hidradenitis suppurativa
Postinflammatory hypopigmentation
Aphthous ulcers (associated with human immunodeficiency virus)

Infectious genital lesions are unique in a number of ways when compared with other infectious processes. Most are communicable and therefore are not only a clinical concern but also a public health concern. Infectious genital lesions can harbor more than one pathogen at a time, making proper diagnosis and management a challenge.[9,10] Morphologic appearance of the ulcer or lesion itself can differ widely from one process to another and even within any single specific pathology. The unpredictable nature of lesion presentation can also make a purely clinical diagnosis unreliable.[11-13] Inflammatory epithelial defects characteristic of these pathologies appear to enhance the transmission of other diseases, most importantly human immunodeficiency virus (HIV). Genital lesions may contribute substantially to the worldwide spread of this disease.[14-18]

This chapter focuses on the broad issues relevant to the assessment and management of genital lesions. For in-depth discussions of individual pathogens, readers are directed to the chapters that address those topics.

HISTORY OF PRESENTATION

Individuals who present with a new genital lesion and who report recent sexual activity, particularly activity with a new partner or someone with a suspected genital infection, are likely to have a sexually transmitted infection. On the other hand, certain clinical circumstances suggest non–sexually transmitted pathology, such as trauma, chemical irritation, or allergic hypersensitivity. A lesion that occurs proximate to sexual exposure (i.e., within hours to 1 or 2 days) may be too early to be accounted for by the incubation period of most infectious pathologies. In the case of a lesion with rapid onset, the nature of the sexual activity, a topic often left unexplored by the clinician and patient, may suggest trauma.[19,20] Traumatic genital lesions may result from sexual assault, questions about which are also often avoided.[21] Recurrent lesions in someone who uses or whose partner uses latex condoms may be attributable to a latex allergy, although allergy typically results in more generalized edema and erythema of the genitals rather than a focal ulcer or papular lesion.[22] Geographic prevalences may be important factors to consider when assessing a genital lesion in a traveler.

A history of recurrent genital lesions with or without dysesthesias preceding the development of lesions usually suggests an infection with HSV. HSV-2, and, less commonly, HSV-1, cause a chronic genital ulcer disease that is characterized by repeated symptomatic or often subclinical outbreaks separated by variable periods of quiescence during which the virus is localized to the dorsal root ganglia. A variety of factors are postulated to precipitate viral shedding, including immunosuppression, other intercurrent illnesses, sun exposure, and menses.[23]

Host factors can be important historical determinants of genital lesion etiology. Patients with preexistent psoriasis or eczema or other noninfectious dermatitides may have a genital lesion related to the underlying dermatologic pathology. Recent history of medication use such as tetracyclines or antineoplastics in someone presenting with a new genital lesion can prompt consideration of a fixed drug eruption. In these cases, lesions may be characterized by pigmentation or superficial ulceration.[24] Candidal balanitis in men has been associated with immunosuppression, contact with a partner who has vaginal candidiasis, and diabetes.[25-28] Vulvovaginal candidiasis is an extremely common problem that may manifest as focal genital lesions.[29] Although it may be more common in women with underlying immunosuppression (e.g., diabetes mellitus, HIV infection), vulvovaginal candidiasis occurs most frequently in women without such risk factors.[30,31] Autoimmune diseases, such as Reiter's syndrome, Crohn's disease, or Behçet's syndrome, may be associated with genital lesions.[32-36] The spectrum of typical and atypical genital lesions associated with HIV infection is broad: Kaposi's sarcoma, giant condyloma acuminatum, chronic nonhealing HSV, and chancroid.[37-41] This reflects both the common occurrence of coinfection with other sexually transmitted diseases and a propensity for HIV immunosuppression to modulate other conditions.

CLINICAL MANIFESTATIONS

Location

In men, lesions associated with infectious or noninfectious processes may be found on or under the prepuce, around the coronal sulcus, on the shaft of the penis, the scrotum, the perianal tissue, the inner thighs, or the rectum. In the female patient, sites of involvement are equally varied. Genital lesions can appear on the mons pubis, the labia, the fourchette, anywhere in the vagina, on the cervix, the inner thighs, or the perianal tissue. As a result of orogenital sex, pathogens such as HSV and syphilis can also cause orolabial lesions. Lesions of chancroid can be disseminated distant from the genitalia and the original site of infection, by a process of autoinoculation, although this is not common.[42,43] In secondary syphilis, spirochetemia causes lesions sometimes widely dispersed from the genitalia that morphologically range from the classic papulosquamid rash of the palms and soles to the moist, raised lesions of condylomata lata (genitals) or mucous patches (orolabial area). *Neisseria gonorrhoeae*, a pathogen not commonly associated with genital lesions, may disseminate and cause tender, necrotic pustules primarily on the distal extremities as part of an arthritis-dermatitis syndrome.[44] Lesions associated with scabies infestation are common in the genital region as well as intertriginous areas elsewhere, including but not limited to the axillary folds and the interdigital spaces. Genital edema can occur after any local inflammatory process.[45]

Pain, Dysesthesias, and Systemic Symptoms

The lesions of syphilis, lymphogranuloma venereum (LGV), scabies, and molluscum contagiosum are ordinarily painless. Herpetic lesions are usually painful, although they may not be noticed until the clinician examines the patient and palpates or abrades the lesion. If herpes lesions are adjacent to or within the urethra, the patient can experience dysuria. Pain or other dysesthesias, including pruritus, may precede the development of a clinically recognizable lesion, particularly during episodes of disease recurrence.[46-48] These "prodromal" symptoms are usually milder than those experienced during a primary outbreak. They may be so characteristic that patients can be reliably instructed to begin antiviral medication before lesions erupt. Chancroid ulcers are typically painful. Genital lesions from immunologically mediated noninfectious causes, such as Behçet's syndrome, genital extensions of Crohn's disease, aphthous ulcers, and vestibulitis, may also be exquisitely tender. Granuloma inguinale (donovanosis), a genital ulcer disease seen primarily in the tropics, is caused by the bacillus *Calymmatobacterium granulomatis*. Although the lesions of this disease are often large and destructive, pain is surprisingly absent. Most patients with exophytic genital warts are asymptomatic; a few may report pain or pruritus.

Pruritus is common only with ectoparasitic infestations such as scabies or lice. The pruritus associated with scabies is often described as intense and worse at night. Although pruritus may be experienced by individuals with herpes or syphilis, it is not characteristic of these conditions. Fever is occasionally seen with secondary syphilis and with primary herpes simplex infection.[48,49] Headaches, fatigue, myalgias, and malaise may also accompany these infections.

Lymphadenopathy

Inguinal lymphadenopathy is a nonspecific finding that is characteristic of inflammatory pathology almost anywhere in the groin or either lower extremity. It may also be a manifestation of systemic disease such as HIV infection, tuberculosis, or lymphoma. It often accompanies genital infection. Although the inguinal and femoral lymph nodes drain the genital region in both men and women, the inner segment of the vagina and the cervix drain into deep pelvic and perirectal lymph nodes. If these lymph nodes are involved in inflammatory genital pathology, pelvic or rectal discomfort may be the most striking symptom.

Bilateral inguinal lymphadenopathy is typical in syphilis. Like the chancre of primary syphilis, it is usually painless. In secondary syphilis, as befitting a systemic process, lymphadenopathy distant from the genital area is common. Typically, the inguinal, axillary, cervical, and epitrochlear nodes are involved.[49] Lymphadenopathy associated with a herpetic genital lesion is usually bilateral and, like the lesion, is also tender. In HSV infection and in syphilis, lymphadenopathy persists for some time after resolution of the lesion.

LGV and chancroid are characterized by expansive, tender lymph nodes called buboes. These may be unilateral or bilateral. A central area of fluctuance often develops; if left untreated, it eventually spontaneously ruptures. Although drainage may be spontaneous, tenderness can become severe enough to warrant intervention and drainage. Lymphadenitis is unusual in granuloma inguinale.

Lesion Morphology

Although the appearance of a genital lesion is not entirely specific, it can implicate an etiologic agent. Herpes infections are characterized by vesicles that evolve into pustules and finally to shallow ulcers on an erythematous base (Fig. 101-1). Multiple lesions are common, and they may erupt in tightly grouped clusters. Sometimes the characteristic evolution of the lesion is not appreciated and the patient or clinician simply observes tender ulcers that assume a wide variety of shapes and sizes because of confluence of evolving vesicles and pustules (Fig. 101-2). In a primary outbreak, lesions can reach considerable size (Fig. 101-3). Immunocompromised individuals, such as transplantation patients, those taking immunosuppressive agents, and those infected with HIV, can also experience extensive herpetic ulceration of the genitals in the setting of either a primary outbreak or a recurrence.[40,50] At the other end of the spectrum, a significant number of patients fail to recognize herpes outbreaks because of mild or absent symptoms.[51] When instructed carefully about these types of outbreaks, most of these individuals can recognize disease.[52]

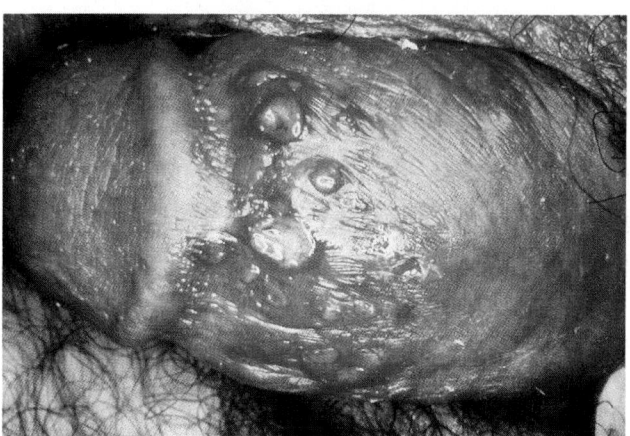

FIGURE 101-1. Genital infection with herpes simplex virus.

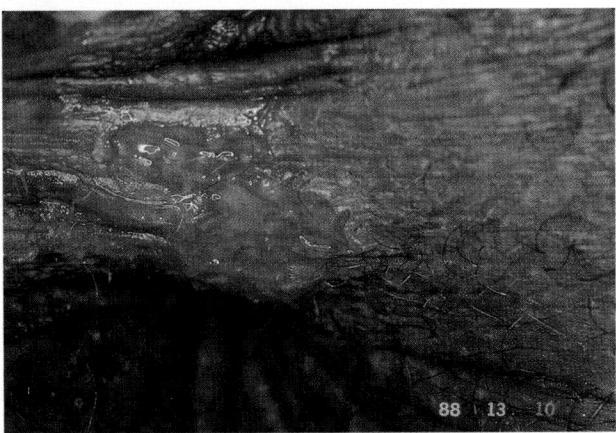

FIGURE 101-2. Irregularly shaped herpes simplex virus ulcer.

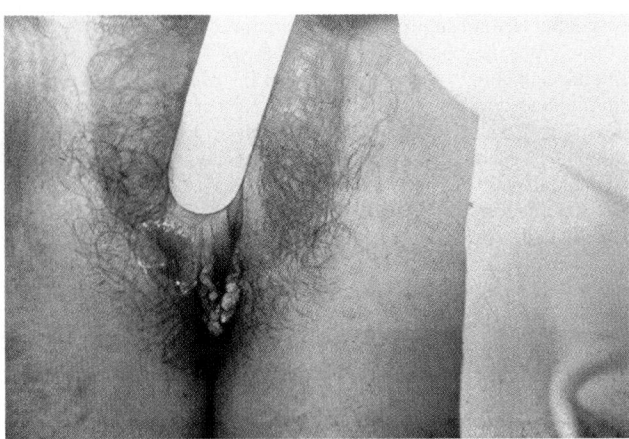

FIGURE 101-4. Chancre of primary syphilis.

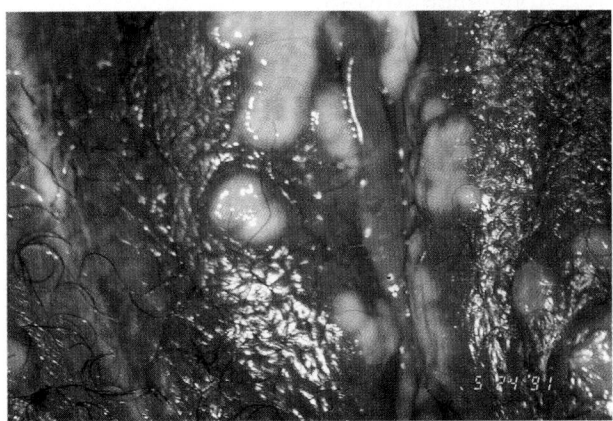

FIGURE 101-5. Condylomata lata of secondary syphilis.

Syphilitic chancres are typically solitary, although they may rarely occur in pairs. They are round and 1 to 2 cm in diameter, with clean margins that are indurated on palpation (Fig. 101-4). The ulcer base usually lacks exudate but occasionally becomes superinfected with other bacteria. The lesions of secondary syphilis are not chancre-like. They may start anywhere as fine macular lesions that evolve into pigmented papules, often with a fine, circumferential scale. In warm, moist areas such as the buttocks and genitals, unique lesions of secondary syphilis known as condylomata lata develop (Fig. 101-5). These are raised, moist nodules or plaques that are teeming with treponemes. They are highly infectious.

Chancroid lesions are similar in size to syphilitic chancres, but their edges are ragged and undermined (Fig. 101-6). The ulcer base is necrotic with a purulent exudate. Compared with the lesions of syphilis, induration of chancroid lesions tends to be less prominent,

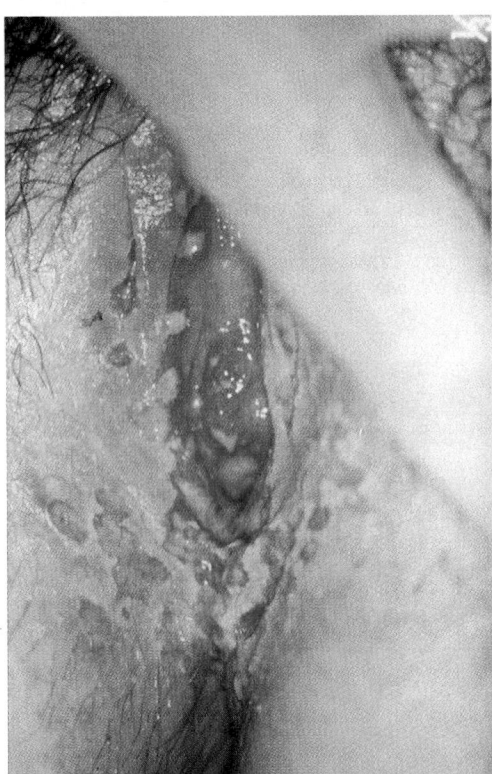

FIGURE 101-3. Severe primary herpes simplex virus infection.

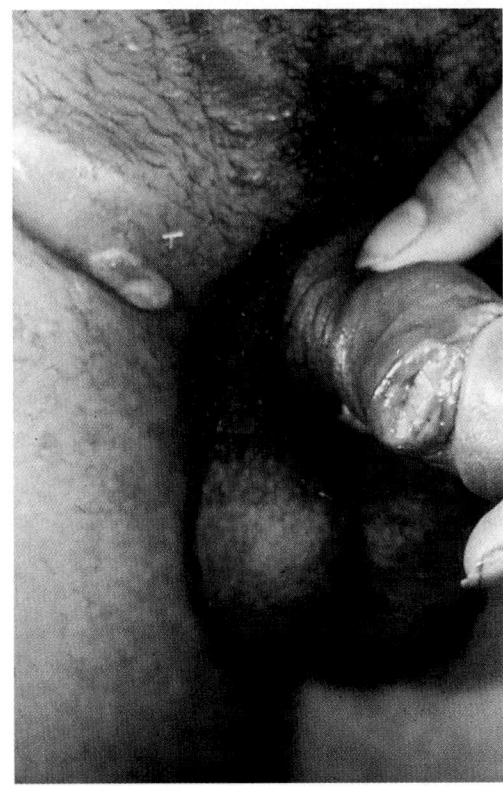

FIGURE 101-6. Genital lesion of chancroid with a draining inguinal lymph node.

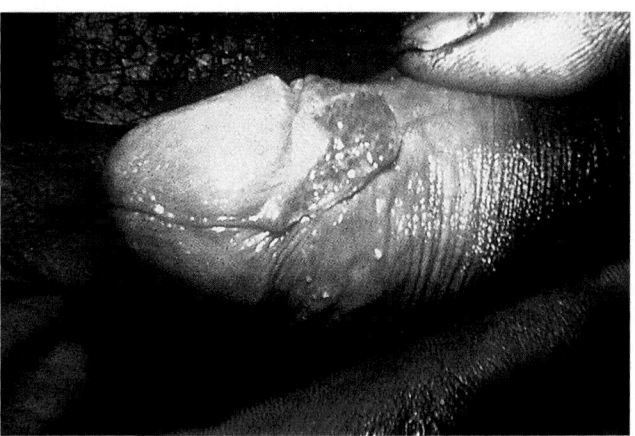

FIGURE 101-7. Granuloma inguinale.

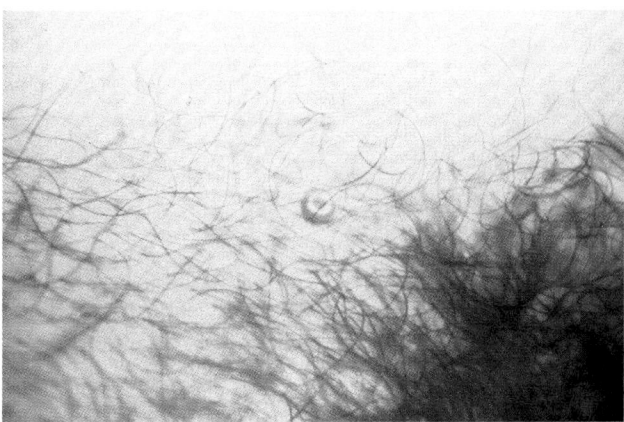

FIGURE 101-9. Lesion of molluscum contagiosum.

accounting for the designation of these ulcers as "soft chancres" *(ulcus molle, chancre mou)*. Despite the obvious tissue damage, adjacent inflammation is absent. Single lesions are the norm, but multiple lesions may be seen.

The lesions of granuloma inguinale start as firm subcutaneous nodules or papules that eventually ulcerate. Typically, this ulcerative process becomes hypertrophic and beefy and bleeds easily (Fig. 101-7).[53] Local tissue destruction may be extensive. Swelling of the vulva and phimosis are common. Variants include deeply necrotic ulcers and dry, "cicatricial" lesions that consist primarily of fibrotic tissue. Occasionally, lesions are confused with squamous cell carcinoma.[54]

LGV (also called Nicholas-Durand-Favre disease) is one of several sexually transmitted diseases caused by *Chlamydia trachomatis* and is attributable specifically to serovars L1, L2, and L3. At its earliest stage, LGV may cause a small papule or herpes-like ulcer. This is usually asymptomatic and resolves before recognition.[55] The patient with LGV then comes to medical attention with tender inguinal lymphadenopathy as the primary process of concern.

Clinically visible lesions of HPV are typically caused by viral types with low oncogenic potential (i.e., types 6 and 11). Most HPV infections are asymptomatic. Lesions can run the gamut from flat or relatively inconspicuous papules to verrucous, pedunculated, or large cauliflower-like masses referred to as condylomata acuminata (Fig. 101-8). Whatever the configuration, these lesions are clinically characteristic and unlikely to be confused with those of other etiologies. Certain HPV types (e.g., 16, 18, 31, 33) have oncogenic potential both on moist mucosal surfaces such as ectocervix and, less commonly, on keratinized epithelium characteristic of the external genitalia. The dysplastic cytologic changes they induce are collectively referred to as

squamous intraepithelial neoplasia (SIL) and may be benign or malignant. Squamous cell carcinoma of the cervix, the vagina, the vulva, the penis, or the anus may arise from previous HPV infection. HPV-associated carcinoma in situ on keratinized epithelium may manifest as multiple papular lesions, referred to as Bowenoid papulosis or, when it occurs as a single plaque, as Bowen's disease. Erythroplasia of Queyrat is a variant of this process that involves the glans of the penis.

Molluscum contagiosum causes benign, wart-like lesions (Fig. 101-9). The etiologic agent of this condition is a member of the poxvirus family. Spread can be sexual or through nonsexual contact in children. Lesions are small, 3 to 5 mm in diameter, multiple, and clustered in the genital or inguinal areas, the perineum, or the inner thighs in adults. They appear pearly with an area of central umbilication, which often can be appreciated only on very close inspection. Lesions of scabies infestation range from papules to nodules with a surrounding crust (Fig. 101-10). With scratching, these lesions are often modified by excoriations or lichenification.

The use of systemic or topical antimicrobial agents before clinical evaluation can have a dramatic effect on lesion morphology.

Duration

Without therapy, herpes ulcers resolve within 3 weeks in cases of primary infection, and a recurrence resolves in 5 to 12 days. Except for some postinflammatory hypopigmentation, there is little scarring. Lesions that heal within days after an outbreak in the absence of therapy are probably not herpetic in nature. On the other hand, lesions proven to be herpetic that persist for longer than 3 to 4 weeks raise the possibility of underlying immunosuppression. Syphilitic chancres and condylomata lata also resolve without therapy, usually between 3 and

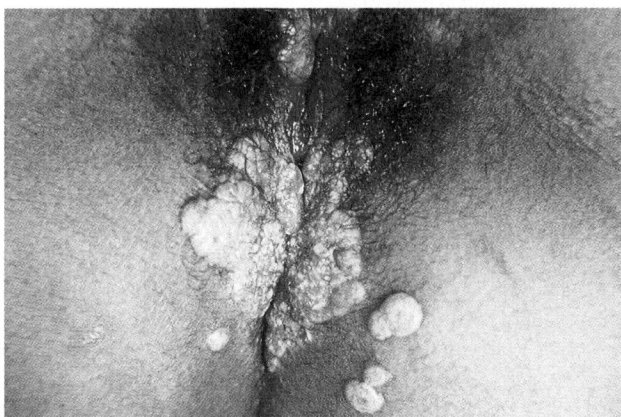

FIGURE 101-8. Genital human papillomavirus lesions.

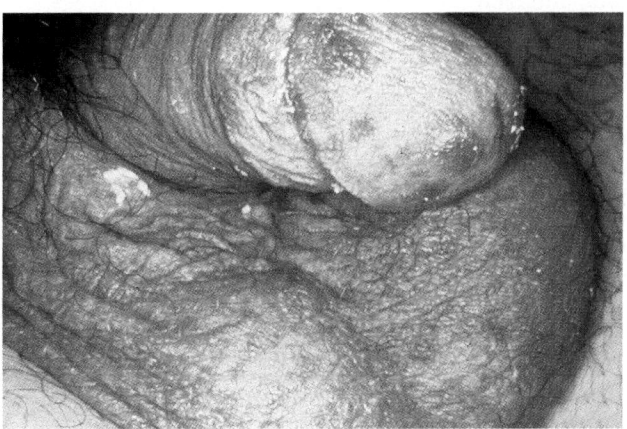

FIGURE 101-10. Infestation with *Sarcoptes scabiei*.

TABLE 101-1 Causes of Genital Ulcer Disease by Region (Percentage of Cases)

Pathogen	Dar es Salaam[4]	South Africa[56]	Los Angeles[5]	St Louis[5]	Thailand[57]	Madagascar[58]
Herpes simplex virus type 2	63	36	76	53	82	10
Haemophilus ducreyi	13	32	0	0	0	33
Treponema pallidum	2	20	0	13	0	29
>1 pathogen	10	9	0	2	2	—
Negative	21	22	24	32	16	32

12 weeks and usually without much scarring. Without therapy, the lesions of chancroid and donovanosis are slowly destructive. Scarring is typical in both of these situations. Lesions caused by HPV or molluscum contagiosum may persist unchanged for a prolonged time, or they may be characterized by brief periods of clinical disease alternating with resolution.

EPIDEMIOLOGY

Understanding of the epidemiology of genital lesions has been hampered by inconsistent access to diagnostic tools in many parts of the world. The probability of a given cause of a genital lesion varies somewhat depending on the region of the world in which the patient lives or acquires infection (Table 101-1). Worldwide, HSV-2 is the most common cause of genital ulcer disease.

In Africa and other tropical and subtropical regions of the world, *H. ducreyi* accounts for a substantial amount of genital ulcer disease. In the developed world, *H. ducreyi* is usually seen only in the context of focal urban outbreaks.[59,60]

In the absence of reliable serologic tests for HPV infection, it has been difficult to accurately determine the prevalence of this organism in different regions of the world. This assessment is further hampered by the asymptomatic nature of most infections. Despite these handicaps, some studies suggest that HPV may be the most common sexually transmitted infection in the United States.[61,62] The incidence of syphilis in the United States declined so precipitously through the 1990s that the U.S. Public Health Service has embarked on an ambitious program to eliminate the disease from the country.[63] Despite these efforts, outbreaks of early-stage syphilis, particularly among men who have sex with men (MSM) and are also infected with HIV, have been reported.[64] Even more dramatic increases in the incidence of syphilis have been seen in the Russian Federation.[65]

LGV occurs primarily in the tropics and subtropics.[55,66] Sporadic cases and outbreaks of LGV do occur in the developed world, and the disease should be considered in travelers returning from endemic areas.[67-69] Donovanosis is endemic in Papua New Guinea but has also been seen in southern Africa, parts of India, the Caribbean, and South America. It is infrequently seen in the United States.[53]

Genital Lesions in Patients with Human Immunodeficiency Virus Infection

Although the majority of HIV-infected individuals with genital lesions manifest disease in a fashion similar to their nonimmunocompromised counterparts, it is clear that some individuals, particularly those with significant immunosuppression, experience more extensive and prolonged disease. Large, persistent, or progressive condylomata acuminata have been well described in this patient population.[70,71] In patients with HIV infection, the lesions of molluscum contagiosum can also vary in size and may number in the hundreds.[72-74] In this population, both primary and recurrent herpetic ulcers may progress to extend over large areas of the perineum.[40,75] The pain associated with such lesions can be so debilitating that it warrants hospitalization. Herpes lesions in HIV-infected individuals may persist well beyond the 2- to 3-week period ordinarily encountered in classic primary or recurrent disease. This finding may serve as an early sign of immunosuppression.[76-78] There has also been concern that HIV-infected patients are more likely to harbor HSV isolates that are resistant to commonly used antiviral agents.[79,80] The lesions of early-stage syphilis probably are

not appreciably altered by HIV infection, although some data suggest that patients present more frequently than usual with multiple chancres. Clinical manifestations of secondary lesions may also develop before the resolution of the syphilitic chancre.[81-83] Anecdotal reports of accelerated disease and failure of routine therapy have not been supported by prospective studies.[81]

Any break in the ordinarily protective barrier of the integument, such as that caused by genital inflammatory lesions, can potentially serve as a conduit through which HIV is more efficiently transmitted from one sexual partner to another. Lesion exudate has been demonstrated to harbor virus.[84-86] There is additional concern that genital HSV-2 may increase local HIV replication, further enhancing the risk of transmission.[86] Syphilis, herpes, and chancroid infections have been associated with a greater likelihood of HIV infection in both retrospective and prospective studies.[87-92]

LABORATORY TESTING

Laboratory tests are critical to the diagnosis and proper management of genital ulcer disease. As previously discussed, although specific pathogens can be linked to well-characterized clinical presentations, there is enough variation to ensure that clinicians relying on educated "guess-work" will be wrong in a significant number of cases. The following discussion is not meant to be exhaustive; for more details, reference should be made to the individual pathogens discussed elsewhere in the text.

There are a number of direct microscopic examinations that can be performed on lesion exudate or a biopsy sample and that help make a diagnosis. Gram staining is not usually helpful in the evaluation of genital lesions. Lesion exudate is typically laden with a variety of nonpathogenic organisms common to genitourinary and perirectal flora. Under ideal circumstances, *H. ducreyi* appears as a gram-negative, slender rod or coccobacillus that aligns in a pattern referred to as "school of fish" (Fig. 101-11). Most clinicians and microbiologists are not experienced enough to recognize this pattern in the welter of other organisms typical of a lesion Gram stain, and its sensitivity and specificity are poor. *H. ducreyi* can be cultivated on special nutrient media using Mueller-Hinton–based chocolate agar, supplemented with 1% IsoVitaleX and 3 μg/mL vancomycin to inhibit the growth of other organisms.[93] The rarity of this organism in the developed world and the expense and limited shelf life of the media make isolation of *H. ducreyi* difficult and uncommon.

Light microscopy of syphilis chancre exudate is not useful. The spirochetes that cause syphilis do not take up standard stains well and are extremely thin. Darkfield microscopy of lesion exudate from either a chancre or condylomata lata can identify spirochetes. Incident light is angled obliquely at the stage by polarizing lenses and then reflected upward through the objective by microbes in the clinical specimen. Spirochetes appear as tightly coiled, white organisms spirally rotating against the black background of the microscopic field.[94] There are nonpathogenic treponemes, particularly in the oral cavity, which cannot be differentiated from *T. pallidum* by darkfield microscopy. In the appropriate clinical setting, a positive darkfield specimen is highly suggestive of syphilis. To perform a proper darkfield examination, ulcers must be cleaned with gauze and saline. Exudate from the lesion is then pressed against a glass slide. The specimen should not be contaminated with too much blood. A cover slip is then applied. Rapid examination of the specimen is essential, because desiccation reduces the viability of organisms. Agar-based methods for the cultivation of

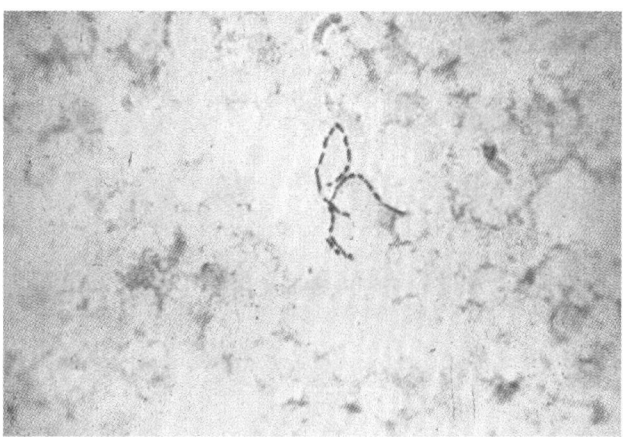

FIGURE 101-11. Gram stain of *Haemophilus ducreyi*.

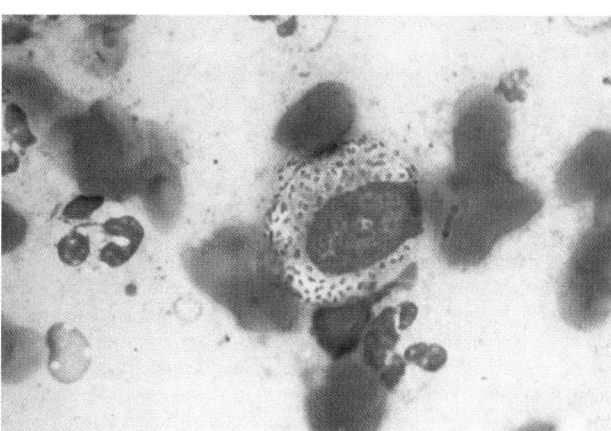

FIGURE 101-12. Biopsy of granuloma inguinale lesion revealing "Donovan bodies" consistent with *Calymmatobacterium granulomatis*.

T. pallidum are not routinely available. Direct fluorescent antibody testing of smears or tissue is available and, unlike darkfield microscopy, can differentiate between pathogenic and nonpathogenic treponemes.[95,96] Silver staining of biopsy material can identify spirochetes but is not commonly performed.

Serologic testing is the most commonly used method for the diagnosis of syphilitic genital lesions. The process requires two steps: a screening test that detects serum antibodies to nontreponemal antigens (e.g., rapid plasma reagin [RPR] test, Venereal Disease Research Laboratory [VDRL] test, unheated serum reagin [USR] test) and then a confirmatory test that detects serum antibody to true treponemal antigens (e.g., fluorescent treponemal antibody absorbed [FTA-ABS] test, *Treponema pallidum* particle agglutination assay [TP-PA]).[97] Early after the appearance of the syphilitic chancre, only the treponemal-specific test may be reactive. Repeat testing with the nontreponemal test should be considered at some time after the ulcer has formed. In rare situations, the nontreponemal test may be falsely nonreactive in secondary syphilis due to the blocking effect of excess antibody; this is known as the prozone phenomenon. Repeat testing should be performed on diluted serum specimens. Ordinarily the nontreponemal serologic test reaches its highest titer in secondary disease and declines with the onset of latency or with effective therapy.

HSV-infected genital lesions can be identified by light microscopy using the Tzanck smear. In this process, epithelial cells are scraped from an ulcer base and stained with Wright-Giemsa stain. Multinucleated giant cells and intranuclear inclusions are characteristic of HSV infections. However, both the sensitivity and the specificity of the Tzanck smear are poor.[98,99] When available, conventional cell culture provides a relatively rapid and accurate diagnosis. Most specimens from a genuine lesion of HSV demonstrate the pathognomonic cytopathic effect (CPE) within 48 hours after collection. Fluorescein conjugated type-specific monoclonal antibody can then be applied to these specimens for confirmation. Serologic tests for herpes antibodies are currently available and can distinguish between antibodies to viral glycoprotein G, which allows for distinction between HSV-1 and HSV-2.[100] Given the prevalent, chronic, and recurring nature of herpes genital infections, these tests are not typically used to establish the role of herpes as a cause of an acute genital lesion. Further modifications now allow for these tests to be performed rapidly in the office or clinic.[101]

C. granulomatis, the cause of granuloma inguinale or donovanosis, can be identified by staining scrapings of a lesion base with either Wright's or Giemsa's stain (Fig. 101-12). Surface cells alone may not harbor the organism, so biopsy is often necessary. Clusters of blue rods, with prominent polar granules and surrounded by pink capsules, are seen within infected epithelial cells and are known as Donovan bodies. Cultivation is difficult.

The diagnosis of LGV is usually based on clinical criteria. Diagnosis on the basis of a genital ulcer or lesion alone is rare. Later,

after the onset of tender unilateral inguinal or femoral adenopathy, the diagnosis is most obvious. Isolation by cell culture or polymerase chain reaction (PCR) of *C. trachomatis* from bubo drainage is diagnostic. When these tests are performed on ulcer exudate, they are considered diagnostic only if an LGV serovar is identified. Testing of serum for *C. trachomatis* antibody can be done with the use of complement fixation or microimmunofluorescence techniques. The latter is the more sensitive and specific serologic study, but it is not widely available outside research centers.

The lesions of HPV are also diagnosed primarily by their clinical appearance. Resort to biopsy of external lesions is infrequent. There is no cell culture system for the cultivation of HPV. The presence of virus in nonkeratinized tissue such as cervical epithelium can be assessed by cytologic methods (e.g., Papanicolaou smear) or biopsy. The cytologic change consistent with HPV is the koilocyte with or without nuclear atypia. Southern blot and in situ hybridization techniques have been limited to a few settings. Application of 3% to 5% acetic acid to suspicious mucosal lesions reveals the characteristic "whitening" of HPV lesions on either female or male genitalia. Serologic tests for HPV are still under development. Their utility in aiding the diagnosis of a chronic, common problem such as HPV will be an issue.

Infestation with ectoparasites such as *Sarcoptes scabiei* is demonstrated by identification of the organism, eggs, or feces under direct light microscopy. This may require the unroofing of the scabies burrow bluntly with a needle or scalpel.

Nucleic acid detection is an increasingly common means of diagnosing infectious diseases. Efforts have been made to apply this technology to the diagnosis of some of the more common genital lesions. Nucleic acid detection can be performed with the use of hybridization techniques, amplification techniques (i.e., PCR, transcription-mediated amplification [TMA], ligase chain reaction [LCR], or some combination of both. PCR tests have been developed for *H. ducreyi*,[102,103] *T. pallidum*,[104,105] and HSV.[106,107] These technologies have also been combined in one "multiplex" platform (M-PCR) to aid in the clinical evaluation of genital lesions.[106,108] The role of such tests in current clinical practice is undefined.

Routine evaluation of genital ulcer disease in the United States should at the very least include viral culture for HSV-2 and serologic tests for syphilis. If darkfield microscopy is readily available, it should be used to identify spirochetes. Unless there is an increase in the prevalence of chancroid, it is difficult to assume that most laboratories will have ready access to media for the cultivation of *H. ducreyi*.

THERAPIES

As frequently as possible, therapy for any genital lesion should be based on an accurate diagnosis. The goals of therapy should include the elimination of the pathogen, resolution of symptoms, reduction in the risk of transmission, and if applicable, a reduction in the frequency of recurrences.

After more than 50 years of use, penicillin remains the treatment of choice for the chancre of primary syphilis and the lesions associated with secondary disease. A single intramuscular injection of 2.4 million units of benzathine penicillin G should result in prompt conversion to darkfield-negative lesions and the onset of healing within 24 to 48 hours. Alternatives to penicillin include a 1-week course of oral doxycycline, 100 mg twice daily; 8 to 10 days of intramuscular ceftriaxone 1 g daily; or 2 g once orally of azithromycin.[8] There are far fewer data and little clinical experience supporting the use of these alternative regimens.[109-112] Regardless of the therapy selected, patients treated for early-stage syphilis require serially repeated serologic tests (nontreponemal) even after lesions heal to verify an adequate response. These can be done at 6-month intervals. Fourfold or two-step dilutional decreases indicate an appropriate response. There is no evidence that HIV-infected patients require additional or different therapies for early syphilis.[81] Serologic tests in these patients should be performed at intervals of less than 6 months.

HSV infections can be treated with a variety of related nucleoside analogues available both orally and intravenously. The goal of therapy may be to hasten the resolution of lesions and reduce infectivity, or to suppress outbreaks in individuals who suffer frequent bouts of disease. Antiviral agents inhibit DNA polymerase and require phosphorylation by viral thymidine kinase to do so. The most commonly used agent, acyclovir, was the first to be marketed. Subsequently, both valacyclovir, a prodrug of acyclovir, and famciclovir, a prodrug of another nucleoside analogue, penciclovir, were introduced for the treatment of herpes. These agents are more bioavailable than acyclovir in oral form and can be dosed less frequently. If necessary, severe herpes genital disease can be treated with intravenous acyclovir. Thymidine kinase–deficient strains of virus have developed that are resistant to this group of antivirals. This phenomenon has been observed primarily, although not exclusively, in immunocompromised hosts.[79,113,114] Disease caused by resistant isolates can be treated with foscarnet, a DNA polymerase inhibitor unrelated to acyclovir and its congeners.[115] Foscarnet is available only for intravenous or topical use. It potentially causes renal dysfunction and hypophosphatemia. Another agent that has activity against herpes is cidofovir, an acyclic nucleoside phosphonate.[116] It is also available intravenously and topically. The adverse effect profile of cidofovir is more favorable than that of foscarnet.

Chancroid may be cured microbiologically with a number of antimicrobial agents, but lesions are often slow to heal and scarring is often long-standing. Although sulfonamides and aminopenicillins were originally used in the treatment of chancroid, microbial resistance has rendered them ineffective. Erythromycin and azithromycin are currently recommended therapies. The latter can be used as a single 1-g dose orally.[8] The third-generation cephalosporin ceftriaxone, given as a single dose of 250 mg intramuscularly, is also effective, but there are concerns about diminished activity in HIV-coinfected individuals.[41,117] Fluoroquinolones effectively treat chancroid but should be administered for at least 3 days and not as single-dose therapy.[118,119] Tender, fluctuant buboes can be aspirated for symptomatic relief.

Although symptomatic HPV infection and molluscum contagiosum may both spontaneously resolve, there is a role for treatment. Therapies include a variety of ablative techniques such as curettage, electrocautery, cryosurgery, and laser. Each of these therapies causes some element of tissue damage. None provides a certain cure, and recurrence is common. Topical agents include podophyllin (from the resin of the mayapple), trichloroacetic acid, and imiquimod (an immune modulator). Podophyllin should not be used on nonkeratinized epithelium. Podophyllin and imiquimod are also available for use as patient-applied preparations. Intralesional interferon injections have been studied but are associated with poor response and significant side effects.[120]

Tetracycline congeners and erythromycin have long been the standard therapy for LGV. The duration of therapy is ordinarily 14 to 21 days. There are no data comparing any particular preparation or, for that matter, satisfactorily defining duration of therapy. Donovanosis can be treated with a variety of antibiotics, including doxycycline, trimethoprim-sulfamethoxazole, fluoroquinolones, and erythromycin. The course of therapy for donovanosis should be 3 weeks or until lesions are healed. Relapse may occur.

OTHER MANAGEMENT ISSUES

Because genital ulcer disease in particular and sexually transmitted diseases in general seem so closely linked to HIV transmission, it is prudent to make HIV counseling and testing services available to all patients who present with venereal genital lesions. It is also necessary for patients with genital lesions to be counseled about the communicable nature of their disease and the need in many of these instances for partner referral. Based on local public health requirements, it may be necessary to report certain infections to the health department. Sexual partners of patients with syphilis and chancroid require evaluation and therapy for those conditions. In the cases of LGV and donovanosis, the treatment of asymptomatic partners is of unclear benefit. The partners of individuals with HSV or HPV need counseling about exposure and the potential for disease. The utility of routine cervical Papanicolaou smears for women should be explained. Finally, methods to avoid future infections (e.g., barrier contraceptives) should be explored with the patient.

NONVENEREAL GENITAL LESIONS

Candida species and other yeasts sometimes cause nonvenereal genital lesions. In women, vaginal colonization with yeast is extremely common, although symptomatic disease occurs in only a fraction of colonized individuals. In a smaller portion still, symptomatic disease may be recurrent. Recent use of antimicrobials is a common predisposing risk factor for candidal infections. Vulvovaginal infection is commonly characterized by a thick, whitish, pruritic vaginal discharge but occasionally manifests solely as vulvar and perineal disease, with an inflammatory vulvitis, erythema, pruritus, superficial excoriations, and ulcerations. Whether this is attributable to the yeast infection itself or to excoriations from itching is unclear. Distinguishing candidal lesions on the external genitalia from those of other common superficial ulcerative processes such as herpes may at times be difficult.

Genital infection with yeast also occurs in men, a condition known as candidal balanitis or balanoposthosis. Rarely, a history of a sexual partner with vulvovaginal infection is elicited, although sexual transmission is not typical. Balanitis usually involves only the glans, which can appear taught and glossy. There may be multiple, discrete, small pustules as well as linear or more substantial erosions. As in women, there is often significant pruritus.[26] A proportion of individuals with candidal balanitis have diabetes mellitus.[28] Skin scrapings or vaginal fluid examined under light microscopy after the addition of potassium hydroxide reveal the pseudohyphae of *Candida* species. Treatment with any of a variety of topical or oral azole antifungal agents is usually effective.

Fixed drug eruptions, which represent a systemic response to medication, may involve the genitalia in either sex. A wide range of agents have been implicated, including antibiotics such as the tetracyclines and the sulfonamides, as well as nonsteroidal anti-inflammatory agents, barbiturates, and oral contraceptives.[121-123] Lesions occur soon after ingestion of the offending agent with the development of erythematous or violaceous, sharply demarcated macules. They may recede with residual hyperpigmentation or evolve to form bullae and erosions. Topical medications applied to the genitals can also cause localized contact dermatitis. Other common dermatologic conditions can involve the genitals, including eczema and psoriasis; they are characterized by the lesions typical of these conditions.[124] In eczema, pruritus leads to scratching, which then results in linear erosions. Chronically, this can cause lichenification or thickening of the skin. In psoriasis, there is epidermal hyperplasia. Lesions are red, well-demarcated, and often scaling. Patients with psoriasis who have been exposed to therapy with ultraviolet light may be at a higher risk for squamous cell carcinoma of the genitals.[125]

Aphthous ulcers of the vagina occur in Behçet's syndrome and in HIV infection.[126-128] The cause of these lesions is unclear, but they are presumably the result of some immune-mediated phenomenon. These lesions are typically small, approximately 1 to 2 mm, but may be quite large in some instances. They may be superficial or deep and often are marked by surrounding erythema. The diagnosis is made by observation, a history of recurrence, and the exclusion of other causes. They are treated with topical or systemic steroids, colchicine, dapsone, or thalidomide.

Genital lesions may also arise from other processes, including trauma[129-132] and folliculitis. Pearly penile papules are anatomic variants characterized by tightly clustered, small, uniform papules exclusively involving the coronal sulcus in a circumferential distribution. These often appear in young adulthood and lead anxious patients to seek clinical care, but they require no intervention. Tuberculosis can cause anogenital fistulas from adjacent, infected genital or gastrointestinal structures or, rarely, primary lesions of the genitals.[133-135] Genital lesions rarely result from systemic infection with other pathogens, such as *Histoplasma capsulatum* and *Entamoeba histolytica*.[136-139]

REFERENCES

1. Oriel JD. The Scars of Venus: A History of Venereology. London: Springer-Verlag; 1994.
2. Quetel C. History of Syphilis. Baltimore: The Johns Hopkins University Press; 1990.
3. Kampmeier R. Herpes genitalis. Sex Transm Dis. 1984;11:41-45.
4. Ahmed HJ, Mbwana J, Gunnarsson E, et al. Etiology of genital ulcer disease and association with human immunodeficiency virus infection in two Tanzanian cities. Sex Transm Dis. 2003;30:114-119.
5. Mertz KJ, Trees D, Levine WC, et al. Etiology of genital ulcers and prevalence of human immunodeficiency virus coinfection in 10 US cities. The Genital Ulcer Disease Surveillance Group. J Infect Dis. 1998;178:1795-1798.
6. Bruisten SM, Cairo I, Fennema H, et al. Diagnosing genital ulcer disease in a clinic for sexually transmitted diseases in Amsterdam, The Netherlands. J Clin Microbiol. 2001;39:601-605.
7. Behets FM, Brathwaite AR, Hylton-Kong T, et al. Genital ulcers: Etiology, clinical diagnosis, and associated human immunodeficiency virus infection in Kingston, Jamaica. Clin Infect Dis. 1999;28:1086-1090.
8. Centers for Disease Control and Prevention. Sexually transmitted diseases: Treatment guidelines, 2002. MMWR Morb Mortal Weekly Rep. 2002;51(RR6):1-80.
9. Dillon SM, Cummings M, Rajagopalan S, McCormack WC. Prospective analysis of genital ulcer disease in Brooklyn, New York. Clin Infect Dis. 1997;24:945-950.
10. Bogaerts J, Ricart CA, Van Dyck E, Piot P. The etiology of genital ulceration in Rwanda. Sex Transm Dis. 1989;16:123-126.
11. Dangor Y, Ballard RC, da L Exposto F, et al. Accuracy of clinical diagnosis of genital ulcer disease. Sex Transm Dis. 1990;4:184-189.
12. DiCarlo R, Martin D. The clinical diagnosis of genital ulcer disease in men. Clin Infect Dis. 1997;2:292-298.
13. Chapel TA, Brown WJ, Jeffres C, Stewart JA. How reliable is the morphological diagnosis of penile ulcerations? Sex Transm Dis. 1977;4:150-152.
14. Hook EW 3rd, Cannon RO, Nahmias AJ, et al. Herpes simplex virus infection as a risk factor for human immunodeficiency virus infection in heterosexuals. J Infect Dis. 1992;165:251-255.
15. Torian LV, Weisfuse IB, Makki HA, et al. Increasing HIV-1 seroprevalence associated with genital ulcer disease, New York City, 1990-1992. AIDS. 1995;9:177-181.
16. Chirgwin K, DeHovitz JA, Dillon S, McCormack WM. HIV infection, genital ulcer disease, and crack cocaine use among patients attending a clinic for sexually transmitted diseases. Am J Public Health. 1991;81:1576-1579.
17. Telzak EE, Chiasson MA, Bevier PJ, et al. HIV-1 seroconversion in patients with and without genital ulcer disease: A prospective study. Ann Intern Med. 1993;119:1181-1186.
18. Greenblatt RM, Lukehart SA, Plummer FA, et al. Genital ulceration as a risk factor for human immunodeficiency virus infection. AIDS. 1988;2:47-50.
19. Rosen T, Conrad N. Genital ulcer caused by human bite to the penis. Sex Transm Dis. 1999;26:527-530.
20. Kaur C, Kaur S, Thami GP. Human bite-induced penile ulceration: Report of a case and review of literature. Int J STD AIDS. 2002;13:852-854.
21. Riggs N, Houry D, Long G, et al. Analysis of 1,076 cases of sexual assault. Ann Emerg Med. 2000;35:358-362.
22. Levy DA, Khouader S, Leynadier F. Allergy to latex condoms. Allergy. 1998;53:1107-1108.
23. Corey L, Spear PG. Infections with herpes simplex viruses. N Engl J Med. 1986;314:686-691, 749-757.
24. Pandhi RK, Kumar AS, Satish DA, Bhutani LK. Fixed drug eruptions on male genitalia: Clinical and etiologic study. Sex Transm Dis. 1984;11:164-166.
25. Morrissey R, Xavier A, Nguyen N, Webb DW. Invasive candidal balanitis due to a condom catheter in a neutropenic patient. South Med J. 1985;78:1247-1249.
26. David LM, Walzman M, Rajamanoharan S. Genital colonisation and infection with candida in heterosexual and homosexual males. Genitourin Med. 1997;73:394-396.
27. Stary A, Soeltz-Szoets J, Ziegler C, et al. Comparison of the efficacy and safety of oral fluconazole and topical clotrimazole in patients with candida balanitis. Genitourin Med. 1996;72:98-102.
28. Waugh MA, Evans EG, Nayyar KC, Fong R. Clotrimazole (Canesten) in the treatment of candidal balanitis in men. With incidental observations on diabetic candidal balanoposthitis. Br J Vener Dis. 1978;54:184-186.
29. Sobel J. Vaginitis. N Engl J Med. 1997;337:1896-1903.
30. Sobel J. Pathogenesis and treatment of recurrent vulvovaginal candidiasis. Clin Infect Dis. 1992;14(Suppl 1):S148-S153.
31. Mardh PA, Rodrigues AG, Genc M, et al. Facts and myths on recurrent vulvovaginal candidosis: A review on epidemiology, clinical manifestations, diagnosis, pathogenesis and therapy. Int J STD AIDS. 2002;13:522-539.
32. Morgan ED, Laszlo JD, Stumpf PG. Incomplete Behcet's syndrome in the differential diagnosis of genital ulceration and postcoital bleeding: A case report. J Reprod Med. 1988;33:844-846.
33. Keat A. Reiter's syndrome and reactive arthritis in perspective. N Engl J Med. 1983;309:1606-1615.
34. Daunt SO, Kotowski KE, O'Reilly AP, Richardson AT. Ulcerative vulvitis in Reiter's syndrome: A case report. Br J Vener Dis. 1982;58:405-407.
35. Acker SM, Sahn EE, Rogers HC, et al. Genital cutaneous Crohn disease: Two cases with unusual clinical and histopathologic features in young men. Am J Dermatopathol. 2000;22:443-446.
36. Cockburn AG, Krolikowski J, Balogh K, Roth RA. Crohn disease of penile and scrotal skin. Urology. 1980;15:596-598.
37. Conley LJ, Ellerbrock TV, Bush TJ, et al. HIV-1 infection and risk of vulvovaginal and perianal condylomata acuminata and intraepithelial neoplasia: A prospective cohort study. Lancet. 2002;359:108-113.
38. Chiasson MA, Ellerbrock TV, Bush TJ, et al. Increased prevalence of vulvovaginal condyloma and vulvar intraepithelial neoplasia in women infected with the human immunodeficiency virus. Obstet Gynecol. 1997;89:690-694.
39. Swierzewski SJ 3rd, Denil J, Ohl DA. The management of meatal obstruction due to Kaposi's sarcoma of the glans. J Urol. 1993;150:193-195.
40. Siegal FP, Lopez C, Hammer GS, et al. Severe acquired immunodeficiency in male homosexuals, manifested by chronic perianal ulcerative herpes simplex lesions. N Engl J Med. 1981;305:1439-1444.
41. Tyndall M, Malisa M, Plummer FA, et al. Ceftriaxone no longer predictably cures chancroid in Kenya. J Infect Dis. 1993;167:469-471.
42. Asin J. Chancroid: A report of 1402 cases. Am J Syph Gon Vener Dis. 1952;36:483-487.
43. Quale J, Teplitz E, Augenbraun M. Atypical presentation of chancroid in a patient infected with the human immunodeficiency virus. Am J Med. 1990;88:43N-44N.
44. Holmes KK, Weisner PJ, Pedersen AH. The gonococcal arthritis-dermatitis syndrome. Ann Intern Med. 1971;75:470-471.
45. Wright RA, Judson FN. Penile venereal edema. JAMA. 1979;241:157-158.
46. Corey L, Holmes KK. Genital herpes simplex virus infections: Current concepts in diagnosis, therapy, and prevention. Ann Intern Med. 1983;98:973-983.
47. Guinan ME, MacCalman J, Kern ER, et al. The course of untreated recurrent genital herpes simplex infection in 27 women. N Engl J Med. 1981;304:759-763.
48. Brookes JL, Haywood S, Green J. Prodromal symptoms in genital herpes simplex infection. Genitourin Med. 1992;68:347-348.
49. Chapel TA. The signs and symptoms of secondary syphilis. Sex Transm Dis. 1980;7:161-164.
50. Whitley R, Barton N, Collins E, et al. Mucocutaneous herpes simplex virus infections in immunocompromised patients: A model for evaluation of topical antiviral agents. Am J Med. 1982;73:236-240.
51. Mertz GJ, Coombs RW, Ashley R, et al. Transmission of genital herpes in couples with one symptomatic and one asymptomatic partner: A prospective study. J Infect Dis. 1988;157:1169-1177.
52. Langenberg A, Benedetti J, Jenkins J, et al. Development of clinically recognizable genital lesions among women previously identified as having "asymptomatic" herpes simplex virus type 2 infection. Ann Intern Med. 1989;110:882-887.
53. Hart G. Donovanosis. Clin Infect Dis. 1997;25:24-30.
54. Barnes R, Masood S, Lammert N, Young RH. Extragenital granuloma inguinale mimicking a soft-tissue neoplasm: A case report and review of the literature. Hum Pathol. 1990;21:559-561.
55. Bauwens JE, Orlander H, Gomez MP, et al. Epidemic lymphogranuloma venereum during epidemics of crack cocaine use and HIV infection in the Bahamas. Sex Transm Dis. 2002;29:253-259.
56. Chen CY, Ballard RC, Beck-Sague CM, et al. Human immunodeficiency virus infection and genital ulcer disease in South Africa: The herpetic connection. Sex Transm Dis. 2000;27:21-29.
57. Beyrer C, Jitwatcharanan K, Natpratan C, et al. Molecular methods for the diagnosis of genital ulcer disease in a sexually transmitted disease clinic population in northern Thailand: Predominance of herpes simplex virus infection. J Infect Dis. 1998;178:243-246.
58. Behets FM, Andriamiadana J, Randrianasolo D, et al. Chancroid, primary syphilis, genital herpes, and lymphogranuloma venereum in Antananarivo, Madagascar. J Infect Dis. 1999;180:1382-1385.
59. Hammond GW, Slutchuk M, Scatliff J, et al. Epidemiologic, clinical, laboratory, and therapeutic features of an urban outbreak of chancroid in North America. Rev Infect Dis. 1980;2:867-879.
60. Blackmore CA, Limpakarnjanarat K, Rigau-Perez JG, et al. An outbreak of chancroid in Orange County, California: Descriptive epidemiology and disease-control measures. J Infect Dis. 1985;151:840-844.

61. Ho GY, Bierman R, Beardsley L, et al. Natural history of cervicovaginal papillomavirus infection in young women. N Engl J Med. 1998;338:423-428.
62. Aral S, Holmes KK. Social and behavioral determinants of the epidemiology of STDs: Industrialized and developing countries. In: Holmes KK, Sparling P, Mardh P, et al., eds. Sexually Transmitted Diseases. 3rd ed. New York: McGraw-Hill; 1999:39-76.
63. Centers for Disease Control and Prevention. Primary and Secondary Syphilis—United States, 2000-2001. MMWR Morb Mortal Wkly Rep. 2002;51:971-973.
64. Centers for Disease Control and Prevention. Primary and Secondary Syphilis Among Men Who Have Sex with Men—New York City, 2001. MMWR Morb Mortal Wkly Rep. 2002;51:853-856.
65. Tichonova L, Borisenko K, Ward H, et al. Epidemics of syphilis in the Russian Federation: Trends, origins, and priorities for control. Lancet. 1997;350:210-213.
66. Fawole OI, Okesola AO, Fawole AO. Genital ulcers disease among sexually transmitted disease clinic attendees in Ibadan, Nigeria. Afr J Med Sci. 2000;29:17-22.
67. Scieux C, Barnes R, Bianchi A, et al. Lymphogranuloma venereum: 27 cases in Paris. J Infect Dis. 1989;160:662-668.
68. McLelland BA, Anderson PC. Lymphogranuloma venereum: Outbreak in a university community. JAMA. 1976;235:56-57.
69. Abrams A. Lymphogranuloma venereum. JAMA. 1968;205:199-202.
70. Palefsky J. Cutaneous and genital HPV-associated lesions in HIV-infected patients. Clin Dermatol. 1997;15:439-447.
71. McMillan A, Bishop PE. Clinical course of anogenital warts in men infected with human immunodeficiency virus. Genitourin Med. 1989;65:225-228.
72. Vozmediano JM, Manrique A, Petraglia S, et al. .Giant molluscum contagiosum in AIDS. Int J Dermatol. 1996;35:45-47.
73. Schwartz JJ, Myskowski PL. Molluscum contagiosum in patients with human immunodeficiency virus infection: A review of twenty-seven patients. J Am Acad Dermatol. 1992;27:583-588.
74. Petersen CS, Gerstoft J. Molluscum contagiosum in HIV-infected patients. Dermatology. 1992;184:19-21.
75. Maier JA, Bergman A, Ross MG. Acquired immunodeficiency syndrome manifested by chronic primary genital herpes. Am J Obstet Gynecol. 1986;155:756-758.
76. Quinnan GV Jr, Masur H, Rook AH, et al. Herpesvirus infections in the acquired immune deficiency syndrome. JAMA. 1984;252:72-77.
77. Bagdades EK, Pillay D, Squire SB, et al. Relationship between herpes simplex virus ulceration and CD4+ cell counts in patients with HIV infection. AIDS. 1992;6:1317-1320.
78. Posavad CM, Koelle DM, Shaughnessy MF, Corey L. Severe genital herpes infections in HIV-infected individuals with impaired herpes simplex virus-specific CD8+ cytotoxic T lymphocyte responses. Proc Natl Acad Sci U S A. 1997;94:10289-10294.
79. Englund JA, Zimmerman ME, Swierkosz EM, et al. Herpes simplex virus resistant to acyclovir: A study in a tertiary care center. Ann Intern Med. 1990;112:416-422.
80. Erlich KS, Jacobson MA, Koehler JE, et al. Foscarnet therapy for severe acyclovir-resistant herpes simplex virus type-2 infections in patients with the acquired immunodeficiency syndrome (AIDS): An uncontrolled trial. Ann Intern Med. 1989;110:710-713.
81. Rolfs RT, Joesoef MR, Hendershot EF, et al. A randomized trial of enhanced therapy for early syphilis in patients with and without human immunodeficiency virus infection. The Syphilis and HIV Study Group. N Engl J Med. 1997;337:307-314.
82. Rompalo AM, Lawlor J, Seaman P, et al. Modification of syphilitic genital ulcer manifestations by coexistent HIV infection. Sex Transm Dis. 2001;28:448-454.
83. Rompalo AM, Joesoef MR, O'Donnell JA, et al.; Syphilis and HIV Study Group. Clinical manifestations of early syphilis by HIV status and gender: Results of the syphilis and HIV study. Sex Transm Dis. 2001;28:158-165.
84. Kreiss JK, Coombs R, Plummer F, et al. Isolation of human immunodeficiency virus from genital ulcers in Nairobi prostitutes. J Infect Dis. 1989;160:380-384.
85. Plummer FA, Wainberg MA, Plourde P, et al. Detection of human immunodeficiency virus type 1 (HIV-1) in genital ulcer exudate of HIV-1-infected men by culture and gene amplification. J Infect Dis. 1990;161:810-811.
86. Schacker T, Ryncarz AJ, Goddard J, et al. Frequent recovery of HIV-1 from genital herpes simplex virus lesions in HIV-1-infected men. JAMA. 1998;280:61-66.
87. Holmberg SD, Stewart JA, Gerber AR, et al. Prior herpes simplex virus type 2 infection as a risk factor for HIV infection. JAMA. 1988;259:1048-1050.
88. Hook EW 3rd, Cannon RO, Nahmias AJ, et al. Herpes simplex virus infection as a risk factor for human immunodeficiency virus infection in heterosexuals. J Infect Dis. 1992;165:251-255.
89. Keet IP, Lee FK, van Griensven GJ, et al. Herpes simplex virus type 2 and other genital ulcerative infections as a risk factor for HIV-1 acquisition. Genitourin Med. 1990;66:330-333.
90. Quinn TC, Glasser D, Cannon RO, et al. Human immunodeficiency virus infection among patients attending clinics for sexually transmitted diseases. N Engl J Med. 1988;318:197-203.
91. Stamm WE, Handsfield HH, Rompalo AM, et al. The association between genital ulcer disease and acquisition of HIV infection in homosexual men. JAMA. 1988;260:1429-1433.
92. Blocker ME, Levine WC, St Louis ME. HIV prevalence in patients with syphilis, United States. Sex Transm Dis. 2000;27:53-59.
93. Trees DL, Morse SA. Chancroid and *Haemophilus ducreyi:* An update. Clin Microbiol Rev. 1995;8:357-375.
94. Larsen S, Pope V, Johnson R, Kennedy E Jr., eds. A Manual for Tests for Syphilis. Washington, DC: American Public Health Association; 1998.
95. Ito F, Hunter EF, George RW, et al. Specific immunofluorescent staining of pathogenic treponemes with a monoclonal antibody. J Clin Microbiol. 1992;30:831-838.
96. Hunter EF, Greer PW, Swisher BL, et al. Immunofluorescent staining of *Treponema* in tissues fixed with formalin. Arch Pathol Lab Med. 1984;108:878-880.
97. Larsen SA, Steiner BM, Rudolph AH. Laboratory diagnosis and interpretation of tests for syphilis. Clin Microbiol Rev. 1995;8:1-21.
98. Solomon AR, Rasmussen JE, Varani J, Pierson CL. The Tzanck smear in the diagnosis of cutaneous herpes simplex. JAMA. 1984;251:633-635.
99. Nahass GT, Goldstein BA, Zhu WY, et al. Comparison of Tzanck smear, viral culture, and DNA diagnostic methods in detection of herpes simplex and varicella-zoster infection. JAMA. 1992;268:2541-2544.
100. Wald A, Ashley-Morrow R. Serological testing for herpes simplex virus (HSV)-1 and HSV-2 infection. Clin Infect Dis. 2002;35(Suppl 2):S173-S182.
101. Ashley RL, Wald A, Eagleton M. Premarket evaluation of the POCkit HSV-2 type-specific serologic test in culture-documented cases of genital herpes simplex virus type 2. Sex Transm Dis. 2000;27:266-269.
102. Johnson SR, Martin DH, Cammarata C, et al. Development of a polymerase chain reaction assay for the detection of *Haemophilus ducreyi.* Sex Transm Dis. 1994;21:13-23.
103. Tekle-Michael T, Van Dyck E, Abdellati S, Laga M. Development of a heminested polymerase chain reaction assay for the detection of *Haemophilus ducreyi* in clinical specimens. Int J STD AIDS. 2001;12:797-803.
104. Liu H, Rodes B, Chen CY, Steiner B. New tests for syphilis: Rational design of a PCR method for detection of *Treponema pallidum* in clinical specimens using unique regions of the DNA polymerase I gene. J Clin Microbiol. 2001;39:1941-1946.
105. Burstain JM, Grimprel E, Lukehart SA, et al. Sensitive detection of *Treponema pallidum* by using the polymerase chain reaction. J Clin Microbiol. 1991;29:62-69.
106. Mertz KJ, Weiss JB, Webb RM, et al. An investigation of genital ulcers in Jackson, Mississippi, with use of a multiplex polymerase chain reaction assay: High prevalence of chancroid and human immunodeficiency virus infection. J Infect Dis. 1998;178:1060-1066.
107. Cone RW, Hobson AC, Palmer J, et al. Extended duration of herpes simplex virus DNA in genital lesions detected by the polymerase chain reaction. J Infect Dis. 1991;164:757-760.
108. Orle KA, Gates CA, Martin DH, et al. Simultaneous PCR detection of *Haemophilus ducreyi, Treponema pallidum,* and herpes simplex virus types 1 and 2 from genital ulcers. J Clin Microbiol. 1996;34:49-54.
109. Verdon MS, Handsfield HH, Johnson RB. Pilot study of azithromycin for the treatment of primary and secondary syphilis. Clin Infect Dis. 1994;19:486-488.
110. Hook E III, Stephans J, Ennis DM. Azithromycin compared with penicillin G benzathine for treatment of incubating syphilis. Ann Intern Med. 1999;131:434-437.
111. Hook EW III, Roddy RE, Handsfield HH. Ceftriaxone therapy for incubating and early syphilis. J Infect Dis. 1988;158:881-884.
112. Moorthy TT, Lee CT, Lim KB, Tan T. Ceftriaxone for treatment of primary syphilis in men: A preliminary study. Sex Transm Dis. 1987;14:116-118.
113. Safrin S, Elbeik T, Phan L, et al. Correlation between response to acyclovir and foscarnet therapy and in vitro susceptibility result for isolates of herpes simplex virus from human immunodeficiency virus-infected patients. Antimicrob Agents Chemother. 1994;38:1246-1250.
114. Barry DW, Lehrman SN, Ellis MN. Clinical and laboratory experience with acyclovir-resistant herpes viruses. J Antimicrob Chemother. 1986;18(Suppl B):75-84.
115. Safrin S, Assaykeen T, Follansbee S, Mills J. Foscarnet therapy for acyclovir-resistant mucocutaneous herpes simplex virus infection in 26 AIDS patients: preliminary data. J Infect Dis. 1990;161:1078-1084.
116. Lalezari JP, Drew WL, Glutzer E, et al. Treatment with intravenous (S)-1-(3-hydroxy-2-(phosphonylmethoxy)propyl)-cytosine of acyclovir-resistant mucocutaneous infection with herpes simplex virus in a patient with AIDS. J Infect Dis. 1994;170:570-572.
117. Bowmer MI, Nsanze H, D'Costa LJ, et al. Single-dose ceftriaxone for chancroid. Antimicrob Agents Chemother. 1987;31:67-69.
118. Naamara W, Plummer FA, Greenblatt RM, et al. Treatment of chancroid with ciprofloxacin: A prospective, randomized clinical trial. Am J Med. 1987;82:317-320.
119. Plourde PJ, D'Costa LJ, Agoki E, et al. A randomized, double-blind study of the efficacy of fleroxacin versus trimethoprim-sulfamethoxazole in men with culture-proven chancroid. J Infect Dis. 1992;165:949-952.
120. Wiley DJ, Douglas J, Beutner K, et al. External genital warts: Diagnosis, treatment, and prevention. Clin Infect Dis. 2002;35:S210-S224.
121. Nussinovitch M, Prais D, Ben-Amitai D, et al. Fixed drug eruption in the genital area in 15 boys. Pediatr Dermatol. 2002;19:216-219.
122. Sehgal VH, Gangwani OP. Genital fixed drug eruptions. Genitourin Med. 1986;62:56-58.
123. Fiumara NJ, Bendetson P. Probable fixed drug eruption from contact with a patient treated with tetracycline. Sex Transm Dis. 1981;8:258-259.
124. Farber EM, Nall L. Genital psoriasis. Cutis. 1992;50:263-266.
125. Stern R. Genital tumors among men with psoriasis exposed to psoralens and ultraviolet A radiation (PUVA) and ultraviolet B radiation. The Photochemotherapy Follow-up Study. N Engl J Med. 1990;322:1093-1097.
126. Schuman P, Christensen C, Sobel JD. Aphthous vaginal ulceration in two women with acquired immunodeficiency syndrome. Am J Obstet Gynecol. 1996;174:1660-1663.
127. Anderson J, Clark RA, Watts DH, et al. Idiopathic genital ulcers in women infected with human immunodeficiency virus. J Acquir Immune Defic Syndr Hum Retrovirol. 1996;13:343-347.
128. Arbesfeld SJ, Kurban AK. Behcet's disease: New perspectives on an enigmatic syndrome. J Am Acad Dermatol. 1988;19:767-779.
129. Rosen T, Conrad N. Genital ulcer caused by human bite to the penis. Sex Transm Dis. 1999;26:527-530.
130. Ball TP Jr, Pickett JD. Traumatic lymphangitis of penis. Urology. 1975;6:594-597.
131. Hinnen U, Elsner P, Barraud M, Burg G. Foreign body granuloma of the penis caused by occupational glass fibre exposure. Genitourin Med. 1997;73:577-578.
132. Fiumara N. Nonvenereal sclerosing lymphangitis of the penis. Arch Dermatol. 1975;111:902-903.
133. Angulo JC, Ramirez JC, Esteban M, Sanchez-Chapado M. Perineal fistulization of genital tuberculosis. J Urol. 1999;161:1576-1577.

134. Price AJ, Bates TS, Deveraj V, Stott MA. An unusual prostatocutaneous fistula. Br J Urol. 1997;80:509-510.

135. Vijaikumar M, Thappa DM, Kaviarasan PK. Papulonecrotic tuberculide of the glans penis. Sex Transm Infect. 2001;77:147.

136. Smith MB, Schnadig VJ, Zaharopoulos P, Van Hook C. Disseminated *Histoplasma capsulatum* infection presenting as genital ulcerations. Obstet Gynecol. 1997;89:842-844.

137. Jayalakshmi P, Goh KL, Soo-Hoo TS, Daud A. Disseminated histoplasmosis presenting as penile ulcer. Aust N Z J Med. 1990;20:175-176.

138. Hejase MJ, Bihrle R, Castillo G, Coogan CL. Amebiasis of the penis. Urology. 1996;48:151-154.

139. Veliath AJ, Bansal R, Sankaran V, et al. Genital amebiasis. Int J Gynaecol Obstet. 1987;25:249-256.

CHAPTER **102**

Urethritis

WILLIAM M. McCORMACK
MICHAEL F. REIN

Urethritis a very common condition that was described in the earliest recorded histories of humankind.[1,2]

The symptoms of urethritis range from the trivial and often overlooked to the disabling. Urethral discharge may be apparent at all times during the day and may be present in sufficient quantity to stain undergarments, or it may be so scanty that it is noted by the patient only on arising as a small bead of moisture or crust at the meatus. It may be completely clear, mucopurulent, or frankly purulent, and it may be white, yellow, green, or brown. Some patients complain only of a deviation of the first morning urine stream. Occasionally, urethral discharge comes to the attention of the patient through the observation of mucus strands in the urine specimen.

The urine stream transiently eliminates most inflammatory discharges; therefore, scanty discharges are best observed on arising, before the passage of any urine. Micturition immediately preceding urethral examination may completely eliminate signs of infection.

The discomfort of urethritis can take several forms. Dysuria is common, and men variously localize it to the meatus, the distal portion of the penis, or anywhere along the shaft. Discomfort is sometimes increased by the acidity or solute content of the urine and therefore may be most marked during the passage of a concentrated first morning urine. Dysuria may be increased in the presence of irritants such as alcohol, which is an observation that sometimes leads the patient to attribute his disease to the ingestion of specific foods or fluids. Discomfort may persist between micturitions and is perceived as pain, itching, frequency, urgency, or a feeling of heaviness in the genitals.

Discomfort experienced only during ejaculation, deep pelvic pain, or pain radiating to the back is infrequent in uncomplicated urethritis and suggests prostatitis or inflammation involving other portions of the urogenital tract, such as the epididymis. Hematuria (particularly if painless) and blood in the ejaculate are uncommon in urethritis. The persistence of hematuria after cure of urethritis demands a thorough urologic evaluation.

EXAMINATION OF THE URETHRA

The genitalia should be examined while the patient is supine. Alternatively, the man can stand before the seated examiner so that the external genitalia are at approximately eye level. A good light source is essential. The patient should remove his trousers and underwear so that the entire genital area can be observed. The underwear may reveal stains of dried discharge, suggesting that it is being produced in large amounts. This observation is particularly useful if the patient has recently urinated.

The patient is preferably examined at least 2 hours after his last micturition. If advised to restrict fluids during the day preceding the examination, he may be able to present for evaluation before passing the first urine of the day, which sometimes permits the recovery of very small amounts of discharge.[3]

The entire genital area should be carefully examined, because other sexually transmitted infections are relatively common in patients with urethritis. Inguinal adenopathy should be sought, and tenderness should be noted. The skin of the entire pubic area, scrotum, groin, and penis should be examined for lesions, and the hair should be examined for nits. The testes, epididymides, and spermatic cords should be palpated for masses or tenderness. The foreskin should be completely retracted and the glans examined. The urethral meatus should be inspected for dried crusts, redness, and spontaneous discharge. If no discharge is present, the urethra should be gently stripped as follows. The examiner places the gloved thumb along the ventral surface of the base of the penis and the forefinger on the dorsum and then applies gentle pressure; the hand is moved slowly toward the meatus. This maneuver frequently expels a discharge that may be collected on a swab for examination (as described later).

If no discharge is delivered by this maneuver, the third and fourth fingers should be used to grip the penis lightly from above, just behind the glans. The thumb and forefinger can then spread open the meatus to examine for urethral redness or the presence of small amounts of discharge. Unless the patient has recently urinated or has been in a state of sexual arousal, virtually no fluid should be expressible from the urethra or observed by spreading the meatus.

If expressed material cannot be collected at the meatus, a specimen must be recovered from inside the urethra. This is best accomplished with a small urethral swab.[4] The swab should be inserted gently at least 2 cm into the urethra, with care taken not to attempt to force the tip past any obstruction. The patient should be warned that the examination is uncomfortable; also, the insertion and removal of the swab should be accomplished as quickly as possible. Patients tolerate the examination better if they are supine. If additional specimens are required for multiple examinations or cultures, separate swabs should be used, and each one should be inserted at least 1 cm deeper than the one preceding it.

Regular cotton swabs should not be used for urethral examination, because their larger diameter makes insertion extremely uncomfortable and because of the possibility that the cotton or the wooden shaft may be toxic to some fastidious pathogens. A small platinum loop is effective, but it must be sterilized in a flame and carefully cooled between uses.

A woman's urethra is best examined while she is in the lithotomy position. The entire genital area should be examined for lesions, and the vagina should be examined as described in Chapter 103. The urethral meatus may be directly visualized, and the urethra may be stripped by placing the gloved finger inside the vagina and gently moving it along the urethra. A small swab may be inserted a short distance into the meatus to obtain a urethral specimen.

EXAMINATION OF THE URETHRAL SPECIMEN

A swab that contains material from the urethra should be rolled across a clean microscope slide. Rolling rather than streaking the swab brings all its surfaces into contact with the slide and better preserves cellular morphologic characteristics. The material may be air-dried and fixed by gentle heating or by rinsing with methanol. Gram staining of urethral material is particularly useful in the workup of urethritis (Box 102-1), and the specimen should be examined with the use of the oil-immersion objective. Specimens obtained from within the urethra usually contain urethral epithelial cells. If recovered from near the meatus, these are typical squamous cells with a very large cytoplasmic-nuclear ratio; if obtained from further within the urethra, they are cuboidal epithelial cells, which are smaller and have relatively larger, less dense nuclei.

Urethral material from patients with acute urethritis contains polymorphonuclear neutrophils (PMNs) (Box 102-2). The area of the smear that contains the most PMNs should be sought. More than

4 PMNs per oil-immersion microscopic field is abnormal and is seen in 60% to 90% of patients with acute symptomatic urethritis.[4,5] However, up to 50% of all men with documented urethral infection do not show 4 PMNs in maximally dense oil-immersion fields.[6-9] The number of PMNs in the smear is reduced by recent micturition; also, there often is considerable observer variation in the number of PMNs detected in a single specimen.[10] Therefore, although purulent discharges may reveal sheets of PMNs, the minimal number of these cells that indicates disease is not known. In general, the presence of even rare PMNs suggests infection, particularly in the patient who has urethral symptoms or who is found to have a small amount of discharge on examination.

The distal centimeter of the urethra is colonized by normal skin or introital flora. The smear usually contains a variety of gram-positive and gram-negative organisms that have no particular significance. Of great diagnostic value, however, is the presence of typical gram-negative, "intracellular" diplococci (Fig. 102-1). These organisms are not randomly distributed among the cells but are seen in large numbers in a few PMNs. They are observed in more than 95% of all symptomatic patients with gonococcal urethritis and in fewer than 2% of all symptomatic men who cannot be shown to have gonorrhea by culture.[11-13] Some strains of *Neisseria gonorrhoeae* are inhibited by the concentrations of vancomycin that usually are employed in selective isolation media; these organisms will not be recovered by standard culture techniques.[14] Extracellular diplococci indicate gonorrhea in only 10% to 29% of all cases, and this predictive value is reduced even further in populations with a low prevalence of gonorrhea.[13] A shortcoming of the Gram-stained smear is that it cannot diagnose coincidental nongonococcal urethritis (NGU) in the presence of gonorrhea. Although a smear containing PMNs that does not reveal gram-negative intracellular diplococci strongly suggests NGU, a smear revealing these organisms does not rule out NGU.

Candida organisms may be recognized as gram-positive or beaded, oval bodies about 3 by 6 µm. The presence of small numbers of yeast cells does not prove a candidal origin for the urethritis, because *Candida* may be recovered from healthy patients, particularly if they are uncircumcised.

Trichomonads are very difficult to identify on Gram-stained smears. Urethral material may be mixed with a small amount of saline and observed as a wet mount with the substage condenser racked down or the substage diaphragm partially closed. Motile trichomonads occasionally are observed but are rarely seen unless the urethral material for examination is obtained before the first voiding. Positive findings on a wet mount are diagnostic of trichomoniasis, but findings on the wet mount are often negative in infected men. Endourethral cultures or cultures of first-void urine sediment in media such as modified Diamond's medium constitute the preferred method for diagnosis of trichomoniasis in men.[15,16]

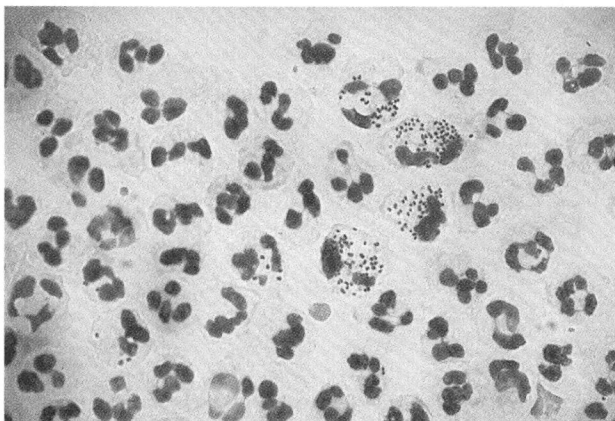

FIGURE 102-1. Gram stain of urethral exudate from a man with gonorrhea. Several neutrophils contain many gram-negative cell-associated diplococci.

After the patient's urethra has been carefully examined, he may be asked to provide a divided urine specimen. The patient delivers the first 10 mL of urine into one container and a midstream urine specimen into a second container. The presence of mucus strands in the first fraction that clear in the second portion suggests urethritis. Equal aliquots of the fractions may be centrifuged and the sediments examined as wet mounts. Observation of more white blood cells in the initial than in the second fraction suggests urethritis, whereas equal numbers of white cells in both fractions suggests cystitis or infection higher in the urinary tract.[3,4] The presence of more than 15 white blood cells × 400 microscopic fields of the sediment from the initial fraction strongly suggests urethritis,[4,6,9] but the minimum significant number of white blood cells is unknown. A PMN count of more than 10 per high-power field is found in 90% of all men with chlamydial urethritis.[6]

The presence of white blood cells in the initial urine fraction provides no clue to the cause of the urethritis. Such a finding, however, may allow an objective diagnosis of urethritis to be made in a man whose Gram-stained smear does not contain PMNs. The first-void urine is more sensitive than the urethral Gram stain for detection of PMNs in men with few or no symptoms of urethritis.

Many men who are infected with *N. gonorrhoeae* or *Chlamydia trachomatis* have no symptoms. Such men often have pyuria that can be detected by examination of the first 10-mL urine sample by either microscopy or leukocyte-esterase "dipstick" testing. This approach provides a noninvasive, inexpensive method for screening men for urethral infection. Men found to have pyuria are candidates for further examination, including examination of endourethral specimens for gonococci and chlamydiae.

If the urine specimen is a first morning micturition, motile trichomonads may be observed in the sediment. In one study, *Trichomonas vaginalis* organisms were recovered by culture of urethral swabs in 80% and first-void urine in 68% of infected patients. When combined, these two cultures detected 49 (98%) of 50 infected men.[15] Trichomonads are recovered less frequently from patients who have already voided during the day.

Culture systems for *C. trachomatis* are not widely available. Nonculture tests such as enzyme-linked immunosorbent assay (ELISA), DNA probes, direct immunofluorescence, and nucleic acid amplification have been developed. Although ELISA, DNA probes, and direct immunofluorescence tests are less sensitive than cultures, nucleic acid amplification tests are more sensitive than chlamydial cultures and retain high specificity.[17,18] Nucleic acid amplification techniques have replaced culture as the test of choice for identification of *C. trachomatis* organisms.[19] Material recovered from the urethra can be cultured with appropriate media for *N. gonorrhoeae*. Nonculture tests are also available for detection of *N. gonorrhoeae* organisms.

These tests offer no significant advantage over culture but can be used in situations in which facilities for culture are not available.

Cultures for *Ureaplasma urealyticum* should not be performed. Their interpretation is complicated by the high prevalence of colonization in asymptomatic, sexually active people. Although they are present in the distal urethra, normal skin organisms (e.g., *Staphylococcus epidermidis,* α-hemolytic streptococci, propionibacteria) and vaginal organisms (e.g., *Candida albicans,* lactobacilli, *Escherichia coli, Gardnerella vaginalis*) are of no diagnostic significance.[20,21]

NONINFECTIOUS URETHRITIS

So psychologically important is the genital tract that trivial symptoms often receive patients' frightened attention. The "worried well" make up a significant fraction of men who are seen in venereal disease clinics and in private practices. Sympathetic questioning as to why the patient thinks he has contracted a genital infection may reveal guilt over masturbation or an extramarital sexual contact. The urethral specimen in these cases usually reveals normal epithelial cells and no white blood cells. Some patients confuse dried remnants of semen with inflammatory discharge. Microscopic examination again fails to reveal inflammatory cells, but spermatozoa may be recognized on the Gram stain as gram-positive ovoids whose coloration fades gradually toward the acrosomal cap. Spermatozoa may also be recognized on the wet mount. However, the clinician must remember that symptoms and signs of true urethritis can be trivial and that microscopic examination may miss minimal inflammation, particularly if the patient has recently voided. Symptomatic patients with negative examination results should have urethral specimens tested for gonococci and chlamydiae and be asked to return in several days, by which time the symptoms may have resolved or examination may provide a diagnosis. Antimicrobial treatment of symptomatic men who have neither objective evidence of urethritis nor positive cultures for urethral pathogens is inadvisable and may serve to reinforce psychosomatic contributions to their symptoms.[22] Occasionally, a patient who complains of a discharge is actually suffering from urinary incontinence.

Chronic irritation of the urethra can elicit a clear, mucoid discharge. Occasionally patients who are concerned that they may have contracted a venereal disease vigorously strip the urethra, looking for a discharge. After several days of this, a clear discharge obligingly appears that may contain a few white blood cells. A history of vigorous urethral stripping is helpful diagnostically. Patients who are receiving treatment for other forms of urethritis should be cautioned not to examine themselves too vigorously for fear that such a traumatic discharge may confuse the clinical picture. Very rarely, patients insert foreign bodies into the urethra and produce a mechanical urethritis.[23]

A heavy precipitation of crystals in the urine can suggest a discharge, and the presence of large amounts of crystalline material or calculous gravel can produce urinary discomfort. The intermittent nature of pain associated with the passage of gravel or the obvious presence of crystals on microscopic examination of the urine sediment usually confirms this diagnosis. White blood cells may be present.

Chemicals can irritate the urethra, and alcohol has long been known to produce mild dysuria. The ingestion of alcohol during treatment for gonorrhea was at one time thought to be responsible for the syndrome of postgonococcal urethritis (discussed later), although it is now known to have an infectious etiology. Occasionally, a patient develops urethral symptoms on contact with vaginal chemicals such as spermicides used by a sexual partner. The history of discomfort immediately after sexual contact may be suggestive. This condition should be diagnosed only after other possible causes have been excluded.

INFECTIOUS URETHRITIS

Gonococcal and Nongonococcal Urethritis

The classic specific etiologic agent of acute urethritis is *N. gonorrhoeae.* Urethral infection of all other causes is referred to collectively as NGU (Box 102-3). As with gonorrhea, most cases of NGU are sex-

---

BOX 102-3

Etiology of Urethritis

Neisseria gonorrhoeae   *Trichomonas vaginalis*
Chlamydia trachomatis   *Mycoplasma genitalium*
Ureaplasma urealyticum   Herpes simplex virus

---

ually acquired. NGU is more common than gonorrhea in the United States and in much of the developed world. In some underdeveloped areas, however, gonorrhea accounts for 80% of the cases of acute urethritis. Like many other sexually transmitted diseases (STDs), gonococcal urethritis and NGU have an increased incidence during the summer months, presumably because of a seasonal increase in sexual activity. The ratio of cases of NGU to those of gonococcal urethritis is greater among groups with higher socioeconomic status in the United States. For example, most of the cases of urethritis seen among college students are nongonococcal in origin, whereas gonorrhea is the most common cause of urethritis in urban STD clinics.[24-26]

Compared with gonococci, the organisms that cause NGU may be relatively less prevalent among homosexual than among heterosexual men with urethritis. In a study of men who had urethritis, Clemens and colleagues[27] recovered gonococci from 45% of men who had sex with men and from 26% of men who had sex with women. Examining consecutive men attending an STD clinic, Stamm and colleagues[8] recovered gonococci from 12% of heterosexual men and 25% of homosexual men; in contrast, chlamydiae were recovered from 14% of heterosexual men but only 5% of homosexual men. Studies have associated fellatio with the acquisition of gonococcal urethritis and NGU in homosexual but not in heterosexual men.[28,29]

Among patients infected with the human immunodeficiency virus (HIV), the quantity of HIV in urethral secretions is increased if the man has concomitant urethritis. Treatment of urethritis reduces the urethral viral load. Recent studies indicate that gonorrhea may facilitate HIV transmission.[30,31]

Historically, there has been considerable interest in the possible role of circumcision in the epidemiology of urethritis. Such studies are difficult to interpret, because certain behavioral factors are associated with circumcision.[32] The presence of a foreskin may mask a urethral discharge and delay presentation for evaluation, but other roles remain speculative.[32]

The clinical spectrum of gonorrhea differs from that of NGU, but there is sufficient overlap that an accurate diagnosis must be based on examination of the urethral specimen. Seventy-five percent of men who acquire urethral gonorrhea develop symptoms within 4 days,[3] and 80% to 90% do so within 2 weeks.[32,33] The incubation period for NGU is much more variable and is often longer. Incubation periods ranging from 2 to 35 days have been described,[24,26,33] but almost 50% of men with NGU developed urethral symptoms within 4 days.[3,24,33] Therefore, an incubation period of less than 1 week is not a reliable factor in the differential diagnosis.[3,24,33] The incubation period of either infection can be prolonged by the ingestion of subcurative doses of antibiotics.

The urethral discharge is described as frankly purulent in three fourths of patients with gonorrhea (Fig. 102-2) but in only 11% to 33% of patients with NGU.[11,26,34] A purulent discharge issuing from the meatus without stripping of the urethra correlates strongly with the diagnosis of gonorrhea but is also seen in 4% of patients with NGU.[11,34] Mucopurulent discharge (Fig. 102-3), consisting of thin, cloudy fluid or mucoid fluid with purulent flecks, is seen in about 50% of the patients with NGU but in only 25% of the patients with symptomatic gonorrhea.[11,34] The discharge is completely clear and moderately viscid in 10% to 50% of patients with NGU, principally those who are minimally symptomatic, but in only 4% of symptomatic patients with gonorrhea.[11,34,35] A diagnosis based on the clinical characteristics of the urethral discharge is unreliable and correctly identifies the causative disorder in only 73% of all cases, even under optimal circumstances.[34] Microscopic examination always should be part of the initial evaluation.

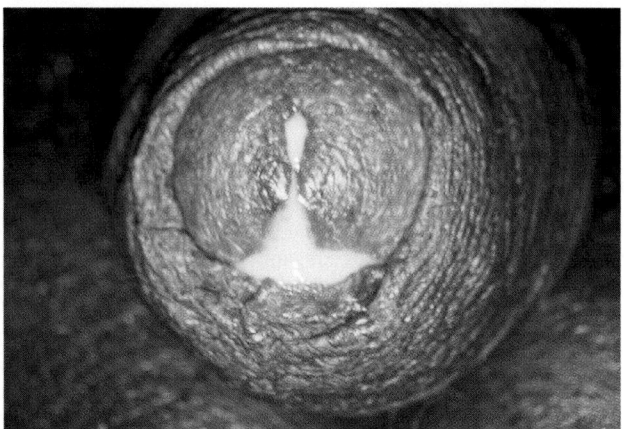

FIGURE 102-2. Purulent urethral discharge from a man with gonococcal urethritis.

Dysuria has been described in 53% to 75% of patients with NGU and in 73% to 88% of patients with symptomatic gonorrhea.[11,36] Only about 10% of patients complaining of dysuria without discharge have gonorrhea; the remainder have NGU.[11] A combination of dysuria and discharge is seen in 71% of patients with gonococcal urethritis but in only 38% of patients with NGU. Therefore, the combination of discharge and dysuria is associated with gonorrhea, whereas the appearance of one without the other is more frequently seen with NGU. The association is insufficiently specific for differentiating these two entities. Urethral discomfort can mimic cystitis in men and women and can result in urinary frequency and urgency.

Symptoms of gonorrhea often begin abruptly, and the patient may remember the specific time of day when they were first noted. NGU usually has a less acute onset, with symptoms increasing over several days. A urethral discharge may appear days in advance of dysuria; the symptoms may wax and wane, even to the point of transiently disappearing before the patient seeks therapy. The mildness and variability of the symptoms may erroneously convince the patient with NGU that he does not have a significant disease; such patients often delay seeking medical attention.[11,36]

In most cases, the symptoms of infectious urethritis resolve even if the causative disorder remains untreated. Ninety-five percent of patients with acute gonococcal urethritis who do not receive treatment are free of symptoms 6 months after contracting the disease,[37] and the symptoms of NGU gradually subside over a period of 1 to 3 months in 30% to 70% of the patients.[38] How many of these asymptomatic patients remain infected and potentially infectious is unknown.

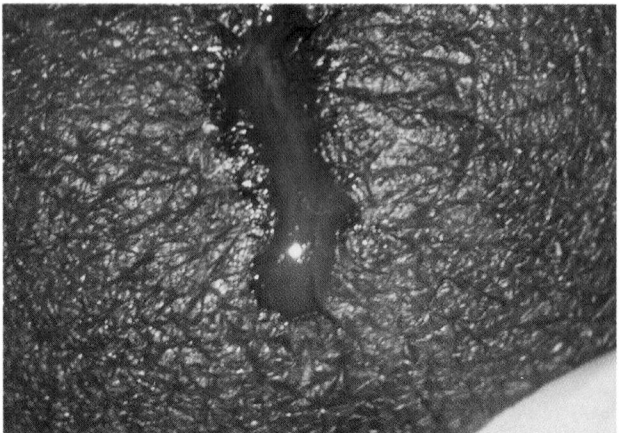

FIGURE 102-3. Mucopurulent urethral discharge from a man with nongonococcal urethritis.

Untreated gonococcal urethritis may subside to a chronic state characterized by little or no urethral discomfort and a small amount of mucoid discharge called *gleet*. This discharge contains small numbers of gonococci and PMNs.

So great is the clinical overlap between NGU and gonococcal urethritis that a diagnosis should not be made on clinical grounds alone. Gram staining of urethral discharge material reveals typical gram-negative, intracellular diplococci in about 95% of cases of symptomatic gonococcal urethritis and is negative in about 97% of the patients with symptomatic NGU.[11-13] Therefore, in a population in which about 50% of the cases of acute urethritis are gonococcal, a positive result on Gram staining suggests gonorrhea, and a negative result suggests NGU with 98% accuracy.[11,13] The finding of typically shaped extracellular diplococci diagnoses gonorrhea with an accuracy of only 10% to 30%.[13] Such results on Gram staining are known as *equivocal* and are found in about 15% of patients with symptomatic urethritis.[11]

The sensitivity of the culture for *N. gonorrhoeae* is less than 100%, partly because some gonococci are inhibited by the vancomycin concentrations used in selective media. The chances of isolating the organism are further reduced if the patient has recently taken antibiotics or if there is a delay in processing the culture. Therefore, it seems likely that most of the few patients with positive findings on Gram staining and negative cultures actually have gonorrhea. In most cases of acute symptomatic urethritis, culture is unnecessary to confirm Gram stain findings diagnostic of gonorrhea. It must be remembered that results on Gram staining are negative in as many as 5% of patients who have gonorrhea, so Gram stain findings suggestive of NGU should be confirmed with a culture for gonococci, although therapy need not be delayed until the results are known. Results on Gram staining cannot be used to make a diagnosis of simultaneous NGU in the presence of gonorrhea. Because of the frequency with which trichomonads are missed with direct microscopic techniques, patients in whom trichomonal urethritis is suspected should be evaluated by culture of urethral and first-void urine specimens.[15]

There is no doubt that urethritis is sexually transmitted. It occurs most frequently during the ages of peak sexual activity and in groups with a high prevalence of other STDs. It is found with increased frequency in persons with a history of other sexually transmitted genital infections.[24,26] It frequently occurs after sexual exposure to a new partner and is almost never seen in virgins except as a part of some systemic conditions. As the etiologic agents of urethritis have been defined, they have been isolated with high frequency from the female and homosexual male sexual partners of infected men—by whom, however, they usually are carried asymptomatically.

Recognition of urethritis as an STD is important for several practical reasons. It allows definition of a population at very high risk for carrying the causative agents, namely, the sexual partners of infected patients. The prevalence of infection with these agents is sufficiently high among sexual partners to justify their treatment on epidemiologic grounds, even if they are asymptomatic. Many episodes of recurrent NGU are terminated only by the treatment of an asymptomatic sexual partner of the infected patient. Because persons with one STD are at increased risk for others, it is important to screen patients with urethritis for other STDs.

Etiology of Nongonococcal Urethritis

The organism most clearly associated with NGU, *C. trachomatis,* is discussed in detail in Chapter 177. This obligate intracellular parasite causes as many as 50% of cases of NGU.[6,20,25,39] Effective *Chlamydia* control programs may reduce the proportion of men with NGU who are infected with *C. trachomatis*. *C. trachomatis* is susceptible to several antimicrobial agents, including the tetracyclines, sulfonamides, erythromycin, and azithromycin. Significantly, it is not reliably eradicated by penicillins, cephalosporins, fluoroquinolones, or spectinomycin in the single doses used to treat uncomplicated gonorrhea.

Chlamydiae are not recovered from at least 50% of men with NGU. Although the clinical features of *Chlamydia*-negative NGU are very similar to those of *Chlamydia*-positive NGU,[24] some workers have suggested that less discharge is produced in patients who are positive for *Chlamydia* than in those who are not, and the mean incubation period may be slightly shorter.[24]

The agents responsible for *Chlamydia*-negative NGU remain, to some extent, unidentified. *Ureaplasma urealyticum*, formerly known as the T-strain mycoplasma, has been recovered from 81% of men with *Chlamydia*-negative NGU, which is significantly higher than the 60% isolation rate from asymptomatic controls.[20,40,42] Furthermore, *U. urealyticum* can be recovered in larger numbers from men with *Chlamydia*-negative NGU than from control subjects.[40,41] Supporting the hypothesis that these agents (see Chapter 180) cause some cases of NGU is the observation that sulfonamides and rifampin, to which the organisms are insensitive, fail to cure most patients with *Chlamydia*-negative NGU.[42,43] Conversely, spectinomycin, which is active against ureaplasmas but inactive against *Chlamydia*, cures patients with NGU from whom only *U. urealyticum* has been isolated.[42] Additional support comes from experiments in which two investigators inoculated themselves with ureaplasmas; both developed NGU.[44] Furthermore, some patients with NGU show rises in immunoglobulin M and immunoglobulin G antibody titers against *U. urealyticum*.[45] Therefore, the weight of evidence favors an etiologic role for *U. urealyticum* organisms in NGU. Accurate assessment of the relative contribution of ureaplasmas is hindered by the ubiquity of the organisms that can be recovered from urethral cultures from many sexually experienced men who have no evidence of urethritis.[46,47] *Mycoplasma hominis* is not a cause of NGU,[46,47] whereas *Mycoplasma genitalium* has been recovered from patients with NGU.[48] Studies in which this fastidious organism was identified with the use of polymerase chain reaction assays identified *M. genitalium* in 16.7% to 33% of men with NGU.[49-54]

Like *Chlamydia*, the ureaplasmas and *M. genitalium* are susceptible to erythromycin, azithromycin, and, usually, tetracyclines—the agents that have been most successful in treating NGU. Some patients, however, are infected with tetracycline-resistant *U. urealyticum*[5,55-57]; such patients may not be cured by tetracycline therapy. A recent study[58] found that azithromycin was considerably more effective than tetracyclines in eradicating *M. genitalium* from men who had urethritis. A significant minority of men with NGU do not carry *C. trachomatis*, *M. genitalium*, or *U. urealyticum*,[42,43,59,60] and it would not be surprising if other agents were in the future identified as causes of NGU. Patients with nonchlamydial, nonureaplasmal NGU have a higher recurrence rate after therapy than do men with chlamydial urethritis.[43,59,60]

Dysuria is described by 83% of women and 44% of men with primary herpes simplex genital infection. Some men notice a clear, mucoid discharge that seems disproportionately mild relative to the degree of dysuria that they experience. Herpes simplex virus (HSV) is recovered from the urethras of about 80% of women and 30% of men with primary infection, and HSV must be regarded as a cause of some cases of NGU. In most such instances, however, the diagnosis of HSV is obvious because of typical genital lesions. Urethral involvement is less common in recurrent disease, and dysuria is described by only 27% of women and 9% of men.[61]

T. vaginalis has been isolated from patients with NGU,[15,16,21] and it causes a small percentage of the cases. The syndrome is not clinically distinguishable from NGU of other causes. With the use of nucleic acid amplification tests, *T. vaginalis* was identified in 2.9% to 19% of men attending urban STD clinics in the United States.[62-64] This organism was associated with signs and symptoms of urethritis, particularly in men older than 28 years of age.

Urethral infection with gram-negative bacilli can be seen in men with diabetes and in those who practice insertive anal intercourse; it may occur in patients with phimosis and in those with urethral trauma after instrumentation or indwelling catheterization.[65] Periurethral abscesses can occur in this setting. Somewhat fewer than 3% of the cases of urethritis are caused by infection higher up in the urinary tract. Syphilis, with an endourethral chancre, and intraurethral condylomata acuminata occasionally cause a urethral discharge. *Neisseria meningitidis* organisms have been isolated from some patients with urethritis.[66]

A few investigators have attributed some cases of NGU to *Clostridium difficile*, *Branhamella catarrhalis*, *Haemophilus influenzae*, corynebacteria, *G. vaginalis*, *Bacteroides urealyticus*, adenoviruses, and schistosomes. Most of these observations, however, were uncontrolled for the presence of such important pathogens as *C. trachomatis* and *U. urealyticum*, and the role of these organisms must be considered unproven. Indeed, other studies have reported the recovery of corynebacteria, *G. vaginalis*, and anaerobes less frequently from patients with NGU than from asymptomatic controls.[20,40,67]

POSTGONOCOCCAL URETHRITIS

Some patients who receive single-dose treatment for acute gonococcal urethritis experience prompt resolution followed, in a few days, by a recurrence of symptoms—usually a mucoid or mucopurulent discharge and sometimes mild dysuria. In other patients, the symptoms never entirely disappear and, after initial rapid improvement, stabilize at a low level. This syndrome is referred to as *postgonococcal urethritis* (PGU); it should be suspected if signs, symptoms, or laboratory evidence of urethritis are found 4 to 7 days after single-dose treatment for gonorrhea.[68,69] PGU is a manifestation of dual urethral infection. Gonococci and the agents of NGU are extremely prevalent in sexually active populations, and they are carried simultaneously and asymptomatically by many women. Male sexual partners of these women may acquire both agents during the same sexual exposure. In the presence of gonorrhea, coincident NGU cannot be diagnosed with Gram staining. Single-dose treatment of gonorrhea with cephalosporins, quinolones, or spectinomycin (no longer available) eradicates the gonococci, eliminating the symptoms of gonorrhea, but it usually spares the agents of NGU. If the incubation period of NGU is exceeded, the patient experiences a recurrence or persistence of milder symptoms that is consistent with the latter infection.

Although PGU was originally thought to result from the consumption of alcohol or other irritants during therapy for gonorrhea, dual infection is now well established as the explanation. *C. trachomatis* has been recovered from 11% to 50% of men with gonorrhea[39]; 75% to 100% of patients with gonorrhea who are also culture-positive for *Chlamydia* will develop PGU if their gonorrhea is treated with an agent that does not eradicate *Chlamydia*.[70-72] *C. trachomatis* can be recovered from almost 50% of patients with PGU, which is similar to the recovery rate in NGU. PGU, however, also develops in 20% to 50% of the patients with gonorrhea from whom chlamydiae are not recovered[71]; some of these cases appear to be associated with ureaplasmal infection. As might be expected, if gonorrhea is treated with a regimen active against the agents of NGU, the incidence of PGU is lower.[72] Accordingly, current treatment schedules for gonorrhea include a second agent such as doxycycline or azithromycin.

Patients with persistence or recurrence of urethral symptoms after therapy for acute gonococcal urethritis may have PGU, but gonococcal reinfection and frank treatment failure are also possible. The patient who is experiencing recurrent urethritis must be evaluated as a new patient to differentiate gonococcal from nongonococcal infection.

ASYMPTOMATIC URETHRAL INFECTION

Patients without specific complaints that are referable to the urethra may be found to have signs of urethritis on physical examination; sexually transmitted pathogens can be recovered from some patients who have neither symptoms nor signs of urethritis. Infected adolescents are less likely to complain of urethral symptoms than are adults.[73]

The importance of asymptomatic urethral gonococcal infection in men is well recognized.[74] Prolonged asymptomatic urethral carriage of gonococci occurs in about 2% to 3% of newly infected men[74]; however, because these men do not seek treatment, the prevalence of asymptomatic urethral gonococcal infections is distinctly higher than 3% and may have considerable epidemiologic significance. Random screening of asymptomatic men is unrewarding[74] except in high-risk populations. Most cases of asymptomatic urethral infection are detected after gonorrhea is diagnosed in female sexual partners or if complications subsequently develop in the infected man. Up to 40% of the asymptomatic sexual partners of women with disseminated gonococcal infection or pelvic inflammatory disease are found to be infected[74]; 60% of the infected men may be asymptomatic. Asymptomatic urethral infection also is prevalent among men with gonococcal dermatitis-arthritis syndrome.[74] Asymptomatic gonorrhea may be diagnosed by examination of Gram-stained urethral material collected on a swab with a sensitivity of only about 70%.[74] Therefore, culture or a nucleic acid amplification test for gonococci is the most appropriate diagnostic test.

Part of the controversy over the etiologic role of *U. urealyticum* is its recovery from 59% of sexually active, asymptomatic men attending venereal disease clinics.[20,40] *C. trachomatis* is recovered from about 3% of such men.[20,40] Many men harboring trichomonads are asymptomatic[16] and represent an important vector of infection.

Asymptomatic urethritis in many cases can be rapidly detected by observing PMNs in material recovered from the urethra with a swab or loop. About 25% of asymptomatic men with four or more PMNs per oil-immersion microscopic field were found to carry *C. trachomatis* in their urethras.[75] Endourethral sampling, however, is uncomfortable and is poorly accepted by asymptomatic men. Examination of first-void urine for leukocytes or leukocyte esterase[17] or for evidence of gonococcal or chlamydial infection with nucleic acid amplification techniques[18] is a more acceptable means of examining men for asymptomatic urethral infection.

Because of the frequency of asymptomatic, sexually transmitted urethral infections in men, asymptomatic sexual partners of infected women or homosexual men should always be evaluated. Because immediate diagnostic techniques are of relatively low sensitivity, such men should receive treatment at the time of their initial presentation (epidemiologic treatment).

URETHRAL SYNDROME AND RELATED DISEASES OF WOMEN

Dysuria, frequency, urgency, and nocturia are common symptoms of bacterial cystitis in women. A similar syndrome occurs in women who do not have classic bacterial infection of the lower urinary tract. Such women are said to have the *acute urethral syndrome*.[76] The usual workup for bacterial urinary tract infection is unrewarding because fewer than 10^5 uropathogens are recovered from each milliliter of urine. If the urine sediment contains PMNs, the symptoms frequently respond to antimicrobial therapy. Some of these patients appear to have bacterial cystitis, although bacteria are recovered from the urine in smaller than usual numbers.[76,77] In other patients, however, the symptoms appear to be related to urethritis rather than cystitis. *E. coli* sometimes causes urethritis in the absence of cystitis.[78] If ordinary bacterial pathogens associated with urinary tract infections are not isolated (even in small numbers), the condition is often caused by sexually transmitted agents.[76,77] If pyuria is absent, cultures for enteric bacteria and agents of STD are less likely to be positive, and antimicrobial treatment is less likely to be effective; a noninfectious explanation for urethral symptoms should be sought in such patients.

N. gonorrhoeae can affect the urethra in women as it does in men, and it occasionally causes the urethral syndrome.[79] Gentle stripping of the urethra may deliver a purulent discharge that on Gram staining reveals typical gram-negative, cell-associated diplococci. The Gram-stained smear from the female urethra has a sensitivity of about 50% for gonorrhea.[80] In about three fourths of affected women, gonococci are recovered from the endocervix as well.[79] The syndrome responds to standard therapy for uncomplicated anogenital gonorrhea (see Chapter 209).

C. trachomatis may be recovered from the urethra in women with dysuria, frequency, and pyuria.[76,77] Indeed, urinary tract symptoms are described by 53% of women in whom *C. trachomatis* is isolated from the urethra.[81,82] This association suggests that in some cases the urethral syndrome is the clinical counterpart of NGU in women. In such patients, if initial drug therapy includes antimicrobial agents that are

active against chlamydiae (e.g., tetracyclines, amoxicillin, fluoroquinolones, sulfonamides, azithromycin), clinical improvement with resolution of symptoms is likely. Relapses, however, are common and may reflect reinfection from an asymptomatic male sexual partner. In most studies, *U. urealyticum* has not been statistically associated with the urethral syndrome,[76,77,81,82] although one group found an association with more than 10^3 organisms per milliliter and pyuria.[83] The acute urethral syndrome, which is associated with pyuria, must be differentiated from the chronic urethral syndrome. The latter is not associated with pyuria and responds poorly to antimicrobial therapy.[84]

Dysuria is a common complaint of women with trichomoniasis. The parasite is recovered from the urethra and periurethral glands in more than 90% of women with the infection (see Chapter 278) and is associated with pyuria.[85] Dysuria also may result from vulvar irritation such as that accompanying vaginal candidiasis, in which case it is often perceived by the patient as being external. It is far less common in patients with bacterial vaginosis.

The urethral syndrome has been treated with steroids[77] or with urethral dilation and other types of instrumentation. Among sexually active women, gonococcal, chlamydial, and trichomonal infection should be ruled out before other therapies are tried.

TREATMENT OF SEXUAL PARTNERS OF MEN WITH NONGONOCOCCAL URETHRITIS

C. trachomatis can be recovered from the endocervix of more than half of the sexual partners of infected men[25,38] and from the urethra alone in about 20% of these women.[81,85] Although infected women usually are asymptomatic, the organism is far from benign (see Chapter 177). *C. trachomatis* is a cause of acute salpingitis. In addition, babies born to infected women may develop chlamydial conjunctivitis or pneumonia, and asymptomatic women undoubtedly are a reservoir for recurrent NGU. The carriage of ureaplasmas has been linked to infertility,[86] although the causal nature of the relationship is controversial.[46,47] These considerations support the routine treatment of female sexual partners of men with NGU, and a negative test for *C. trachomatis* in this setting does not obviate the need for treatment.

COMPLICATIONS OF URETHRITIS

Both *N. gonorrhoeae* and *C. trachomatis* have been identified as causes of acute epididymitis among sexually active men.[87] Epididymitis could conceivably lead to infertility, although an association between infectious epididymitis and infertility in men has not been convincingly demonstrated.[88] In 20% to 30% of men with NGU, prostatic involvement is documented; however, it is usually asymptomatic[5,89] and responds to standard treatments. The role of chlamydiae in the development of chronic nonbacterial prostatitis remains unproven. The organisms have been recovered from some men with chronic nonbacterial prostatitis,[90] and in some patients the condition appeared to respond to treatment with tetracyclines.[90] The role of *U. urealyticum* is even more controversial. The organism was associated with prostatitis in some series but not in others.[46,47] An association with infertility and abnormal semen specimens has been described,[86] but this also is regarded as controversial.[47] Stricture may follow gonococcal urethritis or NGU. *N. gonorrhoeae* and *C. trachomatis* can infect the conjunctiva. Also, an oculogenital syndrome consisting of NGU and conjunctivitis may be seen in about 4% of patients with NGU[91]; it responds to standard therapy with tetracyclines and must be differentiated from Reiter's syndrome (see later discussion).

THERAPY

Specific forms of urethritis, including chlamydial and ureaplasmal infections, gonorrhea, trichomoniasis, and syphilis, should be treated as discussed in the appropriate chapters in Part III of this text. As a syndrome, NGU has been treated with a variety of regimens, but doxycycline and azithromycin are the current drugs of choice.

Tetracyclines are usually prescribed for 7 days; there is little convincing evidence that full-dose regimens exceeding 7 days have any additional benefits.[92,93] Tetracycline hydrochloride is given in doses of 500 mg four times a day.[92,93] The patient should be instructed to take the drug on an empty stomach and not accompanied by milk or antacids. Alternatively, doxycycline can be administered in a dose of 100 mg orally twice daily for 7 days. This drug is highly effective, is well tolerated by patients, and can be taken with food. Twice-daily administration and fewer side effects are probably associated with better compliance.[94] Because inexpensive generic preparations are now available, doxycycline is the tetracycline of choice for treatment of NGU. Administration of doxycycline may be associated with photosensitivity reactions. Minocycline has no apparent advantages over doxycycline, and it produces dizziness in many patients.[60]

Azithromycin is an azalide antimicrobial agent with a prolonged half-life that is active against *C. trachomatis* and *U. urealyticum.* A single 1.0-g oral dose is effective against chlamydial infections[95] and in syndromic NGU.[96]

Both doxycycline and azithromycin are highly effective and well tolerated.[97] Generic doxycycline is inexpensive, but compliance with the 7-day regimen will not be complete in all instances.[98] Azithromycin is more expensive, but compliance can be assured if the drug is given under direct observation.

Erythromycin is as effective as tetracycline in chlamydial infections[7] and is active against tetracycline-resistant ureaplasmas.[5,57] Erythromycin has the additional theoretical advantage of producing higher prostatic levels than those obtainable with tetracycline hydrochloride, and it may be of use in the retreatment of patients whose symptoms are relieved by tetracycline but return after therapy is completed. Such patients may have a prostatic focus of infection that is not cured by tetracycline.[7,99] Gastrointestinal discomfort is a common adverse effect of erythromycin therapy. Patients who cannot tolerate a dose of 500 mg four times daily for 7 days can be given 250 mg four times daily for 14 days, a regimen that is almost as effective in NGU.[7]

Fluoroquinolone antimicrobial agents have been evaluated in chlamydial urethritis and in syndromic NGU. Ciprofloxacin was ineffective,[100] whereas ofloxacin (300 mg twice daily for 7 days) was effective.[101] Newer fluoroquinolones including levofloxacin and gatifloxacin are also effective. Sulfonamides including sulfisoxazole and sulfamethoxazole-trimethoprim (SMX-TMP) can also be used to treat chlamydial infections.

Even if the condition is untreated, the symptoms of NGU resolve within 2 weeks in 14% to 30% of patients[92]; up to 70% of patients have a complete resolution of symptoms within 6 months.[38] Resolution of symptoms does not mean that the infection is cured; asymptomatic patients may remain infected and infectious. Conversely, the inflammatory response accompanying NGU may take some time to resolve, even after the pathogens have been eliminated.[44]

During treatment, the symptoms of NGU frequently resolve before the patient has completed the therapeutic regimen. Patients should be cautioned to complete the entire course of antibiotics, because relapse may be more common if therapy is aborted. To reliably differentiate a relapse from reinfection and to protect sexual partners, patients undergoing treatment for urethritis should refrain from coitus or should use condoms until both partners have completed their medication regimens and their symptoms have resolved.

Because coincident chlamydial infection is very common in men with gonorrhea, the Centers for Disease Control and Prevention has suggested that uncomplicated gonococcal urethritis should be treated with a combined regimen consisting of a single dose of a suitable cephalosporin or fluoroquinolone antibiotic followed by 7 days of doxycycline (100 mg orally twice daily) or by azithromycin (in a single 1.0-g oral dose) (Box 102-4). These regimens have the advantage of providing effective single-dose therapy for gonorrhea and effective therapy for coincident, undiagnosed NGU.[102] Disadvantages include increased cost and the potential for adverse reactions. It is also prudent to use one of these combined regimens to treat urethritis of undetermined origin. Fluoroquinolone-resistant strains of *N. gonorrhoeae* are

---

BOX 102-4

Treatment of Urethritis

Ceftriaxone, 125 mg IM
or
Cefixime, 400 mg PO
or
Ofloxacin, 400 mg PO
or
Ciprofloxacin, 500 mg PO
plus azithromycin, 1.0 g as a single oral dose
or
Doxycycline, 100 mg PO bid for 7 days

---

widespread in many countries in Asia. Increased prevalence of gonococci with decreased susceptibility to fluoroquinolones has been reported in Hawaii and California. In addition, there have been sporadic reports of fluoroquinolone-resistant *N. gonorrhoeae* in other areas of the United States.[103] Patients who have acquired gonococcal infection in Asia, Hawaii, or California should not be treated with fluoroquinolones unless the organism has been shown to be susceptible. Increasing resistance is likely to reduce the utility of quinolones for the treatment of gonorrhea in other areas as well.

Patients who are receiving treatment for urethritis should be examined for other STDs and should be tested serologically for syphilis at the initial visit. An initial workup for trichomoniasis probably is not indicated in most settings, because the infection accounts for a small proportion of cases.[16] Additionally, direct microscopic examination of a urethral specimen for trichomonads usually is unrewarding unless the patient can be seen before the first morning micturition. If the patient's urethritis has not been cured by previous antibacterial therapy, or if symptoms or signs in the sexual partner suggest trichomonal infection, the patient's first-void urine sediment and an endourethral swab sample can be cultured on suitable media.[15] Empirical treatment for trichomoniasis with oral metronidazole may be warranted in some patients.

Syndromic management of urethritis, in which men who have symptoms or signs of urethritis are treated with antimicrobials active against *N. gonorrhoeae* and *C. trachomatis* without any diagnostic studies, has been employed with success in resource-poor settings.

In men whose symptoms and signs do not resolve or in whom clinical manifestations recur after appropriate treatment for urethritis, urethral Gram-stained specimens or first-void urine sediments should be examined to establish the existence of persistent urethritis. Symptoms and signs may persist in the absence of objective evidence of urethritis. Antimicrobial treatment in symptomatic men who do not have objective evidence of urethritis is of questionable value.[22]

Patients who initially receive treatment for NGU but in whom urethritis is not eliminated by doxycycline should be suspected of having infection with *Trichomonas* or doxycycline-resistant *Ureaplasma.*[5,55-57] Because these infections can be impossible to differentiate clinically, such patients may be given empirical treatment with a single 2-g dose of metronidazole followed, after 2 hours (to prevent gastrointestinal upset,) by azithromycin, 1 g orally as a single dose, or erythromycin, 500 mg orally four times daily for 7 days. It is, of course, important that their sexual partners receive the same regimen.

Some men report that their urethral symptoms disappeared while they were taking a tetracycline but reappeared days to weeks after completion of therapy. Such recurrences with objective evidence of urethritis are seen in about 20% of patients with chlamydial NGU and in about 40% of patients with nonchlamydial infection. Among NGU patients from whom neither chlamydiae nor ureaplasmas are isolated, the recurrence rate is greater than 50%.[43,59,60] Eighty percent of cases of recurrent NGU occur in patients in whom neither organism was initially recovered,[60] and 70% to 80% of men with recurrent NGU are culture-negative for both organisms at the time of recurrence.[80] *M. genitalium* has been associated with recurrent or chronic NGU, as have *U. urealyticum* and antibodies to *C. trachomatis* heat-shock protein 60 kDa.[104-106]

Men with recurrent urethritis should be questioned closely about the possibility of reexposure, and attention should be given to ensuring simultaneous treatment of all sexual partners. If reexposure is likely, retreatment with the initial doxycycline or azithromycin regimen may be given. If the patient has not been reexposed, a recurrence of urethritis suggests the possibility that some pathogens remained in a relatively antibiotic-protected site. Prostatic involvement is common in NGU. It is possible that some men have a prostatic focus of infection. In men with repeated relapses, treatment with a 3-week course of erythromycin occasionally succeeds.[107] Patients whose relapses are not eliminated by these maneuvers should be referred for urologic evaluation to rule out anatomic abnormalities.[99] Such men probably are not infected with *Chlamydia* or *Ureaplasma*. About one fourth will be found to have a partial obstruction to urine flow, and about half of these will have urethral strictures.[99] They and their sexual partners do not appear to be at significant risk for infectious complications.[108] Long-term antimicrobial suppression is useful in this setting.[108]

Sexual partners of patients with sexually transmitted urethritis should receive treatment simultaneously. A woman who has been the sexual partner of a man with urethritis of undetermined origin should be given a regimen that is effective against gonococci, chlamydiae, and ureaplasmas. A regimen combining a cephalosporin or a fluoroquinolone with doxycycline, as described previously, is suitable in nonpregnant women. Azithromycin, erythromycin, amoxicillin,[109] or clindamycin[110] may be substituted for doxycycline in pregnancy. Asymptomatic male sexual partners of women known to have gonorrhea, chlamydial infection, or trichomoniasis should receive treatment even in the absence of abnormalities on direct microscopic examination.

REITER'S SYNDROME (REACTIVE ARTHRITIS)

Some cases of NGU appear as one element of Reiter's syndrome, which also includes arthritis, uveitis, and, often, lesions of the skin and mucous membranes.[111] The syndrome complicates 1% to 2% of the cases of NGU[112] and is thought to be the most common peripheral inflammatory arthritis in young men.[113] Its pathogenesis is unclear, but it probably represents an abnormal host response to any of a number of infectious agents.[114] The idiosyncratic nature of the host's response is supported by a strong correlation between the development of Reiter's syndrome and the presence of the HLA-B27 histocompatibility antigen. This antigen has been found in 90% to 96% of patients with Reiter's syndrome,[112,113,115,116] and it also has been related to uveitis and sacroiliitis.[112] Although possibly providing a clue to pathogenesis, the presence of this antigen is not diagnostic.

The inciting infection is of two types.[117] Reiter's syndrome may occur after sexually transmitted urethritis, and most cases in North America and Europe seem to occur in sexually active young people.[118,119] Many cases occur after contact with a new partner, and some cases have been epidemiologically linked.[112] In one series, 9% of cases occurred after gonococcal urethritis, although 50% of affected patients subsequently developed PGU.[120] *C. trachomatis* is strongly implicated in the pathogenesis of Reiter's syndrome. It has been recovered from the urethras of 16% to 44% of patients with Reiter's syndrome and from 69% of those men who had signs of urogenital inflammation at the time of examination.[119,121,122] Antibodies to *C. trachomatis* have been detected in 46% to 67% and *Chlamydia*-specific cell-mediated immunity in 72% of patients with Reiter's syndrome.[114,122,123] Chlamydiae were isolated from synovial biopsies in 15 of 29 patients from a number of small series and from a smaller proportion of synovial fluid specimens.[124] Chlamydial nucleic acids have been identified in the synovial membranes,[125] and chlamydial elementary bodies have been observed in joint fluid.[126] Attempts to isolate or identify mycoplasmas in affected joints have not been successful.[124]

Reiter's syndrome also occurs after bacterial gastroenteritis, and it has been repeatedly described after infection with *Salmonella, Shigella, Yersinia,* or *Campylobacter*.[112,113,115,120,127-130] A few cases suggest that Reiter's syndrome may occur after antibiotic-associated colitis[131] or cryptosporidiosis.[132] Postdysenteric Reiter's syndrome has been reported in 0.24% to 1.50% of patients after epidemics of gastrointestinal infection[128,130]; it is considerably more common among patients who are HLA-B27-positive. Short peptides shared by HLA-B27 and enteric pathogens have raised the question of a contribution of molecular mimicry to pathogenesis.[133] Antibodies reacting with *Yersinia* proteins appear in the sera of many patients with Reiter's syndrome.[134] Synovial fluid lymphocytes react with antigens from enteric pathogens.[135]

Clinically, Reiter's syndrome after genital infection is indistinguishable from that occurring after bacterial gastroenteritis; indeed, 12% to 80% of patients with postdysenteric Reiter's syndrome have genital symptoms.[112,136] The age- and gender-specific attack rates, however, are different; 94% to 99% of the cases of Reiter's syndrome after sexually transmitted infections occur in men. However, up to 10% of the cases of postdysenteric Reiter's syndrome occur in women.[118,130] The syndrome has also been reported in sexually inexperienced children.[118,129]

Reiter's syndrome is encountered with some frequency in HIV-infected persons.[137] It is said to be the most common rheumatologic complication of the acquired immunodeficiency syndrome. The spectrum of clinical manifestations is similar to that in other patients, but the arthritis and mucocutaneous lesions are more severe and may require more intensive therapy.

The syndrome has been observed as a complication of bladder instillation of bacillus Calmette-Guérin.[138] Small numbers of cases suggest the possibility of Reiter's syndrome after respiratory infection with *Chlamydophila psittaci*[139] or *Chlamydophila pneumoniae*.[140]

Clinical Features

NGU is the initial manifestation of Reiter's syndrome in 80% of patients.[112,113] As with other forms of NGU, it usually occurs within 14 days after sexual exposure.[114] The urethritis may be mild and may go unnoticed by the patient, being detectable only by physical examination performed before the first morning micturition. Gonococcal urethritis sometimes precedes Reiter's syndrome,[120] but coinfection with an agent of NGU is difficult to rule out. The urethral discharge may be purulent or mucopurulent, and patients may or may not complain of dysuria. Accompanying prostatitis, usually asymptomatic, has been described by some authors.[113,136,141] Cystitis without urethritis has also been reported and may be a manifestation, particularly in women.[136]

The other features of Reiter's syndrome develop 1 to 5 weeks after the onset of urethritis.[136] Arthritis begins within 4 weeks after the onset of urethritis in four fifths of patients,[112] but it precedes urethritis in about 15%.[118] The knees are most frequently involved, followed by the ankles and small joints of the feet. Sacroiliitis, either symmetrical[136] or, more frequently, asymmetrical,[118,129,141] develops in up to two thirds of patients.[138] It is more common in patients with the HLA-B27 antigen.[129] Ankylosing spondylitis, which occurs in only about 1% of the general population, complicates a significant minority of cases of Reiter's syndrome,[112,116,129,142] and back pain is reported by 60% of all patients.[113] Many patients with Reiter's syndrome and the HLA-B27 antigen develop ankylosing spondylitis,[142] which is rare in patients without the antigen. Calcaneal spurring may be seen in up to one fourth of patients with Reiter's syndrome[118,141] and may produce heel pain. A dactylitis resulting in sausage-shaped swelling of the digits is also characteristic.[118] Arthritis is the most persistent feature of the syndrome; it may last for months to years after other manifestations have disappeared.[118,136]

Mild bilateral conjunctivitis, iritis, keratitis, or uveitis is sometimes present but often lasts for only a few days.[136,141,143] Unlike the conjunctivae in direct infection with *C. trachomatis,* the inflamed conjunctivae in Reiter's syndrome do not manifest follicular hypertrophy. The uveitis is usually anterior, acute, and unilateral.[143]

Dermatologic manifestations occur in up to 50% of patients.[112,113] The initial lesions are waxy papules, which often display a central yellow spot; they occur most frequently on the soles and palms[136] and with decreasing frequency on the nails, scrotum, scalp, and trunk. The papules epithelialize and thicken to produce keratoderma blenorrhagicum in 10% to 25% of the patients.[113] Circinate balanitis is usually painless and occurs in 25% to 40% of all patients.[112,113,136] Circinate and ulcerative vulvitis also are described.[144] Painless erosions on the dorsum of the tongue and fauces occur most commonly with the initial episode and less frequently with recurrence.[133] Incomplete Reiter's syndrome, consisting of urethritis and arthritis or arthritis alone, has been reported.[113,127,145]

The initial episode of Reiter's syndrome usually lasts 2 to 6 months, but episodes lasting for 1 year have been described.[113,136,141] Most patients feel completely well after the attack subsides, but the disease recurs in many cases, at a rate of about 15% in each 5-year period after the initial attack.[112,113,118,126,142,146] During recurrence, the genital symptoms are usually less marked and may be entirely absent.[146-148] More than half of the patients have active disease 15 to 20 years after the initial episode,[113,116,142,146] the risk of residua being somewhat higher among patients with the HLA-B27 antigen.[149] Almost 50% of affected persons develop some degree of permanent disability.[116,142]

Rare complications of Reiter's syndrome include pericarditis, myocarditis, first-degree atrioventricular block, and aortic insufficiency.[116,136,141,150]

Laboratory Features

Anemia is common,[113] and the erythrocyte sedimentation rate is elevated in about 50% of patients.[118] Findings in fluid recovered at the same time from different joints may be dissimilar.[136] Synovial fluid usually contains 1000 to 200,000 white blood cells per mL, more than two thirds of which are PMNs.[136] The glucose level in joint fluid is low in about 50% of affected joints.[136] Synovial biopsy specimens reveal nonspecific inflammatory changes.

Therapy

Treatment of Reiter's syndrome remains controversial. Because of the possibility that the inciting infection may be sexually transmitted NGU, standard antichlamydial treatment is recommended[151] and has been claimed by some authorities to reduce or eliminate urethritis.[152] Others, however, have seen no effect on the arthritis or on the overall course of the disease.[147,151] The relative safety of antichlamydial therapy and the frequency with which chlamydiae are isolated from patients with Reiter's syndrome make such treatment reasonable. Among a population in Greenland with a high prevalence of HLA-B27, treatment of patients who had urethritis or cervicitis with a tetracycline or erythromycin was associated with a lower incidence of subsequent arthritis than was treatment with penicillin or no treatment at all.[153]

Long-term antichlamydial treatment (e.g., with a tetracycline for 3 months) has been suggested, and its use was supported by the results of a double-blind, placebo-controlled trial that demonstrated an ameliorating effect on Chlamydia-associated but not on enteropathogen-associated disease.[154] The effectiveness of long-term tetracycline therapy in other arthritides[155] raises the question of whether the drug is working through an antibacterial effect on persistent, viable microorganisms or through an anti-inflammatory action. That the tetracyclines are more effective in Chlamydia-associated disease than in other reactive arthritides suggests the former.

Administration of nonsteroidal anti-inflammatory drugs (NSAIDs) is the most effective treatment.[113] Indomethacin or tolmetin is favored by some workers,[156] and all of these agents are superior to salicylates or corticosteroids. Sulfasalazine may be beneficial for patients whose symptoms do not respond to an NSAID. Cytotoxic agents such as methotrexate[156] or immunosuppressive agents such as cyclosporine[157] may be of value in recalcitrant cases.

REFERENCES

1. Oriel JD. The history of non-gonococcal urethritis. Genitourin Med. 1996;72:374-379.
2. Taylor-Robinson D. The history of nongonococcal urethritis. Thomas Parran Award Lecture. Sex Transm Dis. 1996;23:86-91.
3. Swartz SL. Diagnosis of nongonococcal urethritis. In: Hobson D, Holmes KK, eds. Nongonococcal Urethritis and Related Infections. Washington, DC: American Society for Microbiology; 1977:15-18.
4. Bowie WR. Comparison of gram stain and first-voided urine sediment in the diagnosis of urethritis. Sex Transm Dis. 1978;5:39-42.
5. Root TE, Edwards LD, Spengler PJ. Nongonococcal urethritis: A survey of clinical and laboratory features. Sex Transm Dis. 1980;7:59-65.
6. Desai K, Robson HG. Comparison of the gram-stained urethral smear and first-voided urine sediment in the diagnosis of nongonococcal urethritis. Sex Transm Dis. 1982;9:21-25.
7. Scheibel JH, Kristensen JK, Hentzer B, et al. Treatment of chlamydial urethritis in men and Chlamydia trachomatis–positive female partners: Comparison of erythromycin and tetracycline in treatment courses of one week. Sex Transm Dis. 1982;9:128-131.
8. Stamm WE, Koutsky LA, Benedetti JK, et al. Chlamydia trachomatis urethral infections in men: Prevalence, risk factors, and clinical manifestations. Ann Intern Med. 1984;100:47-51.
9. Perera SAB. Use of Kova-Slide II with grid and uncentrifuged segmented urine specimens in the diagnosis of nongonococcal urethritis: A quantitative technique. Sex Transm Dis. 1985;12:14-18.
10. Willcox JR, Adler MW, Belsey EM. Observer variation in the interpretation of gram-stained urethral smears. Br J Vener Dis. 1981;57:134-136.
11. Jacobs NF Jr, Kraus SJ. Gonococcal and nongonococcal urethritis in men: Clinical and laboratory differentiation. Ann Intern Med. 1975;82:7-12.
12. Kraus SJ. Semiquantitation of urethral polymorphonuclear leukocytes as objective evidence of nongonococcal urethritis. Sex Transm Dis. 1982;9:52-55.
13. Goodhart ME, Ogden J, Zaidi AA, Kraus SJ. Factors affecting the performance of smear and culture tests for the detection of Neisseria gonorrhoeae. Sex Transm Dis. 1982;9:63-69.
14. Haberberger RL Jr, Mikhail IA, Fox E, et al. Predominance of vancomycin-sensitive strains of Neisseria gonorrhoeae in Djibouti. Lancet 1989;2:683.
15. Krieger JN, Verdon M, Siegel N, et al. Risk assessment and laboratory diagnosis of trichomoniasis in men. J Infect Dis. 1992;166:1362-1366.
16. Krieger JN, Jenny C, Verdon M, et al. Clinical manifestations of trichomoniasis in men. Ann Intern Med. 1993;118:844-849.
17. Puolakkainen M, Hiltunen-Back E, Reunala T, et al. Comparison of performances of two commercially available tests, a PCR assay and a ligase chain reaction test, in detection of urogenital Chlamydia trachomatis infection. J Clin Microbiol. 1998;36:1489-1493.
18. Jaschek G, Gaydos CA, Welsh LE, et al. Direct detection of Chlamydia trachomatis in urine specimens from symptomatic and asymptomatic men by using a rapid polymerase chain reaction assay. J Clin Microbiol. 1993;31:1209-1212.
19. Chernesky M, Jang D, Chong S, et al. Impact of urine collection order on the ability of assays to identify Chlamydia trachomatis infection in men. Sex Transm Dis. 2003;30:345-347.
20. Bowie WR, Pollock HM, Forsyth PS, et al. Bacteriology of the urethra in normal men and men with nongonococcal urethritis. J Clin Microbiol. 1977;6:482-488.
21. Wong JL, Hines PA, Brasher MD, et al. The etiology of nongonococcal urethritis in men attending a venereal disease clinic. Sex Transm Dis. 1977;4:4-8.
22. Augenbraun MH, Cummings M, McCormack WM. Management of chronic urethral symptoms in men. Clin Infect Dis. 1992;15:714-715.
23. Pec J, Straka S, Novomesky F, et al. Mechanical urethritis and ascendent genitourinary infections due to sexual stimulation of the urethra by inserted foreign bodies. Genitourin Med. 1992;68:399-400.
24. McCutchan JA. Epidemiology of venereal urethritis: Comparison of gonorrhea and nongonococcal urethritis. Rev Infect Dis. 1984;6:669-688.
25. Judson FN. Epidemiology and control of nongonococcal urethritis and genital chlamydial infections: A review. Sex Transm Dis. 1981;8:117-126.
26. McChesney JA, Zedd A, King H, et al. Acute urethritis in male college students. JAMA. 1973;226:37-39.
27. Ciemins EL, Flood J, Kent CK, et al. Reexamining the prevalence of Chlamydia trachomatis infection among gay men with urethritis: Implications for STD policy and HIV prevention activities. Sex Transm Dis. 2000;27:249-251.
28. Lafferty WE, Hughes JP, Handsfield HH. Sexually transmitted diseases in men who have sex with men: Acquisition of gonorrhea and nongonococcal urethritis by fellatio and implications for STD/HIV prevention. Sex Transm Dis. 1997;24:272-278.
29. Schwartz MA, Lafferty WE, Hughes JP, Handsfield HH. Risk factors for urethritis in heterosexual men: The role of fellatio and other sexual practices. Sex Transm Dis. 1997;24:449-455.
30. Rotchford K, Strum AW, Wilkinson D. Effect of coinfection with STDs and of STD treatment on HIV shedding in genital-tract secretions: Systematic review and data synthesis. Sex Transm Dis. 2000;27:243-248.
31. Fox KK, del Rio C, Holmes KK, et al. Gonorrhea in the HIV era: A reversal in trends among men who have sex with men. Am J Public Health. 2001;91:959-964.
32. Smith GL, Greenup R, Takafuji ET. Circumcision as a risk factor for urethritis in racial groups. Am J Public Health. 1987;77:452-454.
33. Boyd JT, Csonka GW, Oates JK. Epidemiology of non-specific urethritis. Br J Vener Dis. 1958;34:40-43.
34. Rothenberg R, Judson FN. The clinical diagnosis of urethral discharge. Sex Transm Dis. 1983;10:24-28.
35. Lee Y-H, Rosner B, Alpert S, et al. Clinical and microbiological investigation of men with urethritis. J Infect Dis. 1978;138:798-803.
36. Volk J, Kraus SJ. Nongonococcal urethritis: A venereal disease as prevalent as epidemic gonorrhea. Arch Intern Med. 1974;134:511-514.
37. Holmes KK. Gonococcal infection. Clinical, epidemiologic and laboratory perspectives. Adv Intern Med. 1974;19:259-285.
38. Oriel JD. Treatment of nongonococcal urethritis. In: Hobson D, Holmes KK, eds. Nongonococcal Urethritis and Related Infections. Washington, DC: American Society for Microbiology; 1977:38-42.

39. Johannisson G, Lowhagen G-B, Nilsson S. *Chlamydia trachomatis* and urethritis in men. Scand J Infect Dis. 1982;32(Suppl):87-92.
40. Bowie WR, Wang S-P, Alexander ER, et al. Etiology of nongonococcal urethritis: Evidence for *Chlamydia trachomatis* and *Ureaplasma urealyticum*. J Clin Invest. 1977;59:735-742.
41. Viarengo J, Hebrant F, Piot P. *Ureaplasma urealyticum* in the urethra of healthy men. Br J Vener Dis. 1980;56:169-172.
42. Bowie WR, Floyd JF, Miller Y, et al. Differential response of chlamydial and ureaplasma-associated urethritis to sulphafurazole (sulfisoxazole) and aminocyclitols. Lancet. 1976;2:1276-1278.
43. Coufalik ED, Taylor-Robinson D, Csonka GW. Treatment of nongonococcal urethritis with rifampicin as a means of defining the role of *Ureaplasma urealyticum*. Br J Vener Dis. 1979;55:36-43.
44. Taylor-Robinson D, Csonka GW, Prentice MJ. Human intraurethral inoculation of ureaplasmas. QJM. 1977;46:309-326.
45. Brown MB, Cassell GH, Taylor-Robinson D, et al. Measurement of antibody to *Ureaplasma urealyticum* by an enzyme-linked immunosorbent assay and detection of antibody responses in patients with nongonococcal urethritis. J Clin Microbiol. 1983;17:288-295.
46. Cassell GH, Cole BC. Mycoplasmas as agents of human disease. N Engl J Med. 1981;304:80-89.
47. Taylor-Robinson D, McCormack WM. The genital mycoplasmas. N Engl J Med. 1980;302:1003-1010, 1063-1067.
48. Tully JG, Cole RM, Taylor-Robinson D, et al. A newly discovered mycoplasma in the human urogenital tract. Lancet. 1981;1:1288-1291.
49. Busolo F, Camposampiero D, Bordignon G, Bertollo G. Detection of *Mycoplasma genitalium* and *Chlamydia trachomatis* DNAs in male patients with urethritis using the polymerase chain reaction. New Microbiol. 1997;20:325-332.
50. Keane FE, Thomas BJ, Gilroy CB, et al. The association of *Chlamydia trachomatis* and *Mycoplasma genitalium* with non-gonococcal urethritis: observations on heterosexual men and their female partners. Int J STD AIDS. 2000;11:435-439.
51. Totten PA, Schwartz MA, Sjostrom KE, et al. Association of *Mycoplasma genitalium* with nongonococcal urethritis in heterosexual men. J Infect Dis. 2001;183:269-276.
52. Mena L, Wang X, Mroczkowski TF, Martin DH. *Mycoplasma genitalium* infections in asymptomatic men and men with urethritis attending a sexually transmitted diseases clinic in New Orleans. Clin Infect Dis. 2002;35:1167-1173.
53. Taylor-Robinson D, Jensen JS, Fehler G, et al. Observations on the microbiology of urethritis in black South African men. Int J STD AIDS. 2000;13:323-325.
54. Taylor-Robinson D. *Mycoplasma genitalium:* An update. Int J STD AIDS. 2002;13:145-151.
55. Magalhaes M. Persistent nongonococcal urethritis associated with a minocycline-resistant strain of *Ureaplasma urealyticum:* A case report. Sex Transm Dis. 1983;10:151-152.
56. Arya OP, Pratt BC. Persistent urethritis due to *Ureaplasma urealyticum* in conjugal or stable partnerships. Genitourin Med. 1986;62:329-332.
57. Stimson JB, Hale J, Bowie WR, Holmes KK. Tetracycline-resistant *Ureaplasma urealyticum:* A cause of persistent nongonococcal urethritis. Ann Intern Med. 1981;94:192-194.
58. Falk L, Fredlund H, Jensen JS. Tetracycline treatment does not eradicate *Mycoplasma genitalium*. Sex Transm Infect. 2003;79:318-319.
59. Bowie WR. Urethritis and infections of the lower urogenital tract. Urol Clin North Am. 1980;7:17-28.
60. Bowie WR, Alexander ER, Stimson JB, et al. Therapy for nongonococcal urethritis: Double-blind, randomized comparison of two doses and two durations of minocycline. Ann Intern Med. 1981;95:306-311.
61. Corey L, Adams HG, Brown ZA, et al. Genital herpes simplex virus infection: Clinical manifestations, course, and complications. Ann Intern Med. 1983;98:958-972.
62. Schwebke JR, Hook EW 3rd. High rates of *Trichomonas vaginalis* among men attending a sexually transmitted diseases clinic: Implications for screening and urethritis management. J Infect Dis. 2003;188:465-468.
63. Joyner JL, Douglas JM Jr, Ragsdale S, et al. Comparative prevalence of infection with *Trichomonas vaginalis* among men attending a sexually transmitted diseases clinic. Sex Transm Dis. 2000;27:236-240.
64. Wendel KA, Erbelding EJ, Gaydos CA, Rompalo AM. Use of urine polymerase chain reaction to define the prevalence and clinical presentation of *Trichomonas vaginalis* in men attending an STD clinic. Sex Transm Infect. 2003;79:151-153.
65. Nacey JN, Tulloch AGS, Ferguson AF. Catheter-induced urethritis: A comparison between latex and silicone catheters in a prospective clinical trial. Br J Urol. 1985;57:325-328.
66. Conde-Glez CJ, Calderon E. Urogenital infection due to meningococcus in men and women. Sex Transm Dis. 1991;18:72-75.
67. Woolley PD, Kinghorn GR, Talbot MD, Duerden BI. Microbiological flora in men with non-gonococcal urethritis with particular reference to anaerobic bacteria. Int J STD AIDS. 1990;1:122-125.
68. Arya OP, Mallinson H, Pareek SS, et al. Post-gonococcal cervicitis and postgonococcal urethritis. A study of their epidemiological correlation and the role of *Chlamydia trachomatis* in their aetiology. Br J Vener Dis. 1981;57:395-399.
69. Bowie WR, Alexander ER, Holmes KK. Etiologies of postgonococcal urethritis in homosexual and heterosexual men: Roles of *Chlamydia trachomatis* and *Ureaplasma urealyticum*. Sex Transm Dis. 1978;5:151-154.
70. Terho P. *Chlamydia trachomatis* in gonococcal and postgonococcal urethritis. Br J Vener Dis. 1978;54:326-329.
71. Oriel JD, Ridgway GL, Reeve P, et al. The lack of effect of ampicillin plus probenecid given for genital infections with *Neisseria gonorrhoeae* on associated infections with *Chlamydia trachomatis*. J Infect Dis. 1976;133:568-571.
72. Stamm WE, Guinan ME, Johnson C, et al. Effect of treatment regimens for *Neisseria gonorrhoeae* on simultaneous infection with *Chlamydia trachomatis*. N Engl J Med. 1984;310:545-549.
73. Chambers CV, Shafer M-A, Adger H, et al. Microflora of the urethra in adolescent boys: Relationships to sexual activity and nongonococcal urethritis. J Pediatr. 1987;110:314-321.
74. Handsfield HH, Lipman TO, Harnisch JP, et al. Asymptomatic gonorrhea in men: Diagnosis, natural course, prevalence and significance. N Engl J Med. 1974;290:117-123.
75. Swartz SL, Kraus SJ. Persistent urethral leukocytosis and asymptomatic chlamydial urethritis. J Infect Dis. 1979;140:614-617.
76. Stamm WE. Etiology and management of the acute urethral syndrome. Sex Transm Dis. 1981;8:235-238.
77. Stamm WE, Wagner KF, Amsel R, et al. Causes of the acute urethral syndrome in women. N Engl J Med. 1980;303:409-414.
78. Fihn SD, Johnson C, Stamm WE. *Escherichia coli* urethritis in women with symptoms of acute urinary tract infection. J Infect Dis. 1988;157:196-199.
79. Curran JW. Gonorrhea and the urethral syndrome. Sex Transm Dis. 1977;4:119-121.
80. Goh BT, Varia KB, Ayliffe PF, et al. Diagnosis of gonorrhea by gram-stained smears and cultures in men and women: Role of the urethral smear. Sex Transm Dis. 1985;12:135-139.
81. Paavonen J. *Chlamydia trachomatis*-induced urethritis in female partners of men with nongonococcal urethritis. Sex Transm Dis. 1979;6:69-71.
82. Paavonen J, Vesterinen E. *Chlamydia trachomatis* in cervicitis and urethritis in women. Scand J Infect Dis. 1982;32(Suppl):45-54.
83. Stamm WE, Running K, Hale J, et al. Etiologic role of *Mycoplasma hominis* and *Ureaplasma urealyticum* in women with the acute urethral syndrome. Sex Transm Dis. 1983;10:318-322.
84. Latham RH, Stamm WE. Urethral syndrome in women. Urol Clin North Am. 1984;11:95-101.
85. Feldman RG, Johnson AL, Schober PC, et al. Aetiology of urinary symptoms in sexually active women. Genitourin Med. 1986;62:333-341.
86. Toth A, Lesser ML, Brooks C, et al. Subsequent pregnancies among 161 couples treated for T-mycoplasma genital-tract infection. N Engl J Med. 1983;308:505-507.
87. Berger RE. Acute epididymitis. Sex Transm Dis. 1981;8:286-289.
88. Ness RB, Markovic N, Carlson CL, Coughlin MT. Do men become infertile after having sexually transmitted urethritis? An epidemiologic examination. Fertil Steril. 1997;68:205-213.
89. Holmes KK, Hansfield HH, Wang SP, et al. Etiology of nongonococcal urethritis. N Engl Med. 1975;292:1199-1205.
90. Nilsson S, Johannisson G, Lycke E. Isolation of *Chlamydia trachomatis* from the urethra and from prostatic fluid in men with signs and symptoms of acute urethritis. Acta Dermatol Venereol (Stockh). 1981;61:456-459.
91. Ronnerstam R, Persson K. Chlamydial eye infection in adults. Scand J Infect Dis. 1982;32(Suppl):111-115.
92. Holmes KK, Johnson DW, Floyd TM. Studies of venereal disease: III. Double-blind comparison of tetracycline hydrochloride and placebo in treatment of nongonococcal urethritis. JAMA. 1967;202:474-476.
93. Bowie WR, Yu JS, Fawcett A, et al. Tetracycline in nongonococcal urethritis: Comparison of 2 g and 1 g daily for seven days. Br J Vener Dis. 1980;56:332-336.
94. Jordan WC. Doxycycline vs. tetracycline in the treatment of men with gonorrhea: The compliance factor. Sex Transm Dis. 1981;8:105-109.
95. Martin DH, Mroczkowski TF, Dalu ZA, et al. A controlled trial of a single dose of azithromycin for the treatment of chlamydial urethritis and cervicitis. N Engl J Med. 1992;327:921-925.
96. Stamm WE, Hicks CB, Martin DH, et al. Azithromycin for empirical treatment of the nongonococcal urethritis syndrome in men: A randomized, double-blind study. JAMA. 1995;274:545-549.
97. Lau CY, Qureshi AK. Azithromycin versus doxycycline for genital chlamydial infections: A meta-analysis of randomized clinical trials. Sex Transm Dis. 2002;29:497-502.
98. Augenbraun M, Bachmann L, Wallace T, et al. Compliance with doxycycline therapy in sexually transmitted disease clinics. Sex Transm Dis. 1998;25:1-4.
99. Krieger JN, Hooton TM, Brust PJ, et al. Evaluation of chronic urethritis: Defining the role for endoscopic procedures. Arch Intern Med. 1988;148:703-707.
100. Hooton TM, Rogers ME, Medina TG, et al. Ciprofloxacin compared with doxycycline for nongonococcal urethritis: Ineffectiveness against *Chlamydia trachomatis* due to relapsing infection. JAMA. 1990;264:1418-1421.
101. Mogabgab WJ, Holmes B, Murray M, et al. Randomized comparison of ofloxacin and doxycycline for chlamydia and ureaplasma urethritis and cervicitis. Chemotherapy. 1990;36:70-76.
102. Centers for Disease Control and Prevention. 1998 Guidelines for treatment of sexually transmitted diseases. MMWR Morb Mortal Wkly Rep. 1998;47(No RR-1):1-116.
103. Gordon SM, Carlyn CJ, Doyle LT, et al. The emergence of *Neisseria gonorrhoeae* with decreased susceptibility to ciprofloxacin in Cleveland, Ohio: Epidemiology and risk factors. Ann Intern Med. 1996;125:465-470.
104. Horner P, Thomas B, Gilroy CB, et al. Role of *Mycoplasma genitalium* and *Ureaplasma urealyticum* in acute and chronic nongonococcal urethritis. Clin Infect Dis. 2001;32:995-1003.
105. Maeda SI, Tamaki M, Kojima K, et al. Association of *Mycoplasma genitalium* persistence in the urethra with recurrence of nongonococcal urethritis. Sex Transm Dis. 2001;28:472-476.
106. Horner P, Thomas B, Gilroy C, et al. Antibodies to *Chlamydia trachomatis* heat-shock protein 60 kDa and detection of *Mycoplasma genitalium* and *Ureaplasma urealyticum* are associated independently with chronic nongonococcal urethritis. Sex Transm Dis. 2003;30:129-133.
107. Hooton TM, Wong ES, Barnes RC, et al. Erythromycin for persistent or recurrent nongonococcal urethritis: A randomized placebo-controlled trial. Ann Intern Med. 1990;113:21-26.

108. Berger RE. Recurrent nongonococcal urethritis. JAMA. 1983;249:409.
109. Crombleholme WR, Schachter J, Grossman M, et al. Amoxicillin therapy for *Chlamydia trachomatis* in pregnancy. Obstet Gynecol. 1990;75:752-756.
110. Campbell WR, Dodson MG. Clindamycin therapy for *Chlamydia trachomatis* in women. Am J Obstet Gynecol. 1990;162:343-347.
111. Schneider JM, Matthews JH, Graham BS. Reiter's syndrome. Cutis. 2003;71:198-200.
112. Keat A. Reiter's syndrome and reactive arthritis in perspective. N Engl J Med. 1983;309:1606-1615.
113. Arnett FC Jr. Reiter's syndrome. Johns Hopkins Med J. 1982;150:39-44.
114. Ford DK, deRoza DM, Schulzer M. The specificity of synovial mononuclear cell responses to microbiological antigens in Reiter's syndrome. J Rheumatol. 1982;9:561-567.
115. Lehman DH. Postdysenteric Reiter's syndrome. West J Med. 1977;126:405-407.
116. Sairanen E, Paronen I, Mahonen H. Reiter's syndrome: A follow-up study. Acta Med Scand. 1969;185:57-63.
117. Fendler C, Laitko S, Sorensen H, et al. Frequency of triggering bacteria in patients with reactive arthritis and undifferentiated oligoarthritis and the relative importance of the tests used for diagnosis. Ann Rheum Dis. 2001;60:337-343.
118. Hawkes JG. Clinical and diagnostic features of Reiter's disease: A follow-up study of 39 patients. N Z Med J. 1973;78:347-353.
119. Kousa M, Saikku P, Richmond S, et al. Frequent association of chlamydial infection with Reiter's syndrome. Sex Transm Dis. 1978;5:57-61.
120. Leirisalo M, Skylv G, Kousa M, et al. Followup study on patients with Reiter's disease and reactive arthritis, with special reference to HLA-B27. Arthritis Rheum. 1982;25:249-259.
121. Keat AC, Thomas BJ, Taylor-Robinson D, et al. Evidence of *Chlamydia trachomatis* infection in sexually acquired reactive arthritis. Ann Rheum Dis. 1980;39:431-437.
122. Kousa M. Evidence of chlamydial involvement in the development of arthritis. Scand J Infect Dis. 1982;32(Suppl):116-121.
123. Inman RD, Johnston MEA, Chiu B, et al. Immunochemical analysis of immune response to *Chlamydia trachomatis* in Reiter's syndrome and nonspecific urethritis. Clin Exp Immunol. 1987;69:246-254.
124. Hughes RA, Keat AC. Reiter's syndrome and reactive arthritis: A current view. Semin Arthritis Rheum. 1994;24:190-210.
125. Taylor-Robinson D, Gilroy CB, Thomas BJ, Keat ACS. Detection of *Chlamydia trachomatis* DNA in joints of reactive arthritis patients by polymerase chain reaction. Lancet. 1992;340:81-82.
126. Keat A, Dixey J, Sonnex C, et al. *Chlamydia trachomatis* and reactive arthritis: The missing link. Lancet. 1987;1:72-75.
127. Jones RAK. Reiter's disease after *Salmonella typhimurium* enteritis. BMJ 1977;1:1391.
128. Noer HR. An "experimental" epidemic of Reiter's syndrome. JAMA. 1966;198:693-698.
129. Calin A. Reiter's syndrome. Med Clin North Am. 1977;61:365-376.
130. Paronon I. Reiter's disease. A study of 344 cases observed in Finland. Acta Med Scand. 1948;131(Suppl 212):1-112.
131. Hayward RS, Wensel RH, Kibsey P. Relapsing *Clostridium difficile* colitis and Reiter's syndrome. Am J Gastroenterol. 1990;85:752-756.
132. Cron RQ, Sherry DD. Reiter's syndrome associated with cryptosporidial gastroenteritis. J Rheumatol. 1995;22:1962-1963.
133. Scofield RH, Kurien B, Gross T, et al. HLA-B27 binding of peptide from its own sequence and similar peptides from bacteria: Implications for spondyloarthropathies. Lancet. 1995;345:1542-1544.
134. Kobayashi S, Ogasawara M, Maeda K, et al. Antibodies against *Yersinia enterocolitica* in patients with Reiter's syndrome. J Lab Clin Med. 1985;105:380-389.
135. Ford DK. Lymphocytes from the site of disease in reactive arthritis indicate antigen-specific immunopathology. J Infect Dis. 1991;164:1032-1033.
136. Weinberger HW, Ropes MW, Kulka JP, et al. Reiter's syndrome, clinical and pathologic observations: A long term study of 16 cases. Medicine (Baltimore). 1962;41:35-91.
137. Kaye BR. Rheumatologic manifestations of HIV infections. Clin Rev Allergy Immunol. 1996-7;14:385-416.
138. Saporta L, Gumus E, Karadag H, et al. Reiter syndrome following intracavity BCG administration. Scand J Urol Nephrol 1997;31:211-212.
139. Lanham JG, Doyle DV. Case report: Reactive arthritis following psittacosis. Br J Rheumatol. 1984;23:225-226.
140. Braun J, Laitko S, Treharne J, et al. *Chlamydia pneumoniae*: A new causative agent of reactive arthritis and undifferentiated oligoarthritis. Ann Rheum Dis. 1994;53:100-105.
141. Good AE. Reiter's disease. Postgrad Med. 1977;61:153-158.
142. Marks JS, Holt PJL. The natural history of Reiter's disease: 21 Years of observations. Q J Med. 1986;60:685-697.
143. Lyons JL, Rosenbaum JT. Uveitis associated with inflammatory bowel disease compared with uveitis associated with spondyloarthropathy. Arch Ophthalmol. 1997;115:61-64.
144. Daunt SON, Kotowski KE, O'Reilly AP, et al. Ulcerative vulvitis in Reiter's syndrome: A case report. Br J Vener Dis. 1982;58:405-407.
145. Arnett FC, McClusky OE, Schacter BZ, et al. Incomplete Reiter's syndrome: Discriminating features and HL-A W27 in diagnosis. Ann Intern Med. 1976;84:8-12.
146. Csonka GW. Recurrent attacks in Reiter's disease. Arthritis Rheum. 1960;3:164-169.
147. Catterall RD. The role of microbial infection in Reiter's syndrome. In: Dumont DC, ed. Infection and Immunology in the Rheumatic Diseases. Oxford: Blackwell Scientific Publications; 1976:147-150.
148. Butler MJ, Russell AS, Percy JS, et al. A follow-up study of 48 patients with Reiter's syndrome. Am J Med. 1979;67:808-810.
149. Calin A, Fried JF. An "experimental" epidemic of Reiter's syndrome revisited. Ann Intern Med. 1976;84:564-566.
150. Ruppert GB, Lindsay J, Barth WF. Cardiac conduction abnormalities in Reiter's syndrome. Am J Med. 1982;73:335-340.
151. Bardin T, Schumacher HR. Should we treat postvenereal Reiter's syndrome by antibiotics? (Editorial). J Rheumatol. 1991;18:1780-1781.
152. Ford DK. Reiter's syndrome: Current concepts of etiology and pathogenesis. In: Hobson D, Holmes KK, eds. Nongonococcal Urethritis and Related Infections. Washington, DC: American Society for Microbiology; 1977:64-66.
153. Bardin T, Enel C, Cornelis F, et al. Antibiotic treatment of venereal disease and Reiter's syndrome in a Greenland population. Arthritis Rheum. 1992;35:190-194.
154. Lauhio A, Leirisalo-Repo M, Lähdevirta J, et al. Double-blind, placebo-controlled study of three-month treatment with lymecycline in reactive arthritis, with special reference to *Chlamydia* arthritis. Arthritis Rheum. 1991;34:6-14.
155. Toussirot E, Despaux J, Wending D. Do minocycline and other tetracyclines have a place in rheumatology? Rev Rhum Engl Ed. 1997;64:474-480.
156. Treating Reiter's syndrome (Editorial). Lancet. 1987;2:1125-1126.
157. Kiyohara A, Takamori K, Niizuma N, Ogawa H. Successful treatment of severe recurrent Reiter's syndrome with cyclosporine. J Am Acad Dermatol. 1997;36:482-483.

CHAPTER **103**

Vulvovaginitis and Cervicitis

WILLIAM M. McCORMACK

Vulvovaginal symptoms are common and frequently result in encounters of patients with the health care system, including use of folk remedies, purchase of over-the-counter (OTC) pharmaceuticals, and presentation to health care providers. In one survey[1] of women college graduates with a median age of about 30 years, almost 70% reported at least one lifetime physician-diagnosed and treated vaginal yeast infection; in addition, 29% had been treated for bacterial vaginosis (BV) and 26% for trichomoniasis. More than 20% of the women had been treated for a vaginal yeast infection within the past year.

Genitourinary symptoms in women tend to lack specificity. For example, all women have vaginal secretions, but their ability to discriminate normal from abnormal secretions is often imprecise. Similarly, vulvar discomfort is fairly common and may result from a variety of infectious and noninfectious causes. This chapter discusses vaginal discharge and vulvitis separately, with the understanding that there is considerable overlap between these syndromes and that a presenting patient whose symptoms appear to represent one syndrome may ultimately have a quite different diagnosis.

VAGINAL SECRETIONS

The normal vaginal secretions are a physiologically important biomass. Vaginal cells contain glycogen and are continually shed into the lumen of the vagina. As the cells autolyze, glycogen depolymerizes to glucose, which serves as an energy source for bacteria known as lactobacilli. *Lactobacillus crispatus* and *Lactobacillus jensenii* are the predominant species.[2] Lactobacilli metabolize glucose to lactic acid, which results in a normal vaginal pH of 3.5 to 4.6. Although the vagina is not sterile and many species of bacteria can be isolated from vaginal specimens from healthy women, lactobacilli normally dominate the vaginal flora and comprise more than 95% of the bacteria in the normal vagina. Indeed, the predominant cells in normal vaginal secretions are lactobacilli and vaginal epithelial cells (Fig. 103-1).

In addition to lactic acid, lactobacilli may also produce hydrogen peroxide, which is bactericidal alone and highly bactericidal in combination with physiologic amounts of myeloperoxidase and chloride.[3] Loss of the normal *Lactobacillus*-dominated vaginal flora increases the likelihood of exogenous infection after exposure to sexually transmitted pathogens,[4] as well as the risk of endogenous infection in association with pregnancy and gynecologic surgery.[5]

Therefore, the normal vaginal secretions are a heterogenous suspension of vaginal epithelial cells and lactobacilli in fluid that

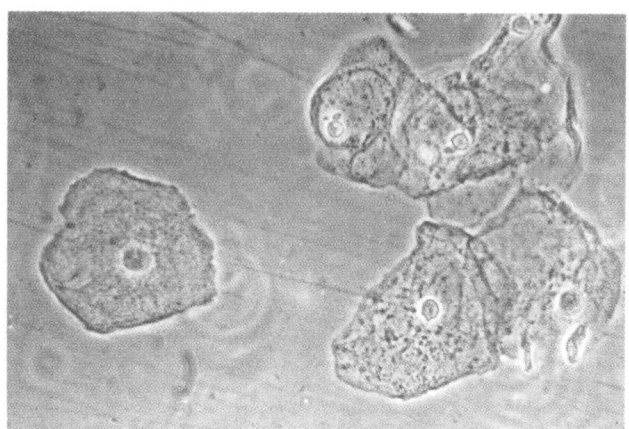

FIGURE 103-1. Normal vaginal secretions as seen in a suspension of vaginal secretions in 0.9% NaCl. Vaginal epithelial cells and lactobacilli are the primary cells seen.

emanates from the cervix and vaginal walls (Fig. 103-2). The secretions have a pH of 3.5 to 4.6, are odorless, and do not cause itching or irritation. The normal secretions are clumpy and tend to remain in the vagina, although in some women egress of normal secretions may require use of a perineal pad. Characteristics of normal vaginal secretions are listed in Box 103-1.

An appreciation of the normal is important in dealing with patients who report an abnormal discharge. A significant minority of such patients have normal secretions. These women may have a large volume of normal secretions; relaxation of the introitus after childbirth that allows outflow of normal volumes of normal secretions; or heightened awareness of a normal amount of physiologic secretions, often as a re-

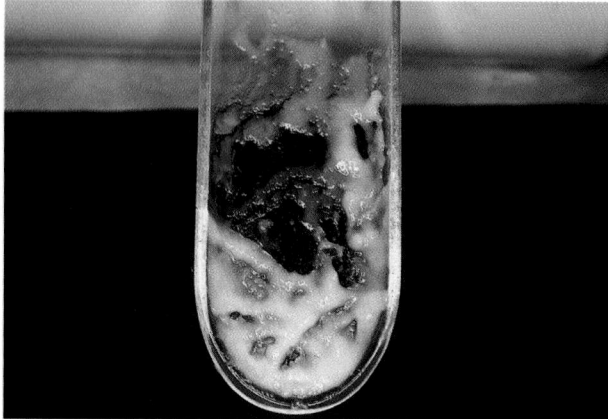

FIGURE 103-2. Normal vaginal secretions on a plastic vaginal speculum. The secretions are off-white in color and heterogenous.

sult of other genitourinary symptoms such as chronic vulvitis. The volume of normal secretions may increase during pregnancy and during use of hormonal contraceptive agents.

Patients with a normal or physiologic vaginal discharge usually have a history of multiple self-directed or clinician-directed treatments with a bewildering array of topical and systemic antibacterial and antifungal agents. Recognition of the normalcy of the secretions is important so that the patient can be reassured that her secretions are normal and so that diagnostic and therapeutic attention can be focused on associated conditions, if any, that may be present.

Box 103-2 lists important characteristics of patients who present with normal vaginal secretions. Notable characteristics include chronicity, absence of odor, absence of vulvar discomfort (unless there is unrelated vulvitis), many unsuccessful visits to a variety of different health care providers, and many ineffective treatments.

On close questioning, a number of these patients do not have sufficient external flow of vaginal secretions to stain their clothing or to require use of a perineal pad. They appreciate what they perceive to be abnormal secretions by extracting normal secretions with use of their index finger. This "finger test" is an important historical clue that the woman has normal secretions.

In addition to normal secretions, the differential diagnosis of vaginal discharge primarily includes three infections (trichomoniasis, vulvovaginal candidiasis, and BV); an idiopathic condition known as desquamative inflammatory vaginitis (DIV); cervicitis (both infectious and noninfectious); and vulvovaginitis associated with estrogen deficiency (Box 103-3).

APPROACH TO THE PATIENT

History

The etiologic diagnosis of vaginitis depends on a careful evaluation of the history, physical examination, and immediate laboratory tests. Historical features are relatively nonspecific,[6] but they may direct clinical suspicion toward certain causes. If at all possible, the history should be obtained with the patient in the sitting position and before she has disrobed.

The medical history (Box 103-4) should include all of the usual gynecologic parameters, including menstrual history, pregnancies, contraception, sexual preference, past and current sexual relationships,

---

BOX 103-4

History from Patients with Vulvovaginal Symptoms

General gynecologic history
    Menstrual history
    Pregnancies
    Sexual preference
    Contraception
    Sexual relationships
    Prior infections
General medical history
    Allergies
    Diabetes
    Malignancies
    Immunodeficiency
Symptoms of vulvovaginitis
    Discharge
    Odor
    Vulvar discomfort
    Dyspareunia

BOX 103-5

Genital Examination of the Patient with Vulvovaginal Symptoms

Adequate illumination
Magnification, if possible
Give the patient a mirror
Inspect the external genitalia
    Lesions
    Mucosal erythema
Examine the vaginal mucosa
    Erythema
    Lesions
    Secretions
Examine the cervix
    Ectropion
    Lesions
    Erythema
    Endocervical secretions
Collect vaginal and cervical specimens
Bimanual examination

---

and prior genitourinary infections. In addition, the patient should be asked about underlying medical conditions such as allergies, diabetes, malignancies, and immunodeficiency syndromes (primarily human immunodeficiency virus [HIV] disease) that might be associated with or influence vulvovaginal disease.

Age. Neonates can acquire trichomonal or candidal vulvovaginitis during passage through an infected birth canal—an argument for treating these infections in pregnant women before term. Neonatal vaginal thrush responds promptly to topical antifungal medications. Neonatal trichomoniasis can be treated with metronidazole.[7] After the neonatal period, a vaginal discharge is abnormal and should prompt a thorough examination. Vaginal candidiasis is rare in prepubescent girls.[8] Prepubescent vaginal epithelium is thin, and the entire vagina is susceptible to infection with *Neisseria gonorrhoeae*. Gonococcal vulvovaginitis often causes profuse vaginal discharge. The diagnosis of a sexually transmitted disease in a young girl should raise the suspicion of child abuse, although some agents have been transmitted to children in the absence of frank sexual contact. Patients in the sexually active years are more likely to have physiologic secretions or infectious vaginitis. Postmenopausal women are more likely to have atrophic vaginitis.

Mode of Onset. An abrupt and identifiable time of onset of symptoms suggests infection. Vaginal discharge associated with neoplasia, estrogen depletion, or a foreign body often has a subacute onset, with symptoms progressing over a period of weeks.

Quantity of Discharge. The amount of discharge is highly variable in all conditions. Patients with vulvovaginal candidiasis often have scanty discharge or note no discharge at all. Atrophic discharges are commonly scanty unless infection has supervened.

External Irritation. Physiologic discharge is rarely associated with vulvar or perineal discomfort. Pruritus with a scant or absent discharge is frequently seen in candidiasis. External discomfort is an infrequent complaint in BV. Severe episodic perineal pain that sometimes prevents urination suggests herpes simplex virus infection, which affects the labia but usually spares the vagina. Chronic discomfort (often interfering with sexual activity) should prompt consideration of a noninfectious vulvitis such as vulvar vestibulitis.

Odor. Vaginal odor in the absence of other symptoms is the initial complaint in many cases of BV. A feculent odor may accompany anaerobic superinfection of genital lesions, or it may be noted in the presence of a foreign body or enterovaginal fistula.

Abdominal Pain. Abdominal discomfort is rare in uncomplicated vulvovaginitis except for some cases of trichomoniasis. Women who complain of abdominal pain should be examined for evidence of urinary tract infection and pelvic inflammatory disease.

Sexual History. Exposure to a new sexual partner increases the likelihood of sexually transmitted disease. A history of genital symptoms in a sexual partner is helpful diagnostically. The commencement of oral contraceptive use may be associated with increased physiologic discharge.

Other Diseases. Diabetes mellitus, acquired immunodeficiency syndrome (AIDS), malignancy and the treatment thereof, and possibly hypoparathyroidism increase the risk of candidal vaginitis. Diseases known to impair host defenses may predispose to otherwise rare infections. Drugs used in the treatment of other diseases may predispose to vaginal infection.

Medications. Systemic or local medications may influence vaginal infection. Antibiotics that are active against the normal bacterial flora of the vagina predispose to candidal vaginitis. Patients who are taking corticosteroids or oral contraceptives are at increased risk for development of vulvovaginal candidiasis. Local medications, including vaginal douches, rarely produce a chemical vaginitis; douching immediately before examination makes diagnosis difficult.

Examination

If the patient has not had recent medical care, a general physical examination can be performed. At the least, the patient's breasts should be examined if she has not had a professional breast examination during the past year. Similarly, a mammogram should be ordered if the patient's age or history dictate that one is indicated.

With the patient supine on the examining table, the pubic hair should be examined for the presence of crab lice or nits. The inguinofemoral areas should be palpated for adenopathy. Suprapubic and lower abdominal tenderness or masses can be sought by palpation.

The gynecologic examination (Box 103-5) requires adequate light. Magnification is helpful and is best provided by a colposcope. Providing the patient with a mirror allows her to participate in the examination and is useful for clarifying the location of symptoms as well as demonstrating important findings to the patient.

With the patient in the lithotomy position, the external genitalia should be carefully inspected. The patient should be asked to point to any areas of external itching, irritation, or other discomfort. Localization of discomfort to vulvar skin or vestibular mucosa provides useful information. The appearance of the vulvar skin and vestibular mucous membranes should be noted, with careful attention to ulcers or other discontinuity of the skin or mucosa, mucosal erythema, and visible secretions. Diffuse perineal erythema may accompany trichomoniasis or candidiasis. Diffuse reddening with small satellite lesions, usually papular or papulopustular, suggests candidiasis. The degree of perineal irritation is quite variable with all infections, but severe perivaginal irritation is uncommon with BV. Labial edema may accompany severe irritation, especially in vulvovaginal candidiasis.

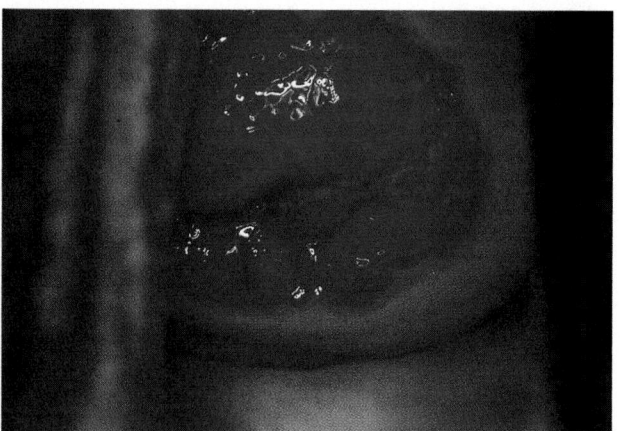

FIGURE 103-3. Normal cervix with a normal ectropion.

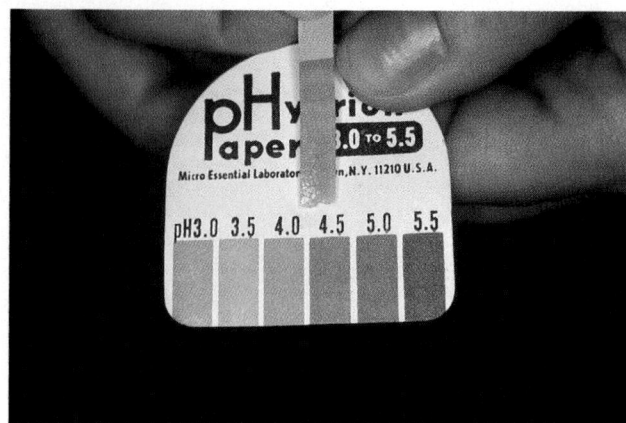

FIGURE 103-4. Examination of vaginal secretions for pH with use of pH paper.

Careful examination of all the extravaginal surfaces may reveal lesions of genital herpes, syphilis, condyloma acuminatum, molluscum contagiosum, scabies, or vulvar vestibulitis.

By spreading the labia with the gloved hand, one may examine the urethral meatus. The urethra may be gently stripped with a finger placed inside the vagina. Urethral discharge is not a common finding, but, if delivered, such material should be examined microscopically and cultured. The introitus and the internal surfaces of the labia minora should be examined for lesions. Vaginal discharge is sometimes observed on the labia or flowing onto the perineum. Such copious discharge is usually associated with trichomoniasis or BV but may accompany other infections.

A speculum is then inserted to expose the cervix and vaginal mucosa. A small-sized speculum is adequate for most patients and minimizes discomfort for patients who have introital lesions. A small amount of lubricant facilitates insertion without compromising the quality of the microbiologic samples to be collected. The vaginal and cervical mucosa should be inspected with attention to erythema and lesions. An ectropion, if present, should be noted (Fig. 103-3). The vaginal secretions should be described, as should any secretions emanating from the endocervical canal or from an ectropion.

Specimens obtained during the examination are listed in Box 103-6. Vaginal pH should be measured. A sample of vaginal material should be collected from the lateral vaginal wall with use of a cotton-tipped applicator. Care should be taken to avoid contamination with endocervical secretions. The collected vaginal secretions are applied to a strip of pH paper and compared with the standard chart provided by the manufacturer (Fig. 103-4).

A sample of vaginal secretions is then examined. The specimen may be prepared in several ways. A swab of vaginal secretions may be agitated in a tube containing about 0.5 mL of normal saline.

Alternatively, a plastic transfer pipette may be used to introduce 2 to 3 mL of normal saline solution into the posterior fornix. The saline solution is mixed with the vaginal secretions by aspiration and reaspiration of the solution, and the resultant suspension of vaginal material is placed into a small tube. The suspension is then examined for odor (whiff test) by placing a drop on a microscope slide, adding a drop of 10% potassium hydroxide (KOH), and smelling the resultant mixture. Normal secretions have no odor. A fishy odor is indicative of BV.

A drop of the suspension of vaginal material is placed on a microscope slide, and a coverslip is added. This "wet mount" can be examined under high power with a bright-field microscope. Phase-contrast microscopy provides an excellent means of evaluating vaginal wet mounts. The relative numbers of epithelial cells and polymorphonuclear neutrophils (PMNs) should be noted. Because PMNs are present in physiologic endocervical discharge that collects in the vagina,[9] small numbers of PMNs may be observed in the vaginal material recovered from healthy women. A finding of many more than one PMN per epithelial cell should raise suspicion of cervical or vaginal inflammation. Observation of relatively few PMNs does not rule out vaginal infection, however. Vaginal candidiasis can produce a discharge that contains only small numbers of PMNs. The relative absence of PMNs is characteristic of the discharge of BV.[10] In fact, the finding of many PMNs in the vaginal discharge of a patient with BV should prompt a search for simultaneous infection, such as trichomoniasis, gonorrhea, or chlamydial cervicitis. Pseudohyphae suggest vaginal candidiasis, but often only moderate or even very small numbers of yeast cells are seen in this condition. Indeed, some patients with vulvovaginal candidiasis have organisms identified only by culture. The wet preparation should be scanned for motile trichomonads.

Normal squamous epithelial cells have transparent cytoplasm and small nuclei. Immature (parabasal) cells are smaller and have larger nuclei. Epithelial cells covered with tiny coccobacillary forms are called *clue cells* and are associated with BV. Clue cells are best recognized by observing the edges of epithelial cells, which may be obscured by the adherent coccobacilli. Some cells are so heavily encrusted that the nuclei are obscured. Trichomonads are best recognized by their characteristic twitching motility. The flagellae and undulating membrane may be observed by careful focusing of the microscope and adjustment of the light source. Trichomonad motility is improved by gentle warming of the preparation. The wet mount is negative in about 30% of the women with trichomoniasis (see Chapter 278), so a negative wet mount does not rule out this infection, particularly in asymptomatic women.

The bacterial flora can be assessed on the wet mount. Normal vaginal flora consists of a sparse population of bacilli. In BV, the predominant flora is tiny coccobacilli. Spermatozoa may be observed as long as 10 days after the last coitus, but motile sperm suggest sexual contact within the preceding 24 hours.[11]

BOX 103-6

Specimens Obtained during the Gynecologic Examination

Vaginal secretions
  pH
  Whiff test
  Saline wet preparation
  Potassium hydroxide (KOH) wet preparation
Endocervical cultures or nonculture tests
  Neisseria gonorrhoeae
  Chlamydia trachomatis
Vaginal cultures
  Candida species
  Trichomonas vaginalis
Cervical cytologic examination (if not documented within the previous 12 months)

Combining a drop of 10% KOH with the vaginal material on a microscope slide and applying a coverslip destroys cellular elements but leaves the bacteria and fungi unscathed. The KOH preparation cannot be used for microscopic diagnosis of trichomoniasis or BV.

A Gram stain of vaginal material is somewhat less useful than the wet mount for differential diagnosis. Although *Candida* spp. are readily recognized on the Gram-stained smear, trichomonads are difficult to identify. Normal vaginal flora consists primarily of gram-positive bacilli, which are mostly lactobacilli. In BV, the normal flora is replaced by sheets of gram-variable coccobacilli, which often overlie the surface of epithelial cells. Women with vulvovaginal candidiasis sometimes have large numbers of budding yeasts and pseudohyphae. The Gram stain is negative in many women from whom *Candida* can be cultured.[12]

Material recovered from the endocervix can be Gram-stained. Cervical discharge usually contains moderate numbers of PMNs, and their presence is not necessarily an indication of infection.[9] The presence of large numbers of PMNs suggests cervicitis. Gram-negative, intracellular diplococci accurately diagnose gonorrhea (see Chapter 209), but extracellular diplococci are less predictive. The cervical Gram stain is positive in only about 60% of women with cervical gonorrhea. Therefore, a negative Gram stain does not rule out this infection.[12]

Before the speculum is removed, endocervical specimens are obtained for examination for *N. gonorrhoeae* and *Chlamydia trachomatis*. Vaginal cultures for yeast are useful to exclude fungal infection, for which the wet preparation is incompletely sensitive.[13] Trichomonads can be sought by inoculating modified Diamond's medium if trichomoniasis is a diagnostic possibility.[14] Finally, a cervical cytologic smear should be obtained if such an examination within the past year cannot be documented. Relying on the patient's history of cervical cytologic examinations is risky, because some women assume that all gynecologic examinations include a "Pap" smear.

Bimanual examination for adnexal tenderness and masses should be a part of the evaluation. Adnexal tenderness is sufficiently uncommon with local vaginal infections that its presence suggests salpingitis.

TRICHOMONIASIS

Etiology and Pathogenesis

Trichomoniasis is caused by the protozoan *Trichomonas vaginalis*. It is a classic exogenous sexually transmitted infection, like gonorrhea and chlamydial infection. The organism is not normally present in the vagina. Transmission almost always occurs through sexual contact. After an incubation period of a few days, patients develop a purulent discharge associated with varying degrees of vulvar irritation, dysuria, and dyspareunia (Box 103-7). An abnormal odor is often present, usually signifying concomitant BV.

Diagnosis

Examination is notable for vulvar, vestibular, and vaginal erythema and a purulent vaginal discharge (Fig. 103-5). A minority of patients manifest characteristic mucosal capillary dilation, which gives the mucosa a "strawberry" appearance.

Vaginal pH is almost always greater than 4.5. A positive whiff test is not unusual. The vaginal wet preparation contains an abundance of leukocytes and motile flagellated trichomonads (Fig. 103-6). In experienced hands, the wet preparation has fairly good sensitivity (70% to 80%) in symptomatic patients.[15] The organism can be cultivated by in-

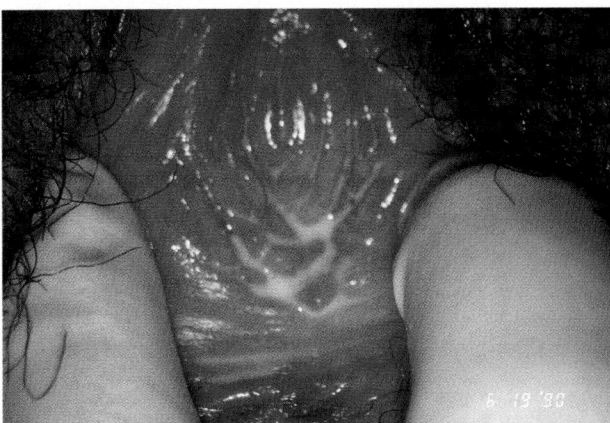

FIGURE 103-5. Trichomoniasis. There are purulent secretions and mucosal erythema.

oculating a liquid medium such as modified Diamond's medium[14] or In Pouch TV.[16] After incubation, aliquots of the liquid medium are examined daily for motile trichomonads. Modified Columbia agar—a solid medium—has also been used.[17] Culture improves the diagnostic yield, especially in asymptomatic patients. Sensitive and specific nucleic acid amplification tests have been developed, but none has been approved by the U. S. Food and Drug Administration (FDA).[18,19]

A wet preparation diagnostic of trichomoniasis is highly specific because of the characteristic motility of the organisms. Diagnostic tests in which the organisms are no longer motile may lack specificity. A common clinical problem is the woman with no epidemiologic evidence for a sexually transmitted condition who has trichomonads visualized on a cervical cytologic examination.[20] In some such cases, the cytologist may have misread the smear. For such a patient, the clinician should obtain confirmation of the diagnosis of trichomoniasis, by wet preparation or culture (or both), before initiating treatment and before embarking on a potentially disruptive epidemiologic investigation.

Treatment

Metronidazole and tinidazole are the only effective agents that are approved by the FDA for the treatment of trichomoniasis. A single 2.0-g oral dose of metronidazole is the treatment of choice.[21] Alternatively, 500 mg can be given twice daily for 7 days. Controlled studies have failed to show any important advantage of the 7-day regimen.[21] The single-dose regimen, if administered under direct observation in the office or clinic, has the obvious advantage of 100% compliance. Because trichomoniasis is almost always sexually transmitted, treat-

BOX 103-7

Symptoms of Trichomoniasis

Purulent vaginal discharge
Vulvar irritation
Dysuria
Dyspareunia
Abnormal vaginal odor

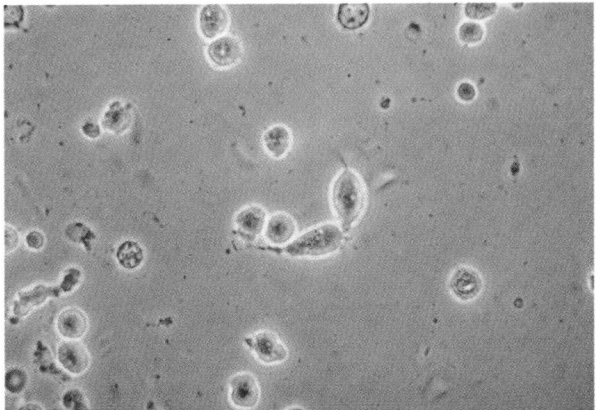

FIGURE 103-6. Trichomoniasis. Suspension of vaginal secretions in 0.9% NaCl. There are leukocytes and flagellated trichomonads.

ment with metronidazole of all recent sexual partners, regardless of their symptoms, is an integral part of management.[21]

The aforementioned regimens containing metronidazole eliminate trichomonads in well over 90% of instances. If this treatment fails (Box 103-8), the diagnosis should be reconfirmed with a wet preparation or culture. Additionally, treatment of all current sexual partners should be assured. Initial retreatment should be with oral metronidazole, 500 mg twice daily for 7 days. If this regimen is not successful, oral metronidazole in a single dose of 2.0 g can be prescribed for 3 to 5 days.[21] If the latter metronidazole regimen fails, the patient can be assumed to have clinically significant metronidazole resistance, and consultation with an expert in the management of trichomoniasis should be sought. Susceptibility testing, available through the Centers for Disease Control and Prevention (telephone 770-488-4115) should be performed.[22] Alternative regimens that include very high doses of metronidazole are usually prescribed. The most widely used regimen is probably that described by Lossick and associates,[23] which consists of both oral (2.5 g daily) and vaginal (0.5 g daily) metronidazole for up to 3 weeks. Antiemetics may be prescribed with this regimen to reduce nausea and vomiting. In Lossick's experience, this regimen was effective in about 90% of cases. Intravenous regimens of metronidazole have also been prescribed.[24] For patients who cannot tolerate metronidazole at this dosage level and for those who do not respond to it, the next choice is usually tinidazole. Recently approved by the FDA for use in trichomoniasis, tinidazole has better in vitro efficacy[25] and is better tolerated than metronidazole, and it has cured most patients with metronidazole-resistant trichomoniasis.[26]

For patients with trichomoniasis who are unresponsive to metronidazole and tinidazole, there are few therapeutic options of proven value. Nonoxynol-9 is active against *T. vaginalis* in vitro and was reported to be effective in one patient.[27] However, in a subsequent study nonoxynol-9 was effective in only 3 of 17 patients.[28] Furazolidone is highly active in vitro against metronidazole-sensitive and metronidazole-resistant isolates of *T. vaginalis*[29] and was effective when given vaginally in a study conducted some years ago.[30] In one study,[31] zinc sulfate douches given in combination with oral metronidazole were effective. In general, however, topical treatments have been disappointing,[14] presumably because of reservoirs of infection in periurethral glands and other areas that are not adequately sterilized by intravaginal medications. Specifically, topical preparations containing metronidazole (e.g., 0.75% metronidazole gel) are ineffective in unselected patients with trichomoniasis[32] and are of no utility in patients with metronidazole resistance except as a possible adjunct to oral treatment.

T. vaginalis organisms have been shown to be estrogen dependent in vitro[33] and in vivo.[34] In one report, discontinuation of estrogen replacement treatment in a postmenopausal woman was associated with resolution of vaginal trichomoniasis.[35] These data suggest that hormonal manipulation should be studied in the management of trichomoniasis that is unresponsive to metronidazole and for women who cannot tolerate metronidazole.

Minor adverse reactions to metronidazole, primarily nausea and a metallic taste, are common, but most patients can tolerate the usual dosage schedules. Metronidazole allergy is unusual. In such instances, desensitization with intravenous[36] or oral[37] incremental dosing protocols has been useful.

Human immunodeficiency virus (HIV) infection has no effect on the incidence or prevalence of trichomoniasis or on persistence or recurrence.[38] Treatment of trichomoniasis decreases the viral load of HIV in vaginal fluid,[39] an observation concordant with the results of studies that show an association of trichomoniasis with HIV acquisition.[19]

Trichomoniasis in pregnancy has been the subject of considerable interest. An association between trichomoniasis and premature rupture of the membranes was reported in 1984.[40] Cotch and colleagues,[41] using data from the Vaginal Infections and Prematurity (VIP) Study, reported in 1997 on the prospective evaluation of 13,816 pregnant women. They found that trichomoniasis was independently associated with a 30% greater likelihood of preterm delivery and low birth weight and a 40% greater likelihood of having a preterm infant of low birth weight. In a more recent study, treatment of trichomoniasis in asymptomatic pregnant women with metronidazole did not prevent preterm delivery.[42] Metronidazole has traditionally been avoided during pregnancy because of largely theoretical concerns about mutagenicity and oncogenicity. However, studies and meta-analyses have not demonstrated a consistent association between metronidazole use during pregnancy and teratogenic or mutagenic effects in infants.[43-45] Therefore, pregnant women who have symptomatic trichomoniasis should be treated with 2.0 g of metronidazole.[21]

VULVOVAGINAL CANDIDIASIS

Etiology and Pathogenesis

Candida albicans and other species of *Candida* can be part of the vaginal flora of asymptomatic women. About 30% of unselected women are colonized. In one study of unselected women,[13] two thirds of colonized women and only 22% of uncolonized women reported symptoms, primarily vulvovaginal itching and irritation. These data suggest that colonization with *Candida* species usually produces symptoms, albeit mild symptoms that do not prompt the patient to seek medical attention.

C. albicans can be isolated from about 80% to 90% of patients with vulvovaginal candidiasis, and other yeasts account for up to 20% of cases.[46] *Candida tropicalis* is isolated from about 1% to 5% and may be associated with a higher rate of recurrence after standard treatments.[47,48] *Candida* (formerly *Torulopsis*) *glabrata* accounts for about 10% of vaginal yeast isolates.[46,47,49-51] Symptomatic vaginitis caused by this organism is associated with less intense itching and dyspareunia[49] than that caused by other *Candida* species, but the organism may be harder to eradicate with standard therapies.[47,51] The relative incidence of vaginitis caused by fungi other than *C. albicans* appears to be increasing.[47] Non-*albicans* infections are associated with recurrent disease (accounting for 21% of recurrent versus 12% of initial infections) and with HIV infection (22% of infections in HIV-positive women versus 12% in HIV-negative women), especially in HIV-infected women who receive prophylaxis with imidazoles or triazoles.[47] It is thought that the widespread use of topical antifungal agents, especially in short courses, may contribute to selection for non-*albicans* yeasts, which are less susceptible to these agents than is *C. albicans*. Cases of vaginitis caused by *Saccharomyces cerevisiae* have been reported and may be associated with baking.[52,53]

Some workers have estimated that 75% of adult women will suffer at least one episode of vulvovaginal candidiasis during their lifetime.[54] Inhibition of normal bacterial flora by antibiotics favors the growth of yeasts,[54,55] although symptomatic cases are seen after the use of antimicrobials that do not suppress lactobacilli.[56] Vulvovaginal candidiasis sometimes occurs after antimicrobial treatment of trichomoniasis or BV.

Growth of yeasts is apparently favored by high estrogen levels, although such levels also promote the growth of lactobacilli.[57-59] The prevalence of vaginal carriage of *Candida* is higher among users of oral contraceptives than among women using other methods of birth control.[46,55,59] The mechanism of this estrogenic predisposition is unclear.

Vulvovaginal candidiasis is associated with poorly controlled diabetes mellitus, and tight glycemic control decreases the frequency of symptomatic infection.[60] However, testing for diabetes in women with recurrent vulvovaginal candidiasis is not cost-effective.[55]

It has been suggested that tight, insulating clothing predisposes to vulvovaginal candidiasis by increasing vulvar warmth and moisture. In prospective studies, a higher prevalence of candidal carriage and higher concentrations of organisms were found in women who wore tight rather than loose clothing.[61-63] Impairment of phagocytic cells or of cell-mediated immunity (e.g., transplantation, chemotherapy) also predisposes to vulvovaginal candidiasis. Some authorities believe that women with HIV infection develop vulvovaginal candidiasis more often than HIV-negative women do, especially if they have low CD4 T-cell counts.[64,65]

The contribution of sexual transmission is poorly defined. Vulvovaginal candidiasis increases in incidence with the onset of sexual activity,[66-68] but the incidence is also increased by the use of oral contraceptives,[46,55,59] the contraceptive sponge,[67] or the intrauterine device,[67] any of which might coincide with sexual activity. Having multiple sexual partners is not associated with a higher incidence of *Candida* infection. Most women who present with vulvovaginal candidiasis have no predisposing illnesses or medications.

The mechanism by which *Candida* produces disease is not well defined. Although it is postulated that differences in virulence must exist,[55] strains isolated from symptomatic women are not demonstrably different from isolates from asymptomatic carriers.[69] Filamentous forms (hyphae and pseudohyphae) are associated with active disease.[70] Pseudohyphae have been observed to penetrate vaginal epithelial cells,[71] and they are more adherent to cells than are budding yeasts (blastospores).[72] Adherence appears to be an important pathogenic feature of *Candida* spp.,[73] and sublethal concentrations of antifungal agents may ameliorate disease by reducing adherence.[74]

The severity of symptoms in vulvovaginal candidiasis is not directly related to the number of yeast cells present. Indeed, very small numbers of yeasts may be present in vaginal material recovered from highly symptomatic women.[55] An immunologic reaction has been

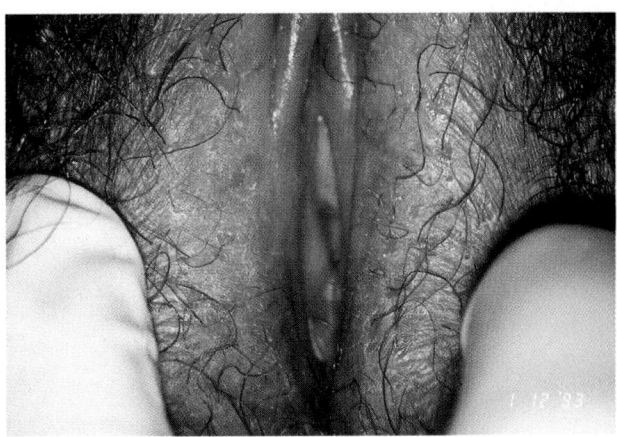

FIGURE 103-8. Vulvovaginal candidiasis. There are excoriations of the skin of the labia majora due to scratching.

suggested as the mechanism for symptomatic disease in such women,[46,75] and one small series suggested that desensitization may decrease the frequency of symptomatic episodes.[76]

Clinical Features

Patients with candidal vulvovaginitis generally complain of perivaginal pruritus, often with little or no discharge (Box 103-9). Dysuria is occasionally noted and is likely to be perceived as vulvar rather than urethral. The labia may be pale or erythematous. Shallow, radial, linear ulcerations (Fig. 103-7), especially on the posterior portion of the introitus, are common. Excoriations caused by scratching are often present (Fig. 103-8). Tiny papules or papulopustules, called satellite lesions, just beyond the main area of erythema are helpful diagnostically. The vaginal walls may be erythematous. Candidal discharge is classically thick and adherent (Fig. 103-9). However, it may be thin and loose, resembling the discharge of other vaginitides.

Diagnosis

Vaginal pH is usually normal. There is no odor when the vaginal secretions are mixed with 10% KOH. Microscopic examination of vaginal material in saline or in 10% KOH may disclose budding yeasts or mycelia (Fig. 103-10). In the symptomatic patient with a diagnostic microscopic examination, fungal cultures are not needed. Microscopic examination of vaginal secretions is incompletely sensitive, however. Accordingly, cultures may be helpful to secure the diagnosis in a patient who has a compatible clinical presentation and a

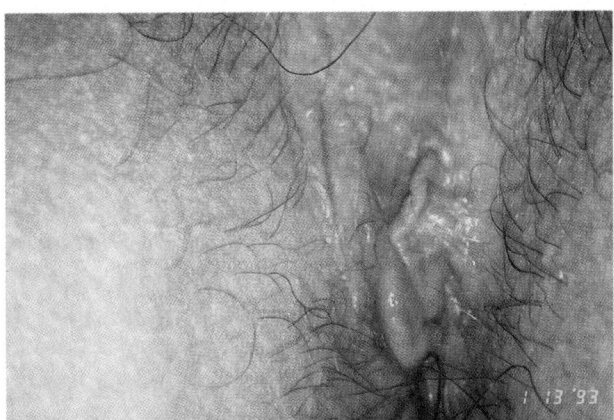

FIGURE 103-7. Vulvovaginal candidiasis. There is a linear ulcer of the perineal skin.

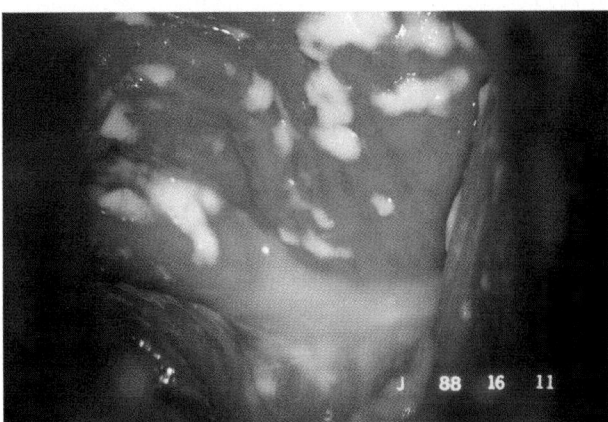

FIGURE 103-9. Vulvovaginal candidiasis. There are adherent white patches with surrounding erythema on the cervical mucosa.

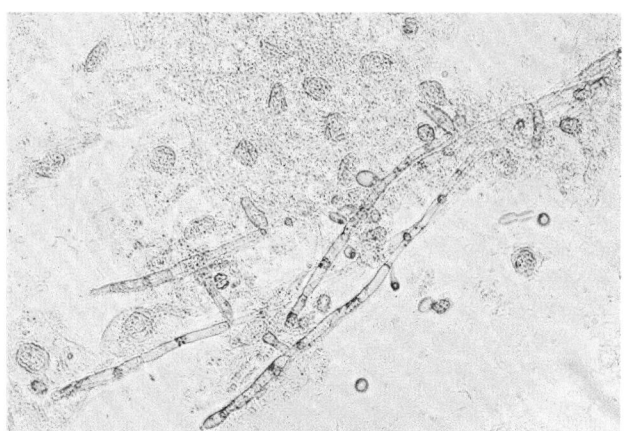

FIGURE 103-10. Vulvovaginal candidiasis. Suspension of vaginal secretions in 0.9% NaCl. Mycelia can be seen.

BOX 103-10

Classification of Patients with Vulvovaginal Candidiasis

Uncomplicated Infection
Sporadic
No underlying disease
Caused by *Candida albicans*
Patient is not pregnant
Mild to moderate severity

Complicated Infection
Underlying illness
   Human immunodeficiency virus disease
   Diabetes mellitus
Recurrent infection (four or more episodes per year)
Caused by non-*albicans* species of *Candida*
Pregnancy
Severe infection

---

negative microscopic examination. It is usually expedient to treat such a patient with antifungal agents while awaiting culture results. Cultures are also useful if empirical treatment produces no response.

Treatment

The treatment of vulvovaginal candidiasis is best approached by classifying the patient as having either uncomplicated or complicated infection (Boxes 103-10 and 103-11).[21]

Uncomplicated vulvovaginal candidiasis is a sporadic infection with C. *albicans,* of mild to moderate severity, in a woman without a

---

BOX 103-11

Treatment of Vulvovaginal Candidiasis

Uncomplicated Infection
Any available topical agent
Fluconazole, 150 mg as a single oral dose

Complicated Infection
Culture confirmation mandatory
Antifungal susceptibility testing may be helpful
Treatment for 10-14 days with vaginal or oral agents
Alternative topical agents
   Boric acid
   5-Flurocytosine
Consider treatment of partners
Long-term suppressive treatment for frequently recurrent disease

---

history of recent candidiasis and without underlying illness such as HIV disease or diabetes mellitus. Most patients have uncomplicated disease, and most cases respond to treatment with short courses of vaginal or oral antifungals. Effective agents include vaginal preparations containing nystatin, miconazole, clotrimazole, butoconazole, terconazole, and tioconazole. All except nystatin and terconazole-containing products are available without a prescription. Self-diagnosis and self-medication with over-the-counter (OTC) antifungal agents should be limited to women who have previously had documented vulvovaginal candidiasis and are experiencing a recurrence of similar symptoms; self-diagnosis in other situations is often erroneous.[77] Failure to respond to self-medication should trigger a visit to a physician. In uncomplicated disease, there does not appear to be any difference in efficiency related to dosage form (vaginal tablets, suppositories, ointments, creams) or to length of treatment (1, 3, 7, or 14 days). Oral fluconazole in a single 150-mg dose is as effective as the aforementioned vaginal medications in the treatment of uncomplicated vulvovaginal candidiasis[78] and has been approved by the FDA for this indication. Oral fluconazole may be less expensive than some topical preparations and is preferred over topical treatments by many women. In this dosage, the side effects are few[78] and systemic toxicity is unlikely. Other oral antifungal agents, such as ketoconazole and itraconazole, are effective but have not been approved by the FDA for the treatment of uncomplicated vulvovaginal candidiasis.

Complicated vulvovaginal candidiasis occurs in patients with underlying conditions that compromise the immune response, such as diabetes, HIV disease, malignancy, or treatment with immunosuppressive agents. Patients who are pregnant or who have severe disease and patients with frequent recurrences (four or more episodes during the past year) should also be considered to have complicated disease, as should women infected with species other than C. *albicans.*

Management of complicated disease should begin with a vaginal culture to confirm the diagnosis and to speciate any isolated yeast. More than half of patients referred because of "chronic fungal vaginitis" have negative yeast cultures and a noninfectious explanation for their symptoms.[79] It is important that these misdiagnosed patients be culled at the outset so that needless and predictably futile antifungal treatment can be avoided and attention directed to establishing an accurate diagnosis. Speciation is important for those patients who do have candidiasis, because infections caused by species of *Candida* other than C. *albicans* are often more difficult to treat.[80]

Pregnant women should be treated with topical agents for at least 7 days. Oral azole antifungal agents should not be used during pregnancy.

Complicated vulvovaginal candidiasis responds poorly to short courses of treatment with oral fluconazole[81] or topical preparations. Treatment for 7 to 14 days or longer is usually required. For patients with recurrent infections, chronic suppressive treatment with an oral antifungal agent may be useful in preventing recurrences once the current infection has responded. A report[82] published in 1986 described the use of 100 mg of ketoconazole daily, but hepatotoxicity can be a problem. More recently, 100 to 200 mg of fluconazole per week has been prescribed. Recurrences are infrequent during chronic suppressive treatment, which is continued for at least 6 months. Once suppressive treatment is discontinued, relapse occurs in about half of the patients within a few weeks, necessitating continued chronic suppression. The remaining patients remain symptom free.

Because a significant minority of healthy women are colonized with *Candida* species, treatment is not indicated for asymptomatic women who have positive vaginal cultures.

Resistance to antifungal agents appears to be increasing. The availability of OTC antifungals and the widespread use of oral agents (ketoconazole, fluconazole, itraconazole), especially in patients with HIV disease, are possible explanations. In any event, an increasing number of cases do not respond to the usual topical and oral agents. Species other than C. *albicans*, especially C. *glabrata*, are more likely to be resistant,[83,84] but nonresponsive C. *albicans* isolates are also beginning to appear.[85,86]

Fungal susceptibility testing is neither widely available nor easy to interrupt. The National Commission for Clinical Laboratory Standards (NCCLS) has published guidelines.[87] Laboratories should offer testing using these guidelines. In vitro resistance predicts treatment failure, whereas in vitro susceptibility to a given agent is more difficult to interpret.

For vulvovaginal candidiasis that does not respond to the available topical and oral agents, intravaginal boric acid has been used with success.[88] Boric acid powder (600 mg) is placed into size 0 gelatin capsules and administered vaginally for 14 days. Treatment of sexual partners has no role in the treatment of sporadic uncomplicated infections, but it may be worth considering for patients who have recurrent infections. Sequential isolates from such patients tend to be identical,[89] suggesting endogenous reactivation or exogenous reinfection from the same partner. Because the responsible organism can often be recovered from male sexual partners,[90] they cannot be ruled out as a possible source of reinfection.

Yogurt has been proposed as a prophylactic agent for recurrent vulvovaginal candidiasis. In a well-done study,[91] oral ingestion of yogurt containing live lactobacilli by patients with documented recurrent vaginal yeast infections was associated with a remarkable reduction in asymptomatic vaginal colonization and symptomatic vaginal infection with *Candida* species. More studies are needed before yogurt can be firmly established as a preventive agent. Patients who wish to try this treatment should be advised to obtain an unpasteurized yogurt product that contains live lactobacilli.

BACTERIAL VAGINOSIS

Many women who present to their physicians with vaginal symptoms have a specific condition, first described by Gardner and Dukes in 1955,[92] that is now referred to as *bacterial vaginosis* (BV).[93,94] Inflammation and perivaginal irritation are considerably milder than in trichomoniasis or candidiasis. Dysuria and dyspareunia are correspondingly rare. Affected women are usually sexually active and often complain of vaginal odor, which frequently is described as "fishy." About 90% of patients also notice a mild to moderate discharge. Abdominal discomfort is occasionally present, but it is usually mild and should prompt evaluation for coincident infections such as salpingitis.

Discharge is often present at the introitus and visible on the labia minora. The labia and vulva are not erythematous or edematous. On speculum examination, the vaginal walls appear uninflamed. The vagina usually contains a grayish, thin, homogenous discharge. A pungent odor may be noted by the examiner.

The endocervix is unaffected by the process, and any cervical discharge should be physiologic. The presence of a purulent cervical discharge may result from coincident gonococcal, chlamydial, or herpetic infection.[95] Abnormalities on bimanual examination are unusual in uncomplicated BV and should prompt a search for other pathologic processes. There is an increased risk of endometritis and salpingitis among women with BV.[96-98]

Other vaginal infections may closely resemble BV; an accurate differential diagnosis depends on laboratory examination. The pH of vaginal fluid is elevated above the normal of 4.6 in about 90% of women with BV.[92,99,100] A vaginal pH of 5 or higher strongly suggests BV.[101] If 10% KOH is added to the vaginal discharge, either on the speculum or on a microscope slide, a distinctively pungent, fishy odor is generated.[99,102] This is a positive "whiff test."

A wet mount of the vaginal fluid from patients with BV reveals clue cells, which are vaginal epithelial cells studded with tiny coccobacilli. These organisms are best appreciated at the edges of the cell and may be dense enough to partially obscure the nucleus. Not all cells in the specimen are clue cells, but some clue cells are seen in more than 90% of patients with BV.[103,104] A finding of increased numbers of PMNs in a patient with BV suggests the presence of a coexisting process, notably cervicitis.[95]

Culture for *Gardnerella vaginalis* can be accomplished on a variety of media (see Chapter 234). The organism can be isolated from virtually all women with BV,[94,102,105] but it is also recovered in smaller numbers from up to 70% of asymptomatic women.[94,105] Therefore, the presence of *G. vaginalis* does not prove that a patient has BV or suggest a need for treatment. The frequency with which *G. vaginalis* organisms can be recovered from healthy women renders a positive culture for this organism uninterpretable. Accordingly, cultures for *G. vaginalis* should not be performed.[103,104]

Epidemiology

BV was initially described in sexually active women, and it is common in populations with a high prevalence of sexually transmitted diseases. The precise contribution of heterosexual transmission to the overall epidemiology of the condition remains controversial. The prevalence is appreciable in lesbians,[106,107] among whom other sexually transmitted diseases are relatively uncommon. Lesbian couples are mostly concordant with regard to vaginal flora (normal or BV), suggesting that BV is sexually transmitted in this setting.[106,107]

Pathophysiology

Microscopic examination of vaginal discharge in BV characteristically reveals a predominant flora of coccobacilli. On the basis of this morphology, the organism most closely associated with BV was originally called *Haemophilus vaginalis*.[92] It has now been given its own genus and is called *Gardnerella vaginalis* in recognition of Dr. Gardner's initial observations (see Chapter 234). Several studies suggest a less than straightforward relationship between *G. vaginalis* and BV. Although Gardner regularly produced BV by inoculating fresh vaginal discharge from patients with BV into the vaginas of healthy volunteers, inoculation of a pure culture of *G. vaginalis* was far less likely to produce disease.[92] In addition, *G. vaginalis* can be isolated from at least 50% of asymptomatic women.[108] Finally, the in vitro sensitivity of *G. vaginalis* to antimicrobial agents does not match the effectiveness of these agents in clinical disease. Metronidazole is highly effective therapy for BV[109] despite the fact that *G. vaginalis* is relatively resistant to the drug in vitro.[99,109]

An explanation for all of these observations is that *G. vaginalis* is not the single cause of BV. BV is actually a synergistic infection involving not only *G. vaginalis* but also other microorganisms. The total number of organisms is dramatically increased in the vaginas of women with BV. Anaerobic gram-negative bacilli such as *Prevotella* spp., *Bacteroides* spp. other than *Bacteroides fragilis,* and various peptococci are involved.

Most cases of BV are also associated with motile, curved anaerobic rods that are gram negative or gram variable. These organisms have been classified into the genus *Mobiluncus.*[110,111] The precise pathogenic role of these organisms remains to be elucidated. *Mycoplasma hominis*[105] and *Ureaplasma urealyticum* can be isolated from the vaginas of many women with BV. Their role as etiologic agents of BV has not been established.

Hydrogen peroxide–producing lactobacilli dominate the normal vaginal flora[2] and appear to protect against exogenous infection. Some workers believe that an undefined change in the vaginal milieu permits the replacement of protective H_2O_2-producing lactobacilli with *G. vaginalis,* anaerobes, and mycoplasmas.

Investigators have linked douching to BV.[112,113] Women who have BV are at increased risk for the development of infection with herpes simplex virus type 2,[114] *N. gonorrhoeae,* and *C. trachomatis.*[4]

BV is more prevalent and more persistent among HIV-infected women, especially among women who have low CD4 T-cell counts.[115,116] In one study, BV was associated with HIV-1 RNA expression in the genital tract of infected women,[117] consistent with the hypothesis that BV predisposes to the acquisition of HIV-1 infection.

Diagnosis

The patient is most likely to complain of odor and of the discharge, which tends to be gray and homogenous (Fig. 103-11). The odor is best described as "fishy" and is caused by the production of amines such as methylamine by *G. vaginalis.* These amines volatilize at increased pH, which explains the propensity of the patient to notice the

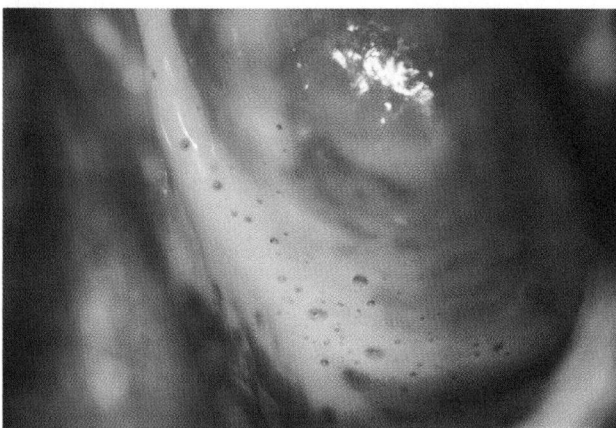

FIGURE 103-11. Bacterial vaginosis. The gray, homogenous discharge that coats the tissues is characteristic.

BOX 103-12

Symptoms Associated with Bacterial Vaginosis

Homogenous vaginal discharge
Fishy vaginal odor
 During menstruation
 After intercourse
Minimal itching or irritation

---

odor when her secretions are more alkaline (e.g., during menses, after intercourse). Vulvovaginal irritation is not usually a prominent symptom—hence, the use of the term "vaginosis" rather than "vaginitis." Box 103-12 details the symptoms usually associated with BV.

Vaginal pH is typically elevated to greater than 4.6. Odor is produced when vaginal secretions are mixed with 10% KOH. Microscopic examination of vaginal secretions suspended in 0.9% NaCl reveals few leukocytes and many small bacilli. The bacilli tend to coat vaginal epithelial cells—the so-called clue cells (Fig. 103-12), so named by Herman Gardner because they provided a "clue" to the diagnosis of this condition.[92]

Criteria for the diagnosis of BV are listed in Box 103-13. Amsel and colleagues[102] suggested that at least three of the four listed criteria (homogenous discharge, positive whiff test, pH >4.6, clue cells) should be present for the diagnosis of BV to be made. Clinicians' de-

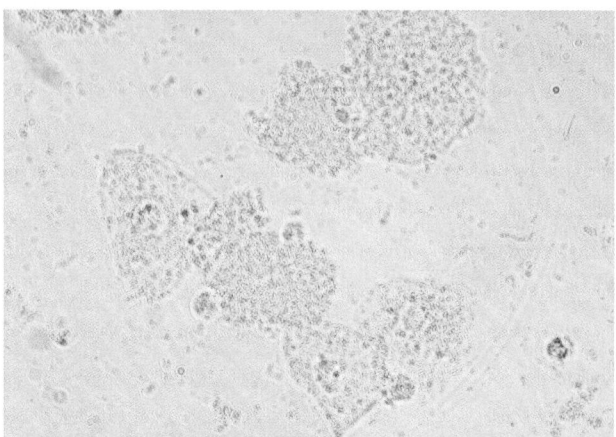

FIGURE 103-12. Bacterial vaginosis. Suspension of vaginal material in 0.9% NaCl. There are many bacteria attached to the vaginal epithelial cells (clue cells).

BOX 103-13

Criteria for the Diagnosis of Bacterial Vaginosis

Homogenous vaginal discharge
Vaginal pH greater than 4.6
Positive whiff test with 10% KOH
Clue cells

---

scriptions of the discharge tend to be poorly reproducible, and some workers prefer to require that all three of the somewhat more objective criteria be present. More recently, criteria have been developed for diagnosis of BV with use of the vaginal Gram stain.[118] This is an objective method of diagnosis that compares well[119,120] with the criteria of Amsel.

Treatment

The primary regimen for the treatment of BV is oral metronidazole, 500 mg twice a day for 7 days. A single 2.0-g dose of metronidazole, such as is used to treat trichomoniasis, is less effective[121] but has the advantage of 100% compliance if taken under direct observation. Vaginal preparations containing 0.75% metronidazole gel[122,123] or 2% clindamycin cream,[124] or ovules containing 100 mg of clindamycin,[125,126] are effective and have few systemic side effects. They are, however, more expensive than generic metronidazole. Oral clindamycin is also effective, but it is not widely prescribed for this indication.

Treatment failures occur fairly commonly with all of these regimens, presumably because a normal *Lactobacillus*-dominated flora fails to become reestablished after the anaerobes and other components of the BV flora have been reduced in number with use of clindamycin or metronidazole. Hallén and associates[127] treated women who had BV with lyophilized hydrogen peroxide–producing *Lactobacillus acidophilus* organisms. Of 28 women treated, 16 had the transient return of a normal vaginal wet preparation. Studies in which antimicrobial agents that reduce the abnormal flora of BV are combined with live lactobacilli are being conducted.

For patients who have BV that is unresponsive to the currently available antimicrobial agents, intravaginal boric acid, 600 mg at bedtime, provides symptomatic relief. Once the symptoms have been controlled, the dosing interval can be increased. Some patients remain symptom free using boric acid capsules once or twice a week.

Recent work has emphasized that BV is far more than a smelly discharge. BV is the result of a major change in the vaginal microbial flora, in which the normal, protective, *Lactobacillus*-dominated flora is replaced with a more complex flora that is composed of large numbers of potentially pathogenic bacteria. Postoperative infections occur more often in women undergoing gynecologic surgery if they have BV than if they have normal flora.[5] In one study,[128] women who had BV and who underwent total abdominal hysterectomy were randomly assigned to receive rectal metronidazole or no treatment. Vaginal cuff infections occurred in none of the treated women but in 27% of the untreated women (*P* <.01). Treatment studies have demonstrated that treatment of BV before induced abortion reduces the risk of subsequent pelvic inflammatory disease.[129,130]

Therefore, it would appear prudent to screen and treat women who have BV before performing induced abortion or hysterectomy. This logic could be extended to women undergoing other invasive gynecologic procedures, although there have been no studies in those areas.

BV during pregnancy is associated with adverse pregnancy outcomes, including premature membrane rupture, early labor, preterm birth, and postpartum endometritis.[131-133] Treatment of pregnant women who have BV and who previously delivered a premature infant reduced the risk of prematurity.[134-136] Accordingly, pregnant women who are at high risk for prematurity should be screened for BV, regardless of symptoms, and treated with oral metronidazole or oral clindamycin.[137] Topical agents do not appear to be as effective as oral agents, and the use of clindamycin cream has been associated with adverse events such as prematurity and neonatal infections.[138-142]

Treatment of pregnant women who have BV and who are at low risk for premature delivery is controversial. One large study showed no reduction in preterm births when such women were given oral metronidazole.[143] A second study[137] showed a reduction in late miscarriages and spontaneous preterm births when oral clindamycin was prescribed to women who had BV early in the second trimester.

BV can be nonsymptomatic. Women without symptoms are not usually treated, although the approach to such patients may change as more is learned about the implications of having abnormal vaginal secretions. Some women who receive treatment may retrospectively notice improvement in vaginal discharge and odor.[144]

There is no evidence to suggest that treatment of male sexual partners has any influence on the restoration of normal vaginal flora in patients with BV.[145,146] Therefore, treatment of sexual partners is not recommended. Some clinicians treat sexual partners of women who have recurrent BV or BV that is poorly responsive to treatment with metronidazole or clindamycin. Although such an approach appears to be reasonable, there is no supporting scientific evidence.

DESQUAMATIVE INFLAMMATORY VAGINITIS

Etiology and Pathogenesis

DIV is an unusual condition of unknown cause. It mimics estrogen deficiency vaginitis and trichomoniasis but usually occurs in women of reproductive age who have normal hormonal function and no evidence of any sexually transmitted conditions.

This disorder sometimes occurs in perimenopausal women or after pregnancy, suggesting a role for changes in the level of estrogen in its etiology.[147] About half of the patients with this condition seen in Brooklyn, New York, are of northern European Ashkenazi Jewish background, and they are more likely than other women of similar background to have the A26 and B35 histocompatibility antigens. This suggests that there may be an inherited susceptibility to this condition in some patients.

Although Gram stains of vaginal material often contain gram positive cocci and Group B streptococci can be recovered from some patients, especially those who are perimenopausal, there is no microorganism that has been clearly associated with this disease.[147]

In a few patients, DIV appears to be a local manifestation of a systemic illness such as systemic lupus erythematosus. Patients with DIV may also have erosive lichen planus involving oral or genital mucous membranes. Some workers[148,149] have suggested that DIV is always part of the lichen planus complex. The paucity of occasions when these two enigmatic conditions coexist does not support this conclusion.

Diagnosis

The patient reports purulent vaginal discharge and varying degrees of vulvar irritation, dysuria, and dyspareunia (Box 103-14). There is of-

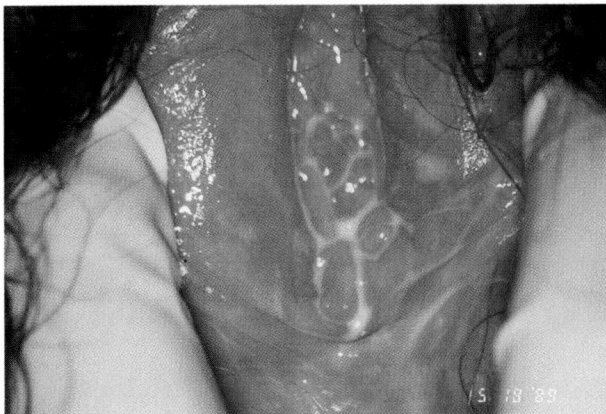

FIGURE 103-13. Desquamative inflammatory vaginitis. There is diffuse mucosal erythema and a purulent vaginal discharge.

ten a history of multiple unsuccessful treatments with a variety of topical and oral antimicrobial agents. Because the disease is most often confused with trichomoniasis, frequently in patients in whom a sexually transmitted condition is highly unlikely, many patients carry the diagnosis of resistant trichomoniasis and have received several courses of metronidazole in various dosage forms and dosages.

The mucosa of the vestibule, vagina, and cervix may show diffuse (Fig. 103-13) or segmental involvement, usually in the proximal vagina. Dilatation of capillary loops (colpitis macularis) may be prominent, and there may be superficial erosions of the mucosa, which are characteristic of this condition (Fig. 103-14).

The vaginal pH is often elevated to greater than 4.6. There is no odor when the vaginal secretions are mixed with 10% KOH. The saline wet preparation contains many leukocytes. Most of the vaginal epithelial cells are immature parabasal cells (Fig. 103-15). Gram-stained smears of vaginal secretions often contain gram-positive cocci. Vaginal cultures may contain a variety of organisms. Group B streptococci can be recovered from vaginal cultures from a significant minority of patients with DIV.[147]

Treatment

Topical corticosteroids and topical boric acid provide symptomatic relief and normalize the appearance of the mucous membranes and vaginal secretions. Relapse is predictable after these agents are discontinued. By far the most effective treatment for this condition is 2% clindamycin vaginal cream: 5 g of the cream (containing 100 mg of clindamycin) is inserted into the vagina at bedtime for 14

BOX 103-14

Characteristics of Desquamative Inflammatory Vaginitis

Symptoms
Purulent discharge
Vulvar discomfort
Dyspareunia

Findings
Mucosal erythema
Purulent secretions
Parabasal cells

Treatment
Clindamycin 2% vaginal cream
Boric acid
Topic corticosteroids

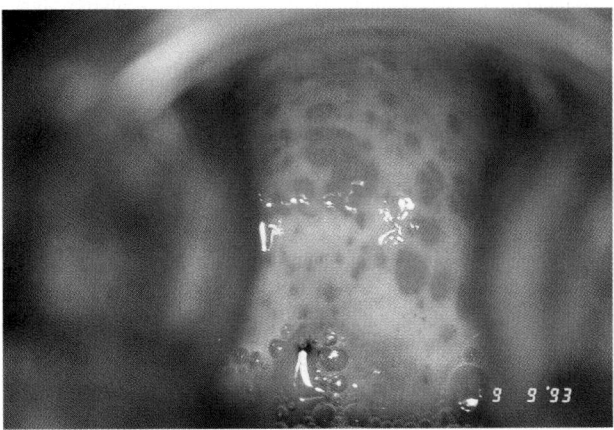

FIGURE 103-14. Desquamative inflammatory vaginitis. There are superficial mucosal erosions.

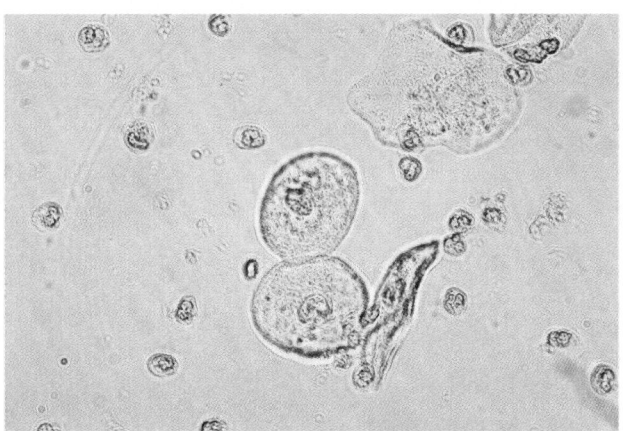

FIGURE 103-15. Desquamative inflammatory vaginitis. The vaginal wet preparation contains many leukocytes and parabasal cells.

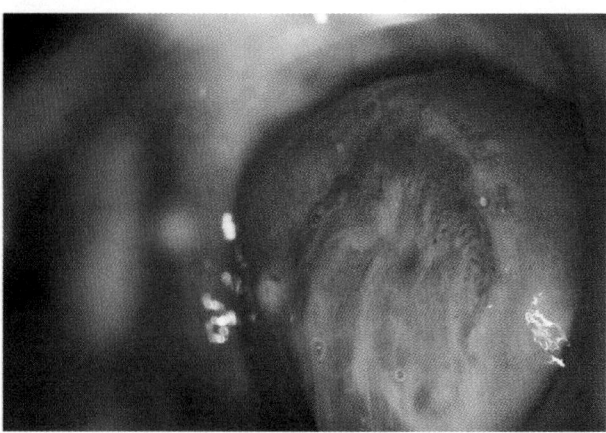

FIGURE 103-16. Noninfectious purulent ectocervicitis. Purulent secretions can be seen to emanate from the ectropion.

days. Most patients have a prolonged remission after this course of treatment. A few patients require a second 14-day course of treatment to induce a remission, but at least 90% of patients with DIV experience a complete remission in association with treatment with topical clindamycin.[147]

Once remission has been induced, it may be lifelong. More commonly, however, relapses occur months to years later. The relapses also respond to retreatment with topical clindamycin. A few patients who have very frequent relapses require continual biweekly intravaginal clindamycin or corticosteroids to remain in remission. Perimenopausal patients who are estrogen deficient may require estrogen replacement as well as topical clindamycin to sustain a remission.

CERVICITIS

Etiology and Pathogenesis

Cervicitis may be infectious or noninfectious. Infectious cervicitis is primarily an endocervicitis caused by *N. gonorrhoeae*, *C. trachomatis*, or both of these sexually transmitted pathogens. Noninfectious cervicitis is usually ectocervicitis in which there is inflammation in an ectropion (Box 103-15). Primary herpes simplex virus infection can cause ectocervicitis, but this seldom occurs without vulvar lesions that make the diagnosis obvious.

Diagnosis

The patient usually complains only of a purulent vaginal discharge. The mucopurulent secretions are not irritating, so there is no vulvar discomfort or introital dyspareunia. Because gonococcal or chlamydial infection can involve the urethra, endometrium, or uterine adnexa, there may be dysuria, abnormal uterine bleeding, lower abdominal pain, or pelvic dyspareunia. With noninfectious cervicitis, dysuria, abdominal pain, and deep (pelvic) dyspareunia are uncommon. There

may be postcoital bleeding due to trauma to the inflamed ectropion during intercourse.

Findings on examination of the vulva and of the vaginal mucosa are usually normal. In infectious endocervicitis, the purulent secretions can be seen to flow from the endocervical canal; in noninfectious ectocervicitis, the purulent secretions can be seen to emanate from the ectropion (Fig. 103-16), often with crystal-clear normal secretions flowing from the endocervix. In some patients with noninfectious endocervicitis, the abnormal secretions are solely endocervical, presumably reflecting the noninfectious endocervicitis. In patients who have gonococcal or chlamydial infection, urethral, uterine, or adnexal tenderness may be present, reflecting infection of these loci. The bimanual examination is usually normal in women who have noninfectious cervicitis.

Vaginal pH may be elevated. There is no odor when the secretions are mixed with 10% KOH. Wet preparations of vaginal secretions contain many leukocytes. The vaginal cells are mature. Gram-stained smears of cervical secretion confirm the presence of many leukocytes and, in gonococcal infection, may contain intracellular cocci. Definitive separation of infectious from noninfectious cervicitis is accomplished by culture or non-culture tests for *N. gonorrhoeae* and *C. trachomatis*.

Treatment

Studies that have attempted to correlate numbers of leukocytes in Gram-stained cervical smears with gonococcal or chlamydial infection have not produced clearcut recommendations as to which patients should be treated for infectious cervicitis without waiting for culture results.[150] Similarly, recommendations that women seen in high-risk settings such as sexually transmitted disease clinics be treated without microbiologic information result in the treatment of many uninfected patients.

Accordingly, patients who have mucopurulent cervicitis should undergo diagnostic testing for the presence of *N. gonorrhoeae* and *C. trachomatis*, but they should not be treated at the initial visit unless there is compelling evidence of sexually transmitted cervicitis, such as a male partner with urethritis, visualization of intracellular gram-negative cocci in cervical Gram staining, or a positive test for the gonococci or chlamydiae in the patient or her sexual partner. It may also be prudent to treat without culture results patients who are considered unlikely to return for follow-up visits.[21]

Patients who have positive tests for sexually transmitted bacteria should be treated with regimens recommended for the specific etiologic agent.[21] If tests for gonococci and chlamydiae are negative, antimicrobial treatment is not likely to be of benefit. If the volume of secretions arising from an ectropion is bothersome, destruction of the ectopic endocervical mucosa of the ectropion with cryotherapy allows

---

BOX 103-15

Cervicitis

Endocervicitis
Sexually transmitted
Neisseria gonorrhoeae, Chlamydia trachomatis, or both
Associated urethritis, endometritis, or salpingitis may be present

Ectocervicitis
Noninfectious
Inflammation in an ectropion
Not associated with urethritis, endometritis, or salpingitis

the ectocervix to become reepithelialized with squamous epithelium, with a resultant diminution in the volume of ectocervical secretions.

ESTROGEN DEFICIENCY VAGINITIS

Etiology and Pathogenesis

Estrogen deficiency vaginitis is seen in postmenopausal women and in younger women who have become estrogen deficient because of disease or because of treatment with pharmaceuticals that interfere with the production or the activity of estrogen.[151] This condition can also be seen during breast-feeding because of an effect of prolactin on estrogen production.[152] Without estrogen, the genital mucosa thins. Glycogen is decreased, and as a result, lactobacilli no longer dominate the vaginal microbial flora. Thinning of the mucosa may result in vulvar discomfort and introital dyspareunia. The thin vaginal mucosa may become infected, presumably by enteric organisms and others that are able to colonize the vagina in the absence of lactobacilli. Frequent urinary tract infections may occur. In some instances, estrogen deficiency vaginitis overlaps with DIV.

Diagnosis

The vestibular and vaginal mucosae are pale, often with patches of erythema. Vaginal secretions, if present, may be purulent. Vaginal pH is elevated. There is no odor when the secretions are mixed with 10% KOH. Microscopic examination of the secretions discloses immature (parabasal) vaginal cells with or without leukocytes. Vaginal cultures contain a variety of enteric and other bacteria.

Treatment

The primary defect is the absence of estrogen. Therefore, definitive treatment involves estrogen replacement or cessation of antiestrogenic drugs or breast-feeding. Topical antibacterial agents containing sulfonamides or clindamycin may improve symptomatic vaginitis, and lubricating agents may relieve vaginal dryness and dyspareunia. Without estrogen replacement, symptoms may recur after cessation of treatment.

VULVITIS AND VESTIBULITIS

External genital discomfort is a very common symptom among women of reproductive age. Usually described as itching or burning, vulvar discomfort may or may not be associated with introital dyspareunia. There are a number of possible causes, few of which are infectious and virtually none of which are sexually transmitted. Nonetheless, the clinician should be aware of these entities in order to rule out infections, prescribe appropriate treatment if the diagnosis is apparent, and refer the patient to a gynecologist or dermatologist who specializes in vulvar disease if an explanation for the patient's symptoms is not readily forthcoming.

The first task in approaching a patient with vulvar symptoms is to attempt to determine whether her discomfort primarily involves the skin of the labia (vulvitis) or the mucous membranes of the vestibule (vestibulitis). An important historical clue is the presence or absence of introital dyspareunia, which is unusual in vulvitis but commonly reported by women who have vestibulitis. During the examination, asking the patient to point to the areas of discomfort may also help to localize the process.

Vulvitis

Etiology and Pathogenesis

Sexually transmitted conditions, including genital ulcers and warts involving the labia majora and labia minora, should be obvious on physical examination. The only infection that commonly causes diffuse vulvitis is vulvovaginal candidiasis, usually in association with involvement of the vestibule and vagina. Most patients with vulvitis are not infected. Rather, they have vulvar dermatitis, for which there are many possible explanations, including topical allergic reactions to products used for personal hygiene, products used to launder underclothing, and particularly topical medications. Lichen sclerosus is an idiopathic chronic inflammatory skin disease that affects primarily vulvar and perianal areas; left untreated, it may lead to chronic vulvar scarring and depigmentation.[153]

Diagnosis

The physical examination should address any discrete lesions that require evaluation, perhaps with biopsy by a specialist in vulvar disease. In most cases, there is diffuse discomfort, usually described as itching, with varying degrees of dermatitis involving the skin of the labia majora and labia minora. Vaginal cultures should be examined for *Candida*.

Treatment

If vaginal cultures contain *Candida* species or other yeasts, a course of treatment with an oral antifungal agent will help to determine whether elimination of the yeast eliminates the patient's symptoms. Oral antifungals are useful in this situation to avoid masking or enhancing of symptoms by topical antifungal drugs. If cultures for *Candida* species are negative, or if eradication of colonizing *Candida* species with oral antifungal treatment does not provide relief of symptoms, the patient can be presumed to have noninfectious vulvitis.

As a first step in the management of noninfectious vulvitis, all topical medications should be discontinued. Sensitization by topical medications, including topical antifungal agents, is a common cause of vulvitis. The patient should be asked whether there have been any changes in products used for personal hygiene or menstrual protection, in soaps used for bathing the genitalia, or in products used to launder underclothing that might have produced a local allergic reaction.

If elimination of potential allergens does not provide relief, topical use of a low-potency corticosteroid, such as 1% hydrocortisone or an oral antihistamine, may provide relief. Lichen sclerosus responds to high-potency corticosteroids.[153] If corticosteroid treatment and removal of potentially sensitizing agents do not result in symptomatic improvement, referral to a specialist in vulvar disease is indicated.

Vestibulitis

Etiology and Pathogenesis

Although the vestibule is involved in most patients who have infectious vaginitis, vestibulitis without associated vaginitis is seldom infectious. Vestibulitis is best characterized as being diffuse or focal. Diffuse vestibulitis is usually part of a process involving other areas, whereas focal vestibulitis is usually localized to the vestibule. The symptoms of vestibulitis include discomfort usually described by the patient as burning and introital dyspareunia.

Vestibular burning is caused primarily by the contact of normally acid vaginal secretions with abnormal vestibular tissue. The burning characteristically increases in intensity during the latter portion of the menstrual cycle, as vaginal secretions become more abundant, and dramatically disappears after menstrual flow begins, presumably because of the increase in vaginal pH associated with menses. The burning is usually temporarily relieved by bathing, which removes acidic vaginal secretions.

Introital dyspareunia is a characteristic symptom of vestibulitis. Pain is noted immediately on penetration, usually increases with continued intercourse, and often requires that relations be discontinued. Sexual dysfunction, including failure to become lubricated and aroused and secondary vaginismus, is predictably associated with dyspareunia.

The most common cause of focal vestibulitis is vulvar vestibulitis,[154] which is also called focal vulvitis,[155] and infection of the minor vestibular glands.[156] Vulvar vestibulitis is fairly common. In one study,[157] 15% of unselected gynecologic patients were found to have this condition. The search for possible infectious causes of vulvar vestibulitis has been unproductive, and the illness is now believed to be noninfectious. The average age at onset is about 25 years. The condition appears to be uncommon in African American women.

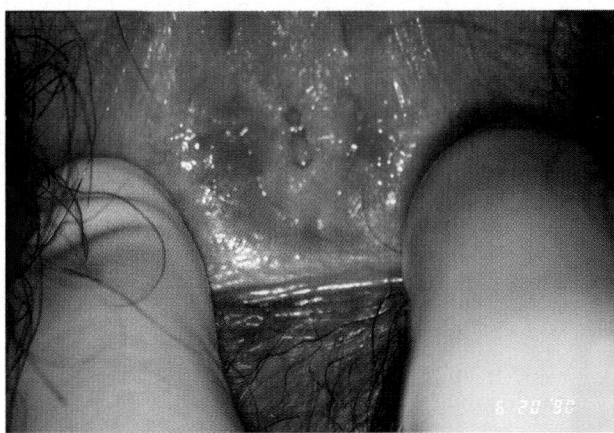

FIGURE 103-17. Vulvar vestibulitis. There are focal, erythematous, tender lesions in the vestibule lateral to the hymen.

Diagnosis

In diffuse vestibulitis, the entire vestibule is inflamed. With focal vulvitis or vulvar vestibulitis, there are erythematous lesions in the vestibule just lateral to the hymen (Fig. 103-17). The usual locations for the lesions are at 4 o'clock and 8 o'clock, near the openings of the Bartholin's ducts. Most patients have two lesions, but there may be a single lesion or several. Palpation of the lesions with a cotton-tipped swab or with the examining finger reproduces the dyspareunia. Cultures for *Candida* and other yeasts should be obtained.

Treatment

Diffuse vestibulitis should be managed as outlined earlier for vulvitis, with oral antifungal treatment for candidiasis if the yeast cultures are positive, avoidance of possible allergens, and use of topical corticosteroids. Vulvar vestibulitis is initially treated symptomatically. Vulvar burning may respond to tap water or baking soda douches to temporarily reduce vaginal acidity. Tepid baths may also provide transient relief. The dyspareunia usually improves with the use of precoital lubricants and topical anesthetic agents. Most patients obtain satisfactory relief of symptoms with these nonoperative measures. For women who do not achieve a satisfactory response, surgical treatment (vestibuloplasty) provides good results in about 75% of patients.[158]

REFERENCES

1. McCormack WM Jr, Zinner SH, McCormack WM. The incidence of genitourinary infections in a cohort of healthy women. Sex Transm Dis. 1994;21:63-64.
2. Vallor AC, Antonio MA, Hawes SE, Hillier SL. Factors associated with acquisition of, or persistent colonization by, vaginal lactobacilli: Role of hydrogen peroxide production. J Infect Dis. 2001;184:1431-1436.
3. Klebanoff SJ, Hillier SL, Eschenbach DA, Waltersdorph AM. Control of the microbial flora of the vagina by H₂O₂-generating lactobacilli. J Infect Dis. 1991;164:94-100.
4. Wiesenfeld HC, Hillier SL, Krohn MA, et al. Bacterial vaginosis is a strong predictor of *Neisseria gonorrhoeae* and *Chlamydia trachomatis* infection. Clin Infect Dis. 2003;36:663-668.
5. Soper DE, Bump RC, Hurt WG. Bacterial vaginosis and trichomoniasis are risk factors for cuff cellulitis after abdominal hysterectomy. Am J Obstet Gynecol. 1990;163:1016-1023.
6. Schaaf VM, Perez-Stable EJ, Borchardt K. The limited value of symptoms and signs in the diagnosis of vaginal infections. Arch Intern Med. 1990;150:1929-1933.
7. Danesh IS, Stephen JM, Gorbach J. Neonatal *Trichomonas vaginalis* infection. J Emerg Med. 1995;13:51-54.
8. Paradise JE, Campos JM, Friedman HM, et al. Vulvovaginitis in premenarcheal girls: Clinical features and diagnostic evaluation. Pediatrics. 1982;70:193-198.
9. Stern JE, Givan AL, Gonzalez JL, et al. Leukocytes in the cervix: A quantitative evaluation of cervicitis. Obstet Gynecol. 1998;91:987-992.
10. Rein MF, Shih LM, Miller JR, Guerrant RL. Use of a lactoferrin assay in the differential diagnosis of female genital tract infections and implications for the pathophysiology of bacterial vaginosis. Sex Transm Dis. 1996;23:517-521.
11. Silverman EM, Silverman AG. Persistence of spermatozoa in the lower genital tracts of women. JAMA. 1978;240:1875-1877.
12. Rothenberg RB, Simon R, Chipperfield E, Catterall, RD. Efficacy of selected diagnostic tests for sexually transmitted diseases. JAMA. 1976;235:49-51.
13. McCormack WM, Starko KM, Zinner SH. Symptoms associated with vaginal colonization with yeast. Am J Obstet Gynecol. 1988;158:31-33.
14. Lossick JG, Kent HL. Trichomoniasis: Trends in diagnosis and management. Am J Obstet Gynecol. 1991;165:1217-1222.
15. DeMeo LR, Draper DL, McGregor JA, et al. Evaluation of a deoxyribonucleic acid probe for the detection of *Trichomonas vaginalis* in vaginal secretions. Am J Obstet Gynecol. 1996;174:1339-1342.
16. Barenfanger J, Drake C, Hanson C. Timing of inoculation of the pouch makes no difference in increased detection of *Trichomonas vaginalis* by the InPouch TV method. J Clin Microbiol. 2002;40:1387-1389.
17. Stary A, Kuchinka-Koch A, Teodorowicz L. Detection of *Trichomonas vaginalis* on modified Columbia agar in the routine laboratory. J Clin Microbiol. 2002;40: 3277-3280.
18. Wendel KA, Erbelding EJ, Gaydos CA, Rompalo AM. *Trichomonas vaginalis* polymerase chain reaction compared with standard diagnostic and therapeutic protocols for detection and treatment of vaginal trichomoniasis. Clin Infect Dis. 2002;35:576-580.
19. Schwebke JR. Update of trichomoniasis. Sex Transm Infect. 2002;78:378-379.
20. Lobo TT, Feijo G, Carvalho SE, et al. A comparative evaluation of the Papanicolaou test for the diagnosis of trichomoniasis. Sex Transm Dis. 2003;30:694-699.
21. Centers for Disease Control and Prevention. Sexually transmitted diseases treatment guidelines, 2002. MMWR Morb Mortal Weekly Rep. 2002;51 (No. RR6).
22. Schmid G, Narcisi E, Mosure D, et al. Prevalence of metronidazole-resistant *Trichomonas vaginalis* in a gynecology clinic. J Reprod Med. 2001;46:545-549.
23. Lossick JG, Muller M, Gorrell TE. *In vitro* drug susceptibility and doses of metronidazole required for cure in cases of refractory vaginal trichomoniasis. J Infect Dis. 1986;153:948-955.
24. Dombrowski MP, Sokol RJ, Brown WJ, Bronsteen RA. Intravenous therapy of metronidazole-resistant *Trichomonas vaginalis*. Obstet Gynecol. 1987;69:524-525.
25. Crowell AL, Sanders-Lewis KA, Secor WE. *In vitro* metronidazole and tinidazole activities against metronidazole-resistant strains of *Trichomonas vaginalis*. Antimicrob Agents Chemother. 2003;47:1407-1409.
26. Sobel JD, Nyirjesy P, Brown W. Tinidazole therapy for metronidazole-resistant vaginal trichomoniasis. Clin Infect Dis. 2001;33:134-136.
27. Livengood CH 3rd, Lossick JG. Resolution of resistant vaginal trichomoniasis associated with the use of intravaginal nonoxynol-9. Obstet Gynecol. 1991;78:954-956.
28. Antonelli NM, Diehl SJ, Wright JW. A randomized trial of intravaginal nonoxynol 9 versus oral metronidazole in the treatment of vaginal trichomoniasis. Am J Obstet Gynecol. 2000;182:1008-1010.
29. Narcisi EM, Secor WE. *In vitro* effect of tinidazole and furazolidone on metronidazole-resistant *Trichomonas vaginalis*. Antimicrob Agents Chemother. 1996;40:1121-1125.
30. Schwartz J. Tricofuron therapy of *Trichomonas* vaginitis. Obstet Gynecol. 1956;7:312-314.
31. Houang ET, Ahmet Z, Lawrence AG. Successful treatment of four patients with recalcitrant vaginal trichomoniasis with a combination of zinc sulfate douche and metronidazole therapy. Sex Transm Dis. 1997;24:116-119.
32. duBouchet L, McGregor JA, Ismail M, McCormack WM. A pilot study of metronidazole vaginal gel versus oral metronidazole for the treatment of *Trichomonas vaginalis* vaginitis. Sex Transm Dis. 1998;24:176-179.
33. Martinotti MG, Savoia D. Effect of some steroid hormones on the growth of *Trichomonas vaginalis*. G Batteriol Virol Immunol. 1985;78:52-59.
34. Azuma T. A study of the parasitizing condition of *Trichomonas vaginalis* with special reference to the relationship between estrogen and the growth of *Trichomonas vaginalis*. J Jap Obstet Gynec Soc. 1968;15:168-172.
35. Sharma R, Pickering J, McCormack WM. Trichomoniasis in a postmenopausal woman cured after discontinuation of estrogen replacement therapy. Sex Transm Dis. 1997;24:543-545.
36. Pearlman MD, Yashar C, Ernst S, Solomon W. An incremental dosing protocol for women with severe vaginal trichomoniasis and adverse reactions to metronidazole. Am J Obstet Gynecol. 1996;174:934-936.
37. Kurohara ML, Kwong FK, Lebherz TB, Klaustermeyer WB. Metronidazole hypersensitivity and oral desensitization. J Allergy Clin Immunol. 1991;88:279-280.
38. Cu-Uvin S, Ko H, Jamieson DJ, et al. Prevalence, incidence, and persistence or recurrence of trichomoniasis among human immunodeficiency virus (HIV)-positive women and among HIV-negative women at high risk for HIV infection. Clin Infect Dis. 2002;34:1406-1411.
39. Wang CC, McClelland RS, Reilly M, et al. The effect of treatment of vaginal infections on shedding of human immunodeficiency virus type 1. J Infect Dis. 2001; 183:1017-1022.
40. Minkoff H, Grunebaum AN, Schwarz RH, et al. Risk factors for prematurity and premature rupture of membranes: A prospective study of the vaginal flora in pregnancy. Am J Obstet Gynecol. 1984;150:965-972.
41. Cotch MF, Pastorek JG II, Nugent RP, et al. *Trichomonas vaginalis* associated with low birth weight and preterm delivery. Sex Transm Dis. 1997;24:353-360.
42. Klebanoff MA, Carey JC, Hauth JC, et al. Failure of metronidazole to prevent preterm delivery among pregnant women with asymptomatic *Trichomonas vaginalis* infection. N Engl J Med. 2001;345:487-493.
43. Caro-Paton T, Carvajal A, Martin de Diego I, et al. Is metronidazole teratogenic? A meta-analysis. Br J Clin Pharmacol. 1997;44:179-182.
44. Burtin P, Taddio A, Ariburnu O, et al. Safety of metronidazole in pregnancy: A meta-analysis. Am J Obstet Gynecol. 1995;172:525-529.
45. Piper JM, Mitchel EF, Ray WA. Prenatal use of metronidazole and birth defects: No association. Obstet Gynecol. 1993;82:348-352.
46. Sobel JD. Candidal vulvovaginitis. Clin Obstet Gynecol. 1993;36:153-165.

47. Spinillo A, Capuzzo E, Gulminetti R, et al. Prevalence of and risk factors for fungal vaginitis caused by non-albicans species. Am J Obstet Gynecol. 1997;176:138-141.
48. Horowitz BJ, Edelstein SW, Lippman L. *Candida tropicalis* vulvovaginitis. Obstet Gynecol. 1985;66:229-232.
49. Geiger AM, Foxman B, Sobel JD. Chronic vulvovaginal candidiasis: Characteristics of women with *Candida albicans*, *C. glabrata* and no *Candida*. Genitourin Med. 1995;75:304-307.
50. Spinillo A, Capuzzo E, Egbe TO, et al. *Torulopsis glabrata* vaginitis. Obstet Gynecol. 1995;85:993-998.
51. Redondo-Lopez V, Lynch M, Schmitt C, et al. *Torulopsis glabrata* vaginitis: Clinical aspects and susceptibility to antifungal agents. Obstet Gynecol. 1990;76:651-655.
52. Sobel JD, Vazquez J, Lynch M, et al. Vaginitis due to *Saccharomyces cerevisiae*: Epidemiology, chemical aspects, and therapy. Clin Infect Dis. 1993;16:93-99.
53. McCullough MJ, Clemons KV, Farina C, et al. Epidemiological investigation of vaginal *Saccharomyces cerevisiae* isolates by a genotypical method. J Clin Microbiol. 1998;36:557-562.
54. Sobel JD. Epidemiology and pathogenesis of recurrent vulvovaginal candidiasis. Am J Obstet Gynecol. 1985;1523:924-935.
55. Sobel JD. Pathogenesis and treatment of recurrent vulvovaginal candidiasis. Clin Infect Dis. 1992;14(Suppl 1):S148-S153.
56. Agnew KJ, Hillier SL. The effect of treatment regimens for vaginitis and cervicitis on vaginal colonization with lactobacilli. Sex Transm Dis. 1995;22:269-273.
57. Larsen B. Vaginal flora in health and disease. Clin Obstet Gynecol. 1993;36:107-121.
58. Sonnex C. Influence of ovarian hormones on urogenital infection. Sex Transm Infect. 1998;74:11-19.
59. Spinillo A, Capuzzo E, Nicola S, et al. The impact of oral contraception on vulvovaginal candidiasis. Contraception. 1995;51:293-297.
60. Anonymous. Adverse events and their association with treatment regimens in the diabetes control and complications trial. Diabetes Care. 1995;18:1415-1427.
61. Elegbe IA, Botu M. A preliminary study on dressing patterns and incidence of candidiasis. Am J Public Health. 1982;72:176-177.
62. Elgebe IA, Elgebe I. Quantitative relationships of *Candida albicans* infections and dressing patterns in Nigerian women. Am J Public Health. 1983;73:450-452.
63. Heidrich FE, Berg AO, Bergman JJ. Clothing factors and vaginitis. J Family Pract. 1984;19:491-494.
64. Sobel JD. Vulvovaginal candidiasis: A comparison of HIV-positive and -negative women. Int J STD AIDS. 2002;13:358-362.
65. Shifrin E, Matityahu D, Feldman J, Minkoff H. Determinants of incident vulvovaginal candidiasis in human immunodeficiency virus-positive women. Infect Dis Obstet Gynecol. 2000;8:176-180.
66. Sobel JD. Vaginitis. N Engl J Med. 1997;337:1896-1903.
67. Gieger AM, Foxman B, Gillespie BW. The epidemiology of vulvovaginal candidiasis among university students. Am J Public Health. 1995;85:1146-1148.
68. Gieger AM, Foxman B. Risk factors in vulvovaginal candidiasis: A case controlled study among university students. Epidemiology. 1996;7:182-187.
69. Odds FC. Genital candidosis. Clin Exp Dermatol. 1982;7:345-354.
70. Odds FC. *Candida* and Candidosis. Baltimore: University Park; 1979:4.
71. Garcia-Tamayo J, Castillo G, Martinez AJ. Human genital candidiasis: Histochemistry, scanning and transmission electron microscopy. Acta Cytol. 1982;26:7-14.
72. Kimura LH, Pearsall NN. Relationship between germination of *Candida albicans* and increased adherence to human buccal epithelial cells. Infect Immun. 1980;28:464-468.
73. King RD, Lee JC, Morris AL. Adherence of *Candida albicans* and other *Candida* species to mucosal epithelial cells. Infect Immun. 1980;27:667-674.
74. Sobel JD, Muller G. Ketoconazole in the prevention of experimental candidal vaginitis. Antimicrob Agents Chemother. 1984;25:281-282.
75. Witkin SS, Jeremias J, Ledger WJ. A localized vaginal allergic response in women with recurrent vaginitis. J Allergy Clin Immunol. 1988;81:412-416.
76. Rigg D, Miller MM, Metzger WJ. Recurrent allergic vulvovaginitis: Treatment with *Candida albicans* allergen immunotherapy. Am J Obstet Gynecol. 1990;162:332-336.
77. Ferris DG, Nyirjesy P, Sobel JD, et al. Over-the-counter antifungal drug misuse associated with patient-diagnosed vulvovaginal candidiasis. Obstet Gynecol. 2002;99:419-425.
78. Sobel JD, Brooker D, Stein GE, et al. Single oral dose fluconazole compared with conventional clotrimazole topical therapy of *Candida* vaginitis. Am J Obstet Gynecol. 1995;172:1263-1268.
79. Weissenbacher S, Witkin SS, Tolbert V, et al. Value of *Candida* polymerase chain reaction and vaginal cytokine analysis for the differential diagnosis of women with recurrent vulvovaginitis. Infect Dis Obstet Gynecol. 2000;8:244-247.
80. Nyirjesy P, Seeney SM, Terry Grody MH, et al. Chronic fungal vaginitis: The valve of cultures. Am J Obstet Gynecol. 1995;173:820-823.
81. Sobel JD, Kapernick PS, Zervos M, et al. Treatment of complicated *Candida* vaginitis: Comparison of single and sequential doses of fluconazole. Am J Obstet Gynecol. 2001;185:363-369.
82. Sobel JD. Recurrent vulvovaginal candidiasis: A prospective study of the efficacy of maintenance ketoconazole therapy. N Engl J Med. 1986;315:1455-1458.
83. Sobel JD. Treatment of vaginal *Candida* infections. Expert Opin Pharmacother. 2002;3:1059-1065.
84. Singh S, Sobel JD, Bhargava P, et al. Vaginitis due to *Candida krusei*: Epidemiology, clinical aspects, therapy. Clin Infect Dis. 2002;35:1066-1070.
85. Sobel JD, Zervos M, Reed BD, et al. Fluconazole susceptibility of vaginal isolates obtained from women with complicated *Candida* vaginitis: Clinical implications. Antimicrob Agents Chemother. 2003;47:34-38.
86. MacNeill C, Weisz J, Carey JC. Clinical resistance of recurrent *Candida albicans* vulvovaginitis to fluconazole in the presence and absence of *in vitro* resistance. J Reprod Med. 2003;48:63-68.
87. National Committee for Clinical Laboratory Standards. Reference method for broth dilution antifungal susceptibility testing of yeasts: Proposed standard M27-T. Wayne, PA: National Committee for Clinical Laboratory Standards; 1995.
88. Sobel JD, Chaim W. Treatment of *Torulopsis glabrata* vaginitis: Retrospective review of boric acid therapy. Clin Infect Dis. 1997;24:649-652.
89. Vazquez JA, Sobel JD, Demitriou R, et al. Karyotyping of *Candida albicans* isolates obtained longitudinally in women with recurrent vulvovaginal candidiasis. J Infect Dis. 1994;170:1566-1569.
90. Horowitz BJ, Edelstein SW, Lippman L. Sexual transmission of *Candida*. Obstet Gynecol. 1987;69:883-886.
91. Hilton E, Isenberg HD, Alperstein P, et al. Ingestion of yogurt containing *Lactobacillus acidophilus* as prophylaxis for candidal vaginitis. Ann Intern Med. 1992;116:353-357.
92. Gardner HL, Dukes CD. *Haemophilus vaginalis* vaginitis: A newly defined specific infection previously classified "nonspecific" vaginitis. Am J Obstet Gynecol. 1955;69:962-976.
93. Huth EJ. Style note: Bacterial vaginosis or vaginal bacteriosis. Ann Intern Med. 1989;111:553-554.
94. Speigel CA. Bacterial vaginosis. Clin Microbiol Rev. 1991;4:485-502.
95. Brunham RC, Paavonen J, Stevens CE, et al. Mucopurulent cervicitis: The ignored counterpart in women of urethritis in men. N Engl J Med. 1984;311:1-6.
96. Eschenbach DA. Bacterial vaginosis and anaerobes in obstetric-gynecologic infections. Clin Infect Dis. 1993;16(Suppl 4):S282-S287.
97. Peipert JF, Mantagno AB, Cooper AS, Sung CJ. Bacterial vaginosis as a risk factor for upper genital tract infection. Am J Obstet Gynecol. 1997;177:1184-1187.
98. Sweet RL. Role of bacterial vaginosis in pelvic inflammatory disease. Clin Infect Dis. 1995;20(Suppl 2):S271-S275.
99. Pheifer TA, Forsyth PS, Durfee MA, et al. Nonspecific vaginitis: Role of *Haemophilus vaginalis* and treatment with metronidazole. N Engl J Med. 1978;298:1429.
100. Chen KC, Forsyth PS, Buchanan TM, Holmes KK. Amine content of vaginal fluid from untreated and treated patients with nonspecific vaginitis. J Clin Invest. 1979;63:828-835.
101. Hanna NF, Taylor-Robinson D, Kalodiki-Karammonoki M, et al. The relation between vaginal pH and the microbiological status in vaginitis. Br J Obstet Gynaecol. 1985;92:1267-1271.
102. Amsel R, Totten PA, Spiegel CA, et al. Nonspecific vaginitis: Diagnostic criteria and microbial and epidemiologic associations. Am J Med. 1983;74:14-22.
103. Bhattacharyya MN, Jones BM. *Haemophilus vaginalis* infection: Diagnosis and treatment. J Reprod Med. 1980;24:71-75.
104. Spiegel CA, Amsel R, Holmes KK. Diagnosis of bacterial vaginosis by direct Gram stain of vaginal fluid. J Clin Microbiol. 1983;18:170-177.
105. Hillier SL, Krohn MA, Rabe LK, et al. The normal vaginal flora, H$_2$O$_2$-producing lactobacilli and bacterial vaginosis in pregnant women. Clin Infect Dis. 1993;16(Suppl 4):S273-S281.
106. Berger BJ, Kolton S, Zenilman JM, et al. Bacterial vaginosis in lesbians: A sexually transmitted disease. Clin Infect Dis. 1995;21:1402-1405.
107. Marrazzo JM, Koutsky LA, Eschenbach DA, et al. Characterization of vaginal flora and bacterial vaginosis in women who have sex with women. J Infect Dis. 2002;185:1307-1313.
108. Ratnam S, Fitzgerald BL. Semiquantitative culture of *Gardnerella vaginalis* in laboratory determination of nonspecific vaginitis. J Clin Microbiol. 1983;18:344-347.
109. Monhanty KC, Deighton R. Comparison of 2 g single dose of metronidazole, nimorazole and tinidazole in the treatment of vaginitis associated with *Gardnerella vaginalis*. J Antimicrob Chemother. 1987;19:393-399.
110. Speigel CA, Roberts M. *Mobiluncus* gen nov, *Mobiluncus curtisii* subspecies *curtisii* sp nov, *Mobiluncus curtisii* subspecies *holmesii* subsp nov, and *Mobiluncus mulieris* sp nov, curved rods from the human vagina. Int J Syst Bacteriol. 1984;34:177-184.
111. Schwebke JR, Lawing LF. Prevalence of *Mobiluncus* spp among women with and without bacterial vaginosis as detected by polymerase chain reaction. Sex Transm Dis. 2001;28:195-199.
112. Holzman C, Leventhal JM, Qiu H, et al. Factors linked to bacterial vaginosis in nonpregnant women. Am J Public Health. 2001;91:1664-1670.
113. Ness RB, Hillier SL, Richter HE, et al. Douching in relation to bacterial vaginosis, lactobacilli, and facultative bacteria in the vagina. Obstet Gynecol. 2002;100:765.
114. Cherpes TL, Meyn LA, Krohn MA, et al. Association between acquisition of herpes simplex virus type 2 in women and bacterial vaginosis. Clin Infect Dis. 2003;37:319-325.
115. Jamieson DJ, Duerr A, Klein RS, et al. Longitudinal analysis of bacterial vaginosis: Findings from the HIV epidemiology research study. Obstet Gynecol. 2001;98:656-663.
116. Warren D, Klein RS, Sobel J, et al. A multicenter study of bacterial vaginosis in women with or at risk for human immunodeficiency virus infection. Infect Dis Obstet Gynecol. 2001;9:133-141.
117. Cu-Uvin S, Hogan JW, Caliendo AM, et al. Association between bacterial vaginosis and expression of human immunodeficiency virus type 1 RNA in the female genital tract. Clin Infect Dis. 2001;33:894-896.
118. Nugent RP, Krohn MA, Hillier SI. Reliability of diagnosing bacterial vaginosis is improved by a standardized method of Gram stain interpretation. J Clin Microbiol. 1991;29:297-301.
119. McCormack WM, Covino JM, Thomason JL, et al. Comparison of clindamycin phosphate vaginal cream with triple sulfonamide vaginal cream in the treatment of bacterial vaginosis. Sex Transm Dis. 2001;28:569-575.
120. Schwebke JR, Hillier SL, Sobel JD, et al. Validity of the vaginal gram stain for the diagnosis of bacterial vaginosis. Obstet Gynecol. 1996;88:573-576.

121. Swedberg J, Steiner JF, Deiss F, et al. Comparison of single-dose vs one-week course of metronidazole for symptomatic bacterial vaginosis. JAMA. 1985;254:1046-1049.

122. Hillier SL, Lipinski C, Briselden AM, Eschenbach DA. Efficiency of intravaginal 0.75% metronidazole gel for the treatment of bacterial vaginosis. Obstet Gynecol. 1993;81:963-967.

123. Hanson JM, McGregor JA, Hillier SL, et al. Metronidazole for bacterial vaginosis: A comparison of vaginal vs. oral therapy. J Reprod Med. 2000;45:889-896.

124. Schmitt C, Sobel JD, Meriwether C. Bacterial vaginosis: Treatment with clindamycin cream versus oral metronidazole. Obstet Gynecol. 1992;79:1020-1023.

125. Sobel J, Peipert JF, McGregor JA, et al. Efficacy of clindamycin vaginal ovule (3-day treatment) vs. clindamycin vaginal cream (7-day treatment) in bacterial vaginosis. Infect Dis Obstet Gynecol. 2001;9:9-15.

126. Paavonen J, Mangioni C, Martin MA, Wajszczuk CP. Vaginal clindamycin and oral metronidazole for bacterial vaginosis: A randomized trial. Obstet Gynecol. 2000;96:256-260.

127. Hallén A, Jarstrand C, Pahlson C. Treatment of bacterial vaginosis with lactobacilli. Sex Transm Dis. 1992;19:146-148.

128. Larsson PG, Carlsson B. Does pre- and postoperative metronidazole treatment lower vaginal cuff infection rate after abdominal hysterectomy among women with bacterial vaginosis? Infect Dis Obstet Gynecol. 2002;10:133-140.

129. Larsson PG, Platz-Christensen J-J, Thejls H, et al. Incidence of pelvic inflammatory disease after first-trimester legal abortion in women with bacterial vaginosis after treatment with metronidazole: A double-blind randomized study. Am J Obstet Gynecol. 1992;166:100-103.

130. Crowley T, Low N, Turner A, et al. Antibiotic prophylaxis to prevent post-abortal upper genital tract infection in women with bacterial vaginosis: Randomized controlled trial. Br J Obstet Gynaecol. 2001;108:396-402.

131. Hillier SL, Nugent RP, Eschenbach DA, et al. Association between bacterial vaginosis and preterm delivery of a low-birth-weight infant. N Engl J Med. 1995;333:1737-1742.

132. Jacobsson B, Pernevi P, Chidekel L, Jorgen Platz-Christensen J. Bacterial vaginosis in early pregnancy may predispose for preterm birth and postpartum endometritis. Acta Obstet Gynecol Scand. 2002;81:1006-1010.

133. Leitich H, Bodner-Adler B, Brunauer M, et al. Bacterial vaginosis as a risk factor for preterm delivery: A meta-analysis. Am J Obstet Gynecol. 2003;189:139-147.

134. Hauth JC, Goldenberg RL, Andrews WW, et al. Reduced incidence of preterm delivery with metronidazole and erythromycin in women with bacterial vaginosis. N Engl J Med. 1995;333:1732-1736.

135. Morales WJ, Schorr S, Albritton J. Effect of metronidazole in patients with preterm birth in preceding pregnancy and bacterial vaginosis: A placebo-controlled, double-blind study. Am J Obstet Gynecol. 1994;171:345-349.

136. Leitich H, Brunauer M, Bodner-Adler B, et al. Antibiotic treatment of bacterial vaginosis in pregnancy: A meta analysis. Am J Obstet Gynecol. 2003;188:752-758.

137. Ugwumadu A, Manyonda I, Reid F, Hay P. Effect of early oral clindamycin on late miscarriage and preterm delivery in asymptomatic women with abnormal vaginal flora and bacterial vaginosis: A randomised controlled trial. Lancet. 2003;361:983-988.

138. McGregor JA, French JI, Jones W, et al. Bacterial vaginosis is associated with prematurity and vaginal fluid mucinase and sialidase: Results of a controlled trial of topical clindamycin cream. Am J Obstet Gynecol. 1994;170:1048-1059.

139. Joesoef MR, Hillier SL, Wiknjosastro G, et al. Intravaginal clindamycin treatment for bacterial vaginosis: Effects on preterm delivery and low birth weight. Am J Obstet Gynecol. 1995;173:1527-1531.

140. Vermeulen GM, Bruinse HW. Prophylactic administration of clindamycin 2% vaginal cream to reduce the incidence of spontaneous preterm birth in women with an increased recurrence risk: A randomised placebo-controlled double-blind trial. Br J Obstet Gynaecol. 1999;106:652-657.

141. Kekki M, Kurki T, Pelkonen J, et al. Vaginal clindamycin in preventing preterm birth and peripartum infections in asymptomatic women with bacterial vaginosis: A randomized, controlled trial. Obstet Gynecol. 2001;97:643-648.

142. Koumans EH, Markowitz LE, Hogan V. Indications for therapy and treatment recommendations for bacterial vaginosis in nonpregnant women: A synthesis of data. Clin Infect Dis. 2002;35(Suppl 2):S152-S172.

143. Carey JC, Klebanoff MA, Hauth JC, et al. Metronidazole to prevent preterm delivery in pregnant women with asymptomatic bacterial vaginosis. N Engl J Med. 2000;342:534-540.

144. Schwebke JR. Asymptomatic bacterial vaginosis: Response to therapy. Am J Obstet Gynecol. 2000;183:1434-1439.

145. Colli E, Landoni M, Parazzini F, et al. Treatment of male partners and recurrence of bacterial vaginosis: A randomized trial. Genitourin Med. 1997;73:267-270.

146. Vejtorp M, Bollerup AC, Vejtorp L, et al. Bacterial vaginosis: A double-blind randomized trial of the effect of treatment of the sexual partner. Br J Obstet Gynaecol. 1988;95:920-926.

147. Sobel JD. Desquamative inflammatory vaginitis: A new subgroup of purulent vaginitis responsive to topical 2% clindamycin therapy. Am J Obstet Gynecol. 1994;171:1215-1220.

148. Edwards L, Friedrich EG Jr. Desquamative vaginitis: Lichen planus in disguise. Obstet Gynecol. 1988;71:832-836.

149. Pelisse M. The vulvo-vaginal-gingival syndrome: A new form of erosive lichen planus. Int J Dermatol. 1989;28:381-384.

150. Kent GP, Harrison HR, Berman SM, Keenlyside RA. Screening for Chlamydia trachomatis infection in a sexually transmitted disease clinic: Comparison of diagnostic tests with clinical and historical risk factors. Sex Transm Dis. 1988;15:51-57.

151. Bachmann GA, Nevadunksy NS. Diagnosis and treatment of atrophic vaginitis. Am Fam Physician. 2000;61:3090-3096.

152. Palmer AR, Likis FE. Lactational atrophic vaginitis. J Midwifery Womens Health. 2003;48:282-284.

153. Nyirjesy P. Lichen sclerosus and other conditions mimicking vulvovaginal candidiasis. Curr Infect Dis Rep. 2002;4:520-524.

154. Friedrich EG Jr. Vulvar vestibulitis syndrome. J Reprod Med. 1987;32:110-114.

155. Peckham BM, Maki DG, Patterson JJ, Hafez G-R. Focal vulvitis: A characteristic syndrome and cause of dyspareunia. Am J Obstet Gynecol. 1986;154:855-864.

156. Woodruff JD, Parmley TH. Infection of the minor vestibular gland. Obstet Gynecol. 1983;62:609-612.

157. Goetsch MF. Vulvar vestibulitis: Prevalence and historic features in a general gynecologic practice population. Am J Obstet Gynecol. 1991;164:1609-1616.

158. McCormack WM, Spence MR. Evaluation of the surgical treatment of vulvar vestibulitis. Eur J Obstet Gynecol Reprod Biol. 1999;86:135-138.

CHAPTER **104**

Infections of the Female Pelvis

DAVID E. SOPER

PHILIP B. MEAD

Infections of the female pelvis constitute a diverse group of both community- and hospital-acquired infections. They are conveniently considered in three categories: infections related to pregnancy, infections occurring after gynecologic surgery, and sexually transmitted pelvic inflammatory disease. Pelvic infections are commonly polymicrobial, with cultures revealing a mixture of both aerobic and anaerobic bacteria.

INTRAPARTUM, POSTPARTUM, AND POSTABORTAL INFECTIONS

Intra-amniotic infection syndrome (IAIS) is a clinically detectable infection of the uterus and its contents during pregnancy.[1] IAIS occurs in up to 10.5% of women in labor.[2] Most cases of IAIS originate after vaginal microorganisms ascend into the intrauterine cavity; this occurs after prolonged rupture of the membranes or labor in patients with multiple vaginal examinations.[3] A few cases, most notably those caused by *Listeria monocytogenes*, result from transplacental hematogenous spread in mothers with bacteremia.[4] The diagnosis is usually made before membrane rupture in these patients. Rare cases have been reported after diagnostic amniocentesis, intrauterine transfusion, or percutaneous umbilical blood sampling. Intrauterine infection also occurs after cervical cerclage in 1% to 2% of patients, and this risk may be as high as 25% if the cerclage is carried out after prolapse of the membranes into the vagina. Risk factors for IAIS include prolonged duration of labor or rupture of membranes, multiple vaginal examinations, young age, low socioeconomic class, nulliparity, and preexisting bacterial vaginosis.[5]

The organisms most commonly isolated from amniotic fluid in cases of IAIS are anaerobes, genital mycoplasmas, group B streptococci, and *Escherichia coli*. The latter two are found most commonly when maternal and neonatal bacteremia complicates intra-amniotic infection.[3] Many of these microorganisms (especially anaerobic bacteria, the mycoplasmas, and *Gardnerella vaginalis*) are associated with bacterial vaginosis. It is presumed that most of the bacteria associated with IAIS arise from a vaginal source.

Maternal manifestations of IAIS are fever, tachycardia, and uterine tenderness. Foul-smelling or grossly purulent amniotic fluid is an uncommon finding. Fetal heart rate abnormalities, primarily tachycardia and decreased variability, are important markers of intrauterine infection. Approximately 5% to 10% of women with preterm labor and intact membranes have symptomatic chorioamnionitis, and another 10% have subclinical infection. In patients with preterm premature rupture of the membranes, the frequency of subclinical infection at the time of admission may be as high as 25%. In full-term pregnancies, IAIS is associated with dysfunctional labor. About 75% of infected women require augmentation of labor with oxytocin, and about 35% require cesarean delivery, usually because of arrest of progress in labor.[6]

Although the diagnosis is based largely on clinical findings, amniotic fluid Gram staining, leukocyte esterase activity, and glucose concentration (<15 mg/dL) have been shown to be useful in supporting the clinical impression. Microbial invasion of the amniotic cavity is accompanied by the presence of high amniotic fluid concentrations of proinflammatory cytokines such as interleukin-1 (IL-1), tumor necrosis factor, IL-6, IL-8, and a gelatinase, matrix metalloproteinase-9 (MMP-9).[7] Measurement of these substances remains expensive and is not readily available.

Antimicrobial therapy for IAIS is aimed at preventing bacteremia in the mother as well as initiating intrapartum treatment of the fetus while awaiting delivery. Gibbs and colleagues[8] documented improved neonatal and maternal outcome when antibiotic therapy is begun intrapartum rather than immediately postpartum. Delivery of the fetus and placenta removes the sites of infection, much like draining an abscess, making this intervention a significant part of therapy. Because group B streptococci and *E. coli* are the most common isolates from infected newborns, a combination of ampicillin plus gentamicin is a reasonable initial regimen for IAIS. This regimen is also sufficient to treat the mother, for women who deliver vaginally. If cesarean delivery is required, up to 15% of operative patients given only ampicillin and gentamicin experience treatment failure by developing postpartum endometritis. These patients probably require better anaerobic coverage, and accordingly a drug such as clindamycin or metronidazole should be added to the treatment regimen to decrease the risk of postpartum endometritis by half.[9] Other broad-spectrum regimens may be equally effective. One additional dose of this broad-spectrum combination of antibiotics is sufficient postpartum therapy for women with IAIS.[10]

Although delivery is essential to cure, no critical diagnosis-to-delivery interval beyond which the frequency of neonatal complications escalates dramatically has been identified. This observation was based primarily on full-term pregnancies in which the majority (80%) delivered within 8 hours.[11] Accordingly, labor must be managed actively, but cesarean delivery should be performed only for accepted obstetric indications.

Postpartum Endometritis

Postpartum infection of the uterus, the most common cause of puerperal fever, is designated endometritis, endomyometritis, or endoparametritis depending on the extent of the disease. Cesarean delivery, particularly after labor or rupture of the membranes of any duration, is the dominant predictor of postpartum endometritis (PPE).[12] The pathogenesis of this infection involves inoculation of the amniotic fluid after membrane rupture or during labor with vaginal microorganisms. The myometrium, leaves of the broad ligament, and the peritoneal cavity are then exposed to this contaminated fluid during surgery (Fig. 104-1). The reported incidence of PPE after cesarean delivery ranges from 10% or less in most private services to 50% or more in large teaching services caring for indigent patients. The incidence after vaginal delivery is only 0.9% to 3.9%. Postulated secondary predictors of postcesarean endometritis include duration of labor or rupture of the membranes, presence of bacterial vaginosis, number of vaginal examinations, and use of internal fetal monitoring.[13,14] Antimicrobial prophylaxis is associated with a 50% reduction in infection in all populations studied. All patients undergoing cesarean delivery, either elective or unscheduled, are candidates for antibiotic prophylaxis.[15] Many patients who develop postcesarean endometritis despite antibiotic prophylaxis have histologic evidence of incipient infection.[16]

Although prolonged membrane rupture, midforceps delivery, anemia, and maternal soft tissue trauma are commonly mentioned as factors predisposing to endometritis after vaginal delivery, these events are not identified in most patients with such infections and are probably relative risk factors. Indigent patients are at substantially higher

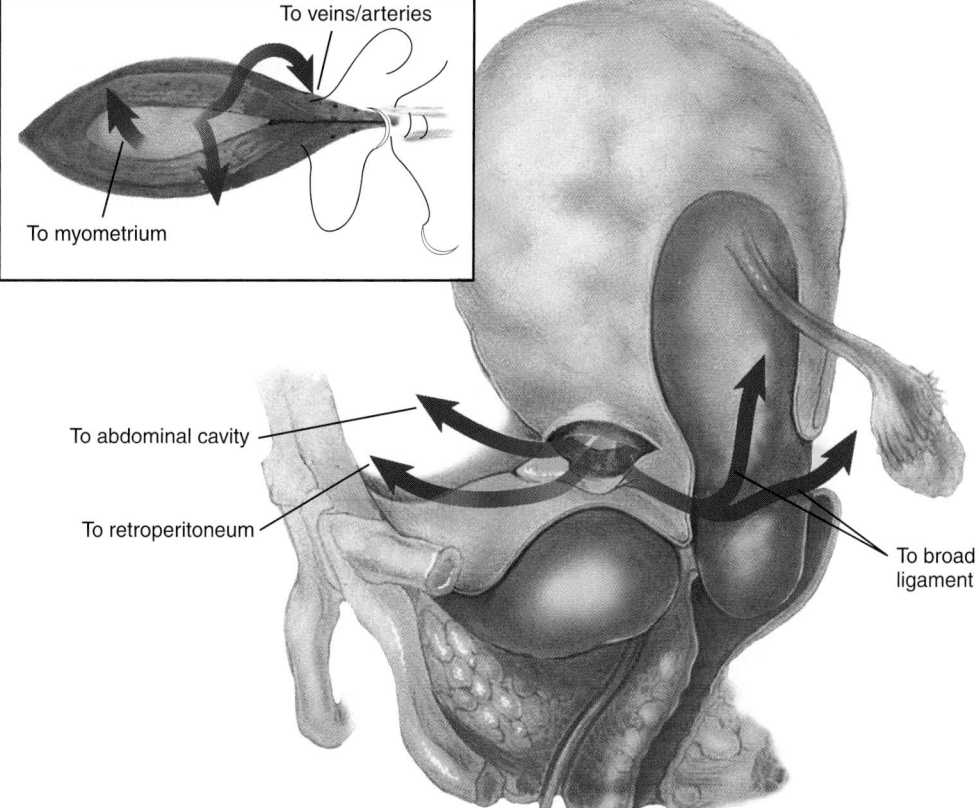

FIGURE 104-1. Pathophysiology of postcesarean endomyometritis. Note the potential pathways for contaminated amniotic fluid to infect the postpartum pelvic tissues.

To veins/arteries

To myometrium

To abdominal cavity

To retroperitoneum

To broad ligament

risk for PPE after either vaginal or abdominal delivery, for reasons that have not been fully delineated.

PPE is a polymicrobial infection caused by a wide variety of bacteria. Group B streptococci, enterococci, other aerobic streptococci, *G. vaginalis*, *E. coli*, *Prevotella bivia*, *Bacteroides* spp., and peptostreptococci are the most common endometrial isolates, with group B streptococci and *G. vaginalis* the most common isolates from the blood.[17-19]

The isolation of *Ureaplasma urealyticum* and *Mycoplasma hominis* from endometrium and blood suggests that these organisms can cause PPE, although good clinical responses have been obtained in patients with mycoplasmas cultured from the blood who were treated with antibiotics not active against these organisms. These organisms have also been reported to be important pathogens associated with abdominal wound infection after cesarean delivery.[20]

Chlamydia trachomatis has been associated with a late form of PPE that occurs more than 2 days to 6 weeks after delivery among women who deliver vaginally.[21] Group A β-hemolytic streptococcal endometritis is rare; it is epidemiologically unique because its source can be exogenous infection (usually in a health care worker), and it is characterized by early onset and rapid progression with few localizing symptoms or physical signs.

The diagnosis of PPE is suggested by the development of fever, usually on the first or second postpartum day. Significant fever is defined as an oral temperature of 38.5° C or higher in the first 24 hours after delivery or 38° C or higher for at least 4 consecutive hours 24 or more hours after delivery. Other consistently associated findings are lower abdominal pain, uterine tenderness, and leukocytosis. These patients may also exhibit a delay of the normally rapid postoperative return of bowel function due to an associated local peritonitis.

Patients with suspected PPE should have the uterus assessed for size, consistency, and tenderness. This requires a bimanual pelvic examination in some patients, whereas in others an abdominal examination is sufficient. The presence of an extrauterine mass suggesting a hematoma, usually involving the space between the lower uterine segment and the bladder, can also be ascertained during bimanual pelvic examination.

The value of transvaginally obtained uterine cultures and the optimal method of obtaining such cultures remain matters of controversy. Although cultures obtained transvaginally are often difficult to interpret because of contaminants, they may be useful for those patients in whom initial therapy fails.[22] Because 10% to 20% of patients have an associated bacteremia, blood cultures are recommended. Bacteremia does not predict the severity of clinical illness or a prolonged recovery, however. A test for *Chlamydia* should be obtained from patients with late-onset PPE, particularly from those at high risk for chlamydial infection (e.g., adolescents).

Clindamycin plus gentamicin has proved to be the most effective regimen in treating PPE, especially if PPE occurs after cesarean delivery.[23] Alternative regimens used for the treatment of PPE include one of the extended-spectrum penicillins or second-generation cephalosporins (e.g., ampicillin/sulbactam, ticarcillin/clavulanic acid, piperacillin/tazobactam, cefotetan, cefoxitin). Failures of those regimens with poor activity against penicillin-resistant anaerobic bacteria (e.g., penicillin and gentamicin without clindamycin) are more likely. For this reason, antimicrobial regimens used in the treatment of postcesarean endometritis should provide satisfactory coverage of penicillin-resistant anaerobic microorganisms (e.g., *P. bivia*). The carbapenems (imipenem/cilastatin, meropenem, ertapenem) have also proved effective in the treatment of these infections but are generally reserved for more resistant infections not usually found on an obstetric service.

Parenteral therapy should be continued until the patient's temperature has remained lower than 37.5° C for 24 hours, the patient is pain free, and the leukocyte count is normal. The use of oral antibiotics after discharge has been shown to be unnecessary.[24] Women with late-onset PPE can be treated as outpatients with oral erythromycin or doxycycline therapy with or without metronidazole depending on whether they have coexistent bacterial vaginosis.

Early-onset PPE should respond to parenteral antimicrobial therapy within 48 hours, with the patient becoming afebrile within 96 hours. Failure to accomplish this goal suggests the presence of an abdominal wound infection in 50% of these patients.[25] Because cephalosporin antibiotic prophylaxis is commonly administered to women undergoing cesarean delivery, enterococcal superinfection is another common explanation for failure to respond or relapse after treatment with regimens that are not effective against enterococci (e.g., extended-spectrum cephalosporins; clindamycin plus gentamicin). This is particularly true if the organism is isolated in pure culture or heavy growth from an endometrial specimen. If an enterococcal superinfection is suspected, one of the following regimens should be employed: clindamycin or metronidazole plus ampicillin plus gentamicin; ampicillin/sulbactam plus gentamicin; cefoxitin or cefotetan plus ampicillin; ticarcillin/clavulanic acid or piperacillin/tazobactam; piperacillin; or mezlocillin. Uncommonly, failure results from lack of coverage of a drug-resistant anaerobe; this can be corrected by a regimen containing either metronidazole or clindamycin. The importance of endometrial cultures for aerobes, anaerobes, and mycoplasmas will increase as antimicrobial resistance to clindamycin grows among isolates of gram-negative anaerobes.[26]

If fever persists despite apparently appropriate antimicrobial therapy, the differential diagnosis includes a wound or pelvic abscess, refractory postpartum fever, and noninfectious fever (e.g., drug fever, breast engorgement).

PPE caused by group A β-hemolytic streptococci has special epidemiologic significance.[27-29] The Centers for Disease Control and Prevention recommends that health care worker screening be undertaken when an episode of postpartum group A streptococcus (GAS) infection is identified. All health care workers present at the delivery and those who performed vaginal examinations before delivery should be screened with cultures of the nares, throat, vagina, rectum, and skin. Any health care worker who is culture positive for GAS should refrain from patient care for the first 24 hours of antimicrobial therapy. If surveillance identifies additional patients or health care workers with positive cultures for GAS, the isolates should be typed by sequencing the variable portion of M-protein gene, serology, or other molecular methods to identify the strain.

Refractory Postpartum Fever of Undetermined Origin

Traditionally, the diagnosis of septic pelvic thrombophlebitis (SPT) was entertained in those patients with PPE refractory to broad-spectrum antimicrobial therapy. Once alternative explanations (wound infection or pelvic abscess) for persistent fever were ruled out, heparin therapy was used to determine whether the diagnosis was SPT or drug fever. Women with SPT responded promptly to therapeutic anticoagulation with heparin and became afebrile within 24 to 48 hours.[30] More recent analysis of this practice has made this therapeutic approach suspect.

Brown and colleagues[31] studied women who had pelvic infection and fever that persisted after 5 days despite adequate antimicrobial therapy with clindamycin, gentamicin, and ampicillin. A diagnosis of SPT was made after computed tomography (CT) revealed uterine vein thrombosis. Women were randomly assigned to one of two management schemes: continuation of antimicrobial therapy, either alone or with the addition of heparin, until the temperature was less than 37.5° C for 48 hours. SPT (1:3000 deliveries) was diagnosed in 22% of women with prolonged infection. There was no significant difference between the responses of women with pelvic infection who were and were not given heparin therapy; in both groups, women required an average of 6 days of therapy before becoming afebrile. These results do not support the common empiric practice of heparin treatment for women with persistent postpartum infection.

Similarly, Witlin and colleagues[32] reviewed the medical records of postpartum women with the diagnosis of SPT for an 8-year period (1986-1994). All patients demonstrated refractory febrile morbidity (mean 5.5 ± 1.9 days before institution of heparin therapy) despite antimicrobial therapy with ampicillin, gentamicin, and clindamycin. Imaging studies (CT, ultrasound, or both) revealed no pelvic pathology. The patients required an average of 4.7 ± 2.1 days (median, 5 days; range, 1-9 days) of heparin therapy before defervescence. Heparin levels were therapeutic at a mean of less than 24 hours (range, 6-24 hours). The authors suggested that currently available imaging studies cannot diagnose the entity we now define as SPT. In addition, their findings do not support the time-honored rule that SPT responds within 24 to 48 hours to therapeutic anticoagulation with heparin.

Taken together, these studies suggest that patients with refractory postpartum fever require more time to resolve their persistent fever than their more responsive counterparts and that anticoagulation does not speed this process along. Antibiotics should be discontinued in patients with persistent fever that look well, have a normal pelvic examination, and have no leukocytosis, considering the diagnosis of drug fever. More prolonged antibiotic therapy (5 to 6 days) with or without adjunct heparin therapy should be anticipated in those patients with persistent fever, continued pelvic organ tenderness, and persistent leukocytosis.

Episiotomy Infections

Infection of the episiotomy site is an uncommon occurrence. Overall, only 0.1% of episiotomies become infected, although this rate increases to 1% to 2% for episiotomies complicated by third- or fourth-degree extensions.

Shy and Eschenbach[33] classified episiotomy infections into four categories, depending on the depth of infection. The simple episiotomy infection is a local infection that is limited to the skin and superficial fascia along the episiotomy incision. In contrast to deeper infection, the associated skin changes of edema and erythema occur only adjacent to the episiotomy. The simple episiotomy infection may initially be treated with broad-spectrum antibiotics with activity against streptococci, staphylococci, Enterobacteriaceae, and anaerobes, including *Bacteroides fragilis*. If therapeutic response is not prompt, the wound should be opened, explored, and débrided under adequate anesthesia to exclude hematoma or previously unrecognized rectovaginal communication. Ramin and colleagues[34] showed that, with proper preoperative care, simple episiotomy infection is not a contraindication to early repair of dehiscence.

Infection of the two layers of the superficial fascia may occur. The more common is *superficial fascia infection without necrosis*, the clinical presentation of which is neither striking nor distinctive. The skin may be erythematous and edematous, but severe systemic manifestations do not occur. If response to broad-spectrum antibiotic therapy does not occur in 24 to 48 hours, or if the clinical condition worsens during antibiotic therapy, then the episiotomy should be surgically explored.

Infection of the superficial fascia with necrosis, most commonly referred to as *necrotizing fasciitis*, is an infection of the subcutaneous tissues (i.e., the superficial fascia) that spreads in the fascial clefts overlying the deep fascia. The deep fascia usually, but not always, is spared; skin involvement results only secondarily, after the nutrient vessels to the skin thrombose. Because the skin is not primarily involved, the episiotomy wound may appear normal, making early recognition difficult and causing fatal delay in treatment. Despite the minimal local findings, patients may appear severely ill, with marked local pain, high fever, and prominent systemic manifestations. Most patients are diabetic. Definitive diagnosis is made at surgery, with the discovery of extensive undermining of surrounding tissues and lack of resistance in the superficial fascial plane to probing with a blunt instrument. Treatment includes broad-spectrum antibiotics (e.g., clindamycin plus ampicillin plus gentamicin) and radical débridement to include removal of all necrotic and pale tissue. It should be emphasized that treatment of this disease is primarily surgical and that less than aggressive resection of all involved tissues will lead to therapeutic failure (see Chapter 86).

In the extremely rare event of infection beneath the deep fascia, muscle may be involved, resulting in the another type of episiotomy infection, myonecrosis. Myonecrosis is commonly caused by *Clostridium perfringens*, although it can occur from a neglected necrotizing fasciitis infection that invades the deep fascia. Myonecrosis of the subgluteal muscles surrounding the hip joint or the psoas muscles can also occur from bacteria introduced into this deep space by a paracervical or pudendal needle during the administration of anesthesia. These patients experience severe hip pain associated with marked limitation of motion.

Both myonecrosis and clostridial infection should be treated with surgical resection and antibiotic therapy. For clostridial infection, high-dose penicillin is the therapy of choice. Radical wide excision may be necessary. Hyperbaric oxygen therapy is at best an adjunctive measure to surgical débridement. Polyvalent gas gangrene antitoxin is probably ineffective.

Soper[35] reported an unusually severe form of clostridial myonecrosis arising from an episiotomy caused by *Clostridium sordellii*. The patient had a distinctive course characterized by the sudden onset of severe and unrelenting hypotension associated with marked, generalized tissue edema and third spacing, with increased hematocrit, marked leukemoid reaction, absence of rash or fever, and a rapid fatal course. This syndrome was subsequently reported in association with retention of a vaginal pack, degeneration of a cervical myoma, and postpartum endometritis.[36]

Postabortal Infections

Infection after abortion is an ascending process that occurs most commonly in the presence of retained products of conception or operative trauma. Risk factors include greater duration of pregnancy, technical difficulties, and the unsuspected presence of sexually transmitted pathogens or bacterial vaginosis.

Symptoms include fever, chills, abdominal pain, and vaginal bleeding, often with the passage of placental tissue. Postabortal infection typically has its onset within 4 days after the procedure.

Physical findings include an elevated temperature, tachycardia, tachypnea, and abdominal tenderness. In the presence of bacteremia, hypotension and frank shock may occur, and the patient may be agitated or disoriented. Pelvic examination reveals a sanguinopurulent discharge and uterine tenderness, with or without adnexal and parametrial tenderness. It is important to look for cervical or vaginal lacerations, especially with a suspected illegal abortion. Transvaginal ultrasonography can assess the intrauterine cavity for the presence of retained products of conception suggesting the need for uterine curettage.

Septic abortion caused by *C. perfringens* has a characteristic clinical presentation. In severe cases, massive intravascular hemolysis produces jaundice, mahogany-colored urine, and severe anemia.

Laboratory evaluation for patients with more than early uncomplicated postabortal endometritis should include a complete blood count, urinalysis, and culture of the endometrial cavity with an endometrial suction curette; blood cultures; anteroposterior radiographs of the abdomen and pelvis; and upright chest roentgenograms.

Simple endometritis, defined as low-grade fever associated with mild uterine tenderness after uncomplicated elective abortion, can be treated with oral regimens recommended for the treatment of pelvic inflammatory disease (see Box 104-3). Patients with established infection, as indicated by fever greater than 38° C, pelvic peritonitis, or tachycardia, should be hospitalized for parenteral antibiotic therapy (see Box 104-1) and prompt uterine evacuation. Stubblefield and Grimes[37] reviewed the management of these cases.

Surgical removal of infected tissue is essential in all but the mildest of postabortal infections. Pelvic ultrasound can be employed to confirm the presence of retained tissue. In most cases, prompt curettage controls the infection. If the uterus is too large to allow suction curettage, oxytocin or vaginal misoprostol administration is often successful. Concurrent laparoscopy may be needed for curettage of a uterus that was perforated at the time of abortion.

Indications for laparotomy and hysterectomy include failure to respond to uterine evacuation and appropriate medical therapy, perforation and infection with suspected bowel injury, pelvic and adnexal abscess, and clostridial necrotizing myonecrosis (gas gangrene). Isolation of *C. perfringens* does not mandate hysterectomy. Initial treatment should include high-dose penicillin (5 million units intravenously every 6 hours), curettage, supportive therapy, and intensive cardiovascular monitoring. Laparotomy is indicated if there is deterioration or no response.

Avoidance of unwanted pregnancies by making contraceptives available is the most important preventive measure. Screening for sexually transmitted diseases (STDs) and bacterial vaginosis before performance of elective abortion is optimal but often impractical. A meta-analysis revealed a substantial protective effect of antibiotics in all subgroups of women undergoing induced abortion, even women in low-risk groups. Routine use of periabortal antibiotics, such as doxycycline, in the United States may prevent up to half of all cases of postabortal infections.[38]

SURGICAL SITE INFECTION AFTER GYNECOLOGIC SURGERY

The identification of surgical site infection (SSI) involves interpretation of clinical and laboratory findings, and it is crucial that surveillance programs use definitions that are consistent and standardized. The SSIs (organ or space) associated with hysterectomy are cuff cellulitis, pelvic cellulitis, and pelvic abscess.

Pathogenesis

Microbial contamination of the surgical site is a necessary precursor of SSI. The risk of SSI can be conceptualized according to the following relationship[39]:

Dose of bacterial contamination × Virulence ÷

Resistance of host patient = Risk of SSI

Quantitatively, it has been shown that if a surgical site is contaminated with more than 10^5 microorganisms per gram of tissue, the risk of SSI is markedly increased.[40] However, the dose of contaminating microorganisms required to produce infection may be much lower if foreign material is present at the site.[41]

Microorganisms may contain or produce toxins and other substances that increase their ability to invade a host, produce damage within the host, or survive on or in host tissue. For example, many gram-negative bacteria produce endotoxin, which stimulates cytokine production. In turn, cytokines can trigger the inflammatory response syndrome that sometimes leads to multiple system organ failure.[42,43] Some bacterial surface components, notably polysaccharide capsules, inhibit phagocytosis, a critical and early host defense response to microbial contamination.[44] Certain strains of clostridia and streptococci produce potent exotoxins that disrupt cell membranes or alter cellular metabolism. A variety of microorganisms, including gram-positive bacteria such as coagulase-negative staphylococci, produce glycocalyx and an associated component call "slime," which physically shields bacteria from phagocytes or inhibits the binding or penetration of antimicrobial agents. Although these and other virulence factors are well defined, their mechanistic relationships to SSI development have not been fully determined.

For SSIs that occur after hysterectomy, the source of pathogens is the endogenous flora of the vagina. The normal vaginal flora consists of lactobacilli, various species of streptococci, *G. vaginalis*, strains of Enterobacteriaceae, and anaerobes. Although anaerobes predominate numerically (10:1), the concentration of lactobacilli in normal women surpasses that of the anaerobic bacteria by a factor of 100 to 1000.[45] Lactobacilli produce both hydrogen peroxide and lactic acid, which play crucial roles in protecting against the overgrowth of pathogens in the vagina. Pathogenic microorganisms such as group B streptococci, *E. coli*, *G. vaginalis*, and anaerobes such as *Prevotella bivia*, are present in increased concentrations in women without this protective flora (e.g., those with bacterial vaginosis).

Other factors alter the vaginal flora as well as bacterial vaginosis and may indirectly predispose to postoperative infection. Ohm and Galask[46,47] showed that *E. coli*, *Klebsiella*, *Proteus*, *Enterobacter*, *B. fragilis*, and enterococci are more common in 5-day postoperative vaginal cultures after abdominal or vaginal hysterectomy than in pre-

operative cultures from the same patients. Although several studies have documented increased enterococcal colonization after perioperative cephalosporin prophylaxis, other factors must be involved, because placebo groups show increased enterococcal colonization as well.

Additional factors that affect the vaginal flora include use of nonoxynol-9–containing vaginal contraceptive preparations, douching, the phase of the menstrual cycle, and menopausal status. The significance of these factors in relation to infection after gynecologic surgery is unknown.

The polymicrobial flora of the vagina remains the source for pathogens causing infection after hysterectomy. Once the vaginal epithelium is breached during excision of the cervix, microorganisms gain entry to the vaginal cuff, paravaginal tissues, and peritoneal cavity. The animal model of intra-abdominal infection devised by Weinstein and colleagues[48] clarified the distinctive roles played by different bacteria in the natural history of pelvic infection. These investigators documented a biphasic response to infection consisting of an initial phase characterized by peritonitis and sepsis, in which gram-negative aerobic bacteria predominate (peritonitis stage), and a secondary phase with abscess formation, in which anaerobes predominate (abscess stage) (Fig. 104-2).

Risk Factors

Several factors, some of which are beyond the surgeon's control, influence the likelihood of development of a postoperative infection. Febrile morbidity is more common after abdominal than after vaginal hysterectomy.[49] The incidence of postoperative infection is higher in patients of lower socioeconomic status, regardless of surgical approach. Age has inconsistently been shown to be a risk factor after hysterectomy, with premenopausal women shown to be at increased risk in some studies, especially after vaginal hysterectomy. Duration of surgery is directly correlated with postoperative infection rates.[50]

Bacterial vaginosis has been associated with an increased risk of infection after abdominal hysterectomy.[51] Patients scheduled for elective hysterectomy should be screened for bacterial vaginosis before the planned procedure. Those found to have bacterial vaginosis should be treated preoperatively or with metronidazole perioperatively for at least 4 days.[52]

Cuff Cellulitis

An inflammatory response at the margins of the vaginal cuff incision is a normal part of the healing process in the early posthysterectomy period. Host defense mechanisms quickly resolve this cellulitis in most patients without need for antibiotic administration. Hemsell[53] observed that 17% of women undergoing vaginal hysterectomy and 35% of those undergoing abdominal hysterectomy had recurrent tempera-

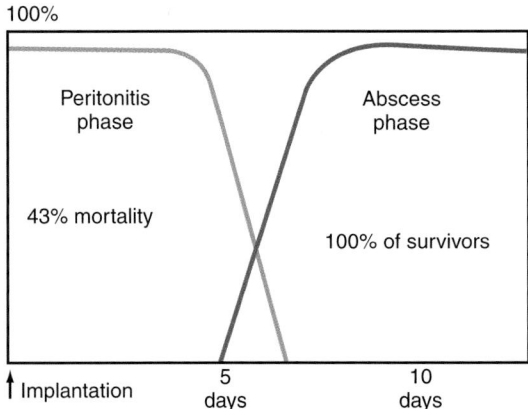

FIGURE 104-2. Biphasic pathophysiology of polymicrobial pelvic infection. *(From Weinstein WM, Onderdonk AB, Bartlett JG, Gorbach SL. Experimental intraabdominal abscesses in rats: Development of an experimental model. Infect Immun. 1974;10:1250-1255.)*

ture elevations on the second or third postoperative day despite normal abdominal and pelvic examinations and no pain. These patients become afebrile without therapy. In a small number of cases, however, cuff cellulitis after hysterectomy requires antibiotic therapy. These women usually present within 10 days after surgery complaining of increasing central lower abdominal and pelvic pain, increased vaginal discharge, and low-grade temperature elevation. Abdominal examination is normal or elicits only slight suprapubic tenderness to deep palpation. On bimanual examination, only the vaginal surgical margin is tender, and no masses are palpable. Women with cuff cellulitis have been treated successfully as outpatients with oral antibiotics, but it is important to choose an antibiotic regimen that includes coverage for anaerobic microorganisms. Examples of such regimens include (1) amoxicillin/clavulanic acid or (2) the combination of a first-generation cephalosporin, a quinolone, or trimethoprim/sulfamethoxazole with metronidazole. Patients should monitor their temperatures at home, and clinical re-evaluation should be considered if improvement in pain and temperature is not noted by 72 hours.

A few patients with cuff cellulitis develop a well-localized collection of pus just above the vaginal cuff (vaginal cuff abscess). In addition to fever, these women may complain of a sense of fullness in the lower abdomen. Bimanual pelvic examination confirms the presence of a vaginal cuff mass, and ultrasound can confirm the presence of an abscess. Vaginal drainage facilitates cure and may be accomplished simply by dilation of the vaginal cuff in a treatment room. Some patients with larger collections may benefit by drainage in the operating room. Any purulent material recovered should be cultured for aerobic and anaerobic pathogens.[54]

Broad-spectrum parenteral antibiotics (Box 104-1) covering both aerobic and anaerobic bacteria should be given until the patient has been afebrile for 24 to 36 hours. Many experts suggest initiating antibiotic therapy with a single broad-spectrum agent, whereas others recommend combination therapy (e.g., clindamycin plus gentamicin) even for clinically milder infections.[55]

BOX 104-1

Intravenous Antibiotic Regimens for Treating Gynecologic Postoperative Infections[54]

Localized Infection with Minimal Systemic Findings
Cefotaxime 1 g q8h
Cefotetan 2 g q12h
Cefoxitin 2 g q6h
Ceftriaxone 2 g, then 1 g q24h
Piperacillin 4 g q6h
Ampicillin/sulbactam 3 g q6h
Mezlocillin 4 g q6h
Ticarcillin/clavulanic acid 3.1 g q4-6h
Piperacillin tazobactam 3.375 g q6h

Extensive Infection with Moderate to Severe Systemic Findings
Clindamycin 900 mg IV q8h
   plus
Gentamicin 2 mg/kg IV, then 1.5 mg/kg q8h (or single daily dose 5 mg/kg)
   with or without
Ampicillin 2 g IV, then 1 g IV q4h
   or
Ampicillin 2 g IV, then 1 g IV q4h
   plus
Gentamicin 2 mg/kg IV, then 1.5 mg/kg q8h (or single daily dose 5 mg/kg)
   plus
Metronidazole 500 mg IV q8h
   or
Imipenem/cilastatin 500-1000 mg IV q6h
   or
Levofloxacin 500 mg IV q24h
   plus
Metronidazole 500 mg IV q8h

Pelvic Abscess

The most serious late postoperative complication is a pelvic abscess. These abscesses may involve one or both residual adnexa (tuboovarian abscess) if the fallopian tubes and ovaries were not removed at surgery. These infections are rare, occur almost exclusively in premenopausal women, occur despite the use of prophylactic antibiotics, and often have a latent period of many weeks between surgery and onset of symptoms.[56]

Patients may have had no apparent infection during their initial hospitalization, or, alternatively, they may have appeared to respond rapidly to the initial selection of antibiotics for presumed pelvic cellulitis, only to relapse after discharge. Typically the fever curve is characterized by a high spike late in the afternoon or early evening. The leukocyte count is often in the range of 20,000/mm³, and the erythrocyte sedimentation rate (ESR) is markedly elevated. Patients with postoperative adnexal abscess often have a palpable mass high in the pelvis.[57] Ultrasonography and CT scans both confirm the presence of a mass and help to determine whether it is loculated, related to an intraperitoneal structure, or drainable percutaneously. Because their location is removed from the vaginal cuff, pelvic/adnexal abscesses cannot be drained through the vaginal cuff unless they extend to the cul-de-sac.

Identification of a postoperative pelvic abscess does not mandate immediate drainage if it is inaccessible, because antibiotic therapy alone is often successful in the treatment of this complication. The frequent isolation of a β-lactamase–producing *Prevotella* species from these abscesses warrants the use of clindamycin, metronidazole, or other agents effective against gram-negative anaerobes. A regimen of clindamycin plus gentamicin is frequently employed. For patients whose infection fails to respond to appropriate antibiotic therapy, drainage is necessary. Ledger and colleagues[58] showed that most such antibiotic failures are caused not by antimicrobial resistance but by the unique environment of the abscess, which inhibits antibiotic effectiveness. Necrosis associated with these types of infections makes surgical exploration necessary in some cases. Associated ovarian vein thrombosis is not uncommon in these women.

If the abscess is located in the posterior cul-de-sac, drainage via colpotomy can be attempted under ultrasound guidance. The abscess cavity should be completely evacuated and a drain placed to prevent reaccumulation of fluid. Abscesses not located in the cul-de-sac may be drained percutaneously if they are located adjacent to the abdominal wall or are determined to be accessible by CT scanning. A pigtail or equivalent catheter should remain in place until drainage ceases, usually 4 to 8 days.[59,60] Patients with suspected postoperative pelvic abscess that fails to respond to antibiotic therapy and cannot be drained by one of the previously mentioned techniques require laparotomy. In most cases, the adnexa are involved and must be removed. Purulent material or tissue should be submitted for aerobic and anaerobic culture.

Parenteral antibiotics should be administered until the patient has remained afebrile for 48 to 72 hours, the leukocyte count is normal, and the signs and symptoms have resolved. Most clinicians choose to treat these patients for 7 days after discharge with oral agents such as amoxicillin/clavulanate or metronidazole. All patients should be reexamined 2 weeks after discharge to ensure that recurrence or reaccumulation of the abscess has not occurred.[61]

Osteomyelitis Pubis

Osteitis pubis has been described as a noninfectious, self-limited inflammatory condition of the symphysis pubis associated with retropubic urologic procedures.[62] It is now recognized that this condition is actually an osteomyelitis of the pubis. It is a rare infection that results from direct inoculation of the bone at the time of surgery or extension of a contiguous focus of infection. Most cases in women occur after urethral suspension or, less commonly, after radical vulvectomy or pelvic exenteration. The diagnosis is based on typical symptoms of suprapubic discomfort; difficulty with ambulation and a wide-based, waddling gait; and changes on radiographic or magnetic resonance images showing irregular bony margins and rarefaction and widening of the symphyseal joint spaces. Wound drainage, low-grade fever, moderate leukocytosis, and an elevated ESR or alkaline phosphatase level may be present.[63]

Patients for whom clinical and radiologic findings are suggestive of this diagnosis should undergo a needle biopsy guided by CT.[64] Specimens should be submitted for histopathologic examination and aerobic and anaerobic culture. If pathogenic microorganisms are recovered and if the interval between onset of symptoms and diagnosis is short, a trial of antimicrobial therapy may be attempted. Patients with a poor response to this management should undergo débridement. If pathogenic microorganisms are not isolated from a needle aspirate, open surgical biopsy with débridement should be undertaken, and specimens of bone or purulent material should be cultured. Common isolates include aerobic gram-negative bacteria as well as staphylococcal and streptococcal species. After débridement, directed antimicrobial therapy should be administered for at least 4 weeks.[65]

Sacral osteomyelitis as a complication of abdominal sacral colpopexy has been reported.[66]

PELVIC INFLAMMATORY DISEASE

Pelvic inflammatory disease (PID) refers to the clinical syndrome that represents a continuum of inflammation from the cervix to the endometrium, fallopian tubes, and contiguous pelvic structures: cervicitis, endometritis, salpingitis, pelvic peritonitis, or tuboovarian abscess.[67] Each year approximately 1 million women in the United States experience an episode of symptomatic PID. Many women with PID have minimal or no symptoms.[68]

PID results from direct canicular spread of microorganisms from the vagina or endocervix to the endometrium and fallopian tube mucosa.[69] Both *Neisseria gonorrhoeae* and *C. trachomatis* commonly cause endocervitis, and 10% to 40% of women with these infections who do not receive adequate treatment develop clinical symptoms of acute PID.[70] In addition to *N. gonorrhoeae* and *C. trachomatis*, a wide variety of bacteria have been isolated from the upper genital tracts of women with acute, symptomatic PID, including anaerobes, gram-negative rods, streptococci, and mycoplasmas.[71,72] Many of these are the same microorganisms that are found in increased concentrations in the vaginas of women with bacterial vaginosis.[73] Moreover, approximately one of every four women with presumed uncomplicated lower genital tract gonococcal or chlamydial infection or bacterial vaginosis, or both, is found to have histologic endometritis (subclinical PID) when evaluated by endometrial biopsy.[69] Uncommonly, respiratory pathogens including *Haemophilus influenzae* and *Streptococcus pyogenes* have also been isolated from the upper genital tracts of women with symptomatic PID.[74,75]

Risk Factors

Age is inversely related to the rate of PID: sexually experienced teenagers are three times more likely to be diagnosed with PID than are women 25 to 29 years of age. A history of multiple sexual partners, an increased rate of acquisition of new partners within the previous 30 days, and frequent sexual intercourse with a single partner are all associated with an increased risk of PID.[76] Women with confirmed PID commonly have concurrent bacterial vaginosis.[77] Contraceptive choice modifies PID risk in a complex manner. Mechanical and chemical barriers decrease risk. Oral contraceptives have a variable effect, decreasing the risk of a clinical diagnosis of PID but having no effect on the rate of infertility or endometrial inflammation. Intrauterine contraceptive devices (IUDs) confer a slightly increased risk of nonsexually transmitted PID in the first months after insertion.[78] Other suggested associations with PID include douching, menses, cigarette smoking, and substance abuse.[79,80]

Although an association between the use of an IUD and increased risk of PID was documented for many years, newer studies suggest that the magnitude of this association was overestimated. Contamination of the endometrial cavity at insertion apparently results in a slightly increased risk of acute PID that is limited to the first 4 months of IUD use. Infections occurring after 4 months are believed to be the result of acquired sexually transmitted pathogens and not the IUD itself.[81]

A unique role for *Actinomyces* organisms in IUD-associated PID has been suggested, but this relationship remains unclear. Although as many as 4% to 8% of IUD users have *Actinomyces*-like organisms identified on Papanicolaou (Pap) smear, their presence has not been equated with pelvic actinomycosis, nor has the risk of subsequent pelvic infection been quantified.[82] In patients with cytology showing *Actinomyces* colonization, Bonacho and associates[83] showed that removal of the IUD was routinely associated with resolution of colonization.

Diagnosis

The clinical diagnosis of acute PID is imprecise. Data indicate that a clinical diagnosis of symptomatic PID has a positive predictive value (PPV) of 65% to 90% compared with laparoscopy. The PPV of a clinical diagnosis of acute PID varies depending on epidemiologic characteristics and the clinical setting, with a higher PPV among sexually active young women (particularly adolescents), among patients attending STD clinics, and in settings in which rates of gonorrhea, chlamydia, and bacterial vaginosis are high.

Many episodes of PID go unrecognized. Although some cases are asymptomatic, others are underdiagnosed because the patient or the health care provider fails to recognize the implications of mild or nonspecific symptoms or signs (e.g., abnormal bleeding, dyspareunia, vaginal discharge). In one study, chlamydial infection was noted in 29% of women experiencing persistent intermenstrual bleeding while taking oral contraceptives, suggesting the presence of endometritis.[84] Given the often subtle presentation of this disease and the significant reproductive sequelae associated with it (infertility, ectopic pregnancy, chronic pelvic pain), clinicians should maintain a low threshold for the diagnosis of PID.

Empiric treatment for PID should be considered in sexually active young women and other women at risk for STDs if the following minimum criteria are present and no other cause for the illness can be identified: (1) pelvic organ tenderness noted on bimanual examination with or without manipulation of the cervix and (2) microscopy showing the presence of white blood cells in the vaginal secretions. Most women with PID have either mucopurulent cervical discharge or evidence of white blood cells on a microscopic evaluation of the vaginal secretions (Fig. 104-3). If cervical discharge appears normal and no white blood cells are found during microscopy, the diagnosis of PID is unlikely, and alternative causes of pain should be investigated.[85] Additional criteria that support a diagnosis of PID include bacterial vaginosis, mucopurulent cervicitis, laboratory documentation of cervical infection with *N. gonorrhoeae* or *C. trachomatis*, oral temperature greater than 38° C, and elevated ESR or C-reactive protein level.

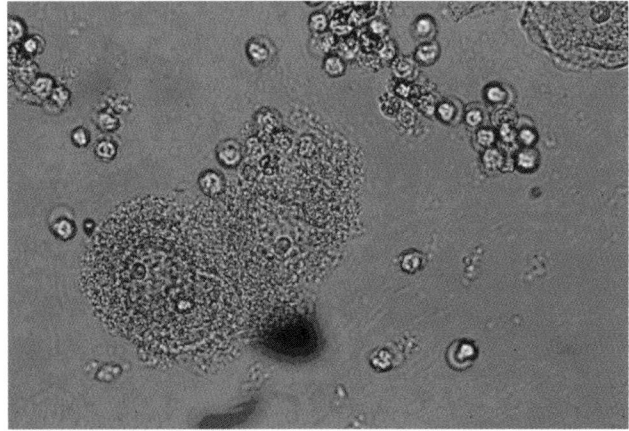

FIGURE 104-3. Microscopy of a wet mount of the vaginal secretions reveals clue cells and inflammatory cells in a patient with pelvic inflammatory disease (×400).

Definitive criteria for PID include histologic evidence of endometritis on endometrial biopsy; transvaginal sonography or other imaging techniques showing thickened, fluid-filled tubes with or without free pelvic fluid or tuboovarian complex; and laparoscopic abnormalities showing tubal purulent exudate, erythema, and edema (Fig. 104-4).

Clinical diagnosis and grading of PID have poor specificity. In fact, women with PID associated with moderate to severe pelvic adhesions or tubal occlusion were found to be less tender on abdominopelvic examination and therefore to appear less ill than women with limited or no adhesions.[86] Diagnostic laparoscopy should be considered in patients for whom empiric therapy has failed and in patients with a history of recurrent PID and negative tests for chlamydia, gonorrhea, and bacterial vaginosis. Endometriosis is a common alternative diagnosis in these women.

Although rare, acute salpingitis can occur in the proximal stump of patients who have undergone surgical sterilization and in women in the first trimester of pregnancy.

Management of Acute Pelvic Inflammatory Disease

In the past, many specialists recommended hospitalization for all patients with PID so that bed rest and supervised treatment with parenteral antibiotics could be initiated. Today, most women with PID are treated as outpatients, reflecting the preponderance of patients with only mild-to-moderate symptoms and signs. A recent prospective, randomized clinical trial compared outpatient treatment, with a single dose of cefoxitin intramuscularly and multidose oral doxycycline, versus inpatient treatment with intravenous cefoxitin and doxycycline in women with clinical symptoms and signs of mild-to-moderate PID. There were no differences in response to therapy or reproductive outcome between inpatient and outpatient regimens.[87] These data suggest that hospitalization can be reserved for those patients with clinically severe disease (severe illness, nausea and vomiting, or high fever), those unable to follow or tolerate an outpatient oral regimen, pregnant women, and women with a clinical diagnosis of tuboovarian abscess.

Treatment consists of pelvic rest and antibiotics. Antibiotic regimens must provide empiric, broad-spectrum coverage of likely pathogens, including *N. gonorrhoeae*, *C. trachomatis*, anaerobes, gram-negative facultative bacteria, and streptococci. Several antimicrobial regimens have been effective in achieving clinical and microbiologic cure in randomized clinical trials with short-term follow-up. The need to eradicate anaerobes from women with PID has not been determined definitively. Moreover, two well-designed clinical trials have confirmed the effectiveness of ofloxacin, an agent with poor anaerobic coverage, in the outpatient treatment of PID. However, anaerobic bacteria associated with bacterial vaginosis have been isolated from the upper reproductive tract of women with PID, and these bacteria have been shown to cause tubal and epithelial destruction. One method of determining the appropriateness of metronidazole therapy in women with PID is to determine the presence of concurrent bacterial vaginosis. The Centers for Disease Control and Prevention has published antibiotic treatment guidelines for acute PID (Boxes 104-2 and 104-3).[88]

Optimal outpatient management includes a follow-up examination performed within 72 hours after the initiation of therapy. Many patients may not return for this visit if they are symptomatically improved. Substantial clinical improvement with lysis of fever, reduction in direct or rebound abdominal tenderness, and reduction in pelvic organ tenderness with bimanual examination should be noted. If there is no response to therapy within 72 hours, patients should be reevaluated and possibly hospitalized to confirm the diagnosis and for consideration of parenteral antibiotic therapy if they are using an oral regimen.

BOX 104-2

Parenteral Treatment Regimens for Pelvic Inflammatory Disease

Parenteral Regimen A
Cefotetan 2 g IV q12h
or
Cefoxitin 2 g IV q6h
plus
Doxycycline 100 mg PO or IV q12h

Parenteral Regimen B
Clindamycin 900 mg IV q8h
plus
Gentamicin 2 mg/kg IV or IM as a loading dose, then 1.5 mg/kg q8h for maintenance; single daily dosing may be substituted.

Alternative Parenteral Regimens
Moxifloxacin 400 mg IV q24h
or
Gatifloxacin 400 mg IV q24h
or
Levofloxacin 500 mg IV once daily
   with or without
Metronidazole 500 mg IV q8h
or
Ampicillin/sulbactam 3 g IV q6h
plus
Doxycycline 100 mg PO or IV q12h

Centers for Disease Control and Prevention. Sexually transmitted diseases treatment guidelines 2002. MMWR Morb Mortal Wkly Rep. 2002;51:48-51.

BOX 104-3

Oral Treatment Regimens for Pelvic Inflammatory Disease

Regimen A
Levofloxacin 500 mg PO once daily for 14 days
or
Moxifloxacin 400 mg PO once daily for 14 days
or
Gatifloxacin 400 mg PO once daily for 14 days
   with or without
Metronidazole 500 mg PO bid for 14 days

Regimen B
Ceftriaxone 250 mg IM in a single dose
or
Cefoxitin 2 g IM in a single dose AND probenecid 1 g orally administered concurrently in a single dose
or
Other parenteral third-generation cephalosporin (e.g., ceftizoxime, cefotaxime)
   plus
Doxycycline 100 mg PO bid for 14 days
   with or without
Metronidazole 500 mg PO bid for 14 days

Centers for Disease Control and Prevention. Sexually transmitted diseases treatment guidelines 2002. MMWR Morb Mortal Wkly Rep. 2002;51:48-51.

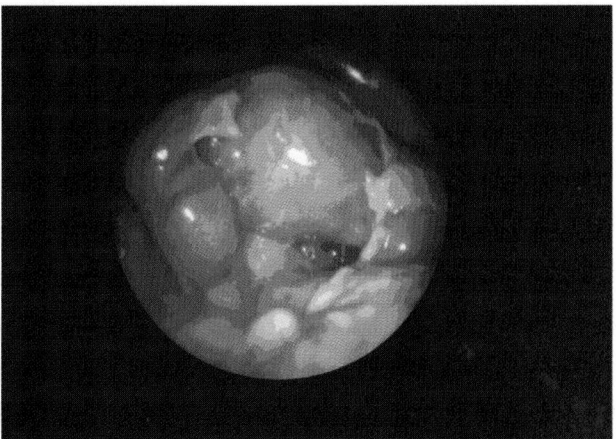

FIGURE 104-4. Laparoscopic confirmation of moderate acute salpingitis, showing patchy fibrin deposits on the serosal surfaces of the fallopian tubes. *(From Soper DE. Cervicitis and endometritis. In: Mandell GL, Sobel JD, eds. Atlas of Infectious Diseases, vol. 9. Philadelphia: Churchill Livingstone; 1997:810, Fig. 8-28.)*

All male sex partners of women with acute PID should be evaluated for sexually transmitted diseases, and those who had sexual contact with the patient during the 60 days preceding the onset of symptoms in the patient should be empirically treated with regimens effective against *C. trachomatis* and *N. gonorrhoeae*. In many circumstances, the male sex partner tests positive for chlamydia or gonorrhea but the patient receiving therapy is negative; such results shed light on the true pathogenesis of infection.[89]

Management of Suspected Tuboovarian Abscess

Patients with suspected tuboovarian abscess should be hospitalized and given broad-spectrum antimicrobial drugs that include adequate coverage for gram-negative anaerobes. Failure of response to medical therapy is suggested by a lack of defervescence within 72 hours or an increase in the size of the mass. Eighty-five percent of abscesses with a diameter of 4 to 6 cm respond to antibiotics alone, but only 40% of those 10 cm or larger respond. Triple-agent therapy with ampicillin, clindamycin, and gentamicin would appear to be the regimen of choice, although other combination regimens have been used effectively.[90,91]

Surgical intervention for a tuboovarian abscess that does not respond to antimicrobial therapy can be carried out laparoscopically, percutaneously, transvaginally, or by laparotomy. A patient with a suspected leaking or ruptured abscess should undergo immediate laparotomy after rapid stabilization and institution of broad-spectrum antibiotics.[92]

Sequelae

After one episode of PID a woman's risk of ectopic pregnancy increases sevenfold. Approximately 13% of women are infertile after a single episode of PID, 25% to 35% after two episodes, and 50 to 75% after three or more episodes. If a true tuboovarian abscess is present, only 7% to 14% of patients are able to conceive after treatment. After treatment for a tuboovarian complex (a less restrictive diagnostic category than tuboovarian abscess), approximately two thirds of women attempting pregnancy are unable to conceive. Other sequelae associated with PID include dyspareunia, pelvic adhesions, and chronic pelvic pain.[93] Screening for cervical chlamydial infection can prevent PID.[94]

REFERENCES

1. Gibbs RS, Duff P. Progress in pathogenesis and management of clinical intra-amniotic infection. Am J Obstet Gynecol. 1991;164:1317-1326.
2. Soper DE, Mayhall CG, Dalton HP. Risk factors for intraamniotic infection: A prospective epidemiologic study. Am J Obstet Gynecol. 1989;161:562-568.
3. Gibbs RS, Blanco JD, St. Clair PF, Castaneda YS. Quantitative bacteriology of amniotic fluid from women with clinical intraamniotic infection at term. J Infect Dis. 1982;145:1-8.
4. Liner RI. Intrauterine *Listeria* infection: Prenatal diagnosis by biophysical assessment and amniocentesis. Am J Obstet Gynecol. 1990;163:1596-1597.
5. Newton ER, Piper J, Peairs W. Bacterial vaginosis and intraamniotic infection. Am J Obstet Gynecol. 1997;176:672-677.
6. Duff P, Sanders R, Gibbs RS. The course of labor in term patients with chorioamnionitis. Am J Obstet Gynecol. 1983;147:391-395.
7. Edwards RK, Clark P, Locksmith GJ, Duff P. Performance characteristics of putative tests for subclinical chorioamnionitis. Infect Dis Obstet Gynecol. 2001;9:209-214.
8. Gibbs RS, Dinsmoor MJ, Newton ER, Ramamurthy RS. A randomized trial of intrapartum versus immediate postpartum treatment of women with intraamniotic infection. Obstet Gynecol. 1988;72:823-828.
9. Hopkins L, Smaill F. Antibiotic regimens for management of intraamniotic infection. Cochrane Database Syst Rev. 2002;(3):CD003254. Review.
10. Edwards RK, Duff P. One additional dose of antibiotics is sufficient postpartum therapy for chorioamnionitis (Abstract). Presented at the 30th Annual Scientific Meeting of the Infectious Disease Society for Obstetrics and Gynecology, Hyannis, Mass, August 7-9, 2003.
11. Sperling RS, Ramamurthy RS, Gibbs RS. A comparison of intrapartum versus immediate postpartum treatment of intra-amniotic infection. Obstet Gynecol. 1987;70:861-865.
12. Seaward PG, Hannah ME, Myhr TL, et al. International multicentre prelabor rupture of membranes study: Evaluation of predictors of clinical chorioamnionitis and postpartum fever in patients with prelabor rupture of membranes at term. Am J Obstet Gynecol. 1997;177:1024-1029.
13. Watts DH, Krohn MA, Hillier SL, Eschenbach DA. Bacterial vaginosis as a risk factor for postcesarean endometritis. Obstet Gynecol. 1990;75:52-58.
14. Chang PL, Newton ER. Predictors of antibiotic prophylactic failure in post-cesarean endometritis. Obstet Gynecol. 1992;80:117-122.
15. Hopkins L, Smaill F. Antibiotic prophylaxis regimens and drugs for cesarean section. Cochrane Database Syst Rev. 2002;(1):CD001067.

16. Gonik B, Shannon RL, Shawar R, et al. Why patients fail antibiotic prophylaxis at cesarean delivery: Histologic evidence for incipient infection for incipient infection. Obstet Gynecol. 1992;79:179-184.
17. Watts DH, Eschenbach DA, Kenny GE. Early postpartum endometritis: The role of bacteria, genital mycoplasmas, and *Chlamydia trachomatis*. Obstet Gynecol. 1989;73:52-60.
18. Eschenbach DA, Rosene K, Tompkins LS, et al. Endometrial cultures obtained by a triple-lumen method from afebrile and febrile postpartum women. J Infect Dis. 1986;153:1038-1045.
19. Watts DH, Hillier SL, Eschenbach DA. Upper genital tract isolates at delivery as predictors of post-cesarean infection among women receiving antibiotic prophylaxis. Obstet Gynecol. 1991;77:287-292.
20. Roberts S, Maccato M, Faro S, Pinell P. The microbiology of post-cesarean wound morbidity. Obstet Gynecol. 1993;81:383-386.
21. Hoyme UB, Kiviat N, Eschenbach DA. The microbiology and treatment of late postpartum endometritis. Obstet Gynecol. 1986;68:226-232.
22. Martens MG, Faro S, Hammil HA, et al. Transcervical uterine cultures with a new endometrial suction curette: A comparison of three sampling methods in postpartum endometritis. Obstet Gynecol. 1989;74:273-276.
23. French LM, Smaill FM. Antibiotic regimens for endometritis after delivery. Cochrane Database Syst Rev. 2000;(2):CD001067.
24. Dinsmoor MJ, Newton ER, Gibbs RS. A randomized, double-blind, placebo-controlled trial of oral antibiotic therapy following intravenous antibiotic therapy for postpartum endometritis. Obstet Gynecol. 1991;77:60-62.
25. Soper DE, Brockwell NJ, Dalton HP. The importance of wound infection in antibiotic failures in the therapy of postpartum endometritis. Surg Gynecol Obstet. 1992;174:265-269.
26. Aldridge KE, Broyles S, Master R. Clindamycin in contemporary ob-gyn: Considerations of antibiotic resistance among beta-hemolytic streptococci and anaerobes (Abstract). Presented at the 30th Annual Scientific Meeting of the Infectious Disease Society for Obstetrics and Gynecology, Hyannis, Mass, August 7-9, 2003.
27. Noronha S, Yue C, Sekosan M. Puerperal group A beta-hemolytic streptococcal toxic shock-like syndrome. Obstet Gynecol. 1996;88:728.
28. Meis JF, Muytjens HC, van den Berg PP, et al. Analysis of an outbreak of puerperal fever due to group A streptococci by random amplified polymorphic DNA fingerprinting. Infect Dis Obstet Gynecol. 1997;5:232-236.
29. Centers for Disease Control and Prevention. Nosocomial group A streptococcal infections associated with asymptomatic health care workers—Maryland and California, 1997. MMWR Morb Mortal Wkly Rep. 1999;48:163-166.
30. Dunn LJ, Van Voorhis LW. Enigmatic fever and pelvic thrombophlebitis. N Engl J Med. 1967;276:265-268.
31. Brown CE, Stettler RW, Twickler D, Cunningham FG. Puerperal septic pelvic thrombophlebitis: Incidence and response to heparin therapy. Am J Obstet Gynecol. 1999;181:143-148.
32. Witlin AG, Mercer BM, Sibai BM. Septic pelvic thrombophlebitis or refractory postpartum fever of undetermined etiology. J Matern Fetal Med. 1996;5:355-358.
33. Shy KK, Eschenbach DA. Fatal perineal cellulitis from an episiotomy site. Obstet Gynecol. 1979;54:292-298.
34. Ramin SM, Ramus RM, Little BB, Gilstrap LC 3rd. Early repair of episiotomy dehiscence associated with infection. Am J Obstet Gynecol. 1992;167:1104-1107.
35. Soper DE. Clostridial myonecrosis arising from an episiotomy. Obstet Gynecol. 1986;68:26S-28S.
36. McGregor JA, Soper DE, Lovell G, Todd JK. Maternal deaths associated with *Clostridium sordellii* infection. Am J Obstet Gynecol. 1989;161:987-995.
37. Stubblefield PG, Grimes DA. Septic abortion. N Engl J Med. 1994;331:310-314.
38. Sawaya GF, Grady D, Kerlikowske K, Grimes DA. Antibiotics at the time of induced abortion: The case for universal prophylaxis based on a meta-analysis. Obstet Gynecol. 1996;87:884-890.
39. Cruise PJ. Surgical wound infection. In: Wonsiewicz MJ, ed. Infectious Diseases. Philadelphia: WB Saunders; 1992:758-764.
40. Krizek TJ, Robson MC. Evolution of quantitative bacteriology in wound management. Am J Surg. 1975;130:579-584.
41. James RC, MacLeod CJ. Induction of staphylococcal infections in mice with small inocula introduced on sutures. Br J Exp Pathol. 1957;38:573-586.
42. Henderson B, Poole S, Wilson M. Microbial/host interactions in health and disease: Who controls the cytokine network? Immunopharmacology 1996;35:1-21.
43. Demling R, LaLonde C, Saldinger P, Knox J. Multiple-organ dysfunction in the surgical patient: Pathophysiology, prevention, and treatment. Curr Probl Surg. 1993;30:345-414.
44. Kasper DL. Bacterial capsule—old dogmas and new tricks. J Infect Dis. 1986;153:407-415.
45. Eschenbach DA, Davick PR, Williams BL, et al. Prevalence of hydrogen peroxide producing *Lactobacillus* species in normal women and women with bacterial vaginosis. J Clin Microbiol. 1989;27:251-256.
46. Ohm MJ, Galask RP. The effect of antibiotic prophylaxis on patients undergoing vaginal operations. Am J Obstet Gynecol. 1975;123:597-604.
47. Ohm MJ, Galask RP. The effect of antibiotic prophylaxis on patients undergoing total abdominal hysterectomy. Am J Obstet Gynecol. 1976;125:448-454.
48. Weinstein WM, Onderdonk AB, Bartlett JG, Gorbach SL. Experimental intraabdominal abscesses in rats: Development of an experimental model. Infect Immun. 1974;10:1250-1255.
49. Dicker RC, Greenspan JR, Strauss, LT, et al. Complications of abdominal and vaginal hysterectomy among women of reproductive age in the United States. Am J Obstet Gynecol. 1982;144:841-848.
50. Shapiro M, Munoz A, Tager IB, et al. Risk factors for infection at the operative site after abdominal or vaginal hysterectomy. N Engl J Med. 1982;307:1661-1666.

51. Soper DE, Bump RC, Hurt WG. Bacterial vaginosis and trichomoniasis vaginitis are risk factors for cuff cellulitis after abdominal hysterectomy. Am J Obstet Gynecol. 1990;163:1016-1023.

52. Larsson P-G, Carlsson B. Does pre- and postoperative metronidazole treatment lower vaginal cuff infection rate after abdominal hysterectomy among women with bacterial vaginosis? Infect Dis Obstet Gynecol. 2002;10:133-140.

53. Hemsell DL. Posthysterectomy infections. In: Faro S, Soper DE. Infectious Diseases in Women. Philadelphia: WB Saunders; 2001:284-292.

54. DeCenzo JA. Cuff abscess after vaginal hysterectomy. Obstet Gynecol. 1968;31:871.

55. Larsen JW, Hager WD, Livengood CH, Hoyme U. Guidelines for the diagnosis, treatment and prevention of postoperative infections. Infect Dis Obstet Gynecol. 2003;11:65-70.

56. Ledger WJ, Campbell C, Wilson JR. Postoperative adnexal infection. Obstet Gynecol. 1968;31:83-89.

57. Livengood CH, Addison WA. Adnexal abscess as a delayed complication of vaginal hysterectomy. Am J Obstet Gynecol. 1982;143:596-597.

58. Ledger WJ, Moore DE, Lowensohn RI, Gee CL. A fever index evaluation of chloramphenicol or clindamycin in patients with serious pelvic infections. Obstet Gynecol. 1977;50:523-530.

59. Harisinghani MG, Gervais DA, Maher MM, et al. Transgluteal approach for percutaneous drainage of deep pelvic abscesses. Radiology 2003;228:701-705.

60. Ryan RS, McGrath FP, Haslam PJ, et al. Ultrasound-guided endocavitary drainage of pelvic abscesses: Technique, results and complications. Clin Radiol. 2003;58:75-79.

61. Corsi PJ, Johnson SC, Gonik B, et al. Transvaginal ultrasound-guided aspiration of pelvic abscesses. Infect Dis Obstet Gynecol. 1999;7:216-221.

62. Lentz SS. Osteitis pubis: A review. Obstet Gynecol Surv. 1995;50:310-315.

63. Kammerer-Doak DN, Cornella JL, Magrina JF, et al. Osteitis pubis after Marshall-Marchetti-Krantz urethropexy: A pubic osteomyelitis. Am J Obstet Gynecol. 1998;179:586-590.

64. Lupovitch A, Elie JC, Wysocki R. Diagnosis of acute bacterial osteomyelitis of the pubis by means of fine needle aspiration. Acta Cytol. 1989;33:649-651.

65. Sexton DJ, Heskestad L, Lambeth WR, et al. Postoperative pubic osteomyelitis misdiagnosed as osteitis pubis: Report of four cases and review. Clin Infect Dis. 1993;17:695-700.

66. Weidner AC, Cundiff GW, Harris RL, Addison WA. Sacral osteomyelitis: An unusual complication of abdominal sacral colpopexy. Obstet Gynecol. 1997;90:689-691.

67. Eckert LO, Hawes SE, Wolner-Hanssen PK, et al. Endometritis: The clinical-pathologic syndrome. Am J Obstet Gynecol. 2002;186:690-695.

68. Patton DL, Moore DE, Spandoni LR, et al. Comparison of the fallopian tube's response to both overt and silent salpingitis. Obstet Gynecol. 1989;63:622-630.

69. Westrom L, Wolner-Hanssen P. Pathogenesis of pelvic inflammatory disease. Genitourin Med. 1993;69:9-17.

70. Wiesenfeld HC, Hillier SL, Krohn MA, et al. Lower genital tract infection and endometritis: insight into subclinical pelvic inflammatory disease. Obstet Gynecol. 2002;100:456-463.

71. Sweet RL, Draper DL, Schachter J, et al. Microbiology and pathogenesis of acute salpingitis as determined by laparoscopy: What is the appropriate site to sample? Am J Obstet Gynecol. 1980;138:985-989.

72. Soper DE, Brockwell NJ, Dalton HP, Johnson D. Observations concerning the microbial etiology of acute salpingitis. Am J Obstet Gynecol. 1994;170:1008-1017.

73. Hillier SL, Kiviat NB, Hawes SE, et al. Role of bacterial vaginosis-associated microorganisms in endometritis. Am J Obstet Gynecol. 1996;175:435-441.

74. Paavonen J, Lehtinen M, Teisala K, et al. *Haemophilus influenzae* causes purulent salpingitis. Am J Obstet Gynecol. 1985;151:338-339.

75. Monif GR, Williams BT, Dase DF. Group A streptococcus as a cause of endometritis/salpingitis/peritonitis in a nongravid female. Obstet Gynecol. 1977;50:509-510.

76. Washington AE, Aral SO, Wolner-Hanssen P, et al. Assessing the risk for pelvic inflammatory disease and its sequelae. JAMA. 1991;266:2581-2586.

77. Sweet RL. Role of bacterial vaginosis in pelvic inflammatory disease. Clin Infect Dis. 1995;20(Suppl 2):S271-S275.

78. Ness RB, Keder LM, Soper DE, et al. Oral contraception and the recognition of endometritis. Am J Obstet Gynecol. 1997;176:580-585.

79. Sweet RL, Blankfort-Doyle M, Robbie MO, Schachter J. The occurrence of chlamydial and gonococcal salpingitis during the menstrual cycle. JAMA. 1986;255:2062-2064.

80. Ness RB, Soper DE, Holley RL, et al. Douching and endometritis: Results from the PID evaluation and clinical health (PEACH) study. Sex Transm Dis. 2000;28:240-245.

81. Grimes DA. Intrauterine device and upper-genital-tract infection. Lancet. 2000;356:1013-1019.

82. Persson E. Genital actinomycosis and *Actinomyces israelii* in the female genital tract. Adv Contracept. 1987;3:115-123.

83. Bonacho I, Pita S, Gomez-Besteiro MI. The importance of removal of the intrauterine device in genital colonization by actinomyces. Gynecol Obstet Invest. 2001;52:119-123.

84. Krettek JE, Arkin SI, Chaisilwattana P, Monif GR. *Chlamydia trachomatis* in patients who used oral contraceptives and had intermenstrual spotting. Obstet Gynecol. 1993;81:728-731.

85. Yudin MH, Hillier SL, Wiesenfeld HC, et al. Vaginal polymorphonuclear leukocytes and bacterial vaginosis as markers for histologic endometritis among women without symptoms of pelvic inflammatory disease. Am J Obstet Gynecol. 2003;188:318-323.

86. Eschenbach DA, Wolner-Hanssen P, Hawes SE, et al. Acute pelvic inflammatory disease: Associations of clinical and laboratory findings with laparoscopic findings. Obstet Gynecol. 1997;89:184-192.

87. Ness RB, Soper DE, Holley RL, et al. Effectiveness of inpatient and outpatient treatment strategies for women with pelvic inflammatory disease: Results from the Pelvic Inflammatory Disease Evaluation and Clinical Health (PEACH) Randomized Trial. Am J Obstet Gynecol. 2002;186:929-937.

88. Centers for Disease Control and Prevention. Sexually transmitted diseases treatment guidelines 2002. MMWR Morb Mortal Wkly Rep. 2002;51:48-51.

89. Gilstrap LC 3rd, Herbert WN, Cunningham FG, et al. Gonorrhea screening in male consorts of women with pelvic infection. JAMA. 1977;238:965-966.

90. Reed SD, Landers DV, Sweet RL. Antibiotic treatment of tuboovarian abscess: Comparison of broad-spectrum beta-lactam agents versus clindamycin-containing regimens. Am J Obstet Gynecol. 1991;164:1556-1561.

91. McNeeley SG, Hendrix SG, Mazzoni MM, et al. Medically sound, cost-effective treatment of pelvic inflammatory disease and tuboovarian abscess. Am J Obstet Gynecol. 1998;178:1272-1278.

92. Weisenfeld HC, Sweet RL. Progress in the management of tuboovarian abscesses. Clin Obstet Gynecol. 1993;36:433-444.

93. Westrom L. Joesoef R, Reynolds G, et al. Pelvic inflammatory disease and fertility: A cohort study of 1,844 women with laparoscopically verified disease and 657 control women with normal laparoscopic results. Sex Transm Dis. 1992;19:185-192.

94. Scholes D, Stergachis A, Heidrich FE, et al. Prevention of pelvic inflammatory disease by screening for cervical chlamydial infection. N Engl J Med. 1996;334:1362-1366.

Prostatitis, Epididymitis, and Orchitis

JOHN N. KRIEGER

ANATOMY AND PHYSIOLOGY OF THE TESTES AND MALE ACCESSORY SEX ORGANS

The testicle has two functional components, seminiferous tubules and interstitial cells. Sperm production is the primary function of the seminiferous tubules. Interstitial cells, located between the seminiferous tubules, are primarily responsible for hormone production. After spermatogenesis, spermatozoa are transported from the testis into the epididymis (Fig. 105-1). Sperm move into the vas deferens, a muscular tube approximately 12 inches long that is easily palpable in the scrotum. Fructose from the seminal vesicles is the major energy source for ejaculated sperm. In addition, the seminal vesicles provide proteins that coagulate the ejaculate. Liquefaction of the semen occurs 5 to 30 minutes after ejaculation due to proteolytic enzymes from the prostate.

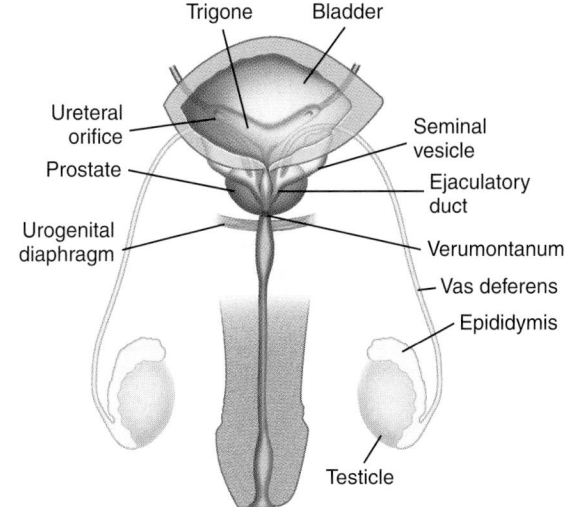

FIGURE 105-1. Anatomy of the male sex organs and lower urinary tract.

HOST DEFENSES OF THE MALE LOWER UROGENITAL TRACT

Organisms that ascend through the urethra cause most infections of the urogenital ducts and accessory sex organs.[1] Mechanical factors, such as the flushing action of micturition and ejaculation, should provide some protection against infection, although the relative significance of these defenses is unclear.

A zinc-containing polypeptide known as the *prostatic antibacterial factor* is the most important antimicrobial substance secreted by the prostate.[1] Men with well-documented chronic bacterial prostatitis have significantly lower levels of zinc in their prostatic fluid than healthy men, but their serum zinc levels are within normal limits. Other findings suggesting that bacterial prostatitis is associated with generalized secretory dysfunction include increased pH of prostatic fluid; reduced calcium, citric acid, and spermine concentrations; and changes in prostatic fluid enzymes. It is unclear whether reduced zinc concentrations precede the development of prostatic infection or represent a secretory dysfunction resulting from such infections. Prostatic secretions of patients with bacterial prostatitis contain high concentrations of immunoglobulins. Several studies have shown antigen-specific antibody coating of bacteria isolated from the lower urinary tracts of patients with prostatitis syndromes. The antigen-specific antibody response in prostatic secretions (predominantly secretory IgA) is significantly greater in magnitude than the serologic response.

The presence of leukocytes is characteristic of many conditions of the male lower urinary tract, including prostatitis. Phagocytosis of abnormal sperm by leukocytes has been observed in infertile men with pyospermia, but the precise role and significance of prostatic fluid leukocytes are uncertain.

PROSTATITIS

Classification

The term *prostatitis* is employed clinically to describe a large group of men with a variety of complaints referable to the lower urogenital tract and perineum. It has been estimated that 50% of men experience symptoms of prostatitis at some time in their lives.[1] Studies suggest that the prevalence of prostatitis is 2% to 16% among men.[2] Among otherwise healthy young men, prostatitis may be the most common urologic diagnosis. A national survey of physician visits found that there were almost 2 million visits annually for prostatitis, accounting for 8% of visits to urologists and 1% of visits to primary care physicians in the United States.[3]

The crucial clinical issue is to distinguish patients with lower urinary tract complaints associated with bacteriuria (i.e., patients who may have acute or chronic bacterial prostatitis) from the larger number of patients without bacteriuria. Further classification of patients with prostatitis depends on careful bacteriologic assessment of the lower urinary tract, which is based on sequential cultures obtained during micturition (Table 105-1). Prostatitis syndromes may be classified into four major groups: acute bacterial prostatitis, chronic bacterial prostatitis, chronic prostatitis/chronic pelvic pain syndrome, and asymptomatic inflammatory prostatitis (Table 105-2).[4] In addition, rare patients develop granulomatous prostatitis.

Bacterial prostatitis is a common diagnosis in clinical practice, but well-documented bacterial infections of the prostate, whether acute or chronic, are uncommon. Most patients with a diagnosis of prostatitis are men with perineal, lower back, or lower abdominal pain or ejaculatory complaints. Most patients have no history of bacteriuria and little objective evidence of bacterial infection of the prostate. Most patients with symptoms of prostatitis may be classified as having chronic prostatitis/chronic pelvic pain syndrome, concerning which there are few firm data on which to base therapeutic decisions.

Acute Bacterial Prostatitis

Acute bacterial prostatitis is seldom a subtle or difficult diagnosis. Patients complain of symptoms associated with lower urinary tract in-

TABLE 105-1 Lower Urinary Tract Localization Using Sequential Urine Cultures[*]

Specimen	Symbol	Description
Voided bladder 1	VB₁	Initial 5-10 mL of urinary stream
Voided bladder 2	VB₂	Midstream specimen
Expressed prostatic secretions	EPS	Secretions expressed from prostate by digital massage
Voided bladder 3	VB3	First 5-10 mL of urinary stream immediately after prostatic massage

[*]Unequivocal diagnosis of bacterial prostatitis requires that the colony count in the VB₃ specimen greatly exceed the count in the VB₁ specimen, preferably by at least 10-fold. Many patients who have chronic bacterial prostatitis harbor only small numbers of bacteria in the prostate, however. In these patients, direct culture of prostatic secretions is particularly useful. Microscopic examination of the EPS is useful for identifying white blood cells and "oval fat bodies"—large lipid-laden macrophages characteristic of the prostatic inflammatory response.

From Stamey T. Pathogenesis and Treatment of Urinary Tract Infections. Baltimore: Williams & Wilkins; 1980.

fection, such as urinary frequency and dysuria. Patients also may experience lower urinary tract obstruction owing to acute edema of the prostate. Signs of systemic toxicity are common. On physical examination, patients may have a high temperature and lower abdominal or suprapubic discomfort due to bladder infection. Findings on rectal examination are frequently impressive, with an exquisitely tender, tense prostate on palpation. Results of urinalysis are abnormal, with pyuria, and cultures are positive. Bacteremia may be present spontaneously or may result from excessively vigorous rectal examinations.

Results of antimicrobial therapy for acute bacterial prostatitis often are dramatic. Many drugs that do not penetrate into the prostate under normal conditions are effective in acute bacterial prostatitis.[1] Drugs that would be appropriate in patients with bacteremia caused by members of the family Enterobacteriaceae, pseudomonads, and enterococci should be administered when specimens have been obtained for urine and blood cultures. Urinary retention is managed best with a suprapubic cystostomy, rather than a transurethral catheter, to avoid obstructing drainage of infected prostatic secretions into the urethra. General measures, including hydration, analgesics, and bed rest, also are indicated. The most important complications of acute bacterial prostatitis are prostatic abscess, prostatic infarction, chronic bacterial prostatitis, and granulomatous prostatitis.

Chronic Bacterial Prostatitis

Chronic bacterial prostatitis is an important cause of bacterial persistence in the male lower urinary tract. Characteristically, patients experience recurrent bacterial urinary tract infections caused by the same organism.[1,4] Patients often are asymptomatic between episodes of bladder bacteriuria. The prostate gland is usually normal on either rectal or endoscopic evaluation. Careful lower urinary tract localization studies constitute the cornerstone on which to base a diagnosis of chronic bacterial prostatitis (see Tables 105-1 and 105-2). Diagnosis of chronic bacterial prostatitis based solely on symptoms, the number of leukocytes in expressed prostatic secretions, or the use of prostate biopsy specimens is inadequate.

Gram-negative rods (members of Enterobacteriaceae or pseudomonads) are the most important pathogens in chronic bacterial prostatitis. Gram-positive cocci, such as *Enterococcus faecalis* or, perhaps, *Staphylococcus saprophyticus,* may be the etiologic organisms in a few cases. Reports implicating many other organisms generally are difficult to evaluate because of methodologic problems with case definition or a lack of documentation of bacteriuria by the alleged pathogen.

Bacteria isolated from patients with chronic bacterial prostatitis, even after multiple episodes of symptomatic bacteriuria and prolonged courses of antibiotics, are generally antibiotic-sensitive strains.[1] *Escherichia coli* strains that cause prostatitis tend, however, to possess

TABLE 105-2   Classification of Prostatitis Syndromes on the Basis of Lower Urinary Tract Localization Studies

Condition	Bacteriuria*	Infection Localized to Prostate†	Inflammatory Response‡	Abnormal Rectal Examination of Prostate§	Systemic Illness∥
Acute bacterial prostatitis	+	+	+	+	+
Chronic bacterial prostatitis	+	+	+	−	−
Chronic prostatitis/chronic pelvic pain syndrome					
Inflammatory subtype¶	−	−	+	−	−
Noninflammatory subtype**	−	−	−	−	−
Asymptomatic inflammatory prostatitis	−	−	+	±	−

*Documented with an identical organism that is shown to localize to a prostatic focus when the midstream urine culture is negative.
†Refer to the text for diagnostic criteria.
‡In expressed prostatic secretions, semen, postmassage urine, or prostate tissue.
§Abnormal findings include exquisite tenderness and swelling that may be associated with signs of lower urinary tract obstruction.
∥Systemic findings frequently include fever and rigors and may include signs of bacteremia.
¶Formerly termed *nonbacterial prostatitis.*
**Formerly termed *prostatodynia.*

urovirulence profiles similar to strains isolated from women with acute pyelonephritis, especially hemolysin and cytotoxic necrotizing factor, with many strains exhibiting multiple virulence factors.[5,6] Several findings can indicate failure of antibiotic therapy in some patients, including poor diffusion of many drugs into the prostatic parenchyma, changes in prostatic fluid pH level associated with infection, and infected calculi, which may serve as persistent foci for bacteria.

Patients with chronic bacterial prostatitis who are not cured may be rendered asymptomatic by long-term, suppressive treatment. Because patients usually are asymptomatic between episodes of bacteriuria, the goal of suppressive therapy is to prevent symptomatic episodes despite the persistence of bacteria in the prostate. Very low doses of agents such as penicillin, tetracycline, nitrofurantoin, nalidixic acid, trimethoprim-sulfamethoxazole, or newer quinolones are remarkably effective in preventing episodes of symptomatic bladder infection in patients with chronic bacterial prostatitis.

Chronic Prostatitis/Chronic Pelvic Pain Syndrome

Patients with chronic prostatitis/chronic pelvic pain syndrome are the largest population of patients with prostatitis, representing more than 90% of patients evaluated. Studies show that chronic prostatitis/chronic pelvic pain syndrome causes substantial morbidity and substantially decreases patients' quality of life.[7] These patients have no history of bacteriuria and lack objective evidence of bacterial infection of their prostatic secretions on careful lower urinary tract localization studies (see Table 105-2). These patients may complain of a variety of perineal and pelvic symptoms, especially pain.[8] Pain or vague discomfort may be perineal, suprapubic, infrapubic, scrotal, or inguinal in location and may be exacerbated by ejaculation. Other complaints include voiding difficulty and erectile dysfunction. The discomfort may be described as either continuous or spasmodic and commonly is described as a "dull ache." Occasional patients complain of increased urinary frequency or dysuria, and ejaculatory complaints are common. Systemic symptoms or signs are usually absent. Physical examination generally is unremarkable. Some patients with chronic prostatitis/chronic pelvic pain syndrome have leukocytes in expressed prostatic secretions, post–prostate massage urine (VB$_3$; see Table 105-1), or semen (in the inflammatory subtype, formerly termed *nonbacterial prostatitis*), whereas others have no objective evidence of inflammation (in the noninflammatory subtype, formerly termed *prostatodynia*; see Table 105-2).[4]

The causes of chronic prostatitis/chronic pelvic pain syndrome are uncertain. Mardh and Colleen[9] and Mardh and associates[10] found no evidence for an etiologic role for *Neisseria gonorrhoeae, Trichomonas vaginalis, Ureaplasma urealyticum, Mycoplasma hominis, Candida albicans,* anaerobic bacteria, *Chlamydia trachomatis,* or viruses in these syndromes. Other researchers have reported, however, that many patients with "subacute or chronic prostatitis" are infected with grampositive bacteria,[11] *C. trachomatis,*[12] or *U. urealyticum.*[13] The techniques, control groups, and findings in these later studies have been questioned by other workers.[1] Molecular studies have shown that pa-

tients with inflammatory chronic prostatitis/chronic pelvic pain syndrome are significantly more likely to have bacterial DNA in prostatic secretions than patients without inflammation[14] or control patients with prostate cancer.[15]

Some authorities have proposed that nonbacterial prostatitis is not an infectious disease. Increased prostaglandins, autoimmunity, psychological abnormalities, neuromuscular dysfunction of the bladder neck or urogenital diaphragm, and allergy to environmental agents all have been suggested as etiologic factors, but supporting data are weak.[16]

Current therapy for symptomatic patients with chronic prostatitis/chronic pelvic pain syndrome is unsatisfactory. The most commonly employed treatments include empirical antimicrobial therapy,[17] α-blockers,[18] and anti-inflammatory therapy.[19] Improving treatment is currently the focus of major research efforts.

Asymptomatic Inflammatory Prostatitis

The new National Institutes of Health consensus classification of prostatitis includes a category for patients who have a diagnosis of prostatitis but who have no genitourinary tract symptoms.[4] These patients have prostate inflammation but have none of the usual symptoms associated with other prostatitis syndromes. It is common for patients with elevated prostate-specific antigen levels to undergo prostate biopsy for evaluation of possible prostate cancer. The most common benign pathologic diagnosis is "prostatitis," based on the histologic finding of inflammatory infiltrates in the prostatic parenchyma. Some clinicians recommend a course of antimicrobial or anti-inflammatory therapy in this situation.[17] These recommendations are based on the observations that acute bacterial prostatitis and exacerbations of chronic bacterial prostatitis are associated with elevations of serum prostate-specific antigen and acid phosphatase. Whether antimicrobial therapy is beneficial for asymptomatic patients with histologic evidence of prostatitis is uncertain. The current consensus is that antimicrobial therapy is not indicated for asymptomatic patients.[20]

Histologic evidence of prostatic inflammation also may be noted in patients with no clinical history of prostatitis who have benign prostate tissue removed during surgical procedures for treatment of bladder outflow obstruction or who have radical prostatectomy for prostate cancer. Asymptomatic inflammatory prostatitis may be diagnosed among men undergoing evaluation for infertility. Many of these men have no genitourinary tract symptoms. On semen analysis, increased numbers of "round cells" may prompt a diagnosis of prostatitis. Other terms used in the infertility literature include *asymptomatic male genital tract infection, male accessory gland infection, prostatoseminal vesiculitis, leukocytospermia,* and *pyosemia (pyospermia).* Some specialists recommend antimicrobial therapy, but the proportion of these patients who have active genital tract infections is poorly defined. It would seem prudent to diagnose a specific genitourinary tract pathogen before recommending antimicrobial therapy for asymptomatic men who present for infertility evaluation.

Animal studies suggest that chronic inflammation may promote prostatic hyperplasia.[21] Epidemiologic studies also suggest that prostatitis may be associated with an increased risk for development of prostate cancer.[22] Confirmation of these potential associations would support efforts to diagnose and treat symptomatic and asymptomatic prostatitis syndromes.

Granulomatous Prostatitis

Granulomatous prostatitis is a characteristic histologic reaction of the prostate to a variety of insults, with granulomas containing lipid-laden histiocytes, plasma cells, and scattered giant cells. In most cases, granulomatous prostatitis follows an episode of acute bacterial prostatitis.[23] There also are many specific infectious causes of granulomatous reaction by the prostate. Tuberculous prostatitis usually is secondary to tuberculosis elsewhere in the genital tract. Most patients have no symptoms referable to prostatic infection. At biopsy, the granulomas may contain typical Langerhans giant cells and exhibit caseous necrosis. These infections are caused most often by *Mycobacterium tuberculosis,* but also have been reported with nontuberculous mycobacteria. Iatrogenic mycobacterial prostatitis may develop in patients who receive intravesicular Calmette-Guérin bacillus for treatment of transitional cell carcinoma of the bladder.[24] Prostatitis may be secondary to systemic involvement with many of the deep mycoses.[25] Most cases of mycotic prostatitis reported have been associated with blastomycosis, coccidioidomycosis, and cryptococcosis. The prostate may be a focus of persistent cryptococcosis in patients with acquired immunodeficiency syndrome (AIDS). Rarely, prostatic histoplasmosis occurs in these patients.

Granulomatous prostatitis is most important in the differential diagnosis for an indurated, firm, or nodular prostate. Findings on rectal examination in these patients raise the suspicion of prostatic carcinoma. Biopsy usually is necessary for diagnosis, and it is important that appropriate stains and culture be used for the detection of specific etiologic agents.

Prostatic Abscess

Prostatic abscess is a rare complication in patients who receive appropriate treatment for acute bacterial prostatitis.[26] Most prostatic abscesses occur in patients with diabetes, in immunocompromised patients, and in patients who have not received appropriate therapy for acute prostatitis. Foreign bodies and urinary tract obstruction are other predisposing factors. In the past, *N. gonorrhoeae* was a common pathogen, but most cases now are caused by the common uropathogens. Infection generally occurs by the ascending route.[26] Occasionally, *S. aureus* is the pathogen, which suggests the possibility of hematogenous infection. Infection with fungi, mycobacteria, and other granuloma-causing organisms is more common in immunocompromised patients.

Patients are usually febrile with irritative and obstructive voiding symptoms, and they may have signs of urosepsis. The clinical presentation closely resembles that of acute bacterial prostatitis. Classically the abscess presents as a fluctuant area in the prostate palpated during rectal examination. The presentation may be subtle, however. Ultrasonography, computed tomography, or magnetic resonance imaging of the pelvis is helpful for confirming the diagnosis or in patients with equivocal clinical findings. Treatment includes draining the abscess, through either a perineal or a transurethral route, and appropriate antimicrobial therapy.

EPIDIDYMITIS

Epididymitis is an inflammatory reaction of the epididymis to a variety of infectious agents or to local trauma. Epididymitis is common, accounting for more than 600,000 visits to physicians per year in the United States. Acute epididymitis is responsible for more days lost from military service than any other disease and is responsible for 20% of urologic hospital admissions in military populations.[27]

Patients with epididymitis usually complain of painful swelling of the scrotum. The onset may be acute over 1 or 2 days or more gradual and often is accompanied by dysuria or irritative lower urinary tract symptoms. Many patients have a urethral discharge. Specific attention should be directed toward eliciting a past history of genitourinary tract disease or sexual exposure. Some patients may have only a nonspecific

finding of fever or other signs of infection. This presentation is particularly common in hospitalized patients who have undergone recent urinary tract manipulation and who may be obtunded by medication.

Tender swelling, frequently accompanied by erythema, generally unilateral, may be noted primarily in the posterior aspect of the scrotum. If the patient is examined early in the course of the disease, the swelling may be localized to one portion of the epididymis. Later, involvement of the ipsilateral testis is common, producing an epididymo-orchitis, and it may be difficult to distinguish the testicle from the epididymis within the inflammatory mass. Scrotal examination commonly reveals the presence of a hydrocele, caused by the secretion of inflammatory fluid between the layers of the tunica vaginalis. Urethral discharge may be apparent on inspection or "stripping" of the urethra.

There are two common types of epididymitis: nonspecific bacterial epididymitis and sexually transmitted epididymitis. Epididymitis also may occur rarely after genital trauma or with disseminated infections.

Nonspecific Bacterial Epididymitis

The most common cause of epididymitis in men older than age 35 years is infection with coliform species or *Pseudomonas* spp.[28] In most series, gram-negative aerobic rods caused more than two thirds of the cases of bacterial epididymitis. Gram-positive cocci also are important pathogens, however, and were the most common organisms in some reports.

Many patients who develop bacterial epididymitis have underlying urologic pathology or have a history of recent genitourinary tract manipulation. Urologic abnormalities are especially common in children who present with epididymitis.[29] The development of epididymitis after surgery or urethral catheterization may occur weeks or rarely months after the manipulation. Epididymitis is particularly likely in patients who undergo urinary tract surgery or instrumentation while they are bacteriuric. Acute and chronic bacterial prostatitis is another important predisposing condition for the development of bacterial epididymitis.

Bacterial epididymitis may be an important focus of organisms causing bacteremia and local morbidity in patients with indwelling transurethral catheters. Genitourinary tract complications of acute bacterial epididymitis include testicular infarction, scrotal abscess, pyocele, a chronic draining scrotal sinus, chronic epididymitis, and infertility.[30]

Tuberculous epididymitis is the most common manifestation of male genital tuberculosis, with orchitis and prostatitis seen less commonly.[31] The usual symptom is a sensation of heaviness or swelling. There is characteristic scrotal swelling with "beadlike" enlargement of the vas deferens. Chronic draining scrotal sinuses may be a feature. The systemic mycoses rarely may cause epididymitis; blastomycetes are the most common pathogen and may cause a draining sinus through the scrotal wall. Iatrogenic cases of epididymitis and orchitis may complicate bacille Calmette-Guérin therapy for transitional cell carcinoma of the bladder.

Medical management is appropriate for most patients with bacterial epididymitis. Initial empirical treatment with agents appropriate for gram-negative rods and gram-positive cocci should be initiated pending urine culture and sensitivity results. Nonspecific measures, such as bed rest, scrotal elevation, analgesics, and local ice packs, are helpful. Surgery may be necessary for management of complications of acute epididymal infections, such as testicular infarction, abscess, or pyocele of the scrotum.

Sexually Transmitted Epididymitis

Sexually transmitted epididymitis is the most common type of epididymitis in young men. *C. trachomatis* and *N. gonorrhoeae* are the major pathogens in this population.[32] Chlamydiae have been identified as the most common cause of epididymitis in younger, sexually active populations. These patients formerly were considered to have "idiopathic," nonspecific epididymitis. Berger and co-workers[33] documented infections with *C. trachomatis* in 17 of 34 cases of epididymitis in patients younger than 35 years old and in only 1 of 16 cases of epididymitis in patients older than 35. Patients with chlamydial epididymitis frequently do not complain of urethral discharge. Eleven of 17 patients with epididymitis caused by chlamydiae had demonstrable discharge, however, usually the scant, watery discharge characteristic of nonspecific urethritis. The median interval from the last sexual exposure was 10 days (range 1 to 45 days). Patients may carry chlamydiae for long periods before the development of overt epididymitis.

Before the availability of penicillin, it was estimated that epididymitis occurred in 10% to 30% of men with gonococcal urethritis. In more recent studies, *N. gonorrhoeae* was identified as the cause of acute epididymitis in 16% of cases in military populations[34] and in 21% of cases in civilians younger than 35 years old.[33] Many patients with gonococcal epididymitis do not have a history of urethral discharge, and a discharge may be demonstrable in only 50% of such patients.

Underlying genitourinary tract abnormalities are uncommon in patients with sexually transmitted epididymitis. Diagnosis depends on a high index of clinical suspicion, evaluation for presence of urethritis (which may be asymptomatic), and appropriate diagnostic tests. Specific antibiotic therapy, generally employing drugs appropriate for chlamydial and gonococcal infections, is the most important aspect of treatment.[32] Patients should be evaluated for other sexually transmitted diseases, and treatment of sexual partners is important. In general, a complete urologic workup is not indicated for patients with uncomplicated sexually transmitted epididymitis. Complications of sexually transmitted epididymitis include abscess formation, testicular infarction, chronic epididymitis, and infertility. Ultrasonography, particularly color-flow Doppler ultrasonography, is useful for the differential diagnosis of complicated cases of epididymitis.[35]

Follow-up

Failure of the signs and symptoms of epididymitis to subside within 3 days requires re-evaluation of the diagnosis and the therapy.[32] Persistent swelling and tenderness after completion of therapy suggest the need for comprehensive evaluation. Considerations in the differential diagnosis include abscess, infarction, testicular cancer, and tuberculous or fungal epididymitis.

ORCHITIS

Orchitis is significantly less common than either prostatitis or epididymitis. Orchitis differs from infections of the male accessory sex glands in two important respects: Blood-borne dissemination is the major route of infection, and viruses are implicated as important pathogens.

Viral Orchitis

Viral infections, particularly mumps, are associated with most cases of orchitis. Although mumps rarely causes orchitis in prepubertal boys, orchitis occurs in approximately 20% of postpubertal patients with mumps.[36] Testicular pain and swelling usually begin 4 to 6 days after the onset of parotitis but may occur without parotid involvement. Orchitis is unilateral in approximately 70% of cases. Contralateral testicular swelling may occur 1 to 9 days after involvement of the first side. The clinical course is variable and ranges from mild testicular discomfort and swelling to severe testicular pain and marked swelling accompanied by nausea, vomiting, prostration, high fever, and constitutional symptoms. Epididymitis and inflammation of the spermatic cord may be noted on physical examination. Resolution of mild cases may occur in 4 to 5 days. More severe cases usually resolve in 3 to 4 weeks. In approximately half of cases, the involved testes undergo some degree of atrophy. In older series, sterility was reported in 25% of patients with bilateral disease. More recent studies have found, however, that mumps orchitis seldom results in infertility.[37] Coxsackie B virus produces a disease that clinically and histologically resembles mumps orchitis.

Infection with lymphocytic choriomeningitis virus occasionally can result in orchitis, which develops 1 to 3 weeks after the onset of the initial fever. Orchitis is usually unilateral and painful. Most cases resolve within 2 weeks.[38]

Bacterial Orchitis

With the exception of viral diseases, acute genitourinary tract infections involving only the testis are distinctly unusual. Pyogenic bacterial orchitis usually occurs because of the contiguous spread from an inflammatory process in the epididymis to cause an epididymoorchitis. Most cases of pyogenic orchitis are caused by *E. coli, Klebsiella pneumoniae, Pseudomonas aeruginosa,* staphylococci, or streptococci. Occasionally, acute orchitis may be caused by other organisms as a result of metastatic seeding. This seeding seems to be a particular risk with brucellosis in endemic areas.[39]

A patient with pyogenic orchitis appears acutely ill, with a high fever and marked discomfort and swelling of the involved testicle. Generally the pain is described as radiating to the inguinal canal, and it frequently is accompanied by nausea and vomiting. On examination, there is usually an acute hydrocele. The testis is swollen and exquisitely tender. The overlying scrotal skin is generally erythematous and edematous. Complications of pyogenic bacterial orchitis include testicular infarction, abscess formation, and pyocele of the scrotum. Surgery usually is required for treatment of these conditions. Orchitis can be caused by tuberculosis and blastomycosis, usually by extension from the epididymis. Involvement of the testicle without palpable abnormality in the adjacent epididymis rarely has been observed with these agents.

PROSTATITIS, EPIDIDYMITIS, AND ORCHITIS IN MEN WITH HUMAN IMMUNODEFICIENCY VIRUS TYPE 1 INFECTION

One study of 140 autopsied AIDS patients found that 2 of 17 cases with systemic toxoplasmosis and 4 of 65 cases of systemic cytomegalovirus infection involved the testes.[40] Other opportunistic infections involving the male genital tract include those due to atypical mycobacteria, cryptococcosis, toxoplasmosis, *Haemophilus parainfluenzae* infections, candidiasis, and *Aspergillus fumigatus* infections. The testes characteristically exhibit azoospermia, marked spermatogenic arrest, germ cell degeneration, peritubular fibrosis, and Leydig cell depletion. These nonspecific findings probably reflect the severe systemic disease in these patients.

Urologic Manifestations

Other urologic manifestations in patients with AIDS and human immunodeficiency virus type 1 (HIV-1) infections reflect involvement of related organ systems. Bladder dysfunction may occur in patients with HIV-1–associated neurologic disorders. This bladder dysfunction increases the risk of urinary tract infection. Urinary tract infections were diagnosed in 14% to 20% of HIV-1–seropositive patients.[41] In another study, bacterial prostatitis was diagnosed in 17 (8%) of 209 men hospitalized for treatment of HIV-1–related infections.[42] The most common presentation of prostatitis was fever plus irritative lower tract symptoms associated with bacteriuria.

Semen as a Vector for Human Immunodeficiency Virus

The relative contributions of behavioral and clinical risk factors to transmission of HIV-1 are incompletely understood, but sexual activity alone provides a limited explanation for transmission of HIV. Expressing risk as a function of frequency and types of sexual contacts has not yielded straightforward patterns; this probably reflects biologic factors that determine infectiousness and the vulnerable partner's susceptibility. Stage of disease and viral load; viral characteristics, such as syncytium-inducing capability; and antiviral treatment have been linked to greater and lesser degrees of infectivity.

Studies suggest that treating other sexually transmitted diseases reduces sexual transmission of HIV.[43] Sexually transmitted infections are believed to increase susceptibility to HIV infection by recruiting target cells and disrupting epithelial barriers. In addition, genital ulcer diseases and urethritis (gonococcal and nongonococcal) increase the HIV viral load in semen. In contrast, sexually transmitted disease treatment reduces HIV shedding.

Epidemiologic studies suggest that direct contact with semen is the most important route for sexual transmission of HIV-1. HIV-1 first was isolated by cocultivation of seminal cells and donor lymphocytes.[44] Shedding of HIV-1 in semen was associated with no significant changes in semen parameters that assess fertility in one study of 50 semen specimens from asymptomatic or minimally symptomatic HIV-1–seropositive men.[45] In contrast, three men with AIDS all had pyospermia and grossly abnormal sperm. Abnormalities in the semen of HIV-1–seropositive men reflect severity of disease and therapies that are toxic to the seminiferous epithelium but do not correlate with seminal shedding of HIV-1.

Semen is composed of cell-free seminal plasma and seminal cells (mature spermatozoa, immature sperm forms, leukocytes, and epithelial cells). Two approaches have been used to determine the likely sources of HIV within the semen. The first approach is to fractionate and analyze ejaculated semen specimens.[46] These studies suggest that most viable (i.e., culturable) HIV in semen is cell associated, particularly with T lymphocytes and macrophages, but not with motile spermatozoa. The second approach is anatomic, based on the observations that vasectomy causes dramatic reductions in seminal cells and eliminates secretions from proximal sites in the male reproductive tract.[47] HIV RNA was assayed in seminal plasma and HIV DNA in seminal cells from 46 asymptomatic, seropositive men before and after vasectomy. Vasectomy produced no significant change in HIV RNA or HIV DNA levels, supporting the conclusion that most seminal HIV is not associated with germinal cells but arises from distal sites in the male reproductive tract.

Several lines of evidence support the idea that the male genital tract may be distinct from the systemic immune compartment.[48] Qualitative and quantitative virologic measurements between blood and genital compartments suggest lack of association between culturability of virus in semen and viral RNA level in blood, discordant distribution of phenotypes, discordant viral RNA levels, a weak correlation between viral RNA level in semen and CD4+ cell count in blood, differences in the biologic variability of viral RNA levels, and differences in the viral load response to antiretroviral therapy.[48] Phylogenetic studies also support the concept of compartmentalization.[49] Some, but not all,[50] studies suggest a weak correlation between HIV-1 RNA levels in the blood plasma and HIV RNA levels in the seminal plasma. Neither HIV-1 RNA blood level nor the CD4+ count reliably predicts either shedding of culturable virus or detection of viral RNA in the semen, however.[48] Factors that may influence the HIV viral load in seminal fluid include systemic illness, antiretroviral therapy, urethritis, male genital tract inflammation, reactivation of genital herpesvirus infection, and seminal shedding of cytomegalovirus or other viruses. If the male reproductive tract is a distinct immunologic compartment, factors determining infectiousness of semen may differ substantially from the factors determining HIV levels in blood, lymphatic tissue, or central nervous system.

REFERENCES

1. Stamey T. Pathogenesis and Treatment of Urinary Tract Infections. Baltimore: Williams & Wilkins; 1980.
2. Cheah P, Liong M, Yuen K, et al. Chronic prostatitis: Symptom survey with follow-up clinical evaluation. Urology. 2003;61:60-64.
3. McNaughton-Collins M, Stafford RS, O'Leary MP, Barry MJ. How common is prostatitis? A national survey of physician visits. J Urol. 1998;159:1224-1228.
4. Krieger JN, Nyberg L Jr, Nickel JC. NIH consensus definition and classification of prostatitis. JAMA. 1999;282:236-237.
5. Andreu A, Fernandez F, Stamm WE. Urovirulence determinants in *Escherichia coli* strains causing prostatitis. J Infect Dis. 1997;176:464-469.
6. Ishitoya S, Yamamoto S, Kanamaru S, et al. Distribution of afaE adhesins in *Escherichia coli* isolated from Japanese patients with urinary tract infection. J Urol. 2003;169:1758-1761.
7. McNaughton-Collins M. The impact of chronic prostatitis/chronic pelvic pain syndrome on patients. World J Urol. 2003;21:86-89.
8. Litwin MS, McNaughton-Collins M, Fowler FJ Jr, et al. The National Institutes of Health chronic prostatitis symptom index: Development and validation of a new outcome measure. Chronic Prostatitis Collaborative Research Network. J Urol. 1999;162:369-375.
9. Mardh PA, Colleen S. Search for uro-genital tract infections in patients with symptoms of prostatitis. Scand J Urol Nephrol. 1975;9:8.
10. Mardh PA, Ripa KT, Colleen S, et al. Role of *Chlamydia trachomatis* in nonacute prostatitis. Br J Vener Dis. 1978;54:330.
11. Nickel JC, Costerton JW. Coagulase-negative staphylococcus in chronic prostatitis. J Urol. 1992;147:398-401.
12. Weidner W, Arens M, Krauss H, et al. *Chlamydia trachomatis* in 'abacterial' prostatitis: Microbiological, cytological and serological studies. Urol Int. 1983;38:146-149.
13. Weidner W, Brunner H, Krause W. Quantitative culture of *Ureaplasma urealyticum* in patients with chronic prostatitis or prostatosis. J Urol. 1980;124:622-625.
14. Krieger JN, Riley DE. Bacteria in the chronic prostatitis-chronic pelvic pain syndrome: Molecular approaches to critical research questions. J Urol. 2002;167:2574-2583.
15. Krieger JN, Riley DE, Vesella RL, et al. Bacterial DNA sequences in prostate tissue from patients with prostate cancer and chronic prostatitis. J Urol. 2000;164:1221-1228.
16. Alexander RB, Brady F, Ponniah S. Autoimmune prostatitis: Evidence of T cell reactivity with normal prostatic proteins. Urology. 1997;50:893-899.
17. Nickel JC, Downey J, Johnston B, et al. Predictors of patient response to antibiotic therapy for the chronic prostatitis/chronic pelvic pain syndrome: A prospective multicenter clinical trial. J Urol. 2001;165:1539-1544.
18. Cheah P, Liong M, Yuen K, et al. Terazocin therapy for chronic prostatitis/chronic pelvic pain syndrome: A prospective randomized clinical trial. J Urol. 2003;169:592-596.
19. Nickel JC, Pontari M, Moon T, et al. A randomized, placebo controlled, multicenter study to evaluate the safety and efficacy of rofecoxib in the treatment of chronic nonbacterial prostatitis. J Urol. 2003;169:1401-1405.
20. Wagenlehner FM, Naber KG. Prostatitis: The role of antibiotic treatment. World J Urol. 2003;21:105-108.
21. Kessler OJ, Keiseri Y, Servadio C, Abramovici A. Role of chronic inflammation in the promotion of prostatic hyperplasia in rats. J Urol. 1998;159:1049-1053.
22. Dennis LK, Lynch CF, Torner JC. Epidemiologic association between prostatitis and prostate cancer. Urology. 2002;60:78-83.
23. Stillwell TJ, Engen DE, Farrow GM. The clinical spectrum of granulomatous prostatitis: A report of 200 cases. J Urol. 1987;138:320-323.
24. LaFontaine PD, Middleman BR, Graham SD Jr, Sanders WH. Incidence of granulomatous prostatitis and acid-fast bacilli after intravesical BCG therapy. Urology. 1997;49:363-366.
25. Schwarz J. Mycotic prostatitis. Urology. 1982;19:1-5.
26. Weinberger M, Cytron S, Servadio C, et al. Prostatic abscess in the antibiotic era. Rev Infect Dis. 1988;10:239-249.
27. Bormel P. Current concepts on the etiology and treatment of epididymitis. Med Bull US Army Europe. 1963;20:332.
28. Berger RE, Alexander ER, Monda GD, et al. *Chlamydia trachomatis* as a cause of acute "idiopathic" epididymitis. N Engl J Med. 1978;298:301-304.
29. Mushtaq I, Fung M, Glasson MJ. Retrospective review of paediatric patients with acute scrotum. Aust N Z J Surg. 2003;73:55.
30. Witherington R, Harper WMT. The surgical management of acute bacterial epididymitis with emphasis on epididymotomy. J Urol. 1982;128:722-725.
31. Ferrie BG, Rundle JS. Tuberculous epididymo-orchitis: A review of 20 cases. Br J Urol. 1983;55:437-439.
32. Centers for Disease Control and Prevention. Sexually transmitted diseases treatment guidelines 2002. MMWR Recomm Rep. 2002;51:1-78.
33. Berger RE, Alexander ER, Harnisch JP, et al. Etiology, manifestations and therapy of acute epididymitis: Prospective study of 50 cases. J Urol. 1979;121:750-754.
34. Watson RA. Gonorrhea and acute epididymitis. Milit Med. 1979;144:785.
35. Yang DM, Kim SH, Kim HN, et al. Differential diagnosis of focal epididymal lesions with gray scale sonographic, color Doppler sonographic, and clinical features. J Ultrasound Med. 2003;22:135-144.
36. Galazka AM, Robertson SE, Kraigher A. Mumps and mumps vaccine: A global review. Bull World Health Organ. 1999;77:3-14.
37. Beard CM, Benson RC Jr, Kelalis PP, et al. The incidence and outcome of mumps orchitis in Rochester, Minnesota, 1935 to 1974. Mayo Clin Proc. 1977;52:3-7.
38. Lewis JM, Utz JP. Orchitis, parotitis and meningoencephalitis due to lymphocytic choriomeningitis virus. N Engl J Med. 1961;265:776-780.
39. Kadikoylu G, Tuncer G, Bolaman Z, Sina M. Brucellar orchitis in Innerwest Anatolia region of Turkey: A report of 12 cases. Urol Int. 2002;69:33-35.
40. Shevchuk MM, Pigato JB, Khalife G, et al. Changing testicular histology in AIDS: Its implication for sexual transmission of HIV. Urology 1999;53:203-208.
41. Miles BJ, Melser M, Farah R, et al. The urological manifestations of the acquired immunodeficiency syndrome. J Urol. 1989;142:771-773.
42. Kaplan MS, Wechsler M, Benson MC. Urologic manifestations of AIDS. Urology. 1987;30:441-443.
43. Cohen MS, Hoffman IF, Royce RA, et al. Reduction of concentration of HIV-1 in semen after treatment of urethritis: Implications for prevention of sexual transmission of HIV-1. Lancet. 1997;349:1868-1873.
44. Ho DD, Schooley R, Rota T, et al. HTLV-III in the semen and blood of a healthy homosexual man. Science. 1984;226:451.
45. Krieger JN, Coombs RW, Collier AC, et al. Fertility parameters in men infected with human immunodeficiency virus. J Infect Dis. 1991;164:464-469.
46. Quayle AJ, Xu C, Mayer KH, Anderson DJ. T lymphocytes and macrophages, but not motile spermatozoa, are a significant source of human immunodeficiency virus in semen. J Infect Dis. 1997;176:960-968.
47. Krieger JN, Nirapathpongporn A, Chaiyaporn M, et al. Vasectomy and human immunodeficiency virus type 1 in semen. J Urol. 1998;159:820-826.
48. Coombs RW, Speck CE, Hughes JP, et al. Association between culturable human immunodeficiency virus type 1 (HIV-1) in semen and HIV-1 RNA levels in semen and blood: Evidence for compartmentalization of HIV-1 between semen and blood. J Infect Dis. 1998;177:320-330.
49. Paranjpe S, Craigo J, Patterson B, et al. Subcompartmentalization of HIV-1 quasispecies between seminal cells and seminal plasma indicates their origin in distinct genital tissues. AIDS Res Hum Retroviruses. 2002;18:1271-1280.
50. Kalichman SC, Cage M, Barnett T, et al. Human immunodeficiency virus in semen and plasma: investigation of sexual transmission risk behavioral correlates. AIDS Res Hum Retroviruses. 2001;17:1695-1703.

CHAPTER **106**

Microbial
Conjunctivitis

SCOTT D. BARNES

DEBORAH PAVAN-LANGSTON

DIMITRI T. AZAR

CONJUNCTIVITIS

Conjunctivitis affects people of all ages and is seen in all geographic locations; it is the most common inflammation of the eye and ocular adnexa.[1] The various forms of conjunctivitis caused by viruses, chlamydia, bacteria, parasites, fungi, and antigens tend to share a number of signs and symptoms, but there are some clinical differences that suggest the appropriate identification and treatment. The patient's history often provides the diagnosis, which may then be confirmed through clinical examination and possibly laboratory evaluation. Different agents cause acute versus chronic conjunctivitis. Onset within 4 weeks before presentation is classified as acute disease.

ANATOMY AND PHYSIOLOGY

The inner surface of the eyelid is covered by a mucous membrane called the conjunctiva. This membrane lining the lids (palpebral conjunctiva) is reflected on itself, forming an inferior and superior cul-de-sac, or fornix, as it then covers the surface of the globe (bulbar conjunctiva) and extends to the edge of the cornea (limbus). These fornices form a physical barrier that prevents a foreign body (e.g., contact lens) from actually becoming "lost" behind the globe. In addition to connecting the lids to the globe, the conjunctiva produces mucus for the tear film and provides protection of the ocular surface from pathogens; the latter is accomplished via resident immune tissue.

The conjunctiva is made up of a superficial epithelial layer overlying the substantia propria. The conjunctival epithelium possesses goblet cells, unique among stratified, nonkeratinized epithelia. These goblet cells are responsible for most of the mucin production in the tear film. Corneal stem cells are known to exist at the limbus, and a similar search for conjunctival stem cells has produced interesting results. Conjunctival cells with stem-like activity have been identified in rabbits, and subdermal injection of clonal cultures of conjunctival epithelium in nude mice has produced cysts with goblet cells and stratified epithelium, suggesting pluripotency that seems to give rise to both cell types.[1a,2] The connective tissue of the substantia propria is loose and highly vascularized, properties that allow for the rather dramatic clinical appearances of significant edema and injection. Abundant numbers of lymphocytes, mast cells, plasma cells, and neutrophils are found throughout the connective tissue.[3] This lymphoid tissue does not form actual lymph nodes; however, its abundance, combined with the phagocytic properties of the conjunctival epithelium, demonstrates the nature of this tissue in dealing with infectious organisms.[4]

CLINICAL PRESENTATION

History and Physical Examination

Particular attention should be paid to the time course of the condition, any inciting events, prior and current medication use, and the patient's own report of the associated symptoms. The physical examination focuses on the appearance of the periorbital skin as well as other mucous membranes (e.g., nasal, oral), unilaterality/bilaterality, the appearance of the conjunctiva, the associated discharge, and any specific facial, lid, and corneal involvement.

Eye Pain

In contrast to keratitis, ocular pain is not common with most forms of conjunctivitis. There is usually some degree of irritation, most commonly described as a foreign body sensation. Although uncommon in most forms of conjunctivitis, the presence of ulcerated lesions in the eyelid and conjunctiva in herpetic, smallpox, and vaccinia conjunctivitis may be quite painful. If the conjunctival process secondarily affects the cornea, eye pain may also become more prominent. Therefore, the presence of significant eye pain should prompt a more thorough search for lid/corneal involvement or intraocular inflammation.

Itching

Almost all patients with conjunctivitis complain of variable ocular burning and itching. However, severe itching tends to be a hallmark of the allergic and toxic causes of conjunctivitis. In addition to the resident lymphoid tissue, the conjunctiva has plentiful immunoglobulin E and mast cells. Degranulation of mast cells and histamine release in response to an inciting antigen are responsible for the significant itching.

Visual Acuity

Visual acuity is usually normal or mildly decreased with conjunctivitis. Unless the cornea has become secondarily involved, vision is preserved. The ocular irritation and discharge may affect the ability to read an eye chart; a topical anesthetic agent and surface irrigation may improve the office examination of vision. A reduction in vision should prompt a search for an associated cause other than the conjunctivitis.

Periocular and Periorbital Skin

Some cases of conjunctivitis have associated skin changes. Skin lesions typical in poxviruses, immune-mediated diseases (Stevens-Johnson syndrome), and herpetic conditions are usually not difficult to recognize; however, a close examination may help identify causes that produce less obvious skin findings. Subtle vesicular changes on the lid margin may be the only sign of an otherwise unimpressive herpetic conjunctivitis. Numerous lesions in molluscum contagiosum provide an easy diagnosis, but small, isolated lesions may be missed if they are buried near the lash margin. Ocular rosacea is quite common and usually bilateral, but caution must be used in unilateral cases, because sebaceous gland carcinoma can manifest in such a fashion. Allergic conjunctivitis incited by antigens such as cosmetics, soaps, lotions, and some medications often has a typical periocular dermal manifestation.

Conjunctival Hyperemia

The rich network of subepithelial vessels that runs throughout the conjunctiva becomes markedly dilated and congested. Against the background of the relatively avascular sclera, this hyperemia appears quite impressive. On closer examination, the hyperemia appears greater near the periphery than in the limbal region (near the corneal border). Saccular aneurysms, petechiae, and subconjunctival or intraconjunctival hemorrhages may be present.

Discharge

Ocular secretion is almost universal in conjunctivitis. Excessive tearing results from either increased lacrimation or impaired lacrimal outflow.

Increased mucin production, especially relative to the aqueous component of the tear film, is a common finding. Exudation from the conjunctival surface contains varying proportions of protein and cellular debris. A serous exudation is mainly proteinaceous; a purulent exudate is more cellular (e.g., leukocytes, fibrin). The combination of proteins, fibrin, mucin, and sloughed epithelial cells can be copious depending on the cause of the inflammation. Significant matting and "sticking together" of the eyelashes is common.

Conjunctival Edema (Chemosis) and Conjunctivochalasis

The loosely adherent subepithelial connective tissue allows the conjunctiva a rather impressive degree of edema. Hemodynamic changes and altered vascular integrity allow transudation through fenestrated capillaries, resulting in chemosis. This edema can be so prominent that the conjunctiva appears to be "bulging" out from between the eyelids, and it may indeed cause exposure if the eyelids cannot adequately close. Depending on the inciting agent, the chemosis may become hemorrhagic. Acute chemosis is often self-limited, but chronic chemosis can lead to conjunctivochalasis, or laxity of the conjunctiva, with resultant redundancy sometimes draping over the lower lid margin.

Conjunctival Papillae

The palpebral conjunctiva contains connective tissue septa that provide anchorage for the tarsus (dense connective tissue providing strength to eyelids). Conjunctival inflammation may result in dilated subepithelial blood vessels that become surrounded by an infiltrate of mixed inflammatory cells (e.g., neutrophils, lymphocytes). This edema produces elevated mounds of conjunctival epithelium, with the septa restricting diffusion beyond the fibrovascular core. The mounds, or "papillae," have a central red dot corresponding to the dilated capillary viewed from above. A mild papillary reaction has a velvety appearance; increasing severity or chronicity may lead to enlarged, cobblestone-like papillae. Mucus and purulent material may collect within the furrows between adjacent papillae. The conjunctiva beyond the tarsus is less likely to reveal papillae, because the septal connections decrease toward the fornices. With prolonged or recurrent inflammation, the septal anchors may weaken to the point at which the papillae appear reduced because of confluence. Although papillae are fairly nonspecific, they appear more commonly in cases of bacterial and allergic conjunctivitis. They are usually much less than 1 mm in size, but giant papillae of 1 to 2 mm may be seen in association with contact lenses, ocular prostheses, or exposed sutures.

Conjunctival Follicles

Lymphoid tissue is normally present within the substantia propria of the conjunctiva except in the neonate, in whom follicles are not visible. Conjunctival follicles are small, elevated clusters of lymphocytes. Small follicles can be observed in the noninflamed conjunctiva, especially in the lower fornix, and clusters of noninflamed follicles have been observed in children and adolescents in a condition called benign lymphoid folliculosis.[5] Follicles associated with conjunctivitis are new, inflamed, and enlarged. There is a similar elevated appearance to conjunctival papillae; however, there is no central vascular core. The vessels surround and peripherally encroach on the raised follicle, with the central lymphocytes and other mononuclear cells often obscuring the vessels. Except in giant papillary conjunctivitis, follicles are larger than papillae. Follicles often have a smooth, glistening surface and are most commonly seen near the tarsus, although their presence has been described on the bulbar and limbal conjunctiva.[6] Like papillae, follicles are a nonspecific sign, but they are most commonly associated with viral, chlamydial, and toxic conjunctivitis.

Membranes and Pseudomembranes

Inflammatory coagulum may coalesce, forming a yellowish-white membrane overlying the palpebral conjunctiva. If the fibrinous layer is intertwined with the conjunctiva via granulation tissue, it is a true membrane and will cause bleeding when removed. Pseudomembranes have a similar appearance but are not as adherent and do not bleed when removed. Viral and bacterial causes of conjunctivitis have an increased likelihood of such membrane formation, although the presence of a membrane does not rule out other causes.

Conjunctival Phlyctenules and Granulomas

A phlyctenule is a whitish, nodular collection of chronic inflammatory cells located at or near the limbus, often in the center of a hyperemic area. This represents a delayed hypersensitivity reaction generally associated with *Staphylococcus* species or tuberculosis. However, it can rarely be associated with coccidioidomycosis, candidiasis, lymphogranuloma venereum, or parasitic conjunctivitis.

Although a granulomatous nodule of chronic inflammatory cells with a fibrovascular proliferation is a classic finding in Parinaud's oculoglandular conjunctivitis, it is not common with most types of conjunctivitis. A conjunctival granuloma is more indicative of an embedded foreign body or a granulomatous disease (e.g., sarcoidosis, tuberculosis), but it may be seen with chlamydial and fungal conjunctivitis.

Corneal Involvement

Because of the close proximity of the conjunctiva to the cornea, it is not surprising to see extension of the conjunctival inflammation. Corneal involvement can be as mild as punctate epithelial erosions or as severe as frank ulceration that may lead to perforation. A number of bacterial agents that can cause conjunctivitis may penetrate an intact corneal epithelium. Foreign body sensation, pain, decreased vision, and photophobia are all signs of corneal involvement; however, many of these signs are present with the inciting conjunctivitis alone. The corneal involvement, especially with viral causes, may quickly improve with the resolution of the conjunctivitis; however, some associations can lead to undesired sequelae. Continued vigilance, a high index of suspicion, and appropriate treatment of corneal involvement are necessary.

Preauricular Adenopathy

The lymphatic vessels of the eyelids drain primarily to the preauricular lymph node. The medial third of the lids and the conjunctiva drain to the submandibular and submental lymph nodes. Preauricular adenopathy is also a nonspecific finding, but it is often present with viral, chlamydial, herpetic, and gonococcal causes of conjunctivitis and may be absent in toxic, allergic, and nongonococcal bacterial conjunctivitis. Submandibular and submental lymphadenopathy are uncommon but are usually present in Parinaud's oculoglandular conjunctivitis.

LABORATORY EVALUATION

Routine laboratory evaluation probably is not performed in most cases of conjunctivitis. Although there is agreement that all cases of suspected ophthalmia neonatorum (conjunctivitis in first month of life) should have laboratory evaluation with cultures and smears for bacterial, chlamydial, and herpetic causes, there is not universal agreement regarding which other cases require laboratory evaluation and which types of evaluation are most appropriate. Because most cases of conjunctivitis are viral, it is expected that most patients will go through a self-limited course, with spontaneous resolution after nothing but supportive therapy. The patient's history and physical examination can often predict the need for laboratory evaluation. Clear cases of viral conjunctivitis may not require conjunctival scraping for stains and cultures, but if bacterial conjunctivitis is suspected, such scrapings are recommended to guide appropriate antibiotic therapy. Indiscriminate use of antibiotics without laboratory identification of a bacterial cause may lead to the emergence of resistant organisms or may aggravate the condition as the result of a toxic or immune-mediated reaction associated with the medication.

The most common procedure involves the use of a calcium alginate swab or culturette device to collect material from the conjunctiva. Material is transferred to slides for appropriate Gram and Giemsa stains and to culture plates (e.g., blood/chocolate agar, fungal media) for further identification and sensitivity testing. Smears from bacterial infections reveal numerous neutrophils along with the standard epithelial and goblet cells. Lymphocytes and monocytes are predominant in viral infections. Herpetic conjunctivitis may reveal multinucleated epithelial cells and eosinophilic, intranuclear inclusion bodies. Chlamydial conjunctivitis often reveals leukocytes, lymphocytes, and epithelial cells with basophilic, intracytoplasmic inclusion bodies; these findings are noted more frequently in children than in adults. Identification of inclusion bodies can be difficult, and suspected cases of herpetic and viral conjunctivitis may be diagnosed with the use of immunofluorescent techniques.

VIRAL CONJUNCTIVITIS

As a group, viral organisms are probably the most common cause of conjunctivitis. Viral conjunctivitis, often called "pink eye," is one of the most frequent reasons for a visit to the emergency room or physician's office. Because the diagnosis can usually be made clinically, viral cultures and laboratory evaluations are not commonly performed.[6] The viral organisms typically produce an acute, unilateral conjunctivitis with involvement of the second eye occurring often within 1 week. The watery discharge and conjunctival hyperemia can be quite impressive. Preauricular adenopathy is often noted on the involved side. Although many health care providers prescribe antibiotics in the mistaken notion that such discharge and hyperemia have a bacterial cause, most cases of viral conjunctivitis spontaneously resolve within days to weeks, usually without adverse sequelae. Numerous viruses can cause conjunctivitis, and many can be identified by slightly differing features of the disease course.

Adenoviral Conjunctivitis

Adenoviruses are responsible for two of the most common types of conjunctivitis. These infections are spread through respiratory fomites or by direct contact with conjunctival secretions. The incubation period varies from 5 to 10 days, with the clinical process lasting 5 to 15 days.[7] Nineteen different serotypes of adenovirus have been reported to cause conjunctivitis.[8] Once the disease course passes, immunocompetent patients are protected from a recurrent adenoviral infection caused by the same serotype.

Pharyngoconjunctival Fever

Pharyngoconjunctival fever (PCF) has been reported to be the most common ocular adenoviral infection[9]; the most commonly implicated serotypes are 3, 4, and 7. The triad of pharyngitis, fever, and subsequent conjunctivitis is the classic clinical presentation. The conjunctivitis is marked by a follicular reaction accompanied by a mild watery discharge, hyperemia, and chemosis (edema of the conjunctiva). The cornea may have very fine, punctate erosions, and preauricular adenopathy is present in about 90% of cases. The condition usually resolves spontaneously within 2 weeks. Supportive treatment with cold compresses and artificial tears is usually sufficient.

Epidemic Keratoconjunctivitis

Epidemic keratoconjunctivitis (EKC) is associated most often with adenovirus serotypes 8, 11, and 19. EKC is more severe than PCF; it lasts 7 to 21 days, with possible corneal sequelae persisting for weeks or months.[10] The mixed papillary and follicular response in the conjunctiva is accompanied by a watery discharge, chemosis, significant hyperemia, and preauricular adenopathy.[7,11] Subconjunctival hemorrhages and conjunctival membranes are found in approximately one third of patients with EKC, especially in the more severe cases.[12] These membranes (and pseudomembranes) are made up primarily of fibrin, leukocytes, and fibroblasts. Removal of the membrane leaves a bleeding conjunctival surface; removal of pseudomembranes is not associated with such bleeding. The presence of either type of membrane can be associated with formation of conjunctival scarring and symblepharon (adhesion of conjunctival surfaces). Corneal involvement

varies from the almost ubiquitous diffuse, punctate epithelial elevations to the subepithelial infiltrates, seen in 20% to 50% of cases, which may persist for months or longer but usually resolve without scarring or neovascularization.[11] Treatment of EKC focuses on relieving the symptoms and minimizing the spread of this highly contagious disease. Patients usually are infectious for 10 to 14 days after onset. Cold compresses, artificial tears, and possibly decongestant eye drops constitute the main treatment. Reduced visual acuity or disabling glare from the subepithelial infiltrates often responds to topical corticosteroids.[13] Removal of the membranes and pseudomembranes, along with administration of topical steroids, often has a significant effect on patient comfort.

Acute Hemorrhagic Conjunctivitis

Also known as Apollo disease, acute hemorrhagic conjunctivitis was initially described in Ghana during the time of the first lunar landing mission in 1969.[14] The disease is associated with coxsackievirus A24 and enterovirus 70.[15] The classic presentation is rapid onset of severe, painful papillary conjunctivitis marked by chemosis, tearing, and small subconjunctival hemorrhages. Although individual hemorrhages are noted at first, these rapidly coalesce to become confluent. The resultant hemorrhagic chemosis can reach alarming proportions. The cornea may have punctate elevations or erosions, but these rarely progress to subepithelial opacities as seen with EKC. The conjunctivitis tends to clear in 4 to 6 days, but the hemorrhages may persist. Epidemics are quite common, especially in developing countries, where up to 50% of the population may be involved. Treatment again is mainly supportive.

Herpes Simplex Conjunctivitis

Primary ocular involvement by herpes simplex virus (HSV) may manifest as an acute follicular conjunctivitis or keratoconjunctivitis with preauricular adenopathy and often with notable vesiculating periocular skin involvement. Pseudomembranes may be present in the fornices. In the absence of frank skin vesiculation, differentiation from adenoviral infection is aided by a careful search of the lid margins for signs of herpetic blistering. In contrast to primary disease, recurrent blepharoconjunctivitis is a much more localized infection. Vesicles are localized rather than diffuse, starting as red papules, which form clear vesicles, break, and scab over to heal without scarring. Virus is present for about 3 days in the lesions, although the lesions themselves take about 1 week to heal. Conjunctivitis is usually diffuse and watery. Occasionally, rose bengal or fluorescein staining reveals a conjunctival dendritic ulcer. As opposed to the host of treatment regimens used when herpetic disease affects the cornea and other ocular components, herpetic manifestations limited to the conjunctiva require minimal supportive treatment. There is no role for antiviral agents or corticosteroids; however, an antibiotic ointment, such as erythromycin, may be used to prevent a bacterial superinfection. Close monitoring for corneal or adnexa involvement is necessary, because this complication would necessitate a change in the treatment regimen.

Varicella and Herpes Zoster Conjunctivitis

Although the follicular conjunctivitis and preauricular adenopathy of herpes zoster virus (HZV) is rarely seen, approximately 4% of patients with chickenpox have conjunctival or corneal findings, or both.[16] Papules may be seen on the lids, conjunctiva, and limbus. Vesicles may be found on the semilunar fold and throughout the conjunctiva. The papules form pustules, which then ulcerate as the disease progresses. Again, there is no indication for antivirals or corticosteroids in this herpetic conjunctivitis. Supportive care, with the possibility of prophylactic antibacterial ointment, is usually sufficient.

Variola (Smallpox) Conjunctivitis

Between 10% and 20% of individuals affected with smallpox develop severe ocular complications.[17] About 5 days after the onset of clinical disease, an exanthematous, watery conjunctivitis may develop, which frequently clears without complication. However, in some patients, pustules then appear on the bulbar conjunctiva. These painful lesions are associated with a great inflammatory reaction and purulent discharge. The lesions often extend to the cornea, leading to inflammation, scarring, and possible perforation with loss of the eye. Specific treatment is currently not established. A promising but unproven treatment is systemic and topical cidofovir; this agent has some activity against variola in vitro and against poxviruses in animal model systems.[18,19] Penicillinase-resistant antimicrobial agents should be used if the skin lesions are secondarily infected or if infection is near or involves the eyes. Daily rinsing of the eyes is important in severe cases. There are no data showing that prophylaxis or treatment of variola conjunctivitis with vaccinia immune globulin (VIG) has any effect, but many experts would use it to reduce the likelihood of spread..

Vaccinia Conjunctivitis

The attention to smallpox as a bioterror hazard has also brought attention to the complications of smallpox vaccine (vaccinia). Lid and conjunctival involvement is the most common form of ocular vaccinia and is similar to that seen on the arm at the site of the intentional vaccination. Initial formation of vesicles progresses to indurated pustules, which then umbilicate to open sores. The resultant scab formation may occasionally scar and leave depigmented marks in the skin. Vaccinia conjunctivitis is characterized by an acute papillary reaction and serous or mucopurulent discharge. Multifocal ulceration of the palpebral and bulbar conjunctiva occurs commonly. Conjunctival ulcers have a whitish center with surrounding injection and edema; they may be covered by a thick, yellowish-gray membrane and may lead to symblepharon formation. Preauricular and submandibular adenopathy commonly accompanies vaccinia conjunctivitis.[20,21] The differential diagnosis of vaccinia lesions of the eyelid or ocular adnexa includes molluscum contagiosum, keratoacanthoma, bacterial blepharitis, and herpes simplex or varicella zoster virus infection.[22]

Treatment of Vaccinia Conjunctivitis

No topical antiviral agents have been approved by the U. S. Food and Drug Administration (FDA) for the treatment of ocular vaccinia, but topical trifluridine, cidofovir, and vidarabine have been shown to be effective in animal and uncontrolled human reports; VIG has been demonstrated to be effective in treatment of lid and conjunctival lesions.[23,24] A recent panel convened by the Centers for Disease Control in Atlanta recommended the treatments shown in Box 106-1 for vaccinia conjunctivitis.[25]

Other Viral Etiologies

Rubella, rubeola, mumps, influenza, Epstein-Barr virus, papillomavirus, molluscum contagiosum, and Newcastle disease virus have all been implicated in conjunctivitis. Rubella produces a catarrhal and/or follicular reaction along with the typical disease findings. Influenza viruses have also been associated with a catarrhal and/or follicular conjunctivitis. Rubeola (measles) produces a catarrhal and/or papillary reaction, often with significant discomfort and photophobia. Pale, avascular spots, similar in appearance to the oral Koplik's spots, can be found in the conjunctiva.[26] Patients with mumps may develop a catarrhal conjunctivitis and punctate epithelial keratitis with severe photophobia and lacrimation but often little discomfort.[27] A follicular conjunctivitis is present in about 5% of patients with Epstein-Barr–induced mononucleosis.[28] Human papillomavirus can produce lesions on the lid margin as well as the conjunctiva; a catarrhal conjunctivitis may follow. Molluscum contagiosum lesions on the lid margin may cause an irritating chronic follicular conjunctivitis with punctate keratitis, superior corneal vascular pannus, and cicatricial punctal occlusion. Lesions may also occur several millimeters away from the lid margins, yet still cause a follicular conjunctivitis culture-positive for virus.[29] Lesions confined only to the cornea or conjunctiva are rare but not unknown. They are usually seen in patients with immune dysfunction.[30] Newcastle disease, seen primarily in poultry workers, veterinarians, and laboratory technicians, typically produces a unilateral, follicular and papillary conjunctivitis with hyperemia, edema, and chemosis usually in the lower fornix, mild tearing, and preauricular adenopathy.[31]

In all of these cases, there is no specific therapy directed toward the conjunctivitis, because it is almost always self-limited. Therapy directed toward the causative agent (e.g., removal of molluscum lesions) may hasten the resolution of the conjunctivitis.

CHLAMYDIAL CONJUNCTIVITIS

Chlamydia trachomatis Infection

Chlamydial infections cause several important acute and chronic eye infections.[32] Studies using monoclonal antibodies to the chlamydial major outer membrane protein have identified several serotypes of *Chlamydia trachomatis*. Serotypes B, Ba, and D through K, which often are sexually transmitted, can cause a follicular conjunctivitis in the adult (inclusion conjunctivitis). The same serotypes can lead to neonatal conjunctivitis if an infected mother transmits the pathogen to the newborn during vaginal delivery. Repeated infections with *C. trachomatis* serotypes A, B, Ba, and C can cause trachoma, a chronic follicular keratoconjunctivitis that remains the most common cause of preventable blindness in the world. *C. trachomatis* infection can also cause Reiter's disease,[33] a triad of urethritis, arthritis, and iridocyclitis frequently seen in sexually active young men who are positive for the HLA-B57 histocompatibility allele. In addition, several cases of Parinaud's oculoglandular syndrome have been reported with lymphogranuloma venereum, a sexually transmitted disease characterized by painful inguinal lymphadenopathy and caused by *C. trachomatis* serotypes L1 through L3.

Chlamydophila pneumoniae Infection

Chlamydophila (formerly *Chlamydia*) *pneumoniae* is a fairly recent addition to the genus *Chlamydia*.[34] The pathogen shares considerable homology with *C. trachomatis* and follows a similar life cycle. However, it is transmitted by aerosol droplets, can target a spectrum of cell types, and is associated with several chronic inflammatory diseases, most notably atherosclerosis.[35] Although *C. pneumoniae* first was isolated from the conjunctiva, there are few studies on its role in ocular disorders. The organism has been detected in conjunctival swabs collected from patients with conjunctivitis,[36] but a clear association with external ocular disease is lacking.

Trachoma

C. trachomatis serotypes A through C are responsible for trachoma. The severely blinding condition is endemic in many developing countries, especially in areas of close overcrowding and poor sanitation. Trachoma is typically the result of multiple untreated infections rather than a one-time event. The initial follicular conjunctivitis begins in the

---

BOX 106-1

Treatment of Vaccinia Conjunctivitis

Mild to Moderate Disease (mild hyperemia and edema, no membranes or focal lesions)
Adults: Trifluridine (Viroptic) drops 9 times daily for 2 wk
Children: Vidarabine 3% ointment (Vira-A) 2 to 5 times daily for 2 wk
A one-time dose of vaccinia immune globulin (VIG), 100 mg/kg IV, is recommended as adjunctive therapy for moderate conjunctivitis

Severe Disease (marked hyperemia, edema, membranes, focal lesions, lymphadenopathy, fever)
A single dose of VIG, 100 mg/kg intravenously, is recommended as adjunctive therapy; repeat in 48 hours if not improved
Adults: Trifluridine (Viroptic) drops nine times daily for 2 wk
Children: Vidarabine 3% ointment (Vira-A) ointment 2 to 5 times daily for 2 wk
Topical antibiotic to the conjunctiva to prevent secondary bacterial infection

From Centers for Disease Control and Prevention. Smallpox: Summary of October 2002 Advisory Committee on Immunization Practices Smallpox Vaccination Recommendations. Atlanta: Centers for Disease Control and Prevention; 2002.

upper palpebral conjunctiva and is followed by limbal follicles. Papillary hypertrophy, mucopurulent discharge, superior corneal pannus (neovascularization), and epithelial keratitis are early features of the disease. Later stages are marked by cicatrization of the conjunctiva, cornea, and eyelids.

Sequelae of Trachoma

The blinding complications of trachoma are the result of corneal exposure and ulceration caused by the conjunctival scarring and lid deformities.[37] Two classic findings are Arlt's line and Hebert's pits. Arlt's line is the horizontal line of conjunctival scarring found along the superior palpebral conjunctiva. Hebert's pits are the sharply demarcated erosions near the limbus that are filled with epithelium after the cicatrization of the limbal follicles. Once regression of the superior pannus occurs, a diffuse corneal haze may be seen. Eyelid deformities are the result of conjunctival scarring. Lids can be turned inward (entropion) or outward (ectropion), and lashes can be directed against the cornea (trichiasis), all of which contribute to an irregular ocular surface. Such irregularities can cause corneal scars, ulcers, neovascularization, and even perforation.

Treatment of Trachoma

Systemic tetracycline or erythromycin has been given for 3 to 4 weeks. Because the clinical response can often take several months, topical tetracycline or erythromycin is often used twice daily for 5 days each month for 6 months.[8] This repeated topical treatment is especially useful in situations in which repeat infection is likely. Loosely based on the smallpox eradication efforts, widespread prophylactic systemic antibiotics have been tried in endemic areas in an attempt to eliminate the disease. A single dose of azithromycin was proposed as a good choice for the eradication theory.[38]

Adult Inclusion Conjunctivitis

C. trachomatis can cause a chronic follicular conjunctivitis in adults and neonates. The adult form is usually sexually transmitted, with an estimated 1 in 300 patients with genital chlamydia developing conjunctivitis,[39] but it can occur with orogenital or hand-to-eye transmission of secretions.[40] The most common presentation is that of a unilateral red eye (although it can be bilateral), preauricular adenopathy, papillary hypertrophy, marked hyperemia, mucopurulent discharge, and a follicular reaction. Men often have a concomitant urethritis; women may have chronic cervicitis. Corneal involvement may quickly follow the conjunctivitis, resulting in punctate keratitis, EKC-like infiltrates, and superior limbal pannus (neovascularization). Corneal scarring and neovascularization are less common with inclusion conjunctivitis than with trachoma, and the upper and lower palpebral conjunctivae are often equally involved, as opposed to the preferentially affected upper conjunctiva in trachoma. However, severe inclusion conjunctivitis may be associated with a chronic, relapsing course leading to characteristics generally seen in trachoma.

Treatment of Adult Inclusion Conjunctivitis

Because of the prominent sexual transmission of this form of conjunctivitis, it is important to simultaneously treat all known partners. Failure to do so often results in more serious sequelae associated with reinfections. Topical antibiotics are relatively ineffective, so systemic therapy is the mainstay of treatment. Tetracycline, doxycycline, or erythromycin is given for 3 weeks, with caution to avoid tetracycline in young children and in pregnant or lactating women.

Lymphogranuloma Venereum

Certain serotypes of *C. trachomatis* (L1, L2, and L3) have been associated with systemic lymphogranuloma venereum. The associated conjunctivitis is often mild and unilateral, producing a scant, watery discharge. Although the conjunctivitis appears mild, there is rather impressive edema in the upper and lower eyelids. In addition to the usual preauricular lymphadenopathy, the nodes in the parotid and submaxillary region are also involved. There is a report of lymphogranuloma venereum conjunctivitis causing a keratitis leading to a corneal perforation in a patient with acquired immunodeficiency syndrome (AIDS).[41] Treatment is similar to that for inclusion conjunctivitis.

BACTERIAL CONJUNCTIVITIS

There is significant disagreement on the actual incidence of bacterial conjunctivitis. Many cases of conjunctivitis are treated as if they were caused by bacterial organisms, but culture-proven bacterial conjunctivitis appears uncommon. The clinical presentation is characterized by a rapid onset of unilateral lid edema, conjunctival injection, and a mucopurulent discharge, followed by involvement of the second eye within 1 to 2 days. *Staphylococcus* and *Corynebacterium* species are the most common organisms to colonize the lids and conjunctiva; consequently, they are prominent causes of infectious conjunctivitis.[42] Although almost any bacterial organism can cause conjunctivitis given the appropriate set of conditions, the most common ones are *Staphylococcus* species, *Streptococcus pneumoniae*, *Haemophilus* species, *Moraxella*, *Corynebacterium diphtheriae*, *Neisseria* species, and enteric gram-negative rods.[43]

Pathogenesis

The pathogenesis of bacterial conjunctivitis usually involves a compromised epithelial surface. Although intact epithelium is an effective barrier to most organisms, *N. gonorrhoeae*, *C. diphtheriae*, *Haemophilus aegyptus* (Koch-Weeks bacillus), and *Listeria monocytogenes* can penetrate such a surface through specialized attachments or toxins, or both.[44] Injured epithelium or specialized attachments allow adhesion, which may result in the entry of various bacterial products and toxins. Enzymatic components such as proteases, coagulases, collagenases, and fibrinolysins, combined with toxins such as those seen in *Staphylococcus* and *Pseudomonas* species, can disrupt underlying tissue, allowing further bacterial entry and possible isolation from host defense mechanisms.[45] Bacterial conjunctivitis can be clinically categorized as acute, hyperacute, or chronic, based on various features.

Acute (Mucopurulent) Bacterial Conjunctivitis

Staphylococcus aureus, Streptococcus pneumoniae, and *Haemophilus influenzae* are the organisms that most commonly cause bacterial conjunctivitis. The acute conjunctivitis is marked by unilateral hyperemia, tearing, mucopurulent discharge, and mattering of the eyelids. *S. aureus* is the most common agent in adults and children; *S. pneumoniae* and *H. influenzae* occur more frequently in children than in adults.[46] *H. influenzae* is often associated with systemic infections, such as upper respiratory tract disease, and its treatment usually requires the administration of systemic antibiotics. Viridans streptococci and *Streptococcus pyogenes* can produce an acute conjunctivitis, often with an associated membranous reaction. Gram-negative rods, other than *Haemophilus* species, rarely cause acute conjunctivitis in the immunocompetent patient.

Treatment of Acute Bacterial Conjunctivitis

Appropriate laboratory confirmation of bacterial conjunctivitis should be attained to guide treatment. Although many mild conjunctival infections resolve on their own, topical antibiotic treatment may speed resolution and reduce severity and morbidity.[47] Treatment with a broad-spectrum agent such as sulfacetamide, trimethoprim-polymixin, or a fluoroquinolone is necessary for 7 to 10 days. Appropriate agents may be selected or altered based on laboratory results.

Hyperacute (Purulent) Bacterial Conjunctivitis

The most frequent cause of hyperacute conjunctivitis is *N. gonorrhoeae*; a less severe form can be seen with *Neisseria meningitidis*.[48] This severe disease is most common in neonates, sexually active adolescents, and young adults. The most impressive characteristic is the copious, thick, yellowish-green, purulent discharge. Marked chemosis, painful hyperemia, and eyelid edema are seen. In contrast to most cases of bacterial conjunctivitis, there is often tender preauricular adenopathy. There may be conjunctival membrane formation, and the condition may rapidly progress to corneal ulceration and perforation, because *Neisseria* species can penetrate an intact corneal epithelium in as little as 24 hours.

Treatment of Hyperacute Bacterial Conjunctivitis

Laboratory evaluation via Gram stain and culture is important, because the treatment of *Neisseria* conjunctivitis is different than that of most bacterial entities. Topical antibiotics can augment treatment, but systemic therapy is the mainstay with *Neisseria* infections. The prevalence of penicillin-resistant organisms has made ceftriaxone the treatment of choice. Gonoccocal conjunctivitis without corneal involvement may be treated with one intramuscular injection of ceftriaxone; corneal involvement usually requires hospitalization for a 3-day course of intravenous treatment. Patients with penicillin allergies may be treated with intramuscular spectinomycin or oral fluoroquinolones. Topical antibiotic ointments and solutions have been considered, but the most important topical therapy is frequent (every 30 to 60 minutes) saline irrigation of the conjunctival surface and fornices to remove the inflammatory cells, proteolytic enzymes, and debris, which may be toxic to the ocular surfaces. Because up to one third of patients with gonococcal conjunctivitis have been reported to have chlamydia, concurrent treatment with tetracycline, doxycycline, or azithromycin may be indicated.

Chronic Bacterial Conjunctivitis

The most common causes of chronic bacterial conjunctivitis are the *Staphylococcus* species.[49] Such infections can be difficult to eradicate, because the eyelid margins and surrounding skin are heavily populated with staphylococci. Associated exotoxins are thought to be responsible for the effect on the conjunctiva, lids, and cornea. A diffuse hyperemia, minimal mucopurulent discharge, and conjunctival thickening with either a follicular or a papillary reaction are common. Eyelid involvement may manifest as redness, telangiectasia, loss of lashes, thickening, or recurrent hordeola ("stye"), and ulceration at the base of the eyelashes may be seen. Maceration and ulceration of the inner and outer canthal angles may be seen in chronic blepharoconjunctivitis caused by *Moraxella* species. Chronic staphylococcal blepharoconjunctivitis may lead to marginal corneal ulceration, most likely as the result of an immune-mediated hypersensitivity reaction. Gramnegative bacteria are more common in chronic than in acute conjunctivitis.[50] Organisms more often associated with the intestinal flora can be associated with chronic conjunctivitis: *Proteus mirabilis* is the most common of these, but *Klebsiella pneumoniae, Escherichia coli,* and *Serratia marcescens* have also been described.

Treatment of Chronic Bacterial Conjunctivitis

Treatment of this type of bacterial conjunctivitis demands appropriate antibiotic therapy combined with aggressive lid hygiene and possible evaluation of the lacrimal system. Laboratory evaluation may guide appropriate antibiotic treatment, often with erythromycin or bacitracin ointment. Lid hygiene involves the use of warm compresses, eyelid scrubs with nontearing shampoo, and gentle lid massage, because the meibomian (sebaceous gland) orifices at the base of the eyelashes may harbor the inciting agents. The lacrimal canaliculus or sac may also serve as a bacterial reservoir requiring antibiotic irrigation and oral antibiotics. The staphylococcal hypersensitivity reaction in the cornea may require mild topical corticosteroid treatment to reduce the associated inflammation. Oral tetracycline or doxycycline may be beneficial in more severe infections.

NEONATAL CONJUNCTIVITIS

Any conjunctivitis occurring within the first 4 weeks of life is classified as neonatal conjunctivitis (ophthalmia neonatorum).[51] Conjunctivitis in the newborn can be bacterial, viral, chlamydial, or toxic (reaction to chemicals). Specific identification of the cause is particularly important, because there is often a potentially serious systemic infection associated with the localized ocular condition.

Chemical Conjunctivitis

In 1881, Credé introduced the use of topical silver nitrate as prophylaxis against neonatal gonococcal infection.[52] The self-limited conjunctivitis, present in approximately 90% of treated newborns, usually begins a few hours after delivery and resolves in 24 to 36 hours.[53] The severity of the symptoms has been reduced with the advent of single-use, buffered ampules; before this innovation, the solution was kept in large, multidose bottles, which allowed for a more concentrated dose when samples were taken from the bottom of the bottle. Although quite effective against *N. gonorrhoeae*, silver nitrate has little effect on bacteria and essentially no effect on chlamydia or viruses.[54] Silver nitrate may injure epithelial cells to such a degree that they are more susceptible to the entry of other microbial agents. Silver nitrate may still be used in some areas, but many hospitals are changing to erythromycin or tetracycline ointment. Betadine is markedly inexpensive and quite effective against many microbial agents; it is becoming more widely used as a prophylactic agent for newborns, especially in developing countries. The associated chemical conjunctivitis is similar in nature and course as that seen with silver nitrate.

Neonatal Chlamydial Conjunctivitis

The most frequent cause of neonatal conjunctivitis in the United States is *C. trachomatis*.[55] Up to 3 million new cases of chlamydial infection occur annually,[56] with 4% to 10% of all pregnant women in the United States being diagnosed with chlamydia.[57] The infant of an untreated mother has a 30% to 40% chance of developing conjunctivitis and a 10% to 20% chance of developing pneumonia.[52] A unilateral or bilateral discharge begins 5 to 14 days after delivery.

Chlamydial conjunctivitis in the neonate differs from that in the adult in a number of ways. No follicular response is seen in the neonate because of the immature immune system's inability to form such a reaction. The amount of mucopurulent discharge is greater in the neonate, as is the propensity to form membranes on the palpebral conjunctiva. The infection in neonates is more responsive to topical medications. Although the typical conjunctivitis is mild and self-limited, severe cases can result in conjunctival scarring with corneal pannus and scarring. If erythromycin or tetracycline ointment is applied to the conjunctival surface within 1 hour after delivery, the chance of developing chlamydial conjunctivitis is reportedly almost zero.[58] However, topical medications cannot treat the pneumonitis and otitis media that may accompany the conjunctivitis. Two weeks of oral erythromycin therapy is given to the newborn with laboratory-proven chlamydia conjunctivitis; a second course may be given if adequate resolution is not achieved with the initial treatment. The mother and her sexual partners must also be treated with oral erythromycin or tetracycline (with caution in breast-feeding mothers) for 1 week.

Gonococcal Conjunctivitis

The incidence of neonatal gonococcal conjunctivitis has dropped dramatically with effective prenatal screening and use of prophylactic antimicrobial agents in newborns. The clinical presentation begins with a hyperacute bilateral conjunctival discharge that appears within the first 24 to 48 hours after delivery. The associated purulent exudate is often so profuse that it reappears immediately after cleaning of the eye. Conjunctival membrane formation is not uncommon. *N. gonorrhoeae* can penetrate an intact epithelial surface and quickly invade the cornea, causing ulceration, perforation, and even endophthalmitis if not promptly treated. Other localized gonococcal infections, such as rhinitis and proctitis, may be present, as well as the rare but more severe disseminated infection with arthritis, meningitis, pneumonia, and septicemia, which could lead to infant death.[56] With resistance emerging against penicillin, tetracycline, and even the fluoroquinolones, a single dose of intramuscular or intravenous ceftriaxone, 125 mg, is the preferred treatment.[59] Hospitalization and hourly saline irrigation of the conjunctival fornices is recommended; if corneal involvement cannot be ruled out because of the copious exudation, topical antibiotics are applied.[60]

Nongonococcal Bacterial Conjunctivitis

Numerous organisms can cause bacterial conjunctivitis in the newborn. The majority of infections are associated with gram-positive organisms such as the *Staphylococcus* and *Streptococcus* species. Gram-negative organisms such as the *Haemophilus* and *Enterobacter* spp., *E. coli*, *P. mirabilis*, *K. pneumoniae*, and *S. marcescens* have been less commonly implicated.[61] Although *Pseudomonas aeruginosa* is a very rare cause of neonatal conjunctivitis, it deserves special consideration because of its ability to rapidly cause corneal ulceration and possible perforation.[62]

Although symptoms can manifest at any time within the first month of life, nongonococcal bacterial conjunctivitis usually manifests 2 to 5 days after delivery. The clinical presentation consists of periorbital edema, chemosis, and conjunctival hyperemia and discharge. There is a higher incidence if obstruction of the nasolacrimal system is present. Conjunctival scrapings for Gram stain and cultures allows for appropriate treatment—usually erythromycin ointment for gram-positive organisms and either gentamicin or tobramycin ointment for gram-negative organisms.

Viral (Herpetic) Conjunctivitis

Herpetic conjunctivitis in the neonate is rare but can be associated with significant morbidity and mortality. HSV types 1 and 2 can be associated with conjunctivitis. In theory, HSV-1 can be transmitted to the infant through oral secretions from an adult or sibling with an active "cold sore," but the more common source is contact with HSV-2 during passage through an infected birth canal. The edema, conjunctival injection, and tearing usually begin within the first 2 weeks of life and may be followed by keratitis or keratouveitis. Diagnosis is commonly made by Giemsa stain but can be confirmed in 24 to 48 hours by viral culture.

PARINAUD'S OCULOGLANDULAR CONJUNCTIVITIS

This classification describes a type of conjunctivitis that has numerous associated causes, including bacterial, viral, parasitic, mycobacterial, syphilitic, leukemic, and fungal agents. The red eye, mucopurulent discharge, and foreign-body sensation are accompanied by one or more granulomatous nodules on the palpebral conjunctiva. There is usually a visibly enlarged preauricular or submandibular lymph node on the involved side. This follicular conjunctivitis is associated with a fever and possible skin rash. *Bartonella henselae*, or cat-scratch disease, is the most common cause, but tularemia, tuberculosis, syphilis, lymphoma, mumps, Epstein-Barr virus, sporotrichosis, and sarcoidosis have all been implicated as potential causes.

Cat-scratch disease often resolves spontaneously, but 1 month of topical and systemic antibiotic therapy has been described. Because of the host of etiologic agents, an extensive workup may be warranted, with the identified cause given the appropriate systemic treatment.

PARASITIC CONJUNCTIVITIS

Leishmaniasis and Microsporidia

A number of parasites may be associated with conjunctivitis, either by primary infection or secondarily as a response to the presence of the parasite. Blepharoconjunctivitis caused by *Leishmania* may begin as simple edema and hyperemia, with eventual progression to superficial phlyctenules in the conjunctiva and at the corneal limbus.[63] These phlyctenules may progress to abscess formation, scarring of the lids and conjunctiva, and even corneal perforation. These parasites are obligate intracellular agents that are transmitted through bites of infected sand flies. Previously uncommon protozoa are now being recovered from the conjunctivae of patients with AIDS.

Microsporidia are ubiquitous obligate intracellular parasites that are found more often in animal hosts, but the related microsporidium, *Encephalitozoon*, has been implicated as the cause of a mild conjunctivitis with punctate epithelial keratitis in immunocompromised patients.[64] Symptoms may be mild and can easily be mistaken for tear film deficiencies or blepharitis; a high index of suspicion is required to make a clinical diagnosis of microsporidial conjunctivitis. Oral albendazole, 400 mg twice daily, has been reported to be effective (see Chapter 282). Topical fumagillin can be obtained as Fumadil B and formulated for human use but is not approved by the FDA; fumagillin has been used to successfully treat microsporidial keratoconjunctivitis (see Chapter 282).[65] In general, medical treatment involves long duration with frequent recurrences after discontinuation of medication.

Other Parasites and Ectoparasites

The tsetse fly can infect humans with the flagellates responsible for African trypanosomiasis or "sleeping sickness." Ocular effects manifest as unilateral conjunctivitis, periorbital edema, and preauricular lymphadenopathy.[66] Cryptosporidia, fly larvae, and nematodes (e.g., *Loa loa*) have also been implicated as parasitic causes of conjunctivitis.[67-69] The lid margin and lashes may be colonized by *Phthirus pubis* (lice) or *Demodex* (mites), with conjunctivitis occurring as a reaction to the organism or its waste products. Treatment for the actual conjunctivitis associated with the parasitic agents is mainly supportive; more aggressive treatment may be necessary for the systemic parasitic condition.

FUNGAL CONJUNCTIVITIS

Although various fungal agents can be recovered from the conjunctiva, fungal conjunctivitis is rarely observed clinically. In comparison to fungal keratitis, relatively few organisms have been implicated in fungal conjunctivitis. *Candida* spp., *Blastomyces* spp., and *Sporothrix schenckii* have been associated with a granulomatous conjunctivitis. These mycoses are treated with systemic antifungal agents. Conjunctival *Rhinosporidium seeberi* infection usually manifests as a fleshy, friable, red, pedunculated mass.[1] Excision of the mass with adequate margins is often curative.

DIFFERENTIAL DIAGNOSIS OF "RED EYE"

Care must be taken with any patient who presents with a "red eye," as there are numerous conditions that can simulate conjunctivitis. As with most conditions, a thorough medical history and physical examination are often helpful in the differential diagnosis. Most cases of conjunctivitis are associated with fairly painless discharge and irritation, essentially normal vision, normally reactive pupil, normal intraocular pressure, essentially clear cornea, and generally diffuse conjunctival injection. Three possible sight-threatening conditions—corneal ulcer, uveitis, and angle-closure glaucoma—often have different signs, which may enable a more proper diagnosis. An attack of angle-closure glaucoma is associated with significant pain, often nausea, usually no discharge, generally markedly decreased vision, mid-dilated nonreactive pupil, markedly elevated intraocular pressure, a cloudy and edematous cornea, and a more localized conjunctival injection in the limbal region. Uveitis is generally associated with mild-to-moderate pain with photophobia, essentially normal to mildly reduced vision, no discharge, a small to normal-sized reactive pupil, normal to low intraocular pressure (elevated in herpetic uveitis and Posner-Schlossman syndrome), a generally clear cornea, and a localized conjunctival injection around the limbus. Corneal ulcers are quite painful and are usually accompanied by moderate to markedly reduced vision, variable mucoid or mucopurulent discharge, normally reactive pupil, normal intraocular pressure, an opaque lesion that is easily visible in the cornea, and usually a generalized conjunctival injection. These generalizations obviously cannot address each specific case of a red eye, but they may serve as guidelines in evaluating the patient who might require treatment beyond that for straightforward conjunctivitis.

REFERENCES

1. O'Brien TP. Conjunctivitis. In: Mandell GL, Bennett JE, Dolin R, eds. Principles and Practice of Infectious Diseases, 5th ed. New York: Churchill Livingstone; 2000:1249-1257.
1a. Wei Z-G, Cotsarelis G, Sun T-T, et al. Label-retaining cells are preferentially located in fornical epithelium: Implications on conjunctival epithelial homeostasis. Invest Ophthalmol Vis Sci. 1995;36:236-246.
2. Wei Z-G, Lin T, Sun T-T, et al. Clonal analysis of the in vivo differentiation potential of keratinocytes. Invest Ophthalmol Vis Sci. 1997;38:753-761.
3. Srinivasan BD, Jakobiec FA, Iwamoto T. Conjunctiva. In: Jakobiec FA, ed. Ocular Anatomy, Embryology and Teratology. Philadelphia: Harper & Row; 1982.
4. Jakobiec FA, Iwamoto T. Ocular adnexa: Introduction to lids, conjunctiva and orbit. In: Jakobiec FA, ed. Ocular Anatomy, Embryology and Teratology. Philadelphia: Harper & Row; 1982.
5. Sutphin JE Jr, Chodosh J, Dana MR, et al. Section 8: External disease and cornea. In: Liesegang TJ, Deutsch TA, Grand MG, eds. Basic and Clinical Science Course. San Francisco: American Academy of Ophthalmology; 2002:24.
6. Thygeson P, Dawson CR. Trachoma and follicular conjunctivitis in children. Arch Ophthalmol. 1966;75:3-12.
7. Dawson CR, Sheppard JD. Follicular conjunctivitis. In: Tasman W, Jaeger EA, eds. Duane's Clinical Ophthalmology, v. 4. Philadelphia: Lippincott Williams & Wilkins; 1991;7.1-7.26.
8. Schmitz H, Wigand R, Heinrich W. Worldwide epidemiology of human adenovirus infections. Am J Epidemiol. 1983;117:455-466.
9. Bell JA, Rowe WP, Engler JI, et al. Pharyngoconjunctival fever: Epidemiological studies of a recently recognized disease entity. JAMA. 1955;157:1083-1092.
10. Dawson CR, Hanna L, Togni B. Adenovirus type 8 infections in the United States: IV. Observations on the pathogenesis of lesions in severe eye disease. Arch Ophthalmol. 1972;87:258-268.
11. Hogan MJ, Crawford JW. Epidemic keratoconjunctivitis (superficial punctate keratitis, keratitis subepithelialis, keratitis maculosa, keratitis nummularis) with a review of the literature and a report of 125 cases. Am J Ophthalmol. 1942;25:1059-1078.
12. Dawson CR, Hanna L, Wood TR, et al. Adenovirus type 8 keratoconjunctivitis in the United States: III. Epidemiologic, clinical, and microbiologic features. Am J Ophthalmol. 1970;69:473-480.
13. Laibson PR, Ortolan G, Dhiri S, et al. The treatment of epidemic keratoconjunctivitis (adenovirus type 8) by corticosteroid therapy. XXI Concilium Ophthalmologicum, Mexico. Amsterdam: Excerpta Medica; 1970:1246-1250.
14. Chatterjee S, Quarcoopome CO, Apenteng A. An epidemic of acute conjunctivitis in Ghana. Ghana Med J. 1970;9:9-11.
15. Yin-Murphy M. Viruses of acute hemorrhagic conjunctivitis (Letter). Lancet. 1973;1:545-546.
16. Stucchi CA, Bianchi G. Complications oculaires graves post-varicelleuses chez l'adulte. Ophthalmologica. 1970;161:108-114.
17. Koplan JP, Hicks JW. Smallpox and vaccinia in the United States—1972. J Infect Dis. 1974;129:224-226.
18. De Clercq E. Cidofovir in the therapy and short-term prophylaxis of poxvirus infections. Trends Pharmacol Sci. 2002;23:456-458.
19. Neyts J, Neyts C. Therapy and short-term prophylaxis of poxvirus infections: Historical background and perspectives. Antiviral Res. 2003;57:25-33.
20. Ruben FL, Lane JM. Ocular vaccinia: An epidemiologic analysis of 348 cases. Arch Ophthalmol. 1970;84:45-48.
21. Semba R. The ocular complications of smallpox and smallpox immunization. Arch Ophthalmol. 2003;121:715-719.
22. Pepose JS, Margolis TP, LaRussa P, Pavan-Langston D. Ocular complications of smallpox vaccination. Am J Ophthalmol. 2003;136:343-352.
23. Hyndiuk RA, Seideman S, Leibsohn JM. Treatment of vaccinial keratitis with trifluorothymidine. Arch Ophthalmol. 1976;94:1785-1786.
24. Pavan-Langston D, Dohlman CH. A double blind clinical study of adenine arabinoside therapy of viral keratoconjunctivitis. Am J Ophthalmol. 1972;74:81-88.
25. Centers for Disease Control and Prevention. Smallpox: Summary of October 2002 Advisory Committee on Immunization Practices Smallpox Vaccination Recommendations. Atlanta: Centers for Disease Control and Prevention; 2002.
26. Deckard PS, Bergstrom TJ. Rubeola keratitis. Ophthalmology. 1981;88:810-813.
27. Mickatavage R, Amdur J. A case report of mumps keratitis. Arch Ophthalmol. 1963;69:758-759.
28. Garau J, Kabins S, DeNosaquo S, et al. Spontaneous cytomegalovirus mononucleosis with conjunctivitis. Arch Intern Med. 1977;137:1631-1632.
29. Asbell P. Viral conjunctivitis. In: Hyndiuk RA, Tabbara KF, eds. Infections of the Eye. Boston: Little, Brown; 1996:453-470.
30. Ingraham HJ, Schoenleber DB. Epibulbar molluscum contagiosum. Am J Ophthalmol. 1998;125:394-396.
31. Wood TR. Newcastle disease. In: Pepose JS, Holland GN, Wilhelmus KR, eds. Ocular Infection and Immunity. St. Louis: Mosby; 1996:873-876.
32. Kalayoglu MV. Ocular chlamydial infections: Pathogenesis and emerging treatment strategies. Curr Drug Targets Infect Disord. 2002;2:85-91.
33. Hughes RA, Keat AC. Reiter's syndrome and reactive arthritis: A current view. Semin Arthritis Rheum. 1994;24:190-210.
34. Grayston JT, Kuo CC, Campbell LA, et al. Chlamydia pneumoniae sp. nov. for Chlamydia sp. strain TWAR. Int J Syst Bacteriol. 1989;39:88-90.
35. Kalayoglu MV, Libby P, Byrne GI. Chlamydia pneumoniae as an emerging risk factor in cardiovascular disease. JAMA. 2002;288:2724-2731.
36. Lietman T, Brooks D, Moncada J, et al. Chronic follicular conjunctivitis associated with Chlamydia psittaci or Chlamydia pneumoniae. Clin Infect Dis. 1998;26: 1335-1340.
37. Dawson CR, Jones BR, Tarizzo M. Guide to trachoma control. Geneva: World Health Organization; 1981:56.
38. Tabbara KF, AbuEl-Asrar AM, Al-Omar O, et al. Single-dose azithromycin in the treatment of trachoma: A randomized, controlled study. Ophthalmology. 1996;103:842-846.
39. Tullo AB, Richmond SJ, Easty PL. The presentation and incidence of paratrachoma in adults. J Hyg (Lond). 1981;87:63-69.
40. Dawson CR. TRIC agent infections of the eye and genital tract. Am J Ophthalmol. 1967;63:1288-1298.
41. Buus DR, Pflugfelder SC, Schachter J, et al. Lymphogranuloma venereum conjunctivitis with a marginal corneal perforation. Ophthalmology. 1988;95;799-802.
42. Perkins RE, Kundsin RB, Pratt MV. Bacteriology of normal and infected conjunctiva. J Clin Microbiol. 1975;1:147-149.
43. Mannis MJ, Plotnick RD. Bacterial conjunctivitis. In: Tasman W, Jaeger EA, eds. Duane's Clinical Ophthalmology, v. 4. Philadelphia: Lippincott Williams & Wilkins; 1998:5.1-5.7.
44. Buchanan TM. Surface antigens pili. In: Roberts RB, ed. The Gonococcus. New York: John Wiley; 1981:256-272.
45. Hyndiuk RA. Experimental Pseudomonas keratitis. Trans Am Ophthalmol Soc. 1981;79:541-624.
46. Foulks GN, Austin R, Knowlton G. Clinical comparison of topical solutions containing trimethoprim in treating ocular surface bacterial infections. J Ocul Pharmacol. 1988;4:111-115.
47. Leibowitz HM. Antibacterial effectiveness of ciprofloxacin 0.3% ophthalmic solution in the treatment of bacterial conjunctivitis. Am J Ophthalmol. 1991;112:29S.
48. Brooke I, Bateman JB, Pettit TH. Meningococcal conjunctivitis. Arch Ophthalmol. 1979;97:890-891.
49. Thygeson P, Kimura SJ. Chronic conjunctivitis. Trans Am Acad Ophthalmol Otolaryngol. 1963;67:494-517.
50. Gutierrez EH. Bacterial infections of the eye. In: Locatcher-Khorazo D, ed. Microbiology of the Eye. St Louis: CV Mosby; 1972:5.
51. Chandler JW. Neonatal conjunctivitis. In: Tasman W, Jaeger EA, eds. Duane's Clinical Ophthalmology, v. 4. Philadelphia: Lippincott-Raven Publishers; 1995; 6.1-6.7.
52. Credé CSF. Die Verhutung der Augenentzundung der Neugenborenen. Arch Gynakk. 1881;17:50-55.
53. Nishida H, Risemberg HM. Silver nitrate ophthalmic solution and chemical conjunctivitis. Pediatrics. 1975;56:368-373.
54. Laga M, Plummer FA, Piot P, et al. Prophylaxis of gonococcal and chlamydial ophthalmia neonatorum: A comparison of silver nitrate and tetracycline. N Engl J Med. 1988;318:653-657.
55. Sutphin JE Jr, Chodosh J, Dana MR, et al. Section 8: External disease and cornea. In: Liesegang TJ, Deutsch TA, Grand MG, eds. Basic and Clinical Science Course. San Francisco: American Academy of Ophthalmology. 2002:161.
56. Centers for Disease Control. Chlamydia trachomatis infections: Policy guidelines for prevention and control. MMWR Morb Mortal Wkly Rep. 1985;34:53S-74S.
57. Holmes KK. The Chlamydia epidemic. JAMA. 1981;245:1718-1723.
58. Harrison HR, English MG, Lee CK, et al. Chlamydia trachomatis infant pneumonitis: Comparison with matched controls and other infant pheumonitis. N Engl J Med. 1978;298:702-708.
59. Centers for Disease Control and Prevention. Sexually transmitted diseases treatment guidelines 2002. MMWR Morb Mortal Wkly Rep.. 2002;51:36-42.
60. Gonococcal infections. In: Pickering LK, ed. 2000 Red Book: Report of the Committee on Infectious Diseases, 25th ed. Elk Grove Village, Ill: American Academy of Pediatrics; 2000:256.
61. Prentice MJ, Hutchinson GR, Taylor-Robinson D. A microbiological study of neonatal conjunctivae and conjunctivitis. Br J Ophthalmol. 1977;61:601-607.
62. Burns RP, Rhodes DH Jr. Pseudomonas eye infection as a cause of death in premature infants. Arch Ophthalmol. 1961;65:517-525.
63. Nandy A, Addy M, Chowdhury AB. Leishmanial blepharoconjunctivitis. Trop Geogr Med. 1991;43:303-306.
64. Friedberg DN, Stenson SM, Orenstein JM, et al. Microsporidial keratoconjunctivitis in acquired immunodeficiency syndrome. Arch Ophthalmol. 1990;108:504-508.
65. Wilkins JH, Joshi N, Margolis TP, et al. Microsporidial keratoconjunctivitis treated successfully with a short course of fumagillin (Letter). Eye. 1994;8:703-704.
66. Neame H. Parenchymatous keratitis in trypanosomiasis in cattle and in dogs, and in man. Br J Ophthalmol. 1927;11:209-216.
67. Green ST, Scott V, McMenamin J, et al. Cryptosporidial enteritis complicated by conjunctivitis (Letter). Ann Rheum Dis. 1991;50:526.
68. Wong D. External ophthalmomyiasis caused by the sheep bot Oestrus ovis L. Br J Ophthalmol. 1982;66:786-787.
69. Ashton N, Cook C. Allergic granulomatous nodules of the eyelid and conjunctiva. The XXXV Edward Jackson Memorial Lecture. Am J Ophthalmol. 1979;87:1-28.

CHAPTER **107**

Microbial Keratitis

SCOTT D. BARNES

DEBORAH PAVAN-LANGSTON

DIMITRI T. AZAR

Keratitis is an inflammation of the cornea produced by infectious organisms or noninfectious agents or stimuli. Microbial keratitis is a potentially vision-threatening event that can be caused by bacteria, viruses, fungi, or parasites.[1] Infectious keratitis is a significant public health problem. The reported incidence ranges from 11 per 100,000 person-years in the United States[2] to 799 per 100,000 person-years in the developing nation of Nepal.[3] Infectious keratitis generally requires prompt diagnosis and expedient treatment in order to prevent blindness or even enucleation. There are few clinical signs that distinguish infectious keratitis from corneal inflammation associated with trauma, hypersensitivity, or immune-mediated conditions. Diagnosis is assisted by the patient's history and ocular examination, focusing on the presence or absence of an epithelial defect and stromal inflammation. The nature of the stromal inflammation, suppurative or nonsuppurative, and its location, focal, multifocal, or diffuse, may serve as important diagnostic clues. Microbiologic tests are needed to establish the etiologic agent and antimicrobial susceptibility, but therapy is often begun before these results are final.

Given the rapid progression and virulent nature of many infectious agents, any corneal inflammation should be considered a threat to vision, requiring prompt evaluation and treatment. Even relatively minor corneal ulcerations may lead to significant reduction in visual acuity should they be located in the visual axis. Corneal perforation can occur in as little as 24 hours with certain virulent organisms; subsequent endophthalmitis (inflammatory process involving the ocular cavity and adjacent structures) leading to loss of vision or even loss of the eye is an ever-present danger in such settings.

ETIOLOGIC AGENTS AND RISK FACTORS

Microbial Agents

The conjunctival surface has been theorized to be the location of hundreds of organisms, any of which might be the origin of a given keratitis. The most commonly encountered organisms involved in microbial keratitis show tremendous geographic variance; some of the more commonly known infectious agents are shown in Table 107-1. Although the climate, vegetation, soil, and individual patient factors tend to favor specific organisms, any known organism can cause microbial keratitis given the appropriate conditions and predisposing risk factors.

Anatomic Protection

The epithelial surface, with its tight junctions formed by desmosomes and hemidesmosomes, is remarkably resistant to the host of virulent organisms found in the surrounding ocular environment. The tear film, containing antimicrobial enzymes, combined with the mechanical action of the blinking eyelids, reduces the likelihood of microbial attachment to and survival on the corneal surface. In general, microbial agents do not cause keratitis in immunocompetent hosts or those without prior epithelial injury. However, there are exceptions in which organisms, such as *Neisseria gonorrhoeae, Listeria monocytogenes, Shigella,* and *Corynebacterium* spp., may invade an intact epithelial surface.

Risk Factors

Predisposing risk factors associated with microbial keratitis usually involve disruption of the corneal epithelium, such as by contact lens

TABLE 107-1 Partial List of Causative Agents in Microbial Keratitis

Bacteria
Gram-positive cocci
  Staphylococcus aureus
  Staphylococcus epidermidis
  Streptococcus pneumoniae, Streptococcus pyogenes, viridans
    streptococci
  Enterococcus faecalis
  Peptostreptococcus spp.
Gram-positive bacilli
  Bacillus coagulans, Bacillus cereus, Bacillus licheniformis
  Brevibacillus (Bacillus) brevis, Brevibacillus (Bacillus) laterosporus
  Corynebacterium diphtheriae
  Clostridium perfringens, Clostridium tetani
Gram-negative coccobacilli
  Neisseria gonorrhoeae
  Moraxella lacunata, Moraxella nonliquefaciens, Moraxella catarrhalis
  Acinetobacter calcoaceticus
  Pasteurella multocida
Gram-negative bacilli
  *Pseudomonas aeruginosa, Pseudomonas stutzeri, Pseudomonas
    fluorescens*
  Burkholderia (Pseudomonas) mallei
  Proteus mirabilis
  Serratia marcescens
  Escherichia coli
  Klebsiella pneumoniae
  Morganella morganii
  Aeromonas hydrophila
  Bartonella henselae
Mycobacteria
  *Mycobacterium tuberculosis, Mycobacterium chelonae, Mycobacterium
    gordonae, Mycobacterium mucogenicum*
Actinomycetes
  Nocardia spp.
Spirochetes
  Treponema pallidum
  Borrelia burgdorferi

Viruses
  Herpes simplex virus
  Varicella-zoster virus
  Adenovirus
  Vaccinia
  Epstein-Barr
  Rubeola
  Enteroviruses
  Coxsackievirus

Fungi
  Fusarium spp.
  Candida spp.
  Aspergillus spp.
  Acremonium spp.
  Alternaria spp.
  Penicillium spp.
  Bipolaris spp.

Chlamydia
  Chlamydia trachomatis

Parasites
  Acanthamoeba polyphaga, Acanthamoeba castellanii
  Onchocerca volvulus
  Leishmania brasiliensis
  Trypanosoma spp.
  Nosema spp.
  Vittaforma (Nosema) corneae
  Encephalitozoon spp.

Table adapted from O'Brien TP. Keratitis. In: Mandell GL, Bennett JE, Dolin R, eds. Principles and Practice of Infectious Diseases. 5th ed. New York: Churchill Livingstone; 2000:1257-1266.

wear, trauma (surgical and nonsurgical), contaminated ocular medications, and altered structure of the corneal surface. Contributing risk factors include diabetes mellitus, systemic immunodeficiency, exposure keratopathy (e.g., Graves' exophthalmopathy, Bell's palsy), surface alteration from or with dysfunctional tear states (e.g., Sjögren's syndrome, neurotrophic cornea, chemical burn, Stevens-Johnson syndrome, medication-related), and anatomic abnormalities (e.g., neoplasia, cicatricial pemphigoid, traumatic lid scarring).

Nonsurgical ocular trauma reportedly accounted for 48% to 65% of all corneal ulcers in some developing countries,[3,4] but such trauma was responsible for only 27% of corneal ulcers reported in 1987 at one large trauma referral center in the United States.[5] In a more recent survey, potential predisposing risk factors were identified in 91% of 300 cases of suspected bacterial keratitis; 50% due to contact lens wear, 21% due to ocular surface disease, 15% due to nonsurgical trauma, and 4% due to corneal surgery.[6]

Contact Lenses

Contact lenses are the most common risk factor for microbial keratitis diagnosed in the United States. The annual incidence of contact lens–associated keratitis is estimated at 0.04% for those using daily-wear soft lenses and 0.21% for those with extended-wear lenses. The risk increases approximately tenfold if the lens users wear their contacts overnight and is also positively correlated with the number of consecutive days lenses are worn without removal.[7] The reported percentage of contact lens–associated corneal ulceration in the general population has increased from 0% in the 1950s and 1960s to 31% in the 1970s and more than 50% of all cases since the 1980s.[2] A similar upward trend in contact lens–associated keratitis was seen in academic referral centers during the 1970s and 1980s, but the trend actually began decreasing to 9% to 18% during the late 1990s.[8-10] Although it is tempting to believe that disposable soft contact lenses have started to decrease the incidence of microbial keratitis, it is more likely that a change in treatment patterns is responsible. The fact that the incidence of contact lens–related keratitis has decreased at academic referral centers while increasing in the community-based population suggests a greater willingness on the part of general practitioners and optometrists to treat such patients rather than refer them to major treatment centers. The introduction of commercially available topical fluoroquinolones in the 1990s parallels the reduction of cases diagnosed in academic centers. The ease of use, low cost, availability, and broad-spectrum coverage against most aerobic gram-negative and gram-positive bacteria make these medications attractive. In a questionnaire-based study, 82% of a random sampling of non–cornea fellowship trained ophthalmologists reported that they would treat less severe cases of suspected bacterial keratitis with a single fluoroquinolone, and 62% indicated they would treat more severe cases in a similar manner.[11]

Laboratory Data and Clinical Response

Clinicians often culture the contact lens and the contact lens case in addition to the patient's cornea. False positives are too frequent to recommend this procedure. In one study, significance of cultures from the lens or case could be confirmed by corneal cultures in only 25% of the cases.[9] Gram-negative organisms, such as *Pseudomonas aeruginosa*, that can be cultured from the lens or case are indeed associated with contact lens–associated microbial keratitis; however, gram-positive organisms, such as *Staphylococcus* and *Streptococcus* spp., have often been shown to be responsible for a majority of these ulcers even when gram-negative organisms have been recovered from the contact lens or storage case. Contact lens use alone can produce sterile inflammatory infiltrates that resolve spontaneously with discontinued use of the lens.

CLINICAL PRESENTATION

Eye Pain

As one of the most richly innervated tissues in the body, inflammation of the cornea generally is accompanied by severe pain. This significant discomfort can greatly affect the physical examination. The continued movement of the eyelids over a corneal lesion further adds to the patient's discomfort. The use of a topical anesthetic in the examination room may greatly facilitate the eye examination; however, continued use of topical anesthetics has been implicated in continued epithelial defects and loss of corneal stroma and should therefore not be prescribed beyond the examination process.

CONJUNCTIVAL INJECTION AND DISCHARGE

The rapid onset of pain is often accompanied by significant conjunctival injection, tearing, photophobia, blepharospasm, and decreased vision. Discharge, so often associated with conjunctivitis, is not usually present other than in some cases of purulent bacterial keratitis. There may be great differences in the presence or absence of injection and, to some degree, tearing and discharge based on the etiologic agent (i.e., viral and parasitic keratitis may have minimal discharge; fungal keratitis may have minimal injection in the early phases).

Corneal Infiltrate

Other than the limbal vessels, the cornea is generally clear. Therefore, corneal inflammation appears quite different than in most other tissues. The invading organism begins a reaction whereby inflammatory cells from the limbal vessels and tear film migrate into the cornea, producing a subtle change in transparency. The resultant inflammatory reaction at the site of a microbial replication is called an "infiltrate."

Epithelial Defect

The infiltrate often has an overlying epithelial defect, because the infectious agent generally enters the cornea through an epithelial defect that can rapidly increase in size with the microbial replication. These epithelial defects can best be visualized using a cobalt blue light after the addition of fluorescein, which will pool in areas of punctate and ulcerative defects. Infections caused by slow-growing, fastidious organisms (i.e., *Mycobacterium*, anaerobic bacteria) may have an intact epithelial surface.

Stromal Suppuration

Microbial keratitis generally produces a sharply demarcated epithelial ulceration and suppurative stromal inflammation. Bacterial organisms generally produce a clearly defined, local inflammation; fungal elements can have a more diffuse or multifocal infiltrate. There is substantial crossover in the presenting characteristics of various microbial agents. Again, a number of slow-growing, fastidious organisms may present without an ulceration or a suppurative infiltrate.

Corneal Edema

The loss of transparency is further affected by the corneal edema that is present in almost all cases of microbial keratitis. The corneal clarity is very specifically maintained through the endothelial cells' ability to maintain a stable level of hydration. The influx of fluid that accompanies the inflammatory cells can overwhelm the endothelium's "pumping" capacity, resulting in varying degrees of edema. This fluid may coalesce under the epithelium, forming uncomfortable bullous elevations. This discomfort can be magnified should the bullae rupture, which then may allow further microbial invasion.

Corneal Neovascularization

Neovascularization of the cornea is a common occurrence with chronic inflammation but can present early in the course of severe keratitis. The presence of neovascularization not only affects the severity of the host inflammatory reaction, but also has long-term consequences. After resolution of the inflammation, the vessels may regress slightly to the point of no longer carrying blood but still remain as empty channels ("ghost vessels"). If the neovascularization does not regress, the vessels not only provide a route for recurrent inflammatory cells but also can directly affect visual acuity and greatly decrease the potential for successful corneal transplantation.

Intraocular Inflammatory Reaction

Intraocular inflammation is not uncommon with microbial keratitis, especially with some of the more virulent gram-negative bacteria. These signs, including cell/flare, hypopyon, synechiae, and glaucoma, are less common with early fungal, viral, and parasitic etiologies, but could present during the course of any case of keratitis. Early, subtle changes may be difficult to detect and are often described as protein ("flare") and leukocytes ("cells") in the anterior chamber on slit-lamp examination. Late changes or signs of more aggressive organisms may be seen in a collection of fibrin and inflammatory white blood cells layering in the inferior portion of the anterior chamber (hypopyon). Adhesive scarring of the pupillary margin (posterior synechiae) or of the peripheral iris (peripheral anterior synechiae) may lead to an irregular pupil or elevated intraocular pressure (glaucoma), which may necessitate urgent medical or surgical treatment. This intraocular inflammation is generally considered sterile unless infection has penetrated Descemet's membrane and entered the anterior chamber.

Stromal Melting (Keratolysis)

Loss of corneal tissue (keratolysis) is a major consequence of the inflammatory reaction seen in microbial keratitis. It is most common with bacterial keratitis. Keratolysis can lead to irregular astigmatism, corneal thinning, a visually significant scar, or even corneal perforation.

LABORATORY EVALUATION

The small amount of specimen to be obtained from the cornea requires careful advance planning and consultation with the microbiology laboratory as to how the specimen should be obtained, transported, and processed.

Collection Methods

The rather small area of active infection and the need to avoid excessive corneal thinning by unnecessary scraping dictate ocular akinesia and patient cooperation. This may be accomplished through use of topical anesthetics (although this may reduce growth of recovered organisms) in patients old enough to cooperate and may necessitate general anesthesia in children. Several studies have shown no statistical difference in organism recovery using sterile surgical blades, blunt platinum spatulas, or calcium alginate swabs (often dipped in trypticase soy broth). Corneal biopsies may be necessary, especially with deeper fungal infections or with *Acanthamoeba* in the later stages. (Earlier stages have organisms in the more superficial layers.) Shave biopsies or partial thickness 1 to 2 mm trephined specimens may be possible at the slit lamp, but may necessitate anesthesia and a minor operating room. Lamellar keratoplasty is not usually necessary, but in cases in which a rapidly progressive, necrotizing keratitis is refractory to treatment or identification is otherwise impossible, or both, a diagnostic and therapeutic penetrating keratoplasty (host corneal removal and transplant) may be necessary.

Stains and Media Inoculation

Material from the scrapings is then transferred directly to glass slides and appropriate culture media (see Chapter 15). The slides should be clean, to avoid artifacts, and sterile, to avoid contaminating the instrument. Multiple slides are desirable in order to permit Gram stain, Calcofluor or other fungal stain, and acid-fast stain. Chlamydia, herpesviruses, mycobacteria, and *Acanthamoeba* require special methods for culture. In addition to culturing the suspected cornea, it may be helpful to culture material from the eyelids, conjunctiva, ocular medication bottles, contact lenses, storage cases, and perhaps the uninvolved eye in order to establish the flora uniquely associated with the patient. If the patient had been treated before evaluation and there is uncertainty as to the diagnosis, it may be wise to consider stopping the medication for 12 to 24 hours and then proceed with culture. Obviously antimicrobials should not be stopped in cases of severe or rapidly progressive ulceration.

Viral Cultures

Viral keratitis is unique among microbial keratitis in that the diagnosis is often possible based on morphology and patient history. Culture for herpes simplex virus and herpes zoster virus is now readily accomplished in most routine diagnostic laboratories (see Chapter 15). Viral transport media must be inoculated and the specimen inoculated

into cell culture the same day. Polymerase chain reaction and immunoassay methods are becoming more widespread, and electron microscopy may be helpful.

BACTERIAL KERATITIS

Most Common Etiology

Several published studies have reported that bacterial pathogens are responsible for 65% to 90% of all cases of microbial keratitis.[12,13] In one large survey, a microbial organism was isolated in 49% of 5845 cases of suspected infectious keratitis; 82% were bacterial, 16% fungal, and 2% parasitic.[14] A more recent, though smaller, survey isolated an organism in 68% of 300 eyes suspected of having bacterial keratitis; 83% were gram-positive, 17% gram-negative, and 2% polymicrobial.[6] The majority of all bacterial keratitis is caused by five major groups: *Staphylococcus* spp., *Streptococcus* spp. (*Streptococcus pneumoniae,* groups A-G streptococci), other gram-positive organisms (*Bacillus* and *Propionibacterium* spp.), gram-negative organisms, such as *Pseudomonas, Haemophilus, Moraxella,* and the Enterobacteriaceae (*Proteus, Serratia, Klebsiella, Enterobacter, Citrobacter)*. The prominence of certain organisms responsible for bacterial keratitis has been changing over many years. *S. pneumoniae* was the most common responsible agent in the past, but other gram-positives, opportunistic commensals, *Pseudomonas,* anaerobes, and protozoa are now increasingly being reported. With the advent of refractive surgery, especially laser assisted in-situ keratomileusis (LASIK), more unusual organisms, such as *Nocardia* and *Mycobacterium* spp., are causing keratitis. The apparent changes in causal organisms could be the result of numerous factors: improved isolation techniques, less frequent culturing as highly effective broad-spectrum single agents (i.e., fluoroquinolones) have been developed, increased use of topical corticosteroids (i.e., refractive and cataract surgery), increased population of systemically immunodeficient patients, and an expansion in the use of soft contact lenses, especially extended-wear and cosmetic lenses.[15,16]

Pathogenesis

The corneal epithelium and Bowman's membrane underneath limit penetration of many organisms into the corneal stroma unless the barrier is breached by trauma. The few organisms that appear to invade in the absence of trauma appear to adhere and elaborate proteolytic enzymes or toxins that lyse the tissue barrier. Migration of leukocytes from the vessels in the corneal limbus into the infected cornea add to tissue destruction.[17]

Geographic Variation

Gram-positive organisms, particularly *Staphylococcus aureus,* continue to be the most common agents causing bacterial keratitis in most series. The order of prevalence in one series from New York City was *S. aureus, Moraxella, Pseudomonas,* and *Streptococcus pneumoniae.*[12] A different order, *S. aureus, S. pneumoniae, Pseudomonas,* and *Moraxella,* was seen in a similar series from London.[18] *Pseudomonas* and *Streptococcus* spp. are the most common bacterial pathogens isolated in previously healthy eyes in the southern United States.[13]

Gram-Positive Bacteria

The strains of staphylococci invading the cornea, usually *S. aureus,* are often resident strains from the patient's own flora.[19,20] *Staphylococcus epidermidis* is not a common infectious agent but this organism, along with *Streptococcus* spp., can cause keratitis in immunodeficient patients and may be associated with chronic dacryocystitis.[21] In these cases of *S. epidermidis* and *Streptococcus* keratitis, ulcers may appear similar to the staphylococcal hypersensitivity keratitis (see later), in which corneal inflammation is thought to be a result of toxins produced by the conjunctiva-based organism or a hypersensitivity reaction to some portion of the bacterial cell wall.

Gram-positive aerobic bacilli do not often cause keratitis in immunocompetent individuals.[22] *Corynebacterium diphtheriae* is one of the organisms reported to invade intact epithelial surfaces. *Bacillus cereus* is a gram-positive rod that can cause severe ulcerative keratitis, often after an injury involving a foreign body.[23] *Nocardia* and *Mycobacterium* spp. are increasingly implicated in bacterial keratitis following refractive surgery (i.e., LASIK).

Staphylococcus hypersensitivity reactions may actually be the most common cause of keratitis. Although it is related to the bacteria, it is a reaction to some exotoxin or antigen rather than direct inoculation or infection. This condition may exist in hosts who may not have any increased bacterial load other than what is considered the normal commensural load in healthy individuals. The punctate epithelial defects, marginal stromal infiltrates, phlyctenules, and peripheral ulcerations are theorized to result from either type III or type IV hypersensitivity reactions. Histologic analysis reveals the presence of plasma cells and lymphocytes in the peripheral cornea but an absence of infectious organisms. Further support for the noninfectious etiology comes from the reduction in pathology when treated with topical steroids alone.

Gram-Negative Bacteria

P. aeruginosa is a particularly virulent and generally most common gram-negative organism implicated in bacterial keratitis. Untreated *P. aeruginosa* keratitis progresses quite rapidly from suppuration to perforation, mainly due to swift corneal destruction from the associated proteolytic enzymes.[24,25] A characteristic inflammatory ring of neutrophilic infiltrate may surround the lesion.[26,27] This "ring infiltrate" is not unique to gram-negative organisms; it can also be seen in fungal, viral, and *Acanthamoeba* keratitis. Patients in burn units and intensive care settings often have altered mental status or anatomic injuries that make ocular exposure and corneal desiccation more common. When this is combined with the frequent colonization of such units with *P. aeruginosa,* this organism can be a significant cause of keratitis.

Less common gram-negative entities have been reported to cause keratitis. Although *Morganella morganii* keratitis may be clinically indistinguishable from *P. aeruginosa* keratitis, Delftia (*Pseudomonas) acidovorans* and *Pseudomonas stutzeri* usually have a more benign course.[28] *Serratia marcescens* has been implicated in contact lens-associated keratitis.[29] *Moraxella* keratitis may be more common in alcoholics and, less commonly, in patients with chronic ocular surface disease.[30,31]

Although *N. gonorrhoeae* is more commonly associated with conjunctivitis, it can penetrate an intact corneal epithelium and cause keratitis. The rather explosive onset and copious purulent exudates may obscure a diagnosis of keratitis. The corneal infiltration may be secondary to the effects of the conjunctival infection. *N. gonorrhoeae* can produce such marked infiltration and edema that the affected conjunctiva may protrude or drape over the corneal surface, exposing the epithelium to numerous proteolytic enzymes; ulceration can quickly result. *Acinetobacter* can produce a keratitis that is clinically indistinguishable from *Neisseria* and can appear morphologically similar on Gram stain.

Mycobacteria

Mycobacterium keratitis had been decreasing in prevalence, paralleling the reduction in systemic tuberculosis. Although primary tuberculous keratitis still is uncommon, an increase in systemic immunodeficient hosts as well as incisional refractive surgery (i.e., LASIK) has been accompanied by an increase in *Mycobacterium* keratitis (*Mycobacterium fortuitum, Mycobacterium chelonae, Mycobacterium gordonae* and *Mycobacterium avium-intracellulare*).[32,33] These nontuberculous species can be quite difficult to isolate and eradicate because they follow a chronic indolent course and are often resistant to conventional antituberculous medications. In the case of refractive surgery, the location under the LASIK flap causes difficulty in obtaining cultures as well as direct application of topical medications. *Mycobacterium* spp. are responsible for eventually producing keratitis in about 15% of patients with tuberculoid leprosy but nearly 100% in those with lepromatous leprosy.[34,35]

TREATMENT OF BACTERIAL KERATITIS

Hospital Admission

An important initial decision in treating keratitis involves hospitalization or outpatient care. Hospitalization may be in order for less compliant patients or in cases with rapid necrosis or thinning. The potential for a rapid downturn and possible perforation should give the clinician a low threshold for admission. The high frequency of antimicrobial administration (perhaps hourly around the clock) and close monitoring may make outpatient care impractical, especially for those living alone, far from the hospital or clinic, or otherwise unable to comply with such demands.

Immediate, Aggressive Therapy

Aggressive antimicrobial therapy is the primary approach with infectious keratitis. Topical administration is the most common route, but subconjunctival injections, parenteral and oral routes, and antibiotic-soaked collagen shields/soft lenses have been, or are currently being, used. The clinician must decide the need to initiate immediate antimicrobial therapy, either directed or broad spectrum, or to wait for laboratory identification of the offending agent. The explosive nature of bacterial keratitis suggests the need for immediate therapy, perhaps guided by results of Gram or Giemsa stains, in all suspicious cases. The rather indolent course of fungal and *Acanthamoeba* keratitis and the significant commitment to months of costly treatment might allow for a delay in therapy until a causative agent is identified. If severe suppurative keratitis is seen, the Gram stain and smear will guide the selection of medication. One specific medication may be selected if only one type of bacterium (gram-positive or gram-negative) can be positively identified and the patient has not previously started an antibiotic. If two or more types of bacteria are identified, if the stain and smears are equivocal, or if the patient has been on any type of antimicrobial, then broad-spectrum therapy is initiated.

Antibiotic Solutions

The route of antibiotic administration should be based on the severity of the disease, but often includes hourly (or more frequent) dosing, especially in cases of severe suppurative keratitis. Although patients may prefer ointments for ease of delivery and the comfort associated with the carrier, topical solutions can actually penetrate ocular tissues and achieve higher concentrations better than antibiotics in ointment formulations. Commercial pharmacies do not often provide concentrated (fortified) antibiotics, but compounding and hospital-based pharmacies can easily formulate fortified antibiotics using most parenteral antibiotic preparations.

Local and Systemic Administration

Subconjunctival injection of antibiotics had been more common in the past and is one way to attain a peak concentration without compliance issues. However, the discomfort and temporary nature make this less attractive, and frequent topical administration of fortified antibiotics can achieve adequate tissue levels. Parenteral administration is uncommon and generally used only in suppurative keratitis with impending or actual perforation or bacterial extension involving the sclera.

Contact Lenses and Collagen Shields

Antibiotics have been administered through the use of collagen shields and soft contact lenses.[36] Although these methods have been used experimentally, there are no controlled clinical studies detailing efficacy and safety. New technologic advances in polymer formation and microspheric packaging of antibiotics have allowed more practical ways to actually impregnate antimicrobials into the contact lens rather than simply soaking the lens or shield in the antibiotic as is done currently. Polymer inserts have been designed to theoretically increase the duration of the drug in the tear film. A rather simple strategy to include drug delivery to the corneal tissue involves placement of temporary punctal plugs to reduce the outflow from the ocular surface.

Unique Pharmacokinetics with Topical Antibiotics

Although laboratory identification is quite helpful, the standard sensitivity testing has its limitations in treating ocular infections. The mean inhibitory concentration (MIC) determinations performed in the laboratory are based on antibiotic concentrations that are achievable through the host's serum. The concentrations achievable through direct topical administration can be many thousands of times greater than that measured in the serum after parenteral administration. This might cause an organism to be labeled "resistant" to testing with an antibiotic at achievable serum concentrations, although it may well be in the process of eradication with that same drug through the highly concentrated topical approach. This highlights the clinical response being the best indicator of actual susceptibility, not to the exclusion of laboratory sensitivities, but within the unique limitations in dealing with the direct approach in eye conditions. The direct application to the infected area may avoid dealing with numerous issues critical with systemic therapy: distribution space, first-pass clearance, absorption characteristics, toxic reaction in nontarget tissues, and impact of renal or hepatic failure.

Initial Therapy

The ideal initial antimicrobial agent should be effective (bactericidal versus bacteriostatic) against the common or suspected corneal pathogens, low rates of resistance, minimal toxicity to ocular tissues, comfort on administration, and rapid penetration into the ocular tissues. Traditionally, broad-spectrum therapy for suspected bacterial keratitis has been the combination of a topical cephalosporin (or vancomycin) and an aminoglycoside (tobramycin or gentamicin), all as fortified concentrations. The main disadvantages of such treatment involve the ocular irritation, difficulty of obtaining noncommercially available solutions, significant cost, and continued refrigeration of some preparations. These inconveniences have led to an increasing interest in initial single-agent therapy using recently developed fluoroquinolones. As single agents or in combination, treatment generally begins with hourly dosing and then is tapered according to the clinical response. The fortified preparations are often continued for 10 to 14 days, after which a broad-spectrum nonfortified antibiotic may be given until resolution.

Many classes of antibiotics have been used for the treatment of specific classes of organisms, often based on Gram stain and eventual identification. The advent of the broad-spectrum fluoroquinolones has altered some of these traditional classes and treatment pathways, but many still hold true. Topical cephalosporin preparations are often used in gram-positive keratitis, especially with *Staphylococcus* spp. Vancomycin is an alternate if resistance is suspected. Gentamicin and tobramycin are the most common therapeutic choices in gram-negative keratitis. Drops are readily available commercially after the clinical improvement warrants a change from the fortified preparation.

Topical Fluoroquinolones

The development of fluoroquinolones has radically altered the previously "standardized" treatment of bacterial keratitis. Cultures were performed on all patients and all were generally started on combination fortified antibiotics. The efficacy of the fluoroquinolones, however, has made some consider monotherapy and question the need for culturing in all cases. The three agents most responsible for this shift are ciprofloxacin, ofloxacin, and levofloxacin. The spectrum of coverage at the high concentrations obtained locally is quite similar for all three, showing activity against most gram-negative aerobes and many gram-positive organisms.[37] These fluoroquinolones have significant activity against *P. aeruginosa*, including strains that may be resistant to other antimicrobials. The three fluoroquinolones are the best commercially available agents with regard to activity against a number of gram-positive species; however, some of the *Streptococcus* and *Enterococcus* species are only somewhat susceptible to these agents. *Haemophilus, Neisseria,* and *Moraxella* spp. are quite susceptible to any of the fluoroquinolones. Ciprofloxacin, ofloxacin, and levofloxacin have reasonable activity topically against some

Mycobacterium and *Chlamydia* species. The greatest gap in coverage appears to be with *Streptococcus* spp. and anaerobic bacteria.

Comparison of Fluoroquinolones and Fortified Antibiotics

Any new medication or alteration in "standard" treatment protocols is best accepted after direct comparison to the gold standard. There are several comparative studies of the fluoroquinolones and the fortified combination therapies. In one randomized, masked comparative study of 122 patients, ofloxacin was found to be as efficacious as fortified gentamicin and fortified cefuroxime.[38] Ofloxacin also compared favorably with fortified tobramycin and fortified cefazolin in another multicenter, randomized study.[39] A similarly designed multicenter study involving 324 patients showed no difference using ciprofloxacin versus fortified cefazolin and fortified tobramycin.[40] In all three studies the patients favored the fluoroquinolone, mainly for greater ocular comfort. The only adverse effect of the fluoroquinolones was the appearance of white crystalline precipitates near the epithelial defect in 16% of patients. This precipitate was seen more frequently with ciprofloxacin than with ofloxacin, consistent with a difference in the pH of the two agents. The precipitates can impair ability to monitor the sub-precipitate infiltrates. The corneal precipitates appear to have no other clinical impact, and they resolve spontaneously after the medication is stopped.

Resistance and Newer-Generation Fluoroquinolones

As the fluoroquinolones have become widely used clinically as well as in animal husbandry, resistance has predictably begun to emerge. Again, laboratory evaluation of "resistance" may not be as clinically relevant given the topical administration; however, clinical resistance is beginning to emerge. Two new fluoroquinolones have recently gained U.S. Food and Drug Administration (FDA) approval for use in ophthalmology. Moxifloxacin and gatifloxacin have been marketed to provide increased gram-positive coverage while still maintaining adequate gram-negative protection, where resistance has not been common. Clinical studies are under way, and the early results appear promising.

Proposed Treatment Guidelines

The spectrum, safety, comfort, cost, and availability of the fluoroquinolones make them a very appealing choice in treating keratitis. Although many practitioners use these medications as first-line agents, fluoroquinolones are still not recommended as empiric therapy in vision-threatening keratitis. Initial treatment, often with combination agents directed toward the likely pathogens, guided by laboratory evaluation, is still essential for such cases. A recent cornea and contact lens congress proposed the following recommendations for managing keratitis. The best approach for corneal ulcers is still not definite.

1. Corneal scrapings are indicated in patients with suspected infectious keratitis when risk factors are present, when there is a large central infiltrate, or after empirical therapy has failed.
2. Culture should be done in all cases of suspected infectious keratitis in community- and hospital-based practices.
3. Fortified cefazolin and aminoglycoside should be used for more severe keratitis.
4. As an alternative, combine a third-generation fluoroquinolone with fortified cefazolin.[14]
5. Monotherapy with a fourth-generation fluoroquinolone can be used for mild keratitis.

Corticosteroids

The use of topical corticosteroids to decrease long-term sequelae of bacterial keratitis is controversial. An intense suppurative inflammatory reaction consisting mainly of polymorphonuclear leukocytes is induced by many bacteria responsible for keratitis. These neutrophils may destroy a significant amount of tissue through free radicals and the liberation of collagenases and gelatinases that dissolve the stroma. The rationale for corticosteroids is to prevent such tissue destruction.

Several studies have shown that concomitant use of topical steroids does not alter or reduce the bactericidal effect of antimicrobials.[41] There is a concern that steroid use may promote a relapse of an organism that appeared to be clinically resolved but still had a low number of active bacteria. This may be the case with virulent organisms that are difficult to eradicate and require only a low inoculum to establish an infection as seen in some gram-negative bacteria such as *P. aeruginosa*.

Supportive Measures

Supportive measures in managing infectious keratitis are numerous. Topical cycloplegics can reduce the discomfort of ciliary spasm, reducing the associated photophobia and preventing synechiae (scarring/adhesions) of the pupil. If corneal ulceration is quite significant, a temporary soft contact lens may act as a bandage to relieve some of the discomfort while allowing repair of the stromal and epithelial surfaces without mechanical disruption from the lid. The contact lens itself can serve as a nidus for infection, but this should not be the case with the temporary nature combined with continued application of antibiotics. The change to commercial-strength antimicrobials is warranted as soon as clinically reasonable because the fortified antibiotics are epitheliotoxic and decrease epithelial healing.

CHLAMYDIAL AND SYPHILITIC KERATITIS

Chlamydiae are small intracellular organisms dependent on their host cell for replication and prolonged survival.[42] Their unique multiphasic life cycle permits the pathogen to establish persistent infections, allowing the organism to escape immune clearance yet express virulence determinants that cause chronic inflammation.[43] In addition, long-lasting protective immunity does not develop following chlamydial infection, and reinfections are common.

Ocular Associations in *Chlamydia*

Chlamydiae cause a spectrum of acute and chronic ocular diseases, ranging from self-limited follicular conjunctivitis to trachoma, often with blinding sequelae.[44] Several serotypes of *Chlamydia trachomatis* can cause a follicular conjunctivitis in the adult, inclusion conjunctivitis. The same serotypes can lead to neonatal conjunctivitis if an infected mother transmits the pathogen to the newborn during vaginal delivery. Repeated infections with certain serotypes can cause trachoma, a chronic follicular keratoconjunctivitis that remains the most common cause of preventable blindness in the world. In developed countries, sexually transmitted *C. trachomatis* rarely causes the sequelae of true trachoma, which is generally marked by repeat infection and chronicity.

The cicatricial phase of trachoma causes lid irregularities leading to exposure or direct trauma from inturned lids or eyelashes which leads to corneal ulceration and opaque scarring, often long after resolution of the infective phase. The resultant effects on the cornea may predispose to bacterial superinfection, further adding to the disease morbidity.

Syphilitic Keratitis (Interstitial Keratitis)

The keratitis associated with syphilis, sometimes termed *interstitial keratitis* (IK), is not often seen in the active phase but is noted in subsequent examinations. The two major categories of IK are associated with syphilis and *Mycobacterium tuberculosis*. IK is rarely associated with acquired primary or secondary syphilis (<3% of all cases), with more than 90% caused by congenital syphilis. The IK usually does not develop until the later phases of congenital syphilis, occurring in about 50% of all untreated patients. The typical presentation is during the early teen years; however, it can develop any time during the first two decades of life. Pain, photophobia, increased tearing, blepharospasm, and decreased vision are common during the acute phase. A severe iridocyclitis is present as the cornea becomes hazy with significant reduction in vision over a few days. Neovascularization progresses centrally over the next months until the vessels coalesce in the central cornea, at which time there is a dramatic change in the disease process.

After resolution of the corneal infiltrates and significant regression of the blood vessels (leaving empty channels or "ghost vessels"), some patients have a surprisingly significant return of visual acuity. Only about 10% have less than 20/200 vision; approximately 70% have between 20/20 and 20/100 vision. Lyme disease has also been implicated as a possible etiology in corneal disease, with *Borrelia burgdorferi* causing an IK similar to that seen with syphilis.[45]

TREATMENT OF CHLAMYDIAL AND SYPHILITIC KERATITIS

Keratitis in patients with trachoma is largely due to the lid scarring or exposure resulting from the conjunctival disease and therefore requires treatment of the associated conditions to reduce the subsequent keratitis. Several generalizations can be made when treating other chlamydial eye infections. First, systemic rather than local therapy is necessary when treating adult inclusion conjunctivitis because the infected individual may harbor the pathogen in the genital tract. Similarly, newborns presenting with neonatal chlamydial conjunctivitis may harbor the organism in the lower respiratory tract and may need to be treated systemically. Individuals treated systemically do not need to be treated locally. Second, all sexual partners must be treated along with the infected patient to prevent primary infection in the partner as well as reinfection in the symptomatic individual. Third, repeat treatment may be necessary because clinical cure rates can be modest, especially for treatment of chronic chlamydial infection. Finally, antibiotics that achieve sustained tissue levels, high intracellular penetration, and low microbial resistance and require an infrequent dosing regimen are generally preferred. To this end, azithromycin is rapidly becoming the mainstay of therapy for many chlamydial infections, including trachoma.

Treatment of Interstitial Keratitis (Syphilitic and Lyme Associated)

Syphilitic interstitial keratitis is an immune phenomenon that may benefit from topical corticosteroids, but antitreponemal therapy has little impact on the corneal process. However, such therapy may be necessary for other systemic manifestations of the disease and does seem to reduce the recurrence rate and likelihood of bilateral involvement. Lyme keratitis may be addressed through the use of corticosteroids with systemic evaluation and treatment following similar reasoning as with syphilis.

VIRAL KERATITIS

Herpes Simplex Virus

Ocular herpes may be classified into three general groups: congenital and neonatal, primary, and recurrent. The vast majority of all ocular herpes infections are caused by herpes simplex virus 1 (HSV-1). Because infection is acquired by passage through an infected birth canal, 80% of neonatal cases are caused by HSV-2.[46,47] Multiple recurrences are far more common with genital and oral herpes than with ocular herpes. Studies have shown an 89% recurrence rate for genital and a 42% recurrence rate for oral HSV over a 1-year period. In contrast, the ocular herpes recurrence rate was 40% over a 5-year period, which is fortunate considering the visual consequences.[48,49] Epithelial ulcers ultimately respond to antiviral therapy, but stromal involvement may not readily clear, leaving a nebulous scar. In the absence of superinfection, the skin lesions heal without scarring.

Primary Herpes Simplex Virus Keratitis

Sixty percent of children are infected with HSV by age 5, all of whom then carry latent virus in their dorsal root ganglions.[50,51] Ocular disease resulting from primary infection or reactivation in the trigeminal ganglion may manifest in many forms, one of which is keratoconjunctivitis. In the absence of skin vesiculation, differentiation from adenoviral infection is aided by a careful search of the lid margins for signs of herpetic blistering.

Primary HSV keratitis is often atypical. Initially, there may be just a nonspecific diffuse punctate keratitis that evolves into multiple scattered microdendritic figures. There may be wandering linear serpiginous ulcers across the entire corneal surface.[48] The diffuse nature of this primary epithelial involvement is probably a function of the host's nonimmune state, which allows more widespread ulceration. Primary disease is, as a rule, confined to the epithelium in terms of clinical findings. Stromal involvement is not usually seen in this phase of the disease, presumably because the host is not immunologically programmed against the virus. Primary ocular herpes should not be confused with "first ocular occurrence." The former is a first encounter with the virus; the latter is the first eye involvement with HSV in a patient who has had a subclinical oral or nasal infection and is immune. First ocular occurrence is, therefore, similar to recurrent ocular herpes as described below.

Recurrent Keratitis

Patients with recurrent herpes have both cellular and humoral immunity against the virus. Herpes simplex–induced eruptions of the corneal epithelium are characteristically thin, branching dendritic ulcers; wider, branching dendrogeographic ulcers; or map-shaped geographic lesions, all caused by live virus. Little inflammatory cell reaction—polymorphonuclear (PMN) leukocytes but no lymphocytes—is seen in this form of ocular herpes, but many free viruses lie in intracellular and extracellular locations, particularly in the basal epithelium.[52] Signs and symptoms include tearing, irritation, photophobia, and often blurring of vision. As the only presenting clinical findings may be a watery conjunctivitis, the patient should be asked about any trauma, previous corneal ulcers, inflammation inside the eye (iritis), nasal or oral cold sore, genital sores, recent use of topical or systemic steroid or immunosuppressive drugs, and immunologic deficiency states, malignancy, organ transplants, or chronic eczema. If corneal examination reveals dendritic or even geographic ulceration, the infectious agent is HSV until proven otherwise. In HSV, corneal sensation is reduced in about 70% of patients,[53] although it is almost never totally absent as often seen in zoster keratitis. The more marked the stromal scarring, found in more chronic cases, the more marked is the decrease in sensitivity. Initially the corneal lesions begin as a fine, transient, punctate keratitis that coalesces to form dendritic, dendrogeographic, or geographic ulcers. In an eye that has had many recurrences or is receiving steroids without antiviral prophylaxis, the more subtle stages may be bypassed and the cornea may simply break down in rapidly forming geographic ulceration. The actual incidence of infectious epithelial HSV keratitis in immunocompetent patients may be much higher than suspected clinically. Kodama and colleagues reported that of 48 eyes with diagnoses of nonherpetic conditions, 19 were culture positive for HSV.[53] Contrary to common opinion, recurrent epithelial infections are not always due to the patient's original HSV strain. Remeijer and associates reported a study on 30 patients in whom sequential corneal HSV-1 isolates revealed that 63% were genotypically the same from recurrence to recurrence, whereas 37% were actually genetically different.[54]

Stromal Inflammation and Intraocular Reaction

Stromal reaction is usually absent or mild and confined to the anterior layers in milder epithelial infections. On occasion, however, even mild epithelial infection may be associated with notable stromal edema and iritis. These eyes are more likely to go on to chronic recurrent immune disease and scarring resulting in visual loss. Concurrent or future stromal disease may be minimized, as well as healing rate enhanced, by gentle débridement of the infected epithelium with a sterile cotton-tipped applicator before instituting antiviral chemotherapy.[55,56] Such débridement is thought to remove much of the immune-inciting antigen that could penetrate to deep stromal layers.

Neurotrophic Keratitis

Occasionally, despite adequate antiviral therapy, epithelial ulcers do not completely heal or, having healed, break down again in an ovoid or dendritiform pattern. This is trophic, or "metaherpetic," keratopathy. Clinically, a trophic ulcer may be distinguished from an actively infected viral ulcer by the appearance of its edge. Trophic ulcers have gray, thickened borders formed by heaped-up epithelium unable to move across or adhere to the damaged ulcer base. In contrast, actively infected ulcers have discrete flat edges that may change their configuration as the ulcer erodes newly infected epithelium. Persistence of trophic ulceration over several weeks or months poses a threat to the integrity of the globe. The longer the ulcer is present, the greater is the chance of collagenolytic activity with subsequent stromal melting (thinning) down to Descemet's membrane, and perforation.

Varicella-Zoster Virus

Contact with the varicella virus in the United States is almost invariable,[57] although the use of varicella-zoster virus (VZV) vaccine as part of the recommended childhood immunizations is now reducing the frequency of chickenpox. Ocular involvement in chickenpox is diagnosed on the basis of an acute or recent history of chickenpox with ocular or periocular involvement with the vesicle-pustules.

VZV infection may involve small phlyctenule-like lesions that may erupt most commonly at the corneal limbus.[48,58,59] It is unclear whether these are due to live virus or to an immune phlyctenule-like reaction, or both. The cornea may develop superficial punctate keratitis, wispy, branching dendritic ulcers without terminal knobs (herpes simplex ulcers have knob-shaped endings on their branches).[60,61] Months after the acute disease, a disciform keratitis similar to that seen in HSV disease may develop.[62] This disciform reaction is steroid responsive but may recur and cause scarring similar to HSV keratitis. Less frequently reported varicella findings in the eye include dendritic keratitis and neurotrophic ulceration with corneal melting.

Herpes Zoster Ophthalmicus

Herpes zoster is a recurrent infection with varicella-zoster virus. Approximately 50% to 72% of patients with periocular zoster have involvement of the ocular structures, develop chronic disease, and possibly suffer a moderate to severe degree of visual loss.[63] Of the three divisions of the fifth (trigeminal) cranial nerve, the first (ophthalmic) is by far the most frequently affected. Herpes zoster ophthalmicus (HZO) occasionally affects the maxillary division, but rarely affects the mandibular division.[64] The first division of the fifth nerve, along with sympathetic branches from the ciliary ganglion, innervate the lids, forehead, tip of the nose, and the majority of the orbit and ocular adnexa.[65]

Clinical Manifestations of Herpes Zoster Ophthalmicus

In Liesegang's study of 94 patients with HZO, two thirds had corneal involvement.[65] This took the form of punctate keratitis (51%), pseudodendrites (51%), anterior stromal infiltrates (41%), sclerokeratitis (1%), keratouveitis-endotheliitis (34%), peripheral ulcerative keratitis (7%), delayed mucous plaques (13%), disciform keratitis (10%), neurotrophic keratitis (25%), and exposure keratitis (11%). A delayed limbal vasculitis with or without anterior ischemic necrosis was also noted on rare occasions. Corneal disease may precede, accompany, or follow the acute disease by months to years and may recur in any of its many forms. The acute epithelial disease is considered infectious and may present as a diffuse superficial punctate keratitis or more commonly as migratory dendritic lesions that at first could be confused with herpes simplex. Piebenga and Laibson also described herpes zoster dendrites that were culture negative but appeared as heaped-up, superficial plaquelike lesions, coarser than herpes simplex dendrites but lacking terminal bulbs (an important differentiating point) and staining poorly with fluorescein.[66] They cause a foreign-body sensation and are elevated, coarse, gray-white, swollen epithelial cells piled in plaques or a dendritiform shape on the corneal surface. They are both migratory and transitory and are usually associated with a neurotrophic keratitis (75%) or previous corneal inflammation (100%). Immune keratitis similar in appearance to HSV stromal disciform edema/

endotheliitis may occur any time after the acute illness, most commonly first appearing after 3 to 4 months.

Corneal Anesthesia

Corneal sensation may be markedly diminished in even the mildest cases of clinically manifest herpes zoster keratitis. Sixty percent of patients have moderate to complete corneal anesthesia (neuroparalysis) secondary to the destructive VZV ganglionitis and to aqueous tear deficiency due to loss of the nasolacrimal reflex.[65,67,68] Anesthetic epithelial breakdown comprises one of the most dangerous aspects of herpes zoster keratitis. One quarter of all HZO patients develop clinical signs of neurotrophic keratitis due to permanent corneal anesthesia. As the corneal epithelium becomes progressively more unhealthy, oval epithelial defects may develop in the palpebral fissure or lower corneal area with subsequent melting and corneal thinning. Neovascularization in these cases is a good sign and should be allowed to take place because healing often accompanies the process. Because many of these eyes are poor surgical risks, it is unlikely that a corneal graft would be successful.

Ocular Complications with Vaccinia (Smallpox) Vaccination

Recent attention to the development and use of a smallpox vaccine has brought about an interest in vaccinia keratitis; the vaccine directed against smallpox is derived from the bovine equivalent, vaccinia.[69] A study by Ruben and Lane indicated that, not only were the ocular complications of vaccination infrequent, they were also not notably vision threatening.[70] Corneal involvement following autoinoculation is uncommon, with reports of approximately 1.2 cases per million primary vaccinations.[70] Other studies indicate postvaccinial keratitis in 6 to 37 percent of vaccinia cases with ocular involvement.[71,72] Keratitis appears more frequently in primary vaccinees than in revaccinees, which is probably a reflection of the immune status of the previously vaccinated patient. Long-term sequelae, such as madarosis (eyelash loss), punctal stenosis, and cicatricial lid changes are more common in cases with corneal manifestations (18%) than in ocular vaccinia without keratitis (2%). However, reexamination of patients with corneal vaccinia after 5 years revealed either no ocular residua or only minor corneal changes, including mild corneal scarring, ghost vessels, and subepithelial opacity with chronic conjunctivitis.[70]

Vaccinia Keratitis

Corneal manifestations of ocular vaccinia range from mild superficial punctate keratitis to interstitial or stromal keratitis, to disciform keratitis with keratic precipitates, to necrosis with perforation. As with epithelial herpes simplex or varicella-zoster keratitis, corneal epithelial vaccinia lesions stain with rose bengal early in the course of the disease and with fluorescein as an epithelial defect evolves. Direct infection of the corneal epithelium with vaccinia may present as multiple punctate lesions, as dendritiform lesions, or in a geographic pattern. All forms of vaccinia epithelial keratitis may closely resemble that seen with herpes simplex. Stromal keratitis due to vaccinia may initially appear as scattered subepithelial opacities similar to that seen in epidemic keratoconjunctivitis. This pattern may evolve to ring infiltrates, ulceration, or stromal necrosis or scarring, which must be differentiated from *Acanthamoeba*, herpes zoster, and herpes simplex stromal keratitis.

Adenoviral Keratitis

Epidemic keratoconjunctivitis (EKC), caused by various adenovirus serotypes, is a highly contagious condition that can have explosive spread in schools, workplaces, and physicians' offices. The keratitis may have an early epithelial component followed by a later subepithelial stage. Active viral replication within epithelial cells marks the early keratitis. The later-developing subepithelial infiltrates (SEIs) probably represent an immune response to viral antigens as microscopic analysis of SEIs reveals lymphocytes, degenerated collagen fibrils, and scarring, but no virus particles. A watery discharge, photophobia, and foreign body sensation is often accompanied by a hemorrhagic conjunctivitis with membrane formation. The keratitis progresses through a fairly orderly process of superficial epithelial keratitis, deep epithelial keratitis, and eventual SEIs.

Differential Diagnosis of Epidemic Keratoconjunctivitis

Pharyngoconjunctival fever is caused by different serotypes of adenovirus with a similar course of conjunctivitis but less commonly leads to epithelial keratitis and SEIs. Pharyngoconjunctival fever may begin in one eye but usually involves both eyes eventually. Enterovirus, molluscum contagiosum, Epstein-Barr virus, and coxsackievirus can be associated with a mild epithelial keratitis similar to the early stages of EKC. Keratitis associated with hemorrhagic conjunctivitis due to enterovirus 70 is discussed in Chapter 169. Keratitis associated with measles (rubeola) generally is similar to that seen in EKC; however, in patients with significant malnutrition and vitamin A deficiency, measles keratitis can become a blinding disease with secondary bacterial infection and possible perforation of the globe.

TREATMENT OF VIRAL KERATITIS

Self-Limited Cases

Many of the cases associated with viral keratitis may not require specific antimicrobial therapy. There may be a twofold reason for this: First, a number of viral conditions are self-limited with relatively minor deleterious effects on the cornea, and second, the research and production of antiviral agents have not led to many viable treatment options, especially as compared to those for bacterial keratitis. However, there are viral organisms that can cause significant visual or ocular morbidity, particularly when combined with the associated inflammatory response.

Treatment of Herpes Simplex Virus and Varicella-Zoster Virus

The management plan for both herpes simplex and herpes zoster has undergone many changes as more antiviral agents and information from basic research and clinical trials become available. Tables 107-2 through 107-4 give the currently recommended treatments. Data in the normal population indicate that the incidence of zoster is much lower in vaccinated healthy children and adults compared with those who have suffered a natural infection.[73] The FDA approval of a live, attenuated VZV vaccine for the immunization of healthy people of all ages who have not had previous varicella, thereby reducing the incidence of varicella and its complications, was hailed as a major step in controlling this disease and a potential key to reducing the incidence of zoster.[74] One question that continues to be raised is, should every patient with herpes zoster receive antiviral treatment? Gnann and

---

TABLE 107-2 Antiviral Medications Used in Herpes Simplex Keratitis

Acute infection: topical or systemic medication. In the immunocompromised, a topical agent may be combined with a systemic agent and continued longer than the indicated period

trifluridine (Viroptic) 1% drops	Nine times daily for 7 days. May decrease dose to 5 times/day after 7 days if ulcer healed
acyclovir (Zovirax) 400 mg PO*	tid for 14-21 days
famciclovir (Famvir) 500 mg PO†	bid for 14-21 days
valacyclovir (Valtrex) 1 g PO†,‡	bid for 14-21 days

Prophylaxis: against recurrent stromal keratitis, high steroid use, and graft rejection/postoperative grafts

acyclovir (Zovirax) 400 mg PO*,†	bid for 12-18 months
famciclovir (Famvir) 250 mg PO†	bid for 12-18 months
valacyclovir (Valtrex) 500 mg PO†,‡	bid for 12-18 months

*Pediatric syrup 200 mg/tsp.
†Not U.S. Food and Drug Administration approved for this specific purpose.
‡For use in immunocompetent hosts only.
Table adapted from Pavan-Langston D. Ophthalmic zoster. In: Watson C, Gershon A, eds. Herpes Zoster and Post-herpetic Neuralgia. 2nd ed. Amsterdam: Elsevier Sciences BV, 2001:119-129. Reprinted with permission from Elsevier.

TABLE 107-3 Management of Herpes Zoster Ophthalmicus (Acute)

Antivirals
Treat for 7 days, preferably starting within 72 hours of onset of rash
famciclovir (Famvir) 500 mg PO tid (immunocompetent or compromised)
valacyclovir (Valtrex) 1 g PO tid (immunocompetent)
acyclovir (Zovirax) 800 mg PO 5 × /day (5 × /d)
Immunocompromised patients: IV acyclovir for 10 days; 10 mg/kg q8h in adults and 500 mg/m² q8h for children younger than 12 years

Pain Prevention and Management
Tricyclic antidepressants, e.g., nortriptyline, desipramine 25-75 mg PO qhs or divided dose for 3 months (or longer PRN) starting lowest dose with antivirals or as early as possible after acute disease onset, increasing over 2-3 weeks PRN. Caution in patients with cardiac disease.
Non-narcotic or short-term narcotic analgesics, e.g., oxycodone, codeine, propoxyphene

Dermatitis Therapy
Cool to tepid wet compresses (if tolerated) to keep dermatitis clean

Ocular Anterior Segment
Exposure keratopathy: topical antibiotic ophthalmic ointment tid
Dendritiform keratopathy: therapy for 2-3 weeks (variably effective)
3% vidarabine ointment, or
1% trifluridine 5 × /day, or
Oral antivirals (see above)
Immune keratopathy, episcleritis, scleritis, or iritis
Topical steroids (1%-0.125% prednisolone, 0.1% dexamethasone, 1% rimexolone, or 0.2%-0.5% loteprednol) q 3-4 hours to qid PRN disease severity
Slow taper. Antibiotic eye drops or gtt/ointment prophylaxis
Oral nonsteroidal anti-inflammatory agents, e.g., ibuprofen 400 mg PO bid-tid
Topical antivirals unnecessary
Cycloplegia PRN iritis (scopolamine qd)

Glaucoma
Topical β-blockers, e.g., timolol or carteolol bid
Add PRN latanoprost qd, brimonidine, or dorzolamide bid
No miotics, e.g., pilocarpine.
Topical steroids if glaucoma due to inflammatory trabeculitis

Table adapted from Pavan-Langston D. Ophthalmic zoster. In: Watson C, Gershon A, eds. Herpes Zoster and Post-herpetic Neuralgia. 2nd ed. Amsterdam: Elsevier Sciences BV, 2001:119-129. Reprinted with permission from Elsevier.

TABLE 107-4 Management of Herpes Zoster Ophthalmicus (Chronic or Recurrent)

Dendritiform or Immune Keratopathy, Episcleritis, Scleritis, Iritis
See Table 107-3

Tenuous, Hazy Epithelium in Anesthetic Cornea
Early lateral tarsorrhaphy and lubrication with artificial tears and tear ointments
Allow vascularization to progress to aid in healing any ulcer
Topical steroids with caution and only at low doses to minimize any inflammation

Exposure Keratopathy or Corneal Ulceration or Thinning
Lateral tarsorrhaphy
Therapeutic soft contact lens, e.g., Permalens or Kontur
Tissue adhesive, e.g., Dermabond, Epidermglu for progressive thinning
Conjunctival flap, transplant, or keratoprosthesis

Glaucoma
See Table 107-3

Postherpetic Neuralgia (PHN) (Drugs Below May Be Used Additively)
Tricyclic antidepressants, e.g., nortriptyline, desipramine, or other tricyclics, 25 mg titrated up to 75 mg qhs or divided dose PRN. Caution if patient has cardiac disease.
Gabapentin (Neurontin): 300 mg PO bid starting dose. Efficacy may not be reached until 600 mg bid-qid. Some may not respond at all.
Slow-release opioids added if tricyclic antidepressants and/or gabapentin not sufficiently effective; oxycodone (OxyContin-SR) 10-40 mg PO q12h
Capsaicin cream one to three times daily to skin as tolerated
Lidocaine skin patches, 12 hours on, 12 hours off painful skin area
Frontal and/or nasal nerve block
Trigeminal ganglion ablation contraindicated

Table adapted from Pavan-Langston D. Ophthalmic zoster. In: Watson C, Gershon A, eds. Herpes Zoster and Post-herpetic Neuralgia. 2nd ed. Amsterdam: Elsevier Sciences BV, 2001:119-129.

Whitley have recommended that treatment be given to those at high risk for complications: older than 50 years of age, immunocompromised, moderately severe to severe pain at presentation, greater degree of skin-surface involvement, and those with HZO.[75] One study of 324 patients compared the effect of antiviral therapy on complications of HZO; the probability of an adverse outcome was 9% in untreated patients and 2% in treated ones.[76]

Treatment of Ocular Vaccinia

During the previous era of routine smallpox vaccination, the treatment of ocular vaccinia was based predominantly on anecdotal reports of the use of vaccinia immune globulin alone or in combination with idoxuridine or topical interferon. Many of these isolated case reports were before the availability of more effective topical antivirals, such as trifluridine and vidarabine. In the absence of masked, controlled clinical trials, a meaningful meta-analysis of the literature is not possible. Because of this limitation, some of the current recommendations, which depart from the previous policy designed in the mid-1960s, were made by the Centers for Disease Control and Prevention after consultation with an outside panel of corneal and external disease and infectious disease specialists.[77] They are based upon principles routinely employed in the treatment of other viral diseases of the ocular surface—treat active viral replication with antivirals followed by cautious use of topical corticosteroids (when appropriate) to prevent inflammatory damage of the cornea and anterior segment. For vaccinia, there is an additional therapeutic agent, intravenous immune globulin (IVIG). Because ocular vaccinia virus

infections are generally self-limited, treatment should be directed toward shortening the course and limiting the severity of the disease. The evaluation and treatment of ocular complications of vaccinia virus should be performed by an ophthalmologist in a timely manner. IGIV should be considered for use in severe ocular disease when keratitis is not present (e.g., severe blepharitis or blepharoconjunctivitis).[77] If keratitis accompanies these conditions, IGIV need not necessarily be withheld, but should be used cautiously (and generally in a single dose) due to a possible increased risk of corneal scar formation. Similarly, if IGIV is indicated based on other criteria (e.g., eczema vaccinatum, progressive vaccinia), its use or dosing need not be withheld if keratitis is also present. For treatment of isolated keratitis, IGIV does not offer added benefit when topical antivirals are used and is not recommended. If IGIV is administered to a patient who has keratitis, informed consent should be obtained after discussion of potential risks and benefits. Although no topical antiviral is licensed by the FDA for the treatment of ocular vaccinia, topical trifluridine drops or vidarabine ointment can be used off-label for this purpose, and is likely more effective and less toxic than topical idoxuridine or cytosine arabinoside.[78,79] Topical vidarabine may be preferable for use in children because it has been available in an ointment preparation that allows less frequent dosing and is associated with less initial stinging than trifluridine. Vidarabine ointment is currently not commercially available but may be obtained through compounding pharmacists. If, however, vidarabine cannot be obtained or the patient would better tolerate drops, trifluridine may be used in children just as it is in ocular herpes simplex. Topical antiviral drugs should be considered for prophylaxis of the conjunctiva and cornea if vaccinia lesions are present on the eyelid, especially if near the lid margin. The use of these drugs for prophylaxis should be balanced against the possible risk of drug toxicity and of introducing virus into the eye by frequent manipulation. Topical trifluridine may possibly have an increased risk of toxicity if used for longer than 14 days. Toxic changes to the ocular surface are almost invariably reversible with discontinuation of the drug.

Treatment of Viral Keratoconjunctivitis

The keratoconjunctivitis associated with EKC (adenoviral mediated) may not require any measures other than artificial tears and possible cycloplegics. There is no effective antiviral for EKC. If, however, the condition is associated with significant pain, photophobia, and visual alteration, a course of mild topical corticosteroids in addition to the cycloplegics may be beneficial. There have been no definitive trials indicating whether topical steroids alter the typical duration of the disease process.

FUNGAL KERATITIS

Although a multitude of genera of molds and yeasts have been identified in fungal keratitis, it is generally much less common than either bacterial or viral keratitis.[13,80] Although there are great differences based on global geography, fungi are generally responsible for less than 5% to 10% of corneal infections in most clinical series reported in the United States. Keratitis due to molds occurs more commonly in areas with a warmer and more humid environment. These fungi are usually inoculated into the cornea by trauma involving plant or vegetable matter. Keratitis due to *Candida albicans* is acquired from the patient's own flora. Corticosteroid use has been implicated in altering the cornea's resistance to fungal infection while certainly potentiating any existing fungal infection. Topical corticosteroids for medical or surgical ocular conditions (i.e., LASIK) as well as the use of soft contact lenses as a "bandage" for postoperative or damaged corneas may increase the likelihood of fungal keratitis.

Numerous fungi can cause keratitis—*Aspergillus, Curvularia, Paecilomyces, Phialophora, Blastomyces, Sporothrix, Exophiala, Pseudallescheria, Scedosporium,* and *Alternaria*—but *Fusarium* spp. appear to be the most commonly isolated.[81,82] *Nocardia* and *Corynebacterium matruchotii* are rare causes of infectious keratitis but give a corneal lesion whose appearance is nearly identical to those seen in fungal keratitis. Because the treatment would be quite different, laboratory evaluation is necessary. A number of fungi have been rarely suspected of causing keratitis but because they are ubiquitous and easily isolated from the environment, their role in true pathogenesis is difficult to ascertain.

Mild Early Clinical Presentation

Patients with fungal keratitis generally have fewer inflammatory signs and symptoms than those with bacterial keratitis. Fungal infections may be mild and indolent, often without suppuration or an ulcerated epithelial surface in the early phases. Molds (most often *Fusarium* or *Aspergillus*) may manifest with gray-white, dry-appearing infiltrates that have a filamentous or feathery edge. The superficial lesions may even appear as strands elevating the corneal surface. Minimal stromal inflammation may be present in a focal or multifocal pattern along with satellite lesions. Larger lesions or deep invasion may be associated with an endothelial plaque or hypopyon. As the keratitis progresses, extensive suppuration may develop, giving the appearance of a bacterial keratitis. A rapidly increasing hypopyon and anterior chamber membranes may be noted. Such rapidly progressive anterior chamber inflammation may herald fungal extension into the anterior chamber.

Candida Keratitis

Major predisposing risk factors for keratitis due to *Candida* spp. are prolonged epithelial ulceration, topical corticosteroid use, recent keratoplasty (corneal transplant), and current corticosteroid use, and current use of a "bandage" soft contact lens (i.e., recurrent erosion, persistent epithelial defect, etc.). *Candida* keratitis is more common in patients with a history of ocular surface disease, previous ocular herpes, exposure keratopathy, and systemic immunosuppression. In contrast to that caused by molds, *Candida* keratitis manifests as an oval epithelial ulceration with an expanding, more sharply demarcated, densely focal suppuration. In this appearance, *Candida* may mimic a gram-positive keratitis, although the inflammatory reaction is generally somewhat less than that seen with bacterial keratitis.

TREATMENT OF FUNGAL KERATITIS

Limited Treatment Options

The development of antifungal preparations has been similar to that for the antivirals, in that there are relatively few treatment options for patients. Most agents must be specially formulated, and a number of the oral and parenteral agents cannot be processed into topical solutions owing to pH or other solubility difficulties. Therapy for fungal keratitis may require a combination of expensive topical and systemic antimicrobials, often for many months. Natamycin suspension, although no longer commercially available in the United States, is the recommended topical treatment for most cases of keratitis due to molds, especially those due to *Fusarium* species. An alternative to natamycin is chlorhexidine gluconate, which was found equally effective when both were compared in a randomized trial with 71 patients in Bangladesh, most of whom had *Aspergillus* or *Fusarium* keratitis.[83] Topical amphotericin B solution, prepared in a pharmacy, is the recommended treatment for *Candida* keratitis and may be an alternative for *Aspergillus* keratitis. Topical preparations of flucytosine, fluconazole, and itraconazole have been used in clinical and experimental situations. Favorable reports of using oral itraconazole for mold keratitis suggest that either this drug or perhaps oral voriconazole may be worth adding to whatever topical therapy is given. Oral fluconazole should be considered for *Candida* keratitis, although experience is limited. Detection of hyphae on wet mounts of corneal scrapings is difficult and mechanical débridement may be necessary as the fungi are often deep within the stroma. The greater sensitivity of Calcofluor white staining of wet mounts recommends this technique for corneal scrapings. Penetration of topical agents into the corneal stroma is usually poor, and the fungal infiltration deep within the stroma is frequently unresponsive to such therapy. Cases with progressive disease unresponsive to maximal oral or topical therapy may ultimately require a penetrating keratoplasty to prevent perforation or loss of the globe due to unchecked fungal extension.

PARASITIC KERATITIS

Acanthamoeba Keratitis

Acanthamoebae are free-living protozoa ubiquitous in fresh water, well water, brackish water, and soil. These protozoa have been increasingly recognized as a worldwide cause of painful keratitis, resistant to many forms of treatment and ultimately responsible for loss of vision or even loss of the eye.[84] They are resistant to killing by freezing, desiccation, and chlorination commonly used in municipal water supplies, swimming pools, and hot tubs. They exist as mobile trophozoites or dormant cysts. The vast majority of reported cases of amoebic keratitis have been associated with contact lens use,[85,86] although corneal trauma involving contaminated water has been implicated. A significant increase in amoebic keratitis was seen when saline tablets were introduced to the general public to enable preparation of homemade saline solutions. A reduction in amoebic keratitis was seen after the tablets were taken off the U.S. market; however, such keratitis persists.

Clinical Signs and Symptoms with Amoebic Keratitis

Patients with amoebic keratitis have photophobia and severe pain, often out of proportion to the clinical appearance. A lengthy and worsening course shows little or no response to a variety of antimicrobial agents. Early infection is often limited to the corneal epithelium, manifesting as a diffuse epithelial keratitis, dendritic lesion, or radial keratitis. At this stage, amoebic keratitis is often misdiagnosed as herpetic keratitis, and attempted treatment is tried with antivirals and corticosteroids. Enlarged corneal nerves have been suggested, but perineural inflammation may be a more appropriate term. This radial keratitis/perineuritis is generally not seen with other types of microbial keratitis. A late finding is the "classic" ring infiltrate after progression of the gray-white superficial nonsuppurative infiltrate generally found in the central or paracentral cornea.

Onchocerciasis

The impact of parasitic keratitis is devastating in some tropical regions. Sclerosing keratitis and corneal opacification can be the result of stromal infestation by microfilariae of *Onchocerca volvulus*.[87] The host for this parasite is the black fly found in Africa and certain areas of Central and South America. The female fly deposits her eggs in vegetation and on rocks in streams and rivers. In spite of the swiftly flowing cool water, the eggs persist. Onchocerciasis, or "river blindness," is one of the leading causes of blindness throughout the world.[88] The ocular lesions are seen after direct invasion of the anterior segment by the microfilaria. Early in the course of the condition, the patient will complain of tearing, photophobia, and redness. Slit lamp examination may reveal microfilariae "swimming" in the anterior chamber or slowly moving through the cornea just under the epithelium.[89] The host tolerates the organism surprisingly well; however, a severe inflammatory reaction begins when the microfilariae die in the cornea.[90] Sclerosing keratitis is the eventual blinding complication following many long-lasting infections.

Leishmaniasis

Leishmania keratitis may appear quite similar to that of onchocerciasis.[91] *Leishmania* parasites are obligate intracellular agents transmitted through bites of infected sand flies. Human infection can take many forms, but cutaneous and mucocutaneous varieties cause edema, ulceration, and scarring of the lids or conjunctivae. Corneal involvement may begin as superficial "bumps" (phlyctenules) that progress to abscess formation and possible corneal perforation.

Microsporidia and Trypanosomes

With the increase in infections due to the human immunodeficiency virus, Microsporidia infections are being more commonly recognized. Microsporidia are ubiquitous obligate intracellular parasites. Except in the immunocompromised patient, they are an unlikely cause of keratitis, generally after traumatic penetration of the stroma. *Vittaforma (Nosema) corneum* has been implicated in a few cases in Africa, India, and Japan.[92] *Nosema ocularum* and *Brachiola (Nosema) algerae* keratitis have also been reported. The ensuing granulomatous inflammation generally leads to necrotizing thinning and perforation. HIV-positive patients may develop mild conjunctivitis with punctate epithelial keratitis caused by the related microsporidium, *Encephalitozoon cuniculi*.[93] Symptoms may be mild and can easily be mistaken for tear film deficiencies or blepharitis, or both; a high index of suspicion is required in such patients to make a clinical diagnosis of microsporidial keratitis. The tsetse fly can infect humans with the hemoflagellates responsible for African trypanosomiasis, or "sleeping sickness." Ocular effects manifest as unilateral conjunctivitis, periorbital edema, and preauricular lymphadenopathy. Interstitial keratitis similar to that seen in syphilitic keratitis has been described.[94]

TREATMENT OF PARASITIC KERATITIS

Early diagnosis of *Acanthamoeba* infection is the single most *predictive* factor in successful treatment. Most cases are initially diagnosed and treated as herpetic keratitis, further delaying proper treatment and usually allowing treatment with corticosteroids, which is proportionally correlated with a poor outcome. Early diagnosis during the epithelial stage may lead to a good visual outcome after débridement and a 3- to 4-month course of antiamebic therapy. If diagnosis is made after stromal infiltrates appear, the prognosis is more guarded because eradication is quite difficult, often requiring up to a year of antiamebic therapy. Numerous agents have been suggested in treating *Acanthamoeba*, likely indicating that the best therapy is uncertain. Diamidines (propamidine, hexamidine), biguanides (polyhexamethylene biguanide, chlorhexidine), aminoglycosides (neomycin, paromomycin), and imidazoles/triazoles (miconazole, clotrimazole, ketoconazole, itraconazole) have all been used in different combinations, depending on availability. Most of these agents are effective against the free-living trophozoite form of the organism but none is particu-

larly effective against the cystic stage. No agreement exists as to the best combination, but successful outcomes have been achieved using a biguanide with or without a diamidine. Similar controversy exists on the use or benefit of corticosteroids, because early use may contribute to persistence of viable cysts. Penetrating keratoplasty may be necessary, medically and therapeutically. However, even in a quiet-appearing eye, such surgery has been associated with a recurrence if performed within the first year of the diagnosis, presumably due to persistent cysts. It may be best to complete a full course of antiamebic therapy followed by a 6-month disease-free course before considering a penetrating keratoplasty.

Onchocerciasis was originally treated with diethylcarbamazine, but ivermectin is equally effective and less toxic.[95] Encephalitozoon conjunctivitis has responded to albendazole 400 mg PO bid (see Chapter 282), suggesting that the drug should be considered for keratitis. Experience with other agents has been discouraging. Penetrating keratoplasty has been used as a last resort.

REFERENCES

1. O'Brien TP. Keratitis. In: Mandell GL, Bennett JE, Dolin R, eds. Principles and Practice of Infectious Diseases. 5th ed. New York: Churchill Livingstone; 2000:1257-1266.
2. Erie JC, Nevitt MP, Hodge DO, et al. Incidence of ulcerative keratitis in a defined population from 1950 through 1988. Arch Ophthalmol. 1993;111:1665-1671.
3. Upadhyay MP, Karmacharya PC, Koirala S, et al. The Bhaktapur eye study: Ocular trauma and antibiotic prophylaxis for the prevention of corneal ulceration in Nepal. Br J Ophthalmol. 2001;85:388-392.
4. Srinivasan M, Gonzales CA, George C, et al. Epidemiology and aetiologic diagnosis of corneal ulceration in Madurai, south India. Br J Ophthalmol. 1997;81:965-971.
5. Ormerod LD, Hertzmark E, Gomez DS, et al. Epidemiology of microbial keratitis in Southern California. A multivariate analysis. Ophthalmology. 1987;94:1322-1333.
6. Bourcier T, Thomas F, Borderie V, et al. Bacterial keratitis: Predisposing factors, clinical and microbiological review of 300 cases. Br J Ophthalmol. 2003;87:834-838.
7. Basic and Clinical Science Course Section 8, External Disease and Cornea. Foundation of the American Academy of Ophthalmology. 2001;169.
8. Jeng BH, McLeod SD. Microbial keratitis (Editorial). Br J Ophthalmol. 2003;87:805-806.
9. Cohen EJ, Fulton JC, Hoffman CJ, et al. Trends in contact lens-associated corneal ulcers. Cornea. 1996;15:566-570.
10. Rattanatam T, Heng WJ, Rapuano CJ, et al. Trends in contact-lens related corneal ulcers. Cornea. 2001;20:290-294.
11. McLeod SD, DeBacker CM, Viana MAG. Differential care of corneal ulcers in the community based on apparent severity. Ophthalmology. 1995;103:479-484.
12. Asbell P, Stenson S. Ulcerative keratitis. Survey of 30 years laboratory experience. Arch Ophthalmol. 1982;100:77.
13. Liesegang TJ, Forster RK. Spectrum of microbial keratitis in South Florida. Am J Ophthalmol. 1980;90:38.
14. Forster RK. Conrad Berens lecture. The management of infectious keratitis as we approach the 21st century. CLAO J. 1998;24:175-180.
15. Schein OD, Poggio EC, Seddon JM, et al. The incidence of ulcerative keratitis among extended contact lens wearers. N Engl J Med. 1989;321:773.
16. Glynn RJ, Schein OD, Seddon JM, et al. The incidence of ulcerative keratitis among aphakic contact lens wearers in New England. Arch Ophthalmol. 1991;109:104-107.
17. Basic and Clinical Science Course Section 8, External Disease and Cornea. Foundation of the American Academy of Ophthalmology. 2001;170.
18. Coster DJ, Wilhelmus KR, Peacock J, et al. Suppurative keratitis in London. In: Trevor-Roper T, ed. European Society of Ophthalmology. The Cornea, Health, and Disease. London: Academic Press; 1981:395.
19. Locatcher-Khorazo D, Gutierrez E. Bacteria typing of *Staphylococcus aureus*. A study of normal, infected eyes in environment. Arch Ophthalmol. 1960;63:774.
20. Locatcher-Khorazo D, Sullivan N, Gutierrez E. *Staphylococcus aureus* isolated from normal and infected eyes. Stage types and sensitivity to antibacterial agents. Arch Ophthalmol. 1967;77:370.
21. Kim HB, Ostler HB. Marginal corneal ulcer due to beta-*Streptococcus*. Arch Ophthalmol. 1977;95:454.
22. vanBusterveld OP, Richards RD. Bacillus infection of the cornea. Arch Ophthalmol. 1965;74:91.
23. O'Day DM, Ho PC, Andrews JS, et al. Mechanism of tissue destruction in ocular *Bacillus cereus* infection. In: Trevor-Roper T, ed. European Society of Ophthalmology. The Cornea, Health, and Disease. London: Academic Press; 1981:403.
24. Brown SI, Bloomfield SE, Wai-Fong IC. The cornea-destroying enzyme of *Pseudomonas aeruginosa*. Invest Ophthalmol. 1974;13:174.
25. Ohman DR, Burns RP, Iglewski BH. Corneal infections in mice with toxin-A and elastase mutants of *Pseudomonas aeruginosa*. J Infect Dis. 1980;142:547.
26. Mondino BJ, Rabin BS, Kessler E, et al. Corneal rings with gram-negative bacteria. Arch Ophthalmol. 1977;95:2222.
27. Belmont JB, Ostler HB, Chandler RD, et al. Non-infectious ring-shaped keratitis associated with *Pseudomonas aeruginosa*: Histopathological and enzymatic characterization. Am J Ophthalmol. 1982;93(3):338-341.

28. Brinser JH, Torczynski E. Unusual *Pseudomonas* corneal ulcers. Am J Ophthalmol. 1977;84:462.
29. Lass JH, Haaf J, Foster CS, et al. Visual outcome in eight cases of *Serratia marcescens* keratitis. Am J Ophthalmol. 1981;92:384.
30. Baum J, Fedukowicz HB, Jordan A. A Survey of *Moraxella* corneal ulcers in a derelict population. Am J Ophthalmol. 1980;90:476.
31. Cobo LM, Coster DJ, Peacock J. Moraxella keratitis in a nonalcoholic population. Br J Ophthalmol. 1981;65:683.
32. Meisler DM, Friedlaender MH, Okumoto M. *Mycobacterium cheloni* keratitis. Am J Ophthalmol. 1982;94:398.
33. Newman PE, Goodman RA, Waring GA, et al. A cluster of cases of *Mycobacterium cheloni* keratitis associated with outpatient office procedures. Am J Ophthalmol. 1984;97:344.
34. Allen JH, Byers JL. The pathology of ocular leprosy. I. Cornea. Arch Ophthalmol. 1960;64:216.
35. Elliott DC. An interpretation of the ocular manifestations of leprosy. Ann N Y Acad Sci. 1951;54:84.
36. O'Brien TP, Sawusch MR, Dick JD, et al. Use of collagen corneal shields versus soft contact lenses to enhance penetration of topical tobramycin. J Cataract Refract Surg. 1988;144:505-507.
37. Bower KS, Kowalski RP, Gordon YJ. Fluoroquinolones in the treatment of bacterial keratitis. Am J Ophthalmol. 1996;121:712-715.
38. Ofloxacin Study Group. Ofloxacin monotherapy for the primary treatment of microbial keratitis: A double-masked, randomized, controlled trial with conventional dual therapy. Ophthalmology. 1997;104:1902-1909.
39. O'Brien TP, Maguire MG, Fink NE, et al. Efficacy of ofloxacin versus cefazolin and tobramycin in the therapy for bacterial keratitis. Report from the Bacterial Keratitis Study Research Group. Arch Ophthalmol. 1995;113:1257-1265.
40. Hyndiuk RA, Eiferman RA, Caldwell DR, et al. Comparison of ciprofloxacin ophthalmic solution 0.3% to fortified tobramycin-cefazolin in treating bacterial corneal ulcers. Ciprofloxacin Bacterial Keratitis Study Group. Ophthalmology. 1996;103:1854-1863.
41. Badenoch PR, Hay GJ, McDonald PJ, et al. A rat model of bacterial keratitis: Effect of antibiotics and corticosteroids. Arch Ophthalmol. 1985;103:718-722.
42. Kalayoglu MV, Byrne GI. *Chlamydia*. In: Dworkin M, ed. Prokaryotes. New York: Springer-Verlag; 2001:1-16.
43. Beatty WL, Morrison RP, Byrne GI. Persistent *Chlamydia:* From cell culture to a paradigm for chlamydial pathogenesis. Microbiol Rev. 1994;58:686-699.
44. Kalayoglu MV. Ocular chlamydial infections: Pathogenesis and emerging treatment strategies. Curr Drug Targets Infect Disord. 2002;2:85-91.
45. Baum J, Bavza M, Weinstein, et al. Bilateral keratitis as a manifestation of Lyme disease. Am J Ophthalmol. 1988;105:107.
46. Nahmias A, Alford C, Korones S. Infection of the newborn with herpesvirus hominis. Adv Pediatr. 1970;17:185.
47. Hutchison D, Smith R, Haughton D. Congenital herpetic keratitis. Arch Ophthalmol. 1975;93:70.
48. Pavan-Langston D. Cornea and external disease. In: Pavan-Langston D, ed. Manual of Ocular Diagnosis and Therapy. Philadelphia: Lippincott Williams & Wilkins; 2002:67-129.
49. Wilhelmus K, Coster DJ, Donovan HC, et al. Prognostic indicators of herpetic keratitis: Analysis of a five year observation period after corneal ulceration. Arch Ophthalmol. 1981;91:1578-1582.
50. Buddingh G, Schrum DI, Lanier JC, Guidry DJ. Studies on the natural history of herpes simplex infections. Pediatrics. 1953;11:595-610.
51. Croen K, Ostrove JM, Dragovic LJ, Straus SE. Patterns of gene expression and sites of latency in human ganglia are different for varicella-zoster and herpes simplex viruses. Proc Natl Acad Science U S A. 1988;85:9773.
52. VanHorn D, Edelhauser H, Schultz R. Experimental Herpes simplex keratitis: Early alterations of corneal epithelium and stroma. Arch Ophthalmol. 1970;84:67.
53. Kodama T, Hayasaka S, Setogawa T. Immunofluorescent staining and corneal sensitivity in patients suspected of having herpes simplex keratitis. Am J Ophthalmol. 1992;113:187.
54. Remeijer L, Maertzdorf J, Bultenwerf J, et al. Corneal herpes simplex virus type 1 superinfection in patients with recrudescent herpetic keratitis. Invest Ophthalmol Vis Sci. 2002;43:358-363.
55. Wilhelmus K. The treatment of herpes simplex virus epithelial keratitis. Trans Am Ophthalmol Soc. 2000;98:505-532.
56. Wilhelmus K. Interventions for herpes simplex virus epithelial keratitis. Review. Cochrane Database Syst Review. 2001;(1):CD002898.
57. Preblud S, D'Angelo LJ. Chicken pox in the United States, 1972-1977. J Infect Dis. 1979;140:257-260.
58. Liesegang T. Varicella-zoster virus eye disease. Review. Cornea. 1999;18:511-531.
59. Wilson FI. Varicella and Herpes zoster ophthalmicus. In: Tabbara K, Hyndiuk R, eds. Infections of the Eye. Boston: Little, Brown; 1996:387-400.
60. Edwards T. Ophthalmic complications of varicella. J Pediatr Ophthalmol. 1965;2:37.
61. deFreitas D, Sato E, Pavan-Langston D, et al. Delayed onset varicella keratitis. Cornea. 1992;11:471-474.
62. Wilhelmus K, Hamill M, Jones D. Varicella disciform stromal keratitis. Am J Ophthalmol. 1991;111:575-580.
63. Miserocchi E, Waheed NK, Dios E, et al. Visual outcome in Herpes simplex virus and Varicella zoster virus uveitis. Ophthalmol. 2002;109:1532.
64. Esiri M, Tomlinson A. Herpes zoster: Demonstration of virus in trigeminal nerve and ganglion by immunofluorescence and electron microscopy. J Neurol Sci. 1972;15:35-38.
65. Liesegang T. Corneal complications from Herpes zoster ophthalmicus. Ophthalmology. 1985;92:316.
66. Piebenga L, Laibson P. Dendritic lesions in Herpes zoster ophthalmicus. Arch Ophthalmol. 1973;90:268.
67. Zaal M, Volker-Dieben H, D'Amaro J. Risk and prognostic factors of postherpetic neuralgia and focal sensory denervation: A prospective evaluation in acute herpes zoster ophthalmicus. Clin J Pain. 2000;16:345-351.
68. Heigle T, Pflugfelder S. Aqueous tear production in patients with neurotrophic keratitis. Cornea. 1996;15:135-138.
69. Semba R. The ocular complications of smallpox and smallpox immunization. Arch Ophthalmol. 2003;121:715-719.
70. Ruben F, Lane J. Ocular vaccinia: Epidemiologic analysis of 348 cases. Arch Ophthalmol. 1970;84:45-51.
71. Ellis P, Winograd L. Current concepts of ocular vaccinia. Trans Proc Coast Otoophthalmol Soc. 1963;44:141-148.
72. Sedan J, Ourgaud A, Guillot P. Les accidents oculaires d'origine vaccinale observes dans le Department des Bouches-du-Rhone au cours de l'epidemie variolique de l'hiver 1952. Ann Oculist. 1953;186:34-61.
73. White C, Letter to the Editor. Pediatrics. 1992;89:354.
74. Pepose J. The potential impact of varicella vaccine and new antivirals on ocular disease related to varicella-zoster virus. Am J Ophthalmol. 1997;123:243-249.
75. Gnann JJ, Whitley R. Clinical practice. Herpes zoster. Review. N Engl J Med. 2002;347:340-346.
76. Severson E, Baratz KH, Hodge DO, Burke JP. Herpes zoster ophthalmicus in Olmsted County, Minn: Have systemic antivirals made a difference? Arch Ophthalmol. 2003;121:386-390.
77. Centers for Disease Control and Prevention. Smallpox vaccination and adverse reactions: Guidance for clinicians. MMWR Dispatch. 2003;52:1-29.
78. Hyndiuk R, Okumoto M, Damiano R, et al. Treatment of vaccinial keratitis with vidarabine. Arch Ophthalmol. 1976;94:1363-1364.
79. Jack MK, Sorenson RW. Vaccinial keratitis treated with IDU. Arch Ophthalmol. 1963; 69:730-732.
80. Jones DB. Opportunistic fungal infections in ophthalmology. Fungal keratitis. In: Chic ED, Balows A, Furcolow ML, eds. Opportunistic Fungal Infections. Springfield, IL: Charles C Thomas; 1975:103.
81. Jones DB, Forster RK, Rebell G. *Fusarium solani* keratitis treated with natamycin (pimaricin): 18 consecutive cases. Arch Ophthalmol. 1972;88:147.
82. Rosa RH Jr, Miller D, Alfonso EC. The changing spectrum of fungal keratitis in South Florida. Ophthalmology. 1994;101:1005-10013.
83. Rahman MR, Johnson GJ, Husain R, et al. Randomised trial of 0.2% chlorhexidine gluconate and 2.5% natamycin for fungal keratitis. Br J Ophthalmol. 1998;82:919-925.
84. Jones DB, Visvesvara GS, Robinson NM. Acanthamoeba polyphagia keratitis and *Acanthamoeba* uveitis associated with fatal meningoencephalitis. Trans Ophthalmol Soc UK. 1975;95:221.
85. Ma P, Willaert E, Juechter KB, et al. A case of keratitis due to *Acanthamoeba* in New York, and features of ten cases. J Infect Dis. 1981;143:662.
86. Mannis NJ, Tamaro R, Roth AM, et al. Acanthamoeba scleral keratitis. Determining diagnostic criteria. Arch Ophthalmol. 1986;104:*1313*-1317.
87. Gibson DW, Heggie C, Connor DA. Clinical and pathologic aspects of onchocerciasis. Pathol Ann. 1980;15:195.
88. Thylefors B. Ocular onchocerciasis. Bull World Health Organ. 1978;56:63.
89. Fuglsang JA. Living microfilaria of Onchocerca volvulus in the cornea. Br J Ophthalmol. 1983;57:712.
90. Rodger FC, Chir M. The pathogenesis and pathology of ocular onchocerciasis. Am J Ophthalmol. 1960;49:104.
91. Roizenblatt J. Interstitial keratitis caused by American (mucocutaneous) leishmaniasis. Am J Ophthalmol. 1979;87:175.
92. Pinnolis M, Egbert PR, Font RL, et al. Nosematosis of the cornea. Arch Ophthalmol. 1981;99:1044.
93. Friedberg DN, Stenson SM, Orenstein JM, et al. Microsporidial keratoconjunctivitis in acquired immunodeficiency syndrome. Arch Ophthalmol. 1990;108:504-508.
94. Neame H. Parenchymatous keratitis in trypanosomiasis in cattle and in dogs and in man. Br J Ophthalmol. 1927;11:209.
95. White AT, Newland HS, Taylor HR, et al. Controlled trial and dose-finding study of ivermectin for treatment of onchocerciasis. J Infect Dis. 1987;156:463-470.

CHAPTER **108**

Endophthalmitis

MARLENE L. DURAND

Endophthalmitis refers to bacterial or fungal infection of the vitreous or aqueous humor or both. Viruses and parasites commonly cause uveitis (e.g., cytomegalovirus retinitis or *Toxoplasma* chorioretinitis) (see Chapter 109), but rarely endophthalmitis. Most cases of endophthalmitis are due to bacteria and present acutely. Acute endophthalmitis is a medical emergency because delayed or inadequate therapy may result in irreversible vision loss.

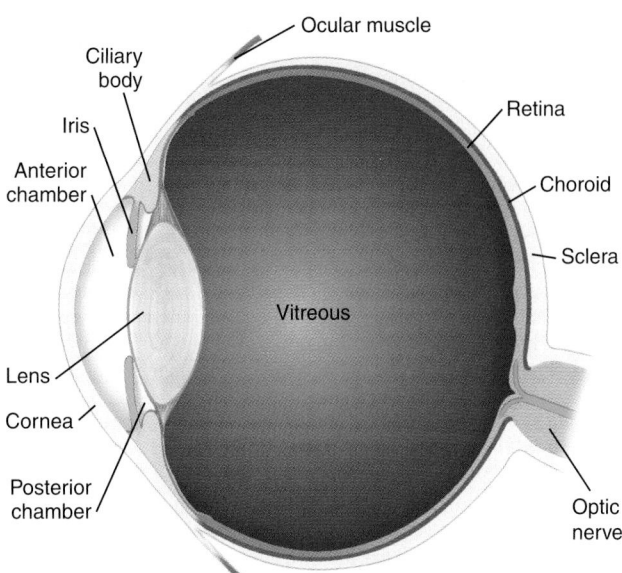

FIGURE 108-1. Cross-sectional diagram of the eye.

ANATOMY AND PATHOGENESIS

The eye is divided into anterior and posterior segments (Fig. 108-1). The anterior segment is divided further into anterior and posterior chambers. The anterior segment is filled with approximately 0.25 mL of aqueous humor, a liquid that is continuously produced and resorbed, with a turnover time of approximately 100 minutes. The vitreous body, in contrast, is a 4-mL gel-like substance that forms in utero and is never regenerated. The vitreous may be removed by vitrectomy surgery and replaced with clear fluids. The lens lies within a fibrous capsule between the anterior and posterior segments, and the posterior lens capsule serves as a barrier between the vitreous and the aqueous. Breaks in this barrier allow vitreous "wicking" into the anterior segment and increase the risk of endophthalmitis after cataract surgery.

Most cases of endophthalmitis are exogenous, in which organisms are introduced into the eye from an external source. This may occur by surgery, trauma, severe corneal infection (keratitis), or through a glaucoma filtering bleb. In exogenous endophthalmitis, the infection is confined to the eye, and there are rarely any systemic symptoms. In endogenous endophthalmitis, organisms seed the eye hematogenously, and patients may have prominent symptoms of the underlying systemic infection (e.g., endocarditis).

ENDOPHTHALMITIS CATEGORIES

It is useful to classify endophthalmitis into six categories (Table 108-1). The first four types discussed here present acutely, whereas the last two usually have a subacute or chronic presentation.

TABLE 108-1 Endophthalmitis Categories and the Most Common Pathogens in Each

Acute postcataract	Coagulase-negative staphylococci
Bleb-related	Viridans streptococci, *Streptococcus pneumoniae, Haemophilus influenzae*
Posttraumatic	*Bacillus cereus*
Endogenous	*Staphylococcus aureus,* streptococci, gram-negative bacilli
Chronic pseudophakic	*Propionibacterium acnes*
Fungal	*Candida, Aspergillus, Fusarium*

Acute Postcataract Endophthalmitis

Acute postcataract endophthalmitis is the most common type of endophthalmitis and an important problem in the United States, where there are more than 2 million cataract surgeries performed annually. Removing a cataract, or opacified lens, requires making an incision through the sclera or cornea, then through the anterior lens capsule to remove the lens. An attempt is made to leave the posterior lens capsule intact. In most cases, an artificial intraocular lens is placed in the residual capsular bag. The incidence of postcataract endophthalmitis is 0.1% to 0.2% in several large series worldwide.[1-3] This incidence has not changed since the 1970s.[4] The pathogenesis of postcataract endophthalmitis has been well established, and in nearly all cases, the source of the bacteria is the patient's own eyelid or conjunctival flora.[5,6] These bacteria contaminate the aqueous at the time of surgery, and many studies have found that aqueous samples taken at the close of surgery often grow bacteria (8% to 43% of cases).[7-10] Endophthalmitis is rare despite this high rate of intraoperative contamination, and rabbit experiments with *Staphylococcus epidermidis* suggest that the immune system can clear small inocula of bacteria of low virulence from the aqueous.[11]

The vitreous is less resistant to infection, and the risk of postcataract endophthalmitis is nearly 14 times higher if a communication with the vitreous occurs during surgery.[12] This communication usually occurs through an inadvertent break in the posterior lens capsule. Other risk factors for postcataract endophthalmitis include diabetes and wound dehiscence or leak.[13,14] Advances in cataract surgery (e.g., phacoemulsification and foldable synthetic intraocular lenses) have allowed incisions so small that they are considered self-sealing. Concerns that this sutureless surgery may increase the risk of postoperative endophthalmitis have not been substantiated with standard "scleral tunnel" incisions.[15] Incisions made through the cornea ("clear cornea incision") have become increasingly popular, although these may carry a higher risk of endophthalmitis than scleral tunnel incisions.[16,17]

Symptoms of endophthalmitis occur within 1 week of surgery in 75% of patients and include eye pain (74%), redness (82%), and decreased vision (94%).[18] The patient often has no symptoms for several days, then symptoms develop rapidly within 24 hours. The pain is often not severe, and patients feel otherwise well. Signs of systemic illness are absent: There is no fever, and the white blood cell count is normal in two thirds of patients and only mildly elevated in the rest. The physical examination is unremarkable except for the involved eye, which is usually injected and has a hypopyon (Fig. 108-2). The hypopyon is a layer of white blood cells in the anterior chamber. Slit-lamp examination reveals white blood cells in the aqueous and vitreous. Inflammation may be so severe that it obscures the funduscopic view of the retina.

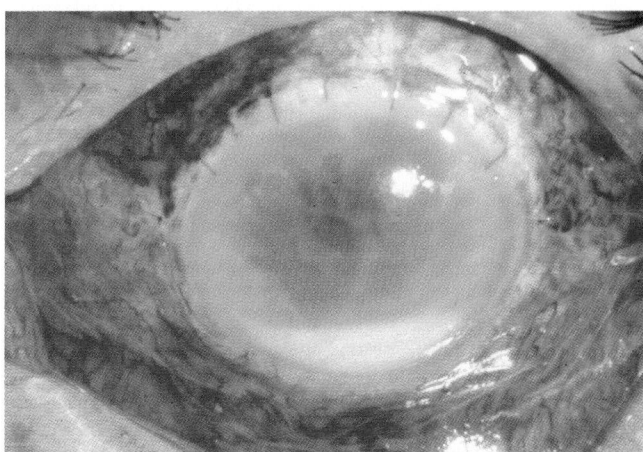

FIGURE 108-2. Eye with endophthalmitis, illustrating a hypopyon. *(Courtesy of Dr. Donald J. D'Amico.)*

Coagulase-negative staphylococci are the major pathogens, causing 70% of culture-positive cases.[18] *Staphylococcus aureus* (10%), streptococci (9%), other gram-positive cocci (5%), and gram-negative bacilli (6%) account for the remaining cases. Streptococci include viridans streptococci, *Streptococcus pneumoniae,* and β-hemolytic streptococci including group A. Thirty percent of patients with clinical evidence of endophthalmitis have negative or equivocal vitreous cultures if strict criteria are used, such as semiconfluent growth or growth on at least two media.[18]

Bleb-Related Endophthalmitis

Bleb-related endophthalmitis occurs in eyes that have a filtering bleb to control glaucoma that is refractory to medical management. A bleb is a surgically created defect in the sclera covered only with conjunctiva that allows excess aqueous to filter out of the eye and into the systemic circulation. Nearly all blebs are created intentionally to reduce intraocular pressure, but a bleb may result as a complication of other eye surgery. The bleb may become infected (blebitis), and bacteria may rapidly enter the eye, resulting in endophthalmitis. Bleb-related endophthalmitis usually occurs abruptly, months to years after bleb surgery. One retrospective review of 49 cases of bleb-related endophthalmitis found that endophthalmitis developed an average of 2 years after bleb placement (range 1 month to 8 years).[19] The incidence of endophthalmitis varies in different series depending on the duration of follow-up, but the follow-up adjusted incidence in one series was 1.3% per patient-year, with a predicted incidence of 7.5% in 5 years.[20] Bleb-related endophthalmitis is typically fulminant because of the bacteria involved. Patients complain of sudden onset of eye pain and decreased vision and on examination have an injected eye, a hypopyon, and often a purulent bleb. In most series, streptococci, including *S. pneumoniae* and viridans streptococci, cause half of the cases; *Haemophilus influenzae* and *Moraxella catarrhalis* are the other major pathogens.[21,22] In contrast, one series found that streptococci caused only 19% of cases, whereas *S. aureus* and *S. epidermidis* caused approximately 30% each.[19]

Posttraumatic Endophthalmitis

Posttraumatic endophthalmitis develops in 4% to 13% of eyes that have sustained penetrating trauma.[23] Endophthalmitis is most likely to follow a lacerating injury with a metal object, whereas glass laceration injuries and blunt trauma rarely lead to endophthalmitis. Lens disruption is another major risk factor and was present in 86% of posttraumatic endophthalmitis cases in one study.[24] Other risk factors include retained intraocular foreign bodies and delay in primary closure of greater than 24 hours.[25,26] *Bacillus cereus* is a major cause of posttraumatic endophthalmitis and the most feared because it produces a fulminant endophthalmitis that usually results in a blind eye.[27] Rare cases of successful therapy have been described.[28] Onset of symptoms in 12 to 24 hours and a ring corneal infiltrate are characteristic of this infection. Other causes of posttraumatic endophthalmitis include coagulase-negative staphylococci, streptococci, and gram-negative bacilli such as *Klebsiella* and *Pseudomonas.*[29,30] Endophthalmitis due to molds occurs rarely and usually has a subacute presentation (see later).

Endogenous Bacterial Endophthalmitis

Endogenous bacterial endophthalmitis results from bacteremic seeding of the eye. Usually a significant focus of bacteremia is identified, such as endocarditis or an intra-abdominal abscess, but transient bacteremia rarely may cause endophthalmitis. Endocarditis was the source in nearly 40% of cases in one U.S. series of 28 patients, whereas one patient developed endophthalmitis 2 days after upper gastrointestinal endoscopy, presumably from transient bacteremia.[31] Patients who are injection drug users also are at risk for endophthalmitis from transient bacteremia. Gastrointestinal or hepatic abscesses, urinary tract infections, meningitis, and infected indwelling catheters are other sources of bacteremia in endogenous endophthalmitis case series.[31-33] In Taiwan, Singapore, and other east Asian nations, pyogenic liver abscess due to *Klebsiella pneumoniae* is preva-

lent[34] and may be complicated by endogenous endophthalmitis in almost 10% of patients.[35]

The bacteria involved in endogenous endophthalmitis (e.g., *S. aureus,* streptococci, gram-negative bacilli) typically cause acute inflammation, and most patients present with acute decrease in vision and eye pain. These may be their only complaints, and the source of bacteremia may not be apparent initially. In one series, half of the patients presented to an ophthalmologist.[31] In a series of 27 patients with fungal or bacterial endogenous endophthalmitis, fewer than 20% of patients had fever on presentation, and more than 40% had an unremarkable general physical examination.[33] A delay in diagnosis is common, but endophthalmitis should be considered in any patient who presents with acute vitritis and hypopyon. Patients with known endocarditis should be monitored for new visual complaints and examined by an ophthalmologist promptly if these develop.

Diagnosis usually is established by culture of vitreous samples or by blood cultures in patients with endophthalmitis whose vitreous cultures fail to grow. Blood cultures are positive in approximately three quarters of patients tested, as are vitreous cultures.[31] Gram-positive organisms are common causes of endogenous endophthalmitis in North America and Europe, whereas gram-negative bacilli (e.g., *Klebsiella, Escherichia coli*) cause most cases in Asia.[32,36] *S. aureus* was the most common organism (approximately 25% of cases) in two U.S. studies,[31,33] whereas *K. pneumoniae* caused 60% of cases in a Singapore study.[36] The U.S. review of 28 cases found that various streptococcal species (e.g., *S. pneumoniae, Streptococcus milleri* group, group B streptococcus) accounted for 32% of cases, whereas *S. aureus* (25%), *E. coli* (18%), and other gram-negative bacilli (14%) were other major pathogens.[31]

Chronic Pseudophakic Endophthalmitis

Chronic pseudophakic endophthalmitis is a rare, indolent infection that is almost always due to *Propionibacterium acnes.* It occurs after standard cataract surgery with artificial intraocular lens (IOL) placement; *pseudophakic* refers to the IOL. Until about 15 years ago, most cases were thought to be due to an immune reaction to the native lens remnant or the IOL ("toxic lens syndrome" or "phakoanaphylactic endophthalmitis").[37] Patients with pseudophakic endophthalmitis typically develop a mild decrease in vision and discomfort in the involved eye weeks to months after cataract surgery. On slit-lamp examination, there are white blood cells and protein in the anterior chamber. A small hypopyon is present in half of patients, and in nearly all patients, there is a white plaque in the residual posterior lens capsule. There also may be white blood cells in the anterior vitreous. Patients often are misdiagnosed as having anterior uveitis and may be treated for months with topical corticosteroids, producing a waxing and waning course of intraocular inflammation. Diagnosis may be difficult because aqueous or vitreous cultures are frequently negative, even in cases in which scanning electron microscopy of the removed IOL or capsule shows bacteria.[38] Biopsy of the posterior lens capsule, including the white plaque, is most likely to yield positive cultures, and capsulectomy is important for successful treatment.[39] Although *P. acnes* has been recovered in almost all culture-positive cases, case reports have described *S. epidermidis,* diphtheroids, and other organisms as etiologies.[40]

Fungal Endophthalmitis

Fungal endophthalmitis cases may be divided into two major categories by incidence and response to therapy: *Candida* endophthalmitis and mold endophthalmitis. In industrialized nations and colder climates, *Candida* endophthalmitis is more common than mold endophthalmitis, whereas the reverse seems to be true in tropical countries. *Candida* endophthalmitis is usually endogenous and responds well to treatment, whereas mold endophthalmitis is almost always exogenous, and successful therapy is rare. Other fungi, such as *Cryptococcus* and the dimorphic fungi, are infrequent causes of endophthalmitis. Endophthalmitis due to these fungi is a result of disseminated disease in nearly all cases.[41-43]

Candida endophthalmitis should be distinguished from *Candida* chorioretinitis; both are included in the term *ocular candidiasis.* In

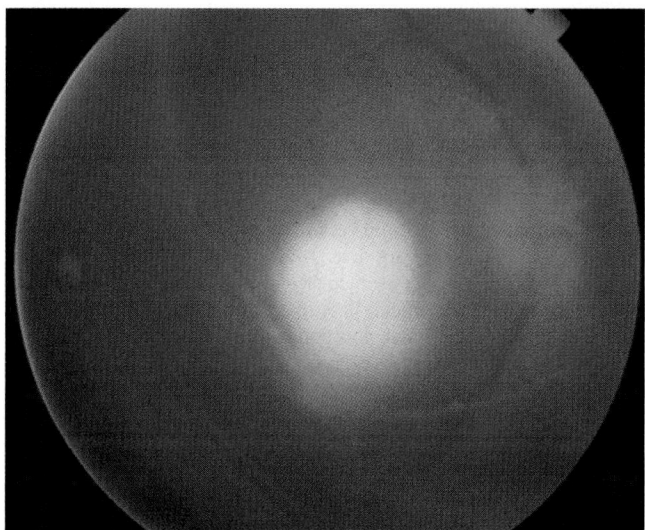

FIGURE 108-3. *Candida* endophthalmitis, with cloudy vitreous and central vitreal "fluff ball."

Candida endophthalmitis, there is significant vitritis, and examination reveals a cloudy vitreous that often contains inflammatory "fluff balls" (Fig. 108-3). In chorioretinitis, there are typically several white chorioretinal lesions but a clear vitreous. The distinction is important because endophthalmitis requires vitrectomy and intravitreal amphotericin in addition to systemic therapy, whereas chorioretinitis usually resolves with systemic therapy alone. Chorioretinitis is much more common than endophthalmitis and is often asymptomatic. In a prospective multicenter study of 118 hospitalized patients with candidemia, 9% were found to have chorioretinitis, almost none had eye symptoms, and none had endophthalmitis.[44] Undiagnosed and untreated chorioretinitis may progress to endophthalmitis, which usually presents as a gradual and painless decrease in vision. This presentation is common in outpatients who have had transient, usually asymptomatic, candidemia from indwelling intravenous lines. Because symptoms are mild and subacute, diagnosis is often delayed. A 10-year retrospective study of 15 patients with endogenous *Candida* endophthalmitis, 11 of whom had an indwelling line, found that the average time from onset of symptoms to treatment of endophthalmitis was 2 months.[45] Diagnosis of *Candida* chorioretinitis is usually presumptive, by clinical appearance of the lesions in the setting of documented candidemia. In contrast, the diagnosis of endophthalmitis is made from vitreous cultures because blood cultures may be negative. *Candida albicans* is the most common organism, although infection with other *Candida* spp. has been reported.[46]

Endophthalmitis due to molds is rare in Western countries. In the United States, it is most common in tropical areas, such as Florida, where 6% of 278 endophthalmitis cases treated between 1996 and 2001 were due to *Aspergillus* and other molds.[47] In tropical countries, such as India, fungal endophthalmitis is a significant problem. Molds accounted for 22% of 124 postcataract endophthalmitis cases in northern India[48] and 21% of 170 postoperative endophthalmitis cases in southern India.[49] Mold endophthalmitis is usually exogenous, with most cases occurring after penetrating eye trauma, eye surgery, or as an extension of keratomycosis. Endogenous mold endophthalmitis has been reported primarily in intravenous drug abusers or immunocompromised patients. The latter are mostly organ transplant patients who have another focus of invasive fungal infection, such as invasive pulmonary aspergillosis.[50] Mold endophthalmitis that develops after surgery usually presents subacutely, 2 to 6 weeks postoperatively. Symptoms include decreased vision and eye pain, and eye examination usually reveals fluffy "cotton ball" vitritis. The surgical corneal or scleral incision may appear normal or may show evidence of wound involvement.[51] Extensive eye involvement (cornea, anterior segment, vitreous) and early presentation (37% within 1 week) characterized

postcataract fungal endophthalmitis in one series from India.[52] In endophthalmitis due to keratomycosis, the infection is seen first in the aqueous, usually as frondlike extensions from the corneal endothelium. *Aspergillus* is the most common cause of mold endophthalmitis, causing 50% to 90% of cases.[49,52]

DIAGNOSIS

The diagnosis of endophthalmitis is suspected from the history and physical examination of the eye and usually is confirmed by culture of the vitreous or, less often, the aqueous. No other laboratory tests can confirm the diagnosis. The endophthalmitis patient is afebrile and has no signs of systemic infection except in two situations: endogenous endophthalmitis, in which there is another focus of infection, and panophthalmitis, in which infection has spread from the globe to the orbit. Panophthalmitis is rare, due to virulent pathogens (e.g., *S. pneumoniae*), and characterized by signs of endophthalmitis plus orbital cellulitis (marked edema and erythema of the eyelids, proptosis, and limitation of extraocular movements). Except for cases of endogenous endophthalmitis and panophthalmitis, blood cultures are negative, and the white blood cell count is normal or only slightly elevated.

Radiologic studies are rarely helpful in acute endophthalmitis and, except for the B-scan, are not warranted before diagnostic vitreous sampling and therapy. The B-scan ("brightness" scan) is an ultrasound of the globe of the eye. It can confirm the presence of vitreous inflammation or show a retinal detachment in cases in which the vitreous cannot be seen (e.g., dense cataract or extensive aqueous inflammation). The normal vitreous is echo-free, whereas multiple vitreous echoes are present when there is vitritis. An initial B-scan showing dense vitreous opacities or membranes, or retinal or choroidal detachment correlated with a poor visual outcome in one report.[53]

The diagnosis of endophthalmitis is made by culturing a sample of the vitreous. The aqueous also may be cultured and is aspirated easily in the ophthalmologist's office, but aqueous cultures rarely add additional information. In one large study in which aqueous and vitreous samples were obtained, aqueous samples yielded the only positive cultures in just 4% of cases.[54] The vitreous may be sampled either by needle aspirate or by vitrectomy (Fig. 108-4). A needle aspirate yields 0.2 to 0.3 mL of vitreous and may be performed in the ophthalmologist's office using a 27-gauge needle and syringe. A vitrectomy is performed in the operating room using a 20-gauge vitrector attached via tubing to a sterile collection bag or canister. Suction is provided by a Venturi-aspiration vitrectomy machine. The vitrector simultaneously cuts and suctions the gel-like vitreous. A separate cannula placed in the vitreous provides continuous infusion of balanced salt solution to maintain eye turgor during the procedure, and this dilutes the vitreous sample. The result is a collection canister containing dilute (20 to 100 mL) vitreous "washings." An undiluted vitreous "biopsy specimen" also may be obtained with the vitrector at the start of the case by attaching a syringe via three-way stopcock.

Gram stains of vitreous samples are positive for organisms in only 40% to 50% of bacterial endophthalmitis cases.[18,31] Positive stains are highly predictive of positive cultures, but negative stains have little predictive value.[54] A unique feature of Gram stains of aqueous or vitreous samples from an inflamed eye is the pigment granule. Pigment granules are most likely melanin released from the iris or retinal pigment epithelium. They appear football shaped or spherical, and the latter may be mistaken for gram-positive cocci. Their true identity is evident when the microscope focus is varied because pigment granules are highly refractile and appear copper-colored with focus modulation, whereas bacteria do not.

Vitreous washings are more likely to yield positive cultures (75% to 90% of cases) than are vitreous aspirates or biopsy specimens (50% to 75% of cases).[18,55] Although aspirate or biopsy samples may be cultured directly on various media (blood agar, chocolate agar, broth, and Sabouraud media), vitreous washings first should be filtered through a 0.45-μm filter. The filter paper is sterilely cut into quarters and placed on the aforementioned media. Before this filtration procedure, a 3-mL

Viterous Aspirate

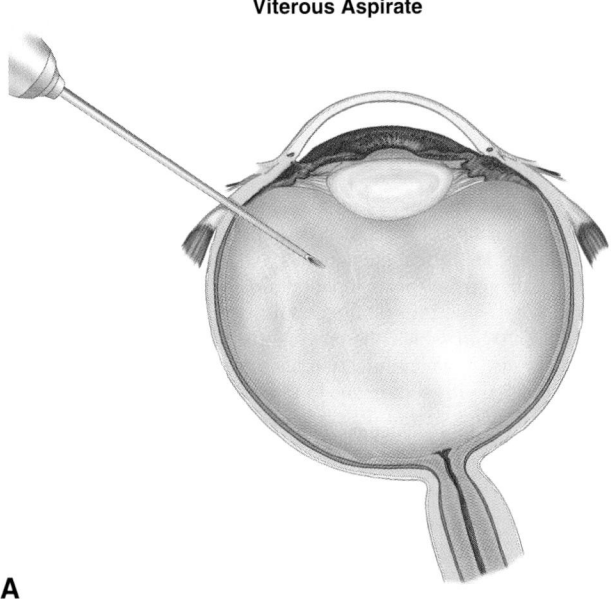

A

Vitrectomy

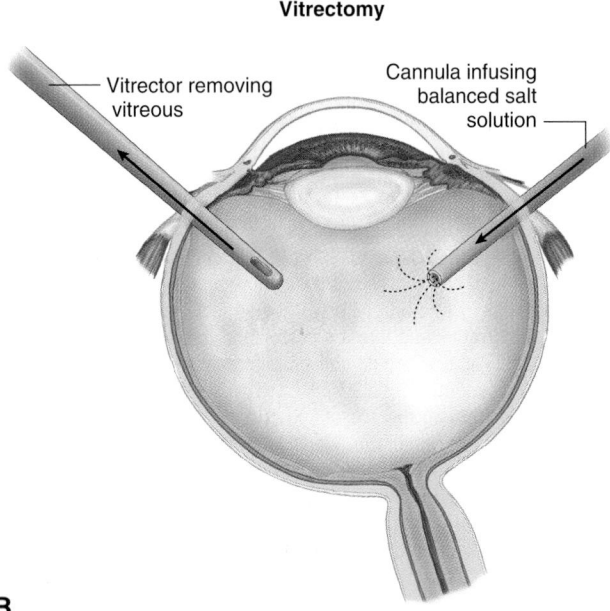

Vitrector removing vitreous

Cannula infusing balanced salt solution

B

FIGURE 108-4. Diagram of vitreous aspirate and vitrectomy.

sample of the washings should be aspirated from the vitrectomy canister and centrifuged to produce a pellet that may be smeared on a slide for Gram stain. A negative culture does not exclude endophthalmitis in the appropriate clinical setting; 18% of 420 patients with postcataract endophthalmitis had negative cultures.[18] The rate of false-positive cultures is unknown but is reduced if positive cultures are counted as those with moderate-to-abundant growth or growth on two media. In a study of 36 patients undergoing vitrectomy for noninfectious indications, one fifth of cultures were positive, but organisms (mostly coagulase-negative staphylococci) grew on only one medium.[56]

Molecular diagnostic techniques, such as polymerase chain reaction, have been applied to vitreous samples but are experimental in endophthalmitis. These seem most promising in diagnosing unusual causes of endophthalmitis (e.g., molds,[57] *Neisseria meningitidis*,[58] *Bartonella henselae*[59]). Organisms common in postcataract endophthalmitis, such as coagulase-negative staphylococci, also are

common in ocular surface flora, so contamination during sampling may limit the diagnostic usefulness of polymerase chain reaction. False-positive rates by polymerase chain reaction of 5% to 14% have been reported in uninfected eyes.[60,61]

TREATMENT

Acute Bacterial Endophthalmitis

Acute bacterial endophthalmitis is a medical emergency because delay in giving appropriate therapy may lead to irreversible loss of vision. Since the 1980s, there has been consensus that injection of antibiotics into the vitreous is an essential component of therapy. The benefit of vitrectomy or of additional antibiotics (subconjunctival, topical, or systemic) remains controversial, however.

Intravitreal antibiotics are injected into the anterior vitreous after a diagnostic vitreous sample is obtained. Standard empirical intravitreal therapy includes vancomycin, 1 mg, plus either ceftazidime, 2.25 mg, or amikacin, 0.4 mg. Each agent is diluted in 0.1 mL of sterile water or normal saline. Ceftazidime is preferred over amikacin by many ophthalmologists because macular infarction has occurred from injected aminoglycosides, although this complication is very rare.[62] Therapeutic levels of injected antibiotics persist in the inflamed aphakic eye for 24 to 48 hours, based on studies in rabbits.[63] In endophthalmitis due to virulent gram-positive organisms (e.g., streptococci), a repeat injection of intravitreal vancomycin may be given after 48 hours if there is little evidence of clinical improvement.

In addition to intravitreal antibiotics, vitrectomy plus intravenous antibiotics (vancomycin plus ceftazidime) was the standard of care for initial therapy of acute endophthalmitis before the 1995 publication of results of the Endophthalmitis Vitrectomy Study (EVS).[18] Since then, this practice has changed, and most ophthalmologists treat endophthalmitis patients as outpatients, with needle aspirate of vitreous, intravitreal antibiotics, and no systemic antibiotic therapy. The EVS was a prospective, multicenter, randomized study of 420 patients with acute postcataract endophthalmitis. The EVS concluded that vitrectomy was necessary only for patients who presented with the worst vision (light perception) and that intravenous antibiotics were not indicated for any patients with postcataract endophthalmitis. These conclusions may have been compromised by design flaws in the study.[64] To answer the question of whether vitrectomy was necessary, patients were randomized to receive either vitrectomy or vitreous "TAP" (aspirate or biopsy). The TAP group was not homogeneous, however, and two thirds had a biopsy rather than a needle aspirate. The vitreous biopsy was performed in the operating room using a vitrector and resembled an abbreviated vitrectomy. Subsequent subgroup analysis confirmed that biopsy and aspirate were not equivalent and that the biopsy subgroup had a better outcome, similar to patients in the vitrectomy arm. Only 11% of the biopsy subgroup were left with severe visual loss versus 24% in the aspirate subgroup.[65] The EVS conclusion that intravenous antibiotics are not helpful also has been criticized.[66,67] The systemic antibiotics used in the study, amikacin plus ceftazidime, have poor activity against coagulase-negative staphylococci, although good activity against gram-negative bacilli. Coagulase-negative staphylococci caused 70% of culture-positive cases in the EVS, whereas gram-negative bacilli caused only 6%. In addition, amikacin penetrates the blood-eye barrier poorly.[68]

Although no definite conclusions can be drawn from the available data, it seems prudent to recommend vitrectomy rather than aspirate in patients with fulminant infections regardless of presenting visual acuity. These patients may be identified by their clinical presentation (rapid worsening of vision and marked intraocular inflammation) or by their category of endophthalmitis. Infections in posttraumatic, bleb-related, or endogenous bacterial endophthalmitis are often due to virulent organisms (e.g., *B. cereus,* streptococci, *H. influenzae, S. aureus*), so vitrectomy is indicated. Vitrectomy, by débriding the vitreous, seems to hasten clearance of pathogens. In the EVS, patients randomized to the vitrectomy group had a lower rate of persistent infection than did patients in the TAP group. Approximately 8% of each group required an early second procedure because of persistent inflammation, and vitreous cultures were repeated. Of these repeat cultures, 71% from the TAP group were still positive versus only 13% from the vitrectomy group.[69] Systemic antibiotics also may be beneficial: The EVS proved only that systemic amikacin plus ceftazidime was not effective in postcataract endophthalmitis. Initial empirical therapy usually includes intravenous vancomycin plus ceftazidime, antibiotics known to cross the blood-eye barrier.[70,71] There is evidence that systemic moxifloxacin and gatifloxacin produce therapeutic vitreous levels even in noninflamed eyes, and these are promising additions to the therapeutic regimen.[72,73] All patients with acute endophthalmitis should receive intravitreal vancomycin plus either amikacin or ceftazidime. Whether intravitreal corticosteroids (dexamethasone, 0.4 mg) also are beneficial is controversial.[74] It is generally accepted that removal of the synthetic IOL is not necessary.

Chronic Pseudophakic Endophthalmitis

Chronic pseudophakic endophthalmitis due to *P. acnes* requires at least vitrectomy and intravitreal vancomycin for treatment, but 50% of cases recur with this therapy alone.[75] The addition of posterior capsulectomy to this regimen reduced the recurrence rate in one study[75] but not in another.[76] Exchanging the IOL for a new one markedly improved success. The combination of total capsulectomy, IOL exchange or removal, vitrectomy, and intravitreal antibiotics cured all cases in both studies, including refractory ones that had failed earlier therapies. Systemic antibiotic therapy is not indicated for this condition.

Fungal Endophthalmitis

Fungal endophthalmitis treatment must include vitrectomy and intravitreal amphotericin, 10 μg. Patients with *Candida* chorioretinitis but no endophthalmitis usually respond to systemic antifungal therapy alone, but endogenous *Candida* endophthalmitis requires vitrectomy and intravitreal amphotericin as well. Patients with endophthalmitis in whom vitrectomy is delayed or withheld may lose vision. A study of 12 patients with *Candida* endophthalmitis (severe vitritis) reported a good outcome in the 7 patients who underwent early vitrectomy, but blindness or scotoma in 4 of 5 patients in whom vitrectomy was delayed more than 1 week or not performed.[77] Regarding systemic therapy, it is unknown whether amphotericin is superior to high-dose fluconazole (≥400 mg orally daily) for fluconazole-sensitive *Candida* spp. Systemic amphotericin has limited penetration of the eye but enough to treat most cases of *Candida* chorioretinitis successfully. Fluconazole achieves vitreous levels that are 50% of plasma levels, and there are many reports of successful fluconazole therapy for ocular candidiasis.[78,79]

All patients with exogenous mold endophthalmitis should have vitrectomy, intravitreal amphotericin, and removal of an IOL if present. If keratomycosis is also present, surgery should include a corneal transplant. An intravitreal injection of amphotericin may be repeated after 1 week if infection persists. Additional injections may be considered, although a safe maximal number of injections is unknown. Systemic antifungal therapy with amphotericin is not warranted because it does not seem to improve visual outcome. Systemic itraconazole does not appreciably cross the blood-eye barrier and so has not been useful. Voriconazole and posaconazole offer great promise, however. Both agents seem to cross the blood-brain barrier and are likely to cross the blood-eye barrier. A case of *Fusarium* endophthalmitis successfully treated with posaconazole and a case of *Paecilomyces* endophthalmitis treated with voriconazole have been reported.[80,81] In addition, we have cared for two patients with exogenous fungal endophthalmitis (*Fusarium* and *Aspergillus*) who responded well to voriconazole. The patient with *Aspergillus* received intravenous caspofungin in addition to voriconazole during initial weeks of therapy.

VISUAL OUTCOME

The final visual outcome after acute bacterial endophthalmitis usually cannot be determined for several months because sequelae of intraocular inflammation resolve slowly. Patients who lose all vision (no light perception) do not regain it, however. Some predictions can be made based on presenting visual acuity and the causative organism, factors that are related.[82] In the EVS, patients who presented with the worst vision, light perception only, were much more likely to have infection from virulent bacteria (streptococci, *S. aureus*, gram-negative bacilli) and a poor visual outcome. Factors that correlated with virulent bacteria in the EVS included presentation with swollen eyelids, afferent pupillary defect, corneal infiltrate, larger hypopyon (≥1.5 mm), or loss of a red reflex.[82] Patients did best if they presented with a mild decrease in vision or had vitreous cultures that were negative or grew coagulase-negative staphylococci. In the EVS, outcome closely correlated with the pathogen recovered.[83] Greater than 80% of eyes with coagulase-negative staphylococci had at least 20/100 vision at follow-up 9 to 12 months later, and only 4% had severe visual loss (<5/200). Results in culture-negative endophthalmitis cases were similar. In contrast, 20/100 or better vision was achieved in only 56% of gram-negative cases, 50% of *S. aureus* cases, and 30% of streptococcal cases. Similar large outcome studies are not available for other types of endophthalmitis, but in general outcomes reflect the virulence of the predominant organisms. The worst outcomes are seen in posttraumatic endophthalmitis due to *B. cereus*, in which salvage of the eye merits a case report.[28] The generally poor visual outcome in bleb-related endophthalmitis reflects the fact that most cases are due to streptococci and *H. influenzae*. Endogenous bacterial endophthalmitis also usually has a poor outcome, although early diagnosis and prompt treatment with vitrectomy and intravitreal antibiotics has saved useful vision even in eyes with virulent organisms.[31]

Visual outcome after chronic *P. acnes* endophthalmitis may depend on the chronicity of the infection. In a review of 36 patients diagnosed with this infection over 22 years, the visual outcome was 20/40 or better in half of the patients, but worse than 20/400 in one fifth of patients.[75]

The visual prognosis for endogenous *Candida* endophthalmitis is difficult to determine because many reviews also include cases of chorioretinitis without vitritis.[33] Patients with chorioretinitis alone usually have excellent visual outcomes. *Candida* endophthalmitis also may have a good outcome if treated with vitrectomy and intravitreal amphotericin in addition to systemic therapy. This treatment resulted in a visual acuity of 20/80 or better in 60% of 17 eyes in one study.[45] In contrast, the prognosis for mold endophthalmitis has been dismal, with rare salvage of useful vision. New antifungals, such as voriconazole and posaconazole, offer hope that this poor prognosis may change.

REFERENCES

1. Montan P, Lundstrom M, Stenevi U, et al. Endophthalmitis following cataract surgery in Sweden: The 1998 national prospective survey. Acta Ophthalmol Scand. 2002;80:258-261.
2. Semmens JB, Li J, Morlet N, et al. Trends in cataract surgery and postoperative endophthalmitis in Western Australia (1980-1998): The Endophthalmitis Population Study of Western Australia. Clin Exp Ophthalmol. 2003;31:213-219.
3. Sandvig KU, Dannevig L. Postoperative endophthalmitis: Establishment and results of a national registry. J Cataract Refract Surg. 2003;29:1273-1280.
4. Allen HF, Mangiaracine AB. Bacterial endophthalmitis after cataract extraction: II. Incidence in 36,000 consecutive operations with special reference to preoperative topical antibiotics. Arch Ophthalmol. 1974;91:3-7.
5. Bannerman TL, Rhoden DL, McAllister SK, et al, for the Endophthalmitis Vitrectomy Study Group. The source of coagulase-negative staphylococci in the Endophthalmitis Vitrectomy Study: A comparison of eyelid and intraocular isolates using pulsed-field gel electrophoresis. Arch Ophthalmol. 1997;115:357-361.
6. Speaker MG, Milch FA, Shah MK, et al. Role of external bacterial flora in the pathogenesis of acute postoperative endophthalmitis. Ophthalmology. 1991;98:639-649.
7. Dickey JB, Thompson KD, Jay WM. Anterior chamber aspirate cultures after uncomplicated cataract surgery. Am J Ophthalmol. 1991;112:278.
8. Sherwood DR, Rich WJ, Jacob JS, et al. Bacterial contamination of intraocular and extraocular fluids during extracapsular cataract extraction. Eye. 1989;3:308-311.
9. Tervo T, Ljungberg P, Kautianinen T, et al. Role of external bacterial flora in the pathogenesis of acute postoperative endophthalmitis. Ophthalmology. 1991;98:639-649.
10. Mistlberger A, Ruckhofer J, Raithel E, et al. Anterior chamber contamination during cataract surgery with intraocular lens implantation. J Cataract Refract Surg. 1997;23:1064-1069.
11. Maxwell DP Jr, Brent BD, Orillac R, et al. A natural history study of experimental *Staphylococcus epidermidis* endophthalmitis. Curr Eye Res. 1993;12:907-912.
12. Menikoff JA, Speaker MG, Marmor M, et al. A case-control study of risk factors for postoperative endophthalmitis. Ophthalmology. 1991;98:1761.

13. Kattan HM, Flynn HW, Pflugfelder SC, et al. Nosocomial endophthalmitis survey: Current incidence of infection after intraocular surgery. Ophthalmology. 1991;98:227-238.

14. Driebe WT Jr, Mandelbaum S, Forster RK, et al. Pseudophakic endophthalmitis: Diagnosis and management. Ophthalmology. 1986;93:442.

15. Turkalj JW, Carlson AN, Manos JP, et al. Is the sutureless cataract incision a valve for bacterial inoculation? J Cataract Refract Surg. 1995;21:472-476.

16. Cooper BA, Holekamp NM, Bohigian G, et al. Case-control study of endophthalmitis after cataract surgery comparing scleral tunnel and clear corneal wounds. Am J Ophthalmol. 2003;136:300-305.

17. Nagaki Y, Hayasaka S, Kadoi C, et al. Bacterial endophthalmitis after small-incision cataract surgery: Effect of incision placement and intraocular lens type. J Cataract Refract Surg. 2003;29:20-26.

18. Endophthalmitis Vitrectomy Study Group. Results of the Endophthalmitis Vitrectomy Study: A randomized trial of immediate vitrectomy and of intravenous antibiotics for the treatment of postoperative bacterial endophthalmitis. Arch Ophthalmol. 1995;113:1479.

19. Waheed S, Ritterband DC, Greenfield DS, et al. New patterns of infecting organisms in late bleb-related endophthalmitis: A ten year review. Eye. 1998;12:910-915.

20. DeBry PW, Perkins TW, Heatley G, et al. Incidence of late-onset bleb-related complications following trabeculectomy with mitomycin. Arch Ophthalmol. 2002;120:297-300.

21. Kangas TA, Greenfield DS, Flynn HW, et al. Delayed-onset endophthalmitis associated with conjunctival filtering blebs. Ophthalmology. 1997;104:746-752.

22. Ciulla TA, Beck AD, Topping TM, et al. Blebitis, early endophthalmitis, and late endophthalmitis after glaucoma-filtering surgery. Ophthalmology. 1997;104:986-995.

23. Duch-Samper AM, Chaques-Alepuz V, Menezo JL, et al. Endophthalmitis following open-globe injuries. Curr Opin Ophthalmol. 1998;9:59-65.

24. Thompson WS, Rubsamen PE, Flynn HW Jr, et al. Endophthalmitis after penetrating ocular trauma: Risk factors and visual acuity outcomes. Ophthalmology. 1995;102:1696-1671.

25. Jonas JB, Budde WM. Early versus late removal of retained intraocular foreign bodies. Retina. 1999;19:193-197.

26. Thompson JT, Parver LM, Enger CL, et al, for the National Eye Trauma System. Infectious endophthalmitis after penetrating injuries with retained intraocular foreign bodies: National Eye Trauma System. Ophthalmology. 1993;100:1468-1474.

27. Davey RT Jr, Tauber WB. Posttraumatic endophthalmitis: The emerging role of *Bacillus cereus* infection. Rev Infect Dis. 1987;9:110-123.

28. Foster RE, Martinez JA, Murray TG, et al. Useful visual outcomes after treatment of *Bacillus cereus* endophthalmitis. Ophthalmology. 1996;103:390-397.

29. Abu el-Asrar AM, al-Amro SA, al-Mosallem AA, et al. Post-traumatic endophthalmitis: Causative organisms and visual outcome. Eur J Ophthalmol. 1999;9:21-31.

30. Alfaro DV, Roth DB, Laughlin RM, et al. Paediatric post-traumatic endophthalmitis. Br J Ophthalmol. 1995;79:888-891.

31. Okada AA, Johnson RP, Liles WC, et al. Endogenous bacterial endophthalmitis: Report of a ten-year retrospective study. Ophthalmology. 1994;101:832-838.

32. Jackson TL, Eykyn SJ, Graham EM, et al. Endogenous bacterial endophthalmitis: A 17-year prospective series and review of 267 reported cases. Surv Ophthalmol. 2003;48:403-423.

33. Binder MI, Chua J, Kaiser PK, et al. Endogenous endophthalmitis: An 18-year review of culture-positive cases at a tertiary care center. Medicine. 2003;82:97-105.

34. Cheng HP, Chang FY, Fung CP, Siu LK. Klebsiella pneumoniae liver abscess in Taiwan is not caused by a clonal spread strain. J. Microbiol Immunol Infect. 2002;35:85-88.

35. Sheu SJ, Chou LC, Hong MC, et al. Risk factors for endogenous endophthalmitis secondary to *Klebsiella pneumoniae* liver abscess. Zhonghua Yi Ziu Za Zhi (Taipei). 2002;65:534-539.

36. Wong JS, Chan TK, Lee HM, et al. Endogenous bacterial endophthalmitis: An east Asian experience and a reappraisal of a severe ocular affliction. Ophthalmology. 2000;107:1483-1496.

37. Piest KL, Apple DJ, Kincaid MC, et al. Localized endophthalmitis: A newly described cause of the so-called toxic lens syndrome. J Cataract Refract Surg. 1987;13:498-510.

38. Busin M, Cusumano A, Spitznos M. Intraocular lens removal from eyes with low-grade endophthalmitis. J Cataract Refract Surg. 1995;21:679-684.

39. Winward KE, Pflugfelder SC, Flynn HW Jr, et al. Postoperative *Propionibacterium* endophthalmitis: Treatment strategies and long-term results. Ophthalmology. 1993;100:447-451.

40. Ficker L, Meredith TA, Wilson LA, et al. Chronic bacterial endophthalmitis. Am J Ophthalmol. 1987;103:745-748.

41. Sheu SJ, Chen YC, Kuo NW, et al. Endogenous cryptococcal endophthalmitis. Ophthalmology. 1998;105:377-381.

42. Cunninham ET Jr, Seiff SR, Berger TG, et al. Intraocular coccidioidomycosis diagnosed by skin biopsy. Arch Ophthalmol. 1998;116:674-677.

43. Gonzales CA, Scott IU, Chaudhry NA, et al. Endogenous endophthalmitis caused by *Histoplasma capsulatum var. capsulatum*: A case report and literature review. Ophthalmology. 2000;107:725-729.

44. Donahue SP, Greven CM, Zuravleff JJ, et al. Intraocular candidiasis in patients with candidemia: Clinical implications derived from a prospective multicenter study. Ophthalmology. 1994;101:1302-1309.

45. Essman TF, Flynn HW, Smiddy WE, et al. Treatment outcomes in a 10-year study of endogenous fungal endophthalmitis. Ophthalmic Surg Lasers. 1997;28:185-194.

46. Joshi N, Hamory BH. Endophthalmitis caused by non-albicans species of *Candida*. Rev Infect Dis. 1991;13:281-287.

47. Benz MS, Scott IU, Flynn HW Jr, et al. Endophthalmitis isolates and antibiotic sensitivities: A 6-year review of culture-proven cases. Am J Ophthalmol. 2004;137:38-42.

48. Gupta A, Gupta V, Gupta A, et al. Spectrum and clinical profile of post cataract surgery endophthalmitis in north India. Indian J Ophthalmol. 2003;139-145.

49. Anand AR, Therese KL, Madhavan HN. Spectrum of aetiological agents of postoperative endophthalmitis and antibiotic susceptibility of bacterial isolates. Indian J Ophthalmol. 2000;48:123-128.

50. Hunt KE, Glasgow BJ. Aspergillus endophthalmitis: An unrecognized endemic disease in orthotopic liver transplantation. Ophthalmology. 1996;103:757-767.

51. Garg P, Mahesh S, Bansal AK, et al. Fungal infection of sutureless self-sealing incision for cataract surgery. Ophthalmology. 2003;110:2173-2177.

52. Narang S, Gupta A, Gupta V, et al. Fungal endophthalmitis following cataract surgery: Clinical presentation, microbiological spectrum, and outcome. Am J Ophthalmol. 2001;132:609-617.

53. Dacey MP, Balencia M, Lee MB, et al. Echographic findings in infectious endophthalmitis. Arch Ophthalmol. 1994;112:1325-1333.

54. Barza M, Pavan PR, Doft BH, et al. Evaluation of microbiological diagnostic techniques in postoperative endophthalmitis in the Endophthalmitis Vitrectomy Study. Arch Ophthalmol. 1997;115:1142-1150.

55. Donahue SP, Kowalski RP, Jewart BH, et al. Vitreous cultures in suspected endophthalmitis: Biopsy or vitrectomy? Ophthalmology. 1993;100:452-455.

56. Mames RN, Friedman SM, Stinson WG, et al. Positive vitreous cultures from eyes without signs of infectious endophthalmitis. Ophthalmic Surg Lasers. 1997;28:365-369.

57. Anand A, Madhavan H, Neelam V, et al. Use of polymerase chain reaction in the diagnosis of fungal endophthalmitis. Ophthalmology. 2001;108:326-330.

58. Kerkhoff FT, van der Zee A, Bergmans AM, et al. Polymerase chain reaction detection of *Neisseria meningitidis* in the intraocular fluid of a patient with endogenous endophthalmitis but without meningitis. Ophthalmology. 2003;110:2134-2136.

59. Goldstein DA, Mouritsen L, Friedlander S, et al. Acute endogenous endophthalmitis due to *Bartonella henselae*. Clin Infect Dis. 2001;33:718-721.

60. Therese KL, Anand AR, Madhavan HN. Polymerase chain reaction in the diagnosis of bacterial endophthalmitis. Br J Ophthalmol. 1998;82:1078-1082.

61. Hykin PG, Tobal K, McIntyre G, et al. The diagnosis of delayed post-operative endophthalmitis by polymerase chain reaction of bacterial DNA in vitreous samples. J Med Microbiol. 1994;40:408-415.

62. Campochiaro PA, Lim JI. Aminoglycoside toxicity in the treatment of endophthalmitis. The Aminoglycoside Study Group. Arch Ophthalmol. 1994;112:48-53.

63. Aguilar HE, Meredith TA, el-Massry A, et al. Vancomycin levels after intravitreal injection: Effects of inflammation and surgery. Retina. 1995;15:428-432.

64. Flynn HW Jr, Meredith TA. The Endophthalmitis Vitrectomy Study (Letter). Arch Ophthalmol. 1996;114:1027-1028.

65. Han DP, Wisniewski SR, Kelsey SF, et al. Microbiologic yields and complication rates of vitreous needle aspiration versus mechanized vitreous biopsy in the Endophthalmitis Vitrectomy Study. Retina. 1999;19:98-102.

66. Haimann MH, Weiss H, Miller J. The Endophthalmitis Vitrectomy Study (Letter). Arch Ophthalmol. 1996;114:1025.

67. Baker AS, Durand M. The Endophthalmitis Vitrectomy Study (Letter). Arch Ophthalmol. 1996;114:1025-1026.

68. El-Massry A, Meredith TA, Aguilar HE, et al. Aminoglycoside concentrations in the vitreous cavity after intravenous administration. Am J Ophthalmol. 1996;122:684-689.

69. Doft BH, Kelsey SF, Wisniewski SR, EVS Study Group. Additional procedures after initial vitrectomy or TAP-biopsy in the Endophthalmitis Vitrectomy Study. Ophthalmology. 1998;105:707-716.

70. Meredith TA, Aguilar HE, Shaarawy A, et al. Vancomycin levels in the vitreous cavity after intravenous administration. Am J Ophthalmol. 1995;119:774-778.

71. Aguilar HE, Meredith TA, Shaarawy A, et al. Vitreous cavity penetration of ceftazidime after intravenous administration. Retina. 1995;15:154-159.

72. Hariprasad SM, Mieler WF, Holz ER. Vitreous and aqueous penetration of orally administered gatifloxacin in humans. Arch Ophthalmol. 2003;121:345-350.

73. Bronner S, Jehl F, Peter JD, et al. Moxifloxacin efficacy and vitreous penetration in a rabbit model of *Staphylococcus aureus* endophthalmitis and effect on gene expression of leucotoxins and virulence regulator factors. Antimicrob Agents Chemother. 2003;47:1621-1629.

74. Das T, Jalali S, Gothwal VK, et al. Intravitreal dexamethasone in exogenous bacterial endophthalmitis: Results of a prospective randomised study. Br J Ophthalmol. 1999;83:1050-1055.

75. Clark WL, Kaiser PK, Flynn HW Jr, et al. Treatment strategies and visual acuity outcomes in chronic postoperative *Propionibacterium acnes* endophthalmitis. Ophthalmology. 1999;106:1665-1670.

76. Aldave AJ, Stein JD, Deramo VA, et al. Treatment strategies for postoperative *Propionibacterium acnes* endophthalmitis. Ophthalmology. 1999;106:2395-2401.

77. Martinez-Vazquez C, Fernandez-Ulloa J, Bordon J, et al. *Candida albicans* endophthalmitis in brown heroin addicts: Response to early vitrectomy preceded and followed by antifungal therapy. Clin Infect Dis. 1998;1130-1133.

78. Akler ME, Vellend H, McNeely DM, et al. Use of fluconazole in the treatment of candidal endophthalmitis. Clin Infect Dis. 1995;20:657-664.

79. Christmas NJ, Smiddy WE. Vitrectomy and systemic fluconazole for treatment of endogenous fungal endophthalmitis. Ophthalmic Surg Lasers. 1996;27:1012-1018.

80. Sponsel WE, Graybill JR, Nevarez HL, et al. Ocular and systemic posaconazole (SCH-56592) treatment of invasive *Fusarium solani* keratitis and endophthalmitis. Br J Ophthalmol. 2002;86:829-830.

81. Garbino J, Ondrusova A, Baglivo E, et al. Successful treatment of *Paecilomyces lilacinus* endophthalmitis with voriconazole. Scand J Infect Dis. 2002;34:701-703.

82. Johnson MW, Doft BH, Kelsey SF, et al. The Endophthalmitis Vitrectomy Study: Relationship between clinical presentation and microbiologic spectrum. Ophthalmology. 1997;104:261-272.
83. The Endophthalmitis Vitectomy Study Group. Microbiologic factors and visual outcome in the Endophthalmitis Vitrectomy Study. Am J Ophthalmol. 1996;122:830-846.

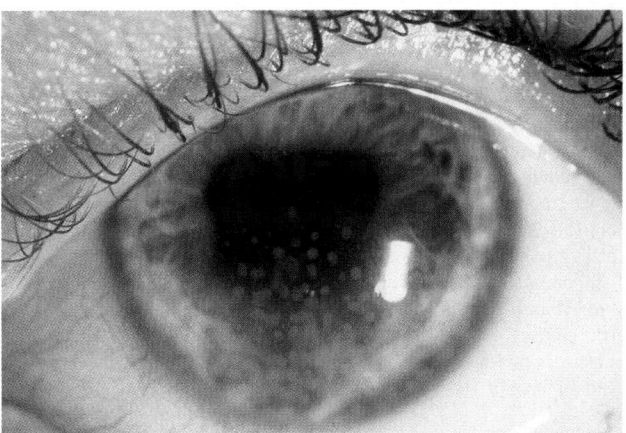

FIGURE 109-1. Granulomatous keratic precipitates, also called "mutton fat keratic precipitates." The white precipitates represent white blood cells that have condensed on the endothelial surface of the cornea in anterior uveitis. They do not represent granulomas. Granular keratic precipitates are similar, but the condensations are much smaller so that the white "dots" appear finer. *(Courtesy of Audrey C. Melanson.)*

Infectious Causes of Uveitis

MARLENE L. DURAND

DEFINITION AND TERMINOLOGY

Uveitis means inflammation of the uvea. The uvea is the pigmented, vascular middle layer of the eye embryologically, sandwiched between the cornea-sclera outer protective layer and the retina. The word *uvea* comes from the Latin word *uva,* meaning "grape," so named by Roman anatomists (Galen, Rufus) because of the appearance of this highly vascular layer when the white sclera was stripped away.[1] The uvea is composed of the iris, ciliary body, and choroid (see Fig. 108-1). The *iris* regulates the amount of light that reaches the retina, the *ciliary body* produces aqueous humor and supports the lens, and the *choroid* helps to nourish the retina.

Retinitis also is included as a type of uveitis even though the retina is not part of the uvea, because the retina is often involved when there is underlying choroidal inflammation. Uveitis is classified by the ocular structures involved. Several anatomic classification schemes exist, but all divide uveitis into anterior, intermediate, posterior, and panuveitis categories (Table 109-1). The International Uveitis Study Group classification is commonly used.[2] In anterior uveitis, inflammation involves the iris (iritis), anterior ciliary body (cyclitis), or both (iridocyclitis). Anterior uveitis is characterized by white blood cells in the aqueous humor. There are often keratic precipitates (cells on the corneal endothelial surface) and iris lesions. Intermediate uveitis refers to inflammation involving the anterior vitreous, ciliary body, and adjacent portion of the retina ("peripheral" retina). Posterior uveitis refers to inflammation involving the choroid (choroiditis), retina (retinitis), both (chorioretinitis), or retinal vessels (retinal vasculitis). There may be inflammation of the posterior vitreous. Panuveitis involves all three parts of the uvea. Uveitis also may extend to involve the cornea (keratouveitis) or sclera (sclerouveitis).

Other terms commonly used in uveitis appear in Figure 109-1. The eye is divided into anterior and posterior segments by the lens. The iris divides the anterior segment further into anterior and posterior chambers. Aqueous humor fills the anterior segment and is produced and re-

sorbed constantly, with a turnover time of 100 minutes. The posterior segment, a term not to be confused with posterior chamber, is filled with the gel-like vitreous. The vitreous is produced in utero and never regenerated, although it may be surgically removed (vitrectomy) and replaced with clear fluids such as saline.

In addition to anatomic location, uveitis is classified as granulomatous or nongranulomatous. *Granulomatous* does not mean there are granulomas on pathology, but describes a type of inflammation in which the white blood cells are condensed into clumps rather than uniformly dispersed. In granulomatous anterior uveitis, "granulomatous" or "mutton fat" keratitic precipitates form on the endothelial surface of the cornea. These are greasy appearing and more yellow than nongranulomatous ("granular") keratitic precipitates (Fig. 109-1). There also may be clusters of white blood cells in the iris, called *Busacca nodules* if in the iris stroma and *Koeppe nodules* if at the pupillary margin. In granulomatous uveitis that involves the posterior segment of the eye, there may be white blood cells in large clusters ("snowballs") in the vitreous, in exudates adjacent to retinal vessels ("candle wax drippings"), or as granulomas within the choroid (e.g., multifocal choroiditis). Granulomatous uveitis is typical of infections such as tuberculosis, syphilis, and toxoplasmosis, although all may have a nongranulomatous presentation. Two types of autoimmune uveitis, sarcoidosis and Vogt-Koyanagi-Harada syndrome, usually produce a granulomatous uveitis. Nongranulomatous inflammation is more characteristic of autoimmune uveitis, such as Behçet's disease, Reiter's syndrome, and ankylosing spondylitis.

TABLE 109-1 **Classification of Uveitis and Major Infectious Etiologies in Each Category**

Category	Ocular Findings	Major Infectious Etiologies (%)*
Anterior (iritis, cyclitis, iridocyclitis)	WBCs in aqueous, keratic precipitates, iris nodules, synechiae	Herpes simplex (10%); syphilis (<1%); TB (<1%); Lyme disease (<1%); leprosy (<1%)
Intermediate	WBCs or "snowballs" in the vitreous, pars plana "snow bank"	Lyme disease (<1%)
Posterior (choroiditis, chorioretinitis, retinitis)	Lesions in choroid, retina, or both; vitritis in some	*Toxoplasma* (25%); CMV (12%)[†]; ARN (6%); *Toxocara* (3%); syphilis (2%); *Candida* (<1%)
Panuveitis	WBCs in aqueous and vitreous	Syphilis (6%); TB (2%); *Candida* (2%)

*Percentage of uveitis cases in each category (not of total uveitis cases). Based on 1237 cases of uveitis seen at Massachusetts Eye & Ear Infirmary, Boston, 1982-1992, by Foster's group (Rodriguez et al[5]).
[†]Series was before use of highly active antiretroviral therapy, and rate for CMV retinitis would be lower now.
ARN, acute retinal necrosis; CMV, cytomegalovirus; TB, tuberculosis; WBC, white blood cells.

EPIDEMIOLOGY

In the United States, uveitis affects 2.3 million people and causes 10% of all cases of blindness.[3] The prevalence in Western countries is 38 per 100,000 population. The prevalence in developing countries is not clear, but a study from West Africa found that uveitis, including that due to onchocerciasis, caused 24% of blindness.[4] Uveitis can occur at any age, but the average age at presentation is approximately 40. The male-to-female ratio is 40:60 in some series[5] and 60:40 in others.[6] Anterior uveitis is much more common and less sight-threatening than other categories of uveitis. It accounts for 90% of uveitis cases in community-based ophthalmology practices but only 60% in university referral centers.[7] Intermediate uveitis, posterior uveitis, and panuveitis each account for 10% to 15% of uveitis cases in university referral centers but only 1% to 5% in community practices.

ETIOLOGY AND PATHOPHYSIOLOGY

Uveitis may be caused by autoimmune conditions, infections, or rarely trauma, but 50% of cases are idiopathic. Some cases of intraocular inflammation "masquerade" as uveitis (masquerade syndromes) but have other causes, such as malignancy (e.g., ocular–central nervous system lymphoma). Infectious uveitis nearly always results from hematogenous spread of infection from another part of the body to the highly vascular uvea. The pathophysiology of uveitis depends on the specific etiology, but in all types there is a breach in the blood-eye barrier. The blood-eye barrier, similar to the blood-brain barrier, normally prevents cells and large proteins from entering the eye. Inflammation causes this barrier to break down, and white blood cells enter the eye. Neutrophils predominate in acute uveitis cases, and mononuclear cells predominate in chronic cases.

The frequency of infectious etiologies varies by category (Fig. 109-2). Most cases of anterior uveitis are idiopathic (40%) or associated with a rheumatologic condition (45%), such as seronegative arthropathies,

ankylosing spondylitis, Reiter's syndrome, and juvenile rheumatoid arthritis. The most common infectious cause is herpes keratouveitis, which accounted for almost 10% of 637 anterior uveitis cases at the Massachusetts Eye and Ear Infirmary in Boston.[5] Syphilis, tuberculosis, and Lyme disease each caused less than 1% of anterior uveitis cases in this series. In 500 cases of anterior uveitis in Madras, India, there were no cases of Lyme disease or syphilis, but tuberculosis and leprosy each caused 0.6% of cases.[6]

Intermediate uveitis most often has an unknown etiology (69%) or is due to sarcoidosis (22%) or multiple sclerosis (8%).[5] Infectious diseases almost never cause intermediate uveitis. In the Boston series, there was only one infectious case (due to Lyme disease) in 162 patients with intermediate uveitis.

Posterior uveitis has the highest rate of infectious etiologies, with more than 40% of cases due to infection. In Boston, Madras, and Paris, toxoplasmosis was the most important cause of posterior uveitis, causing 25% to 39% of cases.[5,6,8] Cytomegalovirus (CMV) retinitis accounted for 12% of cases in the Boston series, but this rate would be much lower now in the era of highly active antiretroviral therapy. Other infectious etiologies in that series included acute retinal necrosis (ARN), a retinitis due to herpesviruses (5.5%); *Toxocara* (2.5%); syphilis (2%); and *Candida* (0.8%), whereas major noninfectious diagnoses were lupus erythematosus, sarcoidosis, and birdshot retinochoroidopathy, an eye disease of unknown etiology (8% each).

Infections cause about 10% of panuveitis cases and include syphilis (6%), tuberculosis (2%), and *Candida* (2%).[5] Sarcoidosis, Behçet's disease, systemic lupus erythematosus, and multifocal choroiditis and panuveitis, an eye disease of unknown etiology, each cause 10% to 15% of cases. About one fifth of panuveitis cases are idiopathic.

GENERAL CLINICAL FEATURES

Because infectious uveitis usually represents a chronic process, patients often present with no systemic complaints. A careful history and physical examination may give clues to the diagnosis, such as a remote history of inadequately treated pulmonary tuberculosis. The findings usually are limited to the eye, however. Patients with anterior uveitis typically present with eye pain in addition to decreased vision in the affected eye. The eye may show a ring of redness near the limbus, or corneal-scleral border, known as a *ciliary flush*. Slit-lamp examination shows cells in the anterior chamber. There may be keratic precipitates, iris nodules, or synechiae (adhesions) between the iris and either the cornea or the lens. The funduscopic examination shows a clear or nearly clear vitreous and a normal retina. Patients with intermediate uveitis present with floaters or blurred vision but no pain or photophobia. The eye is not red. There are few, if any, white blood cells in the aqueous, but there are cells in the vitreous that are often clumped like "snowballs." The dilated, depressed funduscopic examination may show a white exudate or "snow bank" over the pars plana (posterior portion of the ciliary body). In posterior uveitis, patients often have painless loss of vision as their primary symptom. There are few, if any, cells in the anterior chamber, but the funduscopic examination shows lesions in the retina, choroid, or both. There may be retinal vasculitis or periphlebitis (venous sheathing). There may be many cells in the vitreous, typical of toxoplasmosis, or no vitritis, typical of CMV retinitis. Panuveitis is characterized by a combination of the above-mentioned findings.

CLINICAL FEATURES OF COMMON INFECTIOUS ETIOLOGIES

Syphilis

Syphilis may produce anterior uveitis, intermediate uveitis, posterior uveitis, or panuveitis. The uveitis is often granulomatous. Syphilitic anterior uveitis is granulomatous in two thirds of patients[9] and bilateral in half. Interstitial keratitis (corneal inflammation), iris nodules,

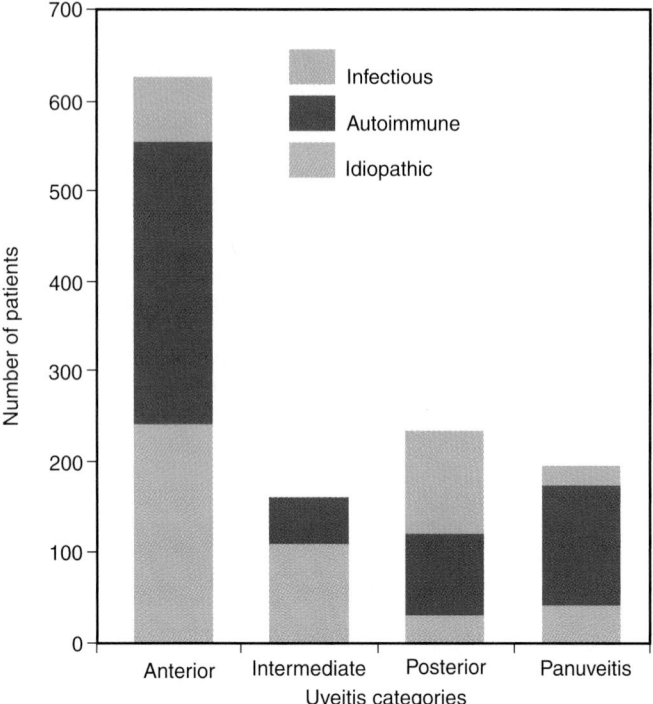

FIGURE 109-2. Bar graph of the etiologies of uveitis by anatomic category (anterior, intermediate, posterior, panuveitis), one bar for each category. Each bar is divided into three colored segments, a different color for each etiology: infectious, autoimmune, (see text) and idiopathic. The height of each bar and each segment are based on data by Rodriguez and colleagues.[5]

dilated iris vessels, and iris atrophy may be seen. The most common form of posterior uveitis is multifocal chorioretinitis, but other manifestations include focal chorioretinitis, pseudoretinitis pigmentosa, retinal necrosis, neuroretinitis, and optic neuritis. Chorioretinitis was the type of uveitis seen in 15 of 20 patients with syphilitic posterior uveitis in one review.[10] Retinal vasculitis may occur, and branch retinal vein occlusions have been described.[11]

Uveitis may occur in either congenital or acquired syphilis. Typical findings in congenital disease include interstitial keratitis and "salt-and-pepper" fundi.[12] Interstitial keratitis does not usually occur until the patient is a teenager or young adult. It may be accompanied by an anterior uveitis. Glaucoma may result from the inflammation.[13] In acquired syphilis, onset of uveitis may occur in secondary or tertiary syphilis. The most common ocular finding in secondary syphilis is iritis, which accounts for more than 70% of eye findings.[11] Symptoms often are acute in onset. In contrast, when ocular syphilis develops in tertiary disease, patients often have slowly progressive decrease in vision as their only symptom. The eye findings are protean and include all of the above-listed findings. In contrast to patients with secondary disease, patients with tertiary disease are often middle-aged or older. They may have no knowledge of prior exposure to syphilis, which likely occurred decades earlier. The diagnosis may be missed if only rapid plasma reagin (RPR) or Venereal Disease Research Laboratory (VDRL) is checked because these tests are often negative in tertiary syphilis. In a series of 50 patients with a reactive absorbed fluorescent treponemal antibody (FTA-Abs) and eye findings consistent with active or inactive ocular syphilis (e.g., chorioretinitis, optic atrophy, iritis, interstitial keratitis), the average age was 59, and the VDRL was reactive in only 24%.[14]

All patients with presumed ocular syphilis should have a lumbar puncture to exclude concomitant neurosyphilis, which may be present in 40% of patients.[14] Patients who test positive for human immunodeficiency virus (HIV) have a higher rate of concurrent ocular syphilis and neurosyphilis.[11,15] HIV-positive patients also are more likely to have acute, bilateral uveitis with more extensive eye involvement (vitreous, retina, and optic nerve involvement simultaneously).[11,16]

It is likely that nearly all cases of uveitis and positive specific syphilis serologies represent infection with *T. pallidum* subsp. *pallidum*. It is possible, however, that some patients from areas endemic for yaws or bejel have positive serologies due to exposure to these nonvenereal *T. pallidum* subspp. in childhood but have uveitis from another etiology. In addition, some authors maintain that uveitis may be a late manifestation of yaws or bejel.[17-19] The eye findings they describe are similar to those seen in ocular syphilis, and the diseases cannot be distinguished from syphilis serologically. The possible distinction would be important to the patient because of social implications, although it would not change therapy.

Tuberculosis

Ocular complications of systemic tuberculosis are rare. Ocular tuberculosis was diagnosed in only 1.4% of the 10,524 patients seen in the eye clinic of a Boston sanatorium between 1940 and 1966.[20] A more recent prospective study of 1005 patients in India with active tuberculosis found evidence of ocular disease in only 14 patients, or 1.4%.[21] Thirteen of these patients had healed ocular disease and so may not have had visual symptoms. In large series of patients seen in uveitis clinics, ocular tuberculosis accounts for only 0.5% to 4% of uveitis cases.[5,6,8] Ocular disease may be more common in HIV-positive patients with tuberculosis. A study of 100 patients hospitalized for tuberculosis in Madrid found presumed ocular tuberculosis in 24% of the 45 HIV-positive patients versus 13% in the 55 HIV-negative patients, although this difference was not statistically significant.[22]

Ocular tuberculosis may present without evidence of systemic disease, so the diagnosis is often presumptive. Most patients have no history of tuberculosis, and half have normal chest radiographs.[23] Eye pathology is rarely available before vision is lost, and the eye is enucleated. Biopsies of the uvea risk vision and are rarely performed. In a review of 40 cases with histologic evidence of intraocular tuberculo-

sis reported between 1869 and 1991, only one case was proved by biopsy, and the rest were proved after loss of the eye.[24] Cultures of the aqueous or vitreous, intraocular samples that may be taken safely, are almost never positive. A rare exception is a report by Biswas and colleagues[25] from India of five cases with positive cultures from the aqueous (three cases), vitreous (one case), or subconjunctival mass (one case). Three of these patients had no other evidence of tuberculosis. Diagnosis by polymerase chain reaction (PCR) of aqueous or vitreous samples has been reported,[26,27] but the sensitivity and specificity of this test is unknown. Most reported cases have no culture confirmation, and many have no evidence of systemic disease.[25,26] A positive purified protein derivative (PPD) skin test may be of little help in determining if a patient with uveitis has ocular tuberculosis, especially when the prevalence of PPD positivity in the general population is high. Rosenbaum and Wernick[28] used Bayes' theorem to calculate that a patient with uveitis and a positive PPD has only a 1% probability of having tuberculosis. Although all patients with uveitis and a positive PPD should not be presumed to have ocular tuberculosis, some factors make the diagnosis much more likely. If the patient has multifocal choroiditis, a history of inadequately treated pulmonary tuberculosis, and a chest radiograph consistent with present or past active disease, ocular tuberculosis should be strongly considered.

Based on studies of patients with systemic tuberculosis and presumed ocular involvement, the spectrum of ocular findings has been described. Tuberculosis can involve any part of the eye, but the most common finding is focal or multifocal choroiditis (Fig. 109-3A). Active or healed choroiditis was found in 78%[21] and 94%[22] of patients with systemic disease and presumed ocular tuberculosis in two reports. In earlier studies, choroidal involvement was seen in 30% to 40% of similar patients.[20,29] Choroidal "tubercles" are usually one quarter to several disk diameters in size and are seen most often in the posterior pole rather than the periphery of the fundus. Most patients have fewer than 5 lesions, but the number ranges from 1 to 60.[24] One or both eyes may be involved. Lesions are yellow, white, or gray.[30] In active disease, overlying vitreous inflammation may be present. Inactive choroidal lesions appear as scars. The appearance of the choroiditis is not pathognomonic for tuberculosis, and similar lesions may be seen in sarcoidosis, syphilis, and rarely metastatic disease.[24] Chronic anterior uveitis, usually granulomatous (i.e., with mutton-fat keratitic precipitates or iris nodules or both), is the next most common manifestation of ocular tuberculosis.[20] There may be an associated vitritis or choroiditis. A third common manifestation is retinal vasculitis or periphlebitis. The mechanism is controversial, with some proponents arguing for direct infection of the vessels and others for immune reaction to tuberculoprotein.[24] In 1880, Eales described recurrent retinal and vitreous hemorrhages in young men, and retinal vasculitis in ocular tuberculosis is often called Eales' disease. In one series of 12 patients with ocular tuberculosis seen in England, 9 had retinal vasculitis.[31] Five of these patients were from India, consistent with other reports that Eales' disease is most common in patients from India, Pakistan, and Afghanistan.[24] Typical features of Eales' disease include vascular sheathing of retinal veins (periphlebitis), vitreous inflammation, and peripheral retinal capillary occlusion. Capillary occlusion leads to neovascularization and subsequent retinal hemorrhages (Fig. 109-3B). Other manifestations of ocular tuberculosis include scleritis, interstitial keratitis, and optic neuritis.

Toxoplasmosis

Ocular toxoplasmosis is the most common cause of posterior uveitis in the United States. It is discussed in detail in Chapter 276.

Cytomegalovirus Retinitis

CMV retinitis affected greater than 30% of patients with acquired immunodeficiency syndrome (AIDS) in the pre–highly active antiretroviral therapy era, but is now rare. Patients with CMV retinitis have painless loss of vision. Eye findings typically include fluffy white retinal infiltrates; retinal vasculitis, which may have a "frosted branch angiitis" pattern; and multiple retinal hemorrhages. An important clinical feature is the absence of significant vitreous inflammation. As a consequence, the view of the retina is clear; this is in contrast to ocular toxoplasmosis, in which vitritis is common. CMV retinitis is discussed further in Chapter 134.

Acute Retinal Necrosis

ARN first was described in 1971 and is a rapidly progressive necrotizing retinitis due to herpesviruses.[32] Herpes simplex virus (HSV) types 1 and 2 and varicella-zoster virus (VZV) cause nearly all cases. Rarely, patients with ARN due to HSV have a history of herpes encephalitis. CMV is a rare cause of ARN and occurs mainly in immunocompro-

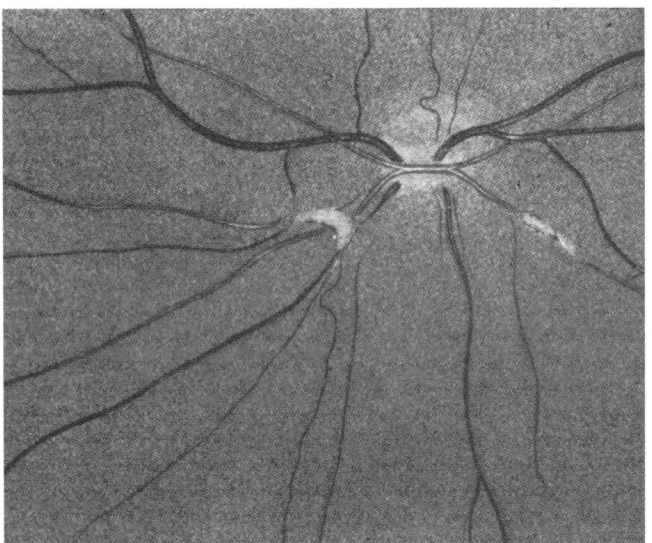

A

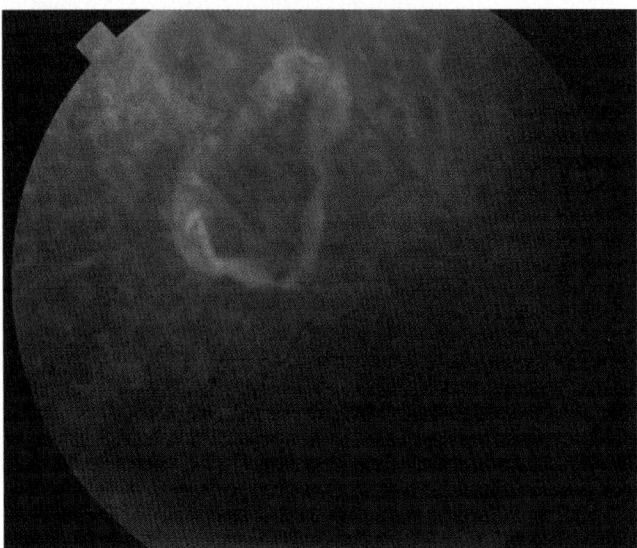

B

FIGURE 109-3. Ocular tuberculosis. **A,** Multifocal choroiditis in a 16-year-old girl with miliary tuberculosis and tuberculous meningitis (color drawing). **B,** Retinal photograph showing signs of Eales' disease in a patient from India: retinal neovascularization surrounded by a large yellow ring of fibrovascular proliferation in the vitreous. *(From Raizman MB, Haas JJ. Case 4-1998—A 32-year-old man with vitreous hemorrhage and mediastinal lymphadenopathy. Case Records of the Massachusetts General Hospital. N Engl J Med. 1998;338:313-319.)*

mised patients. Most patients with ARN are immunocompetent, however. ARN is usually unilateral initially and begins with an anterior uveitis. Patients may have mild eye pain or photophobia, then decreased vision. Funduscopic examination with an indirect ophthalmoscope shows one or more foci of retinal necrosis in the peripheral retina, an area not seen with a direct ophthalmoscope (Fig. 109-4). These foci have sharply demarcated borders. Over the next 3 to 21 days, the retinal necrosis spreads circumferentially and posteriorly.[33] Vascular sheathing develops along with a dense vitritis. Untreated, the disease produces atrophy of the retina and often retinal detachment. Treatment with intravenous acyclovir halts progression. Disease develops in the other eye in 70% of untreated patients but in only 13% of treated patients.[34] A severe variant of ARN occurs in patients with advanced AIDS (CD4+ <100/mm^3), who develop ocular findings typical of ARN, but disease is rapidly progressive.[35] Blindness occurs bilaterally in nearly 60%, and therapy has been disappointing. Nearly all cases are due to VZV, and there is a history of antecedent shingles in most. Another viral retinitis that may occur in advanced AIDS is progressive outer retinal necrosis, so named because of the involvement of the deep layers of the retina. Multiple foci of retinitis develop at the posterior pole, which rapidly coalesce. The cause is VZV, and therapy is rarely successful, with only case reports of success with ganciclovir and foscarnet[36] or ganciclovir and sorivudine.[37]

Herpetic Keratouveitis or Iridocyclitis

HSV is the most common cause of infectious keratitis in the United States, with an estimated 29,000 patients affected annually.[38] Recurrent episodes of keratitis and anterior uveitis are common: 40% of patients with ocular herpetic disease have recurrent episodes of anterior uveitis.[39] Some experts believe that iritis in an eye with previous herpetic keratitis should be considered herpetic until proved otherwise.[40] Patients with herpetic anterior uveitis usually have pain, redness, and photophobia. Eye examination reveals cells in the anterior chamber, and fine or mutton-fat keratitic precipitates. There may be concurrent keratitis. Herpetic iridocyclitis may occur in a patient with no history or findings suggesting herpetic keratitis, but this is uncommon.[41]

Candida Chorioretinitis and Endophthalmitis

Candidemia can lead to fungal seeding of the choroid, then extension into the vitreous as infection progresses. Vitreous infection is called *endophthalmitis* rather than uveitis. *Ocular candidiasis* refers to chorioretinitis, in which there are multiple white chorioretinal lesions but the vitreous is clear, and endophthalmitis, in which the vitreous is cloudy and typically contains a "string of pearls" or "fluff balls." The distinction between chorioretinitis and endophthalmitis is important because therapy differs. Patients with chorioretinitis are often asymptomatic, whereas patients with candidal endophthalmitis usually notice decreased vision. Chorioretinitis is common in candidemia, whereas endophthalmitis is rare. In a prospective study of 118 patients with candidemia, 9% were found to have asymptomatic chorioretinitis, but none had endophthalmitis.[42] Ocular candidiasis also may develop in patients with chronic indwelling intravenous lines who have no symptoms of candidemia and negative blood cultures.[43] Ocular candidiasis is discussed further in Chapter 255.

Toxocara

Ocular toxocariasis usually affects children and either is asymptomatic or causes unilateral decrease in vision. There are three types of ocular manifestations: (1) posterior pole chorioretinal granuloma, (2) peripheral chorioretinal granuloma, and (3) diffuse panuveitis.[44] Ocular toxocariasis is discussed further in Chapter 289.

Rare Infectious Causes of Uveitis

Uveitis rarely may be associated with other infections, including leptospirosis, Lyme disease, brucellosis, Whipple's disease, leprosy, and cat-scratch disease. *Leptospirosis* has been recognized as a cause of uveitis since Weil in 1886 and may occur several months after resolu-

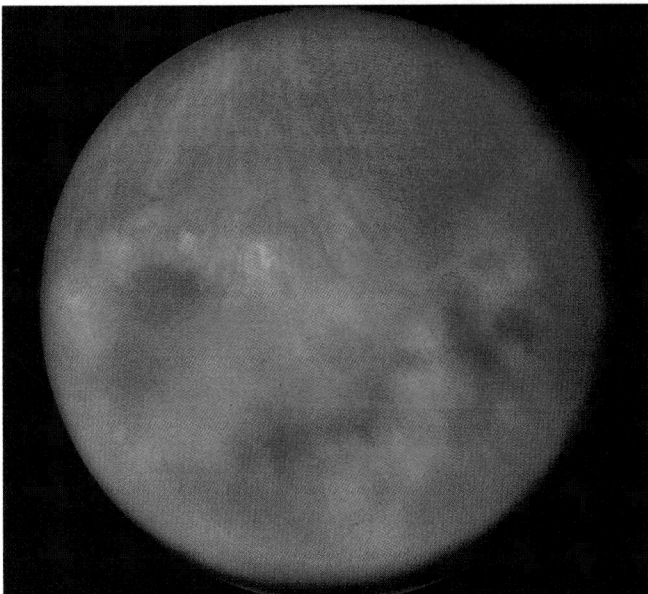

FIGURE 109-4. Funduscopic photograph of acute retinal necrosis showing loss of retinal features in the peripheral retina due to retinal necrosis.

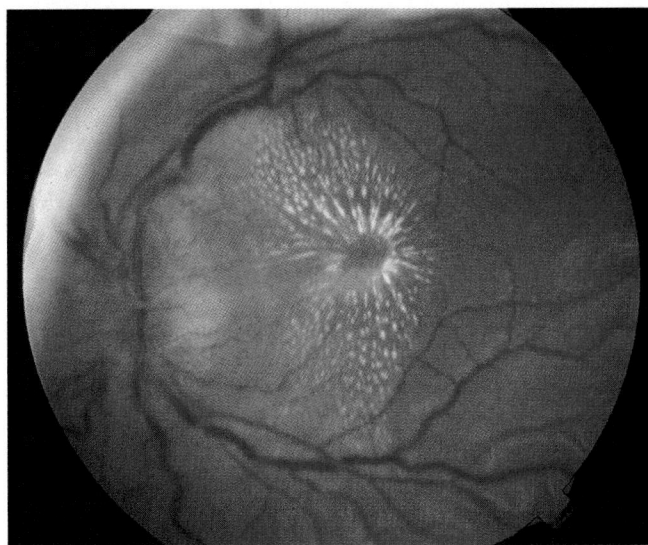

FIGURE 109-5. Funduscopic photograph of cat-scratch disease neuroretinitis, showing macular star in a 9-year-old patient who developed unilateral visual loss after acquiring a kitten. (*Courtesy of Dr. Simmons Lessell.*)

tion of acute illness.[45] An outbreak of uveitis involving 73 patients in southern India occurred in 1994, several months after heavy rains and flooding.[46] The uveitis was bilateral in half of the patients, and 96% had panuveitis. Nearly all patients had had a febrile illness consistent with leptospirosis 1 to 10 months earlier. Leptospiral DNA was detected by PCR in aqueous samples of 80% of patients.[47]

Lyme disease may cause uveitis of any type (e.g., anterior uveitis, intermediate uveitis, neuroretinitis, retinal vasculitis, choroiditis, panuveitis),[48] and manifestations resemble ocular syphilis. Uveitis is usually seen in the late stage of Lyme disease.[49]

Brucellosis may cause uveitis during the acute illness. A prospective study from Turkey of 147 patients with brucellosis found uveitis in 5% (anterior in 6 patients and posterior in 1 patient).[50] The authors noted that osteoarticular complications of brucellosis, such as spondylitis, were more common in patients with ocular involvement. If brucellosis is not diagnosed, uveitis may become chronic and relapsing. Tabbara and Al-Kassimi[51] described a Saudi Arabian patient in whom the diagnosis was missed for 9 years. This patient had a 9-year history of relapsing uveitis treated with corticosteroids and a history of recurrent fevers. A paravertebral abscess due to *Brucella melitensis* eventually was diagnosed and treated, and the uveitis responded to the antibiotic therapy.

Whipple's disease also may produce a chronic uveitis if not diagnosed and treated. Rickman and colleagues[52] described a 59-year-old patient with 4 years of bilateral uveitis that eventually was diagnosed as due to *Tropheryma whipplei* after periodic acid–Schiff stains of vitreous samples showed the organism. The uveitis was granulomatous (iris and retinal "nodules," vitritis, pars planitis) and responded to systemic penicillin and streptomycin. Bodaghi and colleagues[53] in Paris described a patient with apparent ocular Whipple's disease in whom PCR was negative for *T. whipplei* but positive for *Arthrobacter* spp.

In *leprosy,* uveitis occurs mainly in patients with chronic lepromatous leprosy and is nearly always an iridocyclitis.[54] Choroidal involvement is almost never seen. The iridocyclitis is usually bilateral and has a chronic relapsing course.[55] It is often asymptomatic until late stages and is an important cause of blindness in leprosy.[56]

Bartonella henselae, the agent of *cat-scratch disease,* is one cause of neuroretinitis.[57] It may be the most important cause: A study found that 64% of neuroretinitis patients were seropositive for *B. henselae*.[58] Patients present with decreased vision and have characteristic eye findings of optic disk edema and a "macular star," a striking sunburst pattern around the macula (Fig. 109-5). The macular star resolves in 2 to 3 months, and vision spontaneously recovers. The value of antibiotics is unknown.

DIAGNOSIS

Patients with infectious uveitis represent a diagnostic dilemma to ophthalmologists and infectious disease physicians. The diagnosis is nearly always presumptive and cannot be proved by pathology or culture. With rare exceptions, the uvea cannot be biopsied without risking sight, so pathology of the uvea is not available until the eye is lost. The aqueous and vitreous humors may be sampled safely, but these samples rarely yield an infectious organism. The aqueous may be sampled with a 24-gauge needle by the ophthalmologist as an office procedure. The sample taken is usually 0.1 mL because the total volume of aqueous is only 0.2 mL. The vitreous also may be aspirated as an office procedure or by vitrectomy in the operating room. Cytology of vitrectomy samples may be helpful to exclude malignancy (e.g., primary ocular lymphoma or metastatic cancer). Bacterial cultures of the aqueous or vitreous are almost never positive in infectious uveitis, unless the diagnosis is chronic endophthalmitis (e.g., due to *Propionibacterium acnes* or *Candida*) rather than uveitis. In tuberculous uveitis, cultures of the vitreous and aqueous are negative,[59] with rare exceptions as noted earlier. Similarly, viral cultures of aqueous and vitreous samples are rarely positive in herpetic uveitis.

Molecular diagnostic techniques applied to aqueous or vitreous samples eventually may prove helpful in diagnosing infectious causes of uveitis. PCR already seems to be useful in viral uveitis. Yamamoto and co-workers[60] found that PCR tests of aqueous samples from 7 patients with recurrent iridocyclitis of suspected viral etiology were all positive for either HSV (6 samples) or VZV (1 sample), whereas samples from 17 control eyes were negative. In a study of 28 patients with ARN, PCR was positive in 27 (96%) for HSV, VZV, or CMV.[61] The sensitivity and specificity of molecular diagnostic tests for most types of infectious uveitis are unknown, however, making interpretation difficult and results potentially misleading. Often studies that purport to diagnose an infectious uveitis with PCR offer no other support for the diagnosis. Gupta and colleagues[27] reported that 10 of 17 patients

(60%) with presumed ocular tuberculosis had positive aqueous PCR assays for *M. tuberculosis,* but the clinical diagnosis was based on a positive PPD or abnormal chest radiograph (or both) and the absence of another uveitis diagnosis. Their assay also was positive in 23% of the control group of uveitis patients who had a negative PPD and normal chest radiograph. False-negative PCR tests may occur if the assay uses Taq DNA polymerase and if aqueous and vitreous specimens are not pretreated with chloroform extraction to remove PCR inhibitors.[62] This inhibition is not seen in PCR assays using *Thermus thermophilus* HB-8 or *Thermus flavus* DNA polymerases. Most "false-negative" PCR tests may represent truly negative results and signify that the infection in uveitis is in the uvea, not in the aqueous or vitreous.

Positive serologic tests, such as IgG antibodies to *Toxoplasma,* CMV, or HSV, also may be of little help given the high prevalence of such antibodies in the general population. The one serologic test that is always helpful and should be ordered on all patients with uveitis is the specific treponemal test for syphilis (e.g., *T. pallidum* agglutination or FTA-abs). If this test is positive and eye findings are consistent with ocular syphilis, the patient should be treated for ocular syphilis with high-dose intravenous penicillin. Because syphilis can produce almost any ocular manifestation,[63] nearly all patients with uveitis and a positive specific treponemal test require therapy. The *T. pallidum* agglutination test is preferred because the FTA-abs may be falsely positive in some patients, especially patients with rheumatologic conditions.[64] The RPR also should be checked, although false-positive tests are common in autoimmune conditions, and all positive RPR tests must be confirmed with a specific treponemal test. A negative RPR does not exclude ocular syphilis because it is negative in greater than 50% of patients with eye disease due to tertiary syphilis.

Radiologic studies of the eye or orbit sometimes are helpful in uveitis. Magnetic resonance imaging of the brain and orbit may be helpful in suspected cases of ocular–central nervous system lymphoma if brain lesions are found, although eye disease may precede central nervous system lesions by months. Fluorescein angiography of the eye may show retinal vascular patterns consistent with certain diseases, such as viral-induced vasculitis in CMV. Indocyanine green angiography of the eye was found to be useful in detecting and following subclinical choroidal lesions in eight patients with presumed ocular tuberculosis.[65] General radiologic studies (e.g., chest radiograph or computed tomography, gallium scan) may be helpful in distinguishing sarcoidosis from tuberculosis in patients with uveitis because these diseases often produce similar eye findings.

TREATMENT

Treatment for infectious causes of uveitis is usually the same as treatment for the corresponding infection of the central nervous system. *Ocular syphilis* should be treated the same as neurosyphilis, with 10 to 14 days of intravenous penicillin (4 million U every 4 hours, assuming normal renal function). Systemic corticosteroids (e.g., oral prednisone, 80 mg daily) should be started along with the antibiotic therapy, then tapered over several weeks. Many experts follow intravenous penicillin with injections of 2.4 million U of intramuscular benzathine penicillin, once weekly for 3 weeks. All patients with presumed ocular syphilis should be tested for HIV, and all should have a lumbar puncture before starting therapy to exclude concurrent neurosyphilis. If there is evidence of neurosyphilis, antibiotic treatment is the same, but a follow-up lumbar puncture at 6 months is necessary to document resolution of infection.

Ocular tuberculosis should be treated with the same medications and duration of therapy as tuberculous meningitis, although ethambutol is avoided if possible because of potential ocular toxicity. A short course of systemic corticosteroids may be necessary initially if there is sight-threatening inflammation. The treatment of ocular toxoplasmosis, CMV retinitis, and ocular toxocariasis is discussed in Chapters 134, 276, and 289.

ARN is treated with high-dose intravenous acyclovir (10 mg/kg every 8 hours with normal renal function) initially until disease progression stops, followed by valacyclovir or famciclovir for at least 6 weeks. Long-term suppressive antiviral therapy should be considered for immunosuppressed patients.

Herpetic iridocyclitis is treated primarily with topical corticosteroids.[40] Oral acyclovir should be started as well because long-term prophylactic oral acyclovir (400 mg twice daily) seems to be beneficial in preventing recurrences of herpetic stromal keratitis[66] and anterior uveitis.[67]

Ocular candidiasis treatment depends on whether there is endophthalmitis in addition to chorioretinitis. Patients usually develop ocular candidiasis from candidemia, and the prolonged course of systemic amphotericin or high-dose oral fluconazole given for candidemia successfully treats most cases of chorioretinitis. Patients with chorioretinitis should be followed closely, however, because progression to endophthalmitis has occurred despite systemic antifungal therapy.[68,69] Efficacy of newer antifungal agents, such as voriconazole or caspofungin, for candidal endophthalmitis is unknown. Patients with candidal endophthalmitis should undergo vitrectomy and receive an intravitreal injection of amphotericin (10 μg), in addition to systemic therapy. In a study of 12 patients with *Candida albicans* endophthalmitis treated with systemic amphotericin or fluconazole, the 7 patients who also underwent early vitrectomy did well, whereas 4 of 5 patients in whom vitrectomy was delayed (>1 week) or not performed developed visual loss or blindness.[70]

REFERENCES

1. Skinner HA. The Origin of Medical Terms, 2nd ed. Baltimore: Williams & Wilkins; 1961:416.
2. Boch-Michel E, Nussenblatt RB. International Uveitis Study Group recommendations for the evaluation of intraocular inflammatory disease. Am J Ophthalmol. 1987;103:234-235.
3. Suttorp-Schulten MSA, Rothova A. The possible impact of uveitis in blindness: A literature survey. Br J Ophthalmol. 1996;80:844-848.
4. Ronday MJH, Stilma JS, Barbe RF, et al. Blindness from uveitis in a hospital population in Sierra Leone. Br J Ophthalmol. 1994;78:690-693.
5. Rodriguez A, Calonge M, Pedroza-Seres M, et al. Referral patterns of uveitis in a tertiary eye care center. Arch Ophthalmol. 1996;114:593-599.
6. Biswas J, Narain S, Das D, et al. Pattern of uveitis in a referral uveitis clinic in India. Int Ophthalmol. 1996;20:223-228.
7. McCannel CA, Holland GN, Helm CJ, et al. Causes of uveitis in the general practice of ophthalmology. UCLA Community-Based Uveitis Study Group. Am J Ophthalmol. 1996;121:35-46.
8. Bodaghi B, Cassoux N, Wechsler B, et al. Chronic severe uveitis: Etiology and visual outcome in 927 patients from a single center. Medicine. 2001;80:263-270.
9. Barilee GR, Flynn H. Syphilis exposure in patients with uveitis. Ophthalmology. 1997;104:1605-1609.
10. Villanueva AV, Sahouri MJ, Ormerod LD, et al. Posterior uveitis in patients with positive serology for syphilis. Clin Infect Dis. 2000;30:479-485.
11. Becerra LI, Ksiazek SM, Savino PJ, et al. Syphilis uveitis in human immunodeficiency virus-infected and noninfected patients. Ophthalmology. 1989;96:1727-1730.
12. Opremcak EM. Uveitis: A Clinical Manual for Ocular Inflammation. New York: Springer-Verlag; 1995:135.
13. Grant WM. Late glaucoma after interstitial keratitis. Am J Ophthalmol. 1975;79:87-91.
14. Spoor TC, Ramocki JM, Nesi FA, et al. Ocular syphilis 1986: Prevalence of FTA-abs reactivity and cerebrospinal fluid findings. J Clin Neuro-ophthalmol. 1987;7:191-195.
15. Levy JH, Liss RA, Maguire AM. Neurosyphilis and ocular syphilis in patients with concurrent human immunodeficiency virus infection. Retina. 1989;9:175-180.
16. Ormerod LD, Puklin JE, Sobel JD. Syphilitic posterior uveitis: Correlative findings and significance. Clin Infect Dis. 2001;32:1661-1673.
17. Tabbara KF, al Kaff AS, Fadel T. Ocular manifestations of endemic syphilis (bejel). Ophthalmology. 1989;96:1087-1091.
18. Tabbara KF. Brucellosis and nonsyphilic treponemal uveitis. Int Ophthalmol Clin. 1990;30:294-296.
19. Sarangapani S, Benjamin L. Posterior segment changes secondary to late yaws. Eye. 2001;15:664-666.
20. Donahue HC. Ophthalmologic experience in a tuberculosis sanatorium. Am J Ophthalmol. 1967;64:742-748.
21. Biswas J, Badrinath SS. Ocular morbidity in patients with active systemic tuberculosis. Int Ophthalmol. 1996;19:293-298.
22. Bouza E, Merino P, Munoz P, et al. Ocular tuberculosis: A prospective study in a general hospital. Medicine. 1997;76:53-61.
23. Bodaghi B, LeHoang P. Ocular tuberculosis. Curr Opin Ophthalmol. 2000;11:443-448.
24. Helm CJ, Holland GN. Ocular tuberculosis. Surv Ophthalmol. 1993;38:229-256.

25. Biswas J, Madhavan HN, Gopal L, et al. Intraocular tuberculosis: Clinicopathologic study of five cases. Retina. 1995;15:461-468.
26. Sarvananthan N, Wiselka M, Bibby K. Intraocular tuberculosis without detectable systemic infection. Arch Ophthalmol. 1998;116:1386-1388.
27. Gupta V, Arora S, Gupta A, et al. Management of presumed intraocular tuberculosis: Possible role of the polymerase chain reaction. Acta Ophthalmol Scand. 1998;76:679-682.
28. Rosenbaum JT, Wernick R. The utility of routine screening of patients with uveitis for systemic lupus erythematosis or tuberculosis: A Bayesian analysis. Arch Ophthalmol. 1990;108:1291-1293.
29. Massaro D, Katz S, Sachs M. Choroidal tubercles: A clue to hematogenous tuberculosis. Ann Intern Med. 1964;60:231-241.
30. Samson CM, Foster CS. Tuberculosis. In: Foster CS, Vitale AT, eds. Diagnosis and Treatment of Uveitis. Philadelphia: WB Saunders; 2002:268.
31. Rosen PH, Spalton DJ, Graham EM. Intraocular tuberculosis. Eye. 1990;4:486-492.
32. Urayama A, Yamad N, Sasaki T, et al. Unilateral acute uveitis with retinal periarteritis and detachment. Jpn J Clin Ophthalmol. 1971;25:607-619.
33. Heiligenhaus A, Helbig B, Fiedler M. Herpesviruses. In: Foster CS, Vitale AT, eds. Diagnosis and Treatment of Uveitis. Philadelphia: WB Saunders; 2002:318.
34. Paylay DA, Sternberg P, Davis J, et al. Decrease in the risk of bilateral acute retinal necrosis by acyclovir therapy. Am J Ophthalmol. 1991;112:250.
35. Batisse D, Eliaszewicz M, Zazoun L, et al. Acute retinal necrosis in the course of AIDS: Study of 26 cases. AIDS. 1996;10:55-60.
36. Galindez OA, Sabates NR, Whitacre MN, et al. Rapidly progressive outer retinal necrosis caused by varicella zoster virus in a patient infected with human immunodeficiency virus. Clin Infect Dis. 1996;22:149-151.
37. Pinnolis MK, Foxworthy D, Kemp B. Treatment of progressive outer retinal necrosis with sorivudine. Am J Ophthalmol. 1995;119:516-517.
38. Lairson DR, Begley CE, Reynolds TF, et al. Prevention of herpes simplex virus eye disease: A cost-effectiveness analysis. Arch Ophthalmol. 2003;121:108-112.
39. Liesegang T. Ocular herpes simplex infection: Pathogenesis and current therapy. Mayo Clin Proc. 1988;63:1092.
40. Pavan-Langston D. Herpes simplex of the ocular anterior segment. In: Remington JS, Swartz MN, eds. Current Clinical Topics in Infectious Diseases, v. 20. Cambridge, MA: Blackwell Science; 2000:298.
41. Kobashi Y, Hayasaka S, Shibuya Y, et al. Herpes simplex virus iridocyclitis unassociated with keratitis. Ann Ophthalmol. 1996;28:107-109.
42. Donahue SP, Greven CM, Zuravleff JJ, et al. Intraocular candidiaasis in patients with candidemia: Clinical implications derived from a prospective multicenter study. Ophthalmology. 1994;101:1302-1309.
43. Essman TF, Flynn HW, Smiddy WE, et al. Treatment outcomes in a 10-year study of endogenous fungal endophthalmitis. Ophthalmic Surg Lasers. 1997;28:185-194.
44. Lightman S, Towler HMA. Uveitis. London: BMJ Books; 1998:79.
45. Alexander S, Baer A, Fair JR, et al. Leptospiral uveitis. Arch Ophthalmol. 1952;48:292-297.
46. Rathinam SR, Rathnam S, Selvaraz S, et al. Uveitis associated with an epidemic outbreak of leptospirosis. Am J Ophthalmol. 1997;124:71-79.
47. Chu KM, Rathinam R, Namperumalsamy P, et al. Identification of Leptospira species in the pathogenesis of uveitis and determination of clinical ocular characteristics in South India. J Infect Dis. 1998;177:1314-1321.
48. Karma A, Seppala I, Mikkila H, et al. Diagnosis and clinical characteristics of ocular Lyme borreliosis. Am J Ophthalmol. 1995;119:127-135.
49. Mikkila HO, Seppala IJ, Viljanen MK, et al. The expanding clinical spectrum of ocular Lyme borreliosis. Ophthalmology. 2000;107:581-587.
50. Gungur K, Bekir NA, Namiduru M. Ocular complications associated with brucellosis in an endemic area. Eur J Ophthalmol. 2002;12:232-237.
51. Tabbara KF, Al-Kassimi H. Ocular brucellosis. Br J Ophthalmol. 1990;74:249-250.
52. Rickman LS, Freeman WR, Green WR, et al. Brief report: Uveitis caused by *Tropheryma whippelii* (Whipple's bacillus). N Engl J Med. 1995;332:363-366.
53. Bodaghi B, Dauga C, Cassoux N, et al. Whipple's syndrome (uveitis, B27-negative spondylarthropathy, meningitis, and lymphadenopathy) associated with Arthrobacter sp. infection. Ophthalmology. 1998;105:1891-1896.
54. Rawal RC, Kar PK, Desai RN, et al. A clinical study of eye complications in leprosy. Indian J Lepr. 1984;56:232-240.
55. Suryawanshi N. Clinical manifestations of iridocyclitis in leprosy. Indian J Lepr. 1985;57:549-555.
56. Espiritu CG, Gelber R, Ostler HB. Chronic anterior uveitis in leprosy: An insidious cause of blindness. Br J Ophthalmol. 1991;75:273-275.
57. Solley WA, Martin DF, Newman NJ, et al. Cat scratch disease: Posterior segment manifestations. Ophthalmology. 2000;107:817-818.
58. Suhler EB, Lauer AK, Rosenbaum JT. Prevalence of serologic evidence of cat scratch disease in patients with neuroretinitis. Ophthalmology. 2000;107:871-876.
59. Ni C, Papale JJ, Robinson NL, et al. Uveal tuberculosis. Int Ophthalmol Clin. 1982;22:103-124.
60. Yamamoto S, Pavan-Langston D, Kinoshita S, et al. Detecting herpesvirus DNA in uveitis using the polymerase chain reaction. Br J Ophthalmol. 1996;80:465-468.
61. Ganatra JB, Chandler D, Santos C, et al. Viral causes of the acute retinal necrosis syndrome. Am J Ophthalmol. 2000;129:166-172.
62. Wiedbrauk DL, Werner JC, Drevon AM. Inhibition of PCR by aqueous and vitreous fluids. J Clin Microbiol. 1995;33:2643-2646.
63. Margo CE, Hamed LM. Ocular syphilis. Surv Ophthalmol. 1992;37:203-220.
64. Murphy FT, George R, Kubota K, et al. The use of Western blotting as the confirmatory test for syphilis in patients with rheumatic disease. J Rheumatol. 1999;26:2448-2453.
65. Wolfensberger TJ, Piquet B, Herbort CP. Indocyanine green angiographic features in tuberculous chorioretinitis. Am J Ophthalmol. 1999; 127:350-353.
66. Herpetic Eye Disease Study Group. Oral acyclovir for herpes simplex virus eye disease: Effect on prevention of epithelial keratitis and stromal keratitis. Arch Ophthalmol. 2000;118:1030-1036.
67. Rodriguez A, Power WJ, Neves RA, et al. Recurrence rate of herpetic uveitis in patients on long-term oral acyclovir. Doc Ophthalmol. 1995;90:331-340.
68. Virata SR, Kylstra JA, Brown JC, et al. Worsening of endogenous *Candida albicans* endophthalmitis during therapy with intravenous lipid complex amphotericin B. Clin Infect Dis. 1999;28:1177-1178.
69. Feman SS, Nichols JC, Chung SM, et al. Endophthalmitis in patients with disseminated fungal disease. Trans Am Ophthalmol Soc. 2002;100:67-70.
70. Martinez-Vazquez C, Fernandez-Ulloa J, Bordon J, et al. *Candida albicans* endophthalmitis in brown heroin addicts: Response to early vitrectomy preceded and followed by antifungal therapy. Clin Infect Dis. 1998;27:1130-1133.

CHAPTER **110**

Periocular Infections

MARLENE L. DURAND

Periocular infections are infections of the eyelids, lacrimal system, and orbital soft tissues that surround the globe of the eye. These infections may affect vision if not recognized and treated appropriately.

EYELID INFECTIONS

Anatomy

Each eyelid contains a fibrous tarsal plate, which gives the lid its firmness (Fig. 110-1). Within each tarsal plate are 20 to 25 meibomian (or tarsal) glands (Fig. 110-2). These glands may be seen as faint yellow lines on the inner surface of the everted lid, extending perpendicular to the lid margin. Meibomian glands are sebaceous glands that secrete sebum, an oily substance. Sebum prevents the tear film from evaporating too quickly from the ocular surface. At the lid margin, adjacent to the eyelash follicles, are smaller sebaceous glands called *glands of Zeis*.

Hordeolum

A hordeolum is an acute infection of a sebaceous gland of the lid, usually caused by *Staphylococcus aureus*. An internal hordeolum is an infection of a meibomian gland, and patients present with lid swelling, erythema, and tenderness. Internal hordeola may point toward either the skin or the conjunctival surface. An external hordeolum (stye) is an infection of a gland of Zeis, and patients present with a painful pustule, which points to the lid margin. Internal and external hordeola usually respond to frequent warm compresses. Topical bacitracin or erythromycin ointment may be used at night. Incision and drainage of the lesion is rarely required.

Chalazion

A chalazion is a sterile granulomatous reaction to inspissated sebum within an obstructed meibomian gland. It may result from an internal hordeolum or arise de novo.[1] Patients present with a nontender nodule within the lid that points to the conjunctival surface. Chalazia may become large and press on the ocular surface, distorting vision. Most chalazia resolve within 1 month, but recurrences are common in patients with chronic blepharitis. Persistent or recurrent chalazia should be biopsied to exclude sebaceous cell carcinoma of the lid.

Marginal Blepharitis

Marginal blepharitis (Fig. 110-3) is a diffuse inflammation of the lid margins. It is one of the most common conditions seen by ophthalmologists.[2] Marginal blepharitis is usually due to an abnormality of meibomian gland secretion, although superinfection with *S. aureus*

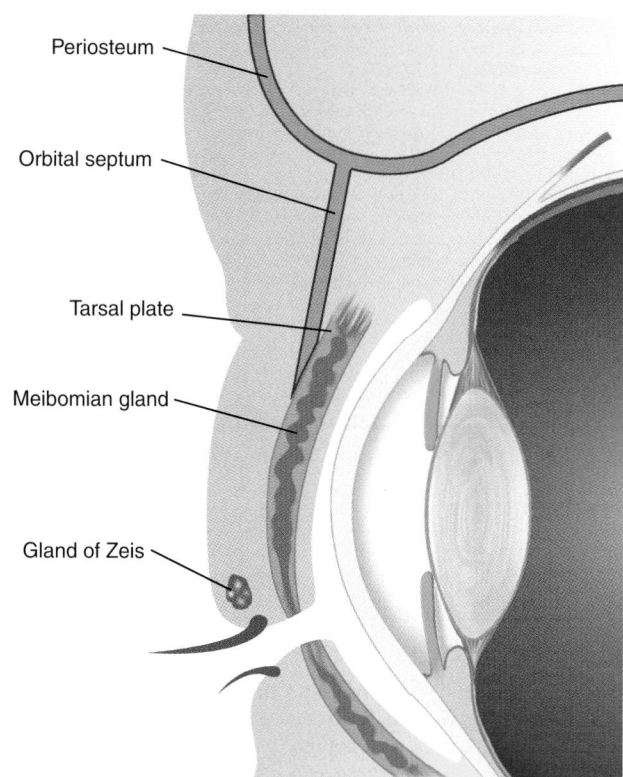

FIGURE 110-1. Diagram of the eye (sagittal section) with uvea highlighted (iris, ciliary body, and choroid, each in different colors). (© *1997 Anthony J. Bron, Ramesh C. Tripathi and Brenda J. Tripathi. Reproduced by permission of Hodder Arnold.)*

may occur. It may be mild, with redness and scaling at the margins (seborrheic blepharitis), or more severe, with small marginal ulcerations and destruction of the hair follicles (ulcerative blepharitis). It is usually chronic and remitting, and it is often associated with seborrheic dermatitis or rosacea. Treatment of the chronic condition is with gentle eyelid scrubs (e.g., twice daily with baby shampoo), with the addition of bacitracin ointment to the lid margins for acute inflammation. Oral tetracycline may be helpful if there is associated rosacea. *Malassezia* yeasts have been associated with seborrheic dermatitis.[3] Dermatitis may respond to antifungal agents, such as a short course of itraconazole.[4]

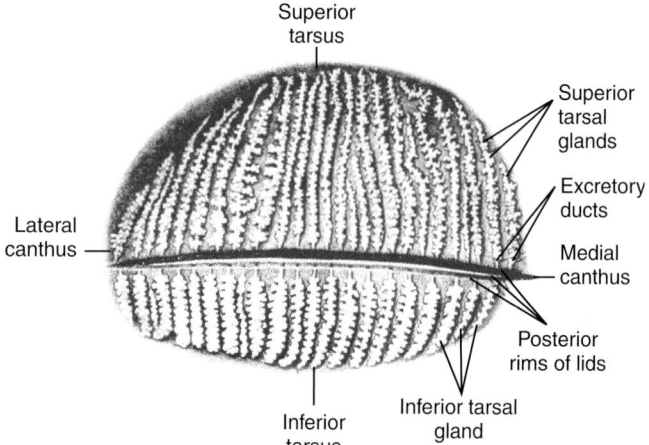

FIGURE 110-2. The meibomian glands. *(From Warwick R. Eugene Wolff's Anatomy of the Eye and Orbit. Philadelphia: WB Saunders; 1976.)*

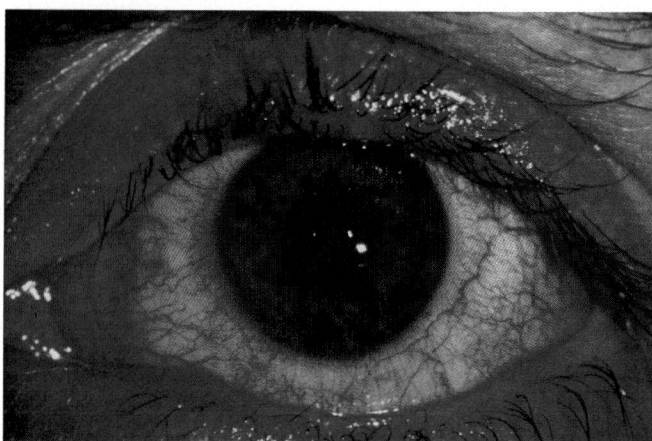

FIGURE 110-3. Photograph of eyelids with marginal blepharitis.

Case reports of rare causes of blepharitis or blepharoconjunctivitis have been published. *Pseudomonas aeruginosa* caused an acute necrotizing blepharoconjunctivitis and subsequent facial cellulitis in a patient with chemotherapy-induced leukopenia.[5] *Leishmania donovani* caused blepharoconjunctivitis in a patient with post–kala-azar dermal leishmaniasis.[6] *Capnocytophaga ochracea* caused a chronic blepharoconjunctivitis in a 70-year-old immunocompetent patient; the organism also was isolated from the gingiva.[7] Phthiriasis palpebrarum is infestation of the eyelashes by crab lice. Patients have pruritus of the lid margins and blepharoconjunctivitis.[8] Herpes simplex blepharitis has been described in adults and children, may be recurrent, and is occasionally bilateral.[9,10]

INFECTIONS OF THE LACRIMAL SYSTEM

Anatomy

The lacrimal gland is located beneath the upper outer orbital rim (Fig. 110-4). It produces tears that flow across the eye, then drain through the puncta, canaliculi, lacrimal sac, and lacrimal duct into the nasal cavity. The only parts of the lacrimal system that are visible on examination are the puncta and sometimes the lacrimal gland. The size of

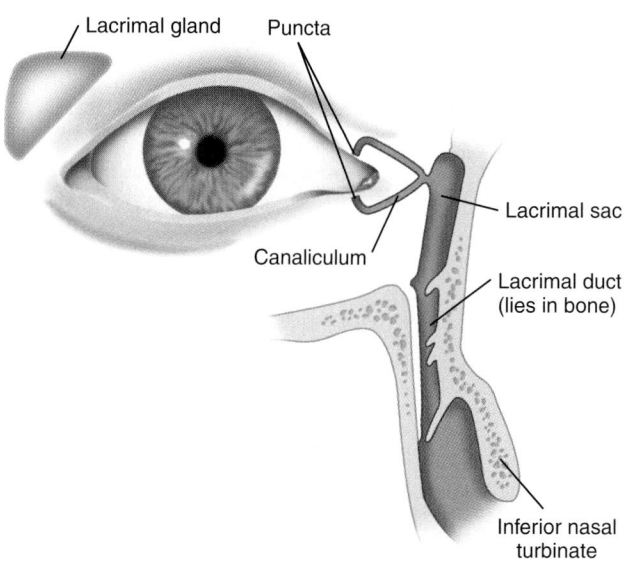

FIGURE 110-4. The lacrimal system. *(Adapted from Barza M, Baum J. Ocular infections. Med Clin North Am. 1983;67:131-152.)*

the lacrimal gland varies, but a portion may be visible in some patients when the upper lid is everted and the patient looks down and in. The gland then appears as a pink mass under the conjunctiva, just under the lateral part of the upper orbital rim.

Dacryoadenitis

Dacryoadenitis is an inflammation of the lacrimal gland. Infections are rare and may be acute or chronic. Acute dacryoadenitis presents with a tender area of erythema and swelling in the lateral part of the upper lid. It may lead to preseptal or orbital cellulitis or may suppurate into an abscess.[11,12] *S. aureus* is the most common pathogen, although streptococci also may be a cause.[13] There are case reports of acute suppurative dacryoadenitis due to *Pseudomonas,* brucellosis, and cysticercosis.[14-16] Epstein-Barr virus may cause acute nonsuppurative dacryoadenitis in mononucleosis, which may be unilateral or bilateral.[17,18] It may result in keratoconjunctivitis sicca.[19] Acute herpes zoster dacryocystitis was described in a patient who, 2 days later, developed iridocyclitis and shingles in the distribution of the first division of the trigeminal nerve.[20] Chronic infectious dacryoadenitis is rare, but most reports describe *Mycobacterium tuberculosis* as the cause.[21,22] Most cases of chronic dacryoadenitis are inflammatory rather than infectious, however. Sjögren's disease and sarcoidosis are the most common associated diseases, although cases of Crohn's disease and Wegener's disease presenting as chronic dacryoadenitis have been described.[23,24] Tumors cause approximately 25% of cases of chronic lacrimal gland enlargement.[13]

Canaliculitis

Canaliculitis may occur spontaneously or develop after placement of silicone in the canaliculi (e.g., punctal plugs to treat dry eyes) or in the nasolacrimal system (tubes for tear drainage).[25,26] Canaliculitis presents as a chronic process, with symptoms of tearing and irritation in the medial portion of the affected eyelid. Examination reveals a swollen, "pouting" punctum and erythema of the adjacent nasal conjunctiva. There may be a unilateral conjunctivitis. The lower canaliculus is affected more often than the upper.[13] A yellow-green exudate and yellowish concretions may be expressed from the involved punctum in many cases of canaliculitis. The concretions represent sulphur granules formed by *Actinomyces israelii,* the organism in nearly all cases. Rare causes include *Propionibacterium propionicum,*[27] *Eikenella corrodens,*[28] *Nocardia asteroides,*[25] *Mycobacterium chelonae,*[29] and *Enterobacter cloacae.*[30] Treatment requires removal of canalicular material and concretions; this usually can be achieved by applying pressure near the nasal corner of the eye or by office curettage of the canaliculus.[31] Occasionally, surgical exploration is required. Some ophthalmologists also infuse penicillin solution through the canaliculus and prescribe penicillin eye drops. These are not available commercially but may be made up as a 100,000 U/mL solution.

Dacryocystitis

Dacryocystitis, or inflammation of the lacrimal sac, is the most common infection of the lacrimal system. It arises because of obstruction of the lacrimal duct, pooling of tears in the lacrimal sac, and subsequent infection. Obstruction may be congenital or may result from trauma, tumors, infection, or inflammation of the duct. Acute dacryocystitis symptoms include pain, swelling, and erythema near the nasal corner of the eye. There is usually epiphora (excessive tearing) and a purulent discharge. Infants often have lacrimal duct obstruction with epiphora, but acute dacryocystitis complicates the obstruction in only 3%.[32] The most common causes of acute dacryocystitis are *S. aureus* and streptococci. Gram-negative bacilli accounted for 25% of isolates in one study, with *Escherichia coli* as the most frequent gram-negative organism isolated.[33] Treatment requires antibiotic therapy (e.g., ampicillin-sulbactam) and occasionally incision and drainage of a lacrimal sac abscess. Chronic or recurrent dacryocystitis usually requires a surgical procedure, dacryocystorhinostomy. One study found that cultures

taken at the time of dacryocystorhinostomy surgery were positive in nearly half of the 114 patients studied, although only one fifth of the patients had a history of dacryocystitis.[34] *Staphylococcus epidermidis* and *S. aureus* were the only organisms isolated in 45% and 24% of culture-positive cases. Whether these reflect nasal flora contamination is unknown. Gram-negative bacilli composed a larger percentage of isolates in patients with a history of dacryocystitis, a finding also noted by others.[35]

PRESEPTAL CELLULITIS AND ORBITAL INFECTIONS

Anatomy

The orbital septum is a thin, fibrous membrane that serves as a barrier between the superficial lids and the orbit. The septum arises from the orbital periosteum at the orbital rim and extends to the tarsal plates of the eyelids (see Fig. 110-1). Infections anterior to the septum are preseptal, and infections posterior to the septum are orbital. *Preseptal cellulitis* involves only the lids and not the orbit, whereas *orbital cellulitis* involves the soft tissues (fat, muscle) contained within the bony orbit (Fig. 110-5). The bony orbit is shaped like a cone placed horizontally, apex tilted medially. It is surrounded by the paranasal sinuses for much of its circumference: the frontal sinus superiorly, the maxillary sinus inferiorly, and the ethmoid medially. The medial orbital wall, the paper-thin lamina papyracea, is also the lateral wall of the ethmoid sinus. It contains multiple foramina for nerves and blood vessels and natural defects called *Zuckerkandl's dehiscences.* For

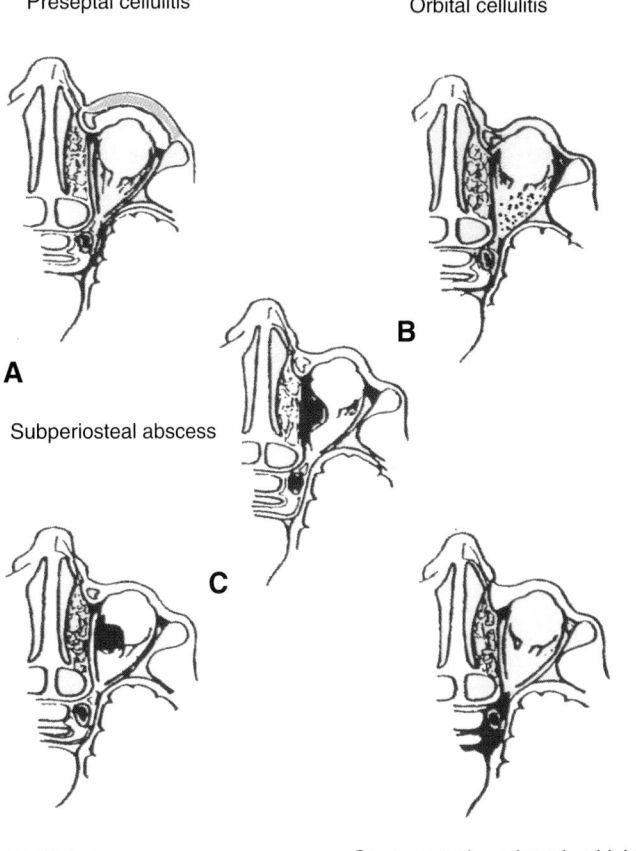

Preseptal cellulitis

Orbital cellulitis

Subperiosteal abscess

A

B

C

Orbital abscess

Cavernous sinus thrombophlebitis

D

E

FIGURE 110-5. Five diagrams illustrating preseptal cellulitis **(A)**, orbital cellulitis **(B)**, subperiosteal abscess **(C)**, orbital abscess **(D)**, and cavernous sinus thrombophlebitis **(E)**. *(Modified from a drawing in Chandler JR, Langenbrunner DJ, Stevens FR. The pathogenesis of orbital complications in acute sinusitis. Laryngoscope. 1970;80:1414.)*

these anatomic reasons, ethmoid sinusitis is the most common cause of sinus-related orbital infection. Periosteum (periorbita) lines the orbit, and infection from the ethmoid sinus may cross the lamina papyracea and collect beneath the periorbita as a *subperiosteal abscess.* Infection may break through the periorbita, or coalesce from an orbital cellulitis, and form an *orbital abscess.* The venous drainage of the middle third of the face and paranasal sinuses is primarily through the valveless orbital veins, which drain inferiorly to the pterygoid plexus and posteriorly to the cavernous sinus.[36] As a consequence, *cavernous sinus thrombophlebitis* may occur as a complication of a sinus or orbital infection (see Chapter 85).

Epidemiology

Preseptal cellulitis is much more common than orbital cellulitis. In a review of 315 pediatric patients (age ≤18 years) with either infection treated in two adjacent Boston hospitals between 1980 and 1998, 94% were preseptal cellulitis cases.[37] Both conditions occur most often in young children: 75% of patients in the Boston study were younger than 5 years old. Children with orbital cellulitis tend to be slightly older than children with preseptal cellulitis. The average age of orbital cellulitis patients in the Boston study was 5 years versus 3 years for preseptal cellulitis patients. A study from New York found similar results, with an average age of 7.6 years for orbital cellulitis and 4.6 years for preseptal cellulitis.[38] The term *orbital cellulitis* often is used in the literature to include cases of subperiosteal and orbital abscess in addition to cellulitis. The distinction is important clinically because abscesses usually require surgical drainage. Subperiosteal abscess occurs almost as often as uncomplicated orbital cellulitis and accounts for 2% to 10% of all cases of preseptal and orbital infections in large inclusive series.[37-41] Orbital abscess is rare, accounting for less than 1% of cases in these series.

Etiology and Bacteriology

Sinusitis causes 80% to 90% of all cases of preseptal and orbital cellulitis.[38] The ethmoid sinus is involved in most of these cases, followed by the maxillary sinus. The frontal sinus, which does not develop until at least age 6, is involved occasionally in older children and adults.[42] Sphenoid sinusitis rarely leads to bacterial orbital infections. The etiology of sinus-related preseptal and orbital cellulitis is usually unknown because blood cultures are often negative. Sinus cultures in these cases reveal typical acute sinusitis pathogens, such as *Streptococcus pneumoniae* and *Haemophilus influenzae.* Some studies show *S. aureus* as a major sinus pathogen.[43] Subperiosteal abscess is caused by ethmoid sinusitis in nearly all cases. Abscess cultures show *S. pneumoniae,* group A streptococcus, nontypable *H. influenzae,* and *S. aureus* as the major pathogens.[44,45] Harris[44] noted that bacteriology varies with age. Greater than 80% (10 of 12) of children younger than age 9 in his study had negative cultures or their infection cleared after intravenous antibiotics without drainage, and the culture-positive cases grew only single aerobes (*S. aureus* or *S. pneumoniae*). Infection in children age 9 or older did not usually clear on intravenous antibiotics alone, and drainage cultures were positive for multiple organisms, usually a mixture of aerobes and anaerobes. Aerobes included *Streptococcus anginosus (milleri)* group, group A and group C streptococci, *S. aureus, H. influenzae,* and *Moraxella catarrhalis,* whereas anaerobes included *Peptostreptococcus, Eikenella, Fusobacterium,* and *Bacteroides* spp. Brook and Frazier[46] found that subperiosteal abscesses in adults also were polymicrobial, with a similar mixture of aerobes and anaerobes. These cultures agreed with maxillary sinus puncture cultures obtained from the same patients.

Preseptal cellulitis may have two other causes besides sinusitis: bacterial superinfection of a rash or break in the eyelid skin and bacteremic seeding. The first may follow trauma, an insect bite, or herpetic lid lesions (herpes simplex or zoster). The pathogens are usually *S. aureus* or group A streptococcus. Preseptal cellulitis that is part of a facial cellulitis or erysipelas is included in this category. Rare cases of group A streptococcal preseptal cellulitis have been complicated by either streptococcal toxic shock syndrome or eyelid necrosis.[47,48]

P. aeruginosa also caused lid necrosis as a complication of blepharitis and preseptal cellulitis in one case.[49] Other unusual causes of preseptal cellulitis include ringworm,[50] atypical mycobacteria,[51] and anthrax.[52] The second cause, bacteremic seeding of the lids, occurs in infants and young children (usually <3 years old). This syndrome has become much less common since the introduction of *H. influenzae* type b (Hib) vaccine. Before the Hib vaccine, preseptal cellulitis was associated with bacteremia in 10% to 33% of cases, with 80% to 100% of these cases due to *H. influenzae.*[53-55] Large studies in the Hib vaccine era found only 4% to 8% of cases were bacteremic, with no cases due to *H. influenzae* type b bacteremia after 1987.[38,39] Streptococci, especially *S. pneumoniae* and group A streptococcus, are the main causes of bacteremia now, although nontypable *H. influenzae* is still an occasional pathogen.[37-39]

Orbital cellulitis and orbital abscess almost always are caused by sinusitis, but rare cases follow penetrating trauma, orbital surgery, peribulbar anesthesia for eye surgery, endophthalmitis, dental abscess, dacryocystitis, or dacryoadenitis.[42,56-58] These nonsinusitis etiologies may be more common in adults than children. In a study from Australia, 91% of children with orbital cellulitis or abscess had sinusitis, whereas only half of adults did.[43] The remaining adults had dacryocystitis, trauma, endophthalmitis, and secondarily infected nasal tumor as etiologies. There was no case of posterior extension of preseptal cellulitis in either children or adults in this study, and the incidence of this is unknown.

Clinical Presentation

Preseptal cellulitis must be distinguished from orbital cellulitis, a much more dangerous infection. The term *periorbital cellulitis,* sometimes used for preseptal cellulitis, should be avoided because it does not make this distinction clear. In preseptal and orbital cellulitis, the lids are red and swollen. The lids may be swollen shut, but it is essential to examine the eye to evaluate visual acuity and extraocular movement. In preseptal cellulitis, vision is normal, there is no afferent pupillary defect, extraocular movements are full and painless, and there is no proptosis. In contrast, patients with orbital cellulitis have some degree of ophthalmoplegia or proptosis or both. There is often deep eye pain and pain with eye movement. Proptosis may not be grossly apparent and should be measured (e.g., with Hertel's exophthalmometer); a difference of 2 mm is significant. Vision may be decreased, and an early warning sign may be an afferent pupillary defect. Fever and leukocytosis are usually present in children with preseptal or orbital cellulitis, but they may be absent in adults. Fever was present in 70% of pediatric cases but only 30% of adult cases in one series.[43]

Patients with subperiosteal abscess usually present with severe ophthalmoplegia, in addition to proptosis, deep eye pain, fever, and marked lid swelling and erythema. Because the abscess is medial in nearly all cases, the eye is typically fixed looking "down and out." Orbital abscesses also are usually medial or superomedial, so physical findings are similar (Fig. 110-6).

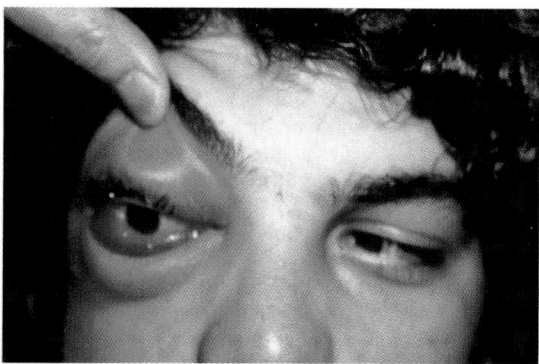

FIGURE 110-6. Patient with orbital abscess (eye looks "down and out").

In orbital cellulitis, signs of marked orbital inflammation usually precede visual loss. In orbital apex syndrome ("posterior orbital cellulitis"), the opposite occurs. Patients present with severe unilateral visual loss and ophthalmoplegia, but with minimal orbital inflammation. Orbital inflammation may worsen subsequently. This syndrome usually is caused by posterior ethmoid or sphenoid sinusitis. These sinuses are adjacent to the orbital apex, through which runs the optic nerve; cranial nerves III, IV, and VI; and the first division of cranial nerve V. Although most cases of orbital apex syndrome are due to the agents of mucormycosis or to *Aspergillus,* rare cases are due to bacteria.[59-61] Visual loss is usually irreversible.

Cavernous sinus thrombophlebitis is also rare and should be suspected in any patient with orbital cellulitis who develops contralateral signs of orbital inflammation (lid swelling, proptosis, ophthalmoplegia). Spread to the opposite eye occurs through the cavernous sinus and usually occurs within 24 to 48 hours of the initial unilateral orbital findings.[62] Patients also may present with bilateral findings, including lid edema, chemosis, proptosis, ptosis, and ophthalmoplegia. There may be decreased sensation over the forehead due to involvement of the first division of cranial nerve V. Visual loss may occur from venous congestion and ischemia. Patients are usually febrile and may be lethargic or obtunded. There is often sphenoid and posterior ethmoid sinusitis. *S. aureus* is the major pathogen, although cases due to streptococci, especially *S. anginosus (milleri)* group; anaerobes; and gram-negative bacilli have been described.[63-65] Two cases with a subacute presentation of cavernous sinus infection were described, one due to *Actinomyces* and the other due to *Actinobacillus actinomycetemcomitans.*[66,67] In both cases, patients initially were misdiagnosed as having Tolosa-Hunt syndrome, an idiopathic, steroid-responsive inflammatory process involving the cavernous sinus.

Laboratory and Radiologic Studies

Laboratory studies (white blood cell count, blood cultures) should be obtained in all patients with preseptal or orbital cellulitis. Leukocytosis with a left shift is present in most patients. Blood cultures are rarely positive in older children and adults but may be positive in 8% of young children, as noted earlier.

The most helpful study in evaluating a patient with orbital infection is computed tomography (CT). A CT scan is not necessary in many cases of preseptal cellulitis because the diagnosis may be made clinically. Some authors advocate CT for all children with preseptal cellulitis, however, and report three cases of subperiosteal abscess that presented similar to preseptal cellulitis, with no proptosis, visual decrease, or ophthalmoplegia.[68] If performed, CT shows lid edema but no proptosis or inflammation ("streaking") of the orbital fat. In patients who present with orbital signs, however, a CT scan should be performed to exclude the presence of a subperiosteal or orbital abscess. Repeat scans also should be obtained in any patient with presumed uncomplicated orbital cellulitis who fails to improve, or worsens, on intravenous antibiotics alone. Findings in orbital cellulitis usually include proptosis, streaking of the intraconal fat, and edema of the medial rectus muscle. In subperiosteal or orbital abscess, there is a low-density mass effect with or without enhancement.[69] An air-fluid level within the mass is even more specific for abscess.[70] Lateral displacement of the medial rectus and displacement of the periosteum away from the lamina papyracea are findings that suggest subperiosteal abscess (Fig. 110-7). CT results alone lead to misdiagnoses, however, and cannot always be relied on to determine the need for surgery. In one study, CT missed the diagnosis for 2 of 10 subperiosteal abscesses and 1 of 5 orbital abscesses.[69] Another review of 159 patients with orbital complications of sinusitis described 4 patients who developed blindness from orbital abscess.[71] The abscess was not diagnosed by CT in any of these four patients before surgery.

If orbital apex syndrome or cavernous sinus thrombosis is suspected, magnetic resonance imaging, magnetic resonance imaging venography, or high-resolution CT with slice thickness of 3 mm or less should be obtained. Findings in cavernous sinus thrombosis include flattening or bowing of the lateral wall of the cavernous sinus

(best viewed on coronal images) and filling defects within the contrast-enhancing cavernous sinus.[62] Dilation of the superior ophthalmic vein due to venous obstruction is an indirect sign of cavernous sinus thrombosis.

The differential diagnosis of bacterial orbital cellulitis includes orbital pseudotumor, tumor, and invasive fungal disease (invasive sinus aspergillosis and mucormycosis). Orbital pseudotumor is an idiopathic disease, more common in adults than children, that often manifests with painful ophthalmoplegia. It may appear with inflammatory proptosis, mimicking orbital cellulitis.[72,73] Tumors of the orbit rarely may manifest with acute inflammation mimicking orbital cellulitis. This has been described in primary ophthalmic rhabdomyosarcoma and retinoblastoma.[74,75] Rhinocerebral mucormycosis, which frequently manifests as an orbital cellulitis, is discussed in Chapter 257. Mucormycosis should be considered in any patient who presents with orbital cellulitis who has risk factors for mucormycosis (e.g., poorly controlled diabetes mellitus, hematologic malignancies, immunosuppression, deferoxamine therapy). In contrast with typical bacterial orbital cellulitis, patients with rhinocerebral mucormycosis may have minimal lid erythema, more pain in the forehead or temple than in the eye, and early onset of decreased sensation in the first and second divisions of cranial nerve V. Invasive sinus aspergillosis usually invades from the sphenoid sinus and may manifest as a subacute orbital apex syndrome. This condition is discussed in Chapter 256.

Treatment

Preseptal cellulitis due to sinusitis should be treated with antibiotics active against *S. aureus, S. pneumoniae,* and *H. influenzae.* Antibiotics should be given intravenously at first in young children because they may be bacteremic. Because penicillin-resistant *S. pneumoniae* is prevalent in many areas, ceftriaxone plus nafcillin would be a reasonable choice for initial therapy. In older children and adults with mild preseptal cellulitis, initial antibiotics may be oral (e.g., amoxicillin-clavulanate).

All patients with orbital cellulitis should be treated with intravenous antibiotics and monitored closely for signs of visual compromise. Clinical worsening should prompt a repeat CT scan and consideration of surgical exploration of the orbit. Sinus drainage surgery also should be considered if sinusitis is present. Nafcillin, metronidazole, and ceftriaxone provide initial broad-spectrum intravenous antibiotic therapy in older children and adults. Nafcillin and ceftriaxone may be sufficient in young children, in whom a mixed aerobe/anaerobe infection is less likely.

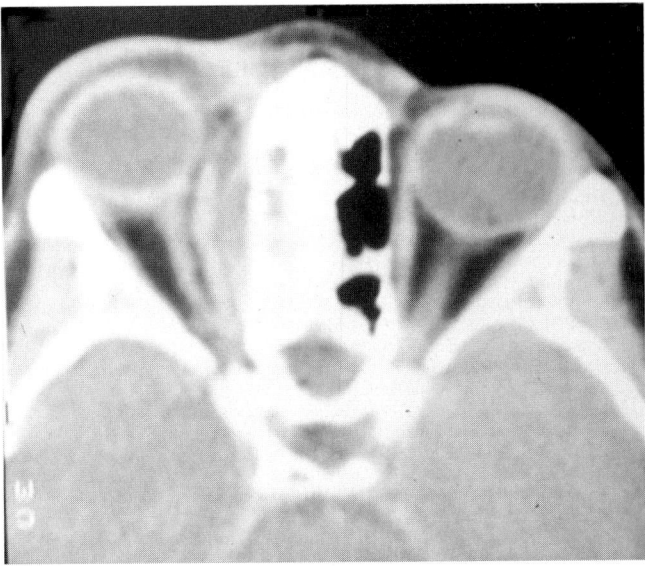

FIGURE 110-7. Computed tomography scan of subperiosteal abscess.

Older children and adults with subperiosteal abscess require prompt surgical drainage in addition to the broad-spectrum antibiotics noted earlier. The need for immediate drainage of subperiosteal abscess in young children is controversial. Some authors recommend a trial of intravenous antibiotics in children younger than age 9 who have a medial subperiosteal abscess that is not large and who do not have frontal sinusitis, visual decrease, chronic sinusitis (e.g., nasal polyps), or infection of dental origin.[76] These authors recommend performing visual and pupillary examinations every 6 hours for at least 48 hours and immediate surgery if the child remains febrile for more than 36 hours, develops visual loss or afferent pupillary defect at any time, worsens after 48 hours, or fails to improve after 72 hours. Other authors advocate immediate surgical drainage in all patients, citing a 10% rate of blindness in this infection without prompt drainage.[77] These authors also note that it may be impossible to obtain frequent and accurate assessments of visual acuity in young, acutely ill children. A third group recommends a trial of intravenous antibiotics only if vision is normal and close monitoring is possible.[68] Surgical drainage does not always require an external incision. A nasal endoscopic approach has proved successful in draining medial subperiosteal abscesses in some patients.[68,77]

All patients with orbital abscesses should have immediate surgical drainage, in addition to initial empirical therapy with nafcillin, metronidazole, and ceftriaxone (or other broad-spectrum agents). Vancomycin should be substituted for nafcillin if methicillin-resistant staphylococci are a possibility.

Nafcillin (or vancomycin), metronidazole, and ceftriaxone also should be used as initial therapy for cavernous sinus thrombosis until culture results are available. Because this infection carries a high risk of intracranial complications (e.g., brain abscess, subdural empyema), any alternative regimen should include antibiotics that cross the blood-brain barrier. In septic cavernous sinus thrombosis, surgical drainage of the primary focus of infection (e.g., sinusitis or dental abscess) should be performed, and patients should be monitored closely for any intracranial extension that may require surgical drainage. The use of anticoagulation has been controversial, but some studies suggested it was beneficial when started early in patients who had no evidence of hemorrhage.[78,79]

REFERENCES

1. Raskin EM, Speaker MG, Laibson PR. Blepharitis. Infect Dis Clin North Am. 1992;6:777-787.
2. McCulley JP, Shine WE. Changing concepts in the diagnosis and management of blepharitis. Cornea. 2000;19:650-658.
3. Gupta AK, Bluhm R, Cooper EA, et al. Seborrheic dermatitis. Dermatol Clin. 2003;21:401-412.
4. Ninomiya J, Nakabayashi A, Higuchi R, et al. A case of seborrheic blepharitis: Treatment with itraconazole. Nippon Ishinkin Gakkai Zasshi. 2002;43:189-191.
5. Giagounidis AA, Meckenstock G, Flacke S, et al. *Pseudomonas aeruginosa* blepharoconjunctivitis during cytoreductive chemotherapy in a woman with acute lymphocytic leukemia. Ann Hematol. 1997;75:121-123.
6. Nandy A, Addy M, Chowdhury AB. Leishmanial blepharoconjunctivits. Trop Geogr Med. 1991;43:303-306.
7. Wasserman D, Asbell PA, Friedman AJ, et al. *Capnocytophaga ochracea* chronic blepharoconjunctivitis. Cornea. 1995;14:533-535.
8. Yoon KC, Park HY, Seo MS, et al. Mechanical treatment of phthiriasis palpebrarum. Korean J Ophthalmol. 2003;17:71-73.
9. Robinson J. Photo quiz: Blepharitis due to herpes simplex virus type 1. Clin Infect Dis. 1997;24:17.
10. Tsao CH, Chen CY, Yeh KW, et al. Monthly recurrent herpes simplex virus blepharitis in a boy for more than 10 years. Infection. 2003;31:257-259.
11. Patel N, Khalil HM, Amirfeyz R, et al. Lacrimal gland abscess complicating acute sinusitis. Int J Pediatr Otorhinolaryngol. 2003;67:917-919.
12. Mirza S, Lobo CJ, Counter P, et al. Lacrimal gland abscess: An unusual complication of rhinosinusitis. ORL J Otorhinolaryngol Relat Spec. 2001;63:379-381.
13. Boruchoff SA, Boruchoff SE. Infections of the lacrimal system. Infect Dis Clin N Am. 1992;6:925-932.
14. Gungur K, Bekir NA, Namiduru M. Ocular complications associated with brucellosis in an endemic area. Eur J Ophthalmol. 2002;12:232-237.
15. Mawn LA, Sanon A, Conlon MR, et al. *Pseudomonas* dacryoadenitis secondary to a lacrimal gland ductule stone. Ophthalm Plast Reconstr Surg. 1997;13:135-138.
16. Sen DK. Acute suppurative dacryoadenitis caused by a cysticercus cellulosa. J Pediatr Ophthalmol Strabismus. 1982;19:100-102.
17. Marchese-Ragona R, Marioni G, Staffieri A, et al. Acute infectious mononucleosis presenting with dacryoadenitis and tonsillitis. Acta Ophthalmol Scand. 2002;80: 345-346.
18. Rhem MN, Wilhelmus KR, Jones DB. Epstein-Barr virus dacryoadenitis. Am J Ophthalmol. 2000;129:372-375.
19. Merayo-Lloves J, Baltatzis S, Foster CS. Epstein-Barr virus dacryoadenitis resulting in keratoconjunctivitis sicca in a child. Am J Ophthalmol. 2001;132:922-923.
20. Obata H, Yamagami S, Saito S, et al. A case of acute dacryoadenitis associated with herpes zoster ophthalmicus. Jpn J Ophthalmol. 2003;47:107-109.
21. van Assen S, Lutterman JA. Tuberculous dacryoadenitis: A rare manifestation of tuberculosis. Neth J Med. 2002;60:327-329.
22. Sardana K, Koranne RV, Langan U, et al. Ocular scrofuloderma with unilateral proptosis. J Dermatol. 2002;29:232-234.
23. Hwang IP, Jordan DR, Acharya V. Lacrimal gland inflammation as the presenting sign of Crohn's disease. Can J Ophthalmol. 2001;36:212-213.
24. Scheilian M, Bagheri A, Aletaha M. Dacryoadenitis as the earliest presenting manifestation of systemic Wegener's granulomatosis. Eur J Ophthalmol. 2002;12:241-243.
25. Lee J, Flanagan JC. Complications associated with silicone intracanalicular plugs. Ophthalm Plast Reconstr Surg. 2001;17:465-469.
26. Rumelt S, Remulla H, Rubin PA. Silicone punctal plug migration resulting in dacryocystitis and canaliculitis. Cornea. 1997;16:377-379.
27. Brazier JS, Hall V. *Propionibacterium propionicum* and infections of the lacrimal apparatus. Clin Infect Dis. 1993;17:892-893.
28. Jordan DR, Agapitos PJ, McCumm PD. *Eikenella corrodens* canaliculitis. Am J Ophthalmol. 1993;115:823-824.
29. Rootman DS, Insler MS, Wolfley DE. Canaliculitis caused by *Mycobacterium chelonae* after lacrimal intubation with silicone tubes. Can J Ophthalmol. 1989;24:221-222.
30. Chumbley LC. Canaliculitis caused by *Enterobacter cloacae*: Report of a case. Br J Ophthalmol. 1984;68:364-366.
31. Pavilack MA, Frueh BR. Thorough curettage in the treatment of chronic canaliculitis. Arch Ophthalmol. 1992;110:200-202.
32. Pollard ZF. Treatment of acute dacryocystitis in neonates. J Pediatr Ophthalmol Strabismus. 1991;28:341-343.
33. Huber-Spitzy V, Steinkogler FJ, Huber E, et al. Acquired dacryocystitis: Microbiology and conservative therapy. Acta Ophthalmol (Copenh). 1992;70:745-749.
34. DeAngelis D, Hurwitz J, Mazzulli T. The role of bacteriologic infection in the etiology of nasolacrimal duct obstruction. Can J Ophthalmol. 2001;36:134-139.
35. Hartikainen J, Lehtonen OP, Saari KM. Bacteriology of lacrimal duct obstruction in adults. Br J Ophthalmol. 1997;81:37-40.
36. Jain A, Rubin PAD. Orbital cellulitis in children. Int Ophthalmol Clin. 2001;41:71-86.
37. Ambati BK, Ambati J, Azar N, et al. Periorbital and orbital cellulitis before and after the advent of *Haemophilus influenzae* type B vaccination. Ophthalmology. 2000;107:1450-1453.
38. Barone SR, Aiuto LT. Periorbital and orbital cellulitis in the *Haemophilus influenzae* vaccine era. J Pediatr Ophthalmol Strabismus. 1997;34:293-296.
39. Donahue SP, Schwartz G. Preseptal and orbital cellulitis in childhood: A changing microbiologic spectrum. Ophthalmology. 1998;105:1902-1905.
40. Sobol SE, Marchand J, Tewfik TL, et al. Orbital complications of sinusitis in children. J Otolaryngol. 2002;31:131-136.
41. Uzcategui N, Warman R, Smith A, et al. Clinical practice guidelines for the management of orbital cellulitis. J Pediatr Ophthalmol Strabismus. 1998;35:73-79.
42. Rumelt S, Rubin PAD. Potential sources for orbital cellulitis. Int Ophthalmol Clin. 1996;36:207-221.
43. Ferguson MP, McNab AA. Current treatment and outcome in orbital cellulitis. Austr N Z J Ophthalmol. 1999;27:375-379.
44. Harris GJ. Subperiosteal abscess of the orbit: Age as a factor in the bacteriology and response to treatment. Ophthalmology. 1994;101:585-595.
45. Skedros DG, Haddad J Jr, Bluestone CD, et al. Subperiosteal orbital abscess in children: Diagnosis, microbiology, and management. Laryngoscope. 1993;103:28-32.
46. Brook I, Frazier EH. Microbiology of subperiosteal orbital abscess and associated maxillary sinusitis. Laryngoscope. 1996;106:1010-1013.
47. Meyer MA. Streptococcal toxic shock syndrome complicating preseptal cellulitis. Am J Ophthalmol. 1997;123:841-843.
48. Stone L, Codere F, Ma SA. Streptococcal lid necrosis in previously healthy children. Can J Ophthalmol. 1991;26:386-390.
49. Prendiville KJ, Bath PE. Lateral cantholysis and eyelid necrosis secondary to *Pseudomonas aeruginosa*. Ann Ophthalmol. 1988;20:193-195.
50. Rajalekshmi PS, Evans SL, Morton CE, et al. Ringworm causing childhood preseptal cellulitis. Ophthalm Plast Reconstr Surg. 2003;19:244-246.
51. Mauriello JA Jr, Atypical Mycobacterial Study Group. Atypical mycobacterial infection of the periocular region after periocular and facial surgery. Ophthalm Plast Reconstr Surg. 2003;19:182-188.
52. Soysal HG Kiratli H, Recep OF. Anthrax as the cause of preseptal cellulitis and cicatricial ectropion. Acta Ophthalmol Scand. 2001;79:208-209.
53. Gellady AM, Shulman ST, Ayoub EM. Periorbital and orbital cellulitis in children. Pediatrics. 1978;61:272-277.
54. Smith TF, O'Day D, Wright PF. Clinical implications of preseptal (periorbital) cellulitis in childhood. Pediatrics. 1978;62:1006-1009.
55. Shapiro ED, Wald ER, Brozanski BA. Periorbital cellulitis and paranasal sinusitis: A reappraisal. Pediatr Infect Dis. 1982;1:91-94.
56. Varma D, Metcalfe TW. Orbital cellulitis after peribulbar anaesthesia for cataract surgery. Eye. 2003;17:105-106.
57. Irvine F, McNab AA. Orbital abscess following uncomplicated phacoemulsification cataract surgery. Clin Exp Ophthalmol. 2002;30:430-431.

58. Allan BP, Egbert MA, Myall RW. Orbital abscess of odontogenic origin: Case report and review of the literature. Int J Oral Maxillofac Surg. 1991;20:268-270.

59. Colson AE, Daily JP. Orbital apex syndrome and cavernous sinus thrombosis due to infection with *Staphylococcus aureus* and *Pseudomonas aeruginosa*. Clin Infect Dis. 1999;29:701-702.

60. Tarazi AE, Shikani AH. Irreversible unilateral visual loss due to acute sinusitis. Arch Otolaryngol Head Neck Surg. 1991;117:1400-1401.

61. Slavin ML, Glaser JS. Acute severe irreversible visual loss with sphenoethmoiditis-"posterior" orbital cellulitis. Arch Ophthalmol. 1987;105:345-348.

62. Ebright JR, Pace MT, Niazi AF. Septic thrombosis of the cavernous sinuses. Arch Intern Med 2001;161:2671-2676.

63. Southwick FS, Richardson EP Jr, Swartz MN. Septic thrombosis of the dural venous sinuses. Medicine. 1986;65:82-106.

64. Watkins LM, Pasternack MS, Banks M, et al. Bilateral cavernous sinus thromboses and intraorbital abscesses secondary to *Streptococcus milleri*. Ophthalmology. 2003;110:569-574.

65. Cannon ML, Antonio BL, McCloskey JJ, et al. Cavernous sinus thrombosis complicating sinusitis. Pediatr Crit Care Med. 2004;5:86-88.

66. Ohta S, Nishizawa S, Namba H, et al. Bilateral cavernous sinus actinomycosis resulting in painful ophthalmoplegia: Case report. J Neurosurg. 2002;96:600-602.

67. Tobias S, Lee JH, Tomford JW. Rare *Actinobacillus* infection of the cavernous sinus causing painful ophthalmoplegia: Case report. Neurosurgery. 2002;51:807-809.

68. Rahbar R, Robson CD, Petersen RA, et al. Management of orbital subperiosteal abscess in children. Arch Otolaryngol Head Neck Surg. 2001;127:281-286.

69. Younis RT, Anand VK, Davidson B. The role of computed tomography and magnetic resonance imaging in patients with sinusitis with complications. Laryngoscope. 2002;112:224-229.

70. Younis RT, Lazar RH, Bustillo A, et al. Orbital infection as a complication of sinusitis: Are diagnostic and treatment trends changing? Ear Nose Throat J. 2002;81:771-775.

71. Patt BS, Manning SC. Blindness resulting from orbital complications of sinusitis. Otolaryngol Head Neck Surg. 1991;104:789-795.

72. Sirbaugh PE. A case of orbital pseudotumor masquerading as orbital cellulitis in a patient with proptosis and fever. Pediatr Emerg Care. 1997;13:337-339.

73. Brown DH, MacRae DL, Allen LH. Orbital pseudotumors. J Otolaryngol. 1988;17:164-168.

74. Shields CL, Shields JA, Honavar SG, et al. Clinical spectrum of primary ophthalmic rhabdomyosarcoma. Ophthalmology. 2001;108:2284-2292.

75. Shields JA, Shields CL, Suvarnamani C, et al. Retinoblastoma manifesting as orbital cellulitis. Am J Ophthalmol. 1991;112:442.

76. Garcia GH, Harris GJ. Criteria for nonsurgical management of subperiosteal abscess of the orbit: Analysis of outcomes 1988-1998. Ophthalmology. 2000;107:1454-1458.

77. Page EL, Wiatrak BJ. Endoscopic and external drainage of orbital subperiosteal abscess. Arch Otolaryngol Head Neck Surg. 1996;122:737-740.

78. Levine SR, Twyman RE, Gilman S. The role of anticoagulation in cavernous sinus thrombosis. Neurology. 1988;38:517-522.

79. Bhatia K, Jones NS. Septic cavernous sinus thrombosis secondary to sinusitis: Are anticoagulants indicated? A review of the literature. J Laryngol Otol. 2002;116:667-676.

CHAPTER **111**

Acute Viral Hepatitis

MICHAEL P. CURRY
SANJIV CHOPRA

HISTORICAL PERSPECTIVE

Hippocrates first described the existence of epidemic jaundice as early as 400 BC. Further outbreaks of jaundice were documented in Europe in the 17th and 18th centuries, notably during periods of conflict. From then until World War II, the existence of viruses as the major cause of liver disease was unknown. The distinction between "infectious" and "serum" hepatitis by Krugman and colleagues in 1967 and the discovery of the Australia antigen by Blumberg and co-workers later that year were landmark events that led to a major increase in our knowledge of viral hepatitis.[1,2] Epidemics of infectious hepatitis acquired from contaminated food and water were linked to hepatitis A virus (HAV) infection. In 1973, Feinstone and associates detected HAV in stool utilizing the technique of immune electron microscopy.[3] Subsequently, HAV was identified as a 27-nm particle resembling an enterovirus, transmission of the infection to marmosets and chimpanzees was recorded, and specific complement fixation and immune adherence antibody tests were developed.[4-6]

The use of the serologic marker, the Australia antigen, provided a means of characterizing the epidemiology of hepatitis B virus (HBV) infection.[2,7,8] Further developments included the identification of the virus as a 42-nm particle (Dane particle) containing an outer coat, the hepatitis B surface antigen (HBsAg), and an inner core, the hepatitis B core antigen; the development of specific tests to detect the hepatitis B antigens and their respective antibodies[9-11]; the transmission of the infection to chimpanzees; and the development of a specific hepatitis B immune serum globulin.[12,13] In 1975, Krugman produced a crude vaccine for HBV infection by boiling the serum of a patient with HBV and was able to prevent transmission of hepatitis B in human subjects.[14] Subsequently, a "new" antigen found in liver specimens from some patients with HBV infection led to the identification of the delta virus or hepatitis D virus (HDV) in 1977.[15] HDV was seen in only a fraction of patients with HBV and was often associated with a more severe or fulminant course of disease. Recognition of an infectious agent distinct from that resulting in hepatitis A or B was now possible, and it became apparent that there existed another or other agents responsible for what was termed non-A, non-B (NANB) hepatitis. In 1974, Prince and Feinstone and their colleagues independently observed that some cases of post-transfusion hepatitis were not caused by HAV or HBV.[16,17]

The development of refined hepatitis B vaccines can be considered one of the major achievements of modern medicine. The initial use of first-generation vaccines derived from plasma HBsAg and subsequent use of recombinant HBV vaccines have resulted in the reduction of HBV carrier rates. Furthermore, the introduction of universal HBV vaccination in Taiwan has resulted in a 75% reduction in the incidence of HBV-related childhood hepatocellular carcinoma, and, hence, the hepatitis B vaccine can truly be called the first "anticancer" vaccine.[18]

In 1978, Alter and colleagues demonstrated the potential for transmission of infection by inoculating chimpanzees with plasma from individuals with NANB hepatitis.[19] Further advances in molecular biology led to the development of tests specific for hepatitis C virus (HCV) by Houghton and colleagues in 1989, and testing of large repositories of stored blood demonstrated that HCV was indeed the subsequent cause of NANB hepatitis.[20]

The existence of another enterically transmitted virus was suspected in 1980 when sera from persons affected by a large waterborne epidemic in Delhi in 1955 were found to lack serologic markers for HAV and HBV infection.[21] Viral particles were recognized in 1983 by immune electron microscopy in the feces of a volunteer infected with fecal material of a person suspected of having enterically transmitted NANB hepatitis, and the virus was named hepatitis E in 1988.[22] The virus was subsequently cloned in 1990, and diagnostic tests were available the following year.[23]

BACKGROUND

The hepatotropic viruses are a group of diverse pathogens that share a common ability to cause inflammation and necrosis of the liver.

The term viral hepatitis generally refers to disease caused by the five well-described hepatotropic viruses, which are divided into enteral and parenteral groups on the basis of their mode of transmission. HAV and hepatitis E virus (HEV) are enterically transmitted by the fecal-oral route and do not exist in a chronic carrier state (Table 111-1). Hepatitis B, C, and D viruses are parenterally transmitted, occur in both acute and chronic forms, and, when they persist in a chronic carrier state, serve as a reservoir for infection. They have the potential to cause chronic hepatitis, cirrhosis, and hepatocellular carcinoma. Other viruses that can cause hepatic inflammation include Epstein-Barr virus (EBV), herpes simplex virus (HSV), mumps, rubella, rubeola, varicella-zoster virus, yellow fever virus, Coxsackie B virus, and adenovirus. Although these agents can cause diagnostic confusion by producing liver inflammation and dysfunction, they are not primary causes of acute or chronic viral hepatitis.

TABLE 111-1 Hepatitis Type and Characteristics of Infection

Characteristic	A	B	C	D	E
Virus family	Picornaviridae	Hepadnaviridae	Flaviviridae	Deltaviridae	Caliciviridae
Nucleic acid	RNA	DNA	RNA	RNA	RNA
Incubation period (days)	15-50	28-160	14-160	Variable	15-45
Mode of transmission:					
Orofecal	Yes	Possible	No	No	Yes
Sexual	Yes	Yes	Rare	Yes	No
Blood	Rare	Yes	Yes	Yes	No
Chronic infection	No	Yes	Yes	Yes	No
Cirrhosis and HCC	No	Yes	Yes	With HBV	No

HBV, hepatitis B virus; HCC, hepatocellular carcinoma.

Novel technologies have further identified other viruses that were initially thought to cause post-transfusion hepatitis, namely, hepatitis G virus (HGV) or GBV-C and the transfusion-transmitted virus (TTV), and SEN viruses, but these are not currently believed to be human pathogens (see Chapter 151). In the case of HAV and HEV, most acute infections result in a self-limited disease with fulminant hepatic failure occurring in only 1% to 2% of infected individuals. However, a significant proportion of patients with acute HCV and HBV infection develop chronic liver disease resulting in cirrhosis, liver failure, and hepatocellular carcinoma. A small number of patients may present with a viral hepatitis–like syndrome without serologic evidence of viral infection. In these seronegative cases, other etiologies including autoimmune hepatitis, drug-induced hepatitis, vascular disease, or viruses not yet identified must be considered in the diagnosis.

Acute viral hepatitis infection is a global public health concern associated with substantial morbidity and mortality. Of the more than 500,000 cases of acute viral hepatitis diagnosed in the United States each year, 32% are caused by HAV, 43% are caused by HBV, 21% are caused by HCV, and 4% are caused by unknown types. During the past decade, an estimated 125,000 to 200,000 HAV infections, 140,000 to 320,000 HBV infections, 35,000 to 180,000 HCV infections, and 6000 to 13,000 HDV infections have occurred each year (based on the estimated annual incidence for these types of viral hepatitis from 1984 to 1994)[24] (Table 111-2). As a result of acute infection with these viruses, approximately 285 deaths from fulminant hepatitis occur annually, 100 from hepatitis A, 150 from hepatitis B, and 35 from HBV-HDV coinfection or superinfection. The number of acute clinical cases of HAV and HBV reported to the National Notifiable Disease Surveillance System (NNDSS) for the year 2001 was 10,609 and 7843, respectively.[24] However, these numbers are almost certainly underestimates of the true number of acute infections. The estimated number of acute clinical cases and the estimated number of new infections reported by the Centers for Disease Control and Prevention (CDC) were 45,000 and 93,000 for HAV and 22,000 and 78,000 for HBV, respectively (Fig. 111-1). Cases of HCV infection are also reported to the NNDSS but are unreliable for monitoring the trends in HCV infection because these reports include cases based only on a positive laboratory test for antibodies to HCV (anti-HCV), most of which may represent chronic infection (Fig. 111-2).

Viruses beyond A to E

Approximately 15% to 17% of hepatitis infections remain unexplained. Acute hepatitis and chronic hepatitis occur sporadically, after transfusion and in organ transplant recipients. Some such cases result in the development of fulminant liver failure. The causative agents for non–A to E hepatitis continue to be sought. Candidate viruses include hepatitis F virus (HFV), HGV, TTV, and SEN virus (see Chapter 151). HFV was initially identified as a putative hepatitis virus spread by the fecal-oral route; however, there is insufficient ev-

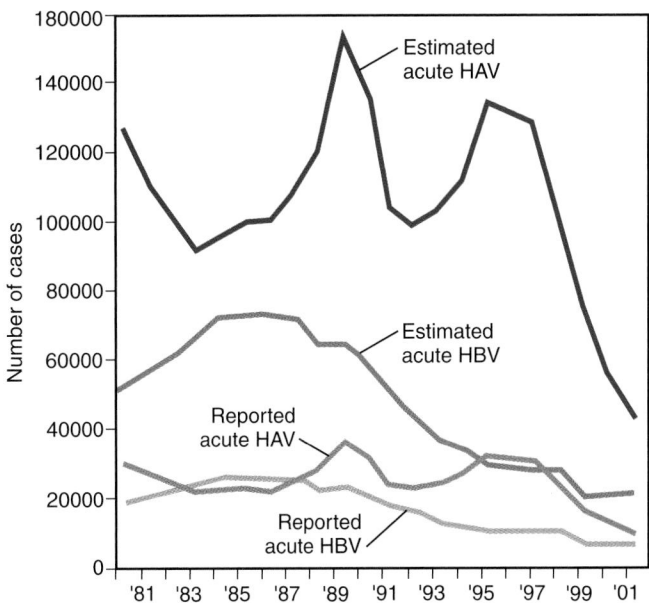

FIGURE 111-1. Incidence of acute hepatitis A virus (HAV) and hepatitis B virus (HBV) infection in the United States from 1980 to 2000. The number of reported cases and the estimated number of cases are shown for HAV and HBV. The ratio of reported acute cases to the total number of newly acquired infections was estimated by catalytic modeling of seroprevalence data from the National Health and Nutrition Examination Survey. Incidence estimates adjusted for underreporting and asymptomatic infections were then calculated by multiplying by the number of cases reported. *(From Summary of Notifiable Diseases—United States, 2000. MMWR Morb Mortal Wkly Rep. 2002;49[53]:I-xxii, 1-100.)*

idence to corroborate this and the identity of HFV is in doubt. HGV is also known as GB virus (so named after the initials of the patient from whom the virus was isolated). There are three related viruses, namely GBV-A, GBV-B, and GBV-C, whose role in human disease, if any, remains unestablished. GBV-B has been shown to cause hepatitis in animal models. GBV-C is closely related to HCV, is found among blood donors and can be transmitted by transfusion, but does not appear to be associated with hepatitis, nor does it worsen the course of concurrent HCV infection.

TABLE 111-2 Estimated Disease Burden of Viral Hepatitis in the United States				
Characteristic	*HAV*	*HBV*	*HCV*	*HDV*
Acute infections (× 1000)/year*	125-200	140-320	35-180	6-13
Fulminant deaths/year	100	150	?	35
Chronic infections	0	1-1.25 million	3.5 million	70,000
Chronic liver disease deaths/year	0	5000	8-10,000	1000

*Range based on estimated annual incidence, 1984 to 1994.

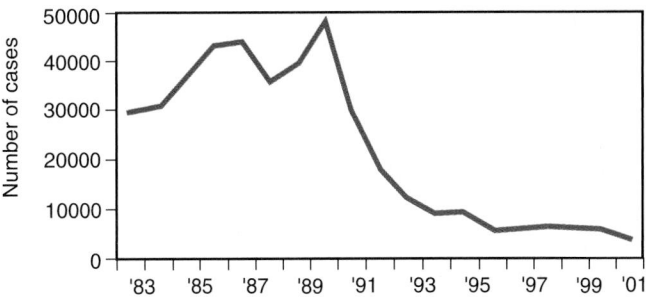

FIGURE 111-2. Estimated number of cases of acute hepatitis C virus (HCV) from 1980 to 2001. Cases of hepatitis C reported to the National Notifiable Disease Surveillance System are unreliable for monitoring trends because these reports include cases based only on a positive laboratory test for anti-HCV; most positive tests are likely to represent chronic HCV infection. *(From Summary of Notifiable Diseases—United States, 2000. MMWR Morb Mortal Wkly Rep. 2002;49[53]:I-xxii, 1-100.)*

Spectrum of Clinical Disease

Acute viral hepatitis may be asymptomatic, marked only by a rise in aminotransferase levels; symptomatic with or without jaundice; subfulminant; or fulminant. Asymptomatic infections are 10 to 30 times more common than symptomatic infections. In addition, there are several different types of illness associated with HAV infection including protracted or cholestatic and relapsing HAV infection.

Asymptomatic hepatitis is recognized by the detection of a rise in liver function tests and the detection of serologic markers of viral infections in an individual often being evaluated for nonspecific constitutional symptoms. Acute asymptomatic infection may also occur with only a minimal rise in liver function tests, as is the case in neonatal HBV infection, in which there appears to be tolerance to the infection. In general, the younger the patient, the milder the clinical form of hepatitis. Asymptomatic HBV infections are detected in 90% of Eskimo children younger than 4 years but are found in only two thirds of adults older than 30 years. The case-fatality rate with acute HAV infection is also directly proportional to the age of the infected individual. The overall case-fatality rate is approximately 0.4%; the lowest case-fatality rate (1.6 per 1000) is seen in individuals 5 to 29 years of age; however, the rate increases to 17.5 per 1000 among persons older than 49 years.[25]

Clinical features of acute symptomatic viral hepatitis are common to all forms of viral hepatitis. There are no clinical features that unequivocally distinguish the individual types of hepatitis from each other; however, there are certain epidemiologic patterns of transmission that may suggest a particular virus. The illness of acute viral hepatitis can be divided into the following broad categories: the incubation period, the preicteric phase, the icteric phase, and the convalescent phase. The incubation period is the time immediately after acquisition of infection to the time of first symptoms and varies from a few weeks to as long as 6 months, depending on the type of the viral infection. During this time, the patient is well and without symptoms. The earliest symptoms are nonspecific and predominantly constitutional. Symptoms include malaise, joint pain, myalgia, fatigue, anorexia, nausea and vomiting, and abdominal or right upper quadrant discomfort. Approximately 25% of patients describe their initial symptoms as an "influenza-like" illness. The symptoms of pharyngitis, cough, coryza, and photophobia generally last only 1 to 3 days and are replaced by the more typical symptoms of malaise and anorexia. Malaise is the most common symptom, occurring in 95% of those with symptomatic disease; it is sometimes profound and may increase later in the day. Anorexia is common but is typically one of the first symptoms to resolve. Patients may give a history of distaste for alcohol and tobacco smoke; however, this dysgeusia is not specific for viral hepatitis and is sometimes seen with other forms of acute hepatitis. Nausea and vomiting are common, are rarely severe, and can increase in severity as the day continues. Abdominal discomfort is experienced by 60% of patients with symptomatic disease. HAV infection is generally associated with an abrupt onset of illness and fever.[26,27]

High temperature and rigors should prompt the physician to look for other causes of liver dysfunction such as cholangitis. Aseptic meningitis and meningoencephalomyelitis are rare complications of acute viral hepatitis.[28] These prodromal symptoms usually last a few days but can persist for 2 to 3 weeks. In the absence of jaundice, these symptoms may be passed off as an influenza-like illness unless a specific exposure or risk is elicited in the history. Jaundice may occur with varying severity and last from a few days to several weeks. It is usually preceded by dark urine reflecting bilirubinuria caused by the rising concentrations of conjugated serum bilirubin. Jaundice is first noted in the sclera and is usually accompanied by pale stool reflecting the absence of bile pigment in the stool. Pruritus, which is reported by 40% of jaundiced patients, is usually mild and transient unless a cholestatic illness is present, as is sometimes the case with HAV infection. At this stage, the low-grade fever may abate. However, anorexia, malaise, and weakness may persist. Complete clinical recovery may take up to 6 months after the onset of symptoms, and fatigue and weakness can persist for some weeks after apparent biochemical recovery. A small percentage of patients develop a "serum sickness–like" illness characterized by fever, urticarial skin rash, and arthritis. These signs, which usually occur at the onset of the illness, are thought to be due to circulating immune complexes and are most common with acute HBV infection.[29] HBV infection in childhood can be associated with a nonrelapsing, nonitching erythematous papular dermatitis involving the face, arms, buttocks, and legs, with enlarged lymph nodes in the axillary and inguinal regions. This is known as Gianotti-Crosti syndrome.[30,31] This presentation is not exclusively caused by HBV infection and can also occur after infection and reactivation of EBV.[32,33]

Relapsing or biphasic hepatitis has been described with HAV infection. The rate of relapse of HAV varies from 1.5% to 11.9%. It occurs at an interval of 4 to 15 weeks after the original illness, and the severity of symptoms and biochemical abnormalities is generally similar to that seen with the initial illness. Rarely, more severe cholestasis is seen with the second episode.[34] One or more relapses may occur. Of note, there is no association between the severity of the initial illness and the development of a relapse. Occasionally, immune-mediated phenomena such as arthritis or cryoglobulinemia occur during a relapse. HAV does not cause chronic liver disease, and liver functions tests invariably return to normal within 12 months.

Cholestatic variants of viral hepatitis have also been described. In acute HAV infection, a protracted cholestatic course of HAV infection with pruritus occurs in 8% of cases. This was first described in 1984 after the advent of diagnostic testing.[35] Severe pruritus, diarrhea, weight loss, and malabsorption may accompany the cholestasis. The pathogenic mechanisms underlying cholestatic hepatitis A are unknown. However, prolonged viral shedding has been noted in patients with persistent elevation of alanine aminotransferase (ALT), indicating that the enterohepatic cycling of HAV may contribute to relapsing or protracted infection. These patients must be considered potentially infectious. As with relapsing HAV infection, all patients recover completely.

Fibrosing cholestatic hepatitis (FCH) is another cholestatic liver injury associated with viral hepatitis. It usually arises acutely in immunosuppressed individuals with chronic viral infection. In 1991, Davies and coauthors described a rapidly progressive and fatal form of recurrent HBV infection occurring in patients undergoing liver transplantation for HBV infection without prophylaxis for reinfection.[36] It is characterized by balloon degeneration of hepatocytes, mild or absent inflammation, sinusoidal fibrosis, and cholestasis. Subsequently, others have demonstrated prominent expression of HBsAg, enhanced HBV transcription, and high levels of HBV DNA. Similar forms of disease have been reported with HCV in both organ transplant recipients and human immunodeficiency virus (HIV)–infected patients.[37,38] Unlike cholestatic HAV infection, FCH caused by HBV or HCV leads to liver failure and death unless successful antiviral therapy is instituted.

Fulminant hepatic failure, defined as severe liver failure that develops within 8 weeks of the onset of symptoms, is the most serious manifestation of viral hepatitis. It is fortunately a rare complication that occurs in only 0.14% to 0.35% of hospitalized cases of HAV infection.[39,40] As the hospitalized cases of HAV infection are only a proportion of all cases of HAV infection, the true prevalence of HAV fulminant hepatic failure is considerably lower. The incidence of fulminant hepatic failure in acute HBV infection is 1% to 4% of hospitalized patients, and the risk increases when there is associated HDV infection.[41] The presence of HBsAg in the blood at the time of presentation does not necessarily implicate HBV as the cause. The risk of acute liver failure as a consequence of acute hepatitis C appears to be very low, but it may be more common in patients with underlying chronic HBV infection.[42] Reports from Japan suggest a higher incidence, but the high rate of positivity in this population may reflect chronic exposure rather than causality. However, the risk of acute liver failure in patients with HCV who become superinfected with HAV is not insignificant. Vento and co-workers prospectively observed patients with chronic

HBV and HCV for acute superimposed HAV infection and found that acute liver failure occurred more frequently in patients with chronic HCV infection than in patients with chronic HBV.[43] Cases such as these have led the National Institutes of Health to recommend that all nonimmune patients with chronic HCV be vaccinated against HAV and HBV. The CDC has made the same recommendation for hepatitis A but is somewhat guarded about vaccination against hepatitis B unless risk factors for HBV infection are present.[44] Acute liver failure secondary to HEV infection varies from 0.6% to 2.8% in men to 20% in pregnant women.[45,46] As HEV infection is common in parts of Asia and Africa, a history of recent travel may be helpful in considering the diagnosis. No evidence has emerged to implicate hepatitis F or G as a causative agent in fulminant hepatic failure.

The term fulminant hepatic failure was introduced in the 1960s to define a disease that is characterized by severe sudden liver cell dysfunction leading to coagulopathy and hepatic encephalopathy in persons with no underlying liver disease. It was defined as fulminant hepatic failure when severe liver failure (defined as the presence of encephalopathy) developed within 8 weeks of the onset of symptoms.[39] Subsequently, nomenclature was proposed to achieve closer alignment with outcome. The term "acute liver failure" is used to describe the onset of encephalopathy within 12 weeks of the onset of jaundice. "Hyperacute" refers to the development within 7 days, and "subacute" refers to an onset between 5 and 12 weeks.[40] The definition excludes patients with preexisting liver disease but allows the inclusion of subclinical disease related to Wilson's disease and some patients with hepatitis B–related liver failure.

There are considerable geographic variations in the etiology of acute liver failure. The most common causes in Japan and Asia are related to viral hepatitis. Hepatitis E is the leading cause in India, and HBV infections are the leading cause in France and Japan. Drug-induced (acetaminophen toxicity) fulminant hepatic failure is most common in the United Kingdom and has become the leading cause of liver failure in the United States.[47] Viral hepatitis was identified in only 12% of cases. HBV and HAV infections accounted for 7% and 4%, respectively, in a multicenter study reported by Lee and colleagues.[48,49]

Physical Findings

The physical findings in acute viral hepatitis are generally nonspecific and are not helpful in differentiating one type from another. Vital signs are usually normal. However, low-grade fever is usually present. Bradycardia, a feature of obstructive jaundice, can occur in acute viral hepatitis if the patient is significantly icteric. The bradycardia correlates with the level of serum bilirubin and is attributed to the effects of bile salts on the sinoatrial node.

Jaundice is more common in adults than children. Pruritus associated with jaundice may lead to excoriations. Features such as spider angiomas are rarely seen in acute liver disease. Urticaria and dermatographism may be seen in patients with an underlying immune-mediated phenomenon. Lymphadenopathy is found in 5%, splenomegaly in approximately 15%, and hepatomegaly in 85% of patients with acute viral hepatitis.[27] Features such as pharyngitis or conjunctival suffusions may provide clues to a specific diagnosis of EBV or leptospirosis.

Histopathology

A liver biopsy is not indicated in patients with acute, self-limited hepatitis. In difficult cases, such as those with protracted or cholestatic disease, liver biopsy may be helpful in establishing the diagnosis, differentiating it from other etiologies, and aiding therapeutic decisions. In cases of fulminant liver failure, liver biopsy is seldom indicated and is often precluded by coagulopathy and thrombocytopenia. The absence of a specific diagnosis does not preclude the performance of liver transplantation in such cases.

The typical histologic findings in acute viral hepatitis include lobular disarray, apoptosis of hepatocytes, mononuclear cell infiltration of the portal and periportal areas, and cholestasis. Hepato-cellular changes range from minor degrees of cell swelling characterized by granular cytoplasm to severe ballooning degeneration and cell death. Hepatocyte nuclei show prominent nucleoli and increased variation in size. Apoptosis, which is thought to be the predominant method of cell death caused by hepatotropic viruses, is evident by shrinking of hepatocytes and the presence of eosinophilic material. Apoptotic bodies may also contain pyknotic nuclear remnants. Hepatocyte loss, liver cell dropout, and anisocytosis coupled with regeneration of hepatocytes result in loss of the orderly pattern of hepatic sinusoidal cords and disarray of the lobule. Cholestasis in the form of bile thrombi in the canaliculi generally correlates with the serum bilirubin level. It is common in acute hepatitis but rare in chronic hepatitis and therefore is of some diagnostic importance. The bile ducts are normal in appearance.

Unlike the findings in classic acute inflammation, the inflammatory components of acute viral hepatitis are characterized predominantly by infiltration of lymphocytes rather than polymorphonuclear inflammatory cells. These lymphocytes are seen in the lobule and the portal tracts. In acute hepatitis, the most conspicuous inflammation is seen in zone 3 of the hepatic acinus. The extent of the inflammation is variable, and portal tracts may be normal or expanded. Inflammatory cells in the lobule give the appearance of "spotty necrosis" and consist of T cells and macrophages. More extensive necrosis between the terminal venule and the portal tract is called bridging necrosis and is a severe manifestation of acute hepatitis. In a minority of patients with acute hepatitis, the necrosis extends throughout the entire lobule or acinus and is referred to as panacinar necrosis. In these cases, the hepatic parenchyma is replaced by collapsed stroma, inflammatory cells, and activated macrophages. Around the surviving portal tracts there is proliferation of bile ducts as a regenerative response.

The hepatitic process may also involve the hepatic sinusoids and central vein. Swelling of the sinusoidal endothelial cells and disruption of the terminal venular cells by lymphocytic infiltration are not uncommon. In contrast to chronic hepatitis, the inflammatory changes in the hepatic lobule usually predominate over those in the portal areas, but portal inflammation is nevertheless present. The density of the inflammatory infiltrate is variable.

With the advent of specific serologic and molecular tests for infectious agents, liver biopsy is neither necessary nor able to differentiate the likely viral agents. However, it may help in suggesting a diagnosis of autoimmune hepatitis or establishing a diagnosis of Wilson's disease.

HEPATITIS A

HAV is the most common cause of viral hepatitis worldwide (see also Chapter 170). It is a member of the picornavirus family and is an icosahedral particle 27 to 32 nm in diameter. Only one serotype exists, but multiple genotypes have been defined on the basis of sequence comparisons. These distinct genotypes can be found in different geographic regions and seven HAV genotypes have been identified worldwide, including four human genotypes (I, II, III, and VII) and three simian strains (IV, V, and VI). The four human genotypes have a nucleotide sequence variation of 15% to 25%.[50,51] However, they are antigenically closely related, and infection with one genotype confers immunity to other strains.

The HAV genome is a single-stranded, positive-sense, linear RNA approximately 7.5 kb in length. It encodes one open reading frame (ORF) that produces a polyprotein 2235 amino acid residues long. The polyprotein is divided into three main functional domains: P1, P2, and P3. P1 encodes the viral capsid proteins and P2 and P3 encode the nonstructural proteins including the RNA helicase, protease, and RNA polymerase. The viral capsid comprises 32 subunits, each of which has four major polypeptides termed VP1 to VP4. The polyprotein is flanked at either end by 5′ and 3′ untranslated regions (UTRs). The 5′ UTR is the most conserved and contains an internal ribosomal entry site for initiation of protein synthesis. It is not known whether infection with different genotypes of the virus has a bearing on the

Unknown	46%
Sexual or household contact	14%
Men who have sex with men	10%
Other contact	8%
Injection drug use	6%
Contact of child or employee in daycare	6%
International traveler	5%
Food- or waterborne infection	4%
Child or employee in daycare	2%

TABLE 111-4 Symptoms and Signs in Epidemic and Sporadic Hepatitis A

Symptoms		Signs	
Anorexia	71-85%	Hepatomegaly	14-78%
Nausea, vomiting	67-79%	Hepatic tenderness	39-46%
Malaise	76-80%	Splenomegaly	3-13%
Fever	18-58%	Jaundice	40-80%
Headache	19-73%	Bradycardia	17%
Abdominal pain	26-54%	Lymphadenopathy	4%
Dark urine	68-94%	Skin rash	14%
Pale stool	52-58%		
Arthralgia	8-19%		

severity or outcome on the clinical illness. Fewer nucleotide substitutions in the 5' UTR have been reported in cases of fulminant and severe hepatitis compared with self-limiting hepatitis.[52]

HAV infection is spread predominantly by direct person-to-person contact by the orofecal route or by the ingestion of contaminated food or water.[53] The source of infection most frequently reported to the CDC in 1999 to 2000 involved personal contact with an infected person. Nevertheless, hepatitis A occurs sporadically in approximately 46% of cases in the United States (Table 111-3). It is highly contagious with a secondary attack rate of 15% to 20% and spreads rapidly between individuals in prolonged close contact, in schools, institutions, and army camps. Infection may also occur by consumption of contaminated ice water or by ingestion of uncooked or undercooked foods that have been washed in contaminated water. Raw shellfish are a particularly common source of infection. Higher seroprevalence rates of HAV infection are seen in men who have sex with men and with oral-anal contact regardless of sexual orientation.[54] Sexual transmission though seminal or vaginal secretions does not appear to be significant. Transmission through blood products is possible, as documented in hemophiliacs who receive products from pooled donors.[55-57] Blood transfusion is rarely associated with transmission.[58] In addition, intravenous drug users are at higher risk for acquiring HAV infection.

Improvements in sanitation and hygiene have resulted in a reduction in the rate of childhood exposure in Sweden and Hong Kong. HAV is a worldwide virus but is highly endemic in developing countries. Patterns of endemicity have been identified as low, medium, and high. In areas of high endemicity, such as Asia, India, the Far East, and parts of South America, infection is almost universal in early childhood and results in a high level of immunity among adults. Within the United States, there is a different epidemiology of HAV infection. The overall seropositivity is 38% and ranges from 11% in children younger than 5 years to 74% in persons older than 50 years. There is considerable variation with geography and ethnicity in the United States, with the highest prevalence rates occurring in Arizona, Alaska, Oregon, New Mexico, Utah, Washington, Oklahoma, South Dakota, Idaho, Nevada, and California. The highest rates of disease are found among Native American and selected Hispanic and migrant populations (Fig. 111-3). The prevalence of HAV infection is also high in the Hasidic Jewish population in New York State, a community that experienced numerous annual outbreaks in a local environment with similarities to daycare centers. Investigators studying the protective efficacy of a formalin-inactivated hepatitis A vaccine with an alum adjuvant used this population of individuals and demonstrated 100% protection in vaccinated subjects.[59]

HAV has an incubation period of 15 to 50 days with a mean period of 30 days. It is excreted in the stools of infected persons for 1 to 2 weeks before and for at least 1 week after the onset of illness. After ingestion, the virus passes through the gastrointestinal mucosa and reaches the liver.[60] The virus enters the hepatocytes through receptors, sheds its capsid, and begins replicating. The virus replicates exclusively in the liver. After replication, the new virions pass into the bile canaliculi and are excreted in the bile. Hepatitis A is an acute self-limiting disease that rarely causes death and is characterized by a spectrum of severity ranging from asymptomatic, inapparent infection to fulminant fatal disease. Jaundice is very unusual in children younger than 4 years, and in the age group from 4 to 6 years, 90% are anicteric. In contrast, jaundice is present in 40% to 70% of those older than 15 years. A prodromal phase of infection is abrupt in onset and develops in 85% of the patients who ultimately become jaundiced (Table 111-4).[26] The development of jaundice is typically associated with improvement in the prodromal symptoms. Jaundice resolves within 2 weeks in the majority of individuals. Extrahepatic manifestations include cutaneous vasculitis involving the buttocks and lower extremities, renal failure, pancreatitis, bradycardia, prolongation of PR and QT intervals, T wave changes, and left axis deviation. Rarely, convulsions, mononeuritis multiplex, Guillain-Barré syndrome, transverse myelitis, and aplastic anemia have been described with acute HAV infection.[61]

The clinical, serologic, and virologic course of an acute HAV infection is shown in Figure 111-4. Antibody to HAV infection is found in the serum at the onset of disease. Initially, the antibody consists of both immunoglobulin G (IgG) and IgM; however, after 3 to 12 months, IgM disappears from the serum and IgG persists, conferring lifelong immunity. A diagnosis of acute HAV is made by finding IgM anti-HAV in an individual with either symptoms or biochemical evidence of hepatitis.

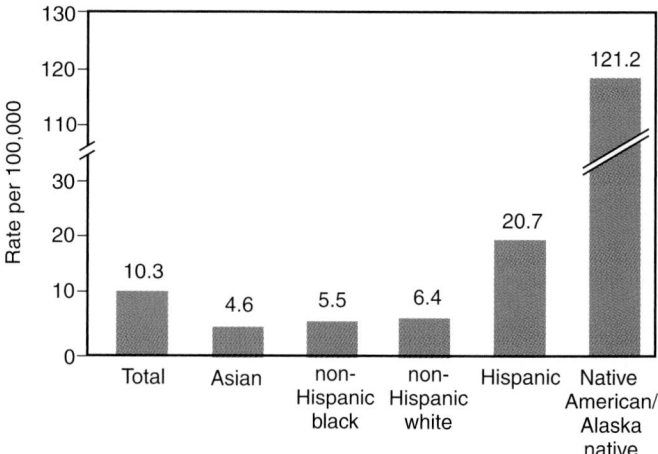

FIGURE 111-3. Hepatitis A rates by race or ethnicity. The highest rates occurred among Native Americans/Alaska Natives and the lowest rates among Asians; rates among Hispanics were higher than among non-Hispanics. Racial or ethnic differences in rates most likely reflected differences in risk factors for infection, such as socioeconomic levels and resultant living conditions and more frequent contact with persons from countries where hepatitis A is endemic.

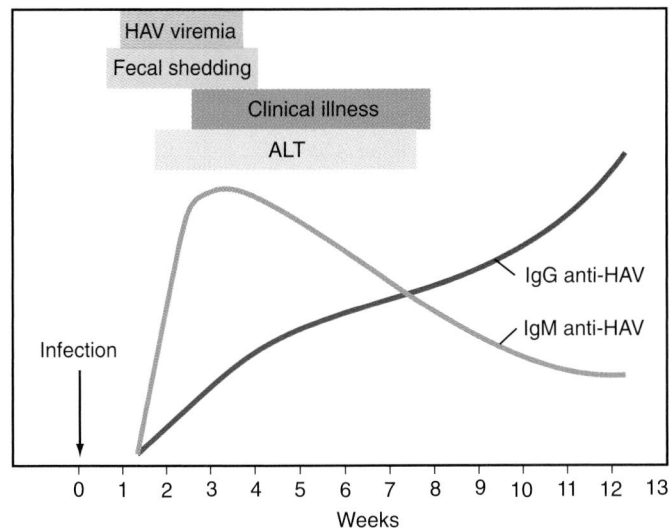

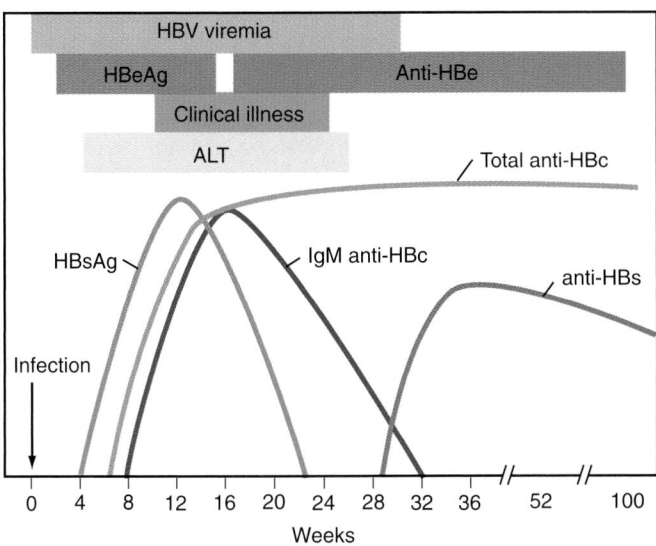

FIGURE 111-4. The clinical, virologic, and serologic course of acute hepatitis A virus (HAV) infection and acute hepatitis B virus (HBV) infection. ALT, alanine aminotransferase; HBc, hepatitis B core; HBsAg, hepatitis B surface antigen; HBeAg, hepatitis B e antigen; IgG, immunoglobulin G.

TABLE 111-5 Endemic Patterns of Hepatitis B Virus Infection			
	Low	*Moderate*	*High*
Carrier rate	<2%	2-7%	>8%
Current or past infection rate	4-6%	20-50%	70-90%
Predominant age at infection	Adult	Adults and children	Neonates and children

largely related to the differences in age at the time of acquisition of infection. In highly endemic areas, most infections occur in the perinatal period or during early childhood, when the rate of progression from acute to chronic HBV infection is approximately 90%.[64] Transmission takes place at the time of birth by maternal-fetal transfusion and exposure to maternal blood in the birth canal as well as in the postpartum period through close contact between mother and baby. Progression to chronic infection for those infected between the ages of 1 and 5 years is 20% to 50%, whereas it is less than 5% for adult-acquired infection (Table 111-5).[65-67]

The prevalence rate in the United States is derived from a study that excluded those at high risk, including incarcerated and homeless individuals, and may represent an underestimation of the actual prevalence rate. An estimated 5% of the civilian, noninstitutionalized U.S. population has serologic evidence of past or present infection; 0.42% have chronic infection and serve as the primary source of infection for others. The overall prevalence of HBV infection differs among racial and ethnic populations and is highest among persons who have emigrated from areas with a high endemicity of HBV infection. The prevalence of infection among blacks is four times that seen in the white population (11.9% versus 2.65%). From 1987 to 1998, reported cases of acute HBV declined by 76%. Disease incidence is highest in blacks, followed by Hispanic Americans and whites.

HBV is transmitted by cutaneous and mucosal exposure to infectious blood or bodily fluids.[68,69] In the United States, hepatitis B occurs in persons exposed to blood through contaminated needles and syringes and through multiple sexual partners.[69] Data from the CDC indicate that the most common risk factor for HBV infection is sexual exposure followed by injection drug use. Employment in health care, receipt of a blood transfusion, and dialysis account for less than 3% of cases. Health care workers, particularly surgeons, pathologists, and hemodialysis staff, have a higher risk for HBV infection.[70] Widespread use of HBV vaccine in this group has reduced the incidence of infection from 9% in 1985 to 0.8% in 1994 to 1995. The risk of HBV infection after a needlestick injury is related to the hepatitis B early antigen (HBeAg) status of the source patient. Several reports document outbreaks in dialysis units in 1994 as a consequence of failure to identify and isolate infected individuals and vaccinate susceptible patients.[71,72] Improved infection control and vaccination of susceptible individuals in dialysis units have reduced the incidence of infection among dialysis patient from 3% in 1980 to 0.1% in 1993. In addition, there are reports of transmission from a cardiothoracic surgeon to patients despite flawless infection control precautions.[73]

With the current screening of blood donors, elimination of those with high-risk behavior from the donor pool, screening for HBsAg and antibodies to the core antigen (anti-HBc), and the use of viral inactivation procedures, the risk of post-transfusion hepatitis B is estimated to be 0.0002 per transfusion recipient.[68] Nearly half of the cases reported to the CDC in 1995 denied a recognized exposure, although approximately 50% of those persons had a history of known risk factors (Fig. 111-5).[74] In endemic areas, horizontal transmission among children may result from close contact leading to transfer of virus across minor skin breaks and mucous membranes. Various bodily fluids have been reported to test positive for HBsAg, and semen and saliva have been consistently shown to harbor infectious virions.[75] Despite this, there is no convincing evi-

HEPATITIS B

HBV (also see Chapter 142) and related viruses are classified in the family of hepadnaviruses. The complete virion or Dane particle is a double-shelled, 42-nm DNA virus.[9] It consists of an envelope composed of virus-encoded proteins, host-derived lipid components, and a core particle made up of nucleocapsid protein, the viral genome, and the polymerase protein. HBV also produces 22-nm spheres and filaments that contain only envelope proteins and are not infectious. The HBV genome is a circular, partially double-stranded DNA approximately 3200 base pairs in length.

HBV infection is a global health problem with an estimated 350 million HBV carriers worldwide and 500,000 deaths each year.[62] Chronic HBV infection is endemic in most parts of sub-Saharan Africa, Southeast Asia, China, and Alaska, with a carrier rate of 8% to 20%. Intermediate prevalence rates (2% to 7%) are seen in Mediterranean countries, Japan, Central Asia, the Middle East, and South America. Low rates of infection (0.1% to 2.0%) are seen in the United States, Canada, western Europe, Australia, and New Zealand.[63] The wide range in the carrier rates in different parts of the world is

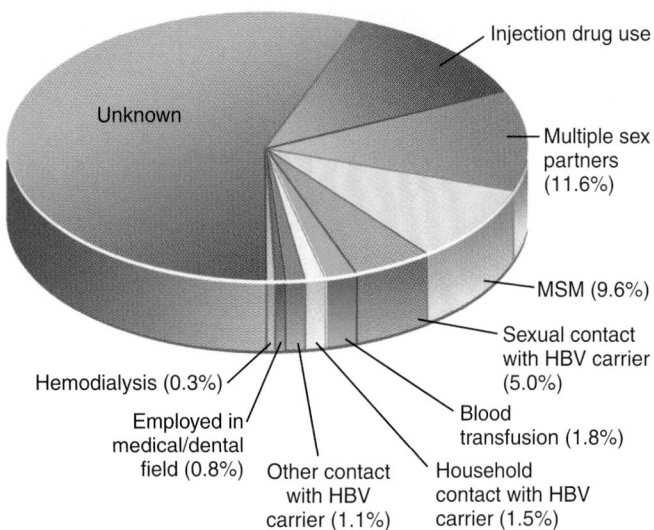

FIGURE 111-5. Risk factors for acute hepatitis B virus (HBV) infection in the United States, 1994 to 1995. Epidemiologic characteristics of patients reported with HBV infection. MSM, men having sex with men. *(From Viral Hepatitis Surveillance Program, Report No. 58, 2003. Centers for Disease Control and Prevention.)*

dence that HBV can be transmitted orally. Similarly, HBsAg and HBV DNA can be found in the breast milk of mothers with chronic HBV infection. In immunized children, there is no increased risk of transmission of HBV related to breast-feeding.[76,77] Because HBV can persist for a long time outside the human body, transmission by contamination of surfaces and tools such as toothbrushes and razors may occur.

The worldwide incidence of HBV infection is decreasing. In 1982, hepatitis B vaccines were licensed in the United States. Despite this, the incidence of acute HBV continued to rise until 1985, when vaccination programs for health care professionals were implemented. Further reductions in the incidence of acute infection were seen with routine infant immunization in 1991 and routine "catch-up" adolescent immunization in 1995. Increased public awareness and education about sexual practices and risk have also contributed to the overall reduction in HBV infection.

The diagnosis of acute HBV infection is based on serologic markers of HBV infection in a clinical setting consistent with an acute hepatitis. HBsAg is the hallmark of HBV infection and appears in the serum during the incubation period, usually 1 to 10 weeks after exposure and 2 to 7 weeks before the onset of symptoms (see Fig. 111-4). Approximately 95% of patients have detectable HBsAg at the onset of jaundice. Most patients who recover from HBV infection clear HBsAg within 6 months, and persistence of HBsAg in the serum beyond this time implies chronic infection. In some patients who demonstrate a vigorous immune response, HBsAg may be cleared rapidly from the serum, and in these cases specific antibody testing provides clues to the diagnosis. HBV infection is associated with the development of anti-HBc before the onset of symptoms and within 1 month after the appearance of HBsAg. HBsAg clearance is usually followed by the development of neutralizing anti-HBs antibodies that confer immunity. In some patients, the anti-HBs antibodies may not appear for several weeks to months. During this period there is no detectable HBsAg or anti-HBs. The presence of an IgM anti-HB$_c$ is the only marker of acute HBV infection during this window period between the disappearance of HBsAg and the appearance of anti-HBs. IgM anti-HBc is usually a marker of recent HBV infection. However, the titer of IgM anti-HBc can increase to detectable levels during exacerbations of chronic HBV infection and therefore be misleading. As the patient recovers from

acute HBV infection, the IgM anti-HBc is replaced by IgG anti-HBc. The presence of anti-HBc and anti-HBs indicates resolved infection.

Early in the course of acute infection, markers of active viral replication (HBeAg and HBV DNA) are also detectable in the serum. During acute HBV infection, HBeAg is rapidly cleared, before the disappearance of HBsAg. In chronic HBV infection, HBeAg may persist for years to decades and seroconversion from HBeAg to anti-HBe is generally associated with a reduction or loss of HBV DNA and can be associated with a flare of hepatitis. A small proportion of patients lose HBeAg but still have active HBV replication and liver damage. These patients generally have a precore mutant that prevents production of HBeAg. Chronic infection develops in a variable proportion of patients depending on the age of exposure. These patients remain positive for HBsAg and anti-HBc, and a variable proportion display HBeAg and HBV DNA positivity.

HEPATITIS D

HDV (also see Chapter 142) is a defective virus of the Deltaviridae family that requires the presence of HBV for virion assembly but not for replication; therefore, HDV infection is closely related to HBV infection.[78] The virus is 35 to 37 nm in diameter with a single-stranded circular RNA and a delta antigen coated with the surface antigen of HBV. There is one recognized serotype and three genotypes with different geographic and disease associations. HDV genotype I prevails in the United States and Europe, where there is an increased risk of a fulminant course or a rapid progressive chronic liver disease. Genotype II, found in East Asia, is less frequently associated with fulminant disease or rapid progression to cirrhosis, and genotype III occurs in South America, where it is associated with outbreaks of fulminant and severe hepatitis among the Yucpa Indians of Venezuela and the Sierra Nevada de Santa Marta in Colombia.[79-81] In the Amazon basin, infection with HDV has been implicated as a cause of Labrea hepatitis or the so-called Amazon black fever. This condition is characterized by viral hepatitis and protein-calorie malnutrition.[82]

It is estimated that about 5% (15 million) of the HBV carriers worldwide are infected with HDV.[83] Despite the fact that HDV is closely associated with HBV, the geographic distribution of HDV does not parallel that of HBV infection. Specific areas that have a high prevalence include the Amazon basin in South America, central Africa, the Mediterranean basin, and the Middle East. It is generally spread by parenteral exposure.[84] However, in some areas, intrafamilial spread has been reported.[85] Infection in western countries is uncommon and predominantly confined to intravenous drug users and multiply transfused individuals. It is endemic in Italy, where it predominantly affects children and young adults and is probably spread through mucosal and parenteral routes. There has been a reduction in the prevalence in Italy because of improvement in socioeconomic conditions, reduction in high-risk sexual behaviors, and HBV vaccination programs.[86] In the Far East, the prevalence varies from 90% in the Pacific Islands to 5% in Japan.

The clinical manifestations of acute HDV infection vary from benign acute hepatitis to fulminant liver failure. In the chronic setting, patients may be asymptomatic carriers or may progress more rapidly to cirrhosis and hepatocellular carcinoma. Acute infection occurs in two clinical scenarios: coinfection with acute HBV infection or superinfection in a patient chronically infected with HBV. Coinfection with HBV results in an acute hepatitis indistinguishable from acute HBV. It is usually severe, with a reported mortality of 2% to 20%. A high incidence of liver failure has been reported among drug addicts.[87,88] Less than 5% of cases of acute coinfection with HDV and HBV result in chronic HDV infection. The disease may be biphasic with two peaks in serum amino transaminases a few weeks apart; the first is related to the peak of HBV replication and the second to the peak of HDV replication. In a small number of patients, HDV superinfection results in clearance of HBsAg. Clearance of HBV results in loss of HDV infection because of the dependence of virion assembly on the HBsAg. In others, this loss is temporary and HBsAg returns when the HDV replication decreases. In cases of superinfection in which HDV and HBV persist, there is usually a significant exacerbation of preexisting HBV liver disease. The disease is severe, and there is an increased risk of fulminant liver failure or progression to cirrhosis. In patients who require liver transplantation for fulminant HDV superinfection, the risk of HBV recurrence is significantly reduced.[89]

The diagnosis of HDV coinfection should be suspected in patients who have a severe fulminant course. Similarly, in patients with chronic HBV who develop an acute hepatitis or have a rapid progression of their liver disease, testing for HDV should be employed. HBsAg must be present to support HDV infection, and IgM anti-HBc should be present to make a diagnosis of acute HBV-HDV coinfection. Total (IgM and IgG) anti-HDV antibody can be detected by enzyme-linked immunosorbent assay (ELISA), and such commercial assays are available in the United States. IgM anti-HDV is present only transiently in acute HDV infection, and commercial testing for clinical diagnosis is not available in the United States. IgG anti-HDV appears late in the course of acute infection and may not be detected unless the test is repeated later in the disease. If chronic disease occurs, high titers of both IgG and IgM anti-HDV are present, and the titer of IgM anti-HDV correlates with the level of HDV replication and the severity of liver disease. Antibody titers of 1:1000 are indicative of ongoing infection. Serum HDV antigen and HDV RNA can be detected during acute infection. HDV antigen is present only transiently, may be missed. HDV RNA is present early, and is readily detectable by polymerase chain reaction (PCR). The U.S. Food and Drug Administration has not approved testing procedures for serum HDV antigen. HDV antigen can be detected by direct immunofluorescence or immunohistochemical staining of liver tissue. However, this is not practical for the diagnosis of acute infection, as few patients undergo liver biopsy for evaluation of acute hepatitis. The detection of intrahepatic HDV antigen has been proposed as the "gold standard" for the diagnosis of HDV infection and is reasonable for consideration in a patient with chronic HBV and suspected HDV superinfection. With prolonged HDV infection, there may be loss of HDV antigen expression in hepatocytes, resulting in a false-negative test.

HEPATITIS C

HCV is an RNA virus of the Flaviviridae family, previously known as NANB hepatitis, which is spread predominantly by parenteral routes (also see Chapter 150). It has a viral genome of 9379 base pairs and is a single-stranded, positive-sense, RNA virus that has a single ORF encoding both structural and nonstructural proteins. An estimated 170 million people are infected worldwide, and HCV infection is now the leading cause for liver transplantation in most transplant centers in the United States because of it propensity to cause chronic liver disease, cirrhosis, and hepatocellular carcinoma. Acute HCV infection accounts for 15% to 16% of cases of acute icteric hepatitis in the United States, ranking below hepatitis A (47% to 49%) and B (33% to 35%). The incidence of acute HCV appears to be falling, with an estimated 36,000 new cases in 1996 compared with 230,000 cases per year in the 1980s.[90] The reasons for this decrease are multiple and include the disappearance of post-transfusion hepatitis, adoption of universal precautions, and a decrease in transmission by injection drug use. The incidence of new infections is highest in young people aged 20 to 39 years with predominance in Hispanic males.[91] At present, the majority of cases of acute HCV occur as a consequence of parenteral exposure through injection drug use.[92] However, in more than 40% of cases reported to the CDC, no recent or readily identifiable risk factor was noted.

The clinical symptoms resemble those of other forms of viral hepatitis, and the disease can be distinguished only by serologic testing. Fewer than 15% to 25% of cases of acute HCV infection result in the development of jaundice, and therefore there is a high rate of subclin-

ical infection.[93] The mean incubation period is 50 days (range 14 to 120). The preicteric phase is defined by nonspecific symptoms of fatigue, poor appetite, right upper quadrant pain, and low-grade fever lasting 2 to 10 days. As with HBV, some patients develop a serum sickness–like syndrome characterized by rash, urticaria, and arthralgias resolving with the onset of jaundice or within a few days. Symptoms of jaundice last 1 to 2 weeks, and patients with a history of jaundice are less likely to progress to chronic disease. Patients with acute, self-limited disease appear to have truly recovered from infection, with normal serum aminotransaminases and absence of HCV RNA and without long-term consequences. After infection with HCV, HCV RNA becomes detectable in the serum within days to 8 weeks.[94] It is usually present in the blood before the development of jaundice, but the titer of the viral RNA may fluctuate greatly and some patients may be intermittently negative for the HCV RNA. The minimal interval after suspected exposure after which a persistently negative HCV PCR test excludes infection has not been definitely established. Anti-HCV ELISA tests become positive as early as 8 weeks after exposure. Approximately one half of patients with symptomatic acute infection have detectable antibodies to HCV detected by ELISA when they first present for care. However, the development of HCV antibodies may be delayed in patients who have subclinical infection. A positive anti-HCV ELISA does not distinguish between those who cleared the infection and those who are chronically infected. The diagnosis of acute HCV relies on a high index of suspicion, and it is necessary to perform an HCV RNA test early in the course of infection or repeated antibody tests later in the disease process. The serum aminotransaminases become elevated approximately 6 to 12 weeks after exposure (range 1 to 26 weeks) and are very variable in concentration. In one series that included 44 patients, the mean ALT was 885 U/L.

Distinction of acute HCV from a newly discovered chronic HCV infection may not always be possible because HCV RNA and anti-HCV antibodies may be present in both situations. A recent exposure history, a negative antibody test with a positive HCV RNA, the presence of symptoms suggestive of an acute hepatitis, and the level of serum amino transaminases may provide some help.

Because of the absence of symptoms associated with acute infection and the high propensity for the development of chronic disease (85%), HCV can persist in an indolent and often silent fashion and arise decades later with manifestations of end-stage liver disease. As a result, periodic screening for infection may be warranted in patients who are at high risk for infection.

Fulminant hepatic failure caused by acute HCV infection is rare but may be more common in patients with underlying chronic HBV infection.[42]

HEPATITIS E

Hepatitis E (also see Chapter 174), previously known as enterically transmitted NANB hepatitis, was first recognized as a distinct clinical entity in the early 1980s when sera from persons affected by a large waterborne epidemic of viral hepatitis in Delhi, India were found to lack serologic markers for HAV and HBV infection.[95] The virus was then identified in the feces of a patient infected with NANB hepatitis.[22] The virus was subsequently cloned in 1990.[23] It is endemic in the Indian subcontinent and Southeast and Central Asia and accounts for a substantial proportion of sporadic hepatitis in both children and adults.[96] Serial epidemics have been reported (Table 111-6); the largest outbreak of HEV was reported in the Xinjiang province of China in 1986 to 1988 and afflicted more than 100,000 people. Sporadic cases are common in areas in which the disease is endemic, such as India, where HEV infection accounts for 50% to 70% of all patients with sporadic hepatitis.[97] Sporadic hepatitis cases are uncommon in nonendemic areas and are generally limited to travelers to endemic areas.[98] However, HEV has been reported in Australia, Italy, and Greece in patients without any such travel history.[99-101] It is transmitted by the

TABLE 111-6 Serial Epidemics of Hepatitis E Virus Infection

Country	Years
India	1955, 1975-1976, and 1991
USSR	1955-1956
Nepal	1973
Burma	1976-1977
Algeria	1980-1981
Ivory Coast	1983-1984
Eastern Sudan and Somalia	1985-1986
Mexico	1986
China	1986-1988
Borneo	1987

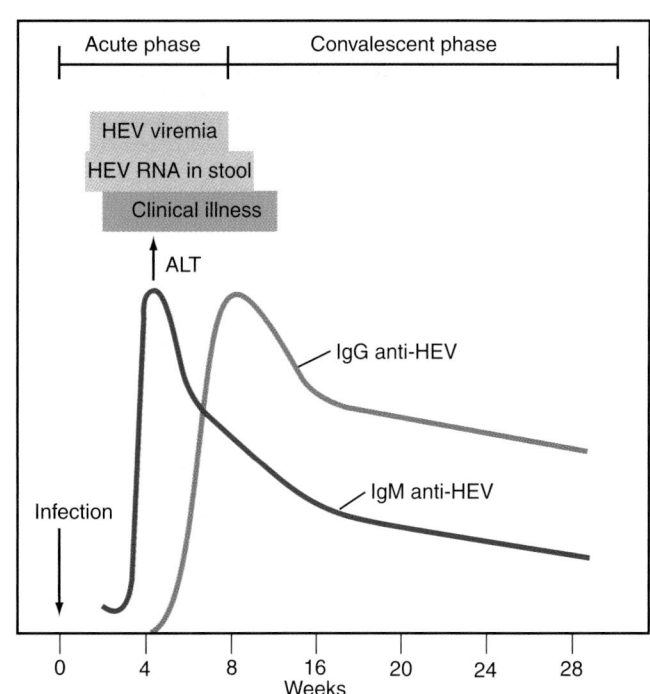

FIGURE 111-6. Time course of clinical and serologic events during acute hepatitis E virus (HEV) infection. ALT, alanine aminotransferase; IgG, immunoglobulin G.

fecal-oral route, and most reported epidemics have been related to the consumption of contaminated drinking water.[95,102] Person-to-person contact does not appear to be an efficient mode of transmission, and secondary attack rates among household contacts are only 0.7% to 2.2%, in contrast to the rate of 15% to 20% seen with HAV. The prevalence of anti-HEV antibodies among multiply transfused patients and injection drug users is similar to that of the general population, and there is no evidence to suggest parenteral or sexual transmission. The highest attack rate ranges from 1% to 15%, and infection occurs more commonly among young adults.

Acute infection during pregnancy is associated with an inordinately high mortality rate for reasons that are unclear. Transmission from mother to baby during pregnancy has been documented to occur with the development of a spectrum of disease ranging from anicteric hepatitis to fulminant hepatic necrosis in the newborn.[46,103]

Studies suggest that HEV can be isolated from several animals including swine and rodents, and molecular sequencing studies indicate that these isolates are phylogenetically related to those resulting in human infection.[104-106] These data suggest that these are reservoirs and that HEV is a zoonotic infection. This may account for sporadic infection among individuals without a travel history.

The incubation period of HEV infection ranges from 15 to 45 days, and the clinical signs and symptoms in patients with typical HEV infection are similar to those seen with other forms of acute viral hepatitis. Malaise, anorexia, nausea, vomiting, abdominal pain, fever, and hepatomegaly usually accompany jaundice. Fulminant liver failure occurs in 0.5% to 3% of patients. However, the figure is approximately 25% in patients with HEV infection who are in the third trimester of pregnancy. Indeed, pregnant women are more frequently affected during HEV outbreaks than nonpregnant women, with attack rates of 8% to 19% from the first to the third trimester compared with 2.8% for nonpregnant women.[46] A cholestatic variant similar to that in HAV infection has been described with HEV infection and usually resolves within 2 to 6 months. The overall mortality rate associated with HEV infection is reported to be 0.5% to 4% in hospitalized patients and 0.07% to 0.6% in population studies.[107,108] HEV infection does not cause chronic liver disease, cirrhosis, or hepatocellular carcinoma. However, hepatic decompensation can occur in patients with underlying liver disease and acute HEV infection.[109]

During acute HEV infection, IgM anti-HEV becomes detectable in the blood during the early phase of the infection and disappears over 4 to 6 months (Fig. 111-6). It is present in 90% of acutely infected patients between 1 and 8 weeks after the onset of illness. IgM precedes the development to IgG and is therefore useful in diagnosing acute HEV infection. The presence of IgG anti-HEV may represent the convalescent phase of an acute illness or previous exposure. In one study, IgG anti-HEV was present 14 years after the initial infection.[110] Reverse transcriptase–PCR (RT-PCR) testing allows detection of viral RNA in serum, stool, and some bodily fluids.

HEPATITIS G

HGV, also called the GB virus C (GBV-C), is an RNA virus belonging to the Flaviviridae family (also see Chapter 151). The virus was initially cloned from the plasma of a surgeon with acute hepatitis and is closely related to HCV. Like HCV infection, it is transmitted by parenteral exposure.[111-113] HGV is distributed globally and has a high prevalence (1.7%) in the volunteer blood donor population in the United States. In a small study of volunteer blood donors with elevated ALT (greater than 120 U), HGV RNA was present in 4% of individuals and anti-HGV antibodies were present in a further 10% of individuals.[114] The prevalence of HGV infection is higher in patients infected with HIV or HCV, patients who have had multiple transfusions or organ transplantation, and patients who are receiving hemodialysis.[115-120]

HGV can be diagnosed by the presence of HGV RNA by PCR techniques. The appearance of anti-HGV appears to be associated with clearance of HGV RNA and with protective immunity.[121]

The clinical significance of HGV infection is unknown, and it has been frequently referred to as the orphan virus. Although HGV RNA has been detected in both acute and chronic liver disease, numerous lines of evidence suggest that it is not pathogenic. Seventy-five percent of patients with detectable HGV RNA have normal liver function tests.[111] In patients who have HCV infection or alcoholic liver disease, HGV infection does not appear to worsen the clinical or histopathologic stage of disease.[122,123] In two studies investigating the cause of liver disease in patients with elevated aminotransferase levels, the prevalence of HGV was not different in the study and control groups.[124,125] In liver transplant recipients with post-transplantation hepatitis of unknown cause, HGV is present in up to 58% of cases. The prevalence is not different from that in a control group of patients without post-transplantation hepatitis.[126] Similarly, the presence of HGV coinfection in patients receiving transplants for HCV does not affect graft survival, the recurrence rate of HCV, or the severity of histologic recurrence of post-transplantation HCV disease.[127] Early reports of HGV-induced fulminant hepatic failure are now controversial. Initial reports from Japan of HGV-associated fulminant hepatic failure have not been substantiated, and it appears that patients may have acquired the HGV after the diagnosis of fulminant hepatic failure through the use of therapeutic blood products.[128-130]

PATHOGENESIS

Viral hepatitis is characterized by a diffuse inflammatory process resulting in acute or chronic liver injury, or both. The precise mechanism by which hepatocytes are injured is not known; however, it is known that antigen-specific and antigen-nonspecific cellular immunities contribute to hepatocyte injury in most types of viral hepatitis. HAV-associated liver injury is not completely understood, although the presence of HAV within hepatocytes before an increase in transaminases and the absence of direct cytopathic injury in cell culture models support a noncytopathic mechanism of injury. Only limited data are available on the immunology of HAV infection, and these studies have typically analyzed only the acute symptomatic phase of the infection in mild icteric cases. Immunohistochemical studies of liver tissue from acutely HAV-infected individuals have demonstrated the presence of CD45RO⁺ memory T cells, CD8⁺ T cells and B cells in the portal areas, and T cells and natural killer cells in the necrotic areas.[131] In vitro cytotoxicity assays demonstrate that peripheral natural killer cells, lymphokine-activated killer cells, and human leukocyte antigen class I–dependent CD8⁺ T cells from HAV-infected individuals are capable of lysing cell lines infected with HAV more efficiently than those cells from HAV antibody–negative individuals, suggesting that hepatocyte injury is immunologically mediated.[132,133]

Similarly, in HBV-associated liver disease, extensive human and animal studies suggest that the liver injury is mediated by a virus-specific cellular and humoral immune response. Acute HBV infection is accompanied by a strong and transient expansion of CD4⁺ T cells directed against multiple epitopes within the HBV. HB$_c$ is the dominant antigen recognized by CD4⁺ T cells in most cases of acute resolving HBV infection. These HBc-specific CD4⁺ cells also contribute to the induction of virus-specific CD8⁺ T cells and help in the production of antibody to HBsAg.[134,135] Individuals who clear HBV infection, either spontaneously or after interferon therapy, maintain these broad and strong peripheral cytotoxic T lymphocyte responses against all HBV epitopes over time.[136]

In contrast, HDV infection may result in hepatocyte cell death through direct cytopathic mechanisms. Hepatocyte cell lines infected with plasmids containing the hepatitis D antigen (HDAg) gene demonstrated impairment of RNA synthesis and cell death, suggesting that HDV might be directly cytopathic to hepatocytes. In addition, microvesicular steatosis of hepatocytes has been observed in association with HDV infection, and recurrence after liver transplantation again suggests a direct cytopathic effect.[137-139]

Elucidation of the mechanisms by which HCV infection results in liver injury has been hampered by the absence of reliable tissue culture and small animal models; however, it is believed that HCV is not directly cytopathic. This premise is based on the following observations: (1) some transgenic animals expressing HCV proteins do not develop cytopathic changes or liver inflammation and (2) cell lines expressing HCV under the control of inducible promoters do not develop cytopathic changes when HCV expression is turned on. Clinical observations suggest that interaction between the virus and the immune response in the first few weeks after the infection may determine the outcome of HCV infection. Resolution of acute HCV infection has been associated with vigorous and polyclonal peripheral blood proliferative responses to multiple HCV antigens, which can persist for many years after resolution of the disease.[140-143] Analysis of the cytokine profile of bulk cultures and peripheral CD4⁺ T-cell clones from individuals with acute self-limiting HCV infection reveals that viral clearance is more common in cases with secretion of interferon-γ and interleukin-2 than in individuals with a predominantly interleukin-10 cytokine profile. Similarly, significant CD8⁺ T-cell responses directed against mul-

tiple class I–restricted HCV epitopes of structural and nonstructural regions of the HCV polyprotein have been shown to correlate with elimination of the virus during the acute illness.[144] There are no data available on the mechanism of liver injury in acute HEV infection.

DIFFERENTIAL DIAGNOSIS

A number of disorders enter into the differential diagnosis of an "acute hepatitis." These include a number of viruses in addition to the classic hepatotropic viruses, nonviral infectious agents, drug-induced liver injury, ischemic hepatitis ("shock liver"), severe autoimmune chronic active hepatitis, acute Budd-Chiari syndrome, Wilson's disease, and syndromes unique to pregnancy such as acute fatty liver of pregnancy and the syndrome of hemolysis, elevated liver enzymes, and low platelets (HELLP) (Table 111-7). Rarely, patients with a common bile duct stone and massive tumor replacement of the liver have a biochemical profile suggesting acute hepatitis. It should also be noted that patients with chronic hepatitis B infection can have an acute hepatitis picture with substantial elevations in aminotransferases in a number of settings. These include superimposed HDV (delta) infection and the phase of hepatitis B e antigen to hepatitis B e antibody seroconversion when spontaneous reactivation occurs.

There is considerable variation in the extent to which other viruses cause hepatitis. EBV is a common cause of acute hepatitis, with subclinical hepatitis noted in 90% of patients with heterophile-positive mononucleosis (see Chapter 135). Most often the serum aminotransferase levels are two to five times the upper limit of normal.[145] Splenomegaly is present in 50% of individuals. Hepatomegaly and jaundice are uncommon. Generally, this syndrome is easily distinguished from acute viral hepatitis. On rare occasions, however, infection with EBV arises as acute icteric hepatitis without the usual telltale signs of fever, lymphadenopathy, and pharyngitis characteristic of mononucleosis. The diagnosis of EBV-induced acute hepatitis is established by the presence of a positive heterophile test and serologic exclusion of other causes of acute viral hepatitis. Fulminant liver failure may occur as a consequence of EBV infection.[146] X-linked lymphoproliferative disease (Duncan's syndrome) is characterized by the development of severe liver failure in young males. This rare disease is characterized by a family history of liver failure, lymphoma, immunoglobulin deficiency, or pancytopenia complicating EBV infection. It is usually fatal.[147]

Cytomegalovirus (CMV) infection is often subclinical in healthy children and adults (see Chapter 134). Among neonates, the infection can be mild and subclinical or fatal. The classic syndrome in neonates consists of hepatomegaly, jaundice, hemolytic anemia, thrombocytopenic purpura, and central nervous system damage with periventricular calcification and microcephaly arising at or shortly after birth.[148] The most common syndrome in immunocompetent adults is CMV "mononucleosis" and is characterized by protracted fever, lassitude, anorexia, malaise, pharyngitis, splenomegaly, and lymphadenopathy. Jaundice is present in less than 10% of patients.[149] Patients characteristically have an absolute

TABLE 111-7 Differential Diagnosis of Acute Hepatitis

Infectious	Noninfectious
Epstein-Barr virus	Drug-induced hepatitis
Cytomegalovirus	Autoimmune hepatitis
Herpes simplex virus	Ischemic hepatitis
Yellow fever	Acute fatty liver of pregnancy
Leptospirosis	Acute Budd-Chiari syndrome
Q fever	Wilson's disease
Human immunodeficiency virus	
Brucellosis	
Lyme disease	
Syphilis	

lymphocytosis with greater than 50% mononuclear cells and greater than 10% atypical lymphocytes. In immunocompromised patients, CMV infection may lead to serious illness. The most common clinical pictures are pneumonia, retinitis, hepatitis, polyradiculopathy, encephalitis, gastrointestinal tract disease, and adrenal involvement; cases of myocarditis, pancreatitis, and genitourinary localizations are less common.[150]

HSV can cause a generalized infection that is usually associated with hepatic dysfunction. It is most common among neonates and immunocompromised children (also see Chapter 132). Most cases of HSV-associated hepatitis in adults also occur in immunosuppressed individuals, often in the post-transplantation setting. Patients present with fever, mild jaundice, and marked elevations in aminotransferases.

Occasionally, patients can develop fulminant hepatic failure associated with HSV infection.[151] Fulminant hepatitis has also been reported in otherwise healthy individuals including pregnant women.[151] In a review of 21 cases of disseminated HSV in pregnancy by Gelven and colleagues,[151a] most patients had nonspecific symptoms and many did not have mucocutaneous lesions. They were usually febrile and anicteric and had markedly elevated aminotransferase values without a corresponding elevation in bilirubin level. Prompt initiation of acyclovir therapy resulted in 100% survival. Delayed or no therapy was associated with a 63% mortality rate.

Yellow fever is enzootic in central Africa, Central America, and South America. More than 90% of cases occur in Africa (see Chapter 149). Yellow fever is characterized by an incubation period (3 to 7 days) much shorter than that of hepatitis A, B, and C viruses. Patients can present with a severe hepatitis. Of note, the serum aspartate aminotransferase (AST) is characteristically higher than the serum ALT, probably because of skeletal or myocardial injury, or both. In severe cases it may be greater than 2000 IU.[152] The serum bilirubin levels are most often in the range of 5 to 10 mg/dL.[153] Yellow fever should be suspected in the recent traveler to enzootic areas who did not receive adequate immunization. The mortality rate in yellow fever approximates 20%.

Patients with leptospirosis infection present with an abrupt onset of fever, chills, myalgias, and headache[154] (see Chapter 237). They may have marked jaundice.[155] At physical examination, prominent conjunctival suffusion is often noted. Leukocytosis, which is uncommon in acute viral hepatitis, may be prominent and together with urinary findings of proteinuria, hematuria, and anuria should raise the suspicion of leptospirosis. The serum creatine phosphokinase is elevated in 50% of patients. Marked jaundice accompanied by renal dysfunction in a febrile patient with leukocytosis should raise the possibility of Weil's syndrome, a severe form of leptospirosis.[155]

Q fever is caused by the rickettsial agent *Coxiella burnetii* and is uncommon in the United States (see Chapter 184). Patients present with fever, chills, and pneumonitis. Mild elevations in ALT and AST (two to five times normal) are noted in 85% of patients. Hyperbilirubinemia and marked elevations of serum alkaline phosphatase can be present. Patients may have a prolonged febrile illness. Epidemiologic features linking exposure to farm or wild animals and the finding of unique hepatic granulomas (fibrin-ring granulomas are suggestive but not pathognomonic) should lead the clinician to suspect Q fever.[156]

A myriad of drugs can cause an acute hepatitis simulating acute viral hepatitis. The spectrum of acute liver injury ranges from mild hepatic dysfunction to fulminant hepatic failure. Common medications associated with severe hepatic toxicity include commonly prescribed analgesics such as acetaminophen and aspirin, antitubercular drugs including isoniazid and rifampin, and the anticonvulsant phenytoin.

In addition, there has been recognition of acute hepatitis caused by a number of herbal agents. These products are aggressively promoted, and many individuals consider these "natural" herbal remedies to be completely devoid of unwanted side effects. Herbal medications documented to produce severe hepatotoxicity including fulminant hepatic

failure include germander (*Teucrium chamaedrys*), chaparral (*Larrea tridentata*), pennyroyal oil (*Mentha pulegium*), mistletoe (*Viscum album*), kava (*Piper methysticum*), jin bu huan (*Lycopodium serratum*), and ma-huang (*Ephedra sinica*). This is by no means a complete list. Patients and their families should be specifically interrogated regarding the use of any unconventional medications, as they are often unaware that over-the-counter medications and herbal agents can have toxic potential.

Alcohol is an important cause of hepatic injury. Patients with severe alcoholic hepatitis (those with hyperbilirubinemia and a marked prolongation of the prothrombin time [PT]) have a mortality rate of 50%. However, even in these severely ill patients the serum aminotransferases are almost always less than 300 IU, and characteristically the serum AST:ALT ratio is greater than 2:1. Patients with acute alcoholic hepatitis may also have prominent leukocytosis, occasionally even a leukemoid reaction. Hence, acute alcoholic hepatitis should seldom be confused with acute viral hepatitis.

Autoimmune hepatitis may arise with an acute hepatitis–like picture with jaundice, marked elevations in serum ALT and AST, and a significant prolongation of the PT. The aminotransferase levels can be in excess of 2000 IU/L. Characteristic laboratory findings include positive antinuclear antibody, smooth muscle antibody, and striking elevations of serum IgG.[157] At histology, the liver biopsy specimens reveal prominent interface hepatitis with or without significant fibrosis. Plasma cells may be prominent. Indeed, this disease has been referred to as plasma cell hepatitis. After exclusion of viral hepatitis by appropriate serologic tests, patients are treated with corticosteroids and usually have a dramatic benefit.

Ischemic hepatitis results from prolonged hypotension or severe left- or right-sided heart failure, and patients may present with a syndrome simulating acute viral hepatitis. Most patients with anoxic liver injury (ischemic hepatitis, shock liver) are admitted to an intensive care unit, trauma unit, or burn unit and have obvious hemodynamic alterations that result in severe centrilobular necrosis of the liver often accompanied by prerenal azotemia. Within the first 12 to 24 hours after the hypotensive episode, patients have dramatic elevations in serum ALT and AST at levels comparable to those seen with acute viral hepatitis. The serum bilirubin may be elevated but is usually less than 10 mg/dL. The correct diagnosis can be confidently made by recognition of the appropriate clinical setting and the characteristic rapid resolution of the dramatic ALT and AST elevations to normal levels within a few days after correction of the underlying hemodynamic insult.[158]

Acute fatty liver of pregnancy and the HELLP syndrome are encountered in women in the third trimester of pregnancy.[159] Preeclampsia is common, and patients may have multiple gestations. Acute fatty liver of pregnancy has an approximate prevalence of 1 in 7000 to 1 in 16,000 deliveries. Affected women may have an inherited defect in mitochondrial beta oxidation of fatty acids that predisposes to this unique disorder. Accumulation of long-chain 3-hydroxyacyl metabolites produced by the fetus or placenta is probably toxic to the liver and the cause of the liver disease. Fetuses of some women affected with the HELLP syndrome also have long-chain 3-hydroxyacyl-coenzyme A dehydrogenase deficiency.[160] Hence, these two syndromes may have a common basis. The differential diagnosis includes acute viral hepatitis and drug-induced hepatic dysfunction because the serum ALT and AST elevations can be greater than 10 times the upper limit of normal. Hepatic failure may occur in both acute fatty liver of pregnancy and the HELLP syndrome. In one series of 46 pregnant women who developed liver disease severe enough to require admission to a liver failure unit, 70% had acute fatty liver and 15% had the HELLP syndrome.[161] Recognition of these syndromes is critically important because the treatment is inducing labor and delivering the newborn, which significantly curtails both maternal and fetal mortality.

Acute Budd-Chiari syndrome (hepatic vein occlusion) can arise as a severe and even fulminant hepatitis with marked elevations in serum ALT and AST, bilirubin, and PT.[162] More than 90% of patients have ascites. The causes of acute Budd-Chiari syndrome include clotting disorders (such as polycythemia vera, paroxysmal nocturnal hemoglobinuria, protein C deficiency, protein S deficiency, antithrombin III deficiency, prothrombin gene mutation, and occult myeloproliferative disorders), primary hepatocellular carcinoma, hypernephroma, the use of contraceptive pills, pregnancy, and congenital webs of the inferior vena cava. A rare and fulminant cause of Budd-Chiari syndrome is Behçet's disease, in which in addition to hepatic vein occlusion there is often accompanying inferior vena cava thrombosis.[163]

Wilson's disease (hepatolenticular degeneration) is a rare autosomal recessive defect of cellular copper export. Reduced biliary excretion of copper leads to accumulation in the liver and other organs, including the brain, kidneys, and eyes. Patients with Wilson's disease can present with an acute and even fulminant hepatitis–like picture with marked elevations in serum ALT, AST, and bilirubin, together with dramatic elevations in the PT.[164] Diagnostic clues to Wilson's disease include low levels of serum uric acid, serum alkaline phosphatase, and serum ceruloplasmin. The diagnosis can be established by documenting the presence of a Kayser-Fleischer ring (a slit-lamp examination by an ophthalmologist is often necessary) in a patient with low serum ceruloplasmin. It is critically important to exclude Wilson's disease in a patient with unexplained acute hepatitis, chronic active hepatitis, liver disease and hemolytic anemia, or liver disease with neurologic manifestations because treatment with D-penicillamine is lifesaving.

MANAGEMENT

There is little specific therapy that can be offered for the treatment of acute viral hepatitis apart from symptomatic management and good supportive care with avoidance of further injuries. One of the most important tasks for the physician is to identify the patient who is likely to experience fulminant hepatic failure and refer for early consultation and assessment. These patients are a minority, and indeed most patients with acute viral hepatitis do not require hospitalization. The latter should be reserved for patients who have dehydration because of inadequate fluid intake related to persistent anorexia or vomiting, patients with a progressive prolongation of the PT, and any patient who displays clinical findings compatible with liver failure such as mental status changes. Patients who have cholestatic hepatitis complicated by ascites, a shrinking liver size, and falling serum albumin levels are at risk for subacute liver failure and may also need access to liver transplantation services. The duration of hospitalization is variable and dependent on the speed of resolution of signs and symptoms. There is no need for patients to remain hospitalized until liver function tests return to normal; most patients can be discharged to recover at home.

Bed rest is generally recommended for patients with acute viral hepatitis. Traditionally, it was recommended for all patients during the symptomatic phase of the illness. These therapeutic precepts were derived from observations of military personnel during the Korean War, and some soldiers with acute HAV infection were assigned to bed rest for 3 months. This concept was challenged by Chalmers and colleagues, who reported that patients returning to duty after a short convalescence period recovered more rapidly than soldiers who had prolonged best rest.[165] Further controlled studies have shown that after symptoms have resolved, normal activity does not slow recovery, induce relapses, or increase the risk of chronic hepatitis.[166]

Dietary manipulation has not been shown to improve symptoms, shorten the duration of the illness, or improve outcome. High-calorie diets (3000 to 4000 kcal/day) and the addition of vitamin supplements have not been shown to enhance recovery. Vitamins are frequently given but none have been shown to affect disease severity. In patients with prolongation in PT, parenteral vitamin K can be administered to distinguish between severe hepatocellular dysfunction and vitamin K deficiency. This is particularly important in patients with prolonged

cholestasis. Well-balanced nutrition is advised, and antinausea medication can be employed in patients with anorexia or nausea to improve a general sense of well-being and prevent dehydration. In patients with mental status changes and those with severe reduction in dietary intake requiring hospitalization, blood sugar should be monitored frequently to treat hypoglycemia. Alcohol should be avoided in the acute illness. There is no evidence that alcohol consumption after recovery leads to relapse or to an increased risk of chronic infection. One study has shown that consumption of up to 26 g of alcohol per day was not harmful to patients with acute HAV infection.[167] It is prudent to advise that alcohol be avoided during the symptomatic phase; however, imposing abstinence for 6 months is unnecessary.

Drug therapy to control symptoms should be judicious, and avoidance of all narcotic and hypnotic medication is advised because of the risk of sedation and coma in those with severe disease. In general, all but clearly necessary medication should be stopped during the course of the acute illness. Pain should be managed with acetaminophen, which should not exceed 2 g/day. Nausea can be managed with metoclopramide, and chlorpromazine should be avoided because it has the potential to cause cholestasis. Pruritus can be managed with cholestyramine. Ursodeoxycholic acid has been used in one pilot study of acute viral hepatitis. Patients were randomly assigned to receive ursodeoxycholic acid or placebo for 3 weeks, with no observed difference in the duration of the illness. However, markers of cholestasis were significantly better in the patients receiving active drug.[168]

Specific Drug Therapy

There are no specific drug therapies available for patients with acute HAV or HEV infection. HAV is resistant to most currently available antiviral drugs. Corticosteroids are helpful in the cholestatic phase of HAV infection in decreasing the serum bilirubin, alleviating itch, and ameliorating the symptoms of fatigue. Prednisone at a dose of 40 mg/day often reduces the serum bilirubin by 40% over 4 days and should be tapered over a period of 2 to 4 weeks. Corticosteroids have not been proved to be of any benefit in fulminant hepatic failure secondary to acute viral hepatitis, and some studies have shown that adverse events outweigh any potential benefits of such therapy.[169]

Studies addressing antiviral therapy for HBV, HDV, and HCV infection have largely involved patients with chronic disease. Pilot studies have addressed the use of interferon alfa in acute HBV infection with resultant liver failure and have shown some benefit in preventing chronic HBV disease. In one study from India, patients with HBV infection for more than 12 weeks were treated with interferon alfa or placebo. Although this study included a small number of patients ($n = 54$), seroconversion (disappearance of HBsAg, HBeAg, and serum HBV DNA and appearance of anti-HBe) was seen more commonly with interferon alfa treatment (80%) than with placebo (53%). Two more patients in the study group seroconverted after treatment stopped, increasing the rate of successful treatment to 90%.[170] In patients who have fulminant hepatic failure related to HBV infection results of interferon alfa therapy are conflicting, with one study from Israel showing survival of 3 of 5 patients treated with interferon alfa whereas only 2 of 12 patients with fulminant HBV or HBV-HDV survived.[171,172] Lamivudine has been studied in one small case series involving three patients with acute HBV infection, with normalization of liver function tests within 1 month and undetectable HBV DNA in all three patients.[173]

Initial studies of treatment in acute HCV infection demonstrated that it was possible to prevent chronic HCV in a significant number of patients. A study by Jaeckel and colleagues from Germany has shown that aggressive treatment of acute HCV infection with interferon alfa resulted in clearance of the HCV infection in 98% of treated patients. No control group was included in the study. However, it is well documented that HCV infection becomes chronic in 50% to 85% of acutely infected individuals, and this study may have demonstrated prevention of the development of chronic HCV infection. Treatment was well tolerated, and only 1 of 44 patients discontinued therapy because of side effects. At the time of discontinuation of therapy in that patient, detectable virus was not present, but it returned later.[174]

Management of Fulminant Hepatic Failure

Patients with acute viral hepatitis rarely develop fulminant hepatic failure. Patients with severe viral hepatitis should be monitored closely with twice-weekly assessment of clinical status, liver function tests, and PT. The development of a rising PT or mental status changes at any juncture should prompt referral to a liver center for evaluation. Management of acute liver failure is best performed in an intensive care unit setting by a multidisciplinary team with access to a transplant center. Supportive care includes intensive care unit observation, optimal management of hemodynamic status with intravenous fluids, central venous access, and Swan-Ganz catheterization. Patients should be assessed frequently for signs of hepatic encephalopathy, and development of grade III encephalopathy should prompt elective intubation for airway protection. Monitoring for raised intracranial pressure by placement of an intracranial pressure monitor or clinical assessment is critical. Systemic infection is common in patients with fulminant hepatic failure, and the clinical features usually associated with infection such as fever and elevated white blood count are frequently absent.[175] The use of prophylactic antibiotics is controversial; however, there are several randomized trials that support their use.[175,176]

The most promising therapy for fulminant liver failure is liver transplantation. Acute liver failure accounts for approximately 5% of all transplantations in the United States and 11% in Europe. The overall success of liver transplantation for fulminant liver failure varies from 59% to 73% depending on the center.

Factors that indicate a poor prognosis without liver transplantation include age younger than 10 or older than 40 years, seronegative or drug-induced hepatitis, serum creatinine greater than 300 μmol/L or 2.3 mg/dL, and a PT greater than 50 seconds. Special consideration needs to be given to patients who receive transplants for acute HBV infection with fulminant liver failure. There is a risk of recurrent HBV infection in the graft with resultant post-transplantation hepatitis and graft loss. The risk is less for patients with HDV coinfection and patients who receive transplants for fulminant liver failure than those who receive transplants for chronic HBV. In these cases, patients need to be treated with hepatitis B immunoglobulin (HBIg) or nucleoside analogues to prevent graft infection and loss.

PREVENTION

Prevention of viral hepatitis relies on improvements in sanitation and vaccination of children for HAV and HBV infection. Prevention measures for specific viruses are discussed in chapters dealing with the individual specific agents

The recommendation regarding prevention of acute hepatitis among close contacts is governed by the type of viral hepatitis and the timing of infection. There is often a delay in the diagnosis of acute viral hepatitis and in determining the causative agent. It is necessary to delay postexposure prophylaxis until the nature of the infection is known. In cases of HAV infection, close contacts should receive immunoglobulin within 2 weeks of coming in contact with the infected patient. The recommended dose of HAV immunoglobulin is 0.02 mL/kg body weight by intramuscular injection (Table 111-8). When administered within 2 weeks after an exposure to HAV, immunoglobulin is more than 85% effective in preventing hepatitis A.[177] Postexposure prophylaxis can safely accompany active immunization for HAV.

Vaccination against HAV is now the mainstay of prevention of HAV infection. Currently two inactivated vaccines are available in the United States, Vaqta and Havrix. Both vaccines are highly immunogenic and efficacious. Within 1 month of the first dose of vaccine, 97% to 100% of children, adolescents, and adults have protective levels of antibody. For prevention of infection in travelers, it is preferable that the first dose be given at least 4 weeks before traveling to the endemic

TABLE 111-8 Dosing Schedule for Immunoglobulin for Pre- and Postexposure Prophylaxis against Hepatitis A Virus Infection

Setting	Duration of Coverage	Immunoglobulin Dose (mL/kg)
Preexposure	Short-term (1-2 mo)	0.02
	Long-term (3-5 mo)	0.06
Postexposure		0.02

area. Havrix is available in two formulations: for persons 2 to 18 years of age, 720 ELISA units (ELU) per dose in a two-dose schedule, and for persons older than 18 years, 1440 ELU per dose in a two-dose schedule. Vaqta is also approved in two formulations: for persons 2 to 17 years of age, 25 IU in a two-dose schedule, and for persons older than 17 years, 50 IU per dose in a two-dose schedule.

Prevention of HBV infection largely relies on vaccination of all children at birth with HBV vaccine. Two types of hepatitis B vaccine have been approved in the United States (Recombivax HB and Engerix-B). The currently available vaccines are produced by recombinant DNA technology. The vaccination schedule most often used for adults is three intramuscular injections, administered at 0, 1, and 6 months (see Chapter 142 for detailed schedules for HBV vaccination in different age groups). The recommended series of three intramuscular doses of hepatitis B vaccine induces a protective antibody response (anti-HB$_s$ greater than 10 mIU/mL in more than 90% of healthy adults and in more than 95% of infants, children, and adolescents).[178,179] Larger vaccine doses or an increased number of doses are required to induce protective antibody in a high proportion of hemodialysis patients and may also be necessary for other immunocompromised persons.[180,181]

For postexposure prophylaxis, appropriate immunoprophylactic treatment can effectively prevent infection. The mainstay of postexposure immunoprophylaxis is hepatitis B vaccine, but in some settings the addition of HBIg provides an increase in protection. Transmission of perinatal HBV infection can be effectively prevented if the HBsAg-positive mother is identified and if her infant receives appropriate immunoprophylaxis. Hepatitis B vaccination and one dose of HBIg, administered to the neonate within 24 hours after birth, are 85% to 95% effective in preventing both HBV infection and the chronic carrier state.[182,183] Hepatitis B vaccine administered alone in either a three-dose or four-dose schedule beginning within 24 hours after birth is 70% to 95% effective in preventing perinatal HBV infections.[184,185]

Prophylaxis for exposure other than perinatal exposure usually combines HBIg and HBV vaccination. HBIg is administered at a dose of 0.06 mL/kg body weight intramuscularly as soon as possible after the exposure (preferably within 24 hours). The effectiveness of HBIg when administered more than 7 days after exposure is unknown. When HBV vaccine is indicated, it should also be administered as soon as possible (preferably within 24 hours) and can be administered simultaneously with HBIg at a separate site.

There are no preventive strategies for acute HDV infection except to prevent HBV infection. Similarly, there is no available postexposure prophylaxis for HCV or HEV infection. Hepatitis C immunoglobulin is currently in development. There is no effective vaccine to prevent HCV infection.

REFERENCES

1. Krugman S, Giles JP, Hammond J. Infectious hepatitis. Evidence for two distinctive clinical, epidemiological, and immunological types of infection. JAMA. 1967;200:365-373.
2. Blumberg BS, Gerstley BJ, Hunderford DA, et al. A serum antigen (Australia antigen) in Down's syndrome, leukemia, and hepatitis. Ann Intern Med. 1967;66:924-931.

3. Feinstone SM, Kapikian AZ, Purceli RH. Hepatitis A: Detection by immune electron microscopy of a viruslike antigen associated with acute illness. Science. 1973;182:1026-1028.
4. Provost PJ, Wolansky BS, Miller WJ, et al. Physical, chemical and morphologic dimensions of human hepatitis A virus strain CR326 (38578). Proc Soc Exp Biol Med. 1975;148:532-539.
5. Kohler H, Lange W, Apodaca J, et al. Demonstration of infectivity in marmosets experimentally infected with hepatitis A. Dev Biol Stand. 1975;30:408-409.
6. Provost PJ, Ittensohn OL, Villarejos VM, Hilleman MR. A specific complement-fixation test for human hepatitis A employing CR326 virus antigen. Diagnosis and epidemiology. Proc Soc Exp Biol Med. 1975;148:962-969.
7. Prince AM. An antigen detected in the blood during the incubation period of serum hepatitis. Proc Natl Acad Sci USA. 1968;60:814-821.
8. London WT, Sutnick AI, Blumberg BS. Australia antigen and acute viral hepatitis. Ann Intern Med. 1969;70:55-59.
9. Dane DS, Cameron CH, Briggs M. Virus-like particles in serum of patients with Australia-antigen-associated hepatitis. Lancet. 1970;1:695-698.
10. Zuckerman AJ, Taylor PE, Almeida JD. Presence of particles other than the Australia-SH antigen in a case of chronic active hepatitis with cirrhosis. Br Med J. 1970;1:262-264.
11. Purcell RH, Gerin JL, Holland PV, et al. Preparation and characterization of complement-fixing hepatitis-associated antigen and antiserum. J Infect Dis. 1970;121:222-226.
12. Barker LF, Chisari FV, McGrath PP, et al. Transmission of type B viral hepatitis to chimpanzees. J Infect Dis. 1973;127:648-662.
13. Roche JK, Stengle JM. Clinical trials of hepatitis B immune globulin. N Engl J Med. 1972;287:251-252.
14. Krugman S. Viral hepatitis type B: Prospects for active immunization. Dev Biol Stand. 1975;30:363-367.
15. Rizzetto M, Canese MG, Arico S, et al. Immunofluorescence detection of new antigen-antibody system (delta/anti-delta) associated to hepatitis B virus in liver and in serum of HBsAg carriers. Gut. 1977;18:997-1003.
16. Prince AM, Brotman B, Grady GF, et al. Long-incubation post-transfusion hepatitis without serological evidence of exposure to hepatitis-B virus. Lancet. 1974;2:241-246.
17. Feinstone SM, Kapikian AZ, Gerin JL, Purcell RH. Buoyant density of the hepatitis A virus-like particle in cesium chloride. J Virol. 1974;13:1412-1414.
18. Chang MH, Chen CJ, Lai MS, et al. Universal hepatitis B vaccination in Taiwan and the incidence of hepatocellular carcinoma in children. Taiwan Childhood Hepatoma Study Group. N Engl J Med. 1997;336:1855-1859.
19. Alter HJ, Purcell RH, Holland PV, Popper H. Transmissible agent in non-A, non-B hepatitis. Lancet. 1978;1:459-463.
20. Choo QL, Kuo G, Weiner AJ, et al. Isolation of a cDNA clone derived from a blood-borne non-A, non-B viral hepatitis genome. Science. 1989;244:359-362.
21. Gupta DN, Smetana HF. The histopathology of viral hepatitis as seen in the Delhi epidemic (1955-56). Indian J Med Res. 1957;45(Suppl):101-113.
22. Balayan MS, Andjaparidze AG, Savinskaya SS, et al. Evidence for a virus in non-A, non-B hepatitis transmitted via the fecal-oral route. Intervirology. 1983;20:23-31.
23. Reyes GR, Purdy MA, Kim JP, et al., Isolation of a cDNA from the virus responsible for enterically transmitted non-A, non-B hepatitis. Science. 1990;247:1335-1339.
24. Summary of Notifiable Diseases—United States, 2000. MMWR Morb Mortal Wkly Rep. 2002;49(53):I-xxii, 1-100.
25. Prevention of hepatitis A through active or passive immunization practices: Recommendations of the advisory committee on immunization practices (ACIP). MMWR Recomm Rep. 1996;45(RR-15):1-30.
26. Lednar WM, Lemon SM, Kirkpatrick JW, et al. Frequency of illness associated with epidemic hepatitis A virus infections in adults. Am J Epidemiol. 1985;122:226-233.
27. Tong MJ, el-Farra NS, Grew MI. Clinical manifestations of hepatitis A: Recent experience in a community teaching hospital. J Infect Dis. 1995;171(Suppl 1):S15-S18.
28. Hodges JR. Hepatitis A and meningo-encephalitis. J Neurol. 1987;234:364-365.
29. Dienstag JL. Hepatitis B as an immune complex disease. Semin Liver Dis. 1981;1:45-57.
30. Gianotti F. Acrodermatitis papulosa infantilis. An Australia antigen disease. Padiatr Padol. 1977;12:58-62.
31. Colombo M, Gerber MA, Vernace SJ, et al. Immune response to hepatitis B virus in children with papular acrodermatitis. Gastroenterology. 1977;73:1103-1106.
32. Hofmann B, Schuppe HC, Adams O, et al. Gianotti-Crosti syndrome associated with Epstein-Barr virus infection. Pediatr Dermatol. 1997;14:273-277.
33. Terasaki K, Koura S, Tachikura T, Kanzaki T. Gianotti-Crosti syndrome associated with endogenous reactivation of Epstein-Barr virus. Dermatology. 2003;207:68-71.
34. Rachima CM, Cohen E, Garty M. Acute hepatitis A: Combination of the relapsing and the cholestatic forms, two rare variants. Am J Med Sci. 2000;319:417-419.
35. Gordon SC, Reddy KR, Schiff L, Schiff ER. Prolonged intrahepatic cholestasis secondary to acute hepatitis A. Ann Intern Med. 1984;101:635-637.
36. Davies SE, Portmann BC, O'Grady JG, et al. Hepatic histological findings after transplantation for chronic hepatitis B virus infection, including a unique pattern of fibrosing cholestatic hepatitis. Hepatology. 1991;13:150-157.
37. Takahashi T, Ashizawa S, Matsumoto H, et al. Fibrosing cholestatic hepatitis developing after liver transplantation: Case report of a patient with HCV-related cirrhosis. Transplant Proc. 2003;35:392-393.
38. Rosenberg PM, Farrell JJ, Abraczinskas DR, et al. Rapidly progressive fibrosing cholestatic hepatitis—Hepatitis C virus in HIV coinfection. Am J Gastroenterol. 2002;97:478-483.
39. Trey C, Davidson L. The management of fulminant hepatic failure. In: Popper H, Shaffner F, eds. Progress in Liver Disease. New York: Grune & Stratton; 1970:282.
40. O'Grady J. Acute liver failure. In: O'Grady JG, Lake JR, Howdle PD, eds. Comprehensive Clinical Hepatology. St. Louis: Mosby; 2000:30.1.
41. Lee W, Schiodt FV. Fulminant liver failure. In: Schiff E, Sorrell MF, Maddrey WC, eds. Schiff's Diseases of the Liver. Philadelphia: JB Lippincott; 1998:879.
42. Chu CM, Yeh CT, Liaw YF. Fulminant hepatic failure in acute hepatitis C: Increased risk in chronic carriers of hepatitis B virus. Gut. 1999;45:613-617.
43. Vento S, Garofano T, Renzini C, et al. Fulminant hepatitis associated with hepatitis A virus superinfection in patients with chronic hepatitis C. N Engl J Med. 1998;338:286-290.
44. Schiff ER. Update in hepatology. Ann Intern Med. 2000;132:460-466.
45. Enterically transmitted non-A, non-B hepatitis—East Africa. MMWR Morb Mortal Wkly Rep. 1987;36:241-244.
46. Khuroo MS, Teli MR, Skidmore S, et al. Incidence and severity of viral hepatitis in pregnancy. Am J Med. 1981;70:252-255.
47. Schiodt FV, Atillasoy E, Shakil AO, et al. Etiology and outcome for 295 patients with acute liver failure in the United States. Liver Transpl Surg. 1999;5:29-34.
48. Ostapowicz G, Fontana RJ, Schiodt FV, et al. Results of a prospective study of acute liver failure at 17 tertiary care centers in the United States. Ann Intern Med. 2002;137:947-954.
49. Schiodt FV, Davem TJ, Shakil AO, et al. Viral hepatitis-related acute liver failure. Am J Gastroenterol. 2003;98:448-453.
50. Robertson BH, Jansen RW, Khanna B, et al. Genetic relatedness of hepatitis A virus strains recovered from different geographical regions. J Gen Virol. 1992;73:1365-1377.
51. Lemon SM, Jansen RW, Brown EA. Genetic, antigenic and biological differences between strains of hepatitis A virus. Vaccine. 1992;10(Suppl 1):S40-S44.
52. Fujiwara K, Yokosuka O, Ehata T, et al. Association between severity of type A hepatitis and nucleotide variations in the 5′ non-translated region of hepatitis A virus RNA: Strains from fulminant hepatitis have fewer nucleotide substitutions. Gut. 2002;51:82-88.
53. Dienstag JL, Routenberg JA, Purcell RH, et al. Foodhandler-associated outbreak of hepatitis type A. An immune electron microscopic study. Ann Intern Med. 1975;83:647-650.
54. Corey L, Holmes KK. Sexual transmission of hepatitis A in homosexual men: Incidence and mechanism. N Engl J Med. 1980;302:435-438.
55. Hollinger FB, Khan NC, Oefinger PE, et al. Posttransfusion hepatitis type A. JAMA. 1983;250:2313-2317.
56. Robertson BH, Friedberg D, Normann A, et al. Sequence variability of hepatitis A virus and factor VIII associated hepatitis A infections in hemophilia patients in Europe. An update. Vox Sang. 1994;67(Suppl 1):39-45; discussion 46.
57. Kedda MA, Kew MC, Cohn RS, et al. An outbreak of hepatitis A among South African patients with hemophilia: Evidence implicating contaminated factor VIII concentrate as the source. Hepatology. 1995;22:1363-1367.
58. Skidmore SJ, Boxall EH, Ala F. A case report of post-transfusion hepatitis A. J Med Virol. 1982;10:223.
59. Werzberger A, Mensch B, Kuter B, et al. A controlled trial of a formalin-inactivated hepatitis A vaccine in healthy children. N Engl J Med. 1992;327:453-457.
60. Mathiesen LR, Moller AM, Purcell RH, et al. Hepatitis A virus in the liver and intestine of marmosets after oral inoculation. Infect Immun. 1980;28:45-48.
61. Schiff ER. Atypical clinical manifestations of hepatitis A. Vaccine. 1992;10(Suppl 1):S18-S20.
62. Maynard JE. Hepatitis B: Global importance and need for control. Vaccine. 1990;8(Suppl):S18-S20; discussion S21-S23.
63. Chan HL, Ghany MG, Lok AS. Hepatitis B. In: Schiff E, Sorrell MF, Maddrey WC, eds. Schiff's Disease of the Liver. Philadelphia: JB Lippincott; 1999:757.
64. Stevens CE, Beasley RP, Tsui J, Lee WC. Vertical transmission of hepatitis B antigen in Taiwan. N Engl J Med. 1975;292:771-774.
65. Beasley RP, Hwang LY, Lin CC, et al. Incidence of hepatitis B virus infections in preschool children in Taiwan. J Infect Dis. 1982;146:198-204.
66. Coursaget P, Yvonnet B, Chotard J, et al. Age- and sex-related study of hepatitis B virus chronic carrier state in infants from an endemic area (Senegal). J Med Virol. 1987;22:1-5.
67. Tassopoulos NC, Papaevangelou GJ, Sjogren MH, et al. Natural history of acute hepatitis B surface antigen-positive hepatitis in Greek adults. Gastroenterology. 1987;92:1844-1850.
68. Dodd RY. The risk of transfusion-transmitted infection. N Engl J Med. 1992;327:419-421.
69. Alter MJ, Hadler SC, Margolis HS, et al. The changing epidemiology of hepatitis B in the United States. Need for alternative vaccination strategies. JAMA. 1990;263:1218-1222.
70. Gerberding JL. The infected health care provider. N Engl J Med. 1996;334:594-595.
71. Outbreaks of hepatitis B virus infection among hemodialysis patients—California, Nebraska and Texas, 1994. MMWR Morb Mortal Wkly Rep. 1996;45:285-289.
72. Fabrizi F, Lunghi G, Martin P. Hepatitis B virus infection in hemodialysis: Recent discoveries. J Nephrol. 2002;15:463-468.
73. Harpaz R, Von Seidlein L, Averhoff FM, et al. Transmission of hepatitis B virus to multiple patients from a surgeon without evidence of inadequate infection control. N Engl J Med. 1996;334:549-554.
74. Goldstein ST, Alter MJ, Williams IT, et al. Incidence and risk factors for acute hepatitis B in the United States, 1982-1998: Implications for vaccination programs. J Infect Dis. 2002;185:713-719.
75. Karayiannis P, Novick DM, Lok AS, et al. Hepatitis B virus DNA in saliva, urine, and seminal fluid of carriers of hepatitis B e antigen. Br Med J (Clin Res Ed). 1985;290:1853-1855.
76. de Martino M, Appendino C, Resti M, et al. Should hepatitis B surface antigen positive mothers breast feed? Arch Dis Child. 1985;60:972-974.

77. Hill JB, Sheffield JS, Kim MJ, et al. Risk of hepatitis B transmission in breast-fed infants of chronic hepatitis B carriers. Obstet Gynecol. 2002;99:1049-1052.

78. Rizzetto M. The delta agent. Hepatology. 1983;3:729-737.

79. Niro GA, Smedile A, Andriulli A, et al. The predominance of hepatitis delta virus genotype I among chronically infected Italian patients. Hepatology. 1997;25:728-734.

80. Wu JC, Choo KB, Chen CM, et al. Genotyping of hepatitis D virus by restriction-fragment length polymorphism and relation to outcome of hepatitis D. Lancet. 1995;346:939-941.

81. Casey JL, Brown TL, Colan EJ, et al. A genotype of hepatitis D virus that occurs in northern South America. Proc Natl Acad Sci USA. 1993;90:9016-9020.

82. Bensabath G, Hadler SC, Soares MC, et al. Hepatitis delta virus infection and Labrea hepatitis. Prevalence and role in fulminant hepatitis in the Amazon Basin. JAMA. 1987;258:479-483.

83. Rizzetto M, Ponzetto A, Forzani I. Epidemiology of hepatitis delta virus: Overview. Prog Clin Biol Res. 1991;364:1-20.

84. Rizzetto M, Ponzetto A, Forzani I. Hepatitis delta virus as a global health problem. Vaccine. 1990;8(Suppl):S10-S14; discussion S21-S23.

85. Rocca G, Poli G, Gerardo P. Familial clustering of the delta infection. Prog Clin Res. 1983;143:133-137.

86. Gaeta GB, Stroffolini T, Chiaramonte M, et al. Chronic hepatitis D: A vanishing disease? An Italian multicenter study. Hepatology. 2000;32:824-827.

87. Smedile A, Farci P, Verme G, et al. Influence of delta infection on severity of hepatitis B. Lancet. 1982;2:945-947.

88. Saracco G, Macagno S, Rosina F, Rizzetto M. Serologic markers with fulminant hepatitis in persons positive for hepatitis B surface antigen. A worldwide epidemiologic and clinical survey. Ann Intern Med. 1988;108:380-383.

89. Samuel D, Muller R, Alexander G, et al. Liver transplantation in European patients with the hepatitis B surface antigen. N Engl J Med. 1993;329:1842-1847.

90. Alter MJ. Epidemiology of hepatitis C. Hepatology. 1997;26(3 Suppl 1):62S-65S.

91. Kim WR. The burden of hepatitis C in the United States. Hepatology. 2002;36(5 Suppl 1):S30-S34.

92. Alter HJ, Conry-Cantelina C, Melpolder J, et al. Hepatitis C in asymptomatic blood donors. Hepatology. 1997;26(3 Suppl 1):29S-33S.

93. Andreone P, Caracceni P, Grazi GL, et al. Lamivudine treatment for acute hepatitis B after liver transplantation. J Hepatol. 1998;29:985-989.

94. Farci P, Alter HJ, Wong D, et al. A long-term study of hepatitis C virus replication in non-A, non-B hepatitis. N Engl J Med. 1991;325:98-104.

95. Vishawanathan R. Infectious hepatitis in Delhi (1955-1956): A critical study: Epidemiology. Indian J Med Res. 1957;45(Suppl 1):1-8.

96. Krawczynski K. Hepatitis E. Hepatology. 1993;17:932-941.

97. Khuroo MS, Rustgi VK, Dawson GJ, et al. Spectrum of hepatitis E virus infection in India. J Med Virol. 1994;43:281-286.

98. Hepatitis E among US travelers, 1989-1992. MMWR Morb Mortal Wkly Rep. 1993;42:1-4.

99. Heath TC, Burrow JN, Currie BJ, et al. Locally acquired hepatitis E in the Northern Territory of Australia. Med J Aust. 1995;162:318-319.

100. Zanetti AR, Dawson GJ. Hepatitis type E in Italy: A seroepidemiological survey. Study Group of Hepatitis E. J Med Virol. 1994;42:318-320.

101. Tassopoulos NC, Krawczynski H, Hatzakis A, et al. Case report: role of hepatitis E virus in the etiology of community-acquired non-A, non-B hepatitis in Greece. J Med Virol. 1994;42:124-128.

102. Wong DC, Purcell RH, Sreenivasan RA, et al. Epidemic and endemic hepatitis in India: Evidence for a non-A, non-B hepatitis virus aetiology. Lancet. 1980;2:876-879.

103. Khuroo MS, Kamili S, Jameel S. Vertical transmission of hepatitis E virus. Lancet. 1995;345:1025-1026.

104. Wu JC, Chen CM, Chiang TY, et al. Clinical and epidemiological implications of swine hepatitis E virus infection. J Med Virol. 2000;60:166-171.

105. Wang YC, Zhang HY, Xia NS, et al. Prevalence, isolation, and partial sequence analysis of hepatitis E virus from domestic animals in China. J Med Virol. 2002;67:516-521.

106. He J, Innis BL, Shrestha MP, et al. Evidence that rodents are a reservoir of hepatitis E virus for humans in Nepal. J Clin Microbiol. 2002;40:4493-4498.

107. Sanyal MC. Epidemic of infectious hepatitis amongst personnel of the armed forces, Delhi (1955-56): Epidemiology. Indian J Med Res. 1957;45(Suppl.):91-99.

108. Naik SR, Aggarwal R, Salunke PN, Mehrotra NN. A large waterborne viral hepatitis E epidemic in Kanpur, India. Bull World Health Organ. 1992;70:597-604.

109. Hamid SS, Atig M, Shehzad F, et al. Hepatitis E virus superinfection in patients with chronic liver disease. Hepatology. 2002;36:474-478.

110. Khuroo MS, Kamili S, Dar MY, et al. Hepatitis E and long-term antibody status. Lancet. 1993;341:1355.

111. Alter HJ. The cloning and clinical implications of HGV and HGBV-C. N Engl J Med. 1996;334:1536-1537.

112. Frey SE, Homan SM, Sokol-Anderson M, et al. Evidence for probable sexual transmission of the hepatitis G virus. Clin Infect Dis. 2002;34:1033-1038.

113. Hinrichsen H, Leimenstoll G, Stegen G, et al. Prevalence of and risk factors for hepatitis G (HGV) infection in haemodialysis patients: A multicentre study. Nephrol Dial Transplant. 2002;17:271-275.

114. Notari EP 4th, Orton SL, Cable RG, et al. Seroprevalence of known and putative hepatitis markers in United States blood donors with ALT levels at least 120 IU per L. Transfusion. 2001;41:751-755.

115. Xiang J, Wunschmann S, Kiekema DJ, et al. Effect of coinfection with GB virus C on survival among patients with HIV infection. N Engl J Med. 2001;345:707-714.

116. Tanaka E, Alter HJ, Nakatsuji Y, et al. Effect of hepatitis G virus infection on chronic hepatitis C. Ann Intern Med. 1996;125:740-743.

117. Murthy BV, Muerhoff AS, Desai SM, et al. GB hepatitis agent in cadaver organ donors and their recipients. Transplantation. 1997;63:346-351.

118. Mauser-Bunschoten EP, Damen M, Zaaijer HL, et al. Hepatitis G virus RNA and hepatitis G virus-E2 antibodies in Dutch hemophilia patients in relation to transfusion history. Blood. 1998;92:2164-2168.

119. De Filippi F. Lampertico P, Soffredini R, et al. High prevalence, low pathogenicity of hepatitis G virus in kidney transplant recipients. Dig Liver Dis. 2001;33:477-479.

120. Masuko K, Mitsui T, Iwano K, et al. Infection with hepatitis GB virus C in patients on maintenance hemodialysis. N Engl J Med. 1996;334:1485-1490.

121. Thomas DL, Vlahov D, Alter HJ, et al. Association of antibody to GB virus C (hepatitis G virus) with viral clearance and protection from reinfection. J Infect Dis. 1998;177:539-542.

122. Bralet MP, Roudot-Thoraval F, Pawlotsky JM, et al. Histopathologic impact of GB virus C infection on chronic hepatitis C. Gastroenterology. 1997;112:188-192.

123. Shimanaka K, Tsutsumi M, Sawada M, et al. Clinicopathological study of chronic hepatitis induced by alcohol with or without hepatitis G virus. Alcohol Clin Exp Res. 1999;23(4 Suppl):29S-32S.

124. Uygun A, Kadayifci A, Kubar A, et al. Insignificant role of hepatitis G virus infection in patients with liver enzyme elevations of unknown etiology. J Clin Gastroenterol. 2000;31:73-76.

125. Berasain C, Betes M, Panizo A, et al. Pathological and virological findings in patients with persistent hypertransaminasaemia of unknown aetiology. Gut. 2000;47:429-435.

126. Pessoa MG, Terrault NA, Ferrell LD, et al. Hepatitis after liver transplantation: The role of the known and unknown viruses. Liver Transpl Surg. 1998;4:461-468.

127. Vargas HE, Laskus T, Radkowski M, et al. Hepatitis G virus coinfection in hepatitis C virus-infected liver transplant recipients. Transplantation. 1997;64:786-788.

128. Yoshiba M, Okamoto H, Mishiro S. Detection of the GBV-C hepatitis virus genome in serum from patients with fulminant hepatitis of unknown aetiology. Lancet. 1995;346:1131-1132.

129. Kanda T, Yokosuka O, Ehata T, et al. Detection of GBV-C RNA in patients with non-A-E fulminant hepatitis by reverse-transcription polymerase chain reaction. Hepatology. 1997;25:1261-1265.

130. Munoz SJ, Alter HJ, Nakatsuji Y, et al. The significance of hepatitis G virus in serum of patients with sporadic fulminant and subfulminant hepatitis of unknown etiology. Blood. 1999;94:1460-1464.

131. Hashimoti E, Kojumahara N, Noguchi S, et al. Immunohistochemical characterization of hepatic lymphocytes in acute hepatitis A, B, and C. J Clin Gastroenterol. 1996;23:199-202.

132. Baba M, Hasegawa H, Nakayabu M, et al. Cytolytic activity of natural killer cells and lymphokine activated killer cells against hepatitis A virus infected fibroblasts. J Clin Lab Immunol. 1993;40:47-60.

133. Vallbracht A, Gabriel P, Maier K, et al. Cell-mediated cytotoxicity in hepatitis A virus infection. Hepatology. 1986;6:1308-1314.

134. Wild J, Grusby MJ, Schirmbeck R, Reimann J. Priming MHC-I-restricted cytotoxic T lymphocyte responses to exogenous hepatitis B surface antigen is CD4+ T cell dependent. J Immunol. 1999;163:1880-1887.

135. Koziel MJ. What once was lost, now is found: Restoration of hepatitis B-specific immunity after treatment of chronic hepatitis B. Hepatology. 1999;29:1331-1333.

136. Rehermann B, Chang KM, McHutchinson JG, et al. Quantitative analysis of the peripheral blood cytotoxic T lymphocyte response in patients with chronic hepatitis C virus infection. J Clin Invest. 1996;98:1432-1440.

137. Macnaughton TB, Gowans EJ, Jilbert AR, Burrell CJ. Hepatitis delta virus RNA, protein synthesis and associated cytotoxicity in a stably transfected cell line. Virology. 1990;177:692-698.

138. Lefkowitch JH, Goldstein H, Yatto R, Berber MA. Cytopathic liver injury in acute delta virus hepatitis. Gastroenterology. 1987;92:1262-1266.

139. David E, Rahier J, Pucci A, et al. Recurrence of hepatitis D (delta) in liver transplants: Histopathological aspects. Gastroenterology. 1993;104:1122-1128.

140. Lechmann M, Ihlenfeldt HG, Braunschweiger I, et al. T- and B-cell responses to different hepatitis C virus antigens in patients with chronic hepatitis C infection and in healthy anti-hepatitis C virus-positive blood donors without viremia. Hepatology. 1996;24:790-795.

141. Missale G, Bertoni R, Lamonaca V, et al. Different clinical behaviors of acute hepatitis C virus infection are associated with different vigor of the anti-viral cell-mediated immune response. J Clin Invest. 1996;98:706-714.

142. Cramp ME, Rossol S, Chokshi S, et al. Hepatitis C virus-specific T-cell reactivity during interferon and ribavirin treatment in chronic hepatitis C. Gastroenterology. 2000;118:346-355.

143. Cramp ME, Carucci P, Rossol S, et al. Hepatitis C virus (HCV) specific immune responses in anti-HCV positive patients without hepatitis C viraemia. Gut. 1999;44:424-429.

144. Gruner NH, Gerlach TJ, Jung MC, et al. Association of hepatitis C virus-specific CD8+ T cells with viral clearance in acute hepatitis C. J Infect Dis. 2000;181:1528-1536.

145. Grotto, I., Mimouni D, Huerta M, et al., Clinical and laboratory presentation of EBV positive infectious mononucleosis in young adults. Epidemiol Infect. 2003;131:683-689.

146. Feranchak AP, Tyson RW, Narkewicz NR, et al. Fulminant Epstein-Barr viral hepatitis: Orthotopic liver transplantation and review of the literature. Liver Transpl Surg. 1998;4:469-476.

147. Seemayer TA, Gross TG, Egeler RM, et al. X-linked lymphoproliferative disease: Twenty-five years after the discovery. Pediatr Res. 1995;38:471-478.

148. Istas AS, Demmler DJ, Dobbins JG, Stewart JA. Surveillance for congenital cytomegalovirus disease: A report from the National Congenital Cytomegalovirus Disease Registry. Clin Infect Dis. 1995;20:665-670.

149. Cohen JI, Corey GR. Cytomegalovirus infection in the normal host. Medicine (Baltimore). 1985;64:100-114.

150. Rubin RH. Cytomegalovirus in solid organ transplantation. Transpl Infect Dis. 2001;3(Suppl 2):1-5.

151. Lee WS, Kelly DA, Tanner MS, et al. Neonatal liver transplantation for fulminant hepatitis caused by herpes simplex virus type 2. J Pediatr Gastroenterol Nutr. 2002;35:220-22.

151a. Gelven PL, Gruber KK, Swiger FK, et al. Fatal disseminated herpes simplex in pregnancy with maternal and neonatal death. South Med J 1996;89:732-734.

152. Oudart JL, Rey M. [Proteinuria, proteinaemia, and serum transaminase activity in 23 confirmed cases of yellow fever]. Bull World Health Organ. 1970;42:95-102.

153. Elton NW, Romero A, Trejos A. Clinical pathology of yellow fever. Am J Clin Pathol. 1955;25:135-146.

154. Sanford JP. Leptospirosis—Time for a booster. N Engl J Med. 1984;310:524-525.

155. Tse KC, Yip PS, Hui KM, et al. Potential benefit of plasma exchange in treatment of severe icteric leptospirosis complicated by acute renal failure. Clin Diagn Lab Immunol. 2002;9:482-484.

156. Fournier PE, Marrie TJ, Raoult D. Diagnosis of Q fever. J Clin Microbiol. 1998;36:1823-1834.

157. Czaja AJ, Manns MP, McFarlane IG, Hoofnagle JH. Autoimmune hepatitis: The investigational and clinical challenges. Hepatology. 2000;31:1194-1200.

158. Fuchs S, Bogomolski-Yahalom V, Psaltiel O, Ackerman Z. Ischemic hepatitis: Clinical and laboratory observations of 34 patients. J Clin Gastroenterol. 1998; 26:183-186.

159. Stone JH. HELLP syndrome: Hemolysis, elevated liver enzymes, and low platelets. JAMA. 1998;280:559-562.

160. Ibdah JA, Bennett MJ, Rinaldo P, et al. A fetal fatty-acid oxidation disorder as a cause of liver disease in pregnant women. N Engl J Med. 1999;340:1723-1731.

161. Pereira SP, O'Donohue J, Wendon J, Williams R. Maternal and perinatal outcome in severe pregnancy-related liver disease. Hepatology. 1997;26:1258-1262.

162. Valla DC. Hepatic vein thrombosis (Budd-Chiari syndrome). Semin Liver Dis. 2002;22:5-14.

163. Bayraktar Y, Balkanci F, Bayraktar M, Aclguneri M. Budd-Chiari syndrome: A common complication of Behçet's disease. Am J Gastroenterol. 1997;92:858-862.

164. Steindl P, Ferenci P, Dienes HP, et al. Wilson's disease in patients presenting with liver disease: A diagnostic challenge. Gastroenterology. 1997;113:212-218.

165. Chalmers T, Eckhardt R, Reynolds W. The treatment of acute infectious hepatitis, controlled studies of the effects of diet, rest and physical activity reconditioning on acute course of the disease and the incidence of relapses and residual abnormalities. J Clin Invest. 1955;34:1163-1235.

166. Repsher LH, Freebern RK. Effects of early and vigorous exercise on recovery from infectious hepatitis. N Engl J Med. 1969;281:1393-1396.

167. Tozun N, Forbes A, Anderson MG, Murray-Lyon IM. Safety of alcohol after viral hepatitis. Lancet. 1991;337:1079-1080.

168. Fabris P, Tositti G, Mazzella G, et al. Effect of ursodeoxycholic acid administration in patients with acute viral hepatitis: A pilot study. Aliment Pharmacol Ther. 1999;13:1187-1193.

169. Gregory PB, Knauer CM, Kempson RL, Miller R. Steroid therapy in severe viral hepatitis. A double-blind, randomized trial of methyl-prednisolone versus placebo. N Engl J Med. 1976;294:681-687.

170. Kundu SS, Kundu AK, Pal NK. Interferon-alpha in the treatment of acute prolonged hepatitis B virus infection. J Assoc Physicians India. 2000;48:671-673.

171. Levin S, Hahn T. Interferon system in acute viral hepatitis. Lancet. 1982;1:592-594.

172. Sanchez-Tapias JM, Mas A, Costa J, et al. Recombinant alpha 2c-interferon therapy in fulminant viral hepatitis. J Hepatol. 1987;5:205-210.

173. Torii N, Hasegawa K, Ogawa M, et al. Effectiveness and long-term outcome of lamivudine therapy for acute hepatitis B. Hepatol Res. 2002;24:34.

174. Jaeckel E, Cornberg M, Wedemeyer H, et al. Treatment of acute hepatitis C with interferon alfa-2b. N Engl J Med. 2001;345:1452-1457.

175. Rolando N, Harvey F, Brahm J, et al. Prospective study of bacterial infection in acute liver failure: An analysis of fifty patients. Hepatology. 1990;11:49-53.

176. Rolando N, Wade JJ, Stanyou A, et al. Prospective study comparing the efficacy of prophylactic parenteral antimicrobials, with or without enteral decontamination, in patients with acute liver failure. Liver Transpl Surg. 1996;2:8-13.

177. Mosley JW, Reisler DM, Brachott D, et al. Comparison of two lots of immune serum globulin for prophylaxis of infectious hepatitis. Am J Epidemiol. 1968;87:539-550.

178. Szmuness W, Stevens CE, Harley EJ, et al. Hepatitis B vaccine: Demonstration of efficacy in a controlled clinical trial in a high-risk population in the United States. N Engl J Med. 1980;303:833-841.

179. Andre FE. Summary of safety and efficacy data on a yeast-derived hepatitis B vaccine. Am J Med. 1989;87(3A):14S-20S.

180. Stevens CE, Alter HJ, Taylor PE, et al. Hepatitis B vaccine in patients receiving hemodialysis. Immunogenicity and efficacy. N Engl J Med. 1984;311:496-501.

181. Collier AC, Corey L, Murphy VL, Handsfield HH. Antibody to human immunodeficiency virus (HIV) and suboptimal response to hepatitis B vaccination. Ann Intern Med. 1988;109:101-105.

182. Stevens CE, Taylor PE, Tong MJ, et al. Yeast-recombinant hepatitis B vaccine. Efficacy with hepatitis B immune globulin in prevention of perinatal hepatitis B virus transmission. JAMA. 1987;257:2612-2616.

183. McMahon BJ, Rhoades ER, Heyward WL, et al. A comprehensive programme to reduce the incidence of hepatitis B virus infection and its sequelae in Alaskan natives. Lancet. 1987;2:1134-1136.

184. Xu ZY, Liu CB, Francis DP, et al. Prevention of perinatal acquisition of hepatitis B virus carriage using vaccine: Preliminary report of a randomized, double-blind placebo-controlled and comparative trial. Pediatrics. 1985;76:713-718.

185. Poovorawan Y, Sanpavat S, Pongpunlert W, et al. Protective efficacy of a recombinant DNA hepatitis B vaccine in neonates of HBe antigen-positive mothers. JAMA. 1989;261:3278-3281.

Chronic Viral Hepatitis

JULES L. DIENSTAG

The term *chronic viral hepatitis* is used to describe protracted hepatocellular necrosis and inflammation, often with fibrosis, lasting longer than 6 months and caused by hepatitis B virus (HBV), hepatitis C virus (HCV), and/or HBV-associated hepatitis D virus (HDV). Nonviral causes of chronic hepatitis that may be confused clinically with chronic viral hepatitis include autoimmune hepatitis, metabolic-genetic disorders (Wilson's disease, hereditary hemochromatosis, α_1-antitrypsin deficiency), alcoholic liver disease, nonalcoholic fatty liver disease, drug-induced liver disease, and granulomatous disorders. The chronic viral hepatitides, however, are readily distinguished from these other forms of chronic hepatitis by serologic/virologic testing. Classified histologically by the degree of hepatocellular necrosis and inflammation (grade) and fibrosis (stage) (Table 112-1),[1-3] chronic viral hepatitis may be mild (even sometimes without liver injury at all, representing an inactive "carrier" state), moderate, or severe. Moreover, chronic viral hepatitis is the most common cause of chronic liver disease; worldwide, as many as 350 to 400 million persons (>5% of the world's population) are infected with HBV[4-6] and 175 million with HCV.[7-9] In the United States alone, 1 to 2 million persons are infected with HBV and 4 million with HCV. With the potential to culminate in cirrhosis, portal hypertension, and even hepatocellular carcinoma, chronic viral hepatitis ranks as the fifth most common cause of human deaths on earth and the tenth most common cause of deaths in the United States, where it has been estimated to result in annual economic losses exceeding $1 billion. Left to follow its natural history, chronic viral hepatitis could account for an even more substantial health and economic burden in coming generations; however, a vaccine to prevent hepatitis B and rapidly evolving antiviral therapies for both hepatitis B and C are likely to reduce the morbidity and mortality of this human scourge.

Neither of the enteric ribonucleic acid (RNA) hepatitis viruses, hepatitis A virus and hepatitis E virus, causes chronic hepatitis; however, acute hepatitis A can be followed by a protracted cholestatic syndrome that may last many months.[10] Similarly, rare instances have been reported in which classical autoimmune hepatitis was initiated by an episode of acute viral hepatitis A, B, or C.[11-13] Both cytomegalovirus

TABLE 112-1   Contemporary Histologic Classification of Chronic Hepatitis According to the Modified Histologic Activity Index of Ishak and Colleagues[1] and the Metavir[3] Scale

Necroinflammatory Activity (Stage)	HAI	Metavir
Periportal necrosis, bridging necrosis	0-4	0-3, 0-1
Intralobular necrosis, confluent	0-6	
Intralobular necrosis, focal	0-4	0-2
Portal inflammation	0-4	0-3
Total	0-18	A0-A3*
Fibrosis (grade)		
None	0	F0
Portal (some)	1	F1
Portal (most)	2	F1
Bridging (few)	3	F2
Bridging (many)	4	F3
Incomplete cirrhosis	5	F4
Cirrhosis	6	F4
Total	6	4

*Necroinflammatory activity: A0, none; A1, mild; A2, moderate; A3, severe. HAI, Histologic Activity Index.

(CMV) and Epstein-Barr virus (EBV) have been implicated as agents of acute hepatitis, primarily in immunocompromised patients, but in immunocompetent patients with systemic acute CMV or EBV infection (e.g., infectious mononucleosis), transient elevations of serum aminotransferase and alkaline phosphatase activities are common. Neither agent is a likely contributor to chronic hepatitis. In the same vein, a series of blood-borne agents described during the 1990s, including "hepatitis G" virus, GB virus C, TTV, and SENV,[14-16] cannot be implicated as causes of acute or chronic hepatitis (see Chapter 151).

In all forms of chronic viral hepatitis, liver injury does not result directly from a cytopathic effect of the virus but, instead, from an ongoing host-mediated, cytolytic T-cell response to virus-infected hepatocytes that is ineffective in achieving adequate clearance of all virus-infected cells.

CHRONIC HEPATITIS B

In persons who fail to clear HBV infection during acute infection (see Chapter 142 for a summary of the virology of HBV infection), chronic infection is characterized serologically by persistence in serum of the HBV envelope protein, hepatitis B surface antigen (HBsAg). Among those with chronic hepatitis B, several important distinctions, based upon levels of HBV replication, epidemiologic considerations, and viral variants, merit attention (Table 112-2).

Distinctions Based on Relative Levels of Hepatitis B Virus Replication

Among those with chronic hepatitis B, a distinction can be drawn between those with highly replicative HBV infection ($>10^5$-10^6 virions/mL) and those with levels of replication below this threshold. In the relatively replicative phase of chronic hepatitis B, levels of HBV deoxyribonucleic acid (DNA) are high (detectable by insensitive hybridization assays or at levels exceeding 10^5 to 10^6 virions/mL by sensitive amplification assays such as those based upon detection by polymerase chain reaction [PCR]); transmissibility of infection to contacts is favored; hepatitis B e antigen (HB_eAg), another serologic marker of HBV replication, is detectable; the expression of HBV nucleocapsid antigens (primarily hepatitis B core antigen [HB_cAg]) in hepatocytes is demonstrable, and clinical markers of liver injury are present. Such patients tend to have moderate to severe chronic hepatitis B.[17,18]

At an annual incidence of approximately 10% to 15%, persons with highly replicative chronic hepatitis B lose markers of high replication and convert spontaneously to a relatively low replicative state characterized by limited infectivity and liver injury, loss of HB_eAg, and loss of detectable hepatocyte expression of HB_cAg.[19-26] Such patients tend to have clinically mild chronic hepatitis or even to be inactive carriers of the virus. Unlike hepatitis C, in which any level of virus replication

can be associated with liver injury, in chronic HBV infection, a threshold exists, on the order of approximately 10^3 to 10^4 virions/mL, below which liver injury is negligible or absent.[27-30] The distinction in level of HBV replication between these two relative phases of chronic HBV infection is reflected by a dramatic difference in infectivity. Babies born to mothers with high-level HBV replication (HB_eAg-reactive, HBV DNA $>10^6$ virions/mL) have a 90% chance of chronic HBV infection, compared with babies born to mothers with low-level HBV replication, whose likelihood of chronic HBV infection is less than or equal to 10%.[31] Similarly, a person sustaining a needlestick contaminated by blood from someone with highly replicative chronic HBV infection has a greater than 30% chance of becoming infected, while the likelihood of infection is only 0.1% if the needlestick derives from a person with low-level HBV replication.[32] Similar distinctions occur between the two groups in sexual transmission. Inactive hepatitis B carriers, who have low-level viremia, absent or negligible histologic activity, normal liver biochemical tests, and minimal infectivity, can undergo HBsAg-to-anti-HBs seroconversion, i.e., the serologic hallmark of recovery from hepatitis B, but at a frequency of only 1% to 2% per year.[33,34] In the setting of immunologic compromise, e.g., cytotoxic chemotherapy, immunosuppression for organ transplantation, human immunodeficiency virus (HIV) infection, inactive carriers and even persons who have recovered from hepatitis B can experience reactivation of hepatitis B, which may be severe.[35,36]

Among the complications of chronic hepatitis B is hepatocellular carcinoma (HCC), postulated to be associated with incorporation of HBV DNA (but not at a recognized, uniform site) into the host genome.[37-41] Ironically, conversion from a state of free episomal HBV DNA to one in which HBV DNA is integrated into the host genome tends to occur, in nature, as HBV infection converts from highly replicative to minimally replicative. In all likelihood, integration of HBV DNA into host DNA does not rely upon this change in replicative status; instead, both integration and reduced replication tend to occur after prolonged HBV infection. Areas of high HCC and HBV prevalence overlap geographically[40]; the relative risk of HCC among persons who harbor HBsAg is 100-fold higher than in those lacking this marker of HBV infection.[37] Recent observations show that among persons with HBsAg, the risk of HCC resides primarily among those with markers of high-level HBV replication.[42] Similarly, severity and progression of chronic hepatitis B are more pronounced in patients with high levels of HBV replication.[22,43-45] Thus the level of HBV replication has a profound influence over the clinical expression of chronic hepatitis B.

Distinctions Based on Epidemiologic Considerations

Chronic hepatitis B follows acute HBV infection in more than 90% of neonates born to mothers with chronic hepatitis B but in only approximately 1% of immunocompetent adults with clinically apparent acute hepatitis B.[46-48] In Asia and sub-Saharan Africa, the prevalence of HBV infection is high, exceeding 10% of the population, whereas in many Western countries, such as the United States, prevalences of 1% to 2% are the rule. These differences in frequency translate into marked distinctions in clinical expression of HBV infection.

In high-prevalence areas, women of childbearing age have the high likelihood of infection characteristic of the population at large; consequently, the risk of perinatal transmission of HBV infection from an infected mother to her baby is high, representing the most common mode of HBV transmission in the population. Acquired in the perinatal period, HBV infection is unlikely to be accompanied by clinically apparent acute hepatitis but almost universally to result in chronic infection, a reflection of tolerance of the virus by the host immune system.[46] Although most such infected persons can have very mild, asymptomatic chronic hepatitis B during childhood and early to middle adulthood, the lifetime risk of succumbing to chronic hepatitis B in such high-HBV-prevalence populations can reach 40% as the result of cirrhosis and HCC.[37]

In contrast, in low-prevalence areas (e.g., the United States, western Europe), the low prevalence of HBV infection in the general pop-

---

TABLE 112-2 Distinctions among Patients with Chronic Hepatitis B

Distinctions Based on Levels of HBV Replication

HBV DNA $\geq 10^5$-10^6 virions/mL versus $\leq 10^3$-10^4 virions/mL
Wild-type HB_eAg-reactive versus HB_eAg-nonreactive

Distinctions Based on Epidemiologic Considerations

High-prevalence areas:	Perinatal acquisition, host tolerance, clinically inapparent acute infection, chronicity >90%, high risk of cirrhosis and hepatocellular carcinoma (HCC)
Low-prevalence areas:	Adolescent/adult sexual/percutaneous acquisition, host intolerance, clinically apparent acute hepatitis, chronicity <1%, low risk of cirrhosis and HCC

Distinctions Based on Viral Variants

Wild-type, HB_eAg-reactive versus precore or core-promoter (HB_eAg-negative) variants

HB_eAg, hepatitis B e antigen; HBV DNA, hepatitis B virus deoxyribonucleic acid.

ulation does not support a large cohort of infected women of child-bearing age; therefore, the frequency of perinatal transmission is low. Instead, most HBV infections in such Western countries occur during adolescence and early adulthood, enhanced by behaviors (e.g., sexual activity, injection-drug use, occupational exposure to blood and contaminated instruments) that foster the spread of blood-borne agents. Such infections result typically in a robust host-immune response to the presence of HBV on hepatocyte membranes, recognized clinically as acute hepatitis, and the cytolytic T-cell response is usually sufficient to eradicate HBV infection. Chronicity of hepatitis B under these circumstances is rare ((1%),[47,49] and, even among those with chronic hepatitis B in such low-HBV-prevalence populations, progression to cirrhosis, and especially to HCC, is much less likely. Therefore, hepatitis B tends to be a chronic, progressive disorder associated with a risk of HCC in high-prevalence populations but an acute, self-limited illness with a low risk of HCC in low-prevalence populations.

What appears to drive the distinction between hepatitis B acquired in infancy and in adulthood is the level of immunologic tolerance to HBV, which is high in the former and low in the latter group. In fact, most persons with chronic hepatitis B do not recall having experienced an acute-hepatitis–like illness (i.e., an episode in which the host-immune system mounted a vigorous attack on HBV-infected liver cells). In this vein, the clinical expression of HBV infection in the immunocompromised host resembles the pattern that occurs in high-prevalence, early-life acquisition areas (high likelihood of chronic infection and its consequences) rather than the pattern of low-prevalence, adulthood-acquired infection.

At least seven genotypes of HBV have been identified, varying in geographic distribution, but our understanding of the impact of genotype on the severity and consequences of chronic hepatitis B is limited.[50-52] Preliminary observations suggest that genotype B is more likely than genotype C to result in severe, progressive chronic hepatitis B and HCC.[53-56]

Distinctions Based on Viral Variants

The distinction between high-replication, HB$_e$Ag-reactive and low-replication HB$_e$Ag-negative chronic hepatitis B has been complicated by the recognition of a variant of chronic hepatitis B, HB$_e$Ag-negative chronic hepatitis B. In this subset of patients with chronic hepatitis B, HB$_e$Ag is undetectable, but other markers of enhanced HBV replication (HBV DNA, intrahepatocytic HB$_c$Ag), elevation of serum aminotransferase activity, and histologic evidence of chronic liver injury are present. Harboring mutations in the precore region of the HBV genome (precore mutations or core-promoter mutations [see Chapter 142]), these patients have HBV infection in which the soluble, nucleocapsid HB$_e$Ag protein cannot be transcribed or translated.[57-63]

Generally, these mutations are acquired later in the natural history of chronic hepatitis B among persons infected early in life, i.e., they follow infection with wild-type HBV infection.[64,65] The exception to this observation are patients with precore-mutant, fulminant hepatitis B in whom HB$_e$Ag-negative infection is transmitted perinatally or horizontally from persons with precore-mutant hepatitis B.[66,67] Still, all patients with these mutations have circulating serum anti-HBe instead of HB$_e$Ag. The precore mutation represents a G-to-A mutation at nucleotide 1896, resulting in a stop codon in the precore gene, where initiation of HB$_e$Ag transcription occurs. In HBV genotype A, the nucleotide at position 1858 is C, adjacent, complementary, and strongly bound to nucleotide 1896 in the loop structure of this part of the viral genome. Because the C_{1858}-G_{1896} bond is so strong, mutations have to occur at both of these sites for a precore mutation to occur, which is very rare; therefore, precore mutations are rarely seen in patients with HBV genotype A. In contrast, in genotypes other than A, the nucleotide at position 1858 is T, adjacent, complementary, and unstably bound to nucleotide 1896 in the HBV genome loop structure. Because the bond between T_{1858} and G_{1896} is so unstable, G_{1896}A mutations can occur readily, without the need for a complementary mutation at position 1858. Therefore, precore mutations occur primarily among persons with HBV genotypes other than A. Consequently, precore muta-

tions and HB$_e$Ag-negative chronic hepatitis are relatively uncommon in parts of the world—the United States—in which genotype A predominates but are very common in other parts of the world—Mediterranean countries, Europe, Asia—in which other genotypes are prevalent.[68,69] Although wild-type chronic hepatitis B predominates in the United States, almost all contemporary cases of chronic hepatitis B in Europe and the Mediterranean are HB$_e$Ag-negative, and in the United States, HB$_e$Ag-negative hepatitis B has begun to emerge, fed by migration from these other countries.[64]

Levels of HBV DNA tend to be lower in patients with HB$_e$Ag-negative chronic hepatitis B, but episodic flares in necroinflammatory activity are common as are severe and progressive chronic hepatitis and its consequences, cirrhosis and HCC.[64] Important distinctions in response to antiviral therapy between wild-type HB$_e$Ag-reactive and mutant HB$_e$Ag-negative chronic hepatitis B are discussed below.

Pathophysiology and Natural History

As noted earlier, like the other human hepatitis viruses, HBV is not cytopathic but instead engenders an endogenous cytolytic T-cell response to virus-infected hepatocytes.[70] Although nucleocapsid HBV antigens appear to be the target for cytolytic T cells, the complex cellular and humoral host factors, and the interaction among them, that determine the severity, duration, and outcome of hepatitis B, are poorly understood. Some authorities have postulated that periods of relative inactivity followed by periods of accelerated liver injury represent an "immune tolerance" phase and an "immune intolerance" phase, respectively, in the natural history of chronic hepatitis B.[29] Such a model, however, is too simplistic and fails to account for low-level or episodic liver injury occurring during periods postulated to represent a tolerance phase; for periods of quiescence that can occur later in the natural history of chronic hepatitis B; for reactivations that can occur at any time during the course of chronic hepatitis B; or for waxing and waning necroinflammatory activity that occurs so commonly in HB$_e$Ag-negative chronic hepatitis B. Currently, the consensus view is that viral proteins are presented by antigen-presenting cells to CD4$^+$ (Th1) lymphocytes and to CD8$^+$ (Th2) lymphocytes. In acute, self-limited HBV infection, the CD4$^+$/Th1 response dominates, supporting cytolytic T-cell destruction of viral antigen–expressing hepatocytes. In chronic hepatitis B, Th2 responses dominate, whereas the weaker cytolytic T-cell response to HBV-infected hepatocytes is insufficient to clear virus-infected cells but sufficient to maintain inefficient but persistent hepatocyte injury. Evidence in experimental chimpanzee infection, however, suggests that this adaptive cellular immune response plays a secondary or "mop-up" role following the innate immune response, which clears 90% of the virus prior to, and without any, liver injury.[71-77]

Clinical Features

In chronic hepatitis B, symptoms run the gamut from absent to severe, debilitating, and life threatening.[44,78] Among inactive hepatitis B carriers and persons with mild to moderate chronic hepatitis B, symptoms are usually absent, although some patients with mild to moderate chronic hepatitis B report fatigue and, less commonly, right upper quadrant discomfort or "fullness." More severe and advanced cases can be associated with fatigue and jaundice, but persons with compensated cirrhosis may have no symptoms at all. Decompensated cirrhosis may be accompanied by fatigue, jaundice, loss of muscle mass (weight loss), ascites, edema, bruising (coagulopathy), gastrointestinal bleeding (gastroesophageal varices or portal hypertensive gastropathy), and/or hepatic encephalopathy. As is the case for acute hepatitis B, chronic hepatitis B may be complicated by immune-complex manifestations, including cutaneous vasculitis, arthritis, glomerulonephritis, and generalized vasculitis.[79]

Viral and laboratory markers of HBV infection are summarized in Chapter 142. The biochemical hallmark of chronic hepatitis B is elevation of serum aminotransferase activity, with normal to near-normal alkaline phosphatase activity. In severe, progressive, and decompensated chronic hepatitis B, bilirubin levels can increase (hepatic excretory dysfunction); albumin can fall and prothrombin time can become prolonged (hepatic synthetic defect); and hypersplenism can occur (primarily thrombocytopenia and leukopenia). Autoantibodies are absent.[78]

Histologic features of chronic viral hepatitis vary from absence of necrosis and inflammation to architectural distortion and fibrosis characteristic of cirrhosis. Generally, histologic injury ("grade") and fibrosis ("stage") are categorized as mild, moderate, or severe. The level of necroinflammatory activity/injury is based upon periportal necrosis, portal inflammation, and intralobular necrosis. Mild activity is confined to portal tracts, whereas necrosis and inflammation spilling beyond the limiting plate of periportal hepatocytes ("interface hepatitis") signify a more severe injury with increased potential for progression. The degree of fibrosis is based upon the localization and extent of scar tissue; fibrosis confined to portal areas is mild, whereas fibrosis that reaches beyond the portal tract (septal or bridging fibrosis), especially that which links portal tracts to other portal tracts or to central veins, connotes a more advanced and progressive process (see Table 112-1).[1,78,80]

Treatment

The goal of antiviral therapy in chronic hepatitis B is to prevent clinical and histologic progression, which in turn can be achieved by eradicating or, more likely, suppressing HBV replication to below the threshold for liver injury (10^3-10^4 virions/mL).[28] In patients with HB_eAg-reactive chronic hepatitis B, HB_eAg-to-anti-HBe seroconversion tends to be associated with a sustained reduction in HBV replication that persists even after therapy is discontinued. Therefore, in HB_eAg-reactive chronic hepatitis B, HB_eAg seroconversion is a potential end point of therapy, after which treatment can be discontinued.[81-84] In patients with HB_eAg-negative chronic hepatitis B, however, HB_eAg seroconversion is not an option, and a sustained response (i.e., maintained even after cessation of treatment) is a less realistic goal; long-term suppressive therapy is usually required.[64,85] Chronic HBV infection is associated with the presence in hepatocytes of covalently closed circular HBV DNA (cccDNA), and whether antiviral therapy can or should affect the level of cccDNA is the subject of debate. Although proponents of one type of therapy over another invoke relative efficacy of the drugs in reducing cccDNA, none have been shown to eradicate this stable form of HBV DNA, but all therapies that reduce HBV replication have been shown to reduce cccDNA as well. Similarly, persons with spontaneous HB_eAg seroconversion experience a concomitant reduction in serum and liver HBV DNA and in hepatic cccDNA. Although demonstrated to date only after interferon therapy,[86-88] successful antiviral therapy with any agent is likely to have a beneficial impact on the natural history of chronic hepatitis B.

Studies of viral kinetics after the initiation of antiviral therapy with any of the available drugs suggest a biphasic decay in viral replication.[89] The short, first phase is related to the viral half-life (approximately 1-2 days), and the second, longer phase is related to the half-life of virus-infected cells (approximately 18-40 days)[90]; however, this simple kinetic model does not account for observations in all patients. In some reports, the second phase is flat for some patients, whereas in others the slope of the decline changed several times, stepwise, during the course of therapy.[91,92] A simple, biphasic decay model is probably too simplistic and does not take into account host-immunologic/cytokine effects, the amount and production of cccDNA, and possible "cure" of infected cells, among other factors.

Candidates for antiviral therapy have HBV DNA levels greater than or equal to 10^5 to 10^6 virions/mL, usually with elevated alanine aminotransferase (ALT) levels, and with histologic evidence of liver injury. Both HB_eAg-reactive (generally with HBV DNA levels (10^5 to 10^6 virions/mL) and HB_eAg-negative (with HBV DNA levels (10^4 to 10^5 virions/mL) chronic hepatitis B are candidates for therapy.[29,30,45,93,94] Successful therapy converts chronic hepatitis B to an inactive carrier state; inactive carriers (characterized by HBsAg reactivity, absence of HB_eAg, HBV DNA <10^4-10^5 virions/mL, persistently normal aminotransferase levels, and absence of, or very limited, necroinflammatory activity [Histologic Activity Index <4] on liver biopsy) are not candidates for therapy with currently available drugs. Patients with decompensated

chronic hepatitis B are not candidates for interferon therapy but may experience therapeutic benefit from nucleoside/nucleotide analogues.

Three antiviral drugs have been approved by the U.S. Food and Drug Administration (FDA) for treatment of chronic hepatitis B: injectable recombinant interferon-alfa[95] and two oral agents, the nucleoside analogue lamivudine[96-100] and the nucleotide analogue adefovir dipivoxil.[101,102] In addition, several other new HBV-specific antiviral drugs are being evaluated in clinical trials, as are long-acting pegylated interferons, developed initially and approved for hepatitis C, and tenofovir disoproxil fumarate, developed initially and approved for HIV infection.[103]

Interferon-alfa

Although reports describing antiviral activity of interferons in patients with chronic hepatitis B date back to the mid-1970s,[104] not until the late 1980s was the convincing efficacy of recombinant interferon-alfa in chronic hepatitis B demonstrated in controlled clinical trials.[95,105,106] Initially, trials focused on patients with HB_eAg-reactive chronic hepatitis B (prior to widespread recognition of HB_eAg-negative chronic hepatitis B). Treatment courses shorter than 3 months were found to be ineffective; interferon-alfa is administered at a dose of 5 million units daily or 10 million units three times a week for 16 weeks.[107-109] A meta-analysis of 15 randomized controlled trials conducted before 1993 and involving 837 subjects showed that interferon-alfa could achieve loss of HB_eAg and of detectable HBV DNA (then measured by insensitive hybridization assays with a detection threshold of $\geq 10^6$ virions/mL) in approximately 30% and loss of HBsAg in just under 10%.[110] The likelihood of HB_eAg seroconversion (loss of HB_eAg and acquisition of anti-HBe) is approximately 20%, and HB_eAg loss after interferon therapy was shown to be associated with histologic improvement. In a more recent meta-analysis of 24 randomized controlled trials involving 1299 patients (including some of the same trials as the 1993 meta-analysis), compared to control subjects, interferon-treated subjects experienced a 25% advantage in normalization of ALT activity, a 25% advantage in HB_eAg loss, a 23% advantage in clearance of HBV DNA by hybridization assay (detection threshold of approximately $\geq 10^5$-10^6 virions/mL), and a 6% advantage in HBsAg loss.[111] Relapse is infrequent after a successful HB_eAg response, and among patients with interferon-associated HB_eAg responses, post-treatment HBsAg seroconversions occur in as many as 80% over the decade following therapy in Western patients,[86,88,111-113] but not in Asian patients.[114,115] In addition, the natural history of chronic hepatitis B is improved after successful interferon therapy; during the decade following successful interferon therapy, both long-term survival and freedom from hepatic decompensation have been reported,[87] and one study from Asia demonstrated a reduction in the frequency of hepatocellular carcinoma.[114] In addition, interferon therapy was found to be cost-effective in patients with chronic hepatitis B.[116,117]

In Asian patients, retrospective studies have shown that hepatic decompensation and hepatocellular carcinoma occur even after spontaneous or interferon-associated HB_eAg responses, and that, by the time these complications occur, most patients have already lost HB_eAg.[114,118] In addition, in Asian patients, the frequency of HB_eAg seroconversion during interferon treatment may be slightly higher than in untreated controls, but, eventually, after treatment, the frequency of HB_eAg seroconversion in the untreated controls increases gradually to the same level as that seen in the interferon-treated group.[119] At first glance, these observations suggest that in Asian cohorts, antiviral drug–associated suppression of HBV replication will not translate into serologic benefit or into improvements in the natural history of chronic hepatitis B, as has already been demonstrated in Western cohorts. These observations, however, do not negate the hypothesis that *early* antiviral therapy could reduce the time during the life of a patient during which high-level HBV replication occurs and that this reduction in HBV-associated liver injury will translate into improvements in the natural history of chronic hepatitis B. Certainly, prospective studies demonstrating the association between baseline HB_eAg reactivity and HCC in untreated Asian patients[42] and reports of reduced HCC among interferon-treated patients in Asian patients[114] support this hypothesis.

In approximately 40% of interferon-treated patients, HB$_e$Ag and HBV DNA responses are accompanied by transient elevations of serum aminotransferase activity,[95,120-122] attributed to a host cytolytic T-cell response to HBV-infected hepatocytes. Similar acute hepatitis–like increases in aminotransferase activity occur during spontaneous HB$_e$Ag seroconversion. Because interferons have immunomodulatory properties, some observers have suggested that the activity of interferon in chronic hepatitis B is a combination of interferon-induced antiviral suppression and immunologic enhancement; others have suggested that the apparent immunologic reactivity is endogenous, occurring in the permissive milieu of sufficient suppression of viremia. Whether the aminotransferase elevations are related directly or indirectly to interferon, patients who are incapable of mounting such a response generally do not respond to interferon. Patients with elevated aminotransferase activity, assumed to have cytolytic T cells already poised to destroy virus-infected hepatocytes, are more likely to respond to interferon than patients with normal or near-normal aminotransferase activity, who, tolerant of the presence of hepatitis B antigens on hepatocyte membranes, do not respond to interferon.[95,120,123,124] Similarly, immunocompromised patients do not respond. In addition to patients with low-level aminotransferase activity and the immunocompromised, patients with very high HBV DNA levels do not respond to interferon, nor do adults who acquired the disease in childhood, common in Asian populations.[95,120,123,125] Attempts to treat very young Asian children with interferon were unsuccessful,[126-129] mostly in children with normal or near-normal ALT activity, but a trial of interferon-alfa in children ages 1 to 17 with elevated aminotransferase activity was just as successful as in adults with comparable biochemical features.[130] Although patients with decompensated cirrhosis can respond, their likelihood of doing so is low, and treatment comes at substantial costs in serious and life-threatening adverse effects and worsening liver disease.[131]

Another variable that appears to influence the response to interferon is the HBV genotype. Preliminary studies suggest that patients with HBV genotypes A or B are more likely to achieve sustained responses to interferon than patients with genotypes C or D[132,133]; however, genotype is not a determinant of interferon response in all studies.[134]

The HBV genome includes a glucocorticoid-responsive element, which is upstream of the promoter region[135,136]; therefore, glucocorticosteroids enhance HBV replication, as had been reported long before a molecular explanation was understood.[137,138] An approach to therapy exploiting this observation was so-called "steroid priming." Theoretically, a short course of corticosteroid therapy can be introduced, resulting in a transient elevation of HBV replication and suppression of cytolytic T-cell activity. Then, when steroid therapy is withdrawn rapidly, presumably, cytolytic T cells recover and are attracted by hepatocytes expressing abundant levels of HBV antigens. What follows is an acute hepatitis–like elevation of aminotransferase activity coinciding with a marked reduction in HBV DNA. Such steroid priming as a prelude to interferon therapy was evaluated in early clinical trials but was found to be no more effective than interferon alone.[95,105,139]

As the recognition of the importance of HB$_e$Ag-negative chronic hepatitis B emerged, interferon therapy was applied to this subgroup of patients. Although aminotransferase and HBV DNA levels were suppressed, relapse was the rule after cessation of short-term (6 months to a year) therapy.[140-143] Several reports suggested that longer-duration (>1 year) therapy could result in sustained responses of approximately 20%.[29,85,144-146]

Because HB$_e$Ag-negative hepatitis B predominates now in Europe, many European authorities consider interferon as first-line therapy for most of their patients with chronic hepatitis B.[93] Moreover, the observations suggesting that interferon stimulates immunologic reactivity to HBV-infected hepatocytes and the almost 10% frequency of HBsAg seroconversion in early clinical trials among HB$_e$Ag-reactive patients have been invoked by some authorities, more commonly in Europe and Asia than in the United States, to adopt interferon as first-line therapy for all patients with chronic hepatitis B.[93,94,147] Now that long-acting, pegylated interferons (see chronic hepatitis C, later) are available, these improved interferons are being tested in clinical trials, alone and in combination with nucleoside analogues, in patients with chronic hepatitis B. In a preliminary trial, peginterferon-alfa-2a at doses of 180 μg and 270 μg weekly appeared to be more effective than standard interferon-alfa-2a at a dose of 4.5 milli-International Units (mIU) three times a week[148]; however, the dose of standard interferon is half that used in registration trials,[95] and the frequency of HB$_e$Ag loss was no greater than that identified in previous clinical trials of standard interferon-alfa-2b.[110] More recent trials do suggest that peginterferon may be more effective than standard interferon,[147] but the superiority of pegylated interferons over standard interferon for chronic hepatitis B remains to be demonstrated. To date, clinical trials of standard interferons plus nucleoside analogues show no benefit over interferon monotherapy or nucleoside analogue monotherapy.[99,100,149-151]

Whether interferon continues to play a role in current treatment of chronic hepatitis B or is eclipsed by more novel therapies, interferon—associated with serologic, virologic, biochemical, histologic, and clinical benefits that persist for years beyond treatment—remains the standard against which new drugs are measured. The most obvious unfavorable features of interferon therapy are its subcutaneous route of administration and its limited tolerability, complicated as therapy is by systemic flulike symptoms, marrow suppression (cytopenias), irritability/depression, and autoimmune events, most commonly thyroiditis. Side effects are usually manageable but limit therapy in those with marked hypersplenism and severe psychiatric disorders. As noted earlier, patients with decompensated cirrhosis are not candidates for interferon therapy.

Lamivudine

Lamivudine, the (−) enantiomer of β-L-2′,3′ dideoxy-3′-thiacytidine and an analogue of deoxycytidine, is a reverse transcriptase inhibitor that results in HBV and HIV ribonucleic acid (RNA) chain termination.[152] The first nucleoside analogue approved for the treatment of chronic hepatitis B, lamivudine, 100 mg daily administered by mouth, reduces HBV DNA replication by a median of 4 logs.[153,154] In HB$_e$Ag-reactive chronic hepatitis B, 1 year of lamivudine treatment, whether in treatment-naïve patients or in those who had failed to respond in the past to interferon, is associated with HB$_e$Ag loss in just under a third, HB$_e$Ag seroconversion in 16% to 20%, histologic improvement in more than 50%, and a return to normal of aminotransferase activity in more than 40%.[97-100] Comparable results have been achieved in children.[155] Suppression of HBV DNA to levels undetectable by hybridization assays (with detectability thresholds of 10^5-10^6 virions/mL) is achieved in almost all patients[97-100] and to levels undetectable by PCR amplification assays (thresholds of 10^2-10^3 virions/mL) in approximately 30%.[153] Unlike interferon, lamivudine is effective in patients with high-level HBV DNA, but like interferon, lamivudine is more likely to result in HB$_e$Ag loss and seroconversion among patients with high baseline aminotransferase levels.[98,120,156] In fact, for the subgroup of patients with ALT levels greater than or equal to five times the upper limit of normal, whether white or Asian, lamivudine therapy achieves HB$_e$Ag seroconversion in approximately 55%. In contrast, for patients with normal aminotransferase activity, common in Asian populations, HB$_e$Ag responses are rarely achieved. HB$_e$Ag seroconversions are more likely if HBV DNA suppression is profound; in one report, all HB$_e$Ag responses were confined to patients whose levels of HBV DNA were suppressed to fewer than 10^4 virions/mL.[28] If HB$_e$Ag responses occur and therapy is stopped after 1 year, the response is durable in more than 80% of cases and, at least in Western cohorts—but not in Asians—may be followed by HBsAg seroconversion (>20% after 2-3 years).[81,82,157,158] Preliminary reports suggest that lamivudine responses are more durable among patients with more protracted treatment duration after HB$_e$Ag response[83,159,160] and among those with HBV genotype B than C infection[160]; in another report, HBV DNA suppression was substantially more profound in lamivudine-treated patients with HBV subtype ayw (genotype D) compared with those with subtype adw (genotype A).[161] If HB$_e$Ag remains detectable during therapy, cessation of therapy results in a return to baseline virologic and biochemical levels; long-term therapy, then, would be indicated to maintain clinical benefit, and HB$_e$Ag seroconversions have been shown to increase over time with duration of therapy, approaching 50% after 5 years.[162] During a year of lamivudine therapy, progression of fibrosis is retarded,[163] and with more protracted therapy, histologic benefit continues. In fact, in patients with compensated cirrhosis treated for 3 years cumulatively, *regression of cirrhosis* has been documented histologically to occur in two-thirds of patients.[164]

In HB$_e$Ag-negative chronic hepatitis B, an HB$_e$Ag serologic response is not a goal; instead, responsiveness is measured by biochemical, virologic, and histologic end points. In this subgroup of patients treated for a year, biochemical responses and suppression of HBV DNA to fewer than 10^4 to 10^5 virions/mL are achieved in three quarters and histologic responses in two thirds.[165] Undetectable HBV DNA as measured by PCR can be achieved in approximately 40% of patients. When therapy is discontinued, a return to baseline is almost invariable; therefore, to maintain benefit in HB$_e$Ag-negative chronic hepatitis B, long-term therapy is required.[145,166,167]

During lamivudine treatment, flares in ALT activity accompany HBV DNA suppression in approximately 40% of patients, and, in the absence of a sustained response (i.e., HB$_e$Ag response), post-treatment ALT flares occur in approximately 20% to 30% of patients.[98,168] Flares in biochemical activity may be no more common in lamivudine-treated patients than in matched placebo recipients, but post-treatment flares are more common in treated patients[158]; usually, post-treatment flares are mild and asymptomatic, but severe, even life-threatening post-treatment flares have been reported, primarily in cirrhotic patients whose hepatic compensation was marginal before treatment.[169,170] Therefore, whenever lamivudine is discontinued, patients should be monitored closely for several months.

Whereas patients with decompensated cirrhosis are not candidates for interferon therapy, they can respond to lamivudine, which can stabilize, retard, or even reverse clinical and laboratory markers of hepatic failure.[171-177] For example, in one report among 23 patients referred to a liver transplantation center after the availability of lamivudine, survival at 4 years was 60%. In contrast, among the 23 patients referred to the same center in the period immediately prior to the availability of lamivudine, all patients for whom donor livers were not available succumbed in just over a year.[174] In addition, a placebo-controlled trial of lamivudine in patients with compensated cirrhosis demonstrated a significantly higher frequency of disease progression ((2-point elevation in Child-Turcotte-Pugh compensation score, life-threatening complication of cirrhosis, emergence of HCC) in the placebo group compared with the lamivudine group, providing proof of principle that nucleoside-analogue maintenance therapy can prevent hepatic decompensation in cirrhotic patients.[178] The observation that lamivudine treatment can retard the clinical progression of cirrhosis suggests that such drug treatment can improve the natural history of chronic hepatitis B, as has been shown in Western patients treated with interferon for chronic hepatitis B.[87] Longer-duration follow-up monitoring will be required before this conclusion can be established.

Besides ALT flares that accompany treatment-related suppression of HBV DNA (similar to those seen during interferon therapy and to those that occur during spontaneous HB$_e$Ag seroconversion) and that accompany cessation of treatment (as viral replication resumes), no adverse effects of therapy were identified in registration trials of lamivudine compared with placebo, nor have adverse events been linked to lamivudine since its approval.[168] Unfortunately, when used as monotherapy, lamivudine is associated with viral resistance.[179] Mutations in the YMDD (tyrosine-methionine-aspartate-aspartate) region of the HBV polymerase emerge in approximately a quarter of patients treated with lamivudine for a year.[28,97-100,165,179-184] The most common of these are methionine-to-valine or methionine-to-isovaline mutations in polymerase domain C at amino acid 204 (M204V, M204I), often accompanied by upstream leucine-to-methionine mutations (L180M) in domain B.[185-187] With each successive year of lamivudine therapy, the frequency of YMDD mutations increases, reaching 70% at 5 years.[162] Initial observations suggested that YMDD-mutant hepatitis B was less "replicatively competent" in vitro,[180,188,189] which corresponded with the biochemical, virologic, and histologic benefit (compared with pretreatment baseline) maintained after transient ALT and HBV DNA elevations accompanying the emergence of the mutations.[179] Although HB$_e$Ag seroconversions continue to occur after the emergence of YMDD mutations, the frequency of HB$_e$Ag responses is lower in YMDD-mutant chronic hepatitis B, and, ultimately, after 2 to 3 years, clinical benefit is lost in some patients[157,162,164,179,190]; this clinical observation may be explained by the emergence of compensatory mutations in other polymerase domains.[186] In immunologically compromised patients, such as those with HIV infection or those receiving immunosuppressive therapy after liver transplantation, the emergence of YMDD variants occurs earlier after the initiation of lamivudine therapy and is more likely to precipitate severe acute hepatitis–like flares and hepatic decompensation[191,192]; severe flares can occur, as reported most frequently in Asian patients,[193] and are also more common in patients with marginally compensated cirrhosis.[170,194] Moreover, in persons with HBV-HIV coinfection, treatment with lamivudine monotherapy results in universal, rapid HIV resistance[195]; therefore, testing for HIV infection should be done prior to the initiation of lamivudine therapy for hepatitis B. When HBV-HIV coinfection is identified, lamivudine monotherapy is contraindicated; instead, combination-drug therapy should be instituted, and if lamivudine is used, the 300-mg HIV dose should be given.

When lamivudine was introduced, no other nucleoside analogues were available (the value of lamivudine-interferon combination therapy was never established in YMDD-variant HBV infection). Because patients tended to do well clinically, certainly compared with their baseline pretreatment status, for at least a year or two after the emergence of YMDD-mutant hepatitis B[157,164,179]; because cessation of lamivudine after YMDD mutations resulted in reversion to wild-type HBV and its attendant higher ALT and HBV DNA levels[181]; and because other antivirals were not available, the general approach was to continue lamivudine after the emergence of YMDD variants unless clinical benefit was lost. Now that other antivirals are available to which YMDD variants are responsive,[185,187,196-199] breakthrough resistance to lamivudine is managed by adding another antiviral drug (see later).

The optimal duration of lamivudine therapy has not been determined. In HB$_e$Ag-reactive chronic hepatitis B, treatment may be stopped several months after HB$_e$Ag seroconversion, and the durability of the response is anticipated to be more than 80%.[81,82] Some authorities suggest treating for another 6 months after seroconversion, and data suggest that Asian patients should be treated even longer before stopping therapy.[83] For patients who have not achieved an HB$_e$Ag response, and for patients with HB$_e$Ag-negative chronic hepatitis B, lamivudine treatment may have to be extended indefinitely.

Adefovir Dipivoxil

Adefovir dipivoxil is the oral prodrug of adefovir, an acyclic phosphonate nucleotide analogue of adenosine monophosphate with antiviral activity against HBV and other hepadnaviruses, retroviruses such as HIV, and herpesviruses. Although doses of greater than or equal to 30 mg daily are associated with nephrotoxicity, at a daily oral dose of 10 mg, adefovir dipivoxil suppresses HBV replication by medians of approximately 3.5 logs in HB$_e$Ag-reactive hepatitis B and 4 logs in HB$_e$Ag-negative hepatitis B, both in treatment-naïve and interferon-failed patients.[101,102] In a phase III clinical trial among HB$_e$Ag-reactive patients, adefovir treatment, 10 mg daily for 48 weeks, resulted in histologic improvement in 53%, return to normal of ALT in 48%, undetectable HBV DNA by PCR (<400 virions/mL) in 21% (median 3.52 log reduction in copies/mL of HBV DNA), loss of HBeAg in 24%, and HBeAg seroconversion in 12%.[102] A 30-mg group included in this study but abandoned because of nephrotoxicity achieved even better results: 59% histologic response, 55% biochemical response, undetectable HBV DNA by PCR in 29% (median 4.76 log reduction in copies/mL of HBV DNA), HBeAg loss in 27%, and HBeAg seroconversion in 14%.[102] As is the case for interferon and lamivudine, adefovir is more likely to result in HBeAg seroconversion in patients with elevated baseline ALT levels; for both the 10- and 30-mg doses of adefovir, the frequency of HBeAg seroconversion increased to 21% for the subset of patients with baseline ALT levels greater than or equal to five times the upper limit of normal.[102] Presumably, HBeAg seroconversion during adefovir therapy will result in a durable response that will allow treatment to be discontinued, but such durability remains to be demonstrated. Certainly, in the absence of an HBeAg response, indefinite continuation of therapy may be required.

In a phase III clinical trial among HBeAg-negative patients, adefovir treatment, 10 mg daily for 48 weeks, resulted in histologic improvement in 64%, return to normal of ALT in 72%, and undetectable HBV DNA by PCR (<400 virions/mL) in 51% (median 3.91 log reduction in copies/mL of HBV DNA).[101] Reactivation is the rule when treatment is discontinued, as observed after short-term interferon or lamivudine therapy. The histologic efficacy of adefovir is similar in patients with both mild and advanced fibrosis. In addition, adefovir appears to reduce $\log_{10}$ HBV DNA levels comparably across all HBV genotypes.[200] Whether cross-genotype activity represents an advantage of adefovir over lamivudine is debatable; HBV genotyping was not available when lamivudine registration trials involving approximately 1000 patients were done, and the number of lamivudine-treated patients in reports of variable responses across genotypes is too small to be conclusive.[160,161] In addition, HBeAg responses to adefovir did differ, ranging from 7% to 20%, among HBV genotypes A through D, but the numbers of HBeAg responses were too small for adequate statistical comparisons.[200] Like lamivudine, adefovir appears to retard progression of fibrosis in patients treated for a year.[101,102] Although reports have appeared in the literature suggesting that adefovir reduces cccDNA in treated patients, in fact cccDNA is reduced (rarely to undetectable levels) in patients who undergo HBeAg seroconversion spontaneously as well as in those achieving seroconversion when treated with interferon, lamivudine, or adefovir.

Adefovir, a flexible acyclic nucleotide that is very similar to its natural substrate, is less likely to be sterically hindered by mutated amino acids in the HBV polymerase YMDD binding site pocket.[185] During courses of adefovir therapy lasting 48 to 60 weeks in immunocompetent, immunocompromised (e.g., HIV-coinfected persons or liver allograft recipients), HBeAg-reactive, and HBeAg-negative patients, no viral resistance was encountered.[201,202] Moreover, lamivudine-resistant YMDD-mutant HBV responds to adefovir.[197-199] In clinical trials of adefovir for lamivudine-resistant YMDD-mutant hepatitis B, adefovir monotherapy (i.e., a switch from lamivudine monotherapy to adefovir monotherapy) reduced HBV DNA by a median of 4 $\log_{10}$ copies/mL and was just as effective as adefovir-lamivudine combination therapy (i.e., the addition of adefovir to lamivudine).[197,198] Based upon this observation, some authorities have recommended switching to adefovir monotherapy in lamivudine-resistant patients; however, when this is done, especially if any delay is introduced between the cessation of lamivudine and the addition of adefovir, ALT flares have been encountered in approximately a third of patients.[198] In addition, in vitro studies indicate that adefovir is actually more effective (lower IC_{50} and reduced resistance) in lamivudine-resistant than in wild-type HBV.[186,187] These observations argue for maintenance of lamivudine when adefovir is added for lamivudine resistance. Furthermore, although no resistance occurs during 48 or 60 weeks of adefovir therapy,[201,202] adefovir resistance does begin to emerge during the second year of treatment. These mutations occur in polymerase domain D, usually an asparagine-to-threonine mutation at residue 236 (N236T)[203]

but also in domain B, an alanine-to-valine mutation at residue 181 (A181V). Preliminary observations during the second year of adefovir treatment indicate that the N236T mutation occurs in 1.7% of patients and the A181V mutation in 0.8% of patients, for a 2.5% frequency of resistance, well below the 40% lamivudine resistance encountered after 2 years of treatment. These adefovir-associated mutations respond to lamivudine.[204]

Safety of adefovir at a dose of 10 mg daily is similar to that of placebo.[101,102] Elevations of ALT occur during and after cessation of therapy, just as was observed in lamivudine-treated patients. At doses of greater than or equal to 30 mg a day of adefovir, however, nephrotoxicity is encountered.[102] A distal renal tubular acidosis occurs, with falling phosphorus and rising creatinine. At a dose of 10 mg, adefovir has a high therapeutic index, and creatinine elevations greater than or equal to 0.5 mg/100 mL were not observed in the registration trials of adefovir.[101,102] At doses of greater than or equal to 30 mg, nephrotoxicity is not encountered before 6 to 8 months of therapy, and, when it occurs, it is reversible. Creatinine monitoring is recommended when adefovir is used, and reductions in dose frequency are mandated for patients with reduced creatinine clearance (C_{Cr}) (for C_{Cr} 20-49 mL/minute, every other day; for C_{Cr} 10-19 mL/minute, every third day; for patients undergoing hemodialysis, once a week after dialysis).

Novel Therapies

Several other drugs were evaluated but not pursued as treatments for chronic hepatitis B, including fialuridine, which had to be abandoned because of severe, irreversible life-threatening mitochondrial toxicity[205-207]; famciclovir[208,209] and ganciclovir, which were not sufficiently effective; and lobucavir,[210] which was abandoned for oncogenicity in experimental animals.[211] The thymidine analogue clevudine appeared promising, reducing HBV DNA levels by approximately 3 logs within a treatment period of 4 weeks and maintaining suppression for more than 6 months after discontinuation of treatment.[29,103,212] In addition, clevudine is the only antiviral drug reported to have activity against HDV. The very long half-life (>40 hours), however, raised concerns about drug accumulation and potential toxicity, and currently, this drug is not being pursued. Also being investigated are immunomodulatory and antifibrotic therapies and agents that, at least in vitro, interfere with HBV replication by interrupting the HBV viral genome directly[29,211,213]; however, none of these approaches is likely to be competitive with the current and new generations of nucleoside/nucleotide analogues developed to treat hepatitis B.[103]

Currently being evaluated in clinical trials is entecavir, a cyclopentyl guanine nucleoside analogue that, at a daily dose of 0.5 mg, reduces HBV DNA by a median of 5 logs[103,210,214]; although cross-resistant with lamivudine, the blood levels achieved with daily doses of 0.5 or 1 mg exceed the increased IC_{50} for YMDD-variant hepatitis B in the vast majority of patients.[186] In this vein, preliminary reports indicate that 1 mg of entecavir suppresses lamivudine-associated YMDD-variant HBV DNA by a mean of more than 4 $\log_{10}$.[212] Entecavir interferes with priming of the HBV polymerase, with reverse transcription of the minus strand of DNA, and with DNA-dependent synthesis of the positive strand of HBV DNA. Phase III trials are nearing completion. To date, entecavir resistance has not been encountered in phase II or phase III clinical trials, but early reports of resistance after liver transplantation have begun to emerge.[215]

The cytosine analogue emtricitabine is very similar in structure and activity to lamivudine. Already approved as therapy for HIV infection, emtricitabine is being studied in patients with chronic hepatitis B. Preliminary results in fewer than 100 patients suggest that at a daily oral dose of 200 mg, its activity is similar to that of lamivudine, suppressing HBV DNA by a median exceeding 3 logs and resulting in HBeAg seroconversion in just over 20% of patients. Resistance, which occurs in the same polymerase YMDD motif as lamivudine, appears to be somewhat less frequent at the end of year 1 (9%) and year 2 (19%) of therapy than lamivudine. Its advantage over lamivudine remains to be defined in adequately sized clinical trials.[103]

Also promising and the subject of current clinical trials are the HBV-specific small-molecule L-nucleosides, LdT (telbivudine) and the valine ester (to increase bioavailability) of LdC (valtorcitabine).[103,216] Telbivudine inhibits HBV (but not HIV or any other viral) polymerase, interfering with plus-strand synthesis of HBV DNA, and in preliminary human trials achieved a median 6 $\log_{10}$ reduction in HBV DNA copies/mL.[217] As an L-nucleoside, telbivudine is cross-resistant with lamivudine but retains activity against the M204V YMDD mutant (not against the M204I or double mutant). In preliminary clinical trials, M204I (but not M204V) resistance emerged in approximately 5% during a year of treatment. The combination of telbivudine plus lamivudine is not additive and achieves no greater inhibition of HBV DNA than telbivudine alone.[103] In fact, none of the currently available nucleos(t)ide analogues provides more profound HBV suppression in combination with any others than the more potent one used alone. In contrast, valtorcitabine, which inhibits HBV DNA by only 2 logs but interferes with both minus-strand and plus-strand HBV DNA synthesis, does appear to have additive activity, at least in the woodchuck model of hepadnavirus infection, with telbivudine. Human trials are anticipated.

Finally, tenofovir disoproxil fumarate, another acyclic nucleotide, approved as an inhibitor of HIV reverse transcriptase, has similar activity in vitro against wild-type and lamivudine-resistant hepatitis B. In preliminary trials among immunocompetent and immunocompromised patients (e.g., HIV-HBV coinfected patients and liver allograft recipients) with lamivudine resistance, tenofovir, 300 mg daily, has been found to reduce lamivudine-resistant HBV replication by 4.5 to more than 6 logs, with negligible nephrotoxicity, a profile that has the potential to be competitive with, or superior to, that of adefovir.[103,218-220]

As more and more potent nucleoside/nucleotide analogues are introduced, predicting what the antiviral therapy landscape will resemble in the coming years is difficult. Clearly, however, the trend has been in the direction of agents with the progressively more profound inhibition of HBV replication.[214,216] In studies of lamivudine monotherapy as well as in studies of lamivudine-telbivudine monotherapy/combination therapy, patients who achieved the most robust inhibition of HBV DNA were the most likely to achieve HB$_e$Ag responses and to avoid drug resistance.[217] For example, among 104 patients with HB$_e$Ag-reactive hepatitis B treated either with lamivudine monotherapy, with telbivudine monotherapy (400 or 600 mg daily) or with combinations of telbivudine plus lamivudine for a full year, for those with HBV DNA suppressed to levels undetectable by PCR, HB$_e$Ag seroconversion occurred in 43%, compared with 35% for those with HBV DNA suppressed to between undetectable and 3 $\log_{10}$ copies/mL, to 10% for those with HBV DNA suppressed to more than 3 $\log_{10}$ copies/mL but fewer than or equal to 4 $\log_{10}$ copies/mL, and to 7% for those with HBV DNA remaining more than 4 $\log_{10}$ copies/mL.[217] Similarly, regardless of the treatment arm, the 1-year incidence of viral breakthrough was zero for those with HBV DNA fewer than 3 $\log_{10}$ copies/mL, 19% for those with more than three but fewer than or equal to 4 $\log_{10}$ copies/mL, and 26% for those with more than 4 $\log_{10}$ copies/mL.[217] Thus the more potent the antiviral in inhibiting HBV replication, the better the outcome is likely to be (Table 112-3).

Inevitably, treatment strategies in the future will take advantage of the relative potencies of available antiviral agents as well as the value of combination therapy, in limiting resistance and yielding treatment synergies, such as improved antiviral kinetics.[211,221-225]

Recommendations for Therapy

Recommendations or guidelines for the treatment of chronic hepatitis B have been issued by the National Institutes of Health,[29] the American Association for the Study of Liver Diseases,[45] the European Association for the Study of the Liver,[93] the Asian Pacific Association for the Study of the Liver,[94] and others (Table 112-4).[30] A consensus among all these recommendations is that patients with normal ALT activity and HBV DNA levels below the threshold associated with liver injury (defined as $<10^5$ virions/mL), i.e., inactive hepatitis B carriers,

are not candidates for antiviral therapy. On the other hand, patients with HBV DNA levels greater than 10^5, ALT levels more than twice the upper limit of normal, and at least moderate necroinflammatory activity and fibrosis on liver biopsy, both those with and without HB$_e$Ag, are considered candidates for therapy. For patients with HB$_e$Ag reactivity, HBV DNA more than 10^5 copies/mL, but with normal or minimally elevated ALT levels less than twice the upper limit of normal, sustained responses are not likely, and treatment is not recommended.

For patients with HB$_e$Ag-reactive chronic hepatitis B who are candidates for therapy, interferon, lamivudine, or adefovir is a potential first-line treatment (Table 112-5). Several authorities recommend interferon as first-line therapy, focusing on its apparent "immunomodulatory" activity, the brief duration of treatment, and the potential for HBsAg seroconversion.[93,147,148,226] In fact, ALT elevations attributed to the immunologic effects of interferon are seen just as commonly during nucleoside/nucleotide analogue therapy,[96,98,102,227] and restoration of endogenous cytolytic T-cell activity/function occurs during nucleoside/nucleotide analogue therapy, as the level of HBV DNA is reduced.[228-230] Some favor interferon for the subgroups most likely to respond, i.e., those with high ALT and low HBV DNA levels; however, these are also the populations most likely to respond to nucleoside/nucleotide analogues. Moreover, HBsAg seroconversions were no more common in interferon-treated than lamivudine-treated patients in a head-to-head trial (although these HBsAg results were not included in the published report).[99] Although interferon requires only limited duration therapy and is not associated clinically with resistance, the need for subcutaneous injections and often intolerable systemic side effects limits its appeal. Lamivudine is safe and administered by mouth, and the subset most likely to respond to interferon is also highly likely to respond to lamivudine; furthermore, lamivudine is effective in a substantial proportion of patients who fail to respond to interferon,[100] including immunocompromised patients[191,192,231,232] and patients with hepatic decompensation.[171-177] On the other hand, the duration of lamivudine therapy is longer than that for interferon, and breakthrough resistance during lamivudine monotherapy is an impediment. Like lamivudine, adefovir is taken by mouth and is effective in prior or predicted interferon nonresponders, including immunocompromised persons,[233] but the frequency of resistance is very low, which represents a compelling advantage. Although adefovir is well tolerated, creatinine monitoring is recommended, and, at an adefovir daily dose of 10 mg, the median $\log_{10}$ reduction in HBV DNA and the frequency of HB$_e$Ag seroconversion—a potential treatment stopping point—appear to be somewhat lower than those achieved with lamivudine. Because patients with HB$_e$Ag-negative chronic hepatitis B require long-duration therapy, adefovir, associated with limited resistance, represents an attractive choice.

For patients with decompensated chronic hepatitis B, interferon is not an option, but either lamivudine or adefovir can be effective. For patients with compensated cirrhosis, lamivudine has been shown to reduce the frequency of decompensation,[178] but the emergence of lamivudine

TABLE 112-3 Relative Potencies of Approved and Novel Antiviral Drugs for Chronic Hepatitis B

	Log_{10} Reduction of HBV DNA
Approved	
Interferon-alfa	?
Lamivudine	4
Adefovir dipivoxil	3.5
Novel	
Entecavir	5
Emtricitabine	3-4
Telbivudine	6
Valtorcitabine	2
Tenofovir disoproxil fumarate	4.5 to >6
Pegylated interferon	3

HBV DNA, hepatitis B virus deoxyribonucleic acid.

TABLE 112-4 Recommendations/Guidelines for Treatment of Chronic Hepatitis B (HBV DNA >10⁶ copies/mL)

	NIH 2000[29]	AASLD 2001[45]	EASL 2002[93]	APASL 2003[94]	U Michigan[30]
ALT normal (<2 × ULN)	No	No	No	No	No
ALT ↑ (≥ 2 × ULN)					
HB$_e$Ag-positive	IFN or LAM	IFN or LAM	IFN	ALT >5 × ULN: LAM	IFN, LAM, or ADV
				ALT <5 × ULN: IFN/LAM	
HB$_e$Ag-negative	LAM	IFN ≥12 months or LAM	IFN 12-24 months	ALT >5 × ULN: LAM	IFN, LAM, or ADV
				ALT <5 × ULN: IFN × 12 months	
Cirrhosis					
Compensated		IFN or LAM	IFN	LAM	IFN, LAM, or ADV
Decompensated	LAM	LAM	LAM or ADV	LAM	LAM or ADV

AASLD, American Association for the Study of Liver Diseases; ADV, adefovir; ALT, alanine aminotransferase; APASL, Asian Pacific Association for the Study of the Liver; EASL, European Association for the Study of the Liver; HB$_e$Ag, hepatitis B e antigen; HBV DNA, hepatitis B virus deoxyribonucleic acid; IFN, interferon; LAM, lamivudine; NIH, National Institutes of Health; ULN, upper limit of normal; U Michigan, University of Michigan.

resistance reduces the anticipated benefit. For patients with lamivudine resistance, the addition of adefovir is recommended.[197,198,223]

Special Patient Populations

Pregnancy. The safety of antiviral drug therapy during pregnancy has not been established. Experience with lamivudine for pregnant women with HIV infection suggests that lamivudine is safe during the end of pregnancy, but data remain limited.[93] Although lamivudine treatment during late pregnancy reduces levels of maternal HBV DNA, studies have not shown that such antiviral therapy reduces the frequency of maternal-fetal transmission of HBV infection below levels achieved with administration of hepatitis B immune globulin and hepatitis B vaccine to newborns.

Liver Transplantation. Antiviral therapy with lamivudine or adefovir in patients with decompensated chronic hepatitis B may delay the need for liver transplantation; however, once liver transplantation is undertaken, HBV reinfection of the new liver occurs universally unless preemptive antiviral measures are instituted.[234-237] Prior to the availability of such antiviral therapy, the majority of patients undergoing liver transplantation could manage well clinically for several years, despite HBV reinfection; however, in an unpredictable proportion, severe allograft-compromising and life-threatening HBV-associated liver injury supervened. The most aggressive form of HBV reactivation, fibrosing cholestatic hepatitis, represents overwhelming expression of HBV in the hepatocyte.[238] Characterized histologically

by fibrosis and cholestasis out of proportion to necroinflammatory activity, this dreaded form of hepatitis B is more reminiscent of direct virus-induced cytopathic injury than indirect cell-mediated cytotoxicity characteristic of virus-associated liver injury in the immunocompetent host. The likelihood of recurrent hepatitis B (i.e., hepatitis associated with HBV infection) correlates with the level of HBV replication prior to transplantation; however, even patients with low-level HBV replication prior to liver transplantation can experience recurrent hepatitis B, because immunosuppression, especially with corticosteroids, enhances HBV replication.[135,136] In fact, even recipients of donor livers from anti–HBs-positive or anti–HB$_c$-positive donors have experienced hepatitis B reactivation after liver transplantation.[239] Patients who undergo liver replacement for fulminant hepatitis B may be an exception to the rule of universal reinfection; in such cases, rapid and overwhelming elimination of HBV-infected hepatocytes depletes the substrate for new HBV replication.

Currently, all centers performing liver transplantation follow a protocol of preemptive prophylaxis with intravenously administered high-dose hepatitis B immune globulin (HBIG) beginning during the anhepatic phase of the procedure and continuing daily for the first week, followed by periodic readministration indefinitely thereafter.[240,241] Rarely, however, HBV envelope (HBsAg) escape mutations emerge during HBIG therapy after liver transplantation.[242-245] The addition of a nucleoside/nucleotide analogue to this regimen has reduced dramatically the risk of recurrent hepatitis B post-

TABLE 112-5 Approved Antiviral Drugs for Chronic Hepatitis B*

	Interferon 5 MU Daily	Lamivudine 100 mg Daily	Adefovir Dipivoxil 10 mg Daily
Route	Subcutaneous	Oral	Oral
Duration	4 months	≥52 weeks	≥48 weeks
Tolerability	Poor	Excellent	Excellent
Nephrotoxicity	None	None	Creatinine monitoring recommended
HB$_e$Ag loss	33%	32%-33%	24%
HB$_e$Ag seroconversion	18%-20%	16%-20%	12%
HB$_e$Ag seroconversion If ALT >5 × ULN	?	55%	21%
Log₁₀ HBV DNA reduction	?	4	3.5-4
HBV DNA PCR negative	Unlikely	~ 30% HB$_e$Ag+	21% HB$_e$Ag+
		39% HB$_e$Ag−	51% HB$_e$Ag−
ALT normalization	HB$_e$Ag responders	>40% HB$_e$Ag+	48% HB$_e$Ag+
		>70% HB$_e$Ag−	72% HB$_e$Ag−
HBsAg loss during treatment	3%-8%	2%-4%	Unlikely
HBsAg loss after treatment	80% over 9 years	23% over 2-3 years	?
Viral resistance	Not recognized	15%-30% at 1 year	None at 1 year
		70% at 5 years	2.5% at 2 years
Cost (US $)	~$5000/4 months	~$1700/year	~$5600/year

*Generally, these comparisons are not head-to-head but are based on results of the drugs tested in registration trials compared with no therapy or placebo.

ALT, alanine aminotransferase; HB$_e$Ag, hepatitis B e antigen; HBsAg, hepatitis B surface antigen; HBV DNA, hepatitis B virus deoxyribonucleic acid; MU, million units; PCR, polymerase chain reaction; ULN, upper limit of normal.

Modified from Braunwald E, Fauci A, Kasper D, et al, eds. Harrison's Principles of Internal Medicine. 16th ed. New York: McGraw-Hill; in press, Table 287-5.

transplantation.[191,192,246,247] Moreover, availability of these potent nucleoside/nucleotide analogue antiviral agents—interferon is not effective—has permitted exploration of strategies to change the route (intramuscular versus intravenous) of administration and to reduce the dose, frequency, and duration of HBIG treatment.[237,248,249] Although the success of post-transplantation lamivudine therapy was hampered by the emergence of resistance,[182-184,191,192] the addition of adefovir, either as rescue therapy or as primary therapy, has overcome the problem of post-transplantation lamivudine resistance and its often dire clinical consequences.[199] Therefore, currently, the outcome of liver transplantation for hepatitis B is comparable to that for patients undergoing the procedure for nonviral types of end-stage liver disease.[237]

Human Immunodeficiency Virus Coinfection. Patients with HIV-HBV coinfection tend to have high levels of HBV DNA and more advanced histologic disease but with relatively limited elevations of aminotransferase activity.[250] Moreover, occasionally, immunologic reconstitution associated with successful highly active antiretroviral therapy (HAART) results in severe exacerbations of hepatitis B in coinfected patients.[251] Interferon is not effective in this subset of immunocompromised patients.[29] Lamivudine, when administered as part of the HAART drug cocktail used to treat patients with HIV infection, is given at a dose of 150 mg twice daily, three times the HBV dose, and is complicated frequently by lamivudine resistance.[252] In HIV-coinfected patients, the emergence of resistance limits the value of lamivudine, but adefovir has been shown to lower HBV DNA levels by 4 or 5 $\log_{10}$ copies/mL and to maintain this effect without resistance even after more than 2 years of treatment.[233,253] Furthermore, tenofovir, effective against both HIV and HBV, and now a popular component of HAART, represents an attractive first-line agent to be used in this population.[218,253]

Immune-Complex Disease. Immune-complex glomerulonephritis and generalized vasculitis (polyarteritis nodosa) can occur in patients with chronic hepatitis B.[79,254] Because these extrahepatic manifestations occur in settings of viral antigen excess, reducing hepatitis B replication can reverse the process. Early trials of interferon demonstrated improvements in nephrotic syndrome and in clinical findings in generalized vasculitis,[255] but oral nucleoside/nucleotide analogues are likely to replace interferon in the management of these patients.

Oncology Patients Requiring Cytotoxic Chemotherapy. When cytotoxic chemotherapy is administered to HBV-infected patients with malignancies, levels of HBV replication are enhanced, whereas cell-mediated immune injury of HBV-infected hepatocytes is suppressed. When cycles of chemotherapy are completed, however, restoration of cytolytic T-cell function occurs at a time of residual high-level HBV antigen expression on hepatocyte membranes, initiating a burst of hepatocytolysis and severe, often fatal, reactivation of hepatitis B.[35,36] Preemptive antiviral therapy with nucleoside/nucleotide analogues, initiated prior to chemotherapy, has been shown to prevent such reactivations of hepatitis B.[231,232,256,257] The optimal duration of antiviral therapy after discontinuation of chemotherapy remains to be defined.

CHRONIC HEPATITIS D

As described in Chapter 142, HDV is a defective agent with a plant-virus-like circular 1700-nucleotide RNA that requires HBV (or hepadnaviruses of other species) to replicate and that depends absolutely on the persistence of HBV to establish chronic infection.[258-260] When acute coinfection with both agents occurs simultaneously, the duration of infection is determined by the duration of HBV infection; therefore, HDV does not increase the frequency of chronicity of acute HBV infection. When HDV superinfection occurs in a person already infected chronically with HBV, chronic hepatitis D follows almost invariably (with rare exceptions), maintained by chronic HBV infection. Clinically, hepatitis D superinfection may be recognized as a flare in aminotransferase activity in a person with chronic hepatitis B, and, generally, chronic hepatitis B is converted to more severe chronic

hepatitis after HDV superinfection; for example, severe, even fatal, chronic hepatitis can follow in an inactive hepatitis B carrier superinfected with HDV.[259,261]

Clinical features of chronic hepatitis D are similar to those of chronic hepatitis B, except for the increased severity and more rapid progression to cirrhosis and end-stage liver disease; in addition, both early mortality and the risk of HCC are increased in patients with hepatitis D.[259-261] When hepatitis D was described originally, the more severe cases attracted clinical attention, and hepatitis D was felt to be invariably severe; however, mild hepatitis, even quiescent liver disease ("inactive carriage") has been recognized, and the disease can become indolent after an early period of severe hepatitis lasting several years.[262] In addition, three genotypes have been identified, with distinct geographic distribution, and genotype 2 has been associated with milder disease.[260] Although focal outbreaks of hepatitis D continue to emerge throughout the world, in Mediterranean countries, where hepatitis D was first recognized, the frequency of hepatitis D declined dramatically during the 1990s, attributed to changes in migration patterns, improvements in socioeconomic conditions, adoption of HIV-avoidance behavior among injection-drug users, and hepatitis B vaccination programs (immunity to hepatitis B protects against infection with hepatitis D).[263]

Although chronic hepatitis D tends to be more severe than, and to require concomitant, chronic hepatitis B, in one clinical situation, these generalizations do not prevail. After liver transplantation for chronic hepatitis D, hepatitis D reinfection can occur without high levels of HBV replication and without liver injury. Even in the absence of maneuvers to prevent the re-establishment of HBV infection (HBIG plus antiviral agents), the outcome of hepatitis D after liver transplantation is comparable to that after nonviral liver disease.[240,264,265] On the other hand, if, after liver transplantation for hepatitis D, high-level HBV infection emerges, severe hepatitis D may follow. Although hepatitis D, like other viral hepatitides, is likely to injure hepatocytes indirectly via cytolytic T-cell activation, and although autoimmune markers (liver-kidney microsomal antibody type 3 [anti-LKM3]) are common in hepatitis D,[266] the mechanism of HDV-associated liver disease has not been defined.

Serologically, the diagnosis of hepatitis D is established by the presence of circulating antibody to HDV (anti-HDV). Unlike anti-HBc in HBV infection, the distinction between IgM and IgG anti-HDV is not useful clinically; although not widely used clinically, testing is available in a limited number of specialized and research laboratories to detect HDV RNA by polymerase chain reaction.[267] Curiously, patients with chronic hepatitis D may harbor liver-kidney microsomal antibody type 3 (anti-LKM3) that recognize uridine diphosphate glucuronosyltransferase and that are distinct from similar LKM antibodies observed in type 2 autoimmune hepatitis and chronic hepatitis C (anti-LKM1) and certain types of drug-induced hepatitis.[266]

Treatment

Neither of the currently available nucleoside/nucleotide analogues active against hepatitis B, lamivudine and adefovir dipivoxil, nor other nucleosides (famciclovir, ribavirin, acyclovir) has been shown to be effective in patients with hepatitis D.[260,268] Interferon-alfa at doses and durations recommended for hepatitis B is ineffective for chronic hepatitis D; however, interferon therapy extended to 12 months and at a dose of 9 million units three times a week can result in clinical improvement (return to normal of aminotransferase activity and an improvement in liver histology) in the more than two thirds of treated patients, despite the fact that therapy has limited impact on HDV replication and that clearance of HDV RNA is unusual.[269] Although, in half of patients treated this way, aminotransferase activity remained normal for 6 months after therapy, ultimately, clinical reactivation followed after cessation of therapy in many patients. On the other hand, biochemical remission was maintained in a proportion of treated patients, even 14 years after completion of therapy, and, in some, clearance of HDV RNA and regression of fibrosis were documented.[260] An anecdotal report of a sustained biochemical, virologic, and histologic response after 12 years of interferon therapy (5 million units daily) in one patient[270] raises the possibility that protracted treatment may be the best approach for patients with chronic hepatitis D. Therefore, some have advocated chronic therapy until eradication of HDV RNA is achieved. Ultimately, novel antiviral approaches for the treatment of chronic hepatitis D will be needed.

As noted earlier, liver transplantation for end-stage chronic hepatitis D has an excellent prognosis; still, the same protocol of HBIG plus a nucleoside/nucleotide analogue used after transplantation for chronic hepatitis B is recommended for patients with chronic hepatitis D to minimize the likelihood of recurrent hepatitis B and its deleterious impact on post-transplantation HDV infection.

CHRONIC HEPATITIS C

In adults with clinically apparent acute hepatitis B, the likelihood of chronic infection is less than 1%.[47,49] In marked contrast, acute hepatitis C is followed by chronic HCV infection in at least 85% of cases.[7,271,272] Contributing to this high frequency of chronic HCV infection are its high replication rate (10^{11}-10^{12} virions/day with a virion half-life of 2-3 hours)[273] without polymerase error proofreading, molecular heterogeneity driven by a high mutation rate (1 mutation per synthesized genome), and, consequently, the virus' ability to change sufficiently and rapidly enough in the face of the evolutionary pressure of host immunity to circumvent neutralizing antibodies.[274,275] In addition to viral genotypes 1 through 6, the nucleotide sequences of which can differ by as much as 30% to 50%, HCV exists as multiple genetically distinct quasispecies, differing in nucleotide sequence by up to 5%.[276-279] Believed to have diverged phylogenetically from related viral agents more than thousands of years ago and to have evolved in humans for this extended period, HCV has established itself firmly among humans, infecting as many as 175 million worldwide.[9] In the United States alone, as many as 1.8% of the population (approximately 4 million) have been infected, and the Public Health Service estimates an annual death toll of 8000 to 10,000.[7,280,281]

The impact of hepatitis C is difficult to minimize. Chronic hepatitis C contributes to approximately 25% to 40% of all chronic liver disease[282] and accounts for up to 40% of all patients undergoing liver transplantation.[283-286] Economic estimates of the annual hepatitis C–related direct medical care costs incurred in the United Stated exceed $1 billion.[284] These statistics may seem surprising in light of the documented decline of acute hepatitis C cases reported over the past several decades. Initially, hepatitis C was recognized in recipients of transfused blood and blood products, but the frequency among transfused persons declined from more than 30% in the 1960s, to approximately 10% in the 1970s (exclusion of "commercial" blood donors),[287] to approximately 5% in the 1980s (adoption of "surrogate" screening tests that identified blood donors with an increased risk of blood-borne viral infections),[288-291] to less than 4% in the early 1990s (adoption of HCV-specific screening tests of donor blood).[292-294] During the 1990s, with progressively increasing sensitivity of donor screening tests for anti-HCV, the frequency of transfusion-associated hepatitis C fell to almost undetectable, effectively imperceptible levels, estimated now to be 1 in 103,000 units transfused.[295] This remarkable reduction in transfusion-associated hepatitis C, however, hardly made a dent in the overall frequency of reported cases, most of which occurred in groups other than blood recipients. In the 1990s, however, the overall frequency of reported cases of acute hepatitis C fell by more than 80% (to its current level of approximately 35,000) mirroring a similar decline among injection-drug users, who adopted behavioral changes designed to minimize acquisition of HIV infection.[296,297]

Despite the fact that the annual incidence of new HCV infections has declined substantially during the last decade of the twentieth century, however, the burden of long-established chronic infections continues to grow and is expected to triple or quadruple over the next generation.[283,284,298] The relatively recent decline in new cases has had no impact on the very large reservoir of chronic infections established, in most instances, two to three decades ago. Of the 4 million people estimated on the basis of serologic surveys to have chronic hepatitis C in the United States, only approximately half a million have come to clinical attention. In the vast majority of cases, hepatitis C is discovered in asymptomatic persons who attempt to donate blood or who have routine laboratory screening during medical evaluations or preinsurance physical examinations. In most such cases, an obvious epidemiologic source is not apparent, but often a percutaneous exposure in the very remote past can be elicited.[299,300] Exposed in adolescence and early adulthood, these patients come to medical attention in their 30s, 40s, and 50s, by which time they may have moderate to advanced liver disease. A more detailed discussion of the distribution and modes of spread of hepatitis C appears in Chapter 150.

Pathophysiology and Natural History

One of the envelope proteins of HCV, E2, contains a binding site for a surface protein on hepatocytes and lymphocytes, CD81, which may represent a cellular receptor for the virus.[301] Like the other hepatitis viruses, HCV is not cytopathic; instead, the presence of virus-infected hepatocytes initiates a cascade of host cellular immunologic events that culminate in clearance of HCV-infected hepatocytes. Early insight has been gleaned from studies of cell-mediated immunity to HCV polypeptides, and the host, genetic, and viral factors that distinguish between the small minority who recover and the large majority who proceed to harbor chronic infection after acute HCV infection are now beginning to be understood. From studies of cell-mediated immunity, a consensus has emerged attributing recovery to a more robust, broadly targeted CD4+ and CD8+ T-cell response to HCV proteins and chronic infection/disease to an absent or minimal and narrowly directed HCV-specific T-cell response.[7,302-307] For spontaneous resolution of hepatitis C, CD4+ T cells, specifically, have been found to be essential for viral clearance.[308,309] In addition, intrahepatic CD4+ and CD8+ responses against a wide spectrum of HCV epitopes have been shown to correlate with viral clearance and recovery from HCV infection, as has the presence of intrahepatic HCV-specific interferon-γ-producing T cells.[310,311] Moreover, genomic analysis of the progression of HCV infection in chimpanzees has revealed transcriptional changes in the interferon-alfa response that correlate with the duration of infection; in addition, genomic signals for antigen processing and presentation and for the adaptive immune response are expressed in association with viral clearance.[312] For HCV infection to be established chronically, as noted above, the host immune response to HCV is usually too limited in impact to contain the infection; in addition, this feeble immunologic response allows superinfection with a different genotype or viral isolate (absence of heterologous immunity) or even, under experimental conditions in chimpanzees, reinfection with the same viral isolate (absence of homologous immunity).[313-316] Accordingly, prospects for an effective hepatitis C vaccine to prevent infection are dim.[317] On the other hand, neutralizing antibodies have been identified against broadly conserved HCV epitopes[318]; potentially, this advance in understanding the humoral immune response to HCV could be exploited to pursue passive immunoprophylaxis with globulin preparations or active immunization with vaccines.

Host factors that have been suggested to correlate with a higher frequency of chronicity after acute infection include male gender, older age (adults more than children), ethnicity (African Americans more than whites), clinically mild/inapparent/anicteric acute infection, certain extended human leukocyte antigen (HLA) haplotypes, and immunologic compromise.[281,319]

The natural history of hepatitis C is variable.[319-329] As noted, as many as 85% of acutely infected persons acquire chronic infection. Progression to cirrhosis among those with chronic hepatitis C has been observed even in patients with asymptomatic and otherwise clinically, biochemically, and histologically mild disease. An analysis of 57 adequately sized and documented published studies showed that among adults (mean age of infection 42) with transfusion-acquired chronic hepatitis C, progression to cirrhosis occurs in approximately 25% over the course of 20 years.[326] A similarly high 20-year, 22% rate of progression to cirrhosis, probably magnified by selection bias, was recorded in cohorts of patients (mean age of infection 29) referred to liver clinics; however, recorded 20-year rates of progression were lower in community-acquired hepatitis C (mean age of infection 26), 7%, and in blood donors (mean age 22), 4%.[326]

Histologic features are perhaps the best predictors of disease progression.[330-333] Among a cohort of Japanese patients who underwent serial liver biopsies over a 20-year period, progression to cirrhosis was limited in those with histologically mild necroinflammatory activity and fibrosis.[334] In contrast, those with moderate and severe hepatitis/fibrosis progressed to cirrhosis almost invariably over 20 to 10 years, respectively.[334] Therefore, baseline liver biopsy is helpful not only to define the degree of liver injury that transpired in the decades before clinical presentation but also to predict the pace of histologic progression over the ensuing one to two decades.[335-337] In a U.S. cohort of 123 untreated patients who underwent paired biopsies a median of almost 4 years apart, histologic progression of fibrosis occurred in 39%, histologic stability in 37%, and improvement in 24%.[338] Whereas some investigators have devised models to assess linear progression of fibrosis in chronic hepatitis C,[331] others have emphasized that the rate of progression is variable, not linear.[336,338,339] In this U.S. cohort, the best predictors of histologic progression of fibrosis were advanced age, the grade of histologic necroinflammatory activity (especially periportal necrosis), and the level of aminotransferase activity.[338] Although a number of anecdotal reports have documented the presence of severe hepatitis and even, rarely, cirrhosis in patients with normal aminotransferase activity,[340-342] such severe histologic changes could have derived from an earlier period of biochemical activity, and in large groups of patients with normal aminotransferase levels, histologic studies have shown that the overwhelming majority of patients, with few exceptions, have mild histologic features.[300,343,344] In addition, in several longitudinal studies of patients with chronic hepatitis C and persistently normal aminotransferase activity, the absence of histologic progression over 5 years or more has been documented.[338,345-348] Therefore, the rationale exists for monitoring patients with persistently normal aminotransferase activity without therapeutic intervention.[349] Still, because as many as a quarter of patients with normal aminotransferase activity followed for several years will ultimately have aminotransferase elevations,[346] even patients with normal aminotransferase levels should be monitored regularly.

Variability in progression of chronic hepatitis C remains a confounding clinical feature of the disease. Yet to be explained are extreme differences in outcome between cohorts of young women who acquired hepatitis C from contaminated anti-D Rh immunoglobulin at the time of childbirth (17- to 20-year progression to cirrhosis of only zero to 2%)[322,325] and cohorts of recipients of HCV-contaminated intravenous globulin (<11-year progression to cirrhosis in 30%).[324] Similarly, the limited progression of transfusion-related chronic hepatitis C in young children compared with that in adults has been described but not explained.[350] For patients who acquired hepatitis C after transfusion in the 1970s, long-duration follow-up studies lasting 20 years (the Transfusion-Transmitted-Viruses Study) showed progression to cirrhosis in approximately 20% but no increase in overall mortality (and only a slight, almost negligible increase in liver-related mortality) compared to a matched, transfused control group in whom hepatitis did not develop.[319-321,328] Therefore, for someone whose perspective is molded by experiences in a blood bank—where asymptomatic, healthy persons with hepatitis C are identified during blood donor screening and where disease progression in transfusion-related hepatitis C is slow and clinically inapparent—hepatitis C appears to be a very slowly progressive and mild disease. In contrast, in a tertiary-care hospital with a liver transplantation program, referrals that funnel in primarily the sickest patients along the spectrum of disease activity[323] bias hepatologists and transplant surgeons to the view that hepatitis C is an invariably progressive and fatal disease. A more balanced reality exists between these

two extremes; in the majority of patients, chronic hepatitis C is a slowly progressive liver disease that may have few clinical consequences over the first two decades; progression to cirrhosis occurs in 2% to 4% of young children and young women, less than 10% of community-based, young adult (<40 years) patient cohorts, but in about 20% to 25% of referral center–based cohorts of older adults.[319,326,336] What is not known is whether, given a sufficiently long time (e.g., three to five decades or more), hepatitis C would be progressive in the majority of patients.

Neither the level of HCV RNA, HCV genotype, nor HCV quasispecies diversity correlates with the degree and rapidity of progression of chronic hepatitis C, but more advanced liver disease is found in patients with higher liver iron levels, almost certainly an indirect reflection of duration of infection.[319] Several factors have been demonstrated to accelerate or to be associated with accelerated progression of fibrosis in chronic hepatitis C, including advanced age at the time of infection; male gender; excessive alcohol use; coinfection with HBV, or, as is common in multitransfused hemophiliacs and injection-drug users, HIV; certain extended HLA haplotypes[351,352]; and concomitant other type of liver disease (e.g., hemochromatosis, steatohepatitis).[300,319,353,354] Fibrosis associated with steatosis has been recognized to be more common in patients with HCV genotype 3,[355] but hepatic steatosis associated with obesity may also be associated with a higher frequency of cirrhosis in patients with chronic hepatitis C.[356] African Americans, in whom acute hepatitis C is more likely to be followed by chronic hepatitis C, are actually less likely to progress to cirrhosis than whites. Severity of chronic hepatitis C is thought to be increased in patients with acute hepatitis A, based primarily on a report of fulminant hepatitis in a group of patients with chronic hepatitis C superinfected with hepatitis A virus.[357] This report, however, documented a unique experience not replicated by other observers.

Among patients with compensated cirrhosis secondary to chronic hepatitis C, long-term studies of the natural history of the disease have demonstrated a very good prognosis, with a 10-year survival of 80%.[358] Once evidence for hepatic decompensation appears, survival falls dramatically to 50%.[358] In cirrhotics, decompensation occurs at an incidence of 4% to 5% per year, mortality at an incidence of 2% to 6% per year, and HCC at an incidence of 1% to 4% (up to 7% in some reports) per year.[358-362] HCC, however, rarely occurs until HCV infection has been established for approximately 20, but more often 30, years, and almost all such patients are already cirrhotic or at the very least have advanced fibrosis.[363-365] Hepatitis C virus is neither a DNA virus nor a retrovirus and therefore does not integrate into the human host genome, as does HBV. In vitro studies suggest that HCV core protein and nonstructural protein NS3 can transform mammalian cells in culture,[366,367] and HCV core protein has been shown to induce HCC in transgenic mice,[368] but the mechanism of hepatocarcinogenesis in chronic hepatitis C is unknown. Like other chronic liver diseases associated with cirrhosis and HCC (e.g., hemochromatosis, autoimmune liver disease, α_1-antitrypsin deficiency, nonalcoholic steatohepatitis, and alcoholic cirrhosis), chronic hepatitis C may lead to liver cancer by promoting endlessly repetitive cycles of hepatocyte regeneration and repair, resulting ultimately in the emergence of malignant clones. Among cirrhotics with hepatitis C, excessive alcohol intake, hepatic iron overload, and concomitant HBV infection appear to increase the risk of HCC.[361] Currently, chronic hepatitis C accounts for approximately a third of all cases of HCC in the United States, where the incidence and mortality of all causes of HCC have doubled over the past 25 years and of HCV-associated HCC tripled during the 1990s.[361,369] In Japan, where HCV infection accounts for 90% of all cases of HCC, the frequency of HCV-associated HCC has tripled over the past four decades.[272,361] As the cohort matures of middle-aged adults who acquired HCV infection in young adulthood—now predominantly otherwise healthy and in the prime of their careers—expectations are that, over the ensuing decade, the frequency of cirrhosis will increase by more than 500%, of

HCC by more than 250%, of liver-related deaths by more than 200%, and of both hepatic decompensation and liver transplantation by more than 60%.[284,298,361,370-372]

Clinical Features

The most typical patient presenting with recently discovered hepatitis C is asymptomatic, but fatigue is one of the more common clinical features in symptomatic persons. Overall, clinical features of chronic hepatitis C, as well as of decompensated cirrhosis associated with hepatitis C, are similar to those of chronic hepatitis B. Similarly, laboratory test abnormalities in chronic hepatitis B and C are similar; the principal abnormality is an elevation of serum aminotransferase activity, usually ALT exceeding aspartate aminotransferase (AST), until cirrhosis supervenes, when, generally, AST exceeds ALT. More characteristic of chronic hepatitis C than other forms of chronic liver disease are episodic fluctuations in aminotransferase activity, postulated to result from bursts of hepatic necroinflammatory activity accompanying the emergence of new quasispecies that overcome host immunologic containment of HCV. With progressive chronic hepatitis C and evolving fibrosis, hypersplenism occurs, and platelet and white blood cell counts fall. In compensated cirrhotics with hepatitis C, laboratory indicators of hepatic synthetic function, prothrombin time and serum albumin, remain normal, but these markers become abnormal in decompensated cirrhosis. Impaired hepatic excretory function tends to be maintained prior to the emergence of severe end-stage cirrhosis, when bilirubin increases.[78,281]

Chronic hepatitis C can be accompanied by circulating autoantibodies, including nuclear antibodies, especially liver kidney microsomal antibody (anti-LKM1), similar to that seen in autoimmune hepatitis type 2.[13,373] Assays for circulating immune complexes (such as those that detect aggregated immunoglobulins or cold-precipitable globulins [cryoprecipitates]) can be detected in as many as half of all patients with chronic hepatitis C,[373,374] but only a small proportion of patients have immune-complex disorders (see later).

Histologic features of chronic hepatitis C are similar to those observed in chronic hepatitis B (see earlier).[375-377] Fibrosis stage 3 in the six-point scale of Ishak (or F2 in the F0-F4 METAVIR staging system) represents septal fibrosis, i.e., scar tissue extending beyond the portal tract and bridging portal-to-portal or portal-to-central zones of the liver lobule.[1,3] Fibrosis stages of 3 or higher are usually progressive and are accepted as histologic criteria for treatment.[335]

Disease manifestations unrelated to the liver have been described in patients with chronic hepatitis C, and HCV RNA has been detected in extrahepatic sites, such as lymphocytes and the spleen.[373,378,379] Among the extrahepatic diseases linked with HCV infection are autoimmune disorders such as Sjögren's (sicca) sydrome and immune-complex disorders such as essential mixed cryoglobulinemia (with a spectrum from mild leukocytoclastic cutaneous vasculitis [palpable purpura, arthralgias] to membranoproliferative glomerulonephritis).[7,281,380-382] In patients with immune-complex disease, HCV RNA and anti-HCV have been found to be concentrated in circulating immune complexes.[383] Essential mixed cryoglobulinemia (EMC) is associated not only with immune-complex diseases but also with lymphoproliferative disorders, such as monoclonal gammopathy of unknown source and B-cell non-Hodgkin's lymphoma, also reported to be more prevalent in patients with hepatitis C (with or without EMC).[373,374,384] Lichen planus and porphyria cutanea tarda have also been linked with chronic hepatitis C[281]; whether hepatitis C can cause neurologic disorders and impaired cognition[281] is controversial.

Hepatitis C Virus–Human Immunodeficiency Virus Coinfection. Because of the common blood-borne routes of acquisition of these two viral agents, approximately a third of patients with HIV infection (three quarters in the subset with injection-drug use) are coinfected with HCV.[385] As the introduction of HAART reduced dramatically the frequency of life-threatening opportunistic infections and malignancies and improved survival, hepatitis C emerged as an important cause of morbidity and mortality in HIV-infected persons. The level of viremia is amplified, the rate of hepatic fibrosis is higher, the course of chronic hepatitis C is accelerated, and the frequency of liver failure more pronounced in HIV-HCV coinfected patients.[386-390] Since the introduction of HAART for HIV infection, mortality secondary to end-stage liver disease caused by HCV infection in this patient population has increased fivefold.[391] Occasionally, an acute hepatitis-like biochemical flare follows the initiation of HAART therapy in HIV-HCV coinfected patients; HAART-related immune recovery resulting in cytolytic T-cell injury of HCV-infected hepatocytes has been invoked to explain this observation.[392]

Treatment

When recombinant interferon-alfa was first approved and introduced in the early 1980s, the duration of therapy (at a dose of 3 million units administered subcutaneously three times a week) was 6 months. The therapeutic end point in early clinical trials was a return to normal of alanine aminotransferase activity (end-treatment response) that occurred in approximately half of all treated patients during therapy but that was sustained 6 months after therapy in less than a quarter.[393-395] When assays were introduced to detect the presence of HCV RNA by reverse-transcription PCR, application of these assays demonstrated that sustained virologic responses (SVRs; i.e., those sustained for at least 6 months after the cessation of therapy), a more stringent end point than biochemical outcome, occurred in less than 10% of patients treated for 6 months.[395] Higher doses, more frequent administration, and different preparations (alfa-2b, alfa-2a, consensus, leukocyte, etc.) of interferon failed to increase the frequency of SVRs, as did induction therapy with higher doses and/or more frequent administration during the early months of therapy.[349,395-404] Doubling the duration of therapy to 12 months, however, doubled the frequency of SVRs to approximately 20%.[395,397,398] The efficacy of therapy was doubled again to approximately 40% when the oral guanine nucleoside ribavirin was added to interferon treatment.[405,406] Ribavirin, active against flaviviruses to which HCV is related, has little demonstrable impact, if any, on HCV replication and is ineffective when used alone[407-409]; however, potentially, this nucleoside analogue could result in immunologic modulation (shift from Th2 response to Th1 response), inhibition of host inosine monophosphate dehydrogenase (IMPDH) activity,[410-413] or induction of viral mutational catastrophe.[414-416] Although the mechanism of ribavirin activity in HCV infection is not known, the addition of ribavirin to interferon, with dose based upon patient weight, reduces the frequency of virologic relapse at the end of therapy, increasing substantially the efficacy of therapy.[404-406,417] Moreover, achievement of SVR after the completion of therapy has been shown to translate into a durable response characterized by maintenance of virologic, biochemical, clinical, and histologic benefit, equivalent to a "cure" in almost all cases.[418,419]

The efficacy of antiviral therapy was improved again by the introduction of pegylated interferons, long-acting interferons bound to polyethylene glycol (PEG). Limiting degradation of circulating interferons, pegylation prolongs the half-life of interferons substantially, permitting once, instead of thrice, weekly injections; pegylated interferon monotherapy doubles the frequency of SVR relative to monotherapy with its nonpegylated interferon counterpart.[420-423] Moreover, the addition of daily oral ribavirin to pegylated interferons increases the frequency of SVR to approximately 55%.[424-426] Two pegylated interferons have been approved, a smaller, linear, 12 kD, partially renally excreted, pegylated interferon-alfa-2b,[421,424] and a larger, branched, 40 kD, nonrenally excreted interferon-alfa-2a (Table 112-6).[420,422,425,426] The two are comparable in efficacy when administered with ribavirin, although the 40 kD molecule has a longer half-life and, because of its large size, a more restricted (8 L) volume of distribution, allowing a common dose (180 μg) to be used over a wide range of patient weights. The smaller, 12 kD molecule has a much larger (20 L) volume of distribution and is administered based upon weight (1.5 μg/kg). Neither pegylated interferon-ribavirin combination has a higher efficacy than nonpegylated interferon–ribavirin combination for patients weighing more than 85 kg.

The side effects of pegylated interferon and ribavirin are similar to those of standard interferon (primarily flulike symptoms, marrow suppression, irritability/depression, and thyroiditis [the most common of potential autoimmune reactions]) plus ribavirin (hemolytic anemia [mean 2-3 g/dL reduction in hemoglobin], nasal/chest congestion, pruritus, drug rashes, gout, etc.); however, neutropenia is more profound, resulting in dose reductions more frequently, in patients treated with pegylated (18%-20%) than with nonpegylated interferons (5%-8%).[424,425,427] Because of the risk of anemia in patients with ischemic cardiovascular or cerebrovascular disease, ribavirin should be avoided in such patients as well as in patients with marked anemia. In addition, teratogenic in animals, ribavirin should not be used in pregnant women or their sexual partners, and contraceptive use should be practiced by women of childbearing age and their sexual partners during and for several months after ribavirin therapy. Excreted by the kidneys, ribavirin is contraindicated in persons with renal insufficiency. The side effects of pegylated interferon plus ribavirin are not inconsequential and require substantial support from those supervising therapy. In the registration trials of combination pegylated interferon-ribavirin therapy, side effects or laboratory abnormalities led to dose reductions in 36% to 45% and drug discontinuation in 10% to 14%.[424,425] Although neutropenia is common, infections are not, even when absolute neutrophil counts fall below 500/mm³; therefore, white blood cell growth factors are rarely required. For patients with ribavirin-associated anemia, options include dose reduction or the addition of erythropoietin injections, which have been shown to improve symptoms of anemia but not necessarily the frequency of SVR.[428] Preliminary assessments among re-treated former nonresponders to standard interferons suggest that maintenance of the ribavirin dose is crucial to achieving SVR during pegylated interferon-ribavirin therapy but only during the first 12 to 20 weeks of therapy; dose reductions thereafter in patients with an early virologic response do not appear to reduce the frequency of ultimate SVR.[429] Whether these observations in re-treated prior nonresponders apply as well to patients being treated for the first time remains to be determined.

In registration trials, both pegylated interferons with ribavirin were tested versus a comparitor arm of standard interferon-alfa-2b with ribavirin; in these combination therapy trials, pegylated interferon-alfa-2b plus ribavirin was comparable in tolerability to standard interferon-alfa-2b plus ribavirin, while pegylated interferon-alfa-2a plus ribavirin was somewhat better tolerated (Table 112-7).[424,425]

In patients with chronic hepatitis C, aminotransferase levels fall during interferon therapy, without the transient ALT flare characteristic of interferon-treated patients with chronic hepatitis B. A two-phase kinetic reduction in HCV RNA follows interferon-based therapy; the first, steep-sloped phase lasts 2 to 3 days and represents inhibition of virus replication and/or release, and the second, less steep-sloped phase lasts weeks to months and is felt to represent turnover of infected hepatocytes.[273,430-432] Studies of standard interferon-ribavirin combination therapy demonstrated convincingly that a 6-month course of therapy suffices for patients with HCV genotypes 2 and 3, whereas a full year is required for optimal benefit in patients with genotype 1.[405,406] The duration of therapy and ribavirin dose were not

assessed equally in registration trials of the two pegylated interferons with ribavirin; however, conclusions from the trials of pegylated interferon-alfa-2a[426] are likely to apply to the use of pegylated interferon-alfa-2b. Therefore, regardless of which pegylated interferon is chosen, most authorities would recommend treating patients who have the more refractory genotype 1 with a full year of combination therapy and daily doses of ribavirin of 1000 mg (for patients weighing <75 kg) or 1200

TABLE 112-7 Comparison of Pegylated Interferon-Alfa-2a and Pegylated Interferon-Alfa-2b in Combination with Ribavirin as Therapy for Chronic Hepatitis C[*]

	PEG IFN-alfa-2a	PEG IFN-alfa-2b
Ribavirin daily dose validated prospectively in clinical trials[†]		
Genotype 1	1000/1200 mg	800 mg
Genotype 2/3	800 mg	800 mg
Duration of therapy in clinical trials[†]		
Genotype 1	48 weeks	48 weeks
Genotype 2/3	48 weeks	24 weeks
Demographics in clinical trials[‡]		
Male	72%	63%
Caucasian	82%	91%
Mean ≥SD age (years)	42.8 ± 10.1	43.9 ± 8
Mean ≥SD weight (kg)	79.8 ± 17.5	82.4 ± 18
± Bridging fibrosis	12%	29%
Genotype 1	65%	68%
HCV RNA (10⁶ copies/mL)	6.0 (mean ± SD)	2.7 (geometric mean)
Sensitivity of HCV RNA assay	100 copies/mL	100 copies/mL
SVR[‡]	56%	54%
Genotype 1[†]	46%-51%	42%
Genotype 2/3[†]	76%-78%	82%
SVR in advanced fibrosis, PEG IFN/ribavirin versus standard IFN/ribavirin[‡§]	44% vs 41%	43% vs 33%
Side effects of PEG IFN/ribavirin versus standard IFN/ribavirin[¶]		
Fever	43% vs 56%	46% vs 33%
Myalgias	42% vs 50%	56% vs 50%
Rigors	24% vs 35%	48% vs 41%
Depression	22% vs 30%	31% vs 34%
Variables associated with SVR[‡]	Non-1 genotype Age ≤40 Weight ≤75 kg	Non-1 genotype Age Weight Baseline HCV RNA No cirrhosis/ bridging fibrosis Ribavirin dose >10.6 mg/kg

[*]Comparisons are based upon studies of each drug tested individually versus other regimens in registration trials and do not represent head-to-head evaluations between the two pegylated interferons. In addition, study populations were not entirely analogous, and methods for determining virologic responsiveness and for recording side effects differed in the studies of the two pegylated interferons. Therefore, conclusions about the relative advantages and disadvantages of the two pegylated interferons should be interpreted cautiously.
[†]Includes all three registration trials.[424-426] In the second of two trials of PEG IFN-alfa-2a, the optimal dose of ribavirin for patients with genotype 1 was found in the treatment arm that was assigned to receive 1000 mg for weight <75 kg or 1200 mg for weight ≥75 kg; the optimal ribavirin dose for patients with genotype 2/3 in that trial was 800 mg.[426]
[‡]Includes data from the first two trials only.[424,425]
[§]In study of PEG IFN-alfa-2b, the comparison was between those with and without cirrhosis or bridging fibrosis,[424] whereas in the trial of PEG IFN-alfa-2a, the comparison was between those with and without cirrhosis.[425]
[¶]These categories of adverse events were the four that were statistically lower in the combination PEG IFN/ribavirin arm versus the standard interferon/ribavirin arm in the trial of PEG IFN-alfa-2a/ribavirin.[425] In the PEG IFN-alfa-2b trial,[424] but not in the PEG IFN-alfa-2a trial,[425] depression was assessed with a validated depression questionnaire.
HCV, hepatitis C virus; IFN, interferon; PEG, polyethylene glycol; RNA, ribonucleic acid; SD, standard deviation; SVR, sustained virologic response.

TABLE 112-6 Comparison of Pegylated Interferon-Alfa-2a and Pegylated Interferon-Alfa-2b for Chronic Hepatitis C

	PEG IFN-alfa-2a	PEG IFN-alfa-2b
PEG	40 kD, branched	12 kD, linear
Mean terminal $T_{1/2}$	80 hours	40 hours
Mean clearance	22 mL/hr/kg	94 mL/hr/kg
Clearance	Hepatic	30% renal
Volume of distribution	8 L	20 L
48-hour trough concentration	16,000 pg/mL	320 pg/mL
Peak:trough ratio	1.3	6
Optimal weekly dose	180 µg	1.5 µg/kg (weight-based)
Storage	Refrigerated	Room temperature
Reconstitution in diluent	No	Yes

IFN, interferon; PEG, polyethylene glycol.

mg (for patients weighing ≥75 kg); for patients with the more favorable genotypes 2 and 3, 6 months of therapy and a daily ribavirin dose of only 800 mg suffice.[337,354,433] The likelihood of SVR is approximately 80% in patients with genotypes 2 and 3[424,425]; although comparable results can be achieved in patients with genotypes 2 and 3 when treated with nonpegylated interferon plus ribavirin,[424,425] improved convenience and tolerability favor pegylated interferon in these patients.

In registration trials of pegylated interferon-alfa-2a and interferon-alfa-2b with ribavirin, ribavirin doses, definitions of response and of adverse effects (e.g., differences in objectivity of recording depression), as well as baseline characteristics (e.g., average weight, percent male, percent with bridging fibrosis/cirrhosis) of the study populations were not entirely equivalent,[424-426,434] and comparisons between the trials of the two pegylated interferons (see Table 112-7) should be interpreted with reservations. Nevertheless, in these trials, among patients with genotype 1, SVR was achieved in 42% of those in the trial of pegylated interferon-alfa-2b (albeit with a suboptimal ribavirin dose)[424] and in 46% to 51% of those in the trials of pegylated interferon-alfa-2a.[425,426]

Genotype is an important predictor of response, as noted above. Other variables that correlate with reduced responsiveness include high-level HCV RNA, advanced histologic grade (necrosis and inflammation) and stage (fibrosis), higher HCV quasispecies diversity, higher hepatic iron levels, age older than 40, obesity, male gender, African American ethnicity,[435] limited adherence (<80% of prescribed interferon, <80% of prescribed ribavirin, <80% of prescribed duration of therapy),[436] and immunologic compromise.[403,424,425,437-443] Patients who fail to achieve a greater than or equal to 2 $\log_{10}$ reduction in HCV RNA during the first 12 weeks of therapy have a less than or equal to 3% likelihood of achieving an SVR, i.e., absence of an early virologic response (EVR) is a strong predictor of nonresponsiveness; in contrast, among patients who achieve an EVR, approximately two thirds will experience an ultimate SVR.[425,444,445] Therefore, the absence of an EVR at 12 weeks has been adopted by some authorities as an important milestone, after which treatment is discontinued, particularly in patients who do not tolerate therapy.[337] If, however, antiviral therapy has other potential benefits besides SVR, e.g., histologic improvement, continuing therapy in the absence of an EVR may be considered. In fact, histologic benefit has been demonstrated in three quarters of interferon-treated patients, including a sizable proportion without virologic response.[395] In addition, in prior nonvirologic responders to interferon monotherapy, a preliminary controlled trial of additional treatment versus no treatment for 2 years demonstrated histologic benefit in the treated group.[446] Therefore, clinical trials are in progress to determine whether maintenance therapy with pegylated interferon can prevent histologic progression in virologic nonresponders.

Successful treatment with interferon-based regimens has been associated with improved survival and with a reduction in complications of chronic hepatitis C in some analyses[447] but not in others.[404] Similarly, antiviral therapy has been calculated to be cost-effective,[448,449] even in patients with mild chronic hepatitis C.[450] In addition, therapy can retard the progression of, and even reverse, fibrosis.[451-454] Many reports have appeared in the literature purporting to show that interferon treatment of cirrhotic patients with hepatitis C can reduce the frequency of HCC.[455-457] These predominantly retrospective studies, however, were potentially flawed by a lead-time bias; treated patients may have had less advanced disease than untreated patients in these trials. Therefore, less advanced disease, not interferon treatment, may have accounted for the reduced frequency of this late neoplastic complication of chronic hepatitis C. Confidence in the conclusions of these studies is minimized as well by other subject selection biases; incomparability of subjects, treatment, and monitoring among trials; inadequately addressed confounding variables (such as alcohol use); and lower publication frequency of studies with negative results.[458] In fact, in other retrospective and prospective studies, interferon treatment had no beneficial impact on the risk of HCC in cirrhotic patients with

chronic hepatitis C.[358,459,460] To determine whether antiviral therapy does reduce the frequency of HCC, investigators have undertaken prospective controlled trials, now in progress, of maintenance pegylated interferon in patients with advanced chronic hepatitis C.

Candidates for Therapy

Patients with chronic hepatitis C, detectable HCV RNA, elevated aminotransferase activity, and histologic evidence of moderate to severe hepatitis and fibrosis (septal or bridging fibrosis, Ishak stage ≥3, METAVIR stage ≥F2) are candidates for antiviral therapy with recommended doses and durations (based upon genotype) of combination pegylated interferon and ribavirin therapy (Table 112-8).[337,354] In patients with histologically milder hepatitis C, progression is sufficiently slow to justify postponement of therapeutic intervention, but continued monitoring is warranted.[337] Because histologic findings predict future progression of chronic hepatitis C, and because treatment is recommended primarily for patients with moderate to severe, but not mild, necroinflammatory activity and fibrosis, a baseline liver biopsy is recommended as a prelude to antiviral therapy.[335,337] Patients with advanced fibrosis and compensated cirrhosis remain candidates for therapy, although their response rates are lower.[337] Whether antiviral therapy with interferon prolongs survival in cirrhotic patients remains the subject of debate, supported by some studies,[359] not by others.[358,460] In the registration trial of pegylated interferon-alfa-2b plus ribavirin versus standard interferon plus ribavirin, analysis of the subset with bridging fibrosis or cirrhosis showed that combination pegylated interferon regimens offered no advantage in SVR (43%-44%) over nonpegylated interferon plus ribavirin (41%).[424,461] Although the nonpegylated interferon-ribavirin combination was as efficacious as the pegylated interferon-ribavirin combination in these patients with advanced fibrosis, the more convenient once-weekly pegylated interferon regimen is more attractive to patients. In patients with decompensated cirrhosis, available antiviral therapy regimens, ineffective and poorly tolerated, are not recommended; instead, such patients should be evaluated as candidates for liver transplantation.[349]

In patients with persistently normal aminotransferase activity, histologic grade and stage do not progress, as documented by serial liver biopsies performed at intervals of up to 5 years[338,345-347]; however, combination therapy with interferon plus ribavirin is just as likely to result in an SVR in patients with normal as with elevated aminotransferase activity.[462] Therefore, this subset of patients may be considered as candidates for therapy or for close monitoring without therapy, depending on such patient variables as motivation, genotype, and histologic stage.[337] Even if a decision is made not to treat patients with such biochemically mild hepatitis C, they should be monitored for biochemical reactivation, which can occur in a quarter of such patients followed for 3 to 5 years.[346]

Patients who have relapsed after a course of standard interferon with or without ribavirin are candidates for re-treatment with the more

TABLE 112-8 Recommendations for Therapy of Chronic Hepatitis C

| | Weekly PEG INF Dose | | | |
	Alfa-2a	Alfa-2b	Daily Ribavirin Dose	Duration
HCV genotype 1	180 μg	1.5 μg/kg	1000/1200 mg*	48 weeks
HCV genotype 2	180 μg	1.5 μg/kg	800 mg	24 weeks

*1000 mg for weight <75 kg, 1200 mg for weight ≥75 kg. In the registration trial of PEG IFN-alfa-2b, the daily dose of ribavirin in the optimal treatment arm was only 800 mg; however, a post-hoc analysis of the data suggested that patients receiving higher doses of ribavirin per kg of body weight had better sustained virologic responses.[424] Most authorities would recommend daily doses of 1000/1200 mg of ribavirin (based upon weight < or ≥75 kg) regardless of which pegylated interferon is used.[337]

HCV, hepatitis C virus; IFN, interferon; PEG, polyethylene glycol.

effective combination of pegylated interferon and ribavirin.[463] For patients who have failed to respond to a prior course of standard interferon, re-treatment with combination standard interferon plus ribavirin yields only a marginal improvement in responsiveness, regardless of the interferon preparation used.[464-466] On the other hand, for such previous nonresponders to interferon, with or without ribavirin, re-treatment with pegylated interferon plus ribavirin can achieve an end-treatment response of up to 40% but a somewhat disappointing low SVR of less than 20%.[429,463] Factors associated with a reduced likelihood of an SVR in such prior nonresponders include genotype 1, a high baseline level of HCV RNA, the inclusion of ribavirin in their prior treatment, African American ethnicity, failure to achieve a substantial reduction in HCV RNA during previous courses of therapy, failure to achieve an EVR during re-treatment, and reductions in ribavirin doses during the first 20 weeks of therapy.[429,463]

In the pivotal registration clinical trials of antiviral therapy for chronic hepatitis C, restrictive entry and exclusion criteria confined the treated population to a narrow subset without co-morbid medical conditions, active alcoholism or other-substance use, uncontrolled neuropsychiatric disorders, etc.[467] Patients with these other conditions can be treated, however, if their other medical conditions can be managed effectively.[337] In most clinical trials, persons with advanced age were not included, and for many elderly patients with chronic hepatitis C, longevity will not be affected by the disease or its treatment. In elderly persons, although treatment should not be precluded automatically, baseline clinical and histologic characteristics, overall health, patient motivation, and anticipated survival independent of hepatitis C should be taken into account in determining whether to embark upon a course of therapy.[349]

In children, progression of chronic hepatitis C tends to be slow, and the disease follows a relatively benign course in most cases. Unfortunately, progression to cirrhosis has been reported in a small proportion of those with childhood-acquired hepatitis C. Clinical trials of antiviral therapy in this population are limited, but efficacy appears to be similar to that achieved in adult populations.[468,469] Antiviral therapy for hepatitis C in this population merits additional study.[337,470]

Special Patient Populations

Acute Hepatitis C. A clinical trial of high-dose, frequent interferon monotherapy (5 million units daily for 4 weeks, then three times weekly for 20 weeks) begun a mean of 89 days after infection in 44 patients demonstrated a 98% SVR 6 months after therapy.[471] Currently many experts recommend treatment of patients with acute hepatitis C with pegylated interferon plus ribavirin at conventional doses, but neither the optimal time to begin therapy nor the duration of therapy has been established in clinical trials.[337,470]

Liver Transplantation. End-stage chronic hepatitis C is the most common indication for liver transplantation.[286,472-475] Recurrent HCV infection is reestablished invariably in the new liver, but clinical progression during the early years after transplantation may be limited and overall early survival unaffected. In contrast, even during the first 5 years after liver transplantation, histologic progression appears to be accelerated, more than half of patients have moderate to severe hepatitis and approximately 10% have advanced fibrosis or cirrhosis,[476,477] and eventually survival is impaired.[478-480] A small proportion of patients with chronic hepatitis C experience early reactivation of hepatitis, and in those with early and difficult to manage rejection, added immunosuppression enhances HCV replication and may amplify HCV-associated liver injury[481]; furthermore, management is confounded by difficulty in distinguishing between rejection and viral liver injury based upon often overlapping clinical and histologic features. The most aggressive form of recurrent hepatitis C after liver transplantation is *fibrosing cholestatic hepatitis,* a rapidly progressive form of liver injury, described above in patients with hepatitis B undergoing liver transplantation, and characterized by progressive fibrosis, cholestasis, and severe jaundice out of proportion with necroinflammatory activity.[482,483] Unfortunately, currently available antiviral therapy for hepatitis C,

whether begun preemptively immediately after transplantation or introduced after the emergence of recurrent HCV-associated liver injury, is disappointingly ineffective after liver transplantation, sometimes suppressing HCV replication but almost never resulting in an SVR.[442,443,484,485] What is more, pegylated interferon and ribavirin are poorly tolerated after liver transplantation, necessitating dose reductions. Because immunosuppression enhances HCV replication,[486,487] attempts are made to minimize the use of immunosuppressive drugs following liver transplantation for chronic hepatitis C.[488]

Human Immunodeficiency Virus Coinfection. If CD4+ T-cell counts are normal, patients with HIV/HCV coinfection can respond to antiviral therapy with standard or pegylated interferon plus ribavirin, but the likelihood of an SVR is approximately half that expected in immunocompetent patients with HCV infections alone.[337,385,489,490] Antiviral therapy of HIV/HCV coinfected patients does not appear to have a deleterious effect on progression of HIV disease, but coinfected patients tolerate pegylated interferon and ribavirin less well than patients with HCV infection alone.[385] Moreover, because ribavirin is an IMPDH inhibitor, its use may potentiate the activity and toxicity of the purine analogue didanosine; therefore, these two drugs should not be used together.[491]

Immune-Complex Disease. The response to antiviral therapy is variable and often disappointing in patients with cutaneous vasculitis or glomerulonephritis resulting from HCV-associated essential mixed cryoglobulinemia. Although some may respond during therapy, SVR is unlikely, and many such patients may require indefinite maintenance of antiviral therapy.[349,492-494] In refractory cases, plasmapheresis and/or cytotoxic therapy may be required.

B-Cell Lymphoma. In patients with B-cell non-Hodgkin's lymphoma associated with chronic HCV infection, antiviral therapy has been reported to achieve disease remission.[495-497]

Future Therapies

Ribavirin enhances, but complicates, interferon therapy for chronic hepatitis C; therefore, second-generation ribavirins and ribavirin prodrugs associated with reduced hematologic toxicity are being developed. Although immune modulators and therapeutic vaccines have been proposed as potential treatments for chronic hepatitis C, precise manipulation of immunologic responses to HCV is not possible, and these approaches are not likely to be practical in the near future. In contrast, interruption of HCV replication with serine protease inhibitors and RNA polymerase inhibitors appears more promising. Several oral protease and polymerase inhibitors have been developed and subjected to early, preliminary clinical trials. Although a 3 log$_{10}$ reduction in HCV RNA has been achieved after only 48 hours of treatment with a prototype protease inhibitor,[498] cardiotoxicity in experimental animals derailed development of this drug. The results of clinical trials with other protease inhibitors and several polymerase inhibitors are awaited eagerly. Because monotherapy with such antivirals is almost certain to result in viral resistance, initially, these specific-enzyme inhibitors will be used in combination with pegylated interferon. Ultimately, interferon-based treatments are likely to be supplanted by combinations of orally administered, small-molecule, oral nucleoside and non-nucleoside HCV inhibitors.

REFERENCES

1. Ishak K, Baptista A, Bianchi L, et al. Histologic grading and staging of chronic hepatitis. J Hepatol. 1995;22:696-699.
2. Desmet VJ, Gerber M, Hoofnagle JH, et al. Classification of chronic hepatitis: Diagnosis, grading, and staging. HEPATOLOGY. 1994;19:1513-1520.
3. Bedossa P, Poynard T, French METAVIR Cooperative Study Group. An algorithm for grading activity in chronic hepatitis C. Hepatology. 1994;24:289-293.
4. Lee WM. Hepatitis B virus infection. N Engl J Med. 1997;337:1733-1745.
5. Kane M. Global programme for control of hepatitis B infection. Vaccine. 1995;13:S47-S49.
6. Alter MJ. Epidemiology of hepatitis B in Europe and worldwide. J Hepatol. 2003;39 (Suppl 1):S64-S69.
7. Lauer GM, Walker BD. Hepatitis C virus infection. N Engl J Med. 2001;345:41-52.

8. Alter MJ, Mast EE. The epidemiology of viral hepatitis in the United States. Gastroenterol Clin North Am. 1994;23:437-455.

9. WHO. Global surveillance and control of hepatitis C. Report of a WHO consultation organized in collaboration with the Viral Hepatitis Prevention Board, Antwerp, Belgium. J Viral Hepat. 1999;6:35-47.

10. Schiff E. Atypical clinical manifestations of hepatitis A. Vaccine. 1992;10(Suppl 1):S18-S23.

11. Vento S, Garofano T, Di Perri G, et al. Identification of hepatitis A virus as a trigger for autoimmune chronic active hepatitis type 1 in susceptible individuals. Lancet. 1991;337:1183-1187.

12. Laskus T, Slusarczyk J. Autoimmune chronic active hepatitis developing after acute type B hepatitis. Digest Dis Sci. 1989;34:1294-1297.

13. Lunel F, Abuaf N, Frangeul L, et al. Liver/kidney microsome antibody type 1 and hepatitis C virus infection. Hepatology. 1992;16:630-636.

14. Simons JN, Leary TP, Dawson GJ, et al. Isolation of novel virus-like sequences associated with human hepatitis. Nat Med. 1995;1:564-569.

15. Linnen J, Wages JJ, Zhang-Keck Z-Y, et al. Molecular cloning and disease association of hepatitis G virus: A transfusion-transmissible agent. Science. 1996;271:505-508.

16. Simmonds P, Davidson F, Lycett C, et al. Detection of a novel DNA virus (TTV) in blood donors and blood products. Lancet. 1998;352:191-195.

17. Seeger C, Ganem D, Varmus HE. Biochemical and genetic evidence for the hepatitis B virus replication strategy. Science. 1986;232:477-484.

18. Lau JYN, Wright TL. Molecular virology and pathogenesis of hepatitis B. Lancet. 1993;342:1335-1340.

19. Bortolotti F, Cadrobbi P, Crivellaro C, et al. Long-term outcome of chronic type B hepatitis in patients who acquire hepatitis B infection in childhood. Gastroenterology. 1990;99:805-810.

20. Hoofnagle JH, Dusheiko GM, Seeff LB, et al. Seroconversion from hepatitis B e antigen to antibody in chronic type B hepatitis. Ann Intern Med. 1981;94:744-748.

21. Liaw Y-F, Chu C-M, Su I-J, et al. Clinical and histological events preceding hepatitis B e antigen seroconversion in chronic type B hepatitis. Gastroenterology. 1983;84:216-219.

22. Fattovich G, Rugge M, Brollo L, et al. Clinical, virologic and histologic outcome following seroconversion from HB$_e$Ag to anti-HBe in chronic hepatitis type B. Hepatology. 1986;6:167-172.

23. Lok ASF, Lai C-L, Wu P-C, et al. Spontaneous hepatitis B e antigen to antibody seroconversion and reversion in Chinese patients with chronic hepatitis B virus infection. Gastroenterology. 1987;92:1839-1843.

24. Perrillo RP, Brunt EM. Hepatic histologic and immunohistochemical changes in chronic hepatitis B after prolonged clearance of hepatitis B e antigen and hepatitis B surface antigen. Ann Intern Med. 1991;115:113-115.

25. Hsu Y-S, Chien R-N, Yeh C-T, et al. Long-term outcome after spontaneous HB$_e$Ag seroconversion in patients with chronic hepatitis B. Hepatology. 2002;35:1522-1527.

26. Realdi G, Alberti A, Rugge M, et al. Seroconversion from hepatitis B e antigen to anti-HBe in chronic hepatitis B virus infection. Gastroenterology. 1980;79:195-199.

27. Di Bisceglie AM, Waggoner JG, Hoofnagle JH. Hepatitis B virus deoxyribonucleic acid in liver of chronic carriers: Correlation with serum markers and changes associated with loss of hepatitis B e antigen after antiviral therapy. Gastroenterology. 1987;93:1236-1241.

28. Gauthier J, Bourne EJ, Lutz MW, et al. Quantitation of hepatitis B viremia and emergence of YMDD variants in patients with chronic hepatitis B treated with lamivudine. J Infect Dis. 1999;180:1757-1752.

29. Lok AS, Heathcote EJ, Hoofnagle JH. Management of hepatitis B: 2000—summary of a workshop. Gastroenterology. 2001;120:1828-1853.

30. Conjeevaram HS, Lok AS-F. Management of chronic hepatitis B. J Hepatol. 2003;38:S90-S103.

31. Stevens CE, Neurath RA, Beasley RP, et al. HB$_e$Ag and anti-HBe detection by radioimmunoassay. Correlation with vertical transmission of hepatitis B virus in Taiwan. J Med Virol 1979;3:237-241.

32. Alter HJ, Seeff LB, Kaplan PM, et al. Type B hepatitis: The infectivity of blood positive for e antigen and DNA polymerase after accidental needlestick exposure. N Engl J Med. 1976;295:909-913.

33. McMahon BJ, Alberts SR, Wainwright RB, et al. Hepatitis B-related sequelae. Prospective study in 1400 hepatitis B surface antigen-positive Alaska native carriers. Arch Intern Med. 1990;150:1051-1054.

34. Liaw Y-F, Sheen I-S, Chen T-J, et al. Incidence, determinants and significance of delayed clearance of serum HBsAg in chronic hepatitis B virus infection: A prospective study. Hepatology. 1991;13:627-631.

35. Hoofnagle JH, Dusheiko GM, Schafer DF, et al. Reactivation of chronic hepatitis B virus infection by cancer chemotherapy. Ann Intern Med. 1982;96:447-449.

36. Lok AS, Liang RH, Chiu EK, et al. Reactivation of B virus replication in patients receiving cytotoxic therapy. Report of a prospective study. Gastroenterology. 1991;100:182-188.

37. Beasley RP, Hwang L-Y, Lin C-C, et al. Hepatocellular carcinoma and hepatitis B virus: A prospective study of 22,707 men in Taiwan. Lancet. 1981;2:1129-1133.

38. Popper H, Shafritz DA, Hoofnagle JH. Relation of the hepatitis B virus carrier state to hepatocellular carcinoma. Hepatology. 1987;7:764-772.

39. Shafritz DA, Shouval D, Sherman HI, et al. Integration of hepatitis B virus DNA into the genome of liver cells in chronic liver disease and hepatocellular carcinoma: Studies in percutaneous liver biopsies and post-mortem tissue specimens. N Engl J Med. 1981;305:1067-1073.

40. Szmuness W. Hepatocellular carcinoma and the hepatitis B virus: Evidence for a causal association. Prog Med Virol. 1978;24:40-69.

41. Bruix J, Llovet JM. Hepatitis B virus and hepatocellular carcinoma. J Hepatol. 2003;39 (Suppl 1):S59-S63.

42. Yang H-I, Lu S-N, Liaw Y-F, et al. Hepatitis B e antigen and the risk of hepatocellular carcinoma. N Engl J Med 2002;347:168-174.

43. Fattovich G, Brollo L, Giustina G, et al. Natural history and prognostic factors for chronic hepatitis type B. Gut. 1991;32:294-298.

44. Fattovich G. Natural history of hepatitis B. J Hepatol. 2003;39(Suppl 1):S50-S58.

45. Lok ASF, McMahon BJ. Chronic hepatitis B. Gastroenterology. 2001;34:1225-1241.

46. McMahon BJ, Alward WL, Hall DB, et al. Acute hepatitis B virus infection: Relation of age to the clinical expression of disease and subsequent development of the carrier state. J Infect Dis. 1985;151:599-603.

47. Tassopoulos NC, Papaevangelou GJ, Sjogren MH, et al. Natural history of acute hepatitis B surface antigen-positive hepatitis in Greek adults. Gastroenterology. 1987;92:1844-1850.

48. McMahon BJ, Holck P, Bulkow L, et al. Serologic and clinical outcomes of 1536 Alaska natives chronically infected with hepatitis B virus. Ann Intern Med. 2001;135:759-768.

49. Seeff LB, Beebe GW, Hoofnagle JH, et al. A serologic follow-up of the 1942 epidemic of post-vaccination hepatitis in the United States Army. N Engl J Med. 1987;316:965-970.

50. Norder H, Courouce AM, Magnius LO. Complete genomes, phylogenetic relatedness, and structural proteins of six strains of the hepatitis B virus, four of which represent two new genotypes. Virology. 1994;198:489-503.

51. Stuyver L, De Gendt S, Van Geyt C, et al. A new genotype of hepatitis B virus: Complete genome and phylogenetic relatedness. J Gen Virol. 2000;81:67-74.

52. Chu C-J, Keeffe EB, Han S-Y, et al. Hepatitis B virus genotypes in the United States: Results of a nationwide study. Gastroenterology. 2003;125:444-451.

53. Kao J-H, Chen P-J, Lai M-Y, et al. Hepatitis B genotypes correlate with clinical outcomes in patients with chronic hepatitis B. Gastroenterology. 2000;118:554-559.

54. Chu C-J, Lok AS. Clinial significance of hepatitis B virus genotypes. Hepatology. 2002;35:1274-1276.

55. Sumi H, Yokosuka O, Seki N, et al. Influence of hepatitis B virus genotypes on the progression of chronic hepatitis B liver disease. Hepatology. 2003;37:19-26.

56. Chu C-J, Hussain M, Lok ASF. Hepatitis B virus genotype B is associated with earlier HB$_e$Ag seroconversion compared with hepatitis B virus genotype C. Gastroenterology. 2002;122:1756-1762.

57. Brunetto MR, Stemler M, Schoedel F, et al. Identification of HBV variants which cannot produce precore derived HB$_e$Ag and may be responsible for severe hepatitis. Ital J Gastroenterol. 1989;21:151-154.

58. Carman WF, Jacyna MR, Hadziyannis S, et al. Mutation preventing formation of hepatitis B e antigen in patients with chronic hepatitis B infection. Lancet. 1989;2:588-591.

59. Brunetto MR, Stemler M, Bonino F, et al. A new hepatitis B virus strain in patients with severe anti-HBe positive chronic hepatitis B. J Virol. 1990;10:258-261.

60. Lok AS, Akarca U, Greene S. Mutations in the pre-core region of hepatitis B virus serve to enhance the stability of the secondary structure of the pre-genome encapsidation signal. Proc Natl Acad Sci U S A. 1994;91:4077-4081.

61. Akarca US, Lok AS. Naturally occurring hepatitis B virus core gene mutations. Hepatology. 1995;22:50-60.

62. Chu CJ, Keeffe EB, Han SY, et al. Prevalence of HBV precore/core promoter variants in the United States. Hepatology. 2003;35:619-628.

63. Okamoto H, Tsuda F, Akahane Y, et al. Hepatitis B virus with mutations in the core promoter for an e antigen-negative phenotype in carriers with antibody to e antigen. J Virol. 1994;68:8102-8110.

64. Hadziyannis SJ, Vassilopoulos D. Hepatitis B e antigen-negative chronic hepatitis B. Hepatology. 2001;34:617-623.

65. Centers for Disease Control and Prevention. Recommendations for prevention and control of hepatitis C virus (HCV) infection and HCV-related chronic disease. MMWR Morb Mortal Wkly Rep. 1998;47:1-39.

66. Liang TJ, Hasegawa K, Rimon N, et al. A hepatitis b virus mutant associated with an epidemic of fulminant hepatitis. N Engl J Med. 1991;324:1705-1709.

67. Omata M, Ehata T, Yokosuka O, et al. Mutations in the precore region of hepatitis B virus DNA in patients with fulminant and severe hepatitis. N Engl J Med. 1991;324:1699-1704.

68. Chan HL, Hussain M, Lok AS. Different hepatitis B virus genotypes are associated with different mutations in the core promoter and precore regions during hepatitis B e antigen seroconversion. Hepatology. 1999;29:976-984.

69. Li JS, Tong SP, Wen YM, et al. Hepatitis B virus genotype A rarely circulates as an HBe-minus mutant: Possible contribution of a single nucleotide in the precore region. J Virol. 1993;67:5402-5410.

70. Chisari FV, Ferrari C. Hepatitis B virus immunopathogenesis. Ann Rev Immunol. 1995;13:29-60.

71. Ferrari C, Penna A, Guiberti T, et al. Intrahepatic, nucleocapsid antigen-specific T cells in chronic active hepatitis B. J Immunol. 1987;139:2050-2058.

72. Guidotti LG, Rochford R, Chung J, et al. Viral clearance without destruction of infected cells during acute HBV infection. Science. 1999;284:825-829.

73. Kakimi K, Guidotti LG, Koezuka Y, et al. Natural killer T cell activation inhibits hepatitis B virus replication in vivo. J Exp Med. 2000;192:921-930.

74. Tsai S-L, Chen M-Y, Lai M-L, et al. Acute exacerbations of chronic type B hepatitis are accompanied by increased T cell responses to hepatitis B core and e antigens. J Clin Invest. 1992;89:87-96.

75. Rehermann B, Ferrari C, Pasquinelli C, et al. The hepatitis B virus persists for decades after patient's recovery from acute viral hepatitis despite active maintenance of cytotoxic T lymphocyte response. Nat Med. 1996;2:1104-1108.

76. Rehermann B. Immune response in hepatitis B virus infection. Semin Liver Dis. 2003;23:21-37.

77. Ferrari C, Missale G, Boni C, et al. Immunopathogenesis of hepatitis B. J Hepatol. 2003;39(Suppl 1):S36-S42.

78. Dienstag J, Isselbacher K. Acute viral hepatitis. In: Braunwald E, Fauci AS, Kasper DL, et al, eds. Harrison's Principles of Internal Medicine. 15th ed. New York: McGraw-Hill; 2001:1721-1737.

79. Dienstag JL. Hepatitis B as an immune complex disease. Semin Liver Dis. 1981;1: 45-57.

80. Desmet VJ. Liver tissue examination. J Hepatol. 2003;39(Suppl 1):S43-S49.

81. Dienstag JL, Schiff ER, Mitchell M, et al. Extended lamivudine retreatment for chronic hepatitis B: Maintenance of viral suppression after discontinuation of therapy. Hepatology. 1999;30:1082-1087.

82. Dienstag JL, Cianciara J, Karayalcin S, et al. Durability of response after lamivudine treatment of chronic hepatitis B. Hepatology. 2003;37:748-755.

83. Ryu S-H, Chung Y-H, Choi M-H, et al. Long-term additional lamivudine therapy enhances durability of lamivudine-induced HBeAg loss: A prospective study. J Hepatol. 2003;39:614-619.

84. van Nunen AB, Hansen BE, Suh DJ, et al. Durability of HBeAg seroconversion following antiviral therapy for chronic hepatitis B: Relation to type of therapy and pretreatment serum hepatitis B virus DNA and alanine aminotransferase. Gut. 2003;52:420-424.

85. Manesis EK, Hadziyannis SJ. Interferon α treatment and retreatment of hepatitis B e antigen-negative chronic hepatitis B. Gastroenterology. 2001;121:101-109.

86. Korenman J, Baker B, Waggoner J, et al. Long-term remission of chronic hepatitis B after alpha-interferon therapy. Ann Intern Med. 1991;114:629-634.

87. Niederau C, Heintges T, Lange S, et al. Long-term follow-up of HBeAg-positive patients treated with interferon alfa for chronic hepatitis B. N Engl J Med. 1996;334:1422-1427.

88. Lau DT-Y, Everhart J, Kleiner DE, et al. Long-term follow up of patients with chronic hepatitis B treated with interferon alfa. Gastroenterology. 1997;113:1660-1667.

89. Nowak MA, Bonhoeffer S, Hill AM, et al. Viral dynamics in hepatitis B virus infection. Proc Nat Acad Sci. 1996;93:4398-4402.

90. Tsiang M, Rooney JF, Toole JJ, et al. Biphasic clearance kinetics of hepatitis B virus from patients during adefovir dipivoxil therapy. Hepatology. 1999;29:1863-1869.

91. Lewin SR, Ribeiro RM, Walters T, et al. Analysis of hepatitis B viral load decline under potent therapy: Complex decay profiles observed. Hepatology. 2001;34: 1012-1020.

92. Perelson AS, Ribeiro RM. Hepatitis B virus kinetics and mathematical modeling. Semin Liver Dis. 2004;24 (Suppl 1):11-16.

93. EASL Jury. EASL international consensus conference on hepatitis B, 13-14 September, 2002, Geneva, Switzerland, consensus statement (long version). J Hepatol. 2003;39 (Suppl 1):S3-S25.

94. Liaw Y-F, Leung NWY, Guan R, et al. Asian-Pacific consensus statement on the management of chronic hepatitis B: An update. J Gastroenterol Hepatol. 2003;18: 239-245.

95. Perrillo RP, Schiff ER, Davis GL, et al. A randomized, controlled trial of interferon alfa-2b alone and after prednisone withdrawal for the treatment of chronic hepatitis B. N Engl J Med. 1990;323:295-301.

96. Dienstag JL, Perrillo RP, Schiff ER, et al. A preliminary trial of lamivudine for chronic hepatitis B infection. N Engl J Med. 1995;333:1657-1661.

97. Lai C-L, Chien R-N, Leung N, et al. A one-year trial of lamivudine for chronic hepatitis B. N Engl J Med. 1998;339:61-68.

98. Dienstag JL, Schiff ER, Wright TL, et al. Lamivudine as initial treatment for chronic hepatitis B in the United States. N Engl J Med. 1999;341:1256-1263.

99. Schalm SW, Heathcote J, Cianciara J, et al. Lamivudine and alpha interferon combination treatment of patients with chronic hepatitis B infection: A randomized trial. Gut. 2000;46:562-568.

100. Schiff ER, Dienstag JL, Karayalcin S, et al. Lamivudine and 24 weeks of lamivudine/interferon combination therapy for hepatitis B e antigen-positive chronic hepatitis B in interferon nonresponders. J Hepatol. 2003;38:818-826.

101. Hadziyannis SJ, Tassopoulos NC, Heathcote EJ, et al. Adefovir dipivoxil for the treatment of hepatitis B e antigen-negative chronic hepatitis B. N Engl J Med. 2003;348:800-807.

102. Marcellin P, Chang T-T, Lim SG, et al. Adefovir dipivoxil for the treatment of hepatitis B e antigen-positive chronic hepatitis B. N Engl J Med. 2003;348: 808-816.

103. Lok ASF. New treatment of chronic hepatitis B. Semin Liver Dis. 2004;24 (Suppl 1): 77-82.

104. Greenberg HB, Pollard RB, Lutwick LI, et al. Effect of leukocyte interferon on hepatitis B virus infection in patients with chronic active hepatitis. N Engl J Med. 1976;295:517-522.

105. Perrillo RP, Regenstein FG, Peters MG, et al. Prednisone withdrawal followed by recombinant alpha interferon in the treatment of chronic type B hepatitis: A randomized, controlled trial. Ann Intern Med. 1988;109:95-100.

106. Hoofnagle JH, Peters M, Mullen KD, et al. Randomized, controlled trial of recombinant human α-interferon in patients with chronic hepatitis B. Gastroenterology. 1988;95:1318-1325.

107. Hoofnagle JH. Therapy of acute and chronic viral hepatitis. Adv Intern Med. 1994;39:241-275.

108. Hoofnagle JH, Di Bisceglie AM. The treatment of chronic viral hepatitis. N Engl J Med. 1997;336:347-356.

109. Manns MP. Current state of interferon therapy in the treatment of chronic hepatitis B. Semin Liver Dis. 2002;22 (Suppl 1):7-13.

110. Wong DKH, Cheung AM, O'Rourke K, et al. Effect of alpha-interferon treatment in patients with hepatitis B e antigen-positive chronic hepatitis B: A meta-analysis. Ann Intern Med. 1993;119:312-323.

111. Craxi A, Di Bona D, Camma C. Interferon-α for HBeAg-positive chronic hepatitis B. J Hepatol. 2003;39 (Suppl 1):S99-S105.

112. Bortolotti F, Jara P, Barbera C, et al. Long term effect of alpha interferon in children with chronic hepatitis B. Gut. 2000;46:715-718.

113. Fattovich G, Giustina G, Sanchez-Tapias J, et al. Delayed clearance of serum HBsAg in compensated cirrhosis B: Relation to interferon alpha therapy and disease prognosis. European Concerted Action on Viral Hepatitis (EUROHEP). Am J Gastroenterol. 1998;93:896-900.

114. Lin S-M, Sheen I-S, Chien R-N, et al. Long-term beneficial effect of interferon therapy in patients with chronic hepatitis B virus infection. Hepatology. 1999;29: 971-975.

115. Lok AS, Chung HT, Liu VW, et al. Long-term follow-up of chronic hepatitis B patients treated with interferon alfa. Gastroenterology. 1993;105:1833-1838.

116. Wong JB, Koff RS, Tine F, et al. Cost-effectiveness of interferon-α2b treatment for hepatitis B e antigen-positive chronic hepatitis B. Ann Intern Med. 1995;122: 664-675.

117. Dusheiko GM, Roberts JA. Treatment of chronic type B and C hepatitis with interferon alfa: An economic appraisal. Hepatology. 1995;22:1863-1873.

118. Yuen MF, Hui CK, Cheng CC, et al. Long-term follow-up of interferon alfa treatment in Chinese patients with chronic hepatitis B infection: The effect on hepatitis B e antigen seroconversion and the development of cirrhosis-related complications. Hepatology. 2001;34:139-145.

119. Yuen M-F, Yuan H-J, Hui C-K, et al. A large population study of spontaneous HBeAg seroconversion and acute exacerbation of chronic hepatitis B infection: Implications for antiviral therapy. Gut. 2003;52:416-419.

120. Perrillo RP, Lai C-L, Liaw YF, et al. Predictors of HBeAg loss after lamivudine treatment for chronic hepatitis B. Hepatology. 2002;36:186-194.

121. Perrillo R. Acute flares in chronic hepatitis B: The natural and unnatural history of an immunologically mediated liver disease. Gastroenterology. 2001;120:1009-1022.

122. Nair S, Perrillo R. Serum alanine aminotransferase flares during interferon treatment of chronic hepatitis B: Is sustained clearance of HBV DNA dependent on levels of pretreatment viremia? Hepatology. 2001;34:1021-1026.

123. Perrillo RP. Factors influencing response to interferon in chronic hepatitis B: Implications for Asian and Western populations (editorial). Hepatology. 1990;12:1433-1435.

124. Perrillo R, Tamburro C, Regenstein F, et al. Low-dose, titratable interferon alfa in decompensated liver disease caused by chronic infection with hepatitis B virus. Gastroenterology. 1995;109:908-916.

125. Brooks MG, Karayiannis P, Thomas HC. Which patients will respond to α interferon therapy? A statistical analysis of predictive factors. Hepatology. 1989;10:761-763.

126. Lai C-L, Lok AS, Lin H-J, et al. Placebo-controlled trial of recombinant alpha 2-interferon in Chinese HBsAg-carrier children. Lancet. 1987;2:877-880.

127. Torre D, Tambini R. Interferon-alpha therapy for chronic hepatitis B in children: A meta-analysis. Clin Infect Dis. 1996;23:131-137.

128. Bortolotti F. Treatment of chronic hepatitis B in children. J Hepatol. 2003;39 (Suppl 1):S200-S205.

129. Broderick AL, Jonas MM. Hepatitis B in children. Semin Liver Dis. 2003;23:59-68.

130. Sokal EM, Conjeevaram HS, Roberts EA, et al. Interferon alfa therapy for chronic hepatitis B in children: A multinational randomized controlled trial. Gastroenterology. 1998;114:988-995.

131. Hoofnagle JH, Di Bisceglie AM, Waggoner JG, et al. Interferon alfa for patients with clinically apparent cirrhosis due to chronic hepatitis B. Gastroenterology. 1993;104:1116-1121.

132. Kao JH, Wu NH, Chen PJ, et al. Hepatitis B genotypes and the response to interferon therapy. J Hepatol. 2000;33:998-1002.

133. Zhang X, Zoulim F, Habersetzer F, et al. Analysis of hepatitis B virus genotypes and pre-core region variability during interferon treatment of HBe antigen negative chronic hepatitis B. J Med Virol. 1996;48:8-16.

134. Erhardt A, Reineke U, Blondin D, et al. Mutations in the core promoter and response to interferon treatment in chronic replicative hepatitis B. Hepatology. 2000;31: 716-725.

135. Tur-Kaspa R, Burk RD, Shaul Y, et al. Hepatitis B virus DNA contains a glucocorticoid-responsive element. Proc Nat Acad Sci. 1986;83:1627-1631.

136. Tur-Kaspa R, Shaul Y, Moore DD, et al. The glucocorticoid receptor recognizes a specific nucleotide sequence in hepatitis B virus DNA causing increased activity of the HBV enhancer. Virology. 1988;167:630-633.

137. Sagnelli E, Manzillo G, Maio G, et al. Serum levels of hepatitis B surface and core antigens during immunosuppressive treatment of HBsAg-positive chronic active hepatitis. Lancet. 1980;2:395-397.

138. Scullard GH, Smith CI, Merigan TC, et al. Effects of immunosuppressive therapy on viral markers in chronic active hepatitis B. Gastroenterology. 1981;81:987-991.

139. Cohard M, Poynard T, Mathurin P, et al. Prednisone-interferon combination in the treatment of chronic hepatitis B: Direct and indirect meta-analysis. Hepatology. 1994;20:1390-1398.

140. Hadziyannis S, Bramou T, Makris A, et al. Interferon alpha-2b treatment of HBeAg negative/serum HBV DNA positive chronic active hepatitis B. J Hepatol. 1990;11(Suppl 1):S133-S136.

141. Lampertico P, Del Ninno E, Manzin A, et al. A randomized, controlled trial of a 24-month course of interferon alfa 2b in patients with chronic hepatitis B who had hepatitis B virus DNA without hepatitis B e antigen in serum. Hepatology. 1997;26:1621-1625.

142. Fattovich G, Farci P, Rugge M, et al. A randomized controlled trial of lymphoblastoid interferon-alpha in patients with chronic hepatitis B lacking HB$_e$Ag. Hepatology. 1992;15:584-589.

143. Pastore G, Santantonio T, Milella A, et al. Anti-HBe-positive chronic hepatitis B with HBV-DNA in the serum: Response to a 6-month course of lymphoblastoid interferon. J Hepatol. 1992;14:221-225.

144. Lampertico P, Del Ninno E, Vigano M, et al. Extended interferon therapy increases hepatitis suppression and reduces liver-related morbidity of hepatitis e antigen negative chronic active hepatitis B. Hepatology. 2003;37:756-763.

145. Hadziyannis SJ, Papatheodoridis GV, Vassilopoulos D. Treatment of HB$_e$Ag-negative chronic hepatitis B. Semin Liver Dis. 2003;23:81-88.

146. Brunetto MR, Oliveri F, Colombatto P, et al. Treatment of HB$_e$Ag-negative chronic hepatitis B with interferon or pegylated interferon. J Hepatol. 2003;39 (Suppl 1):S164-S167.

147. Cooksley WGE. Treatment with interferons (including pegylated interferons) in patients with hepatitis B. Semin Liver Dis. 2004;24 (Suppl 1):45-53.

148. Cooksley WGE, Piratvisuth T, Lee S-D, et al. Peginterferon α-2a (40 kDa): An advance in the treatment of hepatitis B e antigen-positive chronic hepatitis B. J Viral Hepat. 2003;10:298-305.

149. Barbaro G, Zechini F, Pellicelli AM, et al. Long-term efficacy of interferon alpha-2b and lamivudine in combination compared to lamivudine monotherapy in patients with chronic hepatitis B. An Italian multicenter randomized trial. J Hepatol. 2001;35:406-411.

150. Santantonio T, Niro GA, Sinisi E, et al. Lamivudine/interferon combination therapy in anti-HBe positive chronic hepatitis B: A controlled pilot study. J Hepatol. 2002;36:799-804.

151. Yalcin K, Degertekin H, Yildiz F, et al. Comparison of 12-month courses of interferon-α-2b-lamivudine combination therapy and interferon-α-2b monotherapy among patients with untreated chronic hepatitis B. Clin Infect Dis. 2003;36:1516-1522.

152. Doong SL, Tsai CH, Schinazi RF, et al. Inhibition of the replication of hepatitis B virus in vitro by 2',3'-dideoxy-3'-thiacytidine and related analogues. Proc Nat Acad Sci. 1991;88:8495-8499.

153. Honkoop P, de Man RA, Niesters HGM. Quantitative assessment of hepatitis B virus DNA during a 24-week course of lamivudine therapy (letter). Ann Intern Med. 1998;128:697.

154. Honkoop P, de Man RA, Niesters HGM, et al. Quantitative hepatitis B virus DNA assessment by the limiting-dilution polymerase chain reaction in chronic hepatitis B patients: Evidence of continuing viral suppression with longer duration and higher dose of lamivudine therapy. J Hepatol. 1998;5:307-312.

155. Jonas MM, Kelley JA, Mizerski J, et al. Clinical trial of lamivudine in children with chronic hepatitis B. N Engl J Med. 2002;346:1706-1713.

156. Chien R-N, Liaw Y-F, Atkins M, et al. Pretherapy alanine aminotransferase level as a determinant for hepatitis B e antigen seroconversion during lamivudine therapy in patients with chronic hepatitis B. Hepatology. 1999;30:770-774.

157. Liaw YF, Leung NW, Chang TT, et al. Effects of extended lamivudine therapy in Asian patients with chronic hepatitis B. Gastroenterology. 2000;119:172-180.

158. Leung NWY, Lai CL, Chang TT, et al. Extended lamivudine treatment in patients with chronic hepatitis B enhances hepatitis B e antigen seroconversion rates: Results after 3 years of therapy. Hepatology. 2001;33:1527-1532.

159. Song BC, Suh DJ, Lee HC, et al. Hepatitis B e antigen seroconversion after lamivudine therapy is not durable in patients with chronic hepatitis B in Korea. Hepatology. 2000;32:803-806.

160. Chien R-N, Yeh C-T, Tsai S-L, et al. Determinants for sustained HB$_e$Ag response to lamivudine therapy. Hepatology. 2003;38:1267-1273.

161. Zöllner B, Peterson J, Schäfer P, et al. Subtype-dependent response of hepatitis B virus during early phase of lamivudine treatment. Clin Infect Dis. 2002;34:1273-1277.

162. Liaw YF. Results of lamivudine trials in Asia. J Hepatol. 2003;39 (Suppl 1):S111-S115.

163. Kweon Y-O, Goodman ZD, Dienstag JL, et al. Decreasing fibrogenesis: An immunohistochemical study of paired liver biopsies following lamivudine therapy for chronic hepatitis B. J Hepatol. 2001;35:749-755.

164. Dienstag JL, Goldin RD, Heathcote EJ, et al. Histological outcome during long-term lamivudine therapy. Gastroenterology. 2003;124:1-13.

165. Tassopoulos NC, Volpes R, Pastore G, et al. Efficacy of lamivudine in patients with hepatitis B e antigen-negative/hepatitis B virus DNA-positive (precore mutant) chronic hepatitis B. Hepatology. 1999;29:889-896.

166. Hadziyannis S, Papatheodoridis GV, Dimou E, et al. Efficacy of long-term lamivudine monotherapy in patients with hepatitis B e antigen-negative chronic hepatitis B. Hepatology. 2000;32:847-851.

167. Rizzetto M, Marzano A, Lagget M. Treatment of hepatitis B e antigen-negative chronic hepatitis B with lamivudine. J Hepatol. 2003;39(Suppl 1):S168-S171.

168. Lok ASF, Lai C-L, Yao G-B, et al. Long-term safety of lamivudine treatment in patients with chronic hepatitis B. Gastroenterology. 2003;125:1714-1722.

169. Honkoop P, de Man RA, Niesters GM, et al. Acute exacerbation of chronic hepatitis B virus infection after withdrawal of lamivudine therapy. Hepatology. 2000;32:635-639.

170. Liaw Y-F, Chien R-N, Yeh C-T, et al. Acute exacerbation and hepatitis B virus clearance after emergence of YMDD motif mutation during lamivudine therapy. Hepatology. 1999;30:567-572.

171. Villeneuve J-P, Condreay LD, Willems B, et al. Lamivudine treatment for decompensated cirrhosis resulting from chronic hepatitis B. Hepatology. 2000;31:207-210.

172. Kapoor D, Guptan RC, Wakil SM, et al. Beneficial effects of lamivudine in hepatitis B virus-related decompensated cirrhosis. J Hepatol. 2000;33:508-512.

173. Yao FY, Bass NM. Lamivudine treatment in patients with severely decompensated cirrhosis due to replicating hepatitis B infection. J Hepatol. 2000;33:301-307.

174. Yao FY, Terrault NA, Freise C, et al. Lamivudine treatment is beneficial in patients with severely decompensated cirrhosis and actively replicating hepatitis B infection awaiting liver transplantation: A comparative study using a matched, untreated cohort. Hepatology. 2001;34:411-416.

175. Fontana RJ, Hann H-WL, Perrillo RP, et al. Determinants of survival in patients with decompensated chronic hepatitis B treated with antiviral therapy. Gastroenterology. 2002;123:719-727.

176. Fontana RJ. Management of patients with decompensated HBV cirrhosis. Semin Liver Dis. 2003;23:89-100.

177. Fontana RJ, Keeffe EB, Carey W, et al. Effect of lamivudine treatment on survival in 309 North American patients awaiting liver transplantation for chronic hepatitis B. Liver Transpl. 2002;8:433-439.

178. Liaw YF, Chow WC, Shue K, et al. Effects of lamivudine on disease progression and development of liver cancer in advanced chronic hepatitis B: A prospective double-blind placebo-controlled clinical trial (Abstract). Hepatology. 2003;38 (Suppl 1):262A.

179. Lai C-L, Dienstag J, Schiff E, et al. Prevalence and clinical correlates of YMDD variants during lamivudine therapy of patients with chronic hepatitis B. Clin Infect Dis. 2003;36:687-696.

180. Allen MI, Deslauriers M, Andrews CW, et al. Identification and characterization of mutations in hepatitis B virus resistant to lamivudine. Hepatology. 1998;27:1670-1677.

181. Chayama K, Suzuki Y, Kobayashi M, et al. Emergence and takeover of YMDD mutant hepatitis B virus during long-term lamivudine therapy and re-takeover by wild type after cessation of therapy. Hepatology. 1998;27:1711-1716.

182. Ling R, Mutimer D, Ahmed M, et al. Selection of mutations in the hepatitis B virus polymerase during therapy of transplant recipients with lamivudine. Hepatology. 1996;24:711-713.

183. Bartholomew MM, Jansen RW, Jeffers LJ, et al. Hepatitis-B-virus resistance to lamivudine given for recurrent infection after orthotopic liver transplantation. Lancet. 1997;349:20-22.

184. Tipples GA, Ma MM, Fischer KP, et al. Mutation in HBV RNA-dependent DNA polymerase confers resistance to lamivudine in vivo. Hepatology. 1996;24:714-717.

185. Das K, Xiong X, Yang H-I, et al. Molecular modeling and biochemical characterization reveal the mechanism of hepatitis B virus polymerase resistance to lamivudine (3TC) and emtricitabine (FTC). J Virol. 2001;75:4771-4779.

186. Locarnini S. Hepatitis B viral resistance: mechanisms and diagnosis. J Hepatol. 2003;39 (Suppl 1):S124-S132.

187. Chin R, Shaw T, Torresi J, et al. In vitro susceptibilities of wild-type or drug-resistant hepatitis B virus to (-)-β-D-2,6-diaminopurine dioxalane and 2'-fluoro-5-methyl-β-L-arabinofuranosyluracil. Antimicrob Agents Chemother. 2001;45:2495-2501.

188. Melegari M, Scaglioni PP, Wands JR. Hepatitis B virus mutants associated with 3TC and famciclovir administration are replication defective. Hepatology. 1998;27:628-633.

189. Ling R, Harrison TJ. Functional analysis of mutations conferring lamivudine resistance on hepatitis B. J Gen Virol. 1999;80:601-606.

190. Papatheodoridis GV, Dimou E, Laras A, et al. Course of virologic breakthroughs under long-term lamivudine in HB$_e$Ag-negative precore mutant HBV liver disease. Hepatology. 2002;36:219-226.

191. Perrillo RP, Wright T, Rakela J, et al. A multicenter United States–Canadian trial to assess lamivudine monotherapy before and after liver transplantation for chronic hepatitis B. Hepatology 2001;33:424-432.

192. Perrillo R, Rakela J, Dienstag J, et al. Multicenter study of lamivudine therapy for hepatitis B after liver transplantation. Hepatology. 1999;29:1581-1586.

193. Kim JW, Lee HS, Woo GH, et al. Fatal submassive hepatic necrosis associated with tyrosine-methionine-aspartate-aspartate-motif mutation of hepatitis B virus after long-term lamivudine therapy. Clin Infect Dis. 2001;33:403-405.

194. Yuen M-F, Kato T, Mizokami M, et al. Clinical outcome and virologic profiles of severe hepatitis B exacerbations due to YMDD mutations. J Hepatol. 2003;39:850-855.

195. Schuurman R, Nijhuis M, van Leeuwen R, et al. Rapid changes in human immunodeficiency virus type 1 RNA load and appearance of drug-resistant virus populations in persons treated with lamivudine (3TC). J Infect Dis. 1995;171:1411-1419.

196. Ono-Nita SK, Kato N, Shiratori Y, et al. Susceptibility of lamivudine-resistant hepatitis B virus to other reverse transcriptase inhibitors. J Clin Invest. 1999;103:1635-1640.

197. Perrillo R, Hann H-W, Mutimer D, et al. Adefovir dipivoxil added to ongoing lamivudine in chronic hepatitis B with YMDD mutant hepatitis B virus. Gastroenterology. 2004;126:81-90.

198. Peters MG, Hann H-W, Martin P, et al. Adefovir dipivoxil alone or in combination with lamivudine in patients with lamivudine-resistant chronic hepatitis B. Gastroenterology. 2004;126:91-101.

199. Perrillo R, Schiff E, Yoshida E, et al. Adefovir dipivoxil for the treatment of lamivudine-resistant hepatitis B mutants. Hepatology. 2000;32:129-134.

200. Westland C, Delaney W, Yang H, et al. Hepatitis B virus genotypes and virologic response in 694 patients in phase III studies of adefovir dipivoxil. Gastroenterology. 2003;125:107-116.

201. Westland CE, Yang H, Delaney WE, et al. Week 48 resistance surveillance in two phase 3 clinical studies of adefovir dipivoxil for chronic hepatitis B. Hepatology. 2003;38:96-103.

202. Yang H, Westland CE, Delaney WE, et al. Resistance surveillance in chronic hepatitis B patients treated with adefovir dipivoxil for up to 60 weeks. Hepatology. 2002;36:464-473.

203. Angus P, Vaughan R, Xiong S, et al. Resistance to adefovir dipivoxil therapy associated with the selection of a novel mutation in the HBV polymerase. Gastroenterology. 2003;125:292-297.

204. Dusheiko G. Adefovir dipivoxil for the treatment of HBeAg-positive chronic hepatitis B: A review of the major clinical studies. J Hepatol. 2003;39(Suppl 1):S116-S123.

205. Lewis W, Meyer RR, Simpson JF, et al. Mammalian DNA polymerases α, β, γ, δ, and ε incorporate fialuridine (FIAU) monophosphate into DNA and are inhibited competitively by FIAU triphosphate. Biochemistry. 1994;33:14620-14624.

206. McKenzie R, Fried MW, Sallie R, et al. Hepatic failure and lactic acidosis due to fialuridine (FIAU), an investigational nucleoside analogue for chronic hepatitis B. N Engl J Med. 1995;333:1099-1105.

207. Cui L, Yoon S, Schinazi RF, et al. Cellular and molecular events leading to mitochondrial toxicity of 1-(2-deoxy-2-fluoro-1-β-D-arabinofuranosyl)-5-iodouracil in human liver cells. J Clin Invest. 1995;95:555-563.

208. Trepo C, Jezek P, Atkinson G, et al. Famciclovir in chronic hepatitis B: results of a dose-finding study. J Hepatol. 2000;32:1011-1018.

209. de Man RA, Marcellin P, Habal F, et al. A randomized, placebo-controlled study to evaluate the efficacy of 12-month famciclovir treatment in patients with chronic hepatitis B e antigen-positive hepatitis B. Hepatology. 2000;32:413-417.

210. Seifer M, Hamatake RK, Colonno RJ, et al. In vitro inhibition of hepadnavirus polymerases by the triphosphates of BMS-200475 and lobucavir. Antimicrob Agents Chemother. 1998;42:3200-3208.

211. Feld J, Lee J-Y, Locarnini S. New targets and possible new therapeutic approaches in the chemotherapy of chronic hepatitis B. Hepatology. 2003;38:545-553.

212. Buti M, Esteban R. Entecavir, FTC, L-FMAU, LdT and others. J Hepatol. 2003;39(Suppl 1):S139-S142.

213. Klein C, Bock CT, Wedemeyer H, et al. Inhibition of hepatitis B virus replication in vivo by nucleoside analogues and siRNA. Gastroenterology. 2003;125:9-18.

214. Lai C-L, Rosmawati M, Lao J, et al. Entecavir is superior to lamivudine in reducing hepatitis B virus DNA in patients with chronic hepatitis B infection. Gastroenterology. 2002;123:1831-1838.

215. Locarnini S. Molecular virology of hepatitis B virus. Semin Liver Dis. 2004;24 (Suppl 1):3-10.

216. Bryant ML, Bridges EG, Placidi L, et al. Antiviral L-nucleosides specific for hepatitis B virus infection. Antimicrob Agents Chemother. 2001;45:229-235.

217. Lai C-L, Leung NWY, Teo E-K, et al. Results of a one-year international phase IIB comparative trial of telbivudine, lamivudine, and the combination, in patients with chronic hepatitis B (Abstract). Hepatology. 2003;38(Suppl 1):262A.

218. Benhamou Y, Tubiana R, Thibault V. Tenofovir disoproxil fumarate in patients with HIV and lamivudine-resistant hepatitis B virus (letter). N Engl J Med. 2003;348: 177-178.

219. Kuo A, Dienstag JL, Chung RT. Tenofovir disoproxil fumarate for the treatment of lamivudine-resistant hepatitis B. Clin Gastroenterol Hepatol. 2004;2:266-272.

220. Ristig M, Crippin J, Alberg J, et al. Tenofovir disoproxil fumarate therapy for chronic hepatitis B in human immunodeficiency virus/hepatitis B virus-coinfected individuals for whom interferon-α and lamivudine have failed. J Infect Dis. 2002;186: 1844-1847.

221. Richman DD. The impact of drug resistance on the effectiveness of chemotherapy for chronic hepatitis B. Hepatology. 2000;32:866-867.

222. Shaw T, Bowden S, Locarnini S. Chemotherapy for hepatitis B: New treatment options necessitate reappraisal of traditional endpoints. Gastroenterology. 2002;123:2135-2140.

223. Shaw T, Bowden S, Locarnini S. Rescue therapy for drug resistant hepatitis B: Another argument for combination chemotherapy? Gastroenterology. 2004;126: 343-350.

224. Shaw T, Locarnini S. Combination chemotherapy for hepatitis B virus: The final solution? Hepatology. 2000;32:430-432.

225. Lewin SR, Walters T, Locarnini S. Hepatitis B treatment: rational combination chemotherapy based on viral kinetic and animal model studies. Antiviral Res. 2002;55:381-396.

226. Perrillo RP. Overview of treatment of hepatitis B: Key approaches and clinical challenges. Semin Liver Dis. 2004;24 (Suppl 1):23-29.

227. Gilson RJ, Chopra KB, Newell AM, et al. A placebo-controlled phase I/II study of adefovir dipivoxil in patients with chronic hepatitis B virus infection. J Viral Hepat. 1999;6:387-395.

228. Boni C, Bertoletti A, Penna A, et al. Lamivudine treatment can restore T cell responsiveness in chronic hepatitis B. J Clin Invest. 1998;102:968-975.

229. Boni C, Penna A, Ogg GS, et al. Lamivudine treatment can overcome cytotoxic T-cell hyporesponsiveness in chronic hepatitis B: New perspectives for immune therapy. Hepatology. 2001;33:963-971.

230. Boni C, Penna A, Bertoletti A, et al. Transient restoration of anti-viral T cell responses induced by lamivudine therapy in chronic hepatitis B. J Hepatol. 2003;39:595-605.

231. Rossi G, Pelizzari A, Motta M, et al. Primary prophylaxis with lamivudine of hepatitis B virus reactivation in chronic HBsAg carriers with lymphoid malignancies treated with chemotherapy. Br J Haematol. 2001;115:58-62.

232. Liao C, Lee C, Wu H, et al. Lamivudine for the treatment of hepatitis B virus reactivation following chemotherapy for non-Hodgkin's lymphoma. Br J Haematol. 2002;116:166-169.

233. Benhamou Y, Bochet M, Thibault V, et al. Safety and efficacy of adefovir dipivoxil in patients co-infected with HIV-1 and lamivudine-resistant hepatitis B virus: An open label pilot study. Lancet. 2001;358:718-723.

234. Freeman RB, Sanchez H, Lewis WD, et al. Serologic and DNA follow-up data from HBsAg-positive patients treated with orthotopic liver transplantation. Transplantation. 1991;51:793-797.

235. Poterucha JJ, Weisner RH. Liver transplantation and hepatitis B. Ann Intern Med. 1997;126:805-807.

236. Terrault NA, Wright TL. Hepatitis B virus infection and liver transplantation. Gut. 1997;40:568-571.

237. Roche B, Samuel D. Liver transplantation for hepatitis B virus-related liver disease: Indications, prevention of recurrence and results. J Hepatol. 2003;39(Suppl 1): S181-S189.

238. Benner KG, Lee RG, Keeffe EB, et al. Fibrosing cytolytic liver failure secondary to recurrent hepatitis B after liver transplantation. Gastroenterology. 1992;103: 1307-1312.

239. Dickson RC, Everhart JE, Lake JR, et al. Transmission of hepatitis B by transplantation of livers from donors positive for antibody to hepatitis B core antigen. Gastroenterology. 1997;113:1668-1674.

240. Samuel D, Muller R, Alexander G, et al. Liver transplantation in European patients with the hepatitis B surface antigen. N Engl J Med. 1993;329:1842-1847.

241. Pruett TL. Improved clinical outcomes with liver transplantation for hepatitis B-induced chronic liver failure using passive immunization. Ann Surg. 1998;227:841-850.

242. McMahon G, Ehrlich PH, Moustafa ZA, et al. Genetic alterations in the gene encoding the major HBsAg: DNA and immunological analysis of recurrent HBsAg derived from monoclonal antibody-treated liver transplant patients. Hepatology. 1992;15:757-766.

243. Carman WF, Trautwein C, Van Deursen FJ, et al. Hepatitis B virus envelope variation after transplantation with and without hepatitis B immune globulin prophylaxis. Hepatology. 1996;24:489-493.

244. Ghany MG, Ayola B, Villamil FG, et al. Hepatitis B virus S mutants in liver transplant recipients who were reinfected despite hepatitis B immune globulin prophylaxis. Hepatology. 1998;27:213-222.

245. Terrault NA, Zhiou S, McCory RW, et al. Incidence and clinical consequences of surface and polymerase gene mutations in liver transplant recipients on hepatitis B immunoglobulin. Hepatology. 1998;28:555-561.

246. Grellier L, Mutimer D, Ahmed M, et al. Lamivudine prophylaxis against reinfection in liver transplantation for hepatitis B cirrhosis. Lancet. 1996;348:1212-1215.

247. Markowitz JS, Martin P, Conrad AJ, et al. Prophylaxis against hepatitis B recurrence following liver transplantation using combination lamivudine and hepatitis B immune globulin. Hepatology. 1998;28:585.

248. Yao FY, Osorio RW, Roberts JP, et al. Intramuscular hepatitis B immune globulin combined with lamivudine for prophylaxis against hepatitis B recurrence after liver transplantation. Liver Transpl Surg. 1999;5:491-496.

249. Angus PW, McCaughan GW, Gane EJ, et al. Combination low-dose hepatitis B immune globulin and lamivudine therapy provides effective prophylaxis against post-transplantation hepatitis B. Liver Transpl. 2000;6:429-433.

250. Colin JF, Cazals-Hatem D, Loriot MA, et al. Influence of human immunodeficiency virus infection on chronic hepatitis B in homosexual men. Hepatology. 1999;29:1306-1310.

251. Carr A, Cooper D. Restoration of immunity to chronic hepatitis B infection in HIV-infected patients on protease inhibitor. Lancet. 1997;349:995-996.

252. Benhamou Y, Bochet M, Thibault V, et al. Long-term incidence of hepatitis B virus resistance to lamivudine in human immunodeficiency virus-infected patients. Hepatology. 1999;30:1302-1306.

253. Benhamou Y, Poynard T. Treatment of chronic hepatitis B virus infection in patients co-infected with human immunodeficiency virus. J Hepatol. 2003;39(Suppl 1): S194-S199.

254. Dienstag JL, Rhodes AR, Bhan AK, et al. Urticaria associated with acute viral hepatitis type B: Studies of pathogenesis. Ann Intern Med. 1978;88:34-40.

255. Lisker-Melman M, Webb D, Di Bisceglie AM, et al. Glomerulonephritis caused by chronic hepatitis B virus infection: Treatment with recombinant human alpha-interferon. Ann Intern Med. 1989;111:479-483.

256. Lau GKK, He ML, Fong DY, et al. Preemptive use of lamivudine reduces hepatitis B exacerbation after allogeneic hematopoietic cell transplantation. Hepatology. 2002;36:702-709.

257. Tillmann HL, Wedemeyer H, Manns MP. Treatment of hepatitis B in special patient groups: Hemodialysis, heart and renal transplant, fulminant hepatitis, hepatitis B virus reactivation. J Hepatol. 2003;39 (Suppl 1):S206-S211.

258. Rizzetto M, Canese MG, Arico S, et al. Immunofluorescence detection of new antigen-antibody system (d/anti-d) associated to hepatitis B virus in liver and in serum of HBsAg carriers. Gut. 1977;18:997-1003.

259. Rizzetto M. The delta agent. Hepatology. 1983;3:729-737.

260. Farci P, Roskams T, Chessa L, et al. Long-term benefit of interferon α therapy of chronic hepatitis D: Regression of advanced hepatic fibrons. Gastroenterology. 2004;126:1740-1749.

261. Hoofnagle JH. Type D (delta) hepatitis. JAMA. 1989;261:1321-1325.

262. Rosina F, Conoscitore P, Cuppone R, et al. Changing patterns of chronic hepatitis D in southern Europe. Gastroenterology. 1999;117:161-166.

263. Gaeta GB, Stroffolini T, Chiaramonte M, et al. Chronic hepatitis D: A vanishing disease? An Italian multicenter study. Hepatology. 2000;32:824-827.

264. Lerut JP, Donataccio M, Ciccarelli O, et al. Liver transplantation and HBsAg-positive postnecrotic cirrhosis: Adequate immunoprophylaxis and delta virus co-infection as the significant determinants of long-term prognosis. J Hepatol. 1999;30:706-714.

265. Samuel D, Zignego AL, Reynes M, et al. Long-term clinical and virological outcome after liver transplantation for cirrhosis caused by chronic delta hepatitis. Hepatology. 1995;21:333-339.

266. Philipp T, Durazzo M, Trautwein C, et al. Recognition of uridine diphosphate glucuronosyl transferase by LKM-3 antibodies in chronic hepatitis D. Lancet. 1994;344:578-581.

267. Smedile A, Bergmann KF, Baroudy BM, et al. Riboprobe assay for HDV RNA: A sensitive method for the detection of the HDV genome in clinical serum samples. J Med Virol. 1990;30:20-24.

268. Lau DT, Doo E, Park Y, et al. Lamivudine for chronic delta hepatitis. Hepatology. 1999;30:546-549.

269. Farci P, Mandas A, Coiana A, et al. Treatment of chronic hepatitis D with interferon alfa-2a. N Engl J Med. 1994;330:88-94.

270. Lau DT, Kleiner DE, Park Y, et al. Resolution of chronic delta hepatitis after 12 years of interferon alfa therapy. Gastroenterology. 1999;117:1229-1233.

271. Alter MJ, Margolis HS, Krawczynski K, et al. The natural history of community acquired hepatitis C in the United States. N Engl J Med. 1992;327:1899-1905.

272. Alter HJ, Seeff LB. Recovery, persistence, and sequelae in hepatitis C virus infection: a perspective on long-term outcome. Semin Liver Dis. 2000;20:17-35.

273. Neumann AU, Lam NP, Dahari H, et al. Hepatitis C viral dynamics in vivo and the antiviral efficacy of interferon-α therapy. Science. 1998;282:103-107.

274. Farci P, Shimoda A, Coiana A, et al. The outcome of acute hepatitis C predicted by evolution of the viral quasispecies. Science. 2000;288:339-344.

275. Ogata N, Alter HJ, Miller RH, et al. Nucleotide sequence and mutation rate of the H strain of hepatitis C virus. PNAS 1991;88:3392-3396.

276. Simmonds P, Alberti A, Alter HJ, et al. A proposed system for the nomenclature of hepatitis C viral genotypes. Hepatology. 1994;19:1321-1324.

277. Simmonds P. Variability of hepatitis C virus. Hepatology. 1995;21:570-583.

278. Martell M, Esteban JI, Quer J, et al. Hepatitis C virus (HCV) circulates as a population of different but closely related genomes: Quasispecies nature of HCV genome distribution. J Virol. 1992;66:3225-3229.

279. Bukh J, Miller RH, Purcell RH. Genetic heterogeneity of hepatitis C virus: Quasispecies and genotypes. Semin Liver Dis. 1995;15:41-63.

280. Alter MJ, Kruszon-Moran D, Nainan OV, et al. The prevalence of hepatitis C virus infection in the United States, 1988 through 1994. N Engl J Med. 1999;341:556-562.

281. Hoofnagle JH. Course and outcome of hepatitis C. Hepatology. 2002;36 (Suppl 1):S21-S29.

282. Bellentani S, Tiribelli C, Saccoccio G, et al. Prevalence of chronic liver disease in the general population of northern Italy: The Dionysos study. Hepatology. 1994;20:1442-1449.

283. Kim WR, Gross JBJ, Poterucha JJ, et al. Outcome of hospital care of liver disease associated with hepatitis C in the United States. Hepatology. 2001;33:201-206.

284. Kim WR. The burden of hepatitis C in the United States. Hepatology. 2002;36 (Suppl 1):S30-S34.

285. Detre KM, Belle SH, Lombardero M. Liver transplantation for chronic viral hepatitis. Viral Hepat Rev. 1997;2:219-228.

286. Féray C, Gigou M, Sameul D, et al. The course of hepatitis C virus infection after liver transplantation. Hepatology. 1994;20:1137-1143.

287. Alter HJ, Holland PV, Purcell RH, et al. Post-transfusion hepatitis after exclusion of commercial and hepatitis-B antigen-positive donors. Ann Intern Med. 1972;77:691-699.

288. Aach RD, Szmuness W, Mosley JW, et al. Serum alanine aminotransferase of donors in relation to the risk of non-A, non-B hepatitis in recipients: The Transfusion-Transmitted Viruses Study. N Engl J Med. 1981;304:989-994.

289. Alter HJ, Purcell RH, Holland PV, et al. Donor transaminase and recipient hepatitis: Impact of blood transfusion services. JAMA. 1981;246:630-634.

290. Stevens CE, Aach RD, Hollinger FB, et al. Hepatitis B virus antibody in blood donors and the occurrence of non-A, non-B hepatitis in transfusion recipients: An analysis of the Transfusion-Transmitted Viruses Study. Ann Intern Med. 1984;101:733-738.

291. Koziol DE, Holland PV, Alling DW, et al. Antibody to hepatitis B core antigen as a paradoxical marker for non-A, non-B hepatitis agents in donated blood. Ann Intern Med. 1986;104:488-495.

292. Alter HJ, Purcell RH, Shih JW, et al. Detection of antibody to hepatitis C virus in prospectively followed transfusion recipients with acute and chronic non-A, non-B hepatitis. N Engl J Med. 1989;321:1494-1500.

293. Donahue JG, Munoz A, Ness PM, et al. The declining risk of post-transfusion hepatitis C virus infection. N Engl J Med. 1992;327:369-373.

294. Aach RD, Stevens CE, Hollinger FB, et al. Hepatitis C virus infection in post-transfusion hepatitis: An analysis with first- and second-generation assays. N Engl J Med. 1991;325:1325-1329.

295. Schreiber GB, Busch MP, Kleinman SH, et al. The risk of transfusion-transmitted viral infection. N Engl J Med. 1996;334:1685-1690.

296. Williams I. Epidemiology of hepatitis C in the United States. Am J Med. 1999;107:2S-9S.

297. Orland JR, Wright TL, Cooper S. Acute hepatitis C. Hepatology. 2001;33:321-327.

298. Armstrong GL, Alter MJ, McQuillan GM, et al. The past incidence of hepatitis C virus infection: Implications for the future burden of chronic liver disease in the United States. Hepatology. 2000;31:777-782.

299. Conry-Cantilena C, VanRaden M, Gibble J, et al. Routes of infection, viremia, and liver disease in blood donors found to have hepatitis C virus infection. N Engl J Med. 1996;334:1691-1696.

300. Shakil AO, Conry-Cantilena C, Alter HJ, et al. Volunteer blood donors with antibody to hepatitis C virus: Clinical, biochemical, virologic, and histologic features. Ann Intern Med. 1995;123:330-337.

301. Pileri P, Uematsu Y, Campagnoli S, et al. Binding of hepatitis C virus to CD81. Science. 1998;282:938-941.

302. Cooper S, Erickson AL, Adams EJ, et al. Analysis of a successful immune response against hepatitis C virus. Immunity. 1999;10:439-449.

303. Lechner F, Wong DK, Dunbar PR, et al. Analysis of successful immune response in persons infected with hepatitis C virus. J Exp Med. 2000;191:1499-1512.

304. Takaki A, Wiese M, Maertens G, et al. Cellular immune responses persist, humoral responses decrease two decades after recovery from a single source outbreak of hepatitis C. Nat Med. 2000;6:578-582.

305. Koziel MJ, Dudley D, Afdhal N, et al. HLA class I-restricted cytotoxic T lymphocytes specific for hepatitis C virus: Identification of multiple epitopes and characterization of patterns of cytokine release. J Clin Invest. 1995;96:2311-2321.

306. Missale G, Bertoni R, Lamonaca V, et al. Different clinical behaviors of acute hepatitis C virus infection area associated with different vigor of the anti-viral cell-mediated immune response. J Clin Invest. 1996;98:706-714.

307. Rehermann B. Interaction between the hepatitis C virus and the immune system. Semin Liver Dis. 2000;20:127-141.

308. Grakoui A, Shoukry NH, Woolard DJ, et al. HCV persistence and immune evasion in the absence of memory T cell help. Science. 2003;302:659-662.

309. Shoukry NH, Sidney J, Sette A, et al. Conserved hierarchy of helper T cell responses in a chimpanzee during primary and secondary hepatitis C virus infection. J Immunol. 2004;172:483-492.

310. Thimme R, Bukh J, Spangenberg HC, et al. Viral and immunological determinants of hepatitis C virus clearance, persistence, and disease. Proc Nat Acad Sci. 2003;99:15661-15668.

311. Wedemeyer H, He X-S, Nascimbeni M, et al. Impaired effector function of hepatitis C virus-specific CD8+ T cells in chronic hepatitis C virus infection. J Immunol. 2002;169:3447-3458.

312. Su AI, Pezacki JP, Wodicka L, et al. Genomic analysis of the host response to hepatitis C virus infection. Proc Nat Acad Sci. 2002;99:15669-15674.

313. Farci P, Alter HJ, Govindarajan S, et al. Lack of protective immunity against reinfection with hepatitis C virus. Science. 1992;258:135-140.

314. Shimizu YK, Hijikata M, Iwamoto A, et al. Neutralizing antibodies against hepatitis C virus and the emergence of neutralization escape mutant viruses. J Virol. 1994;68:1494-1500.

315. Kao JH, Chen P-J, Wang J-T, et al. Superinfection by homotypic virus in hepatitis C virus carriers: Studies on patients with post-transfusion hepatitis. J Med Virol. 1996;50:303-308.

316. Wyatt CA, Andrus L, Brotman B, et al. Immunity in chimpanzees chronically infected with hepatitis C virus: role of minor quasispecies in reinfection. J Virol. 1998;72:1725-1730.

317. Farci P, Shimoda A, Wong D, et al. Prevention of hepatitis C virus infection in chimpanzees by hyperimmune serum against the hypervariable region 1 of the envelope 2 protein. Proc Nat Acad Sci. 1996;93:15394-15399.

318. Bartosch B, Bukh J, Meunier J-C, et al. In vitro assay for neutralizing antibody to hepatitis C virus: Evidence for broadly conserved neutralization epitopes. Proc Nat Acad Sci. 2003;100:14199-14204.

319. Seeff LB. Natural history of chronic hepatitis C. Hepatology 2002;36(Suppl 1):S35-S46.

320. Seeff LB, Buskell-Bales Z, Wright EC, et al. Long-term mortality after transfusion-associated non-A, non-B hepatitis. N Engl J Med. 1992;327:1906-1911.

321. Seeff LB. Natural history of hepatitis C. Hepatology 1997;26 (Suppl 1):21S-28S.

322. Kenny-Walsh E, Irish Hepatology Research Group. Clinical outcomes after hepatitis C infection from contaminated anti-D immune globulin. N Engl J Med. 1999;340:1228-1233.

323. Tong MJ, El-Farra NS, Reikes AR, et al. Clinical outcomes after transfusion-associated hepatitis C. N Engl J Med. 1995;332:1463-1466.

324. Bjøro K, Frøland SS, Yun Z, et al. Hepatitis C infection in patients with primary hypogammaglobulinemia after treatment with contaminated immune globulin. N Engl J Med. 1994;331:1607-1611.

325. Wiese M, Berr F, Lafrenz M, et al. Low frequency of cirrhosis in a hepatitis C (genotype 1b) single-source outbreak in Germany: A 20-year multicenter study. Hepatology. 2000;32:91-96.

326. Freeman AJ, Dore GJ, Law MG, et al. Estimating progression to cirrhosis in chronic hepatitis C virus infection. Hepatology. 2001;34:809-816.

327. Seeff LB, Miller RN, Rabkin CS, et al. 45-year follow-up of hepatitis C virus infection in healthy young adults. Ann Intern Med. 2000;132:105-111.

328. Seeff LB, Hollinger FB, Alter HJ, et al. Long-term mortality and morbidity of transfusion-associated non-A, non-B, and type C hepatitis: A National Heart, Lung, and Blood Institute collaborative study. Hepatology. 2001;33:455-463.

329. Niederau C, Lange S, Heintges T, et al. Prognosis of chronic hepatitis C: Results of a large, prospective cohort study. Hepatology. 1998;28:1687-1695.

330. Takahashi M, Yamada G, Miyamoto R, et al. Natural course of chronic hepatitis C. Am J Gastroenterol. 1993;88:240-243.

331. Poynard T, Bedossa P, Opolon P, et al. Natural history of liver fibrosis progression in patients with chronic hepatitis C. Lancet. 1997;349:825-832.

332. Fontaine H, Nalpas B, Poulet B, et al. Hepatitis activity index is a key factor in determining the natural history of chronic hepatitis C. Human Pathol. 2001;32:904-909.

333. Matsumara H, Moriyama K, Goto I, et al. Natural course of progression of fibrosis in Japanese patients with chronic liver disease type C—a study of 527 patients at one establishment. J Viral Hepat. 2000;7:268-275.

334. Yano M, Kumada H, Kage M, et al. The long-term pathological evolution of chronic hepatitis C. Hepatology. 1996;23:1334-1340.

335. Dienstag JL. The role of liver biopsy in chronic hepatitis C. Hepatology. 2002;36(Suppl 1):S152-S160.

336. Marcellin P, Asselah T, Boyer N. Fibrosis and disease progression in hepatitis C. Hepatology. 2002;36(Suppl 1):S47-S56.

337. National Institutes of Health Consensus Development Conference statement: management of hepatitis C: 2002—June 10-12, 2002. Hepatology. 2002;36(Suppl 1): S3-S20.

338. Ghany MG, Kleiner DE, Alter H, et al. Progression of fibrosis in chronic hepatitis C. Gastroenterology. 2003;124:97-104.

339. Lagging LM, Westin J, Svensson E, et al. Progression of fibrosis in untreated patients with hepatitis C virus infection. Liver. 2002;22:136-144.

340. Montalto G, Zignego AL, Ruggieri MI, et al. Serum HCV-RNA and liver histologic findings in patients with long-term normal transaminases. Digest Dis Sci. 1997;42:1703-1707.

341. Rossini A, Ravaggi A, Agostinelli E, et al. Virologic characterization and liver histology in HCV positive subjects with normal and elevated ALT levels. Liver. 1997;17:133-138.

342. Alberti A, Noventa F, Benvegnù L, et al. Prevalence of liver disease in a population of asymptomatic persons with hepatitis C virus infection. Ann Intern Med. 2002;137:961-964.

343. Healey CJ, Chapman RW, Fleming KA. Liver histology in hepatitis C infection: a comparison between patients with persistently normal or abnormal transaminases. Gut. 1995;37:274-278.

344. Shiffman ML, Stewart CA, Hofmann CM, et al. Chronic infection with hepatitis C virus in patients with elevated or persistently normal serum alanine aminotransferase levels: Comparison of hepatic histology and response to interferon therapy. J Infect Dis. 2000;182:1595-1601.

345. Mathurin P, Moussalli J, Cadranel J-F, et al. Slow progression rate of fibrosis in hepatitis C virus patients with persistently normal alanine aminotransferase activity. Hepatology. 1998;27:868-872.

346. Persico M, Persico E, Suozzo R, et al. Natural history of hepatitis C virus carriers with persistently normal aminotransferase levels. Gastroenterology. 2000;118: 760-764.

347. Martinon-Peignoux M, Boyer N, Cazals-Hatem D, et al. Prospective study on anti-hepatitis C virus-positive patients with persistently normal serum alanine transaminase with or without detectable serum hepatitis C virus RNA. Hepatology. 2001;34: 1000-1005.

348. Wali M, Lewis S, Hubscher S, et al. Histologic progression during short-term follow-up of patients with chronic hepatitis C virus infection. J Viral Hepat. 1999;6:445-452.

349. National Institutes of Health Consensus Development Conference. Management of hepatitis C. Hepatology 1997;26(Suppl 1):1S-156S.

350. Vogt M, Lang T, Frosner G, et al. Prevalence and clinical outcome of hepatitis C infection in children who underwent cardiac surgery before the implementation of blood-donor screening. N Engl J Med. 1999;341:866-870.

351. Alric L, Fort M, Izopet J, et al. Genes of the major histocompatibility complex class II influence the outcome of hepatitis C virus infection. Gastroenterology. 1997;113:1675-1681.

352. Kuzushita N, Hayashi N, Maribe T, et al. Influence of HLA haplotypes on the clinical course of individuals infected with hepatitis C virus. Hepatology. 1998;27: 240-244.

353. Thomas DL, Astemborski J, Rai RM, et al. The natural history of hepatitis C virus infection: Host, viral, and environmental factors. JAMA. 2000;284:450-456.

354. Alberti A, Benvegnù L. Management of hepatitis C. J Hepatol. 2003;38:S104-S118.

355. Adinolfi LE, Gambardella M, Andreana A, et al. Steatosis accelerates the progression of liver damage of chronic hepatitis C patients and correlates with specific HCV genotype and visceral obesity. Hepatology. 2001;33:1358-1364.

356. Hourigan LF, MacDonald GA, Purdie D, et al. Fibrosis in chronic hepatitis C correlates significantly with body mass index and steatosis. Hepatology. 1999;29: 1215-1219.

357. Vento S, Garofano T, Renzini C, et al. Fulminant hepatitis associated with hepatitis A virus superinfection in patients with chronic hepatitis C. N Engl J Med. 1998;338:286-290.

358. Fattovich G, Giustina G, Degos F, et al. Morbidity and mortality in compensated cirrhosis type C: A retrospective follow-up study of 384 patients. Gastroenterology. 1997;112:463-472.

359. Serfaty L, Aumaitre H, Chazouilleres O, et al. Determinants of outcome of compensated hepatitis C virus-related cirrhosis. Hepatology. 1998;27:1435-1440.

360. Di Bisceglie AM. Hepatitis C and hepatocellular carcinoma. Hepatology. 1997;26(Suppl 1):34S-38S.

361. El-Serag HB. Hepatocellular carcinoma and hepatitis C in the United States. Hepatology 2002;36(Suppl 1):S74-S83.

362. Bruno S, Silini E, Crosignani A, et al. Hepatitis C virus genotypes and risk of hepatocellular carcinoma in cirrhosis: A prospective study. Hepatology. 1997;25:754-758.

363. Kiyosawa K, Akahane Y, Nagata A, et al. Hepatocellular carcinoma after non-A, non-B posttransfusion hepatitis. Am J Gastroenterol. 1984;79:777-781.

364. Ikeda K, Saitoh S, Suzuki Y, et al. Disease progression and hepatocellular carcinogenesis in patients with chronic viral hepatitis: A prospective observation of 2215 patients. J Hepatol. 1998;28:930-938.

365. Kiyosawa K, Sodeyama T, Tanaka E, et al. Interrelationship of blood transfusion, non-A, non-B hepatitis and hepatocellular carcinoma. Analysis by detection of antibody to hepatitis C virus. Hepatology. 1990;12:671-675.

366. Sakamuro D, Furukawa T, Takegami T. Hepatitis C virus nonstructural protein NS3 transforms NIH3T3 cells. J Virol. 1995;69:3893-3896.

367. Ray RB, Lagging LM, Meyer K, et al. Hepatitis C virus core protein cooperates with ras and transforms primary rat embryo fibroblasts to tumorigenic phenotype. J Virol. 1996;70:4438-4443.

368. Moriya K, Fujie H, Shintani Y, et al. The core protein of hepatitis C virus induces hepatocellular carcinoma in transgenic mice. Nat Med. 1998;4:1065-1067.

369. El-Serag HB, Mason AC. Rising incidence of hepatocellular carcinoma in the United States. N Engl J Med. 1999;340:745-750.

370. Wong JB, McQuillan GM, McHutchison JG, et al. Estimating future hepatitis C morbidity, mortality, and costs in the United States. Am J Pub Health. 2000;90: 1562-1569.

371. Kim WR, Brown RS, Jr, Terrault NA, et al. Burden of liver disease in the United States: summary of a workshop. Hepatology. 2002;36:227-242.

372. Davis GL, Albright JE, Cook SE, et al. Projecting future complications of chronic hepatitis C in the United States. Liver Transpl. 2003;9:331-338.

373. Dammacco F, Sansonno D, Piccoli C, et al. The lymphoid system in hepatitis C virus infection: autoimmunity, mixed cryoglobulinemia, and overt B-cell malignancy. Semin Liver Dis. 2000;20:143-157.

374. Lunel F, Musset L, Cacoub P, et al. Cryoglobulinemia in chronic liver diseases: Role of hepatitis C virus and liver damage. Gastroenterology. 1994;106:1291-1300.

375. Dienstag JL. Non-A, non-B hepatitis. I. Recognition, epidemiology, and clinical features. Gastroenterology. 1983;85:439-462.

376. Perrillo RP. The role of liver biopsy in hepatitis C. Hepatology. 2002;26(Suppl 1):57S-61S.

377. Lefkowitch JH, Schiff ER, Davis GL, et al. Pathologic diagnosis of chronic hepatitis C: a multicenter comparative study with chronic hepatitis B. Gastroenterology. 1993;104:595-603.

378. Zignego AL, Macchia D, Monti M, et al. Infection of peripheral mononuclear cells by hepatitis C virus. J Hepatol. 1992;15:382-386.

379. Okuda M, Hino K, Korenaga M, et al. Differences in hypervariable region 1 quasispecies of hepatitis C virus in human serum, peripheral blood mononuclear cells, and liver. Hepatology. 1999;29:217-222.

380. El-Serag HB, Hampel H, Yeh C, et al. Extrahepatic manifestations of hepatitis C among United States male veterans. Hepatology. 2002;36:1439-1445.

381. Marcellin P, Descamps V, Martinot-Peignoux M, et al. Cryoglobulinemia with vasculitis associated with hepatitis C virus infection. Gastroenterology. 1993;104: 272-277.

382. Misiani R, Bellavita P, Fenili D, et al. Hepatitis C virus infection in patients with essential mixed cryoglobulinemia. Ann Intern Med. 1992;117:573-577.

383. Agnello V, Chung RT, Kaplan LM. A role for hepatitis C virus infection in type II cryoglobulinemia. N Engl J Med. 1992;327:1490-1495.

384. Zignego AL, Ferri C, Giannelli F, et al. Prevalence of bcl-2 rearrangement in patients with hepatitis C virus-related mixed cryoglobulinemia with or without B-cell lymphomas. Ann Intern Med. 2002;137:571-580.

385. Thomas DL. Hepatitis C and human immunodeficiency virus infection. Hepatology. 2002;36(Suppl 1):S201-S209.

386. Martin P, Di Bisceglie AM, Kassianides C, et al. Rapidly progressive non-A, non-B hepatitis in patients with human immunodeficiency virus infection. Gastroenterology. 1989;97:1559-1561.

387. Soto B, Sanchez-Quijano A, Rodrigo L, et al. Human immunodeficiency virus infection modifies the natural history of parenterally-acquired hepatitis C with an unusually rapid progression to cirrhosis. J Hepatol. 1997;26:1-5.

388. Rosenberg PM, Farrell JJ, Abraczinskas DR, et al. Rapidly progressive fibrosing cholestatic hepatitis—hepatitis C virus in HIV coinfection. Am J Gastroenterol. 2002;97:478-483.

389. Benhamou Y, Bochet M, DiMartino V, et al. Liver fibrosis progression in human immunodeficiency virus and hepatitis C virus coinfected patients. Hepatology. 1999;30:1054-1058.

390. Graham CS, Baden LR, Yu E, et al. Influence of human immunodeficiency virus infection on the course of hepatitis C virus infection: A meta-analysis. Clin Infect Dis. 2001;33:562-569.

391. Bica I, McGovern B, Dhar R, et al. Increasing mortality due to end-stage liver disease in patients with human immunodeficiency virus infection. Clin Infect Dis. 2001;32:492-497.

392. Chung RT, Evans SR, Yang Y, et al. Immune recovery is associated with persistent rise in HCV RNA, infrequent liver test flares, and is not impaired by HCV in co-infected subjects. AIDS. 2002;16:1915-1923.

393. Davis GL, Balart LA, Schiff ER, et al. Treatment of chronic hepatitis C with recombinant interferon alfa: A multicenter randomized, controlled trial. N Engl J Med. 1989;321:1501-1506.

394. Di Bisceglie AM, Martin P, Kassianides C, et al. Recombinant interferon alfa therapy for chronic hepatitis C: A randomized, double-blind, placebo-controlled trial. N Engl J Med. 1989;321:1506-1510.

395. Carithers RLJ, Emerson SS. Therapy of hepatitis C: Meta-analysis of interferon alfa-2b trials. Hepatology. 1997;26(Suppl 1):83S-88S.

396. Marcellin P, Pouteau M, Martinot-Peignoux M, et al. Lack of benefit of escalating dosage of interferon alfa in patients with chronic hepatitis C. Gastroenterology. 1995;109:156-165.

397. Poynard T, Bedossa P, Chevallier M, et al. A comparison of three interferon alfa-2b regimens for the long-term treatment of chronic non-B hepatitis. N Engl J Med. 1995;332:1457-1462.

398. Poynard T, Leroy V, Cohard M, et al. Meta-analysis of interferon randomized trials in the treatment of viral hepatitis C: Effects of dose and duration. Hepatology. 1996;24:778-789.

399. Lee WM. Therapy of hepatitis C: interferon alfa-2a trials. Hepatology. 1997;26(Suppl 1):89S-95S.

400. Farrell GC. Therapy of hepatitis C: Interferon alfa-n1 trials. Hepatology. 1997;26(Suppl 1):96S-100S.

401. Keeffe EB, Hollinger FB, Consensus Interferon Study Group. Therapy of hepatitis C: consensus interferon trials. Hepatology. 1997;26(Suppl 1):101S-107S.

402. Consensus Statement. EASL international consensus conference on hepatitis C. J Hepatol. 1999;30:956-961.
403. Booth JCL, O'Grady J, Neuberger J, et al. Clinical guidelines on the management of hepatitis C. Gut. 2001;49(Suppl 1):i1-i21.
404. Kjaergard LL, Krogsgaard K, Gluud C. Interferon alfa with or without ribavirin for chronic hepatitis C: Systematic review of randomised trials. BMJ. 2001;323:1151-1155.
405. McHutchison JG, Gordon SC, Schiff ER, et al. Interferon alfa-2b alone or in combination with ribavirin as initial treatment for chronic hepatitis C. N Engl J Med. 1998;339:1485-1492.
406. Poynard T, Marcellin P, Lee SS, et al. Randomized trial of interferon α2b plus ribavirin for 48 weeks or for 24 weeks versus interferon α2b plus placebo for 48 weeks for treatment of chronic infection with hepatitis C virus. Lancet. 1998;352:1426-1432.
407. Dusheiko G, Main J, Thomas H, et al. Ribavirin treatment for patients with chronic hepatitis C: Results of a placebo-controlled study. J Hepatol. 1996;25:591-598.
408. Di Bisceglie AM, Conjeevaram HS, Fried MW, et al. Ribavirin as therapy for chronic hepatitis C: A randomized, double-blind, placebo-controlled trial. Ann Intern Med. 1995;123:897-903.
409. Bodenheimer HC Jr., Lindsay KL, Davis GL, et al. Tolerance and efficacy of oral ribavirin treatment of chronic hepatitis C: A multicenter trial. Hepatology. 1997;26:473-477.
410. Reichard O, Schvarc R, Weiland O. Therapy of hepatitis C: Alpha interferon and ribavirin. Hepatology. 1997;26(Suppl 1):108S-111S.
411. Ning Q, Brown D, Parodo J, et al. Ribavirin inhibits viral-induced macrophage production of tumor necrosis factor, interleukin-1, and procoagulant fg12 prothrombinase and preserves Th1 cytokine production but inhibits Th2 cytokine response. J Immunol. 1998;160:3487-3493.
412. Hong Z. The role of ribavirin-induced mutagenesis in HCV therapy: A concept or a fact? Hepatology. 2003;38:807-810.
413. Lau JY, Tam RC, Liang TJ, et al. Mechanism of action of ribavirin in the combination treatment of chronic HCV infection. Hepatology. 2002;35:1002-1009.
414. Crotty S, Maag D, Arnold JJ, et al. The broad-spectrum antiviral ribonucleoside ribavirin is an RNA virus mutagen. Nat Med. 2000;6:1375-1379.
415. Crotty S, Cameron CE, Andino R. RNA virus error catastrophe: Direct molecular test by using ribavirin. Proc Nat Acad Sci. 2001;98:6895-6900.
416. Contreras AM, Hiasa Y, He W, et al. Viral RNA mutations are region specific and increased by ribavirin in a full-length hepatitis C virus replication system. J Virol. 2002;76:8505-8517.
417. Schalm SW, Hansen BE, Chemello L, et al. Ribavirin enhances the efficacy but not the adverse effects of interferon in chronic hepatitis C. Meta-analysis of individual patient data from European centers. J Hepatol. 1997;26:961-966.
418. Marcellin P, Boyer N, Gervais A, et al. Long-term histologic improvement and loss of detectable intrahepatic HCV RNA in patients with chronic hepatitis C and sustained response to interferon alpha therapy. Ann Intern Med. 1997;127:875-881.
419. Lau DT, Kleiner DE, Ghany MG, et al. 10-year follow-up after interferon-alpha therapy for chronic hepatitis C. Hepatology. 1998;28:1121-1127.
420. Reddy KR, Wright TL, Pockros PJ, et al. Efficacy and safety of pegylated (40-kd) interferon alpha-2a compared with interferon alpha-2a in noncirrhotic patients with chronic hepatitis C. Hepatology. 2001;33:433-438.
421. Lindsay KL, Trepo C, Heintges T, et al. A randomized, double-blind trial comparing pegylated interferon alfa-2b to interferon alfa-2b as initial treatment for chronic hepatitis C. Hepatology. 2001;34:395-403.
422. Zeuzem S, Feinman SV, Rasenack J, et al. Peginterferon alfa-2a in patients with chronic hepatitis C. N Engl J Med. 2000;343:1666-1672.
423. Heathcote EJ, Shiffman ML, Cooksley WG, et al. Peginterferon alfa-2a in patients with chronic hepatitis C and cirrhosis. N Engl J Med. 2000;343:1673-1680.
424. Manns MP, McHutchison JG, Gordon SC, et al. Peginterferon alfa-2b plus ribavirin compared with interferon alfa-2b plus ribavirin for initial treatment of chronic hepatitis C: A randomised trial. Lancet. 2001;358:958-965.
425. Fried MW, Shiffman ML, Reddy KR, et al. Peginterferon alfa-2a plus ribavirin for chronic hepatitis C virus infection. N Engl J Med. 2002;347:975-982.
426. Hadziyannis SJ, Sette H, Morgan T, et al. Peginterferon alfa-2a (40 kilodaltons) and ribavirin combination therapy in chronic hepatitis C: Randomized study of treatment duration and ribavirin dose. Ann Intern Med. 2004;140:346-355.
427. Fried MW. Side effects of therapy of hepatitis C and their management. Hepatology. 2002;36(Suppl 1):S237-S244.
428. Dieterich DT, Spivak JL. Hematologic disorders associated with hepatitis C virus infection and their management. Clin Infect Dis. 2003;37:533-541.
429. Shiffman ML, Di Bisceglie AM, Lindsay KL, et al. Peginterferon alfa-2a and ribavirin in patients with chronic hepatitis C who have failed prior treatment. Gastroenterology. 2004;126:1015-1023.
430. Layden-Almer JE, Ribeiro RM, Wiley T, et al. Viral dynamics and response differences in HCV-infected African American and white patients treated with IFN and ribavirin. Hepatology. 2003;37:1343-1350.
431. Zeuzem S, Schmidt JM, Lee JH, et al. Hepatitis C virus dynamics in vivo: Effect of ribavirin and interferon alfa on viral turnover. Hepatology. 1998;28:245-252.
432. Zeuzem S, Herrmann E, Lee JH, et al. Viral kinetics in patients with chronic hepatitis C treated with standard or peginterferon alfa-2a. Gastroenterology. 2001;120:1438-1447.
433. Di Bisceglie AM, Thompson J, Smith-Wilkaitis N, et al. Combination of interferon and ribavirin in chronic hepatitis C: re-treatment of nonresponders to interferon. Hepatology. 2001;33:704-707.
434. Di Bisceglie AM, Hoofnagle JH. Optimal therapy of hepatitis C. Hepatology. 2002;36(Suppl 1):S121-S127.
435. McHutchison JG, Poynard T, Pianko S, et al. The impact of interferon plus ribavirin on response to therapy in black patients with chronic hepatitis C. Gastroenterology. 2000;119:1317-1323.
436. McHutchison JG, Manns M, Patel K, et al. Adherence to combination therapy enhances sustained response in genotype-1-infected patients with chronic hepatitis C. Gastroenterology. 2002;123:1061-1069.
437. Davis GL, Lau JYN. Factors predictive of a beneficial response to therapy of hepatitis C. Hepatology. 1997;26(Suppl 1):122S-127S.
438. Pagliaro L, Craxi A, Cammaa C, et al. Interferon-a for chronic hepatitis C: An analysis of pretreatment clinical predictors of response. Hepatology. 1994;19:820-828.
439. Davis GL, Lindsay K, Albrecht J, et al. Clinical predictors of response to recombinant alpha interferon-α treatment in patients with chronic non-A, non-B hepatitis (hepatitis C). J Viral Hepat. 1994;1:55-63.
440. Tsubota A, Chayama K, Ikeda K, et al. Factors predictive of response to interferon-α therapy in hepatitis C virus infection. Hepatology. 1994;19:1088-1094.
441. Garson JA, Brillanti B, Whitby K, et al. Analysis of clinical and virological factors associated with response to alpha interferon therapy in chronic hepatitis C. J Med Virol. 1995;45:348-353.
442. Gane EJ, Lo S-K, Riordan SM, et al. A randomized study comparing ribavirin and interferon alfa monotherapy for hepatitis C recurrence after liver transplantation. Hepatology. 1998;27:1403-1407.
443. Wright TL, Combs C, Kim M, et al. Interferon-α therapy for hepatitis C infection after liver transplantation. Hepatology. 1994;20:773-779.
444. Davis GL, Wong JB, McHutchison JG, et al. Early virologic response to treatment with peginterferon alfa-2b plus ribavirin in patients with chronic hepatitis C. Hepatology. 2003;38:645-652.
445. Davis GL. Monitoring of viral levels during therapy of hepatitis C. Hepatology. 2002;36(Suppl 1):S145-S151.
446. Shiffman ML, Hofmann CM, Contos MJ, et al. A randomized, controlled trial of maintenance interferon therapy for patients with chronic hepatitis C virus and persistent viremia. Gastroenterology. 1999;117:1164-1172.
447. Yoshida H, Arakawa Y, Sata M, et al. Interferon therapy prolonged life expectancy among chronic hepatitis C patients. Gastroenterology. 2002;123:483-491.
448. Younossi ZM, Singer ME, McHutchison JG, et al. Cost effectiveness of interferon alpha2b combined with ribavirin for the treatment of chronic hepatitis C. Hepatology. 1999;30:1318-1324.
449. Salomon JA, Weinstein MC, Hammitt JK, et al. Cost-effectiveness of treatment for chronic hepatitis C infection in an evolving patient population. JAMA. 2003;290:228-237.
450. Wong JB, Koff RS. Watchful waiting with periodic liver biopsy versus immediate empirical therapy for histologically mild chronic hepatitis C. A cost-effectiveness analysis. Ann Intern Med. 2000;133:665-675.
451. Shindo M, Di Bisceglie AM, Hoofnagle JH. Long-term follow-up of patients with chronic hepatitis C treated with α-interferon. Hepatology. 1992;15:1013-1016.
452. Poynard T, McHutchison J, Davis GL, et al. Impact of interferon alfa-2b and ribavirin on progression of liver fibrosis in patients with chronic hepatitis C. Hepatology. 2000;32:1131-1137.
453. Shiratori Y, Imazeki F, Moriyama M, et al. Histologic improvement of fibrosis in patients with hepatitis C who have sustained response to interferon therapy. Ann Intern Med. 2000;132:517-524.
454. Sobesky R, Mathurin P, Charlotte F, et al. Modeling the impact of interferon alfa treatment on liver fibrosis progression in chronic hepatitis C: A dynamic view. Gastroenterology. 1999;116:378-386.
455. Nishiguchi S, Kuroki T, Nakatani S, et al. Randomised trial of effects of interferon-α on incidence of hepatocellular carcinoma in chronic active hepatitis C with cirrhosis. Lancet. 1995;346:1051-1055.
456. Mazzella G, Accogli E, Sottili S, et al. Alpha interferon treatment may prevent hepatocellular carcinoma in HCV-related liver cirrhosis. J Hepatol. 1996;24:141-147.
457. Yoshida H, Shiratori Y, Moriyama M, et al. Interferon therapy reduces the risk for hepatocellular carcinoma: National surveillance program of cirrhotic and noncirrhotic patients with chronic hepatitis C in Japan. Ann Intern Med. 1999;131:174-181.
458. Chander G, Sulkowski MS, Jenckes MW, et al. Treatment of chronic hepatitis C: A systematic review. Hepatology 2002;36(Suppl 1):S135-S144.
459. Bernardinello E, Cavalletto L, Chemello L, et al. Long-term clinical outcome after beta-interferon therapy in cirrhotic patients with chronic hepatitis C: TTVH Study Group. Hepatogastroenterology. 1999;46:3216-3222.
460. Fattovich G, Giustina G, Degos F, et al. Effectiveness of inteferon alfa on incidence of hepatocellular carcinoma and decompensation in cirrhosis type C. J Hepatol. 1997;27:201-205.
461. Wright TL. Treatment of patients with hepatitis C and cirrhosis. Hepatology. 2002;36(Suppl 1):S185-S194.
462. Bacon BR. Treatment of patients with hepatitis C and normal serum aminotransferase levels. Hepatology. 2002;36(Suppl 1):S179-S184.
463. Shiffman ML. Retreatment of patients with chronic hepatitis C. Hepatology. 2002;36(Suppl 1):S128-S134.
464. Cummings KJ, Lee SM, West ES, et al. Interferon and ribavirin vs interferon alone in the re-treatment of chronic hepatitis C previously nonresponsive to interferon. JAMA. 2001;285:193-199.
465. Cheng SJ, Bonis PA, Lau J, et al. Interferon and ribavirin for patients with chronic hepatitis C who did not respond to previous interferon therapy: A meta-analysis of controlled and uncontrolled trials. Hepatology. 2001;33:231-240.

466. Camma C, Bruno S, Schepis F, et al. Retreatment with interferon plus ribavirin of chronic hepatitis C non-responders to interferon monotherapy: A meta-analysis of individual patient data. Gut. 2002;51:864-869.

467. Falck-Ytter Y, Kale H, Mullen KD, et al. Surprisingly small effect of antiviral treatment in patients with hepatitis C. Ann Intern Med. 2002;136:288-292.

468. Schwimmer JB, Balistreri WF. Transmission, natural history, and treatment of hepatitis C virus infection in the pediatric population. Semin Liver Dis. 2000;20:37-46.

469. Jonas MM. Children with hepatitis C. Hepatology. 2002;36(Suppl 1):S173-S178.

470. Alberti A, Boccato S, Vario A, et al. Therapy of acute hepatitis c. Hepatology 2002;36(Suppl 1):S195-S200.

471. Jaeckel E, Cornberg M, Wedemeyer H, et al. Treatment of acute hepatitis C with interferon alfa-2b. N Engl J Med. 2001;345:1452-1457.

472. Wright TL. Liver transplantation for chronic hepatitis C viral infection. Gastroenterol Clin North Am. 1993;22:231-242.

473. Féray C, Samuel D, Thiers V, et al. Reinfection of liver graft by hepatitis C virus after liver transplantation. J Clin Invest. 1992;89:1361-1365.

474. Féray C, Gigou M, Samuel D, et al. Influence of the genotype of hepatitis C virus on the severity of recurrent liver disease after liver transplantation. Gastroenterology. 1995;108:1088-1096.

475. Johnson MW, Washburn K, Freeman RB, et al. Hepatitis C viral infection in liver transplantation. Arch Surg. 1996;131:284-291.

476. Gane EJ, Portmann BC, Naoumov NV, et al. Long-term outcome of hepatitis C infection after liver transplantation. N Engl J Med. 1996;334:815-820.

477. Féray C, Caccamo L, Alexander GJM, et al. European collaborative study on factors influencing outcome after liver transplantation for hepatitis C. Gastroenterology. 1999;117:619-625.

478. Forman LM, Lewis JD, Berlin JA, et al. The association between hepatitis C infection and survival after orthotopic liver transplantation. Gastroenterology. 2002;122:889-896.

479. Berenguer M. Natural history of recurrent hepatitis C. Liver Transpl. 2002;8 (Suppl 1):S14-S18.

480. Charlton M. Hepatitis C infection in liver transplantation. Am J Transpl. 2001;1: 197-203.

481. Prieto M, Berenguer M, Rayon JM, et al. High incidence of allograft cirrhosis in hepatitis C virus genotype 1b infection following liver transplantation: Relationship with rejection episodes. Hepatology. 1999;29:250-256.

482. Doughty AL, Spenser JD, Cossart YE, et al. Cholestatic hepatitis after liver transplantation is associated with persistently high serum hepatitis C virus RNA levels. Transpl Surg. 1998;4:15-21.

483. Cotler SJ, Taylor SL, Gretch DR, et al. Hyperbilirubinemia and cholestatic liver injury in hepatitis C-infected liver transplant recipients. Am J Gastroenterol. 2000;95:753-759.

484. Sheiner PA. Hepatitis C after liver transplantation. Semin Liver Dis. 2000;20: 201-209.

485. Gane E. Treatment of recurrent hepatitis C. Liver Transpl. 2002;8(Suppl 1):S28-S37.

486. Fong TL, Valinluck B, Govindarajan S, et al. Short-term prednisone therapy affects aminotransferase activity and hepatitis C virus RNA levels in chronic hepatitis C. Gastroenterology. 1994;107:196-199.

487. Everson GT. Impact of immunosuppressive therapy on recurrence of hepatitis C. Liver Transpl. 2002;8(Suppl 1):S19-S27.

488. Berenguer M, Prieto M, Cordoba J, et al. Early development of chronic active hepatitis in recurrent hepatitis C virus infection after liver transplantation: association with treatment of rejection. J Hepatol. 1998;28:756-763.

489. Soriano V, Sulkowski M, Bergin C, et al. Care of patients with chronic hepatitis C and HIV co-infection: recommendations from the HIV-HCV International Panel. AIDS. 2002;16:813-828.

490. Sulkowski MS. Hepatitis C virus infection in HIV-infected patients. Curr Hepat Rep. 2002;1:16-22.

491. Lafeuillade A, Hittinger G, Chadapaud S. Increased mitochondrial toxicity with ribavirin in HIV/HCV coinfection. Lancet. 2001;357:280-281.

492. Johnson RJ, Gretch DR, Yamabe H, et al. Membranoproliferative glomerulonephritis associated with hepatitis C virus infection. N Engl J Med. 1993;328:465-470.

493. Misiani R, Bellavita P, Fenili D, et al. Interferon alfa-2a therapy in cryoglobulinemia associated with hepatitis C virus. N Engl J Med. 1994;330:751-756.

494. Bonomo L, Casato M, Afeltra A, et al. Treatment of idiopathic mixed cryoglobulinemia with alpha interferon. Am J Med. 1987;83:726-730.

495. Patriarca F, Silvestri F, Fanin R, et al. Long-lasting complete remission of hepatitis C virus (HCV) infection and HCV-associated immunocytoma with alpha-interferon treatment. Br J Haematol. 2001;112:370-372.

496. Hermine O, Lefrère F, Bronowicki J-P, et al. Regression of splenic lymphoma with villous lymphocytes after treatment of hepatitis C virus infection. N Engl J Med. 2002;347:89-94.

497. Mazzaro C, Franzin F, Tulissi T, et al. Regression of monoclonal B-cell expansion in patients affected by mixed cryoglobulinemia responsive to alpha-interferon therapy. Cancer. 1996;77:2604-2613.

498. Lamarre D, Anderson PC, Bailey M, et al. An NS3 protease inhibitor with antiviral effects in humans infected with hepatitis C virus. Nature. 2003;426:186-189.

CHAPTER **113**

Global Perspectives on Human Immunodeficiency Virus Infection and Acquired Immunodeficiency Syndrome

MICHAEL H. MERSON

PETER PIOT

M ore than two decades after the recognition of acquired immunodeficiency syndrome (AIDS) in the United States, the global epidemiologic pattern of human immunodeficiency virus (HIV) infection has changed dramatically. Whereas the disease was originally confined primarily to North America, western Europe, and parts of sub-Saharan Africa, HIV has now spread throughout the world, with major epidemic foci in all continents. In addition, on a worldwide scale, the epidemic has now evolved into a mainly heterosexually transmitted disease of the developing world and, increasingly, of underprivileged populations in the industrialized world. In this aspect, HIV infection now resembles the "classic" infectious diseases, disproportionately affecting those most socially and economically vulnerable.

This chapter focuses on specific features of the epidemiology and impact of HIV infection and AIDS in the developing world as well as the expanding global response to the epidemic. Although two serotypes of HIV are currently recognized, namely, HIV-1 and HIV-2, the term *HIV* is used in this chapter to designate HIV-1, which is the major virus.

SIZE OF THE PROBLEM

As of the end of 2002, the Joint United Nations Programme on HIV/AIDS (UNAIDS) estimated that 42 million adults and children were living with HIV/AIDS, from a cumulative total of well over 70 million persons infected since the beginning of the epidemic. Figure 113-1 shows global estimates of the HIV/AIDS epidemic.[1]

More than 90% of infected persons live in the developing world, and 70% of AIDS cases have occurred in Africa. These figures keep increasing at a staggering rate, with approximately 14,000 new infections per day. In 2002 alone, it is estimated that 5 million people became infected, including 800,000 children younger than 15. The majority of new infections are occurring in sub-Saharan Africa and Asia, although fast-growing epidemics are taking place in eastern Europe and the Caribbean. It is estimated that one third of those currently living with HIV/AIDS are between the ages of 15 and 24.[1,2]

The best current estimates suggest that an additional 45 million people will become infected in 126 low- and middle-income countries between 2002 and 2010 unless prevention efforts are drastically expanded on a global scale.[1] In Nigeria, Ethiopia, Russia, India, and

Number of people living with HIV/AIDS	Total	42 million
	Adults	38.6 million
	Women	*19.2 million*
	Children under 15 years	3.2 million
People newly infected with HIV in 2002	Total	5 million
	Adults	4.2 million
	Women	*2 million*
	Children under 15 years	800,000
AIDS deaths in 2002	Total	3.1 milion
	Adults	2.5 million
	Women	*1.2 million*
	Children under 15 years	610.000

FIGURE 113-1. Global summary of HIV/AIDS epidemic as of December 2002. (Data from UNAIDS and WHO. AIDS Epidemic Update: December 2002. Geneva: UNAIDS, 2002.)

China—five countries that all have early- to middle-stage HIV epidemics and together compose 40% of the world's population—one worst-case scenario projects that there will be 50 million to 75 million infections by 2010.[3] Transmission of HIV in all five of these countries is projected to increase steeply beyond high-risk populations, such as commercial sex workers and injection drug users, to the general population through unsafe heterosexual contact and the movement of migrant or displaced populations. There is little doubt that these growing epidemics have the potential to decimate the social, economic, and political stability of entire regions.

EUROPE

The epidemiology of HIV/AIDS in North America is extensively discussed in Chapter 114; except for this section, this chapter deals mainly with the situation in the developing world. In 2002, a total of 14,439 new HIV infections were reported in western Europe (13,128 of which were reported exclusively in European Union nations)—a 23% increase from 2001.[4] In some countries, HIV incidence has decreased among men who have sex with men. Heterosexual transmission continues to rise, however, in part because of rising infection rates among drug users, who often have sex with noninjectors. In 2002, heterosexual transmission accounted for 44% of all incident HIV infections and 38% of new AIDS cases in western Europe, an increase of 11% from 1998.[4] Injection drug use contributes particularly to HIV transmissions in Spain, Italy, and France. In general, in the industrialized countries of Europe, Australia, and New Zealand, there has been a marked fall or leveling off in AIDS incidence and AIDS mortality in the past decade because of the widespread availability of antiretroviral therapy. However, homosexual and bisexual men still represent a large proportion of AIDS cases in western Europe, reflecting the high incidence of infection in these populations a decade ago.

In previous editions of this textbook, the HIV incidence in eastern Europe was reported to be low but with a potential for an "uncontrolled epidemic." Until the mid-1990s, mass screening of various populations indicated extremely low levels of HIV infection. Since the late 1990s, however, parts of eastern Europe and central Asia have had the fastest growing HIV/AIDS epidemics in the world. Between 1994 and 1997, HIV infections increased sixfold in the former socialist economies, totaling approximately 200,000 adults by the end of 1997 and 1.2 million by the end of 2002 (Fig. 113-2).[1,5] The majority of infections have been identified in injection drug users. In the Russian

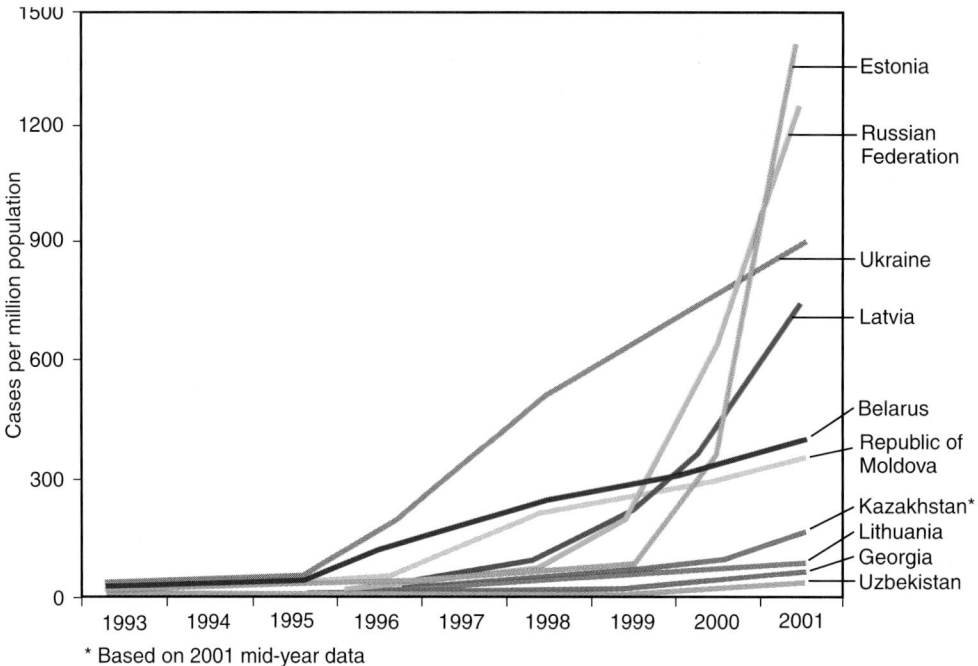

FIGURE 113-2. Cumulative reported HIV infections per million population, eastern European countries, 1993 to 2001. *(Data from UNAIDS and WHO. AIDS Epidemic Update: December 2002. Geneva: UNAIDS, 2002.)*

Federation, where more than three quarters of all HIV infections among the 15 countries of the former Soviet Union are concentrated, approximately 90% of infections are attributed to injection drug use. National adult HIV prevalence now exceeds 1% in the Ukraine. Further, almost 80% of new infections in the Commonwealth of Independent States between 1997 and 2000 have been among people younger than 29.[1] The epidemic continues to grow in Kazakhstan, Azerbaijan, Georgia, Kyrgyzstan, Tajikistan, and Uzbekistan, and transmission has been documented among incarcerated persons throughout the region.

In a few countries in eastern Europe and central Asia, where the epidemic has been larger in scale, such as Belarus and Ukraine, heterosexual contact has begun to eclipse injection drug use as the primary mode of transmission (Fig. 113-3).[1,4] This trend can be expected to occur in other countries in the region, reflecting spread beyond high-risk groups to the general population.[6] This rapid spread of HIV infection in eastern Europe parallels epidemics of other sexually transmitted diseases (STDs) and of injection drug use. Syphilis rates in a number of countries of the region have skyrocketed since the 1990s.[6]

AFRICA

Sub-Saharan Africa remains by far the worst affected region; approximately 70% of HIV-positive persons in the world live here, although it contains only 11% of the global population. Nine percent of all adults younger than 45 years are HIV positive, and in four countries (Botswana, Zimbabwe, Lesotho, and Swaziland) one in three adults is infected. In cities such as Harare, Zimbabwe, and Gaborone, Botswana, as many as 40% of all sexually active adults are infected, and this is even the case now in some rural areas as well. However, the HIV prevalence rate is still well below 1% to 2% in a few countries such as Madagascar, Mali, and Senegal.[1,2,7,8]

In most parts of Africa, the epidemic is still expanding. In general, HIV prevalence is highest in eastern and southern Africa, although in the West African countries of Côte d'Ivoire, Burkina Faso, Cameroon, Nigeria, and Togo it has already exceeded 5%.[2] Figure 113-4 shows the evolution of HIV prevalence among pregnant women in South Africa. Infection rates are rising rapidly in girls and young women, who are often infected by older men and are biologically more vulnerable to sexual acquisition of HIV. For example, in Lusaka, Zambia,

as many as one in four 18-year-old women are infected with HIV, compared with 5% of 18-year-old men.[9] In several countries, it has become the norm for poorer adolescent girls to have relationships with men who are often 6 or more years older, and these relationships are believed to have a transactional basis in which sex is exchanged for material goods or gifts. Increasing age asymmetry in these relationships and risk of HIV infection are positively correlated.[10]

Prevalence rates are generally highest among the most sexually active parts of the population, as illustrated by the age distribution of HIV infections, which peak between the ages of 20 and 40 years; by

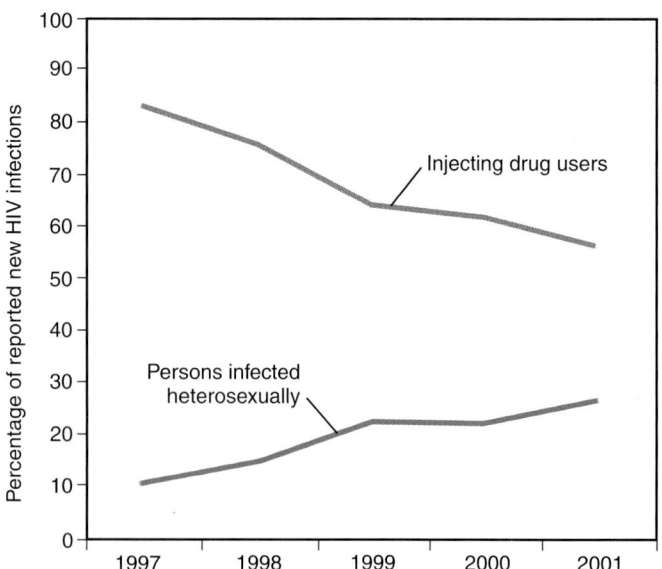

FIGURE 113-3. HIV infections newly diagnosed by transmission group in Ukraine, 1997 to 2001. *(Data from European Centre for the Epidemiological Monitoring of AIDS. HIV/AIDS Surveillance in Europe. End-year report 2002. No. 68. Saint-Maurice, France: Institut de Veille Sanitaire, 2003.)*

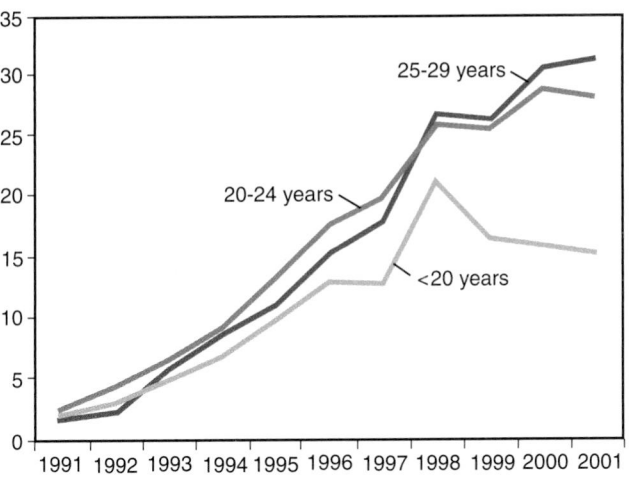

FIGURE 113-4. HIV prevalence (as percentage) by age, South African antenatal clinics, 1991 to 2001. *(Data from UNAIDS and WHO. AIDS Epidemic Update: December 2002. Geneva: UNAIDS, 2002.)*

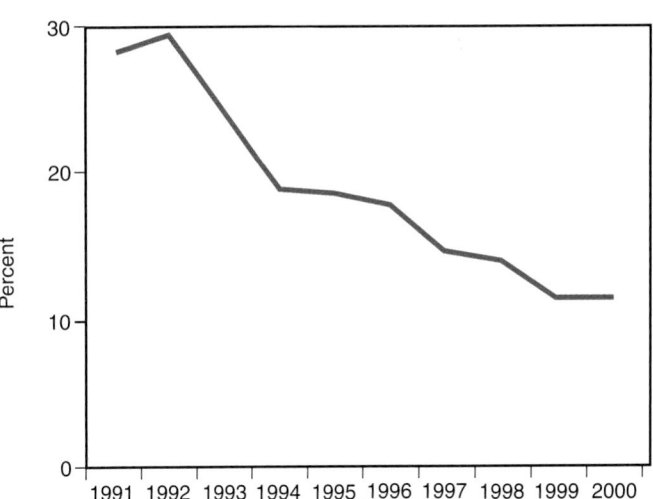

FIGURE 113-5. Trends in HIV prevalence among pregnant women in Kampala, Uganda, 1991 to 2000. *(Data from UNAIDS and WHO. A Global Overview of the Epidemic. Geneva: UNAIDS, July 2002.)*

very high infection rates among men with an STD; and by high rates among sex workers. Even in areas where HIV infection is still relatively uncommon in the population as a whole, prevalence rates well over 10% can be found in these higher risk populations. It is now increasingly common in Africa to find HIV prevalence rates exceeding 80% among sex workers and 50% among STD patients, particularly when the latter have genital ulcers. However, studies in antenatal clinics in Rwanda, Kenya, and Malawi demonstrate that the HIV epidemic is not limited as it was at an earlier stage to people with high-risk sexual behavior.[11-13] They also show that sexual behavior of the partner is an equally important risk factor in HIV infection. This fact is further illustrated by annual HIV incidence rates of 0.3% to as high as 5% in cohorts thought to be representative of the general population.[14] Among highly exposed female sex workers, such incidence rates may be as high as 12% to 50% per year.[15,16]

Mathematical modeling has shown that the sequence and distribution of partnerships can critically affect the transmission of HIV, particularly in the early stages of an epidemic. It is hypothesized that multiple concurrent sexual relationships, in regions such as sub-Saharan Africa where the predominant mode of transmission is heterosexual contact, may amplify rates of HIV infection faster than sequentially monogamous relationships. The implication of these findings is that interventions that emphasize "one partner at a time" messages, in addition to partner reduction and use of condoms, might be more effectively targeted toward sexually active youth and adults.[17]

Although prevention, treatment, and care efforts need to be drastically strengthened in sub-Saharan Africa to lessen the burden of HIV/AIDS, there are the first positive signs of the impact of prevention efforts. This is well documented in urban Uganda, where HIV prevalence rates among antenatal clinic attendees have steadily declined during the past decade, from 25% to 30% in 1991, to 15% in 1996, and to 11% in 2000 (Fig. 113-5).[2,18,19] One key feature of Uganda's approach to prevention has been decentralized information, education, and communication campaigns at the local level that have succeeded in delaying the age of first sexual intercourse, reducing the number of partners, and significantly increasing condom use nationwide among both high-risk groups and the general population.[2] Surveillance in the capital cities of Ethiopia, Rwanda, and Zambia has shown that the prevalence of HIV among young women has significantly declined, paralleling more consistent condom use and less sexual activity among urban adults (Fig. 113-6). In Senegal, an epidemic has been altogether averted by prevention efforts that began early and have maintained the population prevalence of HIV well below 1%.[2,8]

There have also been signs of possible progress in South Africa, where adolescent prevalence rates have dropped since 1998 and condom promotion has increased by a factor of 33 over a 5-year period.[2] However, it should be kept in mind that "stable" prevalence still implies active spread of HIV but at a rate more or less equaling the rate of death from AIDS in that population.[20] Overall, women account for 60% of all HIV infections in sub-Saharan Africa.

The disease burden of HIV infection in sub-Saharan Africa is high and will grow considerably higher. In 2002 alone, 2.4 million Africans died from AIDS, constituting 80% of the global total.[1] In addition, more than half a million children were born with HIV. The enormous impact of AIDS on health services, individuals, and communities is discussed in later sections of this chapter. In southern Africa, in particular, food crises and famine, partly caused by the HIV/AIDS pandemic, have synergistically worsened the impact of the epidemic by further crippling household food security, food production, and labor and fueling political instability and the orphan crisis.[1] It must be kept in mind, however, that AIDS in sub-Saharan Africa is not simply a disease of the poor. The countries of this continent face diverse and complex epidemics, as evidenced by the increased risk for

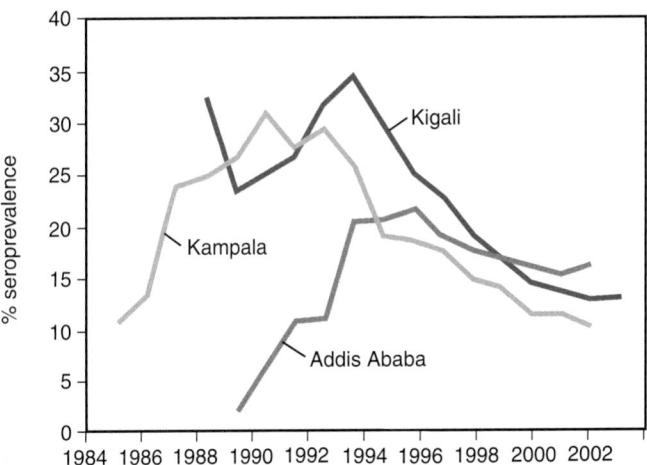

FIGURE 113-6. Declining HIV seroprevalence for pregnant women in selected urban areas of Africa: 1985 to 2002. *(Data from UNAIDS.)*

HIV among well-educated, high-income, and older men and women in rural Tanzania.[21]

A second human immunodeficiency virus, HIV-2, is found in West Africa and rarely in Angola and Mozambique.[22] The highest HIV-2 prevalence rates are found in Guinea-Bissau, where 5% to 10% of the sexually active population are infected, with higher incidence and prevalence of infection in women than men.[23,24] In the other countries where HIV-2 infection is found, prevalence rates are usually lower than 2% among pregnant women.[22]

HIV-2 seems to spread more slowly and the average age of infection appears to be higher than with HIV-1 infection in the same population.[25,26] On the other hand, STD patients and sex workers have the highest risk of HIV-2 infection, indicating that transmission of this virus is also mainly sexual. However, mother-to-child transmission and HIV-2 infection of infants and children are unusual.[27] Overall, the infectivity and risk of transmission of HIV-2 appear to be significantly less than those of HIV-1.[28] Similarly, the rate of disease development is lower after HIV-2 infection compared with HIV-1.[29]

Dually reactive sera for both HIV-1 and HIV-2 antibodies occur frequently in HIV-2–prevalent populations. One third to one half of such cases are caused by concomitant infection with both viruses.[30,31]

MIDDLE EAST AND NORTH AFRICA

Although information is limited and insufficient surveillance has limited accurate monitoring of trends in this region, a handful of countries have documented low-level but growing HIV/AIDS epidemics. The best estimates are that more than 80,000 new infections occurred in 2002, and there are now over half a million people living with HIV/AIDS.[1] In North Africa, transmission of HIV seems to occur mostly through hetero- and homosexual contact; however, in almost all countries in this region, transmission through injection drug use has been documented. Statistics from Iran have shown outbreaks of HIV among vulnerable populations, particularly injection drug users and prisoners, who are predominantly male. In 2001, HIV prevalence among incarcerated drug injectors in the country was 12%. Conservative estimates are that HIV prevalence is 1% among the country's 300,000 drug injectors, half of whom are believed to share injection equipment and more than a third of whom are married.[1] Nascent harm reduction efforts in Iran and surrounding central Asian countries have been spearheaded through the efforts and cooperation of both government and nongovernmental organizations.

Of particular concern in countries such as Djibouti and the Sudan is HIV transmission among mobile or displaced populations, or both. At the end of 2001, data from four sites in the Sudan showed an adult HIV/AIDS population prevalence of nearly 3%, highlighting the potential for a generalized epidemic.[32]

ASIA

HIV continues to spread considerably in Asia and the Pacific, where more than 7.2 million people were living with HIV in 2002; 30% of them were between the ages of 15 and 24.[1] India was the country with the largest number of infected persons at the end of 2002—3.8 million to 4.6 million—which was the second highest figure in the world, after South Africa. China's epidemic also shows no signs of decline, and it is projected that 10 million Chinese will have become infected with HIV by 2010.[1] Even the countries of Southeast Asia that were comparatively unaffected by HIV/AIDS in the 1990s, such as Indonesia, have experienced substantial increases in infections.

The extent of the spread of HIV in Asia is critical for the future of the pandemic because more than half of the world's population lives on this continent. In addition, the full consequences of HIV infection in Asia are just beginning to be seen now that many HIV-positive persons have progressed to AIDS.

HIV-1 spread was first detected in Asia among injection drug users. The virus has spread fulminantly among drug users in selected areas of Thailand, Myanmar, northeast India, Indonesia, and Malaysia,

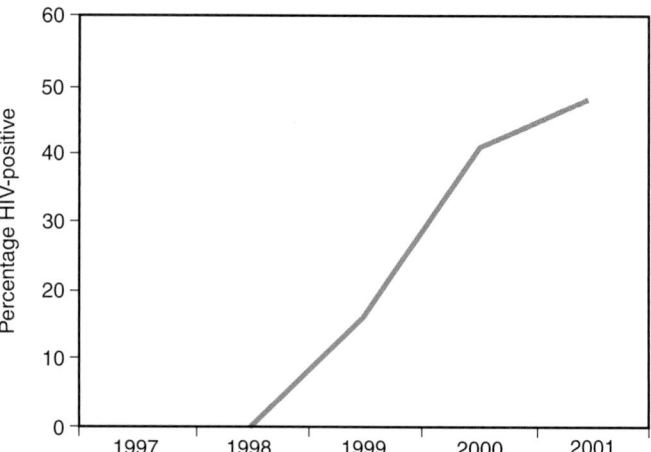

FIGURE 113-7. HIV prevalence among injecting drug users at a drug treatment center in Jakarta, Indonesia, 1997 to 2001. *(Data from UNAIDS and WHO. AIDS Epidemic Update: December 2002. Geneva: UNAIDS, 2002.)*

where HIV seroprevalence levels of 50% are not uncommon in such populations. The situation is similar in some parts of southern China, Malaysia, and Vietnam.[33-36] Figure 113-7 shows the rapid increase in HIV prevalence among injection drug users in Jakarta, Indonesia.

In a simultaneously occurring epidemic, the virus has also been spreading heterosexually, and this is now the main mode of transmission of HIV in Asia. As in Africa, it was initially among female sex workers that HIV infection rates increased most dramatically; in Mumbai, India, for example, HIV seroprevalence rose from zero in 1987 to more than 40% in 1995. However, there is now evidence that groups traditionally considered at low risk, such as married women reporting one lifetime sex partner, can also have high prevalence rates of HIV and STDs. This is especially true for a growing number of women in India and China, where monogamous sexual contact with a spouse remains the most significant risk factor for contracting HIV.[37] In six Indian states, HIV prevalence among women attending antenatal clinics has exceeded 1%, and HIV infections continue to rise in rural areas, suggesting the contribution of migrant labor patterns to the epidemic.[1]

In Thailand, HIV has now spread well beyond the most vulnerable groups, as illustrated by an overall prevalence rate of 1.8% in the adult population at the end of 2001.[38] Molecular and serologic techniques support the separate introduction in Thailand of a different HIV virus subtype among sex workers and injection drug users, among whom HIV prevalence reached as high as 50% in some areas, although it has eventually showed signs of slow decline.[39] Much of Thailand's success, compared with other countries with explosive HIV epidemics, can be attributed to a sustained commitment by its government to public awareness and condom distribution campaigns since the early 1990s. Prevention efforts have resulted in a well-documented decline of HIV incidence among young Thai men, associated with a decrease in commercial sex and increased condom use.[40-42] However, a major proportion of new infections now occur as a result of noncommercial sex, particularly among young people—illustrating the illusion that the HIV pandemic can be controlled simply by "targeted interventions" among those at highest risk. The Thai government has announced that they will make antiretroviral therapy drugs available for less than $US 1 per day.

Cambodia also seems to have begun to succeed in curbing its epidemic; in 2001, the HIV prevalence in pregnant women decreased to 1% to 3% from the peak of 2% to 6% in the late 1990s.[8] Figure 113-8 shows the decrease of HIV prevalence among sex workers in Cambodia with the concurrent increase in consistent condom use.

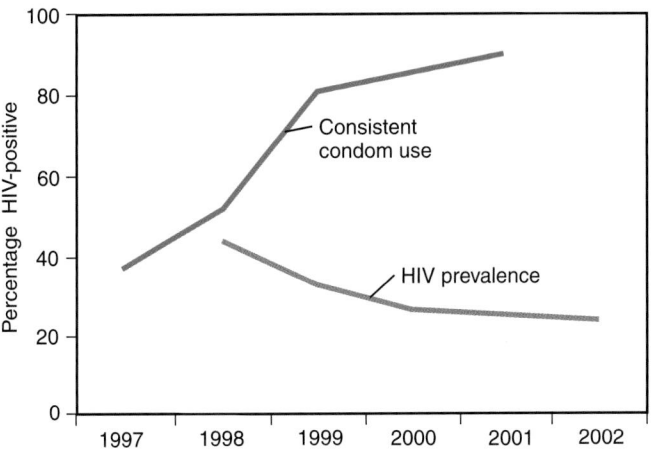

FIGURE 113-8. HIV prevalence and consistent condom use among sex workers in Cambodia, 1997 to 2002. *(Data from UNAIDS and WHO. AIDS Epidemic Update: December 2002. Geneva: UNAIDS, 2002.)*

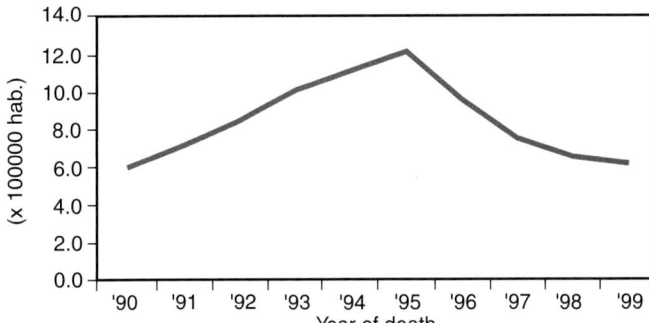

FIGURE 113-9. AIDS deaths in Brazil, 1990 to 1999. *(Data from Levi GC, Vitória MAA. Fighting against AIDS: The Brazilian experience. AIDS. 2002;16:2373-2383.)*

In addition to India, China remains a country of great concern. Currently, there are at least 1.5 million seropositive individuals in the country. HIV has been spreading mainly in three ways: through injection drug use in the southwest; heterosexually, among the more than 100 million migrant laborers nationwide who travel between rural areas and cities to find work; and through contaminated blood supplies. In the last case, blood plasma donors—primarily impoverished rural residents—were reinjected with the blood they donated after it was pooled with other blood to separate out plasma. That practice has resulted in HIV prevalence rates as high as 13% among donors in some areas.[1] Despite these various transmission routes, the crucial question for China remains its vulnerability to a widespread heterosexual HIV epidemic.[43]

LATIN AMERICA AND THE CARIBBEAN

Spread of HIV in the Caribbean and Latin America probably started at about the same time as in the United States. By 2002, 1.9 million adults were infected with HIV in this region, 420,000 of whom lived in the Caribbean.[1] Epidemiologic patterns in the region have been diverse and are changing over time. In general, homosexual and bisexual activity has been the main mode of spread since the beginning of the epidemic, but heterosexual intercourse and injection drug use have become increasingly important routes of transmission since the late 1980s in many countries.[44-46] A large proportion of men who have sex with men often also have sex with women, leading to an increased number of HIV infections among women. Bisexual behavior of their male partners is an important source of HIV infection for women in several Latin American countries.[47] Men who have sex with men throughout the region continue to be at high risk, with prevalence rates as high as 18% in these subgroups. Also, there is clear evidence of increasing infection among impoverished and less educated members of the population.[1,46]

A growing number of governments in Latin America are beginning to provide antiretroviral drugs, an encouraging development despite continued debate over affordable pricing, discussed later in this chapter. Brazil remains one of the world's few success stories in its political determination to secure antiretroviral drugs while also sustaining resources for prevention and care. More than 60% of the 170,000 people receiving antiretroviral drug therapy in Latin America live in Brazil. In the period 1996 to 2001, Brazil's treatment and care program, which guarantees state-funded antiretroviral drug therapy to those who are HIV positive, resulted in an estimated 350,000 avoided hospitalizations with a corresponding savings of more than $US 1 billion.[48] Although it is not exclusively related to antiretroviral therapy, AIDS mortality rates have substantially de-

clined (Fig. 113-9) and median survival time has increased from 5 months for cases diagnosed in the 1980s to 58 months for those diagnosed in 1996.[49] In addition, a large civil society network of nongovernmental and community-based organizations has contributed to the stabilization of the epidemic in Brazil by maintaining prevention efforts, such as needle exchange, condom distribution, and counseling and support programs, throughout the country.[48] Since 1997, HIV prevalence in Brazil has stabilized, with the national adult HIV prevalence at 0.7% by the end of 2001. However, prevalence rates among high-risk groups remain as high as 18% in some regions and the related crisis of 130,000 AIDS orphans has yet to be adequately addressed.[1,2,50]

Certain islands in the Caribbean have some of the highest cumulative incidence rates of AIDS in the world. Haiti remains the most severely affected country, with an adult HIV prevalence rate of more than 6%, followed by the Bahamas with a national prevalence of 3.5%. HIV infection in the Caribbean is a true mosaic of different epidemiologic patterns determined by the local interaction of various risk determinants of HIV transmission.[44] Transmission among men who have sex with men predominates in Trinidad, Tobago, Barbados, Jamaica, and Guyana. Injection drug use and sex for drugs (mainly cocaine and crack) are major risk factors in the Bahamas, Bermuda, Puerto Rico, and Trinidad. Finally, heterosexual transmission is predominant in Haiti and in the neighboring Dominican Republic. Surveillance data from the Dominican Republic in the period 1991 to 2001 show that HIV prevalence among pregnant women has stabilized and that this is positively correlated with increased condom use among sex workers and a reduction in the number of sexual partners among men.[1]

DYNAMICS OF THE SPREAD OF THE HUMAN IMMUNODEFICIENCY VIRUS

There is no difference between modes of transmission of HIV in the developing world and the industrialized countries. Selected aspects of HIV transmission in the developing world and other determinants of HIV spread are reviewed briefly here.

Modes of Transmission

Worldwide, HIV infection is basically a sexually transmitted infection. Unprotected heterosexual intercourse accounts for the large majority of cases of HIV infection in the developing world, but the situation is somewhat different in North America and western Europe.

The low efficiency of penile-vaginal intercourse for transmission of HIV has now been well documented, especially for transmission from women to men. A sustained and fulminant heterosexual epidemic can be explained only by a common occurrence of factors amplifying heterosexual transmission, probably in addition to high-risk sexual behavior patterns.

Factors that may enhance the efficiency of heterosexual transmission of HIV include higher viremia or more advanced immunodeficiency in the infecting partner, receptive anal intercourse, sex during menses, and the presence of other STDs. Viral load of HIV-1 has been shown to be the primary determinant of transmission risk in HIV-discordant couples.[51] Other factors that may increase the risk of heterosexual transmission, but are less well documented, include lack of circumcision in men, the use of various desiccating vaginal agents, traumatic sexual intercourse, and cervical ectopy.[52-54]

Conventional STDs have attracted the most attention as a risk factor because many are curable with relatively inexpensive antibiotics, leading to public health interventions for HIV prevention.[54,55] There is now convincing evidence from prospective studies that particularly genital ulcers (e.g., chancroid, syphilis, genital herpes) but also the more common nonulcerative STDs (e.g., gonorrhea, chlamydial infection) enhance the sexual transmission of HIV. This has been extensively documented in Africa, mainly in Kenya and the Democratic Republic of Congo.[15,56]

Two randomized trials in northern Tanzania and southern Uganda have suggested that community-based treatment of bacterial STDs can reduce the spread of HIV. However, STD treatment as a form of HIV prevention is believed to be more effective early in an epidemic, when HIV-1 prevalence is low (as opposed to moderate or high) and STD prevalence is high. Factors such as viral load and the prevalence of asymptomatic STDs are believed to play a major role in HIV transmission in places with moderate to large HIV/AIDS epidemics.[57,58]

Cohort studies in Nairobi, Kenya, found that the adjusted relative risks of genital ulcers (mainly chancroid) for HIV transmission were 3 to 8, but it is plausible that these lesions increase the risk of HIV transmission during a single sexual act by a factor between 10 and 100.[56] There is also increasing evidence that recent infection with herpes simplex virus type 2 (HSV-2), the most common cause of genital ulcer disease in developed and developing countries, is associated with a high risk of HIV infection, suggesting that antiviral agents that suppress prevalent HSV-2 could have a role in prevention of HIV infection in certain settings.[59] In addition, people with HIV infection with declining immunity have more genital ulcers; this probably increases their infectiousness during sexual intercourse because HIV can often be detected in ulcer material obtained from such persons.

The relative risks of gonorrhea and chlamydial infection for HIV acquisition in women are smaller than those of genital ulcers.[15] However, because these STDs are far more common in most populations than genital ulcers, their contribution to the heterosexual spread of HIV may also be greater.[55] Several studies have found that genital shedding of HIV is greatly enhanced in the presence of urethral, cervical, or vaginal inflammation.[60,61]

Globally, mother-to-child transmission during pregnancy, delivery, or breast-feeding is a second major mode of spread of HIV. Studies on mother-to-child transmission of HIV have found higher rates of transmission in Africa than in North America or Europe (approximately 30% to 40% versus 15% to 20%, respectively).[62,63]

Breast-feeding probably explains most of this higher risk of transmission in Africa.[64] Several studies have shown that the risk of transmission through breast-feeding is approximately 15% but can be as high as 29% for women who acquire HIV infection after delivery.[64-66]

Maternal vitamin A deficiency, high plasma HIV viral load, low CD4+ T-lymphocyte count, chorioamnionitis, prolonged rupture of membranes, biologic phenotype of the virus, and vaginal delivery, rather than cesarean section, have also been associated with increased risk of mother-to-child transmission.[67-71] In contrast to those in high-income countries, pregnant women in most developing countries rarely have access to interventions to prevent mother-to-child transmission of HIV, although the situation is slowly improving as programs to provide antiretroviral drugs to pregnant women and, in some cases, their sexual partners are being initiated.[72,73]

As mentioned, HIV has spread considerably among injection drug users in parts of Asia, eastern Europe, Latin America, and the Caribbean; this has sometimes occurred where injection has replaced smoking and inhaling as a more cost-effective way of administering drugs. Sharing of injection equipment and imprisonment at one point were the strongest predictors of HIV infection in Thailand.[74]

Transfusion with HIV-contaminated blood continues to be a source of HIV infection in some parts of the developing world, particularly in sub-Saharan Africa and China (discussed earlier).[75-77] This illustrates tragically that mere availability of technology (i.e., serologic tests for HIV antibody) is not sufficient to solve a public health problem.

Nosocomial transmission of HIV through injection with nonsterile syringes and needles occurs, but its relative contribution to the spread of HIV in the developing world is not well documented, although it is probably no more than 5%.[78,79] However, outbreaks of injection-associated nosocomial HIV infection in the former Soviet Union and in Romania show that injections for medical purposes may be a source of HIV infection in the community.[80,81]

Factors Influencing the Spread of the Human Immunodeficiency Virus

The HIV/AIDS epidemic is still in a dynamic phase in most parts of the world, with continuing geographic spread and changing epidemiologic patterns. Moreover, there is substantial heterogeneity in the epidemiology of HIV throughout the world.[46]

A multitude of variables influence the spread of HIV. It is the complex mix and interaction of these direct (behavioral) and indirect (demographic) risk and vulnerability factors that determine how and when HIV spreads in the population.[82,83]

Sexual Behavior

Sexual behavior is undoubtedly the most important determinant of HIV spread. Such behavior is very heterogeneous among and within populations. Sexual behavior surveys in Africa and Asia have documented this heterogeneity in terms of number of partners, age of sexual debut, and rates of casual and commercial sex.[82-85] In addition, these studies found that men have generally more partners than women and that in some societies higher socioeconomic status is associated with a higher number of partners. However, according to mathematical models, sexual mixing patterns are equally important in determining the spread of HIV, particularly in early stages of the epidemic.[86] The "core group" concept postulates that a relatively small proportion of the population is contributing to maintenance of the epidemic; this pattern was first described in the 1970s with respect to the epidemiology of gonorrhea in the United States.[87] However, for a chronic viral infection such as HIV, this concept is probably more relevant during the emerging phase of the epidemic than for "mature" epidemics with high levels of HIV infection already occurring among persons at a very young age and with relatively low-risk behavior.

The behavior of one's partner is as relevant for the risk of HIV infection as one's own behavior. This seems particularly true for women, who often become infected by their stable male partner. In some settings, up to 80% of HIV-positive women in long-term stable relationships have been infected by their partner. Data suggest that an increasing proportion of women with HIV infection in Africa, Thailand, Latin America, and India have their husbands as their only sexual contact.[11-13,37,88]

Sexual practices, in particular the frequency of anal intercourse, which is the most efficient mode of sexual transmission of HIV, may also vary among populations. Heterosexual anal intercourse and male bisexual behavior appear to be more frequent in some Latin American countries.[47]

Last, but not least, the rate of condom use plays a major role in the extent of HIV spread. Despite much early skepticism, condoms have become increasingly popular in many parts of the developing world, particularly where social marketing programs are active.[88] The use of condoms has played a role in the significant reduction of HIV incidence among intensively counseled discordant couples in the Democratic Republic of Congo; in large populations of men and women in Thailand, Uganda, and Senegal; and among sex workers in Kenya, the Democratic Republic of Congo, and Bolivia.[19,42,89-93] These "success stories" demonstrate that effective HIV prevention is possible, even under the difficult conditions of resource-poor settings.

Demography and Social Context

There is increasing awareness that personal behavior is critically influenced and conditioned by the sociodemographic, cultural, and legal contexts within a society.[46,94-97]

One of the most striking differences between the industrialized and the developing world is the age structure of the population; a much higher proportion of people in developing countries belong to the sexually most active age group. This by itself often results in higher incidence rates of sexually transmitted infections such as HIV infection.

Traditionally, migration and rapid urbanization have been associated with higher rates of STD. Both rural-to-urban and international migrations occur all over the developing world and have played a major role in the spread of HIV in southern Africa.[98]

An imbalance in numbers between the sexes may be an important determinant of HIV epidemiology because cities with such an imbalance appear to experience more rapid spread of HIV.[85,99] Migration of male labor into the cities of the developing world may create such a situation, but also social constraints on sexual behavior, such as disapproval of premarital and extramarital sex among women and late marriage by men for economic reasons, may be contributing factors. These demographic and social patterns may be associated with a higher rate of sex worker contacts by men.

With the insight that social, political, and economic contexts often contribute to health risk, many HIV prevention programs have begun to focus on structural interventions. Structural interventions have been used extensively in public health policy for a broad range of issues, including injury prevention, smoking cessation, and motor vehicle safety. These interventions address the determinants of health and seek to change the health environment of individuals, communities, and organizations. In HIV prevention, examples of structural interventions include expansion of voluntary HIV counseling and testing services, enactment of laws to prevent HIV discrimination in the workplace, regulations to improve the quality of the blood supply, sex education programs in schools, and syringe exchange programs. There is increasing hope that these prevention methods will complement more individually targeted interventions by addressing the underlying basis of HIV risk.[95,96]

Lastly, poverty is not only a consequence of the HIV/AIDS epidemic but also one of its major driving forces. Poverty is associated with commercial sex work, homeless adults and street children, low rate of literacy, migration and disruption in family patterns, and low status of women, all of which provide fertile ground for an HIV epidemic and make it more difficult for individuals and communities to cope with the consequences of HIV infection. Therefore, programs that concentrate solely on reducing epidemiologic risk factors without addressing simultaneously what makes people vulnerable to HIV are likely to be insufficiently effective.[82,96,97]

Gender

It is now widely recognized that gender inequalities drive the HIV/AIDS epidemic. Among affected populations in diverse regions, a greater percentage of women are HIV positive or face disproportionate risk for infection. In sub-Saharan Africa, for example, more than 12 million women were HIV positive in 2000, compared with 10 million men. This disparity is not confined to the developing world: in the United States, the proportion of all reported AIDS cases among women tripled from 1985 to 1999, the vast majority of them concentrated among black and Hispanic women.[100,101]

Violence against women in homes, schools, and workplaces increases vulnerability to HIV infection. Women with a history of sexual abuse are more likely to engage in unprotected sex, have multiple partners, and exchange sex for money or drugs. In Tanzania, HIV-positive women referred to an urban health center were 2.6 times more likely to have experienced violence from an intimate partner than women who were HIV negative. In Uganda, a higher *perceived* HIV risk for a male partner increased the risk of domestic violence against women by nearly four times compared with men who had a low perceived risk.[102] Violence or fear of violence also

hinders women's ability to discuss sexual health and negotiate condom use with male partners.[103,104]

Economic vulnerability is also a key risk factor for HIV/AIDS for both men and women. Discrimination against women that limits or denies their access to productive resources (i.e., exclusion from employment, education, family income, and property ownership) increases their economic vulnerability and limits their ability to receive health care. Labor and macroeconomic patterns often force men to leave their homes to seek employment in urban areas, where risk of HIV infection through commercial sex is increased. Female-headed households worldwide are also more likely to be economically vulnerable and at risk for sexual exploitation. Worldwide, women continue to bear the disproportionate burden of caregiving for HIV-positive family members and AIDS orphans.[105]

The sociocultural, economic, and political imbalances that endanger the health of women also negatively affect men. Social norms that perpetuate lack of sexual knowledge among women, stigmatize condom use, and reinforce the subordination of women place both sexes at increased risk for HIV infection. In contexts where masculinity must be demonstrated through high-risk behaviors such as substance abuse, unprotected sex with multiple partners, and violence, risk for HIV is concomitantly elevated. In order to address the multifaceted nature of gender disparities in the HIV/AIDS pandemic, prevention and care programs must, at the very least, implement gender-sensitive initiatives that recognize the different needs of women and men, destigmatize discussion and education about sexual health issues, and empower individuals to protect their health.[103]

Stigma and Discrimination

Related, but by no means limited, to gender inequalities, stigmatizing processes also play an important role in HIV risk, transmission, and the quality of life for people living with AIDS. By definition, stigma is more than an attitude or attribute of an individual or a culture; rather, it is a product of a social group's positioning in society and systematically reinforces that group's exclusion and subordination.[106] Stigma is a dynamic process and results in negatively valued differences in families, communities, schools, workplaces, health care systems, and governments. Factors contributing to HIV/AIDS-related stigma include the fatality of AIDS, widespread taboos about the sexual and drug use behaviors that are risk factors for infection, blaming of individuals for infection, and denial that the disease affects one's own community.

The perpetuation of stigma occurs at many levels and undoubtedly worsens the impact of HIV/AIDS. Comparative studies from Uganda and India demonstrate that individuals are more reluctant to seek HIV testing or care for fear of ostracism, humiliation and unemployment, and rejection from family members, colleagues, and their community as a whole.[107] Since the beginning of the pandemic, reports of harassment, scapegoating, and violence against sex workers, AIDS widows, bisexuals and homosexuals, street children, and drug users have been widespread, occurring in countries as diverse as Ethiopia, Thailand, South Africa, Colombia, and India. Stigma within health care systems is also common, resulting in the transfer of HIV-positive individuals to facilities with inferior care or disregard for patients' rights and confidentiality. On a global scale, stigma has discouraged policymakers from prioritizing or even acknowledging HIV and AIDS as urgent national issues.[108]

Now in the third decade of the epidemic, it is clear that HIV/AIDS cannot be associated with one population or region; it is a phenomenon that has stretched across global racial and ethnic, socioeconomic, and cultural strata. The reluctance to discuss what is private behavior perpetuates denial and hinders the dissemination of accurate information and knowledge about the epidemic. Thus far, interventions that have in part succeeded in reducing stigma related to HIV/AIDS have integrated skill building (for example, for caregivers and health care workers) with health information and communication activities, including media campaigns with opinion leaders and role models. Contact with persons living with HIV/AIDS has also shown promise as a way to overcome prejudice and discrimination.[109]

Biologic Variables

As mentioned previously, several studies have documented a higher efficiency of heterosexual transmission of HIV in the presence of more advanced immunodeficiency in the index case owing to higher levels of viremia and virus excretion. In populations that have experienced an HIV epidemic for a longer time, this may imply increased overall efficiency of heterosexual and perinatal transmission of HIV. Such higher rates of transmission have been observed in Africa.

African HIV isolates exhibit a higher degree of genetic variability than American or European isolates.[110,111] It is not known whether such viral variation has implications for the epidemiology of HIV through strain differences in infectivity and cell tropism or in capacity to reach higher levels of viremia. However, it has been shown that differences in these features play a role in the different epidemiologic patterns seen with HIV-1 and HIV-2 infection.

Just as STDs enhance the efficiency of sexual transmission of HIV, their prevalence in a population also partly determines its vulnerability for the spread of HIV. Prevalence rates for various STDs vary widely among populations but are generally higher in the developing world, particularly in urban Africa. They may be particularly high in the populations most vulnerable to STD and HIV infection, such as sex workers and their clients, truck drivers, fishers, and the military. Most important, high levels of STDs are a result not only of unsafe sexual behavior but also of inadequate care for patients with STDs.[112] Lack of circumcision in men has been shown to be a risk factor for HIV infection and may also play a role in the differential spread of HIV because male circumcision is practiced to varying degrees throughout the world.[52]

Impact of Prevention and Care Programs

The most important lesson from the past 15 years is that the spread of HIV can be reversed or prevented on a large scale, including that in some of the poorest countries of the world. The debate over the relative priority of HIV prevention versus treatment and care that has arisen (with the increasing availability of antiretroviral drugs) should be viewed with skepticism. The two complement one another; without one, the other is likely to fail. The most successful responses to the epidemic combine prevention and care strategies to prevent future infections and improve the quality of life for both infected and noninfected individuals. In addition, antiretroviral therapy is essential to alleviate the devastating impact of the HIV/AIDS pandemic on societies as a whole. The effectiveness of national responses to the AIDS pandemic will ultimately determine how extensively HIV will spread. This effectiveness requires, in the first place, political and financial commitment to HIV/AIDS prevention, which to date has often been insufficient. Many countries have needed about 5 to 10 times more financial resources than presently available to control the AIDS epidemic.

The increased availability of rapid tests for diagnosis of HIV infection has the potential to expand the already crucial role of voluntary counseling and testing in prevention and care. Health care centers with adequate resources can provide immediate prevention education or referral to treatment and care services, thus drastically reducing loss to follow-up among patients.

In many developing countries, public health care systems have deteriorated during the past three decades, and the introduction of user fees has resulted in declining access to health services and poorer management of people with STDs. In Nairobi, Kenya, after introduction of user fees at the main STD clinic, the attendance of men decreased significantly, to 40% of what it was before fees were levied.[113] These practices need to be reconsidered in light of the pandemic impact on the health status of poorer populations.

CLINICAL EXPRESSION

The most striking difference in the natural history of HIV infection in adults is the short survival time of AIDS patients in Africa—in general as short as 1 year—compared with patients in the industrialized world.[114] This is obviously a consequence of inadequate medical care and lack of antiretroviral medications for most patients in Africa.

Although all opportunistic diseases may occur in AIDS patients throughout the world, the relative importance of specific diseases may be different in different locations. For instance, major opportunistic diseases in North America, such as *Pneumocystis carinii* pneumonia and Kaposi's sarcoma, are less common in African AIDS patients.[115,116] In contrast, tuberculosis, chronic diarrhea, and bacteremia caused by pathogens such as *Salmonella typhimurium* and *Streptococcus pneumoniae* are common.[117] In southeast Asia, systemic infection with *Penicillium marneffei* is a common opportunistic mycosis in patients with HIV infection. In Chiang Mai, northern Thailand, penicilliosis was diagnosed in 140 (35%) of 400 consecutive AIDS patients and specific prophylaxis with itraconazole was able to prevent development of *P. marneffei*.[118]

Tuberculosis not only is the leading opportunistic infection among adult AIDS patients in Africa but also is itself is greatly affected by the HIV epidemic, with rising incidence rates wherever HIV has become endemic. This rise in incidence is probably entirely attributable to the spread of HIV infection in populations in which 50% to 80% of all adults are infected with *Mycobacterium tuberculosis*. A tuberculosis epidemic is now accompanying the AIDS epidemic in many countries and is one of the major public health consequences of HIV infection in the developing world. In 2000, there were 8.3 million new cases of tuberculosis, the majority of which occurred in sub-Saharan Africa and Southeast Asia, with notable increases among the Commonwealth of Independent States. Further, 11% of all new cases occurred in persons who were HIV positive, and more than 220,000 of the 1.84 million deaths from tuberculosis were attributable to HIV.[119]

In Africa, between 30% and 75% of tuberculosis patients are now infected with HIV. In other developing countries, for the most part, HIV prevalence is still low among tuberculosis patients but usually higher than in the general population. In industrialized countries, the prevalence of HIV in new tuberculosis cases is as high as 14%. However, because pulmonary tuberculosis may develop across a broad spectrum of HIV-associated immunodeficiency in populations in which tuberculosis is endemic, it is of limited use as an AIDS-defining illness.[119,120]

Additional consequences of dual HIV–*M. tuberculosis* infection include a high mortality rate among tuberculosis patients with HIV infection (mostly from HIV-related illness), a growing rate of multidrug resistance of *M. tuberculosis,* and an increase of up to 10-fold in severe skin reactions, including Stevens-Johnson syndrome, during thiacetazone therapy in HIV-positive patients.[121,122]

The cause of death in patients with HIV infection in the developing world is not well studied.[116] In a large study of a representative sample of patients who died during hospitalization in Abidjan, Côte d'Ivoire, tuberculosis, bacteremia with gram-negative rods, and cerebral toxoplasmosis caused 53% of the deaths.[123] Tuberculosis was found in half of the cadavers with an AIDS-defining pathology, compared with only 4% for *P. carinii* pneumonia. In this population, in which both HIV-1 and HIV-2 occur, patients with HIV-2 infection had severe cytomegalovirus infection and HIV-associated encephalitis more often than patients with HIV-1 infection; this finding is compatible with the more prolonged course of disease associated with HIV-2 infection.

IMPACT OF THE HIV/AIDS EPIDEMIC

The impact of the AIDS epidemic on many parts of the developing world is already severe, but it will undoubtedly become worse as the number of people with AIDS and HIV-related illness continues to increase over the next decades. AIDS affects not only individual patients and their relatives but also communities at large, with a long-term impact on households, on the health sector, on demography, and on economic and social systems.[46,124]

Perhaps the most visible aspect of the burden of AIDS is the large number of men and women with AIDS in the hospitals of many

African and Southeast Asian countries, where they now make up at least 50% of all patients. AIDS has also become the major cause of death among hospitalized patients.[97]

With a growing number of persons with HIV infection developing AIDS, the demand for health services will expand rapidly while the supply of health care providers will continue to dwindle. In northern Thailand in 1995, 50% of hospital beds were already occupied by HIV-positive patients, and in Bujumbura, Burundi, that figure reached 70% in the same year.[125] Absorbing this growing burden of patients is a major challenge for health care systems in the developing world.

The long-term demographic impact of AIDS is becoming clearer. As a result of AIDS, life expectancy at birth has declined by 20 to 30 years in the most affected countries in Africa, and overall population growth has slowed (Fig. 113-10). Currently, seven countries in sub-Saharan Africa have life expectancies below 40 years, indicating a tragic reversal of the gains made in the past century. By 2010, five

FIGURE 113-10. Life expectancy at birth with and without AIDS for selected countries, 2010. *(Data from Stanecki KA. The AIDS Pandemic in the 21st Century. Draft Report, July 2002, XIV International Conference on AIDS, Barcelona. Washington, DC: USAID/US Census Bureau, 2002.)*

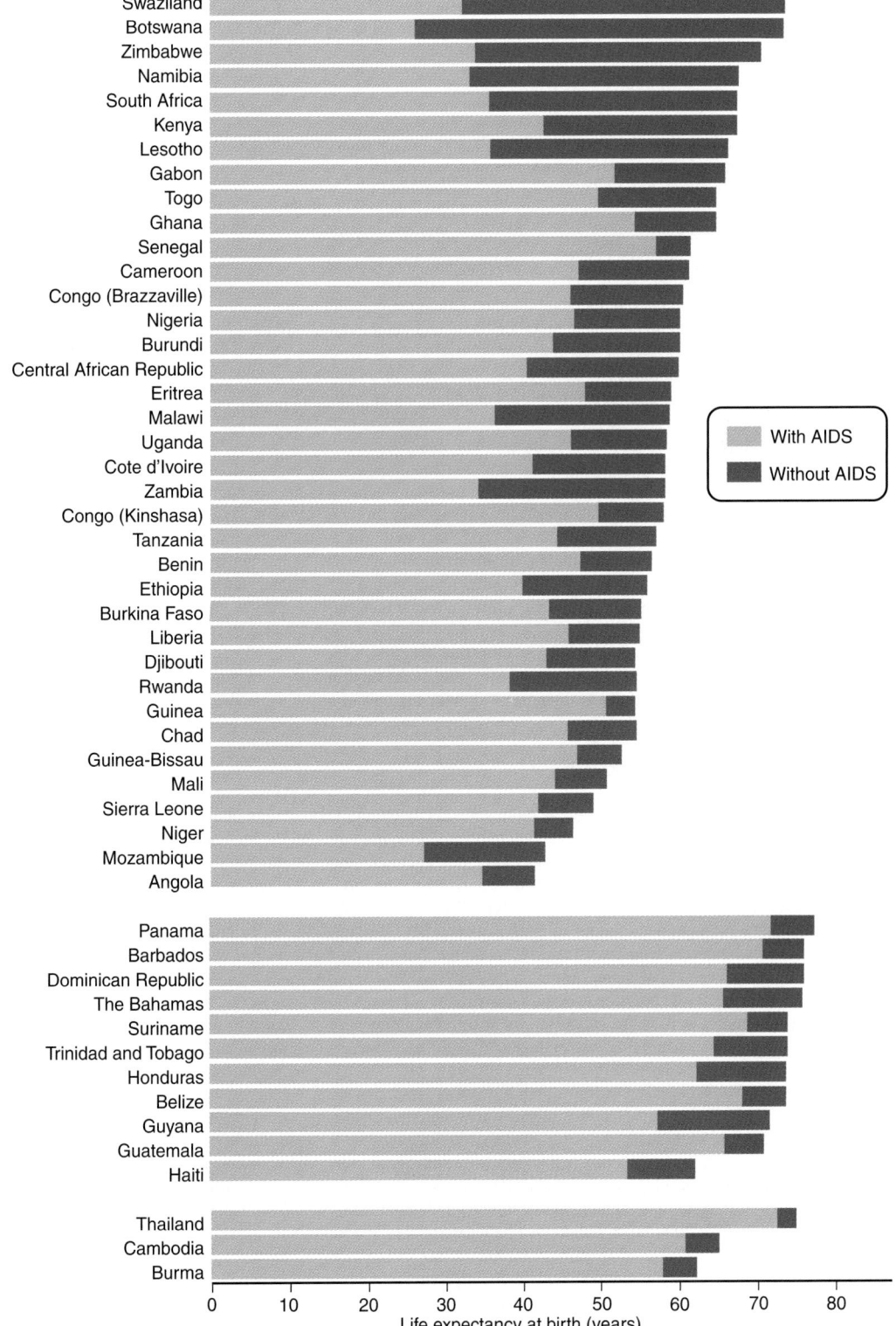

countries (all in sub-Saharan Africa) are expected to have negative population growth rates because of AIDS mortality. In parts of Latin America, the Caribbean, and Southeast Asia, population growth rates have decreased by as much as 50%.[8]

AIDS is now the leading cause of death among adults in many African cities,[126] where the lifetime risk of dying of AIDS exceeds one in three.[127] AIDS is also doubling to quadrupling the mortality rate in children younger than 5 years, leading to a reversal of the benefits of child survival initiatives in many high-prevalence areas. In addition, the number of orphans of parents who died from AIDS is growing at a staggering rate in the worst affected countries, with 14 million AIDS orphans worldwide as of 2002 and an estimated 25 million AIDS orphans by 2010. Increases in the number of orphans have multiple negative impacts, such as decreased enrollment in schools (with girls disproportionately affected), greater risk for starvation and malnutrition, and increased risk of involvement in armed conflict and destabilizing military forces.[128] The educational sector itself has been decimated in many countries because of high rates of teacher absenteeism and death.

In economic terms, AIDS is now the top cause of healthy life lost in urban sub-Saharan Africa. Because HIV infection occurs mostly in adults in their most productive years, it profoundly affects the economic and social sectors.[129,130] Since 1985, 7 million farm workers have died from AIDS, with another 16 million projected to die from AIDS in the next two decades. In general, Africa's per capita income growth has been reduced by 0.7% annually because of HIV/AIDS. In East Africa, absenteeism related to HIV/AIDS accounts for as much as 54% of business costs. The gross domestic product of severely affected countries will continue to decline because of loss of productivity in agriculture, industry, and the service sectors. In Tanzania it is estimated that the real rate of growth of the gross domestic product will decline by 15% to 28% as a result of AIDS between 1995 and 2010.[124,131,132]

Finally, in 2001, the United Nations Security Council declared AIDS a threat to global security. By increasing morbidity and mortality, destroying family and community networks and safety nets, hampering economic growth, and incapacitating health care, police, and military sectors, the epidemic will continue to weaken important regional powers such as Nigeria, Kenya, India, China, and the Russian Federation.

To paraphrase the World Bank's World Development Report 1993, "Historians will look back on the latter half of this century as having had one great medical triumph, the eradication of smallpox, and one great medical tragedy, AIDS."[124]

GLOBAL RESPONSES TO HIV/AIDS

Successful prevention programs worldwide have several key elements in common: they are tailored to the social and economic needs and values of their target populations; they present empowering, accurate, and frank information to those who are unaware of their risk for infection, as well as information on how to protect themselves; they are inclusive of HIV-positive persons and members of civil society; they are supported by a legal and policy framework that protects HIV-positive persons from discrimination in its multiple forms; their programs are multifaceted, multisectoral, and constantly under review for possible change or adaptation; and they are supported by political commitment through effective and accountable leadership at the highest level of government and society at large.[133]

By any standard, current efforts to slow the HIV/AIDS pandemic are inadequate. As of 2003, less than 20% of all people at risk for HIV infection worldwide had access to prevention services. Globally, only 5% of pregnant women at risk for infection had access to antiretroviral therapies to prevent mother-to-child transmission, 24% of people at high risk to AIDS education, and a meager 12% to voluntary HIV counseling and testing services. By 2007, $6.6 billion will be needed for HIV prevention spending, whereas annual spending in 2002 did not even reach one third of that sum.[134] If prevention and treatment programs are simultaneously scaled up, it is estimated that 29 million of the 45 million projected infections by 2010 could be averted (Fig. 113-11).[135]

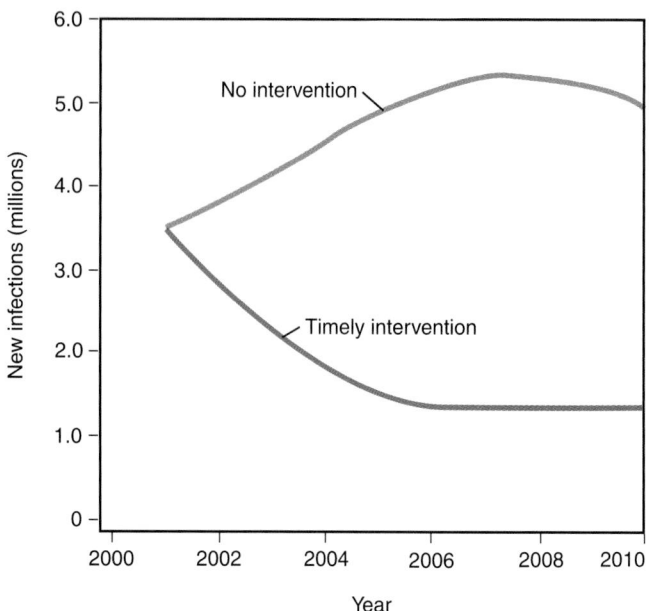

FIGURE 113-11. Projected new adult infections given degree of interventions in 2002 and a timely scale-up of comprehensive prevention, treatment, and care programs. (*Data from Stover J, Walker N, Garnett GP, et al. Can we reverse the HIV/AIDS pandemic with an expanded response? Lancet. 2002;360:73-77.*)

Antiretroviral drugs have succeeded in delaying the onset of illness, reducing mortality from AIDS, and improving the quality of life for people living with HIV. Mother-to-child transmission has been significantly reduced in countries where these drugs are used perinatally, and short-course drug treatment regimens have become the ethical minimum in care.[136] In Brazil, the only developing country with a universal prevention-and-care program, data suggest that HIV incidence has declined with the increase in infected patients taking antiretroviral therapy. Mathematical modeling studies have shown that high usage of these drugs can decrease the overall transmission rate of HIV while keeping transmission of drug-resistant strains low. An important caveat here is that a rise in risky sexual behavior (as has been documented among men who have sex with men in San Francisco and other places in the United States and in western Europe) may undo reductions in HIV prevalence and incidence.[137-139] This reinforces the need for scaling up prevention programs while broadening access to antiretroviral treatment and delivering prevention messages for HIV-positive persons.[140] After years of debate, the dramatic drops in the prices of antiretroviral drugs because of generic manufacturing and differential pricing have made care a reality in poorer nations. By 2005, $4.4 billion will be needed for care and support programs worldwide.[141]

In June 2001, the United Nations General Assembly held a Special Session on HIV/AIDS (UNGASS) at which the Declaration of Commitment on HIV/AIDS was adopted, and it has since served as a blueprint for action against the worsening pandemic. The declaration outlined the key elements of local, regional, and global responses to HIV/AIDS, which included strong leadership, a commitment to human rights principles, treatment and care for HIV-positive persons, and increased resources for prevention and research. Targets were established to reduce HIV prevalence in the most affected countries by 2003, and an overall target expenditure between $7 billion and $10 billion was established for 2005.[142]

After UNGASS, and with the support of the United Nations Secretary General and the G8 countries, the Global Fund for AIDS, Tuberculosis and Malaria (GFATM) was established as a public-private partnership between governments, civil society, and the private sector to raise and dispense resources worldwide to combat these three diseases, with special attention to regions and countries that have been most devastated. By 2003, the Global Fund raised more than $3 billion and completed two rounds of funding for proposals worldwide; 70% of the resources have been devoted to HIV/AIDS prevention and care. In 2003, the World Health Organization launched an initiative to treat 3 million HIV-positive people in developing countries by the end of 2005 (3 by 5) primarily using generic fixed-dose combination anti-retroviral pills certified by its prequalification system. The United States has pledged $15 billion over a 5-year period (known as the Emergency Plan for AIDS Relief) to lessen the impact of HIV/AIDS in 14 countries in Africa and the Caribbean. The plan seeks to prevent 7 million new infections, provide antiretroviral drugs to 2 million persons, and provide care for 10 million infected people. An expedited review process for generic antiretroviral drugs was established by the U.S. Food and Drug Administration in 2004.

The future of the response to HIV/AIDS will also require research and development for new prevention tools, including microbicides and vaccines that can be made available affordably across the world. Although not a panacea, these developments could work synergistically with existing behavioral and structural interventions to mitigate the impact of this most severe pandemic in recorded history.

REFERENCES

1. UNAIDS and WHO. AIDS Epidemic Update: December 2002. Geneva: UNAIDS, 2002.
2. UNAIDS and WHO. AIDS Epidemic Update: December 2001. Geneva: UNAIDS, 2001.
3. National Intelligence Council. The Next Wave of HIV/AIDS: Nigeria, Ethiopia, Russia, India, and China. Washington, DC: NIC, 2002.
4. European Centre for the Epidemiological Monitoring of AIDS. HIV/AIDS Surveillance in Europe. End-year report 2002. No. 68. Saint-Maurice, France: Institut de Veille Sanitaire, 2003.
5. UNAIDS and WHO. Report on the Global HIV/AIDS Epidemic. Geneva: UNAIDS, June 1998.
6. Hamers FF, Downs AM. HIV in central and eastern Europe. Lancet 2003;361: 1035-1044.
7. Laga M, ed. AIDS in Africa. 2nd ed. London: Rapid Science Publishers; 1997.
8. Stanecki KA. The AIDS Pandemic in the 21st Century. Draft Report, July 2002, XIV International Conference on AIDS, Barcelona. Washington, DC: USAID/US Census Bureau, 2002.
9. Fylkesnes K, Kasumba K, Ndhlovu Z, Musonda RM. Comparing sentinel surveillance and population-based HIV prevalence rates in Zambia. In: Laga M, ed. AIDS in Africa. 2nd ed. London: Rapid Science Publishers; 1997:12.
10. Luke N, Kurz KM. Cross-Generational and Transactional Sexual Relations in Sub-Saharan Africa: Prevalence of Behavior and Implications for Negotiating Safer Sexual Practices. Washington, DC: International Center for Research on Women, 2002.
11. Allen S, Lindan C, Serufilira A, et al. Human immunodeficiency virus infection in urban Rwanda: Demographic and behavioral correlates in a representative sample of childbearing women. JAMA. 1991;266:1657-1663.
12. Temmerman M, Mohammed Ali F, Ndinya-Achola JO, et al. Rapid increase of both HIV-1 infection and syphilis among pregnant women in Nairobi, Kenya. AIDS. 1992;6:1181-1185.
13. Dallabetta GA, Miotti PG, Chiphangui JD, et al. High socio-economic status is a risk factor for human immunodeficiency virus type 1 (HIV-1) infection but not for sexually transmitted diseases in women in Malawi: Implications for HIV-1 control. J Infect Dis. 1993;167:36-42.
14. Tarantola D, Schwartländer B. HIV/AIDS epidemics in sub-Saharan Africa: Dynamism, diversity and discrete declines. In: Laga M, ed. AIDS in Africa. 2nd ed. London: Rapid Science Publishers; 1997.
15. Laga M, Manoka A, Kivuvu M, et al. Non-ulcerative sexually transmitted diseases as risk factors for HIV-1 transmission in women: Results from a cohort study. AIDS. 1993;7:95-102.
16. Ngugi EN, Plummer FA, Simonsen JN, et al. Prevention of HIV transmission in Africa: The effectiveness of condom promotion and health education among high-risk prostitutes. Lancet. 1988;2:887-890.
17. Morris M, Kretzschmar M. Concurrent partnerships and the spread of HIV. AIDS. 1997;11:641-648.
18. Asiinwe-Okiroz G, Oppio AA, Musinguzi J, et al. Change in sexual behaviour and decline in HIV infection among young pregnant women in urban Uganda. AIDS. 1997;11:1757-1764.
19. UNAIDS. A Measure of Success in Uganda: The Value of Monitoring both HIV Prevalence and Sexual Behaviour. Geneva: UNAIDS Best Practice Collection, UNAIDS, 1998.
20. Anderson RM, May RM, Boily MC, et al. The spread of HIV-1 in Africa: Sexual contact patterns and the predicted demographic impact of AIDS. Nature. 1991;352: 581-589.
21. Bloom SS, Urassa M, Isingo R, et al. Community effects on the risk of HIV infection in rural Tanzania. Sex Transm Infect. 2002;78:261-266.
22. De Cock KM, Brun-Vézinet F, Soro B. HIV-1 and HIV-2 infections and AIDS in West Africa. AIDS. 1991;5(Suppl 1):S21-S28.
23. Poulsen AG, Aaby P, Gottschau A, et al. HIV-2 infection in Bissau, West Africa, 1987-1989: Incidence, prevalences, and routes of transmission. J AIDS. 1993;6:941-948.
24. Larsen O, da Silva Z, Sandstrom A, et al. Declining HIV-2 prevalence and incidence among men in a community study from Guinea-Bissau. AIDS. 1998;12:1707-1714.
25. Kanki PJ, Travers K, Mboup S, et al. Slower heterosexual spread of HIV-2 than HIV-1. Lancet. 1994;343:943-946.
26. De Cock KM, Adjorlolo G, Ekpini E, et al. Epidemiology and transmission of HIV-2: Why there is no HIV-2 pandemic. JAMA. 1993;270:2083-2086.
27. Andreasson PA, Dias F, Nauclér A, et al. A prospective study of vertical transmission of HIV-2 in Bissau, Guinea-Bissau. AIDS. 1993;7:989-994.
28. Gilbert PB, McKeague IW, Eisen G, et al. Comparison of HIV-1 and HIV-2 infectivity from a prospective cohort study in Senegal. Stat Med. 2003;22:573-593.
29. Marlink R, Kanki P, Thior I, et al. Reduced rate of disease development after HIV-2 infection as compared to HIV-1. Science. 1994;265:1587-1590.
30. George R, Ou C-Y, Parekh B, et al. Prevalence of HIV-1 and HIV-2 mixed infections in Côte d'Ivoire. Lancet. 1992;1:338-339.
31. Peeters M, Gershy-Damet GM, Fransen K, et al. Virological and polymerase chain reaction studies of HIV-1/HIV-2 dual infection in Côte d'Ivoire. Lancet. 1992;1: 339-340.
32. UNAIDS and WHO. Epidemiological Fact Sheet on HIV/AIDS and Sexually Transmitted Infections: Sudan, 2002 Update. Geneva: UNAIDS, 2002.
33. Kaldor JM, ed. AIDS in Asia and the Pacific. 2nd ed. London: Rapid Science Publishers; 1998.
34. Brown T, Chan R, Mugrditchian D, et al, eds. Sexually Transmitted Diseases in Asia and the Pacific. Armidale, Australia: Venereology Publishing; 1998.
35. Des Jarlais DC, Friedman SR, Choopanyq K, et al. International epidemiology of HIV and AIDS among injecting drug users. AIDS. 1992;6:1053-1068.
36. Weinger BG, Limpakarnjanarat K, Ungchusok K, et al. The epidemiology of HIV infection and AIDS in Thailand. AIDS. 1991;5(Suppl 2):S71-S85.
37. Gangakhedkar RR, Bentley ME, Divekar AD, et al. Spread of HIV infection in married monogamous women in India. JAMA. 1997;278:2090-2092.
38. UNAIDS and WHO. Epidemiological Fact Sheet on HIV/AIDS and Sexually Transmitted Infections: Thailand, 2002 Update. Geneva: UNAIDS, 2002.
39. Ou C-Y, Auwanet W, Pan C-P, et al. Wide distribution of two subtypes of HIV-1 in Thailand. AIDS Res Hum Retroviruses. 1992;8:1471-1472.
40. Nelson K, Celentano D, Eiumtrakol S, et al. Changes in sexual behaviour and a decline in HIV infection among young men in Thailand. N Engl J Med. 1996;335: 297-303.
41. Wiput R, Hanenberg R. The 100% condom programme in Thailand. AIDS. 1996;10:1-7.
42. UNAIDS. Connecting Lower HIV Infection Rates with Changes in Sexual Behaviour in Thailand: Data Collection and Comparison. Geneva: UNAIDS Best Practice Collection, UNAIDS, 1998.
43. Beyrer C. Hidden epidemic of sexually transmitted diseases in China: Crisis and opportunity. JAMA. 2003; 289:1303-1305.
44. Hospedales J, White F, Gayle C, et al. Epidemiology of HIV/AIDS in the Caribbean. In: Lamptey P, White F, Figueroa JP, et al, eds. The Handbook for AIDS Prevention in the Caribbean. Research Triangle Park, NC: Family Health International; 1992:1-23.
45. Boletim Epidemiológico AIDS 1992. Brasilia: Programo Nacional de Doencas Sexualmente Transmissiveis/AIDS; 1992.
46. Mann J, Tarantola D, eds. AIDS in the World II. New York: Oxford University Press; 1996.
47. Parker RG, Tawil O. Bisexual behaviour and HIV transmission in Latin America. In: Tielman R, Carballo M, Hendriks A, eds. Bisexuality and HIV/AIDS. New York: Prometheus Press; 1991:59-63.
48. Levi GC, Vitória MAA. Fighting against AIDS: The Brazilian experience. AIDS. 2002;16:2373-2383.
49. Marins JRP, Jamal LF, Chen SY, et al. Dramatic improvement in survival among adult Brazilian AIDS patients. AIDS. 2003;17:1675-1682.
50. UNAIDS and WHO. Epidemiological Fact Sheet on HIV/AIDS and Sexually Transmitted Infections: Brazil, 2002 Update. Geneva: UNAIDS, 2002.
51. Quinn TC, Wawer MJ, Sewankambo N, et al. Viral load and heterosexual transmission of human immunodeficiency virus type 1. N Engl J Med. 2000;342:921-929.
52. Weiss HA, Quigley MA, Hayes RJ. Male circumcision and risk of HIV infection in sub-Saharan Africa: A systematic review and meta-analysis. AIDS. 2000;14:2361-2370.
53. Clemetson DBA, Moss GB, Willerford DM, et al. Detection of HIV DNA in cervical and vaginal secretions: Prevalence and correlates among women in Nairobi, Kenya. JAMA. 1993;269:2860-2864.
54. Wasserheit JN. Epidemiological synergy: Interrelationships between HIV infection and other STDs. Sex Transm Dis. 1992;19:61-77.
55. Laga M, Nzila N, Goeman J. The interrelationship of sexually transmitted diseases and HIV infection: Implications for the control of both epidemics in Africa. AIDS. 1991;5(Suppl 1):S55-S64.
56. Cameron DW, Simonsen JN, D'Costa LJ, et al. Female to male transmission of human immunodeficiency virus type 1: Risk factors for seroconversion in man. Lancet. 1989;2:401-407.
57. Grosskurth H, Gray R, Hayes R, et al. Control of sexually transmitted diseases for HIV-1 prevention: Understanding the implication of the Mwanza and Rakai trials. Lancet. 2000;355:1981-1987.

58. Wawer MJ, Sewankambo NK, Serwadda D, et al. Control of sexually transmitted diseases for AIDS prevention in Uganda: A randomized community trial. Lancet. 1999;353:525-535.

59. Reynolds SJ, Risbud AR, Shepherd ME, et al. Recent herpes simplex virus type 2 infection and the risk of human immunodeficiency virus type 1 acquisition in India. J Infect Dis. 2003;187:1513-1521.

60. Ghys P, Fransen K, Diallo MO, et al. The association between cervicovaginal HIV shedding, sexually transmitted diseases and immunosuppression in female sex workers in Abidjan, Côte d'Ivoire. AIDS. 1997;11:F85-F93.

61. Cohen MS, Hoffman IF, Royce R, et al. Reduction of concentration of HIV-1 in semen after treatment of urethritis: Implications for prevention of sexual transmission of HIV-1. Lancet. 1997;349:1863-1873.

62. The Working Group on Mother-to-Child Transmission of HIV. Rates of mother-to-child transmission of HIV-1 in Africa, America and Europe: Results from 13 perinatal studies. J Acquir Immune Defic Syndr. 1995;8:506-510.

63. Wiktor SZ, Ekpini E, Nduati RW. Prevention of mother-to-child transmission of HIV-1 in Africa. In: Laga M, ed. AIDS in Africa. 2nd ed. London: Rapid Science Publishers; 1997:79-87.

64. Dunn DT, Newell ML, Ades AE, et al. Risk of human immunodeficiency virus type 1 transmission through breast feeding. Lancet. 1992;1:585-588.

65. Ekpini E, Wiktor SZ, Satten GA, et al. Late postnatal transmission of HIV-1 in Abidjan, Côte d'Ivoire. Lancet. 1997;349:1054-1059.

66. Van de Perre P, Simonon A, Msellati P, et al. Postnatal transmission of human immunodeficiency virus in infants born to seropositive mothers. N Engl J Med. 1991;325:593-599.

67. St Louis ME, Kamenga M, Brown C, et al. Risk for perinatal HIV-1 transmission according to maternal immunologic, virologic and placental factors. JAMA. 1993;269:2853-2859.

68. Ryder RW, Nsa W, Hassig SE, et al. Perinatal transmission of the human immunodeficiency virus type 1 to infants of seropositive women in the Democratic Republic of Congo. N Engl J Med. 1989;302:1637-1642.

69. Nduati RW, John GC, Richardson BA, et al. Human immunodeficiency virus type 1-infected cells in breast milk from HIV-1 infected women: Association with immunosuppression and vitamin A deficiency. J Infect Dis. 1995;172:1461-1468.

70. John GC, Nduati RW, Mbori ND, et al. Genital shedding of human immunodeficiency virus type 1 DNA during pregnancy: Association with immunosuppression, abnormal cervical or vaginal discharge, and severe vitamin A deficiency. J Infect Dis. 1997;175:57-62.

71. Semba RD, Miotti PG, Chiphangui JD, et al. Infant mortality and maternal vitamin A deficiency during human immunodeficiency virus infection. Clin Infect Dis. 1995;21:966-972.

72. Global Health Council and Mailman School of Public Health, Columbia University. MTCT-Plus: Spearheading HIV/AIDS Prevention and Care for Mothers and Children. New York, 2002.

73. Mitka M. MTCT-Plus program has two goals: End maternal transmission and treat mothers. JAMA. 2002;288:153-154.

74. Choopanya K, Vanichseni S, Des Jarlais DC, et al. Risk factors and HIV seropositivity among injecting drug users in Bangkok. AIDS. 1991;5:1509-1513.

75. Colebunders R, Ryder R, Francis H, et al. Seroconversion rate, mortality and clinical manifestations associated with the receipt of a human immunodeficiency virus infected blood transfusion. J Infect Dis. 1991;164:450-456.

76. Gershy-Damet GM, Tarantola D. HIV screening of blood donations in sub-Saharan Africa, 1995. In: Laga M, ed. AIDS in Africa. 2nd ed. London: Rapid Science Publishers; 1997:94-95.

77. Jäger H, N'galy B, Perriëns J, et al. Prevention of transfusion-associated HIV transmission in Kinshasa, the Democratic Republic of Congo: HIV screening is not enough. AIDS. 1990;4:571-574.

78. Berkeley S. Parenteral transmission of HIV in Africa. AIDS. 1991;5(Suppl 1):S163-S168.

79. Lepage P, Van de Perre P. Nosocomial transmission of HIV in Africa: What tribute is paid to contaminated blood transfusions and medical injections? Infect Control Hosp Epidemiol. 1989;9:200-203.

80. Pokrovsky VV, Eramone EV. Nosocomial outbreak of HIV infection in Elista, USSR. Abstract WA 05. Fifth International Conference on AIDS, Montreal, June 1989.

81. Hersh BS, Popovici F, Apetrei RC, et al. Acquired immunodeficiency syndrome in Romania. Lancet. 1991;1:645-649.

82. Caraël M, Cleland J, Adeokun L. Overview and selected findings of sexual behaviour surveys. AIDS. 1991;5(Suppl 1):S65-S74.

83. Donovan B, Ross MW. Preventing HIV: Determinants of sexual behavior. Lancet. 2000;355:1897-1901.

84. Anderson RM, May RM. Transmission dynamics of HIV infection. Nature. 1987;26:137-142.

85. Caraël M, Buvé A, Awusabo-Asare K. The making of HIV epidemics: What are the driving forces? In: Laga M, ed. AIDS in Africa. 2nd ed. London: Rapid Science Publishers; 1997:23-32.

86. Boily MC, Anderson RM. Sexual contact patterns between men and women and the spread of HIV-1 in urban centres in Africa. IMA J Math Appl Med Biol. 1991;8:221-247.

87. Yorke JA, Heathcote HW, Nold A. Dynamics and control of the transmission of gonorrhoea. Sex Transm Dis. 1978;5:31-37.

88. Lamptey PR, Kamenga MC, Weir SS. Prevention of sexual transmission of HIV in sub-Saharan Africa: Lessons learned. In: Laga M, ed. AIDS in Africa. 2nd ed. London: Rapid Science Publishers; 1997:63-77.

89. Kamenga M, Ryder RW, Jingu M, et al. Evidence of marked sexual behaviour change associated with low HIV-1 seroconversion in 149 married couples with discordant HIV-1 status: Experiences at an HIV counseling centre in the Democratic Republic of Congo. AIDS. 1991;5:61-67.

90. Trends in HIV Incidence and Prevalence: Natural Course of the Epidemic or Results of Behavioral Change? Geneva: UNAIDS, 1999.

91. Moses S, Plummer FA, Ngugi E, et al. Controlling HIV in Africa: Effectiveness and cost of an intervention in a high-frequency STD transmitter core group. AIDS. 1991;5:407-411.

92. Laga M, Alary M, Nzila N, et al. Condom promotion and STD treatment, and declining incidence of HIV-1 infection in female Zairian sex workers. Lancet. 1994;344:2446-2448.

93. Levine WC, Revallo R, Kaune V, et al. Decline in sexually transmitted disease prevalence in female Bolivian sex workers: Impact of an HIV prevention project. AIDS. 1998;12:1899-1906.

94. UNAIDS. Expanding the Global Response to HIV/AIDS through Focused Action: Reducing Risk and Vulnerability. Definitions, Rationale and Pathways. Geneva: UNAIDS Best Practice Collection, UNAIDS, 1998.

95. Blankership KM, Bray SJ, Merson MH. Structural interventions in public health. AIDS. 2000;14(Suppl 1):11-21.

96. Tawil O, Verster A, O'Reilly KR. Enabling approaches for HIV/AIDS prevention: Can we modify the environment and minimize the risk? AIDS. 1995;9:1299-1306.

97. World Bank. Confronting AIDS: Public Priorities in a Global Epidemic. New York: Oxford University Press; 1997.

98. Hunt CW. Migrant labor and sexually transmitted diseases: AIDS in Africa. J Health Soc Behav. 1989;30:353-373.

99. Larson A. Social context of HIV transmission in Africa: Historical and cultural bases of East and Central African sexual relations. Rev Infect Dis. 1989;11:71-73.

100. UNAIDS and United Nations. Gender and HIV/AIDS. United Nations Special Session on HIV/AIDS, New York, June 25-27, 2001.

101. Centers for Disease Control and Prevention. HIV/AIDS among U.S. Women: Minority and Young Women at Continuing Risk. Atlanta: CDC; 2002.

102. Koenig MA, Lutalo T, Zhao F, et al. Domestic violence in rural Uganda: Evidence from a community-based study. Bull World Health Organ. 2003;81:53-60.

103. Rao Gupta G. Gender, sexuality, and HIV/AIDS: The what, the why, and the how. Plenary Address, XIIIth International AIDS Conference, Durban, South Africa, July 12, 2000.

104. Maman S, Mbwambo JK, Hogan NM, et al. HIV-positive women report more lifetime partner violence: Findings from a voluntary counseling and testing clinic in Dar es Salaam, Tanzania. Am J Public Health. 2002;92:1331-1337.

105. UNAIDS. Gender and HIV/AIDS: Taking Stock of Research and Programmes. Geneva: UNAIDS, March 1999.

106. Parker R, Aggleton P. HIV and AIDS-Related Stigma and Discrimination: A Conceptual Framework and Implications for Action. Rio de Janeiro: ABIA; 2002.

107. UNAIDS, Aggleton P. Comparative Analysis: Research Studies from India and Uganda. HIV and AIDS-Related Discrimination, Stigmatization, and Denial. Geneva: UNAIDS, June 2000.

108. O'Farrell N. Genital ulcers, stigma, HIV, and STI control in sub-Saharan Africa. Sex Transm Infect. 2002;78:143-146.

109. Brown L, Macintyre K, Trujillo L. Interventions to reduce HIV/AIDS stigma: What have we learned? AIDS Educ Prev. 2003;15:49-49.

110. Louwagie J, McCutchan FE, Peeters M, et al. Comparison of *gag* genes from sixty one international HIV-1 isolates provides evidence for multiple genetic subgroups. AIDS. 1993;7:769-780.

111. Janssens W, Buvé A, Nbengason JN. The puzzle of subtypes in Africa. AIDS. 1997;11:705-712.

112. Dallabetta G, Laga M, Lamptey P, ed. Control of Sexually Transmitted Diseases: A Handbook for the Design and Management of Programs. Arlington, Va: Family Health International; 1996.

113. Moses S, Manji F, Bradley JE, et al. Impact of user fees on attendance at a referral centre for sexually transmitted diseases in Kenya. Lancet. 1992;340:463-466.

114. Colebunders RL, Latif AS. Natural history and clinical presentation of HIV-1 infection in adults. AIDS. 1991;5(Suppl 1):S103-S112.

115. Grant AD, Djomand G, De Cock KM. Natural history and spectrum of disease in adults with HIV/AIDS in Africa. In: Laga M, ed. AIDS in Africa. 2nd ed. London: Rapid Science Publishers; 1997:43-54.

116. Lucas SB, Odida M, Wabinga H. The pathology of severe morbidity and mortality due to HIV infection in Africa. AIDS. 1991;5(Suppl 1):S143-S148.

117. Gilks CF, Brindle RJ, Otieno LS, et al. Life-threatening bacteremia in HIV-1 seropositive adults admitted to hospital in Nairobi, Kenya. Lancet. 1990;336:545-549.

118. Supparatpinyo K, Periens J, Nelson KE, Sirisanthana T. A controlled trial of itraconazole to prevent relapse of *Penicillium marneffei* infection in patients infected with the human immunodeficiency virus. N Engl J Med. 1998;339:1739-1743.

119. Corbett EL, Watt CJ, Walker N, et al. The growing burden of tuberculosis: Global trends and interactions with the HIV epidemic. Arch Intern Med. 2003;163:1009-1021.

120. Mukadi Y, Perriëns JH, St Louis ME, et al. Spectrum of immunodeficiency in HIV-1 infected patients with pulmonary tuberculosis in the Democratic Republic of Congo. Lancet. 1993;342:143-146.

121. Raviglione MC, Snider DE Jr, Kochi A. Global epidemiology of tuberculosis: Morbidity and mortality of a worldwide epidemic. JAMA. 1995;275:220-226.

122. De Cock KM, Soro B, Koulibaly IM, et al. Tuberculosis and HIV infection in sub-Saharan Africa. JAMA. 1992;268:1581-1587.

123. Lucas SB, Hounnou A, Peacock C, et al. The mortality and pathology of HIV infection in a West African city. AIDS. 1993;7:1569-1579.

124. World Bank. World Development Report 1993: Investing in Health. New York: Oxford University Press; 1993.
125. De Cock KM, Barrere B, Diaby L, et al. AIDS: The leading cause of adult death in the West African city of Abidjan, Ivory Coast. Science. 1990;249:793-796.
126. World Bank. Intensifying Action against HIV/AIDS in Africa: Responding to a Development Crisis. New York: World Bank; June 1999.
127. UNAIDS, UNICEF, USAID. Children on the Brink 2002: A Joint Report on Orphan Estimates and Program Strategies. Washington, DC: July 2002.
128. Whiteside A, Stover J. The demographic and economic impact of AIDS in Africa. In: Laga M, ed. AIDS in Africa. 2nd ed. London: Rapid Science Publishers; 1997:55-61.
129. Barnett T, Blaikie P. AIDS in Africa: Its Present and Future Impact. London: Bellhaven Press; 1992.
130. World Bank. Tanzania: AIDS Assessment and Planning Study. Washington, DC: The World Bank; 1992.
131. Hecht R, Adeyi O, Semini I. Making AIDS part of the global development agenda. Finance Dev. 2002;39(1).
132. UNAIDS. HIV/AIDS, Human Resources and Sustainable Development. World Summit on Sustainable Development, Johannesburg. Geneva: UNAIDS, 2002.
133. Merson MH. Curtailing the HIV epidemic: The power of prevention. Int AIDS Soc Top HIV Med. 2001;9(6):17-20.
134. Bill and Melinda Gates Foundation, Global HIV Prevention Working Group. Access to HIV Prevention: Closing the Gap. Seattle: Gates Foundation; May 2003.
135. Stover J, Walker N, Garnett GP, et al. Can we reverse the HIV/AIDS pandemic with an expanded response? Lancet. 2002;360:73-77.
136. Nolan ML, Greenberg AE, Fowler MG. A review of clinical trials to prevent mother-to-child HIV-1 transmission in Africa and inform rational intervention strategies. AIDS. 2002;16:1991-1999.
137. Hogg RS, Weber AE, Chan K, et al. Increasing incidence of HIV infections among young gay and bisexual men in Vancouver. AIDS. 2001;15:1321-1322.
138. Del Romero J, Castilla J, Garcia S, et al. Time trend in incidence of HIV seroconversion among homosexual men repeatedly tested in Madrid, 1988-2000. AIDS. 2001;15:1319-1321.
139. Katz MH, Schwarcz SK, Kellogg TA, et al. Impact of highly active antiretroviral treatment on HIV seroincidence among men who have sex with men: San Francisco. Am J Public Health. 2002;92:388-394.
140. Blower S, Farmer P. Predicting the public health impact of antiretrovirals: Preventing HIV in developing countries. AIDScience. 2003;3(11).
141. Schwartländer B, Stover J, Walker L, et al. Resource needs for HIV/AIDS. Science. 2001;292:2434-2436.
142. United Nations General Assembly Special Session on HIV/AIDS. Declaration of Commitment on HIV/AIDS. 25-27 June 2001. New York: United Nations; 2001.

CHAPTER **114**

Epidemiology and Prevention of Acquired Immunodeficiency Syndrome and Human Immunodeficiency Virus Infection

CARLOS DEL RIO

JAMES W. CURRAN

Acquired immunodeficiency syndrome (AIDS) is the most severe manifestation of a clinical spectrum of illness caused by infection with human immunodeficiency virus (HIV). The syndrome is defined by the development of serious opportunistic infections, neoplasms, or other life-threatening manifestations resulting from progressive HIV-induced immunosuppression. AIDS was first recognized in mid-1981, when unusual clusters of *Pneumocystis jirovecii* pneumonia and Kaposi's sarcoma were reported in young, previously healthy homosexual men in New York City, Los Angeles, and San Francisco.[1,2] The subsequent documentation of cases among persons with hemophilia, blood transfusion recipients, and heterosexual injecting drug users and their sex partners suggested that a transmissible agent was the primary cause of the immunologic defects characteristic of AIDS. In 1983,

2 years after the first reports of AIDS, a cytopathic retrovirus was isolated from persons with AIDS and associated conditions such as chronic lymphadenopathy.[3,4] By 1985, serologic tests to detect evidence of infection with HIV had been developed and licensed.

Recent data suggest that HIV originated in Africa. Blood obtained in 1959 from an adult Bantu man in the Democratic Republic of Congo represents the oldest known case of HIV-1 infection in the world.[5] HIV infection has become pandemic, affecting every region of the world, and is a major cause of morbidity and mortality, particularly among young adults. HIV is spread primarily through heterosexual contact, with women accounting now for more than half of new HIV infections in adults.[6] In many developed countries, where transmission through male homosexual contact predominated for the first decade, the number of persons infected through heterosexual contact and injecting drug use is increasing. In contrast, transmission through transfusion of blood and blood products has been virtually eliminated in countries that have systematically instituted HIV antibody screening of donated blood and plasma and heat treatment of clotting factors. In developed countries sharp declines in AIDS incidence and mortality have been noted after the use of highly active antiretroviral therapy (HAART) became widespread in 1996. As a result, the number of people living with HIV infection continues to rise, and preliminary evidence suggests that new infections are also on the increase.[7] In the United States, the HIV epidemic increasingly affects women, minorities, persons infected through heterosexual contact, and the poor.[8] Now more than ever, control and prevention of HIV infection, whether on a global or an individual scale, must be grounded in an understanding of the changing epidemiology of HIV.

HIV AND AIDS SURVEILLANCE IN THE UNITED STATES

All 50 states, the District of Columbia, and all U.S. territories require reporting of AIDS cases to local health authorities by name, and they in turn use a uniform surveillance case definition and case report form to report cases to the Centers for Disease Control and Prevention (CDC).[9] Health department staff members actively survey case reports submitted from physicians, hospitals, and other medical care facilities and from record systems such as death certificates and tumor registries. Along with HIV serologic surveys and HIV infection reporting, the AIDS surveillance system has served as a major resource to monitor and anticipate trends in HIV morbidity.

The initial AIDS surveillance case definition, which was established soon after the first reports of unexplained illnesses associated with cellular immunodeficiency in homosexual or bisexual men, formally listed the opportunistic infections and neoplasms indicative of underlying immunosuppression.[10] In the absence of previously described causes of immunosuppression, a diagnosis of one of these conditions was defined as AIDS. The definition did not include the less severe manifestations of HIV infection and was designed to be highly specific and to provide a standard means to monitor trends of severe immunodeficiency caused by what was then an unknown agent.

One of the initial uses of AIDS surveillance was to search medical records and death certificates retrospectively for previously unrecognized or unreported cases of similar immunodeficiency. This review identified only 125 cases of AIDS diagnosed between 1977 and 1981 and provided evidence that the condition was a new disease in the United States. Although a few isolated cases compatible with AIDS have been retrospectively diagnosed from the 1950s and 1960s, the AIDS epidemic in the United States essentially began in the late 1970s.[11,12]

The AIDS surveillance case definition was modified in 1985, in 1987, and again in 1993.[13-15] These revisions were made to reflect the development of serologic tests to detect HIV in 1985, the recognition of additional clinical illnesses associated with or directly caused by HIV infection, and changes in the clinical management of HIV-infected persons. Each revision to the AIDS surveillance case definition has subsequently resulted in a higher proportion of HIV-infected persons being defined as having AIDS.

The 1985 and 1987 revisions added several new diseases to the AIDS surveillance definition for persons with diagnosed HIV infection. The 1985 revision included disseminated histoplasmosis, chronic isosporiasis, and certain non-Hodgkin's lymphomas. After this revision, the number of AIDS cases reported increased by an estimated 3% to 4%.[16] The 1987 revision incorporated HIV encephalopathy, wasting syndrome, and other AIDS-indicator diseases that are diagnosed presumptively (i.e., without definitive laboratory evidence). As a result of this revision, an estimated additional 10% to 15% of HIV-infected persons became reportable as having AIDS, and AIDS cases increased by as much as 28% in some areas.[17,18] The increase in AIDS case reporting resulting from these revisions was greatest for women, blacks, Hispanic populations, and injecting drug users.[17,18]

In 1993, the AIDS surveillance definition was expanded to include HIV-infected adolescents and adults with severe immunosuppression (<200 CD4+ T lymphocytes/μL or a CD4+ T-lymphocyte percentage of total lymphocytes of <14), pulmonary tuberculosis, recurrent (i.e., two or more episodes in a 12-month period) bacterial pneumonia, and invasive cervical cancer (Table 114-1). The inclusion of measurements of CD4+ T lymphocytes in the 1993 revised case definition was necessary because the results of this test had by then become an integral part of the clinical and therapeutic management of HIV-infected persons. Initiation of antiretroviral therapy was recommended for persons with CD4 T-lymphocyte counts of fewer than 500 cells/μL, and prophylaxis against *P. jirovecii* pneumonia was recommended for all persons with CD4 T-lymphocyte counts of fewer than 200 cells/μL.[19-22] These clinical interventions have delayed or prevented the development of previous AIDS-defining opportunistic illnesses in many HIV-infected patients, which in turn has directly affected the timeliness and representation of AIDS case reporting.[23] Inclusion of these immunologic criteria allows for more accurate representation of the number of persons with severe HIV-related immunosuppression. The clinical conditions added to the 1993 surveillance case definition have been shown to be important health problems for HIV-infected persons. Persons coinfected with HIV and *Mycobacterium tuberculosis* have a much greater likelihood of progression to clinical tuberculosis, and diagnosis and treatment may be more difficult in such patients than in non–HIV-infected persons.[24,25] Other than the conditions in the 1987 surveillance definition, pneumonia is the leading cause of serious illness, hospitalization, and death in HIV-infected persons.[26-28] Cervical dysplasia, a precursor lesion that may progress to cervical cancer, is common among HIV-infected women and increases in severity as immunosuppression worsens.[29-31]

Evaluation studies have shown that AIDS surveillance has provided complete and timely information on diagnosed cases of AIDS in the United States. A national multicenter study published in 1992 used computerized medical records in six areas to determine that 92% of persons with AIDS-defining conditions were reported to local health departments.[32] Of these previously reported cases, 67% were reported to local health departments within 2 months of the date of diagnosis. Studies of state and local death certificate information and national vital statistics found that completeness of reporting of persons with AIDS ranged from 80% to 96% and that 70% to 90% of HIV-related deaths were reported to AIDS surveillance groups.[26,27,33] Thus, completeness of reporting for AIDS in the United States has been among the most complete of all reportable diseases and conditions.[34,35] However, recent advances in HIV treatment have slowed the progression of HIV disease for infected persons and contributed to a decline in AIDS incidence, and as a result many persons infected with HIV may never develop AIDS. Thus, data from the AIDS reporting system, although still important, have become less informative about current trends in HIV transmission. This led public health authorities in 1999 to recommend that all states and territories include surveillance for HIV infection and not just for AIDS.[36] In addition, a revised surveillance case definition for HIV infection that incorporated the reporting criteria for HIV infection and AIDS into a single case definition was recommended by the Council of State and Territorial Epidemiologists at their 1998 annual meeting and published by the CDC in 1999.[37]

By the end of 2003, all states, territories, and cities except Georgia and Philadelphia, have implemented a confidential HIV-case reporting system, However, only 34 states have implemented the same confidential name-based reporting of HIV infection that is used for AIDS case reporting, whereas the others have implemented surveillance using a coded identifier or a name-to-code system rather than using the patient name to report HIV cases. Analysis of data from states that conduct name-based HIV-AIDS surveillance suggests that the reporting of HIV infection in addition to AIDS case surveillance can give a better picture of recent trends in HIV transmission and assist efforts to better plan, implement, and evaluate HIV prevention and medical intervention programs.[39,40] HIV infection reporting provides a minimum estimate of the number of persons known to be infected in a given area as well as information regarding more recently infected persons than those reported with AIDS.[38] In states in which HIV infection is a reportable condition, the number of people reported with HIV infection is on average twice that of those reported with AIDS. In addition, in line with more recent trends in HIV transmission, people reported with HIV infection are more likely than those reported with AIDS to be women, adolescents, and racial and ethnic minorities.[38,41]

Thus, as a result of the increasing effectiveness of antiretroviral therapy to modify the natural history of HIV infection and decrease mortality,[42] AIDS case surveillance data will become less and less useful, making it more appropriate to transition to a surveillance system that emphasizes HIV infection rather than AIDS case reporting.[43]

Concurrent with revision of the AIDS surveillance case definition in 1993, the CDC implemented a revised classification system for HIV-infected adolescents and adults.[15] The system reflected the evolving knowledge about the spectrum and progression of HIV infection and standards of medical care at the time for infected persons. The system is based on a combination of three ranges of CD4 T-lymphocyte counts and three clinical categories (Table 114-2). Dividing the continuum of HIV infection into mutually exclusive and descriptive categories serves many useful purposes, including increased awareness of the spectrum of clinical manifestations of HIV infection; facilitation of surveillance and reporting for AIDS and HIV infection; provision

TABLE 114-1 Conditions Included in the 1993 AIDS Surveillance Case Definition

Bacterial infections, multiple or recurrent*
Candidiasis of bronchi, trachea, or lungs
Candidiasis, esophageal
Cervical cancer, invasive†
Coccidioidomycosis, disseminated or extrapulmonary
Cryptococcosis, extrapulmonary
Cryptosporidiosis, chronic intestinal (>1-month's duration)
Cytomegalovirus disease (other than liver, spleen, or nodes)
Cytomegalovirus retinitis (with loss of vision)
Encephalopathy, HIV related
Herpes simplex, chronic ulcer(s) (>1-month's duration); or bronchitis, pneumonitis, or esophagitis
Histoplasmosis, disseminated or extrapulmonary
Isosporiasis, chronic intestinal (>1-month's duration)
Kaposi's sarcoma
Lymphoid interstitial pneumonia and/or pulmonary lymphoid hyperplasia*
Lymphoma, Burkitt's (or equivalent term)
Lymphoma, immunoblastic (or equivalent term)
Lymphoma, primary, of brain
Mycobacterium avium-intracellulare complex or *Myobacterium kansasii,* disseminated or extrapulmonary
Mycobacterium tuberculosis, any site (pulmonary† or extrapulmonary)
Mycobacterium, other species or unidentified species, disseminated or extrapulmonary
Pneumocystis jirovecii pneumonia
Pneumonia, recurrent†
Progressive multifocal leukoencephalopathy
Salmonella septicemia, recurrent
Toxoplasmosis of brain
Wasting syndrome of HIV infection

*Children younger than 13 years.
†Added in the 1993 expansion of the AIDS surveillance case definition for adolescents and adults.

TABLE 114-2 1993 Revised Classification System for HIV Infection and Expanded AIDS Surveillance Case Definition for Adolescents and Adults*

CD4+ T-Cell Categories	Clinical Categories		
	A	B	C†
	Asymptomatic, Acute (Primary) HIV, or PGL	Symptomatic, Not A or C Conditions	AIDS-Indicator Conditions
1. ≥ 500/μL	A1	B1	C1
2. 200-499/μL	A2	B2	C2
3. <200/μL AIDS-indicator T-cell count*	A3	B3	C3

*Shading indicates conditions included in the 1993 AIDS surveillance case definitions for adolescents and adults.
†Clinical conditions in category C are listed in Table 114–1.
PGL, persistent generalized lymphadenopathy.
From Centers for Disease Control and Prevention. 1993 Revised classification system for HIV infection and expanded surveillance case definition for AIDS among adolescents and adults. MMWR Morb Mortal Wkly Rep. 1992:41:1-19.

of information for designing, standardizing, and evaluating drug and vaccine trials and epidemiologic and natural history studies and for formulating health policy and strategy; and facilitation of scientific communication.[44-46] The public health orientation of the CDC's classification system is complemented by other proposed systems for classifying the natural history of HIV infection, including prognostic staging systems,[46-48] prognostic scoring indices,[49] and systems that can be adapted to settings throughout the world that lack testing for sophisticated laboratory markers.[45]

HIV INFECTION AND AIDS IN ADULTS

Incidence and Prevalence of AIDS and HIV in the United States

In the United States, through December 31, 2002, 859,000 AIDS cases and 501,669 deaths had been reported to the CDC.[50] Since 1981, when the first cases were reported,[1,2] the number of persons with AIDS has increased rapidly. As a result of this rapid growth, the first 100,000 AIDS cases were reported during an 8-year period (1981-1989), whereas the second 100,000 cases were reported in just over 2 years (1989-1991).[51]

In the early 1990s, the number of people reported with AIDS in the United States increased substantially, in part because of expansion of the surveillance definition for AIDS,[15] primarily the inclusion of markers of severe HIV-related immunosuppression. As a result of this expansion, the number of reported AIDS cases increased by more than 100% in 1993 versus 1992.[52] Following the introduction of highly active antiretroviral therapy, the number of deaths and new AIDS cases began to decline for the first time in the history of the epidemic.[42,53] Between 1995 and 1998 the annual number of new AIDS cases fell by 38% (from 69,242 to 42,832) and deaths by 63% (from 51,760 to 18,823). As a result of this dramatic drop in mortality from AIDS, the number of persons living with AIDS in the United States has increased in recent years. At the end of 2002, an estimated 384,906 people were living with AIDS in the United States.

The prevalence of HIV infection is more difficult to determine because many HIV-infected people have never been tested and thus do not know they are infected. In 2002, the CDC estimated that between 850,000 and 950,000 people were infected with HIV in the United States, and 25% did not know that they were infected.[54]

Serologic Monitoring of the HIV Epidemic

Because AIDS is the most advanced manifestation of HIV infection and the period between infection with HIV and the development of AIDS is long, surveillance systems for HIV infection have been used to supplement the information available through AIDS case surveillance. Various methods periodically have been used to estimate the prevalence and incidence of HIV infection over the course of the epidemic. The U.S. Public Health Service has estimated that approximately 850,000 to 950,000 residents are infected with HIV with at least 41,000 new infections occurring annually.[54-57]

HIV seroprevalence surveys describe patterns of current HIV infection. These surveys have been conducted on (1) specimens not linked to personal identifiers and collected for other purposes, (2) name-identified specimens, and (3) specimens collected from populations subject to routine or mandatory HIV screening, such as blood donors or military personnel. In general, the patterns of HIV transmission observed in these studies in the United States are similar to those observed through AIDS case surveillance—higher rates of HIV infection are found among men than women, among blacks and Hispanic populations than whites, and among people 20 to 45 years old than those in other age groups. The highest incidence remains among men who have sex with men, in which incidence peaked in the early 1980s (5-20/100 person-years) and then declined but remained high during the 1990s (2-4/100 person-years).[57] In addition, it is estimated that approximately 0.6% of men and 0.1% of women are infected in the United States. However, the prevalence is much higher for blacks, in whom 2% of men and 0.6% of women are estimated to be infected.[56] Although the number of people who are being tested for HIV has increased in the United States, denial of HIV risk factors and fear of being HIV-positive continue to be major reasons for not being tested for HIV.[58]

Homosexual and bisexual men remain a major population with an increased prevalence of HIV infection. Of surveys conducted primarily in sexually transmitted disease clinics in the early to mid-1980s, HIV seroprevalence rates in homosexual and bisexual men ranged from 10% to 70%, with most rates falling between 20% and 50%.[59] Although the highest rates were found in New York City and San Francisco, areas of high to moderate HIV seroprevalence are dispersed throughout the country.[59] In 1997, a study of unlinked serologic specimens collected from homosexual or bisexual men attending sexually transmitted disease clinics in 17 cities had a median seroprevalence rate of 19.3%, with rates among black men approximately twice those of white men who had sex with men (Fig. 114-1).[60] That same year a probability sample of men who have sex with men in four large US cities demonstrated an overall HIV seroprevalence of 17%; however, the prevalence was 29% among blacks and 42% among those who injected drugs.[61] Among homosexual and bisexual men attending sexually transmitted disease clinics from 1988 to 1992, the overall HIV seroprevalence was 33% (range, 5% to 52%).[62] The HIV seroprevalence rate in this population decreased over time, especially among white homosexual and bisexual men, from 32% in 1989 to 22% in 1992, suggesting a decrease in HIV infection incidence.[63] The incidence of HIV infection among homosexual and bisexual men in some cohort studies dropped in the mid- to late 1980s.[59,64] However, recent studies in young men who have sex with men suggest continued high incidence of HIV. Data from the Young Men's Survey conducted in seven U.S. cities between 1994 and 1998 demonstrated an overall prevalence of HIV infection of 7.2% that ranged from 3.3% among whites to 14.1% among blacks. In that same study, HIV incidence overall was 2.6%, but it was 3.5% among persons ages 20 to 22 years, 4.0% among blacks, and 5.4% among men of mixed races.[65] The increase in the incidence of new HIV infections among homosexual men may be due to continued high-risk behavior in this population.[66,67] The role of HAART in the increase in risk-taking behavior among men who have sex with men is still controversial, but data suggest that people on HAART are more likely to develop sexually transmitted infections, an epidemiologic marker of unsafe sex.[68] In addition, the increase of HIV resistance to antiretroviral drugs among people with

FIGURE 114-1. Comparison of HIV prevalence among men who have sex with men at sexually transmitted disease clinics and drug users entering drug treatment centers, by metropolitan area 1993 to 1997. *(From Centers for Disease Control and Prevention [CDC]. HIV prevalence trends in selected populations in the United States. Results from National Serosurveillance 1993-1997. Atlanta: Centers for Disease Control and Prevention, 2001;1-51.)*

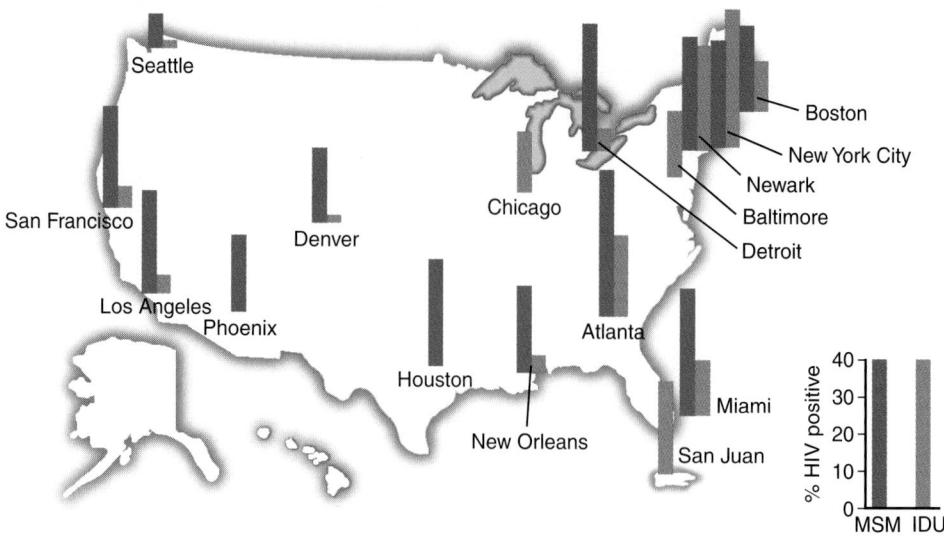

recent infection suggests that their infection is being acquired from people who are known to be HIV infected and receiving therapy.[69]

In contrast to the epidemic among homosexual and bisexual men, the epidemic among injecting drug users has been more concentrated geographically within the United States. Among injecting drug users, the initial HIV seroprevalence studies demonstrated very high rates of HIV infection in the Northeast and along the Atlantic Coast and low rates on the West Coast and in cities in other areas.[59,70,71] Although the highest rates of HIV infection continue to be observed in northeastern cities, the rate of HIV infection among drug users in other cities has increased. Studies conducted in the late 1980s in Atlanta, Chicago, and Baltimore showed an HIV seroprevalence rate greater than 12%.[72-74] Surveys conducted in drug treatment centers in 1997 showed a median HIV seroprevalence rate of 14.8% (range zero to 37.7%) among injecting drug users entering drug treatment programs.[60] Similar findings have been noted in subsequent studies: HIV seroprevalence among injecting drug users admitted to drug treatment centers in Baltimore (25%) and Newark (24%) was high, whereas it was low in San Francisco (7%), Seattle (5%), Denver (2%), and Detroit (1%).[75-77] HIV incidence in the 1990s remained high in the East (1-3/100 person-years) and lower in the West (<0.5/100 person-years).[57]

The reasons for the geographic differences in HIV seroprevalence among injecting drug users remain poorly understood, inasmuch as cities with low prevalence rates have many injecting drug users who practice high-risk behaviors.[77] In addition, the HIV epidemic among injecting drug users is closely related to other risk behaviors such as having unprotected sex, which frequently occurs in the context of illicit substance use.[78] Studies in sexually transmitted disease clinics have also shown elevated rates of HIV infection among heterosexual injecting drug users in comparison with other heterosexual men and women.[62,63] Although heroin injection is typically associated with parenteral transmission of HIV, injectors of cocaine and other drugs also have increased rates of HIV infection.[74-80] Cocaine injection, especially the use of "speedballs" (cocaine or amphetamines with heroin), injection in a "shooting gallery," and sexual risk behavior are associated with HIV infection among injecting drug users.[80,81] Data from New York City suggest that HIV prevalence among drug users declined between 1991 and 1996[82] and suggest that changes in HIV prevalence among sex and needle-sharing partners or changes in risk behavior with such partners might lead to changes in the risk for new infections among drug users.

Certain populations of heterosexual men and women who do not inject drugs also have appreciable rates of HIV infection. From 1988 to 1989, studies conducted in sexually transmitted disease clinics with heterosexual persons who do not inject drugs but have other sexually transmitted diseases found a median seroprevalence of 2.3% with a range of zero to 14%.[63] Although men in these clinics typically had higher rates than women did, in some areas adolescent women had higher rates of HIV infection than adolescent men did. Nearly one third of those infected heterosexually are estimated to have been infected as adolescents.[83]

HIV infection acquired through heterosexual contact is the source of an increasing number of AIDS cases, especially among women.[84] Of persons infected heterosexually, sexual contact with an injecting drug user is the most frequently reported risk. Accordingly, the geographic distribution of HIV rates among persons who acquired their infection through heterosexual contact and among injecting drug users is similar.[85] In addition, persons who use smokable forms of cocaine ("crack" cocaine) and other noninjected illicit drugs have elevated risks for HIV infection as a result of exchanging sex for drugs or money and the presence of other sexually transmitted diseases.[81,86-89] Some people infected through heterosexual contact may not report a risk of HIV infection because they are unaware of the serostatus of their heterosexual partners.[50,63,86] However, the incidence among heterosexual men and women continues to be much lower than among men who have sex with men. In a study conducted among clients of sexually transmitted disease clinics in the United States between 1990 and 1999, the HIV incidence among heterosexual men and women was estimated to be 0.5% compared with 7.1% among men who have sex with men.[90]

Female commercial sex workers (prostitutes) are at increased risk for HIV infection because of injecting drug use and multiple sex partners. In a 1987 multicenter study of prostitutes in various settings in selected cities, 65 (10%) of 670 women tested positive for HIV antibody.[91] Seroprevalence rates for HIV infection ranged from 0% for prescreened prostitutes in Nevada to 69% for prostitutes being treated for drug addiction in New Jersey. Among prostitutes who were studied, the major risk factor was injecting drug use. In a study in south Florida in 1987, 37 (41%) of 90 inner-city sex workers were HIV antibody–positive, including 29 (46%) of 63 women who reported drug use and 8 (30%) of 27 women who denied using drugs.[92] From 1987 to 1991, the prevalence of HIV infection among female sex workers in south Florida remained relatively stable at approximately 24%. However, the incidence of HIV infection among female sex workers in this area who received multiple HIV tests increased from 0.3% per 100 person-years in 1987 to 15% in 1991.[93] Data from a cohort study conducted among drug users in Baltimore, a high-incidence and high-prevalence city, suggest that HIV incidence is doubled among drug-using men who also engage in homosexual sex and among women who have a recent sexually transmitted infection, suggesting that sexual risk behavior is a major determinant of risk even among drug users.[94]

Surveys conducted in some clinical settings indicate that the HIV infection rate is higher than in a more representative sample of the general population.[95-99] In a 1989 to 1991 survey of persons admitted to 20 hospitals, an HIV seroprevalence of 4.7% (range, 0.2% to 14.2%) was observed; in one hospital, 24% of men 15 to 54 years old were infected with HIV.[95] Data from this survey were used to estimate that 225,000 HIV-infected persons were hospitalized in 1990; 72% of them were admitted for conditions other than HIV infection or AIDS. A 1990 to 1992 survey of patients seen in primary care practices revealed an HIV seroprevalence rate of 0.45%, with the seroprevalence among men (0.96%) being higher than the rate among women (0.22%).[96] Voluntary routine HIV counseling and testing among inpatients in a hospital in Boston was able to demonstrate an HIV seroprevalence of 3.8% among patients who otherwise would not have been tested for HIV, suggesting that a substantial number of patients with undiagnosed HIV are being discharged from health care facilities without HIV infection being considered.[97]

In many areas, persons with tuberculosis have high rates of HIV infection, and HIV screening should be provided to all patients diagnosed with tuberculosis.[98] Among 27 tuberculosis treatment clinics in 15 metropolitan areas surveyed between 1988 and 1995, HIV seroprevalence ranged from 0.6% to 42.9%, with a median rate of 8.9%.[99] The highest rates were found in the Northeast and in Atlantic Coast areas and among U.S.-born persons 30 to 39 years old, who had a median seroprevalence of 30.1%. High rates were also noted among those with extrapulmonary disease.

Among patients with syphilis the overall HIV seroprevalence was 15.7%; among men the seroprevalence was 27.5%, and among women it was 12.4%.[100] However, among men who have sex with men and syphilis, the seroprevalence ranged from 64.3% to 90%.

HIV prevalence rates among adolescents attending adolescent medicine clinics in three metropolitan areas (Baltimore, Houston, and New York City) that collected data each year from 1993 to 1997 showed an overall HIV prevalence rate of 0.4% (range, 0.2%-0.5%).[101] Rates were the same for male and female patients (0.4%) and were approximately the same among patients 13 to 19 years of age (0.4%) and those 20 to 24 years of age (0.5%). However, rates were higher among black patients (0.6%) than among Hispanic and white patients (0.1%).

Studies of HIV seroprevalence in entrants to correctional facilities have indicated a wide range of rates, with the highest in areas with a moderate to high incidence of AIDS.[102] From 1991 to 1992, the median HIV seroprevalence was 2.9% (range, zero to 15%) in 35 correctional facilities in 17 metropolitan areas.[73] Rates ranged from 1% to 12.5% for men and zero to 24% for women, which is a reflection of the high rates of drug use in these persons. Among New York state prison entrants between 1987 and 1997, 12% of men and 18% of women were infected with HIV.[103] Between 1992 and 1998, data from nearly 500,000 HIV tests performed in correctional facilities in the United States demonstrated an overall HIV seroprevalence of 3.4%, of which 56% were among persons newly identified as HIV infected.[104]

HIV seroprevalence data are more available for large groups who are routinely tested for HIV infection. These groups include blood donors, applicants for military service, military personnel, and applicants to U.S. Department of Labor Job Corps training programs.[73,101,105-112] These surveys are valuable but are limited in generalizability in that many persons at risk for HIV infection are excluded from some populations (e.g., potential blood donors and military applicants). A study conducted in five blood banks between 1991 and 1996 showed that the prevalence of HIV decreased in first-time donors from 0.030% to 0.015%.[113] Approximately 8 million people voluntarily donate 14 million units of blood annually in the United States. HIV prevalence trends can best be determined from first-time blood donors, who represent approximately 20% of all donations. Since 1985, the American Red Cross, which collects approximately half of the voluntary donations, has provided the CDC with routine HIV screening results for their blood donations. After a slight increase from 1993 to 1994 among men, prevalence then decreased from 0.032% in 1994 to

0.021% in 1997. Among women, prevalence was relatively stable (0.010% to 0.014%) between 1993 and 1997.[101]

The overall prevalence of HIV infection among 2.3 million applicants for military service was 1.31 per 1000 between October 1985 and September 1989.[105] HIV infection rates in this population were higher for men (1.42/1000) than women (0.66/1000), for black non-Hispanic men (3.7/1000) than white men (0.61/1000), and for persons from large metropolitan areas, particularly those with higher rates of AIDS case reporting. The seroprevalence rate among teenage military applicants (0.34/1000) was lower than the median rate for all applicants; the male-to-female ratio was nearly 1:1 and the rate of infection among 17- and 18-year-old females exceeded that of same-age males.[106] Overall, the prevalence of HIV infection in applicants has decreased from approximately 0.15% in 1985 to 0.045% (1 positive for every 2200 applicants tested) in 1997.[60] Rates were particularly high for black male military applicants (0.17%).[101] Because HIV-positive applicants and drug users are not accepted into the military, a self-selection bias among persons in high-risk categories may occur, thus certain populations may be underrepresented among military applicants.[60]

Among U.S. Army active-duty personnel, the HIV incidence rate was 0.17/1000 person-years between 1985 and 1999.[110] The incidence rate for male and female soldiers was 0.18/1000 person-years and 0.08/1000 person-years, respectively. The rate of seroconversion decreased from 0.49 per 1000 person-years from 1985 to 1987 to 0.29 per 1000 person-years from 1988 to 1989.[111] However, a reduction in the seroconversion rate was not observed for black soldiers, thus suggesting a higher rate of continued transmission in this population.

Students who enter Job Corps training programs tend to be economically disadvantaged school-aged youths drawn from racial and ethnic minority communities in both rural and urban areas. For students ages 16 to 21 years who entered training from January 1990 through December 1996, 2.3 per 1000 were infected with HIV, a rate almost 10 times that seen among applicants for military service, with statewide prevalence rates ranging from zero to 0.8% in 1997.[60,112] Among Job Corps applicants, the infection rate increased with age. HIV prevalence was higher for women than for men (2.8 per 1000 versus 2 per 1000). HIV seroprevalence rates were highest for black women (4.9 per 1000). From 1990 through 1996, HIV prevalence rates for women and men declined from 2.8 per 1000 in 1990 to 1.4 per 1000 in 1996. The highest rates were observed in students from large Northeast urban centers and also among students from rural and smaller urban centers in the South. In 1997, HIV prevalence was 0.26% for Job Corps entrants from the South, 0.20% for entrants from the Northeast, 0.11% from the Midwest, and 0.01% from the West.[101]

Another type of broad population survey was the survey of childbearing women, which provided unbiased population-based estimates of HIV infection in women giving birth in the United States. HIV antibody prevalence for childbearing women was ascertained by blinded surveys conducted on residual blood samples collected on filter paper from newborns for routine metabolic screening such as that for phenylketonuria.[114] HIV seroprevalence among childbearing women remained stable nationwide from 1987 through 1994 at values ranging from 1.5 to 1.7 per 1000 women.[115] Seroprevalence decreased over this time in the Northeast and increased in the South. In 1994, HIV seroprevalence rates among black childbearing women were 2 to 20 times higher than for those among white women. The findings of seroprevalence studies of women seeking reproductive care services have also shown the highest HIV rates to be in clinics located along the Atlantic Coast and in Puerto Rico.[60,116] If HIV seroprevalence rates among childbearing women were similar for all women of reproductive age in the United States, in 1994 approximately 84,000 women in this age group would have been infected with HIV.[114] The survey of childbearing women was halted in 1995 in light of congressional concerns about blinded surveys in this population.

Although surveillance for HIV infection has traditionally focused on the incidence of AIDS and the prevalence of HIV, new diagnostic technologies that allow the estimation of incident, HIV infection have become available, including the use the sensitive–less sensitive enzyme immune assay (EIA) test (or serologic testing algorithm for recent HIV seroconversion [STAHRS]) and the measurement of HIV-ribonucleic acid (RNA) by polymerase chain reaction (PCR) in pooled blood specimens that test negative for HIV.[117,118] Having an HIV surveillance system that focuses on incident rather than prevalent infections will allow for better monitoring of the HIV epidemic.[119]

Exposure Categories

Since the first cases of AIDS were reported in 1981, cases in men who have sex with men and heterosexual injecting drug users have consistently represented the largest number of AIDS cases reported. The rate of growth in the total number of AIDS cases and in these two exposure categories was most rapid through 1986.[120,121] In 1987, the rate of increase in AIDS reporting began to slow for homosexual and bisexual men, particularly in cities where AIDS was first recognized. This slowing in case reporting was related to several events, including the increasing use of therapies such as zidovudine and prophylaxis against *P. jirovecii* pneumonia, which delayed the development of AIDS-defining conditions; a decrease in the number of new HIV infections, which in part reflects the impact of prevention programs; and a decline in the completeness of reporting.[55,64,122,123] As a result of this slowing in case reporting, and changes in the dynamics of the HIV epidemic, the proportion of AIDS cases among homosexual and bisexual men has decreased from 65% to 28% of the total cases reported among adults from 1987 to 2002. Cases of AIDS among recipients of blood or blood components and among persons with hemophilia increased dramatically during the mid-1980s, but since 1987 the numbers have declined and these persons represented less than 1% of the AIDS cases reported in 1997. After implementation of HIV antibody testing in March 1985, no more than 5 cases of transfusion-associated HIV infection per year were reported to the CDC during the subsequent years as compared with 714 cases in 1984.[121] Since the initiation of HIV antibody screening of donated blood and plasma and heat treatment of clotting factors, transmission of HIV through blood and blood products has been reported only rarely.[124] Almost all cases of transfusion-associated AIDS diagnosed in 1991 with known transfusion dates were the result of transfusions received before 1986.[121]

Heterosexual contact cases consist of people who report exposure to a person with or at increased risk for HIV infection (e.g., an injecting drug user) or persons born in countries where heterosexual transmission is the major route of HIV infection (e.g., areas of sub-Saharan Africa and some Caribbean countries). AIDS cases associated with heterosexual contact have been increasing steadily and in 2002 represented 29% of all cases reported among adults. Since 1986, the annual percent increase in this group has been higher than that of any other exposure category and has been most striking for women. In 1992, the number of cases diagnosed among women infected through heterosexual contact exceeded the number infected through injecting drug use for the first time and represented 68% of cases among women reported in 2002.[50] Blacks and Hispanic populations account for more than 75% of all persons reported with AIDS attributed to heterosexual contact.[125]

For AIDS cases reported in 2002, 16% of men and 21% of women reported to have acquired HIV through heterosexual contact had a source partner who was an injection drug user. However, this number could be larger because the risk of the partner was not specified for 81% of cases reported as having heterosexually acquired AIDS. In the past, persons with sex partners of unknown HIV infection or risk status were classified in the undetermined category, but as of September 2000, the procedures for investigating cases reported without risk changed from ascertaining risk for all reported cases to estimating risk distributions from statistical models and population-based samples. Selected follow-up and investigation of heterosexual contact cases have identified other sources of exposure to HIV infection for some persons, especially men.[126,127] Nonetheless, it is unlikely that such misclassification bias has significantly influenced national trends.[120]

Of the 42,044 adults and adolescents with AIDS reported in 2002, 4.5% occurred in men who reported having sex with men as well as injecting drugs. Except for this group, people with more than one reported mode of exposure to HIV are counted only once in a hierarchy of exposure categories.[50]

Cases in persons with no reported exposure to HIV through any of the recognized routes are classified as "no risk reported or identified." This category includes cases that are being followed up by local health department officials; cases in persons whose exposure history is incomplete because they died, declined to be interviewed, or were lost to follow-up; and cases in persons who were interviewed or for whom other follow-up information was available and no mode of exposure was identified. Previous studies indicate that when follow-up information is obtained, an established exposure mode can be identified for more than 90% of these persons, and they are subsequently reclassified into the appropriate exposure category.[128] Although surveillance and investigation of cases with an undetermined risk can assist in detecting unusual modes of transmission (e.g., transplantation), such instances remain rare.[129]

AIDS Trends

The 1993 change in the AIDS case definition[15] dramatically changed AIDS incidence trends as a result of a large increase in reported AIDS cases. In 1993, the first year that the new case definition was used, 103,500 AIDS cases were reported to the CDC among persons 13 years or older as compared with 49,016 cases in 1992.[52] In 1994, 1995, and 1996, the number of AIDS cases reported annually decreased in contrast to the artificial peak in the number of cases reported in 1993. Since implementation of the revised case definition, more than half of all cases are reported on the basis of a CD4 T-lymphocyte count of fewer than 200 cells/μL. However, from 1995 to 1996, for the first time in the epidemic, the occurrence of AIDS-defining opportunistic illnesses and death among persons with AIDS decreased 7% and 25%, respectively.[52,130] Declines in AIDS incidence continued from 1998 through 1999, but declines in AIDS incidence began to level and essentially no change occurred from 1999 through 2001. In 2002, AIDS diagnosis increased 2% for a rate of 14.1 per 100,000 population in the United States.[50] In contrast, reported AIDS deaths have continued to decline from 19,005 in 1998 to 16,371 in 2002 (Fig. 114-2).[50] This decrease was largely due to the increasing use of combination antiretroviral therapy.[42]

Demographic Characteristics

Men accounted for 74% of AIDS cases reported in 2002, and AIDS case rates were much higher for men (26.4/100,000) than women (17.3/100,000). However, the number of women reported with AIDS is increasing more rapidly than the number of men, and the proportion of total AIDS cases who are women has increased from 8% in 1988 to 26% in 2002.[50] Most of the increase in AIDS cases among women is due to heterosexual transmission of HIV.

Through December 2002, 64% of reported AIDS cases occurred in persons 25 to 44 years old. Information from HIV infection reporting suggests that adolescents and young adults, particularly young black women, have a high rate of recently acquired infection.[38] Since 1991, 11% of AIDS cases have been reported among people 50 years or older.[131]

In 2002, 28.3% of persons reported with AIDS were white, 50.2% were black non-Hispanic (46% of reported cases among men and 68% among women), and 19.6% were Hispanic (Table 114-3). The rate of AIDS among blacks and Hispanics has increased disproportionately in comparison with whites[132]: In 2002, the rate of AIDS was 108.4 per 100,000 for black non-Hispanic men and 39.7 per 100,000 for Hispanics compared with 12.3 per 100,000 for white non-Hispanic men. Black women had a rate of 76.4 per 100,000; Hispanic women a rate of 26 per 100,000 compared with white women who had a rate of 7 per 100,000.[50] Cases reported among American Indians and Alaskan Natives have significantly increased; however, only 205 cases (0.5% of the total) were reported in 2002 in these populations.[50]

FIGURE 114-2. AIDS cases, deaths, and persons living with AIDS by year, 1985 to 2002, United States. Adjusted for reporting delays. *(From Centers for Disease Control and Prevention. HIV/AIDS Surveillance Report. 2002;14:1-48.)*

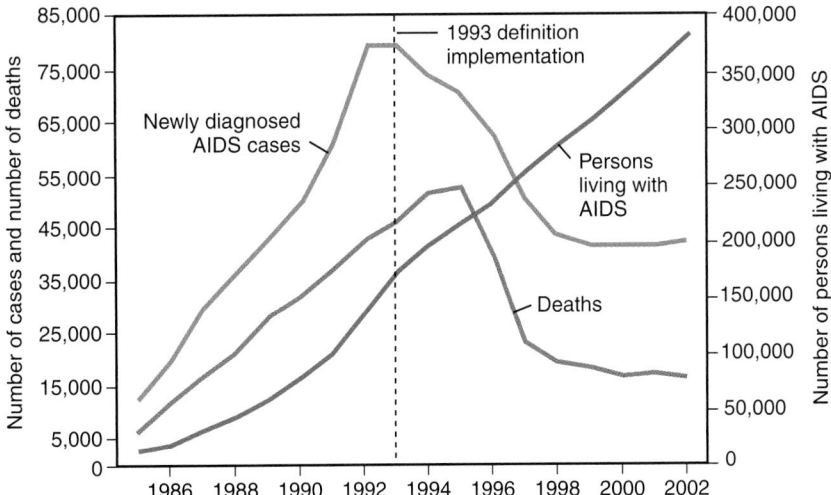

Hispanics with AIDS represent different countries of origin and cultures.[133] Among Hispanic AIDS cases reported in 2002, Puerto Rican–born Hispanics represented 21% and Mexican-born Hispanics 16%. The rate of AIDS is highest for Hispanics in the Northeast and in Puerto Rico. Injecting drug use is the predominant exposure mode in Puerto Rican–born men and women with AIDS residing in either Puerto Rico or the U.S. mainland. The AIDS rate among Hispanics is lowest in the West. Hispanics with AIDS in this area are primarily from Mexico or Central and South America and are less likely to report a history of injecting drug use.

Geographic Distribution of AIDS Cases

The first cases of AIDS reported in the United States were clustered among homosexual and bisexual men and injecting drug users in the major metropolitan areas of the East and West Coasts.[1,2] Since then, AIDS cases have been reported from all 50 states, the District of Columbia, Puerto Rico, the Virgin Islands, and Guam. However, these cases are distributed unevenly across the United States.[37,50] The populous northeastern states and metropolitan areas with more than 1 million persons have the highest rates of AIDS. In 2002, AIDS incidence rates by state varied from 0.5 per 100,000 population in North Dakota to 162.4 per 100,000 population in the District of Columbia (Figs. 114-3 and 114-4).

The geographic distribution of AIDS is changing over time. Five states—New York, California, Florida, Texas, and New Jersey—have reported 56% of all AIDS cases though 2002. However, the proportion of cases from these states had decreased from 54% of the 50,316 cases reported before 1988 to 48% of the 42,651 cases reported in 2002 alone.[50] This change reflects a slowing in case reporting from these areas and a greater increase in the number of persons with AIDS reported from other areas of the United States. The southern region of the United States accounted for 34% of the cases reported through December 1997, and 37% of the cases reported that year alone.[134] In 2001, the rate of AIDS cases reported in metropolitan areas with a population of 500,000 or more was 19 per 100,000. In metropolitan areas with a population of 50,000 to 500,000, the rate was 9.5 per 100,000, whereas in nonmetropolitan areas it was 5.8 per 100,000 population.[135] In 2001, the cities with the highest annual AIDS rates per 100,000 population were New York (65.9), Miami (53.8), Baltimore (50), Jersey City (42.1), Fort Lauderdale (41.3), and West Palm Beach (39.4). Regional variations in AIDS case reporting reflect temporal differences in the introduction of HIV, the rate of new HIV infections over time, migration of HIV-infected persons, and local reporting practices.[122,136] The geographic trends observed in population-based HIV seroprevalence studies are similar to those for AIDS case reporting.[105,107,109-115] With the advent of HIV reporting it is now possible to also monitor trends for HIV infection (not AIDS). In the 30 areas with robust confidential HIV infection reporting, the prevalence rate of HIV infection (not AIDS) among adults was 125.7 per 100,000 at the end of 2002. The rate for adults living with HIV infection (not AIDS) ranged from 12.8 per 100,000 (North Dakota) to 229.7 per 100,000 (Virgin Islands). The prevalence rate of HIV infection (not AIDS) among children was 5.6 per 100,000 population. The rate for children living with HIV infection (not AIDS) ranged from 0.4 per 100,000 in Idaho to 20 per 100,000 in New Jersey.[50]

The geographic distribution of persons with AIDS also varies by the reported mode of HIV transmission and reflects multiple epidemics among different populations in different regions of the country. Men who have sex with men represent a large percentage of AIDS cases in some states, although they are distributed throughout all regions of the United States.[137] Injecting drug use is the second most frequently reported risk behavior for HIV infection in states along the Atlantic Coast of the United States. In 1995, 25,860 (35%) of the AIDS cases reported that year were associated with injecting drug use,[138] but this mode of transmission accounted for greater than 50% of the cases reported from Delaware, Connecticut, Maryland, Rhode Island, and Puerto Rico. Although the highest rates of AIDS associated

TABLE 114-3   Characteristics of Persons Reported with AIDS and Rates by Year of Report, United States, 1997 and 2002

	1997		2002	
	Number (n = 60,634)	*Rate**	*Number (n = 42,136)*	*Rate**
Sex†				
Male	47,312 (78%)	44.0	31,089 (74%)	26.4
Female	13,322 (22%)	11.5	10,955 (26%)	17.3
Race/Ethnicity				
White non-Hispanic	20,197	10.4	11,089	7.0
Black	27,075	83.7	21,169	76.4
Hispanic	12,466	37.7	8,242	26.0
Asian/Pacific Islander	448	4.5	478	4.9
American Indian/ Alaska native	206	10.4	206	11.2

*Per 100,000 population extrapolating from the official 1980 and 1990 census counts (1997 census estimates published in U.S. Bureau of Census Publication PPL-91 and 2002 from the U.S. Census Bureau. Population estimates. Available at http://eire.census.gov/popest/estimates_dataset.php).

†Rates by sex are only for adult/adolescent cases of AIDS.

From Centers for Disease Control and Prevention. HIV/AIDS Surveillance Report. 1997;9(2):1-43; and Centers for Disease Control and Prevention. HIV/AIDS Surveillance Report. 2002;14:1-48.

FIGURE 114-3. Male adolescent/adult AIDS annual rates per 100,000 population, for cases reported in 2001, United States. *(From Centers for Disease Control and Prevention. HIV/AIDS Surveillance Report. 2001;13:1-44.)*

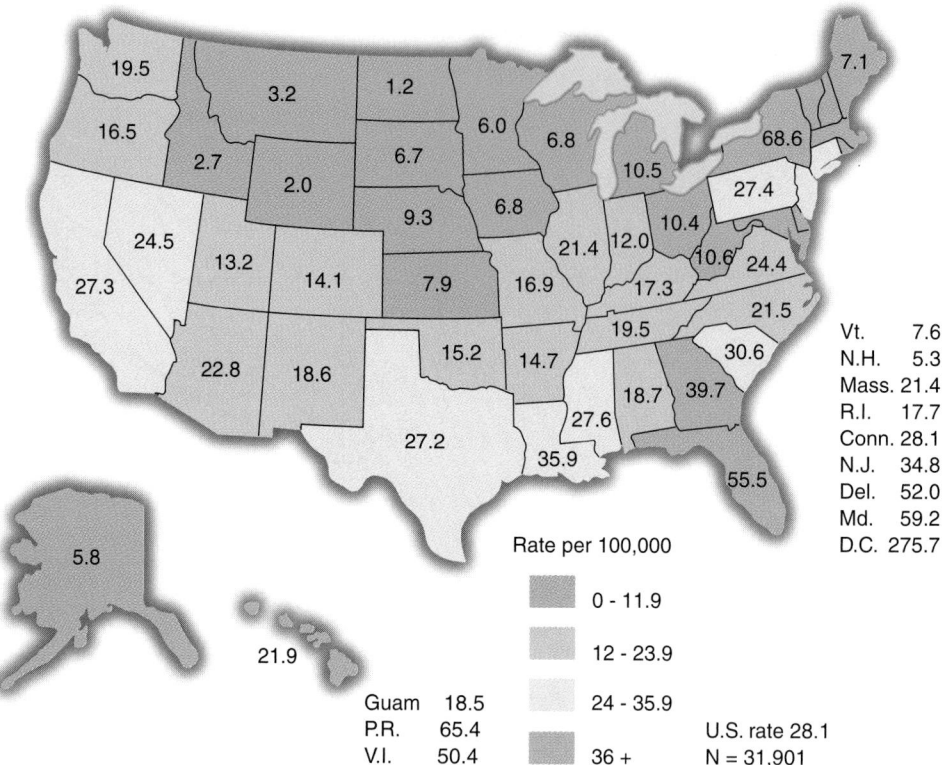

Vt. 7.6
N.H. 5.3
Mass. 21.4
R.I. 17.7
Conn. 28.1
N.J. 34.8
Del. 52.0
Md. 59.2
D.C. 275.7

Rate per 100,000

0 - 11.9
12 - 23.9
24 - 35.9
36 +

Guam 18.5
P.R. 65.4
V.I. 50.4

U.S. rate 28.1
N = 31,901

Clinical Manifestations of HIV Infection

Spectrum and Progression of HIV Infection

with injecting drug use continue to occur in the Northeast, the rate there has slowed down and the number of cases in the South and West has increased at a faster rate. All areas of the country have had an increase in the number of men and women with AIDS reportedly infected through heterosexual contact, but the largest increase in recent years has occurred in the South.

The spectrum of HIV infection ranges from an asymptomatic state to severe immunodeficiency and associated serious secondary infections, neoplasms, and other conditions.[28,140] Initial or primary infection with HIV can be followed by an acute mononucleosis-like illness. Features of this acute illness associated with seroconversion include fever, lymphadenopathy, sweats, myalgia, arthralgia, rash, malaise, lethargy, sore throat, anorexia, nausea, vomiting, diarrhea, headache, photophobia, and mucocutaneous ulcers.[141,142] Less common manifestations have also been reported, including a variety of neurologic conditions (e.g., aseptic meningitis, myelopathy, radiculopathy, peripheral neuropathy, and Guillain-Barré syndrome),[144] *Candida* esophagitis,[145] and mucocutaneous ulcerations (see Chapter 117).

Estimates of the frequency of symptoms among those with primary HIV infection range from 40% to 90%. The signs and symptoms of acute HIV infection are usually manifested days to weeks after exposure.[143,146,147] In a comprehensive review of primary HIV infection, the interval between exposure and symptomatic illness was reported to range on average between 2 and 4 weeks, with the duration of illness lasting from 1 to 2 weeks.[145] However, the diagnosis of acute HIV infection is frequently missed. In a group of 23 persons at risk of HIV infection, 87% were symptomatic and 95% of them sought medical care, yet few had the correct diagnosis made at the first clinic visit.[141] In a prospective study, fever, myalgias, rash, night sweats, and arthralgias occurred more frequently among patients with primary HIV infection but no targeted symptoms allowed for screening for primary infection.[142] Acute HIV infection should therefore be included in the

correct setting in the differential diagnosis of any unexplained febrile illness (see Chapter 117).[143]

The diagnosis of acute HIV infection cannot be made with the standard serologic tests because they detect antibodies and become positive approximately 3 weeks after the initial infection.[148] Studies of homosexual men,[149,150] persons with hemophilia,[149,151] and intravenous drug users[152] have consistently demonstrated the development of detectable HIV antibodies within 3 to 12 weeks after infection. Epidemiologic studies and case reports as well as modeling techniques[149] suggest that seroconversion beyond 6 months is very uncommon. The laboratory diagnosis of primary HIV infection should be made by requesting a plasma HIV-RNA assay which has a sensitivity of 100% and specificity of 97.4%.[142] The presence of detectable p24 antigen test is less sensitive (88.7%) but more specific (100%) than the plasma HIV-RNA assay for the diagnosis of primary infection,[142] and detection of p24 antigen is now used routinely in the screening of blood donors.[153] Thus, the presence of viral p24 antigen or high-titer HIV-RNA in a patient with a negative test for HIV-1 antibodies establishes the diagnosis of acute HIV infection (see Chapter 115). False-positive HIV-RNA tests have been described, but they are not reproducible and have values lower than 3000 copies/mL.[154]

Since 1989, cases of severe cellular immunodeficiency and associated opportunistic conditions in the absence of detectable HIV infection have been reported.[155] A provisional surveillance case definition was subsequently developed and based on the common feature of CD4+ T-lymphocyte depletion; this condition was termed *idiopathic CD4+ T lymphocytopenia.*[156] Extensive laboratory and epidemiologic investigations have determined that these cases do not represent occult HIV infection and do not appear to be etiologically linked, nor is there evidence to support a new transmissible agent.[157]

After primary infection with HIV, the risk for disease progression increases with the duration of infection. Most cohort studies that have evaluated the natural history of HIV infection have been conducted in the United States and Europe and show that AIDS develops in less than 5% of HIV-infected adults within 2 years of infection; without therapy, AIDS develops in approximately 20% to 25% within 6 years

FIGURE   114-4.   Female adult/adolescent AIDS annual rates per 100,000 population, for cases reported in 1997, United States. *(From Centers for Disease Control and Prevention. HIV/AIDS Surveillance Report. 1997;9:39.)*

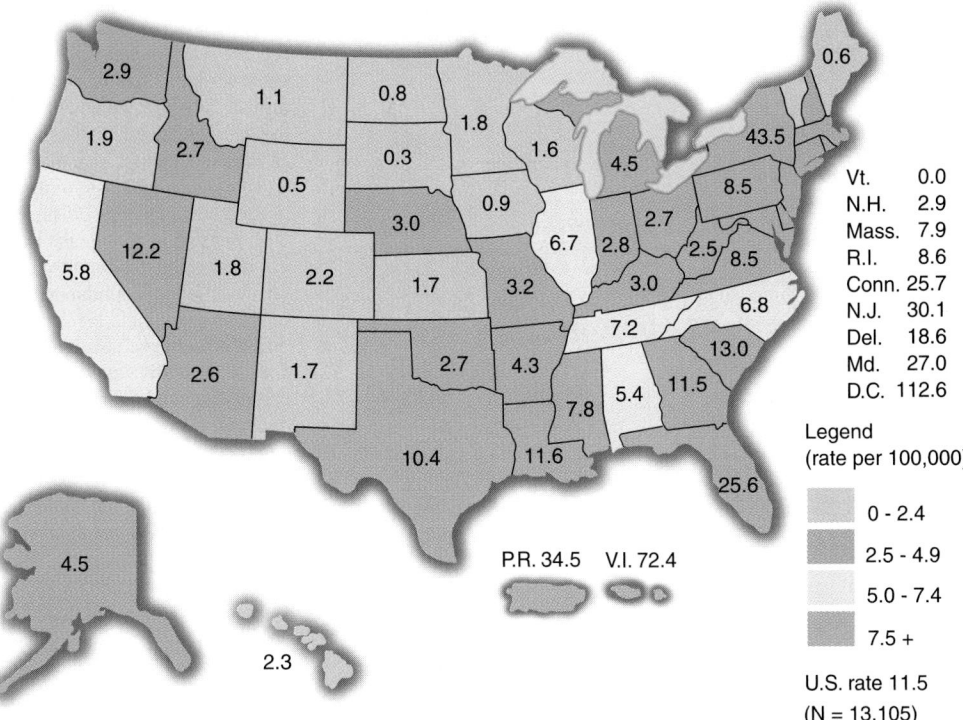

Vt.   0.0
N.H.   2.9
Mass.   7.9
R.I.   8.6
Conn. 25.7
N.J.   30.1
Del.   18.6
Md.   27.0
D.C.   112.6

Legend
(rate per 100,000)

	0 - 2.4
	2.5 - 4.9
	5.0 - 7.4
	7.5 +

U.S. rate 11.5
(N = 13,105)

P.R. 34.5   V.I. 72.4

of infection, and in 50% within 10 years.[158-161] Approximately 5% to 8% of HIV-infected individuals remain clinically asymptomatic with normal CD4 T-lymphocyte counts for more than 8 years after infection. These individuals are called "long-term nonprogressors."[162-164]

Differences in the rate of progression may be due to the route of infection, the size of the viral inoculum, the pathogenicity of the infecting viral strain, or the immunologic status of the host. For example, in one analysis of nearly 700 HIV-infected transfusion recipients, the estimated risk for the development of AIDS was 33% for persons within 5 years of infection and 49% within 7 years of infection.[165] Among recipients infected for similar periods, AIDS developed more rapidly in those who received blood from donors who progressed to AIDS soon after donation (50%) than in those who received blood from other HIV-infected donors (26%). In the same study, recipients in whom AIDS developed had received significantly more units of blood at the time of infection than did HIV-infected recipients without AIDS, which raises the possibility that the underlying clinical status leading to multiple transfusions, particularly the degree of immunosuppression, or exposure to other viral cofactors may also have affected disease progression.

The role of exogenous biologic and behavioral cofactors in the progression to AIDS remains uncertain. Coinfection with other viruses, use of tobacco, and injecting or recreational drug use have not been consistently associated with acceleration of HIV disease.[166-169] Several studies have suggested that the risk of development of AIDS increases significantly with age.[159,169,170] Pregnancy has not been shown to affect the progression of HIV infection.[171]

Because the natural history of HIV infection can vary considerably from person to person, clinical and laboratory predictors of progression are helpful. Oral candidiasis,[172] oral hairy leukoplakia,[173] and severe, recurrent herpes zoster[174] have been associated with an increased likelihood of development of AIDS. Measures of CD4+ T lymphocytes are the most specific laboratory markers of HIV-related immunosuppression and are strongly predictive of disease progression.[175] However, the quantity of HIV-RNA present in serum or plasma (the "viral load") has been found to be the single best predictor of progression to AIDS and death among HIV-infected individuals.[176,177] When both the viral load and CD4 T-cell count are combined, the

prognosis is more accurately defined, and thus both parameters are critically important in the evaluation of HIV-infected persons.[178]

AIDS-Indicator Diseases

The relative frequency of individual AIDS-indicator diseases is most representative for those diseases diagnosed at the time of the initial case report to national AIDS surveillance because subsequent diagnoses are much less completely reported (Table 114-4).

Three clinical conditions accounted for more than 75% of all initial AIDS-indicator conditions reported in 1992: *P. jirovecii* pneumonia (42%), HIV wasting syndrome (20%), and candidiasis of the esophagus (15%). The prevalence of several AIDS-indicator diseases was higher in men who have sex with men than in heterosexual men or women. In general, the reported frequency of AIDS-indicator diseases is similar for men and women with similar modes of exposure to HIV. However, among injecting drug users, esophageal candidiasis, cytomegalovirus disease and retinitis, and herpes simplex virus disease have been reported more frequently for women than men.[179]

Because most AIDS-indicator infections result from the endogenous reactivation of previously acquired pathogens, the frequency of reported opportunistic infections probably reflects in part the geographic-specific prevalence of endemic infections. For example, toxoplasmosis and cryptococcosis are more likely to develop in African and Haitian patients.[180] Similarly, the risk of extrapulmonary tuberculosis among foreign-born persons with AIDS in the United States is highest in those from Haiti, the Philippines, Central America, and Africa.[181] Among U.S.-born persons, those at increased risk for extrapulmonary tuberculosis include residents of the South and Northeast, blacks and Hispanic peoples, and injecting drug users.[182]

Expansion of the surveillance case definition for AIDS in the United States in 1993 to include immunologic criteria (CD4 T-lymphocyte cell count less than 200/µL) caused a substantial distortion in the trend in the incidence of AIDS-defining diseases. Therefore, the CDC developed a procedure for estimating the incidence of AIDS-defining opportunistic infections among persons reported solely on the basis of immunologic criteria; this procedure allowed trends in the incidence of opportunistic infections in persons with AIDS to be estimated as though the case definition had not changed.[182] Changes in incidence

TABLE 114-4 AIDS-Indicator Diseases in Adults/Adolescents and Children Reported in 1997, United States*

AIDS-Indicator Diseases	No. Adults/ Adolescents (%) (n = 60,161)	No. Children (%) (n = 473)
Pneumocystis jirovecii pneumonia		
Definitive diagnosis	5763 (10)	77 (16)
Presumptive diagnosis	3382 (6)	44 (9)
Wasting syndrome	4212 (7)	73 (15)
Kaposi's sarcoma		
Definitive diagnosis	1088 (2)	
Presumptive diagnosis	412 (1)	
Candidiasis, esophageal		
Definitive diagnosis	2057 (3)	30 (6)
Presumptive diagnosis	1255 (2)	20 (4)
Mycobacterium avium-intracellulare complex, extrapulmonary		
Definitive diagnosis	941 (2)	22 (5)
Presumptive diagnosis	183 (<1)	10 (2)
Cytomegalovirus disease	827 (1)	30 (6)
Cytomegalovirus, retinitis		
Definitive diagnosis	551 (1)	4 (1)
Presumptive diagnosis	260 (<1)	5 (1)
HIV encephalopathy	1196 (2)	108 (23)
Herpes simplex disease	1250 (2)	15 (3)
Cryptococcosis, extrapulmonary	1168 (2)	5 (1)
Toxoplasmosis of brain		
Definitive diagnosis	576 (1)	1 (<1)
Presumptive diagnosis	497 (1)	2 (<1)
Cryptosporidiosis, chronic	314 (1)	10 (2)
Lymphoma. immunoblastic	518 (1)	3 (1)
Candidiasis, pulmonary	534 (1)	11 (2)
Mycobacterium tuberculosis		
Extrapulmonary	491 (1)	2 (<1)
Pulmonary	1621 (3)	NA†
Mycobacterial disease, other, extrapulmonary	301 (1)	2 (<1)
Histoplasmosis, extrapulmonary	208 (<1)	1 (<1)
Lymphoma, Burkitt's	162 (<1)	2 (<1)
Progressive multifocal leukoencephalopathy	213 (<1)	1 (<1)
Lymphoma, brain, primary	170 (<1)	1 (<1)
Isosporiasis, chronic	100 (<1)	22 (5)
Coccidioidomycosis, extrapulmonary	74 (<1)	1 (<1)
Salmonella, septicemia	68 (<1)	NA†
Bacterial infections, multiple or recurrent	NA‡	84 (18)
Carcinoma, invasive cervical	144 (<1)	NA†
Histoplasmosis, disseminated or extrapulmonary	208 (<1)	1 (<1)
Lymphoid interstitial pneumonia and/or pulmonary lymphoid hyperplasia	NA‡	80 (17)
Pneumonia, recurrent	1347 (2)	NA†
Immunosuppression, severe, HIV related§	36,634 (61)	NA†

*Percentages exceed 100% because some persons were reported with more than one AIDS-indicator disease.
NA: Not applicable.
†Not applicable as indicator of AIDS in children.
‡Not applicable as indicator of AIDS in adults/adolescents.
§Defined as a CD4 T-lymphocyte count of less than 200 cells/μL or a CD4 percentage less than 14 in adults/adolescents.
From Centers for Disease Control and Prevention. HIV/AIDS Surveillance Report. 1997;9:1-43.

and prevalence trends of AIDS-defining diseases between 1991 and 1996 demonstrated that for homosexual/bisexual men, significant decreasing trends occurred for 11 opportunistic infections, including *Mycobacterium avium-intracellulare* disease, *P. jirovecii* pneumonia, cytomegalovirus retinitis, Kaposi's sarcoma, esophageal candidiasis, cytomegalovirus disease, extrapulmonary cryptococcosis, toxoplasmic encephalitis, tuberculosis, herpes simplex, and disseminated histoplasmosis. In contrast, for injecting drug users, decreasing trends were seen

for only five opportunistic infections (*P. jirovecii* pneumonia, esophageal candidiasis, tuberculosis, chronic herpes simplex, and chronic cryptosporidiosis), and an increase occurred for recurrent pneumonia.[183] The decreasing trend for some AIDS-defining opportunistic infections such as *P. jirovecii* pneumonia is probably related to the increasing use of antiretroviral therapy and prophylaxis against *P. jirovecii* pneumonia. For example, among adults and adolescents with a single AIDS-defining disease reported through 1996, the proportion with *P. jirovecii* pneumonia decreased from 50% in 1988 to 39% in 1996. Although declines were seen in everyone with AIDS during this period, it was most striking for homosexual/bisexual men and persons with hemophilia or a coagulation disorder. Differences in trends for homosexual and bisexual men and injecting drug users may reflect differences in socioeconomic status, access to medical care, or adherence to preventive medications. Increasing use of effective antiretroviral therapy, which began in 1995-1996, had caused, by the end of 1996, a dramatic decrease in the incidence of AIDS-defining opportunistic illnesses,[42] and the incidence of AIDS could no longer be reliably estimated. The decline in AIDS-defining opportunistic illnesses that began in 1996 has continued. With the increasing use of effective antiretroviral therapy, AIDS-defining illnesses are occurring mainly among persons with newly diagnosed HIV infection at the time of AIDS, among those known to be infected but who do not seek or receive care, and among those for whom treatment has failed.[184-187] Among patients who begin antiretroviral therapy, unusual presentation of opportunistic infections can occur as a result of immune reconstitution.[188]

In 1993, three new AIDS-defining illnesses were added to the surveillance case definition: recurrent bacterial pneumonia, invasive cervical carcinoma, and pulmonary tuberculosis.[15] Several studies have shown that persons with HIV-related immunosuppression are at increased risk of bacterial pneumonia,[28,189] which can result in significant morbidity and mortality.[26,27] One study among injecting drug users found that the annual incidence rate of bacterial pneumonia was five times higher in those who were infected with HIV than in those who were seronegative injecting drug users.[189] *Streptococcus pneumoniae* is the most commonly isolated bacterial pathogen and has been reported to precede the onset of other AIDS-defining conditions in 57% to 81% of persons with HIV infection.[190] In a population-based survey in San Francisco, the rate of pneumococcal bacteremia (89% of HIV-infected patients with bacteremia had pneumonia as a major clinical syndrome) among persons with AIDS was nearly 100 times higher than rates reported before the HIV epidemic.[191] The risk of pneumonia in HIV-infected patients is inversely related to their CD4 T-lymphocyte count (see Chapter 118).[28]

Precursor lesions to invasive cervical cancer such as cervical dysplasia, neoplasia, and genital papillomavirus infection are more commonly diagnosed in HIV-infected women than in other women.[29,192] In a prospective clinic-based study of more than 500 women, HIV-infected women were nearly three times more likely to have colposcopy or biopsy-confirmed cervical intraepithelial neoplasia than were HIV-seronegative women.[193] This risk was independent of other potentially confounding factors such as sexual behavior. In this same study, although HIV-infected women had an increased prevalence (52%) of human papillomavirus when compared with uninfected women (22%), human papillomavirus infection was strongly associated with cervical intraepithelial neoplasia in both groups of women.[193,194] The increased risk for human papillomavirus and the development of cervical intraepithelial neoplasia in HIV-infected women was related to the degree of HIV-related immunosuppression.[29,194] Whether the increased frequency of these precursor conditions will translate into a significantly increased frequency of invasive cervical cancer is the subject of current study.

HIV Infection and Tuberculosis

After several decades of declining incidence, the number of new cases of tuberculosis in the United States began to increase in 1986.[195] Many factors contributed to the resurgence of tuberculosis, but the HIV/AIDS epidemic is, in large part, a major cause of these excess cases of tuberculosis.[196] It is estimated that 6000 to 9000 new cases of tuberculosis occur annually in the United States among HIV-infected persons[197]; however, the full spectrum of the overlap between HIV and tuberculosis is not known, and more than 100,000 persons in the United States are thought to be coinfected with HIV and *M. tuberculosis*.[195,196] Comparisons of AIDS and tuberculosis registries conducted by the 50 states and Puerto Rico revealed that 14% of persons with tuberculosis in 1993 and 1994 (27% among those 25-44 years old) also appeared in the AIDS registry.[198] The overlap in demographic and geographic characteristics of the two diseases is evident by surveys of HIV seroprevalence in tuberculosis clinics, as well as by the fact that 80% of those with tuberculosis and AIDS were found in New York, California, Florida, Georgia, New Jersey, Illinois, and Texas. Both tuberculosis and HIV infection disproportionately affect racial and ethnic minorities and the urban poor.[195] In one analysis, black and Hispanic adults who died with AIDS were nearly three times more likely than whites to also have tuberculosis.[199]

HIV infection is a strong risk factor for the development of active tuberculosis in people with latent *M. tuberculosis* infection. In a prospective study of injecting drug users with documented positive tuberculin skin tests, the observed incidence of active tuberculosis was 7.9 per 100 person-years for 49 HIV-infected persons versus no cases among 62 HIV-seronegative persons.[24] The risk of active tuberculosis in HIV-seropositive persons in this study—14% over 2 years[24]—contrasts strikingly with the estimated 10% lifetime risk in HIV-negative persons with latent tuberculosis infection.[200] In addition, HIV-infected persons are at increased risk for the development of active, symptomatic tuberculosis after their initial exposure and subsequent infection with *M. tuberculosis*.[201] Outbreaks of tuberculosis among HIV-infected individuals in correctional facilities, AIDS clinics, and hospital wards suggest that the development of active tuberculosis after exposure is greatly increased among HIV-infected persons. Finally, molecular epidemiology studies conducted in San Francisco and New York suggest that one third of cases in San Francisco and 40% in New York are due to recent transmission rather than reactivation.[202,203]

Drug-resistant tuberculosis is more common in persons with HIV infection than in those with tuberculosis but without HIV infection.[198] In a multivariate analysis conducted by the CDC between 1993 and 1996, being infected with HIV was a risk factor for isoniazid and rifampin monoresistance, as well as multidrug-resistant tuberculosis.[204] In a study conducted in New York City, the proportion of isolates resistant to one or more antituberculosis drugs increased from 10% from 1982 to 1984 to 23% in 1991.[205] Among isolates of *M. tuberculosis* with primary resistance to isoniazid or rifampin, 75% came from patients known to be infected with HIV.[205] The increased risk of drug-resistant tuberculosis among HIV-infected persons may reflect a higher proportion of disease resulting from recently acquired drug-resistant strains,[202,203] as well as other factors such as decreased absorption of oral antimycobacterial drugs among HIV-infected persons.[206] Outbreaks of multidrug-resistant tuberculosis (e.g., resistant to both isoniazid and rifampin and/or other drugs) have been characterized by (1) a high prevalence of HIV infection among the outbreak cases (range, 20%-100%), (2) a high mortality rate among persons infected with resistant strains (range, 72%-89%), (3) a short median interval between diagnosis and death (range, 4-16 weeks), and (4) nosocomial transmission to health care workers.[198,207-209]

Mortality of Persons with HIV Infections and AIDS

Through December 31, 2002, 57% of the 886,575 children, adolescents, and adults in whom AIDS had been diagnosed in the United States were reported to have died.[50] The estimated number of deaths among people with AIDS increased steadily through 1995, when approximately 50,000 persons were estimated to have died of AIDS. In 1996, the estimated number of deaths from AIDS decreased to 37,525 and has continued to drop every year since then to 21,909 in 1997, 17,347 in 2000, and 16,371 in 2002 (see Fig. 114-2).[50] These dramatic declines in AIDS mortality have been largely due to the availability of combination antiretroviral therapy,[42,212,213] and have been more rapid

among whites and among homosexual and bisexual men but have occurred in all populations.[8] The percentage decrease in mortality has been smallest among black women and women in the South.

In 1993, HIV infection became the most common cause of death among persons ages 25 to 44 years.[210] In 1994, 72% of HIV-related deaths occurred in persons ages 25 to 44 years, in whom it was the leading cause of death, accounting for 19% of the deaths in this age group. After 1996, when AIDS mortality began to decline, AIDS was no longer the leading cause of death in this age group. However, in the United States, it continues to be a leading cause of death among black men ages 25 to 44 years.

To put into perspective the impact that AIDS-related mortality had, the years of potential life lost before the age of 65 because of AIDS have been calculated.[211] From 1989 to 1990, the years of potential life lost before the age of 65 years that could be attributed to AIDS and HIV infection increased by 13%. In 1993, AIDS had become the fifth leading cause of years of potential life lost before age 65, and in 1994 it became the fourth. That year it was estimated that approximately 49,500 persons died of AIDS.[210] At a population level, the improvement in survival for AIDS patients as a result of the introduction of HAART in 1996 can be seen in a study conducted in New York City, where the overall cumulative survival at 24 months increased from 43% among patients diagnosed with AIDS from 1990 to 1995 to 76% for patients diagnosed from 1996 through 1998.[212]

AIDS IN CHILDREN

Through December 31, 2002, a total of 9300 cases of AIDS in children younger than 13 years had been reported in the United States.[50] Pediatric cases of AIDS include children who have one of a broad range of "indicator" diseases (see Table 114-1).[15] Although the spectrum of AIDS-defining opportunistic infections and malignancies in children overlaps considerably with those that are included in the surveillance case definition for adults and adolescents, some differences can be noted (see Chapter 123).[214] Three important exceptions for children younger than 13 years are the inclusion of lymphoid interstitial pneumonia and/or pulmonary lymphoid hyperplasia and recurrent bacterial infections and the exclusion of a threshold CD4 T-lymphocyte count (e.g., <200 CD4+ T lymphocytes/μL). Longitudinal evaluations of lymphocyte subsets in both HIV-infected and HIV-uninfected children suggest some measure of prognostic value.[215,216] However, because normal newborns and young infants have a prominent lymphocytosis,[217] moderate declines in CD4+ T lymphocytes by adult standards can represent significant impairment in young children.[215,218]

Pediatric cases are ordered into a hierarchy of mutually exclusive exposure categories, and most children reported with AIDS acquired HIV infection perinatally from their mothers.[219] Of the 473 children reported in 1997, only 1 had hemophilia or another coagulation disorder; 91% were born to mothers either with or at risk for HIV infection; 2 received a transfusion of blood, blood components, or tissue; and 8% had an undetermined risk. As with adults, when follow-up information is available, most children who are initially reported with an undetermined risk are reclassified. In one study, half of the children who were reclassified had mothers who used injecting drugs or were partners of men who used injecting drugs.[220] Of the 90 children reported with AIDS in 2002 who were born to mothers with or at risk for HIV infection, 16% had mothers who reported injecting drugs or having sex with an injecting drug user. The remaining mothers acquired their infection through heterosexual contact with infected men other than injecting drug users (36%) or had an undetermined risk for HIV infection (41%). Because most children acquire HIV infection from their mothers, the racial and ethnic and geographic distribution of children with AIDS parallels that of women with AIDS. Sixty-three percent of pediatric AIDS cases diagnosed in 2002 were black and 26% were Hispanic children. In addition to cases of AIDS, 162 cases of pediatric HIV infection have been reported from states with confidential HIV reporting. The exposure category and race and ethnicity of these cases parallel that of pediatric AIDS cases.

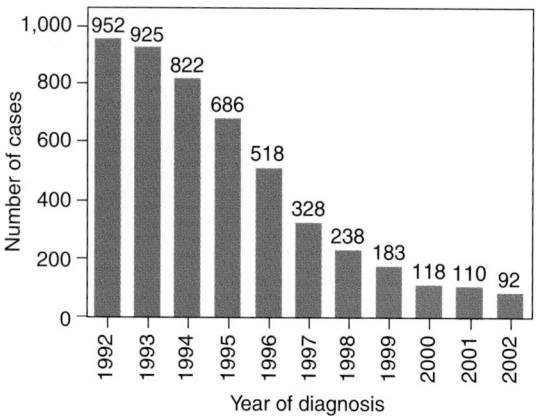

FIGURE 114-5. Estimated pediatric AIDS incidence by year of diagnosis, 1992 to 2002, United States. These numbers do not represent actual cases of children diagnosed with AIDS. Rather, these numbers are point estimates based on cases diagnosed using the 1987 definition, adjusted for reporting delays. The 1993 AIDS surveillance case definition affected only the adult/adolescent cases, not pediatric cases. *(From Centers for Disease Control and Prevention. HIV/AIDS Surveillance Report. 2002; 14:1-48.)*

From 1984 through 1992, the estimated number of children with perinatally acquired AIDS diagnosed each year increased and peaked at 905 in 1992.[219] In 1994, as a result of a clinical trial that demonstrated the efficacy of zidovudine in reducing perinatal HIV transmission by two thirds,[221] the Public Health Service issued recommendations for the use of zidovudine and for counseling and HIV testing of pregnant women in the United States.[222,223] With the implementation of these recommendations, the number of children with perinatally acquired HIV infection has decreased dramatically in the United States, with only 92 cases diagnosed in 2002 (Fig. 114-5).

The relative frequency of certain AIDS-indicator diseases in children younger than 13 years old appears to vary with age. For example, lymphoid interstitial pneumonitis is more common in older children. Of children reported with AIDS in 1991 and 1992 in whom the syndrome was diagnosed before or at 12 months of age, 7% had lymphoid interstitial pneumonitis as compared with 36% of children in whom AIDS was diagnosed at 1 to 4 years of age. In contrast, in children in whom AIDS was diagnosed before or at 12 months of age, 58% had *P. jirovecii* pneumonia versus 14% of those ages 1 to 4 years. This early age at onset, as well as the high mortality rate associated with *P. jirovecii* pneumonia in infants and children, reinforces recommendations that HIV infection in infants should be diagnosed as soon as possible after birth so that prophylaxis can be promptly initiated when indicated.[224]

Overall, 58% of children with AIDS detected through national surveillance are reported to have died. Before the availability of HAART, the survival of HIV-infected children was closely related to age at the initial diagnosis of AIDS and to the specific AIDS-defining condition. The shortest duration of survival, ranging from 1 to 9 months, has been reported for children with an initial AIDS diagnosis of *P. jirovecii* pneumonia.[225-227] In contrast, longer median survival times ranging from 65 to 72 months have been reported for lymphoid interstitial pneumonitis.[225,226] In a longitudinal evaluation of 789 children enrolled in the New York State Medicaid Programs, the proportion of children younger than 6 months at diagnosis who survived 1 year after AIDS was diagnosed (40%-54%) was substantially less than that for children older than 6 months (70%-85%), irrespective of the AIDS-indicator disease.[226] Similar to adults, effective antiretroviral treatment for children, *P. jirovecii* prophylaxis, and intravenous immunoglobulin have had a positive impact on survival by delaying disease progression. Implementation of recommendations by the U.S. Public Health Service for the treatment of HIV-infected women during pregnancy with combination antiretroviral therapy has undoubtedly had a positive impact in further reducing perinatal HIV transmission and may eventually lead to the elimination of perinatal HIV infection in this country.[227]

MODES OF TRANSMISSION

More than a decade after the initial studies were conducted to determine the ways in which HIV is transmitted, surveillance and epidemiologic data throughout the world continue to support only three primary modes of transmission: sexual contact; exposure to blood, largely through injecting drug use and transfusion; and perinatal transmission from infected mothers to their infants.

Sexual Transmission

Sexual contact is the predominant mode of HIV transmission throughout the world. However, the geographic distribution of cases attributable to homosexual and heterosexual transmission varies markedly.[6] Whereas heterosexual transmission is the major mode of spread of HIV infection in Africa, most of South America, and the Caribbean, it accounts for a smaller, albeit growing proportion of AIDS cases in North America and Europe, where male-to-male sexual transmission continues to account for a major proportion of reported cases of AIDS.[228]

The likelihood of acquiring or transmitting HIV infection through a single sexual contact is directly related to certain correlates of exposure, such as the number of partners and the prevalence of HIV infection in the population. Sexual transmission of HIV is relatively inefficient, but behavioral and biologic factors influence the likelihood of HIV transmission in a given sexual encounter. For example, anal sex has been consistently found to be more risky that vaginal sex, which in turn is higher risk than oral sex,[229] and the coexistence of a sexually transmitted infection (most notably the presence of genital ulcerative disease) greatly increases the infectiousness as well as the susceptibility of the individual.[230-232] Carefully performed longitudinal cohort studies conducted in Africa have helped us understand the risk of HIV transmission per coital act. In that study the rate of HIV transmission per coital act was highest in the 5-month period following seroconversion (0.0081/coital act), it declined to 0.0016/coital act at 5-15 months after index seroconversion, stabilized at 0.0010/coital act among HIV-prevalent index partners, and increased before index partner death to as much as 0.0043/coital act.[233] Index partner HIV viral load was the strongest predictor of transmission at each stage of infection. The per-contact risk of acquiring HIV infection from homosexual contacts was estimated in a prospective cohort study of 2189 high-risk homosexual and bisexual men, conducted in San Francisco, Denver, and Chicago. During 2633 person-years of follow-up, 60 seroconversions were observed. The estimated per-contact risk of acquiring HIV from unprotected receptive anal intercourse was 0.82 percent when the partner was known to be HIV infected and 0.27 percent when partners of unknown serostatus were included.[234] The per-contact risk associated with unprotected insertive anal and receptive oral sex with HIV-positive or unknown serostatus partners was 0.06 and 0.04 percent, respectively.

Infectiousness of the Source Partner

Variability in the infectiousness of the source partner has been suggested by observations that some persons appear to be highly efficient transmitters of HIV through sexual contact. Such efficiency is manifested by the infection of a high proportion of an individual's sexual partners,[235] often after only a single contact.[236,237]

Multiple lines of evidence indicate that HIV transmission appears to be more efficient late in the course of HIV infection.[233,238-242] This association was first suggested in a prospective study of infected hemophiliac men and their female sex partners.[239] Subsequent epidemiologic studies have supported the correlation of advanced disease stage, as measured by diseases indicative of AIDS or decreased numbers of peripheral CD4+ T lymphocytes, with an increased likelihood of transmission to sexual partners.[240-243] Furthermore, this association has been observed for male-to-male, male-to-female, and female-to-male transmission. These observations correlate well with laboratory studies demonstrating that both the ability to isolate HIV from semen and the concentration of virus in plasma are inversely proportional to the number of CD4+ T lymphocytes.[244-246] In another study, HIV was isolated more frequently from the cervicovaginal secretions of women with AIDS than from those of women in earlier stages of disease.[247] In addition, primary HIV infection may also be a period associated with increased infectiousness.[248] From a public health point of view, this association could be extremely important because increased infectivity would precede recognition of infection by the individual.[249] With the availability of assays that allow measurement of the quantity of HIV present in plasma, blood, or genital secretions, it is now possible to attempt to correlate infectiousness with the quantity of HIV-RNA present in genital secretions. In general, the higher the plasma viral load, the more likely HIV transmission will occur given similar exposures. In a study conducted in Africa, there were no cases of seroconversion among heterosexual discordant partners when the infected partner had a serum HIV-RNA of fewer than 1500 copies/mL.[250] Similarly, the risk for perinatal transmission of HIV increases as the viral load in the mother increases, and no cases in one study occurred when the maternal viral load in plasma was fewer than 1000 copies/mL, 16.6% when the viral load was between 1001 and 10,000 copies/mL, 21.3% when the viral load was between 10,001 and 50,000 copies/mL, 30.9% for those with viral loads of 50,001 to 100,000 copies/mL, and 40.6% when the viral load was more than 100,000 copies/mL.[251] HIV is more readily detected and also present at higher concentrations in individuals with more advanced disease[252]; however, this correlation is not found in all studies.[247,253] These findings notwithstanding, all infected persons must be presumed to be capable of sexually transmitting HIV, regardless of their stage of infection.

Antiretroviral therapy may influence infectivity and the subsequent risk of transmission through sexual contact. Treatment with zidovudine alone has been associated with decreased detection of HIV in semen,[245] and an epidemiologic study has demonstrated that antiretroviral therapy with zidovudine alone was associated with a 50% reduction in sexual transmission of HIV among discordant heterosexual couples.[254] With the availability of HAART there is significant interest in studying whether the widespread use of HAART results in a reduction of sexually transmitted HIV.[255] However, even with the use of combination antiretroviral therapy and in the presence of suppression of HIV-RNA in plasma, proviral DNA has been detected in the seminal cells of infected men[256] and genital secretions of women.[257] Thus, any protective effect of antiretrovirals on sexual transmission of HIV is likely to be partial and not render an individual completely noninfectious.[258,259]

Because HIV is present in both blood cells and cervicovaginal secretions, sexual contact with an HIV-infected woman during menstruation somewhat increases the risk of female-to-male HIV transmission,[240] as well as the woman's risk of acquiring HIV infection.[241] Nonmenstrual vaginal and penile bleeding have also been reported to be associated with HIV transmission.[260,261]

The probability of saliva from HIV-infected persons transmitting HIV through oral-oral or oral-genital sexual contact is low but real.[262] HIV is found in very low concentrations in the saliva of infected persons,[263,264] and since 1987, 21 case reports of 42 potential instances of oral transmission of HIV have appeared.[262] Such transmissions are difficult to prove or rule out because most persons with HIV and a history of oral sexual contact report genital contact as well.

Epidemiologic and laboratory data indicate that genital ulcer disease in the source partner is an important factor facilitating HIV transmission. The higher rates of heterosexual transmission in Africa may be explained in part by the higher prevalence of genital ulcer disease and other sexually transmitted infections in many developing countries, including ones in Africa, than in countries in North America and Europe.[265] Genital ulcers probably increase the infectiousness of both male and female source partners.[266,267] In a prospective study of more than 400 men who acquired a sexually transmitted disease (including HIV infection) from a group of prostitutes in Nairobi, Kenya, seroconversion to HIV was independently associated with the concurrent acquisition of genital ulcer disease.[268] In a study in Malawi, genital ulcer disease was associated with lower CD4 cell counts and increased plasma HIV-RNA when compared with HIV-infected patients without genital

ulcer disease.[269] Furthermore, a similar study in Uganda suggested that genital ulcers, mainly due to HSV-2, are associated with higher viral loads in both incident and prevalent HIV infected patients.[270] Genital ulcer disease may have augmented the women's infectiousness by increasing viral shedding in the female genital tract through a local inflammatory response mediated by the recruitment and activation of HIV-infected macrophages and lymphocytes to the disrupted mucosal surface.[268,271] The recovery of HIV from genital ulcers in HIV-infected women supports this hypothesis.[272] These data suggest that treatment of genital ulceration and herpes simplex virus (HSV)-2 suppressive therapy may be associated with a reduction in HIV viremia, thus potentially reducing HIV transmission and disease progression.

Nonulcerative sexually transmitted diseases may also enhance sexual transmission of HIV. Among men, urethritis and gonorrhea are associated with increased detection of HIV in semen,[273,274] and appropriate antibiotic treatment diminishes the amount of HIV present in genital secretions.[275]

Susceptibility of the Recipient Partner

As previously mentioned, the presence of genital and anorectal ulceration or mucosal disruption secondary to infection has emerged as one of the most consistent and biologically plausible factors affecting the transmission and acquisition of HIV infection through sexual contact. Although ulcerations that disrupt the genital epithelium can serve simply as a portal of entry for HIV, ulcerations may have a more complex role in HIV transmission. Genital ulcerations cause an inflammatory response that in turn may increase the number of stimulated T lymphocytes at the surface of the ulceration and thus increase the number of susceptible cells.[269,271]

A number of epidemiologic studies have demonstrated that a history of genital ulcer disease in the recipient partner is a risk factor for acquiring HIV in both heterosexual and homosexual men[271,276] and women.[267,276] Although this association may not be surprising, two seroepidemiologic studies of homosexual men have convincingly demonstrated that genital ulcer disease is not simply a marker for increased sexual activity.[271,277] Rather, infection with HIV was independently associated with serologic evidence of prior syphilis or infection with HSV-2, the two most common causes of genital ulcers among homosexual men in the United States. In another study among female prostitutes in Nairobi, 60% of seroconverting women experienced one or more episodes of genital ulcers before seroconverting.[267]

Nonulcerative sexually transmitted diseases such as gonorrhea and chlamydial infection also facilitate the acquisition of HIV infection by causing mucosal disruption of the genital tract.[267] Other nonulcerative sexually transmitted diseases (e.g., urethritis, cervicitis, balanitis, bacterial vaginosis, and genital warts) also increase the risk of acquiring HIV infection.[278-280] The higher frequency of balanitis in uncircumcised men has been postulated as a partial explanation for the increased risk of HIV observed among uncircumcised men in developing countries.[268,281,282]

Noninfectious causes of ulcerations of the genital tract may also pose a risk for sexual transmission of HIV. For example, frequent use of the nonoxynol 9 contraceptive sponge by female prostitutes in Nairobi was associated with increased rates of genital ulcers, vulvitis, and HIV seroconversion in one study.[283] The increased risk for HIV acquisition may be attributable to chemical irritation from the spermicide or to mechanical trauma, both of which can result in inflammation and ulceration.[284] The importance of the treatment of sexually transmitted infections in the HIV epidemic was made evident by a study in Tanzania that showed that prompt management of sexually transmitted infections decreased the incidence of HIV infection by 42%.[285] Certain traumatic sexual practices that result in rectal mucosal disruption and lesions have been associated with HIV infection. Early epidemiologic studies of homosexual men found that receptive anal intercourse, "fisting," and douching increased the risk of HIV transmission.[286-288] Subsequent studies have both supported these findings and extended the association of receptive anal intercourse to heterosexual transmission of HIV.[240,249,261]

Although cases of AIDS have been reported among lesbian and bisexual women, most were infected through injecting drug use practices or through sex with HIV-infected men.[289-291] Female-to-female transmission of HIV appears to be very rare.[292] However, cases of female-to-female transmission of HIV have been reported.[293-295]

No consistent association between oral contraceptive use by women and acquisition of HIV infection has been found. In one study, women who reported taking oral contraceptives had a reduced risk of HIV infection.[241] However, in a longitudinal cohort study of Nairobi prostitutes and a cross-sectional study of sex partners at a sexually transmitted disease clinic in Nairobi, oral contraceptive use was an independent risk factor for HIV seroconversion and for prevalent infection, respectively.[267,296] In contrast, a study of prostitutes in Zaire[276] and a study of pregnant women in a rural U.S. community with a high prevalence of HIV infection[87] found no association between HIV infection and the use of oral contraceptives. The presence of cervical ectopy has been associated with an increased risk of HIV seropositivity among long-term female partners of HIV-positive men in Nairobi.[296] Because oral contraceptives are associated with higher rates of ectopy, the relationship, if any, between oral contraceptives and HIV requires further study.[297]

Although anal and vaginal intercourse are the two sex practices associated with the greatest risk of transmission, other sexual activities involving exposure to semen or blood also carry a potential risk of transmission. For example, seroconversion for HIV antibody has been documented after receptive oral intercourse with ejaculation.[262]

Finally, a mutation in the chemokine receptor gene has been identified that may render the rare homozygous host relatively resistant to HIV infection (see Chapter 166). When this mutation is present in the heterozygous state, it does not prevent infection.[298] The presence of this mutation varies according to race, with 11% and 1.7% homozygosity among whites and blacks, respectively.[248]

Transmission through Injecting Drug Use

Among injecting drug users, HIV is transmitted by parenteral exposure to HIV-infected blood through contaminated needles and other injection equipment. Specific factors that have been associated with HIV infection among injecting drug users include the duration of injecting drug use since 1977, frequency of needle sharing, number of needle-sharing partners, number of injections, median number of injections in "shooting galleries," and prevalence of HIV infection in the area of residence.[59,71,299,300] The rate of HIV infection among injecting drug users varies widely among different geographic areas. In the United States, the rate of HIV infection has been highest in the Northeast.[74,76]

Most studies have found higher rates of HIV infection associated with cocaine and heroin injection than with heroin injection alone, probably because of the greater frequency of cocaine injections.[79,301,302] Another possible explanation is the greater likelihood of exchange of sex for drugs among cocaine users.[303] Among injecting drug users, poor socioeconomic conditions, homelessness, and minority race and ethnicity are associated with an increased frequency of risk behavior and higher rates of HIV infection.[60,81,304,305] Among injecting drug users enrolled in a study in Baltimore from 1988 to 1989, the 703 HIV-infected users were more likely to have a history of syphilis (16.8%) than were the 2218 uninfected injecting drug users (11.3%).[306] The higher rates of sexually transmitted disease among HIV-infected injecting drug users than among uninfected users suggests that some infections are transmitted through unsafe sexual practices rather than injection drug use itself.[94,306,307]

Many injecting drug users have changed their drug use behavior to reduce their risk of HIV infection.[308,309] Drug abuse treatment, street outreach programs, needle and syringe exchange programs, AIDS educational efforts, and HIV counseling and testing programs have all been shown to be effective in reducing, but not eliminating, the risk of HIV transmission in these populations.[310]

Transmission by Blood and Other Tissues

Recipients of unscreened blood or blood products from HIV-infected donors are at high risk for HIV infection. HIV has been transmitted through receipt of whole blood, blood cellular components, plasma, and clotting factors.[311,312] The likelihood of a person becoming infected with HIV after receiving a single-donor blood product documented to be HIV-positive approaches 100%.[313,314] Other blood or plasma products, such as hepatitis B immune globulin, immune serum globulin, Rh(D) immune globulin, and hepatitis B vaccine, are prepared by using one of several fractionation processes that inactivate HIV; use of these products has not been associated with transmission.[315,316]

Before serologic testing for HIV was begun in 1985, 0.04% of 1,200,000 donations in the United States were estimated to be HIV positive.[317] During this time an estimated 29,000 blood or blood product recipients were exposed to HIV; because many died of underlying conditions, 12,000 of these people were estimated to survive long enough for AIDS to develop.[318] Confidential unit exclusion and direct donor deferral, as well as the institution of HIV antibody screening in 1985, followed by additional tests for antibodies to HIV-2 and p24 antigen in 1996, markedly decreased the risk of HIV infection through blood or blood products. With the implementation of p24 antigen testing, the risk of HIV transmission through transfusion of screened blood was estimated to be 1 in 200,000 to 1 in 2,000,000 per unit transfused in the United States.[319,320] Further reduction in the risk of transfusion-transmitted HIV in the United States occurred after the U.S. Food and Drug Administration (FDA) approved the implementation of nucleic acid testing (NAT) of blood units in 2002, which reduces the window period to approximately 12 days.[321] In the clinical trials that led to the approval of NAT by the FDA a total of 7 HIV-1–positive and 88 hepatitis C virus (HCV)–positive donations that would otherwise not have been diagnosed were detected in more than 20 million donations tested. As a result of additional testing, the risk of HIV through transfusion is estimated by the Red Cross in 2001 to be 1 in 2,135,000.[322] The risk of HIV infection for patients with hemophilia who received concentrated clotting factors composed of blood components from potentially thousands of donors was substantial before 1985,[323,324] but now it is exceedingly low. HIV transmission by transplantation of liver, heart, kidney, pancreas, bone, and possibly skin has been reported.[129,325,326] Relatively avascular tissues such as corneas and processed tissues have not been associated with transmission.[129,327,328] AIDS developed in several transplant recipients after receiving a variety of organs from a single HIV-negative cadaver donor. The donor was subsequently found to be HIV infected by culture and PCR.[129]

Perinatal Transmission

Vertical transmission of HIV from an infected woman to her infant can occur during gestation (in utero), at the time of delivery (intrapartum), or postpartum through breast-feeding. Significant progress has been made in elucidating risk factors that influence transmission during these three periods, in detecting infection in the newborn earlier and more reliably, and in the prevention of perinatal transmission with the use of antiretroviral drugs (see Chapter 122).

The occurrence of intrauterine infection is supported by the detection of HIV both in fetal tissue as early as 8 weeks[329] and in placental tissue infected in vivo and in vitro.[330] In addition, the 30% to 50% of infected infants who test positive by PCR or HIV culture at birth[331-333] also suggests intrauterine transmission of HIV. The proportion of infants who become infected in each trimester of pregnancy is unknown, but transmission to the infant early in pregnancy would presumably allow for viral replication to reach a level sufficient for detection by culture or PCR.[334] HIV-infected infants who test negative by PCR or HIV culture at birth may have become infected late in pregnancy or during the intrapartum period. Accumulating information suggests that a sizable proportion of vertical transmission may occur during the intrapartum period.[335,336] Both vaginal and cesarean delivery present frequent and varied opportunities for the infant to be exposed to infected maternal blood and cervicovaginal fluids. Although many studies have found statistically similar rates of transmission for vaginal and cesarean section delivery,[337-340] there are meta-analysis and randomized clinical trials data that elective cesarean section reduces the risk of perinatal HIV transmission even when accounting for the use of antiretrovirals.[341] As a result, the percentage of deliveries performed via elective cesarean section in HIV-infected pregnant women has increased from 20% from 1994 to 1998 to 44% from 1998 to 2000.[342] The isolation of HIV from breast milk,[343] as well as reports of breast-feeding mothers who infected their infants after they had acquired HIV infection through postpartum blood transfusions, provided initial evidence for postnatal HIV transmission.[344] Subsequent evaluation has focused on estimating the added, or attributable, risk of perinatal transmission conveyed by breast-feeding. Several prospective cohort studies that compared breast-fed and bottle-fed infants have detected higher rates of HIV infection in breast-fed children.[336-338,345,346] The attributable risk of transmission through breast-feeding ranges from 14% to 29% and was determined on the basis of data from developing countries where antiretroviral therapy has not been used.[347] Mothers who themselves acquired HIV infection in the postpartum period were more efficient transmitters, presumably because of the increased viral burden associated with primary HIV infection.[348,349] For these reasons, in the United States since 1985, it has been recommended that HIV-infected women abstain from breast-feeding their infants. Epidemiologic studies[346] and mathematic models[350] have evaluated the competing risks of acquiring HIV infection by breast-feeding and the increased morbidity and mortality associated with alternatives to breast-feeding in developing countries. Both approaches have found that for children in many developing countries, the benefits from breast-feeding outweigh the risk of HIV transmission through breast-feeding. However, the risk of not breast-feeding varies greatly between and within developing countries, and thus the situation needs to be considered on an individual basis.

Prospective studies of infants born to women with HIV infection before the use of antiretrovirals have found rates of transmission ranging from 13% to 40%,[337-339,351] with the highest rates of perinatally acquired HIV infection, which approach 40%, reported from Africa.[351] The disparity in these rates most likely reflects differences in the severity of maternal disease stage, nutritional status, rates of breast-feeding, study design, completeness and length of follow-up, and use of different diagnostic criteria.[218] The risk of perinatal transmission appears to vary by the disease stage of the mother. Mothers at both extremes of the clinical spectrum of HIV infection with either acute, primary infection[291,335] or advanced, symptomatic disease[348,351] have been reported to be more likely to transmit HIV to their infants than have asymptomatic seropositive women. The most important risk factor to determine the likelihood that an infant will acquire HIV perinatally is the HIV viral load in the mother.[352,353]

In addition to maternal risk factors, obstetric factors that disrupt the maternal-fetal barrier can increase perinatal transmission. In one study among Zairean women, the presence of histologic chorioamnionitis and funisitis was associated with an overall twofold increase in transmission risk.[354] Preterm delivery, prolonged rupture of membranes (>4 hours), use of illicit drugs during pregnancy, low antenatal CD4 count, and low birth weight are also associated with increased risk for perinatal HIV transmission.[355,356]

Infants born to HIV-infected mothers have passively acquired maternal antibody to HIV that persists for 12 to 18 months. For infants 0 to 6 months of age, PCR and virus culture offer the greatest sensitivity and specificity for detecting HIV infection (see Chapters 115 and 123).[357] Nonetheless, these tests can detect only one half or less of perinatally infected infants, which is a reflection of very low viral burden, sequestration of the virus in other tissues, or recent transmission

to the infant either late in the third trimester or at the time of delivery.[358] Other options for diagnosing HIV infection in infants include HIV-specific IgA assays and an in vitro antibody production assay such as the ELISPOT (a method for quantifying specific and total antibody-secreting cells[359]).[334] However, the overall sensitivity and specificity of these tests are less than those of PCR and viral culture, especially for infants younger than 3 months.

Transmission of HIV in Health Care Settings

Percutaneous, mucous membrane, and cutaneous exposure to blood-contaminated body fluids can occur frequently in the health care setting.[360-362] Such exposure has resulted in occupationally acquired HIV infection in health care workers (see Chapter 304).[363-367] Data from several prospective surveillance projects among health care workers indicate that the average risk of seroconversion after a needlestick injury with HIV-infected blood is approximately 0.3%.[363-365] Percutaneous injury, usually inflicted by a hollow-bore needle, is the most common mechanism of occupational HIV transmission. Transmission of HIV has also been reported after mucous membrane and cutaneous exposure to blood, and in those instances the risk is estimated to be 0.09%.[368] As of December 2001, the CDC had received reports of 57 documented cases of HIV seroconversion temporally associated with occupational exposure to HIV among health care personnel in the United States.[369] In addition, 138 cases of possible occupational transmission of HIV have been reported to the CDC; in these cases, HIV seroconversion temporally associated with an occupational exposure was not documented. In a retrospective study conducted by the CDC, it was found that the risk of transmission of HIV to health care workers was increased when the device causing the injury was visibly contaminated with blood, when the device had been used for insertion into a vein or artery, when the device caused a deep injury, or when the source patient died within 2 months after the exposure.[370]

Because health care workers are more likely than patients to have contact with blood in the health care setting, the risk of HIV transmission from patient to health care worker clearly exceeds that of health care worker to patient.[371,372] Transmission of HIV from a health care worker to patients has been documented in two instances: in a dental practice in Florida[373,374] and from an orthopedic surgeon in France.[375] In the cluster of cases in Florida, the precise events that resulted in the dentist transmitting HIV to 6 of approximately 1100 patients tested for HIV in this practice remain unknown. However, the six patients had no other confirmed exposure to HIV other than receiving treatment from the dentist, and each was infected with a viral strain that was very similar to that of the dentist but dissimilar to those from other HIV-infected persons in the local area.[373,374] The very small risk of a health care worker transmitting HIV to a patient probably depends on several factors, including the type of procedure; the technique, skill, and medical condition of the health care worker; and the titer of circulating virus.[371,376,377] Aside from these two instances, investigation of 22,759 patients of 53 other HIV-infected health care workers has not identified other episodes of health care worker to patient transmission of HIV.[378]

Two patients undergoing nuclear medicine procedures have been reported to have been infected through inadvertent intravenous injections of blood or other material from HIV-infected patients.[379] Also, transmission of HIV through percutaneous or mucocutaneous exposure to blood or other body substances has occurred in homes in which health care has been provided.[380,381] Transmission of HIV from patient to patient through improper sterilization or reuse of contaminated needles and syringes has been reported in Romania and the former Soviet Union.[382,383] Similarly, a report from Australia suggested that a breach in infection control precautions caused HIV to be transmitted from one patient to four other patients during minor surgical procedures performed on the same day by an HIV-negative surgeon.[384] A more detailed review of transmission in the health care setting can be found in Chapter 304.

Other Modes of Transmission

Although HIV has been isolated from a variety of body fluids,[252,264,343,385-387] only blood, semen, other genital secretions, and breast milk have been implicated as sources of infection. HIV infection is acquired through exposure to blood, principally through injecting drug use and receipt of contaminated blood, blood products, organs, and tissues. Exposure of nonintact skin to blood after a motor vehicle accident and a sports injury has been reported to result in HIV infection, but these occurrences are rare.[388,389]

Vaginal and anal intercourse is the predominant way in which persons are exposed to HIV-infected semen and cervicovaginal fluids. However, transmission of HIV through intravaginal insemination with unprocessed donor semen[390,391] and through intrauterine insemination with processed semen[392] has been reported. Although data regarding the magnitude of the risks are conflicting,[390-392] there is no evidence that any procedure can reliably eliminate HIV from semen.[392]

Laboratory and epidemiologic studies indicate that the infectivity of saliva from HIV-infected persons through human bites or occupational contact is extremely low. Furthermore, definitive attribution of HIV transmission to contact with saliva is difficult because saliva is often commingled with blood in these settings. The low risk of saliva-mediated HIV transmission is probably attributable to the very low concentrations of HIV in the saliva of infected persons,[263,264] as well as the presence of HIV inhibitory activity in saliva.[393] One case report of two siblings infected with HIV suggested a bite as the route of transmission for the previously uninfected child.[394] However, because the bite did not break the skin or result in bleeding, the precise mode of transmission remains uncertain. Multiple epidemiologic studies, including occupational and household contact studies, have found no evidence of transmission via a human bite.[395] Similarly, studies of health care workers monitored prospectively after percutaneous, mucous membrane (e.g., during the administration of cardiopulmonary resuscitation), or nonintact skin exposure to saliva from HIV-infected patients have not detected any instances of HIV antibody seroconversion.[364,396]

To examine the risk of HIV transmission through casual contact, studies have evaluated more than 1000 nonsexual household contacts of both adults and children with HIV infection.[395,397-399] In these households, transmission of HIV was found only among sex partners, children born to infected mothers, and persons who themselves had risk factors for HIV infection. However, eight case reports have described household transmission of HIV unassociated with sexual contact, injecting drug use, or breast-feeding. Five of the eight reports were associated with documented or probable blood contact.[381,400-402] Two reports involved nursing care of terminally ill persons with AIDS in which blood exposure might have occurred but was not documented; in both reports, skin contact with other secretions and excretions occurred.[381,403] In the last report, a bite was suggested but not documented to have resulted in transmission.[394]

Laboratory and epidemiologic studies have produced no evidence of replication of HIV within insects, in vitro mechanical transmission of HIV, or transmission through biting or bloodsucking insects.[404-406] The potential role of insect-mediated HIV infection was evaluated in a study of residents in a southern Florida community with a high rate of HIV infection.[407] HIV seropositivity was not associated with either epidemiologic or laboratory evidence of exposure to mosquitoes, as measured by the presence of antibodies to five arboviruses. Additional studies in Africa failed to establish an association between the presence of malaria antibodies and HIV.[408]

HIV INFECTION AND AIDS OUTSIDE THE UNITED STATES

HIV infection is pandemic, affecting almost all countries (see Chapter 113). Through December of 2003, UNAIDS and the World Health Organization (WHO) estimate that approximately 40 (between 34 and 46) million people are living with HIV worldwide, including 2.5 (between 2.1 and 2.9) million children younger than the age of 15. UNAIDS/WHO estimate that every day in 2003, 14,000 people were newly infected with HIV, of which 60% occurred in sub-Saharan Africa, the most severely affected region of the world. More than 95% of all HIV-infected people live in low- and middle-income countries (see Chapter 113). Modes of transmission of HIV are similar throughout the world, but the relative frequency varies considerably between countries and regions. In western Europe, North America, and Australia, as well as some parts of South America and the Caribbean, homosexual and bisexual men and injecting drug users remain the predominantly affected groups.[409] In northern Europe, most AIDS cases have occurred among homosexual and bisexual men, whereas in southern Europe, more than 60% of persons with AIDS are injecting drug users.[410] The sex partners of injecting drug users have been particularly affected by heterosexual transmission of HIV. The proportion of infections attributed to heterosexual transmission has increased over time, particularly in Brazil and other countries in South America, where infection rates among injecting drug users are relatively high.[410-412]

In sub-Saharan Africa and some areas of the Caribbean, heterosexual contact is the most common mode of transmission.[409,413-419] High rates of HIV infection among pregnant women have resulted in a substantial number of children with perinatally acquired HIV.[419] The highest rates of HIV infection in Africa and some Caribbean countries are found among female prostitutes and persons treated for other sexually transmitted diseases.[273,418,420-424] Injecting drug use is less common in developing countries than in some areas of the United States.[409] In contrast, receipt of contaminated blood products remains a major source of HIV transmission in many developing countries, and medical injections with contaminated medical devices continue to result in some HIV infections.[408,409,425]

HIV was introduced later (middle to late 1980s) in Asia, the Middle East, northern Africa, and eastern Europe than in other regions. Progression of the HIV epidemic in southern and Southeast Asia has been quite rapid, with an explosive increase in HIV infection among injecting drug users, prostitutes, and other populations of young adults in Thailand, Myanmar, India, Malaysia, Cambodia, and Vietnam.[410-434] India, China, and the former Soviet republics are now the areas of the world where the epidemic is rapidly expanding. Korea and Japan continue to have low rates of HIV infection among their populations at risk.[435,436]

In eastern Europe and the newly independent states of the former Soviet Union, HIV infections are rapidly increasing, primarily in association with injecting drug use, and the prevalence of HIV among persons who inject drugs is growing. In the Czech Republic, Estonia, and Bulgaria, HIV infections are typically caused by sexual transmission. In the former Soviet Union and Romania, outbreaks of HIV had been related to contaminated blood products and medical equipment; however, rising trends for syphilis and other sexually transmitted infections have given origin to an explosive HIV epidemic in Russia and many of the newly independent states.[437] In 1990, several thousand Romanian children were infected after receiving multiple injections with improperly cleaned needles and syringes and transfusions of unscreened blood.[382] In Russia, a nosocomial outbreak of HIV infection among 152 hospitalized children was associated with the multiple use of unsterilized syringes.[383]

The HIV epidemic is expected to continue to grow in the coming years, with an increasing proportion of infected persons residing in developing countries. A more extensive discussion of AIDS in the developing world is presented in Chapter 113.

HIV-2

A second retrovirus, HIV-2, can result in severe immunosuppression and the development of serious opportunistic diseases that are clinically indistinguishable from those caused by HIV-1. Infection with HIV-2 was first reported in western Africa in 1986.[438] Although cases of HIV-2 infection have since been reported in other parts of Africa, several European countries, Canada, the United States, Brazil, and India,[439] the virus continues to be found mostly among heterosexual persons in western Africa.[440] Differences in the geographic distribution of HIV-1 and HIV-2 may reflect differences in viral load, which in turn can affect transmissibility and the duration of infectiousness.[440] Data from surveillance and serologic surveys indicate that the prevalence of HIV-2 infection in the United States is extremely low.[417,418] In 1992, the FDA recommended that all blood donations be screened with serologic assays for HIV-1 and HIV-2. Serologic testing of more than 24 million blood donations found no HIV-2–infected persons.[418] Similarly, surveys conducted among persons presumably at increased risk of infection with retroviruses through sexual contact and injecting drug use have found very low rates of HIV-2 infection.[439,441] In a survey performed from 1988 to 1990, of 31,533 persons at high risk for HIV infection in the United States, 10% were found to be infected with HIV-1, but only 2 persons (0.006%) were seropositive for HIV-2.[442]

Accumulating information suggests that the modes of transmission for HIV-1 and HIV-2 are similar. Worldwide, HIV-2 infections have been diagnosed predominantly in men and women infected through heterosexual contact and, to a lesser extent, in homosexual men, injecting drug users, transfusion recipients, and persons with hemophilia.[439,443] In general, the patterns of HIV-1 and HIV-2 transmission within a country are similar. Although perinatal transmission of HIV-2 has been reported, numerous studies suggest that HIV-2 is transmitted less efficiently than HIV-1 from mother to child.[443-446] The natural histories of HIV-1 and HIV-2 infection appear similar in that both are characterized by a broad spectrum of disease. However, the incubation period from the time of initial infection to the eventual development of AIDS may be longer for HIV-2.[443,447-449]

HIV-1 and HIV-2 are genetically and immunologically distinct. However, nucleotide sequence analysis indicates that HIV-1 and HIV-2 share a similar genomic organization, thus suggesting a common evolutionary origin.[450] Overall, the nucleotide sequence homology for HIV-1 and HIV-2 is approximately 40%; the *gag* and *pol* genes for the two viruses are approximately 60% homologous.[450] These genetic similarities can result in frequent serologic cross-reactions between HIV-1 and HIV-2. HIV-1 antibody tests using whole virus lysate enzyme immunoassay will detect 41% to 91% of HIV-2-infected persons.[451] Similarly, because the *gag* and *pol* proteins of HIV-1 and HIV-2 are antigenically cross-reactive, HIV-2-infected persons may have an indeterminate HIV-1 Western blot.[452] The available HIV-2 enzyme immunoassay tests have a reported sensitivity of greater than 99%,[439] and criteria for the diagnosis of HIV-2 infection by Western blot have been established.[453] Although dual infection with both HIV-1 and HIV-2 has been reported, in one study among persons in Côte d'Ivoire with antibodies to both retroviruses, PCR and viral isolation results suggested that more than half were probably infected with HIV-1 alone.[454] Preliminary data suggest that HIV-2 infection might protect against subsequent infection with HIV-1.[455]

Currently, blood donations in the United States are tested for evidence of both HIV-1 and HIV-2 antibodies. The very low prevalence of HIV-2 infection in the United States does not warrant routine testing for HIV-2 in settings other than blood centers. The CDC has recommended that tests for both HIV-1 and HIV-2 be performed in two HIV-testing situations: (1) if demographic or behavioral information suggests that HIV-2 infection might be present, for example, sexual or blood contact with a person from a country where HIV-2 is endemic or with a person known to be infected with HIV-2, or (2) when clinical evidence suggests HIV disease in the absence of a positive test for antibodies to HIV-1 or in the presence of an HIV-1 Western blot with only *gag* and *pol* bands.[439] Detailed HIV-2 testing and counseling algorithms have been developed.[439] In general, preventive counseling and medical management for people infected with HIV-2 are similar for those in whom HIV-1 infection is diagnosed.

PREVENTION OF HIV INFECTION IN THE COMMUNITY

Prevention of HIV infection must be based on strategies that interrupt sexual, blood-borne, and perinatal transmission of the virus. Such strategies must be grounded in an understanding of the epidemiology of HIV infection and knowledge of the science of human behavior.

These science-based strategies are the foundation for the design, implementation, and evaluation of prevention efforts. A number of behavioral interventions have been tested and applied to reduce HIV-associated risk behaviors across a variety of populations. In general, these programs are theory driven and emphasize the development of cognitive, social, and technical skills associated with safer sex and drug use practices.[456,457]

As a result of the proven efficacy of HAART and the availability of HIV rapid testing, the CDC recently launched a new prevention initiative that seeks to make HIV testing more widely available, increase the number of people who enter care once diagnosed and thus benefit from medical care and prevention interventions, and further decrease perinatal HIV transmission.[458] Concern about reports of an upsurge in sexually transmitted infections among people known to be HIV infected[459-461] has resulted in new guidelines for the incorporation of HIV prevention into the medical care of HIV-infected persons.[462,463]

Prevention of Sexual Transmission

Strategies for the prevention of sexual transmission of HIV have focused on reducing unsafe sexual behavior (by promoting sexual abstinence or decreasing the number of partners), encouraging condom use, and treating sexually transmitted infections.[464] Consistent use of latex condoms has been shown to be effective for the prevention of HIV transmission at both an individual and population level.[465-467] Multiple epidemiologic studies of heterosexual couples in which one partner is HIV-positive and the other is HIV-negative indicate that the correct and consistent use of condoms can significantly reduce transmission of HIV and other sexually transmitted diseases.[468-471]

In one prospective study of 342 HIV-seronegative women who had no exposure to HIV other than participation in a stable, monogamous relationship with an infected man, 19 seroconversions were detected for an incidence rate of 3.6 per 100 person-years.[470] The risk of acquiring HIV infection was sixfold greater for women whose partners were inconsistent (i.e., never or not always) condom users than for women who reported that their partners always used condoms. A second longitudinal study of heterosexual HIV-serodiscordant couples reported similar findings: No seroconversions occurred among 124 partners who always used condoms, whereas 12 of 121 partners who were irregular condom users seroconverted for an incidence rate of 4.8 per 100 person-years.[471] Deriving precise and consistent estimates of condom efficacy is often hindered by the inability to control for potentially important confounders that may significantly affect transmission, including the presence of other concurrent sexually transmitted diseases, the frequency of sex, the duration of the partnership, anal intercourse, and the source partner's degree of immunosuppression.[469] Two large prospective studies of serodiscordant couples have demonstrated that among partners who do not use condoms regularly, the risk of transmission increases with advanced stages of HIV infection in the index partner and with the presence of a genital tract infection in the HIV-negative partner.[470,471] Such information reinforces the need for ongoing counseling of persons involved in long-term partnerships with infected partners whose clinical condition may change over time.

In Thailand, a program of "100% condom use" in commercial sex establishments led to an enormous increase in condom use and substantial changes in sexual behavior with parallel declines in HIV seroprevalence and sexually transmitted infections.[472-474]

The effectiveness of condoms to prevent heterosexual transmission of HIV has been estimated to be 87%, but it may be as low as 60% or as high as 96%.[475] Many factors can affect the effectiveness of condoms in reducing the risk of HIV transmission such as condom breakage, leakage, and slippage. Although condom breakage can occur, it appears to be uncommon, particularly in developed countries, where studies have found breakage rates of 2% or less for vaginal or anal intercourse.[466,468] Similarly, low rates of slippage (i.e., less than 1%) have been reported.[476] In vitro testing of intact latex condoms to detect leakage of HIV-sized particles suggests that condoms, when properly used, can act as an effective physical barrier and substantially reduce contact with fluid containing HIV-sized particles, even if leakage were to occur.[477]

The effectiveness of condoms during anal intercourse is probably lower as condom breakage and slippage may be considerably higher than during vaginal intercourse.[478]

Intravaginal pouches ("female condoms"), advocated as a "female-controlled" barrier prevention method, also require correct and consistent use.[479,480] The female condom has been shown to be as effective as the male condom for the prevention of sexually transmitted infections,[480-482] and its contraceptive failure rate has ranged from 11% to 26% depending on the consistency and correctness of usage.[481] However, a condom's contraceptive failure rate may not accurately reflect its effectiveness in reducing heterosexual HIV transmission.[466,468]

Currently available spermicides do not protect against transmission of HIV and other sexually transmitted infections, and nonoxynol 9 might increase the risk for HIV sexual transmission. Three randomized controlled trials of the use of nonoxynol 9 by commercial sex workers in Africa failed to demonstrate any protection against HIV infection,[483,484] with one showing an increased risk of HIV transmission with the use of a vaginal sponge containing a high dose of nonoxynol 9.[283] Nonoxynol 9–containing contraceptives also failed to protect against infection with *Neisseria gonorrhoeae* and *Chlamydia trachomatis* in two randomized trials, one among prostitutes in Africa and one among U.S. women recruited from a sexually transmitted disease (STD) clinic.[485,486] The irritative effects of spermicides on the vaginal epithelium may in fact facilitate, rather than reduce HIV transmission.[284] Despite these data, contraceptives containing nonoxynol-9 continue to be commonly used in family planning clinics.[487] Topical microbicides and other female-controlled methods to prevent HIV and sexually transmitted diseases that can be safely and effectively used by women are urgently needed.

Despite the demonstrated benefits of condom use, multiple studies have found relatively low rates of consistent condom use among sexually active homosexual men and heterosexual men and women. Factors that influence condom use are complex.[488] Concern about decreased sexual pleasure or a partner's noncooperation, inadequate communication skills, the temporal effects of drugs or alcohol, use of other methods for contraception, and cultural influences have been correlated with low rates of condom use.[488-491]

Among homosexual and bisexual men, significant reductions in certain high-risk behavior such as sex with nonsteady partners and insertive anal intercourse have been achieved, and reductions in incident HIV infections have been observed.[64,492] However, coincident with these observations is accumulating evidence that such risk-reduction behavior has not been universally adopted and is difficult to maintain over extended periods.[459-461,493] In cross-sectional studies of homosexual and bisexual men, younger men ages 18 to 25 years,[494] blacks,[490] and men from cities with a low AIDS prevalence[495] reported the highest rates of unprotected anal intercourse. Two longitudinal studies of men who adopted safer sexual practices found that 12% of participants in San Francisco[496] and 47% in Chicago[497] acknowledged relapsing to unprotected receptive anal intercourse. One study of men who engaged in receptive anal intercourse found that heavy alcohol ingestion, moderate to heavy drug use, and younger age were associated with subsequent seroconversion.[498] Collectively, these studies highlight the diversity among men who have sex with men, the challenges in preventing new HIV infection, and the need for continued commitment to the development, implementation, and targeting of intervention and education programs suitable for different age, racial and ethnic, socioeconomic, and geographic populations.[498] In the era of effective antiretroviral therapy, new challenges have emerged. Studies suggest that optimism about the effectiveness of HAART and prognosis may be contributing to relapses in high-risk sexual behaviors among HIV-infected persons.[500-502]

The data available suggest that changes in sexual behavior by heterosexual men and women at risk for HIV infection have been limited. In the United States, the HIV epidemic among heterosexual men and women has its roots in injecting drug use, crack cocaine use, and the exchange of sex for drugs.[125,503] Prevention of heterosexually acquired HIV will require efforts to prevent HIV transmission associated with drug use, especially injecting drug use, as well as the prevention and treatment of other sexually transmitted diseases that facilitate HIV transmission.[306,503,504]

Partner notification is another mechanism to assist in the prevention of sexual transmission of HIV. Even though many HIV-infected individuals cooperate in notifying at least some of their sex partners, others do not.[505,506] Although the effectiveness of contact tracing and partner notification has been hotly debated,[507] it is probably an effective prevention strategy,[508,509] particularly when targeted to primary HIV infection. The efficacy of partner notification by the health department appears to be substantially more effective than notification by the infected person or by the patient's physician.[506,510,511]

The control of sexually transmitted infections is also an important intervention to reduce the sexual transmission of HIV. Data from a study in Tanzania in which a syndromic approach was used in the treatment of symptomatic sexually transmitted infections led to a 42% decrease in HIV incidence.[285] In contrast, in the Rakai district of Uganda, a recently completed community-based trial of mass treatment for sexually transmitted infections failed to show a difference between the treated and the control arms.[512] The reasons for the lack of consistency in the results of these two trials are multiple and not yet fully explained.

Based on the rationale that zidovudine treatment decreases the risk of infection after occupational exposure to HIV,[370] the use of antiretrovirals has been proposed as a way to reduce the risk of HIV transmission after sexual exposure.[513] As mentioned, the probability of HIV infection per episode of receptive anal intercourse has been estimated to be 0.82%,[234] whereas the risk after receptive vaginal intercourse is much lower.[233] The most frequently administered treatment, which is based on that used for occupational exposure, is zidovudine (600 mg per day in two or three divided doses) and lamivudine (150 mg orally twice a day) for 4 weeks, with consideration of the addition of a protease inhibitor in selected cases.[514] Most experts do not recommend initiating treatment more than 72 hours after exposure. Feasibility studies have demonstrated that postexposure prophylaxis after sexual and drug use exposure is possible and should be considered in these instances.[515] However, no data exist regarding the efficacy of this preventive therapy, and the possibility of antiretroviral drug resistance in the source partner should be considered when deciding what antiretroviral regimen to prescribe in cases of postexposure prophylaxis.[516]

Prevention of Transmission by Injecting Drug Use

Prevention and treatment of injecting drug use are critical for reducing HIV transmission among injecting drug users,[517] and several studies have documented that significantly lower rates of drug use and related risk behavior are practiced by injecting drug users who are in treatment.[518,519] However, the impact of substance abuse treatment on HIV infections has only been observed for those users who remain in treatment for at least 1 year.[520] For this reason, brief detoxification programs are not considered to be effective strategies for HIV prevention unless they are followed by a longer course of treatment. Furthermore, an estimated 80% of active drug users in the United States are not in treatment because of choice or the unavailability of treatment.[521] This situation has necessitated the development of a creative blend of educational and alternative therapeutic approaches, including the removal of restrictions on the purchase of needles and syringes,[522] needle and syringe exchange programs,[523] proper use of bleach for disinfection of drug injection equipment,[524] and interim methadone maintenance programs.[525] Community outreach-based interventions that include education about HIV transmission and prevention, distribution of condoms and bleach kits have demonstrated significant changes in drug use frequency and drug-related behaviors.[526] Particularly useful have been risk reduction interventions delivered through social networks by peer educators.[527] Improvement in selected drug use behavior has been reported, including a decrease in sharing of drug injecting equipment and an increase in the use of bleach for cleaning equipment,[526-530] although the duration of such behavior has not been studied extensively. Although the overwhelming majority of studies have found that needle exchange programs lead to reductions in sharing of syringes among program participants,[531,532] do not result in increased drug use among participants or in the recruitment of first-time users and that they reduce the transmission of HIV among injecting drug users,[533-535] some studies have been equivocal in their findings,[536] generating controversy surrounding needle exchange programs.[537,538] Because of the difficulties that injection drug users face in the United States in accessing clean needles, interventions via pharmacy sales and physician prescription of syringes for active users are being evaluated.[539,540] Use of bleach was not found to be effective in studies in New York City and Baltimore.[541,542] As mentioned for sexual exposure to HIV, it has also been proposed that antiretroviral therapy should be considered for persons exposed to HIV through injection drug use,[513,514] but no data are available on the effectiveness of this approach for the prevention of HIV infection among injecting drug users.

Prevention of Transmission through Blood and Other Tissues

The first report of transfusion-associated AIDS was in 1982. In 1983, blood banks initiated the voluntary self-exclusion of donors with risks for HIV infection. In 1985, the first serologic assays for HIV antibody became available, and the use of these HIV serologic tests to screen blood donations dramatically decreased the risk of transfusion-associated HIV transmission.[318,319] Serologic identification of repeat donors with HIV infection (including the detection of p24 antigen and nucleic acid testing), screening of blood for hepatitis C and human T-lymphotropic virus types I and II, and reductions in the number of transfusions performed have also lowered transmission risks.[319-322] In addition to HIV antibody testing of plasma donors and deferral procedures for donors with risks for HIV infection, the implementation of viral inactivation procedures such as heat and solvent/detergent treatments and purification with monoclonal antibody has virtually eliminated the risk of HIV transmission through pooled plasma products for persons with hemophilia. In 1993, a recombinant factor VIII product obtained from hamster cells containing the gene for human factor VIII became available as an alternative therapy to pooled human plasma products. Organ and tissue donors should be evaluated and serologically screened in a manner similar to blood donors.[543,544] In addition, donations of semen and bone from a living donor may be quarantined until subsequent testing has definitively ruled out the possibility of delayed seroconversion in the donor. Prompt administration of antiretroviral drugs for postexposure prophylaxis after transfusion of contaminated blood prevented HIV infection in one patient.[545]

Prevention of Transmission in the Health Care Setting

Effective prevention of HIV transmission in the health care setting requires a multifaceted approach to reduce the frequency of occupational blood exposure among health care workers. Such a strategy includes engineering controls that do not rely on worker compliance (e.g., self-sheathing needles), safe work practices and techniques, personal protective equipment, and training.[546,547] In particular, a reduction in percutaneous injuries will require the development of puncture-resistant gloves, the redesign of needles and other sharp instruments, or both. In 1987, the CDC recommended that the principles of "universal precautions" be incorporated in programs for infection control.[548] Under universal precautions, blood and certain other body fluids from *all* patients are considered to be potentially infective. Universal precautions include the appropriate use of hand washing and protective barriers, care in the use and disposal of needles and other sharp instruments, and appropriate disinfection and sterilization of reusable equipment. For occupational exposure to HIV among health care workers, the CDC recommended in 1990 the use of zidovudine for postexposure prophylaxis.[549] This recommendation was further supported by a case-control study involving health care workers from the United States, France, Italy, and the United Kingdom that showed that the risk of HIV seroconversion after occupational exposure was decreased by approximately 81% with the use of zidovudine.[370] Subsequent recommendations have incorporated the newer antiretro-

viral drugs, as well as risk stratification for the type of exposure, in the management of occupational exposure to HIV.[368] A detailed discussion of the prevention of transmission of HIV in the health care setting is presented in Chapter 304.

Prevention of Perinatal Infection

Primary prevention of perinatally acquired HIV infection must center on routine, voluntary counseling and HIV antibody testing and on the availability of reproductive health services for women of reproductive age (see Chapter 122).[550,551] Because a substantial proportion of women may not initially acknowledge high-risk behavior or know the infection status of their partners, routine HIV testing and counseling must be considered a standard of care, especially in areas of high prevalence,[552] and not be reserved only for women with self-reported risk histories. In 1994, results of a randomized, double-blind clinical trial (Pediatric AIDS Clinical Trials Group Protocol 076) found that zidovudine therapy administered to HIV-infected women during pregnancy, at the time of labor, and postpartum to their infants was associated with a 67.5% reduction in the risk of perinatal HIV transmission.[221] Based on these results, a Public Health Service task force issued recommendations for the use of zidovudine for the reduction of perinatal HIV-1 transmission.[222] Several subsequent studies have confirmed the benefits of zidovudine for the prevention of perinatal HIV-1 transmission even when the drug is given for a much shorter period than in the original protocol 076 trial.[553,554] Advances in understanding the pathogenesis of HIV infection and the availability of laboratory tests to monitor the disease (such as HIV-RNA) and better antiretroviral drugs have led to a recent update in the recommendations for the use of antiretroviral drugs in pregnant women.[227] Implementation of these recommendations has resulted in significant public health benefits; for example, the number of children in whom AIDS attributed to perinatal HIV transmission was diagnosed peaked in 1992 at 954 and declined to 92 in 2002.[50] These regimens, however, are not applicable in the vast majority of the developing world where most perinatal HIV transmission occurs, and simpler, shorter, and less costly regimens are urgently needed.[555]

Prevention of postnatal transmission of HIV infection through breast-feeding must take into account the likelihood of competing risks for morbidity and mortality associated with feeding alternatives in developing countries. In 1985, after the first case report implicating HIV transmission from breast milk and the isolation of HIV from breast milk, the CDC recommended that HIV-seropositive women not breast-feed their infants.[556] This recommendation was intended for mothers in the United States, where alternative, safe, and nutritious substitute feeding methods are readily available.[344] In 1992, the WHO and the United Nations International Children's Emergency Fund developed a consensus statement on HIV transmission related to breast-feeding, which stated that "in settings where the primary causes of infant deaths are infectious diseases and malnutrition, breastfeeding should remain the standard advice to pregnant women, including those who are HIV-infected."[557] By 1996, UNAIDS published a revised statement that supported breast-feeding in all populations, irrespective of HIV infection rates, but recommended counseling for women about the risks of HIV transmission through breast-feeding.[558]

When children born to women living with HIV can be ensured uninterrupted access to nutritionally adequate breast-milk substitutes that are safely prepared and fed to them, they are at less risk of illness and death if they are not breast-fed. However, when these conditions are not fulfilled, in particular in an environment where infectious diseases and malnutrition are the primary causes of death during infancy, artificial feeding substantially increases children's risk of illness and death.

The importance of providing safe alternatives to breast-feeding among HIV-infected women has been highlighted by several randomized trials of perinatal transmission prevention in breast-feeding populations. For example, in the PETRA trial the benefits of combination antiretroviral therapy diminished considerably as a result of breast-feeding.[559] In the South African Intrapartum Nevirapine Trial (SAINT), breast-feeding was the most significant risk factor for mother-to-child transmission when antiretroviral therapy was administered to prevent intrapartum and early postpartum HIV transmission.[560]

COUNSELING AND HIV ANTIBODY TESTING

Early recognition of HIV infection through HIV antibody testing has been one of the primary objectives of HIV prevention efforts. However, with the availability of more effective therapies, HIV testing has become an even more important preventive intervention.[458,462] The major benefits of HIV testing programs are (1) referral of HIV-seropositive persons for medical evaluation, treatment, and other social services and (2) counseling to promote the behavior change necessary to reduce HIV transmission.

Physicians have an essential role in this public health effort. As the principal providers of primary health care, they are most frequently named by the general public as the desired source for HIV testing.[561] The number of people who have been tested for HIV antibodies is quite large. Data from the 2001 Behavioral Risk Factor Surveillance System, a random-digit-dialed telephone survey of the civilian, noninstitutionalized population older than the age of 18 years suggests that 45.6% of adults have been tested for HIV in the United States (the range was from 31.5% in South Dakota to 65.3% in the District of Columbia).[562] However, many who are tested for HIV do not return for their results. The CDC estimates that 31% of those who tested HIV-positive in 2000 at CDC-publicly funded testing sites failed to return for their results.[458] The recent approval of rapid HIV tests such as the OraQuick HIV rapid test (OraSure Technologies, Inc., Bethlehem, Pennsylvania) and the subsequent CLIA waiver of this test offers the possibility for more people to be tested for HIV and receive their results on the same day, thus eliminating the need for a second visit.[563]

In an effort to make HIV testing more accessible and available, in 2001 the CDC issued new counseling and referral guidelines.[550] These guidelines recommend offering HIV testing to all patients in all high HIV-prevalence clinical settings.

Indications for HIV Testing

Knowledge of the behavior that places persons at risk for HIV infection, the clinical conditions associated with HIV infection, and the estimated rate of HIV infection in the community served by the health care facility or practitioner is necessary to target HIV counseling and testing effectively. Specific populations or clinical settings in which testing is recommended include the following[550,565,566]:

1. *Persons with behavioral risks for HIV infection.* Those at risk for HIV infection include men who have had sex with other men, people who have injected drugs, male and female prostitutes, sex partners of persons with or at increased risk for HIV infection, and others who consider themselves at risk. To identify risks associated with HIV transmission, physicians should interview patients regarding their sexual and drug use practices. Injecting drug users are at increased risk of HIV infection through contact with contaminated needles or syringes. HIV counseling can provide these people with information on safer sexual and needle-sharing practices that can further reduce HIV transmission, as well as with referrals for substance abuse treatment and preventive services.

2. *Persons with clinical conditions associated with HIV infection.* The HIV antibody test is a useful diagnostic tool for evaluating persons with generalized lymphadenopathy; unexplained weight loss, fever, diarrhea, or dementia; diseases such as tuberculosis, generalized herpes simplex, and chronic candidiasis; and other conditions suggestive of HIV infection.[15]

3. *Persons who received blood or blood products between 1978 and 1985.* Persons who received transfusions of blood or blood components from 1978 to 1985 are at increased risk of transfusion-associated HIV transmission. The risk of transfusion-associated transmission is greatest for persons who received relatively large numbers of units in geographic areas with high rates of AIDS and

HIV infection.[567] Because clotting factor concentrates are derived from many donors nationwide, all persons with hemophilia who received clotting factor concentrate during this time are considered to be at risk for HIV infection.

4. *Persons with other sexually transmitted diseases.* HIV testing should be offered to all persons with other sexually transmitted diseases because many of these persons have probably practiced behaviors that place them at risk for HIV infection.

5. *Women of reproductive age.* Women at risk for HIV infection include those with the behavioral risks outlined earlier and all women living in communities or born in countries where the prevalence of HIV infection among women is known or suspected to be high. Offering HIV testing to all women, especially pregnant women, is particularly important in view of the availability of effective interventions to prevent perinatal transmission.[222,227]

6. *Children born to mothers with HIV infection or at increased risk.* Children born to infected mothers should be evaluated as early as possible after delivery for laboratory and clinical evidence of HIV infection so that appropriate prophylactic and therapeutic interventions can begin. Infected infants often have life-threatening complications of HIV infection in the first few months of life.

7. *Patients 15 to 54 years old in acute health care settings with high rates of unsuspected HIV infection.* High rates of unrecognized HIV infection have been found among patients at some U.S. hospitals and associated clinics.[95,361] In anonymous unlinked serologic surveys, 0.2% to 8.9% of persons receiving care in emergency departments and 0.1% to 7.8% of persons admitted to hospitals were HIV antibody positive. In two studies that collected data on previous HIV testing, many persons were unaware of their HIV infection before hospital admission.[95] Thus, testing on the basis of acknowledged risk behavior or clinical signs and symptoms will recognize only a minority of HIV-infected persons. To address this shortcoming, routine voluntary HIV counseling and testing programs are recommended for hospitals and associated clinics with a high rate of HIV infection, which is defined as an estimated HIV seroprevalence rate of at least 1% or an AIDS diagnosis rate of 1 or higher per 1000 discharges. The AIDS diagnosis rate is the annual number of patients in whom AIDS is diagnosed and reported to the health department divided by the annual number of discharges times 1000. Acute care facilities and other health care institutions such as mental health facilities or private medical practitioners' offices with an HIV prevalence rate greater than 1% should routinely recommend HIV testing.

8. *Persons who sustain occupational exposures that may place them at risk of HIV infection.* Occupational exposures that may place a worker at risk of HIV infection include percutaneous injuries and contact of mucous membranes or skin (especially when the skin is chapped, abraded, or afflicted with dermatitis or the contact is prolonged or involves an extensive area) with blood and other body fluids to which universal precautions apply.

9. *Health care workers who perform exposure-prone procedures.* Health care workers who perform invasive procedures that are considered exposure prone (e.g., procedures that include digital palpation of a needle tip in a body cavity or the simultaneous presence of the health care worker's fingers and a needle or other sharp object in a poorly visualized or highly confined anatomic site) should know their HIV antibody status. Mandatory testing of health care workers for HIV antibody is not recommended.[568]

Guidelines for HIV Counseling and Testing

Testing for HIV infection should be voluntary, with informed consent obtained in accordance with local laws.[550] Confidentiality and the avoidance of discrimination toward persons who test positive must be ensured. Mandatory testing is not recommended except in the limited setting of tissue and organ donation. HIV testing for purposes other than immediate medical care should be deferred until a later time for persons who are too severely ill to give informed consent. Testing patients to reduce the risk of HIV transmission within health care settings has not been shown to be effective and is not a substitute for universal precautions.[360,569]

Although study results have differed, voluntary HIV counseling and testing have been found to reduce the prevalence of high-risk behavior such as unprotected intercourse and is thus an effective intervention that can help reduce HIV transmission.[570-575] Counseling should be performed in accordance with existing CDC recommendations by health care providers knowledgeable about HIV infection.[550,566] HIV testing should be preceded by information about the testing policies of the physician or institution, the medical implications of the test, an assessment of risk, and the opportunity to receive additional information. After testing, HIV-seronegative persons should be informed that continued high-risk sexual or drug use behavior could result in HIV infection. Seronegative persons concerned about a recent exposure should be advised to seek repeated testing at least 6 months after the exposure.

Persons seeking repeat HIV testing may be at particular high risk for HIV infection and are more likely to have a sexually transmitted infection.[576] These patients might benefit from referral to additional HIV prevention and support services as they might view HIV testing as protective. With the availability of HIV rapid tests, HIV post-test counseling can now be done the same day as the HIV test. Persons who test negative can definitively be told that they are not infected unless they have had a recent (within 3 months) known or possible exposure to HIV. Persons who test positive on a rapid test should be told that their preliminary results are positive and that additional testing (EIA and Western blot if the EIA is positive) will be conducted to confirm the diagnosis.[577] A return visit is thus required for those who test HIV-positive using a rapid test.

Counseling of HIV-seropositive people should be tailored for each individual and include an interpretation of the test results and a discussion of the medical, social, and psychological implications of a positive test result. HIV-infected persons should also be instructed to notify sex or needle-sharing partners and to refer them for HIV counseling and testing. If HIV-infected persons are reluctant to inform their partners directly, physicians may offer to inform partners or seek local health department assistance. Confidentiality is very important to protect individuals and not discourage persons from seeking HIV testing.

Persons found to be HIV seropositive should be referred for medical evaluation, including immunologic (CD4 T-lymphocyte cell counts) and virologic (quantitation of HIV-RNA) monitoring, screening for other sexually transmitted diseases, prophylaxis against certain opportunistic illnesses, vaccinations, antiretroviral therapy, and other preventive and therapeutic services.[578]

REFERENCES

1. Centers for Disease Control and Prevention. *Pneumocystis* pneumonia—Los Angeles. MMWR Morb Mortal Wkly Rep. 1981;30:250-252.
2. Centers for Disease Control and Prevention. Kaposi's sarcoma and *Pneumocystis* pneumonia among homosexual men—New York City and California. MMWR Morb Mortal Wkly Rep. 1981;30:305-308.
3. Barre-Sinoussi F, Chermann JC, Rey F, et al. Isolation of a T-lymphotropic retrovirus from a patient at risk for acquired immune deficiency syndrome (AIDS). Science. 1983; 220:868-871.
4. Gallo RC, Sarin PS, Gelmann EP, et al. Isolation of human T-cell leukemia virus in acquired immune deficiency syndrome (AIDS). Science. 1983; 220:865-867.
5. Zhu T, Korber BT, Nahmias AJ, et al. An African HIV-1 sequence from 1959 and implications for the origin of the epidemic. Nature. 1998;391:594-597.
6. UNAIDS. AIDS Epidemic Update, December 2003. Geneva, WHO/UNAIDS.
7. Centers for Disease Control and Prevention. Increases in HIV diagnoses—29 states, 1999-2002. MMWR Morb Mortal Wkly Rep. 2003;53:1145-1148.
8. Karon JM, Fleming PL, Steketee RW, De Cock K. HIV in the United States at the turn of the century: An epidemic in transition. Am J Public Health. 2001;91:1060-1068.
9. Nakashima AK, Fleming PL. HIV/AIDS surveillance in the United States, 1981-2001. J Acquir Immune Defic Syndr. 2003;32(Suppl 1):S68-S85.
10. Centers for Disease Control and Prevention: Update on acquired immune deficiency syndrome (AIDS)—United States. MMWR Morb Mortal Wkly Rep. 1982;31:507-508, 513-514.
11. Garry RF, Witte MH, Gottlieb AA, et al. Documentation of an AIDS virus infection in the United States in 1968. JAMA. 1988;260:2085-2087.
12. Huminer D, Rosenfeld JB, Pitlik SD. AIDS in the pre-AIDS era. Rev Infect Dis. 1987;9:1102-1108.
13. Centers for Disease Control and Prevention. Revision of the case definition of acquired immunodeficiency syndrome for national reporting—United States. MMWR Morb Mortal Wkly Rep. 1985;34:373-375.
14. Centers for Disease Control and Prevention. Revision of the CDC surveillance case definition for acquired immunodeficiency syndrome. MMWR Morb Mortal Wkly Rep. 1987;36(Suppl):S1-S15.
15. Centers for Disease Control and Prevention. 1993 Revised classification system for HIV infection and expanded surveillance case definition for AIDS among adolescents and adults. MMWR Morb Mortal Wkly Rep. 1992;41(RR-17):1-19.
16. Centers for Disease Control and Prevention. Update: Acquired immunodeficiency syndrome—United States, 1981-1988. MMWR Morb Mortal Wkly Rep. 1989;38:229-236.
17. Selik RM, Buehler JW, Karon JM, et al. Impact of the 1987 revision of the case definition of the acquired immunodeficiency syndrome in the United States. J Acquir Immune Defic Syndr. 1990;3:73-82.
18. Payne SF, Rutherford GW, Lemp GF, et al. Effect of the revised AIDS case definition on AIDS reporting in San Francisco: Evidence of increased reporting in intravenous drug users. AIDS. 1990;4:335-339.
19. National Institutes of Health. State-of-the-art conference on azidothymidine therapy for early HIV infection. Am J Med. 1990;89:335-344.
20. Volberding PA, Lagakos SW, Koch MA, et al. Zidovudine in asymptomatic human immunodeficiency virus infection: A controlled trial in persons with fewer than 500 CD4-positive cells per cubic millimeter. The AIDS Clinical Trials Group of the National Institute of Allergy and Infectious Diseases. N Engl J Med. 1990;322:941.
21. Centers for Disease Control and Prevention. Recommendations for prophylaxis against *Pneumocystis carinii* pneumonia for adults and adolescents infected with human immunodeficiency virus. MMWR Morb Mortal Wkly Rep. 1992;41(RR-4):1-11.
22. El Sadr W, Oleshe JM, Agins BD, et al. Evaluation and Management of Early HIV Infection. Clinical Practice Guideline No. 7, Publication No. 940572. Rockville, Md: Agency for Health Care Policy and Research, Public Health Service, U.S. Department of Health and Human Services; 1994:28.
23. Brookmeyer R. Reconstruction and future trends of the AIDS epidemic in the United States. Science. 1991;253:37-42.
24. Selwyn PA, Hartel D, Lewis VA, et al. A prospective study of the risk of tuberculosis among intravenous drug users with human immunodeficiency virus infection. N Engl J Med. 1989;320:545-550.
25. Selwyn PA, Sckell BM, Alcabes P, et al. High risk of active tuberculosis in HIV infected drug users with cutaneous anergy. JAMA. 1992;268:504-509.
26. Buehler JW, Devine OJ, Berkelman RL, et al. Impact of the human immunodeficiency virus epidemic on mortality trends in young men, United States. Am J Public Health. 1990;80:1080-1086.
27. Chu SY, Buehler JW, Berkelman RL. Impact of the human immunodeficiency virus epidemic on mortality in women of reproductive age, United States. JAMA. 1990;264:225-229.
28. Farizo KM, Buehler JW, Chamberland ME, et al. Spectrum of disease in persons with human immunodeficiency virus infection in the United States. JAMA. 1992;267:1798-1805.
29. Schafer A, Friedmann W, Mielke M, et al. The increased frequency of cervical dysplasia-neoplasia in women infected with the human immunodeficiency virus is related to the degree of immunosuppression. Am J Obstet Gynecol. 1991;164:593-599.
30. Feingold AR, Vermund SH, Burk RD, et al. Cervical cytologic abnormalities and papillomavirus in women infected with human immunodeficiency virus. J Acquir Immune Defic Syndr. 1990;3:896-903.
31. Maiman M, Fruchter RG, Serur E, et al. Human immunodeficiency virus infection and cervical neoplasia. Gynecol Oncol. 1990;38:377-382.
32. Rosenblum LS, Buehler JW, Morgan MW, et al. The completeness of AIDS case reporting, 1988: A multisite collaborative surveillance project. Am J Public Health. 1992;82:1495-1499.
33. Buehler JW, Berkelman RL, Stehr-Green JK. The completeness of AIDS surveillance. J Acquir Immune Defic Syndr. 1992;5:257-264.
34. Doyle T, Glynn K, Groseclose S. Completeness of notifiable infectious diseases reporting in the United States: An analytical review. Am J Epidemiol. 2002;155:866-874.
35. Vogt RL, Clark SW, Kappel S. Evaluation of the state surveillance system using hospital discharge diagnoses, 1982-83. Am J Epidemiol. 1986;123:197-198.
36. Centers for Disease Control and Prevention. Guidelines for national human immunodeficiency virus case surveillance, including monitoring for human immunodeficiency virus infection and acquired immunodeficiency syndrome. MMWR Morb Mortal Wkly Rep.1999;48:1-28.
37. Centers for Disease Control and Prevention. Revised surveillance case definition for HIV infection. MMWR Morb Mortal Wkly Rep. 1999;48(RR-13):29-31.
38. Fleming PL, Ward JW, Morgan MW, et al. Mandatory HIV reporting: Characteristics of adults reported with HIV compared to AIDS in the United States. Abstract WSC172. In: Abstracts of the Ninth International Conference on AIDS/Fourth STD World Congress, v. 1. Berlin: 1993:98.
39. Centers for Disease Control and Prevention. Public health uses of HIV-infection reports—South Carolina, 1986-1991. MMWR Morb Mortal Wkly Rep. 1992;41:245-249.
40. Centers for Disease Control and Prevention. Diagnosis and reporting of HIV infection and AIDS in states with HIV/AIDS surveillance—United States, 1994-2000. MMWR Morb Mortal Wkly Rep. 2002;51:595-598.
41. Centers for Disease Control and Prevention. Implementation of named HIV reporting—New York City, 2001. MMWR Morb Mortal Wkly Rep. 2004;52:1248-1252.
42. Palella FJ, Delaney KM, Moorman AC, et al. Declining morbidity and mortality among patients with advanced human immunodeficiency virus infection. N Engl J Med. 1998;338:853-860.

43. Gastin LO, Ward JW, Baker AC. National HIV case reporting in the United States. A defining moment in the history of the epidemic. N Engl J Med. 1997;337:1162-1167.

44. Solomon SL, Curran JW. Public health applications of a classification system for human immunodeficiency virus infection (Editorial). Ann Intern Med. 1987;106:319-321.

45. World Health Organization. Interim proposal for a WHO staging system for HIV infection and diseases. Wkly Epidemiol Rec. 1990;65:221-224.

46. Royce RA, Luckmann RS, Fusaro RE, Winkelstein W Jr. The natural history of HIV-1 infection: Staging classifications of disease. AIDS. 1991;5:355-364.

47. Redfield RR, Wright DC, Tramont EC. The Walter Reed staging classification for HTLV-III/LAV infection. N Engl J Med. 1986;314:131-132.

48. Zolla-Pazner S, DesJarlais DC, Friedman SR, et al. Nonrandom development of immunologic abnormalities after infection with human immunodeficiency virus: Implications for immunologic classification of the disease. Proc Natl Acad Sci U S A. 1987;84:5404-5408.

49. Justice JA, Feinstein AR, Wells CK. A new prognostic staging system for the acquired immunodeficiency syndrome. N Engl J Med. 1989;320:1388-1393.

50. Centers for Disease Control and Prevention. HIV/AIDS Surveillance Report. 2002;14:1-48.

51. Centers for Disease Control and Prevention. The second 100,000 cases of acquired immunodeficiency syndrome—United States, June 1981-December 1991. MMWR Morb Mortal Wkly Rep. 1992;41:28-29.

52. Centers for Disease Control and Prevention. Update: Impact of the expanded AIDS surveillance case distribution for adolescents and adults on case reporting—United States, 1993. MMWR Morb Mortal Wkly Rep. 1994;43:160-161, 167-170.

53. Louie JK, Hsu LC, Osmond DH, et al. Trends in causes of death among persons with acquired immunodeficiency syndrome in the era of highly active antiretroviral therapy, San Francisco, 1994-1998. J Infect Dis. 2002;186:1023-1027.

54. Fleming PL, Byers RH, Sweeney PA, et al. HIV Prevalence in the United States, 2000. Abstract 11. Presented at the Ninth Conference on Retroviruses and Opportunistic Infections, Seattle, Wash., February 24-28, 2002.

55. Karon JM, Rosenberg PS, McQuillan G, et al. Prevalence of HIV infection in the United States, 1984 to 1992. JAMA. 1996;276:126-131.

56. Holmberg SD. The estimated prevalence and incidence of HIV in 96 large US metropolitan areas. Am J Public Health. 1996;86:627-628.

57. Vu MQ, Steketee RW, Valleroy L, et al. HIV incidence in the United States, 1978-1999. J Acquir Immune Defic Syndr. 2002;31:188-201.

58. Kellerman SE, Lehman JS, Lansky A, et al. HIV testing within at-risk populations in the United States and the reasons for seeking or avoiding HIV testing. J Acquir Immune Defic Syndr. 2002;31:202-210.

59. Centers for Disease Control and Prevention. Human immunodeficiency virus infection in the United States: A review of current knowledge. MMWR Morb Mortal Wkly Rep. 1987;36(Suppl 6):S1-S48.

60. Centers for Disease Control and Prevention (CDC). National HIV Prevalence Surveys, 1997 Summary. Atlanta: Centers for Disease Control and Prevention; 1998:1-25.

61. Catania JA, Osmond D, Stall RD, et al. The continuing HIV epidemic among men who have sex with men. Am J Public Health. 2001;91:907-914.

62. Weinstock HS, Sidhu J, Gwinn M, et al. Trends in HIV seroprevalence among persons attending sexually transmitted diseases clinics in the United States. J Acquir Immune Defic Syndr. 1995;9:514-522.

63. McCray E, Onorato IM, the Field Services Branch. Sentinel surveillance of human immunodeficiency virus infection in sexually transmitted disease clinics in the United States. Sex Transm Dis. 1992;19:235-241.

64. Winkelstein W Jr, Wiley JA, Padian N, et al. The San Francisco Men's Health Study: Continued decline in HIV seroconversion rates among homosexual/bisexual men. Am J Public Health. 1988;78:1472-1474.

65. Centers for Disease Control and Prevention. HIV incidence among young men who have sex with men. MMWR Morb Mortal Wkly Rep. 2001;50:440-444.

66. Katz MH, McFarland W, Guillin V, et al. Continuing high prevalence of HIV and risk behaviors among young men who have sex with men: The young men's survey in the San Francisco Bay Area in 1992 to 1993 and in 1994 to 1995. J Acquir Immune Defic Syndr Hum Retrovirol. 1998;19:178-181.

67. Chen SY, Gibson S, Katz MH, et al. Continuing increases in sexual risk behavior and sexually transmitted diseases among men who have sex with men: San Francisco, Calif, 1999-2001, USA. Am J Public Health. 2002;92:1387-1388.

68. Scheer S, Chu PL, Klausner JD, et al. Effect of highly active antiretroviral therapy on diagnoses of sexually transmitted diseases in people with AIDS. Lancet. 2001;357:432-435.

69. Little SJ, Holte S, Routy JP, et al. Antiretroviral-drug resistance among patients recently infected with HIV. New Engl J Med. 2002;347:385-394.

70. Hahn RA, Onorato IM, Jones TS, et al. Prevalence of HIV infection among intravenous drug users in the United States. JAMA. 1989;261:2677-2684.

71. Des Jarlais DC, Friedman SR, Novick DM, et al. HIV-1 infection among intravenous drug users in Manhattan, New York City, from 1977 through 1987. JAMA. 1989;261:1008-1012.

72. Weibel W, Lampinen T, Chene D, et al. HIV-1 seroconversion in a cohort of street intravenous drug users in Chicago. Abstract F.C.556. In: Final Program and Abstracts of the Sixth International Conference on AIDS, v. 2. San Francisco: 1990:220.

73. Centers for Disease Control and Prevention (CDC): National HIV Serosurveillance Summary—Results through 1992. Publication no. HIV/NCID/1193/036. Atlanta: U.S. Department of Health and Human Services, Public Health Service; 1993.

74. Allen DM, Onorato IM, Green TA, et al. HIV infection in intravenous drug users entering drug treatment, United States, 1988 to 1989. Am J Public Health. 1992;82:541-546.

75. Murill C, Weeks HR, Lambert S, et al. Age-specific trends in seroprevalence of HIV and hepatitis B and C virus among injecting drug users admitted to drug treatment in six US cities. Abstract 13224. Presented at the Twelfth International Conference on AIDS, Geneva, June 28-July 3, 1998.

76. Prevosts DR, Allen DM, Lehman JS, et al. Trends in human immunodeficiency virus seroprevalence among injection drug users entering drug treatment centers, United States 1988-1993. Am J Epidemiol. 1996;143:733-742.

77. Battjes RJ, Pickens RW, Brown LS Jr. HIV infection and AIDS risk behaviors among injecting drug users entering methadone treatment: An update. J Acquir Immune Defic Syndr. 1995;10:90-96.

78. Centers for Disease Control and Prevention. HIV diagnoses among injection-drug users in states with HIV surveillance—25 states, 1994-2000. MMWR Morb Mortal Wkly Rep. 2003;52:634-636.

79. Chaisson RE, Bacchetti P, Osmond D, et al. Cocaine use and HIV infection in intravenous drug users in San Francisco. JAMA. 1989;261:561-565.

80. Battjes RJ, Pickens RW, Haverkos HW, Slobada Z. HIV risk factors among injection drug users in five US cities. AIDS. 1994;8:6817.

81. Kral AH, Bluthenthal RN, Booth RE, Watters JK. HIV seroprevalence among street-recruited injection drug and crack cocaine users in 16 US municipalities. Am J Public Health. 1998;88:108-113.

82. DesJarlais DC, Perlis T, Friedman SR, et al. Declining seroprevalence in a very large HIV epidemic: Injection drug users in New York City, 1991 to 1996. Am J Public Health. 1998;88:1801.

83. Byers RH, Lindegren ML, Hanson IC, et al. AIDS patients infected during adolescence, United States. Abstract 284. Presented at the Thirty-second Interscience Conference on Antimicrobial Agents and Chemotherapy, Anaheim, Calif, October 11-14, 1992.

84. Lee LM, Fleming PL. Trends in human immunodeficiency virus diagnoses among women in the United States, 1994-1998. J Am Med Womens Association 2001; 56(3):94-99.

85. Dondero TJ, Allen DM, McCray D, et al. Injected drug use: The driving force for much of the U.S. epidemic. Abstract WC 3356. In: Abstracts of the Seventh International Conference on AIDS, v. 2. Florence, Italy: 1991:385.

86. Chaisson MA, Stoneburner RL, Hildebrandt DS, et al. Heterosexual transmission of HIV-1 associated with the use of smokable freebase cocaine (crack). AIDS. 1991;5:1121-1126.

87. Ellerbrock TV, Lieb S, Harrington PE, et al. Heterosexually transmitted human immunodeficiency virus infection among pregnant women in a rural Florida community. N Engl J Med. 1992;327:1704-1709.

88. Jones D, Irwin KL, Inciardi J, et al. The high-risk sexual practices of crack-smoking sex workers recruited from the streets of three American cities. The Multicenter Crack Cocaine and HIV Infection Study Team. Sex Transm Dis. 1998;25:184-193.

89. Stoneburner RL, Chaisson MA, Weisfuse IB, et al. The epidemic of AIDS and HIV-1 infection among heterosexuals in New York City. AIDS. 1990;4:99-106.

90. Weinstock H, Dale M, Gwinn M, et al. HIV seroincidence among patients at clinics for sexually transmitted diseases in nine cities in the United States. J Acquir Immune Defic Syndr. 2002;29:478-483.

91. Darrow WW, Cohen JB, French J, et al. Multicenter study of HIV antibody in U.S. prostitutes. Abstract W.2.1. Presented at the Third International Conference on AIDS, Washington, D.C., June 1-5, 1987.

92. Fischl MA, Dickinson GM, Flanagan S, et al. Human immunodeficiency virus (HIV) among female prostitutes in south Florida. Abstract W.2.2. Presented at the Third International Conference on AIDS, Washington, D.C., June 1-5, 1987.

93. Onorato IM, Klaskala W, Morgan M. High and rising HIV incidence in female sex workers in Miami, Florida, despite stable HIV prevalence over time. Abstract 285. Presented at the Thirty-second Interscience Conference on Antimicrobial Agents and Chemotherapy, Anaheim, Calif, October 11-14, 1992.

94. Strathdee SA, Galai N, Safaiean M, et al. Sex differences in risk factors for HIV seroconversion among injection drug users: A 10-year perspective. Arch Intern Med. 2001;161:1281-1288.

95. Janssen RS, Satten GA, Stramer SL, et al. HIV infection among patients in U.S. acute care hospitals: Strategies for the counseling and testing of hospital patients. N Engl J Med. 1992;327:445-452.

96. Miller RS, Green LA, Nutting PA, et al. Human immunodeficiency virus seroprevalence in community-based primary care practices, 1990-1992. A report from the Ambulatory Sentinel Practice Network. Arch Fam Med. 1995;4:1042-1047.

97. Walensky RP, Losina E, Steger-Craven KA, Freedberg KA. Identifying undiagnosed human immunodeficiency virus: The yield of routine, voluntary inpatient testing. Arch Intern Med. 2002;162:887-892.

98. Weis SE, Foresman B, Cook PE, Matty KJ. Universal HIV screening at a major metropolitan TB clinic: HIV prevalence and high-risk behaviors among TB patients. Am J Public Health. 1999;89:73-75.

99. Schneider E, McCray E, Onorato IM. HIV seroprevalence among TB clinic patients in the US, 1988-1995. Abstract 145. Presented at the Thirty-sixth Interscience Conference on Antimicrobial Agents and Chemotherapy, New Orleans, La, 1996.

100. Blocker ME, Levine WC, St Louis ME. HIV prevalence in patients with syphilis, United States. Sex Transm Dis. 2000;27:53-59.

101. Centers for Disease Control and Prevention. HIV Prevalence and Trends in Selected Populations in the United States: Results from National Serosurveillance, 1993-1997. Atlanta: Centers for Disease Control and Prevention, 2001;1-51.

102. Withum DG, Guerena-Burgueno F, Gwinn M, et al. High HIV prevalence among female and male prisoners in the United States, 1989-1992: Implications for prevention and treatment strategies. Abstract POC213115. In: Abstracts of the Ninth International Conference on AIDS/Fourth STD World Congress, v. 2. Berlin: 1993:736.

103. Mikl J, Dzierbicki A, Smith PF, et al. Trends in HIV infection rates among New York State prison entrants, 1987-97. Abstract 2356. Presented at the Twelfth International Conference on AIDS, Geneva, June 28-July 3, 1998.

104. Sabin KM, Frey RL Jr, Horsley R, Greby SM. Characteristics and trends of newly identified HIV infections among incarcerated populations: CDC HIV voluntary counseling, testing, and referral system, 1992-1998. J Urban Health. 2001;78:241-255.

105. Brundage JF, Burke DS, Gardner LI, et al. Tracking the spread of the HIV infection epidemic among young adults in the United States: Results of the first four years of screening among civilian applicants for U.S. military service. J Acquir Immune Defic Syndr. 1990;3:1168-1180.

106. Burke DS, Brundage JF, Goldenbaum M, et al. Human immunodeficiency virus infections in teenagers. JAMA. 1990;263:2074-2077.

107. Withers BG, Kelley PW, McNeil JG. A brief review of the epidemiology of HIV in the U.S. Army. Mil Med. 1992;157:80-84.

108. Cowan DN, Pomerantz RS, Wann ZF, et al. Human immunodeficiency virus infection among members of the reserve components of the U.S. Army: Prevalence, incidence, and demographic characteristics. J Infect Dis. 1990;162:827-836.

109. Kelley PW, Miller RN, Pomerantz R, et al. Human immunodeficiency virus seropositivity among members of the active duty U.S. Army 1985-89. Am J Public Health. 1990;80:405-410.

110. Renzullo PO, Sateren WB, Garner RP, et al. HIV-1 seroconversion in United States Army active duty personnel, 1985-1999. AIDS. 2001;15:1569-1574.

111. McNeil JG, Brundage JF, Gardner LI, et al. Trends of HIV seroconversion among young adults in the U.S. Army, 1985 to 1989. JAMA. 1991;265:1709-1714.

112. Valleroy LA, MacKellar DA, Karon JM, et al. HIV infection in disadvantaged out-of-school youth: Prevalence for US Job Corps entrants, 1990 through 1996. J Acquir Immune Defic Syndr Hum Retrovirol. 1998;19:67-73.

113. Glynn SA, Kleinman SH, Schreiber GB, et al. Trends in incidence and prevalence of major transfusion-transmissible viral infections in US blood donors, 1991 to 1996. Retrovirus Epidemiology Donor Study (REDS). JAMA. 2000;284:229-235.

114. Pappaioanou M, George RJ, Hannon WH, et al. HIV seroprevalence surveys of child-bearing women: Objectives, methods, and uses of the data. Public Health Rep. 1990;105:147-152.

115. Fisher-Davis S, Rosen DH, Steinberg S, et al. Trends in HIV prevalence among child-bearing women in the United States, 1989-1994. J Acquir Immune Defic Syndr Hum Retrovirol. 1998;19:158-164.

116. Sweeney PA, Onorato IM, Allen DM, et al. Sentinel surveillance of human immunodeficiency virus infection in women seeking reproductive health services in the United States, 1988-1989. Obstet Gynecol. 1992;79:503-510.

117. Janssen R, Satten G, Stramer S, et al. New testing strategy to detect early HIV-1 infection for use in incidence estimates and for clinical and prevention purposes. JAMA. 1998;280:42-48.

118. Pilcher CD, McPherson JT, Leone PA, et al. Real-time, universal screening for acute HIV infection in a routine HIV counseling and testing population. JAMA. 2002;288:216-221.

119. Rutherford GW, Schwarcz SK, McFarland W. Surveillance for incident HIV infection: new technology and new opportunities. J Acquir Immune Defic Syndr. 2000;25(Suppl 2):S115-S119.

120. Green TA, Karon JM, Nwanyanwu OC. Changes in AIDS incidence trends in the United States. J Acquir Immune Defic Syndr. 1992;5:547-555.

121. Selik RM, Ward JW, Buehler JW. Trends in transfusion-associated acquired immune deficiency syndrome in the United States, 1982 through 1991. Transfusion. 1993;33:890-893.

122. Berkelman R, Karon J, Thomas P, et al. Are AIDS cases among homosexual men leveling. Abstract W.A.O.13. Presented at the Fifth International Conference on AIDS. Montreal: June 4-9, 1989.

123. Gail MH, Rosenberg PS, Goedert JJ. Therapy may explain recent deficits in AIDS incidence. J Acquir Immune Defic Syndr. 1990;3:296-306.

124. Conley LJ, Holmberg SD. Transmission of AIDS from blood screened negative for antibody to the human immunodeficiency virus (Letter). N Engl J Med. 1992;326:1499-1500.

125. Neal JJ, Fleming PL, Green TA, Ward JW. Trends in heterosexually acquired AIDS in the United States, 1988 through 1995. J Acquir Immune Defic Syndr Hum Retrovirol. 1997;14:465-474.

126. Nwanyanwu OC, Conti LA, Ciesielski CA, et al. Increasing frequency of heterosexually transmitted AIDS in southern Florida: Artifact or reality? Am J Public Health. 1993;83:571-573.

127. Klevens RM, Fleming PL, Neal JJ, Li J. Is there really a heterosexual AIDS epidemic in the United States? Findings from a multisite validation study, 1992-1995. Mode of Transmission Validation Study Group. Am J Epidemiol. 1999;149:75-84.

128. Castro KG, Lifson AR, White CR, et al. Investigations of AIDS patients with no previously identified risk factors. JAMA. 1988;259:1338-1342.

129. Simonds RJ, Holmberg SD, Hurwitz RL, et al. Transmission of human immunodeficiency virus type 1 from a seronegative organ and tissue donor. N Engl J Med. 1992;326:726.

130. Centers for Disease Control and Prevention. Update: Trends in AIDS incidence, deaths and prevalence—United States, 1996. MMWR Morb Mortal Wkly Rep. 1997;46:165-173.

131. Centers for Disease Control and Prevention. AIDS among persons aged greater than or equal to 50 years—United States, 1991-1996. MMWR Morb Mortal Wkly Rep. 1998;47:21-27.

132. Centers for Disease Control and Prevention. AIDS among racial/ethnic minorities—United States, 1993. MMWR Morb Mortal Wkly Rep. 1994;43:644-655.

133. Diaz T, Buehler JW, Castro KG, et al. AIDS trends among Hispanics in the United States. Am J Public Health. 1993;83:504-509.

134. Centers for Disease Control and Prevention: Risks for HIV infection among persons residing in rural areas and small cities—selected sites, southern United States, 1995-1996. MMWR Morb Mortal Wkly Rep. 1998;47:974-978.

135. Centers for Disease Control and Prevention. HIV/AIDS Surveillance Report. 2001;13:11.

136. Thomas PA, Hindin R, Greenberg A, et al. Decreased incidence of reported AIDS cases, New York City. Abstract Th.C.707. In: Abstracts of the Sixth International Conference on AIDS, v. 1. San Francisco: 1990:301.

137. Karon J, Berkelman RL. The geographic and ethnic diversity of AIDS incidence trends in homosexual/bisexual men in the United States. J Acquir Immune Defic Syndr. 1991;4:1179-1189.

138. Centers for Disease Control and Prevention. AIDS associated with injecting drug use—United States, 1995. MMWR Morb Mortal Wkly Rep. 1996;45:392-396.

139. Selik RM, Ward JW, Buehler JW. Demographic differences in cumulative incidence rates of transfusion-associated acquired immunodeficiency syndrome. Am J Epidemiol. 1994;140:105-112.

140. Greenberg AE, Thomas PA, Landesman SH, et al. The spectrum of HIV-1-related disease among outpatients in New York City. AIDS. 1992;6:849-859.

141. Schacker T, Collier AC, Hughes J, et al. Clinical and epidemiological features of primary HIV infection. Ann Intern Med. 1996;125:257-264.

142. Daar ES, Little S, Pitt J, et al. Diagnosis of primary HIV-1 infection. Los Angeles County Primary HIV Infection Recruitment Network. Ann Intern Med. 2001;134:25-29.

143. Kahn JO, Walker BD. Current concepts: Acute human immunodeficiency virus type 1 infection. N Engl J Med. 1998;339:33-39.

144. Hardy WD, Daar ES, Sokolov RT Jr, et al. Acute neurologic deterioration in a young man. Rev Infect Dis. 1991;13:745-750.

145. Tindall B, Cooper DA. Primary HIV infection: Host responses and intervention strategies. AIDS. 1991;5:1-14.

146. Fox R, Eldred LJ, Fuchs EJ, et al. Clinical manifestations of acute infection with human immunodeficiency virus in a cohort of gay men. AIDS. 1987;1:35-38.

147. Pedersen C, Lindhardt BO, Jensen BL, et al. Clinical course of primary HIV infection: Consequences for subsequent course of infection. BMJ. 1989;299:154-157.

148. Busch MP, Lee LL, Shatten GA, et al. Time course of detection of viral and serologic markers preceding human immunodeficiency virus type 1 seroconversion: Implications for screening of blood and tissue donors. Transfusion. 1995;35:91-97.

149. Horsburgh CR Jr, Ou CY, Jason J, et al. Duration of human immunodeficiency virus infection before detection of antibody. Lancet. 1989;2:637-640.

150. Pan LZ, Sheppard HW, Winkelstein W, et al. Lack of detection of human immunodeficiency virus in persistently seronegative homosexual men with high or medium risks for infection. J Infect Dis. 1991;164:962-964.

151. Simmonds P, Lainson FAL, Cuthbert R, et al. HIV antigen and antibody detection: Variable responses to infection in the Edinburgh haemophiliac cohort. BMJ. 1988;296:593-598.

152. Yerly S, Chamot E, Deglon JJ, et al. Absence of chronic human immunodeficiency virus infection without seroconversion in intravenous drug users: A prospective and retrospective study. J Infect Dis. 1991;164:965-968.

153. Alter HJ, Epstein JS, Swenson SG, et al. Prevalence of human immunodeficiency virus type 1 p24 antigen in the US blood donors—An assessment of the efficacy of testing in donor screening. The HIV-Antigen Study Group. N Engl J Med. 1990;323:1312-1317.

154. Hecht FM, Busch MP, Rawal B, et al. Use of laboratory tests and clinical symptoms for identification of primary HIV infection. AIDS. 2002;16:1119-1129.

155. Laurence J, Siegal FP, Schattner E, et al. Acquired immunodeficiency syndrome without evidence of infection with human immunodeficiency virus types 1 and 2. Lancet. 1992;340:273-274.

156. Centers for Disease Control and Prevention: Unexplained CD4⁺ T-lymphocyte depletion in persons without evident HIV infection—United States. MMWR Morb Mortal Wkly Rep. 1992;41:541-545.

157. Smith DK, Neal JJ, Holmberg SD, et al. Unexplained opportunistic infections and CD4⁺ T-lymphocytopenia without HIV infection. An investigation of cases in the United States. N Engl J Med. 1993;328:373-379.

158. Centers for Disease Control and Prevention: Projections of the number of persons diagnosed with AIDS and the number of immunosuppressed persons—United States, 1992-1994. MMWR Morb Mortal Wkly Rep. 1992;41(RR-18):1-29.

159. Ragni MV, Kingsley LA. Cumulative risk for AIDS and other HIV outcomes in a cohort of hemophiliacs in western Pennsylvania. J Acquir Immune Defic Syndr. 1990;3:708-713.

160. Kuo JM, Taylor JMG, Detels R. Estimating the AIDS incubation period from a prevalent cohort. Am J Epidemiol. 1991;133:1050-1057.

161. Rutherford GW, Lifson AR, Hessol NA, et al. Course of HIV-1 infection in a cohort of homosexual and bisexual men: An 11 year follow up study. BMJ. 1990;301:1183-1188.

162. Lifson AR, Buchbinder SP, Sheppard HW, et al. Long-term human immunodeficiency virus infection in asymptomatic homosexual and bisexual men with normal CD4⁺ lymphocyte counts: Immunologic and virologic characteristics. J Infect Dis. 1991;163:959-965.

163. Learmont J, Tindall B, Evans L, et al. Long-term symptomless HIV-1 infection in recipients of blood products from a single donor. Lancet. 1992;340:863-867.

164. Ashton JJ, Carr A, Cunningham PM, et al. Predictors of progression in long-term non-progressors. Australian Long-term Nonprogressor Study Group. AIDS Res Hum Retrovirus. 1998;14:117-121.

165. Ward JW, Bush TJ, Perkins HA, et al. The natural history of transfusion-associated infection with human immunodeficiency virus. N Engl J Med. 1989;321:947-952.

166. Selwyn PA, Alcabes P, Hartel D, et al. Clinical manifestations and predictors of disease progression in drug users with human immunodeficiency virus infection. N Engl J Med. 1992;327:1697-1703.

167. Coates RA, Farwell VT, Raboud J, et al. Cofactors of progression to acquired immunodeficiency syndrome in a cohort of male sexual contacts of men with human immunodeficiency virus disease. Am J Epidemiol. 1990;132:717-722.

168. Kaslow RA, Blackwelder WC, Ostrow DG, et al. No evidence for a role of alcohol or other psychoactive drugs in accelerating immunodeficiency in HIV-1 positive individuals. A report from the Multicenter AIDS Cohort Study. JAMA. 1989;261: 3424-3429.

169. Goedert JJ, Kessler CM, Aledort LM, et al. A prospective study of human immunodeficiency virus type 1 infection and the development of AIDS in subjects with hemophilia. N Engl J Med. 1989;321:1141-1148.

170. Mariotto AB, Mariotti S, Pezzotti P, et al. Estimation of the acquired immunodeficiency syndrome incubation period in intravenous drug users: A comparison with male homosexuals. Am J Epidemiol. 1992;135:428-437.

171. Vermund SH, Galbraith MA, Ebner SC, et al. Human immunodeficiency virus/acquired immunodeficiency syndrome in pregnant women. Ann Epidemiol. 1992;2:773-803.

172. Klein RS, Harris CA, Small CB, et al. Oral candidiasis in high-risk patients as the initial manifestation of the acquired immunodeficiency syndrome. N Engl J Med. 1984;311:354-358.

173. Greenspan D, Greenspan JS, Hearst NG, et al. Relation of oral hairy leukoplakia to infection with the human immunodeficiency virus and the risk of developing AIDS. J Infect Dis. 1987;155:475-481.

174. Melbye M, Grossman RJ, Goedert JJ, et al. Risk of AIDS after herpes zoster. Lancet. 1987;1:728-731.

175. Stein DS, Korvick JA, Vermund SH. CD4+ lymphocyte cell enumeration for prediction of clinical course of human immunodeficiency virus disease: A review. J Infect Dis. 1992;165:352-363.

176. Mellors JW, Rinaldo CR, Gupta P, et al. Prognosis in HIV-1 infection predicted by the quantity of virus in plasma. Science. 1996;272:1167-1170.

177. Saag MS, Holodniy M, Kuritzkes DR, et al. HIV viral load markers in clinical practice. Nat Med. 1996;2:625-629.

178. Mellors JW, Muñoz A, Giorgi JV, et al. Plasma viral load and CD4+ lymphocytes as prognostic markers of HIV-infection. Ann Intern Med. 1997;126:946-954.

179. Fleming PL, Ciesielski CA, Byers RH, et al. Gender differences in reported AIDS-indicative diagnoses. J Infect Dis. 1993;168:61-67.

180. Kreiss JK, Castro KG. Special considerations for managing suspected human immunodeficiency virus infection and AIDS in patients from developing countries. J Infect Dis. 1990;162:955-960.

181. Slutsker L, Castro KG, Ward JW, et al. Epidemiology of extrapulmonary tuberculosis among persons with AIDS in the United States. Clin Infect Dis. 1993;16:513-518.

182. Karon JM, Green TA, Hanson DL, Ward JW. Estimating the number of AIDS-defining opportunistic illness diagnoses from data collected under the 1993 AIDS surveillance definition. J Acquir Immune Defic Syndr Hum Retroviral. 1997;16:116-121.

183. Jones JL, Hanson DL, Dworkin MS, et al. Trends in AIDS-related opportunistic infections among men who have sex with men and among injecting drug users, 1991-96. J Infect Dis. 1998;178:114-120.

184. Holtzer CD, Jacobson MA, Hadley WK, et al. Decline in the rate of specific opportunistic infections at the San Francisco General Hospital, 1994-1997. AIDS. 1998;12:1931-1933.

185. Maniar J, Saple DG, Kurimura T. Changing pattern of opportunistic infections. Abstract 13245. Presented at the Twelfth International Conference on AIDS, Geneva, June 28-July 3, 1998.

186. Jacobson MA, Franch M. Altered natural history of AIDS-related opportunistic infections in the era of potent combination antiretroviral therapy. AIDS. 1998;12 (Suppl A):S157-S163.

187. Mouron Y, Alfandari S, Valette M, et al. Impact of protease inhibitors on AIDS-defining events and hospitalizations in 10 French AIDS reference centers. AIDS. 1997;11:F101-F105.

188. Shelburne SA 3rd, Hamill RJ, Rodriguez-Barradas MC, et al. Immune reconstitution inflammatory syndrome: Emergence of a unique syndrome during highly active antiretroviral therapy. Medicine 2002;81:213-227.

189. Selwyn PA, Feingold AR, Hartel D, et al. Increased risk of bacterial pneumonia in HIV-infected intravenous drug users without AIDS. AIDS. 1988;2:167-172.

190. Janoff EN, Breiman RF, Daley CL, et al. Pneumococcal disease during HIV infection. Epidemiologic, clinical, and immunologic perspectives. Ann Intern Med. 1992;117:314-324.

191. Redd SC, Rutherford GW III, Sande MA, et al. The role of human immunodeficiency virus infection in pneumococcal bacteremia in San Francisco residents. J Infect Dis. 1990;162:1012-1017.

192. Laga M, Icenogle JP, Marsella R, et al. Genital papillomavirus infection and cervical dysplasia—opportunistic complications of HIV infection. Int J Cancer. 1992;50:45-48.

193. Ellerbrock T, Wright TC, Chiasson MA, et al. Strong independent association between HIV infection and cervical intraepithelial neoplasia (CIN). Abstract WSB075. In: Abstracts of the Ninth International Conference on AIDS/Fourth STD World Congress, v. 1. Berlin: 1993:50.

194. Wright T, Sun X, Ellerbrock T, et al. Human papillomavirus infections in HIV+ and HIV− women: Prevalence, association with cervical intraepithelial neoplasia, and impact of CD4+ count. Abstract WSB172. In: Abstracts of the Ninth International Conference on AIDS/Fourth STD World Congress, v. 1. Berlin: 1993:60.

195. Barnes PF, Bloch AB, Davidson PT, et al. Tuberculosis in patients with human immunodeficiency virus infection. N Engl J Med. 1991;324:1644-1650.

196. Raviglione MC, Narain JP, Kochi A. HIV-associated tuberculosis in developing countries: Clinical features, diagnosis, and treatment. Bull World Health Organ. 1992;70:515-526.

197. Markowitz N, Harnsen NI, Hopewell PC, et al. Incidence of tuberculosis in the United States among HIV-infected persons. Ann Intern Med. 1997;126:123-132.

198. Centers for Disease Control and Prevention: Prevention of tuberculosis among patients infected with human immunodeficiency virus: Principles of therapy and revised recommendations. MMWR Morb Mortal Wkly Rep. 1998;47(RR-20):1-58.

199. Braun MM, Cote TR, Rabkin CS. Trends in death with tuberculosis during the AIDS era. JAMA. 1993;269:2865-2868.

200. Rieder HL, Snider DE Jr. Tuberculosis and the acquired immunodeficiency syndrome (Editorial). Chest. 1986;90:469-470.

201. Havlir DV, Barnes PF. Tuberculosis in patients with human immunodeficiency virus infection. N Engl J Med. 1998;340:367-373.

202. Small PM, Hopewell PC, Singh SP, et al. The epidemiology of tuberculosis in San Francisco: A population based study using conventional and molecular methods. N Engl J Med. 1994;330:1703.

203. Alland D, Kalbut GE, Moss AR, et al. Transmission of tuberculosis in New York City: An analysis of DNA fingerprinting and conventional epidemiologic methods. N Engl J Med. 1994;330:1710.

204. Moore M, Onorato IM, McCoy E, Castro KG. Trends in drug-resistant tuberculosis in the United States, 1993-1996. JAMA. 1997;278:833-837.

205. Frieden TR, Sterling T, Pablos-Mendez A, et al. The emergence of drug-resistant tuberculosis in New York City. N Engl J Med. 1993;328:521-526.

206. Peloquin C, MacPhee AA, Berning SE. Malabsorption of antimycobacterial medications (Letter). N Engl J Med. 1993;329:1122.

207. Edlin BR, Tokars JI, Grieco MH, et al. An outbreak of multidrug-resistant tuberculosis among hospitalized patients with the acquired immunodeficiency syndrome. N Engl J Med. 1992;326:1514-1521.

208. Pearson ML, Jereb JA, Frieden TR, et al. Nosocomial transmission of multidrug-resistant *Mycobacterium tuberculosis*. A risk to patients and health care workers. Ann Intern Med. 1992;117:191-196.

209. BeckSague C, Dooley SW, Hutton MD, et al. Hospital outbreak of multidrug-resistant *Mycobacterium tuberculosis* infections. Factors in transmission to staff and HIV-infected patients. JAMA. 1992;268:1280-1286.

210. Centers for Disease Control and Prevention: Update: Mortality attributable to HIV-infection among persons aged 25-44 years—United States, 1994. MMWR Morb Mortal Wkly Rep. 1996;45:121-125.

211. Centers for Disease Control and Prevention: Years of potential life lost before age 65—United States, 1990 and 1991. MMWR Morb Mortal Wkly Rep. 1993;42:251-252.

212. Fordyce EJ, Singh TP, Nash D, et al. Survival Rates in NYC in the Era of Combination ART. J Acquir Immune Defic Syndr. 2002;30:111-118.

213. Murphy EL, Collier AC, Kallish LA, et al. Highly active antiretroviral therapy decreases mortality and morbidity in patients with advanced HIV disease. Ann Intern Med. 2001;135:17-26.

214. Turner BJ, Eppes S, McKee LJ, et al. A population-based comparison of the clinical course of children and adults with AIDS. AIDS. 1995;9:65-72.

215. Duliege AM, Messiah A, Blanche S, et al. Natural history of human immunodeficiency virus type 1 infection in children: Prognostic value of laboratory tests on the bimodal progression of the disease. Pediatr Infect Dis J. 1992;11:630-635.

216. McKinney RE Jr, Wilfert CM. Lymphocyte subsets in children younger than 2 years old: Normal values in a population at risk for human immunodeficiency virus infection and diagnostic and prognostic application to infected children. Pediatr Infect Dis J. 1992;11:639-644.

217. Waecker NJ Jr, Ascher DP, Robb ML, et al. Age-adjusted CD4+ lymphocyte parameters in healthy children at risk for infection with human immunodeficiency virus. Clin Infect Dis. 1993;17:123-125.

218. Quinn TC, Ruff A, Modlin J. HIV infection and AIDS in children. Annu Rev Public Health. 1992;13:1-30.

219. Centers for Disease Control and Prevention: AIDS among children—United States, 1996. MMWR Morb Mortal Wkly Rep. 1996;45:1005-1010.

220. Lifson AR, Rogers MF, White C, et al. Unrecognized modes of transmission of HIV: Acquired immunodeficiency syndrome in children reported without risk factors. Pediatr Infect Dis. 1987;6:292-293.

221. Connor EM, Sperling RS, Gelber R, et al. Reduction of maternal-infant transmission of human immunodeficiency virus type 1 with zidovudine treatment. N Engl J Med. 1994;331:1173-1180.

222. Centers for Disease Control and Prevention: Recommendations of the US Public Health Service Task Force on the use of zidovudine to reduce perinatal transmission of human immunodeficiency virus. MMWR Morb Mortal Wkly Rep. 1994;43(RR-11):1-20.

223. Centers for Disease Control and Prevention: US Public Health Service Recommendations for human immunodeficiency virus counseling and testing for pregnant women. MMWR Morb Mortal Wkly Rep. 1995;44(RR-7):1-15.

224. Centers for Disease Control and Prevention: Guidelines for prophylaxis against *Pneumocystis carinii* pneumonia for children infected with human immunodeficiency virus. MMWR Morb Mortal Wkly Rep. 1991;40(RR-2):1-13.

225. Scott GB, Hutto C, Makuch RW, et al. Survival in children with perinatally acquired human immunodeficiency virus type 1 infection. N Engl J Med. 1989;321:1791-1796.

226. Turner BJ, Denison M, Eppes SC, et al. Survival experience of 789 children with the acquired immunodeficiency syndrome. Pediatr Infect Dis J. 1993;12:310-320.

227. Centers for Disease Control and Prevention: Public Health Service recommendations for the use of antiretroviral drugs in pregnant HIV-1 infected women for maternal health and interventions to reduce perinatal HIV-1 transmission in the United States. MMWR Morb Mortal Wkly Rep. 2002;51:1-38.

228. Chin J, Sato PA, Mann JM. Projections of HIV infections and AIDS cases to the year 2000. Bull World Health Organ. 1990;68:1-11.

229. Samuel MC, Hessol N, Shiboski S, et al. Factors associated with human immunodeficiency virus seroconversion in homosexual men in three San Francisco cohorts. J Acquir Immune Defic Syndr. 1993;6:303.

230. Cohen MS. Sexually transmitted diseases enhance HIV transmission: No longer a hypothesis. Lancet. 1998;351(Suppl 3):S5-S7.

231. Quinn TC. Association of sexually transmitted diseases and infection with the human immunodeficiency virus: Biological cofactors and markers of behavioral interventions. Int J STD AIDS. 1996;7(Suppl 2):S17-S24.

232. Fleming DT, Wasserheit JN. From epidemiological synergy to public health policy and practice: The contribution of other sexually transmitted diseases to sexual transmission of HIV infection. Sex Trans Infect. 1999;75:3-17.

233. Wawer MJ, Serwadda D, Li X, et al. HIV-1 Transmission per Coital Act, by Stage of HIV Infection in the HIV+ Index Partner, in Discordant Couples, Rakai, Uganda. Abstract 40. In: Program and Abstracts 10th Conference on Retrovirus and Opportunistic Infections, Boston, Mass, February 2003.

234. Vittinghoff E, Douglas J, Judson F, et al. Per-contact risk of human immunodeficiency virus transmission between male sexual partners. Am J Epidemiol. 1999;150:306-311.

235. Clumeck N, Taelman H, Hermans P, et al. A cluster of HIV infection among heterosexual people without apparent risk factors. N Engl J Med. 1989;321:1460-1462.

236. Peterman TA, Stoneburner RL, Allen JR, et al. Risk of human immunodeficiency virus transmission from heterosexual adults with transfusion-associated infections. JAMA. 1988;59:55-58.

237. Johnson AM, Petherick A, Davidson SJ, et al. Transmission of HIV to heterosexual partners of infected men and women. AIDS. 1989;3:367-372.

238. Seidlin M, Vogler M, Lee E, et al. Heterosexual transmission of HIV in a cohort of couples in New York City. AIDS. 1993;7:1247.

239. Goedert JJ, Eyster ME, Bigger RJ, et al. Heterosexual transmission of human immunodeficiency virus: Association with severe depletion of T-helper lymphocytes in men with hemophilia. AIDS Res Hum Retroviruses. 1987;3:355-361.

240. European Study Group on Heterosexual Transmission of HIV. Comparison of female to male and male to female transmission of HIV in 563 stable couples. BMJ. 1992;304:809-813.

241. Lazzarin A, Saracco A, Musicco M, et al. Man-to-woman sexual transmission of the human immunodeficiency virus. Risk factors related to sexual behavior, man's infectiousness, and woman's susceptibility. Arch Intern Med. 1991;151:2411-2416.

242. Laga M, Taelman H, Van der Stuyft P, et al. Advanced immunodeficiency as a risk factor for heterosexual transmission of HIV. AIDS. 1989;3:361-366.

243. Seage GR III, Mayer KH, Horsburgh CR Jr. Risk of human immunodeficiency virus infection from unprotected receptive anal intercourse increases with decline in immunologic status of infected partners. Am J Epidemiol. 1993;137:899-908.

244. Anderson DJ, Hill JA. CD4 (T4+) lymphocytes in semen of healthy heterosexual men: Implications for the transmission of AIDS (Letter). Fertil Steril. 1987;48:703-704.

245. Anderson DJ, O'Brien TR, Politch JA, et al. Effects of disease stage and zidovudine therapy on the detection of human immunodeficiency virus type 1 in semen. JAMA. 1992;267:2769-2774.

246. Ho DD, Moudgil T, Alam M. Quantitation of human immunodeficiency virus type 1 in the blood of infected persons. N Engl J Med. 1989;321:1621-1625.

247. Hénin Y, Mandelbrot L, Henrion R, et al. Virus excretion in the cervical secretions of pregnant and nonpregnant HIV-infected women. J Acquir Immune Defic Syndr. 1993;6:72-75.

248. Pilcher CD, Eron JJ Jr, Vernazza PL, et al. Sexual transmission during the incubation period of primary HIV infection. JAMA. 2001;286:1713-1714.

249. Cates W Jr, Chesney MA, Cohen MS. Primary HIV infection—A public health opportunity. Am J Public Health. 1997;87:1928-1930.

250. Quinn TC, Wawer MJ, Sewankambo N, et al. Viral load and heterosexual transmission of human immunodeficiency virus type 1. Rakai Project Study Group. N Engl J Med. 2000;342:921-929.

251. Garcia PM, Kalish LA, Pitt J, et al. Maternal levels of plasma human immunodeficiency virus type 1 RNA and the risk of perinatal transmission. Women and Infants Transmission Study Group. N Engl J Med. 1999;341:394-402.

252. Vernazza PL, Eron JJ, Cohen MS, et al. Detection and biologic characterization of infectious HIV-1 in semen of seropositive men. AIDS. 1994;8:1325-1329.

253. Krieger JM, Coombs RW, Collier AC, et al. Recovery of human immunodeficiency virus type 1 from semen: Minimal impact of stage of infection and current antiviral chemotherapy. J Infect Dis. 1991;163:386-388.

254. Musicco M, Lazzarin A, Nicolasi A, et al. Antiretroviral treatment of men infected with human immunodeficiency virus type 1 reduces the incidence of heterosexual transmission: Italian Study Group on HIV Heterosexual Transmission. Arch Intern Med. 1994;154:1971-1976.

255. Hosseinipour M, Cohen MS, Vernazza PL, Kashuba AD. Can antiretroviral therapy be used to prevent sexual transmission of human immunodeficiency virus type 1? Clin Infect Dis. 2002;34:1391-1395.

256. Zhang H, Dornadula G, Beumont M, et al. Human immunodeficiency virus type 1 in the semen of men receiving highly active antiretroviral therapy. N Engl J Med. 1998;339:1803-1809.

257. Rasheed S, Li Z, Xu D, Kovacs A. Presence of cell-free human immunodeficiency virus in cervicovaginal secretions is independent of viral load in the blood in human immunodeficiency virus-infected women. Am J Obstet Gynecol. 1996;175:122-129.

258. Eron JJ, Vernazza PL, Johnston DM, et al. Resistance of HIV-1 to antiretroviral agents in blood and seminal plasma: Implications for transmission. AIDS. 1998;12:F181-F189.

259. Haase AT, Schacker TW. Potential for transmission of HIV-1 despite highly active antiretroviral therapy. N Engl J Med. 1998;339:1846-1848.

260. Padian NS, Shiboski SC, Jewell NP. Female-to-male transmission of human immunodeficiency virus. JAMA. 1991;266:1664-1667.

261. Padian NS, Shiboski SC, Jewell NP. The effect of number of exposures on the risk of heterosexual HIV transmission. J Infect Dis. 1990;161:883-887.

262. Rothenberg RB, Scarlett M, del Rio C, et al. Oral transmission of HIV. AIDS. 1998;12:2095-2105.

263. Goto Y, Yeh CK, Notkins AL, et al. Detection of proviral sequences in saliva of patients infected with human immunodeficiency virus type 1. AIDS Res Hum Retroviruses. 1991;7:343-347.

264. Levy JA, Greenspan D. HIV in saliva (Letter). Lancet. 1988;2:1248.

265. Piot P, Plummer PA. Genital ulcer adenopathy syndrome. In: Holmes KK, Mardh PA, Sparling PF, eds. Sexually Transmitted Diseases. 2nd ed. New York: McGraw-Hill; 1990:711-716.

266. Piot P, Laga M. Genital ulcers, other sexually transmitted diseases, and the sexual transmission of HIV. The first two may be important risk factors for the third. BMJ. 1989;298:623-624.

267. Plummer FA, Simonsen JN, Cameron DW, et al. Cofactors in male-female sexual transmission of human immunodeficiency virus type 1. J Infect Dis. 1991;163:233-239.

268. Cameron DW, Simonsen JN, D'Costa LJ, et al. Female to male transmission of human immunodeficiency virus type 1: Risk factors for seroconversion in men. Lancet. 1989;2:403-407.

269. Dyer JR, Eron JJ, Hoffman IF, et al. Association of CD4 cell depletion and elevated blood and seminal plasma human immunodeficiency virus type 1 (HIV-1) RNA concentrations with genital ulcer disease in HIV-1-infected men in Malawi. J Infect Dis. 1998;177:224-227.

270. Hray RH, Wawer MJ, Li X, et al. Determinants of HIV Viral Load in Incident and Prevalent Infections, Rakai, Uganda. Abstract 908. In: Program and Abstracts 10th Conference on Retrovirus and Opportunistic Infections, Boston, Mass, February 2003.

271. Stamm WE, Handsfield HH, Rompalo AM, et al. The association between genital ulcer disease and acquisition of HIV infection in homosexual men. JAMA. 1988;260:1429-1433.

272. Kreiss KJ, Coombs R, Plummer F, et al. Isolation of human immunodeficiency virus from genital ulcers in Nairobi prostitutes. J Infect Dis. 1989;160:380-384.

273. Moss GB, Overbaugh J, Welch M, et al. Human immunodeficiency virus DNA in urethral secretions in men: Association with gonococcal urethritis and CD4 depletion. J Infect Dis. 1995;172:1469-1474.

274. Atkins MC, Carlin EM, Emery VC, et al. Fluctuations of HIV load in semen of HIV positive patients with newly acquired sexually transmitted diseases. BMJ. 1996;313:341-342.

275. Cohen MS, Hoffman IF, Royce RA, et al. Reduction of concentration of HIV-1 in semen after treatment of urethritis: Implications for prevention of sexual transmission of HIV-1. AIDSCAP Malawi Research Group (Journal Article). Lancet. 1997;349:1868-1873.

276. Greenblatt RM, Lukehart SA, Plummer FA, et al. Genital ulceration as a risk factor for human immunodeficiency virus infection. AIDS. 1988;2:47-50.

277. Holmberg SD, Stewart JA, Gerber AR, et al. Prior herpes simplex virus type 2 infection as a risk factor for HIV infection. JAMA. 1988;259:1048-1050.

278. Laga M, Manoka A, Kivuvu M, et al. Non-ulcerative sexually transmitted diseases as risk factor for HIV-1 transmission in women: Results from a cohort study. AIDS. 1993;7:95-102.

279. Kapiga SH, Shao JF, Lwihula GK, et al. Risk factors for HIV infection among women in Dar-es-Salaam, Tanzania. J Acquir Immune Defic Syndr. 1994;7:301-309.

280. Cohen CR, Duerr A, Pruithithada N, et al. Bacterial vaginosis and HIV seroprevalence among female commercial sex workers in Chaing Mai, Thailand. AIDS. 1995;9:1093-1097.

281. Hira SK, Kamanga J, Macuacua R, et al. Genital ulcers and male circumcision as risk factors for acquiring HIV-1 in Zambia (Letter). J Infect Dis. 1990;161:584-585.

282. Jessamine PG, Plummer FA, Achola JON, et al. Human immunodeficiency virus, genital ulcers and the male foreskin: Synergism in HIV-1 transmission. Scand J Infect Dis. 1990;69(Suppl):S181-S186.

283. Kreiss J, Ngugi E, Holmes K, et al. Efficacy of nonoxynol 9 contraceptive sponge use in preventing heterosexual acquisition of HIV in Nairobi prostitutes. JAMA. 1992;268:477-482.

284. Stone KM, Peterson HB. Spermicides, HIV, and the vaginal sponge (Editorial). JAMA. 1992;268:521-523.

285. Grosskurth H, Mosha F, Todd J, et al. Impact of improved treatment of sexually transmitted diseases on HIV infection in rural Tanzania: Randomized controlled trial. Lancet. 1995;346:530-536.

286. Darrow WW, Echenberg DF, Jaffe HW, et al. Risk factors for human immunodeficiency virus (HIV) infections in homosexual men. Am J Public Health. 1987;77:479-483.

287. Winkelstein W, Lyman DM, Padian N, et al. Sexual practices and risk of infection by the human immunodeficiency virus. The San Francisco Men's Health Study. JAMA. 1987;257:321-325.

288. Kingsley LA, Detels R, Kaslow R, et al. Risk factors for seroconversion to human immunodeficiency virus among male homosexuals. Results from the Multicenter AIDS Cohort Study. Lancet. 1987;1:345-349.

289. Chu SY, Hammett TA, Buehler JW. Update: Epidemiology of reported cases of AIDS in women who report sex only with other women, United States, 1980-1991. AIDS. 1992;6:518.

290. Kral AH, Lorvick J, Bluthenthal RN, Watters JK. HIV risk profile of drug-using women who have sex with women in 19 United States cities. J Acquir Immune Defic Syndr Hum Retrovirol. 1997;16:211-217.

291. Marrazzo JM, Koutsky LA, Handsfield HH. Characteristics of female sexually transmitted disease clinic clients who report same-sex behaviour. Int J STD AIDS. 2001;12:41-46.

292. Petersen LR, Doll L, White C, et al. No evidence for female-to-female HIV transmission among 960,000 female blood donors. J Acquir Immune Defic Syndr. 1992;5:853-855.

293. Marmor M, Weiss LR, Lyden M, et al. Possible female-to-female transmission of human immunodeficiency virus (Letter). Ann Intern Med. 1986;105:969.

294. Monzon OT, Capellan JMB. Female-to-female transmission of HIV (Letter). Lancet. 1987;2:40-41.

295. Rich JD, Buck A, Tuomala RE, et al. Transmission of human immunodeficiency virus infection presumed to have occurred via female-homosexual contact. Clin Infect Dis. 1993;17:1003.

296. Moss GB, Clemetson D, D'Costa L, et al. Association of cervical ectopy with heterosexual transmission of human immunodeficiency virus: Results of a study of couples in Nairobi, Kenya. J Infect Dis. 1991;164:588-591.

297. Stephenson JM. Systematic review of hormonal contraception and risk of HIV transmission: When to resist meta-analysis. AIDS 1998;12:545-553.

298. Dean M, Carrington M, Winkler C, et al. Genetic restriction of HIV-1 infection and progression to AIDS by a deletion allele of the CKR5 structural gene. Science. 1996;273:1856-1862.

299. Schoenbaum EE, Hartel D, Selwyn PA, et al. Risk factors for human immunodeficiency virus infection in intravenous drug users. N Engl J Med. 1989;321:874-879.

300. Lange WR, Synder FR, Lozovsky D, et al. The geographic distribution of human immunodeficiency virus markers in parenteral drug abusers. Am J Public Health. 1988;78:443-446.

301. Anthony JC, Vlahov D, Nelson KE, et al. New evidence on intravenous cocaine use and the risk of infection with human immunodeficiency virus type 1. Am J Epidemiol. 1991;134:1175-1189.

302. Koblin BA, McCusker J, Lewis BF, et al. Racial/ethnic differences in HIV-1 seroprevalence and risky behaviors among intravenous drug users in a multisite study. Am J Epidemiol. 1990;132:837-846.

303. Fernando D, Schilling RF, Fontdevila J, El-Bassel N. Predictors of sharing drugs among injection drug users in the South Bronx: Implications for HIV transmission. J Psychoactive Drugs. 2003;35:227-236.

304. Selik RM, Castro KG, Pappaioanou M, et al. Birthplace and the risk of AIDS among Hispanics in the United States. Am J Public Health. 1989;79:836-839.

305. McCusker J, Koblin B, Lewis BF, et al. Demographic characteristics, risk behaviors, and HIV seroprevalence among intravenous drug users by site of contact: Results from a communitywide HIV surveillance project. Am J Public Health. 1990;80: 1062-1067.

306. Nelson KE, Vlahov D, Cohn S, et al. Sexually transmitted diseases in a population of intravenous drug users: Association with seropositivity to the human immunodeficiency virus (HIV). J Infect Dis. 1991;164:457-463.

307. Rolfs RT, Goldberg M, Sharrar RG. Risk factors for syphilis: Cocaine use and prostitution. Am J Public Health. 1990;80:853-857.

308. Magura S, Grossman JI, Lipton DS, et al. Determinants of needle sharing among intravenous drug users. Am J Public Health. 1989;79:459-462.

309. Guydish JR, Abramowitz A, Woods W, et al. Changes in needle sharing behavior among intravenous drug users: San Francisco, 1986-88. Am J Public Health. 1990;80:995-997.

310. Neaigus A, Sufian M, Friedman SR, et al. Effects of outreach intervention on risk reduction among intravenous drug users. AIDS Educ Prev. 1990;2:253-271.

311. Curran JW, Lawrence DN, Jaffe H, et al. Acquired immunodeficiency syndrome (AIDS) associated with transfusions. N Engl J Med. 1984;310:69-75.

312. Evatt BL, Ramsey RB, Lawrence DN, et al. The acquired immunodeficiency syndrome in patients with hemophilia. Ann Intern Med. 1984;100:499-504.

313. Donegan E, Stuart M, Niland JC, et al. Infection with human immunodeficiency virus type 1 (HIV1) among recipients of antibody-positive blood donations. Ann Intern Med. 1990;113:733-739.

314. Ward JW, Deppe DA, Samson S, et al. Risk of human immunodeficiency virus infection from blood donors who later developed the acquired immunodeficiency syndrome. Ann Intern Med. 1987;106:61-62.

315. Centers for Disease Control and Prevention: Safety of therapeutic immune globulin preparations with respect to transmission of human T-lymphotropic virus type III/lymphadenopathy-associated virus infection. MMWR Morb Mortal Wkly Rep. 1986;35:231-233.

316. Wells MA, Wittek AE, Epstein JS, et al. Inactivation and partition of human T-cell lymphotropic virus, type III, during ethanol fractionation of plasma. Transfusion. 1986;26:210-213.

317. Ward JW, Grindon AJ, Feorino PM, et al. Laboratory and epidemiologic evaluation of an enzyme immunoassay for antibodies to HTL V-III. JAMA. 1986;256:357-361.

318. Peterman TA, Lui KJ, Lawrence DN, et al. Estimating the risks of transfusion-associated acquired immune deficiency syndrome and human immunodeficiency virus infection. Transfusion. 1987;27:371-374.

319. Lackritz EM, Satten GA, Aberle-Grasse J, et al. Estimated risk of transmission of the human immunodeficiency virus by screened blood in the United States. N Engl J Med. 1995;333:1721-1725.

320. Schreiber GB, Bush MP, Kleinman SH, Korelitz JJ. The risk of transfusion-transmitted viral infections. N Engl J Med. 1996;334:1635-1690.

321. FDA Approves First Nucleic Acid Test (NAT) System to Screen Whole Blood Donors for Infections with Human Immunodeficiency Virus (HIV) and Hepatitis C Virus (HCV). Available at: www.fda.gov/bbs/topics/ANSWERS/2002/ANS01140.html.

322. Dodd RY, Notari EP 4th, Stramer SL. Current prevalence and incidence of infectious disease markers and estimated window-period risk in the American Red Cross blood donor population. Transfusion 2002;42:975-979.

323. Stehr-Green JK, Jason JM, Evatt BL, et al. Geographic variability of hemophilia-associated AIDS in the United States: Effect of population characteristics. Am J Hematol. 1989;32:178-183.

324. Eyster ME, Gail MH, Ballard ID, et al. Natural history of human immunodeficiency virus infection in hemophiliacs: Effects of T-cell subsets, platelet counts and age. Ann Intern Med. 1987;107:1-6.

325. Erice A, Rhame FS, Heussner RC, et al. Human immunodeficiency virus infection in patients with solid-organ transplants: Report of five cases and review. Rev Infect Dis. 1991;13:537-547.

326. Clarke JA. HIV transmission and skin grafts. Lancet. 1987;1:983.

327. Pepose JS, McRae S, Quinn TC, et al. Serologic markers after the transplantation of corneas from donors infected with human immunodeficiency virus. Am J Ophthalmol. 1987;103:798-801.

328. Glasser DB. Serologic testing of cornea donors. Cornea. 1998;17:123-128.

329. Lewis SH, Reynolds-Kohler C, Fox HE, et al. HIV-1 in trophoblastic and villous Hofbauer cells, and haematological precursors in eight-week fetuses. Lancet. 1990;335:565-568.

330. Douglas GC, King BF. Maternal-fetal transmission of human immunodeficiency virus: A review of possible routes and cellular mechanisms of infection. Clin Infect Dis. 1992;15:678-691.

331. Krivine A, Firtion G, Cao L, et al. HIV replication during the first weeks of life. Lancet. 1992;339:1187-1189.

332. Rogers MF, Ou CY, Rayfield M, et al. Use of the polymerase chain reaction for early detection of the proviral sequences of human immunodeficiency virus in infants born to seropositive mothers. N Engl J Med. 1989;320:1649-1654.

333. Burgard M, Mayaux MJ, Blanche S, et al. The use of viral culture and p24 antigen testing to diagnose human immunodeficiency virus infection in neonates. N Engl J Med. 1992;327:1192-1197.

334. Rogers MF, Schochetman G, Hoff R. Advances in diagnosis of HIV infection in infants. In: Pizzo PA, Wilfert CM, eds. Pediatric AIDS: The Challenge of HIV Infection in Infants, Children and Adolescents. 2nd ed. Baltimore: Williams & Wilkins; 1994:219-238.

335. Ehrnst A, Lindgren S, Dictor M, et al. HIV in pregnant women and their offspring: Evidence for late transmission. Lancet. 1991;338:203-207.

336. European Collaborative Study. Risk factors for mother-to-child transmission of HIV-1. Lancet. 1992;339:1007-1012.

337. Gabiano C, Tovo PA, de Martino M, et al. Mother-to-child transmission of human immunodeficiency virus type 1: Risk of infection and correlates of transmission. Pediatrics. 1992;90:369-374.

338. Blanche S, Rouzioux C, Moscato MLG, et al. A prospective study of infants born to women seropositive for human immunodeficiency virus type 1. N Engl J Med. 1989;320:1643-1648.

339. Hutto C, Parks WP, Lai S, et al. A hospital-based prospective study of perinatal infection with human immunodeficiency virus type 1. J Pediatr. 1991;118:347-353.

340. Goedert JJ, Duliege AM, Amos CI, et al. High risk of HIV-1 infection for firstborn twins. Lancet. 1991;338:1471-1475.

341. The International Perinatal HIV Group. The mode of delivery and the risk of vertical transmission of human immunodeficiency virus type 1-a meta-analysis of 15 prospective cohort studies. N Engl J Med. 1999;340:977-987.

342. Dominguez KL, Lindegren ML, D'Almada PJ, et al. Increasing trend of cesarean deliveries in HIV-infected women in the United States from 1994 to 2000. J Acquir Immune Defic Syndr. 2003;33:232-238.

343. Thiry L, Sprecher-Goldberger S, Jonckheer T, et al. Isolation of AIDS virus from cell-free breast milk of three healthy virus carriers (Letter). Lancet. 1985;2:891-892.

344. Oxtoby MJ. Human immunodeficiency virus and other viruses in human milk: Placing the issues in broader perspective. Pediatr Infect Dis J. 1988;7:825-835.

345. Phuapradit W. Timing and mechanism of perinatal human immunodeficiency virus-1 infection. Aust N Z J Obstet Gynaecol. 1998;38:293-297.

346. Ryder RW, Manzila T, Baende E, et al. Evidence from Zaire that breastfeeding by HIV-1 seropositive mothers is not a major route for perinatal HIV-1 transmission but does decrease morbidity. AIDS. 1991;5:709-714.

347. Dunn DT, Newell ML, Ades AE, et al. Risk of human immunodeficiency virus type 1 transmission through breastfeeding. Lancet. 1992;340:585-588.

348. Van de Perre P, Simonon A, Msellati P, et al. Postnatal transmission of human immunodeficiency virus type 1 from mother to infant. A prospective cohort study in Kigali, Rwanda. N Engl J Med. 1991;325:593-598.

349. Palasithran P, Ziegler JB, Stewart GJ, et al. Breastfeeding during primary human immunodeficiency virus infection and risk of transmission from mother to infant. J Infect Dis. 1993;167:441.

350. Hu DJ, Heyward WL, Byers RH Jr, et al. HIV infection and breastfeeding: Policy implications through a decision analysis model. AIDS. 1992;6:1505-1513.

351. Ryder RW, Nsa W, Hassig SE, et al. Perinatal transmission of the human immunodeficiency virus type 1 to infants of seropositive women in Zaire. N Engl J Med. 1989;320:1637-1642.

352. Mofenson LM, Lambert JS, Stiehm ER, et al. Risk factors for perinatal transmission of human immunodeficiency virus type 1 in women treated with zidovudine. N Engl J Med. 1999;341:385-393.

353. Jamieson DJ, Sibailly TS, Sadek R, et al. HIV-1 viral load and other risk factors for mother-to-child transmission of HIV-1 in a breast-feeding population in Cote d'Ivoire. J Acquir Immune Defic Syndr. 2003 Dec 1;34:430-436.

354. St. Louis ME, Kamenga M, Brown C, et al. Risk for perinatal HIV-1 transmission according to maternal immunologic, virologic, and placental factors. JAMA. 1993;269:2853-2859.

355. Kuhn L, Steketee RW, Weedon J, et al. Distinct risk factors for intrauterine and intrapartum human immunodeficiency virus transmission and consequences for disease progression in infected children. J Infect Dis. 1999;179:52-58.

356. Landsman SH, Kalish LA, Burns DN, et al. Obstetrical factors and the transmission of human immunodeficiency virus type 1 from mother to child. N Engl J Med. 1996;334:1617-1623.

357. Borkowsky W, Krasinski K, Pollack H, et al. Early diagnosis of human immunodeficiency virus infection in children <6 months of age: Comparison of polymerase chain reaction, culture, and plasma antigen capture techniques. J Infect Dis. 1992;166:616-619.

358. Report of a Consensus Workshop, Siena, Italy, January 17-18, 1992. Early diagnosis of HIV infection in infants. J Acquir Immune Defic Syndr. 1992;5:1169-1178.

359. Nesheim S, Lee F, Sawyer M, et al. Diagnosis of human immunodeficiency virus infection by enzyme-linked immunospot assays in a prospectively followed cohort of infants of human immunodeficiency virus-seropositive women. Pediatr Infect Dis J. 1992;11:635-639.

360. Tokars JI, Bell DM, Culver DH, et al. Percutaneous injuries during surgical procedures. JAMA. 1992;267:2899-2904.

361. Marcus R, Culver DH, Bell DM, et al. Risk of human immunodeficiency virus infection among emergency department workers. Am J Med. 1993;94:363-370.

362. Wong ES, Stotka JL, Chinchilli VM, et al. Are universal precautions effective in reducing the number of occupational exposures among health care workers? A prospective study of physicians on a medical service. JAMA. 1991;265:1123-1128.

363. Tokars JI, Marcus R, Culver DH, et al. Surveillance of HIV infection and zidovudine use among health care workers after occupational exposure to HIV-infected blood. Ann Intern Med. 1993;118:913-919.

364. Henderson DK, Fahey BJ, Willy M, et al. Risk for occupational transmission of human immunodeficiency virus type 1 (HIV 1) associated with clinical exposures. A prospective evaluation. Ann Intern Med. 1990;113:740-746.

365. Gerberding JL. Incidence and prevalence of human immunodeficiency virus, hepatitis B virus, hepatitis C virus and cytomegalovirus among health care personnel at risk for blood exposure: Final report from a longitudinal study. J Infect Dis. 1994;170:1410-1417.

366. Ippolito G, Puro V, De Carli G. The risk of occupational human immunodeficiency virus infection in health care workers. Italian multicenter study. Arch Intern Med. 1993;153:1451-1458.

367. Chamberland ME, Conley LJ, Bush TJ, et al. Health care workers with AIDS. National surveillance update. JAMA. 1991;266:3459-3462.

368. Updated U.S. Public Health Service guidelines for the management of occupational exposures to HBV, HCV, and HIV and recommendations for postexposure prophylaxis. MMWR Morb Mortal Wkly Rep. 2001;50:1-52.

369. Centers for Disease Control and Prevention. HIV/AIDS surveillance report. v. 12. no. 1. Atlanta: Centers for Disease Control and Prevention, 2000:24.

370. Cardo DM, Colver DH, Ciesielski CA, et al. A case-control study of HIV seroconversion in health-care workers after percutaneous exposure. N Engl J Med. 1997;337:1485-1490.

371. Chamberland ME, Bell DM. HIV transmission from health care worker to patient: What is the risk (Editorial)? Ann Intern Med. 1992;116:871-873.

372. Gerberding J. Provider-to-patient HIV transmission: How to keep it exceedingly rare. Ann Intern Med. 1999;130:1-6.

373. Ciesielski C, Marianos D, Ou CY, et al. Transmission of human immunodeficiency virus in a dental practice. Ann Intern Med. 1992;116:798-805.

374. Centers for Disease Control and Prevention: Update: Investigations of patients who have been treated by HIV-infected healthcare workers—United States. MMWR Morb Mortal Wkly Rep. 1993;42:329-337.

375. Lot F, Séguier JC, Fégueux S, et al. Probable transmission of HIV from an orthopedic surgeon to a patient in France. Ann Intern Med. 1999;130:1-6.

376. Ou CY, Ciesielski CA, Myers G, et al. Molecular epidemiology of HIV transmission in a dental practice. Science. 1992;256:1165-1171.

377. Bell DM, Shapiro CN, Gooch BF. Preventing HIV transmission to patients during invasive procedures. J Public Health Dent. 1993;53:170-173.

378. Robert LM, Chamberland ME, Cleveland JL, et al. Investigations of patients of health care workers infected with HIV: the Centers for Disease Control and Prevention database. Ann Intern Med. 1995;122:653.

379. Centers for Disease Control and Prevention. Patient exposures to HIV during nuclear medicine procedures. MMWR Morb Mortal Wkly Rep. 1992;41:575-578.

380. Centers for Disease Control and Prevention. HIV infection in two brothers receiving intravenous therapy for hemophilia. MMWR Morb Mortal Wkly Rep. 1992;41:228-231.

381. Centers for Disease Control and Prevention. Human immunodeficiency virus transmission in household settings—United States. MMWR Morb Mortal Wkly Rep. 1994;43:347, 353-356.

382. Hersh BS, Popovici F, Apetrei RC, et al. Acquired immunodeficiency syndrome in Romania. Lancet. 1991;338:645-649.

383. Pokrovsky VV, Eramova EU. Nosocomial outbreak of HIV infection in Elista, USSR. Abstract W.A.O.5. Presented at the Fifth International Conference on AIDS. Montreal, June 4-9, 1989.

384. Chant K, Lowe D, Rubin G, et al. Patient-to-patient transmission of HIV in private surgical consulting rooms (Letter). Lancet. 1993;342:1548-1549.

385. Fujikawa LS, Salahuddin SZ, Palestine AG, et al. Isolation of human T-lymphotropic virus type III from the tears of a patient with the acquired immunodeficiency syndrome. Lancet. 1985;2:529-530.

386. Ho DD, Rota TR, Schooley RT, et al. Isolation of HTL V-III from cerebrospinal fluid and neural tissues of patients with neurologic syndromes related to the acquired immunodeficiency syndrome. N Engl J Med. 1985;313:1493-1497.

387. Mundy DC, Schinazi RF, Gerber AR, et al. Human immunodeficiency virus isolated from amniotic fluid (Letter). Lancet. 1987;2:459-460.

388. Hill DR. HIV infection following motor vehicle trauma in central Africa. JAMA. 1989;261:3282-3283.

389. Torre D, Sampietro C, Ferraro G, et al. Transmission of HIV-1 infection via sports injury (Letter). Lancet. 1990;335:1105.

390. Stewart GJ, Tyler JPP, Cunningham AL, et al. Transmission of human T-cell lymphotropic virus type III (HTL V-III) by artificial insemination by donor. Lancet. 1985;2:581-585.

391. Chiasson MA, Stoneburner RL, Joseph SC. Human immunodeficiency virus transmission through artificial insemination. J Acquir Immune Defic Syndr. 1990;3:69-72.

392. Centers for Disease Control and Prevention: HIV-1 infection and artificial insemination with processed semen. MMWR Morb Mortal Wkly Rep. 1990;39:249, 255-256.

393. Yeh CK, Handelman B, Fox PC, et al. Further studies of salivary inhibition of HIV-1 infectivity. J Acquir Immun Defic Syndr. 1992;5:898-903.

394. Wahn V, Kramer HH, Voit T, et al. Horizontal transmission of HIV infection between two siblings (Letter). Lancet. 1986;2:694.

395. Rogers MF, White CR, Sanders R, et al. Lack of transmission of human immunodeficiency virus from infected children to their household contacts. Pediatrics. 1990;85:210-214.

396. Saviteer SM, White GC, Cohen MS, et al. HTLV-III exposure during cardiopulmonary resuscitation (Letter). N Engl J Med. 1985;313:1606-1607.

397. Lifson AR. Do alternate modes for transmission of human immunodeficiency virus exist? A review. JAMA. 1988;259:1353-1356.

398. Gershon RRM, Vlahov D, Nelson KE. The risk of transmission of HIV-1 through nonpercutaneous, nonsexual modes—A review. AIDS. 1990;4:645-650.

399. Lusher JM, Operskalski EA, Aledort LM, et al. Risk of human immunodeficiency virus type 1 infection among sexual and nonsexual household contacts of persons with congenital clotting disorders. Pediatrics. 1991;88:242-249.

400. Centers for Disease Control and Prevention: Apparent transmission of human T-lymphotrophic virus type III/lymphadenopathy-associated virus from a child to a mother providing health care. MMWR Morb Mortal Wkly Rep. 1986;35:76-79.

401. Centers for Disease Control and Prevention: HIV transmission between two adolescent brothers with hemophilia. MMWR Morb Mortal Wkly Rep. 1993;42:948-951.

402. Fitzgibbon JE, Gaur S, Frenkel LD, et al. Transmission from one child to another of human immunodeficiency virus type 1 with a zidovudine-resistance mutation. N Engl J Med. 1993;329:1835-1846.

403. Grint P, McEvoy M. Two associated cases of the acquired immunodeficiency syndrome (AIDS). Commun Dis Rep. 1985;42:4.

404. Srinivasan A, York D, Bohan C. Lack of HIV replication in arthropod cells (Letter). Lancet. 1987;1:1094-1095.

405. Miike L. Do Insects Transmit AIDS? Washington, DC: Health Program, Office of Technology Assessment, U.S. Congress; 1987:1-43.

406. Webb PA, Happ CM, Maupin GO, et al. Potential for insect transmission of HIV: Experimental exposure of *Cimex hemipterus* and *Toxorhynchites amboinensis* to human immunodeficiency virus. J Infect Dis. 1989;160:970-977.

407. Castro KG, Lieb S, Jaffe HW, et al. Transmission of HIV in Belle Glade, Florida: Lessons for other communities in the United States. Science. 1988;239:193-197.

408. Greenberg AE, Nguyen-Dinh P, Mann JM, et al. The association between malaria, blood transfusions, and HIV seropositivity in a pediatric population in Kinshasa, Zaire. JAMA. 1988;259:545-549.

409. World Health Organization. Global AIDS surveillance. Part II. Wkly Epidemiol Rec. 1997;72:356-372.

410. Mertens TE, Belsey E, Stoneburner RL, et al. Global estimates of HIV infections and AIDS: Further heterogeneity in spread and impact. AIDS. 1995;9(Suppl 1):S251.

411. Mann JM, Tarantola DJM, eds. AIDS in the World: II. Cambridge: Oxford University Press; 1996:61.

412. Cortes E, Detels R, Aboulafia D, et al. HIV-1, HIV-2, and HTLV-I infection in high risk groups in Brazil. N Engl J Med. 1989;320:953-958.

413. Torrey BB, Way PO. Seroprevalence of HIV in Africa: Winter 1990. CIR staff paper No. 55. Washington, DC: Center for International Research, U.S. Bureau of the Census; 1990.

414. Rwandan HIV Seroprevalence Study Group. Nationwide community based serological survey of HIV-1 and other human retrovirus infections in a central African country. Lancet. 1989;1:941-943.

415. Serwadda D, Wawer MJ, Musgrave SD, et al. HIV risk factors in three geographic strata of rural Rakai District, Uganda. AIDS. 1992;6:983-989.

416. Miotti PG, Dallabetta GA, Ndovi E, et al. HIV-1 and pregnant women: Associated factors, prevalence, estimate of incidence and role in fetal wastage in Central Africa. AIDS. 1990;4:733-736.

417. Allen S, Lindan C, Serufilira A, et al. Human immunodeficiency virus infection in urban Rwanda: Demographic and behavioral correlates in a representative sample of childbearing women. JAMA. 1991;226:1657-1663.

418. N'Galy B, Ryder RW. Epidemiology of HIV infection in Africa. J Acquir Immune Defic Syndr. 1988;1:551-558.

419. Dallabetta GA, Miotti PG, Chiphangwi JD, et al. High socioeconomic status is a risk factor for human immunodeficiency virus type 1 (HIV-1) infection but not for sexually transmitted diseases in women in Malawi: Implications for HIV-1 control. J Infect Dis. 1993;167:36-42.

420. Piot P, Plummer FA, Rey MA, et al. Retrospective seroepidemiology of AIDS virus infections in Nairobi populations. J Infect Dis. 1987;155:1108-1112.
421. Simonsen JN, Plummer FA, Ngugi EN, et al. HIV infection among lower socioeconomic strata prostitutes in Nairobi. AIDS. 1990;4:139-144.
422. Simonsen JN, Cameron W, Gakinya MN, et al. Human immunodeficiency virus infection among men with sexually transmitted diseases. N Engl J Med. 1988;319:274-278.
423. Pape JW, Stanback ME, Pamphile M, et al. Prevalence of HIV infection and high-risk activities in Haiti. J Acquir Immune Defic Syndr. 1990;3:995-1001.
424. Diallo MO, Ackah AN, Lafontaine MF, et al. HIV-1 and HIV-2 infections in men attending sexually transmitted disease clinics in Abidjan, Cote D'Ivoire. AIDS. 1992;6:581-585.
425. Lackritz EM. Prevention of HIV transmission by blood transfusion in the developing world: Achievements and continuing challenges. AIDS. 1998;12(Suppl A):S81.
426. Weniger BG, Limpakarnjanarat K, Ungchusak K, et al. The epidemiology of HIV infection and AIDS in Thailand. AIDS. 1991;5(Suppl 2):S71-S85.
427. Ou CY, Takebe Y, Weniger BG, et al. Independent introduction of two major HIV-1 genotypes into distinct high-risk populations in Thailand. Lancet. 1993;341:1171-1174.
428. Sirisopana N, Torugsa K, Carr J, et al. Prevalence of HIV-1 infection in young men entering the Royal Thai Army. Abstract POCO82778. In: Abstracts of the Ninth International Conference on AIDS/Fourth STD World Congress, v. 2. Berlin: 1993:680.
429. Jain MK, John JT, Keusch GT. Epidemiology of HIV and AIDS in India. AIDS. 1994;8(Suppl 2):S61-S75.
430. Ryan CA, Vathiny OV, Gorbach PM, et al. Explosive spread of HIV-1 and sexually transmitted diseases in Cambodia. Lancet. 1998;351:1175.
431. Singh YN, Malaviya AN, Tripathy SP, et al. HIV serosurveillance among prostitutes and patients from a sexually transmitted diseases clinic in Delhi, India. J Acquir Immune Defic Syndr. 1990;3:287-289.
432. Singh S, Crofts N, Gertig D. HIV infection among IDU's in northeast Malaysia. Abstract POCO82777. In: Abstracts of the Ninth International Conference on AIDS/Fourth STD World Congress, v. 2. Berlin: 1993:680.
433. Zheng X, Thian C, Zhang J, et al. Rapid spread of HIV among drug users and their wives in southwest China. Abstract POCO82766. In: Abstracts of the Ninth International Conference on AIDS/Fourth STD World Congress, v. 2. Berlin: 1993:678.
434. Lindan CP, Lieu TX, Giang LT, et al. Rising HIV infection rates in Ho Chi Minh City herald emerging AIDS epidemic in Vietnam. AIDS. 1997;11(Suppl 1):S513.
435. Oh MD, Choe K, Shin Y, et al. Current status of HIV/AIDS epidemic in South Korea. Abstract POCO82769. In: Abstracts of the Ninth International Conference on AIDS/Fourth STD World Congress, v. 2. Berlin: 1993:678.
436. Soda K, Fukutomi K, Hashimoto S, et al. Temporal trend and projections of HIV/AIDS epidemic in Japan (Abstract POCO82779). In: Abstracts of the Ninth International Conference on AIDS/Fourth STD World Congress, v. 2. Berlin: 1993:680.
437. Gromyko A. Challenge of HIV/AIDS and STD rising trends in Eastern Europe. Abstract 60107. Presented at the Twelfth International Conference on AIDS, Geneva, June 28-July 3, 1998.
438. Clavel F, Guetard D, Brun-Vezinet F, et al. Isolation of a new human retrovirus from West African patients with AIDS. Science. 1986;233:343-346.
439. Centers for Disease Control and Prevention. Testing for antibodies to human immunodeficiency virus type 2 in the United States. MMWR Morb Mortal Wkly Rep. 1992;41(RR-12):1-9.
440. DeCock KM, Adjorlolo G, Ekpini E, et al. Epidemiology and transmission of HIV-2: Why there is no HIV-2 pandemic. JAMA. 1993;270:2083-2086.
441. O'Brien TR, George JR, Holmberg SD. Human immunodeficiency virus type 2 infection in the United States: Epidemiology, diagnosis, and public health implications. JAMA. 1992;267:2775-2779.
442. Onorato IM, O'Brien TR, Schable CA, et al. Sentinel surveillance for HIV-2 infection in high-risk US populations. Am J Public Health. 1993;83:515-519.
443. Markovitz DM. Infection with the human immunodeficiency virus type 2. Ann Intern Med. 1993;118:211-218.
444. Poulsen AG, Kvinesdal BB, Aaby P, et al. Lack of evidence of vertical transmission of human immunodeficiency virus type 2 in a sample of the general population in Bissau. J Acquir Immune Defic Syndr. 1992;5:25-30.
445. Del Mistro A, Chotard J, Hall AJ, et al. HIV-1 and HIV-2 seroprevalence rates in mother-child pairs living in The Gambia (West Africa). J Acquir Immune Defic Syndr. 1992;5:19-24.
446. Adjorlolo-Johnson G, DeCock KM, Ekpini E, et al. Prospective comparison of mother-to-child transmission of HIV-1 and HIV-2 in Abidjan, Ivory Coast. JAMA. 1994;272:462.
447. Dufoort G, Courouce AM, Ancelle-Park R, et al. No clinical signs 14 years after HIV-2 transmission via blood transfusion (Letter). Lancet. 1988;2:510.
448. Pepin J, Morgan G, Dunn D, et al. HIV-2-induced immunosuppression among asymptomatic West African prostitutes: Evidence that HIV-2 is pathogenic, but less so than HIV-1. AIDS. 1991;5:1165-1172.
449. Marlink R, Thior I, Travers K, et al. Reduced virulence of HIV-2 compared to HIV-1. Science. 1994;265:1587.
450. Guyader M, Emerman M, Sonigo P, et al. Genome organization and transactivation of the human immunodeficiency virus type 2. Nature. 1987;326:662-669.
451. George JR, Rayfield MA, Phillips S, et al. Efficacies of US Food and Drug Administration-licensed HIV-1-screening enzyme immunoassays for detecting antibodies to HIV-2. AIDS. 1990;4:321-326.

452. Myers RA, Patel JD, Joseph JM. Identifying HIV-2 seropositive individuals by reevaluating HIV-1 indeterminate sera. J Acquir Immune Defic Syndr. 1992;5:417-423.
453. World Health Organization: Recommendations for interpretation of HIV-2 Western blot results. Wkly Epidemiol Rec. 1990;10:74.
454. Peeters M, Gershy-Damet GM, Fransen K, et al. Virological and polymerase chain reaction studies of HIV-1/HIV-2 dual infection in Cote d'Ivoire. Lancet. 1992;340:339-340.
455. Travers K, Mboup S, Marlink R, et al. Natural protection against HIV-1 infection provided by HIV-2. Science. 1995;268:1612..
456. Centers for Disease Control and Prevention. Compendium of HIV prevention interventions with evidence for effectiveness. Atlanta, GA: CDC, 1999.
457. DiClemente RJ. Looking forward: future directions for HIV prevention research. In: Peterson JL and DiClemente RJ, eds. Handbook of HIV Prevention. New York: Kluwer Academic/Plenum; 2000:311-324.
458. Centers for Disease Control and Prevention. Advancing HIV prevention: New strategies for a changing epidemic—United States, 2003. MMWR Morb Mortal Wkly Rep. 2003;52:329-332.
459. Centers for Disease Control and Prevention. Resurgent bacterial sexually transmitted disease among men who have sex with men—King County, Washington, 1997-1999. MMWR Morbid Mortal Wkly Rep. 1999;48:773-777.
460. Centers for Disease Control and Prevention. Increases in unsafe sex and rectal gonorrhea among men who have sex with men—San Francisco, California, 1994-1997. MMWR Morbid Mortal Wkly Rep. 1999;48:45-48.
461. Erbelding EJ, Stanton D, Quinn TC, et al. Behavioral and biological evidence of persistent high-risk behavior in an HIV primary care population. AIDS 2000; 14:297-301.
462. Janssen RS, Holtgrave DR, Valdiserri RO, et al. The serostatus approach to fighting the HIV epidemic: prevention intervention strategies for infected individuals. Am J Public Health 2001;91:1019-1024.
463. Centers for Disease Control and Prevention. Incorporating HIV prevention into the medical care of persons living with HIV. Recommendations of CDC, the Health Resources and Services Administration, the National Institutes of Health, and the HIV Medicine Association of the Infectious Diseases Society of America. MMWR Morbid Mortal Wkly Rep. 2003;52:1-24.
464. Chen MS, Dellabeta G, Laga M, Holmes KK. A new deal in HIV prevention: Lessons from the global approach. Ann Intern Med. 1994;120:340-341.
465. Johnson AM. Condoms and HIV transmission. N Engl J Med. 1994;331:391-392.
466. Centers for Disease Control and Prevention: Update: Barrier protection against HIV infection and other sexually transmitted diseases. MMWR Morb Mortal Wkly Rep. 1993;42:589-591.
467. National Institute of Allergy and Infectious Diseases. Workshop Summary: Scientific Evidence on Condom Effectiveness for Sexually Transmitted Disease (STD) Prevention. July 20, 2001. Available at www.niaid.nih.gov/dmid/stds/condomreport.pdf.
468. Thompson JL, Yager TJ, Martin JL. Estimated condom failure and frequency of condom use among gay men. Am J Public Health. 1993;83:1409-1413.
469. Weller SC. A metaanalysis of condom effectiveness in reducing sexually transmitted HIV. Soc Sci Med. 1993;36:1635-1644.
470. Saracco A, Musicco M, Nicolosi A, et al. Man-to-women sexual transmission of HIV: Longitudinal study of 343 steady partners of infected men. J Acquir Immune Defic Syndr. 1993;6:497-502.
471. De Vincenzi I. A longitudinal study of human immunodeficiency virus transmission by heterosexual partners. European Study Group on Heterosexual Transmission of HIV. N Engl J Med. 1994;331:341-346.
472. Nelson KE, Celentano DD, Eiumtrakol S, et al. Changes in sexual behavior and a decline in HIV infection among young men in Thailand. N Engl J Med. 1996;335:297-303.
473. Hanenberg RS, Rojanapithayakorn W, Kunasol P, Sokal DC. Impact of Thailand's HIV-control programme as indicated by the decline of sexually transmitted diseases. Lancet. 1994;344:243-245.
474. Rojanapithayakorn W, Hanenberg R. The 100% condom program in Thailand. AIDS 1996; 10(1):1-7.
475. Davis KR, Weller SC. The effectiveness of condoms in reducing heterosexual transmission of HIV. Family Plann Perspect. 1999;31:272-279.
476. Trussell J, Warner DL, Hatcher R. Condom performance during vaginal intercourse: Comparison of TrojanEnz and Tactylon condoms. Contraception. 1992;45:11-19.
477. Carey RF, Herman WA, Retta SM, et al. Effectiveness of latex condoms as a barrier to human immunodeficiency virus-sized particles under conditions of simulated use. Sex Transm Dis. 1992;19:230-234.
478. Silverman BG, Gross TP. Use and effectiveness of condoms during anal intercourse. Sex Transm Dis. 1997;24:11-17.
479. Rosenberg MJ, Gollub EL. Commentary: Methods women can use that may prevent sexually transmitted disease, including HIV. Am J Public Health. 1992;82:1473-1478.
480. French P, Latka M, Gollub EL, et al. Female condoms as effective as male condoms in preventing sexually transmitted diseases. Abstract 60730. Presented at the Twelfth International Conference on AIDS, Geneva, 1998.
481. Fontanet AL, Saba J, Chandelying V, et al. Protection against sexually transmitted diseases by granting sex workers in Thailand the choice of using the male or female condom: Results from a randomized controlled trial. AIDS. 1998;12:1851-1859.
482. French PP, Latka M, Gollub EL, et al. Use-effectiveness of the female versus male condom in preventing sexually transmitted disease in women. Sex Transm Dis. 2003;30:433-439.

483. Roddy R, Zekeng L, Ryan K, et al. A controlled trial of nonoxynol-9-film to reduce male-to-female transmission of sexually transmitted diseases. N Engl J Med. 1998;339:504-510.

484. Van Damme L. Advances in topical microbicides. Presented at the XIII International AIDS Conference, July 9-14, 2000, Durban, South Africa.

485. Louv WC, Austin H, Alexander WJ, et al. A clinical trial of nonoxynol-9 for preventing gonococcal and chlamydial infections. J Infect Dis. 1988;158:513-523.

486. Roddy RE, Zekeng L, Ryan KA, et al. Effect of nonoxynol-9 gel on urogenital gonorrhea and chlamydial infection, a randomized control trial. JAMA. 2002;287: 1117-1122.

487. Centers for Disease Control and Prevention. Nonoxynol-9 spermicide contraception use—United States, 1999. MMWR Morb Mortal Wkly Rep. 2002;51:389-392.

488. Roper WL, Peterson HB, Curran JW. Commentary: Condoms and HIV/STD prevention—clarifying the message. Am J Public Health. 1993;83:501-503.

489. Centers for Disease Control and Prevention: Heterosexual behaviors and factors that influence condom use among patients attending a sexually transmitted disease clinic—San Francisco. MMWR Morb Mortal Wkly Rep. 1990;39:685-689.

490. Peterson JL, Coates TJ, Catania JA, et al. High-risk sexual behavior and condom use among gay and bisexual African-American men. Am J Public Health. 1992;82: 1490-1494.

491. Catania JA, Coates TJ, Kegeles S, et al. Condom use in multiethnic neighborhoods of San Francisco: The population-based AMEN (AIDS in Multiethnic Neighborhoods) study. Am J Public Health. 1991;81:284-287.

492. Osmond DH, Page K, Wiley J, et al. HIV infection in homosexual and bisexual men 18 to 29 years of age: The San Francisco Young Men's Health Study. Am J Public Health. 1994;84:1933-1937.

493. Stall R, Ekstrand M, Polleck L, et al. Relapse from safer sex: The next challenge for AIDS prevention efforts. J Acquir Immune Defic Syndr. 1990;3:1181-1187.

494. Hays RB, Kegeles SM, Coates TJ. High HIV risk-taking among young gay men. AIDS. 1990;4:901-907.

495. St. Lawrence JS, Hood HV, Brasfield T, et al. Differences in gay men's AIDS risk knowledge and behavior patterns in high and low AIDS prevalence cities. Public Health Rep. 1989;104:391-395.

496. Ekstrand ML, Coates TJ. Maintenance of safer sexual behaviors and predictors of risky sex: The San Francisco Men's Health Study. Am J Public Health. 1990;80: 973-977.

497. Adib SM, Joseph JG, Ostrow DG, et al. Relapse in sexual behavior among homosexual men: A 2-year follow-up from the Chicago MACS/CCS. AIDS. 1991;5:757-760.

498. Penkower L, Dew MA, Kingsley L, et al. Behavioral, health and psychosocial factors and risk for HIV infection among sexually active homosexual men: The Multicenter AIDS Cohort Study. Am J Public Health. 1991;81:194-196.

499. Lifson AR. Men who have sex with men: Continued challenges for preventing HIV infection and AIDS (Editorial). Am J Public Health. 1992;82:166-167.

500. Kravcik S, Victor G, Houston S, et al. Effect of antiretroviral therapy and viral load on the perceived risk of HIV transmission and the need for safer sex practices. J Acquir Immune Defic Syndr Hum Retroviral. 1998; 19:124-129

501. DiClemente RJ, Funkhouser E, Wingood GM, et al. Protease inhibitor combination therapy and decreased condom use among gay men. South Med J. 2002;95:421-425.

502. Scheer S, Chu PL, Klausner JD, et al. Effect of highly active antiretroviral therapy on diagnoses of sexually transmitted diseases in people with AIDS. Lancet. 2001;357:425-432.

503. Chirgwin K, DeHovitz JA, Dillon S, et al. HIV infection, genital ulcer disease, and crack cocaine uses among patients attending a clinic for sexually transmitted diseases. Am J Public Health. 1992;81:1576-1579.

504. Centers for Disease Control and Prevention: Condom use among male injecting-drug users—New York City, 1987-1990. MMWR Morb Mortal Wkly Rep. 1992;41: 617-620.

505. Marks G, Richardson JL, Maldonado N. Self-disclosure of HIV infection to sexual partners. Am J Public Health. 1991;81:1321-1323.

506. Landis SE, Schoenbach VJ, Weber DJ, et al. Results of a randomized trial of partner notification in cases of HIV infection in North Carolina. N Engl J Med. 1992;326:101-106.

507. Bayer R, Toomey KE. HIV prevention and the two faces of partner notification. Am J Public Health. 1992;82:1158-1164.

508. Pavia AT, Benyo M, Niler L, et al. Partner notification for control of HIV: Results after 2 years of a statewide program in Utah. Am J Public Health. 1993;83:1418-1424.

509. Golen MR. HIV partner notification: a neglected prevention intervention. Sex Transm Dis. 2002;29:472-475.

510. Macke BA, Maher JE. Partner notification in the United States: An evidence-based review. Am J Prev Med. 1999;17:230-242.

511. Giesecke J, Ramstedt K, Granath F, et al. Efficacy of partner notification for HIV infection. Lancet. 1991;338:1096-1100.

512. Wawer MJ, Sewankambo NK, Serwadda D, et al. Control of sexually transmitted diseases and AIDS prevention in Uganda: A randomized community trial. Lancet. 1999;353:525-535.

513. Centers for Disease Control and Prevention: Management of possible sexual, injecting-drug-use, or other nonoccupational exposure to HIV, including considerations related to antiretroviral therapy. Public Health Service Statement. MMWR Morb Mortal Wkly Rep. 1998;47:1-14.

514. Katz MH, Gerberding JL. Postexposure treatment of people exposed to the human immunodeficiency virus through sexual contact or injection-drug use. N Engl J Med. 1997;336:1097-1100.

515. Kahn JO, Martin JN, Roland ME, et al. Feasibility of postexposure prophylaxis (PEP) against human immunodeficiency virus infection after sexual or injection drug use exposure: The San Francisco PEP Study. J Infect Dis. 2001;183:707-714.

516. Roland ME, Martin JN, Grant RM, et al. Postexposure prophylaxis for human immunodeficiency virus infection after sexual or injection drug use exposure: Identification and characterization of the source of exposure. J Infect Dis. 2001;184:1608-1612.

517. The Twin Epidemics of Substance Use and HIV. Washington, DC: National Commission on AIDS; 1991.

518. Metzger DS, Navaline H, Woody GE. Drug-abuse treatment as AIDS prevention. Public Health Rep. 1998;113(Suppl 1):S97-S106.

519. Gossop M, Marsden J, Stewart D, Treacy S. Reduced injection risk and sexual risk behaviours after drug misuse treatment: Results from the National Treatment Outcome Research Study. AIDS Care. 2002;14:77-93.

520. Metzger DS, Navaline H. HIV prevention among injection drug users: The need for integrated models. J Urban Health. 2003;80:iii59-iii66.

521. Centers for Disease Control and Prevention: Update: Reducing HIV transmission in intravenous-drug users not in drug treatment—United States. MMWR Morb Mortal Wkly Rep. 1990;39:97-101.

522. Groseclose SL, Weinstein B, Jones S, et al. Legal purchase of clean needles and syringes in Connecticut: Do they make a difference? Abstract POD274185. In: Abstracts of the Ninth International Conference on AIDS/Fourth STD World Congress, v. 2. Berlin: 1993:915.

523. U.S. General Accounting Office. Needle Exchange Programs: Research Suggests Promise as an AIDS Prevention Strategy. Washington, D.C.: USGAO, Human Resources Division; 1993. Report to the Chairman, Select Committee on Narcotics Abuse and Control, House of Representatives.

524. Centers for Disease Control and Prevention: Use of bleach for disinfection of drug injection equipment. MMWR Morb Mortal Wkly Rep. 1993;42:418-419.

525. Yancovitz SR, Des Jarlais DC, Peyser NP, et al. A randomized trial of an interim methadone maintenance clinic. Am J Public Health. 1991;81:1185-1191.

526. Coyle SL, Needle RH, Normand J. Outreach-based HIV prevention for injecting drug users: a review of published outcome data. Public Health Rep. 1998;113(Suppl 1):19-30.

527. Latkin CA. Outreach in natural settings: The use of peer leaders for HIV prevention among injecting drug users' networks. Public Health Rep. 1998;113(Suppl 1): 151-159.

528. Stephens RC, Feucht TE, Roman SW. Effects of an intervention program on AIDS-related drug and needle behavior among intravenous drug users. Am J Public Health. 1991;81:568-571.

529. Negigus A, Friedman SR, Curtis R, et al. Relevance of drug injectors' social networks and risk networks for understanding and preventing HIV infection. Soc Sci Med. 1994;38:67.

530. Des Jarlais DC, Friedman SR, Friedman P, et al. HIV/AIDS related behavior change among injecting drug users in different national settings. AIDS. 1995;9:611.

531. Hagan H, McGough JP, Thiede H, et al. Reduced injection frequency and increased entry and retention in substance abuse treatment associated with needle-exchange participation in Seattle drug injectors. J Subst Abuse Treat. 2000;19:247-252.

532. Strathdee SA, Celentano DD, Shah N, et al. Needle exchange attendance and health care utilization promote entry into detoxification. J Urban Health. 1999;76:448-460.

533. The Public Health Impact of Needle Exchange Programs in the United States and Abroad. Summary, Conclusions, and Recommendations. Report prepared for the Centers for Disease Control and Prevention, Atlanta, September 1993.

534. Vlahov D, Junge B. The role of needle exchange programs in HIV prevention. Public Health Rep. 1998;113(Suppl 1):S75-S80.

535. Hurley S, Jolley D, Kaldor J. Effectiveness of needle-exchange programmes for prevention of HIV infection. Lancet. 1997;349:1797.

536. Hagan H, McGough JP, Thiede H, et al. Syringe exchange and risk of infection with hepatitis B and C viruses. Am J Epidemiol. 1999;149:203-213.

537. Moss AR. Epidemiology and the politics of needle exchange. Am J Public Health. 2000;90:1385-1387.

538. Coutinho R. Needle exchange, pragmatism and moralism. Am J Public Health. 2000;90:1387-1388.

539. Rich JD, Macalino GE, McKenzie M, et al. Syringe prescription to prevent HIV infection in Rhode Island: A case study. Am J Public Health. 2001;91:699-700.

540. Burris S, Lurie P, Abrahamson D, Rich JD. Physician prescribing of sterile injection equipment to prevent HIV infection: Time for action. Ann Intern Med. 2000;133: 218-226.

541. Titus S, Marmor M, Des Jarlais DC, et al. Bleach use and HIV seroconversion among New York City injection drug users. J Acquir Immune Defic Syndr. 1994;7:700.

542. Vlahov D, Astemborski J, Soloman L, Nelson KE. Field effectiveness of needle disinfection among injecting drug users. J Acquir Immune Defic Syndr. 1994;7:760.

543. Centers for Disease Control and Prevention: Semen banking, organ and tissue transplantation, and HIV antibody testing. MMWR Morb Mortal Wkly Rep. 1988;37:57-58, 63.

544. Centers for Disease Control and Prevention: Transmission of HIV through bone transplantation: Case report and public health recommendations. MMWR Morb Mortal Wkly Rep. 1988;37:597-599.

545. Katzenstein TL, Dickmeiss E, Aladdin H, et al. Failure to develop HIV infection after receipt of HIV-contaminated blood and postexposure prophylaxis. Ann Intern Med. 2000;133:31-34.

546. Bell DM. Human immunodeficiency virus transmission in health care settings: Risk and risk reduction. Am J Med. 1991;91(Suppl 3B):S294-S300.

547. Do AN, Ciesielski CA, Metler RP, et al. Occupationally acquired human immunodeficiency virus (HIV) infection: National case surveillance data during 20 years of the HIV epidemic in the United States. Infect Control Hosp Epidemiol. 2003;24:86-96.

548. Centers for Disease Control and Prevention: Recommendations for prevention of HIV transmission in healthcare settings. MMWR Morb Mortal Wkly Rep. 1987;36(Suppl 2S):S1-S18.

549. Centers for Disease Control and Prevention: Public Health Service statement on management of occupational exposure to human immunodeficiency virus, including considerations regarding zidovudine postexposure use. MMWR Morb Mortal Wkly Rep. 1990;39:1-14.

550. Centers for Disease Control and Prevention: Revised Guidelines for HIV Counseling, Testing and Referral. MMWR Morb Mortal Wkly Rep. 2001;50:1-58.

551. Institute of Medicine. Reducing the Odds: Preventing Perinatal Transmission of HIV in the United States. Washington DC. National Academy Press, 1998.

552. Lindsay MK, Peterson HB, Feng TI, et al. Routine antepartum human immunodeficiency virus infection screening in an inner-city population. Obstet Gynecol. 1989;74:289-294.

553. Wade NA, Birkhead GS, Warren BL, et al. Abbreviated regimens of zidovudine prophylaxis and perinatal transmission of the human immunodeficiency virus. N Engl J Med. 1998;339:1409-1414.

554. Centers for Disease Control and Prevention: Administration of zidovudine during late pregnancy and delivery to prevent perinatal HIV transmission—Thailand, 1996-1998. MMWR Morb Mortal Wkly Rep. 1998;47:1551-1554.

555. Mofenson LM. Tale of two epidemics—The continuing challenge of preventing mother-to-child transmission of human immunodeficiency virus. J Infect Dis 2003;187:721-724.

556. Centers for Disease Control and Prevention: Recommendations for assisting in the prevention of perinatal transmission of human T-lymphotrophic type III/lymphadenopathy-associated virus. MMWR Morb Mortal Wkly Rep. 1985;34:721-726, 731-732.

557. World Health Organization. Consensus statement from the WHO/UNICEF consultation on HIV transmission and breast-feeding. Wkly Epidemiol Rec. 1992;67:177-179.

558. UNAIDS. HIV and infant feeding: An interim statement. Wkly Epidemiol Rec. 1996;71:289-291.

559. Petra Study Team. Efficacy of three short-course regimens of zidovudine and lamivudine in preventing early and late transmission of HIV-1 from mother to child in Tanzania, South Africa, and Uganda (Petra study): A randomised, double-blind, placebo-controlled trial. Lancet. 2002;359:1178-1186.

560. Moodley D, Moodley J, Coovadia H, et al. A multicenter randomized controlled trial of nevirapine versus a combination of zidovudine and lamivudine to reduce intrapartum and early postpartum mother-to-child transmission of HIV-1. J Infect Dis. 2003;187:725-735.

561. Valdiserri RO, Holtgrave DR, Brackbill RM. American adults' knowledge of HIV testing availability. Am J Public Health. 1993;83:525-528.

562. Centers for Disease Control and Prevention. HIV testing—United States, 2001. MMWR Morbid Mortal Wkly Rep. 2003;52:540-545.

563. Centers for Disease Control and Prevention. Notice to Readers: Approval of a new rapid test for HIV antibody. MMWR Morbid Mortal Wkly Rep. 2002;51:1051-1052.

564. Berrios DC, Hearst N, Cotes TJ, et al. HIV antibody testing among those at risk for infection: The National AIDS Behavioral Surveys. JAMA. 1993;270:1576-1580.

565. Ward J. Testing for retroviral infections: Medical indications and ethical considerations. In: Schochetman G, George JR, eds. AIDS Testing. Methodology and Management Issues. New York: Springer-Verlag; 1992:6-17.

566. Centers for Disease Control and Prevention: Recommendations for HIV testing services for inpatients and outpatients in acute-care hospital settings. MMWR Morb Mortal Wkly Rep. 1993;42:1-17.

567. Centers for Disease Control and Prevention: Human immunodeficiency virus infection in transfusion recipients and their family members. MMWR Morb Mortal Wkly Rep. 1987;36:137-140.

578. Centers for Disease Control and Prevention: Recommendations for preventing transmission of human immunodeficiency virus and hepatitis B virus to patients during exposure-prone invasive procedures. MMWR Morb Mortal Wkly Rep. 1991;40:1-9.

569. Gerberding JL, Littell C, Tarkington A, et al. Risk of exposure of surgical personnel to patients' blood during surgery at San Francisco General Hospital. N Engl J Med. 1990;322:1788-1793.

570. Higgins DL, Galavotti C, O'Reilly KR, et al. Evidence for the effects of HIV antibody counseling and testing on risk behaviors. JAMA. 1991;266:2419-2429.

571. Sangiwa G, Balmer D, Furlonge C, et al. Voluntary HIV counseling and testing reduces risk behavior in developing countries: Results from the voluntary counseling and testing study. Abstract 133/33269. Presented at the Twelfth International Conference on AIDS, Geneva, 1998.

572. Otten MW, Zaidi AA, Wroten JE, et al. Changes in sexually transmitted disease rates after HIV testing and posttest counseling, Miami 1988 to 1989. Am J Public Health. 1993;83:529-533.

573. Zenilman JM, Erickson B, Fox R, et al. Effect of HIV posttest counseling on STD incidence. JAMA. 1992;267:843-845.

574. Holtgrave DR, Valdiserri RO, Gerber AR, et al. Human immunodeficiency virus counseling, testing, referral, and partner notification services: A cost-benefit analysis. Arch Intern Med. 1993;153:1225-1230.

575. Kamb ML, Fishbein M, Douglas JM Jr, et al. Efficacy of risk-reduction counseling to prevent human immunodeficiency virus and sexually transmitted diseases: A randomized controlled trial. JAMA. 1998;280:1161-1167.

576. Leaity S, Sherr L, Wells H, et al. Repeat HIV testing: High-risk behavior or risk reduction strategy? AIDS. 2000;14:547-552.

577. Centers for Disease Control and Prevention. Update: HIV Counseling and Testing Using Rapid Tests—United States, 1995. MMWR Morbid Mortal Wkly Rep. 1998;47:211-215.

578. 2001 USPHS/IDSA Guidelines for the Prevention of Opportunistic Infections in Persons Infected with Human Immunodeficiency Virus. Available at: http://aidsinfo.nih.gov/guidelines/op_infections/OI_112801.html.

Diagnosis of Human Immunodeficiency Virus Infection

FRANK MALDARELLI

Human immunodeficiency virus (HIV) infection results in a progressive immune deficiency that has resulted in more than 22 million deaths worldwide[1] during the past 20 years. By the end of 2003, more than 40 million individuals were living with HIV infection throughout the world, with nearly 14,000 new infections occurring daily.[2] HIV detection methods are a cornerstone of the medical and public health response to track and control the HIV epidemic. Accurate, sensitive, and precise assays have been designed for three general purposes: patient diagnosis, epidemiologic surveillance, and donor screening for blood and tissue products. This chapter will survey the methods, strategies, and circumstances for detection of HIV infection.

Diagnosis of HIV infection is not simply the result of interpretation of a laboratory test, but proceeds from careful history and physical examination to indicated studies; the laboratory aspect of HIV diagnosis is a two-step process that requires sequential use of a highly sensitive *screening* test followed by a highly specific *confirmatory* assay. Evaluation for HIV infection should be conducted in a confidential fashion with voluntary participation, appropriate counseling, and informed consent of the individual. HIV testing is not a static methodology, and methods continue to undergo technologic developments in sensitivity to detect early HIV infection and in new strategies and formats for screening and confirmation. In 2003 the Centers for Disease Control and Prevention (CDC) recommended a change in the approach to HIV detection in the United States and advocated: (1) increasing routine screening of at-risk populations,[3] (2) expanding access to HIV testing outside traditional health care settings, and (3) incorporating real-time HIV screening in appropriate circumstances.[4] As these new approaches are implemented, health care professionals will have more choices and settings for HIV testing, and specialists will evaluate and counsel patients under a variety of circumstances. In addition, because HIV is a worldwide epidemic, physicians may evaluate patients with test results obtained from outside their geographic locale and should be aware that recommendations on the use and interpretation of HIV testing may vary according to governing jurisdiction (CDC, World Health Organization [WHO], other national agencies). Numerous screening and confirmatory tests have been developed, but only a subset have been approved by the U.S. Food and Drug Administration (FDA) or recommended for use by the WHO. Regardless of approval, no assay or test strategy is perfect, and familiarity with assay limitations is essential to ensure accurate identification of HIV infection; misdiagnosis of HIV infection has profound consequences for patients and their contacts; liability issues have been justifiably extreme.[5,6]

BACKGROUND AND PERSPECTIVE

The molecular virology and immune responses to HIV have been extensively characterized (Fig. 115-1.)[7-17] Several standard laboratory procedures used to detect antibodies to HIV proteins including radioimmunoprecipitation, Western blotting, enzyme-linked immunosorbent assays (ELISAs), and immunofluorescence were adapted to form the basis for the earliest HIV detection systems.[18] The first ELISA HIV test kits received FDA approval for use in blood donor screening in the United States in March 1985.[19] All donations reactive in a single test were discarded, and units with repeat reactivity were considered positive for viral antibodies. Within approximately

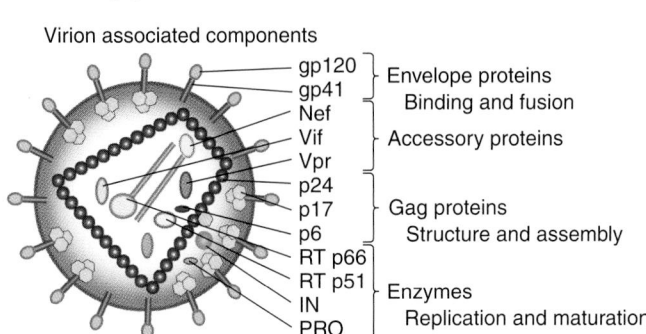

Virion associated components

gp120 ⎤
gp41   ⎦ Envelope proteins
        Binding and fusion

Nef ⎤
Vif ⎥ Accessory proteins
Vpr ⎦

p24 ⎤
p17 ⎥ Gag proteins
p6   ⎦ Structure and assembly

RT p66 ⎤
RT p51 ⎥ Enzymes
IN   ⎥ Replication and maturation
PRO   ⎦

Cell associated components

Rev   Post-transcriptional processing
Tat   Transcriptional activation
Vpu   CD4 degradation, virion production

FIGURE 115-1. Genetic organization of HIV-1. HIV-1 is an enveloped retrovirus with a plus-stranded ribonucleic acid (RNA) genome that contains genes for proteins with structural, enzymatic, and regulatory functions.

3 months, more than 1 million units of donated blood were screened in the United States, with 0.25% reported repeatedly reactive.[19]

After implementation of the first HIV testing procedures, several technical and logistical challenges were identified. Two principal technical issues of the first generation of HIV ELISAs were a high rate of false-positive results arising from a variety of clinical conditions and laboratory artifacts,[20] and a small but ominous number of false-negative results resulting from the inability to detect the presence of HIV antibodies early in infection (so-called window period) before full seroconversion.[21,22]

To address false-positive results, highly specific tests including Western blot (WB), immunofluoresence, and radioimmune precipitation were incorporated as confirmatory assays on all repeat ELISA-reactive samples.[23-25] Although all confirmatory assays are relatively labor intensive, WB procedures proved most useful, efficient, and specific; WB technique was soon established as a widely utilized gold standard test for confirmation, and was FDA approved for use in the United States in 1987.

A second generation of ELISAs decreased false-positive rates by employing recombinant antigens and synthetic peptides instead of infected cell lysates, resulting in greater sensitivity.[26-30] Introduction of an assay to detect the presence of viral antigen (p24) in 1989 was especially useful during early virus infection and improved detection of recent HIV infection.[31-35]

An additional challenge presented by HIV testing was expanding diagnostics beyond blood donation facilities and implementing a public health measure that was confidential, voluntary, and effective. In the United States and elsewhere, so-called alternative sites were es-

tablished, independent of blood centers that were permitted to perform voluntary and confidential HIV testing with pre- and post-test counseling procedures.[36] The logistics of screening at alternative sites[37] were often controversial, but mandatory testing of patient populations was rejected.

In 1986, a second human immunodeficiency virus (HIV-2) was identified in West Africa,[38,39] and shortly thereafter, cases of HIV-2 were detected in the United States, Canada, and Europe[40-45]; changes in ELISAs to include HIV-2 antigens ensued, and combination ELISA kits were introduced in 1991. The number of cumulative cases of HIV-2 in the United States has remained relatively low (<100), and not all ELISAs have been revised to include HIV-2 detection capability for FDA approval.

Rapid testing methods began in the United States with the agglutination assay.[46] Home collection procedures were established in 1996; the first home collection kits contained written pretest counseling, and obtained dried blood spots for shipping and testing; results and post-test counseling were provided by telephone.[47] Practical and safety issues concerning obtaining and processing blood for testing led to development of tests for alternative body fluids, including urine and saliva.[48-52]

As testing procedures for blood donation expanded, variations in laboratories carrying out these evaluations were expected and test kit evaluation procedures were established in the United States with the CDC Model Performance Evaluation Program to evaluate and limit variability,[53,54] and worldwide under WHO auspices.[55] High-performance and quality control measures were documented,[56,57] and guidelines for screening donor organs before transplantation were established by the FDA in 1993.

Inability to detect HIV during early infection (window period) has always been a critical limitation in HIV testing. Methods to detect HIV p24 antigen decreased the window period and were instituted as part of blood donor screening in 1996. Improvements in ELISA approaches using "sandwich" antibody techniques resulted in greater specificity in screening and greater sensitivity in detecting antibody during the window period, and ushered in a new generation of HIV ELISAs.[58,59] Detection of HIV nucleic acid using polymerase chain reaction (PCR), denoted nucleic acid testing (NAT), was developed for diagnosis and found to be more sensitive than third-generation ELISAs in detecting HIV-1 during the window period.[60] NAT was approved for use in screening plasma donors in 2001 and for use in individual blood donors in 2002. As of July 2004, NAT has not been approved for diagnosis of HIV infection in nondonor settings, but careful application of NAT has obvious advantages in specific clinical circumstances. In independent efforts to increase detection of window period infections, fourth-generation assays are in development that employ a combination of third-generation ELISA and sensitive p24 antigen detection.[59,61-63]

HIV testing was developed to detect HIV-subtype (clade) B, the most common subtype in the United States and Europe. The majority of infections worldwide are, however, nonsubtype B. Early generation assays had variable sensitivity to detect these non-B subtypes; inclusion of additional antigens and peptides has improved sensitivity, such that the current versions of ELISA, WB, and NAT assays will detect B and non-B subtypes with indistinguishable sensitivity and specificity.

The development of convenient sampling and ELISA methods has enabled HIV sample collection and HIV testing outside the health care facility, so-called point of care testing. Home sampling programs can be administered to protect anonymity and maintain ethical and regulatory standards. Complete home testing for HIV, however, presents scientific, medical, ethical, and regulatory challenges that preclude routine use at present.

TERMINOLOGY AND PERFORMANCE CHARACTERISTICS

In the United States, the FDA has regulatory oversight for testing, and not all modalities have FDA-approved versions (Table 115-1).[64,65] Serologic tests are broadly divided into screening assays and confirmatory tests (see Table 115-1). Serologic screening assays are available in

TABLE 115-1 Human Immunodeficiency Virus Testing Categories

Testing Categories	Synonyms and Abbreviations	Analyte Detected	Description/Use	Version with FDA Approval for HIV Diagnosis	HIV-2 Detection
Screening serology	Initial testing	IgG and IgM	Presumptive identification of HIV infection		
Enzyme-linked immunosorbent assay	ELISA, RIA	IgG and IgM	Standard screening assay with spectrophotometric reactive result		
Simple	ELISA, RIA	IgG and IgM	Requires no special equipment	No	No
Rapid	ELISA, RIA	IgG and IgM	Results obtained in 10-30 minutes	Yes	No
Simple/rapid	S/R	IgG and IgM	Results obtained in 10-30 minutes, and no special equipment necessary	Yes	No
Particle agglutination	PA	IgG and IgM	ELISA assay with visual readout of clumping particles denoting reactivity	Yes	No
Sensitive/less sensitive/ more sensitive	S/LS, "detuned"	IgG and IgM	Combines a less sensitive ELISA with sensitive ELISA to detect recent HIV infection	No	No
Antigen capture	p24 Antigen detection	p24	Detection of HIV antigen	Yes	Yes (HIV-1 version detects HIV-2)
Immune complex dissociation	ICD	p24	Method to increase p24 detection by disrupting p24 ag-p24 ab complexes, permitting p24 ag capture to occur	No	No
Confirmatory assay	Supplemental testing	IgG	Confirmation of HIV infection		
Western blot	WB	IgG	Confirmation of HIV infection	Yes	Yes but not FDA approved
Immunofluorescence	IFA	IgG	Confirmation of HIV infection	Yes	Yes but not FDA approved
Nucleic acid testing		HIV nucleic acid		Yes	No
NAT	NAT	HIV RNA	Use of PCR techniques to detect HIV nucleic acid in blood donor screening		
HIV RNA detection	HIV RNA, "viral load"	HIV RNA	May be useful in resolving indeterminate or other circumstances	No	Yes but not FDA approved
HIV DNA detection	Proviral DNA load	HIV DNA	PCR technique to detect HIV DNA for use in neonatal diagnosis	No	Yes but not FDA approved
Home collection		IgG	Sample collection performed outside health care facility, testing performed at central location	Yes	No
Home testing		IgG	Sample collection and HIV testing done outside health care facility	No	No

DNA, deoxyribonucleic acid; FDA, U.S. Food and Drug Administration; HIV, human immunodeficiency virus; IgG, immunoglobulin G; IgM, immunoglobulin M; PCR, polymerase chain reaction; RIA, radioimmunoassay; RNA, ribonucleic acid.

a number of ELISA or p24 antigen assay formats for initial testing. Results of screening tests are considered reactive or nonreactive. In the United States, confirmatory tests consist of either WB or immunofluorescence assays; results of confirmatory tests are termed positive, negative, or indeterminate. Home sample collection of dried blood spots for HIV testing is available, but complete home testing is not. Recently, NAT has been introduced (see Table 115-1), with deoxyribonucleic (DNA)– and ribonucleic acid (RNA)–based formats.

Assay limitations are quantified using a number of characteristics: sensitivity, specificity, false-positive rate, and false-negative rate (Table 115-2). For assays of HIV infection, both false-negative and false-positive rates have profound implications. Sensitivity (see Table 115-2) describes the fraction of all patients with infection that are detected by testing. Inadequate sensitivity has great impact in both blood surveillance and individual diagnosis; in both circumstances inability to detect infection potentially exposes others to infection, and misses critical opportunities for counseling and therapy. Specificity (see Table 115-2) describes the proportion of uninfected individuals who test negative for HIV. Decreased specificity results in false-positive findings, prompting profound patient distress and extensive additional evaluation. Decreased specificity compromises HIV testing from a patient diagnosis (fear of positive testing) and public health (inadequate description of the epidemic, unnecessary use of funds) standpoint. To maximize both specificity and sensitivity for detection of HIV infec-

tion, a single test is inadequate. Instead, a sequential strategy has been designed. Testing is initiated with a highly sensitive ELISA screening (>99.5% sensitive); in this phase, false positives may be significant (1%-10%). The screening phase is followed, however, by a highly specific confirmatory test (>99.5% specific); such testing correctly classifies the initial false-positive results. As a consequence, the sequential HIV testing strategy has among the highest levels of sensitivity and specificity for any medical test procedure.

Even at high specificity and sensitivity, positive predictive values and negative predictive values are dependent upon the disease prevalence. As shown in Figure 115-2, in a low-prevalence (0.01%) population, the positive predictive value of a single HIV testing strategy falls dramatically with only a few false-positive results. Populations with higher disease prevalence (0.1%-10%) are also subject to substantial decreases in positive predictive value with introduction of false-positive results (see Fig. 115-2). Using the sequential strategy for HIV detection, the screening assay first identifies specimens that are likely to be positive, and thus the HIV infection prevalence in the population of samples referred for confirmatory testing is already high (90%) and has a positive predictive value that is quite high and remains so even if false positives occur. Thus the combination of repeatedly reactive screening assay followed by a highly specific confirmatory assay yields an effective approach for diagnostic purposes, even in low-prevalence populations.

FIGURE 115-2. Positive predictive value of HIV confirmatory assay is a function of disease prevalence. At very low disease prevalence (0.01%), the positive predictive value of testing declines sharply with any false-positive test results. As the prevalence of infection increases, the positive predictive value improves despite a few false-positive test results. As HIV screening eliminates the majority of HIV-negative individuals for further confirmation, the prevalence of the population of samples referred for confirmatory assay increases dramatically and will be in the range of 90%. The positive predictive value for the sequential strategy remains high despite any false positive.

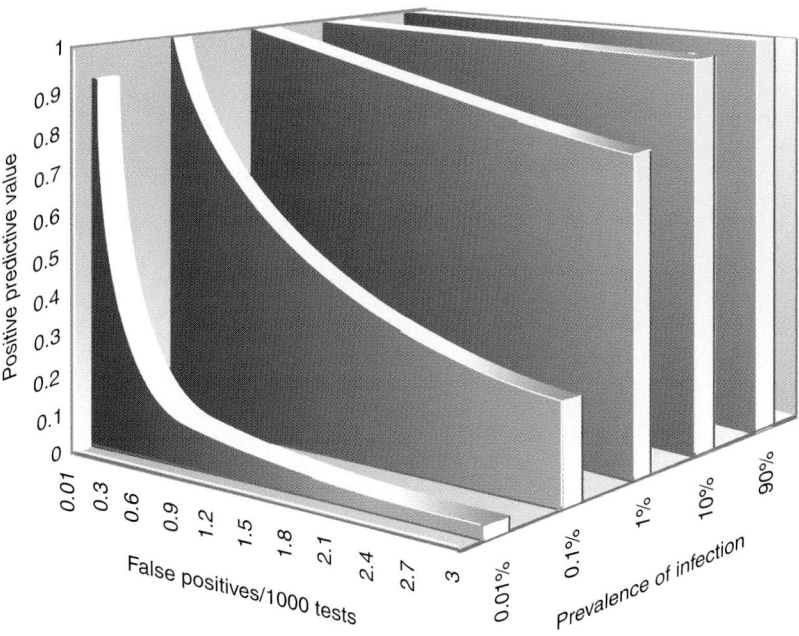

TABLE 115-2   Test Performance Characteristics

Characteristic	Definition	Formula
HIV positive	Number of individuals who are HIV infected and test positive	A
HIV negative	Number of individuals who are HIV uninfected and test negative	B
False HIV positive	Number of individuals who have positive HIV test results but are not infected	C
False HIV negative	Number of individuals who have negative HIV test results but who are HIV infected	D
Total number of individuals with HIV infection	HIV-infected population	A+D
Total number of individuals without HIV infection	HIV-free population	B+C
Total number of positive tests		A+C
Total number of negative tests		B+D
Sensitivity	Number of positive test results/total samples with HIV infection	A/A+D
Specificity	Number of negative test results/total samples without HIV infection	B/B+C
Positive predictive value	Proportion of those with HIV-positive assay who are actually HIV infected	A/A+C
Negative predictive value	Proportion of those with HIV-negative assay who are actually HIV uninfected	B/B+D

HIV, human immunodeficiency virus.

Numerous screening and confirmatory assays have been developed using a variety of patient source materials to determine the presence of HIV infection, but not all test formats are FDA approved for all blood or body fluids (Table 115-3); all testing modalities are available for plasma and serum. HIV test kit names and manufacturers of the FDA-approved assays are available at http://www.fda.gov. In addition, the WHO has evaluated specificity, sensitivity, negative predictive value, positive predictive value, and cost of all test kits the organization supports for distribution throughout the world.[66]

SPECIFIC LABORATORY METHODS FOR DETECTION OF HUMAN IMMUNODEFICIENCY VIRUS INFECTION

Immune Responses to Human Immunodeficiency Virus

Infection with HIV results in virus replication in a variety of cell types expressing surface markers CD4 and a coreceptor such as CXCR4 or CCR5. Viral replication also results in immune processing of viral proteins with display of viral antigen fragments on infected cell surfaces, prompting a cellular and humoral immune reaction (Fig. 115-3). Cellular reactivity represents the earliest detectable immunity to HIV,[67-69] but such responses have not yet been exploited for use in early diagnosis of HIV infection.

Humoral responses represent a reliable method to determine the presence of HIV infection. Antibody production after HIV infection follows a period of intense virus replication, as demonstrated by relatively high viral RNA levels and p24 antigen production preceding development of antibodies (see Fig. 115-3). Precise kinetics of antibody production to individual HIV proteins are incompletely understood, and significant variability has been detected[70]; in general, however, immune responses to HIV-1 appear similar to other infections, with immunoglobulin M (IgM) followed by appearance of immunoglobulin G (IgG) production.[71-75]

TABLE 115-3   Body Fluid for Human Immunodeficiency Virus Testing

Source for HIV Testing	FDA-Approved Testing Modality				
	ELISA	Rapid EIA	Western Blot	IFA	p24 Antigen Capture
Whole blood	X	X			
Dried blood	X				
Plasma	X	X	X	X	X
Serum	X	X	X	X	X
Oral fluid	X		X		
Urine	X		X		
Minipools (donor screen)	X				
Cadaveric serum	X				

EIA, enzyme immunoassay; ELISA, enzyme-linked immunosorbent assay; FDA, U.S. Food and Drug Administration; HIV, human immunodeficiency virus; IFA, indirect immunofluorescence.

The HIV window period (see Fig. 115-3) is the time after infection has occurred but before evidence of HIV infection is detectable. The HIV diagnostic window represents a vulnerable period particularly from a blood safety standpoint, and several major efforts have been launched to minimize its duration. Initial studies with early ELISA and WB assays suggested the HIV window period was on the order of 2.1 months,[76] and progressive improvements in ELISA methodology reduced window periods to no more than 6 weeks (Table 115-4). As shown in Figure 115-3, HIV p24 antigen or HIV RNA is often detectable prior to antibody responses, and use of sensitive HIV antigen and nucleic acid testing has reduced the window period to the current minimum. It is important to note, however, that studies of viral and immune kinetics to estimate the duration of the HIV window period employ seroconversion panels consisting of serial samples obtained from patients with known exposure history.[77] The levels of HIV-1 viremia vary in patients, and the rate of change of HIV RNA levels or production of antibodies during acute HIV infection is unpredictable, thus generalizations regarding the timing of seroconversion in such panels (or in newly infected patients) remain imprecise. Instead, analyses describe only average changes in the window period relative to an established comparator method. In general, the average window period with third-generation antibody tests is 22 days. Standard antigen testing decreases the window period to approximately 16 days, and NAT further reduces this period to 12 days.[78]

Additional serologic assays have been investigated to permit more sensitive HIV detection during the window period. Current assays, especially WB tests, rely largely on recognition of continuous or linear epitopes for diagnosis, because antigen sample preparation for Western blotting destroys conformational epitopes. Several investigators have noted, however, that early immune responses recognize discontinuous conformational epitopes.[71,79,80] B cells reacting to HIV proteins p17 and Nef antibodies have been identified before seroconversion.[81,82] New sensitive assays for HIV-1 p17 IgM have been developed using immune complex transfer technology[83,84] and have, in some cases, detected HIV antibody within 7 days of infection. It is not yet clear that such alternative approaches would significantly shorten the HIV-1 window period in all patients,[83] or represent robust or superior testing procedures compared with current assays, but such serologic techniques may be useful in resource-poor circumstances in which technically detailed PCR assays for early infection may not be feasible.

Once established, HIV seroreactivity is typically lifelong, although several exceptions and observations have been reported:

1. Late in the course of HIV-1 infection in the presence of profound immune deficiency, antibody levels may decline, potentially confusing serodiagnosis. Levels of HIV expression remain relatively high, and detection of HIV RNA is likely to be positive.
2. In rare cases, HIV infection may proceed in the absence of detectable serologic markers.[85-95] Typically, such patients have been characterized by rapid disease progression.
3. Early introduction of antiretroviral therapy may delay the development of full antibody responses to HIV infection.[96] In addition, introduction of antiretroviral therapy may permit humoral immunity such that immunologically silent infection may be detected.[97,98] Therapy may decrease the relative levels of anti-HIV antibodies and may affect detection by certain diagnostic platforms.[99,100]

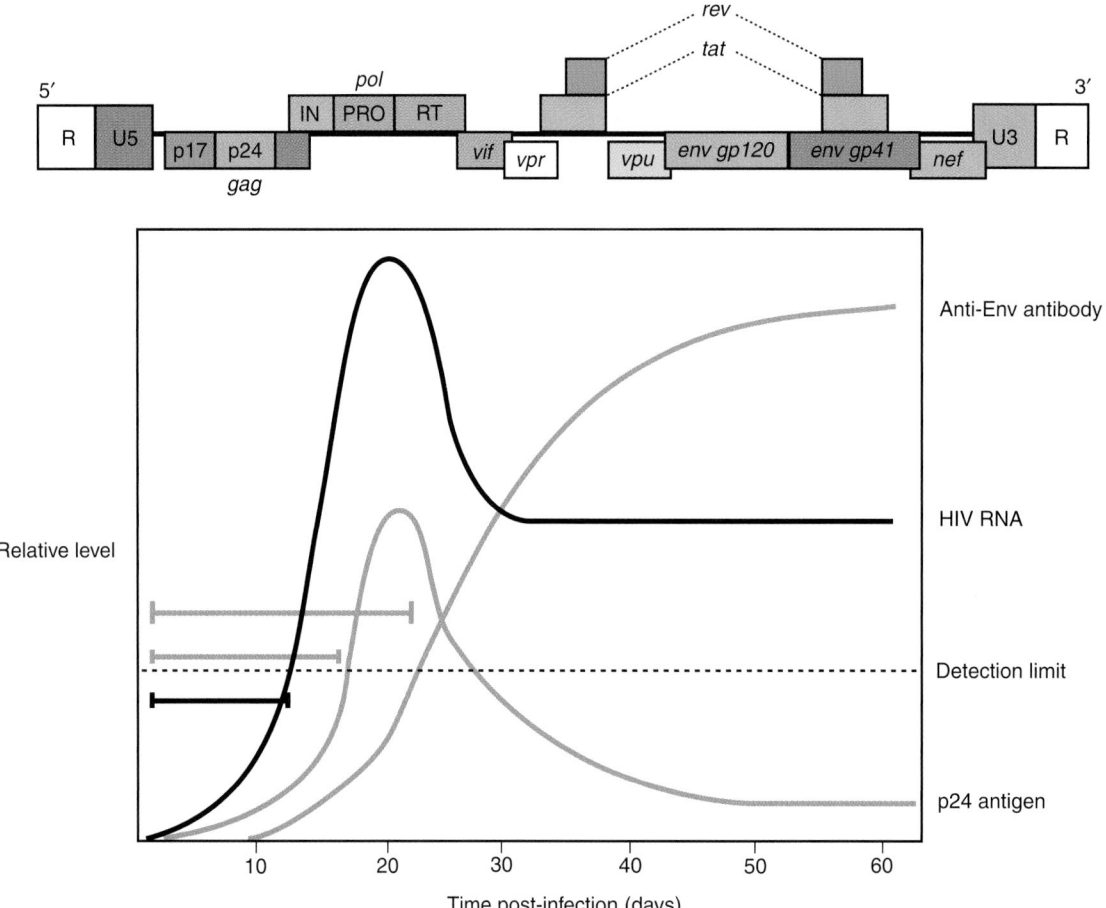

FIGURE 115-3. HIV infection profile. Following HIV infection intense viral replication results in high levels of HIV ribonucleic acid (RNA) and HIV p24 protein in plasma. Increases in anti-HIV antibody are detected. A variable window period (├──┤) is present between the time of infection and the point at which evidence of infection is detected. HIV RNA levels are detected earliest, followed by HIV p24 antigen and finally HIV antibody production.

In these unusual circumstances, it is typically straightforward to reconstruct the clinical course and establish the HIV diagnosis; careful history and judicious use of p24 assays or alternative assays (HIV-1 viral RNA assays or HIV DNA PCR) may be useful for clarification.

HUMAN IMMUNODEFICIENCY VIRUS SCREENING ASSAYS

Serologic Techniques to Detect Anti–Human Immunodeficiency Virus Antibody

Standard Enzyme-Linked Immunosorbent Assays

HIV-1 ELISA tests were the earliest approved serologic tests for HIV infection and remain the most sensitive approved commercial assays for infection. HIV-1/HIV-2 ELISAs have evolved over a number of generations to maximize sensitivity and specificity. All assays capture HIV antibody using immobilized HIV antigens (Fig. 115-4). In their earliest iterations (Table 115-4), whole cell lysates of infected cells were used to coat ELISA wells. Incubation with patient sera permitted anti-HIV antibody to bind to the immobilized antigens, and the bound antibody was identified using enzyme-conjugated antihuman IgG (see Fig. 115-4). Techniques to produce recombinant HIV-1 antigens and chemically synthesized HIV peptides eliminated the use of cell lysates, thereby increasing specificity and sensitivity.[101-103] Third-generation assays employ a sandwich technique using enzyme-coupled HIV antigens (see Fig. 115-4B), and take advantage of the bi- or multivalent nature of antibodies to improve specificity.[104] Sandwich technology expands subtypes of antibodies that can be detected.[105]

Current screening methods are available in various formats with a variety of sources or material (see Table 115-3).

Efforts to improve HIV detection during the HIV-1 seroconversion period have led to combining the standard third-generation ELISA with p24 antigen detection assay (see later). These new fourth-generation assays, though not yet FDA approved, have been reported to reduce the window period by 4.4 to 4.8 days as compared with third-generation assays.[59,106-111] There have been conflicting reports of the presence of a second window period with fourth-generation assays due to a short period when p24 antigen has declined below detection limit but antibody levels have not yet increased above the limit of detection.[112]

Particle Agglutination Assays

HIV antigen antibody reactions have been used to develop relatively rapid, simple assays that do not require equipment to measure a colorimetric readout. Such assays, denoted particle agglutination (PA), are based on the ability of sera containing HIV antibodies to cross link small particles containing HIV antigens on the surface (see Fig. 115-4C). PA has advantages of sensitivity and relatively high inherent specificity, because the presence of bivalent or multivalent reactions is necessary for agglutination to occur. PA assays are relatively easy to perform and require little equipment and as such have important advantages for resource-limited areas.[113-118] Assays based on particle agglutination have been FDA approved[46]; PA assays are subject to reader interpretation, are time sensitive, and have no permanent records of agglutination reactions.[46,118,119] Nevertheless, in large field trials and hospital-based studies, PA platforms performed well for HIV screening.[120-122]

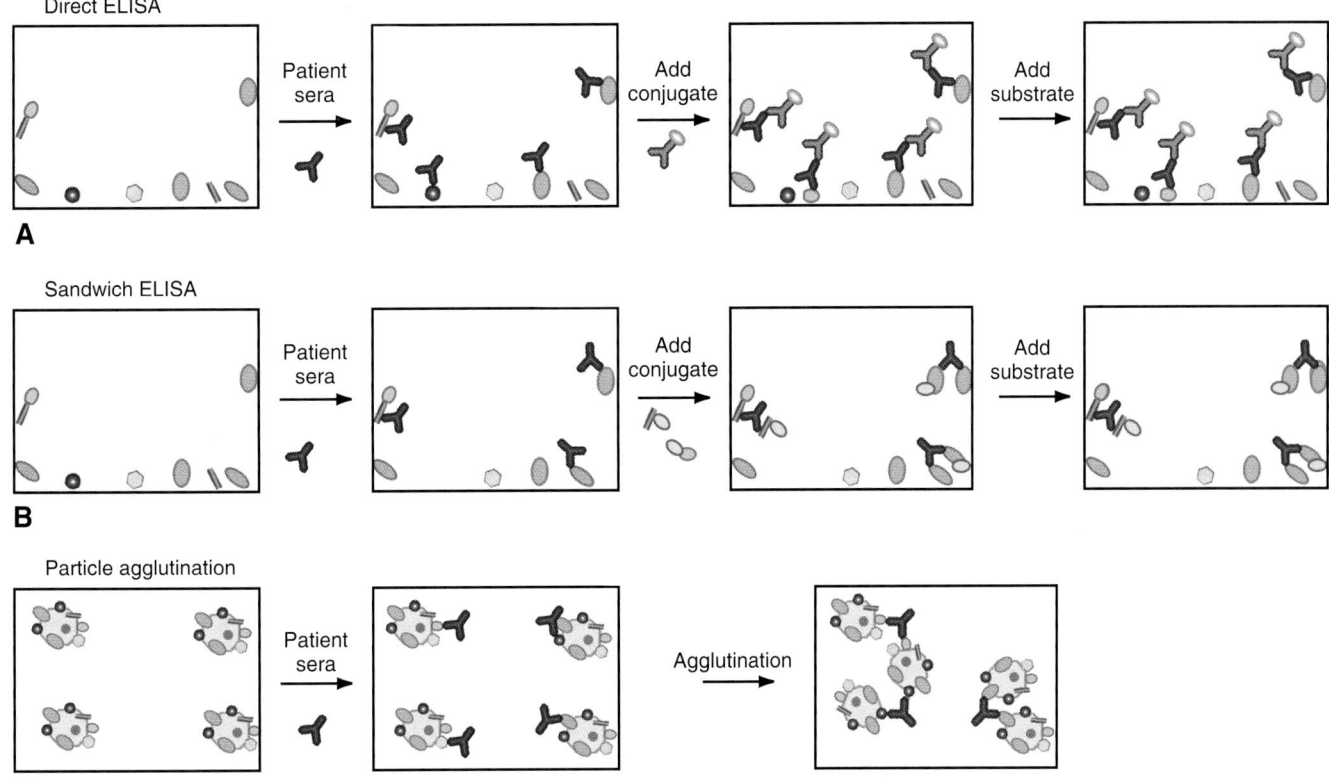

FIGURE 115-4. Comparison of HIV screening techniques. A, Standard enzyme-linked immunosorbent assay (ELISA) technique. ELISA wells coated with HIV viral lysate are incubated with patient sera, permitting binding of specific antibodies to viral proteins. Bound antibody is detected by an anti–immunoglobulin G (IgG) antibody conjugated to assay enzyme, such as horseradish peroxidase or alkaline phosphatase. Conversion of substrate to product is quantitated by spectrophotometry. **B,** Sandwich ELISA. Wells are incubated with patient sera; bound antibodies are detected by purified viral proteins conjugated to detection enzyme; bound enzyme is detected by the addition of substrate. **C,** Agglutination reaction. Patient sera are mixed with small beads coated with viral protein; bivalent or multivalent antibodies cross-link beads, resulting in agglutination. Note that sandwich and agglutination assays may detect multiple antibody classes, whereas in **(A),** only IgG is detected.

TABLE 115-4 Enzyme-Linked Immunosorbent Assay Development

Generation of ELISA Test	Component	Approximate Window Period	Detection of Non-B Subtype	Detection of Group O	Advance
First	Infected cell lysates	63 days	?	?	Laboratory diagnosis of HIV infection
Second	Recombinant protein and peptides	42 days	Not all	±	Decreased false positives
Third	Sandwich with labeled antigen	22 days	+	+	Shortened window substantially
Fourth	Combination p24 antigen detection and sandwich	16 days	+	+	Improved window period

ELISA, enzyme-linked immunosorbent assay; HIV, human immunodeficiency virus.

Alternative Enzyme-Linked Immunosorbent Assay Formats: Simple/Rapid Tests

Despite excellent performance characteristics, there are significant drawbacks of current HIV screening assays, including delays from the time of sample collection to reporting, and the complexity of assay procedure. Simple and rapid tests are manufactured in a variety of formats, and the WHO and CDC differ in details of definition (storage requirements, time required to obtain results). In general these assays employ lateral or capillary flow of sample along a solid support to permit interaction with an embedded antigen; controls are included to identify nonspecific reactivity. Simple tests react with antigen in variable storage requirements at ambient temperature using whole blood as substrate and require little or no equipment. Rapid tests are completed in less than 15 minutes (WHO) or in 30 min or less (CDC). Simple/rapid tests require confirmation, but have been utilized in circumstances of emergency detection (e.g., pregnant women at time of delivery). Sensitivity of rapid testing methods is sufficiently high with non-B HIV subtypes and with group O viruses.[123,124] In seroconversion panels, however, rapid testing may be less sensitive than conventional assays.[123]

Use of rapid HIV testing has resulted in increases in frequency of patient populations receiving test results, including pregnant women[125]; individuals attending sexually transmitted disease (STD) and outpatient clinics[126]; and patients presenting in emergency departments.[127] Modeling studies using the performance characteristics of the Single Use Diagnostic System (SUDS) rapid test kit predicted significant increases in numbers of individuals who would have learned their serostatus if rapid testing had been employed.[64] Rapid HIV testing permits early counseling and discussion of risk reduction and therapy, but is challenged by the consequences of immediately discussing unexpected test results.[128]

Saliva as Source of Patient Material for Enzyme-Linked Immunosorbent Assay

Several investigators noted the presence of anti-HIV antibodies in saliva, which contains little if any infectious virus[49,50,129] and can be obtained safely without the risk of needlestick injury.[130] Oral fluid consists of saliva, bacteria, mucus, debris, and a crevicular transudate containing significant and detectable levels of anti-HIV antibodies in infected individuals.[51,131] The presence of anti-HIV antibody appears to be transudative in origin and generally although not exclusively the result of local synthesis.[132,133] Both immunoglobulin A (IgA)[50] and IgG classes are present, but anti–HIV-1 IgG is present in greater abundance. Even though anti–HIV-1 antibodies in saliva are nearly 1000 times lower in concentration than in serum,[134] IgG levels remain sufficiently high for measurement by both ELISA and WB techniques.[48,135,136] As of 2004, FDA-approved oral based assays detect only HIV-1; there are no FDA-approved oral HIV-2 or HIV-1/2 assays, although methods for oral fluid detection of HIV-2 have been reported (saliva strip[137]).

Oral fluid detection of HIV-1 has excellent performance characteristics comparable to that detected using serum or plasma-based assays.[48,135,136] Recently O'Connell and co-workers[100] reported several false-negative results using oral fluid testing in patients with HIV infection who have undergone antiretroviral therapy early in the course of HIV infection. It is possible that partial resolution of polyclonal gammopathy reduced transudative IgG levels, thereby reducing sensitivity. New assays need to be tested in positive control HIV-infected patients who may be undergoing therapy.[100]

Although little if any infectious HIV is present in saliva, HIV DNA was detected in crevicular fluid samples from patients with gingivitis or periodontitis even in the absence of local bleeding.[138,139] The source of HIV nucleic acid in these circumstances is unclear although oropharyngeal shedding may contribute to the presence of virus at this site.[140]

Saliva IgA has been investigated as source material to diagnose HIV infection in newborns. Early studies in newborns and infants suggested that determining anti-HIV IgA might represent a useful assay to specifically identify HIV-infected infants[141]; more recently, however, several studies have suggested lower sensitivity and greater nonspecific reactivity for saliva IgA detection.[142,143]

Urine as a Source of Patient Material for Enzyme-Linked Immunosorbent Assays

Urine offers relative ease of collection for detection of HIV.[145] Because levels of HIV IgG in urine are relatively low (estimated in the range of 1 mg/L), sensitive techniques are required for detection; ELISAs were developed and were approved in 1996, followed by WB assays in 1998; there were no FDA-approved simple/rapid tests for HIV in urine as of 2004. False-positive results have been identified with urine,[146] although performance characteristics are generally excellent.

Sensitive/Less Sensitive ("Detuned") Assays

The HIV epidemic has been tracked by prevalence using rates of clinical disease (AIDS) and, more recently, by HIV seroprevalence. Estimates of incidence rates of HIV infection have been relatively difficult to obtain but are an important characteristic of epidemics, especially in areas in which infection rates may be changing rapidly. Application of novel ELISA strategy has permitted estimates of HIV-1 incidence rates.[147,148] These assays, denoted sensitive/less sensitive (S/LS) or "detuned" ELISA, employ a dual ELISA strategy. A standard sensitive third-generation ELISA is used to detect all HIV infections and a detuned ELISA that detects only established but not early infections because of the decreased antibody quantity and avidity early in infection. Samples with discordant results, i.e., reactive on the standard assay and nonreactive on the detuned assay, are classified as recent infections. Sensitive/less sensitive assays are not yet approved by the FDA, but appear to be generally applicable in epidemiologic studies of HIV-1 to characterize high risk populations, incidence trends, and peak age incidence of infection[149-151]; if clinical benefits of instituting combination chemotherapy early during the course of HIV-1 infection are clearly demonstrated, such sensitive/less sensitive assays may be especially useful to classify infections[152] and to assist decisions to initiate antiretroviral therapy.

Serologic Techniques to Screen for Human Immunodeficiency Virus Antigens

Acute HIV-1 infection is characterized by relatively high levels of viremia compared with the levels of various anti-HIV antibodies (see Fig. 115-4).[153] As a result, there is a short but significant period in early infection during which p24 antigen is present in the absence of specific anti-p24 antibody. ELISA techniques have been developed to specifically detect p24 using polyclonal patient-derived IgG preparations or monoclonal antibodies to coat ELISA wells. HIV antigen capture assays detect as little as 5 to 20 pg of p24. Assuming that all p24 in blood is from intact virions and that there are approximately 3000 p24 molecules per virion, then the limit of p24 detection is in the range of approximately 40,000 to 200,000 virion particles.

Clinical application of p24 antigens revealed that newly infected patients had transient p24 detectable levels[32,34] and that p24 antigenemia in established disease suggested a poor prognosis.[33] As antibody to p24 develops, complexes of p24 with endogenous antibody interfere with laboratory detection, and p24 sensitivity is reduced.[35] Methods incorporating pH adjustment or heat treatment to dissociate p24 antigen-antibody complexes have resulted in increased p24 detection sensitivity, and immune complex dissociation results in more frequent detection of antigenemia late in disease.[154,155] The combination of heat denaturation and signal amplification using biotinylated tyramide has extended the lower limit of signal detection to 0.5 pg p24 (~4000 virion particles),[156-159] suggesting this assay may be particularly attractive in resource-limited areas without capability to perform quantitative HIV-1 RNA levels.

Gag p24 protein is a relatively well-conserved protein among HIV-1 variants, and commercially available kits have performed consistently well even with diverse HIV-1 subtypes.

False-Positive and False-Negative Results in Screening Tests for Human Immunodeficiency Virus Antibody

HIV screening assays are designed for highest available sensitivity and specificity; sensitivity is a more paramount requirement for screening because the consequences of a false-negative screening test result (which permits HIV infection to proceed undiagnosed) are more profound than those of a false positive result (which will be further evaluated with a confirmatory test). Currently, the false-positive rate in a low-risk population remains low—0.06% to 0.12% in the blood donor population[160]—suggesting that practical test effectiveness is consistent with performance efficacy. Despite high specificity and sensitivity of HIV screening assays, false-negative and false-positive results may occur.

False-negative results from ELISA methodology are rare but may arise from the lack of antibodies of sufficient avidity to generate a colorimetric signal above the assay background threshold. Early HIV infection, as described earlier, represents a common cause of low-level antibody production; rarely immunologically silent HIV infection proceeds without development of antibody response despite HIV replication. Other underlying conditions, such as neoplasms/chemotherapy and common variable immunodeficiency (CVI) represent potential causes of false-negative HIV screening assays, although patients with CVI have had detectable seroconversions.[161] Unusual circumstances, such as extensive transfusion, may sufficiently dilute endogenous antibody in infected individuals to yield false-negative HIV results,[162] and robust antibody reactivity is not universally present.[163]

False-positive screening results are more common than false-negative results and may arise from a number of reasons, generally classified as technical artifacts, chronic medical conditions, multiparity, and unusual circumstances. Reports of false-positive ELISAs are frequent and often occur in the setting of testing patients with low pretest probability for HIV infection; as a result, it is not always certain that the false-positive result was associated with a particular medical condition, or was the result of false-positive rate of the test itself.

Several medical conditions may contribute to a falsely reactive HIV ELISA test, including chronic alcohol use, rheumatic disease, congenital bleeding disorders, syphilis, and neurocysticercosis. In certain rheumatic diseases, polyclonal antibody production has been a persistent source of false-positive HIV ELISA results. Specific reactivity for gp41 has been identified in some cases and p24 reactivity responsible for false positives in Sjögren's syndrome; reactivity is generally of low avidity, and has been eliminated by thiocyanate washing.[164] Recent vaccination with hepatitis B[165] or rabies vaccine[166,167] has been reported to result in false-positive HIV screening results, although the frequency of these events is likely to be quite low.[168] In 1992, influenza vaccination was reported to be associated with increased false-positive HIV testing; an extensive analysis traced increases in false positives to certain ELISA kit lots, and frequent false reactivity after routine influenza vaccination has not been reported because multiparous women also have a higher rate of false-positive screening tests for HIV, although the etiology remains uncertain.

Acute infection may yield false-positive HIV screening assays; recent infection with dengue, malaria, and hepatitis B has been reported to yield false reactivity. False-positive results have been reported in patients with leprosy using early ELISA tests[169,170] with antibodies to lipoarabinomannan of *Mycobacterium leprae* implicated as potential cross-reacting antibody,[171] although a study using double-sandwich ELISA did not reproduce the high rate of false-positive results in this population.[172] Because primary HIV infection may present as an acute viral syndrome with fever, rash, and numerous constitutional symptoms, thoughtful interpretation of any screening assay in patients with such symptoms is warranted. Recent survey of patients with documented acute mononucleosis did not identify positive HIV screening assays.[173] However, several patients with primary HIV infection have been identified during evaluation who had false-positive serologic tests for Epstein-Barr virus (EBV) infection.[174]

The presence of HIV infection may affect serologic detection of other infections; false-positive results for syphilis, Ebola, Marburg, and Lassa fever have been reported in patients with HIV infection; HIV infection has been reported to result in occasional false-negative results in human T-cell leukemia virus (HTLV)-I/II assays.[175]

With time and widespread application, it is possible that new sources of false-positive results may occur. In needlestick circumstances, samples for HIV testing from inpatients may be obtained from indwelling catheters; samples drawn in such fashion may become contaminated with vehicles for drugs administered through the catheter; one diluent, propylene glycol, has been reported to give a false-positive result with HIV ELISAs.[176]

Nonserologic Techniques to Screen for Human Immunodeficiency Virus

Hybridization and Amplification Assays to Detect Human Immunodeficiency Virus Nucleic Acids

Use of NAT is a valuable adjunct to, but not as a replacement for, serologic methods for HIV detection. Various formats can detect HIV-1 RNA with great sensitivity, and new real-time PCR methods have been developed that are capable of detecting a single copy of HIV-1 RNA.[177] Clinical methods for HIV nucleic acid detection for use in monitoring HIV infection have included nucleic acid sequence based amplification (NASBA), branched chain DNA (bDNA), and polymerase chain reaction (PCR) amplification; NASBA formats have detected as low as 22 to 31 copies/mL.[178,179] PCR assays have been developed for use in blood donor screening and have demonstrated utility in identifying patients during the seroconversion period, when HIV RNA levels may be extremely high but anti-HIV antibody is comparatively low. The utility of NAT during early seroconversion has been investigated using either single-donor samples or "minipools" of 16 or 24 plasma samples.

In the United States, trials for FDA approval of NAT screened more than 20 million donations and found 7 HIV-infected samples that scored negative for HIV antibody.[78] NAT systems detected a number of HIV-1 infections that would have been missed by previously licensed test methods, confirming the increased sensitivity of these systems.[180] Similarly, trials in Europe, South Africa, and Japan[181-184] and case reports[185-199] have documented that NAT identified patients in seroconversion windows who had been missed using p24 antigen detection. By contrast, there are also reports of undetected HIV-1 in the setting of relatively low HIV-1 RNA levels, especially in minipools of 16 or 24 plasma samples.[78] Retrospective analysis of a blood transmission case (before NAT) revealed a relatively low viral RNA level (estimated 40 copies/mL)[190]; the benefit of NAT over traditional testing has been estimated to reduce the window period by 2 to 6 days. Using NAT technology, the risk of HIV infection through transfusion was estimated as 1/1,576,000[191]; four cases of p24 antigen–negative blood component were identified in more than 19 million screened units.[192] Consequently, the risk of HIV-1 transmission via blood components is reduced but not completely eliminated by incorporating NAT into screening procedures. The residual risk of HIV infection in the United States is estimated at 1 per 2,135,000[192]; similar or lower risks have been estimated from other reporting countries,[193,194] and although there are concerns regarding subtype sensitivity and sample preparation, many blood centers throughout the world have incorporated NAT as a component of HIV screening. Relative cost-effectiveness of NAT remains a concern.[181,183,195] Nucleic acid testing is approved in the United States for blood donor screening using plasma. Assays must be able to detect 100 copies 95% of the time and several assays are more sensitive than this limit.[179] Standard subtype B virus preparations have been established as quantitative controls.[196] Testing can be performed on single samples or minipools of plasma and may be combined to detect HIV-1 and hepatitis C.

NAT has reported both false-positive and false-negative results in plasma.[197-201] Values exceeding 5000 copies/mL may be useful as cutoff for an HIV-1 RNA level above which is suggestive of HIV infection in a nondonor population.[198] With increasing experience it will be of interest to determine whether NAT will be effective in HIV detection in circumstances in which serologic assays are traditionally less specific (e.g., pregnancy, alcohol, rheumatologic diseases). NAT has not been extensively used for cadaveric specimens; RNA is chemically labile, and delays in sample processing may present particular challenges in detection by this method. NAT is effective in detecting HIV in serum or dried blood spots,[202] and plasma (nonheparinized) is a better starting material, especially for low-copy number detection.

NAT is approved in the United States for use in screening in blood donation services in combination with standard serologic procedures. NAT is not, however, approved by the FDA as a single screening tool under any circumstance or for use in confirmation. Even if performance characteristics were sufficiently robust, groups of HIV-infected individuals would be HIV negative if NAT were used as an exclusive test. As described in Chapter 116, the spectrum of HIV infection includes long-term nonprogressor (LTNP) with persistently high CD4 cell numbers and relatively low HIV-1 RNA levels.[203] Although LTNPs are HIV-1 ELISA reactive and WB positive, screening with current NAT could not be expected to reliably identify such individuals as HIV infected. At present, NAT systems for patient analysis detect only HIV-1; currently, there are no FDA-approved HIV-2 NAT kits. NAT performance characteristics have been established largely with subtype B virus. Although HIV-1 RNA detection assays used to monitor HIV infection have been adapted for use with alternative HIV subtypes, NAT developed for HIV screening has not yet undergone a similar extensive evaluation.

There are obvious potential benefits in employing NAT in HIV detection situations outside of the FDA-approved blood donation indication, especially in helping to identify patients with early HIV infection and in resolving indeterminate WBs or discordant screening results.[204] At present, NAT must be used with caution, close discussion with laboratory experts, and common sense.

HUMAN IMMUNODEFICIENCY VIRUS CONFIRMATORY ASSAYS

Western Blot

The HIV WB represents a specific method to detect the presence of serologic reactivity to individual viral antigens. WB has a specificity of more than 99%, and currently represents the practical gold standard confirmatory test for HIV infection in the United States (Fig. 115-5). Individual HIV proteins are separated by gel electrophoresis, and an-

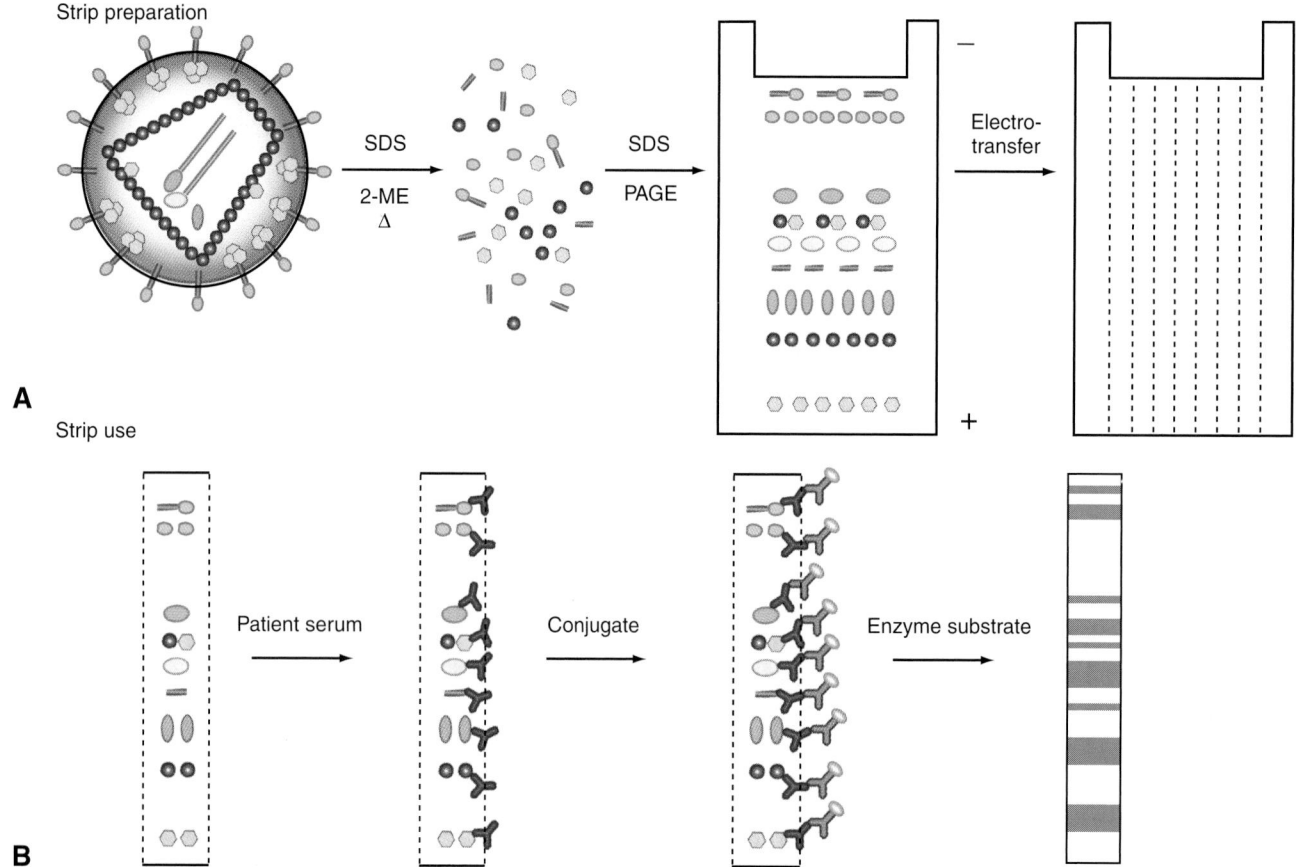

FIGURE 115-5. HIV Western blot. A, Western blot strips are prepared with purified HIV virions that are disrupted with ionic detergent and reducing agent, subjected to sodium dodecyl sulfate–polyacrylamide gel electrophoresis (SDS-PAGE), and electrotransferred to solid strips, typically of nitrocellulose. **B,** Strips are sequentially incubated with patient sample (serum, plasma, saliva, or urine), enzyme conjugated antihuman immunoglobulin G (IgG), and enzyme substrate. The position of enzyme bound identifies the presence of antibody to individual HIV proteins.

tibodies react with the individual proteins. WBs contain only virion proteins incorporated into the virion (Fig. 115-6); gene products confined to the cell (e.g., *vpu, tat, rev,* see Fig. 115-1) are not represented. Other HIV proteins specifically incorporated into virions, such as Vpr, are inconsistently detected in commercial blots, and not included in diagnostic criteria.

WB results are scored as negative, positive, or indeterminate. According to CDC criteria, a negative WB has no reactive bands. The WHO has suggested that a weakly reactive p17 band may be considered negative.[205] Definition of a positive WB has undergone evolution since introduction. Initially, criteria for HIV-positive WB were relatively stringent, and required the presence of antibody to Gag p24, Pol p31, and either Env gp41 or Env gp160/120 (Table 115-5). Under these guidelines, the number of indeterminate blots was high, thereby reducing the efficiency of WB confirmation; the infection status of many patients remained unresolved, but was likely positive. In revising the criteria for positive WBs, different strategies were used by governing agencies (see Table 115-5). Comparison of these approaches[206] in a group of 424 serum samples revealed the CDC/Association of State and Territorial Public Health Laboratory Directors (ASTPHLD) criteria had the fewest number of indeterminate and the greatest number of true positives. Despite revision, the indeterminate rate of HIV-1 WB is too high to permit Western blotting to be used as a screening assay.[207,208]

Indeterminate results may arise from either insensitive detection of true reactivity (window period) or false reactivity with principally single-band reactivity. In general, single-band p24 reactivity remains among the most common reasons for indeterminate WB reactivity[209] and longitudinal studies of persistent single-band p24 reactivity in various populations show that these are consistently not associated with true HIV infection.[210-213] Etiology of false-positive p24 reactivity remains uncertain; analysis by Blomberg of p24 reactivity revealed distinct regions of p24 reactivity in sera from false-positive and true-positive samples.[214] Similarly, Deas and associates and Haist and co-workers[215,216] identified peptides in p24 that were re-

sponsible for false-positive reactivity in patients with systemic lupus erythematosus (SLE) and Sjögren's syndrome. In contrast, Kammerer has reported no specific association with anti-p24 reactivity in rheumatologic patients and HIV false positives.[217] Several autoimmune diseases, notably Hashimoto's thyroiditis and SLE, as well as non-Hodgkin's lymphoma and histiocytosis were associated with p24 reactivity.[88,218] Initial studies of group O viruses with earlier WB versions had variable results,[219] but improvements have resulted in specificity of current WBs that are nearly equivalent for most subtypes. Significant rates of indeterminate results are still reported with samples with elevated bilirubin, SLE, hemolysis, rheumatoid factor, polyclonal gammopathy, hemodialysis, HLA antibodies, and various other infectious diseases, including HTLV-I.[220] Sporadic reports of indeterminate WBs have been cited with schistosomiasis in Brazil,[221] recent tetanus immunization,[222] the presence of heterophile antibodies,[223] or massive proteinuria.[224]

Indeterminate WB results have been reported at higher frequency in Africans.[225-229] Rates of p24 reactivity are particularly high, and although the etiology remains uncertain, it is not likely due to infection with non–subtype B virus. HIV-1 Gag reactivity, particularly p24, was often responsible for indeterminate results, whereas Env reactivity was rarely present.[230] As a consequence, use of alternative criteria for defining HIV infection in African populations has been suggested, including use of the combination of gp160 plus p31.[228,229]

False-positive WBs after repeatedly reactive ELISA have been reported in the presence of rheumatologic disorders, and in extremely rare circumstances, WB may be falsely positive after false-positive enzyme immunoassays (EIAs),[200,231] leading to misdiagnoses of HIV infection. Class II antigens are expressed in certain cell lines (H9) used for large-scale HIV propagation; as class II is incorporated into virions, WB strips may contain low levels of class II, which may the cause of indeterminate results.[232]

Western blotting approaches have been adapted for use with recombinant or peptide proteins in so-called line immunoassays ("INNO-LIA,"

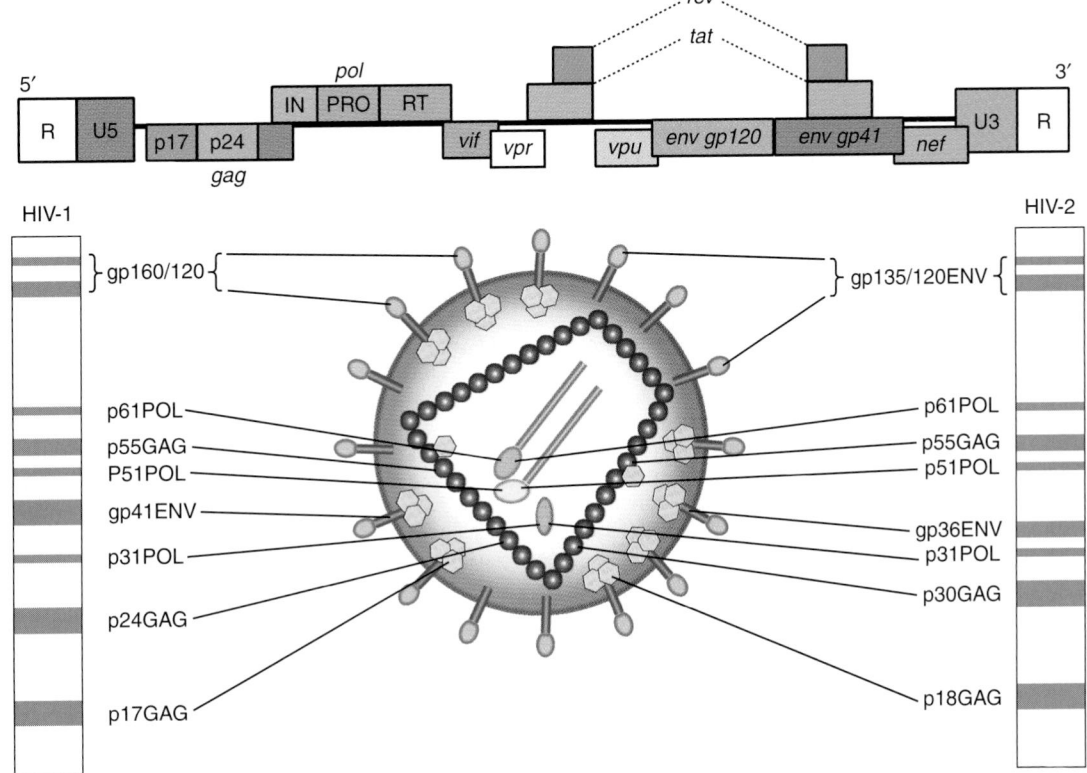

FIGURE 115-6. **Proteins detected by HIV Western blot.** Viral lysates are disrupted, subjected to sodium dodecyl sulfate–polyacrylamide gel electrophoresis (SDS-PAGE), and proteins separated according to molecular size. Positions of viral proteins in typical Western blot strips for HIV-1 and HIV-2 are indicated. The location of each protein in the virion is indicated and the position of the genes encoding relevant proteins is color-coded in the HIV-1 genome map.

TABLE 115-5 Criteria for Positive Western Blot

Version	Criteria
Original criteria	p24 and p31 and gp41 or gp160/120
Current criteria	
ASTPHLD/CDC	Any two bands: p24, gp41, and gp120/160
American Red Cross	Any band from each: Gag, Pol, Env
The Consortium for Retrovirus Serology Standardization	p24 or p31 AND either gp41 or gp160/120

ASTPHLD, Association of State and Territorial Public Health Laboratory Directors; CDC, Centers for Disease Control and Prevention.

"LiaTek,"[233-235] and Pepti-LAV).[236] Because these solid phase assays are constructed without virions, false-positive results stemming from the presence of cellular proteins encapsidated with HIV are eliminated. HIV-1/HIV-2 dually infected individuals may be identified, and such positive WBs[237] may yield fewer indeterminate results.[238,239]

Immunofluorescence

Indirect immunofluorescence (IFA) is a standard virologic technique to identify the presence of antibodies by their specific ability to react with viral antigens expressed in infected cells; bound antibodies are visualized by incubation with fluorescently labeled antihuman antibodies.[240,241] A requirement for antibodies to demonstrate reactivity with characteristic staining patterns provides additional specificity to the interpretation. Indirect immunofluorescence had been used extensively as a confirmatory assay in HIV diagnosis,[241,242] and continues to be utilized in laboratories with extensive experience with the assay. Conditions interfering with immunofluorescence include severe lipemia, hyperbilirubinemia, paraproteinemia, and autoimmune diseases. IFA for HIV-2 has been described,[243] but no such FDA-approved kits are yet available in United States.

Performance characteristics for IFA remain excellent and in good agreement with WB results[244]; in a recent MPEP survey, no false positives were detected, and 14.3% of 215 results were indeterminate. Commercial IFA assays are relatively rapid, straightforward, and inexpensive[245] but require special equipment and expertise; nevertheless they may be particularly suited for programs with limited resources.[246] In the United States, indirect immunofluorescence has largely been replaced by WB.

Radioimmunoprecipitation

Radioimmunoprecipitation assay (RIPA) is a standard technique to identify the presence of antibodies by their ability to react with radiolabeled antigens.[247-249] Radioimmunoprecipitations are highly specific and were used as early confirmatory assays.[248] In some circumstances RIPA may be more sensitive than WB reactivity. Huisman and coworkers detected early Gag p24 reactivity prior to ELISA reactivity, and Saah and associates noted utility of radioimmunoprecipitation in resolving indeterminate WBs early in infection.[79,247] RIPAs were less sensitive than p24 or NAT in seroconversions.[250] Techniques to distinguish HIV-1 and HIV-2 have been reported.[251] Radioimmunoprecipitation assays are relatively labor intensive and have specific equipment and laboratory requirements.

Virologic Techniques to Detect Human Immunodeficiency Virus Infection

Isolation of HIV by in vitro cultivation techniques can be used to establish HIV infection. Although the levels of HIV in plasma may be relatively high, the proportion of circulating viremia that is capable of propagating infection is relatively low, thus the use of serum or plasma for HIV cultivation is relatively insensitive. Use of peripheral blood mononuclear cells (PBMCs) from HIV-infected individuals as a source of HIV has a much higher rate of positive isolation, especially if PBMCs are depleted of CD8+ cells.

Practical Application of Human Immunodeficiency Virus Detection Assays

Several algorithms for HIV detection have been devised depending upon the purpose of the detection (blood surveillance, patient diagnosis, epidemiologic screening). In the United States, the FDA regulates strategies, and worldwide the WHO maintains "best practice" materials, cognizant of the special requirements and limitations of various locations. The advent of rapid testing and point of care or home collection testing complicates such algorithms, but in the United States, regardless of purpose or location, all HIV algorithms used for diagnosis have two distinct stages: a screening phase and a confirmation phase (Fig. 115-7).

Human Immunodeficiency Viruses 1 and 2 Screening Phase

Screening for HIV begins during the patient interview. As described previously, HIV testing is imperfect, with significant false-positive rate in low-prevalence populations. For patient diagnostic purposes, efficient application of HIV testing should be implemented after some risk assessment and with serious consideration of scientific and ethical consequences.[252]

The CDC described populations who should be offered HIV testing (Table 115-6).[253] Epidemiologic and clinical studies have identified certain high-risk populations or medical situations in which HIV testing is recommended, such as for persons visiting STD clinics or any patient presenting for care in areas where the HIV seroprevalence is greater than 1%[144]; individuals presenting to emergency departments may represent patients with early HIV infection,[254] and specific techniques should be considered to detect early HIV infection. HIV testing is recommended for any patient presenting with tuberculosis.

To a large degree, HIV testing is anonymous, voluntary, and confidential; in general, mandatory testing has been rejected because of concerns for patient dignity.[255] In the United States, however, there are notable exceptions. Testing of inmates in federal corrections facilities was mandated beginning in 1998, and 16 states have mandatory testing in state prisons.[256] In certain circumstances, especially sexual offenses, HIV testing has been court ordered; test results are made available to victims and in some cases to prison administrators. In New York, HIV testing of infants is mandatory under the Maternal-Pediatric HIV Prevention and Care Program (1997)[257]; antenatal testing is required in Connecticut except for religious preferences as of 1999; HIV testing of pregnant women in other states is encouraged but not required.[253] Testing as a part of military recruitment is required in the United States and in at least 26 other countries.[255] Testing is mandatory by a number of governments for immigrants entering as workers, students, and temporary or permanent residents; testing performed in U.S. laboratories may or may not be acceptable for this purpose (a list of such countries and whether U.S. testing is accepted is available at http://www.WHO.int). In the face of involuntary HIV testing, governing bodies, such as the WHO, have categorically rejected mandatory HIV testing.[255]

HIV testing guidelines (see Table 115-6) represent minimum recommendations and should not take the place of a careful review of HIV risks. The course of the HIV epidemic in the United States has progressed from standard elevated risk groups; women and older individuals represent two groups in which HIV is spreading; similarly the epidemic has diffused from major metropolitan centers into less densely populated areas. Thoughtful, probing history should accompany the use of any list of standard HIV risks.

Once the decision to offer HIV testing has been made, three specific questions provide useful information to choose the optimum HIV screening test (rapid, routine, or p24 antigen testing) to be performed (see Fig. 115-7A): (1) Is there a risk of acute HIV-1 infection? (2) Is there a risk of HIV-2 infection? (3) Is there a potential patient benefit to use a rapid testing strategy? If there is a significant risk of acute HIV infection, then rapid testing modalities should not be used exclusively for screening because they are slightly less sensitive in this setting. Use of p24 antigen/RNA testing may be considered in this setting in addition to the standard third-generation ELISA. If HIV-2 is a significant consideration (see later), then rapid testing should not be used, because at

FIGURE 115-7. Algorithm for HIV detection in patients at risk for HIV infection. Note that in the absence of documented infection (noted in *blue*), all individuals with HIV risk factors should be monitored and followed as indicated with routine testing. **A,** Screening algorithm. HIV screening should be considered for all patients at elevated risk for infection. The choice of screening test may be guided by clinical circumstances. **B,** Confirmation algorithm. Negative and indeterminate results require discussion and consideration for alternative possibilities, especially the presence of acute HIV infection.

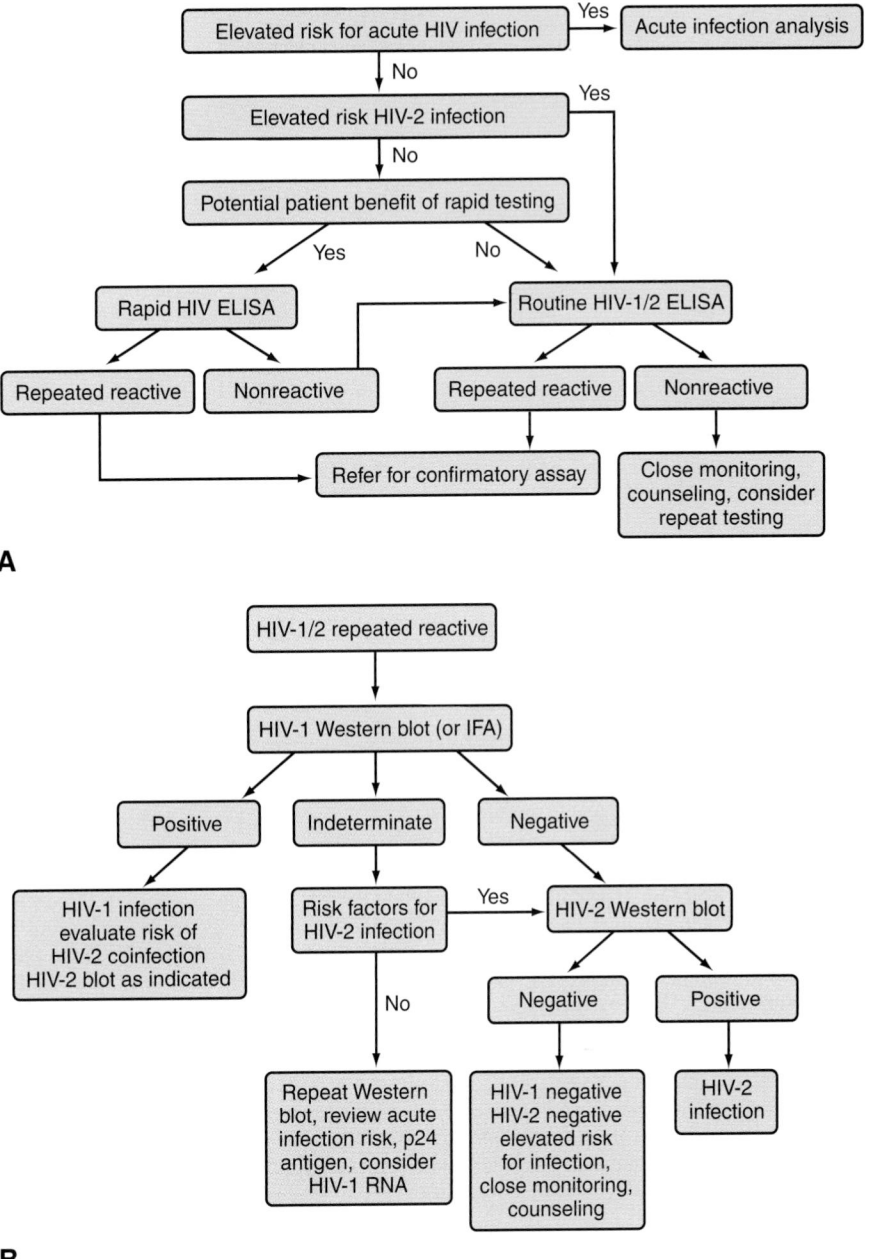

present rapid testing methods only test for HIV-1. If there is a potential patient benefit for rapid diagnosis and the patient is not thought to be at risk for HIV-2 infection or recent HIV-1 infection, then rapid testing should be considered, and advantages and disadvantages discussed. If rapid testing is performed and the result is nonreactive, a standard HIV-1/HIV-2 ELISA should be performed to evaluate the possibility that early infection is present.

All screening ELISA tests with reactive results are automatically repeated in duplicate; repeatedly reactive samples are referred for confirmation. In cases of discordant results, an independent blood sample should be obtained and screening ELISA HIV-1/HIV-2 should be repeated; use of an independent approved HIV-1/HIV-2 ELISA kit using a different detection strategy may be considered. A nonreactive result identifies patients who are at elevated risk but do not have detectable infection. Such individuals represent a critical population that requires continued care and counseling.

Screening Persons with Acute Human Immunodeficiency Virus Infection

Individuals in whom acute HIV infection is strongly considered represent a potentially difficult but important group to diagnose correctly and quickly, especially if early antiretroviral therapy is under consideration. In general, a combination of third-generation HIV-1/HIV-2 ELISA, p24 antigen, and HIV-1 RNA detection may provide useful information in a timely fashion. Either repeated reactivity with HIV-1/HIV-2 ELISA or positive p24 antigen represents a positive screening test for HIV infection, and the presence of positive p24 in the appropriate setting is strongly suggestive of early HIV infection. The time of testing after infection is not always uniform, and p24 antigen may be less sensitive depending upon the emergence of specific anti-p24 antibody. As an alternative, the presence of a high HIV RNA level (>5000-10,000 copies/mL) may represent a useful supporting result. In the early period after infection, HIV-1/HIV-2

TABLE 115-6 Recommendations for Human Immunodeficiency Virus Testing

Recommendations for HIV Testing Categories of Elevated Risk for HIV Infection

Activities
  MSM
  IVDU
  Exchanging sex for drugs or money
  Unprotected sex
  Illness or fever without cause
  Patient request

Specific Exposure
  Occupational
  High risk needle sharing or sexual
  Perinatal

Clinical Circumstances
  Symptoms suggestive of HIV infection
  STD
  Hepatitis
  Confirmed or suspected tuberculosis

Epidemiology
  Geographic areas where HIV prevalence ≥1%

Mandatory Testing
  Federal prisons
  Selected state prisons
  Pregnancy (Connecticut)
  Newborns (New York)
  Court ordered
  Immigration requirement

HIV, human immunodeficiency virus; IVDU, intravenous drug user; MSM, men who have sex with men; STD, sexually transmitted disease.

ELISA may be nonreactive, so a p24 antigen test represents an alternative FDA-approved method to screen for HIV infection. The availability of HIV RNA levels again provides supporting evidence for the presence of early infection.

Exclusive use of HIV-1 RNA measurements in the absence of p24 is somewhat suboptimal. In the case of the ELISA nonreactive early infection patient, with a nonreactive ELISA, an elevated HIV-1 RNA represents the only evidence of infection. Standard HIV RNA assays are not designed for diagnosis, and it is preferable to employ methods designed specifically for screening. In circumstances of discordant results, a repeat specimen should be obtained. In the early infection period, HIV WBs may be negative or indeterminate. Obtaining serial WBs may document evolution of immune reactivity in early infection and document the diagnosis of early infection.

Human Immunodeficiency Viruses 1 and 2 Confirmation Phase

Samples repeatedly reactive in screening assays are referred for confirmation (see Fig. 115-7B). Confirmatory tests approved by FDA include WB and immunofluorescence assays. In practice, WB assays are the most commonly used. As shown in Table 115-4, WBs may be performed in a number of formats and as described above, results may be positive, negative, or indeterminate. Positive WB results of repeatedly reactive ELISA HIV-1/HIV-2 ELISA indicate the presence of HIV-1 infection. Negative WBs indicate the absence of HIV-1 antibodies in sufficient quantities to react with proteins in nitrocellulose strips. In this regard, there should be circumspect consideration for the presence of early (window period) HIV infection. Risk factors for HIV-2 infection should also be reviewed, and HIV-2 WBs should be performed in individuals with opportunistic infections or other AIDS-associated conditions.

Resolving WB indeterminate samples is a critical function of infectious disease specialists in conjunction with clinical laboratories. Indeterminate WBs may represent nonspecific reaction or an early infection, and the pattern of WB reactivity should be evaluated with the perspective of comorbid patient illness and HIV risk factors. Indeterminate blots with single reactivity to gp120/160 or gp41 are less typical for false positives and may suggest early infection.[258] The specific population in which WB indeterminate results are obtained is of importance. Davey and others[259,260] noted numerous indeterminate patterns among high-risk individuals with indeterminate WBs, none of which were predictive of infection. In populations with decreased risk for HIV infection, longitudinal analysis of indeterminate WBs revealed infrequent evolution to infection. Longitudinal studies of blood donors with indeterminate WB did not reveal subsequent full seroconversion.[261,262] Patients who did progress to HIV infection rarely do so in the absence of Env or p24 reactivity.[263] By contrast, Rich and co-workers studied a prison population with HIV risk factors and demonstrated a high rate of full seroconversion in prison inmates with initially indeterminate WBs.[264]

Repeat ELISA/WB using a fresh test specimen is useful in resolving indeterminate WB results. Repeat HIV testing in 4 to 6 weeks is typically indicated to determine whether an indeterminate result represents an evolving immune response to recent HIV infection. For a variety of reasons, the standard wait-and-repeat strategy may introduce unnecessary delay in identifying newly infected patients. p24 Antigen determination is useful in resolving indeterminate blots if p24 is elevated; a negative result represents noncontributory data because early infection may still be present. Use of NAT, although not approved for diagnosis of early HIV infection, may be valuable, especially if the RNA levels obtained are consistent with typical early HIV infection. If so, standard HIV confirmatory assays should still be repeated with time to document antibody reactivity. Although infection with nonsubtype B HIV infection may not result in strong reactions, the performance characteristics of current WBs should be sufficient to detect infection with other subtypes and subtype O infection. Use of additional non–FDA-approved assays cannot be recommended to complete HIV diagnosis as a rule; some line probe assays, however, have reported less nonspecific reactivity with sera containing high anti-DNA antibodies, and may be useful in understanding reactivity in specific circumstances.

Use of alternative confirmatory assays such as RIPA or IFA[265] has been suggested to resolve indeterminate WBs, although the majority remain indeterminate.[266] In regions where HIV-2 is present and PCR technology has become available, Chen and co-workers have suggested nested PCR for *vpu* as a method to detect HIV-1 because the *vpu* gene is present in HIV-1 but not in HIV-2.[267]

Test Counseling

Pre- and post-test counseling sessions represent critical opportunities for health care professionals to affect the rate of HIV transmission and are an integral part of the HIV testing process. Patient counseling is a paramount concern in patient diagnosis, and specially trained counseling should be considered. In general, typical pretest counseling includes a discussion of the importance and limitations of the assays, a discussion of behaviors to reduce risk of contracting HIV, and implications of positive results including effects on employment and insurance. Consent for HIV testing should be documented and some circumstances require written signed consent from patients. Post-test counseling involves a discussion of the results and their accuracy, the implications of negative and positive results, and behavior that may prevent transmission or acquisition, respectively.

Notification strategies are traditionally carried out face to face to permit broad discussion and to address patient concerns. Telephone counseling was found to be surprisingly effective in home collection strategies,[268] and alternatives to face-to-face discussions may be advantageous in certain circumstances. Tsu[269] compared direct (face to face) and telephone notification (patients called to obtain results) in a randomized trial of 351 at-risk and homeless youth. A significantly higher proportion of individuals in the telephone notification group received testing results and post-test counseling compared with those who returned to receive information face to face.

Alternative Strategies for Screening and Confirming Human Immunodeficiency Virus

Although the sequential ELISA/WB is a sensitive and specific approach for HIV detection, it is relatively expensive, is labor intensive, and requires special equipment; alternative strategies are essential for detection of HIV antibodies in resource-poor circumstances. Dual ELISA strategies, using assays with different principles or antigens, have demonstrated 100% sensitivity and specificity in field tests using HIV subtypes appropriate for resource-poor areas.[199,270-277]

The WHO and United Nations Acquired Immunodeficiency Syndrome (UNAIDS)[124,278,279] have proposed three alternative strategies for detection of HIV infection, designed for surveillance of blood supply (strategy I), surveillance and diagnosis (strategy II), and diagnosis (strategy III). In strategy I reactivity in a single screening ELISA or simple/rapid test is reported as HIV positive, and a nonreactive result is HIV negative. This strategy represents a stringent blood safety mechanism, and has been suggested for implementation in areas where HIV seroprevalence exceeds 30% among symptomatic persons, a recommendation that has been supported in field studies.[280] For strategy II, sequential ELISA or simple/rapid tests are utilized. A single positive result prompts use of a second ELISA, and a reactive result with both assays is reported as the presence of HIV infection. Discordant results are repeated, and repeated discordant samples are deemed indeterminate. Strategy II has been suggested for determination of HIV infection in areas where seroprevalence is estimated to be equal to or less than 10% and for diagnosis where seroprevalence is 30% among symptomatic persons and greater than 10% among asymptomatic individuals. Strategy III utilizes two sequential tests, beginning with standard ELISA simple/rapid testing. Samples repeatedly reactive on test one or reactive on tests one and two are tested with an independent test using a different antigen preparation or strategy. Reactivity on all three tests is considered HIV positive. Strategy III has been recommended for diagnosis in asymptomatic patients in areas where HIV seroprevalence is estimated to be equal to or less than 10%.

Testing kits account for a substantial cost of testing.[124,270,275,281] The WHO assists in supplying HIV kits to resource-poor countries using a bulk purchasing strategy and has established standards for performance characteristics and manufacture of individual kits. In addition to technical requirements, the WHO has recommended that any kit marketed internationally should be first approved for use in the home country[124] of manufacture.

SPECIFIC CIRCUMSTANCES AND SPECIAL POPULATIONS

Detection of HIV-2 and HIV-1/HIV-2 Dual Infections

HIV-2 is a retrovirus with a structure and replication program similar to HIV-1 but is distinct from HIV-1 in origin, epidemiology, spread, disease progression, genetic organization, and nucleic acid sequence.[38,39,282] HIV-2 infections originally reported in western Africa are now present in Europe, especially Portugal, and in southern Asia, including India.[283] The CDC reports that African countries with at least 1% HIV-2 prevalence include Angola, Cape Verde, Côte d'Ivoire, The Gambia, Guinea-Bissau, Mali, Mauritania, Mozambique, Nigeria, and Sierra Leone. In addition, Benin, Burkina-Faso, Ghana, Guinea, Liberia, Niger, São Tomé, Senegal, and Togo are reported to have significant numbers of HIV-2 infections. There have been fewer than 100 cases of HIV-2 reported in the United States.[284] Infection with HIV-2 does not prevent infection with HIV-1[285]; sequential HIV-2–HIV-1 infections have been documented,[286] and dual HIV-1/HIV-2 infections are reported in western Africa and India.[283,287,288] The ability to detect HIV-2 infection, discriminate HIV-2 from HIV-1, and identify HIV-1/HIV-2 dual infections has always been important from an epidemiologic and blood safety standpoint, but precise diagnosis has become essential in the era of effective antiretroviral therapy. Specifically, HIV-2 reverse transcriptase is not sensitive to non-nucleotide reverse transcriptase inhibitor (NNRTI) antiretrovirals such as nevirapine, efavirenz, and

delavirdine. As a result, patients with HIV-2 infection (or HIV-1/HIV-2 coinfection) should not be treated with NNRTI-based regimens.

Initially a significant proportion of sera from HIV-2–infected individuals reacted with HIV-1 ELISA kits[289-291]; in the United States, specific screening assays for HIV-2 were not initially developed because of the relatively few number of HIV-2 infections. Screening assays specific for HIV-2 have since been developed; laboratory diagnosis of HIV-2 infection is straightforward and rapid assays are robust in field trials.[292] Typically, screening HIV-1/HIV-2 ELISA results show repeat reactivity, and confirmatory HIV-1 WB is negative, leading to HIV-2 WB. HIV-2 WBs have similar Gag, Pol, and Env proteins, although molecular size (and therefore migration) by sodium dodecyl sulfate–polyacrylamide gel electrophoresis (SDS-PAGE) by these proteins differs from the corresponding HIV-1 proteins (see Fig. 115-6). Some cross-reactivity between relatively well-conserved Gag and Pol proteins may occur, giving rise to unusual indeterminate WB results. Criteria for interpretation of HIV-2 WBs has been reported; initially, significant cross-reactivity of HIV-1 with HIV-2 WBs was reported; requirement for presence of reactivity to both Env proteins gp36 and gp130 reduced the false-positive rate. Resolution of indeterminate WBs is perhaps more problematic with HIV-2 compared with HIV-1. HIV-1 p24 antigen detection assays do detect HIV-2 Gag protein, and there are reports of HIV-2 antigen capture assays with high sensitivity.[293] HIV-2 antigen capture assays are not, however, FDA approved for use in the United States. Methodology for determining HIV-2 RNA levels has not been standardized to the same degree as HIV-1 and no FDA-approved tests are available for this purpose. Indirect immunofluorescence assays have been used to distinguish HIV-1 and HIV-2 infections,[243] but currently there are no FDA-approved HIV-2 IFA test kits. HIV-2 cultivation from infected individuals has been reported,[294] but the frequency of infectious virus recovery was lower than that detected with HIV-1.[294] Use of rapid or line assays containing recombinant antigens has been reported useful in identification of HIV-1/HIV-2 infections.[237,295,296]

As described for HIV-1, alternatives to typical ELISA and WB algorithms have been developed with excellent sensitivity and specificity even in the setting of HIV1/HIV-2 dual infections.[297] Most standard licensed ELISA test kits include HIV-2, and standard algorithms for specific HIV-2 investigation follow from the finding of a positive ELISA and negative HIV-1 WB. With appropriate demographic information (suggesting HIV-2–endemic areas), specific HIV-2 infection should be pursued, especially in the event of a positive ELISA and unusual indeterminate WB reactivity, typically in the absence of Env reactivity.

Little is known regarding the HIV-2 window period, and, unfortunately, third-generation HIV-1/HIV-2 ELISAs are less sensitive in detecting early HIV-2 infection.[298]

Human Immunodeficiency Virus Testing during Pregnancy or at Delivery

Diagnosis of HIV in pregnant women is a public health priority; the advent of effective therapy to reduce the risk of transmission has made such arguments more compelling. Diagnosis in pregnancy may be complicated by increased false-positive rates of ELISA screenings with increased parity. In addition, women may present at delivery without previous evaluation, and rapid tests may be the only available modality to evaluate HIV-infected women expeditiously. In a study of 858 women diagnosed in labor, Constantine and others have suggested that a single screening ELISA at delivery is sufficiently sensitive, although the use of two rapid ELISAs has performance characteristics similar to standard ELISA/WB strategy.[299,300] Studies of HIV detection late in pregnancy or at delivery were ongoing as of June 2004 (Pediatric AIDS Clinical Trial Group [PACTG] P1031).

Perinatal Diagnosis

Diagnosis of HIV infection in the perinatal period is complicated by the prolonged persistence of maternal antibody in newborns following delivery (see Chapters 122 and 123). Standard serologic means for HIV detection are not reliably useful until infants are approximately

18 months of age. Methods for diagnosing true HIV-1 infection in newborns, including serial DNA PCR testing of peripheral blood mononuclear cells, have been developed using whole blood or dried blood spots.[301,302] The National Pediatric HIV Resource Center recommends that in the absence of breast-feeding, two samples be obtained to evaluate the presence of HIV infection: one after 1 month and one after 4 months. Pediatric HIV-1 NAT has disadvantages because infection may take place at parturition, and HIV-1 RNA levels in plasma may be relatively low at delivery even in true infection. Using three sequential DNA PCR assays, none of 224 patients with three sequential negative DNA PCR results were found ultimately to be infected; as a result, the specificity of DNA PCR was greater than 223/224 (>99.95). Use of DNA PCR at birth results in detection of HIV infection in less than 50% of true infections; after to 4 weeks, detection rate increases to 90%. RNA detection is not obviously superior. Delamare and coworkers noted 12 of 48 samples obtained within 10 days of infection were HIV positive using NASBA RNA amplification, whereas 39 of 39 samples taken from day 10 to 3 months were positive.[303] Detection of non-B subtypes by DNA PCR may be suboptimal, with false-negative results documented[304]; more recent versions of RNA PCR assays may be more sensitive in detection.

Alternative techniques to measure the presence of early HIV infection include direct HIV cultivation using techniques standardized by the AIDS Clinical Trials Group,[305] and p24 antigen detection. Antigen detection of p24 may represent an alternative to DNA PCR in developing countries. Although p24 antigen detection has reduced sensitivity as it does in adults,[306] the use of heat-denatured plasma to dissociate p24 from endogenous antibody improves sensitivity in newborns.[158,307]

Several groups have investigated the use of IgA ELISA in diagnosis of HIV-1 infection in newborns.[308,309] Sera were depleted of IgG and assayed for HIV IgA using standard third-generation assays. Sensitivity ranged from 77% to 96% but specificity was 100% in 86 clinic infants or in 141 patients in the AIDS Clinical Trial Group (ACTG) 076 trial of zidovudine (AZT) for prevention of mother-to-child HIV infection. Saliva IgA assay has been investigated but has been suboptimal, with a sensitivity of 80% to 88% in the first 6 months of life, and even lower later.[142]

Maternal-fetal transmission of HIV-2 is much less common than HIV-1 but may occur, especially if women become HIV-2 infected during pregnancy. Diagnosis of HIV-2 infection is similar to that of HIV-1, although Faye and co-workers have reported that assays may be less sensitive than those for HIV-1.[310,311]

Human Immunodeficiency Virus Testing for Blood Donor Screening

Laboratory methods for HIV detection were first implemented in populations as screening tools for blood products, and more than 14,000 individuals who were recipients of blood products as a risk factor for HIV infection have developed AIDS. Since implementation of laboratory screening, cases have decreased markedly. In the United States, 40 adults and adolescents have developed AIDS after receiving blood screened negative for HIV antibody.[312] Improvements in screening ELISA tests and incorporation of p24 antigen detection reduced the window period significantly. Incorporating NAT as a screening tool began in 1999, and has been utilized in minipools of 16 to 128 samples.

Blood surveillance procedures are designed to provide optimum safety of blood products; the screening phase begins with an interview and questionnaire, and donors may be screened out based on history; donors not screened out sign consent for donation and for HIV-1/HIV-2 testing with HIV-1/HIV-2 ELISA and NAT. Any sample reactive on either assay is discarded, and the sample is repeated in both screening assays; if the repeat screen is negative, a second screening assay is performed; if the second screening assay is negative, the sample is considered negative and the donor is not deferred. If the second screening assay is positive, the sample is considered repeatedly reactive and sent for confirmatory WB. Positive WBs are repeated with a separate sample, and the results of ELISA and WB are reported to the

patient with appropriate post-test counseling and referrals. Donor status of screening-reactive/confirmatory test–negative individuals remains under discussion.

A vigilant interview screening process remains essential, especially in times of heightened need for blood products. For instance, following 9/11 terrorist attacks there was a two- to threefold increase in blood donations, and HIV screening noted an increase in the proportion of HIV-reactive units; the estimated potential risk of HIV transmission from an estimated 1 in 1.8 million donations rose to 1 in 1.5 million donations.[313]

Tissue Procurement for Transplantation

HIV transmission from organs transplanted from infected individuals occurred before the availability of sensitive and specific testing. In adults and adolescents there have been 13 cases of AIDS through transplantation or artificial insemination; four of the donors were antibody negative at the time of donation. Not all organs or tissues appear to be equally infectious; HIV transmission by cornea transplants has not been documented,[314] even though several transplants took place using undiagnosed HIV-infected individuals as donors.[315,316] In routine, nonemergency cases of donation (e.g., semen specimens), routine candidate screening and HIV testing of donors are appropriate; alternative specimens for testing, such as semen or aqueous humor, may present technical difficulties,[317] and plasma is favored. False-positive results with postmortem serum have been documented, perhaps due to the effects of autolysis.[318] Even in emergency circumstances of tissue procurement for transplantation, screening by ELISA may be rapid and efficient; rapid assays have been reported to be a useful modality.[319] Both internationally and in the United States, a nonreactive ELISA is used to screen out donors, and no further testing is required. As a result, tissue procurement remains vulnerable owing to the duration of the window period and the sensitivity of the screening assay. (A state-of-the-art report on serologic screening methods for the most relevant microbiologic diseases of organ and tissue donors can be found at http://www.social.coe.int.) Obviously, an accurate history of the organ donor may identify high-risk circumstances.

Human Immunodeficiency Virus Testing in the Setting of Retroviral Syndrome or Other Acute Illness

Primary HIV infection may present as an acute viral syndrome with fever, lymphadenopathy, and rash (see Chapter 117). Diagnosis near the time of infection has obvious social, medical, and public health benefits, but not all screening strategies are equally effective in detecting primary HIV infection. Rapid or simple assays may not be as sensitive as standard third-generation ELISA tests. The window period for HIV infection may vary from patient to patient, and thus the value of a negative screening test must be weighed carefully. Close monitoring, repeat testing, and careful use of NAT may clarify many situations. Viral RNA levels greater than 5000 copies/mL have been associated with true infection.[198] As outlined above, other acute infections may yield false reactivity in HIV screening assays.

Occupational Exposure

HIV-1 infection may be transmitted as an occupational exposure (see Chapter 304) in the hospital setting as a result of needlestick injury, transmission during surgery, in outpatient dental circumstances, or other instances in which contact favoring transmission may occur. It is essential that the serostatus of the potential source of HIV infection be established as expediently as possible. Although testing in these circumstances is time sensitive, it still requires the same elements of counseling, consent, and confidentiality as standard HIV-1 testing. In the United States, in the opinion of the American Medical Association Council of Ethical and Judicial Affairs, involuntary HIV testing is acceptable in the event a health care professional undergoes exposure and the patient refuses to be tested[320]; by contrast, the WHO has unequivocally rejected mandatory HIV testing under any circumstances. In occupational exposures, it is important to test the exposed worker at the time the event took place to establish baseline serostatus. Rapid ELISA testing may be employed, especially if the potential source of HIV is not thought to be acutely HIV-1 infected. In the event of a nonreactive rapid ELISA, it would be prudent to obtain a routine ELISA as well to address the unlikely possibility that the rapid assay was insensitive to an early HIV-1 infection. Judicious use of RNA assays may also be employed. It is essential to carefully scrutinize testing of potential sources of HIV infection in this circumstance because hospitalized or acutely ill patients may have a variety of conditions that may yield a falsely reactive HIV-1/HIV-2 ELISA. In the event the serostatus cannot be established, initiating antiretroviral therapy is an appropriate option (see Chapter 304).

Factitious Human Immunodeficiency Virus Infection

Cases of factitious HIV infection have been reported in the context of psychiatric dysfunction.[321-324] The advent of multiple testing modalities including home collection systems may complicate patient presentation in factitious HIV. Careful history, application of routine algorithms, repeat standard assays, use of appropriate consult services, and common sense may resolve most of these cases.

Point of Care ("Home") Testing

The development of simple or rapid tests presents new opportunities and the possibility of HIV diagnosis outside the traditional testing facility. Two kinds of HIV testing are available outside health care facilities: home collection devices and home testing. Home collection devices are available in the United States and are FDA approved (Home Access, Ab Diagnostics, Inc.). Patients purchasing a home collection kit must contact the distributor using a toll-free telephone number, register a unique identifier contained in the kit, provide demographic data, and receive an educational pretest counseling session. Patients prepare the dried blood spot sample, which is shipped for laboratory testing. After a short (3-7 days) processing time, patients contact the toll-free number for results, which are available through an interactive voice response system or directly from a counselor. All indeterminate and positive results are delivered by trained counselors. Home collection is considered a safe, confidential, and FDA-approved service and has been available in the United States since 1996.

No true home diagnostic kits are FDA approved for private use as of June 2004. Unfortunately, however, rapid or simple HIV kits have become available to individuals through Internet sale. Home sale of HIV test kits may offer ease and, perhaps confidentiality, but is entirely unregulated; private purchase does not ensure any safeguards that pre- and post-test counseling will occur, or that testing will be anonymous or, for that matter, voluntary.

Other Human Retroviral Infections and New Retroviral Zoonoses

Current research indicates HIV-1 and HIV-2 epidemics arose from two independent zoonotic infections from distinct primate species. Infections with HIV-1 type O and N may represent additional independent cross-species events. Although the precise circumstances of these cross-species events remain uncertain, practices and behaviors continue such that new zoonotic retroviral infection remains possible. Evaluation of patients with immune deficiency will undoubtedly involve testing for known retroviruses, and the possibility of novel infections should be considered. Primate hunter/butcherers exposed to animals in which infection with simian immunodeficiency virus (SIV) is endemic may show evidence of exposure using sensitive laboratory-based assays to detect cell-mediated immunity to SIV,[325] but are consistently negative in HIV-1/HIV-2 ELISAs. There are, however, numerous distinct retroviruses in primate species, and the sensitivity of currently approved assays for the detection of more distantly related viruses is uncertain but is likely to be low. Simon and co-workers have reported design of new peptide ELISA screenings using Env gp120 V3 sequences from several HIV-1 M,N,O isolates and from diverse SIV isolates.[326,327] Such assays, which have demonstrated robust performance in field detection of HIV and SIV, may have additional utility in screening potentially contaminated bushmeat and thereby prevent future zoonotic events.[327]

Cross-species transmission of retroviruses has been considered as a consequence of xenotransplantation because candidate species for tissue donation all harbor endogenous retroviruses, e.g., porcine endogenous retrovirus (PERV) in pig species.[328,329] Endogenous retroviruses present in animal genomes may not be expressed in the host species, but may be inducible upon culture in vitro; transmission of PERV to human cells in vitro has been demonstrated by co-cultivation of pig and human cells in vitro.[330] Receptors for PERV are expressed in a variety of tissues,[331] and PERV is resistant to most current antiretrovirals.[332] Thus, one concern is that endogenous retrovirus production may not be detected at time of harvest but may be induced after transplantation. No evidence of PERV transmission to humans has been demonstrated,[333] and studies in nonhuman primates have not detected PERV in experimental xenotransplants,[334] although transmission to SCID or NOD/SCID mice has been reported in pancreatic islet transplants.[334,335] Tacke and co-workers have developed sensitive ELISA and WB assays for PERV expression products; screening recipients of pig tissues and butchers with extensive contact with pigs revealed no evidence of reactivity to PERV.[336] Interestingly, indeterminate WBs have been identified with PERV reagents with patterns similar to HIV WB indeterminates with reactivity to the principal *gag* gene product[336]; none of these indeterminate results represented true infection. Concerns for potential retroviral expression with development of zoonotic disease from other porcine and other tissue have prompted debate, and recommendations on testing of xenotransplanted tissue for the presence of retroviruses have been put forth.[337]

New techniques, including the use of PCR with degenerate primers designed to detect common motifs among retroviruses, have been reported.[338] Clinical studies using sensitive PCR techniques for the detection of novel viral sequences are under way and available for referral.[339]

The presence of additional retroviruses often prompts discussions of potential cross-reaction in HIV-1/HIV-2 assays. Recently Griffiths and co-workers have identified a new exogenous human retrovirus (human retrovirus 5 [HR-5]) in a small number of individuals with rheumatologic diseases.[340] HR-5 is related to a recently described rabbit endogenous virus.[341] Expression products from this virus do not cross react in HIV testing and are not likely responsible for false-positive reaction to HIV in these patient subsets. HTLV-I is an exogenous human retrovirus (see Chapter 165) of the oncoretrovirus family remotely related to HIV. Although early testing procedures detected cross reaction between HIV and HTLV-I, current screening assays for HIV-1/HIV-2 are not likely to be falsely positive because of the presence of HTLV-I, although indeterminate WBs are reported with sera from HTLV-I–infected patients. Humans, like many other mammals and vertebrates, are infected by endogenous retroviruses and are maintained via germline transmission. Endogenous retroviruses in humans are uncommonly, if ever, expressed and do not cross react with serologic or nucleic acid assays for HIV-1 or HIV-2. In certain gene therapy settings, defective retroviral vectors have been utilized to complement patient gene deficiencies; cells from which these defective viruses are propagated include other "helper" viruses and may contribute to development of malignancy in certain situations.[342] Neither the nucleic acids or gene products from the vectors nor the helper cell lines are remotely related to HIV and are not sources of cross reaction. In the future, lentiviral-derived vectors may be available to introduce genes via gene therapy, and would remain integrated in host cells to varying degrees. Depending upon their relatedness to HIV, such vectors may be detected in NAT using cellular DNA as substrate.

CONCLUSION

HIV testing is available for a variety of purposes—epidemiologic surveillance, individual testing, and protection of blood products and tissues for transplantation. Establishing the diagnosis of HIV infection in individuals is a process that optimally requires a coordinated effort among patient, health care, and laboratory personnel. The contribution of infectious disease specialists in diagnosis may be invaluable and should proceed from medical history and physical examination to laboratory diagnostic testing.

ACKNOWLEDGMENTS

I thank J. Coffin, H. Masur, H. C. Lane, J. Mellors, R. T. Davey, J. Falloon, M. A. Polis, J. Kovacs, M. A. Martin, K. Strebel, S. Leitman, J. A. Metcalf, I. Hewlett, and T. Levin for insightful discussions, and I am grateful to NIH Infectious Diseases fellows for useful conversations.

REFERENCES

1. Notice to Readers: The 20th Year of AIDS: A Time to Re-Energize Prevention. MMWR Morb Mortal Wkly Rep. 2001;50:444-445.
2. AIDS epidemic update 2002. Available at: www.UNAIDS.org, 2003.
3. Incorporating HIV prevention into the medical care of persons living with HIV. Recommendations of CDC, the Health Resources and Services Administration, the National Institutes of Health, and the HIV Medicine Association of the Infectious Diseases Society of America. MMWR Recomm Rep. 2003;52(RR-12):1-24.
4. Pilcher CD, McPherson JT, Leone PA, et al. Real-time, universal screening for acute HIV infection in a routine HIV counseling and testing population. JAMA. 2002;288(2):216-221.
5. Gostin LO, Webber DW. HIV infection and AIDS in the public health and health care systems: The role of law and litigation. JAMA. 1998;279(14):1108-1113.
6. Malpractice suit falls within statute of limitations. AIDS Policy Law. 1997;12(16):5.
7. Sarngadharan MG, Popovic M, Bruch L, et al. Antibodies reactive with human T-lymphotropic retroviruses (HTLV-III) in the serum of patients with AIDS. Science. 1984;224(4648):506-508.
8. Safai B, Sarngadharan MG, Groopman JE, et al. Seroepidemiological studies of human T-lymphotropic retrovirus type III in acquired immunodeficiency syndrome. Lancet. 1984;1(8392):1438-1440.
9. Popovic M, Sarngadharan MG, Read E, Gallo RC. Detection, isolation, and continuous production of cytopathic retroviruses (HTLV-III) from patients with AIDS and pre-AIDS. Science. 1984;224(4648):497-500.
10. Gallo RC, Salahuddin SZ, Popovic M, et al. Frequent detection and isolation of cytopathic retroviruses (HTLV-III) from patients with AIDS and at risk for AIDS. Science. 1984;224(4648):500-503.
11. Barre-Sinoussi F, Chermann JC, Rey F, et al. Isolation of a T-lymphotropic retrovirus from a patient at risk for acquired immune deficiency syndrome (AIDS). Science. 1983;220(4599):868-871.
12. Folks T, Benn S, Rabson A, et al. Characterization of a continuous T-cell line susceptible to the cytopathic effects of the acquired immunodeficiency syndrome (AIDS)-associated retrovirus. Proc Natl Acad Sci U S A. 1985;82(13):4539-4543.
13. Gazzard BG, Shanson DC, Farthing C, et al. Clinical findings and serological evidence of HTLV-III infection in homosexual contacts of patients with AIDS and persistent generalised lymphadenopathy in London. Lancet. 1984;2(8401):480-483.
14. Brun-Vezinet F, Rouzioux C, Barre-Sinoussi F, et al. Detection of IgG antibodies to lymphadenopathy-associated virus in patients with AIDS or lymphadenopathy syndrome. Lancet. 1984;1(8389):1253-1256.
15. Fisher AG, Collalti E, Ratner L, et al. A molecular clone of HTLV-III with biological activity. Nature. 1985;316(6025):262-265.
16. Levy JA, Cheng-Mayer C, Dina D, Luciw PA. AIDS retrovirus (ARV-2) clone replicates in transfected human and animal fibroblasts. Science. 1986;232(4753):998-1001.
17. Adachi A, Gendelman HE, Koenig S, et al. Production of acquired immunodeficiency syndrome-associated retrovirus in human and nonhuman cells transfected with an infectious molecular clone. J Virol. 1986;59(2):284-291.
18. Weiss SH, Goedert JJ, Sarngadharan MG, et al. Screening test for HTLV-III (AIDS agent) antibodies. Specificity, sensitivity, and applications. JAMA. 1985;253(2):221-225.
19. Current Trends Update: Public Health Service Workshop on Human T-Lymphotropic Virus Type III Antibody Testing—United States. MMWR Morb Mortal Wkly Rep.1985;34:477-478.
20. Marwick C. Blood banks give HTLV-III test positive appraisal at five months. JAMA. 1985;254(13):1681-1683.
21. Ward JW, Holmberg SD, Allen JR, et al. Transmission of human immunodeficiency virus (HIV) by blood transfusions screened as negative for HIV antibody. N Engl J Med. 1988;318(8):473-478.
22. Steckelberg JM, Cockerill FR, 3rd. Serologic testing for human immunodeficiency virus antibodies. Mayo Clin Proc. 1988;63(4):373-380.
23. De Majo E, Ravina A, Ricciarelli L, et al. Screening and confirmatory tests for antibody to HTLV-III/LAV retrovirus in individuals at risk for AIDS. Ric Clin Lab. 1986;16(3):489-494.
24. Gallo D, Diggs JL, Shell GR, et al. Comparison of detection of antibody to the acquired immune deficiency syndrome virus by enzyme immunoassay, immunofluorescence, and Western blot methods. J Clin Microbiol. 1986;23(6):1049-1051.
25. Kunz C, Heinz FX. Detection of HTLV-III antibodies using ELISA and the western blot. Wien Klin Wochenschr. 1985;97(22):829-832.
26. Hardy CT, Damrow TA, Villareal DB, Kenny GE. Evaluation of viral-lysate enzyme-linked immunosorbent assay kits for detecting human immunodeficiency virus (type 1) infections using human sera standardized by quantitative Western blotting. J Virol Methods. 1992;37(3):259-273.
27. Ng VL, Chiang CS, Debouck C, et al. Reliable confirmation of antibodies to human immunodeficiency virus type 1 (HIV-1) with an enzyme-linked immunoassay using recombinant antigens derived from the HIV-1 gag, pol, and env genes. J Clin Microbiol. 1989;27(5):977-982.
28. Gauthier DK, Turner JG. Anti-HIV antibody testing: procedures and precautions. Am J Infect Control. 1989;17(4):213-225.
29. Hellings JA, Theunissen H, Keur W, Siebelink-Liauw A. New developments in ELISA verification of anti-HIV screening of blood donors. J Virol Methods. 1987;17(1-2):11-17.
30. Weber B, Hess G, Koberstein R, Doerr HW. Evaluation of the automated "Enzymen-Test Anti HIV-1 + 2" and "Enzymen-Test Anti HIV-1/2 selective" for the combined detection and differentiation of anti-HIV-1 and anti-HIV-2 antibodies. J Virol Methods. 1993;44(2-3):251-260.
31. Lee YS. A comparison of reverse transcriptase and antigen capture assays for the detection of HIV. J Virol Methods. 1988;20(1):89-93.
32. Goudsmit J, de Wolf F, Paul DA, et al. Expression of human immunodeficiency virus antigen (HIV-Ag) in serum and cerebrospinal fluid during acute and chronic infection. Lancet. 1986;2(8500):177-180.
33. Allain JP, Laurian Y, Paul DA, et al. Long-term evaluation of HIV antigen and antibodies to p24 and gp41 in patients with hemophilia. Potential clinical importance. N Engl J Med. 1987;317(18):1114-1121.
34. Simmonds P, Lainson FA, Cuthbert R, et al. HIV antigen and antibody detection: Variable responses to infection in the Edinburgh haemophiliac cohort. BMJ (Clin Res Ed). 1988;296(6622):593-598.
35. von Sydow M, Gaines H, Sonnerborg A, et al. Antigen detection in primary HIV infection. BMJ (Clin Res Ed). 1988;296(6617):238-240.
36. Human T-lymphotropic virus type III/lymphadenopathy-associated virus antibody testing at alternate sites. MMWR Morb Mortal Wkly Rep. 1986;35(17):284-287.
37. Shilts R. And the Band Played On: Politics, People and the AIDS Epidemic. New York, Penguin Books; 1988.
38. Clavel F, Guetard D, Brun-Vezinet F, et al. Isolation of a new human retrovirus from West African patients with AIDS. Science. 1986;233(4761):343-346.
39. Clavel F, Guyader M, Guetard D, et al. Molecular cloning and polymorphism of the human immune deficiency virus type 2. Nature. 1986;324(6098):691-695.
40. AIDS due to HIV-2 infection—New Jersey. Can Dis Wkly Rep. 1988;14(12):50-51.
41. Marquart KH, Muller HA, Brede HD. HIV-2 in West Germany. AIDS. 1988;2(2):141.
42. Newmark P. HIV-2 detected in UK. Nature. 1988;332(6162):295.
43. Georgoulias V, Fountouli D, Karvela-Agelakis A, et al. HIV-1 and HIV-2 double infection in Greece. Ann Intern Med. 1988;108(1):155.
44. Neumann PW, Lepine D, Woodside M, et al. HIV-2 infection detected in Canada. Can Dis Wkly Rep. 1988;14(28):125-126.
45. Courouce AM. A prospective study of HIV-2 prevalence in France. AIDS. 1988;2(4):261-265.
46. Starkey CA, Yen-Lieberman B, Proffitt MR. Evaluation of the recombigen HIV-1 latex agglutination test. J Clin Microbiol. 1990;28(4):819-822.
47. Product package insert for Home Access HIV-1 Test System: Summary of Safety and Effectiveness. Available at: www.fda.gov/cber/PMAsumm/P950002S.pdf, 1996.
48. Gallo D, George JR, Fitchen JH, et al. Evaluation of a system using oral mucosal transudate for HIV-1 antibody screening and confirmatory testing. OraSure HIV Clinical Trials Group. JAMA. 1997;277(3):254-258.
49. Archibald DW, Zon LI, Groopman JE, et al. Salivary antibodies as a means of detecting human T cell lymphotropic virus type III/lymphadenopathy-associated virus infection. J Clin Microbiol. 1986;24(5):873-875.
50. Archibald DW, Zon L, Groopman JE, et al. Antibodies to human T-lymphotropic virus type III (HTLV-III) in saliva of acquired immunodeficiency syndrome (AIDS) patients and in persons at risk for AIDS. Blood. 1986;67(3):831-834.
51. Parry JV, Perry KR, Mortimer PP. Sensitive assays for viral antibodies in saliva: An alternative to tests on serum. Lancet. 1987;2(8550):72-75.
52. Tamashiro H, Constantine NT. Serological diagnosis of HIV infection using oral fluid samples. Bull World Health Organ. 1994;72(1):135-143.
53. Valdiserri RO, Taylor RN, Hearn TL, et al. Centers for Disease Control perspective on quality assurance for human immunodeficiency virus type 1 antibody testing. Model Performance Evaluation Program. Arch Pathol Lab Med. 1990;114(3):263-267.
54. Schalla WO, Hearn TL, Taylor RN, et al. CDC's Model Performance Evaluation Program: Assessment of the quality of laboratory performance for HIV-1 antibody testing. Public Health Rep. 1990;105(2):167-171.
55. Snell JJ, Supran EM, Esparza J, Tamashiro H. World Health Organization quality assessment programme on HIV testing. AIDS. 1990;4(8):803-806.
56. Hancock JS, Taylor RN, Johnson CA, et al. Quality of laboratory performance in testing for human immunodeficiency virus type 1 antibody. Identification of variables associated with laboratory performance. Arch Pathol Lab Med. 1993;117(11):1148-1155.
57. Astles JR, Lipman HB, Schalla WO, et al. Impact of quality control on accuracy in enzyme immunoassay testing for human immunodeficiency virus type 1 antibodies. Arch Pathol Lab Med. 1998;122(8):700-707.
58. van Binsbergen J, Keur W, Siebelink A, et al. Strongly enhanced sensitivity of a direct anti-HIV-1/-2 assay in seroconversion by incorporation of HIV p24 ag detection: A new generation vironostika HIV Uni-Form II. J Virol Methods. 1998;76(1-2):59-71.
59. Weber B, Fall EH, Berger A, Doerr HW. Reduction of diagnostic window by new fourth-generation human immunodeficiency virus screening assays. J Clin Microbiol. 1998;36(8):2235-2239.
60. Vargo J, Smith K, Knott C, et al. Clinical specificity and sensitivity of a blood screening assay for detection of HIV-1 and HCV RNA. Transfusion. 2002;42(7):876-885.
61. Brust S, Duttmann H, Feldner J, et al. Shortening of the diagnostic window with a new combined HIV p24 antigen and anti-HIV-1/2/O screening test. J Virol Methods. 2000;90(2):153-165.
62. Saville RD, Constantine NT, Cleghorn FR, et al. Fourth-generation enzyme-linked immunosorbent assay for the simultaneous detection of human immunodeficiency virus antigen and antibody. J Clin Microbiol. 2001;39(7):2518-2524.

63. Weber B, Gurtler L, Thorstensson R, et al. Multicenter evaluation of a new automated fourth-generation human immunodeficiency virus screening assay with a sensitive antigen detection module and high specificity. J Clin Microbiol. 2002;40(6): 1938-1946.
64. Update: HIV counseling and testing using rapid tests—United States, 1995. MMWR Morb Mortal Wkly Rep. 1998;47(11):211-215.
65. Davey RT, Jr., Lane HC. Laboratory methods in the diagnosis and prognostic staging of infection with human immunodeficiency virus type 1. Rev Infect Dis. 1990;12(5):912-930.
66. UNAIDS/WHO Operational Characteristics of Commercially Available Assays to Determine Antibodies to HIV-1 and/or HIV-2 in Human Sera. Report 11. January 1999. Geneva: UNAIDS/WHO. Available at www.UNAIDS.org.
67. Altfeld M, Rosenberg ES, Shankarappa R, et al. Cellular immune responses and viral diversity in individuals treated during acute and early HIV-1 infection. J Exp Med. 2001;193(2):169-180.
68. Wilson JD, Ogg GS, Allen RL, et al. Direct visualization of HIV-1-specific cytotoxic T lymphocytes during primary infection. AIDS. 2000;14(3):225-233.
69. Appay V, Papagno L, Spina CA, et al. Dynamics of T cell responses in HIV infection. J Immunol. 2002;168(7):3660-3666.
70. McRae B, Lange JA, Ascher MS, et al. Immune response to HIV p24 core protein during the early phases of human immunodeficiency virus infection. AIDS Res Hum Retroviruses. 1991;7(8):637-643.
71. Cooper DA, Imrie AA, Penny R. Antibody response to human immunodeficiency virus after primary infection. J Infect Dis. 1987;155(6):1113-1118.
72. Healey DS, Maskill WJ, Gust ID. Detection of anti-HIV immunoglobulin M by particle agglutination following acute HIV infection. AIDS. 1989;3(5):301-304.
73. Gallarda JL, Henrard DR, Liu D, et al. Early detection of antibody to human immunodeficiency virus type 1 by using an antigen conjugate immunoassay correlates with the presence of immunoglobulin M antibody. J Clin Microbiol. 1992;30 (9):2379-2384.
74. Muller F, Muller KH. Detection of anti-HIV-1 immunoglobulin M antibodies in patients with serologically proved HIV-1 infection. Infection. 1988;16(2):115-118.
75. Gaines H, von Sydow M, Parry JV, et al. Detection of immunoglobulin M antibody in primary human immunodeficiency virus infection. AIDS. 1988;2(1):11-15.
76. Horsburgh CR Jr, Ou CY, Jason J, et al. Duration of human immunodeficiency virus infection before detection of antibody. Lancet. 1989;2(8664):637-640.
77. Constantine NT, van der Groen G, Belsey EM, Tamashiro H. Sensitivity of HIV-antibody assays determined by seroconversion panels. AIDS. 1994;8(12):1715-1720.
78. FDA Talk Paper. FDA approves first nucleic acid test (NAT) system to screen whole blood donors for infections with human immunodeficiency virus (HIV and hepatitis C virus (HCV). Available at: www.fda.gov/bbs/topics/ANSWERS/2002/ANS01140.html, 2002.
79. Saah AJ, Farzadegan H, Fox R, et al. Detection of early antibodies in human immunodeficiency virus infection by enzyme-linked immunosorbent assay, Western blot, and radioimmunoprecipitation. J Clin Microbiol. 1987;25(9):1605-1610.
80. Chen J, Wang L, Chen JJ, et al. Detection of antibodies to human immunodeficiency virus (HIV) that recognize conformational epitopes of glycoproteins 160 and 41 often allows for early diagnosis of HIV infection. J Infect Dis. 2002;186(3):321-331.
81. Stramer SL, Heller JS, Coombs RW, et al. Markers of HIV infection prior to IgG antibody seropositivity. JAMA. 1989;262(1):64-69.
82. Ameisen JC, Guy B, Chamaret S, et al. Antibodies to the nef protein and to nef peptides in HIV-1-infected seronegative individuals. AIDS Res Hum Retroviruses. 1989;5(3):279-291.
83. Hashida S, Ishikawa S, Hashinaka K, et al. Earlier detection of human immunodeficiency virus type 1 p24 antigen and immunoglobulin G and M antibodies to p17 antigen in seroconversion serum panels by immune complex transfer enzyme immunoassays. Clin Diagn Lab Immunol. 2000;7(6):872-881.
84. Hashida S, Ishikawa S, Hashinaka K, et al. Optimal conditions of immune complex transfer enzyme immunoassay for p24 antigen of HIV-1. J Clin Lab Anal. 1998;12 (2):115-120.
85. Montagnier L, Brenner C, Chamaret S, et al. Human immunodeficiency virus infection and AIDS in a person with negative serology. J Infect Dis. 1997;175(4):955-959.
86. Persistent lack of detectable HIV-1 antibody in a person with HIV infection—Utah, 1995. MMWR Morb Mortal Wkly Rep. 1996;45(9):181-185.
87. Sullivan PS, Schable C, Koch W, et al. Persistently negative HIV-1 antibody enzyme immunoassay screening results for patients with HIV-1 infection and AIDS: Serologic, clinical, and virologic results. Seronegative AIDS Clinical Study Group. AIDS. 1999;13(1):89-96.
88. Barthel HR, Wallace DJ. False-positive human immunodeficiency virus testing in patients with lupus erythematosus. Semin Arthritis Rheum. 1993;23(1):1-7.
89. Soriano V, Dronda F, Gonzalez-Lopez A, et al. HIV-1 causing AIDS and death in a seronegative individual. Vox Sang. 1994;67(4):410-411.
90. Candotti D, Adu-Sarkodie Y, Davies F, et al. AIDS in an HIV-seronegative Ghanaian woman with intersubtype A/G recombinant HIV-1 infection. J Med Virol. 2000;62(1):1-8.
91. Oka S, Ida S, Shioda T, et al. Genetic analysis of HIV-1 during rapid progression to AIDS in an apparently healthy man. AIDS Res Hum Retroviruses. 1994;10(3): 271-277.
92. Wegner S, Ohl C, DeNobile J, et al. Case report of a woman with seronegative HIV-1 infection. AIDS Res Hum Retroviruses. 1995;11:S173.
93. Ellenberger DL, Sullivan PS, Dorn J, et al. Viral and immunologic examination of human immunodeficiency virus type 1-infected, persistently seronegative persons. J Infect Dis. 1999;180(4):1033-1042.
94. Kopko P, Calhoun L, Petz L. Distinguishing immunosilent AIDS from the acute retroviral syndrome in a frequent blood donor. Transfusion. 1999;39(4):383-386.
95. Michael NL, Brown AE, Voigt RF, et al. Rapid disease progression without seroconversion following primary human immunodeficiency virus type 1 infection—Evidence for highly susceptible human hosts. J Infect Dis. 1997;175(6):1352-1359.
96. Apetrei C, Tamalet C, Edlinger C, et al. Delayed HIV-1 seroconversion after antiretroviral therapy. AIDS. 1998;12(14):1935-1936.
97. Chockalingam M, Clarke L, McCormack WM. HIV infection with negative serological tests: Development of seropositivity in association with highly active antiretroviral therapy. AIDS Patient Care STDS. 2000;14(6):305-308.
98. De Rossi A, Giaquinto C, Del Mistro A, et al. Onset of HIV-1 antibody production after highly active antiretroviral therapy in a seronegative HIV-1-infected child. AIDS. 2000;14(9):1284-1286.
99. Morris L, Binley JM, Clas BA, et al. HIV-1 antigen-specific and -nonspecific B cell responses are sensitive to combination antiretroviral therapy. J Exp Med. 1998;188(2):233-245.
100. O'Connell RJ, Merritt TM, Malia JA, et al. Performance of the OraQuick rapid antibody test for diagnosis of human immunodeficiency virus type 1 infection in patients with various levels of exposure to highly active antiretroviral therapy. J Clin Microbiol. 2003;41(5):2153-2155.
101. Kenealy W, Reed D, Cybulski R, et al. Analysis of human serum antibodies to human immunodeficiency virus (HIV) using recombinant ENV and GAG antigens. AIDS Res Hum Retroviruses. 1987;3(1):95-105.
102. Dawson GJ, Heller JS, Wood CA, et al. Reliable detection of individuals seropositive for the human immunodeficiency virus (HIV) by competitive immunoassays using *Escherichia coli*-expressed HIV structural proteins. J Infect Dis 1988;157(1):149-155.
103. Ragni MV, O'Brien TA, Reed D, et al. Prognostic importance of antibodies to human immunodeficiency virus by recombinant immunoassay and Western blot techniques in HIV antibody-positive hemophiliacs. AIDS Res Hum Retroviruses. 1988;4(3):223-231.
104. Higgins JR, Pedersen NC, Carlson JR. Detection and differentiation by sandwich enzyme-linked immunosorbent assay of human T-cell lymphotropic virus type III/lymphadenopathy-associated virus and acquired immunodeficiency syndrome-associated retroviruslike clinical isolates. J Clin Microbiol. 1986;24(3):424-430.
105. Beelaert G, Vercauteren G, Fransen K, et al. Comparative evaluation of eight commercial enzyme linked immunosorbent assays and 14 simple assays for detection of antibodies to HIV. J Virol Methods. 2002;105(2):197-206.
106. Portincasa P, Grillo R, Pauri P, et al. Multicenter evaluation of the new HIV DUO assay for simultaneous detection of HIV antibodies and p24 antigen. New Microbiol. 2000;23(4):357-365.
107. Chanbancherd P, Limpairojn N, de Souza MS, et al. Evaluation of a new fourth-generation microwell enzyme-linked immunosorbent assay for detection of HIV-1 subtype B and E antibodies. Southeast Asian J Trop Med Public Health. 2001;32(1): 177-179.
108. Weber B, Berger A, Rabenau H, Doerr HW. Evaluation of a new combined antigen and antibody human immunodeficiency virus screening assay, VIDAS HIV DUO Ultra. J Clin Microbiol. 2002;40(4):1420-1426.
109. Polywka S, Feldner J, Duttmann H, Laufs R. Diagnostic evaluation of a new combined HIV p24 antigen and anti-HIV1/2/O screening assay. Clin Lab. 2001;47 (7-8):351-356.
110. Ly TD, Laperche S, Courouce AM. Early detection of human immunodeficiency virus infection using third- and fourth-generation screening assays. Eur J Clin Microbiol Infect Dis. 2001;20(2):104-110.
111. van Binsbergen J, Siebelink A, Jacobs A, et al. Improved performance of seroconversion with a 4th generation HIV antigen/antibody assay. J Virol Methods. 1999;82(1):77-84.
112. Meier T, Knoll E, Henkes M, et al. Evidence for a diagnostic window in fourth generation assays for HIV. J Clin Virol. 2001;23(1-2):113-116.
113. Francis HL, Kabeya M, Kafuama N, et al. Comparison of sensitivities and specificities of latex agglutination and an enzyme-linked immunosorbent assay for detection of antibodies to the human immunodeficiency virus in African sera. J Clin Microbiol. 1988;26(11):2462-2464.
114. Windsor IM, Gomes dos Santos ML, de la Hunt LI, et al. An evaluation of the capillus HIV-1/HIV-2 latex agglutination test using serum and whole blood. Int J STD AIDS. 1997;8(3):192-195.
115. Lepine DG, Neumann PW, Frenette SL, O'Shaughnessy MV. Evaluation of a human immunodeficiency virus test algorithm utilizing a recombinant protein enzyme immunoassay. J Clin Microbiol. 1990;28(6):1169-1171.
116. Elavia AJ, Thomas A, Nandi J, et al. Performance evaluation of a particle agglutination test for antibody to human immunodeficiency virus 1: Comparison with enzyme immunoassay. Vox Sang. 1995;69(1):23-26.
117. Poljak M, Zener N, Seme K, Kristancic L. Particle agglutination test "Serodia HIV-1/2" as a novel anti-HIV-1/2 screening test: comparative study on 3311 serum samples. Folia Biol (Praha). 1997;43(4):171-173.
118. Parry JV, Mortimer PP. An immunoglobulin G antibody capture particle-adherence test (GACPAT) for antibody to HIV-1 and HTLV-I that allows economical large-scale screening. AIDS. 1989;3(3):173-176.
119. Houck JA, Sedmak DD, Grose MP, Neff JC. Sensitivity and interobserver variability of the Recombigen-HIV-1 LA test. Am J Clin Pathol. 1990;93(4):538-540.
120. Louisirirotchanakul S, Kanoksinsombat C, Thongput A, et al. Anti-HIV-1 antibody testing using modified gelatin particle agglutination: A large field study. J Med Assoc Thai. 2001;84(12):1708-1713.
121. Ramalingam S, Kannangai R, Raj AA, et al. Rapid particle agglutination test for human immunodeficiency virus: Hospital-based evaluation. J Clin Microbiol. 2002;40(4):1553-1554.
122. Lien TX, Tien NT, Chanpong GF, et al. Evaluation of rapid diagnostic tests for the detection of human immunodeficiency virus types 1 and 2, hepatitis B surface antigen, and syphilis in Ho Chi Minh City, Vietnam. Am J Trop Med Hyg. 2000;62(2):301-309.
123. Makuwa M, Souquiere S, Niangui MT, et al. Reliability of rapid diagnostic tests for HIV variant infection. J Virol Methods. 2002;103(2):183-190.

124. Meless H, Tegbaru B, Messele T, et al. Evaluation of rapid assays for screening and confirming HIV-1 infection in Ethiopia. Ethiop Med J. 2002;40 (Suppl 1):27-36.

125. Kassler WJ, Dillon BA, Haley C, et al. On-site, rapid HIV testing with same-day results and counseling. AIDS. 1997;11(8):1045-1051.

126. Keenan PA, Keenan JM. Rapid HIV testing in urban outreach: A strategy for improving posttest counseling rates. AIDS Educ Prev. 2001;13(6):541-550.

127. Kelen GD, Shahan JB, Quinn TC. Emergency department-based HIV screening and counseling: Experience with rapid and standard serologic testing. Ann Emerg Med. 1999;33(2):147-155.

128. Malonza IM, Richardson BA, Kreiss JK, et al. The effect of rapid HIV-1 testing on uptake of perinatal HIV-1 interventions: A randomized clinical trial. AIDS. 2003;17(1):113-118.

129. Barr CE, Miller LK, Lopez MR, et al. Recovery of infectious HIV-1 from whole saliva. J Am Dent Assoc. 1992;123(2):36-37, 39-48; discussion 38.

130. Chohan BH, Lavreys L, Mandaliya KN, et al. Validation of a modified commercial enzyme-linked immunoassay for detection of human immunodeficiency virus type 1 immunoglobulin G antibodies in saliva. Clin Diagn Lab Immunol. 2001;8(2):346-348.

131. Connell JA, Parry JV, Mortimer PP, Duncan J. Novel assay for the detection of immunoglobulin G antihuman immunodeficiency virus in untreated saliva and urine. J Med Virol. 1993;41(2):159-164.

132. Raux M, Finkielsztejn L, Salmon-Ceron D, et al. IgG subclass distribution in serum and various mucosal fluids of HIV type 1-infected subjects. AIDS Res Hum Retroviruses. 2000;16(6):583-594.

133. Lu XS, Delfraissy JF, Grangeot-Keros L, et al. Rapid and constant detection of HIV antibody response in saliva of HIV-infected patients; selective distribution of anti-HIV activity in the IgG isotype. Res Virol. 1994;145(6):369-377.

134. Cartry O, Moja P, Quesnel A, et al. Quantification of IgA and IgG and specificities of antibodies to viral proteins in parotid saliva at different stages of HIV-1 infection. Clin Exp Immunol. 1997;109(1):47-53.

135. Martinez PM, Torres AR, Ortiz de Lejarazu R, et al. Human immunodeficiency virus antibody testing by enzyme-linked fluorescent and Western blot assays using serum, gingival-crevicular transudate, and urine samples. J Clin Microbiol. 1999;37(4):1100-1106.

136. Granade TC, Phillips SK, Parekh B, et al. Detection of antibodies to human immunodeficiency virus type 1 in oral fluids: A large-scale evaluation of immunoassay performance. Clin Diagn Lab Immunol. 1998;5(2):171-175.

137. Schramm W, Angulo GB, Torres PC, Burgess-Cassler A. A simple saliva-based test for detecting antibodies to human immunodeficiency virus. Clin Diagn Lab Immunol. 1999;6(4):577-580.

138. Parra B, Slots J. Detection of human viruses in periodontal pockets using polymerase chain reaction. Oral Microbiol Immunol. 1996;11(5):289-293.

139. Maticic M, Poljak M, Kramar B, et al. Proviral HIV-1 DNA in gingival crevicular fluid of HIV-1-infected patients in various stages of HIV disease. J Dent Res. 2000;79(7):1496-1501.

140. Zuckerman RA, Whittington WL, Celum CL, et al. Factors associated with oropharyngeal human immunodeficiency virus shedding. J Infect Dis. 2003;188(1):142-145.

141. Weiblen BJ, Lee FK, Cooper ER, et al. Early diagnosis of HIV infection in infants by detection of IgA HIV antibodies. Lancet. 1990;335(8696):988-990.

142. Morgado de Moura Machado JE, Kayita J, Bakaki P, et al. IgA antibodies to human immunodeficiency virus in serum, saliva and urine for early diagnosis of immunodeficiency virus infection in Ugandan infants. Pediatr Infect Dis J. 2003;22(2):193-195.

143. Jackson S, Prince S, Kulhavy R, Mestecky J. False positivity of enzyme-linked immunosorbent assay for measurement of secretory IgA antibodies directed at HIV type 1 antigens. AIDS Res Hum Retroviruses. 2000;16(6):595-602.

144. George JR, Schochetman G. AIDS testing: A Comprehensive Guide to Medical Social Legal and Management Issues. New York: Springer-Verlag; 1994.

145. Constantine NT, Zhang X, Li L, et al. Application of a rapid assay for detection of antibodies to human immunodeficiency virus in urine. Am J Clin Pathol. 1994;101(2):157-161.

146. Urnovitz HB, Sturge JC, Gottfried TD, Murphy WH. Urine antibody tests: New insights into the dynamics of HIV-1 infection. Clin Chem. 1999;45(9):1602-1613.

147. Janssen RS, Satten GA, Stramer SL, et al. New testing strategy to detect early HIV-1 infection for use in incidence estimates and for clinical and prevention purposes. JAMA. 1998;280(1):42-48.

148. Rutherford GW, Schwarcz SK, McFarland W. Surveillance for incident HIV infection: new technology and new opportunities. J Acquir Immune Defic Syndr. 2000;25(Suppl 2):S115-S119.

149. Gouws E, Williams BG, Sheppard HW, et al. High incidence of HIV-1 in South Africa using a standardized algorithm for recent HIV seroconversion. J Acquir Immune Defic Syndr. 2002;29(5):531-535.

150. Kral AH, Lorvick J, Gee L, et al. Trends in human immunodeficiency virus seroincidence among street-recruited injection drug users in San Francisco, 1987-1998. Am J Epidemiol. 2003;157(10):915-922.

151. McFarland W, Busch MP, Kellogg TA, et al. Detection of early HIV infection and estimation of incidence using a sensitive/less-sensitive enzyme immunoassay testing strategy at anonymous counseling and testing sites in San Francisco. J Acquir Immune Defic Syndr. 1999;22(5):484-489.

152. Constantine NT, Sill AM, Jack N, et al. Improved classification of recent HIV-1 infection by employing a two-stage sensitive/less-sensitive test strategy. J Acquir Immune Defic Syndr. 2003;32(1):94-103.

153. Gaines H, von Sydow M, Sonnerborg A, et al. Antibody response in primary human immunodeficiency virus infection. Lancet. 1987;1(8544):1249-1253.

154. Henrard DR, Wu S, Phillips J, et al. Detection of p24 antigen with and without immune complex dissociation for longitudinal monitoring of human immunodeficiency virus type 1 infection. J Clin Microbiol. 1995;33(1):72-75.

155. Schupbach J. Measurement of HIV-1 p24 antigen by signal-amplification-boosted ELISA of heat-denatured plasma is a simple and inexpensive alternative to tests for viral RNA. AIDS Rev. 2002;4(2):83-92.

156. Sutthent R, Gaudart N, Chokpaibulkit K, et al. p24 Antigen detection assay modified with a booster step for diagnosis and monitoring of human immunodeficiency virus type 1 infection. J Clin Microbiol. 2003;41(3):1016-1022.

157. Schupbach J, Flepp M, Pontelli D, et al. Heat-mediated immune complex dissociation and enzyme-linked immunosorbent assay signal amplification render p24 antigen detection in plasma as sensitive as HIV-1 RNA detection by polymerase chain reaction. AIDS. 1996;10(10):1085-1090.

158. Schupbach J, Boni J, Tomasik Z, et al. Sensitive detection and early prognostic significance of p24 antigen in heat-denatured plasma of human immunodeficiency virus type 1-infected infants. Swiss Neonatal HIV Study Group. J Infect Dis. 1994;170(2):318-324.

159. Ledergerber B, Flepp M, Boni J, et al. Human immunodeficiency virus type 1 p24 concentration measured by boosted ELISA of heat-denatured plasma correlates with decline in CD4 cells, progression to AIDS, and survival: comparison with viral RNA measurement. J Infect Dis. 2000;181(4):1280-1288.

160. Seed CR, Margaritis AR, Bolton WV, et al. Improved efficiency of national HIV, HCV, and HTLV antibody testing algorithms based on sequential screening immunoassays. Transfusion. 2003;43(2):226-234.

161. Morell A, Barandun S, Locher G. HTLV-III seroconversion in a homosexual patient with common variable immunodeficiency. N Engl J Med. 1986;315(7):456-457.

162. Bowen DL, Lane HC, Fauci AS. Immunopathogenesis of the acquired immunodeficiency syndrome. Ann Intern Med. 1985;103(5):704-709.

163. Preiser W, Brink NS, Hayman A, et al. False-negative HIV antibody test results. J Med Virol. 2000;60(1):43-47.

164. Bouillon M, Aubin E, Roberge C, et al. Reduced frequency of blood donors with false-positive HIV-1 and -2 antibody EIA reactivity after elution of low-affinity nonspecific natural antibodies. Transfusion. 2002;42(8):1046-1052.

165. Wai CT, Tambyah PA. False-positive HIV-1 ELISA in patients with hepatitis B. Am J Med. 2002;112(9):737.

166. Pearlman ES, Ballas SK. False-positive human immunodeficiency virus screening test related to rabies vaccination. Arch Pathol Lab Med. 1994;118(8):805-806.

167. Plotkin SA, Loupi E, Blondeau C. False-positive human immunodeficiency virus screening test related to rabies vaccination. Arch Pathol Lab Med. 1995;119(8):679.

168. Henderson S, Leibnitz G, Turnbull M, Palmer GH. False-positive human immunodeficiency virus seroconversion is not common following rabies vaccination. Clin Diagn Lab Immunol. 2002;9(4):942-943.

169. Andrade VL, Avelleira JC, Marques A, et al. Leprosy as cause of false-positive results in serological assays for the detection of antibodies to HIV-1. Int J Lepr Other Mycobact Dis. 1991;59(1):125-126.

170. ShivRaj L, Patil SA, Girdhar A, et al. Antibodies to HIV-1 in sera from patients with mycobacterial infections. Int J Lepr Other Mycobact Dis. 1988;56(4):546-551.

171. Kashala O, Marlink R, Ilunga M, et al. Infection with human immunodeficiency virus type 1 (HIV-1) and human T cell lymphotropic viruses among leprosy patients and contacts: Correlation between HIV-1 cross-reactivity and antibodies to lipoarabinomannan. J Infect Dis. 1994;169(2):296-304.

172. Sterne JA, Turner AC, Fine PE, et al. Testing for antibody to human immunodeficiency virus type 1 in a population in which mycobacterial diseases are endemic. J Infect Dis. 1995;172(2):543-546.

173. Walensky RP, Rosenberg ES, Ferraro MJ, et al. Investigation of primary human immunodeficiency virus infection in patients who test positive for heterophile antibody. Clin Infect Dis. 2001;33(4):570-572.

174. Rosenberg ES, Caliendo AM, Walker BD. Acute HIV infection among patients tested for mononucleosis. N Engl J Med. 1999;340(12):969.

175. Zehender G, De Maddalena C, Gianotto M, et al. High prevalence of false-negative anti-HTLV type I/II enzyme-linked immunosorbent assay results in HIV type 1-positive patients. AIDS Res Hum Retroviruses. 1997;13(13):1141-1146.

176. Ferrer-Canabate J, Agullo-Ortuno T, Garcia-Mancebo ML, et al. Propylene glycol interference in the Vidas HIV DUO assay. Clin Biochem. 2002;35(4):333-334.

177. Palmer S, Wiegand AP, Maldarelli F, et al. New real-time RT-PCR assay with single copy sensitivity for HIV-1 RNA in plasma. J Clin Microbiol. 2003;41:4531-4536.

178. Candotti D, Richetin A, Cant B, et al. Evaluation of a transcription-mediated amplification-based HCV and HIV-1 RNA duplex assay for screening individual blood donations: A comparison with a minipool testing system. Transfusion. 2003;43(2):215-225.

179. Lelie PN, van Drimmelen HA, Cuypers HT, et al. Sensitivity of HCV RNA and HIV RNA blood screening assays. Transfusion. 2002;42(5):527-536.

180. Stramer SL. US NAT yield: Where are we after 2 years? Transfus Med. 2002;12(4):243-253.

181. Tomono T, Murokawa H, Minegishi K, et al. Status of NAT screening for HCV, HIV and HBV: Experience in Japan. Dev Biol (Basel). 2002;108:29-39.

182. Roth WK, Weber M, Buhr S, et al. Yield of HCV and HIV-1 NAT after screening of 3.6 million blood donations in central Europe. Transfusion. 2002;42(7):862-868.

183. Fang CT, Field SP, Busch MP, et al. Human immunodeficiency virus-1 and hepatitis C virus RNA among South African blood donors: estimation of residual transfusion risk and yield of nucleic acid testing. Vox Sang. 2003;85(1):9-19.

184. Jongerius JM, Sjerps M, Cuijpers HT, et al. Validation of the NucliSens Extractor combined with the AmpliScreen HIV version 1.5 and HCV version 2.0 test for application in NAT minipool screening. Transfusion. 2002;42(6):792-797.

185. Aprili G, Gandini G, Piccoli P, et al. Detection of an early HIV-1 infection by HIV RNA testing in an Italian blood donor during the preseroconversion window period. Transfusion. 2003;43(7):848-852.

186. Dreier J, Gotting C, Wolff C, et al. Recent experience with human immunodeficiency virus transmission by cellular blood products in Germany: antibody screening is not sufficient to prevent transmission. Vox Sang 2002;82(2):80-83.

187. Kopko PM, Fernando LP, Bonney EN, et al. HIV transmissions from a window-period platelet donation. Am J Clin Pathol. 2001;116(4):562-566.

188. Toro C, Rodes B, Colino F, et al. Transmission of HIV type 1 through blood transfusion from an antibody-negative/p24 antigen-negative donor. AIDS Res Hum Retroviruses. 2003;19(6):447-448.

189. Suarez AA, Sokol-Anderson ML, Creer M, et al. Case report. Diagnosis of early HIV-1 infection. AIDS Patient Care STDS. 2001;15(5):237-241.

190. Ling AE, Robbins KE, Brown TM, et al. Failure of routine HIV-1 tests in a case involving transmission with preseroconversion blood components during the infectious window period. JAMA. 2000;284(2):210-214.

191. Wang B, Schreiber GB, Glynn SA, et al. Prevalence of transfusion-transmissible viral infections in first-time US blood donors by donation site. Transfusion. 2003;43(6):705-712.

192. Dodd RY, Notari EPt, Stramer SL. Current prevalence and incidence of infectious disease markers and estimated window-period risk in the American Red Cross blood donor population. Transfusion. 2002;42(8):975-979.

193. Seed CR, Cheng A, Ismay SL, et al. Assessing the accuracy of three viral risk models in predicting the outcome of implementing HIV and HCV NAT donor screening in Australia and the implications for future HBV NAT. Transfusion. 2002;42(10):1365-1372.

194. Weusten JJ, van Drimmelen HA, Lelie PN. Mathematic modeling of the risk of HBV, HCV, and HIV transmission by window-phase donations not detected by NAT. Transfusion. 2002;42(5):537-548.

195. Jackson BR, Busch MP, Stramer SL, AuBuchon JP. The cost-effectiveness of NAT for HIV, HCV, and HBV in whole-blood donations. Transfusion. 2003;43(6):721-729.

196. Holmes H, Davis C, Heath A, et al. An international collaborative study to establish the 1st international standard for HIV-1 RNA for use in nucleic acid-based techniques. J Virol Methods. 2001;92(2):141-150.

197. Rich JD, Merriman NA, Mylonakis E, et al. Misdiagnosis of HIV infection by HIV-1 plasma viral load testing: a case series. Ann Intern Med. 1999;130(1):37-39.

198. Hecht FM, Busch MP, Rawal B, et al. Use of laboratory tests and clinical symptoms for identification of primary HIV infection. AIDS. 2002;16(8):1119-1129.

199. Mylonakis E, Paliou M, Lally M, et al. Laboratory testing for infection with the human immunodeficiency virus: established and novel approaches. Am J Med. 2000;109(7):568-576.

200. Mylonakis E, Paliou M, Greenbough TC, et al. Report of a false-positive HIV test result and the potential use of additional tests in establishing HIV serostatus. Arch Intern Med. 2000;160(15):2386-2388.

201. de Mendoza C, Holguin A, Soriano V. False positives for HIV using commercial viral load quantification assays. AIDS. 1998;12(15):2076-2077.

202. Brambilla D, Jennings C, Aldrovandi G, et al. Multicenter evaluation of use of dried blood and plasma spot specimens in quantitative assays for human immunodeficiency virus RNA: Measurement, precision, and RNA stability. J Clin Microbiol. 2003;41(5):1888-1893.

203. Migueles SA, Sabbaghian MS, Shupert WL, et al. HLA B*5701 is highly associated with restriction of virus replication in a subgroup of HIV-infected long term nonprogressors. Proc Natl Acad Sci U S A. 2000;97(6):2709-2714.

204. Ritter D, Taylor J, Walkenbach R, et al. Diagnostic testing for HIV type 1 RNA in seronegative blood. Am J Clin Pathol. 2000;113(1):128-134.

205. Proposed WHO criteria for the interpretation of Western Blot for HIV-1, HIV-2, and HTLV-I/HTLV-II. Wkly Epidemiol Rec. 1990;65:281-283.

206. O'Gorman MR, Weber D, Landis SE, et al. Interpretive criteria of the Western blot assay for serodiagnosis of human immunodeficiency virus type 1 infection. Arch Pathol Lab Med. 1991;115(1):26-30.

207. Midthun K, Garrison L, Clements ML, et al. Frequency of indeterminate western blot tests in healthy adults at low risk for human immunodeficiency virus infection. The NIAID AIDS Vaccine Clinical Trials Network. J Infect Dis. 1990;162(6):1379-1382.

208. Genesca J, Shih JW, Jett BW, et al. What do western blot indeterminate patterns for human immunodeficiency virus mean in EIA-negative blood donors? Lancet. 1989;2(8670):1023-1025.

209. Ramirez E, Uribe P, Escanilla D, et al. Reactivity patterns and infection status of serum samples with indeterminate Western immunoblot tests for antibody to human immunodeficiency virus type 1. J Clin Microbiol. 1992;30(4):801-805.

210. Lefrere JJ, Courouce AM, Lucotte G, et al. Follow-up of subjects with isolated and persistent anti-core (anti-p24 or anti-p17) antibodies to HIV. AIDS. 1988;2(4):287-290.

211. Lee JH. Follow-up investigation of indeterminate western blot results for antibody to human immunodeficiency virus type 1. J Formos Med Assoc. 1994;93(4):283-288.

212. Vardinon N, Yust I, Katz O, et al. Anti-HIV indeterminate western blot in dialysis patients: a long-term follow-up. Am J Kidney Dis. 1999;34(1):146-149.

213. Povolotsky J, Gold JW, Chein N, et al. Differences in human immunodeficiency virus type 1 (HIV-1) anti-p24 reactivities in serum of HIV-1-infected and uninfected subjects: Analysis of indeterminate western blot reactions. J Infect Dis. 1991;163(2):247-251.

214. Blomberg J, Vincic E, Jonsson C, et al. Identification of regions of HIV-1 p24 reactive with sera which give "indeterminate" results in electrophoretic immunoblots with the help of long synthetic peptides. AIDS Res Hum Retroviruses. 1990;6(12):1363-1372.

215. Deas JE, Liu LG, Thompson JJ, et al. Reactivity of sera from systemic lupus erythematosus and Sjogren's syndrome patients with peptides derived from human immunodeficiency virus p24 capsid antigen. Clin Diagn Lab Immunol. 1998;5(2):181-185.

216. Haist S, Marz J, Wolf H, Modrow S. Reactivities of HIV-1 gag-derived peptides with antibodies of HIV-1-infected and uninfected humans. AIDS Res Hum Retroviruses. 1992;8(11):1909-1917.

217. Kammerer R, Burgisser P, Frei PC. Anti-human immunodeficiency virus type 1 antibodies of noninfected subjects are not related to autoantibodies occurring in systemic diseases. Clin Diagn Lab Immunol. 1995;2(4):458-461.

218. Drabick JJ, Horning VL, Lennox JL, et al. A retrospective analysis of diseases associated with indeterminate HIV western blot patterns. Mil Med. 1991;156(2):93-96.

219. Gurtler LG, Zekeng L, Simon F, et al. Reactivity of five anti-HIV-1 subtype O specimens with six different anti-HIV screening ELISAs and three immunoblots. J Virol Methods. 1995;51(2-3):177-183.

220. Insert. Human Immunodeficiency Virus Type 1 (HIV-1) Cambridge Biotech HIV-1 Western Blot Kit. Rockville, Md; 2000.

221. Carneiro-Proietti AB, Cunha IW, Souza MM, et al. HIV-(1/2) indeterminate western blot results: Follow-up of asymptomatic blood donors in Belo Horizonte, Minas Gerais, Brazil. Rev Inst Med Trop Sao Paulo. 1999;41(3):155-158.

222. Celum CL, Coombs RW, Jones M, et al. Risk factors for repeatedly reactive HIV-1 EIA and indeterminate western blots. A population-based case-control study. Arch Intern Med. 1994;154(10):1129-1137.

223. Willman JH, Hill HR, Martins TB, et al. Multiplex analysis of heterophil antibodies in patients with indeterminate HIV immunoassay results. Am J Clin Pathol. 2001;115(5):764-769.

224. Montero A, Ciardi MC, Casella ML, et al. Chronic indeterminate western blot in a patient with AIDS and massive proteinuria. AIDS. 1993;7(5):742-743.

225. Schindzielorz AH, Belshe RB, Mufson MA. Occurrence, characteristics, and patterns of HIV-1 and HIV-2 western blot indeterminate sera in low risk populations in West Virginia and pre-AIDS Africa. Am J Trop Med Hyg. 1990;42(5):460-464.

226. Schoub BD, Lyons SF, Martin DJ, Reinach SG. An analysis of indeterminate western blot patterns of black African subjects. Res Virol. 1990;141(3):397-401.

227. Behets F, Disasi A, Ryder RW, et al. Comparison of five commercial enzyme-linked immunosorbent assays and Western immunoblotting for human immunodeficiency virus antibody detection in serum samples from Central Africa. J Clin Microbiol. 1991;29(10):2280-2284.

228. Meles H, Wolday D, Fontanet A, et al. Indeterminate human immunodeficiency virus Western blot profiles in Ethiopians with discordant screening-assay results. Clin Diagn Lab Immunol. 2002;9(1):160-163.

229. Mahe C, Kaleebu P, Ojwiya A, Whitworth JA. Human immunodeficiency virus type 1 Western blot: Revised diagnostic criteria with fewer indeterminate results for epidemiological studies in Africa. Int J Epidemiol 2002;31(5):985-990.

230. Ayisi NK, Aidoo M. Comparative analysis of HIV-1 and HIV-2 indeterminate western blot patterns. West Afr J Med. 1994;13(3):164-167.

231. Jindal R, Solomon M, Burrows L. False positive tests for HIV in a woman with lupus and renal failure. N Engl J Med. 1993;328(17):1281-1282.

232. Josephson SL, Swack NS, Ramirez MT, Hausler WJ, Jr. Investigation of atypical western blot (immunoblot) reactivity involving core proteins of human immunodeficiency virus type. J Clin Microbiol. 1989;27(5):932-937.

233. Pollet DE, Saman EL, Peeters DC, et al. Confirmation and differentiation of antibodies to human immunodeficiency virus 1 and 2 with a strip-based assay including recombinant antigens and synthetic peptides. Clin Chem. 1991;37(10 Pt 1):1700-1707.

234. Zaaijer HL, van Rixel GA, Kromosoeto JN, et al. Validation of a new immunoblot assay (LiaTek HIV III) for confirmation of human immunodeficiency virus infection. Transfusion. 1998;38(8):776-781.

235. Zaaijer HL, van Rixel T, van Exel-Oehlers P, et al. New anti-human immunodeficiency virus immunoblot assays resolve nonspecific western blot results. Transfusion. 1997;37(2):193-198.

236. Chan EL, Sidaway F, Horsman GB. A comparison of the Genie and western blot assays in confirmatory testing for HIV-1 antibody. J Med Microbiol. 1996;44(3):223-225.

237. Mingle JA. Differentiation of dual seropositivity to HIV 1 and HIV 2 in Ghanaian sera using line immunoassay (INNOLIA). West Afr J Med. 1997;16(2):71-74.

238. Van Kerckhoven I, Vercauteren G, Piot P, van der Groen G. Comparative evaluation of 36 commercial assays for detecting antibodies to HIV. Bull World Health Organ. 1991;69(6):753-760.

239. Mas A, Soriano V, Gutierrez M, et al. Reliability of a new recombinant immunoblot assay (RIBA HIV-1/HIV-2 SIA) as a supplemental (confirmatory) test for HIV-1 and HIV-2 infections. Transfus Sci. 1997;18(1):63-69.

240. Sandstrom EG, Schooley RT, Ho DD, et al. Detection of human anti-HTLV-III antibodies by indirect immunofluorescence using fixed cells. Transfusion. 1985;25(4):308-312.

241. Hedenskog M, Dewhurst S, Ludvigsen C, et al. Testing for antibodies to AIDS-associated retrovirus (HTLV-III/LAV) by indirect fixed cell immunofluorescence: specificity, sensitivity, and applications. J Med Virol. 1986;19(4):325-334.

242. van der Groen G, Vercauteren G, Piot P. Immunofluorescence tests for HIV antibody and their value as confirmatory tests. J Virol Methods. 1987;17(1-2):35-43.

243. Kvinesdal BB, Nielsen CM, Poulsen AG, Hojlyng N. Immunofluorescence assay for detection of antibodies to human immunodeficiency virus type 2. J Clin Microbiol. 1989;27(11):2502-2504.

244. Sullivan MT, Mucke H, Kadey SD, et al. Evaluation of an indirect immunofluorescence assay for confirmation of human immunodeficiency virus type 1 antibody in U.S. blood donor sera. J Clin Microbiol. 1992;30(9):2509-2510.

245. Boshell J, Alvarez C, Marrugo S, et al. Indirect immunofluorescence as a supplementary test for confirming HIV-1 infection: the experience of the National Institutes of Health, 1993-2000. Biomedica (Bogota). 2002;22(1):30-38.

246. Mahony J, Rosenthal K, Chernesky M, et al. Agreement study between two laboratories of immunofluorescence as a confirmatory test for human immunodeficiency virus type 1 antibody screening. J Clin Microbiol. 1989;27(6):1234-1237.

247. Huisman JG, Winkel IN, Lelie PN, et al. Detection of early anti-p24 HIV responses in EIA- and immunoblot-negative individuals. Implications for confirmatory testing. Vox Sang. 1987;53(1):31-36.

248. Pinter A, Honnen WJ. A sensitive radioimmunoprecipitation assay for human immunodeficiency virus (HIV). J Immunol Methods. 1988;112(2):235-241.

249. Resnick L, Shapshak P. Serologic characterization of human immunodeficiency virus infection by Western blot and radioimmunoprecipitation assays. Arch Pathol Lab Med. 1987;111(11):1040-1044.

250. Roberts CR, Longfield JN, Platte RC, et al. Transfusion-associated human immunodeficiency virus type 1 from screened antibody-negative blood donors. Arch Pathol Lab Med. 1994;118(12):1188-1192.

251. Simon F, Cot MC, Lesager C, et al. Differentiation between HIV-1 and HIV-2 infection by radioimmunoprecipitation and synthetic peptides in double reactive sera. AIDS. 1989;3(6):401-402.

252. Grimes DA, Schulz KF. Uses and abuses of screening tests. Lancet. 2002;359(9309):881-884.

253. Revised guidelines for HIV counseling, testing, and referral. MMWR Recomm Rep 2001;50(RR-19):1-57; quiz CE1-19a1-CE6-19a1.

254. Clark SJ, Kelen GD, Henrard DR, et al. Unsuspected primary human immunodeficiency virus type 1 infection in seronegative emergency department patients. J Infect Dis. 1994;170(1):194-197.

255. UNAIDS policy on HIV testing and counseling. Geneva and New York: United Nations; 1997.

256. Braithwaite RL, Arriola KR. Male prisoners and HIV prevention: A call for action ignored. Am J Public Health. 2003;93(5):759-763.

257. Cameron T. Mandatory HIV testing of newborns in New York State: What are the implications? J Health Soc Policy. 2002;14(3):59-78.

258. Downie JC, Howard R, Bowcock B, Cunningham AL. HIV-1 antibody testing strategy: evaluation of ELISA screening and western blot profiles in a mixed low risk/high risk patient population. J Virol Methods. 1989;26(3):291-303.

259. Davey RT, Jr, Deyton LR, Metcalf JA, et al. Indeterminate western blot patterns in a cohort of individuals at high risk for human immunodeficiency virus (HIV-1) exposure. J Clin Immunol. 1992;12(3):185-192.

260. Jackson JB, MacDonald KL, Cadwell J, et al. Absence of HIV infection in blood donors with indeterminate western blot tests for antibody to HIV-1. N Engl J Med. 1990;322(4):217-222.

261. Dock NL, Kleinman SH, Rayfield MA, et al. Human immunodeficiency virus infection and indeterminate western blot patterns. Prospective studies in a low prevalence population. Arch Intern Med. 1991;151(3):525-530.

262. Leitman SF, Klein HG, Melpolder JJ, et al. Clinical implications of positive tests for antibodies to human immunodeficiency virus type 1 in asymptomatic blood donors. N Engl J Med. 1989;321(14):917-924.

263. Kleinman S. The significance of HIV-1-indeterminate western blot results in blood donor populations. Arch Pathol Lab Med. 1990;114(3):298-303.

264. Rich JD, Dickinson BP, Spaulding A, et al. Interpretation of indeterminate HIV serology results in an incarcerated population. J Acquir Immune Defic Syndr Hum Retrovirol. 1998;17(4):376-379.

265. Gastaldello R, Gallego S, Isa MB, et al. Immunofluorescence assay reactivity patterns of serum samples presenting indeterminate Western blot results for antibodies to HIV-1 and HTLV-I/II in Cordoba, Argentina. Rev Inst Med Trop Sao Paulo. 2001; 43(5):277-282.

266. Delaporte E, Peeters M, Simon F, et al. Interpretation of antibodies reacting solely with human retroviral core proteins in western equatorial Africa. AIDS. 1989;3(3):179-182.

267. Chen MY, Lee KL, Hung CC, et al. Strategies for diagnosing HIV-1 infection in atypical Western blots. J Microbiol Immunol Infect. 1997;30(3):135-144.

268. Frank AP, Wandell MG, Headings MD, et al. Anonymous HIV testing using home collection and telemedicine counseling. A multicenter evaluation. Arch Intern Med. 1997;157(3):309-314.

269. Tsu RC, Burm ML, Gilhooly JA, Sells CW. Telephone vs. face-to-face notification of HIV results in high-risk youth. J Adolesc Health. 2002;30(3):154-160.

270. Aidoo S, Ampofo WK, Brandful JA, et al. Suitability of a rapid immunochromatographic test for detection of antibodies to human immunodeficiency virus in Ghana, West Africa. J Clin Microbiol. 2001;39(7):2572-2575.

271. Stetler HC, Granade TC, Nunez CA, et al. Field evaluation of rapid HIV serologic tests for screening and confirming HIV-1 infection in Honduras. AIDS. 1997;11(3):369-375.

272. Downing RG, Otten RA, Marum E, et al. Optimizing the delivery of HIV counseling and testing services: the Uganda experience using rapid HIV antibody test algorithms. J Acquir Immune Defic Syndr Hum Retrovirol. 1998;18(4):384-388.

273. Urassa W, Nozohoor S, Jaffer S, et al. Evaluation of an alternative confirmatory strategy for the diagnosis of HIV infection in Dar Es Salaam, Tanzania, based on simple rapid assays. J Virol Methods. 2002;100(1-2):115-120.

274. Urassa W, Godoy K, Killewo J, et al. The accuracy of an alternative confirmatory strategy for detection of antibodies to HIV-1: Experience from a regional laboratory in Kagera, Tanzania. J Clin Virol. 1999;14(1):25-29.

275. Nkengasong JN, Maurice C, Koblavi S, et al. Evaluation of HIV serial and parallel serologic testing algorithms in Abidjan, Cote d'Ivoire. AIDS. 1999;13(1):109-117.

276. Rehle TM, Mattke P, Liomba GN, et al. Evaluation of a quantitative double ELISA strategy for confirmation and differentiation of HIV infection. J Virol Methods. 1997;66(2):203-209.

277. Constantine NT, Ketema F. Rapid confirmation of HIV infection. Int J Infect Dis. 2002;6(3):170-177.

278. Joint United Nations Programme on HIV/AIDS (UNAIDS)-WHO Revised recommendations for the selection and use of HIV antibody tests. Wkly Epidemiol Rec. 1997;72(12):81-88.

279. Sato PA, Maskill WJ, Tamashiro H, Heymann DL. Strategies for laboratory HIV testing: an examination of alternative approaches not requiring Western blot. Bull World Health Organ. 1994;72(1):129-134.

280. Wilkinson D, Wilkinson N, Lombard C, et al. On-site HIV testing in resource-poor settings: Is one rapid test enough? AIDS. 1997;11(3):377-381.

281. Meda N, Gautier-Charpentier L, Soudre RB, et al. Serological diagnosis of human immuno-deficiency virus in Burkina Faso: Reliable, practical strategies using less expensive commercial test kits. Bull World Health Organ. 1999;77(9):731-739.

282. Lemey P, Pybus OG, Wang B, et al. Tracing the origin and history of the HIV-2 epidemic. Proc Natl Acad Sci U S A. 2003;100(11):6588-6592.

283. Rubsamen-Waigmann H, Maniar J, Gerte S, et al. High proportion of HIV-2 and HIV-1/2 double-reactive sera in two Indian states, Maharashtra and Goa: First appearance of an HIV-2 epidemic along with an HIV-1 epidemic outside of Africa. Zentralbl Bakteriol. 1994;280(3):398-402.

284. CDC Divisions of HIV/AIDS Prevention. Fact sheet. Human immunodeficiency virus type 2. Centers for Disease Control and Prevention. Available at www.cdc.gov/hiv/pubs/facts/hiv2.htm. Accessed June 2004.

285. Norrgren H, Andersson S, Biague AJ, et al. Trends and interaction of HIV-1 and HIV-2 in Guinea-Bissau, west Africa: No protection of HIV-2 against HIV-1 infection. AIDS. 1999;13(6):701-707.

286. van der Loeff MF, Aaby P, Aryioshi K, et al. HIV-2 does not protect against HIV-1 infection in a rural community in Guinea-Bissau. AIDS. 2001;15(17):2303-2310.

287. Alabi AS, Jaffar S, Ariyoshi K, et al. Plasma viral load, CD4 cell percentage, HLA and survival of HIV-1, HIV-2, and dually infected Gambian patients. AIDS. 2003;17(10):1513-1520.

288. Schim van der Loeff MF, Jaffar S, Aveika AA, et al. Mortality of HIV-1, HIV-2 and HIV-1/HIV-2 dually infected patients in a clinic-based cohort in The Gambia. AIDS. 2002;16(13):1775-1783.

289. De Cock KM, Porter A, Kouadio J, et al. Rapid and specific diagnosis of HIV-1 and HIV-2 infections: an evaluation of testing strategies. AIDS. 1990;4(9):875-878.

290. George JR, Rayfield MA, Phillips S, et al. Efficacies of US Food and Drug Administration-licensed HIV-1-screening enzyme immunoassays for detecting antibodies to HIV-2. AIDS. 1990;4(4):321-326.

291. Sazama K, Kuramoto IK, Holland PV, et al. Detection of antibodies to human immunodeficiency virus type 2 (HIV-2) in blood donor sera using United States assay methods for anti-HIV type 1. Transfusion. 1992;32(5):398-401.

292. Koblavi-Deme S, Maurice C, Yavo D, et al. Sensitivity and specificity of human immunodeficiency virus rapid serologic assays and testing algorithms in an antenatal clinic in Abidjan, Ivory Coast. J Clin Microbiol. 2001;39(5):1808-1812.

293. Thorstensson R, Walther L, Putkonen P, et al. A capture enzyme immunoassay for detection of HIV-2/SIV antigen. J Acquir Immune Defic Syndr. 1991;4(4):374-379.

294. Simon F, Matheron S, Tamalet C, et al. Cellular and plasma viral load in patients infected with HIV-2. AIDS. 1993;7(11):1411-1417.

295. Tobler LH, Kaufman E, Gefter N, et al. Use of human immunodeficiency virus (HIV) type 1 and 2 recombinant strip immunoblot assay to resolve enzyme immunoassay anti-HIV-2-repeatedly reactive samples after anti-HIV-1/2 combination enzyme immunoassay screening. Transfusion. 1997;37(9):921-925.

296. Ray CS, Mason PR, Smith H, et al. An evaluation of dipstick-dot immunoassay in the detection of antibodies to HIV-1 and 2 in Zimbabwe. Trop Med Int Health. 1997;2(1):83-88.

297. Andersson S, da Silva Z, Norrgren H, et al. Field evaluation of alternative testing strategies for diagnosis and differentiation of HIV-1 and HIV-2 infections in an HIV-1 and HIV-2-prevalent area. AIDS. 1997;11(15):1815-1822.

298. Christiansen CB, Jessen TE, Nielsen C, Staun-Olsen P. False negative anti-HIV-1/HIV-2 ELISAs in acute HIV-2 infection. Vox Sang. 1996;70(3):144-147.

299. Van Doornum GJ, Buimer M, Gobbers E, et al. Evaluation of an expanded two-ELISA approach for confirmation of reactive serum samples in an HIV-screening programme for pregnant women. J Med Virol. 1998;54(4):285-290.

300. Nogueira SA, Lambert JS, Albuquerque AL, et al. Assessment of a rapid HIV test strategy during labor: a pilot study from Rio de Janeiro, Brazil. J Hum Virol. 2001;4(5):278-282.

301. Cassol S, Butcher A, Kinard S, et al. Rapid screening for early detection of mother-to-child transmission of human immunodeficiency virus type 1. J Clin Microbiol. 1994;32(11):2641-2645.

302. Nielsen K, Bryson YJ. Diagnosis of HIV infection in children. Pediatr Clin North Am. 2000;47(1):39-63.

303. Delamare C, Burgard M, Mayaux MJ, et al. HIV-1 RNA detection in plasma for the diagnosis of infection in neonates. The French Pediatric HIV Infection Study Group. J Acquir Immune Defic Syndr Hum Retrovirol. 1997;15(2):121-125.

304. Cunningham P, Marriott D, Harris C, et al. False negative HIV-1 proviral DNA polymerase chain reaction in a patient with primary infection acquired in Thailand. J Clin Virol. 2003;26(2):163-169.

305. Hollinger FB, Bremer JW, Myers LE, et al. Standardization of sensitive human immunodeficiency virus coculture procedures and establishment of a multicenter quality assurance program for the AIDS Clinical Trials Group. The NIH/NIAID/DAIDS/ACTG Virology Laboratories. J Clin Microbiol. 1992;30(7): 1787-1794.

306. Bremer JW, Lew JF, Cooper E, et al. Diagnosis of infection with human immunodeficiency virus type 1 by a DNA polymerase chain reaction assay among infants enrolled in the Women and Infants' Transmission Study. J Pediatr. 1996;129(2):198-207.

307. Nadal D, Boni J, Kind C, et al. Prospective evaluation of amplification-boosted ELISA for heat-denatured p24 antigen for diagnosis and monitoring of pediatric human immunodeficiency virus type 1 infection. J Infect Dis. 1999;180(4):1089-1095.

308. Liberatore D, Avila MM, Calarota S, et al. Diagnosis of perinatally acquired HIV-1 infection using an IgA ELISA test. Pediatr AIDS HIV Infect. 1996;7(3):164-167.

309. Yasuda S, Iwasaki M, Oka S, et al. Detection of HIV-Gag p24-specific antibodies in sera and saliva of HIV-1-infected adults and in sera of infants born to HIV-1-infected mothers. Microbiol Immunol. 1998;42(4):305-311.

310. Faye A, Burgard M, Crosnier H, et al. Human immunodeficiency virus type 2 infection in children. J Pediatr. 1997;130(6):994-997.

311. Zeichner SR. J Diagnosis and Management of Pediatric HIV Infection; in press.

312. Centers for Disease Control and Prevention/Department of Health and Human Services: HIV/AIDS Surveillance Report. US HIV and AIDS cases reported through June 1997. Atlanta: Centers for Disease Control and Prevention/Department of Health and Human Services; 1997.

313. Glynn SA, Busch MP, Schreiber GB, et al. Effect of a national disaster on blood supply and safety: The September 11 experience. JAMA. 2003;289(17):2246-2253.

314. Glasser DB. Serologic testing of cornea donors. Cornea. 1998;17(2):123-128.

315. Pepose JS, Pardo F, Kessler JA, 2nd, et al. Screening cornea donors for antibodies against human immunodeficiency virus. Efficacy of ELISA testing of cadaveric sera and aqueous humor. Ophthalmology. 1987;94(2):95-100.

316. Schwarz A, Hoffmann F, L'Age-Stehr J, et al. Human immunodeficiency virus transmission by organ donation. Outcome in cornea and kidney recipients. Transplantation. 1987;44(1):21-24.

317. Pepose JS, Pardo FS, Donegan E, Quinn TC. HTLV-III ELISA testing of cadaveric sera to screen potential organ transplant donors. JAMA. 1986;256(7):864.

318. Heim A, Wagner D, Rothamel T, et al. Evaluation of serological screening of cadaveric sera for donor selection for cornea transplantation. J Med Virol. 1999;58(3):291-295.

319. Li L, Constantine NT, Zhang X, Smialek JE. Determination of human immunodeficiency virus antibody status in forensic autopsy cases using a rapid and simple FDA-licensed assay. J Forensic Sci. 1993;38(4):798-805.

320. American Medical Association Council of Ethical and Judicial Affairs. Code of Medical Ethics. E-2.23 HIV Testing 2003.

321. Craven DE, Steger KA, La Chapelle R, Allen DM. Factitious HIV infection: the importance of documenting infection. Ann Intern Med. 1994;121(10):763-766.

322. Sacks M, Burton W, Dermatis H, et al. HIV-related cases among 2,094 admissions to a psychiatric hospital. Psychiatr Serv. 1995;46(2):131-135.

323. Wu AW, Kennedy CJ, Paradise M. Factitious false-positive test for HIV. JAMA. 1988;259(11):1647.

324. Zuger A, O'Dowd MA. The baron has AIDS: A case of factitious human immunodeficiency virus infection and review. Clin Infect Dis. 1992;14(1):211-216.

325. Kalish ML, Ndongmo CB, Wolfe ND, et al. Evidence for continued exposure to and possible infection of humans with SIV. In: HIV Dynamics and Evolution 10th International Workshop; Lake Arrowhead Calif; 2003.

326. Yang C, Dash BC, Simon F, et al. Detection of diverse variants of human immunodeficiency virus-1 groups M, N, and O and simian immunodeficiency viruses from chimpanzees by using generic pol and env primer pairs. J Infect Dis. 2000;181(5):1791-1795.

327. Simon F, Souquiere S, Damond F, et al. Synthetic peptide strategy for the detection of and discrimination among highly divergent primate lentiviruses. AIDS Res Hum Retroviruses. 2001;17(10):937-952.

328. Stoye JP, Le Tissier P, Takeuchi Y, et al. Endogenous retroviruses: A potential problem for xenotransplantation? Ann N Y Acad Sci. 1998;862:67-74.

329. Stoye JP, Coffin JM. The dangers of xenotransplantation. Nat Med. 1995;1(11):1100.

330. Martin U, Kiessig V, Blusch JH, et al. Expression of pig endogenous retrovirus by primary porcine endothelial cells and infection of human cells. Lancet. 1998;352(9129):692-694.

331. Ericsson TA, Takeuchi Y, Templin C, et al. Identification of receptors for pig endogenous retrovirus. Proc Natl Acad Sci U S A. 2003;100(11):6759-6764.

332. Qari SH, Magre S, Garcia-Lerma JG, et al. Susceptibility of the porcine endogenous retrovirus to reverse transcriptase and protease inhibitors. J Virol. 2001;75(2):1048-1053.

333. Birmingham K. FDA subcommittee finds no evidence of PERV transmission. Nat Med. 1999;5(8):855.

334. Switzer WM, Michler RE, Shanmugam V, et al. Lack of cross-species transmission of porcine endogenous retrovirus infection to nonhuman primate recipients of porcine cells, tissues, or organs. Transplantation. 2001;71(7):959-965.

335. van der Laan LJ, Lockey C, Griffeth BC, et al. Infection by porcine endogenous retrovirus after islet xenotransplantation in SCID mice. Nature. 2000;407(6800):90-94.

336. Tacke SJ, Bodusch K, Berg A, Denner J. Sensitive and specific immunological detection methods for porcine endogenous retroviruses applicable to experimental and clinical xenotransplantation. Xenotransplantation. 2001;8(2):125-135.

337. Final Guidance FDA Source Animal, Product, Preclinical and Clinical Issues Concerning the Use of Xenotransplantation Products in Humans, US Department of Health and Human Services, FDA, CBER, April 2003.

338. Gelman IH, Zhang J, Hailman E, et al. Identification and evaluation of new primer sets for the detection of lentivirus proviral DNA. AIDS Res Human Retroviruses. 1992;8(12):1981-1989.

339. Cohen JI. NIAID Clinical Protocol 01-I-0161. Identification of novel viruses. NIH Protocol Office. Tel. 1-800-411-1222.

340. Griffiths DJ, Cooke SP, Herve C, et al. Detection of human retrovirus 5 in patients with arthritis and systemic lupus erythematosus. Arthritis Rheum. 1999;42(3):448-454.

341. Griffiths DJ, Voisset C, Venables PJ, Weiss RA. Novel endogenous retrovirus in rabbits previously reported as human retrovirus 5. J Virol. 2002;76(14):7094-7102.

342. Check E. A tragic setback. Nature. 2002;420(6912):116-118.

CHAPTER **116**

The Immunology of Human Immunodeficiency Virus Infection

MARK DYBUL

MARK CONNORS

ANTHONY S. FAUCI

The interactions between the human immunodeficiency virus (HIV) and the human immune system are extraordinarily complex, as evidenced by the highly variable rates of disease progression observed in HIV-infected individuals. Indeed, even individuals who were infected from a common source may experience widely divergent clinical outcomes.[1] HIV subverts the immune system by infecting CD4+ T cells that normally orchestrate immune responses and by activating the immune system and inducing a cytokine milieu that the virus uses to its own replication advantage. The discovery that certain chemokine receptors function as HIV co-receptors for HIV entry into target cells has expanded the scope of host factors that play a role in the pathogenesis of HIV-induced disease.

The lack of recognizable correlates of protective immunity in HIV infection continues to hamper vaccine development and immunotherapeutic approaches. Robust HIV-specific immune responses, both humoral and cell mediated, are mounted by most infected individuals. It remains unclear why the vast majority of HIV-infected individuals experience inexorable immunodeficiency and disease progression despite the presence of these robust antiviral immune responses. In this regard, qualitative as well as quantitative aspects of virus-specific immune responses may be important in the containment of viral replication.

The progress that has been made to date in understanding the pathogenesis of HIV infection is unparalleled; the recent availability of effective combination antiretroviral therapy (ART) has had extraordinary clinical benefits for patients and has also provided important insights into the immunologic and virologic factors associated with the control of HIV infection and disease progression. However, fundamental questions remain regarding the nature and scope of the precise mechanisms of pathogenesis of HIV disease. It is clear that HIV induces dysfunction of nearly all elements of the immune system and that the pathogenesis of HIV disease is multifactorial.[2] Although mechanisms of CD4+ T-cell depletion and dysfunction in vitro have been elucidated, it remains uncertain which of these mechanisms are responsible for clinically relevant immune deficiency in vivo. Similarly, a great deal is known about HIV-induced dysregulation of the cytokine network; however, any attempt to manipulate this enormously complex and pleiotropic cytokine network for the purpose of inhibiting HIV replication without untoward effects is a daunting task.

HUMAN IMMUNODEFICIENCY VIRUS ENTRY AND DISSEMINATION

Human Immunodeficiency Virus Receptors and Entry into Cells

CD4 was identified as the major cellular receptor for HIV fusion and entry in 1984.[3-5] Transfection of the CD4 gene into CD4-negative (CD4⁻) human cells rendered them infectable with HIV[6]; however, transfection of the human CD4 gene into murine cell lines did not render these cells susceptible to HIV infection despite glycoprotein (gp) 120 binding to CD4, suggesting that other factor(s) were necessary for HIV fusion and entry.[7] These additional factors remained elusive for many years until the recognition of HIV co-receptors.

In late 1995 and early 1996, a series of papers were published that altered our understanding of how HIV enters a target cell. The first report, by Cocchi and co-workers,[8] identified the β or CC chemokines, macrophage inflammatory protein (MIP)-1α, MIP-1β, and RANTES (regulated on activation, normal T cell expressed and secreted) as major components of CD8+ T-cell–derived HIV suppressor factors. They observed that these chemokines in combination could inhibit the infection of activated CD4+ T cells by certain strains of HIV-1, HIV-2, and simian immunodeficiency virus (SIV). Of note, these chemokines did not block infection with HIV-IIIB, the prototypic T-cell line–adapted strain of HIV. Subsequently, the isolation of a gene from an HeLa cell mRNA library was described whose expression allowed gp160-mediated cell fusion in the presence of CD4.[8,9] The protein, called fusin (later renamed CXCR4), is a 7-transmembrane chemokine receptor. This receptor, together with CD4, was required for T-tropic envelope fusion to target cells but was not used by M-tropic strains. The natural ligand for CXCR4 was later determined to be stromal cell–derived factor (SDF)-1[10,11] (Fig. 116-1).

In a separate line of research, Paxton and co-workers[12] studied a population of individuals who had been exposed repeatedly to HIV-infected partners but who remained uninfected. They identified two subjects whose CD4+ T cells were refractory to infection with M-tropic strains of HIV but were easily infectable with T-tropic cell line–adapted strains. In addition, cells from these individuals produced high levels of MIP-1α, MIP-1β, and RANTES, the same chemokines previously identified as suppressors of HIV infection. Subsequently, a new CC chemokine receptor (CCR)-5 was identified; the natural ligands that bind to this receptor were shown to be MIP-1α, MIP-1β, and RANTES.[13-15] In light of the previous work showing that the CCR5 ligands inhibit cellular entry of M-tropic strains of HIV, the obvious question that arose was whether CCR5 might function as a co-receptor for such strains. A series of papers simultaneously showed this to be the case[16-20] (Fig. 116-1). Other chemokine receptors, including CCR1, CCR2b, and CCR3, were also identified in these reports as potential co-receptors for certain HIV strains. Other orphan receptors of the chemokine receptor class have been shown to be potential HIV co-receptors.[19-21]

A mutant allele of the *CCR5* gene has been described that contains a 32–base pair deletion resulting in a truncated nonfunctional co-receptor for HIV entry.[22,23] Because CCR5-utilizing HIV is almost universally responsible for primary infection, individuals homozygous for the *CCR5* mutation are almost completely protected from HIV-1 infection.[22,23] Heterozygosity for the *CCR5* mutation results in reduced expression of CCR5 on the cell surface and diminished infectability of T cells of these patients compared with cells from *CCR5* wild-type individuals.[24] Although heterozygosity for *CCR5* does not appear to afford protection against HIV-1 infection, it may result in slowed progression of disease in HIV-infected individuals.[25-27]

Dissemination of Human Immunodeficiency Virus Infection

It remains unclear which cell type in the blood, lymphoid tissue, spleen, or mucosa is the first to actually become infected with HIV. However, in studies of macaques exposed to SIV intravaginally, bone marrow–derived dendritic cells (DCs) in the vaginal mucosa are the first cells to contain SIV DNA, which is detectable 2 days after exposure. In examinations of lymphoid organs, the pattern of appearance and spread of SIV mirrored the course that DCs take upon migrating from peripheral tissues to lymphoid organs.[28] DCs function by binding antigens in the peripheral tissues, processing them into peptides that are associated with MHC antigens, migrating into the paracortical regions of lymphoid organs via afferent lymphatics and activating T cells. DCs are capable of retaining infectious virus on their surface for extended periods of time. Thus, their role in the initiation of HIV infection likely includes capturing virions at sites of entry, carrying them to the paracortical regions of lymphoid organs, and delivering virus to CD4+ T cells that become activated through their interaction with DCs (Fig. 116-2).

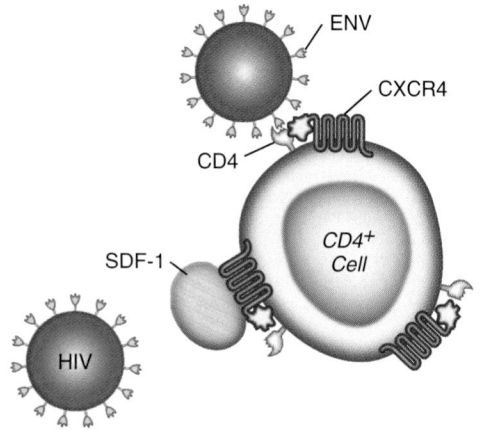

X4 Strain of HIV-1

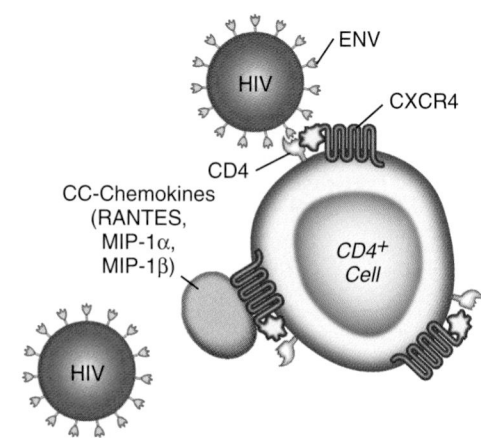

R5 Strain of HIV-1

FIGURE 116-1. Model of CCR5 and CXCR4 use and strain-specific inhibition of HIV binding by co-receptor ligands. Entry of CCR5-utilizing strains of HIV (R5) is blocked by the CCR5 ligands MIP-1α, MIP-1β, and RANTES. Entry of CXCR4-utilizing strains of HIV (X4) is blocked by the CXCR4 ligand SDF-1. *(Adapted with permission from Fauci AS. Host factors and the pathogenesis of HIV-induced disease. Nature. 1996;384:529-534.)*

The precise nature of the early events during primary HIV and SIV infection that lead to viral replication in lymphoid tissue has not been elucidated. DCs express low levels of CD4, and it is generally agreed that these cells can be infected by HIV only at a low level. Although study of DC infection in lymphoid organs has been somewhat limited, in one investigation the frequency of HIV-infected splenic DCs was approximately 2 log less than that observed in CD4+ T cells from the same individuals.[29] In an analysis of lymph node biopsy samples, tissue sections from HIV-infected individuals at various stages of disease were stained for DC markers by immunohistochemistry and for HIV RNA by in situ hybridization. No cells that stained for both DC markers and HIV were observed, suggesting that DCs in these organs were rarely, if ever, infected with HIV at any stage of disease. In vitro studies have demonstrated that DCs and CD4+ T cells form conjugates and that active viral replication takes place within these conjugates.[30] Similar conjugates of DCs and CD4+ T cells containing HIV antigen have been identified in vivo in tonsillar biopsy specimens obtained from individuals infected with HIV,[31] in the peripheral blood at low quantities,[32] and in the submucosal tissue after vaginal exposure to

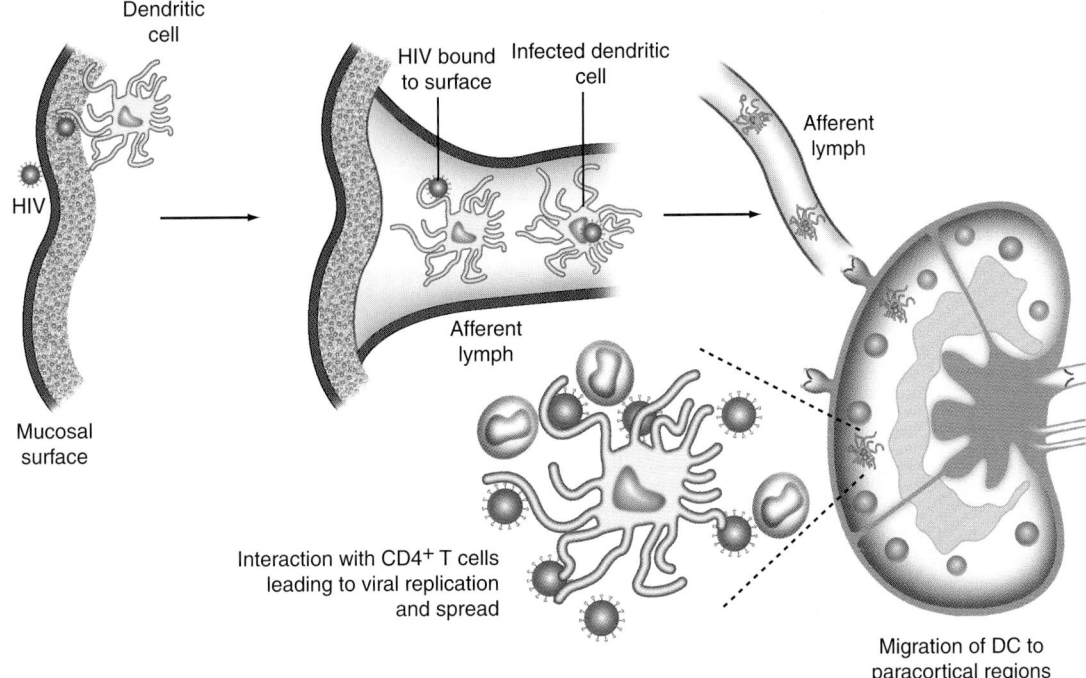

FIGURE 116-2. Initial infection and dissemination of HIV infection. Dendritic cells (DCs) at the site of exposure transport HIV to the paracortical regions of draining lymphoid tissues, leading to infection of CD4+ T cells and dissemination of HIV infection. *(Adapted with permission from Weissman D, Fauci AS. Clin Microbiol Rev. 1997;10:358.)*

SIV.[28] Recently, it has been shown that dendritic cell–specific intracellular adhesion molecule (ICAM)-3–grabbing nonintegrin (DC-SIGN),[33,34] a protein expressed on DCs in the T-cell area of tonsils, lymph nodes, and spleen and in the lamina propria of mucosal tissues, may be important in the attachment of HIV to DCs and may be an important factor in the transmission of HIV from DCs to T cells. It is likely that DCs carry HIV from tissues in which the initial rounds of viral replication occur to the regional lymph nodes, where CD4+ T cells become infected after contact with DCs. This leads to subsequent rounds of virus replication and spread in the absence of HIV-specific immune responses. Thus, lymphoid tissue plays a key role in the initiation and dissemination of HIV infection.

HUMAN IMMUNODEFICIENCY VIRUS–SPECIFIC IMMUNE RESPONSES

Although the immune response to HIV has been extensively studied, a number of fundamental issues remain unresolved. Among the most important of these is that it remains unclear how HIV avoids immunologic control in the majority of infected individuals. New technologies for measuring cellular and humoral immune responses and new models of immune system–mediated protection or control of virus replication permit the dissection of what constitutes an effective immune response against HIV in greater detail than was previously possible. One animal model that has been particularly useful for the study of lentivirus-specific immunity and vaccine development is SIV infection of Rhesus macaques. SIV is closely related to HIV-2 and causes an acute infection that leads to persistent viremia, CD4+ T-cell depletion, immunodeficiency, opportunistic infections, and death in susceptible animals. In addition, the humoral immune response to HIV can be studied in macaques infected with SIV-HIV chimeras (SHIV) that encode the HIV envelope surface glycoprotein. Through passive transfer or depletion studies in experimental animals, and correlative studies in humans, it is now known that humoral immune responses can protect against lentiviral infection and that cellular immune responses can control viral replication. Elucidation of the breadth and magnitude of HIV-specific immune responses, the HIV protein targets of these responses, and the mechanisms by which protection or control occur may provide insights for the development of effective prophylactic or therapeutic vaccines.

Humoral Immune Responses

Antibodies that bind HIV proteins, including the viral surface envelope glycoprotein, can be detected in the plasma within weeks of HIV infection coincident with the decline of plasma viremia.[35,36] In addition, sera of chronically infected patients commonly contain some neutralizing activity against viruses that have undergone laboratory passage. However, high levels of antibodies that are capable of neutralizing viruses that have not undergone laboratory passage (primary isolates) are only rarely detected, typically in long-term nonprogressors.[37,38] Although antibodies that bind HIV proteins or neutralize laboratory isolates are detectable in many individuals, antibodies capable of neutralizing the autologous viral isolate develop well after plasma viremia has declined and are of low magnitude.[39]

In addition to the relatively poor immunogenicity of the envelope glycoprotein, its structure and diversity likely contribute to the lack of antibodies that neutralize broad classes of viral isolates in most chronically infected individuals. Of the antibodies directed against HIV-1–encoded proteins, only those directed against surface envelope glycoprotein are thought to be important in protective immunity. X-ray crystallographic studies and epitope mapping using monoclonal antibodies have permitted detailed study of the envelope glycoprotein structure and antibody binding sites.[40-42] The majority of envelope protein (gp160) is thought to exist in a trimeric structure with six subunits (three gp120s and three gp41s) and is heavily glycosylated. In addition to CD4, HIV envelope protein also binds CC or CXC chemokine receptors as co-receptors to mediate viral entry (see earlier). The CD4 and co-receptor binding sites are located within separate depressions on the gp120 surface.[43] Both the CD4 and co-receptor binding sites are well conserved among known viral isolates and are not glycosylated. For these reasons they are thought to be important targets of neutralizing antibodies. The description of monoclonal antibodies with broadly cross-neutralizing activity that bind to the CD4 binding site has led to the hypothesis that generation of antibodies specific to these sites may be a prerequisite for neutralization.[44] It is thought that these sites remain inaccessible in the native conformation and that binding of antibody to these sites may require the conformational changes induced by CD4 binding.[42,45,46] However, there is not general agreement regarding the absolute necessity to bind these sites for effective neutralization (reviewed in Parren and Burton[47]). In certain studies, antibodies capable of protecting Rhesus macaques against SIV challenge were specific for HLA-DR that is included in the virus envelope on budding from the host cell.[48,49] In addition, the amount of antibody bound to virus particles has been correlated with neutralization regardless of the epitope specificity.[50] Thus, it is possible that antibodies that bind the virus particle but do not bind the CD4 or co-receptor binding site may interfere with virus–cell interactions sufficiently to mediate neutralization of HIV.

The genetic diversity between HIV isolates is also thought to contribute to the difficulty in neutralizing the virus. The level of genetic variation of HIV is high within geographically defined populations and even within a single infected patient. Mutations that occur during the process of reverse transcription and a prolonged duration of infection generate highly diverse viral sequences that coexist in the plasma.[51] The level of diversity of HIV is considerably higher than that of most human RNA viruses and is likely a major contributor to the lack of cross-neutralizing antibodies. For example, it is known for some respiratory viruses that changes in only a few amino acids within the surface glycoproteins can result in loss of cross-neutralization between virus isolates.[52,53] By comparison, HIV viral sequences may vary between 10% and 16% in the plasma of a given individual.[54-56] In addition, recent data suggest that significant levels of antibodies capable of neutralizing autologous virus do arise early during infection, but the virus evolves to escape this neutralization.[57] It is thought that these diverse circulating envelope sequences may represent a constantly evolving target that contributes to the ability of HIV to evade the humoral immune response.

Cellular Immune Responses

Cytotoxic T-Lymphocytes

MHC class I–restricted, HIV-specific, CD8+ cytotoxic T-lymphocyte (CTL) responses are found in the peripheral blood within the first few months of HIV infection and are detected during the chronic phases of infection in the majority of HIV-infected individuals.[58,59] CD8+ T cells specific for each of the known HIV-1 gene products have been detected in the peripheral blood by bulk CTL assays, limiting dilution assays for cytolysis, interferon (IFN)-γ secretion, or tetramer staining. Several lines of evidence suggest that HIV-specific CD8+ T cells play an important role in restriction of virus replication. First, the temporal association of the peak of the HIV-specific CTL response with the decline of viremia during acute infection is thought to represent the effect of virus-specific CTL in restricting HIV replication in humans.[58,60] Further, indirect evidence of an important role of CD8+ T cells in restriction of HIV replication in humans comes from strong associations between restriction of virus replication and certain MHC class I alleles and functional links with epitopes presented by these alleles.[58,60] More direct evidence for the role of CD8+ T cells in restricting lentiviral replication in vivo is provided by several recent studies in experimental animals.[58,60] Last, CD8+ T-cell depletion by exogenous monoclonal antibodies has been shown to abrogate restriction of virus replication in both SHIV-infected as well as SIV-infected monkeys.[61,62] It is now generally accepted that CD8+ T cells are an important component of immune system–mediated restriction of HIV replication. However, although HIV-specific CTL likely exert some control over HIV replication, this restriction is generally incomplete, with viral RNA levels reaching 10^3 to 10^6 copies/mL plasma in the vast majority of HIV-infected individuals during the chronic phase of infection in the absence of ART. Many different mechanisms have been proposed to explain the inability of cell-mediated immunity to control HIV replication. These include viral factors and quantitative and qualitative factors within the HIV-specific CD8+ T-cell pool (Table 116-1).

TABLE 116-1   Proposed Mechanisms by Which Human Immunodeficiency Virus (HIV) Evades Immune System–Mediated Restriction of Virus Replication

Virus mediated
  Broad genetic diversity resulting in CTL "escape" mutations
  MHC downregulation causing diminished recognition of HIV-infected cells
Quantitative defects in CD8+ T-cell responses
  Insufficient numbers of HIV-specific CTL
  Diminished numbers of HIV-specific CTL secondary to loss of "CD4+ T-cell help"
Qualitative defects in CD8+ T-cell responses
  Loss of "CD4+ T-cell help" resulting in CD8+ T-cell dysfunction
  Insufficient maturation of HIV-specific T cells
  Diminished avidity
  Perforin defect

Several viral factors unique to HIV likely contribute to the ability of HIV to evade the cellular immune response. Mutations produced during the reverse transcription process combined with high levels of replication over a prolonged period result in a highly diverse population of viruses that circulate in a given patient. It is thought that this extraordinary level of viral diversity permits development of mutant viruses that escape immune recognition. Selection of "escape" mutations has been documented in HIV-infected humans and SIV-infected macaques. Longitudinal studies of viral sequences and CTL responses to known motifs have shown the appearance of mutations that no longer bind to the MHC class I molecule.[63,64] Some of the best characterized escape mutations have been shown to occur with epitopes presented by HLA-B27.[65,66] Single or clustered mutations cause *gag* peptides to no longer bind to the B27 molecule. These mutants accumulate in the peripheral blood and are associated with diminished responses to the nonmutated sequence. Examples of escape mutations that alter HLA binding and dominant viral sequences have also been observed for HLA-B8, -A3, and -B4.[63,64] However, it should be noted that the interplay of host and viral factors is extraordinarily complex given the large number of viral epitopes targeted by the immune response, timing of gene expression during the viral replication cycle, and complement of MHC class I alleles. The host CTL response is limited by the ability of the MHC class I alleles to bind to various viral epitopes, while viral replication is limited by the degree to which an escape mutation impairs viral replicative capacity or "fitness." In addition, the CD8+ T-cell response to each of the viral proteins in the context of each of a patient's MHC alleles is very broad. Although escape mutations may be found within a single epitope, it is likely that other conserved epitopes within the same gene remain as targets.[67] Thus, it remains uncertain whether these mutations cause true escape from immune system surveillance or whether escape mutations at single epitopes occur in the context of high levels of virus replication. Although escape mutations clearly occur, the relative importance of these mutations in the pathogenesis of HIV infection remains incompletely understood.

In addition to the high levels of diversity generated during HIV infection, other viral factors may contribute to the poor ability of the immune system to control HIV replication. HIV *nef, tat,* and *vpu* are each capable of down-modulating surface expression of MHC class I molecules necessary for recognition of infected cells.[68-70] The effect of *nef* is to diminish cell surface expression of HLA-A and -B molecules, leaving HLA-C and -E unaffected.[71] It has been proposed that these effects may permit infected cells to avoid lysis by HLA-A– or B–restricted T cells, which dominate the cellular immune response, yet also avoid lysis by natural killer (NK) cells that are inhibited by the presence of HLA-C or -E.[71] However, there is no uniform agreement that this is a predominant mechanism by which HIV avoids immunologic control. Several investigators have demonstrated the ability of autologous HIV-infected cells to stimulate cytokine secretion or cytolysis by class I–restricted HIV-specific CD8+ T cells.[72,73] At present, the relative role of MHC downregulation in the loss of restriction of HIV replication remains unclear.

It has also been proposed that HIV avoids immune control because the numbers of HIV-specific CD8[+] T cells may be too low. Inverse correlations were found between the frequency of CD8[+] T cells specific for two putative immunodominant A*0201 restricted HIV epitopes and plasma viral RNA. Others have found associations between higher numbers of HIV-specific CD8[+] T cells and the presence of a CD4[+] T-cell proliferative response to HIV antigens, suggesting that the frequency of HIV-specific CD8[+] T cells falls due to a lack of CD4[+] T-cell help.[74] However, several studies that examined a broad range of HIV epitopes in the context of multiple HLA alleles have not found an inverse correlation between plasma viral RNA and the frequency of HIV-specific CD8[+] T cells.[75-79] In this regard, HIV-specific CD8[+] T cells that respond to a broad array of HIV peptides persist in the range of 1% to 22% in most untreated patients with relatively high-level plasma viremia.[76,77,79,80]

One parameter of the HIV-specific CD8[+] T-cell response that might confer significant restriction of virus replication is the preferential targeting of genes that are expressed early in the virus replication cycle prior to release of mature virions. Several publications have described responses to *tat* or *rev* gene products in infected humans or their SIV homologues in macaques, and certain reports have associated these responses with better outcomes.[81-83] It has been shown previously that several patients with nonprogressive HIV infection have HLA-B*57–restricted responses specific for *tat* or *rev*.[81] However, in other studies the frequency of *tat*- or *rev*-specific CD8[+] T cells did not constitute a large portion of the overall response in patients with progressive or nonprogressive disease.[77,79,80] Although responses to these early genes are of theoretical importance, at present their role in restricting viral replication in infected individuals remains unclear.

Another parameter of the CD8[+] T-cell response that may provide enhanced restriction of virus replication is the breadth or number of HIV peptides to which a patient may respond. During acute infection, expansion of HIV-specific CD8[+] T cells is restricted to a relatively small number of clones. In certain cases these expansions are monoclonal, which carries a poor prognosis.[84] However, several reports describe a narrowly focused CD8[+] T-cell response in nonprogressors or in individuals treated with effective artiretroviral therapy (ART) during acute infection and who have restricted virus replication.[73,80,85] When the total CD8[+] T-cell response has been measured during acute or chronic infection, no relationship has been found between the breadth of the response and levels of plasma HIV viremia.[78,86] Because HIV-specific CD8[+] T cells of most chronically infected patients persist at high frequencies and respond to a broad array of HIV peptides, it does not appear likely that inadequate breadth of the response is a major contributor to poor restriction of virus replication during chronic infection.

Several lines of evidence have suggested that the inability of CD8[+] T cells to control HIV may lie not in the quantity of these cells but rather in qualitative properties of the response. CD3ζ molecules have been shown to be downregulated in the HIV-specific CD8[+] T cells of infected individuals and to have a diminished capacity to lyse autologous infected cells.[87] Progressively diminished secretion of IFN-γ by HIV-specific CD8[+] T cells during late stage disease also has been observed.[88,89] The phenotype of HIV-specific CD8[+] T cells has also been found to be skewed such that they do not express markers consistent with fully mature effector cells.[90] More recently, HIV-infected nonprogressors were differentiated by increased proliferative capacity of HIV-specific CD8[+] T cells linked to enhanced expression of perforin.[79] It is thought that the relative absence of these functions in progressors may represent a mechanism by which HIV avoids immunologic control. Although each of these observations must be confirmed, the persistence of high frequencies of HIV-specific CD8[+] T cells in both nonprogressors and patients with progressive disease strongly suggests that some qualitative parameters likely underlie the vast differences in the abilities of their CD8[+] T cells to restrict viral replication.

Soluble CD8[+] T-Cell–Secreted Factors

In addition to cytolysis, other mechanisms of CD8[+] T-cell–mediated antiviral activities have been described. CD8[+] T cells of HIV-infected patients secrete soluble factors that are able to inhibit viral replication in the absence of cell killing. This noncytolytic antiviral activity was initially described in vitro using CD8[+] T cells from HIV-infected patients.[58,60] Years later the suppressive activity against R5 viruses was shown to be mediated in large part by the CC-chemokines, MIP-1α, MIP-1β, and RANTES.[8] These molecules are natural ligands for CCR5, a co-receptor for R5 strains of HIV-1, and inhibit viral replication primarily by blocking virus entry. In addition to the CC-chemokines, additional, poorly characterized factor(s) act after viral entry to suppress HIV transcription in infected cells.[91-94] These additional factor(s) have been termed CD8[+] T-cell antiviral factors (CAF). Although not required for this suppressive activity, maximal suppression of HIV replication is observed under conditions when cell contact is maintained and cells are HLA matched.[95,96] This suppressive activity has been shown to be greater in peripheral blood mononuclear cells (PBMCs) of HIV-infected patients than in uninfected controls. However, at present, it remains unclear whether these factors are secreted in an antigen-specific manner.[95]

CD4[+] T-Cell Responses

Several animal models of viral pathogenesis have demonstrated that virus-specific CD4[+] T cells are critical in induction or maintenance of an effective CD8[+] CTL response that mediates restriction of virus replication.[97,98] Many viral infections of humans or experimental animals typically result in induction of CD4[+] T-cell responses that can be demonstrated by proliferation to virus antigens in vitro long after elimination or control of infection, which is a reflection of the persistence of these virus-specific memory CD4[+] T cells. Unlike most other infections of humans, HIV infection is characterized by the absence of HIV-specific CD4[+] T-cell proliferative responses in the vast majority of untreated patients.[99] However, these responses have been detected in some cohorts of patients who restrict HIV replication. In this regard, strong HIV-specific CD4[+] T-cell responses are found in relatively rare nonprogressors who restrict HIV replication in the absence of ART.[76,100-102] In addition, proliferative responses to HIV antigens have been found in patients who were treated early during acute infection and who then have restricted HIV replication when ART was withdrawn.[101,103] Because HIV infects CD4[+] T cells, it was believed that the early loss of HIV-specific proliferative responses may be the result of infection and deletion of HIV-specific CD4[+] T cells in the lymphoid tissues on encountering the virus. However, lines of evidence indicate that HIV-specific CD4[+] T cells persist in patients with progressive disease. Although typically absent in untreated patients, there are several recent reports that the prevalence of significant proliferative responses to HIV antigens is as high as 30% to 69% of those receiving effective ART.[104-106] In addition, a number of recent reports in cross-sectional cohorts have documented the persistence of HIV-specific CD4[+] T cells in the majority of patients by intracellular cytokine staining following stimulation with HIV antigens.[77,102,106,107] Furthermore, when both proliferation and frequency have been measured, the absence of HIV-specific CD4[+] T-cell proliferation was not attributable to the complete deletion of HIV-specific CD4[+] T cells.[102,106] In addition, proliferation of HIV-specific CD4[+] T cells was abrogated during an interruption of antiviral therapy, suggesting that diminished proliferation of these cells may be, in part, a result of high levels of HIV antigen, an event that appears similar to that observed during viremia with other human viruses.[108,109] Furthermore, HIV antigen-specific proliferative responses have been demonstrated in vitro after the addition of CD40 ligand and IL-12 or anti-CD28 antibody, indicating that HIV-specific cells with proliferative capacity remain in patients with progressive disease.[102,110] Thus, there is now general agreement that HIV-specific CD4[+] T cells persist in patients with progressive disease; however, the ability of these cells to proliferate in vitro is impaired. It remains unclear at present whether this diminished ability to proliferate in vitro represents a defect contributing to loss of control of viral replication or a normal response to high levels of antigen.

LONG-TERM NONPROGRESSORS

Although rates of disease progression vary widely among HIV-infected individuals, the mean time between infection and development of AIDS is approximately 10 years. In recent years, it has become clear that a small percentage of untreated HIV-infected individuals show no evidence of disease progression despite prolonged infection.[38,111,112] In addition to nonprogressors, other individuals who remain HIV-seronegative despite multiple exposures to HIV have been identified, suggesting that elements of protection exist but may not be readily detected by standard measures of the immune response. This group is likely heterogeneous with regard to the mechanisms of resistance to HIV infection (reviewed in Shearer and co-workers[113]). Studies of nonprogressors and highly exposed seronegative patients have furthered our understanding of the pathogenesis of HIV disease and have increased optimism that some forms of immunologic protection from infection or control of viral replication may exist in HIV infection.

Definitions of *long-term nonprogressors* have varied. One early definition that was commonly used included documented HIV infection for more than 7 years, CD4+ T-cell count greater than 600 cells/μL without significant decline over time, no symptoms of HIV disease, and no history of ART. Because definitions of long-term nonprogressors were created empirically, it is not surprising that such individuals constitute a heterogeneous group. Many individuals that were defined by these clinical criteria have now gone on to progressive disease. However, there remains a small subgroup of untreated long-term nonprogressors that have now been infected for 20 years and maintain normal CD4+ T-cell counts and plasma viral RNA less than 50 copies/mL of plasma.[73,114,115] Mechanisms that may determine a non-progressive course during HIV infection include host genetic factors, effective immunologic control of virus replication, and/or infection with an attenuated strain of HIV (Table 116-2). Compared with individuals with progressive HIV disease, nonprogressors tend to have lower viral loads and more vigorous antiviral humoral and cell-mediated immune responses. Although patients with normal CD4+ T-cell counts and low levels of plasma virus are a heterogeneous group, a small subset of patients with truly nonprogressive HIV infection and control of virus replication in the absence of ART are likely to hold important clues to the basis of an effective immune response to HIV.

Host Genetic Factors

It has been demonstrated that MHC alleles play an important role in determining the rate of disease progression.[116,117] Because definitions of nonprogressors and frequency of these patients have varied between studies, several large population studies have not consistently found associations between HLA alleles and nonprogression.[118-120] However, recent reports, heavily enriched for patients who meet more stringent definitions of nonprogression based upon plasma viral RNA (<50 copies/mL), have found much stronger associations with *HLA-B*5701* or *HLA-B27* alleles.[73,115] In addition, the HIV-specific CD8+ T-cell response in these *B*5701*-positive patients is highly focused on B57-restricted peptides, suggesting that the B57 molecule likely plays a direct role in restriction of virus replication in these individuals.[73,121]

As mentioned (see "Human Immunodeficiency Virus Entry and Dissemination"), the chemokine receptor genotype has an impact on rates of progression of disease. For example, individuals who carry one copy of the mutant *CCR5-Δ32* allele have an increased chance of experiencing a slow rate of disease progression compared with individuals who are homozygous for wild-type alleles.[25,27] In addition, some *CCR2* alleles have been associated with slower rates of disease progression.[122] Despite the association between *CCR5* genotype and nonprogressive HIV infection, this factor does not appear to be a dominant influence in the determination of the state of long-term nonprogression. In this regard, although the frequency of *CCR5* heterozygotes is increased two-fold among nonprogressors compared with HIV-infected controls, fewer than 50% of nonprogressors are *CCR5* heterozygotes (reviewed in Carrington and associates[123]). In a separate study, the immunologic and virologic profile of *CCR5* wild-type and *CCR5* heterozygous nonprogressors was indistinguishable, suggesting that although *CCR5* heterozygotes have an increased chance of becoming nonprogressors, HIV-infected *CCR5* wild-type individuals may arrive at the same phenotype by other means.[25]

Host Immune Response Factors

It is likely that HIV-specific CTLs play a major role in the maintenance of low viral load and the state of nonprogression. In the majority of long-term nonprogressors, neither *CCR5* mutations nor infection with attenuated viruses has been found. In addition, strong MHC class I associations and the likely role of CTLs in reducing levels of plasma viremia during primary HIV infection, as well as the association of progression to AIDS with late viral escape from immunodominant CTL responses, suggest the importance of HIV-specific CTL in restriction of HIV replication.[59,124] Although data from experimental animals and humans strongly suggest that HIV-specific CD8+ T cells likely play an important role in restricting virus replication in long-term nonprogressors, clear and consistent in vitro correlates or mechanisms of such an effect have not been demonstrated. A number of recent studies using more quantitative techniques that examine the response to a broad array of HIV gene products have not found higher frequencies of HIV-specific CD8+ T cells in nonprogressors compared with progressors.[67,73,76-78,80,125] Whether the ability of CD8+ T-cell responses of some long-term nonprogressors to restrict viral replication is due to viral factors (e.g., a lack of escape mutations) or other qualitative aspects of the host response (see "Cytotoxic T Lymphocytes") remains unclear.

The relationship between humoral immune responses to HIV and disease progression remains uncertain.[126] Nonprogressive HIV infection has been associated with maintenance of HIV-specific neutralizing antibodies.[37,38,112,127] Subsequent studies demonstrated that the presence of neutralizing antibodies to primary HIV isolates and to autologous virus was associated with nonprogression.[39,128] Furthermore, viral escape from neutralizing antibody responses is associated with emergence of highly pathogenic HIV and with disease progression.[128,129] Although HIV-infected long-term nonprogressors tend to maintain antibody responses that can neutralize a broad panel of primary isolates and autologous virus isolates, they are a heterogeneous group with regard to these neutralizing antibody responses.[37,39] As is the case with other potential correlates of immunity, it is unclear whether the maintenance of neutralizing antibodies in nonprogressors is simply a marker for a relatively intact immune system or whether these antibodies actually play an active role in determining the state of nonprogression.

TABLE 116-2 Possible Mechanisms of Long-Term Nonprogression with Human Immunodeficiency Virus (HIV) Infection

Host genetic factors
　Slow progressor HLA profile
　Heterozygosity for 32-bp deletion in chemokine receptor CCR5
　Mannose binding lectin alleles
　Tumor necrosis factor c2 microsatellite alleles
　Gc vitamin D–binding factor alleles
Host immune response factors
　Effective CTL responses
　Secretion of CD8 antiviral factor
　Secretion of chemokines that block HIV entry co-receptors CCR5
　　(e.g., MIP-1α, MIP-1β, and RANTES) and CXCR4 (e.g., SDF-1)
　Secretion of interleukin-16
　Effective humoral immune response
　Maintenance of functional lymphoid tissue architecture
Virologic factors
　Infection with attenuated strains of HIV

MIP, macrophage inflammatory protein; RANTES, regulated on activation, normal T-cell expressed and secreted; SDF, stromal cell–derived factor.

Virologic Factors

Infection with attenuated strains of HIV may account for nonprogression in a small subset of individuals. The most extensively characterized association of attenuated viral strains and nonprogression is that of an Australian cohort of nonprogressors who were infected by transfusion from a single nonprogressor donor.[130,131] Viruses from these individuals contained deletions in the *nef* gene and in the U3 region of the long terminal repeat (LTR).[131] Another isolated nonprogressor with viruses containing deletions within the *nef* gene was reported by Kirchhoff and co-workers.[132] Although these cases argue strongly that nonprogression may be due to infection with viral strains containing attenuated *nef* genes, this scenario appears to be a relatively uncommon cause of nonprogression.[133,134] Other anecdotal reports implicate defective *env, gag, rev, vif, vpr, vpu,* and *tat* genes in the pathogenesis of nonprogression,[135-139] although such instances appear to be the exception rather than the rule.[140,141]

RESERVOIRS OF HUMAN IMMUNODEFICIENCY VIRUS INFECTION

There is unequivocal evidence from several lines of investigation that there is ongoing HIV replication despite effective ART. The most powerful demonstration of the inability of ART to eradicate HIV infection comes from in vivo studies of individuals who began ART during the chronic stage of HIV infection, achieved, and maintained suppression of plasma HIV RNA for up to 2 years and subsequently interrupted therapy. Interruption of ART resulted in a rapid rebound of plasma viremia in 95% of individuals.[104] It has been demonstrated that an evolution in HIV envelope and protease genes occurs in individuals who have been effectively treated with ART, indicating persistent HIV replication despite adequate therapy.[142] Finally, it has been demonstrated using ultrasensitive assays with a limit of detection of less than 3 copies/mL that many individuals with "undetectable" (<50 copies/mL) plasma HIV by standard assays have persistent low-level plasma viremia.[143] Thus, there are reservoirs of ongoing HIV replication that persist in the presence of effective ART. Important HIV reservoir sites include lymphoid tissue and resting CD4+ T cells that circulate in the blood. Putative reservoir sites include the reproductive and gastrointestinal tracts, the reticuloendothelial system, bone marrow, peripheral blood dendritic cells and monocytes, and microglial cells of the central nervous system.[144-149] Genetic variability has been demonstrated in HIV isolated simultaneously from the plasma and several reservoir sites, including the reproductive tract and the central nervous system, indicating that there may be compartmentalization of HIV in different sites.[147,149,150] Such compartmentalization may provide a sanctuary for HIV that may be relatively impenetrable by antiretroviral drugs; however, it is unclear if these sanctuary sites contribute significantly to ongoing HIV replication in the presence of ART.

Resting CD4+ T Cells

HIV may enter resting CD4+ T cells, at which point a limited degree of reverse transcription of the HIV genome may occur in these cells.[151,152] This period of preintegration latency may last hours to days; in the absence of an activation signal, unintegrated proviral DNA loses its capacity to initiate a productive infection. If these cells become activated, however, reverse transcription proceeds to completion, followed by nuclear translocation and integration of proviral DNA into cellular DNA.[151,152] Among the total pool of resting CD4+ T cells that harbor viral DNA in infected individuals who are untreated or treated with a less-than-optimal regimen of one or two antiretroviral drugs, only a fraction carry replication-competent HIV.[153] On activation in vitro, these cells can produce high levels of infectious HIV. Shortly after it was established that such a population of latently infected cells exists and may serve as a long-term viral reservoir in infected individuals, this initial observation was extended to patients who were receiving ART. In this regard, it has been clearly demonstrated that the pool of resting CD4+ T cells that carry replication-competent HIV persisted in essentially all infected individuals who were receiving ART

and in whom plasma viremia was suppressed below levels of detectability.[154-156] In addition, this HIV reservoir is established during the earliest stages of HIV infection. The initiation of ART as early as 10 days following infection with HIV does not prevent the establishment of the resting CD4+ T-cell reservoir of HIV.

Cytokines that are naturally produced in the lymphoid tissue microenvironment, particularly IL-2, IL-6, and tumor necrosis factor (TNF)-α, are potent inducers of viral replication in HIV-infected resting CD4+ T cells. In addition, the lymphoid tissue microenvironment may provide subtle activation signals that promote HIV replication in resting CD4+ T cells in the absence of inducing the cells to express classic markers of activation.[157] These data suggest that resting CD4+ T cells that carry replication-competent HIV may contribute in a significant way to ongoing HIV replication in the presence of ART in vivo. In this regard, in certain HIV-infected individuals who had maintained suppression of plasma viremia below the limits of detection while receiving ART and who subsequently interrupted therapy, the rebound plasma HIV RNA was genetically similar to the HIV that was isolated from the resting CD4+ T-cell reservoir prior to treatment interruption. Therefore, the pool of HIV-infected resting CD4+ T cells is a clinically relevant reservoir of HIV.

Lymphoid Tissue

Lymphoid tissue is a major site of HIV replication and plays a role in the progression of disease throughout all stages of infection. In the absence of ART, the early chronic stage of HIV disease is characterized by a dichotomy in viral load between peripheral blood and lymphoid tissue. In this regard, the frequency of infected cells in lymphoid tissue exceeds that in peripheral blood by 5- to 10-fold; differences in levels of viral replication are generally 10- to 100-fold.[158] Embretson and co-workers used in situ polymerase chain reaction to demonstrate that up to 25% of CD4+ T-lymphocytes present in lymph node germinal centers harbor HIV DNA, further emphasizing the role of lymphoid tissue as a critical reservoir for HIV in vivo.[159]

The significant role of lymphoid tissue in ongoing HIV replication during all stages of disease in the absence of ART suggests that this compartment may play a significant role in ongoing HIV replication in the presence of ART. There is a rapid decrease in lymph node viral burden following the initiation of ART; within 24 weeks, the majority of HIV RNA detected by in situ hybridization is eliminated, and it is uncommon to detect HIV RNA in the germinal centers.[160] There is a commensurate decrease in HIV RNA as quantified by reverse transcription–polymerase chain reaction per gram of tissue or in isolated lymph node mononuclear cells. However, it is almost universally possible to detect "burst" cells producing HIV RNA in the subcortical regions of lymph nodes despite prolonged ART; the precise identity of these cells remains unknown.[160] In addition, low-level HIV RNA is detected through a variety of quantification techniques despite prolonged periods of plasma HIV RNA levels less than 50 copies/mL.[160] Lymphoid tissue other than lymph nodes may serve as important reservoirs of HIV infection. Gastrointestinal lymphoid tissue harbors HIV that is not completely cleared with ART. In addition, the variability in the genetic composition of HIV isolated from plasma and gut-associated lymphoid tissue in certain individuals suggests that the latter may serve as a sanctuary site for HIV.[149] However, the precise contribution of non–lymph node lymphoid tissue to persistent HIV replication in the presence of ART remains unknown.

IMMUNE DYSFUNCTION CAUSED BY HUMAN IMMUNODEFICIENCY VIRUS INFECTION

A wide array of immune system deficits are associated with HIV infection. Abnormalities in the function of all limbs of the immune system, including T- and B-lymphocytes, antigen-presenting cells, NK cells, and neutrophils, have been described. Immunodeficiency may become sufficiently profound in the late stages of disease that HIV-specific antibody and CTL responses diminish in the face of high levels of ongoing viral replication.

Lymphoid Tissue

The immunodeficiency induced by HIV can be best appreciated in the context of the microenvironment in which immune responses are generated. Advanced stages of HIV infection are marked by striking disruption of lymphoid tissue architecture.[158,161,162] Follicular involution, hypervascularity, and fibrosis are some of the histopathologic changes evident in lymph nodes from patients with advanced HIV disease. The loss of follicular dendritic cells, which results in follicular involution, has important implications with regard to the pathogenesis of HIV-related immunodeficiency. The ability to mount immune responses against new antigens and the ability to maintain memory responses are severely impaired in the absence of an intact follicular dendritic cell (FDC) network.[163] This loss of functional substrate for the generation and maintenance of immune responses results in loss of containment of HIV replication and enhanced susceptibility to opportunistic infections.

In the advanced stage of disease, there is almost total dissolution of lymphoid tissue architecture. Follicular involution, fibrosis, frank lymphocyte depletion, and fatty infiltration herald complete loss of functional lymphoid tissue, contributing to the state of immunodeficiency and the dramatically enhanced susceptibility to opportunistic infections.

Disruption of the lymphoid microenvironment during the course of HIV infection remains an enigmatic process with considerable implications for future therapeutic interventions. Productive infection of FDCs by HIV may occur, particularly in the late stages of HIV infection; however, the majority of data suggest that productive infection of FDCs is rare during the period of intermediate stage disease when dissolution of the FDC network begins.[164] Direct toxicity to cells by viral gene products may contribute to loss of FDC network integrity. *Tat* and/or gp120 has been shown to be capable of disrupting normal intracellular signaling[165] as well as inducing apoptosis,[166] although these effects have been studied largely in CD4+ T cells and little is known regarding the normal physiology of FDCs and their interactions with HIV proteins. *Tat, nef,* and *vpu* have been found to downregulate MHC class I expression,[70,164] which may interfere with normal cell–cell interactions in the lymphoid microenvironment. Depletion of CD4+ T cells during the course of HIV disease could also lead to withdrawal of a trophic factor necessary for FDC survival. An "innocent bystander" phenomenon is also a possibility, wherein cells such as CD8+ T cells or macrophages infiltrating into hyperplastic lymph nodes elaborate substances such as TNF-α that may be toxic at high, sustained concentrations.

CD4+ T Cells

CD4+ T-cell dysfunction, both quantitative and qualitative, is the hallmark of HIV disease. The opportunistic infections observed with advancing disease are primarily due to defects in T-cell number and function that result directly or indirectly from HIV infection. Direct effects of HIV on CD4+ T-cell function include direct infection of these cells and resultant cytotoxicity with loss of absolute cell numbers. Indirect effects of HIV infection result in decreased CD4+ T-cell proliferation and differentiation, dysregulation and decreased production of IL-2 and other cytokines, decreased IL-2 receptor expression, and defective T-cell colony formation and other precursor defects (reviewed in Pantaleo and Fauci[167]). The loss of immune competence during the course of HIV disease progression can be gauged by the sequential loss of in vitro proliferative responses of peripheral blood lymphocytes to recall antigens, alloantigens, and finally, mitogens.[168]

T cells from HIV-infected individuals manifest a variety of phenotypic abnormalities. In addition to the decrease in IL-2 production and IL-2 receptor expression, the percentage of CD4+ T cells expressing CD28 (i.e., the major costimulatory receptor that is necessary for normal activation of T cells) is reduced during HIV infection in comparison to cells from uninfected individuals.[169] CD28−cells do not respond to activation signals, including anti-CD3 monoclonal antibodies or mitogens, and express markers of terminal activation, including HLA-DR, -CD38, and -CD45RO.[170]

A variety of mechanisms, both directly and indirectly related to HIV infection of CD4+ T cells, are probably responsible for the observed defects in T-cell colony formation, autologous mixed lymphocyte reactions, expression of IL-2 receptors, and IL-2 production. Interference with CD4 expression by HIV gp120,[171] Nef,[172] and Vpu[173] may impair the ability of an infected CD4+ T cell to interact with appropriate MHC class II molecules. Preferential infection by HIV of CD4+CD45RO+ memory cells, the increased susceptibility of these cells to the cytopathic effects of HIV infection, or both may in part explain the loss of memory responses to soluble antigens and the consequent increase in the risk of infection with opportunistic organisms.[174,175] Of note, the CD45RO+ cells appear to be the main source of HIV replication in vivo and produce much more HIV in vitro compared with CD45RA+ cells.[174,175]

An incisive view of the qualitative nature of the immunodeficiency that occurs during the course of HIV infection is provided by study of the CD4+ T-cell receptor Vβ repertoire. Disruptions in the Vβ repertoire are seen with increased frequency in CD4+ T cells from patients with advanced-stage HIV disease, particularly with CD4+ T-cell counts of less than 200 cells/mL[176,177]; these disruptions are caused by severe depletion of cells with various specificities, thus creating "holes" in the immunologic repertoire. Interestingly, increases in CD4+ T-cell counts associated with antiretroviral or IL-2 therapy do not result in restoration of the normal pattern of the disrupted Vβ repertoire.[176]

Mechanisms of CD4+ T-Cell Depletion

There is considerable controversy regarding the relative contribution of various mechanisms for the depletion of CD4+ T cells during the course of HIV infection. As with many other areas of HIV immunopathogenesis, evaluations of patients who initiate, and subsequently withdraw, effective ART have provided fundamental insights into the understanding of the potential contributions of increased destruction, decreased production, and redistribution as mechanisms for CD4+ T-cell depletion in HIV-infected individuals.

Increased Destruction

Direct Infection. The observations that CD4+ T cells are the principal targets of HIV infection in vivo[3-5] and that HIV infection of CD4+ T cells in vitro causes cytopathicity[178-181] led to a reasonable assumption that direct infection of CD4+ T cells in vivo results in their depletion. However, quantitative studies of the frequency of HIV-infected cells in vivo suggest that single cell killing by direct infection with HIV may not be the predominant mechanism of CD4+ T-cell depletion. In this regard, the proportion of HIV-infected peripheral blood CD4+ T cells in individuals in the early asymptomatic stage of HIV infection is typically in the range of 1 in 1000 to 1 in 100,000.[182,183] Although this frequency increases with disease progression, the proportion of HIV-infected peripheral blood CD4+ T cells rarely exceeds 1 in 100 even in patients with AIDS.[183-186] Viral burden and levels of virus expression are far greater in lymphoid tissues than in peripheral blood[158,159,182]; however, these levels, even in lymphoid tissue, do not appear to be sufficiently high to account for CD4+ T-cell depletion solely by direct mechanisms.

Apoptosis. Apoptosis is the morphologic description of a form of programmed cell death critical to physiologic homeostasis in virtually every organ system (reviewed in Thompson[187]). Apoptotic cell death is characterized by plasma membrane blebbing, nuclear condensation, DNA fragmentation, and release of cellular contents in the form of small, dense apoptotic bodies. Ingestion of apoptotic bodies by phagocytes completes the apoptotic death process without the inflammation associated with spillage of cellular contents that occurs in nonphysiologic necrotic cell death. A wide array of physiologic stimuli serve as positive and negative regulators of apoptosis. Important inhibitors of apoptosis include growth factors, extracellular matrix, and CD40 ligand, whereas important activators of apoptosis include CD95 (Fas) ligand, TNF, transforming growth factor-β (TGF-β), neurotransmitters, and withdrawal of growth factor. The discoveries that the *bcl*-2 gene plays an important pathogenic role in lymphomagenesis through its ability to prevent cells from undergoing apoptosis[188,189] and that the *p53* gene is necessary for initiation of apoptosis[190,191] established the paradigm that diseases associated with increased cell survival or increased cell death may result from dysregulation of the normal pathways of apoptosis.

Several investigators suggested that aberrant intracellular signals transduced by HIV might prime CD4+ T cells for apoptosis and thereby result in depletion of these cells during the course of HIV infection.[192] Acute infection of T cells with HIV in vitro was shown to induce apoptosis,[193] and T cells from HIV-infected patients were demonstrated to undergo enhanced rates of apoptosis in vitro when compared with normal T cells, particularly after activation.[194] Cross-linking of CD4 followed by ligation of the T-cell receptor is sufficient to induce apoptosis, which suggests that uninfected CD4+ T cells could be depleted inappropriately upon encountering antigen if CD4 had been cross-linked by gp120. The viral Tat protein can also lead to apoptotic cell death, possibly by upregulating CD95 ligand, by enhancing activation of cyclin-dependent kinases, or both.[195]

It remains uncertain whether HIV-induced apoptosis plays an important role in vivo in CD4+ T-cell depletion. The frequency of apoptotic CD4+ and CD8+ T cells, as well as B cells, is significantly higher in lymphoid tissue from HIV-infected individuals than uninfected controls.[196] The intensity of apoptosis is related to the degree of immune activation and is observed predominantly in uninfected "bystander" cells.[196,197] Although some data support a positive correlation between the stage of HIV disease and susceptibility of peripheral blood T cells to apoptosis,[198] another study found no such correlation[199]; in this regard, it has been reported that the intensity of apoptosis in lymphoid tissue was independent of the peripheral CD4+ T-cell count and level of plasma viremia.[196] Perhaps the most compelling evidence that apoptosis may play a role in HIV pathogenesis is that an increased frequency of apoptosis in CD4+ T cells is seen in HIV-infected humans and in primates infected with pathogenic strains of SIV, but not in primates infected with nonpathogenic strains.[200]

Lymphocyte Turnover. Mathematical models of lymphocyte turnover derived through analysis of immediate changes in circulating CD4+ T-cell counts in individuals following the initiation of HAART led to estimates that approximately 2×10^9 CD4+ T cells are destroyed, and replenished, each day.[201] However, studies using a variety of techniques to measure lymphocyte proliferation, including Ki-67, BrdU, and 2H-glucose, to evaluate the effects of HIV on T-cell turnover have yielded mixed results. Several investigators have demonstrated that there is an increase in CD4+ T-cell proliferation in both HIV and SIV infections (reviewed in Lempicki and associates[202]). In certain studies, the enhanced T-cell proliferation that was observed during active disease was significantly decreased following the initiation of ART, and proliferation increased again in parallel with plasma viremia following the cessation of treatment in these individuals (reviewed in Lempicki and associates[202]). These data suggest that HIV infection results in a high turnover of CD4+ T cells, perhaps as a consequence of destruction of CD4+ T cells through certain of the mechanisms reviewed earlier. However, several investigators have had contrary results and have suggested that HIV replication blocks the ability of new CD4+ T cells to regenerate (reviewed in McCune and co-workers[203]).

Autoimmune Phenomena. Autoimmune phenomena may contribute to CD4+ T-cell depletion in HIV-infected individuals. Autoimmunity may occur as a result of molecular mimicry by viral components, and by abnormal release of nuclear antigens from cells dying by apoptosis. Highly homologous regions exist in the carboxyl terminus of the HIV-1 envelope glycoprotein and the amino terminal domains of different *HLA-DR* and *-DQ* alleles.[204] Monoclonal antibodies generated using the HIV envelope peptide as immunogen can recognize native gp160 and MHC class II molecules.[205] Sera from one-third of HIV-infected individuals were found to react with the gp41 and MHC class II determinants; these sera were capable of inhibiting normal antigen-specific proliferative responses and also eliminated class II–bearing cells by antibody-dependent cellular cy-

totoxicity (ADCC).[205] Similar instances of molecular mimicry between HIV-1 envelope constituents and host proteins that may result in pathogenic autoimmune responses include the collagen-like region of complement component C1q-A[165]; MHC class I heavy chains[206]; *HLA-DR4* and *-DR2* alleles; variable regions of the T-cell receptor alpha-, beta-, and gamma-chains; Fas; functional domains of IgG and IgA; denatured collagen[207]; and a number of nuclear antigens.[208,209]

Bystander Phenomena. Because the frequency of HIV-infected CD4+ T cells is relatively low, investigators have evaluated the destruction of HIV-uninfected cells as a contributory mechanism to the loss of CD4+ T cells during the course of infection. Immune responses that target HIV determinants on infected cells may also contribute to elimination of uninfected cells bearing HIV proteins (e.g., gp120) on their surface. Targeting of such "innocent bystander" cells by antibody and cellular immune responses has been described.[210] In addition, fusion between infected and uninfected cells, resulting in multinucleated giant cells or syncytia, has long been observed in vitro. Other molecules implicated in syncytium formation include LFA-1,[211] CD7,[212] and HLA class I molecules.[213] Syncytia have been observed only rarely in tissues obtained from HIV-infected individuals[31,162]; thus, it is unlikely that syncytium formation is a major pathogenic mechanism of CD4+ T-cell depletion in vivo.

Decreased Production

Decreased production of CD4+ T cells could occur by disruption of the thymic microenvironment[214] and by HIV-induced depletion of thymocytes. Thymic epithelial cells normally secrete IL-6, which can in turn increase HIV replication in infected cells.[215] Subpopulations of thymic CD3−CD4−CD8− cells are susceptible to infection with HIV in vitro,[215] and thymic CD3−CD4+CD8− progenitor cells from HIV-infected patients are infected in vivo. Finally, uninfected thymocytes from HIV-infected individuals are primed for apoptotic death, suggesting that indirect mechanisms of defective thymopoiesis are operative as well. There are in vivo correlates of these deleterious effects of HIV on the thymus. Circulating CD4+ and CD8+ naïve (CD45RA+CD62L+) T cells decrease as a result of HIV infection. In addition, Douek and colleagues[216] demonstrated that recent thymic emigrants in HIV-infected individuals are significantly decreased as a consequence of HIV infection. The percent of circulating and lymph node naïve CD4+ T cells carrying signal-joint TCR excision circle (TREC) gene products, a marker of recent thymic emigration, was significantly reduced in HIV infection compared with age-matched controls. Initiation of effective ART resulted in a significant increase in signal-joint TRECs in CD4+CD45RO−CD27+ naïve T cells in the periphery; the latter finding suggested that the thymus remained functional in these individuals who were past adolescence and may contribute to immune reconstitution. Subsequently, several investigators have demonstrated that, contrary to previously held beliefs, the thymus remains capable of producing substantial quantities of immune-competent cells for decades in many individuals.[217] Zhang and colleagues[218] found similar decreases in TRECs in certain HIV-infected individuals. However, although there was an increase in TRECs in these individuals following the initiation of ART, the numerical increase was not sufficient to account for the rise in levels of naïve CD4+ T cells.

Further upstream from thymic causes of the lack of replenishment of CD4+ T cells, disruption of normal hematopoiesis may contribute to the depletion of CD4+ T cells during HIV infection. A large body of evidence suggests that viral proteins and HIV-induced cytokines can impair the survival and clonogenic potential of CD34+ progenitor cells. CD34+ cells cultured in the presence of HIV exhibit defective clonogenic potential; uninfected CD34+ cells purified from bone marrow of HIV-infected patients also manifest defective clonogenic potential, and are committed to apoptotic death in culture. The HIV envelope gp120 and Tat proteins have been implicated in these effects on CD34+ progenitor cells,[219] possibly due to gp120- and Tat-mediated upregulation of TGF-β or gp120-mediated upregulation of TNF-α.

It has been demonstrated that a subset of CD34+ progenitor cells express CD4 and these cells can be infected with HIV-1 in vitro.[220]

Although several of studies have failed to detect HIV-infected CD34⁺ progenitor cells in most HIV-infected individuals,[221] a large study showed that a substantial minority of HIV-infected patients with severe CD4⁺ T-cell depletion have a reservoir of HIV-infected CD34⁺ progenitor cells.[222] Recent reports demonstrating expression of CXCR4 on CD34⁺ progenitor cells[223] suggest that the CD4⁺ subset of CD34⁺ cells may be susceptible to infection with CXCR4-utilizing strains of HIV (i.e., strains that predominate in the later stages of HIV disease), further substantiating the earlier findings.[222] Nonetheless, the role of direct infection of CD34⁺ progenitor cells in HIV pathogenesis remains controversial.

Redistribution

Although the role of redistribution in the loss of CD4⁺ T cells is unclear, data from both HIV and SIV infections indicate that there is significant trafficking of CD4⁺ T cells from the peripheral blood to lymphoid tissue in acute and chronic infection (reviewed in McCune[203]). The trafficking of lymphocytes is mediated, in part, through the expression of homing receptors, such as CD62L, on CD4⁺ T cells. As circulating T cells expressing homing markers cross-link their ligands on endothelial venule cells, the T cells extravasate from the peripheral blood to the lymph nodes. Because CD62L expression on CD4⁺ T cells is upregulated following HIV infection, it is possible that redistribution contributes to the depletion of circulating CD4⁺ T cells observed during the course of HIV disease. In support of this view, several investigators have suggested that redistribution of CD4⁺ T cells back from lymphoid tissue to the peripheral blood contributes significantly to the increase in CD4⁺ T cells following the initiation of HAART (reviewed in McCune[203]). However, other investigators have developed models in which redistribution is not an important component of the increase in CD4⁺ T cells observed in these patients.[224] In these latter scenarios, CD4⁺ T cells that have trafficked to lymphoid tissues are destroyed by apoptosis or other mechanisms and therefore they are not available for redistribution following the initiation of HAART.

CD8⁺ T Cells

Dysregulation of CD8⁺ T-cell numbers and function is evident throughout the course of HIV disease. After acute primary infection, CD8⁺ T-cell counts usually rebound to supranormal levels and may remain elevated for prolonged periods. Increases in CD8⁺ T cells during all but the late stages of disease may in part reflect the expansion of HIV-specific CD8⁺ CTLs. As with CD4⁺ T cells, as a result of HIV infection there is a significant decrease in naïve CD8⁺ T cells (CD45RA⁺CD62L⁺) carrying signal TRECs compared with age-matched controls.[216]

During HIV disease progression, CD8⁺ T cells assume an abnormal phenotype characterized by the expression of certain activation markers and the absence of expression of the CD25 molecule (IL-2 receptor). Alterations in the phenotype of CD8⁺ T cells in HIV-infected individuals may have prognostic significance. In particular, individuals whose CD8⁺ T cells express HLA-DR but not -CD38 after seroconversion experience a stabilization of their CD4⁺ T-cell counts and a less fulminant disease course, whereas individuals whose CD8⁺ T cells express both HLA-DR and -CD38 experience a more aggressive course with rapid CD4⁺ T-cell depletion and a poorer prognosis.[225,226] CD8⁺ T cells lacking CD28 expression are also increased in HIV disease,[227] possibly reflecting expansion of the CD8⁺CD28⁻CD57⁺ T-cell subset containing in vivo activated CTLs.[228] The loss of CTL activity with disease progression is not restricted to HIV-specific CTLs: a loss of cytotoxic activity to other common antigens including Epstein-Barr virus (EBV) and *Mycobacterium tuberculosis* has also been observed.[229,230]

In addition to CTL activity, other CD8⁺ T-cell functions are impaired during HIV disease progression, including loss of noncytolytic non–MHC restricted CD8⁺ T-cell–derived HIV suppression. Analyses of factors released by CD8⁺ T cells demonstrate that in certain in vitro systems the CD8⁺ T cell–associated suppressor activity termed CAF decreases with disease progression.[231] In contrast, levels of MIP-1α, MIP-1β, and RANTES, factors produced by CD8⁺ T cells that also suppress HIV replication, are not reduced with progression of HIV disease.[232]

B-Lymphocytes

Dysregulation of B-cell activation and the decreased ability of these cells to respond to antigen are likely responsible in part for the increase in certain bacterial infections seen in advanced HIV disease in adults, as well as for the morbidity and mortality associated with bacterial infections in HIV-infected children who cannot mount an adequate humoral response to common bacterial pathogens. The number of circulating B cells may be decreased in primary HIV infection; however, this is usually a transient phenomenon and likely reflects, at least in part, a redistribution of cells into lymphoid tissues. Soon after the resolution of acute HIV infection, hypergammaglobulinemia and B-lymphocyte hyperactivation are noted. The increase in immunoglobulins occurs for all classes of antibody. A large component of the immunoglobulin specificity, at least in early-stage disease, is directed against HIV antigens. It has been suggested that a majority of activated B cells produce antibodies directed against HIV during this stage of infection (reviewed in Amadori and Chieco-Bianchi[233]). B cells isolated from patients with high levels of HIV plasma viremia have been shown to be defective in their proliferative responses to various stimuli.[234] Substantial plasma viremia was also associated with the appearance of a subpopulation of B cells that expressed reduced levels of CD21. Upon fractionation into CD21ʰⁱᵍʰ- and CD21ˡᵒʷ-expressing B cells, the CD21ˡᵒʷ fraction showed dramatically reduced proliferation in response to B-cell stimuli and enhanced secretion of immunoglobulins when compared with the CD21ʰⁱᵍʰ fraction. Electron microscopic analysis of each fraction revealed cells with plasmacytoid features in the CD21ˡᵒʷ B-cell population but not in the CD21ʰⁱᵍʰ population. These results indicate that HIV viremia induces the appearance of a subset of B cells whose function is impaired and that may be responsible for the hypergammaglobulinemia associated with HIV disease. The phenotypic and functional aberrations were reversed upon reduction of HIV plasma viremia by ART, suggesting that control of viremia may contribute to the restoration of the humoral arm of the immune system.

B cells from HIV-infected individuals secrete increased amounts of TNF-α and IL-6, cytokines known to enhance HIV replication[235-237] and express surface-bound TNF-α that can induce the production of HIV from infected CD4⁺ T cells. The secretion of proinflammatory cytokines and the expression of surface-bound TNF-α by B cells in the lymphoid microenvironment may contribute to T-cell activation and HIV replication in these tissues. HIV gp120 has been observed to directly bind to an immunoglobulin variable chain (VH3) and activate these B cells in much the same manner as a superantigen.[238,239] This antigen-independent polyclonal activation may lead in part to the hypergammaglobulinemia and B-lymphocyte hyperactivation of HIV infection. Other portions of HIV, including gp41, directly activate B cells in a non–superantigen-mediated manner.[240] Correlates of B-cell dysfunction observed in HIV-infected individuals include an increase in spontaneous EBV transformation in vitro and may contribute to the observed increased frequency of EBV-induced lymphomas.[241-243]

Several studies have found an overall increase in IgE levels among HIV-infected individuals, likely reflecting a spectrum of IgE regulatory dysfunction. The mechanisms of this increase are unclear but may include B-cell hyperactivation and cytokine dysregulation. Levels of IgE continue to increase with disease progression. An increase in aeroallergen-specific IgE has not been associated with the increase in total IgE; in one study, allergen-specific IgE decreased with HIV disease progression in all but the subgroup with the highest total IgE level.[244] An overall increase in IgE levels was noted in pediatric HIV infection without an increase in allergen-specific IgE, suggesting polyclonal activation. In HIV-infected children, an expanded minor population of B-lymphocytes has been identified that does not express CD23 (IgE receptor) and CD62L (L-selectin) and may be involved in the pathogenesis of IgE dysregulation.[245]

Natural Killer Cells

The presumed role of NK cells is to provide immunosurveillance against virus-infected cells, certain tumor cells, and allogeneic cells. Abnormalities of NK cells are observed throughout the course of HIV disease and these abnormalities increase with disease progression. Most studies report that NK cells are normal in numbers and phenotype in HIV-infected individuals; however, decreases in numbers of the CD16[+]/CD56[+] subpopulation of NK cells with an associated increase in activation markers have been reported.[246] NK cells from HIV-infected individuals are defective in their ability to kill typical NK target cells as well as gp160-expressing cells. In addition, it has recently been demonstrated that HIV viremia is inversely correlated with the ability of NK cells and NK-derived cell supernatants to suppress virus replication.[247] The abnormality in NK cell lysis is thought to occur after binding of the NK cell to its target.[248] NK cells from HIV-infected individuals are able to mediate ADCC.[249] A possible mechanism for defective NK cell activity includes a lack of cytokines necessary for optimal function. Addition of IL-2, IL-12, or IFN-α to cultures enhances the defective in vitro NK cell function of HIV-infected individuals.[250]

NK cells are an important source of HIV inhibitory CC chemokines in HIV-infected individuals.[251] NK cells isolated from HIV-infected individuals produce high constitutive levels of MIP-1α, MIP-1β, and RANTES; high levels of chemokine production are also seen when these cells are stimulated by IL-2, IL-15, or CD16 cross-linking or during lytic killing.[251] Thus, NK cells, like CD8[+] T cells, may inhibit HIV replication by cell-mediated killing, as well as by secretion of soluble HIV inhibitory factors.

Neutrophils

Dysregulation of neutrophil function occurs at all stages of HIV infection. Neutrophils isolated from asymptomatic HIV-infected individuals have an increase in nitroblue tetrazolium reduction, which suggests a state of increased cellular activation.[252] Activation of neutrophils from healthy, uninfected individuals by plasma from HIV-infected individuals indicates the presence of a plasma neutrophil activating factor. In addition, plasma from the same individuals was found to be low in N-acetylcysteine, indicating that depletion of antioxidants may occur as a result of increased oxygen radical production.[253] The oxidative capacity of neutrophils after priming with granulocyte-macrophage colony-stimulating factor is also increased in HIV-infected individuals.[254] Further evidence of neutrophil hyperactivation in HIV infection includes increased expression of adhesion molecules, decreased expression of CD62L, and increased actin polymerization and H_2O_2 production.[252] The opsonizing activity of neutrophils is significantly impaired in HIV infection, and the degree of impairment correlates with disease progression.[255] Neutrophils from AIDS patients undergo apoptosis at an increased rate compared with those from normal controls.[256] Neutrophils from HIV-infected individuals also produce more TNF-α and IL-6 in response to lipopolysaccharide or Candida antigen than do neutrophils from normal donors.[257]

Dysfunction of neutrophils in HIV-infected individuals has several clinical implications. HIV infection, especially in women, is characterized by an increase in the incidence and severity of Candida infections. In a study comparing the ability of neutrophils from HIV-infected patients and normal controls to phagocytize and kill Candida albicans, neutrophils from AIDS patients showed an increased ability to phagocytose the organism, a similar ability to generate reactive oxygen, but a decreased ability to kill Candida, which suggests a defect in nonoxidative killing.[258] A potential mechanism for the decreased ability of neutrophils to kill Candida organisms has been suggested by the finding that IL-10, shown in some studies to be increased in HIV disease, inhibits neutrophil killing of Candida.[259]

Monocyte-Macrophages

Cells of the monocyte-macrophage lineage play key roles in the immunopathogenesis of HIV disease. These cells serve as reservoirs of viral infection and are responsible for a variety of tissue-specific pathologic processes. Dysfunction of these cells contributes to CD4[+] T-cell dysfunction and to impaired host defense against intracellular pathogens.[260]

Monocytic cells express CD4 and numerous HIV co-receptors on their surface, including CCR5, CXCR4, and CCR3,[261,262] and serve as targets of HIV infection. Unlike infection of CD4[+] T cells, HIV is relatively noncytopathic for cells of the monocyte-macrophage lineage, and HIV can replicate extensively in these cells.[144] Chronically infected macrophages may be long lived, and current antiretroviral agents are not capable of targeting chronically infected cells; these cells therefore represent a formidable challenge to eradication of HIV.[263] Circulating monocytes are rarely found to be infected in vivo and are difficult to infect in vitro[144,263,264]; however, infection can readily be demonstrated in tissue macrophages, including resident microglial cells in the brain, pulmonary alveolar macrophages, and mature macrophages derived from blood monocytes in vitro.[146,265-267] Infection of monocytic precursors in bone marrow may be directly or indirectly responsible for certain of the hematologic abnormalities observed in HIV-infected individuals. Lymphoid tissue macrophages can be prolific producers of HIV in the setting of opportunistic infections, during which the cytokine milieu in the tissue favors a highly productive state of HIV infection.[268]

Cells of the monocyte-macrophage lineage are central to the pathogenesis of HIV-induced central nervous system disease. HIV infection of brain microglial cells, derived from the monocytic lineage, may lead to encephalopathy and neuropathy,[269] astrocytosis,[270] and cerebral vasculitis.[271] Levels of monocyte chemotactic protein type 1 (MCP-1) are markedly elevated in the cerebrospinal fluid of AIDS patients with HIV or cytomegalovirus encephalitis.[272] A major source of these high levels of MCP-1 is likely HIV-infected macrophages.[272] MCP-1 in turn recruits and activates monocytes, which elaborate proinflammatory cytokines and thereby enhance HIV replication and induce neuropathologic disease.[273]

Infection of monocyte-macrophages with HIV or exposure of these cells to viral proteins, including envelope glycoproteins and Tat, leads to a number of functional abnormalities. Impaired accessory cell function[274] may result from decreased MHC class II expression, decreased IL-12 secretion, and increased IL-10 secretion[274,275]; this HIV-induced dysregulation of antigen presentation may in turn be a significant cause of hyporesponsiveness of CD4[+] T cells.[276] Defects in the ADCC function of monocyte-macrophages, possibly related to low levels of expression of Fc and complement receptors, have also been observed in HIV infection.[277,278] Finally, HIV-associated abnormalities in antigen uptake, oxidative burst, and chemotaxis have been described in monocyte-macrophages.[275,279,280] As a consequence of these HIV-induced functional abnormalities, monocyte-macrophages exhibit poor intracellular killing of Candida species yeast forms,[281] Toxoplasma gondii,[282] and Histoplasma capsulatum.[283]

Dendritic Cells

DCs are among the first cells to encounter HIV after mucosal exposure and are probably responsible for transporting the virus to lymphoid organs, thus facilitating infection of CD4[+] T cells and viral dissemination (see "Dissemination of Human Immunodeficiency Virus Infection"). DCs express several different chemokine receptors that can be used as HIV co-receptors for entry.[284,285] Studies of DCs from HIV-infected individuals have yielded conflicting results; some authors have found high levels of infection in DCs isolated ex vivo from peripheral blood,[286] whereas others have not. A number of studies have demonstrated that productive infection of tissue DCs with HIV is rare. It is generally agreed that Langerhans cells (DCs resident in the epidermis) from the skin of HIV-infected individuals are occasionally infected; however, such infection occurs at a very low frequency, rarely approaching the level of infection found in peripheral blood CD4[+] T cells and often 10 to 100 times less (reviewed in Zambruno and co-workers[287]). DCs in lymphoid organs also appear to be infrequently infected with HIV in vivo (reviewed in Weissman and Fauci[288]).

It is controversial whether dysfunction of DCs occurs during HIV infection. A number of studies have suggested that HIV infection can impair the ability of DCs to activate T cells[286,289]; however, other studies have found no or minimal HIV-induced DC dysfunction.[290] Interpretation of these studies is complicated by the use of different DC purification techniques, the existence of multiple DC subsets, and differential culture conditions used by investigators. Therefore, further studies are needed to clarify the possible role of DC depletion and dysfunction in the pathogenesis of HIV disease.

ROLE OF CELLULAR ACTIVATION IN THE PATHOGENESIS OF HUMAN IMMUNODEFICIENCY VIRUS INFECTION

The end result of HIV infection is profound immunodeficiency; however, paradoxically, HIV infection is associated with hyperactivation of the immune system through most of the course of disease. HIV subverts the immune system by inducing immune activation and using this milieu toward its own replicative advantage.[192,291,292] The replicative cycle of HIV infection is most efficiently achieved in activated cells.[151,152]

Cytokines that induce T-cell activation can further contribute to viral replication by inducing a state of productive infection in latently infected resting T cells.[293] Several lines of evidence suggest that HIV replication in vivo is dependent on antigen-driven activation of CD4+ T cells. HIV-infected individuals with intercurrent infections experience transient increases in plasma viremia that correlate with the degree of immune activation that was induced; similar observations have been made in SIV-infected macaques and in HIV-infected individuals who received immunizations against various pathogens.[294-297] The amount of viral replication observed after vaccination with influenza vaccine or tetanus toxoid or during active infection with *M. tuberculosis* correlated inversely with the stage of HIV disease.[295-297] Individuals with late-stage HIV disease had a moderate increase in viral replication, whereas individuals with early-stage disease had a much greater increase in plasma viremia over baseline, which suggests a correlation between the ability of the immune system to respond to antigen and the magnitude of viral induction.[295,296] Furthermore, when PBMCs from tetanus toxoid–immunized, HIV-infected individuals were stimulated in vitro with tetanus antigen or when PBMCs from purified protein derivative–positive, HIV-infected individuals were stimulated in vitro with purified protein derivative or live *M. tuberculosis,* subjects with early-stage disease manifested a much stronger proliferative response to the respective antigens and had a larger increase in viral replication in vitro than did individuals with advanced-stage disease.[295-298] These studies suggest that the level of viral replication correlates with the level of immune system activation in response to an antigen.

Analysis of viral quasi-species and immune responses within lymphoid tissue from HIV-infected individuals suggests that HIV replication in vivo may not be driven by sustained high levels of immune activation. Within individual splenic white pulps a restricted number of individual antigen-specific immune responses occurred, and each of the immune responses contained a single or limited number of HIV quasispecies.[54] These data support the theory that within the context of individual antigen-specific immune responses, a single quasi-species of HIV that was present at the initiation of the reaction spread among the newly activated T cells. Thus, it is likely that continuous daily production of HIV occurs in newly activated CD4+ T cells that are being driven by antigen-specific activation.[54,299]

There are numerous potential harmful effects of chronic immune activation. Although activation of the immune system in response to antigenic stimuli is critical for normal immune function, persistent exposure of the immune system to a particular antigen over an extended period of time may lead to a decreased ability to maintain an adequate immune response to the antigen in question. In addition, an aberrantly activated immune system may compromise the functional capability to respond to a broad spectrum of antigens. In terms of virologic effects, although quiescent CD4+ T cells can be infected with HIV, reverse transcription, integration, and virus spread are much more efficient in activated cells.[151,152] In addition, it has been demonstrated that cellular activation induces expression of virus in latently infected CD4+ T cells.[153] These observations highlight the extraordinary capacity of HIV to exploit immune activation for its own replicative advantage.

CYTOKINES AND HUMAN IMMUNODEFICIENCY VIRUS DISEASE: DYSREGULATION OF CYTOKINE PRODUCTION

Chronic immune activation induced by HIV infection and associated opportunistic infections results in dysregulation of the host cytokine network. Many of the observed alterations in cytokine production contribute to HIV pathogenesis by further stimulating viral replication, suppressing the ability of the immune system to mount an efficient antiviral response, and inducing cytokine-mediated cytopathic effects.[291,292,300,301]

HIV infection is associated with increased expression of proinflammatory cytokines, especially during the later stages of disease.[291,301] High levels of TNF-α, IL-1β, and IL-6 are secreted by PBMCs and macrophages from HIV-infected subjects and are found at elevated levels in serum, cerebrospinal fluid, and tissues.[291,301] High levels of expression of these cytokines, as well as IFN-γ[302,303] and IL-10,[303] are particularly evident in lymphoid tissue, a major site of HIV replication throughout the course of disease.[158,159,304] Chronically activated CD8+ T cells[303,305] and macrophages[306] are thought to be major contributors to the elevated cytokine levels observed in HIV-infected subjects.

In addition to alterations in cytokine production caused by chronic immune activation, HIV-specific upregulation of certain cytokines may occur. In this regard, production of proinflammatory cytokines can be upregulated in PBMCs, lymph node mononuclear cells, and macrophages after acute HIV infection in vitro or after treatment with HIV proteins such as envelope gp120 and *tat*.[291,301]

Another major disruption in the cytokine pattern observed in HIV disease is a progressive loss of the ability to produce immunoregulatory cytokines such as IL-2 and IL-12[276,307,308] that are critical for effective cell-mediated immune responses because they stimulate proliferation and lytic activity of CTLs and NK cells. These cell-mediated immune effectors represent the primary mechanism whereby most viral infections are cleared. In addition, IL-12 is essential for stimulating the production of type 1 T-helper (Th1) cytokines, including IL-2 and IFN-γ that favor the development of cell-mediated immune responses (reviewed in Trinchieri[309]). Although it is clear that the Th1 limb of cellular immune responses is impaired during the course of HIV infection,[308,310-312] controversy surrounds the proposed dominance of Th2-like responses (i.e., secretion of IL-4, IL-5, and IL-10) during progression of HIV disease. Clerici and associates[308,310,313] showed that stimulated PBMCs from HIV-infected patients exhibit a preferential Th2 pattern of cytokine secretion with disease progression, and other investigators have found that CD4+ T cells from HIV-infected patients shift their cytokine secretion profile from a Th1-like to a Th2-like pattern during the course of disease progression.[314] However, still other investigators have found a skewing of the cytokine secretion pattern of T cells from HIV-infected patients toward a Th0 state (i.e., secretion of cytokines characteristic of both Th1 and Th2 patterns) rather than toward a Th2 state.[303,312] In either case, the finding that HIV replication is more efficient in Th0 than in Th1 clones[312,315] suggests that depletion of Th1-like cells and a predominance of Th0-like cells may provide more suitable targets for HIV infection and replication during the course of disease progression.[316]

EFFECT OF CYTOKINES ON HUMAN IMMUNODEFICIENCY VIRUS REPLICATION

The effects of cytokines on HIV replication were recognized in early studies wherein activated PBMCs,[317] macrophages,[318] and B cells[319] were shown to produce soluble factors that could dramatically upregulate HIV expression in acutely and chronically infected cells of the lymphocytic and macrophage lineages. These observations led to the identification of numerous cytokines that can directly influence HIV replication in infected cells.[301] Cytokines that have been reported to upregulate HIV replication in vitro include IL-1β, IL-2, IL-3, IL-6, IL-8, IL-12, IL-15, TNF-α, TNF-β, and macrophage and granulocyte-macrophage colony-stimulating factors (see reviews[301,320-323]). IFN-α, IFN-β, and IL-13 are primarily suppressors of HIV production, whereas other cytokines, such as IL-4,[324,325] IL-10,[326,327] IL-13,[324] IFN-γ, and TGF-β reduce or enhance viral replication, depending on the infected cell type and the culture conditions.[301] Many cytokines can influence HIV replication in both T cells and macrophages, such as the interferons and TNF-α, whereas others are cell lineage specific, such as macrophage colony-stimulating factor. The α- and β-chemokines also have profound effects on virus replication. Most of these effects are suppressive; however, under certain circumstances these cytokines can upregulate virus replication (reviewed in Cohen and associates[291]). The effects of a particular cytokine are often greatly influenced by the activity of other cytokines present in the microenvironment. In this regard, certain cytokines have been demonstrated to act in a synergistic[326,328,329] or in an antagonistic[330] manner with other cytokines in regulating HIV replication. Finally, cytokines are pleiotropic, and the overall effects of a particular cytokine on HIV replication often reflect the balance of both HIV-inducing and HIV-inhibiting activities.

Proinflammatory cytokines, particularly TNF-α, are considered the most potent HIV-inducing cytokines, and their mechanism of action is relatively well understood. Both TNF-α and IL-1β activate the cellular nuclear transcription factor NFκB,[331,332] a strong inducer of HIV LTR-mediated transcription. IL-6 increases HIV expression primarily by a post-transcriptional mechanism; however, IL-6 can synergize with NFκB-inducing cytokines to enhance HIV transcription.[328] The role of endogenous proinflammatory cytokines in the regulation of HIV replication has been demonstrated in several cellular systems in vitro. The production of HIV by macrophages or PBMCs stimulated by physiologic inducers of proinflammatory cytokine production such as bacterial endotoxin or IL-2 can be partially or nearly completely abrogated by the addition of antiproinflammatory cytokines,[333,334] neutralizing antibodies to the cytokines, or receptor antagonists such as IL-1ra.[322] In cultures of HIV-infected macrophages, the viral suppressive activity of several cytokines such as IL-10 and TGF-β is largely attributable to their ability to inhibit the secretion or activity of HIV-inducing proinflammatory cytokines.[297,330,334] Thus, HIV production is sensitive to both the antiproinflammatory and the antiproliferative activity of such cytokines.[335]

Although the role of proinflammatory and antiproinflammatory cytokines in the regulation of HIV replication in vivo has not been demonstrated conclusively, several lines of evidence suggest that these cytokines may be involved in regulating viral production. Administration of pentoxifylline, an inhibitor of the secretion and activity of TNF, to HIV-infected individuals was found to reduce HIV viremia in concert with a reduction in plasma levels of TNF-α.[336] The

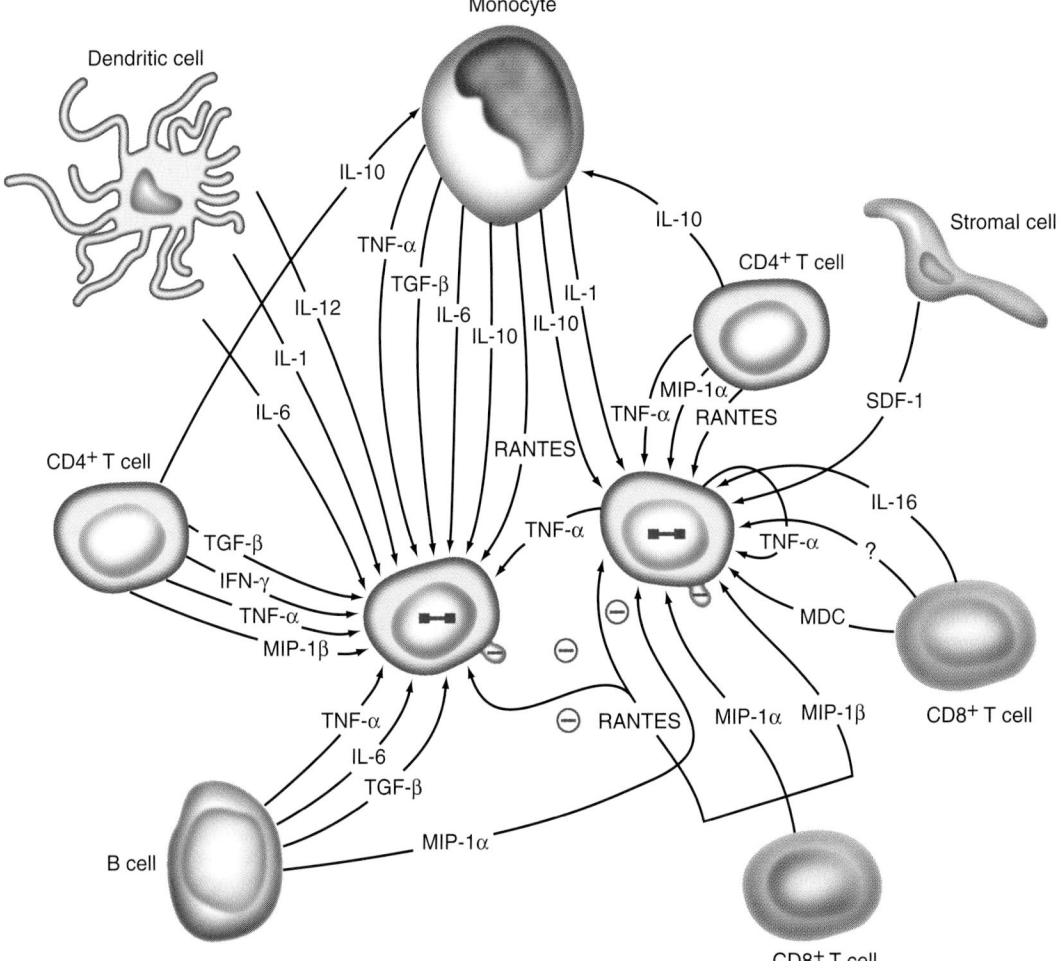

FIGURE 116-3. Cytokine networks that regulate HIV replication. The proinflammatory cytokines TNF-α, IL-1β, and IL-6 strongly enhance viral replication. TGF-β and IL-10 downregulate viral replication; in the case of IL-10 this occurs at least in part owing to downregulation of the proinflammatory cytokines. The CC chemokines inhibit CCR5-utilizing strains of HIV, SDF-1 inhibits CXCR4-utilizing strains, and MDC-1 inhibits both strains. *(Adapted with permission from Fauci AS. Host factors and the pathogenesis of HIV-induced disease. Nature. 1996;384:529-534.)*

kinetics of HIV suppression in vivo correlated with a dramatic reduction in the ability of cells from these subjects to secrete TNF-α and IL-1β in vitro. Furthermore, IL-10 has been found to inhibit acute HIV infection in severe combined immunodeficiency mice engrafted with human fetal thymus and liver.[337]

In addition to the use of immunosuppressive cytokines, which may depress HIV-inducing immune responses, cytokines that stimulate T cells or antigen-presenting cells have been administered to HIV-infected subjects for a number of years. The use of cytokine-based therapies aimed at immune reconstitution in HIV disease has expanded over the past several years, particularly with the development of potent antiretroviral therapies that limit the potential for cytokine-mediated increases in viral replication. In this regard, administration of IL-2 to asymptomatic HIV-infected subjects receiving concomitant ART results in significant and sustained increases in CD4+ T-cell numbers with no concomitant sustained increases in viremia.[338] Similar immune reconstitution therapies are being developed for IL-12, IL-13, and IL-15.[323,339-342] IL-15 is produced by antigen-presenting cells, including monocyte-macrophages and DCs, and uses portions of the IL-2 receptor (the β and γc chains) for signaling. In both HIV-positive and HIV-negative individuals, IL-15 induces many of the same LAK-activating and IFN-γ–enhancing activities as does IL-2. Similarly, both cytokines induce HIV replication in PBMC, although some reports suggest that IL-15 induces less p24 production compared with that induced by IL-2.[323] It has also been suggested that IL-15 plays a role in the hypergammaglobulinemia observed in HIV-infected subjects.[343]

Numerous cell types produce a variety of chemokines,[344] and modulation of the production of these factors may influence HIV replication in a strain-specific manner. Therefore, the overall effect of immune activation and the secretion of proinflammatory or immunoregulatory cytokines on HIV replication must now be considered in the context of potential influences on chemokine production, chemokine co-receptor expression, and the predominant viral quasispecies that is replicating in vivo. Chemokine production, induced during inflammation, is enhanced by several cytokines, including TNF-α, IL-1β, and immunoregulatory cytokines such as IL-2 and IL-15 (reviewed in Weissman and co-workers[345]). Thus, in HIV-infected subjects in the early stages of disease, the ability of TNF-α to stimulate CC chemokine production and thereby suppress CCR5-utilizing viral entry may override its HIV-inducing effects; however, in individuals harboring predominantly CXCR4-utilizing viral quasi-species in the later stages of HIV disease, only the HIV-inducing activity of TNF-α would be influential. In fact, TNF-α–mediated induction of CC-chemokine secretion may actually enhance the entry and replication of CXCR4-utilizing strains of HIV.[346]

Immunoregulatory aspects of chemokine receptor expression may also exert variable strain-dependent effects on HIV replication and spread. In this regard, IL-2 has been shown to upregulate expression of the co-receptor CCR5. In contrast, stimulation of CD4+ T cells through CD3 and CD28 protects cells from HIV infection and potently downregulates HIV replication in infected cells[347]; this effect appears to be due in part to downregulation of CCR5.[348] The puzzling bottleneck in HIV transmission that so heavily favors the emergence of CCR5-utilizing strains of virus in the new host[349] may in part be due to the differential regulatory patterns of the relevant HIV co-receptors.[350] In this regard, CCR5 expression is predominantly seen in previously activated memory T cells (i.e., CD26high, CD45RAlow, CD45RO+), whereas CXCR4 expression is seen in naïve, unactivated cells (i.e., CD26low, CD45RA+, CD45RO−). It is therefore plausible that the profound degree of immune activation that occurs during acute HIV infection may result in high expression of CCR5 and low expression of CXCR4.[351] Similarly, co-infection with various other pathogens may differentially modulate the expression of HIV co-receptors and thereby exert selective pressure on HIV strains that use the co-receptors in question.[352]

Although in vitro culture systems and cell line models have allowed investigators to identify numerous host factors that influence HIV replication and to delineate the mechanisms whereby these factors suppress or enhance viral replication, it is difficult to anticipate how manipulation of these factors will ultimately influence HIV replication in vivo. It is clear that host factors function within the context of an interactive, immunoregulatory cytokine network and can have pleiotropic effects on HIV replication, some of which are viral strain specific. Nevertheless, numerous host factors provide real or potential immunotherapeutic benefit that should be further explored and pursued clinically for the treatment of HIV disease.

CONCLUSIONS

The pathogenesis of HIV infection is a multifactorial process consisting of aberrant cellular activation and dysregulation of nearly every aspect of the immune system. Disease progression is intimately related to virus replication, and the net amount of virus replication reflects a balance among factors that either induce or downregulate virus expression and thereby lead to quantitative and qualitative abnormalities of the immune system by direct and/or indirect mechanisms.

The discovery that certain chemokine receptors function as necessary cofactors for HIV entry into target cells has expanded the scope of host factors critical in the pathogenesis of HIV infection. CCR5 and CXCR4 appear to be the major co-receptors for HIV. Other receptors can function as HIV co-receptors in vitro; however, it remains uncertain to what extent these other receptors are used in vivo. HIV co-receptors represent new potential targets of therapeutic intervention.

Progression of HIV disease in the setting of vigorous anti-HIV immune responses remains a central paradox in the pathogenesis of HIV infection. Elements of both the humoral and cell-mediated immune responses against HIV have been implicated in the partial control of virus replication. However, the lack of correlates of protective immunity in HIV infection continues to be a major obstacle to the rational development of immunotherapeutic approaches and vaccine development. In this regard, studies of the immune responses to HIV mounted by individuals who are exposed to HIV and yet remain uninfected and studies of HIV-infected long-term nonprogressors should provide valuable insight into mechanisms of immune containment of HIV replication.

HIV is the quintessential opportunist, as illustrated by its ability to subvert activation of the immune system to its own replicative advantage. The virus is able to disarm multiple components of the host immune response via both direct and indirect mechanisms. Understanding more about interactions between the virus and host that lead to dysfunction and depletion of the immune system should aid in the development of preventive and therapeutic strategies.

REFERENCES

1. Liu S-L, Schacker T, Musey L, et al. Divergent patterns of progression to AIDS after infection from the same source: Human immunodeficiency virus type 1 evolution and antiviral responses. J Virol. 1997;71:4284-4295.
2. Fauci A. Multifactorial nature of human immunodeficiency virus diseases: Implications for therapy. Science. 1993;262:1011-1018.
3. Dalgleish AG, Beverly PC, Clapham PR, et al. The CD4(T4) antigen is an essential component of the receptor for the AIDS retrovirus. Nature. 1984;312:763-767.
4. Klatzmann D, Barre-Sinoussi F, Nugeyre MT, et al. Selective tropism of lymphadenopathy-associated virus (LAV) for helper-inducer T-lymphocytes. Science. 1984;225:59-63.
5. Klatzmann D, Champagne E, Chamaret S, et al. T-lymphocyte T4 molecule behaves as receptor for human retrovirus LAV. Nature. 1984;312:767-768.
6. Maddon PJ, Dalgleish AG, McDougal JS, et al. The T4 gene encodes the AIDS virus receptor and is expressed in the immune system and the brain. Cell. 1986;47:333-348.
7. Broder CC, Berger EA. Fusogenic selectivity of the envelope glycoprotein is a major determinant of human immunodeficiency virus type 1 tropism for CD4+ T-cell lines vs. primary macrophages. Proc Natl Acad Sci U S A. 1995;92:9004-9008.
8. Cocchi F, DeVico AL, Garzino-Demo A, et al. Identification of RANTES, MIP-1 alpha, and MIP-1 beta as the major HIV-suppressive factors produced by CD8+ T cells. Science. 1995;270:1811-1815.
9. Feng Y, Broder C, Kennedy P, Berger E. HIV-1 entry cofactor: functional cDNA cloning of a seven-transmembrane domain, G-protein coupled receptor. Science. 1996;272:872-877.
10. Bleul CC, Farzan M, Choe H, et al. The lymphocyte chemoattractant SDF-1 is a ligand for LESTR/fusin and blocks HIV-1 entry. Nature. 1996;382:829-833.

11. Oberlin E, Amara A, Bachelerie F, et al. The CXC chemokine SDF-1 is the ligand for LESTR/fusin and prevents infection by T-cell-line-adapted HIV-1. Nature. 1996;382:833-835.

12. Paxton WA, Martin SR, Tse D, et al. Relative resistance to HIV-1 infection of CD4 lymphocytes from persons who remain uninfected despite multiple high-risk sexual exposures. Nat Med. 1996;2:412-417.

13. Samson M, Labbe O, Mollereau C, et al. Molecular cloning and functional expression of a new human CC-chemokine receptor gene. Biochemistry. 1996;35:3362-3367.

14. Combadiere C, Ahuja SK, Tiffany HL, Murphy PM. Cloning and functional expression of CC CKR5, a human monocyte CC chemokine receptor selective for MIP-1(alpha), MIP-1(beta), and RANTES. J Leukoc Biol. 1996;60:147-152.

15. Raport C, Gosling J, Schweickart V, et al. Molecular cloning and functional characterization of a novel human CC chemokine receptor (CCR5) for RANTES, MIP-1beta, and MIP-1alpha. J Biol Chem. 1996;271:17161-17166.

16. Deng H, Liu R, Ellmeier W, et al. Identification of a major co-receptor for primary isolates of HIV-1. Nature. 1996;381:661-666.

17. Dragic T, Litwin V, Allaway G, et al. HIV-1 entry into CD4+ cells is mediated by the chemokine receptor CC-CKR-5. Nature. 1996;381:667-673.

18. Alkhatib G, Combadiere C, Broder C, et al. CC CKR5: A RANTES, MIP-1a, MIP-1b receptor as a fusion cofactor for macrophage-tropic HIV-1. Science. 1996;272:1955-1958.

19. Choe H, Farzan M, Sun Y, et al. The β-chemokine receptors CCR3 and CCR5 facilitate infection by primary HIV-1 isolates. Cell. 1996;85:1135-1138.

20. Doranz B, Rucker J, Yi Y, et al. A dual-tropic primary HIV-1 isolate that uses fusin and the β-chemokine receptors CKR-5, CKR-3, and CKR-2b as fusion cofactors. Cell. 1996;85:1149-1158.

21. Liao F, Alkhatib G, Peden KW, et al. STRL33, a novel chemokine receptor-like protein, functions as a fusion cofactor for both macrophage-tropic and T cell line-tropic HIV-1. J Exp Med. 1997;185:2015-2023.

22. Liu R, Paxton W, Choe S, et al. Homozygous defect in HIV-1 coreceptor accounts for resistance of some multiply-exposed individuals to HIV-1 infection. Cell. 1996;86:367-377.

23. Samson M, Libert F, Doranz B, et al. Resistance to HIV-1 infection in caucasian individuals bearing mutant alleles of the CCR-5 chemokine receptor gene. Nature. 1996;382:722-725.

24. Wu L, Paxton WA, Kassam N, et al. CCR5 levels and expression pattern correlate wtih infectability by macrophage-tropic HIV-1, in vitro. J Exp Med. 1997;185:1681-1692.

25. Cohen O, Vaccarezza M, Lam G, et al. Heterozygosity for a defective gene for CC chemokine receptor 5 is not the sole determinant for the immunologic and virologic phenotype of HIV-infected long term non-progressors. J Clin Invest. 1997;100:1581-1589.

26. Eugen-Olsen J, Iversen AKN, Garred P, et al. Heterozygosity for a deletion in the CKR-5 gene leads to prolonged AIDS free survival and slower CD4 T cell fall in a cohort of HIV seropositive individuals. AIDS. 1997;11:305-310.

27. Huang Y, Paxton WA, Wolinsky SM, et al. The role of a mutant CCR5 allele in HIV-1 transmission and disease progression. Nat Med. 1996;2:1240-1243.

28. Spira AI, Marx PA, Patterson BK, et al. Cellular targets of infection and route of viral dissemination after an intravaginal inoculation of simian immunodeficiency virus into rhesus macaques. J Exp Med. 1996;183:215-225.

29. McIlroy D, Autran B, Cheynier R, et al. Infection frequency of dendritic cells and CD4(+) T lymphocytes in spleens of human immunodeficiency virus-positive patients. J Virol. 1995;69:4737-4745.

30. Pope M, Betjes MG, Romani N, et al. Conjugates of dendritic cells and memory T lymphocytes from skin facilitate productive infection with HIV-1. Cell. 1994;78:389-398.

31. Frankel SS, Wenig BM, Burke AP, et al. Replication of HIV-1 in dendritic cell-derived syncytia at the mucosal surface of the adenoid. Science. 1996;272:115-117.

32. Weissman D, Li Y, Ananworanich J, et al. Three populations of cells with dendritic morphology exist in peripheral blood, only one of which is infectable with human immunodeficiency virus type 1. Proc Natl Acad Sci U S A. 1995;92:826-830.

33. Geijtenbeek TBH, Torensma R, van Vliet SJ, et al. Identification of DC-SIGN, a novel dendritic cell-specific ICAM-3 receptor that supports primary immune responses. Cell. 2000;100:575-585.

34. Geijtenbeek TBH, Kwon DS, Torensma R, et al. DC-SIGN, a dendritic cell-specific HIV-1-binding protein that enhances trans-infection of T cells. Cell. 2000;100:587-597.

35. Lathey JL, Pratt RD, Spector SA. Appearance of autologous neutralizing antibody correlates with reduction in virus load and phenotype switch during primary infection with human immunodeficiency virus type I. J Infect Dis. 1997;175:231-232.

36. Sei Y, Tsang PH, Chu FN, et al. Inverse relationship between HIV-1 p24 antigenemia, anti-p24 antibody and neutralizing antibody response in all stages of HIV-1 infection. Immunol Lett. 1989;20:223-230.

37. Montefiori DC, Pantaleo G, Fink LM, et al. Neutralizing and infection-enhancing antibody responses to human immunodeficiency virus type 1 in long-term nonprogressors. J Infect Dis. 1996;173:60-67.

38. Cao Y, Qin L, Zhang L, et al. Virologic and immunologic characterization of long-term survivors of human immunodeficiency virus type 1 infection. N Engl J Med. 1995;332:201-208.

39. Pilgrim AK, Pantaleo G, Cohen OJ, et al. Neutralizing antibody responses to human immunodeficiency virus type 1 in primary infection and long-term-nonprogressive infection. J Infect Dis. 1997;176:924-932.

40. Kwong PD, Wyatt R, Robinson J, et al. Structure of an HIV gp120 envelope glycoprotein in complex with the CD4 receptor and a neutralizing human antibody. Nature. 1998;393:648-659.

41. McKeating JA, Shotton C, Cordell J, et al. Characterization of neutralizing monoclonal antibodies to linear and conformation-dependent epitopes within the first and second variable domains of human immunodeficiency virus type 1 gp120. J Virol. 1993;67:4932-4944.

42. Saphire EO, Parren PW, Pantophlet R, et al. Crystal structure of a neutralizing human IGG against HIV-1: A template for vaccine design. Science. 2001;293:1155-1159.

43. Rizzuto CD, Wyatt R, Hernandez-Ramos N, et al. A conserved HIV gp120 glycoprotein structure involved in chemokine receptor binding. Science. 1998;280:1949-1953.

44. Trkola A, Purtscher M, Muster T, et al. Human monoclonal antibody 2G12 defines a distinctive neutralization epitope on the gp120 glycoprotein of human immunodeficiency virus type 1. J Virol. 1996;70:1100-1108.

45. Sattentau QJ, Moore JP, Vignaux F, et al. Conformational changes induced in the envelope glycoproteins of the human and simian immunodeficiency viruses by soluble receptor binding. J Virol. 1993;67:7383-7393.

46. Kwong PD, Doyle ML, Casper DJ, et al. HIV-1 evades antibody-mediated neutralization through conformational masking of receptor-binding sites. Nature. 2002;420:678-682.

47. Parren PW, Burton DR. The antiviral activity of antibodies in vitro and in vivo. Adv Immunol. 2001;77:195-262.

48. Stott EJ. Towards a vaccine against AIDS: Lessons from simian immunodeficiency virus vaccines. Curr Top Microbiol Immunol. 1994;188:221-237.

49. Arthur LO, Bess JW Jr, Urban RG, et al. Macaques immunized with HLA-DR are protected from challenge with simian immunodeficiency virus. J Virol. 1995;69:3117-3124.

50. Parren PW, Mondor I, Naniche D, et al. Neutralization of human immunodeficiency virus type 1 by antibody to gp120 is determined primarily by occupancy of sites on the virion irrespective of epitope specificity. J Virol. 1998;72:3512-3519.

51. Coffin JM. HIV population dynamics in vivo: Implications for genetic variation, pathogenesis, and therapy. Science. 1995;267:483-489.

52. Murphy BR, Webster RG. Orthomyxoviruses. Fields Virology. Philadelphia: Lippincott Williams & Wilkins; 1996:1397-1446.

53. Crowe JE, Firestone CY, Crim R, et al. Monoclonal antibody-resistant mutants selected with a respiratory syncytial virus-neutralizing human antibody fab fragment (Fab. 19) define a unique epitope on the fusion (F) glycoprotein. Virology. 1998;252:373-375.

54. Cheynier R, Henrichwark S, Hadida F, et al. HIV and T cell expansion in splenic white pulps is accompanied by infiltration of HIV-specific cytotoxic T lymphocytes. Cell. 1994;78:373-387.

55. Shankarappa R, Margolick JB, Gange SJ, et al. Consistent viral evolutionary changes associated with the progression of human immunodeficiency virus type 1 infection. J Virol. 1999;73:10489-10502.

56. Kuiken CL, Lukashov VV, Baan E, et al. Evidence for limited within-person evolution of the V3 domain of the HIV-1 envelope in the Amsterdam population. AIDS. 1996;10:31-37.

57. Richman DD, Wrin T, Little SJ, Petropoulos CJ. Rapid evolution of the neutralizing antibody response to HIV type 1 infection. Proc Natl Acad Sci U S A. 2003;100:4144-4149.

58. Walker BD, Chakrabarti S, Moss B, et al. HIV specific cytotoxic T lymphocytes in seropositive individuals. Nature. 1987;328:345.

59. Koup RA, Safrit JT, Cao Y, et al. Temporal association of cellular immune responses with the initial control of viremia in primary human immunodeficiency virus type 1 syndrome. J Virol. 1994;68:4650-4655.

60. Walker CM, Moody DJ, Stites DP, Levy JA. CD8+ lymphocytes can control HIV infection in vitro by suppressing virus replication. Science. 1986;234:1563-1566.

61. Schmitz JE, Kuroda MJ, Santra S, et al. Control of viremia in simian immunodeficiency virus infection by CD8+ lymphocytes. Science. 1999;283:857-860.

62. Matano T, Shibata R, Siemon C, et al. Administration of an anti-CD8 monoclonal antibody interferes with the clearance of chimeric simian/human immunodeficiency virus during primary infections of rhesus macaques. J Virol. 1998;72:164-169.

63. Borrow P, Lewicki H, Wei X, et al. Antiviral pressure exerted by HIV-1-specific cytotoxic T lymphocytes (CTLs) during primary infection demonstrated by rapid selection of CTL escape virus. Nat Med. 1997;3:205-211.

64. Goulder PJ, Phillips RE, Colbert RA, et al. Late escape from an immunodominant cytotoxic T-lymphocyte response associated with progression to AIDS. Nat Med. 1997;3:212-217.

65. Nowak MA, May RM, Phillips RE, et al. Antigenic oscillations and shifting immunodominance in HIV-1 infections. Nature. 1995;375:606-611.

66. Goulder PJ, Brander C, Tang Y, et al. Evolution and transmission of stable CTL escape mutations in HIV infection. Nature. 2001;412:334-338.

67. Migueles SA, Laborico AC, Imamichi H, et al. The differential ability of HLA B(*)5701(+) long-term nonprogressors and progressors to restrict human immunodeficiency virus replication is not caused by loss of recognition of autologous viral gag sequences. J Virol. 2003;77:6889-6898.

68. Kerkau T, Bacik I, Bennink JR, et al. The human immunodeficiency virus type 1 (HIV-1) vpu protein interferes with an early step in the biosynthesis of major histocompatibility complex (MHC) class I molecules. J Exp Med. 1997;185:1295-1305.

69. Schwartz O, Marechal V, Gall SL, et al. Endocytosis of major histocompatibility complex class I molecules is induced by the HIV-1 Nef protein. Nat Med. 1996;2:338-342.

70. Howcroft TK, Strebel K, Martin MA, Singer DS. Repression of MHC class I gene promoter activity by two-exon Tat of HIV. Science. 1993;260:1320-1322.

71. Cohen GB, Gandhi RT, Davis DM, et al. The selective downregulation of class I major histocompatibility complex proteins by HIV-1 protects HIV-infected cells from NK cells. Immunity. 1999;10:661-671.

72. Ferrari G, Humphrey W, McElrath MJ, et al. Clade B-based HIV-1 vaccines elicit cross-clade cytotoxic T lymphocyte reactivities in uninfected volunteers. Proc Natl Acad Sci U S A. 1997;94:1396-1401.

73. Migueles SA, Sabbaghian MS, Shupert WL, et al. HLA B*5701 is highly associated with restriction of virus replication in a subgroup of HIV-infected long term nonprogressors. Proc Natl Acad Sci U S A. 2000;97:2709-2714.

74. Kalams SA, Buchbinder SP, Rosenberg ES, et al. Association between virus-specific cytotoxic T-lymphocyte and helper responses in human immunodeficiency virus type 1 infection. J Virol. 1999;73:6715-6720.

75. Dalod M, Dupuis M, Deschemin JC, et al. Broad, intense anti-human immunodeficiency virus (HIV) ex vivo CD8(+) responses in HIV type 1-infected patients: Comparison with anti-Epstein-Barr virus responses and changes during antiretroviral therapy. J Virol. 1999;73:7108-7116.

76. Gea-Banacloche JC, Migueles SA, Martino L, et al. Maintenance of large numbers of virus specific CD8+ T cells in HIV infected progressors and long term nonprogressors. J Immunol. 2000;165:1082-1092.

77. Betts MR, Ambrozak DR, Douek DC, et al. Analysis of total HIV-specific CD4+ and CD8+ T cell responses: Relationship to viral load in untreated HIV infection. J Virol. 2001.

78. Addo MM, Yu XG, Rathod A, et al. Comprehensive epitope analysis of human immunodeficiency virus type 1 (HIV-1)-specific T-cell responses directed against the entire expressed HIV-1 genome demonstrate broadly directed responses, but no correlation to viral load. J Virol. 2003;77:2081-2092.

79. Migueles SA, Laborico AC, Shupert WL, et al. HIV-specific CD8+ T cell proliferation is coupled to perforin expression and is maintained in nonprogressors. Nat Immunol. 2002;3:1061-1068.

80. Migueles SA, Connors M. Frequency and function of HIV-specific CD8(+) T cells. Immunol Lett. 2001;79:141-150.

81. van Baalen CA, Pontesilli O, Huisman RC, et al. Human immunodeficiency virus type 1 Rev- and Tat-specific cytotoxic T lymphocyte frequencies inversely correlate with rapid progression to AIDS. J Gen Virol. 1997;78:1913-1918.

82. Addo MM, Altfeld M, Rosenberg ES, et al. The HIV-1 regulatory proteins Tat and Rev are frequently targeted by cytotoxic T lymphocytes derived from HIV-1-infected individuals. Proc Natl Acad Sci U S A. 2001;98:1781-1786.

83. Allen TM, O'Connor DH, Jing P, et al. Tat-specific cytotoxic T lymphocytes select for SIV escape variants during resolution of primary viraemia. Nature. 2000;407: 386-390.

84. Pantaleo G, Demarest JF, Soudeyns H, et al. Major expansion of CD8+ T cells with a predominant V beta usage during the primary immune response to HIV. Nature. 1994;370:463-467.

85. Altfeld M, Rosenberg ES, Shankarappa R, et al. Cellular immune responses and viral diversity in individuals treated during acute and early HIV-1 infection. J Exp Med. 2001;193:169-180.

86. Cao J, McNevin J, Holte S, et al. Comprehensive analysis of human immunodeficiency virus type 1 (HIV-1)-specific gamma interferon-secreting CD8(+) T cells in primary HIV-1 infection. J Virol. 2003;77:6867-6878.

87. Trimble LA, Shankar P, Patterson M, et al. Human immunodeficiency virus-specific circulating CD8 T lymphocytes have down-modulated CD3zeta and CD28, key signaling molecules for T-cell activation. J Virol. 2000;74:7320-7330.

88. Goepfert PA, Bansal A, Edwards BH, et al. A significant number of human immunodeficiency virus epitope-specific cytotoxic T lymphocytes detected by tetramer binding do not produce gamma interferon. J Virol. 2000;74:10249-10255.

89. Kostense S, Ogg GS, Manting EH, et al. High viral burden in the presence of major HIV-specific CD8(+) T cell expansions: Evidence for impaired CTL effector function. Eur J Immunol. 2001;31:677-686.

90. Champagne P, Ogg GS, King AS, et al. Skewed maturation of memory HIV-specific CD8 T lymphocytes. Nature. 2001;410:106-111.

91. Kinter AL, Ostrowski M, Goletti D, et al. HIV replication in CD4+ T cells of HIV-infected individuals is regulated by a balance between the viral suppressive effects of endogenous beta-chemokines and the viral inductive effects of other endogenous cytokines. Proc Natl Acad Sci U S A. 1996;93:14076-14081.

92. Geiben-Lynn R, Kursar M, Brown NV, et al. Noncytolytic inhibition of X4 virus by bulk CD8(+) cells from human immunodeficiency virus type 1 (HIV-1)-infected persons and HIV-1-specific cytotoxic T lymphocytes is not mediated by beta-chemokines. J Virol. 2001;75:8306-8316.

93. Zhang L, Yu W, He T, et al. Contribution of human alpha-defensin 1, 2, and 3 to the anti-HIV-1 activity of CD8 antiviral factor. Science. 2002;298:995-1000.

94. Chang TL, Francois F, Mosoian A, Klotman ME. CAF-mediated human immunodeficiency virus (HIV) type 1 transcriptional inhibition is distinct from alpha-defensin-1 HIV inhibition. J Virol. 2003;77:6777-6784.

95. Yang OO, Kalams SA, Trocha A, et al. Suppression of human immunodeficiency virus type 1 replication by CD8+ cells: Evidence for HLA class I-restricted triggering of cytolytic and noncytolytic mechanisms. J Virol. 1997;71:3120-3128.

96. Chun TW, Justement JS, Moir S, et al. Suppression of HIV replication in the resting CD4+ T cell reservoir by autologous CD8+ T cells: Implications for the development of therapeutic strategies. Proc Natl Acad Sci U S A. 2001;98:253-258.

97. Matloubian M, Concepcion RJ, Ahmed R. CD4+ T cells are required to sustain CD8+ cytotoxic T-cell responses during chronic viral infection. J Virol. 1994;68:8056-8063.

98. Cardin RD, Brooks JW, Sarawar SR, Doherty PC. Progressive loss of CD8+ T cell-mediated control of a gamma-herpesvirus in the absence of CD4+ T cells. J Exp Med. 1996;184:863-871.

99. Wahren B, Morfeldt-Mansson L, Biberfeld G, et al. Characteristics of the specific cell-mediated immune response in human immunodeficiency virus infection. J Virol. 1987;61:2017-2023.

100. Valentine FT, Paolino A, Saito A, Holzman RS. Lymphocyte-proliferative responses to HIV antigens as a potential measure of immunological reconstitution in HIV disease. AIDS Res Hum Retroviruses. 1998;14 Suppl 2:S161-S166.

101. Rosenberg ES, Billingsley JM, Caliendo AM, et al. Vigorous HIV-1-specific CD4+ T cell responses associated with control of viremia. Science. 1997;278:1447-1450.

102. McNeil AC, Shupert WL, Iyasere CA, et al. High level HIV-1 viremia suppresses viral antigen-specific CD4+ T cell proliferation. Proc Natl Acad Sci U S A. 2001.

103. Rosenberg ES, Altfeld M, Poon SH, et al. Immune control of HIV-1 after early treatment of acute infection. Nature. 2000;407:523-526.

104. Davey RT Jr, Bhat N, Yoder C, et al. HIV-1 and T cell dynamics after interruption of highly active antiretroviral therapy (HAART) in patients with a history of sustained viral suppression. Proc Natl Acad Sci U S A. 1999;96:15109-15114.

105. Al-Harthi L, Siegel J, Spritzler J, et al. Maximum suppression of HIV replication leads to the restoration of HIV-specific responses in early HIV disease. AIDS. 2000;14:761-770.

106. Palmer BE, Boritz E, Blyveis N, Wilson CC. Discordance between frequency of human immunodeficiency virus type 1 (HIV-1)-specific gamma interferon-producing CD4(+) T cells and HIV-1-specific lymphoproliferation in HIV-1-infected subjects with active viral replication. J Virol. 2002;76:5925-5936.

107. Pitcher CJ, Quittner C, Peterson DM, et al. HIV-1-specific CD4+ T cells are detectable in most individuals with active HIV-1 infection, but decline with prolonged viral suppression (see comments). Nat Med. 1999;5:518-525.

108. Boni C, Bertoletti A, Penna A, et al. Lamivudine treatment can restore T cell responsiveness in chronic hepatitis B. J Clin Invest. 1998;102:968-975.

109. Carney WP, Hirsch MS. Mechanisms of immunosuppression in cytomegalovirus mononucleosis. II. Virus-monocyte interactions. J Infect Dis. 1981;144:47-54.

110. Dybul M, Mercier G, Belson M, et al. CD40 ligand trimer and IL-12 enhance peripheral blood mononuclear cells and CD4+ T cell proliferation and production of IFN-gamma in response to p24 antigen in HIV-infected individuals: Potential contribution of anergy to HIV-specific unresponsiveness. J Immunol. 2000;165:1685-1691.

111. Vicenzi E, Bagnarelli P, Santagostino E, et al. Hemophilia and nonprogressing human immunodeficiency virus type 1 infection. Blood. 1997;89:191-200.

112. Pantaleo G, Menzo S, Vaccarezza M, et al. Studies in subjects with long-term nonprogressive human immunodeficiency virus infection. N Engl J Med. 1995;332: 209-216.

113. Shearer GM, Clerici M, Clerici M, et al. Protective immunity against HIV infection: has nature done the experiment for us? HIV-specific T-helper activity in seronegative health care workers exposed to contaminated blood. Immunol Today. 1996;17:21-24.

114. Vesanen M, Stevens CE, Taylor PE, et al. Stability in controlling viral replication identifies long-term nonprogressors as a distinct subgroup among human immunodeficiency virus type 1-infected persons. J Virol. 1996;70:9035-9040.

115. Flores-Villanueva PO, Yunis EJ, Delgado JC, et al. Control of HIV-1 viremia and protection from AIDS are associated with HLA-Bw4 homozygosity. Proc Natl Acad Sci U S A. 2001;98:5140-5145.

116. Ogg GS, Jin X, Bonhoeffer S, et al. Quantitation of HIV-1-specific cytotoxic T lymphocytes and plasma load of viral RNA. Science. 1998;279:2103-2106.

117. Kaslow RA, Duquesnoy R, VanRaden M, et al. A1, Cw7, B8, DR3 HLA antigen combination associated with rapid decline of T-helper lymphocytes in HIV-1 infection. A report from the Multicenter AIDS Cohort Study. Lancet. 1990;335:927-930.

118. Kaslow RA, Carrington M, Apple R, et al. Influence of combinations of human major histocompatibility complex genes on the course of HIV-1 infection. Nat Med. 1996;2:405-411.

119. Hendel H, Caillat-Zucman S, Lebuanec H, et al. New class I and II HLA alleles strongly associated with opposite patterns of progression to AIDS. J Immunol. 1999;162:6942-6946.

120. Carrington M, Nelson GW, Martin MP, et al. HLA and HIV-1: heterozygote advantage and B*35-Cw*04 disadvantage. Science. 1999;283:1748-1752.

121. Goulder PJ, Bunce M, Krausa P, et al. Novel, cross-restricted, conserved, and immunodominant cytotoxic T lymphocyte epitopes in slow progressors in HIV type 1 infection. AIDS Res Hum Retroviruses. 1996;12:1691-1698.

122. Smith MW, Dean M, Carrington M, et al. Contrasting genetic influence of CCR2 and CCR5 variants on HIV-1 infection and disease progression. Hemophilia Growth and Development Study (HGDS), Multicenter AIDS Cohort Study (MACS), Multicenter Hemophilia Cohort Study (MHCS), San Francisco City Cohort (SFCC), ALIVE Study. Science. 1997;277:959-965.

123. Carrington M, Nelson G, O'Brien SJ. Considering genetic profiles in functional studies of immune responsiveness to HIV-1. Immunol Lett. 2001;79:131-140.

124. Borrow P, Lewicki H, Hahn BH, et al. CTL activity associated with control of viremia in primary HIV-1 infection. J Virol. 1994;68:6103-6110.

125. Dyer WB, Ogg GS, Demoitie MA, et al. Strong human immunodeficiency virus (HIV)-specific cytotoxic T-lymphocyte activity in Sydney Blood Bank Cohort patients infected with nef-defective HIV type 1. J Virol. 1999;73:436-443.

126. Zwart G, VanderHoek L, Valk M, et al. Antibody responses to HIV-1 envelope and gag epitopes in HIV-1 seroconverters with rapid versus slow disease progression. Virology. 1994;201:285-293.

127. Sei Y, Tsang PH, Roboz JP, et al. Neutralizing antibodies as a prognostic indicator in the progression of acquired immune deficiency syndrome (AIDS)-related disorders: A double-blind study. J Clin Immunol. 1988;8:464-472.

128. Tsang ML, Evans LA, McQueen P, et al. Neutralizing antibodies against sequential autologous human immunodeficiency virus type 1 isolates after seroconversion. J Infect Dis. 1994;170:1141-1147.

129. Arendrup M, Nielsen C, Hansen J-ES, et al. Autologous HIV-1 neutralizing antibodies: emergence of neutralization-resistant escape virus and subsequent development of escape virus neutralizing antibodies. J Acquir Immune Def Syndr. 1992;5:303-307.

130. Learmont J, Tindall B, Evans L, et al. Long-term symptomless HIV-1 infection in recipients of blood products from a single donor. Lancet. 1992;340:863-867.

131. Deacon NJ, Tsykin A, Solomon A, et al. Genomic structure of an attenuated quasi species of HIV-1 from a blood transfusion donor and recipients. Science. 1995;270:988-991.

132. Kirchhoff F, Greenough TC, Brettler DB, et al. Brief report: Absence of intact nef sequences in a long-term survivor with nonprogressive HIV-1 infection. N Engl J Med. 1995;332:228-232.

133. Huang Y, Zhang L, Ho D. Biological characterization of nef in long term survivors of human immunodeficiency virus type 1 infection. J Virol. 1995;69:8142-8146.

134. Michael NL, Chang G, D'arcy LA, et al. Functional characterization of human immunodeficiency virus type 1 nef genes in patients with divergent rates of disease progression. J Virol. 1995;69:6758-6769.

135. Iversen AKN, Shpaer EG, Rodrigo AG, et al. Persistence of attenuated rev genes in a human immunodeficiency virus type 1-infected asymptomatic individual. J Virol. 1995;69:5743-5753.

136. Michael NL, Chang G, D'arcy LA, et al. Defective accessory genes in a human immunodeficiency virus type 1-infected long-term survivor lacking recoverable virus. J Virol. 1995;69:4228-4236.

137. Huang Y, Zhang L, Ho DD. Characterization of gag and pol sequences from long-term survivors of human immunodeficiency virus type 1 infection. Virology. 1998;240:36-49.

138. Connor RI, Sheridan KE, Lai C, et al. Characterization of the functional properties of env genes from long-term survivors of human immunodeficiency virus type 1 infection. J Virol. 1996;70:5306-5311.

139. Lum JJ, Cohen OJ, Nie Z, et al. Vpr R77Q is associated with long-term nonprogressive HIV infection and impaired induction of apoptosis. J Clin Invest. 2003;111:1547-1554.

140. Cornelissen M, Kuiken C, Zorgdrager F, et al. Gross defects in the vpr and vpu genes of HIV type 1 cannot explain the differences in RNA copy number between long-term asymptomatics and progressors. AIDS Res Hum Retroviruses. 1997;13:247-252.

141. Zhang LQ, Huang YX, Yuan HN, et al. Genetic characterization of vif, vpr, and vpu sequences from long-term survivors of human immunodeficiency virus type 1 infection. Virology. 1997;228:340-349.

142. Furtado MR, Callaway DS, Phair JP, et al. Persistence of HIV-1 transcription in peripheral-blood mononuclear cells in patients receiving potent antiretroviral therapy. N Engl J Med. 1999;340:1614-1622.

143. Dornadula G, Zhang H, VanUitert B, et al. Residual HIV-1 RNA in blood plasma of patients taking suppressive highly active antiretroviral therapy. JAMA. 1999;282:1627-1632.

144. Weinberg JB, Matthews TJ, Cullen BR, Malim MH. Productive human immunodeficiency virus type1 (HIV-1) infection of nonproliferating human monocytes. J Exp Med. 1991;174:1477-1482.

145. Knight SC, Macatonia SE, Patterson S. HIV-1 infection of dendritic cells. Int Rev Immunol. 1990;6:163-175.

146. Koenig S, Gendelman HE, Orenstein JM, et al. Detection of AIDS virus in macrophages in brain tissue from AIDS patients with encephalopathy. Science. 1986;1089-1093.

147. Stingele K, Haas J, Zimmermann T, et al. Independent HIV replication in paired CSF and blood viral isolates during antiretroviral therapy. Neurology. 2001;56:355-361.

148. Barroso PF, Schechter M, Gupta P, et al. Effect of antiretroviral therapy on HIV shedding in semen. Ann Intern Med. 2000;133:280-284.

149. Poles MA, Elliott J, Vingerhoets J, et al. Despite high concordance, distinct mutational and phenotypic drug resistance profiles in human immunodeficiency virus type 1 RNA are observed in gastrointestinal mucosal biopsy specimens and peripheral blood mononuclear cells compared with plasma. J Infect Dis. 2001;183:143-148.

150. Gupta P, Leroux C, Patterson BK, et al. Human immunodeficiency virus type 1 shedding pattern in semen correlates with the compartmentalization of viral Quasi species between blood and semen. J Infect Dis. 2000;182:79-87.

151. Zack JA, Arrigo SJ, Weitsman SR, et al. HIV-1 entry into quiescent primary lymphocytes: Molecular analysis reveals a labile, latent viral structure. Cell. 1990;61:213-222.

152. Bukrinsky M, Stanwick T, Dempsey M, Stevenson M. Quiescent T lymphocytes as an inducible virus reservoir in HIV-1 infection. Science. 1991;254:423-427.

153. Chun TW, Carruth L, Finzi D, et al. Quantification of latent tissue reservoirs and total body viral load in HIV-1 infection. Nature. 1997;387:183-188.

154. Chun TW, Stuyver L, Mizell SB, et al. Presence of an inducible HIV-1 latent reservoir during highly active antiretroviral therapy. Proc Natl Acad Sci U S A. 1997;94:13193-13197.

155. Finzi D, Hermankova M, Pierson T, et al. Identification of a reservoir for HIV-1 in patients on highly active antiretroviral therapy. Science. 1997;278:1295-1300.

156. Wong JK, Hezareh M, Gunthard HF, et al. Recovery of replication-competent HIV despite prolonged suppression of plasma viremia. Science. 1997;278:1291-1295.

157. Kinter AL, Umscheid CA, Arthos J, et al. HIV envelope induces virus expression from resting CD4+ T cells isolated from HIV-infected individuals in the absence of markers of cellular activation or apoptosis. J Immunol. 2003;170:2449-2455.

158. Pantaleo G, Graziosi C, Demarest JF, et al. HIV infection is active and progressive in lymphoid tissue during the clinically latent stage of disease. Nature. 1993;362:355-358.

159. Embretson J, Zupancic M, Ribas J, et al. Massive covert infection of helper T lymphocytes and macrophages by HIV during the incubation period of AIDS. Nature. 1993;362:359-362.

160. Cavert W, Notermans DW, Staskus K, et al. Kinetics of response in lymphoid tissues to antiretroviral therapy of HIV-1 infection. Science. 1997;276:960-963.

161. Fernandez R, Mouradian J, Metroka C, Davies J. The prognostic value of histopathology in persistent generalized lymphadenopathy in homosexual men. N Engl J Med. 1983;309:185-186.

162. Racz P, Tenner-Racz K, Kahl C, et al. Spectrum of morphologic changes of lymph nodes from patients with AIDS or AIDS-related complexes. Prog Allergy. 1986;37:81-181.

163. Tew JG, Burton GF, Kupp LI, Szakal A. Follicular dendritic cells in germinal center reactions. Adv Exp Med Biol. 1993;329:461-465.

164. Schmitz J, van Lunzen J, Tenner-Racz K, et al. Follicular dendritic cells retain HIV-1 particles on their plasma membrane, but are not productively infected in asymptomatic patients with follicular hyperplasia. J Immunol. 1994;153:1352-1359.

165. Hivroz C, Mazerolles F, Soula M, et al. Human immunodeficiency virus gp120 and derived peptides activate protein tyrosine kinase p56lck in human CD4 T lymphocytes. Eur J Immunol. 1993;23:600-607.

166. Li CJ, Friedman DJ, Wang C, et al. Induction of apoptosis in uninfected lymphocytes by HIV-1 Tat protein. Science. 1995;268:429-431.

167. Pantaleo G, Fauci AS. Immunopathogenesis of HIV infection. Annu Rev Microbiol. 1996;50:825-854.

168. Clerici M, Stocks NI, Zajac RA, et al. Detection of three distinct patterns of T helper cell dysfunction in asymptomatic, human immunodeficiency virus-seropositive patients independent of CD4+ cell numbers and clinical settings. J Clin Invest. 1989;84:1892-1899.

169. Choremi-Papadopoulou H, Viglis V, Gargalianos P, et al. Downregulation of CD28 surface antigen on CD4+ and CD8+ T lymphocytes during HIV-1 infection. J Acquir Immune Defic Syndr. 1994;7:245-253.

170. Borthwick NJ, Bofill M, Gombert WM, et al. Lymphocyte activation in HIV-1 infection. II. Functional defects of CD28- T cells. AIDS. 1994;8:431-441.

171. Stevenson M, Meier C, Mann AM, et al. Envelope glycoprotein of HIV induces interference and cytolysis resistance in CD4+ cells: Mechanisms for persistence in AIDS. Cell. 1988;53:483-496.

172. Garcia JV, Miller AD. Serine phosphorylation-independent downregulation of cell-surface CD4 by nef. Nature. 1991;350:508-511.

173. Willey RL, Maldarelli F, Martin MA, Strebel K. Human immunodeficiency virus type 1 Vpu protein induces rapid degradation of CD4. J Virol. 1992;66:7193-7200.

174. Schnittman SM, Lane HC, Greenhouse J, et al. Preferential infection of CD4+ memory T cells by human immunodeficiency virus type 1: Evidence for a role in the selective T-cell functional defects observed in infected individuals. Proc Natl Acad Sci U S A. 1990;87:6058-6062.

175. Spina CA, Prince HE, Richman DD. Preferential replication of HIV-1 in the CD45RO memory cell subset of primary CD4 lymphocytes in vitro. J Clin Invest. 1997;99:1774-1785.

176. Connors M, Kovacs JA, Krevat S, et al. HIV infection induces changes in CD4+ T-cell phenotype and depletions within the CD4+ T-cell repertoire that are not immediately restored by antiviral or immune-based therapies. Nat Med. 1997;3:533-540.

177. Gea-Banacloche JC, Weiskopf EE, Hallahan C, et al. Progression of human immunodeficiency virus disease is associated with increasing disruptions within the CD4+ T cell receptor repertoire. J Infect Dis. 1998;177:579-585.

178. Gallo R, Salahuddin S, Popovic M, et al. Frequent detection and isolation of cytopathic retroviruses (HTLV-III) from patients with AIDS and at risk for AIDS. Science. 1984;224:500-503.

179. Levy JA, Hoffman AD, Kramer SM, et al. Isolation of lymphocytopathic retroviruses from San Francisco patients with AIDS. Science. 1984;225:840-842.

180. Shaw GM, Hahn BH, Arya SK, et al. Molecular characterization of human T-cell leukemia (lymphotropic) virus type III in the acquired immune deficiency syndrome. Science. 1984;226:1165-1171.

181. Popovic M, Sarngadharan M, Read E, Gallo R. Detection, isolation, and continuous production of cytopathic retroviruses (HTLV-III) from patients with AIDS and pre-AIDS. Science. 1984;224:497-500.

182. Pantaleo G, Graziosi C, Butini L, et al. Lymphoid organs function as major reservoirs for human immunodeficiency virus. Proc Natl Acad Sci U S A. 1991;88:9838-9842.

183. Schnittman SM, Greenhouse JJ, Psallidopoulos MC, et al. Increasing viral burden in CD4+ T cells from patients with human immunodeficiency virus (HIV) infection reflects rapidly progressive immunosuppression and clinical disease. Ann Intern Med. 1990;113:438-443.

184. Bagnarelli P, Menzo S, Valenza A, et al. Molecular profile of human immunodeficiency virus type 1 infection in symptomless patients and in patients with AIDS. J Virol. 1992;66:7328-7335.

185. Connor RI, Mohri H, Cao Y, Ho DD. Increased viral burden and cytopathicity correlate temporally with CD4+ T-lymphocyte decline and clinical progression in human immunodeficiency virus type 1-infected individuals. J Virol. 1993;67:1772-1777.

186. Michael NL, Vahey M, Burke RS, Redfield RR. Viral DNA and mRNA expression correlate with the stage of human immunodeficiency virus (HIV) type 1 infection in humans: evidence for viral replication in all stages of HIV disease. J Virol. 1992;66:310-316.

187. Thompson CB. Apoptosis in the pathogenesis and treatment of disease. Science. 1995;267:1456-1462.

188. Vaux DL, Cory S, Adams JM. Bcl-2 gene promotes haemopoietic cell survival and cooperates with c-myc to immortalize pre-B cells. Nature. 1988;335:440-442.

189. Hockenbery D, Nunez G, Milliman C, et al. Bcl-2 is an inner mitochondrial membrane protein that blocks programmed cell death. Nature. 1990;348:334-336.

190. Lowe SW, Schmitt EM, Smith SW, et al. p53 is required for radiation-induced apoptosis in mouse thymocytes. Nature. 1993;362:847-849.

191. Clarke AR, Purdie CA, Harrison DJ, et al. Thymocyte apoptosis induced by p53-dependent and independent pathways. Nature. 1993;362:849-852.

192. Ascher MS, Sheppard HW. AIDS as immune system activation. II. The panergic amnesia hypothesis. J Acquir Immune Defic Syndr. 1990;3:177-191.

193. Laurent-Crawford AG, Krust B, Muller S, et al. The cytopathic effect of HIV is associated with apoptosis. Virology. 1991;185:829-839.

194. Meyaard L, Otto SA, Jonker RR, et al. Programmed death of T cells in HIV-1 infection. Science. 1992;257:217-219.

195. Westendorp MO, Frank R, Ochsenbauer C,, et al. Sensitization of T cells to CD95-mediated apoptosis by HIV-1 Tat and gp120. Nature. 1995;375:497-500.

196. Muro-Cacho C, Pantaleo G, Fauci AS. Analysis of apoptosis in lymph nodes of HIV-infected persons. Intensity of apoptosis correlates with the general state of activation of the lymphoid tissue and not with stage of disease or viral burden. J Immunol. 1995;154:5555-5566.

197. Finkel TH, Tudor-Williams G, Banda NK, et al. Apoptosis occurs predominantly in bystander cells and not in productively infected cells of HIV- and SIV-infected lymph nodes. Nat Med. 1995;1:129-134.

198. Gougeon M-L, Lecoeur H, Dulioust A, et al. Programmed cell death in peripheral lymphocytes from HIV-infected persons. J Immunol. 1996;156:3509-3520.

199. Meyaard L, Otto SA, Keet IP, et al. Programmed death of T cells in human immunodeficiency virus infection. No correlation with progression to disease. J Clin Invest. 1994;93:982-988.

200. Estaquier J, Idziorek T, de Bels F, et al. Programmed cell death and AIDS: significance of T-cell apoptosis in pathogenic and nonpathogenic primate lentiviral infections. Proc Natl Acad Sci U S A. 1994;91:9431-9435.

201. Ho DD, Neumann AU, Perelson AS, et al. Rapid turnover of plasma virions and CD4 lymphocytes in HIV-1 infection. Nature. 1995;373:123-126.

202. Lempicki RA, Kovacs JA, Baseler MW, et al. Impact of HIV-1 infection and highly active antiretroviral therapy on the kinetics of CD4+ and CD8+ T cell turnover in HIV-infected patients. Proc Natl Acad Sci U S A. 2000;97:13778-13783.

203. McCune JM. The dynamics of CD4+ T-cell depletion in HIV disease. Nature. 2001;410:974-979.

204. Golding H, Robey FA, Gates FtD, et al. Identification of homologous regions in human immunodeficiency virus I gp41 and human MHC class II beta 1 domain. I. Monoclonal antibodies against the gp41-derived peptide and patients' sera react with native HLA class II antigens, suggesting a role for autoimmunity in the pathogenesis of acquired immune deficiency syndrome. J Exp Med. 1988;167:914-923.

205. Golding H, Shearer G, Hillman K, et al. Common epitope in human immunodeficiency virus (HIV)1 gp41 and HLA class II elicits immunosuppressive autoantibodies capable of contributing to immune dysfunction in HIV 1-infected individuals. J Clin Invest. 1989;83:1430-1435.

206. Grassi F, Meneveri R, Gullberg M, et al. Human immunodeficiency virus type 1 gp120 mimics a hidden monomorphic epitope borne by class I major histocompatibility complex heavy chains. J Exp Med. 1991;174:53-62.

207. Grant MD, Weaver MS, Tsoukas C, Hoffmann GW. Distribution of antibodies against denatured collagen in AIDS risk groups and homosexual AIDS patients suggests a link between autoimmunity and the immunopathogenesis of AIDS. J Immunol. 1990;144:1241-1250.

208. Muller S, Richalet P, Laurent-Crawford A, et al. Autoantibodies typical of non-organ-specific autoimmune diseases in HIV-seropositive patients. AIDS. 1992;6:933-942.

209. Cassani F, Baffoni L, Raise E, et al. Serum non-organ specific autoantibodies in human immunodeficiency virus 1 infection. J Clin Pathol. 1991;44:64-68.

210. Weinhold KJ, Lyerly HK, Stanley SD, et al. HIV-1 GP120-mediated immune suppression and lymphocyte destruction in the absence of viral infection. J Immunol. 1989;142:3091-3097.

211. Hildreth JE, Orentas RJ. Involvement of a leukocyte adhesion receptor (LFA-1) in HIV-induced syncytium formation. Science. 1989;244:1075-1078.

212. Sato AI, Balamuth FB, Ugen KE, et al. Identification of CD7 glycoprotein as an accessory molecule in HIV-1-mediated syncytium formation and cell free infection. J Immunol. 1994;152:5142-5152.

213. deSantis C, Robbioni P, Longhi R, et al. Role of HLA class I in HIV type 1-induced syncytium formation. AIDS Res Hum Retroviruses. 1996;12:1031-1040.

214. Stanley S, McCune J, Kaneshima H, et al. Human immunodeficiency virus infection of the human thymus and disruption of the thymic microenvironment in the SCID-hu mouse. J Exp Med. 1993;178:1151-1163.

215. Valentin H, Nugeyre MT, Vuillier F, et al. Two subpopulations of human triple-negative thymic cells are susceptible to infection by human immunodeficiency virus type 1 in vitro. J Virol. 1994;68:3041-3050.

216. Douek DC, McFarland RD, Keiser PH, et al. Changes in thymic function with age and during the treatment of HIV infection. Nature. 1998;396:690-695.

217. Jamieson BD, Douek DC, Killian S, et al. Generation of functional thymocytes in the human adult. Immunity. 1999;10:569-575.

218. Zhang L, Lewin SR, Markowitz M, et al. Measuring recent thymic emigrants in blood of normal and HIV-1-infected individuals before and after effective therapy. J Exp Med. 1999;190:725-732.

219. Re MC, Zauli G, Gibellini D, et al. Uninfected haematopoietic progenitor (CD34+) cells purified from the bone marrow of AIDS patients are committed to apoptotic cell death in culture. AIDS. 1993;7:1049-1055.

220. Folks TM, Kessler SW, Orenstein JM, et al. Infection and replication of HIV-1 in purified progenitor cells of normal human bone marrow. Science. 1988;242:919-922.

221. Neal TF, Holland HK, Baum CM, et al. CD34+ progenitor cells from asymptomatic patients are not a major reservoir for human immunodeficiency virus-1. Blood. 1995;86:1749-1756.

222. Stanley SK, Kessler SW, Justement JS, et al. CD34+ bone marrow cells are infected with HIV in a subset of seropositive individuals. J Immunol. 1992;149:689-697.

223. Deichmann M, Kronenwett R, Haas R. Expression of the human immunodeficiency virus type-1 coreceptors CXCR-4 (fusin, LESTR) and CKR-5 in CD34+ hematopoietic progenitor cells. Blood. 1997;89:3522-3528.

224. Hengel RL, Jones BM, Kennedy MS, et al. Cd4+ T cells programmed to traffic to lymph nodes account for increases in numbers of cd4+ T cells up to 1 year after the initiation of highly active antiretroviral therapy for human immunodeficiency virus type 1 infection. J Infect Dis. 2001;184:93-97.

225. Giorgi JV, Ho H-N, Hirji K, et al. CD8+ Lymphocyte activation at human immunodeficiency virus type 1 seroconversion: Development of HLA-DR+ CD38- CD8+ cells is associated with subsequent stable CD4+ cell levels. J Infect Dis. 1994;170:775-781.

226. Mocroft A, Bofill M, Lipman M, et al. CD8+,CD38+ lymphocyte percent: a useful immunological marker for monitoring HIV-1-infected patients. J Acquir Immune Defic Syndr Hum Retrovirol. 1997;14:158-162.

227. Kammerer R, Iten A, Frei PC, Burgisser P. Expansion of T cells negative for CD28 expression in HIV infection. Relation to activation markers and cell adhesion molecules, and correlation with prognostic markers. Med Microbiol Immunol (Berl). 1996;185:19-25.

228. Vingerhoets JH, Vanham GL, Kestens LL, et al. Increased cytolytic T lymphocyte activity and decreased B7 responsiveness are associated with CD28 down-regulation on CD8+ T cells from HIV-infected subjects. Clin Exp Immunol. 1995;100:425-433.

229. Carmichael A, Jin X, Sissons P, Borysiewicz L. Quantitative analysis of the human immunodeficiency virus type 1 (HIV-1)-specific cytotoxic T lymphocyte (CTL) response at different stages of HIV-1 infection: Differential CTL responses to HIV-1 and Epstein-Barr virus in late disease. J Exp Med. 1993;177:249-256.

230. Forte M, Maartens G, Rahelu M, et al. Cytolytic T-cell activity against mycobacterial antigens in HIV. AIDS. 1992;6:407-411.

231. Mackewicz CE, Yang LC, Lifson JD, Levy JA. Non-cytolytic CD8 T-cell anti-HIV responses in primary HIV-1 infection. Lancet. 1994;344:1671-1673.

232. Zanussi S, D'Andrea M, Simonelli C, et al. Serum levels of RANTES and MIP-1a in HIV-positive long-term survivors and progressor patients. AIDS. 1996;10:1431-1432.

233. Amadori A, Chieco-Bianchi L. B-cell activation and HIV-1 infection: Deeds and misdeeds. Immunol Today. 1990;11:374-379.

234. Moir S, Malaspina A, Ogwaro KM, et al. HIV-1 induces phenotypic and functional perturbations of B cells in chronically infected individuals. Proc Natl Acad Sci U S A. 2001;98:10362-10367.

235. Kehrl JH, Rieckmann P, Kozlow E, Fauci AS. Lymphokine production by B cells from normal and HIV-infected individuals. Ann N Y Acad Sci. 1992;651:220-227.

236. Rieckmann P, Poli G, Fox CH, et al. Recombinant gp120 specifically enhances tumor necrosis factor-alpha production and Ig secretion in B lymphocytes from HIV-infected individuals but not from seronegative donors. J Immunol. 1991;147:2922-2927.

237. Rieckmann P, Poli G, Kehrl JH, Fauci AS. Activated B lymphocytes from human immunodeficiency virus-infected individuals induce virus expression in infected T cells and a promonocytic cell line, U1. J Exp Med. 1991;173:1-5.

238. Berberian L, Goodglick L, Kipps TJ, Braun J. Immunoglobulin VH3 gene products: natural ligands for HIV gp120. Science. 1993;261:1588-1591.

239. Goodglick L, Zevit N, Neshat MS, Braun J. Mapping the Ig superantigen-binding site of HIV-1 gp120. J Immunol. 1995;155:5151-5159.

240. Chirmule N, Kalyanaraman VS, Saxinger C, et al. Localization of B-cell stimulatory activity of HIV-1 to the carboxyl terminus of gp41. AIDS Res Hum Retroviruses. 1990;6:299-305.

241. Dolcetti R, Gloghini A, De Vita S, et al. Characteristics of EBV-infected cells in HIV-related lymphadenopathy: Implications for the pathogenesis of EBV-associated and EBV-unrelated lymphomas of HIV-seropositive individuals. Int J Cancer. 1995;63:652-659.

242. Monroe JG, Silberstein LE. HIV-mediated B-lymphocyte activation and lymphomagenesis. J Clin Immunol. 1995;15:61-68.

243. Yao QY, Tierney RJ, Croom-Carter D, et al. Frequency of multiple Epstein-Barr virus infections in T-cell-immunocompromised individuals. J Virol. 1996;70:4884-4894.

244. Goetz DW, Webb EL Jr, Whisman BA, Freeman TM. Aeroallergen-specific IgE changes in individuals with rapid human immunodeficiency virus disease progression. Ann Allergy Asthma Immunol. 1997;78:301-306.

245. Rodriguez C, Thomas JK, O'Rourke S, et al. HIV disease in children is associated with a selective decrease in CD23+ and CD62L+ B cells. Clin Immunol Immunopathol. 1996;81:191-199.

246. Hu PF, Hultin LE, Hultin P, et al. Natural killer cell immunodeficiency in HIV disease is manifest by profoundly decreased numbers of CD16+CD56+ cells and expansion of a population of CD16dimCD56- cells with low lytic activity. J Acquir Immune Defic Syndr Hum Retrovirol. 1995;10:331-340.

247. Kottilil S, Chun TW, Moir S, et al. Innate immunity in human immunodeficiency virus infection: Effect of viremia on natural killer cell function. J Infect Dis. 2003;187:1038-1045.

248. Ahmad A, Menezes J. Defective killing activity against gp120/41-expressing human erythroleukaemic K562 cell line by monocytes and natural killer cells from HIV-infected individuals. AIDS. 1996;10:143-149.

249. Ahmad A, Menezes J. Antibody-dependent cellular cytotoxicity in HIV infections. FASEB J. 1996;10:258-266.

250. Ullum H, Gotzsche PC, Victor J, et al. Defective natural immunity: an early manifestation of human immunodeficiency virus infection. J Exp Med. 1995;182:789-799.

251. Oliva A, Kinter AL, Vaccarezza M, et al. Natural killer cells from human immunodeficiency virus (HIV)-infected individuals are an important source of CC-chemokines and suppress HIV-1 entry and replication in vitro. J Clin Invest. 1998;102:223-231.

252. Elbim C, Prevot MH, Bouscarat F, et al. Impairment of polymorphonuclear neutrophil function in HIV-infected patients. J Cardiovasc Pharmacol. 1995;25(suppl 2):S66-S70.

253. Jarstrand C, Akerlund B. Oxygen radical release by neutrophils of HIV-infected patients. Chem Biol Interact. 1994;91:141-146.

254. Meyer CN, Nielsen H. Priming of neutrophil and monocyte activation in human immunodeficiency virus infection. Comparison of granulocyte colony-stimulating factor, granulocyte-macrophage colony-stimulating factor and interferon-gamma. APMIS. 1996;104:640-646.

255. Tachavanich K, Pattanapanyasat K, Sarasombath S, et al. Opsonophagocytosis and intracellular killing activity of neutrophils in patients with human immunodeficiency virus infection. Asian Pac J Allergy Immunol. 1996;14:49-56.

256. Pitrak DL, Tsai HC, Mullane KM, et al. Accelerated neutrophil apoptosis in the acquired immunodeficiency syndrome. J Clin Invest. 1996;98:2714-2719.

257. Torosantucci A, Chiani P, Quinti I, et al. Responsiveness of human polymorphonuclear cells (PMNL) to stimulation by a mannoprotein fraction (MP-F2) of *Candida albicans;* Enhanced production of IL-6 and tumour necrosis factor-alpha (TNF-alpha) by MP-F2-stimulated PMNL from HIV-infected subjects. Clin Exp Immunol. 1997;107:451-457.

258. Wenisch C, Parschalk B, Zedwitz-Liebenstein K, et al. Dysregulation of the polymorphonuclear leukocyte—*Candida* spp. interaction in HIV-positive patients. AIDS. 1996;10:983-987.

259. Tascini C, Baldelli F, Monari C, et al. Inhibition of fungicidal activity of polymorphonuclear leukocytes from HIV-infected patients by interleukin (IL)-4 and IL-10. AIDS. 1996;10:477-483.

260. Fauci AS. Multifactorial nature of human immunodeficiency virus diseases: Implications for therapy. Science. 1993;262:1011-1018.

261. Cheng-Mayer C, Liu R, Landau NR, Stamatatos L. Macrophage tropism of human immunodeficiency virus type 1 and utilization of the CC-CKR5 coreceptor. J Virol. 1997;71:1657-1661.

262. He J, Chen Y, Farzan M, et al. CCR3 and CCR5 are co-receptors for HIV-1 infection of microglia. Nature. 1997;385:645-649.

263. Perelson AS, Essunger P, Cao Y, et al. Decay characteristics of HIV-1 infected compartments during combination therapy. Nature. 1997;387:188-191.

264. Schnittman SM, Psallidopoulos MC, Lane HC, et al. The reservoir for HIV-1 in human peripheral blood is a T cell that maintains expression of CD4 (published erratum appears in Science. 1989;245:694). Science. 1989;245:305-308.

265. Plata F, Autran B, Martins LP, et al. AIDS virus-specific cytotoxic T lymphocytes in lung disorders. Nature. 1987;328:348-351.

266. Collman R, Hassan NF, Walker R, et al. Infection of monocyte-derived macrophages with human immunodeficiency virus type 1 (HIV-1). J Exp Med. 1989;170.

267. Armstrong J, Horne R. Follicular dendritic cells and virus-like particles in AIDS-related lymphadenopathy. Lancet. 1984;ii:370-372.

268. Orenstein J, Fox C, Wahl S. Macrophages as a source of HIV during opportunistic infections. Science. 1997;276:1857-1861.

269. Britton CB, Miller JR. Neurological complications in acquired immunodeficiency syndrome (AIDS). Neurol Clin. 1984;2:315-339.

270. Neilson SL, Petito CK, Urmacher CD, Posner JB. Subacute encephalitis in acquired immune deficiency syndrome: A postmortem study. Am J Clin Pathol. 1984;82: 678-682.

271. Faulstich M. Acquired immune deficiency syndrome: An overview of central nervous system complications and neuropsychological sequelae. Int J Neurosci. 1986;30: 249-254.

272. Cinque P, Vago L, Mengozzi M, et al. Elevated cerebrospinal fluid levels of monocyte chemotactic protein-1 correlate with HIV-1 encephalitis and local viral replication. AIDS. 1998;12:1327-1332.

273. Giulian D, Vaca K, Noonan CA. Secretion of neurotoxins by mononuclear phagocytes infected with HIV-1. Science. 1990;250:1593-1596.

274. Yoo J, Chen H, Kraus T, et al. Altered cytokine production and accessory cell function after HIV-1 infection. J Immunol. 1996;157:1313-1320.

275. Polyak S, Chen H, Hirsch D, et al. Impaired class II expression and antigen uptake in monocytic cells after HIV-1 infection. J Immunol. 1997;159:2177-2188.

276. Meyaard L, Schuitemaker H, Miedema F. T-cell dysfunction in HIV infection: Anergy due to defective antigen-presenting cell function? Immunol Today. 1993;14:161-164.

277. Bender BS, Augor FA, Quinn TC, et al. Impaired antibody-dependent cell-mediated cytotoxic activity in patients with the acquired immunodeficiency syndrome. Clin Exp Immunol. 1986;64:166-172.

278. Kent SJ, Stent G, Sonza S, et al. HIV-1 infection of monocyte-derived macrophages reduces Fc and complement receptor expression. Clin Exp Immunol. 1994;95:450-454.

279. Poli G, Botazzi B, Acero R, et al. Monocyte function in intravenous drug abusers with lymphadenopathy syndrome and in patients with acquired immunodeficiency syndrome: Selective impairment of chemotaxis. Clin Exp Immunol. 1985;62:136-142.

280. Spear GT, Kessler HA, Rothberg L, et al. Decreased oxidative burst activity of monocytes from asymptomatic HIV-infected individuals. Clin Immunol Immunopathol. 1990;54:184-191.

281. Crowe SM, Vardaxis NJ, Kent SJ, et al. HIV infection of monocyte-derived macrophages in vitro reduces phagocytosis of *Candida albicans.* J Leukoc Biol. 1994;56:318-327.

282. Biggs BA, Hewish M, Kent S, et al. HIV-1 infection of human macrophages impairs phagocytosis and killing of *Toxoplasma gondii.* J Immunol. 1995;154:6132-6139.

283. Chaturvedi S, Newman SL. Modulation of the effector function of human macrophages for *Histoplasma capsulatum* by HIV-1. Role of the envelope glycoprotein gp120. J Clin Invest. 1997;100:1465-1474.

284. Granelli-Piperno A, Moser B, Pope M, et al. Efficient interaction of HIV-1 with purified dendritic cells via multiple chemokine coreceptors. J Exp Med. 1996;184:2433-2438.

285. Rubbert A, Combadiere C, Ostrowski M, et al. Dendritic cells express multiple chemokine receptors used as coreceptors for HIV entry. J Immunol. 1998;160:3933-3941.

286. Macatonia SE, Lau R, Patterson S, et al. Dendritic cell infection, depletion and dysfunction in HIV-infected individuals. Immunology. 1990;71:38-45.

287. Zambruno G, Giannetti A, Bertazzoni U, Girolomoni G. Langerhans cells and HIV infection. Immunol Today. 1995;16:520-524.

288. Weissman D, Fauci AS. Role of dendritic cells in immunopathogenesis of human immunodeficiency virus infection. Clin Microbiol Rev. 1997;10:358-367.

289. Roberts M, Gompels M, Pinching AJ, Knight SC. Dendritic cells from HIV-1 infected individuals show reduced capacity to stimulate autologous T-cell proliferation. Immunol Lett. 1994;43:39-43.

290. Cameron PU, Forsum U, Teppler H, et al. During HIV-1 infection most blood dendritic cells are not productively infected and can induce allogeneic CD4+ T cell clonal expansion. Clin Exp Immunol. 1992;88:226-236.

291. Cohen OJ, Kinter A, Fauci AS. Host factors in the pathogenesis of HIV disease. Immunol Rev. 1997;159:31-48.

292. Fauci AS. Host factors and the pathogenesis of HIV-induced disease. Nature. 1996;384:529-534.

293. Chun TW, Engel D, Mizell SB, et al. Induction of HIV-1 replication in latently infected CD4(+) T cells using a combination of cytokines. J Exp Med. 1998;188:83-91.

294. Fultz PN, Gluckman JC, Muchmore E, Girard M. Transient increases in numbers of infectious cells in an HIV-infected chimpanzee following immune stimulation. AIDS Res Hum Retroviruses. 1992;8:313-317.

295. Staprans S, Hamilton B, Follansbee S, et al. Activation of virus replication after vaccination of HIV-1-infected individuals. J Exp Med. 1995;182:1727-1737.

296. Stanley S, Ostrowski MA, Justement JS, et al. Effect of immunization with a common recall antigen on viral expression in patients infected with human immunodeficiency virus type 1. N Engl J Med. 1996;334:1222-1230.

297. Goletti D, Weissman D, Jackson RW, et al. Effect of *Mycobacterium tuberculosis* on HIV replication. Role of immune activation. J Immunol. 1996;157:1271-1278.

298. Ostrowski MA, Stanley SK, Justement JS, et al. Increased in vitro tetanus-induced production of HIV type 1 following in vivo immunization of HIV type 1-infected individuals with tetanus toxoid. AIDS Res Hum Retroviruses. 1997;13:473-480.

299. Grossman Z, Feinberg MB, Paul WE. Multiple modes of cellular activation and virus transmission in HIV infection: A role for chronically and latently infected cells in sustaining viral replication. Proc Natl Acad Sci U S A. 1998;95:6314-6319.

300. Miedema F. Immunological abnormalities in the natural history of HIV infection: Mechanisms and clinical relevance. Immunodefic Rev. 1992;3:173-193.

301. Poli G, Fauci A. Role of cytokines in the pathogenesis of human immunodeficiency virus infection. In: Aggarwal B, Puri R, eds. Human cytokines: Their role in disease and therapy. Cambridge, MA: Blackwell Science; 1995:421-449.

302. Boyle M, Berger M, Tschuchnigg M, et al. Increased expression of interferon-gamma in hyperplastic lymph nodes from HIV-infected patients. Clin Exp Immunol. 1993;92:100-105.

303. Graziosi C, Pantaleo G, Gantt KR, et al. Lack of evidence for the dichotomy of TH1 and TH2 predominance in HIV-infected individuals. Science. 1994;265:248-252.

304. Pantaleo G, Graziosi C, Butini L, et al. Lymphoid organs function as major reservoirs for human immunodeficiency virus. Proc Natl Acad Sci U S A. 1991;88:9838-9842.

305. Jassoy C, Walker B. HIV-1-specific cytotoxic T lymphocytes and the control of HIV-1 replication. Springer Semin Immunopathol. 1997;18:341-354.

306. Esser R, vonBriesen H, Brugger M, et al. Secretory repertoire of HIV-infected human monocytes/macrophages. Pathobiology. 1991;59:219-222.

307. Lane HC, Depper JM, Greene WC, et al. Qualitative analysis of immune function in patients with the acquired immunodeficiency syndrome: Evidence for a selective defect in soluble antigen recognition. N Engl J Med. 1985;313:79-84.

308. Clerici M, Lucey D, Berzofsky J, et al. Restoration of HIV-specific cell-mediated immune responses by interleukin-12 in vitro. Science. 1993;262:1721-1724.

309. Trinchieri G. Interleukin-12 and its role in the generation of TH1 cells. Immunol Today. 1993;14:335-338.

310. Clerici M, Hakim F, Venzon D, et al. Changes in interleukin-2 and interleukin-4 production in asymptomatic, human immunodeficiency virus-seropositive individuals. J Clin Invest. 1993;91:759-765.

311. Clerici M, Wynn T, Berzofsky J, et al. Role of interleukin-10 in T helper cell dysfunction in asymptomatic individuals infected with the human immunodeficiency virus. J Clin Invest. 1994;93:768-775.

312. Maggi E, Mazzetti M, Ravina A, et al. Ability of HIV to promote a TH1 to TH0 shift and to replicate preferentially in TH2 and TH0 cells. Science. 1994;265:244-248.

313. Clerici M, Shearer G. A TH1-TH2 switch is a critical step in the etiology of HIV infection. Immunol Today. 1993;14:107-111.

314. Klein SA, Dobmeyer JM, Dobmeyer TS, et al. Demonstration of the Th1 to Th2 cytokine shift during the course of HIV-1 infection using cytoplasmic cytokine detection on single cell level by flow cytometry. AIDS. 1997;11:1111-1118.

315. Vyakarnam A, Matear P, Martin S, Wagstaff M. Th1 cells specific for HIV-1 gag p24 are less efficient than Th0 cells in supporting HIV replication, and inhibit virus replication in Th0 cells. Immunology. 1995;86:85-96.

316. Clerici M, Balotta C, Meroni L, et al. Type 1 cytokine production and low prevalence of viral isolation correlate with long term non-progression in HIV infection. AIDS Res Hum Retroviruses. 1996;12:1053-1061.

317. Folks TM, Justement J, Kinter A, et al. Cytokine-induced expression of HIV-1 in a chronically infected promonocyte cell line. Science. 1987;238:800-802.

318. Clouse KA, Robbins PB, Fernie B, et al. Viral antigen stimulation of the production of human monokines capable of regulating HIV1 expression. J Immunol. 1989;143:470-475.

319. Rieckmann P, Poli G, Kerhrl JH, Fauci AS. Activated B lymphocytes from human immunodeficiency virus-infected individuals induce virus expression in infected T cells and a promonocytic cell line, U1. J Exp Med. 1991;173:1-5.

320. Smithgall M, Wong J, Critchett K, Haffar O. IL-7 up-regulates HIV-1 replication in naturally infected peripheral blood mononuclear cells. J Immunol. 1996;156:2324-2330.

321. Bayard-McNeeley M, Doo H, He S, et al. Differential effects of interleukin-12, interleukin-15, and interleukin-2 on human immunodeficiency virus type 1 replication in vitro. Clin Diagn Lab Immunol. 1996;3:547-553.

322. Kinter AL, Poli G, Fox L, et al. HIV replication in IL-2-stimulated peripheral blood mononuclear cells is driven in an autocrine/paracrine manner by endogenous cytokines. J Immunol. 1995;154:2448-2459.

323. Lucey DR, Pinto LA, Bethke FR, et al. In vitro immunologic and virologic effects of interleukin 15 on peripheral blood mononuclear cells from normal donors and human immunodeficiency virus type 1-infected patients. Clin Diagn Lab Immunol. 1997;4:43-48.

324. Naif HM, Li S, Ho-Shon M, et al. The state of maturation of monocytes into macrophages determines the effects of IL-4 and IL-13 on HIV replication. J Immunol. 1997;158:501-511.

325. Valentin A, Lu W, Rosati M, et al. Dual effect of interleukin 4 on HIV-1 expression: Implications for viral phenotypic switch and disease progression. Proc Natl Acad Sci U S A. 1998;95:8886-8891.

326. Weissman D, Poli G, Fauci AS. IL-10 synergizes with multiple cytokines in enhancing HIV production in cells of monocytic lineage. J Acquir Immune Defic Syndr Hum Retrovirol. 1995;9:442-449.

327. Finnegan A, Roebuck KA, Nakai BE, et al. IL-10 cooperates with TNF-alpha to activate HIV-1 from latently and acutely infected cells of monocyte/macrophage lineage. J Immunol. 1996;156:841-851.

328. Poli G, Bressler P, Kinter A, et al. Interleukin 6 induces human immunodeficiency virus expression in infected monocytic cells alone and in synergy with tumor necrosis factor alpha by transcriptional and post-transcriptional mechanisms. J Exp Med. 1990;172:151-158.

329. Poli G, Kinter AL, Fauci AS. Interleukin 1 induces expression of the human immunodeficiency virus alone and in synergy with interleukin 6 in chronically infected U1 cells: Inhibition of inductive effects by the interleukin 1 receptor antagonist. Proc Natl Acad Sci U S A. 1994;91:108-112.

330. Poli G, Kinter AL, Justement JS, et al. Transforming growth factor beta suppresses human immunodeficiency virus expression and replication in infected cells of the monocyte/macrophage lineage. J Exp Med. 1991;173:589-597.

331. Osborn L, Kunkel S, Nabel GJ. Tumor necrosis factor alpha and interleukin 1 stimulate the human immunodeficiency virus enhancer by activation of the nuclear factor kappa B. Proc Natl Acad Sci U S A. 1989;86:2336-2340.

332. Duh EJ, Maury WJ, Folks TM, et al. Tumor necrosis factor alpha activates human immunodeficiency virus type 1 through induction of nuclear factor binding to the NF-kappa B sites in the long terminal repeat. Proc Natl Acad Sci U S A. 1989;86:5974-5978.

333. Goletti D, Kinter AL, Hardy EC, et al. Modulation of endogenous IL-1 beta and IL-1 receptor antagonist results in opposing effects on HIV expression in chronically infected monocytic cells. J Immunol. 1996;156:3501-3508.

334. Weissman D, Poli G, Fauci AS. Interleukin 10 blocks HIV replication in macrophages by inhibiting the autocrine loop of tumor necrosis factor alpha and interleukin 6 induction of virus. AIDS Res Hum Retroviruses. 1994;10:1199-1206.

335. Goletti D, Weissman D, Jackson RW, et al. In vitro induction of human immunodeficiency virus (HIV) replication in purified protein derivative-positive HIV-infected persons by recall antigen response to *Mycobacterium tuberculosis is* the result of a balance of the effects of endogenous interleukin-2 and proinflammatory and antiinflammatory cytokines. J Infect Dis. 1998;177:1332-1338.

336. Clerici M, Piconi S, Balotta C, et al. Pentoxifylline improves cell-mediated immunity and reduces human immunodeficiency virus (HIV) plasma viremia in asymptomatic HIV-seropositive persons. J Infect Dis. 1997;175:1210-1215.

337. Kollmann TR, Pettoello-Mantovani M, Katopodis NF, et al. Inhibition of acute in vivo human immunodeficiency virus infection by human interleukin 10 treatment of SCID mice implanted with human fetal thymus and liver. Proc Natl Acad Sci U S A. 1996;93:3126-3131.

338. Kovacs JA, Vogel S, Albert JM, et al. Controlled trial of interleukin-2 infusions in patients infected with the human immunodeficiency virus. N Engl J Med. 1996;335:1350-1356.

339. Kanai T, Thomas EK, Yasutomi Y, Letvin NL. IL-15 stimulates the expansion of AIDS virus-specific CTL. J Immunol. 1996;157:3681-3687.

340. Lin S, Roberts R, Ank B, et al. Human immunodeficiency virus (HIV) type-1 GP120-specific cell-mediated cytotoxicity (CMC) and natural killer (NK) activity in HIV-infected (HIV+) subjects: Enhancement with interleukin-2 (IL-2), IL-12, and IL-15. Clin Immunol Immunopathol. 1997;82:163-173.

341. McKenzie A, Zurawski G. Interleukin-13: characterization and biologic properties. Cancer Treat Res. 1995;80:367-378.

342. Trinchieri G, Scott P. The role of interleukin 12 in the immune response, disease and therapy. Immunol Today. 1994;15:460-463.

343. Kacani L, Stoiber H, Dierich MP. Role of IL-15 in HIV-1-associated hypergammaglobulinaemia. Clin Exp Immunol. 1997;108:14-18.

344. Baggiolini M, Dewald B, Moser B. Human chemokines: An update. Ann Rev Immunol. 1997;15:675-705.

345. Weissman D, Rabin RL, Arthos J, et al. Macrophage-tropic HIV and SIV envelope proteins induce a signal through the CCR5 chemokine receptor. Nature. 1997;389:981-985.

346. Kinter A, Catanzaro A, Monaco J, et al. CC-chemokines enhance the replication of T-tropic strains of HIV-1 in CD4(+) T cells: Role of signal transduction. Proc Natl Acad Sci U S A. 1998;95:11880-11885.

347. Levine BL, Mosca JD, Riley JL, et al. Antiviral effect and ex vivo CD4+ T cell proliferation in HIV-positive patients as a result of CD28 costimulation. Science. 1996;272:1939-1943.

348. Carroll RG, Riley JL, Levine BL, et al. Differential regulation of HIV-1 fusion cofactor expression by CD28 costimulation of CD4+ T cells. Science. 1997;276:273-276.

349. Zhu T, Mo H, Wang N, et al. Genotypic and phenotypic characterization of HIV-1 in patients with primary infection. Science. 1993;261:1179-1181.

350. Unutmaz D, Littman D. Expression pattern of HIV-1 coreceptors on T cells: Implications for viral transmission and lymphocyte homing. Proc Natl Acad Sci U S A. 1997;94:1615-1618.

351. Ostrowski M, Justement S, Catanzaro A, et al. Expression of chemokine receptors CXCR4 and CCR5 in HIV-1 infected and uninfected individuals. J Immunol. 1998.

352. Moriuchi H, Moriuchi M, Fauci AS. Factors secreted by human T lymphotropic virus type I (HTLV-I)-infected cells can enhance or inhibit replication of HIV-1 in HTLV-I-uninfected cells: Implications for in vivo coinfection with HTLV-I and HIV-1. J Exp Med. 1998;187:1689-1697.

General Clinical Manifestations of Human Immunodeficiency Virus Infection (Including the Acute Retroviral Syndrome and Oral, Cutaneous, Renal, Ocular, and Cardiac Diseases)

TIMOTHY R. STERLING

RICHARD E. CHAISSON

Human immunodeficiency virus (HIV) infection results in a wide range of clinical consequences from asymptomatic carriage to life-threatening opportunistic disease. In persons infected with HIV, ongoing viral replication produces a sequential decline in and ablation of cell-mediated immunity, giving rise to diverse manifestations of opportunistic disease. The acquired immunodeficiency syndrome (AIDS) is the most advanced stage of this illness, in which the infected host can no longer control opportunistic organisms or malignancies that rarely cause illness in immunocompetent individuals. The clinical features of HIV may vary according to the individual's age, sex, race, geographic location, treatment status, and behavioral history. This chapter reviews selected clinical aspects of HIV infection from the acquisition of the virus to death with AIDS and discusses the classification and staging of this important viral infection.

HISTORY

Disease caused by HIV-induced immunosuppression was first described in late 1980 and early 1981, when physicians in Los Angeles, New York, and San Francisco observed opportunistic infections in homosexual men.[1-4] Simultaneously, an outbreak of Kaposi's sarcoma (KS), a previously rare malignancy, was reported in young homosexual men from the same three cities.[5,6] These patients had a selective defect in cell-mediated immunity that was manifested by low numbers of CD4+ T lymphocytes and the development of opportunistic infections.

That opportunistic disease occurred in homosexual men who had previously been healthy suggested that immunodeficiency developed because of an acquired rather than a congenital trait. In 1982, the Centers for Disease Control (CDC) developed a case definition, based on the clinical, immunologic, and epidemiologic features of the first clusters of cases, for what was called the acquired immunodeficiency syndrome (see Chapter 114).[7] AIDS was defined as the occurrence of a reliably diagnosed disease at least moderately indicative of underlying cellular immunodeficiency in a person without a condition known to be associated with an increased incidence of diseases related to cellular immunodeficiency.[6,8] AIDS became a reportable condition in the United States in 1983. Soon after the initial case reports of AIDS, additional cases were observed in persons other than homosexual men. In 1981 and 1982, heterosexual intravenous drug users and immigrants from Haiti were reported to have AIDS.[3,9-12] AIDS cases in hemophiliacs, recipients of blood transfusions, and Africans were soon reported.[13,14]

As the groups of persons at risk for AIDS expanded, clinicians noted an increasing spectrum of clinical manifestations of AIDS-associated immunodeficiency. Unexplained generalized lymphadenopathy, idiopathic thrombocytopenia, oral candidiasis, herpes zoster, and a constitutional wasting syndrome were observed in persons from AIDS risk groups who had deficits in cellular immunity.[15-19] The term *AIDS-related complex* was coined to describe the signs and symptoms of immunodeficiency recognized with increasing frequency in persons at risk for AIDS.[20] In 1982 to 1983, several investigators postulated an asymptomatic carrier state of the AIDS agent in healthy homosexual men, heterosexual partners of intravenous drug users, and Haitians who were noted to have laboratory evidence of impaired cellular immunity.[21] After HIV was first described in 1983 to 1984,[22-24] serologic tests to identify persons infected with HIV were developed that allowed large serologic surveys of at-risk populations to estimate the number of individuals infected with the virus and to delineate the spectrum of HIV-associated diseases.

Retrospective studies of serum and tissue indicate that the virus was present in Africa as early as 1959 and that disease associated with HIV occurred in the United States in 1968.[25,26] The CDC expanded its case definition of AIDS in 1985 and again in 1987 (see Chapter 114) to accommodate the increased number of manifestations of impaired cellular immunity that had become associated with HIV infection.[27,28] The World Health Organization (WHO) also promulgated a case definition for AIDS for use in developing countries that lacked sophisticated diagnostic resource.[29] The AIDS case definition and HIV staging system were revised again in 1993 to include individuals with advanced immunodeficiency and with several other clinical manifestations of HIV disease.[30] New insights into the pathogenesis of HIV disease have emphasized the critical role of viral dynamics in the natural history of HIV infection,[31-33] leading to clinical management schemata based largely on viral load and CD4+ cell levels, as discussed in the following.

CLASSIFICATION OF HUMAN IMMUNODEFICIENCY VIRUS INFECTION

HIV infection represents an ongoing active viral process in a majority of untreated individuals associated with progressive immunodeficiency that is likely to result in serious clinical consequences. Although there may be a prolonged state of clinical latency, during which many patients are unaware of their infection, HIV infection is usually not virologically latent, and infection with the virus should be considered a disease state. Individuals who are infected but asymptomatic may not be ill but do have a chronic and progressive condition that without treatment may ultimately result in a significant impairment and death. Although distinguishing between HIV infection and AIDS has been historically useful for epidemiologic purposes, the distinction is somewhat arbitrary and is less meaningful from a clinical perspective in an era of potent antiretroviral drug therapy. As already noted, current clinical staging approaches favor use of the CD4+ lymphocyte counts and plasma viral load assays.

Several systems for classifying HIV infection and disease have been developed. The 1986 CDC classification system placed HIV-infected persons into four categories: group I, acute infection; group II, asymptomatic infection; group III, persistent generalized lymphadenopathy (PGL); and group IV, symptomatic HIV disease.[34] This system had limited prognostic utility and was supplanted by the 1993 classification system and revised case definition.[30] The 1993 CDC classification system for HIV categorizes HIV-infected individuals according to clinical and CD4+ cell count groupings. The clinical categories are group A, asymptomatic, acute HIV infection, or PGL; group B, symptomatic HIV disease; and group C, AIDS indicator conditions, encompassing the 1987 case definition with the addition of recurrent bacterial pneumonia, pulmonary tuberculosis, and invasive cervical cancer. The CD4+ cell levels are (1) 500/mm³ or greater, (2) 200 to 499/mm³, and (3) less than 200/mm³. CD4+ cell percentages may be used in place of CD4+ cell number. As noted before, patients in all three clinical categories whose CD4+ cell count is less than 200/mm³ or 14% (stages A3, B3, and C3) are now classified as having AIDS by the CDC surveillance definition, along with patients who have AIDS indicator conditions (stages C1, C2, and C3).

The 1993 CDC classification system for HIV infection recognized the prognostic significance of the CD4+ cell count in individuals with HIV infection but was developed before the importance of viral load in the pathogenesis of HIV disease was known. Even so, it is impor-

tant to recognize that there is considerable variation in risk of opportunistic complications and prognosis among individuals with CD4+ cell counts below 200/mm³. Those with CD4+ counts below 50/mm³, for example, are generally considered to have advanced HIV disease and are at much higher risk for death and for development of opportunistic infections such as cytomegalovirus (CMV) disease or disseminated *Mycobacterium avium* complex infection. The CDC classification system was developed at a time when the inevitable course of HIV infection was progression toward advanced immunodeficiency and death and when drug therapy was of limited and transient efficacy in stemming the course of the disease. According to the CDC classification system, HIV-infected individuals are classified on the basis of the most advanced stage they have reached. In the present era, patients treated with combination antiretroviral therapy often experience marked improvement in cellular immune function and have a dramatically lower risk of developing opportunistic disease than they had before receiving treatment. There is no current mechanism for reclassifying patients on the basis of immunologic and clinical improvement resulting from antiretroviral therapy, a situation that understandably curtails use of the CDC and similar staging systems (e.g., the Walter Reed and WHO systems). In areas where combination antiretroviral therapy is not available or widely used, these classification schemes more reliably reflect the maturity and status of the HIV epidemic within populations. The WHO classification system (Table 117-1) is used primarily in developing countries. However, there are limitations

---

TABLE 117-1 World Health Organization Clinical Staging System

Clinical Stage 1
Asymptomatic
Persistent generalized lymphadenopathy (PGL)
Performance scale 1: asymptomatic, normal activity

Clinical Stage 2
Weight loss, <10% of body weight
Minor mucocutaneous manifestations
Herpes zoster, within the last 5 years
Recurrent upper respiratory tract infections (e.g., bacterial sinusitis)
And/or performance scale 2: symptomatic, normal activity

Clinical stage 3
Weight loss, >10% of body weight
Unexplained chronic diarrhea, >1 month
Unexplained prolonged fever (intermittent or constant), >1 month
Oral candidiasis (thrush)
Oral hairy leukoplakia
Pulmonary tuberculosis, within the past year
Severe bacterial infections (e.g., pneumonia, pyomyositis)
And/or performance scale 3: bedridden, >50% of the day during the last month

Clinical stage 4
HIV wasting syndrome, as defined by CDC[30]
Pneumocystis jirovecii pneumonia
Toxoplasmosis of the brain
Cryptosporidiosis with diarrhea, >1 month
Cryptococcosis, extrapulmonary
Cytomegalovirus (CMV) disease of an organ other than liver, spleen, or lymph nodes
Herpes simplex virus (HSV) infection, mucocutaneous >1 month, or visceral any duration
Progressive multifocal leukoencephalopathy (PML)
Any disseminated endemic mycosis (e.g., histoplasmosis, coccidioidomycosis)
Candidiasis of the esophagus, trachea, bronchi, or lungs
Atypical mycobacteriosis, disseminated
Nontyphoid *Salmonella* septicemia
Extrapulmonary tuberculosis
Lymphoma
Kaposi's sarcoma (KS)
HIV encephalopathy, as defined by CDC[30]
And/or performance scale 4: bedridden, >50% of the day during the last month

CDC, Centers for Disease Control and Prevention; HIV, human immunodeficiency virus.

that make it difficult for this staging system to be uniformly implemented. Many of the classifications require the diagnosis of opportunistic infections that cannot be readily confirmed in most resource-poor settings; clinical criteria for establishing presumptive or definitive diagnoses might be useful. Estimates of weight loss and other constitutional symptoms are also quite difficult in such settings.

NATURAL HISTORY OF HUMAN IMMUNODEFICIENCY VIRUS INFECTION

The clinical spectrum of HIV infection includes primary infection (the acute retroviral syndrome), asymptomatic infection, early symptomatic infection, and advanced immunodeficiency with opportunistic complications. Figure 117-1 shows a schematic diagram of the key immunologic, viral, and clinical features of HIV infection in untreated individuals. Viral load or viremia is monitored by measurement of HIV RNA in plasma, and immunologic status is reflected in the absolute number of CD4+ lymphocytes or in the proportion of lymphocytes that express CD4. Primary HIV infection is characterized by a high concentration of HIV RNA in plasma and suppression of the CD4+ cell count. Plasma viremia declines precipitously with antibody seroconversion and the development of an anti-HIV immune response, usually reaching a steady-state level within 6 to 12 months.[35,36] In most untreated asymptomatic patients, the CD4+ cell count declines gradually over several years. The slope of decline is a function of the plasma viral load. Plasma viremia increases, accompanied by a more rapid decline in CD4+ count, before the onset of symptomatic disease. As the viral load rises and CD4+ cell count falls, the risk of opportunistic infections, malignancies, wasting, neurologic complications, and death increases substantially.

There is considerable variation in the progression of HIV disease, with some individuals progressing from infection to AIDS in less than 5 years[37] and so-called long-term nonprogressors remaining asymptomatic without treatment or evidence of immunologic decline for many years.[38,39]

Before the availability of effective antiretroviral therapy, the rate of progression from primary HIV infection to AIDS and from AIDS to death was estimated in a number of studies. Among homosexual men in San Francisco, the median time from seroconversion to AIDS by the 1987 CDC case definition was 9.8 years.[40] Other studies estimated the

period from infection to AIDS (1987 definition) to be 7 years for transfusion recipients, 10 years for hemophiliacs, 10 years for injection drug users, and 8 to 12 years for homosexual men.[41] An important study of the natural history of HIV infection was the study of a cohort of homosexual and bisexual men by the San Francisco Department of Public Health and the CDC beginning early in the AIDS epidemic.[42] These subjects were originally enrolled in a study of hepatitis B vaccine in 1978 and had serologic studies and clinical evaluations that dated from that time. Of the 489 men for whom the time of HIV seroconversion could be reliably estimated, 13% developed AIDS within 5 years, 51% within 10 years, and 54% at 11 years. In addition, of those who had not developed AIDS within 11 years of seroconversion, 19% had symptomatic disease and another 29% had CD4+ cell counts less than 200/mm³. Thus, after 11 years of follow-up, more than three quarters of HIV-infected homosexual men had severe immunodeficiency, had AIDS, or had died. A number of laboratory tests have been correlated with progressive immunodeficiency, the development of AIDS, and mortality. Taken together, however, the CD4+ lymphocyte count and plasma viral load are the best prognostic markers for subsequent disease course in an HIV-infected individual. The CD4+ lymphocyte count, a specific test for cellular immunocompetence, is a sensitive predictor of the development of symptomatic HIV infection and AIDS in the near term, as it reflects current immunologic capacity.[43-47] Conversely, the plasma viral load (HIV-1 RNA) is an extremely useful predictor of disease course over a more extended period of time and is strongly associated with the rate of subsequent CD4+ cell count decline.[48-56] A more rapid decline in CD4+ count, faster clinical progression, and decreased survival are all associated with a higher baseline viral load. In a study of HIV-infected gay or bisexual men enrolled in the Multicenter AIDS Cohort Study, the risk of progression to AIDS and death was highly correlated with plasma viral load at study entry, independent of CD4+ cell count.[51,52] Baseline plasma viral load was a stronger predictor of progression and mortality than CD4+ count. In addition, the average annual decline in the CD4+ count of HIV-infected men varied according to their initial viral load, decreasing by 36 CD4+ cells/year among men with baseline HIV-1 RNA less than 500 copies/mL, and by 77 CD4+ cells/year among men with baseline HIV-1 RNA greater than 30,000 copies/mL.[52] Using the viral load and CD4+ count together, however, gives the best prognostic estimate of subsequent clinical course (Table 117-2). Put in the context of HIV

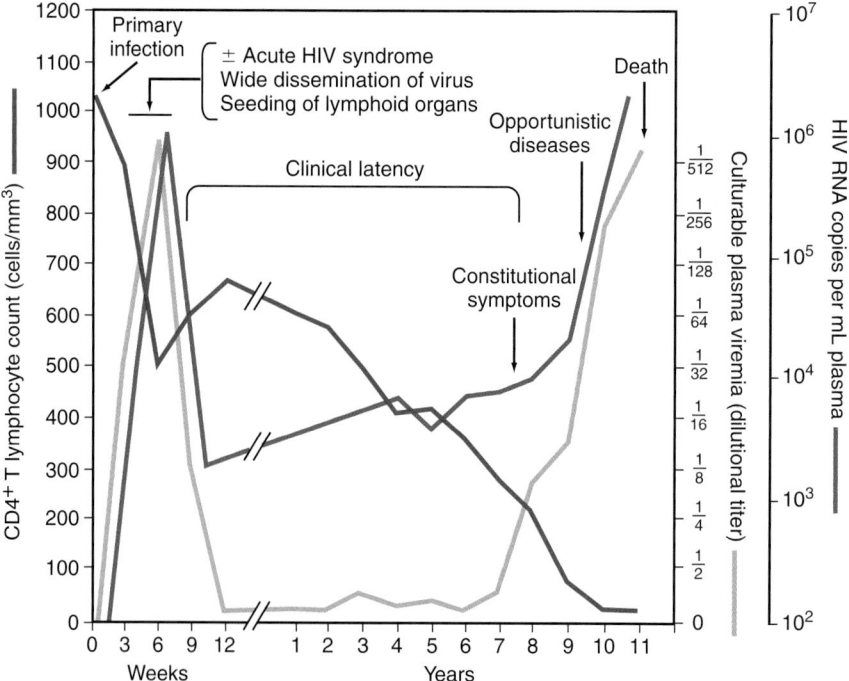

FIGURE 117-1. Natural history of human immunodeficiency virus (HIV) infection in the absence of therapy in a hypothetical patient. *(From Fauci AS, Pantaleo G, Stanley S, Weissman D. Immunopathogenic mechanisms of HIV infection. Ann Intern Med. 1996;124:654-663.)*

pathogenesis, the viral load measures the replicative rate of the infection and its destructive potential for the cellular immune system, and the CD4$^+$ count gauges the extent of immune compromise and the present risk of opportunistic disease. A popular analogy of this situation proposed by John Coffin likens AIDS to an impending train wreck, with the viral load depicting the speed of the train and the CD4$^+$ count reflecting the distance to the disaster.

In the absence of treatment, survival is short after the diagnosis of clinically defined AIDS. A study of survival of the first 505 patients with AIDS in San Francisco found a median survival of 9 months, with most patients dead within 2 years.[57] Patients diagnosed with an opportunistic infection had the most rapid mortality, whereas survival was significantly longer in patients initially diagnosed with KS. Similar results were noted in AIDS patients in New York City, although overall survival was slightly longer (median survival 12 months).[58] Subsequent studies revealed that survival after diagnosis of AIDS was directly related to the CD4$^+$ cell level at diagnosis. In most studies before the availability of combination antiretroviral therapy, median survival after the diagnosis of AIDS was estimated to be between 12 and 18 months.[59] The mean survival time after a CD4$^+$ count of 200/mm^3 was 38 to 40 months.[60,61]

The rate of progression of HIV infection in population-based studies varies depending on age, with older individuals generally having a more rapidly progressive course.[62-66] Whether age differences in the pace of progression of HIV infection are the result of differences in viral setpoints, host immune responses, or both is unclear. Patients who experience more severe or long-lasting symptoms during the acute retroviral syndrome tend to have higher viral loads after seroconversion and progress more rapidly than those who seroconvert without symptoms.[67] Women have approximately one-half log$_{10}$ lower HIV-1 RNA than men after seroconversion, but this difference diminishes with time from seroconversion.[68-70] Although HIV-1 RNA is an important predictor of subsequent disease progression in both women and men,[52,71,72] there is no sex difference in HIV disease progression, particularly when women and men have equal access to care.[73-75] There do not appear to be racial differences in either HIV-1 RNA levels[76] or the natural history of HIV disease progression.[74,77]

Other laboratory studies that predict the development of AIDS in a seropositive individual include a total lymphocyte count less than 1000/mm^3, a total white blood cell count less than 4000/mm^3, a hematocrit less than 40 mL/dL, and a low percentage of CD4$^+$ lymphocytes. Because the CD4$^+$ percentage has a narrower range of variation in most clinical laboratories than the absolute CD4$^+$ cell count, many clinicians favor using this measure for staging and monitoring of patients.[78] Other markers of HIV disease progression that have been validated in clinical studies include the HIV p24 antigen, serum β$_2$-mi-

croglobulin, neopterin, acid-labile interferon-α, anti-p24 antibody, and soluble CD8. These so-called surrogate markers are measures of either viral markers or host immune responses to HIV. Many of these measures do not provide prognostic information independent of the viral load and have therefore been supplanted by quantitative plasma HIV-1 RNA monitoring in developed countries. However, the heat-denatured p24 antigen assay does provide prognostic information independent of HIV-1 RNA and could also be used in lieu of viral load or CD4$^+$ lymphocytes as a marker of subsequent disease progression.[79,80] The low cost of this assay makes it particularly attractive for the developing world. Low-cost alternatives to flow cytometric quantification of CD4$^+$ lymphocytes for application in resource-poor settings are currently under development and include manual assays that utilize enzyme-linked immunosorbent assay or bead-based formats.[81] Other low-cost predictors of disease progression include total lymphocyte count and hemoglobin.[82-84]

The probability of an HIV-infected individual developing opportunistic disease is influenced by several factors. First, immunocompetence is a critical determinant of whether an infected individual can contain a potential pathogen. As discussed later, the CD4$^+$ cell count appears to be the most clinically useful measure of host cellular immunocompetence and plays a central role in the staging of HIV disease. Second, exposure to potential pathogens is required before disease can result. Although some opportunistic pathogens are ubiquitous, resulting in latent or continuous infection in a large proportion of HIV-infected persons (e.g., *Pneumocystis jirovecii*, CMV), others are prevalent in a smaller proportion of individuals and cause disease less often (e.g., *Toxoplasma gondii*, *Mycobacterium tuberculosis*). Other opportunistic pathogens do not appear to be associated with latent reactivation but rather cause disease when a sufficiently immunocompromised host acquires new infection (e.g., *Cryptococcus neoformans*, *M. avium* complex). Third, the relative virulence of a potential pathogen is a factor that may determine which disease is likely to occur. For example, more virulent organisms such as *M. tuberculosis* or *Streptococcus pneumoniae* cause clinical illness in patients with less severe immunodeficiency, whereas less virulent organisms such as P. *jirovecii* or CMV cause illness in those with more severe immunodeficiency.[85-87] Finally, whether a patient is taking chemoprophylactic agents with activity against specific pathogens influences the risk of disease. Figure 117-2 shows CD4$^+$ cell counts at the time of diagnosis of opportunistic diseases in patients with CD4$^+$ cell counts of 300/mm^3 or less evaluated at the Johns Hopkins Hospital before 1996.[88,89] Although the range of CD4$^+$ cell counts for some conditions is broad, most patients with truly opportunistic infections had CD4$^+$ counts less than 100/mm^3.

TABLE 117-2   Probability of Developing Acquired Immunodeficiency Syndrome (1987 Centers for Disease Control Case Definition) in 1604 Men in the Multicenter AIDS Cohort Study*

Baseline Viral Load†	Baseline CD4 Count‡	Number Studied	Number with AIDS	% AIDS at 3 Years	% AIDS at 6 Years	% AIDS at 9 Years
<500	>750	66	3	0	1.7	3.6
	<750	56	13	3.7	9.6	22.3
501-3000	Any	257	90	2.0	16.6	35.4
3001-10,000	>750	93	39	3.2	14.2	59.7
	<750	300	179	8.1	37.7	62.4
10,001-30,000	>750	64	42	9.5	36.7	62.4
	351-750	259	194	16.1	54.9	76.3
	≤350	73	63	40.1	72.9	86.2
>30,000	>500	141	105	32.6	66.8	76.3
	351-500	121	111	47.9	77.7	94.4
	201-350	104	92	64.4	89.3	92.9
	<200	70	67	85.5	97.9	100

*Based on baseline HIV branched-chain DNA viral load and CD4$^+$ cell count.
†HIV RNA copies per milliliter of plasma by branched-chain DNA. Viral load determined by reverse transcriptase–polymerase chain reaction approximately twofold greater.
‡CD4$^+$ cells per cubic millimeter.
AIDS, acquired immunodeficiency syndrome; HIV, human immunodeficiency virus.
From Mellors JW, Munoz A, Giorgi JV, et al. Plasma viral load and CD4$^+$ lymphocytes as prognostic markers of HIV-1 infection. Ann Intern Med. 1997;126:946–954.

FIGURE 117-2. Range of CD4 lymphocyte counts at the time of diagnosis of opportunistic diseases in patients with human immunodeficiency virus (HIV) infection. Boxes represent the 25th to 75th percentiles, bars represent medians, and asterisks represent means. Can, *Candida* esophagitis; CMV, cytomegalovirus; Crp, cryptosporidiosis; Cry, cryptococcosis; Enc, HIV encephalopathy; HSV, herpes simplex virus; Hzos, herpes zoster; KS, Kaposi's sarcoma; MAC, *Mycobacterium avium* complex; NHL, non-Hodgkin's lymphoma; PCP, first episodes of *Pneumocystis jirovecii* pneumonia; PCP2, recurrent *P. jirovecii* pneumonia; PML, progressive multifocal leukoencephalopathy; Tox, toxoplasmosis; WS, wasting syndrome. *(From Moore RD, Chaisson RE. Natural history of opportunistic disease in an HIV-infected urban cohort. Ann Intern Med. 1996;124:633-642.)*

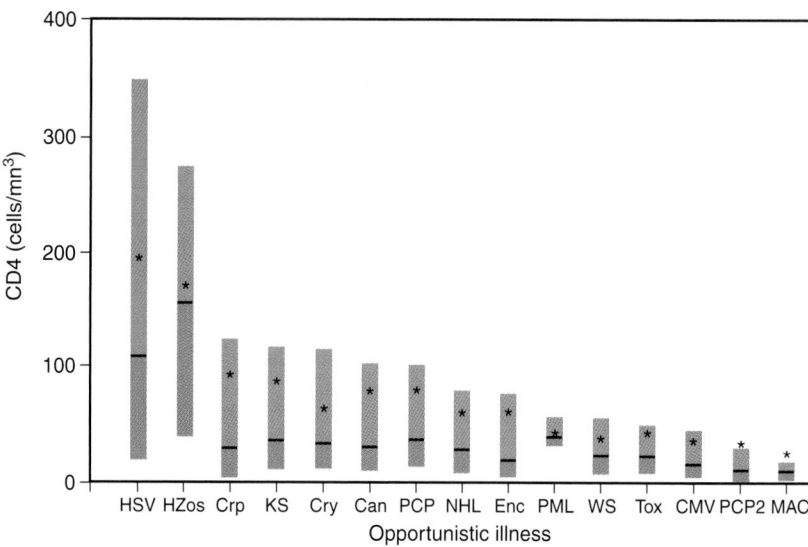

Although the clinical manifestations of HIV infection do not vary according to HIV subtype, the incidence of specific opportunistic infections is profoundly influenced by geography and the prevalence of infectious diseases in particular regions. HIV-1 infection increases susceptibility to tuberculosis, and the incidence of tuberculosis in HIV-infected persons is extremely high in sub-Saharan Africa, where tuberculosis is endemic.[90] Malaria is also endemic in many developing countries and occurs with increased frequency and severity in HIV-infected persons, particularly during pregnancy.[91] Opportunistic infections such as *P. jirovecii* pneumonia, *M. avium* complex disease, CMV retinitis, non-Hodgkin's lymphoma, and HIV encephalopathy that are relatively common in developed countries are uncommon in developing countries, such as those in West Africa.[92] In regions in which it is endemic (e.g., the Mediterranean, Central America, South America, Africa, and Asia), leishmania occurs with increased frequency among HIV-infected persons. Similarly, *T. cruzi* (South America), histoplasmosis (Ohio and Mississippi River valleys, United States), and *Penicillium marneffei* (Thailand, China, Hong Kong) occur with increased frequency in certain regions.

The incidence of specific opportunistic diseases has been determined for several large cohorts of HIV-infected individuals. In the Johns Hopkins study of more than 1200 patients with CD4+ cell counts less than 300/mm³, the 3-year probability of new opportunistic diseases (without highly active antiretroviral therapy [HAART]) was determined. In contrast to findings before the widespread use of prophylaxis, in which the most common opportunistic infection was *P. jirovecii* pneumonia,[65,88] the most common opportunistic infection in this later cohort was *Candida* esophagitis (13.3 cases per 100 person-years). *P. jirovecii* pneumonia, disseminated *M. avium* complex, CMV disease, and the AIDS dementia complex occurred at rates of 5 to 9 cases per 100 person-years. Less common were toxoplasmosis, cryptococcal meningitis, herpes zoster, the wasting syndrome, and KS (2 to 4 cases per 100 person-years). The least common complications were non-Hodgkin's lymphoma, tuberculosis, progressive multifocal leukoencephalopathy, and cryptosporidiosis (1 to 2 per 100 cases person-years). In contrast, other investigators have found a decrease in the incidence of opportunistic conditions but no difference in the spectrum of diagnoses. In a retrospective analysis of 344 AIDS patients enrolled in the British Columbia Drug Treatment Program, declines in the incidence of HIV-related complications were seen between 1994 and 1996, but *P. jirovecii* pneumonia and KS remained the most common AIDS index diagnoses.[93]

Clinical findings may also predict disease progression in seropositive subjects. Oral candidiasis and oral hairy leukoplakia are early clinical markers of immunosuppression and herald the development of AIDS in many patients.[94-96] Generalized lymphadenopathy is also a clinical marker of HIV infection but does not predict progression to AIDS. In one study, the average CD4+ cell count was higher in those with lymphadenopathy than in seropositive individuals without enlarged lymph nodes.[97] Most opportunistic diseases increase the risk of death independently of the CD4+ cell count.[98,99] This may be due not only to morbidity related to the complication itself but also to an increase in immune activation leading to upregulation of HIV replication with acceleration of HIV disease progression. A number of studies have demonstrated increases in HIV viral load in patients with acute opportunistic infections.[100-103]

The Impact of HAART on the Clinical Manifestations of Human Immunodeficiency Virus

Even before the era of HAART, it was clear that antiretroviral therapy and prophylaxis against *P. jirovecii* pneumonia had substantially altered the natural history of AIDS, prolonging the median survival of treated AIDS patients to 2 to 3 years.[104-108] Antiretroviral therapy and prophylaxis against *P. jirovecii* pneumonia and *M. avium* complex also prolonged the time from HIV infection to AIDS, decreased the incidence of opportunistic complications, and improved overall survival.[109-116] Changes in plasma viral and CD4+ cell counts resulting from antiretroviral drug treatment have been shown to be strong predictors of clinical progression (or regression) of HIV disease.[117,118]

The use of combination antiretroviral therapy and the introduction of protease inhibitors in 1995 and 1996 led to a dramatic change in the natural history of treated HIV disease.[119-123] In the HIV Outpatient Study, mortality declined from 29.4 deaths per 100 person-years in 1995 to 8.8 per 100 person-years in the second quarter of 1997 (Fig. 117-3).[124] This decline in mortality was accompanied by marked decreases in the incidence of *P. jirovecii* pneumonia, *M. avium* complex disease, and CMV retinitis; the incidence of any one of those three infections declined from 21.9 per 100 person-years in 1994 to 3.7 per 100 person-years by mid-1997 (Fig. 117-4). The degree of benefit was associated with the intensity of antiretroviral therapy; combination therapy resulted in an improved prognosis compared with monotherapy, and the use of a protease inhibitor in a combination regimen was associated with the greatest benefit. In the United States as a whole, deaths attributed to AIDS decreased by 23% in 1996 and by 44% in 1997.[120,121] Subsequent studies among cohorts of HIV-infected persons have continued to demonstrate the beneficial effect of HAART on clinical disease progression and death (Fig. 117-5).[125] With improved survival rates, death among persons with AIDS is more frequently due to chronic diseases. In a study of persons with AIDS in San Francisco, the proportion of deaths associated with septicemia, non–AIDS-

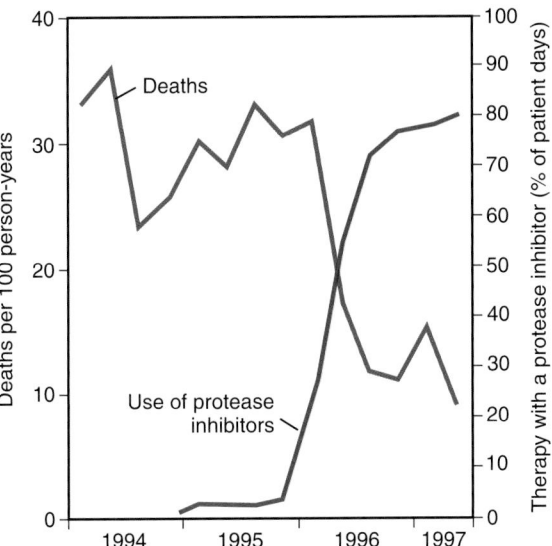

FIGURE 117-3. Incidence of death and use of protease inhibitors in patients with human immunodeficiency virus (HIV) infection and a CD4 count lower than 100/mm³ in the HIV Outpatient Study. *(From Palella FJ, Delaney KM, Moorman AC, et al. Declining morbidity and mortality among patients with advanced human immunodeficiency virus infection. N Engl J Med. 1998:338:853-860. Copyright © 1998 Massachusetts Medical Society. All rights reserved.)*

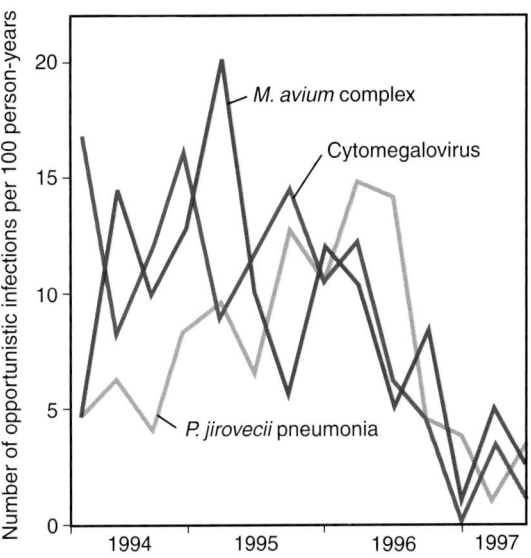

FIGURE 117-4 Incidence of selected opportunistic infections in patients with human immunodeficiency virus (HIV) infection and a CD4 count lower than 100/mm³ in the HIV Outpatient Study in the era before and after the introduction of protease inhibitors. *(From Palella FJ, Delaney KM, Moorman AC, et al. Declining morbidity and mortality among patients with advanced human immunodeficiency virus infection. N Engl J Med. 1998:338:853-860. Copyright © 1998 Massachusetts Medical Society. All rights reserved.)*

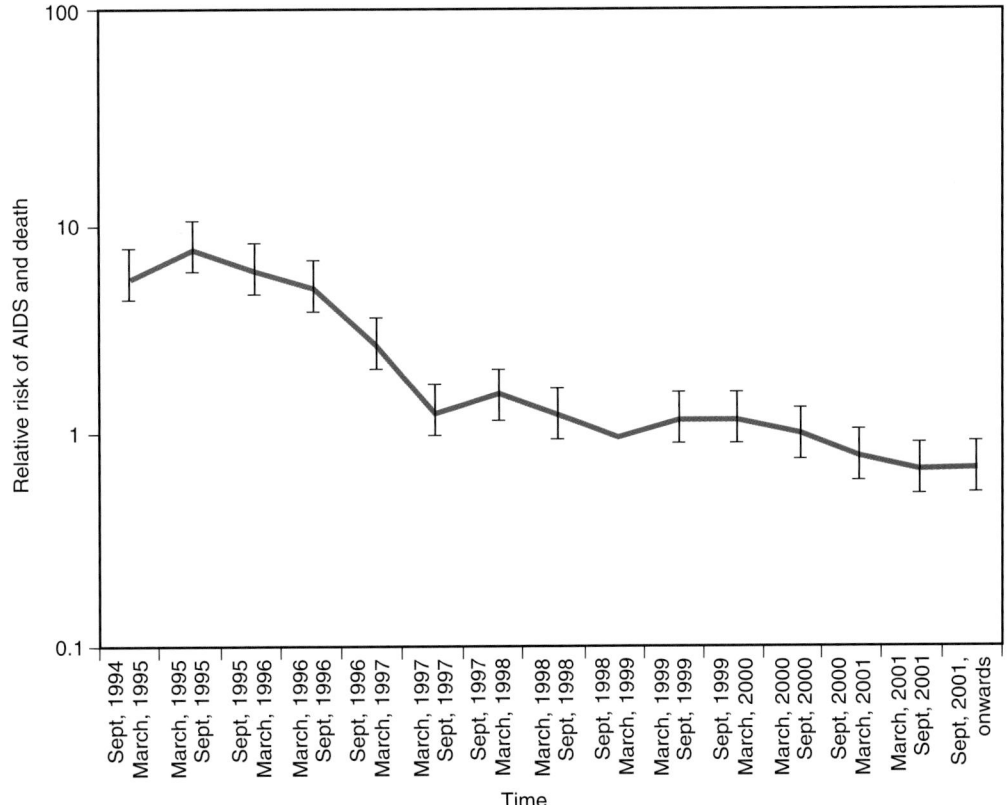

FIGURE 117-5 Relative risk of acquired immunodeficiency syndrome (AIDS) or death since the introduction of highly active antiretroviral therapy (HAART), adjusted for CD4 count at recruitment, age, previous HAART treatment, and AIDS status. Data are from 9803 HIV-infected patients seen at 70 treatment centers in Europe, Israel, and Argentina. Vertical bars represent 95% confidence intervals. *(From Mocroft A, Ledergerber B, Katlama C, et al. Decline in the AIDS and death rates in the EuroSIDA study: An observational study. Lancet. 2003;362:22-29.)*

defining malignancies, chronic liver disease, viral hepatitis, overdose, obstructive lung disease, coronary artery disease, and pancreatitis increased between 1994 and 1998.[126] In a study from Cleveland, 20% to 25% of HIV-infected persons who died between 1997 and 1999 had an undetectable viral load, suggesting that death was due to causes other than HIV.[127] A study from Switzerland indicates that patients receiving effective antiretroviral treatment have a risk of death that is similar to that in patients with cured cancer.[128]

Effective therapy has not only decreased the incidence of new opportunistic infections but also led to the resolution of preexisting conditions.[129] In some cases, the immune restoration resulting from HAART can alter the clinical presentation of specific opportunistic infections, as in the case of focal mycobacterial lymphadenitis or CMV vitritis.[130] It is becoming increasingly clear that the immunologic changes resulting from HAART represent at least a partial immune reconstitution, although the recovery of antigen-specific immunity appears to lag behind CD4+ cell count increases.[131-134] The clinical manifestations of immune reconstitution syndromes are discussed at the end of this chapter. The incidence of new opportunistic infections in patients who have had satisfactory virologic and immunologic responses to HAART is extremely low, even when primary prophylaxis has been discontinued.[135,136] Moreover, reactivation of previously diagnosed opportunistic infections, such as *M. avium* complex infections and CMV retinitis, appears to be uncommon in patients with immune recovery who discontinue maintenance therapy.[137,138]

Thus, over the past two decades the natural history of HIV infection has undergone considerable change, as has our understanding of it. The clinical course of HIV disease in individuals receiving combination antiretroviral therapy is likely to evolve further in the coming years, with additional manifestations and disease trajectories becoming apparent as larger numbers of patients are treated for longer periods of time.

CLINICAL PRESENTATIONS OF HUMAN IMMUNODEFICIENCY VIRUS INFECTION

HIV infection causes disease manifestations of three principal types: an acute viral illness seen in the initial weeks of infection and associated with a high viral load and an intense host immune response, immunologically mediated processes related to host responses to chronic viral infection (e.g., lymphadenopathy, thrombocytopenia, HIV-related dementia), and opportunistic diseases resulting from impaired host responses as the cellular immune system is damaged or ablated. The major clinical syndromes most frequently seen in HIV-infected individuals fall into the last category, that is, opportunistic diseases that arise as a consequence of impaired cellular immunity in late-stage HIV infection. Potent antiretroviral therapy has added two new categories of clinical manifestations that may be commonly encountered in patients with HIV infection: immune reconstitution syndromes with exacerbations of previously silent or adequately treated infections, especially mycobacterial infections,[139] and a syndrome of lipodystrophy with fat loss and redistribution, elevated serum triglycerides and cholesterol, and insulin resistance seen in patients receiving HAART, especially with protease inhibitors.[140] The clinical features of immune reconstitution syndromes are discussed later in this chapter, and the manifestations of drug toxicity related to the treatment of HIV are discussed in Chapter 124.

CLINICAL FINDINGS

Acute Retroviral Syndrome

The initial manifestation of HIV infection in one half to two thirds of recently infected individuals is a mononucleosis-like illness referred to as the acute retroviral syndrome. The syndrome was first described in 1985 by Cooper and colleagues[141] as an acute mononucleosis-like syndrome in 11 of 12 homosexual men who seroconverted for HIV antibodies. In a follow-up study, 36 of 39 (92%) homosexual men with recent HIV infection recalled an illness consistent with the acute retroviral syndrome during the time when their tests showed serocon-

version.[142] Forty percent of a seronegative control group also reported a mononucleosis-like illness, however. Similar descriptions of a characteristic syndrome have been reported in people infected with HIV through parenteral exposures, including health care workers exposed to accidental parenteral inoculation of HIV.[143]

The incidence of the acute retroviral syndrome is not precisely known. Retrospective studies of homosexual men infected with HIV found a low frequency of seroconversion illness.[144,145] A prospective study of homosexual men showed a 55% incidence of a mononucleosis-like illness in 22 subjects who became antibody positive, compared with 21% in 44 nonconverting control subjects.[146] In one study of 378 persons with acute retroviral syndrome, injection drug users had or reported symptoms less frequently than persons who acquired HIV through sexual transmission.[147] Most health care workers with occupationally acquired HIV had the acute retroviral syndrome after exposure.[143,148] Overall, this syndrome is probably underreported and underdiagnosed, as noted in two series of patients, the majority of whom were not initially thought to have acute HIV infection.[149,150]

The clinical features of the acute retroviral syndrome are nonspecific and variable.[151,152] The onset of the illness ranges from 1 to 6 weeks after exposure to the virus but peaks at 3 weeks. Table 117-3 shows the signs and symptoms of the acute retroviral syndrome reported in 209 cases, reviewed by Niu and coworkers.[153] Fever, sweats, malaise, myalgias, anorexia, nausea, diarrhea, and a nonexudative pharyngitis are prominent symptoms.[153-160] Many patients report headaches, photophobia, and meningismus. Two thirds of patients may have a truncal exanthem that may be maculopapular, roseola-like, or urticarial. Skin biopsies are nonspecific, with perivascular lymphocytic infiltrates and dermal mononuclear cell infiltrates.[161] In addition to aseptic meningitis, neurologic symptoms occur in a minority of patients and may include encephalitis, peripheral neuropathy, and an acute, ascending polyneuropathy (Guillain-Barré syndrome). Physical examination frequently reveals cervical, occipital, or axillary lymphadenopathy; rash; and, less commonly, hepatosplenomegaly. Oral aphthous ulcerations (Fig. 117-6) have been reported in several cases; these may involve the esophagus. Oral and esophageal candidiasis during the seroconversion illness has been reported. The remainder of the physical examination is usually unremarkable. Symptoms generally resolve in 10 to 15 days. A wide range of acute opportunistic infections have been reported in patients with the acute retroviral syndrome, including *P. jirovecii* pneumonia, cryptococcal meningitis, and *Candida* esophagitis. Their occurrence is probably due to the depression of the CD4+ cell count that generally accompanies acute HIV infection.

TABLE 117-3 Symptoms and Signs of the Acute Retroviral Syndrome in 209 Patients

Symptom or Sign	Number with Finding	Frequency (%)
Fever	200	96
Adenopathy	154	74
Pharyngitis	146	70
Rash	146	70
Myalgia or arthralgia	112	54
Thrombocytopenia	94	45
Leukopenia	80	38
Diarrhea	67	32
Headache	66	32
Nausea, vomiting	56	27
Elevated transaminases*	38	21
Hepatosplenomegaly	30	14
Thrush	24	12
Neuropathy	13	6
Encephalopathy	12	6

*Based on 178 subjects.

Adapted from Niu MT, Stein DS, Schnittman SM. Primary human immunodeficiency virus type 1 infection: Review of pathogenesis and early treatment intervention in human and animal retrovirus infections. J Infect Dis. 1993;168:1490–1501.

Laboratory evaluation of patients with the syndrome reveals a reduced total lymphocyte count, elevated sedimentation rate, negative heterophile antibody test, and elevated transaminase and alkaline phosphatase levels.[153] When lymphocyte phenotyping is performed, a characteristic pattern is observed.[162] Initially, the total lymphocyte count, including both CD4+ and CD8+ T lymphocytes, decreases with a normal ratio of CD4+ to CD8+ cells. Within several weeks, both the CD4+ and CD8+ cell populations begin to increase. The rise in CD8+ cell numbers is relatively greater than that in CD4+ cells, and the CD4/CD8 ratio is inverted. In the weeks that follow, the CD8+ cell population increases rather markedly because of HIV-specific CD8+ T lymphocytes. The ratio of CD4+ to CD8+ cells usually remains inverted as the acute illness resolves (primarily because of excess numbers of CD8+ cells). In patients with neurologic symptoms, cerebrospinal fluid may show a lymphocytic pleocytosis with normal levels of protein and glucose.[163]

HIV p24 antigen may be detected in the serum and cerebrospinal fluid in about 75% of patients with primary HIV infection within 2 weeks of exposure, often coincidentally with the onset of symptoms.[163,164] Antigenemia can persist for several weeks or months and generally resolves when antibodies to p24 are produced in sufficient quantity to form complexes with free antigen. The most sensitive marker for acute HIV infection, however, is plasma HIV RNA, which is markedly elevated in most patients.[165] Typical RNA levels range from 10^5 to more than 10^6 copies/mL of plasma, and the titers decline as the CD8+ cytotoxic T-cell and antibody responses increase subsequently. Low-level ($<10^4$) false-positive HIV RNA tests may occur, but high-level viremia is virtually diagnostic of acute infection in the absence of anti-HIV antibodies. The enzyme immunoassay for HIV antibodies remains negative for an average of 2 to 6 weeks after the onset of symptoms despite the appearance of specific antibodies on a Western blot of the patient's serum. Anti-p24 appears on the Western blot shortly before seroconversion is detected by enzyme-linked immunosorbent assay and by the appearance of antibodies to other antigens.

The differential diagnosis of the acute retroviral syndrome includes a number of other illnesses: infectious mononucleosis; other viral infections such as influenza, viral hepatitis, measles, rubella, primary herpes simplex virus (HSV) infection; and secondary syphilis. Evaluation of patients presenting with an illness consistent with acute retroviral infection should include a careful history to elicit risks for HIV infection, laboratory tests to rule out mononucleosis and syphilis, HIV antibody and plasma RNA tests, and complete blood counts and differential. There is increasing interest in treating acute HIV with combination antiretroviral therapy, as there is evidence that this may both lower the viral setpoint and lead to enhanced CD4+ and CD8+ HIV-specific responses.[166] However, early treatment does not appear to prevent establishment of reservoirs of latently infected, resting CD4+ cells and may not provide any long-term benefit.[167]

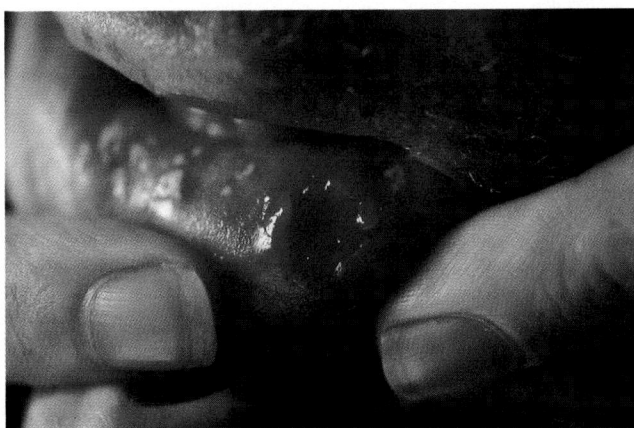

FIGURE 117-6. Aphthous ulcer. *(Courtesy of Stephen Raffanti, MD, MPH.)*

Persistent Generalized Lymphadenopathy

Infection with HIV is associated with a high prevalence of generalized lymphadenopathy, often beginning with the acute retroviral syndrome. In the early 1980s, PGL was recognized as a prodromal state to the development of AIDS in homosexual men who were otherwise healthy.[15,17] The pathogenesis of generalized lymphadenopathy is related to the rapid infection of CD4+ cells in lymph nodes by HIV after initial infection. The syndrome of PGL is defined as the presence of two or more extrainguinal sites of lymphadenopathy for a minimum of 3 to 6 months for which no other explanation can be found. Biopsy specimens of lymph nodes from such patients usually reveal a follicular hyperplasia without specific pathogens.

Approximately 50% to 70% of HIV-infected individuals develop PGL. The most frequently involved node groups are the posterior and anterior cervical, submandibular, occipital, and axillary chains; epitrochlear and femoral nodes may also be enlarged. Physical examination usually reveals symmetrical, mobile, rubbery lymph nodes ranging from 0.5 to 2 cm. Pain and tenderness are uncommon. Localized (i.e., asymmetric) adenopathy and rapid nodal enlargement are not characteristic and suggest an infectious or malignant process. The remainder of the physical examination is often unremarkable, although other complications of HIV infection may be found such as thrush or hairy leukoplakia. Mediastinal and hilar adenopathy is not characteristic of the syndrome; however, abdominal computed tomography often reveals enlarged mesenteric and retroperitoneal adenopathy in HIV-infected persons. The natural history of HIV infection in individuals with PGL does not differ significantly from that of HIV infection without PGL.[97,168] Involution of enlarged lymph nodes, with degeneration of follicular germinal centers and loss of hyperplasia, often accompanies progression of HIV infection to advanced disease.

In patients treated with HAART, previously involuted lymph nodes may again enlarge as HIV-specific and other T cells are replenished. In addition, focal lymphadenitis with constitutional symptoms may occur in patients with previously silent mycobacterial infections 1 to 2 months after starting HAART. These "reversal" reactions or immune reconstitution syndromes are reminiscent of reversal reactions seen in multibacillary forms of leprosy, heralding a return of pathogen-specific T-cell responses.

The differential diagnosis of PGL includes HIV infection and a wide variety of other processes that are associated with generalized lymphadenopathy: sarcoid, secondary syphilis, and Hodgkin's disease, for example. In patients with HIV infection, lymphadenopathy may also be caused by mycobacterial infections, KS, and lymphoma.[169] An unusual cause of lymphadenopathy in patients with HIV infection is Castleman's disease.[170] Castleman's disease is an angioproliferative, hyperplastic process of lymph nodes and other lymphoid tissues showing characteristic histologic findings, with either hyaline vascular or plasma cell variants. In patients with HIV in particular, multicentric Castleman's disease is the most common presentation, with involvement of lymph nodes, liver, spleen, and other organs. Although the etiology of Castleman's disease is not fully understood, infection with human herpesvirus type 8 is thought to underlie a large proportion of cases.[171,172] Unlike PGL, Castleman's disease is associated with constitutional symptoms and multiorgan involvement in most HIV-infected patients. The diagnosis is established histopathologically.

In patients with clinical findings suggesting opportunistic disease, needle aspiration of lymph nodes may help establish a specific diagnosis.[173] Examination of aspirates with cytologic, acid-fast, and Gram stains is valuable in identifying infection or malignancy. If a specific diagnosis is not determined after staining and culture of node aspirates, lymph node biopsy is indicated. Aspiration of lymph nodes in patients with PGL usually reveals benign cells. Biopsy specimens show follicular hyperplasia, with the normal architecture distorted by greatly expanded germinal centers composed of B lymphocytes. It is now known that active viral replication is occurring in these follicular cells and virus is trapped in dendritic cells, although the patient may appear well clinically.[174]

Most patients with PGL require no invasive evaluation and can be managed according to standard guidelines for HIV infection.

Constitutional Disease and Wasting

HIV infection is often completely asymptomatic; however, some patients complain of nonspecific constitutional symptoms in the months or years after primary infection but before opportunistic disease is diagnosed. Patients commonly complain of being easily fatigued and report the need to reduce their normal activities somewhat. Debilitating fatigue is uncommon in the early years of infection. Low-grade fevers (temperature < 38° C), occasional night sweats, and intermittent diarrhea are also reported. Severe wasting with loss of more than 10% of body weight is generally a finding of advanced HIV disease. The exact incidence of constitutional symptoms, fatigue, and weight loss is not known, and the etiology is varied and often multifactorial. The differential diagnosis of these findings includes intercurrent minor illnesses, endocrinologic abnormalities, anemia, and psychological or psychiatric disorders.

Anxiety and depression are common responses to the diagnosis of HIV infection,[175-177] and studies suggest an increased prevalence of affective disorders among HIV-infected individuals. Injection drug users, in particular, have a high prevalence of affective disorders that may result in somatic complaints. Moreover, the physical effects of opiates and withdrawal from stimulants such as cocaine and amphetamines cause fatigue and other constitutional symptoms.

A number of metabolic and endocrinologic disturbances have been identified in patients with HIV.[178-180] Hypogonadism, particularly depression of testosterone or dihydrotestosterone levels, is reported in both men and women with HIV infection and weight loss or wasting.[181,182] Elevated levels of myostatin-immunoreactive protein, a muscle catabolic agent, have been found in men with HIV and wasting.[183] In most clinical studies, however, wasting has been found in association with decreased caloric intake, elevated catabolism caused by opportunistic infections, or chronic diarrhea.[184-187] In advanced HIV, severe wasting, whatever the cause, is strongly associated with the risk of dying.[188] Weight loss has remained an important predictor of mortality even in the era of HAART.[189]

In patients with more advanced HIV disease with high viral loads and severe depletion of CD4+ cells, constitutional disease (fatigue, weight loss, malaise, fever) usually heralds the onset of opportunistic infections or malignancies. In one study of HIV-infected outpatients with fever, a specific etiology could be identified for 83%.[190] Common causes of fever in these patients included *P. jirovecii* pneumonia, *M. avium* complex bacteremia, catheter-related bacteremia, bacterial pneumonia, sinusitis, lymphoma, and drug reactions. Fever of greater than 2 weeks' duration was more often associated with AIDS-defining illnesses.

In African patients with HIV infection, a wasting illness, termed "slim" disease, has been described.[191] These patients have debilitating fatigue, fevers, sweats, protracted diarrhea, and severe weight loss. Opportunistic or conventional pathogens are not found, but the patients waste away and die of severe malnutrition and terminal secondary infections. This illness has been encountered in developed countries as well but far less commonly than in Africa—a pattern that suggests underdiagnosis of opportunistic diseases in Africa. Several studies of African patients with enteropathic slim disease found that most had enteric pathogens or microsporidia when a thorough evaluation was performed.[192,193] In Abidjan, Côte d'Ivoire, 37% of patients who died with a diagnosis of slim disease were found at autopsy to have disseminated tuberculosis,[194] and the presence of tuberculosis at autopsy was strongly associated with the degree of wasting.[195] The definition of wasting syndrome in the United States is the presence of unexplained constitutional disease for more than 1 month with a temperature greater than 38.3° C, diarrhea, and loss of more than 10% of baseline body weight. A thorough evaluation to identify specific pathogens that would explain the symptoms and that might be amenable to treatment is essential before wasting syndrome is diagnosed, and usually a specific cause can be implicated.

Oral Disease

Abnormalities of the oral cavity occur throughout the course of HIV infection. Primary HIV infection has been associated with severe aphthous stomatitis and with oropharyngeal and esophageal candidiasis. As the infection progresses and immunologic impairment proceeds, numerous oral complications arise. In the late stages of disease, oral manifestations are highly prevalent and frequently severe.[196,197] A number of studies have demonstrated that the occurrence of oral lesions such as candidiasis and hairy leukoplakia is associated with an increased risk of progression to AIDS.[198-200]

Oral Candidiasis

Candida infections of the hard and soft palates, buccal mucosa, tongue, pharynx, and hypopharynx are observed frequently. *Candida albicans* is the species most commonly identified, but *Candida tropicalis, Candida glabrata,* and *Candida krusei* infections also occur. Contrary to systemic *Candida* infections, which appear to result from defects in phagocyte function and number, mucosal *Candida* infections result from impaired cellular immunity. The incidence of candidiasis increases with progressive cellular immunodeficiency, particularly as CD4+ lymphocyte counts fall below 200 to 300/mm³.[201] Because oral candidiasis itself is an opportunistic infection, it is predictive of the disease progression and development of other AIDS-related infections.

Several clinical manifestations of candidiasis have been described in HIV-infected patients. The most common form is thrush (pseudomembranous candidiasis). Characteristic "cottage cheese" plaques that can be removed with a tongue blade are seen on the soft palate, tonsils, and buccal mucosa (Fig. 117-7). Less often, thrush involves the lateral and posterior aspects of the tongue, the hard palate, and the hypopharynx. *Candida* infection can produce flat, erythematous plaques distributed in the same way as the pseudomembranous form of the disease but without the characteristic white exudate. This atrophic form of candidiasis is underdiagnosed because many clinicians are unfamiliar with its appearance. Atrophic candidiasis of the tongue also occurs. Less frequently, *Candida* can cause a nonscrapable white plaque similar to that in hairy leukoplakia (see next section). Unlike the corrugated lesions and hairlike projections seen in oral hairy leukoplakia (OHL), candidal lesions are smooth. This hypertrophic form of disease may involve the lateral border of the tongue, the palate, and the buccal mucosa. *Candida* infection of the lateral lip (angular cheilitis) is another common complication. Angular cheilitis can cause pain, fissures, erythema, and difficulty opening the mouth (Fig. 117-8). Physical examination, KOH preparation, and the response to antifungal therapy establish the diagnosis.

The diagnosis of candidiasis is frequently made on the basis of physical examination alone. A KOH preparation of scraped material from a plaque is diagnostic and can be performed easily in most clin-

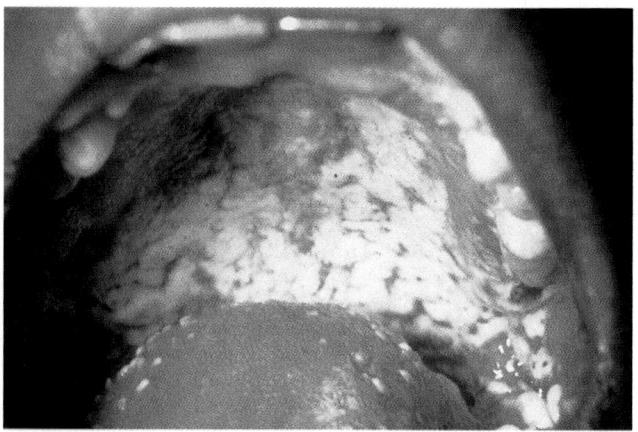

FIGURE 117-7. Oral candidiasis (thrush). (*Courtesy of Stephen Raffanti, MD, MPH.*)

ical settings. Cultures for *Candida* are rarely necessary. A biopsy specimen of oral lesions can be used to distinguish various forms of leukoplakia. A therapeutic trial of antifungal agents can also help to establish a diagnosis. The widespread use of oral triazole antifungal agents has been accompanied by the emergence of disease caused by drug-resistant fungi.[202] Risk factors for fluconazole-resistant candidiasis include an extended duration of prior antifungal therapy and low CD4[+] count.[203] Of note, in patients treated with HAART, rates of fluconazole resistance were relatively low even though many had received several previous courses of fluconazole, suggesting that advanced immunosuppression is the most important risk factor for resistance.[204] In addition, some species of *Candida*, such as *C. krusei* and *C. glabrata*, are frequently less sensitive to fluconazole.

Oral Hairy Leukoplakia

Originally described in 1984 by Greenspan and colleagues,[205] OHL is a raised, white lesion of the oral mucosa that is usually seen on the lateral margin of the tongue. The frequency of occurrence of OHL increases as the CD4[+] count decreases.[201] OHL appears to be caused by the replication of Epstein-Barr virus in the epithelium of keratinized cells on the surface of the tongue and buccal mucosa.[206] Other herpesviruses have also been isolated from cultures of biopsy specimens of lesions; however, their role in the pathogenesis of OHL is unclear. HIV is not routinely cultured from specimens and is not found with DNA probes. The diagnosis of OHL is established by visual inspection, failure to scrape off the lesion with a tongue blade, failure of the lesion to respond to antifungal therapy, and biopsy material or scrapings in which Epstein-Barr virus can be identified. Hairy leukoplakia is usually asymptomatic, although large lesions may impair taste, hinder eating, and cause discomfort. Lesions respond to high-dose acyclovir or ganciclovir, podophyllin, and isotretinoin, but only temporarily.

Gingivitis and Periodontitis

Severe gingivitis (linear gingival erythema) and periodontitis (necrotizing ulcerative periodontitis) have been observed in patients with HIV disease.[207] The onset of symptoms is often insidious but may be abrupt. Pain is often severe; patients may note foul breath, bleeding gums, and loosening of teeth. Physical examination may reveal a bright red marginal line on the gingiva, necrosis and ulceration of interdental papillae, gingival erosion, exfoliation of enamel, and loose teeth. The etiology of gingivitis and periodontitis is unclear. Cigarette smoking may be an important cofactor in the pathogenesis of periodontitis. Mixed cultures of aerobic and anaerobic flora have been obtained from gingival biopsy samples. More severe, ulcerating gingivitis can be caused by infections with gram-negative bacilli, particularly *Klebsiella pneumoniae* and *Enterobacter cloacae.* Infections tend to be chronic, but débridement, irrigation, and topical antiseptic agents or metronidazole therapy may control some cases.

Oral Ulcers

A number of ulcerative lesions may occur in the oral cavity of patients with HIV infection. HSV types 1 and 2 may cause primary or recurrent oral ulcers. These lesions generally appear as small, smooth ulcers on an erythematous base on the lips, buccal mucosa, hard palate, or gums. The ulcers may be single or multiple and are often painful. Episodes may last for several weeks; acyclovir may be beneficial. CMV may rarely cause solitary large ulcers in persons with disseminated CMV infection. Aphthous stomatitis is manifested by single or multiple painful ulcers, often with exudate or necrosis, that may appear on the buccal and labial mucosa and the lateral margin of the tongue (see Fig. 117-6). These ulcers do not occur more commonly than among HIV-seronegative persons, but episodes are more severe and prolonged.[208] They may be treated with topical steroids or thalidomide if persistent.[209-211] The etiology of oral ulcers is best determined by biopsy and viral culture, although minor lesions may be observed without specific therapy in many cases. Several drugs have been reported to cause oral and gastrointestinal ulcers, including zalcitabine, zidovudine, and dapsone.

Other Oral Lesions

The purple-red lesions of KS may occur at any site in the mouth, but the palate is most common. Lesions may become large and nodular. Non-Hodgkin's lymphoma may arise in the mouth as either a swelling or ulcers; biopsy is required for diagnosis. Oral warts caused by human papillomavirus infection may be seen; they are not malignant precursors. Ketoconazole and zidovudine can cause brown oral pigmentation. Salivary glands such as the parotid gland may be enlarged by infiltration with CD8[+] lymphocytes or benign lymphoepithelial cysts. These cysts often respond to antiretroviral therapy.[212]

Musculoskeletal Complications

Polymyositis complicates HIV infection in a small number of patients and can occur at any stage of HIV infection.[213] Clinical features include myalgias, weakness of the proximal muscles, muscle tenderness, wasting, and fatigue.[214] Creatine kinase and other muscle enzyme concentrations are usually elevated, although they do not correlate with disease severity; electrophysiologic studies are consistent with a myopathy.[215,216] The pathogenesis is unknown; most patients respond clinically to a course of corticosteroids. Zidovudine is associated with a polymyositis-like clinical picture in a small proportion of patients who take this drug. The mechanism of this myopathy is inhibition of mitochondrial DNA, which is distinguished on electron microscopy by "ragged red" fibers.[217]

Pyomyositis has been reported in patients with advanced HIV. Skin flora, particularly *Staphylococcus aureus,* are usually recovered from wound cultures, and preexisting skin diseases such as prurigo nodularis are a risk factor.[218,219]

Although rheumatologic findings in patients with HIV disease are not unusual, the extent to which HIV infection is associated with these disorders is not always clear. Defining a specific arthropathy caused by HIV is difficult because many patients with HIV infection are already at increased risk for inflammatory joint disease. Injection drug users, for example, may develop septic arthritis caused by pyogenic bacteria, particularly *S. aureus.* Homosexual men may have an increased risk for gonococcal arthritis or postinfectious reactive arthritis associated with genital or gastrointestinal tract infections (Reiter's syndrome). Immune complex deposition related to hepatitis B or C infection may also be associated with arthritis in patients with HIV infection. Thus, although some animal retroviruses are clearly associated with arthropathies, the situation with HIV remains somewhat clouded.

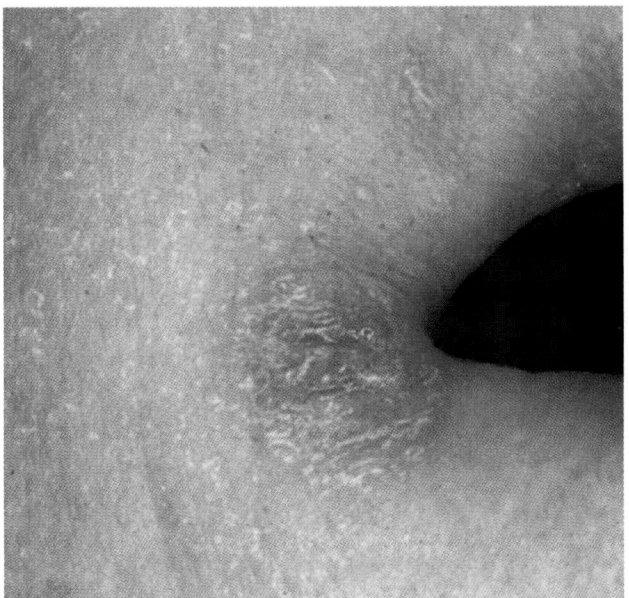

FIGURE 117-8. Angular cheilitis. *(Courtesy of Stephen Raffanti, MD, MPH.)*

Data from three large cohort studies demonstrate that Reiter's syndrome does not occur with increased frequency among HIV-infected persons.[220,221] The clinical course of Reiter's syndrome in HIV-infected persons may be prolonged and severe, however.[222] Patients with this syndrome are usually human leukocyte antigen (HLA)-B27 positive and present with an asymmetric oligoarticular arthritis, primarily of the large joints of the lower extremities, and sacroiliitis. Urethritis, conjunctivitis, keratoderma blennorrhagicum, and circinate balanitis may also be present. An enthesopathy of the Achilles tendon and plantar fascia can result in a characteristic gait in which weight is distributed to the lateral portion of the feet.[223] Aspirated synovial fluid is generally unremarkable, and synovial biopsy specimens show mononuclear cell infiltrates. Management is difficult, as the response to nonsteroidal anti-inflammatory drugs is limited and the use of the high doses of steroids often required further increases the risk of opportunistic infections. Methotrexate and azathioprine should also be avoided because of the resultant exacerbation of immune suppression.

Avascular necrosis of bone occurs at a higher frequency in HIV-infected persons than in HIV-seronegative persons in the general population,[224,225] and the incidence appears to be increasing.[226] Risk factors include corticosteroid therapy, lipid-lowering agents, and testosterone.[225] Although avascular necrosis has been described in persons receiving HAART,[227] such therapy does not appear to affect the risk of avascular necrosis.[228]

Cutaneous Manifestations

Dermatologic consequences of HIV infection include primary cutaneous opportunistic infections and malignancies (which may also disseminate to the viscera) and systemic opportunistic diseases with skin involvement.[229,230]

Viral Infections of the Skin and Mucous Membranes

A wide range of viruses involve the skin in HIV-immunosuppressed patients. The exanthem of acute HIV infection is an erythematous morbilliform eruption of the trunk and upper arms that occurs 2 to 4 weeks after infection and is usually associated with fever, headache, arthralgias, night sweats, pharyngitis, or thrush.[150,231,232] The rash resolves within 5 to 7 days. HSVs (see Chapter 132) frequently cause morbidity in patients with advanced HIV disease.[233] Serology shows previous infection with HSV-2 in more than 90% of homosexual men

with HIV infection; it is less prevalent in other groups. Although HSV-2 recurs frequently even in nonimmunosuppressed hosts, it recurs more frequently and for prolonged periods in patients with HIV infection. HSV-2, a common pathogen of the sacral root dermatomes, often causes outbreaks in the buttocks, perineum, scrotum, or vulva, and shaft and glans of the penis. Characteristic lesions of herpes simplex appear first as painful erythematous papules; later they vesiculate and ulcerate, and pustules may form. Chronic ulcers may become granulated, verrucous, or bloody (Fig. 117-9). Herpes simplex proctitis is associated with severe rectal pain, fever, tenesmus, and obstipation. External lesions may be absent, and the diagnosis is established by anoscopic or sigmoidoscopic examination and cultures. Giant perirectal ulcers and lesions at other sites that yield thymidine kinase–resistant strains of HSV-2 have occurred in patients who were previously treated with acyclovir. HSV infections are diagnosed by the typical appearance and distribution of the lesions and culture. Tzanck preparations may show giant cells, which suggest HSV infection. Some physicians base their diagnosis on how patients respond to an empirical trial of acyclovir. Orolabial HSV infections in HIV-infected persons may be caused by either HSV-1 or HSV-2. Although primary infections may occur after patients acquire HIV, recurrences are the more common manifestation of HSV infection. Often, a prodrome of tingling and pain precedes the appearance of painful vesicles and ulcers. Lesions may be found on the lips, buccal mucosa, gingiva, soft palate, uvula, and tongue. HSV disease may recur chronically in patients with advanced immunosuppression.

In persons with HIV infection varicella-zoster virus (shingles) is often reactivated[234] (see Chapter 133), typically when the CD4+ level is 200 to 500 cells/mm³. There have been reports of herpes zoster after initiation of HAART,[235] suggesting a role of the host immune response in this clinical manifestation. Herpes zoster may occur early in the course of HIV infection, but the incidence in late HIV disease is 5% to 10% annually.[236-240] Dermatomal outbreaks are most common, and a substantial proportion of patients may have several dermatomes involved (Fig. 117-10). Recurrent episodes at the same or different sites, chronic (nonremitting) zoster, and dissemination are often seen.[241] Shingles is often characterized by radicular pain and itching several days before erythematous papules appear, and vesiculation occurs within several days. Lesions are often extremely pruritic, and excoriation with secondary bacterial infection commonly occurs. Over a period of 4 to 7 days, lesions form bullae and crusts and begin to heal, although some patients have zoster chronically. Cranial and thoracic dermatomes, followed by lumbar and sacral roots, are most often involved. Outbreaks along the ophthalmic branch of the trigeminal nerve may result in corneal involvement and lead to scarring and opacification that impair vision. A substantial proportion of patients may experience postherpetic scarring and pain. In patients with HIV infection

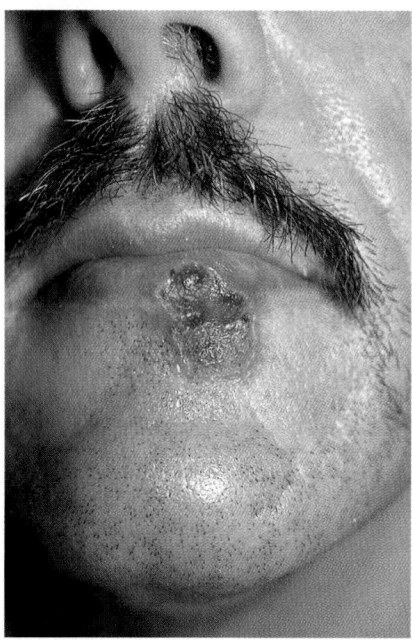

FIGURE 117-9. Herpes simplex. *(Courtesy of Stephen Raffanti, MD, MPH.)*

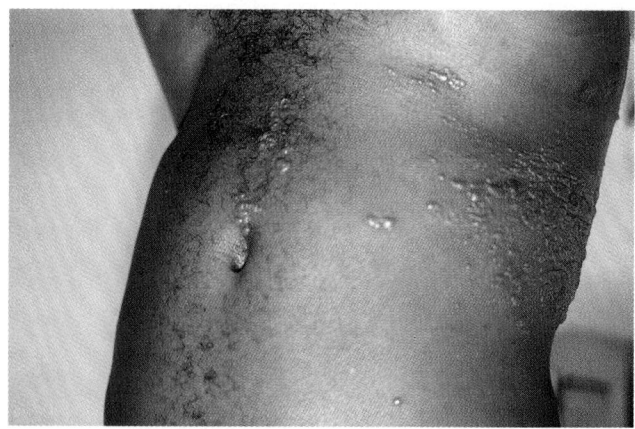

FIGURE 117-10. Herpes zoster in dermatomal distribution. *(Courtesy of Stephen Raffanti, MD, MPH.)*

who acquire primary varicella (chickenpox), the acute infection may progress to a chronic form in a period of weeks to months.

Despite the frequency of disseminated CMV disease in late-stage AIDS, cutaneous manifestations are unusual. Vesicles, bullae, and hyperpigmented indurated plaques have all been described, however. Infections with human papillomavirus, the causative agent of condylomata acuminata, are more prevalent in HIV-infected persons than in the general population. In addition to genital lesions (Chapter 140), warts are often seen in periungual locations, on the feet (plantar warts), and in bearded areas of the face.

Molluscum contagiosum, a cutaneous poxvirus infection, is seen more often in HIV-infected persons than in other populations (see Chapter 130). Most patients have CD4[+] cell counts less than 200/mm[3]. The agent is transmitted by sexual or other close contact; reactivation of remote infection may cause outbreaks in immunosuppressed hosts. Molluscum lesions are small, firm papules with a pearly white umbilicated surface distributed on the face, trunk, or genital areas. The lesions are usually painless and can be differentiated from herpetic lesions by the absence of erythema, smaller size, and resolution of lesions without ulcerating or crusting (Fig. 117-11). Biopsy may be necessary to exclude more serious causes of cutaneous lesions such as cryptococcosis, pyogenic granuloma, and basal cell carcinoma. Liquid nitrogen is used effectively to treat this condition. Lesions may also resolve after initiation of HAART with a resultant increase in CD4[+] level.[242]

Bacillary Angiomatosis

Bacillary angiomatosis is associated with cutaneous and visceral involvement that produces lesions characterized by vascular proliferation, hemorrhage, and necrosis.[243-246] The disease was first described in 1983 in an AIDS patient with subcutaneous nodules with vascular proliferation and evidence of bacterial involvement by electron microscopy.[247] Subsequently, the etiology of bacillary angiomatosis was attributed to the organisms *Bartonella henselae* and *Bartonella quintana* (see Chapter 232). *B. henselae* infection has been associated with cat and flea exposure and *B. quintana* infection with low socioeconomic status, homelessness, and exposure to lice.[248] *Bartonella* organisms have been cultured from skin lesions, blood, liver, bone, and other sites.[243-246]

Patients with bacillary angiomatosis usually present with one or several cutaneous lesions, although disseminated disease is common. The typical skin lesions are purple-red nodules or plaques that can ulcerate and crust. Lesions may be mistaken for cutaneous KS, skin tags, or basal cell carcinoma. Visceral disease may include hepatitis (bacillary peliosis), splenic or osseous lesions, bacillemia, pneumonitis, or, less often, involvement of other organs.[249] Bacillary peliosis is a characteristic illness in which patients present with fever, right upper quadrant pain, hepatomegaly, and elevation of liver enzymes, particularly alkaline phosphatase.[250,251] Imaging studies of the liver may reveal echogenic defects; histologically, lesions have a cystic appearance, with vascular proliferation, hemorrhage, and necrosis.

The diagnosis of bacillary angiomatosis is best made by biopsy of involved sites. Hematoxylin and eosin stains of biopsy specimens from skin lesions show proliferation of small blood vessels in the dermis or cutis, enlarged endothelial cells with abundant cytoplasm, and necrotic and granulomatous changes. Warthin-Starry stains show perivascular accumulations of bacilli; these findings may be confirmed by electron microscopy, although this is not usually necessary. The diagnosis can also be established by culture of the organism in several special media or by detection of *Bartonella* DNA by polymerase chain reaction.[252] Serologic assays for anti-*Bartonella* antibodies are available through the Special Pathogens Branch of the CDC. The natural history of the infection in patients with HIV is for relapses to occur in the absence of prolonged therapy with erythromycin or doxycycline. Fluoroquinolones, other macrolides, and trimethoprim-sulfamethoxazole also have activity against *Bartonella*.

Kaposi's Sarcoma

KS is a vascular neoplastic disorder that in the United States is seen predominantly in HIV-infected homosexual men. Human herpesvirus type 8, which is transmitted sexually, has been implicated in the pathogenesis of KS (see Chapters 121 and 137).[253-255] Although KS also affects visceral organs, the characteristic findings are cutaneous red-purple nodules or plaques (Fig. 117-12). Sites commonly involved include the legs, feet, mucous membranes, hard palate, nose, trunk, and scalp.[256] Lesions of KS are often difficult to distinguish from those of bacillary angiomatosis; biopsy is required for diagnosis.

Other Cutaneous Manifestations

A variety of other skin disorders have been described in HIV-infected patients. Seborrheic dermatitis, an inflammatory condition of sebaceous glands that may be associated with dermatophytic superinfection, is an early complication (Fig. 117-13). Erythema and scaling of midline areas of the forehead, face, and groin are typical findings. Psoriasis occurs in 5% of HIV-infected persons, with scaly reddish plaques, onycholysis, nail pitting, and subungual hyperkeratosis. Associated psoriatic arthritis occurs more frequently than among HIV-seronegative persons with psoriasis. Tinea infections of the scalp, trunk, inguinal and perineal areas, extremities, and feet are also quite common. Onychomycoses, or fungal infections of the fingernails and toenails, are common although usually asymptomatic, causing only cosmetic changes. Bacterial folliculitis may be localized or disseminated in patients with HIV infection, and relapses frequently occur. *S. aureus* is the most common causative pathogen. Eosinophilic folliculitis (Fig. 117-14) is an inflammatory condition associated with raised, pruritic nodules with a pustular head on an erythematous base

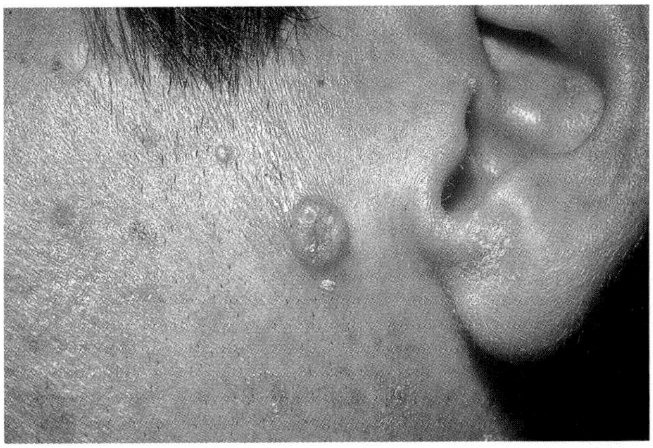

FIGURE 117-11. Molluscum contagiosum. *(Courtesy of Stephen Raffanti, MD, MPH.)*

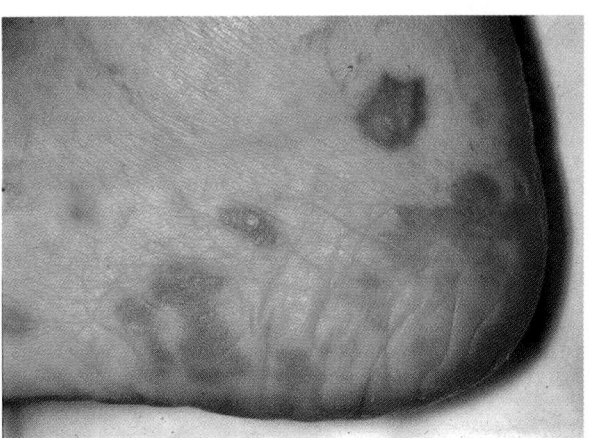

FIGURE 117-12. Kaposi's sarcoma. *(Courtesy of Stephen Raffanti, MD, MPH.)*

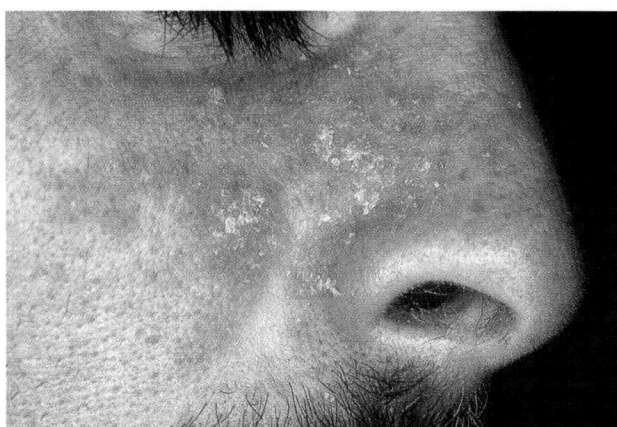

FIGURE 117-13. Seborrheic dermatitis. *(Courtesy of Stephen Raffanti, MD, MPH.)*

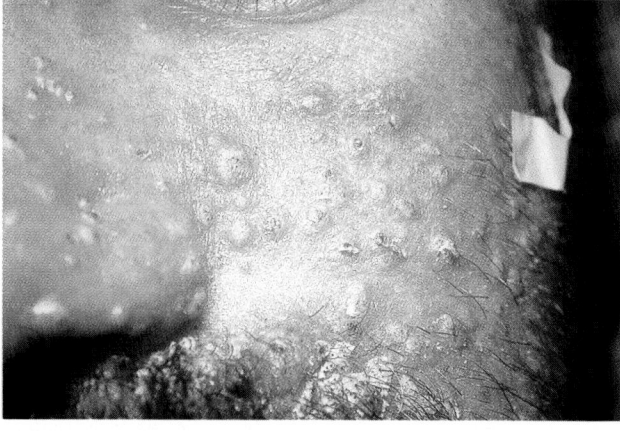

FIGURE 117-15. Cryptococcosis. *(Courtesy of Stephen Raffanti, MD, MPH.)*

and is similar to bacterial folliculitis. Biopsy specimens of these lesions reveal intense infiltration of eosinophils and absence of polymorphonuclear cells and organisms. Xerosis and ichthyosis are also common in patients with more advanced HIV disease and may be refractory to therapy with emollients and anti-inflammatory agents. Prurigo nodularis appears as nodules and papules caused by chronic rubbing and scratching. This is precipitated by one of the many causes of pruritus in HIV-infected persons, such as xerosis, eosinophilic folliculitis, and atopic dermatitis.

Disseminated cryptococcosis and histoplasmosis may cause mucocutaneous papules, nodules, pustules, or ulcers (Figs. 117-15 and 117-16). Biopsy and culture establish the diagnosis. In Thailand and southern China, *P. marneffei* is a common opportunistic fungal infectious agent in AIDS patients.[257] Patients can present with umbilicated papules, subcutaneous nodules, or morbilliform eruptions. Diagnosis is established by identifying the elliptic organism with central septation and characteristic red pigment production when grown in culture. Nontuberculous mycobacteria such as *M. avium* complex and *Mycobacterium haemophilum* may cause cutaneous papules, pustules, abscesses, lymphadenitis, or ulcerations. Culture is required for diagnosis.

Scabies

Sarcoptes scabiei var. *humanus* is the mite responsible for this common ectoparasitic infestation in HIV-infected persons. Scaly pruritic papules or hyperkeratotic plaques may occur on the palms, soles, trunk, or extremities. Characteristic burrows between the fingers and on the wrists

are not always seen. Norwegian (crusted) scabies (Fig. 117-17) is a severe and highly contagious manifestation of this disease, seen particularly with advanced immunosuppression.[258] Permethrin 5% cream and ivermectin are effective therapies.[259]

Renal Disease

A number of renal abnormalities have been described in patients with HIV infection, including a specific HIV-related nephropathy.[260-262] Ascribing renal dysfunction to HIV infection is problematic, however, because some patients with HIV have a high risk for renal disease of other causes. Intravenous drug use, hepatitis B and C infection, hypertension, fluid and electrolyte disorders, and concomitant opportunistic infections and malignancies are all associated with renal dysfunction. In addition, many drugs used to treat HIV infection and its associated opportunistic infections are nephrotoxic. Pentamidine, foscarnet, and the aminoglycosides can cause acute tubular necrosis, and indinavir, sulfadiazine, and intravenous acyclovir can cause intratubular obstruction by crystal formation. Thrombotic thrombocytopenic purpura/hemolytic uremic syndrome has been reported in HIV-infected persons. Hypertension may be a prominent feature, and the prognosis is poor.[263] Immune complex–mediated glomerular diseases, such as those associated with immunoglobulin A nephropathy[264] and hepatitis C virus infection,[265] have also been reported.

HIV-associated nephropathy was first reported in 1984 and occurs in 2% to 10% of HIV-infected persons.[260] Manifestations include proteinuria, mildly elevated serum creatinine levels, and focal and segmental glomerulosclerosis on histopathology. Although this entity is

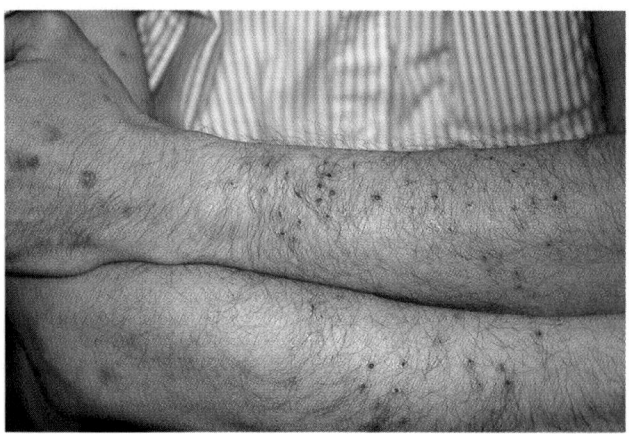

FIGURE 117-14. Eosinophilic dermatitis. *(Courtesy of Stephen Raffanti, MD, MPH.)*

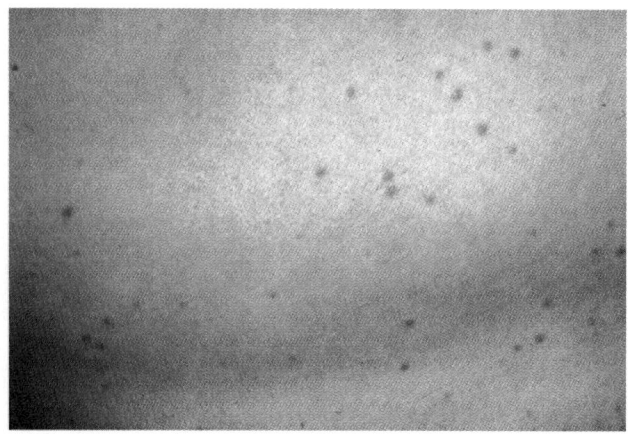

FIGURE 117-16. Histoplasmosis. *(Courtesy of Stephen Raffanti, MD, MPH.)*

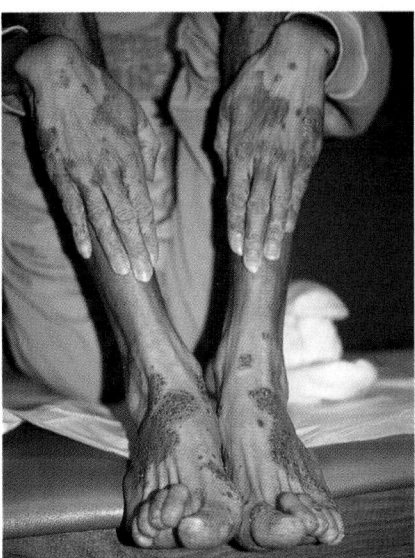

FIGURE 117-17. Norwegian scabies (in a patient with wasting syndrome). (*Courtesy of Stephen Raffanti, MD, MPH.*)

similar to heroin-associated nephropathy, only half of the patients studied had a history of intravenous drug use. In a review of 75 consecutive AIDS patients in Miami, 43% of the patients had proteinuria with more than 0.5 g of proteins per 24 hours; 9% had greater than 3 g per 24 hours.[266] In 36 autopsies, 17 (47%) had renal pathology, 5 had focal glomerulosclerosis, and 12 had mesangial proliferation. A subsequent review of the same population of patients found that patients with a history of intravenous drug use had the highest incidence of renal disease; however, other non–drug-using patients, including children, can develop HIV-related nephropathy. In another series of patients, renal disease was observed in 13 of 32 and included focal glomerulosclerosis, mesangial proliferation, and glomerulonephritis.[267] The pathogenesis of HIV-associated nephropathy is incompletely understood. Human and animal models have demonstrated proliferation of renal epithelial cells and apoptosis[268]; direct HIV-induced damage of glomerular and tubular epithelial cells may be involved. HIV-associated nephropathy is more commonly reported in blacks than in other racial groups, suggesting a biologic or genetic susceptibility to this disorder.[262]

Renal dysfunction in patients with HIV disease is usually diagnosed incidentally when patients present with opportunistic infections and have CD4$^+$ cell counts less than 200/mm^3.[269] Asymptomatic proteinuria, up to 5 g/day, is often the initial finding, and the serum creatinine level is often normal or only mildly elevated. The albumin concentration is almost always low (as is true for most AIDS patients with opportunistic infections), and the blood pressure is usually normal. Renal biopsy most often shows focal and segmental glomerulosclerosis ("collapsing" glomerulosclerosis) with severe tubulointerstitial disease and proliferative microcyst formation. Immunofluorescence studies often reveal deposits of immunoglobulin M and C3, and electron microscopy shows tuboloreticular inclusion bodies.[262]

The clinical course of HIV-related nephropathy progresses quickly, usually because many other opportunistic processes occur simultaneously. Rao and coworkers[260] originally reported death with renal failure in 8 of 11 patients with HIV-related nephropathy in less than 4 months. Because nephropathy is usually diagnosed late in the course of HIV disease, it is difficult to determine the effect of renal dysfunction on survival. Some centers have reported that patients with AIDS respond poorly to maintenance by hemodialysis.[270] There is no proven effective therapy for HIV-associated nephropathy, although reports have suggested a benefit from HAART,[271] corticosteroids,[272] angiotensin-converting enzyme inhibitors,[273] and cyclosporine.[274]

Ocular Complications

Ocular diseases are extremely common manifestations of HIV disease, with a wide variety of causes, ranging from a benign HIV retinopathy to sight-threatening viral opportunistic infections.[275-277] As HIV disease progresses, the risk of ocular complications rises appreciably.

HIV retinopathy occurs in one half to three fourths of all patients with HIV, with the prevalence higher in those with low CD4 counts. The most frequent finding is a cotton-wool spot, a small pale lesion that is thought to represent transient focal retinal ischemia. HIV retinopathy may also produce microaneurysms and retinal hemorrhages. The condition is generally benign, although some patients have developed visual defects attributed to this condition.

The most common and serious ocular complication of HIV disease is retinitis, most often caused by CMV. CMV is ubiquitous in patients with HIV infection and causes serious morbidity in AIDS. CMV is transmitted by the same routes as HIV, and almost all patients with sexually acquired HIV infection are also infected with CMV. Like other herpesviruses, CMV may infect cells latently and be reactivated when host defenses are impaired. Asymptomatic CMV viruria and viremia may be found in one third to one half of patients with advanced HIV disease. The risk of CMV retinitis is determined largely by the CD4$^+$ cell count and CMV DNA level in the peripheral blood. For patients with CD4$^+$ cell counts less than 200/mm^3, the annual risk is 4% to 12%. Further risk stratification is aided by CMV DNA measurements, with aviremic patients having less than 1% risk per year, even at low CD4$^+$ cell counts.[278]

CMV has a unique predilection for the retina, with 90% of end-organ disease in patients with HIV infection being retinitis.[279] Other involved sites include the colon, esophagus, stomach, adrenals, pancreas, brain, and lungs. The onset of CMV retinitis may be insidious or rapid. Patients complain of painless, progressive visual loss, blurring, and "floaters." CMV retinitis usually arises unilaterally, although it may subsequently progress to the contralateral retina. Funduscopic examination of the involved eye typically reveals coalescing white exudates in a vascular pattern with surrounding hemorrhage and edema. Often, lesions are peripheral initially, involve the fovea later, and result in visual loss. Retinal detachment may occur as a late complication.

Fortunately, the advent of combination antiretroviral therapy has resulted in astonishing declines in the incidence of CMV retinitis. Several population-based studies have reported 60% to 90% reductions in the incidence of this disease. Improvement in cell-mediated immunity with antiretroviral therapy results in suppression of CMV DNA in plasma, with a subsequent fall in the risk of disease. Indeed, it appears that patients with treated CMV retinitis who receive HAART may safely discontinue anti-CMV therapy if their CD4$^+$ counts rise to greater than 100 cells/mm^3.[280]

For patients with CD4$^+$ counts less than 50 cells/mm^3, education regarding retinitis symptoms and regular ophthalmologic examinations are recommended. Patients complaining of ocular symptoms should undergo a thorough ophthalmologic examination. Retinal findings may include cotton-wool spots or lesions of infectious retinitis. Less common retinal infections include toxoplasmosis, pneumocystosis, varicella-zoster virus, and ocular syphilis, which is usually a diffuse intraocular process. Cotton-wool spots are prevalent in patients with AIDS but do not appear to predict the development of other retinal disease. The cotton-wool spots are distributed in a vascular pattern similar to that of CMV but do not have the irregular pattern of full retinal exudates and hemorrhages that is characteristic of CMV retinitis. An ophthalmologist or other highly trained observer should examine any patient with signs or symptoms of retinitis promptly, as delay in therapy can result in irreversible visual loss. Cultures of the blood and urine yield CMV in 60% and 80% of cases, respectively, although the diagnosis rarely rests on these results.

Patients who have had CMV retinitis frequently experience acute retinal detachments. Erosion of the retinal border at the site of a necrotic lesion allows the retina to be lifted off underlying tissues. Patients complain of sudden loss of vision, "like a curtain falling" in front of the affected eye. Surgical reattachment is often partially successful in restoring vision, although progressive visual loss may ensue.

Varicella-zoster retinitis is a severe necrotizing retinitis that may occur in patients with advanced HIV disease and low CD4+ cell counts, although some cases occur at earlier stages of HIV disease.[281] Patients most often note rapid visual loss. Funduscopic findings include peripheral necrosis, occlusive vasculopathy, optic neuritis, and vitreal and scleral inflammation, and the syndrome is termed acute retinal necrosis. Varicella-zoster retinitis usually occurs in the absence of zoster at other sites, but a history of varicella-zoster virus disease is common and the virus may be isolated from tissue samples in some patients.[282] Blindness ensues despite therapy in a majority of patients, although responses to acyclovir and foscarnet have been reported.

Ocular toxoplasmosis occurs in patients with advanced immunodeficiency, and many but not all have cerebral toxoplasmosis. *Toxoplasma* retinitis is characterized by discrete, rounded, pale exudates. Lesions are usually discrete foci of retinal inflammation without hemorrhage or vasculopathy. Vitreal inflammation is common. The diagnosis is made by observation by an experienced ophthalmologist.

P. jirovecii may cause a choroiditis that mimics CMV retinitis.[283] The lesions are typically posterior, yellow-orange in appearance, and do not cause vitreal inflammation. Choroidal pneumocystosis occurs most often in patients with previous *P. jirovecii* pneumonia, particularly in those taking aerosolized pentamidine for prophylaxis.

Cardiac Manifestations

Although early clinical observations suggested that HIV infection spared the heart, subsequent experience has shown that cardiac involvement in HIV and AIDS is not unusual.[284,285] Cardiac abnormalities in patients with HIV infection may include opportunistic infections or diseases of the myocardium (e.g., *T. gondii, Trypanosoma cruzi*) or pericardium (e.g., mycobacteria, KS), left ventricular dysfunction and dilated cardiomyopathy, cardiac autonomic abnormalities, and vascular heart disease such as pulmonary hypertension. Infectious endocarditis may also occur in patients with HIV infection, especially injection drug users, but there is little evidence to suggest that the risk is increased after accounting for behaviors. Marantic endocarditis is a manifestation of late-stage HIV disease and is sometimes noted at autopsy. Accelerated atherosclerosis with myocardial infarction has been reported in patients with HIV infection being treated with protease inhibitors and with elevated serum cholesterol and triglyceride levels.[286]

Myocardial disease in HIV-infected individuals is surprisingly common, particularly in late-stage disease. Infectious myocarditis has been reported with a number of opportunistic infections, notably *T. gondii*. In an autopsy-based study in France, for example, 12% of AIDS patients who died were found to have cardiac toxoplasmosis.[287] Most patients with cardiac toxoplasmosis also had cerebral involvement, although several patients had isolated toxoplasmic myocarditis. Myocarditis may be seen in acute *T. gondii* infection, and coincident toxoplasmic pneumonitis may present a clinical picture of diffuse pulmonary infiltrates and cardiac insufficiency. Other opportunistic agents causing myocardial involvement include mycobacteria and fungi.

A more common and underdiagnosed disorder in HIV-infected individuals is cardiomyopathy with left ventricular dysfunction, which may result in congestive heart failure.[288] Several large cohort studies have found that 8% to 12% of patients with HIV infection have echocardiographic evidence of left ventricular dysfunction, and the incidence of dilated cardiomyopathy with severe congestive heart failure (New York Heart Association class III or IV) is 15% to 18% per year.[289,290] Clinical evaluation of patients may reveal only complaints of fatigue and exertional dyspnea, and physical examination may show tachycardia without rales or overt signs of congestive heart failure. Echocardiography shows global hypokinesis and enlargement of all four chambers with a modestly to severely reduced left ventricular ejection fraction and increased end-diastolic volume index. Chest radiography is frequently unhelpful. The etiology of HIV-related cardiomyopathies is multifactorial, with conflicting data on the role of cardiotropic viruses, vitamin deficiencies, and cardiotoxic drugs in causing disease. There is compelling evidence, however, that HIV itself is involved in the pathogenesis of cardiomyopathy in a large proportion of patients.[289,290] HIV has been identified in myocardial tissue by in situ hybridization in several studies and found to be positive in one third to two thirds of patients with myocarditis. In addition, an inflammatory cellular infiltrate composed of major histocompatibility complex class I–expressing CD8+ cells is found in a large proportion of patients, suggesting an autoimmune mechanism in this process. Other viruses also implicated in dilated cardiomyopathy in patients with HIV infection include Epstein-Barr virus, coxsackieviruses, and CMV. Supportive treatment with digoxin, diuretics, and afterload reduction is usually of symptomatic benefit, and some patients with inflammatory myocarditis respond to corticosteroid therapy. Nonetheless, the prognosis for patients with this finding is poor,[291] although combination antiretroviral therapy might change this.

Pericardial effusions have been reported in varying proportions of patients in a number of studies, many of which suffer from selection bias. Among patients with more advanced illness in hospital-based settings, pericardial effusions can be quite common. A Portuguese study found, for example, that 41% of 181 HIV-infected patients had pericardial effusions.[292] Most effusions in this setting are asymptomatic or arise with signs and symptoms of opportunistic disease at other sites. The etiology of pericardial disease in patients with HIV infection is diverse, but opportunistic infections and malignancies are the agents most commonly implicated. Mycobacterial infections, especially tuberculosis, are frequently associated with pericardial involvement in areas where coinfection with HIV and *M. tuberculosis* is common, and nontuberculous mycobacteria may also invade the pericardial space. Other infections seen in the pericardium include bacterial infections, fungal infections (e.g., *Cryptococcus*), and viral cardiopulmonary infections. KS and non-Hodgkin's lymphoma may cause pericardial effusion as well. Cardiac tamponade or cardiac dysfunction resulting from effusions is unusual in most series, and in most cases pericardiocentesis is not necessary as a therapeutic maneuver. One study, however, reported that 40% of patients with an HIV-related pericardial effusion had signs of tamponade.[293]

Hematologic Manifestations

HIV infection can affect all three hematologic cell lines: leukocytes, red blood cells, and platelets. Although neutropenia and anemia are seen primarily in advanced disease, thrombocytopenia can occur in either early-stage disease (e.g., HIV-related thrombocytopenia) or late-stage disease (thrombotic thrombocytopenic purpura [TTP]). Neutropenia may be due to either HIV infection itself or an adverse effect of therapy. In one study, neutropenia was an independent risk factor for bacterial infection after controlling for CD4 count.[294] In another study of 71 patients with an absolute neutrophil count less than 1000 cells/mm^3 for a median of 13 days, only 6 (8%) developed culture-proven infection.[295] The risk of infection increased with decreasing CD4 counts, but most episodes were mild and self-limited.[295] Anemia is common in advanced HIV infection and is an independent risk factor for death.[296,297] HIV-related thrombocytopenia is due to both immune-mediated platelet destruction (as is seen in idiopathic thrombocytopenic purpura) and impaired platelet production.[298] Patients are usually asymptomatic, even with profound thrombocytopenia. The thrombocytopenia usually responds to antiretroviral therapy; this has been best studied with azidothymidine but has also been shown with

HAART.[299,300] TTP in an HIV-infected person was first described by Jokela and colleagues in 1987.[301] The classic diagnostic pentad includes thrombocytopenia, microangiopathic hemolytic anemia, renal failure, fever, and neurologic abnormalities, although not all patients have all of these findings. In addition, given the high frequency of many of these findings in persons with advanced AIDS, such a diagnosis may not always be considered. The incidence of TTP appears to be decreasing in the HAART era.[302]

Immune Reconstitution Syndromes

HAART (regimens that include a HIV protease inhibitor or non-nucleoside reverse transcriptase inhibitor together with nucleoside reverse transcriptase inhibitors) is associated with dramatic reductions in HIV-1 RNA and increases in CD4+ lymphocyte counts. In addition to significantly decreasing HIV-related mortality and the incidence of opportunistic infections (as discussed earlier), the improvement in immune function can be associated with paradoxical worsening of underlying opportunistic infections.[303] The clinical presentation of immune reconstitution syndromes varies according to the pathogen (see later). Not every patient who has immunologic improvement with antiretroviral therapy experiences paradoxical worsening; the risk factors for the development of these syndromes are not well understood.

Mycobacterium tuberculosis

Paradoxical worsening of tuberculosis was initially described in HIV-seronegative tuberculosis patients before the HIV era, but it appears to be more common in HIV-infected patients.[139] Clinical manifestations include fever, adenopathy (e.g., cervical, thoracic, or intra-abdominal), and worsening pulmonary infiltrates. Central nervous system tuberculomas, pleural effusions, and psoas abscesses have also been described.[139,304] Diagnoses such as lymphoma, adverse drug reaction, and tuberculosis treatment failure related to nonadherence, malabsorption, or drug resistance must be excluded before the diagnosis of paradoxical worsening can be established. Receipt of HAART has been associated with an increased risk of paradoxical worsening in some but not all studies; the incidence rate ranges from 7% to 36%.[139,304,305] Persons who experience worsening with HAART usually do so within 2 to 3 weeks of starting therapy. Clinical management includes continuation of antituberculosis and antiretroviral therapy and use of corticosteroids (e.g., prednisone 1 mg/kg per day, then taper as symptoms allow) for symptomatic relief of severe manifestations, such as compromise of the airways or venous return to the heart.

Mycobacterium avium Complex Disease

Focal or diffuse lymphadenitis developing within 2 to 3 months of initiation of HAART has been described in several persons with low baseline CD4+ lymphocyte counts.[130,306] Mycobacteremia is generally not present, but cultures of lymph nodes usually grow *M. avium*. There have also been reports of focal osteomyelitis developing in persons who discontinue either primary or secondary *M. avium* prophylaxis after sustained increases in CD4+ counts during HAART.[307,308] Treatment is the same as that for *M. avium* infection in the absence of immune reconstitution.

Cytomegalovirus

CMV retinitis in the setting of immune reconstitution ("immune recovery uveitis") has been described among persons both with and without a history of CMV retinitis before initiation of HAART.[309-311] Development of CMV disease at extraocular sites (e.g., blood stream, colon, and pancreas) in patients without prior CMV disease has also been described.[312] Among persons with a history of CMV retinitis who subsequently initiate and respond to HAART, 18% to 63% develop immune recovery uveitis.[313,314] The median time of HAART until development of uveitis was 43 weeks in one study.[313] The optimal management is unclear. Oral corticosteroids with or without concomitant anti-CMV therapy are often used.

Varicella-Zoster Virus

There have been several reports of the development of herpes zoster in persons receiving HAART. In two series, herpes zoster developed in 7% to 8% of persons receiving combination antiretroviral therapy and occurred within 17 weeks of initiation of therapy.[315,316] In one report herpes zoster was associated with an increase in CD8+ lymphocytes.[316] The clinical manifestations are usually not severe and respond to acyclovir or famciclovir.

Viral Hepatitis

Persons infected with hepatitis C virus (HCV) can develop acute hepatitis or cirrhosis during HAART.[317,318] It is often difficult to discern whether elevations in hepatic transaminases are due to toxicity of antiretroviral therapy or to immune reconstitution. In a study of 60 persons coinfected with HIV and HCV who completed at least 16 weeks of HAART, immune recovery was associated with a persistent increase in HCV RNA, particularly in persons with baseline CD4 count less than 350 cells/mm^3.[319,320] Other studies have found that hepatotoxicity in coinfected patients who respond to HAART is associated with increased HCV-specific immune responses and T-cell activation.[321] This suggests that at least in some cases, hepatotoxicity is associated with immune reconstitution. There have also been reports of acute hepatitis developing during HAART among persons with prior hepatitis B virus infection, in which increased HBV RNA levels are detected.[322] Management of patients with chronic hepatitis is discussed in Chapter 112.

Other Diseases

Although less commonly reported, paradoxical worsening in the setting of immune reconstitution has also been described after initiation of HAART with *C. neoformans*,[323] *P. jirovecii* pneumonia,[324,325] and progressive multifocal leukoencephalopathy.[326]

REFERENCES

1. Follansbee SE, Busch DF, Wofsy CB, et al. An outbreak of *Pneumocystis carinii* pneumonia in homosexual men. Ann Intern Med. 1982;96:705-713.
2. Gottlieb MS, Schroff R, Schanker HM, et al. *Pneumocystis carinii* pneumonia and mucosal candidiasis in previously healthy homosexual men: Evidence of a new acquired cellular immunodeficiency. N Engl J Med. 1981;305:1425-1431.
3. Masur H, Michelis MA, Greene JB, et al. An outbreak of community-acquired *Pneumocystis carinii* pneumonia: Initial manifestation of cellular immune dysfunction. N Engl J Med. 1981;305:1431-1438.
4. Siegal FP, Lopez C, Hammer GS, et al. Severe acquired immunodeficiency in male homosexuals manifested by chronic perianal ulcerative herpes simplex lesions. N Engl J Med. 1981;305:1439-1444.
5. Centers for Disease Control. Kaposi's sarcoma and *Pneumocystis carinii* pneumonia in homosexual men—New York City and California. MMWR Morb Mortal Wkly Rep. 1982;30:305-308.
6. Centers for Disease Control. Opportunistic infections and Kaposi's sarcoma among Haitians in the United States. MMWR Morb Mortal Wkly Rep. 1982;31:353-361.
7. Centers for Disease Control. Update on acquired immunodeficiency syndrome (AIDS)—United States. MMWR Morb Mortal Wkly Rep. 1982;31:507-514.
8. Centers for Disease Control. Update on immunodeficiency syndrome (AIDS)—United States. MMWR Morb Mortal Wkly Rep. 1985;34:245-248.
9. Centers for Disease Control. *Pneumocystis carinii* pneumonia among persons with hemophilia A. MMWR Morb Mortal Wkly Rep. 1982;31:365-367.
10. Centers for Disease Control. Update on acquired immune deficiency syndrome (AIDS) among patients with hemophilia A. MMWR Morb Mortal Wkly Rep. 1982;31:644-646.
11. Pape JW, Liautaud B, Thomas F, et al. Characteristics of the acquired immunodeficiency syndrome (AIDS) in Haiti. N Engl J Med. 1983;309:945-950.
12. Pape JW, Liautaud B, Thomas F, et al. The acquired immunodeficiency syndrome in Haiti. Ann Intern Med. 1985;103:674-678.
13. Centers for Disease Control. Possible transfusion-associated acquired immune deficiency syndrome AIDS—California. MMWR Morb Mortal Wkly Rep. 1982;31:652-654.
14. Malebranche R, Annoux E, Guerin JM, et al. AIDS with severe gastrointestinal manifestations in Haiti. Lancet. 1983;2:873-878.
15. Abrams DI, Lewis BJ, Beckstead JP, et al. Persistent diffuse lymphadenopathy in homosexual men: Endpoint or prodrome? Ann Intern Med. 1984;100:801-808.
16. Abrams DI, Volberding PA, Linker CA, et al. Immune thrombocytopenic purpura in homosexual men: Clinical manifestations and treatment results (Abstract). Blood. 1984;62:1082.

17. Metroka CE, Cunningham-Rundles S, Pollack MS, et al. Persistent generalized lymphadenopathy in homosexual men. Ann Intern Med. 1983;99:585-591.

18. Morris L, Distenfeld A, Amorosi E, et al. Autoimmune thrombocytopenic purpura in homosexual men. Ann Intern Med. 1982;96:714-717.

19. Walsh CM, Nardi MA, Karpatkin S. On the mechanism of thrombocytopenic purpura in sexually active homosexual men. N Engl J Med. 1984;311:635-639.

20. Abrams DI. AIDS-related conditions. Clin Immunol Allergy. 1986;6:581.

21. Harris C, Small CB, Klein RS, et al. Immunodeficiency in female sexual partners of men with the acquired immunodeficiency syndrome. N Engl J Med. 1984;308:1181-1184.

22. Barre-Sinoussi F, Chermann JC, Rey F, et al. Isolation of a T-lymphotropic retrovirus from a patient at risk for acquired immunodeficiency syndrome (AIDS). Science. 1983;220:868-871.

23. Gallo RC, Saluhudin SZ, Popovic M, et al. Frequent detection and isolation of cytopathic retroviruses (HTLV-III) from patient with AIDS and at risk for AIDS. Science. 1984;224:500-503.

24. Levy JA, Hoffman AD, Kramer SD, et al. Isolation of lymphocytopathic retrovirus from San Francisco patients with AIDS. Science. 1984;225:840-842.

25. Garry RF, Witte MH, Gottlieb AA, et al. Documentation of AIDS virus infection in the United States in 1968. JAMA. 1988;260:2085-2087.

26. Nzilambi N, De Cock KM, Forthal DN, et al. The prevalence of infection with human immunodeficiency virus over a 10-year period in rural Zaire. N Engl J Med. 1988;318:276-279.

27. Centers for Disease Control. Revision of the CDC surveillance case definition for acquired immunodeficiency syndrome. MMWR Morb Mortal Wkly Rep. 1987;36:1S-15S.

28. Selik RM, Buehler JW, Karon JM, et al. Impact of the 1986 revision of the case definition of acquired immunodeficiency syndrome in the United States. J Acquir Immune Defic Syndr. 1990;3:73-82.

29. World Health Organization. Interim proposal for a WHO staging system for HIV infection and diseases. Wkly Epidemiol Rec. 1990;65:221-224.

30. Centers for Disease Control. 1993 revised classification system for HIV infection and expanded surveillance case definition for AIDS among adolescents and adults. MMWR Morb Mortal Wkly Rep. 1992;41:1-19.

31. Ho DD, Neumann AV, Perel AS, et al. Rapid turnover of plasma virions and CD4 lymphocytes in HIV-1 infection. Nature. 1995;373:123-126.

32. Perelson AS, Neumann AV, Markowitz M, et al. HIV-1 dynamics in vivo: Virion clearance rate, infected cell life-span, and viral generation time. Science. 1996;271:1582-1586.

33. Wei X, Ghosh SK, Taylor ME, et al. Viral dynamics in human immunodeficiency virus type 1 infection. Nature. 1995;373:117-122.

34. Centers for Disease Control. Current trends: Classification system for human T lymphotropic virus type III/lymphadenopathy associated virus infections. MMWR Morb Mortal Wkly Rep. 1986;35:334-339.

35. Havlir DV, Richman DD. Viral dynamics of HIV: Implications for drug development and therapeutic strategies. Ann Intern Med. 1996;124:984-989.

36. Henrard DR, Phillips JF, Muenz LR, et al. Natural history of HIV-1 cell-free viremia. JAMA. 1995;274:554-558.

37. Phair J, Jacobson L, Detels R, et al. Acquired immune deficiency syndrome occurring within 5 years of infection with human immunodeficiency virus type 1: The Multicenter AIDS Cohort Study. J Acquir Immune Defic Syndr. 1992;5:490-496.

38. Cao Y, Qin L, Zhang L, et al. Virologic and immunologic characterization of long-term survivors of human immunodeficiency virus type 1 infection. N Engl J Med. 1995;332:201-208.

39. Sheppard HW, Lang W, Ascher MS, et al. The characteristics of non-progressors: Long term HIV-1 infection with stable CD4+ T-cell levels. AIDS. 1993;7:1159-1166.

40. Bacchetti P, Moss AR. Incubation period of AIDS in San Francisco. Nature. 1993;338:251-253.

41. Alcabes P, Munoz A, Vlahov D, Friedland GH. Incubation period of human immunodeficiency virus. AIDS. 1993;15:303-318.

42. Rutherford GW, Lifson AR, Hessol NA, et al. Course of HIV-1 infection in a cohort of homosexual and bisexual men: An 11 year follow-up study. BMJ. 1990;301:1183-1188.

43. Fahey JH, Taylor JM, Detels R, et al. The prognostic value of cellular and serologic markers in infection with human immunodeficiency virus type 1. N Engl J Med. 1990;322:166-172.

44. Goeddert JJ, Biggar RJ, Melbye M, et al. Effect of T4 count and cofactors on the incidence of AIDS in homosexual men: An 11 year follow-up study. JAMA. 1987;257:331-334.

45. Moss AR, Bacchetti P, Osmond D, et al. Seropositivity for HIV and the development of AIDS or AIDS-related condition: Three year follow up of the San Francisco General Hospital Cohort. BMJ. 1988;296:745-750.

46. Munoz A, Schrager L, Bacellar H, et al. Trends in the incidence of outcomes defining acquired immunodeficiency syndrome (AIDS) in the Multicenter AIDS Cohort Study: 1985-1991. Am J Epidemiol. 1993;137:423-438.

47. Polk BF, Fox R, Brookmeyer R, et al. Predictors of the acquired immunodeficiency syndrome developing in a cohort of seropositive homosexual men. N Engl J Med. 1987;316:61-66.

48. Coombs RW, Welles SL, Hooper C, et al. Association of plasma human immunodeficiency virus type 1 RNA level with risk of clinical progression in patients with advanced HIV infection. J Infect Dis. 1996;174:715-712.

49. Lefrere J-J, Roudot-Thoraval F, Mariotti M. The risk of disease progression is determined during the first year of human immunodeficiency virus type 1 infection. J Infect Dis. 1998;177:1541-1548.

50. Mellors JW, Kingsley LA, Rinaldo CR, et al. Quantitation of HIV-1 RNA in plasma predicts outcome after seroconversion. Ann Intern Med. 1995;122:573-579.

51. Mellors JW, Rinaldo CR, Phalguni G, et al. Prognosis in HIV-1 infection predicted by quantity of virus in plasma. Science. 1996;272:1167-1170.

52. Mellors JW, Munoz A, Giorgi JV, et al. Plasma viral load and CD4+ lymphocytes as prognostic markers of HIV-1 infection. Ann Intern Med. 1997;126:946-954.

53. O'Brien TR, Blattner WA, Waters D, et al. Serum HIV-1 RNA levels and time to development of AIDS in the multicenter hemophilia cohort study. JAMA. 1996;276:105-110.

54. Staszewski S, DeMasi R, Hill AM, Dawson D. CD4 cell count and the risk of progression to AIDS and death during treatment with HIV-1 reverse transcriptase inhibitors. AIDS. 1998;12:1991-1997.

55. Welles SL, Jackson JB, Yen-Lieberman B, et al. Prognostic value of plasma human immunodeficiency virus type 1 (HIV-1) disease and with little or no prior zidovudine therapy. J Infect Dis. 1996;174:696-703.

56. Yerly S, Perneger TV, Hirshel B, et al. A critical assessment of the prognostic value of HIV-1 RNA levels and CD4+ cell counts in HIV-infected patients. The Swiss HIV Cohort Study. Arch Intern Med. 1998;158:247-252.

57. Bachetti P, Osmond D, Chaisson RE, et al. Patterns of survival in the acquired immunodeficiency syndrome. J Infect Dis. 1988;157:1044-1047.

58. Rothenberg R, Woelfel M, Stoneburner R, et al. Survival with the acquired immunodeficiency syndrome: Experience with 5833 cases in New York City. N Engl J Med. 1987;317:1297-1302.

59. Mocroft A, Johnson MA, Phillips AN. Factors affecting survival in patients with the acquired immunodeficiency syndrome. AIDS. 1996;10:1057-1065.

60. Osmond D, Harlebois E, Lang W, et al. Changes in AIDS survival time in two San Francisco cohorts of homosexual men, 1983 to 1993. JAMA. 1994;271:1083-1087.

61. Saravolatz L, Neaton J, Sacks L, et al. CD4+ lymphocyte counts and patterns of mortality among patients infected with human immunodeficiency virus who were enrolled in community programs for clinical research on AIDS. Clin Infect Dis. 1996;11:513-520.

62. Ehmann WC, Eyster ME, Wilson SE, et al. Relationship of CD4 lymphocyte counts to survival in a cohort of hemophiliacs infected with HIV. J Acquir Immune Defic Syndr. 1994;7:1095-1094.

63. Eyster ME, Gail MH, Ballard JO, et al. Natural history of human immunodeficiency virus infections in hemophiliacs: Effects of T-cell subsets, platelet counts, and age. Ann Intern Med. 1987;107:1-6.

64. Mariotto AB, Mariotti S, Pezzotti P, et al. Estimation of the acquired immunodeficiency syndrome incubation period in intravenous drug users: A comparison with male homosexuals. Am J Epidemiol. 1992;135:428-437.

65. Moore RD, Keruly J, Richmann DD, et al. Natural history of advanced HIV disease in patients treated with zidovudine. AIDS. 1992;6:671-677.

66. Operskalski EA, Stram DO, Lee H, et al. Human immunodeficiency virus type 1 infection: Relationship of risk group and age to rate of progression to AIDS. J Infect Dis. 1995;172:648-655.

67. Pedersen C, Katzenstein T, Nielsen C, et al. Prognostic value of serum HIV-RNA levels at virologic steady state after seroconversion: Relation to CD4 cell count and clinical course of primary infection. J Acquir Immune Defic Syndr. 1997;16:93-99.

68. Sterling TR, Lyles CM, Vlahov D, et al. Sex differences in longitudinal human immunodeficiency virus type 1 RNA levels among seroconverters. J Infect Dis. 1999;180:666-672.

69. Hubert JB, Rouzioux C, Boufassa F, et al. Gender, disease progression and response to HAART. Abstract 1448.14th International AIDS Conference, Barcelona, Spain, July 7-12, 2002.

70. Gandhi M, Bacchetti P, Miotti P, et al. Does patient sex affect human immunodeficiency virus levels? Clin Infect Dis. 2002;35:313-322.

71. Anastos K, Kalish LA, Hessol N, et al. The relative value of CD4 cell count and quantitative HIV-1 RNA in predicting survival in HIV-1–infected women: Results of the Women's Interagency HIV Study. AIDS. 1999;13:1717-1725.

72. Sterling TR, Vlahov D, Astemborski J, et al. Initial plasma HIV-1 RNA and progression to AIDS in women and men. N Engl J Med. 2001;344:720-725.

73. Melnick SL, Sherer R, Louis TA, et al. Survival and disease progression according to gender of patients with HIV infection. JAMA. 1994;272:1915-1921.

74. Chaisson RE, Keruly JC, Moore RD. Race, sex, drug use, and progression of human immunodeficiency virus disease. N Engl J Med. 1995;333:751-756.

75. Collaborative Group on AIDS Incubation and Survival. Time from HIV-1 seroconversion to AIDS and death before widespread use of highly-active antiretroviral therapy: A collaborative re-analysis. Lancet. 2000;355:1131-1137.

76. Brown AE, Malone JD, Zhou SYJ, et al. Human immunodeficiency virus RNA levels in US adults: A comparison based on race and ethnicity. J Infect Dis. 1997;176:794-797.

77. Pezzotti P, Galai N, Vlahov D, et al. Direct comparison of time to AIDS and infectious disease death between HIV seroconverter injection drug users in Italy and the United States: Results from the ALIVE and ISS studies. AIDS Link to Intravenous Experiences. Italian Seroconversion Study. J Acquir Immune Defic Syndr Hum Retrovirol. 1999;20:275-282.

78. Taylor JM, Fahey JL, Detels R, et al. CD4 percentage, CD4 number, and CD4:CD8 ratio in HIV infection: Which to choose and how to use. J Acquir Immune Defic Syndr. 1989;2:114-124.

79. Schupbach J, Flepp M, Pontelli D, et al. Heat-mediated immune complex dissociation and enzyme-linked immunosorbent assay signal amplification render p24 antigen detection in plasma as sensitive as HIV-1 RNA detection by polymerase chain reaction. AIDS. 1996;10:1085-1090.

80. Sterling TR, Hoover DR, Astemborski J, et al. Heat-denatured human immunodeficiency virus type 1 protein 24 antigen: Prognostic value in adults with early-stage disease. J Infect Dis. 2002;186:1181-1185.

81. Crowe S, Turnbull S, Oelrichs R, Dunne A. Monitoring of human immunodeficiency virus infection in resource-constrained countries. Clin Infect Dis. 2003;37:S25-S35.

82. Badri M, Wood R. Usefulness of total lymphocyte count in monitoring highly active antiretroviral therapy in resource-limited settings. AIDS. 2003;17:541-545.

83. Spacek LA, Griswold M, Quinn TC, Moore RD. Total lymphocyte count and hemoglobin combined in an algorithm to initiate the use of highly active antiretroviral therapy in resource-limited settings. AIDS. 2003;17:1311-1317.

84. Lau B, Gange SJ, Phair JP, et al. Rapid declines in total lymphocyte counts and hemoglobin concentration prior to AIDS among HIV-1-infected men. AIDS. 2003;17:2035-2044.

85. Janoff EN, Breiman RF, Daley CL, et al. Pneumococcal disease during HIV infection. Ann Intern Med. 1992;117:314-324.

86. Masur H, Ognibene FP, Yarchoan R, et al. CD4 counts as predictors of opportunistic pneumonias in human immunodeficiency virus (HIV) infection. Ann Intern Med. 1992;111:223-231.

87. Theuer CP, Hopewell PC, Elias D, et al. Human immunodeficiency virus infection in tuberculosis patients. J Infect Dis. 1990;162:8-12.

88. Gallant JE, Moore RD, Chaisson RE. Prophylaxis for opportunistic infection in patients with HIV infection. Ann Intern Med. 1994;120:932-943.

89. Moore RD, Chaisson RE. Natural history of opportunistic disease in an HIV-infected urban clinical cohort. Ann Intern Med. 1996;124:633-642.

90. Corbett EL, Watt CJ, Walker N, et al. The growing burden of tuberculosis: global trends and interactions with the HIV epidemic. Arch Intern Med. 2003;163:1009-1021.

91. Corbett EL, Steketee RW, ter Kuile FO, et al. HIV-1/AIDS and the control of other infectious diseases in Africa. Lancet. 2002;359:2177-2187.

92. Grant AD, Sidibe K, Domoua K, et al. Spectrum of disease among HIV-infected adults hospitalised in a respiratory medicine unit in Abidjan, Cote d'Ivoire. Int J Tuberc Lung Dis. 1998;2:926-934.

93. Forrest DM, Seminari E, Hogg RS, et al. The incidence and spectrum of AIDS-defining illness in persons treated with antiretroviral drugs. Clin Infect Dis. 1998;27:1379-1385.

94. Carne CA, Weller IVD, Loveday C, et al. From persistent generalized lymphadenopathy to AIDS: Who will progress? Br Med J (Clin Res Ed). 1987;294:868-869.

95. Greenspan D, Greenspan JS, Hearst NG, et al. Relation of oral hairy leukoplakia to infection with the human immunodeficiency virus and risk of developing AIDS. J Infect Dis. 1987;155:475-481.

96. Polk BF, Fox R, Brookmeyer R, et al. Predictors of the acquired immunodeficiency syndrome developing in a cohort of seropositive homosexual men. N Engl J Med. 1993;316:61-66.

97. Murray HW, Godbold JH, Jurica KB, Roberts RB. Progression to AIDS in patients with lymphadenopathy or AIDS-related complex: Reappraisal of risk and predictive factors. Am J Med. 1989;86:533-538.

98. Chaisson RE, Gallant JE, Keruly J, Moore RD. Impact of opportunistic disease on survival in patients with HIV infection. AIDS. 1998;12:29-33.

99. Petruckevitch A, Del Amo J, Phillips AN, et al. Disease progression and survival following specific AIDS-defining conditions: A retrospective cohort study of 2048 HIV-infected persons in London. AIDS. 1998;12:107-113.

100. Bush CE, Donovan RM, Markowitz NP, et al. A study of HIV RNA viral load in AIDS patients with bacterial pneumonia. J Acquir Immune Defic Syndr. 1996;13:23-26.

101. Donovan RM, Bush CE, Markowitz NP, et al. Changes in virus load markers during AIDS-associated opportunistic diseases in human immunodeficiency virus–infected persons. J Infect Dis. 1996;174:401-403.

102. Golletti D, Weissman D, Jackson RW, et al. Effect of *Mycobacterium tuberculosis* on HIV replication. Role of immune activation. J Immunol. 1996;157:1271-1278.

103. Sulkowski M, Chaisson RE, Karp CL, et al. The effect of acute infectious illness on plasma human immunodeficiency virus (HIV) type 1 load and the expression of serologic markers of immune activation among HIV-infected adults. J Infect Dis. 1998;178:1642-1648.

104. Chaisson RE, Keruly J, Richman DD, Moore RD. Pneumocystis prophylaxis and survival in patients with advanced human immunodeficiency virus infection treated with zidovudine. Arch Intern Med. 1992;152:2009-2013.

105. Fischl MA, Richman DD, Greico MH, et al. The efficacy of azidothymidine (AZT) in the treatment of patients with AIDS and AIDS-related complex: A double-blind, placebo-controlled trial. N Engl J Med. 1987;317:185-191.

106. Harris JE. Improved short-term survival of AIDS patients initially diagnosed with *Pneumocystis carinii* pneumonia, 1984 through 1987. JAMA. 1990;263:397-401.

107. Lemp GF, Payne SF, Temelso DN, et al. Survival trends for patients with AIDS. JAMA. 1990;264:402-405.

108. Moore RD, Hidalgo J, Sugland B, et al. Zidovudine and the natural history of the acquired immunodeficiency syndrome. N Engl J Med. 1991;324:1412-1416.

109. Delta Coordinating Committee. Delta: A randomized double-blind controlled trial comparing combinations of zidovudine plus didanosine or zalcitabine with zidovudine alone in HIV-infected individuals. Lancet. 1996;348:283-291.

110. Enger C, Graham N, Peng Y, et al. Survival from early, intermediate, and late stages of HIV infection. JAMA. 1996;275:1329-1334.

111. Fischl MA, Dickinson GM, La Voie L. Safety and efficacy of sulfamethoxazole and trimethoprim chemoprophylaxis for *Pneumocystis carinii* pneumonia in AIDS. JAMA. 1988;259:1185-1189.

112. Graham NM, Zeger SL, Park LP, et al. Effects of zidovudine and *Pneumocystis carinii* pneumonia prophylaxis on progression of HIV-1 infection to AIDS. Lancet. 1991;338:265-269.

113. Graham NM, Zeger SL, Park LP, et al. The effects on survival of early treatment of human immunodeficiency virus infection. N Engl J Med. 1992;326:1037-1042.

114. Hammer S, Katzenstein DA, Hughes MD, et al. A trial comparing nucleoside monotherapy with combination therapy in HIV-infected adults with CD4 cell counts from 200 to 500 per cubic millimeter. N Engl J Med. 1996;335:1081-1090.

115. Pierce M, Crampton S, Henry D, et al. A randomized trial of clarithromycin as prophylaxis against disseminated *Mycobacterium avium* complex infection in patients with advanced acquired immunodeficiency syndrome. N Engl J Med. 1996;335:384-391.

116. Volberding PA, Lagakos SW, Koch MA, et al. Zidovudine in asymptomatic human immunodeficiency virus infection. N Engl J Med. 1990;322:941-949.

117. Delta Coordinating Committee and Delta Virology Committee. HIV-1 RNA response to antiretroviral treatment in 1280 participants in the Delta Trial: An extended virology study. AIDS. 1999;13:57-65.

118. O'Brien WA, Hartigan PM, Martin D, et al. Changes in plasma HIV-1 RNA and CD4+ lymphocyte counts and the risk of progression to AIDS. N Engl J Med 1996;334:426-431.

119. Brodt HR, Kamps BS, Gute P, et al. Changing incidence of AIDS-defining illnesses in the era of antiretroviral combination therapy. AIDS. 1997;11:1731-1738.

120. Centers for Disease Control and Prevention. Update: Trends in AIDS incidence, death, and prevalence—United States, 1996. MMWR Morb Mortal Wkly Rep. 1997;46:861-867.

121. Hogg RS, O'Shaughnessy MV, Gataric N, et al. Decline in deaths from AIDS due to new antiretrovirals (Letter). Lancet. 1997;349:1294.

122. Torres RA, Barr M. Impact of combination therapy for HIV infection on inpatient census. N Engl J Med. 1997;336:1531-1532.

123. Mocroft A, Vella S, Benfield TL, et al. Changing patterns of mortality across Europe in patients infected with HIV-1. EuroSIDA Study Group. Lancet. 1998;352:1725-1730.

124. Palella FJ, Delaney KM, Moorman AC, et al. Declining morbidity and mortality among patients with advanced human immunodeficiency virus infection. N Engl J Med. 1998;338:853-860.

125. Mocroft A, Ledergerber B, Katlama C, et al. Decline in the AIDS and death rates in the EuroSIDA study: an observational study. Lancet. 2003;362:22-29.

126. Louie JK, Hsu LC, Osmond DH, et al. Trends in causes of death among persons with acquired immunodeficiency syndrome in the era of highly active antiretroviral therapy, San Francisco, 1994-1998. J Infect Dis. 2002;186:1023-1027.

127. Valdez H, Chowdhry TK, Asaad R, et al. Changing spectrum of mortality due to human immunodeficiency virus: Analysis of 260 deaths during 1995-1999. Clin Infect Dis. 2001;32:1487-1493.

128. Jaggy C, von Overbeck J, Ledergerber B, et al. Mortality in the Swiss HIV Cohort Study. (SHCS) and the Swiss general population. Lancet 2003;362:877-878.

129. Sepkowitz KA. Effect of HAART on natural history of AIDS-related opportunistic disorders. Lancet. 1998;351:228-229.

130. Race EM, Adelson-Mitty J, Kriegel GR, et al. Focal mycobacterial lymphadenitis following initiation of protease-inhibitor therapy in patients with advanced HIV-1 disease. Lancet. 1998;351:252-255.

131. Autran B, Carcelain G, Li TS, et al. Positive effects of combined antiretroviral therapy on CD4+ T cell homeostasis and function in advanced disease. Science. 1997;277:112-116.

132. Bisset LR, Cone RW, Huber W, et al. Highly active antiretroviral therapy during early HIV infection reverses T-cell activation and maturation abnormalities. AIDS. 1998;12:2115-2123.

133. Pakker NG, Kroon EDMB, Roos MTL, et al. Immune restoration does not invariably occur following long-term HIV-1 suppression during antiretroviral therapy. AIDS. 1999;13:203-212.

134. Powderly WG, Landay A, Lederman MM. Recovery of the immune system with antiretroviral therapy: The end of opportunism? JAMA. 1998;280:72-77.

135. Rodriguez-Guardado A, Maradona JA, Carton JA, et al. *Pneumocystis carinii* prophylaxis can be discontinued after CD4+ cell recovery over 200 × 10(6)/l (Letter). AIDS. 1998;12:2355-2356.

136. Schneider M, Borleffs JC, Stolk RP, et al. Discontinuation of prophylaxis for *Pneumocystis carinii* pneumonia in HIV-1 infected patients treated with highly active antiretroviral therapy. Lancet. 1999;353:201-203.

137. Martinez E, Miro JM, Gonzalez J, et al. Withdrawal of *Mycobacterium avium* complex suppressive therapy in HIV-1 infected patients on highly active antiretroviral therapy. AIDS. 1999;13:147-148.

138. Tural C, Romeu J, Sirera G, et al. Long-lasting remission of cytomegalovirus retinitis without maintenance therapy in human immunodeficiency virus–infected patients. J Infect Dis. 1998;177:1080-1083.

139. Narita M, Ashkin D, Hollender ES, et al. Paradoxical worsening of tuberculosis following antiretroviral therapy in patients with AIDS. Am J Respir Crit Care Med. 1998;158:157-161.

140. Carr A, Samaras SK, Burton S, et al. Peripheral lipodystrophy, hyperlipidaemia and insulin resistance in patients receiving HIV protease inhibitors. AIDS. 1998;12:F51-F58.

141. Cooper DA, Gold J, Maclean P, et al. Acute AIDS retrovirus infection: Definition of a clinical illness associated with seroconversion. Lancet. 1985;1:537-540.

142. Tindall B, Barker S, Donovan B, et al. Characteristics of the acute clinical illness associated with human immunodeficiency virus infection. Arch Intern Med. 1988;148:945-949.

143. Tokars JI, Marcus R, Culver DH, et al. Surveillance of HIV infection and zidovudine use among health care workers after occupational exposure to HIV-infected blood. Ann Intern Med. 1993;118:913-919.

144. Jaffe HW, Hardy AM, Morgan WM, et al. The acquired immunodeficiency syndrome in gay men. Ann Intern Med. 1985;103:622-664.

145. Moss AR, Osmond D, Bachetti P, et al. Risk factors for AIDS and HIV seropositivity in homosexual men. Am J Epidemiol. 1987;125:1035-1047.

146. Fox R, Eldred LJ, Fuchs EJ, et al. Clinical manifestations of acute infection with human immunodeficiency virus in a cohort of gay men. AIDS. 1987;1:35-38.

147. Vanhems P, Routy JP, Hirschel B, et al. Clinical features of acute retroviral syndrome differ by route of infection but not by gender and age. J Acquir Immune Defic Syndr. 2002;31:318-321.

148. Needlestick transmission of HTLV-III from a patient infected in Africa. Lancet. 1984;2:1376-1377.

149. Clark SJ, Kelen GD, Henrard DR, et al. Unsuspected primary human immunodeficiency virus type 1 infection in seronegative emergency department patients. J Infect Dis. 1994;170:194-197.

150. Schacker T, Collier AC, Hughes J, et al. Clinical and epidemiologic features of primary HIV infection. Ann Intern Med. 1996;125:257-264.

151. Kahn JO, Walker BD. Acute human immunodeficiency virus type 1 infection. N Engl J Med. 1998;339:33-39.

152. Quinn TC. Acute primary HIV infection. JAMA. 1997;278:58-62.

153. Niu MT, Stein DS, Schnittman SM. Primary human immunodeficiency virus type I infection: Review of pathogenesis and early treatment intervention in human and animal retrovirus infections. J Infect Dis. 1993;168:1490-1501.

154. Carne CA, Tedder RS, Smith A, et al. Acute encephalopathy coincident with seroconversion for anti-HTLV-III. Lancet. 1985;2:1206-1208.

155. Clark SJ, Saag MS, Decker WD, et al. High titers of cytopathic virus in plasma of patients with symptomatic primary HIV-1 infection. N Engl J Med. 1991;324:954-960.

156. Cooper DA, Imrie AA, Penny R. Antibody response to human immunodeficiency virus after primary infection. Ann Intern Med. 1987;155:1113-1118.

157. Denning DW, Anderson J, Rudge P, et al. Acute myelopathy associated with primary infection with human immunodeficiency virus. Br Med J (Clin Res Ed). 1987;294:143-144.

158. Elder G, Dalakas M, Pezeshkpour G, et al. Ataxic neuropathy due to ganglioneuritis after probable acute human immunodeficiency virus infection. Lancet. 1986;2:1275-1276.

159. Ho DD, Sarngadharan MG, Resnick L, et al. Primary human T-lymphotropic virus type II infection. Ann Intern Med. 1985;103:880-883.

160. Rustin MHA, Ridely CM, Smith MD. The acute exanthem associated with seroconversion to human T-cell lymphotropic virus III in a homosexual man. J Infect Dis. 1986;12:161-163.

161. Balslev E, Thomsen HK, Weismann K. Histopathology of acute human immunodeficiency virus exanthem. J Clin Pathol. 1990;43:201-202.

162. Cooper DA, Tindall B, Wilson E. Characterization of T lymphocyte responses during primary HIV infection. J Infect Dis. 1987;157:889-896.

163. Goudsmit J, De Wolf F, Paul DA, et al. Expression of human immunodeficiency virus antigen (HIV-Ag) in serum and cerebrospinal fluid during acute and chronic infection. Lancet. 1986;2:177-180.

164. Kessler HA, Blaauw B, Spear J, et al. Diagnosis of human immunodeficiency virus infection in seronegative homosexuals presenting with an acute viral syndrome. JAMA. 1987;258:1196-1199.

165. Henrard DR, Phillips J, Windsor I, et al. Detection of human immunodeficiency virus type 1 p24 antigen and plasma RNA: Relevance to indeterminant serologic tests. Transfusion. 1994;34:376-380.

166. Rosenberg ES, Billingsley JM, Caliendo AM, et al. Vigorous HIV-1 specific CD4+ T cell responses associated with control of viremia. Science. 1997;278:1447-1450.

167. Finzi D, Hermankova M, Pierson T, et al. Identification of a reservoir for HIV-1 in patients on highly active antiretroviral therapy. Science. 1997;278:1295-1300.

168. Osmond D, Chaisson RE, Moss A, et al. Lymphadenopathy in asymptomatic patients seropositive for HIV. N Engl J Med. 1987;317:246.

169. Bottles K, McPhaul LW, Volberding P. Fine-needle aspiration biopsy of patients with acquired immunodeficiency syndrome (AIDS): experience in an outpatient clinic. Ann Intern Med. 1988;108:42-45.

170. Oksenhendler E, Duarte M, Soulier J, et al. Multicenter Castleman's disease in HIV infection: A clinical and pathological study of 20 patients. AIDS. 1996;10:61-67.

171. Hengge UR, Ruzicka T, Tyring SK, et al. Update on Kaposi's sarcoma and other HHV8 associated diseases. Part 2: Pathogenesis, Castleman's disease, and pleural effusion lymphoma. Lancet Infect Dis. 2002;2:344-352.

172. Grandadaar M, Dupin N, Calvez V, et al. Exacerbations of clinical symptoms in human immunodeficiency virus type 1–infected patients with multicentric Castleman's disease are associated with a high increase in Kaposi's sarcoma herpes virus DNA load in peripheral blood mononuclear cells. J Infect Dis. 1997;175:198-201.

173. Abrams DI. AIDS related lymphadenopathy: The role of biopsy. J Clin Oncol. 1986;4:126-127.

174. Pantaleo G, Graziosi C, Demarest JF, et al. HIV infection is active and progressive in lymphoid tissue during the clinically latent stage of disease. Nature. 1993;362:355-358.

175. Chuang HT, Devins GM, Hunsley J, Gill MJ. Psychosocial distress and well-being among gay and bisexual men with human immunodeficiency virus infection. Am J Psychiatry. 1989;146:876-880.

176. Miller EN, Selnes OA, McArthur JC, et al. Neuropsychological performances in HIV-1–infected homosexual men. Neurology. 1990;40:197-203.

177. Angelino AF, Treisman GJ. Management of psychiatric disorders in patients infected with human immunodeficiency virus. Clin Infect Dis. 2001;33:847-856.

178. Dobs AS, Dempsey MA, Ladenson PW, et al. Endocrine disorders in men infected with human immunodeficiency virus. Am J Med. 1988;84:611-616.

179. Grunfeld C, Feingold KR. Metabolic disturbances and wasting in the acquired immunodeficiency syndrome. N Engl J Med. 1992;327:329-337.

180. Grinspoon SK, Bilezikian JP. HIV disease and the endocrine system. N Engl J Med. 1992;327:1360-1365.

181. Sattler F, Briggs W, Antonipillai I, et al. Low dihydrotestosterone and weight loss in the AIDS wasting syndrome. J Acquir Immune Defic Syndr Hum Retrovirol. 1998;18:246-251.

182. Mylonakis E, Koutkia P, Grinspoon S. Diagnosis and treatment of androgen deficiency in human immunodeficiency virus–infected men and women. Clin Infect Dis. 2001;33:857-864.

183. Gonzalez-Cadavid NF, Taylor WE, Yarasheski K, et al. Organization of the human myostatin gene and expression in healthy men and HIV-infected men with muscle wasting. Proc Natl Acad Sci U S A. 1998;95:14938-14943.

184. Beaugerie L, Carbonnnel F, Carrat F, et al. Factors of weight loss in patients with HIV and chronic diarrhea. J Acquir Immune Defic Syndr Hum Retrovirol. 1998;19:34-39.

185. Macallan DC, Noble C, Baldwin C, et al. Energy expenditure and wasting in human immunodeficiency virus infection. N Engl J Med. 1995;333:83-88.

186. Strawford A, Hellerstein M. The etiology of wasting in the human immunodeficiency virus and acquired immunodeficiency syndrome. Semin Oncol. 1998;25(2 Suppl 5):76-81.

187. Grinspoon S, Mulligan K. Weight loss and wasting in patients infected with human immunodeficiency virus. Clin Infect Dis. 2003;36:S69-S78.

188. Kotler DP. Wasting syndrome: Nutritional support in HIV infection. J Acquir Immune Defic Syndr. 1994;10:931-934.

189. Tang AM, Forrester J, Spiegelman D, et al. Weight loss and survival in HIV-positive patients in the era of highly active antiretroviral therapy. J Acquir Immune Defic Syndr. 2002;31:230-236.

190. Sepkowitz KA, Telzak EE, Carrow M, et al. Fever among outpatients with advanced human immunodeficiency virus infection. Arch Intern Med. 1993;153:1909-1912.

191. Serwadda D, Mugerwa RD, Sewankambo NK, et al. Slim disease: A new disease in Uganda and its association with HTLV-III infection. Lancet. 1985;2:849-852.

192. Chintu C, Dupont HL, Kaile T, et al. Human immunodeficiency virus–associated diarrhea and wasting in Zambia: Selected risk factors and clinical associations. Am J Trop Med Hyg. 1998;59:38-41.

193. Sewankambo N, Mugerwa R, Goodgame R, et al. Enteropathic AIDS in Uganda: An endoscopic, histologic and microbiologic study. AIDS. 1987;1:9-14.

194. DeCock KM, Soro B, Coulibally IM, et al. Tuberculosis and HIV infection in sub-Saharan Africa. JAMA. 1992;268:1581-1587.

195. Lucas SB, DeCock KM, Hounnou A, et al. Contribution of tuberculosis to slim disease in Africa. BMJ. 1994;308:1531-1533.

196. Greenspan D, Greenspan JS. HIV-related oral disease. Lancet. 1996;348:729-733.

197. Weinert M, Grimes RM, Lynch DP. Oral manifestations of HIV infection. Ann Intern Med. 1996;125:485-496.

198. Feigal DW, Katz MH, Greenspan D, et al. The prevalence of oral lesions in HIV-infected homosexual and bisexual men: Three San Francisco epidemiological cohorts. AIDS. 1991;5:519-525.

199. Klein RS, Harris CA, Small CB, et al. Oral candidiasis in high-risk patients as the initial manifestation of the acquired immunodeficiency syndrome. N Engl J Med. 1984;311:354-358.

200. Royce RA, Luckmann RS, Fusaro RE, Winkelstein W Jr. The natural history of HIV-1 infection: Staging classifications of disease. AIDS. 1991;5:355-364.

201. Lifson AR, Hilton JF, Westenhouse JL, et al. Time from HIV seroconversion to oral candidiasis or hairy leukoplakia among homosexual and bisexual men enrolled in three prospective cohorts. AIDS. 1994;8:73-79.

202. Sanguineti A, Carmichael JK, Campbell K. Fluconazole-resistant *Candida albicans* after long-term suppressive therapy. Arch Intern Med. 1993;153:1122-1124.

203. Maenza JR, Keruly JC, Moore RD, et al. Risk factors for fluconazole-resistant candidiasis in human immunodeficiency virus–infected patients. J Infect Dis. 1996;173:219-225.

204. Barchiesi F, Maracci M, Radi B, et al. Point prevalence, microbiology and fluconazole susceptibility patterns of yeast isolates colonizing the oral cavities of HIV-infected patients in the era of highly active antiretroviral therapy. J Antimicrob Chemother. 2002;50:999-1002.

205. Greenspan D, Greenspan JS, Conant M, et al. Oral "hairy" leucoplakia in male homosexuals: Evidence of association with both papillomavirus and a herpes-group virus. Lancet. 1984;2:831-834.

206. Greenspan JS, Greenspan D, Lennette ET, et al. Replication of Epstein-Barr virus within the epithelial cells of oral "hairy" leukoplakia, an AIDS-associated lesion. N Engl J Med. 1985;313:1564-1571.

207. Rowland RW, Escobar MR, Friedman RB, Kaplowitz LG. Painful gingivitis may be an early sign of infection with the human immunodeficiency virus. Clin Infect Dis. 1993;16:233-236.
208. MacPhail LA, Greenspan D, Greenspan JS. Recurrent aphthous ulcers in association with HIV infection: Diagnosis and treatment. Oral Surg Oral Med Oral Pathol. 1992;73:283-288.
209. Jacobson JM, Greenspan JS, Spritzler J, et al. Thalidomide for the treatment of oral aphthous ulcers in patients with human immunodeficiency virus infection. National Institute of Allergy and Infectious Diseases AIDS Clinical Trials Group. N Engl J Med. 1997;336:1487-1493.
210. Paterson DL, Georghiou PR, Allworth AM, Kemp RJ. Thalidomide as treatment of refractory aphthous ulceration related to human immunodeficiency virus infection. Clin Infect Dis. 1995;20:250-254.
211. Ramirez-Amador VA, Esquivel-Pedraza L, Ponce-de-Leon S, et al. Thalidomide as therapy for human immunodeficiency virus–related oral ulcers: A double-blind placebo-controlled clinical trial. Clin Infect Dis. 1999;28:892-894.
212. Craven DE, Duncan RA, Stram JR, et al. Response of lymphoepithelial parotid cysts to antiretroviral treatment in HIV-infected adults. Ann Intern Med. 1998;128:455-459.
213. Dalakas MC, Pezeshkpour GH, Gnavall M, et al. Polymyositis associated with AIDS retrovirus. JAMA. 1986;256:2381-2383.
214. Kaye BR. Rheumatologic manifestations of infection with human immunodeficiency virus (HIV). Ann Intern Med. 1989;111:158-167.
215. Dalakas MC, Pezeshkpour GH. Neuromuscular diseases associated with human immunodeficiency virus infection. Ann Neurol. 1988;23(Suppl):S38-S48.
216. Johnson RW, Williams FM, Kazi S, et al. Human immunodeficiency virus–associated polymyositis: A longitudinal study of outcome. Arthritis Rheum. 2003;49:172-178.
217. Dalakas MC, Illa I, Pezeshkpour GH, et al. Mitochondrial myopathy caused by long-term zidovudine therapy. N Engl J Med. 1990;322:1098-1105.
218. Schwartzman WA, Lambertus MW, Kennedy CA, Goetz MB. Staphylococcal pyomyositis in patients infected by the human immunodeficiency virus. Am J Med. 1991;90:595-600.
219. Widrow CA, Kellie SM, Saltzman BR, Mathur-Wagh U. Pyomyositis in patients with the human immunodeficiency virus: An unusual form of disseminated bacterial infection. Am J Med. 1991;91:129-136.
220. Clark MR, Solinger AM, Hochberg MC. Human immunodeficiency virus infection is not associated with Reiter's syndrome. Data from three large cohort studies. Rheum Dis Clin North Am. 1992;18:267-276.
221. Hochberg MC, Fox R, Nelson KE, Saah A. HIV infection is not associated with Reiter's syndrome: Data from the Johns Hopkins Multicenter AIDS Cohort Study. AIDS. 1990;4:1149-1151.
222. Winchester R, Bernstein DH, Fischer HD, et al. The co-occurrence of Reiter's syndrome and acquired immunodeficiency. Ann Intern Med. 1987;106:19-26.
223. Kaye BR. Rheumatologic manifestations of HIV infections. Clin Rev Allergy Immunol. 1996;14:385-416.
224. Brown P, Crane L. Avascular necrosis of bone in patients with human immunodeficiency virus infection: Report of 6 cases and review of the literature. Clin Infect Dis. 2001;32:1221-1226.
225. Miller KD, Masur H, Jones EC, et al. High prevalence of osteonecrosis of the femoral head in HIV-infected adults. Ann Intern Med. 2002;137:17-25.
226. Keruly JC, Chaisson RE, Moore RD. Increasing incidence of avascular necrosis of the hip in HIV-infected patients. J Acquir Immune Defic Syndr. 2001;28:101-102.
227. Monier P, McKown K, Bronze MS. Osteonecrosis complicating highly active antiretroviral therapy in patients infected with human immunodeficiency virus. Clin Infect Dis. 2000;31:1488-1492.
228. Glesby MJ, Hoover DR, Vaamonde CM. Osteonecrosis in patients infected with human immunodeficiency virus: A case-control study. J Infect Dis. 2001;184:519-523.
229. Garman ME, Tyring SK. The cutaneous manifestations of HIV infection. Dermatol Clin. 2002;20:193-208.
230. Porras B, Costner M, Friedman-Kien AE, Cockerell CJ. Update on cutaneous manifestations of HIV infection. Med Clin North Am. 1998;82:1033-1080, v.
231. Bollinger RC, Brookmeyer RS, Mehendale SM, et al. Risk factors and clinical presentation of acute primary HIV infection in India. JAMA. 1997;278:2085-2089.
232. Tindall B, Barker S, Donovan B, et al. Characterization of the acute clinical illness associated with human immunodeficiency virus infection. Arch Intern Med. 1988;148:945-949.
233. Quinnan GV Jr, Masur H, Rook AH, et al. Herpesvirus infections in the acquired immune deficiency syndrome. JAMA. 1984;252:72-77.
234. Friedman-Kien AE, Lafleur FL, Gendler E, et al. Herpes zoster: A possible early clinical sign for development of acquired immunodeficiency syndrome in high-risk individuals. J Am Acad Dermatol. 1986;14:1023-1028.
235. Aldeen T, Hay P, Davidson F, Lau R. Herpes zoster infection in HIV-seropositive patients associated with highly active antiretroviral treatment. AIDS. 1998;12:1719-1720.
236. Buchbinder SP, Katz MH, Hessol NA, et al. Herpes zoster and human immunodeficiency virus infection. J Infect Dis. 1992;166:1153-1156.
237. Cohen PR, Beltrani VP, Grossman ME. Disseminated herpes zoster in patients with human immunodeficiency virus infection. Am J Med. 1988;84:1076-1080.
238. Glesby MJ, Moore RD, Chaisson RE. Herpes zoster in patients with advanced human immunodeficiency virus infection treated with zidovudine. Zidovudine Epidemiology Study Group. J Infect Dis. 1993;168:1264-1268.
239. Grossman MC, Grossman ME. Chronic hyperkeratotic herpes zoster and human immunodeficiency virus infection. J Am Acad Dermatol. 1993;28:306-308.
240. Melbye M, Grossman RJ, Goedert JJ, et al. Risk of AIDS after herpes zoster. Lancet. 1987;1:728-731.
241. Gilson IH, Barnett JH, Conant MA, et al. Disseminated ecthymatous herpes varicella-zoster virus infection in patients with acquired immunodeficiency syndrome. J Am Acad Dermatol. 1989;20:637-642.
242. Horn CK, Scott GR, Benton EC. Resolution of severe molluscum contagiosum on effective antiretroviral therapy. Br J Dermatol. 1998;138:715-717.
243. Koehler JE, Quinn FD, Berger TG, et al. Isolation of *Rochalimaea* species from cutaneous and osseous lesions of bacillary angiomatosis. N Engl J Med. 1992;327:1625-1631.
244. Relman DA, Loutit JS, Schmidt TM, et al. The agent of bacillary angiomatosis. An approach to the identification of uncultured pathogens. N Engl J Med. 1990;323:1573-1580.
245. Slater LN, Welch DF, Min KW. *Rochalimaea henselae* causes bacillary angiomatosis and peliosis hepatis. Arch Intern Med. 1992;152:602-606.
246. Tappero JW, Mohle-Boetani J, Koehler JE, et al. The epidemiology of bacillary angiomatosis and bacillary peliosis. JAMA. 1993;269:770-775.
247. Stoler MH, Bonfiglio TA, Steigbigel RT, Pereira M. An atypical subcutaneous infection associated with acquired immune deficiency syndrome. Am J Clin Pathol. 1983;80:714-718.
248. Koehler JE, Sanchez MA, Garrido CS, et al. Molecular epidemiology of bartonella infections in patients with bacillary angiomatosis-peliosis. N Engl J Med. 1997;337:1876-1883.
249. Koehler JE, LeBoit PE, Egbert BM, Berger TG. Cutaneous vascular lesions and disseminated cat-scratch disease in patients with the acquired immunodeficiency syndrome (AIDS) and AIDS- related complex. Ann Intern Med. 1988;109:449-455.
250. Koehler JE, Tappero JW. Bacillary angiomatosis and bacillary peliosis in patients infected with human immunodeficiency virus. Clin Infect Dis. 1993;17:612-624.
251. Mohle-Boetani JC, Koehler JE, Berger TG, et al. Bacillary angiomatosis and bacillary peliosis in patients infected with human immunodeficiency virus: Clinical characteristics in a case-control study. Clin Infect Dis. 1996;22:794-800.
252. Agan BK, Dolan MJ. Laboratory diagnosis of *Bartonella* infections. Clin Lab Med. 2002;22:937-962.
253. Chang Y, Cesarman E, Pessin MS, et al. Identification of herpesvirus-like DNA sequences in AIDS-associated Kaposi's sarcoma. Science. 1994;266:1865-1869.
254. Martin JN, Ganem DE, Osmond DH, et al. Sexual transmission and the natural history of human herpesvirus 8 infection. N Engl J Med. 1998;338:948-954.
255. Antman K, Chang Y. Kaposi's sarcoma. N Engl J Med. 2000;342:1027-1038.
256. Beral V, Peterman TA, Berkelman RL, Jaffe HW. Kaposi's sarcoma among persons with AIDS: A sexually transmitted infection? Lancet. 1990;335:123-128.
257. Supparatpinyo K, Khamwan C, Baosoung V, et al. Disseminated *Penicillium marneffei* infection in southeast Asia. Lancet. 1994;344:110-113.
258. Schlesinger I, Oelrich DM, Tyring SK. Crusted (Norwegian) scabies in patients with AIDS: The range of clinical presentations. South Med J. 1994;87:352-356.
259. Meinking TL, Taplin D, Hermida JL, et al. The treatment of scabies with ivermectin. N Engl J Med. 1995;333:26-30.
260. Rao TK, Filippone EJ, Nicastri AD, et al. Associated focal and segmental glomerulosclerosis in the acquired immunodeficiency syndrome. N Engl J Med. 1984;310:669-673.
261. Rao TK. Acute renal failure syndromes in human immunodeficiency virus infection. Semin Nephrol. 1998;18:378-395.
262. Kimmel PL, Barisoni L, Kopp JB. Pathogenesis and treatment of HIV-associated renal diseases: Lessons from clinical and animal studies, molecular pathologic correlations, and genetic investigations. Ann Intern Med. 2003;139:214-226.
263. Kelleher P, Severn A, Tomson C, et al. The haemolytic uraemic syndrome in patients with AIDS. Genitourin Med. 1996;72:172-175.
264. Kimmel PL, Phillips TM, Ferreira-Centeno A, et al. HIV-associated immune-mediated renal disease. Kidney Int. 1993;44:1327-1340.
265. Stokes MB, Chawla H, Brody RI, et al. Immune complex glomerulonephritis in patients coinfected with human immunodeficiency virus and hepatitis C virus. Am J Kidney Dis. 1997;29:514-525.
266. Pardo V, Aldana M, Colton RM, et al. Glomerular lesions in the acquired immunodeficiency syndrome. Ann Intern Med. 1984;101:429-434.
267. Rao TK, Friedman EA, Nicastri AD. The types of renal disease in the acquired immunodeficiency syndrome. N Engl J Med. 1987;316:1062-1068.
268. Schwartz EJ, Klotman PE. Pathogenesis of human immunodeficiency virus (HIV)–associated nephropathy. Semin Nephrol. 1998;18:436-445.
269. Carbone L, D'Agati V, Cheng JT, Appel GB. Course and prognosis of human immunodeficiency virus–associated nephropathy. Am J Med. 1989;87:389-395.
270. Ortiz C, Meneses R, Jaffe D, et al. Outcome of patients with human immunodeficiency virus on maintenance hemodialysis. Kidney Int. 1988;34:248-253.
271. Szczech LA, Edwards LJ, Sanders LL, et al. Protease inhibitors are associated with a slowed progression of HIV-related renal diseases. Clin Nephrol. 2002;57:336-341.
272. Smith MC, Austen JL, Carey JT, et al. Prednisone improves renal function and proteinuria in human immunodeficiency virus–associated nephropathy. Am J Med. 1996;101:41-48.
273. Burns GC, Paul SK, Toth IR, et al. Effect of angiotensin-converting enzyme inhibition in HIV-associated nephropathy. J Am Soc Nephrol. 1997;8:1140-1146.
274. Inguilli E, Tejani AS, Fikrig S, et al. Nephrotic syndrome associated with acquired immune deficiency syndrome in children. J Pediatr. 1991;119:710-716.
275. Cunningham ET Jr, Margolis TP. Ocular manifestations of HIV infection. N Engl J Med. 1998;339:236-244.

276. Jabs DA. Ocular manifestations of HIV infection. Trans Am Ophthalmol Soc. 1995;93:623-683.
277. Sarraf D, Ernest JT. AIDS and the eyes. Lancet. 1996;348:525-528.
278. Spector SA, Wong R, Hsia K, et al. Plasma cytomegalovirus (CMV) DNA load predicts CMV disease and survival in AIDS patients. J Clin Invest. 1998;101:497-502.
279. Gallant JE, Moore RD, Richman DD, et al. Incidence and natural history of cytomegalovirus disease in patients with advanced human immunodeficiency virus disease treated with zidovudine. The Zidovudine Epidemiology Study Group. J Infect Dis. 1992;166:1223-1227.
280. Whitcup SM, Fortin E, Nussenblatt RB, et al. Therapeutic effect of combination antiretroviral therapy on cytomegalovirus retinitis. JAMA. 1997;277:1519-1520.
281. Margolis TP, Lowder CY, Holland GN, et al. Varicella-zoster virus retinitis in patients with the acquired immunodeficiency syndrome. Am J Ophthalmol. 1991;112:119-131.
282. Bafisse D, Eliaszewicz M, Zazoun L, et al. Acute retinal necrosis in the course of AIDS: Study of 26 cases. AIDS. 1996;10:55-60.
283. Wasserman L, Haghighi P. Otic and ophthalmic pneumocystosis in acquired immunodeficiency syndrome. Report of a case and review of the literature. Arch Pathol Lab Med. 1992;116:500-503.
284. Rerkpattanapipat P, Wongpraparut N, Jacobs LE, Kotler MN. Cardiac manifestations of acquired immunodeficiency syndrome. Arch Intern Med. 2000;160:602-608.
285. Barbarini G, Barbaro G. Incidence of the involvement of the cardiovascular system in HIV infection. AIDS. 2003;17(Suppl 1):S46-S50.
286. Henry K, Melroe H, Huebsch J, et al. Severe premature coronary artery disease with protease inhibitors. Lancet. 1998;351:1328.
287. Hofman P, Melroe H, Heubsch J, et al. Prevalence of *Toxoplasma* myocarditis in patients with the acquired immunodeficiency syndrome. Br Heart J. 1993;70:376-381.
288. Herskowitz A, Wu TC, Willoughby SB, et al. Myocarditis and cardiotropic viral infection associated with severe left ventricular dysfunction in late-stage infection with human immunodeficiency virus. J Am Coll Cardiol. 1994;24:1025-1032.
289. Barbaro G, Di Lorenzo G, Grisorio B, Barbarini G. Incidence of dilated cardiomyopathy and detection of HIV in myocardial cells of HIV-positive patients. Gruppo Italiano per lo Studio Cardiologico dei Pazienti Affetti da AIDS. N Engl J Med. 1998;339:1093-1099.
290. Herskowitz A, Vlahov D, Willoughby S, et al. Prevalence and incidence of left ventricular dysfunction in patients with human immunodeficiency virus infection. Am J Cardiol. 1993;71:955-958.
291. Currie PF, Jacob AJ, Foreman AR, et al. Heart muscle disease related to HIV infection: prognostic implications. BMJ. 1994;309:1605-1607.
292. Silva-Cardoso J, Moura B, Martins L, et al. Pericardial involvement in human immunodeficiency virus infection. Chest. 1999;115:418-422.
293. Chen Y, Brennessel D, Walters J, et al. Human immunodeficiency virus–associated pericardial effusion: Report of 40 cases and review of the literature. Am Heart J. 1999;137:516-521.
294. Moore RD, Keruly JC, Chaisson RE. Neutropenia and bacterial infection in acquired immunodeficiency syndrome. Arch Intern Med. 1995;155:1965-1970.
295. Moore DAJ, Benepal T, Portsmouth S, et al. Etiology and natural history of neutropenia in human immunodeficiency virus disease: A prospective study. Clin Infect Dis. 2001;32:469-476.
296. Moore RD, Keruly JC, Chaisson RE. Anemia and survival in HIV infection. J Acquir Immune Defic Syndr Human Retrovirol. 1998;19:29-33.
297. Mocroft A, Kirk O, Barton SE, et al. Anaemia is an independent predictive marker for clinical prognosis in HIV-infected patients from across Europe. AIDS. 1999;13:943-950.
298. Scaradavou A. HIV-related thrombocytopenia. Blood Rev. 2002;16:73-76.
299. Hymes KB, Greene JB, Karpatkin S. The effect of azidothymidine on HIV-related thrombocytopenia. N Engl J Med. 1988;318:516-517.
300. Caso JAA, Mingo CS, Tena JG. Effect of highly active antiretroviral therapy on thrombocytopenia in patients with HIV infection. N Engl J Med. 1999;341:1239-1240.
301. Jokela J, Flynn T, Henry K. Thrombotic thrombocytopenic purpura in a human immunodeficiency virus (HIV)–seropositive homosexual man. Am J Hematol. 1987;25:341-343.
302. Gervasoni C, Ridolfo AL, Vaccarezza M, et al. Thrombotic microangiopathy in patients with acquired immunodeficiency syndrome before and during the era of introduction of highly active antiretroviral therapy. Clin Infect Dis. 2002;35:1534-1540.
303. DeSimone JA, Pomerantz RJ, Babinchak TJ. Inflammatory reactions in HIV-1–infected persons after initiation of highly active antiretroviral therapy. Ann Intern Med. 2000;133:447-454.
304. Wendel KA, Alwood KS, Gachuhi R, et al. Paradoxical worsening of tuberculosis in HIV-infected persons. Chest. 2001;120:193-197.

305. Navas E, Martin-Davila P, Moreno L, et al. Paradoxical reactions of tuberculosis in patients with the acquired immunodeficiency syndrome who are treated with highly active antiretroviral therapy. Arch Intern Med. 2002;162:97-99.
306. Phillips P, Kwiatkowski MB, Copland M, et al. Mycobacterial lymphadenitis associated with the initiation of combination antiretroviral therapy. J Acquir Immune Defic Syndr Hum Retrovirol. 1999;20:122-128.
307. Currier JS, Williams PL, Koletar SL, et al. Discontinuation of *Mycobacterium avium* complex prophylaxis in patients with antiretroviral therapy-induced increases in CD4+ cell count. A randomized, double-blind, placebo-controlled trial. AIDS Clinical Trials Group 362 Study Team. Ann Intern Med. 2000;133:493-503.
308. Aberg JA, Williams PL, Liu T, et al. A study of discontinuing maintenance therapy in human immunodeficiency virus–infected subjects with disseminated *Mycobacterium avium* complex: AIDS Clinical Trial Group 393 Study Team. J Infect Dis. 2003;187:1046-1052.
309. Karavellas MP, Lowder CY, Macdonald C, et al. Immune recovery vitritis associated with inactive cytomegalovirus retinitis: A new syndrome. Arch Ophthalmol. 1998;116:169-175.
310. Zegans ME, Walton RC, Holland GN, et al. Transient vitreous inflammatory reactions associated with combination antiretroviral therapy in patients with AIDS and cytomegalovirus retinitis. Am J Ophthalmol. 1998;125:292-300.
311. Jacobson MA, Zegans M, Pavan PR, et al. Cytomegalovirus retinitis after initiation of highly active antiretroviral therapy. Lancet. 1997;349:1443-1445.
312. Gilquin J, Piketty C, Thomas V, et al. Acute cytomegalovirus infection in AIDS patients with CD4 counts above $100 \times 10(6)$ cells/l following combination antiretroviral therapy including protease inhibitors. AIDS. 1997;11:1659-1660.
313. Karavellas MP, Plummer DJ, Macdonald JC, et al. Incidence of immune recovery vitritis in cytomegalovirus retinitis patients following institution of successful highly active antiretroviral therapy. J Infect Dis. 1999;179:697-700.
314. Nguyen QD, Kempen JH, Bolton SG, et al. Immune recovery uveitis in patients with AIDS and cytomegalovirus retinitis after highly active antiretroviral therapy. Am J Ophthalmol. 2000;129:634-639.
315. Martinez E, Gatell J, Moran Y, et al. High incidence of herpes zoster in patients with AIDS soon after therapy with protease inhibitors. Clin Infect Dis. 1998;27:1510-1513.
316. Domingo P, Torres OH, Ris J, Vazquez G. Herpes zoster as an immune reconstitution disease after initiation of combination antiretroviral therapy in patients with human immunodeficiency virus type-1 infection. Am J Med. 2001;110:605-609.
317. Zylberberg H, Pialoux G, Carnot F, et al. Rapidly evolving hepatitis C virus–related cirrhosis in a human immunodeficiency virus–infected patient receiving triple antiretroviral therapy. Clin Infect Dis. 1998;27:1255-1258.
318. Puoti M, Torti C, Ripamonti D, et al. Severe hepatotoxicity during combination antiretroviral treatment: Incidence, liver histology, and outcome. J Acquir Immune Defic Syndr. 2003;32:259-267.
319. Chung RT, Evans SR, Yang Y, et al. Immune recovery is associated with persistent rise in hepatitis C virus RNA, infrequent liver test flares, and is not impaired by hepatitis C virus in co-infected subjects. AIDS. 2002;16:1915-1923.
320. Puoti M, Gargiulo F, Roldan EQ, et al. Liver damage and kinetics of hepatitis C virus and human immunodeficiency virus replication during the early phases of combination antiretroviral treatment. J Infect Dis. 2000;181:2033-2036.
321. Stone SF, Lee S, Keane NM, et al. Association of increased hepatitis C virus (HCV)–specific IgG and soluble CD26 dipeptidyl peptidase IV enzyme activity with hepatotoxicity after highly active antiretroviral therapy in human immunodeficiency virus-HCV–coinfected patients. J Infect Dis. 2002;186:1498-1502.
322. Carr A, Cooper DA. Restoration of immunity to chronic hepatitis B infection in HIV-infected patient on protease inhibitor. Lancet. 1997;349:995-996.
323. Woods ML, MacGinley R, Eisen DP, Allworth AM. HIV combination therapy: Partial immune restitution unmasking latent cryptococcal infection. AIDS. 1998;12:1491-1494.
324. Koval CE, Gigliotti F, Nevins D, Demeter LM. Immune reconstitution syndrome after successful treatment of *Pneumocystis carinii* pneumonia in a man with human immunodeficiency virus type 1 infection. Clin Infect Dis. 2002;35:491-493.
325. Wislez M, Bergot E, Antoine M, et al. Acute respiratory failure following HAART introduction in patients treated for *Pneumocystis carinii* pneumonia. Am J Respir Crit Care Med. 2001;164:847-851.
326. Safdar A, Rubocki RJ, Horvath JA, et al. Fatal immune restoration disease in human immunodeficiency virus type 1–infected patients with progressive multifocal leukoencephalopathy: Impact of antiretroviral therapy-associated immune reconstitution. Clin Infect Dis. 2002;35:1250-1257.

CHAPTER **118**

Pulmonary Manifestations of Human Immunodeficiency Virus Infection

PAUL E. SAX

Respiratory complications of human immunodeficiency virus (HIV) infection remain a significant source of morbidity and mortality, even since the introduction of potent combination antiretroviral therapy in 1996.[1] Although the incidence of these complications has declined since then, they are frequently the sentinel event that brings a person unaware of his or her HIV status to medical attention via hospitalization or emergency department visit.

EPIDEMIOLOGY

The Pulmonary Complications of HIV Infection Study followed 1100 HIV-infected patients from 1988 to 1994.[2] The study also included 167 HIV-negative controls. The study preceded the availability of protease inhibitors and the widespread use of triple-combination antiretroviral therapy, but it provided the most accurate data regarding the incidence of specific pulmonary infections among HIV-infected individuals. Importantly, the study included the era after which prophylaxis against *Pneumocystis jirovecii* (formerly *Pneumocystis carinii*) pneumonia (PCP) became standard of care. During the 5 years of follow-up in the study, acute bronchitis was the most common lower airway infection, occurring twice as often among those with HIV infection than in controls. By far the two most common acquired immunodeficiency syndrome (AIDS)-defining complications were bacterial pneumonia and PCP. These occurred with approximately equal frequency, and sequential follow-up showed higher rates of pneumonia with declining CD4 cell counts. Other specific causes of opportunistic infections occurred relatively infrequently and included cases of infection with cytomegalovirus (CMV), *Aspergillus*, cryptococci, and herpes simplex virus.

The use of combination antiretroviral therapy has dramatically diminished the incidence of all of these complications, with some evidence of a greater decline in PCP than in bacterial pneumonia.[1,3] For the former, this decline occurred independent of the frequency of PCP prophylaxis.[4] Long-term administration of antipneumocystis prophylaxis with trimethoprim-sulfamethoxazole (TMP/SMX) in particular and *Mycobacterium avium* complex prophylaxis with macrolide antibiotics likely reduces the incidence of bacterial pneumonia.[5-8] It has been shown, however, that treatment with TMP/SMX increases the rate of colonization with resistant bacteria, especially pneumococci.[9]

DIFFERENTIAL DIAGNOSIS

The differential diagnosis of a person with HIV infection presenting with respiratory symptoms is exceedingly broad and includes infectious, neoplastic, and cardiovascular etiologies (Table 118-1). However, as noted earlier, certain conditions (in particular, PCP and bacterial pneumonia) occur far more commonly than others, and hence the diagnostic evaluation and initial empiric therapy should initially be focused toward these diagnoses.

Certain historical, clinical, and radiographic clues help determine the likelihood of underlying specific opportunistic infections. These include the following:

Clinical or laboratory stage of immunosuppression. The vast majority of cases of PCP occur in individuals with CD4 cell counts less than 200 cells/mm³.[10-12] If the CD4 cell count is unavailable, helpful clinical correlates are the presence or absence of oral candidiasis,

TABLE 118-1 Causes of Pulmonary Disease Associated with Human Immunodeficiency Virus Infection*

Most Common

Bacterial
  Streptococcus pneumoniae
  Haemophilus influenzae
  No organism identified, but responsive to antibacterial therapy

Mycobacterial
  Mycobacteria tuberculosis†

Fungal
  Pneumocystis jirovecii

Less Common but Potentially Clinically Important in Some Settings

Bacterial
  Pseudomonas aeruginosa
  Staphylococcus aureus
  Enterobacteriaceae
  Legionella spp.
  Nocardia spp.
  Rhodococcus equi

Mycobacterial
  Mycobacterium kansasii
  Mycobacterium avium complex

Fungal
  Cryptococcus neoformans
  Histoplasma capsulatum
  Coccidioides spp.
  Aspergillus spp.
  Blastomyces dermatitidis
  Pencillium marneffei

Viral
  Influenza
  Cytomegalovirus
  Herpes simplex virus
  Adenovirus
  Respiratory syncytial virus
  Parainfluenza virus

Parasitic
  Toxoplasma gondii
  Strongyloides stercoralis
  Microsporidia spp.
  Cryptosporidium parvum

Noninfectious
  Kaposi's sarcoma
  Non-Hodgkin's lymphoma
  Lung cancer
  Primary pulmonary hypertension
  Congestive heart failure
  Lymphocytic (or lymphoid) interstitial pneumonitis
  Emphysema
  Abacavir hypersensitivity

*Processes are listed within categories in approximate order of frequency.
†Frequency of *M. tuberculosis* infection is highly dependent on local rates of tuberculosis and the patient's exposure history.

which is known to correlate with advanced HIV-related immunosuppression, or other clinical markers of advanced HIV disease such as weight loss. It should be emphasized that progressive immunosuppression increases the risk of all pulmonary infectious processes, including those that may occur with relatively preserved CD4 cell counts, such as bacterial pneumonia and tuberculosis (TB).

Tempo of the illness. HIV-infected individuals with bacterial pneumonia typically present in much the same way as those without HIV infection—with a relatively acute illness (measured in days) characterized by fever and chills and sometimes also accompanied by pleuritic pain and sputum production.[13] PCP, by contrast, typically manifests as a subacute to chronic illness of several weeks' duration, with the most prominent symptoms being fever and shortness of breath. Other helpful clues to PCP include chest tightness (specifically a sense that it is difficult to take a full breath) and a report that a typical day's activities (climbing stairs, conversing on the telephone) are now associated with dyspnea.

Receipt and type of pneumocystis prophylaxis. Patients receiving TMP/SMX for pneumocystis prophylaxis rarely experience breakthroughs of PCP if they are compliant with therapy. By contrast, second-line prophylaxis such as atovaquone, dapsone, and aerosolized pentamidine are all associated with small but significant rates of treatment failure.[5,14-16] As noted earlier, trimethoprim-sulfamethoxazole reduces the risk of all bacterial infections including pneumonia. However, given the high rates of pneumococcal infection among patients with HIV, as well as the concurrently high rate of pneumococcal resistance to TMP/SMX and macrolides, receipt of these drugs for prophylaxis can only be considered as partially protective at most.

Prior history of opportunistic processes. Some patients with HIV appear to have more prominent B-cell dysfunction and hence are at a much greater risk for the development of encapsulated bacterial infections, in particular those due to *Streptococcus pneumoniae* and *Haemophilus influenzae.* Such individuals frequently have a history of multiple prior visits or hospitalizations for bacterial pneumonia,[8] as well as episodes of otitis media, bronchitis, and other bacterial respiratory infections. In addition, persons with a prior history of pneumocystis are at greater risk for relapse, in particular if they are not receiving antiretroviral therapy or PCP prophylaxis with TMP/SMX.[5]

Injection drug use. Persons with HIV who are active users of injection drugs are more likely to develop invasive bacterial infections, including pneumonia, compared with HIV-positive individuals who acquired HIV from other routes.[17]

Local epidemiology or past residence. The incidence of TB as a complication of HIV infection varies markedly depending on local rates of TB and the patient's prior exposure history. In the United States, a high proportion of TB cases occur in persons who have emigrated from highly TB endemic areas[18]; many of these areas (such as sub-Saharan Africa and parts of the Caribbean) also have high background rates of HIV infection. In addition, homelessness and incarceration both increase the risk of TB exposure and subsequent disease. A person's past residence or travel history may elicit potential exposure not only to TB but also to endemic fungi such as histoplasmosis, coccidioidomycosis, and blastomycosis.

Characteristic radiographic findings. Although no radiographic finding is pathognomonic for a specific microbiologic diagnosis, certain patterns help suggest various diagnoses (Table 118-2). Patients with bacterial pneumonia are more likely to have a focal infiltrate on chest radiography, whereas those with PCP typically show diffuse interstitial infiltrates.[13,19] Importantly, there are many exceptions to these generalizations, including the presence of a normal chest radiograph in up to 10% of those with PCP or TB and the occasional occurrence of diffuse interstitial infiltrates in persons with bacterial pneumonia, in particular, secondary to *H. influenzae.*[20-22] In fact, given the wide range of radiographic findings potentially due to PCP—including cavities, pneumatoceles, pleural effusions, nodules, and pneumothoraces—no radiographic appearance can entirely rule out the diagnosis of PCP in an HIV-infected host.[23]

TRIAGE OF PATIENTS: INFECTION CONTROL ISSUES

Appropriate triage of patients with HIV-related respiratory infections is a frequently encountered dilemma due to the higher rates of TB in this context and the often atypical presentation of the disease. As no clinical or radiographic presentation can entirely exclude TB, practitioners must have a high degree of suspicion and a low threshold to admit such cases to negative airflow rooms until TB has been ruled out or an alternative diagnosis has clearly been established.[24]

We admit patients with HIV and respiratory disease to negative-airflow rooms if any of the following conditions are present:

1. Any clinical presentation highly consistent with TB (cavitary lung disease, subacute course, weight loss)
2. Prior residence in a highly TB endemic area
3. Other risk factors for TB exposure, such as contact with an active case, homelessness, or incarceration
4. History of a positive tuberculin skin test without preventive therapy
5. History of prior TB without documentation that appropriate treatment has been completed

The use of these criteria minimizes, but does not eliminate, the chance that an HIV-infected person is a potential source of a nosocomial exposure to TB.

DIAGNOSTIC TESTS

Diagnostic tests should begin with noninvasive studies, usually while empiric therapy for the most likely diagnoses (bacterial pneumonia, and if suspected, PCP) is started. These include a complete blood count with differential, lactate dehydrogenase (LDH), two sets of blood cultures, and a sputum Gram stain and culture. If TB is being considered, a sputum acid-fast smear and culture should also be obtained and processed at a laboratory that is both experienced in TB diagnostics and can turn around results of acid-fast staining relatively promptly (24 to 48 hours). The purpose of the blood cultures is to facilitate diagnosis of bacterial pneumonia, most notably due to *S. pneumoniae,* where rates of bacteremia in patients with HIV can occur in

---

TABLE 118-2 Radiographic Appearance of Pulmonary Diseases in Human Immunodeficiency Virus Infection

Diffuse Interstitial Infiltrates
Pneumocystis jirovecii
Mycobacterium tuberculosis, especially with advanced human immunodeficiency virus disease
Histoplasma capsulatum
Coccidioides spp.
Cryptococcus neoformans
Toxoplasma gondii
Cytomegalovirus
Influenza
Lymphocytic interstitial pneumonitis
Abacavir hypersensitivity

Focal Consolidation
Pyogenic bacterial pneumonia due to *Streptococcus pneumoniae, Haemophilus influenzae*
Mycobacterium tuberculosis
Legionella spp.
Rhodococcus equi

Hilar Adenopathy
Mycobacterium tuberculosis
Histoplasma capsulatum
Coccidioides spp.
Non-Hodgkin's or Hodgkin's lymphoma
Mycobacterium avium complex

Cavitary Disease
Pyogenic bacterial pneumonia due to *Pseudomonas aeruginosa, Staphylococcus aureus,* Enterobacteriaceae
Mycobacterium tuberculosis
Cryptococcus neoformans
Rhodococcus equi
Histoplasma capsulatum
Aspergillus spp.
Nocardia spp.
Mycobacterium avium complex
Pneumocystis jirovecii

Nodules or Masses
Mycobacterium tuberculosis
Cryptococcus neoformans
Aspergillus spp.
Histoplasma capsulatum
Nocardia spp.
Non-Hodgkin's lymphoma
Kaposi's sarcoma
Lung cancer

Normal Radiograph
Pneumocystis jirovecii
Mycobacterium tuberculosis

up to 60% of cases.[25] Given the low specificity of sputum Gram stain, as well as the low sensitivity of sputum culture, a positive blood culture for a likely organism often is the only method of making a specific etiologic diagnosis in a patient with bacterial pneumonia.

As noted in Chapter 268, LDH levels are generally elevated in patients with PCP, especially when the disease is severe enough to require hospitalization. A normal level suggests an alternative diagnosis, and conversely the level of elevation correlates with the severity of the disease. Because many conditions cause an increase in LDH, the test has a low specificity for PCP but is a helpful adjunctive diagnostic clue pending more definitive tests.[25] In many centers, an induced sputum sample (using hypertonic saline to induce cough) is the initial test of choice for diagnosing PCP and sometimes TB. The sensitivity of this test varies widely based on published reports, with a summary of several analyses citing an overall sensitivity of 55%.[26] Factors that may account for the varying sensitivity include patient cooperation with the test, persistence of the respiratory therapist in obtaining the sample, and experience of the diagnostic lab in identifying the organism. Centers using immunofluorescence staining for diagnosis likely have a higher sensitivity than those using alternative staining methods (Giemsa, toluidine blue).[26,27]

If no definitive diagnosis has been identified, the decision to proceed with other diagnostic tests, both noninvasive and invasive, depends on whether the patient has responded to initial therapy. In clinical practice, a prompt clinical response to empiric antibiotic therapy directed at the most common pathogens in HIV-related pneumonia *(S. pneumoniae* and *H. influenzae)* serves as indirect evidence that alternative processes have not been overlooked.[25] For patients who have not improved clinically, and when the diagnosis is still unknown, expedited referral for fiberoptic bronchoscopy with broncheoalveolar lavage (BAL), with or without a transbronchial biopsy, is recommended. Because BAL alone is highly sensitive for the diagnosis of PCP and because biopsy carries a risk of pneumothorax and pulmonary hemorrhage, many bronchoscopists prefer to perform BAL alone initially, reserving biopsy for a repeat procedure if this is still indicated. The main indication to proceed with a biopsy at the initial procedure is a high likelihood of an alternative diagnosis to PCP; this situation arises when a patient is taking TMP/SMX for PCP prophylaxis, has a relatively high CD4 cell count, or an atypical appearing chest radiograph or if a diagnosis requiring biopsy for identification is highly suspected. Examples of such conditions include CMV, *Aspergillus*, lymphocytic

interstitial pneumonitis, and malignancies other than Kaposi's sarcoma (KS). Additional diagnostic studies depend on the degree of patient immunosuppression, epidemiologic risk factors, the clinical course, and the radiographic appearance. For example, a patient from a histoplasmosis-endemic area with chest imaging showing hilar adenopathy along with diffuse infiltrates should undergo testing for histoplasmosis urinary antigen. Alternatively, someone with a history of neutropenia and receipt of corticosteroids who presents with pleuritic pain and pulmonary nodules may ultimately require video-assisted thorascopic surgery (VATS) for diagnosis of pulmonary aspergillosis. The various diagnostic strategies for patients with HIV-related pulmonary disease are summarized in Table 118-3.

SPECIFIC PATHOGENS

Pneumocystis jirovecii Pneumonia

Early in the HIV epidemic, it was established that the principal risk factor for development of HIV-related PCP was a reduced CD4 cell count. Data from the Multicenter AIDS Cohort Study (MACS) showed that the risk of PCP was markedly increased in patients with CD4 cell counts of less than 200 cells/mm³; thrush and fever were other independent predictors.[10] In the postprophylaxis era, patients with PCP are usually severely immunosuppressed: in one series of patients receiving care at an urban hospital, the median CD4 cell count for a first-time case of PCP was 36 cells/mm³; for a recurrent case, it was 10 cells/mm³.[28]

Care providers need to be aware that PCP remains a frequent sentinel opportunistic infection for patients who are not aware they are HIV positive and that this is also a risk factor for severe disease. In one retrospective series from Baltimore, 77% of patients with diagnosed PCP were not receiving prophylaxis and 33% were not previously known to have HIV infection. Patients not taking preventive therapy accounted for 100% of the deaths, 85% of the hospital days, and 100% of the cases admitted to the ICU.[29] In large part because of this phenomenon, in-hospital mortality from PCP remains significant despite the declining incidence of PCP that began in the early 1990s and continued after the use of potent therapy in 1996.[30]

Risk factors for a poor clinical outcome in PCP include hypoxemia, extensive bilateral pulmonary involvement, concurrent other pulmonary infections, recurrent rather than primary disease, elevated LDH levels, and an alveolar-arterial (A-a) gradient of greater than 30 mm Hg.[31-33] Because of the tendency for PCP to worsen slightly after initiation of

---

TABLE 118-3 Diagnostic Tests Used in Patients with Human Immunodeficiency Virus Infection and Pulmonary Disease

Test	Comment
Indicated in All Patients	
Complete blood count with differential	If neutropenia is present, empiric therapy covering *Pseudomonas aeruginosa* is indicated
Lactate dehydrogenase	Elevated in most patients with PCP; nonspecific
Blood cultures	Helpful for diagnosis of bacterial pneumonia, in particular due to *Streptococcus pneumoniae*
Expectorated sputum	Often not available; Gram stain and culture with low sensitivity and specificity, especially after antibiotics have been started
Induced sputum for PCP stain, AFB stain, and culture	Initial test of choice in most centers for diagnosis of *Pneumocystis jirovecii*, although sensitivity varies widely
Indicated for Patients Not Responding to Initial Empirical Therapy	
Fiberoptic bronchoscopy with broncheoalveolar lavage ± transbronchial biopsy	Broncheoalveolar lavage highly sensitive for diagnosis of PCP; Kaposi's sarcoma often diagnosed by visualizing characteristic purple endobracheal or endobronchial plaques, with no biopsy done due to risk of bleeding. Biopsy often necessary to establish alternative diagnosis such as cytomegalovirus, aspergillus, or lymphocytic interstitial pneumonitis
Video-assisted thoracoscopic biopsy	Useful in diagnosis of peripheral nodules, masses not reachable by bronchoscopic biopsy
Serum cryptococcal antigen	Nearly 100% sensitive for diagnosis of disseminated disease in patients with human immunodeficiency virus infection; if positive, cerebrospinal fluid examination is mandatory to exclude meningitis
Urinary histoplasmosis antigen	Indicated in patients residing in or from histoplasmosis-endemic areas, in particular if imaging demonstrates diffuse or reticulonodular infiltrates
High-resolution computed tomography scan	May help identify abnormalities not evident on chest radiography; a normal test makes PCP highly unlikely
Gallium scan	Negative study rules out PCP; however, positive tests are nonspecific, and other tests (high-resolution computed tomography scan, sputum induction) provide more useful information with greater rapidity

PCP, *Pneumocystis jirovecii* (formerly *Pneumocystis carinii*) pneumonia.

therapy (postulated due to an enhanced inflammatory response to dying organisms), adjunctive corticosteroids are indicated for PO_2 less than 70 mm Hg or an A-a gradient of greater than 35, as this intervention has been shown to reduce the risk of respiratory failure and death.[34,35] Although there has been considerable concern that using adjunctive corticosteroids could worsen concomitant opportunistic infections—in particular, TB and CMV infection—these complications of steroid therapy used in this context have been surprisingly rare.[36] As such, it is not essential to rule out these concurrent infections before the use of steroids for PCP, although naturally one should always remain vigilant for the presence of such processes in a patient at risk.

Since the introduction of potent antiretroviral therapy, studies have identified additional risk factors for poor outcome, including older age, use of treatments other than TMP/SMX, concurrent culture of CMV from BAL fluid, and a $CD4^+$ cell count less than 50/mm[3].[31,37] One retrospective study suggested that when controlling for other factors, receipt of combination antiretroviral therapy at the time of treatment for PCP is associated with improved survival.[38]

Because it is not practical to culture the organism in clinical laboratories, definitive diagnosis relies on visualization of cysts in respiratory secretions. As discussed earlier, induced sputum is often the first diagnostic procedure, followed by BAL obtained by bronchoscopy, which has a sensitivity of 95% to 100%. Identification of cysts on appropriate stains is diagnostic of PCP, as there does not appear to be an asymptomatic carrier state; however, persistence of organisms through and even after therapy is common and does not reflect failure of treatment.[39] Newer diagnostic techniques under investigation include polymerase chain reaction of saliva or sputum, as well as blood tests to measure levels of S-adenosylmethionine, a substance utilized exclusively by P. jirovecii and hence lowered in patients with active disease.[40]

Bacterial Pneumonia

Although most consider HIV-related immunosuppression to be predominantly due to an impairment of cell-mediated immunity, the immune deficits are broader and include both abnormalities in humoral immunity and, in the late stages of disease, neutrophil function.[41-43] As a result, bacterial infections—and particularly bacterial respiratory infections—frequently complicate HIV disease. The rate of bacterial pneumonia among patients with HIV is as much as 100-fold higher than that in HIV-negative controls. Because the encapsulated bacteria (in particular, S. pneumoniae) are more intrinsically virulent than the opportunistic infections of advanced HIV disease, these infections may occur at any stage of HIV disease and hence be the sentinel opportunistic process in a person otherwise unaware that he or she has HIV infection. Among those with HIV infection, risk factors for the development of bacterial pneumonia are progressive immunodeficiency (as measured by the absolute CD4 cell count) and injection drug use.[17] Neither the concomitant use of TMP/SMX for PCP prophylaxis nor a history of having received immunization against S. pneumoniae is sufficiently protective against bacterial pneumonia to warrant a change in empiric therapy when considering this diagnosis.[44] Mortality due to bacterial pneumonia is higher in HIV patients who have a CD4 mm[3] cell count of less than 100 cells/mm[3], radiographic progression of disease on therapy, and shock.[45] As with other opportunistic infections, use of potent combination therapy decreases the risk of bacterial pneumonia.[3]

The most common identified pathogen in HIV-related bacterial pneumonia is S. pneumoniae, generally followed by H. influenzae.[46] Although both typically present with a relatively acute illness and focal consolidation on chest radiography, H. influenzae may rarely cause a more subacute illness with diffuse interstitial infiltrates, suggestive of PCP. Gram-negative bacilli and S. aureus assume increasing importance as immunosuppression worsens, presumably due to both neutrophil dysfunction and selective pressure of other antimicrobials. Pseudomonas aeruginosa infection has been associated with neutropenia, prior treatment with cephalosporins, and CD4 cell counts of less than 50 cells/mm[3]. Another important feature of pseudomonal respiratory infections in HIV-infected patients is their

predilection for relapse; chronic colonization typically ensues, with relapse rates after therapy between 25% and 86%.[47-49] Although pathogens of atypical pneumonia have been identified in HIV-infected hosts, in most published series they occur relatively infrequently if at all.[46] Nocardia spp. are an important cause of pulmonary disease in immunocompromised hosts, including those with HIV infection.[50] The relative rarity of nocardiosis compared with other opportunistic processes may relate to the frequent use of TMP/SMX for PCP prophylaxis, although this does not completely prevent Nocardia infection from occurring. The disease is usually subacute to chronic and limited to the lung, where cavitation may occur; it therefore may present similarly to TB.[51] Dissemination with positive blood cultures is also possible, in particular in patients with advanced immunosuppression.

Rhodococcus equi can cause both localized pulmonary and disseminated disease in HIV-infected hosts, who appear to be particularly susceptible to this pathogen. A gram-positive coccobacillus, R. equi can be mistaken for routine oral flora on sputum smears; a potential clinical clue is that the organism also is weakly acid fast. The typical presentation is one of a chronic pneumonia—with cough, sputum production, and sometime hemoptysis—with radiographs showing cavitary disease and often with associated pleural effusion (Fig. 118-1); however, diverse radiographic findings have been reported.[52] Bacteremia commonly accompanies Rhodococcus pneumonia and may be the most reliable way to make the diagnosis.[53] Because treatment requires prolonged therapy with multiple agents, persistence or recurrence of symptomatic infection is common unless the immune status can be improved with antiretroviral therapy.[52]

HIV infection markedly increases the risk of the development of TB, as either progression of primary disease or reactivation. As noted earlier, the likelihood of a pulmonary process being due to TB is strongly influenced by the exposure history, which is related to the patient's current or past residence and/or the presence of other known risk factors, such as homelessness or incarceration. Areas in the United States with relatively high numbers and rates of TB include the New York metropolitan area (including the cities of northern New Jersey), Florida, California, Chicago, the District of Columbia, Georgia, and Texas.[54] Rates are also high in immigrants from highly TB-endemic regions, such as sub-Saharan Africa, Latin America, Asia, and much of the Caribbean.[18]

The clinical presentation of TB in HIV-infected patients depends on the degree of immunosuppression.[20,24,55,56] Those with higher CD4 cell counts (>400/mm[3]) present similarly to those without HIV, with upper lobe cavitary disease and a low risk of extrapulmonary dissemination; the presence of constitutional symptoms is variable. At more

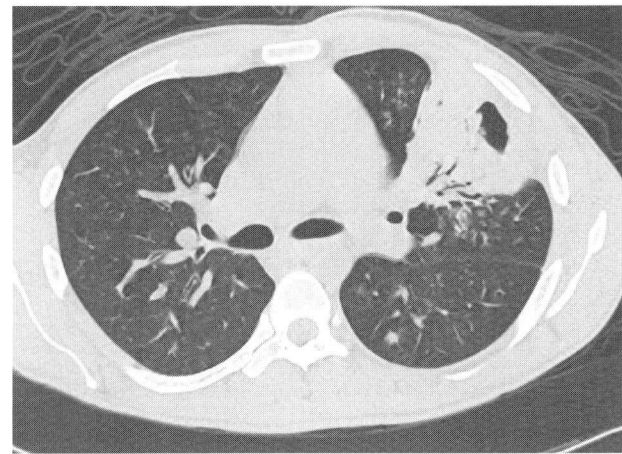

FIGURE 118-1. Chest computed tomography in an HIV-positive patient with pulmonary and disseminated infection due to *Rhodococcus equi*, demonstrating a consolidation with cavitation in the lingula. Sputum and blood cultures were both positive for the organism, which was visualized on both Gram and acid-fast staining of respiratory secretions.

advanced stages of immunosuppression, patients are more likely to have disseminated disease accompanied by prominent constitutional symptoms and unusual pulmonary manifestations such as mediastinal-hilar adenopathy, focal lower lobe or diffuse interstitial infiltrates, and pleural effusions. In these cases, sputum acid-fast smears are less likely to be positive than those with cavitary disease, and diagnosis may ultimately be made by alternative methods such as isolator blood cultures (positive in one fourth to one half of patients) or tissue biopsy of an involved site (lymph node, bone marrow, or liver). Nonetheless, even with negative AFB smears on respiratory secretions, sputum or BAL cultures may ultimately be positive even with relatively subtle parenchymal abnormalities on.

Mycobacteria Other Than *Mycobacterium tuberculosis*

The respiratory tract may act as a portal of entry for *M. avium* complex, but it is rarely a primary cause of respiratory symptoms.[57,58] As a result, recovery of the organism from respiratory secretions may be a marker of colonization and a harbinger of disseminated disease but is not diagnostic of pulmonary infection and does not necessarily warrant treatment.

Among the non-TB mycobacteria, *M. kansasii* is the most likely to cause pulmonary disease in HIV-infected persons. It occurs relatively uncommonly, mostly during advanced HIV disease, and has been associated with a subacute to chronic course that includes constitutional symptoms and cough; radiographic abnormalities include cavities, nodules, or infiltrates.[59,60] Isolation of the organism from sputum or BAL specimens generally warrants therapy, as asymptomatic colonization is unusual.

Fungal Pneumonia

A variety of fungi other than *P. jirovecii* may rarely cause pneumonia in patients with HIV. The most common are *Cryptococcus neoformans;* the endemic fungi *Coccidioides immitis, Histoplasma capsulatum,* and *Blastomyces dermatitidis;* and the mold *Aspergillus fumigatus.*

Each of these organisms rarely causes disease until the patient is severely immunosuppressed (CD4 cell count <100 cells/mm³). They also share the fact that although the lungs act a portal of entry—and may be the initial site of symptoms—hematogenous dissemination commonly occurs to other sites.

Cryptococcal pneumonia typically presents with fever and cough; other associated symptoms may include dyspnea, chest pain, and hemoptysis.[61-63] Nonpulmonary symptoms depend on whether dissemination has occurred, most commonly to the central nervous system, where basilar meningitis can lead to headache, cranial neuropathies, and, in more severe cases, depressed consciousness. On occasion, physical examination reveals white papular lesions on the skin mimicking molluscum contagiosum. A wide range of radiographic abnormalities may occur, including diffuse interstitial infiltrates, focal consolidation, cavitary disease, nodules, adenopathy, and pleural effusions, with more extensive disease seen in those with lower CD4 cell counts. BAL cultures are usually positive, as is the serum cryptococcal antigen; antibody testing has no significant role. Even in the absence of central nervous system symptoms, a cerebrospinal fluid examination is mandatory in patients with AIDS who have cryptococcal pneumonia and a positive serum cryptococcal antigen, as meningitis may be chronic or subacute and produce minimal symptoms. Not surprisingly, HIV patients with higher CD4 cell counts and lower serum cryptococcal antigen titers are more likely to have localized pulmonary disease.[61]

Pulmonary histoplasmosis, coccidioidomycosis, and blastomycosis are generally limited to the geographic regions where these fungi are endemic, although rarely these infections may reactivate many years after travel or residence in one of these areas.[64] *H. capsulatum* is found world wide, most notably in the Mississippi, Ohio, and St. Lawrence River valleys; the Caribbean; southern Mexico; and Central America. In patients with AIDS, pulmonary histoplasmosis presents most commonly as a disseminated disease in an individual with a CD4 cell count of less than 100 cells/mm³, with

fever, wasting, adenopathy, diarrhea, and mucosal lesions accompanying the pulmonary process.[65,66] Cough and dyspnea are the most common pulmonary symptoms; typical radiographic findings are diffuse interstitial or reticulonodular infiltrates. The presence of hilar or mediastinal adenopathy may help distinguish histoplasmosis from *P. jirovecii,* as the clinical presentations in susceptible hosts overlap significantly. The diagnostic test of choice for histoplasmosis is detection of polysaccharide antigen in urine or blood; these tests have reported sensitivities of 93% and 89%, respectively. These tests have supplanted antibody and skin testing, which are rarely indicated. Blood cultures using the lysis-centrifugation method and BAL fluid are also often positive for histoplasmosis in patients with HIV. Because the organism grows relatively slowly, results of histoplasmosis antigen testing are often available before the cultures turn positive.

Coccidioides spp. are endemic to the southwestern United States, northern Mexico, and parts of South and Central America. In endemic areas, they may cause pulmonary disease in HIV-infected individuals, where they predominantly affect those with severe immunosuppression (CD4 cell counts <200 cells/mm³).[67,68] As with histoplasmosis, pulmonary findings are often accompanied by clinical evidence of dissemination, including involvement of the skin, lymph nodes, bone, and meninges. Chest radiographic abnormalities are diverse and may include alveolar infiltrates, nodules, adenopathy, cavities, and pleural effusions. Isolation of the organism in respiratory secretions—usually through bronchoscopy—is generally required to make the diagnosis. A positive isolator blood culture confirms the presence of disseminated disease. Although 80% of HIV-infected patients with pulmonary coccidioidomycosis have positive serologies, these titers have more of a role in monitoring response to therapy than in establishing the diagnosis. Skin testing with coccidioidal antigen has no useful role diagnostically and is no longer commercially available.

Of the endemic fungi, *B. dermatitidis* is the least likely to act as an opportunistic pathogen in patients with HIV.[69] The organism is found in the midwestern and southcentral United States. In a case series of blastomycosis in 15 HIV-infected patients, 12 had evidence of pulmonary involvement and 5 also had disseminated disease at the time of diagnosis. The predominant symptoms at presentation were fever, weight loss, and cough.[70]

Pulmonary aspergillosis in patients with HIV infection occurs almost exclusively in those with advanced HIV-related immunosuppression (CD4 cell count <50/mm³). Frequently other risk factors for aspergillosis are present as well, such as receipt of corticosteroids or neutropenia.[71-74] The specific organism is usually *A. fumigatus* or *Aspergillus niger.* Respiratory tract disease is the most common manifestation; despite the predilection for the organism to invade blood vessel walls and disseminate, focal central nervous system disease due to *Aspergillus* in AIDS patients appears to occur more commonly from contiguous spread from the sinuses, orbits, and ears.[75]

Two types of aspergillus respiratory disease have been described: semi-invasive pseudomembranous tracheitis and invasive pneumonitis. In the former, fever, cough, dyspnea, and wheezing are common symptoms; the diagnosis is established when endoscopic examination reveals an exudative pseudomembrane adherent to the tracheal wall. In invasive pneumonitis, fever and cough may be accompanied by pleuritic pain and hemoptysis. Radiographic abnormalities in both of these forms overlap and can show diffuse infiltrates, cavities, and focal wedge-shaped abnormalities that reflect pulmonary infarction. A definitive diagnosis requires identification of fungal organisms consistent with *Aspergillus* on a biopsy specimen in a patient with the appropriate clinical syndrome. Not uncommonly, a presumptive diagnosis of pulmonary disease is made when *Aspergillus* spp. are cultured from respiratory secretions in a patient with fever, cough, infiltrates, and severe immunosuppression. The diagnosis is especially likely when concomitant risk factors, such as corticosteroid exposure or neutropenia, are present.

Viral Pneumonia

Although patients with HIV infection are at risk for viral pneumonitis, these conditions are rarely diagnosed in clinical practice. Indeed, even when a potential respiratory pathogen is isolated from respiratory secretions, it is often difficult in the absence of specific histopathology to ascribe the pneumonitis solely to the virus identified. An example of this clinical quandary is CMV; isolation of CMV from BAL specimens is relatively common, yet most patients with positive BAL cultures have an alternative diagnosis (especially PCP or bacterial pneumonia) and may improve without specific therapy directed at CMV.[76-78] Nonetheless, in a patient with advanced HIV disease (CD4 cell count <50/mm^3), interstitial infiltrates on chest radiography, and no alternative diagnosis established, CMV may be the sole responsible pathogen. This diagnosis is confirmed when histopathology (samples are usually obtained via transbronchial biopsy or VATS) demonstrates intracellular inclusions typical of CMV; cultures are confirmatory rather than diagnostic. Ganciclovir or valganciclovir therapy is indicated for such cases, or when there is sufficient evidence to suggest that CMV may be acting as a copathogen when treatment of another diagnosis is associated with a suboptimal response.

During influenza season, HIV-infected patients may present with typical symptoms of influenza, consisting of an acute febrile illness associated with cough, myalgias, sore throat, and rigors. Although influenza vaccine is indicated for all HIV-positive individuals, not all patients receive the vaccine, and in addition they may mount a suboptimal response to the vaccine with progressive immunodeficiency.[79] Chest radiographs are typically negative, suggesting that as with HIV-negative patients, primary influenza pneumonia is unusual[80,81]; major complications ensue with bacterial superinfection. The diagnosis of influenza is established either on clinical grounds during influenza season or with use of a rapid influenza diagnostic test on respiratory secretions.

As with other immunosuppressed populations, pneumonitis in HIV patients has been reported due to herpes simplex virus, as well as adenovirus, respiratory syncytial virus, and parainfluenza virus type 3. These are rare causes of pneumonia in HIV-infected patients but should be considered when clinicians cannot identify an alternative diagnosis. For herpes simplex virus, viral isolation in respiratory secretions usually indicates evidence of reactivation in the upper oropharynx rather than primary pneumonitis, but pulmonary or tracheal infection may occur, especially in the context of endotracheal or nasogastric intubation.

Parasitic Pneumonia

Among the various parasitic infections that occur in patients with HIV, none primarily involve the respiratory tract, yet, rarely, they can lead to pulmonary disease as part of generalized dissemination or from focal lung involvement, sometimes without the primary target organ being clinically involved. Pulmonary toxoplasmosis is a rare form of severe pneumonia that occurs predominantly in patients with markedly depressed immune function (CD4 cell count <50/mm^3).[82] Clinical presentation is similar to that of PCP but, unlike PCP, may be accompanied by a sepsis-like syndrome with hypotension. Radiographic abnormalities are diverse, consisting most commonly of a interstitial infiltrates but also potentially nodules, effusions, or a mass lesion; as with PCP, an elevated LDH is a commonly reported laboratory finding.[83] Diagnosis is established by identification of toxoplasma tachyzoites on Giemsa stain of BAL fluid or tissue obtained on biopsy; alternative techniques such as polymerase chain reaction or tissue culture are available in commercial laboratories and research settings.

Despite its association with defects in cell-mediated immunity, disseminated infection to the lung of *Strongyloides stercoralis* is surprisingly rare in HIV-infected individuals, even in areas highly endemic for both HIV and strongyloides. Indeed, many patients with HIV who experience strongyloides superinfection syndrome have other classic risk factors, including receipt of corticosteroids, severe wasting, or human T-cell lymphotrophic virus type I (HTLV-I) coinfection. Clinicians should consider this diagnosis in an HIV-infected patient, especially with the above risk factors, who presents with pneumonitis, gram-negative sepsis, and sometimes associated meningitis.[84,85] Identification of strongyloides larvae on a centrifuged BAL specimen is diagnostic; eosinophilia is variably present, and its absence does not exclude the diagnosis.

Although cryptosporidiosis and microsporidiosis predominantly involve the gastrointestinal tract, both can, rarely, colonize the lung and lead to pulmonary disease.[86,87] Diagnosis is made through direct visualization of the organism on respiratory secretions or histopathology, using appropriate stains—modified acid-fast for cryptosporidiosis and the modified trichrome stain for microsporidiosis. As antimicrobial treatment for these conditions is suboptimal, improving immune function with antiretroviral therapy is the preferred strategy.

Neoplastic and Other Noninfectious Pulmonary Complications of Human Immunodeficiency Virus Infection

The two most common HIV-related neoplasms of the lung are pulmonary KS and non-Hodgkin's lymphoma. Patients with pulmonary KS unusually have evidence of cutaneous and/or mucosal disease; in one series, only 16% had disease limited to the lungs.[88,89] The disease may be asymptomatic even with extensive abnormalities on chest radiograph (Fig. 118-2); these abnormalities are typically nodular infiltrates with or without pulmonary effusions, with chest computed tomography showing a peribronchovascular distribution of infiltrates. Diagnosis is generally made through direct visualization of characteristic purplish plaques on bronchoscopy; because these lesions are highly vascular and quite typical, biopsy is often deferred to avoid the risk of hemorrhage. Treatment with chemotherapy is indicated for symptomatic pulmonary disease (see Chapter 121). However, as with cutaneous KS, potent antiretroviral therapy can induce significant improvement in pulmonary KS, as well as sustained remissions; in some cases, antiretroviral therapy can even obviate the need for chemotherapy at all.[90,91] Conversely, HIV treatment has also rarely been associated with inflammatory worsening of KS as a form of the immune reconstitution syndrome.

The radiographic findings in pulmonary lymphoma are diverse and may consist of nodules, masses, and pleural effusions.[92] Although the diagnosis can sometimes be established through BAL with cytology, transbronchial biopsy, or thoracentesis, these procedures have a low yield and VATS is often required.[93] Nonspecific findings that suggest lymphoma are elevations in LDH and a positive gallium scan corresponding to the area of abnormality on chest imaging.

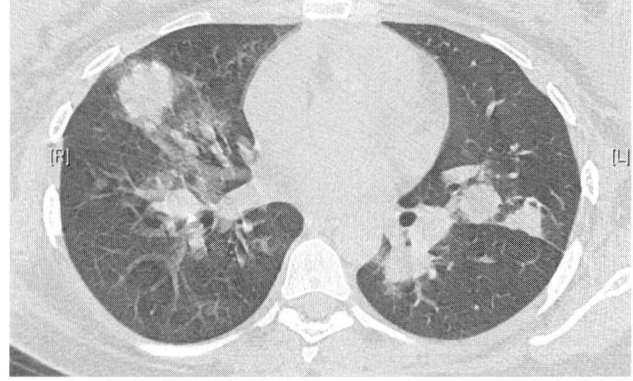

FIGURE 118-2. Chest computed tomography in an HIV-positive patient with biopsy-confirmed pulmonary Kaposi's sarcoma. Despite the extensive bilateral lung nodules evident on this study, the patient's only respiratory symptom was a mild cough. There was nearly complete clearance with chemotherapy and combination antiretroviral therapy.

Although lymphocytic interstitial pneumonitis (LIP) is seen more commonly in HIV-infected children, adults may, rarely, develop this complication as well.[94] It presents similarly to a related condition, nonspecific interstitial pneumonitis, with cough, shortness of breath, and constitutional symptoms. Diffuse reticulonodular or interstitial infiltrates are seen on chest imaging, making differentiation from PCP difficult. However, compared with patients who develop HIV-related opportunistic infections, those with LIP usually have a relatively preserved or even normal CD4 cell counts. Because diagnosis is made through histopathology and exclusion of infectious etiologies, transbronchial or VATS biopsy is indicated. Several case reports have demonstrated that antiretroviral therapy may lead to substantial improvement in LIP.[95,96] For unresponsive cases, corticosteroids may be effective.[94]

HIV infection is a risk factor for the development of pulmonary hypertension.[97] It occurs at all stages of HIV disease, with variable CD4 cell counts and HIV RNA levels at the time of presentation. In some series, women represent a disproportionate number of the cases.[98] The predominant symptom is exertional dyspnea; cough, fatigue, and chest pain may also be present. The key to the diagnosis is recognizing that the symptoms are not related to a primary pulmonary infectious process; physical examination signs consistent with right ventricular hypertrophy or failure are helpful but often not present initially. A cardiac echocardiogram shows evidence of right atrial hypertrophy and elevated pulmonary pressures; this is then confirmed with right heart catheterization. Management of pulmonary hypertension is the same as for HIV-negative hosts, with prostaglandin agonists (epoprostenol), diuretics, and anticoagulation; sildenafil may also have a role, but drug-drug interactions with protease inhibitors can occur. Unfortunately, reports have not shown a consistent beneficial response of this condition to antiretroviral therapy.[97]

There is evidence that patients with HIV are at greater risk for the development of emphysema than are HIV-negative subjects.[99] It is unknown whether effective antiretroviral therapy has offset the increased susceptibility to this condition. Because cigarette smoking is highly prevalent among HIV patients, this is an area of prevention often overlooked among providers.

Abacavir is a nucleoside reverse transcriptase inhibitor that causes a systemic reaction in approximately 5% of individuals, usually within 6 weeks of starting the drug[100] (see Chapter 124). As part of this multisystem reaction, symptoms may include fever, rash, fatigue, malaise, gastrointestinal symptoms, and arthralgias; cough and dyspnea also may occur and may mimic bronchitis or pneumonia.[101] It is critical that clinicians evaluating patients who have recently been started on abacavir be aware that this nucleoside reverse transcriptase inhibitor can cause a systemic hypersensitivity reaction, because continued abacavir treatment in the face of this reaction can be fatal. Symptoms generally resolve slowly after cessation of the drug. Abacavir should never be resumed in such circumstances, as rechallenge can lead to an immediate and life-threatening recurrence of the hypersensitivity reaction. Because abacavir hypersensitivity can mimic other processes, in particular influenza, helpful clinical clues that make hypersensitivity more likely are worsening of symptoms after each dose, gastrointestinal symptoms, and rash.[102]

TREATMENT

Treatment of opprtunistic infections of the lung and other sites is discussed in Chapter 125.

REFERENCES

1. Wolff AJ, O'Donnell AE. Pulmonary manifestations of HIV infection in the era of highly active antiretroviral therapy. Chest. 2001;120:1888-1893.
2. Wallace JM, Hansen NI, Lavange L, et al. Respiratory disease trends in the Pulmonary Complications of HIV Infection Study cohort. Pulmonary Complications of HIV Infection Study Group. Am J Respir Crit Care Med. 1997;155:72-80.
3. Sullivan JH, Moore RD, Keruly JC, Chaisson RE. Effect of antiretroviral therapy on the incidence of bacterial pneumonia in patients with advanced HIV infection. Am J Respir Crit Care Med. 2000;162:64-67.
4. Palella FJ, Jr., Delaney KM, Moorman AC, et al. Declining morbidity and mortality among patients with advanced human immunodeficiency virus infection. HIV Outpatient Study Investigators. N Engl J Med. 1998;338:853-860.
5. Hardy WD, Feinberg J, Finkelstein DM, et al. A controlled trial of trimethoprim-sulfamethoxazole or aerosolized pentamidine for secondary prophylaxis of Pneumocystis carinii pneumonia in patients with the acquired immunodeficiency syndrome. AIDS Clinical Trials Group Protocol 021. N Engl J Med. 1992; 327:1842-1848.
6. Hirschtick RE, Glassroth J, Jordan MC, et al. Bacterial pneumonia in persons infected with the human immunodeficiency virus. Pulmonary Complications of HIV Infection Study Group. N Engl J Med. 1995;333:845-851.
7. Mayer HB, Rose DN, Cohen S, et al. The effect of Pneumocystis carinii pneumonia prophylaxis regimens on the incidence of bacterial infections in HIV-infected patients. Aids. 1993;7:1687-1689.
8. Navin TR, Rimland D, Lennox JL, et al. Risk factors for community-acquired pneumonia among persons infected with human immunodeficiency virus. J Infect Dis. 2000;181:158-164.
9. Rodriguez-Barradas MC, Tharapel RA, Groover JE, et al. Colonization by Streptococcus pneumoniae among human immunodeficiency virus-infected adults: Prevalence of antibiotic resistance, impact of immunization, and characterization by polymerase chain reaction with BOX primers of isolates from persistent S. pneumoniae carriers. J Infect Dis. 1997;175:590-597.
10. Phair J, Munoz A, Detels R, et al. The risk of Pneumocystis carinii pneumonia among men infected with human immunodeficiency virus type 1. Multicenter AIDS Cohort Study Group. N Engl J Med. 1990;322:161-165.
11. Hoover DR, Saah AJ, Bacellar H, et al. Clinical manifestations of AIDS in the era of Pneumocystis prophylaxis. Multicenter AIDS Cohort Study. N Engl J Med. 1993;329:1922-1926.
12. Stansell JD, Osmond DH, Charlebois E, et al. Predictors of Pneumocystis carinii pneumonia in HIV-infected persons. Pulmonary Complications of HIV Infection Study Group. Am J Respir Crit Care Med. 1997;155:60-66.
13. Selwyn PA, Pumerantz AS, Durante A, et al. Clinical predictors of Pneumocystis carinii pneumonia, bacterial pneumonia and tuberculosis in HIV-infected patients. Aids. 1998;12:885-893.
14. Chan C, Montaner J, Lefebvre EA, et al. Atovaquone suspension compared with aerosolized pentamidine for prevention of Pneumocystis carinii pneumonia in human immunodeficiency virus-infected subjects intolerant of trimethoprim or sulfonamides. J Infect Dis. 1999;180:369-376.
15. Bozzette SA, Finkelstein DM, Spector SA, et al. A randomized trial of three antipneumocystis agents in patients with advanced human immunodeficiency virus infection. NIAID AIDS Clinical Trials Group. N Engl J Med. 1995;332:693-699.
16. Torres RA, Barr M, Thorn M, et al. Randomized trial of dapsone and aerosolized pentamidine for the prophylaxis of Pneumocystis carinii pneumonia and toxoplasmic encephalitis. Am J Med. 1993;95:573-583.
17. Afessa B, Green B. Clinical course, prognostic factors, and outcome prediction for HIV patients in the ICU. The PIP (Pulmonary complications, ICU support, and prognostic factors in hospitalized patients with HIV) study. Chest. 2000;118: 138-145.
18. Working Group on Tuberculosis among Foreign-Born Persons. Recommendations for prevention and control of tuberculosis among foreign-born persons. Report of the Working Group on Tuberculosis among Foreign-Born Persons. Centers for Disease Control and Prevention. MMWR Recomm Rep. 1998;47:1-29.
19. Crans CA Jr, Boiselle PM. Imaging features of Pneumocystis carinii pneumonia. Crit Rev Diagn Imaging. 1999;40:251-284.
20. Perlman DC, el-Sadr WM, Nelson ET, et al. Variation of chest radiographic patterns in pulmonary tuberculosis by degree of human immunodeficiency virus-related immunosuppression. The Terry Beirn Community Programs for Clinical Research on AIDS (CPCRA). The AIDS Clinical Trials Group (ACTG). Clin Infect Dis. 1997;25:242-246.
21. Baril L, Astagneau P, Nguyen J, et al. Pyogenic bacterial pneumonia in human immunodeficiency virus-infected inpatients: A clinical, radiological, microbiological, and epidemiological study. Clin Infect Dis. 1998;26:964-971.
22. Cordero E, Pachon J, Rivero A, et al. Haemophilus influenzae pneumonia in human immunodeficiency virus-infected patients. The Grupo Andaluz para el Estudio de las Enfermedades Infecciosas. Clin Infect Dis. 2000;30:461-465.
23. DeLorenzo LJ, Huang CT, Maguire GP, Stone DJ. Roentgenographic patterns of Pneumocystis carinii pneumonia in 104 patients with AIDS. Chest. 1987;91: 323-327.
24. Greenberg SD, Frager D, Suster B, et al. Active pulmonary tuberculosis in patients with AIDS: Spectrum of radiographic findings (including a normal appearance). Radiology. 1994;193:115-119.
25. Janoff EN, Breiman RF, Daley CL, Hopewell PC. Pneumococcal disease during HIV infection. Epidemiologic, clinical, and immunologic perspectives. Ann Intern Med. 1992;117:314-324.
26. Cruciani M, Marcati P, Malena M, et al. Meta-analysis of diagnostic procedures for Pneumocystis carinii pneumonia in HIV-1-infected patients. Eur Respir J. 2002;20:982-989.
27. Kovacs JA, Ng VL, Masur H, et al. Diagnosis of Pneumocystis carinii pneumonia: Improved detection in sputum with use of monoclonal antibodies. N Engl J Med. 1988;318:589-593.
28. Moore RD, Chaisson RE. Natural history of opportunistic disease in an HIV-infected urban clinical cohort. Ann Intern Med. 1996;124:633-642.

29. Gallant JE, McAvinue SM, Moore RD, et al. The impact of prophylaxis on outcome and resource utilization in *Pneumocystis carinii* pneumonia. Chest. 1995;107:1018-1023.

30. Azoulay E, Parrot A, Flahault A, et al. AIDS-related *Pneumocystis carinii* pneumonia in the era of adjunctive steroids: Implication of BAL neutrophilia. Am J Respir Crit Care Med. 1999;160:493-499.

31. Benfield TL, Helweg-Larsen J, Bang D, et al. Prognostic markers of short-term mortality in AIDS-associated *Pneumocystis carinii* pneumonia. Chest. 2001;119:844-851.

32. Brenner M, Ognibene FP, Lack EE, et al. Prognostic factors and life expectancy of patients with acquired immunodeficiency syndrome and *Pneumocystis carinii* pneumonia. Am Rev Respir Dis. 1987;136:1199-1206.

33. Zaman MK, White DA. Serum lactate dehydrogenase levels and *Pneumocystis carinii* pneumonia. Diagnostic and prognostic significance. Am Rev Respir Dis. 1988;137:796-800.

34. Bozzette SA, Sattler FR, Chiu J, et al. A controlled trial of early adjunctive treatment with corticosteroids for *Pneumocystis carinii* pneumonia in the acquired immunodeficiency syndrome. California Collaborative Treatment Group. N Engl J Med. 1990;323:1451-1457.

35. Gagnon S, Boota AM, Fischl MA, et al. Corticosteroids as adjunctive therapy for severe *Pneumocystis carinii* pneumonia in the acquired immunodeficiency syndrome. A double-blind, placebo-controlled trial. N Engl J Med. 1990;323:1444-1450.

36. Gallant JE, Chaisson RE, Moore RD. The effect of adjunctive corticosteroids for the treatment of *Pneumocystis carinii* pneumonia on mortality and subsequent complications. Chest. 1998;114:1258-1263.

37. Dworkin MS, Hanson DL, Navin TR. Survival of patients with AIDS, after diagnosis of *Pneumocystis carinii* pneumonia, in the United States. J Infect Dis. 2001;183:1409-1412.

38. Morris A, Wachter RM, Luce J, et al. Improved survival with highly active antiretroviral therapy in HIV-infected patients with severe *Pneumocystis carinii* pneumonia. Aids. 2003;17:73-80.

39. O'Donnell WJ, Pieciak W, Chertow GM, et al. Clearance of *Pneumocystis carinii* cysts in acute *P. carinii* pneumonia: Assessment by serial sputum induction. Chest. 1998;114:1264-1268.

40. Skelly M, Hoffman J, Fabbri M, et al. S-adenosylmethionine concentrations in diagnosis of *Pneumocystis carinii* pneumonia. Lancet. 2003;361:1267-1268.

41. Parkin JM, Helbert M, Hughes CL, Pinching AJ. Immunoglobulin G subclass deficiency and susceptibility to pyogenic infections in patients with AIDS-related complex and AIDS. Aids. 1989;3:37-39.

42. Lane HC, Masur H, Edgar LC, et al. Abnormalities of B-cell activation and immunoregulation in patients with the acquired immunodeficiency syndrome. N Engl J Med. 1983;309:453-458.

43. Ellis M, Gupta S, Galant S, et al. Impaired neutrophil function in patients with AIDS or AIDS-related complex: A comprehensive evaluation. J Infect Dis. 1988;158:1268-1276.

44. French N, Nakiyingi J, Carpenter LM, et al. 23-Valent pneumococcal polysaccharide vaccine in HIV-1-infected Ugandan adults: Double-blind, randomised and placebo controlled trial. Lancet. 2000;355:2106-2111.

45. Cordero E, Pachon J, Rivero A, et al. Community-acquired bacterial pneumonia in human immunodeficiency virus-infected patients: Validation of severity criteria. The Grupo Andaluz para el Estudio de las Enfermedades Infecciosas. Am J Respir Crit Care Med. 2000;162:2063-2068.

46. Bartlett JG. Pneumonia in the patient with HIV infection. Infect Dis Clin North Am. 1998;12:807-820, xi.

47. Fichtenbaum CJ, Woeltje KF, Powderly WG. Serious *Pseudomonas aeruginosa* infections in patients infected with human immunodeficiency virus: A case-control study. Clin Infect Dis. 1994;19:417-422.

48. Asboe D, Gant V, Aucken HM, et al. Persistence of *Pseudomonas aeruginosa* strains in respiratory infection in AIDS patients. AIDS. 1998;12:1771-1775.

49. Sorvillo F, Beall G, Turner PA, et al. Incidence and determinants of *Pseudomonas aeruginosa* infection among persons with HIV: Association with hospital exposure. Am J Infect Control. 2001;29:79-84.

50. Pintado V, Gomez-Mampaso E, Fortun J, et al. Infection with *Nocardia* species: Clinical spectrum of disease and species distribution in Madrid, Spain, 1978-2001. Infection. 2002;30:338-340.

51. Uttamchandani RB, Daikos GL, Reyes RR, et al. Nocardiosis in 30 patients with advanced human immunodeficiency virus infection: Clinical features and outcome. Clin Infect Dis. 1994;18:348-353.

52. Torres-Tortosa M, Arrizabalaga J, Villanueva JL, et al. Prognosis and clinical evaluation of infection caused by *Rhodococcus equi* in HIV-infected patients: A multicenter study of 67 cases. Chest. 2003;123:1970-1976.

53. Donisi A, Suardi MG, Casari S, et al. *Rhodococcus equi* infection in HIV-infected patients. Aids. 1996;10:359-362.

54. Trends in tuberculosis morbidity—United States, 1992-2002. MMWR Morb Mortal Wkly Rep. 2003;52:217-220, 222.

55. Havlir DV, Barnes PF. Tuberculosis in patients with human immunodeficiency virus infection. N Engl J Med. 1999;340:367-373.

56. Jones BE, Young SM, Antoniskis D, et al. Relationship of the manifestations of tuberculosis to CD4 cell counts in patients with human immunodeficiency virus infection. Am Rev Respir Dis. 1993;148:1292-1297.

57. Chin DP, Hopewell PC, Yajko DM, et al. *Mycobacterium avium* complex in the respiratory or gastrointestinal tract and the risk of *M. avium* complex bacteremia in patients with human immunodeficiency virus infection. J Infect Dis. 1994;169:289-295.

58. Kalayjian RC, Toossi Z, Tomashefski JF Jr, et al. Pulmonary disease due to infection by *Mycobacterium avium* complex in patients with AIDS. Clin Infect Dis. 1995;20:1186-1194.

59. Campo RE, Campo CE. *Mycobacterium kansasii* disease in patients infected with human immunodeficiency virus. Clin Infect Dis. 1997;24:1233-1238.

60. Canueto-Quintero J, Caballero-Granado FJ, Herrero-Romero M, et al. Epidemiological, clinical, and prognostic differences between the diseases caused by *Mycobacterium kansasii* and M*ycobacterium tuberculosis* in patients infected with human immunodeficiency virus: A multicenter study. Clin Infect Dis. 2003;37:584-590.

61. Meyohas MC, Roux P, Bollens D, et al. Pulmonary cryptococcosis: Localized and disseminated infections in 27 patients with AIDS. Clin Infect Dis. 1995;21:628-633.

62. Wasser L, Talavera W. Pulmonary cryptococcosis in AIDS. Chest. 1987;92:692-695.

63. Cameron ML, Bartlett JA, Gallis HA, Waskin HA. Manifestations of pulmonary cryptococcosis in patients with acquired immunodeficiency syndrome. Rev Infect Dis. 1991;13:64-67.

64. Salzman SH, Smith RL, Aranda CP. Histoplasmosis in patients at risk for the acquired immunodeficiency syndrome in a nonendemic setting. Chest. 1988;93:916-921.

65. Nightingale SD, Parks JM, Pounders SM, et al. Disseminated histoplasmosis in patients with AIDS. South Med J. 1990;83:624-630.

66. Wheat LJ, Connolly-Stringfield PA, Baker RL, et al. Disseminated histoplasmosis in the acquired immune deficiency syndrome: Clinical findings, diagnosis and treatment, and review of the literature. Medicine (Baltimore) 1990;69:361-374.

67. Ampel NM. Coccidioidomycosis among persons with human immunodeficiency virus infection in the era of highly active antiretroviral therapy (HAART). Semin Respir Infect. 2001;16:257-262.

68. Ampel NM, Dols CL, Galgiani JN. Coccidioidomycosis during human immunodeficiency virus infection: Results of a prospective study in a coccidioidal endemic area. Am J Med. 1993;94:235-240.

69. Sarosi GA, SF DA. Endemic mycosis complicating human immunodeficiency virus infection. West J Med. 1996;164:335-340.

70. Pappas PG, Pottage JC, Powderly WG, et al. Blastomycosis in patients with the acquired immunodeficiency syndrome. Ann Intern Med. 1992;116:847-853.

71. Pursell KJ, Telzak EE, Armstrong D. *Aspergillus* species colonization and invasive disease in patients with AIDS. Clin Infect Dis. 1992;14:141-148.

72. Minamoto GY, Barlam TF, Vander Els NJ. Invasive aspergillosis in patients with AIDS. Clin Infect Dis. 1992;14:66-74.

73. Denning DW, Follansbee SE, Scolaro M, et al. Pulmonary aspergillosis in the acquired immunodeficiency syndrome. N Engl J Med. 1991;324:654-662.

74. Mylonakis E, Barlam TF, Flanigan T, Rich JD. Pulmonary aspergillosis and invasive disease in AIDS: Review of 342 cases. Chest. 1998;114:251-262.

75. Mylonakis E, Paliou M, Sax PE, et al. Central nervous system aspergillosis in patients with human immunodeficiency virus infection. Report of 6 cases and review. Medicine (Baltimore). 2000;79:269-280.

76. Mann M, Shelhamer JH, Masur H, et al. Lack of clinical utility of bronchoalveolar lavage cultures for cytomegalovirus in HIV infection. Am J Respir Crit Care Med. 1997;155:1723-1728.

77. Miles PR, Baughman RP, Linnemann CC Jr. Cytomegalovirus in the bronchoalveolar lavage fluid of patients with AIDS. Chest. 1990;97:1072-1076.

78. Millar AB, Patou G, Miller RF, et al. Cytomegalovirus in the lungs of patients with AIDS. Respiratory pathogen or passenger? Am Rev Respir Dis. 1990;141:1474-1477.

79. Kroon FP, van Dissel JT, de Jong JC, van Furth R. Antibody response to influenza, tetanus and pneumococcal vaccines in HIV-seropositive individuals in relation to the number of CD4+ lymphocytes. AIDS. 1994;8:469-476.

80. Fine AD, Bridges CB, De Guzman AM, et al. Influenza A among patients with human immunodeficiency virus: An outbreak of infection at a residential facility in New York City. Clin Infect Dis. 2001;32:1784-1791.

81. Skiest DJ, Kaplan P, Machala T, et al. Clinical manifestations of influenza in HIV-infected individuals. Int J STD AIDS. 2001;12:646-650.

82. Rabaud C, May T, Lucet JC, et al. Pulmonary toxoplasmosis in patients infected with human immunodeficiency virus: A French National Survey. Clin Infect Dis. 1996;23:1249-1254.

83. Butt AA, Michaels S, Kissinger P. The association of serum lactate dehydrogenase level with selected opportunistic infections and HIV progression. Int J Infect Dis. 2002;6:178-181.

84. Celedon JC, Mathur-Wagh U, Fox J, et al. Systemic strongyloidiasis in patients infected with the human immunodeficiency virus. A report of 3 cases and review of the literature. Medicine (Baltimore) 1994;73:256-263.

85. Lessnau KD, Can S, Talavera W. Disseminated *Strongyloides stercoralis* in human immunodeficiency virus-infected patients. Treatment failure and a review of the literature. Chest. 1993;104:119-122.

86. Kotler DP, Orenstein JM. Clinical syndromes associated with microsporidiosis. Adv Parasitol. 1998;40:321-349.

87. Meynard JL, Meyohas MC, Binet D, et al. Pulmonary cryptosporidiosis in the acquired immunodeficiency syndrome. Infection. 1996;24:328-331.

88. Huang L, Schnapp LM, Gruden JF, et al. Presentation of AIDS-related pulmonary Kaposi's sarcoma diagnosed by bronchoscopy. Am J Respir Crit Care Med. 1996;153:1385-1390.

89. Aboulafia DM. The epidemiologic, pathologic, and clinical features of AIDS-associated pulmonary Kaposi's sarcoma. Chest. 2000;117:1128-1145.

90. Aboulafia DM. Regression of acquired immunodeficiency syndrome-related pulmonary Kaposi's sarcoma after highly active antiretroviral therapy. Mayo Clin Proc. 1998;73:439-443.

91. Holkova B, Takeshita K, Cheng DM, et al. Effect of highly active antiretroviral therapy on survival in patients with AIDS-associated pulmonary Kaposi's sarcoma treated with chemotherapy. J Clin Oncol. 2001;19:3848-3851.

92. Bazot M, Cadranel J, Benayoun S, et al. Primary pulmonary AIDS-related lymphoma: Radiographic and CT findings. Chest. 1999;116:1282-1286.
93. Eisner MD, Kaplan LD, Herndier B, Stulbarg MS. The pulmonary manifestations of AIDS-related non-Hodgkin's lymphoma. Chest. 1996;110:729-736.
94. Das S, Miller RF. Lymphocytic interstitial pneumonitis in HIV infected adults. Sex Transm Infect. 2003;79:88-93.
95. Dufour V, Wislez M, Bergot E, et al. Improvement of symptomatic human immunodeficiency virus-related lymphoid interstitial pneumonia in patients receiving highly active antiretroviral therapy. Clin Infect Dis. 2003;36:127-130.
96. Ripamonti D, Rizzi M, Maggiolo F, et al. Resolution of lymphocytic interstitial pneumonia in a human immunodeficiency virus-infected adult following the start of highly active antiretroviral therapy. Scand J Infect Dis. 2003;35:348-351.
97. Mehta NJ, Khan IA, Mehta RN, Sepkowitz DA. HIV-related pulmonary hypertension: analytic review of 131 cases. Chest. 2000;118:1133-1141.
98. Opravil M, Pechere M, Speich R, et al. HIV-associated primary pulmonary hypertension. A case control study. Swiss HIV Cohort Study. Am J Respir Crit Care Med. 1997;155:990-995.
99. Diaz PT, King ER, Wewers MD, et al. HIV infection increases susceptibility to smoking-induced emphysema. Chest. 2000;117:285S.
100. Mallal S, Nolan D, Witt C, et al. Association between presence of HLA-B*5701, HLA-DR7, and HLA-DQ3 and hypersensitivity to HIV-1 reverse-transcriptase inhibitor abacavir. Lancet. 2002;359:727-732
101. Abacavir warning: Certain respiratory symptoms can indicate hypersensitivity reaction. AIDS Treat News. 2000:7-8
102. Keiser P, Nassar N, Skiest D, et al. Comparison of symptoms of influenza A with abacavir-associated hypersensitivity reaction. Int J STD AIDS. 2003;14:478-481

CHAPTER **119**

Gastrointestinal and Hepatobiliary Manifestations of Human Immunodeficiency Virus Infection

MARK S. SULKOWSKI
RICHARD E. CHAISSON

Diseases of the gastrointestinal system frequently complicate human immunodeficiency virus (HIV) infection and mark its progression to the acquired immunodeficiency syndrome (AIDS). Many HIV-related gastrointestinal diseases, such as *Candida* esophagitis, biliary cryptosporidiosis, and cytomegalovirus (CMV) colitis, represent opportunistic infections that are the result of advanced immunosuppression, whereas other gastrointestinal processes, such as chronic viral hepatitis and HIV-related medication toxicity, may occur at any stage of HIV disease. The likelihood and nature of gastrointestinal manifestations of HIV depend on both host and environmental factors because infectious complications in particular are a product of both exposure to potential pathogens and immunocompetence. With the advent of highly active antiretroviral therapy (HAART), the incidence and spectrum of HIV-related gastrointestinal manifestations have changed dramatically.[1] HIV-infected patients with advanced immunodeficiency are likely to experience symptomatic gastrointestinal tract disease, and the broad range of diagnostic considerations mandates the systematic evaluation of gastrointestinal complaints among such patients. Conversely, HIV-infected patients with relatively preserved immune function are unlikely to experience gastrointestinal manifestations of opportunistic pathogens but may be at risk for other gastrointestinal disease, such as with hepatitis B and C viruses or adverse effects of antiretroviral therapy.[2]

DISORDERS OF THE ESOPHAGUS

Esophageal disease occurs commonly among HIV-infected persons, affecting up to one third of persons with AIDS (also see Chapter 90).[3] Esophageal abnormalities typically produce symptoms of dysphagia and odynophagia, which may be due to esophageal inflammation or ulceration caused by infectious pathogens or noninfectious processes. Esophagitis is most often due to infection with *Candida albicans* but may also be caused by viruses, such as herpes simplex virus, CMV, and varicella-zoster virus, and less commonly by other infectious agents, such as *Mycobacterium tuberculosis*, nontuberculous mycobacteria, *Histoplasma capsulatum*, *Pneumocystis jirovecii*, and primary HIV infection.[4] Noninfectious processes, such as reflux esophagitis, pill esophagitis (zidovudine, zalcitabine, and doxycycline), and malignancy (carcinoma, lymphoma, and Kaposi's sarcoma), may be characterized by symptoms clinically indistinguishable from those of infections of the esophagus. Esophageal ulcerations are often caused by CMV (45%), idiopathic ulcers (40%), and herpes simplex virus (HSV) (5%) and may involve symptoms of localized pain.[5]

In the era of HAART, the clinical spectrum of esophageal disease has changed substantially; the occurrence of CMV, HSV, and *Candida*-related esophageal disease has decreased significantly.[6] The frequency of idiopathic esophageal ulceration has also decreased with the effective treatment of HIV disease.[7] On the other hand, noninfectious esophageal diseases, such as gastroesophageal reflux disease (GERD) and dysmotility disorders (e.g., achalasia) may account for an increasing proportion of esophageal symptoms.[8]

Regardless of etiology, most esophageal processes are associated with dysphagia or odynophagia, and there may be persistent or intermittent retrosternal pain, nausea, anorexia, and weight loss. The onset of symptoms may be relatively acute but more typically follows an indolent course. Nonesophageal manifestations of disease may be found in patients with odynophagia; for example, oral candidiasis frequently accompanies *Candida* esophagitis, and active CMV infection may be found in other anatomic sites, such as the retina or colon.[9] However, among patients with advanced immunodeficiency, the broad range of disease processes and the possibility of multiple etiologies mandate a methodic approach to the evaluation and management of esophageal symptoms in patients with HIV disease.

During the initial evaluation, medical history may suggest drug-induced esophagitis or GERD, and physical examination may reveal oral candidiasis or CMV retinitis. Patients with relatively high CD4+ T-cell counts who present with symptoms suggestive of GERD may be empirically treated with medications to reduce gastric acid secretion such as proton pump inhibitors or H2 blockers. However, because the absorption of some antiretroviral drugs (e.g., atazanavir) may be reduced in the setting of acid suppression, clinicians should use antacid medications judiciously.[10] Patients with advanced HIV disease with esophageal symptoms, with or without the presence of oral candidiasis should be empirically treated for esophageal candidiasis with antifungal therapy (e.g., fluconazole at 100 to 200 mg/day).[11] Presumptive oral antifungal therapy is highly effective for esophageal candidiasis and is usually preferable to diagnostic upper endoscopy or "blind" brushing of the esophagus via nasogastric tube.[12] If the esophageal symptoms resolve, the diagnosis of candidiasis can be established empirically. However, failure of symptoms to respond to empirical antifungal therapy within 7 to 10 days indicates a need for further evaluation.[13] Most patients with advanced HIV disease (77%) who do not respond to antifungal therapy have esophageal ulceration rather than evidence of persistent esophageal candidiasis.[14] Upper endoscopy with biopsy is a highly sensitive procedure for establishing a specific diagnosis and is the preferred approach to the evaluation of patients with odynophagia or dysphagia who do not respond to empirical antifungal therapy. Upper gastrointestinal contrast radiography may reveal characteristic abnormalities, but these findings are relatively insensitive and nonspecific, whereas the symptom-specific use of upper endoscopy may yield a treatable pathologic diagnosis in as many as 78% of patients.[15]

The endoscopic appearance of esophageal candidiasis resembles cheesy friable plaques that may involve the entire esophagus, whereas viral esophagitis is usually associated with diffuse, erythematous ulceration of the mucosa. CMV esophagitis frequently causes numerous, large, shallow ulcerations, whereas herpes simplex virus esophagitis is typically seen as superficial, confluent ulcers in the distal esophagus and may be associated with concurrent nonesophageal lesions in 38% of patients.[16,17] Idiopathic or aphthous ulcers may have an endoscopic appearance similar to that of CMV ulcers and represent a diagnosis of exclusion. Less commonly, other infectious processes may be observed including those associated with *Mycobacterium avium* complex and *M. tuberculosis* and bacillary angiomatosis. Noninfectious processes, such as drug-induced ulcers and malignancies, may affect the esophagus, with the most common tumors being Kaposi's sarcoma, primary lymphoma, and adenocarcinoma. Persons with HIV infection may also have conventional esophageal pathology, such as reflux esophagitis, achalasia, esophageal strictures, and esophagotracheal fistulas.[8]

For lesions visualized by endoscopy, a biopsy should be performed and tissue sections prepared for histopathologic stains to identify viral inclusion bodies (CMV), multinucleated giant cells (herpes simplex virus or varicella-zoster virus), or invasive fungi. Cultures for fungi and viruses may be helpful, although false-positive results may be seen with CMV and *C. albicans*. Antifungal drug sensitivity testing may be useful if azole-resistant candidiasis is suspected.[18] The yield of endoscopy with biopsy and culture is extremely high and more than one pathologic process may be found; nonetheless, multiple biopsies (more than three) may be needed to exclude the diagnosis of viral esophagitis.[19] Lesions that do not respond to appropriate therapy should be reevaluated by endoscopy with biopsy and culture to confirm the diagnosis and, if indicated, to perform drug sensitivity testing. Additional diagnostic procedures are usually not required but may be useful in special circumstances, such as when there is a clinical suspicion of esophageal dysmotility.

DISORDERS OF THE STOMACH

Gastric disorders in HIV-infected patients may be due to opportunistic infections but are often unrelated to HIV-induced immunodeficiency even among those patients with advanced HIV disease. Patients with gastric disease may present with protean complaints such as nausea, vomiting, early satiety, and anorexia; abdominal pain and hematemesis may also be present. Some disease processes such as CMV gastritis and gastrointestinal Kaposi's sarcoma may be associated with extragastric involvement.

Gastritis and gastroduodenal ulcers may be found in HIV-infected persons with upper gastrointestinal symptoms and may be due to *Helicobacter pylori* infection. However, several studies indicate that the prevalence of *H. pylori*–related disease is lower among HIV-infected persons than among the general population, possibly because of frequent antimicrobial therapy.[20-22] For example, Varsky and co-workers[21] reported that only 5% of 497 HIV-infected patients with upper gastrointestinal complaints had endoscopic evidence of gastroduodenal ulcers, and *H. pylori* infection was found in only one third of these patients. *H. pylori* infection may be detected by serology, urea breath testing, and histologic evaluations, and, more recently, highly accurate noninvasive stool *H. pylori* antigen testing has been developed.[23] HIV-infected patients may also have altered gastric function, including decreased secretion of gastric acid and intrinsic factor.[24] Hypochlorhydria may impair the absorption of some medications, such as ketoconazole, itraconazole, and atazanavir, and may also permit gastric bacterial overgrowth.[10,25,26]

CMV may cause gastric inflammation or ulceration alone or in association with esophageal ulceration. The appearance of gastric CMV may be diverse and includes thickened, edematous gastric folds, erosive gastritis, and superficial or deep ulcerations. The radiographic features may be nonspecific and may even be masslike, suggestive of malignancy.[27] Other gastric infections have been reported, including infection with *Cryptosporidium*, *M. avium* complex infection, histo-plasmosis, cryptococcosis, leishmaniasis, and syphilis. Malignant lesions involving the stomach may also be associated with upper gastrointestinal symptoms. Gastrointestinal Kaposi's sarcoma, associated with human herpesvirus type 8 infection, complicates cutaneous disease in many patients and commonly involves the stomach.[28] Gastric Kaposi's sarcoma lesions may be asymptomatic but can also cause nausea, abdominal pain, and, rarely, severe hemorrhage.[29] AIDS-related lymphomas may also involve the gastrointestinal tract; these lesions tend to be multifocal but are rarely gastric mucosa–associated lymphoid tissue (MALT) lymphomas associated with *H. pylori*.[30]

In light of these diverse diagnostic considerations, patients with persistent upper gastrointestinal symptoms should be evaluated for opportunistic infection and malignancy, particularly those with CD4+ cell counts less than 200/mm³. The definitive diagnosis of upper gastrointestinal pathology often requires endoscopic evaluation with biopsy and cultures. Kaposi's sarcoma lesions typically appear as a violet blue submucosal mass without ulceration or bleeding but may appear as linitis plastica. Biopsies of these lesions may fail to confirm Kaposi's sarcoma in up to two thirds of cases. However, when cutaneous Kaposi's sarcoma has been histologically confirmed, the endoscopic appearance of the lesion may be sufficient to establish the diagnosis.[28] Biopsy and immunohistochemical staining are needed for the diagnosis of gastric lymphoma. Biopsies of gastroduodenal ulcerations should be performed and specimens sent for viral culture and histologic staining for evidence of viral inclusions, fungi, and *H. pylori* infection. Multiple biopsies may be needed to exclude viral pathogens, and additional stains and cultures may be helpful in diagnosing specific infections, such as acid-fast stains and culture for *M. avium* complex.

DISORDERS OF THE BILIARY TREE AND GALLBLADDER

Diseases of the gallbladder and biliary tree affecting HIV-infected persons include non–HIV-associated conditions, such as cholelithiasis, and AIDS-associated conditions, such as acalculous cholecystitis and cholangiopathy. Patients typically present with postprandial pain, fever, right upper quadrant pain and tenderness, and an elevated serum alkaline phosphatase level. Ultrasonographic or computed tomographic imaging studies may reveal evidence of acute cholecystitis or cholangitis related to cholelithiasis, and in patients with advanced immunodeficiency, these studies may suggest acalculous cholecystitis or AIDS-associated cholangitis.[31] During acute or chronic acalculous cholecystitis, the gallbladder generally appears thickened and edematous with obliteration of the gallbladder lumen without evidence of gallstones. Nonvisualization of the gallbladder by radionuclide hepatobiliary scintigraphy is also suggestive of cholecystitis. If a cholecystectomy is performed, operative specimens should be sent for microbiologic and histopathologic evaluation, because before the advent of HAART, opportunistic pathogens were identified in more than 50% of cases.[32] CMV, *Cryptosporidium*, and microsporidia are the pathogens most commonly associated with acalculous cholecystitis; however, multiple organisms or other pathogens, such as *Isospora belli*, may be recovered. However, often no etiologic agent is identified after extensive microbiologic evaluation.[33-35] Although the exclusion of opportunistic infection is critical in the evaluation of HIV-infected patients with signs and symptoms of acute cholecystitis, it is important to note that the incidence of AIDS cholangiopathy is very low in settings where HAART is widely utilized. For example, at one urban hospital in San Francisco only 23 cases of AIDS cholangiopathy were reported between 1993 and 2003.[36] Accordingly, it is likely that noninfectious disorders (e.g., cholelithiasis) will account for an increasing proportion of hepatobiliary disease in HIV-infected patients, particularly among those who undergo cholecystectomy.

If noninvasive, radiographic imaging indicates intra- or extrahepatic biliary ductal dilatation, endoscopic retrograde cholangiopancreatography (ERCP) may be necessary for the diagnosis and management of AIDS-associated cholangiopathy.[37] Cello[38] has described four common patterns of cholangiographic abnormalities revealed by

ERCP: stenosis of the papilla of Vater with dilated extrahepatic biliary tract, sclerosing cholangitis, combination of sclerosing cholangitis and papillary stenosis, and choledochal long stenosis or strictures. ERCP with collection of bile from the common bile duct and duodenal or papillary biopsy may identify an opportunistic pathogen or malignancy. Like acalculous cholecystitis, cholangitis is associated with opportunistic infections by CMV, *Cryptosporidium,* or microsporidia in more than half of cases.[34,39,40] For example, among 82 HIV-infected patients in whom cryptosporidiosis developed during a waterborne outbreak, 24 (29%) had evidence of biliary involvement. Biliary cryptosporidiosis was associated with CD4$^+$ cell counts less than 50/mm^3, and HIV-infected patients were more likely to develop nausea, vomiting, and an elevated alkaline phosphatase level.[40] Other infectious pathogens, such as *Cryptococcus neoformans, I. belli,* and *P. jirovecii,* and biliary tree malignancies, including lymphoma and Kaposi's sarcoma, have also been reported. In addition, bacterial superinfection may complicate any of these disease processes.

If papillary stenosis is present, endoscopic sphincterotomy may produce relief of symptoms and biochemical resolution of cholestasis, although in some case series the clinical effectiveness of this procedure has been disappointing.[41]

DISORDERS OF THE LIVER

Hepatic abnormalities are quite common among HIV-infected persons and are often associated with elevated serum alanine and aspartate aminotransferases and/or alkaline phosphatase levels. Liver disease may be due to acute or chronic viral hepatitis, HIV-related opportunistic infections, or noninfectious processes, such as medication toxicity, alcohol, nonalcoholic fatty liver disease (NAFLD) or malignancy (Table 119-1). Because of shared routes of transmission, chronic hepatitis B virus (HBV) and hepatitis C virus (HCV) infections frequently complicate HIV disease (also see Chapter 112).[42-44]

Approximately 20% of HIV-infected persons who acquire acute HBV infection develop chronic HBV infection, characterized by hepatitis B surface antigenemia (HBsAg) and active viral replication, compared with only 5% of HIV-negative persons.[45,46] In addition, spontaneous reactivation of HBV replication has been reported in anti–hepatitis B surface antibody–positive patients who develop severe immunosuppression.[47-49] To date there is little evidence that HBV infection influences HIV disease progression.[50] Conversely, whereas some early studies suggested that that HBV-related liver disease may be less severe among immunosuppressed patients as a result of attenuated immune-mediated hepatic injury, recent studies indicate an increased risk of liver-related morbidity and mortality among HIV-HBV–coinfected patients compared with those with chronic HBV alone.[43,50,51] For example, among HIV-infected and uninfected men followed longitudinally in the Multicenter AIDS Cohort Study, Thio and colleagues reported that the HIV-HBV coinfected were approximately 19 times more likely to die from liver disease compared with men infected with HBV alone.[43] These data emphasize the importance of prevention, diagnosis, and treatment of hepatitis B among HIV-infected persons.

All HIV-infected persons should be screened for evidence of resolved and active HBV infection.[52] Testing for HBsAg, hepatitis B core antibody, and hepatitis B surface antibody is recommended. Individuals with no evidence of prior infection (i.e., susceptible to HBV) should be vaccinated.[53] Persons with chronic HBV (defined persistent of HBsAg >6 months) should undergo additional evaluation to determine HBV replication status (e.g., hepatitis B e antigen and serum HBV deoxyribonucleic acid [DNA] testing) and liver disease stage (e.g., serum ALT level, liver biopsy).[54] HIV-infected patients with evidence of active HBV replication are at increased risk for the development of cirrhosis, end-stage liver disease, and hepatocellular carcinoma. Accordingly, anti-HBV therapy is recommended for people with an elevated serum ALT level (at least two times the upper limit of normal range), active HBV replication (defined as a positive

TABLE 119-1 Selected Causes of Hepatic Disease in Human Immunodeficiency Virus-Infected Persons

Viruses
  Hepatitis A
  Hepatitis B
  Hepatitis C
  Hepatitis D (with HBV)
  Epstein-Barr
  Cytomegalovirus
  Herpes simplex
  Adenovirus
  Varicella-zoster
Fungi
  Histoplasma capsulatum
  Cryptococcus neoformans
  Coccidioides immitis
  Candida albicans
  Pneumocystis jirovecii
  Penicillium marneffei
Protozoa
  Toxoplasma gondii
  Cryptosporidium parvum
  Microsporida spp.
  Schistosoma
Bacteria
  Mycobacteria
  Mycobacterium avium complex
  Mycobacterium tuberculosis
  Bartonella henselae (peliosis hepatis)
Malignancy
  Kaposi's sarcoma (HHV-8)
  Non-Hodgkin's lymphoma
  Hepatocellular carcinoma
Medications
  Zidovudine
  Didanosine
  Nevirapine
  Ritonavir
  Other HIV-1 protease inhibitors
  Fluconazole
  Macrolide antibiotics
  Isoniazid
  Rifampin
  Trimethoprim-sulfamethoxazole

HBV, hepatitis B virus; HHV-8, human herpesvirus type 8; HIV-1, human immunodeficiency virus type 1.

HBeAg and/or HBV DNA >10^5 copies/mL), and evidence of moderate disease activity and/or fibrosis on liver biopsy.[52-54]

The goals of HBV therapy in HIV-HBV–coinfected patients include sustained suppression of HBV replication, prevention of liver disease, and clearance of HBeAg. Although there is no consensus regarding the most effective anti-HBV regimen for persons with HIV, three antiretroviral drugs approved by the U.S. Food and Drug Administration (FDA) for the treatment of HIV (lamivudine, emtricitabine, tenofovir disoproxil fumarate) also suppress HBV replication by inhibition of the HBV DNA polymerase.[55-59] Notably, to prevent the development of HIV resistance, drugs active against both viruses should be used in combination with other antiretroviral agents. In addition, adefovir dipivoxil is FDA approved for the treatment of chronic HBV infection in HIV-uninfected patients.[60,61] While no anti-HIV activity or HIV resistance has been observed at the 10 mg/day dose of adefovir dipivoxil, some experts remain concerned about remain regarding the potential for emergence of HIV resistance among HBV-HIV–coinfected patients.[62] Interferon or peginterferon-alfa may also be effective in the treatment of chronic HBV; however, there are few data regarding its effectiveness and tolerability in persons coinfected with HIV (see Chapter 112).[63,64] Given the complexity of anti-HBV treatment decisions in persons with HIV and limited data regarding the safety and efficacy of the available anti-HBV drugs, the decision to treat HBV must be individualized.

HCV coinfection is also common. For example, among HIV-infected people with parenteral exposures, such as injection-drug users and recipients of blood products, the prevalence of chronic HCV infection is high, ranging from 60% to 95% worldwide.[42,65] Although the majority of HCV-HIV–coinfected patients have asymptomatic elevations in serum ALT and AST levels, HCV infection may lead to the development of significant hepatic fibrosis or cirrhosis, which may be followed by hepatic decompensation or hepatocellular carcinoma or both.[66,67] HCV-infected patients with end-stage liver disease are profoundly symptomatic with manifestations of portal hypertension, including ascites, esophageal varices, and splenomegaly; decreased hepatic synthetic function, including hypoalbuminemia, thrombocytopenia, and coagulopathy; and hepatic encephalopathy. In addition, extrahepatic manifestations of HCV infection, such as membranous glomerulonephritis, porphyria cutanea tarda, and mixed, type II cryoglobulinemia with or without vasculitis, may occur at any stage of disease.[68]

Studies of the natural history of HCV disease in HIV-infected persons demonstrate enhanced HCV replication and accelerated progression of liver disease, presumably because of HIV-related immunosuppression.[69-72] For example, Darby and colleagues[73] reported a 6-fold higher risk of liver-related mortality among HIV-infected patients with hemophilia who received HCV-positive blood products than in those without HIV infection and a 94-fold higher risk than in the general population. Similarly, among HCV-infected injection-drug users, HIV infection has been shown to be independently associated with the development of cirrhosis.[74] On the other hand, there are conflicting reports on the impact of HCV infection on the natural history of HIV disease. For example, among 1955 patients in a Baltimore HIV clinic, no difference was detected in the progression to AIDS or death, after adjusting for exposure to HAART and HIV suppression.[42] Conversely, among 3111 patients receiving HAART, Greub and colleagues reported that HCV-infected persons had a modestly increased risk of progression to a new AIDS defining event or death, even among the subgroup with continuous suppression of HIV replication.[75] This controversy notwithstanding, with the advent of HAART there has been a marked decline in most opportunistic illnesses, and HCV infection has emerged as an important cause of morbidity and mortality.[76-78] Among HIV-HCV–coinfected patients followed at one urban medical center, hospitalization discharges where a liver-related diagnosis was included as a diagnosis have increased approximately five-fold between 1995 and 2000.[79] Similarly, among HIV-infected patients in France, deaths due to HCV-related end-stage liver disease were more frequent in the HAART era (2001, 14.3%) than in the pre-HAART era (1995, 1.5%).[78] Taken together, these data provide compelling evidence of the increasing importance of HCV disease among HIV-infected patients.

Accordingly, current guidelines recommend that all HIV-infected patients be screened for HCV infection by the detection of anti-HCV antibodies.[80] However, severely immunocompromised patients may have false-negative HCV antibody assays and blood HCV ribonucleic acid (RNA) should be assessed when HCV infection is suspected in persons with negative anti-HCV results (e.g., elevated liver enzymes).[81] Patients with positive HCV antibody results should have further testing to confirm active HCV replication with supplemental testing for HCV RNAase–HIV-infected individuals with chronic HCV infection should be counseled to prevent liver damage and HCV transmission, evaluated for the presence of chronic liver disease and considered for anti-HCV treatment.[2] Because alcohol ingestion may accelerate the progression of liver disease, all HIV-HCV–infected patients should be advised to abstain from alcohol.[82] Assessments of disease severity should include a history and physical examination for signs and symptoms of chronic liver disease, measurement of blood albumin, prothrombin time/International Normalized Ratio (INR), and direct bilirubin, and platelet count. Measurements of the serum alanine aminotransferase and HCV RNA level are important to establish that the infection is ongoing but provide only limited information regarding HCV disease severity.[83] Noninvasive radiographic imaging may reveal hepatic parenchymal abnormalities, mass lesions, or evidence of ascites, splenomegaly, or varices; however, imaging studies cannot reliably exclude the presence of significant histologic liver disease, such as piecemeal necrosis, advanced hepatic fibrosis, or cirrhosis. Histologic evaluation by

liver biopsy provides the best information about HCV-related disease activity and fibrosis stage. In addition, liver biopsy may be useful to exclude other causes of hepatic disease, such as nonalcoholic liver disease, drug toxicity, or opportunistic pathogens.[84]

Current guidelines developed by the National Institutes of Health indicate that treatment of HCV infection in patients with HIV is recommended on a case-by-case basis.[80] However, because there is relatively little published experience treating HIV-HCV–coinfected persons, practice is dictated largely by principles established for the treatment of HIV-uninfected persons. Treatment is currently recommended for patients with chronic hepatitis C who are at the greatest risk for progression to cirrhosis, as characterized by persistently elevated alanine aminotransferase levels, detectable HCV RNA, and histologic findings of portal or bridging fibrosis or at least moderate degrees of inflammation or necrosis (see Chapter 112).

Among HIV-uninfected patients, several randomized, controlled clinical trials have demonstrated that combination therapy with peginterferon-alfa-2a or -alfa-2b plus ribavirin is superior to standard interferon alfa-2b and ribavirin with a similar frequency of adverse events.[85,86] Although studies of PEG interferon-alfa with ribavirin in HIV-infected patients are under way, there are few published data on its safety and effectiveness for the treatment of HCV in HIV-infected persons.[87] Nonetheless, interim analyses of ongoing clinical trials of peginterferon-alfa-2a or -alfa-2b plus ribavirin suggest that combination therapy may be beneficial and reasonably tolerated in some HIV-infected persons.[88] However, many HIV-infected patients may have comorbid conditions, such as major depressive illness, cytopenias, and active illicit drug or alcohol use, which may prevent or complicate peginterferon plus ribavirin therapy.[89] Accordingly, HCV treatment in HIV-infected patients should be coordinated by health care providers with experience in treating both HIV and HCV disease.

Other infectious processes may involve the liver, leading to hepatocellular necrosis or granulomatous inflammation. Viral pathogens, such as CMV, Epstein-Barr virus, herpes simplex virus, and adenovirus, can cause hepatocellular damage, usually in the setting of disseminated disease. Other infectious pathogens, such as mycobacterial and fungal agents, may lead to granulomatous inflammation, characterized by elevated alkaline phosphatase levels and nonspecific hepatic granuloma. *M. avium* complex is the most common opportunistic pathogen affecting the liver and is associated with manifestations of systemic disease, including fever, abdominal pain, and wasting.[84] Extrapulmonary *M. tuberculosis* infection may be associated with hepatic involvement in 5% to 10% of HIV-related cases, and, less commonly, a tuberculosis abscess has been identified.[90] Disseminated fungal infections with organisms including *C. neoformans, H. capsulatum, Coccidioides immitis, Penicillium marneffei,* and *C. albicans* may produce a granulomatous response in liver. *C. neoformans* and *H. capsulatum* may be rapidly detected by evidence of polysaccharide capsular antigenemia; other causes of fungal hepatitis may be diagnosed by histologic and microbiologic evaluation of liver tissue.

P. jirovecii hepatic infection may occur, particularly during aerosolized pentamidine prophylactic therapy. *Bartonella henselae* can cause peliosis hepatis, a vascular proliferative liver infection, in the absence of cutaneous lesions. Peliosis hepatis occurs in patients with advanced immunodeficiency, who may present with fever, weight loss, and hepatosplenomegaly with an elevated serum alkaline phosphatase level. The diagnosis of bartonellosis is made by Warthin-Starry staining of biopsy specimens, culture of the blood or tissue plated on heart infusion agar with 5% rabbit blood, and, more recently, by polymerase chain reaction assay.[91] Blood culture for acid-fast bacilli is usually sufficient to establish the diagnosis of disseminated mycobacterial infection. The evaluation of other potential causes of liver disease may require liver biopsy, which may rapidly yield a treatable diagnosis in more than 60% of HIV-infected patients with unexplained fever and liver abnormalities. Hepatic tissue should be sent for microbiologic evaluation and culture, as well as routine and specific histologic staining for acid-fast bacilli and fungal pathogens.[92,93]

Hepatic mass lesions are commonly due to malignancy, although radiographically, infectious processes may resemble mass lesions. Prior to the use of HAART, the most common hepatic malignancy was Kaposi's sarcoma; hepatic involvement typically occurs in the setting of cutaneous disease and is often associated with hepatomegaly and abdominal pain. Abdominal imaging with contrast-enhanced computed tomography may reveal enhanced lesions located in the capsular, hilar, and portal areas with invasion into the liver parenchyma. The definitive diagnosis of hepatic Kaposi's sarcoma requires biopsy with histologic examination; however, the risk of hemorrhage after a biopsy may be increased because of the vascular nature of the Kaposi's sarcoma lesion. Non-Hodgkin's lymphomas may involve the liver, usually in association with lymph node or visceral involvement, or both, although primary hepatic lymphoma has been reported. Patients may present with "B" symptoms, including weight loss, fever, night sweats, and abdominal pain; jaundice may occur with intra- or extrahepatic bile duct obstruction.[94] Radiographic imaging typically reveals solitary or multiple hepatic mass lesions and involvement of abdominal lymph nodes. Biopsy of the hepatic lesion or involved lymph nodes is needed to confirm the diagnosis of lymphoma. Although the incidence of Kaposi's sarcoma and lymphoma have declined, hepatocellular carcinoma related to chronic HBV or HCV infection has been increasingly recognized in HIV-infected patients, particularly those with cirrhosis; such patients may have evidence of advanced liver disease, elevated serum α-fetoprotein, and radiographic evidence of a mass lesion.[95]

Hepatotoxicity associated with HIV-related medications is a common cause of liver abnormalities, and infection with HIV, HCV, or both may enhance the toxicity of some medications, such as antituberculosis drugs.[96] Patients typically present with elevated serum alanine and aspartate aminotransferase levels, although some drugs, such as macrolide antibiotics (e.g., azithromycin) and trimethoprim-sulfamethoxazole, induce a cholestatic or mixed liver injury pattern. Drug-induced hepatotoxicity is often asymptomatic and detected through routine monitoring of serum liver enzymes. HIV-1 protease inhibitors, particularly ritonavir, and non-nucleoside reverse transcriptase inhibitors, particularly nevirapine, have been associated with severe hepatotoxicity after the initiation of therapy, which may be more common in the setting of concurrent chronic HBV or HCV infection.[97-100] In addition to elevations of serum ALT and AST levels, nucleoside analogue reverse transcriptase inhibitors, such as zidovudine and stavudine, have been associated with mitochondrial toxicity, leading, in some cases, to fatal hepatomegaly with severe steatosis and lactic acidosis.[101-103] More recently, the presence of antiretroviral-associated lipodystrophy has been associated with increased fat accumulation in the liver, suggesting that chronic exposure to HAART may be associated with hepatic steatosis.[104] However, given their role in preventing HIV-related morbidity and mortality, HIV-infected patients who are coinfected with HCV or HBV are candidates for HAART, but should be monitored after initiating treatment with potentially hepatotoxic medications. Treatment should be modified if drug-induced hepatotoxicity is suspected.

DISORDERS OF THE PANCREAS

Diseases involving the pancreas may be caused by processes unrelated to HIV infection, such as alcohol abuse, cholelithiasis, and hyperlipidemia, or may be due to HIV-related opportunistic infections or medication toxicity.[105] AIDS cholangiopathy caused by CMV, *Cryptosporidium*, or microsporidians may involve the juxta-ampullary portion of the pancreatic duct.[106] Mycobacterial infections of the pancreas have been described, including pancreatic abscess related to *M. tuberculosis* and disseminated *M. avium* complex.[107] Fungal

pathogens, such as *C. neoformans* and *Candida* spp., *Toxoplasma gondii*, *P. jirovecii*, and protozoal pathogens may involve the pancreas, typically in the setting of disseminated disease. Pancreatic CMV inclusions are frequently observed in autopsy specimens from patients with disseminated CMV disease, although clinical pancreatitis is infrequently recognized before death.[108]

Drug-induced pancreatic inflammation and dysfunction may also occur in patients with HIV disease. Didanosine may frequently cause asymptomatic hyperamylasemia and clinical pancreatitis has been observed in 1.2% to 6.7% of didanosine recipients, and fulminant pancreatic toxicity has been reported.[109,110] Patients with a prior history of pancreatitis are at higher risk for developing didanosine-related pancreatitis, and the drug should be avoided in this setting. Zalcitabine has also been associated with pancreatitis. Systemic pentamidine therapy for *P. jirovecii* pneumonia is toxic to pancreatic B islet cells and can cause pancreatitis and symptomatic hyperglycemia or hypoglycemia; in contrast, prophylaxis with aerosolized pentamidine rarely leads to pancreatic dysfunction.[111] The risk of pancreatitis in patients receiving intravenous pentamidine is dose related, and most cases occur after 2 weeks of therapy. Other HIV-related medications, including megestrol acetate, have been associated with derangements of glucose homeostasis.[112] More recently, the use of HAART, particularly protease inhibitors, has been linked to the development of hyperglycemia and diabetes mellitus, especially among those with HCV coinfection.[113-115]

DISORDERS OF THE SMALL AND LARGE INTESTINES

Symptomatic disease of the small intestine and colon remains common among HIV-infected individuals with advanced immunodeficiency and may be caused by a diverse range of infectious agents. However, among HIV-infected subjects receiving effective anti-HIV therapy, the incidence of enterocolitis has declined substantially.[116,117] Small bowel diseases generally produce bloating, nausea, cramping, and profuse diarrhea and may be associated with malabsorption and weight loss. In contrast, colitis may produce lower abdominal discomfort and cramping, urgency, and tenesmus and typically causes frequent, small-volume diarrhea. However, the clinical manifestations of small and large bowel infections may be indistinguishable, and some processes may cause panenteritis.[118] In addition, among patients receiving antiretroviral therapy, the incidence of medication-related diarrhea has increased and gastrointestinal adverse effects may lead to discontinuation of antiretroviral medications.[117,119] Furthermore, with prolonged life expectancy, the incidence of colorectal malignancies, such as adenocarcinoma, is expected to increase and colorectal neoplasm should be considered in HIV-infected patients with chronic abdominal symptoms.[120] Rarely, inflammatory bowel disease (e.g., ulcerative colitis, Crohn's disease) has been reported in HIV-infected patients with diarrhea.[121]

The differential diagnosis for enterocolitis in a severely immunocompromised person is extensive and includes bacterial, protozoal, and viral pathogens (Table 119-2). Bacteria that are more common in HIV-infected patients include *Salmonella* spp., *Shigella*, *Campylobacter jejuni*, *Escherichia coli* (enterotoxigenic, enteroadherent, and enteroaggregative), and *Listeria monocytogenes*.[122] Salmonellosis is associated with bacteremia in one half of infections and may be recurrent in HIV-infected persons.[123] Less commonly, bacteremia may occur with *Shigella* and *Campylobacter* infection.[124] *Clostridium difficile* toxin-associated diarrhea may also be more common among individuals with HIV disease, particularly among hospitalized patients and those who have recently received antibiotic therapy.[125,126] Small bowel overgrowth can occur and has been associated with hypochlorhydria and wasting. Other, less common, bacterial causes of enterocolitis include *Aeromonas*, *Plesiomonas*, *Yersinia*, and *Vibrio* spp. Mycobacterial infections of the small bowel are usually associated with late-stage HIV disease and disseminated *M. avium* complex, although enteritis caused by *M. tuberculosis* has been reported.[127,128]

TABLE 119-2 Causes of Lower Gastrointestinal Tract Disease in Patients with Human Immunodeficiency Virus

Causes of Enterocolitis
Bacteria
  Campylobacter jejuni and other spp.
  Salmonella spp.
  Shigella flexneri
  Aeromonas hydrophila
  Plesiomonas shigelloides
  Yersinia enterocolitica
  Vibrio spp.
  Mycobacterium avium complex
  Mycobacterium tuberculosis
  Escherichia coli (enterotoxigenic, enteroadherent)
  Bacterial overgrowth
  Clostridium difficile (toxin)
Parasites
  Cryptosporidium parvum
  Microsporida (*Enterocytozoon bieneusi, Septata intestinalis*)
  Isospora belli
  Entamoeba histolytica
  Giardia lamblia
  Cyclospora cayetanensis
Viruses
  Cytomegalovirus
  Adenovirus
  Calicivirus
  Astrovirus
  Picobirnavirus
  Human immunodeficiency virus
Fungi
  Histoplasma capsulatum

Causes of Proctitis
Bacteria
  Chlamydia trachomatis
  Neisseria gonorrhoeae
  Treponema pallidum
Viruses
  Herpes simplex
  Cytomegalovirus

Parasites infecting the small and large bowel include spore-forming protozoa, *Cryptosporidium*, *Microsporida* spp. (such as *Enterocytozoon bieneusi* and *Septata intestinalis*), *Isospora*, and *Cyclospora*, as well as *Entamoeba histolytica* and *Giardia lamblia*. Amebic infection and giardiasis may occur at any stage of HIV disease and are commonly associated with conventional risk factors, such as sexual practices and travel-related exposures. Disease caused by *Cryptosporidium* is more common and severe in HIV-infected persons with advanced immunosuppression, leading to persistent infection (60%), biliary disease (29%), and even fulminant disease (8%).[129,130] Similarly, microsporidiosis causes diarrhea in patients with advanced HIV disease (CD4+ cell count <50/mm³) and may be associated with cholangiopathy.[131] Less commonly, diarrhea caused by *Isospora* and *Cyclospora* has been reported in persons with advanced immunosuppression.[132,133]

CMV is the most significant viral cause of enterocolitis, leading to fever, abdominal pain and tenderness, bloody diarrhea, and, rarely, intestinal perforation or toxic megacolon. As with its appearance in the esophagus, CMV enterocolitis occurs with severe immunodeficiency and produces mucosal inflammation with superficial ulceration.[134] Other viral pathogens implicated as causes of diarrhea include adenovirus, which may cause a condition that mimics CMV colitis, as well as human herpesvirus 6B, astrovirus, calicivirus, and picobirnavirus (see Chapters 172 and 173).[135]

Proctitis in patients with HIV disease typically reflects sexually transmitted infections, such as herpes simplex virus infection, *Chlamydia trachomatis* infection, syphilis, and gonorrhea, particularly among homosexual men.[135,136] However, advanced immunosuppression may be associated with more severe disease manifestations and

recurrent infection. CMV proctitis is less common but may occur in the setting of extensive CMV colitis.

HIV-infected patients with diarrhea or other symptoms of enterocolitis should be carefully evaluated to identify treatable conditions. Historical assessments should focus on the nature and duration of the symptoms, concomitant medications, travel, and other exposures, such as through food, water, or sexual contact. The standard diagnostic evaluation should include stool leukocyte examination to identify inflammatory causes of diarrhea, such as bacterial pathogens and CMV, and guide empirical therapy; other infectious agents, such as protozoa and *M. avium* complex, are typically not associated with the finding of fecal leukocytes. Stool should be cultured for enteric bacterial pathogens, assayed for *C. difficile* toxin, and examined for ova and parasites.[137] Stool specimens should be examined on at least three occasions with modified acid-fast stain to identify *Cryptosporidium*, *Cyclospora*, and *Isospora*. Special trichrome staining may be useful for the identification of microsporidians.[138]

If noninvasive stool studies are not diagnostic and symptoms persist, endoscopic evolution with biopsy may prove helpful, particularly in patients with chronic diarrhea and severe immunodeficiency (CD4+ cells <100/mm³).[139] Patients with signs and symptoms suggestive of large bowel involvement should undergo colonoscopy and biopsy. The sensitivity of endoscopic biopsy for the diagnosis for CMV disease is high, and colonoscopy may identify disease limited to the right side of the colon, which may be missed during flexible sigmoidoscopy.[140] Upper endoscopy with duodenal biopsy is useful for patients with symptoms of small bowel disease or those with persistent symptoms and negative evaluation of the lower gastrointestinal tract.[141] In addition to hematoxylin and eosin staining, duodenal histologic specimens should be stained with fungal stains and modified acid-fast stain for *Cryptosporidium* as well as undergo electron microscopy for microsporidians. Polymerase chain reaction assay of biopsy specimens may also prove valuable in the diagnosis of some pathogens, such as microsporidians.[142] Small bowel aspirates are generally not useful in the evaluation of unexplained diarrhea.

Approximately 20% to 50% of patients with chronic diarrhea have a negative gastrointestinal tract evaluation.[119,137,143] Patients without an identifiable cause of diarrhea may have HIV-associated enteropathy, the pathology of which is not fully understood. Histologic evaluation of small bowel biopsy specimens may reveal a decrease in villous surface area and crypt cell proliferation in the absence of inflammation.[144] For many pathogens few specific therapies are available, but highly active antiretroviral therapy may effectively control diarrhea in patients with HIV enteropathy, as well as those with microsporidiosis and cryptosporidiosis.[116,117,145] Furthermore, as diagnostic methods improve and additional pathogens are identified, the proportion of patients with unexplained diarrhea may decline.

REFERENCES

1. Monkemuller KE, Call SA, Lazenby AJ, Wilcox CM. Declining prevalence of opportunistic gastrointestinal disease in the era of combination antiretroviral therapy. Am J Gastroenterol. 2000;95:457-462.
2. Sulkowski MS, Thomas DL. Hepatitis C in the HIV infected patient. Ann Intern Med. 2002;138:197-207.
3. Connolly GM, Hawkins D, Harcourt-Webster JN, et al. Oesophageal symptoms, their causes, treatment, and prognosis in patients with the acquired immunodeficiency syndrome. Gut. 1989;30:1033-1039.
4. Rabeneck L, Popovic M, Gartner S, et al. Acute HIV infection presenting with painful swallowing and esophageal ulcers. JAMA. 1990;263:2318-2322.
5. Wilcox CM, Schwartz DA, Clark WS. Esophageal ulceration in human immunodeficiency virus infection. Causes, response to therapy, and long-term outcome. Ann Intern Med. 1995;123:143-149.
6. Ledergerber B, Egger M, Erard V, et al. AIDS-related opportunistic illnesses occurring after initiation of potent antiretroviral therapy: The Swiss HIV Cohort Study. JAMA. 1999;282:2220-2226.
7. Bini EJ, Micale PL, Weinshel EH. Natural history of HIV-associated esophageal disease in the era of protease inhibitor therapy. Dig Dis Sci. 2000;45:1301-1307.
8. Zalar AE, Olmos MA, Piskorz EL, Magnanini FL. Esophageal motility disorders in HIV patients. Dig Dis Sci. 2003;48:962-967.

9. Tavitian A, Raufman JP, Rosenthal LE. Oral candidiasis as a marker for esophageal candidiasis in the acquired immunodeficiency syndrome. Ann Intern Med. 1986;104:54-55.
10. Atazanavir (Reyataz) and emtricitabine (Emtriva) for HIV infection. Med Lett Drugs Ther. 2003;45:90-92.
11. Laine L, Dretler RH, Conteas CN, et al. Fluconazole compared with ketoconazole for the treatment of Candida esophagitis in AIDS. A randomized trial. Ann Intern Med. 1992;117:655-660.
12. Wilcox CM, Alexander LN, Clark WS, Thompson SE, III. Fluconazole compared with endoscopy for human immunodeficiency virus-infected patients with esophageal symptoms. Gastroenterology. 1996;110:1803-1809.
13. Wilcox CM. Short report: Time course of clinical response with fluconazole for Candida oesophagitis in patients with AIDS. Aliment Pharmacol Ther. 1994;8: 347-350.
14. Wilcox CM, Straub RF, Alexander LN, Clark WS. Etiology of esophageal disease in human immunodeficiency virus-infected patients who fail antifungal therapy. Am J Med. 1996;101:599-604.
15. Bashir RM, Wilcox CM. Symptom-specific use of upper gastrointestinal endoscopy in human immunodeficiency virus-infected patients yields high dividends. J Clin Gastroenterol. 1996;23:292-298.
16. Wilcox CM, Diehl DL, Cello JP, et al. Cytomegalovirus esophagitis in patients with AIDS. A clinical, endoscopic, and pathologic correlation. Ann Intern Med. 1990;113:589-593.
17. Genereau T, Lortholary O, Bouchaud O, et al. Herpes simplex esophagitis in patients with AIDS: Report of 34 cases. The Cooperative Study Group on Herpetic Esophagitis in HIV Infection. Clin Infect Dis. 1996;22:926-931.
18. Maenza JR, Keruly JC, Moore RD, et al. Risk factors for fluconazole-resistant candidiasis in human immunodeficiency virus-infected patients. J Infect Dis. 1996;173:219-225.
19. Wilcox CM, Straub RF, Schwartz DA. Prospective evaluation of biopsy number for the diagnosis of viral esophagitis in patients with HIV infection and esophageal ulcer. Gastrointest Endosc. 1996;44:587-593.
20. Edwards PD, Carrick J, Turner J, et al. Helicobacter pylori-associated gastritis is rare in AIDS: Antibiotic effect or a consequence of immunodeficiency? Am J Gastroenterol. 1991;86:1761-1764.
21. Varsky CG, Correa MC, Sarmiento N, et al. Prevalence and etiology of gastroduodenal ulcer in HIV-positive patients: A comparative study of 497 symptomatic subjects evaluated by endoscopy. Am J Gastroenterol. 1998;93:935-940.
22. Fabris P, Bozzola L, Benedetti P, et al. H. pylori infection in HIV-positive patients. A serohistological study. Dig Dis Sci. 1997;42:289-292.
23. Gisbert JP, Pajares JM. Diagnosis of Helicobacter pylori infection by stool antigen determination: A systematic review. Am J Gastroenterol. 2001;96:2829-2838.
24. Lake-Bakaar G, Elsakr M, Hagag N, et al. Changes in parietal cell structure and function in HIV disease. Dig Dis Sci. 1996;41:1398-1408.
25. Lake-Bakaar G, Tom W, Lake-Bakaar D, et al. Gastropathy and ketoconazole malabsorption in the acquired immunodeficiency syndrome (AIDS). Ann Intern Med. 1988;109:471-473.
26. Belitsos PC, Greenson JK, Yardley JH, et al. Association of gastric hypoacidity with opportunistic enteric infections in patients with AIDS. J Infect Dis. 1992;166: 277-284.
27. Teixidor HS, Honig CL, Norsoph E, et al. Cytomegalovirus infection of the alimentary canal: Radiologic findings with pathologic correlation. Radiology. 1987;163:317-323.
28. Friedman SL, Wright TL, Altman DF. Gastrointestinal Kaposi's sarcoma in patients with acquired immunodeficiency syndrome. Endoscopic and autopsy findings. Gastroenterology. 1985;89:102-108.
29. Lew EA, Dieterich DT. Severe hemorrhage caused by gastrointestinal Kaposi's syndrome in patients with the acquired immunodeficiency syndrome: Treatment with endoscopic injection sclerotherapy. Am J Gastroenterol. 1992;87:1471-1474.
30. Cappell MS, Botros N. Predominantly gastrointestinal symptoms and signs in 11 consecutive AIDS patients with gastrointestinal lymphoma: A multicenter, multiyear study including 763 HIV-seropositive patients. Am J Gastroenterol. 1994;89:545-549.
31. Bonacini M. Hepatobiliary complications in patients with human immunodeficiency virus infection. Am J Med. 1992;92:404-411.
32. French AL, Beaudet LM, Benator DA, et al. Cholecystectomy in patients with AIDS: Clinicopathologic correlations in 107 cases. Clin Infect Dis. 1995;21:852-858.
33. Kavin H, Jonas RB, Chowdhury L, Kabins S. Acalculous cholecystitis and cytomegalovirus infection in the acquired immunodeficiency syndrome. Ann Intern Med. 1986;104:53-54.
34. Pol S, Romana CA, Richard S, et al. Microsporidia infection in patients with the human immunodeficiency virus and unexplained cholangitis. N Engl J Med. 1993;328:95-99.
35. Benator DA, French AL, Beaudet LM, et al. Isospora belli infection associated with acalculous cholecystitis in a patient with AIDS. Ann Intern Med. 1994;121:663-664.
36. Ko WF, Cello JP, Rogers SJ, Lecours A. Prognostic factors for the survival of patients with AIDS cholangiopathy. Am J Gastroenterol. 2003;98:2176-2181.
37. Schneiderman DJ, Cello JP, Laing FC. Papillary stenosis and sclerosing cholangitis in the acquired immunodeficiency syndrome. Ann Intern Med. 1987;106:546-549.
38. Cello JP. Acquired immunodeficiency syndrome cholangiopathy: Spectrum of disease. Am J Med. 1989;86:539-546.
39. Benhamou Y, Caumes E, Gerosa Y, et al. AIDS-related cholangiopathy. Critical analysis of a prospective series of 26 patients. Dig Dis Sci. 1993;38:1113-1118.
40. Vakil NB, Schwartz SM, Buggy BP, et al. Biliary cryptosporidiosis in HIV-infected people after the waterborne outbreak of cryptosporidiosis in Milwaukee. N Engl J Med. 1996;334:19-23.
41. Cello JP, Chan MF. Long-term follow-up of endoscopic retrograde cholangiopancreatography sphincterotomy for patients with acquired immune deficiency syndrome papillary stenosis. Am J Med. 1995;99:600-603.
42. Sulkowski MS, Moore RD, Mehta SH, et al. Hepatitis C and progression of HIV disease. JAMA. 2002;288:199-206.
43. Thio CL, Seaberg EC, Skolasky RL, et al. HIV-1, hepatitis B virus, and risk of liver-related mortality in the Multicenter AIDS Cohort Study (MACS). Lancet. 2002;360:1921-1926.
44. Kelen GD, Green GB, Purcell RH, et al. Hepatitis B and hepatitis C in emergency department patients. N Engl J Med. 1992;326:1399-1404.
45. Thio CL. Hepatitis B in the human immunodeficiency virus-infected patient: Epidemiology, natural history, and treatment. Semin Liver Dis. 2003;23:125-136.
46. Kellerman SE, Hanson DL, McNaghten AD, Fleming PL. Prevalence of chronic hepatitis B and incidence of acute hepatitis B infection in human immunodeficiency virus-infected subjects. J Infect Dis. 2003;188:571-577.
47. Hadler SC, Judson FN, O'Malley PM, et al. Outcome of hepatitis B virus infection in homosexual men and its relation to prior human immunodeficiency virus infection. J Infect Dis. 1991;163:454-459.
48. Waite J, Gilson RJ, Weller IV, et al. Hepatitis B virus reactivation or reinfection associated with HIV-1 infection. AIDS. 1988;2:443-448.
49. Vento S, Di Perri G, Garofano T, et al. Reactivation of hepatitis B in AIDS. Lancet. 1989;2:108-109.
50. Gilson RJ, Hawkins AE, Beecham MR, et al. Interactions between HIV and hepatitis B virus in homosexual men: Effects on the natural history of infection. AIDS. 1997;11:597-606.
51. Bodsworth N, Donovan B, Nightingale BN. The effect of concurrent human immunodeficiency virus infection on chronic hepatitis B: A study of 150 homosexual men. J Infect Dis. 1989;160:577-582.
52. Masur Pb PH, Kaplan JE, Holmes KK. Guidelines for preventing opportunistic infections among HIV-infected persons-2002. Recommendations of the U.S. Public Health Service and the Infectious Diseases Society of America. Ann Intern Med. 2002;137:435-478.
53. Rockstroh JK. Management of hepatitis B and C in HIV co-infected patients. J Acquir Immune Defic Syndr. 2003;34(Suppl 1):S59-S65.
54. Lok AS, McMahon BJ. Chronic hepatitis B. Hepatology. 2001;34:1225-1241.
55. Dore GJ, Cooper DA, Barrett C, et al. Dual efficacy of lamivudine treatment in human immunodeficiency virus/hepatitis B virus-coinfected persons in a randomized, controlled study (CAESAR). The CAESAR Coordinating Committee. J Infect Dis. 1999;180:607-613.
56. Haverkamp M, Smit M, Weersink A, et al. The effect of lamivudine on the replication of hepatitis B virus in HIV-infected patients depends on the host immune status (CD4 cell count). AIDS. 2003;17:1572-1574.
57. Benhamou Y, Tubiana R, Thibault V. Tenofovir disoproxil fumarate in patients with HIV and lamivudine-resistant hepatitis B virus. N Engl J Med. 2003;348:177-78.
58. Nelson M, Portsmouth S, Stebbing J, et al. An open-label study of tenofovir in HIV-1 and hepatitis B virus co-infected individuals. AIDS. 2003;17:F7-F10.
59. Gish RG, Leung NW, Wright TL, et al F. Dose range study of pharmacokinetics, safety, and preliminary antiviral activity of emtricitabine in adults with hepatitis B virus infection. Antimicrob Agents Chemother. 2002;46:1734-1740.
60. Hadziyannis SJ, Tassopoulos NC, Heathcote EJ, et al. Adefovir dipivoxil for the treatment of hepatitis B e antigen-negative chronic hepatitis B. N Engl J Med. 2003;348:800-807.
61. Marcellin P, Chang TT, Lim SG, et al. Adefovir dipivoxil for the treatment of hepatitis B e antigen-positive chronic hepatitis B. N Engl J Med. 2003;348:808-816.
62. Benhamou Y, Bochet M, Thibault V, et al. Safety and efficacy of adefovir dipivoxil in patients co-infected with HIV-1 and lamivudine-resistant hepatitis B virus: An open-label pilot study. Lancet. 2001;358:718-723.
63. DiMartino V, Thevenot T, Colin JF, et al. Influence of HIV infection on the response to interferon therapy and the long-term outcome of chronic hepatitis B. Gastroenterology. 2002;123:1812-1822.
64. Cooksley WG, Piratvisuth T, Lee SD, et al. Peginterferon alpha-2a (40 kDa): An advance in the treatment of hepatitis B e antigen-positive chronic hepatitis B. J Viral Hepat. 2003;10:298-305.
65. Brau N, Bini EJ, Shahidi A, et al. Prevalence of hepatitis C and coinfection with HIV among United States veterans in the New York City metropolitan area. Am J Gastroenterol. 2002;97:2071-2078.
66. Tong MJ, El-Farra NS, Reikes AR, Co RL. Clinical outcomes after transfusion-associated hepatitis C. N Engl J Med. 1995;332:1463-1466.
67. Seeff LB. Natural history of hepatitis C. Hepatology. 1997;26:21S-8S.
68. Gumber SC, Chopra S. Hepatitis C: A multifaceted disease—Review of extrahepatic manifestations. Ann Intern Med. 1995;123:615-620.
69. Thomas DL, Shih JW, Alter HJ, et al. Effect of human immunodeficiency virus on hepatitis C virus infection among injecting drug users. J Infect Dis. 1996;174: 690-695.
70. Eyster ME, Diamondstone LS, Lien JM, et al. Natural history of hepatitis C virus infection in multitransfused hemophiliacs: Effect of coinfection with human immunodeficiency virus. The Multicenter Hemophilia Cohort Study. J Acquir Immune Defic Syndr. 1993;6:602-610.
71. Graham CS, Baden LR, Yu E, et al. Influence of human immunodeficiency virus infection on the course of hepatitis c virus infection: A meta-analysis. Clin Infect Dis. 2001;33:562-569.
72. Soto B, Sánchez-Quijano A, Rodrigo L, et al. Human immunodeficiency virus infection modifies the natural history of chronic parenterally-acquired hepatitis C with an unusually rapid progression to cirrhosis. J Hepatol. 1997;26:1-5.

73. Darby SC, Ewart DW, Giangrande PL, et al. Mortality from liver cancer and liver disease in haemophilic men and boys in UK given blood products contaminated with hepatitis C. Lancet. 1997;350:1425-1431.

74. Pol S, Lamorthe B, Thi NT, et al. Retrospective analysis of the impact of HIV infection and alcohol use on chronic hepatitis C in a large cohort of drug users. J Hepatol. 1998;28:945-950.

75. Greub G, Ledergerber B, Battegay M, et al. Clinical progression, survival, and immune recovery during antiretroviral therapy in patients with HIV-1 and hepatitis C virus coinfection: The Swiss HIV Cohort Study. Lancet. 2000;356:1800-1805.

76. Monga HK, Rodriguez-Barradas MC, Breaux K, et al. Hepatitis C virus infection-related morbidity and mortality among patients with human immunodeficiency virus infection. Clin Infect Dis. 2001;33:240-247.

77. Bica I, McGovern B, Dhar R, et al. Increasing mortality due to end-stage liver disease in patients with human immunodeficiency virus infection. Clin Infect Dis. 2001;32:492-497.

78. Rosenthal E, Poiree M, Pradier C, et al. Mortality due to hepatitis C-related liver disease in HIV-infected patients in France (Mortavic 2001 study). AIDS. 2003;17:1803-1809.

79. Gebo KA, Diener-West M, Moore RD. Hospitalization rates differ by hepatitis C status in an urban HIV cohort. J Acquir Immune Defic Syndr. 2003;34:165-173.

80. National Institutes of Health Consensus Development Conference Statement: Management of hepatitis C: 2002—June 10-12, 2002. Hepatology. 2002;36:S3-S20.

81. George SL, Gebhardt J, Klinzman D, et al. Hepatitis C virus viremia in HIV-infected individuals with negative HCV antibody tests. J Acquir Immune Defic Syndr. 2002;31:154-162.

82. Peters MG, Terrault NA. Alcohol use and hepatitis C. Hepatology. 2002;36:S220-S225.

83. Poynard T, Bedossa P, Opolon P. Natural history of liver fibrosis progression in patients with chronic hepatitis C. Lancet. 1997;349:825-832.

84. Poles MA, Dieterich DT, Schwarz ED, et al. Liver biopsy findings in 501 patients infected with human immunodeficiency virus (HIV). J Acquir Immune Defic Syndr Hum Retrovirol. 1996;11:170-177.

85. Manns MP, McHutchison JG, Gordon SC, et al. Peginterferon alfa-2b plus ribavirin compared with interferon alfa-2b plus ribavirin for initial treatment of chronic hepatitis C: A randomised trial. Lancet. 2001;358:958-965.

86. Fried MW, Shiffman ML, Reddy KR, et al. Peginterferon alfa-2a plus ribavirin for chronic hepatitis C virus infection. N Engl J Med. 2002;347:975-982.

87. Perez-Olmeda M, Nunez M, Romero M, et al. Pegylated IFN-alpha 2b plus ribavirin as therapy for chronic hepatitis C in HIV-infected patients. AIDS. 2003;17:1023-1028.

88. Perez-Olmeda M, Nunez M, Romero M, et al. Pegylated IFN-alpha 2b plus ribavirin as therapy for chronic hepatitis C in HIV-infected patients. AIDS. 2003;17:1023-1028.

89. Fried MW. Side effects of therapy of hepatitis C and their management. Hepatology. 2002;36:S237-S244.

90. Chaisson RE, Schecter GF, Theuer CP, et al. Tuberculosis in patients with the acquired immunodeficiency syndrome. Clinical features, response to therapy, and survival. Am Rev Respir Dis. 1987;136:570-574.

91. Koehler JE, Sanchez MA, Garrido CS, et al. Molecular epidemiology of bartonella infections in patients with bacillary angiomatosis-peliosis. N Engl J Med. 1997;337:1876-1883.

92. Poles MA, Dieterich DT. Infections of the liver in HIV-infected patients. Infect Dis Clin North Am. 2000;14:741-759.

93. Cavicchi M, Pialoux G, Carnot F, et al. Value of liver biopsy for the rapid diagnosis of infection in human immunodeficiency virus-infected patients who have unexplained fever and elevated serum levels of alkaline phosphatase or gamma-glutamyl transferase. Clin Infect Dis. 1995;20:606-610.

94. Ziegler JL, Beckstead JA, Volberding PA, et al. Non-Hodgkin's lymphoma in 90 homosexual men. Relation to generalized lymphadenopathy and the acquired immunodeficiency syndrome. N Engl J Med. 1984;311:565-570.

95. Bruno R, Sacchi P, Filice C, et al. Hepatocellular carcinoma in HIV-infected patients with chronic hepatitis: An emerging issue. J Acquir Immune Defic Syndr. 2002;30:535-536.

96. Ungo JR, Jones D, Ashkin D, et al. Antituberculosis drug-induced hepatotoxicity. The role of hepatitis C virus and the human immunodeficiency virus. Am J Respir Crit Care Med. 1998;157:1871-1876.

97. Sulkowski MS, Thomas DL, Chaisson RE, Moore RD. Hepatotoxicity associated with antiretroviral therapy in adults infected with human immunodeficiency virus and the role of hepatitis C or B virus infection. JAMA. 2000;283:74-80.

98. Sulkowski MS, Thomas DL, Mehta SH, et al. Hepatotoxicity associated with nevirapine or efavirenz-containing antiretroviral therapy: role of hepatitis C and B infections. Hepatology. 2002;35:182-189.

99. Wit FW, Weverling GJ, Weel J, et al. Incidence of and risk factors for severe hepatotoxicity associated with antiretroviral combination therapy. J Infect Dis. 2002;186:23-31.

100. den Brinker M, Wit FW, Wertheim-van Dillen PM, et al. Hepatitis B and C virus coinfection and the risk for hepatotoxicity of highly active antiretroviral therapy in HIV-1 infection. AIDS. 2000;14:2895-28902.

101. Freiman JP, Helfert KE, Hamrell MR, Stein DS. Hepatomegaly with severe steatosis in HIV-seropositive patients. AIDS. 1993;7:379-385.

102. Miller KD, Cameron M, Wood LV, et al. Lactic acidosis and hepatic steatosis associated with use of stavudine: Report of four cases. Ann Intern Med. 2000;133:192-196.

103. Ogedegbe AE, Thomas DL, Diehl AM. Hyperlactataemia syndromes associated with HIV therapy. Lancet Infect Dis. 2003;3:329-337.

104. Sutinen J, Hakkinen AM, Westerbacka J, et al. Increased fat accumulation in the liver in HIV-infected patients with antiretroviral therapy-associated lipodystrophy. AIDS. 2002;16:2183-2193.

105. Dutta SK, Ting CD, Lai LL. Study of prevalence, severity, and etiological factors associated with acute pancreatitis in patients infected with human immunodeficiency virus. Am J Gastroenterol. 1997;92:2044-2048.

106. Farman J, Brunetti J, Baer JW, et al. AIDS-related cholangiopancreatographic changes. Abdom Imaging. 1994;19:417-422.

107. Jaber B, Gleckman R. Tuberculous pancreatic abscess as an initial AIDS-defining disorder in a patient infected with the human immunodeficiency virus: Case report and review. Clin Infect Dis. 1995;20:890-894.

108. Wilcox CM, Forsmark CE, Grendell JH, et al. Cytomegalovirus-associated acute pancreatic disease in patients with acquired immunodeficiency syndrome. Report of two patients. Gastroenterology. 1990;99:263-267.

109. Moore RD, Keruly JC, Chaisson RE. Incidence of pancreatitis in HIV-infected patients receiving nucleoside reverse transcriptase inhibitor drugs. AIDS. 2001;15:617-620.

110. Schindzielorz A, Pike I, Daniels M, et al. Rates and risk factors for adverse events associated with didanosine in the expanded access program. Clin Infect Dis. 1994;19:1076-1083.

111. Assan R, Perronne C, Assan D, et al. Pentamidine-induced derangements of glucose homeostasis. Determinant roles of renal failure and drug accumulation. A study of 128 patients. Diabetes Care. 1995;18:47-55.

112. Henry K, Rathgaber S, Sullivan C, McCabe K. Diabetes mellitus induced by megestrol acetate in a patient with AIDS and cachexia. Ann Intern Med. 1992;116:53-54.

113. Mehta SH, Moore RD, Thomas DL, et al. The effect of HAART and HCV infection on the development of hyperglycemia among HIV-infected persons. J Acquir Immune Defic Syndr. 2003;33:577-584.

114. Eastone JA, Decker CF. New-onset diabetes mellitus associated with use of protease inhibitor. Ann Intern Med. 1997;127:948.

115. Brambilla AM, Novati R, Calori G, et al. Stavudine or indinavir-containing regimens are associated with an increased risk of diabetes mellitus in HIV-infected individuals. AIDS. 2003;17:1993-1995.

116. Schmidt W, Wahnschaffe U, Schafer M, et al. Rapid increase of mucosal CD4 T cells followed by clearance of intestinal cryptosporidiosis in an AIDS patient receiving highly active antiretroviral therapy. Gastroenterology. 2001;120:984-987.

117. Call SA, Heudebert G, Saag M, Wilcox CM. The changing etiology of chronic diarrhea in HIV-infected patients with CD4 cell counts less than 200 cells/mm³. Am J Gastroenterol. 2000;95:3142-146.

118. Sharpstone D, Gazzard B. Gastrointestinal manifestations of HIV infection. Lancet. 1996;348:379-383.

119. O'Brien ME, Clark RA, Besch CL, et al. Patterns and correlates of discontinuation of the initial HAART regimen in an urban outpatient cohort. J Acquir Immune Defic Syndr. 2003;34:407-414.

120. Yeguez JF, Martinez SA, Sands DR, et al. Colorectal malignancies in HIV-positive patients. Am Surg. 2003;69:981-987.

121. Shah RJ, Fenoglio-Preiser C, Bleau BL, Giannella RA. Usefulness of colonoscopy with biopsy in the evaluation of patients with chronic diarrhea. Am J Gastroenterol. 2001;96:1091-1095.

122. Angulo FJ, Swerdlow DL. Bacterial enteric infections in persons infected with human immunodeficiency virus. Clin Infect Dis. 1995;21(Suppl 1):S84-S93.

123. Glaser JB, Morton-Kute L, Berger SR, et al. Recurrent *Salmonella typhimurium* bacteremia associated with the acquired immunodeficiency syndrome. Ann Intern Med. 1985;102:189-193.

124. Tee W, Mijch A. *Campylobacter jejuni* bacteremia in human immunodeficiency virus (HIV)-infected and non-HIV-infected patients: Comparison of clinical features and review. Clin Infect Dis. 1998;26:91-96.

125. Barbut F, Meynard JL, Guiguet M, et al. *Clostridium difficile*-associated diarrhea in HIV-infected patients: Epidemiology and risk factors. J Acquir Immune Defic Syndr Hum Retrovirol. 1997;16:176-181.

126. Saddi VR, Glatt AE. *Clostridium difficile*-associated diarrhea in patients with HIV: A 4-year survey. J Acquir Immune Defic Syndr. 2002;31:542-543.

127. Villanueva SE, Martinez Hernandez MP, Fernando Alvarez-Tostado FJ, Valdes OM. Colonic tuberculosis. Dig Dis Sci. 2002;47:2045-2048.

128. Damsker B, Bottone EJ. *Mycobacterium avium-Mycobacterium intracellulare* from the intestinal tracts of patients with the acquired immunodeficiency syndrome: Concepts regarding acquisition and pathogenesis. J Infect Dis. 1985;151:179-181.

129. Navin TR, Weber R, Vugia DJ, et al. Declining CD4+ T-lymphocyte counts are associated with increased risk of enteric parasitosis and chronic diarrhea: Results of a 3-year longitudinal study. J Acquir Immune Defic Syndr Hum Retrovirol. 1999;20:154-159.

130. Manabe YC, Clark DP, Moore RD, et al. Cryptosporidiosis in patients with AIDS: Correlates of disease and survival. Clin Infect Dis. 1998;27:536-542.

131. Rabeneck L, Gyorkey F, Genta RM, et al. The role of Microsporidia in the pathogenesis of HIV-related chronic diarrhea. Ann Intern Med. 1993;119:895-899.

132. DeHovitz JA, Pape JW, Boncy M, Johnson WD, Jr. Clinical manifestations and therapy of *Isospora belli* infection in patients with the acquired immunodeficiency syndrome. N Engl J Med. 1986;315:87-90.

133. Pape JW, Verdier RI, Boncy M, et al. *Cyclospora* infection in adults infected with HIV. Clinical manifestations, treatment, and prophylaxis. Ann Intern Med. 1994;121:654-657.

134. Dieterich DT, Rahmin M. Cytomegalovirus colitis in AIDS: Presentation in 44 patients and a review of the literature. J Acquir Immune Defic Syndr. 1991;4(Suppl 1):S29-S35.

135. Grohmann GS, Glass RI, Pereira HG, et al. Enteric viruses and diarrhea in HIV-infected patients. Enteric Opportunistic Infections Working Group. N Engl J Med. 1993;329:14-20.

136. Rompalo AM. Diagnosis and treatment of sexually acquired proctitis and proctocolitis: An update. Clin Infect Dis. 1999;28(Suppl 1):S84-S90.
137. Datta D, Gazzard B, Stebbing J. The diagnostic yield of stool analysis in 525 HIV-1-infected individuals. AIDS. 2003;17:1711-1713.
138. Goodgame RW. Understanding intestinal spore-forming protozoa: Cryptosporidia, microsporidia, isospora, and cyclospora. Ann Intern Med. 1996;124:429-441.
139. Wilcox CM, Schwartz DA, Cotsonis G, Thompson SE, III. Chronic unexplained diarrhea in human immunodeficiency virus infection: Determination of the best diagnostic approach. Gastroenterology. 1996;110:30-37.
140. Bini EJ, Weinshel EH. Endoscopic evaluation of chronic human immunodeficiency virus-related diarrhea: Is colonoscopy superior to flexible sigmoidoscopy? Am J Gastroenterol. 1998;93:56-60.
141. Bown JW, Savides TJ, Mathews C, et al. Diagnostic yield of duodenal biopsy and aspirate in AIDS-associated diarrhea. Am J Gastroenterol. 1996;91:2289-2292.
142. David F, Schuitema AR, Sarfati C, et al. Detection and species identification of intestinal microsporidia by polymerase chain reaction in duodenal biopsies from human immunodeficiency virus-infected patients. J Infect Dis. 1996;174:874-877.
143. Blanshard C, Francis N, Gazzard BG. Investigation of chronic diarrhoea in acquired immunodeficiency syndrome. A prospective study of 155 patients. Gut. 1996;39:824-832.
144. Greenson JK, Belitsos PC, Yardley JH, Bartlett JG. AIDS enteropathy: Occult enteric infections and duodenal mucosal alterations in chronic diarrhea. Ann Intern Med. 1991;114:366-372.
145. Carr A, Marriott D, Field A, et al. Treatment of HIV-1-associated microsporidiosis and cryptosporidiosis with combination antiretroviral therapy. Lancet. 1998;351:256-261.

CHAPTER **120**

Neurologic Diseases Caused by Human Immunodeficiency Virus-1 and Opportunistic Infections

IGOR J. KORALNIK

Neurologic manifestations are frequent in human immunodeficiency virus (HIV)-1 infection. They constitute the initial presentation in 10% of patients, whereas 30% to 50% develop neurologic complications during the course of the disease.[1,2] Autopsy shows involvement of the nervous system in up to 80% of cases.[3,4]

Diagnosis of neurologic complications in patients with HIV-1 infection poses a particular challenge for the clinicians. Indeed, HIV-infected individuals are often severely debilitated and present with multiple constitutional symptoms related to systemic infections or tumors, which might overshadow or mimic a primary neurologic condition. In addition, HIV-infected individuals are usually treated with a combination of prophylactic drugs and a rapidly growing number of antiretroviral medications. Drug interactions and neurologic side effects of these medications are common, which adds another level of complexity for care providers. However, certain rules can be applied to facilitate the understanding of these challenging cases:

1. The spectrum of neurologic manifestations in HIV-1–infected individuals depends on their degree of immunosuppression, reflected by their CD4+ T-lymphocyte counts, and the speed of disease progression, as estimated by measurement of their plasma HIV-1 viral load.
2. Multiple pathologies may coexist in the context of immunosuppression. The peripheral and central nervous systems are frequently affected concomitantly in HIV-1–infected individuals and opportunistic infections of the brain may be superimposed on primary HIV-1–associated neurologic disorders.

3. Antiretroviral medications and prophylactic drugs taken by HIV-infected individuals often cause neurologic side effects, which must be included in the differential diagnosis of these patients.

PRINCIPAL NEUROLOGIC MANIFESTATIONS OF HUMAN IMMUNODEFICIENCY VIRUS-1 INFECTION

Meningeal Syndrome

Patient Otherwise Asymptomatic, CD4+ T-Lymphocyte Counts Greater Than 200/μL: Aseptic Meningitis

Clinical Presentation. Headache, stiff neck, and fever, associated with nausea and vomiting, can be the first manifestation of HIV-1 infection. It is a self-limited illness that subsides spontaneously after several weeks. In some cases, transient cranial neuropathies may develop, affecting mostly the fifth, seventh, and eight cranial nerves. In addition, patients may present with symptoms of encephalopathy, and postmortem examination of individuals who died from unrelated causes in this early stage showed mild meningeal inflammation, focal cerebral white matter myelin damage, and perivascular inflammatory infiltrates and gliosis.[5,6]

Laboratory Investigations. The cerebrospinal fluid (CSF) analysis shows a moderate lymphocytic pleocytosis (10 to 100 cells/μL), which is typical of viral meningitis.[7] This aseptic meningitis can occur as soon as 1 week after the primary infection, when HIV-1 conventional serology is still negative. HIV-1 RNA, however, should be detectable in the blood and CSF, and the HIV-1 p24 antigen might be detected in the blood. A repeat serology testing after 6 weeks usually helps to clarify this situation.

Treatment. Interestingly, early onset of aseptic meningitis has not been associated with late neurologic manifestations in HIV-1 infection, and patients may remain asymptomatic for many years before developing other symptoms of HIV-1 disease. If they were not properly diagnosed at the time of their acute illness, these patients may therefore unwittingly infect a number of sexual partners. It is therefore crucial to include HIV-1 in the differential diagnosis of aseptic meningitis. This condition might recur at any time throughout the course of the disease, although CSF pleocytosis becomes less common with advanced immunosuppression. Treatment is symptomatic. The decision to start on antiretroviral medications should be based on current guidelines[8] (see Chapter 124).

Patient at Any Stage of Human Immunodeficiency Virus-1 Disease and CD4+ T-Lymphocyte Counts at Any Level: Syphilitic Meningitis

Clinical Presentation. In the United States, as many as 6% of HIV-infected individuals have a history of syphilis. *Treponema pallidum* infection can also occur at any time during HIV-1 infection and mimics neurologic complications of acquired immunodeficiency syndrome (AIDS). Indeed both conditions may cause acute or chronic meningitis, myelopathy, cranial or peripheral neuropathies, cerebrovascular disease, and dementia. Therefore, it is paramount to distinguish neurosyphilis from latent disease with positive serology and normal physical examination in HIV-infected patients, because it has a direct impact on treatment. Neurosyphilis can occur as early as 1 year or as late as 30 years after initial infection. In this chapter, we discuss only syphilitic meningitis; other neurologic complications of this disease are covered in Chapter 235.

Laboratory Investigations. Elevation of protein concentration and leukocyte counts can be found in CSF of approximately 15% of patients with primary syphilis and as many as 40% of patients with secondary syphilis. Some of these patients eventually experience spontaneous cure of this earlier CNS infection, but the persistence of asymptomatic CSF abnormalities for more than 5 years in the untreated patient is highly predictive of the development of clinical neurosyphilis.

A persistent mononuclear pleocytosis and elevated protein concentration can be found in the CSF of HIV-1–infected patients with neurosyphilis,[9] as well as elevated immunoglobulin G (IgG) synthesis rate and oligoclonal bands. This is of no help in establishing the diagnosis of neurosyphilis in the context of HIV-1 infection because these findings occur as well in asymptomatic HIV-1–seropositive patients, especially when they have detectable HIV-1 RNA in their CSF. A positive CSF Venereal Disease Research Laboratories (VDRL) result establishes the diagnosis of neurosyphilis if the tap is not bloody. However, this test may be negative in HIV-1 infection.[10,11] A reactive CSF FTA-ABS test increases the likelihood of *T. pallidum* infection but is less specific because it can result from treated neurosyphilis or from contamination of the CSF with small amounts of blood containing antibody at the time of the lumbar puncture.

Acute symptomatic syphilitic meningitis is usually the earliest clinical manifestation of neurosyphilis, which occurs within the first year of infection and can be associated with cranial nerve palsies, including isolated eighth nerve palsy, and signs and symptoms of hydrocephalus. CSF abnormalities are similar to asymptomatic neurosyphilis, except that CSF VDRL is nearly always positive.

Treatment. HIV-1–infected individuals with a positive serum rapid plasma reagin (RPR) test result, unexplained CSF pleocytosis, and elevated protein concentration as well as symptoms consistent with neurosyphilis should be treated with intravenous penicillin even in the absence of a positive VDRL in the CSF. Treatment consists of intravenous penicillin G (3 to 4 million units intravenously every 4 hours for 10 to 14 days). In case of allergy to penicillin, ceftriaxone (1 g intravenously once daily for at least 10 days) is another option. A careful follow-up of these patients is needed, and a repeat spinal tap 1 month after onset of treatment should show a normalization of the CSF cellularity and protein concentration. Some patients have a transient increase in CSF HIV-1 viral load to greater than 100,000 copies/mL associated with neurosyphilis, which subsides after antibiotic treatment. As it is the case with other opportunistic infections of the brain, this viral burden is likely carried by activated circulating lymphocytes and monocytes coming to combat the CNS infection and should not be interpreted as a manifestation of HIV-1 encephalitis.

Patient with Acquired Immunodeficiency Syndrome, CD4+ T-Lymphocyte Counts of Less Than 200/μL: Cryptococcal Meningitis

Clinical Presentation. This is the most common opportunistic meningitis in AIDS, which affected 10% of patients before the highly active antiretroviral therapy (HAART) era[12] but has decreased in incidence since then[13] (see also Chapter 261). Cryptococcal meningitis differs from aseptic meningitis in that meningismus is present in less than 40% of cases and patients may present with only fever and headache, which become progressively more debilitating. Confusion, blindness, or altered state of consciousness occurs in severe cases.

Laboratory Investigations. The detection of *Cryptococcus neoformans* antigen (Ag) titers by enzyme immunoassay in the CSF provides a rapid diagnosis, which is confirmed subsequently by CSF culture. Other CSF findings include elevated opening pressure, mononuclear pleocytosis, elevated protein and decreased glucose concentration in 50% of the cases, and direct detection of the organism by India ink staining in 70% of the cases. Serum cryptococcal Ag is almost always detected in cryptococcal meningitis, and blood and urine cultures may also be positive.

Brain imaging is usually negative unless an associated abscess or hydrocephalus is present. Poor prognosis factors include altered mental status, absence of CSF pleocytosis, CSF Ag titer greater than 1:1024, a positive blood culture, and hyponatremia.

Treatment. Treatment consists of induction therapy with amphotericin B (0.7-1.0 mg/kg given intravenously daily for 2 weeks) combined with flucytosine (100 mg/kg given orally in 4 divided doses per day). Consolidation therapy then consist of fluconazole (400 mg orally once daily) administered for 8 weeks or until CSF cultures are sterile. Lipid formulations of amphotericin B may be used for patients with

renal insufficiency, and itraconazole may be substituted for fluconazole if patients can tolerate fluconazole but is clearly inferior to the latter. In conjunction with antiretroviral therapy, long-term maintenance antifungal therapy should be administered for life to prevent relapses, using oral fluconazole 200 mg/day.[14]

The outcome is generally favorable within 2 weeks but early mortality still reaches 6%.[15] Complications such as elevated intracranial pressure greater than 200 mm of water occurs in nearly all patients. Such a complication should be recognized and treated aggressively with mechanical drainage, including repeated lumbar punctures, or intraventricular shunts.[16] Corticosteroids, acetazolamide, or mannitol have not been shown to be effective.

Differential Diagnosis of Meningitis

Other central nervous system (CNS) infections in AIDS include tuberculosis, histoplasmosis, aspergillosis, coccidioidomycosis, amoebiasis, *Candida albicans* infection, *Trypanosoma cruzii* infection, herpes simplex and zoster infection, and *Nocardia* asteroides. Geographical differences account for variations in local prevalence. Bacterial meningitis is rare in HIV-infected patients, and the treatment is the same as in immunocompetent individuals

COGNITIVE AND MOTOR SYNDROMES

Human Immunodeficiency Virus-1–Associated Major Cognitive or Motor Disorder

Clinical Presentation

This common CNS complication of HIV-1 infection occur in 15% of patients with AIDS and can be the first manifestation of the disease in 3% to 10%.[17] This condition has also been named AIDS dementia complex or HIV-1 encephalopathy. A less severe entity named HIV-1–associated minor cognitive/motor disorder occurs in an additional 20% to 25%. Risk factors include an AIDS-defining illness or anemia, the latter being a reflection of advanced disease.[18]

The clinical characteristics of this disorder can be subdivided into three main categories: cognitive, behavioral, and motor (Table 120-1).

Initial symptoms are usually subtle. Patients often complain of difficulty with memory and note a slowness of thinking. They have trouble concentrating. Complex mental activities become more time consuming and difficult to perform. A loss of interest for social and professional activities soon follows, and such apathy and social withdrawal may be mistaken for depression. Although cognitive and behavioral symptoms are prominent in most patients, some mainly present with motor dysfunction, which include decreased coordination, altered handwriting, loss of balance, and gait instability.

The mental status examination reveals minor psychomotor slowing, inattention, decreased short-term memory, inability to perform simple calculations, and frontal release signs. Ocular movements testing shows saccadic pursuit. Other frequent findings are brisk reflexes, mild postural tremor, slowing of rapid alternating movements, and gait instability when performing half-turns. If untreated, dementia becomes more global, profoundly impairing orientation, memory, and cognition. Confusional or psychotic episodes have been reported, but seizures are a rare occurrence. Despite the extent of the cerebral involvement, there usually is no aphasia, apraxia, or other signs of discrete cortical dysfunction, except in terminal stages. Therefore, this syndrome has been classified as a frontal-subcortical dementia. A rapid bedside evaluation can be performed with the HIV-1 dementia scale.[19] A more detailed neuropsychologic evaluation should include tests of attention, memory, and psychomotor speed such as trail making, digit span, verbal fluency, grooved pegboard, symbol digit modalities, and Rey auditory verbal learning tests.[20]

Laboratory Investigations

Numerous groups have detected early neurologic dysfunction in HIV-1–infected asymptomatic individuals.[21-23] Subtle electrophysiologic abnormalities can be found in early HIV-1 infection (on electroen-

TABLE 120-1 Clinical Triad in Human Immunodeficiency Virus-1–Associated Cognitive/Motor Disorder

Cognition	*Behavioral*	*Motor*
Forgetfulness	Apathy	Gait instability
Mental slowing	Social withdrawal	Poor coordination
Decreased concentration	Lack of spontaneity	Leg weakness

cephalography, evoked potentials, nerve conduction studies), but they do not seem to have a predictive value for the later onset of AIDS dementia, which occurs generally when the CD4+ T-lymphocyte counts is less than 200/µL. CSF analysis shows mild lymphocytic pleocytosis in 25% and elevated protein in 55%,[24] which can also be found in nondemented patients. Increased CSF levels of nonspecific markers of immune activation (β_2-microglobulin, neopterin, and quinolinic acid) and cytokines (tumor necrosis factor [TNF]-α, interleukin [IL]-1, and IL-6) have been reported, but their use in the clinical setting is limited because these markers are also elevated during opportunistic infections of the CNS and because these assays are not readily available in the clinical setting.

Measurement of the HIV-1 CSF viral load has been evaluated as a surrogate marker in HIV-1–infected individuals with cognitive dysfunction. An elevated CSF HIV-1 viral load greater than 1000 copies/mL was associated with AIDS dementia but only in patients with CD4+ T-lymphocyte counts less than 200 µL,[25-28] whereas plasma HIV-1 viral load was not. However, a wide overlap was found between CSF HIV-1 viral load values of demented and nondemented individuals, and concomitant opportunistic infections of the CNS must be ruled out as they also contribute to transient elevation of HIV-1 viral burden in the CSF.[29] These findings suggest that there may be two phases of HIV-1 infection in the CSF. (1) A transitory infection of the CNS may occur early in the disease via trafficking lymphocytes. These viral strains have a lymphotropic phenotype (using CXCR4 co-receptor) and may respond to therapy in parallel to plasma infection. (2) A more autonomous infection of CNS monocytes/macrophages may take place at a later stage, with macrophage tropic strains (using CCR5 co-receptor).[30] Such patients may need higher drug penetration in the CNS. Whether measurement of the HIV-1 CSF viral load provides an accurate representation of the viral replication occurring within the CNS is unclear. Brain HIV-1 RNA levels are higher than CSF and were found to correlate with CSF values in patients with dementia. However, nondemented patients had identical brain HIV-1 RNA levels as demented patients.[26,31] Sampling differences may account for some of these discrepancies.

Because HIV-1–associated dementia complex is a diagnosis of exclusion, CSF examination is indicated for bacterial, fungal, and acid-fast bacteria cultures, cryptococcal antigen, VDRL, and cytology. In addition, CSF polymerase chain reaction (PCR) for JC virus (JCV), the agent of progressive multifocal leukoencephalopathy (PML), is indicated because this condition is often difficult to distinguish from HIV-1 encephalopathy on brain imaging studies (see later and see Chapter 141).

Imaging Studies

Computed tomography (CT) and magnetic resonance imaging (MRI) may show subcortical greater than cortical atrophy, which is not proportional to the degree of dementia. The MRI may also demonstrate multiple hyperintense signals in T2-weighted images, which are nonenhancing, ill demarcated, and localized bilaterally in the subcortical white matter (Fig. 120-1). MRI is superior to CT scanning to distinguish these abnormalities from confounding illnesses such as PML. Unlike lesions of PML, there is no associated hypointensity in T1-weighted images. However, these MRI findings are not always correlated with decreased performance on neuropsychologic tests and cannot be used to predict the clinical course of patients with dementia.[32]

Finally, metabolic abnormalities have also been detected in the brain of patients with HIV-1[33] and correlate with the severity of AIDS

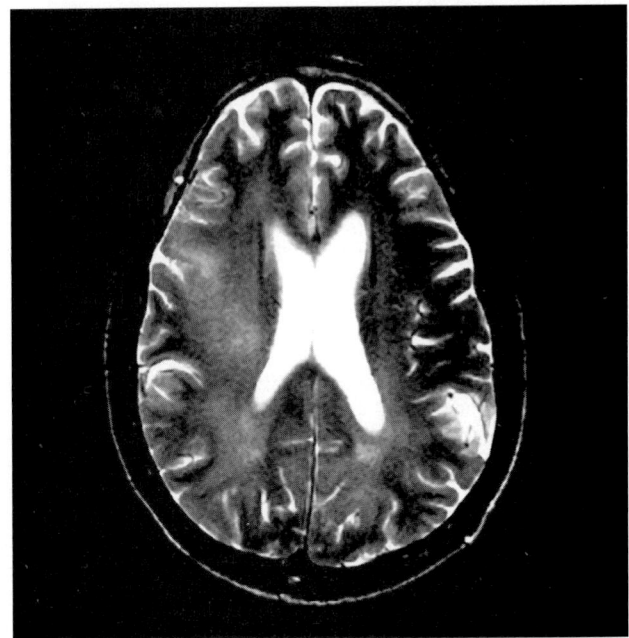

A

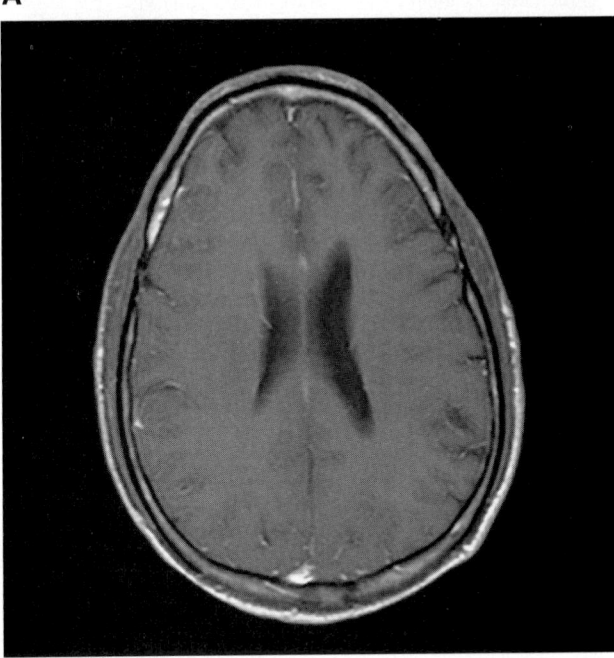

B

FIGURE 120-1. Brain magnetic resonance images of a 42-year-old man with acquired immunodeficiency syndrome dementia. The T2-weighted image **(A)** shows bilateral, ill-defined hyperintense signal in the periventricular white matter and centrum semiovale, which do not enhance with gadolinium injection on the T1-weighted image **(B)**. The ventricles are slightly enlarged, consistent with subcortical atrophy.

dementia using proton magnetic resonance spectroscopy (^{1}H-MRS).[34] These changes were reversible on HAART, paralleling improvement of cognitive functioning in patients with mild dementia.[35] Because cognitive deficits often persist after suppression of HIV-1 replication in the CSF on antiretroviral treatment, ^{1}H-MRS may become a useful surrogate marker of the effect of treatment in HIV-1–infected patients with dementia.

Brain Biopsy and Histologic Analysis

There is no indication to perform a brain biopsy in patients with AIDS dementia, unless imaging studies suggest the presence of another process. Postmortem examination reveals an encephalitis with multinucleated giant cells and microglial nodules, as well as astrocytosis and perivascular mononuclear cell infiltrates. HIV-1 has been found in microglial nodules, perivascular macrophages, and multinucleated giant cells. The latter are the result of the fusion of infected macrophages. HIV-1 has also been found in endothelial cells,[36] and abnormalities of the cerebral microcirculation are characterized by increased cellularity and pleomorphism of endothelial cells, as well as prominent perivascular aggregates of HIV-infected macrophages. These findings are sometimes related to microinfarcts and are postulated to give rise to increased vascular permeability.[37] Indeed, early enhancement has been detected in the basal ganglia in patients with AIDS dementia, suggesting a disruption of the blood-brain barrier (BBB) in these regions.[38] HIV-1 does not infect glial cells in adults, whereas a limited expression of viral regulatory gene products has been demonstrated in glial cells from children with AIDS.[39] White matter pallor involving primarily the centrum semiovale is a hallmark of HIV-1 encephalopathy in adults, which may be caused by seepage of macromolecules and edema fluid in the brain parenchyma through a permeable BBB and may cause injury to the myelinated fibers. Finally, HIV-1 does not infect neurons. Therefore, quantitative neuronal loss, reduction of cell size, or dendritic injury found in the cortex of demented patients[40] must be explained otherwise.

A major pathogenetic mechanisms of AIDS dementia consist of production of cytokines and toxins such as TNF-α, IL2, IL-6, matrix metallo-proteinase-2, -7, and -9, L-cysteine, and neurotoxin by infected microglial cells (see review[41]). Some of these substances are responsible for the activation of the N-methyl-D-aspartate (NMDA) receptors that mediate the excitatory transmission in the brain.[42,43] Indeed, the severity of dementia correlated best with the density of activated macrophages and microglial cells in the brain, rather than the viral burden within these cells.[32,44] Other contributory factors include potential toxicity of the viral proteins gp120[45] or tat.[46] Despite these studies, a unifying explanation of the pathogenesis of AIDS dementia is still lacking, because many laboratory personnel have also observed few neuropathologic changes in some patients with clinical evidence of severe dementia. A summary of the contributing factors to AIDS dementia is shown in Table 120-2.

Treatment

Although the pathophysiology of AIDS dementia is not entirely elucidated, HIV-1 remains the main triggering factor, and it is therefore reasonable to prevent viral replication within the CNS. However, antiretroviral drugs have variable penetration through the BBB, and evaluation of CNS concentration and pharmacokinetics of these medications is incomplete.[47] Zidovudine (AZT) has the highest CSF/plasma ratio of all antiretroviral drugs, and at doses of 1000 to 2000 mg/day, this drug has been shown to induce clear improvement in patients with HIV-1–associated dementia, after 16 weeks of treatment compared with placebo,[48] and a declining incidence of AIDS dementia was documented after its introduction.[49] However, other studies showed that the benefits of AZT monotherapy were time limited (see

---

TABLE 120-2 Pathogenesis of Acquired Immunodeficiency Syndrome Dementia

Microvascular abnormalities with infarcts and alteration of the blood-brain barrier
Productive human immunodeficiency virus (HIV)-1 infection of brain macrophages
Macrophages activation and production of cytokines (TNF-α, IL-l, IL-6)
Synthesis of nitric oxide
Activation of N-methyl-D-aspartate receptors
Neurotoxicity of HIV-1 gp120 and tat proteins

IL, interleukin; TNF, tumor necrosis factor.

---

review[50]). In any event, such high doses are not currently administered to patients because they cause myelosuppression with anemia and leukopenia. Other nucleoside analogue reverse transcriptase inhibitors (NRTIs) with documented penetration through the BBB include stavudine (d4T), which also causes peripheral neuropathy, and abacavir. Abacavir, added to the best background antiretroviral therapy, was not superior to placebo, but these patients were already on HAART and generally had advanced disease.[51]

Among non-nucleoside analogue reverse transcriptase inhibitors (NNRTIs), nevirapine has a better penetration through the BBB than efavirenz, although both improved CNS function as determined by electrophysiologic motor tests in patients with psychomotor slowing, when added to two NRTIs.[52] A trend toward better results with nevirapine compared with efavirenz did not reach statistical significance.

Since 1996, the availability of protease inhibitors (PIs) and the use of three or more drugs in HAART regimens have made a major impact on the incidence of neurologic disease in HIV-1–infected patients.[13,53,54] This is somewhat surprising; PIs in general have very low CSF/plasma ratio because they are highly protein bound. Of all PIs, indinavir has the highest penetration through the BBB and can even be increased by low doses of ritonavir.[55,56] Nevertheless, compared with the early 1990s, the incidence of AIDS dementia has declined by approximately 50%.[13] Because patients on HAART survive longer, the prevalence of AIDS dementia has remained stable, and more cases of AIDS dementia now have CD4+ T-cell counts greater than 200/μL. Therefore, risk factors for AIDS dementia in the HAART era need to be reevaluated.

Although HAART is now the treatment of choice for advanced HIV-1 disease, the optimal drug combination for AIDS dementia has not been established. In a small series of untreated patients who started on HAART, improvement of neuropsychological scores were associated with decrease in CSF HIV-1 viral load at 4 and 8 weeks, and those patients treated with zidovudine and indinavir had a greater improvement in neuropsychologic scores compared to those treated with other drugs.[57] HAART also improves HIV-1–associated motor slowing.[58] Whether regimens containing several drugs with good penetration through the BBB were advantageous has been investigated. However, moderately immunosuppressed patients (CD4+ T-lymphocyte counts around 300/μL) who took either one or multiple CSF-penetrating drugs (zidovudine, stavudine, abacavir, nevirapine, and indinavir) had similar increases in psychomotor speed and CD4+ T-cell counts, and decreases in HIV-1 plasma viral load, although CSF HIV-1 viral loads were not measured.[59] In HAART-experienced patients with CD4+ T-cell counts below 200/μL, those who received multiple CSF penetrating agents had a greater reduction of CSF HIV-1 RNA,[60,61] probably because of the presence of resistant mutants in that compartment.

This hypothesis is confirmed by the analysis of HIV-1 genotypes in paired plasma and CSF samples. Mutations of the reverse transcriptase (RT) and protease genes of CSF strains but not in the corresponding blood isolates were detected in 10 of 23 subjects (43%). Interestingly, mutations conferring resistance to low or high CSF-penetrating agents occurred at similar frequencies.[62] RT mutation patterns differed in 14 of 21 (67%) paired samples from plasma and CSF in one study, and HIV-1 RNA responses and RT genotypes were discordant between CSF and plasma in some subjects.[51,63] In a study of HIV-infected children starting on antiretroviral therapy, 8 of 11 had identical resistance patterns in both CSF and plasma at baseline, whereas at week 48 of treatment, only 1 of 9 children had similar genotypes, suggesting discordant viral evolution in these two compartments.[64] Whether occurrence of drug resistance mutations restricted to CSF strains is associated with an increase of the CSF HIV-1 viral load and worsening of cognitive and motor functioning needs to be studied prospectively. Failure to recognize the occurrence of different genotypic resistance patterns in plasma and CSF may lead to uncontrolled viral replication in the CNS, and worsening neurologic symptoms despite evidence of viral clearance in the periphery. These resistant isolates may, in turn, spill back into the circulation and contribute to the progression of HIV-1 disease. Therefore, genotypic analysis of CSF HIV-1 strains is indicated in patients with cognitive dysfunction who have good virologic response to HAART in the plasma but persistence of an elevated HIV-1 CSF viral load.

In addition to antiretroviral treatment, other experimental compounds have been tested for the treatment of AIDS dementia but so far without evidence of clear benefit. These include a calcium channel blockers (nimodipine), antioxidants (vitamin E, thiotic acid, CPI-1189), a TNF-α antagonist (pentoxifylline), and peptide T. Selegiline, a selective monoamine oxidase type B inhibitor, given at low doses (3.5 mg orally 3 times a week) for its potential antiapoptotic properties, improved scores of verbal memory in one study.[65] Memantine, a noncompetitive NMDA inhibitor, is being evaluated.

CENTRAL NERVOUS SYSTEM MASS LESIONS

Patients with AIDS presenting with change of mental status or an abnormal neurologic examination frequently have brain lesions on CT or MRI. These can be quite extensive and may represent life-threatening emergencies.

Toxoplasma Encephalitis

At the beginning of the AIDS epidemic, *Toxoplasma* encephalitis (TE) was the most common cerebral mass lesion in patients with AIDS. TE is caused by a reactivation of latent infection by the protozoan *Toxoplasma gondii* as a result of progressive loss of cellular immunity. In the United States, where the incidence of seropositivity for *T. gondii* is around 30% in the adult population, TE formerly developed in 3% to 10% of patients with AIDS.[66] In Europe and Africa, where the overall seroprevalence is higher, up to 25% to 50% of patients with AIDS presented with this condition. The incidence of TE has decreased initially thanks to widespread prophylaxis for *Pneumocystis carinii* pneumonia using trimethoprim-sulfamethoxazole, which also prevents CNS toxoplasmosis.[67] Since the era of HAART, there has been a further trend for a decreased incidence of this condition,[13] and it accounted for only 28% of focal brain lesions occurring in patients with AIDS in 1998.[68]

Clinical Presentation

Almost 90% of patients have CD4$^+$ T-lymphocyte counts less than 200/μL, and 75% have CD4$^+$ counts less than 100/μL at the time of clinical presentation. The most common symptoms include headache, confusion, fever, and lethargy. Up to 30% develop seizures.[69] Seventy percent of patients have focal signs on the neurologic examination, such as hemiparesis, cranial nerve palsies, ataxia, and sensory deficits. The clinical presentation is usually subacute, ranging from a few days to a month (see Chapter 276).

Laboratory Investigations

As is the case in the general population, serum anti-*Toxoplasma* IgG antibodies can be detected in patients with TE, whereas IgM antibodies are rarely found, supporting the notion that most cases represent a reactivation of latent infection. Measurement of antibody titers is not helpful to establish the diagnosis. By enzyme-linked immunosorbent assay (ELISA), only 7% of patients known to be seropositive for *T. gondii* had lost their antibodies at the time of presentation.[66] Therefore, a negative serology orients toward another entity, whereas a positive serology is not diagnostic (see Chapter 276).

A mild elevation of CSF protein concentration and a moderate mononucleated pleocytosis (<60 cells/mm³) are common, but nonspecific, and may be due to the underlying HIV-1 infection. A slight decrease of the CSF glucose has been reported but is not a constant finding. The PCR technique has been less useful for detection of *T. gondii* DNA in the CSF compared with other pathogens, with a sensitivity of only 44% to 65% and a specificity of 100%.[70] However, this low sensitivity may be improved by the use of stage-specific PCR primers.[71] CSF analysis is therefore more useful to rule out other infectious processes than to confirm the diagnosis of TE.

Imaging Studies

Neuroimaging by head CT or MRI demonstrates CNS lesions in almost all cases, with the exception of the rare diffuse encephalitic form of toxoplasmosis. Lesions are multiple in two thirds of the cases, and 90% of them display ring enhancement after administration of contrast material. The MRI is more sensitive than the CT to detect multiple lesions. These are generally localized at the corticomedullar junction, in the white matter, or the basal ganglia; and are surrounded by edema; and induce mass effect on surrounding structures (Fig. 120-2). Unfortunately, the neuroradiologic characteristics of TE are not pathognomonic and may be observed in other conditions such as primary CNS lymphoma (PCNSL) (see later).

Brain Biopsy

Because of the good response to therapy, histologic examination is not required for the diagnosis of TE, and an empiric therapeutic trial is recommended, when the clinical and radiologic findings are consistent with this diagnosis. Histologic examination shows mainly necrotic abscesses with blood vessel thrombosis and necrosis. Cysts containing bradyzoites, the dormant form of *T. gondii*, coexist with numerous active tachyzoites.

Treatment

Treatment consists of a combination of pyrimethamine and sulfadiazine, which cause a synergistic and sequential block on the folic acid metabolism necessary for the development of the parasite. Standard acute therapy consist of 200 mg of pyrimethamine orally the first day of treatment, followed by 75 mg/day orally, sulfadiazine 6 g/day orally in four divided doses, and folinic acid 10 to 50 mg/day orally for 6 weeks.

Clindamycin 600 mg intravenously or 450 mg orally 4 times a day is an adequate alternative to sulfadiazine in the previous regimen for patients allergic to sulfonamides. Side effects, which consist of cytopenia, rashes, diarrhea, and elevated liver enzymes, have been reported in 40% to 70% of patients receiving pyrimethamine and sulfadiazine and in 36% of those receiving pyrimethamine and clindamycin. These can cause early discontinuation of therapy. Azithromycin 1200 to 1500 mg orally once a day or atovaquone 750 mg orally 4 times a day can be also combined with pyrimethamine and folinic acid. Although corticosteroids are frequently prescribed to diminish cerebral edema, their use has not been shown to be either beneficial or harmful in TE.[72] Because high doses of steroids also reduce the size of CNS lymphoma lesions, they should be administered only in cases with impending cerebral herniation during the initial medical treatment of presumed TE, to not cloud the diagnosis. Neurologic improvement is clinically apparent in more than half the cases by day 3 of therapy and in most cases by day 7. A failure to improve or a worsening of the symptoms should prompt repeat imaging studies by days 10 to 14, to determine the need of a brain biopsy.

Secondary Prophylaxis

T. gondii is sensitive to treatment only when in tachyzoite form. Because dormant cystic forms may rupture and reinitiate the infectious process at any time, maintenance therapy is necessary to prevent a relapse, which is likely to occur after a delay of 6 to 8 weeks of interruption of treatment. Standard maintenance therapy consists of pyrimethamine 25 to75 mg/day with folinic acid 10 mg daily and either sulfadiazine 2 to 4 g/day in four divided doses or clindamycin 300 mg orally 4 times a day or 450 mg orally 3 times a day. Patients with sustained CD4$^+$ T-cell counts above 200/μL for more than 3 months can discontinue their secondary prophylaxis.[73]

If the diagnosis is made in a timely fashion and the patient does not become intolerant to the treatment, TE is currently an opportunistic infection with a relatively high therapeutic success rate, and death is usually caused by other complications of AIDS.

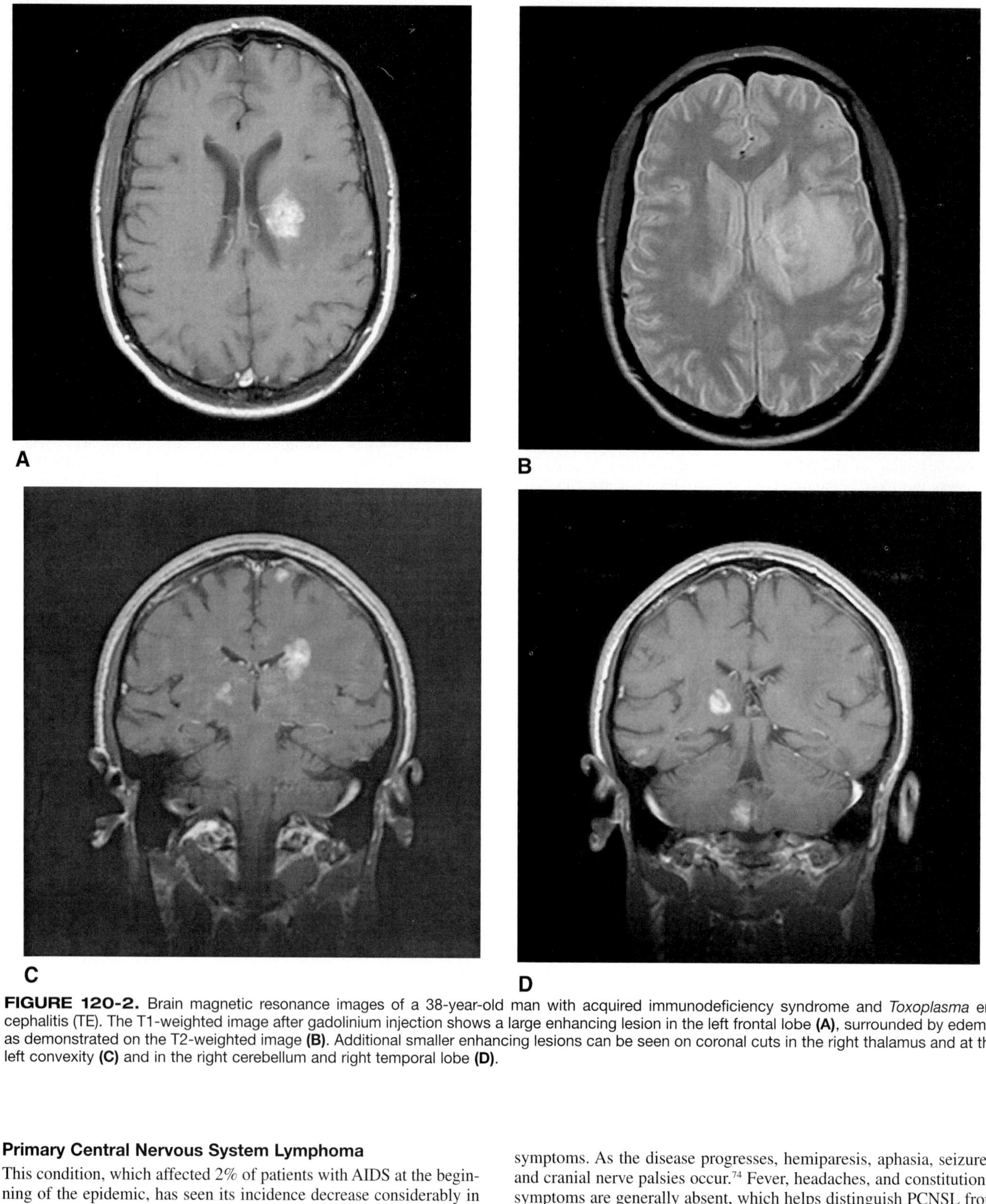

FIGURE 120-2. Brain magnetic resonance images of a 38-year-old man with acquired immunodeficiency syndrome and *Toxoplasma* encephalitis (TE). The T1-weighted image after gadolinium injection shows a large enhancing lesion in the left frontal lobe **(A)**, surrounded by edema, as demonstrated on the T2-weighted image **(B)**. Additional smaller enhancing lesions can be seen on coronal cuts in the right thalamus and at the left convexity **(C)** and in the right cerebellum and right temporal lobe **(D)**.

Primary Central Nervous System Lymphoma

This condition, which affected 2% of patients with AIDS at the beginning of the epidemic, has seen its incidence decrease considerably in the HAART era.[13] In 1998, it accounted for only 12% of AIDS-related focal brain lesions.[68] Its radiographic appearance makes it the principal differential diagnosis of TE.

Clinical Presentation

The onset of symptoms is generally subacute, lasting weeks to months. Confusion, lethargy, and memory loss are the most frequent symptoms. As the disease progresses, hemiparesis, aphasia, seizures, and cranial nerve palsies occur.[74] Fever, headaches, and constitutional symptoms are generally absent, which helps distinguish PCNSL from TE. At the time of diagnosis, the average CD4+ T-lymphocyte counts are usually very low, around 50/μL.

Laboratory Investigations

A mild mononuclear pleocytosis (<30 cells/μL), and elevation of the protein concentration in the CSF is a common finding in patients with PCNSL but is nonspecific and may be due to the underlying HIV-1 infection. High protein levels (up to 590 mg/dL) have been reported in patients with extensive lymphomatous infiltration of both cerebral hemispheres. Hypoglycorrhachia is a rare finding.

It is important to perform cytologic analysis of the CSF because the presence of atypical or malignant lymphomatous cells can establish the diagnosis. Systemic extracerebral lymphomas, which have an increased incidence in AIDS patients, can also cause lymphomatous meningitis but do not generally spread to the brain itself. Similarly, PCNSL do not metastasize systemically. Epstein-Barr virus (EBV) genome can be detected in tumor cells of nearly all primary central nervous system lymphoma, but only in some systemic lymphoma of AIDS patients, and rarely in primary brain lymphoma tissue from patients without immunodeficiency.[75] Detection of EBV DNA by PCR in the CSF has a sensitivity of 80% to 90% and a specificity of 87% to 98% for the diagnosis of PCNSL. Measurement of the EBV CSF viral load by quantified PCR in the CSF may improve the sensitivity of this test and be clinically useful in monitoring responses to treatment.[76]

Imaging Studies

The head CT or MRI usually shows findings consistent with a CNS tumor. Solitary mass lesions are as frequent as multiple lesions.[74] Most lesions display some degree of enhancement, which is usually nodular or patchy. Ring enhancement, identical to that commonly seen in TE, can occur and correlate with central tumor necrosis. Subependymal enhancement seems more specific of CNS lymphoma, but this is a rare feature. Lesions are frequently located in the corpus callosum, the periventricular white matter, or the cortex. Involvement of the posterior fossa occurs only in 10% of cases.[77] Lesions can be surrounded by edema and may induce variable mass effect on neighboring structures[78] (Fig. 120-3). MRI is more sensitive than CT in revealing multiple lesions, which can be useful if a biopsy is being considered. Thallium-201 single photon emission CT (SPECT) shows an accumulation of isotope in the tumor due to increased metabolic activity.[79] However the usefulness of this method in differentiating CNS lymphoma from opportunistic infections may depend heavily on the resolution of the images and appropriate technology may not be available in every center.

Brain Biopsy

If the CSF cytology fails to reveal lymphomatous cells and if EBV PCR is negative in the CSF, an image-guided stereotactic brain biopsy using CT or MRI is the only way to ascertain the diagnosis. The macroscopic appearance of these tumors is generally that of a multifocal, diffusely infiltrating and expanding nonhemorrhagic mass, without well-demarcated borders, simulating the appearance of an infiltrating glioma. However, well-circumscribed, largely necrotic masses can also look like abscesses. Microscopic analysis reveals a variety of patterns, including large cells, small noncleaved cells, immunoblastic, or mixed cellular components. These are generally of B-lymphocyte lineage. EBV is present in tumor cells, suggesting that this virus may has a role in tumorigenesis,[80] as is the case in Burkitt's lymphoma and in nasopharyngeal carcinoma.

Treatment

The response to steroids seen in lymphomas of non-AIDS patients is not always seen in AIDS patients. In patients with altered mental status, debilitating focal symptoms, or impending herniation, dexamethasone 10 mg intravenously or orally followed by 4 mg intravenously or orally every 6 hours can provide a temporary improvement. The treatment of CNS lymphoma in AIDS consists of whole brain irradiation with a total of 3000 cGy of over a 3-week period. Steroids are added to decrease peritumoral edema and mass effect.[77] The palliative response rate before the HAART era was 53%.[81] Combination treatment including radiation and chemotherapy is difficult to tolerate because of high toxicity. A pilot trial using a combination of zidovudine, ganciclovir, and IL-2 showed promising results.[82] In any event, recent data showed that immune recovery induced by HAART leads to dramatic improvement in survival of patients with AIDS-associated PCNSL.[83]

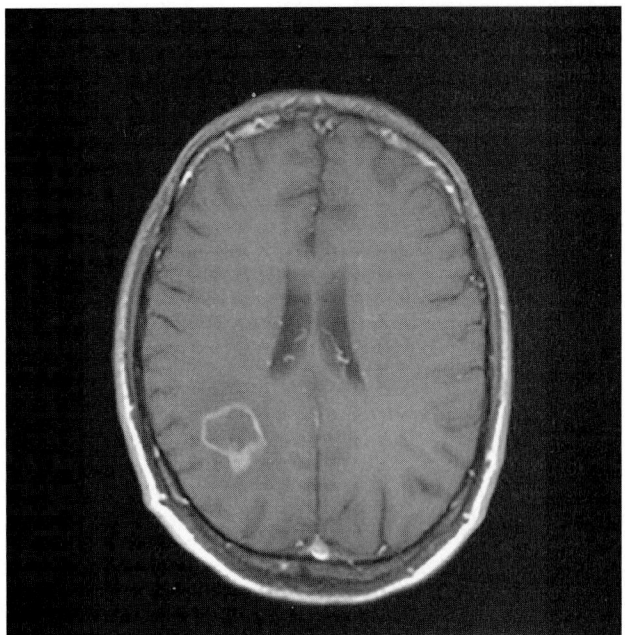

A

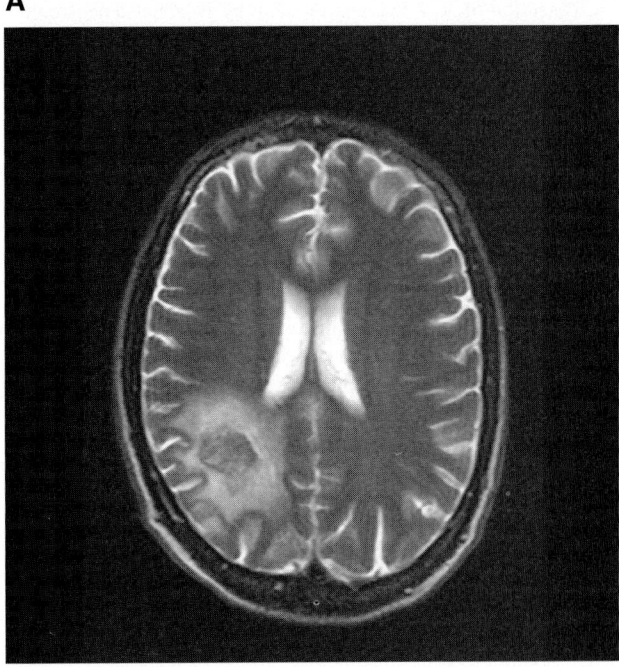

B

FIGURE 120-3. Brain magnetic resonance images of a 50-year-old man with primary central nervous system lymphoma. A 2-cm ring-enhancing lesion is present in the right parietal lobe, surrounded by edema **(A)**. The T2-weighted image shows low signal intensity centrally, which is more consistent with cellular proliferation than with an infectious process **(B)**.

Progressive Multifocal Leukoencephalopathy

Before the AIDS era, PML was a rare disease affecting mainly patients with chronic lymphocytic leukemia, non-Hodgkin's lymphoma or organ transplant recipients.[84] At the beginning of the AIDS epidemic, up to 5% of patients developed PML.[85] Interestingly, the incidence of PML has not decreased since the availability of HAART[13] and has shown even a slight increase. Indeed, up to 28% of focal brain lesions in AIDS were attributed to PML in 1998,[68] which equals cases of TE.

PML is caused by the polyomavirus JCV. This double-stranded DNA virus infects 90% of the normal adult population worldwide and remains quiescent in the kidneys without causing any disease. In the setting of immunosuppression, JCV is reactivated and induces a lytic infection of oligodendrocytes, causing multifocal demyelination of the CNS (see Chapter 141).

Clinical Presentation

PML usually develops when CD4+ T-lymphocyte counts drop below 200/μL.[85] The most common presenting symptoms are limb weakness (hemiparesis or monoparesis), altered mental status, gait ataxia, and visual symptoms, including hemianopsia, diplopia, and third nerve palsy. Approximately 80% of patients have focal neurologic findings.[86] However, PML lesions can occur anywhere in the CNS white matter, particularly at the subcortical level. Because subcortical lesions prevent the transmission of information to and from the cortical areas, presentation implying cerebral cortical dysfunction such as aphasia, apraxia, memory loss, visual agnosia, or seizures does not rule out this diagnosis. Some symptoms can also be attributed to AIDS dementia, which is often superimposed on other CNS pathologies in the end stages of AIDS.

Laboratory Investigations

Conventional CSF analysis either is normal or shows a moderate increase of protein concentration and a mild mononucleated pleocytosis (<25 cells/mm^3), which is nonspecific in the context of HIV-1 infection. Detection of JCV DNA in the CSF by PCR has a sensitivity of 74% to 92% and a specificity of 92% to 96% for the diagnosis of PML.[87,88] Measurement of JCV viral load in the CSF appears to be of value as a correlate of PML disease activity and survival.[88,89,90]

Imaging Studies

The hallmark of PML is patchy or confluent areas of low attenuation on CT or hyperintensity of T2-weighted images on MRI (Fig. 120-4). The MRI is twice as sensitive as CT in distinguishing multiple lesions. These generally do not enhance after administration of contrast material, and they are not surrounded by edema, and hence, substantial mass effect on surrounding structures is absent. However, 8% of lesions can show faint, peripheral, and irregular enhancement. Lesions are usually bilateral, asymmetric, well demarcated, and localized preferentially in the periventricular areas and the subcortical white matter.[91] Involvement of the deep gray structures, including basal ganglia and thalamus, can nevertheless be found in up to 17% of cases. A normal CT or MRI does not rule out PML because microscopic lesions might be smaller than the power of resolution of these tests. One such case showed multiple, small foci of demyelination disseminated among the cortical U fibers at autopsy.[92] HIV-1 encephalopathy can be easily mistaken for PML on brain imaging studies. As in PML, white matter lesions without mass effect or contrast enhancement are the radiologic hallmarks of this disease. However, HIV-1 encephalopathy lesions tend to be symmetric and less clearly demarcated than the lesions of PML, and they are not associated with focal neurologic deficits.[1] H-MRS and magnetization transfer studies have shown a promising potential in differentiating PML lesions from HIV-1 encephalopathy.[93] The typical ^{1}H-MRS pattern in PML lesions include decreased N-acetylaspartate/creatine ratio consistent with axonal compromise, increased choline/creatine ratio, indicating cell membrane breakdown and turnover, and occasional elevation of lipid/lactate and *myo*-inositol.[94-96] In one study, patients who had the longest survival had the highest *myo*-inositol, consistent with glial activity and inflammation in PML lesions.[94] Metabolic alterations consistent with inflammation detected on ^{1}H-MRS in PML lesions are associated with a cellular immune response against JCV. This inflammatory reaction, occurring early after disease onset, appears to be instrumental in the containment of PML.[97]

Brain Biopsy

A brain biopsy may be necessary to establish the diagnosis of PML, when the JC viral load is to low to be detected by PCR in the CSF.[98] Such cases have become more frequent in the era of HAART.[68]

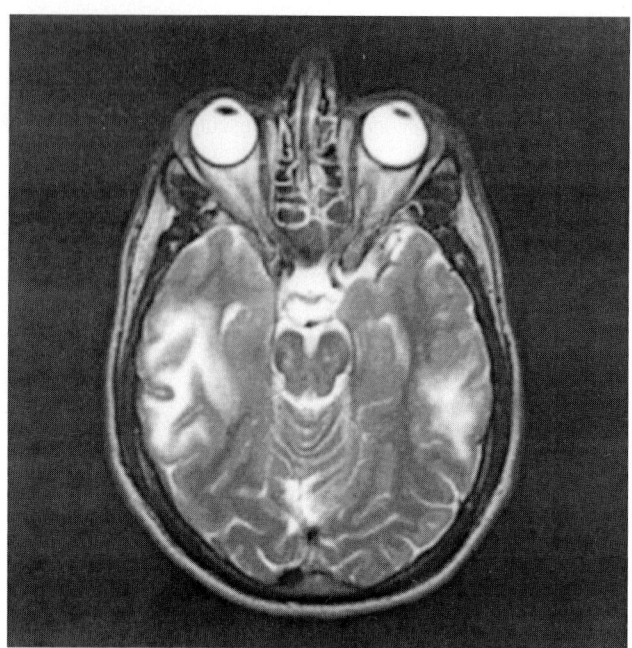

A

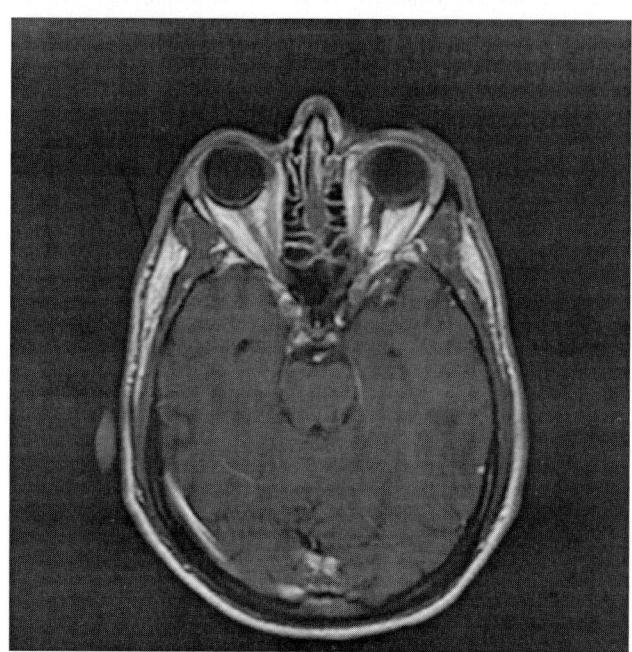

B

FIGURE 120-4. Brain magnetic resonance images of a 43-year-old man with progressive multifocal leukoencephalopathy. Prominent areas of high signal intensity are present in the subcortical white matter of both temporoparietal lobes on T2-weighted images **(A)**. The affected areas are hypointense on T1-weighted images, do not enhance with gadolinium, and are not associated with mass effect or edema **(B)**.

Histologic examination shows areas of demyelination as well as large, hyperchromatic oligodendrocytic nuclei that stain positively for JCV by immunohistochemistry and contain large amounts of JC virions detectable by electron microscopy. Other histologic features of PML include large, bizarre astrocytes with lobulated nuclei and lipid-laden macrophages engaged in removing myelin breakdown products. Rare cases that have a more protracted course may have a detectable perivascular lymphocytic infiltrate.

Treatment

There is no specific treatment for PML. Numerous therapeutic attempts in HIV-infected patients included cytosine arabinoside (Ara-C),[99] interferon-α,[100] topotecan,[101] and cidofovir,[102] but none showed any benefit compared to antiretroviral treatment alone. However, Ara-C, which has been shown to have antiviral effect in vitro,[103] helped stabilize 36% of HIV-negative PML patients in a retrospective study.[104] New systems of drug delivery to the brain[105] might be necessary to improve specific treatment in patients with AIDS and PML.

It is important to realize that there is a large diversity in the natural evolution of PML. In patients with AIDS who are profoundly immunosuppressed, the course of the disease used to be rapidly progressive, leading to death within 2 to 4 months from the time of symptom presentation. However, approximately 10% of patients had a protracted course and survived more than a year. Since the HAART era, median survival has increased to 10.5 months,[106] and half of the patients survive PML, although some have devastating neurologic sequelae. Predictive factors for longer survival include CD4$^+$ T-lymphocyte counts above 300/μL at disease onset, contrast enhancement on brain imaging studies, presence of a mononucleated perivascular inflammatory infiltrate in the PML lesions, absence of brain stem involvement, and PML heralding AIDS.[107] Study of the cellular immune response against JCV showed that detection of JCV-specific cytotoxic T lymphocytes in the peripheral blood mononuclear cells (PBMCs) of HIV-infected patients with PML was associated with long-term survival, whereas those with undetectable cellular immune responses against the virus had a progressive neurologic disease and a fatal outcome.[108-110] Therefore, strategies aimed at boosting this immune response may prove useful for preventing uncontrolled replication of JCV and the spread of PML. For the time being, optimization of HAART and avoidance of immunosuppression remain the best available therapeutic option for patients with PML.

Recently, multiple investigators recognized inflammatory forms of PML, developing shortly after onset of HAART, concomitant to immune recovery. These patients have signs of inflammation in the CNS characterized by contrast-enhancing lesions on neuroimaging studies and/or inflammatory infiltrates on brain biopsy. It has been hypothesized that these inflammatory forms of PML may be a manifestation of HAART-induced immune reconstitution inflammatory syndrome (IRIS), and their outcome is usually favorable.[111] Therefore, clinicians should not disregard the diagnosis of PML in presence of contrast-enhancing brain lesions and should use caution before treating these immunosuppressed individuals with steroids.

Cytomegalovirus Encephalitis

Cytomegalovirus (CMV) may cause necrotizing focal encephalitis and ventriculoencephalitis.[112] It occurs in patients with CD4$^+$ counts of less than 50 cell/μL and is often concomitant with CMV infection of other organs, including retinitis, adrenalitis, and pneumonitis (see Chapter 134). The incidence of CMV disease, including cytomegalovirus encephalitis (CMVE), has decreased considerably since the availability of HAART.[113]

Clinical Presentation

Patients with CMVE show similar features to those with AIDS dementia but tend to have a more acute onset and more prominent confusion/disorientation or apathy/withdrawal. Hyponatremia and cranial nerve involvement, which are usually not present in AIDS dementia, are also helpful for establishing the diagnosis.[114]

Laboratory Investigations

The conventional CSF examination is generally nonspecific, because it is either normal or shows a mild protein elevation and mononucleated pleocytosis. CMV culture often remains negative. However, the detection of CMV DNA by PCR in the CSF is both very sensitive and specific.[115]

Imaging Studies

Focal necrotizing lesions associated with periventricular and meningeal enhancement or hydrocephalus may be seen on brain imaging studies.[116] Although MRI has a better resolution than CT scan, it often lacks sensitivity for diagnosing CMVE.[117]

Brain Biopsy

Microglial nodule encephalitis with CMV inclusions can be readily diagnosed by histologic examination. Interestingly, similar findings can be found at autopsy in 6% to 40% of patients with AIDS and dementia.[112] However, autopsy findings of CMV infection of the brain do not always correlate with the presence of cognitive dysfunction.

Treatment

The management of CMV encephalitis is difficult.[118] In one autopsy-confirmed series, half of the patients were taking maintenance doses of ganciclovir for treatment of CMV retinitis. CMV encephalitis developed in others during first full-dose inductions with ganciclovir or foscarnet for retinitis.[116] Treatment failures might be caused by acquired viral resistance to the medication.

The treatment is similar to that for CMV retinitis, with induction of ganciclovir 5 mg/kg/day intravenously every 12 hours for 14 days, followed by maintenance 5 mg/kg intravenously daily indefinitely, or foscarnet induction 90 mg/kg intravenously every 12 hours for 14 days, followed by maintenance 90 mg/kg/day indefinitely. Blood levels of oral valganciclovir at a dose of 900 mg are equivalent to those of intravenous ganciclovir at a dose of 5 mg/kg. The prognosis is usually poor, with median survival not exceeding 5 weeks. Therefore, combination therapy with ganciclovir and foscarnet at the doses mentioned earlier is justified. Patients who have failed or have become intolerant to these drugs may benefit from cidofovir 5 mg/kg/wk for 2 weeks, followed by 5 mg/kg every 2 weeks. This drug is nephrotoxic and should be given with intravenous hydration and high doses of probenecid before and after cidofovir injection.

Miscellaneous Mass Lesions and Rationale for Brain Biopsy

Brain biopsy used to be considered the gold standard for the diagnosis of CNS mass lesions in AIDS. The biopsy is the most specific, but not always the most sensitive, test. Indeed, sensitivities of 64% to 96% have been reported in AIDS patients. In addition, this procedure is not without significant risks in this patient population. Brain biopsy has a mortality rate of 0% to 3%, a major morbidity rate of 0.5% to 9%, and a minor morbidity rate of 2% to 4%.[119-122]

The brain biopsy is often impractical because of the location of the lesion. In addition, several disease processes can coincide in patients with multiple lesions, and multiple biopsies are rarely performed. Finally, change of therapy indicated by the result of the biopsy are not always possible in patient with advanced AIDS, and overall survival was improved by only a couple of months before the era of HAART.[120,122] The availability of molecular diagnosis by PCR in the CSF has considerably changed the management of these patients.

A decision analysis was performed on 136 consecutive HIV-1 patients presenting with mass lesions between 1991 and 1995.[121] Following 3 weeks of empiric therapy for TE, patients with progressive disease underwent a brain biopsy. CSF PCR amplification for *T. gondii*, EBV, and JCV DNA was performed in 66 patients. The presence or absence of mass effect surrounding the brain lesions, knowledge of the patient serologic status for *T. gondii,* and prophylactic regimen with trimethoprim-sulfamethoxazole, as well as PCR results were used in this analysis. The probability of TE was 0.87 in *Toxoplasma*-seropositive patients with mass effect who were not on trimethoprim-sulfamethoxazole but only 0.59 for those receiving prophylaxis. For *Toxoplasma*-seropositive patients receiving trimethoprim-sulfamethoxazole, the probability of PCNSL was 0.36. Conversely, in *Toxoplasma*-seronegative patients with mass effect, the likelihood of PCNSL was 0.74, which increased to 0.96 if EBV PCR was positive in the CSF. Among focal brain lesions without mass effect, the probability of PML was 0.81, which increased to 0.99 if JCV DNA was detected in the CSF.

Therefore, the brain biopsy is not needed to confirm a diagnosis of PML, and JCV PCR in the CSF is now being used as a diagnostic test and for inclusion of patients in treatment studies.[57] Bypassing the need for tissue diagnosis is more controversial in patients with suspicion of PCNSL, who have positive EBV PCR in the CSF. Because treatment consists of whole brain radiation, the risk of a false-positive PCR result has to be balanced with the risks of the brain biopsy and the fact that this technique does not always yield a definitive diagnosis.

An algorithm for the management of HIV-1–infected patients with CNS mass lesions is shown in Figure 120-5.

SPINAL SYNDROME

Myelopathy is a frequent finding at autopsy in patients with AIDS and is probably underrecognized clinically. It can be primarily HIV-1 associated or caused by other opportunistic infections or tumors.

Vacuolar Myelopathy

Vacuolar myelopathy (VM) is present in 17% to 46% of patients with AIDS at autopsy.[123-125] This disorder occurs with advanced immunosuppression, and the symptoms are often overlooked or attributed to debilitation.

Clinical Presentation

Symptoms are often overshadowed by coexisting central or peripheral nervous system impairment, such as AIDS dementia, which occurs late in the course of the disease.[123] Usually, patients complain of progressive, painless gait disturbance, weakness and sensory disturbances in the legs, as well as impotence in men, and urinary frequency and urgency. The evolution is usually progressive and leads to severe paralysis of the legs and loss of sphincter control. Neurologic signs include spastic paraparesis, hyperreflexia, extensor plantar responses, and mild sensory impairment, with vibratory and position sense being disproportionately affected. There is usually no associated sensory level.

Laboratory Investigations

CSF analysis is either normal or demonstrates mild elevation of protein and lymphocytosis frequently seen in HIV-1 infection.

Opposite to what is observed in AIDS dementia, the CSF HIV-1 viral load is not elevated in patients with VM.[126] CSF examination is however a useful test to rule out other treatable infections (see later).

Imaging Studies

The MRI of the spinal cord is usually normal in patients with VM. However, this examination is useful to rule out an extradural or intradural mass lesion or an epidural abscess.[127]

Histologic Studies

Because an anatomic diagnosis is not possible, VM remains a clinical diagnosis of exclusion. At autopsy, discrete or coalescent 10- to 100-μm vacuoles containing cellular debris or macrophages and, rarely, axonal swelling can be seen in the white matter of the spinal cord, involving principally the posterior and/or lateral columns. These lesions are usually symmetric and more frequent at the middle to lower thoracic levels. Vacuoles appear to be the result of focal swelling within the myelin sheath. Ultrastructural studies indicate both axonal and myelin injury,[128] although axonal destruction is seen only in areas of intense vacuolation. The etiology of VM is still unknown. Consistent with the absence of an elevated HIV-1 CSF viral load, immunohistochemistry studies did not demonstrate an association between HIV-1 antigens and vacuolar myelopathy.[124,129] Therefore, the role of HIV-1 may only be indirect. Because histologic findings are similar to those of subacute combined degeneration of the spinal cord and because patients with VM usually have normal serum levels of vitamin B_{12} and folic acid, it was suggested that abnormal metabolism of the vitamin B_{12}–dependent transmethylation pathway may be important in the pathogenesis of VM. Indeed, S-adenosylmethionine (SAM) and methionine were decreased in the CSF and serum of patients with VM, respectively.[130] The underlying cause of this metabolic disorder is unclear. Macrophage activation might generate substrates that are metabolized by methylation and therefore trigger a local deficit of methyl group donors in the spinal cord, leading to myelin vacuolization.

Treatment

An open-label pilot clinical trial suggested that patients with VM may benefit from supplements of L-methionine 3 g twice per day for 6

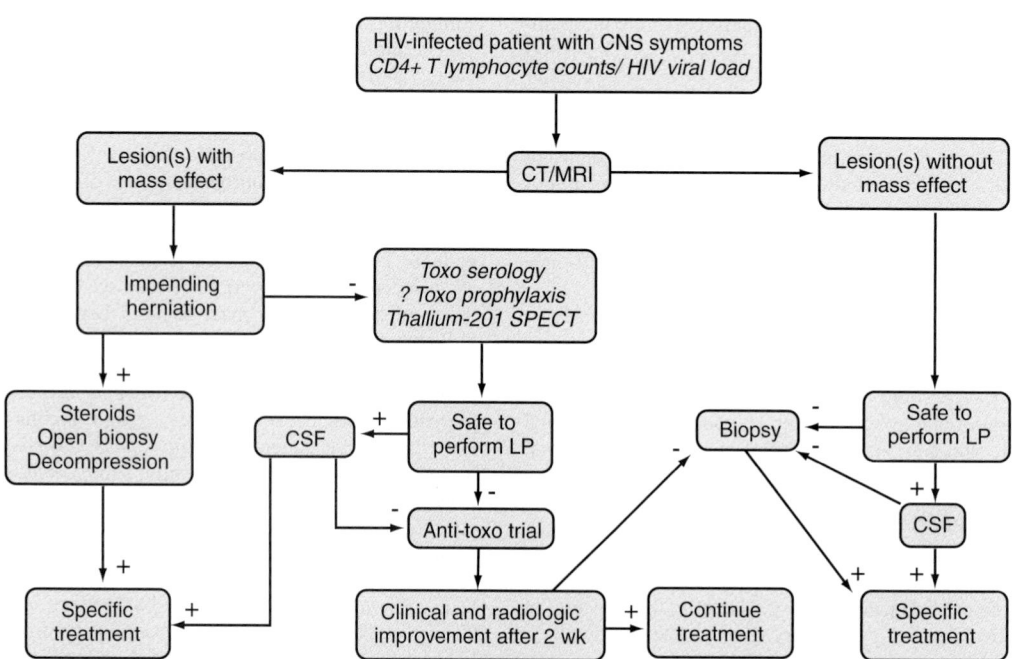

FIGURE 120-5. Management of the human immunodeficiency virus 1-infected patient with central nervous system mass lesions. The elements in italics represent data that contribute to the decision-making process (see text for details). CNS, central nervous system; CSF, cerebrospinal fluid; CT, computed tomography; HIV, human immunodeficiency virus; LP, lumbar puncture; MRI, magnetic resonance imaging; SPECT, single photon emission computerized tomography; toxo, *Toxoplasma* encephalitis.

months.[131] However, there are also reports indicating a role for HAART in the treatment of myelopathy in an antiretroviral-naïve HIV-infected patient,[132] and for the combination of lopinavir/ritonavir in an HAART-experienced patient.[133] Because there is no way to confirm the diagnosis of VM outside of a postmortem examination, it is possible that the patients who responded to various HAART formulations were rather affected by HIV-1 myelitis,[134] which has the same histologic features as HIV-1 encephalitis, and therefore may benefit from antiretroviral treatment.

Differential Diagnosis of a Noncompressive Myelopathy

Other etiologies of noncompressive myelopathy in patients with advanced HIV-1 infection include other viral infections such as CMV, varicella-zoster virus, and HSV types 1 and 2 as well as human T-cell lymphotropic virus type I (HTLV-I). HTLV-I is also transmitted sexually or through transfusion of cellular blood products and is the agent of a chronic spastic paraparesis called HTLV-I–associated myelopathy[135] (see Chapter 165). Syphilitic meningomyelitis and rare fungal or parasitic infections are diagnosed by appropriate serologies and cultures.[136]

PERIPHERAL NERVOUS SYSTEM SYNDROMES

Peripheral neuropathies have become the most common neurologic complication of HIV-infection. Neuropathies include several entities that are thought to be directly associated with HIV and occur at different stages of immunosuppression. Other forms are caused by opportunistic pathogens, such as CMV. Finally, the peripheral nervous system can also be affected by antiretroviral treatment toxicities.

Human Immunodeficiency Virus–Associated Neuropathies

Inflammatory Demyelinating Polyneuropathy

These entities can occur at the time of seroconversion, but are generally diagnosed in seropositive patients who are otherwise asymptomatic and not yet profoundly immunosuppressed although some cases have also been reported in late stages of the disease.[137] Acute inflammatory demyelinating polyneuropathy (AIDP) has clinical features similar to those of Guillain-Barré syndrome (GBS). Sensory symptoms such as paresthesias may precede an acute, progressive weakness of distal and proximal muscles of two or more limbs, associated with areflexia. Respiratory muscles may be involved, and patients sometimes require assisted ventilation.[138] Sensory signs are usually mild, even in the setting of severe weakness. The maximal weakness is usually reached within the first 4 weeks. Patients with a more protracted course are affected by the chronic form of inflammatory demyelinating polyneuropathy (CIDP), which may be monophasic or relapsing.[139] Recently, a severe case of AIDP was observed in a patient with advanced AIDS 4 weeks after starting on HAART, concomitant with immune reconstitution.[140] AIDP should therefore be included in the growing number of HAART-induced immune reconstitution inflammatory syndromes in HIV-infected individuals.

Laboratory Investigations. The CSF analysis often differs from HIV-1–seronegative patients with GBS by the presence of a mononuclear pleocytosis of 20 to 50 cells/μL. The CSF protein concentration is usually elevated to levels up to 250 mg/dL, and a polyclonal gammaglobulinemia can be detected.

Electrophysiologic Studies. Demyelination is demonstrated by reduced motor nerve conduction velocities or prolonged distal latencies and minimum F-wave latencies in two or more nerves. Conduction block is often prominent.

Nerve Biopsy. Sural nerve biopsy generally demonstrates the presence of a perivascular and endoneural mononuclear cell infiltrate with macrophage-mediated segmental demyelination. In severe cases, wallerian-like degeneration of axons can be seen. Similar to GBS occurring in immunocompetent individuals, the etiology of AIDP in HIV-infected patients is thought to be autoimmune. Anti–peripheral nerve myelin antibodies have been found in HIV-1–positive patients with AIDP, as well

as increased level of soluble CD8 and neopterin in the CSF, indicating an abnormal immune activation. CMV was found at autopsy in the peripheral nerves of one patient with AIDS who presented with AIDP.[141]

Treatment. Spontaneous recovery is usually the outcome of AIDP, although HIV-1–infected patients tend to have a more severe course with a slower recovery than immunocompetent individuals with GBS. Plasmapheresis is indicated if the illness is sufficiently severe to warrant treatment. Patients with CIDP benefit from treatment with prednisone or plasmapheresis.[139,142] Prednisone should however be used with great caution in patients with immunosuppression. Other treatments such as intravenous immune globulin have also been used successfully in HIV-1–positive patients with inflammatory demyelinating polyneuropathy, sometimes in combination with plasmapheresis.[143] In cases of AIDP occurring in late stages of the disease, a trial of ganciclovir may be warranted if other treatments are not efficient.[141]

Distal Sensory Polyneuropathy

Human Immunodeficiency Virus Associated. This is the most common cause of peripheral neuropathy in HIV-1 infection, which is symptomatic in 35% of patients and asymptomatic in an additional 20%.[144] Moreover, histologic abnormalities can be detected at autopsy in most patients dying with AIDS.[145] This condition occurs generally in patients with advanced immunosuppression and may be more severe in those with an elevated plasma HIV-1 viral load.[146,147] However, debilitating distal sensory polyneuropathy (DSP) can also occur in patients with undetectable plasma viral load and elevated CD4+ T-cell counts.

Clinical Presentation. DSP is characterized by the progressive onset of symmetric paresthesia, numbness, and painful dysesthesia of the lower extremities. The pain is often described as an aching or burning sensation and is worse on the soles of the feet. Some patients have a lower pain threshold (hyperalgesia) or pain induced by non-noxious stimuli (allodynia), such as the contact with bed covers at night. Symptoms may remain stable or progress over months and ascend in a length-dependent fashion up the legs. Fingertips may become affected when symptoms are up to the knees. Although wearing shoes and walking may exacerbate the pain for some patients, others complain of a maximal discomfort when they are barefoot in bed. Therefore, DSP may have a major negative impact on the patient's ability to ambulate and the quality of their sleep. Perception of noxious stimuli, temperature, and vibrations is usually more affected than light touch and proprioception. DSP may even have several forms, as some patients only have decreased sensation for noxious stimuli and temperature, indicating dysfunction of small unmyelinated sensory fibers; some only have decreased vibration sense and proprioception, consistent with dysfunction of large myelinated fibers; and others have decreased sensation for all modalities. Hyporeflexia of the lower extremities is a very common finding, and gait ataxia with positive Romberg sign is present in severe cases. Weakness is rarely found on the examination or is confined to the intrinsic foot muscles.

Laboratory Investigations. CSF analysis shows only nonspecific findings with mild elevation of protein concentration and mononucleated pleocytosis, which is common in HIV-1 infection.

Electrophysiologic Studies. Nerve conduction studies (NCS) show low-amplitude or absent sural nerve action potentials. Sensory and motor nerve conduction velocities are normal or only mildly reduced. Electromyographic studies demonstrate acute denervation and chronic reinnervation in distal leg muscles. These findings are consistent with an axonal distal symmetric, predominantly sensory, polyneuropathy.

Nerve Biopsy. Sural nerve biopsy confirms the diagnosis of axonal degeneration of myelinated and unmyelinated axons. Punch skin biopsies show evidence of reduced intraepidermal nerve fiber density in the distal leg. A modest dorsal root ganglion (DRG) neuronal loss has also been demonstrated in DSP,[148] as well as selective degeneration of the axons and myelin sheaths in the cervical and upper thoracic level of the gracile tracts. This process therefore represents the degeneration of the centrally directed extension of the sensory neurons.[149]

Inflammatory infiltrates around peripheral nerve fibers and in DRG consists of activated macrophages, with local release of cytokines such as TNF-α, interferon-γ, and IL-6.[145] As it is the case in VM and, to some extent, in HIV encephalitis, productive HIV-1 replication in the peripheral nerves and DRG is sparse and limited to monocyte/macrophages. Therefore, the presence of activated macrophages secreting inflammatory cytokines, rather than the virus itself, seems to account for most of the peripheral nerve damage.[150] How activated macrophages penetrate DRG and peripheral nerve fibers is unclear, and it has been hypothesized that the blood-nerve barrier, like the BBB, may be affected in HIV-infected patients.[145] Finally, experimental models in animals suggest that it is still possible that HIV, or HIV-1 proteins, may have a direct toxic effect in the neuropathic pain of DSP.[151]

Because a similar type of polyneuropathy is common in the HIV-1–seronegative population, other etiologies such as vitamin B_{12} deficiency, neurotoxic medications, alcoholism, or diabetes mellitus should be ruled out.

Nucleoside Neuropathy

Clinical Presentation. Dose-dependent neurotoxicity of NRTIs zalcitabine (ddC), didanosine (ddI), and stavudine (d4T) has been detected in approximately 30% of patients taking these medications.[152] The risk is increased in patients using regimens containing a combination of ddI and d4T.[153] The clinical presentation and electrophysiologic studies are indistinguishable from DSP, and the diagnosis can only be established by a temporal association between initiation of a dideoxynucleoside NRTI and the onset of the symptoms, which occur as early as 1 week. Discontinuation of the offending medication may lead to symptomatic improvement over several weeks in two thirds of patients, although it is often preceded by a transient worsening of symptoms known as "coasting."[154] Because of the widespread use of ddI and d4T in HAART regimens, the prevalence of neuropathy even in relatively immunocompetent HIV-infected individuals with $CD4^+$ T-cell counts greater than 400/μL was as high as 44% in one study.[155]

Laboratory Investigations. The pathogenetic mechanism of nucleoside neuropathy appears to be most likely related to nucleoside-induced mitochondrial dysfunction. Indeed, NRTIs inhibit mitochondrial polymerase in vitro, resulting in tissue-specific injury. Zidovudine (AZT) toxicity affects mainly skeletal muscle (see later), whereas ddI and d4T cause pancreatitis in addition to neuropathy. Consistent with this hypothesis, a recent study showed that raised plasma lactic acid concentration discriminated between d4T nucleoside neuropathy and DSP with 90% sensitivity and specificity.[156] Such common laboratory test may help with the clinical management of HIV-infected patients on NRTI presenting with DSP. Indeed, it is possible that the effect of NRTIs may only be of unmasking a subclinical neuropathy associated with HIV. Nucleoside neuropathy occurs more frequently in individuals with preexisting DSP, and administration of NRTIs to healthy animals does not result in neuropathy.[145] These data suggest that NRTI may only exacerbate an inflammatory process triggered by activated macrophages in peripheral nerve fibers or DRG of HIV-infected individuals. Clinicians should therefore use caution before removing ddI or d4T from successful HAART regimens, unless there is a clear temporal association between the administration of these medications and the onset of the symptoms, or an elevated serum lactate level.[156] Even in these cases, careful review of the patient's HAART exposure and analysis of HIV-1 genotype is required to determine potential treatment alternatives, as maintenance of virologic control is paramount and a risk-benefit analysis may favor the continuation of the NRTIs. A list of neurotoxic medications frequently given to HIV-infected patients is shown in Table 120-3.

Treatment. There is no available therapy that leads to regeneration of nerve fibers and DRG and reversal of symptoms. Suppression of viral replication with HAART is unfortunately not associated with clinical improvement in DSP. Therefore, treatment of neuropathic pain in DSP is purely symptomatic and is aimed primarily at attenuating the painful dysesthesia and improving the quality of life of these patients.

TABLE 120-3 Neurotoxic Medications Used in Human Immunodeficiency Virus-1 Infection

Name	Clinical Presentation
NRTIs	
Zidovudine (AZT)	Myopathy
Zalcitabine (ddC)	DSP
Didanosine (ddI)	DSP
Stavudine (d4T)	DSP
NNRTI	
Efavirenz	Vivid dreams
Antiviral Agent	
Foscarnet	Seizures
Antibacterial Agents	
Isoniazid (INH)	DSP
Dapsone	DSMP
Metronidazole*	DSP
Antineoplastic Agents	
Vincristine	DSMP, CN
Cisplatin	DSP

*High doses only.
CN, cranial neuropathy; DSMP, distal sensory motor polyneuropathy; DSP, distal sensory polyneuropathy; NRTI, nucleoside analogue reverse transcriptase inhibitor; NNRTI, non-nucleoside analogue reverse transcriptase inhibitor.

Treatment should not be administered if numbness and decreased sensation for noxious stimuli and temperature are the only complaints, as they do not improve.

First-line therapies include nonsteroidal anti-inflammatory drugs and acetaminophen, as well as topical application of capsaicin[157] or 5% lidocaine gel.[158] Anticonvulsant medications are the second line of treatment. Medications such as carbamazepine and phenytoin are commonly used in other forms of painful neuropathies are contraindicated because both are metabolized by the liver, which may cause unwanted interactions in patients taking protease inhibitors. Gabapentin is metabolized by the kidneys and is usually well tolerated by HIV-infected individuals.[159] Treatment starts using 300 mg orally at bedtime and is increased to 300 mg orally 3 times daily over 1 week. The extent of symptomatic relief is variable, and some patients may need doses up to 1200 mg 3 times daily for a significant reduction in their discomfort. Fatigue and sleepiness are infrequent but may be limiting in some patients. A recent study using another anticonvulsant, lamotrigine, showed substantial pain reduction in a subgroup of patients receiving neurotoxic NRTIs but no difference compared with placebo in patients with DSP who were not on nucleosides.[160]

Amitriptyline, which is commonly used for the treatment of diabetic neuropathy, is not superior to placebo in HIV-infected patients with DSP.[161] However, adjunction of tricyclics with lower anticholinergic side effects, such as nortriptyline, may benefit patients who remain symptomatic on adequate doses of anticonvulsants. In refractory cases, a combination of anticonvulsant, tricyclic, nonsteroidal anti-inflammatory drug, and topical medications may be necessary to achieve significant relief.

Narcotic analgesics should be kept as last resort because of their addictive potential in the context of a chronic pain syndrome. Tramadol shares properties with opioid analgesics but is less likely to cause dependence and lead to abuse.[162] Long-acting opioid agonists such as fentanyl patches should be preferred to short-acting agents.

Numerous experimental drugs have been disappointing in the treatment of DSP, including mexiletine, peptide T, recombinant human nerve growth factor, plasmapheresis, and acupuncture (see review[163]). Depletion of acetyl carnitine, a substrate in the production of energy during β-oxidation of free fatty acids, was implicated in the pathogenesis of DSP,[164] but this was not confirmed in a larger sample of patients.[165] Potential neuroregenerative agents currently under investigation include neuroimmunophilin ligands and prosaposin.

Mononeuritis Multiplex

Patients with previously asymptomatic HIV-1 infection and CD4$^+$ T-lymphocyte counts above 200/µL, as well as patients with AIDS and profound immunosuppression, can be affected by mononeuritis multiplex (MM).

Clinical Presentation. Patients present with acute onset of sensory or motor deficit limited to one or more peripheral nerve. Involvement of a facial or laryngeal nerve has also been reported. The asymmetric nature of this disorder and the prominent weakness differentiate it from other HIV-associated neuropathies. The course can be self-limited in early HIV-1 infection[166] or more severe in patients with advanced disease.

Laboratory Investigations. CSF analysis is nonspecific and shows only a mild elevation of protein concentration and a mononuclear pleocytosis. Cryoglobulinemia has been reported in one case.[167]

Electrophysiologic Studies. NCS reveal a reduction of the amplitude of sensory nerve action potentials and compound muscle action potentials as well as a mild reduction in nerve conduction velocities in the distribution of single nerves. The electromyographic examination is also consistent with focal or asymmetric multifocal axonal degeneration, although considerable overlap may exist with DSP and IDP.

Nerve Biopsy. Similar to its clinical presentation, the nerve biopsy specimen of patients with MM shows a spectrum of pathologies rather than a single pattern. Axonal degeneration and perivascular inflammatory infiltrates are found in patients with early HIV-1 infection and limited clinical involvement. Patients with AIDS and CMV infection usually have mixed axonal and demyelinating lesions with inflammatory infiltrates containing also polymorphonuclear cells, as well as, sometimes, characteristic cytomegalic inclusion bodies.[168] The most aggressive form consists of a necrotizing arteritis with necrosis of endoneurial or epineurial vessels and might be caused by circulating immune complexes.

Treatment. Mild forms of MM developing in patients who are otherwise asymptomatic might improve without specific treatment. Others might benefit from therapies such as plasmapheresis[167] or IGIV.[169] Corticosteroids and cyclophosphamide should be reserved for aggressive cases of MM with vasculitis proved by nerve biopsy. In late HIV-1 infection, especially in patients with concurrent systemic CMV infection, empiric therapy with ganciclovir for CMV should be considered.[170]

Progressive Polyradiculopathy

Because it occurs late in the course of HIV-1 infection, in patients with low CD4$^+$ T-lymphocyte counts and concurrent systemic illnesses, progressive polyradiculopathy (PP) is often underrecognized.

Clinical Presentation. Patients complain initially of lower extremities and sacral paresthesia and, sometimes, radicular pain in the cauda equina distribution. These symptoms are followed by a rapidly progressive areflexive paraparesis and ascending sensory loss, often accompanied by urinary retention. The upper extremities are relatively spared. A thoracic sensory level, if present, indicates concomitant medullary involvement, but other features indicating upper motor neuron damage such as spasticity and hyperreflexia are usually absent. A prominent infection with CMV, mainly retinitis, oesophagitis, or colitis, is conspicuously present in a majority of cases.

Laboratory Investigations. In contrast to other peripheral nervous system diseases associated with HIV-1 infection, the CSF analysis is useful in establishing the diagnosis. A marked polymorphonuclear cell pleocytosis, elevated protein concentration, and hypoglycorrhachia are the hallmarks of this syndrome.[171] CSF cultures demonstrate the presence of CMV in 60% of the cases.[172] Cultures may take up to 2 weeks to grow, and CSF samples have to be kept on ice immediately after the lumbar puncture. As is the case with CMV encephalitis,[115] CMV DNA may be detectable in the CSF by PCR. Because of the frequent concomitant systemic infection with CMV, blood culture may also be positive for this virus. Urine culture is nonspecific, because many AIDS patients shed CMV in the urine asymp-

tomatically. Cytologic studies can reveal cytomegalic cells with intranuclear and intracytoplasmic CMV inclusions.

Electrophysiologic Studies. The electromyographic examination is useful to differentiate this syndrome from AIDP. Severe and widespread proximal axonal damage in lumbar nerve root distribution is correlated by fibrillation potentials, complex repetitive discharges, and motor unit recruitment patterns in lower extremity muscles. Motor nerve conduction velocities are minimally altered, but affected muscles display prolonged or absent F waves. These findings are consistent with extensive denervation of the lower extremity muscles, which is characteristic in this syndrome.

Nerve Biopsy. Because of the radicular localization of the lesions, a nerve biopsy is not helpful for diagnosis. Autopsy studies reveal a severe inflammation associated with necrosis of the ventral and dorsal nerve roots. Cytomegalic inclusions can be detected within the nucleus and cytoplasm of Schwann, ependymal, and endothelial cells, which are also positive for CMV by in situ hybridization studies. Similar findings have been reported in cranial nerves at the site of exit from the brain stem.

Despite the strong association of polyradiculopathy and CMV in patients with AIDS, other possibilities include neurosyphilis and lymphomatous meningitis, which should be ruled out on the CSF analysis.

Treatment. The treatment of CMV-associated PP is similar to treatment of CMV encephalitis (see earlier). It consists of intravenous ganciclovir and/or foscarnet.[173] Newer anti-CMV medication such as valganciclovir and cidofovir have not been evaluated for PP. Phenotypic and genotypic characterization of viral isolates should be considered in case of resistance to treatment.[174] The clinical response is variable but usually best if therapy is started within days after the onset of symptoms.

Because the results of PCR for CMV DNA in the CSF can take 1 to 2 weeks to obtain, empiric treatment can be justified in this entity, especially if the workup reveals a polymorphonuclear pleocytosis in the CSF or widespread systemic infection with this virus. The rationale is to prevent irreversible necrosis of the nerve roots. In patients who are already paraplegic several weeks after the onset of their symptoms, treatment can achieve stabilization but no real improvement should be expected. Neutropenia is the most common dose-limiting toxicity of ganciclovir and may preclude concomitant use of other myelotoxic drug such as zidovudine. Concomitant treatment with granulocyte colony-stimulating factor (G-CSF) may become necessary in that setting.

Diffuse Infiltrative Lymphocytosis Syndrome–Associated Neuropathy

A small subset of HIV-infected patients develop persistent CD8 hyperlymphocytosis and a Sjögren's syndrome–like syndrome associated with multivisceral CD8 T-cell infiltration, known as the diffuse infiltrative lymphocytosis syndrome (DILS). These individuals generally have higher CD4$^+$ T-lymphocyte counts, fewer opportunistic infections, and longer survival times than do other HIV-infected patients.[175] Some of these patients may develop a primary B-cell lymphoma.

Clinical Presentation

Some of these patients present with an acute or subacute, sensorimotor distal symmetric neuropathy, which is always painful.[176]

Electrophysiologic Studies

Electromyographic and NCS study results are consistent with axonal neuropathy.

Nerve Biopsy

Nerve biopsy shows marked angiocentric CD8 infiltrates without mural necrosis and abundant expression of HIV-1 p24 protein in macrophages. The lymphocytic infiltrate is polyclonal in most patients. The HIV-1 proviral load in peripheral nerve is much higher than in other types of HIV-associated neuropathy.[177]

Treatment

Zidovudine and steroid therapy was associated with improvement in a small group of patients.[176]

Amyotrophic Lateral Sclerosis–Like Syndrome

Several cases of amyotrophic lateral sclerosis (ALS)-like syndromes have been reported in HIV-infected individuals.[178,179] These cases differ from classic ALS because they occurred in younger patients, they were unusually rapidly progressive, and improved after the institution of antiretroviral therapy. The etiology of this syndrome is unclear because HIV-1 does not infect neurons. Obviously, ALS and HIV-1 infection can also be coincidental and, in this case, does not respond to antiretroviral treatment.[180] These data indicate that HIV-1 should be included in the differential diagnosis of ALS.[181] However, one cannot draw the conclusion that classic ALS is caused by an as-yet-unidentified retrovirus, and there is no rationale for administering antiretroviral treatment to these patients.

MUSCULOSKELETAL SYNDROMES

Muscular disorders have been described in HIV-1–infected individuals and can occur at any stages of the disease.

Myopathy

Clinical Presentation

Myopathy occurs in 17% of patients treated with zidovudine for periods over 270 days[182] and in 0.22% of HIV-infected patients who are not taking this medication.[183] The clinical presentation is similar in these two groups. Patients complain principally of lower extremity weakness, characterized by difficulty in rising from a chair or climbing stairs as well as fatigue. Myalgias are present in up to half the cases, and the neurologic examination reveals proximal symmetric weakness, predominant at the level of the hip flexors.[184] This syndrome has to be differentiated from HIV-1 wasting syndrome and may easily be overlooked in a population of debilitated patients who often present with generalized weakness. In addition, it may occur simultaneously with central or peripheral nervous system complications of HIV-1 infection.

Laboratory Investigations

There is a mild elevation of creatine phosphokinase in the serum (median, ≅500 IU/L), although CPK can be as high as 7500 IU/L in some cases.[183] This may be an incidental finding that orients toward a diagnosis in cases where muscle strength is still intact. The creatine phosphokinase level correlates with the degree of myonecrosis seen on muscle biopsy but not with the weakness.

Electrophysiologic Studies

Electromyographic testing may reveal myopathic motor unit potentials with early recruitment and full interference patterns, predominantly in proximal muscles,[184] but it can also be normal in 30% of the cases.[183] Therefore, a normal electromyogram does not rule out this diagnosis.

Muscle Biopsy

The etiology of myopathy in AIDS has been a matter of debate,[185] because both HIV-1 and zidovudine have been incriminated as causative factors. In patients not treated with zidovudine presenting with myopathy, the most common finding is scattered myofiber degeneration, fibrosis, necrosis, and phagocytosis of muscle fibers associated with a variable inflammatory infiltrate similar to that seen in idiopathic polymyositis.[183] HIV-1 does not seem to infect muscle fibers, and opportunistic organisms have been detected only exceptionally. Infiltrating cells are predominantly CD8$^+$ T cells and macrophages.[186] As it is the case for DSP and VM, it is possible that these cells secrete proinflammatory cytokines that may damage muscle fibers, precipitate muscle antigen exposure, and generate an autoimmune response.[187] Interestingly, in a recent series close to half of patients with HIV-1

polymyositis also had DILS. Because both conditions are extremely rare, their association cannot be coincidental.[183]

In zidovudine myopathy, biopsy results reveal numerous ragged-red fibers and abnormal mitochondria.[188] Zidovudine-induced mitochodriotoxicity is mediated through the inhibition of the enzyme γ-DNA polymerase, which is responsible for the replication of mitochondrial DNA. This induces an energy shortage within the muscle, which results in overt myopathy over time.

Treatment

Similar to idiopathic polymyositis, patients with HIV-1 polymyositis have had a favorable response with corticosteroids 60 mg/day during an average of 9 months. However, the risk of long-term immunosuppressive therapy should carefully be considered in this population of patients. Other immune-based therapies such as azathioprine, methotrexate, or IGIV have also been successful.[183] In zidovudine-induced myopathy, treatment consists of zidovudine withdrawal. Objective improvement in muscle strength is expected to occur in most patients after 8 weeks.[189]

Other Musculoskeletal Conditions Associated with Human Immunodeficiency Virus

Rare cases of nemaline rod myopathy, inclusion body myositis, pyomyositis, and cardiomyopathy have also been reported in HIV-infected individuals.[190] More worrisome is the prospect of statin-associated rhabdomyolysis.[191] Indeed, elevated cholesterol and triglyceride values are frequent in HIV-infected patients on HAART, requiring therapy with statins with the aim of preventing cardiovascular complications. Most statins are metabolized by the liver cytochrome P-450 isoenzyme 3A4 (CYP3A4). Similarly, PIs are both substrates for and inhibitors of CYP3A4 and substrates for P-glycoprotein (P-gp), a bidirectional drug transporter that is also inhibited by statins to varying degrees. Pharmacokinetic studies have shown that PIs may greatly increase statins concentrations. Statin-associated rhabdomyolysis occurs within weeks from onset of treatment and may be fatal.[192]

HIV-infected patients on HAART often complain of arthralgias, and cases of frozen shoulder, tendonitis, and temporomandibular joint dysfunction have been described within a year of starting on indinavir. A survey using an anonymous questionnaire answered by 292 HIV-infected patients in Europe indicated that arthralgias were more frequent in patients taking PIs, especially indinavir (40.6%) or ritonavir plus saquinavir (41.9%) compared with NNRTIs (26.5%) or NRTIs (25.3%).[193] Indinavir causes urolithiasis by crystallizing in the urinary tract, and indinavir crystals have been found in the joint fluid of patients with frozen shoulder. Temporary interruption of the PI or replacement with NNRTI should be considered based on the patient's discomfort, HAART history, and HIV-1 genotype studies.

The principal neuromuscular syndromes found in HIV-1 infection are listed in Table 120-4.

Seizures

Seizures are a frequent complication of HIV-1 infection and may occur in as many as 17% of patients. CNS mass lesions and meningitis are the major causes of seizures, but no identifiable cause other than HIV-1 infection can be detected in up to 25% of cases.[194] Unless a reversible cause can be readily identified and treated, anticonvulsant therapy should be initiated after the first seizure.

Clinicians should consider carefully the potential drug-drug interactions between antiepileptic drugs (AEDs) and PIs.[195] As discussed previously, PIs are metabolized in the liver by the isoenzyme CYP3A4. AEDs such as phenytoin, phenobarbital, and carbamazepine increase the activity of this isoenzyme, which may result in insufficient serum PI level, increased viral replication, and selection of resistance mutants.

In addition, protein binding must be considered. Most AEDs and PIs are highly protein bound, as are other medications taken by HIV-infected patients such as trimethoprim-sulfamethoxazole. This may result in competition for available protein binding sites. Valproic acid and phenytoin commonly displace other drugs from albumin and thus

TABLE 120-4 Neuromuscular Syndromes in Human Immunodeficiency Virus-1 Infection

Diagnosis	Disease Stage	Clinical Features	Diagnostic Studies	Treatment
AIDP CIDP	Early > late	Weakness more than sensory loss	CSF: ↑ WBC, ↑↑ protein NCS: demyelination	Early: IGIV, steroids, plasma- pheresis Late: consider ganciclovir/foscarnet
MM	Early Late	Multiple painful mononeuropathies	NCS: multifocal axonal neuropathy. Biopsy: inflammation/ vasculitis CMV	Early: none Late: steroids/cyclophosphamide Ganciclovir/foscarnet
Nucleoside Neuropathy	Any stage	Distal sensory loss Neuropathic pain	NCS: distal axonopathy Increased serum lactate	Nucleoside withdrawal
DSP	Late	Distal sensory loss Neuropathic pain	NCS: distal axonopathy	NSAIDs, capsaicin AED, tricyclics
PP	Late	Progressive flaccid paraparesis, urinary dysfunction, LS pain	CSF: increased WBCs (PMNs), CMV PCR+	Ganciclovir/foscarnet Cidofovir
DILS	Late	Sjögren's syndrome, distal motor and sensory loss, pain	NCS: axonal neuropathy Biopsy: CD8+ T cells, HIV-1	Zidovudine/HAART Steroids
Zidovudine Myopathy	Any stage	Proximal weakness Myalgias	EMG: ± irritative Biopsy: ragged red fibers	Zidovudine withdrawal
Polymyositis	Any stage	Proximal weakness Myalgias	EMG: ± irritative Biopsy: inflammatory infiltrates	Steroids, IGIV Immunosuppressants
ALS-like	Late	Weakness, dysphagia	EMG: neurogenic	HAART

AED, antiepileptic drug; AIDP, acute inflammatory demyelinating polyneuropathy; ALS, amyotrophic lateral sclerosis; CIDP, chronic inflammatory demyelinating polyneuropathy; CMV, cytomegalovirus; CSF, cerebrospinal fluid; DILS, diffuse infiltrative lymphocytosis syndrome; DSP, distal sensory polyneuropathy; EMG, electromyography; HAART, highly active antiretroviral therapy; HIV, human immunodeficiency virus; IGIV, intravenous immunoglobulin; LS, lumbosacral; MM, mononeuritis multiplex; NCS, nerve conduction studies; NSAID, nonsteroidal anti-inflammatory drug; PCR, polymerase chain reaction; PMNs, polymorphonuclear leukocytes; PP, progressive polyradiculopathy; WBCs, white blood cells.

may result in increased free drug levels, side effects, and toxicity. Conversely, PI may also displace AEDs such as carbamazepine from protein binding sites and result in toxicity. Finally, valproic acid may be contraindicated because it has been shown to increase HIV-1 replication in vitro. There have been no studies of the outcome of seizure management in HIV-infected patients on HAART. Until these data are available, clinicians should favor the use of AED that do not affect viral replication and have limited protein binding and no effects on the cytochrome P450 system, such as gabapentin, lamotrigine, levetirac-

etam, tiagabine, and topiramate.[196] The choice of the AED or combination thereof depends on the type of seizure presented by the patient. In the case of status epilepticus or emergencies where intravenous treatment is indicated, traditional AEDs such as phenytoin or phenobarbital should be used temporarily in the acute phase and should then be replaced by medications that have lower interaction potential with PIs once seizure control has been achieved.

A summary of the principal neurologic complications of HIV infection is provided in Figure 120-6.

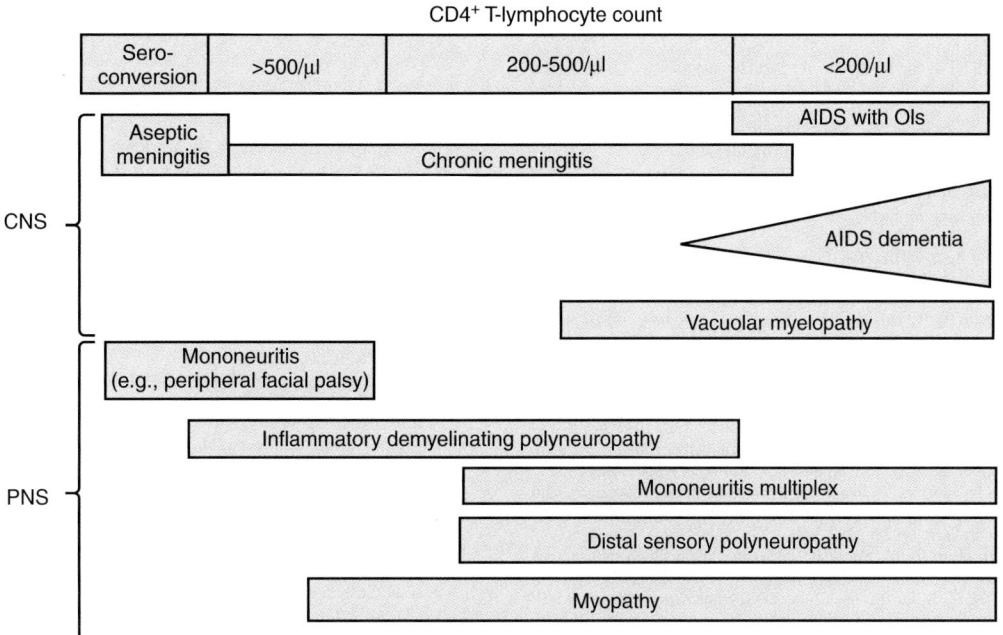

FIGURE 120-6. Occurrence of the principal neurologic complications of human immunodeficiency virus 1 infection according to the degree of immunosuppression as measured by CD4+ T-lymphocyte counts (see text for details). CNS, central nervous system; OIs, opportunistic infections; PNS, peripheral nervous system.

Temporal Trends in Neurologic Manifestations of Human Immunodeficiency Virus Infection

The spectrum of CNS complications of HIV-1 diseases is constantly evolving, and both quantitative and qualitative changes have been noted in recent years.[54,197] Patients are living longer on HAART but they may become resistant to antiretrovirals. The clinical presentation of known diseases such as PML may be altered by HAART-induced immune reconstitution,[111] and new entities, such as severe HIV-associated leukoencephalopathy, have been described in HAART-experienced individuals.[198] Expanded tropism of JCV to cerebellar neurons was demonstrated, which may have implications in the pathogenesis of cerebellar atrophy occurring in HIV-infected individuals.[199] In addition, protease inhibitors are associated with marked increase in serum cholesterol and triglycerides. Therefore, it is possible that long-term HIV-1 survivors are be at increased risk of developing cerebrovascular events.[200] As this population becomes older, age-related entities are expected to overlap with HIV-associated and treatment-associated neurologic conditions and add another layer of complexity to management of these patients.[201] Because of these trends, and the fact that new clinical entities may potentially warrant different treatments, a brain biopsy should be considered in cases where molecular diagnosis cannot be obtained, and postmortem analysis should be discussed for all patients who do not respond to treatment.

REFERENCES

1. Snider WD, Simpson DM, Nielsen S, et al. Neurological complications of acquired immune deficiency syndrome: Analysis of 50 patients. Ann Neurol. 1983;14:403-418.
2. Levy RM, Bredesen DE, Rosenblum ML. Neurological manifestations of the acquired immunodeficiency syndrome (AIDS): Experience at UCSF and review of the literature. J Neurosurg. 1985;62:475-495.
3. Petito CK. Review of central nervous system pathology in human immunodeficiency virus infection. Ann Neurol. 1988;23(suppl):S54-S57.
4. De Girolami U, Smith TW, Henin D, Hauw JJ. Neuropathology of the acquired immunodeficiency syndrome. Arch Pathol Lab Med. 1990;114:643-655.
5. Gray F, Lescs MC, Keohane C, et al. Early brain changes in HIV infection: Neuropathological study of 11 HIV seropositive, non-AIDS cases. J Neuropathol Exp Neurol. 1992;51:177-185.
6. Gray F, Scaravilli F, Everall I, et al. Neuropathology of early HIV-1 infection. Brain Pathol. 1996;6:1-15.
7. Hollander H, McGuire D, Burack JH. Diagnostic lumbar puncture in HIV-infected patients: Analysis of 138 cases. Am J Med. 1994;96:223-228.
8. Dybul M, Fauci AS, Bartlett JG, et al. Guidelines for using antiretroviral agents among HIV-infected adults and adolescents. Ann Intern Med. 2002;137(5 Pt 2):381-433.
9. Johns DR, Tierney M, Felsenstein D. Alteration in the natural history of neurosyphilis by concurrent infection with the human immunodeficiency virus. N Engl J Med. 1987;316:1569-1572.
10. Musher DM, Hamill RJ, Baughn RE. Effect of human immunodeficiency virus (HIV) infection on the course of syphilis and on the response to treatment. Ann Intern Med. 1990;113:872-881.
11. Feraru ER, Aronow HA, Lipton RB. Neurosyphilis in AIDS patients: Initial CSF VDRL may be negative. Neurology. 1990;40(3 Pt 1):541-543.
12. Powderly WG. Cryptococcal meningitis and AIDS. Clin Infect Dis. 1993;17:837-842.
13. Sacktor N. The epidemiology of human immunodeficiency virus-associated neurological disease in the era of highly active antiretroviral therapy. J Neurovirol. 2002;8(suppl 2):115-121.
14. Saag MS, Graybill RJ, Larsen RA, et al. Practice guidelines for the management of cryptococcal disease. Infectious Diseases Society of America. Clin Infect Dis. 2000;30:710-718.
15. van der Horst CM, Saag MS, Cloud GA, et al. Treatment of cryptococcal meningitis associated with the acquired immunodeficiency syndrome. National Institute of Allergy and Infectious Diseases Mycoses Study Group and AIDS Clinical Trials Group. N Engl J Med. 1997;337:15-21.
16. Johnston SR, Corbett EL, Foster O, et al. Raised intracranial pressure and visual complications in AIDS patients with cryptococcal meningitis. J Infect. 1992;24:185-189.
17. McArthur JC, Hoover DR, Bacellar H, et al. Dementia in AIDS patients: Incidence and risk factors. Multicenter AIDS Cohort Study. Neurology. 1993;43:2245-2252.
18. Qureshi AI, Hanson DL, Jones JL, Janssen RS. Estimation of the temporal probability of human immunodeficiency virus (HIV) dementia after risk stratification for HIV-infected persons. Neurology. 1998;50:392-397.
19. Power C, Selnes OA, Grim JA, McArthur JC. HIV Dementia Scale: A rapid screening test. J Acquir Immune Defic Syndr Hum Retrovirol. 1995;8:273-278.
20. Miller EN, Selnes OA, McArthur JC, et al. Neuropsychological performance in HIV-1-infected homosexual men: The Multicenter AIDS Cohort Study (MACS). Neurology. 1990;40:197-203.
21. Smith T, Jakobsen J, Gaub J, et al. Clinical and electrophysiological studies of human immunodeficiency virus-seropositive men without AIDS. Ann Neurol. 1988;23:295-297.
22. Rosenhall U, Hakansson C, Lowhagen GB, et al. Otoneurological abnormalities in asymptomatic HIV-seropositive patients. Acta Neurol Scand. 1989;79:140-145.
23. Koralnik IJ, Beaumanoir A, Hausler R, et al. A controlled study of early neurologic abnormalities in men with asymptomatic human immunodeficiency virus infection. N Engl J Med. 1990;323:864-870.
24. Portegies P, Enting RH, de Gans J, et al. Presentation and course of AIDS dementia complex: 10 Years of follow-up in Amsterdam, the Netherlands. AIDS. 1993;7:669-675.
25. Brew BJ, Pemberton L, Cunningham P, Law MG. Levels of human immunodeficiency virus type 1 RNA in cerebrospinal fluid correlate with AIDS dementia stage. J Infect Dis. 1997;175:963-966.
26. McArthur JC, McClernon DR, Cronin MF, et al. Relationship between human immunodeficiency virus-associated dementia and viral load in cerebrospinal fluid and brain. Ann Neurol. 1997;42:689-698.
27. Ellis RJ, Hsia K, Spector SA, et al. Cerebrospinal fluid human immunodeficiency virus type 1 RNA levels are elevated in neurocognitively impaired individuals with acquired immunodeficiency syndrome. HIV Neurobehavioral Research Center Group. Ann Neurol. 1997;42:679-688.
28. Robertson K, Fiscus S, Kapoor C, et al. CSF, plasma viral load and HIV associated dementia. J Neurovirol. 1998;4:90-94.
29. Ellis RJ, Moore DJ, Childers ME, et al. Progression to neuropsychological impairment in human immunodeficiency virus infection predicted by elevated cerebrospinal fluid levels of human immunodeficiency virus RNA. Arch Neurol. 2002;59:923-928.
30. Price RW. The two faces of HIV infection of cerebrospinal fluid. Trends Microbiol. 2000;8:387-391.
31. Johnson RT, Glass JD, McArthur JC, Chesebro BW. Quantitation of human immunodeficiency virus in brains of demented and nondemented patients with acquired immunodeficiency syndrome. Ann Neurol. 1996;39:392-395.
32. Bouwman FH, Skolasky RL, Hes D, et al. Variable progression of HIV-associated dementia. Neurology. 1998;50:1814-1820.
33. Lopez-Villegas D, Lenkinski RE, Frank I. Biochemical changes in the frontal lobe of HIV-infected individuals detected by magnetic resonance spectroscopy. Proc Natl Acad Sci U S A. 1997;94:9854-9859.
34. Chang L, Ernst T, Leonido-Yee M, et al. Cerebral metabolite abnormalities correlate with clinical severity of HIV-1 cognitive motor complex. Neurology. 1999;52:100-108.
35. Chang L, Ernst T, Leonido-Yee M, et al. Highly active antiretroviral therapy reverses brain metabolite abnormalities in mild HIV dementia. Neurology. 1999;53:782-789.
36. An SF, Groves M, Gray F, Scaravilli F. Early entry and widespread cellular involvement of HIV-1 DNA in brains of HIV-1 positive asymptomatic individuals. J Neuropathol Exp Neurol. 1999;58:1156-1162.
37. Smith TW, DeGirolami U, Henin D, et al. Human immunodeficiency virus (HIV) leukoencephalopathy and the microcirculation. J Neuropathol Exp Neurol. 1990;49:357-370.
38. Berger JR, Nath A, Greenberg RN, et al. Cerebrovascular changes in the basal ganglia with HIV dementia. Neurology. 2000;54:921-926.
39. Tornatore C, Chandra R, Berger JR, Major EO. HIV-1 infection of subcortical astrocytes in the pediatric central nervous system. Neurology. 1994;44(3 Pt 1):481-487.
40. Everall IP, Heaton RK, Marcotte TD, et al. Cortical synaptic density is reduced in mild to moderate human immunodeficiency virus neurocognitive disorder. HNRC Group. HIV Neurobehavioral Research Center. Brain Pathol. 1999;9:209-217.
41. Williams KC, Hickey WF. Central nervous system damage, monocytes and macrophages, and neurological disorders in AIDS. Annu Rev Neurosci. 2002;25:537-562.
42. Giulian D, Vaca K, Noonan CA. Secretion of neurotoxins by mononuclear phagocytes infected with HIV-1. Science. 1990;250:1593-1596.
43. Rostasy K, Monti L, Yiannoutsos C, et al. Human immunodeficiency virus infection, inducible nitric oxide synthase expression, and microglial activation: Pathogenetic relationship to the acquired immunodeficiency syndrome dementia complex. Ann Neurol. 1999;46:207-216.
44. Glass JD, Fedor H, Wesselingh SL, McArthur JC. Immunocytochemical quantitation of human immunodeficiency virus in the brain: Correlations with dementia. Ann Neurol. 1995;38:755-762.
45. Lipton SA, Gendelman HE. Seminars in medicine of the Beth Israel Hospital, Boston. Dementia associated with the acquired immunodeficiency syndrome. N Engl J Med. 1995;332:934-940.
46. Magnuson DS, Knudsen BE, Geiger JD, et al. Human immunodeficiency virus type 1 tat activates non-N-methyl-D-aspartate excitatory amino acid receptors and causes neurotoxicity. Ann Neurol. 1995;37:373-380.
47. Portegies P, Rosenberg NR. AIDS dementia complex: Diagnosis and drug treatment options. CNS Drugs. 1998;9:31-40.
48. Sidtis JJ, Gatsonis C, Price RW, et al. Zidovudine treatment of the AIDS dementia complex: Results of a placebo-controlled trial. AIDS Clinical Trials Group. Ann Neurol. 1993;33:343-349.
49. Portegies P, de Gans J, Lange JM, et al. Declining incidence of AIDS dementia complex after introduction of zidovudine treatment. BMJ. 1989;299:819-821.
50. Simpson DM. Human immunodeficiency virus-associated dementia: Review of pathogenesis, prophylaxis, and treatment studies of zidovudine therapy. Clin Infect Dis. 1999;29:19-34.
51. Lanier ER, Sturge G, McClernon D, et al. HIV-1 reverse transcriptase sequence in plasma and cerebrospinal fluid of patients with AIDS dementia complex treated with Abacavir. AIDS. 2001;15:747-751.
52. von Giesen HJ, Koller H, Theisen A, Arendt G. Therapeutic effects of nonnucleoside reverse transcriptase inhibitors on the central nervous system in HIV-1-infected patients. J Acquir Immune Defic Syndr. 2002;29:363-367.
53. Vago L, Bonetto S, Nebuloni M, et al. Pathological findings in the central nervous system of AIDS patients on assumed antiretroviral therapeutic regimens: Retrospective study of 1597 autopsies. AIDS. 2002;16:1925-1928.

54. Gray F, Chretien F, Vallat-Decouvelaere AV, Scaravilli F. The changing pattern of HIV neuropathology in the HAART era. J Neuropathol Exp Neurol. 2003;62: 429-440.

55. van Praag RM, Weverling GJ, Portegies P, et al. Enhanced penetration of indinavir in cerebrospinal fluid and semen after the addition of low-dose ritonavir. AIDS. 2000;14:1187-1194.

56. Solas C, Lafeuillade A, Halfon P, et al. Discrepancies between protease inhibitor concentrations and viral load in reservoirs and sanctuary sites in human immunodeficiency virus-infected patients. Antimicrob Agents Chemother. 2003;47:238-243.

57. Marra CM, Lockhart D, Zunt JR, et al. Changes in CSF and plasma HIV-1 RNA and cognition after starting potent antiretroviral therapy. Neurology. 2003;60:1388-1390.

58. Sacktor NC, Skolasky RL, Lyles RH, et al. Improvement in HIV-associated motor slowing after antiretroviral therapy including protease inhibitors. J Neurovirol. 2000;6:84-88.

59. Sacktor N, Tarwater PM, Skolasky RL, et al. CSF antiretroviral drug penetrance and the treatment of HIV-associated psychomotor slowing. Neurology. 2001;57:542-544.

60. Antinori A, Giancola ML, Grisetti S, et al. Factors influencing virological response to antiretroviral drugs in cerebrospinal fluid of advanced HIV-1-infected patients. AIDS. 2002;16:1867-1876.

61. De Luca A, Ciancio BC, Larussa D, et al. Correlates of independent HIV-1 replication in the CNS and of its control by antiretrovirals. Neurology. 2002;59:342-347.

62. Stingele K, Haas J, Zimmermann T, et al. Independent HIV replication in paired CSF and blood viral isolates during antiretroviral therapy. Neurology. 2001;56:355-361.

63. Cinque P, Presi S, Bestetti A, et al. Effect of genotypic resistance on the virological response to highly active antiretroviral therapy in cerebrospinal fluid. AIDS Res Hum Retroviruses. 2001;17:377-383.

64. McCoig C, Castrejon MM, Castano E, et al. Effect of combination antiretroviral therapy on cerebrospinal fluid HIV RNA, HIV resistance, and clinical manifestations of encephalopathy. J Pediatr. 2002;141:36-44.

65. Dana Consortium on the Therapy of HIV Dementia and Related Cognitive Disorders. A randomized, double-blind, placebo-controlled trial of deprenyl and thioctic acid in human immunodeficiency virus-associated cognitive impairment. Neurology. 1998;50:645-651.

66. Luft BJ, Hafner R, Korzun AH, et al. Toxoplasmic encephalitis in patients with the acquired immunodeficiency syndrome. Members of the ACTG 077p/ANRS 009 Study Team. N Engl J Med. 1993;329:995-1000.

67. Masur H, Kaplan JE, Holmes KK. Guidelines for preventing opportunistic infections among HIV-infected persons—2002. Recommendations of the U.S. Public Health Service and the Infectious Diseases Society of America. Ann Intern Med. 2002;137(5 Pt 2):435-478.

68. Ammassari A, Cingolani A, Pezzotti P, et al. AIDS-related focal brain lesions in the era of highly active antiretroviral therapy. Neurology. 2000;55:1194-1200.

69. Renold C, Sugar A, Chave JP, et al. Toxoplasma encephalitis in patients with the acquired immunodeficiency syndrome. Medicine (Baltimore) 1992;71:224-239.

70. Schoondermark-van de Ven E, Galama J, Kraaijeveld C, et al. Value of the polymerase chain reaction for the detection of Toxoplasma gondii in cerebrospinal fluid from patients with AIDS. Clin Infect Dis. 1993;16:661-666.

71. Contini C, Cultrera R, Seraceni S, et al. The role of stage-specific oligonucleotide primers in providing effective laboratory support for the molecular diagnosis of reactivated Toxoplasma gondii encephalitis in patients with AIDS. J Med Microbiol. 2002;51:879-890.

72. Haverkos HW. Assessment of therapy for toxoplasma encephalitis. The TE Study Group. Am J Med. 1987;82:907-914.

73. Kaplan JE, Masur H, Holmes KK. Guidelines for preventing opportunistic infections among HIV-infected persons—2002. Recommendations of the U.S. Public Health Service and the Infectious Diseases Society of America. MMWR Recomm Rep. 2002;51(RR-8):1-52.

74. So YT, Beckstead JH, Davis RL. Primary central nervous system lymphoma in acquired immune deficiency syndrome: A clinical and pathological study. Ann Neurol. 1986;20:566-572.

75. MacMahon EM, Glass JD, Hayward SD, et al. Association of Epstein-Barr virus with primary central nervous system lymphoma in AIDS. AIDS Res Hum Retroviruses. 1992;8:740-742.

76. Bossolasco S, Cinque P, Ponzoni M, et al. Epstein-Barr virus DNA load in cerebrospinal fluid and plasma of patients with AIDS-related lymphoma. J Neurovirol. 2002;8:432-438.

77. Forsyth PA, DeAngelis LM. Biology and management of AIDS-associated primary CNS lymphomas. Hematol Oncol Clin North Am. 1996;10:1125-1134.

78. Thurnher MM, Thurnher SA, Schindler E. CNS involvement in AIDS: Spectrum of CT and MR findings. Eur Radiol. 1997;7:1091-1097.

79. Antinori A, De Rossi G, Ammassari A, et al. Value of combined approach with thallium-201 single-photon emission computed tomography and Epstein-Barr virus DNA polymerase chain reaction in CSF for the diagnosis of AIDS-related primary CNS lymphoma. J Clin Oncol. 1999;17:554-560.

80. Knowles DM. Etiology and pathogenesis of AIDS-related non-Hodgkin's lymphoma. Hematol Oncol Clin North Am. 2003;17:785-820.

81. Corn BW, Donahue BR, Rosenstock JG, et al. Performance status and age as independent predictors of survival among AIDS patients with primary CNS lymphoma: A multivariate analysis of a multi-institutional experience. Cancer J Sci Am. 1997;3:52-56.

82. Raez L, Cabral L, Cai JP, et al. Treatment of AIDS-related primary central nervous system lymphoma with zidovudine, ganciclovir, and interleukin 2. AIDS Res Hum Retroviruses. 1999;15:713-719.

83. Hoffmann C, Tabrizian S, Wolf E, et al. Survival of AIDS patients with primary central nervous system lymphoma is dramatically improved by HAART-induced immune recovery. AIDS. 2001;15:2119-2127.

84. Koralnik IJ, Schellingerhavt D, Frosch, MP. Case records of the Massachusetts General Hospital. Weekly clinicopathological exercises. A 66-year-old man with progressive neurologic deficits. N Engl J Med. 2004, 350:1882-1893.

85. Berger JR, Kaszovitz B, Post MJ, Dickinson G. Progressive multifocal leukoencephalopathy associated with human immunodeficiency virus infection. A review of the literature with a report of sixteen cases. Ann Intern Med. 1987;107:78-87.

86. Fong IW, Toma E. The natural history of progressive multifocal leukoencephalopathy in patients with AIDS. Canadian PML Study Group. Clin Infect Dis. 1995;20: 1305-1310.

87. McGuire D, Barhite S, Hollander H, Miles M. JC virus DNA in cerebrospinal fluid of human immunodeficiency virus-infected patients: Predictive value for progressive multifocal leukoencephalopathy [published erratum appears in Ann Neurol. 1995;37:687]. Ann Neurol. 1995;37:395-399.

88. Koralnik IJ, Boden D, Mai VX, et al. JC virus DNA load in patients with and without progressive multifocal leukoencephalopathy. Neurology. 1999;52:253-260.

89. Taoufik Y, Gasnault J, Karaterki A, et al. Prognostic value of JC virus load in cerebrospinal fluid of patients with progressive multifocal leukoencephalopathy. J Infect Dis. 1998;178:1816-1820.

90. Yiannoutsos CT, Major EO, Curfman B, et al. Relation of JC virus DNA in the cerebrospinal fluid to survival in acquired immunodeficiency syndrome patients with biopsy-proven progressive multifocal leukoencephalopathy. Ann Neurol. 1999;45:816-821.

91. Whiteman ML, Post MJ, Berger JR, et al. Progressive multifocal leukoencephalopathy in 47 HIV-seropositive patients: Neuroimaging with clinical and pathologic correlation. Radiology. 1993;187:233-240.

92. Gray F, Geny C, Lescs MC, et al. [AIDS-related progressive multifocal leukoencephalopathy limited to U fibers, responsible for subacute encephalopathy with normal CT scan findings]. Arch Anat Cytol Pathol. 1992;40:132-137.

93. Chang L, Ernst T, Tornatore C, et al. Metabolite abnormalities in progressive multifocal leukoencephalopathy by proton magnetic resonance spectroscopy. Neurology. 1997;48:836-845.

94. Chang L, Miller BL, McBride D, et al. Brain lesions in patients with AIDS: H-1 MR spectroscopy. Radiology. 1995;197:525-531.

95. Simone IL, Federico F, Tortorella C, et al. Localised 1H-MR spectroscopy for metabolic characterisation of diffuse and focal brain lesions in patients infected with HIV. J Neurol Neurosurg Psychiatry. 1998;64:516-523.

96. Iranzo A, Moreno A, Pujol J, et al. Proton magnetic resonance spectroscopy pattern of progressive multifocal leukoencephalopathy in AIDS. J Neurol Neurosurg Psychiatry. 1999;66:520-523.

97. Katz-Brull R, Lenkinski RE, Du Pasquier RA, et al. Elevation of myo-inositol is associated with disease containment in PML. Neurology. In press.

98. Cinque P, Koralnik IJ, Clifford D. The evolving face of progressive multifocal leukoencephalopathy: Towards the definition of a consensus terminology. J Neurovirol. 2003;9(Suppl 1):88-92.

99. Hall CD, Dafni U, Simpson D, et al. Failure of cytarabine in progressive multifocal leukoencephalopathy associated with human immunodeficiency virus infection. AIDS Clinical Trials Group 243 Team. N Engl J Med. 1998;338:1345-1351.

100. Geschwind MD, Skolasky RI, Royal WS, McArthur JC. The relative contributions of HAART and alpha-interferon for therapy of progressive multifocal leukoencephalopathy in AIDS. J Neurovirol. 2001;7:353-357.

101. Royal W 3rd, Dupont B, McGuire D, et al. Topotecan in the treatment of acquired immunodeficiency syndrome-related progressive multifocal leukoencephalopathy. J Neurovirol. 2003;9:411-419.

102. Marra CM, Rajicic N, Barker DE, et al. A pilot study of cidofovir for progressive multifocal leukoencephalopathy in AIDS. AIDS. 2002;16:1791-1797.

103. Hou J, Major EO. The efficacy of nucleoside analogs against JC virus multiplication in a persistently infected human fetal brain cell line. J Neurovirol. 1998;4:451-456.

104. Aksamit AJ. Treatment of non-AIDS progressive multifocal leukoencephalopathy with cytosine arabinoside. J Neurovirol. 2001;7:386-390.

105. Levy RM, Ward S, Schalgeter K, Groothuis D. Alternative delivery systems for antiviral nucleosides and antisense oligonucleotides to the brain. J Neurovirol. 1997;3(suppl 1):S74-S75.

106. Tantisiriwat W, Tebas P, Clifford DB, et al. Progressive multifocal leukoencephalopathy in patients with AIDS receiving highly active antiretroviral therapy. Clin Infect Dis. 1999;28:1152-1154.

107. Berger JR, Levy RM, Flomenhoft D, Dobbs M. Predictive factors for prolonged survival in acquired immunodeficiency syndrome-associated progressive multifocal leukoencephalopathy. Ann Neurol. 1998;44:341-349.

108. Du Pasquier RA, Clark KW, Smith PS, et al. JCV-specific cellular immune response correlates with a favorable clinical outcome in HIV-infected individuals with progressive multifocal leukoencephalopathy. J Neurovirol. 2001;7:318-322.

109. Koralnik IJ, Du Pasquier RA, Kuroda MJ, et al. Association of prolonged survival in HLA-A2+ progressive multifocal leukoencephalopathy patients with a CTL response specific for a commonly recognized JC virus epitope. J Immunol. 2002;168:499-504.

110. Du Pasquier RA, Kuroda MJ, Schmitz JE, et al. Low frequency of cytotoxic T lymphocytes against the novel HLA-A*0201-restricted JC virus epitope VP1p36 in patients with proven or possible progressive multifocal leukoencephalopathy. J Virol. 2003;77:11918-11926.

111. Du Pasquier RA, Koralnik IJ. Inflammatory reaction in progressive multifocal leukoencephalopathy: Harmful or beneficial? J Neurovirol. 2003;9(Suppl 1):25-31.

112. Morgello S, Cho ES, Nielsen S, et al. Cytomegalovirus encephalitis in patients with acquired immunodeficiency syndrome: An autopsy study of 30 cases and a review of the literature. Hum Pathol. 1987;18:289-297.

113. Hammer SM, Squires KE, Hughes MD, et al. A controlled trial of two nucleoside analogues plus indinavir in persons with human immunodeficiency virus infection and CD4 cell counts of. 200 per cubic millimeter or less. AIDS Clinical Trials Group 320 Study Team. N Engl J Med. 1997;337:725-733.
114. Arribas JR, Storch GA, Clifford DB, Tselis AC. Cytomegalovirus encephalitis. Ann Intern Med. 1996;125:577-587.
115. Cinque P, Vago L, Brytting M, et al. Cytomegalovirus infection of the central nervous system in patients with AIDS: Diagnosis by DNA amplification from cerebrospinal fluid. J Infect Dis. 1992;166:1408-1411.
116. Holland NR, Power C, Mathews VP, et al. Cytomegalovirus encephalitis in acquired immunodeficiency syndrome (AIDS). Neurology. 1994;44(3 Pt 1):507-514.
117. Clifford DB, Arribas JR, Storch GA, et al. Magnetic resonance brain imaging lacks sensitivity for AIDS associated cytomegalovirus encephalitis. J Neurovirol. 1996;2:397-403.
118. Whitley RJ, Jacobson MA, Friedberg DN, et al. Guidelines for the treatment of cytomegalovirus diseases in patients with AIDS in the era of potent antiretroviral therapy: Recommendations of an international panel. International AIDS Society-USA. Arch Intern Med. 1998;158:957-969.
119. Levy RM, Russell E, Yungbluth M, et al. The efficacy of image-guided stereotactic brain biopsy in neurologically symptomatic acquired immunodeficiency syndrome patients. Neurosurgery. 1992;30:186-189; discussion, 189-190.
120. Holloway RG, Mushlin AI. Intracranial mass lesions in acquired immunodeficiency syndrome: using decision analysis to determine the effectiveness of stereotactic brain biopsy. Neurology. 1996;46:1010-1015.
121. Antinori A, Ammassari A, De Luca A, et al. Diagnosis of AIDS-related focal brain lesions: A decision-making analysis based on clinical and neuroradiologic characteristics combined with polymerase chain reaction assays in CSF. Neurology. 1997;48:687-694.
122. Antinori A, Ammassari A, Luzzati R, et al. Role of brain biopsy in the management of focal brain lesions in HIV-infected patients. Gruppo Italiano Cooperativo AIDS & Tumori. Neurology. 2000;54:993-997.
123. Petito CK, Navia BA, Cho ES, et al. Vacuolar myelopathy pathologically resembling subacute combined degeneration in patients with the acquired immunodeficiency syndrome. N Engl J Med. 1985;312:874-879.
124. Henin D, Smith TW, De Girolami U, et al. Neuropathology of the spinal cord in the acquired immunodeficiency syndrome. Hum Pathol. 1992;23:1106-1114.
125. Dal Pan GJ, Glass JD, McArthur JC. Clinicopathologic correlations of HIV-1-associated vacuolar myelopathy: An autopsy-based case-control study. Neurology. 1994;44:2159-2164.
126. Geraci A, Di Rocco A, Liu M, et al. AIDS myelopathy is not associated with elevated HIV viral load in cerebrospinal fluid. Neurology. 2000;55:440-442.
127. Thurnher MM, Post MJ, Jinkins JR. MRI of infections and neoplasms of the spine and spinal cord in 55 patients with AIDS. Neuroradiology. 2000;42:551-563.
128. Rottnek M, Di Rocco A, Laudier D, Morgello S. Axonal damage is a late component of vacuolar myelopathy. Neurology. 2002;58:479-481.
129. Shepherd EJ, Brettle RP, Liberski PP, et al. Spinal cord pathology and viral burden in homosexuals and drug users with AIDS. Neuropathol Appl Neurobiol. 1999;25:2-10.
130. Di Rocco A, Bottiglieri T, Werner P, et al. Abnormal cobalamin-dependent transmethylation in AIDS-associated myelopathy. Neurology. 2002;58:730-735.
131. Di Rocco A, Tagliati M, Danisi F, et al. A pilot study of L-methionine for the treatment of AIDS-associated myelopathy. Neurology. 1998;51:266-268.
132. Staudinger R, Henry K. Remission of HIV myelopathy after highly active antiretroviral therapy. Neurology. 2000;54:267-268.
133. Eyer-Silva WA, Couto-Fernandez JC, Caetano MR, et al. Remission of HIV-associated myelopathy after initiation of lopinavir in a patient with extensive previous exposure to highly active antiretroviral therapy. AIDS. 2002;16:2367-2369.
134. Feki I, Belahsen F, Ben Jemaa M, Mhiri C. [Subacute myelitis revealed by human immunodeficiency virus infection]. Rev Neurol (Paris). 2003;159(5 Pt 1):577-580.
135. Gessain A, Gout O. Chronic myelopathy associated with human T-lymphotropic virus type I (HTLV-I). Ann Intern Med. 1992;117:933-946.
136. Berger JR, Sabet A. Infectious myelopathies. Semin Neurol. 2002;22:133-142.
137. Brannagan TH 3rd, Zhou Y. HIV-associated Guillain-Barre syndrome. J Neurol Sci. 2003;208:39-42.
138. Cornblath DR, McArthur JC, Kennedy PG, et al. Inflammatory demyelinating peripheral neuropathies associated with human T-cell lymphotropic virus type III infection. Ann Neurol. 1987;21:32-40.
139. Miller RG, Parry GJ, Pfaeffl W, et al. The spectrum of peripheral neuropathy associated with ARC and AIDS. Muscle Nerve. 1988;11:857-863.
140. Piliero PJ, Fish DG, Preston S, et al. Guillain-Barre syndrome associated with immune reconstitution. Clin Infect Dis. 2003;36:111-114.
141. Morgello S, Simpson DM. Multifocal cytomegalovirus demyelinative polyneuropathy associated with AIDS. Muscle Nerve. 1994;17:176-182.
142. Leger JM, Bouche P, Bolgert F, et al. The spectrum of polyneuropathies in patients infected with HIV. J Neurol Neurosurg Psychiatry. 1989;52:1369-1374.
143. Kiprov D, Pfaeffl W, Parry G, et al. Antibody-mediated peripheral neuropathies associated with ARC and AIDS: Successful treatment with plasmapheresis. J Clin Apheresis. 1988;4:3-7.
144. Schifitto G, McDermott MP, McArthur JC, et al. Incidence of and risk factors for HIV-associated distal sensory polyneuropathy. Neurology. 2002;58:1764-1768.
145. Keswani SC, Pardo CA, Cherry CL, et al. HIV-associated sensory neuropathies. AIDS. 2002;16:2105-2117.
146. Childs EA, Lyles RH, Selnes OA, et al. Plasma viral load and CD4 lymphocytes predict HIV-associated dementia and sensory neuropathy. Neurology. 1999;52:607-613.
147. Simpson DM, Haidich AB, Schifitto G, et al. Severity of HIV-associated neuropathy is associated with plasma HIV-1 RNA levels. AIDS. 2002;16:407-412.
148. Bradley WG, Shapshak P, Delgado S, et al. Morphometric analysis of the peripheral neuropathy of AIDS. Muscle Nerve. 1998;21:1188-1195.
149. Rance NE, McArthur JC, Cornblath DR, et al. Gracile tract degeneration in patients with sensory neuropathy and AIDS. Neurology. 1988;38:265-271.
150. Tyor WR, Wesselingh SL, Griffin JW, et al. Unifying hypothesis for the pathogenesis of HIV-associated dementia complex, vacuolar myelopathy, and sensory neuropathy. J Acquir Immune Defic Syndr Hum Retrovirol. 1995;9:379-388.
151. Herzberg U, Sagen J. Peripheral nerve exposure to HIV viral envelope protein gp120 induces neuropathic pain and spinal gliosis. J Neuroimmunol. 2001;116:29-39.
152. Browne MJ, Mayer KH, Chafee SB, et al. 2′,3′-Didehydro-3′-deoxythymidine (d4T) in patients with AIDS or AIDS-related complex: A phase I trial. J Infect Dis. 1993;167:21-29.
153. Pollard RB, Peterson D, Hardy D, et al. Safety and antiretroviral effects of combined didanosine and stavudine therapy in HIV-infected individuals with CD4 counts of 200 to 500 cells/mm3. J Acquir Immune Defic Syndr. 1999;22:39-48.
154. Berger AR, Arezzo JC, Schaumburg HH, et al. 2′,3′-Dideoxycytidine (ddC) toxic neuropathy: A study of 52 patients. Neurology. 1993;43:358-362.
155. Cherry CL, Costello K, Wooley I, et al. Increasing prevalence of neuropathy in the era of highly active antiretroviral therapy (HHART). In: Ninth Conference on Retroviruses and Opportunistic Infections, Seattle, WA, 2002.
156. Brew BJ, Tisch S, Law M. Lactate concentrations distinguish between nucleoside neuropathy and HIV neuropathy. AIDS. 2003;17:1094-1096.
157. Paice JA, Ferrans CE, Lashley FR, et al. Topical capsaicin in the management of HIV-associated peripheral neuropathy. J Pain Symptom Manage. 2000;19:45-52.
158. Dorfman D, Dalton A, Khan A, et al. Treatment of painful distal sensory polyneuropathy in HIV-infected patients with a topical agent: Results of an open-label trial of 5% lidocaine gel. AIDS. 1999;13:1589-1590.
159. La Spina I, Porazzi D, Maggiolo F, et al. Gabapentin in painful HIV-related neuropathy: A report of 19 patients, preliminary observations. Eur J Neurol. 2001;8:71-75.
160. Simpson DM, McArthur JC, Olney R, et al. Lamotrigine for HIV-associated painful sensory neuropathies: A placebo-controlled trial. Neurology. 2003;60:1508-1514.
161. Kieburtz K, Simpson D, Yiannoutsos C, et al. A randomized trial of amitriptyline and mexiletine for painful neuropathy in HIV infection. AIDS Clinical Trial Group 242 Protocol Team. Neurology. 1998;51:1682-1688.
162. Mendell JR, Sahenk Z. Clinical practice. Painful sensory neuropathy. N Engl J Med. 2003;348:1243-1255.
163. Simpson DM. Selected peripheral neuropathies associated with human immunodeficiency virus infection and antiretroviral therapy. J Neurovirol. 2002;8(suppl 2):33-41.
164. Famularo G, Moretti S, Marcellini S, et al. Acetyl-carnitine deficiency in AIDS patients with neurotoxicity on treatment with antiretroviral nucleoside analogues. AIDS. 1997;11:185-190.
165. Simpson DM, Katzenstein D, Haidich B, et al. Plasma carnitine in HIV-associated neuropathy. AIDS. 2001;15:2207-2208.
166. Simpson DM, Olney RK. Peripheral neuropathies associated with human immunodeficiency virus infection. Neurol Clin. 1992;10:685-711.
167. Stricker RB, Sanders KA, Owen WF, et al. Mononeuritis multiplex associated with cryoglobulinemia in HIV infection. Neurology. 1992;42:2103-2105.
168. Said G, Lacroix C, Chemouilli P, et al. Cytomegalovirus neuropathy in acquired immunodeficiency syndrome: A clinical and pathological study. Ann Neurol. 1991;29:139-146.
169. Schifitto G, Barbano RL, Kieburtz KD, et al. HIV related vasculitic mononeuropathy multiplex: A role for IVIg? J Neurol Neurosurg Psychiatry. 1997;63:255-256.
170. Kolson DL, Gonzalez-Scarano F. HIV-associated neuropathies: Role of HIV-1, CMV, and other viruses. J Peripher Nerv Syst. 2001;6:2-7.
171. So YT, Olney RK. Acute lumbosacral polyradiculopathy in acquired immunodeficiency syndrome: Experience in 23 patients. Ann Neurol. 1994;35:53-58.
172. de Gans J, Portegies P, Tiessens G, et al. Therapy for cytomegalovirus polyradiculomyelitis in patients with AIDS: Treatment with ganciclovir. AIDS. 1990;4:421-425.
173. McCutchan JA. Cytomegalovirus infections of the nervous system in patients with AIDS. Clin Infect Dis. 1995;20:747-754.
174. Smith IL, Shinkai M, Freeman WR, Spector SA. Polyradiculopathy associated with ganciclovir-resistant cytomegalovirus in an AIDS patient: Phenotypic and genotypic characterization of sequential virus isolates. J Infect Dis. 1996;173:1481-1484.
175. Authier FJ, Gheradi RK. Peripheral neuropathies in HIV-infected patients in the era of HAART. Brain Pathol. 2003;13:223-228.
176. Moulignier A, Authier FJ, Baudrimont M, et al. Peripheral neuropathy in human immunodeficiency virus-infected patients with the diffuse infiltrative lymphocytosis syndrome. Ann Neurol. 1997;41:438-445.
177. Gherardi RK, Chretien F, Delfau-Larue MH, et al. Neuropathy in diffuse infiltrative lymphocytosis syndrome: An HIV neuropathy, not a lymphoma. Neurology. 1998;50:1041-1044.
178. Moulignier A, Moulonguet A, Pialoux G, Rozenbaum W. Reversible ALS-like disorder in HIV infection. Neurology. 2001;57:995-1001.
179. MacGowan DJ, Scelsa SN, Waldron M. An ALS-like syndrome with new HIV infection and complete response to antiretroviral therapy. Neurology. 2001;57:1094-1097.
180. Zoccolella S, Carbonara S, Minerva D, et al. A case of concomitant amyotrophic lateral sclerosis and HIV infection. Eur J Neurol. 2002;9:180-182.
181. Jubelt B, Berger JR. Does viral disease underlie ALS? Lessons from the AIDS pandemic. Neurology. 2001;57:945-946.
182. Peters BS, Winer J, Landon DN, et al. Mitochondrial myopathy associated with chronic zidovudine therapy in AIDS. Q J Med. 1993;86:5-15.
183. Johnson RW, Williams FM, Kazi S, et al. Human immunodeficiency virus-associated polymyositis: A longitudinal study of outcome. Arthritis Rheum. 2003;49:172-178.

184. Simpson DM, Citak KA, Godfrey E, et al. Myopathies associated with human immunodeficiency virus and zidovudine: Can their effects be distinguished? Neurology. 1993;43:971-976.
185. Dalakas M. HIV or zidovudine myopathy? Neurology. 1994;44:360-361; author reply, 362-364.
186. Illa I, Nath A, Dalakas M. Immunocytochemical and virological characteristics of HIV-associated inflammatory myopathies: Similarities with seronegative polymyositis. Ann Neurol. 1991;29:474-481.
187. Dalakas MC. Clinical, immunopathologic, and therapeutic considerations of inflammatory myopathies. Clin Neuropharmacol. 1992;15:327-351.
188. Dalakas MC, Illa I, Pezeshkpour GH, et al. Mitochondrial myopathy caused by long-term zidovudine therapy. N Engl J Med. 1990;322:1098-1105.
189. Grau JM, Masanes F, Pedrol E, et al. Human immunodeficiency virus type 1 infection and myopathy: Clinical relevance of zidovudine therapy. Ann Neurol. 1993;34:206-211.
190. Sheikh RA, Yasmeen S, Munn R, et al. AIDS-related myopathy. Med Electron Microsc. 1999;32:79-86.
191. Omar MA, Wilson JP. FDA adverse event reports on statin-associated rhabdomyolysis. Ann Pharmacother. 2002;36:288-295.
192. Hare CB, Vu MP, Grunfeld C, Lampiris HW. Simvastatin-nelfinavir interaction implicated in rhabdomyolysis and death. Clin Infect Dis. 2002;35:e111-112.
193. Florence E, Schrooten W, Verdonck K, et al. Rheumatological complications associated with the use of indinavir and other protease inhibitors. Ann Rheum Dis. 2002;61:82-84.
194. Modi G, Modi M, Martinus I, Saffer D. New-onset seizures associated with HIV infection. Neurology. 2000;55:1558-1561.
195. Romanelli F, Jennings HR, Nath A, et al. Therapeutic dilemma: The use of anticonvulsants in HIV-positive individuals. Neurology. 2000;54:1404-1407.
196. Romanelli F, Ryan M. Seizures in HIV-seropositive individuals: Epidemiology and treatment. CNS Drugs. 2002;16:91-98.
197. Langford TD, Letendre SL, Larrea GJ, Masliah E. Changing patterns in the neuropathogenesis of HIV during the HAART era. Brain Pathol. 2003;13:195-210.
198. Langford TD, Letendre SL, Marcotte TD, et al. Severe, demyelinating leukoencephalopathy in AIDS patients on antiretroviral therapy. AIDS. 2002;16:1019-1029.
199. Du Pasquier RA, Corey S, Margolin DH, et al. Productive infection of cerebellar granule cell neurons by JC virus in an HIV+ individual. Neurology. 2003.
200. Morgello S, Mahboob R, Yakoushina T, et al. Autopsy findings in a human immunodeficiency virus-infected population over 2 decades: Influences of gender, ethnicity, risk factors, and time. Arch Pathol Lab Med. 2002;126:182-190.
201. Goodkin K, Wilkie FL, Concha M, et al. Aging and neuro-AIDS conditions and the changing spectrum of HIV-1-associated morbidity and mortality. J Clin Epidemiol. 2001;54(suppl 1):S35-S43.

CHAPTER **121**

Malignancies in Human Immunodeficiency Virus Infection

AMY GATES

PHOEBE R. TRUBOWITZ

PAUL A. VOLBERDING

Malignancies in the setting of immunodeficiency were well described in the literature long before the advent of the human immunodeficiency virus (HIV) epidemic.[1-3] The incidence of malignancy is increased significantly in the setting of abnormal cell-mediated immunity.[1,3,4] This increase in incidence does not apply, however, to the cancers most commonly seen in the general population. In immunosuppressed individuals, a narrow spectrum of more unusual tumors is observed, such as Kaposi's sarcoma (KS) and non-Hodgkin's lymphoma (NHL).[3,4] HIV infection also produces profound defects in cell-mediated immunity,[5] and patients with HIV infection have a markedly increased risk of developing such neoplasms.

KS was the first cancer to be recognized as related to acquired immunodeficiency syndrome (AIDS)[6,7] and was designated as such by the Centers for Disease Control and Prevention (CDC).[8] The CDC subsequently added primary central nervous system lymphoma (PCNSL), intermediate-grade and high-grade NHL, and invasive cervical cancer to the list of AIDS-defining conditions. The designation of invasive cervical cancer is controversial because its high frequency may reflect individuals' lifestyles and consequently high rates of human papillomavirus (HPV) infection, rather than impaired immunity.[9] Several other cancers have not officially been deemed AIDS-defining by the CDC, but their incidence may be increased in HIV-positive patients.[10] These include anal cancer, Hodgkin's disease (HD), leiomyosarcoma in children, testicular cancer, skin cancer, oral mucosa and head and neck cancer, and possibly lung cancer.[11-13] Regardless of the causal relationship between various malignancies and the underlying immunodeficiency state, the natural history of cancer may be altered in the setting of HIV infection.[14,15] In the era preceding highly active antiretroviral therapy (HAART), patients seemed to present with advanced cancers with unusually aggressive natural histories. Response to therapy in the pre-HAART era was disappointing. Since the widespread implementation of HAART, the incidence, clinical presentation, and response to therapy may be changing.

Management of HIV-infected individuals with a malignancy imposes unique obstacles. The oncologist treating these patients often has to risk further immunocompromise to administer adequate therapy for the treatment of an aggressive neoplasm. Poor bone marrow reserve and the risk of intercurrent opportunistic infections often compromise the delivery of adequate dose intensity in these patients. Toxicities of chemotherapeutic agents, antibiotics, and radiation therapy are often severe, further impairing the effectiveness of treatment.

This chapter focuses on the malignancies most commonly associated with AIDS from primarily a clinical perspective. KS, systemic NHL, PCNSL, and anogenital neoplasia are discussed in detail. The natural history of and various therapeutic options for these malignancies are presented. Brief mention is made of other cancers in the setting of HIV infection.

KAPOSI'S SARCOMA

Epidemiology

Kaposi first described the entity KS in 1872.[16] Before the advent of organ transplantation in the 1950s, KS was a rarely recognized disease, confined largely to persons of Eastern European or Mediterranean descent. This classic variant, usually seen in elderly men, generally has an indolent course and primarily involves the skin over the lower extremities and feet.[17,18] It also can be seen occasionally in homosexual men who are HIV negative.[19] In central Africa, variants of KS can be more aggressive and infiltrating, particularly in children, in whom the lymphadenopathic variant is rapidly fatal.

In the early 1970s, KS was seen occasionally in immunosuppressed allograft recipients.[2] In the early 1980s, cases of KS in young homosexual men helped alert the medical community to the AIDS epidemic. Several aspects of these cases were distinctly unusual. First, they affected a much younger population than prior (classic) KS in the United States. Second, the tumor was much more aggressive. Finally, the patients often had a spectrum of unusual infections diagnosed simultaneously in other homosexual men but had no known reason for immunodeficiency. The combination of these striking findings in similar "risk" populations soon led to the recognition of the common underlying disease, AIDS.

KS is the most common neoplasm affecting HIV-infected individuals. It disproportionately affects HIV-infected homosexual men. In the first several years of the epidemic, 47% of homosexual and bisexual men with newly diagnosed AIDS had KS compared with 3.9% of intravenous drug users.[20] KS is rarely reported in intravenous drug users or other HIV risk groups.[21,22] The proportion of patients with KS as their AIDS-defining illness has changed with the epidemic.[23,24] In New York City, KS was the initial AIDS diagnosis in 50% of homosexual men who were not intravenous drug users diagnosed between 1981 and 1983. Between 1984 and 1987, this proportion decreased to 30%, well before the introduction of effective antiretroviral therapies. Similar trends have been reported in San Francisco.[25] Subsequent data from the Multicenter AIDS Cohort Study indicated a steady decline in the incidence of KS through January 1995 followed by a more precipitous decline from January 1995 to January 1997. This decreased incidence corresponds to the more widespread use of HAART.[26] The number of new KS cases in the cohort decreased from 25.6 per 1000 patient-years in the early 1990s to an average incidence of 7.5 per 1000 patient-years in 1996 to 1997.[26] Numerous other studies have shown a dramatic decline in the occurrence of KS in conjunction with widespread use of HAART.[27,28] A meta-analysis including 47,936 patients found that the incidence of KS declined from 15.2 per 1000 patient-years in the pre-HAART era to 4.9 per 1000 patient-years in the HAART era ($P < .0001$).[29] That translates into a relative risk for KS of 0.32 (99% confidence interval 0.26 to 0.40) in the HAART era compared with the pre-HAART era. Tumor registry data from San Francisco General Hospital showed a decline in the number of newly diagnosed cases of KS from 103 in 1995 to 62 in 1996 to 3 in 2002.

Pathogenesis

The pathogenesis of KS in HIV-infected patients is complex and involves viral processes and dysregulation of cytokine pathways. A sexually transmitted coinfection has long been suspected from the epidemiology of AIDS-related KS.[24,30] In 1994, Chang and co-workers[31] discovered a new herpesvirus, human herpesvirus type 8 (HHV-8), or KS herpesvirus, in KS lesions (see Chapter 137). The virus is found predominantly in a latent form within the endothelial spindle cells of the lesions. It has been identified in all types of KS, including classic KS, African or endemic KS, transplant-associated KS, and AIDS-related KS.[32] The virus also can be found in peripheral blood mononuclear cells in many patients with KS, and this frequently precedes the development of KS in AIDS patients.[33,34] HHV-8 also is associated with rare lymphoproliferative diseases most often seen in HIV-infected individuals, including Castleman's disease and a rare form of NHL called *primary effusion or body cavity lymphoma*.[35]

The transmissibility of HHV-8 is unclear. It has been detected in semen and prostate tissue.[36] More recent data suggest that saliva may be a likely mode of transmission with oropharyngeal entry.[37] Seropositive rates are as expected given the epidemiology of KS[38]; that is, homosexual men with HIV or other active sexually transmitted diseases have the highest seropositivity rates.

The pathogenesis of KS is complex, with multiple putative pathways involving HHV-8, HIV, cytokines, integrins, and altered apoptosis and cell cycle controls.[39,40] The HHV-8 genome encodes many homologues of human cellular gene products that are involved in inflammation, cell cycle regulation, and angiogenesis, such as viral cyclin-D1, vascular endothelial growth factor, basic fibroblast growth factor, and interleukin-6.[41] Cytokines released from spindle cells and inflammatory cells stimulate the growth of the tumors in complex autocrine and paracrine pathways, as does the HIV *tat* gene product.[42] In vivo data show that inoculation of the HIV *tat* gene and basic fibroblast growth factor results in the development of KS-like tumors in nude mice.[42-44] The defective cellular immunity that results from HIV creates a permissive environment for tumor formation.

The histopathology of KS is characterized by a proliferation of abnormal vascular structures. Three histologic variants have been reported: spindle cell, anaplastic, and mixed cell.[45-47] The mixed-cell variant is the most common of the three seen in AIDS patients. Three features characterize this variant: (1) proliferation within the tumor of vascular structures and slits, often lined by abnormally large, malignant-appearing endothelial cells; (2) proliferation of surrounding spindle-shaped cells; and (3) extravasation of erythrocytes. The spindle cell seems to originate from lymphatic endothelium.[48]

Clinical Manifestations

The natural history of AIDS-related KS is variable and difficult to predict. The disease can occur in patients with a wide range of CD4+ cell counts but becomes increasingly common as immune function declines. Although an occasional patient has a spontaneous remission or long interval without disease progression, others have a rapidly progressive course.[49] Patients with limited disease and controlled HIV infection can do reasonably well. In the setting of uncontrolled HIV viral replication, however, KS progresses rapidly.

The skin is the most common first site of presentation. The lesions are generally painless and nonpruritic and appear as firm, slightly raised or nodular tumors. Cutaneous nodules ranging from 0.5 to 2 cm in diameter are observed frequently. In some patients, they may be barely visible or nonpalpable initially; in others, the nodules may have the appearance of small ecchymoses. In more advanced disease, cutaneous lesions can coalesce to form large, plaquelike tumor masses involving extensive cutaneous surfaces, especially over the medial aspect of the upper thigh. In light-skinned individuals, the lesions are typically violaceous in color. In dark-skinned individuals, the lesions appear more brownish or black. Lesions typically appear on the face and in the oral cavity or on the feet and lower extremities, although they may affect almost any site. KS frequently involves the plantar surfaces of the foot but rarely the palms. Other notable sites of disease include the tip of the nose, periorbital area, hard and soft palates, gingival areas of the mouth, external ear, conjunctiva, and penis. At autopsy, almost every organ system can show involvement. Bone marrow disease and parenchymal brain disease are distinctly uncommon, however. KS is a multicentric tumor, and numerous lesions can appear simultaneously in widely scattered areas of the body. KS lesions tend to be circular, but lesions on the back or around the neck can be linear, following cutaneous lymphatic drainage patterns called *Langer's lines*.

The disease may remain quiescent for many months, but this period may be followed by a sudden rapid increase in disease activity with the appearance of numerous new lesions and enlargement of existing ones. Visceral involvement is extremely common, especially as the disease progresses, and may involve almost any site, most commonly the gastrointestinal tract. The head and neck also are sites of typical involvement, and careful inspection of the oral cavity shows evidence of KS lesions in 30% of individuals at the time of initial diagnosis. Oral involvement correlates with KS in the gastrointestinal tract.

KS does not commonly cause death of patients with HIV infection except for patients who develop diffuse pulmonary parenchymal involvement. Despite the relative lack of mortality associated with KS, morbidity associated with more advanced disease can be considerable. Bulky cutaneous lesions may become painful. Large, plaquelike lesions may coalesce and restrict movement. Lymphatic obstruction is common and may result in severe edema, usually involving the lower extremities or the face. Visceral spread of KS involving the gastrointestinal tract is rarely symptomatic. Rare cases of obstruction, perforation, or gastrointestinal bleeding have been reported, however.[50] Finally, the social problems associated with this disfiguring neoplasm in the setting of an already socially stigmatizing disease cannot be overemphasized.

Pulmonary involvement is an ominous complication of KS and merits special attention. In contrast to KS at other visceral sites, pulmonary KS is generally symptomatic. Common symptoms include a barking cough, bronchospasm, and dyspnea. This complication tends to occur in the setting of advanced AIDS, with most individuals having CD4+ cell counts of less than 100/mm³.[51] Pulmonary involvement tends to occur in patients with more extensive cutaneous disease (e.g., with >50 lesions). It can occur, however, in patients with minimal and absent cutaneous KS.[52] The disease is often rapidly progressive when it involves the lungs. Before the HAART era, median survival was 2 to 6 months.[51,53] Several small series indicate that in the setting of aggressive HAART therapy, the outlook for patients with pulmonary KS may be more optimistic.[54-56]

The radiographic appearance is variable, with the characteristic reticulonodular pattern seen in approximately one third of patients.[53] Diffuse interstitial infiltrates are seen more commonly and may be difficult to distinguish from infiltrates in *Pneumocystis carinii* pneumonia.[51,53,57] Pleural effusions, usually cytologically benign, are seen frequently,[51,53,57] and hilar adenopathy is observed in approximately 50% of cases.[51] Respiratory failure resulting in death is common in patients with pulmonary KS.

Careful examination of the skin and oral cavity at each clinic visit is the key to early diagnosis. When lesions are identified, histologic confirmation is essential. This confirmation is particularly important because other cutaneous diseases, some of which can mimic KS, are common in HIV-infected individuals. For cutaneous lesions, a small punch biopsy (2 to 4 mm) is usually adequate.

In the initial evaluation of a patient with KS, tumor extent should be determined by a complete skin examination. The oral cavity also should be examined carefully. Clinically important visceral KS can occur, however, in the absence of cutaneous or oral manifestations in approximately 15% of cases. If unexplained gastrointestinal or pulmonary symptoms are present, a visceral evaluation should be performed. Endoscopically the classic appearance of small submucosal vascular nodules establishes the diagnosis of visceral KS. Biopsies are diagnostic in only a few cases of gastrointestinal KS because the tumors are generally submucosal, but biopsy specimens may exclude other diagnoses. In patients with suspected pulmonary KS, violaceous endobronchial lesions typically are observed on bronchoscopic examination. Endobronchial biopsy is discouraged because of the risk of hemorrhage. Bronchoscopic visualization of typical lesions generally is accepted for the purpose of diagnosis of pulmonary disease in patients who have had KS at other sites.[53] Gallium scanning can be helpful in differentiating KS from pulmonary infection because KS is not gallium avid.[53]

Treatment

With the exception of patients who develop pulmonary involvement, few patients' deaths are due directly to KS. It seems unlikely that therapy directed toward this neoplasm would have a significant impact on survival. A retrospective review of 194 cases of KS by Volberding and colleagues[58] validated this point by showing that there was no significant difference in survival time between a group of patients treated with chemotherapy (or interferon [IFN]-alfa) and patients not treated.

The primary goals of treatment for patients with KS are palliation of symptoms and cosmesis. When to initiate treatment must be decided on a patient-by-patient basis because even disease that seems to be medically uncomplicated may evoke powerful emotions for patients because of the social stigma associated with the disease. Treatments may range from potent HAART to systemic chemotherapy and are discussed next.

Treatment Modalities

KS is a systemic disease mandating a systemic approach to therapy in all patients. Because HIV has direct and indirect roles in the pathogenesis, targeting HIV is a crucial component of therapy. HAART is strongly recommended for all patients with KS. From there, therapeutic options for AIDS-related KS can be divided into local and systemic approaches.

Local Therapy. Radiotherapy has been the mainstay of local therapy for KS. A single dose of 800 cGy or an equivalent fractionated dose can be highly effective in achieving local palliation in selected patients.[59,60] Maximal response to radiotherapy generally is seen over the course of several weeks to months after treatment.[59] Radiotherapy is best suited for patients with a single or a few locally symptomatic areas. Electron-beam radiation applied to the entire face is highly effective in relieving facial edema. Radiotherapy also can be useful for treating dysphagia caused by pharyngeal lesions and tumor masses of the eye or the extremities.[60] Complications such as severe mucositis, radiotherapy fibrosis, loss of skin compliance, and chronic lymphedema are common and may result in significant discomfort after 6 to 12 months. In addition, complete disappearance of lesions is unusual at any site. As a result of the significant oral toxicity that has been observed with x-irradiation, laser surgery has been increasingly employed at San Francisco General Hospital for the treatment of intraoral lesions, with a lower incidence of morbidity.

Small cutaneous lesions can be treated with intralesional chemotherapy for cosmetic purposes.[61] Repeated treatments may be necessary. Intralesional chemotherapy can cause significant pain, and areas of hyperpigmentation frequently remain after treatment.

Cryotherapy using liquid nitrogen and laser therapy have been used successfully for the treatment of isolated, small KS lesions. These modalities have been particularly useful for the treatment of cosmetically unsightly lesions.

Finally, alitretinoin gel (Panretin) is a topical treatment that can be used for limited cutaneous KS. This is a retinoid that binds to retinoic acid and retinoic X receptors to induce differentiation and apoptosis.[62] Its activity also may result from downregulation of interleukin-6 production. Response rates of 49% ($n = 184$) in a phase III study have been reported.[62] Adverse effects include dry skin and light hypersensitivity.

Systemic Therapy. Systemic therapy consisting of antiretroviral therapy alone or in combination with KS-directed therapies is appropriate for most patients. Several antineoplastic agents used alone or in combination are active against KS.

In recent years, single-agent chemotherapy has replaced combination chemotherapy for KS. The liposomal forms of doxorubicin (Doxil) and daunorubicin (DaunoXome) should be considered first-line treatment for relatively advanced KS as a result of their efficacy and low incidence of toxicity. In a large randomized trial, Doxil produced a response rate nearly twice that of doxorubicin (Adriamycin), bleomycin, and vincristine (ABV), the once standard first-line therapy for advanced KS.[64] Liposome-encapsulated doxorubicin also was associated with a lower incidence of toxic effects, such as nausea, fatigue, and alopecia. Neutropenia occurred as frequently with the liposomal agent as with the standard combination regimen.[65] In a similar study, liposomal daunorubicin was compared with Adriamycin, bleomycin, and vinblastine.[66] A lower incidence of alopecia, nausea, and neuropathy was noted with the liposomal agent. Response rates were similar in the two arms.

Paclitaxel (Taxol) has significant antitumor activity in patients with previously untreated[67] and refractory KS.[67,68] Response rates are greater than 50% regardless of prior therapy. Outstanding clinical responses have been seen in patients with advanced refractory symptomatic disease. The most significant side effects are hypersensitivity, myelosuppression, peripheral neuropathy, and alopecia. Most patients in these trials have required adjunctive therapy with colony-stimulating factors (CSFs). This agent should be considered the treatment of choice for refractory KS.

Vinorelbine (Navelbine) is another single agent that can be used as salvage therapy. Response rates of 43% have been reported in phase II studies of heavily pretreated patients.[69] Toxicity is mild and includes myelosuppression and reversible neurotoxicity.

Etoposide (VP-16), Adriamycin, vincristine, and bleomycin all have significant antitumor activity. Combinations such as Adriamycin, bleomycin, and vincristine have resulted in overall response rates of 24% to 60% in patients with pulmonary KS.[70,71] The use of these agents has declined dramatically since the introduction of the aforementioned therapies.

The availability of the myeloid growth factors, granulocyte colony-stimulating factor (G-CSF), and granulocyte-macrophage colony-stimulating factor (GM-CSF) has made it possible to administer myelosuppressive chemotherapy to individuals for whom it might not have been possible in the past. Because many individuals with advanced KS have poor myeloid reserve, these agents can be valuable adjuncts to chemotherapy. For most individuals with KS, however, the use of a CSF is unnecessary. At San Francisco General Hospital, we reserve the use of CSFs for patients who require an anthracycline or paclitaxel as a part of their chemotherapeutic regimen and who have a neutrophil count less than 1500/mm³ before any chemotherapy cycle is initiated. Although no specific guidelines exist, we generally begin administration of CSFs 1 to 4 days after chemotherapy administration. In our experience, a dose of 300 µg (5 µg/kg) administered on alternate days for five doses is often adequate. Therapy should be individualized, however, and frequent neutrophil counts should be obtained during the first cycle of therapy to establish the optimal dosing regimen.

As the pathogenesis of KS is elucidated, targeted therapies, including immunomodulating agents, are intriguing treatment options. IFN-alfa is an attractive agent for the treatment of AIDS-related KS because it has antiproliferative[72] and apparent anti-HIV activity.[73,74] Many clinical trials of IFN-alfa as a single agent have shown significant antitumor activity in AIDS-related KS.[72,75-79] High doses (>20 million U/m²) of IFN-alfa are more effective than lower doses in inducing antitumor responses.[76,77,79,80] Several studies have shown that patients with better immune function (higher CD4⁺ cell counts) and without a prior history of opportunistic infection or systemic symptoms are more likely to respond to IFN-alfa than patients with a more compromised immune status, history of a prior opportunistic infection, or clinical symptoms.[81,82]

Despite objective responses and reports of long disease-free remissions, the use of IFN-alfa in high doses as a single agent has been significantly hampered by its toxicity profile. With long-term administration, many patients experience a flulike syndrome, with low-grade fever, anorexia, malaise, myalgias, and weight loss. Although many develop tachyphylaxis to these symptoms within the first several weeks, they can persist and become disabling. Treatment must be reduced or discontinued altogether.

The combination of IFN-alfa and nucleoside analogues has been investigated in several phase I and phase II trials. The combination of IFN-alfa with a nucleoside analogue is attractive from the standpoint of antiretroviral therapy because these agents seem to inhibit HIV-1 replication at different stages of the viral life cycle. The combination seems to be synergistic in inhibiting HIV-1 replication in vitro.[83] Several studies evaluating zidovudine and IFN-alfa have reported response rates of 40% and greater.[84,85] Combining antiviral therapy with IFN-alfa allows for lower effective dosing of the latter. The use of IFN-alfa in combination with HAART may be considered in patients with relatively intact immune function whose KS is minimally symptomatic. Clinical trials of IFN-alfa with HAART are in progress.

Angiogenesis inhibitors are another class of exciting therapies for KS. Thalidomide and COL-3 are oral agents that have shown activity in mild KS in phase I studies.[86,87] Phase II studies are under way.

Antiviral therapies include anti-HHV-8 therapy and anti-HIV therapy. Therapies directed against HHV-8 have been disappointing. The latent form of HHV-8 predominates in KS lesions, making it a difficult target. Anti-HIV therapy has made a huge impact on the management of patients with KS, however. HAART not only has contributed to the declining incidence of KS, but also may be altering the natural history of the neoplastic process itself. Several anecdotal reports[88-92] exist of anti-KS responses to antiretroviral therapy alone. Gill and colleagues reported a response rate of almost 50% in patients with KS treated with HAART alone.[92a] This phenomenon generally is associated with an effective antiviral response. In addition, HAART may prolong the duration of response to chemotherapy for patients with more advanced KS. Bower and colleagues[93] reported that the time to treatment failure for patients treated with chemotherapy plus HAART was 20.4 months compared with a time to treatment failure of 6 months for patients treated with chemotherapy alone. Holkova and co-workers[54] reported on six patients with pulmonary KS treated with chemotherapy and HAART. All patients responded to treatment, and chemotherapy was stopped when clinical symptoms had resolved and the viral load was undetectable. In contrast to the dismal prognosis of 3- to 5-month median survival in the pre-HAART era, all six patients in this study were well at a median follow-up of 78 weeks.

For patients with asymptomatic KS, a trial of HAART seems warranted and might prove effective enough to eliminate KS-specific therapy altogether. For patients with more advanced KS, HAART seems an integral component of therapy. It is now possible to discontinue KS-specific therapies in patients who show a good virologic response to HAART, eliminating the need for prolonged administration of chemotherapy for some patients.

Treatment

Care of patients with KS should be individually tailored. KS should be thought of as a systemic disease, so in most cases, treatment should be systemic in nature. Systemic therapy may be defined as combination antiretroviral therapy, immunologic therapy, or systemic chemotherapy. Local therapeutic modalities, such as intralesional chemotherapy, radiotherapy, or laser surgery, should be reserved for patients with minimal or locally symptomatic disease. These patients should be concurrently receiving some form of systemic therapy, such as antiviral therapy. Patients with asymptomatic disease should be given combination antiretroviral therapy. If they already are receiving such a regimen, steps should be taken to maximize viral control as determined by viral load measurements. Such intervention alone may be effective therapy for KS in some patients.[94]

For relatively asymptomatic patients whose KS is not responding to antiretroviral therapy alone and for whom the KS is predominantly as issue of cosmesis, enrollment on a clinical trial investigating immunomodulating therapies should be considered. Alitretinoin gel is also an option.

Chemotherapy is recommended for all patients with pulmonary KS and for patients with extensive or symptomatic disease that mandates a rapid response. The liposomal anthracyclines (Doxil and DaunoXome) are considered first-line agents. Paclitaxel and vinorelbine should be used for individuals with refractory disease or contraindications to anthracycline treatment.

SYSTEMIC NON-HODGKIN'S LYMPHOMA

The first cases of NHL in homosexual men were reported in 1982,[95] and increasing numbers have been reported since that time. Overall, HIV-infected individuals have a 200-fold increased risk of NHL compared with HIV-negative individuals. Before HAART, NHL was the initial AIDS diagnosis in 2.5% to 5% of HIV-infected individuals[96] and was estimated to occur in approximately 8% of all HIV-infected individuals. It is controversial whether the incidence of NHL has changed since the introduction of HAART.

The NHLs are a heterogeneous group of malignancies. Their biologic behavior ranges from indolent, requiring no therapy, to aggressive, with few long-term survivors.[97] Although HIV-infected individuals may be at increased risk for all forms of NHL, only intermediate-grade or high-grade lymphomas are considered AIDS-defining.[98] Low-grade lymphomas occur infrequently in individuals with HIV infection and are not AIDS-defining according to the CDC criteria. B-cell phenotype, advanced stage disease, and extranodal disease occur in most patients with HIV NHL. Before HAART, the median survival despite aggressive chemotherapy was 5 to 8 months with most patients dying of intercurrent infection or progressive lymphoma.

Epidemiology

Individuals with impairment of cell-mediated immunity show a marked increase in the incidence of NHL.[1,3] The best described of these groups are immunosuppressed allograft recipients, whose incidence of NHL is 30 to 50 times that of the general population.[3,4,99] Similar trends occur in populations at risk for HIV infection. Harnly and colleagues[100] showed a statistically significant increase in the incidence of NHL among never-married men age 25 to 44 years in San Francisco from 1980 to 1985. The increase in census tracts with a high incidence of AIDS was greater than the increase seen in other San Francisco census tracts. In 1985, the incidence of NHL was five times greater than the rate in 1980. Incidence rates for other neoplasms did not show such increases. The incidence of NHL in New York City follows similar trends.[81]

Several studies have examined the impact of HAART on the incidence of systemic NHL. Most have not shown a significant decline in the incidence of systemic NHL since the widespread use of HAART.[42,101-104] The Multicenter AIDS Cohort Study reported a 21% per year increase in cases of NHL from 1985 to 1997. In contrast, Appleby and associates[29] reported a significant decrease (relative risk of 0.58; 99% confidence interval 0.45 to 0.74) in the incidence of NHL when comparing the HAART era with the pre-HAART era in a meta-analysis including 47,936 patients with systemic lymphoma and central nervous system (CNS) lymphoma.

Pathogenesis

The molecular characteristics of AIDS-related NHL exhibit a great deal of heterogeneity, suggesting that lymphomagenesis may occur by a variety of different mechanisms. Large cell lymphomas, including intermediate-grade large cell lymphomas and high-grade immunoblastic lymphomas, account for about 60% of all lymphomas observed in HIV-infected individuals.[105] Within this histologic subtype, monoclonal and polyclonal malignant lymphoproliferative processes have been shown.[106-109] Autopsy data show these polyclonal processes to be as aggressive as typical monoclonal lymphomas.[81]

In immunosuppressed allograft recipients, Epstein-Barr virus (EBV) is seen in virtually all polyclonal NHLs and has been implicated as a causative agent in the development of this neoplasm.[52,99,110] In contrast, EBV DNA sequences are present in 40% of systemic AIDS-related NHLs.[96,111-113] NHL occurring in HIV-negative individuals is associated with EBV in only 10% to 20% of cases. Another virus has been implicated in a rare type of HIV NHL, primary effusion lymphoma (PEL) or body cavity–based lymphoma. PEL presents as malignant effusions with a paucity of nodal masses. It is aggressive and often refractory to chemotherapy. HHV-8 has been universally found in malignant cells, often in conjunction with EBV.[114-116]

The question of a direct role for HIV in the pathogenesis of HIV-associated lymphomas has been raised by the observation of a clonally integrated HIV genome in tumor-associated macrophages.[118,119] These macrophages have been shown to be activated and proliferating. McGrath and colleagues[120] postulated a sequential pathogenesis model of HIV NHL in which HIV integration into macrophages results in cytokine overexpression and polyclonal B-cell expansion with eventual evolution to a monoclonal process. Support for this model comes from experiments showing that macrophages from the cellular effusions of patients with HIV PEL were capable of inducing the development of murine T-cell lymphomas.[121] Cytokine dysregulation has been well documented, and there is evidence for expression of high levels of the lymphostimulatory cytokines interleukin-6 and interleukin-10 in AIDS-related large cell and immunoblastic lymphomas.[122-124]

The heterogeneity of molecular characteristics, including clonality and the presence or absence of EBV, suggests that lymphomagenesis may occur through several different mechanisms. Although EBV may be involved in the pathogenesis of some HIV NHLs, other viruses, cytokines, and even the underlying immune dysregulation itself may give rise to NHL.

Clinical Characteristics

As in other immunocompromised individuals, most NHLs observed in HIV-infected individuals are classified as B-cell neoplasms.[125-127] A few NHLs of other histologic and immunologic subtypes have been observed, including T-cell lymphoma[96,128,129] and others of uncertain lineage.[130] PEL characteristically has a null phenotype.[115,131] In 327 cases of HIV NHL reported from five centers, 73% of the lymphomas were high grade, 24% were intermediate grade, and 3% were low grade.[96,117,132-134] Most B-cell lymphomas in these patients are classified as diffuse large-cell tumors of intermediate-grade type or high-grade immunoblastic or Burkitt's type.

Systemic NHL occurs in individuals with widely ranging levels of immune function.[96,135,136] Before HAART, a median CD4+ cell count between approximately 100/mm³ and 180/mm³ was reported.[96,137] Of cases, 30% occurred in persons with a CD4+ count greater than 200/mm³.[136] Some data suggest that CD4+ T-cell count at the time of diagnosis of NHL may be increasing in the HAART era.[101] Immune function may vary with histologic subtype. PEL and immunoblastic NHL tend to occur in patients with advanced AIDS, whereas Burkitt's NHL tends to occur in patients with more preserved immune function.[138]

The hallmark of AIDS-related systemic NHL is widespread disease involving extranodal sites. Ziegler and co-workers[139] reported that 95% of patients from several institutions had evidence of extranodal disease, including 42% with CNS involvement and 33% with bone marrow involvement.

Similarly, Knowles and colleagues[117] reported extranodal disease in 87% of a series of 89 patients diagnosed at New York University. The most common sites of extranodal disease were the gastrointestinal tract, CNS, bone marrow, and liver. At San Francisco General Hospital, Kaplan and associates[96] reported that 31% of patients had extranodal disease alone. Several reports described extensive extranodal involvement (stage IV disease) in 60% to 70% of HIV-infected patients at presentation.[96,117,135,139]

Gastrointestinal NHL is common in persons with HIV disease, occurring in 27% of patients. Most of these cases involve the stomach,[140] but virtually any site in the gastrointestinal tract or hepatobiliary tree can be involved. Other unusual sites include the subcutaneous and soft tissue, epidural space, gingiva, paranasal sinus,[117,133,135,139,141] heart, and pericardium.[139,142]

The HAART era has been notable for a change in some of the clinical characteristics of patients with HIV NHL. Matthews and colleagues[101] reported that significantly fewer individuals had a prior AIDS-defining condition or a CD4+ count less than 100/mm³ at the time of NHL diagnosis in the HAART era compared with the pre-HAART era. Age at diagnosis of AIDS-related NHL also was higher in the HAART era compared with the pre-HAART era.[101] It is unclear whether HAART would impact stage of disease at diagnosis or pattern of spread.[143] The effects of HAART on the survival of patients with HIV NHL is unclear and is discussed subsequently.

Prognostic Features

Prognosticators for patients with HIV NHL include host, lymphoma, and AIDS-related factors. Clinical features associated with poor prognosis included age older than 35 years, CD4+ cell count less than 100/mm³, history of intravenous drug use, history of prior AIDS-defining condition, poor performance status, elevated lactate dehydrogenase, and tumor bulk as deemed by stage of disease.[144] Use of HAART has been shown to be a positive prognostic factor.[101]

Treatment

Multiple-agent chemotherapeutic regimens have resulted in a dramatic improvement in the prognosis for non–HIV-infected individuals with aggressive NHL.[145] This success has not been equaled in HIV-infected individuals. Complete response rates of 33% to 56% and survival times of 5 to 8 months were typical before the widespread use of HAART (Table 121-1).[146-148,160]

Pre–Highly Active Antiretroviral Therapy Era

In the pre-HAART era, dose intensity of chemotherapy had been hampered by dose reduction and treatment delays. Cytopenias, related to poor bone marrow reserve, and intercurrent infections were the most common causes of decreased dose intensity.[149-151] This decreased dose intensity likely translated into the poor clinical outcomes observed for patients with HIV NHL.

The substantial toxicity observed with standard-dose chemotherapy led to the investigation of reduced-dose chemotherapy for patients with HIV NHL. Kaplan and colleagues[96] reported the results of a multicenter trial comparing standard-dose m-BACOD (methotrexate, bleomycin, Adriamycin, cyclophosphamide, Oncovin [vincristine], and dexamethasone) with growth factor support (methotrexate, 200 mg/m² day 15; bleomycin, 4 U/m² day 1; doxorubicin, 45 mg/m² day 1; cyclophosphamide, 600 mg/m² day 1; vincristine, 1.4 mg/m² day 1; and dexamethasone, 6 mg/m² days 1 to 5) with low-dose m-BACOD with growth factor support as needed (same dosages except doxorubicin, 25 mg/m² day 1; cyclophosphamide, 300 mg/m² day 1; and dexamethasone, 3 mg/m² days 1 to 5). This study found no significant difference in complete response rate or survival between the two

TABLE 121-1 Response to Chemotherapy and Survival in Human Immunodeficiency Virus–Associated Non-Hodgkin's Lymphoma

Institution*	No.	Treatment Regimen†	Complete Response (%)	Median Survival (mo)
USC	22	m-BACOD and others	45	NA
NYU	83	Various	33	5.0
UCSF	65	Various	54	5.5
MSKCC	30	Various	56	6.0
Pacific Medical Center	31	CHOP MACOP-B	39	7.0
Multicenter	66	Various	53	NA
AIDS Clinical Trials Group	36	m-BACOD‡	42	NA
Italian Cooperative Group	72	Various	35	4.0

*USC, University of Southern California; NYU, New York University; UCSF, University of California, San Francisco; MSKCC, Memorial Sloan-Kettering Cancer Center; Multicenter, UCSF, New York Hospital/Cornell, University of Texas/M.D. Anderson, NYU/Kaplan Cancer Center, MSKCC; AIDS Clinical Trials Group, National Institutes of Health.

†Cyclophosphamide, doxorubicin, vincristine, and prednisone; m-BACOD, methotrexate, bleomycin, doxorubicin (Adriamycin), cyclophosphamide, vincristine (Oncovin), and dexamethasone.

‡Given at reduced doses.

From Ziegler J, Beckstead J, Volberding P, et al. Non-Hodgkin's lymphoma in 90 homosexual men: Relation to generalized lymphadenopathy and the acquired immunodeficiency syndrome. N Engl J Med. 1984;311:565-570.

regimens. Significantly less toxicity (particularly fever and neutropenia) was observed with the use of reduced-dose chemotherapy for patients with HIV NHL. Results were similar for patients with CD4$^+$ cell counts greater or less than 100/mm^3, although overall survival times of patients with CD4$^+$ counts greater than 100/mm^3 were longer in both treatment arms. These data suggested that immune function may be a stronger predictor of clinical outcome than choice of chemotherapy regimen and that most patients did not benefit from higher dose chemotherapy. Before HAART, low-dose therapy was considered appropriate therapy for HIV NHL.

Highly Active Antiretroviral Therapy Era

The dramatic effect on immune reconstitution observed with HAART has renewed interest in an aggressive approach to HIV NHL. The integration of HAART with chemotherapy is considered an essential component of treatment. In addition to standard-dose chemotherapy, infusional chemotherapy, high-dose chemotherapy, and biotherapy are treatment options for patients with HIV NHL.

Integration of Highly Active Antiretroviral Therapy and Chemotherapy

Several groups have explored the feasibility of combining chemotherapy with HAART.[152-156] The AIDS Malignancies Consortium found that although the pharmacokinetics of cyclophosphamide may be altered, there was not an increase in toxicity in patients treated with CHOP (cyclophosphamide, hydroxydaunomycin [doxorubicin], Oncovin [vincristine], and prednisone) and HAART compared with patients treated with CHOP alone.[154] The same group did not observe an adverse effect of chemotherapy on antiretroviral pharmacokinetics. Other authors have reported no significant effects on the pharmacokinetics of select chemotherapies and antiretrovirals that rely on extensive metabolism by the cytochrome P-450 enzyme system when used in combination.[155,156] A potential for significant anemia is recognized in patients treated with chemotherapy plus zidovudine-containing HAART. It is generally recommended that zidovudine be avoided during chemotherapy. In addition, patients treated with HAART and chemotherapy may experience an increased incidence of mucositis and neurotoxicity, but this is not considered a contraindication to HAART.[152,157]

Although the combination of chemotherapy and HAART seems relatively safe, its effects on clinical outcomes are unclear. Several small studies have shown improved survivals in HIV-infected patients treated for NHL with standard-dose chemotherapy in the HAART era compared with the pre-HAART era.[152,153,158,161] Many of these studies are flawed by lack of control for confounding predictors of outcome, such as stage of disease, lactate dehydrogenase, CD4 T-cell count, age,

performance status, and prior AIDS-defining conditions. Matthews reported no significant change in survival among nearly 8000 HIV-infected patients treated for NHL in the HAART era compared with patients treated in the pre-HAART era.[161a]

Given the direct and indirect roles that HIV may play in the pathogenesis of HIV NHL and the improved tolerability of standard chemotherapy dosing in patients treated with HAART, it is considered appropriate to integrate HAART with chemotherapy in approaching these patients.[152,154] Whether this approach will translate into a survival benefit remains to be seen.

Infusional Chemotherapy

Several groups have explored the use of infusional chemotherapy as an approach to HIV NHL. Sparano and colleagues[162] treated 107 previously untreated patients with a 96-hour continuous infusion of cyclophosphamide, doxorubicin, and etoposide (CDE). Antiretroviral therapy was used in all patients, but consisted of didanosine alone in 48 patients and HAART in 59 patients. Growth factor support and opportunistic infection prophylaxis were used in all. This group reported a complete response rate of 44% and a median survival of 14.8 months. The subgroup of patients treated with CDE plus HAART had a median survival of 17.8 months. This compared with a median survival of 8.2 months in patients treated with CDE plus didanosine. These results raise the question of whether improved survival is the result of more effective chemotherapy or improved management of HIV disease.

Little and colleagues[163] reported dramatic results in 39 patients with HIV NHL treated with EPOCH (infusional etoposide, doxorubicin, and vincristine; oral prednisone; and dose-adjusted cyclophosphamide based on CD4 T-cell count). All patients received growth factor support. HAART was held for the duration of chemotherapy. Of patients, 59% had high-risk disease ascertained by adverse risk factors. The median CD4$^+$ count was 198/mm^3. More than one third of patients had CD4$^+$ counts less than 100/mm^3.

This group reported a 74% complete response rate with 60% of patients alive at 53 months. Response rate and survival correlated with immune status. Of patients with CD4$^+$ counts greater than 100/mm^3, 87% achieved a complete response, whereas only 56% of patients with lower CD4$^+$ counts achieved a complete response. At 53 months, 87% of patients with a CD4$^+$ count greater than 100/mm^3 were alive compared with 16% of patients with a CD4$^+$ count less than 100/mm^3. The viral load increased a median of 0.83 log 10 during treatment, but returned to baseline within 3 months of completing chemotherapy and resuming HAART. Similarly the CD4$^+$ count decreased a median of 189/mm^3 during therapy, but returned to baseline within 12 months of completion of chemotherapy.

The results of this single-institution study are promising and have generated further investigation into the use of EPOCH with HAART in HIV NHL. The survival rates for these infusional regimens contrast sharply with prior median survivals of 5 to 8 months observed with standard-dose and reduced-dose chemotherapy in the pre-HAART era. Whether the specific chemotherapy regimen, the mode of delivery, or the integration of HAART is essential to the improved outcomes remains to be determined.

Biotherapy

The anti-CD20+ mouse human chimeric monoclonal antibody rituximab (Rituxan) has emerged as an exciting therapy in HIV-negative NHL. It is an effective agent when used as salvage therapy for refractory NHL.[164,165] Its use in combination with chemotherapy has been shown to improve survival in HIV-negative elderly patients with untreated aggressive NHL.[167] Rituximab recognizes CD20+ cells (B lymphocytes and CD20+ lymphoma cells), binds complement, and induces antibody-dependent cellular cytotoxicity.[168] It also may inhibit cellular proliferation and directly induces apoptosis.[165] Data suggest that rituximab may be synergistic when used in combination with chemotherapy.[169]

The success of rituximab in HIV-negative NHL has generated interest in its use in HIV NHL. The fact that 95% of HIV NHL tumors express CD20+ provides further rationale for its investigation. The AIDS Malignancies Consortium completed a study comparing CHOP with CHOP in combination with rituximab for previously untreated HIV NHL. All patients were treated with growth-colony support factor and *P. carinii* pneumonia prophylaxis. Antiretroviral therapy was required in all patients. Zidovudine therapy was prohibited. A total of 143 patients were treated, 96 with CHOP plus rituximab and 47 with CHOP alone. Approximately one quarter of patients had CD4+ counts less than 50/mm³. Most patients had stage III or stage IV disease, and most had been treated with HAART before their NHL diagnosis.

Preliminary results (L. Kaplan, personal communication) show no significant difference in complete response rate between the two regimens (57% CHOP plus rituximab versus 49% CHOP) and no significant difference in overall survival (109 weeks CHOP plus rituximab versus 165 weeks CHOP; $P = .34$). There was a significantly higher rate of serious infections in the group treated with CHOP plus rituximab. Ten percent of deaths were due to infection in the patients treated with CHOP plus rituximab, whereas only 2% of deaths were due to infection in the patients treated with CHOP alone ($P = .027$). Of all infection-related deaths during the study, 93% of patients had been treated with rituximab, and 61% had CD4+ counts less than 50/mm³. This study raises serious concerns about the use of rituximab in immunocompromised patients in combination with chemotherapy. Further investigation into the use of rituximab in HIV NHL is ongoing.

Salvage Therapy

Historically, recurrent or refractory HIV NHL has had a dismal prognosis with median survivals of 2 to 5 months.[170] Salvage therapies with standard-dose chemotherapies resulted in response rates of 20% to 40% but were of short duration.[170-172] Bi and colleagues[173] reported promising results in 13 patients with refractory HIV NHL treated with ESHAP (etoposide, Solu-Medrol [methylprednisolone sodium, succinate], high-dose ara-C, and Platinol [cisplatin]). This group of heavily pretreated patients had a response rate of 54% with a median survival of 7.1 months. These results were achieved with considerable toxicity, with 100% of patients experiencing profound neutropenia.

The success of high-dose chemotherapy followed by autologous stem cell rescue in HIV-negative patients with recurrent or refractory NHL has raised the question of whether this might be an effective strategy in HIV-positive patients in the HAART era.[174] Krishnan and co-workers[175] reported on seven HIV-infected patients with refractory/recurrent lymphoma treated with high-dose chemotherapy followed by autologous stem cell rescue. All patients were treated with antiretroviral therapy during their chemotherapy. Seven of nine patients were in remission a median of 19 months after transplantation. Infectious-related complications, treatment-related complications, and

time to engraftment were similar to HIV-negative patients. Three patients developed opportunistic infections after transplantation, but all responded to treatment. Effects on immune function were similar to HIV-positive patients treated with standard-dose chemotherapy.

These data have renewed optimism in the use of high-dose chemotherapy as salvage therapy for HIV-infected individuals with refractory NHL. A multicenter study investigating this approach is under way. Other investigational approaches include using EBV cytotoxic T cells as therapy against EBV-positive NHLs, targeting tumor-associated macrophages, and mini-allogeneic bone marrow transplantation.

Treatment Recommendations

For most patients, standard-dose chemotherapy with *P. carinii* pneumonia prophylaxis (regardless of CD4+ T-cell count) and growth factor support is recommended. The use of growth factors results in fewer episodes of febrile neutropenia, fewer hospitalization days, fewer delays in chemotherapy, and fewer dose reductions.[176] Every effort should be made to initiate HAART chemotherapy as early as possible in patients diagnosed with HIV NHL. It is unclear if infusional regimens are superior to CHOP in the treatment of HIV NHL. Enrollment in clinical trials is essential for all potential study candidates. Outside of a clinical trial, CHOP is considered appropriate for most patients with HIV NHL (see later for discussion of Burkitt's histology). The use of rituximab is considered investigational at this time.

Prophylactic, intrathecal chemotherapy is implemented for high-risk patients to decrease the likelihood of meningeal lymphoma. Individuals at risk for meningeal disease, as identified in the nonimmunodeficient population, may have any of the following: small, noncleaved cell histology or other histology with bone marrow, epidural, paranasal sinus, or testicular involvement.

Burkitt's NHL or small, noncleaved NHL merits separate mention. In non-HIV Burkitt's NHL, traditional CHOP-like regimens have had disappointing results. Several groups have published promising results using intensive combination chemotherapy regimens in adults with Burkitt's NHL.[177-179] Few patients with HIV infection were included in these protocols. The optimal treatment of HIV-related Burkitt's NHL is unclear. The decision to use CHOP versus an infusional regimen such as EPOCH versus an intensive leukemia-type regimen is up to the practitioner. Efforts at enrolling such patients in clinical trials are essential.

Similarly, for HIV-infected patients with refractory or recurrent NHL, enrollment in clinical trials is encouraged. Outside of a clinical trial, treatment options include ESHAP or ICE (ifosfamide, mesna, carboplatin, and etoposide). Both regimens have shown significant activity in HIV-negative refractory or recurrent NHL, and, as discussed earlier, ESHAP has been used successfully in HIV-infected patients.[173,180] The use of rituximab is investigational, but given its efficacy as a salvage agent in HIV-negative NHL, it is reasonable to consider its use in HIV NHL.[166]

PRIMARY CENTRAL NERVOUS SYSTEM LYMPHOMA

The incidence of PCNSL in HIV-infected individuals is 1000-fold higher than that in the general population.[105,159,181,182] EBV is identified in virtually all PCNSLs. In one study, 100% of PCNSLs showed evidence of latent EBV infection, as reflected by detection of early antigen (EBER-1) by in situ hybridization.[183] Lymphomas that are seen as primary parenchymal lesions accounted for approximately 20% of all AIDS-related lymphomas before the HAART era.[133,138,184,185] It is exceedingly rare for individuals who present with parenchymal brain lesions to have lymphoma outside the CNS.[105] As is true for many opportunistic infections, PCNSL occurs most often in the advanced stages of AIDS. Before HAART, the median CD4+ cell count of HIV-infected individuals diagnosed with PCNSL was less than 50/mm³.[135,181]

Since the advent of HAART, a significant decline in the number of cases of PCNSL has occurred; this is supported by several large series.[29,186] Appleby and colleagues[29] reported a relative risk of 0.42 (99% confidence interval 0.24 to 0.75) in the risk of CNS lymphoma in HIV-infected individuals in the HAART era compared with the pre-HAART era ($n = 47,936$). Tumor registry data from San Francisco General Hospital show a decline from 18 cases in 1996 to 4 cases in 1997 to 1 case in 2002.

The most common presenting symptoms are confusion, lethargy, personality changes, and memory loss.[105,159,181,186] Other symptoms include hemiparesis, aphasia, seizures, cranial nerve palsies, and headache. Single or multiple, discrete, contrast-enhanced lesions are the most common findings on computed tomography (CT) or magnetic resonance imaging (MRI) of the brain. The radiographic appearance of PCNSL is often difficult to distinguish from that of toxoplasmosis. Solitary lesions are observed in approximately 21% of MRI studies of individuals with toxoplasmosis; solitary lesions are more likely to represent lymphoma. Multiple lesions are present in 50% of cases of PCNSL, however, which creates a diagnostic dilemma.[188] Classic radiographic findings for PCNSL are lesions that are frequently hypodense or isodense and contrast enhanced. Lesions may show central necrosis, and their location is most often periventricular. Lesions can cross the midline, and subependymal involvement is almost pathognomonic.

It is unclear whether HAART has changed the clinical presentation of CNS NHL. Anecdotally, many of these patients present with relatively good performance status, albeit advanced immunosuppression. Similar to the effects of HAART on the approach to systemic NHL, more aggressive strategies are under consideration for patients with PCNSL.

Patients with neurologic symptoms should be evaluated promptly with CT or MRI of the brain. If not contraindicated by the imaging studies, a lumbar puncture should be performed. Meningeal involvement with abnormal findings in the cerebrospinal fluid, including positive cytology for malignancy, is observed in roughly 20% of patients.[159] Serum should be tested for evidence of the cryptococcal antigen and *Toxoplasma* antibody. Toxoplasmosis is rare in patients with negative serologic tests.[189,190] It is prudent for clinicians to perform a brain biopsy in a timely fashion for patients who are seronegative for *Toxoplasma* antibody. Before HAART, the recommendation was that patients with focal intracerebral lesions and positive toxoplasmosis serologic studies could be observed on anti-*Toxoplasma* therapy with subsequent brain biopsy if clinical deterioration or lack of improvement occurred. As is discussed subsequently, HAART has made more aggressive therapies, including high-dose systemic chemotherapy, possible for patients with HIV PCNSL. As such, brain biopsy should be considered essential to the initial approach to these patients.

Two less invasive techniques for diagnosing PCNSL include thallium-201 single-photon emission computed tomography (SPECT) and polymerase chain reaction (PCR) to detect EBV DNA in the cerebrospinal fluid. In one series, thallium scans were negative for all 24 patients with toxoplasmosis and positive for all 12 patients with PCNSL.[25] In another series, nine individuals with PCNSL had positive thallium scans. Positive scans also were obtained for 3 of 10 patients with toxoplasmosis, however.[59] More recent data were not as promising. Licho and colleagues[191] evaluated the sensitivity and specificity of thallium SPECT for differentiating lymphoma from infection in 14 patients with AIDS and focal abnormalities on CT. This group reported a sensitivity and specificity of thallium SPECT no greater than 60% and 55%. The positive predictive value of thallium SPECT for diagnosing lymphoma was 43%, and the negative predictive value was 71%. The conclusion was that thallium SPECT is an unreliable test for differentiating malignancy from infection in patients with AIDS. The role for thallium SPECT in the diagnosis of PCNSL is unclear.

Observations made using PCR to detect EBV DNA in the cerebrospinal fluid have led to the development of an additional, relatively noninvasive means of diagnosing PCNSL. De Luca and co-workers[192] showed that seven of eight individuals with documented PCNSL had positive PCR for EBV in cerebrospinal fluid. Of 11 individuals with brain lesions and no lymphoma, all had negative PCRs. Twenty-one individuals with AIDS but no CNS lesions also were all negative. In a second series, 17 individuals with PCNSL all were found to be positive for EBV by PCR, and 67 of 68 individuals with HIV and no lymphoma were negative.[193] Data from larger studies are confirmatory.[194] Together, these data show the strength of this minimally invasive technique as a diagnostic tool for PCNSL. In conjunction with thallium scanning and *Toxoplasma* serologic studies, EBV detection by PCR may be of particular value.

At present, the standard for diagnosing PCNSL is brain biopsy. Because treatment outcome hinges on early diagnosis and initiation of treatment, early tissue diagnosis should be considered in all HIV-infected patients with focal abnormalities on CT or MRI. When the diagnosis of PCNSL is made, a slit-lamp examination is performed to evaluate for the presence of ocular lymphoma before initiation of therapy. Whether complete staging, including CT of the chest, abdomen, and pelvis and bone marrow biopsy, should be performed is controversial. In HIV-negative individuals, such further staging is not necessary because of the rarity of finding systemic lymphoma in the presence of parenchymal CNS lymphoma. Many practitioners extrapolate this to HIV-infected patients with CNS lymphoma.

Treatment

PCNSL has been a particular therapeutic challenge. Many cases of PCNSL have been diagnosed at autopsy.[139] In the pre-HAART era, most patients presented with PCNSL quite debilitated with advanced AIDS and multiple previous bouts of opportunistic infections.[105]

In the largest published series to date, Baumgartner and co-workers[105] showed significant clinical improvement in 78% of 29 individuals treated with whole-brain irradiation at 4000 cGY; 69% had a complete or partial radiographic response. Other institutions have had similar results with smaller series of patients.[187] Despite good initial response rates, survival times remain short, with median survival times for treated patients 2 to 5 months.[105,181] The most common cause of death in these patients was opportunistic infection.[105,181] In the series of Formenti and associates,[181] 50% of the deaths were due to opportunistic infections with only two deaths resulting from recurrent lymphoma.

Combined-modality therapy (chemotherapy and radiotherapy) also has been investigated.[107,195] In one series published before the advent of HAART, 10 individuals had a complete response rate of 88%. None of these patients' deaths resulted from lymphoma.[195] The median survival of 3.5 months was no better, however, than that in studies with radiotherapy alone.

As with other malignancies, HAART has renewed interest in an aggressive approach to patients with PCNSL. In the HIV-negative population, the median survival of patients with PCNSL has improved dramatically with the use of high-dose methotrexate. Data suggest that the use of single-agent, high-dose methotrexate results in comparable survival times and less neurotoxicity compared with combined chemoradiotherapy.[196] Previously, whole-brain radiotherapy had been used either alone or in conjunction with methotrexate. Patients frequently had leukencephalopathy, a debilitating neurodegenerative complication of treatment seen with increased frequency in patients treated with whole-brain radiotherapy, particularly if combined with high-dose methotrexate.[196] The use of high-dose methotrexate alone results in a much lower incidence of leukencephalopathy.[196] Radiotherapy can be used as salvage treatment if necessary.

Treating HIV PCNSL with high-dose methotrexate is feasible and may result in superior outcomes compared with treatment with radiotherapy alone. Jacomet and colleagues[197] treated 15 patients with PCNSL and HIV with high-dose methotrexate (3 g intravenously every 14 days with leucovorin rescue). The median CD4+ count was 23/mm³. All patients initiated antiretroviral therapy after diagnosis. Growth factor support was uniformly used. Radiation therapy was reserved for patients with refractory or recurrent disease. The overall median survival was 10 months. Patients who achieved a complete response to methotrexate (47%) had a median survival of 19 months. Quality-of-life scores improved, and side effects were tolerable with no cases of cognitive dysfunction. The use of high-dose methotrexate is promising for patients with HIV PCNSL on HAART.

Given the importance of HIV and EBV in the pathogenesis of PCNSL, therapies targeting these viruses are under active investigation. Reports of responses to HAART alone and to hydroxyurea in combination with HAART are intriguing.[198,199] There is evidence that hydroxyurea can induce loss of EBV episomes from lymphoblastoid lymphoma and Burkitt's lymphoma–derived cell lines. Other authors have shown success with intravenous zidovudine (Retrovir), ganciclovir, and interleukin-2.[200,201] This combination is based on in vitro data showing apoptosis of B-cell lymphoma cell lines when exposed to zidovudine and ganciclovir.[202]

Treatment Recommendations

An aggressive approach to HIV-infected patients with PCNSL and relatively good performance status is warranted. Treatment of these patients is investigational, but extrapolation of the treatment of HIV-negative patients with PCNSL to this population should be considered. The use of high-dose methotrexate with leucovorin rescue is a reasonable option. The use of whole-brain radiotherapy can be reserved as salvage therapy for most patients. Every effort should be made to initiate HAART in all HIV patients with PCNSL.

ANOGENITAL NEOPLASIA

Anogenital neoplasia, which includes cervical and anal carcinomas and their likely precursor lesions, cervical and anal squamous intraepithelial lesions (SILs), is an increasingly common problem in HIV-infected patients. Infection with HPV is one of the most important risk factors associated with anogenital neoplasia. HIV and HPV are sexually transmitted with similar risk factors for acquisition. The pathogenesis of anogenital neoplasia in HIV-infected individuals may be related not only to the impairment of cell-mediated immunity caused by HIV, but also to a direct interaction between these two viruses.

Considerable evidence links the development of anogenital carcinoma to HPV infection (see Chapter 140). At least 30 types of HPV have been noted to have a high predilection for the anogenital tract.[203] Specific types, such as HPV-6 and HPV-11, have been associated with benign disease, including condyloma acuminatum, and have been classified as low-risk types. High-risk or oncogenic genotypes (HPV-16, HPV-18, and HPV-31) are associated with high-grade cervical or anal SILs and cervical and anal carcinomas. HPV DNA has been shown in more than 90% of cases of cervical squamous cell carcinoma.[204] Tumor tissues from the anal region also show the presence of HPV DNA, suggesting a similar causative role for this infection in anal carcinoma.[205]

A recognized association exists between anogenital neoplasia and chronic immunodeficiency states. A high prevalence of HPV infection exists in immunosuppressed transplant recipients and probably accounts for their high incidence of anogenital carcinoma. The prevalence of HPV infection is 5 to 17 times greater in immunosuppressed transplant recipients than in the general population.[206]

Histopathology

Currently, most cervical and anal cytologic abnormalities are classified according to the Bethesda system.[207] At the benign end of the spectrum, histopathologic abnormalities secondary to HPV infection include condyloma and HPV-related cellular changes. Condyloma, koilocytosis, mild dysplasia, cervical intraepithelial neoplasia (CIN I), and anal intraepithelial neoplasia (AIN I) all are low-grade SIL (LSIL). At the other end of the spectrum, high-grade SIL (HSIL) encompasses moderate and severe dysplasia, CIN or AIN II, CIN or AIN III, and carcinoma in situ. Almost all of the invasive cancers arise from HSIL, not LSIL. The risk of developing invasive cancer increases with the severity of the dysplasia.

Although it is not clear that an actual increase in cervical or anal cancer exists among HIV-infected individuals, an increase in the prevalence of HPV infection and cervical SIL in HIV-infected women and anal SIL in HIV-infected men and women has been shown.[208-211] It is likely that cervical SIL and anal SIL are precursors of cervical and anal carcinoma, and these cancers are theoretically preventable. The development of adequate screening programs and treatment for precursor lesions are needed.

Cervical Neoplasia

HIV infection has been identified as an important risk factor for HPV infection and the development of HPV-associated neoplasia of the female genital tract. The immunodeficient status that results from HIV infection may increase a woman's susceptibility to HPV infection, and HIV infection may alter the natural history of HPV infection, making the development of anogenital neoplasia more likely.

In a large prospective cohort study,[212] the natural history of HPV infection was compared in HIV-infected and non–HIV-infected women. In the New York City area, 220 HIV-infected and 221 non–HIV-infected women were evaluated at two or more semiannual gynecologic examinations. Each examination included a test of cervicovaginal lavage specimens for HPV DNA. The investigators found that among women without neoplastic lesions identified at their first visit, HPV infection was more common and persistent among HIV-infected women. In addition, the high-risk, oncogenic HIV genotypes were more likely in the HIV-infected women.

In another study comparing HIV-infected and non–HIV-infected women, anal and cervical HPV infection and cytologic abnormalities were described.[213] In this cross-sectional study of 114 women, anal and cervical Papanicolaou smears, dot blot and PCR analysis for HPV, and CD4$^+$ cell counts were performed. Anal HPV infection was twice as common as cervical HPV infection and was more strongly associated with HIV infection. Cervical and anal cytologic abnormalities also were strongly associated with HIV infection and with poor immune status as indicated by a lower CD4$^+$ cell count. The authors concluded that HPV-associated epithelial abnormalities were associated with immunodeficiency among HIV-infected women and that anal HPV infection was at least as common as cervical infection and disease among HIV-infected women.[213]

The importance of a cell-mediated response to HPV is clear. Persistence of HPV infection is thought to be requisite for the development of SILs. In an update concerning the New York cohort, the natural history of cervical HPV infection in HIV-infected women was described.[212] Persistent HPV infection with high-risk types was found in 20% of the seropositive women and 3% of the seronegative women. The likelihood of persistent infection was related to the level of immunosuppression, women with CD4$^+$ counts less than 200/mm^3 being more than twice as likely to have persistence of HPV infection as women with CD4$^+$ counts greater than 500/mm^3.

Maiman and co-workers[214] described a cohort of HIV-infected women in New York with invasive and preinvasive cervical neoplasia. In these women, compared with a group of non–HIV-infected women at the same institution, cervical neoplasia was more advanced at presentation, was more likely to recur, showed perianal involvement more frequently, and was shown more often to have cytologic or histologic evidence of HPV infection. The authors also showed that with standard treatment approaches for advanced cervical cancer in HIV-infected women, there were significantly shorter intervals before disease recurrence and death than for the uninfected women. Maiman and co-workers[215] subsequently confirmed the elevated risk of cervical cancer recurrence in HIV-infected women in New York by examining the New York City cancer and AIDS registries from 1987 to 1995. The registry data indicated that 95% of the HIV-infected women who developed cervical cancer died from their disease.

The CDC added cervical cancer to its list of AIDS-defining conditions in 1993 based on a possible increased risk and unique natural history in patients with HIV infection. Despite the high prevalence of cervical neoplasia in HIV-infected women, only a few cases of invasive cervical cancer have been reported.[214-219] Experience with immunosuppressed transplant recipients suggests that a prolonged period of immunosuppression may be necessary for the development of anogenital carcinoma.[126] In the pre-HAART era, a shorter period of immunodeficiency was common, and survival time may not have been long enough for cervical cancer to develop. With the advent of HAART and other medical therapies that can result in a longer duration of immunodeficiency, the possibility of an increased frequency of cervical cancer is of concern.

Impact of Highly Active Antiretroviral Therapy

It is unclear whether the epidemiology and clinical course of cervical cancer have changed since the widespread use of HAART.[29,220] The long natural history of progression from dysplasia to invasive cancer and the relative infrequency of cervical cancer make changes in its incidence difficult to detect. Appleby and colleagues[29] found no significant decline in the incidence of cervical cancer in the HAART era compared with the pre-HAART era (relative risk of 1.9; 99% confidence interval 0.77 to 4.56; n = 47,936). There are data, however, that the use of HAART may be associated with a decreased incidence of cervical dysplasia, may be associated with a lower likelihood of recurrence after standard therapy, and may result in regression of high-grade lesions to lower grade lesions.[221-224] Whether the use of HAART ultimately translates into a lower incidence of cervical cancer remains to be seen.

Anal Neoplasia

A relationship among HIV infection, HPV infection, and anal neoplasia also exists. The anal and cervical epithelia have similar embryologic origins and histology, ranging from columnar epithelium to a transition zone, an area with increased metaplastic activity, and to a more differentiated squamous epithelium. Papanicolaou smears appear almost identical and are graded using the same criteria. The same HPV genotypes infect the anal and the cervical epithelia, producing similar manifestations ranging from condyloma to SIL to squamous carcinoma.[225] Although anal cancer and its precursor lesion, anal SIL, have not been as well studied as cervical cancer and cervical SIL, similar evidence links HPV to anal cancer.

Palefsky and colleagues[109] assessed the prevalence of anal HPV infection and precancerous abnormalities of the anal epithelium in 97 severely immunodeficient, HIV-infected men. Abnormal anal cytology was found in 39% of the men, and 54% had HPV DNA in their anal cytologic specimens. Abnormalities on anal cytologic smears were significantly associated with the presence of HPV DNA (risk ratio 4.6). Median CD4[+] cell counts in men with abnormal cytologic findings were significantly lower than cell counts in men with normal cytologic findings (P =.05). Similar results have been obtained in subsequent studies.

The natural history of anal HPV infection in homosexual or bisexual men is being characterized by an ongoing prospective study by Palefsky and colleagues[226] in San Francisco. At baseline, 93% of the HIV-infected men and 61% of the non–HIV-infected men had anal HPV infection detected by PCR. Oncogenic subtypes (HPV-16 and HPV-18) were found more commonly in seropositive individuals than seronegative individuals. Similarly, infection with multiple genotypes of HPV was more common in the HIV-infected group. The presence of dysplasia, particularly high-grade dysplasia, was more common in HIV-infected men than HIV-negative men. The relative risk of dysplasia was inversely correlated with CD4[+] cell count.[109,226]

Because anal cancer is thought to develop from HSIL as opposed to LSIL, determining which individuals are at high risk for developing anal HSIL is particularly important. Palefsky and colleagues[227] reported that of 346 HIV-infected men, 61% progressed from LSIL to HSIL over 2 years. Risk factors for progressive disease include CD4[+] counts less than 200/mm[3], infection with multiple HPV genotypes, persistent anal HPV infection, and a high level of infection with high-risk HPV genotypes.[227]

Impact of Highly Active Antiretroviral Therapy

Early data do not show a significant impact of HAART on the natural history of anal dysplasia. Palefsky and colleagues[228] compared the ASIL severity and level of HPV DNA in men with a history of sex with men over a 6-month period before the initiation of HAART with a 6-month period after the initiation of HAART. This group found little effect on HPV DNA levels after 6 months of HAART use. In addition, HAART use was not associated with increased likelihood of regression to a lower severity of ASIL.

Anal Cancer

Anal cancer is a rare malignancy. The incidence is higher in men with a history of anal receptive intercourse than in the general population. The incidence in men with a history of receptive anal intercourse was estimated to be 35 in 100,000 before the AIDS epidemic.[9,229] This rate is similar to the incidence of cervical cancer in women before the introduction of Papanicolaou smear screening and several times higher than current rates of cervical cancer in either HIV-infected or non–HIV-infected women (approximately 8 per 100,000 in the United States).[229] It is not clear whether the incidence of anal cancer is higher in HIV-infected than in non–HIV-infected homosexual men. At the 1998 AIDS Malignancy Conference, Biggar[230] reported that the risk of anal cancer in HIV-infected men doubled from 15-fold to 30-fold as immunosuppression worsened.

Several groups have reported a distinctive clinical course of HIV-related anal cancer in the pre-HAART era. Lorenz and colleagues[231] noted poor treatment outcomes and short survival times of HIV-infected men with anal cancer in their review of the surgical experience with anal carcinoma in HIV-infected men at the University of California San Francisco.

Holland and Swift[232] reported on a retrospective review of the anal cancer treatment outcomes of 7 HIV-infected individuals (pre-HAART) and 55 individuals with negative or unknown serostatus. The individuals were treated with standard radiotherapy with or without adjunctive chemotherapy. Treatment delays and hospitalizations for treatment-related toxicities occurred with much greater frequency in the HIV-infected individuals. This group also had a shorter mean time to treatment failure and higher incidence of relapse.

More recent data suggest a correlation between CD4[+] levels and observed toxicities of treatment of HIV-infected individuals with anal cancer. Hoffman and colleagues[233] reported that patients with CD4[+] counts less than 200/mm[3] were more likely to experience severe skin and bone marrow toxicity and were more likely to die from AIDS-related complications during chemoradiotherapy than patients with CD4[+] counts greater than 200/mm[3]. The same group reported a median survival of 13.5 months for patients with lower CD4[+] counts compared with 24 months in patients with CD4[+] counts greater than 200/mm[3].

It is not yet clear what the impact of HAART will be on the incidence and clinical course of anal cancer. Given the implications of level of immune function on tolerance of combined chemoradiotherapy, HAART use may result in less toxicity and improved outcomes for HIV-related anal cancer.

Clinical Implications of Human Immunodeficiency Virus–Related Anogenital Neoplasia

Because anogenital HPV infection and neoplasia are common in HIV-infected individuals, guidelines are needed for the management of cervical and anal neoplasia in this population. Information on the natural history of these conditions is limited, but it seems that these lesions are precancerous and may evolve into invasive cancer over time. As has been shown with the successful use of the Papanicolaou smear in screening programs in the general population, early detection of preinvasive and minimally invasive cancers of the cervical region can provide the opportunity to cure these diseases. It seems reasonable that some patients with HIV infection, particularly patients with relatively better prognoses, would benefit from early detection and treatment of anogenital neoplasia. Palefsky has proposed guidelines (Table 121-2) for the management of cervical and anal neoplasia in HIV-infected individuals.

Recommendations for Clinical Management

Cervical Squamous Intraepithelial Neoplasia

Abnormal cytology should be followed by colposcopy with biopsy of suspicious areas to determine the grade of lesions. Commonly, women with LSIL are evaluated every 3 to 6 months; lesions may regress spontaneously. Standard treatment should be used for women with HSIL; this

TABLE 121-2 Papanicolaou (Pap) Smears in Human Immunodeficiency Virus–Infected Individuals

Cervical Pap Smears in HIV-Infected Women

When HIV infection is first diagnosed, women *should* have a thorough gynecologic examination, including a Pap smear

If the initial Pap smear is normal, a second Pap smear should be obtained at approximately 6 mos

If both Pap smears are normal, annual Pap smears should follow*

If any Pap smear reveals ASCUS or SIL, refer the individual for colposcopy with biopsy of abnormal area

Anal Pap Smears in HIV-Infected Women and Men Who Have Sex with Men (MSM)

When HIV infection is first diagnosed, an anal Pap smear *could* be part of the initial evaluation

If the initial Pap smear is normal, a second Pap smear could be repeated at approximately 12 mos

If any Pap smear reveals ASCUS or SIL, refer the individual for high-resolution anoscopy (HRA) with biopsy of abnormal area

HIV-infected women and HIV-infected men with no history of anal intercourse may also benefit from anal Pap smears using a schedule similar to the MSM; data, however, are too limited to make firm recommendations.

Anal Pap Smears in Non–HIV-Infected Women and MSM

Men who have had anal warts or have receptive anal intercourse may benefit from an anal Pap smear. Women who have had anal warts, have a history of either cervical or vulvar HSIL or cancer, or have ever had receptive anal intercourse may benefit from an anal Pap smear

If the initial Pap smear is normal, individuals could have a Pap smear every 2 to 3 yr

If any Pap smear reveals ASCUS or SIL, refer the individual for HRA biopsy of abnormal area

*Some clinicians believe that individuals with a CD4+ cell count <500/mm³ should be monitored more frequently.

ASCUS, atypical squamous cells of unknown significance; HSIL, high-grade SIL; SIL, squamous intraepithelial lesion.

From Joel Palefsky, personal communication, 2004.

---

consists of excision or ablation of the lesion with laser ablation, cryotherapy, loop electrosurgical excision procedure, or cone biopsy. Routine, careful follow-up is necessary after therapy because an increased rate of recurrence among HIV-infected women is seen with all of these techniques. The integration of HAART with treatment is encouraged.

Cervical Cancer

Women with invasive cervical cancers should be managed according to the stage of their disease, regardless of their HIV status. Various modalities exist, including cone biopsy, radical hysterectomy, radiation therapy, and combined chemotherapy and radiation. HAART should be initiated or continued in all patients with cervical cancer during treatment.

Anal Squamous Intraepithelial Neoplasia

At this time, there is no universally accepted standard of care for the treatment of anal SIL. As with cervical lesions, only individuals with high-grade disease, particularly patients with severe dysplasia or AIN III, are referred for treatment. For non–HIV-infected and HIV-infected individuals with a good functional status and a reasonable life expectancy, surgical excision or ablation should be considered. Individuals should be referred to an anal surgeon with experience in this setting.

As with cervical lesions, a high rate of recurrence or persistence of high-grade lesions is seen. At present, there are no standard medical therapies for HSIL. A number of protocols designed to investigate new therapies are under way.

Anal Cancer

The integration of HAART with standard treatment for anal cancer is encouraged. It is reasonable to approach HIV-positive patients with anal cancer with the standard treatment offered to HIV-negative patients,

which is combined chemoradiotherapy. Toxicity can be significant, and growth factors and infectious prophylaxis should be used judiciously.

Surgical treatment should be reserved for patients failing chemoradiotherapy because most patients are cured of their disease without a colostomy when treated with radiotherapy and chemotherapy are used as primary therapy. Similarly, excisional biopsies of suspicious anal lesions should be avoided. A nonexcisional biopsy is sufficient. Complications of excisional biopsies include infection and nonhealing ulcers, both of which complicate initiation of chemoradiotherapy.

OTHER NEOPLASMS ASSOCIATED WITH HUMAN IMMUNODEFICIENCY VIRUS

Several malignancies may be AIDS-related but are not considered AIDS-defining. The strongest data exist for leiomyosarcoma in children and HD. Other malignancies that may be seen with increased frequency or have a distinct clinical course in HIV-positive patients include germ cell tumors, nonmelanomatous skin cancer, lung cancer, and plasma cell disorders.[11,59,234-237]

Leiomyosarcoma

The occurrence of leiomyosarcomas and leiomyomas in children with HIV infection has been described in several case reports and small case series.[237-239] Using molecular techniques, one group of investigators who studied these tumors found EBV genomes in all specimens evaluated.[240,241] In individuals with similar tumors but without HIV infection, the viral genome was not found. The authors speculated that in the setting of HIV-induced immunodeficiency, EBV may contribute to the pathogenesis of these smooth muscle tumors in children. It is possible that these tumors some day may be considered AIDS-related.

Hodgkin's Disease

HD currently is not considered an AIDS-defining illness. Controversy exists concerning the precise relationship between Hodgkin's disease and HIV infection. Initial epidemiologic data suggested that no relationship existed. Biggar and colleagues[242,243] compared the rates of HD in San Francisco and New York in the pre-AIDS period (1973 to 1978) with the rates early in the AIDS epidemic. No statistically significant increase in the odds ratio for HD in single young men was observed.

Subsequent epidemiologic studies suggest an increase in the risk of HD among HIV-infected individuals. Hessol and associates[244] reviewed medical records of 6704 homosexual men who participated in the San Francisco City Clinic Cohort Study between 1978 and 1989. The study identified an excess risk attributable to HIV infection of 19.3 cases of HD per 100,000 person-years. Reynolds and associates[245] also found a significantly increased incidence of HD among people with AIDS.

Data from the Multicenter AIDS Cohort Study showed an approximately fourfold increase in the risk of HD in HIV-infected individuals.[246] Several other studies have shown an increased risk of fivefold to ninefold for HD in the HIV-infected population.[247-249] Data from the National AIDS-Cancer Match Registry comparing the risk of HD in the pre-AIDS period with the post-AIDS period in their analysis of 366,000 AIDS cases matched to tumor registries in the United States showed a significant increase in the risk of HD as immune function worsened.[250,251] In the setting of HIV disease, in which the relative risk of HD is markedly lower than the relative risk of NHL, it is not surprising that large numbers of individuals observed over extended periods are required to show a significant increase in the risk of HD.

Clinical observations from the pre-HAART era suggest that HD in HIV-infected individuals may have a different natural history and therapeutic outcome than HD in the general population. In large clinical series of HD in nonimmunodeficient individuals diagnosed in the United States, nodular sclerosis was the most commonly encountered histologic subtype, occurring in 52% to 62% of all cases, with mixed cellularity accounting for approximately 24% and lymphocyte depletion in 3% to 6% of all individuals.[252] In patients with HIV disease, these proportions are significantly shifted, with nearly all reported series indicating a high prevalence of mixed-cellularity disease and a significantly higher frequency of lymphocyte depletion.[253-257]

Advanced HD (stage III or IV) also seems to occur with greater frequency in HIV-infected patients. Various series have shown stage III or stage IV disease in 75% to 95% of HIV-infected patients.[257,258] In comparison, about 33% of non–HIV-infected individuals present with stage III or stage IV disease.[182]

The bone marrow seems to be one of the most common extranodal sites of involvement in HIV-associated HD. Serrano and colleagues[256] identified bone marrow involvement in 10% of non–HIV-infected patients in Spain compared with 50% of HIV-infected individuals.

Considering the multiplicity of unfavorable prognostic factors, including advanced stage of disease, poor histologic subtype, greater extranodal involvement (particularly bone marrow and liver), and presence of B symptoms (unexplained fever >38° C, night sweats, weight loss >10% of body weight within the preceding 6 months), it is not surprising that HIV-infected individuals with HD may be less likely to have durable and complete responses than HIV-negative patients with HD. Before HAART, the outcome of therapy was disappointing.

Among 12 evaluable patients at San Francisco General Hospital, there were 7 complete responders to either MOPP (nitrogen mustard, Oncovorin [vincristine], procarbazine, and prednisone) or MOPP-ABVD (MOPP alternating with Adriamycin, bleomycin, vinblastine, and dacarbazine).[258] Six of the complete responders subsequently had relapses. Eight patients (62%) developed *P. carinii* pneumonia during treatment. There were no long-term survivors. Half of the patients died with advanced HD, and the remaining patients died as a result of opportunistic infections. Median survival time was less than 1 year in this population compared with 12 years in the control population. The mean dose intensity of chemotherapy delivered to the patients was only 41% of the planned therapeutic dose. Poor bone marrow reserve and intercurrent opportunistic infections resulted in frequent dose reductions and delays in chemotherapy administration. These factors may account for the high relapse rate observed in complete responders.

The Italian cooperative group for AIDS-related tumors reported similar trends.[254] Seventeen patients were treated with MOPP, ABVD, ABV, or MOPP-ABVD. Only eight patients (30%) achieved complete remission. Of 13 patients who died, 7 (54%) died of opportunistic infections, 3 died of progression of HD, and 2 died of disseminated intravascular coagulopathy. The median survival of the 17 patients who were treated was 15 months.

It does not seem that the use of HAART has altered the epidemiology of HD in HIV-infected patients. Appleby and colleagues[29] did not find a significant change in the incidence of HD when comparing the HAART era with the pre-HAART era in a meta-analysis including more than 20 case-control or cohort series. The outcome for patients with HIV-related HD may be better, however, since the implementation of HAART. Gerard and colleagues[259] reported the results of a retrospective single-institution study comparing the characteristics of HIV-related HD in the pre-HAART era (*n* = 61) with the post-HAART era (*n* = 47). This group found a slightly higher complete response rate in the pre-HAART era. In addition, the survival of patients with HIV HD in the HAART era was significantly superior to survival in the pre-HAART era. The 2-year estimated survival in the HAART era patients was 62% versus 45% in the pre-HAART patients (*P* = .03).

The use of HAART has renewed interest in an aggressive approach to patients with HIV and HD. It is recommended to treat patients with HIV HD identically to patients without HIV, using opportunistic infection prophylaxis (*P. carinii* pneumonia) and growth colony factors in all. ABVD or ABVD-MOPP hybrids seem to be better tolerated in HIV-infected patients compared with MOPP.[249]

The use of the Stanford V regimen (mechlorethamine, doxorubicin, vinblastine, vincristine, bleomycin, etoposide, and prednisone) in HIV-infected patients with HD seems feasible. Spina and colleagues[260] reported the results of 59 patients with HIV and HD treated with the Stanford V regimen and HAART. With a median follow-up of 17 months, 56% of patients were alive and disease-free. The estimated 3-year overall survival was 51%. This contrasts with a pre-HAART median survival of 12 to 15 months for patients with HIV HD.[261,262]

CONCLUSIONS

To date, all AIDS-defining malignancies have been associated with a virus other than HIV. Although a direct link has not been identified, evidence is mounting in favor of a strong relationship between immune dysfunction; the presence of latent viruses, including EBV, HHV-8, and HPV; and the development of neoplasms in HIV-positive patients.

It is crucial for HIV-infected patients and physicians to understand that most malignancies arising in the setting of HIV infection tend to occur at a more advanced stage; behave more aggressively; and although often responsive to medical intervention, recur more frequently. In addition, the patient's immune status presents a difficult baseline from which to initiate and maintain an intensive chemotherapeutic regimen. Integrating HAART with standard therapy offered to HIV-negative patients is essential to optimizing outcomes. In addition, judicious use of OI prophylaxis and growth colony factors is needed to support these patients through difficult therapy. Enrollment in clinical studies is crucial to furthering the understanding of the optimal treatment of HIV-infected patients with malignancies.

REFERENCES

1. Frizzera G, Rosai J, Dehner L, et al. Lymphoreticular disorders in primary immunodeficiencies: New findings based on an up-to-date histologic classification of 35 cases. Cancer. 1980;46:692-699.
2. Harwood A, Osoba D, Hofstader S, et al. Kaposi's sarcoma in recipients of renal transplants. Am J Med. 1979;67:759-765.
3. Hoover R, Fraumeni J. Risk of cancer in renal transplant recipients. Lancet. 1973;2:55-57.
4. Penn I. The incidence of malignancies in transplant recipients. Transplant Proc. 1975;7:323-326.
5. Pinching A. The immunology of AIDS and HIV infection. Clin Immunol Allergy. 1986;6:645.
6. Ziegler J, Templeton AC, Vogel CL. Kaposi's sarcoma: A comparison of classical, endemic, and epidemic forms. Semin Oncol. 1984;11:47-52.
7. Friedman-Kien A, Laubenstein LJ, Rubinstein P, et al. Disseminated Kaposi's sarcoma in homosexual men. Ann Intern Med. 1982;96:693-700.
8. Centers for Disease Control. Revision of the Case Definition of AIDS Used by CDC for National Reporting (CDC Reportable AIDS), 1985. Atlanta: Department of Health and Human Services; 1985.
9. Biggar RJ, Rabkin CS. The epidemiology of AIDS-related neoplasms. Hematol Oncol Clin North Am. 1996;10:997-1010.
10. Melbye M, Rabkin C, Frisch M, et al. Changing patterns of anal cancer incidence in the United States, 1940-1989. Am J Epidemiol. 1994;139:772-780.
11. Lyter DW, Bryant J, Thackeray R, et al. Incidence of human immunodeficiency virus-related and nonrelated malignancies in a large cohort of homosexual men. J Clin Oncol. 1995;13:2540-2546.
12. Remick S. Non-AIDS-defining cancers. Hematol Oncol Clin North Am. 1996;10:1203-1213.
13. Volm M, Von Roenn J. Non-AIDS-defining malignancies in patients with HIV infection. Curr Opin Oncol. 1996;8:386-391.
14. Ravalli S, Chabon A, Khan A. Gastrointestinal neoplasia in young HIV-positive patients. Am J Clin Pathol. 1989;91:458-461.
15. Tirelli U, Vaccher E, Sinicco A, et al. Forty-nine unusual HIV-related malignant tumors. Program of the 5th International Conference on AIDS, Montreal, 1989.
16. Braun M. Classics in oncology: Idiopathic multiple pigmented sarcoma of the skin by Kaposi. CA Cancer J Clin. 1982;32:340-347.
17. Kaposi M. Zur Nomenclatur des idiopathischen Pigmentsarkom Kaposi. Arch Dermatol Syph (Berl) 1894;29:164.
18. Koebner H. Kranken Vorstellung (idiopathisches multiples sarcoma Hemorrhagicum der Extremitaten). Arch Dermatol Syph (Berl) 1909;94:121.
19. Moore PS, Chang Y. Detection of herpes-like DNA sequences in Kaposi's sarcoma in patients with and without HIV infection. N Engl J Med. 1995;332:1181-1185.
20. DeJarlais D, Marmor M, Thomas P, et al. Kaposi's sarcoma among four different AIDS risk groups. Lancet. 1988;1:1119.
21. Mitsuyasu R, Groopman J. Biology and therapy of Kaposi's sarcoma. Semin Oncol. 1984;11:53-59.
22. Safai B. Pathophysiology and epidemiology of epidemic Kaposi's sarcoma. Semin Oncol. 1987;2(Suppl 3):7-12.
23. Des Jarlais D, Stoneburner R, Thomas P. Declines in proportion of Kaposi's sarcoma among cases of AIDS in multiple risk groups in New York City. Lancet. 1987;2:1024-1025.

24. Beral V, Peterman T, Berkelman R, et al. Kaposi's sarcoma among persons with AIDS: A sexually transmitted infection? Lancet. 1990;335:123-128.

25. Ruiz A, Ganz WI, Post MJ, et al. Use of thallium-201 brain SPECT to differentiate cerebral lymphoma from toxoplasma encephalitis in AIDS patients. AJNR Am J Neuroradiol. 1994;15:1885-1894.

26. Jacobson L. Impact of highly effective antiretroviral therapy on recent trends in cancer among HIV-infected individuals. Abstract S5. Presented at the Second National AIDS Malignancy Conference, Bethesda, MD, April 6-8, 1998.

27. Buchbinder S, Vittinghoff E, Colfax G, et al. Declines in AIDS incidence associated with highly active antiretroviral therapy (HAART) are not reflected in KS and lymphoma incidence. Abstract S7. Presented at the Second National AIDS Malignancy Conference, Bethesda, MD, April 6-8, 1998.

28. Jones J, Hanson D, Ward J. Effect of antiretroviral therapy on recent trends in cancer among HIV-infected persons. Abstract S3. Presented at the Second National AIDS Malignancy Conference, Bethesda, MD, April 6-8, 1998.

29. Appleby P, Beral V, Newton R, et al. Highly active antiretroviral therapy and incidence of cancer in human immunodeficiency virus-infected adults. J Natl Cancer Inst. 2000;92:1823-1830.

30. Jacobson L, Armenian H. An integrated approach to the epidemiology of Kaposi's sarcoma. Curr Opin Oncol. 1995;7:450-455.

31. Chang Y, Cesarman E, Pessin MS, et al. Identification of herpesvirus-like DNA sequences in AIDS-associated Kaposi's sarcoma. Science. 1994;266:1865-1869.

32. Schalling M, Ekman M, Kaaya EE, et al. A role for a new herpes virus (KSHV) in different forms of Kaposi's sarcoma. Nat Med. 1995;1:707-708.

33. Whitby D, Howard MR, Tenant-Flowers M, et al. Detection of Kaposi sarcoma associated herpesvirus in peripheral blood of HIV-infected individuals and progression to Kaposi's sarcoma. Lancet. 1995;346:799-802.

34. Humphrey RW, O'Brien TR, Newcomb FM, et al. Kaposi's sarcoma (KS)-associated herpesvirus-like KNA sequences in peripheral blood mononuclear cells: Association with KS and persistence in patients receiving anti-herpesvirus drugs. Blood. 1996; 88:297-301.

35. Soulier J, Grothet L, Oksenhendler E, et al. Kaposi's sarcoma-associated herpesvirus-like DNA sequences in multicentric Castleman's disease. Blood. 1995;86:1276-1280.

36. Monini P, de Lellis L, Fabris M, et al. Kaposi's sarcoma-associated herpesvirus DNA sequences in prostate tissue and human semen. N Engl J Med. 1996;334:1168-1172.

37. Pauk J, Huang ML, Brodie SJ, et al. Mucosal shedding of human herpesvirus 8 in men. N Engl J Med. 2000;343:1369-1377.

38. Kedes DH, Operskalski E, Busch M, et al. The epidemiology of human herpesvirus 8 (Kaposi's sarcoma-associated herpesvirus): Distribution of infection in KS risk groups and evidence for sexual transmission. Nat Med. 1996;2:918-924.

39. Miles SA. Pathogenesis of AIDS-related Kaposi's sarcoma: Evidence of a viral etiology. Hematol Oncol Clin North Am. 1996;10:1011-1021.

40. Nickloff B, Foreman K. Charting a new course through the chaos of KS (Kaposi's sarcoma). Am J Pathol. 1996;148:1323-1329.

41. Cannon M, Cesarman E. Kaposi's sarcoma-associated herpesvirus and acquired immunodeficiency syndrome-related malignancy. Semin Oncol. 2000;27:409-419.

42. Dezube B. Acquired immunodeficiency syndrome-related Kaposi's sarcoma: Clinical features, staging and treatment. Semin Oncol. 2000;27:424-430.

43. Albini A, Barillari G, Benelli R, et al. Angiogenic properties of human immunodeficiency virus type 1 tat protein. Proc Natl Acad Sci U S A. 1995;92:4838-4842.

44. Ensoli B, Barillari G, Salahuddin SZ, et al. Tat protein of HIV-1 stimulates growth of cells derived from Kaposi's sarcoma lesions of AIDS patients. Nature. 1990;345:84-86.

45. Green TL, Beckstead JH, Lozada-Nur F, et al. Histopathologic spectrum of oral Kaposi's sarcoma. Oral Surg Oral Med Oral Pathol. 1984;58:306-314.

46. Dorfman R. Kaposi's sarcoma revisited. Hum Pathol. 1984;15:1013-1017.

47. McNeil C. HIV infection with Hodgkin's disease: The virus makes a difference (News). J Natl Cancer Inst. 1997;89:754-755.

48. Beckstead JH, Wood GS, Fletcher V. Evidence for the origin of Kaposi's sarcoma from lymphatic endothelium. Am J Pathol. 1985;119:294-300.

49. Conant MA, Opp KM, Poretz D, et al. Reduction of Kaposi's sarcoma lesions following treatment of AIDS with ritonavir. AIDS. 1997;11:1300-1301.

50. Friedman SL. Gastrointestinal hepatobiliary neoplasms in AIDS. Gastroenterol Clin North Am. 1988;17:465-486.

51. Gill P, Akil B, Colletti P, et al. Pulmonary Kaposi's sarcoma: Clinical findings and results of therapy. Am J Med. 1989;87:57-61.

52. Hanto D, Gajl-Peczalkska K, Frizzera G, et al. Clinical spectrum of lymphoproliferative disorders in renal transplant recipients and evidence for the role of Epstein-Barr virus. Cancer Res. 1981;41:4253-4261.

53. Kaplan L, Hopewell P, Jaffe H. Kaposi's sarcoma involving the lung in patients with the acquired immunodeficiency syndrome. J Acquir Immune Defic Syndr. 1988;1:23-30.

54. Holkova B, Takeshita K, Cheng D, et al. Effect of highly active antiretroviral therapy on survival in patients with AIDS-associated Kaposi's sarcoma treated with chemotherapy. J Clin Oncol. 2001;19:3848-3851.

55. Aboulafia DM. Regression of acquired immunodeficiency-related Kaposi's sarcoma after highly active antiretroviral therapy. Mayo Clin Proc. 1998;73:439-443.

56. Kaobayashi M, Takaori-Kondot K, Shindo K, et al: Successful treatment with Paclitaxel of advanced acquired immunodeficiency-associated Kaposi's sarcoma. Intern Med. 2002;41:1209-1212.

57. Davis S, Henschke C, Chamides B, et al. Intrathoracic Kaposi sarcoma in AIDS patients: Radiographic-pathologic correlation. Radiology. 1987;163:495-500.

58. Volberding P, Kusick P, Feigal D. Effects of chemotherapy for HIV-associated Kaposi's sarcoma on long-term survival (Abstract 11). Proc Am Soc Clin Oncol. 1989;8:3.

59. Chak L, Gill P, Levine A, et al. Radiation therapy for AIDS-related Kaposi's sarcoma. J Clin Oncol. 1988;6:863-867.

60. Hill D. The role of radiotherapy for epidemic Kaposi's sarcoma. Semin Oncol. 1987;14(Suppl 3):1207.

61. Newcomer VD. Human immunodeficiency virus infection and acquired immunodeficiency syndrome in the elderly (Letter). Arch Dermatol. 1997;133:1311-1312.

62. Walmsley S, Northfelt D, Melosky B, et al. Treatment of AIDS-related cutaneous Kaposi's sarcoma with topical Alitretinoin (9-cis-retinoic acid) gel. J Acquir Immune Defic Syndr. 1999;22:235-246.

63. Bernstein Z, Wilson D, Summers K, et al. Pilot/phase I study—photodynamic therapy (PDT) for treatment of AIDS-associated Kaposi's sarcoma (AIDS/KS). Proc Am Soc Clin Oncol. 1995;14:289.

64. Northfelt DW, Dezube BJ, Thommes JA, et al. Pegylated-liposomal doxorubicin versus doxorubicin, bleomycin, and vincristine in the treatment of AIDS-related Kaposi's sarcoma: Results of a randomized phase III clinical trial. J Clin Oncol. 1998;16:2445-2451.

65. Northfelt DW, Dezube BJ, Thommes JA, et al. Efficacy of pegylated-liposomal doxorubicin in the treatment of AIDS-related Kaposi's sarcoma after failure of standard chemotherapy. J Clin Oncol. 1997;15:653-659.

66. Gill P, Wernz J, Scadden D, et al. Randomized phase III trial of liposomal daunorubicin versus doxorubicin, bleomycin, and vincristine in AIDS-related Kaposi's sarcoma. J Clin Oncol. 1996;14:2353-2364.

67. Gill P, Hadienberg J, Espina B, et al. Low dose paclitaxel (Taxol) every two weeks over 3 hours is safe and effective in the treatment of advanced AIDS-related Kaposi's sarcoma. Abstract 1516. Presented at the American Society of Hematology (ASH), Thirty-ninth Annual Meeting, Seattle, December 2-5, 1995.

68. Saville M, Lietzau J, Pluda J, et al. Activity of placlitaxel (Taxol) as therapy for HIV-associated Kaposi's sarcoma. Lancet. 1995;346:26-28.

69. Nasti G, Errante D, Talamini R, et al. Vinorelbine is an effective and safe drug for AIDS-related Kaposi's sarcoma: Results of a phase II study. J Clin Oncol. 2000; 18:1550-1557.

70. Gill PS, Wernz J, Scadden DT, et al. Randomized phase III trial of liposomal daunorubicin versus doxorubicin, bleomycin and vincristine in AIDS-related Kaposi's sarcoma. J Clin Oncol. 1996;14:2353-2364.

71. Ireland-Gill A, Espina B, Akil B, et al. Treatment of acquired immunodeficiency syndrome-related Kaposi's sarcoma using bleomycin-containing combination chemotherapy regimens. Semin Oncol. 1992;2(Suppl 5):32-36.

72. Krown S. The role of interferon in the therapy of epidemic Kaposi's sarcoma. Semin Oncol. 1987;14(Suppl 3):27-33.

73. Kovacs J, Lance H, Masur H, et al. A phase III, placebo-controlled trial of recombinant alpha-interferon in asymptomatic individuals seropositive for the acquired immunodeficiency syndrome. Clin Res. 1987;35:479A.

74. Lane H, Feinberg J, Davery V, et al. Anti-retroviral effects of interferon-alpha in AIDS-associated Kaposi's sarcoma. Lancet. 1988;2:1218-1222.

75. deWit R, Schatenkerk J, Boucher C, et al. Clinical and virological effects of high-dose recombinant interferon-alpha in disseminated AIDS-related Kaposi's sarcoma. Lancet. 1988;2:1214-1217.

76. Groopman J, Gottlieb M, Goodman J, et al. Recombinant alpha-2 interferon therapy for Kaposi's sarcoma associated with the acquired immunodeficiency syndrome. Ann Intern Med. 1984;100:671-676.

77. Real F, Oettgen H, Krown S. Kaposi's sarcoma and the acquired immunodeficiency syndrome: Treatment with high and low doses of leukocyte A interferon. J Clin Oncol. 1986;4:544-551.

78. Volberding P, Mitsuyasu R. Recombinant interferon alpha in the treatment of acquired immune deficiency syndrome-related Kaposi's sarcoma. Semin Oncol. 1985;2(Suppl 5):2-6.

79. Volberding P, Mitsuyasu R, Golando J, et al. Treatment of Kaposi's sarcoma with interferon alfa-2 (Intron A). Cancer. 1987;59:620-625.

80. Rios A, Mansell P, Newell G, et al. Treatment of acquired immunodeficiency syndrome-related Kaposi's sarcoma with lymphoblastoid interferon. J Clin Oncol. 1985;3:506-512.

81. Kristal A, Nasca P, Burnett W, et al. Changes in the epidemiology of non-Hodgkin's lymphoma associated with epidemic human immunodeficiency virus (HIV) infection. Am J Epidemiol. 1988;128:711-718.

82. Vaccher E, Tirelli U, Spina M, et al. Age and serum lactate dehydrogenase level are independent prognostic factors in human immunodeficiency virus-related non-Hodgkin's lymphomas: A single-institute study of 96 patients. J Clin Oncol. 1996; 14:2217-2223.

83. Hartshorn K, Vogt M, Chou T, et al. Synergistic inhibition of human immunodeficiency virus in vitro by azidothymidine and recombinant alpha A interferon. Antimicrob Agent Chemother. 1987;31:168-172.

84. Fischl M, Finkelstein D, He W, et al. A phase II study of recombinant human interferon-alpha 2a plus zidovudine in patients with AIDS-related Kaposi's sarcoma. J Acquir Immunodefic Syndr. 1996;11:379-384.

85. Mauss S, Jablonski H. Efficacy, safety and tolerance of low-dose, long-term interferon alpha 2b and zidovudine in early-stage AIDS-associated Kaposi's sarcoma. J Acquir Immunodefic Syndr. 1995;10:157-162.

86. Little RF, Wyvill KM, Pluda JM, et al. Activity of thalidomide in AIDS-related Kaposi's sarcoma. J Clin Oncol. 2000;18:2593-2602.

87. Cianfrocca M, Cooley T, Lee J, et al. Matrix metalloproteinase inhibitor COL-3 in the treatment of acquired immunodeficiency syndrome-related Kaposi's sarcoma: A phase I AIDS Malignancy Consortium study. J Clin Oncol. 2002;20:153-159.

88. Aboulafia D. Regression of acquired immunodeficiency syndrome-related pulmonary Kaposi's sarcoma after highly active antiretroviral therapy. Mayo Clin Proc. 1998;73:439-443.

89. Henry K, Worley J, Sullivan C, et al. Documented improvement in late stage manifestations of AIDS after starting ritonavir in combination with two reverse transcriptase inhibitors. Abstract 356. Presented at the Fourth Conference of Retroviruses and Opportunistic Infections, Chicago, January 22-26, 1997.

90. Parra R, Leal M, Delgrado J, et al. Regression of invasive AIDS-related Kaposi's sarcoma following antiretroviral therapy. Clin Infect Dis. 1998;26:218-219.

91. Wit FW, Sol CJ, Renwick N, et al. Regression of AIDS-related Kaposi's sarcoma associated with clearance of human herpesvirus-8 from peripheral blood mononuclear cells following initiation of antiretroviral therapy (Letter). AIDS. 1998;12:218-219.

92. Workman C, Lewis C, Smith D. Resolution of Kaposi's sarcoma associated with saquinavir therapy-case report. Abstract Tu.B.2217. Presented at the International Conference on AIDS, Vancouver, British Columbia, Canada, July 7-12, 1996.

92a. Gill J, Bourboulia D, Wilkinson J, et al. Prospective study of the effects of antiretroviral therapy on Kaposi sarcoma–associated herpesvirus infection in patients with and without Kaposi sarcoma. J Acquir Immune Def Syndr. 2002;31:384-390.

93. Bower M, Fox P, Fife K, et al. Highly active anti-retroviral therapy (HAART) prolongs time to treatment failure in Kaposi's sarcoma. AIDS. 1999;13:2105-2111.

94. Volm M, Wernz J. Patients with advanced AIDS-related Kaposi's sarcoma (KS) no longer require systemic therapy after introduction of effective antiretroviral therapy. Abstract 162. Presented at the Thirty-third Annual ASCO Meeting, Denver, May 17-20, 1997.

95. Ziegler J, Drew W, Miner R, et al. Outbreak of Burkitt's-like lymphoma in homosexual men. Lancet. 1982;2:631.

96. Kaplan LD, Abrams DI, Feigal E, et al. AIDS-associated non-Hodgkin's lymphoma in San Francisco. JAMA. 1989;261:719-724.

97. National Cancer Institute. NCI-sponsored study of classifications of non-Hodgkin's lymphoma: Summary and description of a working formulation for clinical usage. The Non-Hodgkin's Lymphoma Pathologic Classification Project. Cancer. 1982; 49:2112-2135.

98. Centers for Disease Control. Revision of the case definition of acquired immunodeficiency syndrome for national reporting-United States. MMWR Morb Mortal Wkly Rep. 1985;4:373-374.

99. Penn I. Lymphomas complicating organ transplantation. Transplant Proc. 1983;15(Suppl 1):2790-2797.

100. Harnly M, Swan S, Holly E, et al. Temporal trends in the incidence of non-Hodgkin's lymphoma and selected malignancies in a population with a high incidence of acquired immunodeficiency syndrome (AIDS). Am J Epidemiol. 1988;128:261-267.

101. Matthews G, Bower M, Mandalia S, et al. Changes in acquired immunodeficiency syndrome-related lymphoma since the introduction of highly active antiretroviral therapy. Blood. 2000;96:2730-2734.

102. Ledergerber B, Telenti A, Egger M. Risk of HIV-related Kaposi's sarcoma and non-Hodgkin's lymphoma with potent antiretroviral therapy: prospective cohort study. BMJ. 1999;319:23-24.

103. Rabkin CS, Testa MA, Huang J, et al. Kaposi's sarcoma and non-Hodgkin's lymphoma incidence trends in AIDS Clinical Trial Group study participants. J Acquir Immune Defic Syndr. 1999;21(Suppl 1):S31-S33.

104. Buchbinder S. Combination antiretroviral therapy and incidence of AIDS-related malignancies. J Acquir Immune Defic Syndr. 1999;21:S23-26.

105. Baumgartner J, Rachlin J, Beckstead J, et al. Primary central nervous system lymphomas: Natural history and response to radiation therapy in 55 patients with acquired immunodeficiency syndrome. J Neurosurg. 1990;73:206-211.

106. Bais C, Santomasso B, Coso O, et al. G-protein-coupled receptor of Kaposi's sarcoma-associated herpesvirus is a vital oncogene and angiogenesis activator. Nature. 1998;391:86-89.

107. Chamberlain MC. Long survival in patients with acquired immune deficiency syndrome-related primary central nervous system lymphoma. Cancer. 1994;73:1728-1730.

108. Palefsky J. Human papillomavirus infection among HIV-infected individuals. Hematol Oncol Clin North Am. 1991;5:357-370.

109. Palefsky J, Gonzales J, Greenblatt R, et al. Anal intraepithelial neoplasia and anal papillomavirus infection among homosexual males with group IV HIV disease. JAMA. 1990;263:2911-2916.

110. Shearer W, Ritz J, Finego M, et al. Epstein-Barr virus-associated B-cell proliferations of diverse clonal origins after bone marrow transplantation in a 12-year-old patient with severe combined immunodeficiency. N Engl J Med. 1985;312:1151-1159.

111. Meeker T, Shiramizu B, Kaplan L, et al. Evidence for molecular subtypes of HIV-associated lymphoma: Division into peripheral monoclonal, polyclonal and central nervous system lymphoma. AIDS. 1991;5:669-674.

112. Shiramizu B, Herndier B, Meeker T, et al. Molecular and immunophenotypic characterization of AIDS-associated EBV-negative polyclonal lymphoma. J Clin Oncol. 1992;10:383-389.

113. Subar M, Neri A, Inghirami G, et al. Frequent c-myc oncogene activation and infrequent presence of Epstein-Barr virus genome in AIDS-associated lymphoma. Blood. 1988;72:667-671.

114. Gaidano G, Capello D, Carbone A. The molecular basis of acquired immunodeficiency syndrome-related lymphomagenesis. Semin Oncol. 2000;27:431-441.

115. Komanduri K, Luce J, McGrath M, et al. The natural history and molecular heterogeneity of HIV-associated primary malignant lymphomatous effusions. J Acquir Immune Defic Syndr. 1996;13:215-226.

116. Cesarman E, Chang Y, Moore P, et al. Kaposi's sarcoma-associated herpesvirus-like DNA sequences in AIDS-related body-cavity-based lymphomas. N Engl J Med. 1995;332:1186-1191.

117. Knowles D, Chamulak G, Subar M, et al. Lymphoid neoplasia associated with the acquired immunodeficiency syndrome (AIDS). Ann Intern Med. 1988;108:744-753.

118. Herndier B, Shiramizu B, Jewett N, et al. Acquired immunodeficiency syndrome-associated T-cell lymphoma: Evidence for human immunodeficiency virus type 1-associated T-cell transformation. Blood. 1992;79:1768-1774.

119. Shiramizu B, Herndier BG, McGrath MS. Identification of a common clonal human immunodeficiency virus integration site in human immunodeficiency virus-associated lymphomas. Cancer Res. 1994;54:2069-2072.

120. McGrath M, Shiramizu B, Herndier B. Clonal HIV in the pathogenesis of AIDS-related lymphoma: Sequential pathogenesis. In: Goedert JJ, ed. Infectious Causes of Cancer: Targets for Intervention. Totowa, NJ: Humana Press; 2000:231-242.

121. Zenger E, Abbey N, Weinstein M, et al. Injection of primary effusion lymphoma cells or associated macrophages into severe combined immunodeficient mice causes murine lymphomas. Cancer Res. 2002;62:5536-5542.

122. Emilie D, Coumbaras J, Raphael M, et al. Interleukin-6 production in high-grade B lymphomas: Correlation with the presence of malignant immunoblasts in acquired immunodeficiency syndrome and in human immunodeficiency virus-seronegative patients. Blood. 1992;80:498-504.

123. Emilie D, Touitou R, Raphael M, et al. In vivo production of interleukin-10 by malignant cells in AIDS lymphomas. Eur J Immunol. 1992;22:2937-2942.

124. McGrath M, Marsh J, Nolan T, et al. Lymphokine gene expression and effects on cell proliferation in AIDS-associated NHL (Abstract). J Cell Biochem. 1993;17E (Suppl):270.

125. Kaplan L, Kahn J, Jacobson M, et al. Primary bile duct lymphoma in the acquired immmunodeficiency syndrome (AIDS). Ann Intern Med. 1989;110:162.

126. Penn I. Cancers of the anogenital region in renal transplant recipients: Analysis of 65 cases. Cancer. 1986;58:611-616.

127. Rogo K, Kavoo-Linge R. Human immunodeficiency virus seroprevalence among cervical cancer patients. Gynecol Oncol. 1990;37:87-92.

128. Nasr S, Brynes R, Garrison C, et al. Peripheral T-cell lymphoma in a patient with acquired immunodeficiency syndrome. Cancer. 1988;61:947-951.

129. Presant C, Gala K, Wiseman C, et al. Human immunodeficiency virus-associated T-cell lymphoblastic lymphoma in AIDS. Cancer. 1987;60:1459-1461.

130. Cannon M, Cesarman E. Kaposi's sarcoma-associated herpesvirus and acquired immunodeficiency syndrome-related malignancy. Semin Oncol. 2000;27:409-419.

131. Knowles D, Inghirami G, Ubraico A, et al. Molecular genetic analysis of three AIDS-associated neoplasms of uncertain lineage demonstrates their B-cell derivation and the possible pathogenic role of Epstein-Barr virus. Blood. 1989;73:792-799.

132. Gill P, Levine A, Krail M, et al. AIDS-related malignant lymphoma: Results of prospective treatment trials. J Clin Oncol. 1987;5:1322-1328.

133. Lowenthal D, Straus D, Campbell S, et al. AIDS-related lymphoid neoplasia: The Memorial Hospital experience. Cancer. 1988;61:2325-2337.

134. Bermudez M, Grant K, Rodvien R, et al. Non-Hodgkin's lymphoma in a population with or at risk for acquired immunodeficiency syndrome: Indications for intensive chemotherapy. Am J Med. 1989;86:71-76.

135. Levine A, Sullivan-Halley J, Pike M, et al. Human immunodeficiency virus-related lymphoma: Prognostic factors predictive of survival. Cancer. 1991;68:2466-2472.

136. Northfelt D, Volberding P, Kaplan L. Degree of immunodeficiency at diagnosis of AIDS-associated non-Hodgkin's lymphoma. Proceedings of American Society of Clinical Oncology, San Diego, May 17-19, 1992.

137. Levin RJ, Henick DH, Cohen AF. Human immunodeficiency virus-associated non-Hodgkin's lymphoma presenting as an auricular perichondritis. Otolaryngol Head Neck Surg. 1995;112:493-495.

138. Knowles D. Etiology and pathogenesis of AIDS-related non-Hodgkin's lymphoma. Hematol Oncol Clin North Am. 1996;10:1081-1109.

139. Ziegler J, Beckstead J, Volberding P, et al. Non-Hodgkin's lymphoma in 90 homosexual men: Relation to generalized lymphadenopathy and the acquired immunodeficiency syndrome. N Engl J Med. 1984;311:565-570.

140. Burkes R, Meyer P, Gill P, et al. Rectal lymphoma in homosexual men. Arch Intern Med. 1986;146:913-915.

141. Kaplan L, Straus D, Testa M, et al. Randomized trial of standard-dose vs. low-dose mBACOD chemotherapy for HIV-associated non-Hodgkin's lymphoma. N Engl J Med. 1997;336:1641-1648.

142. Tirelli U, Vaccher E, Rezza G, et al. Hodgkin's disease and infection with the human immunodeficiency virus in Italy. Ann Intern Med. 1988;108:309.

143. Gerard L, Galicier L, Maillard A, et al. Systemic non-Hodgkin lymphoma in HIV-infected patients with effective suppression of HIV replication: Persistent occurrence but improved survival. J Acquir Immune Defic Syndr. 2002;30:478-484.

144. Straus DJ, Huang J, Testa MA, et al. Prognostic factors in the treatment of human immunodeficiency virus-associated non-Hodgkin's lymphoma: Analysis of AIDS Clinical Trials Group protocol 142—Low-dose versus standard-dose m-BACOD plus granulocyte-macrophage colony-stimulating factor. National Institute of Allergy and Infectious Diseases. J Clin Oncol. 1998;16:3601-3606.

145. De Vita V, Hubbard S, Young R, et al. The role of chemotherapy in diffuse aggressive lymphomas. Semin Hematol. 1988;25(Suppl 2):2-10.

146. Biggar RJ, Rabkin CS. The epidemiology of AIDS-related neoplasms. Hematol Oncol Clin North Am. 1996;10:997-1010.

147. Kaplan LD, Straus DJ, Testa MA, et al. Low-dose compared with standard-dose m-BACOD chemotherapy for non-Hodgkin's lymphoma associated with human immunodeficiency virus infection. National Institute of Allergy and Infectious Diseases AIDS Clinical Trials Group. N Engl J Med. 1997;336:1641-1648.

148. Sandler AS, Kaplan LD. Diagnosis and management of systemic non-Hodgkin's lymphoma in HIV disease. Hematol Oncol Clin North Am. 1996;10:1111-1124.

149. Hessol N, Katz M, Liu J, et al. Increased incidence of Hodgkin's disease in homosexual men with HIV infection. Ann Intern Med. 1992;117:309-311.

150. Porter C. Biological properties of N4-spermidine derivatives and their potential in anticancer chemotherapy. Cancer Res. 1982;42:4072-4078.

151. Boulanger E, Agbalika F, Maarek O, et al. A clinical, molecular and cytogenetic study of 12 cases of human herpesvirus-8 associated primary effusion lymphoma. Presented at American Society of Hematology Annual Meeting, San Francisco, 2000.

152. Vaccher E, Spina M, di Gennaro G, et al. Concomitant CHOP chemotherapy and highly active antiretroviral therapy in patients with HIV-related non-Hodgkin's lymphoma. Cancer. 2001;91:155-163.

153. Romeu J, Navarro T, Tural C. Effect of HAART on response to therapy and survival in patients with AIDS-related non-Hodgkin's lymphoma (NHL). Presented at XIII International AIDS Conference, Durban, South Africa, 2000.
154. Ratner L, Lee J, Tang S, et al. Chemotherapy for human immunodeficiency virus-associated non-Hodgkin's lymphoma in combination with highly active antiretroviral therapy. J Clin Oncol. 2001;19:2171-2178.
155. Vinodh R, Nannan P, Richard M, et al. Paclitaxel in the treatment of human immunodeficiency virus 1-associated Kaposi's sarcoma-drug-drug interactions with protease inhibitors and a nonnucleoside reverse transcriptase inhibitor: a case report study. Cancer Chemother Pharm. 1999;43:516-519.
156. Fumagalli L, Zucchetti M, Parisi I, et al. The pharmacokinetics of liposomal encapsulated daunorubicin are not modified by HAART in patients with HIV-associated Kaposi's sarcoma. Cancer Chemother Pharm. 2000;45:495-501.
157. Sparano J, Wiernik P, Hu X, et al. Infusional cyclophosphamide, doxorubicin and etoposide in HIV-associated non-Hodgkin's lymphoma. Med Oncol. 1998;15:50-57.
158. Besson C, Goubar A, Gabarre J, et al. Changes in AIDS-related lymphoma since the era of highly active antiretroviral therapy. Blood. 2001;98:2339-2344.
159. Gill P, Levine A, Meyer R, et al. Primary central nervous system lymphoma in homosexual men: Clinical, immunologic and pathologic factors. Am J Med. 1985;78:742-748.
160. Gill P, Levine A, Krailo M, et al. AIDS-related malignant lymphoma: Results of prospective treatment trials. J Clin Oncol. 1987;5:1322.
161. Gerard L, Galicier L, Maillard A, et al. Systemic non-Hodgkin lymphoma in HIV-infected patients with effective suppression of HIV replication: Persistent occurrence but improved survival. J Acquir Immune Defic Syndr. 2003;32:347-348.
161a. Matthews GV, Bower M, Mandalia S, et al. Changes in acquired immunodeficiency syndrome–related lymphoma since the introduction of highly active antiretroviral therapy. Blood. 2002;96:2730-2734.
162. Sparano JA, Wiernik PH, Hu X, et al. Pilot trial of infusional cyclophosphamide, doxorubicin, and etoposide plus didanosine and filgrastim in patients with human immunodeficiency virus-associated non-Hodgkin's lymphoma. J Clin Oncol. 1996;14:3026-3035.
163. Little RF, Pittaluga S, Grant N, et al. Highly effective treatment of acquired immunodeficiency syndrome-related lymphoma with dose-adjusted EPOCH: Impact of antiretroviral therapy suspension and tumor biology. Blood 2003;101:4653-4654.
164. Maloney D, Grillo-Lopez A, White C, et al. IDEC-C2B8 (rituximab) anti-CD20 monoclonal antibody therapy in patients with relapsed low-grade non-Hodgkin's lymphoma. Blood. 1997;90:2188-2195.
165. McLaughlin P, Grillo-Lopez A, Link B, et al. Rituximab chimeric anti-CD20 monoclonal antibody therapy for relapsed indolent lymphoma: Half of patients respond to a 4-dose treatment program. J Clin Oncol. 1998;16:2825-2833.
166. Coiffier B, Haioun C, Ketterer N, et al. Rituximab (anti-CD20 monoclonal antibody) for the treatment of patients with relapsing or refractory aggressive lymphoma: A multicenter phase II study. Blood. 1998;92:1919-1927.
167. Coiffier B, Lepage E, Herbrecht R, et al. Rituximab plus CHOP is superior to CHOP alone in elderly patients with diffuse large B-cell lymphoma (DLCL): Interim results of a randomized GELA study. Abstract 950. Presented at the American Society of Hematology Conference, San Francisco, December 2000.
168. Reff M, Carner K, Chambers K, et al. Depletion of B cells in vivo by a chimeric mouse human monoclonal antibody to CD20. Blood. 1994;83:435-445.
169. Demiden A, Lam T, Alas S, et al. Chimeric anti-CD20 monoclonal antibody sensitizes a B cell lymphoma cell line to cell killing by cytotoxic drugs. Cancer Biother Radiopharm. 1997;12:177-186.
170. Tirelli U, Errante D, Spina M, et al. Second line chemotherapy in HIV-related non-Hodgkin's lymphoma. Cancer. 1996;77:2127-2131.
171. Kaplan LD, Moran T, Song L, et al. Continuous-infusions ifosfamide/mesna with daily etoposide for refractory HIV-associated non-Hodgkin's lymphoma (NHL). Abstract 185. Presented at the American Society of Clinical Oncology meeting, 1998.
172. Tulpule A, Dezube B, Doweiko J, et al. A phase II trial of liposomal daunorubicin in relapsed and refractory AIDS-related lymphomas. Abstract MoPpB1087. Program and abstracts of the XII International AIDS Conference, Durban, South Africa, July 9-14, 2000.
173. Bi J, Espina B, Tulpule A, et al. High-dose cytosine-arabinoside and cisplatin regimens as salvage therapy for refractory or relapsed AIDS-related non-Hodgkin's lymphoma. J Acquir Defic Syndr. 2001;28:416-421.
174. Philip T, Guglielmi C, Hagenbeck A, et al. Autologous bone marrow transplantation as compared with salvage chemotherapy in relapses of chemotherapy-sensitive non-Hodgkin's lymphoma. N Engl J Med. 1995;333:1540-1545/
175. Krishnan A, Molina A, Zaia J, et al. Autologous stem cell transplantation for HIV-associated lymphoma. Blood. 2001;98:3857-3859.
176. Kaplan L, Kahn J, Crowe S, et al. Clinical and virologic effects of recombinant human granulocyte-macrophage colony-stimulating factor in patients receiving chemotherapy for human immunodeficiency virus-associated non-Hodgkin's lymphoma: Results of a randomized trial. J Clin Oncol. 1991;9:929-940.
177. Soussain C, Patte C, Ostronoff M, et al. Small noncleaved cell lymphoma and leukemia in adults: A retrospective study of 65 adults treated with the LMB Pediatric Protocols. Blood. 1995;85:664-674.
178. McMaster M, Greer J, Greco A, et al. Effective treatment of small-noncleaved-cell lymphoma with high-intensity, brief-duration chemotherapy. J Clin Oncol. 1991;9:941-946.
179. Magrath I, Adde M, Shad A, et al. Adults and children with small non-cleaved-cell lymphoma have a similar excellent outcome when treated with the same chemotherapy regimen. J Clin Oncol. 1996;14:925-934.
180. Moskowitz C, Bertino J, Glassman J, et al. Ifosfamide, carboplatin and etoposide: A highly effective cytoreductive and peripheral-blood-progenitor-cell mobilization regimen for transplant-eligible patients with non-Hodgkin's lymphoma. J Clin Oncol. 1999;17:3776-3785.
181. Formenti S, Gill P, Rarick M, et al. Primary central nervous system lymphoma in AIDS: Results of radiation therapy. Cancer. 1989;63:1101-1107.
182. So Y, Beckstead J, Davis R. Primary central nervous system lymphoma in acquired immunodeficiency syndrome: A clinical and pathological study. Ann Neurol. 1986;20:566-572.
183. MacMahon E, Glass J, Hayward S, et al. Epstein-Barr virus in AIDS-related primary central nervous system lymphoma. Lancet. 1991;338:969.
184. Beral V, Peterman T, Berkelman R, et al. AIDS-associated non-Hodgkin's lymphoma. Lancet. 1991;337:805.
185. Levine A. Acquired immunodeficiency syndrome-related lymphoma. Blood. 1992;80:8.
186. Jones J, Hanson D, Dworkin M, et al. Effect of antiretroviral therapy on recent trends in selected cancers among HIV-infected persons. J Acquir Immune Defic Syndr. 1999;21:S11-S17.
187. Goldstein J, Dickson D, Moser F, et al. Primary central nervous system lymphoma in acquired immunodeficiency syndrome: A clinical and pathologic study with results of treatment with radiation. Cancer. 1991;67:2756.
188. Ciricillo S, Rosenblum M. Use of CT and MRI imaging to distinguish intracranial lesions and to define the need for biopsy in AIDS patients. J Neurosurg. 1990;73:Z 720-724.
189. Grant I, Gold J, Armstron D. Risk of CNS toxoplasmosis in patients with acquired immune deficiency syndrome. Abstract 441. Program of the Interscience Conference on Antimicrobial Agents and Chemotherapy, New Orleans, September 28-October 1, 1986.
190. Porter S, Sande M. Toxoplasmosis of the central nervous system in the acquired immunodeficiency syndrome. N Engl J Med. 1992;327:1643-1648.
191. Licho R, Litofsky NS, Senitko M, et al. Inaccuracy of Tl-201 brain SPECT in distinguishing cerebral infections from lymphoma in patients with AIDS. Clin Nucl Med. 2002;27:81-86.
192. De Luca A, Antinori A, Cingolani A, et al. Evaluation of cerebrospinal fluid EBV-DNA and IL-10 as markers for in vivo diagnosis of AIDS-related primary central nervous system lymphoma [Erratum published in Br J Haematol. 1995;91:1035]. Br J Haematol. 1995;90:844-849.
193. Cinque P, Brytting M, Vago L, et al. Epstein-Barr virus DNA in cerebrospinal fluid from patients with AIDS-related primary lymphoma of the central nervous system. Lancet. 1993;342:398-410.
194. Cingolani A, De Luca A, Larocca LM, et al. Minimally invasive diagnosis of acquired immunodeficiency syndrome-related primary central nervous system lymphoma. J Natl Cancer Inst. 1998;90:364-369.
195. Forsyth PA, Yahalom J, DeAngelis LM. Combined-modality therapy in the treatment of primary central nervous system lymphoma in AIDS. Neurology. 1994;44:1473-1479.
196. Ferreri A, Reni M, Villa E. Therapeutic management of primary central nervous system lymphoma: Lessons from prospective trials. Ann Oncol. 2000;11:927-937.
197. Jacomet C, Girard P, Lebrette M, et al. Intravenous methotrexate for primary central nervous system non-Hodgkin's lymphoma in AIDS. AIDS. 1997;11:1725-1730.
198. Corales R, Taege A, Rehm S. Regression of AIDS-related CNS lymphoma with HAART. Presented at XIII International AIDS Conference, Durban, South Africa, 2000.
199. Frieberg A, Slobod K, Taylor G, et al. EBV-targeted therapy for AIDS-related primary central nervous system lymphoma. Presented at American Society of Hematology Meeting, San Francisco, 2000.
200. Levine A. Acquired immunodeficiency syndrome-related lymphoma: Clinical aspects. Semin Oncol. 2000;27:442-453.
201. Raez L, Cabral L, Cai J. Antivirals induce apoptosis and tumor regression in AIDS-related primary central nervous system lymphoma. Presented at Third National AIDS Malignancy Conference, Bethesda, MD, 1999.
202. Baiocchi R, Peng R, Schmalbrock P. An in vivo preclinical model to evaluate an effective antiviral regimen in Epstein-barr virus-associated primary central nervous system lymphoma. Presented at International Conference on Malignant Lymphoma, Lugano, Switzerland, 1999.
203. Vernon S, Holmes K, Reeves W. Human papillomavirus infection and associated disease in persons infected with human immunodeficiency virus. Clin Infect Dis. 1995;(21 Suppl 1):S121-S124.
204. Pfister H. The role of human papillomavirus in anogential cancer. Obstet Gynecol Clin North Am. 1996;23:579-595.
205. Gal A, Saul S, Stoer M. In situ hybridization analysis of human papillomavirus in anal squamous cell carcinoma. Mod Pathol. 1989;2:439-443.
206. Sillman F, Sedlis A. Anogenital papillomavirus infection and neoplasia in immunodeficient women. Obstet Gynecol Clin North Am. 1987;14:537-538.
207. Committee TBSE. The Bethesda system for reporting cervical/vaginal cytologic diagnoses: Report of the 1991 Bethesda workshop. Hum Pathol. 1992;23:719-721.
208. Hillemans E, Ellerbrock T, McPhillips S. Prevalence of anal human papillomavirus infection and anal cytologic abnormalitites in HIV-seropositive women. AIDS. 1996;10:1641-1647.
209. Cardillo M, Hagan R, Abadi J, et al. CD4 T cell count, viral load and squamous intraepithelial lesions in women infected with human immunodeficiency virus. Cancer. 2001;92A:111-114.
210. Hocke C, Leroy V, Morlet P, et al. Cervical dysplasia and HIV infection in women: Prevalence and associated factors. Eur J Obstet Gynecol Reprod Biol. 1998;81:69-76.
211. Palefsky J, Holly E, Ralston M, et al. High incidence of anal and high-grade squamous intra-epithelial lesions among HIV-positive and HIV-negative homosexual and bisexual men. AIDS. 1998;12:495-503.
212. Sun X, Kuhn L, Ellerbrock T, et al. Human papillomavirus infection in women infected with the human immunodeficiency virus. N Engl J Med. 1997;337:1343-1349.

213. Wright A, Darragh T, Vranizan K, et al. Anal and cervical papillomavirus infection and risk of anal and cervical epithelial abnormalities in human immunodeficiency virus-infected women. Obstet Gynecol. 1997;89:76-80.

214. Maiman M, Fructer R, Serur E, et al. Human immunodeficiency virus infection and cervical neoplasia. Gynecol Oncol. 1990;38:377-382.

215. Maiman M, Fructer R, Clark M, et al. Cervical cancer as an AIDS-defining illness. Obstet Gynecol. 1997;89:76-80.

216. Maiman M, Fructer R, Guy L, et al. Human immunodeficiency virus infection and invasive cervical cancer. Cancer. 1993;71:402-406.

217. Monfardini S, Vaccher E, Pizzocaro G, et al. Unusual malignant tumors in 49 patients with HIV infection. AIDS. 1989;3:499-452.

218. Rellihan M, Dooley D, Burke T, et al. Rapidly progressing cervical cancer in a patient with human immunodeficiency virus infection. Gynecol Oncol. 1990;36:435-438.

219. Saccucci P, Mastrone M, Are P, et al. Rapidly progressive squamous cell carcinoma of the cervix in a patient with acquired immunodeficiency syndrome: Case report. Eur J Gynaecol Oncol. 1996;17:306-308.

220. Dorrucci M, Suligoi B, Serraino D, et al. Incidence of invasive cervical cancer in a cohort of HIV-seropositive women before and after the introduction of highly active antiretroviral therapy. J Acquir Immune Defic Syndr. 2001;26:377-380.

221. Robinson W. Invasive and preinvasive cervical neoplasia in human immunodeficiency virus-infected women. Semin Oncol. 2000;27:463-470.

222. Delmas MC, Agarossi A, Bergeron C, et al. Incidence of squamous intraepithelial lesions (SIL) in HIV-infected women (Abstract 623/22306). Int Conf AIDS. 1998;12:324.

223. Heard I, Schmitz V, Costagliola D, et al. Early regression of cervical lesions in HIV-seropositive women receiving highly active antiretroviral therapy. AIDS. 1998;12:1459-1464.

224. Heard I, Tassie J, Kazachkine M, et al. Highly active antiretroviral therapy enhances regression of cervical intraepithelial neoplasia in HIV-seropositive women. AIDS. 2002;16:1799-1802.

225. Zbar A, Fenger C, Efron J, et al. The pathology and molecular biology of anal intraepithelial neoplasia: Comparisons with cervical and vulvar intraepithelial carcinoma. Int J Colorectal Dis. 2002;17:203-215.

226. Palefsky JM, Holly EA, Ralston ML, et al. Prevalence and risk factors for human papillomavirus infection of the anal canal in human immunodeficiency virus (HIV)-positive and HIV-negative homosexual men. J Infect Dis. 1998;177:361-367.

227. Palefsky J, Holly E, Hogeboom C, et al. Virologic, immunologic, and clinical parameters in the incidence and progression of anal squamous intraepithelial lesions in HIV-positive and HIV-negative homosexual men. J Acquir Immun Defic Syndr. 1998;17:314-319.

228. Palefsky J, Holly E, Ralston M, et al. Effect of highly active antiretroviral therapy on the natural history of anal squamous intraepithelial lesions and anal human papillomavirus infection. J Acquir Immun Defic Syndr. 2001;28:422-428.

229. Berry J, Palefsky J. Pathogenesis and clinical manifestations of HIV-associated anogenital neoplasia. AIDS Knowledge Base, HIV InSite, November 1998; available at: http://hivinsite.ucsf.edu.

230. Biggar R. Cancers in AIDS: What types and what clues to etiology? Presented at the 1998 National AIDS Malignancy Conference, sponsored by the National Cancer Institute, Bethesda, MD, April 6-8, 1998.

231. Lorenz HP, Wilson W, Leigh B, et al. Squamous cell carcinoma of the anus and HIV infection. Dis Colon Rectum. 1991;34:336-338.

232. Holland J, Swift P. Tolerance of patients with human immunodeficiency virus and carcinoma to treatment with combined chemotherapy and radiation therapy. Radiology. 1994;193:251-254.

233. Hoffman R, Welton ML, Klencke B, et al. The significance of pretreatment CD4 count on the outcome and treatment tolerance of HIV-positive patients with anal cancer. Int J Radiat Oncol Biol Phys. 1999;44:127-131.

234. Remick S. Non-AIDS-defining cancers. Hematol Oncol Clin North Am. 1996;10:1203-1213.

235. Grulich A, Wan X, Lau M, et al. Risk of cancer in people with AIDS. AIDS. 1999;13:839-843.

236. Goedert J. The epidemiology of AIDS malignancies. Semin Oncol. 2000;27:390-401.

237. Rabkin C. Association of non-AIDS-defining cancer with HIV infection. J Natl Cancer Inst Monogr. 1998;23:23-25.

238. Polluck B, Jenson G, Leach C, et al. Risk factors of pediatric HIV-related malignancies. JAMA. 2003;289:2393-2399.

239. Rabkin C, Biggar R, Horm J. Increased incidence of cancers associated with the human immunodeficiency virus epidemic. Int J Cancer. 1991;47:692-696.

240. McClain L, Leach C, Jenson H, et al. Association of Epstein-Barr virus with leiomyosarcomas in children with AIDS. N Engl J Med. 1995;332:12-18.

241. Timmerman J, Northfelt D, Small E. Malignant germ cell tumors in men infected with human immunodeficiency virus: Natural history and results of therapy. J Clin Oncol. 1995;13:1391-1397.

242. Biggar R, Horm J, Goedert J, et al. Cancer in a group at risk of acquired immunodeficiency syndrome (AIDS) through 1984. Am J Epidemiol. 1987;126:578.

243. Biggar R, Burnett W, Mikl J, et al. Cancer among New York men at risk of acquired immunodeficiency syndrome. Int J Cancer. 1989;43:979.

244. Hessol N, Katz M, Liu J, et al. Increased incidence of Hodgkin's disease in homosexual men with HIV infection. Ann Intern Med. 1992;117:309.

245. Reynolds P, Saunders L, Layefsky M, et al. The spectrum of acquired immunodeficiency syndrome (AIDS)-associated malignancies in San Francisco, 1980-1987. Am J Epidemiol. 1993;37:19.

246. Lyter D, Kingsley L, Rinaldo C, et al. Malignancies in the Multicenter AIDS Cohort Study (MACS), 1984-1994. Presented at the American Society of Clinical Oncology, Thirty-second Annual Meeting, Philadelphia, May 18-21, 1996.

247. Biggar RJ, Rabkin CS. The epidemiology of AIDS-related neoplasms. Hematol Oncol Clin North Am. 1996;10:997-1010.

248. Hessol NA, Katz MH, Liu JY, et al. Increased incidence of Hodgkin's disease in homosexual men with HIV infection. Ann Intern Med. 1992;117:309-311.

249. Spina M, Vaccher E, Nasti G, et al. Human immunodeficiency virus-associated Hodgkin's disease. Semin Oncol. 2000;27:480-488.

250. Biggar RJ, Frisch M, Engels EA, et al. The National AIDS-Cancer Match Registry (Abstract S3). Abstracts of the Fourth International AIDS Malignancy Conference, May 16-18, 2000, Bethesda, MD. J Acquir Immune Defic Syndr. 2000;23:A8.

251. Biggar R, Rabkin C. The epidemiology of AIDS-related neoplasms. In: Krown S, von Roenn JH, eds. Hematologic and Oncologic Aspects of HIV Infection. Philadelphia: WB Saunders; 1996:997-1010.

252. Davis S, Dahlberg S, Nyers M, et al. Hodgkin's disease in the United States: A comparison of patient characteristics and survival in the centralized cancer patient data system and the surveillance, epidemiology, and end results program. J Natl Cancer Inst. 1987;78:471.

253. Monfardini S, Tirelli U, Vaccher E, et al. Hodgkin's disease in 63 intravenous drug users infected with human immunodeficiency virus. Ann Oncol. 1991;2(Suppl 2):201.

254. Ree H, Strauchen J, Hkan A, et al. Human immunodeficiency virus-associated Hodgkin's disease: Clinicopathologic studies of 24 cases and preponderance of mixed cellularity typed characterized by the occurrence of fibrohistiocytoid stromal cells. Cancer. 1991;67:1614.

255. Rubio R. Hodgkin's disease associated with human immunodeficiency virus infection: A clinical study of 46 cases. Cooperative Study Group of Malignancies Associated with HIV Infection of Madrid. Cancer. 1994;73:2400-2407.

256. Serrano M, Bellas C, Campo E, et al. Hodgkin's disease in patients with antibodies to human immunodeficiency virus: A study of 22 patients. Cancer. 1990;65:2248.

257. Tirelli U, Errante D, Vaccher E, et al. High frequency of Epstein-Barr virus genome detection in Hodgkin's disease of HIV positive patients. Int J Cancer. 1990;46:581.

258. Gold J, Altarac D, Ree H, et al. HIV associated Hodgkin's disease: A clinical study of 18 cases and review of the literature. Am J Hematol. 1991;36:93.

259. Gerard L, Galicier L, Boulanger E, et al. Improved survival in HIV-related Hodgkin's lymphoma since the introduction of highly active antiretroviral therapy. AIDS. 2003;17:81-87.

260. Spina M, Gabarre J, Rossi G, et al. Stanford V regimen and concomitant HAART in 59 patients with Hodgkin disease and HIV infection. Blood. 2002;100:1984-1988.

261. Kaplan L, Kahn J, Northfelt D, et al. Novel combination chemotherapy for Hodgkin's disease (HD) in HIV-infected individuals (Abstract 7). Proceedings of the American Society of Clinical Oncology, Houston, May 19-21, 1991.

262. Levine A, Cheung T, Tulpule A, et al. Preliminary results of AIDS Clinical Trials Group (ACTG) study # 149: Phase II trial of ABVD chemotherapy with G-CSF in HIV infected patients with Hodgkin's disease (HD) (Abstract S7). Presented at the National AIDS Malignancy Conference, Bethesda, MD, April 28-30, 1997.

CHAPTER **122**

Human Immunodeficiency Virus Infection in Women

SUSAN E. COHN

REBECCA A. CLARK

Human immunodeficiency virus (HIV) infection has had a profound impact on the health of women worldwide, and by the end of 2002, 46% of the more than 42 million people living with HIV infection, or 19.2 million, were women.[1] Women constitute the fastest growing segment of the population with HIV infection in the United States and represent 7% of all cases of acquired immunodeficiency syndrome (AIDS) reported as of 1985; this proportion increased to 26% of all AIDS cases newly diagnosed in 2001.[2] This chapter discusses the epidemiology of HIV infection in women, transmission of HIV to women, pregnancy and risk of perinatal transmission, clinical manifestations of HIV infection in women, and management issues for women with HIV infection.

EPIDEMIOLOGY OF HUMAN IMMUNODEFICIENCY VIRUS INFECTION AND ACQUIRED IMMUNODEFICIENCY SYNDROME IN WOMEN

United States

When AIDS first was recognized in 1981, it was considered to be a disease of men who have sex with men and of persons who used injection drugs. With the rapid increase in the number of women infected with HIV has come an increased understanding of the potential for heterosexual transmission of HIV infection in the United States. Between 1990 and 1994, the incidence of AIDS reported in women increased by 89%, which is three times the reported 29% increase in men.[3] By 2001, women accounted for 26% of new AIDS diagnoses (11,164/43,158 cases), 18% of the 816,149 cumulative AIDS cases, and 32% of newly reported HIV diagnoses (11,394/35,575 cases).[2] Overall, AIDS rates continue to be lower in women than in men: 9.1 per 100,000 women compared with 28.1 per 100,000 men in 2001.[2]

Increasingly, women are acquiring HIV infection through heterosexual contact, with a slowing of injection drug use (IDU)–associated cases since 1992. Since 1995, heterosexual contact has become the predominant mode of exposure for women in the United States.[4] By 2001, most AIDS cases due to heterosexual transmission were attributed to sex with an injection drug user (38%) or sex with an HIV-infected partner of risk not specified (54%).[2] Bisexually active men also may be contributing to the spread of HIV infection to women because, at least in a Boston cohort, they were more likely to have unprotected sex with their female partners than with their male partners.[5,6]

The AIDS epidemic has had a major impact on morbidity and mortality among young women. By 1992, AIDS was the fourth leading cause of death among women 25 to 44 years old in the United States and was the leading cause of death among women in the same age group in 15 primarily East Coast cities.[7] By 1995, HIV infection was the third leading cause of death in women in this age group and the leading cause of death among African-American women.[8] Deaths from AIDS peaked in 1994 and 1995, then began decreasing in 1996.[9] The percentage decrease in mortality was smallest among African-American women and women from the South; the highest death rates were among the population below the poverty level.[3] In 1999, death rates were highest among African Americans (32.5 per 100,000, almost 11 times higher than among whites).[3] Decreased mortality has been attributed to improved combination antiretroviral regimens, including protease inhibitors, rather than to advances in prevention of HIV transmission. These potent antiretroviral medication regimens also have been associated with decreased progression to AIDS, fewer opportunistic infections, fewer hospitalizations, and prolonged survival.[10,11] Women have not benefited to the same degree as noted for men who acquired HIV infection through male-to-male sexual contact, presumably because women as a group have had less access to medical care and potent antiretroviral agents (see section on "Sex Differences in Viral Load and Human Immunodeficiency Virus Disease Progression").

HIV disproportionately affects women of color; black and Hispanic women accounted for 80% of reported AIDS cases in 2001.[2] AIDS is predominantly a disease of childbearing women; 87% of affected women were diagnosed between 20 and 50 years of age. Women older than 50 have accounted for only 9% of all reported cases; however, underrecognition may be common, and older women typically present for medical attention with advanced disease and are unaware of their risk for HIV infection.[2,12,13] A study of women older than 50 with AIDS found that they were more likely than younger women to live alone (24% versus 11%), to have not completed high school (63% versus 37%), to be tested for HIV infection while hospitalized (51% versus 32%), and to have never used a condom before diagnosis of HIV infection (86% versus 67%).[14]

The epidemiology of drug use affects the epidemiology of HIV infection among American women. In 1996, after exclusion of the 24% of women whose initial mode of transmission was not reported, two thirds of HIV-infected women reported IDU (45%) or heterosexual contact with an injection drug user (18%).[15] By 2001, after excluding the 42% of women without a reported risk behavior, only one third of women with newly diagnosed AIDS reported IDU, and 14% reported heterosexual contact with an injection drug user.[2] Since the mid-1980s, heroin has become less popular, whereas cocaine and other drugs have been used increasingly. When used intravenously, these newer drugs typically are injected more frequently and are associated with increased needle sharing.[7,16] The use of smokable freebase ("crack") became widespread after its first appearance in New York City in 1985 because of its low cost and high addictive potential. Although smoking crack cocaine itself does not transmit HIV, the tendency of persons who use crack to engage in unsafe behaviors, such as increased sexual activity with multiple partners and exchange of sex for drugs, has resulted in the increased spread of HIV infection and other sexually transmitted diseases (STDs), including syphilis.[17,18]

Only five potential incidences of female-to-female sexual transmission of HIV have been documented in the literature.[7] In a review of 164 women with AIDS who reported having sexual contact only with women, 93% injected drugs and 7% had received a blood transfusion; no cases were attributable to female-to-female sexual transmission.[7,19] In a study of 498 lesbian and bisexual women frequenting public venues in San Francisco and Berkeley, California, 6 (1.2%) were HIV infected.[20] This population showed high rates of high-risk behaviors (10% reported IDU, and 40% reported unprotected sex with men, some of whom were bisexual men and male injection drug users), and no evidence for sexual transmission between women was found. These data and others suggest that the frequency of female-to-female HIV transmission remains very low.[21]

HIV transmission through intravaginal insemination of donor semen has been reported.[22-24] Use of assisted reproductive technologies, which include sperm washing and intracytoplasmic sperm injection, seems to have an extremely low risk for horizontal transmission from an HIV-infected man to an HIV-negative woman or vertical transmission to children born from these procedures.[25-27] Although these techniques seem to be promising, they are presently not available in the United States outside of a research setting, require specialized laboratories, and are quite costly. These expensive assisted reproductive procedures often are not covered by insurance and are not accessible to most couples.

Worldwide

New estimates from the World Health Organization (WHO) indicate that HIV infection is far more prevalent worldwide than previously thought.[1] As of December 2001, there were an estimated 42 million people living with HIV/AIDS, 46% of whom were women.[1] In 2001, there were almost 14,000 new HIV infections a day; 6600 (48%) were in women, and 2100 were in children. Worldwide, HIV infection is spread primarily through heterosexual contact, although IDU and its contribution to exposure to HIV vary geographically. Because female drug users have sexual partners who are at high risk of HIV infection, and because IDU can lead to exchange of sex for drugs or money, there may be underrecognition and underreporting of cases spread through heterosexual contact.

The geographic region with the highest number of HIV-infected women is sub-Saharan Africa, where in 2002, 29.4 million people were living with HIV, and more than half of these were women.[1] In four southern African countries, national adult HIV prevalence was greater than 30% by the end of 2002. In 2001, an estimated 6% to 11% of young African women age 15 to 24 were living with HIV/AIDS. Heterosexual transmission continues to be the predominant mode of HIV transmission in Africa. Concomitant with poor access to information and services for prevention of mother-to-child transmission in sub-Saharan Africa, 720,000 HIV-infected children were born there in 2002, representing about 90% of the new pediatric HIV infections in the world.[1] As in the United States, AIDS initially was concentrated in urban areas, but now has spread outward to smaller towns and rural areas, primarily along highways and truck routes.[28,29] There have been some hopeful signs that the epidemic could be brought under control in sub-Saharan Africa. In South Africa, HIV prevalence rates for pregnant women younger than 20 decreased from 21% in 1998 to 15.4% in 2001. In Addis Abada, Ethiopia, HIV infection rates among women 15 to 24 attending antenatal clinics decreased from 24.2% in 1995 to 15.1% in 2001. Despite more recent positive trends, these countries all face massive challenges not only to sustain and expand prevention efforts, but also to provide adequate treatment (including antiretroviral therapy), care, and support to the millions of people living with HIV/AIDS or orphaned by the epidemic.[1]

The area with the largest growth in the HIV epidemic probably will be in Asia, where the epidemic is newer than in Africa.[1] In 2002, an estimated 7.2 million people were living with HIV in Asia and the Pacific, and about 1 million were newly infected with HIV.[1] High rates of HIV infection are seen among injecting drug users, sex workers, and men who have sex with men in countries throughout Asia. Seroprevalence rates vary greatly, often with concurrent epidemics within a country; genetic analyses in China suggest little overlap between HIV epidemics among injection drug users and commercial sex workers.[1] HIV also is spreading heterosexually among people who became infected when they sold their blood to collecting centers that improperly adhered to safety procedures.[1] Few countries in Asia have sophisticated systems for adequately monitoring the epidemic, and small differences in rates can alter estimates of numbers of infected persons greatly, given the enormous size of the combined population of China, India, and Southeast Asia.[1] More recent economic and social unrest in Indonesia seems to be associated with a sharp increase in IDU and with it a significant increase in HIV infections. After an initial explosion in seroprevalence rates among female commercial sex workers in Thailand, government-sponsored prevention efforts have resulted in dramatically decreasing incidences.[1] Half of the new HIV infections in Thailand now seem to be occurring in the sexual partners (and wives) of men who were infected by sex workers in the 1990s.[1]

The HIV epidemic is well established in Latin America and the Caribbean and continues to be concentrated in neglected populations living on the social and economic margins of society.[1] In Brazil, HIV seroprevalence is increasing among women and heterosexuals as the rates among drug users and their partners increase. Twelve countries in Latin America and the Caribbean have estimated HIV seroprevalence rates of 1% or more in pregnant women, making this the second most affected region in the world after sub-Saharan Africa.[1] Haiti remains the worst affected with an estimated national adult HIV prevalence of greater than 6%.[1] Some of these countries (especially Brazil) have started to provide antiretroviral medications to persons with HIV/AIDS. Access to HIV medications is unequal across the region, partly due to varying drug prices.

The high mortality rate for HIV/AIDS has had a major impact on families. At the end of 2001, an estimated 14 million children and adolescents worldwide had been orphaned by AIDS, by loss of their mother or both parents to AIDS.[1] More than 80% of children orphaned as a result of AIDS were in sub-Saharan Africa.[30] Saving lives of parents through access to antiretroviral therapies in resource-poor countries and helping to alleviate poverty and improve education are central to the global response to the orphan crisis.[30]

TRANSMISSION OF HUMAN IMMUNODEFICIENCY VIRUS TO WOMEN

Heterosexual Transmission

Efficiency of Heterosexual Transmission of Human Immunodeficiency Virus

Globally, heterosexual transmission accounts for the spread of HIV infection in approximately 90% of persons living with AIDS and is the fastest growing mode of HIV transmission in the United States.[31] Mechanisms of heterosexual transmission remain poorly understood, however.[7] HIV has been isolated from semen of HIV-infected men and from cervicovaginal secretions of HIV-infected women. Although heterosexual transmission seems more efficient from men to women than

from women to men, HIV-infected women can spread HIV to their uninfected sexual partners.[32-34] The most likely explanation for this difference in ease of HIV spread from men to their partners relates to the larger volume of semen compared with cervicovaginal secretions and to the higher concentration of HIV on average in seminal fluid.

HIV is not transmitted consistently by sexual contact. Although some persons become infected after a single sexual exposure or artificial insemination with HIV-infected semen,[23] others remain uninfected despite hundreds of exposures.[35-37] This lack of transmission may be due to the amount of virus, the host immune response, the relative virulence of HIV isolates, or some combination thereof.

The efficiency of heterosexual transmission of HIV between women and men has not been characterized fully. The efficiency of transmission of gonorrhea, a well-studied STD, is approximately 25% after a single male contact with an infected woman and close to 90% for transmission by infected men to uninfected female partners.[38,39] HIV is much less efficiently transmitted; however, the extremely long incubation period of HIV disease has hindered specific inferences about the relative rates and efficiency of sexual transmission because many persons do not learn of their infection until years after the relevant exposure. Estimates of infectivity for each sexual contact have ranged from 3 per 100 for the most efficient transmitters in a male homosexual cohort study[40] to less than 1 per 10,000 contacts in studies of heterosexual couples discordant for HIV serostatus.[32,35,41] In a California study of heterosexual HIV serostatus–discordant couples, the risk of male-to-female transmission was 17 times higher than the risk of female-to-male transmission.[33] An Italian study of 730 discordant heterosexual couples found the transmission of HIV from men to women to be twice as efficient as from women to men.[42] More recent studies of monogamous HIV-discordant partners in Uganda suggest that the efficiency of HIV spread may be more similar between men and women than was appreciated initially.[41]

Factors Associated with Heterosexual Transmission

Factors that have been associated with greater likelihood of transmitting HIV between heterosexual partners include viremia of greater magnitude or more advanced immunodeficiency in the infecting partner, the presence of any STD including ulcerative and nonulcerative disease, sexual activity during menses, receptive anal sex, unprotected vaginal sex, traumatic sex, increased number of sexual contacts, and infectivity of the HIV-infected partner.[40,43-45] Other less well-documented factors that are thought to increase the risk of heterosexual transmission include lack of circumcision in men[46]; cervical ectopy; certain contraceptive practices, such as hormonal contraception or use of nonoxynol 9; and higher viral load in genital secretions (Table 122-1). The chemokine receptor gene mutation (32-base-pair deletion in *CCR5*) seems to confer resistance to HIV in persons who are homozygous for this trait.[44] Although persons with more advanced disease are more likely to transmit HIV, consistent with their increased viral burden, the data are incomplete. In some men receiving potent antiretroviral therapy, HIV was cleared successfully from the blood to below the level of detection of some laboratories (e.g., <400 copies/mL), but the men still were able to transmit HIV, suggesting a compartmentalization of HIV between semen and plasma.[47] Some investigators have found that treatment-induced changes in HIV viral load generally are associated with a corresponding change in the amounts of seminal and cervicovaginal HIV RNA, supporting the hypothesis that potent antiretroviral therapy may reduce the spread of HIV.[48-52]

STDs, particularly diseases associated with genital ulcers, increase the efficiency of HIV transmission and the susceptibility to HIV infection.[51] Genital ulcerative diseases, which include syphilis, chancroid, and genital herpes, are thought to enhance the access of HIV to mucosal tissues, lymphatic drainage, and systemic lymphocytes.[52,53] HIV also may be transmitted through intact mucosal membranes, presumably by infecting dendritic cells within the mucous membranes of the genital tract.[54] Epidemiologic studies suggest that ulcerative and nonulcerative STDs increase the susceptibility to HIV infection; female sex workers in Zaire had an increased risk of HIV seroconversion

TABLE 122-1 Risk Factors Associated with Sexual Transmission of Human Immunodeficiency Virus

Sexually transmitted infections
  Ulcerative/nonulcerative diseases
Genital tract inflammation
HIV disease
  Higher viral loads
  Lower CD4$^+$ levels
  Acute HIV infection
  Lack of effective antiretroviral therapy
  Lack of heterozygosity or homozygosity for the inactivating 32-base-pair deletion in the chemokine receptor gene (*CCR5*)
Anatomic factors
  Lack of circumcision
  Cervical ectopy
  Leukocytospermia
  ?Hormonal contraception
Sexual practices
  Sexual activity during menses
  Receptive anal intercourse
  Bleeding during intercourse (disruption of vaginal mucosa through trauma)
  Lack of barrier protection
HIV viral features
  Syncytium formation
  Certain viral clades

  HIV, human immunodeficiency virus.

if they had nonulcerative STDs,[55] and among HIV serostatus–discordant sex partners, seroconversion was more likely if the previously HIV-negative sex partner had ulcerative and nonulcerative STDs.[56] Nonulcerative STDs, such as gonorrhea, chlamydial infection, and trichomoniasis, seem to increase the number of lymphocytes, monocytes, and Langerhan's cells in the endocervix in susceptible seronegative women and provide more potential targets for HIV infection.[51] Similarly, nonulcerative STDs may increase the number of HIV-infected cells in the genital tracts of HIV-positive transmitters. Cohen and associates[57] found that HIV-infected men with urethritis had seminal plasma HIV-1 RNA eight times the levels in seropositive men without urethritis. Treatment of urethritis was associated with significant decreases in HIV-1 concentration in semen, suggesting a decrease in infectivity with successful STD treatment.

The introduction of highly active antiretroviral therapy (HAART) has led to significant reductions in morbidity and mortality due to HIV infection. Epidemiologic data suggest that HAART has contributed to a resurgence of unsafe sexual practices, especially among some men who have sex with men.[58] HAART use is thought to be associated with a loss of fear of acquiring and transmitting HIV; decreased use of condoms; and more unsafe sex among HIV-discordant and HIV-concordant couples, especially if they have responded well to HAART. Other current factors associated with potential increases in sexual transmission of HIV include use of the Internet to identify potential sex partners, increased use of Viagra (Pfizer, New York, NY) as a recreational drug, and increased desire of HIV-infected persons to have children.[58-60]

Human Immunodeficiency Virus Infection of the Genital Tract. Much research has been dedicated to isolation, identification, and quantification of the amount of HIV present within cervicovaginal secretions. The presence of HIV in the female genital tract is crucial for heterosexual transmission of HIV and for perinatal transmission of HIV during labor and delivery. HIV-1 has been isolated from cervical and cervicovaginal secretions obtained using cervicovaginal lavage (CVL) and vaginal or cervical swabs or wicks.[61]

It is controversial how well plasma HIV viral load correlates with genital tract HIV levels. Some more recent studies have suggested that elevated plasma HIV-1 viral levels and lower CD4$^+$ cell counts are strong predictors of genital HIV-1 levels,[49,62-64] whereas other studies have failed to document a clear association between the two compartments.[65,66] A study of four HIV-infected women, using amino acid sequence analysis of cell-free HIV RNA in plasma and CVL virus, found CVL virus to be genotypically distinct from plasma HIV.[67]

Other studies have found strong similarities, however, between virus genotypes from blood and cervical swab samples.[68] Cervicovaginal and seminal HIV viral loads are more likely to be high during acute HIV seroconversion and late in the course of HIV infection. Although viral loads in genital secretions tend to be lower after initiation of effective antiretroviral medications, detectable HIV in genital secretions has been reported in men and women with undetectable plasma HIV levels.[63,66] Patients with a low plasma virus burden still potentially may transmit HIV to a sexual partner or perinatally to an infant, although the risk is low.

HIV has been detected in menstrual blood, and having intercourse during menses increases the risk of infecting the male partner.[7] Menstruation introduces about 80 mL of blood into the genital tract over a 3- to 5-day period.[69] This menstrual blood is likely to contain HIV-infected cells and free virus, reflecting the HIV viral load of peripheral blood. Menstrual blood raises the pH in the vagina to the neutral range, improving the viability of HIV shed in menses and HIV in semen deposited in the vagina during intercourse.[70] Higher levels of HIV in the genital tract may be seen with conditions that raise the vaginal pH, such as blood in the vagina, bacterial vaginosis, menopause, intercourse, and possibly the use of some forms of birth control.[71,72] More recent studies confirmed that although plasma HIV-1 viral load remained constant during the menstrual cycle, genital viral loads were lower in the periovulatory phase and highest during menses.[73,74] These results suggest that local factors may affect the genital viral load compartment independent of plasma viral load.[73,74]

Research currently is under way to develop intravaginal microbial agents capable of reducing the heterosexual and perinatal transmission of HIV-1.[75] Although nonoxynol 9, a commonly used spermicidal agent, has anti-HIV activity in vitro, there have been safety concerns after reports of vaginal ulceration and inflammation during clinical studies.[76,77] Preliminary results from a placebo-controlled study of 400 women in Cameroon found similar rates of HIV seropositivity among women who inserted nonoxynol 9 or placebo in advance of and during sexual relations.[78] A placebo-controlled trial of nonoxynol 9 in sex workers in four countries did not show a protective effect of nonoxynol 9 on HIV-1 transmission.[79] The risk of acquiring HIV was higher in the nonoxynol 9 group that used a mean of 3.5 applicators or more per working day compared with women who used fewer administrations per day or the placebo. Nonoxynol 9 may cause toxic effects enhancing HIV-1 infection, and its use no longer is recommended as a potential HIV-1 prevention method. Assessment of other microbicides is under way.[75] Cleansing the birth canal with chlorhexidine has been studied in Malawi; it did not reduce perinatal HIV transmission[80] but did reduce early neonatal and maternal postpartum infectious problems.[81]

One early study showed that cervical shedding of HIV was associated with oral contraceptive pill use, cervical ectopy, and pregnancy.[82] Women with genital infection or cervicovaginal dysplasia have higher levels of proinflammatory cytokines in CVL fluid, which may affect local HIV replication and may influence the risk of acquisition or transmission of HIV.[83] Data from a community-based cohort in Rakai, Uganda, did not find an association between hormonal contraception use and HIV acquisition after adjusting for behavioral confounding.[84] More research is needed to identify risk factors associated with genital shedding of HIV, including the role of hormonal contraceptive use and of potent antiretrovirals in decreasing HIV viral loads within the genital tract.

Risk of female-to-male transmission is likely to be associated with the presence of HIV in cervicovaginal secretions of HIV-infected women.[67,85] In a study of 1201 female sex workers, cervicovaginal shedding of HIV-1 was more frequent in immunosuppressed women, in women with *Neisseria gonorrhoeae* or *Chlamydia trachomatis* infection, and in women with a cervical or vaginal ulcer.[86] HIV-1 shedding decreased from 42% to 21% in women whose STDs were cured, theoretically decreasing the infectivity of their secretions.[86] As understanding of the relationship between peripheral HIV viral load and HIV viral load within genital secretions broadens, so will the ability to assess more fully the infectivity of genital secretions.

Strategies to Prevent Heterosexual Transmission

Treatment of STDs is likely to decrease transmission of HIV and susceptibility to HIV infection. In a Tanzanian clinical trial conducted among persons in rural communities, universal STD screening and treatment of symptomatic cases of STD resulted in a 40% reduction in HIV incidence compared with that in a village in which no STD screening or treatment was available.[87]

Barrier contraceptives constitute an effective means of preventing HIV transmission. De Vincenzi[56] found no heterosexual transmission among 124 HIV serostatus–discordant couples who used condoms consistently but a seroconversion rate of 4.8 per 100 person-years for the 121 discordant couples who used condoms inconsistently. The use of barrier contraceptives such as condoms should be promoted as a means of contraception and as partial protection against HIV and other STDs.

The Centers for Disease Control and Prevention (CDC) has expanded its prevention activities to include the Serostatus Approach to Fighting the Epidemic (SAFE), a program that especially targets HIV-infected persons.[88] SAFE encourages people to know their HIV status and, if infected, encourages them to seek high-quality care and prevention services, helps them adhere to treatment regimens, and supports them in adopting and sustaining HIV risk reduction behavior. By ensuring quality HIV care and focusing on behavioral interventions to prevent HIV, it is hoped that the close to 1 million persons living in the United States with HIV will limit their spread of HIV to others.

Perinatal Transmission

Understanding of factors associated with increased perinatal transmission has increased greatly, and advances have led to earlier, more reliable detection of HIV infection in newborns. Although antiretroviral medications used during pregnancy and delivery have resulted in dramatic decreases in perinatal transmission, much still is poorly understood about mechanisms and pathogenesis of mother-to-child transmission.

Before the use of antiretroviral medications, estimates of the frequency of perinatal transmission ranged from a low of 13% in Europe to a high of more than 60% in Africa, with frequencies of 14% to 33% reported in the United States.[89,90] As the number of women who become HIV infected during their childbearing years increases, so will the number of children who contract HIV perinatally without effective intervention. Practical, cost-effective strategies to reduce perinatal transmission while preserving the mother's health and future treatment options are urgently needed.

Timing of Transmission

HIV can be transmitted from an HIV-infected woman to her child during intrauterine gestation, at delivery, or in the postpartum period through breast-feeding. HIV-1 has been isolated from fetal blood samples taken before elective terminations[91] and from fetal tissues at 8 weeks of gestation.[92-95] In addition, in fetuses lost early in pregnancy, one study found that half had thymic tissue heavily infected with HIV, resulting in lymphoid depletion, epithelial injury, and precocious involution.[96] In half of the infants who eventually are proven to be HIV infected, HIV-1 can be identified by culture, polymerase chain reaction assay, or p24 antigen detection at or shortly after birth, which suggests that they were infected in utero before delivery.[97] HIV-infected infants who test negative for HIV by polymerase chain reaction assay or culture at birth may have been infected late in pregnancy or during the birthing process. The differences in onset and progression of HIV infection in infants may reflect timing of infection, whereas infants infected earlier in pregnancy typically present with more rapid progression to AIDS than do infants infected at birth, who present with asymptomatic HIV infection and have prolonged survival.[98,99]

Perinatal transmission is thought to occur near or during delivery in most cases.[89,90,100,101] The French Collaborative Study, using virologic and serologic data, applied mathematical modeling to estimate the timing of perinatal transmission in non–breast-feeding women.[90,102] The investigators estimated that 92% of all instances of transmission occurred during the last 2 months of pregnancy, and 65%

(95% confidence interval 22% to 92%) occurred during the intrapartum period.[102]

Twin studies have been used to further understanding of the timing of perinatal HIV transmission. Goedert and co-workers[103] studied 22 pairs of HIV seropositivity–discordant twins, and in 18 of the 22 pairs, the presenting twin was the infected sibling. Data from the International Registry of HIV-Exposed Twins suggest that the risk of infection in the twin who is born first is twice that in the second-born twin (26% and 13%).[90,103,104] The greater infection rates of first-born twins may be linked to increased contact with maternal secretions during birth.

Risk Factors for Increased Perinatal Transmission

Perinatal transmission is a multifactorial process, influenced by viral, immune, and clinical factors in the mother and the infant (Table 122-2). Maternal plasma viral load is the strongest predictor of the risk of transmitting HIV perinatally.[100,105] Coll and associates[106] studied 67 HIV-1-infected mothers during pregnancy and labor and their 69 newborns (including two sets of twins) and found a strong relationship between plasma viral RNA concentrations of greater than 10^5/mL (odds ratio 22, 95% confidence interval 4.4 to 119.2, $P < .00001$) and CD4$^+$ cell counts of fewer than 400/mm^3 (odds ratio 4.1, 95% confidence interval 1.1 to 15.4, $P = .01$) and transmission of HIV. Women with more advanced HIV disease and lower CD4$^+$ and higher CD8$^+$ T-cell counts are at increased risk to transmit HIV perinatally.[89,107-109] In a nested case-control study within a prospectively followed cohort of HIV-in-

---

TABLE 122-2 Potential Factors Influencing Mother-to-Child Transmission of Human Immunodeficiency Virus

Maternal Factors
Advanced HIV disease, as measured by
   Clinical staging
   Low CD4$^+$lymphocyte count
   Higher viral loads
   p24 antigenemia
Primary HIV infection
Viral phenotype: syncytium-inducing
Viral genotype: virulent mutant strain of HIV
Coinfection with other sexually transmitted diseases
Firstborn twins
Obstetric events
   Vaginal delivery
   Invasive procedures or fetal monitoring during labor
   Prolonged premature rupture of membranes (>4 hr)
Older maternal age
Cigarette smoking and illicit drug use during pregnancy
Breast-feeding
Unprotected sexual intercourse with multiple partners
Fetal or Placental Factors
Chorioamnionitis
Prematurity
Low birth weight
Labor or Birth Canal Factors
Cervicovaginal viral load
Local HIV-specific immune response
Maternal-fetal transfusion of blood
Immune Factors
Humoral
   Neutralizing antibody
   Antibody-dependent cellular cytotoxicity
   gp120 V3 loop antibody
   MHC concordance
   Other
Cell-mediated
   Cytotoxic T lymphocytes
   CD8 suppression
Mucosal immunity

HIV, human immunodeficiency virus; MHC, major histocompatibility complex.
Adapted from Sprecher S, Soumenkoff G, Puissant F, et al. Vertical transmission in a 15 week fetus. Lancet. 1986;2:228, © by The Lancet Ltd, 1986; and Bryson YJ. Perinatal HIV-1 transmission: Recent advances and therapeutic interventions. AIDS. 1996;3:533–542.

fected women, Thea and colleagues[110] found that high maternal viral load increased the likelihood of perinatal transmission in women without AIDS. Primary HIV infection in pregnancy or during breast-feeding associated with acute high-titer HIV viremia also seems to be associated with increased rates of transmission. No threshold has been observed below which transmission does not occur; women with undetectable plasma HIV RNA have transmitted HIV perinatally.[105,111] In a collaboration of studies, Ioannidis and co-workers[112] identified 44 cases of perinatal HIV-1 transmission among 1202 women with HIV-1 RNA viral loads less than 1000 copies/mL at delivery or at the measurement closest to delivery. The transmission rate was about 1% for women on antiretroviral therapy, which was significantly lower than the 9.8% rate for untreated mothers. Multiple RNA measurements were obtained during pregnancy or at the time of delivery in 12 cases, 10 of whom had a mean viral load greater than 500 copies/mL. Perinatal HIV-1 transmission may be almost eliminated with antiretroviral prophylaxis accompanied by suppression of maternal viremia.[112]

Use of antiretroviral regimens for perinatal prophylaxis that may not be completely suppressive (e.g., zidovudine [ZDV] or nevirapine monotherapy) may result in the development of resistance mutations and possibly increase the risk for perinatal transmission or progression in infected infants. Perinatal transmission of HIV with mutations associated with ZDV resistance have been described.[113] A study from the Women and Infants Transmission Study (WITS) of women who received ZDV during pregnancy found that 25% (34/142) of maternal isolates had at least one ZDV-associated resistance mutation; a lower CD4+ count and higher HIV-1 viral load were associated with having a ZDV resistance mutation at delivery. In multivariate analyses, the presence of any ZDV mutations was associated independently with perinatal transmission.[114] Others studies have not found a correlation between maternal ZDV resistance and perinatal transmission.[115,116] The association of other resistance mutations (e.g., to non-nucleoside reverse transcriptase inhibitors) with perinatal transmission is still unclear. The decision whether to obtain HIV resistance testing during pregnancy is controversial and must be individualized based on the woman's risk for having acquired or developed HIV mutations.

Many reports have correlated perinatal transmission to virologic factors, including p24 antigenemia,[89,108] syncytium-inducing versus non–syncytium-inducing phenotype,[89] and persistently positive HIV-1 cultures.[107] Although production of autologous neutralizing antibody seems to be protective, with low levels associated with increased transmission, more recent studies have reported conflicting results.[90] MacDonald and associates[117] found that maternal-child major histocompatibility complex discordance was associated with decreased perinatal transmission of HIV.

Vitamin A deficiency in pregnant HIV-infected women has been associated with increased vaginal HIV-1 shedding[118] and increased perinatal transmission in nonindustrialized countries.[119] In a cohort of HIV-infected women in Malawi, low maternal levels of vitamin A during pregnancy were common; in a multivariate logistic regression analysis, vitamin A deficiency was an independent predictor of perinatal transmission.[119] Vitamin A helps promote epithelial cell regeneration, and low vitamin A levels may be associated with mucosal breaks and increased HIV shedding into genital secretions.[90,120] Vitamin A deficiency also is associated with impaired immunity and increased susceptibility to infection. Given the possibility of teratogenicity of vitamin A when administered early in gestation,[121] and the finding that few pregnant women in the United States have vitamin A deficiency, vitamin A supplementation beyond that present in prenatal vitamins is not recommended at present. Many of the world's pregnant women may be at risk for vitamin A deficiency, however, and may benefit from supplementation.

Viral biologic phenotypes may influence transmission. Monocyte-macrophage–tropic or non–syncytium-inducing viral isolates may be more likely to be transmitted than maternal T cell–tropic or syncytium-inducing isolates.[90] Isolates obtained from infected infants tend to be of non–syncytium-inducing phenotype,[122] and neonatal macrophages preferentially are infected by non–syncytium-inducing monocyte-macrophage–tropic viral isolates.[90,123]

HIV-1 can be classified into at least nine different genotypes (clades) based on differences in the envelope region of the viral genome.[90] The distribution of subtypes differs around the world: Subtype B predominates in the United States and Europe; subtypes A, C, and D predominate in Africa; and subtypes B and E predominate in Thailand.[90] The role of subtypes in perinatal transmission is as yet undefined, but some epidemiologic studies have suggested that subtype E may be transmitted sexually more efficiently than subtype B, perhaps accounting for at least some of the differences in transmission rates seen between countries.[90,124]

Sociodemographic and lifestyle factors also seem to influence the risk of perinatal transmission. Maternal drug and tobacco use, especially after the first trimester, may modify the risk of perinatal HIV-1 transmission.[121,125] Several studies have suggested that the rate of perinatal transmission is increased with a higher frequency of unprotected vaginal intercourse after the first trimester of pregnancy even after controlling for maternal CD4+ counts, ZDV use, and higher frequency of STDs diagnosed during pregnancy.[121,125,126]

Obstetric factors also are thought to be associated with increased perinatal HIV-1 transmission. These include chorioamnionitis; placenta previa; preterm delivery; and invasive interventions, such as scalp monitoring, chorionic villus sampling, amniocentesis, cord blood sampling, and placental biopsy.[127,128]

Several studies done before combination antiretroviral therapy and viral load testing became a routine part of clinical practice consistently showed that elective cesarean delivery performed before the onset of labor and rupture of membranes significantly reduces the risk of perinatal transmission of HIV-1 by 55% to 80%.[100] The protective benefit of elective cesarean section was shown in two studies: (1) a large meta-analysis of 15 prospective North American and European cohort studies consisting of 8533 mother-child pairs[129] and (2) a prospective randomized clinical trial of elective cesarean section versus vaginal delivery among 370 mother-child pairs.[130] In the meta-analysis, after adjustment for receipt of antiretroviral therapy, maternal stage of disease, and infant birth weight, an elective cesarean section decreased the risk of perinatal transmission of HIV-1 by 50% (adjusted odds ratio 0.43; 95% confidence interval 0.33% to 0.56%).[129] The transmission rate in the randomized prospective clinical trial within the cesarean section arm was only 1.8% (3 of 170 infants) compared with 10.5% (21 of 200 infants) in the vaginal delivery arm.[130] Although the data clearly show a protective benefit of elective cesarean section, these studies were performed in populations not receiving HAART with protease inhibitors or non-nucleoside reverse transcriptase inhibitors and in which patients did not have HIV viral loads monitored.

The degree of protective efficacy that cesarean section offers to patients on HAART or with undetectable plasma viral loads is unknown. Among 366 women in four studies, there has been only 1 documented case of HIV transmission among women on antiretroviral medications with viral loads less than or equal to 500 copies/mL late in pregnancy.[100] Scheduled cesarean section is unlikely to reduce this low transmission rate further among treated women with undetectable viral loads, and it would not prevent in utero transmssion.[100] For HIV-positive women, cesarean section may be associated with increased risk of infection and other postoperative morbidity, especially in women with advanced HIV disease.[131] The morbidity from cesarean section was low in the prospective randomized trial, but postpartum fever was significantly more frequent in the women who delivered by elective cesarean section versus vaginal delivery (6.7% versus 1.1%, $P = .002$).[130] Current national guidelines recommend that women with HIV-1 RNA levels greater than 1000 copies/mL be counseled regarding the benefit of scheduled cesarean delivery in reducing the risk of perinatal transmission. Women should be informed of the risks associated with cesarean delivery, and these risks to the mother should be balanced with potential benefits expected for the neonate. Women should be counseled about the limitations of the current data, and the woman's informed decision about mode of delivery should be respected and honored.[100]

HIV transmission through breast milk is supported by detection of HIV-1 in the cellular and acellular compartments of breast milk and reports of transmission from mothers infected with HIV-1 during the postnatal period.[89,132-135] A study in Rwanda found that 36% to 60% of breast-fed infants born to postnatally infected women became infected with HIV and that seroconversion in infant and mother occurred during the same 3-month period.[133] These infants presumably were exposed to high viral titers, and no maternal HIV-1-specific humoral or cellular immune response was detected. A meta-analysis of studies published before 1992 suggested an attributable risk of transmission through breast milk by women who were infected before pregnancy of 14% and by postnatally infected women of 26%.[133,136] Breast-feeding now is thought to play a significant role in perinatal HIV transmission, and in many international settings, transmission of HIV during lactation accounts for one third to one half of all HIV transmission from mothers to infants.[137]

Transmission of HIV via breast-feeding can occur throughout lactation. A study quantified breast milk HIV-1 RNA levels in serial samples collected from 275 women for 2 years after delivery.[138] Higher maternal plasma virus load, lower maternal CD4$^+$ T-cell count, and detection of HIV-1 DNA in maternal genital secretions were significantly associated with elevated breast milk HIV-1 RNA. The median viral load in colostrum/early milk was significantly higher than that in mature breast milk collected 14 days after delivery. Breast-feeding mothers who transmitted HIV-1 to their infants had significantly higher breast milk viral RNA throughout lactation and more consistent viral shedding compared with mothers who did not transmit HIV-1.[138] They found a 2-fold increased risk of transmission was associated with every 10-fold increase in breast milk virus load. The risk of transmission is highest early after delivery when HIV levels in breast milk are highest, and increased duration of breast-feeding increases risk.[138,139] In areas of the world where adequate sanitary replacement feeding is not available, the decision to withhold breast-feeding so as to decrease HIV transmission may lead to increased rates of child morbidity and mortality from diarrheal and respiratory diseases and malnutrition.[140] Ideally, women should be counseled about the risks of breast-feeding transmission of HIV, the risks of morbidity and mortality among non-breastfed infants, and the availability of adequate formula feeding. Women in the United States and other areas where access to nutritionally adequate formula feeding can be ensured should be counseled not to breastfeed their infants.[100]

A variety of factors may increase the risk of perinatal transmission of HIV. Some of these factors may be amenable to modification, such as lowering viral load with antiretroviral agents or limiting the amount of time the infant is exposed to the genital secretions of the infected mother by delivery by cesarean section, shortening the labor process, decreasing the exposure to ruptured membranes, or limiting invasive procedures such as scalp monitoring.[128] Promotion of safer sexual practices, including condom use and limiting sexual partners, and abstaining from drug, tobacco, and alcohol use also may reduce the risk of perinatal transmission.

Impact of Pregnancy on Human Immunodeficiency Virus Infection

Although pregnancy and HIV infection are immunosuppressive conditions, large studies in the United States and Europe have failed to show that pregnancy accelerates HIV replication or disease progression.[141-144] Data from developing countries suggest that there may be a progression of HIV disease in pregnancy under certain conditions.[145] Differences in the impact of pregnancy on HIV infection across geographic areas may reflect differences in potential confounding issues, such as poverty and nutrition, greater likelihood of advanced HIV disease at the time of pregnancy, and the impact of additional infectious diseases.[96] Pregnancy does not seem to result in acceleration of HIV disease in most HIV-infected women; however, women with more advanced disease tend to experience disease progression over a shorter period than that typical of women with less advanced disease, suggesting that the pregnancy may enhance progression of HIV disease in such cases.[146]

Conflicting data exist regarding the effects of HIV infection and pregnancy on T-cell function and phenotype.[146] Cellular immunity and CD4$^+$ lymphocyte levels are expected to decline during pregnancy but eventually return to baseline.[96,146] In HIV-positive and HIV-negative pregnant women, the number of CD4$^+$ cells decreases, reaching their lowest levels in the third trimester, whereas the CD4$^+$ percentage remains relatively stable.[147] CD4$^+$ percentage, rather than absolute number, may be a more accurate measure of immune function in HIV-infected pregnant women. It is still unclear whether these CD4$^+$ declines are due to the HIV infection, to pregnancy, or to hemodilution. HIV viral loads remain relatively stable throughout pregnancy in the absence of treatment.[148] Determination of whether immunologic changes in HIV-positive women result in progression of HIV disease during pregnancy requires additional prospective, longitudinal studies.

Impact of Human Immunodeficiency Virus Infection on Pregnancy Outcome

Maternal HIV infection has not been associated with fetal anomalies, premature delivery, low birth weight, or specific pregnancy-related abnormalities in studies from industrialized countries.[96,146,149] A dysmorphic syndrome associated with HIV infection first was reported in 1986. The clinical features included growth retardation, microcephaly, flattened nasal bridge, prominent forehead, obliquely placed eyes, and patulous lips.[150,151] Subsequent reports have not found an association between congenital anomalies and HIV serostatus, however.[152,153] The original observations now are thought to be due to confounding variables, such as drug and alcohol use. Because infection with HIV early in pregnancy appears to be uncommon, embryopathy does not seem to be a major problem in pregnancies in women with HIV infection. Reports from various developing areas have noted an increased incidence of preterm deliveries and low-birth-weight infants.[96,154] HIV infection does not seem to be a cause of spontaneous abortion; however, most published reports suggest a trend in that direction. In a large study from Malawi that tested 6605 consecutive women for HIV, HIV-seropositive women were more likely than HIV-seronegative women to have reported a history of spontaneous abortion (15% versus 7%).[155] Additional studies with adequate numbers of women are needed to elucidate more fully the impact of HIV infection on pregnancy outcome.

Use of Antiretroviral Drugs in Pregnancy for Maternal Health and to Reduce Perinatal Transmission

Advances in antiretroviral therapy have reduced the risk of perinatal HIV transmission greatly. Studies have shown that the most important determinant of perinatal HIV transmission is maternal viral load. If the viral load is less than 1000 copies/mL in pregnancy, the HIV perinatal transmission rate is estimated to be 2% or less. Among women with a viral load less than 1000 copies/mL, antiretroviral therapy provides additional protection (1% perinatal transmission risk among women on treatment and 10% transmission among women on no antiretroviral therapy) (see earlier section).

The goals of antiretroviral therapy in pregnancy are to optimize maternal health, to provide maximal suppression of the viral load, to prevent perinatal HIV transmission, and to avoid potential maternal or fetal toxicity. This section reviews data on use of antiretroviral medications in pregnancy and the current guidelines for antiretroviral chemoprophylaxis to reduce perinatal HIV-1 transmission. The subsequent section addresses use of antiretroviral medications in pregnancy and the optimal management of pregnant HIV-infected women.

Use of Antiretroviral Drugs in Pregnancy to Reduce Perinatal Transmission

Zidovudine. Numerous studies are currently under way, in the United States and globally, to evaluate the use of antiretroviral agents to reduce perinatal transmission. ZDV was the first such agent studied, and in February 1994, the landmark study AIDS Clinical Trials Group Protocol 076 (ACTG 076) showed that ZDV given to pregnant women after the first trimester and during labor and to newborns during their first 6 weeks could reduce perinatal transmission by 67.5%.[111,156] Women with CD4$^+$ cell counts greater than 200/mm^3 were assigned randomly to a ZDV treatment group or to a control group in which placebo was given. The women in the treatment group received 100 mg of ZDV five times a day starting between 14 and 34 weeks of gestation and continued throughout pregnancy, followed by intrapartum ZDV (given as an intravenous loading dose of 2 mg/kg over 1 hour during labor, then a continuous intravenous infusion of 1 mg/kg/hr until delivery), with oral administration of ZDV to the infant (syrup 2 mg/kg every 6 hours) for 6 weeks. The rate of perinatal transmission was reduced to 8.3% in the 205 women who received ZDV, from a rate of 25.5% in the 204 women who received no antiretroviral therapy ($P =$ .00006).[156] In August 1994, the U.S. Public Health Service Task Force issued recommendations for the use of ZDV for reduction of perinatal HIV-1 transmission,[157] followed in July 1995 by recommendations for universal prenatal HIV-1 counseling and HIV-1 testing with informed consent for all pregnant women in the United States.[158] Subsequent epidemiologic studies in the United States and France showed successful use of the ACTG 076 ZDV regimen in the "real" world to achieve dramatic reductions in perinatal transmission rates.[159-161]

The ZDV regimen chosen for ACTG 076 was well tolerated, and there were no significant differences in adverse events between the women receiving ZDV and women receiving placebo. The only evidence of toxicity observed more frequently in the treatment group was a lower hemoglobin concentration in neonates, which was not clinically significant; hemoglobin levels returned to levels measured in infants born to mothers in the placebo group by week 12 postpartum. Prolonged exposure of adult rodents to high doses of ZDV has been associated with the development of noninvasive squamous epithelial vaginal tumors in 3% to 12% of females.[100] In humans, ZDV is extensively metabolized, and most of the drug excreted in urine is in the glucuronide form. In mice, however, ZDV excreted in the urine is mostly unmetabolized. The vaginal tumors are thought to form as a result of chronic exposure of the vaginal epithelium of rodents to unmetabolized ZDV, resulting from reflux of urine containing high concentrations of ZDV into the vaginal vault. This hypothesis was tested by administering 5 mg or 20 mg of ZDV per mL of saline into the vaginas of female mice; vaginal squamous cell carcinomas were documented at the higher concentration.[100] A National Institutes of Health panel reviewed the data on ZDV toxicity in 1997 and concluded that the proven benefit of ZDV in reducing the risk for perinatal transmission outweighs the hypothetical concerns of carcinogenesis raised in the rodent studies.[162] No ZDV-associated tumors have been reported to date in studies of nearly 1000 children exposed to ZDV over an average follow-up period of 3 years.[162] Similar rates of congenital abnormalities occurred among infants in ACTG 076 with and without in utero ZDV exposure. Data from the Antiretroviral Pregnancy Registry also have not shown an increased risk for congenital abnormalities among infants born to mothers who receive ZDV during pregnancy compared with the general population.[100] Because little is known about the long-term effects of antiretroviral medication, all exposed children, regardless of HIV serostatus, should receive careful long-term follow-up evaluation.[163]

A more recent study evaluated the long-term postpartum clinical, immune, and viral parameters between women enrolled to receive ZDV versus placebo in ACTG 076.[164] Of 474 eligible women, 226 (48%) enrolled in the study (mean follow-up of 4.1 years). There were no significant differences in HIV progression, time to AIDS or death, or CD4+ count or HIV viral load levels. Genotypic ZDV resistance also did not differ between groups, and mutations were seen in 10% of 156 women (9% of ZDV group women and 11% of placebo group women).[164] The mechanism by which ZDV reduces perinatal transmission is undefined. The effect of ZDV on maternal HIV viral load is insufficient to explain fully its efficacy, especially when it is given to pregnant women with extensive prior ZDV experience.[111,165] Pre-exposure prophylaxis of the fetus or infant may be important, and ZDV may be unique because, in contrast to didanosine or zalcitabine, it is metabolized to the active triphosphate form within the placenta. The efficacy of ZDV chemoprophylaxis was evaluated in pregnant women with more advanced HIV disease than that which affected the women in ACTG 076 (i.e., ACTG 185), 23% of whom had received ZDV previously. All women received the same three-part ZDV regimen

as outlined previously, combined with infusions of either hyperimmune HIV-1 immunoglobulin containing high levels of HIV-1 antibodies or standard intravenous immune globulin. The study was stopped prematurely when women in the treatment and the placebo groups were found to have similar low rates of perinatal transmission of 4.8%.[100]

The use of ZDV in accordance with the ACTG 076 regimen by HIV-infected pregnant women in the United States and Europe has resulted in marked declines in perinatal transmission rates, typically to 3% to 4%. Because of the complexity of the regimen and the cost of the drug, ZDV has not been used in most resource-poor countries where most perinatal HIV-1 infection is occurring. Results from a study in Thailand indicate that a short-term antenatal regimen of ZDV can reduce the risk for perinatal HIV transmission by approximately 50%.[166,167] HIV-infected women were assigned randomly to receive either 300 mg of ZDV twice a day from 36 weeks of gestation until onset of labor, plus 300 mg every 3 hours from onset of labor until delivery, or a placebo. All women were given a supply of infant formula and counseled against breast-feeding, consistent with national guidelines for HIV-infected women in Thailand. Of 392 infants born, 55 tested HIV-positive on polymerase chain reaction assay (18 in the ZDV group and 37 in the placebo group), all by the second-month visit. The HIV transmission rate was 9.4% (95% confidence interval 5.2% to 13.5%) in the ZDV group compared with 18.9% (95% confidence interval 13% to 24%) in the placebo group.[166] Data from New York State indicated that the rate of perinatal HIV transmission among 939 HIV-exposed infants varied depending on when ZDV prophylaxis was begun. When treatment was begun prenatally, the rate of HIV transmission was 6.1% (95% confidence interval 4.1% to 8.9%); when treatment was begun intrapartum, the rate was 10% (95% confidence interval 3.3% to 21.8%); when treatment was begun within 48 hours of life, the rate was 9.3% (95% confidence interval 4.1% to 17.5%); and when treatment was begun on day 3 of life or later, the rate was 18.4% (95% confidence interval 7.7% to 34.3%).[168] Without ZDV prophylaxis, the rate of HIV transmission was 26.6% (95% confidence interval 21.1% to 32.7%).[168] Because it is not known precisely when ZDV confers efficacy, and because of theoretical benefits of ZDV administration during any of the three time periods, administration of partial ZDV regimens is preferred over no administration.

Concerns have been raised that ZDV use during pregnancy and delivery may be ineffective if the mothers have developed ZDV resistance. Although none of the women participating in ACTG 076 had high-level genotypic resistance to ZDV, low-level resistance was not associated with an increase in perinatal transmission, after adjusting for HIV RNA levels.[115] Frenkel and colleagues[169] studied the HIV-1 viral isolates from 16 pregnant women who received ZDV and found 2 of 16 to be highly resistant to ZDV, with mutations at codons 41 and 215. Two additional isolates had mutations at codon 70 (one susceptible and one moderately resistant to ZDV). One of the women with a highly resistant strain transmitted HIV to her infant, and the infant's isolate was also highly resistant to ZDV.[169] Development of alternative antiretroviral strategies may mitigate these concerns.

ZDV monotherapy in pregnant women has been the minimal standard of care since the release of results from ACTG 076 in 1994. Several additional studies suggest that use of combination antiretroviral regimens during pregnancy may reduce transmission further. In an open-label, nonrandomized study in France, lamivudine was added at 32 weeks' gestation to standard ZDV prophylaxis; lamivudine also was given to the infant in addition to ZDV for 6 weeks.[100,170] The transmission rate in the ZDV-lamivudine group was 1.6% compared with 6.8% in the historical control group. In a longitudinal prospective study conducted in the United States started in 1990, after 10 years, HIV transmission rates were 20% in women on no antiretroviral treatment during pregnancy, 10.4% in women who received ZDV alone, 3.8% in women on combination therapy without protease inhibitors, and 1.2% in women who received combination therapy with protease inhibitors.[171]

An African trial (PETRA) assessed the efficacy of three short-course regimens of ZDV and lamivudine in preventing early and late transmission of HIV-1 among breast-feeding, HIV-1-infected women. The investigators found that combination therapy with ZDV and lamivudine administered starting at 36 weeks' gestation, orally intrapartum, and for 1 week postpartum to mother and infant reduced transmission at 6 weeks from 15.3% in the placebo group to 5.7%.[100,172] Starting ZDV/lamivudine intrapartum and continuing it for 1 week postpartum in the mother and infant reduced transmission at 6 weeks to 8.9% compared with 15.3 % in the placebo group. In this trial, giving ZDV/lamivudine only during the intrapartum period was not effective in lowering HIV transmission.[100,172]

Another study in Uganda (HIVNET 012) showed that a single 200-mg oral dose of nevirapine given to the mother at onset of labor combined with a single oral dose of 2 mg/kg given to the infant at age 48 to 72 hours reduced transmission among breast-feeding mothers by 47% compared with a short course of ZDV given orally during labor and to the infant for 1 week up to age 14 to 16 weeks.[173] A South African study compared a short course of nevirapine (one dose in labor and a second dose 48 hours postpartum to the mother, and a single dose to the infant at age 48 hours) with oral ZDV/lamivudine in labor and for 1 week after delivery to the mother and infant.[100,174] The overall estimated HIV-1 infection rates in 1307 infants by 8 weeks were 12.3% (95% confidence interval 9.7% to 15%) for nevirapine and 9.3% (95% confidence interval 7% to 11.6%) for ZDV/lamivudine ($P = .11$).[174]

A study in the United States, Europe, Brazil, and the Bahamas (ACTG 316) evaluated whether adding a two-dose intrapartum/newborn nevirapine regimen (HIVNET 012 regimen) to non–breast-feeding women on standard antiretroviral therapy (including the full three-part ZDV regimen) would reduce HIV transmission rates further.[175] Transmission was not significantly different between women receiving antiretroviral therapy only (77% were combination regimen), 1.6% (10/617 births), versus women receiving additional nevirapine, 1.4% (9/631 births). The risk of perinatal HIV transmission is low among women who receive prenatal care, antenatal antiretroviral therapy, and access to elective cesarean section; no benefit from additional intrapartum/newborn nevirapine was shown in this population.

Combination antiretroviral regimens are far superior to ZDV monotherapy in reducing HIV viral load and in prolonging survival.[10,11] In mid-1997, two different panels convened by the U.S. Department of Health and Human Services, the National Institutes of Health, and the International AIDS Society issued draft principles and guidelines on the use of antiretroviral agents in HIV-infected adults.[176,177] Although there are no controlled clinical trials showing safety or efficacy of most antiretrovirals during pregnancy, both panels recommended that antiretroviral therapy in pregnant women generally should be the same as for nonpregnant adults, unless clear fetal or maternal contraindications exist.

The CDC revise their recommendations for the use of antiretroviral drugs in pregnant women infected with HIV-1 on an ongoing basis, and the recommendations are fully accessible online at http://aidsinfo.nih.gov/guidelines/.[100] The CDC has concluded that pregnancy is not a reason to defer standard therapy and outlines unique considerations for combination therapy use, including the potential need to alter dosing as a result of physiologic changes associated with pregnancy, the potential for adverse short-term or long-term effects on the fetus and newborn, and efficacy in reducing the risk of perinatal transmission. Women who are offered antiretroviral medication during pregnancy should be informed about the known and unknown short-term and long-term benefits and risks of therapy for infected women and their infants. The current pharmacokinetic and safety data for the different antiretroviral agents are listed in Table 122-3.

Nucleoside and Nucleotide Reverse Transcriptase Inhibitors. Of the seven currently approved nucleoside reverse transcriptase inhibitors, ZDV, lamivudine, didanosine, and stavudine have been evaluated in clinical trials in pregnant women.[100,178,179] Zalcitabine, abacavir, and emtricitabine have not been studied in pregnant women. ZDV is well tolerated and does not require dose modification for use in pregnant women. The pharmacokinetics of lamivudine do not seem to be altered by pregnancy, and no dose modification is indicated except in

young children, in whom the dose is decreased because of the reduced clearance of lamivudine in infants 1 week old. Although a study of 12 pregnant women found the clearance of intravenous and oral didanosine given antepartum was greater than that observed at 6 weeks postpartum, no dose modifications currently are recommended.[178] A phase I/II safety and pharmacokinetic study of combination stavudine and lamivudine in pregnant HIV-infected women and their infants was conducted (PACTG 332); both drugs were well tolerated, with pharmacokinetics similar to those in nonpregnant adults.[180] Cases of lactic acidosis, in some cases fatal, have been described in pregnant women receiving didanosine/stavudine along with other antiretroviral agents. The U.S. Food and Drug Administration (FDA) and Bristol Myers Squibb have issued a warning to health care professionals that pregnant women may be at increased risk of fatal lactic acidosis when prescribed didanosine and stavudine concomitantly. The combination of these two drugs should be prescribed for pregnant women only when the potential benefit clearly outweighs the potential risk.[179]

All of the nucleoside analogue antiretroviral drugs are classified by the FDA as FDA pregnancy category C agents except for didanosine and emtricitabine, which are classified as FDA pregnancy category B drugs.[100] Although most of the nucleoside analogues are thought to cross the placenta in primates, didanosine and zalcitabine undergo less placental transfer than is noted for ZDV, stavudine, and lamivudine.[100] Emtricitabine has not been studied in pregnant women. According to a report from the Antiretroviral Pregnancy Registry, there were no increases in birth defects associated with use of ZDV, lamivudine, or stavudine in pregnancy.[179]

Tenofovir disoproxil fumarate, the first nucleotide analogue reverse transcriptase inhibitor, is classified as an FDA pregnancy category B drug. There are no data on whether tenofovir crosses the placenta or is excreted in breast milk in humans. Tenofovir has not yet been studied prospectively in pregnant women or neonates.

Use of Nucleoside Analogue Drugs and Mitochondrial Toxicity. The major toxicity of the nucleoside reverse transcriptase inhibitor class is related to effects on mitochondrial DNA synthesis; these drugs have varying affinity for mitochondrial gamma DNA polymerase, resulting in depletion and dysfunction of mitochondrial DNA. Clinical disorders linked to mitochondrial toxicity may be subtle (mild peripheral neuropathy or myopathy) or fulminant (hepatic steatosis, lactic acidosis, and liver failure). The relative potency of the nucleosides in inhibiting mitochondrial gamma DNA polymerase in vitro is highest for zalcitabine, followed by didanosine, stavudine, lamivudine, ZDV, and abacavir.[179] These toxicities may be of particular concern for pregnant women and for infants with in utero exposure to nucleoside analogue drugs. It is unclear whether mitochondrial toxicity and lactic acidosis/hepatic steatosis syndromes are more common in pregnancy. Their clinical presentation can mimic some of the adverse effects of pregnancy, such as nausea, vomiting, and malaise. Abacavir can cause a rare, but potentially fatal, hypersensitivity reaction. Patients who start abacavir must be counseled thoroughly about symptoms of hypersensitivity, and patients who stop abacavir because of suspected hypersensitivity should never be rechallenged with this drug. Providers who manage women with HIV during pregnancy should be alert to the early diagnosis of these potentially fatal syndromes.

Non-nucleoside Reverse Transcriptase Inhibitors. The safety and pharmacokinetics of nevirapine, a non-nucleoside reverse transcriptase inhibitor, were studied in HIV-1-infected pregnant women, who received a single 200-mg oral dose at the onset of labor and whose newborns received a single dose of 2 mg/kg at 2 to 3 days of age.[100] The drug was well tolerated by mothers and infants with prolonged half-life and elimination in both populations. Pharmacokinetic parameters in pregnant women receiving intrapartum nevirapine were similar, although more variable than in nonpregnant adults. This single dose of nevirapine was sufficient to maintain levels associated with antiviral activity for the first week of life.[100]

Nevirapine pharmacokinetics also were studied in HIV-infected pregnant women beginning long-term therapy late in the third

TABLE 122-3   Preclinical and Clinical Data Relevant to Use of Antiretrovirals in Pregnancy

Antiretroviral Drug	FDA Category[*]	Placental Passage (newborn:maternal drug ratio)	Long-Term Animal Carcinogenicity Studies	Rodent Teratogenicity
Nucleoside and Nucleotide Analogue RTIs				
Abacavir	C	Yes, in rats	Not completed	Positive (rodent, anasarca and skeletal malformations at high dose; not seen in rabbits)
Didanosine (ddI)	B	Yes, in humans (0.5)	Negative (no tumors, lifetime rodent study)	Negative
Emtricitabine (FTC)	B	Unknown	Not completed	Negative
Lamivudine (3TC)	C	Yes, in humans (~1.0)	Negative (no tumors, lifetime rodent study)	Negative
Stavudine (d4T)	C	Yes, in rhesus monkeys (0.76)	Not completed	Negative (decreased sternal bone calcium in rodents)
Tenofovir DF (TDF)	B	Yes, in rats and monkeys	Not completed	Negative (osteomalacia when given to juvenile animals at high doses)
Zalcitabine (ddC)	C	Yes, in rhesus monkeys (0.30-0.50)	Positive (rodent, thymic lymphomas)	Positive (rodent, hydrocephalus at high dose)
Zidovudine (ZDV, AZT)	C	Yes, in humans (0.85)	Positive (rodent, noninvasive vaginal epithelial/gynecologic tumors)	Positive (rodent, near lethal dose)
Non-nucleoside Analogue RTIs				
Delavirdine	C	Unknown	Not completed	Positive (rodent, ventral septal defect)
Efavirenz	C	Yes, in cynomolgus monkeys, rats, rabbits (~1.0)	Not completed	Positive (anencephaly, anophthalmia, microphthalmia in monkeys)
Nevirapine	C	Yes, in humans (~1.0)	Not completed	Negative
Protease Inhibitors				
Amprenavir	C	Unknown	Not completed	Negative (deficient ossification of bones, thymic elongation in rats and rabbits)
Atazanavir	B	Unknown	Not completed	Negative
Fosamprenavir	C	Unknown	Positive (increased benign and malignant liver tumors in male rodents)	Negative (deficient ossification with amprenavir but not fosamprenavir)
Indinavir	C	Minimal (human)	Not completed	Negative (extra ribs in rodents)
Lopinavir-Ritonavir	C	Unknown	Not completed	Negative (delayed skeletal ossification and increase in skeletal variations in rats at maternally toxic doses)
Nelfinavir	B	Minimal (human)	Not completed	Negative
Ritonavir	B	Minimal (human)	Positive (rodent, liver tumors)	Negative (cryptorchidism in rodents)
Saquinavir	B	Minimal (human)	Not completed	Negative
Fusion Inhibitors				
Enfuvirtide	B	Unknown	Not completed	Negative

[*]FDA Pregnancy categories are as follows:

A—Adequate and well-controlled studies of pregnant women fail to demonstrate a risk to the fetus during the first trimester of pregnancy (and there is no evidence of risk during later trimesters).

B—Animal reproduction studies fail to demonstrate a risk to the fetus and adequate but well-controlled studies of pregnant women have not been conducted.

C—Safety in human pregnancy has not been determined, animal studies either are positive for fetal risk or have not been conducted, and the drug should not be used unless the potential benefit outweighs the potential risk to the fetus.

D—Positive evidence of human fetal risk exists based on adverse reaction data from investigational or marketing experiences, but the potential benefits from the use of drug in pregnant women may be acceptable despite its potential risks.

X—Studies in animals or reports of adverse reactions have indicated that the risk associated with the use of the drug for pregnant women clearly outweighs any possible benefit.

RTIs, reverse transcriptase inhibitors.

Adapted from the U.S. Public Health Service Task Force. Recommendations for use of antiretroviral drugs in pregnant women infected with HIV-1 for maternal health and interventions to reduce perinatal HIV-1 transmission in the United States. Accessible online at http://www.aidsinfo.nih.gov/guidelines/ Updated November 26, 2003. Accessed June 3, 2004; and U. S. Public Health Service Task Force. Supplement: Safety and toxicity of individual antiretroviral agents in pregnancy. Updated March 23, 2004. Accessible online at: http://www.aidsinfo.nih.gov/guidelines/perinatal\st_032304.html.

trimester and their infants.[181] Initial-dose pharmacokinetics profiles in pregnant women were similar to the profiles seen in nonpregnant adults. Serum nevirapine concentrations declined to less than the target concentration by day 7 of life in 4 of 8 infants, suggesting that nevirapine elimination is accelerated in infants whose mothers received long-term nevirapine compared with newborns whose mothers received only a single intrapartum nevirapine dose.[179]

According to a report from the Antiretroviral Pregnancy Registry, there were no increases in birth defects associated with use of nevirapine in pregnancy.[179] Nevirapine resistance can be induced by a single mutation. Single-dose nevirapine for prevention of mother-to-child transmission (MTCT) selects for non-nucleoside RTI (NNRTI)-resistant mutations, with rates as high as 75% using composite (bulk) genotyping.[179a,179b] Nevirapine-resistance mutations were detected at 6

weeks postpartum in 19% of antiretroviral-naive women in HIVNET 012 and in 15% (14 of 95) of a subset of women particpating in ACTG 316 who received a single dose of nevirapine intrapartum. The most common mutation was K103N, which was present in 10 of the latter 14 women.[179,182] Nevirapine mutations were also detected in 11 out of 24 (46%) evaluable infants who were HIV infected by 6 to 8 weeks of age. The most common nevirapine-resistance mutation detected in infants was Y181C. These mutations faded from detection by 12 months of age in all seven evaluable infants. Of nine evaluable infants with late HIV-1 infection, only one had evidence of nevirapine resistance.[179,183] The implications of perinatal selection of NNRTI-resistant viruses by single-dose nevirapine prophylaxis for subsequent pregnancies have not been delineated. Prior selection of NNRTI-resistant virus in the setting of therapeutic use compromises the subsequent response to NNRTI-based regimens.[183a] This is demonstrable whether or not there is still circulating NNRTI-resistant virus when bulk sequencing techniques are used.[183a] It is not yet known whether archived NNRTI-resistant virus selected by short-course MTCT NNRTI-based regimens will also compromise the subsequent response to therapeutic use of NNRTI-based regimens, although preliminary data from Thailand suggest that this may be the case.[183b]

Severe, life-threatening, and in some cases fatal hepatotoxicity, including fulminant and cholestatic hepatitis, hepatic necrosis, and hepatic failure, has been reported in HIV-infected patients receiving nevirapine in combination with other drugs for treatment of HIV disease and in a small number of individuals receiving nevirapine as part of a combination regimen for postexposure prophylaxis of nosocomial or sexual HIV exposure.[179] Women with CD4 counts greater than 250 cells/mm[3] are at considerably higher risk of hepatotoxicities.[179,183c] In addition, severe, life-threatening hypersensitivity skin reactions, including Stevens-Johnson syndrome, have been reported in HIV-infected individuals receiving nevirapine for treatment. Patients should be monitored intensively during the first 18 weeks to detect potentially life-threatening hepatotoxicity or skin reactions.

Delavirdine and efavirenz have not been studied in phase I pharmacokinetic and safety trials in pregnant women. Of seven women who inadvertently became pregnant while on clinical trials of antiviral regimens containing delavirdine, three had ectopic pregnancies, three had healthy infants, and one woman delivered a premature infant with a muscular ventricular septal defect.[100] Delavirdine is known to be teratogenic in rodents when administered in high doses. Studies using efavirenz in pregnant monkeys at doses similar to those being studied in humans showed newborn abnormalities at birth. Three of 20 monkeys were born with birth defects, including one with a cleft palate, one with microphthalmia, and another with anencephaly and anophthalmia.[184] There has been a case report of myelomeningocele in a human infant born to a woman who was receiving efavirenz at the time of conception and during the first trimester.[185] Because of the potential for teratogenicity, pregnancy should be avoided in women receiving efavirenz.[179] Teratogenicity studies for delavirdine or nevirapine have not been conducted in primates.[179] These three FDA-approved non-nucleoside reverse transcriptase inhibitors are classified as FDA pregnancy category C agents.

Protease Inhibitors. No data are available regarding drug dosage, safety, and tolerance of any of the protease inhibitors in pregnant women or in neonates, although phase I studies of several of these agents—indinavir, ritonavir, nelfinavir, and saquinavir in combination with ZDV and lamivudine—in HIV-1-infected pregnant women and their infants are currently under way in the United States. Amprenavir, lopinavir/ritonavir, and atazanavir, three of the more recently approved protease inhibitors, have not yet been studied in pregnant women or infants. Preliminary data on combination therapy with indinavir (800 mg three times daily), saquinavir (1200 mg three times daily), and nelfinavir (750 mg three times daily) in pregnancy suggest that the plasma area under the curve of these protease inhibitors may be lower than observed in nonpregnant HIV-infected individuals.[179] Some preliminary data are available on placental passage in animals (see Table 122-3), but long-term animal carcinogenicity studies are not yet completed.

Indinavir and atazanavir have been associated with infrequent side effects (i.e., hyperbilirubinemia) that could be problematic for a newborn if transplacental passage occurs and the drug is administered near the time of delivery.[100] Neonates may have immature hepatic metabolic enzymes, which may result in prolonged drug half-life and possibly exacerbation of the physiologic hyperbilirubinemia observed in newborns. In addition, neonates may be at higher risk of renal stone formation secondary to crystallization of indinavir because of their immature renal function and inability to ensure adequate hydration voluntarily.[100]

Protease inhibitors have been associated with onset of diabetes, hyperglycemia, diabetic ketoacidosis, and exacerbation of existing diabetes mellitus.[186-188] Because pregnancy is a risk factor for hyperglycemia, and because it is unknown whether protease inhibitors would exacerbate the risk for pregnancy-associated hyperglycemia, HIV-1-infected pregnant women receiving these agents should be aware of the risk of hyperglycemia and taught to recognize the early manifestations of hyperglycemia to ensure prompt medical care if the signs and symptoms develop. Pregnant women on protease inhibitors should have glucose levels monitored closely. Ritonavir, nelfinavir, saquinavir, and atazanavir are classified as FDA pregnancy category B agents, and indinavir, amprenavir, and lopinavir/ritonavir are classified as pregnancy category C drugs.

Fusion Inhibitors. Enfuvirtide is the first antiretroviral drug in the fusion inhibitor class to be approved and is classified as an FDA pregnancy category B drug. It is a 36-amino acid peptide that inhibits binding or fusion of HIV to host target cells; enfuvirtide must be administered subcutaneously. Enfuvirtide was approved for use in HIV-infected adults and children 6 years old or older for use in combination with other antiretroviral drugs for the treatment of individuals with ongoing HIV replication despite ongoing therapy (salvage). No studies of enfuvirtide have been conducted in pregnant women or infants.[100]

Management of Pregnant Human Immunodeficiency Virus–Infected Women

With the improved clinical outlook of persons with HIV, increasingly HIV-infected women are interested in having children. In a national survey of HIV-infected persons in care in the United States, 28% to 29% desired children in the future, and among persons desiring children, 69% of women and 59% of men expected to have one or more children in the future.[189] Preconceptual counseling should include a thorough discussion of the woman's health, including HIV status, optimal treatment strategies for her health, and, if she were to become pregnant, strategies for preventing perinatal transmission and potential harm to her infant. If the potential father is HIV infected, his antiretroviral therapy also should be optimized. If the potential father is HIV negative, the safest approach to conception is to perform intravaginal or intrauterine inseminations during the periovulatory period. Couples comprising a woman who is HIV negative and a man who is HIV infected have limited options for conception without putting the woman at risk for HIV infection. (See earlier discussion of use of assisted reproductive technologies.)

An HIV-infected pregnant woman should be managed closely by her obstetrician and the HIV specialist caring for her when she is not pregnant.[190] A thorough history should be taken and physical examination done to document baseline findings and to allow for early detection of abnormalities. The history should identify any factors known to be associated with enhanced perinatal transmission, such as a history of STDs, drug and alcohol use, tobacco use, and high-risk sexual activity including lack of condom use, because altering these practices may reduce perinatal transmission risk without the use of pharmacologic agents. A complete physical examination including a pelvic examination can reveal concurrent conditions that may warrant therapy. The woman's HIV-1 disease status should be evaluated at presentation and at least every trimester with lymphocyte marker studies (i.e., CD4[+]/CD8[+] subsets) and viral load assessment. Ongoing routine obstetric care and decisions about initiating, continuing, or adjusting antiretroviral therapy should be the same as for non–HIV- infected women. Viral load testing also should be repeated 2 to 4 weeks after changing antiretroviral medications to provide feedback on the effectiveness of the antiretroviral regimen. The U.S. Public Health Service recommends that infected women in the United States refrain from breast-feeding to avoid postnatal transmission of HIV-1 to infants through breast milk.[158]

The woman should make decisions about antiretroviral medication in pregnancy after discussion with her health care provider about the known and unknown benefits and risks of therapy. Because the risk of teratogenicity is greatest during the first trimester, many health care providers advocate waiting until the end of the first trimester before starting new medications. The clinical, immunologic, and virologic status of the mother must be weighed against the potential effect on the fetus. An HIV-infected woman who is already receiving antiretroviral therapy and who discovers she is pregnant may choose either to continue her therapy or discontinue it temporarily until 14 weeks' gestation.[100] If therapy is discontinued, all drugs should be stopped appropriately and reintroduced simultaneously to avoid the development of antiretroviral drug resistance. Discontinuing antiretroviral medications may result in a rebound of viral load, however, which may have an impact on HIV transmission and the subsequent ability to obtain rapid virologic control.

Given the data on maternal viral load and perinatal HIV transmission, current guidelines recommend consideration of potent combination therapy (at least three drugs) for pregnant women with a viral load greater than 1000 copies/mL, regardless of CD4[+] count. Because ZDV is the only antiretroviral agent that has been shown to reduce perinatal transmission, independent of its effect on reducing maternal viral load, the addition of ZDV or substitution of ZDV for another nucleoside analogue antiretroviral is recommended after 14 weeks' gestation.[100] If a pregnant woman is on stavudine, the option of replacing stavudine with ZDV should be considered. Stavudine and ZDV are competitive antagonists and should not be given together. Women with a viral load less than 1000 copies/mL and a CD4[+] count in the normal range may consider the option of ZDV monotherapy because antiretroviral medication would be indicated primarily to prevent perinatal transmission.[100] Dual combination therapy (i.e., ZDV plus lamivudine) should be avoided because the combination is less likely to suppress HIV replication fully and may lead to development of lamivudine resistance, most commonly the M184V mutation. The combination of didanosine and stavudine should be avoided if possible because of rare case reports of fulminant hepatitis and lactic acidosis in late pregnancy among women on these drugs.[179] Efavirenz should be avoided in pregnancy, particularly in the first trimester, because of teratogenic effects in primate studies.

The standard ZDV dosing regimen for adults is 200 mg three times a day or 300 mg twice daily, but because the mechanism by which ZDV reduces perinatal transmission is unknown, the regimen of ZDV taken two or three times daily may not be equivalent to that observed in ACTG 076. Maternal adherence is expected to be enhanced, however, with this simpler regimen. ZDV administration is recommended for pregnant women during labor and for newborns regardless of the antepartum antiretroviral regimen.[100] Likewise, the 6-week neonatal ZDV component of the ZDV chemoprophylactic regimen should be initiated as soon as possible after delivery, preferably within 12 to 24 hours of birth, even if ZDV was not given during pregnancy or labor. Discussion of treatment options and recommendations should not be coercive, however, and the decision regarding whether to take antiretroviral drugs ultimately resides with the pregnant woman. Practitioners who provide health care for HIV-1-infected pregnant women and their newborns should report prospectively all cases of prenatal exposure to any antiretroviral medication (either alone or in combination) to the Antiretroviral Pregnancy Registry (Research Park, 1011 Ashes Drive, Wilmington, NC 28405; telephone: 1-800-258-4263; fax: 1-800-800-1052; Internet access: www.APRegistry.com).[100,179] Treatment and prophylaxis of opportunistic infections during pregnancy should follow guidelines similar to those for nonpregnant women.[191] Pregnant women who develop active opportunistic infections, including tuberculosis, should receive a drug regimen developed by obstetric and infectious diseases specialists. As with antiretroviral medications, the potential benefits of prophylactic agents must be weighed against their potential risks. Pneumococcal, hepatitis B, and inactivated influenza vaccines may be given if indicated during pregnancy. Live vaccines, such as rubella, measles, mumps, and varicella, are contraindicated during pregnancy and labor and in the early postpartum period.

Guidelines for the prevention of perinatal HIV transmission now include use of potent combination therapy, as clinically indicated, with inclusion of ZDV in the regimen when possible.[192] Information on management of HIV during pregnancy is changing rapidly. The reader is encouraged to obtain the most current information about HIV and women from up-to-date sources on the Internet. One of the best sources on HIV/AIDS is AIDS Info, a web-based service of the U.S. Department of Health and Human Services (www.aidsinfo.nih.gov/) that offers current information on research, clinical trials, and treatment for patients and health care providers. There are links to the most current guidelines for management of women during pregnancy[100] and for information on the safety and toxicity of antiretrovirals in pregnancy.[179] The U.S. government also has published *A Guide to the Clinical Care*

with Women with HIV/AIDS, 2001 First Edition, which is fully accessible online at http://hrsa.gov/publications/womencare.htm and available free of charge by mail.[147] Because optimal HIV care must be individualized and incorporate rapidly changing knowledge, consultation with an HIV/AIDS expert is strongly recommended.

CLINICAL MANIFESTATIONS AND NATURAL HISTORY OF HUMAN IMMUNODEFICIENCY VIRUS INFECTION IN WOMEN

In the beginning of the HIV epidemic, initial data on the natural history of HIV infection was derived from predominantly male cohorts. Subsequent data on the clinical manifestations of HIV infection in women suggested few sex differences in nongynecologic opportunistic processes and HIV disease progression. Women can present with gynecologic disease, however, that is influenced by their HIV-induced immune suppression.

Initial Manifestations and Human Immunodeficiency Virus–Related Symptoms

Recurrent vulvovaginal candidiasis (VVC) historically was a frequent presenting HIV-related symptom in women. In one study describing clinical manifestations among HIV-infected women, recurrent VVC occurred in 38% and was the most prevalent initial complaint.[193] Serious bacterial infections were another common initial diagnosis signaling HIV infection. In two early descriptive studies, 9% to 13% of women were diagnosed with at least one serious bacterial infection. The etiologic agent often was not identified, but *Streptococcus pneumoniae* and *Haemophilus influenzae* were implicated in most patients for whom culture results were known.[193,194] There have been conflicting data regarding whether or not HIV-infected women are at higher risk than men for serious bacterial infections,[195,196] but it is probable that an IDU history and degree of immune compromise are important risk factors.[196] Other HIV-related, nongynecologic signs and symptoms occurring in women that were described in the pre-HAART era were similar to those noted in men,[193-195] but at least one study found women were more likely to be diagnosed with oral candidiasis compared with men.[195]

In recent years, recognition of the association between HIV infection and abnormal Papanicolaou (Pap) smears has prompted HIV testing among women with squamous intraepithelial lesions (SIL) or cervical intraepithelial neoplasia (CIN). SIL or CIN is often the first HIV-related symptom today. Currently, many asymptomatic women also are diagnosed with HIV during prenatal screening.

Acquired Immunodeficiency Syndrome–Defining Opportunistic Processes

In 1993, the most frequent 1987 CDC AIDS-defining opportunistic processes[197] among men and women were *Pneumocystis jirovecii* (formerly *Pneumocystis carinii*) pneumonia, *Candida* esophagitis, and wasting syndrome. *Candida* esophagitis accounted for a larger proportion of the AIDS-defining events in women (19.6%) compared with events in heterosexual men (14.6%) or homosexual/bisexual men (12.3%).[198] Using the 1993 CDC data, multivariate analyses adjusted for race, age, and geographic region showed female injection drug users were more likely than heterosexual male injection drug users to be identified with *Candida* esophagitis, cytomegalovirus (CMV) disease, and herpes simplex virus (HSV) disease and less apt to be diagnosed with either Kaposi's sarcoma (KS) or extrapulmonary tuberculosis.[198]

Nongynecologic Malignancies

Among 1950 women (1554 HIV-infected, 391 non–HIV-infected) enrolled into the Women's Interagency HIV Study (WIHS), 45 incident cancers were diagnosed during the median follow-up of 5.04 years. In addition to cervical cancer, other malignancies that were significantly higher among HIV-infected women included KS (standardized incidence ratio 275.8), non-Hodgkin's lymphoma (standardized incidence ratio 27.4), and lung cancer (standardized incidence ratio 10.2). Cancers were more frequent before 1997 (or in the pre-HAART era).[199] The incidence of lung cancer also was increased among HIV-infected women in the HIV Epidemiology Research Study (HERS) cohort. HIV-infected women with lung cancer were typically young smokers (mean age 40 years) with stage IV adenocarcinoma. All died within 6 months of diagnosis.[200]

Although KS is an infrequent complication, there is evidence that this malignancy may have a different presentation in women than in men. In a review of 15 women with KS, the median CD4+ count was only 13/mm3, and the median crude survival time was 8.9 months compared with 23.3 months observed in men.[201] This evidence implies that women with KS may have a highly aggressive disease course. Women with KS also have been noted to have an increased incidence of noncutaneous disease, lymphedema, lymph node disease, and visceral disease.[202] A review of seven women with intrathoracic KS noted a median CD4+ count of 18/mm3 and a variety of radiographic findings, including nodular opacities, peribronchovascular opacities, thickened interlobular septa, pleural effusions, and lymphadenopathy.[203] Women also may have gynecologic involvement. There is at least one case report of KS presenting as a vulvar mass[204] and two cases of KS diagnosed by cervical biopsy.[205]

The review of incident malignancies occurring in the WIHS cohort did not find an excess of breast cancers among HIV-infected or non–HIV-infected women. Early data from the WIHS cohort on seven women showed unusual pathologic types of breast cancer and a relatively young median age (47 years).[206] A summary of subsequent case reports of women not enrolled into the WIHS showed that most women presented with a palpable breast mass and had not undergone mammography. Of the nine women whose ages were available, only one was older than 40. The remaining eight were between 23 and 38 years old. Eight of 10 women had metastatic disease at the time of diagnosis, and the available histopathology results uniformly described poorly differentiated or undifferentiated tumors.[207-212] There are no specific recommendations for mammogram screening of HIV-infected women, and these women should follow guidelines established for the general population.

Gynecologic Infections and Disease

Cervicovaginal Human Immunodeficiency Virus–1 RNA Shedding. Several studies have focused on the genital tract as a separate compartment, particularly because there is evidence that the genital tract may harbor different quasispecies of HIV.[213,214] Genital tract HIV RNA levels are associated with plasma HIV-1 RNA levels, CD4+ cell count, hormonal contraceptive use, pregnancy, cervical ectopy, various cervical or vaginal infections, and vitamin A deficiency.[215-224] HIV RNA suppression in the genital tract rapidly occurs after institution of HAART and is correlated strongly with plasma HIV-1 RNA levels.[222] Decreased cervicovaginal HIV shedding also is correlated with resolution of sexually transmitted infections[224] and treatment of *Trichomonas* vaginitis and VVC.[225] Phase of menstrual cycle and serum estradiol or progesterone levels are not associated with genital tract HIV RNA levels.[218,226]

Vaginal Infections

Bacterial Vaginosis. Bacterial vaginosis has been the most frequent vaginal infection in some U.S. cohorts of HIV-infected women, occurring in 35% to 47% of women.[227,228] Factors associated with bacterial vaginosis among U.S. HIV-infected women include alcohol use, smoking, and multiple sex partners.[227] HIV infection and induced immune suppression may modify the course of bacterial vaginosis. Bacterial vaginosis is more persistent among HIV-infected women compared with non–HIV-infected women, particularly women with lower CD4+ counts. Women with low CD4+ counts are more likely to have severe symptoms from bacterial vaginosis.[229] Although HIV-infected women may have more severe or persistent bacterial vaginosis infections, there are no unique treatment recommendations.

Vulvovaginal Candidiasis. Although one study has shown that recurrent VVC occurs early in the disease process (median CD4+ count 506/mm3),[230] this finding has not been substantiated in other studies. Other investigators have found that the frequency of VVC noticeably increases only when the CD4+ count decreases to less than 100 to 200/mm3.[231,232] The first description of VVC among HIV-infected women characterized this infection as frequent and chronic, often persistent, and poorly responsive to antifungal therapy.[233] More recent data have shown that although VVC may be more frequent among HIV-infected women, the symptoms are similar to those experienced by non–HIV-infected women.[234]

Limited data on the molecular epidemiology of mucosal candidiasis in HIV-infected women reveal that the dominant strains of *Candida* colonizing the oropharynx and vagina are different, suggesting that the development of disease in these body sites may be disassociated.[235] Although *Candida albicans* is the cause of greater than 95% of oropharyngeal candidiasis, it accounts for only 75% to 85% of the cases of VVC, and mixed fungal infections with two or more *Candida* spp. are more common in the oropharynx.[234]

Fluconazole at a dose of 200 mg weekly for the prevention of mucosal candidiasis among HIV-infected women has been shown to be safe and efficacious and did not precipitate resistance to vaginal *C. albicans* isolates.[236] In one study, this dose of fluconazole did reduce vaginal colonization with *C. albicans*, however, and non-*albicans* spp., particularly *Candida glabrata*, rapidly supervened.[237] There was a trend toward more in vitro azole resistance in *C. glabrata* isolates from women who received fluconazole.[238] For this reason, long-term azole prophylaxis should be considered only for women at high risk for developing recurrent symptomatic VVC. Recommendations for treatment currently are based on whether VVC is uncomplicated versus complicated (defined as recurrent VVC, severe VVC, non-*albicans* candidiasis, or having selected conditions including immune suppression).[239] Therapy for VVC in HIV-infected women should not differ from therapy for non–HIV-infected women (CDC), but prolonged (i.e., 7 to 14 days) courses of conventional antimycotic treatments may be necessary for women with severe VVC; very low CD4+ counts; or additional immunocompromising conditions, such as diabetes or receipt of corticosteroid treatment.

Trichomoniasis Vaginitis. Trichomoniasis vaginitis is one of the most common sexually transmitted infections (STIs) among HIV-infected and non–HIV-infected women. Proportions of HIV-infected women diagnosed with *Trichomonas* vaginitis have ranged from 6% to 27% in various U.S. cohorts.[193,194,227,240,241] Women with IDU[194,227,241] and women with more than two sexual partners[240] are at increased risk for *Trichomonas* vaginitis. Reinfection is common, occurs in 36% of HIV-infected women, and is associated with a history of another STI (relative risk 1.52, 95% confidence interval 1.08 to 2.14).[242] Becoming pregnant may be protective (relative risk 0.59, 95% confidence interval 0.39 to 0.87).[242] There is no evidence that the presentation or response to treatment is associated with either HIV infection or HIV-induced immune suppression. HIV-infected women should receive the same treatment as non–HIV-infected women.

Mucopurulent Cervicitis and Pelvic Inflammatory Disease. Positive cervical cultures and mucopurulent cervicitis due to *Neisseria gonorrhoeae* and *C. trachomatis* are relatively frequent among HIV-infected women, particularly adolescents. Four cohort U.S. studies found the proportions of HIV-infected women diagnosed with *N. gonorrhoeae* or *C. trachomatis* cervical infections were 4.2% to 12% and 0.8% to 7%.[193-195,227] *N. gonorrhoeae* was the most common STI in a cohort of 91 HIV-infected adolescent girls.[243]

Several studies performed in the United States or Africa compared the presentation and course of pelvic inflammatory disease (PID) between HIV-infected and non–HIV-infected women. Four studies[244-247] found HIV-infected women had a lower admission white blood cell count, and five studies[244,245,247-249] noted HIV-infected women were more likely to have tubo-ovarian abscesses or require surgical intervention. HIV-infected women were more likely to have persistent fevers refractory to antibiotics in one study[244] and higher temperatures and mean clinical severity scores in another study.[248] Barbosa and colleagues[246] noted HIV-infected women were more likely to remain febrile 48 hours after initiation of antimicrobial therapy. By day 5 or 6 of therapy, however, there was no statistically significant difference in the presence of fever.

The microbiology of PID in these studies is similar to that described in non–HIV-infected women with PID, although the frequency of *N. gonorrhoeae* and *C. trachomatis* may be lower among HIV-infected women.[245,250] One study showed *Mycoplasma* spp. and *Streptococcus* spp. were more likely to be isolated in endometrial biopsy specimens of HIV-infected women ($P <.05$).[247] Another study of Kenyan women with PID found the prevalence of bacterial vaginosis significantly higher among HIV-infected women with low CD4$^+$ counts,[250] and a South African study noted *Trichomonas* vaginitis infection of the lower genital tract was significantly associated with a clinical PID diagnosis in HIV-infected women ($P = .002$).[251]

Very rare causes of PID among HIV-infected women may include CMV and tuberculosis. There has been one report of a case of silent oophoritis due to CMV in a woman with advanced HIV disease found at autopsy.[252] In addition, there are a few reports of HIV-infected women with clinically diagnosed PID who failed to respond to conventional regimens but seemed to have benefited from ganciclovir therapy after CMV was found in genital secretions.[253] There is one report of a young African patient with isolated acute PID due to tuberculosis diagnosed by laparotomy and salingo-oophorectomy.[254]

Taken together, these studies suggest HIV infection may influence the morbidity of PID and possibly have some effect on the microbiology. There does not seem to be a difference, however, in response to therapy. HIV-infected women should receive conventional recommended antibiotic regimens.[239]

Human Papillomavirus Infections and Disease. HIV-infected women are two to three times more likely than non–HIV-infected women to have detectable levels of human papillomavirus (HPV) DNA in cervicovaginal specimens[255-260] and approximately five times as likely to have SIL, vulvovaginal condylomata acuminata, or anal intraepithelial neoplasia.[260-263] The prevalence of SIL among HIV-infected women is high and has been reported to range between approximately 12% and 40%.[193,194,264,265] Adolescent women are particularly prone to HPV infection and disease with high prevalence rates of HPV infection (77.4%)[266] and SIL (55%).[243]

Among HIV-infected women, HPV disease, as manifested by findings of SIL or CIN on cervical studies, is influenced by HIV-induced immune suppression. SIL and clinically evident HPV infections have been associated with a declining CD4$^+$ count.[194,265,267,268] In addition, women with high plasma HIV RNA levels are at increased risk for cervical HPV infection with high-risk types and cervical cytologic abnormalities.[265,269,270] Vitamin A may play a protective role. In one study, HIV-infected women with low serum retinol levels (<1.05 (mol/L) were more likely to have cervical SIL (multivariate odds ratio 1.75; $P = .02$) even after adjustment for HPV status, nutritional status, and HIV disease stage.[271]

Although most HIV-infected women with SIL present with low-grade lesions,[255,256,261] SIL has been reported to be more severe and extensive in HIV-infected women compared with non–HIV-infected women and can present as multifocal extensive cervical and lower genital tract lesions.[272] The increased incidence of HPV-related disease among HIV-infected women may be due to the high rate of persistent HPV infections, particularly among women with advanced immune suppression, with the oncogenic HPV types associated with the development of high-grade lesions and cervical cancer.[273,274]

The risk of cervical disease progression among HIV-infected women with either low-grade SIL or type 1 CIN is relatively low. Observational studies have shown about 14% to 22% of women have cervical disease progression annually,[275-278] and only 20.6% of HIV-infected women with low-grade cervical dysplasia experienced progression to high-grade SIL in a randomized, observation-controlled clinical trial evaluating treatment with isotretinoin (median follow-up was 65 weeks for subjects on oral isotretinoin and 49 weeks for subjects on observation, $n = 102$). The difference between the two arms was not significant.[279] In observational studies, progression of low-grade SIL has been associated with lower CD4$^+$ counts and presence of HPV types 16, 18, and 33.[278,280] Time to cervical disease progression was slightly associated with CD4$^+$ count in the randomized clinical trial, but the only significantly associated covariate was age. Subjects younger than 30 had a shortened time to progression than subjects older than 30, independent of treatment with isotretinoin ($P = .046$).[279]

The results from the one clinical trial and few observational studies suggest that observation without excisional therapy may be appropriate for HIV-infected women with low-grade SIL or type 1 CIN.

In contrast to low-grade lesions, the risk of recurrent disease after treatment among HIV-infected women with type 2 CIN or type 3 CIN approaches 40% to 60% annually. Cervical disease progression and recurrent disease after treatment are correlated to low CD4$^+$ counts.[267,278,280-282] One study showed that nearly 50% of HIV-infected women had positive cone biopsy margins, suggesting this population may need more aggressive management than merely close follow-up colposcopies.[283] A clinical trial evaluating the efficacy of 5-fluorouracil treatment for prevention of recurrent cervical disease after ablative therapy for type 2 CIN or type 3 CIN in 101 HIV-infected women found 5-fluorouracil treatment to be significantly protective, reducing the recurrence rate from 47% to 28% in the 5-fluorouracil arm.[284]

Invasive cervical carcinoma became an AIDS-defining diagnosis in 1993. The incidence is low among HIV-infected women, although the prevalence of SIL and CIN is high. Invasive cervical carcinoma is an important AIDS-defining illness, however, and may be the most common AIDS-related malignancy among HIV-infected women in areas with a high prevalence of HPV infection.[285] Compared with non–HIV-infected women, HIV-infected women with invasive cervical carcinoma were likely to present with advanced clinical disease, have persistent or recurrent disease at follow-up, have a short time to recurrence, have a short survival after diagnosis, and die of cervical cancer.[286] In the pre-HAART era, the median CD4$^+$ count was relatively higher (153/mm^3 versus 50/mm^3) among women with invasive cervical carcinoma compared with women diagnosed with other opportunistic illnesses,[287] but women with low CD4$^+$ counts have a particularly poor prognosis.[288] Limited data on women with invasive cervical carcinoma in the post-HAART era have shown a better outcome. A review of malignancies in the HERS cohort found that women diagnosed with invasive cervical carcinoma had a higher mean CD4$^+$ count (443/mm^3) and, at time of publication, only one of four women had died of metastatic disease 55 months after diagnosis.[200]

Studies to date conducted in the United States, France, Italy, and Canada have had conflicting results regarding the impact of HAART on the persistence of HPV infection and cervical disease. There was no association between HAART and persistence of HPV infection in the French and Italian cohorts after a mean follow-up of 17.7 and 15.4 months.[289,290] Luque and co-workers[291] found U.S. women who received antiretroviral therapy were less likely to have HPV DNA detected in cervical samples than women not on any antiretroviral therapy. The regression rate of CIN was twofold higher among women receiving HAART in the French cohort,[289] but there was no association between HAART and cervical disease progression or regression in the Italian cohort ($n = 163$),[290] a second U.S. cohort ($n = 602$, follow-up 12 months),[292] and a Canadian cohort ($n = 99$).[293] Some studies have shown that antiretroviral therapy seems to have a beneficial effect on the incidence of HPV infection and disease.[267,291]

Because of the increased risk for cervical disease, in 1993 the CDC recommended HIV-infected women should have a Pap smear performed when found to be HIV infected; if normal, the Pap should be repeated in 6 months. Women who have never had an abnormal Pap smear and have had at least two normal Pap smears can undergo Pap screening every 12 months.[239] Although the risk for cervical HPV disease is lower among women with repeated normal Pap smears, one study showed 20% of HIV-infected women with no history of cervical disease developed biopsy-confirmed incident SIL within 3 years, highlighting the importance of relatively frequent cervical cancer screening in this population.[294] If inflammation/atypia is present, the Pap smear should be repeated in 3 months.[295] Routine baseline colposcopy screening is not recommended, but women with SIL, HPV findings, and persistent atypia should be referred to colposcopy.[239,295] Among HIV-infected women, mild cytologic atypia[296] and atypical cells of undetermined significance[297] are often associated with CIN.

Although most studies have focused on cervical disease, HPV also can cause genital warts and anal or vulvar SIL. Anal HPV infections seem to be more prevalent than cervical infections and have similar risk factors, including CD4$^+$ counts less than 200 cells/mm^3 and age younger than 45 years.[298] The characteristic course of HPV anal infection among HIV-infected women is unclear, and the optimal management is unknown. HIV infection and induced immune suppression seem to increase the risk for HPV vulvovaginal lesions.[299] These observations suggest HIV-infected women should have a thorough inspection of the vulva and perianal region during each gynecologic examination.

Genital Ulcer Disease. The most common causes of genital ulcer disease among HIV-infected women are HSV and syphilis. Proportions of women diagnosed with these two infections in U.S. cohorts have ranged from 3% to 22% for syphilis and 4% to 18% for HSV.[193-195,227,240,241] Injection drug users and women who exchange sex for drugs or money are at higher risk for syphilis.[194,227] Women with lower CD4$^+$ counts are more likely to have active and severe genital ulcer disease due to HSV.[194,300] Because HIV seems to modify the course of HSV, the CDC has specific recommendations regarding treatment for episodic infections or suppression for HIV-infected persons. In general, doses of acyclovir, famciclovir, and valacyclovir are higher, and duration of treatment is longer (see Chapter 132).[239] Persistent large ulcerations recalcitrant to HSV treatments may herald either acyclovir resistance or the presence of idiopathic aphthous ulcerations, described subsequently.

In women with advanced HIV disease, idiopathic vulvar or vaginal ulcers are a rare manifestation[194,301-305]; the ulcers can be intractable, progress to fistula formation, and cause severe bleeding. In a national retrospective review of 29 women with idiopathic genital ulcers (defined by either negative HSV and syphilis testing or a nondiagnostic ulcer biopsy), the median CD4$^+$ count was only 50/mm^3, and 68% had a prior AIDS-defining event. In 37% of patients, oral ulcers coexisted, and in 19%, genital ulcers progressed to fistula formation. Although the numbers were small, there was often a good response to either corticosteroid treatment (topical, intralesional, or systemic) or initiation of antiretroviral treatment among antiretroviral-naive women.[303] Thalidomide also is an effective treatment.[306]

CMV rarely can cause disease in the lower female genital tract. Women present with labial, vulvar, and cervical ulcerations and typically are severely immunocompromised. They often have coexistent CMV retinal or gastrointestinal tract disease. In addition to painful genital ulcers, some women have had fevers and significant cervical bleeding. Women with this manifestation generally responded to intravenous ganciclovir (see Chapter 134).[305,307-309]

Sex Hormones, Ovulation, and Menstrual Function

There is little information pertaining to sex hormones in HIV-infected women. One study evaluated hormonal levels in 16 HIV-infected women with normal menstrual cycles (in whom the stage of disease was unknown) and found the mean serum progesterone, estradiol, and cortisol levels during each phase of the cycle were similar to literature values historically seen.[310] Although these findings suggest that HIV infection does not influence the reproductive endocrine system, some studies evaluating menstrual function imply that there may be an effect on pituitary-gonadal functioning by the virus or subsequent immune dysfunction.

In one study of 248 HIV-infected women and 82 non–HIV-infected controls, HIV-infected women were more likely to experience amenorrhea or intervals greater than 6 weeks without menstrual bleeding and were less likely to have typical premenstrual symptoms, suggesting that anovulatory cycles may be more common in this population.[311] A second study of 797 HIV-infected women and 205 non–HIV-infected controls found the prevalence of amenorrhea, defined as no menstrual periods for greater than 90 days, was 7% among HIV-infected women and 5% among non–HIV-infected controls. On multivariate analysis, HIV infection, heroin use, low albumin, and live births in the past year each were independently associated with amenorrhea. Amenorrhea also was more common among women with low CD4$^+$ counts (<50/mm^3), and the etiology of amenorrhea was associated with hypothalamic dysfunction, with low or normal levels of follicle-

stimulating hormone and low levels of estradiol in approximately 80% of HIV-infected women.[312] Later information on this cohort showed there also was a significant association between high viral loads and lower CD4$^+$ counts and cycle length (short and long) and cycle variability.[312] In contrast to these studies, two additional studies did not find that HIV infection status or CD4$^+$ count was associated with menstrual dysfunction.[313,314]

Dysfunctional bleeding often occurs in women who are anovulatory or perimenopausal. HIV infection may have minimal influence on the prevalence of anovulation and the age at which menopause occurs. One study of HIV-infected women with regular menses ($n = 14$) found that 4 (29%) did not ovulate during a single cycle,[315] which is similar to comparable HIV-negative women (5% to 31% are anovulatory).[316,317] The HIV-infected anovulatory women tended to be older (38 years old versus 31 years old) and to have higher CD4$^+$ counts (632/mm^3 versus 392/mm^3) compared with women who ovulated. A second study of HIV-infected women with normal and abnormal menses ($n = 33$) found that 48% of women did not ovulate.[318]

Clinicians should look for potential causes in HIV-infected women presenting with dysfunctional uterine bleeding. In addition to cervical or endometrial cancer, other malignancies may present with bleeding. One case report described an HIV-infected woman diagnosed with high-grade, immunoblastic, non-Hodgkin's lymphoma originating in the endometrium who presented with intractable menometrorrhagia requiring a hysterectomy.[319] Although there have not been reports from either clinical trial or observational cohort studies to suggest any influence of antiretroviral therapies on menstrual cycling, one series of case reports described four women taking ritonavir who had significant hypermenorrhea.[320]

A small survey study of HIV-infected women suggested menopause may occur relatively early (mean 47 years by recall).[321] A second study of 24 HIV-infected women age 20 to 42 years found 2 (8%), age 35 and 42 years, had presumed early menopause, defined by elevated follicle-stimulating hormone levels and cessation of menses.[318] The safety and benefits of hormone replacement therapy have not been studied in HIV-infected women.

Metabolic Complications and Antiretroviral-Associated Adverse Events

Several metabolic complications, including fat maldistribution, hyperglycemia, and dyslipidemias, thought to be adverse events associated with or influenced by antiretroviral therapies have been described. Although early reports described primarily HIV-infected men, studies of HIV-infected women have shown similar results. A comprehensive comparison of 75 HIV-infected women (age 25 to 46 years) and 30 weight-matched, non–HIV-infected controls found HIV-infected women were significantly more likely to have truncal adiposity, hyperinsulinemia, and hypertriglyceridemia compared with control subjects, independent of protease inhibitor use.[322] A second study of HIV-infected women compared 21 women with self-reported body shape changes on HAART with 21 women without changes also on HAART. The most frequent complaints were increased abdominal girth, increased breast size, increased body weight, and peripheral fat wasting. No covariates were found to be significant predictors of fat maldistribution, although women with body shape changes had a lower mean CD4$^+$ count compared with women without reported changes (322/mm^3 versus 500/mm^3, $P = .07$). Serum lipid abnormalities also were significantly increased in both groups after institution of HAART.[323] A third study of HIV-infected women ($n = 306$) determined 10.5% experienced fat maldistribution. Women with fat redistribution had significantly more truncal fat and less leg fat and clinically were characterized by breast and abdominal fat accumulation accompanied by wasting of the glutei and lower limbs. Significant factors associated with fat maldistribution in multivariate analyses included receipt of antiretroviral therapy for longer than 1000 days and initial viral load greater than 10,000 copies.[324] A comparison study of HIV-infected men ($n = 27$) and women ($n = 13$) found adverse effects on lipid and insulin levels either more marked or occurring only in women. The metabolic changes that occurred during HAART eliminated the advantageous sex difference for atherosclerosis risk usually seen in women.[325]

Women seem to be at increased risk for the syndrome of lactic acidosis and hepatic steatosis with or without pancreatitis that is associated with nucleoside/nucleotide analogue reverse transcriptase inhibitors.[326] This complication also has been described in later stage pregnant or postpartum women whose antiretroviral regimen included stavudine and didanosine.[327]

Bone complications that have been described include avascular necrosis, osteopenia, and osteoporosis. Decreased bone density seems to be more common among persons receiving protease inhibitor therapies[328,329] and may be linked to impaired fasting glucoses.[330] In one study, the prevalence of osteopenia was 50% among HIV-infected postmenopausal women and 25% among HIV-infected perimenopausal women. Of women prescribed protease inhibitor therapies, 60% had osteopenia compared with 13% of women not on these therapies ($P = .04$).[331]

In addition to metabolic complications, women may experience a higher frequency of ARV-associated hepatotoxicity and rash events. In a retrospective cohort, female sex was one covariate significantly associated with development of elevated aminotransferase levels even after analyses were adjusted for confounders, such as coexistent hepatitis B or C infection and selected concomitant medications.[332] Women also may be at increased risk for nevirapine associated hepatotoxicity[333,334] and have a sevenfold higher risk for developing severe skin rashes compared with men.[335,336]

Sex Differences in Viral Load and Human Immunodeficiency Virus Disease Progression

Although initial observations of survival in HIV infection implied that women possibly had a worse prognosis than men,[337,338] more recent data generally have not supported sex differences in the rate of HIV disease progression.[339-343] This observation possibly reflects the fact that in the early years of the epidemic, women often had delayed access to health care, perhaps because of delayed recognition of HIV infection or because of family and child care obligations.[344] One study that evaluated the association of sex on disease-free survival time with the introduction of protease inhibitors after 1995 found that the gain in women was significantly less than in men, suggesting that there is a sex difference in the benefit derived from HAART.[345] Several reasons could explain this finding, including sex differences in use of HAART regimens, adherence to complex regimens, and antiretroviral-associated adverse events. At least one study has shown that women were significantly less likely than men to start HAART regimens in an area that provided free access to antiretroviral therapies. Female sex remained significant in multivariate models adjusted for potential confounders, including risk group, age, history of antiretroviral treatments, CD4+ cell count levels, and education.[342]

Studies have had conflicting results as to whether there is a sex difference in HIV-1 RNA viral loads. In a cross-sectional study of an IDU cohort, there was a consistent trend toward lower viral load levels in women compared with men after adjustment for CD4+ cell count, race, and drug use within the prior 6 months. There was no difference, however, in HIV disease progression to AIDS.[346] Additional analyses of seroconverters in the IDU cohort found that the sex difference was present at the time of seroconversion but disappeared after 5 to 6 years because women had more rapid viral load increases.[347] This study again confirmed that the rates of HIV disease progression to AIDS did not differ.[348] Another small longitudinal study showed similar results: An initial small sex difference in HIV-1 RNA viral loads was present, which diminished over time.[349]

Two other large cohort studies (the Swiss HIV Cohort and the ICONA studies) found modest sex differences (0.13 $\log_{10}$) among selected subgroups.[350,351] Two additional studies (a Johns Hopkins cohort and comparison between the WIHS and MAC study) found either no sex difference[352] or a minimal difference only at higher CD4+ cell count levels.[353] Taken together, the studies suggest that there may be a mild sex influence on viral load levels, but the difference is seen predominantly at higher CD4+ cell count levels.

Studies that evaluated selected demographic, epidemiologic, clinical, and laboratory features for determination of HIV disease progression among cohorts of HIV-infected women in the pre-HAART and post-HAART era have shown that predictive markers are similar to the markers identified in men. These include high HIV RNA values; low CD4+ cell counts; rapid CD4+ cell count declines; a baseline CDC AIDS-defining opportunistic process; a low body mass index; and illness attributable to HIV infection, such as chronic diarrhea, herpes zoster, and oral candidiasis.[354-357] As discussed earlier, pregnancy does not seem to be an independent risk factor for disease progression in most studies.[358-361]

Management Issues

Several studies have shown HIV-infected women are less likely than men to receive health care services, including medications.[344,363] This finding reflects the fact that delivery of health care to HIV-infected women can be a challenge. Barriers specific for this population have been identified in several studies and include child care responsibilities and the need for several services, such as gynecologic or obstetric care, which can necessitate multiple visits to different locations.[363-365] In addition, IDU has been shown to interfere with access to health care and compliance with treatment,[366] and a substantial proportion of women reported to the CDC with a diagnosis of AIDS have had a history of IDU.[367]

Strategies shown to improve accrual and retention of HIV-infected women into health care include combining clinics for mothers and their children, integrating gynecologic/colposcopy services on site into primary care clinics, daily availability of health care provider services, and provision of on-site child care and transportation services.[368] In young HIV-infected women or infected adolescents, several specific management issues should be addressed. The frequency of STIs has been shown to be disturbingly high among adolescent women. In a New Orleans cohort of HIV-infected girls age 13 to 18 years, 75% were diagnosed with an STI at clinic entry or during follow-up.[369] There is also a high prevalence of psychosocial problems, including a history of sexual abuse,[370,371] substance abuse,[370,371] and psychiatric diagnoses[370] among HIV-infected adolescents. These findings emphasize the importance of discussing optimal methods for contraception and STI protection and incorporating psychosocial management into the comprehensive care for this population.

Reproductive and contraceptive options need to be discussed with all premenopausal women. Condoms are universally recommended for STI protection. Women who choose not to become pregnant may wish to employ an additional method. Preferred reversible contraceptive methods are hormonal therapies (either combined estrogen/progesterone regimens or progestin-only regimens). Selected protease inhibitor and non-nucleoside reverse transcriptase inhibitor therapies are known to have significant interactions with estrogen, which may interfere with the hormonal contraceptive therapy efficacy.[372] Concurrent use of a barrier method adds a second contraceptive method in addition to providing STI protection. There currently is no information on potential interactions between antiretroviral therapies and progestin treatments, but a pharmacokinetic study of depomedroxyprogesterone acetate (or Depo-Provera) and selected protease inhibitors and non-nucleoside reverse transcriptase inhibitors is ongoing.

Intrauterine devices are an acceptable alternative for women at low risk for STIs.[373] Women should be counseled, however, about the known association of this method and PID. Periodic screening for *N. gonorrhoeae* and *C. trachomatis* should be considered. Spermicidal agents offer pregnancy protection, but not adequate STI protection and may increase the risk of vaginal irritation or ulceration if used frequently.[374]

Older HIV-infected women are unique because they are at risk for various medical conditions due to their age and should receive routine recommended health maintenance screening examinations, such as mammography. Underlying medical conditions, including but not limited to hypertension, diabetes, coronary artery disease, angina, chronic obstructive pulmonary disease, asthma, and arthritis, are common.[375] HIV-infected women at least 40 years old also are more likely to be diagnosed with psychiatric illnesses, such as substance abuse, anxiety, depression, psychosis, and dementia, compared with younger HIV-infected women.[376]

Provider experience in the management of advanced HIV infection has been shown to be associated significantly with the outcome of HIV-infected women. A retrospective cohort study of women with a diagnosis of AIDS who attended 117 New York State clinics found that provider experience, as measured by number of HIV-infected patients being followed, was a predictor for survival. After adjustment for demographic and clinic variables, 71% of patients who received care in the high-experience clinics were alive compared with 53% in the low-experience clinics after 21 months.[377]

Offering enrollment into clinical trials also is an advantageous management option for HIV-infected women. At least one study has shown women who participate in antiretroviral therapy clinical trials have significantly longer survival.[378] Historically a relatively low proportion of HIV-infected women were enrolled into clinical trials. It has been difficult to study the influence of sex on the toxicity or efficacy of antiretroviral therapies. In recent years, investigators have become more cognizant of the importance of studying sex differences, particularly since at least one antiretroviral clinical trial showed a unique toxicity and efficacy profile for women.[379] Today, many ongoing and planned clinical trials have objectives addressing sex or gender issues, which would broaden understanding of women with HIV infection.

REFERENCES

1. UNAIDS/WHO. AIDS epidemic update: December, 2002. Available at: http://www.unaids.org/worldaidsday/2002/press/Epiupdate.html. Accessed July 7, 2003.
2. Centers for Disease Control and Prevention. HIV/AIDS Surveillance Report. 2001;13:2-44. Available at: http://www.cdc.gov/hiv/stats/hasrlink.htm.
3. Karon JM, Fleming PL, Steketee RW, et al. HIV in the United States at the turn of the century: An epidemic in transition. Am J Public Health. 2001;91:1060-1068.
4. Hader SL, Smith DK, Moore JS, et al. HIV infection in women in the United States: Status at the millennium. JAMA. 2001;285:1186-1192.
5. Wold C, Seage GR III, Lenderking WR, et al. Unsafe sex in men who have sex with both men and women. J Acquir Immune Defic Syndr Hum Retrovirol. 1998;17:361-367.
6. Kahn JG, Gurvey J, Pollack LM, et al. How many HIV infections cross the bisexual bridge? An estimate from the United States. AIDS. 1997;11:1031-1037.
7. Wortley PM, Chu SY, Berkelman RL. Epidemiology of HIV/AIDS in women and the impact of the expanded 1993 CDC surveillance definition of AIDS. In: Cotton D, Watts DH, eds. The Medical Management of AIDS in Women. New York: Wiley-Liss; 1997:3-14.
8. Centers for Disease Control and Prevention. Update: Mortality attributable to HIV infection among persons aged 25-44 years-United States, 1994. MMWR Morb Mortal Wkly Rep. 1996;45:121-125.
9. Palella FJ Jr, Deloria-Knoll M, Chmiel JS, et al. Survival benefit of initiating antiretroviral therapy in HIV-infected persons in different CD4+ cell strata. Ann Intern Med. 2003;138:620-626.
10. Palella F, Delaney KM, Moorman AC, et al. Declining morbidity and mortality among patients with advanced human immunodeficiency virus infection. N Engl J Med. 1998;338:853-860.
11. Hogg RS, Heath KV, Yip B, et al. Improved survival among HIV-infected individuals following initiation of antiretroviral therapy. JAMA. 1998;279:450-454.
12. Centers for Disease Control and Prevention. AIDS among persons aged 50 years—United States, 1991-1996. MMWR Morb Mortal Wkly Rep. 1998;47:21-27.
13. Clark RA, Bessinger R. Clinical manifestations and predictors of survival in older women infected with HIV. J Acquir Immune Defic Syndr Hum Retrovirol. 1997;15:341-345.
14. Schable B, Chu SY, Diaz T. Characteristics of women 50 years of age or older with heterosexually acquired AIDS. Am J Public Health. 1996;86:1616-1618.
15. Centers for Disease Control and Prevention. HIV/AIDS Surveillance Report. 1996;8:2-39.
16. Chaisson RE, Bacchetti P, Osmond D, et al. Cocaine use and HIV infection in intravenous drug users in San Francisco. JAMA. 1989;261:561-565.
17. Edlin BR, Irwin KL, Faruque S, et al. Intersecting epidemics—crack cocaine use and HIV infection among inner-city young adults. Multicenter Crack Cocaine and HIV Infection Study Team. N Engl J Med. 1994;331:1422-1427.
18. Fullilove RE, Fullilove MT, Bowser BP, et al. Risk of sexually transmitted disease among black adolescent crack users in Oakland and San Francisco, Calif. JAMA 1990;263:851-855.
19. Chu SY, Hammett TA, Buehler JW. Update: Epidemiology of reported cases of AIDS in women who report sex only with other women, United States, 1980-1991. AIDS. 1992;6:518-519.
20. Lemp GF, Jones M, Kellogg TA, et al. HIV seroprevalence and risk behaviors among lesbians and bisexual women in San Francisco and Berkeley, California. Am J Public Health. 1995;85:1549-1552.
21. Rich JD, Buck A, Tuomala RE, et al. Transmission of human immunodeficiency virus infection presumed to have occurred via female homosexual contact. Clin Infect Dis. 1993;17:1003-1005.
22. Centers for Disease Control and Prevention. HIV-1 infection and artificial insemination with processed semen. MMWR Morb Mortal Wkly Rep. 1990;39:249.
23. Stewart GL, Typer JP, Cunningham AL, et al. Transmission of human T-cell lymphotropic virus type III by artificial insemination by donor. Lancet. 1985;2:581-584.
24. Chiasson MA, Stoneburner RL, Joseph SC. Human immunodeficiency virus transmission through artificial insemination. J Acquir Immune Defic Syndr. 1990;3:69-72.
25. Sauer MV, Chang PL. Establishing a clinical program for human immunodeficiency virus 1-seropositive men to father seronegative children by means of in vitro fertilization with intracytoplasmic sperm injection. Am J Obstet Gynecol. 2002;186:627-633.
26. Al-Khan A, Colon J, Palta V, et al. Assisted reproductive technology for men and women infected with human immunodeficiency virus type 1. Clin Infect Dis. 2003;36:195-200.
27. Ohl J, Partisani M, Wittemer C, et al. Assisted reproduction techniques for HIV serodiscordant couples: 18 months of experience. Hum Reprod. 2003;18:1244-1249.
28. Cohn SE, Klein JD, Mohr JE, et al. The geography of AIDS: Patterns of urban and rural migration. South Med J. 1994;87:599-606.
29. Fowler MG, Melnick SL, Mathieson BJ. Women and HIV: Epidemiology and global overview. Obstet Gynecol Clin North Am. 1997;24:705-729.
30. Shetty AK, Powell G. Children orphaned by AIDS: A global perspective. Semin Pediatr Infect Dis. 2003;14:25-31.
31. Neal JJ, Fleming PL, Green TA, et al. Trends in heterosexually acquired AIDS in the United States, 1988 through 1995. J Acquir Immune Defic Syndr Hum Retrovirol. 1997;14:465-474.
32. Padian N, Marquis L, Francis DP, et al. Male-to-female transmission of human immunodeficiency virus. JAMA. 1987;258:788-790.
33. Padian NS, Shiboski SC, Jewell NP. Female-to-male transmission of human immunodeficiency virus. JAMA. 1991;266:1664-1667.
34. Fowler MG. Update: Transmission of HIV-1 from mother to child. Curr Opin Obstet Gynecol. 1997;9:343-348.
35. Peterman TA, Stoneburner RL, Allen JR, et al. Risk of human immunodeficiency virus transmission from heterosexual adults with transfusion-associated infections. JAMA. 1988;259:55-58.
36. Padian NS, Shiboski SC, Jewell NP. The effect of number of exposures on the risk of heterosexual HIV transmission. J Infect Dis. 1990;161:883-887.
37. Fowke KR, Nagelkerke NJ, Kimani J, et al. Resistance to HIV-1 infection among persistently seronegative prostitutes in Nairobi, Kenya. Lancet. 1996;348:1347-1351.
38. Holmes KK, Johnson DW, Trostle HJ. An estimate of the risk of men acquiring gonorrhea by sexual contact with infected females. Am J Epidemiol. 1970;91:170-174.
39. Platt R, Rice PA, McCormack WM. Risk of acquiring gonorrhea and prevalence of abnormal adnexal findings among women recently exposed to gonorrhea. JAMA. 1983;250:3205-3209.
40. DeGruttola V, Seage GR III, Mayer KH, et al. Infectiousness of HIV between male homosexual partners. J Clin Epidemiol. 1989;42:849-856.
41. Gray RH, Wawer MJ, Brookmeyer R, et al. Probability of HIV-1 transmission per coital act in monogamous, heterosexual, HIV-1-discordant couples in Rakai, Uganda. Lancet. 2001;357:1149-1153.
42. Nicolosi A, Correa Leite ML, Musicco M, et al. The efficiency of male-to-female and female-to-male sexual transmission of the human immunodeficiency virus: A study of 730 stable couples. Italian Study Group on HIV Heterosexual Transmission. Epidemiology. 1994;5:570-575.
43. Quinn TC, Wawer MJ, Sewankambo N, et al. Viral load and heterosexual transmission of human immunodeficiency virus type 1. Rakai Project Study Group. N Engl J Med. 2000;342:921-929.
44. Skurnick JH, Kennedy CA, Perez G, et al. Behavioral and demographic risk factors for transmission of human immunodeficiency virus type 1 in heterosexual couples: Report from the Heterosexual HIV Transmission Study. Clin Infect Dis. 1998;26:855-864.
45. Guimaraes MD, Vlahov D, Castilho EA. Postcoital vaginal bleeding as a risk factor for transmission of the human immunodeficiency virus in a heterosexual partner study in Brazil. Rio de Janeiro Heterosexual Study Group. Arch Intern Med. 1997;157:1362-1368.
46. Gray RH, Kiwanuka N, Quinn TC, et al. Male circumcision and HIV acquisition and transmission: Cohort studies in Rakai, Uganda. Rakai Project Team. AIDS. 2000;14:2371-2381.
47. Liuzzi G, Chirianni A, Clementi M, et al. Analysis of HIV-1 load in blood, semen and saliva: Evidence for different viral compartments in a cross-sectional and longitudinal study. AIDS. 1996;10:F51-F56.
48. Vernazza PL, Gilliam BL, Flepp M, et al. Effect of antiviral treatment on the shedding of HIV-1 in semen. AIDS. 1997;11:1249-1254.
49. Cu-Uvin SC, Caliendo AM. Cervicovaginal human immunodeficiency virus secretion and plasma viral load in human immunodeficiency virus-seropositive women. Obstet Gynecol. 1997;90:739-743.
50. Gupta P, Mellors J, Kingsley L, et al. High viral load in semen of human immunodeficiency virus type 1-infected men at all stages of disease and its reduction by therapy with protease and nonnucleoside reverse transcriptase inhibitors. J Virol. 1997;71:6271-6275.
51. Levine WC, Pope V, Bhoomkar A, et al. Increase in endocervical CD4+ lymphocytes among women with nonulcerative sexually transmitted diseases. J Infect Dis. 1998;177:167-174.
52. Wasserheit JN. Epidemiological synergy: Interrelationships between human immunodeficiency virus infection and other sexually transmitted diseases. Sex Transm Dis. 1992;19:61-77.
53. Wasserheit JN. STD-HIV interactions: From epidemiological synergy to patient management and public health. Abstract P31. Presented at the Thirty-fifth Annual Meeting of the Infectious Diseases Society of America, Chicago, Ill, September 13-16, 1997.
54. Mayer KH, Anderson DJ. Heterosexual transmission of HIV. In: Minkoff H, DeHovitz JA, Duerr A, eds. HIV Infection in Women. New York: Raven; 1995:73-85.
55. Laga M, Manoka A, Kivuvu M, et al. Non-ulcerative sexually transmitted diseases as risk factors for HIV-1 transmission in women: Results from a cohort study. AIDS. 1993;7:95-102.

56. de Vincenzi I. A longitudinal study of human immunodeficiency virus transmission by heterosexual partners. European Study Group on Heterosexual Transmission of HIV. N Engl J Med. 1994;331:341-346.
57. Cohen MS, Hoffman IF, Royce RA, et al. Reduction of concentration of HIV-1 in semen after treatment of urethritis: Implications for prevention of sexual transmission of HIV-1. AIDSCAP Malawi Research Group. Lancet. 1997;349:1868-1873.
58. Ciesielski CA. Sexually transmitted diseases in men who have sex with men: An epidemiologic review. Curr Infect Dis Rep. 2003;5:145-152.
59. Klein J, Pena JE, Thornton MH, et al. Understanding the motivations, concerns, and desires of human immunodeficiency virus 1-serodiscordant couples wishing to have children through assisted reproduction. Obstet Gynecol. 2003;101(5 Pt 1):987-994.
60. Tashima KT, Alt EN, Harwell JI, et al. Internet sex-seeking leads to acute HIV infection: A report of two cases. Int J STD AIDS. 2003;14:285-286.
61. Coombs RW, Wright DJ, Reichelderfer PS, et al. Variation of human immunodeficiency virus type 1 viral RNA levels in the female genital tract: Implications for applying measurements to individual women. J Infect Dis. 2001;184:1187-1191.
62. Goulston C, McFarland W, Katzenstein D. Human immunodeficiency virus type 1 RNA shedding in the female genital tract. J Infect Dis. 1998;177:1100-1103.
63. Cu-Uvin S, Caliendo AM, Reinert S, et al. Effect of highly active antiretroviral therapy on cervicovaginal HIV-1 RNA. AIDS. 2000;14:415-421.
64. Xu C, Politch JA, Tucker L, et al. Factors associated with increased levels of human immunodeficiency virus type 1 DNA in semen. J Infect Dis. 1997;176:941-947.
65. Rasheed S, Li Z, Xu D, Kovacs A. Presence of cell-free human immunodeficiency virus in cervicovaginal secretions is independent of viral load in the blood of human immunodeficiency virus-infected women. Am J Obstet Gynecol. 1996;175:122-129.
66. Coombs RW, Speck CE, Hughes JP, et al. Association between culturable human immunodeficiency virus type 1 (HIV-1) in semen and HIV-1 RNA levels in semen and blood: Evidence for compartmentalization of HIV-1 between semen and blood. J Infect Dis. 1998;177:320-330.
67. Wright TC Jr, Subbarao S, Ellerbrock TV, et al. Human immunodeficiency virus 1 expression in the female genital tract in association with cervical inflammation and ulceration. Am J Obstet Gynecol. 2001;184:279-285.
68. Shaheen F, Sison AV, McIntosh L, et al. Analysis of HIV-1 in the cervicovaginal secretions and blood of pregnant and nonpregnant women. J Hum Virol. 1999;2:154-166.
69. Rybo G. Menstrual blood loss in relation to parity and menstrual pattern. Acta Obstet Gynecol Scand. 1966;45:25-45.
70. Tevi-Benissan C, Belec L, Levy M, et al. In vivo semen-associated pH neutralization of cervicovaginal secretions. Clin Diagn Lab Immunol. 1997;4:367-374.
71. Moller BR, Kasperson P. Acidity of the vagina. In: Horowitz BJ, Mardh P-A, eds. Vaginitis and Vaginosis. New York: Wiley-Liss; 1991:63-67.
72. Cu-Uvin S, Hogan JW, Caliendo AM, et al. Association between bacterial vaginosis and expression of human immunodeficiency virus type 1 RNA in the female genital tract. Clin Infect Dis. 2001;33:894-896.
73. Reichelderfer PS, Coombs RW, Wright DJ, et al. Effect of menstrual cycle on HIV-1 levels in the peripheral blood and genital tract. WHS 001 Study Team. AIDS. 2000;14:2101-2107.
74. Money DM, Arikan YY, Remple V, et al. Genital tract and plasma human immunodeficiency virus viral load throughout the menstrual cycle in women who infected with ovulatory human immunodeficiency virus. Am J Obstet Gynecol. 2003;188:122-128.
75. Turpin JA. Considerations and development of topical microbicides to inhibit the sexual transmission of HIV. Expert Opin Investig Drugs. 2002;11:1077-1097.
76. Kreiss JK, Kiviat NB, Plummer FA, et al. Human immunodeficiency virus, human papillomavirus, and cervical intraepithelial neoplasia in Nairobi prostitutes. Sex Transm Dis. 1992;19:54-59.
77. Stafford MK, Ward H, Flanagan A, et al. Safety study of nonoxynol-9 as a vaginal microbicide: Evidence of adverse effects. J Acquir Immune Defic Syndr Hum Retrovirol. 1998;17:327-331.
78. Wainberg MA. The need for vaginal microbicides with antiviral specificity. AIDS. 1998;12:4-6.
79. Van Damme L, Ramjee G, Alary M, et al. Effectiveness of COL-1492, a nonoxynol-9 vaginal gel, on HIV-1 transmission in female sex workers: A randomised controlled trial [Erratum in: Lancet. 2002 Dec 7;360(9348):1892]. Lancet. 2002;360:971-7.
80. Biggar RJ, Miotti PG, Taha TE, et al. Perinatal intervention trial in Africa: Effect of a birth canal cleansing intervention to prevent HIV transmission. Lancet. 1996;347:1647-1650.
81. Taha TE, Biggar RJ, Broadhead RL, et al. Effect of cleansing the birth canal with antiseptic solution on maternal and newborn morbidity and mortality in Malawi: Clinical trial. BMJ. 1997;315:216-219.
82. Clemetson DB, Moss GB, Willerford DM, et al. Detection of HIV DNA in cervical and vaginal secretions: Prevalence and correlates among women in Nairobi, Kenya. JAMA. 1993;289:2860-2864.
83. Sha BE, D'Amico RD, Landay AL, et al. Evaluation of immunologic markers in cervicovaginal fluid of HIV-infected and uninfected women: Implications for the immunologic response to HIV in the female genital tract. J Acquir Immune Defic Syndr Hum Retrovirol. 1997;16:161-168.
84. Kiddugavu M, Makumbi F, Wawer MJ, et al. Hormonal contraceptive use and HIV-1 infection in a population-based cohort in Rakai, Uganda. AIDS. 2003;17:233-240.
85. Critchlow CW, Kiviat NB. Detection of human immunodeficiency virus type 1 and type 2 in the female genital tract: Implications for the understanding of virus transmission. Obstet Gynecol Surv. 1997;52:314-324.
86. Ghys PD, Fransen K, Diallo MO, et al. The associations between cervicovaginal HIV shedding, sexually transmitted diseases and immunosuppression in female sex workers in Abidjan, Cote d'Ivoire. AIDS. 1997;11:F85-F93.
87. Grosskurth H, Mosha F, Todd J, et al. Impact of improved treatment of sexually transmitted diseases on HIV infection in rural Tanzania: Randomised controlled trial. Lancet. 1995;346:530-536.
88. Janssen RS, Holtgrave DR, Valdiserri RO, et al. The serostatus approach to fighting the HIV epidemic: Prevention strategies for infected individuals. Am J Public Health. 2001;91:1019-1024.
89. European Collaborative Study. Risk factors for mother-to-child transmission of HIV-1. Lancet. 1992;339:1007-1012.
90. Mofenson LM. Mother-child HIV-1 transmission: Timing and determinants. Obstet Gynecol Clin North Am. 1997;24:759-784.
91. Viscarello RR, Cullen MT, DeGennaro NJ, et al. Fetal blood sampling in HIV-seropositive women before elective midtrimester termination of pregnancy. Am J Obstet Gynecol. 1992;167:1075-1079.
92. Lewis SH, Reynnolds-Kohler C, Fox HE, et al. HIV-1 in trophoblastic and villous Hofbauer cells, and haematological precursors in eight-week fetuses. Lancet. 1990;335:565-568.
93. Maury W, Potts BJ, Rabson AB. HIV-1 infection of first-trimester and term human placental tissue: A possible mode of maternal-fetal transmission. J Infect Dis. 1989;160:583-588.
94. Jovius E, Koch MA, Schafer A, et al. LAV/HTLV-III in a 20 week fetus. Lancet. 1985;2:1129.
95. Sprecher S, Soumenkoff G, Puissant F, et al. Vertical transmission in a 15 week fetus. Lancet. 1986;2:288.
96. Levine AM. HIV disease in women: Clinical care options for HIV. Healthcare Communications Group LLC. 1997;9:3-24.
97. Kalish LA, Pitt J, Lew J, et al. Defining the time of fetal or perinatal acquisition of human immunodeficiency virus type 1 infection on the basis of age at first positive culture. Women and Infants Transmission Study (WITS). J Infect Dis. 1997;175:712-715.
98. Quinn TC, Ruff A, Modlin J. HIV infection and AIDS in children. Annu Rev Public Health. 1992;13:1-30.
99. Blanche S, Tardieu M, Duliege A-M, et al. Longitudinal study of 94 symptomatic infants with perinatally acquired human immunodeficiency virus infection: Evidence for a bimodal expression of clinical and biological symptoms. Am J Dis Child. 1990;144:1210-1215.
100. Public Health Service Task Force. Recommendations for the use of antiretroviral drugs in pregnant women infected with HIV-1 for maternal health and interventions to reduce perinatal HIV-1 transmission in the United States. Available at: http://www.aidsinfo.nih.gov/guidelines/. Updated November 26, 2003. Accessed June 3, 2004.
101. Ehrnst A, Lindgren S, Dictor M, et al. HIV in pregnant women and their offspring: Evidence for late transmission. Lancet. 1991;338:203-207.
102. Rouzioux C, Costagliola D, Burgard M, et al. Estimating timing of mother-to-child human immunodeficiency virus type-1 (HIV-1) transmission by use of a Markov model. The HIV Infection in Newborns French Collaborative Study Group. Am J Epidemiol. 1995;142:1330-1337.
103. Goedert JJ, Duliege AM, Amos CI, et al. High risk of HIV-1 infection for first-born twins. The International Registry of HIV-Exposed Twins. Lancet. 1991;338:1471-1475.
104. Duliege A-M, Amos CI, Felton S, et al. Birth order, delivery route, and concordance in the transmission of human immunodeficiency virus type-1 from mothers to twins. J Pediatr. 1995;126:625-632.
105. Mayaux MJ, Dussaix E, Isopet J, et al. Maternal virus load during pregnancy and mother-to-child transmission of human immunodeficiency virus type 1: The French perinatal cohort studies. SEROGEST Cohort Group. J Infect Dis. 1997;175:172-175.
106. Coll O, Hernandez M, Boucher CA, et al. Vertical HIV-1 transmission correlates with a high maternal viral load at delivery. J Acquir Immune Defic Syndr Hum Retrovirol. 1997;4:26-30.
107. Pitt J, Brambilla D, Reichelderfer P, et al. Maternal immunologic and virologic risk factors for infant human immunodeficiency virus type 1 infection: Findings from the Women and Infants Transmission Study. J Infect Dis. 1997;175:567-575.
108. St. Louis ME, Kamenga M, Brown C, et al. Risk for perinatal HIV-1 transmission according to maternal immunologic, virologic, and placental factors. JAMA. 1993;269:2853-2859.
109. Report of a Consensus Workshop, Siena, Italy, January 17-18, 1992. Maternal factors involved in mother-to-child transmission of HIV-1. J Acquir Immune Defic Syndr Hum Retrovirol. 1992;5:1019-1029.
110. Thea DM, Steketee RW, Pliner V, et al. The effect of maternal viral load on the risk of perinatal transmission of HIV-1. New York City Perinatal HIV Transmission Collaborative Study Group. AIDS. 1997;11:437-444.
111. Sperling RS, Shapiro DE, Coombs RW, et al. Maternal viral load, zidovudine treatment, and the risk of transmission of human immunodeficiency virus type 1 from mother to infant. Pediatric AIDS Clinical Trials Group Protocol 076 Study Group. N Engl J Med. 1996;335:1621-1629.
112. Ioannidis JP, Abrams EJ, Ammann A, et al. Perinatal transmission of human immunodeficiency virus type 1 by pregnant women with RNA virus loads <1000 copies/ml. J Infect Dis. 2001;183:539-545.
113. Colgrove RC, Pitt J, Chung PH, et al. Selective vertical transmission of HIV-1 antiretroviral resistance mutations. AIDS. 1998;12:2281-2288.
114. Welles SL, Pitt J, Colgrove R, et al. HIV-1 genotypic zidovudine drug resistance and the risk of maternal-infant transmission in the Women and Infants Transmission Study. The Women and Infants Transmission Study Group. AIDS. 2000;14:263-271.
115. Eastman PS, Shapiro DE, Coombs RW, et al. Maternal viral genotypic zidovudine resistance and infrequent failure of zidovudine therapy to prevent perinatal transmission of human immunodeficiency virus type 1 in pediatric AIDS. AIDS Clinical Trials Group Protocol 076. J Infect Dis. 1998;177:557-564.
116. Palumbo P, Holland B, Dobbs T, et al. Perinatal AIDS Collaborative Transmission Study. Antiretroviral resistance mutations among pregnant human immunodeficiency virus type 1-infected women and their newborns in the United States: Vertical transmission and clades. J Infect Dis. 2001;184:1120-1126.
117. MacDonald KS, Embree J, Njenga S, et al. Mother-child class I HLA concordance increases perinatal human immunodeficiency virus type 1 transmission. J Infect Dis. 1998;177:551-556.

118. John GC, Nduati RW, Mbori-Ngacha D, et al. Genital shedding of human immunodeficiency virus type 1 DNA during pregnancy: Association with immunosuppression, abnormal cervical or vaginal discharge, and severe vitamin A deficiency. J Infect Dis. 1997;175:57-62.
119. Semba RD, Miotti PG, Chiphangwi JD, et al. Maternal vitamin A deficiency and mother-to-child transmission of HIV-1. Lancet. 1994;343:1593-1597.
120. Mostad SB, Overbaugh J, DeVange DM, et al. Hormonal contraception, vitamin A deficiency, and other risk factors for shedding of HIV-1 infected cells from the cervix and vagina. Lancet. 1997;350:922-927.
121. Rodriguez EM, Mofenson LM, Chang BH, et al. Association of maternal drug use during pregnancy with maternal HIV culture positivity and perinatal HIV transmission. AIDS. 1996;10:273-282.
122. Van't Wout AB, Kootstra NA, Mulder-Kampinga GA, et al. Macrophage-tropic variants initiate human immunodeficiency virus type 1 infection after sexual, parenteral, and vertical transmission. J Clin Invest. 1995;94:2060-2067.
123. Reinhardt PP, Reinhardt B, Lathey JL, et al. Human cord blood mononuclear cells are preferentially infected by non-syncytium inducing macrophage-tropic human immunodeficiency virus type 1 isolates. J Clin Microbiol. 1995;33:292-297.
124. Kunanusont C, Foy HM, Kreiss JK, et al. HIV-1 subtypes and male-to-female transmission in Thailand. Lancet. 1995;345:1078-1083.
125. Bulterys M, Landesman S, Burns DN, et al. Sexual behavior and injection drug use during pregnancy and vertical transmission of HIV-1. J Acquir Immune Defic Syndr. 1997;15:76-82.
126. Matheson PB, Thomas PA, Abrams EJ, et al. Heterosexual behavior during pregnancy and perinatal transmission of HIV-1. New York City Perinatal HIV Transmission Collaborative Study Group. AIDS. 1996;10:1249-1256.
127. Landesman SH, Kalish LA, Burns DN, et al. Obstetrical factors and the transmission of human immunodeficiency virus type 1 from mother to child. N Engl J Med. 1996;334:1617-1623.
128. Zorrilla CD. Obstetric factors and mother-to-infant transmission of HIV-1. Infect Dis Clin North Am. 1997;11:109-118.
129. International Perinatal HIV Group. The mode of delivery and the risk of vertical transmission of human immunodeficiency virus type 1: A meta-analysis of 15 prospective cohort studies. N Engl J Med. 1999;340:977-987.
130. European Mode of Delivery Collaboration. Elective caesarean-section versus vaginal delivery in prevention of vertical transmission: A randomized clinical trial. Lancet. 1999;353:1035-1039.
131. Landers DV, Sweet RL. Reducing mother-to-infant transmission of HIV-the door remains open. N Engl J Med. 1996;334:1664-1665.
132. Oxtoby MJ. Human immunodeficiency virus and other viruses in human milk: Placing the issues in broader perspective. Pediatr Infect Dis J. 1988;7:825-835.
133. Van de Perre P, Simonon A, Msellati P, et al. Postnatal transmission of human immunodeficiency virus type 1 from mother to infant: A prospective cohort study in Kigali, Rwanda. N Engl J Med. 1991;325:593-598.
134. Lewis P, Nduati R, Kreiss JK, et al. Cell-free human immunodeficiency virus type 1 in breast milk. J Infect Dis. 1998;177:34-39.
135. Nduati RW, John GC, Richardson BA, et al. Human immunodeficiency virus type 1-infected cells in breast milk: Association with immunosuppression and vitamin A deficiency. J Infect Dis. 1995;172:1461-1468.
136. Dunn DT, Newell ML, Ades AE, et al. Risk of human immunodeficiency virus type 1 transmission through breastfeeding. Lancet. 1992;340:585-588.
137. Fowler MG, Newell ML. Breast-feeding and HIV-1 transmission in resource-limited settings. J Acquir Immune Defic Syndr. 2002;30:230-239.
138. Rousseau CM, Nduati RW, Richardson BA, et al. Longitudinal analysis of human immunodeficiency virus type 1 RNA in breast milk and of its relationship to infant infection and maternal disease. J Infect Dis. 2003;187:741-747.
139. Miotti PG, Taha TE, Kumwenda NI, et al. HIV transmission through breastfeeding: A study in Malawi. JAMA. 1999;282:744-749.
140. Weinberg GA. The dilemma of postnatal mother-to-child transmission of HIV: To breastfeed or not? Birth. 2000;27:199-205.
141. Berrebia A, Kobuch WE, Puel J, et al. Influence of pregnancy on human immunodeficiency virus disease. Eur J Obstet Gynecol Reprod Biol. 1990;37:211-217.
142. Weisser M, Rudin C, Battegay M, et al. Does pregnancy influence the course of HIV infection? Evidence from two large Swiss cohort studies. J Acquir Immune Defic Syndr Hum Retrovirol. 1998;17:404-410.
143. Minkoff HL, Henderson C, Mendez H, et al. Pregnancy outcomes among mothers infected with HIV and uninfected control subjects. Am J Obstet Gynecol. 1990;163: 1598-1604.
144. Bessinger R, Clark R, Kissinger P, et al. Pregnancy is not associated with the progression of HIV disease in women attending an HIV outpatient program. Am J Epidemiol. 1998;147:434-440.
145. Deschamps MM, Papa JW, Desvarieux M, et al. A prospective study of HIV-seropositive asymptomatic women of childbearing age in a developing country. J Acquir Immune Defic Syndr. 1993;6:446-451.
146. Landers DV, Martinez de Tejada B, Coyne BA. Immunology of HIV and pregnancy: The effects of each on the other. Obstet Gynecol Clin North Am. 1997;24:821-831.
147. A Guide to the Clinical Care of Women with HIV: 2001. First edition published by the HIV/AIDS Bureau, HRSA. Available at: http://hab.hrsa.gov/womencare.htm.
148. Burns DN, Landesman S, Minkoff H, et al. The influence of pregnancy on human immunodeficiency virus type 1 infection: Antepartum and postpartum changes in human immunodeficiency virus type 1 viral load. Am J Obstet Gynecol. 1998;178:355-359.
149. Tuomala RE, Shapiro DE, Mofenson LM, et al: Antiretroviral therapy during pregnancy and the risk of an adverse outcome. N Engl J Med. 2002;346:1863-1870.
150. Marion RW, Wiznia AA, Hutcheon G, et al. Human T cell lymphotrophic virus type embryopathy: A new dysmorphia syndrome. Am J Dis Child. 1986;140:638-640.
151. Marion RW, Wiznia AA, Hutcheon RG, et al. Fetal AIDS syndrome score: Correlation between severity of dysmorphism and age at diagnosis of immunodeficiency. Am J Dis Child. 1987;141:429-431.
152. Nicholas SW. Is there an HIV associated facial dysmorphism? Pediatr Ann. 1988;17:353.
153. Qazi QH, Sheikh TM, Fikrig S. Lack of evidence for craniofacial dysmorphism in perinatal HIV infection. J Pediatr. 1988;112:7-11.
154. Temmerman M, Chomba EN, Ndinya-Achola J, et al. Maternal human immunodeficiency virus-1 infection and pregnancy outcome. Obstet Gynecol. 1994;83:495-501.
155. Miotti PG, Dallabetta G, Ndovi E, et al. HIV-1 and pregnant women: Associated factors, prevalence, estimate of incidence and role in fetal wastage in central Africa. AIDS. 1990;4:733-736.
156. Connor EM, Sperling RS, Gelber R, et al. Reduction of maternal-infant transmission of human immunodeficiency virus type 1 with zidovudine treatment. Pediatric AIDS Clinical Trials Group Protocol 076 Study Group. N Engl J Med. 1994;331:1173-1180.
157. Centers for Disease Control and Prevention. Recommendations of the U.S. Public Health Service Task Force on the use of zidovudine to reduce perinatal transmission of human immunodeficiency virus. MMWR Morb Mortal Wkly Rep. 1994;43:1-20.
158. Centers for Disease Control and Prevention. U.S. Public Health Service recommendations for human immunodeficiency virus counseling and voluntary testing for pregnant women. MMWR Morb Mortal Wkly Rep. 1995;44:1-14.
159. Fiscus SA, Adimora AA, Schoenbach VJ, et al. Perinatal HIV infection and the effect of zidovudine therapy on transmission in rural and urban counties. JAMA. 1996;275: 1483-1488.
160. Cooper ER, Nugent RP, Diaz C, et al. After AIDS clinical trial 076: The changing pattern of zidovudine use during pregnancy, and the subsequent reduction in the vertical transmission of human immunodeficiency virus in a cohort of infected women and their infants. Women and Infants Transmission Study Group. J Infect Dis. 1996;174: 1207-1211.
161. Forbes J, Burdge D, Money D. Impact of antiretroviral therapy (ART) on the outcome of infants born to HIV seropositive mothers in British Columbia. Abstract 248. Presented at the Fifth Conference on Retroviruses and Opportunistic Infections, Chicago, Ill, February 1-5, 1998.
162. National Institute of Allergy and Infectious Disease, National Institutes of Health. Summary of a meeting of a panel to review studies of transplacental toxicity of AZT. NIAID Fact Sheet. 1997.
163. Khalsa AM, Currier J. Women and HIV: A review of current epidemiology, gynecologic manifestations, and perinatal transmission. Prim Care. 1997;24:617-641.
164. Bardeguez AD, Shapiro DE, Mofenson LM, et al. Effect of cessation of zidovudine prophylaxis to reduce vertical transmission on maternal HIV disease progression and survival. Pediatrics AIDS Clinical Trials Group 288 Protocol Team. J Acquir Immune Defic Syndr. 2003;32:170-181.
165. Aleixo LF, Goodenow MM, Sleasman JW: Zidovudine administered to women infected with human immunodeficiency virus type 1 and to their neonates reduces pediatric infection independent of an effect on levels of maternal virus. J Pediatr. 1997; 130:906-914.
166. Centers for Disease Control and Prevention. Administration of zidovudine during late pregnancy and delivery to prevent perinatal HIV infection—Thailand, 1996-98. MMWR Morb Mortal Wkly Rep. 1998;4:151-154.
167. Shaffer N, Chuachoowong R, Mock PA, et al. Short-course zidovudine for perinatal HIV-1 transmission in Bangkok, Thailand: A randomised controlled trial. Bangkok Collaborative Perinatal HIV Transmission Study Group. Lancet. 1999;353:773-780.
168. Wade NA, Birkhead GS, Warren BL, et al. Abbreviated regimens of zidovudine prophylaxis and perinatal transmission of the human immunodeficiency virus. N Engl J Med. 1998;339:1409-1414.
169. Frenkel LM, Wagner LE 2nd, Demeter LM, et al. Effects of zidovudine use during pregnancy on resistance and vertical transmission of human immunodeficiency virus type 1. Clin Infect Dis. 1995;20:1321-1326.
170. Mandelbrot L, Landreau-Mascaro A, Rekacewicz C, et al. Lamivudine-zidovudine combination for prevention of maternal-infant transmission of HIV-1. JAMA. 2001;285:2083-2093.
171. Cooper ER, Charurat M, Mofenson L, et al. Combination antiretroviral strategies for the treatment of pregnant HIV-1-infected women and prevention of perinatal HIV-1 transmission. Women and Infants' Transmission Study Group. J Acquir Immune Defic Syndr. 2002;29:484-494.
172. Petra Study Team. Efficacy of three short-course regimens of zidovudine and lamivudine in preventing early and late transmission of HIV-1 from mother to child in Tanzania, South Africa, and Uganda (Petra study): A randomised, double-blind, placebo-controlled trial. Lancet. 2002;359:1178-1186.
173. Guay LA, Musoke P, Fleming T, et al. Intrapartum and neonatal single-dose nevirapine compared with zidovudine for prevention of mother-to-child transmission of HIV-1 in Kampala, Uganda: HIVNET 012 randomised trial. Lancet. 1999;354:795-802.
174. Moodley D, Moodley J, Coovadia H, et al. A multicenter randomized controlled trial of nevirapine versus a combination of zidovudine and lamivudine to reduce intrapartum and early postpartum mother-to-child transmission of human immunodeficiency virus type 1. South African Intrapartum Nevirapine Trial (SAINT) Investigators. J Infect Dis. 2003;187:725-735.
175. Dorenbaum A, Cunningham CK, Gelber RD, et al. Two-dose intrapartum/newborn nevirapine and standard antiretroviral therapy to reduce perinatal HIV transmission: A randomized trial. International PACTG 316 Team. JAMA. 2002;288:189-198.
176. Centers for Disease Control and Prevention. Report of the NIH panel to define principles of therapy of HIV infection and guidelines for the use of antiretroviral agents in HIV-infected adults and adolescents. MMWR Morb Mortal Wkly Rep. 1998;47:1-82.
177. Carpenter CC, Fischl MA, Hammer SM, et al. Antiretroviral therapy for HIV infection in 1997: Updated recommendations of the International AIDS Society-USA panel. JAMA. 1997;277:1962-1969.

178. Wang Y, Livingston E, Patil S, et al. Pharmacokinetics of didanosine in antepartum and postpartum human immunodeficiency virus-infected pregnant women and their neonates: An AIDS Clinical Trials Group study. J Infect Dis. 1999;180:1536-1541.
179. U.S. Public Health Service Task Force. Supplement: Safety and toxicity of individual antiretroviral agents in pregnancy. Updated March 23, 2004. Available at: http://www.aidsinfo.nih.gov/guidelines/adult/ST032304.html.
179a. Schooley R. Single-dose nevirapine for MTCT prevention and women's health: Proposed studies. Presented at the Adult AIDS Clinical Trials Group Women's Health Committee Business Meeting, Baltimore, Md, December 2003.
179b. Mellors J, Palmer S, Nissley D, et al. Low-frequency NNRTI-resistant variants contribute to failure of efavirenz-containing regimens in NNRTI-experienced patients in ACTG Study 398. Presented at the Adult AIDS Clinical Trials Group Virology Symposium; Crystal City, Va, August 2003.
180. Wade N, Unadkat J, Huang S, et al. Pharmacokinetics and safety of d4T and 3TC in HIV-infected pregnant women and their infants (PACTG 332). Abstract 886. Presented at Tenth Conference on Retroviruses and Opportunistic Infections, Boston, Mass, February 10-14, 2003.
181. Mirochnick M, Siminski S, Fenton T, et al. Nevirapine pharmacokinetics in pregnant women and in their infants after in utero exposure. Pediatr Infect Dis J. 2001;20:803-805.
182. Cunningham CK, Chaix ML, Rekacewicz C, et al. Development of resistance mutations in women receiving standard antiretroviral therapy who received intrapartum nevirapine to prevent perinatal human immunodeficiency virus type 1 transmission: A substudy of pediatric AIDS clinical trials group protocol 316. J Infect Dis. 2002;186:181-188.
183. Eshleman SH, Mracna M, Guay LA, et al. Selection and fading of resistance mutations in women and infants receiving nevirapine to prevent HIV-1 vertical transmission (HIVNET 012). AIDS. 2001;15:1951-1957.
183a. Antinori A, Zaccarelli M, Cingolani A, et al. Cross-resistance among nonnucleoside reverse transcriptase inhibitors limits recycling efavirenz after NVP failure. AIDS Res Hum Retroviruses. 2002;18:835-838.
183b. Jourdain G, Ngo-Giang-Huong N, Tungyai P, et al. Exposure to intrapartum single-dose nevirapine and subsequent maternal 6-month response to NNRTI-based regimens. Abstract 41LB. Presented at the Eleventh Conference on Retroviruses and Opportunistic Infections, San Francisco, Calif, February 2004.
183c. Hitti J, Frenkel L, Stek A, et al. Maternal toxicity with continuous nevirapine in pregnancy: Results from PACTG 1022. J Acquir Immun Defic Syndr 2004;36:772-776.
184. National Institute of Allergy and Infectious Disease, National Institutes of Health. Safety information of DMP-266. 1998.
185. Fundaro C, Genovese O, Rendeli C, et al. Myelomeningocele in a child with intrauterine exposure to efavirenz. AIDS. 2002;16:299-300.
186. FDA Public Health Advisory. Reports of diabetes and hyperglycemia in patients receiving protease inhibitors for the treatment of human immunodeficiency virus (HIV). JAMA. 1997;278:379.
187. Dube M, Johnson D, Currier J, et al. Protease inhibitor-associated hyperglycaemia (Letter). Lancet. 1997;350:713-714.
188. Visnegarwala F, Krause K, Musher D. Severe diabetes associated with protease inhibitor therapy (Letter). Ann Intern Med. 1997;127:947.
189. Chen JL, Philips KA, Kanouse DE, et al. Fertility desires and intentions of HIV-positive men and women. Fam Plann Perspect. 2001;33:144-152, 165.
190. Watts DH. Management of human immunodeficiency virus infection in pregnancy. N Engl J Med. 2002;346:1879-1891.
191. Centers for Disease Control and Prevention. 1997 USPHS/IDSA guidelines for the prevention of opportunistic infections in persons infected with human immunodeficiency virus. USPHS/IDSA Prevention of Opportunistic Infections Working Group. MMWR Morb Mortal Wkly Rep. 1997;46:1-46.
192. Bryson YJ. Perinatal HIV-1 transmission: Recent advances and therapeutic interventions. AIDS. 1996;3:S33-S42.
193. Carpenter CJC, Mayer KH, Stein MD, et al. Human immunodeficiency virus infection in North American women: Experience with 200 cases and a review of the literature. Medicine. 1991;70:307-325.
194. Clark RA, Brandon W, Dumestre J, et al. Clinical manifestations of infection with the human immunodeficiency virus in women in Louisiana. Clin Infect Dis. 1993;17: 173-177.
195. Greenberg AE, Thomas PA, Landesman SH, et al. The spectrum of HIV-1-related disease among outpatients in New York City. AIDS. 1992;6:849-859.
196. Clark RA, Kissinger P. Is gender associated with serious pyogenic infections diagnosed in HIV infected persons? Am J Epidemiol. 1995;141:176.
197. Centers for Disease Control. Revision of the CDC surveillance case definition for acquired immunodeficiency syndrome. MMWR Morbid Mortal Wkly Rep. 1987;36:3S-11S.
198. Fleming PJ, Ciesielski CA, Byers RH, et al. Gender differences in reported AIDS-indicative diagnoses. J Infect Dis. 1993;168:61-67.
199. Hessol NA, Preston-Martin S, Seaberg EC, et al. Increased incidence of cancer among participants in the women's interagency HIV study. Abstract ThPeC7482. Presented at Fourteenth International AIDS Conference, Barcelona, Spain, July 2002.
200. Phelps RM, Smith DK, Heilig CM, et al. Cancer incidence in women with or at risk for HIV. Int J Cancer. 2001;94:753-757.
201. Blair JM, Kovacs A, Beall G, et al. Kaposi's sarcoma in women with AIDS (abstract no. 106.4). Natl Conf Women HIV. 1997:109.
202. Cooley TP, Hirschhorn LR, O'Keane JC. Kaposi's sarcoma in women with AIDS. AIDS. 1996;10:1221-1225.
203. Haramati LB, Wong J. Intrathoracic Kaposi's sarcoma in women with AIDS. Chest. 2000;117:410-414.
204. Macasaet MA, Duerr A, Thelmo W, et al. Kaposi's sarcoma presenting as a vulvar mass. Obstet Gynecol. 1995;86:695-697.
205. Darai E, Vlastos G, Madelenat P. Acquired immunodeficiency syndrome-related Kaposi's sarcoma: Two cervical cases. Am J Obstet Gynecol. 1995:173:979.
206. Levine AM, Preston-Martin S, Fruchter R, et al. Unusual cases of breast cancer in HIV-infected women: Data from Women's Interagency HIV Study (WIHS) (abstract no. 123.1). Natl Conf Women HIV. 1997;123.
207. Rose PG, Fraire AE. Multiple gynecologic neoplasms in a young HIV-positive patient. J Surg Oncol. 1993;53:269-272.
208. Remick SC, Harper GR, Abdullah MA, et al. Metastatic breast cancer in a young patient seropositive for human immunodeficiency virus. J Natl Cancer Inst. 1991;83:447-448.
209. Spina M, Nasti G, Simonelli C, et al. Breast cancer in a woman with HIV infection: A case report. Ann Oncol. 1994;5:661-662.
210. Gachupin-Garcia A, Selwyn PA, Budner NS. Population-based study of malignancies and HIV infection among injecting drug users in a New York City methadone treatment program: 1985-1991. AIDS. 1992;6:843-848.
211. Mayer AP, Greenberg ML. FNB diagnosis of breast carcinoma associated with HIV infection: A case report and review of HIV-associated malignancy. Pathology. 1996;28: 90-95.
212. Guth AA. Breast cancer and HIV: What do we know? Am Surg. 1999;65:209-211.
213. Overbaugh J, Anderson RJ, Ndinya-Achola JO, et al. Distinct but related human immunodeficiency virus type 1 variant populations in genital secretions and blood. AIDS Res Hum Retroviruses. 1996;12:107-115.
214. Poss M, Martin HL, Kreiss JK, et al. Diversity in virus populations from genital secretions and peripheral blood from women recently infected with human immunodeficiency virus type 1. J Virol. 1995;69:8118-8122.
215. Monstad SB, Kreiss JK. Shedding HIV-1 in the genital tract. AIDS. 1996;10:1305-1315.
216. Monstad SB, Overbaugh J, DeVange DM, et al. Hormonal contraception, vitamin A deficiency, and other risk factors for cervical and vaginal shedding of HIV-1 infected cells. Lancet. 1997;350:922-927.
217. Mostad SB, Jackson S, Overbaugh J, et al. Cervical and vaginal shedding of human immunodeficiency virus type 1-infected cells throughout the menstrual cycle. J Infect Dis. 1998;178:983-991.
218. Clemetson DBA, Moss GB, Willerford D, et al. Detection of HIV DNA in cervical and vaginal secretions: Prevalence and correlates among women in Nairobi, Kenya. JAMA. 1993;269:2860-2864.
219. Kreiss J, Willerford D, Hensel M, et al. Association between cervical inflammation and cervical shedding of human immunodeficiency virus DNA. J Infect Dis. 1994;170:1597-1601.
220. Henin Y, Mandelbrot L, Henrion R, et al. Virus excretion in the cervicovaginal secretions of pregnant and nonpregnant HIV-infected women. J Acquir Immun Defic Syndr. 1993;6:72-75.
221. John GC, Nduati RW, Mbori-Ngacha D, et al. Genital shedding of human immunodeficiency virus type 1 DNA during pregnancy: Association with immunosuppression, abnormal cervical or vaginal discharge, and severe vitamin A deficiency. J Infect Dis. 1997;175:57-62.
222. Cu-Uvin S, Caliendo AM, Reinert S, et al. Effect of highly active antiretroviral therapy on cervicovaginal HIV-1 RNA. AIDS. 2000;14:415-421.
223. Kovacs A, Chan LS, Chun Chen Z, et al. HIV-1 RNA in plasma and genital tract secretions in women infected with HIV-1. J Acquir Immune Defic Syndr. 1999;22:124-131.
224. Ghys PD, Fransen K, Diallo MO, et al. The associations between cervicovaginal HIV shedding, sexually transmitted diseases and immunosuppression in female sex workers in Abidjan, Cote d'Ivoire. AIDS. 1997;11:F85-F93.
225. Wang CC, McClelland RS, Reilly M, et al. The effect of treatment of vaginal infections on shedding of human immunodeficiency virus type 1. J Infect Dis. 2001;183: 1017-1022.
226. Money D, Arikan Y, Remple V, et al. Genital tract and plasma HIV viral load throughout the menstrual cycle. Abstract 716. Presented at Eighth Conference on Retroviruses and Opportunistic Infections, Chicago, Ill, February 2001.
227. Cu-Uvin S, Hogan JW, Warren D, et al. Prevalence of lower genital tract infections among human immunodeficiency virus (HIV)-seropositive and high-risk HIV-seronegative women. Clin Infect Dis. 1999;29:1145-1150.
228. Warren D, Klein RS, Sobel J, et al. A multicenter study of bacterial vaginosis in women with or at risk for human immunodeficiency virus infection. Infect Dis Obstet Gynecol. 2001;9:133-141.
229. Jamieson DJ, Duerr A, Klein RS, et al. Longitudinal analysis of bacterial vaginosis: Findings from the HIV epidemiology research study. Obstet Gynecol. 2001;98:656-663.
230. Imam N, Carpenter CC, Mayer KH, et al. Hierarchical pattern of mucosal candida infections in HIV-seropositive women. Am J Med. 1990;89:142-146.
231. Duerr A, Sierra MF, Feldman J, et al. Immune compromise and prevalence of *Candida* vulvovaginitis in human immunodeficiency virus-infected women. Obstet Gynecol. 1997;90:252-256.
232. Shifrin E, Matityahyu D, Feldman J, et al. Determinants of incident vulvovaginal candidiasis in human immunodeficiency virus-positive women. Infect Dis Obstet Gynecol. 2000;8:176-180.
233. Rhoads JL, Wright DC, Redfield RR, et al. Chronic vaginal candidiasis in women with human immunodeficiency virus infection. JAMA. 1987;257:3105-3107.
234. Sobel JD. Vulvovaginal candidiasis: A comparison of HIV-positive and -negative women. Int J STD AIDS. 2002;13:358-362.
235. Dahl KM, Keath EJ, Powderly WG. Molecular epidemiology of mucosal candidiasis in HIV-positive women. AIDS Res Hum Retroviruses. 1997;13:485-491.
236. Schuman P, Capps L, Peng G, et al. Weekly fluconazole for the prevention of mucosal candidiasis in women with HIV infection. Ann Intern Med. 1997;126:689-696.
237. Vazquez JA, Sobel JD, Peng G, et al. Evolution of vaginal *Candida* species recovered from human immunodeficiency virus-infected women receiving fluconazole prophylaxis: The emergence of *Candida glabrata*? Clin Infect Dis. 1999;28:1025-1031.
238. Vazquez JA, Peng G, Sobel JD, et al. Evolution of antifungal susceptibility among *Candida* species isolates recovered from human immunodeficiency virus-infected women receiving fluconazole prophylaxis. Clin Infect Dis. 2001;33:1069-1075.

239. Centers for Disease Control. Sexually transmitted diseases treatment guidelines 2002. MMWR Morbid Mortal Wkly Rep. 2002;51:1-80.
240. Greenblatt RM, Bacchetti P, Barkan S, et al. Lower genital tract infections among HIV-infected and high-risk uninfected women. Sex Transm Dis. 1999;26:143-151.
241. Capps L, Peng G, Doyle M, et al. Sexually transmitted infections in women infected with the human immunodeficiency virus. Sex Transm Dis. 1998;25:443-447.
242. Niccolai LM, Kopicko JJ, Kassie A, et al. Incidence and predictors of reinfection with *Trichomonas vaginalis* in HIV-infected women. Sex Transm Dis. 2000;27:284-288.
243. Fuller C, Clark RA, Kissinger P, et al. Clinical manifestations of infection with human immunodeficiency virus among adolescents in Louisiana. J Adolesc Health. 1996;18:422-428.
244. Hoegsberg B, Abulafia O, Sedlis A, et al. Sexually transmitted diseases and human immunodeficiency virus infection among women with pelvic inflammatory disease. Am J Obstet Gynecol. 1990;163:1135-1139.
245. Korn AP, Landers DV, Green JR, et al. Pelvic inflammatory disease in human immunodeficiency virus-infected women. Obstet Gynecol. 1993;82:765-768.
246. Barbosa C, Macasaet M, Brockmann S, et al. Pelvic inflammatory disease and human immunodeficiency virus infection. Obstet Gynecol. 1997;89:65-70.
247. Irwin KL, Moorman AC, O'Sullivan MJ, et al. Influence of human immunodeficiency virus inflection on pelvic inflammatory disease. Obstet Gynecol. 2000;95:525-534.
248. Kamenga MC, De Cock KM, St. Louis ME, et al. The impact of human immunodeficiency virus infection on pelvic inflammatory disease: A case-control study in Abidjan, Ivory Coast. Am J Obstet Gynecol. 1995;172:919-925.
249. Cohen CR, Sinei S, Reilly M, et al. Effect of human immunodeficiency virus 1 infection upon acute salpingitis in a laparoscopic study. J Infect Dis. 1998;178:1352-1358.
250. Bukesi EA, Cohen CR, Stevens CE, et al. Effects of human immunodeficiency virus 1 infection on microbial origins of pelvic inflammatory disease and on efficacy of ambulatory oral therapy. Am J Obset Gynecol. 1999;18:1374-1381.
251. Moodley P, Wilkinson D, Connolly C, et al. *Trichomonas vaginalis* is associated with pelvic inflammatory disease in women infected with human immunodeficiency virus. Clin Infect Dis. 2002;15:519-522.
252. Manfredi R, Alampi G, Talo S, et al. Silent oophoritis due to cytomegalovirus in a patient with advanced HIV disease. Int J STD AIDS. 2000;11:410-412.
253. Shah PN, Barton SE. Vaginal cytomegalovirus infection in a woman with AIDS. Int J STD AIDS. 1993;4:346-347.
254. Giannacopoulos KCh, Hatzidaki EG, Papanicolaou NC, et al. Genital tuberculosis in a HIV-infected women: A case report. Eur J Obstet Gynecol Reprod Biol. 1998;80: 227-229.
255. Sun XW, Ellerbrock TV, Lungu O, et al. Human papillomavirus infection in human immunodeficiency virus-seropositive women. Obstet Gynecol. 1995;85:680-686.
256. Vermund SH, Kelley KF, Klein RS, et al. High risk of human papillomavirus infection and cervical squamous intrepithelial lesions among women with symptomatic human immunodeficiency virus infection. Am J Obstet Gynecol. 1991;165:392-400.
257. Hillemanns P, Ellerbrock TV, McPhillips S, et al. Prevalence of anal human papillomavirus infection and anal cytologic abnormalities in HIV-seropositive women. AIDS. 1996;10:1641-1647.
258. Laga M, Icenogle JP, Marsella R, et al. Genital papillomavirus infection and cervical dysplasia—opportunistic complications of HIV infection. Int J Cancer. 1992;50:45-48.
259. Chaisson MA, Ellerbrock TV, Bush TJ, et al. Increased prevalence of vulvovaginal condyloma and vulvar intraepithelial neoplasia in women infected with the human immunodeficiency virus. Obstet Gynecol. 1997;89:690-694.
260. Kreiss JK, Kiviat NB, Plummer FA, et al. Human immunodeficiency virus, human papillomavirus, and cervical intraepithelial neoplasia in Nairobi prostitutes. Sex Transm Dis. 1992;19:54-59.
261. Wright TC, Ellerbrock TV, Chiasson MA, et al. Cervical intraepithelial neoplasia in women infected with human immunodeficiency virus: Prevalence, risk factors, and validity of Papanicolaou smears. New York Cervical Disease Study. Obstet Gynecol. 1994;84:591-597.
262. Williams AB, Darragh TM, Vranizan K, et al. Anal and cervical human papillomavirus infection and risk of anal and cervical abnormalities in human immunodeficiency virus-infected women. Obstet Gynecol. 1994;83:205-211.
263. Korn A, Landers DV. Gynecological disease in women infected with human immunodeficiency virus type 1. J Acquir Immune Defic Syndr. 1995;9:361-370.
264. Sha BE, Benson CA, Pottage JC, et al. HIV infection in women: An observational study of clinical characteristics, disease progression, and survival for a cohort of women in Chicago. J Acquir Immune Defic Syndr. 1995;8:486-495.
265. Massad LS, Riester KA, Anastos KM, et al. Prevalence and predictors of squamous cell abnormalities in Papanicolaou smears from women infected with HIV-1. J Acquir Immune Defic Syndr. 1999;21:33-41.
266. Moscicki AB, Ellenberg JH, Vermund SH, et al. Prevalence of and risks for cervical human papillomavirus infection and squamous intrepithelial lesions in adolescent girls: Impact of infection with human immunodeficiency virus. Arch Pediatr Adolesc Med. 2000;154:127-134.
267. Delmas MC, Larsen C, Van Benthem B, et al. Cervical squamous intraepithelial lesions in HIV-infected women: Prevalence, incidence and regression. European Study Group on Natural History of HIV Infection in Women. AIDS. 2000;18:1775-1784.
268. Maiman M, Tarricone N, Vieira J, et al. Colposcopic evaluation of HIV infected women. Obstet Gynecol. 1991;78:84-88.
269. Luque A, Demeter L, Reichman R. Association of human papillomavirus infection and disease with magnitude of human immunodeficiency virus type 1 (HIV-1) RNA plasma level among women with HIV-1 infection. J Infect Dis. 1999;179:1405-1409.
270. Massad LS, Riester KA, Anastos KM, et al. Prevalence and predictors of squamous cell abnormalities in Papanicolaou smears from women infected with HIV-1. Women's Interagency HIV Study Group. J Acquir Immune Defic Syndr. 1999;21: 33-41.
271. French AL, Kirstein LM, Massad LS, et al. Association of vitamin A deficiency with cervical squamous intraepithelial lesions in human immunodeficiency virus-infected women. J Infect Dis. 2000;182:1084-1089.
272. Centers for Disease Control: Risk for cervical disease in HIV infected women—New York City. MMWR Morbid Mortal Wkly Rep. 1990;39:846-849.
273. Sun XW, Kuhn L, Ellerbrock TV, et al. Human papillomavirus infection in women infected with human immunodeficiency virus. N Engl J Med. 1997;337:1343-1349.
274. Ahdieh L, Klein RS, Burk R, et al. Prevalence, incidence, and type-specific persistence of human papillomavirus in human immunodeficiency virus (HIV)-positive and HIV-negative women. J Infect Dis. 2001;184:682-690.
275. Belafsky P, Clark RA, Kissinger P, et al. Natural history of low-grade squamous intraepithelial lesions in women infected with human immunodeficiency virus. J Acquir Immune Defic Syndr. 1996;11:511-512.
276. Biggers SD, LaGuardia KD. The natural history of low grade squamous intraepithelial lesions of the cervix in women with human immunodeficiency virus infection: Evidence for an algorithm for management. Abstract no. Th.B.4138. Presented at Eleventh International Conference on AIDS. Vancouver, Canada, 1996.
277. Olaitan A, Mocroft A, McCArthy K, et al. Cervical abnormality and sexually transmitted disease screening in human immunodeficiency virus-positive women. Obstet Gynecol. 1997;89:71-75.
278. Six C, Heard I, Bergeron C, et al. Comparative prevalence, incidence and short-term prognosis of cervical squamous intraepithelial lesions amongst HIV-positive and HIV-negative women. AIDS. 1998;12:1047-1056.
279. Robinson WR, Andersen J, Darragh TM, et al. Isotretinoin for low-grade cervical dysplasia in human immunodeficiency virus-infected women. Obstet Gynecol. 2002;99:777-784.
280. Massad LS, Ahdieh L, Benning L, et al. Evolution of cervical abnormalities among women with HIV-1: Evidence from surveillance cytology in the women's interagency HIV study. J Acquir Immune Defic Syndr. 2001;27:432-442.
281. Wright TC, Koulos J, Schnoll F, et al. Cervical intrepithelial neoplasia in human immunodeficiency virus-seropositive women. Obstet Oncol. 1994;55:253-258.
282. Maiman M, Fruchter RG, Serur E, et al. Recurrent cervical intraepithelial neoplasia in human immunodeficiency virus-seropositive women. Obstet Gynecol. 1993;82:170-174.
283. Boardman LA, Peipert JE, Hogan JW, et al. Positive cone biopsy specimen margins in women infected with the human immunodeficiency virus. Am J Obstet Gynecol. 1999;181:1395-1399.
284. Maiman M, Watts DH, Andersen J, et al. Vaginal 5-fluorouracil for high-grade dysplasia in human immunodeficiency virus infection: A randomized trial. Obstet Gynecol. 1999;94:954-961.
285. Maiman M, Fuchter RG, Clark M, et al. Cervical cancer as an AIDS-defining illness. Obstet Gynecol. 1997;89:76-80.
286. Maiman M, Fruchter RG, Serur E, et al. Human immunodeficiency virus infection and cervical neoplasia. Gynecol Oncol. 1990;38:377-382.
287. Klevens RM, Fleming PL, Mays MA, et al. Characteristics of women with AIDS and invasive cervical cancer. Obstet Gynecol. 1996;88:269-273.
288. Maiman M, Fruchter RG, Guy L, et al. Human immunodeficiency virus infection and invasive cervical carcinoma. Cancer. 1993;71:402-406.
289. Heard I, Schmitz V, Costagliola D, et al. Early regression of cervical lesions in HIV-seropositive women receiving highly active antiretroviral therapy. AIDS. 1998;12:1459-1464.
290. Lillo FB, Ferrari D, Veglia F, et al. Human papillomavirus infection and associated cervical disease in human immunodeficiency virus-infected women: Effect of highly active antiretroviral therapy. J Infect Dis. 2001;184:547-551.
291. Luque AE, Li H, Demeter LM, et al. Effect of antiretroviral therapy on human papillomavirus infection and disease among HIV-infected women (abstract no. 724). Conf Retroviruses Opportunistic Infect. 2001;8:262.
292. Duerr A, Jamieson D, Cu-Uvin S, et al. Effect of highly active antiretroviral therapies on Pap smear abnormalities. Abstract no. MoPeB2245. Presented at the Thirteenth International Conference on AIDS, Durban, South Africa, July 9-14, 2000.
293. Money D, Hankins C, Rachlis A, et al. HAART and evolution of abnormal cervical cytology in women with HIV. Abstract WePeB5969. Presented at Fourteenth International AIDS Conference, Barcelona, Spain, 2002.
294. Ellerbrock TV, Chiasson MA, Bush TJ, et al. Incidence of cervical squamous intraepithelial lesions in HIV-infected women. JAMA. 2000;283:1031-1037.
295. Centers for Disease Control. 1993 Sexually transmitted diseases treatment guidelines. MMWR Morbid Mortal Wkly Rep. 1993;42(RR14):14.
296. Wright TC, Moscarelli RD, Dole P, et al. Significance of mild cytologic atypia in women infected with human immunodeficiency virus. Obstet Gynecol. 1996;87:515-519.
297. Holcomb K, Abulafia O, Matthews RP, et al. The significance of ASCUS cytology in HIV-positive women. Gynecol Oncol. 1999;75:118-121.
298. Palefsky JM, Holly EA, Ralston ML, et al. Prevalence and risk factors for anal human papillomavirus infection in human immunodeficiency virus-positive and high-risk HIV-negative women. J Infect Dis. 2001;183:383-391.
299. Conley LJ, Ellerbrock T, Bush TJ, et al. HIV-1 infection and risk of vulvovaginal and perianal condylomata acuminata and intraepithelial neoplasia in women infected: A prospective study. Lancet. 2002;359:108-113.
300. Sobel JD. Gynecologic infections in human immunodeficiency virus-infected women. Clin Infect Dis. 2000;31:1225-1233.
301. Schuman P, Christensen C, Sobel J. Aphthous vaginal ulceration in two women with AIDS. Am J Obstet Gynecol. 1990;14:1660-1663.
302. Covino JM, McCormack WM. Vulvar ulcer of unknown etiology in a human immunodeficiency virus-infected woman: Response to treatment with zidovudine. Am J Obstet Gynecol. 1990;153:116-118.

303. Anderson J, Clark RA, Watts H, et al. Idiopathic genital ulcers in women infected with human immunodeficiency virus. J Acquir Immune Defic Syndr. 1996;13:343-347.

304. Schuman P, Sobel JD, Christensen C. Aphthous vaginal ulceration in two women with acquired immunodeficiency syndrome. Am J Obstet Gynecol. 1996;174:1660-1663.

305. LaGuardia KD, White M, Saigo PE, et al. Genital ulcer disease in women infected with human immunodeficiency virus infection. Am J Obstet Gynecol. 1995;172:553-562.

306. Verberkmoes A, Boer K, Wertheim PM, et al. Thalidomide for genital ulcer in HIV-positive women. Lancet. 1996;347:974.

307. Friedmann W, Schafer A, Kretschmer R, et al. Disseminated cytomegalovirus infection of the female genital tract. Gynecol Obstet Invest. 1991;31:56-57.

308. Walker N. Cervical cytomegalovirus infection in a women with AIDS. Clin Infect Dis. 1997;25:930-931.

309. Sewell CA, Anderson JR. Cytomegalovirus disease in the lower female genital tract. AIDS Patient Care STDs. 2001;15:459-462.

310. Shelton M, Adams J, Gugino L, et al. Menstrual cycle hormone patterns in HIV-infected women. Presented at Third Conference on Retroviruses and Opportunistic Infections, Washington, DC, 1996.

311. Chirgwin KD, Feldman J, Muneyyirci-Delale O, et al. Menstrual function in human immunodeficiency virus-infected women without acquired immunodeficiency syndrome. J Acquir Immune Defic Syndr. 1996;12:489-494.

312. Harlow SD, Schuman P, Cohen M, et al. Effect of HIV infection on menstrual cycle length. J Acquir Immune Defic Syndr. 2000;24:68-75.

313. Ellerbrock TV, Wright TC, Bush T, et al. Characteristics of menstruation in women infected with human immunodeficiency virus. Obstet Gynecol. 1996;87:1030-1034.

314. Shah PN, Smith JR, Wells C, et al. Menstrual symptoms in women infected by the human immunodeficiency virus. Obstet Gynecol. 1994;83:397-400.

315. Greenblat RM, Ameli N, Grant RM, et al. Impact of the ovulatory cycle on virologic and immunologic markers in HIV-infected women. J Infect Dis. 2000;181:82-90.

316. Bakos O, Lundkvist O, Wide L, et al. Ultrasonographical and hormonal description of the normal ovulatory menstrual cycle. Acta Obstet Gynecol Scand. 1994;73:790-796.

317. Waller K, Swan S, Windham G, et al. Use of urine biomarkers to evaluate menstrual function in healthy premenopausal women. Am J Epidemiol. 1998;147:1071-1080.

318. Clark RA, Mulligan K, Stamenovic E, et al. Frequency of anovulation and early menopause among women enrolled in selected AIDS clinical trials group studies. J Infect Dis. 2001;184:1325-1327.

319. Gates EJ, Diaz-Arrastia C, DiMaio T, et al. Non-Hodgkin lymphoma of the endometrium in human immunodeficiency virus infection. Obstet Gynecol. 1997;90:697-699.

320. Nielsen H. Hypermenorrhoea associated with ritonavir. Lancet. 1999;353:811-812.

321. Clark RA, Cohn S, Jarek C, et al. Perimenopausal symptomatology among HIV-infected women at least 40 years of age. J Acquir Immune Defic Syndr. 2000;23:99-100.

322. Hadigan C, Miller K, Corcoran C, et al. Fasting hyperinsulinemia and changes in regional body composition in human immunodeficiency virus-infected women. J Clin Endocrinol Metab. 1999;84:1932-1937.

323. Dong KL, Bausserman LL, Flynn MM, et al. Changes in body habitus and serum lipid abnormalities in HIV-positive women on highly active antiretroviral therapy (HAART). J Acquir Immune Defic Syndr. 1999;21:107-113.

324. Gervasoni C, Ridolfo AL, Trifiro G, et al. Redistribution of body fat in HIV-infected women undergoing combination antiretroviral therapy. AIDS. 1999;13:465-471.

325. Pernerstorfer-Schoen H, Jilma B, Perschler A, et al. Sex differences in HAART-associated dyslipidaemia. AIDS. 2001;15:725-734.

326. Boxwell DE, Styrt BA. Lactic acidosis in patients receiving nucleoside reverse transcriptase inhibitors. Abstract 1284. Presented at Thirty-ninth Interscience Conference on Antimicrobial Agents and Chemotherapy, San Francisco, Calif, 1999.

327. Bristol Myers Squibb Company. Healthcare provider important drug warning letter. January 5, 2001.

328. Tebas P, Powderly WG, Claxton S, et al. Accelerated bone mineral loss in HIV-infected patients receiving potent antiretroviral therapy. AIDS. 2000;14:F63-67.

329. McDermott AY, Shevitz A, Knox T, et al. Effect of highly active antiretroviral therapy on fat, lean, and bone mass in HIV-seropositive men and women. Am J Clin Nutr. 2001;74:679-686.

330. Brown T, Timpone J, Ruppe M, et al. Bone loss associated with abnormalities in glucose metabolism in HIV patients on protease inhibitors. Abstract 317-T. Presented at Ninth Conference on Retroviruses and Opportunistic Infections, Seattle, Wash, 2000.

331. Arnsten JH, Freeman R, Santoro N, et al. Bone mineral density and protease inhibitor use in older HIV-infected women. Abstract 717-T. Presented at Ninth Conference on Retroviruses and Opportunistic Infections, Seattle, Wash, 2000.

332. Wit FW, Weverling GJ, Weel J, et al. Incidence of and risk factors for severe hepatotoxicity associated with antiretroviral combination therapy. J Infect Dis. 2002;186:23-31.

333. Sanne I. Severe liver toxicity in patients receiving two nucleoside analogues and a non-nucleoside reverse transcriptase inhibitor. AIDS. 2000;14(Suppl 4):S12.

334. Barlett J. Severe liver toxicity in patients receiving two nucleoside analogues and a non-nucleoside reverse transcriptase inhibitor. Abstract 19. Presented at Eighth Conference on Retroviruses and Opportunistic Infections, Chicago, Ill, February 2001.

335. Bersoff-Matcha SJ, Miller WC, Aberg JA, et al. Sex difference in nevirapine rash. Clin Infect Dis. 2001;32:124-129.

336. Antinori A, Baldini F, Girardi E, et al. Female sex and the use of anti-allergic agents increase the risk of developing cutaneous rash associated with nevirapine therapy. AIDS. 2001;15:1579-1581.

337. Friedland GH, Saltzman B, Vileno J, et al. Survival differences in patients with AIDS. J Acquir Immun Defic Syndr. 1991;4:144-153.

338. Rothenberg R, Woelfel M, Stoneburner R, et al. Survival with the acquired immunodeficiency syndrome. N Engl J Med. 1997;317:1297-1302.

339. Chaisson RE, Keruly JC, Moore RD. Race, sex, drug use, and progression of HIV disease. N Engl J Med. 1995;333:751-756.

340. Melnick S, Shere R, Louis TA, et al. Survival and disease progression according to gender of patients with HIV infection. JAMA. 1993;272;1915-1921.

341. Flanigan TP, Imam N, Lange N, et al. Decline of CD4 lymphocyte counts from the time of seroconversion in HIV-positive women. J Women Health. 1992;1:231-234.

342. Mocroft A, Gill MJ, Davidson W, et al. Are there gender differences in starting protease inhibitors, HAART, and disease progression despite equal access to care? J Acquir Immune Defic Syndr. 2000;24:475-482.

343. Moore AL, Sabin CA, Johnson MA, et al. Gender and clinical outcomes after starting highly active antiretroviral treatment: A cohort study. Aquir Immune Defic Syndr. 2002;29:197-202.

344. Hellinger FJ. The use of health services by women with HIV infection. Health Serv Res. 1993;28:543-561.

345. Poundstone KE, Chaisson RE, Moore RD. Differences in HIV disease progression by injection drug use and by sex in the era of highly active antiretroviral therapy. AIDS. 2001;15:1115-1123.

346. Farzadegan H, Hoover DR, Astemborski J, et al. Sex differences in HIV-1 viral load and progression to AIDS. Lancet. 1998;352:1510-1514.

347. Sterling TR, Lyles CM, Vlahov D, et al. Sex differences in longitudinal human immunodeficiency virus type 1 RNA levels among seroconverters. J Infect Dis. 1999;180:666-672.

348. Sterling TR, Vlahov D, Atemborski J, et al. Initial HIV-1 RNA level and progression to AIDS in women and men. N Engl J Med. 2001;334:720-725.

349. Evans JS, Nims T, Cooley J, et al. Serum levels of virus burden in early-stage human immunodeficiency virus type 1 disease in women. J Infect Dis. 1997;175:795-800.

350. Junghans C, Ledergerber B, Chan P, et al. Sex differences in HIV-1 viral load and progression to AIDS. Swiss HIV Cohort Study. Lancet. 1999;353:589.

351. Moroni M: Sex differences in HIV-1 viral load and progression to AIDS. ICONA Study Group. Italian Cohort of HIV-1 positive individuals. Lancet. 1999;353:589-590.

352. Moore RD, Cheever L, Keruly JC, et al. Lack of sex difference in CD4 to HIV-1 RNA viral load ratio. Lancet. 1999;353:464.

353. Anastos K, Gange SJ, Lau B, et al. Gender specific differences in quantitative HIV-1 RNA levels. Abstract 274. Presented at Sixth Conference on Retroviruses and Opportunistic Infections, Chicago, Ill, 1999.

354. Clark RA, Brandon W, Rice J, et al. Predictors of HIV disease progression in women. J Acquir Immune Defic Syndr. 1995;9:43-50.

355. Lindan CP, Allen S, Serufilira A, et al. Predictors of mortality among HIV infected women in Kigali, Rwanda. Ann Intern Med. 1992;116:320-328.

356. Anastos K, Kovacs A, Kalish L, et al. Quantitative HIV-1 RNA and other factors associated with survival in the Women's Interagency HIV Study (WIHS). Abstract no. 207. Presented at Fifth Conference on Retroviruses and Opportunistic Infections, Chicago, Ill, 1998.

357. Anastos K, Barron Y, Miotti P, et al. Risk of progression to AIDS and death in women infected with HIV-1 initiating highly active antiretroviral treatment at different stages of disease. Arch Intern Med. 2002;162:1973-1980.

358. Bessinger R, Clark R, Kissinger P, et al. Pregnancy is not associated with the progression of HIV disease in women attending an HIV outpatient program. Am J Epidemiol. 1998;147:434-440.

359. Dunn DT, Newell ML, Ades AE, et al. Risk of human immunodeficiency virus type 1 transmission through breastfeeding. Lancet. 1992;340:585-588.

360. Berrebia A, Kobuch WE, Puel J, et al. Influence of pregnancy on human immunodeficiency virus disease. Eur J Obstet Gynecol Reprod Biol. 1990;37:211-217.

361. Weisser M, Rudin C, Bettegay M, et al. Does pregnancy influence the course of HIV infection? Evidence from two large Swiss cohort studies. J Acquir Immune Defic Syndr Hum Retrovirol. 1998;17:404-410.

362. Minkoff HL, Henderson C, Mendez H, et al. Pregnancy outcomes among mothers infected with HIV and uninfected control subjects. Am J Obstet Gynecol. 1990;163:1598-1604.

363. Stein MD, Liebman B, Waachtel TJ, et al. HIV-positive women: Reasons they are tested for HIV and their clinical characteristics on entry into health care system. J Gen Intern Med. 1991;6:286-289.

364. Hogan AJ, Soloman DJ, Boukight RR, et al. Under-utilization of medical care services by HIV-infected women? Some preliminary results from Michigan Medicaid Program. AIDS. 1991;5:338-339.

365. Butz AM, Hutton N, Joyner M, et al. HIV-infected women and infants: Social and health factors impeding utilization of health care. J Nurse Midwifery. 1993;38:103-109.

366. Lowinson JH, Ruiz P, Millman RB, et al. Substance Abuse. Baltimore: Williams & Wilkins; 1992:734-788.

367. Centers for Disease Control. Summary of all the reports on HIV and AIDS. Available at: http://www.cdc.gov/hiv/pubs/facts.htm. Accessed July 11, 2003.

368. Kissinger P, Clark RA, Rice J, et al. Evaluation of a program to remove barriers to public health care for women with HIV infection. South Med J. 1995;88:1121-1125.

369. Fuller C, Clark RA, Kissinger P, et al. Clinical manifestations of infection with human immunodeficiency virus among adolescents in Louisiana. J Adolesc Health. 1996;18:422-428.

370. Kissinger P, Fuller C, Clark RA, et al. Psychosocial characteristics of HIV-infected adolescents in New Orleans. J Adolesc Health. 1997;20:258.

371. Hein K, Dell R, Futterman D, et al. Comparison of HIV+ and HIV− adolescents: Risk factors and psychosocial determinants. Pediatrics. 1995;95:96-104.

372. Flexner C. HIV-protease inhibitors. N Engl J Med. 1998;338:1281-1282.

373. Sinei SK, Morrison CS, Sekadde-Kigondu S, et al. Complications of use of intrauterine devices among HIV-1-infected women. Lancet. 1998;351:1238-1241.

374. Stafford MK, Ward H, Flanagan A, et al. Safety study of nonoxynol 9 as a vaginal microbicide: Evidence of adverse effects. J Acquir Immune Defic Syndr Hum Retrovirol. 1998;17:327-331.

375. Schneider DJ, Kloser P. HIV disease in the older inner-city women. Presented at Eighth International Conference on AIDS, Amsterdam, The Netherlands, 1992.

376. Clark RA, Bessinger R. Clinical manifestations and predictors of survival in older women infected with HIV. J Acquir Immune Defic Syndr. 1997;15:341-345.

377. Laine C, Markson LE, McKee LJ, et al. The relationship of clinic experience with advanced HIV and survival of women with AIDS. AIDS. 1998;12:417-424.

378. Sha BE, Benson CA, Pottage JC, et al. HIV infection in women: An observational study of clinical characteristics, disease progression, and survival for a cohort of women in Chicago. J Acquir Immune Defic. 1995;8:486-495.

379. Currier JS, Spino C, Grimes J, et al. Differences between women and men in adverse events and CD4+ responses to nucleoside analogue therapy for HIV infection. The Aids Clinical Trials Group 175 Team. J Acquir Immune Defic Syndr. 2000;24:316-324.

CHAPTER **123**

Pediatric Human Immunodeficiency Virus Infection

GEOFFREY A. WEINBERG

SANDRA K. BURCHETT

The epidemic of acquired immunodeficiency syndrome (AIDS) was first recognized in adults in the United States in 1981, although sporadic cases in the United States and Europe had occurred since at least the mid-1970s.[1-5] In retrospect, it is known that pediatric cases occurred almost as early as adult cases.[6-9] The infection has now reached pandemic proportions in many areas of the world.[10] In the United States, human immunodeficiency virus (HIV) infection and AIDS occur primarily (99%) in adults; globally, pediatric HIV infections were responsible for at least 6% of prevalent infections, 14% of incident infections, and 17% of deaths in calendar year 2003.[10-12]

Although the pathogenesis of HIV infection and the general virologic and immunologic principles underlying the use of antiretroviral therapy are similar for HIV-infected children and adults, unique considerations apply to infants, children, and adolescents. These include (1) the acquisition of infection through perinatal exposure for the vast majority of children (i.e., a primary infection acquired in the context of an immature immune system); (2) in utero exposure to antiretroviral medications; (3) differences in immunologic markers, viral load, and serologic diagnostic strategies in young infants; (4) changes in pharmacokinetic parameters with age; (5) considerations related to the formulation and palatability of medications; and (6) issues of adherence in infants and young children dependent on others for medication administration, and in adolescents facing adherence challenges from developmental issues including peer pressure. This chapter addresses the salient pediatric-specific issues in the epidemiology, diagnosis, clinical manifestations, and treatment of pediatric HIV infection.

EPIDEMIOLOGY

The Joint United Nations Programme on HIV/AIDS (UNAIDS) and the World Health Organization (WHO) estimated that, as of December 2003, there were 2.5 million children younger than 15 years of age living with HIV/AIDS worldwide. Additionally, it is estimated that 700,000 children became infected with HIV, and 500,000 children died of AIDS in 2003.[12] It is hoped that the lessons learned in the United States and the industrialized world, where newly acquired pediatric HIV infection has become infrequent, will help to turn the tide of the global pandemic.

United States

In most states, only pediatric AIDS, as opposed to HIV infection, is reportable. From the beginning of reporting efforts in 1981 through 2002, a total of 9300 cases of AIDS in children younger than 13 years of age were reported to the Centers for Disease Control and Prevention (CDC), most among children of color (59% blacks, 23% Hispanic, 17% white),[11] and most in New York, New Jersey, Florida, California, and Texas. The mode of infection for 93% of the cases of pediatric AIDS in 2002 was vertical: mother-to-child transmission (MTCT). The remaining 7% of cases were accounted for by transfusion of blood components, sexual abuse or assault, and, very rarely, household, school, child care, hospital or clinic exposure.[13-15] Breast-feeding remains a possible mode of transmission; hence, the recommendation contraindicating the use of breast milk from HIV-infected mothers in countries where infant formula is easily available.[12,16,17] Fewer than 1% of cases have been reported to have no identifiable risk factor.[11]

To prevent MTCT, it is important to understand the epidemiology of HIV infection in women of childbearing age so that appropriate preventive or treatment strategies can be designed. As reported by the CDC in 2000, 45% of mothers of children with AIDS reported heterosexual contact as the primary risk behavior for their own HIV acquisition, consistent with the general rise worldwide in heterosexual transmission. In the 5 years after antenatal and neonatal zidovudine prophylaxis[18] was implemented as the standard of care in the United States for HIV-seropositive pregnant women, the number of pediatric AIDS cases reported in the United States decreased by 86% among infants younger than 1 year of age, and by 78% in children aged 1 to 5 years.[19] These changes reflected a clear success in decreasing perinatal transmission as well as better antiretroviral therapy and prophylactic medications to prevent progression of HIV infection to AIDS. Only 50 infants younger than 1 year of age were reported with AIDS in 2002,[11] an affirmation that the combination of clinical investigation, public health policy implementation, and continued antiretroviral drug development has in fact sharply curtailed the rate of perinatally acquired pediatric HIV/AIDS in the United States (Fig. 123-1). Domestic preventive efforts continue to focus on offering HIV counseling and testing as part of routine prenatal care, with rapid initiation of antiretroviral therapy for seropositive women (see Chapter 122). A retrospective review of New York state data showed that preventive prophylactic benefit can still be seen if the perinatal zidovudine regimen is not begun until labor and delivery or even as late as within the first postnatal 48 hours.[20] Programs in other states have dramatically reduced

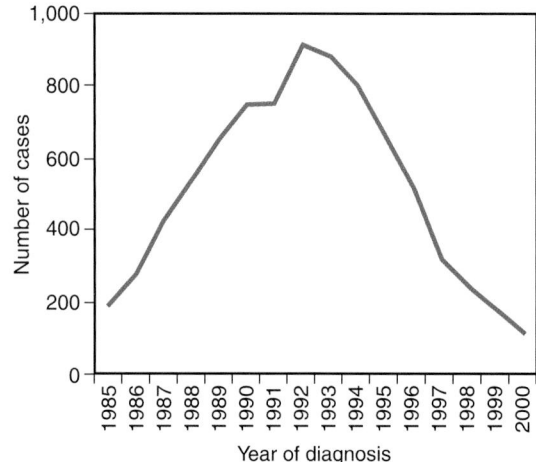

FIGURE 123-1. Perinatally acquired AIDS cases in the United States, by year of diagnosis, 1985-2000. Note: Data adjusted for reporting delays and for estimated proportional redistribution of cases reported without a risk; data reported through December 2001.

the numbers of infected infants as well.[21] Although early identification of asymptomatic infected infants enables initiation of treatment that can avert progression to AIDS, prevention of MTCT is clearly preferred. In order not to miss any opportunities for prevention of MTCT, antenatal counseling must routinely be offered, and it must be made easy to request and to obtain. Antenatal counseling allows antiretroviral therapy to be initiated in all seropositive pregnancies, regardless of HIV viral load or CD4$^+$ T-lymphocyte count, and leads to the prevention of transmission of HIV from otherwise undiagnosed seropositive women via breast-feeding.

Worldwide

Western Europe has seen a pattern of pediatric HIV/AIDS similar to that of the United States: an eventual rise in the proportion of children infected via MTCT occurred after both the increase in HIV prevalence in the heterosexual population and the initiation of screening of blood products. Eastern Europe has a very different epidemiologic pattern, with as many as 80% of HIV-infected persons being younger than 30 years of age, predominately in the injection drug–using group, in whom lack of condom use is prominent. In the latter situation, there was a more dramatic and immediate rise in pediatric HIV/AIDS due to MTCT, simultaneous with the spread of HIV through heterosexual transmission.

Similarly, in some Asian countries such as India and China, a rapidly increasing seroprevalence among commercial sex workers and injection drug users was quickly followed by an increase in pediatric HIV infection via MTCT. In China, there also have been isolated pockets of infection in which unsafe blood collection practices have contributed more significantly to pediatric HIV infection. The seroprevalence among young adults in Cambodia, Myanmar, and Thailand approaches 1% to 3%.

The estimates of the numbers of children younger than 15 years of age with HIV/AIDS in the African countries are staggering. These cases are almost exclusively caused by MTCT, with some contribution from transfusion with contaminated blood products. MTCT is particularly problematic in sub-Saharan Africa, where the epidemic has three patterns. First, in the countries affected earliest by HIV, seropositivity in antenatal clinics has reached a plateau: 40% in Botswana, 18% in Mozambique, and 25% in South Africa. A second pattern is represented by Uganda, the only sub-Saharan African country in which seroprevalence has clearly declined (from as much as 30% to as low as 8%), most likely in part because of intense efforts at prevention of MTCT. Finally, a few countries still exhibit a relatively low seroprevalence (e.g., 1% in Senegal); these countries began preventive efforts in the antenatal clinics at a time when the nationwide seroprevalence was low.[12]

Mother-to-Child Transmission

The reader is referred to Chapter 122 for further discussion of perinatal transmission including timing of infection; however, a few essential points are reiterated here. The MTCT rate is estimated to range from 13% to 39% for infants born throughout the world to HIV-seropositive women who did not receive antiretroviral therapy during pregnancy or intrapartum.[22,23] In the United States, the transmission rate decreased from 25% to 8% in 1995, after incorporation of an antenatal, intrapartum, and neonatal regimen of zidovudine (PACTG 076) into standard-of-care guidelines.[18,24] Currently, the rate of MTCT in the United States is less than 2%.[15,25] Correlates of MTCT include HIV viral load greater than 1000 copies/mL, low CD4$^+$ T-cell count, prolonged rupture of membranes, preterm delivery, delivery after initiation of labor or ruptured membranes, concomitant genital ulcerative disease, and seroconversion during pregnancy.[22,23,26-29] In vaginal deliveries, a firstborn twin is at greater risk for HIV infection than is a secondborn twin, although this relationship may not hold true in developing countries.[30-32] Prevention of transmission by cesarean section has been suggested by several, but not all, studies.[33-36] It is clear that vertical transmission is most significantly reduced by the use of antiretroviral therapy (including zidovudine) in pregnant women and their newborn infants (see Chapter 122).[18,22,24]

Despite this knowledge, many large pediatric HIV treatment centers continue to diagnose cases of pediatric HIV, almost exclusively in children whose mothers were not known to be HIV infected antenatally or at delivery, highlighting the difficulty of obtaining universal antenatal testing.

The majority of MTCT occurs at or just before delivery (50%), with an additional 25% occurring antenatally and 25% postnatally through breast-feeding.[16,23,26] Preventive therapies and other measures have differential effects depending on the stage of pregnancy in which they are applied. Table 123-1 summarizes salient features of several completed national and international trials of MTCT prevention. Most trials of zidovudine with or without other agents such as nevirapine or lamivudine have shown an efficacy of at least 50%, compared with placebo, in the reduction of MTCT among non–breast-feeding women. Appropriately designed antenatal antiretroviral therapy attempts to both optimize maternal health and target antenatal and intrapartum transmission.[15,22,25,37-39] Therefore, where the funding and infrastructure for early diagnosis and initiation of maternal antiretroviral treatment of prophylaxis exist, this should become the standard of care. Interventions held until delivery have no effect on those infants already infected in utero but can reduce the rate of intrapartum transmission.[38,40]

Finally, the rate of infection among infants of seropositive women who breastfeed is greater than that among infants of non–breast-feeding women, despite MTCT prophylaxis.[14,16,17] HIV has been detected in both the cellular and the cell-free fractions of human breast milk, and breast-feeding has been implicated in the transmission of HIV infection.[16,17,41-43] A high maternal plasma viral concentration (load) may also be a factor in the frequency of transmission by breast-feeding.[16,17,29,42,43] Women should be strongly encouraged to choose an alternative to breast-feeding if safe and nutritionally replete formulas are available. At present, active research is focused on defining safer practices (e.g., early weaning) in developing countries without these alternatives.[14,16,17]

Although the majority of data suggest that there are no immediate adverse outcomes in the fetus or newborn after MTCT prophylaxis, research continues to evaluate the long-term effects of antiretroviral exposure in these infants. Blanche and co-workers[44] reported on eight infants, two of whom died, who were thought to have mitochondrial toxicity caused by exposure to MTCT antiretroviral prophylaxis. This preliminary report prompted an intensive review of larger databases from five cohorts.[45] Among more than 20,000 children born to HIV-infected women—of whom more than half received prophylactic nucleoside analogue reverse transcriptase inhibitors (NRTIs)—223 children died. Only three of these deaths were thought to be possibly related to a mitochondrial abnormality, and none was highly suggestive of such an etiology.[45] At present, the proven benefit of antiretroviral prophylaxis in preventing an as yet incurable infection would seem to outweigh the risks entailed by in utero or neonatal exposure to antiretroviral drugs.

Adolescents

Although there has been remarkable success in reducing new perinatal HIV infections through aggressive MTCT prevention programs, the total number of reported cases of AIDS in adolescents continues to increase, and the acquisition of HIV infection during adolescence significantly contributes to the large number of cases in young adults. If the average incubation period of adult AIDS is 5 to 10 years, then all of the roughly 40,000 individuals diagnosed with AIDS between the ages of 15 to 24 years (4% of the total U.S. case number), and a large portion of those with AIDS at ages 25 to 31 years (34% of the U.S. case number), may be assumed to have initially acquired their HIV infection as adolescents. Routes of transmission of HIV in adolescents are similar to those in adults: sexual contact or injection drug use. It is imperative to focus preventive efforts on this population in the United States.

TABLE 123-1 Design and Results of Completed Trials of Antiretroviral Prophylaxis for Prevention of Mother-to-Child HIV Transmission (MTCT)

| Trial (Location) | Breast-feeding | Antiretroviral Therapy | | | | Point Estimates of MTCT (%) | Relative Efficacy vs Placebo (%) |
		Antepartum (Initiation Date, Wk of Pregnancy)	Intrapartum	Postpartum, Maternal (Duration)	Postpartum, Infant (Duration)		
PACTG 076 (United States, France)	No	ZDV (14-34)	ZDV	None	ZDV (6 wk)	ZDV: 8.3 Placebo: 25.5	68
Bangkok/CDC (Thailand)	No	ZDV (36)	ZDV	None	None	ZDV: 9.4 Placebo: 18.9	50
Thailand Perinatal Trial (Thailand)	No	Long-long arm: ZDV (28)	ZDV	None	ZDV (6 wk)	Long-long arm: 6.5	NA
		Long-short arm: ZDV (28)	ZDV	None	ZDV (3 days)	Long-short arm: 4.7	
		Short-long arm: ZDV (35)	ZDV	None	ZDV (6 wk)	Short-long arm: 8.6	
		Short-short arm: ZDV (35)	ZDV	None	ZDV (3 days)	Short-short arm: 10.5	
PACTG 316 (United States, Europe, Brazil, Bahamas)	No	Arm A: Nonstudy therapy (14-34)	ZDV	All women continued their previous nonstudy therapy	ZDV (6 wk)	Arm A: 1.6	NA
		Arm B: Nonstudy therapy (14-34)	ZDV + NVP		ZDV (6 wk) + NVP (1 dose)	Arm B: 1.4	
Retro-CI (Ivory Coast)	Yes	ZDV (36)	ZDV	None	None	ZDV: 15.7 Placebo: 24.9	37
DITRAME/ANRS (Ivory Coast, Burkina Faso)	Yes	ZDV (36-38)	ZDV	ZDV (1 wk)	None	ZDV: 18.0 Placebo: 27.5	38
PETRA (South Africa, Uganda, Tanzania)	Yes	Arm A: ZDV + 3TC (36)	ZDV + 3TC	ZDV + 3TC (1 wk)	ZDV + 3TC (1 wk)	8.6	50
		Arm B: None	ZDV + 3TC	ZDV + 3TC (1 wk)	ZDV + 3TC (1 wk)	10.8	37
		Arm C: None	ZDV + 3TC	None	None	17.7 Placebo: 17.2	0
HIVNET 012 (Uganda)	Yes	Arm A: None	ZDV	None	ZDV (4 wk)	Arm A: 25.1	NA
		Arm B: None	NVP (1 dose)	None	NVP (1 dose)	Arm B: 13.1	
SAINT (South Africa)	Yes	Arm A: None	ZDV + 3TC	ZDV + 3TC (1 wk)	ZDV + 3TC (1 wk)	9.3	NA
		Arm B: None	NVP (1 dose)	NVP (1 dose)	NVP (1 dose)	12.3	

3TC, lamivudine; NVP, nevirapine; ZDV, zidovudine; NA, not applicable.

CLINICAL MANIFESTATIONS

General

HIV-infected infants usually are asymptomatic during the first few months of life. In the era before highly active antiretroviral therapy (HAART), the mean age at onset of symptoms was estimated to be about 1 year for perinatally infected infants (Fig. 123-2); with antiretroviral therapy and opportunistic infection prophylaxis, increasing numbers of children are remaining asymptomatic for more than 5 years, and increasing numbers are surviving through adolescence.[46-54] Before the availability of HAART, two categories of infection based on incubation period and progression of symptoms were recognized. Approximately 10% to 15% of children died before 4 years of age, most before 18 months of age; the majority of children, however, survived beyond 5 years of age.[46-51,55-59] These two patterns may reflect in utero (rapid progressor) and peripartum (slow progressor) infection.

HIV infection in children causes a varied clinical course. AIDS represents the most severe end of the clinical spectrum, as with adult AIDS infection. The CDC surveillance definitions and classification scheme for pediatric HIV infection are given in Tables 123-2 and 123-3, respectively. Although the pediatric classification system was established for surveillance of HIV infection, its clinical categories (Table 123-4) are used to help define progression of the disease.[14,60,62]

Infants younger than 2 years of age may present with *Pneumocystis jirovecii* pneumonia (PCP), generalized adenopathy, hepatomegaly, splenomegaly, failure to thrive, and, if unimmunized, recurrent invasive bacterial infections (*Streptococcus pneumoniae, Haemophilus influenzae,* and *Salmonella* spp.). School-aged children may begin to show progressive cognitive delay, recurrent otitis media, pneumonia, sinusitis, and lymphoid interstitial pneumonitis. Finally, the oldest children present with opportunistic infections suggestive of very low CD4+ T-cell counts, such as oral candidiasis, recurrent diarrhea, cardiomyopathy, HIV encephalopathy, and malignancies.[26,63,64] In the present era, with earlier diagnosis and more common use of HAART, many of these manifestations are becoming less common.[54,64-66]

PCP is the most common serious opportunistic infection in children with HIV infection and is associated with a high mortality.[11,67-70] PCP occurs most frequently in infants between 3 and 6 months of age, but it can occur in younger infants, beginning as early as 4 to 6 weeks of age Fig. 123-3).[70] Infants and children characteristically develop a subacute, diffuse pneumonitis with dyspnea at rest, tachypnea, oxygen desaturation, nonproductive cough, and fever.[70] However, the magnitude of these signs is variable. The chest roentgenogram often shows bilateral diffuse interstitial disease; rarely, lobar, miliary, and nodular lesions occur as well (Fig. 123-4). Occasionally, the chest roentgenogram at the time of diagnosis appears normal. Without a heightened awareness of PCP as a potential diagnosis, the disease may be far advanced before it is diagnosed. In these cases, the mortality rate is high, ranging from 5% to 40% with treatment, and almost 100% if untreated.[63,64,70]

Other common opportunistic infections that occur as a presentation in children with AIDS include *Candida* esophagitis, disseminated cy-

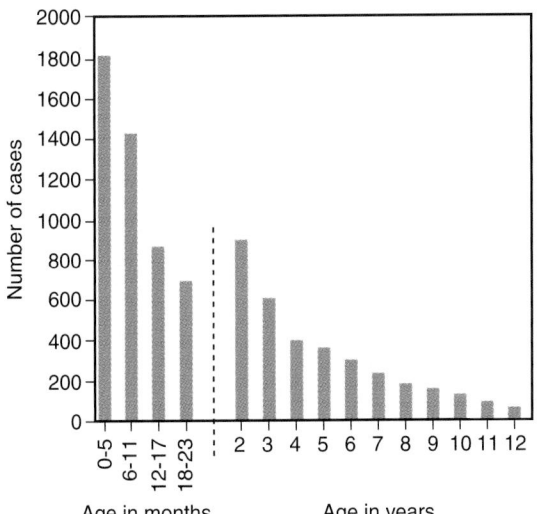

FIGURE 123-2. Perinatally acquired AIDS cases in the United States, by age at diagnosis, 1982-2001.

tomegalovirus infection, and chronic or disseminated herpes simplex virus and varicella-zoster virus infections. Infections with *Mycobacterium tuberculosis* or *Mycobacterium avium* complex, chronic enteritis caused by *Cryptosporidium* or other agents, and disseminated or central nervous system cryptococcal or *Toxoplasma gondii* infections are distinctly less common in children than in adults. Fewer than 14% of HIV-infected children have *M. avium* complex infection and fewer than 1% have *Cryptococcus* infection, compared with 18% to 36% and 5% to 15%, respectively, in adults.[26,64,71-73] Similarly, coexisting infection with hepatitis C virus and HIV in children is less common than in adults (2% versus 33%, respectively), as is coinfection with hepatitis G (GB virus C) and HIV (6% versus 17% to 43%).[74,75] However, in perinatally infected children with known HIV, opportunistic infections are more common as the immune system wanes, and disseminated *M. avium* infection may be the ultimate cause of death.

The development of opportunistic infections, particularly PCP, progressive neurologic disease, and severe wasting, is associated with a poor prognosis.[26,46,48,63] If these diagnoses herald a new diagnosis of HIV/AIDS and are not reversible with aggressive treatment and HAART, the prognosis remains poor. However, many infants who present with PCP recover and reconstitute to normal numbers of CD4+ T-lymphocytes on HAART, living many years with a good quality of life. The prognosis for survival before HAART was also poor in children infected perinatally in whom virus was detected early (i.e., by 7 days of life) and in those who become symptomatic within the first year of life.[27,46-51,55,57-59] With earlier and more effective treatment, survival of HIV-infected children is likely to continue to improve.

Clinical Manifestations in Children and Adults

Although many aspects of adult HIV infection apply to children, a number of presentations of clinical syndromes are unique to children. In the absence of HAART, the overall progression of illness in young children is more rapid than in adults, perhaps because of the relative immaturity of the child's immune system and end organs (e.g., under-myelinated central nervous system) and the expansion of target cells (e.g., a functioning thymus and higher CD4+ T-cell counts than in adults).[64]

Abnormalities in growth were among the first manifestations of HIV infection to be recognized in children, and wasting syndrome is an AIDS-defining condition. Growth abnormalities have been established as independent risk factors for death.[76,77] Progressive stunting (decreased height for age), underweight (decreased weight for age), and, to a lesser extent, wasting (decreased weight for height) are the most common abnormalities in postnatal growth.[63,78-86] Growth retardation is often apparent within 3 to 4 months after birth, and the magnitude of height and weight impairment increases with age.[63,78-86] In the pre-HAART era, at least one third of HIV-infected children experienced severe growth delay.[77] Reduction in food intake, increased metabolic needs, impaired nutrient absorption, and diarrhea may all be factors in growth faltering.[82-86] HIV-infected children may require a greater number of calories to grow than are provided by the recommended daily allowance for healthy children of the same age; this increased requirement may be delivered by high-calorie-density supplements or by nasogastric or gastrostomy tube feeding. Gastrostomy tube supplementation has been shown to be useful in improving weight and fat mass.[87] HAART has also been shown to cause increased growth in height, weight, and muscle mass, although not all studies have been consistent in this regard.[88-91] Appetite stimulants such as megestrol acetate have been used to improve dietary intake, although the adverse effect of potential life-threatening adrenal suppression has dampened enthusiasm for this drug.[92] The roles of dronabinol, oxandrolone, and recombinant human growth hormone in combating growth failure are uncertain because of their potential adverse effects and lack of data on their efficacy. With the advent of HAART, it is hoped that HIV-induced growth abnormalities will lessen in importance.

Recurrent invasive bacterial infections historically were more prominent in pediatric versus adult HIV disease, but such infections have declined with the use of antiretroviral agents and trimethoprim-sulfamethoxazole for prophylaxis against PCP.[93,94] Rates of invasive pneumococcal infection among HIV-infected children were three times those of controls in one study[93]; in another study, pneumococcal infection rates among HIV-infected children approached 100 to 300 times those in non–HIV-infected controls.[94] With the implementation of universal infant pneumococcal conjugate vaccination in the United States, disease rates may fall in HIV-infected children over time.[95]

Pulmonary complications of pediatric HIV infection are notable for the frequency of lymphocytic interstitial pneumonitis, a chronic lymphoproliferative disorder that affects 30% to 40% of these children but is rare in HIV-positive adults.[96,97] Lymphocytic interstitial pneumonitis is characterized by diffuse infiltration of the alveoli and small airways by lym-

TABLE 123-2   1994 Revised Human Immunodeficiency Virus Pediatric Classification System: Immune Categories Based on Age-Specific CD41+ T-Cell Count (Cells/mm³) and Percentage http://www.aidsinfo.nih.gov/guidelines/pediatric/ - table1fn1 of Total Lymphocytes

	Age <12 mo		Age 1-5 yr		Age 6-12 yr	
Immune Category	No.	%	No.	%	No.	%
Category 1: No suppression	≥1500	≥25	≥1000	≥25	≥500	≥25
Category 2: Moderate suppression	750-1499	15-24	500-999	15-24	200-499	15-24
Category 3: Severe suppression	<750	<15	<500	<15	<200	<15

Modified from Centers for Disease Control and Prevention. 1994 revised classification system for human immunodeficiency virus infection in children less than 13 years of age; official authorized addenda: Human immunodeficiency virus infection codes and official guidelines for coding and reporting ICD-9-CM. MMWR Morb Mortal Wkly Rep. 1994;43(RR-12):1-19.

Category N: Not Symptomatic
Children who have no signs or symptoms considered to be the result of HIV infection or who have only one of the conditions listed in category A.

Category A: Mildly Symptomatic
Children with 2 or more of the following conditions but none of the conditions listed in categories B and C:
Lymphadenopathy (≥0.5 cm at more than two sites; bilateral nodes at one anatomic level [e.g., neck] do not count as two sites
Hepatomegaly
Splenomegaly
Dermatitis
Parotitis
Recurrent or persistent upper respiratory infection, sinusitis, or otitis media

Category B: Moderately Symptomatic
Children who have symptomatic conditions, other than those listed for category A or category C, that are attributed to HIV infection. Examples of conditions in clinical category B include but are not limited to the following:
Anemia (<8 g/dL), neutropenia (<1000/mm^3, or thrombocytopenia (<100,000/mm^3) persisting ≥30 days
Bacterial meningitis, pneumonia, or sepsis (single episode)
Candidiasis, oropharyngeal (i.e., thrush) persisting for >2 mo in children aged >6 mo
Cardiomyopathy
Cytomegalovirus infection with onset before age 1 mo
Diarrhea, recurrent or chronic
Hepatitis
Herpes simplex virus (HSV) stomatitis, recurrent (i.e., more than two episodes within 1 year)
HSV bronchitis, pneumonitis, or esophagitis with onset before age 1 mo
Herpes zoster (i.e., shingles) involving at least two distinct episodes or more than one dermatome
Leiomyosarcoma
Lymphoid interstitial pneumonia (LIP) or pulmonary lymphoid hyperplasia complex
Nephropathy
Nocardiosis
Fever lasting >1 mo
Toxoplasmosis with onset before age 1 mo
Varicella, disseminated (i.e., complicated chickenpox)

Category C: Severely Symptomatic
Children who have any condition listed in the 1987 surveillance case definition for AIDS, with the exception of LIP (which is a category B condition).

From Centers for Disease Control and Prevention. 1994 revised classification system for human immunodeficiency virus infection in children less than 13 years of age; official authorized addenda: Human immunodeficiency virus infection codes and official guidelines for coding and reporting ICD-9-CM. MMWR Morb Mortal Wkly Rep. 1994;43(RR-12):1-19.

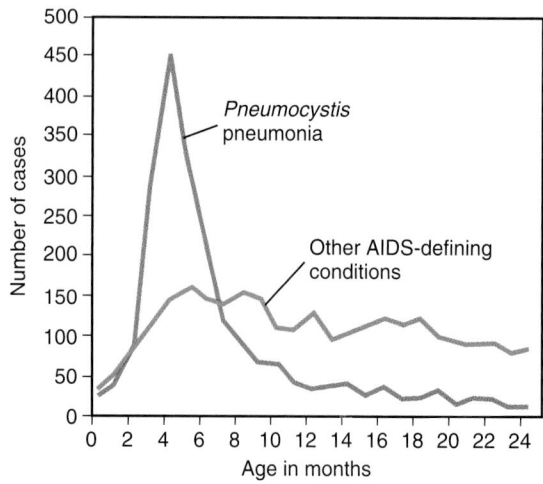

FIGURE 123-3. AIDS-defining conditions, by age at diagnosis for perinatally acquired AIDS cases reported through 2001.

phocytes and plasma cells. Clinically, the child may have a nonproductive cough and the insidious onset of hypoxia, bronchiectasis, and pulmonary decompensation during otherwise minor upper or lower respiratory tract infections; some children exhibit clubbing of the digits.[96,97] Radiographs show interstitial infiltrates and reticulonodular patterns that are easily confused with tuberculosis or PCP. Lymphocytic interstitial pneumonitis has responded to both antiretroviral therapy and corticosteroids.[96,97] The cause of lymphocytic interstitial pneumonitis is unclear, although it is speculated that an exaggerated local response to Epstein-Barr virus or HIV, or both, may be causative.[96,97] Lymphocytic interstitial pneumonitis, although contained within clinical category B, is nevertheless considered an AIDS-defining condition (see Table 123-3).

Central nervous system complications in pediatric HIV infection are frequent, and encephalopathy is an AIDS-defining condition. In the early years of the epidemic, 50% to 60% of children with advanced HIV infection exhibited progressive encephalopathy; more recent estimates from cohorts including asymptomatic, mildly symptomatic, and symptomatic children range from 20% to 40%. Pediatric HIV encephalopathy is manifested in either a progressive form, which is characterized by impaired brain growth, acquired microcephaly, progressive motor dysfunction, and loss of developmental milestones, or a static form, in which children acquire skills and abilities at a continued but subnormal rate, with varied degrees of

TABLE 123-4 Likelihood of Developing AIDS or Death within 12 Months, by Age and CD41⁺ T-Cell Percentage of Total Lymphocytes or Log10 HIV-1 RNA Copy Number in HIV-Infected Children Receiving No Therapy or Zidovudine Monotherapy

Age	*CD4+ T-Cell Percentage*				*Log₁₀ HIV RNA Copy Number*		
	10%	*20%*	*30%*	*40%*	*6.0*	*5.0*	*4.0*
Percent Developing AIDS (95% Confidence Interval)							
6 Mo	51 (45-57)	31 (27-35)	20 (18-23)	16 (14-17)	24 (16-27)	14 (10-16)	11 (7-16)
1 Yr	40 (45-57)	21 (18-23)	13 (12-14)	9.9 (8.5-11.4)	21 (12-24)	11 (8-12)	7.8 (4.4-12.1)
2 Yr	29 (26-31)	12 (11-14)	7.2 (6.4-8.2)	5.9 (4.9-7.1)	19 (8-22)	8.1 (6.5-9.3)	5.3 (3.2-8.5)
5 Yr	15 (12-18)	4.7 (3.9-5.7)	3.1 (2.5-4.0)	2.9 (2.1-3.8)	17 (5-21)	6.0 (4.5-8.0)	3.2 (2.1-4.9)
10 Yr	7.4 (5.0-10.8)	2.2 (1.6-2.8)	1.8 (1.2-3.0)	1.7 (1.1-3.1)	16 (3-20)	5.1 (3.0-7.7)	2.2 (1.4-3.2)
Percent Mortality (95% Confidence Interval)							
6 Mo	30 (26-35)	12 (10-15)	6.4 (5.3-7.8)	4.6 (3.8-5.5)	9.7 (8.1-12.0)	4.1 (2.9-5.4)	2.7 (0.9-4.1)
1 Yr	20 (18-23)	6.8 (5.6-8.4)	3.3 (2.8-3.9)	2.5 (2.0-3.1)	8.8 (7.2-11.0)	3.1 (2.4-4.0)	1.7 (0.8-2.8)
2 Yr	12 (11-14)	3.1 (2.6-3.7)	1.5 (1.2-1.9)	1.2 (0.9-1.6)	8.2 (6.4-10.4)	2.5 (1.8-3.1)	1.1 (0.6-1.8)
5 Yr	4.9 (3.8-5.9)	0.9 (0.7-1.2)	0.5 (0.3-0.7)	0.5 (0.3-0.7)	7.8 (5.9-10.2)	2.1 (1.4-2.9)	0.7 (0.4-1.0)
10 Yr	2.1 (1.3-3.0)	0.3 (0.2-0.5)	0.2 (0.1-0.4)	0.2 (0.1-0.4)	7.7 (5.7-10.0)	2.0 (1.2-2.9)	0.6 (0.3-0.9)

Modified from Dunn D, HIV Paediatric Prognostic Markers Collaborative Study Group. Short-term risk of disease progression in HIV-1-infected children receiving no antiretroviral therapy or zidovudine monotherapy: A meta-analysis. Lancet. 2003;362:1605-1611.

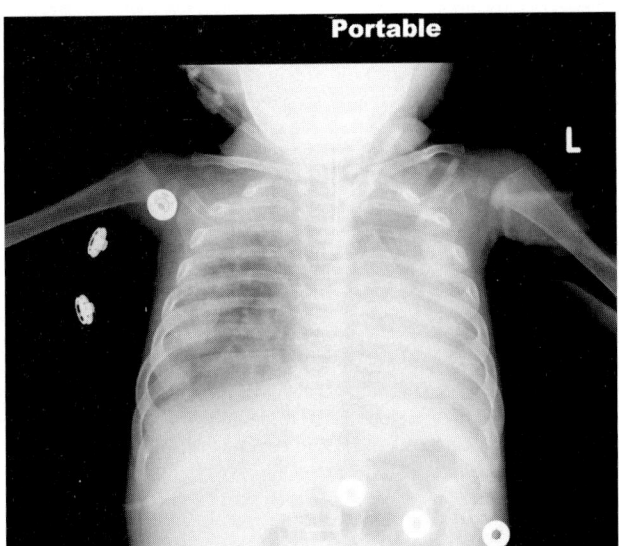

FIGURE 123-4. Chest radiograph of a 4-month-old child with *Pneumocystis* pneumonia.

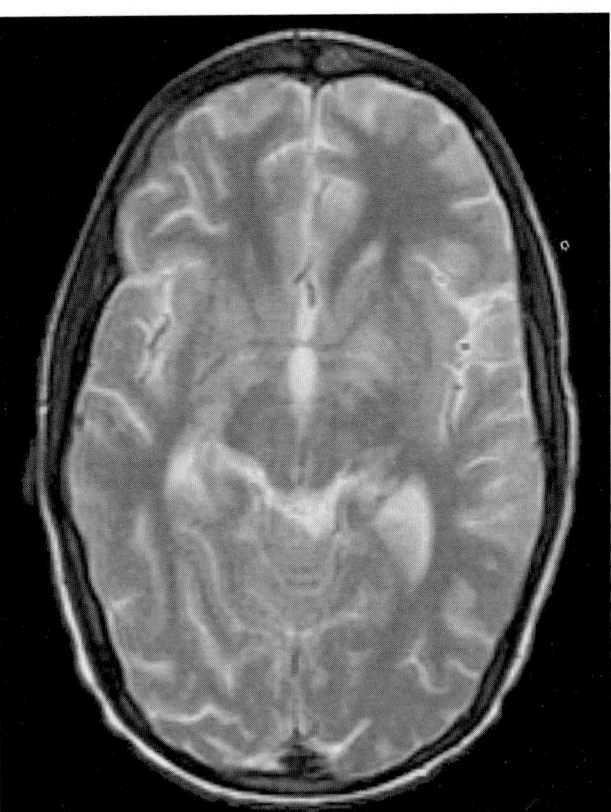

FIGURE 123-5. Magnetic resonance image of the brain of a 14-year-old child with perinatal HIV infection and HIV encephalopathy, showing cortical atrophy, asymmetrical enhancement.

motor involvement.[98-100] A middle "plateau" form has also been described, with retention of previously acquired developmental milestones but no further development after some point in time.[99] Pure dementia is more commonly seen in adults, not children. A delay in early language development may be seen in the absence of other abnormalities.[101] Neuroimaging findings in pediatric HIV encephalopathy commonly include variable degrees of cerebral atrophy and bilateral symmetric calcification of the basal ganglia and frontal white matter (Fig. 123-5).[99,102,103] Pediatric HIV encephalopathy is associated with greater mortality; antiretroviral therapy can prevent cognitive decline and prolong survival.[104-106]

Chronic diarrhea, wasting, and gastrointestinal *Candida* infections are common in both adults and children infected with HIV. Esophagitis from *Candida,* cytomegalovirus, or herpes simplex virus occurs in children as in adults, as do bacterial enteritis and, to a lesser extent, cryptosporidiosis, aphthous ulcers, and pancreatitis.[85,107]

Oral manifestations of HIV are common in both adults and children, but the spectrum of conditions varies.[108-112] In children, recurrent candidiasis, herpes simplex virus infections, recurrent aphthous ulcers, parotid enlargement, linear gingival erythema, and delayed tooth eruption are all commonly associated with symptomatic HIV infection. However, lesions commonly seen in adults (e.g., hairy leukoplakia, Kaposi's sarcoma, non-Hodgkin's lymphoma and, to a large extent, necrotizing gingivitis/periodontitis), are rarely seen in children.

Cardiologic manifestations of HIV infection in children have been recognized.[64,113] Although generally not clinically significant, left ventricular dysfunction and dilated cardiomyopathy are detected frequently by echocardiography and may be related to the occurrence of congestive heart failure and arrhythmias and sudden cardiorespiratory arrests.[114-116] Cardiomyopathy appears to be associated with HIV encephalopathy.[100,117] A large ongoing pediatric study has been designed to understand the clinical role of cardiologic manifestations of pediatric HIV infection.[118] Some of the results from this study to date indicate that there is little to no cardiac toxicity of zidovudine in infants and no unusual increase in cardiac congenital anomalies in HIV-exposed children.[119,120]

The kidney is also affected by HIV infection, in both adults and children.[121-123] Rarely, nephritis can be the presenting symptom complex suggestive of an HIV/AIDS diagnosis. Both glomerulonephropathy and tubular lesions are noted.[121-123]

Hematologic complications such as leukopenia, anemia, and thrombocytopenia occur in both children and adults infected with HIV.[124] Circulating antineutrophil antibodies are common but do not appear to cause neutropenia.[125] Newborns may be more susceptible than adults and older children to bone marrow suppression by antiretroviral agents.[126]

Malignancies in pediatric HIV infection have been relatively uncommon, but leiomyosarcomas and certain lymphomas, including those of the central nervous system and non-Hodgkin's B-cell lymphomas of the Burkitt's type, occur much more frequently in children with HIV infection than in nonimmunocompromised children.[127-132]

A number of complications commonly seen in adult HIV infection occur only rarely in children; these include cerebral toxoplasmosis, cryptococcal meningitis and pneumonia, progressive multifocal leukoencephalopathy (PML), all forms of Kaposi's sarcoma, bacillary angiomatosis, cytomegalovirus retinitis, and hypersensitivity to trimethoprim-sulfamethoxazole.[63,64,70,99] Peripheral neuropathy and myopathy appear to be rarer in children than in adults, although symptoms may be missed in preverbal children.[99] However, as children and adolescents survive longer, perhaps with low CD4+ T-cell counts after years of antiretroviral therapy, it will not be unexpected if the incidence of "adult-type" complications (e.g., PML, Kaposi's sarcoma, central nervous system lymphoma) increases in children.

Metabolic complications of HIV and its treatment by HAART include lactic acidemia, hyperglycemia, osteopenia, avascular necrosis, and fat redistribution ("lipodystrophy"). Lactic acidemia, perhaps resulting from NRTI-induced mitochondrial dysfunction, has been reported most commonly in adults but can occur in children.[133] Whether this syndrome occurs in HIV-exposed infants after in utero exposure is controversial.[44,45,134] Similarly, definitive studies of insulin resistance and hyperglycemia in children are not available. Osteonecrosis and avascular necrosis of the femoral heads (equivalent to Legg-Calvé-Perthes disease) has been reported to be 5 to 9 times more common in HIV-infected children than in children not infected.[135] The mechanisms by which other factors such as glucocorticosteroid usage, sickle cell anemia, or hypercoagulable states may interact with HIV infection or HAART in causing avascular necrosis of bone are unclear. Lipodystrophy—including peripheral lipoatrophy or central fat accumulation (or both), gynecomastia, cervical fat pad accumulation (buffalo hump), and hyperlipidemia—occurs in perhaps 18% to 29% of HIV-infected children, less commonly than reported in adults.[136,137] Because of limited data on the pathophysiology and long-term cardiologic risks of lipodystrophy, no guidelines on the management of lipodystrophy in children are available (as of January, 2004) beyond those published for HIV-infected adults or for children without HIV infection.[138-141]

LABORATORY FINDINGS

The most notable finding in pediatric HIV infection, particularly as the disease progresses, is an increasing loss of cell-mediated immunity, similar to that observed in adults with HIV infection.[142] The peripheral blood lymphocyte count initially can be normal, but eventually lymphopenia develops because of a decrease in the total number of circulating T lymphocytes. The cells most affected are the CD4+ helper T lymphocytes. The CD8+ suppressor T lymphocytes usually increase in number initially and are not depleted until late in the course of the infection. These changes in cell populations result in a decrease of the normal CD4+/CD8+ cell ratio. The normal values for peripheral CD4+ T-cell counts and percentages in children are distinctly different from those in adults and are directly related to age.[60,143-145] The lower limits of normal values for children are actually slightly higher than those used as breakpoints in Table 123-2, confirming the utility of the breakpoints listed. Responses of T lymphocytes to plant lectin mitogens (phytohemagglutinin, concanavalin A, and particularly pokeweed) are decreased or absent, and HIV-infected children may be anergic to skin test antigens such as mumps, *Candida, Trichophyton,* tetanus, and tuberculin (purified protein derivative), similar to HIV-infected adults.[64,142]

Although B-lymphocyte numbers remain normal or are somewhat increased, humoral immune dysfunction accompanies cellular dysfunction. Serum immunoglobulin concentrations, particularly immunoglobulin G (IgG) and IgA, frequently are elevated in HIV-infected children and have been used as surrogate diagnostic markers for pediatric HIV infection.[146] Some children develop panhypogammaglobulinemia. Specific antibody responses to antigens to which the patient has not previously been exposed can be abnormal.[64,142]

Circulating concentrations of virus (viral load) in children younger than 12 months of age are very high (mean, approximately 200,000 RNA copies/mL).[147-149] By 24 months of age, viral concentrations decrease, to a mean of approximately 40,000 RNA copies/mL. Data suggest that plasma viral concentration determinations in conjunction with CD4+ T-cell counts are more accurate predictors than each marker alone of the prognosis and of survival.[61,148-150] However, there appears to be considerable overlap in RNA levels in infants and children with or without rapid disease progression, making RNA levels less predictive than in adults.[147,148] In general, high levels of HIV RNA (>300,000 copies/mL in infants younger than 12 months of age; >100,000 copies/mL in young children) are associated with higher long-term risk for death, especially if the CD4+ T-cell percentage is less than 15%.[148] The predictive quartiles of baseline HIV RNA associated with risks for disease progression or death in children are much wider than those reported in adult studies.[61,149] In resource-poor settings, complete blood counts and levels of serum albumin may serve as alternative surrogate markers of disease progression.[151]

The diurnal variation in HIV RNA levels appears to be greater in infants and young children also. For this reason, only fivefold or greater ($0.7 \log_{10}$) changes may be significant in children younger than 2 years of age, as opposed to threefold ($0.5 \log_{10}$) or greater changes in older children and adults.[62,152]

DIAGNOSTIC TESTS

Proper use of diagnostic tests for pediatric HIV infection is heavily dependent on the age of the child (also see Chapter 115). Beyond the age of 18 months, standard serologic evaluations with enzyme immunoassay (EIA) and confirmatory Western blot assay may be performed as for an adult. However, infants born to HIV-seropositive women pose a special diagnostic challenge; they are seropositive at birth, whether or not they are infected, as a result of the transplacental passage of maternal antibody to HIV, which is detectable in the infant for as long as 18 months after birth. Because IgG antibody tests for HIV are not useful for diagnosis in children younger than 18 months of age, tests that detect the presence of the virus itself must be performed. These include HIV DNA polymerase chain reaction (PCR), culture, RNA PCR, and acid-dissociated p24 antigen. However, if an infant younger than 18 months who has a positive serologic test for HIV develops an AIDS-defining illness (category C; see Table 123-3), the diagnosis of HIV infection is established even if virologic tests are negative.

DNA Polymerase Chain Reaction

The preferred test for HIV diagnosis in the infant younger than 18 months of age is the detection of HIV DNA by use of PCR, which is the most sensitive and specific test to detect HIV infection in children born to HIV-infected women.[14,15,60,62,146,153-155] This assay is performed on whole blood so that the genomic DNA present in peripheral blood monocytes and macrophages is detected. A benefit of detecting HIV DNA in the host cell genome is that the test is not influenced by antiretroviral therapy. An additional benefit of this technique is that it can be performed on whole blood collected on dried filter paper ("Guthrie cards"), enabling easy and safe transportation from a variety of point-of-care testing sites, including those in developing countries.[156-161] Consistent with the concept that as many as 70% of perinatally infected infants acquire infection at or around the time of birth, DNA PCR testing is not positive in the first few days of life despite its extraordinary sensitivity, but almost 100% of infected infants can be diagnosed by 4 to 6 months of age with this technique.[15,162-165] Many authorities now suggest that HIV DNA PCR testing be performed within the first 2 or 3 days of life and again during the first 4 weeks.[14,15,62] At minimum, in the absence of any clinical illness, HIV infection can reasonably be excluded in the infant who has had two negative PCR tests at 1 month of age or older, including one at 4 months of age.[14,15,62,67]

It should be recalled that non–subtype B viruses predominate in some parts of the world, such as central Africa, southeast Asia, and India. Currently available HIV DNA PCR (and RNA PCR) assays may have lower sensitivity for non–subtype B strains (especially group O strains), yielding false-negative results.[155,166,167]

Human Immunodeficiency Virus Culture

HIV culture is also a sensitive diagnostic tool, especially in infants not exposed to antiretroviral therapy, and it is specific, but it is not generally widely available. It is being replaced in most areas by DNA PCR.[14,15,60,62,146]

RNA Assay

Detection of HIV RNA ("viral load" assay) is probably as sensitive and specific as DNA PCR in infants not exposed to antiretroviral therapy.[153,154,166,168,169] However, at present it is recommended that the HIV RNA assay not be used as a primary diagnostic test because of questions about the specificity of low levels of positivity in some laboratories. HIV RNA PCR testing may be used as a confirmatory test for diagnosis if the RNA level is greater than 10,000 copies/mL plasma. Because plasma specimens must undergo centrifugation and must be kept frozen to prevent degradation, the HIV RNA PCR assay for diagnosis is less useful in many point-of-care sites.

Acid-Dissociated P24 Antigen

Dissociation of immune complexes by acid treatment, followed by assay for HIV p24 antigen, may also be used to confirm the presence of HIV infection. The assay is technically less difficult to perform than PCR, but it is also much less sensitive, even with recent improvements.[14,15,60,164,170,171]

Serologic Testing

EIAs are used most widely to screen for serum HIV antibody in older children and adolescents. These tests are highly sensitive and specific, but false-positive results occur in a small percentage of cases. As in the testing of adults, repeat EIA testing of initially reactive specimens from children is required to reduce the likelihood of laboratory error; repeatedly reactive tests are highly reliable. Western blot or immunofluorescent antibody tests should be used for confirmation. A positive HIV-antibody test in a child 18 months of age or older usually indicates infection.[14,60] Serum antibodies to HIV are present eventually in virtually all infected children, although rarely a child with HIV infection lacks HIV antibody because of hypogammaglobulinemia or the inability to produce antibody in very advanced disease.[146]

Rapid HIV Testing

Rapid testing methodology will have its biggest impact in the prevention of MTCT. Women who present for delivery and do not have a documented HIV test antenatally can be offered rapid testing so that prophylactic therapy can be offered to prevent MTCT. Point-of-care testing sites (e.g., labor and delivery suites) have been shown to obtain a result and institute therapy more quickly than sites using a clinical laboratory. Point-of-care sites may have Clinical Laboratories Improvement Act (CLIA) certification waived after completion of the waiver program. As an example, the OraQuick Rapid HIV-1 Antibody Test is easy to use and can be performed on oral fluid, serum, or whole blood; it is said to approach 100% sensitivity and 99.9% specificity. The turnaround time is 20 minutes, and the CLIA waiver is applicable. However, it should be recalled that the positive predictive value (PPV) of any test varies with the prevalence of the condition tested (Bayes' theorem). For example, if the HIV prevalence among women in labor is 10%, the PPV of OraQuick testing (using the earlier figures for sensitivity and specificity) will be 99%. If the prevalence of HIV infection among women in labor is only 0.5% (as in many obstetric wards in the United States), the PPV of OraQuick will be only 83%.

Perinatal HIV Serologic Testing Algorithm

Prenatal testing of pregnant women is critically important in identifying opportunities to prevent MTCT. For those women not presenting for prenatal care, rapid testing during labor and delivery, or, at the very latest, testing of the newborn infant may also provide information allowing the interruption of MTCT.

Optimal testing of infants born to HIV-infected women includes two or three HIV DNA PCR assays, performed during the first days to weeks of life, at 1 month of age, and at 4 months of age. A positive assay constitutes presumptive evidence of HIV infection; a second diagnostic test should be performed immediately, using either the same assay or one of the confirmatory assays (i.e., culture or RNA PCR) to confirm the diagnosis. Two or more negative PCR tests (minimally, at 1 month and 4 months of age) constitute evidence of presumed absence of infection. Follow-up serologic tests should be performed to confirm the exclusion of HIV infection (seroreversion). Such tests include either two negative EIA tests performed between 6 and 18 months of age or one negative EIA test after 18 months of age.[14,67] Some experts still recommend that the final EIA test be performed at 24 months of age, especially if PCR assays were not performed.

The American Academy of Pediatrics has recommended, on the basis of advances in therapy to reduce the rate of perinatal HIV transmission and the continued occurrence of life-threatening illness in young infants with unrecognized HIV infection, that documented, routine HIV education and routine testing with consent for all pregnant women in the United States should be carried out.[14] Documented consent for maternal or newborn HIV testing, or both, may be obtained in a variety of ways, including by right of refusal (documented patient education, with testing to take place unless re-

jected in writing by the patient). Similar statements have been published by the American College of Obstetrics and Gynecology and the National Academy of Science's Institute of Medicine. In addition, it is recommended that routine education about HIV infection and testing should become part of a comprehensive program of health care for women, particularly for women of childbearing age, and that all testing programs for the detection of HIV infection should evaluate periodically the proportion of women who refuse HIV testing after HIV education.[14] Those programs in which a proportionately low number of women receive HIV testing should be examined as to the reasons for poor acceptance, with appropriate program modifications made as needed.[14]

For women who are seen by a health care professional for the first time in labor and who either have not received prenatal care or who previously tested negative but have not been tested for HIV infection during the current pregnancy, education about HIV infection and maternal HIV testing are recommended during labor or in the immediate postpartum period. For newborns whose mothers' HIV serostatus was not determined during the recent pregnancy or in the postpartum period, the infant's health care provider should educate the mother concerning the potential benefits of HIV testing for her infant, and the possible risks and benefits to herself of knowing the child's serostatus, and then recommend HIV testing for the newborn. In some jurisdictions, perinatal testing is mandated by law (see later discussion). Finally, the health care provider for the infant needs to be informed of the mother's HIV serostatus so that appropriate care and testing of the infant can be accomplished. Similarly, if the infant is found to be seropositive and the serostatus of the mother is unknown, the health care provider for the child should ensure that information about the serostatus and its significance is provided to the mother and, with her consent, to her health care provider. The mother should receive appropriate referral to adult HIV-related services.

Health care providers should be aware of local regulations regarding prenatal and perinatal HIV testing. For example, in the state of New York, HIV testing (with consent) of all pregnant women, as well as routine HIV testing of all newborns, is mandated as the standard of care (guidelines are available on the World Wide Web at www.hivguidelines.org). In addition, if information about the HIV status of a woman in labor is not available from testing during that pregnancy, rapid testing of either the mother (with consent) or the newborn (consent not required) must be performed to guide initiation of antiretroviral therapy to prevent vertical transmission. Other states (e.g., Connecticut) have employed enhanced surveillance of HIV-exposed infants. The role of rapid HIV testing of women in labor is under investigation by the CDC and the Pediatric AIDS Clinical Trials Group (MIRIAD study).

Informed Consent for HIV Serologic Testing

Testing for HIV infection can carry substantial psychosocial risks.[14] Counseling of the parents or other primary caregivers (and of the patient if he or she is old enough to comprehend the possible risks and benefits of testing and the consequences of HIV infection) is mandatory before testing of an infant or child. Written or oral consent, consistent with state and local laws and hospital regulations, must be obtained and recorded in the patient's chart. The necessity for counseling and consent should not deter efforts to undertake appropriate diagnostic testing for HIV infection. The parents' or patient's refusal to give consent does not relieve physicians of their professional and legal responsibilities to their patients. If the physician believes that testing is essential to the child's health, authorization for testing needs to be obtained by other means (e.g., court order). The results of serologic tests should be discussed in person with the family or primary caregiver and, if appropriate according to age, with the patient; if the result is positive, appropriate counseling and subsequent follow-up care must be provided. Maintenance of confidentiality in all cases is essential to preserving the patient's and parents' trust and consent.

TREATMENT

General Considerations

The overall goal of treatment of HIV in children is to maintain or achieve a normal CD4+ T-cell count and percentage. This is attained by suppression of HIV viral load with antiretroviral therapy. The decisions of how and when to initiate treatment, and even what treatment to give, depend on multiple factors, including age and clinical status at presentation, CD4+ T-cell percentage, and HIV RNA viral load. Although HIV viral load does not correlate absolutely with prognosis, data suggest that infants with more than 100,000 copies/mL may have rapid disease progression. At any given RNA level, the prognosis is worse for children younger than 1 year of age (see Table 123-4).[62] Even if the laboratory parameters would suggest that therapy be

TABLE 123-5 Pediatric Dosages for Antiretroviral Medications

Drug Name [Trade Name]	Formulation	Oral Dosage, by Age and Body Weight (BW)
Nucleoside Reverse Transcriptase Inhibitors (NRTIs)		
Zidovudine (ZDV, AZT, azidothymidine) [Retrovir]	100 mg capsules, 300 mg tablets 10 mg/mL syrup	0-6 wk: 2 mg/kg q6h 3 mo-13 yr: 160 mg/m² q8h to 180 mg/m² q12h ≥13 yr: 200 mg q8h or 300 mg q12h
Didanosine (ddI, dideoxyinosine) [Videx; sustained release *Videx EC*]	25, 50, 100, 150, 200 mg chewable tablets 100, 167, 250 mg buffered powder 10 mg/mL pediatric solution *Videx EC*: 125, 200, 250, 400 mg capsules	0-3 mo: 50 mg/m² q12h 3 mo-13 yr: 120 mg/m² q12h (90-150 mg/m² q12h) ≥13 yr, BW <60 kg: tablets, 125 mg q12h [or buffered powder, 167 mg q12h; or *Videx EC*, 250 mg q24h] ≥13 yr, BW ≥60 kg: tablets, 200 mg q12h [or buffered powder, 250 mg q12h; or *Videx EC*, 400 mg q24h]
Zalcitabine (ddC, dideoxycytidine) [Hivid]	0.375, 0.75 mg tablets	<13 yr: 0.01 mg/kg q8h ≥13 yr: 0.75 mg q8h
Stavudine (d4T) [Zerit; sustained release *Zerit XR*]	15, 20, 30, 40 mg capsules 1 mg/mL syrup *Zerit XR*: 37.5, 50, 75, 100 mg capsules	0-1 mo: 0.5 mg/kg q12h 1 mo-13 yr: 1 mg/kg q12h ≥13 yr, BW 30-60 kg: 30 mg q12h [or *Zerit XR*, 75 mg q24h] ≥13 yr, BW >60 kg: 40 mg q12h [or *Zerit XR*, 100 mg q24h]
Lamivudine (3TC) [Epivir]	150, 300 mg tablets 10 mg/mL syrup	0-3 mo: 2 mg/kg q12h 3 mo-13 yr: 4 mg/kg q12h ≥13 yr: 150 mg q12h or 300 mg q24h
Abacavir (ABC, 1592U89) [Ziagen]	300 mg tablets 20 mg/mL syrup	<13 yr: 8 mg/kg q12h ≥13 yr: 300 mg q12h (≤5% hypersensitivity all ages—do NOT rechallenge!)
Emtricitabine (FTC) [Emtriva]	200 mg hard gel capsules	<18 yr: Unknown ≥18 yr: 200 mg q24h
Combination NRTI tablets	Combivir = ZDV/3TC (300/150) Trizivir = ZDV/3TC/ABC (300/150/300)	≥13 yr: 1 tablet q12h ≥13 yr: 1 tablet q12h
Nucleotide Reverse Transcriptase Inhibitor (NtRI)		
Tenofovir [Viread]	300 mg tablets	<18 yr: Unknown ≥18 yr: 300 mg q24h
Non-Nucleoside Reverse Transcriptase Inhibitors (NNRTIs)		
Nevirapine (NVP) [Viramune]	200 mg tablets 10 mg/mL syrup	<13 yr: 120-200 mg/m2 q12h ≥13 yr: 200 mg q12h (14-day dose escalation lead-in period reduces complications at all ages)
Delavirdine (DLV) [Rescriptor]	100, 200 mg tablets	<13 yr: Unknown ≥13 yr: 400 mg q8h
Efavirenz (DMP266) [Sustiva]	50, 100, 200 mg capsules 600 mg tablets	<13 yr: 200-400 mg q24h (BW 10-14 kg, 200 mg; 15-19 kg, 250 mg; 20-24 kg, 300 mg; 25-32 kg, 350 mg; 33-40 kg, 400 mg) ≥13 yr: 600 mg q24h
Protease Inhibitors (PIs)		
Saquinavir (SQV) [Invirase, Fortovase]	Invirase: 200 mg hard gel capsules Fortovase: 200 mg soft gel capsules	<13 yr: 50 mg/kg q8h ≥13 yr: Invirase 600 mg q8h, or Fortovase 1200 mg q8h
Indinavir (IDV) [Crixivan]	200, 400 mg capsules	<13 yr: Unknown (350-500 mg/m² q8h under study) ≥13 yr: 800 mg q8h
Ritonavir (RTV) [Norvir]	100 mg soft gel capsules 80 mg/ml elixir	<13 yr: 350-400 mg/m² q12h (dose escalation lead-in period reduces complications at all ages) ≥13 yr: 600 mg q12h [lower dosage when used in dual PI therapy]
Nelfinavir (NFV) [Viracept]	50 mg/level scoop powder 250, 625 mg tablets	<13 yr: 50-55 mg/kg q12h ≥13 yr: 1250 mg q12h preferred (alternatively, 750 mg q8h)
Amprenavir (APV) [Agenerase]	50, 150 mg soft gel capsules 15 mg/mL syrup	4-13 yr: 20 mg/kg q12h (Note: syrup has high propylene glycol and vitamin E content; capsules also have high vitamin E content. Not suitable for children <4 yr of age.)
FosAmprenavir (fosAPV) [Lexiva]	*Lexiva*: 700 mg tablets	≥13 yr: 1200 mg q12h [*Lexiva 1400*] mg bid (700 mg bid if RTV 100 mg bid-boosted)
Lopinavir/ritonavir (LPVr) (ABT378r) [Kaletra]	133.3/33.3 mg soft gel capsules 80/20 mg/mL elixir	<13 yr: 10-12 mg/kg q12h (BW 7-14 kg, 12 mg/kg; 15-40 kg, 10 mg/kg) ≥13 yr: 400 mg q12h
Atazanavir (ATZ) [Reyataz]	100, 150, 200 mg capsules	<13 yr: Unknown ≥13 yr: 400 mg q24h
Fusion Inhibitor		
Enfuvirtide (T20) [Fuzeon]	Lyophilized single-use vial; resuspension supplies 90 mg/mL for SC injection	6-16 yr: 2 mg/kg SC q12h (maximum, 90 mg q12h)

From Working Group on Antiretroviral Therapy and Medical Management of HIV-Infected Children. Guidelines for the use of antiretroviral agents in pediatric HIV infection. Table revised February 2004. Not all doses listed are approved by the U.S. Food and Drug Administration. Updated guidelines are available at http://AIDSinfo.nih.gov and should be consulted.

TABLE 123-6 Indications for Initiation of Antiretroviral Therapy in Children Younger Than 12 Months of Age Infected with Human Immunodeficiency Virus (HIV)

Clinical Category		CD4⁺ T-Cell Percentage	Plasma HIV RNA Copy Number*	Recommendation
Symptomatic (Clinical category A, B, or C)	*or*	<25% (Immune category 2 or 3)	Any value	Treat
Asymptomatic (Clinical category N)	*and*	≥25% (Immune category 1)	Any value	Consider treatment†

*Plasma HIV RNA levels are higher in HIV-infected infants than in older infected children and adults. Levels may be difficult to interpret in infants <12 mo of age, because overall HIV RNA levels are high and because there is overlap in HIV RNA levels between infants who have and do not have rapid disease progression.

†Because HIV infection progresses more rapidly in infants than in older children or adults, some experts would treat all HIV-infected infants <6 mo or <12 mo of age, regardless of clinical, immunologic, or virologic parameters.

From Working Group on Antiretroviral Therapy and Medical Management of HIV-Infected Children. Guidelines for the use of antiretroviral agents in pediatric HIV infection. Updated guidelines are available at http://AIDSinfo.nih.gov and should be consulted.

started or changed, adherence to the selected regimen is a key concern because of lack of palatability, other side effects, pill burden, frequency of dosing, unwillingness to disclose the child's infection status to others, and so on. Factors that may become barriers to adherence should be addressed before initiation of the antiretroviral regimen. Other factors that must be considered include history of HIV-related or AIDS-defining illnesses, availability of palatable drug formulations, dosing complications (e.g., food restrictions), coinfections that may alter the risks or benefits of a particular regimen (e.g., hepatitis C), and drug-drug interactions.

An increasing number of studies are examining the pharmacokinetics of antiretroviral agents in infants, children, and adolescents, because drug distribution in these patient groups may differ from that in adults. Current guidelines are based on age, but many experts believe that dosage of medications for adolescents should be prescribed according to Tanner's staging of puberty in addition to age.[62] Adolescents in early puberty (i.e., Tanner stages I and II) should be administered doses based on the pediatric schedules given in Table 123-5, whereas those in late puberty (Tanner stage V) may require adult dosing schedules.[152] Adolescents in their growth spurt (Tanner stages III and IV) may require dose modification to ensure efficacy and minimize toxicity.[62]

Adherence to complex drug regimens can be especially difficult for children who depend on others for the administration of medication. In addition, not all necessary antiretroviral medications for the prevention of opportunistic infections are available as palatable liquids suitable for administration to infants and children. Other barriers, such as variable absorption of medicines by infants who require frequent feeding, difficulty in providing midday doses if the child is at school, and the reluctance of parents to have antiretroviral medications in the home while maintaining secrecy, can all act to reduce compliance. Adolescents may have further challenges because of developmental issues, such as not wanting to be different from peers or not understanding why medications are required during asymptomatic periods, and social issues, such as a lack of family support, distrust of the medical establishment, and denial and fear of HIV infection. All of these issues need to be addressed if medications are to be prescribed for a child or adolescent.[62,172-175]

Guidelines for Treatment of Pediatric HIV Infection

The reader is referred to the Working Group on Antiretroviral Therapy and Medical Management of HIV-Infected Children, available at http://aidsinfo.nih.gov.[62] This document is continuously updated as new information accrues. Tables 123-5 through 123-9 have been excerpted from these Guidelines (January 20, 2004, version) to provide a framework for pediatric dosages of medications, when such medications are initiated, and considerations for when changes should be made. Primary care physicians are encouraged to participate actively in the care of HIV-infected patients in consultation with specialists who have expertise in the treatment of pediatric HIV infection.[14,62] Expert opinions and knowledge about diagnostic and therapeutic strategies are changing rapidly. In areas of the United States in which enrollment of HIV-infected children into clinical trials is possible, it should be encouraged. Adverse effects of antiretroviral medications in children are similar to those experienced by adults, in general, although the Working Group Guidelines should be consulted.[62,152]

TABLE 123-7 Indications for Initiation of Antiretroviral Therapy in Children 1 Year of Age or Older Infected with Human Immunodeficiency Virus (HIV)

Clinical Category		CD4⁺ T-Cell Percentage		Plasma HIV RNA Copy Number	Recommendation
AIDS (Clinical category C)	*or*	<15% (Immune category 3)		Any value	Treat
Mild-to-moderate symptoms (Clinical category A or B)	*or*	15-25%* (Immune category 2)	*or*	≥100,000 copies/mL†	Consider treatment
Asymptomatic (Clinical category N)	*and*	>25% (Immune category 1)	*and*	<100,000 copies/mL†	Many experts would defer therapy and closely monitor clinical, immune, and viral parameters

*Many experts would initiate therapy in children with CD4⁺ T-cell percentages between 15% and 20% of total lymphocytes and defer therapy with increased monitoring frequency in children with CD4⁺ T-cell percentages between 21% and 25%.

†There is controversy among pediatric HIV experts regarding the plasma HIV RNA threshold that warrants consideration of therapy in children in the absence of clinical or immune abnormalities; some experts would consider initiation of therapy in asymptomatic children with plasma HIV RNA levels between 50,000 and 100,000 copies/mL.

From Working Group on Antiretroviral Therapy and Medical Management of HIV-Infected Children. Guidelines for the use of antiretroviral agents in pediatric HIV infection. Updated guidelines are available at http://AIDSinfo.nih.gov and should be consulted.

TABLE 123-8   Summary of Recommended Antiretroviral Regimens for Initial Therapy for Human Immunodeficiency Virus (HIV) Infection in Children

Protease Inhibitor (PI)–Based Regimens

Strongly recommended
Two nucleoside reverse transcriptase inhibitors (NRTIs) *plus* lopinavir/ritonavir *or* nelfinavir *or* ritonavir
Alternative recommendation
Two NRTIs *plus* amprenavir (children ≥4 yr) *or* indinavir

Non-nucleoside Reverse Transcriptase Inhibitor (NNRTI)–Based Regimens

Strongly recommended
For children >3 yr, two NRTIs *plus* efavirenz (with or without nelfinavir)
For children ≤3 yr and those who cannot swallow capsules, two NRTIs *plus* nevirapine
Alternative recommendation
Two NRTIs *plus* nevirapine (children >3 yr)

Nucleoside Analogue–Based Regimens

Strongly recommended
None
Alternative recommendation
Zidovudine *plus* lamivudine *plus* abacavir
Use in special circumstances
Two NRTIs

Regimens That Are Not Recommended

Monotherapy
Certain two NRTI combinations
Two NRTIs *plus* saquinavir soft or hard gel capsule as a sole PI

Insufficient Data to Recommend

Two NRTIs *plus* delavirdine
Dual PIs, including saquinavir soft or hard gel capsule with low-dose ritonavir, with the exception of lopinavir/ritonavir
One NRTI *plus* NNRTI *plus* PI
Tenofovir-containing regimens
Enfuvirtide (T-20)–containing regimens
Emtricitabine (FTC)–containing regimens
Atazanavir-containing regimens
Fosamprenavir-containing regimens

From Working Group on Antiretroviral Therapy and Medical Management of HIV-Infected Children. Guidelines for the use of antiretroviral agents in pediatric HIV infection. Revised February 2004. Updated guidelines are available at http://AIDSinfo.nih.gov and should be consulted

TABLE 123-9   Selected Considerations for Changing Antiretroviral Therapy for Human Immunodeficiency Virus (HIV)–Infected Children

Virologic Considerations

Less than a minimally acceptable virologic response after 8-12 wk of therapy. For children receiving aggressive antiretroviral therapy, such a response is defined as a less than tenfold (1.0 $\log_{10}$) decrease from baseline HIV RNA levels, after at least two measurements.
HIV RNA not suppressed to undetectable levels after 4-6 mo of antiretroviral therapy (for those children who began with very high RNA levels, failure to maintain RNA levels suppressed to at least 1.5 to 2.0 $\log_{10}$ below initial baseline).
Repeated detection of HIV RNA in children who initially had undetectable levels in response to antiretroviral therapy.
A reproducible increase in HIV RNA copy number among children who have had a substantial HIV RNA response but still have low levels of detectable HIV RNA. Such an increase would warrant change in therapy if, after achieving a virologic nadir, a greater than threefold (>0.5 $\log_{10}$) increase in copy number is observed for children aged ≥2 yr, or a greater than fivefold (>0.7 $\log_{10}$) increase for children aged <2 yr.

Immunologic Considerations

Change in immunologic classification (see Table 123-2).
For children with CD4$^+$ T-cell percentages <15% of total lymphocytes (i.e., Immune category 3), a persistent decline of ≥ 5 percentage points in CD4$^+$ T-cell percentage (e.g., from 15% to 10%).
A rapid and substantial decrease in absolute CD4+ T-cell count (e.g., >30% decline in <6 mo).

Clinical Considerations

Progressive neurodevelopmental deterioration.
Growth failure, defined as persistent decline in weight-growth velocity despite adequate nutritional support and without other explanation.
Disease progression, defined as advancement from one pediatric clinical category to another (e.g., from Clinical category A to Clinical category B).

From Working Group on Antiretroviral Therapy and Medical Management of HIV-Infected Children. Guidelines for the use of antiretroviral agents in pediatric HIV infection. Revised February 2004. Updated guidelines are available at http://AIDSinfo.nih.gov and should be consulted.

Other new antiretroviral drugs, immunomodulators, and vaccines for therapeutic use are under evaluation. Further information on therapeutic trials in HIV-infected children can be obtained from the websites listed in Table 123-10.

The value of intravenous immune globulin (IGIV) in children with HIV infection has been evaluated in several trials. IGIV therapy in combination with antiviral agents may be given for children with humoral immunodeficiency, including (1) children with hypogammaglobulinemia (IgG level <250 mg/dL); (2) children with recurrent, serious bacterial infections (defined as two or more serious bacterial infections such as bacteremia, meningitis, or pneumonia in a 1-year period); (3) children who fail to form antibodies to common antigens; and (4) children living in areas where measles is highly prevalent who have not developed an antibody response after two doses (1 month or more apart) of measles-mumps-rubella (MMR) vaccine.[14] The dose of IGIV is 400 mg/kg given every 4 weeks. IGIV may also be useful in the treatment of HIV-associated thrombocytopenia in a dose of 500 to 1000 mg/kg per day for 3 to 5 days.[14] In addition, children with bronchiectasis despite treatment with the standard medical regimen of cyclic antibiotics and aggressive respiratory therapy may benefit from adjunctive IGIV therapy at 600 mg/kg per dose, given monthly.[14]

TABLE 123-10   Useful Websites for Information on Pediatric HIV/AIDS

Website	*Sponsor*	*Comments*
Http://www.cdc.gov/hiv/hivinfo.htm	CDC	Compendium of information, websites, telephone and FAX numbers; Spanish language links
Http://www.aidsinfo.nih.gov	NIH/CDC/FDA	Continuously updated guidelines
Http://www.hivguidelines.org	New York State AIDS Institute	Updated guidelines and chapters
Http://www.unaids.org	UNAIDS/WHO/UNICEF	Guidelines relevant to developing countries
Http://www.niaid.nih.gov/daids/	NIAID/NIH	Summary of NIH activities; information on HIV/AIDS topics
Http://www.iasusa.org	International AIDS Society—USA	Updated therapy and antiretroviral resistance information
Http://www.pedhivaids.org and Http://www.womenchildrenhiv.org	François-Xavier Bagnoud Center and National Pediatric & Family HIV Resource Center at the University of Medicine and Dentistry of New Jersey	Pediatric-specific information, links, presentations

CDC, Centers for Disease Control and Prevention; FDA, U.S. Food and Drug Administration; NIH, National Institutes of Health; UNAIDS, Joint United Nations Programme on HIV/AIDS; UNICEF, United Nations Children's Fund; WHO, World Health Organization.

Controlled Clinical Trials of Pediatric HIV Antiretroviral Therapy

Substantial improvements in neurodevelopment, growth, immunologic status, and virologic status have been demonstrated in studies of zidovudine (ZDV), didanosine (ddI), lamivudine, and stavudine monotherapy[176-181]; therapy with two NRTIs[182,183]; and combination therapy with one or two NRTIs plus a protease inhibitor or two NRTIs plus the non-nucleoside reverse transcriptase inhibitor, nevirapine.[184-188] The results of Pediatric AIDS Clinical Trials Group (PACTG) study 152 showed that the combination of ZDV and ddI was more effective than ZDV or ddI therapy alone (although ddI alone had some beneficial effects in children older than 3 years of age).[183] Subsequently, the results from PACTG study 300 showed that combination therapy with ZDV plus lamivudine, or ZDV plus ddI, was superior to ddI alone when analyzed by either clinical or virologic end points.[182] PACTG study 338 showed that combination therapy including a protease inhibitor is more effective in suppressing viral replication than is dual NRTI therapy. A study of aggressive early therapy of HIV-infected infants aged 2 to 3 months administered ZDV, ddI, and nevirapine reported impressive levels of viral suppression.[186] After the introduction of HIV protease inhibitors in palatable formulations suitable for use in children, many clinical trials reporting virologic, immunologic, and clinical success were published (and only selected ones are cited here).[62,65,88,90,104,106,150,152,185-190,189-196] As noted earlier, the increased survival of children with HIV in the HAART era provides clear evidence of therapeutic success, much as in studies of adults given HAART.[54,66]

Prophylaxis against Opportunistic Infections

Early diagnosis and aggressive treatment of opportunistic infections may prolong survival (see Chapter 125).[14,68,69] Prophylaxis against a first episode of PCP is indicated for most patients with significant immunocompromise, including those with HIV infection and those with primary or acquired immunodeficiency, such as from chemotherapy or other immunosuppressive therapy. Lifelong chemoprophylaxis, regardless of the CD4+ T-cell count, is strongly recommended for any HIV-infected persons, including children of any age, who already have had an episode of PCP.

Because half of all cases of PCP in children with perinatally acquired HIV occur in infants 3 to 6 months of age, early identification of infants who have been perinatally exposed to HIV is essential so that prophylaxis can be initiated before they are at risk. The most effective means to implement this recommendation is by diagnosing maternal HIV infection before or during pregnancy. Prophylaxis for PCP is recommended for all infants born to HIV-infected women, beginning at 4 to 6 weeks of age and regardless of the CD4+ T-cell counts. Prophylaxis for PCP should be discontinued for children in whom HIV infection has been excluded. Children whose HIV infection status has not yet been determined should continue prophylaxis throughout the first year of life.

Prophylaxis should be continued after 1 year of age for HIV-infected children who have had any CD4+ T-cell determination in the first 12 months of life indicating severe immunosuppression (i.e., CD4+ T lymphocytes less than 750 cells/μL or less than 15% of total circulating lymphocytes). Prophylaxis may be discontinued at 1 year of age if CD4+ T-cell monitoring has been appropriate and counts have remained greater than these threshold values that define immunosuppression.

For HIV-infected children aged 1 to 5 years, PCP prophylaxis should be administered if (1) any CD4+ T-cell count is less than 500 cells/μL or the CD4+ T-cell percentage is less than 15% of total lymphocytes; (2) a rapidly declining CD4+ T-cell count occurs; or (3) severely symptomatic HIV disease (category C) is present. Criteria are the same for older children and adolescents, except for different, age-specific definitions of low absolute CD4+ T-cell counts. For children 6 years of age or older, any CD4+ T-cell count of less than 200 cells/μL is an indication for chemoprophylaxis. For adolescents or adults, PCP prophylaxis is indicated if the CD4+ T-cell count is less than 200 cells/μL or the patient has unexplained fever for 2 or more weeks or a history of oropharyngeal candidiasis.

HIV-infected children older than 1 year of age, not previously receiving PCP prophylaxis (e.g., those children not previously identified or whose PCP prophylaxis was discontinued), should begin prophylaxis if at any time their CD4+ T-cell counts indicate severe immunosuppression.

The recommended drug regimen for prophylaxis in all immunocompromised patients (whether from HIV infection, malignancy, or other causes) is trimethoprim-sulfamethoxazole (150 mg trimethroprim/m²/day with 750 mg sulfamethoxazole/m²/day) administered orally in divided doses twice a day three times per week on consecutive days (e.g., Monday-Tuesday-Wednesday); alternative dosing schedules include administering the same total dose once daily, 3 days per week, or dividing the dose and giving it every day of the week or on alternate days. For patients who cannot tolerate trimethoprim-sulfamethoxazole, aerosolized pentamidine (300 mg via Respirgard II inhaler monthly) is considered to be an alternative for those children 5 years of age or older; daily oral dapsone (2 mg/kg, not to exceed 100 mg) is another alternative drug for prophylaxis in children, especially those younger than 5 years. Intravenous pentamidine has also been used, but it appears to be less effective and potentially more toxic than other prophylactic regimens.

Other drugs with potential for prophylaxis include pyrimethamine with dapsone, pyrimethamine-sulfadoxine, and oral atovaquone. Experience with these drugs in both adults and children is limited. These agents should be considered only in unusual situations in which the recommended regimens are not tolerated or cannot be used.

Although prophylaxis substantially reduces the risk of PCP, pulmonary and extrapulmonary *P. jirovecii* infections have occurred in HIV-infected adults and children receiving prophylaxis. The drug of choice for treatment of *P. jirovecii* infections in children is trimethoprim-sulfamethoxazole; parenterally administered pentamidine is an alternative. In children, experience with other agents such as atovaquone, trimetrexate with leucovorin, dapsone with trimethoprim, and clindamycin with primaquine is limited.[70] Corticosteroids may be a useful adjunctive therapy for moderate to severe PCP in children, as has proved to be the case in adults.[70,197-201]

Chemoprophylaxis is also suggested to prevent *M. avium* complex infections in children older than 6 years of age who have CD4+ T-cell counts lower than 50 cells/μL; azithromycin (weekly) or clarithromycin (daily) is the drug of choice, with daily rifabutin as an alternative.[68,69] Younger children are given prophylactic drugs at higher CD4+ T-cell counts, in accordance with age-adjusted normal values.[68,69]

Other opportunistic infections such as cytomegalovirus infections, fungal disease, and toxoplasmic encephalitis may also warrant chemoprophylaxis in children, but data are lacking to provide clear indications.[68,69]

Immunization Recommendations

Published guidelines regarding recommended immunizations for children with HIV infection are available and should be consulted.[14,68,69] The specific comments that follow are grouped according to whether the child is symptomatic, asymptomatic, or a seronegative contact of a person with HIV infection.[14,68,69]

Children with Symptomatic HIV Infection

In general, live-viral vaccines (e.g., varicella) and live-bacterial vaccines (e.g., Calmette-Guérin bacillus [BCG]) should not be given to patients with AIDS or other clinical manifestations of advanced HIV infection indicative of immunosuppression.

Routinely recommended inactivated vaccines—namely, diphtheria and tetanus toxoids and acellular pertussis (DTaP) (or, where still used, diphtheria and tetanus toxoids and pertussis [DTP]), hepatitis B, *H. influenzae* type b conjugate, pneumococcal conjugate, and inactivated poliovirus vaccines—should be given according to the usual immunization schedule. Pneumococcal polysaccharide vaccine (at 2 years of age) and inactivated influenza vaccine (yearly, beginning at the age of 6 months) also are recommended. No adverse effects beyond those seen in non–HIV-infected children are to be expected from these inactivated vaccines.[14,68,69]

Because of the occurrence of severe measles in symptomatic HIV-infected children and the lack of reported serious or unusual reactions to immunization with MMR, measles immunization of HIV-infected children (given as MMR) is recommended unless there is severe immunocompromise. This is an exception to the general rule against use of live vaccines in children with symptomatic HIV infection. If possible, vaccine should be given at 12 months of age (i.e., before deterioration of the immune system) to enhance the likelihood of an immune response. The second dose may be administered as soon as 1 month (4 weeks) later in an attempt to induce seroconversion as early as possible. If the risk of exposure to measles is increased (e.g., during an outbreak), the vaccine should be given at an earlier age, such as 6 to 9 months. However, MMR vaccine is contraindicated in severely immunocompromised persons with HIV infection (immune category 3; see Table 123-2), because of the rare occurrence of fatal pneumonitis with vaccine strain measles virus.[202,203]

In general, children with symptomatic HIV infection have poor immunologic responses to vaccines. Such children, when exposed to a vaccine-preventable disease such as measles or tetanus, should be considered susceptible regardless of the history of vaccination and should receive, if indicated, passive immunoprophylaxis. Immune globulin should also be given to any unimmunized household member who is exposed to measles infection.

Children with Asymptomatic HIV Infection

Children with asymptomatic HIV infection should receive DTaP or DTP, inactivated poliovirus, *H. influenzae* type b and pneumococcal conjugate, hepatitis B, and MMR vaccines, according to the usual immunization schedules. No adverse effects beyond those seen in non–HIV-infected children are to be expected from these vaccines.[14]

Varicella vaccine (live, attenuated) is safe and recommended for children with early HIV infection (CDC categories N1 and A1).[14,68,69]

Pneumococcal polysaccharide vaccination is indicated for HIV-infected children 2 years of age and older, because they are at increased risk for invasive pneumococcal infection. Revaccination once after 3 to 5 years is recommended. Yearly influenza vaccinations should be given to asymptomatic HIV-infected children 6 months of age or older. The inactivated (killed) influenza vaccine should be used, rather than the nasal spray live-attenuated vaccine (FluMist), until further data regarding safety of the latter accrue. Other inactivated vaccines (e.g., hepatitis A vaccine) may be given to those living in areas with high risk of disease.

In the United States and in areas of low prevalence of tuberculosis, BCG is not recommended. However, in developing countries where the prevalence of tuberculosis is high, the WHO recommends that BCG vaccine be given to all infants at birth if they are asymptomatic, regardless of maternal HIV infection status.

Seronegative Children Residing in the Household of a Patient with Symptomatic HIV Infection

MMR may be given to HIV-uninfected children who are living in the household of a patient with symptomatic HIV infection, because MMR vaccine viruses are not transmitted. To reduce the risk of transmission of influenza to patients with symptomatic HIV infection, yearly influenza vaccination is indicated for their household contacts.

Although person-to-person transmission of the varicella vaccine virus has been reported rarely, varicella vaccination of siblings and susceptible adult caregivers of patients with HIV infection is strongly encouraged, to prevent acquisition of the wild-type varicella-zoster infection, which can cause severe disease in immunocompromised hosts.

Passive Immunization of Children with HIV Infection

Measles. Symptomatic HIV-infected children who are exposed to measles should receive immune globulin prophylaxis (0.5 mL/kg, maximum 15 mL), regardless of vaccination status. Exposed, asymptomatic HIV-infected patients who are susceptible should also receive immune globulin; the recommended dose is 0.25 mL/kg. Children who have received IGIV within 2 weeks of exposure do not require additional passive immunization.

Tetanus. In the management of wounds classified as tetanus prone, children with HIV infection should receive tetanus immune globulin regardless of their vaccination status.

Varicella. Children infected with HIV who are exposed to varicella or herpes zoster and who are susceptible should receive varicella-zoster immune globulin. Children who have received IGIV or varicella-zoster immune globulin within 2 weeks of exposure do not require additional passive immunization.

HIV INFECTION IN ADOLESCENTS

Information regarding HIV infection and AIDS should be regarded as an important component of the anticipatory guidance provided by physicians to their adolescent patients.[14] This guidance should include information about transmission, implications of infection, and strategies for prevention including abstinence from behaviors that place adolescents at risk and safer sex practices for those who decide to be sexually active. Diagnostic testing should be available and offered. Parental involvement in adolescent health care is a desirable goal; however, the consent of the adolescent alone should be sufficient to provide evaluation and treatment for suspected or confirmed HIV infection.[14] Particular efforts should be targeted at those adolescents who are without an identified health care provider. HIV-infected adolescents should be counseled as to ways in which they can inform sexual partners of their seropositive status and advised to use barrier protection for all sexual activity. If the provider believes that disclosure to a sexual partner without the consent of the patient must be made, several factors should be considered, including relevant laws that may prohibit or require such disclosure, the effects on future provider-patient relationships, and the safety of the patient.

HIV-infected adolescents who require therapy face a complicated set of issues. They are frequently inexperienced with medication regimens and health care provision systems; they may fear or deny their HIV infection; and they may distrust any information given to them by the medical establishment.[62] Adolescents may also have complex biopsychosocial issues such as low self-esteem, chaotic and unstructured lifestyles, peer pressures not to be singled out with illness, and a lack of family support, all of which may reduce adherence. The concrete thought processes of adolescents might make it difficult for them to understand why medications are necessary during periods of asymptomatic infection, especially if they have experienced any adverse effects of medication. Therefore, treatment regimens for adolescents must balance the goal of prescribing a maximally potent antiretroviral regimen with a realistic assessment of existing and potential support systems for the adolescent to adhere to such a regimen.[62,152]

SCHOOL ATTENDANCE, CHILD CARE, AND FOSTER CARE OF CHILDREN WITH HIV INFECTION

With the current standard of care, pediatric HIV infection has become a chronic condition that requires daily medication but should not prevent the infected child from participating in routine activities of daily life, including school attendance. In the absence of blood exposure, HIV infection is not acquired through the types of contact that usually occur in a school setting, including contact with saliva or tears. Hence, children with HIV infection should not be excluded from school for the protection of other children or personnel.[13,14] Most school-aged children and adolescents infected with HIV should be allowed to attend school without restrictions, provided the child's physician gives approval.[14] The need for a more restricted school environment for some infected children should be evaluated on a case-by-case basis with consideration of conditions that may pose an increased risk to others, such as aggressive biting behavior or the presence of exudative, weeping skin lesions that cannot be covered. This risk should be assessed regularly by the child's physician. Only the child's parents or other guardians and the child's physician have an absolute need to know that the child is HIV infected.[13,14] The number of personnel who are aware of the child's condition should be kept to the minimum needed to ensure proper care of the child. The family has the right to inform the school, if they so choose. Persons involved in the care and education of an infected student must respect the student's right to confidentiality. Similarly, there is no reason to restrict foster care, adoption, or child care placement of HIV-infected children to protect the health of other family members or personnel.[14] All schools and child care settings should adopt routine procedures for handling blood or blood-contaminated fluids, including disposal of sanitary napkins, regardless of whether students with HIV infection are known to be in attendance.[14]

As the life expectancy of HIV-infected children and adolescents increases, the school population of HIV-infected children and adolescents will also increase. An understanding of the effects of chronic illness and recognition of neurodevelopmental problems in these children are essential to provide appropriate educational programs.

PEDIATRIC SEXUAL ABUSE AND SEXUAL ASSAULT

After the discovery of sexual abuse or assault by a person who has or is at risk for HIV infection, counseling of the abused child or adolescent and the family must be provided, and consideration of HIV postexposure prophylaxis (PEP) must be entertained. Serologic evaluation of the perpetrator for HIV infection should be performed whenever possible in accordance with local laws. The child or adolescent should be tested for sexually transmitted infections at the time of the assault and serologically for HIV at the time of sexual exposure and at 6 weeks, 3 months, and 6 months after sexual contact.[14]

Guidelines for PEP for pediatric and adolescent survivors of sexual assault or abuse have been published and are similar to those recommended for adults[14,204-206] (also see Chapter 124). Such guidelines are based on expert opinion and analogy to PEP for occupational exposure among health care workers. Clinical trials evidence exists only for occupational PEP, however, and the published guidelines for all forms of PEP (i.e., sexual assault or occupational exposure) vary in both the exact indications for PEP and in whether two or three antiretroviral agents should be used if PEP is prescribed.[204] The U.S. Public Health Service recommends consideration of PEP after sexual assault in which the risk for HIV exposure is likely to be high, as judged by the local prevalence of HIV/AIDS, the HIV risk behaviors of the assailant, and whether penetration or ejaculation occurred during the assault; if PEP is recommended, it is recommended that the regimen contain zidovudine (ZDV) and lamivudine (3TC) and that it be initiated within 72 hours after sexual exposure.[207] In contrast, The New York State Department of Health AIDS Institute recommends basing initiation of PEP only on the characteristics of the assault and suggests beginning a three-drug HAART regimen (ZDV, 3TC and nelfinavir or tenofovir) in all cases, within 36 hours after exposure[204] (see guidelines available at http://www.hivguidelines.org/public_html/center/clinical-guidelines/clinical-guidelines.shtml [accessed April 2, 2004]). Consultation with an expert in pediatric HIV infection is advised, and practitioners should be aware of local regulations concerning standards of care (e.g., official New York, California, and Rhode Island state treatment guidelines). Survivors of sexual assault or abuse should be serologically tested at baseline and at 1, 3, and 6 months after the assault, whether PEP is prescribed or not. Additionally, some experts would recommend use of an HIV RNA test if the assault victim develops an illness consistent with primary HIV infection syndrome (e.g., fever, malaise, rash, adenopathy).

CHILDREN WITH ACCIDENTAL HIV EXPOSURE

Injuries from hypodermic needles and syringes discarded in public places, usually by injection drug users, are perceived by victims as a significant risk for transmission of HIV infection, although these injuries pose less of a risk than that resulting from needlestick injuries in health care settings.[14,205] The risk of HIV transmission from a discarded needle in public places appears to be low, and data on the efficacy of PEP in such cases are not available. Consultation with a spe-

cialist in HIV infection should be obtained when deciding whether to give a child postexposure chemoprophylaxis (see Chapter 304).[14,205] The schedule of testing for serum HIV antibody is identical to that described for child victims of sexual assault. If PEP is recommended, it seems reasonable to follow the pediatric sexual assault guidelines.

Additional information on a variety of HIV-related topics can be found on the websites listed in Table 123-10.

REFERENCES

1. Centers for Disease Control and Prevention. *Pneumocystis* pneumonia—Los Angeles. MMWR Morb Mortal Wkly Rep. 1981;30:250-252.
2. Centers for Disease Control and Prevention. Kaposi's sarcoma and *Pneumocystis* pneumonia among homosexual men—New York City and California. MMWR Morb Mortal Wkly Rep. 1981;30:305-308.
3. Gottlieb MS, Schroff R, Schanker HM, et al. *Pneumocystis carinii* pneumonia and mucosal candidiasis in previously healthy homosexual men: Evidence of a new acquired cellular immunodeficiency. N Engl J Med. 1981;305:1425-1431.
4. Masur H, Michelis MA, Greene JB, et al. An outbreak of community acquired *Pneumocystis carinii* pneumonia: Initial manifestation of cellular immune dysfunction. N Engl J Med. 1981;305:1431-1438.
5. Huminer D, Rosenfeld JB, Pitlik SD. AIDS in the pre-AIDS era. Rev Infect Dis. 1987;9:1102-1108.
6. Ammann AJ, Cowan MJ, Wara DW, et al: Acquired immunodeficiency in an infant: Possible transmission by means of blood products. Lancet. 1983;1:956-958.
7. Oleske J, Minnefor A, Cooper R Jr, Thomas K, et al. Immune deficiency syndrome in children. JAMA. 1983;249:2345-2349.
8. Rubinstein A, Sicklick M, Gupta A, et al. Acquired immunodeficiency with reversed T4/T8 ratios in infants born to promiscuous and drug-addicted mothers. JAMA. 1983;249:2350-2356.
9. Scott GB, Buck BE, Leterman JG, et al. Acquired immunodeficiency syndrome in infants. N Engl J Med. 1984;310:76-81.
10. Mertens TE, Low-Beer D. HIV and AIDS: Where is the epidemic going? Bull World Health Organ. 1996;74:121-129.
11. Centers for Disease Control and Prevention. HIV/AIDS Surveillance Report. 2002;14:1-40.
12. AIDS epidemic update: 2003. UNAIDS/WHO Document 0.339E, December, 2003. Available at: http://www.unaids.org. Accessed April 2, 2004.
13. Simonds RJ, Chanock S. Medical issues related to caring for human immunodeficiency virus-infected children in and out of the home. Pediatr Infect Dis J. 1993;12:845-852.
14. American Academy of Pediatrics. Human immunodeficiency virus infection. In: Pickering LK, ed. 2003 Red Book: Report of the Committee on Infectious Diseases. 26th ed. Elk Grove Village, Ill: American Academy of Pediatrics; 2003:360-382.
15. Mofenson LM, the Committee on Pediatric AIDS. Technical report: Perinatal human immunodeficiency virus testing and prevention of transmission. Pediatrics 2000;106:e88.
16. Read JS, American Academy of Pediatrics Committee on Pediatric AIDS. Human milk, breastfeeding, and transmission of human immunodeficiency virus type 1 in the United States. Pediatrics 2003;112:1196-1205.
17. Weinberg GA. The dilemma of postnatal mother-to-child transmission of HIV: To breastfeed or not? Birth. 2000;27:199-205.
18. Connor EM, Sperling RS, Gelber R, et al. Reduction of maternal-infant transmission of human immunodeficiency virus type 1 with zidovudine treatment. N Engl J Med. 1994;331:1173-1180.
19. Lindegren ML, Byers RH Jr, Thomas P, et al. Trends in perinatal transmission of HIV/AIDS in the United States. JAMA. 1999;282:531-538.
20. Wade NA, Birkhead GS, Warren BL, et al. Abbreviated regimens of zidovudine prophylaxis and perinatal transmission of the human immunodeficiency virus. N Engl J Med. 1998;339:1409-1414.
21. Fiscus SA, Adimora AA, Funk ML, et al. Trends in interventions to reduce perinatal human immunodeficiency virus type 1 transmission in North Carolina. Pediatr Infect Dis J. 2002;21:664-668.
22. Centers for Disease Control and Prevention. Public Health Services Task Force recommendations for the use of antiretroviral drugs in pregnant women infected with HIV-1 for maternal health and interventions to reduce perinatal HIV-1 transmission in the United States. November 26, 2003. Available at: http://aidsinfo.nih.gov. guidelines. Accessed June 14, 2004.
23. Tudor-Williams G, Lyall EGH. Perinatal transmission of HIV. Curr Opin Infect Dis. 1997;10:239-245.
24. Centers for Disease Control and Prevention. Recommendations of the Public Health Service Task Force on use of zidovudine to reduce perinatal transmission of human immunodeficiency virus. MMWR Morb Mortal Wkly Rep. 1994;43(RR-11):1-21.
25. Dorenbaum A, Cunningham CK, Gelber RD, et al. Two-dose intrapartum/newborn nevirapine and standard antiretroviral therapy to reduce perinatal HIV transmission: A randomized trial. JAMA. 2002;288:189-198.
26. Scarlatti G. Pediatric HIV infection. Lancet. 1996;348:863-868.
27. Kuhn L, Steketeern RW, Weedon J, et al: Distinct risk factors for intrauterine and intrapartum human immunodeficiency virus transmission and consequences for disease progression in infected children. J Infect Dis. 1997;179:52-58.

28. Ioannidis JP, Abrams EJ, Ammann A, et al. Perinatal transmission of human immunodeficiency virus type 1 by pregnant women with RNA virus loads <1000 copies/ml. J Infect Dis. 2001;183:539-545.

29. John GC, Nduati RW, Mbori-Ngacha DA, et al. Correlates of mother-to-child human immunodeficiency virus type 1 (HIV-1) transmission: Association with maternal plasma HIV-1 RNA load, genital HIV-1 DNA shedding, and breast infections. J Infect Dis. 2001;183:206-212.

30. Goedert JJ, Duliege AM, Amos CI, et al. High risk of HIV-1 infection for first-born twins. The International Registry of HIV-Exposed Twins. Lancet. 1991;338:1471-1475.

31. Duliege AM, Amos CI, Felton S, et al. Birth order, delivery route, and concordance in the transmission of HIV-1 from mothers to twins. J Pediatr. 1995;126:625-632.

32. Biggar RJ, Cassol S, Kumwenda N, et al. The risk of human immunodeficiency virus-1 infection in twin pairs born to infected mothers in Africa. J Infect Dis. 2003;188:850-855.

33. European Mode of Delivery Collaboration. Elective Caesarian section versus vaginal delivery in prevention of vertical HIV-1 infection: A randomised clinical trial. Lancet. 1999;353:1035-1039.

34. Landesman SH, Kalish CA, Burns DN, et al. Obstetrical factors and the transmission of human immunodeficiency virus type 1 from mother to child. N Engl J Med. 1996;334:1617-1623.

35. Mandelbrot L, Le Chenadec J, Berrebi A, et al. Perinatal HIV-1 transmission: Interaction between zidovudine prophylaxis and mode of delivery in the French Perinatal Cohort. JAMA. 1998;280:55-60.

36. The International Perinatal HIV Group. The mode of delivery and the risk of vertical transmission of human immunodeficiency virus type 1-a meta-analysis of 15 prospective cohort studies. N Eng J Med. 1999;340:977-987.

37. Mofenson LM. Mother-child HIV-1 transmission: Timing and determinants. Obstet Gynecol Clin North Am. 1997;24:759-784.

38. Guay LA, Musoke P, Fleming T, et al. Intrapartum and neonatal single-dose nevirapine compared with zidovudine for prevention of mother-to-child transmission of HIV-1 in Kampala, Uganda: HIVNET 012 randomised trial. Lancet. 1999;354:795-802.

39. Lallemant M, Jourdain G, Le Coeur S, et al. A trial of shortened zidovudine regimens to prevent mother-to-child transmission of human immunodeficiency virus type 1. Perinatal HIV Prevention Trial (Thailand) Investigators. N Engl J Med. 2000;343:982-991.

40. PETRA Study Team. Efficacy of three short-course regimens of zidovudine and lamivudine in preventing early and late transmission of HIV-1 from mother to child in Tanzania, South Africa, and Uganda (Petra study): A randomised, double-blind, placebo-controlled trial. Lancet. 2002;359:1178-1186.

41. Leroy V, Newell M-L, Dabis F, et al. International multicentre pooled analysis of late postnatal mother-to-child transmission of HIV-1 infection. Lancet. 1998;352:597-600.

42. Nduati R, John G, Mbori-Ngacha D, et al. Effect of breastfeeding and formula feeding on transmission of HIV-1: A randomized clinical trial. JAMA. 2000;283:1167-1174.

43. Nduati R, Richardson BA, John G, et al. Effect of breastfeeding on mortality among HIV-1 infected women: A randomised trial. Lancet. 2001;357:1651-1655.

44. Blanche S, Tardieu M, Rustin P, et al. Persistent mitochondrial dysfunction and perinatal exposure to antiretroviral nucleoside analogues. Lancet. 1999;354:1084-1089.

45. The Perinatal Safety Review Working Group. Nucleoside exposure in the children of HIV-infected women receiving antiretroviral drugs: Absence of clear evidence for mitochondrial disease in children who died before 5 years of age in five United States cohorts. J Acquir Immune Defic Syndr. 2000;25:261-268.

46. Morris CR, Araba-Owoyele L, Spector SA, Maldonado YA. Disease patterns and survival after acquired immunodeficiency syndrome diagnosis in human immunodeficiency virus-infected children. Pediatr Infect Dis J. 1996;15:321-328.

47. Bamji M, Thea DM, Weedon J, et al. Prospective study of human immunodeficiency virus 1-related disease among 512 infants born to infected women in New York City. Pediatr Infect Dis J. 1996;15:891-898.

48. Italian Register for HIV Infection in Children. Features of children perinatally infected with HIV-1 surviving longer than 5 years. Lancet. 1994;343:191-195.

49. Galli L, de Martino M, Pier-Angelo T, et al. Onset of clinical signs in children with HIV-1 perinatal infections. AIDS. 1995;9:455-461.

50. Grubman S, Gross E, Lerner-Weiss N, et al. Older children and adolescents living with perinatally acquired human immunodeficiency virus infection. Pediatrics. 1995;95:657-663.

51. Barnhart HX, Caldwell MB, Thomas P, et al. Natural history of human immunodeficiency virus disease in perinatally infected children: An analysis from the Pediatric Spectrum of Disease Project. Pediatrics. 1996;97:710-716.

52. Abrams EJ, Weedon J, Bertolli J, et al. Aging cohort of perinatally human immunodeficiency virus-infected children in New York City. New York City Pediatric Surveillance of Disease Consortium. Pediatr Infect Dis J. 2001;20:511-517.

53. Frederick T, Thomas P, Mascola L, et al. Human immunodeficiency virus-infected adolescents: A descriptive study of older children in New York City, Los Angeles County, Massachusetts and Washington, DC. Pediatr Infect Dis J. 2000;19:551-555.

54. Gibb DM, Duong T, Tookey PA, et al. Decline in mortality, AIDS, and hospital admissions in perinatally HIV-1 infected children in the United Kingdom and Ireland. BMJ. 2003;327:1019.

55. Mayaux M-J, Burgard M, Teglas J-P, et al. Neonatal characteristics in rapidly progressive perinatally acquired HIV-1 disease. JAMA. 1996;275:606-610.

56. Rosenberg PS, Biggar RJ. Trends in HIV incidence among young adults in the United States. JAMA. 1998;279:1894-1899.

57. Scott GB, Hutto C, Makuch RW, et al. Survival in children with perinatally acquired human immunodeficiency virus type 1 infection. N Engl J Med. 1989;321:1791-1796.

58. Turner BJ, Denison M, Eppes SC, et al. Survival experience of 789 children with the acquired immunodeficiency syndrome. Pediatr Infect Dis J. 1993;12:310-320.

59. Abrams EJ, Matheson PB, Thomas PA, et al. Neonatal predictors of infection status and early death among 332 infants at risk of HIV-1 infection monitored prospectively from birth. Pediatrics. 1995;96:451-458.

60. Centers for Disease Control and Prevention. 1994 Revised classification system for human immunodeficiency virus infection in children less than 13 years of age; official authorized addenda: Human immunodeficiency virus infection codes and official guidelines for coding and reporting ICD-9-CM. MMWR Morb Mortal Wkly Rep. 1994;43(RR-12):1-19.

61. Dunn D, HIV Paediatric Prognostic Markers Collaborative Study Group. Short-term risk of disease progression in HIV-1-infected children receiving no antiretroviral therapy or zidovudine monotherapy: A meta-analysis. Lancet. 2003;362:1605-1611.

62. Working Group on Antiretroviral Therapy and Medical Management of HIV-Infected Children. Guidelines for the use of antiretroviral agents in pediatric HIV infection. January 20, 2004. Available at: http://aidsinfo.nih.gov.guidelines. Accessed June 14, 2004.

63. Domachowske J. Pediatric human immunodeficiency virus infection. Clin Microbiol Rev. 1996;9:448-468.

64. Hanson IC, Shearer WT. Lentiviruses (human immunodeficiency virus type 1 and acquired immunodeficiency syndrome). In: Feigin RD, Cherry JD, DemmlerGJ, Kaplan SL, eds. Textbook of Pediatric Infectious Diseases. 5th ed. Philadelphia: WB Saunders; 2004:2455-2481.

65. Saulsbury F. Resolution of organ-specific complications of human immunodeficiency virus infection in children with use of highly active antiretroviral therapy. Clin Infect Dis. 2001;32:464-468.

66. Gortmaker SL, Hughes M, Cervia J, et al. Effect of combination therapy including protease inhibitors on mortality among children and adolescents infected with HIV-1. N Engl J Med. 2001;345:1522-1528.

67. Centers for Disease Control and Prevention. 1995 Revised guidelines for prophylaxis against *Pneumocystis carinii* pneumonia for children infected with or perinatally exposed to human immunodeficiency virus. MMWR Morb Mortal Wkly Rep. 1995;44(RR-4):1-11.

68. Kaplan JE, Masur H, Holmes KK. Prevention of opportunistic infections in persons infected with human immunodeficiency virus. Clin Infect Dis. 2000;30(Suppl 1):S1-S93.

69. Centers for Disease Control and Prevention. Guidelines for preventing opportunistic infections among HIV-infected persons—2002. MMWR Morb Mortal Wkly Rep. 2002;51(RR-8):1-52.

70. Weinberg GA, White AC Jr, Rathore MH. Other infectious agents (*Pneumocystis carinii, Legionella pneumophila,* and protozoan and helminthic pulmonary infections). In: Taussig L, Landau L, LeSouëf PN, et al, eds. Pediatric Respiratory Medicine. St. Louis: Mosby; 1999:762-784.

71. Gonzalez CE, Shetty D, Lewis L, et al. Cryptococcosis in human immunodeficiency virus-infected children. Pediatr Infect Dis J. 1996;15:796-800.

72. Abadi J, Nachman S, Kressel AB, Pirofski L. Cryptococcosis in children with AIDS. Clin Infect Dis. 1999;28:309-313.

73. Hoyt L, Oleske J, Holland B, Connor E. Nontuberculous mycobacteria in children with acquired immunodeficiency syndrome. Pediatr Infect Dis J. 1992;11:354-360.

74. Schuval S, Van Dyke R, Lindsey J, et al. GB virus C prevalence in perinatally-infected HIV-positive children (Abstract 682). In: Program and Abstracts of the 41st Annual Meeting of the Infectious Diseases Society of America, San Diego, Calif, October 9-12, 2003. Alexandria, Va: Infectious Diseases Society of America, pp 143-144.

75. Schuval S, Van Dyke R, Lindsey J, et al. Hepatitis C prevalence in perinatally-infected HIV-positive children (Abstract 683). In: Program and Abstracts of the 41st Annual Meeting of the Infectious Diseases Society of America, October 9-12, 2003. Alexandria, Va: Infectious Diseases Society of America, San Diego, Calif, p 144.

76. Chantry CJ, Byrd RS, Englund JA, et al. Growth, survival and viral load in symptomatic childhood human immunodeficiency virus infection. Pediatr Infect Dis J. 2003;22:1033-1039.

77. McKinney RE, Wilfert C, and the AIDS Clinical Trials Group Protocol 043 Study Group. Growth as a prognostic factor in children with human immunodeficiency virus infection treated with zidovudine. J Pediatr. 1994;125:728-733.

78. McKinney RE, Robertson JW, Duke Pediatric AIDS Clinical Trials Unit. Effect of human immunodeficiency virus infection on the growth of young children. J Pediatr. 1993;123:579-582.

79. Miller TL, Evans SJ, Orav EJ, et al. Growth and body composition in children with human immunodeficiency virus-1 infection. Am J Clin Nutr. 1993;57:588-592.

80. Arpadi SM, Horlick MNB, Wang J, et al. Body composition in prepubertal children with human immunodeficiency virus type 1 infection. Arch Pediatr Adolesc Med. 1998;152:688-693.

81. Newell ML, Borja MC, Peckham C. Height, weight, and growth in children born to mothers with HIV-1 infection in Europe. Pediatrics. 2003;111:e52-e60.

82. Saavedra J, Henderson RA, Perman JA, et al. Longitudinal assessment of growth in children born to mothers with human immunodeficiency virus infection. Arch Pediatr Adolesc Med. 1995;149:497-502.

83. Moye Jr. J, Rich KC, Kalish LA, et al. Natural history of somatic growth in infants born to women infected by human immunodeficiency virus. J Pediatr. 1996;128:58-69.

84. Arpadi SM, Cuff PA, Kotler DP, et al. Growth velocity, fat-free mass, and energy intake are inversely related to viral load in HIV-infected children. J Nutr. 2000;130:2498-2502.

85. Miller TL, Garg S. Gastrointestinal and nutritional problems in pediatric HIV disease. In: Pizzo PA, Wilfert CM, eds. Pediatric AIDS: The Challenge of HIV Infection in Infants, Children, and Adolescents. 3rd ed. Baltimore: Lippincott Williams & Wilkins; 1998:363-382.

86. McKinney RE Jr. Abnormalities in growth and development. In: Pizzo PA, Wilfert CM, eds. Pediatric AIDS: The Challenge of HIV Infection in Infants, Children, and Adolescents. 3rd ed. Baltimore: Lippincott Williams & Wilkins; 1998:417-426.

87. Miller TL, Awnetwant EL, Evans S, et al. Gastrostomy tube supplementation for HIV infected children. Pediatrics. 1995; 96:696-702.

88. Dreimane D, Nielsen K, Deveikis A, et al. Effect of protease inhibitors combined with standard antiretroviral therapy on linear growth and weight gain in human immunodeficiency virus type 1-infected children. Pediatr Infect Dis J. 2001;20:315-316.
89. Miller TL, Mawn BE, Orav EJ, et al. The effect of protease inhibitor therapy on growth and body composition in human immunodeficiency virus type-1 infected children. Pediatrics. 2001;107:e77-e82.
90. Buchacz K, Cervia JS, Lindsey JC, et al. Impact of protease inhibitor-containing combination antiretroviral therapies on height and weight growth in HIV-infected children. Pediatrics. 2001;108:e72-e78.
91. Nachman SA, Lindsey JC, Pelton S, et al. Growth in human immunodeficiency virus-infected children receiving ritonavir-containing antiretroviral therapy. Arch Pediatr Adolesc Med. 2002;156:497-503.
92. Stockheim JA, Daaboul JJ, Yogev R, et al. Adrenal suppression in children with the human immunodeficiency virus treated with megestrol acetate. J Pediatr. 1999;134:368-370.
93. Andiman WA, Mezger J, Shapiro E. Invasive bacterial infections in children born to women infected with human immunodeficiency virus type 1. J Pediatr. 1994;124:846-852.
94. Mao C, Harper M, McIntosh K, et al. Invasive pneumococcal infections in human immunodeficiency virus-infected children. J Infect Dis. 1996;173:870-876.
95. Nachman S, Kim S, King J, et al. Safety and immunogenicity of a heptavalent pneumococcal conjugate vaccine in infants with human immunodeficiency virus type 1 infection. Pediatrics. 2003;112:66-73.
96. Andiman WA, Shearer WT. Lymphoid interstitial pneumonitis. In: Pizzo PA, Wilfert CM, eds. Pediatric AIDS: The Challenge of HIV Infection in Infants, Children, and Adolescents. 3rd ed. Baltimore: Lippincott Williams & Wilkins; 1998:323-334.
97. Pitt J. Lymphocytic interstitial pneumonia. Pediatr Clin North Am. 1991;38:89-95.
98. Epstein LG, Sharer LR, Oleske JM, et al. Neurologic manifestations of HIV infection in children. Pediatrics. 1986;78:678-687.
99. Browers P, Wolters P, Civitello L. Central nervous system: Manifestation and assessment. In: Pizzo PA, Wilfert CM, eds. Pediatric AIDS: The Challenge of HIV Infection in Infants, Children, and Adolescents. 3rd ed. Baltimore: Lippincott Williams & Wilkins; 1998:323-334.
100. Cooper ER, Hanson C, Diaz C, et al. Encephalopathy and progression of human immunodeficiency virus disease in a cohort of children with perinatally acquired human immunodeficiency virus infection. J Pediatr. 1998;132:808-812.
101. Coplan J, Contello KA, Cunningham CK, et al. Early language development in children exposed to or infected with human immunodeficiency virus. Pediatrics. 1998;102:1. Available at: http://www.pediatrics.org/cgi/content/full/102/1/e8. Accessed April 2, 2004.
102. Belman AL, Diamond G, Dickson D, et al. Pediatric acquired immunodeficiency syndrome: Neurologic syndromes. Am J Dis Child. 1988;142:29-35.
103. Scarmatov V, Frank Y, Rozenstein A. Central brain atrophy in childhood AIDS encephalopathy. AIDS. 1996;10:1227-1231.
104. McCoig C, Castrejon MM, Castano E, et al. Effect of combination antiretroviral therapy on cerebrospinal fluid HIV RNA, HIV resistance, and clinical manifestations of encephalopathy. J Pediatr 2002;141:36-44.
105. Llorente A, Brouwers P, Charurat M, et al. Early neurodevelopmental markers predictive of mortality in infants infected with HIV-1. Dev Med Child Neurol. 2003;45:76-84.
106. Lindsey JC, Hughes MD, McKinney RE, et al. Treatment-mediated changes in human immunodeficiency virus (HIV) type 1 RNA and CD4 cell counts as predictors of weight growth failure, cognitive decline, and survival in HIV-infected children. J Infect Dis. 2000;182:1385-1393.
107. Miller TL, Winter HS, Luginbuhl LM, et al. Pancreatitis in pediatric human immunodeficiency virus infection. J Pediatr. 1992;120:223-227.
108. Hauk MJ, Moss ME, Weinberg GA, Berkowitz RJ. Delayed tooth eruption: Association with severity of HIV infection. Pediatr Dent. 2001;23:260-262.
109. Hauk M, Berkowitz RJ, Moss M, et al. Hospitalizations associated with oral lesions in perinatally HIV-infected children. Pediatr Dent. 1997;19:484-485.
110. Greenspan D, Greenspan JS. HIV-related oral disease. Lancet. 1996;348:729-733.
111. Patton LL, Phelan JA, Ramos-Gomez FJ, et al. Prevalence and classification of HIV-associated oral lesions. Oral Dis. 2002;8:98-109.
112. Greenspan JS, Greenspan D. The epidemiology of the oral lesions of HIV infection in the developed world. Oral Dis. 2002;8:34-39.
113. Lipshultz SE, Bancroft EA, Boller SMA. Cardiovascular manifestation (sic) of HIV infection in children. In: Pizzo PA, Wilfert CM, eds. Pediatric AIDS: The Challenge of HIV Infection in Infants, Children, and Adolescents. 3rd ed. Baltimore: Lippincott Williams & Wilkins; 1998:335-362.
114. Lipshultz SE, Chanock S, Sanders SP, et al. Cardiovascular manifestations of human immunodeficiency virus in infants and children. Am J Cardiol. 1989;63:1489-1497.
115. Luginbuhl LM, Orav EJ, McIntosh K, Lipshultz SE. Cardiac morbidity and related mortality in children with HIV infection. JAMA. 1993;269:2869-2875.
116. Langston C, Cooper ER, Goldfarb J, et al. Human immunodeficiency virus-related mortality in infants and children: Data from the pediatric pulmonary and cardiovascular complications of vertically transmitted HIV (P(2)C(2)) Study. Pediatrics. 2001;107:328-338.
117. Lipshultz SE, Orav EJ, Sanders SP, et al. Cardiac structure and function in children with human immunodeficiency virus infection treated with zidovudine. N Engl J Med. 1992;327:1260-1265.
118. P^2C^2 HIV Study Group. The pediatric pulmonary and cardiovascular complication of vertically transmitted human immunodeficiency virus (P^2C^2 HIV) infection study: Design and methods. J Clin Epidemiol. 1996;49:1285-1294.
119. Lipshultz SE, Easley KA, Orav EJ, et al. Absence of cardiac toxicity of zidovudine in infants. Pediatric Pulmonary and Cardiac Complications of Vertically Transmitted HIV Infection Study Group. N Engl J Med. 2000;343:759-766.
120. Starc TJ, Lipshultz SE, Easley KA, et al. Incidence of cardiac abnormalities in children with human immunodeficiency virus infection: The prospective P2C2 HIV study. J Pediatr. 2002;141:327-334.
121. Strauss J, Abitol C, Zilleruelo G, et al. Renal problems. In: Pizzo PA, Wilfert CM, eds. Pediatric AIDS: The Challenge of HIV Infection in Infants, Children, and Adolescents. 3rd ed. Baltimore: Lippincott Williams & Wilkins; 1998:395-402.
122. Strauss J, Zilleruelo G, Abitbol C, et al. Human immunodeficiency virus nephropathy. Pediatr Nephrol. 1993;7:220-225.
123. Strauss J, Abitbol C, Zilleruelo G, et al. Renal disease in children with the acquired immunodeficiency syndrome. N Engl J Med. 1989;321:625-630.
124. Mueller BU. Hematological problems. In: Pizzo PA, Wilfert CM, eds. Pediatric AIDS: The Challenge of HIV Infection in Infants, Children, and Adolescents. 3rd ed. Baltimore: Lippincott Williams & Wilkins; 1998:427-442.
125. Weinberg GA, Gigliotti F, Stroncek DF, et al. Lack of relation of granulocyte antibodies (antineutrophil antibodies) to neutropenia in children with human immunodeficiency virus infection. Pediatr Infect Dis J. 1997;16:881-884.
126. Watson WJ, Stevens TP, Weinberg GA. Profound anemia in a newborn infant of a mother receiving antiretroviral therapy. Pediatr Infect Dis J. 1998;17:435-436.
127. Goedert JJ, Coté TR, Virgo P, et al. Spectrum of AIDS-associated malignant disorders. Lancet. 1998;351:1833-1839.
128. Mueller BU, Pizzo PA. Malignancies in pediatric AIDS. Curr Opin Pediatr. 1996;8:45-49.
129. Chadwick EG, Connor EJ, Hanson ICG, et al. Tumors of smooth-muscle origin in HIV-infected children. JAMA. 1990;263:3182-3184.
130. Granovsky M, Mueller BU. Malignancies in children with HIV infection. In: Pizzo PA, Wilfert CM, eds. Pediatric AIDS: The Challenge of HIV Infection in Infants, Children, and Adolescents. 3rd ed. Baltimore: Lippincott Williams & Wilkins; 1998:443-462.
131. Pollock BH, Jenson HB, Leach CT, et al. Risk factors for pediatric human immunodeficiency virus-related malignancy. JAMA. 2003;289:2393-2399.
132. Biggar RJ, Frisch M, Goedert JJ. Risk of cancer in children with AIDS. AIDS-Cancer Match Registry Study Group. JAMA. 2000;284:205-209.
133. Church JA, Mitchell WG, Gonzalez-Gomez I, et al. Mitochondrial DNA depletion, near-fatal metabolic acidosis, and liver failure in an HIV-infected child treated with combination antiretroviral therapy. J Pediatr. 2001;138:748-751.
134. European Collaborative Study. Exposure to antiretroviral therapy in utero or early life: The health of uninfected children born to HIV-infected women. J Acquir Immune Defic Syndr. 2003;32:380-387.
135. Gaughan DM, Mofenson LM, Hughes MD, et al. Osteonecrosis of the hip (Legg-Calvé-Perthes disease) in human immunodeficiency virus-infected children. Pediatrics. 2002;109:e74-e81.
136. Amaya RA, Kozinetz CA, McMeans A, et al. Lipodystrophy syndrome in human immunodeficiency virus-infected children. Pediatr Infect Dis J. 2002;21:405-410.
137. Arpadi, SM, Cuff PA, Horlick M, et al. Lipodystrophy in HIV-infected children is associated with high viral load and low CD4+-lymphocyte count and CD4+-lymphocyte percent at baseline and use of protease inhibitors and stavudine. J Acquir Immun Defic Syndr. 2001;27:30-34.
138. Schambelan M, Benson CA, Carr A, et al. Management of metabolic complications associated with antiretroviral therapy for HIV-1 infection: Recommendations of an International AIDS Society-USA panel. J Acquir Immune Defic Syndr. 2002;31:257-275.
139. Dube MP, Stein JH, Aberg JA, et al. Guidelines for the evaluation and management of dyslipidemia in human immunodeficiency virus (HIV)-infected adults receiving antiretroviral therapy: Recommendations of the HIV Medical Association of the Infectious Disease Society of America and the Adult AIDS Clinical Trials Group. Clin Infect Dis. 2003;37:613-627.
140. Kavey RE, Daniels SR, Lauer RM, et al. American Heart Association guidelines for primary prevention of atherosclerotic cardiovascular disease beginning in childhood. J Pediatr. 2003;142:368-372.
141. American Academy of Pediatrics Committee on Nutrition. Cholesterol in childhood. Pediatrics. 1998;101:141-147.
142. Palumbo P, Burchett SK. Diagnosis of HIV infection and markers of disease progression in infants and children. In: Pizzo PA, Wilfert CM, eds. Pediatric AIDS: The Challenge of HIV Infection in Infants, Children, and Adolescents. 3rd ed. Baltimore: Lippincott Williams & Wilkins; 1998:67-88.
143. Comans-Bitter WM, de Groot R, van den Beemd R, et al. Immunophenotyping of blood lymphocytes in childhood: Reference values for lymphocyte subpopulations. J Pediatr. 1997;130:388-393.
144. European Collaborative Study. Age-related standards for T lymphocyte subsets based on uninfected children born to human immunodeficiency virus 1-infected women. Pediatr Infect Dis J. 1992;11:1018-1026.
145. Shearer WT, Rosenblatt HM, Gelman RS, et al. Lymphocyte subsets in healthy children from birth through 18 years of age: The Pediatric AIDS Clinical Trials Group P1009 study. J Allergy Clin Immunol. 2003;112:973-980.
146. Committee on Pediatric AIDS, American Academy of Pediatrics. Evaluation and medical treatment of the HIV-exposed infant. Pediatrics. 1997;99:909-917.
147. Shearer WT, Quinn TC, LaRussa P, et al. Viral load and disease progression in infants infected with human immunodeficiency virus type 1. N Engl J Med. 1997;336:1337-1342.
148. Mofenson LM, Korelitz J, Meyer WA, et al. The relationship between serum human immunodeficiency virus type 1 (HIV-1) RNA level, CD4 lymphocyte percent, and long-term mortality risk in HIV-1-infected children. J Infect Dis. 1997;175:1029-1038.
149. Palumbo PE, Raskino C, Fiscus S, et al. Predictive value of quantitative plasma HIV RNA and $CD4^+$ lymphocyte count in HIV-infected infants and children. JAMA. 1998;279:756-761.
150. Palumbo PE, Raskino C, Fiscus S, et al. Virologic and immunologic response to nucleoside reverse transcriptase inhibitor therapy among human immunodeficiency virus-infected infants and children. J Infect Dis. 1999;179:576-583.

151. Mofenson LM, Harris DR, Moye J, et al. Alternatives to HIV-1 RNA concentration and CD4 count to predict mortality in HIV-1-infected children in resource-poor settings. Lancet. 2003;362:1625-1627.

152. Panel on Clinical Practices for Treatment of HIV Infection. Guidelines for the use of antiretroviral agents in HIV-infected adults and adolescents. March 23, 2004. Available at: http://aidsinfo.nih.gov.guidelines. Accessed June 14, 2004

153. Cunningham CK, Charbonneau TT, Song K, et al. Comparison of human immunodeficiency virus 1 DNA polymerase chain reaction and qualitative and quantitative RNA polymerase chain reaction in human immunodeficiency virus 1-exposed infants. Pediatr Infect Dis J. 1999;18:30-35.

154. Reisler RB, Thea DM, Pliner V, et al. Early detection of reverse transcriptase activity in plasma of neonates infected with HIV-1: A comparative analysis with RNA-based and DNA-based testing using polymerase chain reaction. J Acquir Immune Defic Syndr. 2001;26:93-102.

155. Kline NE, Schwarzwald H, Kline MW. False negative DNA polymerase chain reaction in an infant with subtype C human immunodeficiency virus 1 infection. Pediatr Infect Dis J. 2002;21:885-886.

156. Biggar RJ, Miley W, Miotti P, et al. Blood collection on filter paper: A practical approach to sample collection for studies of perinatal HIV transmission. J Acquir Immune Defic Syndr Hum Retrovirol. 1997;14:368-373.

157. Brambilla D, Jennings C, Aldrovandi G, et al. Multicenter evaluation of use of dried blood and plasma spot specimens in quantitative assays for human immunodeficiency virus RNA: Measurement, precision, and RNA stability. J Clin Microbiol. 2003;41:1888-1893.

158. Beck IA, Drennan KD, Melvin AJ, et al. Simple, sensitive, and specific detection of human immunodeficiency virus type 1 subtype B DNA in dried blood samples for diagnosis in infants in the field. J Clin Microbiol. 2001;39:29-33.

159. Comeau AM, Hsu HW, Schwerzler M, et al. Identifying human immunodeficiency virus infection at birth: Application of polymerase chain reaction to Guthrie cards. J Pediatr. 1993;123:252-258.

160. Comeau AM, Pitt J, Hillyer GV, et al. Early detection of human immunodeficiency virus on dried blood spot specimens: Sensitivity across serial specimens. Women and Infants Transmission Study Group. J Pediatr. 1996;129:111-118.

161. Panteleeff DD, John G, Nduati R, et al. Rapid method for screening dried blood samples on filter paper for human immunodeficiency virus type 1 DNA. J Clin Microbiol. 1999;37:350-353.

162. Dunn DT, Brandt CD, Kirvine A, et al. The sensitivity of HIV-1 DNA polymerase chain reaction in the neonatal period and the relative contributions of intra-uterine and intrapartum transmission. AIDS. 1995;9:F7-F11.

163. McIntosh K, Pitt J, Brambilla D, et al. Blood culture in the first 6 months of life for diagnosis of vertically transmitted human immunodeficiency virus infection. J Infect Dis. 1994;170:996-1000.

164. Nesheim S, Lee F, Kalish ML, et al. Diagnosis of perinatal human immunodeficiency virus infection by polymerase chain reaction and p24 antigen detection after immune complex dissociation in an urban community hospital. J Infect Dis. 1997;175:1333-1336.

165. Bryson YJ, Luzuriaga K, Sullivan JL, Wara DW. Proposed definitions for in utero versus intrapartum transmission of HIV-1. N Engl J Med. 1993;327:1246-1247.

166. Young NL, Shaffer N, Chaowanachan T, et al. Early diagnosis of HIV-1-infected infants in Thailand using RNA and DNA PCR assays sensitive to non-B subtypes. J Acquir Immune Defic Syndr. 2000;24:401-407.

167. Cunningham P, Marriott D, Harris C, et al. False negative HIV-1 proviral DNA polymerase chain reaction in a patient with primary infection acquired in Thailand. J Clin Virol. 2003;26:163-169.

168. Simonds RJ, Brown TM, Thea DM, et al. Sensitivity and specificity of a qualitative RNA detection assay to diagnose HIV infection in young infants. Perinatal AIDS Collaborative Transmission Study. AIDS. 1998;12:1545-1549.

169. Nesheim S, Palumbo P, Sullivan K, et al. Quantitative RNA testing for diagnosis of HIV-infected infants. J Acquir Immune Defic Syndr. 2003;32:192-195.

170. Schupbach J. Measurement of HIV-1 p24 antigen by signal-amplification-boosted ELISA of heat-denatured plasma is a simple and inexpensive alternative to tests for viral RNA. AIDS Rev. 2002;4:83-92.

171. Sutthent R, Gaudart N, Chokpaibulkit K, et al. p24 Antigen detection assay modified with a booster step for diagnosis and monitoring of human immunodeficiency virus type 1 infection. J Clin Microbiol. 2003;41:1016-1022.

172. Gigliotti F, Murante BL, Weinberg GA. Short course directly observed therapy to monitor compliance with antiretroviral therapy in human immunodeficiency virus-infected children. Pediatr Infect Dis J. 2001;20:716-718.

173. Van Dyke RB, Lee S, Johnson GM, et al. Reported adherence as a determinant of response to highly active antiretroviral therapy in children who have human immunodeficiency virus infection. Pediatrics. 2002;109:e61.

174. Watson DC, Farley JJ. Efficacy of and adherence to highly active antiretroviral therapy in children infected with human immunodeficiency virus type 1. Pediatr Infect Dis J. 1999;18:682-689.

175. Murphy DA, Sarr M, Durako SJ, et al. Barriers to HAART adherence among human immunodeficiency virus-infected adolescents. Arch Pediatr Adolesc Med. 2003;157:249-255.

176. Pizzo PA, Eddy J, Falloon J, et al. Effect of continuous intravenous infusion of zidovudine (AZT) in children with symptomatic HIV infection. N Engl J Med. 1988;319:889-896.

177. McKinney RE, Maha MA, Connor EM, et al. A multicenter trial of oral zidovudine in children with advanced human immunodeficiency virus disease. N Engl J Med. 1991;324:1018-1025.

178. Butler KM, Husson RN, Balis FM, et al. Dideoxyinosine in children with symptomatic human immunodeficiency virus infection. N Engl J Med. 1991;324:137-144.

179. Lewis LL, Venzon D, Church J, et al. Lamivudine in children with human immunodeficiency virus infection: A phase I/II study. J Infect Dis. 1996;174:16-25.

180. Kline MW, Dunkle LM, Church JA, et al. A phase I/II evaluation of stavudine (d4T) in children with human immunodeficiency virus infection. Pediatrics. 1995;96:247-252.

181. Kline MW, Van Dyke RB, Lindsey JC, et al. A randomized comparative trial of stavudine (d4T) versus zidovudine (ZDV, AZT) in children with human immunodeficiency virus infection. Pediatrics. 1998;101:214-220.

182. McKinney RE Jr., Johnson GM, Stanley K, et al. A randomized study of combined zidovudine-lamivudine versus didanosine monotherapy in children with symptomatic therapy-naive HIG-1 infection. The Pediatric AIDS Clinical Trials Group Protocol 300 Study Team. J Pediatr. 1998;133:500-508.

183. Englund JA, Baker CJ, Raskino C, et al. Zidovudine, didanosine or both as the initial treatment for symptomatic HIV-infected children. N Engl J Med. 1997;336:1704-1712.

184. Krogstad P, Wiznia A, Luzuriaga K, et al. Treatment of human immunodeficiency virus 1-infected infants and children with the protease inhibitor nelfinavir mesylate. Clin Infect Dis. 1999;28:1109-1118.

185. Yogev R, Lee S, Wiznia A, et al. Stavudine, nevirapine and ritonavir in stable antiretroviral therapy-experienced children with human immunodeficiency virus infection. Pediatr Infect Dis J. 2002;21:119-125.

186. Luzuriaga K, Bryson Y, Krogstad P, et al. Combination treatment with zidovudine, didanosine and nevirapine in infants with human immunodeficiency virus type 1 infection. N Engl J Med. 1997;336:1343-1349.

187. Mueller BU, Nelson RP Jr, Sleasman J, et al. A phase I/II study of the protease inhibitor ritonavir in children with human immunodeficiency virus infection. Pediatrics. 1998;101:335-343.

188. Mueller BU, Sleasman S, Nelson RP Jr, et al. A phase I/II study of the protease inhibitor indinavir in children with HIV infection. Pediatrics. 1998;102:101-109.

189. Wiznia A, Stanley K, Krogstad P, et al. Combination nucleoside analog reverse transcriptase inhibitor(s) plus nevirapine, nelfinavir, or ritonavir in stable antiretroviral therapy-experienced HIV-infected children: Week 24 results of a randomized controlled trial—PACTG 377. Pediatric AIDS Clinical Trials Group 377 Study Team. AIDS Res Hum Retroviruses. 2000;16:1113-1121.

190. Nachman SA, Stanley K, Yogev R, et al. Nucleoside analogs plus ritonavir in stable antiretroviral therapy-experienced HIV-infected children: A randomized controlled trial. Pediatric AIDS Clinical Trials Group 338 Study Team. JAMA. 2000;283:492-498.

191. Nachman SA, Lindsey JC, Pelton S, et al. Growth in human immunodeficiency virus-infected children receiving ritonavir-containing antiretroviral therapy. Arch Pediatr Adolesc Med. 2002;156:497-503.

192. Borkowsky W, Stanley K, Douglas SD, et al. Immunologic response to combination nucleoside analogue plus protease inhibitor therapy in stable antiretroviral therapy-experienced human immunodeficiency virus-infected children. J Infect Dis. 2000;182:96-103.

193. Krogstad P, Lee S, Johnson G, et al. Nucleoside-analogue reverse-transcriptase inhibitors plus nevirapine, nelfinavir, or ritonavir for pretreated children infected with human immunodeficiency virus type 1. Clin Infect Dis. 2002;34:991-1001.

194. Floren LC, Wiznia A, Hayashi S, et al. Nelfinavir pharmacokinetics in stable human immunodeficiency virus-positive children: Pediatric AIDS Clinical Trials Group Protocol 377. Pediatrics. 2003;112:e220-e227.

195. Comparison of dual nucleoside-analogue reverse-transcriptase inhibitor regimens with and without nelfinavir in children with HIV-1 who have not previously been treated: The PENTA 5 randomised trial. Lancet. 2002;359:733-740.

196. Soh CH, Oleske JM, Brady MT, et al. Long-term effects of protease-inhibitor-based combination therapy on CD4 T-cell recovery in HIV-1-infected children and adolescents. Lancet. 2003;362:2045-2051.

197. Sleasman JW, Hemenway C, Klein AS, Barrett DJ. Corticosteroids improve survival of children with AIDS and Pneumocystis carinii pneumonia. Am J Dis Child. 1993;147:30-34.

198. Bye MR, Cairas-Bazarian C, Ewig JM. Markedly reduced mortality associated with corticosteroid therapy of Pneumocystis carinii pneumonia in children with acquired immunodeficiency syndrome. Arch Pediatr Adolesc Med. 1994;148:638-641.

199. Barone SR, Aiuto LT, Krilov LR. Increased survival of young infants with Pneumocystis carinii pneumonia and acute respiratory failure with early steroid administration. Clin Infect Dis. 1994;19:212-213.

200. McLaughlin GE, Virdee SS, Schleien CL, et al. Effect of corticosteroid on survival of children with acquired immunodeficiency syndrome and Pneumocystis carinii-related respiratory failure. J Pediatr. 1995;126:821-824.

201. National Institutes of Health-University of California Expert Panel for Corticosteroids as Adjunctive Therapy for Pneumocystis Pneumonia. Consensus statement on the use of corticosteroids as adjunctive therapy for Pneumocystis pneumonia in the acquired immunodeficiency syndrome. N Engl J Med. 1990;323:1500-1504.

202. Centers for Disease Control and Prevention. Measles pneumonitis following measles-mumps-rubella vaccination of a patient with HIV infection, 1993. MMWR Morb Mortal Wkly Rep. 1996;45:603-606.

203. Angel JB, Walpita P, Lerch RA, et al. Vaccine-associated measles pneumonitis in an adult with AIDS. Ann Intern Med. 1998;129:104-106.

204. Weinberg, GA. Concise reviews of pediatric infectious diseases: Post-exposure prophylaxis against HIV infection following sexual assault. Pediatr Infect Dis J. 2002;21:959-960.

205. Havens PL, Committee on Pediatric AIDS. Postexposure prophylaxis in children and adolescents for nonoccupational exposure to human immunodeficiency virus. Pediatrics. 2003;111:1475-1489.

206. Olshen E, Samples CL. Postexposure prophylaxis: An intervention to prevent human immunodeficiency virus infection in adolescents. Curr Opin Pediatr. 2003;15:379-384.

207. Centers for Disease Control and Prevention. Updated U. S. Public Health Service guidelines for the management of occupational exposures to HBV, HCV, and HIV and recommendations for postexposure prophylaxis. MMWR Morb Mortal Wkly Rep. 2001;50(No. RR-11):1-52.

Antiretroviral Therapy for Human Immunodeficiency Virus Infection

GEORGE J. HANNA

MARTIN S. HIRSCH

The treatment of human immunodeficiency virus type 1 (HIV-1) infection has evolved at a rapid pace. In 1987, less than 4 years after HIV-1 was identified as the agent that causes the acquired immunodeficiency syndrome (AIDS), zidovudine was approved for treatment of HIV-1 infection. In the next 8 years, three other nucleoside analogues that also inhibit the HIV-1 enzyme reverse transcriptase (RT) were introduced. Between 1995 and 2003, fifteen new antiretroviral agents were approved, including HIV-1 protease inhibitors, non-nucleoside reverse transcriptase inhibitors (NNRTIs), and a fusion inhibitor. Concurrently, a better understanding of the dynamics of HIV-1 replication and drug resistance mechanisms caused a shift from single- to combination-drug therapy. In addition, technologic advances in quantifying HIV-1 RNA led to a reliance on plasma HIV-1 RNA levels, also known as *viral load*, for monitoring infection. The treatment of HIV-1 infection today requires an understanding of viral replication dynamics, antiviral potency, pharmacokinetics and toxicities of individual drugs, and interactions among drugs used in combination. Moreover, appropriate therapeutic strategies require a knowledge of the limitations imposed by failure of one drug on the future use of the same or related drugs.

ANTIRETROVIRAL AGENTS

HIV-1 is an enveloped virus that contains two copies of genomic RNA.[1,2] Through its gp120 surface glycoprotein, the virus binds to cellular receptors, most commonly CD4, in association with a chemokine receptor.[3] This binding induces conformational changes in gp120 so as to uncover and cause other conformational changes in the underlying viral transmembrane protein gp41. These changes in gp41 bring the viral and cellular envelopes into closer proximity, allow their fusion, and permit entry of the viral capsid into the cellular cytoplasm. The first U.S. Food and Drug Administration (FDA)–approved antiretroviral agent that interferes with viral entry, enfuvirtide, inhibits the ability of gp41 to mediate fusion of viral and cellular envelopes.

Once inside the cytoplasm, the viral RT, along with other viral proteins and possibly cellular proteins, converts the viral genomic RNA into a double-stranded DNA molecule by sequential steps, first using the viral RNA as a template to polymerize DNA and form an RNA:DNA hybrid, then degrading the RNA with the RNase H activity associated with the enzyme.[4] The resulting single-stranded DNA is then used as a template to polymerize the second DNA strand. Once double-stranded viral DNA is formed, it is transported to the nucleus, where it is integrated into the cellular genome with the aid of the viral integrase enzyme. Most of the currently available antiretroviral drugs are specific inhibitors of the viral RT.

After integration, HIV-1 DNA is transcribed and translated using predominantly cellular transcription and protein synthesis machinery, although several HIV-1 regulatory genes may influence these processes. Certain viral proteins, including those that form the protein components of the viral core, are synthesized as precursor polyproteins (gag and gag-pol) and require cleavage by a viral protease to yield mature proteins.[1] Immature viral structural proteins, genomic RNA, and replicative enzymes assemble initially as an immature viral core particle in the cytoplasm. This particle associates with envelope glycoproteins at the plasma membrane and buds out as an enveloped viral particle. During the process of budding, the viral protease cleaves the polyproteins in the core, converting the immature viral particle into an infectious virion. Drugs that inhibit the viral protease enzyme prevent cleavage of the polyproteins so that the viral particles remain immature and replication-defective.

Nucleoside and Nucleotide Analogue Reverse Transcriptase Inhibitors

Several drugs inhibit viral replication by acting as nucleoside analogues and interfering with the DNA polymerase function of the viral RT (Fig. 124-1, Table 124-1). After uptake by host cells, nucleoside analogues are converted to their triphosphate forms by cellular kinases.[5] Phosphorylation by nucleoside kinases is crucial for rendering the drugs active in suppressing viral replication. Because nucleoside kinase activity varies in different cell types and in different cell activation states, the ability of nucleoside analogues to inhibit RT in different compartments may vary as well. For instance, the nucleoside kinase activity of macrophages or monocytes at rest may be insufficient to yield adequate intracellular levels of zidovudine triphosphate, whereas the levels of the triphosphate form of didanosine appear to be adequate in resting cells.[6] The triphosphate forms of the drugs have high affinity for the HIV-1 RT and compete with the natural enzyme substrates (deoxynucleoside triphosphates) for binding to the RT. They are incorporated into the growing DNA chain, leading to premature chain termination (because they lack a 3′-hydroxyl group to form a phosphodiester bond with the incoming nucleotide). Nucleoside analogue RT inhibitors generally have activity against a broad range of retroviruses, including HIV-1, HIV-2, and human T-lymphotropic virus type 1 (HTLV-1).[5,7]

Because the expression of the nucleoside kinase responsible for the first phosphorylation step of the nucleoside analogues varies in different tissues and in cells during different states of activation, the ability of some cells to activate nucleoside analogue RT inhibitors may be limited. Nucleotide (or nucleoside monophosphate) analogues, in contrast, require only the last two phosphorylation steps. Because enzymes responsible for these steps are ubiquitous, nucleotide RT inhibitors may have antiviral activity in a broader range of tissues and cell types. Once converted intracellularly to its diphosphate form, the nucleotide analogue competes with the natural substrates of RT and can function as a chain terminator.

Besides having a similar mechanism of antiviral activity, nucleoside and nucleotide RT inhibitors may also share associations with certain adverse effects. All may be associated with asymptomatic hyperlactatemia and, more rarely, symptomatic lactic acidosis and severe hepatomegaly with steatosis, which can be fatal.[8,9] These and other adverse effects of nucleoside and nucleotide analogues may be related to their ability to inhibit DNA-polymerase γ, which is involved in mitochondrial DNA replication. In vitro nucleoside analogues differ in their ability to inhibit DNA-polymerase γ, with zalcitabine, didanosine, stavudine, and zidovudine being associated with greater mitochondrial toxicity than emtricitabine, lamivudine, and tenofovir.[10,11] However, for any specific nucleoside RT inhibitor, the occurrence and severity of adverse effects putatively related to DNA-polymerase γ inhibition varies markedly in different patients, suggesting that factors other than DNA-polymerase γ inhibition must play an important role as well.[12]

Zidovudine

Zidovudine (3′-azido-2′,3′-dideoxythymidine; AZT or ZDV) is an analogue of the nucleoside thymidine. It is available in both oral and parenteral formulations. In its oral formulation, it is well absorbed, with an average bioavailability of 63%.[5,13] Although its plasma half-life is only 1.1 hours, the half-life of the intracellular biologically active triphosphate form is 3 to 4 hours, allowing twice-daily dosing. Zidovudine is metabolized primarily in the liver by glucuronidation to an inactive compound, and 90% of the absorbed dose is excreted in

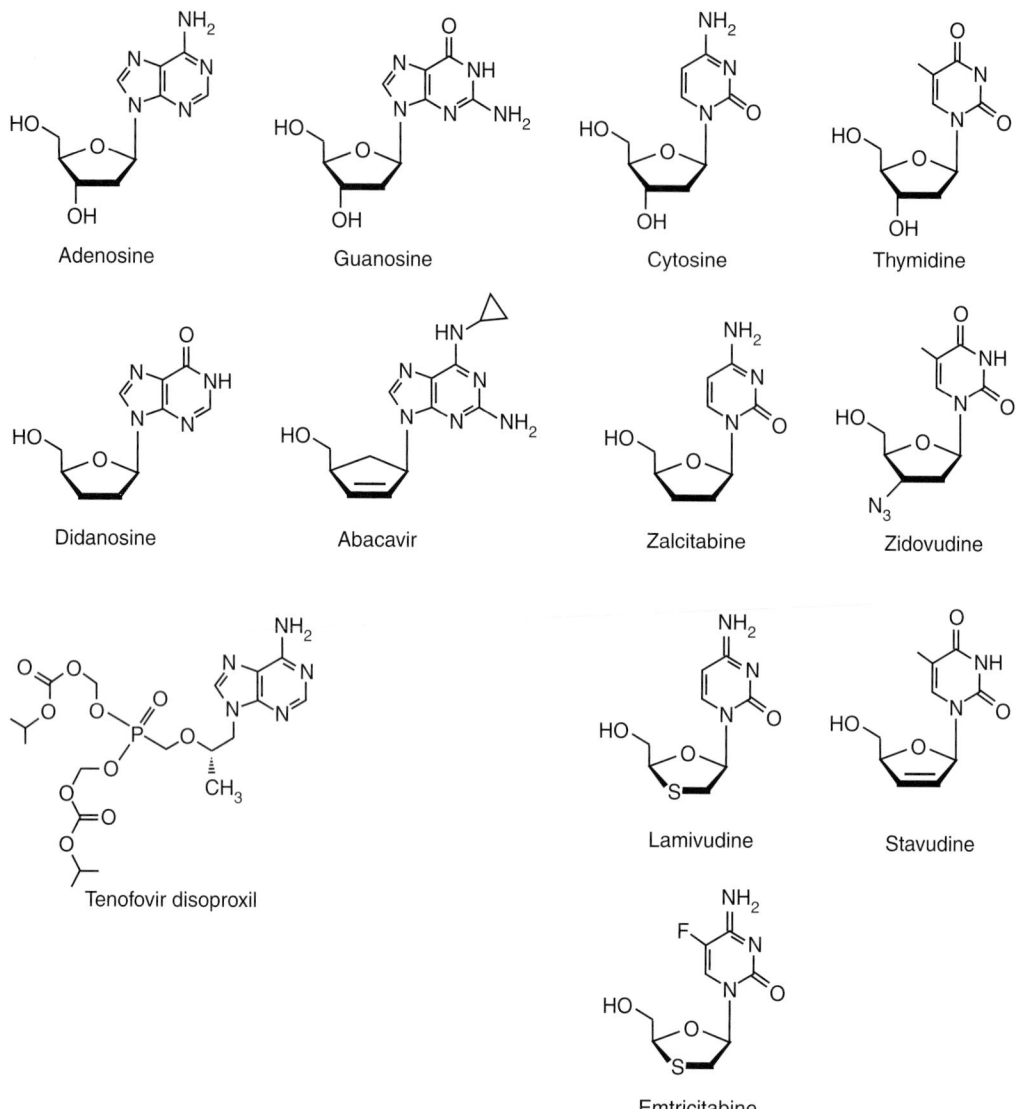

FIGURE 124-1. Nucleoside or nucleotide analogue reverse transcriptase inhibitors. Shown on top are the naturally occurring nucleosides (adenosine, guanosine, cytosine, and thymidine); below each of them are shown the respective analogues used in antiretroviral therapy.

urine. Current adult dosing for zidovudine is usually 300 mg orally every 12 hours. In severe renal failure and hemodialysis dependence, dosing should be adjusted to 100 mg orally every 6 to 8 hours. The parenteral formulation of zidovudine is used primarily peripartum to decrease maternal transmission of HIV-1.

The first blinded, placebo-controlled trial of an antiretroviral compound was a monotherapy study of zidovudine in adults with AIDS or advanced AIDS-related complex (ARC).[14] The 6-month trial compared zidovudine at 1500 mg/day with placebo and was terminated early when it showed significantly lower rates of opportunistic infections and death in the zidovudine-treated group. However, longer follow-up of all patients on open-label zidovudine monotherapy suggested decreasing clinical benefits of zidovudine within 1 year after initiation of therapy.[15] Subsequent studies of zidovudine monotherapy in adults with earlier HIV disease showed only small and transient clinical benefits lasting less than 2 years.[16-18] These studies provided compelling evidence of the limitation of antiretroviral monotherapy. Only recently has the intrinsic antiviral activity of zidovudine in terms of viral load changes been reported. A 2-week study of zidovudine monotherapy with zidovudine 300 mg twice daily resulted in a maximal decline in plasma HIV-1 RNA of 0.9 $\log_{10}$ on day 9.[19]

Soon after its introduction into clinical use, zidovudine was noted to have in vitro additive or synergistic antiviral effects with other nucleoside RT inhibitors (including didanosine and lamivudine), several NNRTIs, and protease inhibitors.[20-22] These observations suggested the possibility of combining zidovudine with other antiretroviral agents in combination therapy. Indeed, combination antiretroviral therapy has demonstrated that zidovudine, when administered as part of a regimen that includes other nucleoside RT inhibitors and either an NNRTI or a protease inhibitor can have an important role in inducing and maintaining long-term suppression of viremia and permitting immunologic reconstitution.[23-25] In contrast, zidovudine and stavudine display antagonistic in vitro antiviral effects.[22] A clinical trial showed that a combination of zidovudine and stavudine failed to produce better antiviral activity compared with stavudine alone, and therefore this combination is not recommended for antiretroviral therapy.[26]

At the time of its introduction, zidovudine was used at doses of 1000 to 1500 mg/day, which caused significant toxicity. Later studies confirmed that zidovudine at doses of 500 to 600 mg/day has benefits equivalent to those seen at higher doses, but with reduced toxicity.[16,27] Adverse effects of zidovudine are also seen more commonly in patients with more advanced disease.[28] The most serious toxicity of zi-

TABLE 124-1   Approved Nucleoside and Nucleotide Reverse Transcriptase Inhibitors (NRTIs)

Agent	Trade Name	Oral Bioavailability (%)	Serum Half-Life (h)	Intracellular Half-Life of Triphosphate (h)	Elimination	Adult Dose*	Availability
Zidovudine	Retrovir	63	1.1	3-4	Hepatic glucuronidation Renal excretion	300 mg PO q12h or 200 mg PO q8h	300-mg tablets 100-mg capsules 10-mg/mL syrup 10-mg/mL solution for IV infusion
Didanosine	Videx Videx EC	40 fasted	1.5	8-24	Cellular metabolism	≥60 kg: enteric-coated tablets 400 mg PO qd; buffered tablets 200 mg PO q12h or 400 mg PO qd; buffered powder 250 mg PO q12h <60 kg: enteric-coated tablets 250 mg PO qd; buffered tablets 125 mg PO q12h or 250 mg PO qd; buffered powder 167 mg PO q12h	125-, 200-, 250-, and 400-mg enteric-coated tablets 25-, 50-, 100-, 150-, and 200-mg buffered chewable tablets 100-, 167-, and 250-mg buffered powder packets 10-mg/mL solution
Zalcitabine	Hivid	87	1.2	2.6	Renal excretion	0.75 mg PO q8h	0.375- and 0.75-mg tablets
Stavudine	Zerit Zerit XR	86	1.1	3	Renal excretion	≥60 kg: immediate-release capsules 40 mg PO q12h; extended-release tablets 100 mg PO qd <60 kg: immediate-release capsules 30 mg PO q12h; extended-release tablets 75 mg PO qd	15-, 20-, 30-, and 40-mg immediate-release capsules 37.5-, 50-, 75-, and 100-mg extended-release tablets 1-mg/mL solution
Lamivudine	Epivir	86	2.5	11-14	Renal excretion	300 mg PO qd or 150 mg PO q12h	150- and 300-mg tablets 10-mg/mL solution
Abacavir	Ziagen	83	1.5	3.3	Hepatic glucuronidation and carboxylation	300 mg PO q12h	300-mg tablets 20-mg/mL solution
Tenofovir	Viread	39 with meal	12-14	>12[†]	Renal excretion	300 mg PO qd	300-mg tablet
Emtricitabine	Emtriva	93	10	>24	Renal excretion	200 mg PO qd	200-mg capsules
Zidovudine + lamivudine	Combivir[‡]					One tablet PO q12h	300-mg zidovudine/ 150-mg lamivudine tablets
Zidovudine + lamivudine + abacavir	Trizivir[‡]					One tablet PO q12h	300-mg zidovudine/ 150-mg lamivudine/300-mg abacavir tablets

*For pediatric dose see Chapter 123.
[†]Diphosphate.
[‡]Pharmacokinetic properties are similar to those of the component drugs used separately.

dovudine is bone marrow suppression. Although macrocytosis not related to vitamin deficiency is seen in virtually all patients who are taking therapeutic doses of zidovudine, severe anemia or neutropenia can also develop, especially in situations in which bone marrow reserves are poor secondary to vitamin B_{12} deficiency or opportunistic infections.[28] The incidence of granulocytopenia (neutrophil count <750 cells/mm[3]) has ranged from 1.8% in asymptomatic individuals receiving 500 mg/day of zidovudine to 47% in persons with AIDS receiving 1500 mg/day.[16,28] Similarly, severe anemia (hemoglobin levels <8 g/dL) was seen in 1.1% of asymptomatic individuals receiving 500 mg/day but in at least 29% of persons with AIDS receiving 1500 mg/day. Less commonly, chronic zidovudine use can cause myopathy and myositis, which improve after zidovudine discontinuation, unlike primary HIV-1 myopathy.[29] Less serious but more common adverse reactions include headache, insomnia, myalgia, fatigue, nail pigmentation, nausea, bloating, and dyspepsia. Although there is tachyphylaxis to many of these effects in most patients, some remain intolerant to zidovudine. Mild elevations in serum hepatic enzyme levels may also be

seen, although these occur usually with the concomitant administration of other potential hepatotoxins.[15] Hematologic indices should be monitored while zidovudine is being used, especially if it is taken with other potentially myelosuppressive drugs (e.g., ganciclovir) or drugs that decrease the clearance of zidovudine (e.g., methadone, probenecid).

Didanosine

Didanosine (2′,3′-dideoxyinosine; ddI) is a purine dideoxynucleoside that is phosphorylated to dideoxyadenosine triphosphate in cells. Because didanosine is inactivated by gastric acid, it must be administered as a buffered solution or tablet or as an enteric-coated tablet. The buffer in the buffered formulations may in turn interfere with the absorption of several medications, including delavirdine, indinavir, atazanavir, ketoconazole, itraconazole, and fluoroquinolones. Didanosine absorption in its current formulations is best when the drug is taken in a fasting state, with an oral bioavailability of 40%. Although didanosine's plasma half-life is approximately 1.5 hours, the relatively long intracellular half-life of its triphosphate form (8 to 24 hours) makes once-daily dosing possible. Didanosine is eliminated both by metabolism in cells of diverse tissues, with hypoxanthine as an intermediate, and by renal excretion. For an adult weighing 60 kg or more, the usual dosage of didanosine is one 400-mg tablet orally once daily. For an adult weighing less than 60 kg, the dose should be decreased to one 250-mg tablet orally once daily. In severe renal failure and hemodialysis dependence, dosing should be adjusted. Coadministration of didanosine and tenofovir in the same regimen causes a significant increase in didanosine blood levels and requires a decrease of the dose of didanosine (from 400 mg to 250 mg daily for an adult weighing 60 kg or more).[30]

Initial studies of didanosine compared its efficacy with that of zidovudine in trials of single-drug therapy. In individuals with previous zidovudine experience, switching to didanosine decreased the rate of new AIDS-defining events or death, but no statistically significant difference in mortality alone could be detected, and the benefit of didanosine monotherapy appeared to be transient.[31-33] In adults with little or no prior zidovudine experience, the advantages of didanosine monotherapy over zidovudine were less evident.[34,35]

When used as part of a combination regimen, didanosine provides more pronounced and more durable clinical benefits than it does when used as a single-drug regimen. These benefits are most pronounced in antiretroviral-naive individuals, in whom the combination of didanosine and zidovudine resulted in greater increases in CD4+ T-lymphocyte counts and more profound decreases in disease progression and mortality compared with zidovudine alone.[35-37] However, the potency of combination therapy is less if didanosine is added to zidovudine therapy in individuals with a considerable history of prior zidovudine monotherapy.[35,37-39] Regimens that include didanosine with two other antiretroviral drugs have demonstrated longer-term suppression of viremia and considerably greater immunologic reconstitution than is seen with the two-drug regimen of zidovudine and didanosine.[40,41]

The most serious toxicity associated with didanosine is pancreatitis. Although up to 20% of individuals treated with didanosine may develop increases in serum amylase levels, the rate of clinical pancreatitis may approach 7%.[31,34] The risk of pancreatitis is higher with more advanced immunosuppression and if didanosine is taken with other agents that increase the risk of pancreatitis (e.g., ethanol, intravenous pentamidine). Although pancreatitis often resolves after didanosine therapy is discontinued, fatalities have been observed. Pancreatitis as well as hepatotoxicity occurs more frequently when didanosine is used with stavudine or hydroxyurea. A peripheral neuropathy, predominantly sensory and characterized by distal numbness, tingling, or pain, has been noted in up to 13% of persons taking didanosine.[31,34] Neuropathy occurs more commonly in patients with a prior history of neuropathy or previous neurotoxic drug therapy, and it usually resolves if didanosine is stopped promptly. Asymptomatic hyperuricemia and hypertriglyceridemia have also been noted.[42] Diarrhea, abdominal discomfort, and nausea are less serious but common adverse effects of the buffered formulations; they are considerably less common with the enteric-coated tablets.

Zalcitabine

Zalcitabine (2′, 3′-dideoxycytidine; ddC) is a cytidine nucleoside analogue that is well absorbed orally (bioavailability of 87%), but its absorption diminishes significantly when it is administered with food.[5] Its plasma half-life is 1.2 hours, and the intracellular half-life of its triphosphate form is 2.6 hours. Zalcitabine is excreted largely unchanged in the urine, and dosing may need to be modified in patients with decreased creatinine clearance. The adult dose is 0.75 mg orally every 8 hours.

Initial studies of zalcitabine monotherapy found that it had efficacy comparable to that of zidovudine or didanosine.[43-45] Although the clinical benefits of monotherapy with all three nucleosides are limited and transient, the combination of zidovudine with zalcitabine produced more lasting benefits in individuals with no prior antiretroviral experience.[35,37,39] In contrast, the efficacy of zalcitabine with zidovudine was

less in zidovudine-experienced subjects. Current use of zalcitabine has been limited by the necessity for frequent dosing and the frequent incidence of adverse effects.

A major toxicity of zalcitabine is peripheral neuropathy, which is seen more frequently than with didanosine therapy.[45] The incidence of neuropathy increases with higher doses of the drug, lower creatinine clearance, and lower CD4+ T-cell counts; up to one third of patients with advanced disease may be affected.[43] Neuropathy is generally reversible if the drug is discontinued promptly. Pancreatitis has also been observed in 1% to 2% of all patients taking zalcitabine; it is seen more commonly in patients who also have other risks for pancreatitis.[37] Other reactions include oral ulcers, which may be severe in 3% of patients, and fixed drug eruptions.

Stavudine

Stavudine (2′,3′-didehydro-2′,3′-dideoxythymidine; d4T) is a thymidine nucleoside analogue that is well absorbed after oral administration, with oral bioavailability of 86%. Its plasma half-life is approximately 1.1 hours, and the intracellular half-life of its triphosphate form is approximately 3 hours.[46] Approximately 40% of an oral dose is eliminated through the kidneys, and the dose should be reduced in patients with renal insufficiency.[47] The metabolic fate of 60% of an oral dose is unknown, but the pharmacokinetics of the drug do not appear to be altered in patients with hepatic impairment.[48] The adult dose of stavudine is 40 mg orally twice a day for a patient weighing 60 kg or more and 30 mg orally twice a day if the weight is less than 60 kg. An extended-release formulation allows once-daily dosing with 100 mg for a person weighing 60 kg or more, or 75 mg if the weight is less than 60 kg.

Initial studies of stavudine involved monotherapy comparisons with zidovudine. In adults with prior zidovudine use, changing therapy to stavudine was beneficial compared with continuing zidovudine in terms of CD4+ T-cell response and frequency of clinical end points.[49] However, stavudine monotherapy appeared to be inferior to didanosine monotherapy in zidovudine-experienced individuals in its ability to decrease HIV-1 RNA levels and increase CD4+ T-cell counts, suggesting that zidovudine and stavudine may share a greater cross-resistance profile.[26] In vitro, stavudine has shown additive to synergistic antiviral activity against HIV-1 in combination with lamivudine.[22] The combination of stavudine and lamivudine (with a protease inhibitor) for the treatment of antiretroviral-naive patients resulted in potent, durable suppression of HIV-1 RNA.[50,51] In contrast, stavudine in combination with zidovudine in vitro showed antagonistic activity against HIV-1.[22] In clinical trials, the combination of zidovudine and stavudine failed to demonstrate improved antiviral activity compared with stavudine alone.[26]

Stavudine's major adverse effect is a sensory peripheral neuropathy, similar to that seen with didanosine and zalcitabine.[52] Neuropathy develops in approximately 13% of stavudine-treated patients.[49] The incidence is increased in patients with advanced disease (up to 25%) and in those with other current or prior risk factors for neuropathy. Neuropathy is generally reversible if the drug is discontinued promptly. If symptoms resolve completely, stavudine may be restarted at half the recommended dose. Compared with other nucleosides, stavudine is more likely to be associated with lactic acidosis.[53-55] Rarely, motor weakness has been observed in association with stavudine therapy, usually accompanied by lactic acidosis. When used as part of a protease inhibitor–containing regimen, stavudine was associated with an increased risk of lipoatrophy, compared with zidovudine.[56] Fatal cases of pancreatitis and hepatotoxicity have been observed when stavudine was used with didanosine. Although macrocytosis can be seen in many patients, there does not appear to be an increased rate of anemia associated with stavudine in adults.[57]

Lamivudine

Lamivudine ((−)-β-enantiomer of 2′,3′-dideoxy-3′-thiacytidine; 3TC) is a cytidine nucleoside analogue that is absorbed well orally, with a bioavailability of 86%. Its serum half-life is 2.5 hours, and the intracellular half-life of the biologically active triphosphate form is 11 to 14 hours.[58] Approximately 70% of a dose is excreted unchanged in urine, and lamivudine dosing should be adjusted in patients with renal impairment. The dose in adults is 150 mg orally every 12 hours or 300 mg orally once daily.

If lamivudine is used alone, it causes a decrease in plasma viral RNA levels and an increase in CD4+ T-cell counts, but these effects are largely transient, with a return of both measures toward baseline by 8 weeks of therapy.[59] Lamivudine has shown synergistic activity when combined with either zidovudine or stavudine in vitro.[22] Two clinical trials evaluated the combination of lamivudine and zidovudine in antiretroviral-naive individuals and demonstrated the advantages of combination therapy over monotherapy.[60,61] Trials that examined the combination of zidovudine with lamivudine in zidovudine-experienced subjects showed antiviral and immunologic benefits that were better than monotherapy, but these benefits were less than those seen in antiretroviral-naive subjects.[62,63] Nevertheless, the addition of lamivudine to previous treatment regimens of zidovudine alone or zidovudine with didanosine or zalcitabine in adults with CD4+ T-cell counts of 25 to 250 cells/mm[3] was still associated with a 60% decrease in mortality and a 57% decrease in clinical progression to a new AIDS-defining illness or death.[64]

Several studies of the combination of lamivudine with zidovudine and a protease inhibitor or an NNRTI showed potent and durable decreases in viremia and progressive immune reconstitution.[23-25] The use of lamivudine in combinations that do not include zidovudine is also associated with potent and durable antiviral activity. For instance, the combination of lamivudine and stavudine can provide potent and durable viral suppression and CD4+ T-cell increases in antiretroviral-naive individuals, comparable to what is seen with zidovudine and lamivudine.[50,51,65] Similar benefits of this combination, although less pronounced, can still be seen in persons with prior experience with zidovudine, didanosine, or zalcitabine.[66] Lamivudine with tenofovir has also shown potent and durable antiviral activity, comparable to stavudine with lamivudine.[67] Other combinations, such as lamivudine with didanosine, have been less well studied.[65,68]

Lamivudine is generally very well tolerated in adults.[60-64] The most frequent adverse events have been headache, dizziness, malaise, and fatigue.

Abacavir

Abacavir is a guanosine nucleoside analogue that is well absorbed orally, with a bioavailability of 83%. Although the plasma half-life of abacavir is less than 2 hours, the intracellular half-life of its biologically active form, carbovir triphosphate, is 3.3 hours. Abacavir is metabolized primarily by glucuronidation and carboxylation. The adult dose is 300 mg orally every 12 hours.

Abacavir produces a median drop of 1.1 $\log_{10}$ in HIV-1 RNA levels and a median increase of 92 CD4+ T cells/mm[3] at week 4 of therapy when used alone.[69] If combined with zidovudine and lamivudine, it can provide a drop in HIV-1 RNA levels of approximately 2.0 $\log_{10}$, which lasts at least 24 weeks.[70] However, a combination of zidovudine, lamivudine, and abacavir provides inferior efficacy, in terms of durable viral load reduction, compared with some regimens that contain a protease inhibitor or an NNRTI. For example, in antiretroviral-naive individuals with baseline HIV-1 RNA levels greater than 5.0 $\log_{10}$ who received zidovudine, lamivudine, and either abacavir or indinavir, the proportion of patients achieving undetectable viral load (<50 copies/mL) at week 48 was 45% in the indinavir group but 31% in the abacavir group.[71] Also, regardless of whether the baseline HIV-1 RNA level was less than or greater than 5.0 $\log_{10}$, the rate of virologic failure was higher in those who received abacavir with zidovudine and lamivudine than in those who received efavirenz with zidovudine and lamivudine.[72] The use of abacavir in other combinations is a subject of ongoing studies. In one study, the combination of abacavir administered once daily with lamivudine and tenofovir was noted to result in poorer efficacy than expected, and this combination is not currently recommended.[73]

Abacavir has been generally well tolerated, with the most common adverse effects being nausea, headache, weakness, insomnia, and abdominal pain. Its most serious adverse effect is a hypersensitivity reaction, which occurs in 3% to 5% of treated individuals.[74] Symptoms appear 1 to 4 weeks after initiation of therapy and include fever and malaise, often with nausea, vomiting, diarrhea, myalgia, arthralgia, respiratory symptoms (cough, sore throat, or shortness of breath), and rash, although rash may be absent. Laboratory abnormalities have included acute lymphopenia, elevated results on liver function tests, and elevated creatine phosphokinase levels. Symptoms resolve within 1 to 2 days after discontinuation of abacavir. Rechallenge with the drug, even at a decreased dose, may cause the return of symptoms within hours with increased severity and often with life-threatening hypotension and facial or throat swelling. Therefore, individuals with suspected hypersensitivity reactions to abacavir should not be rechallenged with the drug.

Tenofovir

Tenofovir (9-[-(R)-2-(phosphonomethoxy)propyl]adenine; PMPA) is an analogue of the nucleotide adenine that requires only two phosphorylation steps to render it biologically active as tenofovir diphosphate. In its native form, tenofovir is poorly absorbed orally. However, a prodrug of tenofovir, tenofovir disoproxil fumarate, increases the bioavailability of tenofovir to 25% in the fasted state.[75] Taking tenofovir disoproxil fumarate with a meal increases bioavailability further to 39%. The plasma half-life of tenofovir is approximately 12 to 14 hours, and the intracellular half-life of the biologically active diphosphate is usually well over 12 hours, allowing for once-daily dosing.[76] The drug is excreted through the kidneys. Coadministration of tenofovir with didanosine in the same regimen causes a significant increase in didanosine blood levels and requires a decrease of the dose of didanosine.[30] Tenofovir has also been noted to decrease blood levels of some protease inhibitors, including lopinavir, ritonavir, and atazanavir, and certain protease inhibitors (e.g., atazanavir, ritonavir-boosted lopinavir) cause an increase in blood levels of tenofovir.[77] The clinical significance of these observations is currently unknown.

Tenofovir administration caused plasma HIV-1 RNA levels to decline by 1.5 $\log_{10}$ copies/mL over 21 days of monotherapy.[78] In highly treatment-experienced patients with HIV-1 RNA levels between 400 and 100,000 copies/mL, the addition of tenofovir to an existing regimen caused a decrease in HIV-1 RNA of approximately 0.6 $\log_{10}$ copies/mL, which was sustained through week 48 of therapy.[79] A larger placebo-controlled trial confirmed similar findings.[80] In antiretroviral-naive individuals, the combination regimen of tenofovir, lamivudine, and efavirenz had similar efficacy to a regimen of stavudine, lamivudine, and efavirenz, with less toxicity (e.g., lipid abnormalities, peripheral neuropathy).[67] However, the combination of tenofovir with abacavir and lamivudine (in a once-daily regimen) was noted to result in poorer efficacy than expected in antiretroviral-naive subjects and is not currently recommended.[73]

Tenofovir is generally well tolerated, and the most common adverse effects have been nausea, diarrhea, vomiting, and flatulence. Long-term toxicity of tenofovir use is being studied. Renal impairment in patients receiving tenofovir has been reported, but a causal relationship with tenofovir has not been established.[81] More profound decreases in bone mineral density were noted for tenofovir (compared with stavudine) when used in combination with lamivudine and efavirenz, but the clinical relevance of this observation is unknown.

Emtricitabine

Emtricitabine ([−]-2′,3′-dideoxy-5-fluoro-3′-thiacytidine; FTC) is a cytidine nucleoside analogue that is structurally similar to lamivudine. It is well absorbed orally, with oral bioavailability of 93%. Its plasma half-life is approximately 10 hours, and the intracellular half-life of its biologically active triphosphate form at steady state is greater than 24 hours, allowing for once daily-dosing.[82] Emtricitabine is not extensively metabolized, and it is excreted primarily by the kidneys. In patients with renal impairment, an increase in the dosing interval is required. In vitro, emtricitabine triphosphate has lower inhibitory effects on mitochondrial DNA polymerase γ, compared with the triphosphate forms of several approved nucleoside RT inhibitors.[10] Whether this will result in fewer adverse events during clinical use remains unknown.

A monotherapy study of 200 mg emtricitabine daily in antiretroviral-naive adults demonstrated a decrease in HIV-1 RNA of 1.9 $\log_{10}$ copies/mL at 14 days.[83] Emtricitabine interacts additively to synergistically in vitro with several other nucleoside RT inhibitors, NNRTIs, and protease inhibitors. Combination therapy that includes emtricitabine has potent antiviral activity. Forty antiretroviral-naive adults with a median CD4+ T-cell count of 373 cells/mm^3 and a plasma HIV-1 RNA level of 4.77 $\log_{10}$ copies/mL were treated with a once-daily regimen of emtricitabine, didanosine, and efavirenz.[41] At 24 weeks of therapy, plasma HIV-1 RNA had decreased by a median of 3.5 $\log_{10}$ copies/mL, and 93% of subjects had undetectable plasma HIV-1 RNA (<50 copies/mL). CD4+ T-cell counts increased by a median of 159 cells/mm^3. A larger clinical trial compared emtricitabine with stavudine, each in combination with didanosine and efavirenz in antiretroviral-naive adults for 60 weeks.[84] Patients in the emtricitabine arm had a lower rate of virologic failure than those in the stavudine arm. However, it is important to note that regimens based on a combination of stavudine and didanosine (as used in this study) are generally not recommended based on their decreased tolerability. In two randomized clinical trials, emtricitabine (200 mg daily) appeared to have antiviral activity and safety equivalent to lamivudine (150 mg twice daily).[85] Adults who switched from lamivudine to emtricitabine after achieving plasma viral load suppression (<400 copies/mL) on a lamivudine-containing regimen had a similar likelihood of continued virologic suppression at week 48 as those who continued receiving lamivudine. In another trial, antiretroviral-naive subjects who started emtricitabine, stavudine, and an NNRTI also had a rate of virologic suppression at week 24 similar to that of subjects who started lamivudine, stavudine, and an NNRTI.

Emtricitabine appears to be well tolerated. Adverse effects related to emtricitabine have included nausea, headache, and hyperpigmentation of the palms and soles. Reported hepatotoxicity in subjects taking combinations including emtricitabine with nevirapine appears to be related to the nevirapine component, although a potential contribution by emtricitabine cannot be ruled out.[86] Nevertheless, among patients taking emtricitabine without NNRTIs, hepatic toxicity does not appear to be a significant problem.

Mechanisms of Resistance

A major determinant of antiretroviral drug failure is viral genotypic variation conferring drug resistance.[87,88] HIV-1 infection is a dynamic process, with high rates of replication and a great potential for genetic variation.[89-91] Given that HIV-1 RT lacks a proofreading function and is estimated to have an in vivo forward mutation rate of about 10^{-5} mutations per base pair per cycle, a mutation may occur on average at each nucleotide position as often as 10^4 times a day in an untreated individual.[92] HIV-1 genetic variants conferring resistance to single antiretroviral agents may exist in the infected individual before any therapy is begun. When a patient starts a drug regimen, the regimen selects for preexisting mutations as well as additional mutations that appear in different genetic backgrounds. Mutations continue to accumulate unless replication is slowed enough to curtail genetic diversification. Genotypic resistance has been reported for each of the antiretroviral agents in current use.

Viral isolates with reduced sensitivity to zidovudine were documented within 3 years after its introduction.[93] In HIV-1–infected individuals receiving zidovudine monotherapy, the first mutation to arise in RT is usually a change in codon 70 from Lys to Arg (Lys70→Arg), which is seen transiently and is usually replaced by Thr215→Tyr after a few months of therapy.[94-96] During ongoing therapy, other mutations (including Met41→Leu, Asp67→Asn, Leu210→Trp, Thr215→Phe, Lys219→Glu or Gln, and reappearance of Lys70→Arg) accumulate and confer augmented resistance to zidovudine.[95-99] Although single-

codon mutations confer only minimal resistance to zidovudine, a highly zidovudine-resistant virus with a 100-fold increase in the 50% inhibitory concentration (IC$_{50}$) arises after three or four substitutions.[93,97,98,100] The same mutations also arise during suboptimal therapy with stavudine.[101,102] Because these mutations can be selected by the thymidine analogues zidovudine and stavudine, they are sometimes referred to as thymidine-associated mutations (TAMs). However, although zidovudine-resistant mutants may appear susceptible to other RT inhibitors in some in vitro assays, a large study of viral isolates from individuals receiving chronic zidovudine monotherapy found that each 10-fold decrease in zidovudine susceptibility was accompanied by a 2-fold decrease in susceptibility to either didanosine or zalcitabine.[103] Furthermore, these same mutations have been associated with virologic failure of several nucleoside or nucleotide RT inhibitors other than zidovudine or stavudine, including didanosine, abacavir, and tenofovir.[104-107] For this reason, they are often referred to in general as nucleoside-associated mutations (NAMs).

Resistance dynamics for lamivudine and emtricitabine are similar. In individuals treated with lamivudine alone, high-level resistance (>100-fold increase in IC$_{50}$) appears within 4 to 8 weeks, conferred by mutations at RT codon 184.[59,108] Met184→Ile is observed initially, followed by Met184→Val. Emtricitabine failure also commonly selects for the same mutations.[109] Met184→Val by itself confers low-level cross-resistance to didanosine, zalcitabine, and abacavir but no cross-resistance to zidovudine, stavudine, or tenofovir.[108,110] At least for didanosine, the low-level phenotypic resistance conferred by Met184→Val does not preclude a virologic response to salvage therapy that includes didanosine.[111,112]

Resistance to didanosine or zalcitabine arises slowly in patients during monotherapy. Mutations in RT associated with decreased susceptibility include Lys65→Arg and Thr69→Asp for zalcitabine and Lys65→Arg and Leu74→Val for didanosine; these mutations confer a 4-fold to 10-fold increase in IC$_{50}$ relative to wild-type virus.[113-116] Resistance to abacavir is also slow to arise and has been associated with RT mutations Lys65→Arg, Leu74→Val, Tyr115→Phe, and Met184→Val, which, in combination, may increase the IC$_{50}$ of the drug by up to 10-fold.[117] However, virus with multiple zidovudine resistance mutations often displays decreased susceptibility to abacavir.[106,118,119] Resistance to tenofovir arises slowly and is often conferred by Lys65→Arg. However, certain NAMs also cause a diminished response to tenofovir.[107,120]

Interactions among various drug-selected substitutions may be important in the virologic activity of multidrug combinations. For example, the lamivudine resistance mutation RT Met184→Val may suppress the resistance to zidovudine, stavudine, or tenofovir conferred by several NAMs.[121,122] Similarly, the didanosine resistance RT mutation Leu74→Val and the substitution Lys65→Arg, associated with resistance to tenofovir, didanosine, zalcitabine, and abacavir, each suppress the phenotypic increase in IC$_{50}$ to zidovudine seen with some NAMs.[115,123] The clinical relevance of these mutational interactions has not yet been established. In contrast, Met184→Val increases the phenotypic resistance to abacavir conferred by NAMs, and the presence of Met184→Val with NAMs results in poorer virologic response to abacavir than the presence of NAMs alone.[106]

Mutations that individually confer resistance to various drugs in a particular combination play an important role in the development of resistance during therapy with that combination, but new patterns of genotypic resistance may evolve with combination therapy. For the combination of zidovudine and lamivudine, the RT Met184→Val mutant virus emerges rapidly, whereas zidovudine resistance mutations develop at a slower rate than during zidovudine monotherapy; this virus is resistant to lamivudine but remains sensitive to zidovudine for some time after zidovudine-selected mutations evolve.[121] However, a virus resistant to both zidovudine and lamivudine emerges after long-term failing combination therapy through one of several pathways. Resistance may involve complex selection for newly recognized substitutions in RT (including substitutions at codon 333), in addition to persistent zidovudine resistance mutations and the lamivudine resistance mutation at codon 184.[124] The virus may accumulate additional NAMs, thereby abrogating the reversal of zidovudine resistance conferred by Met184→Val.[125] Finally, newly recognized mutations (e.g., RT Asp44→Glu, Val118→Ile) can confer lower-level resistance to lamivudine (approximately 10-fold, compared with more than 100-fold with Met184→Val).[126] However, unlike Met184→Val, these mutations do not reverse zidovudine resistance.

Other novel combinations of unexpected mutations conferring multidrug resistance have been described in viruses from patients receiving multiple nucleoside regimens. A multinucleoside-resistant virus with several novel mutations in RT (Ala62→Val, Val75→Ile, Phe77→Leu, Pro116→Tyr, and Gln151→Met) has been described in some patients receiving long-term therapy with nucleosides.[127,128] This virus is resistant to zidovudine, didanosine, zalcitabine, stavudine, abacavir, and, to some degree, lamivudine. Insertion of two extra amino acids at codon 69 has been seen in several individuals with extensive treatment with nucleoside RT inhibitors.[129] This insertion, in the context of zidovudine resistance mutations, confers decreased susceptibility to all currently approved nucleoside and nucleotide RT inhibitors.

The determinants of phenotypic resistance to the effects of antiretroviral agents may not reside solely in viral genes. Alterations in cells of individuals exposed to a drug may allow an otherwise susceptible virus to replicate despite the presence of adequate serum levels of the antiretroviral agent. For instance, chronic zidovudine exposure may alter cellular phosphorylation mechanisms, rendering cells inefficient in phosphorylating nucleoside analogue RT inhibitors to their biologically active triphosphate forms.[130] Although this mechanism may be partly responsible for the poorer virologic and clinical response of zidovudine-experienced individuals to other nucleoside RT inhibitors, its role in antiretroviral failure remains to be clarified.[131]

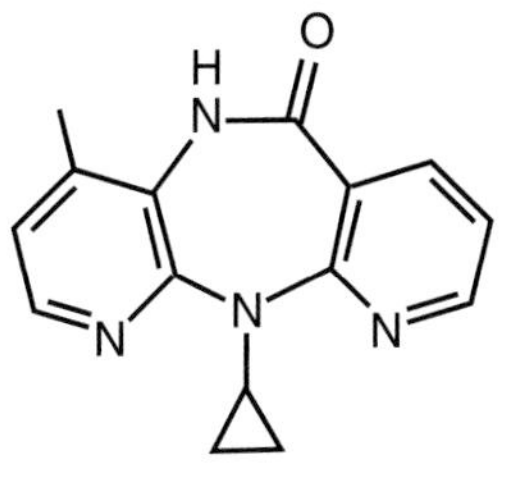

Non-nucleoside Reverse Transcriptase Inhibitors

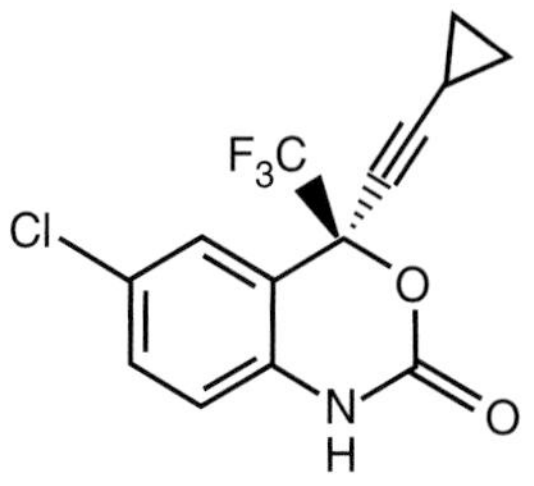

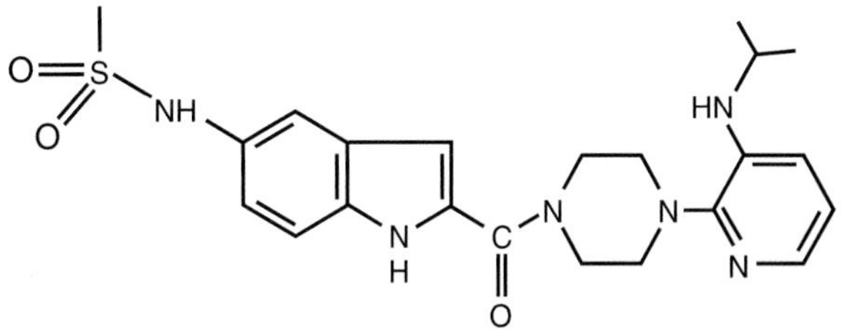

NNRTIs (Fig. 124-2, Table 124-2) include compounds with widely divergent chemical structures. They do not require phosphorylation or intracellular processing to become activated.[132] They are noncompetitive inhibitors of RT and cause allosteric inhibition of enzyme function by binding at sites distinct from the nucleoside-binding site. All have excellent activity against HIV-1 but none against HIV-2.

Nevirapine

Nevirapine is well absorbed orally with a bioavailability of greater than 90%, which is not altered by taking the drug with meals or antacid. Its plasma half-life is longer than 24 hours.[133] Nevirapine is metabolized extensively in the liver through the cytochrome P-450 (CYP) enzyme complex, primarily the CYP3A family. Nevirapine induces its own metabolism and causes a twofold increase in its apparent oral clearance in the first 2 to 4 weeks of therapy. For this reason, and to decrease the incidence of drug-induced rash, the initial adult dose is 200 mg once a day for the first 2 weeks, followed by 200 mg twice a day thereafter. Nevirapine also induces the metabolism, and thereby decreases the blood levels, of other drugs that are metabolized by cytochrome P-450, including oral contraceptive agents, methadone, rifampin, rifabutin, ketoconazole, and some protease inhibitors (saquinavir, indinavir, and lopinavir). Other inducers of CYP3A, such as rifampin and rifabutin, may decrease blood levels of nevirapine, whereas inhibitors, such as ketoconazole, may increase nevirapine concentrations.

Used alone, nevirapine produces a drop in viral RNA of 1 to 2 $\log_{10}$ by 2 weeks of therapy.[134] However, these values return to baseline by 4 weeks of therapy, in conjunction with the emergence of virus resistant to nevirapine.[135] In vitro, nevirapine has additive to synergistic activity against HIV-1 when used in combination with several nucleoside RT inhibitors or protease inhibitors. In antiretroviral-naive adults with a CD4+ T-cell count of 200 to 600 cells/mm³, the combination of nevirapine with zidovudine and didanosine produced maximal decreases in HIV-1 RNA of 2.2 $\log_{10}$ at week 8 that were sustained through the first year of therapy.[40] After 1 year of treatment, the mean CD4+ T-cell

FIGURE 124-2. Non-nucleoside reverse transcriptase inhibitors (NNRTIs).

count had increased by 139 cells/mm³, and 45% of subjects had levels of plasma HIV-1 RNA that were undetectable (<20 copies/mL). In contrast, decreases in HIV-1 RNA were transient, and improvements in CD4+ T-cell counts were smaller for combinations of zidovudine with didanosine or zidovudine with nevirapine. In antiretroviral-naive adults with more advanced disease (i.e., those with AIDS or a CD4+ T-cell count <200 cells/mm³), the combination of nevirapine, zidovudine, and didanosine had similarly greater virologic and immunologic benefits compared with the combination of zidovudine and didanosine.[136] However, the efficacy of nevirapine in combination with zidovudine and didanosine may be limited by prior antiretroviral use. In adults who had extensive prior use of nucleoside analogue RT inhibitors (almost all with zidovudine, with or without didanosine or zalcitabine, for a median of 25 months), the three-drug combination of nevirapine, zidovudine, and didanosine produced a maximal HIV-1 RNA drop of 1.1 $\log_{10}$ at 4 weeks, but by week 48, the HIV-1 RNA levels were not different from baseline.[137]

Nevirapine has also been studied in combination with stavudine and lamivudine in antiretroviral-naive subjects; the virologic success rate was 56% at week 48, compared with 62% with a regimen of efavirenz, stavudine, and lamivudine.[138] In patients with suppressed viremia on a protease inhibitor–containing regimen, a switch from the protease inhibitor to nevirapine was associated with maintenance of viral suppression and with amelioration of certain metabolic adverse effects of the protease inhibitors.[139,140]

The most frequent adverse effect of nevirapine has been rash, usually an erythematous maculopapular eruption sparing the palms and soles.[40] It has occurred in approximately 22% of patients during the first 1 to 8 weeks of therapy. Generally mild and self-limited, the rash can be monitored on a stable dose of nevirapine, with escalation of the dose after the first 2 weeks of therapy, when the rash dissipates. However, in up to 9% of patients, severe rash can develop, possibly leading to Stevens-Johnson syndrome.[137] If the rash is severe or extensive or involves the mucous membranes, nevirapine should be discontinued.

TABLE 124-2   Approved Non-nucleoside Reverse Transcriptase Inhibitors (NNRTIs)

Agent	Trade Name	Oral Bioavailability (%)	Serum Half-Life (hr)	Elimination	Adult Dose*	Availability
Nevirapine	Viramune	>90	>24	Hepatic cytochrome P-450	200 mg PO qd for 14 days, then 200 mg PO q12h if no rash develops	200-mg tablets 10-mg/mL solution
Delavirdine	Rescriptor	85	5.8	Hepatic cytochrome P-450	400 mg PO q8h	100- and 200-mg tablets
Efavirenz	Sustiva Stocrin		>40	Hepatic cytochrome P-450	600 mg PO qd	50-, 100-, and 200-mg capsules 600-mg tablets

*For pediatric dose see Chapter 123.

Elevated hepatic enzyme levels are seen frequently (up to 22% of subjects), and occasionally there may be progression to life-threatening clinical hepatitis.[40]

Delavirdine

Delavirdine is well absorbed orally, with bioavailability of 85%.[141] It requires an acidic environment for optimal absorption. The use of antacids within 1 hour of delavirdine administration or the use of histamine type 2 (H_2) blockers or proton pump inhibitors may reduce its absorption. The half-life of delavirdine is 5.8 hours. It is highly protein bound (98%). Delavirdine is metabolized primarily by the hepatic cytochrome P-450 enzyme complex. Several drugs may induce hepatic metabolism of delavirdine and thereby decrease its plasma levels; these include nelfinavir, amprenavir, rifabutin, rifampin, and several anticonvulsant agents. Conversely, unlike the other NNRTIs, delavirdine inhibits the hepatic metabolism of several drugs. Significant increases in plasma levels of saquinavir, ritonavir, indinavir, nelfinavir, amprenavir, clarithromycin, and rifabutin have been documented, and potentially serious adverse events have been predicted for dihydropyridine calcium channel blockers (e.g., nifedipine), cisapride, warfarin, quinidine, methadone, sildenafil, certain 3-hydroxy-3-methylglutaryl coenzyme A (HMG-CoA) reductase inhibitors (e.g., atorvastatin, cerivastatin), ergot derivatives, some nonsedating antihistamines (e.g., terfenadine, astemizole), and several benzodiazepines. The usual adult dose of delavirdine is 400 mg three times a day.

In a group of mostly antiretroviral-naive adults, the combination of delavirdine with zidovudine and lamivudine produced a greater decrease in HIV-1 RNA levels (2.25 $\log_{10}$ at 24 weeks of therapy) than either zidovudine with lamivudine (1.32 $\log_{10}$) or zidovudine with delavirdine (0.55 $\log_{10}$).[142] Viral RNA levels became undetectable (<400 copies/mL) by week 24 in 71% of individuals receiving the three-drug regimen, and CD4+ T-cell counts increased by 105 cells/mm³.

As with nevirapine, rash may occur, in up to 38% of patients receiving delavirdine, during the first 1 to 3 weeks of therapy.[141] This is usually an erythematous, maculopapular, mildly pruritic eruption that is often confluent. In most cases, the rash is transient, peaks over 2 to 3 days, and then resolves gradually. Although the rash is usually mild and does not require discontinuation of delavirdine, it may be severe in 3% to 4% of patients, necessitating discontinuation of therapy. Other adverse effects have included nausea, fatigue, and headache.

Efavirenz

Efavirenz is well absorbed orally, and its bioavailability is increased if it is taken with food. Efavirenz should be taken on an empty stomach, because the increased concentrations that result when it is taken with food may increase the frequency of adverse effects. Its half-life is longer than 40 hours, allowing once-daily dosing. Efavirenz is highly protein bound (99.5%). It is metabolized primarily by the hepatic cytochrome P-450 enzyme complex (principally CYP3A4 and CYP2B6). Inhibitors of these enzymes (e.g., ritonavir) are likely to increase efavirenz levels, whereas inducers (e.g., rifampin) may decrease them. Efavirenz itself is an inducer as well as an inhibitor of cytochrome P-450 enzymes and may alter the hepatic metabolism of several drugs significantly. For example, it decreases plasma levels of saquinavir, indinavir, amprenavir, lopinavir, atazanavir, methadone, rifabutin, and clarithromycin but increases levels of ritonavir. The adult dose is 600 mg once daily.

The combination of efavirenz with zidovudine and lamivudine in antiretroviral-naive patients provided potent and durable viral load suppression in three large studies. In an open-label comparison with a regimen of indinavir, zidovudine, and lamivudine, the efavirenz regimen provided greater viral load suppression (<50 copies/mL in 64%, compared with 43% for indinavir in the intent-to-treat analysis) at 48 weeks of therapy.[24] Both regimens were associated with marked increases in CD4+ T-cell counts (201 cells/mm³ for efavirenz and 185 cells/mm³ for indinavir). The second study compared efavirenz with nelfinavir, each in combination with zidovudine and lamivudine, and showed superiority of the efavirenz regimen in terms of virologic efficacy over 48 weeks of therapy.[143] The third investigation was a large, six-arm, randomized study involving 980 subjects that allowed comparison of efavirenz with nelfinavir, or with the combination of efavirenz and nelfinavir, when combined with a nucleoside backbone of either zidovudine with lamivudine or stavudine with didanosine.[25,144] Subjects who received a three-drug regimen and experienced virologic failure or drug toxicity were switched to the regimen containing the other three study drugs. Subjects were monitored for a median of 2.3 years, and the primary end point was time to second regimen failure of the three-drug regimens or to first failure of the four-drug regimen. Starting therapy with efavirenz, zidovudine, and lamivudine appeared to delay sequential regimen failure compared to starting either with nelfinavir, zidovudine, and lamivudine or efavirenz, stavudine, and didanosine.[25] Furthermore, no differences in time to first regimen failure were apparent when the three-drug regimen of efavirenz, zidovudine, and lamivudine was compared with the four-drug regimen of efavirenz, nelfinavir, zidovudine, and lamivudine.[144]

Similar results were reported when efavirenz combined with two nucleoside analogues was compared with either a single protease inhibitor or ritonavir plus saquinavir in combination with nucleoside analogues in antiretroviral-naive subjects.[145] The combination of efavirenz with stavudine and lamivudine in antiretroviral-naive patients resulted in a therapeutic success rate of 62%.[138] Efavirenz in combination with didanosine and emtricitabine also conferred potent antiviral activity.[146] In subjects with undetectable HIV-1 RNA (<400 copies/mL) on a regimen that included a protease inhibitor, switching to a once-daily regimen of efavirenz, emtricitabine, and didanosine resulted in more subjects retaining undetectable HIV-1 RNA (95% with <50 copies/mL) than did continuing on the same protease inhibitor–based regimen (87% with <50 copies/mL) at 48 weeks after the switch.

Combinations of efavirenz with antiretroviral agents other than nucleoside or nucleotide analogues have been the subjects of several recent trials. A regimen containing both efavirenz and nevirapine failed to show superior efficacy when compared with efavirenz or nevirapine alone.[138] Combinations of efavirenz and protease inhibitors appear to be promising. An early study showed that a combination of efavirenz and indinavir (at 1000 mg every 8 hours) produced undetectable HIV-

1 RNA (<50 copies/mL) in 47% of antiretroviral-naive subjects at 48 weeks of therapy in an intent-to-treat analysis. Although this result was inferior to that seen in the efavirenz with zidovudine and lamivudine arm (64% undetectable), it was comparable to the indinavir with zidovudine and lamivudine arm (43% undetectable).[24] More recent studies suggested good antiviral activity of efavirenz in combination with ritonavir-boosted protease inhibitors.[147-149] In antiretroviral-experienced subjects who had previously had heavy exposure to nucleoside analogues (but were naive to NNRTIs and protease inhibitors), salvage with nucleoside analogues and efavirenz caused a higher rate of viral suppression than did salvage with a regimen containing nucleoside analogues and nelfinavir or efavirenz alone.[150] However, in antiretroviral-naive subjects, the addition of nelfinavir to a three-drug regimen of zidovudine, lamivudine, and efavirenz provided no additional benefit compared with the three-drug regimen alone.[144]

The most frequent adverse effects have been central nervous system complaints including lightheadedness, dizziness, a sense of disengagement, sleep disturbances (insomnia, somnolence, or abnormal dreams), and headache. These often diminish with continued therapy, and dosing at bedtime may improve the tolerability of these symptoms. Psychiatric symptoms, including depression, mania, and psychosis, have also been observed; if severe, they may necessitate discontinuation of efavirenz. Rash has also been observed, but it usually was not severe or did not require drug discontinuation. Elevations in total cholesterol (of 10% to 20%) as well as occasional increases in hepatic transaminases have been observed with efavirenz treatment.

Mechanisms of Resistance

Mutations that confer high-level resistance to nevirapine (most commonly RT Lys101→Glu, Lys103→Asn, Gly106→Ala, Tyr181→Cys, and Gly190→Ala) are selected rapidly during suboptimal nevirapine therapy.[135,151] A similar pattern has been observed for delavirdine, with resistance mutations that include RT Lys103→Asn, Tyr181→Cys, and Pro236→Leu.[152,153] Efavirenz resistance in treated patients has been most commonly caused by RT Lys103→Asn, although other substitutions (including Tyr188→Leu and Gly190→Ser) have also been seen.[154,155] Mutations that confer resistance to one NNRTI often confer cross-resistance to several other NNRTIs. The considerable overlap in the resistance profile of these drugs makes broad cross-resistance to the currently available drugs in this class likely after virologic failure of one of them. In fact, clinical studies suggest decreased efficacy of efavirenz in individuals with prior NNRTI experience.[156]

Cross-resistance does not occur between nucleoside analogue RT inhibitors and NNRTIs, allowing the potential use of NNRTIs in individuals in whom a nucleoside analogue–resistant virus is suspected. Furthermore, nucleoside analogue–resistant viruses often display increased susceptibility (hypersusceptibility) to NNRTIs.[157] Some studies have suggested that NNRTI hypersusceptibility is associated with a better clinical virologic response to a regimen that includes efavirenz.[158-160]

Protease Inhibitors

The HIV protease (or proteinase) enzyme is an aspartyl protease that is essential for post-translational cleavage of gag and gag-pol polyprotein.[1] Several viral proteins, including those that form the protein components of the viral core, as well as protease itself, RT, and integrase, are synthesized as polyproteins that require cleavage by the viral protease to produce mature proteins. Protease inhibitors appear to block the necessary cleavage of these polyproteins in the late stages of the viral replicative cycle, causing the production of immature, defective viral particles.[161,162] Unlike nucleoside analogue RT inhibitors, protease inhibitors do not need intracellular processing to be activated. Protease inhibitors are active against HIV-1 and HIV-2.

Currently available protease inhibitors (Fig. 124-3, Table 124-3) are extensively metabolized by the hepatic cytochrome P-450 enzyme complex, primarily through the isoenzyme CYP3A4. Protease inhibitors may interfere, to varied degrees, with the hepatic metabolism of other drugs by acting as cytochrome P-450 inducers or inhibitors.[163-165] Although these effects are most prominent with ritonavir, the use of any protease inhibitor should prompt a careful review of concurrently used medications to avoid potential adverse effects, including review of appropriate product monographs. For instance, protease inhibitors may increase plasma levels of the antihistamines terfenadine and astemizole, or the gastrointestinal motility agent cisapride, which may decrease the threshold for life-threatening arrhythmias. These agents should be avoided when using currently available protease inhibitors. Other drugs may alter blood levels of protease inhibitors by altering their metabolism. Inhibitors of cytochrome P-450 (e.g., ketoconazole) may increase levels markedly, whereas inducers (e.g., rifampin, rifabutin, St. John's wort) may decrease levels significantly.

Several metabolic adverse effects have been associated with the chronic use of protease inhibitors.[166] Most protease inhibitors induce significant increases in blood levels of triglycerides and cholesterol.[167] Hyperglycemia and new onset or exacerbation of previous diabetes mellitus have been noted.[168-170] Hyperglycemia and hyperlipidemia may in turn be associated with an increased risk of myocardial infarction.[171,172] Body habitus changes due to either lipoatrophy or lipohypertrophy were ascribed initially to protease inhibitors but now are recognized to be multifactorial in etiology.[173,174] A lipoatrophy syndrome with symmetrical loss of subcutaneous fat from the face and extremities was seen soon after the introduction of protease inhibitor therapy.[175] Abnormal fat deposits at the posterior base of the neck and in the abdominal viscera, often with elevated serum triglyceride levels, have also been reported.[176,177] Osteopenia, osteoporosis, and osteonecrosis have been observed in patients treated with protease inhibitor–containing regimens, although their specific relationship to protease inhibitors (rather than HIV infection or antiretroviral therapy in general) remains to be established.[178] Guidelines for the management of several of these metabolic complications are available.[179-181] Protease inhibitors have also been associated with increased bleeding episodes in persons with hemophilia.

Saquinavir

Two formulations of oral saquinavir have been developed, a hard capsule and a soft gel capsule. Although the bioavailability of the hard capsule formulation has been low (average of 4%), the newer soft gel capsule has substantially improved bioavailability. Saquinavir should preferably be taken with meals with a high fat content to maximize absorption. It is highly protein bound (97%). Several drugs, including nevirapine, efavirenz, rifampin, rifabutin, and many anticonvulsants (phenobarbital, phenytoin, carbamazepine) induce metabolism of saquinavir and may decrease its plasma concentration considerably. In contrast, drugs such as ritonavir, indinavir, nelfinavir, delavirdine, ketoconazole, and clarithromycin inhibit the metabolism of saquinavir and may increase its levels markedly. Saquinavir may inhibit the metabolism of sildenafil, cisapride, ergot derivatives, many benzodiazepine sedatives (e.g., triazolam, midazolam), and several nonsedating antihistamines (e.g., terfenadine, astemizole), potentially causing dangerously high levels of these drugs. The usual adult dose of the soft gel capsule formulation of saquinavir is 1200 mg orally every 8 hours, but lower doses should be used in combination with some protease inhibitors.

Initial studies of saquinavir in the hard capsule formulation showed that, when used alone, its benefits in terms of viral load decrease and CD4+ T-cell increase were transient.[182,183] Studies of saquinavir in combination with nucleoside analogue RT inhibitors have shown more durable responses. In adults with an extensive prior history of zidovudine use, the combination of a saquinavir hard capsule at 600 mg three times daily with zidovudine and zalcitabine was superior to zidovudine with zalcitabine or to zidovudine with saquinavir in terms of maximal decrease in HIV-1 RNA levels and increase in CD4+ T-cell counts.[184] Nevertheless, the response to therapy was poor in comparison with other protease inhibitor–containing regimens, probably because of the low saquinavir bioavailability from the hard capsule and the extensive prior nucleoside analogue experience of the subjects. Studies of the soft gel capsule formulation have produced better

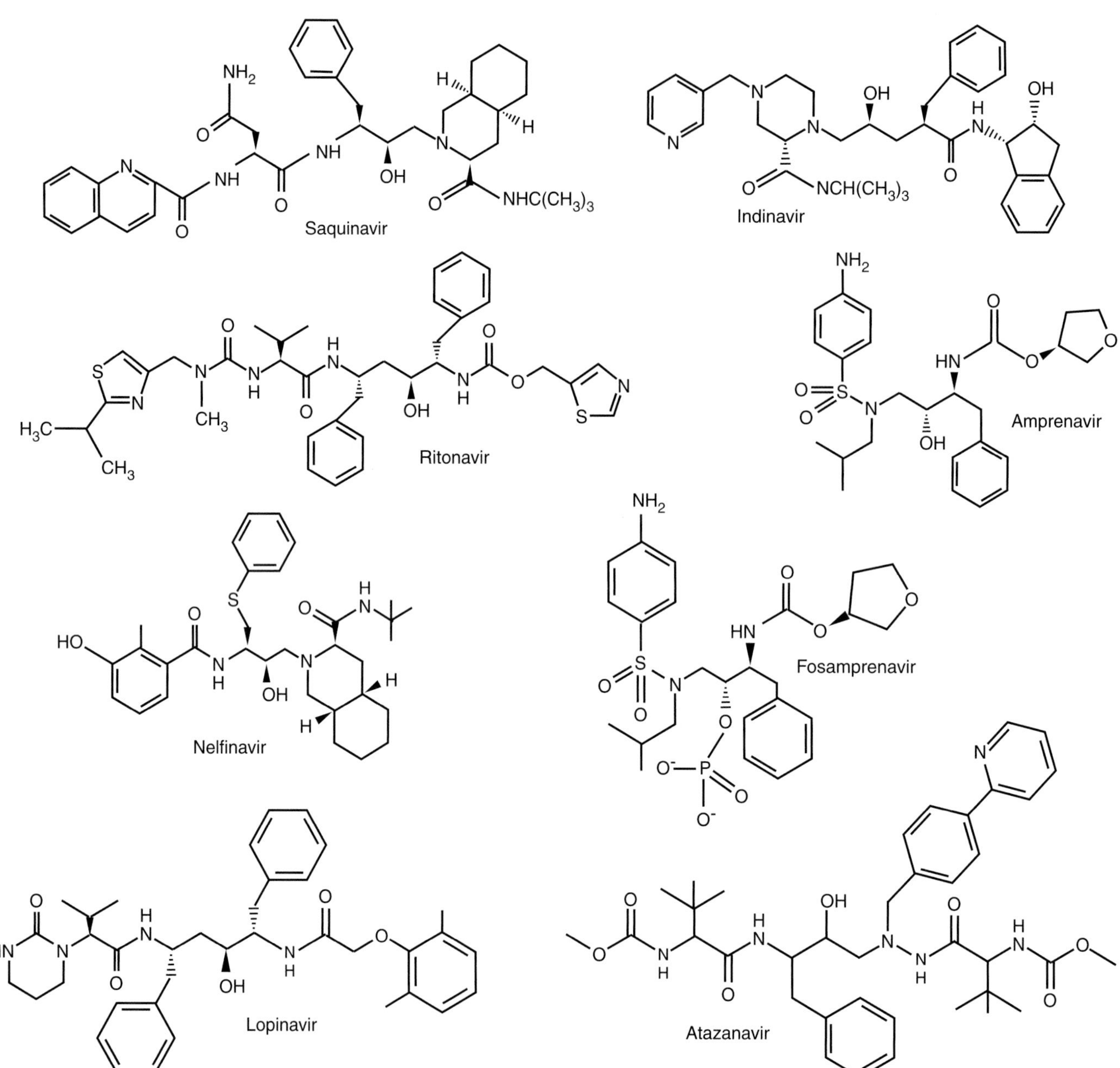

FIGURE 124-3. Protease inhibitors.

results. In antiretroviral-naive adults, the saquinavir soft gel capsule administered at 1200 mg three times daily was compared with the hard capsule formulation at 600 mg three times daily, each in combination with two nucleoside analogue RT inhibitors.[185] At 16 weeks of therapy, combinations with the soft gel formulation produced a mean reduction in plasma viral RNA of 2.0 $\log_{10}$, whereas those with the hard capsule formulation resulted in 1.6 $\log_{10}$ reduction. Furthermore, 80% of subjects taking the soft gel form had undetectable HIV-1 RNA levels (<400 copies/mL), whereas only 43% of those taking the hard capsule achieved similar levels of viral suppression. Another study demonstrated that soft gel saquinavir in combination with zidovudine and lamivudine had antiviral efficacy similar to that of a regimen of indinavir, zidovudine, and lamivudine in antiretroviral-naive patients.[186]

Taking advantage of ritonavir's marked inhibitory effects on saquinavir metabolism, the combination of saquinavir and ritonavir, which causes at least a 20-fold increase in saquinavir levels compared with saquinavir used alone, has been shown to have potent antiretro-

viral activity.[187,188] The benefits in viral suppression were more prominent in individuals who were protease inhibitor–naive. When used with ritonavir, saquinavir can be given twice daily. In protease inhibitor–naive subjects, the combination of ritonavir and hard capsule saquinavir (each at 400 mg twice a day) with two nucleoside analogues resulted in greater virologic suppression (<200 copies/mL) than either indinavir or ritonavir with two nucleoside analogues.[189]

Adverse reactions to saquinavir have included diarrhea, nausea, abdominal discomfort, and dyspepsia. These reactions have been infrequent with the hard capsule formulation but appear to be more frequent and more severe with the soft gel capsule.[190] Elevated triglyceride levels and asymptomatic elevations in liver enzyme and creatine phosphokinase levels have also been noted.

Ritonavir

Ritonavir is well absorbed orally, with a bioavailability of approximately 70%. It is highly protein bound in plasma (>98%), and has a

TABLE 124-3 Approved Protease Inhibitors

Agent	Trade Name	Oral Bioavailability (%)	Serum Half-Life (hr)	Elimination	Adult Dose*	Availability
Saquinavir (soft gel capsule)	Fortovase	—	1-2	Hepatic cytochrome P-450	1200 mg PO q8h	200-mg soft gel capsules
Saquinavir (hard capsule)	Invirase	4	1-2	Hepatic cytochrome P-450	When used in combination with ritonavir, 400 mg PO q12h	200-mg hard capsules
Ritonavir	Norvir	70	3-5	Hepatic cytochrome P-450	300 mg PO q12h with escalation over 1-2 wk to 600 mg PO q12h; when used in combination with saquinavir, dose often decreased to 400 mg PO q12h	100-mg capsules 80-mg/mL solution
Indinavir	Crixivan	60-65	1.8	Hepatic cytochrome P-450	800 mg PO p8h	100-, 200-, 333-, and 400-mg capsules
Nelfinavir	Viracept	70-80	3.5-5	Hepatic cytochrome P-450	1250 mg PO q12h or 750 mg PO q8h	250- and 625-mg tablets 50-mg/g powder
Amprenavir	Agenerase	—	7-11	Hepatic cytochrome P-450	Capsules 1200 mg PO q12h Solution 1400 mg PO q12h	50- and 150-mg capsules 15-mg/mL solution
Fosamprenavir	Lexira	—	7-11	Hepatic cytochrome P-450	1400 mg PO q12h	700-mg tablets
Lopinavir + ritonavir	Kaletra	—	5-6	Hepatic cytochrome P-450	Three capsules PO q12h Solution 5 ml PO q12h	133.3-mg lopinavir/ 33.3-mg ritonavir capsules 80-mg lopinavir/20-mg ritonavir per mL solution
Atazanavir	Reyataz	—	7	Hepatic cytochrome P-450	400 mg PO qd	100-, 150-, and 200-mg capsules

*For pediatric dose see Chapter 123. Consult product monograph for appropriate dose when low-dose ritonavir is used for pharmacokinetic enhancement.

half-life of 3 to 5 hours.[191,192] Other drugs may alter the metabolism of ritonavir, thereby either increasing its serum levels (as observed with clarithromycin, ketoconazole, fluconazole, and fluoxetine) or decreasing its levels (as observed with rifampin and some anticonvulsant agents). Conversely, ritonavir itself can cause marked alterations in the metabolism of other drugs. It induces hepatic metabolism of several drugs as well as itself, thereby decreasing the bioavailability of ethinyl estradiol in oral contraceptive agents, theophylline, and possibly atovaquone and some analgesic agents (including morphine, methadone, codeine, naproxen, and ketoprofen). Ritonavir may also inhibit the metabolism of other drugs, potentially causing serious adverse effects when used with rifabutin, several antiarrhythmic agents (amiodarone, quinidine, flecainide, encainide, and quinidine), some nonsedating antihistamines (astemizole and terfenadine), cisapride, meperidine, propoxyphene, ergot derivatives, and several benzodiazepines. It may also cause large increases in plasma levels of saquinavir, indinavir, nelfinavir, amprenavir, atazanavir, erythromycin, clarithromycin, ketoconazole, itraconazole, sildenafil, quinine, carbamazepine, calcium channel blockers, warfarin, analgesic agents (including methadone, fentanyl, and piroxicam), antidepressants (including desipramine, bupropion, sertraline, trazodone, and fluoxetine), some neuroleptics, several hypolipidemic agents, corticosteroids, and others. Because the liquid formulation of ritonavir contains alcohol, patients taking metronidazole or disulfiram may have severe reactions if they take liquid ritonavir concomitantly. The usual adult dose of ritonavir is 600 mg orally every 12 hours, although lower doses may be used in combination with some other protease inhibitors. Ritonavir should be stored in a refrigerator and shielded from light.

Used alone, ritonavir produced a maximal decrease in HIV-1 RNA levels of at least 1.0 $\log_{10}$ at weeks 2 to 4 of therapy.[192,193] Although HIV-1 RNA levels subsequently rose, they remained significantly lower than baseline by week 32 of therapy. In one study, mean increases in CD4+ T-cell counts of up to 230 cells/mm³ (above a baseline

mean of 130 cells/mm³) were sustained through the 32 weeks of observation.[192] In combination therapy, ritonavir has shown potent and durable clinical benefits. Among adults with advanced HIV disease (CD4+ T-cell count <100 cells/mm³) whose median length of prior antiretroviral therapy was 3 years (although protease inhibitor naive), the addition of ritonavir to the nucleoside analogue RT inhibitor regimen resulted in a decreased viral RNA level of 0.6 $\log_{10}$ from baseline and a mean increase in CD4+ T-cell counts of more than 50 cells/mm³ after 1 year of therapy.[194] In the ritonavir-treated group, the rate of clinical progression was 42% lower and the death rate was 30% lower during the first year of therapy, compared with controls. Ritonavir has also shown potent antiviral activity in combination with other protease inhibitors, including saquinavir, indinavir, and nelfinavir.

The ability of ritonavir to inhibit cytochrome P-450 metabolism, coupled with the observation that currently available protease inhibitors are metabolized by this enzyme system, has prompted its use as a pharmacokinetic enhancer of several other protease inhibitors. Often, a low dose of ritonavir (100 to 200 mg given up to twice daily) is used to increase the blood levels of the other protease inhibitor, allowing lower and less frequent dosing.[195] In the treatment of virus with protease inhibitor resistance, such increased blood levels may inhibit an otherwise resistant virus. Several ritonavir-boosted protease inhibitor regimens have been described, including saquinavir, indinavir, amprenavir, and atazanavir.[147,189,195-198] The current lopinavir formulation is available only in combination with low-dose ritonavir.

Adverse reactions to ritonavir have included gastrointestinal disturbances (nausea, vomiting, or diarrhea in up to 52% and, less frequently, anorexia and abdominal pain), weakness, circumoral or peripheral paresthesias, altered taste, and headache.[192,194] Adverse effects appear to be more common in patients with more advanced disease. They are also related to plasma levels of ritonavir and are greatest at the beginning of therapy, before ritonavir induces an increase in its own metabolism. Toxicities often improve with continued therapy and may be less severe if ritonavir is taken with meals. Also, starting the dosage at 300 mg orally every 12 hours and escalating over 1 to 2 weeks to the full adult dose of 600 mg orally every 12 hours decreases the severity of adverse effects. Most patients experience some elevations in cholesterol levels (30% to 40%) and in triglyceride levels (200% to 300%), and many also develop elevated levels of liver transaminases and creatine phosphokinase.[192,194]

Indinavir

Indinavir requires an acidic environment for optimal solubility, and food with high protein or fat content interferes with its absorption. Therefore, indinavir should be taken in a fasting state (1 hour before a meal or 2 hours after a meal) or with a light, low-fat snack for optimal bioavailability of 60% to 65%. Indinavir has a half-life of 1.8 hours and exhibits less protein binding (60%) in blood than other protease inhibitors do. Certain drugs inhibit indinavir's metabolism, increasing its plasma concentration. These include ritonavir, nelfinavir, delavirdine, ketoconazole, itraconazole, and clarithromycin. Other drugs, including nevirapine, efavirenz, rifampin, rifabutin, and fluconazole, may increase the metabolism of indinavir, thereby decreasing its plasma concentration. In turn, indinavir inhibits the metabolism of saquinavir, nelfinavir, clarithromycin, ketoconazole, and rifabutin and may similarly affect rifampin, some nonsedating antihistamines (terfenadine, astemizole), ergotamines, cisapride, and several benzodiazepines. The usual adult dose of indinavir is 800 mg orally every 8 hours.

Indinavir provides potent and durable benefits, especially when used as part of a combination regimen. In adults with a median CD4+ T-cell count of 144 cells/mm³ who were previously treated with zidovudine, treatment with indinavir monotherapy or with zidovudine and lamivudine resulted in a transient decrease in plasma HIV-1 RNA levels that diminished with increasing time on therapy.[199] However, treatment with zidovudine, lamivudine, and indinavir produced a decrease in HIV-1 RNA levels of 2.0 log₁₀ that persisted over more than 1 year of therapy. At week 24 of therapy, 90% of subjects receiving the three-drug regimen had undetectable HIV-1 RNA levels (<500 copies/mL) whereas only 43% of those receiving indinavir monotherapy and 30% of those receiving zidovudine with lamivudine had equivalent viral suppression. Long-term follow-up of subjects who initially received the triple-drug regimen showed sustained suppression of plasma viral RNA and persistent CD4+ T-cell increases for up to 3 years.[200,201]

A larger study with adults who were zidovudine experienced and had more advanced disease (mean CD4+ T-cell count, 87 cells/mm³) demonstrated a durable antiviral effect with the combination regimen of zidovudine, lamivudine, and indinavir.[23] The three-drug regimen provided a decrease in viral RNA levels of 2.8 log₁₀ at week 24, with 60% of subjects having undetectable HIV-1 RNA levels (<500 copies/mL). In contrast, the combination of zidovudine and lamivudine without a protease inhibitor produced a decrease in viral RNA levels of 1.0 log₁₀ at week 24, with only 9% of subjects having undetectable plasma HIV-1 RNA. By week 40, CD4+ T-cell counts had increased by 121 cells/mm³ in the three-drug arm and by 40 cells/mm³ in the two-drug arm. With a median duration of follow-up of only 38 weeks, the study showed a 47% decrease in the rate of clinical progression to a new AIDS-defining diagnosis or death in the protease inhibitor–containing arm.

A third study compared indinavir monotherapy with the combination of zidovudine and lamivudine and with the combination of all three drugs in adults with advanced HIV disease (CD4+ T-cell counts ≤50 cells/mm³) who were zidovudine experienced.[202] After 24 weeks, the median decreases in plasma viral RNA were 2.2 log₁₀ in patients in the three-drug arm but only 0.17 log₁₀ in those in the indinavir-monotherapy arm and 0.16 log₁₀ in those taking two nucleoside analogue RT inhibitors. The proportion of individuals with undetectable plasma viral RNA levels (<500 copies/mL) was 65% for the three-drug regimen, 4% for indinavir monotherapy, and 0% for zidovudine combined with lamivudine. Median increases in CD4+ T-cell counts

were 86 cells/mm³ in those on the three-drug regimen, 61 cells/mm³ with indinavir monotherapy, and zero cells/mm³ in the two-drug arm. In a 192-week extension of this study in 108 subjects initially randomly assigned to the three-drug arm, long-term virologic and immunologic benefits continued to be observed in a small, but substantial, number of individuals.[203]

Combinations of indinavir with other protease inhibitors or with NNRTIs have been studied less well, although several have resulted in substantial antiviral potency.[24,196,204] The use of ritonavir as a pharmacokinetic enhancer of indinavir may allow less frequent dosing of indinavir.[195]

The most serious adverse effect of indinavir has been nephrolithiasis, with stones consisting of crystallized indinavir causing symptoms in 4% to 9% of treated individuals.[23,205] The frequency of nephrolithiasis can be reduced with high oral fluid intake (at least 1.5 L/day) throughout the day. Indinavir-associated nephrolithiasis is treated supportively with hydration and analgesia, and interruption of indinavir therapy usually is not necessary. Gastrointestinal irritation (abdominal discomfort and nausea) is commonly observed if indinavir is taken in a fasting state. To improve tolerability, the drug may be taken with a small, low-fat, low-protein meal without significantly compromising its absorption. Other adverse reactions include insomnia, dry throat, and dry skin. An indirect hyperbilirubinemia is often observed (at least 10% of individuals) but does not lead to clinically significant liver disease.

Nelfinavir

Nelfinavir has good bioavailability, and its absorption (70% to 80%) is optimal when it is administered with food.[206] It is highly protein bound in plasma (>98%) and has a half-life of 3.5 to 5 hours. Drugs that decrease nelfinavir's metabolism and increase its levels include delavirdine, ritonavir, indinavir, and ketoconazole. Rifampin and rifabutin increase nelfinavir's metabolism and reduce its plasma levels. Nelfinavir affects the metabolism of several drugs. It decreases levels of delavirdine and of ethinyl estradiol and norethindrone in oral contraceptive agents and may markedly increase levels of saquinavir, indinavir, rifabutin, cisapride, ergot derivatives, some nonsedating antihistamines (terfenadine, astemizole), and several antiarrhythmics and benzodiazepines. The usual adult dose of nelfinavir is 1250 mg orally every 12 hours.

In a population of antiretroviral-naive adults, the combination of zidovudine, lamivudine, and nelfinavir (750 mg three times daily) resulted in a mean increase in CD4+ T-cell counts of 127 cells/mm³ and a decrease in plasma HIV-1 RNA of 2.9 log₁₀ at 12 months of therapy.[207] By 6 months of therapy, 55% of subjects receiving the three-drug regimen had undetectable HIV-1 RNA levels (<50 copies/mL), and this response was maintained through 1 year of therapy. However, compared with regimens that contain some other protease inhibitors or NNRTIs, the efficacy of nelfinavir-containing regimens appears to be lower. In antiretroviral-naive subjects, the combination of nelfinavir with zidovudine and lamivudine resulted in less sustainable viral load suppression than did efavirenz with zidovudine and lamivudine.[25] In subjects who were nucleoside RT inhibitor experienced but protease inhibitor and NNRTI naive, salvage therapy with efavirenz and two nucleoside RT inhibitors was more likely than salvage with nelfinavir plus two nucleoside RT inhibitors to lead to durable viral suppression.[143] In antiretroviral-naive subjects, lopinavir/ritonavir, in combination with stavudine and lamivudine, also resulted in greater and more durable viral load suppression, compared with a regimen of nelfinavir with the same nucleoside RT inhibitors.[208] In protease inhibitor–experienced individuals, the efficacy of nelfinavir is significantly compromised compared with salvage with other protease inhibitors.[209]

Nelfinavir is generally well tolerated. Gastrointestinal complaints are common and include flatulence and mild to moderate diarrhea that can usually be controlled with antidiarrheal medications such as loperamide.

Amprenavir

Amprenavir is well absorbed orally and may be taken with or without food, although taking it with a high-fat meal may decrease blood levels of amprenavir and is not recommended. It has a half-life of 7 to 11 hours. Amprenavir is metabolized by the hepatic cytochrome P-450 enzyme system. Inducers of this enzyme system (e.g., efavirenz, rifampin) are likely to decrease amprenavir blood levels, whereas inhibitors (including indinavir, ritonavir, ketoconazole, and clarithromycin) may increase its levels. Amprenavir is also an inhibitor of cytochrome P-450 and can cause significant increases in blood levels of certain coadministered drugs, such as ketoconazole and rifabutin. The oral solution contains propylene glycol and should not be used by patients who are also taking metronidazole or disulfiram. The usual adult dose of amprenavir is 1200 mg every 12 hours. When given with low-dose ritonavir (100 mg), amprenavir (1200 mg) may be given once daily.

A study comparing amprenavir alone with the combination of amprenavir with zidovudine and lamivudine found that 63% of subjects taking the combination regimen had undetectable viral RNA levels (<500 copies/mL) at week 24 of therapy.[210] Amprenavir has also shown potency when used with other protease inhibitors. A pilot study of combinations of amprenavir with each of saquinavir, indinavir, and nelfinavir demonstrated median decreases in HIV-1 RNA levels of 1.7 to 3.4 $\log_{10}$ at week 48 of therapy, similar to the antiviral effects of amprenavir with zidovudine and lamivudine.[211] In salvage settings involving protease inhibitor–experienced subjects, a combination of amprenavir with another protease inhibitor (saquinavir, indinavir, or nelfinavir) together with efavirenz, abacavir, and a nucleotide RT inhibitor resulted in undetectable plasma HIV-1 RNA levels (<200 copies/mL) in approximately 35% of subjects at 24 weeks of therapy.[212]

Amprenavir is usually well tolerated. The most frequent side effects have been headache, gastrointestinal complaints (nausea and diarrhea), and rash. A new formulation of a prodrug of amprenavir, called fosamprenavir, has recently been approved. Fosamprenavir is associated with a smaller pill burden and appears to have improved tolerability compared with amprenavir.

Lopinavir

Lopinavir is currently co-formulated with ritonavir, which inhibits the metabolism of lopinavir and consequently results in adequately high levels of the drug. It should be taken with food to enhance its bioavailability. Lopinavir is highly protein bound (98% to 99%). Its half-life is 5 to 6 hours. Because lopinavir is metabolized by cytochrome P-450 enzymes, enzyme inducers such as efavirenz, nevirapine, and rifampin may decrease its blood levels, and enzyme inhibitors (most notably ritonavir) may increase its levels substantially. The combination of lopinavir and ritonavir in the current formulation inhibits several hepatic metabolizing enzymes and increases the levels of some. When co-administered with lopinavir/ritonavir, increases in blood levels of several protease inhibitors, rifabutin, ketoconazole, atorvastatin, and other drugs (as listed in the earlier section on ritonavir) may be seen, whereas decreases in levels of methadone, ethinyl estradiol, and norethindrone may occur. Because the liquid formulation contains alcohol, patients taking metronidazole or disulfiram may have severe reactions if taking liquid lopinavir/ritonavir concomitantly. The usual dose of lopinavir/ritonavir is 400/100 mg every 12 hours.

In antiretroviral-naive patients, lopinavir/ritonavir in combination with stavudine and lamivudine resulted in undetectable levels of HIV-1 RNA (<50 copies/mL) in 67% of patients at 48 weeks.[208] This virologic response was superior to that observed with the combination of nelfinavir, stavudine, and lamivudine, which resulted in undetectable viral load in 52% of patients. Lopinavir/ritonavir has also been studied in antiretroviral-experienced subjects, in whom, despite prior failure of some protease inhibitors, it was associated with significant and durable virologic responses.[213] In a study comparing lopinavir/

ritonavir to ritonavir-boosted fosamprenavir in protease inhibitor–experienced subjects, 50% of those receiving lopinavir/ritonavir had undetectable viral load (<50 copies/mL) at week 48, compared with 46% of those receiving fosamprenavir/ritonavir twice daily.[214]

The most frequent adverse effects of lopinavir/ritonavir have included nausea, vomiting, and diarrhea. Elevations in serum cholesterol and triglyceride levels are common.

Atazanavir

Atazanavir has good oral bioavailability, and its absorption is increased if it is taken with a light meal. Its half-life is approximately 7 hours, allowing for once-daily dosing. Atazanavir undergoes metabolism primarily by hepatic cytochrome P-450 enzyme CYP3A4. Administration of atazanavir with ritonavir (which inhibits atazanavir metabolism) increases concentrations of atazanavir by several-fold. On the other hand, inducers of cytochrome P-450 metabolism (e.g., efavirenz) can decrease atazanavir levels considerably. Atazanavir may inhibit the metabolism of other drugs, including saquinavir, rifabutin, clarithromycin, and diltiazem, raising their blood levels significantly. The dose of atazanavir is 400 mg once daily.

In antiretroviral-naive patients, the combination of atazanavir with zidovudine and lamivudine showed antiviral activity and CD4+ T-cell increases equivalent to those observed with the combination of efavirenz, zidovudine, and lamivudine at 48 weeks of therapy.[215] In protease inhibitor–experienced patients, however, atazanavir showed inferior antiviral activity (decrease in HIV-1 RNA of 1.67 $\log_{10}$ copies/mL) compared with lopinavir/ritonavir (decrease of 2.11 $\log_{10}$ copies/mL) after 24 weeks of salvage therapy with two nucleoside analogues.[216] However, ritonavir-boosting of atazanavir (100 mg ritonavir with 300 mg atazanavir) appeared to render it equally potent to lopinavir/ritonavir in combination with tenofovir and a nucleoside analogue for salvage therapy of protease inhibitor–experienced patients up to 24 weeks of therapy.[198]

The most frequent adverse effects of atazanavir have been diarrhea and nausea, although these have been noted less commonly than with other protease inhibitors in comparative trials. The most common laboratory abnormality associated with treatment has been asymptomatic elevation of serum unconjugated bilirubin, seen in the majority of subjects treated with 400 mg daily. Although it was usually mild, unconjugated hyperbilirubinemia caused jaundice in approximately 7% to 8% of subjects; however, few subjects discontinued the drug because of jaundice. Hyperbilirubinemia has not been associated with elevations of hepatic transaminase levels or hepatic injury, and it is reversible on discontinuation of atazanavir. Unlike other protease inhibitors, atazanavir has caused very little adverse change in blood lipids to date.

Mechanisms of Resistance

Resistance mutations in protease are often classified as primary or secondary. A primary resistance mutation is often the initial resistance mutation that arises during selection with a protease inhibitor; it confers significant in vitro resistance to the inhibitor and is often unique to the particular inhibitor used. Primary resistance mutations are not found as naturally occurring polymorphisms in HIV-1 strains. A virus that contains only the initial primary resistance mutation to a particular protease inhibitor may have little cross-resistance to other protease inhibitors. However, with longer therapy, a highly resistant virus can evolve that contains many other mutations that are common to several protease inhibitors and that confer broad cross-resistance to the entire class. These secondary resistance mutations by themselves confer either very little or no resistance to protease inhibitors. However, when seen on a background of primary resistance mutations, they confer higher levels of resistance than are observed with the primary mutations alone. Different protease inhibitors have largely overlapping spectra of secondary mutations, and the accumulation of several secondary mutations on a background of a primary mutation often leads to cross-resistance to several other protease inhibitors. Unlike primary protease resistance mutations, secondary mutations may be observed as naturally occurring polymorphisms, and their detection (without a primary mutation) does not necessarily imply drug selection.

For saquinavir, one or two primary mutations in the protease (most commonly Leu90→Met, less often Gly48→Val, or rarely both) are enough to increase the IC_{50} significantly and are associated with increased plasma viral RNA levels.[217,218] One or two mutations selected by ritonavir (the first usually being Val82→Ala or Phe) are needed to reduce drug susceptibility, and the accumulation of further mutations (including Lys20→Arg, Leu33→Phe, Met36→Ile or Leu, Met46→Ile or Leu, Ile54→Val, Ala71→Val or Thr, Val82→Thr or Ser, Ile84→Val, and Leu90→Met) confers increasing levels of resistance.[219] For indinavir, a large number of mutations are selected in various combinations and sequential orders in different patients. Most commonly, these include Val82→Ala or Phe or Thr, or Met46→Ile or Leu; other changes include Leu10→Ile or Val or Arg, Lys20→Met or Arg, Leu24→Ile, Ile54→Val or Ala, Leu63→Pro, Ala71→Val or Thr, Ile84→Val, and Leu90→Met.[220,221] Single or double substitutions do not appear to decrease in vitro susceptibility to indinavir significantly, but an increased number of resistance substitutions are associated with a greater magnitude of phenotypic resistance to the drug.

Resistance to nelfinavir often arises first in conjunction with Asp30→Asn.[222] This primary mutation does not (by itself) confer cross-resistance to other protease inhibitors. Compared with some other primary protease inhibitor resistance mutations, the presence of Asp30→Asn was associated with an improved and more durable virologic response to a salvage regimen containing saquinavir and ritonavir.[223] However, if nelfinavir-containing therapy is continued in the setting of continued viremia, mutations other than Asp30→Asn (such as Glu35→Asp, Met36→Ile, Met46→Ile, Ala71→Val or Thr, Val77→Ile, and Asn88→Asp or Ser) accumulate and may render the virus cross-resistant to protease inhibitors other than nelfinavir.[222] Amprenavir-selected substitutions in the protease have included Leu10→Phe, Val32→Ile, Met46→Ile or Leu, Ile47→Val, Ile50→Val, Ile54→Leu or Met, and Ile84→Val.[224,225] For lopinavir, no signature primary mutation has been identified. The accumulation of several mutations appears to be required for significant resistance to lopinavir.[226] In protease inhibitor–naive subjects, the primary resistance mutation for atazanavir appears to be Ile50→Leu, which does not confer resistance to other protease inhibitors.[227] However, in patients with previous protease inhibitor experience who have protease inhibitor–resistant virus, subsequent failure of atazanavir only rarely selects for Ile50→Leu; instead, it usually selects for mutations that confer broader protease inhibitor cross-resistance.

Although certain protease inhibitor–resistant mutants may have decreased protease enzymatic function and replicative capacity, compensatory mutations in the protease region (secondary resistance mutations) or in the *gag* region (including protease cleavage sites) may at least partially restore viral replicative fitness.[228-230]

Entry Inhibitors

The process of HIV-1 entry into host cells is complex and consists of several distinct steps, each of which forms a separate target for entry inhibition.[3,231] The first step, viral attachment to the host cell, is accomplished through binding of the viral envelope glycoprotein complex gp160 to its cellular receptor CD4. The gp160 complex consists of an external glycoprotein gp120 and a transmembrane glycoprotein gp41 that anchors gp120 to the enveloped virus. The gp120 binds with high affinity to cell surface CD4 molecules of the host cell. This binding induces conformational changes in gp120 so as to uncover a previously hidden site that is capable of binding to another host cell receptor. This second receptor (called a co-receptor, to distinguish it from the initial receptor CD4) is usually the chemokine receptor CCR5 or CXCR4.[232] Macrophage-tropic clinical isolates of HIV-1, which are found commonly early after infection, use CCR5; T-cell–tropic clinical isolates, which are sometimes seen after long-term HIV-1 infection and are capable of inducing syncytia, use CXCR4. Several small molecules that inhibit the binding of gp120 to either co-receptor are being investigated as potential antiretroviral drugs.

This second step in HIV-1 entry, co-receptor binding, causes further conformational changes in HIV-1 gp120. These changes allow exposure of the gp41 portion of the envelope glycoprotein, previously covered by gp120, and lead to the third step in HIV-1 entry, fusion of viral envelope to host cell membrane. Fusion is mediated by progressive conformational changes of gp41 that bring the viral and cellular envelopes together and allow entry of the viral core into the cellular cytoplasm. Fusion can be prevented by polypeptides that bind specifically to gp41 and inhibit the conformational changes necessary for fusion.

Enfuvirtide

Enfuvirtide (T-20) is a 36–amino-acid synthetic peptide that is administered as a subcutaneous injection (Table 124-4).[233] It appears to be similarly active against HIV-1 strains that use different co-receptors, but it has no activity against HIV-2. It has a bioavailability (compared with intravenous injection) of 84% and a half-life of 3.8 hours. It is metabolized most likely through catabolism to its constituent amino acids. Enfuvirtide is available as a powder in single-use vials, each containing 108 mg of the drug. It must be reconstituted with 1.1 mL of sterile water before injection of 1 mL of the solution to deliver 90 mg of enfuvirtide into the subcutaneous space of the abdomen, thigh, or arm. The dose of enfuvirtide is 90 mg every 12 hours.

Two large prospective, randomized trials examined the efficacy of enfuvirtide when added to an optimized salvage regimen in heavily antiretroviral-experienced patients.[234,235] At 24 weeks of therapy, the addition of enfuvirtide was associated with a significantly greater decrease in viral load compared with an optimized regimen that did not include enfuvirtide (1.70 versus 0.76 $\log_{10}$ copies/mL in one study, 1.43 versus 0.65 $\log_{10}$ copies/mL in the other). The mean increases in CD4+ T-cell counts were also greater in the enfuvirtide arms of these studies.

The most common adverse effects of enfuvirtide have been local injection site reactions, which have occurred in most patients. Reactions have included pain, induration, erythema, nodules, cysts, pruritus, and ecchymosis. In prospective studies, an increased rate of bacterial pneumonia was observed in patients receiving enfuvirtide. Hypersensitivity reactions, manifested as rash, fever, nausea, vomiting, chills, hypotension, elevated hepatic transaminase levels, or some combination of these, have also been noted rarely.

TABLE 124-4 Approved Entry Inhibitors						
Agent	Trade Name	Bioavailability (%)	Serum Half-Life (hr)	Elimination	Adult Dose*	Availability
Enfuvirtide	Fuzeon	84	3.8	Catabolism to constituent amino acids	90 mg SC q12h	108-mg single-use vials, for reconstitution with 1.1 mL sterile water

*For pediatric dose see Chapter 123.

After passage of virus in increasing concentrations of enfuvirtide in vitro, mutations in gp41codons 36-38 have been noted.[236] These mutations appear to confer decreased susceptibility to the drug in vitro. Mutations within and near that region have also been noted in HIV-1 from patients who received suboptimal dosing of enfuvirtide monotherapy.[237]

CLINICAL ISSUES

In untreated HIV-1 infection, ongoing viral replication leads to progressive damage to the immune system, ultimately resulting in opportunistic infections or neoplasms and death.[238] Although the rate of disease progression varies widely, exceptions to this principle are rare. The ultimate goals of antiretroviral therapy are to prevent and possibly reverse immunologic deterioration, avert opportunistic infections and other morbidity related to HIV-1 disease, and thereby prolong survival. Antiretroviral therapy itself is accompanied by risks for adverse effects and the possibility of virologic failure, viral drug resistance, and limitations of future therapeutic options. Therefore, before starting therapy, the risks and benefits of antiretroviral therapy need to be weighed carefully.[239-241]

Assays for Monitoring Infection

The widespread use of plasma HIV-1 RNA levels to monitor HIV-1 infection and antiretroviral therapy has transformed the clinical care of HIV-1–infected individuals. The level of HIV-1 RNA reflects the magnitude of viral replication. It correlates with the rate of CD4+ T-cell decline, the relative risk of clinical disease progression, and the time to death.[242-245] On antiretroviral therapy, the magnitude of the decrease in HIV-1 RNA levels is related to the relative risk of disease progression and death.[38,246-248] Baseline HIV-1 RNA levels should be checked before antiretroviral therapy is initiated to estimate the risk of progression and to guide subsequent therapy.[249] Ideally, this should be done when the patient is clinically stable, because HIV-1 RNA levels may be transiently elevated for several weeks after the initial HIV-1 infection, during an intercurrent illness, and for up to 1 month after an immunization. Two measurements separated by 1 to 4 weeks minimize the effects of technical and biologic variance that can cause HIV-1 RNA levels to vary by up to threefold ($0.5 \log_{10}$).[246]

With potent antiretroviral therapy capable of halting detectable viral replication, the viral load usually decreases by 1 to 2 $\log_{10}$ within 2 weeks of therapy and reaches a nadir by 12 weeks, although up to 16 to 24 weeks may be required to reach a nadir in situations in which initial plasma HIV-1 RNA levels are very high. After therapy is initiated or changed, it is prudent to check HIV-1 RNA levels at least monthly until the nadir is reached, and then at least every 3 to 4 months. A consistent increase in viral load of more than $0.5 \log_{10}$ suggests a failing antiretroviral regimen. If antiretroviral therapy is deferred, periodic HIV-1 RNA measurements are useful for monitoring progression of the infection; increases in HIV-1 RNA levels above baseline may herald a more rapid immunologic or clinical decline. For an individual patient, it is important to monitor HIV-1 RNA levels using the same assay each time, because different methods of quantifying viral RNA levels do not always give directly comparable values (see Chapter 115).

The CD4+ T-cell count reflects the extent of immune damage that has already occurred because of HIV-1 infection. CD4+ T-cell counts correlate with the risk of developing opportunistic infections or neoplasms and with the time to death. Baseline CD4+ T-cell counts should be obtained before antiretroviral therapy is initiated, to assess the prognosis and to guide the prophylactic therapy against opportunistic infections. Two measurements separated by 1 to 4 weeks reduce the effects of biologic and technical variance that may alter the cell counts by up to 30%.[250] After therapy is initiated, CD4+ T-cell count should be measured periodically, at least every 3 to 4 months, to monitor immunologic improvement. If antiretroviral therapy is deferred, CD4+

T-cell counts should be obtained regularly to monitor the progression of the disease and to institute appropriate prophylaxis against opportunistic infections.

Initiating Therapy

The decision to start antiretroviral therapy must be individualized, taking into account the relative risks and benefits of therapy. Guidelines for such decisions from the U.S. Department of Health and Human Services and from professional societies have recently been published.[239-241,251] The CD4+ T-cell count and the HIV-1 RNA level can serve as powerful predictors of disease progression and survival in untreated patients. For both measurements, there is a continuum of increasing risk of disease progression and death associated with decreasing CD4+ T-cell counts and increasing HIV-1 RNA levels. [241-244,252] Current understanding of the pathogenesis of AIDS suggests that therapy may be beneficial for patients with any detectable plasma HIV-1 RNA level regardless of the CD4+ T-cell count. Furthermore, higher CD4+ T-cell counts and lower plasma viral load are associated with an increased likelihood of control of viremia with the first antiretroviral regimen.[253-255] Therefore, initiation of therapy earlier in the disease course may be more likely to lead to durable suppression of viremia. However, because of the adverse effects associated with current antiretroviral therapy and the possibility of therapeutic failure with selection of drug-resistant viruses, the risks and benefits of antiretroviral therapy need to be assessed throughout the course of HIV-1 infection.

Antiretroviral therapy should be offered to HIV-1–infected individuals who have significantly decreased CD4+ T-cell counts (<350 cells/mm^3) or symptomatic disease, regardless of their plasma HIV-1 RNA levels. In contrast, untreated individuals with relatively preserved CD4+ T-cell counts (>350 cells/mm^3) and relatively low HIV-1 RNA levels (<50,000 copies/mL) appear to be at low risk for disease progression in the short run. For these individuals, and for any persons who choose to defer treatment, CD4+ T-cell counts and HIV-1 RNA levels should be monitored and the need to start therapy reassessed regularly. Plasma HIV-1 RNA values greater than 100,000 copies/mL also seem to be an adverse risk factor for progression and should prompt consideration of therapy.[252,256]

The potential benefit of antiretroviral therapy must be balanced against possible adverse effects as well as against the inconvenience of taking multiple drugs several times a day, often in a strict regimen around meals.[251] In that regard, the recent introduction of regimens that can be administered once or twice daily and have minimal food effects may improve adherence to therapy. Patients must be committed to antiretroviral therapy for an indefinite period in order to realize its full benefits. Given the potential for drug resistance and for extensive cross-resistance within a class of antiretrovirals, the haphazard use of these drugs may render current as well as later antiretroviral therapy ineffective. Therefore, deferral of antiretroviral therapy to a time when a patient is able to take medications consistently is preferable to use of suboptimal therapy. A thorough and informed discussion between the health care provider and the patient is essential for successful long-term therapy.

Drugs in a combination should be started simultaneously; the sequential addition of drugs over an extended period results in an increased risk of development of resistance. Close attention should be paid to dosing schedules. Adherence often requires extensive education and is enhanced by a continuing collaboration between the health care providers and the patient. If it is necessary to stop one drug temporarily, it is usually preferable to stop the entire combination, to avoid selection of resistance to the rest of the drugs in the regimen at a time when antiretroviral potency is suboptimal.

Once the decision to start antiretroviral therapy has been made, the aim of treatment should be the suppression of plasma HIV-1 RNA to below detectable limits of the most sensitive available HIV-1 RNA assay. Less profound suppression of viral replication may be associated with the evolution of resistant virus that will result in continuing immune system damage and may compromise current and future antiretroviral therapy options. Inability of a regimen to produce viral suppression to less than 50 copies/mL in the first 6 months of therapy has been associated with failure to control viremia at 1 year and at later time points.[257,258] Predictors of failures also include advanced immunodeficiency, high baseline viral load or low CD4+ T-cell count, prior antiretroviral therapy, poor virologic or immunologic response by 8 weeks of therapy, and nonadherence to a regimen.[23,199,202,253,254,259-261] If successful in suppressing viral replication completely, treatment with the full regimen should be continued indefinitely. Replication-competent virus can be isolated from individuals receiving combination therapy even if HIV-1 RNA levels have been undetectable (<50 copies/mL) for up to several years.[262,263]

Design of Combination Therapy

Several considerations are important in the design of combination regimens. First, the drugs in the combination should offer additive or synergistic antiviral activity. Such interactions have been documented for several commonly used combinations, including zidovudine with didanosine or lamivudine, stavudine with lamivudine, nucleoside analogue RT inhibitors with NNRTIs, and nucleoside analogue RT inhibitors with protease inhibitors.[22,264] However, some combinations, notably zidovudine and stavudine, can be antagonistic in vitro and may offer relatively poor efficacy when used together clinically.[22,26]

Second, pharmacokinetic interactions among the drugs in a combination may lead to clinically significant alterations in absorption or metabolism of the drugs. The buffered formulation of didanosine cannot be taken simultaneously with antiretrovirals that require an acidic environment for adequate absorption, such as delavirdine, indinavir, or atazanavir. Some antiretroviral agents (e.g., tenofovir, atazanavir) should ordinarily be taken with food to enhance absorption, whereas others (e.g., didanosine, indinavir) are best taken on an empty stomach, making for potentially complicated regimens with a combination of these drugs. Delavirdine and ritonavir increase plasma levels of certain protease inhibitors through the inhibition of hepatic metabolism. In contrast, nevirapine and efavirenz may increase the metabolism of several protease inhibitors and decrease their plasma level, necessitating increased dosage or ritonavir boosting if any of these protease inhibitors is used with either of these NNRTIs.

Third, different drugs may be able to target cells at different levels of activation or in different tissue reservoirs.[265] For example, because of different phosphorylation dynamics, didanosine, zalcitabine, and lamivudine are active in quiescent cells, whereas zidovudine and stavudine are more active in replicating cells.[6] Combinations that include one drug from each category may provide broader antiretroviral coverage, although this has not been demonstrated clinically. The central nervous system penetration of zidovudine, stavudine, and nevirapine is good, whereas that of didanosine, lamivudine, and delavirdine is relatively poor; for most protease inhibitors, the issue remains to be studied carefully. However, the relationship between the ratio of drug concentrations in cerebrospinal fluid and in plasma and antiretroviral activity within the central nervous system has not been established. The use of a combination regimen capable of suppressing HIV-1 replication in all body compartments may be necessary for long-term efficacy.

Fourth, care must be taken when combining drugs with overlapping toxicities. The use of didanosine and zalcitabine in combination increases the risk of peripheral neuropathy to unacceptable levels. Similarly, the use of stavudine and didanosine has been associated with increased adverse effects of pancreatitis and lactic acidosis. Whereas combination therapy offers the theoretical advantage that toxicity may be reduced if doses of individual drugs can be decreased, suboptimal dosing may promote the development of drug resistance.

Fifth, the likelihood of adherence to the regimen should be taken into account. A regimen involving multiple pills taken many times during the course of a day in association with a regimented meal schedule poses major challenges. A regimen involving few pills taken once or twice a day regardless of meals is far more likely to foster adherence.

Sixth, antiretroviral drugs should be combined with attention to the ability of HIV-1 to develop drug resistance to the individual components. Genotypic resistance may be expected to arise for any new antiretroviral regimen that incompletely inhibits viral replication.[92] Combination regimens that produce more potent inhibition of viral replication may delay or prevent resistance by limiting the opportunity for new mutations to occur or accumulate.[266] Regimens that are not expected to provide complete suppression of HIV-1 RNA should not contain agents for which high-level resistance develops rapidly, such as lamivudine or NNRTIs. In contrast, combinations should be designed to create significant hurdles for the evolution of viral resistance. For instance, a multidrug combination in which significant resistance to all drugs can arise with only one or two mutations may have less durable efficacy compared with an equipotent combination that requires many more mutations for the virus to escape from the suppression of replication. The possibility of preexisting virus resistant to one or more drugs must also be kept in mind, especially in patients with a prior history of antiretroviral therapy. A broader antiretroviral coverage, especially with agents that do not share cross-resistance patterns with previously experienced drugs, is more likely to produce lasting benefits. An antiretroviral agent may give rise to a specific resistance mutation that resensitizes a virus that was previously resistant to another drug used in the same combination. An example of this phenomenon is the lamivudine resistance mutation in RT codon 184; in a background of some NAMs, the mutation resensitizes the virus to zidovudine.[121] This may explain why the combination of zidovudine and lamivudine confers some long-term benefits, as measured by levels of HIV-1 RNA and CD4+ T-cell counts, in previously heavily zidovudine-treated patients despite the development of the mutation of RT codon 184. Finally, a choice in regimens should be made based in part on preserving future therapeutic options in case the initial combination fails. Once resistant virus arises in an infected individual, it may persist indefinitely, at least as a minority population. Therefore, choices for current and previous therapies significantly influence future therapeutic options.

Seventh, when choosing a regimen for a specific patient, consideration should be given to patient-specific factors that could affect selection of the regimen. These factors include the patient's predisposition to potential drug toxicity, interactions of antiretrovirals with other drugs used by the patient, and the patient's ability to adhere to the regimen. These issues are particularly relevant for patients with opportunistic infections or malignancies, who may require several other medications.

Clinical Experience with Combination Therapy

HIV-1 therapeutics has evolved rapidly from antiretroviral monotherapy to combination therapy—initially with two nucleoside analogue combinations, and later with three-drug regimens. Benefits have been most clearly demonstrated in antiretroviral-naive individuals. Currently, most patients on their initial antiretroviral regimen or first salvage regimen are taking a combination of two nucleoside analogue RT inhibitors with either a protease inhibitor or an NNRTI.

Nucleoside or Nucleotide Analogue Reverse Transcriptase Inhibitors

Several nucleoside combinations have been demonstrated to produce potent and durable benefits in combination with either a protease inhibitor or an NNRTI. Well-studied combinations include zidovudine with lamivudine,[23-25] stavudine with lamivudine,[51] tenofovir with lamivudine,[67] zidovudine with didanosine,[40] and didanosine with lamivudine.[68,267] Emtricitabine may substitute for lamivudine in these combinations, but experience with it is limited.[84,85] Comparative trials have demonstrated that the antiretroviral activities of several pairs of these combinations (e.g., zidovudine with lamivudine versus stavudine with lamivudine,[51] stavudine with lamivudine versus tenofovir with lamivudine[67]) appear to be similar, although the adverse effect and resistance profiles may differ. Trials have also found that some combinations are less effective than others. For example, zidovudine with lamivudine was found to have better overall efficacy than stavudine with didanosine, in part because of increased toxicity of the latter combination.[144]

Protease Inhibitors

Combinations of two nucleoside analogue RT inhibitors with a potent protease inhibitor (e.g., indinavir, ritonavir, nelfinavir, atazanavir, soft gel capsule formulation of saquinavir) have shown clinical efficacy or virologic activity, or both, in protease inhibitor–naive subjects without pharmacokinetic enhancement with low-dose ritonavir.[23,186,207,215] However, even in antiretroviral-naive patients, lopinavir/ritonavir had greater efficacy, in terms of more potent and durable virologic suppression, than did unboosted nelfinavir.[208] In protease inhibitor–experienced subjects, a regimen containing either a ritonavir-boosted protease inhibitor or dual protease inhibitors may be necessary to suppress plasma HIV-1 RNA optimally.[212,216]

Non-nucleoside Reverse Transcriptase Inhibitors

Combinations of two nucleoside RT inhibitors with an NNRTI may produce viral suppression and immunologic improvements that are equivalent to those seen in combinations that include protease inhibitors. Immunologic and virologic benefits of a combination of nevirapine, zidovudine, and didanosine in antiretroviral-naive individuals were not substantially inferior to those observed with protease inhibitor–containing regimens.[40] Efavirenz has been more clearly demonstrated to have efficacy at least equivalent to that of several protease inhibitors. The combination of efavirenz with zidovudine and lamivudine in antiretroviral-naive patients provided greater viral load suppression at 48 weeks of therapy than did the combination of indinavir, zidovudine, and lamivudine.[24] Studies have also demonstrated efavirenz's superior efficacy compared with nelfinavir when combined with zidovudine and lamivudine.[25,143]

Few direct comparisons of NNRTIs are available. In the largest trial to compare two NNRTIs, the virologic success rate of nevirapine in combination with stavudine and lamivudine in antiretroviral-naive subjects was 56% at week 48, compared with 62% for a regimen of efavirenz, stavudine, and lamivudine.[138]

Other Therapeutic Regimens

Initial studies of regimens that contain only nucleoside or nucleotide RT inhibitors appeared promising, particularly for abacavir, zidovudine, and lamivudine in antiretroviral-naive patients whose plasma HIV-1 RNA levels were less than 100,000 copies/mL.[71] More recent direct comparisons of this regimen with efavirenz, zidovudine, and lamivudine demonstrated that its potency and durability were inferior to those of the efavirenz-based regimen.[72] Another protease inhibitor– and NNRTI-sparing regimen, consisting of abacavir, tenofovir, and lamivudine, also appeared to have poorer efficacy than expected.[73] Currently, regimens without either protease inhibitors or NNRTIs cannot be recommended as first-line therapy.[241]

Other combinations, such as ones containing two protease inhibitors or ones that include both a protease inhibitor and an NNRTI, are less well studied and cannot be recommended currently. However, combinations of two protease inhibitors, with or without nucleoside analogue RT inhibitors, have resulted in potent and durable viral suppression, as demonstrated by saquinavir with ritonavir or by amprenavir with other protease inhibitors.[189,211] Combinations that include a protease inhibitor and an NNRTI can similarly show potent viral suppression, as demonstrated by efavirenz with ritonavir-boosted or unboosted protease inhibitors.[147-149,212]

Predictors of Success

The patient's history of antiretroviral drug experience has a large impact on the likelihood of success of a given combination regimen.

For example, although the combination of didanosine and zidovudine decreased the rate of disease progression or death compared with zidovudine alone in zidovudine-experienced adults, the clinical benefits were less than those observed in zidovudine-naive subjects.[35,37] Similar observations can be made for three-drug combinations. Although the addition of ritonavir to a stable regimen of nucleoside analogue RT inhibitors in heavily nucleoside analogue–experienced individuals with advanced HIV disease significantly reduced the rate of clinical progression and death in the first year of therapy, the decrease in viral load at 1 year of therapy was only 0.6 log$_{10}$, far less than that usually observed in antiretroviral-naive individuals receiving combination therapy.[194] In individuals with advanced disease and considerable prior exposure to nucleoside analogue RT inhibitors, the combination of nevirapine with zidovudine and didanosine, although better than zidovudine with didanosine alone, produced only a transient benefit in viral suppression, in contrast to durable benefits obtained in antiretroviral-naive individuals.[40,137] Even short periods (<2 months) of suboptimal nucleoside RT inhibitor therapy may increase the risk of virologic failure of a new combination antiretroviral regimen.[268]

In addition to the history of antiretroviral drug use, other baseline factors are predictive of antiretroviral therapy failure. These include advanced immunodeficiency, high baseline viral load, and low baseline CD4+ T-cell count.[23,199,202,253,254] Virologic responses during the early phase of therapy are also predictive of long-term success. Poor virologic response by 8 weeks of therapy (and possibly as early as 1 week of therapy) is associated with poor long-term virologic control.[260,261] Inability of a regimen to produce viral suppression to less than 50 copies/mL in the first 6 months of therapy is also associated with failure to control viremia at 1 year and at later time points.[257,258]

Some general principles can be deduced from these trials. First, the long-term efficacy of a regimen is related to the overall potency of the combination. Combinations that produce a greater nadir in viral load are more likely to have durable benefits. Second, the antiviral potency of a combination is not related simply to the type or number of drugs in the combination, but to how they are combined. Third, the most impressive benefits from a particular combination are usually seen in individuals who are antiretroviral naive and in those who have higher CD4+ T-cell counts. Fourth, in antiretroviral-experienced individuals, the results of addition of a single drug to a failing regimen are inferior to those obtained with a change to a regimen with at least two new drugs to which cross-resistance is unlikely.

Changing Therapy

Clinical assessment of the patient along with the HIV-1 RNA levels and CD4+ T-cell counts should be used to assess the need to change therapy.[239,241] If the patient experiences drug toxicity or intolerance or is unable to adhere to therapy, a change in therapy is required. In these situations, it may be appropriate simply to replace the offending drug by another that is better tolerated and exhibits similar potency in the combination. For instance, if an effective protease inhibitor regimen is associated with clinically significant lipid abnormalities, switching the protease inhibitor to either nevirapine or efavirenz may cause an improvement in the lipid profiles without compromising virologic efficacy.[269]

A change in therapy should also be contemplated if a patient is receiving suboptimal therapy, such as monotherapy with any antiretroviral agent or a combination of two or three nucleoside analogue RT inhibitors, because these regimens are associated with a high risk of failure to suppress viral replication.[72,73] If the patient has undetectable HIV-1 RNA with these regimens, an option is simply to add other drugs to form a regimen that is more likely to produce long-term viral suppression.

The plasma HIV-1 RNA level is the most sensitive indicator of viral replication, and a persistently detectable level during therapy indicates suboptimal control of viral infection. If viral RNA levels are elevated due to immunization or intercurrent infection, they should return to baseline within 2 to 4 weeks after immunization or recovery from the illness. The HIV-1 RNA level may also be high secondary to incomplete adherence to the drug regimen, decreased absorption of drugs, or altered metabolism. Addressing the cause of the elevation in these cases may return the viral load to undetectable levels without necessarily changing the drug regimen.

Clinical situations that should prompt consideration for changing therapy include (1) a poor early virologic response to therapy, defined as a decrease in viral RNA of less than 1.0 log$_{10}$ by 2 months of therapy; (2) failure to suppress plasma HIV-1 RNA to undetectable levels by 4 to 6 months after starting therapy; (3) repeated detection of virus in plasma after initial suppression to undetectable levels, suggesting the development of resistance; (4) a reproducible and significant increase ($\geq$0.5 log$_{10}$ or threefold) in viral RNA levels from the nadir, not secondary to a self-limited or correctable cause; (5) a persistent and significant decline in the CD4$^+$ T-cell count; (6) clinical deterioration while on a stable regimen.[239,240] Although it may be ideal to change therapy for any persistently detectable HIV-1 RNA level, this suggestion is tempered by the frequent limitations on remaining treatment options, especially in the heavily pretreated patient. Nevertheless, the consideration for change is more urgent with higher rebound in plasma HIV-1 RNA levels.

When considering changing therapy, an assessment of the likelihood of resistance to each previously used drug should be made, because this may limit the use of drugs that share cross-resistance patterns. Assays are available for determining genotypic resistance (by assessing the presence of mutations associated with resistance to specific drugs) or phenotypic susceptibility (by testing the isolate's susceptibility in vitro to different drugs).[88,270] Several retrospective studies have suggested that response to salvage therapy is influenced by baseline susceptibility of the virus to the drugs in the salvage regimen.[271] Prospective clinical trials assessing the utility of HIV-1 drug-resistance testing have shown significant but modest improvements in virologic outcomes with genotypic assays.[271] A major difficulty with genotypic assays is the interpretation of often complex combinations of resistance mutations. One study demonstrated that the provision of expert advice to aid the interpretation of genotypic resistance test results further increased the likelihood of virologic suppression beyond that provided by obtaining a genotypic resistance assay without expert consultation.[272] Some, but not all, trials of phenotypic resistance testing have demonstrated improved virologic outcomes. A major problem with interpreting phenotypic resistance assays is that the IC$_{50}$ increases that are clinically significant in limiting virologic response are often unknown, although this is an area of active research. Resistance testing is currently recommended for patients who have virologic failure or who do not respond to an antiretroviral regimen, in cases of recent acquisition of HIV-1 infection (because the prevalence of transmission of drug-resistant HIV-1 appears to be increasing[273]), and for pregnant women with detectable plasma HIV-1 RNA.[88]

There are few clinical data to guide changes in therapy in individuals with failing multidrug regimens.[239-241] A failing regimen of two nucleoside analogues and an NNRTI may be replaced by two new nucleoside analogues and a protease inhibitor, or by a combination of two protease inhibitors with one or two new nucleoside analogues. Alternatives for a failing regimen of two nucleoside analogues and a protease inhibitor depend in part on the particular protease inhibitor in the failing combination and its pattern of cross-resistance. Salvage regimens are often complicated and are evolving at a rapid pace. Consultation with a physician who is experienced with antiretroviral therapy should be considered.

The aim of treatment after changing therapy should still be to suppress the plasma HIV-1 RNA levels to below detectable limits of the most sensitive available HIV-1 RNA assay. If complete suppression of viral replication cannot be attained with any regimen, the goal should be modified to attaining as low a plasma HIV-1 RNA level as possible for as long as possible. Minimizing viral replication is likely to slow further immune deterioration. There is a continuum of increasing clinical benefits (in terms of disease progression and survival) with decreasing HIV-1 RNA levels, and regimens that produce

only a 0.6 log$_{10}$ mean decrease in HIV-1 RNA levels still can result in lower rates of clinical progression and death.[194] Furthermore, even though stopping therapy in patients with multiple-drug–resistant virus caused the predominant viral population to change genotype and revert to wild type, there was a sharp increase in viral load and a significant decrease in the CD4$^+$ T-cell count soon after cessation of therapy in most patients.[274]

SPECIAL CIRCUMSTANCES

Postexposure Prophylaxis

Certain occupational exposures to HIV-1 may lead to infection. Blood, tissue, semen, vaginal secretions, cerebrospinal fluid, serosal fluids, amniotic fluid, any bodily fluids contaminated with visible blood from infected individuals, and concentrated HIV-1 in a laboratory are potential sources of infectious virus, whereas sweat, tears, and nonbloody saliva, urine, and feces are unlikely to cause occupational transmission[275] (also see Chapter 304). The average risk for percutaneous exposure to blood from an infected person is estimated to be 0.2% to 0.5%, whereas mucous membrane exposure carries a risk of approximately 0.1% and exposure through intact skin carries a negligible risk in the majority of situations.[275] However, several factors relating to the viral inoculum alter the actual risk in specific cases.[276] For instance, if the source patient has advanced AIDS and a high level of plasma HIV-1 RNA, the risks are likely to be substantially higher. Similarly, exposure to a large volume of infected fluid can also increase the risk, as noted for deep penetrating injuries, for injuries caused by a sharp device covered with visible blood, or for injuries caused by needles used to enter a blood vessel of the source patient.

A case-control study demonstrated that the administration of zidovudine in the immediate postoccupational exposure period decreased the odds of transmission by approximately 80%.[276] The ability of combination therapy to suppress viral replication better than monotherapy has prompted consideration of its use in postexposure prophylaxis. Furthermore, concern over the presence and transmissibility of virus resistant to zidovudine or other antiretroviral agents argues for both broader coverage and flexibility in designing the prophylaxis regimen. However, data on the efficacy of prophylaxis with a multidrug regimen are lacking. The fact that an average of more than 99.5% of occupational exposures to HIV-1–containing blood do not result in transmission of the virus suggests the need to use agents with minimal toxicity and high tolerability.

Guidelines on the use of chemoprophylaxis after occupational exposures have been published (see Chapter 304).[277-280] For each case of exposure, both the source and the patient should be assessed for the presence of HIV-1 infection before the incident and for the likelihood of a high plasma HIV-1 RNA level and drug resistance in any source known to have HIV-1 infection. The basic prophylaxis regimen is a combination of two nucleoside analogue RT inhibitors with or without a potent protease inhibitor. If drug resistance in the source patient is a concern, alternative antiretroviral regimens should be considered. Chemoprophylaxis should be initiated as soon as possible, preferably within a few hours after the incident, because its efficacy is expected to wane with time. The optimal duration of chemoprophylaxis is unknown, although current guidelines recommend 4 weeks of therapy. Exposed individuals should be monitored with antibody testing for HIV-1 infection at baseline and at 6 weeks, 12 weeks, and 6 months after exposure.

The evidence that antiretroviral treatment can decrease the rate of HIV-1 transmission in occupational exposure has led to its consideration for individuals with recent sexual exposures to HIV-1.[281-283] There are very limited data on the efficacy of this intervention or on the optimal drug regimen or timing of therapy.[284] Situations should be assessed individually for the risk of transmission and for the potential risks and benefits of prophylaxis with an antiretroviral regimen. Like occupational chemoprophylaxis, prophylaxis with two nucleoside analogue RT inhibitors, with or without a protease inhibitor, for 4 weeks may be considered in specific situations in which there is a significant risk of transmission.

Acute HIV-1 Infection

Although acute infection with HIV-1 mimics several viral syndromes, it can be diagnosed by the detection of an elevated plasma concentration of HIV-1 RNA in the context of a negative or indeterminate HIV-1 antibody test (see Chapter 115).[285] Several unique considerations favor treatment during this phase of infection. Treatment may limit the extent of viral dissemination throughout the body, possibly into compartments that may be difficult to treat during chronic infection. In addition, early treatment may limit the likelihood of transmission to others, because some of the highest virus titers in genital secretions are observed during primary infection syndromes. Treatment may also attenuate the progress of HIV-1 disease, both acutely and later by producing a lower plasma viral RNA setpoint. Early treatment may also limit the extent of viral genetic variability that accumulates with time and that may allow resistance to drugs to occur readily. It may also allow salvage of a CD4+ T cell–specific immune response, which may be important in the immune control of HIV-1 infection.[286,287]

There are, however, no controlled studies to show a long-range benefit of early therapy for primary HIV-1 syndromes. Furthermore, it is unclear whether therapy, once started, must continue indefinitely or can be discontinued after a finite period (e.g., 1 year). The principles of therapy in acute infection are similar to those for chronic infection, and studies are underway to determine the value of treatment interruptions after varying durations of antiretroviral therapy.

FUTURE DIRECTIONS

Several novel nucleoside and non-nucleoside analogue RT inhibitors, protease inhibitors, and entry inhibitors are under development.[3,231] New compounds that inhibit the binding of HIV-1 to co-receptors or inhibit fusion have been developed and have been shown to have antiviral activity in vivo.[288-290] Entry inhibitors may be particularly useful against HIV-1 strains that are resistant to RT and protease inhibitors. Furthermore, entry inhibitors that target different steps of entry (e.g., co-receptor binding inhibitors and fusion inhibitors) may demonstrate synergistic antiviral activity in vitro,[291,292] suggesting that combination antiretroviral therapy conceivably could include several entry inhibitors, each targeting different steps of entry.

The HIV-1 integrase enzyme is crucial for HIV-1 proviral DNA integration into the host genome and for the establishment of infection. Integrase inhibitors are expected to inhibit viral replication, and several candidate agents are in clinical development.[293] The viral nucleocapsid protein is important for RNA encapsidation and virus maturation and may also serve as a promising target for therapy. A recently described compound appears to specifically inhibit gag cleavage and viral maturation and is reported to have good antiviral activity in vitro.[294]

REFERENCES

1. Greene WC. The molecular biology of human immunodeficiency virus type 1 infection. N Engl J Med. 1991;324:308-317.
2. Greene WC, Peterlin BM. Charting HIV's remarkable voyage through the cell: Basic science as a passport to future therapy. Nat Med. 2002;8:673-680.
3. D'Souza MP, Cairns JS, Plaeger SF. Current evidence and future directions for targeting HIV entry: Therapeutic and prophylactic strategies. JAMA. 2000;284:215-222.
4. Goff SP. Retroviral reverse transcriptase: Synthesis, structure, and function. J Acquir Immune Defic Syndr. 1990;3:817-831.
5. Yarchoan R, Mitsuya H, Myers CE, Broder S. Clinical pharmacology of 3'-azido-2',3'-dideoxythymidine (zidovudine) and related dideoxynucleosides [published erratum appears in N Engl J Med. 1990 Jan 25;322(4):280]. N Engl J Med. 1989;321:726-738.
6. Gao WY, Shirasaka T, Johns DG, et al. Differential phosphorylation of azidothymidine, dideoxycytidine, and dideoxyinosine in resting and activated peripheral blood mononuclear cells. J Clin Invest. 1993;91:2326-2333.
7. Palmer S, Alaeus A, Albert J, Cox S. Drug susceptibility of subtypes A,B,C,D, and E human immunodeficiency virus type 1 primary isolates. AIDS Res Hum Retroviruses. 1998;14:157-162.
8. Lonergan JT, Behling C, Pfander H, et al. Hyperlactatemia and hepatic abnormalities in 10 human immunodeficiency virus-infected patients receiving nucleoside analogue combination regimens. Clin Infect Dis. 2000;31:162-166.
9. Carr A. Lactic acidemia in infection with human immunodeficiency virus. Clin Infect Dis. 2003;36:S96-S100.
10. Cui L, Schinazi RF, Gosselin G, et al. Effect of beta-enantiomeric and racemic nucleoside analogues on mitochondrial functions in HepG2 cells: Implications for predicting drug hepatotoxicity. Biochem Pharmacol. 1996;52:1577-1584.
11. Birkus G, Hitchcock MJ, Cihlar T. Assessment of mitochondrial toxicity in human cells treated with tenofovir: Comparison with other nucleoside reverse transcriptase inhibitors. Antimicrob Agents Chemother. 2002;46:716-723.
12. Bonnet F, Bonarek M, Morlat P, et al. Risk factors for lactic acidosis in HIV-infected patients treated with nucleoside reverse-transcriptase inhibitors: A case-control study. Clin Infect Dis. 2003;36:1324-1328.
13. Connolly KJ, Hammer SM. Antiretroviral therapy: Reverse transcriptase inhibition. Antimicrob Agents Chemother. 1992;36:245-254.
14. Fischl MA, Richman DD, Grieco MH, et al. The efficacy of azidothymidine (AZT) in the treatment of patients with AIDS and AIDS-related complex: A double-blind, placebo-controlled trial. N Engl J Med. 1987;317:185-191.
15. Fischl MA, Richman DD, Causey DM, et al. Prolonged zidovudine therapy in patients with AIDS and advanced AIDS-related complex. AZT Collaborative Working Group. JAMA. 1989;262:2405-2410.
16. Volberding PA, Lagakos SW, Koch MA, et al. Zidovudine in asymptomatic human immunodeficiency virus infection: A controlled trial in persons with fewer than 500 CD4-positive cells per cubic millimeter. The AIDS Clinical Trials Group of the National Institute of Allergy and Infectious Diseases. N Engl J Med. 1990;322:941-949.
17. Volberding PA, Lagakos SW, Grimes JM, et al. The duration of zidovudine benefit in persons with asymptomatic HIV infection: Prolonged evaluation of protocol 019 of the AIDS Clinical Trials Group. JAMA. 1994;272:437-442.
18. Concorde: MRC/ANRS randomised double-blind controlled trial of immediate and deferred zidovudine in symptom-free HIV infection. Concorde Coordinating Committee. Lancet. 1994;343:871-881.
19. Ruane PJ, Richmond GJ, DeJesus E, et al. Pharmacodynamic effects of zidovudine 600 mg once/day versus 300 mg twice/day in therapy-naive patients infected with human immunodeficiency virus. Pharmacotherapy 2004;24:307-312.
20. Johnson VA, Merrill DP, Videler JA, et al. Two-drug combinations of zidovudine, didanosine, and recombinant interferon-alpha A inhibit replication of zidovudine-resistant human immunodeficiency virus type 1 synergistically in vitro. J Infect Dis. 1991;164:646-655.
21. Johnson VA, Merrill DP, Chou TC, Hirsch MS. Human immunodeficiency virus type 1 (HIV-1) inhibitory interactions between protease inhibitor Ro 31-8959 and zidovudine, 2',3'-dideoxycytidine, or recombinant interferon-alpha A against zidovudine-sensitive or -resistant HIV-1 in vitro. J Infect Dis. 1992;166:1143-1146.
22. Merrill DP, Moonis M, Chou TC, Hirsch MS. Lamivudine or stavudine in two- and three-drug combinations against human immunodeficiency virus type 1 replication in vitro. J Infect Dis. 1996;173:355-364.
23. Hammer SM, Squires KE, Hughes MD, et al. A controlled trial of two nucleoside analogues plus indinavir in persons with human immunodeficiency virus infection and CD4 cell counts of 200 per cubic millimeter or less. AIDS Clinical Trials Group 320 Study Team. N Engl J Med. 1997;337:725-733.
24. Staszewski S, Morales-Ramirez J, Tashima KT, et al. Efavirenz plus zidovudine and lamivudine, efavirenz plus indinavir, and indinavir plus zidovudine and lamivudine in the treatment of HIV-1 infection in adults. Study 006 Team. N Engl J Med. 1999;341:1865-1873.
25. Robbins GK, De Gruttola V, Shafer RW, et al. Comparison of sequential three-drug regimens as initial therapy for HIV-1 infection. N Engl J Med. 2003;349:2293-2303.
26. Havlir DV, Tierney C, Friedland GH, et al. In vivo antagonism with zidovudine plus stavudine combination therapy. J Infect Dis. 2000;182:321-325.
27. Fischl MA, Parker CB, Pettinelli C, et al. A randomized controlled trial of a reduced daily dose of zidovudine in patients with the acquired immunodeficiency syndrome. The AIDS Clinical Trials Group. N Engl J Med. 1990;323:1009-1014.
28. Richman DD, Fischl MA, Grieco MH, et al. The toxicity of azidothymidine (AZT) in the treatment of patients with AIDS and AIDS-related complex: A double-blind, placebo-controlled trial. N Engl J Med. 1987;317:192-197.
29. Dalakas MC, Illa I, Pezeshkpour GH, et al. Mitochondrial myopathy caused by long-term zidovudine therapy N Engl J Med. 1990;322:1098-1105.
30. Kaul S, Damle B, Bassi K, et al. Pharmacokinetic evaluation of reduced doses of didanosine enteric coated capsules (ddI-EC) in combination with tenofovir disoproxil fumarate (TDF) and food for a once-daily antiretroviral regimen (Abstract 8.1). In: Fourth International Workshop on Clinical Pharmacology of HIV Therapy, Cannes, France, March 27-29, 2003.
31. Kahn JO, Lagakos SW, Richman DD, et al. A controlled trial comparing continued zidovudine with didanosine in human immunodeficiency virus infection. The NIAID AIDS Clinical Trials Group. N Engl J Med. 1992;327:581-587.
32. Spruance SL, Pavia AT, Peterson D, et al. Didanosine compared with continuation of zidovudine in HIV-infected patients with signs of clinical deterioration while receiving zidovudine: A randomized, double-blind clinical trial. The Bristol-Myers Squibb AI454-010 Study Group. Ann Intern Med. 1994;120:360-368.
33. Montaner JS, Schechter MT, Rachlis A, et al. Didanosine compared with continued zidovudine therapy for HIV-infected patients with 200 to 500 CD4 cells/mm³: A double-blind, randomized, controlled trial. Canadian HIV Trials Network Protocol 002 Study Group. Ann Intern Med. 1995;123:561-571.

34. Dolin R, Amato DA, Fischl MA, et al. Zidovudine compared with didanosine in patients with advanced HIV type 1 infection and little or no previous experience with zidovudine. AIDS Clinical Trials Group. [Published erratum appears in Arch Intern Med. 1995;155:2255.] Arch Intern Med. 1995;155:961-974.

35. Hammer SM, Katzenstein DA, Hughes MD, et al. A trial comparing nucleoside monotherapy with combination therapy in HIV-infected adults with CD4 cell counts from 200 to 500 per cubic millimeter. AIDS Clinical Trials Group Study 175 Study Team. N Engl J Med. 1996;335:1081-1090.

36. Collier AC, Coombs RW, Fischl MA, et al. Combination therapy with zidovudine and didanosine compared with zidovudine alone in HIV-1 infection. Ann Intern Med. 1993;119:786-793.

37. Delta: A randomised double-blind controlled trial comparing combinations of zidovudine plus didanosine or zalcitabine with zidovudine alone in HIV-infected individuals. Delta Coordinating Committee. [Published erratum appears in Lancet. 1996;348:834.] Lancet. 1996;348:283-291.

38. Katzenstein DA, Hammer SM, Hughes MD, et al. The relation of virologic and immunologic markers to clinical outcomes after nucleoside therapy in HIV-infected adults with 200 to 500 CD4 cells per cubic millimeter. AIDS Clinical Trials Group Study 175 Virology Study Team. [Published erratum appears in N Engl J Med. 1997;337:1097.] N Engl J Med. 1996;335:1091-1098.

39. Saravolatz LD, Winslow DL, Collins G, et al. Zidovudine alone or in combination with didanosine or zalcitabine in HIV-infected patients with the acquired immunodeficiency syndrome or fewer than 200 CD4 cells per cubic millimeter. Investigators for the Terry Beirn Community Programs for Clinical Research on AIDS. N Engl J Med. 1996;335:1099-1106.

40. Montaner JS, Reiss P, Cooper D, et al. A randomized, double-blind trial comparing combinations of nevirapine, didanosine, and zidovudine for HIV-infected patients: The INCAS Trial (Italy, The Netherlands, Canada and Australia Study). JAMA. 1998;279:930-937.

41. Molina JM, Ferchal F, Rancinan C, et al. Once-daily combination therapy with emtricitabine, didanosine, and efavirenz in human immunodeficiency virus-infected patients. J Infect Dis. 2000;182:599-602.

42. Yarchoan R, Pluda JM, Thomas RV, et al. Long-term toxicity/activity profile of 2′,3′-dideoxyinosine in AIDS or AIDS-related complex. Lancet. 1990;336:526-529.

43. Fischl MA, Olson RM, Follansbee SE, et al. Zalcitabine compared with zidovudine in patients with advanced HIV-1 infection who received previous zidovudine therapy. Ann Intern Med. 1993;118:762-769.

44. Fischl MA, Stanley K, Collier AC, et al. Combination and monotherapy with zidovudine and zalcitabine in patients with advanced HIV disease. The NIAID AIDS Clinical Trials Group. Ann Intern Med. 1995;122:24-32.

45. Abrams DI, Goldman AI, Launer C, et al. A comparative trial of didanosine or zalcitabine after treatment with zidovudine in patients with human immunodeficiency virus infection. The Terry Beirn Community Programs for Clinical Research on AIDS. N Engl J Med. 1994;330:657-662.

46. Dudley MN, Graham KK, Kaul S, et al. Pharmacokinetics of stavudine in patients with AIDS or AIDS-related complex. J Infect Dis. 1992;166:480-485.

47. Grasela DM, Stoltz RR, Barry M, et al. Pharmacokinetics of single-dose oral stavudine in subjects with renal impairment and in subjects requiring hemodialysis. Antimicrob Agents Chemother. 2000;44:2149-2153.

48. Schaad HJ, Petty BG, Grasela DM, et al. Pharmacokinetics and safety of a single dose of stavudine (d4T) in patients with severe hepatic impairment. Antimicrob Agents Chemother. 1997;41:2793-2796.

49. Spruance SL, Pavia AT, Mellors JW, et al. Clinical efficacy of monotherapy with stavudine compared with zidovudine in HIV-infected, zidovudine-experienced patients: A randomized, double-blind, controlled trial. Bristol-Myers Squibb Stavudine/019 Study Group. Ann Intern Med. 1997;126:355-363.

50. Foudraine NA, de Jong JJ, Jan Weverling G, et al. An open randomized controlled trial of zidovudine plus lamivudine versus stavudine plus lamivudine. AIDS. 1998;12:1513-1519.

51. Joly V, Flandre P, Meiffredy V, et al. Efficacy of zidovudine compared to stavudine, both in combination with lamivudine and indinavir, in human immunodeficiency virus-infected nucleoside-experienced patients with no prior exposure to lamivudine, stavudine, or protease inhibitors (Novavir Trial). The Novavir Study Group. Antimicrob Agents Chemother. 2002;46:1906-1913.

52. Browne MJ, Mayer KH, Chafee SB, et al. 2′,3′-didehydro-3′-deoxythymidine (d4T) in patients with AIDS or AIDS-related complex: A phase I trial. J Infect Dis. 1993;167:21-29.

53. Mokrzycki MH, Harris C, May H, et al. Lactic acidosis associated with stavudine administration: A report of five cases. Clin Infect Dis. 2000;30:198-200.

54. Miller KD, Cameron M, Wood LV, et al. Lactic acidosis and hepatic steatosis associated with use of stavudine: Report of four cases. Ann Intern Med. 2000;133:192-196.

55. Boubaker K, Flepp M, Sudre P, et al. Hyperlactatemia and antiretroviral therapy: The Swiss HIV Cohort Study. Clin Infect Dis. 2001;33:1931-1937.

56. Joly V, Flandre P, Meiffredy V, et al. Increased risk of lipoatrophy under stavudine in HIV-1-infected patients: Results of a substudy from a comparative trial. AIDS. 2002;16:2447-2454.

57. Martin GJ, Blazes DL, Mayers DL, Spooner KM. Stavudine-induced macrocytosis during therapy for human immunodeficiency virus infection. Clin Infect Dis. 1999;29:459-460.

58. van Leeuwen R, Lange JM, Hussey EK, et al. The safety and pharmacokinetics of a reverse transcriptase inhibitor, 3TC, in patients with HIV infection: A phase I study. AIDS. 1992;6:1471-1475.

59. Schuurman R, Nijhuis M, van Leeuwen R, et al. Rapid changes in human immunodeficiency virus type 1 RNA load and appearance of drug-resistant virus populations in persons treated with lamivudine (3TC). J Infect Dis. 1995;171:1411-1419.

60. Eron JJ, Benoit SL, Jemsek J, et al. Treatment with lamivudine, zidovudine, or both in HIV-positive patients with 200 to 500 CD4+ cells per cubic millimeter. North American HIV Working Party. N Engl J Med. 1995;333:1662-1669.

61. Katlama C, Ingrand D, Loveday C, et al. Safety and efficacy of lamivudine-zidovudine combination therapy in antiretroviral-naive patients: A randomized controlled comparison with zidovudine monotherapy. Lamivudine European HIV Working Group. JAMA. 1996;276:118-125.

62. Staszewski S, Loveday C, Picazo JJ, et al. Safety and efficacy of lamivudine-zidovudine combination therapy in zidovudine-experienced patients: A randomized controlled comparison with zidovudine monotherapy. Lamivudine European HIV Working Group. JAMA. 1996;276:111-117.

63. Bartlett JA, Benoit SL, Johnson VA, et al. Lamivudine plus zidovudine compared with zalcitabine plus zidovudine in patients with HIV infection: A randomized, double-blind, placebo-controlled trial. North American HIV Working Party. Ann Intern Med. 1996;125:161-172.

64. Randomised trial of addition of lamivudine or lamivudine plus loviride to zidovudine-containing regimens for patients with HIV-1 infection: The CAESAR trial. Lancet. 1997;349:1413-1421.

65. Kuritzkes DR, Marschner I, Johnson VA, et al. Lamivudine in combination with zidovudine, stavudine, or didanosine in patients with HIV-1 infection: A randomized, double-blind, placebo-controlled trial. National Institute of Allergy and Infectious Disease AIDS Clinical Trials Group Protocol 306 Investigators. AIDS. 1999;13:685-694.

66. Katlama C, Valantin MA, Matheron S, et al. Efficacy and tolerability of stavudine plus lamivudine in treatment-naive and treatment-experienced patients with HIV-1 infection. Ann Intern Med. 1998;129:525-531.

67. Staszewski S, Gallant JE, Pozniak AL, et al. Favourable metabolic profile for tenofovir disoproxil fumarate (TDF) versus stavudine (d4T) when used in combination with lamivudine and efavirenz in antiretroviral naive patients: 96-Week interim results (Abstract 562). Antiviral Ther. 2003;8:S336.

68. de Mendoza C, Soriano V, Perez-Olmeda M, et al. Efficacy and safety of didanosine and lamivudine both once daily plus indinavir in human immunodeficiency virus-infected patients. J Hum Virol. 2000;3:335-340.

69. Saag MS, Sonnerborg A, Torres RA, et al. Antiretroviral effect and safety of abacavir alone and in combination with zidovudine in HIV-infected adults. Abacavir Phase 2 Clinical Team. AIDS. 1998;12:F203-F209.

70. Staszewski S, Katlama C, Harrer T, et al. A dose-ranging study to evaluate the safety and efficacy of abacavir alone or in combination with zidovudine and lamivudine in antiretroviral treatment-naive subjects. AIDS. 1998;12:F197-F202.

71. Staszewski S, Keiser P, Montaner J, et al. Abacavir-lamivudine-zidovudine vs indinavir-lamivudine-zidovudine in antiretroviral-naive HIV-infected adults: A randomized equivalence trial. CNAAB3005 International Study Team. JAMA. 2001;285:1155-1163.

72. Gulick RM, Ribaudo HJ, Shikuma CM, et al. Triple-nucleoside regimens versus efavirenz-containing regimens for the initial treatment of HIV-1 infection. N Engl J Med 2004;350:1850-1861.

73. Farthing C, Khanlou H, Yeh V. Early virologic failure in a pilot study evaluating the efficacy of abacavir, lamivudine and tenofovir in the treatment naive HIV-infected patients (Abstract 43). Antiviral Ther. 2003;8:S195.

74. Kessler HA, Johnson J, Follansbee S, et al. Abacavir expanded access program for adult patients infected with human immunodeficiency virus type 1. Clin Infect Dis. 2002;34:535-542.

75. Barditch-Crovo P, Deeks SG, Collier A, et al. Phase I/II trial of the pharmacokinetics, safety, and antiretroviral activity of tenofovir disoproxil fumarate in human immunodeficiency virus-infected adults. Antimicrob Agents Chemother. 2001;45:2733-2739.

76. Fung HB, Stone EA, Piacenti FJ. Tenofovir disoproxil fumarate: A nucleotide reverse transcriptase inhibitor for the treatment of HIV infection. Clin Ther. 2002;24:1515-1548.

77. Kaul S, Bassi K, Damle B, et al. Pharmacokinetic (PK) evaluation of the combination of atazanavir (ATV), enteric coated didanosine (ddI-EC), and tenofovir disoproxil fumarate (TDF) for a once-daily antiretroviral regimen (Abstract A-1616). In: Program and Abstracts of the 43d Interscience Conference on Antimicrobial Agents and Chemotherapy, September 14-17, 2003. Washington: American Society for Microbiology; 2003:36.

78. Louie M, Hogan C, Hurley A, et al. Determining the antiviral activity of tenofovir disoproxil fumarate in treatment-naive chronically HIV-1-infected individuals. AIDS. 2003;17:1151-1156.

79. Schooley RT, Ruane P, Myers RA, et al. Tenofovir DF in antiretroviral-experienced patients: Results from a 48-week, randomized, double-blind study. AIDS. 2002;16:1257-1263.

80. McColl DJ, Miller MD. The use of tenofovir disoproxil fumarate for the treatment of nucleoside-resistant HIV-1. J Antimicrob Chemother. 2003;51:219-223.

81. Karras A, Lafaurie M, Furco A, et al. Tenofovir-related nephrotoxicity in human immunodeficiency virus-infected patients: Three cases of renal failure, Fanconi syndrome, and nephrogenic diabetes insipidus. Clin Infect Dis. 2003;36:1070-1073.

82. Wang LH, Delehanty J, Hulett L, et al. High levels of intracellular FTC-triphosphate correlate with the potent antiviral activity of FTC in vitro (Abstract LB-2). In: Program and Abstracts of the 38th Interscience Conference on Antimicrobial Agents and Chemotherapy, September 24-27, 1998. Washington, DC: American Society for Microbiology; 1998.

83. Rousseau FS, Kahn JO, Thompson M, et al. Prototype trial design for rapid dose selection of antiretroviral drugs: An example using emtricitabine (Coviracil). J Antimicrob Chemother. 2001;48:507-513.

84. Raffi F, Saag M, Cahn P, et al. A randomized, double-blind, multicentre comparison of emtricitabine QD to stavudine BID in treatment-naive HIV-infected patients (Abstract 38). Antiviral Ther. 2003;8:S193-S194.

85. Van Der Horst C, Sanne I, Wakeford C, et al. Two randomized, controlled, equivalence trials of emtricitabine (FTC) to lamivudine (3TC) (Abstract 18). In: Program and Abstracts of the Eighth Conference on Retroviruses and Opportunistic Infections, February 4-8, 2001. Alexandria, Va: Foundation for Retrovirology and Human Health; 2001:48.

86. Bartlett J. Severe liver toxicity in patients receiving two nucleoside analogues and a non-nucleoside reverse transcriptase inhibitor (Abstract 19). In: Program and Abstracts of the Eighth Conference on Retroviruses and Opportunistic Infections, February 4-8, 2001. Alexandria, Va: Foundation for Retrovirology and Human Health; 2001:48.

87. Hanna GJ, D'Aquila RT. Antiretroviral drug resistance in HIV-1. Curr Infect Dis Rep. 1999;1:289-297.

88. Hirsch MS, Brun-Vezinet F, Clotet B, et al. Antiretroviral drug resistance testing in adults infected with human immunodeficiency virus type 1: 2003 Recommendations of an International AIDS Society-USA Panel. Clin Infect Dis. 2003;37:113-128.

89. Ho DD, Neumann AU, Perelson AS, et al. Rapid turnover of plasma virions and CD4 lymphocytes in HIV-1 infection. Nature. 1995;373:123-126.

90. Wei X, Ghosh SK, Taylor ME, et al. Viral dynamics in human immunodeficiency virus type 1 infection. Nature. 1995;373:117-122.

91. Perelson AS, Neumann AU, Markowitz M, et al. HIV-1 dynamics in vivo: Virion clearance rate, infected cell life-span, and viral generation time. Science. 1996;271:1582-1586.

92. Coffin JM. HIV population dynamics in vivo: Implications for genetic variation, pathogenesis, and therapy. Science. 1995;267:483-489.

93. Larder BA, Kemp SD. Multiple mutations in HIV-1 reverse transcriptase confer high-level resistance to zidovudine (AZT). Science. 1989;246:1155-1158.

94. Boucher CA, Tersmette M, Lange JM, et al. Zidovudine sensitivity of human immunodeficiency viruses from high-risk, symptom-free individuals during therapy. Lancet. 1990;336:585-590.

95. Boucher CA, O'Sullivan E, Mulder JW, et al. Ordered appearance of zidovudine resistance mutations during treatment of 18 human immunodeficiency virus-positive subjects. J Infect Dis. 1992;165:105-110.

96. Loveday C, Kaye S, Tenant-Flowers M, et al. HIV-1 RNA serum-load and resistant viral genotypes during early zidovudine therapy. Lancet. 1995;345:820-824.

97. Larder BA, Kellam P, Kemp SD. Zidovudine resistance predicted by direct detection of mutations in DNA from HIV-infected lymphocytes. AIDS. 1991;5:137-144.

98. Kellam P, Boucher CA, Larder BA. Fifth mutation in human immunodeficiency virus type 1 reverse transcriptase contributes to the development of high-level resistance to zidovudine. Proc Natl Acad Sci U S A. 1992;89:1934-1938.

99. Hooker DJ, Tachedjian G, Solomon AE, et al. An in vivo mutation from leucine to tryptophan at position 210 in human immunodeficiency virus type 1 reverse transcriptase contributes to high-level resistance to 3'-azido-3'-deoxythymidine. J Virol. 1996;70:8010-8018.

100. Larder BA, Coates KE, Kemp SD. Zidovudine-resistant human immunodeficiency virus selected by passage in cell culture. J Virol. 1991;65:5232-5236.

101. Pellegrin I, Izopet J, Reynes J, et al. Emergence of zidovudine and multidrug-resistance mutations in the HIV-1 reverse transcriptase gene in therapy-naive patients receiving stavudine plus didanosine combination therapy. STADI Group. AIDS. 1999;13:1705-1709.

102. Coakley EP, Gillis JM, Hammer SM. Phenotypic and genotypic resistance patterns of HIV-1 isolates derived from individuals treated with didanosine and stavudine. AIDS. 2000;14:F9-F15.

103. Mayers DL, Japour AJ, Arduino JM, et al. Dideoxynucleoside resistance emerges with prolonged zidovudine monotherapy. The RV43 Study Group. Antimicrob Agents Chemother. 1994;38:307-314.

104. Shulman NS, Machekano RA, Shafer RW, et al. Genotypic correlates of a virologic response to stavudine after zidovudine monotherapy. J Acquir Immune Defic Syndr. 2001;27:377-380.

105. D'Aquila RT, Johnson VA, Welles SL, et al. Zidovudine resistance and HIV-1 disease progression during antiretroviral therapy. AIDS Clinical Trials Group Protocol 116B/117 Team and the Virology Committee Resistance Working Group. Ann Intern Med. 1995;122:401-408.

106. Brun-Vezinet F, Descamps D, Ruffault A, et al. Clinically relevant interpretation of genotype for resistance to abacavir. AIDS. 2003;17:1795-1802.

107. Miller MD, Margot N, Lu B, et al. Genotypic and phenotypic predictors of the magnitude of response to tenofovir disoproxil fumarate treatment in antiretroviral-experienced patients. J Infect Dis. 2004;189:837-846.

108. Gao Q, Gu Z, Parniak MA, et al. The same mutation that encodes low-level human immunodeficiency virus type 1 resistance to 2',3'-dideoxyinosine and 2',3'-dideoxycytidine confers high-level resistance to the (−) enantiomer of 2',3'-dideoxy-3'-thiacytidine. Antimicrob Agents Chemother. 1993;37:1390-1392.

109. Tisdale M, Kemp SD, Parry NR, Larder BA. Rapid in vitro selection of human immunodeficiency virus type 1 resistant to 3'-thiacytidine inhibitors due to a mutation in the YMDD region of reverse transcriptase. Proc Natl Acad Sci U S A. 1993;90:5653-5656.

110. Gu Z, Gao Q, Li X, et al. Novel mutation in the human immunodeficiency virus type 1 reverse transcriptase gene that encodes cross-resistance to 2',3'-dideoxyinosine and 2',3'-dideoxycytidine. J Virol. 1992;66:7128-7135.

111. Winters MA, Bosch RJ, Albrecht MA, Katzenstein DA. Clinical impact of the M184V mutation on switching to didanosine or maintaining lamivudine treatment in nucleoside reverse-transcriptase inhibitor-experienced patients. J Infect Dis. 2003;188:537-540.

112. Pozniak A, Gazzard BG, Peeters M, et al. Influence of the M184V mutation on virologic outcome of highly active antiretroviral therapy with or without ddI (Abstract 152). Antiviral Ther. 2002;7:S124.

113. Fitzgibbon JE, Howell RM, Haberzettl CA, et al. Human immunodeficiency virus type 1 pol gene mutations which cause decreased susceptibility to 2',3'-dideoxycytidine. Antimicrob Agents Chemother. 1992;36:153-157.

114. Zhang D, Caliendo AM, Eron JJ, et al. Resistance to 2',3'-dideoxycytidine conferred by a mutation in codon 65 of the human immunodeficiency virus type 1 reverse transcriptase. Antimicrob Agents Chemother. 1994;38:282-287.

115. St Clair MH, Martin JL, Tudor-Williams G, et al. Resistance to ddI and sensitivity to AZT induced by a mutation in HIV-1 reverse transcriptase. Science. 1991;253:1557-1559.

116. Eron JJ, Chow YK, Caliendo AM, et al. Pol mutations conferring zidovudine and didanosine resistance with different effects in vitro yield multiply resistant human immunodeficiency virus type 1 isolates in vivo. Antimicrob Agents Chemother. 1993;37:1480-1487.

117. Tisdale M, Alnadaf T, Cousens D. Combination of mutations in human immunodeficiency virus type 1 reverse transcriptase required for resistance to the carbocyclic nucleoside 1592U89. Antimicrob Agents Chemother. 1997;41:1094-1098.

118. Miller V, Sturmer M, Staszewski S, et al. The M184V mutation in HIV-1 reverse transcriptase (RT) conferring lamivudine resistance does not result in broad cross-resistance to nucleoside analogue RT inhibitors. AIDS. 1998;12:705-712.

119. Walter H, Schmidt B, Werwein M, et al. Prediction of abacavir resistance from genotypic data: Impact of zidovudine and lamivudine resistance in vitro and in vivo. Antimicrob Agents Chemother. 2002;46:89-94.

120. Harrigan PR, Miller MD, McKenna P, et al. Phenotypic susceptibilities to tenofovir in a large panel of clinically derived human immunodeficiency virus type 1 isolates. Antimicrob Agents Chemother. 2002;46:1067-1072.

121. Larder BA, Kemp SD, Harrigan PR. Potential mechanism for sustained antiretroviral efficacy of AZT-3TC combination therapy. Science. 1995;269:696-699.

122. Miller MD, Anton KE, Mulato AS, et al. Human immunodeficiency virus type 1 expressing the lamivudine-associated M184V mutation in reverse transcriptase shows increased susceptibility to adefovir and decreased replication capability in vitro. J Infect Dis. 1999;179:92-100.

123. Bazmi HZ, Hammond JL, Cavalcanti SC, et al. In vitro selection of mutations in the human immunodeficiency virus type 1 reverse transcriptase that decrease susceptibility to (−)-beta-D-dioxolane-guanosine and suppress resistance to 3'-azido-3'-deoxythymidine. Antimicrob Agents Chemother. 2000;44:1783-1788.

124. Kemp SD, Shi C, Bloor S, et al. A novel polymorphism at codon 333 of human immunodeficiency virus type 1 reverse transcriptase can facilitate dual resistance to zidovudine and L-2',3'-dideoxy-3'-thiacytidine. J Virol. 1998;72:5093-5098.

125. Nijhuis M, Schuurman R, de Jong D, et al. Lamivudine-resistant human immunodeficiency virus type 1 variants (184V) require multiple amino acid changes to become co-resistant to zidovudine in vivo. J Infect Dis. 1997;176:398-405.

126. Hertogs K, Bloor S, De Vroey V, et al. A novel human immunodeficiency virus type 1 reverse transcriptase mutational pattern confers phenotypic lamivudine resistance in the absence of mutation 184V. Antimicrob Agents Chemother. 2000;44:568-573.

127. Shirasaka T, Kavlick MF, Ueno T, et al. Emergence of human immunodeficiency virus type 1 variants with resistance to multiple dideoxynucleosides in patients receiving therapy with dideoxynucleosides. Proc Natl Acad Sci U S A. 1995;92:2398-2402.

128. Shafer RW, Kozal MJ, Winters MA, et al. Combination therapy with zidovudine and didanosine selects for drug-resistant human immunodeficiency virus type 1 strains with unique patterns of pol gene mutations. J Infect Dis. 1994;169:722-729.

129. Winters MA, Coolley KL, Girard YA, et al. A 6-basepair insert in the reverse transcriptase gene of human immunodeficiency virus type 1 confers resistance to multiple nucleoside inhibitors. J Clin Invest. 1998;102:1769-1775.

130. Medina DJ, Tung PP, Lerner-Tung MB, et al. Sanctuary growth of human immunodeficiency virus in the presence of 3'-azido-3'-deoxythymidine. J Virol. 1995;69:1606-1611.

131. Hoggard PG, Sales SD, Phiboonbanakit D, et al. Influence of prior exposure to zidovudine on stavudine phosphorylation in vivo and ex vivo. Antimicrob Agents Chemother. 2001;45:577-582.

132. De Clercq E. Antiviral therapy for human immunodeficiency virus infections. Clin Microbiol Rev. 1995;8:200-239.

133. Cheeseman SH, Hattox SE, McLaughlin MM, et al. Pharmacokinetics of nevirapine: Initial single-rising-dose study in humans. Antimicrob Agents Chemother. 1993;37:178-182.

134. Havlir DV, Eastman S, Gamst A, Richman DD. Nevirapine-resistant human immunodeficiency virus: Kinetics of replication and estimated prevalence in untreated patients. J Virol. 1996;70:7894-7899.

135. Richman DD, Havlir D, Corbeil J, et al. Nevirapine resistance mutations of human immunodeficiency virus type 1 selected during therapy. J Virol. 1994;68:1660-1666.

136. Floridia M, Bucciardini R, Ricciardulli D, et al. A randomized, double-blind trial on the use of a triple combination including nevirapine, a nonnucleoside reverse transcriptase HIV inhibitor, in antiretroviral-naive patients with advanced disease. J Acquir Immune Defic Syndr Hum Retrovirol. 1999;20:11-19.

137. D'Aquila RT, Hughes MD, Johnson VA, et al. Nevirapine, zidovudine, and didanosine compared with zidovudine and didanosine in patients with HIV-1 infection: A randomized, double-blind, placebo-controlled trial. National Institute of Allergy and Infectious Diseases AIDS Clinical Trials Group Protocol 241 Investigators. Ann Intern Med. 1996;124:1019-1030.

138. van Leth F, Phanuphak P, Ruxrungtham K, et al. Comparison of first-line antiretroviral therapy with regimens including nevirapine, efavirenz, or both drugs, plus stavudine and lamivudine: A randomised open-label trial, the 2NN Study. Lancet. 2004;363:1253-1263.

139. Martinez E, Conget I, Lozano L, et al. Reversion of metabolic abnormalities after switching from HIV-1 protease inhibitors to nevirapine. AIDS. 1999;13:805-810.

140. Dieleman JP, Sturkenboom MC, Wit FW, et al. Low risk of treatment failure after substitution of nevirapine for protease inhibitors among human immunodeficiency virus-infected patients with virus suppression. J Infect Dis. 2002;185:1261-1268.

141. Scott LJ, Perry CM. Delavirdine: A review of its use in HIV infection. Drugs. 2000;60:1411-1444.

142. Sargent S, Green S, Para M, et al. Sustained plasma viral burden reductions and CD4 increases in HIV-1 infected patients with Rescriptor (DLV) + Retrovir (ZDV) + Epivir (3TC) (Abstract 699). In: Fifth Conference on Retroviruses and Opportunistic Infections, Chicago, 1998. Chicago: Feb. 1-5, 1998:209.

143. Albrecht MA, Bosch RJ, Hammer SM, et al. Nelfinavir, efavirenz, or both after the failure of nucleoside treatment of HIV infection. N Engl J Med. 2001;345:398-407.

144. Shafer RW, Smeaton LM, Robbins GK, et al. Comparison of four-drug and sequential three-drug regimens as initial therapy for HIV-1 infection. N Engl J Med. 2003;349:2304-2315.

145. Lucas GM, Chaisson RE, Moore RD. Comparison of initial combination antiretroviral therapy with a single protease inhibitor, ritonavir and saquinavir, or efavirenz. AIDS. 2001;15:1679-1686.

146. Molina JM, Ferchal F, Journot V, et al. Emtricitabine, didanosine and efavirenz once-daily (OD) versus continued PI-based HAART (C) in HIV-infected adults with undetectable plasma HIV-RNA: 48-Week results of a prospective randomized multicentre trial (ALIZE-ANRS 99) (Abstract 37). Antiviral Ther. 2003;8:S193.

147. Lopez-Cortes LF, Ruiz-Valderas R, Viciana P, et al. Once-daily saquinavir-sgc plus low-dose ritonavir (1200/100 mg) in combination with efavirenz: Pharmacokinetics and efficacy in HIV-infected patients with prior antiretroviral therapy. J Acquir Immune Defic Syndr. 2003;32:240-242.

148. Ferre V, Allavena C, Poizot-Martin I, et al. BIKS Study (lopinavir/ritonavir-efavirenz combination): Complete 24-week results (Abstract 36). Antiviral Ther. 2003;8:S193.

149. Stek M, Hirschel B, Benetucci J, et al. Comparison of PI-boosted indinavir with efavirenz plus stavudine regimens in EASIER (European and South American Study of Indinavir, Efavirenz, and Ritonavir) (Abstract 39). Antiviral Ther. 2003;8:S194.

150. Albrecht MA, Bosch RJ, Hammer SM, et al. Nelfinavir, efavirenz, or both after the failure of nucleoside treatment of HIV infection. N Engl J Med. 2001;345:398-407.

151. Hanna GJ, Johnson VA, Kuritzkes DR, et al. Patterns of resistance mutations selected by treatment of human immunodeficiency virus type 1 infection with zidovudine, didanosine, and nevirapine. J Infect Dis. 2000;181:904-911.

152. Demeter LM, Shafer RW, Meehan PM, et al. Delavirdine susceptibilities and associated reverse transcriptase mutations in human immunodeficiency virus type 1 isolates from patients in a phase I/II trial of delavirdine monotherapy (ACTG 260). Antimicrob Agents Chemother. 2000;44:794-797.

153. Joly V, Moroni M, Concia E, et al. Delavirdine in combination with zidovudine in treatment of human immunodeficiency virus type 1-infected patients: Evaluation of efficacy and emergence of viral resistance in a randomized, comparative phase III trial. The M/3331/0013B Study Group. Antimicrob Agents Chemother. 2000;44:3155-3157.

154. Bacheler LT, Anton ED, Kudish P, et al. Human immunodeficiency virus type 1 mutations selected in patients failing efavirenz combination therapy. Antimicrob Agents Chemother. 2000;44:2475-2484.

155. Bacheler L, Jeffrey S, Hanna G, et al. Genotypic correlates of phenotypic resistance to efavirenz in virus isolates from patients failing NNRTI combination therapy. J Virol. 2001;75:4999-5008.

156. Shulman NS, Zolopa AR, Passaro DJ, et al. Efavirenz- and adefovir dipivoxil-based salvage therapy in highly treatment-experienced patients: Clinical and genotypic predictors of virologic response. J Acquir Immune Defic Syndr. 2000;23:221-226.

157. Whitcomb JM, Huang W, Limoli K, et al. Hypersusceptibility to non-nucleoside reverse transcriptase inhibitors in HIV-1: Clinical, phenotypic and genotypic correlates. AIDS. 2002;16:F41-F47.

158. Shulman N, Zolopa AR, Passaro D, et al. Phenotypic hypersusceptibility to non-nucleoside reverse transcriptase inhibitors in treatment-experienced HIV-infected patients: Impact on virological response to efavirenz-based therapy. AIDS. 2001;15:1125-1132.

159. Hammer SM, Vaida F, Bennett KK, et al. Dual vs single protease inhibitor therapy following antiretroviral treatment failure: A randomized trial. JAMA 2002;288:169-180.

160. Katzenstein DA, Bosch RJ, Hellmann N, et al. Phenotypic susceptibility and virological outcome in nucleoside-experienced patients receiving three or four antiretroviral drugs. AIDS. 2003;17:821-830.

161. Deeks SG, Smith M, Holodniy M, Kahn JO. HIV-1 protease inhibitors: A review for clinicians. JAMA. 1997;277:145-153.

162. McDonald CK, Kuritzkes DR. Human immunodeficiency virus type 1 protease inhibitors. Arch Intern Med. 1997;157:951-959.

163. Piscitelli SC, Flexner C, Minor JR, et al. Drug interactions in patients infected with human immunodeficiency virus. Clin Infect Dis. 1996;23:685-693.

164. Flexner C. HIV-protease inhibitors. N Engl J Med. 1998;338:1281-1292.

165. Piscitelli SC, Gallicano KD. Interactions among drugs for HIV and opportunistic infections. N Engl J Med. 2001;344:984-996.

166. Tsiodras S, Mantzoros C, Hammer S, Samore M. Effects of protease inhibitors on hyperglycemia, hyperlipidemia, and lipodystrophy: A 5-year cohort study. Arch Intern Med. 2000;160:2050-2056.

167. Smith JH, Martin GJ, Decker CF. Hyperlipidemia associated with the use of protease inhibitors. Clin Infect Dis. 2000;31:207-208.

168. Dube MP, Johnson DL, Currier JS, Leedom JM. Protease inhibitor-associated hyperglycaemia. Lancet. 1997;350:713-714.

169. Eastone JA, Decker CF. New-onset diabetes mellitus associated with use of protease inhibitor. Ann Intern Med. 1997;127:948.

170. Dube MP. Disorders of glucose metabolism in patients infected with human immunodeficiency virus. Clin Infect Dis. 2000;31:1467-1475.

171. Passalaris JD, Sepkowitz KA, Glesby MJ. Coronary artery disease and human immunodeficiency virus infection. Clin Infect Dis. 2000;31:787-797.

172. Holmberg SD, Moorman AC, Williamson JM, et al. Protease inhibitors and cardiovascular outcomes in patients with HIV-1. Lancet. 2002;360:1747-1748.

173. Carr A. HIV protease inhibitor-related lipodystrophy syndrome. Clin Infect Dis. 2000;30:S135-S142.

174. Sattler F. Body habitus changes related to lipodystrophy. Clin Infect Dis. 2003;36:S84-S90.

175. Viraben R, Aquilina C. Indinavir-associated lipodystrophy. AIDS. 1998;12:F37-F39.

176. Lo JC, Mulligan K, Tai VW, et al. "Buffalo hump" in men with HIV-1 infection. Lancet. 1998;351:867-870.

177. Miller KD, Jones E, Yanovski JA, et al. Visceral abdominal-fat accumulation associated with use of indinavir. Lancet. 1998;351:871-875.

178. Monier P, McKown K, Bronze MS. Osteonecrosis complicating highly active antiretroviral therapy in patients infected with human immunodeficiency virus. Clin Infect Dis. 2000;31:1488-1492.

179. Dube MP, Sprecher D, Henry WK, et al. Preliminary guidelines for the evaluation and management of dyslipidemia in adults infected with human immunodeficiency virus and receiving antiretroviral therapy: Recommendations of the Adult AIDS Clinical Trial Group Cardiovascular Disease Focus Group. Clin Infect Dis. 2000;31:1216-1224.

180. Schambelan M, Benson CA, Carr A, et al. Management of metabolic complications associated with antiretroviral therapy for HIV-1 infection: Recommendations of an International AIDS Society-USA panel. J Acquir Immune Defic Syndr. 2002;31:257-275.

181. Dube MP, Stein JH, Aberg JA, et al. Guidelines for the evaluation and management of dyslipidemia in human immunodeficiency virus (HIV)-infected adults receiving antiretroviral therapy: Recommendations of the HIV Medical Association of the Infectious Disease Society of America and the Adult AIDS Clinical Trials Group. Clin Infect Dis. 2003;37:613-627.

182. Kitchen VS, Skinner C, Ariyoshi K, et al. Safety and activity of saquinavir in HIV infection. Lancet. 1995;345:952-955.

183. Schapiro JM, Winters MA, Stewart F, et al. The effect of high-dose saquinavir on viral load and CD4+ T-cell counts in HIV-infected patients. Ann Intern Med. 1996;124:1039-1050.

184. Collier AC, Coombs RW, Schoenfeld DA, et al. Treatment of human immunodeficiency virus infection with saquinavir, zidovudine, and zalcitabine. AIDS Clinical Trials Group. N Engl J Med. 1996;334:1011-1017.

185. Mitsuyasu RT, Skolnik PR, Cohen SR, et al. Activity of the soft gelatin formulation of saquinavir in combination therapy in antiretroviral-naive patients. NV15355 Study Team. AIDS. 1998;12:F103-F109.

186. Cohen Stuart JW, Schuurman R, Burger DM, et al. Randomized trial comparing saquinavir soft gelatin capsules versus indinavir as part of triple therapy (CHEESE study). AIDS. 1999;13:F53-F58.

187. Merry C, Barry MG, Mulcahy F, et al. Saquinavir pharmacokinetics alone and in combination with ritonavir in HIV-infected patients. AIDS. 1997;11:F29-F33.

188. Rhone SA, Hogg RS, Yip B, et al. The antiviral effect of ritonavir and saquinavir in combination amongst HIV-infected adults: Results from a community-based study. AIDS. 1998;12:619-624.

189. Kirk O, Katzenstein TL, Gerstoft J, et al. Combination therapy containing ritonavir plus saquinavir has superior short-term antiretroviral efficacy: A randomized trial. AIDS. 1999;13:F9-F16.

190. Gill MJ. Safety profile of soft gelatin formulation of saquinavir in combination with nucleosides in a broad patient population. NV15182 Study Team. AIDS. 1998;12:1400-1402.

191. Kempf DJ, Marsh KC, Denissen JF, et al. ABT-538 is a potent inhibitor of human immunodeficiency virus protease and has high oral bioavailability in humans. Proc Natl Acad Sci U S A. 1995;92:2484-2488.

192. Danner SA, Carr A, Leonard JM, et al. A short-term study of the safety, pharmacokinetics, and efficacy of ritonavir, an inhibitor of HIV-1 protease. European-Australian Collaborative Ritonavir Study Group. N Engl J Med. 1995;333:1528-1533.

193. Markowitz M, Saag M, Powderly WG, et al. A preliminary study of ritonavir, an inhibitor of HIV-1 protease, to treat HIV-1 infection. N Engl J Med. 1995;333: 1534-1539.
194. Cameron DW, Heath-Chiozzi M, Danner S, et al. Randomised placebo-controlled trial of ritonavir in advanced HIV-1 disease. The Advanced HIV Disease Ritonavir Study Group. Lancet. 1998;351:543-549.
195. Cooper CL, van Heeswijk RP, Gallicano K, Cameron DW. A review of low-dose ritonavir in protease inhibitor combination therapy. Clin Infect Dis. 2003;36: 1585-1592.
196. Mole L, Schmidgall D, Holodniy M. A pilot trial of indinavir, ritonavir, didanosine, and lamivudine in a once-daily four-drug regimen for HIV infection. J Acquir Immune Defic Syndr. 2001;27:260-265.
197. Duval X, Lamotte C, Race E, et al. Amprenavir inhibitory quotient and virological response in human immunodeficiency virus-infected patients on an amprenavir-containing salvage regimen without or with ritonavir. Antimicrob Agents Chemother. 2002;46:570-574.
198. Badaro R, DeJesus E, Lazzarin A, et al. Efficacy and safety of atazanavir (ATV) with ritonavir (RTV) or saquinavir (SQV) versus lopinavir/ritonavir (LPV/RTV) in combination with tenofovir (TFV) and one NRTI in patients who have experienced virologic failure to multiple HAART regimens: 16-Week results from BMS AI424-045 (Abstract 118). Antiviral Ther. 2003;8:S212-S213.
199. Gulick RM, Mellors JW, Havlir D, et al. Treatment with indinavir, zidovudine, and lamivudine in adults with human immunodeficiency virus infection and prior antiretroviral therapy. N Engl J Med. 1997;337:734-739.
200. Gulick RM, Mellors JW, Havlir D, et al. Simultaneous vs sequential initiation of therapy with indinavir, zidovudine, and lamivudine for HIV-1 infection: 100-Week follow-up. JAMA. 1998;280:35-41.
201. Gulick RM, Mellors JW, Havlir D, et al. 3-Year suppression of HIV viremia with indinavir, zidovudine, and lamivudine. Ann Intern Med. 2000;133:35-39.
202. Hirsch M, Steigbigel R, Staszewski S, et al. A randomized, controlled trial of indinavir, zidovudine, and lamivudine in adults with advanced human immunodeficiency virus type 1 infection and prior antiretroviral therapy. J Infect Dis. 1999;180:659-665.
203. Hirsch MS, DiNubile MJ, Harvey CM, et al. Long-term efficacy, safety, and tolerability of indinavir-based therapy in protease inhibitor-naive adults with advanced HIV infection. Clin Infect Dis. 2003;37:1119-1124.
204. Gulick RM, Smeaton LM, D'Aquila RT, et al. Indinavir, nevirapine, stavudine, and lamivudine for human immunodeficiency virus-infected, amprenavir-experienced subjects: AIDS Clinical Trials Group Protocol 373. J Infect Dis. 2001;183:715-721.
205. Kopp JB, Miller KD, Mican JA, et al. Crystalluria and urinary tract abnormalities associated with indinavir. Ann Intern Med. 1997;127:119-125.
206. Bardsley-Elliot A, Plosker GL. Nelfinavir: An update on its use in HIV infection. Drugs. 2000;59:581-620.
207. Saag MS, Tebas P, Sension M, et al. Randomized, double-blind comparison of two nelfinavir doses plus nucleosides in HIV-infected patients. Agouron Study 511. AIDS. 2001;15:1971-1978.
208. Walmsley S, Bernstein B, King M, et al. Lopinavir-ritonavir versus nelfinavir for the initial treatment of HIV infection. N Engl J Med. 2002;346:2039-2046.
209. Lawrence J, Schapiro J, Winters M, et al. Clinical resistance patterns and responses to two sequential protease inhibitor regimens in saquinavir and reverse transcriptase inhibitor-experienced persons. J Infect Dis. 1999;179:1356-1364.
210. Murphy RL, Gulick RM, DeGruttola V, et al. Treatment with amprenavir alone or amprenavir with zidovudine and lamivudine in adults with human immunodeficiency virus infection. AIDS Clinical Trials Group 347 Study Team. J Infect Dis. 1999;179:808-816.
211. Eron JJ, Haubrich R, Lang W, et al. A phase II trial of dual protease inhibitor therapy: Amprenavir in combination with indinavir, nelfinavir, or saquinavir. J Acquir Immune Defic Syndr. 2001;26:458-461.
212. Hammer SM, Vaida F, Bennett KK, et al. Dual vs single protease inhibitor therapy following antiretroviral treatment failure: A randomized trial. JAMA. 2002;288: 169-180.
213. Benson CA, Deeks SG, Brun SC, et al. Safety and antiviral activity at 48 weeks of lopinavir/ritonavir plus nevirapine and 2 nucleoside reverse-transcriptase inhibitors in human immunodeficiency virus type 1–infected protease inhibitor–experienced patients. J Infect Dis. 2002;185:599-607.
214. Lexiva (fosamprenavir calcium) prescribing information. GlaxoSmithKline, Research Triangle Park, NC. 2003.
215. Squires KE, Thiry A, Giordano M, et al. Atazanavir (ATV) QD vs efavirenz (EFV) QD with fixed-dose ZDV + 3TC BID: Comparison of antiviral efficacy and safety (Abstract xxx). In: Program and Abstracts of the 42nd Interscience Conference on Antimicrobial Agents and Chemotherapy, September 27-30, 2002. San Diego, Calif: American Society for Microbiology; 2002:xxx.
216. Nieto-Cisneros L, Zala C, Fessel WJ, et al. Antiviral efficacy, metabolic changes and safety of atazanavir (ATV) versus lopinavir/ritonavir (LPV/RTV) in combination with two NRTIs in patients who have experienced virological failure with prior PI-containing regimen(s): 24 Week results from BMS AI424-043 (Abstract 117). Antiviral Ther. 2003;8:S212.
217. Jacobsen H, Hanggi M, Ott M, et al. In vivo resistance to a human immunodeficiency virus type 1 proteinase inhibitor: Mutations, kinetics, and frequencies. J Infect Dis. 1996;173:1379-1387.
218. Schapiro JM, Lawrence J, Speck R, et al. Resistance mutations to zidovudine and saquinavir in patients receiving zidovudine plus saquinavir or zidovudine and zalcitabine plus saquinavir in AIDS clinical trials group 229. J Infect Dis. 1999;179: 249-253.
219. Molla A, Korneyeva M, Gao Q, et al. Ordered accumulation of mutations in HIV protease confers resistance to ritonavir. Nat Med. 1996;2:760-766.
220. Condra JH, Schleif WA, Blahy OM, et al. In vivo emergence of HIV-1 variants resistant to multiple protease inhibitors. Nature. 1995;374:569-571.
221. Condra JH, Holder DJ, Schleif WA, et al. Genetic correlates of in vivo viral resistance to indinavir, a human immunodeficiency virus type 1 protease inhibitor. J Virol. 1996;70:8270-8276.
222. Patick AK, Duran M, Cao Y, et al. Genotypic and phenotypic characterization of human immunodeficiency virus type 1 variants isolated from patients treated with the protease inhibitor nelfinavir. Antimicrob Agents Chemother. 1998;42:2637-2644.
223. Zolopa AR, Shafer RW, Warford A, et al. HIV-1 genotypic resistance patterns predict response to saquinavir-ritonavir therapy in patients in whom previous protease inhibitor therapy had failed. Ann Intern Med. 1999;131:813-821.
224. Partaledis JA, Yamaguchi K, Tisdale M, et al. In vitro selection and characterization of human immunodeficiency virus type 1 (HIV-1) isolates with reduced sensitivity to hydroxyethylamino sulfonamide inhibitors of HIV-1 aspartyl protease. J Virol. 1995;69:5228-5235.
225. Maguire M, Shortino D, Klein A, et al. Emergence of resistance to protease inhibitor amprenavir in human immunodeficiency virus type 1-infected patients: Selection of four alternative viral protease genotypes and influence of viral susceptibility to coadministered reverse transcriptase nucleoside inhibitors. Antimicrob Agents Chemother. 2002;46:731-738.
226. Kempf DJ, Isaacson JD, King MS, et al. Identification of genotypic changes in human immunodeficiency virus protease that correlate with reduced susceptibility to the protease inhibitor lopinavir among viral isolates from protease inhibitor-experienced patients. J Virol. 2001;75:7462-7469.
227. Colonno R, Rose R, McLaren C, et al. Identification of I50L as the signature atazanavir (ATV) resistance mutation in treatment-naive HIV-1-infected patients receiving ATV-containing regimens. J Infect Dis. 2004;189:1802-1810.
228. Martinez-Picado J, Savara AV, Sutton L, D'Aquila RT. Replicative fitness of protease inhibitor-resistant mutants of human immunodeficiency virus type 1. J Virol. 1999;73:3744-3752.
229. Doyon L, Croteau G, Thibeault D, et al. Second locus involved in human immunodeficiency virus type 1 resistance to protease inhibitors. J Virol. 1996;70:3763-3769.
230. Zhang YM, Imamichi H, Imamichi T, et al. Drug resistance during indinavir therapy is caused by mutations in the protease gene and in its Gag substrate cleavage sites. J Virol. 1997;71:6662-6670.
231. Kilby JM, Eron JJ. Novel therapies based on mechanisms of HIV-1 cell entry. N Engl J Med. 2003;348:2228-2238.
232. Cairns JS, D'Souza MP. Chemokines and HIV-1 second receptors: The therapeutic connection. Nat Med. 1998;4:563-568.
233. Moyle G. Stopping HIV fusion with enfuvirtide: The first step to extracellular HAART. J Antimicrob Chemother. 2003;51:213-217.
234. Lalezari JP, Henry K, O'Hearn M, et al. Enfuvirtide, an HIV-1 fusion inhibitor, for drug-resistant HIV infection in North and South America. TORO 1 Study Group. N Engl J Med. 2003;348:2175-2185.
235. Lazzarin A, Clotet B, Cooper D, et al. Efficacy of enfuvirtide in patients infected with drug-resistant HIV-1 in Europe and Australia. N Engl J Med. 2003;348:2186-2195.
236. Rimsky LT, Shugars DC, Matthews TJ. Determinants of human immunodeficiency virus type 1 resistance to gp41-derived inhibitory peptides. J Virol. 1998;72:986-993.
237. Wei X, Decker JM, Liu H, et al. Emergence of resistant human immunodeficiency virus type 1 in patients receiving fusion inhibitor (T-20) monotherapy. Antimicrob Agents Chemother. 2002;46:1896-1905.
238. Report of the NIH Panel to Define Principles of Therapy of HIV Infection. MMWR Morb Mortal Wkly Rep. 1998;47:1-41.
239. Yeni PG, Hammer SM, Carpenter CC, et al. Antiretroviral treatment for adult HIV infection in 2002: Updated recommendations of the International AIDS Society-USA Panel. JAMA. 2002;288:222-235.
240. European guidelines for the clinical management and treatment of HIV-infected adults in Europe. AIDS. 2003;17(Suppl 2):S3-S26.
241. Guidelines for the use of antiretroviral agents in HIV-1-infected adults and adolescents. Department of Health and Human Services, 2003. 2003 Jul 14.
242. Mellors JW, Rinaldo CR Jr, Gupta P, et al. Prognosis in HIV-1 infection predicted by the quantity of virus in plasma [Published erratum appears in Science. 1997;275:14]. Science. 1996;272:1167-1170.
243. Mellors JW, Munoz A, Giorgi JV, et al. Plasma viral load and CD4+ lymphocytes as prognostic markers of HIV-1 infection. Ann Intern Med. 1997;126:946-954.
244. Vlahov D, Graham N, Hoover D, et al. Prognostic indicators for AIDS and infectious disease death in HIV-infected injection drug users: Plasma viral load and CD4+ cell count. JAMA. 1998;279:35-40.
245. Engels EA, Rosenberg PS, O'Brien TR, Goedert JJ. Plasma HIV viral load in patients with hemophilia and late-stage HIV disease: A measure of current immune suppression. Multicenter Hemophilia Cohort Study. Ann Intern Med. 1999;131:256-264.
246. Hughes MD, Johnson VA, Hirsch MS, et al. Monitoring plasma HIV-1 RNA levels in addition to CD4+ lymphocyte count improves assessment of antiretroviral therapeutic response. ACTG 241 Protocol Virology Substudy Team. Ann Intern Med. 1997;126:929-938.
247. O'Brien WA, Hartigan PM, Daar ES, et al. Changes in plasma HIV RNA levels and CD4+ lymphocyte counts predict both response to antiretroviral therapy and therapeutic failure. VA Cooperative Study Group on AIDS. Ann Intern Med. 1997;126:939-945.

248. Marschner IC, Collier AC, Coombs RW, et al. Use of changes in plasma levels of human immunodeficiency virus type 1 RNA to assess the clinical benefit of antiretroviral therapy. J Infect Dis. 1998;177:40-47.

249. Saag MS, Holodniy M, Kuritzkes DR, et al. HIV viral load markers in clinical practice. Nat Med. 1996;2:625-629.

250. Sax PE, Boswell SL, White-Guthro M, Hirsch MS. Potential clinical implications of interlaboratory variability in CD4+ T-lymphocyte counts of patients infected with human immunodeficiency virus. Clin Infect Dis. 1995;21:1121-1125.

251. Gallant JE. Strategies for long-term success in the treatment of HIV infection. JAMA. 2000;283:1329-1334.

252. Egger M, May M, Chene G, et al. Prognosis of HIV-1-infected patients starting highly active antiretroviral therapy: A collaborative analysis of prospective studies. Lancet. 2002;360:119-129.

253. Chaisson RE, Keruly JC, Moore RD. Association of initial CD4 cell count and viral load with response to highly active antiretroviral therapy. JAMA. 2000;284: 3128-3129.

254. Bratt G, Karlsson A, Leandersson AC, et al. Treatment history and baseline viral load, but not viral tropism or CCR-5 genotype, influence prolonged antiviral efficacy of highly active antiretroviral treatment. AIDS. 1998;12:2193-2202.

255. Palella FJ Jr, Deloria-Knoll M, Chmiel JS, et al. Survival benefit of initiating antiretroviral therapy in HIV-infected persons in different CD4+ cell strata. Ann Intern Med. 2003;138:620-626.

256. Wood E, Hogg RS, Yip B, et al. Higher baseline levels of plasma human immunodeficiency virus type 1 RNA are associated with increased mortality after initiation of triple-drug antiretroviral therapy. J Infect Dis. 2003;188:1421-1425.

257. Raboud JM, Rae S, Hogg RS, et al. Suppression of plasma virus load below the detection limit of a human immunodeficiency virus kit is associated with longer virologic response than suppression below the limit of quantitation. J Infect Dis. 1999;180:1347-1350.

258. Rizzardi GP, De Boer RJ, Hoover S, et al. Predicting the duration of antiviral treatment needed to suppress plasma HIV-1 RNA. J Clin Invest. 2000;105:777-782.

259. Paterson DL, Swindells S, Mohr J, et al. Adherence to protease inhibitor therapy and outcomes in patients with HIV infection [Published erratum appears in Ann Intern Med. 2002;136:253]. Ann Intern Med. 2000;133:21-30.

260. Demeter LM, Hughes MD, Coombs RW, et al. Predictors of virologic and clinical outcomes in HIV-1-infected patients receiving concurrent treatment with indinavir, zidovudine, and lamivudine. AIDS Clinical Trials Group Protocol 320. Ann Intern Med. 2001;135:954-964.

261. Polis MA, Sidorov IA, Yoder C, et al. Correlation between reduction in plasma HIV-1 RNA concentration 1 week after start of antiretroviral treatment and longer-term efficacy. Lancet. 2001;358:1760-1765.

262. Finzi D, Hermankova M, Pierson T, et al. Identification of a reservoir for HIV-1 in patients on highly active antiretroviral therapy. Science. 1997;278:1295-1300.

263. Wong JK, Hezareh M, Gunthard HF, et al. Recovery of replication-competent HIV despite prolonged suppression of plasma viremia. Science. 1997;278:1291-1295.

264. Caliendo AM, Hirsch MS. Combination therapy for infection due to human immunodeficiency virus type 1 [Published erratum appears in Clin Infect Dis. 1994;19:379]. Clin Infect Dis. 1994;18:516-524.

265. Schrager LK, D'Souza MP. Cellular and anatomical reservoirs of HIV-1 in patients receiving potent antiretroviral combination therapy. JAMA. 1998;280:67-71.

266. Havlir DV, Richman DD. Viral dynamics of HIV: Implications for drug development and therapeutic strategies. Ann Intern Med. 1996;124:984-994.

267. Staszewski S, Haberl A, Gute P, et al. Nevirapine/didanosine/lamivudine once daily in HIV-1-infected intravenous drug users. Antiviral Ther. 1998;3(Suppl 4):55-56.

268. Phillips AN, Staszewski S, Lampe F, et al. Human immunodeficiency virus rebound after suppression to <400 copies/mL during initial highly active antiretroviral therapy regimens, according to prior nucleoside experience and duration of suppression. J Infect Dis. 2002;186:1086-1091.

269. Negredo E, Cruz L, Paredes R, et al. Virological, immunological, and clinical impact of switching from protease inhibitors to nevirapine or to efavirenz in patients with human immunodeficiency virus infection and long-lasting viral suppression. Clin Infect Dis. 2002;34:504-510.

270. Hanna GJ, Caliendo AM. Testing for HIV-1 drug resistance. Mol Diagn. 2001;6: 253-263.

271. Hanna GJ, D'Aquila RT. Clinical use of genotypic and phenotypic drug resistance testing to monitor antiretroviral chemotherapy. Clin Infect Dis. 2001;32:774-782.

272. Tural C, Ruiz L, Holtzer C, et al. Clinical utility of HIV-1 genotyping and expert advice: The Havana trial. AIDS. 2002;16:209-218.

273. Little SJ, Holte S, Routy JP, et al. Antiretroviral-drug resistance among patients recently infected with HIV. N Engl J Med. 2002;347:385-394.

274. Deeks SG, Wrin T, Liegler T, et al. Virologic and immunologic consequences of discontinuing combination antiretroviral-drug therapy in HIV-infected patients with detectable viremia. N Engl J Med. 2001;344:472-480.

275. Gerberding JL. Management of occupational exposures to blood-borne viruses. N Engl J Med. 1995;332:444-451.

276. Cardo DM, Culver DH, Ciesielski CA, et al. A case-control study of HIV seroconversion in health care workers after percutaneous exposure. Centers for Disease Control and Prevention Needlestick Surveillance Group. N Engl J Med. 1997;337:1485-1490.

277. Gerberding JL. Prophylaxis for occupational exposure to HIV. Ann Intern Med. 1996;125:497-501.

278. Public Health Service guidelines for the management of health-care worker exposures to HIV and recommendations for postexposure prophylaxis. MMWR Morb Mortal Wkly Rep. 1998;47:1-34.

279. Updated U.S. Public Health Service guidelines for the management of occupational exposures to HBV, HCV, and HIV and recommendations for postexposure prophylaxis. MMWR Morb Mortal Wkly Rep 2001;RR-50:1-52.

280. Gerberding JL. Occupational exposure to HIV in health care settings. N Engl J Med. 2003;348:826-833.

281. Katz MH, Gerberding JL. The care of persons with recent sexual exposure to HIV. Ann Intern Med. 1998;128:306-312.

282. Management of possible sexual, injecting-drug-use, or other nonoccupational exposure to HIV, including considerations related to antiretroviral therapy. Public Health Service statement. Centers for Disease Control and Prevention. MMWR Morb Mortal Wkly Rep. 1998;47:1-14.

283. Lurie P, Miller S, Hecht F, et al. Postexposure prophylaxis after nonoccupational HIV exposure: Clinical, ethical, and policy considerations. JAMA. 1998;280:1769-1773.

284. Kahn JO, Martin JN, Roland ME, et al. Feasibility of postexposure prophylaxis (PEP) against human immunodeficiency virus infection after sexual or injection drug use exposure: The San Francisco PEP Study. J Infect Dis. 2001;183:707-714.

285. Kahn JO, Walker BD. Acute human immunodeficiency virus type 1 infection. N Engl J Med. 1998;339:33-39.

286. Rosenberg ES, Billingsley JM, Caliendo AM, et al. Vigorous HIV-1-specific CD4+ T cell responses associated with control of viremia. Science. 1997;278:1447-1450.

287. Rosenberg ES, Altfeld M, Poon SH, et al. Immune control of HIV-1 after early treatment of acute infection. Nature. 2000;407:523-526.

288. Reynes J, Rouzier R, Kanouni T, et al. SCH C: Safety and antiviral effects of a CCR5 receptor antagonist in HIV-1 infected subjects (Abstract 1). In: Program and Abstracts of the Ninth Conference on Retroviruses and Opportunistic Infections, February 24-28, 2002. Alexandria, Va: Foundation for Retrovirology and Human Health; 2002:53.

289. Schols D, Claes S, De Clercq E, et al. AMD-3100, a CXCR4 antagonist, reduced HIV viral load and X4 virus levels in humans (Abstract 2). In: Program and Abstracts of the Ninth Conference on Retroviruses and Opportunistic Infections, February 24-28, 2002. Alexandria, Va: Foundation for Retrovirology and Human Health; 2002:53.

290. Eron JJ, Gulick RM, Bartlett J, et al. Short-term safety and antiretroviral activity of T-1249, a second-generation fusion inhibitor of HIV. J Infect Dis. 2004;189: 1075-1083.

291. Tremblay CL, Kollmann C, Giguel F, et al. Strong in vitro synergy between the fusion inhibitor T-20 and the CXCR4 blocker AMD-3100. J Acquir Immune Defic Syndr. 2000;25:99-102.

292. Tremblay CL, Giguel F, Kollmann C, et al. Anti-human immunodeficiency virus interactions of SCH-C (SCH 351125), a CCR5 antagonist, with other antiretroviral agents in vitro. Antimicrob Agents Chemother. 2002;46:1336-1339.

293. Hazuda DJ, Felock P, Witmer M, et al. Inhibitors of strand transfer that prevent integration and inhibit HIV-1 replication in cells. Science. 2000;287:646-650.

294. Li F, Goila-Gaur R, Salzwedel K, et al. PA-457: A potent HIV inhibitor that disrupts core condensation by targeting a late step in Gag processing. Proc Natl Acad Sci. U S A 2003;100:13555-13560.

Management of Opportunistic Infections Associated with Human Immunodeficiency Virus Infection

HENRY MASUR

The quality and duration of survival for patients with human immunodeficiency virus (HIV) infection has improved remarkably since the acquired immunodeficiency disease (AIDS) was first recognized in the early 1980s.[1-6] Much of the early improvement in prognosis was the result of anti-*Pneumocystis* prophylaxis, improved management of acute opportunistic infections, and nucleoside antiretroviral therapy.[7-10] Since 1995, an increasing number of patients have received antiretroviral regimens that combine two or more antiretroviral agents: for patients who respond in terms of a significantly reduced HIV viral burden and a stable or increased circulating CD4+ T-lymphocyte cell count, there has been a dramatic decrease in clinical complications.[1-6] This sharp reduction in the number of AIDS-associated opportunistic infections has redirected the focus of management to maximizing the potency, durability, and tolerability of antiretroviral therapy (ART).

HIV-infected patients continue to develop opportunistic infections. This occurs because many patients are unaware of their HIV status until they present with an opportunistic infection and because patients fail ART because of nonadherence, poor drug absorption, unfavorable pharmacokinetic interactions, or development of resistant virus.[4,10,11]

For patients who do not receive sustained benefit from ART, and for those who do not take ART for various reasons, health care providers need to be cognizant that a substantial contribution to improved prognosis can be made by more effective management of the opportunistic processes that complicate the immunosuppression caused by HIV.[7-12] Management of opportunistic infections has become more successful because of advances in several convergent areas: understanding unique features of the natural history of HIV-associated opportunistic infections; being able to measure the course of immunologic decline and being able to relate these measurements to the occurrence of opportunistic processes; developing new diagnostic techniques; identifying more effective therapies; designing more effective and comprehensive preventive strategies; and vastly improving the education of health care workers and patients.

The range and diversity of new approaches to the management of opportunistic infections in patients with HIV infection present problems as well as opportunities. Many patients have difficulty affording the cost of medical care or cannot take time from work or family responsibilities to obtain optimal management. Most patients find it difficult to adhere to highly complex schedules of assessments and medications, especially considering the multiple-drug regimens associated with ART. When patients initiate ART, familiar pathogens such as cytomegalovirus (CMV) and *Mycobacterium avium* complex (MAC) may be associated with less familiar manifestations.[12-17] Some pathogens are increasingly resistant to the most widely used agents. In addition, pathogens that were previously unrecognized or seldom identified in patients with HIV infection, such as *Enterocytozoon, Cyclospora,* human herpesvirus-6, oxacillin-resistant *Staphylococcus aureus, Aspergillus,* and *Penicillium* are now producing clinical disease as patients live longer, travel, or reside in diverse geographic areas and receive preventive management for the more frequently recognized pathogens.

Aggressive preventive, diagnostic, and therapeutic management strategies for opportunistic infections in patients with HIV infection are crucial elements of the increasingly successful efforts to improve the prognosis for this patient population. Health care resources used to manage opportunistic infections are unequivocally well spent if applied with a strategy that emphasizes prevention and that provides aggressive recognition of and therapy for acute syndromes.[18]

PROSPECTIVE MONITORING

Prospective clinical and laboratory assessment is vital to the effective management of opportunistic infections in patients with HIV infection, just as it is important for management of ART.

The CD4+ T-cell count is a valuable marker to determine when patients are at increased risk for development of a specific opportunistic infection.[19-23] For example, *Pneumocystis jirovecii* pneumonia (PCP) occurs rarely in patients who have CD4+ T-cell counts higher than 200 to 250 cells/mm^3,[19-21] and disseminated MAC occurs rarely in patients with counts higher than 50 cells/mm^3.[24,25] This information is very helpful for focusing a diagnostic evaluation. If a patient with a CD4+ T-cell count of 700 cells/mm^3 develops cough and fever, for instance, the likelihood that this syndrome is caused by PCP is slim (but not zero). Therefore, sputum examination for *Pneumocystis* is not initially indicated, and most attention, when processing respiratory secretions, should be directed at common bacterial and viral pathogens. In contrast, if the CD4+ T-cell count is 25 cells/mm^3, the search for *Pneumocystis* in sputum or bronchoalveolar lavage is a very important focus because PCP is so common in this patient population.[19,20]

Although CD4+ T-cell counts provide a useful estimate of susceptibility to infections, they are not perfect predictive tools. For example, although more than 90% of cases of PCP occur in patients with CD4+ T-cell counts lower than 200 cells/mm^3, some cases occur in patients with counts in the range of 200 to 300 cells/mm^3, and a few occur in those with counts greater than 300 cells/mm^3.[19-21] For some patients, errors have been caused by inaccurate laboratory measurements. In others, a high viral load or a rapidly falling CD4+ T-cell count means that a value obtained 2 to 4 weeks previously is not a true reflection of the patient's current immunologic status.

A frequent concern is that CD4+ T-cell counts in patients receiving ART may not accurately reflect the clinical susceptibility to opportunistic infections. Evaluation of several large databases[5] demonstrated that ART does not alter the relationship between CD4+ T-cell counts and the occurrence of opportunistic infections in any substantial manner, regardless of how low the nadir CD4+ T-cell count was before initiation of ART.[4,26-28] There has also been concern that the phenotype or functional capacity of lymphocytes in patients responding to ART may not be identical to the phenotype or functional capacity of cells in patients with similar CD4+ T-cell counts who have never received ART.[26] Although differences in laboratory characteristics have been documented, there is no evidence that differences in laboratory markers other than the CD4+ T-cell number and percentage are clinically useful for predicting the occurrence of opportunistic infections.[29,30]

CD4+ T-cell counts are not the only laboratory predictors of opportunistic infection. HIV viral load in the circulation is an independent predictor: with each log increase in titer, the likelihood of occurrence of an opportunistic infection increases.[22,27,31-34] The CMV viral load is also an independent predictor of the occurrence of AIDS-defining events, although CMV viral loads are currently used only for research purposes.[35]

Specific blood or urine tests for individual pathogens may also be useful predictors of the occurrence (or relapse) of opportunistic infections. Serum cryptococcal antigen, urine histoplasma antigen, and serum CMV polymerase chain reaction (PCR) are examples of such assays.[35-37]

Clinical findings can be useful predictors of susceptibility to supplement the information derived from CD4+ T-cell counts and HIV viral loads. For example, the development of otherwise unexplained oropharyngeal candidiasis, oral hairy leukoplakia, previous PCP (and presumably other opportunistic infections), wasting, or any type of pneumonia is a good indicator of current susceptibility to PCP and the need to consider prophylaxis, independent of the CD4$^+$ T-cell count and the HIV viral load.[27,31-34]

MANAGEMENT OF ANTIRETROVIRAL THERAPY FOR PATIENTS WITH ACUTE OPPORTUNISTIC INFECTION

If a patient develops acute PCP, severe microsporidial diarrhea, or some other acute or severe opportunistic infection, the question often arises whether to initiate or continue ART.[11,12] Unquestionably, the immune augmentation that ART produces is likely to be beneficial ultimately in clearing the offending pathogen. However, the potential benefit of ART must be weighed against other factors. For ART-naive patients, the initiation of ART may produce an enhanced inflammatory response that could be detrimental in the short term. For example, ART-related immune-reactivation retinitis or lymphadenitis and pulmonary exacerbation after initial improvement in PCP have been reported.[13-17] Some of these syndromes can be life-threatening. In addition, initiation of ART at a time when adherence is poor or oral absorption less than optimal may diminish the effectiveness of ART and enhance the likelihood of emergence of drug-resistant HIV strains. For acutely ill patients with changing drug regimens, drugs could alter pharmacokinetics and result in suboptimal or, alternatively, toxic serum drug concentrations.[38] Suboptimal levels enhance the likelihood of development of HIV resistance to antiretroviral agents. Therefore, in some circumstances, withholding of all ART until an acute opportunistic infection resolves might be the most prudent course.

For some opportunistic infections, ART is the only intervention currently available that has the potential to ameliorate the clinical syndrome. For example, in many cases, ART should be initiated for patients with cryptosporidiosis, certain forms of microsporidiosis, or progressive multifocal leukoencephalopathy.[39-41]

SPECTRUM OF OPPORTUNISTIC PATHOGENS

Patients with HIV infection are highly susceptible to a unique constellation of pathogens. The opportunistic infections that an individual patient develops are heavily influenced by the degree of immunosuppression and by environmental exposures, as well as other factors.

Traditionally, most HIV-associated opportunistic infections were thought to be caused by reactivation of latent infection, but this conclusion was based primarily on speculation rather than data. Some episodes of opportunistic infection, such as outbreaks of multidrug-resistant *Mycobacterium tuberculosis*, clearly represent primary infection. Exogenous reinfection with new strains of tuberculosis, identified by molecular typing systems, has been described.[42,43] As techniques to identify strain variants for various microorganisms become more widely applied, additional information will be forthcoming about how often episodes of *Pneumocystis, Candida,* or CMV infection, for example, represent primary infection or reinfection rather than reactivation.[44,45] Such information will influence strategies for preventing subsequent episodes of opportunistic processes.

The infectious complications of HIV-induced immunosuppression vary geographically because of different exposure patterns. Histoplasmosis, for example, is very common as a cause of pulmonary infiltrates in the Ohio River Valley[46]; *Trypanosoma cruzi* can cause fever and cerebral mass lesions in Brazil[47,48]; *M. tuberculosis* is common in certain parts of New York City, Miami, Africa, and Haiti[42,43,49,50]; *Penicillium marneffei* is well recognized in southern China and Thailand[51]; and isosporiasis is common in Haiti.[52] Specific behavior patterns also influence exposure and, consequently, the infectious manifestations of HIV-induced immunosuppression. For example, homosexual men are much more likely to develop Kaposi's sarcoma or ulcerative perirectal herpes simplex than are patients with other behavioral risk factors.[53]

Many of the opportunistic infections that characterize HIV-induced immunosuppression occur in patients with HIV infection much more frequently than in almost any other patient group. For example, without prophylaxis or effective ART, PCP ultimately develops in at least 80% of HIV-infected patients in North America.[10,20] The annual attack rate for patients with CD4$^+$ T-cell counts lower than 100 cells/mm^3 is probably twice that for patients with severe combined immunodeficiency syndrome and more than 10 times the rate for patients with organ transplants, solid tumors, or most hematologic malignant neoplasms.[54] Disseminated MAC was rarely recognized in humans before the advent of HIV infection, yet it occurs in 30% to 50% of patients with advanced HIV infection in the absence of ART and specific chemoprophylaxis.[24,25,55]

Tuberculosis, cerebral toxoplasmosis, cryptosporidiosis, microsporidiosis, and Kaposi's sarcoma are examples of other processes that cause disease much more commonly in patients with HIV infection than in those with other immunodeficiencies; indeed, their presence should strongly suggest that HIV testing be performed. If a routine enzyme-linked immunosorbent assay (ELISA) or Western blot HIV test result is negative but the CD4$^+$ T-cell count is low, consideration should be given to an unusual strain of HIV that might be missed by the assay kit being used (e.g., HIV-1 type O, HIV-2) or to an immunoglobulin synthetic defect. In such cases, which are uncommon with current testing techniques, the utility of an alternative serologic technique or a plasma viral load assay for HIV should be explored (see Chapter 115).

INFECTIONS DUE TO PATHOGENS THAT ARE NOT OPPORTUNISTIC

Patients with HIV infection develop nonopportunistic as well as opportunistic infections; they are not immune to common, community-acquired, or hospital-acquired pathogens. Therefore, if a patient with HIV infection develops a respiratory syndrome, influenza, *Mycoplasma pneumoniae,* or *Legionella* infection must be considered in the differential diagnosis, although these processes do not occur with increased frequency or severity in patients with HIV infection. Similarly, patients with HIV infection can develop ventilator-associated pneumonia or intravascular access–associated bacteremia or fungemia, and such processes should not be overlooked when assessing fever or new-onset organ dysfunction.

Infections related to patient behavior or exposure must also be considered when evaluating the cause for an infectious syndrome. For example, homosexual men may develop urethral or rectal gonorrhea that does not differ from syndromes seen in HIV-negative patients. Intravenous drug abusers may develop skin infections or bacteremia as a result of their injection drug use. Nonopportunistic pathogens must remain a prominent aspect of the differential diagnosis of infections in this population.

DRUG INTERACTIONS

Some drugs used for treatment or prevention of opportunistic infections can interact with each other or with other drugs such as antiretroviral agents.[38] Such interactions can alter the efficacy and toxicity of prescribed drugs. This most often occurs with drugs that share the same hepatic cytochrome metabolic pathway. Protease inhibitors and non-nucleoside reverse transcriptase inhibitors, as well as rifampin, rifabutin, azoles, and quinolones, need special attention because they are all metabolized by these hepatic enzymes. The interaction of rifampin with saquinavir or ritonavir, for example, can result in very low serum protease inhibitor levels, increasing the likelihood that retroviral resistance will develop. The interaction of fluconazole or a quinolone with rifabutin can augment rifabutin serum levels, increasing the likelihood of rifabutin-related uveitis.[56] The influence of newly introduced drugs on the pharmacokinetics of concurrent drugs needs to be carefully considered.

Drug interactions can occur because of interactions related to absorption or metabolism.

Health care providers must be cognizant that clinically important interactions can be caused by newly prescribed medications or nutritional supplements. Before initiating any new drug, prescription or nonprescription, the implications for the pharmacokinetics of the existing regimen must be considered.

GENERAL PRINCIPLES OF MANAGEMENT

Opportunistic infections commonly seen in HIV-infected patients can be categorized into two groups in terms of response to therapy: those that may respond to conventional or investigational drugs but have a high likelihood of recurring after therapy is discontinued (unless ART substantially increases the CD4+ T-cell count) and those that do not respond to available drugs. (Tuberculosis is one of the few opportunistic infections that rarely recurs after one of the recommended courses of therapy.) The successful management of those opportunistic infections that are treatable depends on (1) prompt diagnosis, (2) initiation of therapy before the clinical syndrome is severe, (3) recognition that a poor response to therapy may indicate that a pathogen other than the one initially identified is present or that the pathogen is resistant to the therapeutic agent employed, and (4) recognition that most therapies must be continued lifelong to prevent relapses or recurrences (unless ART is able to substantially increase the CD4+ T-cell count).

The management of opportunistic infections in HIV-infected patients differs from management in other patient populations because the natural history of specific processes such as PCP or cryptococcosis[57,58] is different in patients with HIV compared with other causes of immunosuppression. HIV-infected patients have a higher frequency of intolerances for therapeutic agents such as trimethoprim-sulfamethoxazole (TMP-SMX) or clindamycin compared with other patient groups.[10,12,57-59] Consideration must also be given to interactions between drugs directed against opportunistic pathogens and the multiplicity of prescription and nonprescription drugs directed against other concomitant processes and HIV itself.[12,38] Such interactions can reduce drug efficacy or augment drug toxicity. The success of long-term management of opportunistic infections is highly dependent on the degree of immunosuppression caused by the underlying disease. In HIV infection, improving the degree of the immunosuppression must be a major focus of management if the opportunistic infection is to be managed or prevented over the long term with maximum efficacy and success.

An issue that frequently arises is whether to use empirical antimicrobial regimens or to withhold therapy until a specific diagnosis is established.[60-64] For some clinical scenarios, such as esophagitis, the presence of a central nervous system (CNS) mass lesion,[62,63] or the presence of active retinitis,[64] empirical therapy is usually reasonable because clinical features, immune profiles, and other noninvasive laboratory tests make correct diagnosis highly likely. In other situations, such as meningitis, fever and wasting, or chronic diarrhea, the clinical presentation is so nonspecific or the consequences of erroneous diagnosis so severe that a definitive diagnosis should be sought.

Frequently, cost is an issue that increases the attractiveness of empirical diagnosis and therapy, especially in situations involving mild presentations (e.g., a patient with fever, cough, and pulmonary infiltrates but a partial pressure of oxygen greater than 85 mm Hg on room air). The empirical approach should be influenced by the CD4+ T-cell count and HIV viral load, because these factors influence which organisms are most likely to be causing the syndrome. In some settings with certain clinical presentations and appropriate strategic considerations, a clinical rather than a laboratory diagnosis is appropriate.

Patients who respond to ART, as manifested by sustained increases in CD4+ T-cell counts, appear to derive substantial protection against opportunistic infection.[65-82] There are sufficient data to recommend that for patients who have raised CD4+ T-cell counts above the thresholds suggested in well-established, evidence-based guidelines,[10] primary prophylaxis (preventing a first episode of disease) or secondary prophylaxis (preventing relapse or recurrence) can be discontinued. (However, histoplasmosis and coccidioidomycosis may be exceptions, in that data are not yet available to convincingly confirm the safety of this approach with these specific pathogens.) Prophylaxis should be restarted if the CD4+ T-cell count subsequently falls below the threshold indicated in the guidelines.[10]

Tables 125-1 through 125-4 summarize current recommendations from the United States Public Health Service and the Infectious Disease Society of America for prophylaxis to prevent first episodes (Table 125-1) or recurrence (Table 125-2) of opportunistic infections; starting, discontinuing, and restarting prophylaxis (Table 125-3); and treatment of acute opportunistic infections (Table 125-4).

Text continues on p. 1684

TABLE 125-1 Prophylaxis to Prevent a First Episode of Opportunistic Disease in Adults and Adolescents Infected with Human Immunodeficiency Virus

| | | Preventive Regimens*† | |
Pathogen	Indication	First Choice	Alternatives
Strongly Recommended as Standard of Care			
Pneumocystis jirovecii	CD4 count <200 or oropharyngeal candidiasis	TMP-SMX, 1 double-strength tablet PO qd [AI], *or* TMP-SMX, 1 single-strength tablet PO qd [AI]	Dapsone, 50 mg PO bid or 100 mg PO qd [BI] Dapsone, 50 mg PO qd, plus pyrimethamine, 50 mg PO every wk, plus leucovorin 25 mg PO every wk [BI] Dapsone, 200 mg PO, plus pyrimethamine, 75 mg PO, plus leucovorin, 25 mg PO every wk [BI] Aerosolized pentamidine, 300 mg every mo via Respirgard II nebulizer [BI] Atovaquone, 1500 mg PO qd [BI] TMP-SMZ, 1 double-strength tablet PO three times per wk [BI]
Mycobacterium tuberculosis (isoniazid-sensitive)	TST reaction ≥5 mm or prior positive TST result without treatment, or contact with case of active TB regardless of TST result [BIII]	Isoniazid, 300 mg PO, plus pyridoxine, 50 mg PO qd × 9 mo [AII], *or* Isoniazid, 900 mg PO, plus pyridoxine, 100 mg PO twice weekly × 9 mo [BII]	Rifampin, 600 mg PO qd × 4 mo [BIII] Rifabutin, 300 mg PO qd × 4 mo [CIII]
M. tuberculosis (isoniazid-resistant)	Same as for isoniazid-sensitive organism; high probability of exposure to isoniazid-resistant TB	Rifampin, 600 mg PO qd × 4 mo [AIII], *or* rifabutin, 300 mg PO qd × 4 mo [BIII]	Pyrazinamide, 15-20 mg/kg PO qd, plus *either* rifampin, 600 mg PO qd × 2 mo [BI], or rifabutin, 300 mg PO qd × 2 mo [CIII]
M. tuberculosis (MDR)	Same as for isoniazid-sensitive organism; high probability of exposure to multidrug-resistant TB	Choice of drugs requires consultation with public health authorities and depends on susceptibility of isolate from source patient	

Continued

TABLE 125-1 Prophylaxis to Prevent a First Episode of Opportunistic Disease in Adults and Adolescents Infected with Human Immunodeficiency Virus—cont'd

		Preventive Regimens*†	
Pathogen	**Indication**	**First Choice**	**Alternatives**
Strongly Recommended as Standard of Care—cont'd			
Toxoplasma gondii	Immunoglobulin G antibody to *Toxoplasma* and CD4 count <100	TMP-SMX, 1 double-strength tablet PO qd [AII]	TMP-SMX, 1 single-strength tablet PO qd [BIII] Dapsone, 50 mg PO qd, plus pyrimethamine, 50 mg PO every wk, plus leucovorin, 25 mg PO every wk [BI] Dapsone, 200 mg PO every wk, plus pyrimethamine, 75 mg PO every wk, plus leucovorin, 25 mg PO every wk [BI] Atovaquone, 1500 mg PO qd with or without pyrimethamine, 25 mg PO qd, plus leucovorin, 10 mg PO qd [CIII]
Mycobacterium avium complex	CD4 count <50	Azithromycin, 1200 mg PO every wk [AI], *or* Clarithromycin, 500 mg PO bid [AI]	Rifabutin, 300 mg PO qd [BI] Azithromycin, 1200 mg PO every wk, plus rifabutin, 300 mg PO qd [CI]
Varicella-zoster virus (VZV)	Significant exposure to chickenpox *or* shingles for patients who have no history of either condition or, if available, negative antibody to VZV	Varicella-zoster immune globulin (VZIG), 5 vials (1.25 mL each) IM, administered ≤96 hr after exposure, ideally within 48 hr [AIII]	None
Generally Recommended			
Streptococcus pneumoniae	CD4 count ≥200	23-Valent polysaccharide vaccine, 0.5 mL IM [BII]	None
Hepatitis B virus	All susceptible (anti-HBc–negative) patients	Hepatitis B vaccine: 3 doses [BII]	None
Influenza virus	All patients (annually, before influenza season)	Inactivated trivalent influenza virus vaccine: 1 annual dose (0.5 mL) IM [BIII]	Oseltamivir, 75 mg PO qd (influenza A or B) [CIII] Rimantadine, 100 mg PO bid (influenza A only) [CIII] Amantadine, 100 mg PO bid (influenza A only) [CIII]
Hepatitis A virus (HAV)	All susceptible (anti-HAV–negative) patients who are at increased risk for HAV infection (e.g., illicit drug users, men who have sex with men, hemophiliacs) or who have chronic liver disease, including chronic hepatitis B or hepatitis C	Hepatitis A vaccine: 2 doses [BIII]	None
Evidence for Efficacy but Not Routinely Indicated			
Bacteria	Neutropenia	G-CSF, 5-10 μg/kg SC qd × 2-4 wk, *or* GM-CSF, 250 μg/m² SC or IV × 2-4 wk [CII]	None
Cryptococcus neoformans	CD4 count <50	Fluconazole, 100-200 mg PO qd [CI]	Itraconazole capsule, 200 mg PO qd [CIII]
Histoplasma capsulatum	CD4 count <100, endemic geographic area	Itraconazole capsule, 200 mg PO qd [CI]	None
Cytomegalovirus	CD4 count <50 and CMV antibody positivity	Oral ganciclovir, 1 g PO tid [CI]‡	None

*Rating strength of the recommendation (in brackets):

 A = Both strong evidence for efficacy and substantial clinical benefit support recommendation for use; should always be offered.

 B = Moderate evidence for efficacy, or strong evidence for efficacy but only limited clinical benefit, supports recommendation for use; should generally be offered.

 C = Evidence for efficacy is insufficient to support a recommendation for or against use, or evidence for efficacy might not outweigh adverse consequences (e.g., drug toxicity, drug interactions) or cost of the chemoprophylaxis or alternative approaches; optional.

 D = Moderate evidence for lack of efficacy or for adverse outcome supports a recommendation against use; should generally not be offered.

 E = Good evidence for lack of efficacy or for adverse outcome supports a recommendation against use; should never be offered.

†Quality of evidence supporting the recommendation (in brackets):

 I = Evidence from at least one properly randomized, controlled trial.

 II = Evidence from at least one well-designed clinical trial without randomization, from cohort or case-controlled analytic studies (preferably from more than one center), or from multiple time-series studies; or, dramatic results from uncontrolled experiments.

 III = Evidence from opinions of respected authorities based on clinical experience, descriptive studies, or reports of expert committees.

‡Since oral ganciclovir is not available in the United States, oral valganciclovir could logically be used, although it has not been extensively studied for primary prophylaxis.

 Anti-HBc, antibody to hepatitis B core antigen; CD4 count, CD4⁺ T-lymphocyte count (cells/mm³); G-CSF, granulocyte colony-stimulating factor; GM-CSF, granulocyte-macrophage colony-stimulating factor; MDR, multidrug-resistant (isoniazid and rifampin); TB, tuberculosis; TMP-SMX, trimethoprim-sulfamethoxazole; TST, tuberculin skin test.

 From U.S. Public Health Service/Infectious Disease Society of America Prevention of Opportunistic Infections Working Group. USPHS/IDSA Guidelines for the Prevention of Opportunistic Infections in Persons Infected with Human Immunodeficiency Virus. 2001. Available at www.aidsinfo.nih.gov. Accessed June 12, 2004.

TABLE 125-2 **Prophylaxis to Prevent Recurrence of Opportunistic Disease (after Chemotherapy for Acute Disease) in Adults and Adolescents Infected with Human Immunodeficiency Virus**

Pathogen	Indication	Preventive Regimens*† First Choice	Alternatives
Recommended as Standard of Care			
Pneumocystis jirovecii	Prior *P. jirovecii* pneumonia (PCP)	TMP-SMX, 1 double-strength tablet PO qd [AI], *or* TMP-SMX, 1 single-strength tablet PO qd [AI]	Dapsone, 50 mg PO bid or 100 mg PO qd [BI] Dapsone, 50 mg PO qd, plus pyrimethamine, 50 mg PO every wk, plus leucovorin, 25 mg PO every wk [BI] Dapsone, 200 mg PO every wk, plus pyrimethamine, 75 mg PO every wk, plus leucovorin, 25 mg PO every wk [BI] Aerosolized pentamidine, 300 mg every mo via Respirgard II nebulizer [BI] Atovaquone, 1500 mg PO qd [BI] TMP-SMZ, 1 double-strength tablet PO three times per wk [CI]
Toxoplasma gondii	Prior toxoplasmic encephalitis	Sulfadiazine, 500-1000 mg PO qid, plus pyrimethamine, 25-50 mg PO qd, plus leucovorin, PO qd [AI]	Clindamycin, 300-450 mg PO q6-8h, plus pyrimethamine, 25-50 mg PO qd, plus leucovorin, 10-25 mg PO qd [BI] Atovaquone, 750 mg PO q6-12h, with or without pyrimethamine, 25 mg PO qd, plus leucovorin, 10 mg PO qd [CIII]
Mycobacterium avium complex	Documented disseminated disease	Clarithromycin, 500 mg PO bid [AI] plus ethambutol, 15 mg/kg PO qd [AII] with or without rifabutin, 300 mg PO qd [CI]	Azithromycin, 500 mg PO qd [AII], plus ethambutol, 15 mg/kg PO qd [AII], with or without rifabutin, 300 mg PO qd [CI]
Cytomegalovirus	Prior end-organ disease	Ganciclovir, 5-6 mg/kg/day IV 5-7 days/wk or 1000 mg PO tid [AI], or foscarnet, 90-120 mg/kg IV qd [AI], *or (for retinitis)* ganciclovir sustained-release implant q6-9mo, plus ganciclovir, 1.0-1.5 g PO tid [AII]‡	Cidofovir, 5 mg/kg IV every other wk, with probenecid, 2 g PO 3 hr before the cidofovir dose followed by 1 g PO 2 hr after the dose and 1 g PO 8 hr after the dose (total of 4 g) [AI] Fomivirsen, 1 vial (330 µg) injected into the vitreous, then repeated q2-4 wk [AI] Valganciclovir, 900 mg PO qd [BI]
Cryptococcus neoformans	Documented disease	Fluconazole, 200 mg PO qd [AI]	Amphotericin B, 0.6-1.0 mg/kg IV once to three times per wk [AI] Itraconazole capsule, 200 mg PO qd [BI]
Histoplasma capsulatum	Documented disease	Itraconazole capsule, 200 mg PO bid [AI]	Amphotericin B, 1.0 mg/kg IV every wk [AI]
Coccidioides immitis	Documented disease	Fluconazole, 400 mg PO qd [AI]	Amphotericin B, 1.0 mg/kg IV every wk [AI] Itraconazole capsule, 200 mg PO bid [AII]
Salmonella species (non-typhi)	Bacteremia	Ciprofloxacin, 500 mg PO bid for several months [BII]	Antibiotic chemoprophylaxis with another active agent [CIII]
Recommended Only If Subsequent Episodes Are Frequent or Severe			
Herpes simplex virus	Frequent/severe recurrences	Acyclovir, 200 mg PO tid or 400 mg PO bid [AI], *or* famciclovir, 250 mg PO bid [AI]	Valacyclovir, 500 mg PO bid [CIII]
Candida (oropharyngeal or vaginal)	Frequent/severe recurrences	Fluconazole, 100-200 mg PO qd [CI]	Itraconazole solution, 200 mg PO qd [CI]
Candida (esophageal)	Frequent/severe recurrences	Fluconazole, 100-200 mg PO qd [BI]	Itraconazole solution, 200 mg PO qd [BI]

*Rating strength of the recommendation (in brackets):

A = Both strong evidence for efficacy and substantial clinical benefit support recommendation for use; should always be offered.

B = Moderate evidence for efficacy, or strong evidence for efficacy but only limited clinical benefit, supports recommendation for use; should generally be offered.

C = Evidence for efficacy is insufficient to support a recommendation for or against use, or evidence for efficacy might not outweigh adverse consequences (e.g., drug toxicity, drug interactions) or cost of the chemoprophylaxis or alternative approaches; optional.

D = Moderate evidence for lack of efficacy or for adverse outcome supports a recommendation against use; should generally not be offered.

E = Good evidence for lack of efficacy or for adverse outcome supports a recommendation against use; should never be offered.

†Quality of evidence supporting the recommendation (in brackets):

I = Evidence from at least one properly randomized, controlled trial.

II = Evidence from at least one well-designed clinical trial without randomization, from cohort or case-controlled analytic studies (preferably from more than one center), or from multiple time-series studies; or, dramatic results from uncontrolled experiments.

III = Evidence from opinions of respected authorities based on clinical experience, descriptive studies, or reports of expert committees.

‡Because oral ganciclovir is no longer available in the United States, oral valganciclovir should be used, although it has not been studied as extensively in this setting. TMP-SMX, trimethoprim-sulfamethoxazole.

From U. S. Public Health Service/Infectious Disease Society of America Prevention of Opportunistic Infections Working Group. USPHS/IDSA Guidelines for Therapy of Opportunistic Infections in Persons Infected with Human Immunodeficiency Virus. 2003. Available at www.aidsinfo.nih.gov. In press.

TABLE 125-3 Criteria for Starting, Discontinuing, and Restarting Opportunistic Infection Prophylaxis in Adults Infected with Human Immunodeficiency Virus*†

Pathogen	Primary Prophylaxis			Secondary Prophylaxis		
	Initiating	*Discontinuing*	*Restarting*	*Initiating*	*Discontinuing*	*Restarting*
Pneumocystis jirovecii pneumonia (PCP)	CD4 count <200 or oropharyngeal candidiasis [AI]	CD4 count >200 for ≥3 mo [AI]	CD4 count <200 [AIII]	Prior PCP [AI]	CD4 count >200 for ≥ 3 mo [BII]	CD4 count <200 [AIII]
Toxoplasmosis	Immunoglobulin G antibody to *Toxoplasma* and CD4 count <100 [AI]	CD4 count >200 for ≥3 mo [AI]	CD4 count <100-200 [AIII]	Prior toxoplasmic encephalitis [AI]	CD4 count >200 sustained (e.g., ≥ 6 mo) + initial MAC therapy completed + asymptomatic for toxoplasmosis [CIII]	CD4 count <200 [AIII]
Disseminated *Mycobacterium avium* complex (MAC)	CD4 count <50 [AI]	CD4 count >100 for ≥3 mo [AI]	CD4 count <50-100 [AIII]	Documented disseminated disease [AII]	CD4 count >100 sustained (e.g., ≥6 mo) + 12 mo of MAC therapy completed + asymptomatic for MAC [CIII]	CD4 count <100 [AIII]
Cryptococcosis	None	NA	NA	Documented disease [AI]	CD4 count >100-200 sustained (e.g., ≥6 mo) + initial therapy completed + asymptomatic for cryptococcosis [CIII]	CD4 count <100-200 [AIII]
Histoplasmosis	None	NA	NA	Documented disease [AI]	No criteria recommended for stopping	NA
Coccidioidomycosis	None	NA	NA	Documented disease [AI]	No criteria recommended for stopping	NA
Cytomegalovirus retinitis	None	NA	NA	Documented end-organ disease [AI]	CD4 count >100-150 sustained (e.g., ≥6 mo) + no evidence of active disease + regular ophthalmic examination [BII]	CD4 count <100-150 [AIII]

*Rating strength of the recommendation (in brackets):

    A = Both strong evidence for efficacy and substantial clinical benefit support recommendation for use; should always be offered.

    B = Moderate evidence for efficacy, or strong evidence for efficacy but only limited clinical benefit, supports recommendation for use; should generally be offered.

    C = Evidence for efficacy is insufficient to support a recommendation for or against use, or evidence for efficacy might not outweigh adverse consequences (e.g., drug toxicity, drug interactions) or cost of the chemoprophylaxis or alternative approaches; optional.

    D = Moderate evidence for lack of efficacy or for adverse outcome supports a recommendation against use; should generally not be offered.

    E = Good evidence for lack of efficacy or for adverse outcome supports a recommendation against use; should never be offered.

†Quality of evidence supporting the recommendation (in brackets):

    I = Evidence from at least one properly randomized, controlled trial.

    II = Evidence from at least one well-designed clinical trial without randomization, from cohort or case-controlled analytic studies (preferably from more than one center), or from multiple time-series studies; or, dramatic results from uncontrolled experiments.

    III = Evidence from opinions of respected authorities based on clinical experience, descriptive studies, or reports of expert committees.

    CD4 count, CD4+ T-lymphocyte count (cells/mm³); NA, not applicable.

From U.S. Public Health Service/Infectious Disease Society of America Prevention of Opportunistic Infections Working Group. USPHS/IDSA Guidelines for the Prevention of Opportunistic Infections in Persons Infected with Human Immunodeficiency Virus. 2001. Available at www.aidsinfo.nih.gov. Accessed April 12, 2004.

OPPORTUNISTIC INFECTIONS

Pneumocystis jirovecii Pneumonia

PCP continues to be a common complication of HIV infection in North America and western Europe, although in some areas of the world it is much less commonly recognized (see Chapter 268).[2,4,10,12,83] Although specific prophylaxis and ART have reduced the number of cases, many patients do not recognize that they have HIV infection until they present with PCP. Other patients fail to take prophylactic medications; some develop PCP despite prophylaxis, especially if the regimen does not include TMP-SMX; and some do not have a sustained response to ART.[57,84-88] Therefore, PCP continues to be a substantial cause of morbidity and mortality.

Pneumocystis disease most often manifests as pulmonary dysfunction in patients with HIV infection. Patients may have chest tightness or exercise intolerance as very early symptoms, before chest radiography results are abnormal and before arterial blood gases reveal hypoxemia.[57] If therapy is to have the greatest chance to succeed, patients and clinicians must be trained to initiate diagnostic evaluation at this stage, before pulmonary dysfunction is severe.[83-90] Even with very mild manifestations of disease, organisms can be recovered readily from sputum or bronchoalveolar lavage, allowing initiation of therapy on an outpatient basis at a stage when prognosis is excellent.[91,92]

In large series of patients, PCP can be distinguished from bacterial pneumonia or tuberculosis by the duration of symptoms, the character of the sputum, and the radiologic manifestations. However, in individual cases, it is much more difficult to reliably distinguish PCP from a variety of other infectious and noninfectious processes, including tuberculosis, histoplasmosis, and nonspecific interstitial pneumonitis.[46,61,93,94] Therefore, it is important to establish a specific diagnosis to ascertain that the correct pathogen is being treated and to avoid the toxicities, cost, and inconvenience of unnecessary drugs. Establishing a specific diagnosis also has epidemiologic implications in terms of ascertaining the isolation precautions or contact tracing that is needed. However, given the cost of a diagnostic evaluation, in some settings it may be necessary to treat mild cases of presumptive PCP empirically.[61] If patients do not improve, the yield of a diagnostic evaluation of *Pneumocystis* infection should not be diminished substantially

Text continues on p. 1692

TABLE 125-4 Treatment of AIDS-Associated Opportunistic Infections in Adults*†

Opportunistic Infections	Preferred Therapy and Duration	Alternative Therapy	Other Options and Issues*
Pneumocystis jirovecii pneumonia (PCP)	*Acute Therapy:* • Trimethoprim-sulfamethoxazole (TMP/SMX): [15-20 mg TMP + 75-100 mg SMX]/kg/day IV given q6h or q8h (AI); *or* • Same daily dose of TMP/SMX PO in 3 divided doses (AI); *or* • TMP-SMX DS 2 tablets tid (AI) Total duration = 21 days (AII); *Chronic Maintenance Therapy:* (Secondary prophylaxis) *First choice:* • TMP-SMX 1 double-strength tablet (DS) PO daily (AI); *or* • TMP-SMX 1 single-strength tablet (SS) PO daily (AI) *Alternatives:* • Dapsone 50 mg PO twice daily or 100 mg daily (BI); *or* • Dapsone 50 mg PO daily plus pyrimethamine 50 mg weekly PO plus leucovorin 25 mg PO weekly (BI); *or* • Dapsone 200 mg PO plus pyrimethamine 75 mg PO plus leucovorin 25 mg PO weekly (BI); aerosolized pentamidine 300 mg every month via Respirgard II nebulizer (manufactured by Marquest, Englewood, CO) (BI); *or* • Atovaquone 1500 mg PO daily (BI); *or* • TMP-SMX 1 DS PO three times weekly (CI)	*For Severe PCP:* Pentamidine 4 mg/kg IV qd infused over at least 60 min (AI); some experts reduce dose to 3 mg/kg IV qd because of toxicities (BI) *For Mild to Moderate PCP:* • Dapsone 100 mg PO qd + TMP 15 mg/kg/day PO (3 divided doses) (BI); *or* • Primaquine 15-30 mg (base) PO qd + clindamycin 600-900 mg IV q6h to q8h or clindamycin 300-450 mg PO q6h to q8h (BI); *or* • Atovaquone 750 mg PO bid with food (BI); *or* • Trimetrexate 45 mg/m² or 1.2 mg/kg IV qd with leucovorin 20 mg/m² or 0.5 mg/kg IV or PO q6h (leucovorin must be continued for 3 days after the last trimetrexate dose) (BI); addition of dapsone or SMX or sulfadiazine may improve efficacy (CIII)	Indications for corticosteroids (AI): Pao₂ <70 mm Hg at room air; *or* alveolar-arterial O₂ gradient >35 mm Hg Prednisone doses (beginning as early as possible and within 72 h of PCP therapy) (AI): 40 mg bid days 1-5, 40 mg qd days 6-10, then 20 mg qd days 11-21 IV methylprednisolone can be given as 75% of prednisone dose *Chronic Maintenance Therapy* (Secondary prophylaxis) should be discontinued if CD4⁺ T lymphocyte count increases in response to ART from <200 to >200 cells/μL for >3 months (BII)
Toxoplasma gondii encephalitis	*Acute Therapy:* Pyrimethamine 200 mg PO × 1, then 50 mg (<60 kg) to 75 mg (≥60 kg) PO qd + sulfadiazine 1000 (<60 kg) to 1500 mg (≥60 kg) PO q6h + leucovorin 10-20 mg PO qd (can increase up to 50 mg or higher) (AI) Total duration for acute therapy = at least 6 wk (BII) *Chronic Maintenance Therapy:* (Secondary prophylaxis) *First choice:* • Sulfadiazine 500-1000 mg PO four times daily + pyrimethamine 25-50 mg PO qd + leucovorin 10-25 mg (AI) *Second choice:* • Clindamycin 300-450 mg PO every 6-8 hr + pryimethamine 25-50 mg PO qd + leucovorin 10-25 PO qd (BI); *or* • Atovaquone 750 mg PO every 6-12 hr with or without pyrimethamine 25 mg PO qd + leucovorin 10 mg PO qd (CIII) • Continue with 50% of acute dose for patients on pyrimethamine + sulfadiazine or clindamycin (AI) or those receiving TMP-SMX (BII); *or* • [Pyrimethamine 50 mg qd + leucovorin 15 mg qd + sulfadiazine 1 gm q12h] given tiw (AI); *or* • Full dose of alternative regimens continued indefinitely (CIII)	• Pyrimethamine (leucovorin)‡ + clindamycin 600 mg IV or PO q6h (AI); *or* • TMP-SMX (5 mg/kg TMP + 25 mg/kg SMX) IV or PO bid (BI); *or* • Atovaquone 1500 mg PO bid with meals (or nutritional supplement) + pyrimethamine (leucovorin)‡ (BII); *or* • Atovaquone 1500 mg PO bid with meals (or nutritional supplement) + sulfadiazine 1000-1500 mg PO q6h (BII); *or* • Atovaquone 1500 mg PO bid with meals (BII); *or* • Pyrimethamine (leucovorin)‡ + azithromycin 900-1200 mg PO qd (BII) *For severely ill patients who cannot take oral meds:* TMP-SMX IV + pyrimethamine PO (CIII) For other regimens with limited experience (CIII), see text.	Adjunctive corticosteroids (e.g., dexamethasone) should be given when clinically indicated for treatment of mass effect due to focal lesions or associated edema (BIII) and discontinued as soon as clinically feasible Anticonvulsants should be administered to patients with a history of seizures (AIII) *Secondary prophylaxis may be discontinued if:* • Free of *Toxoplasma* encephalitis signs and symptoms; and sustained CD4⁺ T lymphocyte count of >200 cells/μL for ≥6 months of ART (CIII)

Continued

*Rating strength of the recommendation (in brackets):

    A = Both strong evidence for efficacy and substantial clinical benefit support recommendation for use; should always be offered.

    B = Moderate evidence for efficacy, or strong evidence for efficacy but only limited clinical benefit, supports recommendation for use; should generally be offered.

    C = Evidence for efficacy is insufficient to support a recommendation for or against use, or evidence for efficacy might not outweigh adverse consequences (e.g., drug toxicity, drug interactions) or cost of the chemoprophylaxis or alternative approaches; optional.

    D = Moderate evidence for lack of efficacy or for adverse outcome supports a recommendation against use; should generally not be offered.

    E = Good evidence for lack of efficacy or for adverse outcome supports a recommendation against use; should never be offered.

†Quality of evidence supporting the recommendation (in brackets):

    I = Evidence from at least one properly randomized, controlled trial.

    II = Evidence from at least one well-designed clinical trial without randomization, from cohort or case-controlled analytic studies (preferably from more than one center), or from multiple time-series studies; or, dramatic results from uncontrolled experiments.

    III = Evidence from opinions of respected authorities based on clinical experience, descriptive studies, or reports of expert committees.

‡Pyrimethamine and leucovorin doses—same as in "preferred therapy" for toxoplasmosis.

§Pyrazinamide dose: <55 kg = 1000 mg; 56-75 kg = 1500 mg; ≥76 kg = 2000 mg; ethambutol dose: <55 kg = 800 mg; 56-75 kg = 1200 mg; ≥76 kg = 1600 mg.

∥In HIV-HBV coinfected patients who do not need HIV therapy but who have HBeAg⁺ chronic hepatitis B and ALT higher than twice normal, some authorities would recommend treating HBV with interferon-alfa provided there is no evidence of hepatic decompensation. This strategy spares the patient from developing HIV and HBV resistance to lamivudine therapy and from the toxicity of ART.

ART, antiretroviral therapy; HAART, highly active antiretroviral therapy; IM, intramuscular; IV, intravenous; PO, oral; SQ, subcutaneous; qd, daily; bid, twice a day; tid, three times daily; qid, four times a day; tiw, three times weekly; wk, weeks, q'n'h, every 'n' hour.

From U.S. Public Health Service/Infectious Disease Society of America. USPHS/IDSA Guidelines for Therapy of Opportunistic Infections in Persons Infected with Human Immunodeficiency Virus. 2004. Available at www.aidsinfo.nih.gov. In press.

TABLE 125-4 Treatment of AIDS-Associated Opportunistic Infections in Adults*†—cont'd

Opportunistic Infections	Preferred Therapy and Duration	Alternative Therapy	Other Options and Issues*
Cryptosporidiosis	Symptomatic treatment of diarrhea (AIII) Effective ART therapy (to increase CD4+ count to >100 cells/μL) can result in complete sustained clinical, microbiologic, and histologic resolution of HIV-associated cryptosporidiosis (AII)	Nitazoxanide 500 mg PO bid Paromomycin 25-35 mg/kg PO in 2 to 4 divided doses	Supportive care including hydration, nutritional support
Microsporidiosis	Initiate or optimize ART with immune reconstitution to CD4 >100 cells/μL (AII) *For disseminated (not ocular) and intestinal infection due to microsporidia other than Enterocytozoon bienuesi:* • Albendazole 400 mg PO bid (AII), continue until CD4 >200 cells/μL (AIII) *For ocular infection:* • Fumidil B 3 mg/mL in saline (final conc. = fumagillin 70 μg/mL) eye drops continued indefinitely (not available in US) (BII) + albendazole 400 mg PO bid for management of systemic infection (BIII) *For gastrointestinal infections due to Enterocytozoon bienuesi:* • Fumagillin 60 mg PO qd (not available in US) (BII)	*Disseminated disease:* Itraconazole 400 mg PO qd + albendazole for disseminated disease due to *Trachipleistophora* or *Brachiola* (CIII)	Fluid support in patients with diarrhea resulting in severe dehydration (AIII) Nutritional supplement for patients with severe malnutrition and wasting (AIII) Treatment for ocular infection should be continued indefinitely (BIII). With immune reconstitution, it is possible that this treatment can be discontinued (CIII) Chronic maintenance therapy may be discontinued if patients (CII): • Remain asymptomatic with regard to signs and symptoms of microsporidiosis • Sustained CD4+ T-lymphocyte counts >200 cells/μL for ≥6 months on ART
Mycobacterium tuberculosis (MTB)	**For Drug-Sensitive MTB** *Initial Phase (8 weeks, AI):* Isoniazid (INH) 5 mg/kg (max 300 mg) PO qd + [rifampin 10 mg/kg (max 600 mg) PO qd or rifabutin 300 mg PO qd (or dose adjusted based on concomitant meds‡)] + pyrazinamide (PZA) (dose based on wt§) PO qd + ethambutol (EMB) (dose based on wt§) PO qd *Continuation Phase (18 weeks, AI)* • INH 5 mg/kg (max 300 mg) PO qd + [rifampin 10 mg/kg (max 600 mg) or rifabutin 300 mg PO or qd]; *or* • INH 15 mg/kg (max 900 mg) PO biw or tiw + [rifampin 10 mg/kg (max 600 mg) or rifabutin 300 mg PO or tiw] In patients with delayed clinical or microbiologic response to initial therapy (e.g., sputum culture [+] after 2 months or if cavitary pulmonary lesions are present), total duration up to 9 months (BII)	**Treatment for Drug-Resistant MTB:** *Resistant to INH:* • Discontinue INH (and streptomycin, if used) • Rifamycin, PZA, and EMB × 6 months (BII); *or* • Rifamycin + EMB × 12 months (preferably with PZA during at least first 2 months) (BII) *Resistant to rifamycin:* • INH + PZA + EMB + a fluoroquinolone (e.g., levofloxacin 500 mg/day) for 2 months, followed by 10-16 additional months with INH + EMB + fluoroquinolone (BIII) *Multidrug resistant (MDR) TB—both INH and rifamycin resistant:* • Therapy should be individualized based on resistance pattern and with close consultation with experienced specialist (AIII) **TB Treatment in Patients with Liver Disease** *If AST >3× normal prior to treatment initiation:* • Standard therapy with frequent monitoring; *or* • Rifamycin + EMB + PZA × 6 months • INH + rifamycin + EMB × 2 months, then INH + rifamycin × 7 months (BII) *For patients with severe liver disease:* • Rifamycin + EMB × 12 months (preferably with another agent such as fluoroquinolone for first 2 months) (CII)	Treatment by Directly Observed Therapy (DOT) is strongly recommended for all HIV patients (AII) Rifabutin has less drug interaction potential and can be used in place of rifampin Rifapentine given once weekly can result in development of resistance; it is not recommended in HIV patients (EI) Twice weekly intermittent regimen containing rifamycin may lead to rifamycin resistance, particularly in advanced HIV patients with CD4 cell count <100 cells/μL; in this situation, therapy must be given as daily or three times weekly For paradoxical reaction that is not severe: may be treated with nonsteroidal anti-inflammatory drugs (NSAIDs) without change in TB or HIV medications (BIII)

*Rating strength of the recommendation (in brackets):

    A = Both strong evidence for efficacy and substantial clinical benefit support recommendation for use; should always be offered.

    B = Moderate evidence for efficacy, or strong evidence for efficacy but only limited clinical benefit, supports recommendation for use; should generally be offered.

    C = Evidence for efficacy is insufficient to support a recommendation for or against use, or evidence for efficacy might not outweigh adverse consequences (e.g., drug toxicity, drug interactions) or cost of the chemoprophylaxis or alternative approaches; optional.

    D = Moderate evidence for lack of efficacy or for adverse outcome supports a recommendation against use; should generally not be offered.

    E = Good evidence for lack of efficacy or for adverse outcome supports a recommendation against use; should never be offered.

†Quality of evidence supporting the recommendation (in brackets):

    I = Evidence from at least one properly randomized, controlled trial.

    II = Evidence from at least one well-designed clinical trial without randomization, from cohort or case-controlled analytic studies (preferably from more than one center), or from multiple time-series studies; or, dramatic results from uncontrolled experiments.

    III = Evidence from opinions of respected authorities based on clinical experience, descriptive studies, or reports of expert committees.

‡Pyrimethamine and leucovorin doses—same as in "preferred therapy" for toxoplasmosis.

§Pyrazinamide dose: <55 kg = 1000 mg; 56-75 kg = 1500 mg; ≥76 kg = 2000 mg; ethambutol dose: <55 kg = 800 mg; 56-75 kg = 1200 mg; ≥76 kg = 1600 mg.

‖In HIV-HBV coinfected patients who do not need HIV therapy but who have HBeAg+ chronic hepatitis B and ALT higher than twice normal, some authorities would recommend treating HBV with interferon-alfa provided there is no evidence of hepatic decompensation. This strategy spares the patient from developing HIV and HBV resistance to lamivudine therapy and from the toxicity of ART.

ART, antiretroviral therapy; HAART, highly active antiretroviral therapy; IM, intramuscular; IV, intravenous; PO, oral; SQ, subcutaneous; qd, daily; bid, twice a day; tid, three times daily; qid, four times a day; tiw, three times weekly; wk, weeks, q'n'h, every 'n' hour.

From U.S. Public Health Service/Infectious Disease Society of America. USPHS/IDSA Guidelines for Therapy of Opportunistic Infections in Persons Infected with Human Immunodeficiency Virus. 2004. Available at www.aidsinfo.nih.gov. In press.

TABLE 125-4 Treatment of AIDS-Associated Opportunistic Infections in Adults*†—cont'd

Opportunistic Infections	Preferred Therapy and Duration	Alternative Therapy	Other Options and Issues*
Mycobacterium avium complex disease	At least two drugs as initial therapy: Clarithromycin 500 mg PO bid (AI) + ethambutol 15 mg/kg PO qd (AI) Consider adding third drug for patients with advanced immunosuppression (CD4 <50), high mycobacterial loads, or in the absence of effective ART: Rifabutin 300 mg PO qd (AI) (dosage may be adjusted based on drug-drug interactions) (CIII) *Duration (chronic maintenance therapy):* Lifelong therapy unless in patients with sustained immune recovery on ART (AII). *Chronic Maintenance Therapy:* (Secondary prophylaxis) *First choice:* • Clarithromycin 500 mg PO bid (AI) plus ethambutol 15 mg/kg body weight PO qd (AII); with or without rifabutin 300 mg PO qd (CI) *Second choice:* • Azithromycin 500 mg PO qd (AII) plus ethambutol 15 mg/kg body weight PO qd (AII); with or without rifabutin 300 mg PO qd (CI)	*Alternative to clarithromycin:* Azithromycin 500-600 mg PO qd (AII) *Alternative third or fourth drug for patients with more severe symptoms or disseminated disease (CIII):* • Ciprofloxacin 500-750 mg PO bid; *or* • Levofloxacin 500 mg PO qd; *or* • Amikacin 10-15 mg/kg IV qd	NSAIDs may be used for patients who experience moderate to severe symptoms due to ART-associated immune reconstitution syndrome (CIII) If symptoms persist, short term (4-8 wk of systemic corticosteroid) (20-40 mg of prednisone) can be used. (CIII) Maintenance therapy can be discontinued in patients who (CIII): • Completed ≥12 months therapy, and • Remain asymptomatic, and • Have sustained (>6 months) CD4 count >100 cells/μL
Bacterial pneumonia	*Empiric therapy (targeting toward* Streptococcus pneumoniae *and* Haemophilus influenzae*):* • Extended spectrum cephalosporin (e.g., cefotaxime or ceftriaxone) (AIII); *or* • Fluoroquinolone with enhanced activity against pneumococcus (e.g., gatifloxacin, levofloxacin, or moxifloxacin) (AIII) *Empiric therapy in patients with severe illness:* • Extended-spectrum cephalosporin + a macrolide (AIII)	*For high-level penicillin-resistant isolates (MIC ≥4.0 μg/mL):* • Consider adding vancomycin or a fluoroquinolone (CIII) • *Empiric therapy in patients with severe immunodeficiency (CD4 <100), a known history of prior Pseudomonas infection, bronchiectasis, or relative or absolute neutropenia (BIII):* Broaden empiric coverage to include antimicrobials with activities against *P. aeruginosa* and other gram-negative bacilli—e.g., ceftazidime, cefepime, piperacillin-tazobactam, a carbapenem, or high-dose ciprofloxacin or levofloxacin • If ceftazidime or ciprofloxacin is used, addition of another antibacterial with optimal coverage for gram-positive infection is recommended • TMP-SMX PO or IV (BIII) • Third-generation cephalosporin—such as ceftriaxone (IV) or cefotaxime (IV) (BIII)	Patients with CD4+ T-lymphocyte count of ≥200 cells/μL should receive a single dose of 23-valent polysaccharide pneumococcal vaccine (if not received in the past 5 yr) (BII) Yearly influenza vaccine may be useful in preventing pneumococcal superinfection after influenza respiratory infection (BII) Antibiotic prophylaxis may be considered in patients with frequent recurrences (CIII); caution should be taken for the risks of development of drug resistance and drug toxicities
Salmonellosis	*Salmonella gastroenteritis:* • Ciprofloxacin 500 mg-750 mg PO bid (or 400 mg IV bid) (AIII) *Duration:* • Mild gastroenteritis without bacteremia: 7-14 days (BIII) • Advanced HIV (CD4 <200) and/or bacteremia: at least 4-6 wk (BIII) *Chronic Suppressive Therapy:* • For patients who relapse after cessation of therapy—to be given for several months or until ART-induced immune reconstitution (BIII) • For patients with *Salmonella* bacteremia—ciprofloxacin 500 mg bid (BII)		Treatment is recommended in HIV patients owing to high risk of bacteremia in this population (BIII) Newer fluoroquinolones (e.g., levofloxacin, gatifloxacin, or moxifloxacin) may also be effective (BIII)
Campylobacter jejuni infections	*For mild disease*—may withhold therapy unless symptoms persist for > several days Optimal therapy—not well defined; options include • Ciprofloxacin 500 mg PO bid (BIII); *or* • Azithromycin 500 mg PO qd (BIII) • Consider addition of an aminoglycoside in bacteremic patients (CIII) *Duration:* • Mild to moderate disease: 7 days • Bacteremia: at least 2 wk		There is an increasing rate of quinolone resistance Antimicrobial therapy should be modified based on susceptibility reports Role of aminoglycoside is unclear
Shigellosis	Fluoroquinolone IV or PO × 3-7 days (AIII) Duration for bacteremia: 14 days (AIII)	• TMP-SMX DS 1 tab PO bid 3-7 days; *or* (BIII) • Azithromycin 500 mg PO on day 1, then 250 mg PO qd × 4 days (BIII) Duration for bacteremia: 14 days (AIII)	Therapy is indicated both to shorten the duration of illness and to prevent spread of infection (AIII) *Shigella* infections acquired outside of US have high rates of TMP-SMX resistance
Bartonella infections	*Non-CNS infections* • Erythromycin 500 mg PO qid (or IV at same dose if unable to take PO) (AII); *or* • Doxycycline 100 mg PO or IV q12h (AII) *CNS infections:* • Doxycycline 100 mg PO or IV q12h (AIII) *Duration:* At least 3 months (AII) Life-long therapy for patients with relapse (AIII)	• Azithromycin 600 mg PO qd (BIII) • Clarithromycin 500 mg PO bid (BII) • Fluoroquinolones have variable activity in case reports and in vitro; may be considered as alternative (CIII)	

Continued

TABLE 125-4 Treatment of AIDS-Associated Opportunistic Infections in Adults*†—cont'd

Opportunistic Infections	Preferred Therapy and Duration	Alternative Therapy	Other Options and Issues*
Treponema pallidum infection (syphilis)	*Early Stage (primary, secondary, and early latent syphilis):* • Benzathine penicillin G 2.4 MIU IM × 1 (AII) *Late-Latent Disease (>1 yr or of unknown duration, without CNS involvement)* • Benzathine penicillin G 2.4 MIU IM weekly × 3 (AIII) *Late-Stage (Aortitis and gummata)* • Infectious diseases consultation (AIII) *Neurosyphilis (CNS involvement including otic and ocular disease)* • Aqueous crystalline penicillin G 3-4 MIU IV q4h or total dose by continuous IV infusion × 10-14 days (AII) +/− benzathine penicillin G 2.4 MIU IM weekly × 3 after completion of IV therapy (CIII)	*Early Stage (primary, secondary, and early latent syphilis)—treatment with close clinical monitoring (BIII)* • Doxycycline 100 mg PO bid × 14 days; or • Ceftriaxone 1 gm IM or IV qd × 8-10 days; or • Azithromycin 2 gm PO × 1 dose *Late-Latent Disease (without CNS involvement)* • Doxycycline 100 mg PO bid × 28 days (BIII) *Neurosyphilis* • Procaine penicillin 2.4 MIU IM qd + probenecid 500 mg PO qid × 10-14 days (BII) +/− benzathine penicillin G. 2.4 MIU IM weekly × 3 after completion of above (CIII); or • *For penicillin-allergic pts—*Ceftriaxone 2 g IM or IV qd × 10-14 days (CIII)	Desensitization to penicillin may be a better option than ceftriaxone in penicillin-allergic patients with neurosyphillis (BIII) Combination of procaine penicillin + probenecid is not recommended for patients with history of sulfa allergy, as these patients may be at risk of hypersensitivity reactions to probenecid
Candidiasis (mucosal)	*Oropharyngeal Candidiasis:* *Initial episodes (7-14 day treatment):* • Fluconazole 100 mg PO qd (AI); or • Itraconazole oral solution 200 mg PO qd (AI); or • Clotrimazole troches 10 mg PO 5 × qd (BII); or • Nystatin suspension 4-6 mL qid or 1-2 flavored pastilles 4-5 × qd (BII) *Esophageal Candidiasis (14-21 days):* • Fluconazole 100 mg (up to 400 mg) PO or IV qd (AI); or • Itraconazole oral solution 200 mg PO qd (AI) *Vulvovaginitis:* • Topical azoles (clotrimazole, butoconazole, miconazole, tionazole, or terconazole) × 3-7 days (AII) • Topical nystatin × 14 days (AII) • Oral itraconazole 200 mg bid × 1 day or 200 mg qd × 3 days (AII) • Oral fluconazole 150 mg × 1 dose (AII)	*Fluconazole-Refractory Oropharyngeal Candidiasis:* • Itraconazole oral solution ≥200 mg PO qd (BII); or • Amphotericin B suspension 100 mg/mL (not available in US)—1 mL PO qid (BII); or • Amphotericin B deoxycholate 0.3 mg/kg IV qd (BII); or • Caspofungin 50 mg qd (AII) • Voriconazole 200 mg PO bid (BII) *Fluconazole-Refractory Esophageal Candidiasis:* • Caspofungin 50 mg qd (AII); or • Voriconazole 200 mg PO or IV bid (AII) • Amphotericin B 0.3-0.7 mg/kg IV qd (CIII); or • Amphotericin liposomal or lipid complex 3-5 mg/kg IV qd (CIII) *C. glabrata and other non-albicans Candida:* • Caspofungin (BII); or • Amphotericin B preparations (BIII)	*Suppressive therapy: generally not recommended (DIII) unless patients have frequent or severe recurrences* • *Oropharyngeal candidiasis—*fluconazole or itraconazole oral solution may be considered (CI) • *Vulvovaginal candidiasis—*daily topical azole for recurrent cases (CII) • *Esophageal candidiasis—*fluconazole 100-200 mg qd (BI) Chronic or prolonged use of azoles may promote development of resistance
Cryptococcus neoformans meningitis	*Acute Infection:* • Amphotericin B deoxycholate 0.7 mg/kg IV qd ± flucytosine 25 mg/kg PO qid × 2 wk (AI); or • Liposomal amphotericin B 4 mg/kg IV qd ± flucytosine 25 mg/kg PO qid × 2 wk (AI) *Consolidation Therapy:* • Fluconazole 400 mg PO qd × 8 wk or until CSF cultures are sterile (AI) *Chronic Maintenance Therapy:* (Secondary prophylaxis) *First choice:* • Fluconazole 200 mg PO qd (AI); *Second choice* • Amphotericin B 0.6-1.0 mg/kg body weight intravenously weekly-three times (AI); or • Itraconazole 200 mg capsule PO qd (BI)	*Acute Infection (Alternative):* • Amphotericin B 0.7 mg/kg/day IV × 2 wk (BI); or • Fluconazole 400-800 mg/day (PO or IV) for less severe disease • Fluconazole 400-800 mg/day (PO or IV) + flucytosine 25 mg/kg PO qid for 4-6 wk (BII) *Consolidation Therapy (alternative):* • Itraconazole 200 mg PO bid (BI) *Maintenance Therapy (alternative):* • Amphotericin B 1 mg/kg IV per week—for patients with multiple relapse on azole(s) or intolerant of azole(s) (CI); or • Itraconazole 200 mg PO qd—for patients intolerance of or failed fluconazole (BI)	Repeated lumbar puncture may be indicated as adjunctive therapy for patients with increased intracranial pressure (AII) Discontinuation of antifungal therapy can be considered in patients who remain asymptomatic, with CD4+ T-lymphocyte count >100-200 cells/μL for >6 months (CIII) Some may consider performing a lumbar puncture before discontinuation of maintenance therapy

*Rating strength of the recommendation (in brackets):

A = Both strong evidence for efficacy and substantial clinical benefit support recommendation for use; should always be offered.

B = Moderate evidence for efficacy, or strong evidence for efficacy but only limited clinical benefit, supports recommendation for use; should generally be offered.

C = Evidence for efficacy is insufficient to support a recommendation for or against use, or evidence for efficacy might not outweigh adverse consequences (e.g., drug toxicity, drug interactions) or cost of the chemoprophylaxis or alternative approaches; optional.

D = Moderate evidence for lack of efficacy or for adverse outcome supports a recommendation against use; should generally not be offered.

E = Good evidence for lack of efficacy or for adverse outcome supports a recommendation against use; should never be offered.

†Quality of evidence supporting the recommendation (in brackets):

I = Evidence from at least one properly randomized, controlled trial.

II = Evidence from at least one well-designed clinical trial without randomization, from cohort or case-controlled analytic studies (preferably from more than one center), or from multiple time-series studies; or, dramatic results from uncontrolled experiments.

III = Evidence from opinions of respected authorities based on clinical experience, descriptive studies, or reports of expert committees.

‡Pyrimethamine and leucovorin doses—same as in "preferred therapy" for toxoplasmosis.

§Pyrazinamide dose: <55 kg = 1000 mg; 56-75 kg = 1500 mg; ≥76 kg = 2000 mg; ethambutol dose: <55 kg = 800 mg; 56-75 kg = 1200 mg; ≥76 kg = 1600 mg.

∥In HIV-HBV coinfected patients who do not need HIV therapy but who have HBeAg+ chronic hepatitis B and ALT higher than twice normal, some authorities would recommend treating HBV with interferon-alfa provided there is no evidence of hepatic decompensation. This strategy spares the patient from developing HIV and HBV resistance to lamivudine therapy and from the toxicity of ART.

ART, antiretroviral therapy; HAART, highly active antiretroviral therapy; IM, intramuscular; IV, intravenous; PO, oral; SQ, subcutaneous; qd, daily; bid, twice a day; tid, three times daily; qid, four times a day; tiw, three times weekly; wk, weeks, q'n'h, every 'n' hour.

From U.S. Public Health Service/Infectious Disease Society of America. USPHS/IDSA Guidelines for Therapy of Opportunistic Infections in Persons Infected with Human Immunodeficiency Virus. 2004. Available at www.aidsinfo.nih.gov. In press.

TABLE 125-4 Treatment of AIDS-Associated Opportunistic Infections in Adults*†—cont'd

Opportunistic Infections	Preferred Therapy and Duration	Alternative Therapy	Other Options and Issues*
Histoplasma capsulatum infections	**Severe Disseminated:** *Acute Phase (3-10 days or until clinically improved):* • Amphotericin B deoxycholate 0.7 mg/kg IV qd (AI); *or* • Liposomal amphotericin B 4 mg/kg IV qd (AI) *Continuation Phase (12 wk):* • Itraconazole 200 mg cap PO bid (AII) **Less Severe Disseminated:** • Itraconazole 200 mg cap PO tid × 3 days, then 200 mg PO bid × 12 wks (AII) **Meningitis:** • Amphotericin B deoxycholate or liposomal × 12-16 wk (AII) *Chronic Maintenance Therapy (chronic suppression):* • Itraconazole 200 mg cap PO bid (AI) *Chronic Maintenance Therapy:* (Secondary prophylaxis) *First choice:* • Itraconazole capsule 200 mg PO bid (AI) *Second choice:* • Amphotericin B 1 mg/kg body weight intravenously weekly (AI); *or* • Itraconazole 200 mg capsule PO bid (AII)	**Severe Disseminated:** *Acute Phase (alternative):* • Itraconazole 400 mg IV qd (BIII) *Continuation Phase Alternatives:* • Itraconazole oral solution • Fluconazole 800 mg qd (CII) **Mild Disseminated:** • Fluconazole 800 mg PO qd (CII)	Acute pulmonary histoplasmosis in HIV-1–infected patients with CD4+ T-lymphocye count >500 cells/µL— may require no therapy (AIII) Some experts would consider discontinuing chronic maintenance therapy (secondary prophylaxis) (CIII) in patients who are: • In remission • Completed 1 yr itraconazole • CD4 cells count >100 cells/µL
Coccidiodomycosis	**Nonmeningeal Infection:** *Acute Phase (diffuse pulmonary or disseminated disease):* • Amphotericin B deoxycholate 0.5-1.0 mg/kg IV qd continue until clinical improvement, usually 500-1,000 mg total dose (AII) *Acute Phase (milder disease):* • Fluconazole 400-800 mg PO qd (BIII); *or* • Itraconazole 200 mg PO bid (BIII) **Meningeal Infections:** • Fluconazole 400-800 mg IV or PO qd (AII) *Chronic Maintenance Therapy (AII):* • Fluconazole 400 mg PO qd; *or* • Itraconazole 200 mg PO bid *Chronic Maintenance Therapy* (Secondary prophylaxis) *First choice:* • Fluconazole 400 mg PO qd (AII) *Second choice:* • Amphotericin B 1 mg/kg body weight intravenously weekly (AI); *or* • Itraconazole 200 mg capsule PO bid (AII)	**Nonmeningeal Infection:** *Acute Phase (diffuse pulmonary or disseminated disease):* • Some experts add azole to amphotericin B therapy (BIII) **Meningeal Infections:** • Intrathecal amphoterin B (CI)	Not enough data to recommend discontinuation of chronic maintenance therapy at this point
Invasive aspergillosis	Voriconazole 400 mg IV or PO q12h × 2 days, then 200 mg q12h (AIII) *Duration of therapy:* based on clinical response	• Amphotericin B deoxycholate 1 mg/kg/day IV (AIII); *or* • Lipid formulations of amphotericin B 5 mg/kg/day IV (AIII) • Voriconazole + caspofungin (CIII)	Not enough data to recommend chronic suppression or maintenance therapy (CIII)
Cytomegalovirus (CMV) disease	**CMV Retinitis:** *For immediate sight-threatening lesions:* Ganciclovir (GCV) intraocular implant + valganciclovir 900 mg PO qd (AI) *For peripheral lesions:* Valganciclovir 900 mg PO bid × 14-21 days, then 900 mg PO qd (AII) *Duration of chronic maintenance therapy:* • Implant—replace every 6 to 8 months until immune recovery on ART • Systemic therapy—continue for life (AI) or until immune recovery on ART (BII) *Chronic Maintenance Therapy:* (Secondary prophylaxis) *First choice:* • Ganciclovir 5-6 mg/kg body weight/day intravenously 5-7 days weekly or 1000 mg PO tid (AI); *or* • Foscarnet 90-120 mg/kg body weight intravenously qd (AI); *or* • For retinitis, ganciclovir sustained-release implant every 6-9 months plus ganciclovir 1.0-1.5 gm PO tid (AI) *Second choice:* • Cidofovir 5 mg/kg body weight intravenously every other week with probenecid 2 gm PO 3 hours before the dose followed by 1 gm PO 2 hours after the dose, and 1 gm PO 8 hours after the dose (total of 4 gm) (AI); *or*	**CMV Retinitis:** • Valganciclovir 900 mg PO bid × 14-21 days, then 900 mg PO qd (BII) • Ganciclovir intraocular implant + valganciclovir 900 mg PO qd (AI): *or* • Ganciclovir 5 mg/kg IV q12h × 14-21 days, then 5 mg/kg IV qd (AI); *or* • Ganciclovir 5 mg/kg IV q12h × 14-21 days, then valganciclovir 900 mg PO qd (AI); *or* • Foscarnet 60 mg/kg IV q8h or 90 mg/kg IV q12h × 14-21 days, then 90-120 mg/kg IV q24h (AI); *or* • Cidofovir 5 mg/kg IV × 2 wk, then 5 mg/kg every other week; each dose should be given with IV saline hydration and oral probenecid (AI); *or* • Repeated intravitreal injections with fomivirsen (for relapses only, not as initial therapy) (AI)	Choice of initial therapy for CMV retinitis should be individualized, based on location and severity of the lesion(s), level of immunosuppression, and other factors such as concomitant medications and ability to adhere to treatment (AIII) Initial therapy in patients with CMV retinitis, esophagitis, colitis, and pneumonitis should include optimization of ART (BIII) Some experts suggest delaying ART in patients with CMV neurologic disease owing to concerns of worsening of condition as a result of immune recovery inflammatory reaction (CIII) Preemptive treatment of patients with CMV viremia without evidence of organ involvement is generally not recommended (DIII)

Continued

TABLE 125-4 Treatment of AIDS-Associated Opportunistic Infections in Adults*†—cont'd

Opportunistic Infections	Preferred Therapy and Duration	Alternative Therapy	Other Options and Issues*
Cytomegalovirus (CMV) disease, cont'd	• Fomivirsen 1 vial (330 μg) injected into the vitreous, then repeated every 2-4 wk (AI); *or* • Valganciclovir 900 mg PO qd (BI) **CMV Esophagitis or Colitis:** • Ganciclovir IV or foscarnet IV × 21-28 days or until signs and symptoms have resolved (BII); oral valganciclovir may be used if symptoms are not severe enough to interfere with oral absorption (BII) • Maintenance therapy is generally not necessary, but should be considered after relapses (BII) **CMV Pneumonitis:** • Treatment should be considered in patients with histologic evidence of CMV pneumonitis who do not respond to treatment of other pathogens (AIII) • The role of maintenance therapy is not yet established (CIII) **CMV Neurologic Disease:** • GCV IV + foscarnet IV continue until symptomatic improvement (BII) • Maintenance therapy should be continued for life (AI)		Maintenance therapy for CMV retinitis can be safely discontinued in patients with inactive disease and sustained CD4$^+$ T-lymphocyte (>100-150 cells/mm^3 for >6 months)—consultation with ophthalmologist is advised (BII) Patients with CMV retinitis who discontinued maintenance therapy should undergo regular eye examination for early detection of relapse (AIII) Immune recovery uveitis (IRU) may develop in the setting of immune reconstitution Treatment of IRU: Periocular corticosteroid or short courses of systemic steroid Because of its poor oral bioavailability and with the availability of valganciclovir, oral ganciclovir should no longer be used (DIII)
Herpes simplex virus (HSV) disease	*Orolabial lesions and initial or recurrent genital HSV:* Famciclovir 500 mg PO bid or valaciclovir 1 gm PO bid or acyclovir 400 mg PO tid × 7 days (AII) *Moderate to severe mucocutaneous HSV infections:* • Initial therapy acyclovir 5 mg/kg IV q8h (AII) • After lesions began to regress, change to famciclovir 500 mg PO bid or valacyclovir 1 gm PO bid or acyclovir 400 mg PO tid (AII) Continue therapy until lesions have completely healed *HSV keratitis:* • Trifluridine 1% ophthalmic solution, one drop onto the cornea every 2 hr, not to exceed 9 drops per day, for no longer than 21 days (AII) *HSV encephalitis:* • Acyclovir 10 mg/kg IV q8h × 14-21 days (AII)	*Acyclovir-resistant HSV:* • Foscarnet 120-200 mg/kg/day IV in 2-3 divided doses until clinical response (AI) • Cidofovir 5 mg/kg IV weekly until clinical response (AI) *Alternative for acyclovir-resistant HSV infections:* • Topical trifluridine • Topical cidofovir *Note:* Both of the above preparations are not commercially available. Extemporaneous compounding of these topical products can be prepared using trifluridine ophthalmic solution and cidofovir for intravenous administration.	Chronic suppressive therapy with oral acyclovir, famciclovir, or valacyclovir may be indicated in patients with frequent or severe recurrences
Varicella zoster virus (VZV) disease	*Primary VZV infection (chicken pox):* • Acyclovir 10 mg/kg IV q8h × 7-10 days (AII) • Switch to oral therapy (acyclovir 800 mg PO qid or valacyclovir 1 g tid or famciclovir 500 mg tid) after defervescent if there is no evidence of visceral involvement (AII) *Local dermatomal herpes zoster:* • Famciclovir 500 mg or valacyclovir 1 gm PO tid × 7-10 days (AII) *Extensive cutaneous lesion or visceral involvement:* • Acyclovir 10 mg/kg q8h, continue until cutaneous and visceral disease clearly resolved (AIII) *Progressive outer retinal necrosis (PORN):* • Acyclovir IV 10 mg/kg q8h + foscarnet 60 mg/kg IV q8h (AIII)		

*Rating strength of the recommendation (in brackets):

A = Both strong evidence for efficacy and substantial clinical benefit support recommendation for use; should always be offered.

B = Moderate evidence for efficacy, or strong evidence for efficacy but only limited clinical benefit, supports recommendation for use; should generally be offered.

C = Evidence for efficacy is insufficient to support a recommendation for or against use, or evidence for efficacy might not outweigh adverse consequences (e.g., drug toxicity, drug interactions) or cost of the chemoprophylaxis or alternative approaches; optional.

D = Moderate evidence for lack of efficacy or for adverse outcome supports a recommendation against use; should generally not be offered.

E = Good evidence for lack of efficacy or for adverse outcome supports a recommendation against use; should never be offered.

†Quality of evidence supporting the recommendation (in brackets):

I = Evidence from at least one properly randomized, controlled trial.

II = Evidence from at least one well-designed clinical trial without randomization, from cohort or case-controlled analytic studies (preferably from more than one center), or from multiple time-series studies; or, dramatic results from uncontrolled experiments.

III = Evidence from opinions of respected authorities based on clinical experience, descriptive studies, or reports of expert committees.

‡Pyrimethamine and leucovorin doses—same as in "preferred therapy" for toxoplasmosis.

§Pyrazinamide dose: <55 kg = 1000 mg; 56-75 kg = 1500 mg; ≥76 kg = 2000 mg; ethambutol dose: <55 kg = 800 mg; 56-75 kg = 1200 mg; ≥76 kg = 1600 mg.

‖In HIV-HBV coinfected patients who do not need HIV therapy but who have HBeAg$^+$ chronic hepatitis B and ALT higher than twice normal, some authorities would recommend treating HBV with interferon-alfa provided there is no evidence of hepatic decompensation. This strategy spares the patient from developing HIV and HBV resistance to lamivudine therapy and from the toxicity of ART.

ART, antiretroviral therapy; HAART, highly active antiretroviral therapy; IM, intramuscular; IV, intravenous; PO, oral; SQ, subcutaneous; qd, daily; bid, twice a day; tid, three times daily; qid, four times a day; tiw, three times weekly; wk, weeks, q'n'h, every 'n' hour.

From U.S. Public Health Service/Infectious Disease Society of America. USPHS/IDSA Guidelines for Therapy of Opportunistic Infections in Persons Infected with Human Immunodeficiency Virus. 2004. Available at www.aidsinfo.nih.gov. In press.

TABLE 125-4 Treatment of AIDS-Associated Opportunistic Infections in Adults*†—cont'd

Opportunistic Infections	Preferred Therapy and Duration	Alternative Therapy	Other Options and Issues*
	Treatment of Condyloma Acuminata (Genital Warts)		
Human papillomavirus disease	**Patient-Applied Treatment:** Podofilox 0.5% solution or 0.5% gel: apply to all lesions bid × 3 consecutive days, repeat weekly × up to 4 wk (BIII): *or* Imiquimod 5% cream: apply to lesion at bedtime and remove in the morning on 3 nonconsecutive nights weekly, up to 16 wk (BII)	**Provider-Applied Treatment:** • Liquid nitrogen cryotherapy: apply until each lesion is thoroughly frozen, repeat every 1-2 wk for up to 3-4 times (BIII) • Trichloroacetic acid or bichloroacetic acid cauterization: 80-95% aqueous solution, apply to each lesion, repeat weekly for 3-6 wk (BIII) • Surgical excision (BII) or laser surgery (CIII) • Cidofovir topical (CIII): not commercially available • Podophyllin resin 10-25% suspension in tincture of benzoin: apply to area and wash off in a few hours, repeat weekly for up to 3-6 wk (CIII) • Intralesional interferon-α is an option, but is generally not recommended	Intralesional interferon-α: generally not recommended due to high cost, difficult administration, and potential for systemic side effects (DIII) The rate of recurrence of genital warts is high despite treatment There are limited data on the responses to treatment in HIV-1 infected patients
	Treatment of Cervical Intraepithelial Neoplasia (CIN) or Anal Intraepithelial Neoplasia (AIN)		
	CIN 1: • Pap smears and/or colposcopy every 4-6 months *CIN 2 or 3:* • Loop electrosurgical excision procedure (LEEP) (BIII) *AIN:* Insufficient data to recommend specific treatment. Treatment decision based on size, location of lesion, and grade of histology (CIII)	*CIN 2 or 3:* • Cryotherapy (BIII) • Laser therapy (BIII) • Cone biopsy (BIII)	Low-dose intravaginal 5-fluorouracil (2 gm twice weekly × 6 months) for CIN may reduce short-term risk for recurrence (CIII) Efficacy of treatment of AIN 2 or 3 in preventing anal cancer is unknown
Hepatitis C virus disease	Combination therapy (AI) [Peginterferon alfa-2b (1.5 μg/kg) SQ weekly; or peginterferon alfa-2a (180 μg) SQ weekly] + Ribavirin PO (weight-based dosing: if <75 mg, 400 mg in AM + 600 mg in PM: if >75 kg, 600 mg bid) *Duration of Therapy:* *For genotype 1:* • 48 wk—For patients who demonstrate an early virologic response (≥2 log decrease in HCV viral load at 12 wk) (AI) • 12 wk—For patients who failed to achieve early virologic response at 12 wks (BI); therapy beyond 12 wk is almost always futile for achieving virologic cure *For genotype 2 or 3:* • 24 wk—based on data in non–HIV-1 infected patients (BII) • Some experts suggest 48 wk (CIII)	*When ribavirin is contraindicated (e.g., unstable cardiopulmonary disease, preexisting anemia, or hemoglobinopathy):* Peginterferon alfa-2b 1.5 μg/kg or peginterferon alfa-2a 180 μg SQ weekly (AII)	All patients should be counseled to avoid alcohol consumption because of increased risk of fibrosis progression Preliminary data suggest that responses to HCV therapy correlate with CD4+ cell count. • Some suggest treating HCV before CD4+ drops below 500 cells/μL (BIII) • Conversely, if patient has CD4+ <500 cells/μL some suggest initiating ARV before treatment of HCV (BIII)
Hepatitis B virus disease	Owing to the lack of controlled trial data on the use of antiviral agents against HBV in HIV/HBV coinfected patients, none of the current therapies can be recommended as preferred regimens In patients with HIV/HBV/HCV coinfection, consideration for antiretroviral therapy should be the first priority. If antiretroviral therapy is not required, then treatment for HCV should be considered before HBV, as interferon treatment for HBV may also treat HBV infection (CIII)	*Lamivudine-naïve patients requiring ART:* • Lamivudine 150 mg PO bid should be used as part of an ART regimen (BIII) for a minimum of 1 yr or 6 months after seroconversion from HBeAg (+) to HbeAg (−) and anti-e positive (BIII) • Adefovir 10 mg/day in addition to ART for a minimum of 1 year or 6 months after seroconversion from HBeAg (+) to HbeAg (−) and anti-e positive (BIII); • Some experts advise adding adefovir 10 mg/day or tenofovir 300 mg/day to lamivudine (CIII) *or* • Interferon-alfa-2a or -2b 5 million units (MU) SQ qd or 10 MU SQ tiw may be considered in patients who do not require anitretroviral therapy (CIII)‖ or PEG IFN 180 μg SQ q wk *Duration of interferon alfa therapy:* HBeAg (+) patients: 16-24 wk (BII) HBeAg (−) patients: minimum of 12 months (BIII) *Lamivudine-naïve patients in whom ART is not indicated:* • Adefovir 10 mg PO qd (CIII) or PEG IFN 180 μg SQ q wk *Use for treatment of both HIV and HBV infection:* Tenofovir 300 mg PO qd as part of an ART regimen +/− lamivudine (CIII)	All patients should be advised to avoid or limit alcohol consumption (AII) Patients should receive 2 doses of hepatitis A vaccine, preferably before CD4+ T-cell count drops below 200 cells/μL (BIII) Interferon should not be used in patients with decompensated liver diseae (EII) Discontinuation of therapy for HBV infection risks flare of liver disease in ≈15% of patients and loss of anti-HBV benefit HAART should always include HBV treatment to minimize immune reconstitution flares

TABLE 125-4 Treatment of AIDS-Associated Opportunistic Infections in Adults*†—cont'd

Opportunistic Infections	Preferred Therapy and Duration	Alternative Therapy	Other Options and Issues*
Penicilliosis	*Acute infection in severely ill patients:* Amphotericin B 0.6 mg/kg/day IV × 2 wk; followed by itraconazole oral solution 400 mg daily × 10 wk (AII) *Chronic suppressive therapy:* Itraconazole 200 mg PO qd (AI)		ART should be administered according to standard of care in the community (CIII)
Leishmaniasis	Pentavalent antimony (or sodium stibogluconate) = 20 mg/kg IV or IM qd (AI) × 3-4 wk depending on initial response (CIII) *Secondary prophylaxis:* Single dose of the initial therapy every 4 wk, especially in patients with CD4 <200 cells/μL (AI)	• Amphotericin B deoxycholate (AI) 0.5-1.0 mg/kg IV qd (maximum of 50 mg qd) for total dose of 1.5-2.0 gm (BII); *or* • Amphotericin B lipid formulation (AI) 3-5 mg/kg IV qd × 10 days (BII); there is less experience with shorter regimens (see text); *or* • Pentamidine isethionate 3-4 mg/kg IV tiw × 3-4 wk followed by monthly maintenance therapy (BII) *Secondary prophylaxis:* Single dose of the initial therapy every 4 wk, especially in patients with CD4 <200 cells/μL (AI) • Ketoconazole 200-400 PO qd • Sulfonamide	Severely neutropenic patients with visceral leishmaniasis may benefit from short course of granulocyte macrophage colony stimulating factor (GM-CSF) 5 μg/kg/day SQ × 5 days (CII) *Other regimens—generally not recommended:* • Miltefosine 100 mg/day for 30 days (CIII). Schedule for secondary prophylaxis is unknown.
Paracoccidioidomycosis	Amphotericin B for severely ill (BII) Itraconazole 100-200 mg PO qd for less ill (BII)		Potent ART should be initiated in accordance with standards of care in the community (AIII)
Isospora belli infection	TMP 160 mg + SMX 800 mg PO (or IV) qid × 10 days (AII) *or* TMP 320 mg + SMX 1600 mg PO (or IV) bid × 10-14 days (AIII) *Secondary prophylaxis:* In patients with CD4 <200, TMP 320 mg + SMX 1600 mg PO qd or tiw (AII)	• Pyrimethamine 50-75 mg PO qd + leucovorin 5-10 mg PO qd (BII); *or* • Ciprofloxacin 500 mg PO bid (BII) • Other fluoroquinolones (BII) *Alternative secondary prophylaxis:* Pyrimethamine 25 mg PO qd + leucovorin (BII)	Fluid management in patients with dehydration (AIII) Nutritional supplementation for malnutrition and wasting (AIII) Immune reconstitution with ART may result in fewer relapses (AIII) Discontinuation of secondary prophylaxis may be considered in patients with sustained CD4⁺ T-cell count < 200 cells/mL for >3 months (BIII)
Chagas' disease (American trypanosomiasis)	Benznidazole 5-8 mg/kg/day in 2 divided doses × 30-60 days (AIII) Lifelong secondary prophylaxis probably indicated (CIII)	Nifurtimox (currently not available) 10 mg/kg/days (BIII)	

*Rating strength of the recommendation (in brackets):
   A = Both strong evidence for efficacy and substantial clinical benefit support recommendation for use; should always be offered.
   B = Moderate evidence for efficacy, or strong evidence for efficacy but only limited clinical benefit, supports recommendation for use; should generally be offered.
   C = Evidence for efficacy is insufficient to support a recommendation for or against use, or evidence for efficacy might not outweigh adverse consequences (e.g., drug toxicity, drug interactions) or cost of the chemoprophylaxis or alternative approaches; optional.
   D = Moderate evidence for lack of efficacy or for adverse outcome supports a recommendation against use; should generally not be offered.
   E = Good evidence for lack of efficacy or for adverse outcome supports a recommendation against use; should never be offered.
†Quality of evidence supporting the recommendation (in brackets):
   I = Evidence from at least one properly randomized, controlled trial.
   II = Evidence from at least one well-designed clinical trial without randomization, from cohort or case-controlled analytic studies (preferably from more than one center), or from multiple time-series studies; or, dramatic results from uncontrolled experiments.
   III = Evidence from opinions of respected authorities based on clinical experience, descriptive studies, or reports of expert committees.
‡Pyrimethamine and leucovorin doses—same as in "preferred therapy" for toxoplasmosis.
§Pyrazinamide dose: <55 kg = 1000 mg; 56-75 kg = 1500 mg; ≥76 kg = 2000 mg; ethambutol dose: <55 kg = 800 mg; 56-75 kg = 1200 mg; ≥76 kg = 1600 mg.
‖In HIV-HBV coinfected patients who do not need HIV therapy but who have HBeAg⁺ chronic hepatitis B and ALT higher than twice normal, some authorities would recommend treating HBV with interferon-alfa provided there is no evidence of hepatic decompensation. This strategy spares the patient from developing HIV and HBV resistance to lamivudine therapy and from the toxicity of ART.
ART, antiretroviral therapy; HAART, highly active antiretroviral therapy; IM, intramuscular; IV, intravenous; PO, oral; SQ, subcutaneous; qd, daily; bid, twice a day; tid, three times daily; qid, four times a day; tiw, three times weekly; wk, weeks, q'n'h, every 'n' hour.
From U.S. Public Health Service/Infectious Disease Society of America. USPHS/IDSA Guidelines for Therapy of Opportunistic Infections in Persons Infected with Human Immunodeficiency Virus. 2004. Available at www.aidsinfo.nih.gov. In press.

within the first several days or even 2 weeks after initiation of therapy. Empirical diagnoses by definition preclude the possibility of screening for tuberculosis, eliminating the potential for early identification of tuberculosis and reduction of transmission. The availability of induced sputum examination provides a very sensitive, relatively low-cost method for diagnosis of PCP and detection of tuberculosis.[92,95] Nucleic acid detection systems that use oral washes or gargles offer promise for outpatient assessments, but their utility remains to be established.[96]

The likelihood that an AIDS patient will survive an episode of PCP depends on the severity of pulmonary dysfunction at the time of initiation of therapy, the patient's ability to tolerate available regimens, the

presence of concomitant pathology, and the severity of the patient's immunologic dysfunction. A poor prognosis correlates best with an alveolar-arterial gradient greater than 30 mm Hg, a severely abnormal chest radiography result, or a large number of organisms detected on lavage or biopsy.[86,89,90] Any drug therapy is more likely to be successful if it is started at a time when pulmonary dysfunction is mild and if other severe opportunistic infections or neoplasms are absent. Second, third, or subsequent episodes of PCP do not carry a worse prognosis than the first episode.[97]

Oral TMP-SMX is the treatment of choice for acute PCP because of its convenience of administration, high degree of efficacy, and manageability of associated toxicities (see Table 125-4).[12,98,99] No agent has been shown to have a higher efficacy for PCP than TMP-SMX. There is no clear reason to prefer intravenous over oral TMP-SMX in adherent patients without obvious gastrointestinal dysfunction. Patients usually improve clinically within 4 to 8 days, in terms of fever, respiratory rate, arterial-alveolar gradient, and dyspnea, although there may be an initial worsening during the first 8 to 72 hours of therapy if adjunctive corticosteroid therapy is not given.[57,98-104]

Survival for mild episodes treated with TMP-SMX has improved steadily over the past 2 decades. For patients with an initial room air partial pressure of oxygen (Po$_2$) higher than 70 mm Hg, survival has improved from between 85% and 90% to between 95% and 99% in optimal circumstances.[98,105] Nonadherent patients and patients with significant concomitant disorders do not have such good results. This improvement presumably reflects the better understanding that TMP-SMX can be continued despite non–life-threatening toxicities In addition, better alternative agents are available for patients who truly have treatment failure with TMP-SMX or who are unable to tolerate the drug.[12,105-108]

Microbiologic resistance of *Pneumocystis* to TMP-SMX was not described until recently because the organism isolated from humans cannot be grown in vitro. Reports document that some human isolates contain mutations in their dihydropteroate synthase enzyme, the target for sulfonamides. When this mutation occurs in other organisms (e.g., *Streptococcus pneumoniae, Plasmodia* spp.), it produces microbiologic and clinical resistance. Further information is needed to determine whether these mutations in fact confer sulfonamide resistance to *Pneumocystis* that is clinically significant, and whether the frequency of such resistance will become sufficient to warrant new therapeutic and prophylactic strategies.[109,110]

Common adverse reactions to TMP-SMX include rash, nausea, vomiting, granulocytopenia, transaminase elevations, nephritis, and hyperkalemia.[58,59,111] These reactions do not invariably require discontinuation of TMP-SMX therapy. The rashes, which commonly occur between days 8 and 12 of therapy, may be limited in extent and associated with a degree of pruritus that the patient can tolerate for 21 days. They are more frequent in patients with higher CD4$^+$ T-cell counts. Life-threatening desquamating processes (e.g., Stevens-Johnson syndrome) are rare in AIDS patients, although a few fatal cases have been reported. Severe febrile, hypotensive episodes that resemble septic shock in terms of hemodynamics have also been reported. Granulocytopenia is most often a dose-related phenomenon that may resolve partially or completely if the dose of TMP-SMX is reduced by 25%.[98] Granulocytopenia responds to leucovorin administration only rarely. A report that leucovorin administration can diminish the likelihood of therapeutic response to TMP-SMX was intriguing but not conclusive.[112] Nausea and vomiting can be troublesome complications of TMP-SMX therapy. Severe nausea may result from very high sulfonamide levels and may resolve if the dose is reduced. Transaminase levels may fluctuate until therapy is stopped; they usually return promptly to baseline values if they were caused by TMP-SMX rather than another drug or a coexisting process such as a viral hepatitis.

Overall, adverse reactions in the past required discontinuation of TMP-SMX therapy in about 25% of cases.[58,59,105,108,111] Although it has not been proved by a prospective study, adverse reactions can probably be reduced without sacrificing efficacy by lowering the recommended dose of TMP-SMX, from TMP 20 mg/kg/day (with SMX 100 mg/kg/day) to TMP 15 mg/kg/day (with SMX 75 mg/kg/day).[98] About 70% to 80% of sulfonamide-intolerant individuals can tolerate dapsone for significant periods.[113] TMP-dapsone has potency comparable to that of TMP-SMX.[99] Gradual dose escalation of TMP-SMX can reduce the impact of adverse effects, but this approach is appropriate in selected patients for prophylaxis, not as therapy in patients with acute illness.[114,115]

Parenteral pentamidine is effective therapy for PCP.[12,98] This regimen is inconvenient to administer, however, and the adverse reactions associated with it can be life-threatening. Renal dysfunction, hypoglycemia, hyperglycemia, granulocytopenia, and hypotension are reported in 10% to 50% of patients.[12,98,116] For many years, pentamidine

was administered intramuscularly because early reports described fatal hypotension when the drug was given intravenously.[117] However, intramuscular administration of pentamidine is no longer recommended except in unusual circumstances, because the intramuscular injections are often associated with painful sterile abscesses that can become superinfected. Moreover, the hypotension originally associated with intravenous pentamidine was related to the rate of infusion. If pentamidine is administered over a period of at least 60 minutes in 100 to 150 mL of dextrose in water, clinically important hypotension is unusual.[118] The renal dysfunction associated with pentamidine can be severe. If the serum creatinine level rises by more than 1.0 to 2.0 mg/dL, strong consideration should be given to withholding therapy for a few days or changing to an alternative agent. Hypoglycemia can be a life-threatening complication of pentamidine therapy; it can occur at any juncture during therapy or for many weeks after therapy has been completed.[119] Hypoglycemia occurs more frequently in patients who have pentamidine-induced renal dysfunction. The unpredictability of the hypoglycemia adds an element of risk to the inpatient or outpatient use of this drug. Life-threatening hypoglycemia is sufficiently uncommon, however, that this effective agent is still recommended for patients with severe disease who cannot tolerate TMP-SMX or TMP-dapsone. Lowering the dose of parenteral pentamidine from 4 to 3 mg/kg/day has been advocated to reduce toxicity; whether this also reduces efficacy is unknown.[120]

Dapsone (100 mg orally every day) plus TMP (5 mg/kg orally every 8 hours or 300 mg orally every 8 hours) appears to be as effective as TMP-SMX but less toxic.[12,99,121] Skin rashes are very common among HIV-infected patients treated with dapsone, but a 21-day course of therapy can usually be completed without interruption. Oral dapsone alone has some efficacy when 100 mg is administered every day for 21 days, but there is probably not enough activity to warrant use of this agent as single-drug therapy.[122] Higher doses are not well tolerated.

Atovaquone is a hydroxynaphthoquinone that appears to affect mitochondrial electron transport in microorganisms and therefore has a mechanism of action distinct from that of TMP-SMX or pentamidine.[105] Atovaquone is available as an oral suspension but is not available in a parenteral form. For patients with mild or moderate PCP, it has a high degree of efficacy and is extremely well tolerated. A large, prospective, double-blind study demonstrated that atovaquone, although very effective and much better tolerated than TMP-SMX, is associated with more treatment failures.[105] Because atovaquone, unlike TMP-SMX, has no antibacterial activity, it is possible that patients in the atovaquone-treated groups were more likely to die of unrecognized, concurrent bacterial processes. Atovaquone is better tolerated than intravenous pentamidine.[123] The absorption of atovaquone suspension can be erratic, especially in patients who cannot consume fatty foods with this medication. Atovaquone takes several days to reach steady-state levels. It should not be given to patients with significant gastrointestinal dysfunction. Mutations that could confer atovaquone resistance have been identified in human isolates,[124] but their clinical relevance remains to be determined. The primary toxicity associated with atovaquone is skin rash. Atovaquone is a reasonable treatment option for patients with mild or moderate PCP who cannot tolerate TMP-SMX and who are good candidates for oral therapy.

Clindamycin plus primaquine is also effective therapy for PCP.[99,107] Despite the fact that primaquine can be given only orally, this regimen has been used successfully in patients with mild, moderate, and severe disease. Clindamycin plus primaquine is associated with considerable toxicity, including rash, serum transaminase elevation, diarrhea, and hemolysis. It is a reasonable oral regimen for patients who are unable to tolerate other regimens.

Trimetrexate is a potent inhibitor of dihydrofolate reductase that is effective therapy against PCP when used either alone (4.5 mg/m^2 intravenously every day) or in combination with a sulfonamide.[12,108,125] Because trimetrexate inhibits the dihydrofolate reductase of human cells as well as the enzyme of *Pneumocystis*, it must be given in conjunction with high-dose leucovorin (20 mg q6h intravenously or orally every 6 hours), which rescues mammalian cells without diminishing the anti-*Pneumocystis* effect of the drug. Trimetrexate is well tolerated when given with leucovorin. Leukopenia is its major adverse effect. Trimetrexate has a high degree of efficacy and has the advantage of being available as a parenteral agent. However, a large, multicenter, double-blind study demonstrated that trimetrexate therapy is associated with a higher rate of poor response and death than is therapy with TMP-SMX.[108] The relapse rate after trimetrexate therapy is high: 60% of patients experience relapse within the first 60 days if prophylaxis is not given. This relapse rate is probably much lower if a few days of sulfonamide therapy are given concurrently; the most convenient method is to administer TMP-SMX with the trimetrexate.

Regardless of which specific agent is chosen as the initial therapy for PCP, adjunctive corticosteroid therapy is indicated for any patient whose initial room air PO_2 is lower than 70 mm Hg.[12,100-104] Three prospective trials demonstrated that the frequencies of ventilatory failure and mortality can be reduced substantially by the prompt use of corticosteroids.[100-102] The precise mechanism by which corticosteroids provide benefit is not well delineated. Physiologically, adjunctive corticosteroids appear to prevent much of the decline in oxygenation that characteristically occurs during the first 3 days of treatment.[104] This decline may be caused by the inflammatory response elicited by dying organisms. Adjunctive corticosteroids may also provide benefit for patients with an initial room air PO_2 higher than 70 mm Hg. There is physiologic evidence that indicates improved lung function in such patients, but so few patients with mild PCP develop respiratory failure or die that it is difficult to substantiate a survival benefit. The safety of the 21-day regimen is well substantiated: reactivation of tuberculosis, CMV, or Kaposi's sarcoma is unusual.[126] Whether such short courses of corticosteroids could predispose patients to osteonecrosis of the hip is not clear.[127] Interestingly, the frequency of TMP-SMX–related rash is not diminished by corticosteroids.[128]

If an HIV-infected patient with PCP fails to improve while receiving conventional therapy, there are no controlled data to indicate which modifications in therapy are optimal.[12,106] The mean time to improvement for HIV-infected patients treated with conventional therapy is 4 to 8 days,[57,98] so therapeutic failure probably should not be diagnosed until patients have received 4 to 8 days of therapy. Clinicians often feel compelled to alter therapy earlier, however, especially if the patient is deteriorating rapidly. If a patient has not improved after 5 to 10 days of therapy, a repeat diagnostic procedure should be considered to determine whether another treatable pathogen is present. Bronchoalveolar lavage is the procedure of choice. Transbronchial biopsy often can be performed to assess for the presence of CMV and can be very helpful in establishing the presence of fungal or mycobacterial processes, which are the major diagnostic considerations. *Pneumocystis* is often present in lavage or tissue for at least 3 to 4 weeks after initiation of therapy, even in patients who respond promptly, so its presence after 7 to 10 days of therapy does not necessarily imply that therapy is ineffective.[129] A decision regarding therapeutic efficacy should be based on clinical and laboratory parameters such as oxygenation, ventilation, and fever. The presence of extensive intra-alveolar exudate or extensive fibrosis after 7 to 10 days of therapy is probably a more ominous sign. Open lung biopsy is rarely necessary to establish a diagnosis of PCP, but it can be useful for identifying other processes. Kaposi's sarcoma of the lung is usually apparent on bronchoscopy because of endobronchial lesions that are obvious to the bronchoscopist.[130] However, if such lesions are not seen on bronchoscopy, Kaposi's sarcoma of the lung is one treatable process that is difficult or impossible to diagnose reliably from cytology or from transbronchial biopsy specimens. Nodular lesions on chest computed tomography (CT) scans, extensive intrabronchial lesions, and the presence of a bloody pleural effusion may be helpful clues that Kaposi's sarcoma is the cause of pulmonary dysfunction. CMV and lymphoma are other processes that may be identified by cytology or by some form of biopsy more readily than by sputum assessment.

If *Pneumocystis* infection is the only identifiable cause of the pulmonary dysfunction after 7 to 10 days of therapy and no improvement has been observed, there are several therapeutic alternatives: (1) switch from TMP-SMX to parenteral pentamidine or vice-versa, (2) add corticosteroids to conventional therapy if they have not already been added, (3) switch to intravenous trimetrexate (with or without parenteral sulfonamide in the form of TMP-SMX), (4) switch to intravenous clindamycin with oral primaquine, or (5) use two specific therapies concurrently (e.g., TMP-SMX plus pentamidine). Each of these approaches has been associated with a successful outcome in some cases. A controlled trial is needed to determine the best approach, but such trials are difficult to perform because of the large size, complexity, and cost of a valid study. Whether AIDS patients with PCP should be supported aggressively with intensive care, mechanical ventilation, or other interventions depends on issues specific to each individual patient. The most reasonable approach would be to individualize each management plan in terms of the days of therapy that have been completed, the therapeutic alternatives that are available, and the concomitant processes that may be present. The patient's wishes and the availability of resources need to be taken into account. Published data indicate that some AIDS patients with PCP can survive intubation and mechanical ventilation and lead independent lives for many months after hospital discharge.[86,89,90,131,132] The best candidates for intensive care and mechanical ventilation are patients who have presented with no other serious opportunistic processes, those who have received fewer than 7 days of specific therapy, and those who have clearly articulated a desire for aggressive support.

Prevention of PCP is a major priority in the management of HIV infection.[10,20,54] Prevention of PCP is logical because episodes are frequent (at least 80% to 90% of HIV-infected patients in North America develop an episode at some point if they have received neither anti-*Pneumocystis* prophylaxis nor ART), morbidity and mortality due to PCP can be substantial, low-cost drugs are available that are effective, and the period of high susceptibility can be defined.[10,20,54] Prospective and retrospective studies have shown that most primary episodes of PCP occur in patients with CD4+ T-cell counts lower than 200 cells/mm³ or in patients with otherwise unexplained oropharyngeal candidiasis, regardless of their CD4+ T-cell count.[10,20,54] Therefore, these are the indications for primary prophylaxis. Other documented predictors of the occurrence of PCP, independent of the CD4+ T-cell count, are high HIV viral load,[19,22] wasting syndrome, previous AIDS-defining event, and prior pneumonia of any type.[27] These parameters should probably be added to the list of factors encouraging primary prophylaxis. A few cases of PCP occur in patients with CD4+ T-cell counts higher than 200 cells/mm³ who do not have fever or mucocutaneous candidiasis, and for this reason clinicians may prefer to initiate prophylaxis at somewhat earlier time points. However, such a strategy results in prophylactic therapy for a relatively larger patient population to prevent a relatively small incremental number of treatable cases. Secondary prophylaxis (the prevention of second or subsequent episodes of PCP) is conventionally indicated for everyone who has had a documented PCP episode, because the 1-year recurrence rate is approximately 65% for patients who receive no prophylaxis.[10] As mentioned earlier, there is considerable evidence suggesting that discontinuation of prophylaxis is reasonable for patients who respond to ART and who manifest CD4+ T-cell counts that are persistently about 200 cells/mm³, especially if the other listed risk factors are absent and if patients can be trained to seek medical care promptly if symptoms suggestive of PCP develop (see Table 125-3).[67-83]

TMP-SMX is the preferred prophylactic regimen for any HIV-infected patient who can tolerate it (see Tables 125-1 and 125-2).[10,54] If it is administered at a dose of 160 mg TMP plus 800 mg SMX (i.e., one double-strength tablet once daily), episodes of PCP are extremely uncommon among patients who adhere to the regimen. Trials have demonstrated that TMP-SMX is much more effective for either primary or secondary prophylaxis than aerosolized pentamidine or dapsone-containing regimens.[133-144] TMP-SMX also has the benefit, based on retrospective analyses, of reducing the frequency of toxoplasmosis,[136,143] and it may have a beneficial effect on reducing the frequency of pneumococcal and *Haemophilus* infections when daily regimens are used.[136]

Comparative trials have confirmed that TMP-SMX is not nearly as well tolerated as aerosolized pentamidine. About 20% to 40% of patients cannot tolerate TMP-SMX because of the side effects of rash, pruritus, fever, granulocytopenia, thrombocytopenia, anemia, hepatitis, nephritis, nausea, or vomiting. Reducing the dose of TMP-SMX by 50% (i.e., a single-strength tablet daily) or reducing the frequency to two or three times weekly lowers the toxicity.[137] In a study comparing TMP-SMX at a dose of one double-strength tablet daily with TMP-SMX at one double-strength tablet three times weekly, there was no difference in efficacy when the data were evaluated based on an intent-to-treat analysis.[144] However, when occurrences of PCP were analyzed based on the regimen patients were actually taking at the time that PCP was diagnosed, there were more failures on the intermittent regimen. This finding has suggested to some investigators that the intermittent regimen is less effective.

Because TMP-SMX is the preferred regimen, strategies to increase patient tolerance of this regimen are important. Gradual dose escalation of TMP-SMX at the time at which prophylaxis is restarted was shown in two controlled studies to increase tolerability.[114,115]

For patients who cannot tolerate TMP-SMX, there are several alternatives. Daily dapsone or weekly dapsone-pyrimethamine has an efficacy comparable to that of aerosolized pentamidine (i.e., not as effective as daily TMP-SMX when used as prophylaxis for PCP). Dapsone-containing regimens, especially dapsone-pyrimethamine regimens, are effective as prophylaxis against toxoplasmosis.[138,139] Dapsone or dapsone-pyrimethamine, like TMP-SMX, is poorly tolerated by a substantial number of patients; fever, rash, pruritus, and hemolysis occur. About 20% of patients who cannot tolerate TMP-SMX also cannot tolerate dapsone-containing regimens.[113] Aerosolized pentamidine, although not as effective as TMP-SMX, has a definite ability to reduce the frequency of PCP when used for primary or secondary prophylaxis. The manner in which aerosolized pentamidine is delivered to the patient is a major determinant of efficacy and safety.[145,146] Because different nebulizers deliver different spectra and different densities of particle sizes, they deliver different amounts of drug to the lung. For this reason, the dosing regimens for the Respirgard II nebulizer and the Fisons nebulizer are quite different. Only the Respirgard II jet nebulizer and the Fisons ultrasonic nebulizer have been studied in large, well-controlled trials with clinical end points. Aerosolized pentamidine is well tolerated by most patients. Coughing and wheezing can be ameliorated or prevented by nebulized albuterol. A bitter taste is often reported. Cases of pancreatitis and renal dysfunction have been attributed to aerosolized pentamidine, but it is not certain that aerosolized pentamidine was the cause. A major concern related to the use of aerosolized pentamidine is environmental contamination with drug and respiratory aerosols, which is created when patients cough or become disconnected from the nebulizer. Health care workers and patients may inhale enough pentamidine to develop detectable urine levels of the drug.[146] The clinical importance of this effect is unknown. More important, if the patient has pulmonary tuberculosis, the environmental contamination produced by dispersed respiratory particles has considerable potential to spread tuberculosis.[147] Patients need to be carefully screened for pulmonary tuberculosis before aerosolized pentamidine prophylaxis is initiated.

Atovaquone has been assessed as prophylaxis in trials comparing it with either dapsone alone or aerosolized pentamidine.[148,149] In both situations, atovaquone was equally effective as the alternative, and it was better tolerated than dapsone.

If patients cannot tolerate TMP-SMX and have an excessive number of breakthroughs while receiving dapsone-containing regimens, aerosolized pentamidine, or atovaquone, there are several poorly studied options. The best option for intolerant patients is to try to maximize the patient's ability to tolerate TMP-SMX by using a dose escalation strategy (to standard doses) and perhaps attempt an intermittent (three times weekly) regimen. Aerosolized pentamidine can be administered by employing doses higher than the approved regimen (300 mg twice monthly or 600 mg once monthly), perhaps with dapsone or azithromycin in addition.[150] Results with clindamycin-primaquine have been disappointing. Whether the need for alternative regimens will grow substantially remains to be seen and depends on the clinical relevance of sulfonamide resistance and the long-term success of ART.

Patients who experience breakthrough while receiving prophylactic therapy are usually those who are not receiving TMP-SMX, who are not adherent, or who have very low CD4$^+$ T-cell counts.[151,152] For such patients, education to reinforce adherence to prophylactic regimens, the use of strategies to enhance tolerability of TMP-SMX, and efforts to augment CD4$^+$ T-cell counts by ART are recommended.

Toxoplasma gondii

In most cases, *Toxoplasma gondii* (see Chapter 276) causes disease in patients with HIV infection by reactivation rather than by primary infection.[153] Patients almost always have immunoglobulin G antibodies against *Toxoplasma*, have fairly advanced disease (CD4$^+$ T-cell counts lower than 100 cells/mm^3), and have not been receiving TMP-SMX prophylaxis.[153,154] Because the seroprevalence of toxoplasmosis is much higher in some areas, such as western Europe and South America, than in the United States (i.e., there is a higher incidence of latent infection), those areas have much higher frequencies of AIDS-associated toxoplasmosis.

In patients with HIV infection, toxoplasmosis manifests most often as cerebral disease. Retinochoroiditis, pneumonitis, disseminated disease, and a sepsis-like syndrome have all been reported, but these are not as frequent as focal lesions of the CNS. If an HIV-infected patient with a CD4$^+$ T-cell count of less than 100 cells/mm^3 presents with a space-occupying cerebral lesion that involves gray matter, the differential diagnosis primarily includes toxoplasmosis and lymphoma. Fungal, mycobacterial, and viral processes manifest as space-occupying lesions infrequently, and progressive multifocal leukoencephalopathy should manifest differently because it affects primarily white matter.

In the era of ART, CNS lymphoma appears to be increasing in frequency compared with CNS toxoplasmosis. In large groups of patients, clinical or imaging characteristics distinguish lymphoma from toxoplasmosis.[155-158] There is some diagnostic utility for immunoglobulin or PCR tests of cerebrospinal fluid,[155] for single photon emission computed tomography (SPECT) or positron emission tomography (PET) scanning,[156] or for magnetic resonance imaging (MRI) scanning.[157] A positive cerebrospinal fluid PCR assay for Epstein-Barr virus appears to be highly specific for primary CNS lymphoma.[158] In individual cases, establishing a diagnosis with confidence requires a definitive biopsy or, in the case of toxoplasmosis, a response to empirical therapy. Therapy for toxoplasmosis is highly successful, and an empirical approach focusing initially on toxoplasmosis is usually considered reasonable. A definitive diagnostic study (i.e., brain biopsy) has some morbidity associated with it, and the diagnostic yield may be only 50% if toxoplasmosis is the cause. The cysts and tachyzoites of *T. gondii* can be very difficult to recognize in fragments of necrotic brain tissue, and even several small needle biopsy samples may miss the area that has abundant organisms. Because toxoplasmosis is the most common cause of gray matter lesions that benefits from therapy, and because needle biopsy has diagnostic limitations, empirical therapy with pyrimethamine (200 mg orally on day 1, followed by 50 to 100 mg orally every day) plus sulfadiazine (1 to 1.5 g orally every 6 hours) is reasonable (see Table 125-4). If a lumbar puncture can be performed safely and a PCR test for Epstein-Barr virus is available, a positive result would be suggestive of primary CNS lymphoma and could prompt either immediate biopsy or therapy directed at the neoplastic process.

Regarding sulfadiazine and pyrimethamine, some clinicians use higher doses of both drugs, but there is no clear evidence that higher doses are more effective, and they almost certainly produce more toxicity. If unequivocal improvement based on clinical and radiologic criteria does not occur within 10 to 21 days, a biopsy should be performed to establish whether the cause is an infectious or a neoplastic process other than toxoplasmosis.[62,63,159-160] Corticosteroids to reduce inflammation may be necessary in patients with substantial or progressive neurologic dysfunction or signs of increased intracranial pressure. The administration of corticosteroids can make early evaluation of the clinical and radiologic response to specific therapy difficult, because the observed improvement may be solely the result of corticosteroid therapy and unrelated to the anti-*Toxoplasma* regimen employed. Long-term antiseizure medication may be necessary. Although some clinicians institute this prophylactically, it is reasonable to initiate it only if a seizure occurs. For patients who have a response, anti-*Toxoplasma* therapy should be continued lifelong, in the absence of an ART-induced rise in the CD4+ T-cell count, because relapses occur in the same sites manifesting initially if therapy is discontinued, even after 8 to 12 months of treatment.[62,159,160] Whether the long-term suppressive regimen will be as effective if both pyrimethamine and sulfadiazine are not included at full doses remains to be demonstrated. If the CD4+ T-cell count rises dramatically (e.g., to levels higher than 200 cells/mm³), anti-*Toxoplasma* therapy can be safely discontinued after 6 months of therapy, provided that the lesion has largely resolved on cerebral imaging and the patient is neurologically stable (see Table 125-3).[12]

Treatment failures are unusual for patients with toxoplasmosis who are able to tolerate both pyrimethamine and sulfadiazine. Radiologically proven failures in patients who are adhering to their drug regimen should raise the possibility that toxoplasmosis is not the correct or the only diagnosis. Adverse reactions to sulfadiazine (leukopenia, rash, elevated levels of transaminases, nausea, nephritis) and to pyrimethamine (leukopenia, thrombocytopenia) are common. The leukopenia often does not respond to leucovorin therapy, although a short course of leucovorin (10 to 20 mg orally or intravenously every 6 hours) should be administered.

For patients unable to tolerate sulfadiazine, clindamycin plus pyrimethamine is also effective (see Table 125-1).[159,160] Atovaquone plus pyrimethamine is another reasonable alternative.[161,162] Clarithromycin plus pyrimethamine,[163] doxycycline,[164] or dapsone plus pyrimethamine[165] may also be useful regimens. Pyrimethamine by itself does not appear efficacious,[166,167] nor is trimetrexate[168] alone effective for long periods of time. Immunotherapy with interferon-γ or interleukin-12 might also be useful.

TMP-SMX offers considerable protection as primary prophylaxis.[143] Dapsone-pyrimethamine also has substantial efficacy.

Herpes Simplex and Varicella-Zoster Virus

Herpes simplex (see Chapter 132) is a frequent cause of genital and perirectal ulcerations in patients with HIV infection. Oral acyclovir (200 mg every 4 hours), valacyclovir, or famciclovir is effective therapy for herpes simplex virus genital lesions, perirectal lesions, proctitis, oral lesions, digital lesions, and esophagitis.[169-173] Disseminated herpes simplex viral infections and focal visceral manifestations are unusual in HIV-infected patients. Intravenous therapy is rarely necessary unless the patient has a major gastrointestinal disorder that prevents oral absorption. Topical acyclovir has not been demonstrated to be highly effective in patients with HIV infection.

The response of acyclovir-sensitive herpes simplex lesions is usually prompt and occurs within 3 to 10 days. Famciclovir or valacyclovir are probably as effective and safe as acyclovir and are more convenient because they can be given twice or three times daily. Therapy should continue until the lesions are crusted over or epithelialized. Relapses occur with high frequency. If relapses occur quickly or often, long-term suppression may be necessary. A regimen of oral acyclovir, 400 mg twice daily or 200 mg three or four times per day, is often used, although valacyclovir or famciclovir is more convenient. Acyclovir-resistant isolates occur.[174-176] Foscarnet and cidofovir are active against herpes simplex and have been used successfully against acyclovir-resistant strains.[174-176] Foscarnet-resistant herpes simplex virus has also been reported.[177] Favorable experience has been reported with topical preparations of trifluridine, foscarnet, or cidofovir.[177-180] If lesions recur, the causative virus may be a drug-susceptible strain even if the prior episode was caused by a drug-resistant stain.

Dermatomal herpes zoster lesions are usually similar in extent and distribution to those seen in immunocompetent patients (see Chapter 133). About 20% to 30% of HIV-infected patients have at least one recurrence. Dissemination of the varicella-zoster virus is an unusual event; if dissemination does occur, lesions may be atypical.[181-183] A high index of suspicion should be maintained that hyperkeratotic, verrucous, or ecthymatous lesions could be caused by varicella-zoster virus infection. However, clinically apparent visceral disease has rarely been documented, even in cases in which extensive disseminated cutaneous lesions have been observed. If organ involvement occurs, organs of the CNS, including the retina, are those most commonly affected. Varicella-zoster virus may produce characteristic retinal lesions, including a manifestation designated as "progressive outer retinal necrosis" and one designated "acute retinal necrosis."

For dermatomal disease, acyclovir, valacyclovir, or famciclovir therapy can have a role in hastening the crusting of lesions, in preventing postherpetic neuralgia, and in preventing recurrences in HIV-infected patients (see Table 125-4). Therapy appears to be indicated if the initial lesion occurred within the last 72 hours or new vesicles have recently appeared, or if evidence of dissemination or ophthalmic involvement is apparent. Treatment should probably continue until all lesions are scabbed or crusted, even if this requires more than 7 to 10 days. Patients with zoster ophthalmicus might be logical candidates for high-dose intravenous acyclovir (10 mg/kg every 8 hours). The use of corticosteroid therapy to prevent postherpetic neuralgia is controversial, and concern regarding the immunosuppressive effects of corticosteroids remains.[184,185] Acyclovir-resistant isolates do occur,[186-188] and some of these cases have been treated successfully with foscarnet or cidofovir.

About 5% of patients with HIV infection do not have detectable antibodies to varicella-zoster virus. If they are exposed to this virus, primary varicella can be severe.[188] Intravenous acyclovir therapy is probably beneficial for such patients.

Cytomegalovirus

CMV infection, as assessed by serology, is almost universal among HIV-infected patients who have acquired disease through homosexual contact (see Chapter 134). In contrast, only about 75% of patients who are heterosexual are seropositive for CMV.[189,190]

Historically, before either specific anti-CMV prophylaxis or ART was available, 21% to 44% of patients developed CMV-associated disease at some point during their illness.[9,191] HIV-infected patients with circulating CD4+ T-cell counts lower than 50 cells/mm³ are often viremic and viruric with CMV.[192] The likelihood of development of CMV-associated disease is related to both the degree of immunosuppression and the quantity of circulating CMV. The latter can be assessed by a variety of quantitative systems that detect antigen or nucleic acid in circulating blood.[35,193] A strategy to intervene in high-risk patients (i.e., those with low CD4+ T-cell counts and detectable CMV above some defined threshold) is logical because oral agents are available, but such an approach has yet to be definitively evaluated and shown to be both useful and cost-effective.

Retinitis is the most commonly recognized disease caused by CMV.[9,191,194,195] CMV retinitis has the potential to involve and rapidly damage the macula and optic disk, to cause retinal detachments, and to result in visual impairment and ultimately in blindness. Therefore, therapy is urgent when disease is recognized unless the lesions are small and peripheral. A variety of approaches can be used employing intravenous ganciclovir, intravenous foscarnet, intravenous cidofovir, oral valganciclovir, or ganciclovir ocular implants. For extensive retinitis, for vision-threatening retinitis, and for extraocular manifestations, intravenous therapy is usually preferred until there is clear clinical response; intraocular implants may be useful in addition to intravenous or oral therapy. CMV retinitis responds to either ganciclovir, administered intravenously at a dose of 5 mg/kg every 12 hours, or foscarnet, administered intravenously at 60 mg/kg every 8 hours (see Table 125-4).[64] Empirical therapy without a specific histologic or virologic diagnosis is reasonable, because obtaining retinal or vitreous material for examination is risky (detached retinas or secondary infections may result), the appearance of CMV retinitis is quite characteristic to an experienced ophthalmologist, and CMV causes most cases of retinitis that occur in HIV-infected patients.[196]

Intravenous ganciclovir and intravenous foscarnet are equally effective in terms of inducing remission of retinitis. Intravenous cidofovir is also effective.[197,198] New lesions or progressive disease may be identified during the first 7 days of therapy, and these do not necessarily imply a poor response. Considerable improvement in inflammation, edema, and hemorrhage will be recognized in responders before the end of 21 days of therapy. For patients treated with a 21-day course of intravenous therapy but no maintenance therapy, relapse at the same site as the initial lesions and at new sites almost invariably occurs within a few weeks or months unless ART results in a substantial rise in the CD4$^+$ T-cell count. Maintenance regimens using intravenous ganciclovir, 5 to 6 mg/kg daily on 5 to 7 days per week, or intravenous foscarnet, 90 mg daily, are often administered, but these regimens only prolong the interval until relapse by several weeks: the mean time to progression for patients receiving ganciclovir or foscarnet maintenance regimens is 50 to 59 days.[64]

Oral valganciclovir is an attractive alternative to intravenous therapy.[199,200] Oral valganciclovir has similar but not identical pharmacokinetics to intravenous ganciclovir. Its oral bioavailability is quite predictable for patients with normal gastrointestinal function, but the oral route is not preferred as the sole initial therapy for patients with severe or vision-threatening disease. Oral ganciclovir is no longer used since the advent of oral valganciclovir.

The major toxicity of ganciclovir and valganciclovir is bone marrow suppression with neutropenia and thrombocytopenia. Confusion, nausea, vomiting, transaminase elevation, and inhibition of spermatogenesis also occur. If patients with sight-threatening CMV lesions become neutropenic while receiving ganciclovir or valganciclovir, other infectious, neoplastic, immunologic, and drug-related causes of the neutropenia should be sought. Granulocyte colony-stimulating factor (G-CSF) may be useful to permit continued ganciclovir or valganciclovir therapy. Alternatively, another therapy, such as a ganciclovir implant[201,202] or parenteral foscarnet, may be tried. Foscarnet is nephrotoxic and can cause nausea, vomiting, anorexia, seizures, hypocalcemia, and hypomagnesemia.[64] Foscarnet generally must be infused over 60 minutes, after salt loading with a 60-minute infusion of normal saline, and therefore requires more infusion time than ganciclovir therapy. Cidofovir has the advantage that it can be given once every 2 weeks after two consecutive weekly doses, obviating the need for permanent intravenous access. Cidofovir is nephrotoxic, and each dose should be administered with probenecid after hydration with 1 L of normal saline. The long half-life can be a disadvantage if toxicity occurs.

Local instillation into the globe of an agent active against CMV is a logical approach to therapy for CMV retinitis. Local instillation of ganciclovir, foscarnet, or antisense nucleic acid (fomivirsen) has been tried with some success.[199,201-204] The most widely used approach is surgical implantation of an intraocular device impregnated with ganciclovir, which has a very high success rate.[201,202] Current implants fail after about 6 months due to depletion of the drug and must be replaced. The implantation of these devices can be associated with retinal detachments or endophthalmitis. Obviously, these implants provide local therapy only; their use is associated with a high rate of CMV disease in the contralateral eye and at extraocular loci, unless the patient has had a sustained immunologic response to ART. Oral valganciclovir should be given to patients with these implants to prevent ocular and extraocular disease.[200-203]

Esophagitis, enteritis, colitis, pneumonitis, and encephalitis are life-threatening syndromes caused by CMV that have been documented to respond to therapy.[205-207] A specific diagnosis for these syndromes should be established by histology or cytology, because they are indistinguishable from syndromes caused by other pathogens on the basis of clinical criteria alone. Culture of CMV from tissue, secretions, or excretions is insufficiently specific for CMV-caused disease to be used as a basis for therapy except in the case of neurologic disease. Detection of CMV by culture or, more often, by PCR in cerebrospinal fluid is highly suggestive that CMV is the cause of a compatible neurologic syndrome.

For patients with esophagitis, colitis, or rectal ulcers, improvement in clinical symptoms is usually noted during the first week of therapy with valganciclovir, ganciclovir, or foscarnet.[207] Improved performance status and increased weight are often noted, especially if ther-

apy results in reduced dysphagia or reduced diarrhea. There is considerably less experience with ganciclovir therapy for CMV pneumonia.[205] No consensus exists regarding the specific criteria for establishing this diagnosis, and many patients with no response to ganciclovir therapy had very severe and advanced lung damage before ganciclovir treatment was started. Therapy for bone marrow transplant recipients with ganciclovir is usually given concurrently with immune serum globulin or hyperimmune globulin.[206] However, there are no convincing data that immune or hyperimmune globulin enhances efficacy. As a result of this experience, immune serum globulin is often administered to patients with HIV infection and suspected CMV pneumonia as an adjunct to ganciclovir or foscarnet.

Recurrence of CMV retinitis is extremely unusual if the CD4$^+$ T-cell count rises to more than 50 to 100 cells/mm^3 after institution of ART. It is reasonable to stop maintenance therapy if the CD4$^+$ T-cell count has been higher than 50 to 100 cells/mm^3, the lesion is inactive, the lesion is not vision-threatening, and regular ophthalmologic follow-up is possible.[10] Clinicians need to distinguish between the recurrence of CMV retinitis or extraocular disease and immune reconstitution vitreitis, because management of these syndromes is quite different from management of CMV retinitis.[15,16]

Ganciclovir-resistant and foscarnet-resistant isolates are being recognized with increasing frequency by laboratories, especially in patients receiving oral valganciclovir.[208-211] Ganciclovir-resistant isolates usually have mutations in the *UL97* gene and maintain susceptibility to foscarnet or cidofovir. Some CMV isolates have mutations in the DNA polymerase gene, which can confer resistance to both foscarnet and cidofovir.[211] There is some evidence that ganciclovir in combination with foscarnet may be synergistic.[212,213]

Because CMV frequently causes specific organ damage in patients with HIV infection and may contribute to the febrile wasting syndromes associated with HIV disease, prevention of CMV disease is a logical goal. Strategies based on intervention with intravenous or oral regimens when CMV is detected by a nucleic acid or antigen assay of serum or peripheral white blood cells are logical but not validated. Patients might also wish to consider methods to reduce infection or reinfection by practicing safe sex, avoiding infected needles, and receiving only blood products that have been determined to be CMV free or have been filtered. Oral ganciclovir has been used to prevent primary CMV disease: studies suggest that this drug was probably effective.[214-215] Few clinicians used oral ganciclovir as primary prophylaxis because of the cost, toxicity, and inconvenience of this drug. Oral valganciclovir has not been studied for primary prophylaxis. Oral valganciclovir is not recommended by most clinicians for primary prophylaxis.[10]

Epstein-Barr Virus and Human Herpesvirus-6 and -7

Epstein-Barr virus (see Chapter 135) has been implicated in the pathogenesis of oral hairy leukoplakia and primary CNS lymphoma and may have a role in the pathogenesis of some cases of nonspecific pneumonitis, lymphadenopathy, lymphoma, fever, or wasting. There is insufficient evidence to warrant specific therapy for Epstein-Barr virus at this point, and no drug is clearly effective. Detection of Epstein-Barr virus by qualitative PCR in the cerebrospinal fluid of a patient with a CNS mass lesion is suggestive of primary CNS lymphoma but is not unequivocally specific.

Human herpes virus-6 and -7 (see Chapter 136) can be isolated from some patients with HIV infection. It is not clear how often they cause clinically important syndromes such as fever, rash, pneumonitis, or cerebritis in this patient population. If there is a strong suspicion that they could be the cause of a clinical syndrome, foscarnet therapy is a logical approach based on in vitro studies. Cidofovir and ganciclovir also have activity.

Progressive Multifocal Leukoencephalopathy

Progressive multifocal leukoencephalopathy is a unifocal or multifocal demyelinating process caused by the JC virus (see Chapter 141).[216,217] This disorder produces characteristic white matter lesions. It must be distinguished from AIDS dementia complex and cerebral infarction. Detection of JC virus in the cerebrospinal fluid by nucleic acid amplification is helpful diagnostically.[216,217] Specific therapy has not been effective.[218] Examples of dramatic clinical and radiologic improvement after institution of ART have been reported, although some patients worsen after institution of ART due to an immune reactivation syndrome.[41,219]

Candida Species

Stomatitis, esophagitis, vaginitis, and proctitis caused by *Candida* species infection are common and often respond to topical therapy (nystatin or clotrimazole), oral therapy (itraconazole or fluconazole), or intravenous therapy (fluconazole, voriconazole, caspofungin, or one of several amphotericin B preparations).[220-227] Fluconazole (50 to 200 mg orally every 24 hours) is the most convenient regimen and is therefore preferred unless there is a strong suspicion that the pathogen is fluconazole resistant. For oropharyngeal disease, single-dose therapy with 400 mg may be adequate, but a variety of daily doses (50 to 400 mg) and durations of therapy (1 to 28 days) have been studied, and most have reasonable response rates: 100 mg orally every day for 7 to 14 days is often recommended. If esophagitis is present, a longer course (14 to 21 days) is often employed. Itraconazole and voriconazole are also effective. For vulvovaginal candidiasis, one oral dose of fluconazole (150 mg) is equivalent in efficacy to a 7-day course of topical therapy. Fluconazole, itraconazole, and voriconazole all inhibit certain hepatic enzymes of the cytochrome P-450 class, resulting in elevated levels of drugs such as protease inhibitors and non-nucleoside reverse transcriptase inhibitors.

There is usually no urgency to institute antifungal therapy for any of these candidal mucosal disorders: esophagitis is rarely associated with bleeding, perforation, fungemia, or disseminated fungal disease. Stomatitis, esophagitis, and proctitis often recur after therapy is discontinued if CD4+ T-cell counts remain low. Fluconazole administration may have to be continued for life if recurrences are frequent or severe and the CD4+ T-cell counts remain low (see Table 125-2). Patients with no response to topical or oral azole therapy after 2 weeks usually have CD4+ T-cell counts lower than 50 cells/mm³ and extensive prior exposure to fluconazole.[45] The reasons for therapeutic failure need to be assessed, focusing on adherence to dosage regimens and drug interactions, as well as resistance of organisms to fluconazole. If there is no response to a 7-day course of oral fluconazole (200 mg or more every day), higher doses of fluconazole are rarely effective. Other options include itraconazole, cyclodextrin solution, voriconazole, caspofungin, and intravenous amphotericin B.[223-226,228] Patients with refractory candidiasis almost universally require lifelong therapy unless they manifest substantial immunologic and virologic response to ART. *Candida* isolates that are clinically and microbiologically resistant to fluconazole are being described with increasing frequency (see Chapter 255).

Disseminated candidiasis is not a common occurrence in HIV-infected patients unless they are receiving drug therapy that makes them neutropenic (especially cytotoxic antineoplastic therapy) or have an infected intravenous catheter. Treatment is similar to that in other patient populations, with particular attention directed at removing contaminated intravenous lines or discontinuing therapies that may be producing neutropenia.

Cryptococcus neoformans, Histoplasma capsulatum, and Coccidioides immitis

Meningitis is the most common manifestation of cryptococcal disease in patients with HIV infection. Most of the experience with treatment of cryptococcal disease in patients with HIV is derived from patients with meningitis.[229,230] Patients with factors predicting a poor outcome require more aggressive therapy than those with mild disease do. Baseline factors predicting a poor therapeutic response in patients with meningitis include altered mental status (e.g., confusion, lethargy, obtundation), cerebrospinal fluid antigen titer greater than 1:32 to 1:1024, decreased cerebrospinal fluid leukocyte count (fewer than 20 cells/mm³), age younger than 35 years, positive blood cultures

for *Cryptococcus*, and perhaps hyponatremia and positive CNS cultures for *Cryptococcus*.[231-234] As for other opportunistic infections, early recognition and institution of therapy are important for maximizing the likelihood of a favorable response. Diagnosis is readily established by culture and cryptococcal antigen testing of blood and cerebrospinal fluid.

The best studied therapy for cryptococcal meningitis is amphotericin B, 0.7 to 1.0 mg/kg/day (with or without flucytosine) given intravenously for at least 2 weeks; followed by fluconazole, 400 mg orally every day for 8 weeks; followed by fluconazole, 200 mg orally every day for life (see Table 125-4).[231-234] In early trials, there was a suggestion that amphotericin B was comparable in efficacy to fluconazole, but these trials used low doses of amphotericin B. Subsequent experience with initial fluconazole or itraconazole therapy was less promising. Currently, many clinicians are reluctant to use either azole as initial therapy, although some physicians might use such a regimen for a patient with very mild disease. Flucytosine is associated with potential bone marrow suppression and hepatotoxicity. For maintenance therapy, prospective data document that fluconazole is more effective than itraconazole in patients monitored for at least 24 weeks.[233] Using the recommended regimen of amphotericin B plus flucytosine followed by fluconazole maintenance therapy, a large prospective trial showed an acute mortality rate of 6%.[231-233]

Cryptococcus rarely becomes resistant to amphotericin B or fluconazole.[235,236] Susceptibility testing is available only as a research procedure.

There is considerable interest in using alternative drugs to amphotericin B to improve convenience, reduce toxicity, and further improve efficacy. Liposomal amphotericin preparations are effective therapies for cryptococcal meningitis, although it is not unequivocally established that they are as effective as the nonlipid formulation.[237]

The condition of patients with cryptococcal disease may deteriorate because of the consequences of increased intracranial pressure.[238] Clinical signs of increased pressure need to be sought, especially at presentation and during acute induction therapy. The baseline opening pressure should be measured at the time of the initial lumbar puncture in patients with focal neurologic findings or altered mental status. An imaging study of the CNS may be useful before the initial lumbar puncture and subsequently if the clinical status deteriorates. If the opening pressure is high (>25 cm H_2O), consideration should be given to reducing the pressure by repeated lumbar punctures or by insertion of a cerebrospinal fluid drain or shunt.

Patients being treated successfully for cryptococcal meningitis should demonstrate a decline in the cerebrospinal fluid cryptococcal antigen titer. There is no well-defined utility to serial monitoring of serum antigen titers, and such titers do not correlate closely with outcome.[36]

Maintenance fluconazole therapy can be stopped for patients who are asymptomatic, have completed 6 months of therapy, and have had a sustained increase in CD4+ T-cell counts with ART to more than 100 to 200 cells/mm³ for at least 6 months (see Table 125-3).[10,239-241] Some clinicians would repeat the lumbar puncture before stopping therapy, to assess the antigen titer and the presence of viable organisms, but there is no evidence that this is necessary.

Histoplasmosis is a particularly common, life-threatening, opportunistic infection in patients with HIV infection in certain geographic areas such as Indianapolis, Kansas City, and Puerto Rico.[37,46] Diagnosis is often established by direct microscopy or culture of bronchoalveolar lavage, bone marrow, or blood. Antigen detection in an appropriate reference laboratory is also highly sensitive for identification of disease. Although a sensitive and specific assay is available only from specialized laboratories, the sensitivity of the test is high in urine (95%), serum (80%), bronchoalveolar lavage (70%), and cerebrospinal fluid (50%).[37,141,242,243] Acute therapy should consist of intravenous amphotericin B, 0.5 to 1.0 mg/kg daily for 3 to 14 days, for most patients.[37,46,243-247] Itraconazole (200 mg orally twice a day) is also effective but should probably be reserved as initial therapy for patients with very mild disease (see Table 125-4).[37,46,243] Liposomal amphotericin B has been used successfully for long-term maintenance therapy; either itraconazole (200 mg orally twice daily to maintain serum levels higher than 1 μg/mL) or amphotericin B (0.5 to 0.8 mg/kg intravenously every week) is adequate.[247] Serum and urine *Histoplasma capsulatum* polysaccharide antigens are useful for monitoring both the initial and the long-term phases of treatment; they predict treatment failure or relapse.[46,242,243]

Maintenance therapy should probably be continued lifelong until there are more data confirming the safety of discontinuing it. Stopping such therapy in patients who are asymptomatic, have received a long course of therapy, and have negative urinary antigen levels is reasonable, but there is yet insufficient experience to warrant confidence that this approach is safe.[10]

Coccidioidomycosis is a complication of HIV infection in the southwestern United States.[248,249] The diagnosis can be established by direct microscopy or culture of bronchoalveolar lavage, blood, or cerebrospinal fluid. Serum immunoglobulin G titers can be helpful; they are usually positive in the presence of active disease. For patients with diffuse pulmonary infiltrates and CD4+ T-cell counts lower than 50 cells/mm³, therapy should consist of amphotericin B, 1.0 to 1.5 mg/kg/day. If meningeal involvement is present, either intrathecal amphotericin B (0.3 to 0.5 mg via intrathecal reservoir) twice weekly or fluconazole is a necessary addition to systemic amphotericin B. Focal pneumonia in patients with CD4+ T-cell counts higher than 50 cells/mm³ and relatively mild disease can probably be treated adequately with fluconazole alone, 400 mg orally every day. Lifelong maintenance therapy with either fluconazole or itraconazole is recommended.[10] The maintenance dose of azole therapy can be adjusted based on clinical status, and anti-*Coccidioides* antibody titer.

As with histoplasmosis, there is too little clinical experience with stopping of maintenance therapy in patients with an ART-induced rise in CD4+ T-cell counts to determine whether this approach is safe.

Aspergillosis is recognized as a cause of pseudomembranous tracheobronchitis, pneumonia, sinusitis, and disseminated disease.[250] Diagnosis is difficult to confirm without visualization of hyphae in tissue. Therapy is often unsuccessful because of both poor host immune function (patients often have a CD4+ T-cell count lower than 50 cells/mm³ or a neutrophil count lower than 500 cells/mm³) and the presence of extensive disease at the time of diagnosis. Strong consideration should be given to surgical resection of the most obviously affected tissue as an adjunct to medical therapy. Treatment with voriconazole or high-dose amphotericin B (1.0 to 1.5 mg/kg) is the standard approach. Whether lipid formulations of amphotericin B offer any advantage in terms of efficacy remains to be determined. Itraconazole has activity against *Aspergillus* but is not the preferred choice for single-agent therapy. Whether any combination therapy offers improved efficacy over variconazole or amphotericin B monotherapy remains to be determined.

Streptococcus pneumoniae, Haemophilus influenzae, and Other Bacterial Processes

Patients with HIV infection report a higher incidence of respiratory infections than do patients without HIV infection.[251-253] The frequency of these infections is inversely related to the CD4+ T-cell count. These respiratory infections include upper tract diseases (sinusitis, otitis, and bronchitis) and lower tract disease (pneumonia). *S. pneumoniae* and *Haemophilus influenzae* are common causes. Diagnosis and therapy do not differ from the approaches established for patients who are not infected with HIV.

The frequency of bacterial infections can be reduced by prophylactic regimens employing TMP-SMX,[136] clarithromycin,[254] or azithromycin.[255] These drugs are rarely prescribed specifically for their prophylactic antibacterial effect against pneumococci and *Haemophilus,* but they reduce such bacterial infections when prescribed to prevent PCP (TMP-SMX) or disseminated MAC (clarithromycin or azithromycin). G-CSF can reduce the frequency of bacterial infections in severely neutropenic patients with cancer, and it has been used for neutropenic patients with HIV infection. Because pneumococcal disease can be reduced by the administration of pneumo-

coccal vaccine to patients with CD4+ T-cell counts higher than 200 cells/mm³, routine immunization to such patients should be given.[10] Immunization should probably be repeated once after 5 years, and it should probably be repeated if the initial vaccine was administered when the CD4+ T-lymphocyte count was lower than 200 cells/mm³ and later rose to more than 200 cells/mm³ due to ART. Patients with HIV have been given the conjugated polysaccharide pneumococcal vaccine, but it is not yet clear whether the vaccine offers this patient population any clinical advantage over the 23-valent vaccine.

Other bacterial processes have also been described to occur with increased frequency among patients with HIV infection. Some are caused by the use of intravascular devices that, when contaminated, have the potential to cause bacteremias (or fungemias). Some are related to neutropenia, which can complicate advanced HIV disease or occur as a complication of the use of certain drugs (e.g., ganciclovir, pentamidine, pyrimethamine, sulfonamides, antineoplastic agents). Infections with other bacteria (e.g., *Rhodococcus equi*) appear to occur with increased frequency or virulence for unclear reasons.

Mycobacterium Species Infection

Mycobacterium tuberculosis

Tuberculosis most often manifests in patients with HIV infection as a pulmonary process. Radiographic appearances are diverse. Extrapulmonary manifestations are more likely to occur in patients infected with HIV than in immunocompetent patients.[256-258] Diagnosis is established by identification of *M. tuberculosis* in respiratory secretions, tissue, blood, or any other material, using culture, nucleic acid probes, or demonstration of suggestive organisms by staining. Therapy for tuberculosis is reviewed in Chapter 248. For patients with HIV infection, initial therapy generally consists of daily oral isoniazid (300 mg every day), rifampin (600 mg every day), and pyrazinamide (15 to 25 mg/kg every day) (see Table 125-1).[258] Ethambutol (15 to 25 mg/kg every day) should be added to the initial regimen if there is any reason to suspect drug resistance: from a practical perspective, most clinicians always add ethambutol to their initial regimen. In most areas in the United States, therefore, a four-drug initial regimen is appropriate. If the organism is susceptible to all drugs being used, isoniazid and pyrazinamide and rifampin should be continued to complete an initial 2 months of therapy; isoniazid plus rifampin should then be continued for a minimum of 4 additional months. Longer courses must be considered for patients with cavitary disease and for those whose sputum culture does not convert to negative at 2 months. Once-weekly isoniazid-rifapentine regimens should not be used for HIV-infected patients, and twice-weekly isoniazid-rifampin regimens should not be used for HIV-infected patients with CD4+ T-cell counts lower than 100 cells/mm³. Peripheral neuropathy is a major concern in patients with HIV infection. Pyridoxine, 50 mg PO every day, should be administered concurrently with isoniazid.

The optimal duration of therapy is controversial. Some experts prefer a 9- or 12-month regimen rather than a 6-month regimen (6 months is routinely recommended by the Centers for Disease Control and Prevention [CDC] for sensitive isolates being treated with daily regimens, starting with isoniazid, rifabutin, ethambutol, and pyrazinamide). A study of HIV-infected patients showed a lower relapse or recurrence rate for patients treated for 12 months (1.9%) than for patients treated for 6 months (9%).[259] It is not certain whether this difference was caused by relapses or by reinfections. If patients have a delayed response to therapy (e.g., they are still symptomatic or still have positive cultures after 2 months), or if they have extensive disease (e.g., pulmonary cavities), treatment for 9 to 12 months is preferred. Whatever regimen is chosen, directly observed therapy (DOT) should be considered for every patient. If response to therapy is not optimal based on clinical or microbiologic grounds after 8 weeks of therapy, chest radiography and drug susceptibility testing should be repeated. Measurement of serum drug levels may also be helpful, although such tests are not widely available. Secondary prophylaxis is not recommended, although its use may be reasonable in highly endemic areas to prevent reinfection.

A well-described syndrome associated with treatment of tuberculosis in non–HIV-infected patients is "paradoxical response."[13-16,258,260] After initiation of antituberculosis therapy, areas that are clinically involved may worsen (e.g., clinical disease may worsen in terms of oxygenation, cough, or fever in patients with recognized lung involvement). Subclinically involved areas, such as the meninges, pericardium, or lymph nodes, may also become clinically involved, because there is a more intense inflammatory response. This syndrome also occurs in HIV-infected patients who start antituberculosis therapy.[13-16] It appears to be especially pronounced when patients newly recognized to have tuberculosis and HIV start both ART and antituberculosis therapy simultaneously. The resulting fever, lymphadenopathy, pulmonary exacerbation, and other extrapulmonary manifestations can be marked. Many clinicians do not initiate ART until at least 6 to 8 weeks after starting antituberculosis therapy, but such an approach is based on anecdotal experience.[12,258]

A major problem associated with antituberculosis therapy is management of drug interactions between antituberculosis and antiretroviral medications, especially the interactions among rifamycins, protease inhibitors, and non-nucleoside reverse transcriptase inhibitors. The CDC has made dosing recommendations for patients receiving ART that includes protease inhibitors and non-nucleoside reverse transcriptase inhibitors.[258] For regimens that include a rifamycin, oral rifabutin (150 mg every day) rather than rifampin should be used with soft gel saquinavir, nelfinavir mesylate, indinavir, amprenavir, or nevirapine. If efavirenz is used, the dose of rifabutin should be increased to 450 mg daily or twice weekly.[258] Rifamycins should not be used with hard gel saquinavir, ritonavir, or delavirdine; in those cases, therapy for at least 9 months with a regimen that includes streptomycin (or another injectable antituberculosis drug) along with isoniazid, pyrazinamide, and ethambutol should be considered (see also Chapter 124).[258] Drug interactions often involve more than two drugs that are affected by the cytochrome P-450 systems; in such cases, pharmacokinetics are not easily predictable unless the particular drug combination has been studied.

Treatment of drug-resistant tuberculosis is discussed in Chapter 248. Drug-resistant strains have been particular problems in primary tuberculous infections associated with outbreaks at health care facilities and other institutional settings.[42,43] Therapy is chosen based on prior drug exposure and drug susceptibility patterns.

Chemoprophylaxis should be administered to any HIV-infected patient with a tuberculin skin test induration that is 5 mm in diameter or larger if that patient has never received adequate prophylaxis or therapy.[258] In addition, HIV-infected patients should receive chemoprophylaxis regardless of tuberculin skin test status if they have had close contact with a patient with infectious tuberculosis.

Nine months of isoniazid prophylaxis is preferred over a 6-month regimen (see Table 125-2).[258] Isoniazid can be administered either daily or twice weekly at appropriate doses. Alternative regimens not employing isoniazid should be considered in patients with severe liver disease. It is important to recognize that in areas such as Haiti, where tuberculosis is endemic, isoniazid prophylaxis can have a major impact on survival.[49] Rifampin (600 mg every day) is an alternative regimen, although it is not as well studied as isoniazid. A combination of pyrazinamide plus rifampin administered for 2 months is also probably effective for prophylaxis in patients with HIV infection.[261] It has the advantage of a shorter duration than the isoniazid regimen. However, there has been sufficient toxicity associated with this regimen that few clinicians currently use this approach. Protease inhibitors should not be used concurrently with rifampin. Another option for prophylaxis is a 3-month course of isoniazid plus rifampin. Any regimen that includes a rifamycin may produce drug interactions with protease inhibitors, non-nucleoside reverse transcriptase inhibitors, and other drugs metabolized by the cytochrome P-450 system.

In addition to considering chemoprophylaxis, patients with HIV infection should reduce their likelihood of exposure to tuberculosis. Employment in homeless shelters, correctional facilities, or respiratory disease health care facilities, for example, should be considered with caution.

Mycobacterium avium Complex

MAC disease has been much less common since the widespread use of ART.[3,4,261] MAC most often manifests as a systemic process characterized by fever, weight loss, elevated serum alkaline phosphatase levels, and substantial anemia.[261,262] Wasting, diarrhea, or lymphadenopathy may be seen. Diagnosis is most readily established by blood culture or by biopsy of affected tissue. Culture of organisms from respiratory secretions, stool, or urine does not unequivocally establish the presence of invasive disease or the need for therapy. Patients colonized with MAC do not necessarily develop disease due to MAC; therefore, a positive culture of sputum or stool or urine is not necessarily an indication for therapy.

Studies to date have demonstrated that several specific chemotherapies can reduce or eliminate mycobacteria over a period of weeks or months.[263-266] Most patients with a favorable microbiologic response experience an improvement in symptoms and signs. Drugs that have microbiologic activity and satisfactory toxicity profiles include clarithromycin, azithromycin, rifabutin, ethambutol, amikacin, and several quinolones.

Initial treatment regimens usually include either clarithromycin or azithromycin plus ethambutol (see Table 125-4). Because there is more experience with clarithromycin than with azithromycin, the former drug is usually preferred. The recommended dose of clarithromycin is 500 mg orally twice daily; higher doses have been associated with higher mortality rates,[10] for reasons that are unclear. There is little experience regarding MAC therapy with the extended-release preparation of clarithromycin. If clarithromycin or azithromycin is used as monotherapy, relapse occurs in most patients in less than 1 year. If other drugs are added to the macrolide, especially ethambutol, the relapse rate and time to relapse are improved substantially.[267] Therefore, clarithromycin plus ethambutol is the recommended regimen unless there is reason to suspect that the isolate is macrolide resistant.[12]

Although many clinicians recommend initial therapy consisting of clarithromycin plus ethambutol, additional drugs such as rifabutin or amikacin or ciprofloxacin may be added if the disease is severe or extensive. Some experts advocate a three-drug regimen of clarithromycin, ethambutol, and rifabutin for patients with extensive disease or prior opportunistic infections. However, the evidence that rifabutin adds to efficacy is weak, and rifabutin adds complexity to the issue of pharmacokinetic interactions.[266] Clofazimine is no longer recommended because of an association with increased mortality.[10] Susceptibility testing of isolates is not performed routinely unless the likelihood of drug resistance is high. Susceptibility testing might be appropriate if a patient has developed bacteremia while receiving macrolide therapy. Susceptibility testing has been best validated for clarithromycin, azithromycin, and perhaps rifabutin. However, many isolates recovered from patients receiving prophylaxis are still macrolide sensitive for reasons that are not entirely clear.

Most patients demonstrate defervescence and lower quantities of circulating MAC within 2 to 4 weeks after initiation of therapy unless the disease is extensive, drug adherence is poor, or absorption or pharmacokinetic issues result in suboptimal serum tissue concentrations of drug. In such cases, MAC susceptibility testing and serum drug level monitoring are likely to be useful.

If MAC bacteremia reoccurs after a period of clinical and mycobacterial improvement, organisms are often resistant to the drugs used in the treatment regimen. It is logical to choose a new regimen based on susceptibility results, although, as noted, such testing has not been validated as clinically useful for most drugs. A multidrug regimen employing rifabutin and other agents to which the patient has not been exposed is often recommended. Whether the macrolide should be continued despite clinical or in vitro resistance is controversial.

Regarding the optimal duration of therapy for patients demonstrating sustained clinical and microbiologic response, guidelines and recommendations have emphasized the need for lifelong therapy. Evidence suggests that therapy does not need to be lifelong in patients who are asymptomatic, have received at least 12 months of therapy, and have had an ART-induced increase in CD4$^+$ T-cell counts to greater than 100 cells/mm^3 for at least 6 months.[268-270]

Chemoprophylaxis for MAC disease is a logical management strategy, because this disease is frequent, severe, and difficult to treat in the long term and because there are parameters for identifying patients who are at highest risk. Patients at risk include those with a CD4$^+$ T-cell count lower than 50 cells/mm^3, especially those with a previous opportunistic infection (especially CMV disease), or a respiratory or gastrointestinal tract that is colonized with MAC.[25,271,272] Clarithromycin, azithromycin, and rifabutin are each effective chemoprophylactic agents in terms of reducing the incidence of disease and reducing mortality.[267,270,271] Clarithromycin (500 mg orally twice daily) or azithromycin (1200 mg once per week) is more effective than rifabutin and produces fewer important drug interactions (see Table 125-2). The combination of rifabutin plus azithromycin is more effective than either drug alone, but few clinicians employ this regimen because of the adverse effects and cost associated with this combination regimen. There is little experience with the clarithromycin extended-release preparation. If breakthrough occurs during clarithromycin prophylaxis, some isolates will be clarithromycin resistant; this is less often the case for breakthroughs that occur during rifabutin or azithromycin prophylaxis.

The risk of disseminated *Mycobacterium avium-intracellulare* is markedly reduced in patients with low CD4$^+$ T-cell counts in whom highly active ART produces a sustained immunologic and virologic response.[269,270] Current guidelines from the U.S. Public Health Service and the Infectious Disease Society of America recommend that prophylaxis can be discontinued if patients have a sustained rise in CD4$^+$ T-cell count after initiation of ART.[10]

Enteric Pathogens: *Salmonella, Shigella,* and *Campylobacter* Species, *Entamoeba histolytica,* and *Giardia lamblia*

Enteric disease due to *Salmonella, Shigella,* or *Campylobacter* is common. Bacteremia appears to occur more commonly in HIV-infected patients than in HIV-uninfected patients. Amoebiasis and giardiasis also occur, but their manifestations are not necessarily different from those in immunocompetent patients.

Initial therapy for *Salmonella, Shigella, Campylobacter, Entamoeba,* and *Giardia* infections follows standard guidelines. Infections with *Salmonella,* and perhaps *Shigella* and *Campylobacter,* tend to relapse if long-term suppressive therapy is not administered.

Cryptosporidium, Isospora, Cyclospora, and Microsporidia

The four types of protozoa—cryptosporidia, isospora, cyclospora, and microsporidia—are often recognized as causes of chronic diarrheal syndromes. Each can cause biliary and pancreatic disease by infecting the biliary-pancreatic ducts as well. Microsporidia (see Chapter 282) can also cause systemic disease and can produce keratitis. These pathogens can be identified in stool by appropriate direct microscopic techniques or by tissue biopsy. For corneal disease, microsporidia can be identified by corneal scrapings.

Therapy for cryptosporidiosis (see Chapter 280) has been disappointing. Symptomatic therapy employing antimotility drugs and dietary alterations is often helpful. Octreotide offers little benefit beyond that achievable with more readily available antimotility agents.[273] Some early results with immunoglobulin preparations such as hyperimmune bovine colostrum were promising.[274,275] Many clinicians reported some transient benefit from paromomycin, but a controlled trial of this agent showed no substantial difference between the effects of this drug and those of placebo.[276] Several reports suggested that, for

some patients who respond favorably to ART, dramatic improvement in cryptosporidial diarrhea and nutritional status can occur.[277,278]

Prevention of cryptosporidiosis should focus on environmental control, because no drugs are known to be effective for prevention.[10] In some areas where outbreaks have been linked to the local drinking water supply or where contamination of water is likely, water should be boiled for 1 minute or filtered through a device capable of removing particles as small as 1 μm in diameter. Whether all individuals infected with HIV should drink bottled or filtered water exclusively is controversial. Individuals at risk should also avoid contact with farm animals, infected humans, or pets that are at high risk (e.g., dogs and cats younger than 6 months of age, stray animals, animals with diarrhea).[10]

Isospora and *Cyclospora* (see Chapter 281) can each be treated effectively with TMP-SMX.[279,280] Patients usually respond symptomatically within 7 to 10 days, but the relapse rate is high unless TMP-SMX is continued lifelong for patients whose CD4$^+$ T-cell counts remain low. If patients respond to ART with sustained increases in CD4$^+$ T-cell counts and sustained suppression of HIV viral loads, it is logical to presume that long-term maintenance therapy for isosporiasis or cyclosporiasis can be discontinued. Ciprofloxacin is also active against *Cyclospora.*[281]

Both albendazole and fumagillin have activity in vitro and in vivo against some microsporidia. There are numerous reports that albendazole can have a beneficial effect on diarrhea caused by *Encephalitozoon intestinalis,* disseminated disease caused by *Encephalitozoon hellem* or *Encephalitozoon cuniculi,* and disease caused by *Nosema* or *Tachipleistophora.*[282-286] Albendazole has not been as effective in treating the major cause of microsporidial diarrhea: *Enterocytozoon bieneusi.* Some patients with *E. bieneusi* diarrhea experience transient symptomatic improvement after albendazole therapy, but there is little evidence for microbiologic improvement or improvement in D-xylose absorption, and relapse often occurs promptly after drug therapy is discontinued. Oral fumagillin,[287] an investigational agent, as well as octreotide[288] and thalidomide,[289] have been reported to decrease diarrhea due to *E. bieneusi* in small series.

Microsporidial keratitis has been treated successfully with lifelong topical fumagillin.[283] Patients with microsporidial keratitis should be assessed for systemic microsporidiosis, and systemic therapy with albendazole should be considered.

Because little is known about the transmission of microsporidia to humans, no specific recommendations for prevention can be made. It is logical to presume that prevention of food and water contamination by animals decreases transmission of this organism.

Treponema pallidum

Syphilis is often recognized in HIV-infected patients either because of characteristic lesions of primary or secondary disease or because a screening serology result for *Treponema pallidum* is positive. With the resurgence of syphilis in HIV-infected patients in many areas, treponemal disease is likely to become increasingly important as a cause of disease in this patient population. The clinical manifestations of syphilis, as well as its diagnosis and treatment, do not differ dramatically in HIV-infected and -uninfected patients.[290-292] Syphilis can have diverse manifestations of primary, secondary, and tertiary disease. Especially among those HIV-infected individuals who are in population groups experiencing a resurgence in syphilis, *T. pallidum* should enter into the differential diagnosis of dermatologic, ocular, and neurologic syndromes. Infected patients can be diagnostically and therapeutically approached similarly to HIV-uninfected individuals. There is concern that HIV-infected patients may have an increased incidence of neurosyphilis. There is no clear consensus concerning the need to perform lumbar punctures for asymptomatic patients with late latent syphilis. It is becoming increasingly apparent that CNS involvement is relatively common in patients with primary and secondary syphilis (see Chapter 235). If careful diagnostic studies are employed, as many as 40% of patients with primary or secondary syphilis will have serologic or microbiologic evidence of *T. pallidum* in their cerebrospinal fluid regardless of their HIV status. A single dose of 2.4 million units (MIU) benzathine penicillin may be inadequate to cure the CNS involvement or to prevent systemic relapses, as measured by subsequent rises in serum Venereal Disease Research Laboratory (VDRL) titers. The optimal treatment for HIV-infected patients with early or latent syphilis has not been established: procaine penicillin (1.2 MIU daily for 10 to 14 days) may have advantages over serial doses of benzathine penicillin (2.4 MIU every week for 3 or 4 weeks) in terms of preventing relapses.[12]

Bartonella

Bartonella henselae and *Bartonella quintana* (see Chapter 232) have been described as the causes of a spectrum of clinical syndromes in patients with HIV infection.[293-295] These syndromes include cutaneous and subcutaneous angiomatous papules, which can be confused with Kaposi's sarcoma, and angiomatous masses in the liver (peliosis hepatis), bone, lymph nodes, lungs, and CNS, which appear to be mass lesions. Bartonellosis can also manifest as fever and bacteremia. The diagnosis is usually established by Warthin-Starry stain of tissue or by culture of blood or tissue using enriched agar. Most experience with therapy has been with either erythromycin or doxycycline. At least 2 g daily of erythromycin should be given for at least 8 to 12 weeks for patients with cutaneous disease.[12] Doxycycline should be given at a dose of 100 mg every 12 hours. Clinical response may be seen during the first week. Cutaneous lesions may require 1 to 2 months to resolve; hepatic lesions may require 2 to 3 months. Hepatic and osseous lesions should be treated initially with intravenous erythromycin. Rifampin may be useful as an adjunct to the primary drug. A Jarisch-Herxheimer reaction may be seen in response to the first few drug doses. Treatment failures and relapses occur.

Prevention of bartonellosis should focus on reducing exposure to the vectors, namely, the body louse (for *B. quintana*) and cats and cat fleas (for *B. henselae*).

Kaposi's Sarcoma

The presence of Kaposi's sarcoma does not necessarily mandate institution of specific therapy, especially if lesions are few in number and inconspicuous. Lesions may regress in patients who respond to ART. Local measures can be useful, including excision, radiation, and intralesional injection with chemotherapy.[296-298] When lesions in the oropharynx are irradiated, mucositis seems to be especially common.

If cutaneous Kaposi's sarcoma is extensive, recombinant interferon-γ therapy (10 to 30 million units/m^2 given intramuscularly, intravenously, or subcutaneously every day) can be useful, especially for patients with circulating CD4$^+$ T-cell counts greater than 100 to 200 cells/mm^3.[298] Objective tumor responses may be seen in 4 to 8 weeks, with maximal responses in 12 to 24 weeks. Late initial responses after many months of therapy occasionally occur. Because the tumor response is not rapid, interferon-γ therapy is not desirable for urgent, life-threatening situations such as laryngeal or extensive pulmonary involvement. Adverse effects of interferon-γ include confusion, fatigue, myalgia, leukopenia, thrombocytopenia, hepatitis, and cardiomyopathy.

Kaposi's sarcoma can cause life-threatening disease by obstructing a vital structure such as the larynx, bronchus, biliary tract, or bowel. Kaposi's sarcoma can occasionally infiltrate a vital organ such as the lung and cause fatal hypoxemia. In these life-threatening situations, either radiation therapy or cytotoxic chemotherapy is necessary to produce a rapid and substantial response. The optimal mode of therapy depends on the location and extent of the tumor. A variety of chemotherapeutic regimens have been used with some success, including liposomal vinblastine; etoposide; vincristine; vincristine and vinblastine; vinblastine and bleomycin; and doxorubicin, bleomycin, and vincristine.[28] The optimal drug regimens for specific situations have not been determined. Preliminary evidence suggests that ganciclovir or foscarnet therapy may reduce the risk of Kaposi's sarcoma.

Lymphoma and Other Neoplastic Diseases

Lymphomas of the Hodgkin's, non-Hodgkin's, and Burkitt's types are often recognized as patients with HIV infection survive longer (see Chapter 121). The risk of lymphoma is not confined to specific CD4$^+$ T-cell count ranges. After a diagnosis is established by tissue biopsy, a staging workup is appropriate. Chemotherapy and radiation therapy each have potential therapeutic value. Long-term remissions are being reported, especially for patients who have none of the following risk factors: CD4$^+$ T-cell count lower than 100 cells/mm^3, bone marrow involvement, Karnofsky performance status less than 70%, stage IV disease, or prior AIDS-defining illness.[299] The optimal therapeutic approach is controversial: chemotherapy and radiation therapy can each have beneficial roles, and long-term remission should be the goal.[300] ART is an important part of optimal management, although drug interactions between antiretroviral and antineoplastic agents should be carefully managed. Primary effusion cell lymphomas, multicentric Castleman's disease, cervical and anal squamous cell carcinomas, and certain solid tumors also occur with increased frequency among patients with HIV infection.

REFERENCES

1. Palella FJ, Delaney KM, Moorman AC, et al. Declining morbidity and mortality among patients with advanced immunodeficiency virus infection. N Engl J Med. 1998;338:853-860.
2. Mocroft A, Ledergerber B, Katlama C, et al. Decline in the AIDS and death rates in the Eurosida Study: An observational study. Lancet. 2003;362:22-27.
3. Mocroft A, Brettle R, Kirk O, et al. Changes in the cause of death among HIV positive subjects across Europe: Results from the Eurosida Study. AIDS. 2002;16:1663-1671.
4. Jones JL, Hanson DL, Dworken MS, et al. Surveillance for AIDS-defining opportunistic illnesses, 1992-1997. MMWR Morb Mortal Wkly Rep. 1999;48(SS-2):1-22.
5. Egger M, May M, Chene G, et al. Prognosis of HIV-1 infected patients starting highly active antiretroviral therapy: A collaborative analysis of prospective studies. Lancet. 2002;360:119-129.
6. Lemp GF, Payne SF, Neal D, et al. Survival trends for patients with AIDS. JAMA. 1990;263:402-406.
7. Chaisson RE, Keruly J, Richman DD, et al. *Pneumocystis* prophylaxis and survival in patients with advanced HIV infection treated with zidovudine. Arch Intern Med. 1992;152:2009-2013.
8. Graham NM, Zeger SL, Park LP, et al. Effect of zidovudine and *Pneumocystis carinii* pneumonia prophylaxis on progression of HIV-1 infection to AIDS. Lancet. 1991;338:265-269.
9. Moore RD, Chaisson RE. Natural history of opportunistic disease in an HIV-infected urban clinical cohort. Ann Intern Med. 1996;124:633-642.
10. U.S. Public Health Service/Infectious Disease Society of America Prevention of Opportunistic Infections Working Group. USPHS/IDSA Guidelines for the Prevention of Opportunistic Infections in Persons Infected with Human Immunodeficiency Virus. 2001. Available at www.aidsinfo.nih.gov. Accessed April 12, 2004.
11. Panel on Clinical Practices for Treatment of HIV Infection, Department of Health and Human Services. Guidelines for the use of antiretroviral agents in HIV-infected adults and adolescents. March 23, 2004. Available at www.aidsinfo.nih.gov. Accessed April 12, 2004.
12. U.S. Public Health Service/Infectious Disease Society of America. USPHS/IDSA Guidelines for Therapy of Opportunistic Infections in Persons Infected with Human Immunodeficiency Virus. Available at www.aidsinfo.nih.gov. In press.
13. Race EM, Adelson-Mitty J, Kriegel GR, et al. Focal mycobacterial lymphadenitis following initiation of protease-inhibitor therapy in patients with advanced HIV-1 disease. Lancet. 1998;351:252-255.
14. Navas E, Martin-Davila P, Moreno L, et al. Paradoxical reactions of tuberculosis in patients with the acquired immunodeficiency syndrome who are treated with highly active antiretroviral therapy. Arch Intern Med. 2002;162:97-99.
15. Shelborne SA, Hamill RJ, Rodriguez-Barradas MC, et al. Immune reconstitution syndrome. Medicine (Baltimore). 2002;81:213-227.
16. DeSimone JA, Pomerantz RJ, Babinchak TJ, et al. Inflammatory reactions in HIV-1 infected persons after initiation of highly active antiretroviral therapy. Ann Intern Med. 2000;133:447-454.
17. Sepkowitz KA. Effect of HAART on natural history of AIDS-related opportunistic disorders. Lancet. 1998;351:228-230.
18. Freedberg KA, Scharfstein JA, Seage GR III, et al. The cost-effectiveness of preventing AIDS-related opportunistic infections. JAMA. 1998;279:130-136.
19. Masur H, Ognibene FP, Yarchoan R, et al. CD4$^+$ T lymphocyte counts as predictors of opportunistic pneumonias in human immunodeficiency virus (HIV) infection. Ann Intern Med. 1989;111:223-231.
20. Phair J, Munoz A, Detels R, et al. The risk of *Pneumocystis carinii* pneumonia among men infected with human immunodeficiency virus type 1. N Engl J Med. 1990;322:161-165.
21. Chu SY, Hanson DL, Ciesielski C, et al. Prophylaxis against *Pneumocystis carinii* pneumonia at higher CD4$^+$ T lymphocyte counts (Letter). JAMA. 1995;273:848.
22. Mellors JW, Munoz A, Giorgi JV, et al. Plasma viral load and CD4$^+$ T lymphocytes as prognostic markers of HIV-1 infection. Ann Intern Med. 1997;126:946-954.

23. Yarchoan R, Venzon DJ, Pluda JM, et al. CD4+ T lymphocyte count and the risk for death in patients infected with HIV receiving antiretroviral therapy. Ann Intern Med. 1991;115:188-189.
24. Havlik JA Jr, Horsburgh CR Jr, Metchock B, et al. Disseminated *Mycobacterium avium* complex infection: Clinical identification and epidemiologic trends. J Infect Dis. 1992;165:577-580.
25. Nightingale SD, Cameron DW, Gordin FM, et al. Two controlled trials of rifabutin prophylaxis against *Mycobacterium avium* complex infection in AIDS. N Engl J Med. 1993;329:828-833.
26. Connors M, Kovacs JA, Krevat S, et al. HIV infection induces changes in CD4+ T lymphocyte cell phenotype and depletions within the CD4+ T lymphocyte cell repertoire that are not immediately restored by antiviral or immune-based therapies. Nat Med. 1997;3:533-540.
27. Kaplan JE, Hanson DL, Jones JL, et al. Viral load as an independent risk factor for opportunistic infections in HIV-infected adults and adolescents. AIDS. 2001;15:1831-1836.
28. Miller V, Mocroft A, Reiss P, et al. Relations among CD4+ T lymphocyte count nadir, antiretroviral therapy, and HIV-1 disease progression: Results from the Eurosida Study. Ann Intern Med. 1999;130:570-577.
29. Lederman HM, Willams PL, Wu JW. Incomplete immunologic reconstitution after initiation of highly active antiretroviral therapy in human immunodeficiency virus-infected patients with severe CD4+ cell depletion. J Infect Dis. 2003;188:1794-1803.
30. Hengel RL, Kovacs JA. Surrogate markers of immune function in human immunodeficiency virus-infected patients: What are they surrogates for? J Infect Dis. 2003; 188:1791-1793.
31. Tierney C, Lathey JL, Christopherson C, et al. Prognostic value of baseline human immunodeficiency virus type 1 DNA measurement for disease progression in patients receiving nucleoside therapy. J Infect Dis. 2003;187:144-148.
32. Saag MS, Holodniy M, Kuritzkes DR, et al. HIV viral load markers in clinical practice. Nat Med. 1996;2:625-629.
33. Press N, Tyndall MW, Wood E. Virologic and immunologic response, clinical progression, and highly active antiretroviral therapy adherence. J Acquir Immune Defic Syndr. 2002;31:5112-5117.
34. Katzenstein DA, Hammer SM, Hughes MD, et al. The relation of virologic and immunologic markers to clinical outcomes after nucleoside therapy in HIV-infected adults with 200 to 500 CD4+ T lymphocyte cells per cubic millimeter. N Engl J Med. 1996;335:1091-1098.
35. Spector SA, Wong R, Hsia K, et al. Plasma cytomegalovirus (CMV) DNA load predicts CMV disease and survival in AIDS patients. J Clin Invest. 1998;101:497.
36. Powderly WG, Cloud GA, Dismukes WE, Saag MS. Measurement of cryptococcal antigen in serum and cerebrospinal fluid: Value in the management of AIDS-associated cryptococcal meningitis. Clin Infect Dis. 1994;18:789-792.
37. Wheat LJ, Connolly-Stringfield P, Blair R, et al. Histoplasmosis relapse in patients with AIDS: Detection using *Histoplasma capsulatum* variety capsulatum antigen levels. Ann Intern Med. 1991;115:936-941.
38. Piscitelli SC, Gallicano KD. Interactions among drugs for HIV and opportunistic infections. N Engl J Med. 2001;344:984-996.
39. Carr A, Marriott D, Field A. et al. Treatment of HIV-1 associated microsporidiosis and cryptosporidiosis with combination antiretroviral therapy. Lancet. 1998;351:256-261.
40. Mrudaca G, Campelli A, Setti M, et al. Complete remission of AIDS/Kaposi sarcoma after treatment with a combination of two nucleoside reverse transcription inhibitors and one non-nucleoside reverse transcriptase inhibitor. AIDS. 2002;16:304-305.
41. Cinque P, Bossolasco S, Brambilla AM, et al. The effect of highly active antiretroviral therapy-induced immune reconstitution on development and outcome of progressive multifocal leukoencephalopathy: Study of 43 cases with review of the literature. J Neurovirol. 2003;9(Suppl):73-80.
42. Small PM, Shafer RW, Hopewell PC, et al. Exogenous reinfection with multidrug-resistant *Mycobacterium tuberculosis* in patients with advanced HIV infection. N Engl J Med. 1993;328:1137-1144.
43. Daley CL, Small PM, Schecter GF, et al. An outbreak of tuberculosis with accelerated progression among persons infected with human immunodeficiency virus: An analysis using restriction-fragment-length polymorphisms. N Engl J Med. 1992;326:231-235.
44. Nimri LF, Moura IN, Huang L, et al. Genetic diversity of *Pneumocystis carinii* f. sp. hominis based on variations in nucleotide sequences of internal transcribed spacers of rRNA genes. J Clin Microbiol. 2002;40:1146-1151.
45. Maenza JR, Keruly JC, Moore RD, et al. Risk factors for fluconazole-resistant candidiasis in human immunodeficiency virus-infected patients. Clin Infect Dis. 1996;173:219.
46. Wheat LJ, Connolly-Stringfield PA, Baker RL, et al. Disseminated histoplasmosis in the acquired immunodeficiency syndrome: Clinical findings, diagnosis and treatment, and review of the literature. Medicine (Baltimore). 1990;69:361-374.
47. Silva N, O'Bryan L, Medeiros E, et al. *Trypanosoma cruzi* meningoencephalitis in HIV infected patients. J Acquir Immune Defic Syndr Hum Retrovirol. 1999;20: 342-349.
48. Ferreira MS, Nishioka SA, Silvestre MT, et al. Reactivation of Chagas' disease in patients with AIDS: Report of three new cases and review of the literature. Clin Infect Dis. 1997;25:1397-1400.
49. Pape JW, Jean Simone S, Ho JL, et al. Effect of isoniazid prophylaxis on incidence of active tuberculosis and progression in HIV infection. Lancet. 1993;342:268-272.
50. Mukadi Y, Perriens JH, St. Louis ME, et al. Spectrum of immunodeficiency in HIV-1 infected patients with pulmonary tuberculosis in Zaire. Lancet. 1993;342:143-146.
51. Duong TA. Infection due to *Penicillium marneffei*, an emerging pathogen: Review of 155 reported cases. Clin Infect Dis. 1996;23:125-130.
52. Pape JW, Verdier R, Johnson WD, et al. Treatment and prophylaxis of *Isospora belli* infection. N Engl J Med. 1989;320:1044-1047.
53. Kahn JO, Northfelt DW, Miles SA. AIDS associated Kaposi's sarcoma. AIDS Clin Rev. 1992;261-280.
54. Masur H. Prevention and treatment of *Pneumocystis* pneumonia. N Engl J Med. 1992;327:1853-1860.
55. Masur H (Chairman) and the U.S. Public Health Service Task Force on Prophylaxis and Therapy for *Mycobacterium avium* Complex. Recommendations on prophylaxis and therapy for disseminated *Mycobacterium avium* complex disease in patients infected with the human immunodeficiency virus. N Engl J Med. 1993;329:898-890.
56. Shafran SD, Deschenes J, Miller M, et al. Uveitis and pseudojaundice during a regimen of clarithromycin, rifabutin and ethambutol. N Engl J Med. 1994;10:438-439.
57. Kovacs JA, Hiemenz JW, Macher AM, et al. *Pneumocystis carinii* pneumonia: A comparison between patients with the acquired immunodeficiency syndrome and patients with other immunodeficiencies. Ann Intern Med. 1998;100:663-671.
58. Kovacs JA, Kovacs AA, Polis M. Cryptococcosis in the acquired immunodeficiency syndrome. Ann Intern Med. 1985;103:533-538.
59. Gordin FM, Simon GL, Wofsy CB, et al. Adverse reactions to trimethoprim-sulfamethoxazole in patients with the acquired immunodeficiency syndrome. Ann Intern Med. 1984;100:495-499.
60. Tu JV, Biem J, Detsky AS. Bronchoscopy versus empirical therapy in HIV-infected patients with presumptive *Pneumocystis carinii* pneumonia. Am Rev Respir Dis. 1993;18:370-377.
61. Masur H, Shelhamer JS. Empiric outpatient management of HIV related pneumonia: Economical or unwise? (Editorial). Ann Intern Med. 1996;12:51-53.
62. Luft BJ, Hafner R, Korzun AH. Toxoplasmic encephalitis in patients with the acquired immunodeficiency syndrome. N Engl J Med. 1993;329:995-1000.
63. Mathews C, Barba D, Fullerton SC. Early biopsy versus empiric treatment with delayed biopsy of non-responders in suspected HIV associated cerebral toxoplasmosis: A decision analysis. AIDS. 1995;9:1243.
64. Jacobson MA. Treatment of cytomegalovirus retinitis in patients with the acquired immunodeficiency syndrome. N Engl J Med.1997;337:105.
65. MacDonald JC, Torriani FJ, Morse LS, et al. Lack of reactivation of cytomegalovirus (CMV) retinitis after stopping CMV maintenance therapy in AIDS patients with sustained elevations in CD4+ T lymphocyte cells in response to highly active antiretroviral therapy. J Infect Dis. 1998;177:1182-1187.
66. Tural C, Romeu J, Sirera G, et al. Long-lasting remission of cytomegalovirus retinitis without maintenance therapy in human immunodeficiency virus-infected patients. J Infect Dis. 1998;177:1080-1083.
67. Schneider MME, Borleffs JCC, Stolk RP, et al. Discontinuation of *Pneumocystis carinii* pneumonia prophylaxis in HIV-1 infected patients treated with highly active antiretroviral therapy. Lancet. 1999;353:201-203.
68. Furrer H, Egger M, Opravil M, et al. Discontinuation of primary prophylaxis against *Pneumocystis carinii* pneumonia in HIV-1-infected adults treated with combination antiretroviral therapy. N Engl J Med. 1999;340:1301-1306.
69. Weverling GJ, Mocroft A, Ledergerber B, et al. Discontinuation of *Pneumocystis carinii* pneumonia prophylaxis after start of highly active antiretroviral therapy in HIV-1 infection. Lancet. 1999;353:1293-1298.
70. Yangco BF, VonBargen JC, Moorman AC, Holmberg SD. Discontinuation of chemoprophylaxis for *Pneumocystis carinii* pneumonia in patients with HIV infection. Ann Intern Med. 2000;132:201-205.
71. Kirk O, Lundgren JD, Pederson C, et al. Can chemoprophylaxis against opportunistic infections be discontinued after an increase in CD4 cells induced by highly active antiretroviral therapy? AIDS. 1999;13:1647-1651.
72. Lopez JC, Miro JM, Pena JM, Podzamczer D, and the GESIDA 04/98 Study Group. A randomized trial of the discontinuation of primary and secondary prophylaxis against *Pneumocystis carinii* pneumonia after HAART in patients with HIV infection. N Engl J Med. 2001;344:159-167.
73. Mussini C, Pezzotti P, Govoni A, et al. Discontinuation of primary prophylaxis for *Pneumocystis carinii* pneumonia and toxoplasmic encephalitis in human immunodeficiency virus type I-infected patients: The changes in opportunistic prophylaxis study. J Infect Dis. 2000;181:1635-1642.
74. Furrer H, Opravil M, Rossi M, et al. Discontinuation of primary prophylaxis in HIV infected patients at high risk of *Pneumocystis* pneumonia: A prospective multicentre study. AIDS. 2001;15:501-507.
75. Ledergerber B, Mocroft A, Reiss P, et al. Discontinuation of secondary prophylaxis against *Pneumocystis carinii* pneumonia in patients with HIV infection who have a response to antiretroviral therapy. N Engl J Med. 2001;344:168-174.
76. Abgrall S, Matheron S, LaMoing V, et al. *Pneumocystis carinii* pneumonia recurrence in HIV patients on highly active antiretroviral therapy: Secondary prophylaxis. J Acquir Immune Defic Syndr 2001;26:1518.
77. Jubault V, Pacanowski J, Rabian C, Viard J-P. Interruption of prophylaxis for major opportunistic infections in HIV-infected patients receiving triple combination antiretroviral therapy. Ann Intern Med. 2000;151:163.
78. Furrer H, Opravil M, Rossi M, et al. Stop Cox 2: Is it safe to discontinue secondary PCP prophylaxis? Experience of the Swiss Cohort Study. Presented at the Conference on Retroviral Disease and Opportunistic Infection, San Francisco, Calif, 2000.
79. Soriano V, Dona C, Rodriguez-Rosado R, et al. Discontinuation of secondary prophylaxis for opportunistic infections in HIV-infected patients receiving highly active antiretroviral therapy. AIDS. 2000;14:383-386.
80. Mussini C, Pazzoti P, Borghi V. An open, controlled, randomized study of discontinuation of prophylaxis for PCP in patients with AIDS (#MOPeB2275). Presented at the Seventh Conference on Retroviruses and Opportunistic Infections, San Francisco, Calif, 2000.
81. Zeller V, Joulian M, Truffaut C, et al. Discontinuing maintenance treatment for *Pneumocystis* pneumonia, toxoplasmic encephalitis, and disseminated *Mycobacterium avium* complex infection (Abstract 737). Program and abstracts of the First IAS Conference on HIV Pathogenesis and Treatment, Buenos Aires, Argentina, July 8-11.

82. Masur H, Kaplan J. Does *Pneumocystis carinii* prophylaxis still need to be lifelong? N Engl J Med. 1999;340:1356-1357.

83. Kaplan JE, Hanson D, Dworkin MS, et al. Epidemiology of human immunodeficiency virus-associated opportunistic infections in the United States in the era of highly active antiretroviral therapy. Clin Infect Dis. 2000;30(Suppl 1):S5-S14.

84. Stansell JD, Osmond DH, Charlebois E, et al, and the Pulmonary Complications of HIV Infection Study Group. Predictors of *Pneumocystis carinii* pneumonia in HIV-infected persons. Am J Respir Crit Care Med. 1997;155:60.

85. Kaplan JE, Hanson D, Navin TR, Jones JL. Risk factors for primary *Pneumocystis carinii* pneumonia in HIV infected adolescents and adults in the United States: Reassessment of indications for chemoprophylaxis. J Infect Dis. 1998;178:1126-1132.

86. Morres A, Creasman J, Turner J, et al. Intensive care of human immunodeficiency virus infected patients during the era of highly active antiretroviral therapy. Am J Respir Crit Care Med. 2002;166:262-267.

87. Lundgren JD, Barton SE, Lazzarin A, et al, and the AIDS in Europe Study Group. Factors associated with the development of *Pneumocystis carinii* pneumonia in 5,025 European patients with AIDS. Clin Infect Dis. 1995;21:106.

88. Saah AJ, Hoover DR, Peng Y, et al, for the Multicenter AIDS Cohort Study. Predictors for failure of *Pneumocystis carinii* pneumonia prophylaxis. JAMA. 1995;273:1197.

89. Brenner M, Ognibene FP, Lack EE. Prognostic factors and life expectancy of acquired immunodeficiency syndrome patients with *Pneumocystis carinii* pneumonia. Am Rev Respir Dis.1987;136:1199-1206.

90. el Sadr WM, Simberkoff MS. Survival and prognostic factors in severe *Pneumocystis carinii* pneumonia requiring mechanical ventilation. Am Rev Respir Dis. 1988;137:1264-1267.

91. Ognibene FP, Shelhamer J, Gill V, et al. The diagnosis of *Pneumocystis carinii* pneumonia in patients with the acquired immunodeficiency syndrome using subsegmental bronchoalveolar lavage. Am Rev Respir Dis.1984;129:933-937.

92. Kovacs JA, Ng VL, Leoung G, et al. Diagnosis of *Pneumocystis* pneumonia: Improved detection in sputum with use of monoclonal antibodies. N Engl J Med. 1988;318:589-593.

93. Barnes PF, Steele MA, Young SMM, Vachon LA. Tuberculosis in patients with human immunodeficiency virus infection: How often does it mimic *Pneumocystis carinii* pneumonia? Chest. 1992;102:428-432.

94. Ognibene FP, Masur H, Rogers P, et al. Nonspecific interstitial pneumonitis without evidence of *Pneumocystis carinii* in asymptomatic patients infected with human immunodeficiency virus (HIV). Ann Intern Med. 1988;109:874-879.

95. Ng VL, Geaghan SM, Leoung G, et al. Lack of effect of prophylactic aerosolized pentamidine on the detection of *Pneumocystis carinii* in induced sputum or bronchoalveolar lavage specimens. Arch Pathol Lab Med. 1993;117:493-496.

96. Larsen HH, Huang L, Kovacs JA, et al. A prospective, blinded study of quantitative touch-down polymerase chain reaction using oral-wash samples for diagnosis of *Pneumocystis* pneumonia in HIV-infected patients. J Infect Dis. 2004;189: 1679-1683.

97. Dohn MN, Baughman RP, Vigdorth EM, Frame D. Equal survival rates for first, second and third episodes of *Pneumocystis carinii* pneumonia in patients with AIDS. Arch Intern Med. 1992;152:2465-2470.

98. Sattler FR, Cowan R, Nielsen DM, et al. Trimethoprim-sulfamethoxazole versus pentamidine for therapy of *Pneumocystis* pneumonia: A prospective non-crossover study in patients with AIDS. Ann Intern Med. 1988;109:280-287.

99. Safrin S, Finkelstein DM, Feinberg J, et al. Comparison of three regimens for treatment of mild to moderate *Pneumocystis carinii* pneumonia in patients with AIDS: A double blind, randomized trial of oral trimethoprim-sulfamethoxazole, dapsonetrimethoprim, and clindamycin-primaquine. ACTG 108 Study Group. Ann Intern Med. 1996;124:792-802.

100. Bozzette SA, Sattler FR, Chiu J, et al. A controlled trial of early adjunctive treatment with corticosteroids for *Pneumocystis carinii* pneumonia in the acquired immunodeficiency syndrome. N Engl J Med. 1990;323:1451-1457.

101. Gagnon S, Boota AM, Fischl MA, et al. Corticosteroids as adjunctive therapy for severe *Pneumocystis carinii* pneumonia in the acquired immunodeficiency syndrome: A double-blind, placebo-controlled trial. N Engl J Med. 1990;323:1444-1450.

102. Nielsen TL, Eeftinck Schattenkerk JK, Jensen BN, et al. Adjunctive corticosteroid therapy for *Pneumocystis carinii* pneumonia in AIDS: A randomized European multicenter open label study. J Acquir Immune Defic Syndr. 1992;5:726-731.

103. Consensus statement on the use of corticosteroids as adjunctive therapy for *Pneumocystis* pneumonia in the acquired immunodeficiency syndrome. The National Institutes of Health, University of California Expert Panel for Corticosteroids as Adjunctive Therapy for *Pneumocystis* Pneumonia. N Engl J Med. 1990;323:1500-1504.

104. Montaner JSG, Lawson LM, Levitt N, et al. Oral corticosteroids prevent early deterioration in patients with moderately severe AIDS-related *Pneumocystis carinii* pneumonia. Ann Intern Med. 1990;113:14-20.

105. Hughes W, Leoung G, Kramer F, et al. Comparison of atovaquone (566C80) with trimethoprim-sulfamethoxazole to treat *Pneumocystis carinii* pneumonia in patients with AIDS. N Engl J Med. 1993;328:1521-1527.

106. Smego RA, Nagar S, Maloha B, et al. A meta-analysis of salvage therapy for *Pneumocystis carinii* pneumonia. Arch Intern Med. 2001;161:1529-1533.

107. Noskin GA, Murphy RL, Black JR, Phair JP. Salvage therapy with clindamycin/primaquine for *Pneumocystis carinii* pneumonia. Clin Infect Dis. 1992;14:183-188.

108. Sattler FR, Frame P, Davis R, et al. Trimetrexate with leucovorin versus trimethoprim-sulfamethoxazole for moderate to severe episodes of *Pneumocystis carinii* pneumonia in patients with AIDS: A prospective, controlled multicenter investigation of the AIDS Clinical Trials Group Protocol 029/031. J Infect Dis. 1994;170:165-172.

109. Mei Q, Gurunathan S, Masur H, Kovacs J. Failure of co-trimoxazole in *Pneumocystis carinii* infection and the mutations in dihydropteroate synthase gene. Lancet. 1998;351:1631-1632.

110. Nahimana A, Rabodonirina M, Helwig-Larsen J, et al. Sulfa resistance and dihydropteroate synthase mutants in recurrent *Pneumocystis carinii* pneumonia. Emerg Infect Dis. 2003;9864-9867.

111. Neuman MG, Malkiewicz IM, Phillips EJ, et al. Monitoring adverse drug reactions to sulfonamide antibiotics in human immunodeficiency virus infected individuals. Ther Drug Monit 2002;24:728-736.

112. Safrin S, Lee BL, Sande MA. Adjunctive folinic acid with trimethoprim-sulfamethoxazole for *Pneumocystis carinii* pneumonia in AIDS patients is associated with an increased risk of therapeutic failure and death. J Infect Dis. 1994;170:912-917.

113. Holtzer CD, Flaherty JF Jr, Coleman RL. Cross-reactivity in HIV-infected patients switched from trimethoprim-sulfamethoxazole to dapsone. Pharmacotherapy. 1998;18:831-835.

114. Para MF, Finkelstein D, Becker S, et al. Reduced toxicity with gradual initiation of trimethoprim-sulfamethoxazole as primary prophylaxis for *Pneumocystis carinii* pneumonia: AIDS Clinical Trials Group 268. J Acquir Immune Defic Syndr. 2000;24:337-343.

115. Leoung GS, Stanford JF, Giordano MF, et al. Trimethoprim-sulfamethoxazole (TMP-SMZ) dose escalation versus direct rechallenge for *Pneumocystis carinii* pneumonia prophylaxis in human immunodeficiency virus-infected patients with previous adverse reaction to TMP-SMZ. J Infect Dis. 2001;184:992-997.

116. O'Brien JG, Dong BJ, Coleman RL, et al. A 5-year retrospective review of adverse drug reactions and their risk factors in human immunodeficiency virus-infected patients who were receiving intravenous pentamidine therapy for *Pneumocystis carinii* pneumonia. Clin Infect Dis. 1997;24:854-859.

117. Navin TR, Fontaine RE. Intravenous versus intramuscular administration of pentamidine. N Engl J Med. 1984;311:1701-1702.

118. Mallory DL, Parrillo JE, Bailey KR, et al. Cardiovascular effects and safety of intravenous and intramuscular pentamidine isethionate. Crit Care Med. 1987;15:503-505.

119. Waskin H, Stehr-Green JK, Helmick CG, et al. Risk factors for hypoglycemia associated with pentamidine therapy for *Pneumocystis* pneumonia. JAMA. 1988;260:345-347.

120. Conte JE, Chernoff D, Feigal DW, et al. Intravenous or inhaled pentamidine for treating *Pneumocystis carinii* pneumonia in AIDS. Ann Intern Med. 1990;113:203-209.

121. Medina I, Mills J, Leoung G, et al. Oral therapy for *Pneumocystis carinii* pneumonia in the acquired immunodeficiency syndrome: A controlled trial of trimethoprim-sulfamethoxazole versus trimethoprim-dapsone. N Engl J Med. 1990;323:776-782.

122. Mills J, Leoung G, Medina J, et al. Dapsone treatment of *Pneumocystis carinii* pneumonia in the acquired immunodeficiency syndrome. Antimicrob Agents Chemother. 1988;32:1057-1060.

123. Dohn MN, Weinberg WG, Torres RA, et al. Oral atovaquone compared with intravenous pentamidine for *Pneumocystis carinii* pneumonia in patients with AIDS. Ann Intern Med. 1994;121:174-180.

124. Walker DJ, Wakefield AE, Dohn MN, et al. Sequence polymorphism in the *Pneumocystis carinii* cytochrome b gene and association with atovaquone failure. J Infect Dis. 1998;178:1767-1775.

125. Allegra CJ, Chabner BA, Tuazon CU, et al. Trimetrexate for the treatment of *Pneumocystis carinii* pneumonia in patients with the acquired immunodeficiency syndrome. N Engl J Med. 1987;317:978-985.

126. Jones BD, Taikwel EK, Mercado AL, et al. Tuberculosis in patients with HIV infection who receive corticosteroids for presumed *Pneumocystis carinii* pneumonia. Am J Respir Crit Care Med. 1994;49:1686-1688.

127. Miller K, Masur H, Jones EC, et al. High prevalence of osteonecrosis of the femoral head in HIV-infected adults. Ann Intern Med. 2002;137:17-25.

128. Caumes E, Roudier C, Rogeaux O, et al. Effect of corticosteroids on the incidence of adverse cutaneous reactions to trimethoprim-sulfamethoxazole during treatment of AIDS-associated *Pneumocystis carinii* pneumonia. Clin Infect Dis. 1994;18:319-323.

129. Shelhamer JH, Ognibene FP, Macher AM, et al. Persistence of *Pneumocystis carinii* in lung tissue of acquired immunodeficiency syndrome patients treated for *Pneumocystis* pneumonia. Am Rev Respir Dis. 1984;130:1161-1166.

130. Ognibene FP, Steis R, Macher AM, et al. Kaposi's sarcoma-causing infiltrates and respiratory failure in the acquired immunodeficiency syndrome. Ann Intern Med. 1985;102:471-475.

131. Morris A, Wachter RM, Luce J, et al. Improved survival with highly active antiretroviral therapy in HIV-infected patients with severe PCP. AIDS. 2003;17:73-80.

132. Wachter RM, Luce JM, Hopewell PC. Critical care of patients with AIDS. JAMA. 1992;267:541-547.

133. Rosen MJ, Clayton K, Schnieder RF, et al. Intensive care of patients with HIV infection: Utilization, critical illnesses, and outcomes. Am J Respir Crit Care Med. 1997; 155:67-71.

134. Schneider MME, Hoepelman AIM, Eeftinck Schattenkerk JKM, et al. A controlled trial of aerosolized pentamidine or trimethoprim-sulfamethoxazole as primary prophylaxis against *Pneumocystis carinii* pneumonia in patients with human immunodeficiency virus infection. N Engl J Med. 1992;327:1836-1841.

135. Leoung GS, Feigal DW Jr, Montgomery AB, et al. Aerosolized pentamidine for prophylaxis against *Pneumocystis carinii* pneumonia: The San Francisco Community Prophylaxis Trial. N Engl J Med. 1990;323:769-775.

136. Hardy WD, Feinberg J, Finkelstein DM, et al. A controlled trial of trimethoprim-sulfamethoxazole or aerosolized pentamidine for secondary prophylaxis of *Pneumocystis carinii* pneumonia in patients with the acquired immunodeficiency syndrome: AIDS Clinical Trials Group Protocol 021. N Engl J Med. 1992;327:1842-1848.

137. Schneider MME, Nielsen TL, Nelsing S, et al. Efficacy and toxicity of two doses of trimethoprim-sulfamethoxazole as primary prophylaxis against *Pneumocystis carinii* pneumonia in patients with human immunodeficiency virus. J Infect Dis. 1995;171:1632-1636.

138. Girard P-M, Landman R, Gaudebout C, et al. Dapsone-pyrimethamine compared with aerosolized pentamidine as primary prophylaxis against *Pneumocystis carinii* pneumonia and toxoplasmosis in HIV infection. N Engl J Med. 1993;328:1514-1520.

139. Blum RN, Miller LA, Gaggini LC, Cohn DL. Comparative trial of dapsone vs. trimethoprim-sulfamethoxazole for primary prophylaxis of *Pneumocystis carinii* pneumonia. J Acquir Immune Defic Syndr. 1992;15:341-347.

140. Kemper CA, Tucker RM, Lang DS, et al. Low dose dapsone prophylaxis of *Pneumocystis carinii* pneumonia in AIDS and AIDS-related complex. AIDS. 1990;4:1145-1148.

141. Montaner JSG, Lawson LM, Gervais A, et al. Aerosol pentamidine for secondary prophylaxis of AIDS-related *Pneumocystis carinii* pneumonia: A randomized, placebo-controlled study. Ann Intern Med. 1991;114:948-953.

142. Hirschel B, Lazzarin A, Chopard P, et al. A controlled study of inhaled pentamidine for primary prevention of *Pneumocystis carinii* pneumonia. N Engl J Med. 1991; 324:1079-1083.

143. Carr A, Tindall B, Brew BJ, et al. Low-dose trimethoprim-sulfamethoxazole prophylaxis for toxoplasmic encephalitis in patients with AIDS. Ann Intern Med. 1992;117:106-111.

144. El-Sadr WM, Luskin-Hawk R, Yurik TM, et al. A randomized trial of daily and thrice-weekly trimethoprim-sulfamethoxazole for the prevention of *Pneumocystis carinii* pneumonia in human immunodeficiency virus-infected persons. Clin Infect Dis. 1999;29:775-783.

145. O'Doherty MJ, Thomas S, Page C, et al. Differences in relative efficacy of nebulizers for pentamidine administration. Lancet. 1988;2:1283-1286.

146. O'Riordan TG, Smaldone GC. Exposure of health care workers to aerosolized pentamidine. Chest. 1992;101:1494-1499.

147. Centers for Disease Control and Prevention. *Mycobacterium tuberculosis* transmission in a health clinic—Florida, 1988. MMWR Morb Mortal Wkly Rep. 1988;38:256-258, 263-264.

148. El-Sadr WM, Murphy RL, Yurik TM, et al. Atovaquone compared with dapsone for the prevention of *Pneumocystis carinii* pneumonia in patients with HIV infection who cannot tolerate trimethoprim, sulfonamides, or both. N Engl J Med. 1998;339:1889-1895.

149. Chan C, Montaner J, Lefebure E, et al. Atovaquone suspension compared with aerosolized pentamidine for prevention of *Pneumocystis carinii* pneumonia in human immunodeficiency virus-infected subjects intolerant of trimethoprim or sulfonamides. J Infect Dis. 1999;180:369-376.

150. Golden JA, Katz MH, Chernoff DN, et al. A randomized comparison of once monthly or twice monthly high dose aerosolized pentamidine prophylaxis. Chest. 1993; 104:743-750.

151. Moorman AC, Von Bargen JC, Palella FJ, et al. *Pneumocystis carinii* pneumonia incidence and chemoprophylaxis failure in ambulatory HIV-infected patients. J Acquir Immune Defic Syndr Hum Retrovirol. 1998;19:182-188.

152. Stansell JD, Osmond DH, Charlebois E, et al. Predictors of *Pneumocystis carinii* pneumonia in HIV-infected persons. Am J Respir Crit Care Med. 1997;155:60-66.

153. Porter SB, Sande MA. Toxoplasmosis of the central nervous system in the acquired immunodeficiency syndrome. N Engl J Med. 1992;327:1643-1648.

154. Israelski DM, Chmiel JS, Poggenser L, et al. Prevalence of *Toxoplasma* infection in a cohort of homosexual men at risk of AIDS and toxoplasmic encephalitis. J Acquir Immune Defic Syndr. 1993;6:414-418.

155. Cingolani A, De Luca A, Ammassari A, et al. PCR detection of *Toxoplasma gondii* DNA in CSF for the differential diagnosis of AIDS-related focal brain lesions. J Med Microbiol. 1996;45:472.

156. Barker DE, Trepashko D, DeMarais P, et al. Utility of thallium brain SPECT in the exclusion of CNS lymphoma in AIDS (Abstract No. 708). In: Abstracts of the Fourth Conference on Retroviruses and Opportunistic Infections, Washington, DC, January 22-26, 1996.

157. Jarvik JG, Hesselink JR, Kennedy C, et al. Acquired immunodeficiency syndrome: Magnetic resonance patterns of brain involvement with pathologic correlation. Arch Neurol. 1998;45:731-736.

158. Antinori A, Ammassari A, DeLuca A, et al. Diagnosis of AIDS-related focal brain lesions: A decision making analysis based on clinical and neurological characteristics combined with polymerase chain reaction assays in CSF. Neurology. 1997;48:687.

159. Dannemann B, McCutchan JA, Israelski D, et al. Treatment of toxoplasmic encephalitis in patients with AIDS: A randomized trial comparing pyrimethamine plus clindamycin to pyrimethamine plus sulfonamides. Ann Intern Med. 1992;116:33-43.

160. Katlama C, De Wit S, O'Doherty E, et al. Pyrimethamine-clindamycin vs. pyrimethamine-sulfadiazine as acute and long-term therapy for toxoplasmic encephalitis in patients with AIDS. Clin Infect Dis. 1996;22:268.

161. Kovacs JA, O'Neill D, Feuerstein I, et al. Efficacy of atovaquone in treatment of toxoplasmosis in patients with AIDS. Lancet. 1992;340:637-638.

162. Torres RA, Winberg W, Stansell J, et al. Atovaquone for salvage treatment and suppression of toxoplasmic encephalitis in patients with AIDS. Clin Infect Dis. 1997;24:422.

163. Fernandez-Martin J, Leport C, Morlat P, et al. Pyrimethamine-clarithromycin combination for therapy of acute *Toxoplasma* encephalitis in patients with AIDS. Antimicrob Agents Chemother. 1991;35:2049.

164. Morris JT, Kelly JW. Effective treatment of cerebral toxoplasmosis with doxycycline. Am J Med. 1992;93:107.

165. Derouin F, Piketty C, Chastang C, et al. Antitoxoplasma effects of dapsone alone and combined with pyrimethamine. Antimicrob Agents Chemother. 1991;35:252-255.

166. Leport C, Chene G, Morlat P, et al. Pyrimethamine for primary prophylaxis of toxoplasmic encephalitis in patients with human immunodeficiency virus infection: A double-blind, randomized trial. ANRS 005-ACTG 154 Group Members. Agence Nationale de Recherche sur le SIDA. J Infect Dis. 1996;173:91-97.

167. de Gans J, Portegies P, Reiss P, et al. Pyrimethamine as maintenance therapy for central nervous system toxoplasmosis in 38 patients with AIDS. J Acquir Immune Defic Syndr. 1992;5:137-142.

168. Masur H, Polis MA, Tuazon CU, et al. Salvage trial of trimetrexate-leucovorin for the treatment of cerebral toxoplasmosis in patients with AIDS. J Infect Dis. 1993;167:1422-1426.

169. Kalb RE, Grossman ME. Chronic perianal herpes simplex in immunocompromised hosts. Am J Med. 1986;80:486-490.

170. Stewart JA, Reef SE, Pellett PE, et al. Herpes virus infection in persons with HIV. Clin Infect Dis. 1995;21(Suppl):S114.

171. LaGuardia RD, White MH, Saigo PE, et al. Genital ulcer disease in women infected with human immunodeficiency virus. Am J Obstet Gynecol. 1995;172:553.

172. Sacks SL, Aoki FY, Diaz-Mitoma F, et al. Patient initiated, twice-daily oral famciclovir for early recurrent genital herpes: A randomized double blind multicenter trial. JAMA. 1996;276:44.

173. Mertz GJ, Loveless MO, Levin MJ, et al. Oral famciclovir for suppression of recurrent genital herpes simplex virus infection in women: A multicenter, double blind placebo controlled study. Arch Intern Med. 1997;157:343.

174. Lalezari JP, Drew WL, Glutzer E, et al. Treatment with intravenous (s)-1-(3-hydroxy-2-phosphonylmethoxypropyl) cytosine of acyclovir-resistant mucocutaneous infection with herpes simplex virus in a patient with AIDS. J Infect Dis. 1994;170:550.

175. Reyes M, Shaik NS, Graber JM, et al. Acyclovir-resistant genital herpes among persons attending sexually transmitted disease and human immunodeficiency virus clinics. Arch Intern Med. 2003;163:76-80.

176. Chatis PA, Miller CH, Schrager LE, et al. Successful treatment with foscarnet of an acyclovir-resistant mucocutaneous infection with herpes simplex virus in a patient with acquired immunodeficiency syndrome. N Engl J Med. 1989;320:297.

177. Safrin S, Kemmerly S, Plotkin B, et al. Foscarnet-resistant herpes simplex virus infection in patients with AIDS. J Infect Dis. 1994;169:193.

178. Birch CJ, Tyssen DP, Tacheddjian G, et al. Clinical effects and in vitro studies of trifluorothymidine combined with interferon-α for treatment of drug resistant and sensitive herpes simplex virus infections. J Infect Dis. 1992;166:108.

179. Kessler HA, Hurwitz C, Farthing C, et al. Pilot study of topical trifluridine for the treatment of acyclovir-resistant mucocutanous herpes simplex disease in patients with AIDS (ACTG 172). J Acquir Immune Defic Syndr. 1996;12:147.

180. Lalezari J, Schacker T, Feinberg J, et al. A randomized, double blind, placebo-controlled study of cidofovir gel for the treatment of acyclovir-unresponsive mucocutaneous herpes simplex virus infections in patients with AIDS. J Infect Dis. 1997;17:862.

181. LeBoit PE, Limova M, Yen TSB, et al. Chronic verrucous varicella zoster infection in patients with the acquired immunodeficiency syndrome (AIDS): Histologic and molecular biologic findings. Am J Dermatopathol. 1992;12:1.

182. Hoppenjans WB, Bibler MR, Orme RL, et al. Prolonged cutaneous herpes zoster in acquired immunodeficiency syndrome. Arch Dermatol. 1990;126:1048-1050.

183. Janier M, Hillion B, Baccard M, et al. Chronic varicella zoster infection in acquired immunodeficiency syndrome. J Am Acad Dermatol. 1988;18:584-585.

184. Whitley RJ, Weiss J, Gnann JW, et al. A randomized placebo-controlled trial of acyclovir with and without steroids for the treatment of herpes zoster. Ann Intern Med. 1996;125:376-383.

185. Wood MJ, Johnson RW, McKendrick MW, et al. A randomized trial of acyclovir for 7 days or 21 days with and without prednisone for treatment of acute herpes zoster. N Engl J Med. 1994;330:896-900.

186. Boivin G, Edelman CK, Pedneault L, et al. Phenotypic and genotypic characterization of acyclovir resistant varicella zoster viruses isolated from persons with AIDS. J Infect Dis. 1994;170:68.

187. Lyall EGH, Ogilvie MM, Smith NM, et al. Acyclovir resistant varicella zoster and HIV infection. Arch Dis Child. 1994;70:133.

188. Perronne C, Lazamas M, Leport C, et al. Varicella in patients infected with the human immunodeficiency virus. Arch Dermatol. 1990;126:1033.

189. Collier AC, Meyers JD, Corey L, et al. Cytomegalovirus infection in homosexual men: Relationship to sexual practices, antibody to human immunodeficiency virus, and cell-mediated immunity. Am J Med. 1987;23:593.

190. Drew WL, Miner RC, Ziegler JL, et al. Cytomegalovirus and Kaposi's sarcoma in young homosexual men. Lancet. 1982;1:125.

191. Hoover DR, Saah AJ, Bacellar H, et al. Clinical manifestations of AIDS in the era of *Pneumocystis* prophylaxis. N Engl J Med. 1993;329:1922.

192. Zurlo JJ, O'Neill D, Polis MA, et al. Lack of clinical utility of cytomegalovirus blood and urine cultures in patients with HIV infection. Ann Intern Med. 1993;118:12-17.

193. Wetherill PE, Landry ML, Alcabes P, et al. Use of a quantitative cytomegalovirus (CMV) antigenemia test in evaluation of HIV⁺ patients with and without CMV disease. J Acquir Immune Defic Syndr. 1996;12:33.

194. Jacobson MA, Mills J. Serious cytomegalovirus disease in the acquired immunodeficiency syndrome (AIDS). Ann Intern Med. 1988;108:585-594.

195. Drew WL. Cytomegalovirus infection in patients with AIDS. Clin Infect Dis. 1992;14:608-615.

196. Bloom JN, Palestine AG. The diagnosis of cytomegalovirus retinitis. Ann Intern Med. 1988;109:963-969.

197. Studies of the Ocular Complications of AIDS Research Group, AIDS Clinical Trials Group. Mortality in patients with the acquired immunodeficiency syndrome treated with either foscarnet or ganciclovir for cytomegalovirus retinitis. N Engl J Med. 1992;326:213-220.

198. Rahal FM, Arevalo JF, Chavez de la Paz E, et al. Treatment of cytomegalovirus retinitis with intravitreous cidofovir in patients with AIDS: A preliminary report. Ann Intern Med. 1996;125:98.

199. Vitravene Study Group. Safety of intravitreous fomivirsen for treatment of cytomegalovirus retinitis in patients with AIDS. Am J Ophthalmol 2002;133:484-498.

200. Martin DF, Kupferman BD, Welitz RA, et al. Oral ganciclovir for patients with cytomegalovirus treated with ganciclovir implant. N Engl J Med. 1999;340:1063-1070.

201. Musch DC, Martin DF, Gordon JF, et al. Treatment of cytomegalovirus retinitis with a sustained release intraocular ganciclovir implant. N Engl J Med. 1997;337:83.

202. Marx JL, Kapusta MA, Patel SS, et al. Use of the ganciclovir implant in the treatment of recurrent cytomegalovirus retinitis. Arch Ophthalmol. 1996;114:815.

203. Martin DF, Sierra-Madero J, Walmsely S, et al. A controlled trial of valganciclovir as induction therapy for cytomegalovirus retinitis. N Engl J Med. 2002;346:1119-1126.

204. Kirsch LS, Arevalo JF, DeClercq E, et al. Phase I/II study of intravitreal cidofovir for the treatment of cytomegalovirus retinitis in patients with the acquired immunodeficiency syndrome. Am J Ophthalmol. 1995;119:466.

205. Uberti-Foppa C, Lazzerin A, Gianolti N, et al. Cytomegalovirus pneumonia in AIDS patients: Value of cytomegalovirus culture from BAL fluid and correlation with lung disease. Chest. 1998;113:919-923.

206. Emanuel D, Cunningham I, Jules-Elysee K, et al. Cytomegalovirus pneumonia after bone-marrow transplantation successfully treated with the combination of ganciclovir and high-dose intravenous immune globulin. Ann Intern Med. 1988;109:777-782.

207. Parente F, Bianchi-Porro G. Treatment of cytomegalovirus esophagitis in patients with AIDS: A randomized controlled study of foscarnet versus ganciclovir. Am J Gastroenterol. 1998;93:317-322.

208. Erice A, Gil-Roda C, Perez JL, et al. Antiviral susceptibilities and analysis of UL97 and DNA polymerase sequences of clinical cytomegalovirus isolates from immunocompromised patients. J Infect Dis. 1997;175:1087.

209. Drew WL, Stempien MJ, Andrews J, et al. Cytomegalovirus (CMV) resistance in patients with CMV retinitis and AIDS treated with oral or intravenous ganciclovir. J Infect Dis. 1999;179:1352-1355.

210. Jabs DA, Martin BK, Forman MS, et al. Cytomegalovirus resistance to ganciclovir and clinical outcomes of patients with cytomegalovirus retinitis. Am J Opthalmol. 2003;135:26-34.

211. Sullivan V, Coen DM. Isolation of foscarnet-resistant human cytomegalovirus: Patterns of resistance and sensitivity to other antiviral drugs. J Infect Dis. 1991;164:781-784.

212. Studies of the Ocular Complications of AIDS Research Group in Collaboration with the AIDS Clinical Trials Group. Combination foscarnet and ganciclovir therapy vs. monotherapy for the treatment of relapsed cytomegalovirus retinitis in patients with AIDS. Arch Ophthalmol. 1996;114:23.

213. Studies of Ocular Complications of AIDS Research Group, in collaboration with the AIDS Clinical Trials Group. Foscarnet-ganciclovir for cytomegalovirus retinitis trial 4: Visual outcomes. Ophthalmology. 1994;101:1250.

214. Spector SA, McKinley GF, Lalezari JP, et al. Oral ganciclovir for the prevention of cytomegalovirus retinitis in persons with AIDS. N Engl J Med. 1996;334:1491.

215. Brosgart CL, Torres RA, Thompson MA, et al. A randomized, placebo controlled trial of the safety and efficacy of oral ganciclovir for prophylaxis of cytomegalovirus disease in HIV infected individuals. AIDS. 1998;12:269-277.

216. Major EO, Amemiya K, Tornatore CS, et al. Pathogenesis and molecular biology of progressive multifocal leukoencephalopathy, the JC virus-induced demyelinating disease of the human brain. Clin Microbiol. Rev. 1992;5:49-73.

217. Matsiota-Bernard P, De Truchis P, Gray F, et al. JC virus detection in the cerebrospinal fluid of AIDS patients with progressive multifocal leucoencephalopathy and monitoring of the antiviral treatment by a PCR method. J Med Microbiol. 1997;46:256.

218. Hall C, Dafni U, Simpson D, et al. Failure of cytosine arabinoside therapy for human immunodeficiency virus-1 associated progressive multifocal leukoencephalopathy. N Engl J Med. 1998;338:1345-1351.

219. Baldeweg T, Catalan J. Remission of progressive multifocal leucoencephalopathy after antiretroviral therapy. Lancet. 1997;349:1554.

220. De Wit S, Goosens H, Weerts D, et al. Comparison of fluconazole and ketoconazole for oropharyngeal candidiasis in AIDS. Lancet. 1989;1:746.

221. Koletar SL, Russell JA, Fass RJ, et al. Comparison of oral fluconazole and clotrimazole troches as treatment for oral candidiasis in patients infected with human immunodeficiency virus. Antimicrob Agents Chemother. 1990;34:2267.

222. Laine L, Dretler RH, Conteas CN, et al. Fluconazole compared with ketoconazole for the treatment of Candida esophagitis in AIDS. Ann Intern Med. 1992;117:655.

223. de Repentigny L, Ratelle J. Comparison of itraconazole and ketoconazole in HIV-positive patients with oropharyngeal or esophageal candidiasis. Chemotherapy. 1996;42:374.

224. Van Huesden AM, Merkus HM, Corbeij RS, et al. Single-dose oral fluconazole versus single-dose topical miconazole for the treatment of acute vulvovaginal candidiasis. Acta Obstet Gynecol Scand. 1990;69:417.

225. Wooley PD, Higgins SP. Comparison of clotrimazole, fluconazole and itraconazole in vaginal candidiasis. Br J Clin Pract. 1995;49:65.

226. Fichtenbaum CJ, Zackin R, Rajicic N, et al. Amphotericin B oral suspension for fluconazole-refractory oral candidiasis in persons with HIV infection. AIDS. 2000;14:845-852.

227. Sobel JD, Brooker D, Stein GE, et al. Single oral dose fluconazole compared with conventional clotrimazole topical therapy of Candida vaginitis. Am J Obstet Gynecol. 1995;172:1263.

228. Saag MS, Fessel WJ, Kaufman CA, et al. Treatment of fluconazole-refractory oropharyngeal candidiasis with itraconazole oral solution in HIV-positive patients. AIDS Res Hum Retroviruses. 1999;15:1413-1417.

229. Zuger A, Louis E, Holzman RS, et al. Cryptococcal disease in patients with the acquired immunodeficiency syndrome: Diagnostic features and outcome of treatment. Ann Intern Med. 1986;104:234-240.

230. Chuck SL, Sande MA. Infections with Cryptococcus neoformans in the acquired immunodeficiency syndrome. N Engl J Med. 1989;321:794-799.

231. Van der Horst CM, Saag MS, Cloud GA, et al. Treatment of cryptococcal meningitis associated with the acquired immunodeficiency syndrome. N Engl J Med. 1997;337:15.

232. Powderly WG, Saag MS, Clud GA, et al. A controlled trial of fluconazole or amphotericin B to prevent relapse of cryptococcal meningitis in patients with the acquired immunodeficiency syndrome. N Engl J Med. 1992;326:793.

233. Saag MS, and the NIAID Mycoses Study Group. Comparison of fluconazole versus itraconazole as maintenance therapy of AIDS-associated cryptococcal meningitis. Clin Infect Dis. 1999;28:291-296.

234. Aberg J, Powderly WG. Cryptococcosis. In: Dolin R, Masur H, Saag M, eds. AIDS Therapy. 2nd ed. New York: Churchill Livingstone; 2003:498-510.

235. Paugam A, Dupouy-Camet J, Blanche P, et al. Increased fluconazole resistance of Cryptococcus neoformans isolated from a patient with AIDS and recurrent meningitis. Clin Infect Dis. 1994;19:975.

236. Armengou A, Porcar C, Mascaro J, et al. Possible development of resistance to fluconazole during suppressive therapy for AIDS-associated cryptococcal meningitis. Clin Infect Dis. 1996;23:1337.

237. Leenders AC, Reiss P, Portegies P, et al. Liposomal amphotericin B (AmBisome) compared with amphotericin B both followed by oral fluconazole in the treatment of AIDS-associated cryptococcal meningitis. AIDS. 1997;11:1463-1471.

238. Denning DW, Armstrong RW, Lewis BH, et al. Elevated cerebrospinal fluid pressures in patients with cryptococcal meningitis and acquired immunodeficiency syndrome. Am J Med. 1991;91:267.

239. Aberg JA, Price RW, Heeren DM, Bredt B. A pilot study of the discontinuation of antifungal therapy for disseminated cryptococcal disease following immunologic response to antiretroviral therapy. J Infect Dis. 2002;185:1179-1182.

240. Mussini C, Cossarizza A, Oezzotti P, et al. Discontinuation or continuation of maintenance therapy for cryptococcal meningitis in patients with AIDS treated with HAART (Abstract 546). In: Progress and Abstracts of the Eighth Conference on Retroviruses and Opportunistic Infections, Chicago, February 2001.

241. Martinez E, Garcia-Viejo MA, Marcos MA. Discontinuation of secondary prophylaxis for cryptococcal meningitis in HIV-infected patients responding to highly active antiretroviral therapy. AIDS. 2000;14:2615.

242. Williams B, Fojtasek M, Connolly-Stringfield P, et al. Diagnosis of histoplasmosis by antigen detection during an outbreak in Indianapolis, Ind. Arch Pathol Lab Med. 1994;118:1205-1208.

243. Wheat LJ, Hafner R, Wulfsohn M, et al. Prevention of relapse of histoplasmosis with itraconazole in patients with the acquired immunodeficiency syndrome. The National Institute of Allergy and Infectious Diseases Clinical Trials and Mycoses Study Group Collaborators. Ann Intern Med. 1993;118:610-616.

244. Wheat J, Hafner R, Korzun AH, et al. Itraconazole treatment of disseminated histoplasmosis in patients with the acquired immunodeficiency syndrome. Am J Med. 1995;98:336.

245. Wheat J, MaWhinney S, Hafner R, et al. Treatment of histoplasmosis with fluconazole in patients with acquired immunodeficiency syndrome. Am J Med. 1997;103:223-232.

246. Hecht FM, Wheat J, Korzun AH, et al. Itraconazole maintenance treatment for histoplasmosis in AIDS: A prospective, multicenter trial. J Acquir Immune Defic Syndr Hum Retrovirol. 1997;16:100-107.

247. Johnson P, Wheat LJ, Cloud G, et al. A multicenter randomized trial comparing amphotericin B (AmB) and liposomal amphotericin B (AmBisome, LAmB) as induction therapy of disseminated histoplasmosis (DH) in AIDS patients. Ann Intern Med. 2002;137:154.

248. Singh VR, Smith KD, Lawrence J, et al. Coccidioidomycosis in patients infected with human immunodeficiency virus: Review of 91 cases at a single institution. Clin Infect Dis. 1996;23:563.

249. Chiller TM, Galgiani JN, Stevens DA. Coccidiomycosis. Infect Dis Clin North Am. 2003;17:41-57.

250. Mylonakis E, Barlam TF, Flanigan T, et al. Pulmonary aspergillosis and invasive disease in AIDS: Review of 342 cases. Chest. 1998;114:251-262.

251. Wallace JM, Hansen NI, LaVange L, et al. Respiratory disease trends in the Pulmonary Complications of HIV Infection Study cohort. Am J Respir Crit Care Med. 1997;155:72.

252. Hirschtick RE, Glassroth J, Jordan MC, et al. Bacterial pneumonia in persons infected with the human immunodeficiency virus. N Engl J Med. l995;333:845.

253. Mundy LM, Auwaerter PG, Oldach D, et al. Community-acquired pneumonia: Impact of immune status. Am J Respir Crit Care Med. 1995;152:1309-1315.

254. Pierce M, Crampton S, Henry D, et al. A randomized trial of clarithromycin as prophylaxis against disseminated Mycobacterium avium complex infection in patients with advanced acquired immunodeficiency syndrome. N Engl J Med. 1996;335:392.

255. Currier JS, Williams P, Feiberg J, et al. Impact of prophylaxis for Mycobacterium avium complex on bacterial infections in patients with advanced human immunodeficiency virus disease. Clin Infect Dis. 2001;32:1615-1622.

256. Barnes PF, Bloch AB, Davidson PT, Snider DE. Tuberculosis in patients with human immunodeficiency virus infection. N Engl J Med. 1991;324:1644-1650.

257. Barnes PR, Barrows SA. Tuberculosis in the 1990's. Ann Intern Med. 1993;119:400-410.

258. American Thoracic Society, Centers for Disease Control and Prevention, and Infectious Diseases Society of America. Treatment of tuberculosis. MMWR Recomm Rep. 2003;52(RR-11):1-77.

259. Perriens JH, St. Louis ME, Mukadi YB, et al. Pulmonary tuberculosis in HIV-infected patients in Zaire. N Engl J Med. 1995;332:779.

260. Huang L, Beard CB, Creasman J, et al. Sulfa or sulfone prophylaxis and geographic region predict mutations in the *Pneumocystis carinii* dihydropteroate synthase gene. J Infect Dis 2000;182:1192-1198.

261. Gordin FM, Cohn DL, Sullam PM, et al. Early manifestations of disseminated *Mycobacterium avium* complex disease: A prospective evaluation. J Infect Dis. 1997;176:126.

262. Chaisson RE, Benson CA, Dube MP, et al. Clarithromycin therapy for bacteremic *Mycobacterium avium* complex disease in patients with AIDS. Ann Intern Med. 1994;121:905.

263. Kemper CA, Meng RC, Nussbaum J, et al. Treatment of *Mycobacterium avium* complex bacteremia in AIDS with a four-drug oral regimen. Ann Intern Med. 1992;116:466.

264. Shafran SD, Singer J, Zarowney DP, et al. A comparison of two regimens for the treatment of *Mycobacterium avium* complex bacteremia in AIDS: Rifabutin, ethambutol, and clarithromycin versus rifampin, ethambutol, clofazimine, and ciprofloxacin. N Engl J Med. 1996;335:377.

265. May T, Brel F, Beuscart C, et al. Comparison of combination therapy regimens for treatment of human immunodeficiency virus-infected patients with disseminated bacteremia due to *Mycobacterium avium*. Clin Infect Dis. 1997;25:621.

266. Gordin FM, Sullam PM, Shafran SD, et al. A randomized, placebo-controlled study of rifabutin added to a regimen of clarithromycin and ethambutol for treatment of disseminated infection with *Mycobacterium avium* complex. Clin Infect Dis. 1999;28:1080-1085.

267. Dube MP, Sattler F, Torriani F, et al. A randomized evaluation of ethambutol for prevention of relapse and drug resistance during treatment of *Mycobacterium avium* complex bacteremia with clarithromycin-based combination therapy. J Infect Dis. 1997;176:1225.

268. Aberg JA, Yajko DM, Jacobson MA. Eradication of AIDS-related disseminated *Mycobacterium avium* complex infection after 12 months of antimycobacterial therapy combined with highly active antiretroviral therapy. J Infect Dis. 1998;178:1446.

269. Aberg JA, Williams PL, Liv T, et al. A study of discontinuing maintenance therapy in human immunodeficiency virus infected subjects with disseminated *Mycobacterium avium* complex. AIDS Clinical Trial Group 393 Study Team. J Infect Dis. 2003;187:1046-1052.

270. Shafran SD, Gill MJ, Lalonde RG, et al. Successful discontinuation of MAC therapy following effective HAART (Abstract 547). In: Abstracts of the Eighth Conference on Retroviruses and Opportunistic Infections, Chicago. Alexandria, Va: Foundation for Retrovirology and Human Health; 2001:208.

271. Benson CA, Williams PL, Cohn DL, et al. Clarithromycin or rifabutin alone or in combination for primary prophylaxis of *Mycobacterium avium* complex disease in-patients with AIDS: A randomized, double-blind, placebo-controlled trial. J Infect Dis. 2000;181:1289-1297.

272. Havlir DV, Dube MP, Sattler FR, et al. Prophylaxis against disseminated *Mycobacterium avium* complex with weekly azithromycin, daily rifabutin, or both. N Engl J Med. 1996;335:392.

273. Simon DM, Cello JP, Valenzuela J, et al. Multicenter trial of octreotide in patients with refractory acquired immunodeficiency syndrome-associated microsporidiosis and cryptosporidiosis with combination antiretroviral therapy. Lancet. 1998;351:256.

274. Ungar BLP, Ward DJ, Fayer R, et al. Cessation of *Cryptosporidium*-associated diarrhea in an acquired immunodeficiency syndrome patient after treatment with hyperimmune bovine colostrum. Gastroenterology. 1990;98:486.

275. Rossignol JF, Hidalgo H, Feregrino M. A double-'blind' placebo-controlled study of nitazoxanide in the treatment of cryptosporidial diarrhea in AIDS patients in Mexico. Trans R Soc Trop Med Hyg. 1998;92:663-666.

276. Hewitt RG, Yiannoutsos CT, Higgs ES, et al. Paromycin: No more effective than placebo for treatment of cryptosporidiosis in patients with advanced human immunodeficiency virus infection. Clin Infect Dis. 2000;31:1084.

277. Grube H, Ramratnam B, Ley C, et al. Resolution of AIDS associated cryptosporidiosis after treatment with indinavir. Am J Gastroenterol. 1997;92:726.

278. Lafaurie M, Sarfati C, Menotti J, Molina JM. Remission of disseminated infection caused by *Encephalocytozoon intestinalis* with highly active antiretroviral therapy. AIDS. 2003;17:640-641.

279. Pape JW, Verdier RI, Johnson WD Jr. Treatment and prophylaxis of *Isospora belli* infection in patients with the acquired immunodeficiency syndrome. N Engl J Med. 1989;320:1044.

280. Pape JW, Verdier RI, Boncy M, et al. *Cyclospora* infection in adults infected with HIV: Clinical manifestations, treatment, and prophylaxis. Ann Intern Med. 1994;121:654.

281. Verdier RI, Fitzgerald DW, Johnson WD, Pope JW. Trimethoprim-sulfamethoxazole compared with ciprofloxacin for treatment and prophylaxis of *Isospora belli* and *Cyclospora cayetanensis* infection in HIV infected patients: A randomized controlled trial. Ann Intern Med. 2000;132:885-888.

282. Dore GJ, Marriott DJ, Hing MC, et al. Disseminated microsporidiosis due to *Septata intestinalis* in nine patients infected with the human immunodeficiency virus: Response to therapy with albendazole. Clin Infect Dis. 1995;21:70.

283. Diesenhouse MC, Wilson LA, Corrent GF, et al. Treatment of microsporidial keratoconjunctivitis with topical fumagillin. Am J Ophthalmol. 1993;115:293.

284. Lecuit M, Oksenhendler E, Sarfati C. Use of albendazole for disseminated microsporidian infection in a patient with AIDS. Clin Infect Dis. 1994;19:332.

285. Dieterich DT, Lew EA, Kotler DP, et al. Treatment with albendazole for intestinal disease due to *Enterocytozoon bieneusi* in patients with AIDS. J Infect Dis. 1994;169:178.

286. Molina JM, Oksenhendler E, Beauvais B, et al. Disseminated microsporidiosis due to *Septata intestinalis* in patients with AIDS: Clinical features and response to albendazole therapy. J Infect Dis. 1995;171:245.

287. Molina JM, Tourneur M, Sarfati C, et al. Fumagillin treatment of intestinal microsporidiosis. N Engl J Med. 2002;346:1963-1969.

288. Cello JP, Grendell JH, Basuk P, et al. Effect of octreotide on refractory AIDS-associated diarrhea. Ann Intern Med. 1991;115:705.

289. Sharpstone D, Rowbotton A, Nelson M, et al. The treatment of microsporidial diarrhea with thalidomide. AIDS. 1995;9:658.

290. Quinn TC, Cannon RO, Glasser D, et al. The association of syphilis with risk of human immunodeficiency virus infection in patients attending sexually transmitted disease clinics. Arch Intern Med. 1990;150:1297.

291. Hutchinson CM, Hook EW III, Shepherd M, et al. Altered clinical presentations and manifestations of early syphilis in patients with human immunodeficiency virus infection. Ann Intern Med. 1994;121:94.

292. Gourevitch M, Selwyn PA, Davenny K, et al. Effects of HIV infection on the serologic manifestations and response to treatment of syphilis in intravenous drug users. Ann Intern Med. 1993;118:350.

293. Koehler JE, Sanchez MA, Tye S, et al. Prevalence of *Bartonella* infection among human immunodeficiency virus-infected patients with fever. Clin Infect Dis 2003;37:559-566.

294. Regnery RL, Childs JE, Koehler JE. Infections associated with *Bartonella* species in persons infected with human immunodeficiency virus. Clin Infect Dis 1995;21(Suppl 1):S94-S98.

295. Koehler JE. Bartonellosis. In: Dolin R, Masur H, Saag MS, eds. AIDS Therapy. 2nd ed. New York: Churchill Livingstone; 2003:491-497.

296. Berson AM, Quivey JM, Harris JW, et al. Radiation therapy for AIDS-related Kaposi's sarcoma. Int J Radiat Oncol Biol Phys. 1993;27:1057.

297. Boudreaux AA, Smith LL, Cosby CD, et al. Intralesional vinblastine for cutaneous Kaposi's sarcoma associated with acquired immunodeficiency syndrome: A clinical trial to evaluate efficacy and discomfort associated with injection. J Am Acad Dermatol. 1993;28:61.

298. Krown SE, Gold JWM, Niedzwiecki D, et al. Interferon-α with zidovudine: Safety, tolerance, and clinical and virologic effects in patients with Kaposi's sarcoma associated with the acquired immunodeficiency syndrome (AIDS). Ann Intern Med. 1990;112:812.

299. Levine AM, Sullivan-Halley J, Pike MC, et al. HIV-related lymphoma: Prognostic factors predictive of survival. Cancer. 1991;68:2466.

300. Scadden D. Non-Hodgkin's lymphoma. In: Dolin R, Masur H, Saag MS, eds. AIDS Therapy. 2nd ed. Philadelphia: WB Saunders; 2003:696-705.

CHAPTER **126**

Vaccines for Human Immunodeficiency Virus-1 Infection

DAN H. BAROUCH

LINDSEY R. BADEN

RAPHAEL DOLIN

The development of safe and effective vaccines against human immunodeficiency virus-1 (HIV-1) infection or associated disease, or both, is the object of intensive research efforts throughout the world. It is becoming increasingly clear that effective vaccination offers the best hope for containing the epidemic of HIV-1 infection, particularly where extraordinarily rapid spread is being observed (see Chapter 113). The effects of highly active antiretroviral therapy (HAART) remain of uncertain duration and present serious problems of toxicity. In any case, because of high cost and limited availability, HAART is beyond the reach of most individuals at risk for HIV infection. Attempts to modify high-risk behavior to control the spread of HIV-1 have met with variable success, although in some areas extensive implementation of such efforts is just now getting underway. For these reasons, national and international public health agencies have afforded the highest priority to efforts to develop HIV vaccines. The explosive spread of acquired immunodeficiency syndrome (AIDS) in the developing world has imparted a particular sense of urgency to these efforts.

The development of vaccines against HIV-1 presents formidable scientific, logistic, and social challenges, and these have been the subject of several recent reviews.[1-4] Among the most important problems is a current lack of understanding of the critical parameters of immunity that might protect against HIV infection or disease, or both. Additionally, substantial genotypic variation occurs among HIV-1 strains, along with high frequencies of mutation and recombination in the replication of individual isolates. The relationship of these genotypic variations to the expression of antigens that might induce protective immunity remains poorly defined. However, it appears likely that an effective vaccine will have to stimulate broadly directed immune responses (i.e., those that are able to inhibit antigenically diverse strains of HIV-1).

Historically, investigation of these types of questions has been greatly facilitated by the use of animal model systems. Nonhuman primate models of infection with simian immunodeficiency virus (SIV) and chimeric HIV-SIV (SHIV) viruses have provided important information. However, because nonhuman primates do not represent a fully satisfactory model for HIV infection, carefully conducted studies of candidate HIV-1 vaccines in human volunteers have been undertaken and have provided important data regarding responses to HIV-1 immunogens. Data from these studies and from studies of immune responses in HIV-1–infected patients are reviewed in this chapter.

IMMUNE RESPONSES TO HIV-1 INFECTION

The molecular virology and antigenic characteristics of HIV-1 have now been elucidated in extraordinary detail (see Chapters 116 and 166). In humans infected with HIV-1, humoral and cell-mediated immune responses directed at a variety of viral antigens have been described. However, as noted earlier, the correlation of specific immune responses with protection from infection or disease, or both, has not yet been accomplished. The existence of naturally acquired immunity, the cornerstone on which the development of many viral vaccines has been based, remains a controversial concept in HIV-1 infections. Evidence to support this concept has emerged from studies of commercial sex workers who have remained uninfected despite repeated exposure to HIV-infected individuals and who have developed cell-mediated immune responses to HIV.[5,6] Studies of uninfected newborns born to HIV-positive mothers have also described HIV-specific cell-mediated immune responses.[7] In addition, studies of HIV-infected individuals in whom HIV virus replication and associated disease has not progressed over long periods (long-term nonprogressors) have also suggested that protective cell-mediated immune responses may develop.[8] Levels of circulating HIV-specific cytotoxic T lymphocytes (CTLs) have been inversely correlated with levels of virus in blood,[9,10] and the concept that such CTL activity inhibits virus replication is consistent with the results of experiments in humans.[11] The importance of such CTL activity is also supported by findings from challenge studies of SIV in macaques, in which depletion of CD8+ T lymphocytes resulted in markedly increased virus loads.[12,13]

The generation of neutralizing antibodies has been the major in vitro immunologic parameter on which the development of virtually all viral vaccines has been based. However, evidence for the role of neutralizing antibodies as a protective immune response against HIV-1 infection or disease is less compelling than that noted earlier for cell-mediated immune responses. Nonetheless, studies in chimpanzees and in macaques have indicated that passive administration of neutralizing antibodies can provide some protection against HIV or SIV infection, provided that such antibodies have appropriate specificity and sufficiently high titers are maintained.[14-20]

The relationship between immune responses to HIV and possible vaccine-induced protection are discussed in more detail in the following sections.

Neutralizing Antibodies

The measurement of neutralizing antibody activity is highly dependent on the passage history of the HIV-1 employed in the test. T-cell line–adapted (TCLA) viruses are considerably "easier" to neutralize than non–laboratory-adapted (primary) isolates, and they also have differences in antibody specificities. Neutralizing epitopes are present in a variety of HIV-1 proteins, most extensively on the envelope proteins, gp120 and gp41. In TCLA viruses, neutralizing antibodies are directed against a 35–amino-acid stretch of the third variable region of gp120 (V3 loop) and to the CD4 binding domain of the envelope protein.[21,22] The latter is a discontinuous and highly conformation-dependent site. Neutralizing antibodies directed against the V3 loop are generally more narrow (strain specific) in their activity than are the more broadly active antibodies directed against the CD4 binding domain.[23,24] Additional epitopes for neutralizing antibodies have been described on the V2 region of gp120[25] and on gp41.[26] Neutralizing antibodies have also been detected against Gag, Pol, and various regulatory proteins, but they most likely play minor roles in neutralizing activity against HIV-1.[27,28]

For primary isolates (R5 viruses), the V3 loop does not appear to represent a primary neutralization epitope. However, recently generated monoclonal antibodies with specificity against conformation-dependent epitopes mapping to the V3 loop have been reported to neutralize primary isolates, including some antibodies with apparent cross-clade activity.[29] Antibodies generated by vaccine candidates studied in phase I/II trials thus far have not been able to neutralize primary isolates consistently, even if high titers of neutralizing activity against laboratory-adapted strains are present. The reasons for these observations are currently unclear, but they suggest that neutralization epitopes differ between primary and laboratory-adapted isolates or perhaps are differentially expressed or presented in TCLA viruses and primary isolates. The elucidation of the three-dimensional structure of the HIV-1 envelope indicates that it has a highly dynamic configuration, with important differences depending on the state of activation and binding to cellular receptors.[30] Factors such as glycosylation, protein folding, and oligomerization may also be important to the antigenic properties of HIV envelope proteins.

Various levels of neutralizing antibodies are present throughout the course of HIV-1 infection. They can be detected within weeks after the onset of symptoms in primary HIV-1 infection and may play a role in the early reduction of plasma viremia, although they are clearly inadequate over time to clear the HIV infection.[31] The reasons for the relative lack of effectiveness of the neutralizing response are not fully understood. In part, it may be related to the generation of "escape mutants" during active virus replication, which leads to viruses that are less susceptible to neutralization by the initial immune responses to infection.[32] Recent evidence has indicated that initial neutralization-sensitive viruses are replaced by successive populations of resistant escape viruses with mutations in the *env* gene.[33] Many of these result in modifications in N-linked glycosylation sites, which may lead to "glycan shielding" as a neutralization escape mechanism.[34] Overall, a consistent correlation between levels of neutralizing antibodies and the clinical course of HIV-associated disease has not been found, although some studies have indicated that the presence of broadly neutralizing antibodies is a favorable prognostic indicator.[35]

In addition to neutralization activity, antibody-dependent cellular cytotoxicity against HIV-1 can be detected in HIV-infected patients. Antibody-dependent cellular cytotoxicity is directed primarily against sites on the viral envelope, including the V3 loop[36] and the extracellular domain of gp41.[37] The significance of antibody-dependent cellular cytotoxicity as a host defense against HIV-1 infection remains undefined.

Considerable research is underway to develop more complex envelope vaccine immunogens that might prove more immunogenic than monomeric gp120. Examples of these strategies include construction of envelope trimers that may more closely resemble the native envelope spike on viral surfaces,[38-40] deletion of variable loops or other structural regions of the envelope protein,[40,41] and stabilization of envelope conformations that may resemble intermediate structures in the membrane fusion process in which conserved epitopes are exposed.[42,43] These approaches are in the early stages of development and in preclinical evaluation in animal models, and the extent to which they will increase the breadth of clinically significant neutralizing antibody responses is not clear.

Cell-Mediated Immune Responses

Cell-mediated responses are considered to be important in the restriction of virus replication and therefore in the resolution of a number of viral infections. In particular, CTL activity, mediated by CD8$^+$ T lymphocytes in the context of major histocompatibility (MHC) class I restriction, is an important mechanism for elimination of virus-infected host cells. CTL activity against HIV antigens has been detected in HIV-1–seropositive individuals and appears to wane as HIV-1 disease progresses.[44-46] CD4$^+$ and CD8$^+$ T-lymphocyte activities have also been detected in humans immunized with candidate HIV-1 vaccines (see later discussion). CTL activity is directed against antigens on a variety of HIV-1 proteins, including envelope glycoproteins, particularly Gag internal structural proteins (p17, p24, p15), as well as against the products of regulatory genes.[44,47-51] In recipients of candidate HIV-1 vaccines, CD8$^+$ CTLs have been detected after administration of live-virus vector vaccines.[52-55] The administration of subunit vaccines alone has generated only CD4$^+$ CTLs to date.[1]

CTLs are capable of lysis of cells infected with primary isolates of HIV-1 and demonstrate broad-based activity against isolates from different clades.[56-58] As noted earlier, several lines of evidence suggest that CD8$^+$ CTL activity may be important in the control of HIV-1 replication in vivo, both in humans and in primate models. Patients with stable, low levels of HIV-1 viremia (nonprogressors) have been noted to have high levels of HIV-1–specific lymphoproliferative responses,[8] and it has been suggested that this is a marker for the ability of the immune response to control viral replication. The means by which lymphoproliferative responses might exert an inhibitory effect on HIV infection, by providing helper functions to CD8$^+$ CTLs or through another effector mechanism, are not well defined.

Potentially Deleterious Immune Responses

The possibility that HIV-1 infection or immunization may induce immune responses that are deleterious to the host has been an ongoing concern in efforts to develop HIV-1 vaccines. Antibody-dependent enhancement of in vitro infection with HIV-1, by either complement-mediated or Fc-mediated mechanisms, has been reported.[59,60] This apparently occurs through the interaction of virus–antibody complexes, with or without complement, with cells that bear Fc or complement receptors. This interaction may facilitate (enhance) entry of virus into cells that otherwise might not be infected by the virus. Such enhancing antibodies have been detected in vitro in serum specimens from patients with HIV-1 infection, as well as after immunization with recombinant HIV-1 envelope glycoproteins.[61,62] Complement-mediated antibody-dependent enhancement of epitopes has been detected on gp41,[63,64] and an Fc-mediated conformational epitope has been identified on gp120.[65] However, enhancement of infection has not been observed in vivo, and the biologic significance of enhancing antibodies is not known.

As is the case with proteins contained in other viruses, HIV-1 proteins have areas of homology with naturally occurring host regulatory and structural proteins. These include areas of homology between gp120 and interleukin-2 (IL-2),[66] neuroleukin,[67] chemokines, and β-chains of MHC class II molecules[68]; between gp41 and human leukocyte antigen (HLA) DR molecules[69]; and between Gag protein and thymosin-α1.[70] The significance of these observations is unknown. Although the potential for deleterious immune responses remains a consideration in the development of HIV-1 vaccines, it should be noted that autoimmunity, immunosuppression, enhancement of infection, and other deleterious effects have not been detected in studies of candidate HIV vaccines in humans or in animal models to date (see later discussion).

TYPES OF CANDIDATE HIV-1 VACCINES

Because of the uncertainty regarding the optimal type of immune responses that should be generated by an HIV-1 vaccine, a variety of different approaches to candidate HIV-1 vaccines has been proposed. Some of these are currently at various stages of preclinical development, whereas others have entered or completed phase I and II trials in humans (Table 126-1). Two candidate vaccines, consisting of recombinant gp120 proteins, have recently completed phase III efficacy trials (see later discussion). The major types of candidate vaccines under development or consideration are discussed in the following sections.

Whole Virus Vaccines

Traditionally, the initial approach to the development of virus vaccines has been to generate an inactivated or "killed" whole virus preparation. This may be particularly advantageous when the parameters of immunity are not defined and, therefore, the critical antigenic components of a vaccine are difficult to predict. Compared with a subunit preparation, a whole virus vaccine offers inclusion of a larger number of potentially relevant antigens. In HIV-1 vaccine development, this approach has received relatively little emphasis, primarily because of considerations of safety. The chief concern is related to the potential hazard of retained genetic material in such a vaccine (i.e., the potential risk of transmission of infectious HIV-1). Whole virus vaccines can now be prepared by techniques that render any remaining nucleic acid extremely unlikely to be infectious, and such vaccines can be ascertained to be free of nucleic acids by techniques of extraordinarily high sensitivity. However, the lack of an entirely appropriate animal model in which to demonstrate that a vaccine preparation is free of infectious HIV-1 still poses a significant problem.

Early studies of whole virus preparations of HIV in animal models used formalin inactivation of virus preparations, which clearly denatured some native proteins. More recently, milder methods of inactivation have been studied. These include removal of essential Zn^{2+} ions from Gag and integrase proteins through the use of Aldithriol,[105] and ultraviolet irradiation and psoralen treatment of viral particles.[106] The immunogenicity of virus particles inactivated by these methods is currently being evaluated in animal models.

Envelope Proteins

Vaccines composed of HIV-1 envelope proteins have undergone the most extensive study in humans. As noted earlier, important neutralizing epitopes, as well as T-cell epitopes, have been identified on HIV-1 envelope proteins. Envelope HIV-1 vaccines studied in humans have been generated through recombinant DNA expression systems, which provide an efficient means to prepare large quantities of purified proteins and also bypass concerns about possible contamination with other HIV-1 components. These recombinant proteins have been generated from laboratory-adapted HIV strains with a number of different vectors and cell systems, including insect,[107] yeast,[108] and mammalian cell cultures.[109-111] Depending on the vector and cell system employed, as well as on the purification procedures, these recombinant proteins may have important differences when compared with their naturally occurring analogues, including differences in tertiary structure, glycosylation, and oligomerization. Envelope protein vaccine candidates that have been evaluated in human trials include an rgp160 generated via a baculovirus vector and produced in insect cells (LAI strain)[62-71,105-111]; a fully glycosylated rgp160 made via a vaccinia vector in Vero cells (LAI and MN strains)[111]; a nonglycosylated rgp120 made in yeast cells (SF-2 strain)[112]; an rgp120 generated in Chinese hamster ovary cells (SF-2 strain)[81]; and an rgp120 generated in Chinese hamster

TABLE 126-1 Phase I Studies of Candidate HIV-1 Vaccines in HIV-1-Seronegative Volunteers

Vaccine Type	Cell Type, Production Method	HIV-1 Strains	Sponsor	Reference or Protocol No.
Envelope Proteins				
rgp160	Insect (baculovirus)	LAI	MicroGeneSys	62, 71, 72
rgp160	Vero (vaccinia)	LAI, MN	ImmunoAG	73-76
rgp120 (Env 2-3)	Yeast	SF-2	Chiron/Biocine	77, 78
rgp120	CHO cells	LAI/MN	Genentech	79, 80
rgp120	CHO cells	SF-2	Chiron/Biocine	81, 82
rgp120 + *nef-tat*	CHO cells	ACH320	GlaxoSmithKline	HVTN 041
Peptides				
gp120-V3 loop peptides	Synthetic octameric peptides	MN, 15 strains	United Biomedical Inc.	83, 84
p14HGP-30	Synthetic linear peptide (p17)	LAI	Viral Technologies Inc.	85-87
Gag lipopeptide P3C541b	Synthetic linear peptide		United Biomedical Inc.	AVEG 021
p14/p24:Ty-VLP	VLP, yeast transposon	LAI	British Biotech PLC	88, AVEG 019
HIV-1 gp120 C4-V3 peptides	Hybrid synthetic peptides	MN, EV91, RF, CANO	Wyeth-Lederle, Haynes	AVEG 020
V3 loop peptides	Chemical synthesis	MN	Swiss Serum and Vaccine	3
Gag-Pol-Nef-Env lipopeptides	Chemical synthesis and lipid conjugation	Clade B	Aventis Pasteur/ANRS	3
CLTB-36; V3-p24 peptide	Chemical synthesis	Clade B	Aventis Pasteur/ANRS	3
V3 multi-peptides	Chemical synthesis	Clade B	CIGB-Cuba	3
Live Vectors				
HIVAC-1e	Vaccinia construct with gp160	LAI	Bristol-Myers-Squibb (Oncogen)	89, 90
Vaccinia-HIV (TBC-3B)	Vaccinia construct with gp160, Gag, Pol	IIIB	Theron Biologics	91
Canarypox vCP 125	Canarypox construct with gp160	MN	Aventis Pasteur	92-94
Canarypox vCP 205	Canarypox with gp120, TM gp41, Gag, protease	MN/LAI	Aventis Pasteur	95, 96
Canarypox vCP 300	Canarypox with gp120, TM gp41, Gag, protease, CTL epitopes in POL and Nef	MN/LAI	Aventis Pasteur	97
Canarypox vCP 1433	Canarypox with gp120, TM gp41, Gag, protease CTL epitopes in POL and Nef	MN/LAI	Aventis Pasteur	AVEG 034
Canarypox vCP 1452	Canarypox as 1433 with two vaccinia virus coding sequences	MN/LAI	Aventis Pasteur	AVEG 034
Canarypox vCP 1521	Canarypox with gp120 from clade E, Gag, protease from clade B	Clade E, LAI	Aventis Pasteur	RV 144
MVA construct	p24, p17 inserts, CTL epitopes	Clade A	IAVI-MRC-UK-U Nairobi-IDT	185
Adenovirus MRK Ad5 HIV-1 *gag*	Replication-defective adenovirus 5	Clade B	Merck	HVTN 050
VEE VX101	VEE with *gag* insert AVX101	Clade C	Alphavax	HVTN 040
Salmonella typhi CVD 908 VVG 203	*Salmonella typhi* vector expressing gp120	LAI	University of Maryland Center for Vaccine Development	AVEG 028
Live Vector + Subunit Boost				
HIVAC-1e + rgp160 (baculovirus)	—*	LAI	Oncogen/MicroGenSys	52, 98, 99
HIVAC-1e + gp160	—	LAI + MN	Oncogen/ImmunoAG	100
HIVAC-1e + rgp120 (CHO)	—	LAI + SF-2	Oncogen/Chiron	100
HIVAC-1e + rgp120 (CHO)	—	LAI + LAI or MN	Oncogen/Genentech	100
TBC-3B + rgp120 (CHO)	—	+ MN	Therion/VaxGen	91
vCP125 + rgp120 (CHO)	—	MN + SF-2	AP/Chiron	92
vCP205 + rgp120 (CHO)	—	MN + SF-2	AP/Chiron	95
vCP300 + rgp120 (CHO)	—	MN + SF-2	AP/Chiron	97
vCP1452 + AIDSVAX B/B	—	MN + GNE8	AP/VaxGen	101
DNA Vaccines				
HIV-1 *env/rev* (APL 400-003)	GeneVax-HIV DNA plasmid backbone	MN	Wyeth-Lederle	102
HIV-1 *gag/pol* (APL 400-047)	GeneVax-HIV DNA plasmid backbone	HXB2 (LAI)	Wyeth-Lederle	103
HIV-1 *gag* + minigenes	Plasmid	Clade A	IAVI-MRC-UK Nairobi Cobra	3
HIV-1 *gag*	Plasmid	Clade B	Merck	104
HIV-1 *env, gag, pol, nef*	Plasmids VRC HIV-DNA-009	Clades A, B, C	VRC	VRC 004
HIV-1 *env, gag, pro,* RT, Tat, Vpu, Rev	Plasmids pGA2, JS2	Clade B	Emory University	HVTN 045
HIV-1 polyepitopes	Plasmids coding for CTL epitopes	EP HIV-1090	Epimmune	HVTN 048

*As noted above.
AVEG, AIDS Vaccine Evaluation Group; CHO, Chinese hamster ovary; CTL, cytotoxic T lymphocytes; HVTN, HIV Vaccine Trial Network; MVA, modified vaccinia virus Ankara; VEE, Venezuelan equine encephalitis; VRC, Vaccine Research Center.

ovary cells (IIIB and MN strains).[79,80] These rgp120 vaccines have been derived from TCLA viruses. However, rgp120 subunit candidate vaccines have been generated from primary isolates from clade B (GNE8) and clade E (CM244) viruses and have been studied in phase III efficacy trials (see later discussion).

Synthetic Peptides

Another approach to the development of envelope vaccines is the generation of synthetic peptides that include only epitopes of immunologic interest. This affords the opportunity to include only those epitopes that are most important for a protective response in the vaccine and to exclude minor or even potentially deleterious epitopes, such as ones that might be associated with enhancement of infection or immunopathogenesis. Conversely, a potential disadvantage of this approach is that synthetic peptides may not stimulate immune responses to noncontiguous or conformation-dependent epitopes. In addition, synthetic peptides are generally not as immunogenic as whole or native proteins. However, this problem might be overcome by coupling peptides to protein carriers or by the addition of more potent adjuvants, or both. An example of this approach is a vaccine candidate that consists of synthetically produced peptides from the V3 loops of multiple strains of HIV-1, linked to an oligolysine backbone.[113] Another example is a hybrid linear peptide that consists of multiple epitopes that are recognized by B cells, helper T cells, and CTLs.[114,115] The combination of a lipophilic membrane-anchoring moiety such as tripalmitoyl glyceryl cysteine with synthetic peptides resulted in the formation of liposomes that could be used to generate CD8+ CTL responses.[116]

Internal or Core Proteins

Vaccine candidates composed of HIV-1 internal proteins, either entirely or in part, have received relatively less attention. As noted earlier, it is believed that core proteins are particularly important in the generation of cell-mediated immune responses and especially CTLs, although neutralizing antibodies against internal proteins have been reported as well. Examples of vaccine candidates based on internal proteins include a 30–amino-acid peptide of p17 of HIV-1 (HGP-30)[117]; a portion of p17/p24 proteins formulated as a virus-like particle by introduction into the yeast retrotransposon Ty (Ty-Gag)[118]; a p24 protein generated via a baculovirus vector or via Chinese hamster ovary cells; and p55 particulate proteins.[68]

Live Vectors

Considerable interest exists in the development of live vector vaccines for HIV-1. Such vaccines have the potential to present HIV-1 antigens in the context of a replicating microbial system; in addition, in the case of an obligate intracellular organism such as a virus, the antigens are expressed by host cells. Presentation of antigen to the host in this manner may result in a more efficient immune response, particularly with respect to the generation of MHC class I–restricted CD8+ CTLs. The development of an efficiently replicating, genetically stable, live vector also offers important advantages for the large-scale production of vaccines. Some live vectors, such as vaccinia virus, are also resistant to environmental inactivation, which is of practical importance for the use of vaccines in field conditions in developing countries. However, live vectors need to be selected carefully, because they can contribute morbidity of their own in certain clinical settings (e.g., administration of a vaccinia vector to individuals with eczema or depressed cell-mediated immune defenses). An additional limitation of live vector vaccines is the development of immunity to the vector after initial immunization, so that repeated doses (boosts) with the vector may not be possible, at least over the short term. However, it may be possible to boost with the protein product of the HIV-1 gene inserted in the vector (e.g., with gp160) rather than with the live vector itself, as discussed later.

The most extensively studied live vectors for HIV-1 vaccine development are the poxvirus vectors vaccinia[119] and canarypox.[120] These vectors are well characterized, contain large DNA genomes into which multiple genes can be inserted, and infect multiple cell types. Stable constructs have been generated that contain various combinations of HIV-1 *env, gag, pol,* and regulatory genes, and these have undergone or are undergoing evaluations in clinical trials (see later discussion). As noted earlier, vaccinia vectors have the potential to cause serious illness in immunosuppressed subjects and those with eczematoid skin disorders, either as a result of vaccination or by spread from vaccinees. Further attenuated vaccinia vectors are being developed to address this concern.[121,122] Modified vaccinia Ankara (MVA) is a highly host-restricted virus with multiple genetic deletions after passage in chick embryo fibroblasts. A variety of HIV-1 MVA constructs that have been generated have undergone animal studies and are now beginning phase I studies in humans.[123,124] Both MVA and canarypox have the advantage of undergoing a single-cycle, nonproductive infection in mammalian cells; they do not cause disease in humans and cannot be transmitted from person to person. However, canarypox vectors appear considerably less immunogenic overall than vaccinia vectors in humans (see later discussion).

Considerable interest exists in the use of adenoviruses as live vectors for HIV-1 vaccines. The most extensively studied construct has been an adenovirus serotype 5 (Ad5) vector that has been made replication incompetent through deletion of the E1 gene.[125] Ad5 vectors expressing *gag* appear to be stable and well tolerated, and they are currently under evaluation for immunogenicity in humans. A major limitation in the use of such vectors is the presence of pre-existing immunity to adenovirus 5 in the general population; seroprevalence rates of 40% to 60% in the developed world and greater than 90% in parts of the developing world have been noted. This limitation is being addressed by the development of adenovirus vectors to which immunity is much less common, such as adenovirus serotype 35.

Another vector of particular interest is Venezuelan equine encephalitis (VEE) virus.[126] This virus has a predilection for infection of dendritic cells and can stimulate high levels of both systemic immunoglobulin G (IgG) and local IgA production. Replicons of VEE with HIV-1 inserts are now undergoing phase I trials in humans. Other alphaviruses being studied as candidate HIV vectors include Sindbis virus[127] and Semliki Forest virus.[128]

Other viral vectors based on adeno-associated viruses,[129] vesicular stomatitis virus,[130] and polioviruses[131] are at various stages of development. Bacterial vectors are also being developed, including ones based on *Salmonella*[132] and Calmette-Guérin bacillus.[133]

Nucleic Acid Vaccination

The observation that segments of nucleic acid genomes or plasmids ("naked DNA") administered intramuscularly undergo transcription and express proteins has led to the use of this technique as a means to deliver antigens for immunization. The technique permits construction of a vaccine that consists only of the components of immunologic interest. The proteins are presented through the MHC class I–restricted pathway, thus stimulating CTLs. Initial studies of DNA vaccination in humans generated low levels of immunogenicity, primarily because of inefficient expression of the native genes that were used. The use of codon-optimized synthetic genes resulted in more efficient expression of gene products. Immunogenicity was also improved by adsorbing DNA to microparticles and, in animal studies, by the use of cytokines such as IL-2, IL-12, and granulocyte-macrophage colony-stimulating factor (GM-CSF) as adjuvants. DNA vaccination is being studied for a variety of potential viral vaccines, including phase I studies with HIV-1 vaccines (see Table 126-1).[134,135]

Live-Attenuated Virus Vaccines

The use of live-attenuated virus vaccines has been highly successful in the control of several important viral diseases, including measles, rubella, and polio. These vaccines present in a manner that most closely resembles naturally occurring infection and that also stimulates a broad array of humoral and cell-mediated immune responses. With some live-attenuated virus vaccines, immunity is particularly long-lasting. Depending on the site of immunization, live-attenuated viruses may be highly efficient in the stimulation of local (mucosal) immunity, which may be especially important for prevention of HIV-1 infection transmitted by the sexual route. Boosting by repeated mucosal immunizations may also be possible, depending on the intensity and duration of local immune responses stimulated by initial immunization.

Clearly, the major concern in the development of live-attenuated HIV-1 vaccine candidates is safety. The problem of devising adequate safety tests, particularly given the lack of an entirely suitable animal model for HIV-1 disease, was noted earlier. The incomplete understanding of the pathogenesis of HIV-1–associated disease, and the associated difficulty of identification of virulence factors, has also inhibited attempts to develop live-attenuated viruses. HIV-1 is known to have a number of regulatory genes that affect different points of the virus replicative cycle (see Chapter 166). One approach to the development of a live-attenuated virus vaccine has been to delete one or more regulatory genes, which can result in a mutant virus that has lost pathogenicity. Because such a virus has a genetic deletion, it would appear to be less likely to revert to its pathogenic parent, at least by reconstruction of the deleted gene. The attenuated mutant virus would nonetheless have to replicate sufficiently well to stimulate humoral and cell-mediated immunity. One such live-attenuated SIV vaccine, in which the *nef* gene was deleted,[136] provided impressive protection against virulent SIV challenge in macaques. The precise mechanism of protection for the *nef*-deleted vaccine is unclear but may depend on the continued presence of replicating virus in various cellular compartments. As with other live virus vaccines, attenuation is a relative term and is highly dependent on host factors. *Nef*-deleted SIV viruses that are nonpathogenic in adult monkeys have caused disease when administered to neonatal animals.[137,138] Even in adult monkeys, *nef*-deleted mutants have been observed to undergo repair with restoration of virulence, illustrating the risks inherent in such an approach.[139] As a result, the development of live-attenuated HIV-1 vaccine is proceeding cautiously.

ANIMAL MODELS

The availability of an appropriate and practical animal model is of great importance to studies of the pathogenesis of HIV-1 disease and to the development of vaccines and chemotherapeutic agents. For the development of vaccines, an animal model offers the opportunity to conduct experimental virus challenges and thereby to study the protective effects of candidate vaccines directly. Despite the fact that considerable progress has been made in this area, there is as yet no perfect animal model of HIV-1 infection. Chimpanzees are the only established animal model system in which experimental infection with HIV-1 can be consistently achieved. After infection, chimpanzees mount immune responses to HIV-1, and virus can be isolated from peripheral blood mononuclear cells, although this becomes increasingly difficult as time passes. HIV-1–infected chimpanzees do not show consistent evidence of HIV-related disease, although HIV-1 strains have been adapted to cause disease to some degree in chimpanzees.[140,141] In addition, chimpanzees are extraordinarily expensive and in short supply, so only small numbers are available for experimental studies of candidate vaccines.

The most extensively developed primate model is the macaque, most frequently *Macaca mulatta,* or rhesus macaque, which can be infected with SIV.[142] This model has the advantage that SIV causes disease in macaques, and macaques are much more readily available and less expensive than chimpanzees. After an incubation period that is considerably shorter than that seen in humans infected with HIV, SIV infection results in immunosuppression and in the development of opportunistic infections. Death often results within 3 to 5 months. A particularly virulent strain, SIV_{pbj}, can cause overwhelming disease 1 to 2 weeks after infection.[143] Although differences in the frequency and type of opportunistic processes exist between SIV-induced disease in macaques and HIV-1–induced disease in humans, overall the disease patterns have many features in common. SIV and HIV-1 are also similar in genetic structure and organization, although some differences exist.[144,145] The inability to infect macaques with HIV-1 has prevented candidate HIV-1 vaccines from being directly examined in that animal model. However, chimeric viruses (SHIV) have been developed that have an envelope derived from HIV-1 and internal proteins from SIV; these viruses can infect macaques and induce disease.[146] SHIVs offer promise of great utility in studies of candidate HIV-1 vaccines in macaques.

Preclinical Vaccine Studies

Numerous studies of candidate vaccines have been carried out in primate models. As noted earlier, there are SIV strains that have a broad range of virulence, ranging from persistent infection with little or no disease to rapid, lethal infection. As might be anticipated, candidate vaccines have been generally more effective in inducing protection against less virulent experimental infections, such as $SIVmac_{Bk28}$ or HIV-1 in chimpanzees, than against a more virulent challenge such as $SIVsm_{pbj14}$.[136] In addition to the virulence of the challenge strain of virus, important variables to be considered in the interpretation of primate challenge studies are the dose of the challenge virus, the route of administration of virus (intravenous versus intrarectal or intravaginal), the homology between the immunizing virus and the challenge strain, and the type of end point that was used for evidence of efficacy. The heterogeneity of experimental conditions under which primate challenge studies have been carried out has resulted in apparent inconsistencies of results among some studies and difficulty in generalizing conclusions from others. Overall, a definition of the critical in vitro correlates of protection has not yet emerged from these studies. However, the importance of

virus-specific cellular immune responses has been clearly demonstrated by studies showing that in vivo depletion of CD8$^+$ T lymphocytes in SIV-infected rhesus macaques leads to dramatic increases in plasma viral RNA levels.[12,147] Moreover, major expansions of SIV-specific CD8$^+$ CTLs were shown to occur during acute SIV infection and were maintained during chronic infection.[148,149] These and other studies have provided a convincing rationale that HIV-1 vaccines should elicit potent virus-specific cellular immune responses.

The importance of humoral immune responses was illustrated by studies in rhesus macaques demonstrating that passive infusions of HIV-1–specific neutralizing monoclonal antibodies afforded complete protection against infection with pathogenic SHIV isolates.[18,19] Humoral immune responses also appear to contribute to the control of viral replication in chronic SIV infection.[13] Although vaccine-elicited antibody responses have been shown to provide a degree of protection against homologous viral challenges in certain settings,[150-152] it has proved extraordinarily difficult to generate broadly reactive neutralizing antibodies by vaccination. As noted earlier, this problem is related in part to the extraordinary diversity of envelope genes worldwide and to viral immune evasion strategies.

Whole inactivated virus vaccines and recombinant monomeric gp120 subunit vaccines both exhibited early apparent successes in nonhuman primate challenge studies.[153,154] However, subsequent studies revealed that the apparent protection afforded by these approaches could be explained either by experimental artifacts or by the use of nonpathogenic challenge models.[154,155] A major limitation of these approaches is their inability to elicit virus-specific CTL responses as well as their inability to generate broadly reactive neutralizing antibodies.

Injection of plasmid DNA vaccines expressing a wide variety of antigens has proved immunogenic in animal models of a number of diseases.[156-159] In particular, DNA vaccines were shown to elicit potent HIV/SIV-specific cellular immune responses that reduced viral replication after SIV and SHIV challenges in rhesus monkeys.[160,161] Moreover, DNA vaccines augmented by plasmid IL-2 constructs were able to protect monkeys against SHIV-induced disease progression.[161] However, relatively high doses of DNA have been required to generate potent immune responses in nonhuman primates. Most importantly, DNA vaccines have proved only marginally immunogenic in humans to date, as described earlier. Therefore, it is likely that plasmid DNA vaccines will require either effective adjuvants or boosts with heterologous vector-based vaccines to augment their immunogenicity.

Poxviruses have been explored extensively as candidate HIV-1 vaccine vectors in animal model studies. Recombinant, replication-competent vaccinia virus was initially shown to elicit potent immune responses in nonhuman primates.[162,163] However, substantial safety risks associated with vaccinia in immunosuppressed individuals have led to the development of attenuated poxviruses that undergo little or no replication in the host. Recombinant modified vaccinia Ankara (rMVA) vaccines have also been shown to elicit potent HIV/SIV-specific CTL responses in nonhuman primates. Moreover, both rMVA vaccines alone and DNA prime/rMVA boost regimens reduced viral replication after SIV and SHIV challenges and protected against SHIV-induced disease progression.[164-168]

Canarypox (ALVAC) vectors have also been studied in nonhuman primates, but the immunogenicity of these vectors has been generally disappointing. The potential utility of combining ALVAC vectors with protein subunits or other live vectors is still under investigation.

E1-deleted, replication-incompetent, recombinant adenovirus serotype 5 (rAd5) vectors have been shown to elicit impressive immune responses in nonhuman primates. Moreover, these vaccines have afforded effective control of viral replication after SHIV challenges and protection against SHIV-induced disease progression.[156] Clinical trials using rAd5 vaccines as well as DNA prime/rAd5 boost regimens are currently in progress (see later discussion).

Implications and Limitations

Nonhuman primate challenge studies have demonstrated that certain plasmid DNA vaccines and recombinant live vector–based vaccines elicit high-frequency virus-specific cellular immune responses and significantly attenuate viral replication and clinical disease progression after SIV and SHIV challenges.[94,160,161,168] However, several important limitations of these CTL-based vaccines have become apparent. First, none of these vaccine approaches has afforded sterilizing immunity (i.e., complete protection against infection). Although this may reflect in part the high virus inoculum typically used in experimental challenge studies, it is also possible that vaccine-elicited CTL responses function only by suppressing viral replication after infection of host cells and do not have any intrinsic capability to block primary infection. Supporting this hypothesis is the observation that vaccine-elicited CTL responses failed to augment the partial protection afforded by a suboptimal dose of passively transferred neutralizing antibodies in rhesus macaques.[169]

A second important limitation with CTL-based vaccines is their inability to eradicate the virus after infection. It is clear that vaccine-elicited CTL responses effectively control viral replication to very low levels after viral challenges in nonhuman primates. However, the constant immune selection pressure and inability to eradicate the virus can lead to the eventual emergence of a virus population carrying mutations in dominant CTL epitopes. Such mutant viruses may then escape from recognition by dominant epitope-specific CTLs, resulting in breakthrough viral replication and clinical disease progression. Viral escape from dominant CTLs has in fact been observed in vaccinated, infected rhesus macaques at a time when plasma virus was effectively controlled to undetectable levels. Such viral escape resulted in rapid loss of control of viral replication, clinical disease progression, and eventual AIDS vaccine failure.[170] Thus, the partial protection afforded by CTL-based AIDS vaccines can be undermined by viral immune evasion strategies. These data suggest that broad vaccine-elicited CTL responses against multiple epitopes will be required to afford durable control of viral replication.

HUMAN TRIALS

More than 50 candidate HIV-1 vaccines were studied in more than 13,000 HIV-1–uninfected normal volunteers between 1990 and 2003. The study of candidate HIV-1 vaccines in humans poses several unique problems beyond those encountered in studies of other experimental vaccines. Volunteers need to be fully informed of the potential hazards of immunization and of the limitations of our knowledge regarding the pathogenesis of HIV-1–associated disease. Volunteers must be made aware that they may become seropositive for HIV-1 by conventional "screening assays" and of the possible difficulties of employment, eligibility for insurance, and immigration that might result. Volunteers must also be counseled not to abandon behaviors aimed at reducing acquisition of HIV-1 infection because of a hope that the vaccine under study will provide protection against such infection. A detailed description of the procedures employed in the conduct of phase I studies of HIV-1 candidate vaccines in humans, including measures taken to address the preceding issues, has been published.[62]

The purpose of the initial trials (phase I studies) that have been undertaken is to examine the immunogenicity and safety of various vaccine candidates in humans. Because studies in primates have not clearly established the superiority of one vaccine approach over another, several different types of vaccine candidates are being evaluated in humans (see Table 126-1). Studies directed at the development of preventive vaccines have been carried out in healthy, HIV-1–seronegative volunteers. For most phase I studies, these are individuals who have

been determined to be at low risk for acquisition of HIV-1 infection, to avoid the potentially confounding effects of an intercurrent HIV-1 infection. Phase II studies have been carried out in subjects who were generally at higher risk for the acquisition of HIV-1 infection (Table 126-2). Vaccines intended for immunotherapy have been studied in HIV-1–seropositive subjects (see later discussion).

Phase I Studies

Recombinant Envelope Proteins

Recombinant envelope proteins (rgp160 and rgp120) have undergone extensive study in humans. The viruses from which the envelope proteins were derived were mostly from clade B (LAI, SF-2, and MN strains) and were from TCLA-adapted X4 viruses. Exceptions were the more recently generated rgp120 from a primary isolate of clade B (GNE8) and rgp120 from a primary isolate from clade E (CM244). Combinations of these latter rgp120s were used in recently completed phase III efficacy trials (see later discussion).

The majority of studies with the preceding vaccines were phase I studies of safety and immunogenicity carried out in relatively small numbers of volunteers who were at low risk for acquisition of HIV-1 infection.[62,73,74,78-82,112,172,173] These studies also examined the effects of varying dosages and schedules of immunization. The recombinant envelope vaccines were administered intramuscularly in multiple-dose schedules, combined with various adjuvants.

Overall, the recombinant envelope HIV-1 candidate vaccines were very well tolerated. Vaccinees experienced mild local reactions comparable in frequency and magnitude to those seen with administration of licensed vaccines. An exception was the combination of rgp120 with MTP-PE, a synthetic lipophilic muramyl tripeptide adjuvant, which had a significantly higher rate of local and systemic reactions.[172] The use of QS21 as an adjuvant was also associated with significant reactogenicity.[173]

Immunization with at least three doses of these recombinant envelope proteins resulted in high rates (>90%) of binding antibodies to specific HIV-1 proteins, as determined by Western blot or enzyme-linked immunosorbent assay. High rates of neutralizing antibodies were also induced by the rgp120 immunogens, particularly those generated in Chinese hamster ovary cells.[79-82] In general, rgp120 immunogens induced greater neutralizing antibodies, but less binding antibodies, than did the rgp160 immunogens.

Neutralizing antibodies were generally restricted to type-specific activity against the homologous isolate. Perhaps most troubling was the unanticipated observation that serum neutralizing activity from the vaccinees was effective only against laboratory-adapted viruses grown in T-cell lines; non–laboratory-adapted HIV-1 viruses (primary isolates) were not neutralized.[174-176] Subsequent discoveries of HIV coreceptors and structural definition of the HIV envelope have helped to explain why the immune responses to T-cell line–adapted viruses might be different from those to primary isolates (see earlier discussion and Chapter 166).

In addition to circulating antibodies, the recombinant immunogens also readily induced T-cell proliferative responses to HIV-1–specific antigens.[177,178] However, as might be predicted from the known pathway for processing of peptide antigens that results in an association with MHC class II molecules, recombinant protein immunogens did not induce CD8+ CTLs, although some CD4+ cytolytic activity was detected.[179]

VaxGen conducted a phase I/II trial of their bivalent gp120 B/B vaccine, which consists of gp120 (MN) and gp120 (GNE8), a clade B

TABLE 126-2 Phase II Studies of Candidate HIV-1 Vaccines in HIV-1-Seronegative Volunteers

Vaccine	Cell Type, Production Method	HIV-1 Strains	Sponsor	Reference
rgp120	CHO cells	SF-2 + MN	Chiron/Biocine, Aventis Pasteur	125
vCP 205 + rgp120	Canarypox-gp120, TM gp41, Gag, protease; CHO cells	MN/LAI, SF-2	Aventis Pasteur, Chiron/Biocine	171
vCP 1452 + AIDSVAX B/B	Canarypox-gp120, TM gp41, Pol, CTL epitopes from *nef* and *pol*; CHO cells	MN/LAI, MN + GNE8	Aventis Pasteur, VaxGen	101

CHO, Chinese hamster ovary; CTL, cytotoxic T lymphocytes.

primary isolate. This vaccine was administered at 0, 1, 6, and 12 months to 122 subjects in the United States, at doses of 100, 300, and 600 μg. The vaccine was well tolerated and was reported to induce MN-specific antibodies in 76% of subjects and GNE8-specific antibodies in 91% of subjects at the 300-μg dose. A similar study was conducted of a gp120 B/E vaccine, which included a primary clade E isolate (CM244), in 92 subjects in Thailand; 83% of subjects developed antibody activity against MN, and 100% against CM244.

Synthetic Peptides

Synthetic peptides that have undergone phase I studies in humans include peptides from envelope or Gag proteins derived from clade B viruses or from multiple other clades (see Table 126-1). Several techniques have been employed for the presentation of immunogens in these vaccine formulations, including conjugation with an oligolysine backbone or with a lipopeptide, encapsulation in polylactide copolymers, and as a fusion protein particle in a self-assembling yeast protein, Ty. In general, these peptide vaccines have been poorly immunogenic, whether administered intramuscularly or by rectal or oral routes.[83,85-87,180-182] Low levels of binding antibodies and little or no neutralizing activity were seen. More complex peptides containing epitopes of neutralizing antibodies, CTLs, and helper T-cell activity are currently under development.

Live Virus Vector Vaccines

Vaccinia and canarypox vector constructs with inserts of HIV-1 genes have also undergone extensive phase I studies in humans (see Table 126-1). Vaccinia virus vectors that express gp160 alone or multiple HIV-1 proteins (gp160, Gag, and Pol) have been administered to normal volunteers in studies similar to those previously carried out with the recombinant envelope immunogens.[89-91,98,183,184] The vaccinia constructs were administered by scarification and resulted in local lesions indistinguishable in character from those seen with the vaccinia parent. The vaccinia vectors induced only low levels of humoral antibody. The neutralizing activity that was seen was also relatively restricted, was directed at the homologous virus strain, and was active only against TCLA viruses and not against primary isolates. However, induction of CD8+ CTLs directed against HIV-1–infected target cells regularly developed.[52,54,183] The presence of preexisting immunity to vaccinia reduced immunogenicity of the vector constructs, and initial immunization with the vaccinia vector provided solid immunity against subsequent infection or "takes" with the vector.[52,89,90]

Although the vaccinia constructs were generally well tolerated, the possibility exists of serious problems if vaccinia were inadvertently administered or spread to immunosuppressed patients or to those with eczematoid skin disorders. For this reason, vectors were sought that might carry less of a risk in this regard. Canarypox is an avian poxvirus that undergoes an abortive replicative cycle in mammalian cells. Because administration of canarypox to humans does not result in the production of infectious virus, it provides a greater margin of safety than does vaccinia. Canarypox constructs have been generated that express gp160, gp120/gp41 (transmembrane protein)/Gag/protease, with and without the addition of epitopes in *nef/pol.* In several phase I studies and two phase II studies, intramuscularly administered canarypox was very well tolerated and did not result in detectable lesions.[92-94,97] Relatively weak humoral antibody responses were observed, but HIV-1–specific CD8+ CTL responses were seen in 15% to 30% of subjects at any single point in time, and at least once in 35% to 65% of subjects over the duration of the study.[92-94,97] Vectors that express multiple HIV antigens appear to induce CTLs with higher frequency than do those that express only one antigen. The kinetics and duration of the CTL responses are not fully defined, but they may last for at least 6 months. CTLs induced by the canarypox vectors killed cells infected with primary isolates, as well as cells infected with viruses from clades other than the homologous clade B.[56] MVA constructs expressing several HIV-1 proteins, including proteins p24 and p17, and CTL epitopes from a clade A virus have undergone a phase I study and demonstrated induction of HIV-specific CTLs.[185] Clinical studies of another MVA construct with clade B *env, gag, tat, ref, nef,* and *pol* inserts are planned.

Adenoviral HIV-1 vectors have also undergone phase I studies in HIV-1–uninfected subjects. Dose escalation studies have been conducted with MRK Ad5, a vector rendered replication incompetent through deletions in the E1 gene, in which the *gag* gene was inserted. Doses ranged from 10^9 to 10^{11} viral particles per dose and were occasionally associated with side effects such as fevers, chills, and myalgias within 24 to 48 hours after vaccination, although these generally were not of sufficient severity to require withdrawal from the study. Preliminary reports indicated that 44% to 56% of vaccinated subjects developed HIV-1–specific cell-mediated immune responses, as measured by enzyme-linked immunospot (ELISPOT) assays, and some responses were directed at cross-clade antigens from clades A and C viruses.[104] As discussed previously, the presence of preexisting immunity to Ad5 significantly inhibited immunogenicity to the construct. A large-scale phase II study of MRK Ad5-*gag* construct at doses of 10^9 or 10^{10} viral particles per dose involving 435 subjects (HIV Vaccine Trial Network, HVTN 050) began in early 2004.

Nucleic Acid Vaccines

Phase I studies of DNA-based HIV-1 vaccines have been conducted in relatively small numbers of HIV-1–uninfected subjects, and the vaccines appear to be nonreactogenic. An *env-* and *rev-* encoding DNA vaccine was given intramuscularly to 12 subjects in doses of either 100 or 300 μg at 0, 1, 2, and 6 months, and modest HIV-1 specific T-cell responses were noted sporadically at the higher dose.[102] The AIDS Vaccine Evaluation Group (AVEG) conducted a study of a DNA *gag-pol* vaccine in 52 subjects in doses ranging from 100 μg to 3 mg at 0, 1, 2, and 6 months and generated low levels of T-lymphocyte responses.[103] DNA *gag* vaccines also have been tested in doses up to 5 mg in studies conducted by Merck, although cell-mediated immune responses appeared to be less robust with their DNA vaccines than with their adenoviral-based vaccines.[104]

A multi-clade DNA vaccine has been developed by the National Institute of Allergy and Infectious Diseases (NIAID) Vaccine Research Center (VRC) in Bethesda, Maryland. It consists of plasmids encoding *env* from clades A, B, and C and *gag-pol-nef* plasmids from clade B. Phase I trials of this candidate vaccine are underway at the VRC[186] and through the HVTN (HVTN 052). A phase I trial of this DNA vaccine, in combination with a plasmid encoding a fusion protein of IL-2/Ig as an adjuvant, began in early 2004 (HVTN 044).

Prime-Boost Vaccination Approaches

Studies from animal models have suggested that administration of a "boost" with a heterologous immunogen may augment the humoral and cellular responses observed after administration of the vector used for priming. This was seen in trials in humans, in which administration of two booster doses of rgp120 after priming with vaccinia vectors resulted in high titers of neutralizing antibodies, similar to those seen after three or four doses of rgp120 alone.[52,187] However, the neutralizing antibodies induced were still relatively type specific, and they neutralized TCLA viruses but not primary isolates of HIV-1. Boosting with a gp120 subunit did increase lymphoproliferative responses and antibody-dependent cytotoxicity but did not appear to affect lymphoproliferative response. Prime boost strategies have also been employed in phase I studies, by priming with live vectors followed by boosting with protein vaccines and by priming with DNA vaccines followed by boosting with live vectors. The prime boost strategy has also been evaluated in phase II studies (described later).

Phase II Clinical Studies

Three phase II studies of candidate HIV-1 vaccines have been performed: two by the AVEG and one by the HVTN (see Table 126-2). In AVEG 201, two recombinant gp120 subunit vaccines were studied in 296 HIV-seronegative subjects in six demographic groups: four with higher risk behavior and two with lower risk behavior.[104] After three immunizations, more than 87% of subjects had neutralizing antibodies to the homologous isolate, and they persisted for at least 2 years in 57% of subjects who were tested. However, the study showed somewhat lower neutralizing and other antibody responses to one of the vaccines (HIV-1$_{SF-2}$ gp120) in the intravenous drug user group and, to a lesser extent, in heterosexual partners of HIV-infected individuals. The reasons for this observation have not been explained, but it illustrates the importance of assessing immunogenicity in diverse groups other than simply low-risk subjects.

The second phase II study was a collaboration between AVEG and HIV Network for Prevention (HIVNET) (AVEG 202–HIVNET 014).[171] This study examined a prime-boost regimen consisting of a canarypox/HIV-1 construct, vCP 205, with an rgp120 (SF-2) boost in 435 subjects, of whom 60 were lower risk and 375 were higher risk. The vaccines were generally well tolerated in these groups. More than 90% of subjects who received the prime-boost regimen developed neutralizing antibodies against the homologous TCLA virus, and one third of those who received regimens containing vCP 205 developed anti-HIV CTL responses. There appeared to be no significant difference in immune responses between the higher- and lower-risk groups in this study.

The HVTN recently completed a phase II study of a canarypox vector ALVAC-HIV (vCP 1452) that contained inserts of gp120, the transmembrane portion of gp41, *gag,* a portion of *pol,* and several CTL epitopes from *nef* and *pol.* Boosts were administered with AIDSVAX B/B. The vector was administered at a dose of $10^{7.26}$ median tissue culture infective dose (TCID$_{50}$) at 0, 1, 3, and 6 months to 330 subjects. The vaccine was well tolerated, but the overall immunogenicity was disappointing. Vaccinees developed HIV-1–specific CTL at a cumulative frequency of less than 30% at any point throughout the study, and less than 15% at any single time point.[101] Why vCP1452 was less immunogenic in this phase II study than other canarypox constructs in phase I studies is not clear. Raising the dose of vCP 1452 to $10^{8.0}$ significantly increased reactogenicity but did not augment immunogenicity.[188]

Efficacy Trials of Candidate HIV-1 Vaccines

Determination of the efficacy of a candidate HIV vaccine requires the conduct of large-scale, rigorously controlled clinical trials. Such trials present formidable scientific, logistic, and social challenges and require extensive resources. The appropriate criteria to determine that a candidate HIV vaccine has sufficient promise to proceed to an efficacy trial remain a matter of substantial controversy. This is particularly so because of the lack of understanding of the critical parameters of immunity noted previously and the limitations of information that can be obtained from animal model systems. Nonetheless, it is increasingly appreciated that properly conducted efficacy trials themselves may provide important information regarding correlates of protection that cannot be obtained otherwise, even if the candidate vaccine is only minimally effective. This information could then be "fed back" to investigators for appropriate modification or revision of vaccine development efforts.

The first phase III (efficacy) trial of a candidate vaccine (AIDSVAX B/B) was recently completed by VaxGen, Inc.[189] (Table 126-3). The vaccine candidate consisted of two rgp120 proteins from clade B isolates (MN and GNE8) in alum; it was administered at 0, 1, 6, 12, 18, 24, and 30 months in a multicenter study. The experimental design was a double-blind, randomly allocated, placebo-controlled study (vaccine:placebo = 2:1) conducted in 5417 subjects, of whom 5109 were men who have sex with men and 308 were women at heterosexual risk for HIV infection. At the end of the 3-year period of observation, the rates of the major study end point (HIV-1 infection) were virtually the same in the vaccine group (5.7%) and the placebo group (5.8%).

VaxGen also recently completed a second phase III study in Thailand, of a similar rgp120 vaccine (AIDSVAX B/E), from a clade B isolate (MN) and a primary clade E isolate (A244). The experimental design was similar to that described previously, except that the vaccine-to-placebo ratio was 1:1, and the study population consisted of 2546 injection drug users. The annualized rate of infection was 3.1% in both placebo and vaccine recipients.[190]

A phase III trial of a prime-boost regimen consisting of ALVAC vCP 1521 boosted by AIDSVAX B/E as a collaborative study by the U.S. and Thai governments began in late 2003.

TABLE 126-3 Phase III Studies of Candidate HIV-1 Vaccines in HIV-1–Seronegative Volunteers

Vaccine	Cell Type	HIV-1 Strains	Sponsor	Reference
AIDSVAX B/B	CHO cells	MN, GNE8	VaxGen	189
AIDSVAX B/E	CHO cells	MN, A244	VaxGen	190

CHO, Chinese hamster ovary.

Vaccine Studies in HIV-1–Infected Persons (Immunotherapy)

The goal of vaccination of HIV-1–seropositive persons (immunotherapy) is to induce immune responses in the host that may retard progression of disease, either through inhibition of virus replication or spread or by other, as yet undefined mechanisms. Several preliminary studies in nonhuman primates have suggested possible benefits of therapeutic vaccination. Recombinant poxvirus vaccines were shown to augment cellular immune responses in SIV-infected rhesus monkeys receiving antiretroviral therapy and to improve control of viral replication after withdrawal of antiretroviral therapy.[191,192] In addition, autologous dendritic cells pulsed with inactivated whole virus particles similarly produced augmented immune responses and lowered viral loads in SIV-infected monkeys.[193]

Data suggesting that functional immunity to HIV-1 can be augmented in HIV-1–infected humans has come from clinical studies involving structured treatment interruptions (STIs) in patients treated with antiretroviral therapy during acute infection. Treatment early during acute infection has been shown to preserve HIV-1–specific CD4$^+$ T-cell responses.[194,195] In addition, STIs in these individuals were demonstrated to expand virus-specific immune responses and led to effective, albeit transient, control of viral replication.[196] In rhesus macaques treated with antiretroviral therapy early in acute SIV infection, serial STIs similarly resulted in enhanced virus-specific immunity and effective control of viral replication.[197] However, in contrast to STIs in acutely treated individuals, no beneficial effects were observed after STIs in individuals treated with antiretroviral therapy during chronic infection.[198-201] In fact, in certain studies, individuals treated during chronic infection who underwent STIs developed drug resistance mutations and exhibited accelerated disease progression, compared with those who remained on antiretroviral therapy. Therefore, enthusiasm for STIs in patients treated during chronic infection is waning. It is hoped that therapeutic vaccines may provide a safer and perhaps more effective method to enhance virus-specific immune responses, compared with the "autovaccination" that results from the burst of viral replication that occurs after STIs.

Approximately 50 therapeutic vaccine studies have been conducted to date with candidate HIV-1 vaccines in HIV-1–seropositive individuals. These include the inactivated virus preparation of Salk,[202,203] recombinant gp160 and gp120 proteins,[204-208] p24 preparations,[209] synthetic peptides, DNA vaccines,[210] ALVAC vectors, and peptide-pulsed dendritic cell vaccines.[211] These candidate vaccines have been studied primarily in asymptomatic individuals with CD4 counts of 400 cells/mm^3 and greater, although some studies in patients with lower CD4 counts have also been carried out. Available results from phase I studies indicate that these vaccines are generally well tolerated and that they induce a variety of humoral and cellular immune responses to the immunogen that either were previously undetectable or were present at low levels only. These responses have included rises in serum antibody to specific epitopes on the immunogen, increased T-cell proliferative responses, and increased CTL activity. However, no convincing effects on virus loads, CD4 counts, or clinical disease progression have been shown in these studies.

A controlled trial of this approach was conducted by the AIDS Clinical Trials Group (ACTG 214),[212] which investigated the effect of four rgp120 vaccines: a CHO-derived rgp120 (LAI) in an alum adjuvant, a CHO-derived rgp120 (MN) in alum, a CHO-derived rgp120

(SF-2) in MF59, and a yeast-derived rgp120 from SF-2 (Env 2-3) in MF59. These were studied under a double-blind, placebo (adjuvant only)–controlled experimental design in HIV-1–infected patients with CD4 counts greater than 500/mm³ who were not receiving antiretroviral therapy. The vaccines were very well tolerated, and the LAI- and MN-derived rgp120s induced HIV-specific lymphoproliferative responses in 29% and 24% of subjects, respectively. The SF-2–derived vaccines were less immunogenic. No effects on CD4 counts were noted in the treatment arms. A companion trial was conducted in subjects who had CD4 counts of less than 500/mm³ on entry; it showed overall lower rates of induction of HIV-specific lymphocyte responses,[212,213] and no effects on CD4 counts or on disease progression were noted. Other studies using rgp160 or rgp120 vaccines in HIV-1–infected subjects also failed to demonstrate an effect on decline of T cells or on disease progression.[208,214]

A major caveat in the interpretation of these therapeutic vaccine studies is that they used early-generation vaccine candidates with variable immunogenicity. Whether therapeutic vaccination with more immunogenic vaccines can provide meaningful benefits to HIV-1–infected individuals remains to be tested. In any case, it is likely that enhancing immune control of HIV-1 in most individuals treated during chronic infection with impaired immune function may prove far more difficult than augmenting immune control in the small numbers of individuals treated early during acute infection. Nevertheless, therapeutic vaccine studies using the current generation of vaccines are in progress in both acutely and chronically treated patients.

SUMMARY

A large body of information has been generated concerning the immune responses to HIV-1 infection and to administration of candidate HIV-1 vaccines in phase I, II, and III studies in humans. Multiple vaccine approaches have been undertaken, the most extensive of which have used recombinant envelope proteins (rgp120s) and poxvirus vector constructs. Overall, the vaccines have been well tolerated and without serious toxicities. The rgp120s administered in multiple-dose regimens induce binding and neutralizing antibodies that are type specific. Neutralizing antibodies are active against laboratory-adapted viruses but not against primary isolates. Lymphocyte proliferative responses are seen, but rgp120s do not induce CD8⁺ CTLs. Two phase III studies of rgp120 vaccines developed by VaxGen failed to demonstrate efficacy in prevention of HIV-1 infection. Phase I and II studies have been undertaken of poxvirus vectors, which appear to induce CD8⁺ CTLs that can kill cells infected by virus from multiple clades. Vaccinia vectors appear to be most immunogenic, but concerns exist regarding their reactogenicity in immunosuppressed patients. Canarypox vectors were poorly immunogenic in the largest (phase II) study carried out. Pox vectors are poor inducers of humoral antibodies but could be boosted with rgp120 proteins, although these antibodies were still active only against laboratory-adapted strains. Adenovirus, MVA, and alphavirus vectors are in early stages of clinical study, and other novel vectors are at various stages of preclinical development. DNA vaccines are undergoing phase I trials. The ability of immunogens to generate broadly active neutralizing antibodies that are effective against primary isolates is a major unmet need in the field.

REFERENCES

1. Dolin R. HIV vaccines for prevention of infection and disease in humans: HIV/AIDS 2000. KH Mayer, Guest Editor. Infect Dis Clin North Am. 2000;14:1001-1016.
2. Elizaga ML, McElrath MJ. Progress in the development of a preventive HIV-1 vaccine. Clin Lab Med. 2002;22:963-980.
3. Girard MP, Mastro TD, Koff WC. Human immunodeficiency virus vaccines. In: Plotkin SA, Orenstein WAS, eds. Vaccines. 4th ed. Philadelphia: Elsevier; 2004:1219-1258.
4. Letvin NL, Barouch DH, Montefiori DC. Prospects for vaccine protection against HIV-1 infection and AIDS. Annu Rev Immunol. 2002;20:73-99.
5. Fowke KR, Nagelkerke NJ, Kimani J, et al. Resistance to HIV-1 infection among persistently seronegative prostitutes in Nairobi, Kenya. Lancet. 1996;348:1347-1351.
6. Rowland-Jones S, Sutton J, Ariyoshi K, et al. HIV-specific cytotoxic T cells in HIV-exposed but uninfected Gambian women. Nat Med. 1995;1:59-64.
7. Rowland-Jones SL, Nixon DF, Aldhous MC, et al. HIV-specific cytotoxic T-cell activity in an HIV-exposed but uninfected infant. Lancet. 1993;341:860-861.
8. Rosenberg ES, Billingsley JM, Caliendo AM, et al. Vigorous HIV-1-specific CD4⁺ T cell responses associated with control of viremia. Science. 1997;278:1447-1450.
9. Musey L, Hughes J, Schacker T, et al. Cytotoxic T-cell responses, viral load, and disease progression in early human immunodeficiency virus type 1 infection. N Engl J Med. 1997;337:1267-1274.
10. Ogg GS, Jin X, Bonhoeffer S, et al. Quantitation of HIV-1 specific cytotoxic T lymphocytes and plasma load of viral RNA. Science 1998;279:2103-2106.
11. Brodie SJ, Lewinsohn DA, Patterson BK, et al. In vivo migration and function of transferred HIV-1 specific cytotoxic T cells. Nat Med 1999;5:34-41.
12. Jin X, Bauer DE, Tuttleton SE, et al. Dramatic rise in plasma viremia after CD8⁺ T cell depletion in simian immunodeficiency virus-infected macaques. J Exp Med. 1999;189:991-998.
13. Schmitz JE, Kuroda MJ, Santra S, et al. Effect of humoral immune responses on controlling viremia during primary infection of rhesus monkeys with simian immunodeficiency virus. J Virol. 2003;77:2165-2173.
14. Berman PW, Gregory TJ, Riddle L, et al. Protection of chimpanzees from infection by HIV-1 after vaccination with recombinant glycoprotein gp120 but not gp160. Nature. 1990;345:622-625.
15. Bruck C, Thiriart C, Fabry L, et al. HIV-1 envelope-elicited neutralizing antibody titres correlate with protection and virus load in chimpanzees. Vaccine. 1994;12:1141-1148.
16. Emini EA, Schlief WA, Nunberg JH, et al. Prevention of HIV-1 infection in chimpanzees by gp120 V3 domain-specific monoclonal antibody. Nature. 1991;355:728-730.
17. Igarashi T, Brown C, Azadegan A, et al. Human immunodeficiency virus type 1 neutralizing antibodies accelerate clearance of cell-free virions from blood plasma. Nat Med. 1999;5:211-216.
18. Mascola JR, Lewis MG, Stiegler G, et al. Protection of macaques against pathogenic simian/human immunodeficiency virus 89.6PD by passive transfer of neutralizing antibodies. J Virol. 1999;73:4009-4018.
19. Mascola JR, Stiegler G, VanCott TC, et al. Protection of macaques against vaginal transmission of a pathogenic HIV-1/SIV chimeric virus by passive infusion of neutralizing antibodies. Nat Med. 2000;6:207-210.
20. Schmitz JE, Kuroda MJ, Santra S, et al. Effect of humoral immune responses on controlling viremia during primary infection of rhesus monkeys with simian immunodeficiency virus. J Virol. 2003;77:2165-2173.
21. Javaherian K, Langlois AJ, McDanal CB, et al. Principal neutralizing domain of the human immunodeficiency virus type 1 envelope protein. Proc Natl Acad Sci U S A. 1989;86:6768-6772.
22. Moore JP, Nara PL. The role of the V3 loop of gp120 in HIV infection. AIDS. 1991;5(Suppl 2):S21-S33.
23. Ho DD, McKeating JA, Li XL, et al. Conformational epitope on gp120 important in CD4 binding and human immunodeficiency virus type 1 neutralization identified by a human monoclonal antibody. J Virol. 1991;65:489-493.
24. Thali M, Furman C, Ho DD, et al. Discontinuous, conserved neutralization epitopes overlapping the CD4-binding region of human immunodeficiency virus type 1 gp120 envelope glycoprotein. J Virol. 1992;66:5635-5641.
25. McKeating JA, Shotton C, Cordell J, et al. Characterization of neutralizing monoclonal antibodies to linear and conformation-dependent epitopes within the first and second variable domains of human immunodeficiency virus type 1 gp120. J Virol. 1993;67:4932-4944.
26. Muster T, Steindl F, Purtscher M, et al. A conserved neutralizing epitope on gp41 of human immunodeficiency virus type 1. J Virol. 1993;67:6642-6647.
27. Papsidero LD, Sheu M, Ruscetti FW. Human immunodeficiency virus type 1 neutralizing monoclonal antibodies which react with p17 core protein characterization and epitope mapping. J Virol. 1989;63:267-272.
28. Sano K, Lee MH, Morales F, et al. Antibody that inhibits human immunodeficiency virus reverse transcriptase and association with inability to isolate virus. J Clin Microbiol. 1987;25:2415-2417.
29. Gorny MK, Williams C, Volsky B, et al. Human monoclonal antibodies specific for conformation-sensitive epitopes of V3 neutralize human immunodeficiency virus type 1 primary isolates from various clades. J Virol 2002;76:9035-9045.
30. Wyatt R, Sodroski J. The HIV-1 envelope glycoproteins: Fusogens, antigens, and immunogens. Science. 1998;280:1884-1888.
31. Clark SJ, Saag MS, Decker WD, et al. High titers of cytopathic virus in plasma of patients with symptomatic primary HIV-1 infection. N Engl J Med. 1991;324:954-960.
32. Arendrup M, Nielsen C, Hansen JE, et al. Autologous HIV-1 neutralizing antibodies: Emergence of neutralization-resistant escape virus and subsequent development of escape virus neutralizing antibodies. J Acquir Immune Defic Syndr. 1992;5:303-307.
33. Richman DD, Wrin TL, Little SJ, Petropoulos CJ. Rapid evolution of the neutralizing antibody response to human immunodeficiency virus (HIV) type 1 infection. Proc Nat Acad Sci U S A. 2003;100:4144-4149.
34. Wei X, Decker JM, Wang S, et al. Antibody neutralization and escape by HIV-1. Nature. 2003;422:307-312.
35. Montefiori DC, Pantaleo G, Fink LM, et al. Neutralizing and infection-enhancing antibody responses to human immunodeficiency virus type 1 in long term nonprogressors. J Infect Dis. 1996;173:60-67.
36. Baum LL, Cassutt KJ, Knigge K, et al. HIV-1 gp120-specific antibody-dependent cell mediated cytotoxicity correlates with rate of disease progression. J Immunol. 1996;157:2168-2173.
37. Tyler DS, Stanley SD, Zolla-Pazner SB, et al. Identifications of sites within gp41 that serve as targets for antibody-dependent cellular cytotoxicity by using human monoclonal antibodies. J Immunol. 1990;145:3276-3282.

38. Binley JM, Sanders RW, Clas B, et al. A recombinant human immunodeficiency virus type 1 envelope glycoprotein complex stabilized by an intramolecular disulfide bond between the gp120 and gp41 subunits is an antigenic mimic of the trimeric virion-associated structure. J Virol. 2000;74:627-643.
39. Yang X, Florin L, Farzan M, et al. Modifications that stabilize human immunodeficiency virus envelope glycoprotein trimers in solution. J Virol. 2000;74: 4746-4654.
40. Chakrabarti BK, Kong WP, Wu BY, et al. Modifications of the human immunodeficiency virus envelope glycoprotein enhance immunogenicity for genetic immunization. J Virol. 2002;76:5357-5368.
41. Barnett SW, Lu S, Sravastava I, et al. The ability of an oligomeric human immunodeficiency virus type 1 (HIV-1) envelope antigen to elicit neutralizing antibodies against primary HIV-1 isolates is improved following partial deletion of the second hypervariable region. J Virol. 2001;75:5526-5540.
42. Fouts TR, Tuskan R, Godfrey K, et al. Expression and characterization of a single-chain polypeptide analogue of the human immunodeficiency virus type 1 gp120-CD4 receptor complex. J Virol. 2000;74:11427-11436.
43. Fouts T, Godfrey K, Bobb K, et al. Crosslinked HIV-1 envelope-CD4 receptor complexes elicit broadly cross-reactive neutralizing antibodies in rhesus macaques. Proc Natl Acad Sci U S A. 2002;99:11842-11847.
44. Plata F. Implications of HIV-specific cytotoxic T lymphocytes in AIDS. Biotherapy. 1992;5:31-45.
45. Takahashi H, Germain RN, Moses B, et al. An immunodominant class I-restricted cytotoxic T lymphocyte determinant of human immunodeficiency virus type 1 induces CD4 class II-restricted help for itself. J Exp Med. 1990;171:571-576.
46. Rosenberg ZF, Fauci AS. The immunopathogenesis of HIV infection. Adv Immunol. 1989;47:377-431.
47. Langlade-Demoyen P, Michel F, Hoffenbach A, et al. Immune recognition of AIDS virus antigens by human and murine cytotoxic T lymphocytes. J Immunol. 1988;141:1949-1957.
48. Riviere Y, Tanneau-Salvadori F, Regnault A, et al. Human immunodeficiency virus-specific cytotoxic responses of seropositive individuals: Distinct types of effector cells mediate killing of targets expressing gag and env proteins. J Virol. 1989;63:2270-2277.
49. Walker BD, Flexner C, Paradis TJ, et al. HIV-1 reverse transcriptase is a target for cytotoxic T lymphocytes in infected individuals. Science. 1988;240:64-66.
50. Chenciner N, Michel F, Dadaglio G, et al. Multiple subsets of HIV-specific cytotoxic T lymphocytes in humans and mice. Eur J Immunol. 1989;19:1537-1544.
51. Walker BD, Flexner C, Birch-Limberger K, et al. Long-term culture and fine specificity of human cytotoxic T-lymphocyte clones reactive with human immunodeficiency virus type 1. Proc Natl Acad Sci U S A. 1989;86:9514-9518.
52. Cooney EL, McElrath MJ, Corey L, et al. Enhanced immunity to human immunodeficiency virus (HIV) envelope elicited by a combined vaccine regimen consisting of priming with vaccinia recombinant expressing HIV envelope and boosting with gp160 protein. Proc Natl Acad Sci U S A. 1993;90:1882-1886.
53. Hammond SA, Bollinger RC, Stanhope PE, et al. Comparative clonal analysis of human immunodeficiency virus type 1 (HIV-1)-specific $CD4^+$ and $CD8^+$ cytolytic T lymphocytes isolated from seronegative humans immunized with candidate HIV-1 vaccines. J Exp Med. 1992;176:1531-1542.
54. El-Daher N, Keefer MC, Reichman RC, et al. Persisting human immunodeficiency virus type 1 gp160-specific human T lymphocyte responses including $CD8^+$ cytotoxic activity after receipt of envelope vaccines. J Infect Dis. 1993;168:306-313.
55. Graham BS, Keefer MC, McElrath MJ, et al. Safety and immunogenicity of a candidate HIV-1 vaccine in healthy adults: Recombinant glycoprotein (rgp)120, a randomized, double-blind trial. Ann Intern Med. 1996;125:270-279.
56. Ferrari G, Humphrey W, McElrath MJ, et al. Clade B-based HIV-1 vaccines elicit cross-clade cytotoxic T lymphocyte reactivities in uninfected volunteers. Proc Natl Acad Sci U S A. 1997;94:1396-1401.
57. Cao H, Kanki P, Sankale JL, et al. Cytotoxic T-lymphocyte cross-reactivity among different human immunodeficiency virus type 1 clades: Implications for vaccine development. J Virol 1997;71:8615-8623.
58. Bertoletti A, Cham F, McAdam S, et al. Cytotoxic T cells from human immunodeficiency virus type 2-infected patients frequently crossreact with different human immunodeficiency virus type 1 clades. J Virol. 1998;72:2439-2448.
59. Robinson WE Jr, Montefiori DC, Mitchell WM. Antibody-dependent enhancement of human immunodeficiency virus type 1 infection. Lancet. 1988;1:790-794.
60. Takeda A, Tuazon CU, Ennis FA. Antibody-enhanced infection by HIV-1 via Fc receptor-mediated entry. Science. 1988;242:580-583.
61. Montefiori DC, Lefkowitz LB Jr, Keller RE, et al. Absence of a clinical correlation for complement mediated, infection-enhancing antibodies in plasma or sera from HIV-1 infected individuals. AIDS. 1991;5:413-417.
62. Dolin R, Graham B, Greenberg S, et al. and the AIDS vaccine Clinical Trials Network. Safety and immunogenicity of an HIV-1 recombinant gp160 candidate vaccine in humans. Ann Intern Med. 1991;114:119-127.
63. Robinson WE Jr, Gorny MK, Xu JY, et al. Two immunodominant domains of gp41 bind antibodies which enhance human immunodeficiency virus type 1 infection in vitro. J Virol. 1991;65:4169-4176.
64. Jiang SB, Lin K, Neurath AR. Enhancement of human immunodeficiency virus type 1 infection by antisera to peptides from the envelope glycoproteins gp120/gp41. J Exp Med. 1991;174:1557-1563.
65. Takeda A, Robinson JE, Ho DD, et al. Distinction of human immunodeficiency virus type 1 neutralization and infection enhancement by human monoclonal antibodies to glycoprotein 120. J Clin Invest. 1992;89:1952-1957.
66. Reiher WE, Blalock JE, Brunck TK. Sequence homology between acquired immunodeficiency syndrome virus envelope protein and interleukin-2. Proc Natl Acad Sci U S A. 1986;83:9188-9192.
67. Lee MR, Ho DD, Gurney ME. Functional interaction and partial homology between human immunodeficiency virus and neuroleukin. Science. 1987;237:1047-1051.
68. Pugliese O, Viora M, Camponeschi B, et al. A gp120 HIV peptide with high similarity to HLA class II beta chains enhances PPD-specific and autoreactive T cell activation. Clin Exp Immunol. 1992;90:170-174.
69. Golding H, Robey FA, Gates FT, et al. Identification of homologous regions in human immunodeficiency virus 1 gp41 and human MHC class II beta I domain. J Exp Med. 1988;167:914-923.
70. Sarin PS, Sun DK, Thornton AH, et al. Neutralization of HTLV-III/LAV replication by antiserum to thymosin α-1. Science. 1986;232:1135-1137.
71. Keefer MC, Graham BS, Belshe RB, et al. Studies of high doses of a human immunodeficiency virus type 1 recombinant glycoprotein 160 candidate vaccine in HIV-1 seronegative humans. AIDS Res Hum Retroviruses. 1994;10:1713-1723.
72. Kovacs JA, Vasudevachari MB, Easter M, et al. Induction of humoral and cell-mediated anti-human immunodeficiency virus (HIV) responses in HIV sero-negative volunteers by immunization with recombinant gp160. J Clin Invest. 1993;92:919-928.
73. Gorse GJ, McElrath MJ, Matthews TJ, et al. Modulation of immunologic responses to HIV-1 recombinant gp160 vaccine by dose and schedule of administration. Vaccine. 1998;16:493-506.
74. Gorse GJ, Corey L, Patel GB, et al. HIV_{MN} recombinant glycoprotein 160 vaccine-induced cellular and humoral immunity boosted by HIV-1_{MN} recombinant glycoprotein 120 vaccine. AIDS Res Hum Retroviruses. 1999;2:115-132.
75. Belshe RB, Clements ML, Dolin R, et al. Safety and immunogenicity of a fully glycosylated recombinant gp160 human immunodeficiency virus type 1 vaccine in subjects at low risk of infection. J Infect Dis. 1993;168:1387-1395.
76. Gorse GJ, Schwartz DH, Graham BS, et al. HIV-1 recombinant gp160 vaccine given in accelerated dose schedules. Clin Exp Immunol. 1994;98:178-184.
77. Casimiro DR, Chen L, Fu TM, et al. Comparative immunogenicity in rhesus monkeys of DNA plasmid, recombinant vaccinia virus, and replication-defective adenovirus vectors expressing a human immunodeficiency virus type 1 gag gene. J Virol. 2003; 77:6305-6313.
78. Keefer MC, Graham BS, Belshe RB, et al. Studies of high doses of a human immunodeficiency virus type 1 recombinant glycoprotein 160 candidate vaccine in HIV-1 seronegative humans. AIDS Res Hum Retroviruses. 1994;10:1713-1723.
79. Schwartz DH, Gorse G, Clements ML, et al. Induction of HIV-1 neutralising and syncytium-inhibiting antibodies in uninfected recipients of HIV-IIIB rgp120 subunit vaccine. Lancet. 1993;342:69-73.
80. Belshe RB, Graham BS, Keefer MC, et al. Neutralizing antibodies to HIV-1 in seronegative volunteers immunized with recombinant gp120 from the MN strain of HIV-1. JAMA. 1994;272:475-480.
81. Kahn JO, Sinangil F, Baenziger J, et al. Clinical and immunologic responses to human immunodeficiency virus (HIV) type 1 SF2 gp120 subunit vaccine combined with MF59 adjuvant with or without muramyl tripeptide dipalmitoyl phosphatidylethanolamine in non-HIV-infected human volunteers. J Infect Dis. 1994;170:1288-1291.
82. Graham BS, Keefer MC, McElrath MJ, NIAID AIDS Vaccine Evaluation Group. Safety and immunogenicity of a candidate HIV-1 vaccine in healthy adults: Recombinant glycoprotein (rgp)120. A randomized, double-blind trial. Ann Intern Med. 1996;125:270-279.
83. Gorse GJ, Keefer MC, Belshe RB, et al. A dose-ranging study of a prototype synthetic HIV-1 V3 branched peptide vaccine. J Infect Dis. 1996;173:330-339.
84. Keefer ML, Lambert JS, Koff W, et al. A phase I study of a multivalent HIV-1 peptide vaccine in HIV-1 uninfected subjects. Abstract #403. Thirty-third Infectious Disease Society of America Annual Meeting, San Francisco, Calif, September 16-18, 1995.
85. Sarin PS, Mora CA, Naylor PH, et al. HIV-1 p17 synthetic peptide vaccine HGP-30: Induction of immune response in human subjects and preliminary evidence of protection against HIV challenge in SCID mice. Cell Mol Biol. 1995;41:401-407.
86. Kahn JO, Stites DP, Scillian J, et al. A phase I study of HGP-30, a 30 amino acid subunit of the human immunodeficiency virus (HIV) p17 synthetic peptide analogue subunit vaccine in seronegative subjects. AIDS Res Hum Retroviruses. 1992;8:1321-1325.
87. Naylor PH, Sztein MB, Wada S, et al. Preclinical and clinical studies on immunogenicity and safety of the HIV-1 p17 based synthetic peptide AIDS vaccine: HGP-30-KLH. Int J Immunopharmacol. 1991;13(Suppl 1):117-127.
88. Martin S, Weber J, Rott I, et al. Recombinant HIV-1 gag p24-Ty virus-like-particles (VLPs) induce HIV-1 p24 specific T helper cells in seronegative subjects vaccinated with these particles. Abstract POA2194. Presented at the Eighth International Conference on AIDS/III STD World Congress, Amsterdam, July 1992.
89. Cooney EL, Collier AC, Greenberg PD, et al. Safety and immunologic response to a recombinant vaccinia virus vaccine expressing HIV envelope glycoprotein. Lancet. 1991;337:567-572.
90. Graham BS, Belshe RB, Clements ML, et al. Vaccination of vaccinia-naive adults with human immunodeficiency virus type 1 gp160 recombinant vaccinia virus in a blinded, controlled randomized clinical trial. J Infect Dis. 1992; 166:244-252.
91. Keefer MC, McElrath MJ, Weinhold K, et al. A phase I trial of vaccinia-env/gag/pol (TBC-3B) given by alternative routes, boosted with rgp120MN [AVEG 014C]. Poster presentation. Twelfth World AIDS Conference, Geneva, Switzerland, June 28-July 3, 1998.
92. Clements-Mann ML, Weinhold K, Matthews TJ, et al. Immune responses to human immunodeficiency virus (HIV) type 1 induced by canarypox expressing HIV-1_{MN} gp120, HIV-1_{SF-2} recombinant gp120, or both vaccines in seronegative adults. J Infect Dis. 1998;177:1230-1246.
93. Pialoux G, Excler JL, Riviere Y, et al. A prime-boost approach to HIV preventive vaccine using a recombinant canarypox virus expressing glycoprotein 160 (MN/LAI). AIDS Res Hum Retroviruses. 1995;11:373-381.

94. Fleury B, Janvier G, Pialoux G, et al. Memory cytotoxic T lymphocyte responses in human immunodeficiency virus type I (HIV-1)-negative volunteers immunized with a recombinant canarypox expressing gp160 of HIV-1 and boosted with a recombinant gp160. J Infect Dis. 1996;174:734-738.

95. Belshe RB, Gorse GJ, Mulligan MJ, et al. Induction of immune responses to HIV-1 by canarypox (ALVAC) HIV-1 and gp120 SF-2 recombinant vaccines in uninfected volunteers. AIDS. 1998;12:2407-2415.

96. Corey L, Weinhold K, McElrath J, et al. Safety and immunogenicity of live recombinant canarypox vector containing the envelope, gag and protease genes of HIV-1 in seronegative adult volunteers. Oral Abstract [Mo.A.282]. Presented at the Eleventh International Conference on AIDS, Vancouver, Canada, July 7-12, 1996.

97. Evans TG, Keefer MC, Weinhold KJ, et al. A canarypox vaccine expressing multiple human immunodeficiency virus type 1 genes given alone or with rgp120 elicits broad and durable CD8+ cytotoxic T lymphocyte responses in seronegative volunteers. J Infect Dis. 1999;180:290-298.

98. Graham BS, Gorse GJ, Schwartz DH, et al. Determinants of antibody response after recombinant gp160 boosting in vaccinia-naive volunteers primed with gp160-recombinant vaccinia virus. J Infect Dis. 1994;170:782-786.

99. Graham BS, Matthews TJ, Belshe RB, et al. Augmentation of human immunodeficiency virus type 1 neutralizing antibody by priming with gp160 in vaccinia and boosting with rgp160 in vaccinia naïve adults. J Infect Dis. 1993;167:533-537.

100. Corey L, McElrath MJ, Weinhold K, et al. (AIDS Vaccine Evaluation Group). Cytotoxic T cell and neutralizing antibody responses to human immunodeficiency virus type 1 envelope with a combination vaccine regimen. J Infect Dis. 1998;177:301-309.

101. HIV Vaccine Trial Network, Protocol HVTN 203, results submitted 2004.

102. Boyer JD, Cohen AD, Vogt S, et al. Vaccination of seronegative volunteers with a human immunodeficiency virus type 1 env/rev DNA vaccine induces antigen specific proliferation and lymphocyte production of B chemokines. J Infect Dis. 2000;181:476-483.

103. Mulligan M, Goepfert P, Corey L, et al. AVEG 031: Phase 1 evaluation of a *gag-pol* facilitated DNA vaccine for HIV-1 prevention. Poster presentation. Twelfth World AIDS Conference, Geneva, Switzerland, June 28-July 3, 1998.

104. Emini E. A potential HIV vaccine using a replication defective adenoviral vaccine vector. Presented at the Ninth Conference on Retroviruses and Opportunistic Infections, session 12. Seattle, Wash, February 24-28, 2002.

105. Arthur LO, Bess JW Jr, Chertova EN, et al. Chemical inactivation of retroviral infectivity by targeting nucleocapsid protein zinc fingers: A candidate SIV vaccine. AIDS Res Hum Retrovirus. 1998;14(Suppl 3):S311-S319.

106. Lin L, Cook DN, Wiesehahn GP, et al. Photochemical inactivation of viruses and bacteria in platelet concentrates by use of a novel psoralen and long-wavelength ultraviolet light. Transfusion. 1997;37:423-435.

107. Cochran MA, Ericson BL, Knell JD, et al. Use of baculovirus recombinants as general method for the production of subunit vaccines. In: Ginsberg H, Brown F, Lerner RA, et al, eds. Vaccines 87. Cold Springs Harbor, NY: Cold Springs Harbor Press; 1987:384-388.

108. Steimer KS, van Nest G, Dina D, et al. Genetically engineered human immunodeficiency virus envelope glycoprotein gp 120 produced in yeast is the target of neutralizing antibodies. In: Ginsberg H, Brown F, Lerner RA, et al, eds. Vaccines 87. Cold Springs Harbor, NY: Cold Springs Harbor Press; 1987;236-241.

109. Haigwood NL, Nara PL, Brooks E, et al. Native but not denatured recombinant human immunodeficiency virus type 1 gp120 generates broad-spectrum neutralizing antibodies in baboons. J Virol. 1992;66:172-182.

110. Lasky LA, Groopman JE, Fennie CW, et al. Neutralization of the AIDS retrovirus by antibodies to a recombinant envelope glycoprotein. Science. 1986;233:209-212.

111. Barrett N, Mitterer A, Mundt W, et al. Large scale production and purification of a vaccinia derived HIV-1 gp160 and analysis of its immunogenicity. AIDS Res Hum Retroviruses. 1989;25:159-171.

112. Wintsch J, Chaignat CL, Braun DG, et al. Safety and immunogenicity of a genetically engineered human immunodeficiency virus vaccine. J Infect Dis. 1991;163:219-225.

113. Defoort NP, Nardelli B, Huang W, et al. Macromolecular assemblage in the design of a synthetic AIDS vaccine. Proc Natl Acad Sci U S A. 1992;89:3879-3883.

114. Palker TJ, Matthews TJ, Langlois A, et al. Polyvalent human immunodeficiency virus synthetic immunogen comprised of envelope gp120 T helper cell sites and B cell neutralization epitopes. J Immunol. 1989;142:3612-3619.

115. Ahlers JD, Dunlop N, Pendleton CD, et al. Candidate HIV type 1 multideterminant cluster peptide-P18MN vaccine constructs elicit type 1 helper T cells, cytotoxic T cells, and neutralizing antibody, all using the same adjuvant immunization. AIDS Res Hum Retroviruses. 1996;12:259-272.

116. Deprez B, Sauzet JP, Boutillon C, et al. Comparative efficiency of simple lipopeptide constructs for in vivo induction of virus-specific CTL. Vaccine. 1996;5:375-382.

117. Naylor PH, Sztein MB, Wada S, et al. Preclinical and clinical studies on immunogenicity and safety of the HIV-1 p17 based synthetic peptide AIDS vaccine: HGP-30-KLH. Int J Immunopharmacol. 1991;13(Suppl):117-127.

118. Adams SE, Dawson KM, Gull K, et al. The expression of hybrid HIV: Ty virus-like particles in yeast. Nature. 1987;329:68-70.

119. Hu SL, Kosowski SG, Dalrymple JM. Expression of AIDS virus envelope in recombinant vaccinia viruses. Nature. 1986;320:537-540.

120. Tartaglia J, Cox WI, Taylor J, et al. Highly attenuated poxvirus vectors. AIDS Res Hum Retroviruses. 1992;8:1445-1447.

121. Tartaglia J, Perkus ME, Taylor J, et al. NYVAC: A highly attenuated strain of vaccinia virus. Virology. 1992;188:217-232.

122. Paoletti E. Applications of pox virus vectors to vaccination: An update. Proc Natl Acad Sci U S A. 1996;93:11349-11353.

123. Robinson HL, Montefiori DC, Johnson RP, et al. Neutralizing antibody-independent containment of immunodeficiency virus challenge by DNA priming and recombinant pox virus booster immunization. Nat Med. 1999;5:526-534.

124. Robinson HL. New hope for an AIDS vaccine. Nat Rev Immunol. 2002;2:239-250.

125. Shiver JW, Fu TM, Chen L, et al. Replication-incompetent adenoviral vaccine vector elicits effective anti-immunodeficiency-virus immunity. Nature 2002;415: 331-335.

126. Davis NL, Caley IJ, Brown KW, et al. Vaccination of macaques against pathogenic simian immunodeficiency virus with Venezuelan equine encephalitis virus replicon particles. J Virol. 2000;74:371-378.

127. Gardner JP, Frolov I, Perri S, et al. Infection of human dendritic cells by a Sindbis virus replicon vector is determined by a single amino acid substitution in the E2 glycoprotein. J Virol. 2000;74:11849-11857.

128. Morris-Downes MM, Phenix KV, Smyth J, et al. Semliki Forest virus based vaccines: Persistence, distribution, and pathological analyses in two animal systems. Vaccine. 2001;19:1978-1988.

129. Liu XL, Clark KR, Johnson PR. Production of recombinant adeno-associated virus vectors using a packaging cell line and a hybrid recombinant adenovirus. Gene Ther. 1999;6:293-299.

130. Rose NF, Roberts A, Buonocore L, Rose JK. Glycoprotein exchange vectors based on vesicular stomatitis virus allow effective boosting and generation of neutralizing antibodies to a primary isolate of human immunodeficiency virus type 1. J Virol. 2000;74:10903-10910.

131. Dedieu JF, Ronco J, van der Werf S, et al. Poliovirus chimaeras expressing sequences from the principal neutralization domain of human immunodeficiency virus type 1. J Virol. 1992;66:3161-3167.

132. Fouts TR, Tuskan RG, Chada S, et al. Construction and immunogenicity of *Salmonella typhimurium* vaccine vectors that express HIV-1 gp120. Vaccine. 1995; 13:1697-1705.

133. Aldovini A, Young RA. Humoral and cell-mediated immune responses to live recombinant BCG-HIV vaccines. Nature. 1991;351:479-482.

134. Klinman DM, Takeno M, Icheno M, et al. DNA vaccines: Safety and efficiency issues. Springer Semin Immunopathol. 1997;19:245-256.

135. Donnelly JJ, Ulmer JB, Shiver JW, Liu MA. DNA vaccines. Annu Rev Immunol. 1997;15:617-648.

136. Daniel MD, Kirchhoff F, Czajak SC, et al. Protective effects of a live attenuated SIV vaccine with a deletion in the *nef* gene. Science. 1992;258:1938-1941.

137. Ruprecht RM, Baba TW, Liska V. Attenuated HIV vaccine: Caveats. Science. 1996;271:1790-1792.

138. Baba TW, Liska V, Khimani AH, et al. Live attenuated multiply deleted simian immunodeficiency virus causes AIDs in infants and adult macaques. Nat Med. 1999;5:194-203.

139. Whatmore AM, Cook N, Hall GA, et al. Repair and evolution of *nef* in vivo modulates simian immunodeficiency virus virulence. J Virol. 1995;69:5117-5123.

140. Villinger F, Brar SS, Brice GT, et al. Immune and hematopoietic parameters in HIV-1 infected chimpanzees during clinical progression toward AIDS. J Med Primatol. 1997;26:11-18.

141. Novembre FJ, Saucier M, Anderson DC, et al. Development of AIDS in a chimpanzee infected with human immunodeficiency virus type 1. J Virol. 1997;71:4086-4091.

142. Letvin NL, King NW. Immunologic and pathologic manifestations of the infection of rhesus monkeys with simian immunodeficiency virus of macaques. J Acquir Immune Defic Syndr. 1990;3:1023-1040.

143. Fultz PN, McClure HM, Anderson DC, et al. Identification and biologic characterization of an acutely lethal variant of simian immunodeficiency virus from sooty mangabeys (SIV/SMM). AIDS Res Hum Retroviruses. 1989;5:397-409.

144. Desrosiers RC. The simian immunodeficiency viruses. Annu Rev Immunol. 1990;8:557-578.

145. Kodama T, Wooley DP, Naidu YM, et al. The significance of premature stop codons in env of SIV. J Virol. 1989;63:4709-4714.

146. Pialoux G, Excler JL, Riviere Y, et al. A prime-boost approach to HIV preventive vaccine using a recombinant canarypox virus expressing glycoprotein 160 (MN/LAI). AIDS Res Hum Retroviruses. 1995;11:373-381.

147. Schmitz JE, Kuroda MJ, Santra S, et al. Control of viremia in simian immunodeficiency virus infection by CD8+ lymphocytes. Science. 1999;283:857-860.

148. Kuroda MJ, Schmitz JE, Barouch DH, et al. Analysis of Gag-specific cytotoxic T lymphocytes in simian immunodeficiency virus-infected rhesus monkeys by cell staining with a tetrameric major histocompatibility complex class I-peptide complex. J. Exp. Med. 1998;187:1373-1381.

149. Kuroda MJ, Schmitz JE, Charini WA, et al. Emergence of CTL coincides with clearance of virus during primary simian immunodeficiency virus infection in rhesus monkeys. J Immunol. 1999;162:5127-5133.

150. Letvin NL, Montefiori DC, Yasutomi Y, et al. Potent, protective anti-HIV immune responses generated by bimodal HIV envelope DNA plus protein vaccination. Proc Natl Acad Sci U S A. 1997;94:9378-9383.

151. Earl PL, Sugiura W, Montefiori DC, et al. Immunogenicity and protective efficacy of oligomeric human immunodeficiency virus type 1 gp140. J Virol. 2001;75:645-653.

152. Cho MW, Kim YB, Lee MK, et al. Polyvalent envelope glycoprotein vaccine elicits a broader neutralizing antibody response but is unable to provide sterilizing protection against heterologous simian/human immunodeficiency virus infection in pigtailed macaques. J Virol. 2001;75:2224-2234.

153. Murphey-Corb M, Martin LN, Davison-Fairburn B, et al. A formalin-inactivated whole SIV vaccine confers protection in macaques. Science. 1989;246:1293-1297.

154. Berman PW, Gregory TJ, Riddle L, et al. Protection of chimpanzees from infection by HIV-1 after vaccination with recombinant glycoprotein gp120 but not gp160. Nature. 1990;345:622-625.

155. Stott EJ. Anti-cell antibody in macaques. Nature. 1991;353:393.

156. Wolff JA, Malone RW, Williams P, et al. Direct gene transfer into mouse muscle *in vivo*. Science. 1990;247:1465-1468.

157. Tang DC, Devit M, Johnson SA. Genetic immunization is a simple method for eliciting an immune response. Nature. 1992;356:152-154.

158. Ulmer JB, Donnelly JJ, Parker SE, et al. Heterologous protection against influenza by injection of DNA encoding a viral protein. Science. 1993;259:1745-1749.

159. Donnelly JJ, Ulmer JB, Shiver JW, Liu MA. DNA vaccines. Annu Rev Immunol. 1997;15:617-648.

160. Egan MA, Charini WA, Kuroda MJ, et al. Simian immunodeficiency virus (SIV) *gag* DNA-vaccinated rhesus monkeys develop secondary cytotoxic T-lymphocyte responses and control viral replication after pathogenic SIV infection. J Virol. 2000;74:7485-7495.

161. Barouch DH, Santra S, Schmitz JE, et al. Control of viremia and prevention of clinical AIDS in rhesus monkeys by cytokine-augmented DNA vaccination. Science. 2000;290:486-492.

162. Shen L, Chen ZW, Miller MD, et al. Recombinant virus vaccine-induced SIV-specific CD8+ cytotoxic T lymphocytes. Science. 1991;252:440-443.

163. Hu S-L, Abrams K, Barber GN, et al. Protection of macaques against SIV infection by subunit vaccines of SIV envelope glycoprotein gp160. Science. 1992;255:456-459.

164. Seth A, Ourmanov I, Schmitz JE, et al. Immunization with a modified vaccinia virus expressing simian immunodeficiency virus (SIV) Gag-Pol primes for an anamnestic Gag-specific cytotoxic T-lymphocyte response and is associated with reduction of viremia after SIV challenge. J Virol. 2000;74:2502-2509.

165. Ourmanov I, Brown CR, Moss B, et al. Comparative efficacy of recombinant modified vaccinia virus Ankara expressing simian immunodeficiency virus (SIV) Gag-Pol and/or Env in macaques challenged with pathogenic SIV. J Virol. 2000;74:2740-2751.

166. Amara RR, Villinger F, Altman JD, et al. Control of a mucosal challenge and prevention of clinical AIDS in rhesus monkeys by a multiprotein DNA/MVA vaccine. Science. 2001;292:69-74.

167. Amara RR, Villinger F, Staprans SI, et al. Different patterns of immune responses but similar control of a simian-human immunodeficiency virus 89.6P mucosal challenge by modified vaccinia virus Ankara (MVA) and DNA/MVA vaccines. J Virol. 2002;76:7625-7631.

168. Barouch DH, Santra S, Kuroda MJ, et al. Reduction of simian-human immunodeficiency virus 89.6P viremia in rhesus monkeys by recombinant modified vaccinia virus Ankara vaccination. J Virol. 2001;75:5151-5158.

169. Mascola JR, Lewis MG, VanCott TC, et al. Cellular immunity elicited by human immunodeficiency virus type 1/simian immunodeficiency virus DNA vaccination does not augment the sterile protection afforded by passive infusion of neutralizing antibodies. J Virol. 2003;77:10348-10356.

170. Barouch DH, Kunstman J, Kuroda MJ, et al. Eventual AIDS vaccine failure in a rhesus monkey by viral escape from cytotoxic T lymphocytes. Nature. 2002;415:335-339.

171. Belshe RB, Stevens C, Gorse G, et al (NIAID AVEG, HIVNET Vaccine Development Groups). Safety and immunogenicity of a canarypox vectored HIV-1 vaccine with or without gp120 in higher and lower risk volunteers. J Infect Dis. 2001;183:1343-1352.

172. Keefer MC, Graham BS, McElrath MJ, NIAID AIDS Vaccine Evaluation Group. Safety and immunogenicity of ENV 2-3, a human immunodeficiency virus type 1 candidate vaccine, in combination with a novel adjuvant, MTP-PE/MF59. AIDS Res Hum Retroviruses. 1996;12:683-693.

173. Evan TG, McElrath MJ, Matthews T, et al. QS-21 promotes a dose-sparing adjuvant effect during HIV-1 subunit immunization. Vaccine. 2001;19:2080-2091.

174. Mascola JR, Snyder SW, Weislow OS, et al. Immunization with envelope subunit vaccine products elicits neutralizing antibodies against laboratory-adapted but not primary isolates of human immunodeficiency virus type-1. J Infect Dis. 1996;173:340-348.

175. Moore JP, Cao Y, Qing L, et al. Primary isolates of human immunodeficiency virus type 1 are relatively resistant to neutralization by monoclonal antibodies to gp120 and their neutralization is not predicted by studies with monomeric gp120. J Virol. 1995;69:101-109.

176. Burton DR. A vaccine for HIV type-1: The antibody perspective. Proc Natl Acad Sci U S A. 1997;94:10018-10023.

177. Keefer MC, Bonnez W, Roberts NJ Jr, et al. Human immunodeficiency virus (HIV-1) gp160-specific lymphocyte proliferative responses of mononuclear leukocytes from HIV-1 recombinant gp160 vaccine recipients. J Infect Dis. 1991;163:448-453.

178. Gorse GJ, Belshe RB, Newman FK, et al. Lymphocyte proliferative responses following immunization with human immunodeficiency virus recombinant gp160. Vaccine. 1992;10:383-388.

179. Orentas RJ, Hildreth JEK, Obah E, et al. Induction of CD4+ human cytolytic T cells specific for HIV-infected cells by a gp160 subunit vaccine. Science. 1990;248:1234-1237.

180. Li D, Forrest BD, Li Z, et al. International clinical trials of HIV vaccines: II. Phase I trial of an HIV-1 synthetic peptide vaccine evaluating an accelerated immunization schedule in Yunnan, China. Asian Pac J Allergy Immunol. 1997;15:105-113.

181. Kelleher AD, Emery S, Cunningham P, et al. Safety and immunogenicity of UBI HIV-1 (MN) octameric V3 peptide vaccine administered by subcutaneous injection. AIDS Res Hum Retroviruses. 1997;13:29-32.

182. Phanuphak P, Teeratakulpixarn S, Sarangbin S, et al. International clinical trials of HIV vaccines: I. Phase I trial of an HIV-1 synthetic peptide vaccine in Bangkok, Thailand. Asian Pac J Allergy Immunol. 1997;15:41-48.

183. Zagury D, Bernard J, Cheynier R, et al. A group specific anamnestic immune reaction against HIV-1 induced by a candidate vaccine against AIDS. Nature. 1988;332:728-731.

184. Stanhope PE, Clements ML, Siliciano RF. Human CD4+ cytolytic T lymphocyte responses to a human immunodeficiency virus type 1 gp160 subunit vaccine. J Infect Dis. 1993;168:92-100.

185. Hauke T, McMichael A. Design and construction of an experimental HIV-1 vaccine for a year 2000 clinical trial in Kenya. Nat Med. 2000;6:951-955.

186. Graham B, Tavel J, Koup R, et al. Phase I clinical studies of DNA vaccines for HIV. Abstract 50. Presented at AIDS Vaccine Conference 2003, New York, NY.

187. Graham BS, Matthews TJ, Belshe RB, et al. Augmentation of human immunodeficiency virus type 1 neutralizing antibody by priming with gp160 recombinant vaccinia and boosting with rgp160 in vaccinia naïve adults. J Infect Dis. 1993;167:533-537.

188. Goepfert P, Horton H, McElrath J, et al. Safety, tolerability and CD8+ T-cell immunogenicity of high dose liver recombinant canarypox AVAC-HIV vaccine (vCP1452) in healthy, HIV-1 uninfected adults. Abstract 82. Tenth Conference on Retroviruses and Opportunistic Infections, Boston, Mass, February 10-14, 2003.

189. VaxGen, Data presented, February 24, 2003.

190. VaxGen, Data presented, November 12, 2003.

191. Hel Z, Venzon D, Poudyal M, et al. Viremia control following antiretroviral treatment and therapeutic immunization during primary SIV251 infection of macaques. Nat Med. 2000;6:1140-1146.

192. Tryniszewska E, Nacsa J, Lewis MG, et al. Vaccination of macaques with long-standing SIVmac251 infection lowers the viral set point after cessation of antiretroviral therapy. J Immunol. 2002;169:5347-5357.

193. Lu W, Wu X, Lu Y, et al. Therapeutic dendritic-cell vaccine for simian AIDS. Nat. Med. 2003;9:27-32.

194. Rosenberg ES, Billingsley JM, Caliendo AM, et al. Vigorous HIV-1-specific CD4+ T cell responses associated with control of viremia. Science. 1997;278:1447-1450.

195. Oxenius A, Price DA, Easterbrook PJ, et al. Early highly active antiretroviral therapy for acute HIV-1 infection preserves immune function of CD8+ and CD4+ T lymphocytes. Proc Natl Acad Sci U S A. 2000;97:3382-3387.

196. Rosenberg ES, Altfeld M, Poon SH, et al. Immune control of HIV-1 after treatment of acute infection. Nature. 2000;407:523-526.

197. Lori F, Lewis MG, Xu J, et al. Control of SIV rebound through structured treatment interruptions during early infection. Science. 2000;290:1591-1593.

198. Ortiz GM, Nixon DF, Trkola A, et al. HIV-1-specific immune responses in subjects who temporarily contain virus replication after discontinuation of highly active antiretroviral therapy. J Clin Invest. 1999;104:677-678.

199. Oxenius A, Price DA, Gunthard HF, et al. Stimulation of HIV-specific cellular immunity by structured treatment interruption fails to enhance viral control in chronic HIV infection. Proc Natl Acad Sci U S A. 2002;99:13747-13752.

200. Ruiz L, Ribera E, Bonjoch A, et al. Role of structured treatment interruption before a 5-drug salvage antiretroviral regimen: The Retrogene Study. J Infect Dis. 2003;188:977-985.

201. Lawrence J, Mayers DL, Hullsiek KH, et al. Structured treatment interruption in patients with multidrug-resistant human immunodeficiency virus. N Engl J Med. 2003;349:837-846.

202. Salk J. Prospects for the control of AIDS by immunizing seropositive individuals. Nature. 1987;327:473-476.

203. Levine AM, Groshen S, Allen J, et al. Initial studies on active immunization of HIV-infected subjects using a gp120-depleted HIV-1 immunogen: Long-term follow-up. J Acquir Immune Defic Syndr Hum Retrovirol. 1996;114:351-364.

204. Redfield RR, Birx DL, Ketter N, et al. A phase I evaluation of the safety and immunogenicity of recombinant gp160 in patients with early human immunodeficiency virus infection. N Engl J Med. 1991;324:1677-1684.

205. Valentine FT, Kundu S, Haslett PAJ, et al. A randomized, placebo-controlled study of the immunogenicity of human immunodeficiency virus (HIV) rgp160 vaccine in HIV-infected subjects with ≥400/mm³ CD4 T lymphocyte (AIDS Clinical Trial Group Protocol 137). J Infect Dis. 1996;143:1336-1346.

206. Eron JJ, Ashby MA, Giordano MF, et al. Randomised trial of MN rgp120 HIV-1 vaccine in symptomless HIV-1 infection. Lancet. 1996;348:1547-1551.

207. Kahn JO, Cherng DW, Mayer K, et al. Evaluation of HIV-1 immunogen, an immunologic modifier, administered to patients infected with HIV having 300 to 549 × 10⁶/L CD4 cell counts: A randomized control trial. JAMA. 2000;284:2193-2202.

208. Sandstrom E, Wahren B. Therapeutic immunisation with recombinant gp160 in HIV-1 infection: A randomised double-blind placebo-controlled trial. Nordic VAC-04 Study Group. Lancet. 1999;353:1735-1742.

209. Blick G, Crook S, Buchanan S, et al. A phase I/II study of the toxicity, immunogenicity and efficacy of recombinant gp160 and p24 vaccines (Vax-Syn) in HIV-infected individuals regardless of CD4 ± cell count. Abstract TuB0562. Eighth International Conference on AIDS/III STD, World Congress, Amsterdam, July 1992.

210. MacGregor RR, Boyer JD, Ugen KE, et al. First human trial of a DNA-based vaccine for treatment of human immunodeficiency virus type 1 infection: Safety and host response. J Infect Dis. 1998;178:92-100.

211. Dhodapkar MV, Steinman RM, Sapp M, et al. Rapid generation of broad T-cell immunity in humans after a single injection of mature dendritic cells. J Clin Invest. 1999;104:173-180.

212. Schooley RT, Spino C, Chiu S, et al. Poor immunogenicity of HIV-1 envelope vaccines with alum or MF59 adjuvant in HIV infected individuals: Results of two randomized trials. Abstract 756. Presented at the Fourth Conference on Retroviruses and Opportunistic Infections, Washington, DC, January 22-26, 1997.

213. Kuritzkes DR, Spino C, Valentine F, et al. Associations of plasma HIV-1 RNA, CD4 count, and immune response in patients with 50-500 CD4 cells/μL. Abstract 757. Presented at the Fourth Conference on Retroviruses and Opportunistic Infections, Washington, DC, January 22-26, 1997.

214. Birx DL, Davis C, Ruiz N, et al. Results of a phase II double-blinded multicenter placebo controlled HIV therapeutic vaccine trial. Abstract Tu.A.275. Presented at the Eleventh International Conference on AIDS, Vancouver, Canada, 1996.

CHAPTER **127**

Chronic Fatigue Syndrome

N. CARY ENGLEBERG

TABLE 127-1 Proposed Infectious Causes of Chronic Fatigue Syndrome

Proposed Etiologic Agent	Suggestive Studies	Negative Studies
Epstein-Barr virus	6,7,118	12,14,15,38,119,120
Cytomegalovirus	121,122	12,38,119,120
Human herpesvirus 6	39,40,123,124	12,38,120,125,126
Human herpesvirus 7	—	40,120,123,126
Human herpesvirus 8	—	40,120,127
Enteroviruses	128-130	12,38,131-134
Parvovirus	35	120,135,136
Human spumavirus	137	—
Human retrovirus	138	139-141
Bornavirus	142	143
Borrelia burgdorferi	144	145,146
Brucella spp.	147	3
Mycoplasma spp.	148,149	150
Candida albicans	151,152	153

Chronic fatigue syndrome (CFS) refers to an illness that consists of profound, prolonged fatigue associated with other somatic or neuropsychological symptoms. The diagnosis is based on the patient's subjective report of a compatible symptom cluster and the absence of any medical or psychiatric condition that might account for the complaints. Attempts to ascribe CFS to a single, coherent cause have been fruitless. The available evidence favors the notion that the syndromal definition identifies a heterogeneous population of patients in whom fatigue, pain, cognitive complaints, and viral-like symptoms, such as low-grade fever, sore throat, and tender lymph nodes, are the final common pathophysiologic consequences of a variety of different causes.

Other names for this disorder include *myalgic encephalomyelitis* (in Great Britain and Canada) and *chronic fatigue and immune dysfunction syndrome* (in the United States). Most authorities in the United States prefer the name *chronic fatigue syndrome* because there is no convincing evidence that either inflammation of the central nervous system (CNS) or immune system dysfunction is responsible for the symptoms of the disorder. *Postviral fatigue* and *postinfectious fatigue* are less strictly defined designations for chronic idiopathic fatigue when it is perceived to be induced by an infectious disease and persists after resolution of the infection.

HISTORY

Although popular interest in CFS has been a relatively recent phenomenon, a historical perspective suggests that the illness is not new.[1] For several centuries, an illness resembling CFS has been described repeatedly in the medical literature by different names. The illness has been attributed variously to neurologic, cardiovascular, endocrine, and infectious causes. The proximate association of infections, especially influenza, with chronic fatigue (i.e., neurasthenia) was appreciated in the late 19th century.[2] In the 1950s, Spink[3] found that nearly 20% of patients with serologic evidence of brucellosis developed lingering symptoms of fatigue, weakness, myalgic pain, mental confusion, and depression in the absence of evidence for continued, active infection, whether or not they had received treatment. He hypothesized that the development of "chronic brucellosis" involved an infection and a psychological predisposition. Later studies by Imboden and co-workers[4] confirmed this impression by showing that patients with chronic brucellosis scored unfavorably on the Minnesota Multiphasic Personality Inventory relative to patients who had recovered from acute brucellosis. To test the hypothesis that a psychological propensity precedes the chronic fatigue illness, these authors conducted a retrospective cohort analysis of military personnel and dependents in Maryland after an outbreak of Asian influenza during the winter of 1957-1958.[5] All subjects had completed the Minnesota Multiphasic Personality Inventory in August 1957, just before the epidemic. Prolonged convalescence from influenza was correlated with preexisting, unfavorable scores on certain subscales of this test. The typical Minnesota Multiphasic Personality Inventory profile associated with prolonged postinfluenzal symptoms was nearly identical to that observed in patients with chronic brucellosis.[5]

In 1985, two large series of patients with prolonged fatigue and other symptoms were reported to have elevated antibody titers against Epstein-Barr virus (EBV) compared with healthy controls.[6,7] In the same year, a large outbreak of chronic fatigue with associated symptoms and serologic tests suggesting chronic EBV infection occurred in the area of Lake Tahoe, Nevada.[8] It was proposed that idiopathic chronic fatigue might be due to "chronic mononucleosis." This hypothesis was appealing because it had long been observed that persistent fatigue may follow documented acute mononucleosis in a small proportion of cases.[9-11] Several subsequent investigations failed to confirm a role for active EBV replication in the persistence of this clinical syndrome, however.[12-16] Numerous other infectious agents have been proposed as the cause of CFS, including *Candida albicans, Borrelia burgdorferi,* enteroviruses, cytomegalovirus, human herpesvirus 6, spumavirus, retroviruses, and *Bornavirus* (Table 127-1). The evidence that active infection with any of these agents causes a significant proportion of chronic fatigue cases is either inconclusive or refuted by subsequent investigations.

In addition to stimulating a search for alternate causes, the definition of a common clinical syndrome with no apparent cause led to a series of conferences sponsored by the National Institutes of Health and the Centers for Disease Control and Prevention (CDC) from 1985 to 1994. The purpose of these conferences was to arrive at a consensus definition of the clinical syndrome that could be applied uniformly by investigators studying the epidemiology, clinical features, etiology, and treatment of the disorder (Table 127-2).

TABLE 127-2 CDC/NIH Consensus Conference Definition of Chronic Fatigue Syndrome

Clinically evaluated, unexplained chronic fatigue for >6 mo duration, which is not lifelong or the result of ongoing exertion and is not alleviated substantially by rest. Fatigue is associated with a significant reduction in occupational, educational, social, or personal activities

Plus

≥ 4 of the following concurrent symptoms
  Impaired memory or concentration
  Sore throat
  Tender cervical or axillary lymph nodes
  Muscle pain
  Multijoint pain
  New headaches
  Unrefreshing sleep
  Postexertion malaise

CDC, Centers for Disease Control and Prevention; NIH, National Institutes of Health.

Adapted from Fukuda K, Straus SE, Hickie I, et al. The chronic fatigue syndrome: A comprehensive approach to its definition and study. International Chronic Fatigue Syndrome Study Group. Ann Intern Med. 1994;121:953-959.

EPIDEMIOLOGY

Fatigue is one of the most common complaints encountered in general medical practice. In most patients, the complaint eventually is attributed to a diagnosable medical condition or is short-lived. According to the most recent consensus conference definition, severe fatigue that remains unexplained after baseline physical and laboratory examinations and persists for more than 6 months is designated as *idiopathic chronic fatigue*. Patients with idiopathic chronic fatigue who also complain of four or more of the associated symptoms listed in Table 127-2 may be considered to have CFS.[17]

Because the case definition requires a medical evaluation, it can be applied only to study the prevalence of CFS in populations who seek medical attention. In a general medical practice in Boston, idiopathic chronic fatigue was reported by 8.5% of patients, but only 0.3% could be diagnosed with CFS.[18] The CDC ascertained the national prevalence of CFS by conducting case finding through a network of physicians in four cities. The prevalence, age, and sex distribution were remarkably similar in the four cities. The prevalence ranged from 3 to 11 per 100,000 population. Patients were predominantly women (7:1) and clustered in the 30 to 50 year age group.[19] Similar estimates of prevalence were reported from studies in Australia and the United Kingdom.[20,21] The characteristic predominance of upper middle class white women in their 30s and 40s resulted in the pejorative term "yuppie flu." These and other observations are biased, however, by reliance on clinic-based case ascertainment. When a random telephone survey was conducted in the San Francisco area, a different epidemiologic pattern emerged.[22] The overall prevalence of subjects reporting a CFS-like illness was 0.2% of the population, and the female predominance was less dramatic (2.9:1). The age distribution was the same as that seen in clinic-based studies, but the distribution of cases by income showed higher rates in persons with family incomes less than $40,000, suggesting that the perception of "yuppie flu" is an artifact of health care use by the affected populations. The rates of CFS-like illness were higher in African Americans and Hispanics than in whites and Asian Americans, and there was no preponderance of cases in any individual occupational group. Similar findings have been reported in other community-based studies.[23,24]

Outbreaks of idiopathic illness consistent with CFS have been reported occasionally since the 1940s.[25] In many of these outbreaks, the involvement of an infectious agent is unlikely because certain subgroups of the population at risk were affected disproportionately. Large hospital outbreaks in Los Angeles and London affected the professional staff, but not the hospitalized patients or nonprofessional staff.[26,27] An acute outbreak of neuromyasthenia in New Zealand resulted in CFS in many of the affected individuals. A 10-year follow-up of these cases indicated that most patients had recovered partially or completely.[28]

ETIOLOGY AND PATHOGENESIS

Attempts to elucidate the pathophysiology of CFS have been hampered by several methodologic problems. Foremost among these is the problem of selecting a homogeneous group of subjects for study from among patients identified by the working definition. In a symptom cluster analysis of patients meeting the CDC criteria, at least two distinct subgroups emerged—one having numerous syndromal and nonsyndromal symptoms with high severity scores and a second, larger group with limited symptoms and only moderate severity.[29] Similarly, some patients have an acute onset that sometimes is associated with an infectious disease or other definable stressor, whereas others describe an insidious and progressive onset. Most patients have past or current psychiatric disorders,[30-32] whereas some have no past or present psychiatric symptoms. There is no reason to assume a priori that patients with these diverse clinical circumstances have the same disorders simply because they meet the CDC criteria at the time of presentation.

Infectious causes of CFS have been proposed (see Table 127-1), but there is no reproducible evidence that any single agent is responsible for any significant proportion of these illnesses. A relatively small proportion of all CFS cases immediately follow a diagnosed infection (e.g., EBV infection, influenza, brucellosis), including some that are highly localized geographically (e.g., Lyme disease, Q fever, Ross River virus infection).[5,33-35] The occurrence of clinically indistinguishable "postinfectious" fatigue states after several unrelated infections supports the concept that CFS may be a nonspecific sequela to a variety of illnesses rather than a disease with a specific infectious cause. Controversy persists about whether chronic fatigue can be triggered by any infectious or traumatic event or whether only a particular type of infection or trauma is necessary. In either case, postinfectious and idiopathic cases have indistinguishable clinical and psychosocial features.[36] Patients seen in general practice for common infections do not have an increased frequency of prolonged fatigue relative to patients seen for other medical problems.[37]

Because some cases of chronic fatigue have an onset immediately after a specific infectious disease, chronic persistent infection frequently has been invoked as one possible pathogenesis. Prolonged convalescence from infectious mononucleosis is a well-recognized phenomenon.[9-11] Although there was never any direct virologic evidence favoring chronic EBV infection as a cause of CFS, a significant body of negative research has accumulated to reject this hypothesis. These studies showed no significant differences in serologic titers,[12,38] shedding of virus in saliva,[16] blood lymphocyte-transforming activity,[15,16] or EBV-specific cytotoxic lymphocytes[15] between patients and healthy controls. In addition, a large treatment study compared intravenous and oral acyclovir with placebo in CFS patients and failed to show any benefit.[14] Similarly, negative microbiologic data have been collected for other specific infectious agents (see Table 127-1). The possibility that CFS patients may reactivate latent viruses more frequently than healthy individuals has been proposed,[39,40] but it is not clear how or whether viral reactivation affects the ongoing symptom complex.[41]

To investigate a possible genetic predisposition to chronic fatigue illnesses, family history and twin studies have been conducted. In one study, CFS patients reported higher rates of fatigue illness in family members than medical control patients.[42] Similarly, twin studies in Australia and Great Britain suggest that disabling fatigue of greater than 1 month's duration occurs more frequently in monozygotic than in dizygotic twins.[43,44] Applying the CDC criteria for CFS, a study in the United States showed a concordance of 38% in monozygotic twins versus 11% in dizygotic twins.[45] These findings support the existence of a familial and genetic predisposition for CFS and the emerging concept of CFS as a complex and multifactorial process with predisposing and perpetuating factors.

Some of the proposed inciting and perpetuating factors involve disruptions in various biologic systems (e.g., the immune system, skeletal muscle, heart, CNS). Although subtle alterations in some of these systems have been identified in patients, similar changes are observed in individuals without symptoms. Differences in various measures of immune function (e.g., cytokine levels, in vitro lymphocyte function, flow cytometry) have been observed by comparing CFS patients and healthy persons; however, many of the studies are inconsistent with one another or have not been reproduced. The most consistent immune alterations have included an increase in T lymphocytes expressing activation markers[46] (e.g., in the number of lymphocytes bearing the CD45RA differentiation marker).[47] These findings suggest mild activation of the cellular immune system, but the relevance of these alterations is unclear, given the inconsistent immunologic differences among monozygotic twin pairs that are discordant for CFS.[48] It is not clear that a change in lymphocyte subsets occurs in conjunction with clinical improvement.[49]

Another immunologic finding more common in CFS patients than in healthy controls is a reduction in natural killer cell function and in number of lymphocytes bearing the CD16 marker.[50,51] This finding raised the concern that malignancies might occur at an increased rate in CFS. Analysis of cancer registries following the large 1985 Lake Tahoe outbreak did not support this notion, however.[52] The potential consequences of reduced natural killer cell function are unknown; however, this phenomenon is not specific, and experimental data suggest that similar reductions may follow a variety of other physical and emotional stresses. Although immunologic studies eventually may provide some insight into the pathophysiology of CFS, no significant functional deficiencies in any arm of the immune system have been identified.

More recent research has focused on possible dysregulation of an innate antiviral pathway as a common feature of CFS. In this system, interferons activate expression of the enzyme 2',5'-oligoadenylate synthetase. The 2',5'-adenylate oligonucleotides resulting from the activity of this enzyme bind to and activate RNase L, which degrades viral and other RNAs. CFS patients are purported to have increased levels of 2',5'-adenylate oligonucleotides and RNase L activity.[53,54] In addition, a low-molecular-weight RNase L molecule has been detected more frequently in CFS patients than in healthy controls (88% versus 32%).[55,56] The significance of alterations in this pathway remains to be determined.

Because idiopathic chronic fatigue usually includes neuropsychological symptoms and subtle alterations of hormones regulated at the hypothalamic level (see later), the hypothesis that the CNS is the principal site of the pathophysiology has gained support in recent years. Accumulating data from CNS imaging studies support this notion, but the significance of these findings still is unclear.[39,57-60] Investigators have observed regions of reduced cerebral blood flow in CFS patients relative to healthy controls[60,61]; however, these findings were not confirmed in a study of single-photon emission computed tomography scanning in monozygotic twins discordant for CFS.[62]

In any multifactorial hypothesis of CFS pathogenesis, psychological and psychosocial factors play a determinant role. As in the earlier studies of brucellosis and influenza by Imboden and co-workers,[5] contemporary investigators have found that psychosocial factors also are important determinants of persistent symptoms 6 months after onset of infectious mononucleosis.[63] In a study of "viral illnesses" in general practice, psychiatric morbidity, belief in vulnerability to viruses, and attributional style at initial presentation were more important predictors of fatigue at 6 months than were "viral" symptoms during the initial infection.[64] Several studies have reported that a prior history of depression frequently is present in chronic fatigue states and may represent an important predisposing condition.[65-68] Psychiatric morbidity is a common accompaniment of CFS, along with the infectious, neurohormonal, and immune alterations mentioned earlier. It is unclear to what extent each of these factors contributes to the pathogenesis of the illness or is a direct consequence of it.

CLINICAL MANIFESTATIONS

CFS occasionally develops in the aftermath of an identifiable infectious disease, such as infectious mononucleosis or influenza. More often, however, an infectious triggering event is not confirmed. Flulike symptoms may persist or develop de novo after the acute onset. These symptoms include sore throat, low-grade fever, tender adenopathy, generalized myalgia, migratory arthralgia, and headache. In contrast, objective physical findings corresponding to these subjective complaints, such as pharyngitis, a temperature greater than 100.5° F, and palpable adenopathy, are rare after the resolution of the initial illness. The presence of significant objective muscle weakness or frank arthritis should suggest an alternative diagnosis.

Persistent, disabling fatigue is the cardinal symptom of CFS. Patients often report that they have a limited allotment of energy each day and cannot function when it is depleted. Consequently, exhausting fatigue that lasts hours to a few days may follow even modest exertion.

Fatigue often is accompanied by neurocognitive difficulties and disturbances of sleep. Patients may describe difficulty with concentration and memory, although actual deficits are not consistently demonstrable using neuropsychological testing. Either insomnia or excessive sleep may be reported. A thorough sleep history helps to determine

whether formal polysomnography is indicated to rule out a primary sleep disorder. Sleep disorders are common among patients who present with fatigue, even among patients who meet symptomatic criteria for CFS.[69-71] Any or all of the symptoms may occur persistently or occur with striking seasonality. Some cases of CFS have seasonal variation comparable to that seen with seasonal affective disorder.[72]

Most patients who meet symptom criteria for CFS also have a past or current history of a psychiatric disorder (e.g., depression or anxiety disorder).[30-32] The treating physician must determine whether a preexisting psychiatric disorder accounts for all of the patient's complaints. If so, CFS should not be diagnosed. In contrast, altered mood states that occur in the context of the CFS often are transient and reactive to the physical disability and discomfort.

LABORATORY FINDINGS

No laboratory tests are diagnostic for CFS. Laboratory evaluation requires testing only for the purpose of ruling out unrecognized medical conditions that account for the symptoms. The minimal evaluation consists of a complete blood count, serum chemistry profile, urinalysis, and thyroid function testing.[17] Additional tests may be indicated when the history or the quality of the patient's symptoms suggest specific alternate diseases (e.g., chronic infection, collagen vascular disease, neurologic disorder, or neoplasm). A low-titer antinuclear antibody test is found in 15% to 54% of patients with CFS.[73,74] Antibodies against DNA and extractable nuclear antigens typically are absent. Instead, antibodies directed against insoluble nuclear matrix proteins are responsible for the nuclear fluorescence.[74,75] The significance of these autoantibodies is unknown.

When groups of patients with CFS are compared with control groups, significant differences have been found in many laboratory or radiologic results (e.g., in hormone levels, CNS radiologic tests, measures of cellular immunity, autonomic function). These findings may provide some insight into the pathophysiology of chronic fatigue states, but they have no diagnostic value in individual patients. In all of these examples, there is significant overlap between the fatigued and normal groups, and the tests cannot be used as a reliable marker for the disorder in an individual.

Urinary free cortisol levels have been shown to be lower in patients with CFS than in age-matched and sex-matched healthy controls, although the means of both groups are within the defined normal range.[76,77] Exaggerated adrenal responsiveness to corticotropin infusions in these patients suggests that a subtle defect in hypothalamic-pituitary-adrenal (HPA)–axis activity may exist at the pituitary level or above.[78] Similarly reduced HPA-axis activity has been observed in fibromyalgia and in post-traumatic stress disorder, whereas the opposite is found in major depressive disorder (i.e., an increased HPA-axis activity driven from the hypothalamus).[79] In contrast, gonadotropin levels are not affected by either CFS or fibromyalgia.[80] These findings suggest the presence of a common pathophysiology in CFS and other stress-related disorders that is centered in the CNS. Cortisol levels are not sufficiently discriminatory to be of value in diagnosis, however. Levels should be obtained only when clinical findings indicate a need to rule out frank adrenal insufficiency.

Small areas of localized increased signal intensity have been reported more frequently in brain magnetic resonance imaging studies of CFS patients than in those of healthy controls.[39] Similarly, changes in the perfusion of certain areas of the brain are suggested by studies using single photon emission computed tomography,[58-60] although different research groups have reported different anatomic findings. The causes of these findings are unknown, and their relationship to symptoms is not clear. Because the findings are not specific for CFS, CNS imaging should be used only when it is medically indicated to rule out a structural abnormality.

Because immunologic tests (e.g., flow cytometry, cytokine levels, in vitro lymphocyte function) have no diagnostic or prognostic significance, they are of value only in the context of a research study and should not be ordered as part of the routine evaluation for idiopathic chronic fatigue. Laboratory evaluation of the 2′,5′-oligoadenylate synthetase pathway[54] is not sufficiently specific to be helpful in diagnosis.

MANAGEMENT

General Principles

CFS is defined as an idiopathic disorder (see Table 127-2). Specific medical or psychiatric therapy is rational only when an alternate or coexisting diagnosis is present. Antimicrobial therapy is not indicated unless there is clear evidence of a specific, active infection producing disease manifestations. Failed trials of antimicrobial therapy have been cited as evidence that conventional infectious agents are not a perpetuating factor in CFS.

Conservative therapy for idiopathic fatigue syndromes is appropriately nonspecific and should be focused on remediation of symptoms and physical rehabilitation instead of specific, presumed causes.[81] There is no general consensus about which nonspecific therapies are most appropriate, and the existing adequately controlled studies often have reported inconsistent results.[82,83] Because CFS is a heterogeneous disorder, the outcomes of treatment studies are influenced heavily by the method of selecting patients. Also, noncontrolled treatment observations are of minimal value in these disorders because most controlled trials have shown a robust placebo effect.

The treatment of individual patients is empirical. It is useful to objectify the symptoms as much as possible so that the response to any intervention can be assessed independently. Medications should be evaluated in an additive or sequential manner so that there can be no confusion about their efficacy or adverse effects. With the large range of symptoms with which these patients present, physicians are faced with a variety of treatments from which to choose, and patients may inquire about unconventional or alternative therapies. In the absence of evidence for efficacy, empirical treatment choices should be guided by a concern for safety and cost.

Pharmacologic Therapy

Medications may be useful for the treatment of symptoms, including non-narcotic pain relievers for myalgia, arthralgia, or headache; non-addictive sleep aids for sleep disruption; and psychoactive agents for depression or anxiety. Various vitamins and "nutritional supplements" have no proven, consistent benefit and may be costly.[84-88] Costly "immune-enhancing" therapies, such as intravenous immune globulin, immunostimulants, and cytokines, have failed to provide benefit in controlled studies.[89-94]

Carefully controlled treatment trials do not show a consistent benefit from any single pharmacologic agent. It has been useful to extrapolate from more conclusive studies of fibromyalgia patients because this idiopathic condition has significant overlap with CFS. Although the diagnosis of fibromyalgia is based on subjective pain and musculoskeletal tenderness, symptoms of profound fatigue, sleep disruption, and cognitive or emotional difficulties are common accompaniments. In addition, fibromyalgia and CFS share certain biologic features (e.g., autonomic and neuroendocrine findings). Tricyclic antidepressants and other drugs with serotoninergic activity are beneficial in fibromyalgia, and common experience suggests that chronic fatigue patients with pain and sleep disorder may respond in a similar fashion.[95,96] One large placebo-controlled trial of fluoxetine therapy for CFS failed to show benefit; however, this study was criticized because the treated subjects already had experienced disabling symptoms for many years.[97] A subsequent trial showed a favorable effect on symptoms associated with depression accompanying CFS.[98] Studies evaluating treatment with monoamine oxidase inhibitors have yielded conflicting results.[99-101] Newer antidepressants are safe and relatively inexpensive, however, and a large body of evidence suggests they may have favorable effects on symptoms of depression, pain, and insomnia in other groups of patients.

Researchers at the Johns Hopkins University reported that chronic fatigue patients had abnormal responses to a 45-minute tilt-table test protocol.[102] Virtually all of the patients had syncope or re-production of fatigue symptoms, whereas only about one third of healthy controls had an abnormal response. These investigators proposed that the persistent fatigue may be attributable to neurally mediated hypotension and treatable as such. They used combinations of fludrocortisone, atenolol, and sertraline with increased salt intake and reported a favorable durable response in 39% of patients. Two subsequent controlled trials failed to show any benefit using this approach to therapy.[103,104]

The finding of depressed HPA-axis activity as a feature of chronic fatigue illnesses motivated a study at the National Institutes of Health in which patients received either replacement hydrocortisone or placebo for 3 months. This study and a subsequent trial suggest that there was minor improvement in the hydrocortisone group during treatment.[105,106] There was also profound and sustained suppression of the HPA axis and loss of bone density, however, which prompted investigators to recommend against the use of steroids for treatment.[106,107]

Nonpharmacologic Therapy

All patients should be counseled regarding exercise and sleep hygiene. Exercise traditionally has been advocated in the treatment of fibromyalgia. Several studies of CFS patients have confirmed the widely held view that light aerobic exercise is beneficial.[98,108,109] In contrast, there is no evidence to support the prescription of bed rest. Continuous inactivity may reinforce illness behavior and lead to complicating myofascial pain syndromes. Because physical activity induces symptoms in many patients, exercise must be introduced gradually.

Many patients have significant disruptions in their sleep patterns that should be corrected gradually. Daytime napping should be limited or avoided altogether because this behavior may disrupt nighttime sleep further. Melatonin is a popular over-the-counter sleep remedy used by many patients; however, the rationale for this therapy is unclear, given that CFS patients have normal levels and timing of endogenous melatonin secretion.[110]

Although occasional patients report relief of symptoms with dietary alterations, there is no reliable experimental evidence to inform changes in diet. Highly restrictive diets that may impair general nutrition should be discouraged.

Discussions about the "reality" of CFS are decidedly unhelpful and often insulting to patients. Similarly, framing the illness in a manner that is inconsistent with the patient's perceptions (e.g., as "depression" in the absence of formal psychiatric criteria) is likely to evoke resistance and nonadherence. The best approach is the one that is most consistent with current understanding of CFS: to recognize and to validate the patient's symptoms as part of an idiopathic syndrome. In doing so, it is essential to educate the patient about the unexplained nature of the fatiguing illness and to correct any misinformation that the patient may have about its cause or treatment. This approach allows the physician to enlist the patient's support in pursuing the rational management agenda previously described. Along similar lines, several studies have shown the value of formal cognitive-behavioral therapy.[111-115] This approach involves a restructuring of the patient's beliefs concerning the causes of the illness and an objective assessment of the symptoms and disabilities. Individual counseling provided in general medical practice may serve the same functions and seems to be as effective as formal cognitive-behavioral therapy.[116,117] Classic insight-oriented psychotherapy rarely is indicated but may be helpful in patients who experience significant, ongoing emotional stress at home or work.

SUMMARY

Prolonged idiopathic fatigue states may arise spontaneously or during the convalescence from an infectious disease. When associated with other symptoms, the diagnostic criteria for CFS may be met, although the distinction between syndromal and nonsyndromal chronic fatigue may be artificial. There are no laboratory tests that confirm or exclude the diagnosis of CFS. Various infections have been proposed as occult causes of the syndrome, but none has been implicated in any significant proportion of the patients who meet the clinical definition. In contrast, most experimental evidence points to a reversible derangement of certain CNS functions, and treatment modalities such as exercise, cognitive-behavioral therapy, and medications that act in the CNS seem to provide the most benefit.

REFERENCES

1. Straus SE. History of chronic fatigue syndrome. Rev Infect Dis. 1991;13 (Suppl 1):S2-S7.
2. Wessely S. The history of chronic fatigue syndrome. In: Straus SE, ed. Chronic Fatigue Syndrome. New York: Marcel Dekker; 1994:3-44.
3. Spink WW. What is chronic brucellosis? Ann Intern Med. 1951;35:358-374.
4. Imboden JB, Canter A, Cluff LE, et al. Brucellosis: III. Psychological aspects of delayed convalescence. Arch Intern Med. 1959;103:406-414.
5. Imboden JB, Canter A, Cluff LE. Convalescence from influenza: A study of the psychological and clinical determinants. Arch Intern Med. 1961;108:393-399.
6. Jones J, Ray C, Minnich L, et al. Evidence for active Epstein-Barr virus infection in patients with persistent, unexplained illnesses: Elevated anti-early antigen antibodies. Ann Intern Med. 1985;102:1-7.
7. Straus SE, Tosato G, Armstrong G, et al. Persisting illness and fatigue in adults with evidence of Epstein-Barr virus infection. Ann Intern Med. 1985;102:7-16.
8. Holmes GP, Kaplan JE, Stewart JA, et al. A cluster of patients with a chronic mononucleosis-like syndrome. JAMA. 1987;257:2297-2302.
9. Isaacs R. Chronic infectious mononucleosis. Blood. 1948;3:858-861.
10. Thompson D, Godleski J, Herman S. Prognosis of post infectious mononucleosis. J Am Coll Health Assoc. 1969;17:453-457.
11. White P, Grover S, Kangro H, et al. The validity and reliability of the fatigue syndrome that follows glandular fever. Psychol Med. 1995;25:917-924.
12. Buchwald D, Ashley R, Pearlman T, et al. Viral serologies in patients with chronic fatigue and chronic fatigue syndrome. J Med Virol. 1996;50:25-30.
13. Mawle AC, Nisenbaum R, Dobbins JG, et al. Seroepidemiology of chronic fatigue syndrome: A case-control study. Clin Infect Dis. 1995;21:1386-1389.
14. Straus SE, Dale JK, Tobi M, et al. Acyclovir treatment of the chronic fatigue syndrome. N Engl J Med. 1988;319:1692-1698.
15. Swanink C, van der Meer J, Vercoulen J, et al. Epstein-Barr virus (EBV) and the chronic fatigue syndrome: Normal virus load in blood and normal immunologic reactivity in the EBV regression assay. Clin Infect Dis. 1995;20:1390-1392.
16. Sumaya C. Serologic and virologic epidemiology of Epstein-Barr virus: Relevance to chronic fatigue syndrome. Rev Infect Dis. 1991;13(Suppl 1):S19-S25.
17. Fukuda K, Straus SE, Hickie I, et al. The chronic fatigue syndrome: A comprehensive approach to its definition and study. International Chronic Fatigue Syndrome Study Group. Ann Intern Med. 1994;121:953-959.
18. Bates DW, Schmitt W, Buchwald D, et al. Prevalence of fatigue and chronic fatigue syndrome in a primary care practice. Arch Intern Med. 1993;153:2759-2765.
19. Gunn WJ, Connell DB, Randall B. Epidemiology of chronic fatigue syndrome: The Centers for Disease Control Study. Ciba Found Symp. 1993;173:83-93.
20. Price RK, North CS, Wessely S, et al. Estimating the prevalence of chronic fatigue syndrome and associated symptoms in the community. Public Health Rep. 1992; 107:514-522.
21. Lloyd A, Hickie I, Boughton C, et al. Prevalence of chronic fatigue syndrome in an Australian population. Med J Aust. 1990;153:522-528.
22. Steele L, Dobbins JG, Fukuda K, et al. The epidemiology of chronic fatigue in San Francisco. Am J Med. 1998;105(3A):83S-90S.
23. Jason LA, Richman JA, Rademaker AW, et al. A community-based study of chronic fatigue syndrome. Arch Intern Med. 1999;105:2129-2137.
24. Buchwald D, Umali P, Umali J, et al. Chronic fatigue and the chronic fatigue syndrome in a Pacific Northwest health care system. Ann Intern Med. 1995;123:81-88.
25. Briggs NC, Levine PH. A comparative review of systemic and neurological symptomatology in 12 outbreaks collectively described as chronic fatigue syndrome, epidemic neuromyasthenia, and myalgic encephalomyelitis. Clin Infect Dis. 1994;18(Suppl 1):S32-S42.
26. Crowley N, Nelson M, Stovin S. Epidemiological aspects of an outbreak of encephalomyelitis at the Royal Free Hospital. J Hyg. 1957;55:102-122.
27. Stevans G. The 1934 epidemic of poliomyelitis in Southern California. Am J Public Health. 1934;12:1213-1214.
28. Levine P, Snow P, Ranum B, et al. Epidemic neuromyasthenia and chronic fatigue syndrome in west Otago, New Zealand: A 10-year follow-up. Arch Intern Med. 1997;157:750-754.
29. Hickie I, Lloyd A, Hadzi Pavlovic D, et al. Can the chronic fatigue syndrome be defined by distinct clinical features? Psychol Med. 1995;25:925-935.
30. Manu P, Matthews DA, Lane TJ. The mental health of patients with a chief complaint of chronic fatigue: A prospective evaluation and follow-up. Arch Intern Med. 1988;148:2213-2217.
31. Pawlikowska T, Chalder T, Hirsch SR, et al. Population based study of fatigue and psychological distress. BMJ. 1994;308:763-766.
32. Kroenke K, Wood DR, Mangelsdorff AD, et al. Chronic fatigue in primary care: Prevalence, patient characteristics and outcome. JAMA. 1988;260:929-934.
33. Ayres JG, Smith EG, Flint N. Protracted fatigue and debility after Q fever (Letter). Lancet 1996;347:978-979.
34. Gaudino E, Coyle P, Krupp L. Post-Lyme syndrome and chronic fatigue syndrome: Neuropsychiatric similarities and differences. Arch Neurol. 1997;54:1372-1376.
35. Jacobson S, Daly J, Thorne G, et al. Chronic parvovirus B19 infection resulting in chronic fatigue syndrome: Case history and review. Clin Infect Dis. 1997;24: 1048-1051.
36. Buchwald D, Umali J, Pearlman T, et al. Postinfectious chronic fatigue: A distinct syndrome? Clin Infect Dis. 1996;23:385-387.
37. Wessely S, Chalder T, Hirsch S, et al. Postinfectious fatigue: Prospective cohort study in primary care. Lancet. 1995;345:1333-1338.
38. Mawle A, Nisenbaum R, Dobbins J, et al. Seroepidemiology of chronic fatigue syndrome: A case-control study. Clin Infect Dis. 1995;21:1386-1389.
39. Buchwald D, Cheney P, Peterson D, et al. A chronic illness characterized by fatigue, neurologic and immunologic disorders, and active human herpesvirus type 6 infection. Ann Intern Med. 1992;116:103-113.
40. Ablashi DV, Eastman HB, Owen CB, et al. Frequent HHV-6 reactivation in multiple sclerosis (MS) and chronic fatigue syndrome (CFS) patients. J Clin Virol. 2000;16:179-191.
41. Linde A, Andersson B, Svenson SB, et al. Serum levels of lymphokines and soluble cellular receptors in primary Epstein-Barr virus infection and in patients with chronic fatigue syndrome. J Infect Dis. 1992;165:994-1000.
42. Walsh CM, Zainal NZ, Middleton SJ, et al. A family history study of chronic fatigue syndrome. Psychiatr Genet. 2001;11:123-128.
43. Hickie IB, Bansal AS, Kirk KM, et al. A twin study of the etiology of prolonged fatigue and immune activation. Twin Res. 2001;4:94-102.
44. Farmer A, Scourfield J, Martin N, et al. Is disabling fatigue in childhood influenced by genes? Psychol Med. 1999;29:279-282.
45. Buchwald D, Herrell R, Ashton S, et al. A twin study of chronic fatigue. Psychosom Med. 2001;63:936-943.
46. Klimas NG, Salvato FR, Morgan R, et al. Immunologic abnormalities in chronic fatigue syndrome. J Clin Microbiol. 1990;28:1403-1410.
47. Straus SE, Fritz S, Dale JK, et al. Lymphocyte phenotype and function in the chronic fatigue syndrome. J Clin Immunol. 1993;13:30-40.
48. Sabath DE, Barcy S, Koelle DM, et al. Cellular immunity in monozygotic twins discordant for chronic fatigue syndrome. J Infect Dis. 2002;185:828-832.
49. Peakman M, Deale A, Field R, et al. Clinical improvement in chronic fatigue syndrome is not associated with lymphocyte subsets of function or activation. Clin Immunol Immunopathol. 1997;82:83-91.
50. Caliguri M, Murray C, Buchwald D, et al. Phenotypic and functional deficiency of natural killer cells in patients with chronic fatigue syndrome. J Immunol. 1987; 139:3303-3313.
51. Barker E, Fujimura SF, Fadem MB, et al. Immunologic abnormalities associated with chronic fatigue syndrome. Clin Infect Dis. 1994;18(Suppl 1):S136-S141.
52. Levine PH, Atherton M, Fears T, et al. An approach to studies of cancer subsequent to clusters of chronic fatigue syndrome: Use of data from the Nevada State Cancer Registry. Clin Infect Dis. 1994;18(Suppl 1):S49-S53.
53. Suhadolnik RJ, Reichenbach NL, Hitzges P, et al. Upregulation of the 2-5A synthetase/RNase L antiviral pathway associated with chronic fatigue syndrome. Clin Infect Dis. 1994;18(Suppl 1):S96-S104.
54. De Meirleir K, Suhadolnik RJ, Lebleu B, et al. Antiviral pathway activation in chronic fatigue syndrome and acute infection. Clin Infect Dis. 2002;34:1420-1422.
55. De Meirleir K, Bisbal C, Campine I, et al. A 37 kDa 2-5A binding protein as a potential biochemical marker for chronic fatigue syndrome. Am J Med. 2000;108:99.
56. Suhadolnik RJ, Peterson DL, O'Brien K, et al. Biochemical evidence for a novel low molecular weight 2-5A-dependent RNase L in chronic fatigue syndrome. J Interferon Cytokine Res. 1997;17:377-385.
57. Natelson BH, Cohen JM, Brassloff I, et al. A controlled study of brain magnetic resonance imaging in patients with the chronic fatigue syndrome. J Neurol Sci. 1993;120:213-217.
58. Fischler B, D'Haenen H, Cluydts R, et al. Comparison of 99m Tc HMPAO SPECT scan between chronic fatigue syndrome, major depression and healthy controls: An exploratory study of clinical correlates of regional cerebral blood flow. Neuropsychobiology. 1996;34:175-183.
59. Costa D, Tannock C, Brostoff J. Brainstem perfusion is impaired in chronic fatigue syndrome. QJM. 1995;88:767-773.
60. Schwartz RB, Komaroff AL, Garada BM, et al. SPECT imaging of the brain: Comparison of findings in patients with chronic fatigue syndrome, AIDS dementia complex, and major unipolar depression. AJR Am J Roentgenol. 1994;162:943-951.
61. Ichise M, Salit I, Abbey S, et al. Assessment of regional cerebral perfusion by 99Tcm-HMPAO SPECT in chronic fatigue syndrome. Nucl Med Commun. 1992;13: 767-772.
62. Lewis DH, Mayberg HS, Fischer ME, et al. Monozygotic twins discordant for chronic fatigue syndrome: Regional cerebral blood flow SPECT. Radiology. 2001;219: 766-773.
63. Katon W, Russo J, Ashley RL, et al. Infectious mononucleosis: Psychological symptoms during acute and subacute phases of illness. Gen Hosp Psychiatry. 1999;21: 21-29.
64. Cope H, David A, Pelosi A, et al. Predictors of chronic "postviral" fatigue. Lancet. 1994;344:862-868.
65. Manu P, Matthews DA, Lane TJ. Depression among patients with a chief complaint of chronic fatigue. J Affect Disord. 1989;17:165-172.
66. Katon WJ, Buchwald D, Simon G, et al. Psychiatric illness in patients with chronic fatigue and those with rheumatoid arthritis. J Gen Intern Med. 1991;6:277-285.
67. Wood GC, Bentall RP, Gopfert M, et al. A comparative assessment of patients with chronic fatigue syndrome and muscle diseases. Psychol Med. 1991;21:618-628.

68. Wessely S, Chalder T, Hirsch S, et al. Psychological symptoms, somatic symptoms, and psychiatric disorder in chronic fatigue and chronic fatigue syndrome: A prospective study in the primary care setting. Am J Psychiatry. 1996;153:1050-1059.

69. Whelton CL, Salit I, Moldofsky H. Sleep, Epstein-Barr virus infection, musculoskeletal pain, and depressive symptoms in chronic fatigue syndrome. J Rheumatol. 1992;19:939-943.

70. Morriss R, Sharpe M, Sharpley A, et al. Abnormalities of sleep in patients with the chronic fatigue syndrome. BMJ. 1993;306:1161-1164.

71. Buchwald D, Pascualy R, Bombardier C, et al. Sleep disorders in patients with chronic fatigue. Clin Infect Dis. 1994;18(Suppl. 1):S68-S72.

72. Zubieta J, Engleberg N, Yargic L, et al. Seasonal symptom variation in patients with chronic fatigue: Comparison with major mood disorders. J Psychiatr Res. 1994; 28:13-22.

73. Bates D, Buchwald D, Lee J, et al. Clinical laboratory test findings in patients with chronic fatigue syndrome. Arch Intern Med. 1995;155:97-103.

74. Konstantinov K, von Mikecz A, Buchwald D, et al. Autoantibodies to nuclear envelope antigens in chronic fatigue syndrome. J Clin Invest. 1996;98:1888-1896.

75. von Mikecz A, Konstantinov K, Buchwald D, et al. High frequency of autoantibodies to insoluble cellular antigens in patients with chronic fatigue syndrome. Arthritis Rheum. 1997;40:295-305.

76. Demitrack M. Neuroendocrine correlates of chronic fatigue syndrome: A brief review. J Psychiatr Res. 1997;31:69-82.

77. Scott LV, Dinan TG. Urinary free cortisol excretion in chronic fatigue syndrome, major depression and in healthy volunteers. J Affect Disord. 1998;47:49-54.

78. Scott LV, Medbak S, Dinan TG. The low dose ACTH test in chronic fatigue syndrome and in health. Clin Endocrinol. 1998;48:733-737.

79. Crofford L, Engleberg NC, Demitrack MA. Neurohormonal perturbations in fibromyalgia. In: Chikanza IC, ed. Bailliere's Clinical Rheumatology. Philadelphia: Bailliere Tindall; 1996:365-378.

80. Korszun A, Young EA, Engleberg NC, et al. Follicular phase hypothalamic-pituitary-gonadal axis function in women with fibromyalgia and chronic fatigue syndrome. J Rheumatol. 2000;27:1526-1530.

81. Engleberg NC. Medically-oriented therapy for chronic fatigue syndrome and related conditions. In: Demitrack MA, Abbey SE, eds. Chronic Fatigue Syndrome: An Integrative Approach to Evaluation and Treatment. New York: Guilford; 1996: 287-307.

82. Whiting P, Bagnall AM, Sowden AJ, et al. Interventions for the treatment and management of chronic fatigue syndrome: A systematic review. JAMA. 2001;286: 1360-1368.

83. Afari N, Buchwald D. Chronic fatigue syndrome: A review. Am J Psychiatry. 2003;160:221-236.

84. Martin RWY, Ogston SA, Evans JR. Effects of vitamin and mineral supplementation on symptoms associated with chronic fatigue syndrome with coxsackie B antibodies. J Nutr Med. 1994;4:11-23.

85. Kaslow JE, Rucker L, Onishi R. Liver extract-folic acid-cyanocobalamin vs placebo for chronic fatigue syndrome. Arch Intern Med. 1989;149:2501-2503.

86. Behan PO, Behan WMH, Horrobin D. Effect of high doses of essential fatty acids on the postviral fatigue syndrome. Acta Neurol Scand. 1990;82:209-216.

87. Warren G, McKendrick M, Peet M. The role of essential fatty acids in chronic fatigue syndrome: A case-controlled study of red-cell membrane essential fatty acids (EFA) and a placebo-controlled treatment study with high dose of EFA. Acta Neurol Scand. 1999;99:112-116.

88. Forsyth LM, Preuss HG, MacDowell AL, et al. Therapeutic effects of oral NADH on the symptoms of patients with chronic fatigue syndrome. Ann Allergy Asthma Immunol. 1999;82:185-191.

89. Straus SE. Intravenous immunoglobulin treatment for the chronic fatigue syndrome. Am J Med. 1990;89:551-553.

90. Peterson P, Shepard J, Macres M, et al. A controlled trial of intravenous immunoglobulin G in chronic fatigue syndrome. Am J Med. 1990;89:554-560.

91. Lloyd A, Hickie I, Brockman A, et al. Immunologic and psychologic therapy for patients with chronic fatigue syndrome: A double-blind, placebo-controlled trial. Am J Med. 1993;94:197-203.

92. Lloyd A, Hickie I, Wakefield D, et al. A double-blind, placebo-controlled trial of intravenous immunoglobulin therapy in patients with chronic fatigue syndrome. Am J Med. 1990;89:561-568.

93. Vollmer Conna U, Hickie I, Hadzi Pavlovic D, et al. Intravenous immunoglobulin is ineffective in the treatment of patients with chronic fatigue syndrome. Am J Med. 1997;103:38-43.

94. De Vinci C, Levine PH, Pizza G, et al. Lessons from a pilot study of transfer factor in chronic fatigue syndrome. Biotherapy. 1996;9:87-90.

95. Goldenberg DL. A review of the role of tricyclic medications in the treatment of fibromyalgia syndrome. J Rheumatol. 1989;169(Suppl 19):S137-S139.

96. Gracious B, Wisner KL. Nortriptyline in chronic fatigue syndrome: A double blind, placebo-controlled single case study. Biol Psychiatry. 1991;30:405-408.

97. Vercoulen J, Swanink C, Zitman F, et al. Randomised, double-blind, placebo-controlled study of fluoxetine in chronic fatigue syndrome. Lancet. 1996;347:858-861.

98. Wearden AJ, Morriss RK, Mullis R, et al. Randomised, double-blind, placebo-controlled treatment trial of fluoxetine and graded exercise for chronic fatigue syndrome. Br J Psychiatry. 1998;172:485-490.

99. Natelson B, Cheu J, Pareja J, et al. Randomized, double blind, controlled placebo-phase in trial of low dose phenelzine in the chronic fatigue syndrome. Psychopharmacology. 1996;226:230.

100. Natelson BH, Cheu J, Hill N, et al. Single-blind, placebo phase-in trial of two escalating doses of selegiline in the chronic fatigue syndrome. Neuropsychobiology. 1998;37:150-154.

101. Hickie IB, Wilson AJ, Wright JM, et al. A randomized, double-blind placebo-controlled trial of moclobemide in patients with chronic fatigue syndrome. J Clin Psychiatry. 2000;61:643-648.

102. Bou-Holaigah I, Rowe P, Kan J, et al. The relationship between neurally mediated hypotension and the chronic fatigue syndrome. JAMA. 1995;274:961-967.

103. Rowe PC, Calkins H, DeBusk K, et al. Fludrocortisone acetate to treat neurally-mediated hypotension in chronic fatigue syndrome: A randomized controlled trial. JAMA. 2001;285:52-59.

104. Peterson PK, Pheley A, Schroeppel J, et al. A preliminary placebo-controlled crossover trial of fludrocortisone for chronic fatigue syndrome. Arch Intern Med. 1998;158:908-914.

105. Cleare AJ, Heap E, Malhi GS, et al. Low-dose hydrocortisone in chronic fatigue syndrome: A randomised crossover trial. Lancet. 1999;353:455-458.

106. McKenzie R, O'Fallon A, Dale J, et al. Low-dose hydrocortisone treatment of chronic fatigue syndrome: Results of a placebo controlled study of its efficacy and safety. JAMA. 1998;280:1061-1066.

107. McKenzie R, Reynolds JC, O'Fallon A, et al. Decreased bone mineral density during low dose glucocorticoid administration in a randomized, placebo-controlled trial. J Rheumatol. 2000;27:2222-2226.

108. Fulcher K, White P. Randomised controlled trial of graded exercise in patients with the chronic fatigue syndrome. BMJ. 1997;314:1647-1652.

109. Powell P, Bentall RP, Nye FJ, et al. Randomised control trial of patient education to encourage graded exercise in chronic fatigue syndrome. BMJ. 2001;322:1-5.

110. Korszun A, Sackett-Lundeen L, Papadopoulos E, et al. Melatonin levels in women with fibromyalgia and chronic fatigue syndrome. J Rheumatol. 1999;26:2675-2680.

111. Friedberg F, Krupp LB. A comparison of cognitive behavioral treatment for chronic fatigue syndrome and primary depression. Clin Infect Dis. 1994;18(Suppl 1): S105-S110.

112. Deale A, Chalder T, Marks I, et al. Cognitive behavior therapy for chronic fatigue syndrome: A randomized controlled trial. Am J Psychiatry. 1997;157:408-414.

113. Sharpe M, Hawton K, Simkin S, et al. Cognitive behaviour therapy for the chronic fatigue syndrome: A randomized controlled trial. BMJ. 1996;312:22-26.

114. Sharpe MC. Cognitive-behavioral therapy for patients with chronic syndrome—how? In: Demitrack MA, Abbey SE, eds. Chronic Fatigue Syndrome: An Integrative Approach to Evaluation and Treatment. New York: Guilford; 1996:240-262.

115. Prins JB, Bleijenberg G, Bazelmans E, et al. Cognitive behaviour therapy for chronic fatigue syndrome: A multicenter randomised controlled trial. Lancet. 2001;357: 841-847.

116. Ridsdale L, Godfrey E, Chalder T, et al. Chronic fatigue in general practice: Is counselling as good as cognitive behaviour therapy? Br J Gen Pract. 2001;51:19-24.

117. Chisolm D, Godfrey E, Ridsdale L, et al. Chronic fatigue in general practice: Economic evaluation of counseling versus cognitive behaviour therapy. Br J Gen Pract. 2001;51:15-18.

118. Natelson BH, Ye N, Moul DE, et al. High titers of anti-Epstein-Barr virus DNA polymerase are found in patients with severe fatiguing illness. J Med Virol. 1994;42: 42-46.

119. Wray B, Gaughf C, Chandler F Jr, et al. Detection of Epstein-Barr virus and cytomegalovirus in patients with chronic fatigue. Ann Allergy. 1993;71:223-226.

120. Koelle DM, Barcy S, Huang ML, et al. Markers of viral infection in monozygotic twins discordant for chronic fatigue syndrome. Clin Infect Dis. 2002;35:518-525.

121. Lerner AM, Zervos M, Dworkin HJ, et al. A unified theory of the cause of chronic fatigue syndrome. Infect Dis Clin Pract. 1997;6:239-243.

122. Lerner AM, Zervos M, Dworkin HJ, et al. New cardiomyopathy: Pilot study of intravenous ganciclovir in a subset of the chronic fatigue syndrome. Infect Dis Clin Pract. 1997;6:110-117.

123. Di Luca D, Zorzenon M, Mirandola P, et al. Human herpesvirus 6 and human herpesvirus 7 in chronic fatigue syndrome. J Clin Microbiol. 1995;33:1660-1661.

124. Patnaik M, Komaroff A, Conley E, et al. Prevalence of IgM antibodies to human herpesvirus 6 early antigen (p41/38) in patients with chronic fatigue syndrome. J Infect Dis. 1995;172:1364-1367.

125. Cuende J, Civeira P, Diez N, et al. [High prevalence without reactivation of herpes virus 6 in subjects with chronic fatigue syndrome]. Anales Med Int. 1997;14:441-444.

126. Reeves WC, Stamey FR, Black JB, et al. Human herpesviruses 6 and 7 in chronic fatigue syndrome: A case-control study. Clin Infect Dis. 2000;31:48-52.

127. Pauk J, Buchwald D, Corey L. Letter to the editor. J Clin Virol. 2001;21:103-104.

128. Yousef GE, Bell EJ, Mann GF, et al. Chronic enterovirus infection in patients with postviral fatigue syndrome. Lancet. 1988;1:146-150.

129. Cunningham L, Bowles N, Lane R, et al. Persistence of enteroviral RNA in chronic fatigue syndrome is associated with the abnormal production of equal amounts of positive and negative strands of enteroviral RNA. J Gen Virol. 1990;71:1399-1402.

130. Gow J, Behan W, Clements G, et al. Enteroviral RNA sequences detected by polymerase chain reaction in muscle of patients with postviral fatigue syndrome. BMJ. 1991;302:692-696.

131. McArdle A, McArdle F, Jackson M, et al. Investigation by polymerase chain reaction of enteroviral infection in patients with chronic fatigue syndrome. Clin Sci. 1996;90:295-300.

132. Gow JW, Behan WMH, Simpson K, et al. Studies on enterovirus in patients with chronic fatigue syndrome. Clin Infect Dis. 1994;18(Suppl 1):S126-S129.

133. Lindh G, Samuelson A, Hedlund K, et al. No findings of enteroviruses in Swedish patients with chronic fatigue syndrome. Scand J Infect Dis. 1996;28:305-307.

134. Naim C, Galbraith DN, Clements GB. Comparison of coxsackie B neutralisation and enteroviral PCR in chronic fatigue patients. J Med Virol. 1995;46.

135. Berg AM, Naides SJ, Simms RW. Established fibromyalgia syndrome and parvovirus B19 infection. J Rheumatol. 1993;20:1941-1943.

136. Ilaria R Jr, Komaroff A, Fagioli L, et al. Absence of parvovirus B19 infection in chronic fatigue syndrome. Arthritis Rheum. 1995;38:638-641.

137. Martin W. Severe stealth virus encephalopathy following chronic-fatigue-syndrome-like illness: Clinical and histopathological features. Pathobiology. 1996.

138. DeFreitas E, Hilliard B, Cheney P, et al. Retroviral sequences related to human T-lymphotropic virus type II in patients with chronic fatigue immune dysfunction syndrome. Proc Natl Acad Sci U S A. 1991;88:2922-2926.

139. Heneine W, Woods T, Sinha S, et al. Lack of evidence for infection with known human and animal retroviruses in patients with chronic fatigue syndrome. Clin Infect Dis. 1994;18(Suppl 1):S121-S125.

140. Khan A, Heneine W, Chapman L, et al. Assessment of a retrovirus sequence and other possible risk factors for the chronic fatigue syndrome in adults. Ann Intern Med. 1993;118:241-245.

141. Gelman IH, Unger ER, Mawle AC, et al. Chronic fatigue syndrome is not associated with expression of endogenous retroviral p15E. Mol Diagn. 2000;5:155-156.

142. Kitani T, Kuratsune H, Fuke I, et al. Possible correlation between Borna disease virus infection and Japanese patients with chronic fatigue syndrome. Microbiol Immunol. 1996;40:459-462.

143. Bode L, Komaroff AL, Ludwig H. No serologic evidence of Borna disease virus in patients with chronic fatigue syndrome. Clin Infect Dis. 1992;15:1049.

144. Asch ES, Bujak DI, Weiss M, et al. Lyme disease: An infectious and postinfectious syndrome. J Rheumatol. 1994;21:454-461.

145. Dinerman H, Steere AC. Lyme disease associated with fibromyalgia. Ann Intern Med. 1992;117:281-285.

146. Lightfoot R Jr, Luft B, Rahn D, et al. Empiric parenteral antibiotic treatment of patients with fibromyalgia and fatigue and a positive serologic result for Lyme disease: A cost-effectiveness analysis. Ann Intern Med. 1993;119:503-509.

147. Evans AC. Chronic brucellosis. JAMA. 1934;103:665-667.

148. Vojdani A, Choppa PC, Tagle C, et al. Detection of *Mycoplasma* genus and *Mycoplasma fermentans* by PCR in patients with chronic fatigue syndrome. FEMS Immunol Med Microbiol. 1998;22:355-365.

149. Nijs J, Nicolson GL, DeBecker P, et al. High prevalence of *Mycoplasma* infections among European chronic fatigue patients: Examination of four *Mycoplasma* species in blood of chronic fatigue patients. FEMS Immunol Med Microbiol. 2002;34:209-214.

150. Komaroff AL, Bell DS, Cheney PR, et al. Absence of antibody to *Mycoplasma fermentans* in patients with chronic fatigue syndrome. Clin Infect Dis. 1993;17:1074-1075.

151. Crook WG. The Yeast Connection: A Medical Breakthrough. 3rd ed. Jackson, Tenn: Professional Books; 1983.

152. Truss CO. The role of *Candida albicans* in human illness. Orthomol Psychiatry. 1981;10:228-238.

153. Dismukes WE, Wade JS, Lee JY, et al. A randomized, double-blind trial of nystatin therapy for the candidiasis hypersensitivity syndrome. N Engl J Med. 1990;323:1717-1723.

INDEX

Note: Page numbers followed by f indicate figures; those followed by t indicate tables.

A

A-B model, of toxins, 24
Abacavir, 1657t, 1659
  dosage of, 684t-685t
  drug interactions with, 686t
  for perinatal HIV transmission prevention, 1625t
  formulations of, 649t
    pediatric, 1646t
  prophylactic, after occupational exposure to HIV, 3402, 3402t
  side effects of, 1573
  structure of, 1656f
Abdomen. *See also under* Intra-abdominal.
  anatomy of, 927-929, 927f, 928f
  in severe sepsis, 913, 913f
Abdominal wall, in secondary peritonitis, 935
Abiotrophia spp.
  blood culture of, 210, 210t
  cardiovascular device infections from, 1023
  prosthetic valve endocarditis from, 1025, 1026, 1027
Abiotrophia adjacens (Granulicatella adiacens), 2440
Abiotrophia defectiva, 2440
  vancomycin for, 418
ABO blood groups, in infection susceptibility, 44t, 46
Abortion
  septic, 1375-1376
    from *Campylobacter jejuni,* 2552
  spontaneous
    from *Brucella,* 2671
    from *Chlamydia trachomatis,* 2249
    from hepatitis E virus, 2210
    from parvovirus B19, 1895, 1896
Abscess, 1188t, 1191. *See also specific sites.*
  actinomycotic, 2925-2929, 2925f
  brain. *See* Brain abscess.
  Brodie's, 1330
  colonic, 2813, 2813f
  cutaneous. *See also* Skin infections.
    from *Cryptococcus neoformans,* 3003t, 3004-3005, 3004f
    in injection drug users, 3463
  epidural, 1165-1168, 1166f, 1167f, 1326-1327, 1326f
    clinical features of, 1079-1080
    in injection drug users, 3471-3472
  from *Candida,* 2940
  in melioidosis, 2624-2625, 2626f-2628f
  internal, in melioidosis, 2625, 2627f, 2628f
  intra-abdominal
    from *Bacteroides fragilis,* 2814
    from *Candida,* 2947, 2947f
      treatment of, 2950
    in transplant recipients, 3505
    vs. enteric fever, 1274t
  laboratory studies for, 213
    specimen collection and transport for, 205t
  liver. *See* Liver abscess.

Abscess *(Continued)*
  lung, 853-856, 854t, 855f, 2624, 2625f, 2626f
    from *Entamoeba histolytica,* 3103
    from *Nocardia,* 1151t, 1152, 2916f, 2917-2918
    in melioidosis, 2624, 2625f, 2626f
  muscle, 1194-1202, 1195t
  orbital, 1421-1424, 1421f-1423f. *See also* Orbital abscess/cellulitis.
    in mucormycosis, 1423, 2975-2977, 2976f
  paraspinal
    from *Coccidioides immitis,* 3044, 3046f
    tuberculous, 2879
  Pautrier's, 2108
  pelvic, 1377
  perinephric, 895-896, 896f
  periodontal, 791. *See also* Odontogenic infections.
  peritoneal, 943-944, 944f
  peritonsillar, 754, 756
  prostatic, 894, 894f, 1383t, 1384
    in melioidosis, 2625, 2628, 2628f
  psoas, 1200-1201
    in melioidosis, 2625, 2627f
  renal, 875, 895-896, 896f
    in endocarditis, 981
  soft tissue. *See* Soft tissue infections.
  spinal. *See* Abscess, epidural; Abscess, paraspinal.
  splenic, 967-968, 967t
    in endocarditis, 982
    in injection drug users, 3470-3471
    in melioidosis, 2627f
  subcutaneous, 1187-1191, 1188t
  subhepatic, 928
  subperiosteal, 1003, 1421-1424, 1421f, 1423f
  subphrenic space, 928
  tubo-ovarian, 1378, 1379t, 1380
  vaginal cuff, postoperative, 1377, 1377t
Absidia spp., morphology of, 2974, 2974f
Absorption, of drugs, 271t, 272
Absorption rate constant, 272
Acanthamoeba [spp.]
  characteristics of, 3112, 3112f
  disseminated infections from, 3114
  keratitis from, 1398, 1404, 1405, 3111-3119. *See also* Keratitis, from *Acanthamoeba.*
  meningoencephalitis from, 1088, 1101, 1104-1105, 1106t, 1115, 3111-3119. *See also* Granulomatous amebic encephalitis.
  treatment of, 576t-577t
Acanthamoeba glebae, 3112f
Accessory gene regulator, 2324-2325, 2324f
Acedapsone, for leprosy, 499
Acetaminophen
  for fever, 713-715
  for hepatitis, 1437
Acetazolamide, for altitude illness, 3644
N-Acetyl muramyl-L-alanine amidase, 35

Acetylcholine, botulinum toxin effect on, 2823-2824, 2824f
Achlorhydria, gastrointestinal infections and, 1217
Achromobacter spp., 2751t, 2757-2758
  laboratory identification of, 221t
Acid-fast stain
  for aerobic actinomycetes, 228
  for *Mycobacterium tuberculosis,* 2853, 2854t
Acidity, of skin, 35
Acidosis, in malaria, 3125
Acinetobacter [spp.], 2632-2635
  bacteremia from, 2634
  cardiovascular device infections from, 1023
  clinical manifestations of, 2633-2634
  endocarditis from, 992
  epidemiology of, 2633
  genitourinary infections from, 2634
  history of, 2632, 2633t
  in peritoneal dialysis, 941
  laboratory identification of, 220, 221t
  meningitis from, 1114, 2634
  microbiology of, 2632
  multidrug-resistant, 2634-2635
    prior-authorization program for, 615
  pathogenesis of, 2633
  peritonitis from, 938
  pneumonia from, nosocomial, 3367t, 3368
  respiratory tract infections from, 2634
  soft tissue infections from, 2634
  treatment of, 2634-2635
    with aminoglycosides, 334t-335t
    with penicillins, 284t, 288t
    with quinolones, 455t
    with rifamycin, 374t
Acinetobacter anitratus, carbapenems for, 313t
Acinetobacter baumannii, aminoglycoside susceptibility to, 332-333, 332t
Acinetobacter calcoaceticus–Acinetobacter baumannii complex, 2632, 2633
Acne vulgaris
  clindamycin for, 411
  erythromycin for, 401t
  topical antibacterials for, 483
Acquired immunodeficiency syndrome (AIDS). *See* AIDS entries; Human immunodeficiency virus infection.
Acquired pellicle, 789
Acremonium spp., 3073
  mycetoma from, 2991-2995, 2992t, 2993f
  nail infections from, 3060
Acridine orange, 214t
Acrodermatitis chronica atrophicans, in borreliosis, 738-739
ACTH, in acute-phase response, 40
Actinobacillus [spp.], 2751t, 2752-2753
Actinobacillus actinomycetemcomitans, 2752
  cardiovascular device infections from, 1023
  endocarditis from, 991
    prosthetic valve, treatment of, 1028, 1029t
  laboratory identification of, 220
  odontogenic infections from, 788, 788f, 789

Actinobacillus equuli, 2752-2753
Actinobacillus hominis, 2753
Actinobacillus lignieresii, 2752-2753
Actinobacillus suis, 2752-2753
Actinobaculum [spp.], 2924
Actinomadura [spp.], laboratory tests for, 228-229
Actinomadura madurae, mycetoma from, 2991-2995, 2992t
Actinomyces [spp.] *See also* Actinomycosis.
    characteristics of, 2924-2925, 2930, 2930f
    classification of, 2924
    companion microbes of, 2924, 2925
    endocarditis from, 992
    identification of, 2929-2931, 2930f
    in oral cavity, 787, 787t, 2924
    laboratory identification of, 219-220, 219t
    pathogenicity of, 2924-2925
Actinomyces europeus, laboratory identification of, 219t, 220
Actinomyces israelii
    abdominal, vs. enteric fever, 1274t, 1278
    Actinobacillus actinomycetemcomitans with, 2752
    laboratory identification of, 219, 219t
    penicillins for, 288t
    sclerosing mediastinitis from, 1075
Actinomyces naeslundii, laboratory identification of, 219, 219t
Actinomyces odontolyticus, laboratory identification of, 219, 219t
Actinomyces radingae, laboratory identification of, 219t, 220
Actinomyces turicensis, laboratory identification of, 219t, 220
Actinomyces viscosus
    laboratory identification of, 219, 219t
    transient bacteremia from, 978
Actinomycetes
    aerobic
        collection and transport of, 228
        direct detection of, 228
        epidemiology of, 229
        identification of, 228-229
        laboratory tests for, 228-229
        processing and planting of, 228
        susceptibility testing of, 229
    aerobic nocardiform, 2916
Actinomycetoma, 2916, 2917, 2929, 2991-2995
Actinomycosis, 2924-2931
    abdominal, 2926-2928, 2928f
    brain abscess in, 1158t, 2929
    central nervous system disease in, 1158t, 2929
    cervicofacial, 797t, 2925-2926
    clinical features of, 2925-2929
    copathogens in, 2924
    course of, 2925
    diagnosis of, 2929-2931, 2930f
    disseminated, 2929
    epidemiology of, 2924
    etiology of, 2924
    mediastinal, 2926
    musculoskeletal, 2929
    odontogenic infections in, 788, 788f, 2925
    osteomyelitis in, 2926, 2929
    pathogenesis and pathophysiology of, 2924-2925
    pelvic, 1378, 2928-2929, 2928f
    pleuropulmonary, 847
    risk factors for, 2925
    subcutaneous abscess in, 1191
    thoracic, 2926, 2927f
    treatment of, 2931, 2931t
        with quinupristin-dalfopristin, 425
        with tetracyclines, 358
    vs. nocardiosis, 2931

Actinomycotic granuloma, 2929
Acupuncture, immune effects of, 610
Acute disseminated encephalomyelitis, 2053
Acute fatty liver of pregnancy, 1436
Acute hemorrhagic conjunctivitis, 1389, 2136, 2137, 2155-2156, 2156f
Acute laryngotracheobronchitis. *See* Laryngotracheobronchitis.
Acute lymphonodular pharyngitis, 2151
Acute necrotizing ulcerative gingivitis, 754, 756, 791
    treatment of, 796, 796t
Acute phase response, muscle proteolysis in, 1202
Acute poststreptococcal glomerulonephritis. *See* Glomerulonephritis, poststreptococcal.
Acute respiratory disease, 753
Acute respiratory distress syndrome (ARDS)
    complement in, 86-87
    corticosteroids for, 559
    fatty acid diet in, 144
    from herpes simplex virus, 1770, 1774t
    in leptospirosis, 2792
    in malaria, 3125, 3132
Acute retinal necrosis, 1416, 1417f, 1418
Acute urethral syndrome, 2248, 2250
Acute-phase response, 709-710, 710t
Acyclovir, 515t, 516-520
    activity spectrum of, 516, 517t
    dosage of, 680t-681t
    drug interactions with, 518, 686t
    for acute retinal necrosis, 1418
    for cytomegalovirus, 520
    for genital herpes, 1344, 1773, 1773t
    for herpes B virus, 1833-1834, 1834t
    for herpes simplex keratitis, 1402t, 1773t
    for herpes simplex virus, 518-519, 1773, 1773t-1774t
        in HIV infection, 1683t, 1686t
    for herpes zoster, 1784
    for herpes zoster ophthalmicus, 1403t
    for herpesviruses, 1760t, 1761, 1773, 1773t-1774t
    for herpetic encephalitis, 1770, 1773t
    for herpetic iridocyclitis, 1418, 1773t
    for herpetic meningitis, 1767, 1773t
    for human herpesvirus 6, 1823
    for human immunodeficiency virus, 520
    for infectious mononucleosis, 520
    for neonatal herpes, 1771, 1773t
    for varicella-zoster virus, 519-520, 1784
        in HIV infection, 1686t-1687t
        in stem cell transplant, 3494
    for X-linked lymphoproliferative disease, 1815
    formulations of, 649t
    mechanism of action of, 516
    pharmacokinetics of, 517-518, 518t
    prophylactic, for transplant recipients, 3482, 3494
    resistance to, 516-517, 517t
    structure of, 516, 517f
    toxicity of, 518
Adefovir, 515t, 520-521
    dosage of, 680t-681t
    for hepatitis B virus
        in chronic infections, 1446-1447, 1448, 1448t, 1449, 1449t, 1450, 1881, 1882
        in HIV infection, 1691t
    formulations of, 649t
    in renal insufficiency, 521, 521t
    structure of, 520, 520f
Adenitis. *See* Lymphadenitis/lymphadenopathy.
Adeno-associated viruses, 1840
Adenosine deaminase deficiency, 150t

Adenoviruses, 1835-1840
    appendicitis from, 969
    bronchiolitis from, 813, 813t
    central nervous system infections from, 1839
    characteristics of, 1835-1837, 1836f, 1836t
    classification of, 183t6t, 1835-1837
    clinical manifestations of, 1837-1839, 1837t
    colds from, 747-750, 747t
    collection of, 233t
    conjunctivitis from, 1389
    croup from, 761
    discovery of, 1835
    disease spectrum of, 1837-1839, 1837t
    epidemiology of, 1837
    gastroenteritis from, 1239, 1239t
    gastrointestinal infections from, 235
    genome of, 1837
    hemorrhagic cystitis from, 1838
    host defenses against, 126
    immune response to, 1837, 1837f
    in HIV vaccine testing, 1712
    in stem cell transplant, 3494
    infantile diarrhea from, 1838
    intussusception from, 1838-1839
    keratitis from, 754, 1398, 1402, 1404, 1838, 1839
    keratoconjunctivitis from, 754, 1402, 1404, 1838
    laboratory tests for, 234, 235
    laryngitis from, 758, 759t
    latency of, 1837
    myocarditis from, 1052
    noninflammatory diarrhea from, 1239
    oncogenicity of, 183t6t, 1835, 1837
    pancreatic infections from, 959t, 960
    pathogenesis of, 1837
    pharyngitis from, 754
    pharyngoconjunctival fever from, 1838
    receptors for, 1732t
    respiratory infections from, 1838, 1839
    sinusitis from, 776, 776t
    structure of, 1835, 1836f
    urinary tract infections from, 882
    vaccines for, 1839-1840
        in myocarditis prevention, 1058
Adenylate cyclase toxin, 25t, 27
    of *Bordetella pertussis,* 2702, 2703
Adherence, 14-22
    altered receptor expression and, 20
    biofilms in, 21-22, 21t
    in cardiovascular device infections, 1022
    in endocarditis, 1045
    of *Bacillus,* 2494
    of enteric pathogens, 1221-1222
    of enteropathogenic *Escherichia coli,* 2575
    of *Streptococcus agalactiae* (group B), 2425
    of *Streptococcus pneumoniae,* 2394
    P fimbriae in, 19-20, 19f
    species specificity of, 15
Adhesins, 3
    conformation of, 16, 16f
    fimbriate, in *Escherichia coli* adherence, 1221
    identification of, 14-15, 15t
    immune response to, 17
    in adherence mediation, 14, 14f
    microbial synergy and, 20
    of Enterobacteriaceae, 2571
    of *Haemophilus influenzae,* 2662, 2662t
    of *Pseudomonas aeruginosa,* 2594
    of *Staphylococcus aureus,* 2326-2327, 2326f, 2326t
    of *Streptococcus pyogenes* (group A), 2363
    of uropathogenic *Escherichia coli,* 877, 877t
    proteolytic fragmentation of, 16, 16f, 16t

Adhesins (Continued)
  receptors for
    identification of, 15-16, 15t
    interactions with, 16-17, 16f, 16t
    therapy with, 20-21, 20t
Adipsin, 69t
Adolescents, HIV infection in, 1481, 1639, 1650
Adrenal glands
  histoplasmosis of, 3020
  insufficiency of
    in sepsis, 915-916
    in septic shock, 918
    Paracoccidioides brasiliensis of, 3065
    tuberculosis of, 2883
Adrenaline (epinephrine), nebulized
  for bronchiolitis, 817
  for croup, 763-764
α-Adrenergic blockade, for tetanus, 2820
Adrenocorticotropic hormone, in acute-phase
    response, 40
Adult inclusion conjunctivitis, 1391, 1392, 2245,
    2247t, 2250
Adult T-cell leukemia/lymphoma, 2108-2110,
    2108f-2111f, 2108t. *See also* Hematologic
    malignancies.
  treatment of, 2112
Aedes [spp.]
  alphavirus infections from, 1915, 1916
  California encephalitis from, 2086-2089, 2086t
  control measures for, 1943
  dengue from, 178, 235t
  dengue/dengue hemorrhagic fever from, 1929
  distribution of, 179, 179f
  flavivirus infections from, 1926-1945, 1945t
  geographic distribution of, 1927f, 1930f
  hantavirus infections from, 2086t, 2087-2089
  hemorrhagic fever with renal syndrome from,
    2086t, 2087-2089
  Rift Valley fever from, 2086t, 2087-2089
  yellow fever from, 1929
Aedes aegypti, distribution of, 179, 179f
Aerobic infections, from gram-negative bacilli,
    laboratory identification of, 220-221
Aeromonas [spp.], 2751t, 2753-2754
  Act toxin of, 1221
  aminoglycosides for, 334t-335t
  laboratory detection of, 212
  quinolones for, 455t
  traveler's diarrhea from, 1242
  weanling diarrhea from, 1238
Aeromonas hydrophila
  carbapenems for, 313t
  myonecrosis from, 1200
  pore-forming toxin of, 30
Afipia [spp.], 739-740
Afipia felis, 739-740
  cat-scratch disease from, 2736
  identification of, 2742, 2743t
Aflatoxin, hepatocellular carcinoma and, 1873
Africa, HIV infection in, 1466-1468, 1467f
  among women, 1617-1618
African histoplasmosis, 3021
African tick-bite fever, 2090t, 2285t, 2287t, 2292-
    2293, 3653f
  vs. malaria, 3133
African trypanosomiasis, 3165-3169. *See also*
    Trypanosomiasis, African.
Agammaglobulinemia, 65
  immunoglobulin G replacement in, 67
  X-linked, 65, 150t, 153
    chronic meningoencephalitis in, 2154-2155
Age
  immune response to vaccines and, 3558
  immunity and, 40
  in antimicrobial agent selection, 243-244

Age (Continued)
  in gastrointestinal infections, 1216
  temperature and, 705, 707
Agent, 167-168
  host relationship with, 166-167
Agglutination, 58
  antigen detection by, 214-215, 214t
Agglutinin, 2636
Agr, 2324-2325, 2324f
Agranulocytosis, infantile genetic, 104
Agrobacterium tumefaciens, toxin secretion in, 26
AIDS. *See also* Human immunodeficiency virus
    infection.
AIDS case definition, 1482, 1483f
AIDS dementia complex, 1584-1587, 1585f,
    1585t, 1586t
  pathogenesis of, 2129-2130
AIDS-defining opportunistic processes, in
    women, 1627-1630
Air conditioning, in legionnaires' disease, 2711,
    2712, 2713, 2720
Air sampling, for bioterrorist attacks, 3598-3599
Air travel. *See also* Travelers.
  health problems in, 3644
Airborne precautions, 3327-3329, 3327t, 3328t,
    3330t
Airway defense mechanisms, 820, 820t
Airway hyperreactivity, from respiratory syncytial
    virus, 2015t, 2016t, 2019
Al Khurma virus, 1945t
  as biological weapon, 3627-3629, 3628t
Alagoas virus, 2045, 2045t
Albendazole
  adverse effects of, 581t
  for ascariasis, 571t, 3263
  for capillariasis, 571t, 3298
  for cutaneous larva migrans, 571t, 3296
  for cysticercosis, 3290
  for encephalitozoon conjunctivitis, 1405
  for enterobiasis, 572t, 3265
  for fluke infections, 572t
  for giardiasis, 3202t, 3203
  for gnathostomiasis, 3297
  for helminthic disease, 569t, 570t
  for hookworms, 3264
  for hydatid cyst, 3291
  for intestinal nematodes, 592-593
  for isosporiasis, in HIV infection, 1689t
  for liver flukes, 3277t, 3282
  for loiasis, 3273
  for microsporidiosis, 574t, 3247-3249, 3248t
    in HIV infection, 1690t
    of eye, 1393, 3248t, 3249
  for strongyloidiasis, 3265
  for tapeworms, 575t
  for trichinosis, 576t, 3269
  for *Trichostrongylus,* 576t
  for *Trichuris trichiura,* 576t
  for visceral larva migrans, 576t
  for *Wuchereria bancrofti,* 577t
  structure of, 592f
Albumin, nutritional status and, 140, 140t
Albuterol, for chronic obstructive pulmonary
    disease, 810t
Albuterol-ipratropium, for chronic obstructive
    pulmonary disease, 810t
Alcaligenes spp., 2751t, 2757
  endocarditis from, 992
Alcaligenes faecalis, 2757
  laboratory identification of, 221t
Alcaligenes xylosoxidans, pulmonary infections
    from, in cystic fibrosis, 871
Alcaligenes xylosoxidans subsp. *xylosoxidans,*
    2757
Alcohol, as disinfectant, 479, 3333-3334

Alcohol use/abuse
  cirrhosis from, 930
  HCV-related hepatic fibrosis and, 1960
  in hepatitis A, 2180
  metronidazole and, 393t
Alcoholic hepatitis, 1436
  from hepatitis C, 1436
Alexandrium spp., 3255, 3256t
Alexin, 69
Algal blooms, 3255-3256, 3255f, 3256t
Alitretinoin gel, for Kaposi's sarcoma, 1603
Allergic bronchopulmonary aspergillosis, 2962,
    2963t
  in cystic fibrosis, 871-872, 873
Allergic fungal sinusitis, 3070-3072, 3071f
  from *Aspergillus,* 2962
Alloiococcus spp., laboratory identification of,
    217t, 218
Allopurinol, for leishmaniasis, in HIV infection,
    1692t
Alma-Arasan virus, 1945t
Alopecia
  differential diagnosis of, 3056-3057
  from arenaviruses, 2095
  from *Candida,* 2944
  from dermatophytes, 3056-3057, 3057f
Alphaviruses, 1913-1919
  arthritis from, 1317
  characteristics of, 1913-1914, 1914t
  classification of, 1914, 1914t
  clinical manifestations of, 1914t
  course of, 1917f
  disease spectrum of, 1914t
  encephalitis from, 1914t, 1915-1916
  epidemiology of, 1914t
  fever from, 1916
  historical perspective on, 1913-1919
  New World, 1913
  Old World, 1913
  polyarthritis from, 1916
  rash from, 1916
  replication of, 1913-1914
  structure of, 1913
  transmission of, 1914, 1914t, 1915f
Alternaria spp., sinusitis from, 3070-3071, 3076t
Alternative and complementary therapies, 603-
    610, 604t. *See also specific therapy.*
  for colds, 604t, 608, 750
  for diarrhea, 604t, 606-607
  for urinary tract infections, 20, 21, 604t
  hepatitis from, 1436
Alternative pathway, 69t
  deficiencies in, 151t
  generation of, 72-73
Altitude illness, 3644
Aluminum, metronidazole interactions with, 393t
Alveolar cyst disease, 3286t, 3290, 3291-3292
Alveolar hemorrhage, in stem cell transplant,
    3488
Alveolar macrophages, 820
Amanita spp., poisoning from, 1290, 1291t
Amantadine, 515t, 521-523
  activity spectrum of, 521
  dosage of, 680t-681t
  drug interactions with, 522-523, 686t
  for hepatitis C, 523
  for influenza, 523, 805, 2072-2073, 2072t
    for prophylaxis, 2078
    in HIV infection, 1682t
  for renal insufficiency, 522t
  formulations of, 649t
  mechanism of action of, 522
  pharmacokinetics of, 522
  resistance to, 522, 2073
  side effects of, 2072t, 2073

Amantadine *(Continued)*
 structure of, 521f
 toxicity of, 523
Amazon black fever, 1432
Amblyomma americanum, 2312, 2315, 3312-3314, 3313t
Amblyomma cajennense, 2288
Amblyomma maculatum, 3312-3314, 3313t. *See also* Tick(s).
Ambocepto, 69
AMD-070, 20, 20t
AMD-3100, 20, 20t
Amdinocillin, dosage of, 650t-651t
Amebae, *Legionella pneumophila* growth in, 2712, 2712f
Amebiasis. *See Entamoeba histolytica.*
Amebic colitis, 3102-3106
 diagnosis of, 3104-3105
 sigmoidoscopy of, 1264
 treatment of, 3105-3106, 3106t
Amebic infections
 acquired immunity to, 18-19
 antiparasitics for, 568t-569t
 central nervous system, 1088, 1101, 1104-1105, 1106t, 1115
 extraintestinal, 3103-3107
 from *Acanthamoeba,* 3111-3119. *See also Acanthamoeba* spp.
 from *Balamuthia mandrillaris,* 3111-3119. *See also Balamuthia mandrillaris.*
 from *Entamoeba histolytica,* 3097-3107. *See also Entamoeba histolytica.*
 from free-living amebas, 3111
 from *Naegleria,* 3111-3119. *See also Naegleria* spp.
 from *Sappinia diploidea,* 3111-3119. *See also Sappinia diploidea.*
 hepatic abscess from, 951-955. *See also* Liver abscess.
 intestinal, 3102-3107
 ocular, 1398, 1404-1405
 perianal, 3103
 pleuropulmonary, 3103
 treatment of, 571t, 576t-577t, 582-583, 583f
 vs. enteric fever, 1275t, 1278
Amebic keratitis, 1404, 1405
Amebic liver abscess
 clinical features of, 3103
 diagnosis of, 3105
 pleural effusion in, 847, 849
 treatment of, 3105, 3106, 3106t
Amebomas, 3105
Amenorrhea, in HIV infection, 1630
American cutaneous leishmaniasis, 3145t, 3149-3152, 3149f, 3150f. *See also* Leishmaniasis.
American dog tick, 3312-3314, 3313f, 3313t
American Indians, hepatitis A in, 2170, 2170f, 2179, 2179f
American mucocutaneous leishmaniasis, 3145t, 3150f, 3152, 3153. *See also* Leishmaniasis.
American trypanosomiasis, 3156-3163. *See also* Trypanosomiasis, American.
Amikacin
 antimicrobial activity of, 333, 334t-335t
 dosage of, 660t-661t
 for actinomycetoma, 2995
 for brain abscess, 1159t
 for endophthalmitis, 1410-1411
 for febrile neutropenia, 3450-3452, 3451t, 3453, 3453f, 3453t
 for meningitis, 1106t, 1107t
 for *Mycobacterium avium* complex, 2903-2906, 2904t
  in HIV infection, 1687t
 for *Mycobacterium tuberculosis,* 494, 495

Amikacin *(Continued)*
 for nocardiosis, 2920-2921, 2920t
 for nontuberculous mycobacterial infections, 497
 for nontuberculous mycobacterial pulmonary disease, 2911, 2913t
 for peritonitis, 939
 for *Pseudomonas aeruginosa* bacteremia, 2601
 for shunt infections, 1129t
 for staphylococcal endocarditis, 998
 formulations of, 647t
 names and sources of, 329t
 once-daily dosage regimens for, 348t
 structure of, 329f, 330
 susceptibility of, 332-333, 332t
Aminocyclitol, 328
Aminoglycoside phosphotransferase, 261, 261t
Aminoglycosides, 328-350
 administration of, 337-338
 adverse reactions to, 339t
 antimicrobial activity of
  combination therapy and, 336, 337t
  dosing regimen in, 336
  energy-dependent phase of, 331
  in vitro, 333-335, 334t-335t
  mechanism of, 331
  microbiology of, 333, 334t-335t
  postantibiotic effect in, 334
  structure and, 330, 330f
  synergy in, 334-335, 336t
  time course of, 333-334
 beta-lactam, for streptococcal endocarditis, 995
 biologic activity of, 330
 chemical families of, 330, 330t
 chemistry of, 330-331
 cochlear toxicity from, 341-343
 distribution of, 338
 dosage of, 345-350, 660t-661t
  in cystic fibrosis, 349-350
  in endocarditis, 350
  individualized, 346
  multiple daily
   in dialysis, 346, 346t
   loading dose in, 345, 345t
   maintenance dose in, 345-346, 345t
   renal function and, 345-346, 345t, 346t
  once-daily, 346-347
   regimens for, 347-348, 347t, 348t
   serum level monitoring with, 348-349
  pediatric, 349, 349t
 drug interactions with, 686t
 enzymatic inactivation of, 331
 excretion of, 338
 for acute pyelonephritis, 889
 for dialysis-related peritonitis, 942
 for Enterobacteriaceae endocarditis, 999
 for experimental endocarditis, 1048
 for intra-abdominal peritonitis, 337
 for nontuberculous mycobacterial infections, 496-497
 for nutritionally variant streptococci, 2425
 for penicillin-resistant enterococcal endocarditis, 996-997
 for peritonitis, in continuous ambulatory peritoneal dialysis, 350, 350t
 for *Pseudomonas aeruginosa* bacteremia, 2600-2601
 for pulmonary infections, in cystic fibrosis, 872
 for secondary peritonitis, 937t, 939
 for sepsis, 918
 for *Streptococcus agalactiae* (group B), 2429
 for tuberculosis, 334t-335t, 344t
 formulations of, 647t
 in pregnancy, 245
 indications for, 343-345, 344t

Aminoglycosides *(Continued)*
 metabolism of, 338
 names and sources of, 328, 329t
 nephrotoxicity of, 339-341, 339f, 340t, 341t
 neuromuscular blockade after, 343
 ototoxicity of, 341-343, 872
 pharmacokinetics of, 338
 pharmacology of, 337-338
 prophylactic, 344-345
 resistance to
  acquired, 331-332
  enzymes in, 261, 261t
  epidemiology of, 332-333, 332t
  in enterococci, 332
  inner membrane permeability in, 262
  intrinsic, 331
  prevention of, 336-337
  ribosomal binding alteration in, 263-264
 structure of, 328, 329t, 330
 susceptibility of, 332, 332t
 toxicity of, 338-343, 338t
 types of, 328, 329t
 vestibular toxicity from, 341, 343
δ-Aminolevulinic acid, 216t
Aminopenicillin, 290-291, 291f
 minimal inhibitory concentration of, 283
 uses of, 287, 288t
Aminoquinolines, for malaria, 584-585, 584f, 585f
Aminosalicylic acid
 dosage of, 676t-677t
 drug interactions with, 686t
 formulations of, 649t
Amithiozone, for *Mycobacterium tuberculosis,* 496
Amnesic shellfish poisoning, 3255f, 3256, 3256t
Amniotic fluid infections, 1372-1373
Amniotic membranes, premature rupture of, *Chlamydia trachomatis* and, 2249
Amodiaquine, for malaria, 3134, 3134t
 in pregnancy, 3135
Amorolfine, for onychomycosis, 3058
Amoxicillin, 291
 allergy to, 323
 dosage of, 650t-651t
 for actinomycosis, 2931, 2931t
 for acute pyelonephritis, 889
 for anaerobes, 284t
 for bacilli, 284t
 for chronic *Salmonella* carriage, 2650
 for COPD exacerbations, 811t
 for endocarditis prophylaxis, 1050t
 for Enterobacteriaceae, 284t
 for experimental endocarditis, 1048
 for *Helicobacter pylori* infections, 2563
 for leptospirosis, 2793t
 for lower urinary tract infections, 890
 for lung abscess, 856
 for Lyme disease, 2806, 2806t
 for lymphadenitis, 1211
 for lymphangitis, 1212
 for odontogenic infections, 797t, 798
 for otitis media, 768-769, 769
  for prevention, 769
 for *Pasteurella,* 2690
 for pneumococcal pneumonia, 2404
 for pneumonia, 837-839, 837t, 838t
 for *Pseudomonas,* 284t
 for relapsing urinary tract infections, 891
 for sinusitis, 779-780, 779t
 for *Streptococcus pneumoniae* otitis media, 2404
 for *Streptococcus pneumoniae* sinusitis, 2404
 for syphilis, 2782

Amoxicillin (Continued)
  for urogenital chlamydial infections, in
      pregnancy, 2250
  for viridans streptococcal endocarditis, 2438
  formulations of, 646t
  minimal inhibitory concentration of, 284t
  pneumococcal resistance to, 837, 837t
  prophylactic, for anthrax, 3621
Amoxicillin-clavulanate
  antibacterial activity of, 315t
  dosage of, 650t-651t
  for bites, 3554t
  for cellulitis, 1180
  for febrile neutropenia, 3450-3452, 3451t,
      3453t
  for nocardiosis, 2920, 2920t, 2921
  for Streptococcus pneumoniae otitis media,
      2404
  formulations of, 646t
  prophylactic, in cancer-related febrile
      neutropenia, 3444, 3445f
  uses of, 316
Amoxicillin-sulbactam, for pneumonia, 837-839,
      838t
Amphotericin B, 502-506
  activity spectrum of, 502
  candidiasis, of eye, 1418
  combination therapy with, 248
  dosage of, 678t-679t
  drug interactions with, 686t-687t
  for amebic meningitis, 1115
  for aspergillosis, 2967-2968, 2968t
      for prophylaxis, 2970
      in HIV infection, 1699
  for blastomycosis, 3036-3037, 3036t
  for brain abscess, 1159t, 1160
  for cancer-related febrile neutropenia, 3454-3455
  for candidiasis, 2949-2951
      in esophagitis, 1234
      in HIV infection, 1687t
      in stem cell transplant, 3495
  for catheter-related urinary tract infections, 3377
  for coccidioidomycosis, 3047-3048
      in HIV infection, 1683t, 1687t, 1699
  for cryptococcal infections, in HIV infection,
      1683t, 1688t, 1698
  for cryptococcal meningitis, 1584, 3007, 3008
  for dialysis-related peritonitis, 942, 942t
  for endophthalmitis, 1411
  for fungal endocarditis, 1000, 1001
      prosthetic valve, 1028-1029
  for fusariosis, 3073
  for histoplasmosis, 3023, 3024
      in HIV infection, 1683t, 1698-1699
  for mucormycosis, 2979
  for naegleria, 571t
  for paracoccidioidomycosis, 3065
  for penicilliosis, in HIV infection, 1689t
  for shunt infections, 1129t, 1130
  for sporotrichosis, 2987
  for suppurative thrombophlebitis, 1005
  for urinary tract infections, 892
  for visceral leishmaniasis, 3152, 3153
  formulations of, 502-505, 649t, 2949
  indications for, 569t
  lipid complex, 505
      formulations of, 649t
  lipid-associated, 505-506
  lipid-encapsulated, for visceral leishmaniasis,
      578t
  liposomal, 505-506
      for aspergillosis, 2968-2969, 2968t
      for leishmaniasis, 592
          in HIV infection, 1692t
      formulations of, 649t

Amphotericin B (Continued)
  liposome-encapsulated, for Trypanosomatidae,
      569t
  mechanism of action of, 502, 504f
  preemptive, for pancreatic infections, 963t
  renal toxicity of, 2967
  resistance of, 502
  structure of, 502, 503f
Amphotericin B cholesteryl sulfate complex
  for leishmaniasis, in HIV infection, 1692t
  formulations of, 649t
Amphotericin B colloidal dispersion, 505
Amphotericin B deoxycholate, 502-505
  administration of, 504
  adverse reactions to, 504
  dosage of, 504-505
  for American trypanosomiasis, in HIV
      infection, 1692t
  for cryptococcosis, in HIV infection, 1688t
  for fungal arthritis, 1318
  for histoplasmosis, in HIV infection, 1688t
  for leishmaniasis, 592
  for Trypanosomatidae, 569t
  nephrotoxicity of, 502-504
  pharmacology of, 502
  vs. lipid-associated formulations, 505-506
Ampicillin, 290-291, 291f
  allergy to, 323
  dosage of, 650t-651t
  for anaerobes, 284t
  for bacilli, 284t
  for biliary tract infections, 957
  for brain abscess, 1159, 1159t
  for clostridial cellulitis, 1189
  for COPD exacerbations, 811t
  for dialysis-related peritonitis, 942t
  for diphtheroid prosthetic valve endocarditis,
      1028
  for endocarditis prophylaxis, 1050t
  for Enterobacteriaceae, 284t
      in endocarditis, 999
  for enterococcal endocarditis, 997, 2416, 2416t
      penicillin-resistant, 996, 997
      prosthetic valve, 1027-1028, 1027t-1029t
  for Enterococcus, 2416
  for experimental endocarditis, 1048
  for hepatic abscess, 954t
  for infectious mononucleosis, rash from, 1806,
      1806f, 1806t
  for intra-amniotic infection syndrome, 1372
  for leptospirosis, 2793t
  for listeriosis, 2482-2483
  for meningitis, 1106t, 1107t, 1112, 1113
      for perinatal prophylaxis, 1118
  for nocardiosis, 2920, 2920t
  for osteomyelitis, 1324t
  for peritonitis, 938
  for pneumococcal pneumonia, 2405
  for postoperative gynecologic infections, 1377t
  for Pseudomonas, 284t
  for rat-bite fever, 2710
  for streptococcal prosthetic valve endocarditis,
      1027t
  for streptococcus group B, 2429, 2429t, 2430
  for streptococcus group G, 2445
  for Yersinia pseudotuberculosis, 2700
  formulations of, 646t
  minimal inhibitory concentration of, 284t
  uses of, 287, 288t
Ampicillin-chloramphenicol, for meningitis, 249
Ampicillin-sulbactam
  for acute necrotizing ulcerative gingivitis, 796,
      796t
  for acute pyelonephritis, 889
  for brain abscess, 1159t, 1159t

for deep fascial space infections, 797t
  for epiglottitis, 786
  for experimental endocarditis, 1048
  for Lemierre's disease, 756
  for odontogenic infections, 797t
  for penicillin-resistant enterococcal
      endocarditis, 996
  for peritonitis, 938
  for peritonsillar abscess, 756
  for secondary peritonitis, 937t
Ampicillin-sulbactam
  dosage of, 650t-651t
  for cellulitis, 1180
  for pelvic inflammatory disease, 1379t
  for postoperative gynecologic infections, 1377t
  formulations of, 646t
Amplicon, in false-positive reactions, 215
Amprenavir, 1665t, 1667
  dosage of, 684t-685t
  formulations of, 649t
  pediatric, 1646t
  resistance to, 1668
  structure of, 1663f
Amyotrophic lateral sclerosis–like syndrome,
      in HIV infection, 1596, 1597t
Anabolic steroids, for weight loss, 145
Anaerobes
  collection and transport of, 205t
  definition of, 2811
  facultative, in secondary peritonitis, 933, 934,
      936-937
  in normal flora, 2811
  in susceptibility testing, 224
  obligate, in secondary peritonitis, 932, 933-
      934, 936-937
Anaerobic bacterial infections, 2810-2816
  anaerobe definition in, 2811
  antibiotic resistance in, 2816
  bacteremia in, 2813
  beta-lactamase production by, 256-257
  bone, 2813
  central nervous system, 2813, 2813f
  clinical manifestations of, 2812-2813, 2812f,
      2812t, 2813f
  diagnosis of, 2815
  endocarditis from, 992
      treatment of, 1000
  etiology of, 2811-2812
  from gram-negative bacilli, 2838-2845
      clinical manifestations of, 2840-2843
      colonization in, 2839
      facultative, laboratory identification of, 220-
          221
      immunity to, 2840
      microbiology of, 2839, 2839t
      pathogenesis of, 2839-2840
      treatment of, 2843-2845, 2844t
      virulence factors in, 2840, 2840t
  from gram-positive cocci, 2847-2849
      clinical isolates in, 2847-2848, 2848f
      taxonomy of, 2847
      treatment of, 2848-2849
      vancomycin for, 418
  from gram-positive nonsporulating bacilli,
      2849-2852
      clinical isolates in, 2850-2851
      normal flora and, 2850
      taxonomy in, 2849-2850, 2850f
      treatment of, 2851-2852
  intra-abdominal, 2812-2813, 2813f
  joint, 2813
  laboratory identification of, 221
  Melaney's gangrene from, 2812, 2812f
  metronidazole for, 393
  of mouth, head, neck, 2812

Anaerobic bacterial infections *(Continued)*
  organisms in, 2811, 2811t
  pathogenesis of, 2814-2815, 2814t
  pelvic, 2813
  penicillins for, 288t
  pleuropulmonary, 2812
  skin, 2813
  soft tissue, 2813
  treatment of, 367t, 2815-2816, 2815t
  virulence factors in, 2814, 2814t
Anal disease. *See under* Anus; Perianal.
Anal intraepithelial neoplasia, in HIV infection,
  1609
  treatment of, 1691t
Analgesics
  for herpes zoster ophthalmicus, 1403t
  for rheumatic fever, 2385, 2385t
  for urinary tract infections, 888
Anaphylactoid reactions, 65
Anaphylatoxin inactivator, 70t
Anaphylatoxins, 65, 76
Anaphylaxis, 65
  rifamycin and, 377
Anaplasma [spp.]
  characteristics of, 2311t, 2312
  classification and taxonomy of, 2284,
    2310-2312, 2311t
  vector of, 2285t
Anaplasma marginale, 2311, 2311t, 2312
Anaplasma phagocytophilum, 2311, 2311t, 2312
  Borrelia burgdorferi with, 2803
  characteristics of, 2311t, 2312
  human granulocytic anaplasmosis from, 2312-
    2313, 2315
  transmission of, 2312-2313
Anaplasma platys, 2311, 2311t, 2312
Anaplasmataceae, classification and taxonomy of,
  2310-2312, 2311t
Anaplasmosis. *See also* Ehrlichiosis.
  human granulocytic, 740, 2311-2313, 2311t,
    2315, 3312, 3313t, 3314
Ancylostoma braziliense, 3294t, 3295-3296
Ancylostoma caninum
  eosinophilic gastroenteritis from, 3294t, 3297
  treatment of, 571t
Ancylostoma duodenale, 3261t, 3264
  treatment of, 573t, 592
Anemia
  aplastic
    from chloramphenicol, 368-369
    hepatitis-associated, 1981, 1985
  from *Mycobacterium avium* complex, 2901,
    2901t
  from parvovirus B19, 1894, 1896
  hemolytic
    from cytomegalovirus, 1790
    from Epstein-Barr virus, 1806
    from sulfonamides, 442
  in endocarditis, 985
  in malaria, 3125, 3132
  iron deficiency, 142-143. *See also* Iron.
    from hookworm infections, 3264
  sickle cell. *See* Sickle cell disease/trait.
Aneurysms
  coronary artery, in Kawasaki disease, 3317,
    3318
  mycotic, 1005-1009. *See also* Mycotic
    aneurysms.
Angina
  Ludwig's, 754, 756, 793, 793f, 2841. *See also*
    Odontogenic infections.
    mediastinitis from, 1070
    treatment of, 793, 797, 797t
  Vincent's, 754, 756, 791, 2841

Angioedema
  complement replacement in, 88
  hereditary, C1 inhibitor deficiency in, 85
Angiogenesis inhibitors, for Kaposi's sarcoma,
  1604
Angiomatosis, bacillary. *See* Bacillary
  angiomatosis.
Angioplasty, percutaneous transluminal coronary,
  infections in, 1039-1040
Angiostrongyliasis, abdominal, 3294t, 3297
Angiostrongylus cantonensis
  meningitis from
    acute, 1088, 1101, 1105, 1115-1116, 1117
    chronic, 1138
    eosinophilic, 3294t, 3296
  treatment of, 577t
Angiostrongylus costaricensis, 3294t, 3297
  syndrome of abdominal pain, diarrhea, and
    eosinophilia from, 1281t, 1282
  treatment of, 577t
Angular cheilitis
  from *Candida,* 2941, 2951
  in HIV infection, 1554, 1555f
Anichkov myocytes, in rheumatic fever, 2381
Anidulafungin, 511
  for aspergillosis, 2968t, 2969
Animal(s). *See* Zoonosis(es) *and specific types.*
  rabies vaccine for, 2053
Animal bites, 3552-3553, 3552t, 3553t
  laboratory studies for, 213
  of head and neck, 800
  rabies from, 2050
Anisakiasis, 3294t, 3295
Anisakis marina
  syndrome of abdominal pain, diarrhea, and
    eosinophilia from, 1281t, 1282
  treatment of, 571t
Anogenital warts, 1341-1344, 1842-1843, 1845-
  1846, 1846f. *See also* Human
  papillomavirus(es).
  clinical features of, 1845-1847, 1846f
  diagnosis of, 847-848
  epidemiology of, 1842-1843
  pathogenesis of, 1843-1845
  prevention of, 1850
  treatment of, 848-1850
Anopheles spp., 3127-3128, 3128f
  alphavirus infections from, 1916
  malaria from, 3127-3128
Anorectal cancer, from human papillomavirus,
  1843, 1846
Anoscopy, in human papillomavirus infection,
  1847
Antacids
  metronidazole interactions with, 393t
  quinolones with, 458
Antagonism, drug, 274
  in combination antimicrobial therapy, 248-249
Anthrax, 2485-2490. *See also Bacillus anthracis.*
  antibiotic prophylaxis against, 2489
  as biological weapon, 2487, 2488, 3592-3593,
    3618-3623
    clinical presentation of, 3618-3620, 3619f
    diagnosis of, 3620-3621
    emergency preparedness for, 3621t
    environmental decontamination for, 3622-
      3623
    historical perspective on, 3618
      potential impact of, 3594
    incubation period for, 3618
    post-exposure prophylaxis for, 3621-3622,
      3623t
    staging of, 3618-3620, 3619f
    treatment of, 3621, 3622t

Anthrax *(Continued)*
  clinical manifestations of, 2486-2488
  cutaneous, 1176-1177, 1176f, 1177t, 2486,
    2487f, 3653f
    from bioterrorism, 3620, 3623t
    inguinal buboes in, 1208
    post-exposure prophylaxis for, 3623t
    treatment of, 2489-2490, 2490t
  disinfection/sterilization and, 3342
  epidemiology of, 2486
  gastrointestinal, 2486-2487, 2487f
    from bioterrorism, 3620
    vs. enteric fever, 1274t, 1277
  hemorrhagic meningoencephalitis in, 2488
  historical perspective on, 2485
  history in, 823t
  inhalational, 2487-2488
    clinical features of, 3619-3620
    from bioterrorism, 3619-3620
    hemorrhagic mediastinitis in, 1073
    staging of, 320t, 3619
    treatment of, 2489-2490, 2489t, 3621, 3622t
  isolation precautions for, 3329, 3330t
  meningitis from, 3618-3619, 3619f
  pathogenesis of, 2485-2486
  prevention of, 2488-2489
    post-exposure, 3621-3622, 3623t
    pre-exposure, 3622, 3623t
  treatment of, 2489-2490, 2489t
    with erythromycin, 401t
    with mupirocin, 485t
    with penicillins, 288t
    with quinolones, 464
    with sulfonamides, 441t
  vaccines for, 2488-2489, 3561-3562, 3562t,
    3622-3623, 3623t
Anthrax toxin, 27, 2485
Anthrax toxin receptor, 26
Antibacterial agents. *See* Antimicrobial agents.
Antibiotics. *See* Antimicrobial agents.
Antibody(ies), 52-67. *See also* B cell(s);
    Immunoglobulin(s).
  adherence inhibition by, 15, 15t
  affinity of, 53-54
  after pneumococcal vaccination, 2405-2406
  anticapsular, to *Streptococcus pneumoniae,*
    2396-2397
  antigen binding with, 53-54
  antigen-specific, 59
  anti-idiotypic, 63
  autoreactive, 59, 60, 64
  avidity of, 53-54
  blocking function of, 55
  circulating, in endocarditis, 981
  cleavage fragments of, 53, 54f
  cytotoxic, 319-320, 319t
  definition of, 52
  effector functions mediated by, 55-56, 56t
  functional, 57-59, 58f
  heart-reactive
    in myocarditis, 1054
    in rheumatic fever, 2381
  heavy chains of, 53, 53f
  in alternate pathway activation, 72-73
  in complement activation, 55, 71
  in endocarditis, 980-981
  in urinary tract infections, 880
  laboratory measurement of, 56-59, 58f
  light chains of, 52, 53f
  monoclonal. *See* Monoclonal antibodies.
  natural, 40-41
  neutralizing, 55
    in HIV infection, 1708-1709
    in HIV vaccine testing, 1714

Antibody(ies) (Continued)
  nomenclature for, 53, 54f
  opsonic, in streptococcal pyoderma, 2369
  preformed, in endocarditis, 980
  primary response of, 56, 57f
  production of, 56, 57f
    downregulation of, 63
  secondary response of, 56, 57f
  structure of, 52-53, 53f, 53t, 57, 58f
  therapeutic uses of, 66-67
  to fungi, 231-232
  to Legionella pneumophila, 2718, 2718t
Antibody-dependent cellular cytotoxicity, 56
Anticapsular antibody, to Streptococcus
    pneumoniae, 2396-2397
Anticoagulants
  for suppurative intracranial thrombosis, 1170
  rifamycin interaction with, 376t
  tetracycline with, 364t
Anticonvulsants
  for central nervous system infections, 1083
  for toxoplasmic encephalitis, 3189
  protease inhibitor interaction with, 1596-1597
  rifamycin interaction with, 376t
Anticytokine therapy
  for weight loss, 145
  infection risk in, 560
Antidepressants, for herpes zoster ophthalmicus,
    1403t
Antiepileptics. See Anticonvulsants.
Antifimbrial antibodies, in urinary tract
    infections, 880
Antifungal agents, 502-511. See also specific
    drugs.
  azole, 507-510
  dosage of, 678t-679t
  echinocandin, 510-511
  empiric, for febrile neutropenia, 3439
  for cancer-related febrile neutropenia, 3454-
    3455
  in prevention, 3445-3447, 3446f, 3447t
  formulations of, 649t
  prophylactic, for transplant recipients, 3482,
    3482t, 3483
  rifamycin interaction with, 376t
Antigen(s)
  from penicillins, 286, 287f
  measurement of, 59
  presentation, 37
  stimulation of, 60-61
  T-cell–independent, 62-63
Antigen binding, 53-54
  sites for, DNA rearrangement and, 60, 60f,
    60t
Antigen challenge, of humoral immunity, 154
Antigen detection, 214-215, 214t
  in coccidiodomycosis, 3046-3047
  in pneumonia, 828
Antigen presentation, 61-62, 132-133
  by CD1, 129-130
  MHC class I molecules in, 125, 125f
  to T cells, 125
Antigen processing
  by CD1, 129
  MHC class I pathway for, 126-127, 127f
  MHC class II pathway for, 127-128, 128f
  transporter associated with, 126
Antigenic variation, 8
Antigenicity, 168
Antigen-specific memory, 134
Anti-HB$_c$, 1871-1872, 1871f, 1878, 1878t,
    1879
Anti-HB$_e$, 1876, 1878-1879, 1878t
Anti-HB$_s$, 1871-1872, 1871f, 1878

Antihistamines
  for colds, 749-750
  for otitis media, 769
  for sinusitis, 780
Anti–human immunodeficiency virus antibody,
    serologic detection of, 1511-1512, 1511f,
    1512t
  false results in, 1513
Anti-immunoglobulins, 65
Anti-infectives, tetracycline with, 364t
Anti-inflammatory agents
  for meningitis, 1116
  for sepsis, 920-921
Anti-inflammatory response, 909
Antilymphocyte serums, for transplant
    immunosuppression, infections and, 3478-
    3479
Antimicrobial agents, 242-250. See also specific
    agent.
  adverse reactions to, 243
  age and, 243-244
  beta-lactam antibiotics. See Beta-lactam
    antibiotics.
  clinical trials for, 619-627
    goals for, 620-621
    interpretation of, 619-620, 620t
  commensal flora effects of, 40
  drug concentrations for, 888
  empiric
    for febrile neutropenia, 3439
    for immunocompromised host, 3439
  for febrile neutropenia
    for prevention, 3442-3444, 3443f-3445f,
      3451t2
    for treatment, 3450-3454, 3450t, 3451f,
      3453f, 3453t, 3454f, 3454t
  gastrointestinal flora effects on, 1217
  genetic abnormalities and, 244
  hepatic function and, 245
  host factors and, 243-247
  in combination, 247-249
    adverse effects of, 249
    antagonism from, 248-249, 274
    cost of, 249
    disadvantages of, 248-249
    efficacy of, 247, 247f
    for polymicrobial infections, 247
    indications for, 247
    resistance prevention with, 247
    synergism between, 248, 274
    toxicity of, 248
  in pregnancy, 244-245
  in renal insufficiency, 888-889
  in spinal cord injury, 3513
  indifference to, 274
  infections site and, 245-247
  interactions between
    antagonistic, 248-249, 274
    synergistic, 248, 274
  metabolic abnormalities and, 244
  mucosal injury from, 3424
  online resources for, 3661
  organism identification for, 242
  organism susceptibility to, 242-243
  outpatient parenteral, 629-632
    agent use in, 630-631, 630t
    devices in, 631
    infections amenable to, 629-630, 629t
    models of, 629, 629t
    monitoring in, 632
    patient selection for, 631-632, 631t, 632t
  P fimbriae in, 19
  pharmacodynamics of, 274-279. See also
    Pharmacodynamics.

Antimicrobial agents (Continued)
  pharmacokinetics of, 271-274. See also
    Pharmacokinetics.
  prophylactic
    for transplant recipients, 3482, 3482t
    preoperative, 3538-3544, 3543t
      cost-benefit analysis for, 3544
      novel approaches to, 3542
      regimens for, 3542, 3543t
      selection of, 3541
      side effects of, 3542-3544
      timing and duration of, 3541-3542
  renal function and, 245
  resistance to, 184-185
    auxotrophs in, 265
    biofilms in, 21-22
    by anaerobes, 2816
    cell wall precursor target alteration in, 264,
      264t
    control of, 265-266, 266f
    efflux promotion in, 262-263, 263t
    enzymatic inhibition in, 255-261
    enzymes in, 261-262, 261t
    genetics of, 253-255, 254f, 255f, 265-266
    integrons in, 255, 255f
    mechanisms of, 255-265, 256t-257t
    membrane permeability in, 262
    molecular mechanisms of, 253-266
    plasmids in, 253
    prevention of, 247, 615, 616
    ribosomal binding site alteration in, 263-264,
      263t
    surveillance for, 164
    target enzyme alteration in, 264-265
    target overproduction in, 265
    target site protection in, 265
    transposable genetic elements in, 253-255,
      254f
  susceptibility testing for, 222-224. See also
    Susceptibility testing.
  nosocomial infections and, 3324
  therapy with, 611-618
    administration route in, 249-250
    agent selection in, 242-247
    antibiotic rotation in, 616
    computer programs in, 614
    dosing regimens in, 250, 650t-675t
    educational programs in, 612
    formulary restriction in, 612-613
    funding for, 617
    homogeneity from, 615-616
    multidisciplinary approaches to, 614, 614f
    outcomes in, 614-615, 615t
    philosophy of, 611-612
    principles of, 242-250
    prior-approval programs in, 613
    program design for, 616-617, 616t, 617f
    resistance prevention in, 615, 616
    response monitoring in, 250
    restricted formulary in, 615-616
    strategies of, 612-614, 612t, 613f, 614f
    substitution and streamlining programs in,
      613-614
    usage diversity in, 613f
  tissue concentrations of, 888-889
  topical. See Topical antibacterial therapy.
  urinary concentration of, 888
Antimicrobial systems, oxygen-independent, 102
Antimony
  for visceral leishmaniasis, 3152
  pentavalent
    for American mucocutaneous leishmaniasis,
      3153
    for cutaneous leishmaniasis, 3153

Antimony *(Continued)*
for *Leishmania*, 591
in HIV infection, 1692t
for visceral leishmaniasis, 3152
Antimotility agents, for *Clostridium difficile*–associated colitis, 1258
Antimycobacterial agents, 489-499. *See also* Antituberculous agents.
for nontuberculous infections, 496-497
formulations of, 649t
Antiparasitics, 568-596
activity spectrum of, 568t-570t
adverse effects of, 581t-582t
Antipicornaviral drugs, 20t, 21
Antipruritics
for cholestasis, 383
for lice, 3303-3304
for mites, 3311
Antipyretics, 712-713
indications for, 714-715
response to, diagnostic implications of, 713-714
types of, 713
Antiretroviral therapy, 1655-1673
agents for, 1655-1669. *See also specific class or drug.*
anal dysplasia and, 1610
antibody responses in, 1510
CD4+ counts in, 1679
cervical cancer and, 1610
changing regimens in, 1671-1672
clinical impact of, 1550, 1551f, 1552
combination, 1670-1671
cryptococcal meningitis and, 3004
dosage of, 684t-685t
drug interactions in, 1680
entry inhibitors in, 20-21, 20t, 1668-1669, 1668t
for acute HIV infection, 1673
for acute HIV-1 infections, 1673
for AIDS dementia, 1586-1587
for cytomegalovirus, 1561
for gastroenteritis, 1241
for hepatitis B virus, 1577
for Kaposi's sarcoma, 1604
for opportunistic infections, 1679
for postexposure prophylaxis, 1672-1673
adverse reactions to, 3403
in pregnancy, 3403-3404
occupational, 3400-3405, 3402t, 3403t
formulations of, 649t
hepatitis C virus and, 1578
hepatotoxicity of, 1579, 1970
HIV replication in, 1533
HIV transmission effect of, 1489, 1494, 1619
Hodgkin's disease and, 1612
human papillomavirus and, 1629
immune reconstitution syndrome in, 1561, 2901
in cryptococcosis, 3004, 3007, 3008
in *Mycobacterium avium* complex infections, 2901, 2901f, 2902f
in toxoplasmosis, 3004, 3007, 3008
in perinatal HIV transmission suppression, 1621, 1622-1626, 1625t
in pregnancy, 1626-1627
in women, 1630
initiation of, 1669-1670
interleukin-2 in, 557
lymphadenopathy from, 1553
lymphoma effects of, 1605
neurotoxicity of, 1594, 1594t
non-nucleoside reverse transcriptase inhibitors in, 1661-1663, 1662t. *See also* Non-nucleoside reverse transcriptase inhibitors.

Antiretroviral therapy *(Continued)*
nucleoside reverse transcriptase inhibitors in, 1655-1661, 1656f, 1657t. *See also* Nucleoside reverse transcriptase inhibitors.
pediatric, 1646t-1648t, 1647-1649
perinatal prophylaxis with, 1639, 1640t
pharmacodynamics of, 278-279
primary central nervous system lymphoma and, 1607-1608
protease inhibitors in, 1663-1668, 1664f, 1665t. *See also* Protease inhibitors.
RNA assay monitoring during, 1669
with chemotherapy, for non-Hodgkin's lymphoma, 1606
with cryptococcal meningitis, 3004, 3007, 3008
with hepatitis C coinfection, 1970
Antiseizure agents. *See* Anticonvulsants.
Antiseptics
device-related infections and, 3356
in endocarditis prevention, 1045
topical. *See* Topical antibacterial therapy.
Antisera, microorganism identification by, 221
Antistreptolysin O, in rheumatic fever, 2382, 2384
Antithymocyte globulins, for transplant immunosuppression, infections and, 3478-3479
Antitoxin, 52
for botulism, 2826
for gas gangrene, 2834
Antituberculous agents, 489-494, 2867-2875. *See also specific agents.*
combination, 2868
course of, 2869
directly observed therapy with, 2868, 2868t
first-line agents in, 489-494, 490t
for multidrug resistant infections, 2869
in childhood, 2872
in HIV infection, 2870-2872, 2871t
in liver disease, 2872
in pericarditis, 1062
in pregnancy, 2872
in renal failure, 2872
mutational resistance in, 492t
regimens for, 2868-2869
four-drug, 2868, 2868t
in latent infections, 2872-2874, 2872t
three-drug, 2868
resistance to, 2867, 2867t
re-treatment with, 2869
second-line agents in, 494-496, 2868
treatment algorithm for, 2869, 2870f
with immunosuppressive drugs, 2872
Antivenin, 66
Antiviral agents, 514-542, 515t. *See also* Antiretroviral therapy *and specific agents.*
administration of, 516
dosage of, 680t-683t
for colds, 750
formulations of, 649t
immune response to, 514
mechanism of action of, 514, 1734-1735
prophylactic
for cancer patients, 3448
for transplant recipients, 3482, 3482t
resistance to, 238, 514, 516
Anus. *See also under* Perianal.
cancer of, 1610, 1611
disorders of, in HIV infection, 1610, 1691t
human papillomavirus of, 1691t
intraepithelial neoplasia of, in HIV infection, 1609
neoplasia of, 1610
in HIV infection, 1609
treatment of, 1691t

Aorta
abdominal, aneurysm of
mycotic, 1007-1008
secondary infections of, 1007
tuberculosis of, 2882-2883
Aortic valve, endocarditis of, 976, 977. *See also* Endocarditis.
Aphthous ulcers
esophageal, 1233, 1233t
in acute retroviral syndrome, 1552, 1553f
oral, 798. *See also* Ulcer(s), oral.
differential diagnosis of, 754, 756
in immunocompromised host, 798-799
in Marshall's syndrome, 1208
vs. herpetic pharyngitis, 756
vaginal, 1345
Apicomplexa spp., 3121-3122
Aplastic anemia
from chloramphenicol, 368-369
hepatitis-associated, 1981, 1985
Aplastic crisis, from parvovirus B19, 1894, 1896
Apnea, from respiratory syncytial virus, 2018-2019
Apodemus agrarius, hantavirus pulmonary syndrome from, 2086t, 2087-2089
Apoi virus, 1945t
Apollo disease, 1389
Apophysomyces spp., mucormycosis from, 2974, 2978
Apoptosis
by pathogens, 10
complement in, 76-77
Appendicitis, 968-970
actinomycotic, 2926-2927, 2928f
computed tomography of, 969-970, 970f
intraperitoneal abscess in, 943
pain in, 969, 970t
pinworms and, 3266
vs. primary peritonitis, 930
Appetite stimulants, 145
Ara-C, for progressive multifocal leukoencephalopathy, 1861
Arachidonic acid, 143, 143f
Arboviruses
collection of, 233t
in elderly, 3521
laboratory studies for, 235-236, 235t
meningitis from, 1085
Arcanobacterium [spp.], 2924
Arcanobacterium bernardiae, 2471
Arcanobacterium haemolyticum, 2470
pharyngitis from, 755, 756, 2365
Arcanobacterium pyogenes, 2470-2471
Arcobacter [spp.], 2548, 2549t
Arcobacter butzleri, 2548
Arcobacter skirrowi, 2548
ARDS. *See* Acute respiratory distress syndrome (ARDS).
Arenaviruses, 2090-2096, 2092t
characteristics of, 2091f, 2091t, 2092
clinical manifestations of, 2091t, 2094-2095
diagnosis of, 2095-2096
disinfection/sterilization and, 3342
epidemiology/epizootology of, 2091t, 2092-2094
isolation precautions for, 3330t
pathogenesis of, 2091t, 2094
prevention of, 2096, 3330t, 3342
treatment of, 2096
Argentine hemorrhagic fever, 2090-2096, 2091t. *See also* South American hemorrhagic fevers.
as biological weapon, 3627-3629, 3627t
Arginine vasopressin, antipyretic effects of, 710
Arizona spp., mycotic aneurysm from, 1008

ArlS, 2325
Arrhythmias
  erythromycin and, 400
  in endocarditis, 994
  in myocarditis, 1056
Artemether
  adverse effects of, 581t
  for malaria, 574t, 604t, 3134t, 3135, 3136
  for schistosomiasis, 3279
Artemisia annua, for malaria, 605, 605f
Artemisinin(s)
  for malaria, 586-587, 605, 3134t, 3135, 3136
  structure of, 606f
Artemisinin derivatives, 569t
Arterial blood gases, in peritonitis, 940
Arterial monitoring lines, infections of, 3355, 3356t
Arterial wall infections, 1006
Arteritis. *See also* Endarteritis.
  salmonellosis in, 2647t
  temporal
    empirical corticosteroids for, 725
    fever in, 725, 726-727
Artesunate
  adverse effects of, 581t
  for malaria, 573t, 578t, 3134t, 3135, 3136
Artesunic acid, 606f
Arthritis, 1311-1320. *See also* Arthropathy.
  bacterial, 1311-1316
    differential diagnosis of, 1315
    patient approach in, 1315
    predisposing factors in, 1311, 1311t
    treatment of, 1316, 1316f
  chronic infectious, 1317-1318, 1317t
  from *Actinomyces,* 2929
  from alphaviruses, 1916
  from anaerobic gram-negative bacilli, 2843
  from *Blastomyces dermatitidis,* 1318, 3033, 3033f
  from *Candida,* 1317-1318, 2946-2947, 2951
  from *Coccidioides immitis,* 1318, 3044
  from *Cryptococcus neoformans,* 1318
  from *Escherichia coli,* 1312, 1312t
  from *Haemophilus influenzae,* 1312, 1312t
  from *Histoplasma capsulatum,* 1318
  from HTLV, 2111
  from *Kingella kingae,* 1312, 1312t
  from lymphocytic choriomeningitis virus, 2095
  from mumps virus, 2005
  from *Mycoplasma pneumoniae,* 2275
  from nontuberculous mycobacteria, 2910t, 2912
  from parvovirus B19, 1894
  from *Pseudallescheria boydii,* 3068-3069
  from *Pseudomonas aeruginosa,* 1312, 1312t
  from rubella, 1922
  from *Scedosporium prolificans,* 3069, 3069f
  from *Sporothrix schenckii,* 1318, 2985, 2985f, 2986, 2987
  from *Staphylococcus aureus,* 1312, 1312t, 2347
  from *Streptococcus* [spp.], 1312, 1312t
  from *Streptococcus agalactiae* (group B), 2427
  from streptococcus group C, 2443
  from streptococcus group G, 2443
  fungal, 1317-1319
  gonococcal, 1313-1315
    clinical features of, 1314-1315, 1315f
    disseminated, 2522
    pathogenesis of, 1314
  in elderly, 3521
  in injection drug users, 3464-3465
  in Lyme disease, 35, 2800, 2805
  in Reiter's syndrome, 1354-1355, 2247-2248
  in rheumatic fever, 2383
  infectious, 1311-1320
  juvenile rheumatoid, fever in, 727

Arthritis *(Continued)*
  Lyme. *See* Lyme disease.
  mycobacterial, 1319
  nongonococcal, 1311-1313
    clinical features of, 1312t, 1313, 1313f
    epidemiology of, 1312t
    imaging of, 1313, 1314f
    microbiology of, 1312, 1312t
    pathophysiology of, 1311-1312
  poststreptococcal, 2383
  quinolones for, 463
  reactive, 1354-1355, 2247-2248
    from *Chlamydia trachomatis,* 1354-1355, 2247-2248
    urethritis and, 1354-1355, 1414, 2247-2248
    uveitis and, 1354-1355, 1414
  rheumatoid, pleural effusion and, 847, 849
  septic, 1311-1316
  sternoclavicular, from *Pseudomonas aeruginosa,* 2603
  viral, 1316-1317, 1316f
Arthrobacter spp., 2471
Arthroderma spp., 3052
Arthropathy. *See also* Arthritis.
  from parvovirus B19, 1894
  from quinolones, 466
  in Whipple's disease, 1308
  reactive, 35
Arthropods, 3301-3302
  diseases transmitted by, 3301t
Arthus reaction, 319t, 320
Artificial heart, infections of, 1035
Arua virus, 1913-1919, 1914t
Ascariasis, 3260-3263, 3261f, 3261t, 3262f, 3264
  acute pancreatitis in, 959, 959t
  biliary tract infections in, 956
  pulmonary infiltrates with eosinophilia in, 835
  syndrome of abdominal pain, diarrhea, and eosinophilia in, 1281-1282, 1281t
  treatment of, 571t, 592, 594
Aschoff nodule, in rheumatic fever, 2381
Ascites, peritonitis in, 929. *See also* Peritonitis.
Ascorbic acid, 141-142
Aseptic meningitis, 16-17, 1084-1085, 1101, 2148-2149. *See also* Meningitis, from viruses.
Asia, HIV infection in, 1468-1469, 1468f, 1469f
  among women, 1618
Aspergillomas, 2962-2963
Aspergillus [spp.], 229, 2958-2970
  acute pancreatitis from, 959, 959t
  allergic bronchopulmonary, 2962, 2963t
    in cystic fibrosis, 871-872, 873
  allergic responses to, 1963t, 2962
  antimicrobial therapy for, 504, 505, 506, 508, 510, 511
  appearance of, in tissue, 2936f, 2938t, 2959-2960, 2959f-2960f
  brain abscess from, 1152, 1155, 1157, 1158t, 1160
  cardiovascular device infections from, 1023
  characteristics of, 2958-2960, 2958t
  chest film in, 866f
  chronic granulomatous disease from, 155, 156
  clinical manifestations of, 2962-2966
  culture of, 2958-2959, 2959f-2960f, 2966-2967
  diagnosis of, 2966-2967
  direct detection of, 230
  disseminated, 2963-2966, 2964f
  empyema from, 2963
  endocarditis from, 993
    prosthetic valve, 1030
    treatment of, 1001
  endophthalmitis from, 1409, 1411
  epidemiology of, 2960-2961
  fungus balls from, 2962-2963

Aspergillus [spp.] *(Continued)*
  identification of, 2966-2967
  immune response to, 2961-2962
  in cancer patients, 3436
    prevention of, 3446-3447
  in dialysis patients, 941
  in HIV infection, 1699
  in transplant recipients, 2960-2961, 2961f, 3495-3496, 3507
  invasive, 2963-2966
  isolation of, 231
  keratitis from, 1404
  mortality in, 2967, 2967t
  mycotic aneurysm from, 993
  myocarditis from, 1053
  of bone, 2966, 2966f
  of central nervous system, 1152, 1155, 1157, 1158t, 1160
    in immunocompromised host, 3437-3438, 3507
  of ear, 766, 2963
  of eye, 1404, 1409, 1411, 2963, 2966
    in injection drug users, 3472
  of gastrointestinal tract, 2966
  of heart, 993, 1001, 1030, 1053, 1059, 2966
  of lung
    chronic, 2963
    invasive, 2963-2964, 2964f, 2966-2967
  of nails, 2963, 3060
  of sinuses, 2964-2965, 3070-3071
  of skin, 2966, 2966f
  outcome in, 2967, 2967t
  pathogenesis of, 2961-2962
  pathogenicity of, 2961-2962
  pericarditis from, 1059
  prevention of, 2969-27970
  risk factors for, 2960-2961
  saprophytic colonization by, 2962-2963
  sclerosing mediastinitis from, 1075
  sinusitis from, 777, 777t, 778, 2962, 2964-2965
  splenic abscess from, 967, 967t
  superficial, 2962-2963
  susceptibility testing for, 2966
  toxins produced by, 2962
  tracheobronchitis from, 2964
  transmission of, 2961
  treatment of, 2967-2969, 2968t
Aspergillus amstelodami, 2958, 2960
Aspergillus flavus, characteristics of, 2958-2959, 2958t, 2959f
Aspergillus fumigatus
  characteristics of, 2958-2959, 2958t, 2959f
  in peritoneal dialysis, 941
  pathogenicity of, 2962
  pneumonia from
    chest film in, 866f
    in chronic granulomatous disease, 155, 156f
    in cystic fibrosis, 871-872, 873
    in HIV infection, 1571
Aspergillus nidulans, 2958, 2960
  chronic granulomatous disease from, 156
Aspergillus niger, characteristics of, 2958, 2958t, 2959-2960, 2960f
Aspergillus terreus
  antimicrobial resistance of, 2967
  characteristics of, 2958, 2958t, 2959-2960, 2960f
  chest film in, 866f
Aspiration. *See also* Drainage.
  of amebic liver abscess, 3106
  of vitreous, 1409, 1410, 1410f
  sinus
    in acute sinusitis, 776, 776t
    in chronic sinusitis, 781, 782t
  specimen collection and transport in, 206t
  transtracheal, for sputum collection, 826

Aspiration pneumonia, 834-835. *See also* Pneumonia, nosocomial.
  chest film in, 829
  from anaerobic infections, 2812
  lung abscess and, 853-856
Aspirin
  for fever, 713
  for Kawasaki disease, 3318
  for rheumatic fever, 2385, 2385t
Asplenia, 3524-3530
  antimicrobial prophylaxis in, 3529
  associated pathogens of, 3421t
  babesiosis and, 3528
  bartonellosis and, 3528
  causes of, 3524, 3524t
  congenital, 3525
  diagnosis of, 3525-3526, 3525f
  ehrlichiosis and, 3528
  evaluation in, 3525-3526
  HIV infection and, 3528
  immunization and, 3529-3530, 3530t, 3644
  malaria and, 3528
  postoperative infections and, 3528
  postsplenectomy sepsis and, 734, 3526-3528, 3526f-3528f, 3526t, 3530
  sepsis and, 734
  spleen-sparing therapy and, 3530
Asthma, 815
  bronchial, eosophils in, 110-111
  bronchiolitis and, 815, 816
  from human metapneumovirus, 2028-2029, 2028t, 2029t
  from rhinoviruses, 2190
  hepatitis A and, 2172
  infectious. *See* Bronchiolitis.
Asthmatic bronchitis. *See* Bronchiolitis.
Astrakhan fever, 2287t
Astroviruses, 2201-2202
  gastrointestinal infections from, 1239, 1239t
  laboratory studies for, 235
Ataxia-telangiectasia, 150t
  immunodeficiency in, 66
  T-cell function in, 153
Atazanavir, 1663f, 1665t, 1667
  dosage of, 684t-685t
  pediatric, 1646t
Atherosclerosis
  from *Chlamydia pneumoniae,* 2263-2266, 2264t
  mycotic aneurysms in, 1006
Athlete's foot (tinea pedis), 3054.
Atopobium spp., 2850
Atovaquone
  adverse effects of, 581t
  for babesiosis, 571t, 3213
  for brain abscess, 1159t
  for malaria, 587
  for *Pneumocystis jirovecii,* 575t, 1681t, 1683t, 1685t, 1693, 1695, 3088
    for prophylaxis, 3447, 3447t
  for toxoplasmosis, 1682t, 1683t, 1685t
    in immunocompromised host, 3189, 3189t, 3190
  indications for, 569t
  structure of, 587f
Atovaquone-proguanil, 587
  for malaria, 573t, 574t, 578t, 3129, 3133, 3134t, 3135
    for prophylaxis, 3137-3138, 3137t
      for travelers, 3641-3642, 3641t
    resistance to, 3129. *See also* Malaria, drug-resistant.
  indications for, 569t
Atrioventricular valves, in endocarditis, 981
Atrophic vaginitis, 1369

Attachment inhibitors, 20
Atypical pneumonia. *See* Pneumonia, atypical.
Auchmeromyia senegalensis, myiasis from, 3308-3310, 3308t
Aum Shinrikyo cult, 3591, 3624
Aura virus, 1913-1919, 1914t. *See also* Alphaviruses.
Australian bat lyssavirus, 2047t
  laboratory studies for, 238
Autoantibodies, in systemic lupus erythematosus, 79
Autoclaves, 3338. *See also* Sterilization.
Autoimmune hepatitis, 1436
Autoimmune uveitis, 1414
Autoimmunity, 65
Autolysin, from *Streptococcus pneumoniae,* 2396, 2396t
Autolysis-related locus sensor, 2325
Autonomic nervous system, in sepsis, 915
Autotransporters, in toxin secretion, 26
Auxotrophs, in antibiotic resistance, 265
Avascular necrosis, in HIV infection, 1556
Avian pneumovirus, 2026-2027, 2027f
Avihepadnaviruses, 1864
Axetil, 305, 305t
Axillary lymphadenitis, 1205. *See also* Lymphadenitis/lymphadenopathy.
Axillary temperature, 704-705. *See also* Temperature.
Azathioprine
  for transplant immunosuppression, infections and, 3478
  in cytomegalovirus reactivation, 1794-1795
Azelaic acid, 484t
Azithromycin, 402-406
  adverse reactions to, 404
  antimicrobial activity of, 402-403
  chemistry of, 402, 403f
  dosage of, 664t-665t
  drug interactions with, 400t, 404, 687t
  for babesiosis, 571t, 3213
  for bacillary angiomatosis, 1185
  for *Bartonella,* 1691t
  for *Bordetella pertussis,* 2706
  for brain abscess, 1159t
  for *Campylobacter jejuni,* 1689t
  for chancroid, 1344
  for *Chlamydia trachomatis,* 2525
  for chlamydial pneumonia, 2263
    atherosclerosis after, 2265
  for COPD exacerbations, 811, 811t
  for cryptosporidiosis, 3222
  for experimental endocarditis, 1048
  for *Haemophilus ducreyi,* 2667
  for *Legionella pneumophila,* 2719t
  for meningitis, 1118
  for *Mycobacterium avium* complex, 1682t, 1683t, 1687t, 1700, 2903-2906, 2904t
    for prophylaxis, 2906
  for *Mycoplasma pneumoniae,* 2278
  for *Neisseria gonorrhoeae,* 2524t, 2525
  for neonatal conjunctivitis, 2247t
  for pneumonia, 837-839, 837t, 838t
  for protozoa, 589
  for pulmonary infections, in cystic fibrosis, 872
  for respiratory infections, 462
  for scrub typhus, 2310
  for *Shigella,* 1689t, 2659t
  for streptococcal pharyngitis, 2368
  for syphilis, 1344
  for *Toxoplasma,* in immunocompromised host, 3189, 3189t
  for *Toxoplasma* encephalitis, 1587
  for trachoma, 2244
  for traveler's diarrhea, 1243

Azithromycin *(Continued)*
  for urethritis, 1207
  for urogenital chlamydial infections, 2247t, 2249
  formulations of, 648t
  in vitro susceptibilities to, 397t
  mechanism of action of, 402
  pharmacology of, 403-404
  resistance to, 402
    pneumococcal, 837, 837t
  uses of, 404-406
Azlocillin, 292, 292f
  dosage of, 650t-651t
  for anaerobes, 284t
  for bacilli, 284t
  for Enterobacteriaceae, 284t
  for peritonitis, 938
  for *Pseudomonas,* 284t
  formulations of, 646t
  minimal inhibitory concentration of, 284t
Azoles, 507-510. *See also specific agents.*
Azotemia, amphotericin B deoxycholate and, 503-504
Aztreonam, 314-315
  antibacterial activity of, 314, 315t
  dosage of, 658t-659t
  drug interactions with, 687t
  for acute pyelonephritis, 889
  for bacterial arthritis, 1316t
  for brain abscess, 1159t
  for meningitis, 1106t, 1107t, 1114
  for peritonitis, 939
  for *Pseudomonas aeruginosa* bacteremia, 2601
  for secondary peritonitis, 937t
  formulations of, 648t
  resistance to, beta-lactamases in, 256, 258t
  structure of, 314, 314f
Azuricidin, 102

B

B cell(s). *See also* Lymphocyte(s).
  antibody production by, 59-64
  antigen-activated, 61-62
  autoreactive antibody production by, 60
  defects in, 66, 153-154
  DNA rearrangement in, 60, 60f
  dysregulation of, in HIV infection, 1536
  Epstein-Barr virus in, 1802-1803. *See also* Epstein-Barr virus.
  in conjugate vaccines, 62, 63f
  in immunodeficiency, 150t
  in primary immune response, 56, 57f
  in T-cell defects, 152-153, 153t
  lymph node entry of, 121
  pulmonary, 821
  signals for, 60-61, 62f
  surface molecules of, 60, 61t
  T cell activation by, 61-62, 63f
  T cell interactions with, 61, 62f
  T cell–independent antigens and, 63-64
  Toll-like receptor distribution in, 38, 39t
B cell coreceptor complex, 61
B cell follicles, 120, 121f
B cell lymphoma. *See also* Lymphoma.
  chronic hepatitis C and, 1456
  HIV-related, 2130
B cell receptor, 61
B1 cells, 63-64
B7 molecules, 61t
  in T cell activation, 62
Babanki virus, 1914-1919
Babesia [spp.], 568. *See also* Babesiosis.
  complement receptors and, 78
  specimen collection and transport in, 205t

Babesia [spp.] *(Continued)*
    treatment of, 571t, 577t
    vs. enteric fever, 1275t
Babesia bigemina, 3209
Babesia divergens, 3209, 3211
Babesia microti, 3209
    antimicrobial therapy for, 401t, 405-406
    Borrelia burgdorferi with, 2803
    classification of, 3211
    host range of, 3211
    morphology of, 3211
    tick-host interactions and, 3210-3211, 3210f
    transmission of, 3210-3211, 3210f
Babesiosis, 3209-3214
    clinical features of, 3212
    diagnosis of, 3213, 3213f
    etiology of, 3209-3210
    historical perspective on, 3209
    pathogenesis of, 3212-3213
    pathogen-host interactions in, 3210-3211,
        3210f
    postsplenectomy, 3528
    prevention of, 3214
    transmission of, 3210-3211, 3210f
    treatment of, 3213-3214
Bacampicillin
    dosage of, 650t-651t
    formulations of, 646t
Bacillary angiomatosis, 739-740
    cutaneous, 2735, 2735f
    from *Bartonella,* 2735-2736, 2735f-2737f
    histology of, 2736, 2737f
    in HIV infection, 1185, 1557
    internal, 2735, 2736f
Bacille Calmette-Guérin vaccine, 2320, 2875,
    3562, 3562t
    parenteral exposure through, 123
Bacillus [spp.], 2493-2495
    adherence of, 2494
    central nervous system infections from, 2495
    commercial uses of, 2494
    contamination by, 2493
    endocarditis from, 992
    epidemiology of, 2493
    eye infections from, 2495
    food poisoning from, 2494, 2495
    laboratory identification of, 218, 219t
    microbiology of, 2493
    muscle infections from, 2495
    pseudoinfections from, 2493
    soft tissue infections from, 2495
    systemic infections from, 2494-2495, 2495t
    toxins of, 2494
    treatment of, 2495
        with daptomycin, 428
        with linezolid, 437, 437t
        with quinolones, 456t
        with quinupristin-dalfopristin, 425
        with vancomycin, 418, 2495
Bacillus anthracis, 2485-2490, 2493. *See also*
    Anthrax.
    chancriform lesions from, 1176-1177, 1176f,
        1177t
    disinfection/sterilization and, 3342
    drug-resistant, 2490
    edema factor of, 2485, 2486
    evolution of, 6
    hemorrhagic meningoencephalitis from, 2488
    history of, 2485
    immunization for, 3561-3562, 3562t
    isolation precautions for, 3329, 3330t
    laboratory detection of, 213-214, 218
    lethal factor of, 2485
    mediastinitis from, 1073
    meningitis from, 2490

Bacillus anthracis (Continued)
    microbiology of, 2485-2486
    plasmid-encoded, 6t
    toxins of, 27, 2485
    virulence factors of, 2485
Bacillus badius, 2493
Bacillus cereus, 2493, 2495t
    endophthalmitis from, 1408-1411
    foodborne disease from, 1219, 1287-1288,
        1291, 1294, 1294t, 2494
    in pathogenic studies, 10
    keratitis from, 1398-1400
    noninflammatory diarrhea from, 1239
    skin infections from, 1184
Bacillus circulans, 2495t
Bacillus licheniformis, 2493, 2495t
    food poisoning from, 2494
Bacillus megaterium, 2493, 2495t
Bacillus mycoides, 2493
Bacillus pumilus, 2493
    cardiac occlusion device infections from, 1036
    clinical manifestations of, 2495t
    food poisoning from, 2494
    in meningococcus immunity, 2501
Bacillus sphaericus, 2493, 2495t
Bacillus stearothermophilus, 2493
Bacillus subtilis, 2493
    clinical manifestations of, 2495t
    food poisoning from, 2494
    mupirocin for, 485t
    Staphylococcus aureus and, 2321, 2332
Bacillus thuringiensis, 2493
Bacitracin, 484, 484t
    drug interactions with, 687t
    for *Clostridium difficile*–associated colitis,
        1257-1258, 1258t
    prophylactic
        for wound infections, 480
        intravascular devices and, 3356
    streptococcal group G sensitivity to, 2442
Bacitracin (A) disk, 216t
Bacterascites, in primary peritonitis, 929
Bacteremia, 906t. *See also* Septicemia.
    after invasive nonsurgical cardiologic
        procedures, 1039-1040
    Bartonella, 739-740
    catheter-related, 209-210, 2618. *See also*
        Catheter-related infections.
    definition of, 906t
    from *Acinetobacter,* 2634
    from *Aeromonas,* 2754
    from anaerobic infections, 2813, 2842
    from *Bacillus,* 2494
    from *Bacteroides fragilis,* 2842
    from *Campylobacter jejuni,* 2552
    from *Clostridium,* 2929-2830
    from *Clostridium perfringens,* 2830
    from *Clostridium septicum,* 2830, 2929
    from *Clostridium tertium,* 2830
    from coagulase-negative *Staphylococcus* spp.,
        pediatric, 2357
    from dental procedures, 1045-1046, 1046t
    from *Enterococcus,* 2412-2413
    from *Erysipelothrix rhusiopathiae,* 2497-2498
    from *Kingella,* 2534
    from *Listeria monocytogenes,* 2481
    from *Moraxella (Branhamella) catarrhalis,*
        2531
    from mucositis, laboratory diagnosis of, 3428
    from *Neisseria meningitidis,* 2502
    from non-bacilliformis *Bartonella,* 2734-2735
    from nontypeable *Haemophilus influenzae,*
        2663
    from nutritionally variant streptococci, 2441
    from *Pseudomonas aeruginosa,* 2598-2600

Bacteremia *(Continued)*
    ecthyma gangrenosum in, 2600, 2600f
    treatment of, 2600-2601
    from *Salmonella,* 2646
        in HIV infection, 2649-2650
    from *Staphylococcus aureus,* 2342
    from *Staphylococcus epidermidis,* in
        immunocompromise, 2356
    from *Streptococcus agalactiae* (group B), 2441
    from *Streptococcus anginosus* group, 2454
    from streptococcus group C, 2444-2445
    from streptococcus group G, 2445
    from *Streptococcus pyogenes* (group A), 2375
    from type b *Haemophilus influenzae,* 2664
    from viridans streptococci, 2436, 2437, 2438
    in children, fever in, 713, 724
    in cirrhosis, 929
    in complement deficiency, 158
    in disseminated gonococcal infections, 2522-
        2523
    in elderly, 3520
    in hypotension, 913-914
    in immunocompromised host, 3432-3434
    in multiorgan dysfunction, 913-914
    in primary peritonitis, 929
    in staphylococcal endocarditis, 999
    in suppurative thrombophlebitis, 1004
    in transplant recipients, 3506
    incidence of, 978t
    intravascular device-related, 3347-3358. *See*
        also specific devices.
    nosocomial
        from coagulase-negative staphylococci,
            2353-2354
        from *Staphylococcus aureus,* 2342
    pseudomonal, 736
    subcutaneous abscess in, 1191
    surgical procedures and, 1046, 1047b
    transient, in endocarditis, 977-978, 978t
    treatment of, with quinolones, 464-465
    vs. malaria, 3132
Bacteria
    antibody neutralization of, 55
    biochemical tests for, 216t
    cell wall of, 281-282, 282f
    classification of, 2319
    clonal organization and, 5
    collection and transport of, 205t, 206t, 207t
    commensal. *See also* Microbial flora.
        in bacteremia, 913
    evolution of, 2320
    extracellular replication of, 123
    host defense avoidance by, 102-103
    intracellular, 122-123
    microaerophilic, 2811
    therapeutic use of, 2320
    translocation of, in primary peritonitis, 929
Bacterial antigen tests, in central nervous system
    infections, 211
Bacterial endocarditis. *See* Infective endocarditis.
Bacterial flora. *See* Microbial flora.
Bacterial infections, 2320
    antibiotic resistance in, 253-266. *See also*
        Antimicrobial agents, resistance to.
    arthritis from, 1311-1316, 1311t, 1312t, 1316t
    complement deficiency and, 81
    endocarditis from, 992
    enteric, in primary peritonitis, 929-930
    genital tract, 212
    in diarrhea, 212
    in pediatric HIV infection, 1641
    in pericarditis, 1059, 1059t
    in vaginitis, 212
    mechanism of, 2319, 2319t
    neutropenia in, 154

Bacterial infections *(Continued)*
  polymorphism and, 2319-2320
  respiratory, 175
    diagnosis of, 209t
  time course in, 2319, 2320t
  urinary tract, 881-882
  variation in, 2319
  vs. enteric fever, 1274t
Bacterial lipopolysaccharide
  in bacterial sepsis, 712, 714
  in febrile response, 708, 710, 711
Bacterial overgrowth syndrome, 1226, 1243-1244
Bacterial tracheitis, 764
Bacterial vaginosis, 1365-1367, 1366f, 1366t
  anaerobic, 2813
  clue cells in, 1360
  from gram-negative bacilli, 2842
  in HIV infection, 1628
  laboratory studies for, 212
  pelvic inflammatory disease and, 1378
Bactericidal activity, testing for, 223
Bactericidal mechanisms, oxygen-dependent,
  101-102
Bactericidal titration (test), serum, 223
Bactericidal/permeability-increasing protein, for
  meningitis, 1116
Bacteriophages, in virulence-associate gene
  exchange, 5
Bacteriuria. *See also* Urinary tract infections.
  antimicrobial therapy for, 889
  asymptomatic, 891
  catheterization and, 883
  definitions in, 875
  epidemiology of, 883
  gestational, 892-893
  in elderly, 883, 887, 3517-3518
  in hypertension, 887
  in spinal cord injury, 3513-3514
  nosocomial, 883, 887
  pediatric, 882-883, 882f
    recurrent, 477
  treatment of, 887-888
  true, 885
Bacteroides [spp.], 2811
  antibiotic resistance of, 390, 2815, 2844-2845
  antimicrobial therapy for
    quinolones in, 456t
    tetracyclines in, 360t
  biliary tract infections from, 956
  diverticulitis from, 972
  in colon, 2839
  mediastinitis from, 1072
  peritonitis from
    primary, 929
    secondary, 932, 933
    treatment of, 938
  suppurative thrombophlebitis from, 1004
  virulence factors of, 2840, 2840t
Bacteroides distasonis, metronidazole for, 389t
Bacteroides forsythus, odontogenic infections
  from, 788, 788f
Bacteroides fragilis, 2811-2812
  antimicrobial therapy for, 2843-2844, 2844,
    2844t
    aminoglycosides in, 334t-335t
    azithromycin in, 397t
    carbapenems in, 313t
    cephalosporins in, 298t, 937
    chloramphenicol in, 367t
    clarithromycin in, 397t
    clindamycin in, 409t, 937
    erythromycin in, 397t, 398
    mupirocin in, 485t
    penicillins in, 284t, 288t, 938
    quinolones in, 456t

Bacteroides fragilis (Continued)
    telithromycin in, 397t
    trimethoprim in, 444t
  appendicitis from, 969
  bacteremia from, 2842
  beta-lactamase production by, 256-257
  Bft toxin of, 1221
  brain abscess from, 1153, 1154, 1157, 1158t
  empyema from, 846
  endocarditis from, 992, 2843
    treatment of, 1000
  enterotoxigenic, 29
  immunity to, 2840
  intra-abdominal infections from, 2841-2842
  lipopolysaccharide of, 2814
  microbiology of, 2839, 2839t
  mycotic aneurysm from, 1008
  pathogenesis of, 2814, 2814t
  secondary peritonitis from, 936, 937
    treatment of, 389t, 937, 938, 939
  typhlitis from, 973
  virulence factors of, 2814, 2814t, 2840, 2840t
Bacteroides melaninogenicus, clindamycin for,
  409t
Bacteroides oralis, endocarditis from, 992
Bacteroides ovatus
  metronidazole for, 389t
  virulence factors of, 2840, 2840t
Bacteroides theataiotaomicron, metronidazole for,
  389t
Bacteroides vulgatus, metronidazole for, 389t
Balamuthia mandrillaris, 3111-3119. *See also*
  Granulomatous amebic encephalitis.
  characteristics of, 3112, 3113f
  treatment of, 577t
Balanitis
  from *Candida,* 2943
  in Reiter's syndrome, 1354-1355
Balantidiasis, 3232-3233, 3233f
Balantidium coli, 3232-3233, 3233f
  dysentery from, 1266
  treatment of, 571t
    antiparasitics in, 568t-569t
    metronidazole in, 393
Balloon pump, intra-aortic, infections of, 1039
Balyisascaris procyonis, 3294, 3294t
  ocular infections from, 3295
  visceral infections from, 3294, 3294t, 3295
Bancroftian filariasis, 3270-3272, 3270f-3272f
  lymphangitis in, 1208, 1212, 3271, 3271f
Banna virus, 1900
Banzi virus, 1945t
Barbiturates
  for intracranial hypertension, 1117
  tetracycline with, 364t
Barchiola (Nosema) algerae, keratitis from, 1405
Bare lymphocyte syndrome, 125
Barmah Forest virus, 238, 1913-1919, 1914,
  1914t. *See also* Alphaviruses.
Barotrauma, hyperbaric oxygen and, 564
Bartholinitis, from *Chlamydia trachomatis,* 2248
Bartonella [spp.], 739-740, 2733-2744
  antimicrobial susceptibility testing for, 2742-2743
  blood culture of, 210, 210t
  cardiovascular device infections from, 1023
  classification of, 2284, 2733, 2733t
  clinical manifestations of, 2733-2740
  collection and transport of, 205t
  culture of, 2741-2742
  direct examination of, 2741
  epidemiology of, 2733
  identification of, 2742, 2742f, 2743t
  in HIV infection
    bacillary angiomatosis from, 2735-2736,
      2735f, 2736f

Bartonella [spp.] *(Continued)*
    bacteremia from, 2734
    treatment of, 1691t-1692t, 1702
  laboratory diagnosis of, 221, 2741-2744
  pathogenesis of, 2740-2741
  polymerase chain reaction assay for, 2743
  postsplenectomy, 3528
  prosthetic valve endocarditis from, 1026
  serologic testing of, 2743-2744
  skin lesions from, 739-740
  treatment of, 2744
Bartonella bacilliformis, 739-740, 2733, 3653t
  identification of, 2742, 2743t
  Oroya fever from, 2733-2734
  pathogenesis of, 2741
  postsplenctomy, 3528
  prevention of, 2744
  treatment of, 2744
  verruga peruana from, 2733-2734, 2734f
  vs. enteric fever, 1274t, 1277
Bartonella clarridgeiae, 739-740
  cat-scratch disease from, 2736
  epidemiology of, 2733
  identification of, 2742, 2743t
  prevention of, 2744
Bartonella elizabethae
  bacteremia from, 2734
  epidemiology of, 2733
  identification of, 2742, 2743t
Bartonella henselae, 739-740
  antimicrobial susceptibility testing for, 2742
  azithromycin for, 401t
  bacillary angiomatosis from, 1185, 2735-2736,
    2736f
  bacillary peliosis from, 2736
  bacteremia from, 2734
  Borrelia burgdorferi coinfection with, 2739
  cat-scratch disease from, 1207, 1211, 2736-2740,
    2737f-2740f. *See also* Cat-scratch disease.
  culture of, 2741, 2742, 2742f
  epidemiology of, 2733
  erythromycin for, 401t
  identification of, 2742, 2743t
  in HIV infection, 1702, 2740
  Parinaud's oculoglandular syndrome from,
    1207, 1391
  pathogenesis of, 2740-2741
  postsplenectomy, 3528
  prevention of, 2744
  serologic testing for, 2743
  skin lesions from, 739-740
  splenic abscess from, 967, 967t
  treatment of, 2744
  uveitis from, 1417, 1417f
Bartonella koehlerae, 2733
Bartonella quintana, 739-740, 2733
  antimicrobial susceptibility testing for, 2742-
    2743
  bacillary angiomatosis from, 1185, 2735-2736
  bacillary peliosis from, 2736
  bacteremia from, 2734
  culture of, 2742
  identification of, 2742, 2743t
  in HIV infection, 1702
  pathogenesis of, 2741
  prevention of, 2744
  serologic testing for, 2743
  treatment of, 401t, 2744
  trench fever from, 2734
Bartonella vinsonii, bacteremia from, 2735
Basidiobolomycosis, 2974t, 2980-2981
Basilar skull fractures, cerebrospinal fluid leak in
  chemoprophylaxis for, 1103
  radiography of, 1103
  surgery for, 1117

Bathing, for fever, 713, 714, 715
Bats, *Histoplasma capsulatum* and, 3013-3014
Baylisascaris procyonis
  meningitis from, 1088
  treatment of, 577t
Bcg, in tuberculosis immunity, 2860
Bebaru virus, 1913-1919, 1914t. *See also* Alphaviruses.
Bedpans, decontamination of, 3333
Beef tapeworm, 3286t, 3288. *See also*
  Tapeworms.
Behçet's disease
  meningitis in, 1139
  vaginal aphthous ulcers in, 1345
Bejel, 2787
Bell's palsy, 1766
Benzathine penicillin. *See* Penicillin G.
Benznidazole
  adverse effects of, 581t
  for trypanosomiasis, 569t, 576t, 591, 3162
  in HIV infection, 1692t
Benzodiazepines, for tetanus, 2820
Benzonatate, for chronic obstructive pulmonary
  disease, 810t
Benzoyl peroxide, 484t
  for acne vulgaris, 483
Bergeyella spp., 2751t, 2762
Berne virus, 1990
Beta-carotene, in lung cancer prevention, 141
Beta-lactam antibiotics, 311-317
  allergy to, 318-325
    classification of, 318-320, 319f, 319t, 320t
    clinical manifestations of, 320, 320t
    diagnosis of, 322-323
    idiopathic, 320
    Levine's classification of, 320, 320t
    major determinants in, 320
    minor determinants in, 322
    risk factors for, 322
  combination, 249
  cross-reactivity among, 324-325
  desensitization to, 323-324, 324t
  development of, 257
  dosage of, 658t-659t
  for *Bacillus,* 2495
  for *Mycobacterium tuberculosis,* 496
  for nontuberculous mycobacteria, 497
  for *Pseudomonas aeruginosa,* 2601, 2603
  for secondary peritonitis, 938-939
  for *Streptococcus pneumoniae* meningitis, 2405
  for viridans streptococci, 2440
  immune response to, 320f, 322
  immunochemistry of, 320, 321f, 322
  mechanism of action of, penicillin-binding
    protein inactivation in, 282
  resistance to
    by *Staphylococcus aureus,* 2333, 2334t
    efflux in, 263
    beta-lactamase in, 260-261
    mechanisms of, 260-261, 261t
    target enzyme alteration in, 264-265
  semisynthetic, allergy to, 323
  structure of, 320, 321f
Beta-lactamase
  anaerobic bacterial producers of, 256-257
  broad spectrum, 256, 258t
  CAZ-7, 260
  chromosomally determined, 260
  class A, 256, 258t-259t
  class C, 256, 259t
  classes of, 255
  classification of, 256, 256t, 257f, 282-283, 283t
  clinical isolates of, 257, 260
  CTX-1, 257
  extended-spectrum, 256, 257, 258t-259t, 260, 299
    in susceptibility testing, 224

Beta-lactamase *(Continued)*
  gram-negative producers of, 256, 258t-259t
  gram-positive producers of, 256
  in anaerobe antibiotic resistance, 2816
  in antibiotic resistance, 255-257, 260-261
  in aztreonam resistance, 256, 258t
  in beta-lactam antibiotic resistance, 260-261
  in cephalosporin resistance, 256, 258t, 259t,
    299
  in imipenem resistance, 256, 259t
  in meropenem resistance, 256, 259t
  in penicillin resistance, 282-283
  IRT, 260
  of *Klebsiella pneumoniae,* 938
  plasmid encoding of, 256, 258t-259t
  SHV-1, 257
  SHV-2, 257
  TEM-1, 257
  TRI, 260
Beta-lactamase inhibitors, 315-317
Bichloroacetic acid
  for genital warts, 1849
  for human papillomavirus, in HIV infection,
    1691t
Bifidobacterium spp., 2850-2851, 2850f
Bifoconazole, for onychomycosis, 3058
Bile
  in *Campylobacter jejuni* colonization, 2551
  in secondary peritonitis, 933
Bile duct, common, inflammation of, 955
Bile solubility, 216t
Biliary atresia, orthoreoviruses and, 1899
Biliary disease. *See also* Gallbladder disease.
  in cryptosporidiosis, 3220, 3221
  in microsporidiosis, 3238t, 3242
Biliary tract, drainage of, 957
Biliary tract infections, 955-957
  clinical presentation of, 955-956
  diagnosis of, 956
  from *Clostridium,* 2830
  imaging of, 956, 956f
  in HIV infection, 1576-1577
  microbiology of, 956-957
  pathogenesis of, 955, 955f
  pyogenic liver abscess from, 951, 952t
  treatment of, 957
BILN 1061, for hepatitis C, 1969
Bilophila [spp.], antimicrobial therapy for, 2844t
Bilophila wadsworthia, 2812
  appendicitis from, 969
  intra-abdominal infections from, 2842
  secondary peritonitis from, 932
Bioassays, of enterotoxins, 1220
Bioavailability, 272
Biochemical methods, 215-221, 215t, 216t, 218t-
  221t
Biofilms, 21-22, 21t
Biologic gradient, 167
Biologic response modifiers. *See*
  Immunomodulators.
Biologic therapeutics. *See* Immunomodulators.
Biological weapons. *See* Bioterrorism.
Biological Weapons Convention, 3591, 3594
Biopsy
  brain. *See* Brain biopsy.
  liver
    in acute viral hepatitis, 1429, 2175
    in chronic hepatitis C, 1452, 1963, 1963t
    in hepatitis C, 1452, 1961-1962, 1963, 1963t
      chronic, 1452, 1963, 1963t
    in hepatitis E, 2209, 2209f
  lung
    for *Pneumocystis,* 3087
    in acute pneumonia, 827
    in chronic pneumonia, 863-864

Biopsy *(Continued)*
  in paracoccidioidomycosis, 3064-3065,
    3065f
  specimen collection and transport for, 205t
Bioterrorism
  agents of, 196t, 3592-3593
    of greatest concern, 3595-3597
  air sampling for, 3598-3599
  anthrax in, 1176-1177, 1176f, 1177t, 2487,
    2488, 3592-3593, 3618-3623
    treatment of, 2489-2490, 2489t, 2490t
    vaccine for, 3561
  biological weapons programs and, 3591-3592
  botulinum toxin in, 2825, 3624-3625
  Burkholderia pseudomallei in, 2630
  changing attitudes toward, 3591-3592
  data mining for, 3598
  detection and diagnosis of, 3598-3599
  disinfection/sterilization and, 3342
  emergency preparedness for, 192-201, 3593,
    3595-3600, 3598t. *See also* Emergency
    preparedness.
  foodborne disease in, 1292
  historical perspective on, 3591-3592, 3593
  infections caused by, laboratory studies for,
    213-214
  information sources for, 3611, 3611t
  isolation precautions and, 3329-3330, 3330t
  legislation for, 3600
  overview of, 3591-3600
  plague in, 2691, 2696, 2697, 3601-3604
  production of, 3596
  public health response to, 3599
  research and development for, 3599-3600
  Rickettsia rickettsii in, 2288
  risk assessment for, 3595
  smallpox in, 3592-3593, 3612-3617
  sources of, 3596
  syndromic surveillance for, 3598
  tularemia in, 3607-3611
  viral hemorrhagic fevers in, 3626-3629, 3626t-
    3629t
  viral, laboratory studies for, 237
  vs. chemical terrorism, 3595, 3595t
  weaponizing of, 3596-3597
Biotherapy, for HIV-related non-Hodgkin's
  lymphoma, 1607
Biotransformation, 273
Biphasic milk fever, 1928
Bipolaris spp.
  brain abscess from, 3070, 3076t
  mycotic aneurysm from, 993
  sinusitis from, 3070-3071, 3071f, 3076t
Birds. *See also* Zoonosis(es).
  Chlamydia psittaci and, 2251, 2256-2258,
    2336-2338
  Cryptococcus neoformans and, 2998-2999
  Histoplasma capsulatum and, 3013-3014
Bisexual men
  hepatitis A in, 2171, 2178
  HIV infection in, 1479-1480, 1480f. *See also*
    Human immunodeficiency virus (HIV).
Bismuth salts, for *Helicobacter pylori* infections,
  2563
Bismuth subsalicylate
  for rotavirus, 1909
  for traveler's diarrhea, 1242
  tetracycline with, 364t
Bites. *See also* Wound infections.
  animal, 3552-3553, 3552t, 3553t
    Capnocytophaga canimorsus from, 2731-2732
    laboratory studies for, 213
  of head and neck, 800
  human, 800, 3554-3555
    HIV and, 3398

Bites. *See also* Wound infections.
  of head and neck, 800
    Pasteurella in, 800, 2687, 3552
  rabies from, 2050
  snake, 3553-3554
    antivenin for, 66
  spider, 3653f
  tick, 3313
Bithionol
  adverse effects of, 581t
  for *Fasciola hepatica,* 596
  for fluke infections, 572t
  for helminthic disease, 570t
BK virus, 1856-1861
  characteristics of, 1857
  clinical manifestations of, 1858-1859, 1859t
  diagnosis of, 1859-1861
  epidemiology of, 1857, 1859t
  in pregnancy, 1858-1859, 1859t
  laboratory studies for, 237
  pathogenesis of, 1857-1858
  prevention of, 1861
  renal disease from, 1858
    in transplant recipients, 3509
  treatment of, 1861
  ureteral stenosis from, 1858
Black dots, in chromoblastomycosis, 2989, 2990f
Black piedra, 3061
Black-dot ringworm, 3056
Bladder
  defense mechanisms of, 879-880
  schistosomiasis of, 3279
Bladder catheterization. *See also* Catheter-related
    infections.
  in spinal cord injury, 3512-3514
Bladder worm, 3286t
Blastocystis hominis, 3233-3234, 3234f
  traveler's diarrhea from, 1242
  treatment of, 577t
Blastocystosis, 3233-3234
Blastomyces [spp.]
  gastrointestinal, 1269
  sclerosing mediastinitis from, 1075
  treatment of, 504, 507, 508
Blastomyces dermatitidis, 3026-3037
  appearance of in tissue, 2938t
  arthritis from, 1318
  central nervous system infections from, 3029t,
    3033, 3034f
  characteristics of, 3026
  chest film in, 867f, 3030, 3030f-3032f, 3031
  chronic/recurrent infections from, 3029-3030,
    3031-3033
  clinical manifestations of, 3029-3034, 3029t,
    3030t
  course of, 3030f, 3031
  culture of, 3035
  diagnosis of, 3034-3036
  ecology of, 3027
  epidemiology of, 3026-3027, 3027f
  extrapulmonary infections from, 3029-3030,
    3029t, 3030t
  fever from, 726
  genitourinary infections from, 3033
  historical perspective on, 3026
  identification of, 231
  immune response to, 3027-3029
  in children, 3033-3034
  in immunocompromised host, 3034
  in pregnancy, 3034
  laboratory tests for, 229
  laryngitis from, 759
  multiorgan involvement in, 3029t, 3030t, 3033
  musculoskeletal infections from, 3033, 3033f
  mycelial form of, 3026

Blastomyces dermatitidis (Continued)
  pathogenesis and pathology of, 3027
  prostatitis from, 894
  pulmonary infections from
    acute, 3030
    as primary infections, 3027, 3030
    chronic/recurrent, 3031, 3031f, 3032f
    in HIV infection, 1571
  risk factors for, 3027
  serology of, 3035-3036
  serotypes of, 3026
  skin lesions from, 3027, 3031-3032, 3032f,
    3033f
  subcutaneous nodules from, 3033
  treatment of, 3036-3037, 3036t
  W-1 antigen and, 3028, 3029
  yeast form of, 3026, 3026f
Blastomycosis
  European. *See Cryptococcus neoformans.*
  keloidal, 3075, 3075f, 3076t
Blastoschizomyces capitatus, 3074, 3076, 3076t
Bleb-related endophthalmitis, 1407t, 1408-1411
Bleomycin, for HIV-related non-Hodgkin's
    lymphoma, 1605
Blepharitis, 1419-1420, 1420f
Blepharoconjunctivitis, 1420. *See also*
    Conjunctivitis.
Blindness. *See River blindness;* Vision loss.
Blister, necrotic, in sepsis, 917-918
Blood
  culture of, 209-210, 210t, 3428
    collection and transport protocol for, 205t
    in catheter-related infections, 3351
    in endocarditis, 985-986
    in pneumonia, 828
      pneumococcal, 2400, 2401t
  HIV infection transmission through, 1492
Blood flow, in severe sepsis, 911
Blood patch, 1080
Blood transfusions. *See* Transfusions.
Blood vessels. *See also under* Arteritis;
    Endarteritis; Vascular; Vasculitis.
  endothelium of, injury to, in severe sepsis, 911
Blood-brain barrier, in AIDS dementia, 1586
Blowflies, myiasis from, 3307-3310, 3308t
BMS-806, 20
Body fluids
  drug concentrations in, 635, 650t-685t
  infections in, laboratory tests for, 211
Body lice, 3302-3304, 3302f, 3303f
Body mass index, 140, 140t
  in elderly patient, 146
Body temperature. *See* Temperature.
Boerhaave syndrome, 1070
Bolivian hemorrhagic fever, 2090-2096, 2091t.
    See also South American hemorrhagic fevers.
  as biological weapon, 3627-3629, 3627t
Bombesin, antipyretic effects of, 711
Bone infections. *See also* Osteomyelitis.
  anaerobic, 2813
    from gram-negative bacilli, 2843
  complications of, in HIV-infected women, 1631
  from *Bacillus,* 2495
  from *Enterococcus,* 2413
  from *Kingella,* 2533
  from *Pasteurella,* 2688
  from *Pseudomonas aeruginosa,* 2602-2603
  from *Salmonella,* 2647t
  laboratory studies for, 213
  quinolones for, 463
Bone marrow
  chloramphenicol effects on, 368
  laboratory studies for
    in chronic failure, 234-235
    specimen collection and transport in, 205t

Bone marrow failure
  granulocyte-macrophage colony-stimulating
    factor after, 554
  in hepatitis, 1981, 1985
  neutropenic enterocolitis in, 973
Bone marrow transplantation. *See also*
    Hematopoietic stem cell transplantation;
    Transplantation.
  adenovirus in, 1839
  cytomegalovirus in, 1795
    prevention of, 1793-1794
  enterovirus in, 2155
  esophagitis in, 1234t
  for chronic granulomatous disease, 109
  granulocyte-macrophage colony-stimulating
    factor in, 554
  immunosuppression in, 3422t
  infections in, 3422t
  intravenous immune globulin therapy in, 558
  parainfluenza virus in, 2000
Bone scans
  for osteomyelitis, 1323, 1324f
  for prosthetic joint infections, 1333-1334
Bone, tetracycline effects on, 363, 363t
Bordetella [spp.], 2701-2706
  characteristics of, 2701-2703
  endocarditis from, 992
  laboratory identification of, 220-221
  tetanus toxin in, 26
Bordetella avium, 2701
Bordetella bronchiseptica, 2701, 2702
  evolution of, 6
  laboratory identification of, 221t
  tetanus toxin in, 26
Bordetella hinzii, 2701
Bordetella holmesii, 2701
Bordetella parapertussis, 2701, 2702
  tetanus toxin in, 26
Bordetella pertussis, 2701-2705. *See also*
    Pertussis.
  acute bronchitis from, 747-749
  adenylate cyclase toxin of, 27
  antisera identification of, 221
  characteristics of, 2701, 2702
  clones of, 5
  epidemiology of, 2703
  evolution of, 6
  genetic regulation of, 7
  laboratory culture of, 208
  lipopolysaccharide of, 2702
  pertussis from, 748
  pneumonia from, 2704
  polymerase chain reaction assay for, 2704-2705
  regulation of, 7t
  tetanus toxin in, 26
  toxins of, 27-28, 2702
  treatment of, 367t, 397t, 398, 401t, 405, 485t
  vaccines for, 2705-2706
  virulence factors of, 2702-2703
Bordetella-Alcaligenes complex, 2701
Boric acid
  for bacterial vaginosis, 1366
  for desquamative inflammatory, 1367
  for vulvovaginal candidiasis, 1365
Borrelia [spp.], 2795-2797
  relapsing fever from, 3314
Borrelia afzelii, 2798
  ehrlichiosis from, 3312
Borrelia burgdorferi, 738, 2798-2807. *See also*
    Lyme disease.
  animal model of, 2800-2801
  antibodies to, 2802, 2804, 2804f
  characteristics of, 2798, 2799f
  coinfection with, 2803
    from *Bartonella henselae,* 2739

Borrelia burgdorferi (Continued)
  detection of, 2803-2804, 2804f
  dissemination of, 2800
  electron micrography of, 2799f
  encephalitis from, 1145, 1146
  enzyme-linked immunosorbent assay for, 2804, 2804f
  erythema migrans from, 738
  fever from, 723f
  hosts for, 2798-2799
  immune response to, 2800
  in joints, 2800
  meningitis from
    acute, 1088, 1100, 1104, 1106t, 1115
    chronic, 1137
  myocarditis from, 1055
  pathogenesis of, 2800
  pericarditis from, 1059
  treatment of, 358, 401t, 403
  uveitis from, 1417
  Western blotting for, 2804, 2805f
Borrelia garinii, 2798
  ehrlichiosis from, 3312
Borrelia lonestari, 3314
Borrelia recurrentis, 2795
Borreliosis, Lyme. See Borrelia burgdorferi; Lyme disease.
Boston exanthem, 2150
Botflies, myiasis from, 3307-3310, 3308t
Botryomyces caespitosus, chromoblastomycosis from, 2988-2991
Botryomycosis, in immunocompromised host, 1185
Bottle flies, myiasis from, 3308-3310, 3308t
Botulinum antitoxin, 2837
Botulinum toxin(s), 1219, 2822-2823
  action of, 28
  as biological weapons, 2825, 3624-3625
  cell entry by, 27
  mechanism of, 2823-2824, 2824f
  therapeutic uses of, 30-31
Botulism, 1147-1148, 2822-2826
  clinical manifestations of, 28, 2824-2825, 2825t
  diagnosis of, 2825
  differential diagnosis of, 2825, 2826f
  disinfection/sterilization and, 3342
  epidemiology of, 2823
  foodborne, 2823, 2824
  history of, 2823
  infant, 28, 2823, 2824
  inhalational, 2823, 2825
  isolation precautions for, 3330t
  muscle contraction in, 28
  of undetermined etiology, 2823
  pathogenesis of, 2823-2824, 2824f
  prevention of, 2826
  treatment of, 2825-2826
  wound, 2823, 2824-2825
    in injection drug users, 3472
Boutonneuse fever, 2090t, 2292
Bovine anti-Cryptosporidium immune globulin, 3222
Bovine ephemeral fever, 2047
Bovine immunodeficiency virus, 2119
Bovine leukemia virus, 2119
Bovine spongiform encephalopathy, new variant Creutzfeldt-Jakob disease and, 2227-2228, 3630
Bowel. See also Colon; Small intestine.
  preoperative, 3543t
Bowenoid papulosis, 1341, 1846, 1846f
Bowen's disease, 1341, 1846, 1846f
BPI, neutrophil bactericidal activity, 102

Brachiola algerae, 3237, 3238t. See also Microsporidia.
Brachiola vesicularum, treatment of, 574t
Brain abscess, 1150-1161
  bacterial
    antimicrobial therapy for, 1157-1160, 1158t, 1159t
    etiology of, 1151
    surgery for, 1160
  clinical features of, 1079-1080, 1154-1155, 1154t
  diagnosis of, 1155-1157, 1156f
  epidemiology of, 1151
  etiology of, 1151-1152, 1151t
  from Actinomyces, 1158t, 2929
  from anaerobic infections, 2813, 2813f, 2841
  from Aspergillus spp., 1152, 1155, 1157, 1158t, 1160
  from Bacteroides fragilis, 1153, 1154, 1157, 1158t
  from Blastomyces dermatitidis, 3033, 3034f
  from Candida spp., 1152, 1158t, 1160
  from Cryptococcus neoformans, 1158t
  from dark-walled fungi, 3070, 3070f, 3071f
  from Entamoeba histolytica, 3103
  from Enterobacteriaceae, 1158t
  from Fusobacterium, 1158t
  from Haemophilus spp., 1158t
  from Listeria monocytogenes, 1151, 2481
  from meningitis, 1153
  from Mucorales, 1152, 1155, 1158t, 1160, 2976-2977, 2978
  from Mycobacterium tuberculosis, 1158t
  from Nocardia spp., 1151, 1158, 1158t, 1160, 2918, 2921
  from Prevotella melaninogenica, 1157, 1158t
  from protozoa and helminths, 1152, 1155, 1157, 1158, 1158t
  from Pseudallescheria boydii, 1152, 1155, 1158t, 1160, 3068-3069
  from Pseudomonas aeruginosa, 1151, 1157, 1158t
  from Scedosporium apiospermum, 1152
  from Staphylococcus spp., 1151, 1153, 1154, 1157, 1158t
  from Streptococcus spp., 1151, 1154, 1157, 1158t
  from Streptococcus anginosus group, 2454
  from Toxoplasma gondii, 1152, 1155, 1157, 1158, 1158t, 3175-3176, 3175f
  fungal
    antimicrobial therapy for, 1159t, 1160-1161
    etiology of, 1151-1152
    surgery for, 1160-1161
  host defense mechanisms in, 1154
  hyperbaric oxygen for, 566-567
  in immunocompromised host, 1137, 1151t, 1152, 1157
  in injection drug users, 3471
  in mucormycosis, 1152, 1155, 1158t, 1160, 2976-2977, 2978
  in neonate, 1153
  initial management of, 1157-1159, 1158t
  initiation of infections in, 1153
  mortality from, 1151
  natural history of, 1153-1154
  pathogenesis of, 1152-1153
  predisposing conditions for, 1151t
  protozoal and helminthic
    etiology of, 1152
    treatment of, 1152, 1157, 1158, 1158t
  treatment of
    antimicrobial, 1159-1160, 1159t
    empiric, 1157-1159, 1158t
    surgical, 1160

Brain biopsy
  in AIDS dementia, 1586
  in brain abscess, 1135
  in Creutzfeldt-Jakob disease, 2225
  in HIV infection, 1591-1592
  in meningitis, 1135
  in primary central nervous system lymphoma, 1589
  in progressive multifocal leukoencephalopathy, 1590, 1860, 1860f
  in toxoplasmosis, 3186
Brain herniation, from lumbar puncture, 1080
Brain stem encephalitis, from Listeria monocytogenes, 2481, 2482f
Brainerd diarrhea, 1242, 1291
Brazil, HIV infection in, 1469, 1469f
Brazilian hemorrhagic fever, 2090-2096, 2091t. See also South American hemorrhagic fevers.
Breast, tuberculosis of, 2883
Breast cancer, in HIV infection, 1628
Breast-feeding
  antibiotics in, 245
  HIV transmission via, 1490-1491, 1620, 1622
    prevention of, 1495-1496
  human T-cell lymphotrophic virus transmission via, 2104-2105, 2104t, 2111-2112, 2113
  in enteric infections protection, 1218
  in Shigella control, 2659
  rotavirus infections and, 1908, 1909
  tetracycline in, 361
Breda virus, 1990
Brevibacillus [spp.], 2493
  laboratory identification of, 218, 219t
Brevibacillus brevis, 2493, 2495t
Brevibacillus laterosporus, 2493, 2495t
Brevibacterium spp., 2471
Brill-Zinsser disease, vs. enteric fever, 1275t
Brivudin, 540, 541f
Brodie's abscess, 1330
Brompheniramine, for cough, 805
Bronchial cleft cysts, infected, 799-800
Bronchial wash, specimen collection and transport from, 207t
Bronchiectasis
  brain abscess from, 1151t, 1152
  bronchiolitis obliterans and, 817
  from Mycobacterium avium complex, 2899-2901, 2900f
Bronchiolitis, 812-818
  asthma and, 815, 816
  clinical manifestations of, 815
  complications of, 816
  course of, 815
  diagnosis of, 816
  differential diagnosis of, 816
  epidemiology of, 813-814, 813f
  etiology of, 812-813, 813t
  from adenoviruses, 813, 813t, 1838
  from human metapneumovirus, 2028-2029, 2028t, 2029t
  from microsporidia, 3238t, 3244
  from parainfluenza viruses, 812-813, 813t, 2000, 2000t
  from respiratory syncytial virus, 812-813, 813t, 2011-2012, 2014-2016
  laboratory findings in, 816
  pathophysiology of, 814-815, 814f, 815f
  prevention of, 817
  treatment of, 816-817
Bronchiolitis obliterans, 817-818
Bronchiolitis obliterans organizing pneumonia (BOOP), chest film in, 860f
Bronchitis
  acute, 803-805
  asthmatic. See Bronchiolitis.

Bronchitis *(Continued)*
  chronic, 806-811. *See also* Chronic obstructive
    pulmonary disease (COPD).
  exacerbation of, *Streptococcus pneumoniae* in,
    2400
  from adenoviruses, 1838
  from *Chlamydia pneumoniae*, 2262
  from *Moraxella (Branhamella) catarrhalis*,
    2531f
  from respiratory syncytial virus, 2014-2016,
    2015t
  infectious, 803-805
  postinfectious, 803-805, 804t
  treatment of, 407, 462
Bronchoalveolar lavage
  for acute pneumonia, 827
  for chronic pneumonia, 863
  for nosocomial pneumonia, 3362, 3365, 3365t,
    3366-3367
  specimen collection and transport from, 207t
Bronchodilators
  for bronchiolitis, 817
  for chronic obstructive pulmonary disease, 810t
  for croup, 763-764
  for cystic fibrosis, 872
  for respiratory syncytial virus, 2020
Bronchopleural fistula, tuberculous, 2878
Bronchoscopy
  for acute pneumonia, 826-827
  for chronic pneumonia, 863, 867
  for lung abscess, 856
  for nosocomial pneumonia, 3366
  for tuberculosis, 2867
  laboratory culture in, 208
Bronchus-associated lymphoid tissue (BALT),
  821
Broviac catheter, infections of, 3353-3355, 3354t
Brown recluse spider bites, 3653f
Brucella [spp.], 2669-2672. *See also* Brucellosis.
  blood culture of, 210, 210t
  characteristics of, 2669-2670
  chronic fatigue from, 1270
  collection and transport of, 205t
  endocarditis from, 992
    prosthetic valve, 1026
  enteric fever from, 1274t
  history of, 2669
  immunity to, 2670
  infections from, 2671-2672
  isolation precautions for, 3330t
  laboratory detection of, 213-214, 220-221
  mycotic aneurysm from, 1008
  pathogenesis of, 2670
  uveitis from, 1417
  vaccines for, 2672
Brucella abortus, aminoglycosides for, 344t
Brucellosis, 2669-2672. *See also Brucella* [spp.]
  clinical manifestations of, 2670-2671
  complications of, 2671-2672
  diagnosis of, 2672
  epidemiology of, 2670, 2670f
  history in, 823t
  prevention of, 2672
  treatment of, 2672
    with chloramphenicol, 367t
    with quinolones, 465
    with rifamycin, 382
Brudzinski's sign, 1099
Brugia malayi
  treatment of, 572t, 578t, 594
  tropical pulmonary eosinophilia and, 3274-
    3275
Brugia timori, treatment of, 572t, 578t, 594
Brugian filariasis, 3270-3272, 3270f-3272f
  lymphangitis in, 1208, 1212, 3271, 3271f

Bruton tyrosine kinase, 65
Buboes, 2245. *See also*
    Lymphadenitis/lymphadenopathy.
  in plague, 2693-2694, 2694f
  inguinal, 1209t, 1210
    differential diagnosis of, 2245
    in cutaneous anthrax, 1208
    in filariasis, 1208, 1212
    in plague, 1208, 2693-2694, 2694f
    in sexually transmitted diseases, 1207-1208
Bubonic plague, 2693-2694, 2693t, 2694f. *See
    also* Plague.
  inguinal buboes in, 1208
  treatment of, 1211
Buccal spaces
  anatomy of, 790, 790f
  infections of, 792. *See also* Odontogenic
    infections.
Budd-Chiari syndrome, hepatitis in, 1436
Budesonide, for croup, 2001
Buffered charcoal–yeast extract, for *Legionella*
    diagnosis, 2727
Buggy Creek virus, 1914-1919
Bulbar paralytic poliomyelitis, 2143. *See also*
    Poliomyelitis.
Bullae, 730t, 731, 733. *See also* Rash.
  causes of, 733-734
Bullous erysipelas, 1177
Bullous impetigo, 737, 1174, 2330, 2330f. *See
    also* Impetigo.
  from *Streptococcus aureus*, 2369
Bull's eye lesion, in erythema multiforme, 732
Bundle-forming pilus, of enteropathogenic
    Escherichia coli, 2575
Bunyaviridae, 2086-2089, 2086t
Bur hole drainage, for subdural empyema, 1165
Burkholderia [spp.]
  isolation precautions for, 3330t
  laboratory identification of, 220, 220t, 221t
  pyomyositis from, 1196
Burkholderia ambifaria, 2615
Burkholderia anthina, 2615
Burkholderia cepacia, 2615-2620
  after lung transplantation, 871, 2618, 2619f
  carbapenems for, 313t
  clinical manifestations of, 2618-2619
  epidemiology of, 2617-2618
  identification of, 2615-2616
  in chronic granulomatous disease, 155, 156
  iron acquisition in, 2617
  laboratory identification of, 220t
  microbiology of, 2615-2616
  pathogenesis of, 2616-2617
  pneumonia from, 2618, 2618f
    in cystic fibrosis, 871
    nosocomial, 3367t
  prevention of, 2619-2620
  taxonomy of, 2615, 2616f
  treatment of, 2619
    with aminoglycosides, 334t-335t
    with quinolones, 455t
    with rifamycin, 382
    with trimethoprim-sulfamethoxazole, 444,
      444t
  virulence factors of, 2616-2617
Burkholderia mallei, 2630-2631, 2630f
Burkholderia multivorans, 2615
Burkholderia pseudomallei, 2622-2630. *See also*
    Melioidosis.
  characteristics of, 2622
  colonization by, 2625
  history of, 2622
  laboratory diagnosis of, 2628
  latency of, 2628
  natural history of, 2623, 2623f

Burkholderia pseudomallei (Continued)
  pathogenesis of, 2623-2624
  pulmonary infections from, in cystic fibrosis, 871
  splenic abscess from, 967, 967t
  transmission of, 2623, 2623f
  treatment of, 444, 2628-2629, 2629t
Burkholderia pyrrocinia, 2615
Burkholderia stabilis, 2615
Burkholderia vietnamiensis, 2615
Burkitt's lymphoma, 1808-1809, 1808t. *See also*
    Hematologic malignancies; Lymphoma.
Burn infections, 349f, 3547-3551, 3550f. *See also*
    Wound infections.
  from *Pseudomonas aeruginosa*, 2589-2590,
    2605-2606
  prevention of, topical antibacterial therapy for,
    482
Bursitis
  from nontuberculous mycobacteria, 2910t, 2913
  septic, 1319-1320
    from *Staphylococcus aureus*, 2347
Buruli ulcer, 2911
Buschke-Löwenstein tumors, 1846
Bush yaws, 3145t, 3149, 3150
Bussuquara virus, 1945t
Butoconazole, for vulvovaginal candidiasis, 1364
N-Butyldeoxynojirimycin, 20
Bypass procedures, for prosthetic vascular graft
    infections, 1038

C

C1
  deficiency of, 80t
  regulation of, 73
C1 inhibitor, 73, 74t
  deficiency of, 79, 80t
    in hereditary angioedema, 85
    in endotoxic shock, 86
C1q, 55, 69t
  activation of, 71
  autoantibodies to, in systemic lupus
    erythematosus, 79
  deficiency of, 79, 83, 151t
  measurement of, 59
C1qR, 74t, 75
C1r, 69t, 71, 75
C1r deficiency, 151t
C1s, 69t, 71, 75
C1s deficiency, 151t
C2, 69t, 75
  deficiency of, 79, 80t, 83
C2 deficiency, 151t
C3, 69t, 75
  and vascular disease, 82-83
  deficiency of, 80t, 151t
    molecular basis of, 83
    primary, 81-82
    replacement therapy for, 88
    secondary, 82
    vaccines in, 88
  in adaptive immunity, 76
  in complement cascade, 73
  in neutrophil ingestion, 99
  measurement of, 59
C3 convertase
  in alternate pathway activation, 72-73, 72f
  in classic pathway activation, 71-72, 72f
  in complement activation, 74-75
  regulation of, 73-74
C3 nephritic factors, deficiency of, 80t
C3a, 55
C3a/C4aR, 74t
C3b, 55, 74
  as opsonin, 55-56

C3b receptors, 76
C3b/C4b receptor, 75
C4, 71, 75
  deficiency of, 79, 80t, 83, 151t
  measurement of, 59
C4 nephritic factors, deficiency of, 80t
C4bBP, 74t, 75
C5, 69t, 73, 75
  deficiency of, 80t, 83, 151t
C5 convertase, 73
C5a, 55
  in septic shock, 86-87
  in severe sepsis, 912
C5a receptor, 74t, 75
C5b-7 complex, 74
C6, 69t, 73
  deficiency of, 80t, 83-84
C6 deficiency, 151t
C7, 69t, 73
  deficiency of, 80t, 83-84, 151t
C8, 69t, 73, 74
  deficiency of, 80t, 83-84, 151t
C9, 69t, 73, 74
  deficiency of, 80t, 83-84, 151t
C14, 69t
Caffeic acid test, 231
Caffeine, quinolone effects on, 458-459
Cag, 2558, 2559
Calamus masculinus, South American
    hemorrhagic fevers from, 2093
Calciphylaxis, 1182
Calcium hypochlorite, disinfection with, 3334
Calcofluor white stain, 214t
  of fungi, 230
Calculi
  biliary. *See* Cholecystitis.
  in urinary tract infections, 881, 881f
    catheter-related, 3373
Caliciviruses, 2194-2199
  characteristics of, 2195-2196, 2195f, 2196f
  classification of, 2196
  clinical manifestations of, 2198, 2198f
  diagnosis of, 2198-2199
  epidemiology of, 2196-2197
  gastroenteritis from, 1239, 1239t
    laboratory studies for, 235
  historical perspective on, 2195
  immune response to, 2198
  incidence of, 2197
  outbreaks of, 2197
  pathogenesis of, 2197-2198, 2197f
  prevention of, 2199
  transmission of, 2196
  treatment of, 2199
  vaccine for, 2199
California encephalitis virus, 1146-1147, 2086-
    2089, 2086t
Calliphora spp., myiasis from, 3307-3310, 3308t
Calymmatobacterium granulomatis, 2579, 2748-
    2450. *See also* Granuloma inguinale.
  biology of, 2748
  detection of, 2749-2750, 2750f
  diagnosis of, 1343, 1343f
  Klebsiella and, 2750
Cambodia, HIV infection in, 1468, 1469f
Campylobacter [spp.], 2548-2555
  appendicitis from, 969
  blood culture of, 210, 210t
  clinical manifestations of, 2548, 2549t
  enteritis from, azithromycin for, 405
  epidemiology of, 2549-2550
  in HIV infection, treatment of, 1701
  infections from, 2553
  laboratory identification of, 221
  microbiology of, 2548-2549

Campylobacter [spp.] *(Continued)*
  pathogenesis of, 2551
  pathogenicity of, 2548, 2549t
  quinolone-resistant, 465, 1243
  tetracyclines for, 358
  toxins of, 1221
  traveler's diarrhea from, 1242, 1243
  treatment of, 1226
Campylobacter cinaedi, 2548
Campylobacter coli, 2553, 2555
  diarrhea from, 178
Campylobacter fennelliae, 2548
Campylobacter fetus
  bacteriologic studies for, 2553-2554
  clinical manifestations of, 2552-2553, 2553t
  endocarditis from, 991
  enteric fever from, 1274t
  enteric fever–like syndrome from, 1276-1277
  immunity in, 2552
  in primary peritonitis, 929
  mycotic aneurysm from, 1008
  pathogenesis of, 2551, 2551f
  treatment of, 2555
Campylobacter fetus subsp. *venerealis,* 2553
Campylobacter hyointestinalis, 2553
Campylobacter jejuni
  bacteriologic studies for, 2553
  biochemistry of, 2558t
  clinical manifestations of, 2552, 2553t
  colitis from, 2551
  culture of, 1224, 2549, 2550f
  diarrhea from, 178
  enteritis from, 1265-1266
  epidemiology of, 2550
  foodborne disease from, 1288, 1289
  gastroenteritis from, quinolones for, 461
  immunity to, 2551-2552
  in HIV infection, 1689t
  laboratory identification of, 221
  neuritis from, 1148
  pathogenesis of, 2551
  prognosis of, 2555
  quinolone-resistant, 465, 1243
  transmission of, 2550
  treatment of, 313t, 397t, 401t, 455t, 2554
Campylobacter parvum, diarrhea from, 178
Campylobacter sputorum subsp. *bubulus,* 2553
Campylobacter sputorum subsp. *sputorum,* 2553
Campylobacter upsaliensis, 2553
Canarypox vectors, in HIV vaccine testing, 1712,
    1714
Cancer. *See also* Immunocompromised host *and*
    specific types.
  antibody deficiency in, 66
  bacterial toxins for, 30
  cellulitis in, 1179, 3438
  chemoprophylaxis in
    antibacterial, 3442-3445, 3443f-3445f
    antifungal, 3445-3447, 3446f, 3447t
    antiviral, 3448
    for *Pneumocystis jirovecii,* 3447
  chemotherapy for. *See* Chemotherapy.
  chronic hepatitis C and, 1456
  Clostridium difficile in, 3438
  cryptococcosis in, 2999t, 3000, 3437-3438
  cytomegalovirus infections in, 3436
  diarrhea in, 3438
  fever in, 713-714, 719, 723, 723f, 726
    with neutropenia, 3448-3457. *See also*
        Febrile neutropenia, in cancer.
    without neutropenia, 3448
  genitourinary infections in, 3438
  hematologic
    chronic hepatitis C and, 1456
    cryptococcosis in, 3000

Cancer *(Continued)*
  immunosuppression in, 3432
  infections in, 3432-3439. *See also* Cancer,
      infections in.
  herpes simplex virus in, 3439
  HIV-related, 1601-1612, 2119, 2130. *See also*
      Kaposi's sarcoma; Lymphoma, HIV-
      related.
    in children, 1643
  human papillomavirus and, 1843
  immunotherapy for, 3457-3458
  infections in, 3342-3358, 3432-3439. *See also*
      Febrile neutropenia.
    catheter-related, 3433-3434, 3434f, 3455-
        3457
    clinical presentation of, 3432-3439
    management of, 3439
    prevention of, 3442-3448
  influenza in, 3435-3436
  intestinal decontamination in, 3442
  meningitis in, 1138-1139
  mucormycosis in, 2975-2977
  mucositis in, 3457
  neutropenic enterocolitis in, 3438, 3457
  pulmonary infiltrates in, 3434-3437, 3457
  pyoderma grangrenosum in, 3439
  sinusitis in, 3437
  skin infections in, 3438-3439
  solid-tumor, infections in, 3432t
  syndrome of abdominal pain, diarrhea, and
      eosinophilia from, 1281t, 1283
  tuberculosis in, 3436-3437
  varicella-zoster virus in, 3439
  viruses in, 1738
  vs. enteric fever, 1275t
Cancrum oris, 798
Candida [spp.], 2938-2951. *See also specific*
    pathogen.
  alopecia from, 2944
  appearance of in tissue, 2936f, 2938t, 2940
  arthritis from, 1317-1318, 2946-2947, 2951
  brain abscess from, 1152, 1158t, 1160
  cardiac, 979, 992-993, 1001, 1030, 1053, 2945-
      2946
  cardiovascular device infections from, 1023
  catheter-related, 2948-2949, 2950, 3353
  central nervous system, 1138, 1152, 1158t,
      1160, 2945, 2950
  characteristics of, 2938-2939
  chorioretinitis from, 1408-1409, 1411, 1417
  clinical manifestations of, 2939-2940
  cutaneous, 2942-2944
    chronic, 2944, 2944f
    generalized, 2942, 2942f
    in disseminated disease, 1187, 2943, 2943f
    interdigital, 2943, 2943f
  diaper rash from, 2944, 2944f, 2951
  disseminated, 2948-2949
    in hematologic cancer, 3433
    pathogenesis of, 2940
    skin lesions in, 739, 1187, 2943, 2943f
  drunken disease from, 2949
  ecology of, 2939
  empyema from, 847
  endocarditis from, 979, 992-993, 2945-2946
    prosthetic valve, 1030
    treatment of, 1001
  endophthalmitis from, 1408-1409, 1409f, 1411,
      1417, 2947-2948f, 2951
  epidemiology of, 2939
  esophagitis from, 1231-1232, 1232f, 2941-
      2942, 2941f
    chronic, 2944
    in HIV infection, 1550, 1575
    treatment of, 1233-1234, 1233t, 2951

Candida [spp.] *(Continued)*
folliculitis from, 1175, 2942, 2943f
gallbladder, 2947
gastric, 2941f, 2942
gastrointestinal ulcers from, 1269
granuloma from, 2944, 2945f
hepatic, 952, 2947, 2947f
hepatosplenic, in hematologic cancer, 3433
histopathology of, 2936f, 2938t, 2940
historical perspective on, 2938
iatrogenic factors in, 2940
identification of, 231
immune response to, 2939-2940
in cancer patients, prevention of, 3444-3447, 3446f, 3447t
in HIV infection
oral, 1554-1555, 1554f
pediatric, 1643
treatment of, 1683t, 1687t, 1698
vulvovaginal, 1628
in immunocompromised host, 2944, 2945f, 3479
prevention of, 3444-3447, 3446f, 3447t, 3483
in neonates, 2949
in peritoneal dialysis, 941
in transplant recipients, 3479, 3495
prevention of, 3483
intestinal, 2942
isolation of, 231
keratitis from, 1404
laryngitis from, 2951
liver abscess from, 952
mediastinitis from, 1072
meningitis from, 1138, 2945, 2950
mucocutaneous
acute, 2940-2944
chronic, 2944, 2945f, 2951
mucositis from, 2940-2942
musculoskeletal, 1317-1318, 2946-2947, 2947f
mycotic aneurysm from, 993
myocarditis from, 1053
myositis from, 2947
ocular, 1404, 1409, 1411, 1417, 2947-2948, 2948f, 2951
in injection drug users, 3472
of nails, 2943, 2943f
chronic, 2944, 2945f
of scalp, chronic, 2944
oropharyngeal, 2940-2941, 2940f, 2941f
chronic, 2944
in immunocompromised host, 798-799, 2944, 3437, 3483
prevention of, in transplant recipients, 3483
treatment of, 2950-2951
osteomyelitis from, 2946
otitis externa from, 766
pancreatic infections from, 959t, 960, 961
pathogenesis and pathophysiology of, 2939-2940
pathogenic, 2939
perianal, 2944, 2944f
pericarditis from, 1059
peritoneal, 932, 937, 2947
pneumonia from, 2945
portal of entry for, 2940
prevention of, 2949
prostatitis from, 894
pseudomembranous colitis from, 1250
public health burden of, 2938
pyomyositis from, 1196
renal, 2946, 2947f
respiratory tract, 2945
nosocomial, 3365, 3365t
risk factors for, 2940
sepsis from, 907

Candida [spp.] *(Continued)*
shunt infections from, 1127, 1127t, 1129
splenic, 967, 967t, 2947, 2947f
suppurative thrombophlebitis from, 1004
total parenteral nutrition catheter infections from, 3352-3354
treatment of, 504, 506, 509, 511, 2949-2951
typhlitis from, 973
urethritis from, 1348
urinary tract, 2946
catheter-related, 3372
treatment of, 3376-3377
in cancer, 2946
virulence factors in, 2940
vulvovaginitis from, 212, 1344, 1362-1365, 1363f, 1364f, 1364t, 1369
genital herpes and, 1768
Candida albicans. See *Candida* [spp.].
Candida dubliniensis, 231, 2939
Candida glabrata, 2949
appearance of in tissue, 2936f, 2938t
pancreatic infections from, 961
vulvovaginitis from, 1362-1365, 1363f, 1364f, 1364t
Candida krusei, 2949
Candida parapsilosis
endocarditis from, 992-993
in peritoneal dialysis, 941
Candida, pneumonia from, 2945
nosocomial, 3365, 3365t
Candida tropicalis, 2949
endocarditis from, 992
vulvovaginitis from, 1362-1365, 1363f, 1364f, 1364t
Candidemia, 2948-2949, 2950
catheter-related, 2948-2949, 2950, 3353
pathogenesis of, 2940
Candiduria, 2946
pathogenesis of, 2940
treatment of, 892, 2950, 3376-3377
Canine space, 790, 790f
infections of, 792. *See also* Odontogenic infections
Canaliculitis, 1421
from *Actinomyces,* 2926
from *Propionibacterium propionicum,* 2924
Cannulation. *See also* Catheter-related infections.
suppurative thrombophlebitis prevention in, 1005
Canyon hypothesis, 16
Capillaria philippinensis
syndrome of abdominal pain, diarrhea, and eosinophilia from, 1281t, 1282
treatment of, 571t
Capillariasis, 3294t, 3298
Capnocytophaga [spp.], 2730-2732
diseases from, 2731-2732
laboratory identification of, 221
microbiology of, 2730
odontogenic infections from, 788, 788f, 789
taxonomy of, 2730
treatment of, 2731-2732
Capnocytophaga canimorsus, 2730, 2731-2732
bite wound infections from, 3552
postsplenectomy sepsis from, 3528
rash in, 738
vs. *Dysgonomonas capnocytophagoides,* 2756
Capnocytophaga cynodegmi, 2730, 2731-2732
Capnocytophaga granulosa, 2731
Capnocytophaga haemolytica, 2730, 2731
Capnocytophaga ochracea, 2731
Capnocytophaga sputigena, 2731

Capreomycin
dosage of, 676t-677t
drug interactions with, 687t
for tuberculosis, 495
formulations of, 649t
Capsid, viral, 1730-1731, 1731f
Captopril, for myocarditis, 1057
Carbamazepine, tetracycline with, 364t
Carbapenems, 311-314. *See also* Beta-lactam antibiotics.
adverse reactions of, 314
antibacterial activity of, 312-313, 313t
chemistry of, 311-312
clinical uses of, 314
cross-reactivity among, 325
for peritonitis, 938-939
for preemptive pancreatic infection treatment, 965t
for sepsis, 918
mechanism of action of, 312
pharmacology of, 313-314
resistance of, 312
structure of, 312f, 320f
Carbenicillin, 291, 292f
dosage of, 650t-651t
for *Pseudomonas aeruginosa* bacteremia, 2600
formulations of, 646t
uses of, 287, 288t
Carbenicillin indanyl sodium
dosage of, 650t-651t
formulations of, 646t
Carbenicillinase, 256, 258t
Carboxypenicillin, 291-292, 292f
susceptibility to, 283-284
Carboxypeptidase, 74t
Carboxypeptidase N, 70t
Carbuncles, 1175-1176
staphylococcal, 2340
Carcinoma erysipeloides, 1179, 1180
Cardiac arrhythmias
erythromycin and, 400
in myocarditis, 1056
Cardiac catheterization
in endocarditis, 986-987
infections in, 1036
Cardiac fluid, collection and transport of, 206t
Cardiac occlusion devices, infections of, 1036
Cardiac pacemakers, infections of, 1033-1034
Cardiac tamponade
in HIV infection, 1560
in pericarditis, 1060
Cardiac valves
diseases of, in rheumatic fever, 2382-2383, 2383f, 2386
in endocarditis, 976, 977
replacement of, for endocarditis, 1001-1002
streptococci susceptibility of, 2436
Cardiobacterium [spp.], 2751t, 2754-2755
Cardiobacterium hominis
cardiovascular device infections from, 1023
endocarditis from, 991
prosthetic valve, treatment of, 1028, 1029t
laboratory identification of, 220
Cardiomyopathy
dilated
after enteroviral myopericarditis, 2153
myocarditis in, 1052-1057
from *Trypanosoma cruzi,* 3160, 3160f
left ventricular dysfunction with, in HIV infection, 1560
Cardiopulmonary bypass, postoperative infections and, 3538
Cardiothoracic surgery, mediastinitis from, 1071-1072
treatment of, 1074

Cardiotoxicity
    of BILN 2061, 1969
    of quinidine gluconate, 3135-3136
Cardiovascular agents, rifamycin interaction with, 376t
Cardiovascular device infections, 1022-1034, 1022t
    clinical manifestations of, 1023
    diagnosis of, 1023
    epidemiology of, 1022
    from *Staphylococcus epidermidis*, 2357
    microbiology of, 1023
    pathogenesis of, 1022-1023
    prevention of, 1024
    treatment of, 1023-1024
Cardiovascular disease, atherosclerotic, from *Chlamydia pneumoniae*, 2263-2266
Cardiovascular system
    Brucella infections of, 2671
    in secondary peritonitis, 934-935
    syphilis of, 2776
    viral infections of, specimen collection in, 233t
Carditis
    from *Candida*, 2945, 2950
    from *Chlamydia psittaci*, 2257
    from enteroviruses, 2152-2153
    in Kawasaki disease, 3317
    rheumatic, 2381, 2382
Caribbean, HIV infection in, 1469
    among women, 1618
Caries. *See* Dental caries.
L-Carnitine, for lipodystrophy, 609
β-Carotene, in lung cancer prevention, 141
Carotid artery erosion, in odontogenic infections, 794
Carotid artery, synthetic patches for, infections of, 1040-1041
Carrión's disease, 2733
Casaba virus, 1913-1919, 1914t. *See also* Alphaviruses.
Case series, 164-165
Case-control studies, 165
Case-fatality rate, 167
Caspofungin, 511
    dosage of, 678t-679t
    drug interactions with, 687t
    for aspergillosis, 2968t, 2969
    for cancer-related febrile neutropenia, 3455
    for *Candida* esophagitis, 1234
    for candidiasis, 2949-2951
    for fusariosis, 3073
    formulations of, 649t
    structure of, 503f
Castleman's disease
    human herpesvirus type 8 in, 1602
    multicentric, 1830, 1830f
Cat(s), as toxoplasmosis vector, 3181, 3191
Cat bites, 3552-3553, 3552t, 3553t
    Pasteurella infections in, 2687-2688
Cat flea, as *Bartonella henselae* vector, 2733
Catalase test, 216t, 217, 217t
Cataract, removal of, endophthalmitis after, 1407-1411, 1407f, 1408f
CATCH 22, 150t
Catecholamines, 909
Cathelicidins, 102
Catheterization
    cardiac. *See* Cardiac catheterization.
    urine collection by, 885
Catheter-related infections, 3347-3358, 3424. *See also* Percutaneous intravascular devices.
    anti-infective equipment and, 3357-3358
    diagnosis of, 3350-3351, 3350t
    epidemiology of, 3348
    from *Candida*, 2948-2949, 2950
    from femoral artery catheterization, 1040

Catheter-related infections *(Continued)*
    from infusate contamination, 3347-3348
    from insertion site contamination, 3348
    from junction contamination, 3348
    from nontuberculous mycobacteria, 2910t, 2913
    from *Staphylococcus aureus*, 3349
    from *Stenotrophomonas maltophilia*, 2618
    in arterial lines, transducers, and transducer domes, 3355-3356, 3356t
    in cancer patients, 3433-3434, 3434f, 3455-3457
    in central venous access, 2618, 3352-3355, 3353t, 3354t, 3357-3358
    in elderly, 3518
    in peripheral intravenous cannulization, 3351-3352
    in pulmonary artery catheterization, 3355
    in spinal cord injury, 3513-3514
    in total parenteral nutrition, 3352-3355, 3353t, 3354t
    laboratory diagnosis of, 3428
    microbiology of, 3349-3350, 3350t
    pathogenesis of, 3347-3348, 3347f
    pathogens in, 3421t
    prevention of, 3356-3358, 3356t
    risk factors for, 3348-3349, 3349t
    urinary tract, 3370-3377. *See also* Urinary tract infections, catheter-related.
Catheters
    bacteremia from, 209-210
    bacteriuria in, 883
    central venous, *Stenotrophomonas maltophilia* infections of, 2618
    femoral artery, infections of, 1040
    for intraperitoneal abscess drainage, 944
    infections from
        in endocarditis risk, 1044-1045
        methenamine for, 477
        topical antibacterial therapy for, 481
        vancomycin for, 423
    intravenous, tip cultures of, 210
    Ochrobactrum anthropi infections of, 2759
    peritoneal dialysis
        peritonitis from, 942
        Staphylococcus epidermidis infections of, 2355
    specimen collection and transport from, 205t
    Staphylococcus epidermidis infections of, 2354-2355
    suppurative thrombophlebitis prevention with, 1005
Cationic antimicrobial protein, 102
Cat-scratch disease, 1207
    ciprofloxacin for, 465
    computed tomography of, 2737, 2739f
    diagnosis of, 2740
    differential diagnosis of, 2740
    encephalopathy in, 2738-2739
    from *Bartonella henselae*, 2736-2740, 2737f-2740f
    lymphadenopathy in, 2736-2737, 2737f, 2738f
    neuroretinitis in, 2739-2740, 2740f
    papule in, 2736, 2737f
    Parinaud's oculoglandular syndrome in, 1207, 1391, 2737, 2739f
    treatment of, 1211
    uveitis in, 1417, 1417f
Cavernous sinus thrombosis, 794, 795f, 797t, 1168-1170, 1169f, 1421-1424, 1421f. *See also* Odontogenic infections.
    treatment of, 797t
CCAAT/enhancer binding protein epsilon, 108
CCL19, 121
CCL21, 121

CCR2, in human immunodeficiency virus infection susceptibility, 45, 45t, 47
CCR5, 1528, 1528f
    blockade of, 20
    in HIV replication, 1540
CCR5
    in HIV nonprogression, 1532
    in human immunodeficiency virus infection susceptibility, 45, 45t, 47, 48
    mutation of, 1528
CCR5 chemokine receptor, 35
CCR7, 121
CD1, 128-130
    antigen presentation by, 129
    antigen processing by, 129, 130f
    isoforms of, 129, 130f
    mycobacteria presentation to, 129-130
    proteins of, 129
    structure of, 129, 129f
CD4, 133
    apoptosis of, 1534-1535
    CD8+ T cells and, 134
    decreased production of, 1535-1536
    depletion of, in HIV infection, 1534-1536
    in acute retroviral syndrome, 1553
    in antiretroviral therapy, 1669, 1679
    in HIV infection, 1527-1528, 1528f, 1531-1532, 1709
        pregnancy and, 1622
    in HIV infection–related lymphoma, 1605
    in leprosy, 2888, 2889
    in opportunistic infections, 1549, 1550f, 1679-1680
        prophylaxis indications and, 1684t
    in *Pneumocystis jirovecii* pneumonia, 1679
    in *Pseudomonas aeruginosa* resistance, 2591
    in sepsis, 916
    in tuberculosis response, 2859-2860
    redistribution of, 1536
    resting, as HIV reservoir, 1533
    soluble, 20, 20t
    thymic selection of, 131
CD4 receptors, human immunodeficiency virus binding to, 17, 17f
CD5, 63
CD8, 133
    effector functions of, 133-134
    in acute retroviral syndrome, 1553
    in HIV infection, 1530-1531, 1530t, 1536, 1709
    in HIV nonprogression, 1532
    in sepsis, 916
    in viral infections, 122
    thymic selection of, 131
CD8+ T-cell antiviral factors, in HIV infection, 1531
CD14, 907, 907f
CD18 deficiency, 154
CD19, 61, 75
CD21, 61
    in HIV infection, 1536
CD22, 61t
CD28, in T cell activation, 62
CD32, in infections susceptibility, 46
CD36, in malaria susceptibility, 44t
CD40, deficiency of, 153
CD40 ligand, 61
CD46, 82-83
CD47, in neutrophil migration, 98
CD55, 74t
CD59, 74, 74t
    deficiency of, 80t
    in paroxysmal nocturnal hemoglobinuria, 86
    serum resistance and, 77
    in T cell activation, 62-63

CD81, 61
CD86, in T cell activation, 63
CD154, 61
Cefaclor
    dosage of, 654t-655t
    formulations of, 647t
    structure of, 295f
    uses of, 305, 305t
Cefadroxil
    dosage of, 654t-655t
    for cellulitis, 1180
    for impetigo, 1173
    formulations of, 647t
    structure of, 294f
    uses of, 304, 305t
Cefamandole
    dosage of, 654t-655t
    formulations of, 647t
    prophylactic, perioperative, 3543t
    structure of, 295f
    uses of, 304, 305, 305t
Cefazolin
    dosage of, 654t-655t
    for bacterial arthritis, 1316t
    for cellulitis, 1180
    for dialysis-related peritonitis, 942t
    for endocarditis prophylaxis, 1050t
    for osteomyelitis, 1324t, 1325
    for peritonitis, 938
    for Staphylococcus aureus endocarditis,
        2344t
    for streptococcal endocarditis, 995
    for Streptococcus agalactiae (group B)
        infections, 2430
    formulations of, 647t
    prophylactic, perioperative, 3543t
    structure of, 294f
    uses of, 304, 305t
Cefdinir
    dosage of, 656t-657t
    for otitis media, 769
    for sinusitis, 779-780, 779t
    for streptococcal pharyngitis, 2368
    for Streptococcus pneumoniae otitis media,
        2404
    formulations of, 647t
    structure of, 296f
    uses of, 305t, 306
Cefditoren
    dosage of, 656t-657t
    drug interactions with, 687t
    formulations of, 647t
    structure of, 296f
    uses of, 305t, 306
Cefepime
    chemistry of, 295, 297f, 297t
    clinical uses of, 305t, 307
    dosage of, 658t-659t
    for acute pyelonephritis, 889
    for asplenia, 3529
    for bacterial arthritis, 1316t
    for brain abscess, 1157, 1159t
    for febrile neutropenia, 3450-3452,
        3451t
    for meningitis, 1106t, 1107t, 1112
    for osteomyelitis, 1324t
    for pneumonia, 837-839, 837t, 838t
    for Pseudomonas aeruginosa bacteremia,
        2601
    for sepsis, 919t
    formulations of, 647t
    uses of, 305t, 306
Cefixime
    dosage of, 656t-657t

    for febrile neutropenia, 3450-3452,
        3451t
    for Shigella, 2659t
    for streptococcal pharyngitis, 2368
    for urethritis, 1207
    formulations of, 647t
    structure of, 296f
    uses of, 305t, 306
Cefmetazole
    dosage of, 654t-655t
    formulations of, 647t
    prophylactic, perioperative, 3543t
    structure of, 295f
    uses of, 305-306, 305t
Cefonicid
    dosage of, 654t-655t
    formulations of, 647t
    structure of, 295f
    uses of, 304, 305, 305t
Cefoperazone
    dosage of, 656t-657t
    for peritonitis, 938
    formulations of, 647t
    structure of, 296f
    uses of, 305t, 306
Cefotaxime
    dosage of, 656t-657t
    for brain abscess, 1157, 1159, 1159t
    for epiglottitis, 786
    for Lyme borreliosis, 1115
    for meningitis, 1106t, 1107t, 1112-1115
    for nocardiosis, 2921
    for pneumococcal pneumonia, 2405
    for postoperative gynecologic infections,
        1377t
    for primary peritonitis, 931
    for sepsis, 919
    for streptococcus group G, 2445
    formulations of, 647t
    prophylactic, nosocomial pneumonia and, 3368
    structure of, 296f
    uses of, 305t, 306
Cefotetan
    dosage of, 654t-655t
    for odontogenic infections, 797, 797t
    for pelvic inflammatory disease, 1379t
    for peritonitis, 938
    for postoperative gynecologic infections, 1377t
    formulations of, 647t
    prophylactic, perioperative, 3543t
    resistance to, cephamycinases in, 259t
    structure of, 295f
    uses of, 305-306, 305t
Cefoxitin
    dosage of, 656t-657t
    for nontuberculous mycobacterial infections,
        2911, 2913t
    for odontogenic infections, 797, 797t
    for pelvic inflammatory disease, 460, 1379t,
        2525, 2525t
    for peritonitis, 937t, 938
    for postoperative gynecologic infections, 1377t
    formulations of, 647t
    prophylactic, perioperative, 3543t
    resistance to, cephamycinases in, 259t
    structure of, 295f
    uses of, 305-306, 305t
Cefpirome, 305t, 306
Cefpodoxime
    dosage of, 656t-657t
    for Neisseria gonorrhoeae infections, 2524,
        2524t
    for pneumonia, 837-839, 838t
    for sinusitis, 779-780, 779t

Cefpodoxime (Continued)
    for streptococcal pharyngitis, 2368
    for Streptococcus pneumoniae otitis media,
        2404
    formulations of, 647t
    structure of, 296f
    uses of, 305t, 306
Cefprozil
    dosage of, 656t-657t
    for pneumonia, 837-839, 838t
    formulations of, 647t
    structure of, 295f
    uses of, 305, 305t
Cefsulodin
    dosage of, 656t-657t
    formulations of, 647t
Ceftazidime
    dosage of, 656t-657t
    for acute pyelonephritis, 889
    for bacterial arthritis, 1316t
    for dialysis-related peritonitis, 942t
    for endophthalmitis, 1410-1411
    for febrile neutropenia, 3453f
    for melioidosis, 2629t
    for meningitis, 1106t, 1107t, 1114, 2604
    for Pseudomonas aeruginosa bacteremia, 2601
    for Pseudomonas aeruginosa burn infections,
        2606
    for Pseudomonas aeruginosa meningitis, 2604
    formulations of, 647t
    in preemptive pancreatic infection treatment,
        963, 963t
    structure of, 296f
    uses of, 305t, 306-307
Ceftibuten
    for streptococcal pharyngitis, 2368
    formulations of, 647t
    structure of, 296f
    uses of, 305t, 307
Ceftizoxime
    dosage of, 658t-659t
    for brain abscess, 1159, 1159t
    for odontogenic infections, 797, 797t
    for peritonitis, 938
    formulations of, 647t
    structure of, 296f
    uses of, 305t, 306
Ceftriaxone
    dosage of, 658t-659t
    for asplenia, 3529
    for bacterial arthritis, 1316t
    for brain abscess, 1157, 1159, 1159t
    for cavernous sinus thrombosis, 1424
    for chancroid, 1344
    for culture-negative endocarditis, 1001
    for disseminated gonococcal infections, 2526
    for epiglottitis, 786
    for febrile neutropenia, 3450-3452, 3451t,
        3453t
    for gonococcal epididymitis, 2526
    for gonococcal pelvic inflammatory disease,
        2525, 2525t
    for Haemophilus ducreyi, 2667
    for leptospirosis, 2793t
    for Lyme disease, 1115, 2806, 2806t
    for lymphangitis, 1212
    for meningitis, 1106t, 1107t, 1112-1115, 2405,
        2507, 2507t
    for prevention, 1118
    for Neisseria gonorrhoeae, 2524, 2524t
    for Neisseria meningitidis, 2507, 2507t, 2509
    for neonatal conjunctivitis, 1392-1393
    for neurosyphilis, 1115
    for nocardiosis, 2920t, 2921

Ceftriaxone (Continued)
  for orbital/preseptal cellulitis, 1423-1424, 1423f
  for osteomyelitis, 1324t, 1325
  for otitis media, 769
  for pediatric gonorrhea, 2526
  for pelvic inflammatory disease, 1379t
  for pneumococcal pneumonia, 2405
  for pneumonia, 837-839, 837t, 838t
  for postoperative gynecologic infections, 1377t
  for primary peritonitis, 931
  for prosthetic valve endocarditis, 1029
  for sepsis, 919t
  for *Shigella,* 2659t
  for streptococcal endocarditis, 995
    prosthetic valve, 1027t
  for *Streptococcus pneumoniae* meningitis, 2405
  for syphilis, 1344
  for *Treponema pallidum,* in HIV infection, 1690t
  for typhoid fever, 2648, 2649t
  for urethritis, 1207
  for urogenital chlamydial infections, 2247t, 2250
  for viridans streptococcus endocarditis, 2437t, 2438
  for Whipple's disease, 1309, 1310t
  formulations of, 647t
  pneumococcal resistance to, 837, 837t
  resistance to
    by *Neisseria gonorrhoeae,* 2519
    by *Salmonella,* 2640
  structure of, 296f
  uses of, 305t, 306, 307
Cefuroxime
  dosage of, 656t-657t
  for COPD exacerbations, 811t
  for Lyme disease, 2806, 2806t
  for meningitis, 1112
  for *Neisseria gonorrhoeae,* 2524-2525, 2524t
  for nocardiosis, 2921
  for otitis media, 769
  for peritonitis, 938
  for pneumonia, 837-839, 837t, 838t
  for respiratory infections, 462
  for sinusitis, 779-780, 779t
  for streptococcal pharyngitis, 2368
  for *Streptococcus pneumoniae* otitis media, 2404
  formulations of, 647t
  in preemptive pancreatic infection treatment, 965, 965t
  in preemptive pancreatic infections treatment, 963, 963t, 964
  pneumococcal resistance to, 837, 837t
  prophylactic, perioperative, 3543t
  resistance to, beta-lactamases in, 259t
  structure of, 295f
  uses of, 304-305, 305t
Cell membrane permeability, in antibiotic resistance, 262
Cell membrane proteins, in complement regulation, 74t
Cellubrevin, in botulism, 2823
Cellular tropism, 34-35
Cellulitis, 1178-1180. *See also* Soft tissue infections.
  after saphenous vein resection, 1178, 1180
  anaerobic
    clostridial, 1187-1189, 1188t
    nonclostridial, 1188t, 1189
  clinical findings in, 1178-1180
  diagnosis of, 1179
  differential diagnosis of, 1179-1180, 1180t

Cellulitis, 1178-1180 (Continued)
  eosinophilic, 1180
  etiology of, 1178-1180, 1178t
  from *Aeromonas hydrophila,* 1179
  from *Clostridium* spp., 1187-1189, 1188t
    crepitant, 2831
    vs. gas gangrene, 1199
  from *Cryptococcus neoformans,* 3003t, 3004-3005, 3005f
  from *Erysipelothrix rhusiopathiae,* 1179
  from *Haemophilus influenzae,* 1178-1179, 1186
  from *Helicobacter cinaedi,* 1186
  from *Streptococcus iniae,* 1184
  from *Streptococcus pyogenes* (group A), 2370-2371, 2371f
  from type b *Haemophilus influenzae,* 2664
  from *Vibrio vulnificus,* 1179, 2546
  gangrenous, 1181-1182, 1181f, 1183t, 1186
  in cancer, 1179, 3438
  in elderly, 3520
  in immunocompromised host, 1179, 3438
  in injection drug users, 3463
  in neonates, 1178-1179
  in sepsis, 917
  of scalp, 1179
  orbital, 1421-1424, 1421f-1423f
    in mucormycosis, 1423, 2975-2977, 2976f
  pelvic, from herpes simplex virus, 1768
  perianal, from *Streptococcus pyogenes* (group A), 2375
  pneumococcal, 1179
  predisposing factors in, 1178t
  preseptal, 1421-1424, 1421f-1423f
  quinolones for, 463-464
  recurrent, 1180
  staphylococcal, 1179, 1180, 2341, 2341f
  streptococcal, 1178, 1179, 1180, 1184, 1189
  synergistic necrotizing, 1183t, 1188t, 1191, 1200
  treatment of, 1180
  types of, 1178t
  vaginal cuff, postoperative, 1376-1377, 1377t
Centers for Disease Control and Prevention
  Gilardi rod group 1, 2762
  group EF-4, 2751t, 2756
  group NO-1, 2762
  group WO-1, 2762
  group WO-2, 2762
  groups O-1,2,3, 2762
Central European encephalitis, 1928, 1929. *See also* Tick-borne encephalitis.
Central nervous system
  cephalosporin effects on, 304
  isoniazid effects on, 490
  metronidazole effects on, 391
  penicillin effects on, 287
  quinolone effects on, 466
  tetracycline effects on, 363t, 364-365
  trimethoprim effects on, 445
  tuberculosis of, 2877-2878, 2877f
Central nervous system infections, 1079-1083. *See also specific sites and types.*
  anaerobic, 2813, 2813f
  brain abscess in, 1150-1161
  cerebrospinal fluid analysis in, 1080-1082, 1081t, 1082t
  clinical manifestations of, 1079-1080
  diagnosis of, 1080-1082
  differential diagnosis of, 3437
  encephalitis in, 1132t, 1143-1147
  focal lesions in, 1079-1080, 1132t
  from *Bacillus,* 2495
  from *Bartonella henselae,* 2739
  from *Bordetella pertussis,* 2704

Central nervous system infections (Continued)
  from *Brucella,* 2671
  from *Campylobacter fetus,* 2553
  from *Clostridium,* 2830
  from HIV
    complications of, 1583-1598
    masses in, 1591-1592, 1592f
    pediatric, 1642-1643
  from *Listeria monocytogenes,* 2480, 2481
  from lumbar puncture, 1080
  from *Mycobacterium tuberculosis,* 2877-2878, 2877f
  from *Pasteurella,* 2688
  from *Pseudomonas aeruginosa,* 2603-2604
  from *Salmonella,* 2647t
  from *Schistosoma,* 3279
  from *Streptococcus anginosus* group, 2454
  in cancer, 3437-3438
  in elderly, 3521
  in endocarditis, 982, 984
  in immunocompromised host, 3437-3438
  in Lyme disease, 2802, 2802t
  in syphilis, 2774-2776
  in systemic response regulation, 908
  in Whipple's disease, 1308-1309
  intracranial pressure monitoring in, 1083
  laboratory diagnosis of, 210-211
  lumbar puncture in, 1080-1082
  management of, 1082-1083
    adjunctive therapy in, 1082-1083
    antimicrobial therapy in, 1082
    surgery in, 1082-1083
  meningitis in
    acute, 1083-1119. *See also* Meningitis, acute.
    chronic, 1132-1140. *See also* Meningitis, chronic.
  myelitis in, 1143-1147
  neuritis in, 1143-1147
  neuroimaging studies in, 1082
  route of entry in, 1144
  shunt-related, 1035, 1126-1130
  viral, specimen collection in, 233t
Central nervous system lymphoma, HIV-related, 1588-1589, 1589f, 1607-1609, 1695, 1813
  treatment of, 1608-1609
Central venous catheter infections, 3352-3355, 3353f, 3354t. *See also* Catheter-related infections.
  anti-infective equipment and, 3357-3358
  from *Stenotrophomonas maltophilia,* 2618
Cepacia syndrome, 2618, 2618f
Cephadrine, dosage of, 654t-655t
Cephalexin
  dosage of, 654t-655t
  for cellulitis, 1180
  for impetigo, 1173, 1174
  for lymphadenitis, 1211
  for lymphangitis, 1212
  for relapsing urinary tract infections, 891
  for skin infections, 463-464
  formulations of, 647t
  structure of, 294f
  uses of, 304, 305t
Cephalosporins, 294-307. *See also* Beta-lactam antibiotics *and specific agents.*
  activity spectrum of, 297, 298t-299t, 300
  adverse reactions to, 303-304, 303t
  chemistry of, 294-296, 294f-297f
  classification of, 296-297, 297t
  cross-reactivity among, 324-325
  distribution of, 302
  dosage of, 305t, 654t-659t
    in renal insufficiency, 302t, 303
  drug interactions with, 687t

Cephalosporins (Continued)
first-generation
chemistry of, 294-295, 294f, 297t
clinical uses of, 304, 305t
dosage of, 654t-655t
formulations of, 647t
for acute pyelonephritis, 889
for biliary tract infections, 957
for brain abscess, 1157, 1158t, 1159, 1159t
for disseminated gonococcal infections, 2526
for Enterobacteriaceae endocarditis, 999
for enterococcal endocarditis, 997
for *Haemophilus* endocarditis, 1000
for liver abscess, 954t
for Lyme borreliosis, 1115
for meningitis, 1112-1114
for *Neisseria gonorrhoeae*, 2524t, 2525
for *Neisseria meningitidis,* 2507, 2507t
for neurosyphilis, 1115
for nocardiosis, 2920t, 2921
for otitis media, 769
for peritonitis
primary, 931
secondary, 938
for pneumococcal pneumonia, 2405
for staphylococcal endocarditis, 998
prosthetic valve, 1026t, 1027
for streptococcal pharyngitis, 2367t, 2368
for streptococcal pyoderma, 2370
for *Streptococcus agalactiae* (group B), 2429
for *Streptococcus anginosus* group, 2455
for suppurative thrombophlebitis, 1005
for typhoid fever, 2648, 2649t
for urogenital chlamydial infections, 2247t, 2250
formulations of, 647t
fourth-generation. *See also* Cefepime.
chemistry of, 295, 297f, 297t
clinical uses of, 305t, 307
formulations of, 647t
in preemptive pancreatic infection treatment,
965t
mechanism of action of, 297
nucleus of, 294, 294f
pharmacokinetics, 301, 301t
pharmacology of, 301-303, 301t, 302t
prophylactic, perioperative, 3543t
resistance to
by *Neisseria gonorrhoeae,* 186
by *Salmonella,* 2640
mechanisms of, 299-300
postoperative infections and, 3539-3540
second-generation
chemistry of, 295, 295f, 297t
clinical uses of, 304-306, 305t
dosage of, 654t-657t
formulations of, 647t
structure of, 320f
third-generation
chemistry of, 295, 296f, 297t
clinical uses of, 305t, 306-307
dosage of, 656t-659t
formulations of, 647t
uses of, 304-307
Cephalothin
dosage of, 654t-655t
for penicillin-resistant enterococcal
endocarditis, 996
formulations of, 647t
structure of, 294f
uses of, 304, 305t
Cephamycin, 297t, 304, 305t
Cephamycin C, 294
Cephapirin
dosage of, 654t-655t
formulations of, 647t

Cephapirin (Continued)
structure of, 294f
uses of, 304, 305t
Cephradine
for cellulitis, 1180
formulations of, 647t
structure of, 294f
uses of, 304, 305t
Cercarial dermatitis, 3278, 3294t, 3298
Cercopithecine herpesvirus. *See also* Herpes B
virus.
laboratory studies for, 238
valacyclovir for, 520
Cerebellar ataxia, from varicella zoster virus,
1782
Cerebral amebiasis, 3103
Cerebral cryptococcomas, 3004, 3004f, 3007
Cerebral edema. *See also* Intracranial
hypertension.
in cryptococcal meningitis, 3008
Cerebral function, in sepsis, 915
Cerebral malaria, 3122, 3123-3125. *See also*
Malaria.
sickle cell anemia and, 3126
Cerebral mucormycosis, 2978
brain abscess in, 1152, 1155, 1158t, 1160,
2976-2977
in injection drug users, 2978, 3471
Cerebrospinal fluid
bactericidal activity in, 1111
collection and transport of, 206t, 1080
in HIV infection, 1585
in primary central nervous system lymphoma,
1588-1589
in progressive multifocal leukoencephalopathy,
1590
vancomycin in, 420
viridians streptococci in, 2439
Cerebrospinal fluid analysis, 1080-1082
appearance of, 1080-1081
cell count in, 1081
culture in, 3-4, 1080t
for brain abscess, 1157
glucose concentration in, 1081
in Creutzfeldt-Jakob disease, 2224
in cryptococcosis, 3002-3003
in encephalitis, 1145
in meningitis, 1080-1082, 1081t, 1101-1103
acute, 1080-1082, 1081t, 1101-1103
aseptic, 2148-2149
chronic, 1134-1135, 1134t
in myelitis, 1145-1146
in neuritis, 1147-1148
in progressive multifocal leukoencephalopathy,
1860
in shunt infections, 1129. *See also*
Cerebrospinal fluid shunt infections.
in subdural empyema, 1164
in suppurative intracranial thrombosis, 1169
in toxoplasmosis, 3185
India ink smear in, 2937
latex agglutination test in, 1081-1082
lumbar puncture for, 1080
opening pressure in, 1080-1081
polymerase chain reaction in, 1082
protein concentration in, 1081
specimen collection and transport for, 1080
tests in, 3-4, 1080t
Cerebrospinal fluid hypoglycorrhacia, 1081,
1081t
Cerebrospinal fluid leak
in skull fractures
chemoprophylaxis for, 1103
radiography of, 1103
surgery for, 1117

Cerebrospinal fluid leak (Continued)
radiography of, 1103
surgery for, 1117
Cerebrospinal fluid shunt infections, 1035, 1126-
1130
bacterial virulence factors in, 1128
clinical features of, 1128
diagnosis of, 1128-1129
epidemiology of, 1126-1127
etiology of, 1127, 1127t
from *Coccidioides immitis,* 3048
host defense mechanisms in, 1128
incidence of, 1126-1127
pathogenesis of, 1127-1128
pathophysiology of, 1127-1128
risk factors for, 1126-1127, 1127t
shunt reimplantation after, 1130
shunt removal in, 1130
treatment of, 1129-1130, 1129t
Cerebrospinal fluid VDRL test, for neurosyphilis,
2779-2780
Cerebrovascular accident, fever of unknown
origin in, 721
Cervical cancer, 1611
Chlamydia trachomatis and, 2248
human papillomavirus and, 1843, 1850-1851,
1851t
in HIV infection, 1486, 1610, 1611t
screening for, 1850-1851, 1851t
in HIV infection, 1610, 1611t
Cervical discharge, examination of, 1361
Cervical intraepithelial neoplasia, 1610-1611
in HIV infection, 1609
treatment of, 1691t
Cervical lymphadenitis, 799, 1205, 1208, 1209t.
See also Lymphadenitis/lymphadenopathy.
from nontuberculous mycobacteria, 2897,
2899, 2902, 2902f, 2903-2905, 2904t,
2906, 2910t, 2911
tuberculous, 1206-1207
Cervicitis, 1368-1369
examination in, 1361
from *Chlamydia trachomatis,* 1368-1369,
2247t, 2248, 2249t, 2250
from cytomegalovirus, in pregnancy, 1796-
1798, 1797t
from herpes simplex virus, 1766, 1767f. *See
also* Herpes simplex virus, genital.
from human papillomavirus, 1609
in HIV infection, 1629, 1691t
from *Mycoplasma genitalium,* 2281, 2281t
from *Neisseria gonorrhoeae,* 1368-1369, 2520,
2520f
quinolones for, 460
in pelvic inflammatory disease, 1378-1380,
1379t
mucopurulent, in HIV infection, 1628
Cervicofacial infections. *See* Neck infections;
Orofacial infections.
Cervicovaginal lavage, for HIV, 1619
Cesarean delivery, antibiotic prophylaxis for,
1373, 1374
Cestodes. *See* Tapeworms.
CFTR gene, 869-870
CH$_{50}$, in complement evaluation, 87
Chaetomium spp., brain abscess from, 3070
Chagas' disease, 3156-3163. *See also*
Trypanosomiasis, American.
Chagoma, 3158
Chalazion, 1419
Chancre, syphilitic, 733, 1340-1344
characteristics of, 1339-1340, 1340f
duration of, 1341-1342
presentation of, 1338-1339

Chancriform lesions, etiology of, 1173t, 1176
Chancroid, 1338-1344, 1340f, 1342t
  ciprofloxacin for, 460
  clinical features of, 1340-1341, 1340f
  diagnosis of, 1342
  duration of, 1342
  epidemiology of, 1342
  from *Haemophilus ducreyi,* 2666-2667
  in HIV infection, 1342
  inguinal buboes in, 1207
  laboratory tests for, 1342, 1343f
  presentation of, 1338-1339
  treatment of, 1344
Chandipura virus, 1939, 2045, 2045t
Changuinola virus, 1899
Chaperones, 8
Chédiak-Higashi syndrome, 151t, 154
  impaired chemotaxis in, 105, 105f
  laboratory studies in, 149
Cheilitis, angular
  from *Candida,* 2941, 2951
  in HIV infection, 1554, 1555f
Chemical conjunctivitis, in neonate, 1392
Chemical sterilants, 3331. *See also* Sterilization.
Chemoattractants, in neutrophil migration, 98
Chemokine(s)
  acute-phase response and, 38, 38t
  CD8⁺ T-cell production of, 134
  chemotaxis and, 39
  in HIV replication, 1540
  in neutrophil migration, 98
  in *Pseudomonas aeruginosa* resistance, 2590-2591
  innate immunity and, 38, 38t
  lymphocyte mediation by, 121
Chemokine receptor(s)
  HIV binding to, 17, 17f
  in infections susceptibility, 47-48
Chemokine receptor gene, HIV transmission and, 1489
Chemokine/co-receptor inhibitors, 20-21
Chemotaxis
  chemokines and, 39
  defective, 105-106, 105f
    extrinsic, 105
    intrinsic, 105-106, 105f
Chemotherapy. *See also* Cancer.
  enterocolitis from, 3438, 3457
  febrile neutropenia and, 3432-3439, 3442-3458. *See also* Febrile neutropenia, in cancer.
  for HIV-related lymphoma, 1605-1607, 1606t
  for Hodgkin's disease, 1612
  for Kaposi's sarcoma, 1603
  for primary central nervous system lymphoma, 1608
  immunosuppression from, 3432
  in chronic hepatitis B, 1450
  in stem cell transplant, 3486
  mucositis from, 3438, 3457
  specimen collection before, 204
  thymic effects of, 132
Chest films. *See* Radiography, chest.
Chest tube, for pleural effusion/empyema, 850-851
Cheyletiella spp., 3311
Chicken, *Salmonella* infections from, 2639-240, 2639f
Chickenpox. *See* Varicella.
Chiclero's ulcer, 3145t, 3149, 3150
Chiggers, 3310-3311, 3311f
  as scrub typhus vector, 2285t, 3311
Chikungunya virus, 1913-1919, 1914t. *See also* Alphaviruses.
  laboratory studies for, 238

Child care centers
  diarrhea in, 1241
  hepatitis A outbreaks in, 2171, 2171f, 2178
  rhinovirus outbreaks in, 2188
Children
  acute respiratory infections in, 174-175
  aminoglycoside dosage in, 349, 349t
  anthrax in, post-exposure prophylaxis for, 3622t
  appendicitis in, vs. primary peritonitis, 930
  bacteriuria in, 882-883, 882f
  blastomycosis in, 3033-3034
  chloramphenicol in, 368
  cholera in, 2540
  cryptosporidiosis in, 3217, 3219
    malnutrition and, 3219-3220
  diarrhea in, 176-177
    mortality rates from, 1215
  drug dosages for, 650t-685t
  endocarditis prophylaxis in, 1049
  fever in
    bacteremia and, 713, 724
    fever of unknown origin in, 713, 720, 724
    seizures in, 712-713
  giardiasis in, 3201
  HIV exposure in, accidental, 1651
  HIV infection in, 1487-1488, 1488f, 1638-1651
    antiretroviral therapy for, 1646t-1648t, 1647-1649
      prophylaxis with, 1639, 1640t
    bacterial infections in, 1641
    Candida infections in, 1643
    cardiac manifestations of, 1643
    central nervous system complications in, 1642-1643
    classification of, 1640, 1641t, 1642t
    clinical categories of, 1640, 1641t, 1642t
    clinical manifestations of, 1640-1644
    complications of, 1643
    culture in, 1644
    daily life management in, 1650-1651
    diagnosis of, 1644-1645
    encephalopathy in, 1642-1643, 1643f
    epidemiology of, 1638-1639
    from accidental exposure, 1651
    growth abnormalities in, 1641
    hematologic complications in, 1643
    immunizations in, 1649-1650
    in United States, 1638-1639, 1638f
    informed consent in, 1645
    intravenous immune globulin in, 1648
    kidney in, 1643
    laboratory findings in, 1644
    lymphocytic interstitial pneumonitis in, 1641
    malignancies in, 1643
    metabolic complications of, 1643-1644
    opportunistic infections in, 1640-1641
      prophylaxis against, 1649
    p24 antigen in, 1644-1645
    Pneumocystis jirovecii pneumonia in, 1640, 1643f
      prophylaxis against, 1649
    polymerase chain reaction assay in, 1644
    prevention of, perinatal, 1639, 1640t
    rapid testing in, 1645
    RNA assay in, 1644
    serologic testing in, 1645
    symptom onset in, 1640, 1641f
    transmission of, perinatal, 1638f, 1639, 1640t
    treatment of, 1646-1650
    Web sites for, 1648t
    worldwide, 1639
  Kawasaki disease in, 755, 1179, 3316-3318, 3316f, 3317f

Children *(Continued)*
  legionnaires' disease in, 2715
  leukemia in, chloramphenicol and, 369
  meningitis in
    combination therapy for, 249
    glucocorticosteroids for, 559
    treatment of, 1107t
  mycotic aneurysms in, 1006
  Neisseria gonorrhoeae infections in, 2523
    treatment of, 2526
  nitrofurantoin in, 475-476
  respiratory tract infections in, from nontypeable *Haemophilus influenzae,* 2663
  rheumatic fever in, 2381
  rotavirus infections in, 178, 1904
  sexual abuse/assault of, HIV infection in, 1651
  Shigella treatment in, 2659, 2659t
  Staphylococcus epidermidis infections in, 2357
  Streptococcus agalactiae (group B) infections in, 2426-2427
  syphilis in, 2777, 2777t
  temperature in, 707
  tuberculosis in, 2862, 2863-2864
    treatment of, 2872
  urinary tract infections in, 886-887
    imaging of, 899-900, 900f
  vaccines for
    adverse effects of, 3580t-3581t
    DPT, 2464
    pneumococcal, 175
    schedule of, 3563f, 3564f, 3574-3575
    standards for, 3582t
  viral infections in, laboratory studies for, 234-235, 235t
  Yersinia enterocolitica infections in, 2698
Chimpanzee, as HIV reservoir, 2119
Chimpanzee coryza agent, 2009
China, HIV infection in, 1469
  among women, 1618
Chinese restaurant syndrome, 1290
Chiropractic therapy, 604
Chlamydia [spp.]
  biology of, 2236
  characteristics of, 2236-2238, 2237t
  classification of, 2236, 2256
  clinical manifestations of, 2237t, 2238
  collection and transport of, 207t
  complications of, 2237t, 2238
  course of, 2237t, 2238
  elementary body of, 2236, 2237f, 2238, 2239-2240, 2240f
  endocarditis from, treatment of, 1001
  genital infections from, quinolones for, 460
  genome of, 2237-2238
  host range of, 2237t, 2238
  inclusions of, 2236, 2237f
  life cycle of, 2236, 2239-2240, 2240f
  persistence of, 2238
  prevention of, 2237t
  reinfections with, 2238
  replication of, 2236
  respiratory, laboratory culture of, 208
  reticulate body of, 2236, 2237f, 2238, 2239-2240, 2240f
  rifamycin for, 382
  strains of, 2237t, 2238
  structure of, 2236, 2237, 2237f
  transmission of, 2237t, 2238, 2245-2246, 2245f
  tropism of, 2237t, 2238
Chlamydia pecorum, 2227t, 2236-2238

Chlamydia pneumoniae. See Chlamydophila pneumoniae.

Chlamydia psittaci. See Chlamydophila psittaci.

Chlamydia trachomatis, 2239-2253
  acute urethral syndrome from, 2248
  antigenic composition of, 2237t, 2240-2241
  biovars of, 2236
  cervical cancer and, 2248
  characteristics of, 2236-2238, 2237t
  clinical manifestations of, 2244-2251, 2247t
  conjunctivitis from, 1390-1391, 2245, 2247t, 2249
    in adults, 1391, 1392, 2245, 2247t, 2250
    in neonates, 1392-1393, 2247t, 2249t, 2250-2251, 2252-2253
    pathogenesis of, 1390, 2245, 2247t
  culture of, 2242, 2243t
  diagnosis of, 1343, 1348
  endocarditis from, 993
  endometritis from, 2248
    postpartum, 1374
  epidemiology of, 2237t, 2239, 2239f
  epididymitis from, 1384-1385, 2246, 2247t
  genome of, 2241
  HIV infection and, 2248
  immune response to, 2241-2242
  incidence of, 2239, 2239f
  infertility from, 2249
  keratitis from, 1400
  laboratory diagnosis of, 213, 2242-2243, 2243t, 2247t
  life cycle of, 2239-2240, 2240
  lymphogranuloma venereum from, 1338-1344, 2244-2245
  mucopurulent cervicitis from, 1628
  Neisseria gonorrhoeae coinfection and, 2246, 2524, 2525
  ocular infections from, 1390-1391, 2245, 2245f, 2247t. *See also* Conjunctivitis, from *Chlamydia trachomatis;* Trachoma.
    in neonate, 2247t, 2250-2251
    treatment of, 2247t, 2249
  otitis media from, 768
  partner notification for, 2251
  pathogenesis of, 2241
  pelvic inflammatory disease from, 1378-1380, 1378f, 1379f, 1379t, 2247t, 2248-2250, 2249t, 2250-2251
  perinatal infections from, 2247t, 2250-2251
  pneumonia from, 834, 2247t, 2249, 2250-2251, 2251f
    in neonates, 2247t, 2249, 2250-2251, 2251f
    sputum in, 826
  pregnancy in
    complications from, 2249
    perinatal transmission in, 2250-2251, 2447t
  prevalence of, 2236
  prevention of, 2251
  proctitis/proctocolitis from, 2246, 2247t
  prostatitis from, 2246, 2247t
  public health impact of, 2239
  reactive arthritis from, 1354-1355, 2247-2249
  Reiter's syndrome from, 1354-1355, 2247
  salpingitis from, 2248, 2447t
  screening for, 2251
  serovars of, 2240-2241
  strains of, 2236, 2237t, 2238
  trachoma from, 405, 1390-1391, 1400, 2244, 2244t. *See also* Trachoma.
  transmission of, 2237t, 2238, 2245-2246, 2245f
  treatment of, 2247t, 2249-2251
    with azithromycin, 397t, 401t, 403
    with clarithromycin, 397t, 403
    with erythromycin, 397t, 398, 401t, 402
    with quinolones, 455t

Chlamydia trachomatis (Continued)
    with sulfonamides, 441t
    with telithromycin, 397t
    with trimethoprim, 444t
    with trimethoprim-sulfamethoxazole, 446
  tropism of, 2237t, 2240
  urethral syndrome from, 1352
  urethritis from, 1347-1355, 2245f, 2246, 2247t, 2248. *See also* Urethritis.
  urogenital infections from, 2245-2250, 2245f, 2247t
    treatment of, 2247t, 2249-2250

Chlamydophila [spp.], rifamycin for, 382

Chlamydophila pneumoniae, 2258-2266
  acute bronchitis from, 747-749
  asymptomatic, 2261
  atherosclerosis from, 2259, 2263-2266, 2264t
  characteristics of, 2236-2238, 2237t, 2258-2259, 2259f
  chronic, 2259, 2262
  clinical manifestations of, 2262-2263
  conjunctivitis from, 1390
  COPD exacerbations from, 809
  culture of, 2259
  endocarditis from, 993
  epidemics of, 2262
  epidemiology of, 2260-2262, 2261f, 2261t, 2262f
  historical perspective on, 2258
  laboratory diagnosis of, 2259-2260
  laryngitis from, 758, 759t
  myocarditis from, 1053
  otitis media from, 2262
  PCR assay for, 826
  pharyngitis from, 755, 2262
  pneumonia from
    atypical, 833, 834
    community-acquired, 831-833
    diagnosis of, 826, 828
    sputum in, 826
    treatment of, 836-839, 837t, 838t, 2263
  prevalence of, 2236
  quinolones for, 455t
  respiratory infections from, 209t, 2262-2263
  sinusitis from, 776, 776t
  treatment of, 360t, 397t, 398, 401t, 403, 406
  vaccines for, 2263
  vascular, 2263-2266

Chlamydophila psittaci, 2251, 2256-2258
  characteristics of, 2236-2238, 2237t
  endocarditis from, 993
  isolation precautions for, 3330t
  myocarditis from, 1053
  pneumonia from, 833

Chloramphenicol, 366-370
  activity of, 366-367, 367t
  dosage of, 666t-667t
  drug interactions with, 369-370, 369t, 687t-688t
  for brain abscess, 1159t
  for epidemic typhus, 2305
  for *Francisella tularensis,* 2682
  for *Listeria monocytogenes,* 2483
  for Lyme borreliosis, 1115
  for meningitis, 1106t, 1107t, 1112, 1113
  for murine typhus, 2308
  for *Neisseria meningitidis,* 2507
  for plague, 3603
  for rickettsial diseases, 2293
  for Rocky Mountain spotted fever, 2091
  for scrub typhus, 2310
  for secondary peritonitis, 937
  for tularemia, in bioterrorism attack, 3610t, 3611

Chloramphenicol *(Continued)*
  for typhoid fever, 2648, 2649t
  for *Yersina pestis,* 2697
  formulations of, 648t
  gray baby syndrome from, 369
  hepatic function and, 245
  in children, 368
  in liver failure, 368
  in metabolic disorders, 244
  in renal insufficiency, 368
  indications for, 370
  mechanism of action of, 366-367
  metabolism of, 368
  monitoring of, 368
  neutropenia from, 103
  optic neuritis from, 369
  pharmacology of, 367-368, 368f
  preparations of, 366
  resistance to, 261, 366-367, 1112
    by *Staphylococcus aureus,* 2334t
  serum levels of, 367, 368f
  side effects of, 369
  structure of, 366, 366f
  toxicity of, 368-369

Chloramphenicol acetyltransferase, 261

Chlorhexidine, skin disinfection with, 479

Chlorhexidine oral rinse, 780, 796t

Chlorine (chlorination), disinfection with, 3334
  emerging pathogens and, 3340, 3341

Chlornchiasis, 3277t, 3279f, 3281-3282, 3281f

Chloroguanide, 587

Chloroquine, 584-585
  adverse effects of, 581t
  drug interactions with, 688t
  for malaria, 573t, 574t, 3129, 3133-3135, 3134t
  for prophylaxis, 3137-3138, 3137t
    in travelers, 3641-3642, 3641t
  resistance to, 3129. *See also* Malaria, drug-resistant.
  indications for, 569t
  structure of, 584f

Chlorpheniramine
  for colds, 749-750
  for cough, 805

7-Chlortetracycline, 357f

Cholangiopancreatography, endoscopic retrograde
  for acute cholangitis, 957
  for HIV infection, 1576-1577

Cholangiopathy, in HIV infection, 956-957, 1576-1577, 1579

Cholangitis, 955. *See also* Gallbladder disease.
  from *Cryptosporidium,* 3220, 3221
  from microsporidia, 3238t, 3242, 3245
  in transplant recipients, 3505
  pyogenic liver abscess in, 951
  sclerosing
    HIV-related, 956-957
    in cryptosporidiosis, 3220, 3221
  treatment of, 957

Cholecystitis
  acalculous, 955, 956
    in HIV infection, 1576-1577
  acute (ascending), 956
  antibiotics for, 957
  from *Cryptosporidium,* 3220, 3221
  from cytomegalovirus, 1792
  from microsporidia, 3238t, 3242, 3245
  pathogenesis of, 955, 955f
  ultrasonography of, 956f

Cholelithiasis, in HIV infection, 1576-1577

Cholera, 1223, 2536-2542. *See also Vibrio cholerae.*
   clinical manifestations of, 2539-2540, 2539f
   dehydration in, 2539, 2540t
   diarrhea in, 2539
      electrolyte concentration of, 2537, 2537t
   epidemics of, 2536, 2538
   epidemiology of, 2537-2539, 2538t
   history of, 2536
   pandemic of, 2536
   pathophysiology of, 2537, 2537t
   pediatric, 2540
   prevention, 2541-2542
   treatment of, 461, 2540-2541, 2540t, 2541f, 2541t
      with chloramphenicol, 367t
      with trimethoprim, 444t
   vaccines for, 1226, 2542, 3562
      for travelers, 3639t, 3641
Cholera toxin, 1219
   action of, 29
   cell entry by, 26
Cholestasis, pruritus of, 383
Cholestatic hepatitis
   fibrosing, 1449
   from erythromycin, 400
   from hepatitis A, 2173, 2174t
      post-transplant, 1449, 1456
   from hepatitis E, 2173, 2174t, 2209
Cholestyramine, for *Clostridium difficile*–associated colitis, 1258, 1258t
Chorea, Sydenham's, in rheumatic fever, 2383-2384
Chorioamnionitis, 1372-1373
Chorioretinitis. *See also* Retinitis.
   from *Candida* spp., 1408-1409, 1411, 1417
   from cytomegalovirus, 1416, 1790-1791, 1791f
   from herpes simplex virus, 1769
   from *Onchocerca volvulus,* 3273-3274
   from *Toxoplasma gondii,* 3176, 3177, 3179-3180, 3179f
      diagnosis of, 3186
      in pregnancy, 3191
      treatment of, 3186, 3190
   in injection drug users, 3472
Chromatography, of mycobacteria, 226-227
Chromobacterium violaceum, 2751t, 2755
   in chronic granulomatous disease, 155-156
Chromoblastomycosis, 2988-2991, 3070t
   histopathology of, 2938t, 2989
   ketoconazole for, 507
Chronic bronchitis, 806-811. *See also* Chronic obstructive pulmonary disease (COPD).
Chronic fatigue syndrome, 1270-1274, 1807-1808
   from human herpesvirus 6 infections, 1823
   vs. Lyme disease, 2805-2806
Chronic granulomatous disease. *See* Granulomatous disease, chronic.
Chronic lymphocytic meningitis, 1139-1140
Chronic mucocutaneous candidiasis, 2944, 2945f, 2951
Chronic nondysenteric syndrome, in amebic colitis, 3103
Chronic nonspecific lung diseases, 806
Chronic obstructive pulmonary disease (COPD), 806-811
   airway pathology in, 807
   antimicrobial therapy for, 810-811, 811t
      prophylactic, 810
   classification of, 806-807
   clinical definitions of, 806
   clinical features of, 807
   diagnostic criteria for, 807
   Dutch hypothesis for, 806
   etiology of, 807

Chronic obstructive pulmonary disease (COPD) (Continued)
   exacerbations of, 807-811
      definition of, 807-808
      from influenza virus, 2071
      from rhinoviruses, 2190
      implications of, 808
      infections and, 808-810
      management of, 810-811, 810t, 811t
      microbiology of, 809-810
      severity of, 808
   Haemophilus influenzae in, 2661, 2662, 2663
   impact of, 807
   management of, 810
   Moraxella (Branhamella) catarrhalis in, 2530-2531
   pneumonia and, 822
   prevalence of, 807
   stable
      bacteria in, 808
         atypical, 809
      viruses in, 808
   zanamivir toxicity in, 539
Chronic pelvic pain syndrome, 894
Chronic pneumonia syndrome. *See* Pneumonia, chronic.
Chronic progressive myelopathy, 2108t, 2110-2111
   transfusion-related, 2106
   treatment of, 2112-2113
Chronic wasting disease, 2230
Chryseobacterium [spp.], 2751t, 2757-2758
   vancomycin for, 418
Chryseobacterium indologenes, 2757-2758
Chryseobacterium meningosepticum, 2758, 2758f
Chrysomyia bezziana, myiasis from, 3308-3310, 3308t
Chyluria, in filariasis, 3271-3272
Cidofovir, 515t, 523-525
   activity spectrum of, 517t, 523-524
   dosage of, 680t-681t
   drug interactions with, 524-525, 688t
   for adenovirus infections, 1839
   for cytomegalovirus encephalitis, 1591
   for cytomegalovirus infections, 1793
      in HIV infection, 1683t, 1686t, 1697
   for genital herpes, 1344
   for genital warts, 1850
   for herpesvirus infections, 1760t, 1761, 1774
   for human herpesvirus 6 infections, 1823
   for molluscum contagiosum, 1754
   for orf, 1753
   for poxvirus infections, 1749
   for progressive multifocal leukoencephalopathy, 1861
   formulations of, 649t
   mechanism of action of, 524
   pharmacokinetics of, 524
   resistance of, 524
   structure of, 524f
   toxicity of, 525
   uses of, 525
Ciguatera fish poisoning, 1290, 1290t, 3255, 3255f, 3256t
   treatment of, 1296
Ciliary neurotropic factor, as pyrogen, 708-709
Ciliates, treatment of, 582-583, 583f
Cimetidine
   chloramphenicol interactions with, 369t
   for cutaneous warts, 1848
   metronidazole interactions with, 393t
   tetracycline with, 364t
Cinchonism, quinine and, 585
Cinoxacin, 451, 452f
   dosage of, 672t-673t
   formulations of, 648t

Ciprofloxacin
   antimicrobial activity of, 455t, 456t
   dosage of, 458t, 672t-673t
   for acute pyelonephritis, 889
   for anthrax, 1177t, 2489, 2489t, 2490t
   for *Bacillus,* 2495
   for bacterial arthritis, 1316t
   for bacterial gastroenteritis, 460-461
   for brain abscess, 1159t
   for *Campylobacter jejuni,* in HIV infection, 1689t
   for cellulitis, 1180
   for chancroid, 460
   for cholera, 461
   for chronic *Salmonella* carriage, 2650
   for community-acquired pneumonia, 462
   for enteric fever, 461
   for febrile neutropenia, 3450-3452, 3451t, 3453t
   for *Francisella tularensis,* 2683
   for genital chlamydial infections, 460
   for gonococcal urethritis, 460
   for *Haemophilus ducreyi,* 2667
   for hospital-acquired pneumonia, 462-463
   for *Isospora belli,* in HIV infection, 1689t
   for keratitis, 1399
   for lower urinary tract infections, 890
   for meningitis, 465, 1106t, 1107t, 1113, 1114
      for prevention, 1118
   for mycobacterial infections, 464
   for *Mycobacterium avium* complex, in HIV infection, 1687t
   for *Neisseria gonorrhoeae,* 2524t
   for *Neisseria meningitidis,* 2507, 2507t, 2509
   for neutropenia, 464
   for nocardiosis, 2920t
   for osteomyelitis, 463, 1324t
      from *Pseudomonas aeruginosa,* 2603
      of jaw, 797t
   for pelvic inflammatory disease, 460
   for peritonitis, 461, 939
   for plague, 3603
   for prostatitis, 895
   for psittacosis, 2257
   for relapsing urinary tract infections, 891
   for respiratory infections, 462
   for rickettsial diseases, 2293
   for *Salmonella,* in HIV infection, 1683t, 1689t
   for sepsis, 919t
   for *Shigella,* 2659t
      in HIV infection, 1689t
   for skin infections, 463-464
   for *Streptococcus agalactiae* (group B), 2429
   for traveler's diarrhea, 1243
   for tularemia, in bioterrorism attack, 3610t, 3611, 3611t
   for typhoid fever, 2648, 2649t
   for urethritis, 1207
   for urinary tract infections, 459, 460
   formulations of, 648t
   in preemptive pancreatic infection treatment, 965t
   kill curves for, for *Pseudomonas aeruginosa,* 275, 275f
   metronidazole with, for intra-abdominal infections, 461
   pharmacology of, 457t
   prophylactic
      for anthrax, 3621, 3622t
      for tularemia, 3609-3610, 3609t
   resistance to, 465
      by *Neisseria gonorrhoeae,* 186, 2519
      by *Salmonella typhi,* 2638
   side effects of, 3609t
Ciprofloxacin-rifampin, for *Staphylococcus aureus* osteomyelitis, 2346-2347

Circulation, in severe sepsis, 911
Cirrhosis. *See also* Peritonitis.
  alcoholic, 930
  hepatocellular carcinoma and, 1961
  in hepatitis B, 1876-1877
  in hepatitis C, 1452, 1453, 1959-1961, 1959f,
    1960t
  in hepatitis D, 1877
  primary peritonitis in, 929
Cisapride, metronidazole interactions with, 393t
Cisplatin, neurotoxicity of, 1594t
Citrate, in viral collection, 232
Citrobacter [spp.], 2580
  endocarditis from, 991
  enterotoxigenic, 1237
  peritonitis from, treatment of, 938
  treatment of
    with aminoglycosides, 334t-335t
    with nitrofurantoin, 473
    with quinolones, 455t
  weanling diarrhea from, 1238
Citrobacter amalonaticus, 2580
Citrobacter diversus, 2580
  brain abscess from, 1151, 1153
  carbapenems for, 313t
  penicillins for, 284t
  rifamycin for, 374t
Citrobacter freundii, 2580
  carbapenems for, 313t
  cephalosporins for, 298t
  mupirocin for, 485t
  mycotic aneurysm from, 1008
  penicillins for, 284t, 288t
  rifamycin for, 374t
  trimethoprim for, 444t
Citrus red mite, 3311
Cladophialophora bantiana
  appearance of in tissue, 2936f, 2938t
  brain abscess from, 3070, 3070f, 3071f, 3076t
Cladophialophora (Cladosporium) carrionii,
  chromoblastomycosis from, 2988-2991
Cladosporium bantianum, brain abscess from,
  3070, 3070f, 3076t
Cladosporium trichoides, brain abscess from,
  3070, 3070f, 3076t
Clam digger's itch, 3278, 3294t, 3298
Clara cells, 1998
Clarithromycin, 402-406
  adverse reactions to, 404
  antimicrobial activity of, 402-403
  chemistry of, 402, 403f
  dosage of, 664t-665t
  drug interactions with, 400t, 404, 688t
  for bartonellosis, in HIV infection, 1691t
  for *Bordetella pertussis*, 2706
  for chlamydial pneumonia, 2263
  for cryptosporidiosis, 3222
  for disseminated *Mycobacterium avium*
    complex prophylaxis, 2906
  for endocarditis prophylaxis, 1050t
  for experimental endocarditis, 1048
  for *Helicobacter pylori*, 2563
  for *Legionella pneumophila*, 2719t
  for leprosy, 499
  for *Mycobacterium avium* complex, 2903-2906,
    2904t, 2905t
    in HIV infection, 1682t, 1683t, 1687t, 1700
  for nocardiosis, 2920t
  for nontuberculous mycobacterial infections,
    496, 2910, 2911, 2912, 2913t
  for pneumonia, 837-839, 837t, 838t
  for respiratory infections, 462
  for streptococcal pharyngitis, 2368
  for toxoplasmosis, in immunocompromised
    host, 3189, 3189t

Clarithromycin *(Continued)*
  formulations of, 648t
  in vitro susceptibilities to, 397t
  mechanism of action of, 402
  pharmacology of, 403
  resistance to, 402
    pneumococcal, 837, 837t
  uses of, 404-406
Classic pathway, 69t
  activation of, 71-72, 72f
Clavicle, osteomyelitis of, 1329
Clavulanate, 316, 316f
Clavulanic acid, for *Pasteurella*, 2690
Clean wound, 3534, 3534t
Clean-contaminated wound, 3534, 3534t
Clenched fist injuries, 3555
Clethrionomys glareolus, hemorrhagic fever with
  renal syndrome from, 2086t, 2087-2089
Clevudine, 540
  for chronic hepatitis B, 1447, 1881
Clindamycin, 408-411, 484t
  adverse reactions to, 410
  antimicrobial activity of, 408-409, 409t
  chemistry of, 408, 409f
  dosage of, 411, 666t-667t
  drug interactions with, 410, 688t
  for acne vulgaris, 483
  for actinomycosis, 2931, 2931t
  for acute necrotizing ulcerative gingivitis, 796,
    796t
  for babesiosis, 571t, 3213
  for *Bacillus*, 2495
  for bacterial arthritis, 1316t
  for bacterial vaginosis, 1366-1367
  for brain abscess, 1159t
  for carbuncles, 1175
  for cervicofacial actinomycosis, 797t
  for clostridial cellulitis, 1189
  for deep fascial space infections, 797t
  for desquamative inflammatory, 1367-1368
  for dialysis-related peritonitis, 942t
  for endocarditis prophylaxis, 1050t
  for experimental endocarditis, 1048
  for gas gangrene, 1199
  for Lemierre's disease, 756
  for lung abscess, 855-856
  for lymphadenitis, 1211
  for malaria, 573t
  for odontogenic infections, 797t, 797t
  for osteomyelitis of jaw, 797t
  for parotitis, 797t
  for pelvic inflammatory disease, 460, 1379t,
    2247t, 2250
  for peritonsillar abscess, 756
  for *Pneumocystis*, 3088
    for prophylaxis, 3090
  for *Pneumocystis jirovecii*, 575t
    in HIV infection, 1693
  for pneumonia, 806t, 837-839
  for postoperative gynecologic infections,
    1377t
  for protozoa, 589
  for secondary peritonitis, 937, 937t, 938
  for sepsis, 919, 919t
  for sialadenitis, 797t
  for staphylococcal endocarditis, 999
  for *Staphylococcus aureus* nasal carriage, 1176
  for streptococcal necrotizing myositis, strep
  for streptococcal toxic shock syndrome, 2374
  for suppurative thrombophlebitis, 1005
  for *Toxoplasma gondii*, 3188
    for chorioretinitis, 3190
    for encephalitis prophylaxis, 3190
    in encephalitis, 1587
    in HIV infection, 1683t, 1685t, 1696

Clindamycin *(Continued)*
  in immunocompromised host, 3188-3190,
    3189t
  for urogenital chlamydial infections, 2250
  formulations of, 648t
  hepatic function and, 245
  in preemptive pancreatic infection treatment,
    965t
  indications for, 569t
  mechanism of action of, 408
  pharmacology of, 409-410
  pseudomembranous colitis from, 1265f
  resistance to, 408-409
    by *Streptococcus agalactiae* (group B), 2429
  uses of, 410-411
Clindamycin-benzoyl peroxide, 483, 484t
Clinical Pulmonary Infection Score (CPIS), 3362,
  3363t, 3366
Clinical trials, 166
  analysis of, 624-626, 626f
  bias in, 623
  blinding in, 621-622
  conclusions of, 626-627, 626t
  control regimen in, 623
  design of, 621-623
  effectiveness in, 621
  efficacy in, 621
  end points in, 623-624
  equivalence, 620
  error types in, 622-623
  exclusion criteria in, 621
  explanatory, 621
  hypothesis testing in, 622-623
  inclusion criteria in, 621
  management (strategy), 621
  noninferiority, 620
  randomization in, 621-622
  sample size in, 622-623
  stratification in, 621-622
  superiority, 620
Clofazimine
  dosage of, 676t-677t
  drug interactions with, 688t
  for leprosy, 498, 2893, 2894
  for nontuberculous mycobacteria, 497
  formulations of, 649t
Clones, of microbial pathogens, 5
Clonorchis sinensis
  biliary tract infections from, 956
  in stem cell transplant, 3496
  pancreatic infections from, 959t, 960
  syndrome of abdominal pain, diarrhea, and
    eosinophilia from, 1281t, 1282
  treatment of, 572t
Clostridium [spp.], 2811, 2828-2837
  bacteremia from, 2929-2830
  biliary tract infections from, 2830
  cellulitis from, 1187-1189, 1188t
    vs. gas gangrene, 1199
  central nervous system infections from, 2830
  endocarditis from, 992
  enteric infections from, 2834-2837, 2835t
  female genitourinary tract infections from,
    2830
  histotoxic syndromes from, 2828, 2829t
  intra-abdominal infections from, 2830
  microbiology of, 2828, 2929t
  myonecrosis from. *See* Gas gangrene.
  neutropenic enterocolitis from, 2834, 2835t,
    2836
  prevention of, 2837
  pulmonary infections from, 2830
  secondary peritonitis from, 937
    treatment of, 938
  soft tissue infections from, 2830-2831

Clostridium [spp.] *(Continued)*
  subcutaneous tissue infections from, 1187-1189, 1188t
  treatment of, 2837
    with metronidazole, 389t
    with penicillins, 288t
    with quinolones, 456t
Clostridium baratii, 2823
Clostridium botulinum, 2822-2826. *See also* Botulism.
  characteristics of, 2823
  disinfection/sterilization and, 3342
  foodborne disease from, 1289, 1292, 1295, 2823, 2834
  isolation precautions for, 3330t
  microbiology of, 2828
  neuritis from, 1147-1148
  phage-encoded, 6t
  therapeutic use of, 2320
  toxins of, 2822-2824
    action of, 28
    as biological weapons, 2825, 3624-3625
    cell entry by, 27
    clinical manifestations and, 2824, 2825t
    mechanism of, 2823-2824, 2824f
    therapeutic use of, 30-31
    treatment of, 1296
Clostridium butyricum, 2823
Clostridium difficile
  age effects on, 1216
  contact precautions for, 3329
  culture of, 1256
  epidemic strains of, 1253
  in cystic fibrosis, 870, 872
  in hospitals, environmental disinfection for, 3334
  in immunocompromised host, 3438
  institutional diarrhea from, 1241
  laboratory detection of, 212
  microbiology of, 1251-1252
  pseudomembranous colitis from. *See* Pseudomembranous colitis, from *Clostridium difficile.*
  reservoirs of, 1253
  toxins of, 1221
    action of, 29
    collection and transport of, 207t
    noninflammatory diarrhea from, 1239
    treatment of
      with carbapenems, 313t
      with mupirocin, 485t
      with quinolones, 456t
      with quinupristin-dalfopristin, 425
      with rifamycin, 382-383
      with tetracyclines, 360t
  typhlitis from, 973
Clostridium freundii, toxins of, 29
Clostridium haemolyticum, 2828
Clostridium histolyticum, 2828
Clostridium novyi, 2828
Clostridium perfringens
  bacteremia from, 2830
  enterotoxin of, 1220
  foodborne disease from, 1288, 1291, 1294, 1294t, 2834, 2835t, 2836-2837
  gas gangrene from, 2831-2834, 2833f. *See also* Gas gangrene.
  isolation precautions for, 3330t
  microbiology of, 2828-2829
  mouse model of, 2832
  myocarditis from, 1053
  myonecrosis from. *See* Gas gangrene.
  necrotizing enteritis from, 1268
  noninflammatory diarrhea from, 1239
  peritonitis from

Clostridium perfringens (Continued)
  primary, 929
  secondary, 938
  pseudomembranous colitis from, 1250
  pulmonary infections from, 2830
  septic abortion from, 1375, 1377t
  subcutaneous tissue infections from, 1187-1189, 1188t, 1198-1200
  toxins of, 2829, 2831, 2831t
  treatment of
    with carbapenems, 313t
    with chloramphenicol, 367t
    with clindamycin, 409t, 411
    with daptomycin, 428
    with macrolide antibiotics, 397t
    with penicillins, 284t
    with quinolones, 456t
    with tetracyclines, 360t
    with trimethoprim, 444t
  type A, 2836
  type C, 1220-1221
    enteritis necroticans from, 2834-2835, 2835t
Clostridium ramosum, 2828
Clostridium septicum
  bacteremia from, 2830, 2929
  microbiology of, 2828
  mycotic aneurysm from, 1008
  myonecrosis from. *See* Gas gangrene.
  neutropenic enterocolitis from, 2834, 2835t, 2836
  subcutaneous tissue infections from, 1187-1189, 1188t
  typhlitis from, 973
Clostridium sporogenes, 2828
  mupirocin for, 485t
Clostridium tertium, 2828
  bacteremia from, 2830
  laboratory identification of, 218, 219t
Clostridium tetani, 2817-2821. *See also* Tetanus.
  characteristics of, 2817-2818, 2817f
  culture of, 2819
  neuritis from, 1147-1148
  plasmid-encoded, 6t
  toxins of, 28, 2817, 2818
Clotrimazole
  for candidiasis, 2949-2951
    in HIV infection, 1687t
  formulations of, 649t
Cloxacillin, 290, 290f
  dosage of, 650t-651t
  for staphylococcal endocarditis, 998
  for *Staphylococcus aureus* osteomyelitis, 2346
  formulations of, 646t
  minimal inhibitory concentration of, 284t
Clozapine, methadone with, 459
Clue cells
  in bacterial vaginosis, 1360, 1378f
  in pelvic inflammatory disease, 1378f
Clusterin, 70t, 74t
Coagulase test, 216t, 217, 217t
Coagulation, inflammation-activated, 910, 910f
Coagulopathy, in sepsis, 912, 916
Cocaine abuse, endocarditis in, 984
Cocal virus, 2045, 2045t
Cocci
  gram-negative
    laboratory identification of, 220
    mediastinitis from, 1072b
    penicillins for, 288t
  gram-positive
    aerobic, 217, 217t
      aminoglycosides for, 344t
    anaerobic
      carbapenems for, 313t
      metronidazole for, 389t
      quinolones for, 456t

Cocci *(Continued)*
  facultatively anaerobic, 217, 217t
  laboratory studies for, 216-220, 217t, 219t
  mediastinitis from, 1072b
  penicillins for, 284t, 288t
  taxonomic changes in, 217t
Coccidian protozoa, 3228-3232
Coccidioides [spp.]
  appearance of in tissue, 2936f, *2937f,* 2938t, *2938t*
  identification of, 231
  laboratory tests for, 229
  meningitis from, 1137
Coccidioides immitis, 3040-3049
  arthritis from, 1318
  characteristics of, 3040-3041
  clinical manifestations of, 3042-3045, 3043f-3046f
  culture of, 3046
  diagnosis of, 3045-3047
  disseminated infections from, 3043-3045, 3045f, 3046f
  endemicity of, 3040, 3041f
  epidemiology of, 3040-3042, 3041f
  fever from, 726
  histopathology of, 3041
  immune response to, 3041
  in HIV infection, treatment of, 1683t, 1684t, 1687t-1688t, 1699
  in immunocompromised host, 3043-3045, 3045f, 3046f
  incidence of, 3041
  laryngitis from, 759
  meningitis from, 1137, 3044-3045
  mycelial form of, 3041
  mycotic aneurysm from, 993
  pancreatic infections from, 959t, 960
  pathogenesis of, 3041
  pericarditis from, 1059
  prevention of, 3049
  pulmonary infections from, 3042-3043, 3043f-3045f
    in HIV infection, 1571
  sclerosing mediastinitis from, 1075
  serology of, 3046
  shunt infections from, 3048
  spherulic form of, 3041, 3041f
  strains of, 3041
  transmission of, 3041
  treatment of, 504, 507, 508, 3047-3049
  vaccine for, 3049
Coccidioides posadasii, 3041
Coccidioidomycosis
  chest film in, 864f
  history in, 823t
Cochlea, aminoglycoside-induced injury of, 341-343
Cochliomyia homnivorax, myiasis from, 3308-3310, 3308t
Coenurosis, 3286t, 3292
Cogan's syndrome, 1899
Cognitive impairment, from shellfish poisoning, 3256, 3256t
Cohort studies, 165
Cold agglutinin test, for *Mycoplasma pneumoniae,* 2276-2278, 2277f
Cold therapy. *See* Cryotherapy.
Colds. *See* Common cold.
Colestipol, for *Clostridium difficile*–associated colitis, 1258, 1258t
Colistimethate, 435-436
  dosage of, 668t-669t
  drug interactions with, 688t
  formulations of, 648t

Colistin, 435-436
  for meningitis, 1114
  for *Pseudomonas aeruginosa*, 2608
  for shunt infections, 1129t, 1130
  in preemptive pancreatic infection treatment,
    963t
Colitis. *See also* Enterocolitis.
  amebic, 3102-3103
    diagnosis of, 3104-3105
    sigmoidoscopy of, 1264
    treatment of, 3105-3106, 3106t
  antibiotic-associated, 1249-1259. *See also*
    Pseudomembranous colitis.
  chemotherapy-induced, 3438, 3457
  cytomegalovirus, 1791-1792
  fecal leukocytes in, 1263-1264, 1264f
  from *Campylobacter jejuni*, 2551, 2552
  from *Clostridium difficile. See*
    Pseudomembranous colitis.
  from cytomegalovirus, 530, 1580, 1791-1792
  inflammatory, 1263
    cytotoxins in, 1220-1221
  pseudomembranous. *See* Pseudomembranous
    colitis.
  ulcerative postdysenteric, 3103
Collagen vascular disease, vs. enteric fever, 1275t
Collectins
  in phagocytosis, 37
  in *Pseudomonas aeruginosa* resistance, 2590
Colon. *See also under* Gastrointestinal; Intestinal.
  abscess of, from anaerobic infections, 2813,
    2813f
  anaerobic colonization of, 2839
  Bacteroides infections of, 2839
  cancer of, *Streptococcus bovis* in, 2417
  flora of, in secondary peritonitis, 932
  in HIV infection, 1579-1580, 1580t
  in tropical sprue, 1304
Colonic dilation
  in amebic colitis, 3103
  in American trypanosomiasis, 3158, 3163
Colonization, 3, 167
Colonoscopy, in HIV infection, 1580
Colony-stimulating factors, 94, 551-554
  for Kaposi's sarcoma, 1603
  for neutropenia, 104
    in cancer, 3457-3458, 3458
  granulocyte, 552-554, 552t, 908
    adverse effects of, 553-554
    after hematopoietic stem cell transplantation,
      552, 553
    dosage of, 553
    for community-acquired pneumonia, 553
    for HIV-related neutropenia, 1682t
    for neutropenia, 552-553
    for postoperative infections, 553
    pegylated, 552t
  granulocyte-macrophage, 552t, 554
    adverse effects of, 554
    dosage of, 554
    for HIV-related neutropenia, 1682t
    uses of, 554
  macrophage, 554
Colorado tick fever, 235t, 1900-1901, 1900f
Colorectal surgery, infection prevention in, 401t
Colposcopy, in human papillomavirus infection,
  1847
Coltiviruses, 1900-1901
Commensals. *See* Microbial flora.
Common cold, 747-750, 2189-2190, 2190f. *See*
  also Respiratory tract infections.
  attack rates in, 748
  clinical features of, 749, 2189
  complications of, 2189-2190

Common cold *(Continued)*
  cough in, 750, 803-804, 803t, 804f, 804t, 805,
    2189
  course of, 2189, 2190f
  diagnosis of, 749
  Echinacea for, 604t
  Echinacea for, 604t, 608, 750
  Echinacea for, 608
  etiology of, 747, 747t
  from coronaviruses, 1990-1996
  from rhinoviruses, 2185-2192. *See also*
    Rhinoviruses.
  in chronic bronchitis, 2190
  interferon-alpha for, 555
  laryngitis in, 758-759
  nose blowing in, 774, 775f
  otitis media and, 2189
  pathogenesis of, 748-749, 2188, 2188t, 2189
  pharyngitis in, 753. *See also* Pharyngitis.
  prevention of, 750, 2192
  seasonal incidence of, 747-748, 2187
  sinusitis and, 772-780, 774f, 2189. *See also*
    Sinusitis.
  transmission of, 748, 2187-2188
  treatment of, 749-750, 2192
  vitamin C for, 142, 604t, 608-609
  zinc for, 142, 608
Common variable immunodeficiency syndrome,
  65, 66
Common warts, 1842, 1845. *See also* Human
  papillomavirus(es).
Community intervention trials, 166
Community-acquired infections
  from *Corynebacterium*, 2466, 2466t
  from *Legionella*, 2715, 2726
  from methicillin-resistant *Staphylococcus
    aureus*, 184, 2334
  from *Pseudomonas aeruginosa*, 2588
  pneumonia in. *See* Pneumonia, acute,
    community-acquired.
Complement, 69-88
  activation of, 36, 69-70, 70f
    antibodies in, 55
    by alternative pathway, 72-73, 72f
    by classic pathway, 71-72, 72f
    by *Streptococcus pneumoniae*, 2396
    cell surface, 72
    fluid-phase, 72
    host vs. microbial cell surfaces in, 74-75
    in severe sepsis, 912
    regulation of, 73-75, 74t
  alternative pathway for
    activation by, 72-73, 72f
    deficiency in, 81, 82t, 83, 151t
  catabolism of, 71
  classic pathway for
    activation by, 71-72, 72f
    deficiency in, 79-81, 83
  deficiency of, 78-86, 80t, 151t, 158, 158f
    evaluation of, 87-88
    frequency of, 78-79, 78f
    in alternative pathway, 81, 82t, 83
    in bacterial infections, 81
    in classic pathway, 79-81, 83
    in gonococcal bacteremia, 2522
    in meningococcal disease, 83, 84-85, 2506
    in paroxysmal nocturnal hemoglobinuria, 85-
      86
    in *Streptococcus pneumoniae* infections, 2398
    in systemic lupus erythematosus, 79-81
    inherited, 83
    late, 83-85
    molecular basis of, 83
    treatment of, 88

Complement *(Continued)*
  distribution of, 71
  functions mediated by, 76-77
  in acute-phase response, 710, 710t
  in apoptosis, 76-77
  in immune complexes, 76
  in immune response, 76
  in infectious diseases, 86-87
  in inflammation, 76, 86
  in local host response, 908
  in microorganism elimination, 76
  in phagocytosis, 99
  in *Pseudomonas aeruginosa* resistance, 2590
  in renal disorders, 87
  in rheumatologic disorders, 87
  in self-nonself distinction, 76
  in *Streptococcus agalactiae* (group B)
    infections, 2426
  measurement of, 59
  microbial interactions with, 77-78
  plasma proteins of, 69-70, 69t, 70t
  synthesis of, 71
Complement cascade, 36, 69-70, 70f
  C3 in, 73
Complement fixation, 58
Complement proteins, 75. *See also* C1 *and
  related entries.*
Complement receptors, 16, 74t, 75, 76, 78
  deficiency of, 80t
  in systemic lupus erythematosus, 87
Complement regulatory-acquiring proteins, 77
Complementarity defining regions, 55
Complementary therapies, 603-610, 604t. *See
  also specific therapy.*
  for colds, 604t, 608, 750
  for diarrhea, 604t, 606-607
  for urinary tract infections, 20, 21, 604t
  hepatitis from, 1436
Computed tomography. *See also* Radiography.
  for appendicitis, 969-970, 970f
  for brain abscess, 7f, 1155-1157
  for cat-scratch disease, 2737, 2739f
  for central nervous system infections, 1082,
    1103, 1103f
  for cholecystitis, 956
  for Creutzfeldt-Jakob disease, 2224
  for cryptococcosis, 3004f, 3007
  for diverticulitis, 972
  for emphysematous pyelonephritis, 890, 890f
  for epidural abscess, 1167
  for glanders, 2630, 2630f
  for intraperitoneal abscess, 944
  for intrarenal abscess, 895, 896f
  for mediastinitis, 1073, 1073f
  for melioidosis, 2625f, 2627f, 2628f
  for meningitis
    acute, 1082, 1103
    chronic, 1082, 1135
  for mesenteric adenitis, 1280
  for *Mycobacterium avium* complex pulmonary
    disease, 2899f, 2900f
  for mycotic aneurysm, 1008
  for nasopharyngeal cancer, 1813, 1814t
  for nocardiosis, 2918, 2918f
  for odontogenic infections, 780, 795f
  for orbital infections, 1423, 1423f
  for osteomyelitis, 1323
  for pediatric pyelonephritis, 900, 900f
  for percutaneous liver abscess aspiration, 954,
    954f
  for perinephric abscess, 895, 896f
  for pleural effusion/empyema, 848, 848f,
    849f
  for pneumonia, 830

Computed tomography *(Continued)*
  for primary central nervous system lymphoma, 1589
  for progressive multifocal leukoencephalopathy, 1590, 1860
  for prosthetic vascular graft infections, 1037
  for pyomyositis, 1197
  for rabies, 2052, 2052f
  for secondary peritonitis, 935
  for septic arthritis, 1313, 1314f
  for sinusitis, 778
  for splenic abscess, 968
  for subdural empyema, 1164-1165
  for suppurative intracranial thrombosis, 1169
  for suppurative thrombophlebitis, 1004
  for toxoplasmic encephalitis, 3183-3185, 3184f
  for urinary tract infections, 897-898, 897f, 898f
  for xanthogranulomatous pyelonephritis, 899, 899f
Computers. *See* Digital resources.
Concentration vs. time plot, 272, 272f
Condoms
  in HIV infection prevention, 1470, 1493-1494
    in women, 1631
  in *Neisseria gonorrheae* infections prevention, 2527
Condylomata acuminata, 846f, 1341-1344, 1841-1846. *See also* Human papillomavirus(es).
  clinical features of, 1845-1847, 1846f
  diagnosis of, 847-848
  epidemiology of, 1842-1843
  imiquimod for, 559
  in HIV infection, 1609, 1691t
  interferon-alfa for, 555
  oral, 1847, 1850
  pathogenesis of, 1843-1845
  prevention of, 1850
  treatment of, 515t, 555, 559, 1848-1850
Condylomata lata, 733, 1340-1342, 1340f, 2773
Congenital heart disease
  brain abscess from, 1151t, 1152
  respiratory syncytial virus in, 2017t, 2018
Congenital infections. *See also* Neonates; Pregnancy.
  from cytomegalovirus, 1796-1797
  from measles virus, 2035
  from *Toxoplasma gondii,* 3170, 3180-3181
    diagnosis of, 3187-3188
    treatment of, 3191
Congenital varicella, 1782-1783
Congestive heart failure
  blood stream infections in, 1040
  endocarditis in, 983, 994
    treatment of, 1001-1002
  in prosthetic valve endocarditis, 1030
  in rheumatic fever, 2382
  leptospirosis in, 2792
Congo floor maggot, myiasis from, 3308-3310, 3308t
Conidiobolomycosis, 2974t, 2980-2981, 2981f
Conjunctival papillomas, 1847
Conjunctival petechiae, 736
Conjunctivitis, 1387-1394. *See also* Keratitis; Keratoconjunctivitis; Ocular infections.
  acute hemorrhagic, 1389, 2136, 2137, 2155-2156, 2156f
  adult inclusion, 1391, 1392, 2245, 2247t, 2250
  anatomic aspects of, 1387
  chemical, in neonate, 1392
  clinical presentation of, 1387-1388
  differential diagnosis of, 1393-1394
  epidemic, 1389
  filarial, 3272-3273, 3272f
  from adenoviruses, 754, 1389, 1838

Conjunctivitis *(Continued)*
  from bacteria, 1391-1392
    acute (mucopurulent), 1391
    chronic, 1392
    hyperacute (purulent), 1391-1392
    in neonate, 1392-1393
  from *Candida,* 2947-2948, 2948f, 2951
  from *Chlamydia pneumoniae,* 1390
  from *Chlamydia trachomatis,* 1390-1391, 2245, 2247t, 2249
    in adults, 1391, 1392, 2245, 2247t, 2250
    in neonates, 1392-1393, 2247t, 2249, 2250-2251, 2252-2253
    pathogenesis of, 1390, 2245, 2247t
  from *Corynebacterium diphtheriae,* 1391
  from filaria, 3272-3273, 3272f
  from *Haemophilus influenzae,* 1391, 2663
  from *Leishmania,* 1393
  from microsporidia, 1393, 1405, 3238t, 3243-3244, 3248t, 3249
  from *Neisseria gonorrhoeae,* 2521, 2521f
  from respiratory syncytial virus, 2015t
  from varicella zoster virus, 1401-1403, 1402t, 1782, 1783
  fungal, 1393
  gonococcal, 1391-1392
    in neonate, 1392-1393
  herpes simplex, 1389, 1773t
    in neonate, 1393
  herpes zoster, 1389
  history in, 1387
  in Kawasaki disease, 3316, 3316f
  in Parinaud's oculoglandular syndrome, 2737, 2739f
  in pharyngoconjunctival fever, 754, 1389, 1402
  in Reiter's syndrome, 1354-1355
  inclusion
    adult, 1391, 1392, 2245, 2247t, 2250
    neonatal, 1392-1393, 2247t, 2250
    pathogenesis of, 1390, 2245, 2247t
  laboratory findings in, 1388-1389
  lymphogranuloma venereum and, 1390, 1391
  neonatal, 1392-1393, 2247t, 2249, 2250-2253
  parasitic, 1393
  Parinaud's oculoglandular, 1207, 1393
  physical examination in, 1387
  vaccinia, 1390, 1390t
  varicella, 1389
  variola, 1389-1390
  viral, 1389-1390, 1390t
    in neonate, 1393
Connective tissue disease, meningitis in, 1139
Consciousness, vancomycin effects on, 421
Constitutional disease, in HIV infection, 1554
Contact lenses
  culture of, 1396
  drug administration via, 1398-1399
  keratitis from, 1396, 1404, 3114
Contact precautions, 3327t, 3328t, 3329, 3330t
Contagious ecthyma, 1753
Contaminated wound, 3534, 3534t
Continuous ambulatory peritoneal dialysis. *See also* Dialysis.
  aminoglycoside dosing in, 346, 346t
  peritonitis in, 941-942, 942t
    aminoglycosides for, 350, 350t
    vancomycin in, 420
Contraceptives. *See also* Condoms; Intrauterine devices.
  for HIV-infected women, 1631
  pelvic inflammatory disease and, 1378
  urinary tract infections and, 876
Cooling methods, for fever, 713, 714, 715
Coombs classification, 64

Copper penny bodies, 2989, 2990f
Coquillettidia spp., alphavirus infections from, 1915
Cordylobia anthropophaga, myiasis from, 3307-3310, 3308t
Cordylobia rodhaini, myiasis from, 3308-3310, 3308t
Core temperature, 704, 705. *See also* Temperature.
Cornea
  biopsy of, 1397
  infections of. *See* Keratitis; Keratoconjunctivitis.
  Pseudomonas aeruginosa spread in, 2598
  scraping of, 1397
Corneal transplantation
  Creutzfeldt-Jakob disease from, 2223
  rabies transmission via, 2050
Corneal ulcers, 1388. *See also* Keratitis.
  from microsporidia, 1405, 3238t, 3243-3245, 3248t, 3249
  vs. conjunctivitis, 1393
Coronary artery aneurysms, in Kawasaki disease, 3317, 3318
Coronary artery bypass
  cellulitis in, 1178, 1180, 2371
  mediastinitis in, 1071
Coronary artery disease
  from *Chlamydia pneumoniae,* 2263-2266
  in myocarditis, 1055
Coronary artery stents, infections of, 1040
Coronaviridae, 1990
Coronaviruses, 1990-1996
  characteristics of, 1991-1992
  classification of, 1991
  clinical manifestations of, 1994-1995, 1994t
  colds from, 747-750, 747t. *See also* Common cold.
  collection of, 233t
  culture of, 1992
  discovery of, 1990
  disinfection/sterilization and, 3341
  epidemiology of, 1992-1994, 1993f
  gastroenteritis from, 1239, 1239t
    laboratory studies for, 235
  genome of, 1991-1992, 1991f
  laboratory diagnosis of, 1995-1996
  laryngitis from, 758, 759t
  multiple sclerosis and, 1995
  pathogenesis of, 1994
  receptors for, 1732t
  replication of, 1991
  structure of, 1991, 1992f
  vaccines for, 1996
Coronavirus-like particles, 1992
Corticosteroids, 558-559. *See also* Prednisone.
  aerosol, thrush from, 2941
  as aspergillosis risk factor, 2961, 2962
  as mucormycosis risk factor, 2975, 2977
  for allergic bronchopulmonary aspergillosis, 2963t
  for bacterial keratitis, 1399-1400
  for *Bordetella pertussis,* 2706
  for brain abscess, 1157
  for bronchiolitis, 817
  for central nervous system infections, 1083
  for chronic obstructive pulmonary disease, 810t
  for chronic pneumonia, 867
  for cough, 805
  for cryptococcosis, 3008
  for cystic fibrosis, 872
  for disseminated *Mycobacterium avium* complex disease, 2906
  for endophthalmitis, 1411

Corticosteroids *(Continued)*
  for fever, 713
  for hepatitis, 1437
  for herpes zoster, 1784
  for herpes zoster ophthalmicus, 1403t
  for HIV-related myopathy, 1596
  for infections, 909
  for infectious mononucleosis, 1814
  for inflammation, 40
  for leprosy drug reactions, 499
  for meningitis
    acute, 1107-1111, 1108t-1110t, 1116, 1117
    chronic, 1135, 1140
  for myocarditis, 1058
  for ocular syphilis, 1418
  for otitis media, 769
  for pericarditis, 1062
  for *Pneumocystis jirovecii,* 3089
    in HIV infection, 1694
  for pulmonary tuberculosis, 2870
  for respiratory syncytial virus, 2020
  for SARS, 1996
  for toxoplasmic encephalitis, 3189
  for toxoplasmosis, in HIV infection, 1695-1696
  for transplant immunosuppression, infections
    and, 3478, 3478t
  for tuberculous pericarditis, 2879
  for typhoid fever, 2649
  in cytomegalovirus reactivation, 1794-1795
  nebulized, for croup, 764, 2001
  topical, for sinusitis, 780
Corticotropin-releasing hormone, antipyretic
    effects of, 710
Corynebacteria JK, aminoglycoside combination
    therapy for, 336t
Corynebacterium [spp.], 2465-2467, 2466t
  biochemical testing of, 2467
  cardiovascular device infections from, 1023
  community-acquired infections from, 2466,
    2466t
  COPD exacerbations from, 809
  endocarditis from, 991, 992
  identification of, 219, 219t
  in injection drug users, 992
  laboratory tests for, 228-229
  lipophilic, 2469-2470
  microbiology of, 2466-2467
  mycotic aneurysm from, 1008
  nonlipophilic fermentative, 2467-2469
  nonlipophilic nonfermentative, 2469
  nosocomial infections from, 2466, 2466t
  otitis externa from, 766
  prosthetic vascular graft infections from, 1037
  sinusitis from, 782t
  susceptibility testing of, 2467
  taxonomy of, 2466, 2467t
  treatment of
    with daptomycin, 428
    with linezolid, 437, 437t
    with quinolones, 456t
    with quinupristin-dalfopristin, 425
    with vancomycin, 418
Corynebacterium accolens, 2470
Corynebacterium afermentans subsp.
    afermentans, 2469
Corynebacterium afermentans subsp. *lipophilum,*
    2470
Corynebacterium amycolatum, 2468
Corynebacterium argentoratense, 2468
Corynebacterium auris, 2469
Corynebacterium bovis, 2470
Corynebacterium confusum, 2468
Corynebacterium diphtheriae, 2457-2464. *See
    also* Diphtheria.
  characteristics of, 2458

Corynebacterium diphtheriae (Continued)
  conjunctivitis from, 1391
  culture of, 208
  exotoxin production by, 2458
  identification of, 219, 219t, 2462-2463
  invasive disease from, 2462
  membranous ulcers from, 1180
  myocarditis from, 1053, 2461-2462
  neurotoxicity of, 1148, 2462
  nontoxigenic, endocarditis from, 991
  pathogenesis of, 2460-2461, 2460f
  phage-encoded, 6t
  pharyngitis from, 2365
  prevention of, 2463-2464
  reservoir for, 2458
  respiratory tract infections from, 2460, 2460f,
    2461-2462, 2461f
  skin infections from, 2462
  toxins of, 26-28, 1055
  treatment of, 2463-2464
    with macrolide antibiotics, 397t, 398
    with penicillins, 284t, 288t
    with sulfonamides, 441t
    with trimethoprim, 444t
  virulence of, 2460
Corynebacterium glucuronolyticum, 2468
Corynebacterium hofmannii, mupirocin for, 485t
Corynebacterium jeikeium, 2469
  identification of, 219, 219t
  mupirocin for, 485t
  shunt infections from, 1035
Corynebacterium kroppenstedtii, 2470
Corynebacterium lipophiloflavum, 2470
Corynebacterium macginleyi, 2470
Corynebacterium matruchotii, 2468
Corynebacterium minutissimum, 2468
  erythrasma from, 1182, 4828-483
  identification of, 219, 219t
  pitted keratolysis from, 1182
Corynebacterium propinquum, 2469
Corynebacterium pseudodiphtheriticum, 2469
  endocarditis from, 991
Corynebacterium pseudotuberculosis, 2467
  lymphadenitis from, 1207
Corynebacterium riegelii, 2468
Corynebacterium striatum, 2468
Corynebacterium tuberculostearicum, 2470
Corynebacterium ulcerans, 2467
  pharyngitis from, 755
Corynebacterium urealyticum, 2468, 2469-2470
  identification of, 219, 219t
  urinary tract infections from, 882
Corynebacterium xerosis, 2467-2468
  endocarditis from, 991
  mupirocin for, 485t
Cough
  etiology of, 803t, 804t, 2016
  from human metapneumovirus, 2028-2029,
    2028t, 2029t
  from respiratory syncytial virus, 2014, 2015,
    2015t, 2016
  in acute bronchitis, 803-804, 804t
  in bronchiolitis, 815
  in chronic obstructive pulmonary disease, 804
  in colds, 750, 803-804, 803t, 804f, 804t, 805
  in croup, 761
  management of, 805
  whooping. *See* Pertussis.
Cowpox, 740-741, 1749
Coxiella [spp.], classification of, 2284
Coxiella burnetii
  cardiovascular device infections from, 1023
  characteristics of, 2296-2297, 2296f
  endocarditis from, 993
  hepatitis from, 1436

Coxiella burnetii (Continued)
  isolation precautions for, 3330t
  meningoencephalitis from, 2300
  mycotic aneurysm from, 993
  pneumonia from, 833, 2297-2299, 2298f
  Q fever from, 2296-2301. *See also* Q fever.
  transmission of, 2297
  vaccine for, 2301
Coxsackieviruses, 2146. *See also* Enterovirus(es).
  acute hemorrhagic conjunctivitis from, 1389,
    2136, 2137, 2155-2156, 2156f
  classification of, 2133, 2134t
  communicability period for, 2137
  conjunctivitis from, 1389
  culture of, 2137-2138
  diabetes mellitus and, 2157
  encephalitis from, 2149
    in immunocompromised host, 2154-2155
  epidemic pleurodynia from, 2151-2152
  epidemiology of, 2136-2137, 2136t
  exanthems from, 2149-2150
  gastrointestinal disease from, 2156-2157
  genome of, 2134
  group B
    epidemic pleurodynia from, 1201
    myocarditis from, 1052, 1053, 1053t, 1054,
      1054f
    pericarditis from, 1058
  hand-foot-mouth disease from, 2150, 2157
  hepatitis from, 2156
    in neonate, 2154
  herpangina from, 754, 2151
  host range of, 2133, 2134t
  immune response to, 2135-2136
  in neonates, 2153-2154
  in pregnancy, 2137, 2153
  incidence of, 2136t, 2137
  incubation period for, 2137
  laboratory diagnosis of, 235, 2137-2138
  meningitis from, 1085, 2148-2149
    in immunocompromised host, 2154-2155
  minor/major viremia in, 2135
  mutation of, 2135
  myopericarditis from, 2152-2153
    in neonate, 2154
  myositis from, 2151-2152
  noninflammatory diarrhea from, 1239
  orchitits from, 2156-2157
  pancreatitis from, 959, 959t
  paralysis from, 2149, 2156, 2157
  pneumonia from, in neonates, 2154
  prevention of, 2138
  proteins of, 2134
  receptors for, 1732t, 2134, 2134t
  replication of, 2135
  respiratory infections from, 2150-2151
  transmission of, 2137
  treatment of, 2138
Cranberry juice
  for urinary tract infections, 20t, 21, 604t,
    605-606
  urinary pH and, 888
Cranial nerves
  in neurosyphilis, 2776
  tetanus of, 2819, 2819f
Craniectomy
  for subdural empyema, 1165
  of epidural abscess, 1167-1168
Craniotomy, for subdural empyema,
    1165
C-reactive protein
  in acute-phase response, 709
  in bacterial meningitis, 1103
  in local host response, 908
  in pneumonia, 828

Creatinine clearance, in aminoglycoside dosing, 345-346, 345t
Creatinine kinase, in myocarditis, 1056
Creatinine, nutritional status and, 140, 140t
Creeping eruption, 3294t, 3295-3296
Crepitant myositis, 1200
Creutzfeldt-Jakob disease, 48, 2222-2228, 2222t
    clinical features of, 2222, 2222t, 2223-2224
    diagnosis of, 2224-2226
    discovery of, 2222
    epidemiology of, 2222-2223, 2222t
    familial, 2222, 2222t
    genetics of, 2226-2227
    iatrogenic, 2222-2223, 2222t
    infection control measures for, 2230-2231, 3341
    new variant, 2227-2228, 3630
    prevention of, 2230-2231
    risk factors for, 2223
    sporadic, 2222-2223, 2222t
    transmission of, 2222-2223, 2222t, 3388
Crimean-Congo hemorrhagic fever, 2086-2089, 2086t
    as biological weapon, 3627-3629, 3627t
    clinical features of, 3629t
    ribavirin for, 538
Crohn's disease, metronidazole for, 394
Cross-sectional surveys, 165
Crotamiton
    adverse effects of, 581t
    for scabies, 575t
Croup. See Laryngotracheobronchitis.
Crush injuries, from animal bites, 3552
Crusted scabies, 3305-3307, 3306, 3306f, 3307
    in HIV infection, 1558, 1559f
Cryogens, endogenous, 710-711, 711f
Cryoglobulinemia, 65
Cryoglobulins, in endocarditis, 981
Cryotherapy
    for chromoblastomycosis, 2990, 2991
    for cutaneous warts, 1848
    for genital warts, 1849
    for Kaposi's sarcoma, 1603
Cryptococcemia, 3005
Cryptococcomas, cerebral, 3004, 3004f, 3007
Cryptococcus albidus, classification and taxonomy of, 2997-2998
Cryptococcus laurentii, classification and taxonomy of, 2997-2998
Cryptococcus neoformans, 2997-3009
    antigen testing for, 211
    appearance of in tissue, 2936f, 2938t
    arthritis from, 1318
    body temperature and, 3001
    brain abscess from, 1158t
    capsule of, 3000-3001
    central nervous system infections from, 3002-3004, 3003t, 3004f, 3007-3009
        in transplant recipients, 3508
    characteristics of, 2997-2998, 3000-3001
    classification and taxonomy of, 2997-2998
    clinical manifestations of, 3002-3005, 3003t
    coinfection in, 3002
    culture of, 2998, 3006, 3006f
    direct detection of, 230-231
    disseminated, 3005
    ecology of, 2998-2999
    endocarditis from, 1001
    epidemiology of, 2999-3000
    genome of, 2997, 3000
    histopathology of, 2998
    historical perspective on, 2997
    identification of, 231, 2998
    immune reconstitution syndrome and, 3004, 3007

Cryptococcus neoformans (Continued)
    immune response to, 3000, 3001-3002
    in cancer, 2999t, 3000, 3437
    in HIV infection, 1558, 1558f, 2999-3005, 2999t
        treatment of, 1682t, 1683t, 1684t, 1688t, 1689t, 1698
    in transplant recipients, 2999t, 3000, 3508
    laboratory diagnosis of, 3005-3007, 3005f
    laryngitis from, 759
    life cycle of, 2997
    melanin production in, 3001
    meningitis from, 1136-1137, 1584
        amphotericin B for, 504, 505
        clinical features of, 3002-3004, 3003f, 3004f
        diagnosis of, 3005-3007
        fluconazole for, 509
        in HIV infection, 1682t, 1683t, 1684t, 1688t, 1698
        in immunocompromised host, 1140
        prognosis of, 3008-3009
        treatment of, 3007-3008
        with pulmonary coinfection, 3002-3003
    nonmeningeal, 507
    ocular infections from, 3003t, 3005
    osteomyelitis from, 3005
    pancreatic infections from, 959-960, 959t
    pathogenesis of, 3002
    pathogenicity of, 3000-3001, 3002
    pericarditis from, 1059
    peritonitis from, 3005
    pneumonia from, in HIV infection, 1571
    prevention of, 3009
    prognosis of, 3008-3009
    prostatitis from, 894, 3005
    pulmonary infections from, 3002-3003, 3003f, 3003t, 3007
        radiography in, 3002-3003, 3003f, 3007
    risk factors for, 2999t
    serology of, 3006-3007
    serotypes of, 2997-2999
        prevalence of, 2999-3000
    skin infections from, 3003t, 3004-3005, 3004f
    staining of, 3005-3006, 3005f, 3006f
    susceptibility testing for, 3007
    transmission of, 3000
    treatment of, 506, 507
    vaccine for, 3009
Cryptococcus neoformans var. bacillisporas, 2998
Cryptococcus neoformans var. gatti, 2997, 2998, 2999, 3000, 3004
Cryptococcus neoformans var. grubii, 2997-2999, 3001, 3004
Cryptococcus neoformans var. neoformans, 2997-2999, 3001, 3004
Cryptosporidiosis, 3215-3223
    clinical features of, 3219-3220
    diagnosis of, 3220-3221, 3221f
    epidemiology of, 3215-3217, 3219
    etiology of, 3215, 3216f
    immune response in, 3217, 3218-3219
    in children, 3217, 3219
        malnutrition and, 3219-3220
    in immunocompromised host, 3217, 3220, 3223
    infectious dose in, 3216
    management of, 3221-3222
    pathology and pathogenesis of, 3217-3218
    prevention of, 3222
    risk factors for, 3217
    transmission of, 3215-3216, 3216f
Cryptosporidium [spp.], 3215-3223. See also Cryptosporidiosis.
    acute pancreatitis from, 959, 959t
    characteristics of, 3215

Cryptosporidium [spp.] (Continued)
    classification and taxonomy of, 2997-2998, 3215
    culture of, 1224
    diarrhea from, inflammatory, 1240, 1242, 1270
    in HIV infection, 1241
        cholangitis from, 957
        treatment of, 406, 1701
    infectious dose of, 3216
    laboratory detection of, 212
    life cycle of, 3215, 3216f
    nosocomial, 1241
    oocysts of, 3216f, 3217
    pneumonia from, in HIV infection, 1572
    treatment of, 571t
    virulence of, 1216-1217
Cryptosporidium felis, 3215
Cryptosporidium hominis, 3215
Cryptosporidium meleagridis, 3215
Cryptosporidium muris, 3215
Cryptosporidium parvum, 568, 584, 3215
    aminoglycosides for, 344t
    diarrhea from, 1215
    disinfection/sterilization and, 3340
    invasiveness of, 1222
    isolation precautions for, 3330t
    nitazoxanide for, 583
    rifamycin for, 383
    transmission of, 177
    traveler's diarrhea from, 1242
CSCL12, 121
CT. See Computed tomography.
Ctenocephalides felis, 2293, 2306
    as Bartonella henselae vector, 2733
Cuff cellulitis, postoperative, 1376-1377, 1377t
Culex spp.
    alphaviruses and, 1915, 1916
    coltiviruses and, 1900
    flaviviruses and, 1928, 1932-1934, 1934f, 1945t
Culiseta spp.
    alphavirus infections from, 1915, 1916
    Jamestown Canyon virus from, 2089
Culture, 215. See also specific pathogen.
    blood
        in catheter-related infections, 3351
        in pneumonia, 828
    catheter, 3350-3351
    cerebrospinal fluid, 1081-1082, 1081t, 1101. See also Cerebrospinal fluid analysis.
    media used for, 215, 216t
    sinus, 776, 776t
    sputum, 825-826, 862
    throat, 755
Cunninghamella spp., mucormycosis from, 2974, 2974f, 2977f
Currant-jelly sputum, 824, 824f
Curvularia [spp.], 231
Curvularia geniculata, mycetoma from, 2991-2995, 2992t, 2994f
    sinusitis from, 3070-3071, 3076t
Cutaneous disorders. See under Skin.
Cutaneous larva migrans, 3294t, 3295-3296
Cutaneous leishmaniasis, 3145t, 3149-3152, 3149f, 3150f. See also Leishmaniasis.
Cuterebra spp., myiasis from, 3307-3310, 3308t
CXCL13, 121
CXCR4, 121, 1528, 1528f
    blockade of, 20
    in HIV replication, 1540
    in HIV susceptibility, 47
CXCR5, 121
Cyclacillin
    dosage of, 650t-651t
    formulations of, 646t

Cyclooxygenase, antipyretic effects of, 713
Cyclophosphamide
  chloramphenicol interactions with, 369t
  for HIV-related non-Hodgkin's lymphoma, 1605
  for transplant immunosuppression, infections and, 3478
  in cytomegalovirus reactivation, 1794-1795
Cycloserine
  dosage of, 676t-677t
  drug interactions with, 688t
  for *Mycobacterium tuberculosis,* 495
  formulations of, 649t
Cyclospora [spp.], 568, 1290-1291, 3229, 3230f
  culture of, 1224
  diarrhea from, 1270
  in HIV infection, 1701
  laboratory detection of, 212
  treatment of, 569t, 572t
Cyclospora cayetanensis, 177, 584
  traveler's diarrhea from, 1242
  treatment of, 577t, 578t
Cyclosporine
  chloramphenicol interactions with, 369t
  for transplant immunosuppression, infections and, 3478
  in cytomegalovirus reactivation, 1794-1795
  metronidazole interactions with, 393t
CYP3A4, 273
Cyst(s)
  alveolar, 3286t, 3290, 3291-3292
  bronchial cleft, infected, 799-800
  echinococcal, hepatic, 953
  epidermal, infected, 1185
  hydatid, 575t, 580t, 3286t, 3290-3291, 3291f, 3292
  infected embryologic, 799-800
Cystic fibrosis, 869-873
  allergic bronchopulmonary aspergillosis in, 2962, 2963t
  aminoglycoside dosage in, 349-350
  Burkholderia cepacia in, 871, 2617, 2618, 2619f
  clinical manifestations of, 869
  Clostridium difficile in, 870, 872
  diagnosis of, 869
  genetic susceptibility to, 48
  hypergammaglobulinemia in, 65
  lung transplant for, 871, 873
  Mycobacterium avrum complex in, 2900
  nontuberculous mycobacterial infections in, 2910-2911, 2910t, 2913t
  pathogenesis of, 869-870
  Pseudomonas aeruginosa in, 870-871, 2591-2592, 2593f, 2598
  pulmonary infections in
    exacerbations of, 463
    microbiology of, 870-872
    treatment of, 872-873, 892
  respiratory syncytial virus in, 2017-2018
  typhoid resistance in, 46
Cystic fibrosis transmembrane conductance regulator, 48
  in *Pseudomonas aeruginosa* infections, 2591, 2592, 2593f
Cystic hygroma, infected, 799-800
Cysticercosis, 1202, 3286t, 3289-3290, 3289f, 3292. *See also* Tapeworms.
  meningitis in, 1137, 3289-3290
  myositis in, 1202
  racemose, 3290
Cysticercus cellulosae, 3286t. *See also* Tapeworms.
  treatment of, 575t, 580t

Cystitis, 875. *See also* Urinary tract infections.
  from *Candida,* 2946, 2950
  from microsporidia, 3243
  hemorrhagic
    from adenoviruses, 1838, 1839
    in stem cell transplant, 3487
  in elderly, 3518
  in spinal cord injury, 3513-3514
  nitrofurantoin for, 474
  urethral syndrome from, 1352
Cystourethrography, voiding
  in pediatric urinary tract infections, 899, 900f
  of vesicoureteral reflux, 899, 900f
Cytarabine, for progressive multifocal leukoencephalopathy, 1861
Cytidine deaminase deficiency, autosomal recessive activation-induced, 153
Cytochrome P-3A4, quinolone effects on, 459
Cytochrome P-450
  in fusidic acid interactions, 327
  in pharmacokinetics, 273-274
  quinupristin-dalfopristin effects on, 427
Cytochrome-b_{558}, in oxidative burst, 100
Cytokines
  acute-phase response and, 38, 38t
  CD8$^+$ T-cell production of, 134
  immunomodulation with, 551, 552t
  in acute-phase response, 39, 709-710, 710t
  in AIDS dementia, 1586
  in fever, 708-709, 711
  in HIV infection, 1536, 1538
  in HIV replication, 1538-1540, 1539f
  in HIV treatment, 1540
  in infection susceptibility, 47
  in leprosy, 2889
  in mycobacterial resistance, 157f
  in pneumonia, 828
  in *Pseudomonas aeruginosa* resistance, 2590-2591
  in secondary peritonitis, 934
  in sepsis syndrome, 712
  in septic shock, 913
  in severe sepsis, 911-912
  in streptococcal toxic shock syndrome, 2372-2373
  in *Streptococcus agalactiae* (group B) infections, 2426
  in *Streptococcus pneumoniae* disease, 2396
  in systemic response, 908
  in viral meningitis, 1089
  innate immunity and, 38, 38t
  neutrophil life span and, 101
  proinflammatory, in ascites, 929-930
  pyrogenic
    in acute-phase response, 709-710, 710t
    in febrile response, 708-709, 711
    in sepsis syndrome, 712
  receptors for, 61t
  Toll-like receptors and, 38, 38f, 39
Cytomegalovirus, 1786-1798
  AIDS cholangiopathy from, 957
  appendicitis from, 969
  cervical carriage of, 1796-1798, 1797t
  characteristics of, 1787
  cidofovir-resistant, 524
  clinical features of, 1758, 1758t, 1760t
  colitis from, 530, 1580, 1791-1792
  collection of, 232, 233t
  congenital infections from, 1796-1797
  culture of, 1788-1789
  diagnosis of, 1761
  drug resistance in, 1793-1794, 1794f, 1796
    in transplant recipients, 1796
  encephalitis from, 1591

Cytomegalovirus *(Continued)*
  epidemiology of, 1759, 1759t
  esophagitis from, 1232, 1233t, 1234, 1791
  foscarnet-resistant, 527
  ganciclovir-resistant, 529
  gastric, 1576
  genome of, 1787, 1794f
  Guillain-Barré syndrome from, 1790
  hemolytic anemia from, 1790
  hepatitis from, 1435
    in transplant recipients, 1795-1796
  immune response to, 126, 1759
  in adrenal insufficiency, 915
  in hematologic cancer, 3436
  in HIV infection, 172, 1234, 1550, 1556-1557, 1576, 1591, 1790-1792
    colitis from, 1791-1792
    polyradiculopathy from, 1791
    prevention of, 1793-1794
    retinitis from, 1559-1560, 1790-1791, 1791f
    treatment of, 1682t-1686t, 1696-1697, 1792-1793
  in neonates, 1797
  in pregnancy, 1789, 1796-1798, 1797t
  in transplant recipients, 1793-1796, 3477, 3478t, 3479t, 3480, 3501-3502, 3502t, 3508-3509
    drug resistance in, 1796
    from donor organ, 1795-1796
    ganciclovir for, 530
    in heart transplants, 3478t, 3502t4
    in kidney transplants, 1796, 3478t, 3502t
    in liver transplants, 1795-1796, 3478t, 3502t.
      See also Liver transplantation, cytomegalovirus in.
    in lung transplants, 3477, 3478t, 3502t
    in stem cell transplants, 1793-1794, 1795, 3492-3494, 3493t
    late-onset, 1795
    monitoring for, 3481
    preoperative tests for, 3481
    prevention of, 1793-1796, 3482-3483
  infectious mononucleosis from, 1789, 1812
  isolation of, 1787
  laboratory diagnosis of, 236, 1787-1788
  laryngitis from, 759
  latency of, 1787
  meningoencephalitis from, 1085, 1091, 1790
  myocarditis from, 1052, 1053t, 1790
  nosocomial infections from, 3414-3416
  oncogenicity of, 1759
  overview of, 1786-1787
  pancreatitis from, 959, 959t
  pneumonia from, 1572, 1789, 1790f
    in transplant recipients, 1795
  prevention of, 1760t, 1761, 1793
  rash from, 1790
  reactivation of, 1794-1795
  receptors for, 1732t
  replication of, 1787
  retinitis from, 1415-1416, 1559-1560, 1790-1793, 1791f
    antiviral drugs for, 515t
    cidofovir for, 525
    fomivirsen for, 527
    foscarnet for, 528
    in HIV infection, 1684t-1686t, 1696-1697
    treatment of, 527-528, 530
  structure of, 1756-1757, 1756t, 1787
  susceptibility testing for, 238
  teratogenicity of, 1789
  thrombocytopenia from, 1790
  transfusion-related, 1789, 3387
  transmission of, 1759-1761, 1759t, 1789, 3387

Cytomegalovirus *(Continued)*
   treatment of, 515t, 520, 1760t, 1761, 1792-1793
     antiretroviral agents in, 1561
      drug resistance in, 1792-1793
      maribavir for, 541
    uveitis from, 1415-1416
    variants of, 1787
Cytomegalovirus hyperimmune globulin, 558
Cytomegalovirus immune serum, 66
Cytomegalovirus syndrome, 1796
Cytoplasm, pathogens in, 123
Cytosine arabinoside, for progressive multifocal
   leukoencephalopathy, 1861
Cytotoxic drugs. *See* Chemotherapy.
Cytotoxicity, antibody-dependent cellular, 56
Cytotoxins, 30, 1220-1221, 1220t
   of *Pseudomonas aeruginosa,* 2596

D

Dacron carotid patches, infections of, 1040-1041
Dacryoadenitis, 1421
Dacryocystitis, 1421
Dactylaria gallopava, brain abscess from, 3070
DAF, 75
   in paroxysmal nocturnal hemoglobinuria, 86
Dalfopristin
   for pneumonia, 837-839, 837t, 838t
   for shunt infections, 1129t, 1130
   pneumococcal resistance to, 837, 837t
Dane particle, 1864
Danger space, 790, 790f
   infections of, 793. *See also* Odontogenic
     infections.
Dapsone
   adverse effects of, 581t
   dosage of, 670t-671t
   drug interactions with, 689t
   for brain abscess, 1159t
   for leprosy, 498, 2893, 2894
   for *Pneumocystis,* 3088
     for prophylaxis, 3090
   for *Pneumocystis jirovecii,* 569t, 575t, 1681t,
     1683t, 1685t, 1693, 1695
     for prophylaxis, 3447, 3447t
   for pneumocystosis, 588
   for *Toxoplasma gondii,* 1682t, 1696
     for encephalitis prophylaxis, 3190
     in immunocompromised host, 3189, 3189t
   formulations of, 648t
   neurotoxicity of, 1594t
Daptomycin, 427-428
   for osteomyelitis, 1325
   for secondary peritonitis, 937
   for *Staphylococcus aureus,* 2337
   for vancomycin-resistant enterococcal
     endocarditis, 997
Darbrand, 1268-1269
Darkfield examination, for syphilis, 2778, 2778f
Dark-walled fungi, 3070-3072, 3070f-3072f,
   3070t, 3076t
Data mining, for bioterrorist attacks, 3598
Day care centers
   diarrhea in, 1241
   hepatitis A outbreaks in, 2171, 2171f, 2178
   rhinovirus outbreaks in, 2188
Deafness
   from erythromycin, 400
   from Lassa fever virus, 2095
   from mumps virus, 2005
   from otitis media, 768
Deamidating toxins, 25t
Decay-accelerating factor, 74t
   deficiency of, 80t

Decongestants
   for colds, 750
   for otitis media, 769
   for sinusitis, 780
Decontamination. *See also* Disinfection.
   definition of, 3331
   in hospitals, 3331-3333, 3332t
Decubitus ulcers
   in elderly, 3519-3520
   infected, 1184
     in spinal cord injury, 3515-3516
Deep fascial space infections, 754, 756, 791-793,
   792f, 793f. *See also* Odontogenic infections.
   treatment of, 797-798, 797t
Deep venous thrombosis. *See also* Suppurative
   thrombophlebitis.
   in airplane passengers, 3643-3644
Deer, in Lyme disease transmission, 2798
DEET, in Lyme disease prevention, 2807
Defensins, neutrophil bactericidal activity, 102
Deferoxamine
   bacterial infections with, 158
   mucormycosis and, 2975, 2977
Defibrillators, implantable, infections of, 1033-
   1034
Dehydration
   in cholera, 2539, 2540t
   in diarrhea, 1223-1224
Dehydroemetine, for amebiasis, 3106, 3106t
Dehydroepiandrosterone, for HIV infection, 609
Deinocerites spp., Venezuelan equine encephalitis
   from, 1915
Delavirdine, 1662, 1662t
   dosage of, 684t-685t
   drug interactions with, 689t
   for perinatal HIV transmission prevention,
     1625t, 1626
   formulations of, 649t
     pediatric, 1646t
   resistance to, 1663
   structure of, 1661f
Delivery
   cesarean
     antibiotic prophylaxis for, 1373, 1374
     endometritis and, 1373-1376, 1373f
     in HIV transmission prevention, 1621-1622
     maternal herpes and, 1771, 1772
   episiotomy infections from, 1375, 1377t
   HIV transmission in, 1490-1491, 1620
Delta agent. *See* Hepatitis D virus.
Deltaretroviruses, 2098. *See also* Human T-cell
   lymphotropic virus (HTLV).
Dematiaceous fungi, 3070-3072, 3070f-3072f,
   3070t, 3076t
Demeclocycline, 358t
   dosage of, 662t-663t
   formulations of, 647t
   nephrogenic diabetes insipidus from, 364
Dementia, AIDS, 1584-1587, 1585f, 1585t, 1586t
   pathogenesis of, 2129-2130
Demodex mites, 3310, 3311
Dendritic cells, 120
   in antigen presentation, 132-133
   in HIV infection, 1528, 1529, 1537-1538
   in innate inflammatory response, 132-133
   in intestinal tissues, 122
   in phagocytosis, 37
   in T-cell priming, 132-133
   pulmonary, 820-821
Dengue fever, 178-179, 179f, 235t
   as biological weapon, 3627-3629, 3628t
   classification of, 1936f
   clinical features of, 1936f, 1938-1939, 3629t,
     3653f

Dengue fever *(Continued)*
   diagnosis of, 1942
   differential diagnosis of, 1939
   epidemiology of, 1929-1930
   geographic distribution of, 3640f
   historical perspective on, 1927
   in travelers, 3647t, 3648t, 3649
   pathogenesis of, 1936-1937, 1936f
   prevention of, 1943-1944
   skin lesions in, 739
   treatment of, 1943
   vs. enteric fever, 1274t, 1277, 1278
   vs. malaria, 3133
Dengue hemorrhagic fever, 178
   classification of, 1936f
   clinical features of, 1936f, 1938-1939
   diagnosis of, 1942
   differential diagnosis of, 1939
   epidemiology of, 1929-1930
   historical perspective on, 1927
   pathogenesis of, 1936-1937, 1936f
   prevention of, 1943-1944
   skin lesions in, 739
   treatment of, 1943
Dengue shock syndrome, 178, 739, 1936-1937
   treatment of, 1943
Dental caries, 788, 788f, 790
   dentoalveolar infections and, 790. *See also*
     Odontogenic infections.
   from *Streptococcus mutans,* 788-789
   pathogenesis of, 788-789, 790
   prevention of, 781
Dental discoloration, from tetracycline, 363-364
Dental history, in immunodeficiency, 149
Dental infections. *See* Odontogenic infections.
Dental plaque, anaerobes in, 2839
Dental procedures
   antibiotic prophylaxis for, 793-794
   bacteremia after, 793-794
   endocarditis from, 1045-1046, 1046t
     antibiotic prophlaxis for, 1044
   HIV transmission during, prevention of, 3397
Dentoalveolar infections, 790-791. *See also*
   Odontogenic infections.
Denture sore mouth, 2941, 2951
Deoxyguanosine, 517f
Deoxyribonucleic acid. *See* DNA.
Depression, St. John's wort for, 609
Dermabacter hominis, 2471
Dermacentor spp., 3312-3314, 3313f, 3313t. *See
   also* Tick(s).
   Colorado tick fever from, 1900-1901, 1900f
   ehrlichiosis from, 2312
   Omsk hemorrhagic fever from, 1945
   Rickettsia slovaca infections from, 2285t,
     2287t, 2293
   Rocky Mountain spotted fever from, 2288-
     2289, 2289f
Dermanyssus gallinae, 3311
Dermatitis. *See* Skin infections.
Dermatitis herpetiformis, diarrhea in, 1243
Dermatobia hominis, myiasis from, 3307-3310,
   3308t
Dermatopathic lymphadenitis, 1204-1205. *See
   also* Lymphadenitis/lymphadenopathy.
Dermatophagoides spp., 3311
Dermatophilus spp., laboratory tests for, 228-229
Dermatophyte(s)
   characteristics of, 3052-3053, 3052t
   classification and taxonomy of, 3051-3052,
     3052t
   historical perspective on, 3051
   pathogenicity of, 3052, 3053-3054
   species of, 3052-3053, 3052t

Dermatophyte(s) *(Continued)*
  specimen collection and transport for, 207t
  strains of, 3052
  streptococcal cellulitis from, 2371
  vs. dimorphic molds, 229, 230t
Dermatophyte mycetoma, 2991
Dermatophytoses, 3051-3059. *See also under*
    Tinea.
  age and, 3053
  anthropophilic, 3052-3053, 3052t
  clinical features of, 3054-3057
  deep, 3057, 3057f
  diagnosis of, 3058
  epidemiology of, 3052-3053
  etiology of, 3051-3052, 3052t, 3053t. *See also*
    Dermatophyte(s)
  geophilic, 3052, 3052t
  id reactions in, 3058
  immune response to, 3054, 3058
  of hair, 3056-3057, 3061
  of nails, 3057, 3058, 3059, 3095t
  pathogenesis of, 3053-3054
  treatment of, 3058-3059, 3059t
  zoophilic, 3052, 3052t
Dermonecrotic toxin, 28
  of *Bordetella pertussis,* 2702, 2703
Desert Shield virus, 2196. *See also* Caliciviruses.
Desipramine, for herpes zoster ophthalmicus,
    1403t
Desquamative inflammatory vaginitis, 1367-1368,
    1367f, 1367t, 1368f
Dexamethasone
  for croup, 2001
  for endophthalmitis, 1411
  for HIV-related non-Hodgkin's lymphoma,
    1605
  for meningitis, 1107-1111, 1108t-1110t, 1116
    in children, 559
  for primary central nervous system lymphoma,
    1589
  nebulized, for croup, 764
Dextran, in endocarditis, 978-979
Diabetes mellitus
  antimicrobial therapy in, 244
  bacteriuria in, 883
  congenital mumps and, 2006
  coxsackieviruses and, 2157
  foot ulcers in, 1184
  mucormycosis in, 2974-2980
  osteomyelitis in, 1327-1328, 1327t
  urinary tract infections in, 887
Dialister granuliformans, endocarditis from, 992
Dialysis
  aminoglycoside dosing in, 346, 346t
  catheter-related infections in. *See also*
    Catheter-related infections.
      from *Staphylococcus epidermidis,* 2355
      prophylaxis for, 481-482
  for streptococcal toxic shock syndrome, 2374
  hepatitis B virus transmission in, 3382
  hepatitis C virus transmission in, 3384
  osteomyelitis in, 1329
  penicillin dosage in, 285, 285t
  peritonitis in, 941-943, 942t, 2355
  prosthetic vascular graft infections in, 1038-
    1039
  quinolone dosage in, 458, 458t
  respiratory disease in, 87
Diaper rash, from *Candida,* 2944, 2944f, 2951
Diarrhea, 3217. *See also under* Dysentery;
    Gastroenteritis; Gastrointestinal.
  antibiotic-associated, 1249-1250. *See also*
    Pseudomembranous colitis.
  antimicrobial resistant bacteria in, 185-186
  bacterial adherence in, 1221-1222

Diarrhea *(Continued)*
  bacterial overgrowth in, 1244
  Brainerd, 1242, 1291
  causes of, 177-178
  chemotherapy-induced, 3438
  childhood mortality in, 1215
  chronic, bacterial overgrowth with, 1244
  clindamycin therapy and, 938
  complementary and alternative medicine for,
    604t, 606-607
  diagnosis of, 1223-1234, 1225f, 1226
  emergence of, 176-178
  epidemic, in newborn nurseries, 1236-1237,
    1237t
  from *Aeromonas,* 2753-2754
  from anaerobic gram-negative bacilli, 2842
  from *Bacillus,* 2494
  from *Bacteroides fragilis,* 2813, 2842
  from *Balantidium coli,* 3232-3233
  from *Blastocystis hominis,* 3233-3234
  from caliciviruses, 2194-2199
  from *Campylobacter jejuni,* 2552
  from *Clostridium difficile,* 938, 1221
  from coccidian protozoa, 3228-3232
  from coronaviruses, 1990-1996
  from *Cryptosporidium,* 1270, 3218, 3219,
    3221-3222
  from *Cyclospora,* 1270, 3229
  from cytomegalovirus, 1791-1792
  from enteroviruses, 2156
  from *Escherichia coli,* 1218, 1219t. *See also*
    specific pathotypes under *Escherichia coli.*
      enteroaggressive, 2577-2578
      enteroinvasive, 2578
      enteropathogenic, 2575-2576
      enterotoxigenic, 1220, 2574-2575
  from *Giardia lamblia,* 3201, 3201t
  from *Isospora belli,* 3230-3232
  from microsporidia, 3238t, 3242-3245, 3244,
    3248t, 3249
  from non-O1 *Vibrio cholerae,* 2547
  from nontyphoidal *Salmonella,* 2644
  from *Plesiomonas shigelloides,* 2756
  from rotaviruses, 178, 1904-1910. *See also*
    Rotaviruses.
  from *Sarcocystis,* 3232
  from *Vibrio cholerae,* 2537, 2537t
  from *Vibrio mimicus,* 2547
  from *Vibrio parahaemolyticus,* 2545
  homeopathy for, 607-608
  in cancer, 3438
  in cholera, 2539
  in day care centers, 1241
  in elderly, 3521
  in HIV infection, 1240-1241, 1240t
  in immunocompromised host, 3438
  in institutions, 1241
  in long-term care facilities, 1241
  in stem cell transplant, 3488
  infantile, from adenoviruses, 1838
  laboratory tests for, 212
  malnutrition and, 1215
  noninflammatory, 1239-1240
    chronic, 1243
      vs. bacterial overgrowth, 1244
    differential diagnosis of, 1243
  nosocomial, 1241
  parenteral, vs. epidemic infantile diarrhea,
    1236
  traveler's, 1241-1243, 1242t, 1243t, 3642,
    3643f, 3652
    antimicrobial therapy for, 1226
    from enterotoxigenic *Escherichia coli,* 2575
    prevention of, 3642
    quinolones for, 460

Diarrhea *(Continued)*
    self-treatment for, 3643, 3643f
    treatment of, 1226, 1243
      with quinolones, 460
  treatment of, 1226
  viral, 235
  weanling, 1237-1238
  zinc for, 607
Diarrhetic shellfish poisoning, 3255f, 3256, 3256t
Dibekacin, names and sources of, 329t
Dichlorobenzene, for cutaneous warts, 1848
Diclazuril, for *Isospora belli,* 1689t
Dicloxacillin, 290, 290f
  dosage of, 650t-651t
  for carbuncles, 1175
  for cellulitis, 1180
  for impetigo, 1173, 1174
  for lymphadenitis, 1211
  for lymphangitis, 1212
  formulations of, 646t
  minimal inhibitory concentration of, 284t
Didanosine, 1657-1658, 1657t
  dosage of, 684t-685t
  drug interactions with, 690t
  formulations of, 649t
  neurotoxicity of, 1594t
  pancreatitis from, 1579
  pediatric, 1646t
  prophylactic
    after occupational exposure to HIV, 3402, 3402t
    in pregnancy, 3404
  for perinatal HIV transmission, 1624, 1625t
  resistance to, 1660
  structure of, 1656f
Dientamoeba fragilis
  syndrome of abdominal pain, diarrhea, and
    eosinophilia from, 1281t, 1283
  treatment of, 572t, 583
    with metronidazole, 393
Diet. *See also* Nutrition *and specific dietary
    components, e.g.,* Fish oil.
  urinary pH and, 888
Diethylcarbamazine
  adverse effects of, 581t
  for filariasis, 572t, 3271-3272
  for helminthic disease, 570t
  for loiasis, 572t, 577t, 3273
  for onchocerciasis, 3274
  for systemic nematodes, 594
  for tropical pulmonary eosinophilia, 572t, 3275
  for *Wuchereria bancrofti,* 577t
  structure of, 594f
N,N-Diethylmetatoluamide, in Lyme disease
    prevention, 2807
Differential fluorescence induction, 10
Diffuse alveolar hemorrhage, in stem cell
    transplant, 3488
Diffuse unilateral subacute neuroretinitis, 3295
DiGeorge's syndrome, 150t
  T-cell function in, 132, 153
Digital herpes, 1769, 1769f, 1773t
Digital resources, 3656-3661
  electronic medical records, 3660-3661
  for biological weapons, 3611, 3611t
  for travel medicine, 3638t
  Internet, 3656-3658, 3658t, 3659t
  personal digital assistants, 3658-3660, 3660t,
    3661t
  practice tools, 3660-3661, 3661t
Dihydroartemisinin, 606f
Dihydrofolate reductase inhibitors, 587
Dihydropteroate reductase, in trimethoprim
    resistance, 265
Dihydropteroate synthase, in sulfonamide
    resistance, 265

Dihydroqinghaosu, 606f
Diiodohydroxyquin, for amebiasis, 3106, 3106t
Dilated cardiomyopathy. *See also*
    Cardiomyopathy.
    after enteroviral myopericarditis, 2153
    myocarditis in, 1052-1057
Diloxanide furoate
    adverse effects of, 581t
    for amebiasis, 571t, 3106, 3106t
    for luminal protozoa, 583
    indications for, 568t
7-Dimethylamino-demethyl-6-deoxy-tetracycline,
    357f
Dimethylglycytamido-6-demethyl-6-
    deoxytetracycline, 357f
Dimethylsulfoxide, idoxuridine in, 531
Dinophysis spp., 3256, 3256t
Diphenoxylate-atropine
    for *Clostridium difficile*–associated colitis,
        1258
    for traveler's diarrhea, 1242
Diphtheria, 1147-1148. *See also*
    Corynebacterium diphtheriae.
    cardiac toxicity in, 2461-2462
    cutaneous, 1180-1181, 2462
    diagnosis of, 2462-2463, 2463f
    differential diagnosis of, 2463
    epidemiology of, 2458-2460, 2459f
    history of, 2457-2458
    invasive, 2462
    myocardial involvement in, 1053
    neuropathy in, 2462
    pathogenesis of, 2460-2461, 2460f
    pharyngitis in, 755, 756
    prevention of, 2464
    respiratory, 2460, 2460f, 2461-2462, 2461f
    treatment of, 2463-2464
    vs. epiglottitis, 785
    wound, 1180-1181
Diphtheria antitoxin, 2463
    for cutaneous diphtheria, 1181
Diphtheria, tetanus, pertussis (DTP) vaccine,
    2464, 3562, 3563, 3563f, 3564t
    contraindications to, 3583t
    immunization rate for, 2460
    schedule for children, 3564t
Diphtheria toxin, 26
    action of, 28
    cell entry by, 27
    immunization schedule for, 2464
    in myocarditis, 1055
Diphtheria vaccine, 3562-3564. *See also*
    Diphtheria, tetanus, pertussis (DTP) vaccine.
    for adults, 3576f, 3577f
Diphtheroids
    in peritoneal dialysis, 941
    prosthetic valve endocarditis from, 1024, 1025
    treatment of, 1028
Diphyllobothrium [spp.], 3286t, 3287, 3288. *See
    also* Tapeworms.
Diphyllobothrium latum
    syndrome of abdominal pain, diarrhea, and
        eosinophilia from, 1281t, 1283
    treatment of, 575t
Dipylidium caninum, 3288
    treatment of, 575t
Direct fluorescent antibody tests, for sputum, 826
Dirithromycin, 408
    dosage of, 664t-665t
    drug interactions with, 690t
    formulations of, 648t
Dirofilaria repens, ocular infections from, 3273
Dirofilariasis, 3294t, 3297-3298
Disease(s). *See also* Infectious disease(s).
    definition of, 167

Disease surveillance, 164
Disinfection. *See also* Infection control.
    bioterrorism and, 3342
    definition of, 3331
    emerging pathogens and, 3340-3342
    in hospitals, 3331-3333, 3332t
        environmental, 3334
    OSHA blood-borne pathogen standard and,
        3340
    resistance to, 3340-3342
    with alcohol, 3333-3334
    with chlorine compounds, 3334
    with glutaraldehyde, 3334-3335, 3335t
    with hydrogen peroxide, 3335t, 3336-3337
    with iodophors, 3335t
    with *ortho*-phthalaldehyde, 3335t
    with pasteurization, 3338
    with peracetic acid, 3335t, 3336
    with peracetic acid/hydrogen peroxide, 3335t,
        3336-3337
    with phenolics, 3337
    with quaternary ammonium compounds, 3337-
        3338
Disk diffusion susceptibility testing, 223
Disseminated gonococcal infections, skin lesions
    in, 736
Disseminated granulomatosis, fever in, 726
Disseminated intravascular coagulation, 735
    in meningococcal disease, 2508
    in sepsis, 916
Disseminated *Mycobacterium avium* disease,
    2897, 2898-2899, 2899f, 2901, 2901f, 2901t,
    2903-2906
Distributional clearance, 272. *See also* Drug
    distribution.
Disulfiram, metronidazole interactions with, 393t
Diuretics, tetracycline with, 364t
Diverticulitis, 971-973
    actinomycotic, 2927
    intraperitoneal abscess in, 943
DNA
    of *Mycobacterium tuberculosis,* 2854t, 2855
    polymorphic, random amplification of, 222
    rearrangement of, in immunoglobulin
        production, 60, 60f, 60t
DNA gyrase, quinolone inhibition of, 265, 451, 453
DNA probes, for pneumonia, 828
DNA viruses, 2098. *See also* Human T-cell
    lymphotropic virus (HTLV).
DNases, 2364
Dobrava virus, 2086-2089, 2086t
Docosahexaenoic acid, 143
Docosanol, 515t, 525
Döderlein's bacilli, 36
Dog(s)
    bites of, 3552-3553, 3552t, 3553t
        Capnocytophaga canimorsus in, 2731-2732
        laboratory studies for, 213
        of head and neck, 800
        Pasteurella in, 2687
        rabies from, 2050
    heartworm in, dirofilariasis from, 3294t, 3297-
        3298
    mites of, 3311
    sarcoptic mange in, 3305
    Toxocara canis infections in, 3293-3294
Dog ticks, 3312-3314, 3313f, 3313t. *See also*
    Tick(s).
Dolosicoccus spp., laboratory identification of,
    217t, 218
Dolosigranulum spp., laboratory identification of,
    217t, 218
Donovan bodies, 1343, 1343f, 2749, 2750f
Donovanosis. *See* Granuloma inguinale.
Dosage guidelines, 635, 650t-685t

Dot/Icm, 2714
Doxorubicin, for HIV-related non-Hodgkin's
    lymphoma, 1605
Doxycycline, 358t
    dosage of, 662t-663t
    food interactions with, 364t
    for actinomycosis, 2931, 2931t
    for anthrax, 1177t, 2489t, 2490t
    for bacillary angiomatosis, 1185
    for bartonellosis, 1691t, 1692t, 2744
    for brucellosis, 2672
    for cellulitis, 1180
    for cervicofacial actinomycosis, 797t
    for *Chlamydia trachomatis*, 2525
    for chlamydial pneumonia, 2263
        atherosclerosis after, 2265
    for COPD exacerbations, 811t
    for ehrlichiosis, 2315
    for epidemic typhus, 2305
    for epididymitis, 2526
    for legionellosis, 2719t
    for leptospirosis, 2793t
    for Lyme disease, 2806, 2806t
        for prophylaxis, 3315
    for lymphogranuloma venereum, 2245
    for malaria, 573t, 574t, 3129, 3133, 3134t, 3135
        for prophylaxis, 3137-3138, 3137t
            in travelers, 3641-3642, 3641t
    for melioidosis, 2629t
    for meningitis, 1106t, 1107t
    for murine typhus, 2308
    for *Mycoplasma pneumoniae,* 2278
    for *Neisseria gonorrhoeae,* 2524t, 2525, 2525t,
        2526
    for neonatal conjunctivitis, 2247t
    for parasites, 589
    for pelvic inflammatory disease, 460, 1379t,
        2247t, 2525, 2525t
    for periodontitis, 796, 796t
    for plague, 2696, 3603
    for pneumonia, 806t, 837-839
        pneumococcal, 2404
    for psittacosis, 2257
    for Q fever endocarditis, 1001, 2300
    for rickettsial diseases, 2287, 2293
    for rickettsialpox, 2296
    for Rocky Mountain spotted fever, 2091-2292
    for scrub typhus, 2310
    for sepsis, 919
    for syphilis, 1344, 1690t, 2781t, 2782
    for toxoplasmosis, 1696
        in immunocompromised host, 3189
    for tularemia, 2682
        in bioterrorism attack, 3610t, 3611, 3611t
    for urethritis, 1207, 2247t, 2249
    for urogenital chlamydial infections, 1207,
        2247t, 2249, 2250
    for Whipple's disease, 1309, 1310t
    formulations of, 647t
    indications for, 569t
    pharmacology of, 362t
    prophylactic
        for anthrax, 3621, 3622t
        for travelers, 3643
        for tularemia, 3609-3610, 3609t
    side effects of, 363t, 3609t
Dracunculiasis, 3269-3270, 3270f
    metronidazole for, 572t
Drainage. *See also* Aspiration.
    of amebic liver abscess, 3106
    of brain abscess, 1160
    of epidural abscess, 1167-1168
    of lung abscess, 856
    of pleural effusion/empyema, 850-851
    of subdural empyema, 1165

DRB1*1501, in tuberculosis, 2858
DRB1*1502, in tuberculosis, 2858
Droplet precautions, 3327t, 3328t, 3329, 3330t
Drug(s). See also specific drugs and drug families.
  absorption of, 271t, 272
  acute pancreatitis from, 959, 959b
  antimicrobial. See Antimicrobial agents.
  body fluid concentrations of, 635, 650t-685t
  chronic pulmonary disease from, 859, 862f
  dosage of
    guidelines for, 635, 650t-685t
    in renal failure, 635, 651t-685t
    in spinal cord injury, 3513
  elimination of, 271t, 274
  fever from, 727
  hepatitis from, 1436
  immunodeficiency from, 158
  injection of, subcutaneous abscess from, 1191
  intraventricular administration of, 1129-1130
  protein binding of, 273
  rash from, 731
    in HIV infection, 742
  steady-state concentration of, 274
  Stevens-Johnson syndrome from, 732, 733
  toxic epidermal necrolysis from, 732, 733
    vs. staphylococcal scalded skin syndrome, 726
  trade names for, 635t-646t
Drug abuse. See Injection drug users.
Drug distribution, 271t, 272-273, 272f
  concentration vs. time plot in, 272, 272f
  volume of, 272
Drug eruptions, 731. See also Rash.
  in HIV infection, 742
  in infectious mononucleosis, 1806, 1806f, 1806t
Drug interactions, 686t-700t
  antagonistic, 274
    in combination antimicrobial therapy, 248-249
Drug resistance. See specific drugs.
Drunken disease, 2949
Duct tape, for cutaneous warts, 1848
Duffy antigen, malaria and, 3127
Duffy blood group, malaria susceptibility and, 44t, 46
Dumb rabies, 2051, 2051t
Duncan's syndrome, 150t, 153, 1435, 1807
  Epstein-Barr virus infections in, 66
Duodenal ulcers. See Peptic ulcers.
Dust mites, 3311
Dutch hypothesis, 806
Duvenhage virus, 2047t
Dwarf tapeworm, 3286t, 3287-3288. See also Tapeworms.
Dwarfism, nutritious, 140
Dysentery. See also Diarrhea; Gastroenteritis.
  acute, 1263-1269
  bacillary, 1264, 1265f, 2655-2660. See also Shigella [spp.]
    cyclic epidemics of, 2657
    diagnosis of, 2657-2658, 2658f
    epidemiology of, 2656-2657
    laboratory findings in, 2658, 2658f
    pathogenesis of, 2656, 2656f
    treatment of, 2658-2659, 2659t
  causes of, 1264t
  diagnosis of, 1267-1269
  epidemiology of, 1263
  fecal leukocytes in, 1263-1264, 1264f
  from Balantidium coli, 1266
  from Campylobacter jejuni, 1265-1266
  from Entamoeba, 1266
  from Escherichia coli, 1265, 1265t

Dysentery (Continued)
  from Salmonella, 1266-1267
  from Schistosoma, 1266
  from Spirillum, 1267
  from Treponema hyodysenteriae, 1267
  from trichinosis, 1266
  from Vibrio, 1266
  from Yersinia enterocolitica, 1267
  history of, 2655
  treatment of, 1267-1269
Dysgenesis, reticular, 150t, 152
Dysgonomonas [spp.], 2751t, 2755-2756
Dysgonomonas capnocytophagoides, 2755-2756
Dysrhythmias
  erythromycin and, 400
  in myocarditis, 1056
Dystroglycans, 9
Dystrophin, in myocarditis, 1055
Dysuria, 886, 886f, 891

E

Eales' disease, 1416
Ear infections. See Otitis.
East African trypanosomiasis. See also Trypanosomiasis, African.
  vs. malaria, 3133
Eastern equine encephalitis, 235t, 1146, 1913-1919, 1914t. See also Alphaviruses.
  isolation precautions for, 3330t
Eastern Europe, HIV infection in, 1465-1466, 1466f
Eaton-Lambert myasthenic syndrome, vs. botulism, 2825, 2826f
Ebola virus, 739, 2057-2059, 2057f
  as biological weapon, 3627-3629, 3628t
  clinical features of, 3629t
  disinfection/sterilization and, 3342
Echinacea, 610
  for colds, 604t, 608, 750
Echinocandins, 510-511
  for candidiasis, 2949
  prophylactic, for cancer patients, 3446, 3447t
Echinococcus [spp.], 3290-3292, 3292t. See also Tapeworms.
  albendazole for, 592
Echinococcus granulosus, 3286t, 3290-3291, 3293
  pancreatic infections from, 959t, 960
  treatment of, 575t
Echinococcus multilocularis, 3286t, 3290-3291
  treatment of, 575t, 580t
Echinococcus vogeli, 3290-3291
Echinostoma spp., syndrome of abdominal pain, diarrhea, and eosinophilia from, 1281t, 1283
Echocardiography
  for endocarditis, 986-987
    prosthetic valve, 1030
    treatment duration and, 999
  for myocarditis, 1056
  for pericarditis, 1060-1061, 1061
Echoviruses. See also Enterovirus(es).
  arthritis from, 2156-2157
  classification of, 2133, 2134t
  communicability period for, 2137
  culture of, 2137-2138
  encephalitis from, 2149
    in immunocompromised host, 2154-2155
  epidemic pleurodynia from, 2151-2152
  epidemiology of, 2136-2137, 2136t
  exanthems from, 2149-2150
  gastrointestinal disease from, 2156
  genome of, 2134
  hand-foot-mouth disease from, 2150, 2157

Echoviruses (Continued)
  hepatitis from, 2156
    in neonate, 2154
  herpangina from, 754, 2151
  host range of, 2133, 2134t
  immune response to, 2135-2136
  in neonates, 2153-2154
  in pregnancy, 2137, 2153
  incidence of, 2136t, 2137
  incubation period for, 2137
  laboratory diagnosis of, 235, 2137-2138
  meningitis from, 1085, 2148-2149
    in immunocompromised host, 2154-2155
  minor/major viremia in, 2135
  mutation of, 2135
  myopericarditis from, 2152-2153
    in neonate, 2154
  myositis from, 2151-2152
  orchitis from, 2156-2157
  paralysis from, 2149, 2156, 2157
  pathogenesis of, 2135
  pneumonia from, in neonates, 2154
  prevention of, 2138
  proteins of, 2134
  receptors for, 1732t, 2134, 2134t
  respiratory infections from, 2150-2151
  transmission of, 2137
  treatment of, 2138
Econazole, formulations of, 649t
ECRF3, 98
Ecthyma, 1176
  streptococcal, 2369
Ecthyma gangrenosum, 733, 736, 1186
  from Pseudomonas aeruginosa bacteremia, 2600, 2600f
  in cancer, 3438-3439
  in sepsis, 917-918
Ectodermal dysplasia, X-linked, with immunodeficiency, 153
Ectoparasites, 3301-3302, 3301t. See also specific types.
Ectopic pregnancy, after pelvic inflammatory disease, 2249
Ectothrix infections, 3056, 3057f
Eczema, genital lesions in, 1344
Eczema herpeticum, 1766
Eczema vaccinatum, 741, 1745
Edema
  cerebral. See also Intracranial hypertension.
    in cryptococcal meningitis, 3008
  pulmonary, in malaria, 3125
Edema factor, of Bacillus anthracis, 2485, 2486
Edge Hill virus, 1945t
Edwarsiella tarda, 2580
Efavirenz, 1662-1663, 1662t
  dosage of, 684t-685t
  drug interactions with, 690t
  neurotoxicity of, 1594t
  pediatric, 1646t
  prophylactic
    after occupational exposure to HIV, 3402, 3402t
    for perinatal HIV transmission, 1625t, 1626
  resistance to, 1663
  structure of, 1661f
Efflux
  in multidrug resistance, 454
  in Staphylococcus aureus resistance, 2335-2336, 2336t
Eflornithine
  adverse effects of, 581t
  for African trypanosomiasis, 591, 3168, 3168t, 3169
  for Trypanosomatidae, 569t, 576t, 580t

Eggs, *Salmonella enteritidis* infections from, 2639-240, 2639f
Ehrlichia [spp.]
　characteristics of, 2311t, 2312
　classification and taxonomy of, 2284, 2310-2312, 2311t
　historical perspective on, 2284-2286, 2285t
　skin lesions from, 740
　target cells of, 2287t, 2311t
　vectors of, 2285t, 2311t
　veterinary diseases from, 2310-2312, 2311t
Ehrlichia canis, 2310-2311, 2311t
Ehrlichia chaffeensis, 740, 2310-2313, 2311t, 3312, 3313t, 3314
　human monocytotropic ehrlichiosis from, 2313
Ehrlichia equi, 740
Ehrlichia ewingii, 2311, 2311t, 3312, 3313t, 3314
Ehrlichia muris, 2311, 2311t
Ehrlichia phagocytophila, 740
Ehrlichia ruminatum, 2311, 2311t
Ehrlichiosis
　canine, 2311, 2311t
　from *Anaplasma phagocytophilum,* 2311-2313, 2315
　from *E. chaffeensis,* 2285t, 2287t, 2311-2315, 2311t, 3312, 3313t, 3314
　from *E. ewingii,* 2315, 3312, 3313t, 3314
　from *E. muris,* 2315
　human granulocytic, 740, 2285t, 2287t, 2311-2313, 2311t, 2313t, 2315, 3312, 3313t, 3314
　human monocytotropic, 740, 2285t, 2287t, 2311-2315, 2311t, 3312, 3313t, 3314
　postsplenectomy, 3528
　rifamycin for, 382
　vs. enteric fever, 1275t, 1278
Eicosanoids, 143, 143f
Eicosapentaenoic acid, 143, 143f
Eikenella [spp.], 2751t, 2758-2759
Eikenella corrodens, 2758-2759
　bite infections from, 800
　cardiovascular device infections from, 1023
　endocarditis from, 991
　　prosthetic valve, 1028, 1029t
　in clenched fist injuries, 3555
　laboratory identification of, 220
El Niño, in cholera transmission, 2538
Elderly
　antimicrobial agent selection for, 244
　bacteremia in, 3520
　bacteriuria in, 883, 887
　diarrhea in, 1241
　drug therapy for, 3522
　fever of unknown origin in, 719, 720, 720t, 3521-3522
　human metapneumovirus and, 2029, 2029t
　immunizations for, 3522
　infections in, 3517-3522
　infectious diarrhea in, 3521
　infective endocarditis in, 3520-3521
　malnutrition in, 146-147, 146t
　meningitis in, 3521
　pneumonia in, 832, 3518-3519
　　chronic, 858
　　from *Moraxella (Branhamella) catarrhalis,* 2531
　pressure sores in, 3519-3520
　respiratory syncytial virus in, 2016-2017
　septic arthritis in, 3521
　skin infections in, 3519-3520
　Streptococcus agalactiae (group B) infections in, 2427
　temperature in, 705, 707
　tuberculosis in, 2863, 3519
　　lower lung field, 2865

Elderly *(Continued)*
　urinary tract infections in, 3517-3518
　　catheter-related, 3373
　West Nile virus in, 3521
Electrocardiography, for myocarditis, 1056
Electroencephalography, for Creutzfeldt-Jakob disease, 2225, 2226
Electronic medical records, 3660-3661
Electrophysiologic studies, in botulism diagnosis, 2825, 2826f
Electrosurgery
　for cutaneous warts, 1848
　for genital warts, 1849
Elephantiasis, 3271, 3271f
Elephantiasis nostras, 1211
ELISA. *See* Enzyme-linked immunosorbent assay.
ELISPOT assays, 117, 118f
Embolism
　in endocarditis, 981, 984
　　from *Staphylococcus aureus,* 2343
　　prosthetic valve, 1030
　pulmonary
　　fever from, 726
　　in airplane passengers, 3644
　　in spinal cord injury, 3514-3515
　　pleural effusion and, 847, 849
Embryologic cysts, infected, 799-800
Emergency preparedness, 192-201
　ambulatory care in, 201
　communication plan in, 193, 195f
　education in, 198
　electronic resources for, 193, 193t
　emergency department in, 201
　exposure management in, 198
　for bioterrorism, 3595-3600, 3598t
　health care worker surveillance in, 198
　infection control in, 193-195
　　diagnosis and detection in, 193-194, 196t
　　policies for, 194-195, 196t
　　syndromic surveillance for, 194
　infrastructural, 199-200, 199f, 200t
　isolation technique in, 195-198
　media management in, 201
　patient transport in, 200, 200f
　plans for, 193, 194f
　respiratory isolation precautions in, 197, 197f
　screening procedures in, 198-199, 199f
　surge capacity in, 193
　visitors in, 200
Emerging diseases
　convergence model of, 174, 174f
　definition of, 739
　emergency preparedness for, 192-201. *See also* Emergency preparedness.
　newly identified, 174, 174t
Emetine, for amebic liver abscess, 3106
Emphysema, 806-811. *See also* Chronic obstructive pulmonary disease (COPD).
　in HIV infection, 1573
Empirical therapy, 620
Empyema. *See also* Pleural effusion.
　brain abscess from, 1151t, 1152
　clinical features of, 847
　etiology of, 846-847
　from anaerobic infections, 2812
　from *Aspergillus,* 2963
　from *Haemophilus influenzae,* 2664
　from *Staphylococcus aureus,* 2345
　imaging of, 847-849, 848f
　in pneumococcal pneumonia, 2402
　laboratory findings in, 849-850
　microbiology of, 846-847
　pathophysiology of, 846
　risk assessment for, 850t

Empyema *(Continued)*
　subdural, 1164-1165
　thoracic, from *Candida,* 2945
　treatment of, 850-851, 850t
　tuberculous, 2878
Emtricitabine, 541, 541f, 1657t, 1659-1660
　dosage of, 684t-685t
　for chronic hepatitis B, 1447, 1448t, 1881
　pediatric, 1646t
　resistance to, 1660
　structure of, 1656f
ENA-78, 846
Enanthems, 731, 734. *See also* Rash.
Encephalitis, 1143-1147. *See also* Central nervous system infections; Meningoencephalitis.
　California, 1146-1147, 2086-2089, 2086t
　Central European, 1928, 1929
　chronic, from enteroviruses, 2154-2155
　clinical features of, 1079-1080, 1144-1145
　Eastern equine, 235t, 1146, 1913-1919, 1914t
　　isolation precautions for, 3330t
　etiology of, 1146-1147, 1146t, 1147t
　European tick-borne, 1934
　Far Eastern, 1934, 1941
　fever from, 1822, 1822f, 1822t
　from adenoviruses, 1839
　from alphaviruses, 1146t, 1913-1919, 1914t. *See also* Alphaviruses.
　from Colorado tick fever, 1900-1901, 1900f
　from coltiviruses, 1899
　from *Coxiella burnetii,* 2300
　from *Cryptococcosis,* 3003-3004
　from cytomegalovirus, 1790
　from enteroviruses, 2149
　from Epstein-Barr virus, 1807
　from flaviviruses, 1926-1945. *See also* Japanese encephalitis; St. Louis encephalitis; Tick-borne encephalitis; West Nile encephalitis.
　from Hendra virus, 1146
　from herpes B virus, 1833-1834, 1833f
　from herpes simplex virus, 519, 1145, 1146, 1769-1770, 1773t
　　vs. herpes simplex meningitis, 1085
　from human herpesvirus 7, 1824
　from Jamestown Canyon virus, 2086t, 2089
　from La Crosse virus, 235t, 1146, 2086-2089, 2086t, 2951
　　ribavirin for, 538
　from *Listeria monocytogenes,* 2481, 2482f
　from measles, 2032, 2034
　from microsporidia, 3238t, 3243, 3245
　from mumps virus, 2005
　from *Mycoplasma pneumoniae,* 2274f, 2275
　from Nipah virus, 1146, 2039t, 2040f, 2041-2042, 2043f
　from orbiviruses, 1899
　from parvovirus B19, 1895
　from polioviruses, 2143
　from rabies virus, 2049-2051
　from rubella, 1922
　from *Toxoplasma gondii,* 443, 1587, 1588f, 3175-3176, 3175f, 3179-3180, 3184f, 3192f
　　diagnosis of, 3183-3186, 3184f, 3192f
　　prevention of, 3190
　　treatment of, 3188-3190, 3189t
　from varicella zoster virus, 1782
　granulomatous amebic, 1088, 1101, 1104-1105, 1106t, 1115, 3111-3119. *See also* *Acanthamoeba* spp.; Granulomatous amebic encephalitis.
　granulomatous microsporidial, 3243
　isolation precautions for, 3330t

Encephalitis (Continued)
Japanese. See Japanese encephalitis.
laboratory findings in, 1145-1146
Murray Valley, 1929
nonviral, 1147, 1147t
pathogenesis and pathophysiology of, 1144
Rocio, 1945
Russian spring-summer, 1928, 1929
St. Louis, 235t, 1146, 1940-1941. See also St.
  Louis encephalitis.
Siberian tick-borne, 1934
specimen collection in, 233t
tick-borne, 1145, 1146, 1926-1945, 1927f. See
  also Tick-borne encephalitis.
treatment of, 1147
  antiviral, 515t
Venezuelan equine, 235t, 1913-1919, 1914t
  isolation precautions for, 3330t
viral, 538
West Nile. See West Nile encephalitis.
Western equine, 235t, 1913-1919, 1914t
  isolation precautions for, 3330t
Encephalitozoon [spp.], 3237, 3238t, 3245. See
  also Microsporidia.
  in HIV infection, 1701
  treatment of, 574t, 592
Encephalitozoon hellem, 579t
Encephalitozoon intestinalis, 568
  in HIV infection, 1701
Encephalomyelitis, 1143-1147
  acute disseminated, 2053
  clinical features of, 1144-1145
  etiology of, 1146-1147, 1146t
  from vaccinia virus, 1745
  in melioidosis, 2628, 2628f
  laboratory findings in, 1145-1146
  pathogenesis and pathophysiology of, 1144
  postvaccinial, 2053
  treatment of, 1147
Encephalopathy
  from vaccinia virus, 1745
  in cat-scratch disease, 2738-2739
  in HIV infection, 1584
    in children, 1643
  in sepsis, 915
Encystation, 18
Endarterectomy, carotid artery, infections of,
  1040-1041
Endarteritis, 1005-1009. See also Arteritis.
  clinical manifestations of, 1007-1008
  epidemiology of, 1006
  etiology of, 1008-1009
  mycotic aneurysms in. See Mycotic aneurysms.
  obliterative, in syphilis, 2771, 2771f
  pathogenesis of, 1006
  pathology of, 1006-1007
  treatment of, 1009
Endocardial fibroelastosis, congenital mumps
  and, 2006
Endocarditis, 975-1002. See also Myocarditis;
  Pericarditis.
  adherence in, 978-979
  age onset in, 975
  antibodies in, 980-981
  bacterial, 975, 992
  blood culture in, 985-986
  cardiac valves in, 976, 977
  central nervous system in, 982
  classification of, 975
  clinical manifestations of, 982-988
  coagulase-negative staphylococcal, 2354
  conditions predisposing to, 1044
  congestive heart failure in, 983
  culture-negative, 985-986, 993
    treatment of, 1001

Endocarditis (Continued)
  definitions in, 975
  dental procedures and, 1045-1046, 1046t
  diagnosis of
    criteria for, 987-988, 988t
    tests in, 985-987
  echocardiography in, 986-987
  epidemiology of, 975-977
  etiology of, 988-994, 988t
  experimental, 1047-1048
  eyes in, 982, 983f
  fever in, 983
  from Actinobacillus actinomycetemcomitans,
    2752, 2753
  from anaerobic bacilli, 1000, 2842-2843
  from anaerobic bacteria, 992
  from Aspergillus, 993, 1030
  from Bacillus, 2495
  from Bacteroides, 992
  from Bacteroides fragilis, 1000, 2843
  from Bartonella, 1026, 2734-2735
  from Brucella, 992, 1026
  from Candida, 979, 992-993, 1030
  from Cardiobacterium hominis, 2754
  from Chlamydia, 1001
  from Chlamydia trachomatis, 993
  from Chlamydophila psittaci, 993
  from Chlamydophila pneumoniae, 993
  from Corynebacterium, 991, 992
  from Coxiella burnetii, 993
  from diphtheroids, 1024, 1025, 1028
  from Enterobacteriaceae, 990-991, 999-1000
  from Enterococcus, 989, 2412-2413
    penicillin-resistant, 996-998
    treatment of, 248, 425, 996-998, 1027-1028,
      1027t, 1028t, 2416-2417, 2416t
    vancomycin-resistant, 997
  from Enterococcus faecalis, 979
  from Erysipelothrix rhusiopathiae,
    2497-2498
  from gram-negative bacilli, 990-991, 1025,
    1028, 2842-2843
  from gram-negative bacteria, 991
  from HACEK organisms, 991, 1025, 1026
    treatment of, 1000, 1028, 1029t
  from Haemophilus, 991, 1000
  from Kingella, 991, 2533
  from Legionella, 1026
  from Listeria, 991
  from Listeria monocytogenes, 2481
  from Neisseria, 991
  from Neisseria gonorrhoeae, 1000, 2523
  from nutritionally variant streptococci, 2440
  from oral infections, 1044
  from Pseudomonas, 991, 999-1000
  from Pseudomonas aeruginosa, 1030, 2606
  from Q fever, 993, 1001
  from Salmonella, 990-991, 2647t
  from Spirillum minus, 993
  from Staphylococcus, 990
    coagulase-negative, 2354
    treatment of, 998-999, 1026-1027, 1026t
  from Staphylococcus aureus. See
    Staphylococcus aureus, endocarditis from.
  from Staphylococcus epidermidis, 380, 1024,
    1025, 1030, 2354
  from Staphylococcus lugdunensis, 990, 2354
  from Streptococcus, 978, 988-990, 1027
    penicillin-resistant, 996-998
    penicillin-sensitive, 995-996
    treatment of, 995-998, 1027, 1027t
    vaccination for, 1045
  from Streptococcus adjacens, 979
  from Streptococcus agalactiae (group B), 2427
  from Streptococcus anginosus group, 2454

Endocarditis (Continued)
  from Streptococcus defectivus, 979
  from Streptococcus gordonii, 979
  from streptococcus group C, 2444
  from streptococcus group G, 2444
  from Streptococcus mutans, 978
  from Streptococcus pyogenes (group A),
    978
  from Streptococcus sanguis, 978, 979-980
  from Tropheryma whipplei, 993, 1026
  from viridans streptococci, 2436-2438, 2436t,
    2437t
  fungal, 992-993
    treatment of, 1000-1001
  heart disease in, 976-977, 981, 983, 994
  hemodynamic factors in, 977
  hypergammaglobulinemia in, 65
  immunopathologic factors in, 980-981
  in drug addiction, 984-985, 990, 992
  in HIV infection, 981, 984-985, 1560
  incidence of, 975
  kidney in, 981-982, 984
  lung in, 982
  medical procedures and, 1046, 1046b
  meningococcal, 1000
  microorganisms in, 2344t
  mycotic aneurysms in, 982
  native valve, 1024-1025
  nonbacterial thrombotic, 977, 978-980, 978t
  nosocomial, 975-976
  pathogenesis of, 977, 977f
  pathology of, 981-982, 982f
  pathophysiology of, 977
  pericarditis with, 1060
  peripheral manifestations of, 983-984
  platelets in, 979-980
  pneumococcal, 1000
  polymicrobial, 994
  prevention of, 1044-1045, 1048-1049
    after cardiotomy, 1048-1049
    antibiotics in, 1045
    bacterial adherence and, 1045
    chemoprophylaxis in, 1044-1050
      efficacy of, 1047-1048
      malpractice issues in, 1049-1050
      recommendations for, 1049t, 1050, 1050t
      vancomycin in, 420, 423
    immunization in, 1045
    infections control in, 1044
  prosthetic valve, 976, 990, 1024-1032
    clinical manifestations of, 1025
    complicated, 1029-1030
    culture-negative, 1026
    diagnosis of, 1025
    echocardiography of, 1026, 1030
    epidemiology of, 1024
    extension of, 1029-1030
    fungal, 1024, 1025
      treatment of, 1028-1029
    incidence of, 1024
    laboratory studies for, 1025
    microbiology of, 1025
    microorganisms in, 1024-1027, 1030, 2354,
      2752
    pathogenesis of, 1024-1025
    pathology of, 1025
    prevention of, 1032
    prognosis of, 1032
    relapse of, 1030
    treatment of
      anticoagulants in, 1032
      antimicrobials in, 1026-1029, 1026t-
        1029t, 1032
      surgery in, 1029-1032, 1031t
  rheumatoid factor in, 980

Endocarditis *(Continued)*
  risk for, 1045-1047, 1046b, 1046t, 1047b
    cardiac conditions and, 1046, 1046b
    surgical procedures and, 1046, 1047b
  skin infections and, 982, 983f, 984, 1044
  spleen in, 982, 984
  surgical procedures and, 1046, 1046b
  symptoms and signs of, 982-983, 983t
  thrombocidins in, 980
  transient bacteremia in, 977-978, 978t
  treatment of, 994-1002, 2344t
    antimicrobials in, 994-1001
      agent selection in, 246
      monitoring of, 994-995
    fusidic acid in, 327
    outpatient parenteral antimicrobial therapy
      in, 629, 629t
    surgery in, 1001-1002
    with aminoglycosides, 350
    with quinolones, 465
    with vancomycin, 422
  underlying cardiac disease in, 1046-1047,
    1047b
Endocervix. *See also under* Cervical.
  Neisseria gonorrhoeae infections of, 2520,
    2520f
Endocrine system, tetracycline effects on, 363t
Endocrine-related agents, rifamycin interaction
  with, 376t
Endocrinopathy, diarrhea in, 1243
Endocytosis, bacteria-mediated, by *Salmonella,*
  2642, 2642f
Endometritis
  from *Chlamydia trachomatis,* 2247t, 2248
  from *Mycoplasma genitalium,* 2281, 2281t
  in pelvic inflammatory disease, 1378-1380,
    1379t
  postabortal, 1375-1376, 1377t
  postpartum, 1373-1376, 1373f
Endomyometritis, postpartum, 1373-1376, 1373f
Endoparametritis, postpartum, 1373-1376, 1373f
Endophthalmitis, 1406-1411, 1408. *See also*
  Ocular infections.
  acute postcataract, 1407-1408, 1407f, 1408f
  anatomic aspects of, 1407, 1407f
  bleb-related, 1407t, 1408
  chronic pseudophakic, 1407t, 1408
  classification of, 1407, 1407t
  diagnosis of, 1409-1410
  endogenous bacterial, 1407, 1408
  etiology of, 1407t
  exogenous, 1407
  from *Aspergillus,* 1409, 1411
  from *Bacillus,* 2495
  from bacteria, 1407-1408
  from *Candida,* 1408-1409, 1409f, 1411, 1417,
    2947-2948, 2947-2948f, 2951
  from fungi, 1407t, 1408-1409
  from *Fusarium,* 1409, 1411
  from *Klebsiella pneumoniae,* 1408
  from *Propionibacterium acnes,* 1408,
    1411
  from *Pseudomonas aeruginosa,* 2604
  from *Sporothrix schenckii,* 2986
  from *Staphylococcus epidermidis,* 2357
  fungal, amphotericin B for, 505
  in injection drug users, 3472
  pathogenesis of, 1407
  posttraumatic, 1407t, 1408
  treatment of, 1410-1411
    vancomycin in, 420, 423
  visual outcome in, 1411
Endoscopic retrograde cholangiopancreatography
  for acute cholangitis, 957
  for HIV infection, 1576-1577

Endoscopy
  for *Candida* esophagitis, 1231, 1232f
  for *Helicobacter pylori* infections, 2562, 2562t
  for HIV infection, 1580
  for pseudomembranous colitis, 1256
  for Whipple's disease, 1309
Endosomes, bacterial pathogens in, 123
Endothelial cells, neutrophil adherence to, 96, 97
Endothelial injury, in severe sepsis, 911
Endothelial venules, high, 120, 120f
Endothrix infections, 3056
Endotoxemia, systemic inflammation from, 914
Enfuvirtide, 21, 1668-1669, 1668t
  dosage of, 684t-685t
  for perinatal HIV transmission prevention, 1626
  formulations of, 649t
  pediatric, 1646t
Enoxacin
  dosage of, 672t-673t
  formulations of, 648t
Entamoeba [spp.]
  in HIV infection, 1701
  metronidazole for, 389
Entamoeba coli, 3097
Entamoeba dispar, 3097-3098
  characteristics of, 3097-3098, 3101
  colonization with, 951
  diagnosis of, 3104
  dysentery from, 1266
  epidemiology of, 3099
  treatment of, 3105
  vaccine for, 3107
  vs. *Entamoeba histolytica,* 3097-3098, 3099,
    3101, 3104
Entamoeba dysentereae, 3097
Entamoeba gingivalis, 3097
Entamoeba hartmanni, 3097
Entamoeba histolytica, 3097-3107
  adherence of, 16, 17
  antigens of, 3097-3098
  characteristics of, 3097-3100
  classification of, 3097
  clinical manifestations of, 3012t, 3102-3104
    in extraintestinal disease, 3103-3104
    in intestinal disease, 3012t, 3102-3103
  cysts of, 3098, 3098f
  diagnosis of
    in extraintestinal disease, 3105
    in intestinal disease, 3104-3105
  differential diagnosis of, 3104-3105
  dysentery from, 1266
  epidemiology of, 3098-3100
  Gal/GalNAc adherence lectin of, 18-19, 18f
  gangrene from, 1182
  genome of, 3097, 3098
  hepatic abscess from, 951, 953
  historical perspective on, 3097
  immune response to, 3101-3102
  in travelers, 3099
  invasiveness of, 1222
  life cycle of, 3098
  pancreatic infections from, 959t, 960
  pathology and pathogenesis of, 3100-3102,
    3100f
  prevention of, 3107
  risk factors for, 3099-3100, 3099t
  treatment of, 344t, 571t, 582, 583, 3016t, 3105-
    3106, 3106t
  vs. *Entamoeba dispar,* 3097-3098, 3099, 3101,
    3104
Entamoeba invadens, 3098
  encystation in, 18
Entamoeba moshkovskii, 3098
Entamoeba polecki, 3097
  metronidazole for, 572t, 582

Entamoeba terrapinae, 3098
Entecavir, 540-541, 541f
  for chronic hepatitis B, 1447, 1448t, 1881
Enteral nutrition, 144
  in pancreatic infections prevention, 962
Enteric fever, 1273-1279
  differential diagnosis of, 1274t-1275t, 1276-
    1278
  epidemiology of, 1274t, 1276
  etiology of, 1273, 1274t
  from *Salmonella,* 2644-2646
  history of, 2636
  laboratory findings in, 1273, 1274t, 1275-1276
  pathogenesis of, 1273
  physical findings in, 1273, 1276t
  symptoms of, 1273, 1274t, 1276t
  treatment of, 1278-1279
    with quinolones, 461
  vs. enteric fever–like syndromes, 1276-1277
  vs. malaria, 3132
  vs. systemic infections, 1277-1278
Enteric flora. *See* Microbial flora, of
  gastrointestinal tract.
Enteritis. *See also* Gastrointestinal tract
  infections.
  chronic inflammatory, 1269-1270
  from *Campylobacter,* 405, 2553, 2554f
  from *Campylobacter jejuni,* 1265-1266, 2552
  from *Salmonella,* 1266-1267
  from *Yersinia enterocolitica,* 1267
  parasitic, 1270
Enteritis necroticans, from *Clostridium*
  perfringens type C, 2834-2835, 2835t
Enterobacter [spp.], 2579. *See also*
  Enterobacteriaceae.
  biliary tract infections from, 956
  endocarditis from, 991
  in peritoneal dialysis, 941
  beta-lactamase production by, 260
  mycotic aneurysm from, 1008
  osteomyelitis from, 1324
  percutaneous intravascular device infections
    from, 3356
  peritonitis from, 938, 939
    secondary, 937
  pneumonia from, 836
  prostatitis from, 894
  suppurative thrombophlebitis from,
    1004
  treatment of
    with aminoglycosides, 334t-337t
    with chloramphenicol, 367t
    with nitrofurantoin, 473
    with penicillins, 284t, 288t
  urinary tract infections from, 881, 882
Enterobacter aerogenes, 2579
  aminoglycosides for, 344t
  carbapenems for, 313t
  cephalosporins for, 298t
  meningitis from, 1114
  mupirocin for, 485t
  quinolones for, 455t
  rifamycin for, 374t
Enterobacter agglomerans, rifamycin
  for, 374t
Enterobacter cloacae, 2579
  carbapenems for, 313t
  cephalosporins for, 298t
  mupirocin for, 485t
  quinolones for, 455t
  rifamycin for, 374t
  tetracyclines for, 359t
  vancomycin for, 359t
Enterobacter faecium, meningitis from, 1114
Enterobacter sakazakii, 2579

Enterobacteriaceae, 2567-2581, 2567t. *See also specific genus.*
  adhesins of, 2571
  aminoglycosides for
    combination therapy with, 336t, 337t
    susceptibility of, 332-333, 332t
  appendicitis from, 969
  brain abscess from, 1158t
  capsules of, 2572
  diverticulitis from, 972
  endocarditis from, 990-991
    treatment of, 999-1000
  epidemiology of, 2567-2568
  fimbriae of, 2569-2570, 2570f, 2571
  flagellae of, 2569, 2570f
  inner membrane of, 2568, 2568f
  iron acquisition by, 2572
  keratitis from, 1397-1400
  laboratory identification of, 220
  lipopolysaccharide of, 2569, 2572
  outer membrane of, 2568f, 2569
  peptidoglycan cell wall of, 2568f, 2569
  periplasmic space of, 2568f, 2569
  pili of, 2571
  plasmids of, 2572-2573
  pneumonia from, nosocomial, 3367t
  secretion systems of, 2571-2572
  serine protease autotransporters of, 2571
  structure of, 2568-2570, 2568f
  surface polysaccharides of, 2569
  toxins of, 2571-2572
  typhlitis from, 973
  urinary tract infections from, female, 880
  virulence factors of, 2570-2573
Enterobacterial common antigen, 2569
Enterobactin, 2572
Enterobius vermicularis, 592, 3261t, 3266
  treatment of, 572t, 592
Enterococcus [spp.], 2411-2417
  aminoglycoside-resistant, 332
  antimicrobial susceptibility of, 2414-2415, 2414t
  bacteremia from, 2412-2413
  beta-lactamase production by, 256
  cardiovascular device infections from, 1023
  diverticulitis from, 972
  drug-resistant, 263t, 2414-2415, 2414t
    contact precautions and, 3329
    treatment of, 1028, 1028t, 1029t
  endocarditis from, 989, 2412-2413
    prosthetic valve, treatment of, 1027-1028, 1027t, 1028t
    treatment of, 248, 425, 996-998, 2416-2417, 2416t
  epidemiology of, 2412
  intra-abdominal infections from, 2413
    peritoneal, 337
  laboratory identification of, 217, 217t, 218
  liver abscess from, 952
  meningitis from, 1088, 2413
  microbiology of, 2411, 2411t
  mycotic aneurysm from, 1008
  neonatal sepsis from, 2413-2414
  osteomyelitis from, 1324
  pancreatic infections from, 961
  pathogenicity of, 2411-2412
  pelvic infections from, 2413
  penicillin-resistant, 996-998
  quinupristin-dalfopristin–resistant, 426
  respiratory tract infections from, 2413
  secondary peritonitis from, 936, 937
  suppurative thrombophlebitis from, 1004
  susceptibility testing for, 224
  tissue infections from, 2413
  tolerance in, 2414

Enterococcus [spp.] *(Continued)*
  treatment of, 2415-2417, 2416t
    for drug-resistant strains, 1028, 1028t, 1029t
    with aminoglycoside combination therapy, 336t
    with chloramphenicol, 367t
    with clindamycin, 409t
    with combination antimicrobial therapy, 248
    with daptomycin, 428
    with macrolides, 397t
    with rifamycin, 381
  typhlitis from, 973
  urinary tract infections from, 2412
    catheter-related, 3372
  vancomycin-resistant, 185, 264, 264t, 418-419, 2335, 2415, 2417
    contact precautions for, 3329
    disinfection/sterilization and, 3341-3342
    in pseudomembranous colitis, 1252
    linezolid for, 438
    metronidazole for, 392-393
  wound infections from, 2413
Enterococcus faecalis
  aminoglycosides for, 344t
    in combination therapy, 337t
  antimicrobial susceptibility of, 2414, 2414t
  carbapenems for, 313t
  endocarditis from, 979
  laboratory identification of, 218
  linezolid for, 437, 437t
  mupirocin for, 485t
  nitrofurantoin for, 473
  penicillin-resistant, treatment of, 996
  penicillins for, 284t, 288t
  quinolones for, 456t
  quinupristin-dalfopristin–resistant, 425, 426
  rifamycin for, 374t
  sulfonamides for, 441t
  telithromycin for, 407
  tetracyclines for, 359t
  trimethoprim for, 444t
  vancomycin for, 359t
  vancomycin-resistant, 185
Enterococcus faecium
  antimicrobial susceptibility of, 2414, 2414t
  beta-lactamase–producing, 2415, 2417
  treatment of
    with aminoglycoside combination therapy, 337t
    with linezolid, 437, 437t
    with mupirocin, 485t
    with nitrofurantoin, 473
    with quinolones, 456t
    with quinupristin-dalfopristin, 425, 426
    with telithromycin, 407
    with tetracyclines, 359t
    with vancomycin, 359t, 2417
  vancomycin-resistant, 185
    chloramphenicol for, 370
    quinupristin-dalfopristin for, 427
Enterococcus raffinosus, penicillin-resistant, 996
Enterocolitis. *See also* Colitis.
  causes of, 1264t
  eosinophilic, treatment of, 571t
  from cytomegalovirus, 1580
  from *Yersinia enterocolitica,* 2699
  in HIV infection, 1579-1580, 1580t
  neutropenic, 973, 3457
    chemotherapy-induced, 3438, 3457
    etiology of, 3421t
    from *Clostridium* spp., 2834, 2835t, 2836
    in stem cell transplant, 3421t
Enterocytozoon [spp.], 3237, 3238t, 3243. *See also* Microsporidia.
  clinical manifestations of, 3238t, 3243-3244, 3245

Enterocytozoon [spp.] *(Continued)*
  life cycle of, 3243
  pathogenicity of, 3242-3243
Enterocytozoon bieneusi, 568, 579t
  AIDS cholangiopathy from, 957
Enterotoxins, 1219-1220, 1220t. *See also* Toxin(s).
  actions of, 28-29
  of *Bacteroides fragilis,* 29
  of *Staphylococcus aureus,* 29, 2330
  of *Vibrio,* 29, 1220, 2537
Enterovirus(es), 2133-2138. *See also specific types.*
  acute hemorrhagic conjunctivitis from, 1389, 2136, 2137, 2155-2156, 2156f
  arthritis from, 2156-2157
  bronchiolitis from, 813t
  characteristics of, 2133
  classification of, 2133, 2134t
  communicability period for, 2137
  conjunctivitis from, 1389
  croup from, 761
  culture of, 2137-2138
  diabetes mellitus and, 2157
  encephalitis from, 2149
    in immunocompromised host, 2154-2155
  epidemic infantile diarrhea from, 1237
  epidemic pleurodynia from, 2151-2152
  epidemic/pandemic outbreaks of, 2136
  epidemiology of, 2136-2137, 2136t
  exanthems from, 2149-2150
  gastroenteritis from, 1239
  genome of, 2134
  genotyping of, 2136-2137
  hand-foot-mouth disease from, 2150, 2157
  hepatitis from, 2156
    in neonate, 2154
  herpangina from, 2151
  host range of, 2133, 2134t
  immune response to, 2135-2136
  in bone marrow transplant recipients, 2155
  in immunocompromised host, 2154-2155
  in neonates, 2153-2154
  in pregnancy, 2137, 2153
  incidence of, 2136t, 2137
  incubation period for, 2137
  laboratory diagnosis of, 235, 2137-2138
    specimen collection and transport for, 232, 233t
  meningitis from, 1084-1085, 1098-1099, 1101, 2137, 2148-2149
    in immunocompromised host, 2154-2155
  minor/major viremia in, 2135
  molecular biology of, 2134-2135
  mutation of, 2135
  myocarditis from, 1052, 1053t, 1054-1055, 2152-2153
  myositis from, 2151-2152
  newly discovered, 2157
  orchitis from, 2156
  pancreatitis from, 2156
  paralysis from, 2149, 2156, 2157
  pathogenesis of, 2135
  pericarditis from, 1058, 2152-2153
    in neonate, 2154
  pneumonia from, in neonates, 2154
  prevention of, 2138
  proteins of, 2134
  receptors for, 2134, 2134t
  replication of, 2135
  respiratory infections from, 2150-2151
  Reye's syndrome and, 2149
  rhinoviruses and, 2185
  shedding of, 2135, 2137
  transmission of, 2137
  treatment of, 2138

Enterovirus(es) *(Continued)*
  tropism of, in neonate, 2153
  types 68-71, 2157
Enterovirus 68, 2157
Enterovirus 69, 2157
Enterovirus 70, 2157
Enterovirus 71, 2157
Entomophthorales, 2974, 2974t
Entomophthoramycosis, 2974, 2980-2981, 2981f
Entry inhibitors, 20-21, 20t, 1668-1669, 1668t
Env, 1708
Environmental hygiene, nosocomial infections
    and, 3324
Enzyme(s)
  as toxins, 24
  drug-metabolizing, allosteric activation of, 273
Enzyme-linked immunosorbent assay, 57, 58f,
    214-215, 214t, 242
  for *Aspergillus,* 2967
  for *Bartonella,* 2743
  for *Borrelia burgdorferi,* 2804, 2804f
  for coccidioidomycosis, 3047
  for cytomegalovirus, 237
  for endemic treponematoses, 2787
  for Epstein-Barr virus, 237
  for hepatitis virus, 237
  for HIV infection, 1506-1507, 1508t, 1511-
    1513, 1511f, 1512t, 1519
  for human herpesvirus 6, 237
  for pediatric HIV infection, 1644
  for respiratory viruses, 234
  for rotavirus, 235
  for *Yersina pestis,* 2696
Enzymopathy, lymphocyte, 152
Eosinophil(s), 109-111, 110f
  circulating, 110
  development of, 110
  granules in, 110, 110f
Eosinophilia
  from quinolones, 467
  in endocardial lesions, 110
  in helminthic infections, 110, 3258-3259, 3293
  in travelers, 3652, 3654
  pulmonary, 835
  tropical pulmonary, 3274-3275, 3274f
    diethylcarbamazine for, 572t
Eosinophilia-myalgia syndrome, 1202
Eosinophilic cellulitis, 1180
Eosinophilic gastroenteritis, 3294t, 3297
Eosinophilic meningitis, 3294t, 3296
Eperezolid, 436, 436f, 438
Eperythrozoon spp., classification of, 2284
Ephemeroviurses, 2047t
Epidemic(s). *See also specific infections.*
  host-parasite relationship in, 4
Epidemic keratoconjunctivitis, 754, 1398, 1402,
    1404, 1435, 1807
  from adenoviruses, 1838
Epidemic pleurodynia, 1201, 2151-2152
Epidemic typhus, 2285t, 2286, 2287t, 2303-2305,
    2308
Epidemiology, 161-171
  agent in, 167-168
  antigenicity in, 168
  biologic gradient in, 167
  case-fatality rate, 167
  clinical trials in, 166
  community intervention trials in, 166
  definition of, 161
  disease prevention in, 169-171
    primary, 170-171
    risk assessment in, 169-170
    secondary, 171
    strategies for, 169
    tertiary, 171

Epidemiology *(Continued)*
  epidemiologic studies in, 161-164
    biology in, 162-163
    disease in, 161-162
    enrollment criteria for, 162
    goals of, 161
    incidence in, 162
    infections in, 161-162
    methods in, 163
    population in, 161, 162
    prevalence in, 162
    risk in, 162-163, 162f
    statistics in, 162-163, 162f
    types of, 163-164, 163t
  experimental studies in, 166
  gradient of infections in, 167
  host in, 168, 168t
  host-agent relationship in, 166-167
  immunogenicity in, 168
  infectivity in, 167
  observational studies in, 164-166
    case series, 164-165
    case-control, 165
    cohort, 165
    cross-sectional surveys in, 165
    disease surveillance, 164
    outbreak investigations in, 165-166
  pathogenicity in, 167
  secondary attack rate in, 167
  transmission routes in, 168-169
  virulence in, 167
Epidermal cysts, infected, 1185
Epidermodysplasia verruciformis, 1842, 1845,
    1850. *See also* Human papillomavirus(es).
Epidermophyton [spp.], 3051-3052. *See also*
    Dermatophyte(s).
Epidermophyton floccosum, 3052t, 3053, 3053t
  tinea cruris from, 3054-3055
  tinea pedis from, 3054
Epididymitis, 1384-1386
  from *Blastomyces dermatitidis,* 3029t, 3033, 3033f
  from *Candida,* 2951
  from *Chlamydia trachomatis,* 1352, 1384-
    1385, 2246, 2247t
    treatment of, 2247t, 2250
  from *Mycobacterium tuberculosis,* 1384
  from *Neisseria gonorrhoeae,* 1352, 1384, 1385,
    2519-2520, 2526
  in HIV infection, 1385-1386
  nonspecific bacterial, 1384
  sexually transmitted, 1384-1385
Epididymo-orchitis. *See also* Orchitis.
  from mumps virus, 2005
Epidural abscess, 1165-1168, 1166f, 1167f, 1326-
    1327, 1326f
  clinical features of, 1079-1080
  spinal, 1165-1168
    in injection drug users, 3471-3472
Epiglottitis, 784-786
  from *Haemophilus influenzae,* 784-786, 2664
  fulminant meningococcal, 2506
  vs. croup, 763, 785
  vs. diphtheria, 785
Epinephrine, nebulized
  for bronchiolitis, 817
  for croup, 763-764, 2001
Episiotomy infections, 1375, 1377t
Epithelial cells, respiratory, 820
Epitope, 53-54, 55
Epitrochlear lymphadenitis, 1205-1206
Epstein-Barr virus, 1801-1815
  adherence of, 17
  antibodies to, 1811-1812, 1811t
  appendicitis from, 969
  Burkitt's lymphoma from, 1808-1809, 1808t

Epstein-Barr virus *(Continued)*
  central nervous system lymphoma from, 1808t,
    1813
  characteristics of, 1802-1803, 1802t
  chronic fatigue syndrome from, 1270-1274,
    1807-1808
  chronic/persistent, 1807-1808
  clevudine for, 540
  clinical manifestations of, 1758, 1758t, 1760t,
    1805-1810, 1805t, 1806f, 1806t
  collection of, 233t
  complement receptor usage by, 78
  conjunctivitis from, 1390
  culture of, 1812
  diagnosis of, 1761
  differential diagnosis of, 1812-1813
  epidemiology of, 1759, 1759t, 1803-1804
  hepatitis from, 1435, 1812
  histopathology of, 1805
  historical perspective on, 1801-1802
  Hodgkin's disease from, 1808t, 1809-1810,
    1809f
  host range of, 1802
  human herpesvirus 8 and, 2130
  hypergammaglobulinemia in, 65
  immune response in, 1758, 1804-1805
  in HIV infection, 1697
  in transplant recipients, 3509-3510
  incidence of, 1803-1804
  infectious mononucleosis from, 1789, 1801-
    1815
  interleukin-10 in, 122
  isolation of, 1802
  laboratory diagnosis of, 236, 1810-1812, 1810t,
    1811t
  latency of, 1802-1803, 1802t, 1803t
  lymphocytosis from, 1810-1811, 1810t, 1811t
  lymphoma from, 1605, 1808-1810, 1808t, 1809f
    primary central nervous system, 1589, 1607
  lymphoproliferative disease from, 66, 1808-
    1810, 1808t, 1809f
    in transplant recipients, 3510
    X-linked, 1435, 1807, 1814-1815
  lytic infections from, 1803
  meningitis from, 1085
  myocarditis from, 1052-1053, 1053t
  nasopharyngeal cancer from, 1808t, 1810,
    1810f, 1813, 1813f, 1814f
  neutropenia from, 1811
  oncogenicity of, 1759
  oral hairy leukoplakia from, 1808
  pancreatic infections from, 959t, 960
  pathogenesis of, 1802-1803, 1804-1805
  pharyngitis from, 755
  prevention of, 1760t, 1761
  receptor for, 1732t
  replication of, 1802
  shedding of, 1802, 1802t, 1803t
  strains of, 1803
  structure of, 1756-1757, 1756t, 1802
  thrombocytopenia from, 1811
  transfusion-related, 1789, 3387
  transmission of, 1759-1761, 1759t, 1789, 1802,
    1804, 3387
    nosocomial, 3416
  treatment of, 1760t, 1761
  vaccine for, 1815
Equine rabies immune globulin, 2053
Erm
  in quinupristin-dalfopristin resistance, 426
  in *Staphylococcus aureus* resistance, 2335
Erosio interdigitalis blastomycetica, 2942, 2943f
Ertapenem
  antibacterial activity of, 313
  chemistry of, 312, 312f

Ertapenem *(Continued)*
  clinical uses of, 314
  dosage of, 658t-659t
  drug interactions with, 690t
  for acute pyelonephritis, 889
  for peritonitis, 939
  for pneumonia, 837-839, 838t
  formulations of, 648t
  pharmacology of, 313-314
Erwinia spp., 2581
Erysipelas, 1177-1178, 1177f
  from *Staphylococcus,* 2341
  from *Streptococcus pyogenes* (group A), 2370,
    2371f
Erysipeloid, 1179
Erysipeloid of Rosenbach, 2370, 2497, 2497f
Erysipelothrix [spp.], penicillins for, 288t
Erysipelothrix rhusiopathiae, 2496-2498
  cellulitis from, 1179
  clinical manifestations of, 2497-2498, 2497f
  endocarditis from, 992
  epidemiology of, 2497
  laboratory identification of, 219, 219t
  microbiology of, 2496-2497
  pathogenesis of, 2497
  prevention of, 2498
  treatment of, 2498
    with linezolid, 437, 437t
    with mupirocin, 485t
    with quinupristin-dalfopristin, 425
Erythema, 731-732. *See also* Rash.
  blanching/nonblanching, 731-732
  diffuse, 733
    in sepsis, 918
Erythema induratum, 733
Erythema infectiosum, 732, 1893-1894, 1893f.
    See also Parvovirus B19.
  pediatric, 234-235
Erythema marginatum, 733
  in rheumatic fever, 2383, 2383f
Erythema migrans, 734
  in Lyme disease, 734, 738, 2798, 2801-2802,
    2801f, 2802t, 3314f
Erythema multiforme, 732, 733
  from *Coccidioides immitis,* 3043
  from herpes simplex virus, 732, 1765-1766,
    1766f, 1774t
    acyclovir for, 519
  from *Mycoplasma pneumoniae,* 2274, 2274f
Erythema nodosum, 733, 733t
  from *Coccidioides immitis,* 3043
  from *Yersinia enterocolitica,* 2699
Erythema nodosum leprosum, 2892, 2893f
  thalidomide for, 499, 560
  treatment of, 2895
Erythrasma, 1182-1184
  topical antibacterial therapy for, 482-483
Erythrocyte band 3, in malaria susceptibility, 44t
Erythrocyte transfusion
  for sepsis, 920
  in chronic granulomatous disease, 109
Erythroderma, in sepsis, 918
Erythromycin, 396-402, 483, 484t
  adverse reactions from, 400
  antimicrobial activity of, 396-399, 397t
  base of, 396, 396f
  chemistry of, 396
  dosage of, 664t-665t
  drug interactions with, 400, 400t, 690t-691t
  for acne vulgaris, 483
  for actinomycosis, 2931, 2931t
  for bacillary angiomatosis, 1185
  for *Bartonella,* 1691t, 2744
  for *Bordetella pertussis,* 2706
  for *Calymmatobacterium granulomatis,* 2750

Erythromycin *(Continued)*
  for carbuncles, 1175
  for cellulitis, 1180
  for chancroid, 1344
  for *Chlamydia trachomatis,* 2525
  for chlamydial infections, in neonates, 2247t,
    2250-2251
  for chlamydial pneumonia, 2263
  for conjunctivitis, in neonate, 1392, 2247t,
    2250
  for *Corynebacterium diphtheriae,* 2463-2464
  for cutaneous diphtheria, 1181
  for *Enterococcus,* 2416
  for erysipelas, 1178
  for erythrasma, 1182-1184
  for experimental endocarditis, 1048
  for *Haemophilus ducreyi,* 2667
  for impetigo, 1173
  for *Legionella,* 2719t, 2727
  for Lyme disease, 2806, 2806t
  for lymphadenitis, 1211
  for *Mycoplasma pneumoniae,* 2278
  for nocardiosis, 2920t
  for pneumonia, 837-839, 837t, 838t
    for neonate, 2247t, 2250-2251
  for Q fever pneumonia, 2299
  for relapsing fever, 2797
  for streptococcal pharyngitis, 2367t, 2368
  for streptococcal pyoderma, 2370
  for streptococcus group G, 2445
  for trachoma, 1391
  for urethritis, 1207
  for urogenital chlamydial infections, in
    pregnancy, 2250
  formulations of, 648t
  in vitro susceptibilities to, 397, 397t
  inactivation of, 398
  mechanism of action of, 396
  pharmacology of, 399-400, 399t
  prophylactic, perioperative, 3543t
  resistance to, 397-398
    by *Streptococcus agalactiae* (group B), 2429
    pneumococcal, 837, 837t
  serum levels of, 399, 399t
  uses of, 400, 401t, 402
Erythromycin estolate, formulations of, 648t
Erythromycin ethyl succinate
  dosage of, 664t-665t
  formulations of, 648t
Erythromycin etolate, dosage of, 664t-665t
Erythromycin gluceptate
  dosage of, 664t-665t
  formulations of, 648t
Erythromycin lactobionate
  dosage of, 664t-665t
  formulations of, 648t
Erythromycin stearate, dosage of, 664t-665t
Erythromycin stearate, formulations of, 648t
Erythromycin-benzoyl peroxide, 484, 484t
Erythroplasia of Queyrat, 1341, 1846
Eschar
  in ehrlichioses, 2287t
  in rickettsioses, 2287t
Escherichia albertii, 2580
Escherichia blattae, 2578
Escherichia coli, 2573-2578
  adherence by, 14f
  adherence of, 1218, 1219t
  antisera identification of, 221
  appendicitis from, 969
  arthritis from, 1312, 1312t
  bacillary dysentery from, 2655, 2655f
  biliary tract infections from, 956
  classification of, 1236-1237, 1237t
  clonal analysis of, 5

Escherichia coli (Continued)
  culture of, 1224
  cystitis from, 474
  diarrheogenic, 178
    adherence capacity of, 1221-1222
    pathogenesis of, 1218, 1219t
  diffusely adherent, 1218, 1219t, 1221, 2573t
  disinfection/sterilization and, 3340
  endocarditis from, 991
  enteroaggregative, 1218, 1219t, 1220, 2573t,
    2577-2578
    adherence of, 1221
    diarrhea from, 1215
      chronic, 1269
    toxin of, 1220
    tropical sprue from, 1302
  enterohemorrhagic, 1218, 1219t, 1220, 1265,
    2573t, 2576-2577, 2577f
    infantile epidemic diarrhea from, 1237,
      1237t
    laboratory detection of, 212
    O26, 1221
    O157, 1265
    O157:H7, 1221, 1265
    phage-encoded, 6t
    serotypes of, 1237, 1237t, 1265
    spread of, 1217
    toxin of, 1220
  enteroinvasive, 1218, 1219t, 1220, 1265, 1265t,
    2573t, 2578
    plasmids of, 6t, 2572
    toxin of, 1220
  enteropathogenic, 1218, 1219t, 2573t, 2575-
    2576, 2575f, 2576f
    adherence of, 1221
    attaching and effacing effect of, 2575, 2575f,
      2576f
    chronic diarrhea from, 1269
    epidemic infantile diarrhea from, 1236-1237,
      1237t
    pedestal (pseudopod) formation by, 9, 9f
    serotypes of, 1237, 1237t
    toxin of, 1220
  enterotoxigenic, 1218, 1219-1220, 1219t,
    2573t, 2574-2575
    age effects on, 1216
    foodborne disease from, 1288
    inflammatory diarrhea from, 1240
    plasmid-encoded, 6t
    species specificity of, 1216
    toxins of, 1219-1220
      vaccine for, 1226
    traveler's diarrhea from, 1242, 1242t, 1243t
    weanling diarrhea from, 1237-1238
  extended-spectrum beta-lactamase–producing
    strains of, in susceptibility testing, 224
  extraintestinal, 6t, 2573-2574
  heat-labile enterotoxin of, 29, 1220, 1237, 1240
  heat-stable enterotoxin of, 29, 1220, 1240
  hemolysins of, 2571
  in peritoneal dialysis, 941
  intra-amniotic infection syndrome from, 1372-
    1373
  invasiveness of, 1222
  beta-lactamase production by, 260
  meningitis from, 1087
  mycotic aneurysm from, 1008
  neonatal bacteremia from, 2574
  nitrofurantoin-resistant, 473
  O78, epidemic infantile diarrhea from,
    1237
  O157, 1224
  O157:H7, 177-178, 1220, 2577
    bacillary dysentery from, 2655
    epidemiologic studies of, 161

Escherichia coli (Continued)
foodborne disease from, 1288, 1289, 1291, 1294-1295, 1294t
O159, epidemic infantile diarrhea from, 1237
osteomyelitis from, hyperbaric oxygen for, 566
P fimbriae of, 19-20, 19f
adherence of, cranberry juice for, 20t, 21
adhesin-based therapies for, 20t, 21
pancreatic infections from, 961, 962
peritonitis from, 929
secondary, 936, 937
treatment of, 938, 939
pneumonia from, 836
prostatitis from, 893, 894
pyogenic liver abscess from, 952
quinolone-resistant, 453, 454, 465-466
regulation of, 7t
secretion system of, 2571-2572
Shiga toxin–producing, 2573t, 2576-2577, 2577f
foodborne disease from, 1289
splenic abscess from, 967, 967t
suppurative thrombophlebitis from, 1004
toxins of, 26, 29
transient bacteremia from, 978
treatment of
with aminoglycosides, 334t-335t, 337t
with carbapenems, 313t
with cephalosporins, 298t
with chloramphenicol, 367t
with linezolid, 437, 437t
with mupirocin, 485t
with nitrofurantoin, 473
with penicillins, 284t, 288t
with quinolones, 455t
with rifamycin, 374t
with sulfonamides, 441t
with tetracyclines, 359t
with trimethoprim, 444t
with trimethoprim-sulfamethoxazole, 444
with vancomycin, 359t
urinary tract infections from, catheter-related, 3372
uropathogenic, 876-878, 877t, 2356, 2573, 2574
vaginal secretion effects on, 880
Escherichia coli K1 antigen, in meningococcus immunity, 2501
Escherichia fergusonii, 2578
Escherichia vulneris, 2578
Esophageal dilation, in American trypanosomiasis, 3158, 3160, 3161f, 3163
Esophagitis, 1231-1234
clinical manifestations of, 1231
etiology of, 1231t
from Candida, 1231-1232, 1232f, 1550, 2941-2942, 2941f, 2951
chronic, 2944
from cytomegalovirus, 1232, 1791
from Helicobacter pylori, 2562
from herpes simplex virus, 1232-1233, 1233f, 1770
in HIV infection, 1232-1233, 1232f, 1233f, 1234t, 1550, 1575-1576
in immunocompromised host, 3437, 3438
treatment of, 1233-1234, 1233t
Esophagography, of Candida esophagitis, 1232, 1232f
Esophagus
aphthous ulceration of, 1233, 1233t
perforation of, mediastinitis from, 1070, 1072-1074
Espundia, 3145t, 3152, 3153

Essential mixed cryoglobulinemia, hepatitis C–related, 1453, 1962
Estrogen deficiency vaginitis, 1369
Estrogen, immune effects of, 40
Estrogen replacement therapy, urinary tract infections incidence with, 892
Eta, 2329
Etb, 2329
Ethambutol
dosage of, 676t-677t
for brain abscess, 1159t
for Mycobacterium avium complex, 2903-2906, 2904t
for nontuberculous mycobacterial infections, 496-497, 2910, 2911, 2913t
for tuberculosis, 492-493, 2867, 2868, 2869
in children, 2872
in HIV infection, 1687t, 1699, 2870, 2871t
isoniazid with, 2869
formulations of, 649t
Ethanol, tetracycline with, 364t
Ethionamide
dosage of, 676t-677t
drug interactions with, 691t
for leprosy, 499
for Mycobacterium tuberculosis, 495-496
formulations of, 649t
Ethmoid sinus
anatomy and physiology of, 773, 773t
infections of. See Sinusitis.
Ethyl alcohol, disinfection with, 3333-3334
Ethylene oxide, sterilization with, 3337t, 3339
Ethylenediaminetetraacetic acid, in viral collection, 232
Ethylhydrocupreine hydrochloride, 216t
Eubacterium [spp.], 2850, 2851
actinomycosis from, 2924
in oral cavity, 787, 787t
metronidazole for, 389t
Eubacterium lentum
chloramphenicol for, 367t
secondary peritonitis from, 937
Euglycemia, 909
Eugonic fermenter-4, 2751t, 2756
Eumycetoma, 2916, 2917, 2991-2995
from dark-walled fungi, 3070t
Europe, HIV infection in, 1465-1466, 1466f
European bat lyssaviruses, 2047t
European tick-borne encephalitis virus, 1934
Everglades virus, 1913-1919, 1914t. See also Alphaviruses.
Evernimicin, dosage of, 668t-669t
Evolutionary aspects, of infectious disease susceptibility, 48-49
Ewingella americana, 2580-2581
Exanthem(s), 731. See also Rash.
Boston, 2150
from enteroviruses, 2149-2150
herpetiform, 2150
in HIV infection, 1556
morbilliform, 2150
petechial, 2150
purpuric, 2150
reseoliform, 2150
rubelliform, 2150
specimen collection in, 233t
Exanthem subitum
from human herpesvirus 6, 739, 1822, 1822f, 1824
from human herpesvirus 7, 1824
laboratory studies for, 237
Exercise, for weight loss, 145
Exo Y toxin, 27
Exocytosis, 101
Exoenzymes, of Pseudomonas aeruginosa, 2596

Exophiala [spp.], chromoblastomycosis from, 2988-2991
Exophiala dermatitidis, in chronic granulomatous disease, 155
Exophiala (Wangiella) jeanselmei, 3074, 3076t
Exophiala spinifera, 3070, 3071t, 3072
Exophiala wernickii, tinea nigra from, 3061
Exotoxins
of Pseudomonas aeruginosa, 2595-2596
pyogenic, 29-30
streptococcal, 29
Experimental studies, 166
Exserohilum spp., sinusitis from, 3070-3071, 3076t
Eyach virus, 1900, 1901
Eye. See also under Ocular.
red, differential diagnosis of, 1393-1394
Eyelid infections, 1419-1420, 1420f

F

F(ab′)₂, 53, 54f
Fab, 53, 54f
Facial infections. See also Orofacial infections.
from dermatophytes, 3056, 3056f
from diphtheria, 2461, 2461f
from Streptococcus, 2370, 2370f
Facklamia spp., laboratory identification of, 217t, 218
Factitious fever, 727
Factor B, 75
in host vs. microbial cell surface discrimination, 74
Factor D, 75
deficiency of, 80t
Factor H, 70t, 74t, 75
deficiency of, 80t, 82, 83, 151t
in host vs. microbial cell surface discrimination, 74
Factor H, MCP, and vascular disease, 82-83
Factor I, 70t, 74t, 75
deficiency of, 80t, 83, 151t
Factor P, deficiency of, 80t
Facultative organisms, 2811
Falciform ligament, 927-928
Falcon assay, for schistosomiasis, 3280
Fallopian tubes, 927. See also Salpingitis.
Neisseria gonorrhoeae in, 2514, 2515f
Famciclovir, 515t, 525-526
dosage of, 680t-681t
for hepatitis B, 1881, 1882
for herpes genitalis, 1344
for herpes simplex keratitis, 1402t
for herpes simplex virus, 1686t, 1773t-1774t, 1774
for herpes zoster ophthalmicus, 1403t
for herpesviruses, 1760t, 1761, 1773t-1774t, 1774
for varicella-zoster virus, 1686t
formulations of, 649t
in renal insufficiency, 526t
uses of, 526
Familial Creutzfeldt-Jakob disease, 2222, 2222t
Far Eastern encephalitis, 1934, 1941. See also Tick-borne encephalitis.
Fascial spaces
anatomy of, 790, 790f
infections of, 754, 756
deep, 791-793, 792f, 793f. See also Odontogenic infections.
treatment of, 797-798, 797t
Fasciitis
at episiotomy site, 1375, 1377t
necrotizing. See Necrotizing fasciitis.

Fasciola hepatica, 3277t, 3279f, 3281-3282, 3281f
  biliary tract infections from, 956
  syndrome of abdominal pain, diarrhea, and
      eosinophilia from, 1281t, 1282-1283
  treatment of, 572t
Fasciolopsis buski, 3277t, 3282-3283
  syndrome of abdominal pain, diarrhea, and
      eosinophilia from, 1281t, 1283
  treatment of, 572t
FAST-ELISA, for schistosomiasis, 3280
Fat, dietary, in tropical sprue, 1303
Fatal familial insomnia, 2222t, 2229, 2230
Fatigue
  chronic, 1270-1274, 1807-1808
    from human herpesvirus 6 infections, 1823
    vs. Lyme disease, 2805-2806
  HIV-related, hyperbaric oxygen for, 566
Fatty acids, 143-144
  polyunsaturated, 143
Favus, 3051, 3053, 3056
Fc, 53, 54f
Fc receptors, 56, 56t, 61t
FcγR, in opsonization, 56
FcγRIIa receptor, in meningococcal disease, 85
FcγRIIB, 61
¹⁸F-FDG-PET, for brain abscess, 1158-1159
Febrile neutropenia, 719t, 721-722, 722t, 725,
    3427-3428. *See also* Fever;
    Immunocompromised host; Neutropenia.
  bacteremic, 3432-3434
  catheter-related, 3433-3434, 3434f, 3455-3457
  chemoprophylaxis for
    against *Pneumocystis jirovecii,* 3447, 3447t
    antibacterial, 3442-3445, 3443f-3445f
    antifungal, 3445-3447, 3447t-3446t
    antiviral, 3448
  clinical evaluation in, 3448, 3448t
  etiology of, 3427f
  from *Pseudomonas aeruginosa,* 2606-2607
  immunoprophylaxis for, 3457-3458
  immunotherapy for, 3458
  in cancer, 3432-3439, 3448-3458. *See also*
      Cancer.
    bone marrow colony-stimulating factors for,
        3457-3458
    classification of, 3448
    epidemiology of, 3448-3449
    etiology of, 3449, 3449f
    fungemic, 3432-3434
    granulocyte transfusion for, 3458
    immune globulin for, 3458
    prevention of, 3442-3448, 3457-3458
    treatment of, 3439, 3449-3558
    with abdominal symptoms, 3457
    with pulmonary infiltrates, 3457
  in catheter-related infections, 3455-3457
  in transplant recipients, 3483-3484
  initial evaluation in, 3448, 3448t
  mortality trends in, 3448
  natural history of, 3448-3449, 3450t
  risk assessment for, 3449, 3450t
  standard workup for, 3432
  transfusion-related, 3433
  treatment of, 3449-3455
    empirical antibiotic, 3450-3454, 3451t2
    empirical antifungal, 3454-3455
    empirical anti–gram-positive, 3453–3454,
        3454f
    for catheter-related infections, 3455-3457
    for persistent infections, 3452-3455, 3454t
    in low-risk patients, 3452
    in non–low-risk patients, 3450-3452
    intravenous vs. oral therapy in, 3452, 3453t
    outpatient, 3452, 3453t
  vancomycin for, 423

Febrile neutrophilic dermatosis. *See* Sweet
    syndrome.
Febrile response, 703, 708-709. *See also* Fever.
  acute-phase response and, 709-710, 710t
  definition of, 703
  endogenous cryogens in, 710-711, 711f
  endogenous pyrogens in, 708-709, 711, f
    immune response and, 711-712
  events in, 709f
  evolutionary perspective on, 711-712, 712f
  exogenous pyrogens in, 708
Febrile seizures, 712-713
  prevention of, 714
Febrile urinary tract infections, catheter-related, 3373
Fecal testing, 1224
Fecal-oral transmission
  of hepatitis A virus, 3381
  of hepatitis E virus, 3382
Feet. *See* Foot.
Feline immunodeficiency virus, 2119
Feline leukemia virus, 2119
FemA, 2328, 2329f
Female condom, in HIV infection prevention,
    1494
Females. *See* Gender; Women.
FemB, 2328, 2329f
FemC, 2328, 2329f
Femoral artery catheterization, infections in, 1040
Fetal demise
  from *Chlamydia trachomatis,* 2249
  from hepatitis E virus, 2210
  from parvovirus B19, 1895, 1896
Fetal hydrops
  from parvovirus B19, 1895, 1896
  laboratory studies for, 234-235
Fetal membranes, premature rupture of,
    Chlamydia trachomatis and, 2249
Fever. *See also under* Febrile; Temperature.
  adaptive role of, 711-712, 712f
  ascending phase of, 709
  beneficial effects of, 711-712, 714
  detrimental effects of, 712-713
  evaluation of, themometry in, 703-707
  febrile response and, 703, 708-709, 709f. *See
      also* Febrile response
  historical perspective on, 703
  in cancer, 713-714, 719, 723, 723f
  in liver abscess, 953
  in neutropenia, 3427-3428, 3427f
  in pneumonia, 823
  in spinal cord injury, 3513
  in travelers, 3646-3652
  induction phase of, 709
  infantile, from human herpesvirus 6, 1822,
      1822f, 1822t
  of unknown origin, 718-727, 3427-3428
    biopsy in, 725
    classic, 718-721, 719t
    clinical definitions of, 719t
    clinical evaluation of, 722-725, 722t, 3439
    definition of, 718, 719t
    drug-induced, 727
    empiric therapy for, 3439
    etiology of, 718-719, 719t, 720t, 726-727
    factitious, 727
    fever patterns in, 722-724, 723f
    history in, 722
    imaging studies in, 724-725
    in children, 713, 720, 724
    in disseminated granulomatoses, 726
    in elderly, 719, 720, 3521-3522
    in endocarditis, 726
    in HIV infection, 719t, 721-722, 722t
      fever in, 719t, 721-722, 722t
    in lymphoma, 726

Fever *(Continued)*
    in polymyalgia rheumatica, 726-727
    in Still's disease, 726-727
    in temporal arteritis, 725, 726-727
    in thromboembolic disease, 726
    in transplant recipients, 3483-3484
    in travelers, 720-721, 3646-3648, 3647t
    laboratory findings in, 724
    laparotomy in, 725
    management of, 3439
    neutropenic, 719t, 721-722, 722t. *See also*
        Febrile neutropenia.
    nosocomial, 719t, 721
    physical findings in, 724, 724t
    postpartum, 1374-1375
    prognosis of, 725-726
    subtypes of, 719t
    treatment of, *725*
      risks and benefits of, 713-714
    upper limit of, 710
  patterns of, 722-724, 723f
  periodic
    in Marshall's syndrome, 1208
    with aphthous ulcers, pharyngitis and
        adenitis, 1208
  plateau phase of, 709
  postoperative, 719t, 721
  relapsing, 722, 723f
  seizures from, 712-713, 714
  terminology of, 703, 722
  treatment of, 712-715
    drugs in, 713
    indications for, 714-715
    physical measures in, 713, 714, 715
    rationale for, 712-713
    response to, diagnostic implications of, 713-
        714
  with rash, 729-742. *See also* Rash.
FhmB, 2328, 2329f
Fiber, dietary, diverticulitis and, 972
Fiberoptic bronchoscopy. *See* Bronchoscopy.
Fibrinolytics, for pleural effusion/empyema, 851
Fibromyalgia, vs. Lyme disease, 2805-2806
Fibronectin, 37
Fibronectin receptor, in phagocytosis, 99
Fibronectin-binding proteins, in *Staphylococcus
    aureus* endocarditis, 2343
Fibrosing cholestatic hepatitis, 1449, 1456
Fibrosis, periglomerular, 876
Fifth disease, 732, 1893-1894, 1893f. *See also*
    Parvovirus B19.
Filariasis
  bancroftian, 3270-3272, 3270f-3272f
  brugian, 3270-3272, 3270f-3272f
  diethylcarbamazine for, 572t
  in dirofilariasis, 3294t, 3297-3298
  in loiasis, 3272-3273, 3272f
  in *Mansonella* infections, 3274
  in onchocerciasis, 3273-3274
  in tropical pulmonary eosinophilia, 3274-3275,
      3274f
  lymphangitis in, 1208, 1212, 3271, 3271t
  ocular, 3272-3274, 3272f
  Wolbachia in, 2286, 3271, 3273
Filgrastim, for leishmaniasis, 1692t
Filariasis, specimen collection and transport in,
    205t
Filobasidiella [spp.], 2998
Filobasidiella bacillospora, 2998
Filobasidiella neoformans, 2998
Filoviruses, 739, 2057-2059, 2057f
  disinfection/sterilization and, 3342
  isolation precautions for, 3330t
Fim, 878
FimA, endocarditis from, 979

Fimbriae
  of Enterobacteriaceae, 2569-2570, 2570f, 2571
  P, of *Escherichia coli,* 19-20, 19f
Finger(s)
  herpetic whitlow of, 1769, 1769f, 1773t
  human bites of, 3554
  in endocarditis, 983-984
Fingernails. *See* Nails.
Fish
  capillariasis from, 3294t, 3298
  poisonous, 1289-1290, 1290t, 1292, 3255,
    3255f, 3256t
  skin infections from, 1184
Fish oil, immune effects of, 143-144
Fish tapeworm, 3286t, 3287. *See also* Tapeworms.
Fistulas
  bronchopleural, tuberculous, 2878
  pharyngocutaneous, postradiation, 800
Fite staining, for *Mycobacterium leprae,* 2891-
    2892, 2892f, 2893f
Fitz-Hugh–Curtis syndrome, 2521-2522
Flagellates
  antiparasitics for, 568t-569t
  of Enterobacteriaceae, 2569, 2570f
  treatment of, 582-583, 583f
Flash sterilization, 333
Flat warts, 1842, 1845, 1848. *See also* Human
    papillomavirus(es).
Flatworms
  cestode, 3285-3292
  trematode, 3276-3284
Flaviviruses, 1926-1945
  characteristics of, 1928-1929
  classification of, 1929
  clinical features of, 1938-1942
  epidemiology of, 1929-1935
  geographic distribution of, 1927-1928, 1927f
  historical perspective on, 1927-1928
  host range for, 1928-1929
  laboratory diagnosis of, 1942
  less common, 1944-1945, 1945t
  pathogenesis of, 1935-1938
  prevention of, 1943-1944
  public health burden of, 1926
  replication of, 1928
  structure of, 1928
  treatment of, 1943-1944
Flavobacterium spp., 2751t, 2759
  endocarditis from, 992
Flea-borne infection(s), 2286
  murine typhus as, 2306-2308
  plague as, 2697
Fleas, sand, 3310
Flesh flies, myiasis from, 3308-3310, 3308t
Flies, myiasis from, 3307-3310, 3308t
Flinder's Island spotted fever, 2285t, 2287t, 2292-
    2293
Flora. *See* Microbial flora.
Flow cytometry, 117, 118f
Flu. *See also* Influenza virus(es).
  intestinal, 1238-1239, 1239t
Flucloxacillin, 290, 290f
  dosage of, 650t-651t
  for *Staphylococcus aureus* endocarditis, 2344t
  for *Staphylococcus aureus* osteomyelitis, 2346
  formulations of, 646t
Fluconazole, 509
  dosage of, 678t-679t
  drug interactions with, 691t
  for blastomycosis, 3036-3037, 3036t
  for brain abscess, 1159t, 1160
  for cancer-related febrile neutropenia
    for prophylaxis, 3446, 3447t
    in empiric therapy, 3455
  for candidiasis, 1683t, 1687t, 1698, 2949-2951

Fluconazole *(Continued)*
  esophageal, 1234, 1575
    in stem cell transplant, 3495
    vulvovaginal, 1364
  for catheter-related infections, 3377
  for coccidioidomycosis, 1683t, 1688t, 3047-
    3048
  for cryptococcal meningitis, 3007, 3008
    for prophylaxis, 3009
  for *Cryptococcus neoformans,* 1584, 1682t,
    1683t, 1688t, 1698
  for dermatophytosis, 3050t, 3058-3059
  for endophthalmitis, 1411
  for eumycetoma, 2995
  for fungal arthritis, 1318
  for histoplasmosis, 1688t, 3023, 3024
  for meningitis, 1135, 1584
  for paracoccidioidomycosis, 3065
  for sporotrichosis, 2987
  for suppurative thrombophlebitis, 1005
  for urinary tract infections, 892
    catheter-related, 3377
  formulations of, 649t
  prophylactic, for transplant recipients, 3483
  structure of, 503f
Flucytosine, 506-507
  dosage of, 678t-679t
  for brain abscess, 1159t
  for cryptococcal meningitis, 3007, 3008
  for *Cryptococcus neoformans,* 1584, 1688t,
    1698
  for dialysis-related peritonitis, 942
  for meningitis, 1584, 3007, 3008
  formulations of, 649t
5-Flucytosine, for brain abscess, 1160
Fluid balance, gastrointestinal, 1222-1223,
    1222f
Fluid management
  in central nervous system infections, 1083
  in dengue/dengue hemorrhagic fever, 1943
  in peritonitis, 940
  in rotavirus infections, 1909
  in sepsis, 919-920
  in streptococcal toxic shock syndrome, 2374
  in urinary tract infections, 888
Fluids, collection and transport of, 206t
Flukes. *See* Trematodes.
Fluorescent treponemal antibody absorption,
    2778t, 2779, 2780
  for endemic treponematoses, 2787
Fluoride, for dental prophylaxis, 781-782, 796t
5-Fluorocytosine
  for fungal endocarditis, 1001
  for suppurative thrombophlebitis, 1005
  structure of, 503f
^{18}F-Fluorodeoxyglucose positron emission
    tomography, for brain abscess, 1158-1159
Fluoroquinolones. *See* Quinolones.
5-Fluorouracil, for genital warts, 1849
Flying squirrels, as typhus reservoir, 2304, 2305
Focal vulvitis, 1369-1370, 1370f
Folate
  deficiency of, in tropical sprue, 1303
  trimethoprim/sulfonamide effects on, 443,
    443f, 445
Folate antagonists, formulations of, 648t
Folinic acid
  for *Toxoplasma* encephalitis, 1587
  with pyrimethamine, for toxoplasmosis,
    3188
    in congenital infections, 3191
    in pregnancy, 3190
Follicle mites, 3311
Follicular dendritic cell network, in HIV
    infection, 1534

Folliculitis, 1175
  eosinophilic, in HIV infection, 1557-1558,
    1558f
  from *Candida,* 1175, 2942, 2943f
  from *Malassezia,* 1175, 3060-3061
  from *Pseudomonas aeruginosa,* 733, 736,
    1175, 2605
  nodular, from *Trichophyton rubrum,* 3055
  staphylococcal, 2340
Fomivirsen, 515t, 526-527
  for cytomegalovirus prophylaxis, 1683t
Fonsecaea spp., chromoblastomycosis from,
    2988-2991
Food handling, in infection prevention, 1296-
    1297
Foodborne disease, 1286-1297
  bacterial toxins in, 1286-1289, 1287t
  botulism as, 2823, 2824
  causes of, 1286, 1287t
  clinical features of, 1286-1291
  cryptosporidiosis as, 3217
  epidemiology of, 1291-1293, 1292t, 1293t
  fatalities from, 1295t
  foods in, 1291-1292, 1292t
  from *Bacillus,* 2494, 2495
  from *Bacillus cereus,* 1219, 1287-1288, 1291,
    1294, 1294t, 2494
  from caliciviruses, 2197
  from *Campylobacter jejuni,* 1288, 1289
  from *Clostridium botulinum,* 1289, 1292, 1295,
    2823, 2834
  from *Clostridium perfringens,* 1288, 1291,
    1294, 1294t, 2834, 2835t, 2836-2837
  from *Escherichia coli,* 1288
  from *Escherichia coli* O157:H7, 1288, 1289,
    1291, 1294-1295, 1294t
  from *Escherichia coli* Shiga toxin, 1289
  from fish, 1289-1290, 1290t, 1292
  from heavy metals, 1289, 1292
  from hepatitis E virus, 2207, 2207f, 2208
  from *Listeria monocytogenes,* 2479, 2481-
    2482, 2483, 2483t
  from mushrooms, 1290, 1291t
  from noroviruses, 1288-1289, 1292
  from *Salmonella,* 1288, 1291-1292, 2639-2640,
    2639f, 2650
  from shellfish, 1289-1290, 1290t
  from *Shigella,* 1288, 2657, 2659
  from *Staphylococcus,* 1219, 2332
  from *Staphylococcus aureus,* 1286-1287, 2339
  from *Vibrio cholerae,* 1288, 1292, 2538
  from *Vibrio parahaemolyticus,* 1288, 2544,
    2545
  from *Yersinia enterocolitica,* 1289, 1292, 2698
  geography in, 1292t, 1293
  giardiasis as, 3200
  hepatitis A as, 2166, 2171, 2171f, 2172
  hospitalization in, 1295t
  intentional, 1292
  laboratory diagnosis of, 1293-1295, 1294t
  nonbacterial toxins in, 1289-1291, 1290t,
    1291t
  outbreak investigations of, 165-166
  pathogenesis of, 1286-1291
  population changes in, 1293
  postinfection syndromes from, 1289
  prevention of, 1296-1297, 1297t
    in travelers, 3642
  relative rates of, 1286, 1287f
  seasonality in, 1292t, 1293
  surveillance of, 1296
  systemic illness in, 1289
  toxoplasmosis as, 3172-3173
  treatment of, 1295-1296
  typhoid fever as, 2638

Foot
  chromoblastomycosis of, 2989, 2989f
  diabetic ulcers of, 1184
  fungal infections of, 3054
  mycetoma of. See Mycetoma.
  osteomyelitis of, from *Pseudomonas aeruginosa*, 2603
  plantar warts of, 1842, 1845, 1848. See also Human papillomavirus(es).
Foramen of Winslow, 928
Foreign bodies
  antimicrobial selection and, 246
  infections from
    from *Staphylococcus epidermidis*, 2357-2358
    rifamycin for, 381
Formaldehyde, urinary, methenamine and, 476, 477
Fort Morgan virus, 1913-1919, 1914t. See also Alphaviruses.
FosAmprenavir, pediatric, 1646t
Foscarnet, 515t, 527-528
  dosage of, 680t-681t
  drug interactions with, 691t-692t
  for cytomegalovirus, 1591, 1683t, 1686t, 1696-1697, 1793
    for polyradiculopathy, 1791
    in stem cell transplant, 3493t
  for encephalitis, 1591
  for genital herpes, 1344, 1774
  for herpes simplex virus, 1686t
  for herpesviruses, 1760t, 1761, 1774
  for human herpesvirus 6, 1823
  for varicella-zoster virus, 1687t
  formulations of, 649t
  in renal insufficiency, 527, 528t
  neurotoxicity of, 1594t
  structure of, 524f
Fosfomycin
  for *Enterococcus*, 2416
  for staphylococcal endocarditis, 999
  formulations of, 648t
Fournier's gangrene, 1190, 1191, 2813
  hyperbaric oxygen for, 566
Fractures
  microbial contamination of, osteomyelitis from, 1325-1326, 1325f
  skull, cerebrospinal fluid leak in, 1103, 1117
Francisella [spp].
  characteristics of, 2674-2676, 2675t
  laboratory identification of, 220-221
Francisella novicida, 10
Francisella philomiragia, 2676, 2681
Francisella tularensis, 2674-2683. See also Tularemia.
  as biological weapon, 3607-3611
  characteristics of, 2674-2676, 2675t
  chemoprophylaxis against, 2683
  clinical manifestations of, 2678-2681
  culture of, 3609
  diagnosis of, 2681-2682
  disinfection/sterilization and, 3342
  history of, 2674
  isolation precautions for, 3330t
  laboratory detection of, 213-214
  lymphadenopathy from, 2679, 2680f
  pathogenesis of, 2677-2678
  pharyngeal infections from, 2680
  pneumonia from, 2677, 2680-2681, 2681f
  polymerase chain reaction assay for, 2682
  serologic studies for, 2682
  skin infections from, 2681
  transmission of, 2676

Francisella tularensis (Continued)
  treatment of, 2682-2683
    with aminoglycosides, 334t-335t, 344t
  typhoid fever from, 2680
  ulcers from, 2679, 2679f
  vaccines for, 2683
  vectors of, 2676-2677
Francisella tularensis subsp. *holarctica*, 2674, 2675, 2675t
Francisella tularensis subsp. *mediaasiatica*, 2674, 2675t
Francisella tularensis subsp. *novicida*, 2674, 2675, 2675t, 2681
Francisella tularensis subsp. *tularensis*, 2674, 2675, 2675t
Frequency
  acute onset, 886, 886f
  treatment of, 891
Fresh-frozen plasma. See also Plasma.
  complement replacement via, 88
Friedlander's pneumonia, 824, 824f
Frontal sinus
  anatomy and physiology of, 773, 773t
  infections of. See Sinusitis.
Fruits, *Salmonella* in, 2640
Fulminant hepatic failure. See Hepatic failure, fulminant.
Fumagillin, for microsporidiosis, 574t, 1690t, 3247-3249, 3248t
  of eye, 1393, 3248t, 3249
Fumidil B, for *Microsporidia*, 1690t
Functional hyposplenism, 3525, 3525t. See also Asplenia.
Fungal aneurysms. See Mycotic aneurysms.
Fungal empyema thoracis, 2945
Fungal infections, 2944, 2945f. See also specific fungi and diseases.
  antifungal agents for, 502-511
  epidemiology of, 231, 2937-2938
  fluconazole for, 509
  genetic susceptibility to, 46
  hepatic, 1578
  in HIV infection, 509, 1558, 1578
  in immunocompromised host, 2944, 2945f
    prevention of, 3445-3447, 3446f, 3447t
    treatment of, 3454-3455
  in neutropenia, macrophage colony-stimulating factor for, 554
  itraconazole for, 508
  laboratory diagnosis of, 229-232, 230t, 232f, 2935-2937, 2936f-2937f
    safety issues in, 229-230
  neutropenia in, 154
  of cardiovascular devices, 1023
  of urinary tract, 882
  rifamycin for, 383
  transmission of, 2937-2938
  voriconazole for, 510
Fungal pneumonia, in immunocompromised host, 3436. See also Pneumonia.
Fungal prostatitis, 1383t, 1384
Fungemia
  in immunocompromised host, 3432-3434
  skin lesions in, 1187
Fungi. See also specific species.
  appearance of in tissue, 2936f, 2937, 2937f, 2938t
  characteristics of, 2935-2937, 2936f, 2938t
  classification of, 2935-2937
  collection and transport of, 205t, 206t, 207t, 230, 230t
  dark-walled (dematiaceous), 3070-3072, 3070f-3072f, 3070t, 3076t
  dimorphic, 2935

Fungi *(Continued)*
  direct stains for, 214
  identification of, 231, 232f
  isolation of, 231
  laboratory tests for, 229-232, 230t, 232f, 2935-2937
    safety issues in, 229-230
  life cycle of, 2935-2934
  melanin production by, 3001
  mycotoxin-producing, 2937
  processing and planting of, 231
  serology of, 231-232
  staining of, 2836f-2937f, 2937, 2938t
  structure of, 2836f-2937f, 2935-2938
  susceptibility testing of, 231
  taxonomy of, 2935
  telemorphic, 2937
  terminology for, 229, 230t, 2935t
  transmission of, 2937-2938
  yeast vs. mold, 2935
Fungus balls, of lung, 2962-2963
Fur, in iron acquisition, 2572
Furazolidone, 569t
  adverse effects of, 581t
  drug interactions with, 692t
  for giardiasis, 3202t, 3203
  for luminal protozoa, 583
Furious rabies, 2041t, 2050-2051
Furuncles, 1175-1176
  staphylococcal, 2340
Furunculoid myiasis, 3307-3310, 33108t
Fusarium spp., 229, 3072-3073, 3076t
  disseminated infections from, 3072-3073
    in transplant recipients, 3496
  endophthalmitis from, 1409, 1411
  identification of, 231
  in peritoneal dialysis, 941
  in stem cell transplant, 3496
  keratitis from, 1404
  nail infections from, 3060, 3072
  pulmonary infections from, in immunocompromised host, 3436
  skin lesions from, 3072-3073, 3072f
Fusidic acid, 326-328, 484t, 487
  adverse reactions to, 327
  antimicrobial activity of, 326-327, 326t
  dosage of, 327t, 668t-669t
  drug interactions with, 327
  for *Clostridium difficile*–associated colitis, 1258, 1258t
  for impetigo, 1173
  formulations of, 648t
  mechanism of action of, 326
  pharmacology of, 327
  Staphylococcus aureus resistance to, 2334t
  structure of, 326
  uses of, 327-328
Fusion inhibitors, 20-21
  for perinatal HIV transmission prevention, 1626
  pediatric, 1646t
Fusobacterium [spp.], 2811, 2812
  biliary tract infections from, 956
  brain abscess from, 1158t
  in oral cavity, 787, 787t
  mediastinitis from, 1072
  microbiology of, 2839, 2839t
  pericarditis from, 1059
  secondary peritonitis from, 937
    treatment of, 938
  treatment of, 2844, 2844t
    with chloramphenicol, 367t
    with clindamycin, 409t
    with metronidazole, 389t

Fusobacterium [spp.] *(Continued)*
　with penicillins, 288t
　with quinolones, 456t
　with tetracyclines, 360t
　virulence factors of, 2840, 2840t
Fusobacterium necrophorum
　endocarditis from, 992
　lung abscess from, 854
　pharyngitis from, 754
　suppurative jugular thrombophlebitis from, 794, 854
　virulence factors of, 2814, 2814t
Fusobacterium nucleatum, 2730
　empyema from, 846
　endocarditis from, 992
　noma (gangrenous stomatitis) from, 798
　odontogenic infections from, 788
　penicillins for, 284t

G

G6PD deficiency. *See* Glucose-6-phosphate-dehydrogenase deficiency.
Gabapentin, for herpes zoster ophthalmicus, 1403t
Galactomannan, blood detection of, 231
Gal/GalNAc adherence lectin
　active immunization with, 19
　of *Entamoeba histolytica*, 18-19, 18f
Gallbladder disease, 955, 1576-1577
　from *Candida*, 2947, 2950
　from *Cryptosporidium*, 3220, 3221
　from microsporidia, 3238t, 3242, 3245
　in HIV infection, 1576-1577
　in transplant recipients, 3505
　pyogenic liver abscess from, 951
　sclerosing, AIDS-related, 956-957
　treatment of, 957
Gambierdiscus toxicus, 1290
Gammopathy, monoclonal, serum protein electrophoresis for, 57
Ganciclovir, 528-530
　activity spectrum of, 517t, 528
　dosage of, 680t-681t
　drug interactions with, 529, 692t
　for cytomegalovirus, 530, 1791-1793
　　in colitis, 1791-1792
　　in encephalitis, 1591
　　in HIV infection, 1682t, 1683t, 1685t-1686t, 1696-1697
　　in polyradiculopathy, 1791
　　in retinitis, 1790-1791, 1792-1793
　　in transplant recipients, 1793-1796, 3482, 3493, 3493t, 4394
　　resistance to, 1792-1793, 1796
　for herpes B virus, 520, 1833-1834, 1834t
　for herpesviruses, 1760t, 1761, 1774, 1790-1791, 1791f
　for human herpesvirus 6, 1823
　for myocarditis, 1058
　for X-linked lymphoproliferative disease, 1815
　formulations of, 649t
　in renal insufficiency, 529t
　mechanism of action of, 528-529
　myelotoxicity of, 1791, 1796
　pharmacokinetics of, 529
　resistance of, 529
　structure of, 517f
　toxicity of, 529-530
Ganglioside receptors, 27
Gangosa, of yaws, 2786-2787, 2787f
Gangrene
　differential diagnosis of, 1183t
　etiology of, 1183t

Gangrene *(Continued)*
　Fournier's, 1190, 1191, 2813
　　hyperbaric oxygen for, 566
　gas. *See* Gas gangrene.
　hemolytic streptococcal, 1188t, 1189-1191
　infected vascular, 1188t
　infectious, 1181-1182, 1181f, 1183t
　Melaney's, 2812, 2812f
　progressive bacterial synergistic, 1181-1182, 1181f, 1183t
　pseudomonal, 1181, 1183t, 1186
　streptococcal, 1181, 1183t, 1187, 1188t, 1189-1191
　symmetric peripheral, 735
Gangrenous cellulitis, 1181-1182, 1181f, 1183t, 1186
Gangrenous stomatitis, 798
Gardnerella [spp.], in vaginosis, 212
Gardnerella vaginalis, 2762-2763
　asymptomatic colonization with, 1365
　bacterial vaginosis from, 1365-1367, 1366f, 1366t
　diagnosis of, 1365
　in urinary tract infections, 882
　metronidazole for, 389
Garenoxacin, 451
　dosage of, 672t-673t
　for meningitis, 1113
Garissa virus, 2089
Garlic, 610
　for hypercholesterolemia, 609
Gas gangrene, 1183t, 1188t, 1198-1200, 1199f, 2831-2834
　at episiotomy site, 1375, 1377t
　clinical findings in, 1198-1199, 1199f
　clinical manifestations of, 2832, 2833f
　Clostridium perfringens toxins in, 2831, 2831t
　diagnosis of, 1199, 2832-2833
　differential diagnosis of, 1199
　epidemiology of, 2831-2832
　etiology of, 1198, 1199
　history of, 2831
　noninfectious, 1188t
　pathogenesis and pathophysiology of, 1198
　prognosis for, 2834
　treatment of, 564-566, 1199-1200, 2833-2834, 2834f
Gasterophilus spp., myiasis from, 3308-3310, 3308t
Gastric acid
　antimicrobial agent selection and, 243
　as host defense, 1217
　in secondary peritonitis, 933
Gastric candidiasis, 2942
Gastric carcinoma, from *Helicobacter pylori*, 2561
Gastric disease, in HIV infection, 1576
Gastric flora. *See* Gastrointestinal flora.
Gastric lymphoma, from *Helicobacter pylori*, 2562
Gastric mucosa, injury of, 3424-3426
Gastric reservoir hypothesis, nosocomial pneumonia and, 3364
Gastric surgery, gastrointestinal infections and, 1217
Gastric ulcers
　blood group O–associated, 46
　clarithromycin for, 405
　from *Candida albicans*, 1269
　from *Helicobacter pylori*, 2561
　in HIV infection, 1576
Gastrin, in *Helicobacter pylori* infections, 2559
Gastritis
　in HIV infection, 1576
　laboratory tests for, 211-212

Gastroenteritis. *See also under* Diarrhea; Dysentery; Gastrointestinal.
　bacterial, quinolones for, 460-461
　definition of, 1215
　eosinophilic, 3294t, 3297
　　syndrome of abdominal pain, diarrhea, and eosinophilia from, 1281t, 1283
　erythromycin for, 402
　febrile, from *Listeria monocytogenes*, 2481-2482
　from adenoviruses, 1839
　from algal blooms, 3255-3256, 3255f, 3256t
　from astroviruses, 2201-2202, 2202f, 2202t
　from caliciviruses, 2194-2199
　from coronaviruses, 1990-1996
　from enteroviruses, 2156
　from nontyphoidal *Salmonella*, 2644
　from picobirnaviruses, 2203
　from rotaviruses, 3341
　from *Vibrio parahaemolyticus*, 2545
　in elderly, 3521
　in travelers, 3642, 3652
　Reiter's syndrome and, 1354-1355
　viral, 1238-1239, 1239t
Gastroesophageal reflux disease, in HIV infection, 1575
Gastroesophageal reflux, nephropathy from, 886
Gastrointestinal flora, 36, 1217-1218, 3423f, 3424-3426, 3425f
　as host defense, 36, 1217-1218
　in secondary peritonitis, 932
Gastrointestinal tract
　anthrax of, 2486-2487, 2487f
　bacterial overgrowth of, metronidazole for, 393-394
　cephalosporin effects on, 304
　disorders of
　　in HIV infection, 1575-1580
　　in sepsis, 917
　　penicillins and, 287
　flora of, 36, 1217-1218, 3423f, 3424-3426, 3425f
　　as host defense, 36, 1217-1218
　　in secondary peritonitis, 932
　fluid balance in, 1222-1223, 1222f
　in chronic granulomatous disease, 156
　in plague, 2695
　in secondary peritonitis, 934
　in tropical sprue, 1304
　metronidazole effects on, 392
　motility of, 1217
　mucosa of, 122
　nitrofurantoin effects on, 475
　non-Hodgkin's lymphoma of, in HIV infection, 1605
　quinolone effects on, 466
　rifamycin effects on, 377
　strangulation of, in secondary peritonitis, 933
　tetracycline effects on, 363t, 364
　ulcers of. *See* Peptic ulcers.
Gastrointestinal tract infections. *See also specific infections and pathogens.*
　adherence in, 1221-1222
　age in, 1216
　control of, 1226
　cytotoxins in, 1220-1221, 1220t
　diagnosis of, 211-212, 1223-1234, 1225f, 1226, 3429
　enterotoxins in, 1219-1220, 1220t
　environmental factors in, 1215-1216, 1216t
　epidemiology of, 1215-1216, 1216t
　from *Brucella*, 2671
　from *Candida albicans*, 1269
　from coronaviruses, 1990-1996

Gastrointestinal tract infections *(Continued)*
  from *Escherichia coli,* 1218, 1219t
  from microsporidia, 3238t, 3242-3245, 3247-
    3249, 3248t
  from mucormycosis, 2978
  from *Mycobacterium avium* complex, 2898,
    2898f, 2899f
  from *Salmonella,* 2642-2643, 2642f
  from *Shigella,* 2656
  from *Streptococcus agalactiae* (group B), 2424
  from syphilis, 1269, 2774
  from tuberculosis, 1269, 2881
  gastric acidity in, 1217
  genotype in, 1216
  host factors in, 1216-1218, 1216t
  human milk protection in, 1218
  hygiene in, 1216-1217, 1217t
  immunity in, 1218
  in immunocompromised host, laboratory
    diagnosis of, 3429
  intestinal motility in, 1217
  invasiveness in, 1222
  microbial factors in, 1218-1222, 1219t, 1220t
  neurotoxins in, 1219, 1220t
  occurrence of, 1215
  physical barriers in, 1217
  physiologic derangements in, 1222-1223, 1222f
  prevention of, 1226
  principles of, 1215-1226
  scope of, 1215
  serum factors in, 1218
  toxins in, 1219, 1220t
  treatment of, 1226
    with quinolones, 460-462
    with trimethoprim-sulfamethoxazole, 446
  types of, 1223, 1223t
  viral, laboratory studies for, 233t, 235
  virulence factors in, 1222
  water-related, 1215-1216, 1216t
Gastrospirillum hominis, 2563
Gatifloxacin
  antimicrobial activity of, 455t, 456t
  dosage of, 458t, 672t-673t
  for community-acquired pneumonia, 462
  for deep fascial space infections, 797t
  for *Enterococcus,* 2416
  for gonococcal urethritis, 460
  for keratitis, 1399
  for legionellosis, 2719t
  for meningitis, 1113
  for odontogenic infections, 797t
  for osteomyelitis of jaw, 797t
  for pelvic inflammatory disease, 1379t
  for peritonitis, 939
  for pneumonia, 837-839, 838t
  for respiratory infections, 462
  for sinusitis, 779-780, 779t
  for skin infections, 463-464
  for urinary tract infections, 459
  formulations of, 648t
  pharmacology of, 457t
Gay men
  hepatitis A in, 2171, 2178
  HIV infection in, 1479-1480, 1480f. *See also*
    Human immunodeficiency virus infection.
  sexually transmitted diseases in. *See* Sexually
    transmitted diseases.
  syphilis in, 2770
GB virus, 1981-1982. *See also* Hepatitis G virus.
GBV-A, 1982
GBV-B, 1982
GBV-C, 1982. *See also* Hepatitis G virus.
Gell and Coombs classification, in beta-lactam
  allergy, 319-320, 319t

Gell classification, 64
Gemella haemolysans
  endocarditis from, 990
  laboratory identification of, 217t, 218
Gemella morbillorum, 2435
  prosthetic valve endocarditis from, 1027
Gemifloxacin
  antimicrobial activity of, 455t, 456t
  dosage of, 458t, 672t-673t
  for community-acquired pneumonia, 462
  for meningitis, 1113
  for pneumonia, 837-839, 838t
  for respiratory infections, 462
  formulations of, 648t
  pharmacology of, 457t
Gender. *See also* Women.
  in HIV infection transmission, 1471
  temperature and, 705, 706
Gene therapy, for neutrophil defects, 109
Genes(s)
  candidate, 43
  polymorphisms in, in infection susceptibility,
    913
  susceptibility, 43
Genetics
  in bacterial infections, 2319-2320
  of aminoglycoside-induced cochlear toxicity,
    342
  of antibiotic resistance, 253-255, 254f, 255f,
    265-266
  of hepatitis, 45
  of HIV infection, 45, 45t
  of infectious disease, 42-49, 43t
  of malaria, 43-44, 44t
  of microbial pathogenicity, 5
  of mycobacterial disease, 44-45, 44t
Genital(s)
  in primary peritonitis, 930
  normal flora of, 212
  syphilitic chancre of, 2772-2773, 2772f,
    2773f
  ulcers of
    from *Haemophilus ducreyi,* 2667
    from HIV infection, 1630
Genital lesions, 1338-1386, 1339-1341, 1339f-
  1341f. *See also specific types and infections.*
  clinical features of, 1339-1341, 1339f-1341
  duration of, 1341-1342
  epidemiology of, 1342
  etiology of, 1342t
    infectious, 1338t, 1342t
    noninfectious, 1338t, 1344-1345
  history of, 1338-1339
  in fixed drug eruptions, 1344
  in HIV infection, 1342
  laboratory testing for, 1342-1343, 1343f
  morphology of, 1339-1341, 1339f-1341
  nonvenereal, 1338t, 1344-1345
  presentation of, 1338-1339
  treatment of, 1343-1344
  venereal, 1338-1344, 1338t. *See also* Sexually
    transmitted diseases.
Genital warts, 1341-1344, 1842-1843, 1845-1846,
  1846f. *See also* Human papillomavirus(es).
  clinical features of, 1845-1847, 1846f
  diagnosis of, 1847-1848
  epidemiology of, 1842-1843
  imiquimod for, 559
  in HIV infection, 1609, 1691t
  interferon-alfa for, 555
  pathogenesis of, 1843-1845
  prevention of, 1850
  treatment of, 515t, 555, 559, 848-1850, 1848-
    1850

Genitourinary tract infections
  female, 876, 886, 886f, 887
    anaerobic, 2813
    from gram-negative bacilli, 2842
    from *Clostridium,* 2830
    from HIV, 1619. *See also* Women, HIV
     infection in.
    from *Mycobacterium tuberculosis,* 2880-2881
    from *Streptococcus agalactiae* (group B), 6,
     2428
    sexually transmitted. *See* Sexually
     transmitted diseases.
  from *Acinetobacter,* 2634
  from *Brucella,* 2671
  from chronic granulomatous disease, 156
  from *Entamoeba histolytica,* 3103-3104
  from *Salmonella,* 2647t
  from *Schistosoma,* 3279
  host defenses in, 36
  in cancer, 3438
  laboratory studies for, 212-213
    specimen collection and transport for, 206t,
     233t
  male, 1382-1386
    anatomic aspects of, 1381, 1381f
    from tuberculosis, 2880
    host defenses in, 1381, 1381f, 1382
  metronidazole for, 392
  sexually transmitted. *See* Sexually transmitted
    diseases.
Genome
  of pathogens, 3
  of viruses, 1729-1730, 1730t
Genotype
  in gastrointestinal infections, 1216
  in viral susceptibility testing, 238-239
Gentamicin
  antimicrobial activity of, 333, 334t-335t
  chemical family of, 330t
  dosage of, 660t-661t
  for acute pyelonephritis, 889
  for bacterial arthritis, 1316t
  for biliary tract infections, 957
  for brain abscess, 1159t
  for *Calymmatobacterium granulomatis,* 2750
  for culture-negative endocarditis, 1001
  for diphtheroid prosthetic valve endocarditis,
    1028
  for Enterobacteriaceae endocarditis, 999
  for enterococcal endocarditis, 997, 998, 2416,
    2416t
    penicillin-resistant, 996
    prosthetic valve, 1027-1028, 1027t, 1028t,
     1029
  for febrile neutropenia, 3450-3452, 3451t
  for *Francisella tularensis,* 2682
  for intra-amniotic infection syndrome, 1372
  for liver abscess, 954t
  for Meniere's disease, 343
  for meningitis, 1106t, 1107t
  for osteomyelitis, 1324t
  for pelvic inflammatory disease, 1379t
  for peritonitis, 939
    dialysis-related, 942t
    secondary, 937
  for plague, 3603
  for postoperative gynecologic infections, 1377t
  for shunt infections, 1129t, 1130
  for *Staphylococcus aureus* endocarditis, 998,
    2344t
    prosthetic valve, 1026t, 1027
  for streptococcal endocarditis, 995
    prosthetic valve, 1027t
  for streptococcus group C, 2445

Gentamicin (Continued)
  for suppurative thrombophlebitis, 1005
  for tularemia, in bioterrorism attack, 3610t,
    3611
  for viridans streptococcal endocarditis, 2437t,
    2438
  for *Yersina pestis,* 2696
  formulations of, 647t
  names and sources of, 329t
  once-daily dosage regimens for, 347, 347t
  resistance to
    by *Staphylococcus aureus,* 2334t
    by streptococcus group G, 2446
  structure of, 329f, 330
  susceptibility of, 332-333, 332t
German measles. *See* Rubella.
Germicides
  definition of, 3331
  sterilization with, 3331-3333, 3332t
Gerstmann-Sträussler-Scheinker syndrome, 2222t,
  2228-2229, 2230
Getah virus, 1913-1919, 1914t. *See also*
  Alphaviruses.
Gianotti-Crosti syndrome, 1428, 1877, 2150
Giant cell arteritis
  empirical corticosteroids for, 725
  fever in, 725, 726-727
Giardia [spp.]
  classification of, 3198-3199
  culture of, 1224
  in HIV infection, 1701
  laboratory detection of, 212
  metronidazole for, 389
    resistance to, 390
  treatment of, 578t
Giardia lamblia, 3198-3203
  characteristics of, 3198-3199, 3199f
  clinical manifestations of, 3201, 3201f
  diagnosis of, 3202
  diarrhea from, 1215, 1242
  epidemiology of, 3199-3200
  immune response to, 3200-3201
  in pregnancy, 3203
  pathogenesis of, 3200-3201
  prevention of, 3203
  risk factors for, 3201
  small intestinal disease from, 1270
  transmission of, 3200
  treatment of, 573t, 3202-3203, 3202t
    with albendazole, 592
    with nitazoxanide, 583
Gingivitis. *See also* Odontogenic infections;
  Periodontal disease/periodontitis.
  acute necrotizing ulcerative, 754, 756, 791
    treatment of, 796, 796t
  clinical features of, 791
  from herpes simplex virus, 1765-1766
  in HIV infection, 1555
  in immunocompromised host, 3437
  lung abscess and, 787
  microbiology of, 788
  pathogenesis of, 789
Gingivostomatitis. *See* Gingivitis; Stomatitis.
Glanders, 2630-2631, 2630f
Glaucoma, vs. conjunctivitis, 1393
Glaucomys volans, as typhus reservoir, 2304
Globicatella spp., laboratory identification of,
  217t, 218
Globin, in malaria susceptibility, 44t
Glomerulonephritis. *See also* Nephritis.
  immune complex, in endocarditis, 981-982
  membranoproliferative
    hepatitis C–related, 1962
    type II, 82

Glomerulonephritis (Continued)
  poststreptoccocal, 2380, 2386-2389
    clinical features of, 2387
    epidemiology of, 2387, 2387t
    etiology of, 2386
    history of, 2386
    laboratory findings in, 2387-2388
    pathogenesis of, 2386-2387
    pathology of, 2387
    pharyngitis in, 2387t
    prevention of, 2388
    prognosis of, 2388-2389
    pyoderma in, 2387t
    treatment of, 2388
Gloves, health care personnel use of, 3327, 3327t,
  3329
  HIV and, 3397
Glucocorticosteroids. *See* Corticosteroids.
Glucose
  in cerebrospinal fluid, 1081, 1081t
  in infections, 909
  in sepsis, 916
  quinolone effects on, 459
Glucose-6-phosphate dehydrogenase deficiency,
  108
  antimicrobial therapy in, 244
  dapsone in, 2894
  malaria and, 43, 44, 44t, 46, 3126-3127
  primaquine toxicity in, 108
Glucosylating toxins, 25t
Glutaraldehyde, disinfection with, 3334-3335,
  3335t
Glycerol, for intracranial hypertension, 1116
Glycopeptides, 417-425. *See also* Teicoplanin;
  Vancomycin.
  Staphylococcus aureus resistance to, 2334t, 2335
Glycophorin C, in malaria susceptibility, 44t
Glycoprotein (gp) 120/41 adhesin, of human
  immunodeficiency virus, 17-18, 17f, 20
Glycoprotein, viral adherence, 17
Glycosylphosphatidylinositol, in paroxysmal
  nocturnal hemoglobinuria, 86
Gnathostomiasis, 3294t, 3296-3297, 3653f
  treatment of, 573t
Gongylonema spp., treatment of, 573t
Gonococcal infections. *See also* Neisseria
  gonorrhoeae.
  conjunctivitis in, 1391-1392
    in neonate, 1392-1393
  disseminated, skin lesions in, 736
  etiology of, 1349
  in females, 1352
  rash in, 736
  skin lesions in, 1186
  treatment of, 1352-1354
  urethritis in
    clinical features of, 1347, 1349-1350
    complications of, 1352
    diagnosis of, 1350
    etiology of, 1349
    in females, 1352
    quinolones for, 460
    treatment of, 1352-1354
Gonococcal urethritis, 2519, 2520f
Gonorrhea. *See* Gonococcal infections; *Neisseria*
  gonorrhoeae.
Gonyaulax spp., 1290
Gordonia [spp.], laboratory tests for, 228-229
Gordonia bronchialis, 2473
Gordonia rubripertinctus, 2473
Gowns, health care personnel use of, 3327t, 3329
Grafts. *See also* Transplantation.
  prosthetic vascular, infections of, 1036-1039
  Staphylococcus infections of, 2357

Graft-versus-host disease, 152
  in stem cell transplant, 3487
Grahamella, 2733
Grains. *See also* Granules.
  in actinomycosis, 2930-2931, 2930f
  in dermatophytosis, 3057
  in mycetoma, 2991-2992, 2992t, 2993-2994,
    2994f, 2995f
Gram stain, 214, 214t, 242
  of cerebrospinal fluid, 1081
    in meningitis, 1081, 1102
  of *Lactobacillus,* 2850, 2850f
  of *Neisseria gonorrhoeae,* 1350
  of *Propionibacterium,* 2849, 2850f
  of sputum, 823-825, 824f, 825f
Gram-negative bacilli infections, 2751-2763
  aerobic, aminoglycosides for, 344t
  brain abscess from, 1151
  characteristics of, 2811, 2811t, 2839, 2839t
  classification of, by infections site, 2752, 2752t
  endocarditis from, 990-991
    prosthetic valve, 1025, 1028
  in glucose fermenters, 2751t
  in glucose nonfermenters, 2751t, 2757-2762
  mediastinitis from, 1072b
  meningitis from, 1087, 1106t, 1114
  nomenclature for, 2751t
  nonfermentative with nonpigmented colonies,
    220-221, 220t
  nosocomial pneumonia from, 3364
  nosocomial pneumonia in, 836
  penicillins for, 288t
  taxonomic changes in, 217t
Gram-negative bacterial infections
  antimicrobial therapy for, 2815, 2815t
  beta-lactamase production in, 256, 256t, 258t-259t
  chloramphenicol for, 367t
  complement interactions in, 77, 78
  endocarditis from, 991
  in severe sepsis, 913
  keratitis from, 1397-1400
  penicillins for, 291-292, 292f
  shunt, 1127, 1127t
Gram-negative cocci. *See* Cocci, gram-negative.
Gram-positive bacilli infections, 991-992
  laboratory identification of, 218-220, 219t
  mediastinitis from, 1072b
  penicillins for, 288t
  taxonomic changes in, 217t
Gram-positive bacterial infections
  beta-lactamase production by, 256
  chloramphenicol for, 367t
  in severe sepsis, 913
  vancomycin-resistant, 419
Gram-positive cocci. *See* Cocci, gram-positive.
Granules. *See also* Grains.
  eosinophilic, 110, 110f
  neutrophilic
    azurophilic, 94, 94t
    deficiency of, 108, 155
    primary, 94, 94t
    specific, 94, 94t, 108
Granulicatella [spp.], blood culture of, 210, 210t
Granulicatella adiacens, vancomycin for, 418, 2440
  endocarditis from, 979
Granulicatella balaenopterae, 2440
Granulocyte(s). *See also* Eosinophil(s);
  Neutrophil(s).
  release of, 95-96
Granulocyte colony-stimulating factors, 552-554,
  552t, 908
  adverse effects of, 553-554
  after stem cell transplantation, 552, 553
  dosage of, 553

Granulocyte colony-stimulating factors *(Continued)*
    for community-acquired pneumonia, 553
    for neutropenia, 552-553
        in cancer, 3457-3458
        in HIV infection, 1682t
    for postoperative infections, 553
    pegylated, 552t
Granulocyte transfusions
    for febrile neutropenia, in cancer, 3458
    for granulocytopenia, 109
Granulocyte-macrophage colony-stimulating
        factors, 552t, 554
    adverse effects of, 554
    dosage of, 554
    for febrile neutropenia, in cancer, 3457-3458
    for HIV-related neutropenia, 1682t
    uses of, 554
Granulocytopenia, 3421-3422. *See also*
        Immunocompromised host.
    associated pathogens of, 3421t
Granulocytosis
    in inflammation, 96
    in leukocyte adhesion deficiency syndromes, 104
Granuloma
    in actinomycosis, 2929
    in candidiasis, 2944
    in chronic granulomatous disease, 156
    in histoplasmosis, 3016, 3016f
        mediastinal, 3017-3018
    in paracoccidioidomycosis, 3064
    swimming pool, 1212, 1213
Granuloma inguinale, 1341, 1341f
    clinical features of, 1339, 1341, 1341f
    duration of, 1342
    epidemiology of, 1342
    presentation of, 1338-1339
    pseudobuboes in, 1208
    treatment of, 1344
Granulomatosis infantiseptica, 2480
Granulomatous amebic encephalitis, 1088, 1101,
        1104-1105, 1106t, 1115, 3111-3119
    clinical features of, 3116, 3116t, 3117
    diagnosis of, 3117, 3118
    epidemiology of, 3114
    etiology of, 3111-3112, 3112f, 3113f
    pathogenesis and pathophysiology of, 3113f,
        3115, 3115f
    treatment of, 3118-3119
Granulomatous angiitis, meningitis in, 1139
Granulomatous disease(s). *See also* Granuloma.
    chronic, 150t, 155-156, 155f, 156f
        assays for, 107
        autosomal recessive, 150t
        bone marrow transplantation for, 109
        Chromobacterium violaceum in, 2755
        gene therapy for, 109
        hepatic abscess in, 154
        infections in, 107
        inheritance patterns in, 106, 106t
        interferon-gamma for, 556
        lymphangitis in, 1210, 1212
        neutrophil defects in, 106-108
        prophylactic antibiotics for, 108-109
        treatment of, 107-108
        X-linked, 150t, 156
    disseminated, fever in, 726
    vs. enteric fever, 1275t
Granulomatous microsporidial encephalitis, 3243
Granulomatous prostatitis, 1383t, 1384
Granulomatous uveitis, 1413, 1413f
Granulysin, 134
Gray baby syndrome, chloramphenicol and, 369
Grepafloxacin
    for pneumonia, 837-839, 837t, 838t
    pneumococcal resistance to, 837, 837t

Griseofulvin
    dosage of, 678t-679t
    drug interactions with, 692t
    for dermatophytosis, 3050t, 3058-3059
    formulations of, 649t
Groin
    dermatophytosis of, 3054-3055. *See also* Tinea
        cruris.
    Fournier's gangrene of, 1190, 1191
    fungal infections of, differential diagnosis of,
        3054-3055
    pediculosis of, 3302-3304, 3302f, 3303f
Ground itch, 3264
Growth factor(s)
    for cancer-related febrile neutropenia, 3458
    receptors for, 9
Growth hormone, for weight loss, 145
Guanarito virus, 2090-2096, 2092t
    as biological weapon, 3627-3629, 3627t
    Venezuelan hemorrhagic fever from, 2090-
        2096, 2091t. *See also* South American
        hemorrhagic fevers.
Guanoside triphosphate, in oxidative
        burst, 101
Guanosine, structure of, 537f
Guillain-Barré syndrome, 1148
    from *Campylobacter jejuni*, 2552, 2555
    from cytomegalovirus, 1790
    from enteroviruses, 2149
    from influenza virus, 2071
        postvaccination, 2075
Guinea worm, 3269-3270, 3270f
Gulf Coast tick, 3312-3314, 3313f, 3313t
Gumma, 2776-2777
Gummatous neurosyphilis, 1088
Gymnodinium breve, 1290, 3255-3256, 3255f,
        3256t
Gynecologic disorders. *See* Genitourinary tract
        infections; Sexually transmitted diseases *and
        specific disorders*.
Gynecologic surgery, surgical site infections after,
        1376-1378, 1377t
GyrA, in quinolone resistance, 454

H

HACEK organisms, 1038-1039, 2668, 2752, 2758
Haemagogus spp.
    alphavirus infections from, 1916
    yellow fever from, 1929
Haemaphysalis [spp.], Kyasanur Forest disease
        from, 1945
Haemobartonella [spp.], classification of, 2284
Haemophilus [spp.], 2667-2668, 2667t
    brain abscess from, 1158t
    conjunctivitis from, 1391
        in neonate, 1393
    endocarditis from, 991
        treatment of, 1000
    keratitis from, 1397-1400
    laboratory identification of, 220-221
    penicillins for, 283, 284t, 288t
Haemophilus aegyptius, endocarditis from, 991
Haemophilus aphrophilus, 2667, 2667t
    cardiovascular device infections from, 1023
    laboratory identification of, 220
    prosthetic valve endocarditis from, 1028, 1029t
Haemophilus ducreyi, 2666-2667
    genital lesions from, 1338-1344. *See also*
        Chancroid.
    laboratory examination of, 1342, 1343f
    treatment of, 401t
Haemophilus influenzae, 2661-2666
    adhesins of, 2662, 2662t
    antisera identification of, 221

Haemophilus influenzae (Continued)
    arthritis from, 1312, 1312t
    beta-lactamase production by, 260
    biogroup aegyptius, 2666
    cellulitis from, 1178-1179, 1186
        preseptal, 1422
    characteristics of, 2661
    chloramphenicol-resistant, 370
    complement deficiency in, 79
    conjunctivitis from, 1391, 2663
    empyema from, 846
    epidemiology of, 2661-2662
    epiglottitis from, 784-786, 2664
    genome of, 6
    H5N1, 186, 186f
    in chronic obstructive pulmonary disease,
        2661, 2662
        in exacerbations, 809
        in stable disease, 808
    in HIV infection, 1699
    in sputum, 824f, 825
    laryngitis from, 759
    meningitis from, 1085, 1086-1087, 1112
        glucocorticoids for, 559
        laboratory tests for, 211
        prevention of, 1117, 1118
        rifamycin for, 381-382
        treatment of, 1106t, 1112
    nontypeable, 2662t
        bacteremia from, 2663
        community-acquired pneumonia from, 2663
        conjunctivitis from, 2663
        diagnosis of, 2664-2665
        immunity to, 2662-2663
        in chronic obstructive pulmonary disease,
            2663
        invasive infections from, 2663
        neonatal sepsis from, 2663
        otitis media from, 2663
        pediatric respiratory infections from, 2663
        sinusitis from, 2663
        treatment of, 2665
    otitis media from, 767, 767t, 769, 2662
    pericarditis from, 1059
    pneumonia from, 1570, 2664
        aspiration, 835
        community-acquired, 831-833
        diagnosis of, 824f, 825, 829
        in HIV infection, 1570
        nosocomial, 836, 3365, 3365t, 3367t, 3368
        treatment of, 836-839, 837t, 838t
    postsplenectomy sepsis from, 3527-3528
    respiratory tract colonization by, 2661-2662
    serotypes of, 175
    sinusitis from, 775, 776, 776t, 779, 780, 782t,
        2663
    treatment of
        with adhesin-based therapies, 20t
        with aminoglycosides, 334t-335t
        with carbapenems, 313t
        with cephalosporins, 298t
        with chloramphenicol, 367t
        with clindamycin, 409t
        with linezolid, 437, 437t
        with macrolides, 397t, 401t, 403
        with mupirocin, 485t
        with penicillins, 284t
        with quinolones, 455t
        with quinupristin-dalfopristin, 425
        with rifamycin, 374t
        with sulfonamides, 441t
        with tetracyclines, 358, 359t
        with trimethoprim, 444, 444t
        with trimethoprim-sulfamethoxazole, 446
        with vancomycin, 359t

Haemophilus influenzae (Continued)
  type b, 2662, 2662t
    bacteremia from, 2664
    cellulitis from, 2664
    chemoprophylaxis for, 2665-2666
    diagnosis of, 2665
    empyema from, 2664
    epiglottitis from, 2664
    immunity to, 168, 2663
    immunization for, 2666, 2666t
    meningitis from, 2664
    pneumonia from, 2664
    treatment of, 2665
    vaccine for, 1118, 2666, 2666t, 3563f, 3564-3565, 3564t
      in complement deficiency, 88
      schedule for children, 3564t
Haemophilus parainfluenzae, 2667, 2667t
  cardiovascular device infections from, 1023
  endocarditis from, 991
    prosthetic valve, 1028, 1029t
Haemophilus paraphrophilus, 2667, 2667t
Haemophilus sengis, endocarditis from, 991
Hafnia alvei, 2578, 2580
Hair, nits in, 3302-3304, 3303f
Hair infections
  ectothrix, 3056, 3057f
  endothrix, 3056
  from dermatophytes, 3056-3057, 3057f, 3061
  from *Piedraia hortae,* 3056-3057, 3061
  from *Trichosporon,* 3056-3057, 3061
Hair loss
  differential diagnosis of, 3056-3057
  from arenaviruses, 2095
  from *Candida,* 2944
  from dermatophytes, 3056-3057, 3057f
Hair removal, preoperative, 3540
Hairy leukoplakia, 1808
  in HIV infection, 1555
  treatment of, 1815
Half-life, drug clearance and, 274
Halofantrine
  adverse effects of, 581t
  drug interactions with, 692t
  for malaria, 573t, 586
Hand. *See also* Finger(s); Nails.
  bites of, 3552-3555
  clenched fist injuries of, 3555
  dermatophytosis of, 3056
Hand hygiene, of health care personnel, 3326-3327, 3327t
  and device-related bacteremia, 3356
Hand-foot-mouth disease, 2150, 2157
Hansen's disease. *See* Leprosy; *Mycobacterium leprae.*
Hantaan virus, 2086-2089, 2086t
  as biological weapon, 3627-3629, 3628t
Hantaviruses
  as biological weapon, 3627-3629, 3628t
  hantavirus pulmonary syndrome from, 2086-2089, 2086t
    chest film in, 830
    clinical features of, 3629t
  hemorrhagic fever with renal syndrome from, 2086-2089, 2086t, 3629t
  historical perspective on, 823t
  laboratory studies for, 238
  rash from, 739
Haptenization, in beta-lactam allergy, 320, 321f
Hartmann procedure, for diverticulitis, 973
Harvest mite, 3310-3311, 3311f
Haverhillia multiformis, 2708
Hawaii virus, 2195, 2196, 2197. *See also* Caliciviruses.
Haycocknema perplexum, 3269

HB$_c$Ag, 1431, 1432, 1864, 1865f, 1866, 1867, 1871-1872, 1871f, 1878
HB$_e$Ag, 1431, 1443, 1865f, 1866, 1867, 1871f, 1872, 1876, 1878, 1878t, 1879
HB$_s$Ag-negative hepatitis B virus, 1876
HB$_s$Ag, 1431-1432, 1864-1865, 1864f, 1865f, 1866, 1867, 1871-1872, 1873, 1878, 1878t, 1879
HB$_s$Ag escape mutants, vaccine-associated, 1885
HBx, 1865f, 1866, 1868
  in hepatocellular carcinoma, 1872
HDAg, 1870, 1870f
Head and neck. *See also* Orofacial infections.
  cancer of.
    radiation-related complications in, 800
    wound infections in, 800
  irradiation of, complications of, 800
Head lice, 3302-3304, 3302f, 3303f
Headache, after lumbar puncture, 1080
Health care workers
  Creutzfeldt-Jakob disease in, 2223
  cytomegalovirus exposure in, 3415-3416
  hepatitis A in, 2171-2172
  hepatitis B transmission by, 1883, 3382
  hepatitis B transmission to, 3382
  hepatitis C transmission by, 3384
  herpes simplex virus exposure of, 3410
  HIV infection in
    diagnosis of, 1520-1521
    prevention of, 1495
    transmission of, 1491
  HIV transmission by, 3394-3395, 3395t
  HIV transmission to, 3392-3394, 3392f, 3393t
    management of occupational exposures and, 3397-3399
    prevention of, 3396-3397
      postexposure prophylaxis in, 3400-3405, 3402t, 3403t
  HIV-infected, management of, 3399-3400
  needlestick injuries in, hepatitis C from, 1961, 1965, 1969
  nosocomial infections and, 3324. *See also* Nosocomial infections.
  tuberculosis exposure in, treatment of, 2873f, 2874
Hearing loss
  from erythromycin, 400
  from Lassa fever virus, 2095
  from mumps virus, 2005
  from otitis media, 768
Heart. *See also under* Cardiac; Cardiovascular.
  artificial, infections of, 1035
  in Lyme disease, 2802, 2802t
  in pediatric HIV infection, 1643
  in sepsis, 916
  in Whipple's disease, 1308
  surgery on
    endocarditis prophylaxis in, 1048-1049
    suture line infections in, 1035-1036
  vegetations of, in endocarditis, 981
Heart disease
  brain abscess from, 1151t, 1152
  congenital
    brain abscess from, 1151t, 1152
    respiratory syncytial virus in, 2017t, 2018
    from *Trypanosoma cruzi,* 3158, 3158f, 3160, 3160f
  in endocarditis, 976-977, 1046-1047, 1047b
  in HIV infection, 1560
  rheumatic, 2382-2383, 2383f
Heart failure
  blood-stream infections in, 1040
  endocarditis in, 983, 994
    treatment of, 1001-1002
  in prosthetic valve endocarditis, 1030

Heart failure *(Continued)*
  in rheumatic fever, 2382
  leptospirosis in, 2792
Heart murmur, in endocarditis, 983
Heart transplantation. *See also* Transplantation.
  cytomegalovirus in, 3477, 3478t
  for Chagas' disease, 3160-3161
  infections in, 3502t, 3503-3504. *See also* Transplantation, infections in.
  mediastinitis in, 1071
  survival in, 3501t
  toxoplasmosis after, 3177-3178, 3177t
Heart-lung transplantation. *See also* Transplantation.
  cytomegalovirus in, 3477, 3478t
  infections in, 3502t, 3504. *See also* Transplantation, infections in.
  survival in, 3501t
Heart-reactive antibodies, in rheumatic fever, 2381
Heat therapy, for chromoblastomycosis, 2990
Heating systems, in legionnaires' disease prevention, 2720
Heavy metal poisoning, 1292, 1295
  diarrhea from, 1243
  foodborne, 1289
  treatment of, 1296
Heck's disease, 1847
Helcococcus spp., laboratory identification of, 217t, 218
Helicobacter [spp.]
  blood culture of, 210, 210t
  clinical manifestations of, 2548, 2549t
  laboratory identification of, 221
  pathogenicity of, 2548, 2549t
Helicobacter cinaedi, 2553, 2558
  cellulitis from, 1186
Helicobacter felis, 2558t
Helicobacter fennelliae, 2553, 2558
Helicobacter heilmanii, 2558, 2563
Helicobacter mustelae, 2558t
Helicobacter pylori, 187, 2557-2563
  acute acquisition of, 2560
  biochemistry of, 2558, 2558t
  blood group type associated with, 46
  clones of, 5
  colonization with, 2560-2562
  diagnosis of, 211-212, 221, 2562, 2562t
  disease from, 2320
  disinfection/sterilization and, 3340-3341
  duodenal ulceration from, 2560-2561, 2561f
  epidemiology of, 2558-2559, 2559f
  esophageal disease from, 2562
  evolution of, 6
  gastric carcinoma from, 2561
  gastric infections from, in HIV infection, 1576
  gastric lymphoma from, 2562
  gastric ulceration from, 2561
  gastrointestinal lesions from, 2560-2562, 2560t
  genetic regulation of, 7
  genome of, 11
  metronidazole-resistant, 390
  microbiology of, 2557-2558
  pathogenesis of, 2559-2560
  pathology of, 2559-2560
  toxin secretion in, 26
  treatment of, 2563
    with furazolidone, 583
    with macrolides, 397t, 401t
    with metronidazole, 389, 393
    with quinolones, 461
    with rifamycin, 382
Helicobacter (Flexispira) rappini, 2553
5-Helix, 21

Helminthic infections, 568, 3258-3259. *See also specific types.*
  biology of, 3258
  brain abscess from, 1152
  clinical features of, 3294t
  diagnosis of, 3259, 3259t, 3293
  eosinophilia in, 110, 3258-3259, 3293
  epidemiology of, 3258
  geographic distribution of, 3258
  host-parasite relationship in, 3258-3259, 3293
  immune response in, 39
  life cycle of, 3258
  meningitis from, 1084t, 1088
    clinical features of, 1101
    diagnosis of, 1104-1105
    treatment of, 1106t, 1115-1116, 1117
  pathogenesis of, 3258, 3293
  pathogenicity of, 3258
  prevention of, 3260
    eradication programs in, 3259
  structure of, 3258
  treatment of, 569t-570t, 3259
  vs. enteric fever, 1278
HELPP syndrome, hepatitis in, 1436
Hemagglutination assay
  for endemic treponematoses, 2787
  for *Treponema pallidum,* 58, 2778t, 2779
Hemagglutination inhibition test, for measles, 2031, 2036
Hemagglutinin, 14-15
  proteolytic fragmentation of, 16, 16f
Hematologic malignancies. *See also* Cancer; Leukemia; Lymphoma.
  infections in, 3432-3439
Hematologic system
  Brucella infections of, 2671
  in pediatric HIV infection, 1643
Hematologic toxicity
  of chloramphenicol, 368-369
  of linezolid, 438
  of nitrofurantoin, 475
  of rifamycin, 377
  of tetracyclines, 363t
Hematopoiesis, cyclic, 154
Hematopoietic growth factors, for cancer-related febrile neutropenia, 3458
Hematopoietic malignancy, 158. *See also* Hematologic malignancies.
Hematopoietic stem cell transplantation. *See also* Bone marrow transplantation; Transplantation.
  adenovirus in, 3494
  aspergillosis in, 2960-2961, 3495-3496
  candidiasis in, 3495
  chemotherapy in, 3486
  cytomegalovirus in, 3492-3494, 3493t
  diarrhea in, 3488
  Epstein-Barr virus in, 3495
  for HIV-related non-Hodgkin's lymphoma, 1607
  graft-versus-host disease in, 3487
  granulocyte colony-stimulating factor after, 552, 553
  hemorrhagic cystitis in, 3487
  hepatitis in, 3487-3488
  herpes simplex virus in, 3492
  HLA matching in, 3487
  human herpes virus 6 in, 3495
  immune globulin for, 3497
  immune system reconstitution in, 3496-3497, 3497t
  immunization and, 3496-3497, 3497t
  infections in, 3486-3497
    bacterial, 3492
    clinical features of, 3491-3496
    fungal, 2960-2961, 3495-3496

Hematopoietic stem cell transplantation *(Continued)*
    natural history of, 3491-3496
    parasitic, 3496
    prevention of, 3487, 3491
    risk periods for, 3488-3491, 3489f
    types of, 3487-3488
    viral, 3492-3495, 3493t
  legionellosis in, 3492
  mycobacteria in, 3492
  nocardiosis in, 3492
  nonmyeloablative, 3487, 3491
  osteomyelitis in, 3488
  parvovirus in, 3495
  Pneumocystis jirovecii in, 3495
  pneumonia in, 3488, 3494-3495
  rash in, 3488
  respiratory infections in, 3494, 3495
  techniques of, 3486-3487
  toxoplasmosis in, 3177t, 3178-3179
  varicella-zoster virus in, 1783, 3494
  veno-occlusive disease in, 3487
  viridans-group streptococci in, 3492
Hemodialysis. *See also* Dialysis.
  aminoglycoside dosing in, 346, 346t
  catheter infections in, prophylaxis for, 481-482
  hepatitis B virus transmission in, 3382
  hepatitis C virus transmission in, 3384
  osteomyelitis in, 1329
  prosthetic vascular graft infections in, 1038-1039
Hemodynamic monitoring, transducers in, infections of, 3355-3356, 3356t
Hemoglobin C, malaria and, 43, 3126
Hemoglobin E, malaria and, 43, 3126
Hemoglobin F, malaria and, 3126
Hemoglobin gene, in thalassemia susceptibility, 46
Hemoglobin S, malaria and, 43, 3126
Hemoglobinuria, paroxysmal nocturnal, complement deficiency in, 85-86
Hemolysins, 30
  of Enterobacteriaceae, 2571
Hemolytic anemia
  from cytomegalovirus, 1790
  from Epstein-Barr virus, 1806
  from sulfonamides, 442
Hemolytic disease, pediatric, laboratory studies for, 234-235
Hemolytic streptococcal gangrene, 1188t, 1189-1191. *See also* Necrotizing fasciitis.
Hemolytic-uremic syndrome, 2156
  atypical, factor H deficiency in, 82
  diarrhea in, 1243
  from enterohemorrhagic *Escherichia coli,* 2576, 2577
Hemoperfusion, for streptococcal toxic shock syndrome, 2374
Hemorrhage
  diffuse alveolar, in stem cell transplant, 3488
  intracranial, in mycotic aneurysms, 1007
  subconjunctival, in acute hemorrhagic conjunctivitis, 1389, 2136, 2137, 2156
Hemorrhagic cystitis
  from adenoviruses, 1838, 1839
  in stem cell transplant, 3487
Hemorrhagic fever(s)
  Crimean-Congo, 2086-2089, 2086t
  disinfection/sterilization and, 3342
  isolation precautions for, 3329, 3330t
  South American, 2090-2096. *See also* South American hemorrhagic fevers.
  with renal syndrome, 2086-2089, 2086t
Hemorrhagic fever with renal syndrome, 739, 3629t
  as biological weapon, 3627-3629, 3628t
  ribavirin for, 538

Hemorrhagic fevers, 2057-2059
  rash in, 739
Hendra virus, 180, 2038-2041, 2039f, 2039t
  encephalitis from, 1146
  laboratory studies for, 238
Hepacivirus spp., 1950
Hepadnaviruses, 1864
  clevudine for, 540
Heparin
  for septic pelvic thrombophlebitis, 1375
  for suppurative thrombophlebitis, 1005
  in viral collection, 232
Heparnavirus, 2162
HEPAT, 1434
Hepatic actinomycosis, 2927-2928
Hepatic artery, in pyogenic liver abscess, 951, 952t
Hepatic candidiasis, 2947, 2947f, 2950
Hepatic failure
  acute, 1428-1429
    definition of, 1429
    etiology of, 1429
  classification of, 1429
  fulminant, 1427, 1428-1429. *See also* Hepatitis, fulminant.
    from hepatitis A, 2173-2174, 2174t
    from hepatitis B, 1428-1429, 1875
    from hepatitis C, 1428-1429, 1433, 1961
    from hepatitis E, 1428-1429, 2209-2210
    from hepatitis G, 1981, 1985
    in neonate, 2154
    treatment of, 1437
  hyperacute, 1429
  subacute, 1429
Hepatic fibrosis, from hepatitis C, 1959-1961, 1959f, 1960t
  diagnosis of, 1963-1964
Hepatitis. *See also specific etiologies.*
  acute viral, 1426-1438
    alcohol avoidance in, 1437
    asymptomatic, 1428
    bed rest in, 1437
    cholestatic variants of, 1428
    clinical features of, 1428-1429
    diet in, 1437
    differential diagnosis of, 1435-1436, 1435t
    disease spectrum of, 1427-1429
    epidemiology of, 1427, 1427f, 1427t
    fibrosing cholestatic, 1428
    from cytomegalovirus, 1435
    from enteroviruses, 2156
      in neonates, 2154
    from Epstein-Barr virus, 1435, 1812
    from HAV, 1429-1430. *See also* Hepatitis A virus.
    from HBV, 1430-1432. *See also* Hepatitis B virus.
    from HCV, 1433. *See also* Hepatitis C virus.
    from HDV, 1432-1433. *See also* Hepatitis D virus.
    from HEV, 1433-1434. *See also* Hepatitis E virus.
    from HGV, 1434. *See also* Hepatitis G virus.
    fulminant, 1428-1429. *See also* Hepatitis, fulminant.
  alcoholic, 1436
  aplastic anemia in, 1981, 1985
  autoimmune, 1436
  cholestatic
    fibrosing, 1449, 1456
    from erythromycin, 400
    from HAV, 2173, 2174t
      post-transplant, 1449, 1456
    from HEV, 2173, 2174t, 2209

Hepatitis *(Continued)*
  chronic, 1441-1456
    acute liver failure in, 1428-1429
    classification of, 1441-1442, 1441t
    etiology of, 1441-1442
    from HBV, 1442-1450. *See also* Hepatitis B
      virus.
    from HCV, 1451-1456. *See also* Hepatitis C virus.
    from HDV, 1450-1451. *See also* Hepatitis D
      virus.
    fulminant, 1428-1429. *See also* Hepatitis,
      fulminant.
    hepatitis vaccine for, 1428-1429
    non-ABC, 1981. *See also* Hepatitis G.
    prevention of, 1437
  drug-induced, 1436. *See also* Hepatotoxicity.
  from adenovirus, 1839
  from *Coxiella burnetii,* 1436, 2300
  from cytomegalovirus, 1435, 1789
    in transplant recipients, 1795-1796
  from dengue fever, 1938
  from enteroviruses, in neonate, 2154
  from Epstein-Barr virus, 1807
  from herbal agents, 1436
  from herpes simplex virus, 1435, 1770, 1774t
  from human herpesvirus 6, 1823
  from human herpesvirus 7, 1824
  from isoniazid, 490
  from *Leptospira,* 1436
  from measles virus, 2034, 2035
  from microsporidia, 3238t, 3243
  from mumps virus, 2005
  from parvovirus B19, 1895
  from rifampin, 491
  from rifamycin, 377
  from trimethoprim, 445
  from TT virus, 1987-1988
  fulminant, 1427, 1428-1429
    from HAV, 1428-1429, 1437, 2173-2174, 2174t
    from HBV, 1428-1429, 1875
    from HCV, 1428-1429, 1433, 1961
    from HEG, 1981, 1985
    from HEV, 1428-1429, 2209-2210
    in neonate, 2154
    management of, 1437
  histopathology of, 1429
  historical perspective on, 1426
  in Budd-Chiari syndrome, 1436
  in HELPP syndrome, 1436
  in pregnancy, 1433-1434, 1436
  in transplant recipients, 1449-1450, 1877-1878,
    1881-1882, 1986, 3487-3488, 3507
  in travelers, 3647t, 3648t, 3649
  in Wilson's disease, 1436
  in yellow fever, 1435
  incidence of, 1427, 1427f, 1427t
  ischemic, 1436
  laboratory studies for, 237, 237t
  Labrea, 1432
  management of, 1436-1437
  milk thistle for, 609
  non-ABC, 1981, 1985. *See also* Hepatitis G.
  noninfectious, 1435t, 1436
  nosocomial, 3381, 3381t, 3383t
    blood-borne transmission of, 3382-3384
    fecal-oral transmission of, 3381-3382
  overview of, 1426-1429
  pathogenesis of, 1434-1435
  physical findings in, 1429
  prevention of, 1438, 1438t
  relapsing/biphasic, 1428
  syphilitic, 2774
  vs. enteric fever, 1274t
  vs. infectious mononucleosis, 1812
  with schistosomiasis, 3280

Hepatitis A immune globulin, 1438, 1438t
Hepatitis A vaccine, 1438, 2175-2176, 2177-
    2178, 2177t, 2178t, 3563f, 3565
  for adults, 3576f, 3577f
  for chronic hepatitis, 1428
  for elderly, 3522
  for HIV infection, 1682t
  for travelers, 3638, 3639, 3639t
  in chronic hepatitis B, 1882
Hepatitis A virus, 1429-1430, 2162-2180. *See
    also* Hepatitis, acute viral.
  antibody to, 1430
  antigenic composition of, 2164f, 2165
  asthma and, 2172
  biology of, 2165
  cell entry mechanisms of, 2165
  characteristics of, 1426t, 1429, 2162-2166
  classification of, 2162
  clinical manifestations of, 1430, 1430t, 2173,
    2174t
    extrahepatic, 2173
  community-wide epidemics of, 2171, 2179
  complications of, 2173-2174
  course of, 1430, 1431f, 2173
  culture of, 2165
  diagnosis of, 1430, 2165, 2166, 2174-2175
  discovery of, 1426
  endemicity of, 2167-2168
  epidemiology of, 1430, 1430f, 1430t, 2166-2172
    in United States, 2168-2171, 2168f
    trends in, 2179, 2179f
    worldwide patterns in, 2167-2168, 2167f
  fecal excretion of, 266f, 2166, 2172
  foodborne, 2166, 2171, 2171f, 2172
  fulminant, 1428-1429, 1437, 2173-2174, 2174t
  genome of, 2162-2165, 2163f
  genotypes/serotypes of, 1429
  geographic distribution of, 3640f
    in United States, 2170-2171, 2171f, 2171t
    worldwide, 2167-2168, 2167f
  historical perspective on, 2162
  hospitalization for, 2173, 2174t, 2180
  host range of, 2166
  immune response to, 2172, 2175
  immunization for. *See* Hepatitis A vaccine.
  in child-care centers, 2171, 2171f, 2178
  in health care workers, 2172, 2178
  in HIV infection, prophylaxis against, 1682t
  in injection drug users, 2171, 2171f, 2178, 3470
  in men who have sex with men, 2171, 2171f,
    2178
  in Native Americans, 2170, 2170f, 2179, 2179f
  in neonates, 2173
  in pregnancy, 2173
  in schools and institutions, 2171, 2171f, 2178
  in travelers, 2171f, 2172, 2178
  incidence of, 2168-2171, 2168f, 2179-2180,
    2179f
    age and, 2169-2170, 2169f
    race and, 2170, 2170f
    regional variations in, 2171, 2170f,
      2170t
    trends in, 2179, 2179f, 2180f
  incubation period for, 2172
  liver transplant for, 2179
  management of, 1436-1437, 2179-2180
  morality from, 2173, 2174t
  nosocomial, 2172, 3381
  pathogenesis of, 1434, 2172
  pathophysiology of, 1430
  prevention of, 1438, 1438t, 2175-2179
    disease control strategies in, 2178
    for high-risk groups, 2178-2179
    immune globulin in, 2175, 2176-2177, 2177t
    vaccines for. *See* Hepatitis A vaccine.

Hepatitis A virus *(Continued)*
  proteins of, 2162-2165, 2163f
  relapsing, 2173
  replication of, 2165
    sites of, 2172
  resistance of to physical/chemical agents, 2162
  risk factors for, 1429t, 2171-2172, 2171f
  serologic markers of, 1430, 1431f
  shedding of, 2166, 2172
  strains of, 2164f, 2165
  structure of, 2162, 2163f
  transfusion-related, 2166-2167, 2171, 2171f,
    2178
  transmission of, 1429-1430, 2166-2167, 2166f
    from transfusion, 3386
    intrauterine, 2173
  tropism of, 2165, 2172
  waterborne, 2166, 2171, 2171f, 2172
Hepatitis B core antigen (HB$_c$Ag), 1431, 1432,
    1864, 1865f, 1866, 1867, 1871-1872, 1871f,
    1878
Hepatitis B early antigen (HB$_e$Ag), 1431, 1443,
    1865f, 1866, 1867, 1871f, 1872, 1876, 1878,
    1878t, 1879
Hepatitis B immune globulin, 1438, 3573-3574
  for postexposure prophylaxis, 1883, 3382-3383
  for post-transplant prophylaxis, 1449-1450,
    1882
Hepatitis B, in transplant recipients, 1449-1450,
    1877-1878, 1881-1882, 3507
Hepatitis B surface antigen (HB$_s$Ag), 1431-1432,
    1864-1865, 1864f, 1865f, 1866, 1867, 1871-
    1872, 1873, 1878, 1878t, 1879
Hepatitis B surface antigen (HB$_s$Ag) escape
    mutants, vaccine-associated, 1885
Hepatitis B surface antigenemia, in HIV
    infection, 1577
Hepatitis B vaccine, 1438, 1873, 1883-1885,
    1884f, 3563f, 3564t, 3565-3566
  dosage of, 1883-1884, 1884t
  durability of response to, 1885
  efficacy of, 1884
  for adults, 3576f, 3577f
  for chronic hepatitis, 1428
  for contacts, 1882-1883
  for elderly, 3522
  for HIV infection, 1682t
  for neonates, 1884, 1884t
  for postexposure prophylaxis, 1883
  for travelers, 3638-3639, 3639t
  HB$_s$Ag escape mutants and, 1885
  indications for, 1883
  schedule for children, 3564t
  under development, 1884
Hepatitis B virus
  acute infections from, 1430-1432. *See also*
    Hepatitis, acute viral.
    antibodies in, 1432
    asymptomatic, 1428
    clinical manifestations of, 1874-1875
    course of, 1431f, 1871, 1871f, 1875
    diagnosis of, 1431-1432, 1875, 1878, 1878t
    epidemiology of, 1430-1431, 1431t, 1432f,
      1873-1874, 1874f
    laboratory findings in, 1875, 1878, 1878t
    management of, 1436-1437
    pathogenesis of, 1434-1435, 1871-1872, 1871f
    post-transfusion, 1431
    post-transplantation, 1877-1878
    prevalence of, 1431, 1431t
    prevention of, 1438, 1438t, 1883-1885, 1884f
    prognosis of, 1875
    risk factors for, 1431, 1432f, 1874, 1874t
    serologic markers of, 1431-1432, 1431f
    treatment of, 1879, 1879t

Hepatitis B virus (Continued)
  acute pancreatitis from, 959, 959t
  antiretroviral therapy effect on, 1561
  arthritis from, 1317
  biology of, 1864-1865
  characteristics of, 1426t, 1430, 1442, 1864-1870
  chronic infections from, 1442-1450. See also
      Hepatitis, chronic.
    acute liver failure in, 1428-1429
    cirrhosis in, 1876-1877
    classification of, 1442-1443, 1442t
    clinical features of, 1443-1444, 1875
    contact screening in, 1882-1883
    course of, 1443, 1871f, 1872, 1876
    diagnosis of, 1443-1444, 1875, 1878-1879,
        1878t
    epidemiology of, 1442-1443, 1873-1874,
        1873t
    extrahepatic disease and, 1450
    HBₑAg-reactive, 1443, 1444
    hepatitis A vaccine in, 1882
    histopathology of, 1444
    in HIV infection, 1450, 1882
    pathophysiology of, 1443
    post-transplant reactivation of, 1449-1450,
        1881-1882
    prevention of, 1883-1885, 1884f
    prognosis of, 1876-1877
    risk factors for, 1874, 1874t
    treatment of, 1444-1450, 1879-1883, 1879t
      adefovir in, 1446-1447, 1448, 1449t,
          1881, 1882
      after liver transplant, 1449-1450, 1881-
          1882
      clevudine in, 1447, 1881
      emtricitabine in, 1447, 1448t, 1881
      entecavir in, 1447, 1448t, 1881
      famciclovir in, 1881, 1882
      in pregnancy, 1449
      interferon in, 1444-1445, 1448, 1448t,
          1449t, 1880, 1882
      lamivudine in, 1445-1446, 1448-1449,
          1448t, 1449t, 1450, 1880-1881, 1882
      patient selection for, 1879-1880, 1879t
      recommendations for, 1448-1449
      telbivudine in, 1448, 1448t
      tenofovir in, 1448, 1448t, 1881
      valtorcitabine in, 1448, 1448t
      with cancer chemotherapy, 1450
      with HIV coinfection, 1450, 1882
      with immune-complex disease, 1450
  classification of, 1864
  discovery of, 1426
  epidemiology of, 1873-1874, 1873t, 1874f,
      3382
  extrahepatic manifestations of, 1865, 1877
  fulminant, 1428-1429, 1875
  genetic susceptibility to, 45
  genome of, 1865-1867, 1865f
  genotypes of, 1431, 1443
  geographic distribution of, 3640f
  HBₑAg-negative, 1876
  HBx and, 1868
  hepatitis C coinfection and, 1878
    cirrhosis and, 1960
    hepatocellular carcinoma and, 1961
  hepatitis D coinfection and, 1432, 1450, 1870,
      1877, 1882
  hepatotropism of, 1865
  historical perspective on, 1864
  immune response to, 1871-1872, 1871f
  immunization for. See Hepatitis B vaccine.
  in HIV infection, 1561, 1577
    prophylaxis against, 1682t
    treatment of, 1690t-1691t

Hepatitis B virus (Continued)
  in injection drug users, 3469-3470
  in transplant recipients, 3487-3488, 3507
  life cycle of, 1865, 1865f
  morphogenesis and assembly of, 1868-1870
  mutations in, 1443, 1876, 1878t
    vaccination and, 1885
  nosocomial, 3382-3383, 3383t
  penciclovir-resistant, 526
  perinatal, 1874, 1884, 1884t
    prevention of, 1884, 1884t
  postexposure immunoprophylaxis for, 1883
  prevalence of, 1873-1874, 1874f, 1874t
  previous infections from, diagnosis of, 1878
  replication of, 1442, 1867-1868, 1867f, 1869f
    measurement of, 1879
  resistance to, vitamin D receptor in, 48
  structure of, 1864, 1864f
  susceptibility to, tumor necrosis factor in, 47
  transcription of, 1867
  translation of, 1867, 1868f
  transmission of, 1431, 1873t, 1874, 3382
    by infected health care workers, 1883, 3382
    from transfusion, 3385-3386, 3385f, 3386,
        3386t
  treatment of, 3382-3383, 3383t
    with adefovir dipivoxil, 521
    with antiviral drugs, 515t
    with clevudine, 540
    with emtricitabine, 540
    with entecavir, 540-541
    with famciclovir, 526
    with interferons, 533-534, 555
    with lamivudine, 535
    with tenofovir, 542
    with thymosin-alpha₁, 560
  variants of, 1443
Hepatitis B virus early antigen, 237
Hepatitis B virus polymerase protein, 1867, 1868f
Hepatitis C vaccine, 1969
Hepatitis C virus, 1433, 1950-1972
  acute infections from. See also Hepatitis, acute
      viral.
    clinical features of, 1433, 1961
    course of, 1433
    diagnosis of, 1433
    epidemiology of, 1433
    interferon alfa prophylaxis in, 1437
    pathogenesis of, 1435
    serologic markers of, 1433
    transfusion-related, 1451, 1452, 1453
    treatment of, 1437, 1968-1969
    vs. chronic infections, 1433
  acute liver failure in, 1428-1429
  alcohol use and, 1960
  antiretroviral therapy effect on, 1561
  as sexually transmitted disease, 1965
  characteristics of, 1426t, 1433, 1451, 1950-
      1957
  chronic infections from, 1451-1456. See also
      Hepatitis, chronic.
    acute liver failure in, 1428-1429
    cirrhosis in, 1452, 1453
    clinical features of, 1453, 1961-1962
    course of, 1451-1453, 1961
    diagnosis of, 1451, 1453
    epidemiology of, 1451
    extrahepatic disease and, 1453
    hepatitis G coinfection in, 1434
    hepatocellular carcinoma in, 1452-1453
    histopathology of, 1452, 1453
    impact of, 1451
    in HIV infection, 1453
    incidence of, 1451
    pathophysiology of, 1451

Hepatitis C virus (Continued)
  post-transplant, 1456
  prevention of, 1437
  prognostic factors in, 1452, 1455
  transfusion-related, 1451
  treatment of, 1453-1456, 1966-1969
    adjunctive, 1968
    adverse reactions to, 1968
    agents for, 1969
    candidates for, 1455-1456
    for persistent infections, 1969
    future directions in, 1456
    initial, 1968
    interferon in, 1453-1455, 1454t
    liver transplant in, 1456
    patient selection for, 1968
    response to, 1966, 1966f, 1967-1968, 1968f
    ribavirin in, 1453-1455, 1454t
    with B-cell lymphoma, 1456
    with HIV coinfection, 1456
    with immune-complex disease, 1456
  cirrhosis from, 1959-1961, 1959f, 1960t
  clinical features of, 1961-1962
  complications of, 1959-1961, 1959f, 1960t
  course of, 1957-1958, 1957-1960, 1958f, 1959f
  culture of, 1957
  diagnosis of, 1962-1964, 1963-1964
  discovery of, 1426
  disinfection/sterilization and, 3340
  enzyme immunoassays for, 1962, 1963
  epidemiology of, 1964-1966, 3383
  essential mixed cryoglobulinemia and, 1962
  experimental models of, 1956-1957, 1957f
  extrahepatic manifestations of, 1962
  fulminant, 1428-1429, 1433, 1961. See also
      Heptatitis, fulminant.
  genetic diversity of, 1955-1956, 1955f, 1956f
  genetic susceptibility to, 45
  genome of, 1950-1951, 1951f, 1952f
  genotypes of, 1955-1956, 1955f, 1956f
    identification of, 1962
  hepatic fibrosis in, 1959-1961, 1959f
    diagnosis of, 1963-1964
    noninvasive markers of, 1963-1964
  hepatitis B coinfection and, 1878
    cirrhosis and, 1960
    hepatocellular carcinoma and, 1961
  hepatitis G coinfection and, 1985
  hepatocellular carcinoma and, 1452-1453,
      1961, 1962
  immune response to, 1955, 1958-1959
  in HIV infection, 1561, 1577-1578, 1960,
      1960t, 1969-1972
    aniretroviral agents and, 1970
    course of, 1970
    diagnosis of, 1970-1971
    epidemiology of, 1970
    pathogenesis of, 1970
    synergy between, 1970
    treatment of, 1691t, 1971-1972, 1971f
  in injection drug users, 1961, 3470
  in pregnancy, 1965-1966
  in transplant recipients, 3488, 3507
  incidence and prevalence of, 1964
  laboratory findings in, 1962-1964
  liver biopsy in, 1452, 1961-1962, 1963, 1963t
  membranoproliferative glomerulonephritis and,
      1962
  neonatal, 1965-1966
  nosocomial, 1965, 3383-3384
  pathogenesis of, 1957-1961
  persistence of, 1957-1959, 1958f
  porphyria cutanea tarda and, 1962
  pretreatment evaluation of, 1963
  prevention of, 1969

Hepatitis C virus (Continued)
  proteins of, 1951-1954
  quasispecies variation in, 1055
  replication of, 1954-1955, 1954f
    experimental models of, 1956-1957, 1957f
    sites of, 1955, 1956
  ribavirin-resistant, 537
  RNA tests for, 1962, 1963
  screening for, indications for, 1963t
  serology of, 1962
  structure of, 1950, 1951f
  transfusion-related, 1451, 1452, 1453, 1965,
    3385-3386, 3385f, 3386-3387, 3386t
    prevention of, 1969
  transmission of, 1964-1966, 3384-3387
  treatment of, 1966-1969, 3384
    with amantadine, 523
    with antiviral drugs, 515t
    with interferons, 534, 555
    with ribavirin, 538, 555
    with viramidine, 541
  tropism of, 1956
  vaccine for, 1969
Hepatitis D antigen, 1870, 1870f
Hepatitis D virus, 1426, 1870-1871
  acute infections from, 1432-1433. See also
    Hepatitis, acute viral.
  characteristics of, 1426t, 1432, 1450
  chronic infections from, 1450-1451. See also
    Hepatitis, chronic.
    cirrhosis in, 1877
    clinical features of, 1450, 1877
    course of, 1877
    diagnosis of, 1450, 1872
    epidemiology of, 1450, 1874
    pathogenesis of, 1872
    post-transplant, 1450
    prognosis of, 1877
    serologic markers of, 1450
    treatment of, 1450-1451
  clinical manifestations of, 1432, 1450, 1877
  course of, 1432, 1877
  diagnosis of, 1432-1433
  discovery of, 1426
  epidemiology of, 1432, 1874
  genome of, 1870-1871, 1870f
  genotypes/serotypes of, 1432, 1870
  hepatitis B coinfection and, 1432, 1450, 1870,
    1877, 1882
  host range of, 1871
  in injection drug users, 3470
  life cycle of, 1870-1871
  nosocomial, 3384
  pathogenesis of, 1435, 1872
  replication of, 1870-1871, 1870f
  risk factors for, 1432
  serologic markers of, 1433
  structure of, 1870, 1870f
  transmission of, from transfusion, 3386
Hepatitis E virus, 1433-1434, 1434, 2204-2212
  antigenic composition of, 2205-2206
  characteristics of, 1426t, 2204-2206
  classification of, 2205
  clinical manifestations of, 1433, 2210, 2210f
  clinical relevance of, 1434
  complications of, 2209-2210, 2210, 2210f
  course of, 1434, 1434f
  discovery of, 1426, 1433, 2204
  endemicity of, 2007f, 2207
  epidemic, 2206-2208, 2207f
  epidemiology of, 2206-2209
  fulminant, 1428-1429
  genome of, 2204-2205, 2205f
  geographic distribution of, 2205
  historical perspective on, 1426, 1433, 2204

Hepatitis E virus (Continued)
  host range of, 2208
  immune response to, 2210, 2211
  in animals, 2208-2209
  in pregnancy, 2209-2210, 2210f
  incubation period for, 2208, 2209
  laboratory diagnosis of, 2210-2211, 2211f
  mortality in, 2209
  nosocomial, 3382
  pathogenesis of, 2209-2210
  pathology of, 2209-2210, 2209f
  prevention of, 2211-2212
  replication of, 2209
  serologic markers of, 1434, 1434f
  seroprevalence of, 2207, 2207f
  severity of, 2209-2210, 2210f
  shedding of, 2208
  strains of, 2205, 2206f
  structure of, 2204, 2204f
  transmission of, 2208
  vaccine for, 2212
Hepatitis early antigen (HB$_e$Ag)-negative hepatitis
  B virus, 1876
Hepatitis F virus, 1427, 1982
Hepatitis G virus, 1426-1427, 1434, 1981-1987
  characteristics of, 1982, 1987t
  clinical relevance of, 1983-1984, 1987, 1987t
  diagnosis of, 1434, 1982
  discovery of, 1981-1982
  epidemics of, 1433, 1433t
  epidemiology of, 1433, 1983
  fulminant, 1985
  future perspectives on, 1987
  genome of, 1982
  genotypes of, 1982
  hepatitis C coinfection and, 1985
  hepatocellular carcinoma and, 1985-1986
  HIV coinfection and, 1986-1987, 1986f
  in injection drug users, 3470
  in pregnancy, 1433-1434
  in transplant recipients, 1986
  persistence of, 1983
  prevalence of, 1982-1983
  replication of, 1986
  serologic markers of, 1433, 1434
  structure of, 1982
  transfusion-related, 1984, 1984f, 1985f,
    3387
  transmission of, 1433, 1983, 3387
  tropism of, 1986, 1987
Hepatobiliary system infections
  from *Brucella*, 2671
  from *Salmonella*, 2647t
Hepatocellular carcinoma
  clinical features of, 1962
  etiology of, 1872-1873
  hepatitis B–related, 1442, 1872, 1873-1874,
    1877, 1883
    surveillance for, 1883
  hepatitis C–related, 1452-1453, 1961-1962
  hepatitis G–related, 1985-1986
Hepatolenticular degeneration, 1436
Hepatosplenic candidiasis, 2947, 2947f,
  2950
  in hematologic cancer, 3433
Hepatosplenic schistosomiasis, 3279
Hepatotoxicity, 1436
  of antiretroviral agents, 1579, 1970
  of isoniazid, 490, 2873
  of nitrofurantoin, 475
  of tetracycline, 363t, 364
Hepatoxoxicity, of rifamycin, 377
Herbal medicine. See Complementary therapies.
Heroin users. See Injection drug users.
Herpangina, 754, 2151

Herpes B virus, 1832-1834
  biology of, 1833-1834
  classification of, 1833
  clinical features of, 1758t, 1760t, 1832f, 1833
  diagnosis of, 1761, 1833
  epidemiology of, 1759, 1759t
  historical perspective on, 1833
  immune response in, 1758
  laboratory studies for, 238
  prevention of, 1760t, 1761
  structure of, 1756-1757, 1756t
  transmission of, 1759-1761, 1759t
  treatment of, 1760t, 1761, 1833-1834, 1834t
    ganciclovir in, 530
    valacyclovir in, 520
  vaccine for, 1834
Herpes gladiatorum, 1769
Herpes labialis. See Herpes simplex virus,
  orolabial.
Herpes simplex virus, 1762-1774
  acute retinal necrosis from, 1416, 1417f
  acyclovir-resistant, 516-517, 1774
    cidofovir for, 525
    foscarnet for, 528
    treatment of, 517
  ARDS from, 1770
  Bell's palsy from, 1766
  characteristics of, 1762-1763
  clinical features of, 1758t, 1760t, 1765-1770
  collection of, 233t
  conjunctivitis from, 1389, 1773t
    in neonate, 1393
  croup from, 761
  cutaneous, 1769, 1773t
  diagnosis of, 236, 1342, 1343, 1761, 1772-
    1773
  disseminated, 1768, 1774t
  encephalitis from, 1145, 1146, 1769-1770,
    1773t
    acyclovir for, 519
    vs. herpes simplex meningitis, 1085
  epidemiology of, 1759, 1759t, 1763-1764,
    1764t
  erythema multiforme from, 732, 1765-1766,
    1766f, 1774t
  esophagitis from, 1232-1233, 1233f, 1770, 1774t
    in HIV infection, 1234
    treatment of, 1233-1234, 1233t
  foscarnet-resistant, 527
  ganciclovir-resistant, foscarnet for, 528
  genital, 1766-1768, 1766f, 1767f
    acyclovir for, 518-519
    clinical features of, 1339, 1339f-1441f,
      1341, 1766-1767, 1766f, 1767f
    diagnosis of, 1342-1343, 1772-1773
    duration of, 1341
    extragenital lesions in, 1768
    famciclovir for, 526
    superinfections in, 1768
    treatment of, 1773-1774, 1773t
  genome of, 1763
  gingivostomatitis from, 1765-1766, 1766f, 1773t
    in immunocompromised host, 3437
  hepatitis from, 1435, 1770, 1774t
  HIV infection and, 1342, 1556, 1556f, 1759,
    1769
    treatment of, 1683t, 1686t, 1696
  host defenses against, 126
  immune response in, 1758, 1765
  in immunocompromised host, 1342, 1758,
    1759, 1765, 1768, 1769, 1770-1771, 3439
    treatment of, 1773t
  in pregnancy, 1771-1772, 1773t-1774t
    peripartum care and, 3410, 3410t
  in transplant recipients, 3492, 3508

Herpes simplex virus (Continued)
  incidence of, 1764
  inguinal buboes in, 1207-1208
  iridocyclitis from, 1416, 1773t
  keratitis from, 1400-1403, 1402t, 1416,
    1773t
    idoxuridine for, 531
  laryngitis from, 759
  latency of, 1763, 1765, 1768-1769
  lesions in, 1338-1344, 1339-1344, 1339f,
    1340f, 1342t
  meningitis from, 1085, 1101, 1111, 1767-1768,
    1773t
    Mollaret's, 1085, 1101, 1138
  mucocutaneous, acyclovir for, 519
  myocarditis from, 1053, 1053t
  neonatal, 1771-1772, 1771t, 1773t
  nosocomial, 3409-3410, 3410t
  occupational exposure to, 3410
  ocular, 1389, 1393, 1400-1403, 1402t, 1416-
    1417, 1769, 1770f, 1773t
  of finger, 1769, 1769f
  oncogenicity of, 1759
  orofacial, 754, 756, 1765-1766, 1766f, 1773t
    diagnosis of, 1772-1773
    in immunocompromised host, 1773-1774,
      1773t
    reactivation of, 1768-1769
    recurrent, 1768
    treatment of, 1773-1774, 1773t
  orolabial
    acyclovir for, 519
    penciclovir for, 526
  pathogenesis of, 1764-1765
  pelvic inflammatory disease from, 1768
  penciclovir-resistant, 526
  pharyngitis from, 754, 756, 1770, 1774t
  pneumonitis from, 1770, 1774t
  presentation of, 1338-1339
  prevention of, 1760t, 1761
  proctitis from, 1766-1767, 1773t
  reactivation of, 1763, 1765, 1768-1769
    in pregnancy, 1771
    prevention of, 1773t
  receptors for, 1732t
  replication of, 1763
  sacral radiculopathy from, 1766-1767, 1767f,
    1773t
  seroprevalence of, 1763-1764, 1764t
  skin lesions from, in HIV infection, 742
  structure of, 1762-1763
  susceptibility testing for, 238
  transmission of, 1759-1761, 1759t, 1764
  treatment of, 1344, 1760t, 1761, 1773-1774,
    1773t-1774t
    with acyclovir, 518-519
    with antiviral drugs, 515t
    with idoxuridine, 531
    with interferon-alpha, 555
    with valacyclovir, 519, 519t
  type 1
    clinical manifestations of, 1758, 1758t
    collection of, 233t
    complement effects on, 77
    laboratory studies for, 236
    seroprevalence of, 1763-1764, 1764t
    structure of, 1756-1757, 1756t
  type 2
    acute pancreatitis from, 959, 959t
    clinical manifestations of, 1758, 1758t
    collection of, 233t
    laboratory studies for, 236
    seroprevalence of, 1763-1764, 1764t
    structure of,1756-1757, 1756t
  uveitis from, 1416

Herpes simplex virus (Continued)
  variants of, 1763
  vesiculobullous eruptions from, 734
  visceral, 1770, 1774t
  vs. syphilis, 2772-2773
Herpes zoster ophthalmicus, 1389, 1401-1403,
  1402t, 1416, 1417f, 1782, 1783
Herpes zoster virus. See also Varicella-zoster
  virus.
  clinical manifestations of, 1783-1784, 1783f
  conjunctivitis from, 1389. See also Herpes
    zoster ophthalmicus.
  diagnosis of, 1784
  epidemiology of, 1781-1782
  etiology of, 1781
  historical perspective on, 1781
  in HIV infection, 1556, 1556f
  in transplant recipients, 1783, 3494, 3508
  meningitis from, 1085, 1101
  ocular complications of, 1389, 1401-1403,
    1402t, 1416, 1417f, 1782, 1783
  pathogenesis of, 1782
  postherpetic neuralgia and, 1783
  prevention of, 1785
  treatment of, 1784-1785
    with antiviral drugs, 515t
    with brivudin, 540
    with famciclovir, 526
    with valacyclovir, 519t
Herpesvirus [spp.], 2205
Herpesvirus simiae. See Herpes B virus.
Herpesvirus 6. See Human herpesvirus 6.
Herpesviruses. See also specific viruses.
  alpha, 1762
  beta, 1762
  classification of, 1756-1757, 1756t, 1762
  clinical features of, 1758t, 1760t
  clinical manifestations of, 1758, 1758t
  congenital infections from, 1759
  diagnosis of, 1761
  epidemiology of, 1759, 1759t
  gamma, 1762
  genome of, 1756-1757, 1756t, 1757f
  host range of, 1757
  immune response in, 1758
  in immunocompromised host, 1758, 1758t
  interactions among, 1758
  laboratory studies for, 236-237
  latency of, 1757-1758, 1758t
  meningitis from, 1085, 1099, 1101
  oncogenicity of, 1759
  overview of, 1756-1761
  pathogenesis of, 1757
  prevention of, 1760t, 1761
  recurrent infections from, 1758, 1758t
  replication of, 1757
  structure of, 1756-1757, 1756t, 1757f
  transmission of, 1759-1761, 1759t
    nosocomial, 3409-3417
  treatment of, 1760t, 1761
    with interferons, 534
    with vidarabine, 539
  tropism of, 1757
  variants of, 1756-1757, 1756t, 1757f
Herpetic whitlow, 1769, 1769f, 1773t
Heterophyes heterophyes, 3277t, 3283
  syndrome of abdominal pain, diarrhea, and
    eosinophilia from, 1281t, 1283
  treatment of, 572t
Heterotopic ossification, in spinal cord injury, 3516
Hexachlorophene, skin disinfection with, 479
Hickman catheter, infections of, 3353-3355,
  3354t
Hidradenitis suppurativa, 1185
  staphylococcal, 2340

Highlands J virus, 1913-1919, 1914t. See also
  Alphaviruses.
Highly active antiretroviral therapy. See
  Antiretroviral therapy.
High-mobility group box-1, in severe sepsis, 911
Hippurate hydrolysis, 216t
Hippuric acid, in urine, 888
Histamine fish poisoning, 1289, 1292
Histiocytic necrotizing lymphadenitis, 1210
Histiocytosis, sinus, with lymphadenopathy, 1210
Histoplasma [spp.]
  antigen of, collection and transport of, 207t
  direct detection of, 231
  gastrointestinal, 1270
Histoplasma capsulatum, 3012-3025
  African histoplasmosis from, 3021
  amphotericin B for, 504
  appearance of in tissue, 2936f, 2938t
  arthritis from, 1318
  characteristics of, 3014-3015
  classification of, 3014
  clinical manifestations of, 3016-3021, 3016t
  culture of, 3022
  direct detection of, 230-231
  disseminated, 3016t, 3019-3021
    acute progressive, 3019-3020, 3020f, 3024
    chronic progressive, 3020-3021, 3024
    subacute progressive, 3020, 3024
    treatment of, 3024
    vs. enteric fever, 1275t
  ecology of, 3013-3014, 3013f
  endocarditis from, 993
    treatment of, 1001
  epidemiology of, 3013-3014, 3013f
  fever from, 726
  genome of, 3014
  granulomas from, 3016-3018, 3016f
    mediastinal, 3017-3018
  historical perspective on, 3013
  identification of, 231
  immune response to, 3015-3016
  in HIV infection, 1558, 1558f
    prophylaxis against, 1682t, 1683t, 1684t
    treatment of, 1688t, 1698-1699
  isolation of, 230
  laboratory diagnosis of, 229, 3022-3023
  laryngeal infections from, 759
  mediastinal fibrosis from, 3018, 3018f, 3023
  mediastinal granulomas from, 3017-3018,
    3023
  meningitis from, 1134-1135, 1137, 3020, 3021,
    3024
  mycelial phase of, 3014, 3014f, 3015
  ocular infections from, 3021
  pancreatic infections from, 959t, 960
  pathogenesis of, 3015-3016
  pericarditis from, 1059
  prevention of, 3024, 3025
  prostatitis from, 894
  pulmonary infections from
    acute primary, 3016-3017, 3016t, 3017f,
      3023
    acute reinfections, 3016-3017, 3016t,
      3017f
    cavitary, 3016t, 3018-3109, 3018f, 3023-
      3024
    chest film in, 863f
    histoplasmoma in, 3017
    history in, 823t
    in HIV infection, 1571
  sclerosing mediastinitis from, 1075
  serology of, 863, 3022
  skin test for, 3022-3023
  staining of, 3022
  strains of, 3014

Histoplasma capsulatum (Continued)
　treatment of, 3023-3025
　　with itraconazole, 508, 509
　　with ketoconazole, 507
　　with liposomal amphotericin B, 505
　vaccine for, 3025
　yeast phase of, 3014-3015, 3014f
Histoplasma capsulatum var. *duboisii,* 3021
Histoplasmoma, 3017, 3020
　treatment of, 3023
HLA-B
　in HIV susceptibility, 45, 45t
　in malaria susceptibility, 44t
HLA-B27
　in HIV nonprogression, 1532
　reactive arthropathy and, 35
HLA-B53, in malaria resistance, 47
HLA-DR
　in hepatitis B susceptibility, 45
　in HIV susceptibility, 45, 45t
　in malaria resistance, 47
　in malaria susceptibility, 44t
　in mycobacterial disease susceptibility, 44, 44t
HLA-DR2
　in leprosy susceptibility, 47
　in tuberculosis, 2858
HLA-DR11, in hepatitis C resistance, 47
HLA-DRB1*1302
　in hepatitis B resistance, 47
　in malaria resistance, 47
Hoarseness
　in croup, 761
　in laryngitis, 758-759
Hobbies, pneumonia and, 823t, 858
Hodgkin's disease, 1808t, 1809-1810, 1809f. *See also* Cancer; Lymphoma.
　fever in, 723, 723f, 726, 3432-3434
　in HIV infection, 1611-1612
　infections in, 3432-3439
Homeless shelters, tuberculosis spread in, 2858
Homeopathy, for diarrhea, 607-608
Homologous restriction factor, deficiency of, 80t
Homosexual men
　hepatitis A in, 2171, 2178
　HIV infection in, 1479-1480, 1480f. *See also* Human immunodeficiency virus infection.
　sexually transmitted diseases in. *See* Sexually transmitted diseases.
　syphilis in, 2770
Hookworms, 3261t, 3264
　cutaneous larva migrans from, 3294t, 3295-3296
　treatment of, 573t
Hordeolum, 1419
Hormones
　immune effects of, 40
　in commensal flora, 40
Hortaea (Exophiala) wernickii, tinea nigra from, 3061
Hospital(s)
　disinfection in, 3331-3338, 3332t, 3335t
　infections acquired in, 3323-3417. *See also* Nosocomial infections.
　infectious waste management in, 3342, 3343t
　isolation in, 3326-3330, 3327t, 3328t, 3330t
　quality assessment in, 3324-3325
　standard precautions in, 3326-3327
　sterilization in, 3331-3333, 3332t
Hospital epidemiologist, 3325
Hospital epidemiology programs, 3323, 3324-3326, 3324t
Hospital preparedness. *See* Emergency preparedness.
Hospital waste
　control of, 3342, 3343t
　definition of, 3342

Host, 168, 168t
　adhesion receptors of
　　identification of, 15-16, 15t
　　interactions in, 16-17, 16f, 16t
　genetics of, in disease susceptibility, 42-43, 43t
　pathogen access to, 3-4
Host defenses, 4
　acute-phase response in, 34, 164f, 908-910
　　innate immunity and, 37-39, 37t-39t, 38f
　　Toll-like receptor signaling and, 39
　against *Salmonella,* 2644
　against *Streptococcus agalactiae* (group B), 2425-2426
　against *Streptococcus pneumoniae,* 2396-2397
　anti-infective, 908
　anti-inflammatory, 909
　antimicrobial drug effects on, 247
　complement-mediated bactericidal activity in, 77-78
　cutaneous, 35
　enteric, 36, 1216-1218, 1216t
　in eye, 36
　in gastrointestinal tract, 36
　in genitourinary tract, 36, 879, 879t
　in HIV nonprogression, 1532
　in mucous membranes, 35-36
　in prosthetic joint infections, 1333
　in *Pseudomonas aeruginosa* infections, 2589-2592, 2594-2595
　in respiratory tract, 36
　in sepsis, 922
　in *Staphylococcus aureus* endocarditis, 2343
　innate, 34-41
　local, 907-908, 907f, 908t
　metabolic, 39, 909-910
　microbial defenses against, 102-103
　natural antibodies in, 40-41
　nonspecific, 36-37
　normal, 907-910, 907f, 908t, 909t, 910f
　normal flora in, 40
　pathologic, to infections, 910-913
　physical, 35-36
　procoagulant, 910, 910f
　subversion of, 9-10
　systemic, 908, 909t
　thermoregulatory, 910
Host-agent relationship, 166-167
Hot tub lung disease, 2900-2901, 2901f, 2905
Hourglass sign, in croup, 762, 762f
Howell-Jolly bodies, 3525-3526, 3525f
Human bites, 3554-3555
　HIV and, 3398
　of head and neck, 800
Human botulinum immune globulin, 2826
Human ehrlichioses. *See* Ehrlichiosis.
Human endogenous retrovirus, 2119
Human globulin, in pneumococcal infections prevention, 2406
Human granulocytic anaplasmosis (ehrlichiosis), 740, 2285t, 2287t, 2311-2313, 2311t, 2313t, 2315
Human growth hormone, Creutzfeldt-Jakob disease from, 2222-2223
Human herpesvirus 4. *See* Epstein-Barr virus.
Human herpesvirus 6
　biology of, 1821
　central nervous system disorders from, 1822
　chronic fatigue syndrome from, 1823
　clinical manifestations of, 1758, 1758t, 1760t, 1822
　collection of, 233t
　diagnosis of, 1761, 1823
　encephalitis from, 1822
　epidemiology of, 1759, 1759t, 1821, 1821f
　exanthem subitum from, 1822, 1822f

Human herpesvirus 6 *(Continued)*
　fever from, 1822, 1822f, 1822t
　immune response in, 1758, 1821-1822
　in HIV infection, 1697
　in immunocompromised host, 1823
　in transplant recipients, 3495, 3508
　infections from, 739
　infectious mononucleosis from, 1822-1823
　laboratory studies for, 236-237
　pathogenesis of, 1821
　prevention of, 1760t, 1761
　rash from, 739
　skin diseases from, 1823
　structure of, 1756-1757, 1756t
　transmission of, 1759-1761, 1759t, 3416
　treatment of, 1760t, 1761, 1823
Human herpesvirus 7, 739, 1823-1824, 1824f
　biology of, 1823
　clinical manifestations of, 1758t, 1760t, 1824
　diagnosis of, 1761, 1823-1824
　epidemiology of, 1759, 1759t, 1823, 1824f
　immune response in, 1758, 1823
　in HIV infection, 1697
　laboratory studies for, 237
　pathogenesis of, 1823
　prevention of, 1760t, 1761
　structure of, 1756-1757, 1756t
　transmission of, 1759-1761, 1759t, 3416
　treatment of, 1760t, 1761, 1824
Human herpesvirus 8, 739
　antiviral therapy for, 1604
　biology of, 1756-1757, 1756t, 1827-1828
　classification of, 1827
　clinical manifestations of, 1758, 1758t, 1760t, 1828-1831
　diagnosis of, 1761
　epidemiology of, 1759, 1759t, 1828
　Epstein-Barr virus and, 2130
　immune response in, 1758
　immune response to, 126-127
　in transplant recipients, 3509
　Kaposi's sarcoma from, 1602, 1759, 1827-1831, 2130. *See also* Kaposi's sarcoma.
　laboratory studies for, 237
　multicentric Castleman's disease from, 1830, 1830f
　oncogenicity of, 1759
　pathogenesis of, 1828
　prevention of, 1760t, 1761
　primary effusion lymphoma from, 1830
　structure of, 1756-1757, 1756t, 1827
　transmission of, 1759-1761, 1759t, 3387, 3417
　treatment of, 1760t, 1761
Human immunodeficiency virus (HIV), 181-182, 181f, 2119-2130, 3528. *See also* Retroviruses.
　accidental exposure to, pediatric, 1651
　adherence of, 17
　antigens of, serologic detection of, 1512-1513
　as lentiretrovirus, 2120
　blood product screening for, 1520
　cellular integration of, 2122 , 2124f, 2126, 2126f, 2129, 2130f
　chemokines and, 2128
　classification of, 2119-2120
　complement interactions with, 77, 78
　culture of, pediatric, 1645
　detection of, 1506-1507, 1519
　entry inhibitors for, 20-21, 20t, 1668-1669, 1668t
　envelope glycoproteins in, 2123t, 2124, 2125
　false-positive ELISA for, after rabies vaccination, 2054
　foscarnet-resistant, 527
　fusion-active state of, 2126, 2126f

Human immunodeficiency virus (HIV) *(Continued)*
  Gag proteins in, 2123t, 2124, 2125
  genes of, 2123-2124, 2123t
    expression of, 2127-2128, 2128f
    regulatory/accessory, 2123t, 2126-2127
    structural, 2123t, 2125-2128
  genetics of, 1472, 1507f
  genome of, 2120-2121, 2120f, 2123-2124,
    2123t, 2124f
  gp 120/41 adhesin of, 17-18, 17f, 20
  host interactions with, 2128-2129
  HTLV and, 1521, 2112, 2113
  immune response to, 1509-1511, 1510f, 2121,
    2128-2129
  in HIV-associated lymphoma, 1605
  in vitro cultivation of, 1516
  integrase in, 2123t, 2125, 2130f
  laboratory studies for, 237
  latency of, 2128-2129
  life cycle of, 2120f, 2121-2122
  long terminal repeats in, 2127-2128, 2128f
  mobile DNA elements in, 2120-2121, 2120f
  Nef protein in, 2123t, 2126-2127
  non–syncytia-forming, 2121
  occupational exposure to, prophylaxis after,
    1672-1673
  oncogenicity of, 2119, 2130
  origin of, 2119
  persistence of, 2128-2129
  Pol protein in, 2123-2124, 2123t, 2125
  protease in, 2123t, 2125
  proteins of, 2122-2123, 2123t
    regulatory/accessory, 2123t, 2126-2127
    structural, 2123t, 2125-2128
  rapid tests for, pediatric, 1645
  receptors for, 1527-1528, 1528f, 1732t, 2128
  replication of, 2120f, 2122
    chemokines in, 1540
    cytokines in, 1538-1540, 1539f
  reservoirs for, 1533
  resistance to, genetic factors in, 35
  Rev protein in, 2123t, 2126-2127
  reverse transcriptase in, 2119, 2123t, 2125,
    2130f
  RNA assay of, during antiretroviral therapy,
    1669, 1671-1672
  serologic tests for, pediatric, 1645
  shedding of, cervicovaginal, 1628
  strains of, 2125-2126, 2129
    attenuated, in infection nonprogression, 1533
    variant, 2129
  structure of, 2120, 2120f, 2122-2123, 2123t
  subtypes of, 1621
  syncytia-inducing, 2121
  Tat protein in, 2123t, 2126-2127
    Kaposi's sarcoma and, 2130
  transcription/translation in, 2127-2128, 2128f,
    2130f
  transmission of, 1488-1492
    antiretroviral therapy and, 1619
    biologic variables in, 1472
    demography in, 1471
    gender in, 1471
    heterosexual, 1618-1619, 1619t
      prevention of, 1620
    in developing world, 1469-1472
    in health care workers, 1491, 1520-1521
    modes of, 1469-1470
    perinatal, 1490-1491, 1620-1627
      antiretroviral therapy for, 1621, 1622-
        1626, 1625t
      cesarean delivery and, 1621-1622
      prevention of, 1495-1496
      risk factors for, 1620-1622, 1620t
      through breast-feeding, 1622

Human immunodeficiency virus (HIV) *(Continued)*
    timing of, 1620
    viral load in, 1620-1621
    vitamin A deficiency in, 1621
    prevention of, 1472
    recipient partner susceptibility in, 1489-1490
    risk factors in, 1619t
    sexual behavior in, 1470-1471, 1488-1490
    sexually transmitted diseases in, 1470, 1472,
      1618-1619
    source partner infectiousness in, 1488-1489
    stigmatizing processes in, 1471
    through blood products, 1490
    through bodily fluids, 1492
    through intravenous drug use, 1490
    transplantation in, 1520
  tropism of, 2128
  type 1, 182, 1492-1493, 2119
    cell tropism of, 17-18
  type 2, 182, 1492-1493, 2119
    detection of, 1507, 1519
    in West Africa, 1468
    previous infections with, 1556
  type N, 1521
  type O, 1521
  Vif protein in, 2123t, 2126-2127
  viral loads of, sex differences in, 1631
  viral-cell fusion in, 2126, 2130f
  Vpr protein in, 2123t, 2126-2127
  Vpu protein in, 2123t, 2126-2127
  Western blot testing for, 58
  within cervicovaginal secretions, 1619
Human immunodeficiency virus infection, 158.
  See also Immunocompromised host.
  acute liver failure in, 1428-1429
  acute retroviral syndrome in, 1552-1553,
    1552f, 1553f
  acute stage of, 2121
  adenovirus infection, 1839
  AIDS case definition in, 1482, 1483f
  amebiasis in, 3099
  American trypanosomiasis in, 3160-3161
  amyotrophic lateral sclerosis–like syndrome in,
    1596, 1597t
  angular cheilitis in, 1554, 1555f
  anogenital neoplasia in, 1609-1611
  arthritis in, 1317
  aspergillosis in, 1699
  asplenia and, 3528
  avascular necrosis in, 1556
  bacillary angiomatosis in, 740, 1185, 1557
  bacterial infections in, pulmonary, 1568
  bacteriuria in, 883
  bartonellosis in, 740
    bacillary angiomatosis from, 2735-2736,
      2735f, 2736f
    bacillary peliosis from, 2736
    bacteremia from, 2734
    neurologic complications of, 2740
    treatment of, 1691t-1692t, 1702
  blastomycosis in, 3034
  B-lymphocytes in, 1536
  brain abscess from, 1137, 1151t, 1152, 1157,
    1158
  cancer in, 1601-1612, 2130. *See also* Human
    immunodeficiency virus infection,
    lymphoma in; Kaposi's sarcoma.
  candidasis in
    oral disease from, 1554-1555, 1554f
    treatment of, 1683t, 1687t, 1698
    vulvovaginal, 1628
  cardiac manifestations of, 1560
  $CD4^+$ response in, 1531-1532, 1534-1536
  $CD8^+$ response in, 1530-1531, 1530t, 1536
  cell-mediated immunity in, 1709

Human immunodeficiency virus infection
  (Continued)
  central nervous system lesions in, 1583-1598,
    1592f
  cervical neoplasia in, 1609
  chlamydial cervicitis in, 2248
  cholangiopathy in, 956-957
  classification of, 1547-1548, 1547t
  clinical manifestations of, 1484-1487, 1552-
    1561
    antiretroviral therapy impact on, 1550,
      1551f, 1552
    in developing world, 1472
  Clostridium difficile colitis in, 1252
  coccidioidomycosis in, 3043-3044, 3044f,
    3045f
    treatment of, 1683t, 1684t, 1687t-1688t,
      1699
  cognitive/motor disorders in, 1584-1587
    biopsy in, 1586, 1586t
    clinical presentation of, 1584, 1585t
    imaging of, 1585, 1585f
    laboratory studies for, 1584-1585, 1585t
    pathogenesis of, 1586t, 2129-2130
    treatment of, 1586-1587
  colonic disorders in, 1579-1580, 1580t
  complementary and alternative medicine for,
    609
  constitutional symptoms in, 1554
  counseling for, 1496-1497
  course of, 2121
  cryptococcosis in, 1558, 1558f, 2999-3005,
    2999t
    treatment of, 1682t, 1683t, 1684t, 1688t,
      1698
  cryptosporidiosis in, 1241, 3217, 3220, 3223
    treatment of, 1701
  cutaneous manifestations of, 1556-1558,
    1556f-1559f
  Cyclospora in, 1701
  cytokine dysregulation in, 1538
  cytomegalovirus in, 172, 1234, 1556-1557,
    1561, 1576, 1790-1792
    colitis from, 1791-1792
    encephalitis from, 1591
    polyradiculopathy from, 1791
    prevention of, 1792-1793
    retinitis from, 1559-1560, 1790-1791,
      1791f
    treatment of, 1682t-1686t, 1696-1697
  cytotoxic T-lymphocytes in, 1530-1531, 1530t
  delayed-type hypersensitivity in, 152-153
  dementia in, 1584-1587, 1585f, 1585t, 1586t
    pathogenesis of, 2129-2130
  demography of, 1482-1483, 1483t
  dendritic cells in, 1537-1538
  diagnosis of, 1484, 1496-1497, 1506-1522
    after occupational exposure, 1520-1521
    algorithm for, 1516, 1517f
    alternative strategies in, 1519
    body fluid tests in, 1509, 1509t
    confirmatory assays in, 1514-1519
    counseling in, 1518
    enzyme-linked immunosorbent assays in,
      1508t, 1511-1513, 1511f, 1512t
    in dual infections, 1519
    in pregnancy, 1519
    indirect immunofluorescence in, 1516
    laboratory methods in, 1509-1511, 1510f
    nonserologic assays in, 1513-1514
    nosocomial infection prevention and, 3399-
      3400
    nucleic acid testing in, 1508t, 1513-1514
    perinatal, 1519-1520
    point of care (home) testing in, 1508t, 1521

Human immunodeficiency virus infection,
  (Continued)
    positive predictive value in, 1508, 1509f
    radioimmunoprecipitation in, 1516
    recommendations in, 1516-1517, 1518t
    screening phase in, 1516-1517, 1518t
    serologic assays in, 1507-1508, 1508t,
        1509t, 1511-1513, 1511f, 1512t
    test performance in, 1508, 1509t
    Western blot in, 1514-1516, 1514f, 1515f,
        1516t
    window period in, 1510, 1510f
  diarrhea in, 1240-1241, 1240t
  diffuse infiltrative lymphocytosis
      syndrome–associated neuropathy in, 1595-
      1596, 1597t
  disinfection/sterilization and, 3340
  dissemination of, 1528-1529, 1529f
  distal sensory polyneuropathy in, 1593-1594
  drug reactions in, 742
  ELISA for, 1508t, 1511-1513, 1511f, 1512t
  empyema in, 847
  emtricitabine for, 540
  Encephalitozoon in, 1701
  endocarditis in, 981, 984-985, 1560
  enteric pathogens in, 1701
  epidemic of, 181-182, 181f
  epidemiologic studies for, 161
  epididymitis in, 1385-1386
  epiglottitis in, 785
  Epstein-Barr virus in, 1697
  esophageal disorders in, 1232-1234, 1232f,
      1233, 1233f, 1234t, 1575-1576
  exposure categories in, 1482
  factitious, 1521
  fatigue in, 566
  fever in, 719t, 721-722, 722t
  fungal infections in, 1558, 1578
    fluconazole prophylaxis for, 509
  gastric disorders in, 1576
  gastrointestinal disorders in, 1575-1580
  genetic susceptibility to, 45, 45t
  genital herpes and, 1769
  genital infections in, 1342
  geographic distribution of, 1483-1484, 1484f,
      1485f
  gingivitis in, 1555
  global perspectives on, 1465-1475, 1492
  Haemophilus influenzae in, 1699
  hematologic manifestations of, 1560-1561
  hepatic disorders in, 1577-1579, 1578t
  hepatitis B in, 1561, 1577, 1877, 1882
    chronic, 1450
    treatment of, 1682t, 1690t-1691t
  hepatitis C in, 1561, 1577-1578, 1960, 1960t,
      1969-1972
    antiretroviral agents and, 1970
    chronic, 1453, 1456
    course of, 1970
    diagnosis of, 1970-1971
    epidemiology of, 1970
    pathogenesis of, 1970
    synergy between, 1970
    treatment of, 1691t, 1971-1972, 1971f
  hepatitis G in, 1986-1987, 1986f
  herpes simplex virus in, 1556, 1556f, 1759,
      1770-1771
    acyclovir-resistant, 517
    skin lesions from, 742
    treatment of, 1683t, 1686t, 1696
  herpes zoster in, 1556, 1556f, 1783
  herpesviruses in, 1697
  histoplasmosis in, 1558, 1558f, 3013-3025
    treatment of, 1682t, 1683t, 1684t, 1688t,
        1698-1699

Human immunodeficiency virus infection,
  (Continued)
    historical perspective on, 2119
  history of, 1546-1547
  Hodgkin's disease in, 1611-1612
  human herpesvirus 6 in, 1823
  human papillomavirus in, 1609-1610, 1844-
      1845
  idiopathic CD4+ T lymphocytopenia in, 1484
  immune reconstitution syndrome in, 1561,
      2901
    in cryptococcosis, 3004, 3007
    in Mycobacterium avium complex, 2901,
        2901f, 2902f
    in toxoplasmosis, 3180
  immune response to, 1533-1538, 1708-1709
    cellular, 1530-1532, 1530t
    humoral, 1529-1530
  immunizations in, 3644
  immunology of, 1527-1540
  in adolescents, 1639
  in Africa, 1466-1468, 1467f
  in Asia, 1468-1469, 1468f, 1469f
  in Caribbean, 1469
  in children, 1487-1488, 1488f, 1638-1651. See
      also Children, HIV infection in.
  in developing world, 1472-1474, 1473f
  in immunocompromised host, 1844-1845, 1850
  in injection drug users. See Injection drug
      users, HIV infection in.
  in Latin America, 1469, 1469f
  in Middle East, 1468
  in North Africa, 1468
  in pregnancy, 1622. See also Human
      immunodeficiency virus (HIV),
      transmission of, perinatal.
    treatment of, 1626-1627
  in women, 1616-1632. See also Women, HIV
      infection in.
  incidence of, 1479
  indicator diseases in, 1485-1486, 1486t
  inflammatory demyelinating polyneuropathy in,
      1593, 1597t
  influenza virus in, 2070
  isosporiasis in, 1701
  Kaposi's sarcoma in, 1557, 1557f, 1601-1604,
      1702, 1759, 1827-1831, 2129-2130. See
      also Kaposi's sarcoma.
  leiomyosarcoma in, 1611
  leprosy in, 2891
  long-term nonprogression in, 1532-1533, 1532t
  lymphadenitis in, 1206, 1207, 1210-1211
  lymphadenopathy in, 1553-1554
  lymphoid tissue response in, 1534
  lymphoma in, 1702
    central nervous system, 1588-1589, 1589f,
        1607-1609, 1813
    Hodkin's, 1611-1612
    non-Hodgkin's, 1604-1607
    primary effusion, 1810, 1830, 1830f
  measles in, 2034
    immunization for, 2007, 2036
  measles-mumps-rubella vaccine in, 2007, 2036
  meningitis in, 1085, 1099, 1101-1102, 1111,
      1583-1584
  molluscum contagiosum in, 1557, 1557f
  monocyte-macrophage response in, 1537
  mononeuritis multiplex in, 1595, 1597t
  mortality in, 1487
  mucormycosis in, 2979
  multicentric Castleman's disease in, 1830, 1830f
  musculoskeletal complications of, 1555-1556
  myalgias in, 1201
  Mycobacterium avium complex in, 489, 1550,
      1561, 1571, 2897-2906

Human immunodeficiency virus infection,
  (Continued)
    treatment of, 1682t, 1683t, 1684t, 1687t,
        1700-1701
    Mycobacterium tuberculosis in. See
        Tuberculosis, in HIV infection.
  myocarditis in, 1053
  myopathy in, 1596, 1597t
  natural history of, 1548-1550, 1548f, 1549t,
      1550f, 1551f, 1552
  natural killer cells in, 1537
  neurologic disease in, 1583-1598
    in bartonellosis, 2740
    pathogenesis of, 2129
  neuromuscular syndromes in, 1596, 1597t
  neurosyphilis in, 1088, 1115, 1140
  neutralizing antibodies in, 1708-1709
  neutropenia in, 1560
    colony-stimulating factors for, 553, 554
    prophylaxis against, 1682t
  neutrophils in, 1537
  nonopportunistic infections in, 1680
  nontuberculous mycobacterial pulmonary
      disease in, 2910-2911, 2910t, 2913t
  nosocomial, 3391-3405
    prevention of, 3395-3397
      HIV testing in, 3399-3400
    risk factors for, 3393-3394, 3393t, 3395
    transmission of
      from health care worker to patient, 3394-
          3395, 3395t
      from patient to health care worker, 3392-
          3394, 3392f, 3393t, 3396-3397
      from patient to patient, 3395
  nucleoside therapy–related neuropathy in,
      1594, 1594t, 1597t
  nutrition in, 145
  occupational exposure to, 3392-3394, 3392f,
      3393t, 3400-3405
    management of, 3397-3399
  ocular disease in, 1559-1560
  opportunistic infections in, 1486, 1549-1550,
      1550f
    antiretroviral therapy impact on, 1550,
        1551f, 1552
    in developing world, 1472
    monitoring during, 1679-1680
    organisms in, 1680
    prophylaxis for, 1681t-1684t
    treatment of, 1679-1702, 1681, 1685t-1691t
  oral disease in, 1554-1555, 1554f
    hairy leukoplakia in, 1555
    ulcerative, 1555
  orchitis in, 1385-1386
  pancreatitis in, 960, 1579
  Pap smear in, 1610, 1611t, 1627
  parvovirus B19 in, 1894, 1896
  pathogenesis of, 1538
    T-cell depletion in, 2128-2129
    viral load and, 2128-2129
  Penicillium marneffei in, 3074-3075, 3074f
  pericardial effusion in, 1059, 1560
  perinatal. See Human immunodeficiency virus
      (HIV), transmission of, perinatal.
  periodontitis in, 1555
  pharyngitis in, 753
  Pneumocystis infections in, 3080-3090. See
      also under Pneumocystis.
  pneumonia in, 822-823, 832-833, 1570-1572,
      3080-3090. See also Human
      immunodeficiency virus infection,
      pulmonary complications of; Pneumonia.
    bacterial, 1570-1571, 1570f
    from Pneumocystis, 1684, 1692-1693, 3080-
        3090. See also Pneumocystis jirovecii.

Human immunodeficiency virus infection
(Continued)
from Streptococcus pneumoniae, 1486,
1682t, 1699, 2398
fungal, 1571
HIV-related, 822-873
parasitic, 1572
polymyositis in, 1555, 1597t
population groups affected by, 1465, 1465t
prevalence of, 1479
prevention of, 1493-1496. See also Human
immunodeficiency virus vaccines.
in blood products, 1495
in health care setting, 1495
in intravenous drug users, 1494-1495
in travelers, 3642
sexual behavior modification in, 1493-1494
progression of, 1484-1485, 1548-1549
genetic factors in, 35
sex differences in, 1631
progressive multifocal leukoencephalopathy in, 525,
1589-1591, 1590f, 1697-1698, 1856-1861
progressive polyradiculopathy in, 1595, 1597t
prostatitis in, 1384, 1385-1386
protozoal infections in, 1701
Pseudomonas aeruginosa in, 2607
pulmonary complications of, 1567-1573
diagnosis of, 1568-1569
differential diagnosis of, 1567-1568, 1567t
epidemiology of, 1567
neoplastic, 1572-1573, 1572f
noninfectious, 1572-1573, 1572f
radiography for, 1568, 1568t
triage in, 1568
pulmonary hypertension in, 1573
pyomyositis in, 1195
Reiter's syndrome in, 1354, 1555-1556
renal disease in, 1558-1559
respiratory syncytial virus in, 2018
rheumatologic findings in, 1555
Rhodococcus equi in, 1570, 1570f, 2472
salmonellosis in, 2646, 2649-2650
treatment of, 1683t, 1689t, 1701
scabies in, 1558, 1559f
screening for, 1516-1517, 1518t
seborrheic dermatitis in, 1557, 1558f
seizures in, 1596-1597, 1597f
semen as vector of, 1385-1386
serologic monitoring of, 1479-1482, 1480f
skin lesions in, 741-742, 741t
small intestinal disorders in, 1579-1580,
1580t
spectrum of, 1484-1485
sporotrichosis in, 2986, 2987
sulfonamides in, 442
surveillance case definition for, 1477-1479,
1478t, 1479t
susceptibility testing in, 238
susceptibility to, 47
syphilis in, 742, 1690t, 1701-1702, 2782,
2783
neurologic complications of, 1088, 1115
thymic function in, 132
toxoplasmosis in, 1695, 3177, 3179-3180. See
also Toxoplasma gondii, in
immunocompromised host.
encephalitis from, 1587, 1588f
pneumonia from, 1572
prophylaxis against, 1682t-1684t
retinitis from, 1560
treatment of, 580t, 1685t, 1695-1696
transfusion-related, 3385-3386, 3385f, 3386t
transmission of, 2120f, 2121
transplantation and, 3480
travel and, 3644

Human immunodeficiency virus infection
(Continued)
treatment of
cytokine-based, 1540
hepatotoxicity in, 1579, 1970
neurotoxicity in, 1594, 1594t
outpatient parenteral antimicrobial therapy
in, 629t, 630
with acyclovir, 520
with adhesin-based therapies, 20t
with antiretroviral therapy. See Antiretroviral
therapy.
with dehydroepiandrosterone, 609
with immunotherapy, 1715-1716
with interferons, 534
with interleukin-2, 557
with intravenous immune globulin therapy,
557-558
with rifamycin, 376, 376t
with tenofovir, 542
with trimethoprim, 445
tuberculin testing in, 2861
tuberculosis in. See Tuberculosis, in HIV
infection.
urethritis in, 1349
urinary tract infections in, 1385-1386
vaccines for. See Human immunodeficiency
virus vaccines.
vaginal aphthous ulcers in, 1345
varicella-zoster virus in, 1556, 1561
retinitis from, 1560
treatment of, 1682t, 1683t, 1686t-1687t, 1696
vascular myelopathy in, 1592-1593
viral infections in, cutaneous, 1556-1557,
1556f, 1557f
viral load in, 1548-1549
viral pneumonia in, 1572
visceral leishmaniasis in, 3148
vitamin A deficiency in, 141
vs. infectious mononucleosis, 1813
vulvovaginal candidiasis in, 1362, 1363
wasting in, 145-146, 1554
weight loss in, 145-146
Human immunodeficiency virus vaccines,
1707-1716
animal models for, 1712-1713
candidate, 1709-1712, 1710t
cytotoxic T-lymphocyte–based, 1712-1713
envelope protein, 1709-1710, 1710t, 1713-1714
humoral immunity in, 1712
internal protein, 1710t, 1711
live attenuated, 1710t, 1711-1712
live vector, 1710t, 1711, 1712-1713
live virus, 1714
nucleic acid, 1710t, 1711, 1712, 1714
prime-boost approaches in, 1714
recommendations for, 3577-3578, 3578t
synthetic peptide, 1710-1711, 1710t, 1714
testing of
in humans, 1713-1716, 1713t, 1715t
in primates, 1712-1713
in seropositive persons, 1715-1716
phase studies for, 1713-1715, 1713t, 1715t
whole virus, 1709, 1710t, 1712
Human leukocyte antigen (HLA). See also under
HLA.
alleles of, 131
in HIV susceptibility, 47
in infection susceptibility, 47
in malaria susceptibility, 43, 44
Human metapneumovirus, 175, 2009, 2026-2030
characteristics of, 2026-2027, 2026f, 2027f,
2030f
clinical manifestations of, 2028-2029, 2028t,
2029t

Human metapneumovirus (Continued)
culture of, 2029-2030, 2030f
diagnosis of, 2029-2030
epidemiology of, 2027-2028, 2027t, 2028t
laboratory studies for, 238
laryngitis from, 758, 759t
prevention of, 2030
transmission of, 2030
treatment of, 2030
vaccine for, 2030
Human milk. See Breast-feeding.
Human monocytotropic ehrlichiosis, 740, 2285t,
2287t, 2311-2315, 2311t, 2313t
Human papillomavirus(es), 1841-1851
anal, 1610
carcinogenicity of, 1843, 1846, 1850-1851,
1851t
cervicovaginal, 1609
in HIV infection, 1629
characteristics of, 1841-1842
clinical manifestations of, 1845-1847, 1848f
collection of, 233t
conjunctivitis from, 1390, 1847
cutaneous warts from, 1842, 1845
diagnosis of, 1343, 1842, 1847-1848
disease spectrum of, 1842, 1842t
disinfection/sterilization and, 3341
epidemiology of, 1342, 1842-1843
epidermodysplasia verruciformis from, 1842,
1845, 1850
genital lesions from, 1341-1344, 1842-1851
genital warts from, 1341-1344, 1341f, 1842-
1843, 1845-1846, 1846f
clinical features of, 1341, 1341f
diagnosis of, 1343
duration of, 1342
presentation of, 1338-1339
genome of, 1841-1842
host response to, 1844-1845
in HIV infection, 1609-1610, 1629
treatment of, 1691t
in immunocompromised host, 1844-1845, 1850
in neonates, 1843
in pregnancy, 1843
laboratory studies for, 238
oral lesions from, 1847, 1850
pathogenesis of, 1843-1845, 1844f
prevalence of, 1842-1843
recurrent respiratory papillomatosis from,
1843, 1847, 1850
replication of, 1841-1842
serologic markers for, 1845
structure of, 1841
transmission of, 1843
treatment of, 1848-1850
types of, 1842, 1842t
vaccine for, 1851
Human parvovirus B19. See Parvovirus B19.
Human polyomavirus, 233t
Human rabies immune globulin, 2053
Human retrovirus, 1521
laboratory studies for, 237
Human T-cell lymphotropic virus (HTLV), 2098-
2113, 2123-2124, 2123t, 2124f. See also
Retroviruses.
adult T-cell leukemia/lymphoma from, 2108-
2110, 2108f-2111f, 2108t
treatment of, 2112
age and, 2106-2107
arthritis from, 1317
arthropathy from, 2111
biology of, 2101-2102, 2101f
chronic progressive myelopathy from, 2110-
2111
treatment of, 2112-2113

Human T-cell lymphotropic virus (HTLV)
    (Continued)
    classification of, 2119
    clinical manifestations of, 2108f-2111f,
        2108-2112, 2108t
    culture of, 2102
    discovery of, 2098, 2119
    epidemiology of
        molecular, 2103-2104, 2104f
        serologic, 2103
    genome of, 2098, 2099f, 2099t, 2120f, 2124f
    geographic distribution of, 2103-2104, 2104f
    HIV and, 1521, 2112, 2113
    immune response to, 2107-2108, 2107f
    in children, 2111-2112
    infective dermatitis syndrome from, 2111
    laboratory diagnosis of, 237, 2102-2103, 2102f
    myelopathy from, 2108t, 2110-2111, 2112
        transfusion-related, 2106
        treatment of, 2112-2113
    ocular complications from, 2111
    origin of, 2103, 2119
    parasitic infections and, 2109, 2111
    persistent lymphadenopathy syndrome from,
        2112
    polymyositis from, 2111
    prevention of, 2113
    proteins of, 2098-2100, 2099t, 2102
    receptor for, 1732t
    replication of, 2099f, 2101-2102, 2101f
    structure of, 2098-2101, 2098f, 2099f
    subtypes of, 2103
    transfusion-related, 2104t, 2106, 3385, 3386
        prevention of, 2113
    transmission of, 2104-2107, 2104t
        demographic patterns of, 2104t, 2106-2107,
            2106f
        mother-to-child, 2104-2105, 2104t, 2105f,
            2111-2112, 2113
        parenteral, 2104t, 2106
            prevention of, 2113
        sexual, 2104t, 2105-2106
            prevention of, 2113
    treatment of, 2112-2113
    type I, 2098, 2119
    type II, 2098, 2119
    vaccines for, 2113
Human tetanus immune globulin, 2820, 2837
Humidification, for croup, 763
Hyalohyphomycoses, 3073
Hyalomma spp., Crimean-Congo hemorrhagic
    fever from, 2086t, 2087-2089
Hyaluronidase, 2364
Hybridization
    in microorganism identification, 222
    subtractive, 11
Hydatid cyst, 575t, 580t, 3286t, 3290-3291,
    3291f, 3292
Hydration. See Fluid management.
Hydrocephalus
    in cryptococcal meningitis, 3007, 3008
    shunt infections in, 1126-1130, 3048. See also
        Cerebrospinal fluid shunt infections.
Hydrocortisone, for sepsis, 920
Hydrogen peroxide
    disinfection with, 3335t, 3336-3337
    in neutrophil bactericidal activity, 102
    lyophilized, for bacterial vaginosis, 1366
Hydrogen peroxide gas plasma, sterilization with,
    3337t, 3339-3340
Hydrophobia, in rabies, 2050-2051
Hydrops fetalis, laboratory studies for, 234-235
Hydroxychloroquine
    drug interactions with, 692t
    for Q fever endocarditis, 1001, 2300

Hydroxyl radical, in neutrophil bactericidal
    activity, 102
Hydroxyzine
    for lice, 3303-3304
    for mites, 3311
Hygiene, in gastrointestinal infections, 1216-
    1217, 1217t
Hymenolepis diminuta, 3288
Hymenolepis nana, 3286t, 3287-3288. See also
    Tapeworms.
    syndrome of abdominal pain, diarrhea, and
        eosinophilia from, 1281t, 1283
    treatment of, 575t
Hyperbaric oxygen, 563-567
    adverse effects of, 564, 565t
    equipment for, 564, 565f
    for anaerobic gram-negative bacilli, 2843
    for clostridial myonecrosis, 564-566
    for Fournier's gangrene, 566
    for gas gangrene, 1199-1200, 2833, 2834
    for mucormycosis, 566
    for necrotizing fasciitis, 566
    for osteomyelitis of jaw, 798
    for peritonitis, 940
    for refractory osteomyelitis, 566
    indications for, 564, 564t
    physiologic effects of, 564
Hypercholesterolemia, garlic for, 609
Hypergammaglobulinemia, 65
    in endocarditis, 985
Hyperglycemia, prevention of, in sepsis, 921-922
Hyperimmunoglobulin E syndrome, 151t, 157-
    158, 157f
    interferon-gamma for, 556
    pneumatoceles in, 157, 157f
Hyperimmunoglobulin M syndrome, 65-66, 153
Hyperimmunoglobulinemia E, with impaired
    chemotaxis, 105-106
Hyperkalemia, from trimethoprim, 445
Hypersensitivity pneumonitis. See also
    Pneumonitis.
    from Ascaris lumbricoides, 3262
    from Mycobacterium avium complex, 2900-
        2903, 2905
Hypersensitivity reactions
    cell-mediated, 319t, 320
    Coombs classification of, 64
    cytotoxic antibodies in, 319-320, 319t
    delayed-type, 152-153, 153t
    Gell and Coombs classification of, 319-320, 319t
    Gell classification of, 64
    immediate, 319, 319t
    immune complexes in, 319t, 320
    to antimicrobial agents, 244
    to cephalosporins, 303
    to chloramphenicol, 369
    to erythromycin, 400
    to isoniazid, 490
    to penicillins, 286, 286t
    to quinolones, 466
    to rifampin, 491
    to sulfonamides, 442
    to teicoplanin, 424
    to tetracyclines, 362, 363t
    type I, 64, 110
    type II, 64
    type III, 64-65
Hypertension
    bacteriuria in, 887
    in poststreptoccocal acute glomerulonephritis,
        2387
    intracranial. See Intracranial hypertension.
Hyperthermia
    definition of, 703
    vs. fever, 703

Hyperventilation, for intracranial hypertension,
    1116
Hyphae, 229, 230t
Hypochlorites, disinfection with, 3334
    emerging pathogens and, 3340, 3341
Hypochlorous acid, in neutrophil bactericidal
    activity, 102
Hypocomplementemia, in endocarditis, 985
Hypoderma bovis, myiasis from, 3308-3310,
    3308t
Hypogammaglobulinemia, 151t
    immunoglobulin G replacement in, 67
    of infancy, 153
Hypoglycemia
    in malaria, 3125
    quinolones and, 467
Hypoglycorrhachia, cerebrospinal fluid, 1081,
    1081t
Hypokalemia, penicillins and, 286
Hypophosphatemia, neutrophil defects in, 106
Hyposplenism, functional, 3525, 3525t. See also
    Asplenia.
Hypotension
    bacteremia and, 913-914
    definition of, 906t
    in streptococcal toxic shock syndrome, 2374
Hypothalamic-pituitary-adrenal axis, in sepsis,
    915
Hypothalamus, in thermoregulation, 6f, 707-708
Hypovitaminosis E, 141
Hypoxemia, in croup, 762, 763
Hypoxia, cytopathic, in severe sepsis, 911
Hysterectomy, surgical site infections after, 1376-
    1377, 1377t

I

IB4 monoclonal antibody, 1383t, 1384-1385
Ibuprofen
    for colds, 750
    for cough, 805
    for fever, 713-715
Id reactions, 3058
Idiopathic pneumonia syndrome, in stem cell
    transplant, 3488
Idoxuridine, 524f, 530-531
Ig (immunoglobulin). See under Immunoglobulin.
Ignavigranum spp., laboratory identification of,
    217t, 218
Ikari syndrome, 2659
Ilhéus virus, 1945t
Iliac artery, external, mycotic aneurysm of, 1007
Iliac lymphadenitis, 1206
Imidazoles, 507. See also specific agents.
Imipenem
    antibacterial activity of, 312-313, 313t
    chemistry of, 312, 312f
    clinical uses of, 314
    dosage of, 658t-659t
    drug interactions with, 692t
    for acute pyelonephritis, 889
    for brain abscess, 1159, 1159t
    for Erysipelothrix rhusiopathiae, 2498
    for hospital-acquired pneumonia, 462-463
    for melioidosis, 2629t
    for nocardiosis, 2920-2921, 2920t
    for pneumonia, 837-839, 837t, 838t
    for preemptive pancreatic infection treatment,
        963, 963t
    for secondary peritonitis, 937t
    for Streptococcus agalactiae (group B), 2429
    formulations of, 648t
    pharmacology of, 313-314
    pneumococcal resistance to, 837, 837t
    resistance to, carbapenemases in, 256, 259t

Imipenem-cilastatin
for febrile neutropenia, 3450-3452, 3451t
for multidrug-resistant *Enterococcus*, 1028, 1029t
for postoperative gynecologic infections, 1377t
for preemptive pancreatic infection treatment, 965, 965t
for sepsis, 919t
Imiquimod, 515t, 531
for cutaneous warts, 1848
for genital warts, 559, 1849
for human papillomavirus, 1691t
Immune complex(es)
complement in, 76
in endocarditis, 981, 985
in hypersensitivity reactions, 64-65, 319t, 320
in systemic lupus erythematosus, 80-81
measurement of, 59
Immune complex disease
chronic hepatitis B in, 1450
chronic hepatitis C in, 1453, 1456
Immune complex glomerulonephritis, in endocarditis, 981-982
Immune globulin(s), 557-558, 557t, 3573
bovine anti-*Cryptosporidium*, 3222
for cryptosporidiosis, 3222
currently available, 3562t
for *Campylobacter jejuni*, 2552
for enterovirus infections, in immunocompromised host, 2155
for febrile neutropenia, in cancer, 3458
for *Helicobacter pylori* infections, 2562
for hepatitis A, 1438, 1438t
for hepatitis B, post-transplant prophylactic, 1449-1450
for hepatitis C, 1969
for hepatitis E, 2211-2212
for Kawasaki disease, 3318
for measles, 2035
for mumps, 2007
for nontyphoidal *Salmonella*, 2649
for ocular vaccinia, 1403
for parvovirus B19, 1896
for rabies, 2053
for respiratory syncytial virus, 2021
in immunocompromised host, 2018
for rotavirus, 1909
for streptococcal necrotizing myositis
for streptococcal toxic shock syndrome, 2374
for vaccinia, 1745, 3574
for conjunctivitis, 1390t
for eczema vaccinatum, 1745
for poxvirus infections, 1749
for progressive vaccinia, 1745
for varicella-zoster, 1785
for viral meningitis, 1116
for viral myocarditis, 1058
in pediatric HIV infection, 1648
in stem cell transplant, 3497
indications for, 557-558, 557t
production of, 59-64
prophylactic, for transplant-related cytomegalovirus infections, 3482
replacement, 66-67
respiratory syncytial virus, 2021, 3574
for immunocompromised host, 2018
for otitis media, 770
Rh, 3574
structure of, 52-55
tetanus, 66, 3574
in pediatric HIV infection, 1650
total, 56-57
varicella-zoster, 1785, 3574
for HIV infection, 1682t
for pediatric HIV infection, 1650

Immune plasma, varicella-zoster, 1785
Immune reconstitution syndrome, 2901
in antiretroviral therapy, 1561, 2901
in cryptococcosis, 3004, 3007
in *Mycobacterium avium* complex, 2901, 2901f, 2902f
in toxoplasmosis, 3180
Immune system
cephalosporin effects on, 303-304
compartmentalization of, 119
in HIV infection, 1533-1538
in sepsis, 917
intracellular bacteria detection by, 122-123
physical barriers in, 3423-3426
platelets in, 3427
spleen in, 3423
Immunity
acquired, 94, 908, 908t
to amebiasis, 18-19
acupuncture effects on, 610
adaptive, 34, 34t, 1218
C3 modulation of, 76
innate immunity and, 123, 124
Toll-like receptors signaling in, 38-39
aging effects on, 40
cell-mediated, 117-135
defects in, 3422
in HIV infection, 1530-1532, 1530t, 1709
in malnutrition, 140
in tuberculosis, 2859-2860
in urinary tract infections, 880-881
in viral infections, 122
microbial pathogenesis in, 122
to *Bacteroides fragilis*, 2840
to *Bordetella pertussis*, 2706
to *Listeria monocytogenes*, 2480
to *Pseudomonas aeruginosa*, 2591
commensal flora effects on, 40
complement-mediated. *See also* Complement.
deficiencies in, 158, 158f
dysregulation of, 40
fatty acids and, 143-144
fever and, 711-712
hormone effects on, 40
humoral
antigen challenge of, 154
defects in, 3422-3423
in HIV infection, 1509, 1529-1530
in HIV nonprogression, 1532
in HIV vaccines, 1712
in urinary tract infections, 880, 881
intestinal, 1218
to *Bacteroides fragilis*, 2840
in leprosy, 2888
in vitamin deficiencies, 141-143, 143f
innate, 34, 34t, 908, 908t, 1218
acute-phase response and, 37-39, 37t-39t, 38f
alterations in, 39-41
components of, 93-94
in myocarditis, 1055
receptors of, 123-128
to *Pseudomonas aeruginosa*, 2590-2591
to *Salmonella*, 2644
intestinal, 1218
massage effects on, 609
natural antibodies in, 40-41
nonspecific, 34, 34t
alterations in, 39-41
steady-state components of, 36-37
nutrition and, 139-147, 3427
pathogen-specific, 117-119, 118f, 119f
postoperative, 3537-3538
primary, 56, 57f
protein-energy malnutrition and, 140-141

Immunity *(Continued)*
pulmonary, 821
rifampin effects on, 491
secondary, 56, 57f
stress effects on, 40
T cell–mediated, 124
to adhesin, 17
to human immunodeficiency virus, 1509-1511, 1510f, 1708-1709
with antiviral drugs, 514
with beta-lactam antibiotics, 320f, 322
Immunizations, 3557-3585. *See also* Vaccine(s) *and specific diseases or vaccines.*
active, 3557
for elderly, 3522
for endocarditis prevention, 1045
for travelers, 3560-3561, 3560t, 3561t, 3637-3641, 3639t
interactions among, 3641
spacing of, 3641
in HIV infection, 3644
in children, 1649-1650
in immunocompromised host, 3644
in myocarditis prevention, 1058
in pregnancy, 3575, 3577, 3644
in spinal cord injury, 3514-3515
in transplant recipients, 3481-3482, 3496-3497
passive, 66, 3557
recommendations for, 3637-3641, 3639t
Immunocompromised host. *See also* Asplenia; Cancer; Human immunodeficiency virus infection; Immunodeficiency; Transplantation.
acyclovir-resistant herpes simplex virus in, 516-517
adenovirus infections in, 1839
American trypanosomiasis in, 3160-3161
aspergillosis in, 2960-2961, 2961f, 3436
bacteremia in, 3432-3434
Bartonella bacillary peliosis in, 2736
Bartonella infections in, 739-740
BK virus in, 1857-1861
blastomycosis in, 3034
botryomycosis in, 1185
brain abscess in, 1137, 1151t, 1152, 1157
candidiasis in, 2944, 2945f, 2948-2949, 2951
chronic mucocutaneous, 2944, 2945f
prevention of, 3444-3447, 3446f, 3447t
cellulitis in, 1179, 3438
gangrenous, 1182
Clostridium difficile in, 3438
coccidioidomycosis in, 3043-3044, 3044f, 3045f
combination antimicrobial therapy in, 248
common pathogens in, 3421t
concurrent illnesses in, 3427
cryptococcosis in, 2999, 2999t
cryptosporidiosis in, 3217, 3220, 3223
cytomegalovirus in, 1790-1796, 1793-1794
diarrhea in, 3438
empiric therapy for, 3439
empyema in, 847
enteroviruses in, 2154-2155
epiglottitis in, 785
Epstein-Barr virus in, 1808-1809, 1808t
febrile neutropenia in. *See* Febrile neutropenia.
fever of unknown origin in, 719t, 721-722
fungal infections in, 2944, 2945f
prevention of, 3444-3447, 3446f, 3447t
treatment of, 3454-3455
fungemia in, 3432-3434
genitourinary infections in, 3438
granulocytopenia in, 3421-3422
granulomatous amebic encephalitis in, 3116, 3117

Immunocompromised host *(Continued)*
  hepatitis B in, 1877-1878
  herpes simplex virus in, 1765, 1766, 1768,
      1770-1771, 3439
    acyclovir for, 519
    treatment of, 1773t
  herpes zoster in, 1783-1784
  herpesviruses in, 1758, 1758t, 1783
  HIV infection in, 1844-1845, 1850. *See also*
      Human immunodeficiency virus infection.
  human herpesvirus 6 in, 1823
  human papillomavirus in, 1844-1845, 1850
  immunodeficiencies in, 3318, 3421-3427
    granulocytopenia, 3421-3422, 3421t
  infections in
    etiology of, 3421t
    laboratory diagnosis of, 3428-3429, 3439
    management of, 3439
    overview of, 3421-3430
    pathogenesis of, 3421-3428
    sequence of events in, 3422t, 3429-3430,
        3429f
  influenza virus in, 2070
  JC virus in, 1857-1861
  Legionella infections in, 2726
  lung abscess in, 854
  measles in, 2034
    prevention of, 2035, 2036
  mechanical ventilation in, 3437
  meningitis in, 1140
  mucocutaneous disease in, 2944, 2945f
    antiviral drugs for, 515t
  mucormycosis in, 2975-2980
  mucositis in, 798-799, 3424-3426, 3426f
  Mycoplasma pneumoniae in, 2275
  nocardiosis in, 2917
  nutritional status of, 3427
  odontogenic infections in, 3437
  parvovirus B19 in, 1894, 1896
  Pneumocystis jirovecii in, 829, 3436
    prevention of, 3447, 3447t
  pneumonia in, 835-836
    diagnosis of, 208
  poliomyelitis in, 2145
  polyomaviruses in, 1857-1861
  progressive multifocal leukoencephalopathy in,
      1856-1861, 1859t
  prophylactic trimethoprim-sulfamethoxazole
      for, 447
  pyoderma grangrenosum in, 3439
  respiratory syncytial virus in, 2018, 2019t
  Rhodococcus equi in, 2473
  risk factors in, 3421-3427
  rotavirus in, 1904
  sepsis in, from *Capnocytophaga*, 2731
  sinusitis in, 3437
  skin disorders in, 741-742, 741t, 1184, 3438-
      3439
  Staphylococcus epidermidis bacteremia in, 2356
  stomatitis in, 798-799
  tetanus prophylaxis in, 2821
  thrombocytopenia in, 3427
  toxoplasmosis in, 3177-3180
  travel by, 3644
  vaccines for, 3577-3578, 3578t
  varicella in, 1782, 1783
  varicella-zoster virus in, 3439
    acyclovir for, 520
Immunodeficiency, 65-66. *See also*
    Immunocompromised host;
    Immunosuppression.
  acquired, 158
  common variable, 65, 66, 150t, 153-154
  congenital, 150t-151t
  evaluation of, 149-158

Immunodeficiency *(Continued)*
  history in, 149
  humoral, clinical evaluation of, 66
  in *Pseudomonas aeruginosa* infections, 2591
  index of suspicion in, 149, 149t
  laboratory studies for, 149, 152t
  pathogens associated with, 149, 149t
  physical examination in, 149
  prophylaxis in, intravenous immune globulin
      for, 558
  screening of, 149, 152t
  selective, 66
  severe combined, 66, 150t
  with hyper-IgM, 150t
  X-linked, 150t
Immunodiffusion tests, for coccidioidomycosis,
    3047
Immunogenicity, 168
  vaccines and, 3557-3558
Immunoglobulin(s), 52-53, 3573-3574
  classes of, 54-55
  congenital defects in, 153-154
  definition of, 3557
Immunoglobulin A, 52, 53t, 54-55
  against Gal/GalNAc lectin, 18-19
  antibodies to, tests for, 3183
  blocking function of, 55
  deficiency of, 57, 65, 150t
    in enteric infections, 1218, 1302-1303
  Fc receptors for, 56, 56t
  for *Campylobacter jejuni,* 2552
  for *Helicobacter pylori,* 2562
  in complement activation, 56
  in urinary tract infections, 880, 881
  secretory, 35
Immunoglobulin alpha, 61t
Immunoglobulin beta, 61t
Immunoglobulin D, 53t, 55, 60-61, 61t
Immunoglobulin E, 52, 53t, 55
  antibodies to, tests for, 3183
  beta-lactam–specific, 319
  Fc receptors for, 56, 56t
  in beta-lactam allergy, 320, 321f, 322
  in HIV infection, 1536
  in Job's syndrome, 157-158
  measurement of, 57
Immunoglobulin G, 52, 53t, 54
  after pneumococcal vaccination, 2405-2406
  antibodies to, tests for, 3182-3183
  as opsonin, 55-56
  beta-lactam–specific, 320
  deficiency of, in immunoglobulin A deficiency,
      65
  Fc receptors for, 56, 56t
  for *Helicobacter pylori* infections, 2562
  for parvovirus B19, 1896
  in complement activation, 55, 71
  in endocarditis, 990
  in phagocytosis, 99
  in secondary immune response, 57
  in urinary tract infections, 880
  intramuscular, 557
  nonhuman, antibody response to, 54
  secretory, 35
  subclasses of
    deficiency of, 66
    measurement of, 57
Immunoglobulin M, 52, 53t, 54, 61t
  antibodies to, tests for, 3183
  beta-lactam–specific, 320
  for *Helicobacter pylori* infections, 2562
  in complement activation, 55, 71
  in primary immune response, 56, 57f
  membrane, 60-61
  production of, 60-61

Immunoglobulin M anti-HB$_c$, 1878, 1878t
Immunohistochemistry, 58-59
Immunologic synapse, 132
Immunologic techniques, 117-120
Immunomodulators, 551-560. *See also specific
    agent.*
  classification of, 551
  cytokine, 551, 552t
  in fungal infections, 511
    for sepsis, 920
  in viral infections, 514
Immunonutrition, 144
Immunoreceptor tyrosine-based activation motif,
    61
Immunoreceptor tyrosine-based inhibitory motif,
    61
Immunosenescence, 40
Immunosorbent assay
  enzyme-linked, 57, 58f
  solid-phase, 57, 58f, 59
Immunosuppression. *See also* Immuno-
    compromised host;
    Immunodeficiency.
  for myocarditis, 1058
  in septic shock, 86
  in severe sepsis, 912
  in transplantation, infections and, 3477-3479
  Legionella infections in, 2726, 2727f, 2728f
  pulmonary tuberculosis in, treatment of, 2872
  rifamycin and, 376t, 378
Immunotherapy
  for HIV infection, 1715-1716
  for *Pseudomonas aeruginosa*, 2599
  for toxoplasmosis, 3188
Immunotoxin BL22, 30
Impetigo, 1172-1174
  bullous, 737, 1174, 2330, 2330f
    from *Streptococcus aureus*, 2369
  staphylococcal, 2339-2340, 2341f
  streptococcal, 2339-2340, 2368-2370, 2369f
  topical antibacterials for, 482
  vs. varicella, 1784
Impetigo contagiosa, from *Streptococcus
    pyogenes* (group A), 2368-2370, 2369f
Implant infections, outpatient parenteral
    antimicrobial therapy for, 629t, 630
In vivo expression technology, 10
Inclusion conjunctivitis. *See also* Conjunctivitis.
  adult, 1391, 1392, 2245, 2247t, 2250
  neonatal, 1392, 2247t, 2250-2251
  pathogenesis of, 1390, 2245, 2247t
Increased intracranial pressure. *See* Intracranial
    hypertension.
India ink smear, of cerebrospinal fluid, 2937
  for *Cryptococcus neoformans,* 3005-3006,
      3005f
Indifference, to antimicrobial agents, 274
Indinavir, 1665t, 1666
  dosage of, 684t-685t
  formulations of, 649t
  musculoskeletal complications of, 1596
  pediatric, 1646t
  prophylactic
    after occupational exposure to HIV, 3402,
        3402t
    for perinatal HIV transmission, 1625t, 1626
  resistance to, 1668
  structure of, 1663f
Indole, 216t
Indole-3-carbinol (IC3), for recurrent respiratory
    papillomatosis, 1850
Indolicin, 102
Indonesia, HIV infection in, 1468, 1468f
Inducible nitric oxide synthase, in malaria
    susceptibility, 44t

Induction, differential fluorescence, 10
Infants. *See also* Neonates.
  diarrhea in, from adenoviruses, 1838
  fever of unknown origin in, 720
  meningitis in, treatment of, 1107t
  pneumonia in, from *Chlamydia trachomatis,* 2247t, 2249
  respiratory syncytial virus in, 2011-2015, 2017-2018
Infection control. *See also* Nosocomial infections.
  for postoperative infections, 3540, 3540t
  for prion diseases, 2230-2231, 3341
  hospital employee health and, 3324
  in transplantation, 3483, 3483t, 3491
  organization of, 3323-3326
Infection-control committee, 3325
Infection-control professionals, 3325
Infectious asthma. *See* Bronchiolitis.
Infectious bronchitis, 803-805, 804t
Infectious disease(s), 151t
  acute-phase responses to, 164f, 908-910
  bloodstream, laboratory diagnosis of, 209-210, 210t
  causes of death in, 173, 173f, 174t
  chain of, 167
  complement in, 86-87
  definitions of, 3, 161-162, 167, 906t
  diagnosis of, 203, 204f
  emerging, 173-187, 739. *See also specific infections, e.g.,* Severe acute respiratory syndrome (SARS).
    convergence model of, 174, 174f
    emergency preparedness for, 192-201. *See also* Emergency preparedness.
    newly identified, 174, 174t
  endogenous, 167
  evolutionary effects of, 35
  exogenous, 167
  genetics of, 42-49
    evolutionary aspects of, 48-49
    magnitude of, 42-43, 43t
  gradient of, 167
  highly contagious
    agents of, 196t
    hospital preparedness for. *See* Emergency preparedness.
  immunoglobulin M release in, 56
  in anticytokine therapy, 560
  in infection response, 908
  inflammatory response to, 909
  local response to, 907-908, 907f, 908t
  malnutrition and, 39-40
  molecular techniques for, 11-12
  mortality from, hereditary factors in, 34, 35f
  pathologic response to, 910-913
  prevention of
    in complement deficiency, 88
    intravenous immune globulin in, 558
  secondary, prevention of, in sepsis, 921
  site of, antimicrobial choice and, 245-247
  susceptibility to
    gene polymorphisms in, 913
    human leukocyte antigens in, 47
  systemic response to, 908, 909t
  thermoregulatory response to, 910
  transmission routes in, 168-169
Infectious gangrene, 1181-1182, 1181f, 1183t
Infectious mononucleosis
  acyclovir for, 520
  central nervous system involvement in, 1807, 1807t
  clinical features of, 1789, 1805-1806, 1805-1807, 1805t, 1806f, 1806t
  complications of, 1789-1790, 1806-1807
  conjunctivitis in, 1390

Infectious mononucleosis *(Continued)*
  course of, 1807
  diagnosis of, 1789
  epidemiology of, 1803-1804
  etiology of, 1789, 1812
  from cytomegalovirus, 1789-1790, 1812
  from Epstein-Barr virus, 1789-1815
  hemolytic anemia in, 1806
  heterophile-negative, 1812
  incidence of, 1803-1804
  laboratory diagnosis of, 237, 1810-1812, 1810t, 1811t
  mortality in, 1807
  pathogenesis of, 1804-1805
  pharyngitis in, 755
  prevention of, 1815
  public health impact of, 1804
  rash in, 1806, 1806f, 1806t
  renal dysfunction in, 1807
  splenic rupture in, 1806-1807
  thrombocytopenia in, 1806
  transmission of, 1804
  treatment of, 1813-1815
  vs. enteric fever, 1274t
Infectious waste
  definition of, 3342
  management of, 3342, 3343t
Infective dermatitis syndrome, from HTLV, 2111
Infective endocarditis
  brain abscess from, 1151t, 1152
    in injection drug users, 3471
  fever in, 726
  from *Actinomyces,* 2926
  from *Aspergillus,* 2966
  from *Bartonella,* 739-740
  from *Candida,* 2945-2946, 2950
  from *Chlamydophila psittaci,* 2257
  from *Coxiella burnetii,* 2299-2300, 2299f, 2300f
  from *Histoplasma capsulatum,* 3020, 3024
  in elderly, 3520-3521
  in injection drug users, 3465-3467
    central nervous system infections from, 3471-3472
  Janeway lesions in, 736, 1187
  myalgias in, 1201
  Osler nodes in, 736, 1187
  skin lesions in, 736, 1186-1187
  subcutaneous abscess in, 1191
  urinary tract, 2946
Infectivity, 167
Infertility
  after pelvic inflammatory disease, 1380, 2249
  from *Chlamydia trachomatis,* 1380, 2247t, 2249
  from mumps virus, 2005
Inflammation
  complement in, 76, 86
  granulocytosis in, 96
  immune globulin for, 67
  in secondary peritonitis, 934
  innate, dendritic cells in, 132-133
  local, 907
  mediators of, 120
  neutrophils in, 96-101. *See also* Neutrophil(s).
  procoagulant response to, 910, 910f
  systemic, prevention of, 908, 909t
  zinc levels in, 142
Inflammatory bowel disease, vs. amebiasis, 3105
Inflammatory myositis, 1201
Influenza virus(es), 2060-2078
  adherence of, 16f
  antigenic drift in, 2064
  antigenic shift in, 2064-2065, 2064f
  antigenic variation in, 2064

Influenza virus(es) *(Continued)*
  avian, 2064-2065
  bronchiolitis from, 813, 813t
  CD8$^+$ T-cell responses in, 122
  chemoprophylaxis for, 2078
  classification of, 2060, 2060t
  clinical manifestations of, 2069-2071
  colds from, 747-750, 747t
  collection of, 233t
  complications of
    nonpulmonary, 2071
    pulmonary, 2067, 2070-2071, 2070t
  croup from, 760t, 761
  diagnosis of, 2071-2072
  epidemic outbreaks of, 2063, 2063f, 2064f
  epidemiology of, 2061-2065
  genome of, 2061, 2061t
  histopathology of, 2066-2067, 2067f
  historical perspective on, 2060
  hospitalization for, 2016, 2016t, 2062-2063
  host range of, 2064-2065
  immune response to, 2066f, 2068-2069
  in hematologic malignancies, 3435-3436
  in HIV infection, 1682t
  in transplant recipients, 3494, 3509
  isolation of, 2071
  laboratory tests for, 234
  laryngitis from, 758, 759t
  morbidity and mortality from, 2061-2062, 2062t
  myalgias in, 1201
  pandemic outbreaks of, 264f, 265f, 2063-2064
  pathogenesis of, 2065-2069
  pathogenicity of, 2067-2068
  pathophysiology of, 2067, 2067f
  persistent bronchitis from, 750, 803-804, 803t, 804t
  pharyngitis from, 754
  pneumonia from, 831, 2067, 2070-2071
  prevention of, 2075-2078. *See also* Influenza virus(es), vaccine for.
    chemoprophylaxis in, 2078
    family prophylaxis in, 2078
    outbreak prophylaxis in, 2078
    seasonal prophylaxis in, 2078
  public health impact of, 2061-2063, 2062t
  rapid tests for, 2071-2072
  receptor for, 1732t
  replication of, 2067-2068
  secondary bacterial pneumonia after, 20
  shedding of, 2066, 2066f
  sinusitis from, 776, 776t
  strains of, 2063, 2064-2065
  structure of, 1732f, 2060-2061, 2061f
  transmission of, 2065
    interspecies, 2064-2065
  treatment of, 515t, 805, 2072-2075, 2072t
    with interferons, 534
    with oseltamivir, 536-537
    with ribavirin, 538
    with zanamivir, 539-540
  type A
    myocarditis from, 1052, 1053, 1053t
    outbreaks of, 186-187, 186f
    susceptibility testing for, 238
  types of, 2078, 2078t
  vaccine for, 770, 839, 2075-2078, 2076f, 2077t, 3557, 3563f, 3564-3565, 3566-3567
    for adults, 3576f, 3577f
    for otitis media, 770
    for travelers, 3639, 3639t
    in HIV infection, 1682t
  virulence of, in selenium deficiency, 142
  vs. malaria, 3132
Influenza-like syndrome, rifamycin and, 378
Information technology. *See* Digital resources.

Informed consent, for pediatric HIV testing, 1645
Infundibulum, 773, 778f
Inguinal lymphadenitis, 1207-1208, 1209t, 1210.
    See also Lymphadenitis/Lymphadenopathy.
  filarial, 1208, 1212, 3271, 3271f
  in bubonic plague, 1208
  in cutaneous anthrax, 1208
  in sexually transmitted diseases, 1207-1208,
    1210, 1339
Injection drug users, 3462-3473
  cellulitis in, 2371
  central nervous system infections in, 3471-
    3472
  cerebral mucormycosis in, 2978
  endocarditis in, 984-985, 990, 992
    treatment of, 998, 2343-2344
  hepatitis A in, 2171, 2178, 3470
  hepatitis B in, 3469-3470
  hepatitis C in, 1961, 1965, 3470
  hepatitis D in, 3470
  hepatitis G in, 3470
  HIV infection in, 182, 1482, 3472-3473
    prevention of, 1494-1495
    serologic monitoring of, 1480, 1480f
    transmission of, 1468, 1468f, 1470, 1490
    tuberculosis with, 2874
  host defenses in, 3462-3463
  HTLV in, 2106
  infective endocarditis in, 3465-3467
    central nervous system complications of,
      3471-3472
  musculoskeletal infections in, 3464-3465
  mycotic aneurysms in, 3467-3468, 3468f, 3471
  ocular infections in, 3472
  osteomyelitis in, 1329
  pulmonary infections in, 859, 3468-3469,
    3469f
  septic thrombophlebitis in, 3467
  sexually transmitted diseases in, 3472-3473
  skin and soft tissue infections in, 1191, 3463-
    3464
  splenic abscess in, 3470-3471
  tetanus in, 3472
  wound botulism in, 3472
Injection site abscesses, 1191
Insect(s). *See also* Zoonosis(es).
  in HIV transmission, 1492
Insect control
  for babesiosis, 3214
  for flavivirus infections, 1943
  for leishmaniasis, 3154
  for Lyme disease, 2807
  for malaria, 1943, 3138
  for travelers, 3642
  methods of, 1901
Insertion sequences, in antibiotic resistance, 253,
  254-255
Insomnia, in prion diseases, 2220, 2229
Institutional outbreaks, of hepatitis A, 2171,
  2171f
Integrin(s), 9, 37
  adherence of, 16
  in antibiotic resistance, 255, 255f
  in inflammatory response, 96-97
  lymphocyte mediation by, 121
Integrin-associated protein, 97
Intensive care unit, streptococcal toxic shock
  syndrome management in, 2374
Intensive care unit patients, fever of unknown
  origin in, 719t, 721
Intercellular adhesion molecule-1, 15, 15t,
  61, 97
  in malaria susceptibility, 44t
  of rhinoviruses, 21
Intercellular adhesion molecule-2, 97

Intercellular adhesion molecule-3, 97
Interferon(s), 531-535, 555
  as pyrogens, 708-709, 709f, 711-712
  classification of, 531, 532t
  drug interactions with, 533
  for chronic hepatitis B, 1444-1445, 1448,
    1448t, 1449t, 1880, 1881, 1882
  for chronic hepatitis C, 1453-1455, 1454t
  for genital warts, 1849-1850
  for myocarditis, 1058
  mechanism of action of, 531-532
  pharmacokinetics of, 532-533
  toxicity of, 533
  uses of, 533-535
Interferon-alfa
  drug interactions with, 692t
  for acute hepatitis, 1437
    for prevention, 1437
    for treatment, 1437
  for chronic hepatitis B, 1444-1445, 1448t,
    1449t, 1880, 1881, 1882
  for colds, 2192
  for hepatitis C
    in acute infections, 1968-1969
    in chronic infections, 197t, 1453-1455,
      1454t, 1966-1968, 1966f
    with HIV coinfection, 1971-1972, 1971f
  for hepatitis D, 1450-1451
  for hepatitis, in HIV infection, 1691t
  for herpesvirus infections, 1760t, 1761
  for Kaposi's sarcoma, 1604
  for recurrent respiratory papillomatosis, 1850
  pegylated, 552t
    with ribavirin, 1578
  toxicity of, 1968
Interferon-alfa-2a
  dosage of, 680t-681t
  formulations of, 649t
Interferon-alfa-2b
  dosage of, 680t-681t
  for colds, 750
  formulations of, 649t
Interferon-alfa-2b/ribavirin, dosage of, 680t-681t
Interferon-alfacon-1, dosage of, 682t-683t
Interferon-alfa-n3, dosage of, 682t-683t
Interferon-alpha, 38, 38t, 515t, 552t, 555-556
Interferon-alpha receptor, in malaria
  susceptibility, 44t
Interferon-beta, 38, 38t
Interferon-gamma, 38, 38t, 552t, 556
  defects in, 157, 157f
  for chronic granulomatous disease, 107, 156
  for melioidosis, 2624
  for *Mycobacterium avium* complex, 2905
  for toxoplasmosis, 3188
  in mycobacterial disease susceptibility, 44t, 45,
    123
  in sepsis prevention, 922
  in viral meningitis, 1089
Interferon-gamma receptor, deficiency of, 151t
Interleukin, in leprosy, 2888
Interleukin-1, 38, 38t, 556
  as pyrogen, 708-709, 711-712
  fish oil effects on, 144
  in acute-phase response, 39
  in HIV infection, 1538, 1539, 1539f
  in meningococcal disease, 2508
  in *Pseudomonas aeruginosa* resistance, 2590
  in systemic response, 908
Interleukin-1 receptor–associated kinase-4
  deficiency, 151t, 156
Interleukin-2, 38, 38t, 557
  deficiency of, 150t
  fish oil effects on, 144
  in HIV infection, 1538, 1539

Interleukin-3, in HIV replication, 1539
Interleukin-4, 38, 38t
  in infection susceptibility, 46
Interleukin-5, in eosinophil production, 110
Interleukin-6, 38, 38t
  in acute-phase response, 39, 709
  in HIV infection, 1536, 1538, 1539, 1539f
  in meningococcal disease, 2508
  in severe sepsis, 911
  in systemic response, 908
  in viral meningitis, 1089
Interleukin-8, 38t
  in HIV replication, 1539
  in urinary tract infections, 879
Interleukin-9, in infection susceptibility, 46
Interleukin-10, 38, 38t, 557
  Epstein-Barr virus expression of, 122
  in HIV replication, 1539, 1539f
  in infection susceptibility, 46
Interleukin-12, 38, 38t, 557
  defects in, 151t, 157
  in HIV infection, 1538, 1539
  in melioidosis, 2624
Interleukin-13, 38t
  in infection susceptibility, 46
Interleukin-15, 38, 38t
  in HIV replication, 1539
Interleukin-18, 38t
  poxvirus expression of, 122
Intermediate, definition of, 223
Internet. *See* Digital resources.
Interstitial keratitis, 1400
Interstitial macrophages, 820-821
Interstitial pneumonitis. *See* Pneumonia;
  Pneumonitis.
Intertrigo, 2943, 2951
Interventricular septal hypertrophy, endocarditis
  in, 976
Intervertebral disk, osteomyelitis of, 1326-1327,
  1326f
Intestinal amebiasis, 3097-3107. *See also*
  Entamoeba histolytica.
Intestinal candidiasis, 2942
Intestinal decontamination, for cancer patients,
  3442
Intestinal flora, 1217-1218, 3423f, 3424-3426,
  3425f. *See also* Microbial flora.
  normal, 36
Intestinal flukes, 3277t, 3279f, 3282-3283
Intestinal nematodes, 3259t, 3260-3266
Intestinal roundworms, 3259t, 3260-3266
Intestinal tapeworms. *See* Tapeworms.
Intimin, of Enterobacteriaceae, 2571
Intra-abdominal abscess
  from *Bacteroides fragilis,* 2814
  from *Candida,* 2947, 2947f
    treatment of, 2950
  in transplant recipients, 3505
  vs. enteric fever, 1274t, 1278
Intra-abdominal actinomycosis, 2926-2928, 2928f
Intra-abdominal angiostrongyliasis, 3294t, 3297
Intra-abdominal infections
  anaerobic, 2812-2813, 2813f
    from gram-negative bacilli, 2841-2842
    treatment of, 2816
  from *Clostridium,* 2830
  from *Enterococcus,* 2413
  from *Pasteurella,* 2689
  from *Streptococcus anginosus* group, 2454-
    2455
  treatment of, with quinolones, 460-462
Intra-amniotic infection syndrome, 1372-1373
Intra-aortic balloon counterpulsation, infections
  of, 1039
Intracellular cytokine staining, 117-118, 118f

Intracranial abscess. *See* Brain abscess.
Intracranial hypertension
  in meningitis, 1095-1096, 1116-1117
    from *Cryptococcus,* 3007, 3008
  monitoring for, 1083
  tetracyclines and, 364
  treatment of, 1116-1117
Intracranial pressure monitoring, 1083
Intrathecal *Treponema pallidum* antibody index, 2779
Intrauterine devices
  for HIV-infected women, 1631
  pelvic inflammatory disease and, 1378
    from *Actinomyces,* 2925-2928, 2928f
Intrauterine transfusion, for hydrops fetalis, 1896
Intravascular devices. *See also specific devices.*
  percutaneous, infections due to, 3347-3358.
    See also Catheter-related infections.
  diagnosis of, 3350-3351, 3350t
  epidemiology of, 3348
  from infusate contamination, 3347-3348
  from insertion site contamination, 3348
  from junction contamination, 3348
  microbiology of, 3349-3350, 3350t
  pathogenesis of, 3347-3348, 3347f
  prevention of, 3356-3358, 3356t
  risk factors for, 3348-3349, 3349t
Intravenous drug use. *See* Injection drug users.
Intravenous immune globulin. *See* Immune globulin(s).
Intravenous lines, infection of. *See* Catheter-related infections.
Intravenous therapy. *See* Fluid management.
Intussusception
  from adenoviruses, 1838-1839
  rotavirus vaccine and, 1909-1910
Invasin, of Enterobacteriaceae, 2571
Iodochlorhydroxyquin, for traveler's diarrhea, 1242
Iodophor disinfectants, 3336
  for intravascular device insertion sites, 3356
  for skin, 479
Iodoquinol
  adverse effects of, 581t
  for amebiasis, 571t, 3106, 3106t
  for balantidiasis, 571t
  for *Blastocystis hominis,* 577t
  for *Dientamoeba fragilis,* 572t
  for luminal protozoa, 583
  indications for, 568t
Ipecac fluid, diarrhea from, 1243
Ippy virus, 2093
IRAK-4 deficiency, 38
Iridocyclitis, herpetic, 1416, 1773t
Iris lesion, in erythema multiforme, 732
Iron
  acquisition of
    by *Burkholderia cepacia,* 2617
    by Enterobacteriaceae, 2572
    by *Pseudomonas aeruginosa,* 2595
  in acute-phase response, 39
  in enteric infections, 1218
  in *Listeria monocytogenes* virulence, 2480
Iron deficiency, 142-143
  from hookworm infections, 3264
Ischemia, in sepsis, 918
Ischemic hepatitis, 1436
Isepamicin
  dosage of, 660t-661t
  names and sources of, 329t
Isohemagglutinins, 154

Isolation precautions, 3326-3330
Isoniazid, 489-491
  adverse reactions to, 490
  dosage of, 490-491, 490t, 676t-677t
  drug interactions with, 692t
  for brain abscess, 1159t
  for nontuberculous mycobacteria, 497
    in pulmonary disease, 2910, 2913t
  for tuberculosis, 489-491, 490t, 2867
    ethambutol with, 2869
    in children, 2872
    in HIV infection, 1681t, 1687t, 1699, 1700, 2870, 2871t, 2872
    latent, 2873-2874
    regimens for, 2868, 2868t, 2869
  formulations of, 649t
  hepatic function and, 245
  neurotoxicity of, 1594t
  prophylaxis with
    for quiescent tuberculosis, 2874
    in HIV infection, 1681t
Isopropyl alcohol, disinfection with, 3333-3334
Isospora [spp.], 3230-3232, 3231f
  in HIV infection, 1689t-1690t, 1701
Isospora belli, 568, 584
  AIDS cholangiopathy from, 957
  in HIV infection, 1689t-1690t, 1701
  small intestinal, 1270
  syndrome of abdominal pain, diarrhea, and eosinophilia from, 1281t, 1283
  traveler's diarrhea from, 1242
  treatment of, 569t, 577t, 578t
    with pyrimethamine, 588
    with trimethoprim-sulfamethoxazole, 573t
Israeli spotted fever, 2287t
Itching. *See* Antipruritics.
ITPA index, 2779
Itraconazole, 508-509
  dosage of, 678t-679t
  drug interactions with, 693t
  for allergic fungal sinusitis, 3072
  for aspergillosis, 2968t, 2969
    for prophylaxis, 2970
    in cystic fibrosis, 873
  for *Aspergillus* endocarditis, 1001
  for bacterial pneumonia, in HIV infection, 1689t
  for blastomycosis, 3036-3037, 3036t
  for brain abscess, 1159t, 1160
  for candidiasis, 2949-2951
    esophageal, 1234
    in HIV infection, 1683t, 1687t
  for chromoblastomycosis, 2990-2991
  for coccidioidomycosis, 3047-3048
    in HIV infection, 1683t, 1687t, 1688t
  for cryptococcosis, meningeal, 3007-3008
  for cryptococosis, in HIV infection, 1682t, 1683t, 1688t
  for dark-walled fungal infections, 3072
  for dermatophytosis, 3050t, 3058-3059
  for eumycetoma, 2995
  for fungal arthritis, 1318
  for histoplasmosis, 3023, 3024
    in HIV infection, 1682t, 1683t, 1688t, 1698
  for leishmaniasis, 592
  for microsporidiosis
    in HIV infection, 1690t
    ocular, 3249
  for paracoccidioidomycosis, 3065
  for pityriasis versicolor, 3060
  for sporotrichosis, 2987
  formulations of, 649t
  prophylactic, for cancer patients, 3445-3446, 3447t
  structure of, 503f
Ivemark's syndrome, 3525

Ivermectin
  adverse effects of, 581t
  for cutaneous larva migrans, 571t, 3296
  for filariasis, 3272
  for gnathostomiasis, 3297
  for helminthic disease, 570t
  for loiasis, 3273
  for nematodes
    intestinal, 595
    systemic, 594-595
  for onchocerciasis, 572t, 577t, 3274
  for scabies, 575t, 3306
  for strongyloidiasis, 575t, 3265
  for *Wuchereria bancrofti,* 577t
Ixodes spp., 1900-1901, 1900f, 3312-3315, 3313f, 3313t. *See also* Tick(s).
  babesiosis from, 3209-3211, 3210f
  biology and ecology of, 3312, 3313t
  ehrlichiosis from, 235, 2312
  encephalitis from, 1928, 1935, 1945t. *See also* Tick-borne encephalitis.
  Eyach virus from, 1901
  Lyme disease from, 1935, 2798-2799, 2800f, 3313t, 3314

J

Jamestown Canyon virus, 2086t, 2089
Janeway lesions, 736, 1187
  in endocarditis, 982, 983f
Japanese encephalitis, 1145, 1146
  clinical features of, 1939-1940
  diagnosis of, 238, 1942
  differential diagnosis of, 1939
  epidemiology of, 1927f, 1930-1932, 1931t, 1935f
  geographic distribution of, 1927f, 1930-1932, 1931t, 3640f
  historical perspective on, 1927
  pathogenesis of, 1937-1938
  prevention of, 1927-1928, 1944
  treatment of, 1944
  vaccine for, 1944, 3567
    for travelers, 3639t, 3640-3641
Japanese spotted fever, 2285t, 2287t, 2292-2293
Jarisch-Herxheimer reaction
  in relapsing fever treatment, 2797
  in syphilis treatment, 2782-2783
Jaundice
  in acute viral hepatitis, 1428, 1429, 1430
  in sepsis, 917
Jaw
  actinomycosis of, 2925-2926, 2925f
  fractures of, 800
  osteomyelitis of, 797t, 798
  radionecrosis of, 800
JC virus, 1856-1861
  characteristics of, 1857
  clinical manifestations of, 1858-1859, 1859f
  diagnosis of, 1859-1861
  epidemiology of, 1857, 1859t
  in pregnancy, 1858-1859, 1859t
  in transplant recipients, 3509
  laboratory studies for, 237
  pathogenesis of, 1857-1858
  prevention of, 1861
  progressive multifocal leukoencephalopathy from, 3509
  treatment of, 1861
Jet lag, 3644
Job's syndrome, 151t, 157-158, 157f
  dental history in, 149
  impaired chemotaxis in, 105-106
  pneumatoceles in, 157, 157f

Jock itch, 3054-3055, 3058-3059, 3059t
Joint Commission on Accreditation of Healthcare
    Organizations (JCAHO), 3325
Joint infections. *See also* Arthritis.
    anaerobic, 2813
        from gram-negative bacilli, 2843
    from *Brucella*, 2671
    from *Pasteurella*, 2688
    from *Pseudomonas aeruginosa*, 2602-2603
    from *Salmonella*, 2647t
    in rheumatic fever, 2383
    treatment of, with quinolones, 463
Josamycin, dosage of, 664t-665t
Journals, online, 3659t
Jugular thrombophlebitis, suppurative, 754, 754f,
    794, 794f
    lung abscess and, 854
    treatment of, 797t
Junin virus, 2090-2096, 2092t
    Argentine hemorrhagic fever from, 2090-2096,
        2091t. *See also* South American
        hemorrhagic fevers.
    as biological weapon, 3627-3629, 3627t
Juvenile diabetes mellitus, congenital mumps and,
    2006
Juvenile rheumatoid arthritis. *See also*
    Rheumatoid arthritis.
    fever in, 727
Juvenile warts, 1842, 1845. *See also* Human
    papillomavirus(es).

K

Kala-azar, 3145t, 3147, 3148, 3152-3153. *See
    also* Leishmaniasis, visceral.
Kanamycin
    antimicrobial activity of, 333, 334t-335t
    chemical family of, 330t
    dosage of, 660t-661t
    for *Mycobacterium tuberculosis*, 494, 495
    formulations of, 647t
    names and sources of, 329t
    once-daily dosage regimens for, 348t
    structure of, 329f, 330
Kaolin, tetracycline with, 364t
Kaolin-pectin, for traveler's diarrhea, 1242
Kaposi's sarcoma, 1601-1604, 1602, 1759, 1827-
    1831, 1830f, 2130. *See also* Human
    herpesvirus 8.
    clinical features of, 1602-1603, 1828-1830,
        1829f, 1830f
    epidemiology of, 1601-1602, 1828
    etiology of, 1759
    hepatic, 1579
    in HIV infection, 1557, 1557f, 1601-1604
    in transplant recipients, 1829-1830, 3509
    in women, 1627-1628
    pathogenesis of, 1602, 1828
    pulmonary, 1602, 1702
    treatment of, 1603-1604, 1702, 1831
    variants of, 1828-1830
Karshi virus, 1945t
Kartagener's syndrome, 106
Katayama fever, 3133, 3278
    vs. enteric fever, 1275t
    vs. malaria, 3133
Kato-Katz technique, for schistosomiasis,
    3280
Kawasaki disease, 3316-3318, 3316f, 3317f
    pharyngitis in, 755, 3316
    rash in, 732, 733, 3316, 3317f
    toxins in, 29-30
    vs. cellulitis, 1179
Kell antigen system, 109
Keloidal blastomycosis, 3075, 3075f, 3076t

Keratitis, 1395-1405. *See also*
    Keratoconjunctivitis; Ocular infections.
    anatomic aspects of, 1395
    clinical features of, 1396-1397
    conjunctival injection and discharge in, 1396-
        1397
    contact lens–related, 1396, 1404, 3111-3119.
        See also Keratitis, from *Acanthamoeba*.
    etiology of, 1395, 1395t
    from *Acanthamoeba*, 576t, 1398, 1404, 1405
        clinical features of, 3116-3117, 3116t, 3117f
        diagnosis of, 3117-3118
        epidemiology of, 3114
        etiology of, 3112
        pathogenesis and pathophysioloy of, 3115
        treatment of, 3117
    from adenoviruses, 754, 1389, 1402, 1404,
        1838, 1839
    from *Aspergillus*, 1404, 2963, 2966
    from *Bacillus*, 1398-1400, 2495
    from bacteria, 1397-1400
        etiology of, 1397-1398
        laboratory findings in, 1397-1400
        pathogenesis of, 1397
        treatment of, 1398-1400
    from *Candida*, 1404, 2947-2948, 2948f, 2951
    from *Chlamydia trachomatis*, 1400
    from Enterobacteriaceae, 1397-1400
    from fungi, 1404
    from *Fusarium*, 1404
    from *Haemophilus influenzae*, 1397-1400
    from herpes simplex virus, 531, 1400-1403,
        1402t, 1416, 1769, 1770f, 1773t
    from *Leishmania*, 1405
    from measles virus, 1402
    from microsporidia, 1405, 3238t, 3243-3245,
        3244f, 3248t, 3249
    from *Moxarella*, 1397-1400
    from *Mycobacterium*, 1398-1400
    from *Neisseria gonorrhoeae*, 1397-1400
    from *Nocardia*, 1398-1400
    from *Onchocerca volvulus*, 1405, 3273-3274
    from parasites, 1404-1405
    from *Pseudomonas*, 1397-1400, 2604
    from *Staphylococcus*, 1397-1400
    from *Treponema pallidum*, 1400
    from trypanosomes, 1405
    from vaccinia, 1402, 1403
    from varicella-zoster virus, 1401-1403, 1402t,
        1782, 1783
    from viruses, 1400-1404
        differential diagnosis of, 1402
        etiology of, 1400-1402
        treatment of, 1402-1404, 1402t, 1403t
    interstitial, 1400
    keratolytic, 1397
    laboratory findings in, 1396, 1397
    LASIK-related, 1398
    neurotrophic, 1401
    risk factors for, 1395-1396
Keratoconjunctivitis. *See also* Conjunctivitis;
    Ocular infections.
    epidemic, 754, 1389, 1402, 1404
    from adenoviruses, 1838
    from herpes simplex virus, 538
    from microsporidia, 1405, 3238t, 3243-3244,
        3243-3245, 3248t, 3249
    in pharyngoconjunctival fever, 754, 1398, 1402
    neonatal, antiviral drugs for, 515t
Keratolysis, pitted, 1182
Keratolytics
    for cutaneous warts, 1848
    for dermatophytosis, 3058
Keratouveitis, from herpes simplex virus, 1416-
    1417

Kereovo virus, 1899
Kerion, 3056
Kernig's sign, 1099
Ketoconazole, 507-508
    dosage of, 678t-679t
    drug interactions with, 693t
    for AIDS-related esophagitis, 1234
    for blastomycosis, 3036-3037, 3036t
    for candidiasis, 2949-2951
    for coccidioidomycosis, 3047-3048
    for conidiobolomycosis, 2981
    for eumycetoma, 2995
    for histoplasmosis, 3023, 3024
    for leishmaniasis, 592
        cutaneous, 3153
        in HIV infection, 1692t
    for paracoccidioidomycosis, 3065
    for pityriasis versicolor, 3060
    for sporotrichosis, 2987
    for vulvovaginal candidiasis, 1364
    formulations of, 649t
    structure of, 503f
Ketolides, 406-408. *See also* Telithromycin.
Kidney(s). *See also under* Renal.
    abscess of, 875, 895
        diagnosis of, 895-896, 896f
        in endocarditis, 981
        treatment of, 896
    cephalosporin effects on, 303-304
    disease of
        complement in, 87
        from BK virus, 1858-1861
        in endocarditis, 981-982
        in HIV infection, 1558-1559
        penicillin dosage in, 285, 285t
    drug-related injury of
        from aminoglycosides, 339-341, 339f, 340t,
            341t
        from amphotericin B, 2967
        from penicillins, 286
    function of
        aminoglycoside dosing and, 345-346, 345t,
            346t, 347t, 348, 348t
        in antimicrobial therapy, 243, 245
        tetracyclines and, 362, 363t, 364
    in pediatric HIV infection, 1643
    in secondary peritonitis, 935
    in sepsis, 917
    in urinary tract infections, 884, 887
    tuberculosis of, 2880, 2880t
Kidney transplantation. *See* Renal transplantation;
    Transplantation.
Kikuchi's disease, 1210
Kingella [spp.], 2529
    bacteremia from, 2534
    endocarditis from, 991, 2533
    epidemiology of, 2533
    history of, 2532-2533
    microbiology of, 2532-2533, 2533t, 2633t
    respiratory tract colonization by, 2533
    skeletal infections from, 2533
    treatment of, 2534
Kingella kingae, 2533
    arthritis from, 1312, 1312t
    cardiovascular device infections from, 1023
    laboratory identification of, 220
    prosthetic valve endocarditis from, treatment
        of, 1028, 1029t
Kirby-Bauer procedure, 223
Kissing bugs, Chagas' disease from, 3157-3158,
    3158f
Klebsiella [spp.], 2578-2579
    biliary tract infections from, 956
    Calymmatobacterium granulomatis and, 2750
    endocarditis from, 991

Klebsiella [spp.] *(Continued)*
   enterotoxigenic, 1237
   in peritoneal dialysis, 941
   mycotic aneurysm from, 1008
   prostatitis from, 894
   secondary peritonitis from, 937
   suppurative thrombophlebitis from, 1004
   treatment of
      with aminoglycosides, 334t-335t, 337t, 344t
      with nitrofurantoin, 473
      with penicillins, 284t, 288t
      with sulfonamides, 441t
      with trimethoprim, 444t
   urinary tract infections from, 881, 882
   weanling diarrhea from, 1238
Klebsiella oxytoca, 2579
   carbapenems for, 313t
   extended-spectrum beta-lactamase–producing
      strains of, in susceptibility testing, 224
Klebsiella pneumoniae, 2578
   beta-lactamase–producing, 257, 260, 938
      in susceptibility testing, 224
   endophthalmitis from, 1408
   meningitis from, 1087
   multidrug-resistant, 2578
   pancreatic infections from, 961
   peritonitis from, 929, 937
      treatment of, 938, 939
   pneumonia from
      chest film in, 829
      community-acquired, 832
      nosocomial, 836
      sputum in, 824, 824f, 825f
   pyogenic liver abscess from, 952
   quinolone-resistant, 454
   treatment of
      with aminoglycoside combination therapy,
         337t
      with carbapenems, 313t
      with cephalosporins, 298t
      with chloramphenicol, 367t
      with mupirocin, 485t
      with quinolones, 455t
      with rifamycin, 374t
      with tetracyclines, 359t
      with vancomycin, 359t
   urinary tract infections from, catheter-related,
      3372
Klebsiella pneumoniae subsp. *ozaenae,* 2579
Klebsiella pneumoniae subsp. *rhinoscleromatis,*
   2578-2579
Kluyvera spp., 2581
Koch's postulates, 11
Koilocytosis, in HIV infection, 1609
Kokobera virus, 1945t
Koplik spots, 734, 2033
Kostmann's syndrome, 104, 149
Koutango virus, 1945t
Kunjin virus, 1928, 1929, 1945t
Kuru, 2219, 2221-2222, 2222t, 2230
Kwashiorkor, 140
Kyasanur Forest disease, 1929, 1945
   as biological weapon, 3627-3629, 3628t
Kyzylagach virus, 1913-1919, 1914t. *See also*
   Alphaviruses.

L

La Crosse virus, 235t, 1146, 2086-2089, 2086t,
   2951
   ribavirin for, 538
Labial herpes. *See* Herpes simplex virus,
   orolabial.
Labor, preterm. *See also* Prematurity.
   from *Chlamydia trachomatis,* 2249

Laboratory tests. *See also specific tests,
      infections, and pathogens.*
   antimicrobial susceptibility, 222-224
   detection methods in, 214-222
   for aerobic actinomycetes, 228-229
   for central nervous system infections, 210-211
   for fungi, 229-232, 230t, 232f
   for gastrointestinal tract infections, 211-212
   for genital tract infections, 212-213
   for mycobacteria, 224-228
   for respiratory tract infections, 208, 209t
   for skin, skeletal, soft tissue infections, 213
   for sterile body fluid infections, 211
   for urinary tract infections, 211
   for viruses, 232-239
   in bioterrorism, 213-214
   specimen collection and transport in, 204, 205t-
      207t, 208
   specimen selection for, 204
Labrea hepatitis, 1432
Lacazia loboi, 3075, 3075f, 3076t
Lacrimal infections, 1420-1421, 1420f
   from *Actinomyces,* 2926
   from *Propionibacterium propionicum,* 2924
β-Lactam antibiotics. *See* Beta-lactam antibiotics.
Lactate dehydrogenase, in *Pneumocystis jirovecii*
   pneumonia, 1569
Lactate, in sepsis, 916
Lactation. *See* Breast-feeding.
Lactic acid, in stool, 1224
Lactic acidosis
   in HIV-infected women, 1630-1631
   in malaria, 3125
Lactobacillus [spp.]
   for rotavirus, 1909
   for vulvovaginal candidiasis, 1365
   Gram stain of, 2850, 2850f
   in oral cavity, 787, 787t
   infections from, 2851
   laboratory identification of, 219, 219t
   treatment of
      with daptomycin, 428
      with quinupristin-dalfopristin, 425
Lactobacillus acidophilus, vancomycin for, 418
Lactococcus spp., laboratory identification of,
   217t, 218
Lactoferrin, 908
   fecal, 1224
   in neutrophil-specific granule deficiency, 155
   neutrophil bactericidal activity, 102
Lactose intolerance, acidic stool in, 1224
Lady Windemere syndrome, 2899-2900, 2900f
Lagos bat virus, 2047t
Lagoviruses, 2196
Lamina propria, T cells in, 122
Laminin receptor, in phagocytosis, 99
Lamivudine, 515t, 535, 1657t, 1658-1659
   dosage of, 684t-685t
   drug interactions with, 693t
   for hepatitis, 1437
   for hepatitis B
      chronic, 1445-1446, 1448-1449, 1448t,
         1449t, 1450, 1880-1881, 1882
      in HIV infection, 1691t
   for perinatal HIV transmission prevention,
      1624, 1625t, 1640t
   formulations of, 649t
   pediatric, 1646t
   prophylactic, after occupational exposure to
      HIV, 3402, 3402t
   resistance to, 1660, 1881
   structure of, 520, 520f, 1656f
Langat virus, 1945t
Langer's lines, in Kaposi's sarcoma, 1602
Large intestine. *See* Colon.

Larva migrans
   cutaneous, 571t, 3294t, 3295-3296
   ocular, 3294-3295, 3294t
   visceral, 576t, 3293-3294, 3294t
Laryngeal diphtheria, 2461
Laryngitis, 758-759
   diagnosis of, 759
   etiology of, 758-759, 759t
   in blastomycosis, 759
   in candidiasis, 2951
   in histoplasmosis, 759
   in immunocompromised host, 3437
   in streptococcal pharyngitis, 759
   in tuberculosis, 759, 2882
   treatment of, 759
Laryngotracheobronchitis, 760-764
   bacterial tracheitis and, 764
   clinical features of, 762
   diagnosis of, 763
   differential diagnosis of, 763
   epidemiology of, 761
   etiology of, 760-761, 760t
   from influenza, 2070, 2071
   from respiratory syncytial virus, 2014, 2015t
   historical perspective on, 760
   incidence of, 760
   laboratory findings in, 763
   outcome in, 764
   pathophysiology of, 761-762, 762f
   prevention of, 764, 2001
   radiographic findings in, 762, 762f
   recurrent, 764
   spasmodic croup in, 760
   treatment of, 763-764, 2001
   vs. epiglottitis, 785
Laser surgery
   for cutaneous warts, 1848
   for genital warts, 1849
   for recurrent respiratory papillomatosis, 1850
   refractive, keratitis from, 1398
Lassa fever, 2090-2096
   as biological weapon, 3627-3629, 3627t
   characteristics of, 2092, 2092f
   clinical manifestations of, 2095, 3629t
   diagnosis of, 2095-2096
   disinfection/sterilization and, 3342
   epidemiology/epizootology of, 2091t, 2093
   in pregnancy, 2095
   nosocomial, 2096
   pathogenesis of, 2091t, 2094
   prevention of, 2091t, 2096
   ribavirin for, 538
   treatment of, 2091t, 2096
Lassa fever virus, receptor for, 1732t
Lateral pharyngeal space, 790, 790f
   infections of, 792, 793, 797, 797t. *See also*
      Odontogenic infections.
Lateral sinus thrombosis, 1168-1170
Latex agglutination, 242
   antigen detection by, 214-215, 214t
   for coagulase-positive vs. coagulase-negative
      gram-positive cocci, 217
   for cytomegalovirus, 237
   for pediatric viral infections, 234
   for rotavirus, 235
Latin America, HIV infection in, 1469, 1469f
   among women, 1618
Lavage
   bronchoalvelolar. *See* Bronchoalveolar lavage.
   sinus, 780, 781
Lebomo virus, 1899
Lectin
   in host receptor identification, 15, 15t
   mannose-binding. *See* Mannose-binding lectin.
   specific for Gal/GalNAc, 18-19, 18f

Lectin-binding pathway, 72
Leeches, *Aeromonas* infections from, 2754
Left ventricular assist device–related infections, 1034-1035, 3503-3504
Legionella [spp.], 2711, 2725-2728, 2725t
    acute pancreatitis from, 959, 959t
    aerosolization of, 2713, 2726
    antigen of, collection and transport of, 207t
    antisera identification of, 221
    blood culture of, 210, 210t
    cardiovascular device infections from, 1023
    characteristics of, 2711, 2725
    clinical manifestations of, 2726-2727, 2727f
    collection and transport of, 207t
    community outbreaks of, 2726
    culture of, 208
    diagnosis of, 2727
    environmental cultures for, 2720-2721
    epidemiology of, 2725-2726
    identification of, 220-221, 2711, 2712f
    in immunosuppression, 2726, 2727f, 2728f
    in stem cell transplant, 3492
    in transplant recipients, 3506
    microbial ecology of, 2712, 2712f
    myocarditis from, 1053
    pathogenesis of, 2712-2714
    pneumonia from, 209t, 2725-2726
    Pontiac fever from, 2713-2714, 2717
    prevention of, 2728
    prosthetic valve endocarditis from, 1026
    specimen selection for, 204
    treatment of, 2727-2728
        with azithromycin, 401t
        with erythromycin, 401t, 402
        with quinolones, 455t
        with quinupristin-dalfopristin, 425
        with rifamycin, 374t, 382
    vs. enteric fever, 1274t, 1278
Legionella anisa, 2725
Legionella bozemanii, 2725t, 2726
Legionella dumoffii, 2725, 2726
Legionella feeleii, 2725, 2726
Legionella longbeachae, 2726
Legionella maceachernii, 2725
Legionella micdadei, 2725, 2726, 2727f
    cutaneous infections from, 2726
Legionella pneumophila, 2711-2721, 2718, 2718t
    aerosolization of, 2716
    amebae and, 2712, 2712f
    antigen detection for, 828
    atypical disease from, 834
    chest film in, 830
    clinical presentation of, 2716-2717
    coinfection in, 2720
    community-acquired, 831-833, 2715
    complement receptors and, 78
    contagiousness of, 2714
    culture of, 208, 2718, 2718t
    detection of, 2717-2718, 2718t
    engineering modifications for, 2720
    environmental culture in, 2720-2721
    environmental decontamination in, 2716
    epidemics of, 2714-2715
    epidemiology of, 2714-2716
    history in, 823t
    history of, 2711
    identification of, 2711, 2712f
    immunofluorescent microscopy of, 2718, 2718t
    in sputum, 825, 826
    incubation period for, 2714
    investigation of, 2716
    laboratory diagnosis of, 825-830, 2717-2718, 2718t
    metastatic infections in, 2717
    mortality rates in, 2715

Legionella pneumophila (Continued)
    nosocomial, 836, 2715
    pathogenesis of, 2712-2714
    patterns of, 2714-2715
    pediatric, 2715
    pericarditis from, 1059
    pleural effusion from, 847
    prevention of, 2720-2721
    primary infections in, 2717
    risk factors for, 2715-2716
    serogroup 1, 2711
    specimen selection for, 204
    survival of, 9
    transmission of, 2716
    treatment of, 403, 836-839, 837t, 838t, 2718-2720, 2719t
        with macrolides, 397t, 398
    virulence factors of, 2714
    within macrophages, 2713, 2713f
Legionella sainthelensis, 2726
Legionella-like amebal pathogens, 2725
Leifsonia aquatica, 2471-2472
Leiomyosarcoma, in HIV infection, 1611
Leishmania [spp.], 3145-3154
    blepharoconjunctivitis from, 1393
    characteristics of, 3146-3147
    classification of, 3145t, 3146-3147
    clinical syndromes from, 3145t. *See also* Leishmaniasis.
    complement receptors and, 78
    genetic susceptibility to, 46
    in HIV infection, 1692t
    Old World, ketoconazole for, 507
    splenic abscess from, 967, 967t
    treatment of, 569t, 573t, 578t, 590, 591-592
    vectors of, 3146
Leishmania aethiopica, cutaneous leishmaniasis from, 3145t, 3150
Leishmania amazonensis
    cutaneous leishmaniasis from, 3145t, 3150
    visceral leishmaniasis from, 3145t, 3147
Leishmania braziliensis, 590
    cutaneous leishmaniasis from, 3145t, 3150, 3151
    mucocutaneous leishmaniasis from, 3145t, 3151
Leishmania chagasi, visceral leishmaniasis from, 3145t, 3147, 3148
Leishmania donovani
    miltefosine for, 578t
    pancreatic infections from, 959t, 960
    post–kala-azar dermal leishmaniasis from, 3145t, 3148
    treatment of, 590
    visceral leishmaniasis from, 3145t, 3147, 3148
Leishmania guyanensis, cutaneous leishmaniasis from, 3145t, 3150, 3151
Leishmania infantum, visceral leishmaniasis from, 3145t, 3147, 3148
Leishmania major, cutaneous leishmaniasis from, 3145t, 3150, 3151
Leishmania mexicana, cutaneous leishmaniasis from, 3145t, 3150
Leishmania panamensis, cutaneous leishmaniasis from, 3145t, 3150
Leishmania peruviana, cutaneous leishmaniasis from, 3145t, 3150
Leishmania tropica
    cutaneous leishmaniasis from, 3145t, 3150, 3151
    leishmaniasis recidivans from, 3151
    mucocutaneous leishmaniasis from, 3145t, 3151
    visceral leishmaniasis from, 3145t, 3147
    viscerotropic leishmaniasis from, 3145t, 3148

Leishmaniasis, 3146-3154
    American mucocutaneous, 3145t, 3150f, 3152, 3153
    cutaneous, 3145t, 3149-3152, 3149f, 3150f
        clinical features of, 3150f, 3151
        diagnosis of, 3151
        diffuse, 3145t, 3151
        disseminated, 3145t, 3151
        epidemiology of, 3149
        etiology of, 3149-3150
        immune response to, 3150-3151
        New World (American), 3145t, 3149-3152, 3149f, 3150f
        Old World, 3145t, 3149-3152
        pathogenesis of, 3150-3151
        relapsing, 3145t, 3151
    etiology of, 3145t, 3146-3147
    mucosal, 3145t, 3150f, 3152, 3153
    overview of, 3145-3154
    post–kala-azar dermal, 3145t, 3148-3149
    prevention of, 3154
    treatment of, 3145t, 3152-3153
    visceral, 3145t, 3147-3149, 3152-3153
        clinical features of, 3148-3149
        diagnosis of, 3149
        differential diagnosis of, 3149
        epidemiology of, 3147
        immune response to, 3147-3148
        pathogenesis of, 3147-3148
    viscerotropic, 3145t, 3148
Leishmaniasis recidivans, 3145t, 3151
Lemierre's disease, 754, 754f, 756, 794, 794f, 2841. *See also* Odontogenic infections.
    from *Arcanobacterium haemolyticum,* 2470
    lung abscess and, 854
    mediastinitis from, 1070
    treatment of, 797t
Lentiretroviruses, 2119-2120
Leprosy, 2886-2895
    borderline, 2888, 2890, 2892f
        lepromatous, 2888, 2890, 2891f
        tuberculoid, 2888, 2890, 2892f
    classification of, 2888
    clinical manifestations of, 2890-2891, 2890f-2892f
    complications of, 2893
    cytokines in, 2889
    diagnosis of, 2890-2891, 2890f-2892f
    differential diagnosis of, 2891
    epidemiology of, 2886
    erythema nodosum leprosum in, 2892, 2893f, 2895
    genetic susceptibility to, 44, 44t, 47, 2888-2889, 2889t
    histopathology of, 2891-2892, 2892f, 2983f
    history of, 2886-2887
    HIV infection in, 2891
    hypoesthesia in, 2890-2891
    immunity in, 2888, 2889
    lepromatous, 1147-1148, 2888, 2890, 2890f, 2891f
        treatment of
            with fusidic acid, 327
            with interferon-gamma, 556
    Lucio's phenomenon in, 2892, 2893f, 2895
    nerve damage in, 2889
    peripheral neuropathy in, 2891
    prevention of, 2895
    rehabilitation in, 2895
    resistance to, 48
    reversal reactions in, 2892, 2893f, 2895
    treatment of, 497-499
        adverse reactions to, 499
        in relapse, 2894-2895
        regimens for, 2894
    tuberculoid, 1147-1148, 2888

Leptomyxid ameba. *See Balamuthia mandrillaris.*
Leptospira spp., 2789-2794
  acute pancreatitis from, 959, 959t
  biphasic nature of, 2790, 2791f
  blood culture of, 210, 210t
  characteristics of, 2789, 2789f
  classification of, 2789, 2790f, 2790t
  clinical manifestations of, 2790-2792, 2791f,
    2792t
  collection and transport of, 205t, 207t
  epidemiology of, 2790
  etiology of, 2789-2790, 2789f, 2789t, 2790t
  hepatitis from, 1436
  history of, 2789
  laboratory diagnosis of, 2792-2793, 2793f
  pathogenesis of, 2790
  prevention of, 2793-2794
  transmission of, 2790
  treatment of, 2793, 2793t
  vaccine for, 2793-2794
  vs. enteric fever, 1274t, 1277
Leptospires, 2789, 2789f
  classification of, 2789, 2790f, 2790t
  direct detection of, 2792
  histology of, 2792, 2793f
  indirect detection of, 2792-2793
  isolation of, 2792
Leptospirosis
  history in, 823t
  in travelers, 3643, 3647t, 3648t, 3651
  prevention of, 3643
  uveitis in, 1416-1417
  vs. malaria, 3133
Leptotrichia spp., in oral cavity, 787, 787t
Lesbians, HIV transmission in, 1489
Lesser sac, 928
Lethal factor, of *Bacillus anthracis,* 2485
Leuconostoc spp., 2418
  laboratory identification of, 217t, 218
  linezolid for, 437, 437t
  quinupristin-dalfopristin for, 425
Leucovorin
  for *Pneumocystis jirovecii,* in HIV infection,
    1681t, 1683t, 1685t
  for *Toxoplasma gondii,* in HIV infection,
    1682t, 1683t, 1685t, 1696
Leukemia. *See also* Cancer.
  adult T-cell, 2108-2110, 2108f-2111f, 2108t
    treatment of, 2112
  Capnocytophaga infections in, 2731
  chloramphenicol and, 369
  infections in, 3432-3439
  mucormycosis in, 2975-2977
Leukocyte(s)
  in cerebrospinal fluid, 1081, 1081t
  in *Pseudomonas aeruginosa* resistance, 2591
  transfusion of, for granulocytopenia, 109
Leukocyte adhesion deficiency, 104, 154-155
  type 1, 104, 151t, 154
    periodontal disease in, 149, 152f
  type 2, 104, 151t, 155
Leukocyte function-associated antigen-1, 97
Leukocyte transfusions
  for chronic granulomatous disease, 109
  for granulocytopenia, 109
Leukocytosis
  acute, 908
  in endocarditis, 985
  neutrophilic, in sepsis, 916
Leukopenia
  from quinolones, 467
  in endocarditis, 985
Leukotrienes, in neutrophil migration, 98
Levine's classification, of beta-lactam allergy,
    320, 320t

Levofloxacin
  antimicrobial activity of, 455t, 456t
  dosage of, 458t, 672t-673t
  for bacterial arthritis, 1316t
  for *Chlamydia,* 460
  for COPD exacerbations, 811, 811t
  for deep fascial space infections, 797t
  for *Enterococcus,* 2416
  for keratitis, 1399
  for *Legionella pneumophila,* 2719t
  for *Mycobacterium avium* complex, in HIV
    infection, 1687t
  for *Neisseria gonorrhoeae,* 2524t
    in epididymitis, 2526
    in pelvic inflammatory disease, 2525
    in urethritis, 460
  for odontogenic infections, 797t
  for osteomyelitis, 1324t
  for pelvic inflammatory disease, 1379t
  for peritonitis, 461, 939
  for pneumonia, 837-839, 837t, 838t
    community-acquired, 462
    from *Legionella,* 2719t
    nosocomial, 463
  for postoperative gynecologic infections, 1377t
  for sepsis, 919t
  for *Shigella,* 2659t
  for sinusitis, 779-780, 779t
  for skin infections, 463-464
  for traveler's diarrhea, 1243
  for urinary tract infections, 460
  for urogenital chlamydial infections, 2247t,
    2249, 2250
  formulations of, 648t
  pharmacology of, 457t
  pneumococcal resistance to, 837, 837t
  structure of, 451, 452f
Levovirin, 541
Lice, 573t, 3302-3304, 3302f, 3303f
  typhus from, 2285t, 2286, 2287t, 2303-2305,
    2308
Lichen sclerosus, vulvar, 1369
Ligands
  cellular tropism and, 35
  of Toll-like receptors, 37t
Limax flavus agglutinin, 16
Limulus amebocyte lysate, 914
Lincomycin, 408-411
  adverse reactions to, 410
  antimicrobial activity of, 408-409
  chemistry of, 408, 409f
  dosage of, 666t-667t
  formulations of, 648t
  mechanism of action of, 408
  pharmacology of, 409-410
Lincosamide, resistance to, 261-262, 263, 263t
  by *Staphylococcus aureus,* 2334t, 2335-2336
Lindane
  for lice, 3303-3304
  for scabies, 3306
Linezolid
  adverse effects of, 438-439
  antimicrobial activity of, 437, 437t
  dosage of, 668t-669t
  drug interactions with, 693t
  for brain abscess, 1160
  for cellulitis, 1180
  for *Enterococcus,* 2417
    multidrug-resistant, 1028, 1029t
    vancomycin-resistant, 438
  for nocardiosis, 2920t, 2921
  for nontuberculous mycobacteria, 497
  for osteomyelitis, 1324t, 1325
  for pneumonia, 438, 837-839, 837t, 838t
  for *Staphylococcus aureus,* 438, 2336-2337

Linezolid *(Continued)*
  for *Streptococcus pneumoniae,* 438
  for tuberculosis, 494, 495
  formulations of, 648t
  pharmacology of, 437
  resistance to, 438
    by enterococci, 438, 1028, 1029t
    by pneumococci, 837, 837t
    by *Staphylococcus aureus,* 2334t
  structure of, 436, 436f
α-Linolenic acid, 143
Lipids, in sepsis, 916
Lipocortin-1, antipyretic effects of, 710
Lipodystrophy, 609
Lipolysis, 909
Liponyssoides sanguineus, 3311
  as rickettsialpox vector, 2295-2296
Lipo-oligosaccharide
  in *Moraxella (Branhamella) catarrhalis,* 2530
  in *Neisseria gonorrhoeae,* 2514, 2516
  in *Neisseria meningitidis,* 2500, 2503-2504
Lipopeptides, 427-428. *See also* Daptomycin.
Lipopolysaccharide, 907, 907f
  composition of, 77
  in bacterial sepsis, 712, 714
  in febrile response, 708, 710, 711
  of *Bacteroides fragilis,* 2814
  of *Bordetella,* 2702
  of Enterobacteriaceae, 2569, 2572
  of *Helicobacter pylori,* 2559
  of *Legionella,* 2714
  of *Pseudomonas aeruginosa,* 2588, 2588f,
    2595
Lipopolysaccharide receptor, 34
Lipopolysaccharide-binding protein, 907, 907f
Lipoprotein, in sepsis, 916
Lipoprotein receptors, 75
Liposomal amphotericin B. *See also*
    Amphotericin B.
  for aspergillosis, 2968-2969, 2968t
    for prophylaxis, 2970
  for brain abscess, 1159t
  for mucormycosis, 2979
Lipoteichoic acid
  in *Staphylococcus aureus,* 2327
  in *Streptococcus pyogenes* (group A), 2363
Lipovnic virus, 1899
Liquid nitrogen, for human papillomavirus, 1691t
Lisofylline, 560
Listeria [spp.]
  endocarditis from, 991
  laboratory differentiation of, 2478, 2479t
Listeria monocytogenes, 2478-2483
  bacteremia from, 2481
  brain abscess from, 1151, 1158t, 2481
  brain stem encephalitis from, 2481, 2482f
  cellular immunity to, 2480
  central nervous system infections from, 2480,
    2481
  cytoplasmic replication of, 123
  diagnosis of, 2482, 2482t
  endocarditis from, 991, 2481
  epidemiology of, 2478-2479
  febrile gastroenteritis from, 2481-2482
  foodborne disease from, 2479, 2481-2482
    prevention of, 2483, 2483t
  in neonates, 2480
  in pregnancy, 2480
  intra-amniotic infection syndrome from, 1372
  laboratory identification of, 219, 219t
  meningitis from, 1087, 1106t, 1113, 2481,
    2481t, 2483
    in transplant recipients, 3507
  microbiology of, 2478
  mycotic aneurysm from, 1008

Listeria monocytogenes (Continued)
  pathogenesis of, 2479-2480
  prevention of, 1297t, 2483, 2483t
  survival by, 9
  treatment of, 2482-2483
    with aminoglycoside combination therapy,
      336t, 337t
    with carbapenems, 313t
    with linezolid, 437, 437t
    with macrolides, 397t, 398
    with mupirocin, 485t
    with penicillins, 284t, 288t
    with quinolones, 456t
    with quinupristin-dalfopristin, 425
    with rifamycin, 374t
    with sulfonamides, 441t
    with trimethoprim, 444t
    with trimethoprim-sulfamethoxazole, 444
    with vancomycin, 418
Lithium, metronidazole interactions with, 393t
Liver. *See also under* Hepatic.
  antimicrobial therapy and, 244, 245
  complement synthesis in, 71
  cystic lesions of, 953, 3290-3291, 3291f
    differential diagnosis of, 3105
  echinococcal cyst of, 953
  hydatid cyst of, 3290-3291, 3291f
  in infection response, 908
  in leptospirosis, 2792
  in primary peritonitis, 929-930
  in sepsis, 917
  schistosomiasis of, 3279
  shock, 1436
  steatosis of, in HIV-infected women, 1630-1631
  trematode infections of, 595
  tuberculosis of, 2881
Liver abscess, 943, 951-955
  actinomycotic, 2927-2928
  amebic, 951-955
    clinical features of, 3103
    diagnosis of, 3105
    pleural effusion in, 847, 849
    treatment of, 3105, 3106, 3106t
  antibiotics for, 954-955, 954t
  clinical presentation of, 952-953, 952t
  CT-guided aspiration of, 954, 954f
  diagnosis of, 953
  epidemiology of, 951
  etiology of, 951
  in chronic granulomatous disease, 155, 156f
  in neutrophil disorders, 154
  in transplant recipients, 3505
  microbiology of, 952, 952t
  pathogenesis of, 951-952
  pathophysiology of, 951-952
  pyogenic, 951
  routes of, 952t
  treatment of, 953-955, 954f, 954t
Liver biopsy
  in acute viral hepatitis, 1429, 2175
  in chronic hepatitis C, 1452, 1963, 1963t
  in hepatitis C, 1452, 1961-1962, 1963, 1963t
  in hepatitis E, 2209, 2209f
Liver disease. *See also under* Hepatic;
  Hepatitis.
  alcoholic, 1436
  autoimmune, 1436
  differential diagnosis of, 1435-1436, 1435t
  drug-related
    from chloramphenicol, 368
    from isoniazid, 490, 2873
    from nitrofurantoin, 475
    from rifamycin, 377
    from tetracycline, 363t, 364
  in HIV infection, 1579

Liver disease *(Continued)*
  in Budd-Chiari syndrome, 1436
  in HIV infection, 1577-1579, 1578t
  in pregnancy, 1436
  in Wilson's disease, 1436
  ischemic, 1436
  quinolone dosage in, 458, 458t
  tuberculosis in, 2872
Liver enzymes, in hepatic fibrosis, 1964
Liver failure. *See* Hepatic failure.
Liver flukes, 3277t, 3279f, 3281-3282, 3281f
Liver transplantation. *See also* Transplantation.
  cytomegalovirus in, 1436, 1795-1796, 3502t,
    3508-3509
    from donor organ, 1794
    ganciclovir for, 530
    prevention of, 1793-1794
  fibrosing cholestatic hepatitis after, 1449, 1456
  for chronic hepatitis C, 1456
  for fulminant liver failure, 1437
  for hepatitis A, 2179
  hepatitis B after, 1449-1450, 1877-1878, 1881-
    1882
    prophylaxis for, 1449-1450
  infections in, 2502t, 3502f, 3502t, 3504-3505.
    See also Transplantation, infections in.
  surgical factors in, 3477, 3477f
  prognostic indicators in, 1436
  survival in, 3501, 3501t
  toxoplasmosis after, 3177t, 3178
Loa loa, 3272-3273, 3272f
  treatment of infection with, 572t, 577t, 595
Loboa loboi, laboratory studies of, 229
Lobomycosis, 3075, 3075f, 3076t
Lobo's disease, 3075, 3075f, 3076t
Lockjaw, 2818, 2818f
Locus of enterocyte effacement island, in
  Escherichia coli, 2575
Lomefloxacin
  dosage of, 672t-673t
  formulations of, 648t
Lone Star tick, 3312-3314, 3313f, 3313t
Long-term care facilities, diarrhea in, 1241
Loperamide
  for *Clostridium difficile*–associated colitis,
    1258
  for traveler's diarrhea, 1243, 3643f
Lopinavir, 1665t, 1667
  drug interactions with, 696t-697t
  resistance to, 1668
  structure of, 1663f
Lopinavir-ritonavir
  dosage of, 684t-685t
  drug interactions with, 696t-697t
  formulations of, 649t
  pediatric, 1646t
Loracarbef
  dosage of, 658t-659t
  formulations of, 648t
  structure of, 295f
  uses of, 305, 305t
Lordsdale virus, 2196. *See also* Caliciviruses.
Louping ill virus, 1929
Louse-borne typhus, 2285t, 2286, 2287t, 2303-
  2305, 2308
Loxosceles laeta bites, 3653f
LPXTG, in *Staphylococcus aureus,* 2326,
  2327t
Lucilia spp., myiasis from, 3308-3310, 3308t
Lucio's phenomenon, 2892, 2893f
  treatment of, 2895
Ludwig's angina, 754, 756, 793, 793f, 2841. *See
  also* Odontogenic infections.
  mediastinitis from, 1070
  treatment of, 793, 797, 797t

Lumbar puncture, 1080-1082. *See also*
  Cerebrospinal fluid analysis.
  for subdural empyema, 1164
Lumefantrine, for malaria, 3134t, 3135
Lund's fly, myiasis from, 3308, 3308t
Lung. *See also under* Pulmonary; Respiratory.
  acute injury to, in sepsis, 917
  cavitary lesions of, differential diagnosis of,
    854t, 855, 860, 861t
  diseases of, in endocarditis, 982
  fungus balls of, 2962-2963
  host defenses in, 820-822
    impairment of, 821-822
  hydatid cyst of, 3290-3292
  in Kaposi's sarcoma, 1602
  in severe sepsis, 913, 913f
  indigenous flora of, 808
  nitrofurantoin effects on, 475
Lung abscess, 853-856, 854t, 855f, 2624, 2625f,
  2626f
  from *Entamoeba histolytica,* 3103
  from *Nocardia,* 1151t, 1152, 2916f, 2917-2918
  in melioidosis, 2624, 2625f, 2626f
Lung biopsy
  for *Pneumocystis,* 3087
  in acute pneumonia, 827
  in chronic pneumonia, 863-864
  in paracoccidioidomycosis, 3064-3065, 3065f
Lung cancer
  in female HIV infections, 1627
  tuberculosis in, 2867
Lung flukes, 3277t, 3279f, 3283
Lung transplantation
  aspergillosis in, 2961, 2961f
  Burkholderia cepacia in, 871, 2618, 2619f
  cytomegalovirus in, 3477, 3478t
  in cystic fibrosis
    outcome of, 873
    pulmonary infections and, 871
  infections in, 3502t, 3504. *See also*
    Transplantation, infections in.
  parainfluenza virus in, 2000
  survival in, 3501t
Lupus. *See* Systemic lupus erythematosus.
Lupus-like syndrome, rifamycin and, 378
Lutzomyia spp., leishmaniasis from, 3146
Lyme disease, 1935, 2798-2807. *See also
  Borrelia burgdorferi.*
  animal hosts for, 2798-2799
  animal model of, 2800-2801
  arthritis in, 2800, 2805
  cardiac involvement in, 2802, 2802t
  clinical manifestations of, 2801-2803
  coinfection in, 2803
  congenital, 2803
  differential diagnosis of, 2804-2806
  disseminated, 2801-2802, 2802t
  encephalitis in, 1145, 1146, 1935
  epidemiology of, 2799
  erythema migrans in, 734, 738, 2798, 2801-
    2802, 2801f, 2802t, 3314f
  from *Ixodes* spp., 1935
  laboratory diagnosis of, 2803-2804, 2804f, 2805f
  localized, 2801, 2801f, 2802t
  meningitis in
    acute, 1088, 1100, 1104, 1106t, 1115
    chronic, 1137
  myocarditis from, 1053
  neurologic abnormalities in, 2802, 2802t
  ocular infections in, 2802, 2802t
  pathogenesis of, 2800
  persistent, 2800, 2803
  prevention of, 2807
  stages of, 2801-2803, 2802t
  tick vectors of, 2798-2799, 2800f

Lyme disease *(Continued)*
    transmission of, 2798-2799, 2800f
    treatment of, 405-406, 2806-2807, 2806t
    uveitis in, 1417
    vaccine for, 3315
    vs. tick-borne encephalitis, 1942
Lymph nodes
    anatomy of, 119-120, 120f
    B cells in, 121
    blood flow in, 120, 120f
    drainage of, cellulitis and, 2371
    renal, in pyelonephritis, 876
    T cells in, 121
Lymphadenitis/lymphadenopathy, 1204-1211. *See also* Lymphangitis.
    axillary, 1205
    cervical, 799, 1205, 1208, 1209t
        in HIV infection, 1206
        tuberculous, 1206-1207
    chronic, 1204-1205
    clinical features of, 1205
    dermatopathic, 1204-1205
    differential diagnosis of, 1208-1210, 1209t
    epitrochlear, 1205-1206
    etiology of, 1208-1210, 1209t
    from adenoviruses, 1838
    from filaria, 1208, 1212, 3271, 3271f
    from *Mycobacterium avium* complex, 2897, 2899, 2902, 2902f, 2903-2905, 2904t, 2906
    from *Mycobacterium tuberculosis,* 2881-2882, 2882f
    from nontuberculous mycobacteria, 1206-1207, 2910t, 2911
    from *Paracoccidioides brasiliensis,* 3065
    from rickettsiae, 2287t
    from *Sporothrix,* 1211-1213, 2984-2985, 2985f
    from *Toxoplasma gondii,* 1210, 3175f, 3176, 3177
    generalized, 1208, 1209t, 1210
        in HIV infection, 1210-1211
    granulomatous, from nondiphtheria *Corynebacterium,* 1207
    histiocytic necrotizing, 1210
    iliac, 1206
    in cat-scratch disease, 1207
    in chronic granulomatous disease, 1210
    in HIV infection, 1206, 1207, 1210-1211
    in infectious mononucleosis, 1806
    in Marshall's syndrome, 1208
    in oculoglandular syndrome, 1207
    in Rosai-Dorfman disease, 1210
    in sexually transmitted diseases, 1207-1208
    inguinal, 1207-1208, 1209t, 1210, 1339
        differential diagnosis of, 2245
        filarial, 1208, 1212, 3271, 3271f
        in bubonic plague, 1208
        in cutaneous anthrax, 1208
        in sexually transmitted diseases, 1207-1208, 1210, 1339
    mediastinal, 1205, 1207
        in inhalational anthrax, 1073
    mesenteric, 1279-1280
        from *Yersinia pseudotuberculosis,* 2699
    nonpyogenic, 1206-1208
    pathogenesis and pathology of, 1204-1205
    preauricular, 1207
    pyogenic, 1205-1206
    recurrent, 1208
    subpectoral, 1205
    suppurative, 1205-1206
    treatment of, 122, 1211
    tuberculous, 2881-2882, 2882f
    with sinus histiocytosis, 1210

Lymphangioleiomyomatosis, chest film in, 863f
Lymphangioma, infected, 799-800
Lymphangitis, 1211-1213, 1212t. *See also* Lymphadenitis/lymphadenopathy.
    chronic granulomatous, 1210, 1212
    filarial, 1208, 1212
    from cat-scratch disease, 2736-2737, 2737f, 2738f
    from *Francisella tularensis,* 2679, 2680f
    from *Mycobacterium tuberculosis,* 2882
    from *Streptococcus pyogenes* (group A), 2375
    mediastinal, tuberculous, 2882
    persistent generalized, in HIV infection, 1553-1554
Lymphedema, chronic, 1213
Lymphocutaneous sporotrichosis, 1211-1213, 2984-2985, 2985f
Lymphocyte(s). *See also* B cell(s); T cell(s).
    chemokine mediation of, 121
    defects in, 152-154, 157-158
    in cerebrospinal fluid, 1081, 1081t
    integrin mediation of, 121
    intraepithelial, 122
    on mucosal surface, 122
    pulmonary, 821
    turnover of, in HIV infection, 1535
Lymphocyte count, 152
    in malnutrition, 140
Lymphocyte function–associated molecule 1, 61
Lymphocytic choriomeningitis virus, 2090-2096
    characteristics of, 2092
    clinical manifestations, extrameningeal, 2095
    clinical manifestations of, 2091t, 2094-2095
    collection of, 233t
    diagnosis of, 2095-2096
    epidemiology/epizootology of, 2091t, 2092-2093
    in pregnancy, 2095
    meningitis from, 19, 1085, 1099, 1101, 2090-2096, 2091t
    pathogenesis of, 2093, 2093t
    prevention of, 2091t, 2096
    receptor for, 1732t
    treatment of, 2091t, 2096
Lymphocytopenia, 152
    idiopathic CD4$^+$ T, 1484
Lymphocytosis
    from Epstein-Barr virus, 1810-1811, 1810t, 1811t
    HIV-related, neuropathy in, 1595-1596, 1597f
Lymphogranuloma venereum, 1341
    clinical manifestations of, 1339, 1341
    conjunctivitis and, 1390, 1391
    epidemiology of, 1342
    from *Chlamydia trachomatis,* 1338-1344, 2244-2245
    inguinal buboes in, 1207
    laboratory diagnosis of, 2242
    pathogenesis of, 2241
    presentation of, 1338-1339
    treatment of, 1344, 2245
        with erythromycin, 401t
Lymphoid tissue
    anatomy of, 119
    in HIV infection, 1533, 1534
Lymphoid tumors
    immune dysfunction in, 158
    mucosa-associated, *Helicobacter pylori* in, 2562
Lymphoma. *See also* Cancer.
    adult T-cell, 2108-2110, 2108f-2111f, 2108t
        treatment of, 2112

Lymphoma *(Continued)*
    B-cell
        chronic hepatitis C and, 1456
        in HIV infection, 1605
    Burkitt's, 1808-1809, 1808t
    central nervous system, in HIV infection, 1588-1589, 1589f, 1607-1609, 1813
    Epstein-Barr virus–related, 1808-1810, 1808t, 1809f, 1813
    fever in, 723, 723f, 726
    gastric, from *Helicobacter pylori,* 2562
    HIV-related, 1588-1589, 1589f, 1702, 1813, 2130
    Hodgkin's, 1808t, 1809-1810, 1809f
    infections in, 3432-3439
    non-Hodgkin's. *See* Non-Hodgkin's lymphoma.
    primary effusion (body cavity), 1602, 1605, 1810, 1830, 1830f
        from Epstein-Barr virus, 1810
        from human herpesvirus 8, 1830, 1830f
Lymphopenia, idiopathic CD4$^+$, 158
Lymphoproliferative disease
    from Epstein-Barr virus, 66, 1808-1810, 1808t, 1809f
    in transplant recipients, 3510
    X-linked, 150t, 1435, 1807, 1814-1815
        treatment of, 1814-1815
Lymphostatin, 1221
Lyophilized hydrogen peroxide, for bacterial vaginosis, 1366
Lysozyme, 35
    neutrophil bactericidal activity of, 102
Lyssaviruses, 2047-2048, 2047t. *See also* Rabies.
    characteristics of, 2047-2048, 2047t, 2048f, 2048t
    classification of, 2047, 2047t
    replication of, 2048

M

M protein, in group A *Streptococcus,* 2363, 2363f
M2 inhibitors, for influenza, 2072-2073, 2072t
Mac-1, 97
Macaca monkeys
    hepatitis B virus from, 1832-1834, 1832f
    in HIV vaccine testing, 1712
Macacanema flormosana, ocular infections from, 3273
Machupo virus, 2090-2096, 2092t
    as biological weapon, 3627-3629, 3627t
    Bolivian hemorrhagic fever from, 2090-2096, 2091t. *See also* South American hemorrhagic fevers.
Macroevolutionary change, in antibiotic resistance, 253
Macroglobulins, in endocarditis, 981
Macrolides, 396-402. *See also* Azithromycin; Clarithromycin; Erythromycin.
    for *Legionella,* 2727-2728
    for nontuberculous mycobacterial infections, 496
    for pneumococcal pneumonia, 2404
    for streptococcal pharyngitis, 2368
    indications for, 397t, 401t
    resistance to, 263t
        by *Staphylococcus aureus,* 2334t, 2335-2336
        enzymes in, 261-263
        rifamycin interaction with, 376t
Macrophage(s), 56
    in HIV infection, 1537
    in phagocytosis, 37
    in *Pseudomonas aeruginosa* resistance, 2591
    in tuberculosis response, 2859-2860
    Legionella pneumophila of, 2713, 2713f

Macrophage(s) (Continued)
  pulmonary, 820
  Salmonella of, 2643-2644
Macrophage infectivity potentiator, 2714
Macrophage migration-inhibiting factor, in severe
  sepsis, 911
Macules, 730t, 731
Maculopapular rash. *See also* Rash.
  causes of, 732-733
Mad cow disease. *See* Bovine spongiform
  encephalopathy.
Madura foot, 2916, 2917, 2991-2995, 2992t
Madurella spp., mycetoma from, 2916, 2917,
  2991-2995, 2992t
Maduromycosis, 2916, 2917, 2991-2995
Mafenide, 441, 484t
  for burns, 3548-3549, 3550
Maggots, myiasis from, 3307-3310, 3308t
Magnetic resonance cholangiography, 956
Magnetic resonance imaging. *See also*
  Radiography.
  for AIDS dementia, 1585, 1585f
  for brain abscess, 7f, 1155-1157
  for central nervous system infections, 1082,
    1103, 1104f, 1135
  for Creutzfeldt-Jakob disease, 2224-2225, 2226
  for epidural abscess, 1167, 1167f
  for intraperitoneal abscess, 944
  for lymphadenitis, 2738f
  for meningitis
    acute, 1082, 1103, 1104f
    chronic, 1082, 1135
  for mycotic aneurysm, 1008
  for myocarditis, 1056
  for odontogenic infections, 780
  for osteomyelitis, 1323, 2346, 2347f
  for pleural effusion/empyema, 849
  for Pott's disease, 2879f
  for primary central nervous system lymphoma,
    1589, 1589f
  for progressive multifocal leukoencephalopathy,
    1590, 1590f, 1860, 1860f
  for prosthetic vascular graft infections, 1037
  for pyomyositis, 1197
  for rabies, 2052, 2052f
  for septic arthritis, 1313, 1314f
  for sinusitis, 778
  for splenic abscess, 968
  for subdural empyema, 1164-1165, 1166f
  for suppurative intracranial thrombosis, 1169, 1169f
  for vertebral osteomyelitis, 1326, 1326f
Major histocompatibility complex (MHC),
  polymorphism of, vaccines and, 3558
Major histocompatibility complex (MHC)
  molecules, 75
  alleles of, in HIV nonprogression, 1532
  class I, 131
    antigen processing by, 126-127, 127f
    cross-priming by, 127
    in antiviral defense, 126-127
    structure of, 125, 125f
  class II
    antigen processing by, 127-128, 128f
    structure of, 125-126, 125f
  defective, 150t
  immunogenetics of, 131-135
  in phagocytosis, 37
  in T-cell activation, 61-62, 132
  in viral infections, 122
Major histocompatibility complex (MHC)
  tetramers, 118-119, 119f
Malabsorption
  bacterial overgrowth with, 1244
  from *Giardia lamblia,* 3201
  in tropical sprue, 1303-1304

Malaria, 3121-3138. *See also under Plasmodium*
  [spp.].
  anemia in, 3125, 3132
  cerebral, 3122, 3123
  clinical presentation of, 3129
  control of, 3121, 3121f, 3128
  course of, 3129-3130
  diagnosis of, 3129-3132
    blood smears in, 3130-3131
    in severe disease, 3131-3132, 3131t
    rapid diagnostic tests in, 3131
    specimen collection and transport for, 205t
  diarrhea in, 1242
  differential diagnosis of, 3132-3133, 3132t
  drug-resistant
    geographic distribution of, 3128-3129, 3128f
    mechanisms of resistance in, 3129
    mortality trends and, 3121, 3121f
  Duffy antigen and, 3127
  emergence of, 183-184, 183f
  epidemiology of, 3127-3128, 3128f
  fever in, 723, 723f
  from *Plasmodium falciparum,* 3123-3125
  from *Plasmodium malariae,* 3126
  from *Plasmodium ovale,* 3125-3126
  from *Plasmodium vivax,* 3125-3126
  genetic resistance to, 3126-3127
  genetic susceptibility to, 43-44, 44t
  geographic distribution of, 3127-3128, 3128f
  glucose-6-phosphate dehydrogenase deficiency
    and, 43, 44, 44t, 46, 3126-3127
  hemoglobin C and, 3126
  hemoglobin E and, 3126
  hemoglobin F and, 3126
  hemoglobin S and, 3126
  historical perspective on, 3121-3122
  history in, 3129-3130
  hyperbilirubinemia in, 3132
  hypergammaglobulinemia in, 65
  hyperparasitemia in, 3132
  hypoglycemia in, 3125, 3132
  immunology of, 3127, 3127f
  in pregnancy, 3125, 3127
  in sub-Saharan Africa, 3121, 3121f
  in travelers, 3128, 3129, 3647t, 3649,
    3648t
    prevention of, 3641-3642, 3641t
  insect control for, 1943, 3138
  late-onset (recrudescent), 3129-3132
  metabolic acidosis in, 3125
  mortality in
    causes of, 3133
    trends in, 3121, 3121f
  mosquito control for, 3138
  paroxysms in, 3122, 3129-3130
  pathogenesis and pathophysiology of, 3122-
    3126, 3123f
  physical examination in, 3129-3130
  placental, 3125
  postsplenectomy, 3528
  prevention of, 184, 1943, 3136-3138, 3138
    in travelers, 3641-3642, 3641t
  prostration in, 3132
  public health impact of, 3121, 3123
  pulmonary edema in, 3125
  rash in, 734
  resistance to, 47
  respiratory distress in, 3125, 3132
  risk assessment for, 3136-3137
  severe, clinical/laboratory criteria for, 3131-
    3132, 3131t
  shock in, 3132
  sickle cell disease and, 35, 43, 44, 46, 3126
  sickle cell trait and, 35, 43, 44, 46
  Southeast Asian ovalocytosis and, 3127

Malaria (Continued)
  splenic rupture in, 3126
  susceptibility to, 47
  thalassemia and, 3126
  transfusion-related, 3388
  transmission of, 183
  treatment of, 573t-574t, 578t-579t, 584-588,
    584f, 585f, 605, 605f, 606f, 3133-3136,
    3135
    CDC Hotline for, 3135
    complementary and alternative medicine in,
      604t
    drug resistance in. *See* Malaria, drug-
      resistant.
    for infants, 3135
    for travelers, 3135
    general principles of, 3133
    in *falciparum* malaria, 3133
    in non-*falciparum* malaria, 3134t, 3136
    in pregnancy, 3135
    in severe malaria, 3134t, 3135-3136
    in uncomplicated malaria, 3133-3135, 3134t
    insecticide-treated bed nets in, 184
  vomiting in, 3132
  vs. enteric fever, 1275t, 1277, 1278
Malaria Hotline, 3135
Malassezia [spp.]
  folliculitis from, 1175, 3060-3061
  pityriasis versicolor from, 3060
  seborrheic dermatitis from, 3061
  species of, 3060
Malassezia furfur, 3060, 3073-3074, 3076t
  folliculitis from, 1175, 3060-3061
  suppurative thrombophlebitis from, 1004
Malassezia globosa, 3074
Malassezia obtusa, 3074
Malassezia restricta, 3074
Malassezia slooffiae, 3074
Malassezia sympodialis, 3074
Malathion
  adverse effects of, 581t
  for lice, 3303-3304
Malayan filariasis, 3270-3272, 3270f-3272f
Malignant disease. *See* Cancer.
Malignant otitis externa, 766
Malnutrition
  bacterial overgrowth with, 1226, 1244
  cryptosporidiosis and, 3219-3220
  diagnosis of, 140, 140t
  diarrhea and, 1215
  epidemiology of, 140
  immunosuppression in, 3427
  in elderly, 146-147, 146t
  in HIV infection, 144-145
  infections in, 39-40
  protein-energy, 140-141, 146, 146t
  treatment of, 144, 146-147, 146t
Malpractice, endocarditis prophylaxis and, 1049-
  1050
Mandible
  actinomycosis of, 2925, 2925f
  fractures of, 800
  osteomyelitis of, 794-795, 797t, 798
  radionecrosis of, 800
Mange
  red, 3311
  sarcoptic, 3305
Mannose receptor, 124
  in phagocytosis, 37
Mannose-associated serum proteases, 71, 75
Mannose-binding lectin, 36-37, 69t
  deficiency of, 80t
  gene polymorphisms in, 913
  in hepatitis B susceptibility, 45
  in infection susceptibility, 48

Mannose-binding lectin (Continued)
in local host response, 908
in mycobacterial disease susceptibility, 44t
in Pseudomonas aeruginosa resistance, 2590
Mannose-binding lectin–associated serine
protease, deficiency of, 80t, 81, 83
Mannose-binding protein, 69t, 70
deficiency of, 81, 83
in abnormal phagocytosis, 106
in bronchial asthma, 110-111
in complement activation, 71
in mycobacterial infections, 78
Mansonella [spp.], 3274
Mansonella ozzardi, 572t, 577t
Mansonella perstans, 572t
Mansonella streptocerca, 572t
Mansonia spp., Venezuelan equine encephalitis
from, 1915
MAP 19, 75
Marasmus, 140
Marburg virus, 739, 2057-2059
as biological weapon, 3627-3629, 3628t
clinical features of, 3629t
disinfection/sterilization and, 3342
Marginal blepharitis, 1419-1420, 1420f
Maribavir, 541
Marine biotoxins, 3255-3256, 3255f, 3256t
Marshall's syndrome, 1208
Masks, health care personnel use of, 3327t, 3328,
3329
Massage, immune effects of, 609
Masseteric space, 790, 790f
infections of, 791-792. See also Odontogenic
infections.
Mast cells, degranulation of, 319, 319f
Masticator spaces, 790, 790f
infections of, 791-792, 792f. See also
Odontogenic infections.
Mastitis, staphylococcal, 2340
Mastoiditis, 771
suppurative intracranial thrombophlebitis from,
1168-1170
Mastomys spp., Lassa virus from, 2093, 2094
Matrix proteins, viral, 1730-1731, 1731f
Maxillary actinomycosis, 2925-2926
Maxillary fractures, 800
Maxillary osteomyelitis, 794-795, 797t, 798
Maxillary ostium, 773, 778f
Maxillary sinus, anatomy and physiology of, 773,
773t, 778f
Maxillary sinusitis, 794. See also Odontogenic
infections; Sinusitis.
Maxillofacial trauma, 800
Maximal serum concentration:minimum
inhibitory concentration ratio, 276-277, 276f
Mayaro virus, 1913-1919, 1914t. See also Alphaviruses.
MbtB, 2887
MC virus, 2195. See also Caliciviruses.
MCP, 75
MD-2, 907, 907f
Measles, mumps, rubella (MMR) vaccine, 1117,
1921-1924, 2007, 2032, 2035-2036, 3563f,
3564t, 3567-3568
autism and, 2036
complications of, 2036
for adults, 346f, 347f
in pediatric HIV infection, 1650
schedule for children, 3564t
Measles immune globulin, 2035
Measles virus, 2031-2036
atypical, 2034
characteristics of, 2031-2032
clinical manifestations of, 2033-2034
collection of, 233t
complications of, 2033-2034

Measles virus (Continued)
congenital, 2034-2035
conjunctivitis from, 1390
croup from, 761
culture of, 2031-2032
diagnosis of, 2035
encephalitis from, 2032, 2034
epidemiology of, 2032
hepatitis from, 2034, 2035
immune response to, 2033
in adults, 2035
in immunocompromised host, 2034
prevention of, 2035, 2036
in neonate, 2035
in pregnancy, 2034-2035
in tuberculosis, 2035
keratitis from, 1402
Koplik spots from, 734, 2033
modified, 2034
otitis media from, 2035
pancreatic infections from, 959t, 960
pathogenesis of, 2032-2033
pneumonia from, 2034
prevention of, 2035-2036
rash from, 2033, 2033f
receptors for, 1732t
sinusitis from, 2035
subacute sclerosing panencephalitis from, 2032
transmission of, 2032
treatment of, 2036
vaccine for, 2032, 2035-2036, 3567-3568. See
also Measles, mumps, rubella (MMR)
vaccine.
atypical measles after, 2034
vitamin A for, 141
Mebendazole
adverse effects of, 581t
drug interactions with, 693t
for ascariasis, 571t, 3263
for capillariasis, 571t, 3298
for enterobiasis, 572t, 3266
for helminthic disease, 570t
for hookworms, 3264
for hydatid cyst, 3291
for intestinal nematodes, 593
for trichinosis, 576t, 3269
for Trichomonas vaginalis, 576t
for Trichostrongylus, 576t
for Trichuris trichiura, 576t
for visceral larva migrans, 576t
structure of, 593f
MecA, 2333
Mechanical ventilation
for botulism, 2825-2826
in immunocompromised host, 3437
pneumonia and, 835-836, 3362-3363. See also
Pneumonia, nosocomial.
diagnosis of, 827
pneumonia from. See also Pneumonia,
nosocomial.
lung abscess from, 854
MecI, 2333
MecRI, 2333
Media, culture, 215, 216t
Mediastinal actinomycosis, 2926
Mediastinal histoplasmosis, 3017-3018, 3018f
treatment of, 3023
Mediastinal lymphadenitis, 1205, 1207
Mediastinitis, 1070-1075
antibiotics for, 1074
bacteriology of, 1072, 1072b
cardiothoracic surgery and, 1071-1072, 1073
treatment of, 1074
causes of, 1071b
clinical manifestations of, 1072-1073

Mediastinitis (Continued)
complications of, 1074
computed tomography of, 1073, 1073f
diagnosis of, 1072-1073, 1072f, 1073f
epidemiology of, 1070
esophageal perforation and, 1070, 1072-1073
treatment of, 1073-1074
in heart transplant recipients, 3503
odontogenic infections and, 1070-1071
pathogenesis of, 1070
patient flora and, 1071-1072
pharyngeal infections and, 1070-1071
prognosis of, 1074
radiography of, 1072, 1072f
sclerosing (fibrosing, granulomatous), 1074-
1075, 1075b
treatment of, 1073-1074
tuberculous fibrosing, 2882
Mediastinum, anatomy of, 1070, 1070f
Medical devices, indwelling. See also Catheter-
related infections.
microorganisms associated with, 21, 21t
Medical records, electronic, 3660-3661
Medical waste
control of, 3342, 3343t
definition for, 3342
Mediterranean spotted fever, 2287t
quinolones for, 465
rifamycin for, 382
Medlar bodies, 2989, 2990f
Medullary hypotonia, as host defense, 36
Mefloquine
adverse effects of, 581t
for malaria, 573t, 574t, 578t, 579t, 586, 3129,
3134t, 3135
for prophylaxis, 3137-3138, 3137t
in travelers, 3641-3642, 3641t
resistance to, 3129. See also Malaria, drug-
resistant.
indications for, 569t
structure of, 586f
Megacolon
in amebic colitis, 3103
in American trypanosomiasis, 3158, 3160,
3163
Megaesophagus, in American trypanosomiasis,
3158, 3160, 3161f, 3163
Meglumine antimoniate
adverse effects of, 581t
for leishmaniasis, 591, 3153
for Trypanosomatidae, 569t
Meibomian glands, 1419, 1420f
Melaney's gangrene, 2812, 2812f
Melanin, as fungal protective factor, 3001
α-Melanocyte–stimulating hormone, antipyretic
effects of, 710
Melarsoprol
adverse effects of, 581t
for trypanosomiasis, 569t, 576t, 590-591,
3168-3169, 3168t
Melioidosis, 2622-2630
chronic, 2624-2625, 2626f
clinical manifestations of, 2624-2628, 2625t
cutaneous, 2625, 2626f, 2627f
encephalomyelitis in, 2628, 2628f
epidemiology of, 2622-2623
fatal septicemic, 2624, 2625f
historical perspective on, 2622
history in, 823t
internal abscesses in, 2625, 2627f, 2628f
osteomyelitis in, 2625, 2627f
pneumonia in, 2624, 2625f, 2626f
prevention of, 2629-2630
prostatic abscess in, 2625, 2628, 2628f
psoas abscess in, 2625, 2627f

Melioidosis *(Continued)*
  pulmonary abscess in, 2624, 2625f, 2626f
  rainfall and, 2623
  risk factors for, 2624, 2624t
  septicemic, vs. enteric fever, 1274t, 1277
  treatment of, 2628-2629, 2629t
Membrane attack complex, 69t
  assembly of, 73, 76
  in paroxysmal nocturnal hemoglobinuria, 86
  regulation of, 74
Membrane-damaging toxins, 30
Membranoproliferative glomerulonephritis
  hepatitis C–related, 1962
  type II, 82
Membranous ulcers, 1180
Memory impairment, from shellfish poisoning,
    3256, 3256t
Men who have sex with men
  hepatitis A in, 2171, 2178
  HIV infection in, 1479-1480, 1480f. *See also*
      Human immunodeficiency virus infection.
  sexually transmitted diseases in. *See* Sexually
      transmitted diseases.
  syphilis in, 2770
Menangle virus, 2038-2039, 2039f, 2039t, 2042-
    2044
  laboratory studies for, 238
Meniere's disease, gentamicin for, 343
Meningeal biopsy, in meningitis, 1135
Meningitis. *See also* Central nervous system
    infections; Meningoencephalitis.
  acute, 1083-1119
  adhesive, in chronic leptomeningeal infections,
      1144
  aseptic, 1084-1085, 1098-1099, 1101, 2148-
      2149. *See* Meningitis, from viruses.
  chemoprophylaxis for, rifamycin in, 381-382
  chronic, 1132-1140
    benign, 1140
    corticosteroids for, 1140
    differential diagnosis of, 1132, 1133t, 1135-
        1140, 1136t
    empiric therapy for, 1135
    from *Angiostrongylus antonensis*, 1138,
        1140
    from *Blastomyces*, 1140
    from *Borrelia burgdorferi*, 1137
    from *Candida*, 1138
    from *Coccidioides* spp., 1137, 1140, 3044-
        3045, 3048
    from *Cryptococcus neoformans*, 1136-1137,
        1140
    from cytomegalovirus, 1140
    from enteroviruses, 2154-2155
    from fungi, 1138
    from *Histoplasma capsulatum*, 1134-1135,
        1137, 1140
    from *Sporothrix schenckii*, 1134, 1134f,
        1135, 1138
    from *Toxoplasma gondii*, 1140
    from *Treponema pallidum*, 1138, 1140
    history in, 1132-1133, 1133t
    in Behçet's disease, 1139
    in connective tissue disease, 1139
    in cysticercosis, 1137, 3289-3290
    in granulomatous angiitis, 1139
    in HIV infection, 1140
    in immunocompromised host, 1140
    in polyarteritis nodosa, 1139
    in sarcoidosis, 1138-1139
    in Sjögren's syndrome, 1139
    in systemic lupus erythematosus, 1139
    in Vogt-Koyanagi-Harada syndrome, 1139
    in Wegener's granulomatosis, 1139
    initial evaluation in, 1133t

Meningitis *(Continued)*
    laboratory evaluation in, 1134-1135, 1134t
    lymphocytic, 1139-1140
    neoplastic, 1138-1139
    noninfectious causes of, 1138-1140
    physical examination in, 1133-1134, 1133f
    rare causes of, 1138, 1140
    skin lesions in, 1186
    steroid-responsive, 1140
    tuberculous, 1135, 1136, 1140
    types of, 1132t
    vs. acute meningitis, 1132
    vs. recurrent meningitis, 1132
  eosinophilic, 3294t, 3296
  from *Acanthamoeba*, 1088, 1104-1105, 1115,
      3111-3119. *See also Acanthamoeba* [spp.].
  from *Acinetobacter*, 2634
  from *Acinetobacter baumannii*, 1114
  from *Actinomyces*, 2929
  from adenoviruses, 1839
  from aerobic gram-negative bacilli, 1087
  from anaerobic gram-negative bacilli, 2840-
      2841
  from *Angiostrongylus cantonensis*, 1088, 1101,
      1105, 1115-1116, 1118
  from arboviruses, 1085
  from *Bacillus anthracis*, 2490, 3618-3619,
      3619f
  from bacteria
    antimicrobial selection in, 246
    blood-brain barrier alterations in, 1095
    brain abscess from, 1153
    cerebral blood flow alterations in,
        1096-1097
    cerebrospinal fluid analysis in, 1080-1082,
        1081t
    clinical features of, 1079-1080, 1098-1101,
        1099t
    C-reactive protein in, 1103
    diagnosis of, 211, 1085, 1101-1105,
        1102-1103
    differential diagnosis of, 1084t, 1085-1088
    epidemiology of, 1084-1088
    etiology of, 1084-1088, 1084t, 1086t
    in elderly, 1100
    in infants and children, 1100, 1107t
    in neonates, 1087, 1100, 1106t, 1107t, 1114,
        1118
    increased intracranial pressure in, 1095-
        1096, 1116-1117
    initial management of, 1105-1111, 1105t-
        1110t
    intravascular survival in, 1091
    meningeal invasion in, 1091-1092
    mucosal colonization and systemic invasion
        in, 1090-1091
    neuronal injury in, 1097-1098
    noninfectious causes of, 1084t
    pathogenesis and pathophysiology of, 1089-
        1098
    prevention of, 1117-1119
    procalcitonin in, 1103
    rash in, 735-736, 1186
    recurrent, 1132
    shunt-related. *See* Cerebrospinal fluid shunt
        infections.
    skin lesions in, 735-736, 1186
    subarachnoid space inflammation in, 1093-
        1094, 1093t
    subarachnoid space survival in, 1092-1093
    treatment of, 246, 249, 1105-1117,
        1105t-1110t
    vs. aseptic meningitis, 2149
    vs. chronic meningitis, 1132
  from *Baylisascaris procyonis*, 1088

Meningitis *(Continued)*
  from *Blastomyces dermatitidis*, 3033
  from *Borrelia burgdorferi*, 1088, 1100, 1104,
      1106t, 1115
  from *Candida*, 1138, 2945, 2950
  from *Chryseobacterium meningosepticum*, in
      neonate, 2757-2758
  from *Citrobacter diversus*, 1151, 1153
  from *Coccidioides*, 1137, 1140, 3044-3045,
      3048
  from *Coxiella burnetii*, 2300
  from *Cryptococcus neoformans*, 1136-1137, 1584
    amphotericin B for, 504, 505
    clinical features of, 3002-3004, 3003t, 3004f
    diagnosis of, 3005-3007
    fluconazole for, 509
    in HIV infection, 1682t, 1683t, 1684t, 1688t,
        1698
    in immunocompromised host, 1140
    prognosis of, 3008-3009
    treatment of, 3007-3008
    with pulmonary coinfection, 3002-3003
  from dark-walled fungi, 3070, 3070f, 3071f
  from enterobacteria, 1106t
  from *Enterococcus*, 2413
  from enteroviruses, 16-17, 1084-1085, 1101,
      2137, 2138, 2148-2149
  from Epstein-Barr virus, 1807
  from gram-negative bacilli, 1087, 1106t, 1114
  from *Haemophilus influenzae*, 1085, 1086-
      1087, 1106t, 1112, 1117, 1118, 2664. *See
      also Haemophilus influenzae*, meningitis
      from.
    rifamycin for, 381-382
  from Hendra virus, 2041
  from herpes simplex virus, 1085, 1101, 1111,
      1767-1768, 1773t
  from herpesviruses, 1085, 1767-1768
  from *Histoplasma capsulatum*, 1134-1135,
      1137, 3020, 3021, 3024
  from HIV, 1085
  from *Leptospira*, 2791-2792
  from *Listeria monocytogenes*, 1087, 1106t,
      1113, 2481, 2481t, 2483
  from lymphocytic choriomeningitis virus, 19,
      1085, 1099, 2090-2096, 2091t
  from mumps virus, 1085, 1099, 1099t, 2004-
      2005
  from *Mycobacterium tuberculosis*, 2877-2878,
      2877f
    glucocorticosteroids for, 558-559
    spinal, 2878
  from *Mycoplasma pneumoniae*, 2274f, 2275
  from *Naegleria fowleri*, 1088, 1101, 1104-
      1105, 1106t, 1115, 3111-3119. *See also*
      Primary amebic meningoencephalitis.
  from *Neisseria meningitidis*, 1087, 1106t,
      1112, 1117-1119. *See also* Meningitis,
      meningococcal.
  from parvovirus B19, 1895
  from protozoa and helminths, 1084t, 1088
    clinical features of, 1101
    diagnosis of, 1104-1105
    treatment of, 1106t, 1115-1116, 1117
  from *Pseudomonas aeruginosa*, 1087, 1106t,
      1114, 2604
  from rickettsiae, 1084t
  from St. Louis encephalitis virus, 1085
  from *Salmonella*, 1087, 1114
  from *Sappinia diploidea*, 3112, 3113f, 3114,
      3117, 3118, 3119
  from spirochetes, 1084t, 1088, 1100, 1106t
    clinical features of, 1100
    diagnosis of, 1085, 1103-1104
    treatment of, 1115

Meningitis *(Continued)*
  from *Sporothrix schenckii,* 2985-2986,
      2987
  from *Staphylococcus aureus,* 1088, 1106t,
      1114, 2345
  from *Staphylococcus epidermidis,* 1088, 1106t
  from *Stenotrophomonas maltophilia,* 1114
  from *Streptococcus agalactiae* (group B),
      1087, 1106t, 1114, 1118, 2428
  from streptococcus group C, 2444
  from streptococcus group G, 2444
  from *Streptococcus pneumoniae,* 1087, 1106t,
      1112-1113, 1118, 1119, 2399-2400, 2437-
      2439
    antibiotic susceptibility in, 2403t
    prevention of, 1118, 1119
    treatment of, 1106t, 1112-1113, 2405
    vancomycin for, 422-423
  from *Toxoplasma gondii,* 3175-3176, 3175f
  from *Treponema pallidum,* 1088, 1100, 1103-
      1104, 1106t, 1115, 1583-1584
  from varicella-zoster virus, 1085, 1101, 1783
  from viridans streptococci, 15-17
  from viruses, 16-17, 1084-1085, 1101, 1583,
      2148-2149.
    adjunctive therapy for, 1116-1117
    clinical features of, 1098-1099
    diagnosis of, 1101-1102
    differential diagnosis of, 1084t
    epidemiology of, 1084-1085, 1084t
    etiology of, 1084-1085, 1084t
    initial management of, 1105-1111
    pathogenesis and pathophysiology of, 1089-
        1090
    prevention of, 1117
    treatment of, 1111
  in cancer, 3437-3438
  in children, glucocorticosteroids for, 559
  in complement deficiency, 158
  in elderly, 3521
  in HIV infection, 1583-1584
  in immunocompromised host, 3437-3438
  in injection drug users, 3471
  in Lyme disease, 2802
  in neonates, from *Chryseobacterium
      meningosepticum,* 2757-2758
  in plague, 2695
  in shunt infections, 1127, 1127t
  in transplant recipients, 3507-3508
  meningococcal, 381, 1087, 1106t, 1112, 1117-
      1118. *See also* Meningococcal infections;
      Neisseria meningitidis.
    clinical manifestations of, 2503-2504
    geographic distribution of, 3640f
    prevention of, 1117-1118
    treatment of, 1106t, 1112, 2507t
    vaccine for, for travelers, 3639t, 3640
  Mollaret's, 1085, 1101, 1138
  rash in, 1100, 1186
  recurrent
    differential diagnosis of, 1133t
    vs. chronic meningitis, 1132
  specimen collection in, 233t
  treatment of
    adjunctive, 1116-1117
    antimicrobials in, 1105t-1107t,
        1111-1116
    dexamethasone in, 26t-28t,
        1106-1111
    empiric, 1105-1111, 1105t-1107t
    initial, 1105-1111
    outpatient parenteral antimicrobial therapy
        in, 629, 629t
    with cephalosporins, 306
    with chloramphenicol, 366, 370

Meningitis *(Continued)*
  with quinolones, 465
  with vancomycin, 422-423
Meningococcal infections, 735. *See also
    Neisseria meningitidis.*
  capsular polysaccharides in, 2499-2500, 2499t
  cell wall antigens in, 2500
  clinical manifestations of, 2502-2506, 2503f-2505f
  complement in, 86
    deficiency of, 78-79, 78f, 83, 84-85
    disseminated. *See* Meningococcemia.
  endocarditis from, 1000
  epidemiology of, 2502
  geographic distribution of, 3640f
  myocardium in, 2504
  prevention of, 88
  properdin deficiency in, 81, 82t, 87
  protection against, cytokines in, 47
  recurrent, 84
  relapse of, 84
  serotypes in, 2500
  tetracyclines for, 358
Meningococcal vaccine, 3568
  for adults, 346f, 347f
  for meningitis, 1118-1119
  for travelers, 3639t, 3640
  indications for, 1118-1119
Meningococcemia, 912, 2502. *See also*
    Meningococcal infections; *Neisseria
    meningitidis.*
  bacteremia in, 913
  chronic, 735-736, 1186, 2505-2506
  clinical manifestations of, 2503, 2503f
  complement deficiency in, 2506
  fulminant, endotoxemia in, 914
  rash in, 730, 731t, 732-733, 735-736
  skin lesions in, 1186
  treatment of, 2507t
Meningococci, penicillin-resistant, 1112
Meningoencephalitis, 1143. *See also* Central
    nervous system infections; Encephalitis;
    Meningitis.
  amebic, 571t, 576t-577t, 3111-3119. *See also*
      Primary amebic meningoencephalitis.
  chronic, from enteroviruses, 2154-2155
  from *Acanthamoeba,* 1088, 1101, 1104-1105,
      1106t, 1115, 3111-3119. *See also
      Acanthamoeba* [spp.]; Granulomatous
      amebic encephalitis.
  from *Balamuthia mandrillaris,* 3111-3119. *See
      also* Granulomatous amebic encephalitis.
  from *Brucella,* 1138
  from *Campylobacter fetus,* 2553
  from *Cryptococcosis,* 3003-3004
  from cytomegalovirus, 1790
  from *Entamoeba histolytica,* 3103
  from mumps virus, 2005
  from *Naegleria fowleri,* 3111-3119. *See also*
      Primary amebic meningoencephalitis.
  from *Neisseria meningitidis,* 2502
  from St. Louis encephalitis virus, 1085
  from *Sappinia diploidea,* 3112, 3113f, 3114,
      3117, 3118, 3119
  from *Schistosomes,* 3279
  hemorrhagic, 2488
  in immunocompromised host, 3437-3438
Meningoencephalomyelitis, 1143
Meningovascular meningitis, 1088
Menopause, in HIV infection, 1630
Menstruation, in HIV infection, 1489, 1619, 1630
Meropenem
  antibacterial activity of, 312-313, 313t
  chemistry of, 312, 312f
  clinical uses of, 314
  dosage of, 658t-659t

Meropenem *(Continued)*
  drug interactions with, 693t
  for acute pyelonephritis, 889
  for bacterial arthritis, 1316t
  for brain abscess, 1159, 1159t
  for *Burkholderia cepacia,* 2619
  for febrile neutropenia, 3450-3452, 3451t
  for melioidosis, 2629t
  for meningitis, 1106t, 1107t, 1113
  for nocardiosis, 2921
  for peritonitis, 938
  for pneumonia, 837-839, 837t, 838t
  for *Pseudomonas aeruginosa* bacteremia, 2601
  for sepsis, 919t
  for *Streptococcus agalactiae* (group B), 2429
  formulations of, 648t
  pharmacology of, 313-314
  resistance to, 312
    by pneumococci, 837, 837t
    carbapenemases in, 256, 259t
Mesenteric artery, superior, mycotic aneurysm of,
    1007
Mesocolon, transverse, 927, 927f
Metabolic acidosis, in malaria, 3125
Metabolic defects, congenital, metronidazole for,
    394
Metabolism, 909-910
  in female HIV infection, 1630-1631
  in host defense, 39
  in pediatric HIV infection, 1643-1644
  in secondary peritonitis, 935
  of drugs, 271t, 273
Metagonimus yokogawai, 3277t, 3283
  syndrome of abdominal pain, diarrhea, and
      eosinophilia from, 1281t, 1283
  treatment of, 572t
Metalloprotease toxins, 25t
Metapneumovirus. *See* Human metapneumovirus.
Methacycline
  dosage of, 662t-663t
  formulations of, 647t
Methadone, clozapine with, 459
Methenamine, 476-477, 476f
  drug interactions with, 693t
  urinary pH and, 888
Methenamine hippurate, dosage of, 674t-675t
Methenamine mandelate
  dosage of, 674t-675t
  formulations of, 648t
Methenamine silver stain, of fungi, 230
Methicillin, 289-290, 290f
  dosage of, 652t-653t
  formulations of, 646t
  minimal inhibitory concentration of, 284t
  resistance to. *See Staphylococcus aureus,*
      methicillin-resistant
L-Methionine, for vascular myelopathy, 1592-
    1593
Methotrexate
  for HIV-related non-Hodgkin's lymphoma,
      1605
  for primary central nervous system lymphoma,
      1608
  for transplant immunosuppression, infections
      and, 3478
Methoxyflurane, tetracycline with, 364t
Methylobacterium spp., 2751t, 2761
Metorchis conjunctus, 3281
  syndrome of abdominal pain, diarrhea, and
      eosinophilia from, 1281t, 1282
  treatment of, 572t
Metrionate, for schistosomiasis, 3280
Metronidazole, 388-394, 484t, 582-583
  activity spectrum of, 389, 389t
  administration of, 391, 391t

Metronidazole (Continued)
 adverse reactions to, 391-392, 581t
 dosage of, 391, 391t, 666t-667t
 drug interactions with, 392, 393t, 693t-694t
 fecal flora effects of, 392
 food interactions with, 393t
 for acute necrotizing ulcerative gingivitis, 796, 796t
 for amebiasis, 571t, 3106, 3106t
 for amebiosis, 953
 for anaerobic infections, 393
 for bacterial vaginosis, 1366-1367
 for Bacteroides, 2815
 for balantidiasis, 571t
 for Blastocystis hominis, 577t
 for brain abscess, 1157, 1158t, 1159, 1159t
 for cavernous sinus thrombosis, 1424
 for chlamydial pneumonia, atherosclerosis after, 2265
 for clostridial cellulitis, 1189
 for Clostridium difficile–associated colitis, 1257, 1258, 1258t
 for deep fascial space infections, 797t
 for Dientamoeba fragilis, 572t
 for dracunculiasis, 572t, 3269-3270, 3270f
 for Entamoeba polecki, 572t
 for giardiasis, 3202, 3202t
 for Helicobacter pylori infections, 2563
 for Lemierre's disease, 756
 for liver abscess, 953, 954, 954t
 for luminal protozoa, 582
 for lung abscess, 855-856
 for microsporidiosis, 3248
 for Neisseria gonorrhoeae, 2525, 2525t
 for odontogenic infections, 797t, 798
 for orbital/preseptal cellulitis, 1423-1424, 1423f
 for parasitic infections, 393
 for parotitis, 797t
 for pelvic inflammatory disease, 1379t, 2247t, 2250, 2525, 2525t
 for periodontitis, 796, 796t
 for peritonsillar abscess, 756
 for postoperative gynecologic infections, 1377t
 for secondary peritonitis, 938
 for sialadenitis, 797t
 for suppurative thrombophlebitis, 1005
 for trichomoniasis, 1361-1362, 3207-3208
 for urethritis, 1207
 for vancomycin-resistant enterococci, 392-393
 formulations of, 648t
 in preemptive pancreatic infection treatment, 965t
 indications for, 393-394, 568t
 mechanism of action of, 388-389
 mutagenic properties of, 392
 neurotoxicity of, 1594t
 pharmacokinetics of, 390-391, 390t
 prophylaxis with, 394
 resistance to, 389-390
 structure of, 583f
 topical, 391
Mezlocillin, 292, 292f
 antimicrobial activity of, 333, 334t-335t
 dosage of, 652t-653t
 for anaerobes, 284t
 for bacilli, 284t
 for Enterobacteriaceae, 284t
 for peritonitis, 938
 for postoperative gynecologic infections, 1377t
 for Pseudomonas, 284t
 formulations of, 646t
Micafungin, 511
 dosage of, 678t-679t
 for aspergillosis, 2968t, 2969
 prophylactic, for cancer patients, 3446

Mice
 hantavirus pulmonary syndrome from, 2086-2089, 2086t
 lymphocytic chorioretinitis virus from, 2092
 mites of, 3311
Michaelis-Menten kinetics, 273
Miconazole
 dosage of, 678t-679t
 drug interactions with, 694t
 for brain abscess, 1159t
 for candidiasis, 2949-2951
  vulvovaginal, 1364
 formulations of, 649t
Microbacterium spp., 2471
Microbial flora, 3423-3426, 3423f
 anaerobes in, 2811
 drug effects on, 3424
 endogenous, 3
 fecal, in secondary peritonitis, 934
 hand hygiene and, 3327
 in host protection, 40
 in opportunistic infections, 4
 normal bowel, 36
 of gastrointestinal tract, 36, 1217-1218, 3423f, 3424-3426, 3425f
  as host defense, 36, 1217-1218
  in secondary peritonitis, 932
 of lungs, 808
 of oral cavity, 787-788, 787t, 789, 3423f, 3424-3425, 3424-3426, 3425f
  lung abscess from, 854
 of skin, 3423-3424, 3423f
  postoperative infections and, 3535, 3544
 of vagina, 1360-1361
  assessment of, 1360-1361
  in secondary peritonitis, 932-933
  Mycoplasma spp. in, 2281
Microbial surface component reacting with adherence matrix molecules, on Staphylococcus aureus, 2326, 2327t
Microbicides, in Neisseria gonorrheae infection prevention, 2527
Microbiology laboratory, 203-239. See also Laboratory tests.
Microcirculation, in severe sepsis, 911
Micrococcus [spp.]
 endocarditis from, 992
 laboratory identification of, 217
 linezolid for, 437, 437t
Micrococcus luteus, mupirocin for, 485t
Microevolutionary change, in antibiotic resistance, 253
Microfilariae. See Filariasis.
Microscopy, direct stains with, 214, 214t
Microsporidia, 3237-3249
 characteristics of, 3237-3238
 classification of, 3240
 clinical manifestations of, 3238t, 3244-3246
  in immunocompetent host, 3244-3245
  in immunocompromised host, 3244-3245
 cutaneous infections from, 3238t, 3244, 3247-3249, 3248t
 diagnosis of, 3242f, 3246-3247, 3246t
 encephalitis from, 3238t, 3243, 3245
 epidemiology of, 3240-3241
 gastrointestinal infections from, 3242-3245, 3242f, 3247-3249, 3248t
 genitourinary infections from, 3238t, 3243, 3247-3249, 3248t
 genome of, 3240
 host range of, 3237, 3238t
 immune response to, 3241-3242
 in HIV infection, 1572, 1690t
 in travelers, 3244
 life cycle of, 3240, 3243

Microsporidia (Continued)
 musculoskeletal infections from, 3238t, 3244, 3247-3249, 3248t
 myositis from, 3238t, 3244, 3245-3246, 3247-3249, 3248t
 ocular infections from, 1393, 1405, 3238t, 3243-3245, 3248t, 3249
 pathogenic, 3238t
 pathology and pathogenesis of, 3242-3244, 3242f
 phylogeny of, 3240
 pneumonia from, 1572
 polar tube of, 3237-3238, 3239f
 prevention of, 3249
 respiratory infections from, 3238t, 3244, 3247-3249, 3248t
 sinusitis from, 3238t, 3244, 3247-3249, 3248t
 species of, 3237
 structure of, 3237-3238, 3238, 3239f
 transmission of, 3249
 treatment of, 574t, 3247-3249, 3248t
Microsporidium spp., 3237, 3238t
Microsporum [spp.], 3051-3059. See also Dermatophyte(s).
 blepharoconjunctivitis from, 1393
Microsporum audouinii, 3052t, 3053, 3053t
Microsporum canis, 3052, 3052t, 3053, 3053t
 tinea corporis from, 3055
Microsporum ferrugineum, 3052t, 3053, 3053t
Microsporum gypseum, 3052, 3052t, 3055
Microsporum nanum, 3052, 3052t
Microsporum persicolor, 3052, 3052t
Microsporum rivalieri, 3052, 3052t
Middle East, HIV infection in, 1468
Middleburg virus, 1914
Military service, HIV infection in, 1481
Milk, human. See Breast-feeding.
Milk thistle, for hepatitis, 609
Miltefosine
 adverse effects of, 581t
 for leishmaniasis, 578t, 592, 3153
 for Trypanosomatidae, 569t
Minimal bactericidal concentration, 242
Minimal inhibitory concentration, 242, 245-246
 for bacteria, 274
 in dosing, 250
 in time-dependent killing curve, 275, 276f
 maximal serum concentration to, 276-277, 276f
 pharmacodynamic relationships and, 275, 275f
 tests for, 223
Minimal lethal concentration, 242
Minocycline, 358t. See also Tetracycline(s).
 dosage of, 662t-663t
 food interactions with, 364t
 for actinomycosis, 2931, 2931t
 for leprosy, 499, 2893
 for Neisseria meningitidis carriage, 2509
 for nocardiosis, 2920t, 2921
 for nontuberculous mycobacterial skin infections, 2911, 2913t
 for periodontitis, 796, 796t
 formulations of, 647t
 pharmacology of, 362t
 side effects of, 363t
 structure of, 357f
 vertigo from, 364
Miscarriage
 from Chlamydia trachomatis, 2249
 from hepatitis E virus, 2210
 from parvovirus B19, 1895, 1896
Mite-borne disease(s). See also Scabies.
 rickettsialpox as, 2295-2296
Mites, 3310-3311, 3311f
Mitochondria, nucleoside analogue toxicity in, 1624

Mitral valve
  endocarditis of, 976, 977
  prolapse of, in endocarditis, 976, 1046-1047
  Staphylococcus aureus endocarditis of, 2342, 2343f
MMF, for transplant immunosuppression, infections and, 3478
MMR vaccine. *See* Measles, mumps, rubella (MMR) vaccine.
Mo-1, 97
Mobala virus, 2093
Mobile DNA elements, in retroviruses, 2120-2121, 2120f
Mobiluncus spp., 2850, 2851, 2763
Modoc virus, 1945t
Mogibacterium spp., 2850
Mokola virus, 2047t
Molds, 229, 230t. *See also* Fungi.
  anamorph, 229
  appearance of in tissue, 2936f-2937f, 2938t
  dematiaceous, 229, 230t
  dimorphic, 229
  hyaline, 229
  teleomorph, 229
  vs. yeast, 2935
Molecular assays, 11-12, 215, 221-222
  false-positives in, 215
  for susceptibility determination, 224
Molecular mimicry, 65
Molecular typing, of *Mycobacterium tuberculosis*, 227
Mollaret's meningitis, 1085, 1101, 1138
Molluscum contagiosum, 10, 1338-1344, 1753-1754
  clinical features of, 1339, 1341, 1341f, 1754, 1754f
  conjunctivitis from, 1390
  diagnosis of, 1754
  duration of, 1342
  epidemiology of, 1342, 1754
  in HIV infection, 1342
  ocular, 1390
  pathogenesis and pathophysiology of, 1753-1754
  presentation of, 1338-1339
  treatment of, 1344, 1754
  vs. anogenital warts, 1847
Moniliformis moniliformis, pyrantel pamoate for, 574t
Monkey(s)
  hepatitis B virus in, 1832-1834, 1832f
  hepatitis E virus in, 2208
  herpes B virus in. *See* Herpes B virus.
  HIV in, 2119
Monkeypox, 180-181, 740-741, 1747-1749, 1748f
  specimen collection in, 233t
Monoamine oxidase, inhibition of, 438
Monobactams, 314-315. *See also* Beta-lactam antibiotics.
  cross-reactivity among, 325
  structure of, 320f
Monoclonal antibodies
  for meningitis, 1116
  for transplant immunosuppression, infections and, 3478-3479
  in host receptor identification, 15, 15t
  therapeutic uses of, 67, 88
Monocytes, 56
  activation of, 39
  complement synthesis in, 71
  in HIV infection, 1537
  in phagocytosis, 37
  Toll-like receptor distribution in, 38, 39, 39t
Mononeuritis multiplex, in HIV infection, 1595, 1597t

Mononucleosis. *See* Infectious mononucleosis.
Montelukast, for chronic obstructive pulmonary disease, 810t
Mopeia virus, 2093
Moraxella [spp.], 2529
  conjunctivitis from, 1391, 1392
  endocarditis from, 992
  identification of, 220, 221t, 2532, 2533t
  in oral cavity, 787, 787t
  keratitis from, 1397-1400
  microbiology of, 2633t
Moraxella (Branhamella) catarrhalis, 2529-2532
  bacteremia from, 2531
  beta-lactamase of, 2531
  biochemical characteristics of, 2532, 2532t
  COPD from, 809, 2530-2531
  epidemiology of, 2530
  growth characteristics of, 2532, 2532t
  history of, 2529
  laboratory identification of, 220
  laryngitis from, 759
  microbiology of, 2529
  nosocomial respiratory infections from, 2531
  otitis media from, 767, 767t, 769, 2530, 2531f
  pathogenesis of, 2530
  pneumonia from, 832
    in elderly, 2531
    nosocomial, 3365, 3365t
  respiratory tract colonization with, 2530
  sinusitis from, 776, 776t, 779, 782t, 2531
  surface antigens of, 2530
  treatment of, 2531-2532
    with cephalosporins, 298t
    with macrolides, 397t, 401t, 403
    with mupirocin, 485t
    with quinolones, 455t
    with quinupristin-dalfopristin, 425
    with trimethoprim-sulfamethoxazole, 444
Morganella [spp.], 2580
  peritonitis from, 938
  treatment of
    with aminoglycosides, 334t-335t
    with cephalosporins, 298t
    with penicillins, 284t
Morganella morganii, 2580
  treatment of
    with carbapenems, 313t
    with mupirocin, 485t
    with quinolones, 455t
    with rifamycin, 374t
Morison's pouch, 927, 927f
Mosquito-borne infections
  from alphaviruses, 1913-1919
  from *Brugia* spp., 3270-3272
  from Bunyaviridae, 2086-2089, 2086t
  from coltiviruses, 1900
  from flaviviruses, 1926-1945
  from *Plasmodium* spp. *See* Malaria.
  from *Wucheria bancrofti*, 3270-3272
  prevention of, 1943, 3138
    in travelers, 3642
Motion sickness, 3644
  in travelers, 3644
Mouse. *See* Mice.
Moxalactam
  dosage of, 658t-659t
  formulations of, 647t
  structure of, 296f
  uses of, 305t, 306

Moxifloxacin
  antimicrobial activity of, 455t, 456t
  dosage of, 458t, 672t-673t
  for *Enterococcus*, 2416
  for keratitis, 1399
  for *Legionella pneumophila*, 2719t
  for meningitis, 1113
  for *Mycobacterium avium* complex, 2905
  for nocardiosis, 2920t
  for odontogenic infections, 797t
  for osteomyelitis of jaw, 797t
  for pelvic inflammatory disease, 1379t
  for peritonitis, 939
  for pneumonia, 462, 837-839, 838t
  for psittacosis, 2257
  for respiratory infections, 462
  for sepsis, 919t
  for sinusitis, 779-780, 779t
  formulations of, 648t
  pharmacology of, 457t
MRI. *See* Magnetic resonance imaging.
MSCRAMM, on *Staphylococcus aureus*, 2326, 2327t
Mucocutaneous candidiasis. *See* Candida [spp.].
Mucocutaneous disease, in immunocompromised host, antiviral drugs for, 515t
Mucocutaneous herpes. *See* Herpes simplex virus.
Mucocutaneous lymph node syndrome. *See* Kawasaki disease.
Mucopolysaccharides, in complement activation, 74
Mucor hiemalis, cutaneous mucormycosis from, 2978
Mucorales, 2973-2974, 2974f
  appearance of in tissue, 2979, 2979f
  characteristics of, 2974-2975, 2974f
  classification of, 2974, 2974t
  immune response to, 2975
  species of, 2974, 2974t
  terminology of, 2973
Mucormycosis, 2973-2981
  AIDS-related, 2979
  appearance of in tissue, 2938t
  central nervous system, 2978
  cerebral, 1152, 1155, 1158t, 1160, 2976-2977, 2978
    in injection drug users, 2978, 3471
  clinical features of, 2975-2979, 2976f-2978f
  cutaneous, 2977-2978
    necrotizing, 1184t
  diagnosis of, 2579f, 2979
  differential diagnosis of, 2579f, 2979
  epidemiology of, 2974-2975
  etiology of, 2974, 2974t
  gastrointestinal, 2978
  in transplant recipients, 2975
  orbital cellulitis in, 1423, 2975-2977, 2976f, 2977f
  outcome in, 2980
  pathogenesis of, 2975-2980
  prevention of, 2980
  pulmonary, 2977, 2978f, 2979f
  rhinocerebral, 1423, 2975-2977, 2976f, 2977f
  risk factors for, 2975-2979, 2976f-2978f
  splenic abscess from, 967, 967t
  transmission of, 2974
  treatment of, 1160, 2979-2980
    with amphotericin B, 504
    with hyperbaric oxygen, 566
Mucosa
  barrier functions of, 3423
    impairment of, 3424-3426
  in host defense, 35-36
  in *Pseudomonas aeruginosa* infections, 2590
  surface, lymphocytes on, 122

Mucositis, 3424-3246
  associated pathogens of, 3421t
  bacteremia from, laboratory diagnosis of, 3428
  gastrointestinal, 3424-3426
  in cancer patients, 3457
  in immunocompromised host, 798-799, 3424-3426
  oral. *See* Stomatitis.
Multicentric Castleman's disease, 1830, 1830f
Multidrug resistance. *See specific drugs and pathogens.*
Multilocus sequence typing, 222
Multiorgan failure, bacteremia and, 913-914
Multiple myeloma. *See* Hematologic malignancies.
Multiple sclerosis
  coronaviruses and, 1995
  vs. chronic progressive myelopathy, 2110-2111
Multivitamins, for elderly patient, 146, 146t
Mumps immune globulin, 2007
Mumps virus, 2003-2007
  acute pancreatitis from, 959, 959t
  characteristics of, 2003
  clinical manifestations of, 2004-2005, 2004t
  collection of, 233t
  complications of, 2005-2006
  congenital, 2005-2006
  conjunctivitis from, 1390
  diagnosis of, 2006
  differential diagnosis of, 2006-2007
  epidemiology of, 2003
  historical perspective on, 2003
  immune response to, 2006
  meningitis from, 1085, 1099, 1099t, 1101, 1117
  orchitis from, 1385
  parotitis from, 799
  pathogenesis of, 2003-2004
  pathology of, 2004
  prevention of, 2007
  transmission of, 2003-2004
  treatment of, 2007
  vaccine for, 1117, 2007, 3568-3569. *See also* Measles, mumps, rubella (MMR) vaccine.
Mupirocin, 484t, 485-487
  adverse effects of, 486-487
  antibacterial activity of, 485-486, 485t
  catheter infections prophylaxis with, 481-482
  for dialysis-related peritonitis, 942
  for impetigo, 1173
  for *Staphylococcus aureus,* 1039
    in nasal carriage, 480, 481, 483-484, 3540
  for *Staphylococcus aureus* nasal carriage, 1176
  pharmacokinetics of, 486
  preoperative, 3540
  prophylaxis with, 480
  structure of, 485, 485f
  uses of, 486
Muriform cells, 2989, 2990f
Murine typhus, 2287t, 2306-2308
Murray Valley encephalitis, 1929, 1944-1945
Mus spp. *See* Mice.
Musca domestica, myiasis from, 3307-3310, 3308t
Muscle. *See also* Myositis *and related entries.*
  in botulism, 28
Muscle biopsy, in HIV-related myopathy, 1596
Muscle necrosis, in burn patients, 3551
Muscle proteolysis, in acute-phase response, 1202
Musculoskeletal system, in endocarditis, 984
Mushroom poisoning, 1290, 1291t
  treatment of, 1296
Mutagenesis, signature-tagged, 10
Mutant prevention concentration, 274
Mutant selection window, 274

MX virus, 2196. *See also* Caliciviruses.
Myalgia, 1195t, 1201-1202
  from rifabutin, 493
  in endocarditis, 1201
  in influenza, 1201
  in toxoplasmosis, 1201
  parasitic, 1202
Myasthenia gravis
  telithromycin effects on, 407
  vs. botulism, 2825
Mycetoma, 2916, 2917, 2929, 2975-2977, 2976f, 2977f, 2991-2995, 2993f-2995f
  from *Coccidioides immitis,* 3043, 3045f
  from dark-walled fungi, 3070t
  from *Pseudallescheria boydii,* 3068-3069, 3076t
Mycobacteria
  antigen presentation to, 129-130
  categories of, 226
  characteristics of, 2897-2898
  complement receptors and, 78
  genetic susceptibility to, 44-45, 44t, 123
  identification of, 226-227
    mycolic acid analysis in, 226-227
    NAP test in, 227
    nucleic acid–based methods of, 225, 226
  in stem cell transplant, 3492
  isolation of, 226, 227, 227t
  keratitis from, 1398-1400
  laboratory tests for, 224-228
    safety issues in, 224
  nontuberculous, 157, 2909-2914. *See also* *Mycobacterium avium* complex.
    catheter-related, 2910t, 2913
    clinical manifestations of, 2910-2913, 2910t
    culture of, 2913
    disinfection/sterilization and, 3340
    disseminated disease from, 2910t, 2912, 2913t
    environmental niches of, 2910
    in cystic fibrosis, 871, 873
    intermediately growing, 2910
    laboratory diagnosis of, 2913-2914
    lymphadenitis from, 1206-1207, 2910t, 2911
    musculoskeletal infections from, 2910t, 2912
    pulmonary disease from, 2910-2911, 2910t, 2911t, 2913t
    rapidly growing, 2909
    rifamycin for, 379
    skin infections from, 2910t, 2911-2912, 2913t
    slowly growing, 2909-2910
    soft tissue infections from, 2910t, 2911-2912, 2913t
    susceptibility testing for, 2913
    treatment of, 496-497, 2910-2912, 2913t
  resistance in, 157f
  respiratory, 209t
  specimens containing
    collection and transport of, 205t, 206t, 207t, 224-225
    direct detection of, 225
    processing and planting of, 225-226
  splenic abscess from, 967, 967t
  stains for, 214t, 225
  susceptibility testing of, 47, 227
Mycobacterium [spp.]
  cardiovascular device infections from, 1023
  laboratory tests for, 228-229
  nontuberculous, treatment of, 496-497
  speciation for, 2854t, 2855
  treatment of
    with clarithromycin, 405
    with linezolid, 437, 437t
    with quinolones, 464

Mycobacterium abscessus
  pulmonary disease from, 2910, 2911, 2911t, 2913t
  skin and soft tissue infections from, 2911-2912
  treatment of, 359t, 496
Mycobacterium asiaticum, 2909-2914, 2910t
Mycobacterium aurum, 2909-2914, 2910t
Mycobacterium avium complex, 2897-2906, 2910t. *See also* Mycobacteria, nontuberculous.
  AIDS cholangiopathy from, 957
  antiretroviral therapy effect on, 1561
  characteristics of, 2897-2899
  chest film in, 864f, 2899f, 2900f
  clinical manifestations of, 2899-2902, 2899f-2902f, 2901t
  culture of, 2902
  diagnosis of, 2902-2903
  direct detection of, 225
  disseminated disease in, 2897, 2898-2899, 2899f, 2901, 2901f, 2901t, 2903-2906
    with pulmonary disease, 2901
  epidemiology of, 2897
  immune response to, 2899
  in HIV infection, 489, 1550, 1561, 1571
    treatment of, 1682t, 1683t, 1684t, 1687t, 1700-1701
  interferon-gamma defects in, 157
  lymphadenitis from, 1206-1207, 2897, 2899, 2902, 2902f, 2903-2905, 2904t, 2906
  macrolide-resistant, 2905
  pancreatic infections from, 959, 959t
  pericarditis from, 1059
  prevention of, 2906
  pulmonary disease from, 2897, 2898, 2899-2901, 2900f, 2901f, 2901t, 2902, 2903-2905, 2906
  splenic abscess from, 967, 967t
  treatment of, 405, 2903-2906, 2904t, 2905t
    with aminoglycosides, 334t-335t, 344t, 496-497
    with macrolides, 397t, 401t, 403, 496, 1682t, 1700
    with quinolones, 456t
    with rifabutin, 493-494, 1700
    with rifampin, 496
    with rifamycin, 379
Mycobacterium bohemicum, 2910-2914, 2910t
Mycobacterium bonickei, 2909-2914, 2910t
Mycobacterium bovis, 2853, 3562
  spread of, 2857
  chemotherapy in, 2857-2858
Mycobacterium branderi, 2910-2914, 2910t
Mycobacterium celatum, 2910-2914, 2910t
Mycobacterium chelonae, 2909-2914, 2910t
  in peritoneal dialysis, 941
  skin and soft tissue infections from, 2911-2912
  treatment of
    with macrolides, 496
    with quinolones, 456t
    with rifamycin, 374t
    with tetracyclines, 359t
    with vancomycin, 359t
Mycobacterium conspicuum, 2910-2914, 2910t
Mycobacterium elephantis, 2909-2914, 2910t
Mycobacterium flavescens, 2909-2914, 2910t
Mycobacterium fortuitum
  in peritoneal dialysis, 941
  treatment of
    with aminoglycosides, 496-497
    with quinolones, 456t
    with rifamycin, 374t
    with tetracyclines, 359t
    with vancomycin, 359t
Mycobacterium fortuitum complex, 2909-2914

Mycobacterium fortuitum/chelonae complex, treatment of, 401t
Mycobacterium fortuitus, 2909-2914, 2910t
  skin and soft tissue infections from, 2911-2912
Mycobacterium genavense, 2909-2914, 2910t
Mycobacterium goodii, 2909-2914, 2910t
Mycobacterium gordonae, 2910-2914, 2910t
  isolates of, 226
Mycobacterium haemophilum, 2909-2914, 2910t
  skin and soft tissue infections from, 2912
  treatment of, 496
Mycobacterium heckeshornense, 2910-2914, 2910t
Mycobacterium houstonense, 2909-2914, 2910t
Mycobacterium immunogenum, 2909-2914, 2910t
Mycobacterium interjectum, 2910-2914, 2910t
Mycobacterium intracellulare, 2897, 2909-2914, 2910t. *See also Mycobacterium avium* complex.
Mycobacterium kansasii, 2909-2914, 2910t
  cutaneous infections from, 2912
  direct detection of, 225
  disseminated disease from, 2912-2913, 2913t
  ethambutol for, 497
  in HIV infection, 1571
  pericarditis from, 1059
  pulmonary disease from, 2910-2911, 2911t, 2913t
  rifampin-resistant, sulfonamides for, 443
  treatment of
    with quinolones, 456t
    with rifabutin, 493-494
Mycobacterium lentiflavum, 2909-2914, 2910-2914, 2910t
Mycobacterium leprae, 497, 2886-2895
  arthritis from, 1319
  discovery of, 2886
  evolution of, 6
  Fite staining of, 2891-2892, 2892f, 2893f
  genome of, 2887-2888
  immune response to, 2888
  microbiology of, 2887-2888
  nerve damage from, 2889
  neuritis from, 1147-1148
  transmission of, 2886
  treatment of, 498-499
    with interferon-gamma, 556
    with macrolides, 403
    with rifamycin, 379
Mycobacterium leprae laminin-binding protein, 2889
Mycobacterium mageritense, 2909-2914, 2910t
Mycobacterium malmoense, 496, 2909-2914, 2910t
Mycobacterium marinum, 2910-2914, 2910t
  skin infections from, 2911, 2913t
  treatment of, 496, 497
Mycobacterium mucogenicum, 2909-2914, 2910t
Mycobacterium neoaurum, 2909-2914, 2910t
Mycobacterium neworleansense, 2909-2914, 2910t
Mycobacterium nonchromogenicum, 2909-2914, 2910t
Mycobacterium novocastrense, 2909-2914, 2910t
Mycobacterium palustre, 2910-2914, 2910t
Mycobacterium peregrinum, 2909-2914, 2910t
Mycobacterium phlei, 2909-2914, 2910t
Mycobacterium porcinum, 2909-2914, 2910t
Mycobacterium scrofulaceum, 2909-2914, 2910t
  treatment of, 496-497
Mycobacterium senegalense, 2909-2914, 2910t
Mycobacterium septicum, 2909-2914, 2910t
Mycobacterium shottsii, 2910-2914, 2910t
Mycobacterium simiae, 2909-2914, 2910t
Mycobacterium smegmatis, 2909-2914, 2910t

Mycobacterium szulgai, 2909-2914, 2910t
Mycobacterium terrae, 2909-2914, 2910t
Mycobacterium triplex, 2909-2914, 2910t
Mycobacterium tuberculosis, 2852-2883. *See also* Tuberculosis.
  acid-fast staining of, 2853, 2854t
  antigens of, 2860, 2861
  antimicrobial susceptibility testing for, 2854t, 2855
  antiretroviral therapy effect on, 1561
  arthritis from, 1319
  brain abscess from, 1158t
  bronchoalveolar lavage for, 825, 825f, 826
  cervical lymphadenitis from, 1206-1207
  culture of, 2853, 2854t
  direct detection of, 225
  DNA of, 2854t, 2855
  drug-resistant, 489, 2867, 2867t
  epididymitis from, 1384
  evolution of, 6
  granulomatous prostatitis from, 1383t, 1384
  immunity to, 2859-2860
  in HIV infection. *See* Tuberculosis, in HIV infection.
  in peritoneal dialysis, 941
  in sputum, 825, 825f, 826
  isolation of, 226
  keratitis in, 1400
  laboratory tests for, 227, 228t
  latent, assays for, 227-228, 2861
  microbiology of, 2853-2855, 2854t
  molecular typing of, 227
  multidrug-resistant, disinfection/sterilization and, 3340
  mycotic aneurysm from, 993
  nosocomial infections from, 3327-3329
  nucleic acid amplification of, 2853-2855, 2854t
  osteomyelitis from, 1329-1330
  pancreatic infections from, 959, 959t
  pericarditis from, 1059
  prostatitis from, 894
  restriction fragment length polymorphism of, 2854t, 2855
  splenic abscess from, 967, 967t
  spread of, 2857
  susceptibility to, 123
  treatment of, 2867-2875. *See also* Antituberculous agents *and specific agents.*
    first-line antimycobacterial drugs in, 378, 489-494, 490t-492t
    second-line antimycobacterial drugs in, 456t, 494-496
  tuberculin test for, 2860-2861, 2861t
  uveitis from, 1415, 1416f, 1418
  vs. *Mycobacterium leprae,* 2887
Mycobacterium tuberculosis complex, susceptibility testing of, 227
Mycobacterium tusciae, 2910-2914, 2910t
Mycobacterium ulcerans, skin and soft tissue infections from, 2912
Mycobacterium vaccae, 2909-2914, 2910t
Mycobacterium wolinskyi, 2909-2914, 2910t
Mycobacterium xenopi, 2909-2914, 2910t
  treatment of, 496, 497
Mycolic acid analysis, mycobacteria identification by, 226-227
Mycology. *See under* Fungal; Fungi.
Mycoplasma [spp.], 2269-2271
  acute pancreatitis from, 959, 959t
  as culture contaminants, 2270-2271
  characteristics of, 2269-2270, 2269f, 2269t, 2276t
  classification of, 2270, 2270f
  culture of, 208
  genital, 2280-2282, 2281t
    extragenital infections by, 2271

Mycoplasma [spp.] *(Continued)*
  pathogenesis of, 2270-2271
  quinupristin-dalfopristin for, 425
Mycoplasma arginini, in immunocompromised host, 2271
Mycoplasma fermentans, 2270, 2271, 2280-2282, 2281t
Mycoplasma genitalium, 2280-2282, 2281t, 2282f
  urethritis from, 1351. *See also* Urethritis, nongonococcal.
Mycoplasma hominis, 2280-2282, 2281t
  in urinary tract infections, 882
  postpartum endometritis from, 1374
  quinolones for, 455t
Mycoplasma incognitus, 2270, 2271
Mycoplasma penetrans, 2270, 2271, 2280-2282, 2281t
Mycoplasma pirum, 2270, 2271
Mycoplasma pneumoniae, 2271-2278
  acute bronchitis from, 747-749
  characteristics of, 2272
  clinical manifestation(s) of, 2272-2275
    cardiac, 2275
    dermatologic, 2274, 2274f
    extrapulmonary, 2274-2275
    musculoskeletal, 2275
    neurologic, 2275
    Raynaud's phenomenon as, 2274-2275, 2274f, 2276
    renal, 2275, 2276
  COPD exacerbations from, 809
  croup from, 760, 760t, 761
  culture of, 2277
  diagnosis of, 209t, 2276-2278
  epidemiology of, 2272
  erythema multiforme from, 2274, 2274f
  historical perspective on, 2271-2272
  immune response to, 2275-2276
  in immunocompromised host, 2275
  in sickle cell disease, 2274f, 2275
  laryngitis from, 759
  myocarditis from, 1053
  otitis media from, 768
  pathology and pathophysiology of, 2276
  pericarditis from, 1059
  pharyngitis from, 755, 2365
  pneumonia from, 2273-2274, 2273f
    atypical, 833-834
    chest film in, 830
    community-acquired, 831-833
    serum antibody assays for, 828
    sputum in, 826
    treatment of, 836-839, 837t, 838t
  prevention of, 2278
  risk factors for, 2275
  sinusitis from, 776, 776t
  transmission of, 2272-2273
  treatment of, 2278
    with clindamycin, 409t
    with linezolid, 437, 437t
    with macrolides, 397t, 398, 401t, 402, 403
    with quinolones, 455t
    with tetracyclines, 360t
  vs. enteric fever, 1278
Mycoplasma primatum, 2280-2282, 2281t
Mycoplasma spermatophilum, 2280-2282, 2281t
Mycoses. *See under* Fungal.
Mycotic aneurysms, 1005-1009
  classification of, 1006t
  clinical manifestations of, 1007-1008
  epidemiology of, 1006
  etiology of, 1008-1009
  in endocarditis, 982, 2343
  in injection drug users, 3467-3468, 3471
  intracranial, 1007

Mycotic aneurysms (Continued)
  laboratory findings in, 1008
  pathogenesis of, 1006
  pathology of, 1006-1007
  treatment of, 1009
Myelitis, 1143-1147
  clinical features of, 1144-1145
  etiology of, 1146-1147, 1146t
  from herpes B virus, 1833-1834
  in injection drug users, 3472
  in schistosomiasis, 3279
  in toxoplasmosis, 3179
  laboratory findings in, 1145-1146
  pathogenesis and pathophysiology of, 1144
  treatment of, 1147
Myelokathexis, 151t
Myelopathy
  noncompressive, differential diagnosis of, 1593
  vascular, in HIV infection, 1592-1593
Myeloperoxidase
  deficiency of, 108, 151t, 155
  in oxygen-dependent bactericidal mechanisms,
    101-102
Myelosuppression. See also Immunosuppression.
  granulocyte-macrophage colony-stimulating
    factor after, 554
  in hepatitis, 1981, 1985
  neutropenic enterocolitis in, 973
Myelotoxicity, of ganciclovir, 1791
Myiasis, 3307-3310, 3308t, 3309f, 3310f
Myocardial conduction system, in prosthetic
    valve endocarditis, 1030
Myocardial infarction
  in endocarditis, 981
  pleural effusion after, 847, 849-850
Myocarditis, 1052-1058. See also Endocarditis;
    Pericarditis.
  clinical manifestations of, 1055-1056
  diagnosis of, 1056-1057
  etiology of, 1052-1053, 1053t
  from Actinomyces, 2926
  from Candida, 2945
  from Chlamydophila psittaci, 2257
  from Corynebacterium diphtheriae, 1053,
    2461-2462
  from coxsackievirus B, 1054, 1054f
  from cytomegalovirus, 1790
  from enteroviruses, 2152-2153
    in neonate, 2154
  from influenza virus, 2071
  from lymphocytic choriomeningitis virus, 2095
  from mumps virus, 2005
  from parvovirus B19, 1895
  from polioviruses, 2143
  from Toxoplasma gondii, 3175f, 3176, 3177
  from Trypanosoma cruzi, 3158, 3158f, 3160
  in endocarditis, 994
  in HIV infection, 1053, 1560
  in Kawasaki disease, 3317
  in primary amebic meningoencephalitis, 3114
  noninfectious causes of, 1057, 1057t
  pathology of, 1054-1055, 1054f, 1055f
  prevention of, 1058
  treatment of, 1057-1058
  viral causes of, 1052-1054, 1053t, 1054f
Myonecrosis
  anaerobic
    streptococcal, 1200
    synergistic nonclostridial, 1188t, 1191,
      1200
    at episiotomy site, 1375, 1377t
    clostridial. See Gas gangrene.
    from Aeromonas hydrophila, 1200
    from Streptococcus pyogenes (group A), 2372
    nonclostridial, 1200

Myopathy
  in HIV infection, 1596
  in sepsis, 915
Myopericarditis, from enteroviruses, 2152-2153.
    See also Myocarditis; Pericarditis.
  in neonate, 2154
Myositis, 1194-1197, 1194-1202
  anaerobic streptococcal, 1188t
  classification of, 1195t
  clostridial. See Gas gangrene.
  cysticercus cellulosal, 1202
  etiology of, 1195t
  from Bacillus, 2495
  from Candida spp., 2947
  from Clostridium, 2831
  from enteroviruses, 2151-2152
  from HTLV, 2111
  from influenza virus, 2071
  from microsporidia, 3238t, 3244, 3245-3246,
    3247-3249, 3248t
  from Streptococcus pyogenes (group A), 2372,
    2372f
  from Toxoplasma gondii, 3175f, 3176, 3177
  in HIV infection, 1201, 1555
  in injection drug users, 3464
  inflammatory, 1201
  nonclostridial (crepitant), 1200
  nonpyogenic, 1195t, 1201-1202
  psoas abscess, 1200-1201
  pyogenic, 1194-1202, 1195t
  pyomyositis, 1195-1197
  streptococcal necrotizing, 1197-1198
Myringotomy, 770-771
Myroides spp., 2751t, 2759

N

Nacheromyia senegalensis, myiasis from, 3308-
    3310, 3308t
Naegleria [spp.]
  amphotericin B for, 571t, 592
  meningitis from, 1088
Naegleria aerobia. See Naegleria fowleri.
Naegleria australiensis, 3112
Naegleria fowleri, 3111-3119
  characteristics of, 3112, 3112f
  meningitis from, 1088, 1101, 1104-1105,
    1106t, 1115, 3111-3119. See also Primary
    amebic meningoencephalitis
Naegleria gruberi, 3115
Naegleria invadens. See Naegleria fowleri.
Naegleria italica, 3112
Nafcillin, 290, 290f
  dosage of, 652t-653t
  for bacterial arthritis, 1316t
  for brain abscess, 1157, 1159, 1159t
  for cavernous sinus thrombosis, 1424
  for cellulitis, 1180
  for infectious gangrene, 1182
  for lymphangitis, 1212
  for meningitis, 1106t, 1107t, 1114
  for orbital/preseptal cellulitis, 1423-1424
  for osteomyelitis, 1324t
    of jaw, 797t
  for parotitis, 797t
  for sialadenitis, 797t
  for staphylococcal endocarditis, 998, 999,
    2344t
    prosthetic valve, 1026t, 1027
  for staphylococcal osteomyelitis, 2346
  for staphylococcal scalded skin syndrome, 1174
  for suppurative thrombophlebitis, 1005
  formulations of, 646t
  minimal inhibitory concentration of, 284t
  prophylactic, perioperative, 3543t

Nails
  aspergillosis of, 2963
  dermatophytosis of, 3057, 3058, 3059, 3095t
  fungal infections of. See Onychomycosis.
Nairovirus spp., Crimean-Congo hemorrhagic
    fever from, 2086-2089, 2086t
Nalidixic acid, 451
  antimicrobial activity of, 455t, 456t
  dosage of, 672t-673t
  drug interactions with, 694t
  formulations of, 648t
  resistance to, outer membrane permeability in,
    262
  structure of, 451, 452f
Nannizzia spp., 3052
Nanophyetiasis, 3294t, 3298
Nanophyetus salmincola, syndrome of abdominal
    pain, diarrhea, and eosinophilia from, 1281t,
    1283
NAP test, for mycobacteria, 227
Naproxen, for fever, in cancer, 713-714, 725
Narcotics
  abuse of. See Injection drug users.
  rifamycin interaction with, 376t
Nasal cavity
  diphtheria of, 2461
  Staphylococcus aureus carriage in, 2322,
    2338-2339
    eradication of, 1176, 3540
  tuberculosis of, 2883
Nasal polyposis, from microsporidia, 3244
Nasojejunal tube, in pancreatic infections, 962
Nasolabial coccidioidomycosis, 3044, 3045f
Nasopharynx
  cancer of, 1808t, 1810, 1810f
    diagnosis of, 1813, 1813f, 1814f
  Moraxella (Branhamella) catarrhalis
    colonization of, 2530
  Neisseria meningitidis carriage in, 2500, 2501
National Committee for Clinical Laboratory
    Standards
  for biochemical methods, 216
  for molecular assays, 215
  for susceptibility testing, 222
Native Americans, hepatitis A in, 2170, 2170f,
    2179, 2179f
Natural antibodies, 40-41
Natural killer cells, 129, 135
  in HIV infection, 1537
  in sepsis, 916
  Toll-like receptor distribution in, 38, 39t
Natural resistance-associated macrophage
    protein-1
  in infection susceptibility, 48
  in mycobacterial disease susceptibility, 44-45,
    44t
Nausea, 1238-1239, 1239t
Nduma virus, 1914
Nebraska calf diarrhea virus, 1238
Necator americanus, 3261t, 3264
  albendazole for, 592
  treatment of, 573t
Neck infections
  anaerobic, 2812
  cystic, 799-800
  from Streptococcus anginosus group, 2454
  mediastinitis from, 1070-1071
Necrosis, papillary, pyelonephritis and, 875, 876,
    876f
Necrotizing enteritis, 1268-1269
Necrotizing enterocolitis, in newborn, 1267-1268
Necrotizing fasciitis, 1188t, 1189-1191
  at episiotomy site, 1375, 1377t
  clinical features of, 1188t, 1189-1190
  diagnosis of, 1190

Necrotizing fasciitis *(Continued)*
differential diagnosis of, 1188t, 1197
etiology of, 1188t, 1189, 1190
from *Streptococcus pyogenes,* 1188t, 1189-1191, 2371-2372
hyperbaric oxygen for, 566
in injection drug users, 3464
staphylococcal, 2341-2342
treatment of, 1190-1191
type I, 1188t, 1189
type II, 1188t, 1189
Necrotizing pneumonia, 853-856
from anaerobic infections, 2812
Necrotizing ulcerative gingivitis, 754, 756, 791
treatment of, 796, 796t
Needle exchange programs, in HIV infection prevention, 1494-1495
Needlestick injuries
hepatitis C from, 1961, 1965, 1969
HIV from, 3392, 3398
prevention of, 3396, 3397
Nef, in HIV nonprogression, 1533
Negishi virus, 1945t
Negri bodies, 2049, 2050f
Neisseria [spp.], 2529
biochemical characteristics of, 2532, 2532t
complement deficiency in, 79
COPD exacerbations from, 809
endocarditis from, 991
in narcotic addicts, 992
growth characteristics of, 2532, 2532t
laboratory identification of, 220
microbiology of, 2633t
susceptibility to, 56
treatment of
with linezolid, 437, 437t
with penicillins, 283, 284t
Neisseria cinerea, 2532, 2532t
Neisseria gonorrhoeae, 2514-2527. *See also*
Gonococcal infections.
adaptation by, 4
antibiotic resistant, 186, 1314, 2519
arthritis from, 1313-1315, 1315f, 2522
biochemical characteristics of, 2532, 2532t
cervicitis from, 1368-1369, 2520, 2520f
Chlamydia trachomatis coinfection and, 2246, 2524, 2525
clinical manifestations of, 2519-2523
clones of, 5
collection and transport of, 207t
complement deficiency from, 78-79
complications of, 2519-2520
conjunctivitis from, 1391-1392, 2521, 2521f
in neonate, 1392-1393
control measures for, 2526-2527
culture of, 1350, 2514, 2523
description of, 2514
diagnosis of, 2523-2524
disseminated, 1313-1314, 2522-2523, 2522f
treatment of, 2526
endocarditis from, 991
treatment of, 1000
endocervical infections from, 1368-1369, 2520, 2520f
epidemiology of, 2517-2519
epididymitis from, 1384, 1385
genetics of, 2516
genital infections from
in men, 2519, 2519f, 2520f
in women, 2520
Gram stain of, 1350, 2524
growth of, 2514
identification of, 220, 1315
in pregnancy, 2522
incidence of, 2517, 2517f, 2518f, 2518t

Neisseria gonorrhoeae (Continued)
incubation period for, 2519, 2519f, 2520
keratitis from, 1397-1400
laboratory studies for, 213
local infections from, 2521
mucopurulent cervicitis from, 1628
mupirocin for, 485t
neonatal infections with, 2523
nucleic acid amplification tests of, 2523-2524
outer membrane of, 2514-2516
pathology of, 2517, 2517t
pediatric infections from, 2523
treatment of, 2526
pelvic inflammatory disease from, 1378-1380, 1378f, 1379f, 1379t, 2521
treatment of, 2525-2526, 2525t
pericarditis from, 1059
perihepatitis from, 2521-2522
pharyngitis from, 754, 2365, 2521
pili of, 2514, 2515f
prevention of, 2526-2527
proctitis from, 1267, 2520
prostatitis from, 893
quinolone-resistant, 465
rash from, 736
respiratory infections from, 208
secondary peritonitis from, 933
sialylation of, 77
skin lesions from, 1186
strain typing of, 2516
surface structure of, 2514, 2515f
transmission of, 2517-2519
treatment of, 2524-2526, 2524t, 2525t
sex partner management in, 2526
with aminoglycosides, 334t-335t, 344t
with carbapenems, 313t
with cephalosporins, 298t
with chloramphenicol, 367t
with clindamycin, 409t
with macrolides, 397t, 398
with penicillins, 284t, 287, 288t
with quinolones, 455t
with quinupristin-dalfopristin, 425
with rifamycin, 374t
with spectinomycin, 350
with sulfonamides, 441t
with tetracyclines, 358
with trimethoprim, 444t
with trimethoprim-sulfamethoxazole, 444, 446
uncomplicated infections with, treatment of, 2524-2525, 2524t
urethral syndrome from, 1352
urethritis from, 460, 2519, 2520f
vaccine for, 2527
virulence factors of, 1314
Neisseria lactamica, 2532, 2532t
Neisseria meningitidis, 2498-2510. *See also under* Meningococcal.
antigenic structure of, 2499-2500
antisera identification of, 221
bacteremia from, 2502, 2506
bactericidal antibody activity against, 2500-2501
biochemistry of, 2499-2500, 2499t, 2532, 2532t
capsular polysaccharides of, 2499-2500, 2499t
carriage of, 2501-2502
chemoprophylaxis for, 2509
cell wall antigens of, 2500
clinical manifestations of, 2502-2506, 2503f-2505f
clones of, 5
collection and transport of, 210
conjunctivitis from, 1391-1392

Neisseria meningitidis (Continued)
diagnosis of, 2506-2507
epidemiology of, 2502
history of, 2498-2499
identification of, 220
infections from, 2502-2510
inflammation from, 914
meningitis from, 381, 1087, 1106t, 1112, 1117-1118. *See also* Meningococcal infections; *Neisseria meningitidis.*
clinical manifestations of, 2503-2504
geographic distribution of, 3640f
prevention of, 1117-1118
treatment of, 1106t, 1112, 2507t
vaccine for, for travelers, 3639t, 3640
meningococcemia from, 2502, 2503, 2503f-
meningoencephalitis from, 2502
pathogenesis of, 2500
pericarditis from, 1059
pharyngitis from, 2365
postsplenectomy sepsis from, 3528
rash from, 735-736, 1186
respiratory infections from, 2506
sepsis from, 907
serotypes of, 2502
skin lesions from, 735-736, 1186
transmission of, 2501
treatment of, 2507-2510, 2507t
with carbapenems, 313t
with cephalosporins, 298t, 2507, 2507t
with chloramphenicol, 367t
with clindamycin, 409t
with macrolides, 397t, 398
with mupirocin, 485t
with penicillins, 284t, 287, 288t
with quinolones, 455t
with quinupristin-dalfopristin, 425
with rifamycin, 374t, 381
with sulfonamides, 441t, 443
with trimethoprim, 444t
vaccine for, 1118-1119, 2507t, 2509-2510
W135, epidemic disease from, 2502
Neisseria sicca, 2532, 2532t
Neisseria subflava, 2532, 2532t
Neisseria weaveri, 2532, 2532t
Neisseriaceae, 2633t
Nelfinavir, 1665t, 1666
dosage of, 684t-685t
for perinatal HIV transmission prevention, 1625t, 1626
formulations of, 649t
pediatric, 1646t
resistance to, 1668
structure of, 1663f
Nematodes
intestinal, 3259t, 3260-3266
treatment of, 569t-570t, 592-594
syndrome of abdominal pain, diarrhea, and eosinophilia from, 1281t
systemic, treatment of, 594-595
tissue, 3267-3275
treatment of, 569t-570t
Neomycin, 484-485, 484t
chemical family of, 330t
dosage of, 660t-661t
formulations of, 647t
names and sources of, 329t
prophylactic
for wound infections, 480
perioperative, 3543t
structure of, 329f, 330
Neomycin-bacitracin-polymyxin, for wound infection prophylaxis, 480

Neonates. *See also* Children; Congenital
    infections; Infants.
    bacteremia in, from *Escherichia coli,* 2574
    brain abscess in, 1153
    Campylobacter jejuni in, 2552
    candidiasis in, 2949
    cellulitis in, 1178-1179
    chlamydiae in, 1392, 2247t, 2250-2251
    conjunctivitis in, 1189, 1392-1393, 2247t,
        2250-2251
    cytomegalovirus, 1797-1798
    dengue fever in, 1938
    enteroviruses in, 2153-2154
    group G streptococcal sepsis in, 2444
    hepatitis in
        from enteroviruses, 2154
        from hepatitis A virus, 2173
        from hepatitis B virus, 1874
            prevention of, 1884, 1884t
    herpes simplex virus in, 1759, 1771-1772,
        1771t
        keratitis from, 1189, 1400, 1402-1403, 1402t
    herpesviruses in, 1759
    HTLV in, 2103-2104, 2111-2112, 2113
    human papillomavirus in, 1843
    keratoconjunctivitis in, antiviral drugs for, 515t
    listeriosis in, 2480
    Lyme disease in, 2803
    measles in, 2035
    meningitis in, 1087, 1100, 1106t, 1114, 1118
        from *Chryseobacterium meningosepticum,*
            2757-2758
        prevention of, 1118
        treatment of, 1107t, 1114
    necrotizing enterocolitis in, 1267-1268
    necrotizing fasciitis in, 1189
    Neisseria gonorrhoeae in, 2523
    nosocomial epidemic diarrhea in, 1236-1237,
        1237t
    penicillin dosage in, 289t
    pneumonia in, from *Chlamydia trachomatis,*
        2247t, 2249, 2250-2251, 2251f
    sepsis in
        from *Enterococcus,* 2413-2414
        from nontypeable *Haemophilus influenzae,*
            2663
    Streptococcus agalactiae (group B) infections
        in, 2424-2427
    sulfonamides in, 244
    syphilis in, 2777, 2777t
    tetanus in, 2819, 2819f
    toxoplasmosis in
        diagnosis of, 3187-3188
        treatment of, 3191
    tuberculosis in, 2862
    varicella in, 1782-1783
        prevention of, 1785
    viral infections in, specimen collection for,
        233t
    vulvovaginitis in, 1359
Neoplastic meningitis, 1138-1139
Neorickettsia [spp.]
    classification and taxonomy of, 2284, 2310-
        2312, 2311t
    sennetsu neorickettsiosis from, 2315-2316
Neorickettsia helminthoeca, 2311, 2311t, 2312
Neorickettsia risticii, 2311, 2311t, 2312
Neorickettsia sennetsu, 2311, 2311t, 2312
Neosporin, prophylactic, intravascular devices
    and, 3356
Neotestudina rosatii, mycetoma from, 2991-2995,
    2992t, 2994f
Nephritis. *See also* Glomerulonephritis.
    acute focal bacterial, 895
    from *Aspergillus,* 2966

Nephritis *(Continued)*
    from *Candida,* 2946
    from microsporidia, 3243
    in elderly, 3517-3518
    in spinal cord injury, 3514
    in transplant recipients, 3503, 3509
    interstitial
        chronic, 876
        tuberculous, 2880
    shunt, 1128
Nephronia, lobar, 895
Nephropathia epidemica, 2086t, 2088-2089
Nephropathy
    HIV-associated, 1558-1559
    reflux, 886
Nephrotic syndrome, from hepatitis B, 1877
Nephrotoxicity
    of adefovir dipivoxil, 521
    of aminoglycosides, 339-341, 339f, 340t, 341t
    of amphotericin B deoxycholate, 502-504
    of cidofovir, 525
    of foscarnet, 527-528
    of teicoplanin, 424
    of vancomycin, 421
Nerve stimulation, for botulism diagnosis, 2825,
    2826f
Netilmicin
    antimicrobial activity of, 333, 334t-335t
    dosage of, 660t-661t
    formulations of, 647t
    names and sources of, 329t
    once-daily dosage regimens for, 348t
    structure of, 329f, 330
Neuraminidase inhibitors, 20, 20t
    for influenza, 2072t, 2073-2075
Neuraminidase, *Streptococcus pneumoniae*
    production of, 2396, 2396t
Neuritis, 1147-1148
Neurocysticercosis, 1137, 3289-3290
Neuromuscular blockade, after aminoglycoside
    administration, 343
Neuropathy
    distal sensory, in HIV infection, 1593-1594,
        1597t
    from *Corynebacterium diphtheriae,* 2462
    from ethambutol, 493
    in sepsis, 915
    inflammatory demyelinating, in HIV infection,
        1593, 1597t
Neuropsychiatric agents, rifamycin interaction
    with, 376t
Neuroretinitis. *See also* Retinitis.
    diffuse unilateral subacute, 3295
    in cat-scratch disease, 1417, 1417f, 2739-2740,
        2740f
Neurosyphilis. *See also* Syphilis.
    asymptomatic, 2775
    chronology of, 2774-2776, 2775f
    classification of, 1088, 2774, 2775t
    clinical features of, 1100, 2775, 2775t
    cranial nerves in, 2776
    encephalomyelitis in, 4, 1145
    etiology of, 1088
    gummatous, 1088
    in HIV infection, 1140
    late, 2774-2776
    meningitis in
        acute, 1088, 1100, 1103-1104, 1106t, 1115
        chronic, 1138, 1140
    meningovascular, 2775
    ocular inflammation in, 2776
    otitis in, 2776
    parenchymatous, 1088, 2775-2776
    tests for, 2779-2780
    treatment of, 1115, 2782

Neurotoxic shellfish poisoning, 3255-3256,
    3255f, 3256t
Neurotoxicity, 1219, 1220t
    clostridial, 28
    of amantadine, 523
    of foscarnet, 528
    of ganciclovir, 530
    of isoniazid, 490
    of tetracyclines, 363t, 364-365
Neurotoxins, of *Corynebacterium diphtheriae,*
    2462
Neutropenia, 103-104, 103t, 154. *See also*
    Immunocompromised host.
    acquired, 103-104
    associated pathogens of, 3421t
    cyclic, 104, 151t, 154
    febrile. *See* Febrile neutropenia.
    from vancomycin, 421
    fungal infections with
        macrophage colony-stimulating factor for,
            554
        prophylaxis for, 509, 510
    granulocyte colony-stimulating factor for, 552-
        553
    hereditary, 104
    in HIV infection, 1560
        colony-stimulating factors for, 553, 554
        prophylaxis against, 1682t
    infections in
        pathogenesis of, 3421-3428, 3426f
        sequence of events in, 3422t, 3429-3430,
            3429f
    mucormycosis in, 2974-2980
    Pseudomonas aeruginosa infections with, 2591
    quinolones for, 464
    severe chronic, 151t
    Streptococcus pneumoniae infections with,
        2398
    with cidofovir, 525
    with ganciclovir, 530
    with penicillins, 286
    X-linked, Wiskott-Aldrich syndrome protein in,
        153
Neutropenic enterocolitis (typhlitis), 973, 3457
    chemotherapy-induced, 3438, 3457
    etiology of, 3421t
    from *Clostridium* spp., 2834, 2835t, 2836
    in stem cell transplant, 3421t
Neutrophil(s), 56, 94-109
    apoptosis of, 101
    circulating, 96
    defects in, 103-109, 103t, 154-156, 155f, 156f
        antimicrobial prophylaxis for, 108-109
        bone marrow transplantation for, 109
        chemotaxic, 105-106, 105f
        gene therapy for, 109
        granulocyte transfusions for, 109
        intracellular killing, 106
    degranulation of, 101
    development of, 94
    evaluation of, 109, 110t
    exocytosis of, 101
    in HIV infection, 1537
    in inflammation, 96-101
    in leukocyte adhesion deficiency syndromes,
        104
    in local host response, 908
    ingestion by, 99, 99f
    kinetics of, 95-96
    life span of, 101
    microbial defenses against, 102-103
    microbicidal mechanisms of
        oxygen-dependent, 101-102
        oxygen-independent, 102
    migration of, 96-98, 97f, 98f

Neutrophil(s) (Continued)
mobilization of, 95-96
morphology of, 94-95, 94t, 95f
oxidative burst in, 99-101, 100f
abnormalities of, 106-108
in chronic granulomatous disease, 155, 155f
phagosome disposition by, 99-101, 100f
polymorphonuclear, 95-96
priming of, 96
pulmonary, 821
receptors of, 95
recruitment of, 96-98, 97f, 98f
resolution of, 101
structure of, 94-95, 94t, 95f
tissue, 96
Neutrophil elastase, 154
Neutrophil-specific granule deficiency, 151t, 155
Nevirapine, 1661-1662, 1662t
dosage of, 684t-685t
drug interactions with, 694t
for AIDS dementia, 1586
for perinatal HIV transmission prevention,
1624-1625, 1625t, 1640t
formulations of, 649t
pediatric, 1646t
resistance to, 1663
structure of, 1661f
New and emerging diseases, definition of, 739
New World cutaneous leishmaniasis, 3145t, 3149-
3152, 3149f, 3150f. See also Leishmaniasis.
New York virus, 2087
Newborns. See Neonates.
Newcastle disease, conjunctivitis in, 1390
Neytrtu, 3457-3458
Niacin poisoning, 1290
Nicholas-Durand-Favre disease. See
Lymphogranuloma venereum.
Niclosamide
for cestodes, 596
for helminthic disease, 570t
for intestinal flukes, 3277t
for tapeworms, 575t, 3289
structure of, 596f
Nifurtimox
adverse effects of, 581t
for African trypanosomiasis, 576t
for trypanosomiasis, 569t, 591, 3162
Nikkomycins, 511
Nipah virus, 180, 238, 1939, 2038-2039, 2039f,
2039t, 2040f, 2041-2042, 2043f
encephalitis from, 538, 1146
Nitazoxanide, 568t
adverse effects of, 581t
for amebiasis, 576t
for cryptosporidiosis, 571t, 3221-3222
for giardiasis, 3202-3203, 3202t
for helminthic disease, 570t
for isosporiasis, in HIV infection, 1689t
for luminal protozoa, 583
Nitric oxide, Salmonella resistance to, 2643-2644
Nitrofurantoin, 473-476
adverse effects of, 475
antimicrobial activity of, 473-474
dosage of, 474, 674t-675t
drug interactions with, 694t
for complicated urinary tract infections,
474
for Enterococcus, 2416
for uncomplicated cystitis, 474
for uncomplicated pyelonephritis, 474
formulations of, 648t
in children, 475-476
in pregnancy, 475-476
mechanism of action of, 473
pharmacology of, 474

Nitrofurantoin (Continued)
prophylactic, for recurrent urinary tract
infections, 475, 892
resistance to, 473
structure of, 473, 473f
urinary pH and, 888
Nitroimidazoles, for amebic liver abscess, 953
Nits, 3302-3304, 3303f
Nitzschia pungens, 1290
Nocardia [spp.], 2916-2922
blood culture of, 210, 210t
brain abscess from, 1151, 1158, 1158t, 1160,
2918
central nervous system infection from, 1088,
2918
characteristics of, 2916-2917, 2916f
classification of, 2916
clinical manifestations of, 2917-2918, 2918f
culture of, 2919
disseminated infections from, 2918, 2919f
ecology of, 2916
epidemiology of, 2916
identification of, 228-229, 2918-2919
in chronic granulomatous disease, 155
in immunocompromised host, 3436-3437
in transplant recipients, 3492, 3508
keratitis from, 1398-1400
laboratory diagnosis of, 228-229, 2916, 2918-
2919
lung abscess from, 1151t, 1152, 2916f, 2917-
2918
meningitis from, 1088, 2918
mycetoma from, 2917, 2991-2995, 2992t,
2995f
pathology and pathogenesis of, 2916
pleural effusion in, 847
pneumonia from, in HIV infection, 1570
prevention of, 2921
prognosis of, 2921-2922
pulmonary disease from, 1151t, 1152, 2916f,
2917-2918, 2918f
respiratory infections from, 209t
sclerosing mediastinitis from, 1075
skin infections from, 2917
splenic abscess from, 967, 967t
stains for, 214t
structure of, 2916-2917
taxonomy of, 229
transient colonization by, 2918
treatment of, 2919-2922, 2920t
with concurrent immunosuppression, 2921,
2922
with quinolones, 456t
virulence of, 2916-2917
vs. Actinomyces, 2931
Nocardia asteroides
in peritoneal dialysis, 941
pancreatic infections from, 959, 959t
sulfonamides for, 441t, 443
trimethoprim for, 444t
Nocardiopsis spp., laboratory tests for, 228-229
Nod protein receptors, 124
Nodular folliculitis, from Trichophyton rubrum,
3055
Nodular scabies, 3305, 3305f, 3306f
Nodules, 733. See also Rash.
causes of, 733, 733t
in rheumatic fever, 2383
pulmonary
differential diagnosis of, 861t
in coccidioidomycosis, 3043, 3044f
radiographic appearance of, 861t
subcutaneous, in blastomycosis, 3029t,
3033
Noma, 798

Non-A, non-B hepatitis, 1950. See also Hepatitis
C virus.
Non-ABC hepatitis, 1981
Non–A–E hepatitis, 1981, 1983-1984
Nongonococcal urethritis. See Urethritis,
nongonococcal.
Non-Hodgkin's lymphoma. See also Cancer;
Hematologic malignancies.
HIV-related, 1604-1607, 2130
antiretroviral therapy for, 1606
biotherapy for, 1607
chemotherapy for, 1605-1606, 1606t
clinical manifestations of, 1605
epidemiology of, 1604-1605
in women, 1627
liver in, 1579
pathogenesis of, 1605
prognosis of, 1605
pulmonary, 1572
salvage therapy for, 1607
treatment of, 1605-1607, 1606t
Non-nucleoside reverse transcriptase inhibitors,
1661-1663, 1662t
combination therapy with, 1672
for perinatal HIV transmission prevention,
1624-1626, 1625t
pediatric, 1646t, 1648t
resistance to, 1663
rifamycin interaction with, 376t
structures of, 1661f
Nonoxynol 9
for Chlamydia trachomatis prophylaxis, 2251
for Neisseria gonorrheae prophylaxis, 2527
in HIV transmission, 1494, 1619
in urinary tract infections, 876
Nonphyetus salmincola, 572t
Nonrenal clearance, 274
Nonsteroidal anti-inflammatory drugs
for colds, 749-750
for fever, 713-715
in myocarditis, 1054
quinolone effects on, 459
Nontuberculous mycobacteria. See Mycobacteria,
nontuberculous.
Norfloxacin, 457t
antimicrobial activity of, 455t, 456t
dosage of, 458t, 672t-673t
for bacterial gastroenteritis, 460-461
for cholera, 461
for genital chlamydial infections, 460
for gonococcal urethritis, 460
for Shigella, 2659t
for urinary tract infections, 459
formulations of, 648t
in preemptive pancreatic infection treatment,
963t
pharmacology of, 457t
Noroviruses, 2194-2199, 2195f, 2196f. See also
Caliciviruses.
collection of, 233t
diarrhea from, 178
disinfection/sterilization and, 3341
foodborne disease from, 1288-1289, 1292
gastroenteritis from, 1239, 1239t
laboratory studies for, 235
North Africa, HIV infection in, 1468
Nortriptyline, for herpes zoster ophthalmicus,
1403t
Norwalk virus, 2194-2199, 2195f, 2196f. See also
Caliciviruses.
Norwalk-like viruses
collection of, 233t
noninflammatory diarrhea from, 1239
Norwegian scabies, 3305-3307, 3306f
in HIV infection, 1558, 1559f

Nose blowing, sinusitis and, 774, 775f
Nosema [spp.], 3240. *See also* Microsporidia.
  in HIV infection, 1701
Nosema algerae, keratitis from, 1405
Nosema ocularum, keratitis from, 1405
Nosocomial infections, 3323-3417. *See also*
    Postoperative infections; Wound infections.
  antimicrobial utilization and, 3324
  bacteremia in
    from coagulase-negative staphylococci,
      2353-2354
    from *Staphylococcus aureus,* 2342
  bacteriuria in, 883
    treatment of, 887
  catheter-related, 3347-3358. *See also* Catheter-
    related infections.
  control of, 3323-3326
  decontamination against, 3331
  diarrhea in, 1241
  disinfection against, 3331-3333, 3332t
  education on, 3324
  employee health and, 3324
  endocarditis in, 975-976
  environmental hygiene and, 3324
  fever of unknown origin in, 719t, 721
  from arenaviruses, 2096
  from *Corynebacterium,* 2466, 2466t
  from *Cryptosporidium,* 1241
  from cytomegalovirus, 3414-3416
  from Epstein-Barr virus, 3416
  from hepatitis, 3381-3384, 3381t, 3383t
  from hepatitis A, 2171-2172
  from hepatitis C, 1965
  from herpesviruses, 3409-3417
  from HIV, 3391-3405
  from human herpesvirus 6, 3416
  from human herpesvirus 7, 3416
  from human herpesvirus 8, 3417
  from Lassa virus, 2096
  from *Legionella,* 2715, 2726, 2727f
  from methicillin-resistant *Staphylococcus
    aureus,* 2333
  from *Moraxella (Branhamella) catarrhalis,*
    2531
  from *Mycobacterium tuberculosis,* 2858-2859,
    3327-3329
  from *Pseudomonas aeruginosa,* 2588-2589
  from respiratory syncytial virus, 2017
    prevention of, 2020-2021
  from *Salmonella,* 2650
    nontyphoidal, 2640-2641
  from SARS, 3330
  from *Staphylococcus epidermidis,* 2353
  from *Stenotrophomonas maltophilia,* 2616-
    2617
  from transfusions, 3385-3388, 3385f, 3386t,
    3387t
  from varicella-zoster virus, 3410-3414, 3412f,
    3413f
  future challenges of, 3326
  HIV infection transmission in, 1470
  hospital epidemiology program organization
    and, 3325
  hospital waste and, control of, 3342, 3343t
  infectious waste and, management of, 3342,
    3343t
  isolation and, 3326-3330, 3327t, 3328t, 3330t
  JCAHO standards and, 3325
  new-product evaluation and, 3324
  of respiratory tract, 835-836, 3362-3368. *See
    also* Pneumonia, nosocomial.
    from *Moraxella (Branhamella) catarrhalis,*
      2531
    from respiratory syncytial virus, 2017, 2020-
      2021

Nosocomial infections *(Continued)*
  of urinary tract, 3370-3377
  outbreak investigation and, 3323, 3324t
  percutaneous intravascular devices and, 3347-
    3358
  pneumonia in
    from *Staphylococcus aureus,* 2345
    in sepsis, 921
    quinolones for, 462-463
  policy development and, 3324
  sterilization against, 3331-3333, 3332t, 3338-
    3340
  surveillance and, 3323
  tetracycline resistance in, 359
  treatment of, with cephalosporins, 306
  urinary tract, 882
NOX gene family, in oxidative burst, 101
NRAMP1
  in infection susceptibility, 48
  in mycobacterial disease susceptibility, 44-45,
    44t
Nuclear factor κB essential modulator, defects in,
    156-157
Nuclear medicine studies. *See* Radionuclide
    scanning.
Nucleic acid amplification, 11-12
  for HIV infection, 1508t, 1513-1514
  for mycobacteria, 225, 226
  for *Mycobacterium tuberculosis,* 2853-2855,
    2854t
  for *Neisseria gonorrhoeae,* 2523-2524
  microorganism identification with, 221-222
Nucleic acid hybridization techniques, in sputum
    examination, 826
Nucleocapsid, viral, 1730-1731, 1731f
Nucleoside reverse transcriptase inhibitors, 1655-
    1661, 1656f, 1657t
  combination therapy with, 1671-1672
  for Kaposi's sarcoma, 1604
  neurotoxicity of, 1594, 1594t, 1597t
  pediatric, 1646t, 1648t
  perinatal HIV transmission prevention with,
    1624, 1625t
  resistance to, 1660-1661
  structures of, 1656f
Nursing homes, tuberculin positivity in, 2875
Nutrition, 139-147. *See also* Malnutrition *and
    specific nutrients.*
  assessment of, 140, 140t
  immunity and, 139-147, 3427
  in HIV infection, 145
  in sepsis, 921
Nutritional support, 144
  catheter-related infections in, 3352-3355,
    3353t, 3354t
  for elderly patients, 146-147, 146t
  in pancreatic infection prevention, 962
  total parenteral nutrition in, 1035
Nystatin
  dosage of, 678t-679t
  for candidiasis, 1687t, 2949-2951
  for vulvovaginal candidiasis, 1364
  formulations of, 649t

O

Obesity, chronic disease in, 140
Observational studies, 164-166
Obstetric delivery. *See* Delivery; Labor.
Occupational exposures. *See also* Health care
    workers; Nosocomial infections.
  immunizations for, 3575
  pneumonia and, 823t, 858
  to cytomegalovirus, 3415-3416
  to disinfectants, 3333

Occupational exposures *(Continued)*
  to Epstein-Barr virus, 3416
  to herpes simplex virus, 3410
  to HIV, 3392-3394, 3392f, 3393t, 3397-3399
    chemoprophylaxis after, 3400-3405, 3402t,
      3403t
  to varicella-zoster virus, 3413-3414
Occupational Safety and Health Administration
    (OSHA), blood-borne pathogen standard of,
    disinfection and, 3340
Ochrobactrum [spp.], 2751t, 2759
Ochrobactrum anthropi, 2759
Ochroconis gallopavum, brain abscess from, 3070
Ockelbo virus, 1914-1919
Ocular infections
  from *Aspergillus,* 1404, 1409, 1411, 2963,
    2966
  from *Bacillus,* 2495
  from *Borrelia burgdorferi,* 2802, 2802t
  from *Brucella,* 2671-2672
  from *Candida,* 1404, 1408-1409, 1411, 1417,
    2947-2948, 2948f, 2951
    in injection drug users, 3472
  from *Cryptococcus neoformans,* 3003t, 3005
  from *Dirofilaria repens,* 3273
  from *Histoplasma capsulatum,* 3021, 3025
  from *Macacanema formosana,* 3273
  from microsporidia, 1393, 1405, 3238t, 3243-
    3245, 3248t, 3249
  from *Mycobacterium tuberculosis,* 1415-1416,
    1416f
  from myiasis, 3310
  from *Onchocerca lupi,* 3273
  from *Pseudomonas aeruginosa,* 1397-1400,
    2604
  from *Setaria labiatopapillosa,* 3273
  from *Sporothrix schenckii,* 2986
  from *Staphylococcus epidermidis,* 2357
  from *Toxocara canis,* 3294-3295, 3294t
  from *Toxoplasma gondii,* 3176
  host defenses in, 36
  in endocarditis, 982, 983f
  in HIV infection, 1559-1560
  in injection drug users, 3472
  in mucormycosis, 2975-2977, 2976f
  in neonates, 1189, 1392-1393, 1400, 1402-
    1403, 1402t, 2247t, 2250-2251
  in Reiter's syndrome, 1354-1355
  specimen collection and transport in, 206t
  viral, 519, 520
    specimen collection in, 233t
Ocular larva migrans, 3294-3295, 3294t
Oculogenital infections, from *Chlamydia
    trachomatis,* 2245, 2245f, 2247t, 2249-2250
Oculogenital syndrome, nongonococcal urethritis
    and, 1207
Oculoglandular syndrome, 1207, 1390, 1393
  in cat-scratch disease, 2737, 2739f
  lymphadenitis in, 1207
Odocoileus virginianus, in Lyme disease
    transmission, 2798
Odontogenic infections, 787-798
  anatomic considerations in, 789-790, 789f,
    790f
  brain abscess from, 1151t, 1152
  carotid artery erosion in, 794
  clinical presentation of, 790-793
  complications of, 793-795
  deep fascial space, 754, 756, 791-793, 792f
  dentoalveolar, 790-791
  diagnosis of, 795
  from anaerobic gram-negative bacilli, 2841
  from *Streptococcus mutans,* 2436
  gingival, 791

Odontogenic infections *(Continued)*
  host defenses against, 789
  imaging of, 795, 796f
  in immunocompromised host, 3437
  lung abscess and, 787
  microbiology of, 787-788, 787t, 788f
  periodontal, 791
  septic cavernous sinus thrombosis in, 794, 795f
  sinusitis from, 778
  spread of, 789-790, 789f-791f
  suppurative, treatment of, 797-798, 797t
  treatment of, 795-798, 796t, 797t
Oerskovia spp., 2471
Oesophagostomum bifurcum, 579t
Oestridae, myiasis from, 3307-3310, 3308t
Oestrus ovis, myiasis from, 3308-3310, 3308t
Ofloxacin
  antimicrobial activity of, 455t, 456t
  dosage of, 458t, 672t-673t
  for bacterial gastroenteritis, 460-461
  for community-acquired pneumonia, 462
  for enteric fever, 461
  for genital chlamydial infections, 460
  for hospital-acquired pneumonia, 463
  for keratitis, 1399
  for leprosy, 499
  for mycobacterial infections, 464
  for *Neisseria gonorrhoeae,* 2524t
    in epididymitis, 2526
    in pelvic inflammatory disease, 2525, 2525t
    in urethritis, 460
  for *Neisseria meningitidis* carriage, 2509
  for neutropenia, 464
  for pelvic inflammatory disease, 460, 2247t,
      2250
  for peritonitis, 461
  for psittacosis, 2257
  for respiratory infections, 462
  for septic arthritis, 463
  for skin infections, 463-464
  for typhoid fever, 2648, 2649t
  for urethritis, 1207
  for urinary tract infections, 459, 460
  for urogenital chlamydial infections, 2247t,
      2249, 2250
  formulations of, 648t
  in preemptive pancreatic infection treatment,
      963-964, 963t
  pharmacology of, 457t
  structure of, 451, 452f
OKT3, in cytomegalovirus reactivation, 1795
Old World cutaneous leishmaniasis, 3145t, 3149-
    3152. *See also* Leishmaniasis.
Older adults. *See* Elderly.
Oligella [spp.], 2751t, 2759
Oligella ureolytica, 2759
Oligella urethralis, 2759
Oligosaccharides, for otitis media prevention, 769
Omega-3 fatty acid, 143
Omentum, greater, 927, 927f
Omphalitis, necrotizing fasciitis from, 1189
Omsk hemorrhagic fever, 1929, 1945
  as biological weapon, 3627-3629, 3628t
Onchocerca [spp.], 3273-3274
  ocular infections from, 1405, 3273
  skin lesions from, 3653f
Onchocerca volvulus
  diethylcarbamazine for, 594
  ivermectin for, 572t, 577t, 594
Oncogenic viruses, 1738
Online resources. *See* Digital resources.
Onychomycosis
  differential diagnosis of, 3057
  etiology of, 3060
  from *Acremonium,* 3060

Onychomycosis *(Continued)*
  from *Aspergillus,* 2963, 3060
  from *Candida,* 2943, 2943f
    chronic, 2944, 2945f
  from dermatophytes, 3057
    treatment of, 3058, 3059
  from *Fusarium,* 3060
  from *Scopulariopsis brevicaulis,* 3060
  from *Scytalidium,* 3058, 3059, 3060f
  superficial white, 3057
O'nyong-nyong virus, 1913-1919, 1914t. *See also*
    Alphaviruses.
Opa, 2515
Opacity factor, in group A *Streptococcus,* 2363
Ophthalmia neonatorum, 1189, 1392-1393, 1400,
    1402-1403, 1402t, 2247t, 2250-2251
  gonococcal, 2523
Ophthalmomyiasis, 3310
Opioids
  abuse of. *See* Injection drug users.
  rifamycin interaction with, 376t
Opisthorchis [spp.], 3277t, 3281-3282, 3281f
Opisthorchis felineus, biliary tract infections
    from, 956
Opisthorchis viverrini
  biliary tract infections from, 956
  syndrome of abdominal pain, diarrhea, and
      eosinophilia from, 1281t, 1282
  treatment of, 572t
Opisthotonus, from tetanus, 2818, 2819f
Opportunism, 3
Opportunistic infections. *See also*
    Immunocompromised host *and specific*
    diseases and pathogens.
  CD4 in, 1549, 1550f, 1679-1680
    prophylaxis indications and, 1684t
  commensals in, 4
  etiology of, 3421t
  in HIV infection, 1486, 1549-1550, 1550f
    antiretroviral therapy impact on, 1550,
        1551f, 1552, 1679
    in developing world, 1472
    in women, 1627-1630
    monitoring during, 1679-1680
    organisms in, 1680
    pediatric, 1640-1641
      prophylaxis against, 1649
    prophylaxis for, 1681t-1684t
    treatment of, 1679-1702, 1681, 1685t-1691t
  laboratory diagnosis of, 3428-3429, 3439
  management of, 3439
  overview of, 3421-3430
  pathogenesis of, 3421-3428
  pathogens in, 3, 4
  sequence of events in, 3422t, 3429-3430, 3429f
Opsonins, 56, 99
Opsonization, 55-56, 56t, 70, 106
  complement-mediated, 76
  of *Streptococcus agalactiae* (group B)
      infections, 2426
Optic neuritis
  from chloramphenicol, 369
  from ethambutol, 493
Optochin, 216t
Oral cavity. *See also* Stomatitis.
  anaerobic infections of, 2812, 2839
    from gram-negative bacilli, 2841
  candidiasis of, 2490f, 2940-2941, 2940f, 2941f,
      2950-2951
    chronic, 2944
    in immunocompromised host, 798-799,
        2944, 3483
    prevention of, in transplant recipients, 3483
    treatment of, 2950-2951
  Capnocytophaga in, 2731

Oral cavity *(Continued)*
  enanthems of, 731, 734
  flora of, 787-788, 787t, 789, 3423f, 3424-3426,
      3425f
    lung abscess from, 854
  host defenses in, 789
  in HIV infection, 1554-1555, 1554f, 1555f
  in pediatric HIV infection, 1643
  lesions of, in immunocompromised host, 3437
  leukoplakia of
    from *Candida,* 2941
    hairy
      in HIV infection, 1555, 1808
      treatment of, 1815
  portals of entry in, 3425f
  specimen collection and transport from, 206t-5t
  ulcers of, 754, 798
    differential diagnosis of, 754, 756
    from herpes simplex virus, 1765-1766,
        1766f, 1773-1774, 1773t. *See also*
        Herpes simplex virus, orofacial.
    from *Paracoccidioides brasiliensis,* 3064-
        3065, 3065f
    in acute retroviral syndrome, 1552, 1553f
    in hand-foot-mouth disease, 798-799, 2150
    in histoplasmosis, 3021, 3021f
    in HIV infection, 1555
    in immunocompromised host, 798-799
    in Marshall's syndrome, 1208
    vs. herpetic pharyngitis, 756
  verrucous lesions of, 1847, 1850
Oral contraceptives
  in HIV transmission, 1489, 1619
  tetracycline with, 364t
Oral hairy leukoplakia, 1808
  treatment of, 1815
Oral health, in endocarditis prevention, 1044
Oral mucositis, in immunocompromised host,
    798-799
Oral rehydration therapy, 1226. *See also* Fluid
    management.
  for rotavirus, 1909
Orbital abscess/cellulitis, 1421-1424, 1421f-1423f
  in mucormycosis, 1423, 2975-2977, 2976f
Orbital apex syndrome, 1423
Orbiviruses, 1899
Orchitis, 1385
  from *Candida,* 2951
  from lymphocytic choriomeningitis virus,
      2095
  from mumps virus, 2005, 2007
  in HIV infection, 1385-1386
  in melioidosis, 2628f
Orf, 1753
Oriental sore, 3149
Orientia [spp.], 2311
  classification of, 2284
Orientia tsutsugamushi, 2284, 2309-2310,
    2309f
  vector of, 2285t, 3311
Ornidazole
  adverse effects of, 581t
  for luminal protozoa, 582-583
Ornithodoros spp., 3312-3314, 3313t
  in relapsing fever transmission, 2795
Ornithonyssus bacoti, 3311
Orofacial fascial spaces, 790, 790f
Orofacial infections, 787-800
  anaerobic, 2812
  from *Actinomyces,* 797t, 2925-2926
  from herpes simplex virus. *See* Herpes simplex
      virus, orofacial.
  from *Streptococcus anginosus* group, 2454
  mediastinitis from, 1070-1071
  nonodontogenic, 798-799

Orofacial infections (Continued)
  odontogenic, 787-798. See also Odontogenic infections.
Oropharyngeal infections. See also Oral cavity; Pharyngitis.
  from Candida, 2940-2941, 2940f, 2941f
    chronic, 2944
    in immunocompromised host, 798-799, 2944, 3437, 3483
    prevention of, in transplant recipients, 3483
    treatment of, 2950-2951
Oropouche virus, 2089
Oroya fever, 739-740
  from Bartonella bacilliformis, 2733-2734
  postsplenectomy, 3528
  vs. enteric fever, 1277
Ortho-benzyl-para-chlorophenol, disinfection with, 3337
Orthohepadnaviruses, 1864
Orthopedic implant infections
  rifamycin for, 380-381
  teicoplanin for, 425
Ortho-phenylphenol, disinfection with, 3337
Ortho-phthalaldehyde (OPA), disinfection with, 3335t, 3336
Orthopoxviruses
  characteristics of, 1742-1744, 1743f
  classification of, 1742-1749
  pathogenesis of, 1744
  treatment of, 1749
  vaccinia virus, 740-741, 1744-1746
  variola virus, 740-741, 1389-1390, 1746-1747
Orthoreoviruses, 1899
Orungo virus, 1899
Oseltamivir, 515t, 535-536
  dosage of, 682t-683t
  for influenza, 805, 2072t, 2073-2075
    for prophylaxis, 1682t, 2078
  formulations of, 649t
  side effects of, 2072t, 2074
  structure of, 535, 536f
Osler nodes, 736, 1187
  in endocarditis, 984
Osteitis pubis, 1328-1329
Osteochondritis, ciprofloxacin for, 463
Osteomyelitis, 1322-1330
  after contaminated open fracture, 1325-1326, 1325f
  anaerobic, 2813
    from gram-negative bacilli, 2843
  antimicrobial therapy for, 246, 1324-1325, 1324t
    outpatient parenteral, 629-630, 629t
    with quinolones, 463
    with vancomycin, 423
  bone scans of, 1323, 1324f
  classification of, 1322-1323, 1322t, 1323t
  complications of, in HIV-infected women, 1631
  culture-negative, 1330
  diagnosis of, 1323
  experimental models of, 1323
  from Actinomyces, 2926, 2929
  from anaerobic gram-negative bacilli, 2843
  from Aspergillus, 2966, 2966f
  from Bacillus, 2495
  from Blastomyces dermatitidis, 3033, 3033f
  from Candida, 2946
  from Coccidioides immitis, 3044, 3045f
  from Cryptococcus neoformans, 3005
  from Enterococcus, 2413
  from Kingella, 2533
  from Mycobacterium tuberculosis, 1329-1330
  from nontuberculous mycobacteria, 2910t, 2912

Osteomyelitis (Continued)
  from Pasteurella, 2688
  from Pseudomonas aeruginosa, 2602-2603, 2603
  from Salmonella, 2647t
  from Sporothrix schenckii, 2985, 2985f, 2986, 2987
  from Staphylococcus aureus, 2345-2347, 2345t, 2347f
    rifamycin for, 380-381
  from Staphylococcus epidermidis, 2356-2357
  from Streptococcus agalactiae (group B), 2427
  from streptococcus group C, 2443
  from streptococcus group G, 2443
  fungal, 1330
  hematogenous, 1328
  in diabetes mellitus, 1327-1328, 1327t
  in hemodialysis, 1329
  in injection drug users, 1329, 3464-3465
  in melioidosis, 2625, 2627f
  in sickle cell disease, 1329
  in sinusitis, 781, 781f
  in spinal cord injury, 3515-3516
  in stem cell transplant, 3488
  laboratory studies for, 213
  magnetic resonance imaging of, 2346, 2347f
  microbiology of, 1323t, 2345t
  of clavicle, 1329
  of jaw, 794-795. See also Odontogenic infections.
    treatment of, 797t, 798
  of sacroiliac joint, 1329
  of vertebrae, 1326-1327, 1326f
    from Aspergillus, 2966, 2966f
    from Candida, 2946, 2947f
    from Coccidioides immitis, 3044, 3045f
    from Pseudomonas aeruginosa, 2602-2603
    in injection drug users, 3465
  quinolones for, 463
  refractory, hyperbaric oxygen for, 566
  subcutaneous abscess in, 1191
  surgery for, 1325t
Osteomyelitis pubis, 1377-1378
Otitis, 766-771
  from anaerobic gram-negative bacilli, 2841
  from Pseudomonas aeruginosa, 2604-2605
  syphilitic, 2776
    treatment of, 2782
  tuberculous, 2882
Otitis externa, 766
  ciprofloxacin for, 463
  from Actinomyces, 2926
  from Aspergillus, 766, 2963
  in immunocompromised host, 3437
  malignant (necrotizing), from Pseudomonas aeruginosa, 2604-2605
Otitis media, 766-771
  azithromycin for, 404
  bacterial, 767, 767t
  brain abscess from, 1151t, 1152
  chemoprophylaxis for, 769-770
  chronic suppurative, from Pseudomonas aeruginosa, 2605
  clarithromycin for, 404
  colds and, 2189-2190
  course of, 768
  diagnosis of, 768
  epidemiology of, 767
  from Actinomyces, 2926
  from anaerobic infections, 2812
  from Chlamydophila pneumoniae, 2262
  from Chlamydia trachomatis, 768
  from Haemophilus influenzae, 767, 767t, 769, 2662, 2663

Otitis media (Continued)
  from measles virus, 2035
  from Moraxella (Branhamella) catarrhalis, 2530, 2531f
  from parainfluenza virus, 2-3, 2000
  from respiratory syncytial virus, 2014-2015, 2015t, 2016, 2016t
  from rhinoviruses, 2189-2190
  from Streptococcus pneumoniae, 2399
    treatment of, 2404
  immunology of, 768
  management of, 768-769
  mastoiditis from, 771
  microbiology of, 767-768, 767t
  pathogenesis of, 767
  prevention of, 770-771
  suppurative intracranial thrombophlebitis from, 1168-1170
  tympanostomy tubes for, 770-771
  vaccines for, 770, 770t
  viral, 767-768
Ototoxicity
  of aminoglycosides, 341-343, 872
  of erythromycin, 400
  of teicoplanin, 424
  of vancomycin, 421
Otr, in tetracycline resistance, 358, 360t
Outbreak investigations, 165-166
  nosocomial infections and, 3323, 3324t
Ova and parasite examination, 3202. See also Stool examination.
  specimen collection and transport for, 207t
Ovulation, in HIV infection, 1630
Oxacillin, 290, 290f
  dosage of, 652t-653t
  for anaerobes, 284t
  for bacilli, 284t
  for bacterial arthritis, 1316t
  for brain abscess, 1159, 1159t
  for Enterobacteriaceae, 284t
  for meningitis, 1106t, 1107t, 1114
  for osteomyelitis, 1324t
  for Pseudomonas, 284t
  for staphylococcal endocarditis, 2344t
    prosthetic valve, 1026t, 1027
  formulations of, 646t
  minimal inhibitory concentration of, 284t
  prophylactic, perioperative, 3543t
Oxacillinase, 256, 258t
Oxamniquine, for schistosomiasis, 575t, 580t, 596, 3280
Oxazolidinones, 436-439
  adverse effects of, 438-439
  antimicrobial activity of, 437, 437t
  mechanism of action of, 436
  pharmacology of, 437
  resistance to, 438
  structure of, 436, 436f
  uses of, 437-438, 437t
Oxidase, 216t
Oxidative burst
  abnormalities of, 106-108
    in chronic granulomatous disease, 155, 155f
  in neutrophils, 99-101, 100f
Oxolinic acid, 451, 452f
  dosage of, 672t-673t
Oxygen administration
  for bronchiolitis, 817
  for peritonitis, 940
  hyperbaric. See Hyperbaric oxygen.
  postoperative infections and, 3537-3538

Oxytetracycline, 358t. *See also* Tetracycline(s).
  dosage of, 662t-663t
  formulations of, 647t
Oysters, *Vibrio vulnificus* in, 2545, 2546

P

P fimbriae
  of *Escherichia coli,* 19-20, 19f, 877-878
    purified, 19-20
P15s, 102
P22*phox,* 100
P24 antigen
  in acute retroviral syndrome, 1553
  in HIV testing, 1512-1513
  in pediatric HIV infection, 1645
P47*phox,* 100-101
  deficiency of, 106-107
P67*phox,* 100-101
  deficiency of, 107
P150,95, 97
Pacemakers, infections of, 1033-1034
Paclitaxel, for Kaposi's sarcoma, 1603
Paecilomyces spp., 3073
  in chronic granulomatous disease, 155
Paenibacillus [spp.], 218, 219t
Paenibacillus alvei, 2493
Pain
  in appendicitis, 969, 970t
  muscle. *See* Myalgia.
PAIR procedure, for hydatid cyst, 3291
Palivizumab, 3574
  dosage of, 682t-683t
  for otitis media, 770
  for respiratory syncytial virus, 558, 2021
    in immunocompromised host, 2018
  formulations of, 649t
Palm pilots, 3658-3660, 3660t, 3661t
Panbronchiolitis, erythromycin for, 402
Pancreatic enzymes, in secondary peritonitis, 933
Pancreatic infections, 959-965
  abscess in, 960, 961t
  definitions in, 960, 961t
  diagnosis of, 960-961
  enteral feeding for, 962
  flora in, 961
  in acute pancreatitis, 960-965
  in HIV infection, 1579
  necrosis in, 960, 961t
  preemptive antibiotics for, 962-965, 963t, 965t
  prevention of, 962-965
  pseudocyst in, 960, 961t
  selective gut decontamination for, 962
  treatment of, 961-962
  tuberculosis in, 2881
Pancreatic transplantation
  infections in, 3505. *See also* Transplantation, infections in.
  survival in, 3501t
Pancreatitis, 961t
  acute, pleural effusion and, 847, 849
  drug-induced, 959, 959b, 1579
  fluid collection in, 960, 961t
  from cytomegalovirus, 1792
  from enteroviruses, 2156
  from mumps virus, 2005
  fungal infections in, 961
  in cryptosporidiosis, 3220, 3221
  in HIV infection, 960, 1579
  infectious causes of, 959-960, 959b. *See also* Pancreatic infections.
  severe, 960, 961t
Pancriolauryl test, for tropical sprue, 1303
Panonychus citri, 3311
Pantoea agglomerans, 2579, 2581

Pap, 877
Papanicolaou smear, 1850-1851, 1851t
  in HIV infection, 1610, 1611t, 1627
  of fungi, 230
Papillary necrosis, pyelonephritis and, 875, 876, 876f
Papillomatosis. *See also* Human papillomavirus(es).
  conjunctival, 1847
  oral, 1847, 1850
  respiratory, 525
Papillomaviruses, 1841-1851. *See also* Human papillomavirus(es).
  antiviral agents for, 515t
  interferons for, 534, 555
Papua New Guinea, enteritis necroticans in, 2835
Papular-purpuric gloves-and-socks syndrome, 732
  pediatric, 234-235
Papules, 730t, 731. *See also* Rash.
  causes of, 732-733
  from cat-scratch disease, 2736, 2737f
  in syphilis, 2773
  of yaws, 2786-2787, 2786f, 2787f
Para-aminobenzoic acid, 440, 440f
Paracentesis, in secondary peritonitis, 935
Paracoccidioides brasiliensis, 3062-3066
  adrenal infections from, 3065
  appearance of in tissue, 2938t, 3062, 3063f
  characteristics of, 3062
  chronic adult form of, 3063, 3064
  clinical manifestations of, 3063-3065, 3064f, 3065f
  culture of, 3062, 3063f, 3066
  differential diagnosis of, 3065
  ecology of, 3062-3063
  epidemiology of, 3062-3063
  gastrointestinal involvement from, 1269
  geographic distribution of, 3062-3063
  histopathology of, 3065-3066
  immune response to, 3063-3064
  in HIV infection, 1688t
  itraconazole for, 508
  juvenile form of, 3063, 3064
  ketoconazole for, 507
  laboratory diagnosis of, 229, 3065-3066
  latency of, 3063
  lymphadenopathy from, 3065
  mucosal lesions from, 3064, 3065f
  pancreatic infections from, 959t, 960
  pathogenesis of, 3063-3064
  pulmonary infections from, 3064, 3064f, 3065f
  serology of, 3066
  skin lesions from, 3064-3065, 3065f
  transmission of, 3063
  treatment of, 3066
Paracolic gutter, 927, 928, 928f
Paracolon spp., endocarditis from, 992
Paragonimus spp., 3277t, 3281f, 3283
  praziquantel for, 595
  pulmonary infections from, triclabendazole for, 577t
Paragonimus westermani
  pancreatic infections from, 959t, 960
  treatment of, 572t
Parainfluenza virus(es), 1998-2001
  bronchiolitis from, 812-813, 813t, 2000, 2000t
  characteristics of, 1998
  classification of, 1998
  clinical manifestations of, 2000, 2000t
  colds from, 747-750, 747t
  collection of, 233t
  croup from, 760-761, 760t, 2000
  diagnosis of, 2000-2001
  epidemiology of, 1999-2000
  immune response to, 1998-1999, 1999f

Parainfluenza virus(es) *(Continued)*
  in bone marrow transplant recipients, 2000
  in stem cell transplant recipients, 3494
  laboratory tests for, 234
  laryngitis from, 758, 759t
  otitis media from, 2000
  pathogenesis of, 1998
  replication of, 1998
  sinusitis from, 776, 776t
  treatment of, 2001
  tropism of, 1998
  vaccines for, 2001
Paralysis
  acute motor, in acute hemorrhagic conjunctivitis, 2156
  from enteroviruses, 2149, 2156, 2157
  from nonpolio enteroviruses, 2150-2151
  from polioviruses, 2141-2144
  infections in, 3512-3516
  tick, 3313t, 3314
Paralytic rabies, 2051, 2051t
Paralytic shellfish poisoning, 3255, 3255f, 3256t
Paramyxoviruses, 2003, 2009
  vitamin A for, 141
  zoonotic, 2038-2044
    classification of, 2038, 2039f
    Hendra virus, 2038-2041
    Menangle virus, 2038-2039, 2042-2044
    Nipah virus, 2038-2039, 2041-2042
    structure of, 2039, 2040f
Parapneumonic effusion. *See* Pleural effusion.
Parapoxviruses, 1753
Parasitic infections. *See also specific parasites.*
  biliary tract, 956
  conjunctivitis from, 1393
  enteritis from, 1270
  eosinophilia in, 110, 3258-3259, 3293
  gastrointestinal, in HIV infection, 1580
  geographic distribution of, 3654t
  helminthic, 568, 3258-3259. *See also* Helminthic infections.
  HTLV and, 2109, 2111
  in transplant recipients, 3506-3507
  in travelers, 3652, 3654
  keratitis from, 1404-1405
  laboratory detection of, 212
  pericarditis from, 1059, 1059t
  pneumonia from, in HIV infection, 1572
  protozoal, 3095, 3095t, 3096t. *See also* Protozoal infections.
  pulmonary infiltrates with eosinophilia from, 835
  specimen collection and transport for, 206t, 207t
  taxonomy of, 568
  treatment of, 568-596
    adverse effects of, 581t-582t
    drug activity spectrum in, 568t-570t
  vs. enteric fever, 1275t, 1278
Paraspinal abscess
  from *Coccidioides immitis,* 3044, 3046f
  tuberculous, 2879
Paratyphoid fever
  from *Salmonella paratyphi,* 2644-2645
  in travelers, 3647t, 3648t, 3649
ParC, in quinolone resistance, 454
Parenchymatous neurosyphilis, 1088, 2775-2776
Parenteral nutrition. *See also* Nutritional support.
  in pancreatic infections, 962
Parinaud's syndrome, 1207, 1390, 1393
  in cat-scratch disease, 2737, 2739f
  lymphadenitis in, 1207
Paromomycin
  adverse effects of, 581t
  for amebiasis, 571t, 3106, 3106t

Paromomycin *(Continued)*
　for cryptosporidiosis, 3222
　for *Dientamoeba fragilis,* 572t
　for giardiasis, 3202t
　for *Leishmania,* 578t
　for luminal protozoa, 583
　indications for, 568t
　names and sources of, 329t
　structure of, 329f, 330
Paronychia
　from self-inoculation, 3554
　fungal. *See* Onychomycosis.
Parotid space, 790, 790f
　infections of, 792. *See also* Odontogenic
　　infections.
Parotitis
　chronic bacterial, 799
　differential diagnosis of, 2006-2007
　etiology of, 2006-2007
　from anaerobic gram-negative bacilli, 2841
　from mumps virus, 2004, 2006-2007
　suppurative, 797t, 799
　viral, 799
Particle agglutination assays, for HIV infection,
　1511, 1511f
Partner notification, for *Chlamydia trachomatis,*
　2251
Parvovirus(es), 233t
　adeno-associated viruses and, 1840
　in stem cell transplant, 3495
　receptor for, 1732t
Parvovirus B19, 1891-1896
　arthritis from, 1316-1317, 1316f
　arthropathy from, 1894
　central nervous system involvement in, 1895
　characteristics of, 1891-1892, 1891f, 1892f
　clinical manifestations of, 1891-1892, 1891t,
　　1893-1895, 1893f
　course of, 1892-1893, 1892f
　diagnosis of, 1896
　epidemiology of, 1893
　erythema infectiosum from, 732, 1893-1894,
　　1893f
　fetal infections with, 1895
　hepatitis from, 1895
　immune response to, 1895
　in imunocompromised host, 1894, 1896
　myocarditis from, 1052, 1053, 1053t, 1895
　pathogenesis of, 1892-1893
　pediatric, laboratory studies for, 234-235
　prevention of, 1896
　pure red cell aplasia from, 1894, 1896
　rash from, 732
　receptor for, 1732t
　transient aplastic crisis from, 1894, 1896
　transmission of, 1893, 3387
　treatment of, 1896
　vaccine for, 1896
　vasculitis from, 1895
　virus-associated hemophagocytic syndrome
　　from, 1894-1895
Pasteurella [spp.], 2687-2690
　bone and joint infections from, 2688
　central nervous system infections from,
　　2688
　characteristics of, 2687, 2687t
　classification of, 2687, 2687t, 3552
　endocarditis from, 2688-2689
　epidemiology of, 2687-2688
　from animal bites, 800, 2687, 2688, 3552
　intra-abdominal infections from, 2689
　laboratory identification of, 221
　pathogenesis of, 2688
　respiratory tract infections from, 2689
　septicemia from, 2688-2689

Pasteurella [spp.] *(Continued)*
　skin and soft tissue infections from, 2688
　treatment of, 2689-2690
Pasteurella haemolytica, toxin secretion in, 26
Pasteurella multocida
　beta-lactamase–producing, 2689
　bite infections from, 800, 2687, 2688, 3552
　history in, 823t
　laboratory identification of, 221
　mupirocin for, 485t
　penicillins for, 288t
Pasteurization, of equipment, 3338
Pathogen-associated molecular patterns, 37, 56,
　62, 124
Pathogenicity, 167
　clonal analysis of, 5
　detection of, 11-12
　evolution of, 6
　genetic organization of, 5
　genomics of, 6
　islands of, 6
　Koch's postulates and, 11
　molecular perspective on, 3-12
　regulation of, 6-8, 7t
　virulence genes in, 5, 6t, 10-11
Pathogens
　as intracellular parasites, 8-9, 9f
　attributes of, 3-4
　definition of, 3
　host and, 3-4
　host subversion mechanisms of, 9-10
　molecular biology of, 3
　multiplication of, 4
　phagosomal, 123
　primary vs. opportunistic, 3, 4
　principal, 3
　replication of, 9
　survival strategy of, 4, 9
Patriot Act, 3600
Pattern recognition receptors, 56, 63
Pautrier's microabscess, 2108
PCV 7 vaccine, for otitis media, 770,
　770t
Pearly penile papules, 1345
Pectin, tetracycline with, 364t
Pediculosis, 3302-3304, 3302f, 3303f
Pediculus capitis, 573t
Pediculus humanus, 573t, 2733
Pediococcus spp., 2446
　laboratory identification of, 217t, 218
　linezolid for, 437, 437t
　quinupristin-dalfopristin for, 425
Pefloxacin
　antimicrobial activity of, 455t, 456t
　dosage of, 458t, 674t-675t
　for leprosy, 499
　for meningitis, 465, 1113, 1114
　for nontyphoidal *Salmonella,* 2649
　in preemptive pancreatic infection treatment,
　　963t, 964
　pharmacology of, 457t
Peginterferon alfa, for hepatitis C
　in acute infections, 1969
　in chronic infections, 1967-1968, 1967f, 1968f
　with HIV coinfection, 1971-1972, 1971f
Peginterferon alfa-2b, dosage of, 682t-683t
Peginterferon alfa-2b/ribavirin, formulations of,
　649t
Pel-Ebstein fever, 723, 723f, 726
Peliosis, 739-740
　bacillary, from *Bartonella,* 2736
Pellicle, acquired, 789
Pelvic abscess, 1377
Pelvic cellulitis, from herpes simplex virus,
　1768

Pelvic infections, 1372-1380
　after gynecologic surgery, 1376-1378, 1377t
　anaerobic, 2813
　clindamycin for, 410-411
　from *Enterococcus,* 2413
　from herpes simplex virus, 1768
　intra-amniotic infection syndrome and, 1372-
　　1373
　intrapartum, 1372-1373
　postabortal, 1375-1376
　postpartum, 1373-1375
　suppurative thrombophlebitis in, 1003-1004
Pelvic inflammatory disease, 1378-1380, 1378f,
　　1379f, 1379t, 2247t, 2248-2250
　ectopic pregnancy after, 2249
　from *Actinomyces,* 2925, 2928-2929, 2928f
　from anaerobic vaginosis, 2813
　from *Chlamydia trachomatis,* 1378-1380,
　　1378f, 1379f, 1379t, 2247t, 2248-2250
　from herpes simplex virus, 1768
　from *Mycoplasma genitalium,* 2281, 2281t
　from *Neisseria gonorrhoeae,* 1378-1380,
　　1378f, 1379f, 1379t, 2521
　treatment of, 2525-2526, 2525t
　in HIV infection, 1628-1629
　IUD-associated, 1378, 2925, 2928-2929, 2928f
　quinolones for, 460
　treatment of, 2247t, 2250
Pelvic recess, 927, 927f
Pemphigus neonatorum, 1174, 1174f
Penciclovir, 515t, 525-526
　activity spectrum of, 517t
　for genital herpes, 1344
　for herpesvirus infections, 1760t, 1761
　structure of, 517f
　uses of, 526
Penicillin(s), 281-293, 650t-651t. *See also* Beta-
　　lactam antibiotics.
　absorption of, 285, 285t
　adverse reactions to, 286-287, 286t, 287f
　allergy to, 322, 2782
　antigens from, 286, 287f
　chemistry of, 281
　classification of, 283-284, 284t
　cross-reactivity with, 324-325
　dosage of, 289t, 650t-653t
　　in children, 650t, 652t
　　in newborns, 650t, 652f
　　in renal disease, 285, 285t
　excretion of, 285
　extended-spectrum, 333, 334t-335t
　for actinomycosis, 2931, 2931t
　for acute necrotizing ulcerative gingivitis, 796,
　　796t, 797t, 836-837, 837t
　for anaerobes, 284t
　for anthrax, 2490
　for bacilli, 284t
　for botulism, 2826
　for brain abscess, 1157, 1158, 1158t, 1159t
　for cervicofacial actinomycosis, 797t
　for chronic lymphedema, 1213
　for clostridial cellulitis, 1189
　for *Clostridium,* 2837
　for *Clostridium perfringens,* 2833
　for cocci, 284t
　for *Corynebacterium diphtheriae,* 2463
　for culture-negative endocarditis, 1001
　for deep fascial space infections, 797t
　for diphtheroid prosthetic valve endocarditis,
　　1028
　for endemic treponematoses, 2788
　for Enterobacteriaceae, 284t
　for enterococcal endocarditis, 997, 998, 999,
　　2416, 2416t
　　penicillin-resistant, 997

Penicillin(s) *(Continued)*
prosthetic valve, 1027-1028, 1027t, 1028t
streptomycin-resistant, 997
for *Erysipelothrix rhusiopathiae,* 2498
for experimental endocarditis, 1048
for febrile neutropenia, 3450-3452, 3451t
for gonococci endocarditis, 1000
for impetigo, 1172-1173
for infectious gangrene, 1182
for Lemierre's disease, 756
for leptospirosis, 2793t
for *Leuconostoc,* 2418
for lung abscess, 855
for Lyme disease, 2806, 2806t
for lymphangitis, 1212, 1213
for mediastinitis, 1074
for meningitis, 1106t, 1107t, 1112-1115
for *Neisseria meningitidis,* 2507, 2507t, 2508, 2509
for neurosyphilis, 1115
for nutritionally variant streptococci, 2440-2441
for ocular syphilis, 1418
for odontogenic infections, 797-798, 797t
for osteomyelitis, 1324t
for *Pasteurella,* 2689
for peritonitis
primary, 931
secondary, 938
for peritonsillar abscess, 756
for pneumococcal endocarditis, 1000
for pneumococcal pneumonia, 2404-2405
for pneumonia, 836-839, 837t, 838t
for postabortal infections, 1375-1376
for postpartum endometritis, 1374
for poststreptoccocal acute glomerulonephritis, 2388
for *Pseudomonas,* 284t
for *Pseudomonas* endocarditis, 1000
for rat-bite fever, 2710
for rheumatic fever prophylaxis, 2385-2386, 2385t
for sepsis, 918
for staphylococcal endocarditis, 998
for staphylococcal osteomyelitis, 2346
for staphylococcal scalded skin syndrome, 1174
for streptococcal cellulitis, 2371
for streptococcal endocarditis, 995-996
prosthetic valve, 1027t
for streptococcal meningitis, 2405
for streptococcal pharyngitis, 756, 2367-2368, 2367t
for streptococcal toxic shock syndrome, 2374
for streptococci group C, 2445
for *Streptococcus agalactiae* (group B), 2429, 2430, 2430t
for *Streptococcus anginosus* group, 2455
for *Streptococcus bovis,* 2417
for streptococcus group G, 2445
for suppurative thrombophlebitis, 1005
for syphilis, 2780-2781, 2781t, 2782
in HIV infection, 1690t
for viridans streptococcal endocarditis, 2437-2438, 2437t
for viridians streptococcal meningitis, 2439
formulations of, 646t-647t
isoxazolyl, 290, 290f
major determinants of, 320
mechanism of action of, 281-282, 282f
minor determinants of, 320
penicillinase-resistant, 288t, 289-290, 290f, 2370
pharmacology of, 285-286, 285t

Penicillin(s) *(Continued)*
pneumococcal resistance to, 836-837, 837t
prophylactic, 288
renal function and, 245
resistance to, 282-283, 283t
by anaerobic gram-negative bacilli, 2843-2844
by *Neisseria gonorrhoeae,* 2519
by *Staphylococcus aureus,* 2333, 2334t
by *Streptococcus pneumoniae,* 185
by viridans streptococci, 2439-2440
meningococcal, 1112
semisynthetic, allergy to, 323
structure of, 281, 281f, 320, 321f
susceptibility to, 262, 283-284, 284t
tetracycline with, 365
uses of, 287-288, 288t
Penicillin G, 289, 290f
dosage of, 652t-653t
for brain abscess, 1157, 1158, 1159t
for cellulitis, 1180
for cutaneous diphtheria, 1181
for erysipelas, 1178
for gas gangrene, 1199
for impetigo, 1173
for infectious gangrene, 1182
for Lyme borreliosis, 1115
for lymphadenitis, 1211
for lymphangitis, 1212
for meningitis, 1112, 1113
for perinatal prophylaxis, 1118
for streptococcal necrotizing myositis, 1197-1198
for syphilis, 1344
ocular, 1418
formulations of, 646t
Penicillin G benzathine
dosage of, 652t-653t
formulations of, 646t
Penicillin G procaine
dosage of, 652t-653t
formulations of, 646t
Penicillin V, 289, 290f
for erysipelas, 1178
for impetigo, 1173
for lymphadenitis, 1211
for lymphangitis, 1212
Penicillin V potassium
dosage of, 652t-653t
formulations of, 646t
Penicillinase, *Staphylococcus aureus* resistance to, 2334t
Penicillin-binding protein, 2328, 2329f
in beta-lactam resistance, 264
in cephalosporin action, 297
in methicillin-resistant *Staphylococcus aureus,* 2334-2335
in penicillin action, 282, 282f
in penicillin resistance, 283
in *Streptococcus pneumoniae* susceptibility, 2402-2403
Penicillin-streptomycin, 248
Penicilliosis, in HIV infection, 1689t
Penicillium [spp.], isolation of, 231
Penicillium marneffei, 3074-3075, 3074f, 3076t
appearance of in tissue, 2936f, 2938t
laboratory tests for, 229
vs. enteric fever, 1275t
Penicilloyl
in beta-lactam allergy, 320
skin testing with, 322-323
Penis
candidiasis of, 2943
lesions of. *See* Genital lesions.
pearly papules of, 1345

Penis *(Continued)*
urethral gonorrhea complications of, 2520
verrucous lesions of, 1341, 1841-1850, 1846f.
See also Genital warts; Human papillomavirus(es).
Pentamidine
adverse effects of, 581t
drug interactions with, 694t
for *Balamuthia mandrillaris,* 577t
for leishmaniasis
in HIV infection, 1692t
visceral, 3153
for *Pneumocystis,* 3088-3089
for *Pneumocystis jirovecii,* 569t, 575t, 1681t, 1685t, 1693, 1695
for prophylaxis, 3447, 3447t
for protozoa, 589-590
for trypanosomiasis, 569t, 576t, 3168, 3168t
structure of, 589f
Pentatrichomonas hominis, 3205
Pentavalent antimony, for leishmaniasis, 591
cutaneous, 3153
for American mucocutaneous, 3153
in HIV infection, 1692t
visceral, 3152
Pentobarbital, for intracranial hypertension, 1117
Pentoxifylline, 560
for meningitis, 1116
Peptic ulcers
blood group O–associated, 46
clarithromycin for, 405
from *Candida albicans,* 1269
from *Helicobacter pylori,* 2561
in HIV infection, 1576
Peptides
in MHC class I antigen presentation, 125, 125f
in MHC class II antigen presentation, 125-126, 125f
Peptidoglycan
in bacterial cell wall, 282, 282f
in *Staphylococcus aureus,* 2327-2328, 2328f
in *Streptococcus pneumoniae,* 2393
Peptococcus [spp.]
chloramphenicol for, 367t
clindamycin for, 409t
in peritonitis
primary, 929
secondary, 937, 938
macrolides for, 397t
Peptococcus niger, 2848
Peptococcus (Anaerococcus) prevotii, mupirocin for, 485t
Peptostreptococcus [spp.]
appendicitis from, 969
diverticulitis from, 972
empyema from, 846
in oral cavity, 787, 787t
infection sites for, 2848-2849, 2849f
lung abscess from, 854
odontogenic infections from, 788, 788f
osteomyelitis from, 1324
pericarditis from, 1059
peritonitis from
primary, 929
secondary, 937
taxonomy of, 2848
treatment of
with chloramphenicol, 367t
with clindamycin, 409t
with daptomycin, 428
with macrolides, 397t
with penicillins, 284t, 288t
with quinupristin-dalfopristin, 425

Peptostreptococcus anaerobius, mupirocin for, 485t
Peptostreptococcus magnus, 2849
Peracetic acid
    disinfection with, 3335t, 3336-3337
    sterilization with, 3336, 3337t, 3340
Percutaneous intravascular devices. *See also* Catheter-related infections *and specific devices.*
    infections due to, 3347-3358
        diagnosis of, 3350-3351, 3350t
        epidemiology of, 3348
        from infusate contamination, 3347-3348
        from insertion site contamination, 3348
        from junction contamination, 3348
        microbiology of, 3349-3350, 3350t
        pathogenesis of, 3347-3348, 3347f
        prevention of, 3356-3358, 3356t
        risk factors for, 3348-3349, 3349t
Percutaneous transluminal coronary angioplasty, infections in, 1039-1040
Perforin, CD8+ T-cell release of, 134
Perianal actinomycosis, 2927
Perianal amebiasis, 3103
Perianal candidiasis, 2944, 2944f
Perianal cellulitis, in cancer, 3438
Perianal warts. *See* Anogenital warts.
Periarteriolar sheath, 120
Pericardial effusion, in HIV infection, 1059, 1560
Pericardial friction rub, in pericarditis, 1060
Pericardiocentesis, in pericarditis, 1061, 1062
Pericardiotomy
    in pericarditis, 1061
    pleural effusion after, 847, 849-850
Pericarditis, 1058-1062. *See also* Endocarditis; Myocarditis.
    bacterial, 1059, 1059t
    clinical manifestations of, 1060-1061
    constrictive, 1060
        in tuberculosis, 1062
    diagnosis of, 1061
    endocarditis with, 1060
    etiology of, 1058-1059, 1059t
    from *Actinomyces,* 2926
    from *Aspergillus,* 2966
    from *Candida,* 2945
    from *Chlamydia psittaci,* 2257
    from enteroviruses, 2152-2153
    from *Haemophilus influenzae,* 1059
    from *Histoplasma capsulatum,* 3017, 3020, 3024
    from influenza virus, 2071
    from *Staphylococcus aureus,* 2345
    fungal, 1059, 1059t
    in Kawasaki disease, 3317
    in meningococcal disease, 2504
    infectious causes of, 1059t
    noninfectious causes of, 1061t
    parasitic, 1059, 1059t
    pathogenesis of, 1059-1060
    pathology of, 1059-1060
    pathophysiology of, 1059-1060
    purulent, 1059, 1060
    tamponade in, 1060
    treatment of, 1061-1062
    tuberculous, 1059, 1060, 1060f, 1062, 2878-2879
    viral, 1058-1059, 1059t
Pericoronitis, 791. *See also* Odontogenic infections.
Perifolliculitis capitis, 1179
Periglomerular fibrosis, 876
Perihepatitis. *See also* Hepatitis.
    from *Neisseria gonorrhoeae,* 930, 2521-2522

Perimandibular actinomycosis, 2925-2926, 2925f
Perinatal infections. *See also* Neonates; Pregnancy.
    viral, specimen collection in, 233t
Perinephric abscess, 895
    diagnosis of, 895-896, 896f
    treatment of, 896
Periodic acid–Schiff stain, of fungi, 230
Periodic fever
    aphthous ulcers, pharyngitis and adenitis (PFAPA) syndrome, 1208
    in Marshall's syndrome, 1208
    of unknown origin, 723, 723f, 726, 727
Periodontal abscess, 791. *See also* Odontogenic infections.
Periodontal disease/periodontitis, 790, 791. *See also* Gingivitis; Odontogenic infections.
    clinical features of, 791
    from *Actinobacillus actinomycetemcomitans,* 2752, 2753
    from anaerobic infections, 2812
        with gram-negative bacilli, 2841
    from *Capnocytophaga,* 2731
    in HIV infection, 1555
    in leukocyte adhesion deficiency-1, 149, 152f
    lung abscess and, 853
    microbiology of, 788
    pathogenesis of, 789
    treatment of, 796-797, 796t, 797t
Peripheral compartment, volume of, 272
Peripheral nervous system, in sepsis, 915
Peripheral neuropathy
    in leprosy, 2889, 2891, 2893
    isoniazid and, 490
    nitrofurantoin and, 475
Peripheral vascular stents. *See also* Percutaneous intravascular devices.
    infections of, 1036
Perirectal actinomycosis, 2927
Peritoneal abscess, 943-944, 944f
Peritoneal cavity, 928
    anatomy of, 927-928, 927f
    rupture of, in secondary peritonitis, 933
Peritoneal dialysis. *See also* Dialysis.
    aminoglycoside dosing in, 346, 346t
    catheter-related infections in. *See also* Catheter-related infections.
        from *Staphylococcus epidermidis,* 2355
    prophylaxis for, 481-482
    penicillin dosage in, 285, 285t
    peritonitis in, 941-943, 942t
        from *Staphylococcus epidermidis,* 2355
Peritoneal fluid, collection and transport of, 206t
Peritoneal membrane, 928-929
Peritoneal reflections, 927, 927f
Peritoneal surgery, peritonitis prevention in, 940-941
Peritoneum, parietal, 928
Peritonitis, 929-943
    after gynecologic surgery, 1376-1377, 1376f, 1377t
    chemical, 933
    dialysis-related, 941-943, 942t, 2355
    eosinophilic, 941
    from *Candida,* 933, 2947, 2950
    from *Cryptococcus neoformans,* 3005
    fungal, 942
    in pelvic inflammatory disease, 1378-1380, 1379t
    in transplant recipients, 3505
    postoperative, prevention of, 940-941
    primary, 929-931
        bacteriologic characteristics of, 929

Peritonitis *(Continued)*
    clinical manifestations of, 930
    diagnosis of, 930-931
    etiology of, 929
    laboratory findings in, 930
    pathogenesis of, 929-930
    prevention of, 931
    prognosis of, 931
    treatment of, 931
    quinolones for, 461-462
    secondary, 931-941
        antimicrobial therapy for, 936-940, 937t
        clinical manifestations of, 935
        diagnosis of, 935-936
        etiology of, 931
        fluid replacement in, 940
        gastrointestinal drainage for, 940
        hyperbaric oxygen for, 940
        microbiologic characteristics of, 931-933
        pathogenesis of, 933-934
        pathophysiology of, 934-935
        physical findings in, 935
        prognosis for, 936
        respiratory support for, 940
        surgery for, 940
        symptoms of, 935
        transfusion in, 940
        treatment of, 936-940, 937t
    shunt-related, 1128
    spontaneous bacterial, 929
    treatment of
        with aminoglycosides, 337
        with vancomycin, 423
    tuberculous, 930, 2881
Peritonsillar abscess, 754, 756
Permethrin
    adverse effects of, 581t
    for lice, 2305, 3303-3304
    for scabies, 575t, 3306
Peromyscus leucopus, 2312
    in Lyme disease transmission, 2798
    New York virus from, 2086t, 2087-2089
Peromyscus maniculatus, Sin Nombre virus from, 2086t, 2087-2089
Peroxynitrite, in bacterial meningitis, 1098
Persistent lymphadenopathy syndrome, from HTLV, 2112
Personal digital assistants, 3658-3660, 3660t, 3661t
Pertussis, 2701-2706. *See also Bordetella pertussis.*
    cell-mediated immunity in, 2706
    clinical manifestations of, 2704
    complications of, 2704
    diagnosis of, 2704-2705
    epidemiology of, 2703
    erythromycin for, 402
    from adenoviruses, 1838
    persistent bronchitis and, 748
    prevention of, 2705-2706
    treatment of, 2706
Pertussis toxin, 27, 2702, 2703
Pertussis vaccine, 3569. *See also* Diphtheria, tetanus, pertussis (DTP) vaccine.
    acellular, 2705-2706
    whole-cell, 2705
Pestiviruses, gastroenteritis from, 1239
PET (positron emission tomography), for brain abscess, 1158-1159
Petechiae, 730t, 731, 732, 734. *See also* Rash.
    conjunctival, 736
    in endocarditis, 736, 982, 982f, 984
    in meningococcal sepsis, 2503, 2503f-2505f
    in sepsis, 917

PFAPA syndrome, 1208
Pfiesteria-associated syndrome, 3256, 3256t
PGG-glucan, 560
PH
  in antimicrobial selection, 246
  urinary, in urinary tract infection treatment, 888
Phaeohyphomycosis, 3070-3072, 3070f-3072f,
    3070t, 3072t, 3076t
  itraconazole for, 508
Phage-encoded virulence factors, 5, 6t
Phagocytes, 56. *See also* Eosinophil(s);
    Neutrophil(s).
  defects in, 154-158, 155f, 156f
  evaluation of, 109, 110t
  gene polymorphisms in, 913
  granulocytic, 93-111
  in immunodeficiency, 150t-151t
  in local host response, 908
  microbial defenses against, 102-103
  mononuclear, 37
  signaling defects in, 156-157
Phagocytosis, 37
  abnormal, 106
  acute-phase response in, 34
  ingestion in, 99
  of *Streptococcus pneumoniae*, 2395
  opsonin-independent, 37
  pulmonary, 820
Phagosomes, 56
  bacterial pathogens in, 123
Pharmacodynamics, 274-279
  abbreviations/definitions in, 271t
  animal models of, 274
  concentration-dependent killing agents in, 275,
    275f
  human trials in, 275, 275f
  in vitro models of, 274
  indices of, 279
  maximal serum concentration to minimum
    inhibitory concentration ratio in, 276-277,
    276f
  of antiretroviral agents, 278-279
  of bactericidal agents, 274
  of bacteriostatic agents, 274
  pharmacokinetics and, 271f
  postantibiotic effect in, 278
  study methodology for, 274-279
  time above minimal inhibitory concentration in,
    278
  time-dependent killing agents in, 275-276,
    275f, 276f
  24-hour area under serum concentration curve
    to minimal inhibitory concentration ratio
    in, 277-278, 277f
Pharmacokinetics, 271-274
  abbreviations/definitions in, 271t
  absorption in, 271t, 272
  biotransformation in, 273
  cytochrome P-450 system in, 273-274
  distribution in, 271t, 272-273, 272f
  dose-dependent (saturation, zero-order), 273
  elimination in, 274
  metabolism in, 273
  models for, 271-272
  pharmacodynamics and, 271f
Pharyngeal cleft cysts, infected, 799-800
Pharyngitis, 752-757
  acute lymphonodular, 2151
  anaerobic, 2812
  clinical features of, 753-755
  diagnosis of, 755-756
  epidemiology of, 753
  etiology of, 2t, 752-753
  exudative, 755
  from adenoviruses, 754, 756-757, 1838

Pharyngitis *(Continued)*
  from anaerobic gram-negative bacilli, 2841
  from arcanobacteria, 755, 756, 2365, 2470
  from *Candida*, 2940-2941, 2940f, 2941f
    chronic, 2944
    in immunocompromised host, 798-799,
      2944, 3437, 3483
    prevention of, in transplant recipients, 3483
    treatment of, 2950-2951
  from *Chlamydia pneumoniae*, 755, 2262
  from corynebacteria, 755, 2365
  from enteroviruses, 754, 2151
  from Epstein-Barr virus, 1805, 1807
  from *Francisella tularensis*, 2680
  from *Fusobacterium necrophorum*, 754, 755,
    756
  from herpes simplex virus, 754, 756-757,
    1765-1766, 1770, 1774t
  from *Mycoplasma pneumoniae*, 755, 2365
  from *Neisseria gonorrhoeae*, 2365, 2521
    diagnosis of, 755
  from *Neisseria meningitidis*, 2365, 2506
  from orthoreoviruses, 1899
  from respiratory syncytial virus, 2015t
  from viruses, 2365-2366
  from *Yersinia*, 755, 2365, 2699
  gingivostomatitis from, 1765-1766
  in colds, 750, 753
  in diphtheria, 755, 2461, 2461f
  in HIV infection, 753
  in immunocompromised host, 3437
  in infectious mononucleosis, 755
  in influenza, 754
  in Kawasaki disease, 755, 3316
  in Lemierre's disease, 754, 756
  in Ludwig' angina, 754, 756
  in Marshall's syndrome, 1208
  in plague, 2695
  in poststreptoccocal acute glomerulonephritis,
    2387t
  in Vincent's angina, 754, 756
  laboratory tests of, 208
  mediastinitis from, 1070-1071
  noninfectious, 755, 756
  pathogenesis of, 753
  peritonsillar abscess and, 754, 756
  prevention of, 757
  streptococcal, 1t, 737-738, 752-753, 753-754
    azithromycin for
    clinical features of, 753-754
    diagnosis of, 755
    from *Streptococcus zooepidemicus*, 2443
    group A–associated, 738, 753-754, 2364-2368
      clinical manifestations of, 2365
      diagnosis of, 2365-2367
      epidemiology of, 2364-2365, 2364f
      nonsuppurative complications for, 2365
      rapid antigen detection tests for, 2366-
        2367
      rheumatic fever after, 2382
      suppurative complications for, 2365
      throat culture for, 2366, 2368
      treatment of, 407, 2367-2368, 2367t
      vs. nonstreptococcal sore throat, 2366
    group C–associated, 20-21, 754, 2442-2443
    group G–associated, 754, 2442-2443
    laryngitis in, 759
    rheumatic fever from, 756, 757
    treatment of, 411
    vaccines for, 757
    vs. infectious mononucleosis, 1813
  treatment of, 756-757
  vs. common cold, 755
Pharyngoconjunctival fever, 754, 1389, 1402
  from adenoviruses, 1838

Pharyngocutaneous fistulas, postradiation, 800
Pharyngomaxillary space. *See* Lateral pharyngeal
    space.
Phenazopyridine, 441
  for urinary tract infections, 888
Phenobarbital
  chloramphenicol interactions with, 369t
  for febrile seizures, 714
Phenols, disinfection with, 3337
Phenotypic assays, in viral susceptibility testing,
    238
Phenytoin
  chloramphenicol with, 369t
  metronidazole with, 393t
  tetracycline with, 364t
Phialophora verrucosa, chromoblastomycosis
    from, 2988-2991
Phlebitis. *See* Thrombophlebitis.
Phlebotomus spp., leishmaniasis from, 3146
Phlebovirus spp., 2086t, 2089
PhoP/PhoQ regulatory system, 2644
Phormia regina, myiasis from, 3308-3310, 3308t
Phosphoglycolipid-1, in *Mycobacterium leprae*,
    2889
Phospholipase, of *Pseudomonas aeruginosa*,
    2596
Phospholipid antibodies, in systemic lupus
    erythematosus, 80
Photodynamic therapy, for cutaneous warts, 1848
Photorhabdus spp., 2581
Photosensitivity, from tetracycline, 362
Phrenicocolic ligament, 927
Phthirus pubis, 573t, 3302-3304, 3302f, 3303f
Phycomycetes spp.
  gastrointestinal infections from, 1269-1270
  pancreatic infections from, 959t, 960
Phycomycosis, 2973. *See also* Mucormycosis.
Physical barriers, to microorganisms, 35-36
Pian bois, 3145t, 3149, 3150
Pichia (Hansenula) anomala, 3074
Picobirnaviruses, 2203
Picornaviruses, 2133, 2162. *See also*
    Enterovirus(es); Hepatitis A virus;
    Rhinoviruses.
  adherence of, 16, 16f
  adhesin-based therapies for, 20t, 21
  antibody blocking of, 55
  gastroenteritis from, 1239
  pleconaril for, 542
  rhinoviruses, 2185-2192
Piedra
  black, 3061
  white, 3061, 3073
Piedraia hortae, 3061
Pig-bel, 1268-1269
Pigmentary changes, from tetracycline, 362-363
Pili
  molecular mechanisms of, 8
  of Enterobacteriaceae, 2571
  of *Neisseria gonorrhoeae*, 2514, 2515f
  of *Pseudomonas aeruginosa*, 2593-2594
Pink eye. *See* Conjunctivitis, viral.
Pinta, 2787
Pinworms, 592, 3261t, 3266
  treatment of, 592
Piperacillin, 292-293, 292f, 837-839, 837t, 838t
  antimicrobial activity of, 333, 334t-335t
  dosage of, 652t-653t
  for anaerobes, 284t
  for bacilli, 284t
  for Enterobacteriaceae, 284t
  for febrile neutropenia, 3450-3454, 3451t
  for peritonitis, 938
    for dialysis-related, 942t
    secondary, 937t

Piperacillin *(Continued)*
for postoperative gynecologic infections, 1377t
for *Pseudomonas,* 284t
formulations of, 646t
minimal inhibitory concentration of, 284t
uses of, 287, 288, 288t
Piperacillin-tazobactam, 317, 837-839, 837t, 838t
dosage of, 652t-653t
for acute pyelonephritis, 889
for bacterial arthritis, 1316t
for febrile neutropenia, 3450-3454, 3451t
for *Pseudomonas aeruginosa* bacteremia, 2601
for sepsis, 919t
formulations of, 646t
Piperazine
drug interactions with, 694t
for ascariasis, 3263
for intestinal nematodes, 594
Piperazinyl, with quinolones, 451
Piperonyl butoxide, adverse effects of, 582t
Piry virus, 2045, 2045t
Pitted keratolysis, 1182
Pittsburgh Pneumonia Agent, 2725
Pityriasis rosea, from human herpesvirus 7, 1824
Pityriasis versicolor, 3060
Pivmecillinam, formulations of, 646t
Pivoxyl, 305t, 306
Pixuna virus, 1913-1919, 1914t. *See also*
Alphaviruses.
Placenta, tetracycline crossing of, 361
Placental malaria, 3125, 3127
Plague, 2691-2697. *See also Yersinia pestis.*
as biological weapon, 3601-3604
clinical features of, 3602
historical perspective on, 3601
infection control for, 3604
laboratory diagnosis of, 3602-3603
prophylaxis for, 3603-3604, 3603t
surveillance and decontamination for, 3604
transmission of, 3602
treatment of, 3603t, 3604
bubonic, 2693-2694, 2693t, 2694f
inguinal buboes in, 1208
treatment of, 1211
clinical manifestations of, 2693-2695, 2693t
diagnosis of, 2695-2696
epidemiology of, 2691-2693, 2692f, 2693f
gastrointestinal tract in, 2695
geographic distribution of, 2691, 2692f, 2693
historical perspective on, 2691, 3601
history in, 823t
laboratory findings in, 2695, 2695f
meningitis in, 2695
pandemics of, 3601
pathogenesis of, 2693
peripatetic, 2691
pharyngitis in, 2695
pneumonic, 2693t, 2694-2695
disinfection/sterilization and, 3342
isolation precautions for, 3329-3330, 3330t
precaution protocols for, 2697
prophylaxis against, 2697
reservoirs for, 2697
septicemic, 2693t, 2694, 2695f
vs. enteric fever, 1277
treatment of, 2696-2697
with aminoglycosides, 334t-335t, 344t
vaccines for, 2697, 3569, 3603-3604
vector control for, 2697
vs. enteric fever, 1274t
Plaque, dental, anaerobes in, 2839
Plaques, cutaneous, 731. *See also* Rash.
Plasma
complement in, 71
in sepsis, 916

Plasma *(Continued)*
transfusion of
complement replacement via, 88
in peritonitis, 940
Plasma proteins, in complement regulation, 74t
Plasmacytoid dendritic cells
in adaptive immunity, 39
Toll-like receptor distribution in, 38, 39t
Plasmid(s)
in antibiotic resistance, 253
of Enterobacteriaceae, 2572-2573
of *Neisseria gonorrhoeae,* 2516
Plasmid-encoded virulence factors, 5, 6t
Plasmodium [spp.], 568, 584. *See also* Malaria.
antigenic variation in, 3127, 3127f
characteristics of, 3121-3122, 3122f
erythrocyte invasion by, 3122, 3122f, 3123
immune response to, 3127, 3127f
life cycle of, 3121-3122, 3122f
treatment of, 569t, 584, 586-588
Plasmodium falciparum, 183, 584. *See also*
Malaria.
characteristics of, 3121-3122, 3122f, 3124f
chloroquine-resistant, 584
treatment of, 573t
with azithromycin, 406
with sulfadoxine-pyrimethamine, 441
geographic distribution of, 3127
immune response to, 43
life cycle of, 3121-3122, 3122f
microvascular sequestration of, 3123-3125,
3123f
morphology of, 3124f
multidrug-resistant, treatment of, 578t-579t
prophylaxis against
with primaquine, 585
with proguanil, 587
quinine-resistant, 585
resistance of, 184
treatment of
with atovaquone-proguanil, 587
with clindamycin, 411
with doxycycline, 589
with halofantrine, 586
with sulfonamides, 443
with tetracycline, 589
zinc supplementation in, 142
Plasmodium malariae, 183, 3122, 3126. *See also*
Malaria.
geographic distribution of, 3127
treatment of, 573t
Plasmodium ovale, 183, 3122, 3126
geographic distribution of, 3127
treatment of, 573t, 579t
with atovaquone-proguanil, 587
with primaquine, 585
Plasmodium vivax, 183, 584, 3122, 3125. *See
also* Malaria.
chloroquine-resistant, treatment of, 574t
Duffy blood group and, 46
geographic distribution of, 3127
resistance of, 184
treatment of, 573t, 579t
with atovaquone-proguanil, 587
with halofantrine, 586
with primaquine, 585
Platelet(s)
defects in, 3427
in endocarditis, 979-980
in *Staphylococcus aureus* endocarditis,
2343
Platelet microbicidal proteins, in endocarditis,
980
Platelet–endothelial cell adhesion molecule, 97
Platyhelminths, treatment of, 595-596

Pleconaril, 541-542
for colds, 750, 2192
for enterovirus infections, 2138, 2149, 2153
for meningitis, 1111, 2138, 2149
for myocarditis, 1058
for rhinoviruses, 20t, 21
Pleistophora spp., 574t, 3237, 3238t. *See also*
Microsporidia.
Plesiomonas shigelloides, 2580-2581, 2751t,
2756-2757
Pleural effusion, 845-851. *See also* Empyema.
clinical features of, 847
etiology of, 846-847
exudative vs. transudative, 849t
imaging of, 847-849, 848f, 862f
in pneumonia, 827-828
laboratory findings in, 849-850
microbiology of, 846-847
noninfectious causes of, 847, 849-850
pathophysiology of, 846
risk assessment for, 850t
treatment of, 850-851, 850t
tuberculous, 2878
Pleural fluid, collection and transport of, 206t
Pleural mesothelial cells, 846
Pleurisy, tuberculous, 847, 2878
diagnosis of, 849
Pleuritis, shunt-related, 1128
Pleurodynia, 1201
epidemic, 2151-2152
Pleuropulmonary amebiasis, 3103
Pneumatic otoscopy, 768
Pneumatocele
in pneumonia, 829, 830f
multifocal postinflammatory, in Job's
syndrome, 157, 157f
Pneumococcal pneumonia, 1570, 2400-2402,
2401f, 2401t
antibiotic susceptibility in, 2403t
chest film in, 829, 829f
clinical findings in, 2400
community-acquired, 831-833
complications of, 2402
diagnosis of, 828, 829
in HIV infection, 1570
laboratory findings in, 2400-2402, 2401f, 2401t
nosocomial, 836, 3365, 3365t, 3367t
pathogenesis of, 2400
pneumatocele in, 829
predisposing factors in, 2398
radiographic findings in, 2400
risk factors for, 831
sputum in, 824-825, 824f, 826
treatment of, 836-839, 837t, 838t, 2404-2405
vaccine for, 839
Pneumococcal surface protein A, 2395-2396, 2396t
Pneumococcal vaccine, 839, 1119, 2405-2407,
2406t, 3563f, 3564t, 3569-3570
antibody levels after, 2405-2406
capsular polysaccharide, 2405
for adults, 346f, 347f
for otitis media, 770
heptavalent protein-polysaccharide conjugate,
175
in complement deficiency, 88
in HIV infection, 1682t, 1683t
polyvalent conjugate, 185
polyvalent polysaccharide, 175
protection after, 2406, 2406t
protein conjugate, 2405-2406
schedule for children, 3564t
Pneumococcus. *See Streptococcus pneumoniae.*
Pneumocystis [spp.], 3080-3090
antigens of, 3081
characteristics of, 3080-3081

Pneumocystis [spp.] *(Continued)*
  classification and taxonomy of, 3080
  course and prognosis of, 3087-3088
  culture of, 3080, 3081
  epidemiology of, 3081-3082
  extrapulmonary disease from, 3085
  health care burden of, 3087
  histopathology of, 3081, 3081f, 3084f
  historical perspective on, 3080
  host range of, 3080
  immune response to, 3082-3084, 3084f
  in immunocompromised host, 3436
  laboratory studies of, 229
  life cycle of, 3080-3081, 3080f
  molecular detection of, 231
  pathology and pathogenesis of, 3082-3084
  pneumonia from, 65, 66, 208, 231
  pulmonary infections from, 3082-3085
  respiratory, diagnosis of, 209t
  strains of, 3080
  transmission of, 3082
  treatment of, 3085, 3088-3090
Pneumocystis carinii. See *Pneumocystis jirovecii.*
Pneumocystis jirovecii, 584
  appearance of in tissue, 2938t
  bronchoalveolar lavage for, 827
  chest film in, 829
  classification of, 568
  direct detection of, 230
  in HIV infection, 832-833, 1486, 1550, 1567-1570
    CD4+counts in, 1679, 1694-1695
    choroiditis from, 1560
    diagnosis of, 1684, 1692-1693
    hepatic involvement in, 1578-1579
    lactate dehydrogenase in, 1569
    pediatric, 1488, 1640, 1643f
      prophylaxis against, 1649
    pneumonia from, 1567-1570
    prophylaxis against, 1681t, 1683t, 1684t, 1694-1695
    treatment of, 1685t, 1693-1694
  in immunocompromised host, 3436
    prevention of, 3447, 3447t
  in sputum, 825, 826
  in stem cell transplant, 3495
  in transplant recipients, 3479, 3495
    prevention of, 3482
  pancreatic infections from, 959t, 960
  prophylaxis against, 585
  splenic abscess from, 967, 967t
  treatment of, 569t, 575t, 580t
    with clindamycin, 411, 589
    with dapsone, 498, 588
    with glucocorticosteroids, 558
    with pentamidine, 589
    with primaquine, 585
    with pyrimethamine, 588
    with trimethoprim-sulfamethoxazole, 444, 447, 580t
Pneumolysin, *Streptococcus pneumoniae*
  production of, 2395, 2396, 2396t
Pneumonia. *See also* Pulmonary infections;
  Respiratory tract infections.
  acute, 819-839
    clinical features of, 822, 823
    colonization vs. infections in, 825-826
    community-acquired, 830-833
      classification of, 831
      clinical features of, 831
      course of, 833
      diagnosis of, 831
      epidemiology of, 831
      etiology of, 831-832

Pneumonia *(Continued)*
      from nontypeable *Haemophilus influenzae,* 2663
      HIV-related, 832-833
      in elderly, 832
      mild, 832
      severe, 833
      slowly resolving, 833
      treatment of, 306, 404-405, 407, 462, 553
    diagnostic difficulty in, 823
    diagnostic procedures in, 823-830
    epidemiology of, 822
    history in, 822-823
    pathogenesis of, 821-822
    physical examination in, 823
    predisposing factors in, 822
    prevention of, 839
    treatment of, 836-839, 837t, 838t
      duration and route of, 839
      empirical, 836-839, 837t, 838t
      with complementary and alternative medicine, 604t
      with erythromycin, 402
  aspiration, 834-835. *See also* Pneumonia, nosocomial.
    chest film in, 829
    from anaerobic infections, 2812
    lung abscess and, 853-856
  atypical, 833-834, 2297
    etiology of, 1838, 2272
    from *Coxiella burnetii,* 2297-2299, 2298f
    from *Mycoplasma pneumoniae,* 2272-2278
    radiographic findings in, 2272
  blind endotracheal suctioning in, 827
  blind protected brush specimens in, 827
  blood culture in, 828
  bronchiolitis obliterans organizing, chest film in, 860f
  bronchoalvelolar lavage in, 827
  chest radiography in, 828-830, 829f
  chronic, 857-867. *See also specific infections.*
    chest films in, 860, 860f-867f, 861t
    clinical features of, 859
    diagnosis of, 859-864
    eosinophilic, 835
    epidemiology of, 858-859
    etiology of, 857-858, 857t
    noninfectious causes of, 857, 857t
    risk factors for, 858-859
    treatment of, 867
  computed tomography in, 830
  COPD and, 822
  cytokines in, 828
  diagnosis of, in immunocompromised host, 208
  empyema and, 845-851
  eosinophilic, 835
  fiberoptic bronchoscopy in, 826-827
  Friedlander's, 824, 824f
  from *Actinomyces.* See Actinomycosis.
  from adenoviruses, 1838, 1839
  from *Aspergillus.* See under Aspergillus.
  from *Bordetella pertussis,* 2704
  from *Burkholderia cepacia,* 2618, 2618f
    in cystic fibrosis, 871
    nosocomial, 3367t
  from *Candida,* 2945
    nosocomial, 3365, 3365t
  from *Chlamydia pneumoniae,* 209t, 2262-2263
  from *Chlamydia psittaci,* 833, 2251, 2256-2258
  from *Chlamydia trachomatis,* 834, 2249, 2447t
    in neonates, 2247t, 2249, 2250-2251, 2251f, 2447t
  from *Coccidioides,* 3042-3043, 3043f-3045f
  from coronaviruses, 1990-1996
  from *Coxiella burnetii,* 833, 2297-2299, 2298f

Pneumonia *(Continued)*
  from *Cryptococcus neoformans,* 3002-3003, 3003f, 3007
  from cytomegalovirus, 530, 1789, 1790f
    in transplant recipients, 1795
  from *Enterobacter* spp., 836
  from enteroviruses, 2150
    in neonates, 2154
  from Epstein-Barr virus, 1807
  from *Escherichia coli,* 836
  from *Francisella tularensis,* 2677, 2680-2681, 2681f, 3607-3608, 3608f
  from *Haemophilus influenzae,* 1570, 2664
    aspiration, 835
    community-acquired, 831-833
    diagnosis of, 824f, 825, 829
    in HIV infection, 1570
    nosocomial, 836, 3365, 3365t, 3367t
    treatment of, 836-839, 837t, 838t
  from hantaviruses, 2086-2089, 2086t
    chest film in, 830
    clinical features of, 3629t
  from influenza virus, 2067, 2070-2071
  from *Klebsiella pneumoniae,* 2578. *See also Klebsiella pneumoniae.*
    chest film in, 829
    nosocomial, 836
    sputum in, 824, 824f, 825f
  from *Legionella pneumophila,* 2725-2726
    atypical, 833-834, 834
    chest film in, 830
    community-acquired, 831-833
    diagnosis of, 825-830
    history in, 823t
    nosocomial, 836
    treatment of, 405
  from measles, 2034
  from *Moraxella (Branhamella) catarrhalis,* 832, 2531
  from *Mycobacterium tuberculosis.* See Tuberculosis, pulmonary.
  from *Mycoplasma pneumoniae,* 2273-2274, 2273f
    atypical, 833-834
    community-acquired, 831-833
    diagnosis of, 826, 828, 830
    treatment of, 836-839, 837t, 838t
  from *Neisseria meningitidis,* 2506
  from *Pneumocystis,* 208, 231, 3080-3090. *See also under Pneumocystis.*
    clinical features of, 3084-3085
    course and prognosis of, 3087-3088
    diagnosis of, 3085-3086
    epidemiology of, 3081-3082
    etiology of, 3080-3081
    pathology and pathogenesis of, 3082-3084
    prevention of, 3089-3090
    treatment of, 3085, 3088-3090
  from *Pseudallescheria boydii,* 3068-3069
  from *Pseudomonas aeruginosa,* 2598, 2601-2602. *See also Pseudomonas aeruginosa.*
    aspiration, 835
    chest film in, 829
    chronic, 2602
    community-acquired, 831-833
    diagnosis of, 829
    in cystic fibrosis, 870, 872
    in HIV infection, 1570
    nosocomial, 835-836, 3367t
    treatment of, 836-839, 837t, 838t
  from respiratory syncytial virus, 2011-2012, 2014-2017
  from *Rhodococcus equi,* 1570, 1570f, 2472
  from *Serratia marcescens,* 836
  from *Staphylococcus aureus,* 20, 2345

Pneumonia *(Continued)*
aspiration, 835
chest film in, 829, 830f
community-acquired, 831-833
diagnosis of, 825, 825f, 829, 830f
in cystic fibrosis, 870
methicillin-resistant, 423
nosocomial, 836, 3364, 3365, 3365t, 3367t, 3368
treatment of, 836-839, 837t, 838t
from *Stenotrophomonas maltophilia,* 2618
from *Streptococcus agalactiae* (group B), 2428
from S*treptococcus pneumoniae. See* Pneumococcal pneumonia.
from *Streptococcus pyogenes* (group A), 2375
from viridans streptococci, 2438, 2439
fungal, 1571
in immunocompromised host, 3436
hospitalization for, 2016, 2016t
impaired pulmonary defenses and, 821-822
in burn patients, 3550
in cancer patients, 3434-3437, 3457
in complement deficiency, 158
in elderly, 3518-3519
in hematologic malignancies, 3434-3437
in HIV infection, 822-823, 832-833, 1486, 1570-1571, 1570-1572, 1570f, 1682t, 1689t, 1699, 2398, 3080-3090. *See also* Human immunodeficiency virus infection, pneumonia in.
in immunocompromised host, 835-836
diagnosis of, 208
in injection drug users, 3468-3469, 3468f
in measles, vitamin A for, 604t, 606-607
in melioidosis, 2624, 2625f, 2626f
in plague, 2693t, 2694-2695
in spinal cord injury, 3514-3515
in transplant recipients, 3488, 3493-3495, 3494-3495, 3506
in travelers, 3647t, 3648t, 3651
intestinal, vs. enteric fever, 1277
laboratory culture in, 208
lung biopsy in, 827
microbiology of, 819t
necrotizing, 853-856
from anaerobic infections, 2812
nonrespiratory symptoms of, 822
nosocomial, 835-836, 3362-3368
definition of, 3362-3363, 3363t
diagnosis of, 3366-3367
epidemiology of, 3363
etiology of, 3365-3366, 3365t
from respiratory syncytial virus, 2017
prevention of, 2020-2021
from *Staphylococcus aureus,* 2345
in sepsis, 921
lung abscess and, 854
pathogenesis of, 3364-3365
prevention of, 3368, 3368t
quinolones for, 462-463
risk factors for, 3363-3364, 3364t
treatment of, 3367-3368, 3367t
ventilator-associated, 827, 835-836
overview of, 819-820
parasitic, 1572
pleural effusion and, 845-851
pleural fluid analysis in, 827-828
pneumatocele in, 829, 830f
pneumococcal. *See* Pneumococcal pneumonia.
postinfluenza, 831
pulmonary defense systems and, 820-822, 820t
radioisotope scanning in, 830

Pneumonia *(Continued)*
recurrent, 822
risk factors for, 823t, 831
secondary bacterial, after influenza infections, 20
serologic studies in, 828
sputum examination in, 823-826, 824f, 825f
transtracheal aspiration in, 826
underlying respiratory disease and, 822
urinalysis in, 828
ventilator-associated, 835-836, 3362-3368. *See also* Pneumonia, nosocomial.
diagnosis of, 827
lung abscess from, 854
viral, 1572
vs. enteric fever, 1274t
walking, 2273
with respiratory syncytial virus coinfection, 2019
Pneumonia from, *pseudomonas aeruginosa,* 2598
Pneumonic plague, 2693t, 2694-2695. *See also* Plague.
disinfection/sterilization and, 3342
isolation precautions for, 3329-3330, 3330t
Pneumonitis
from *Ascaris lumbricoides,* 3262
from cytomegalovirus, 1789, 1790f
in transplant recipients, 1795
from herpes simplex virus, 1770, 1774t
from respiratory syncytial virus, 2011-2012, 2014-2016
from *Toxoplasma gondii,* 3176, 3179
from varicella zoster virus, 1782
hemorrhagic, in leptospirosis, 2792
hypersensitivity, from *Mycobacterium avium* complex, 2900-2903, 2905
lymphocytic interstitial
in HIV infection, 1573
in pediatric HIV infection, 1641
lymphoid interstitial, pediatric, 1488
Pneumothorax, from *Coccidioides immitis,* 3043, 3045f
Pneumovirinae, 2009
Pneumovirus, 2009
Podofilox, for human papillomavirus, 1691t
Podophyllin resin
for genital warts, 1849
for human papillomavirus, 1691t
Podophyllotoxin, for genital warts, 1849
Poliomyelitis
abortive, 2142
asymptomatic, 2142
bulbar paralytic, 2143
clinical features of, 1242f, 2142-2143
complications of, 2143
differential diagnosis of, 2143
endemic, 2141
eradication of, 2141, 2146
etiology of. *See* Polioviruses.
geographic distribution of, 3640f
historical perspective on, 2141
in immunocompromised host, 2145
in pregnancy, 2137, 2143
incidence of, 2141
incubation period for, 2137, 2142
laboratory diagnosis of, 2143
mortality from, 2144
nonparalytic, 2142
paralysis in, 2142-2143
pathogenesis of, 2142
postpoliomyelitis syndrome and, 2144
prevention of, 2144-2146. *See also* Polioviruses, vaccines for.
prognosis of, 2143-2144

Poliomyelitis *(Continued)*
respiratory paralysis in, 2144
spinal paralytic, 2142-2143, 2142f
surveillance for, 2146
vaccine-associated, 2145, 2146
Polioviruses, 2141-2146. *See also* Enterovirus(es).
characteristics of, 2141-2142
classification of, 2133, 2134t
clinical manifestations of. *See* Poliomyelitis.
communicability period for, 2137
culture of, 2137-2138
endemic, 2141
epidemiology of, 2136-2137
genome of, 2134, 2142
genotyping of, 2136-2137
historical perspective on, 2141
host range of, 2133, 2134t
immune response to, 2135-2136
incubation period for, 2137, 2142
laboratory diagnosis of, 2137-2138, 2143
minor/major viremia from, 2135, 2142, 2143
molecular biology of, 2134-2135, 2134t
mutation of, 2135
myocarditis from, 2143
pathogenesis of, 2135
prevention of, 2138
proteins of, 2134
receptors for, 1732t, 2134-2135, 2134t
replication of, 2135
serotypes of, 2142
shedding of, 2135, 2137
structure of, 1731f
transmission of, 2137
treatment of, 2138
vaccine-derived, 2141-2142, 2145.2146
vaccines for, 2144-2146
for travelers, 3639t, 3641
in developing world, 2145
inactivated, 2144, 3563f, 3564t, 3570-3571
live attenuated, 2144-2145, 3570, 3571
poliomyelitis from, 2145, 2146
schedule for children, 3564t
wild-type, 2136, 2142
Poloxamer-iodine, disinfection with, 3336
Polyarteritis nodosa
from hepatitis B, 1877
meningitis in, 1139
Polyarthritis. *See also* Arthritis.
in rheumatic fever, 2382
reactive, from *Yersinia enterocolitica,* 2699
Polyclonal antilymphocyte serums, for transplant immunosuppression, infections and, 3478-3479
Polycystic kidney disease, renal infections in, 890
Polymerase chain reaction assay, 11-12, 215, 242
false-negatives in, 215
for adenovirus, 235
for *Bartonella* spp., 2743
for *Bordetella pertussis,* 2704-2705
for *Borrelia burgdorferi,* 2804
for cerebrospinal fluid. *See also* Cerebrospinal fluid analysis.
in brain abscess, 1157
in meningitis, 1082, 1101
in progressive multifocal leukoencephalopathy, 1860-1861
for *Chlamydia pneumoniae,* 826, 2259
for cytomegalovirus, 1788
for enteroviruses, 235, 2138
for *Francisella tularensis,* 2682
for hepatitis B, 1879, 1879t
for herpesviruses, 237
for *Histoplasma capsulatum,* 3022
for HIV infection, pediatric, 1645
for HTLV, 2102

Polymerase chain reaction assay *(Continued)*
for influenza virus, 2072
for *Legionella pneumophila,* 826
for leptospirosis, 2792
for *Mycobacterium tuberculosis,* 828, 2854t
for *Mycoplasma pneumoniae,* 826
for *Neisseria gonorrhoeae,* 1315
for parvovirus B19, 1896
for *Pneumocystis,* 3082-3084, 3084f
for primary central nervous system lymphoma, 1608
for rickettsial diseases, 2286
for *Staphylococcus aureus,* 2324
for *Streptococcus pneumoniae,* 826, 828
for syphilis, 2780
for *Toxoplasma gondii,* 3182
for *Tropheryma whipplei,* 1309
for *Trypanosoma cruzi,* 3162
in sputum examination, 826
real-time, 215
Polymethylmethacrylate, in prosthetic joint infections, 1333
Polymorphisms, 273
in bacterial infections, 2319-2320
Polymorphonuclear leukocytes, in *Pseudomonas aeruginosa* resistance, 2591
Polymorphonuclear neutrophils, in phagocytosis, 37
Polymyalgia. *See also* Myalgia.
from rifabutin, 493
Polymyalgia rheumatica, fever in, 726-727
Polymyositis, 1194-1197. *See also* Myositis.
from HTLV, 2111
in HIV infection, 1201, 1555
Polymyxin B, 435-436, 484t, 485
dosage of, 668t-669t
drug interactions with, 694t
for shunt infections, 1129t, 1130
prophylactic, intravascular devices and, 3356
Polymyxin B-bacitracin-neomycin, 484t
Polymyxin B-neomycin-hydrocortisone, 484t
Polymyxin E, for *Pseudomonas aeruginosa,* 2608
Polyneuropathy
distal sensory, in HIV infection, 1593-1594, 1597t
in sepsis, 915
inflammatory demyelinating, in HIV infection, 1593, 1597t
Polyomaviruses, 1856-1861
characteristics of, 1857
clinical manifestations of, 1858-1859, 1858t, 1859t
culture of, 1859
diagnosis of, 1859-1861, 1860f
epidemiology of, 1857, 1859t
in pregnancy, 1858-1859
in transplant recipients, 3509
pathogenesis of, 1857-1858
prevention of, 1861
treatment of, 1861
Polyps, nasal, from microsporidia, 3244
Polyradiculopathy
cytomegalovirus, 1791
progressive, in HIV infection, 1595, 1597t
Polyribitol ribose phosphate antibodies, in *Haemophilus influenzae* infections, 2663
Polysaccharide antigen, in conjugate vaccines, 62, 63f
Polysaccharide(s), capsular
complement interaction with, 77-78
of meningococcus, 2499-2500, 2499t
of *Staphylococcus aureus,* 2321, 2322t
Polystyrence superantigen absorbing device, for streptococcal toxic shock syndrome, 2374

Polytetrafluoroethylene, in prosthetic vascular graft infections, 1039
Pontiac fever, 2711, 2726. *See also Legionella* [spp.].
clinical presentation of, 2717
pathogenesis of, 2713-2714
Population, definition of, 161, 162
Porcine endogenous retrovirus, cross-species transmission of, 1521
Pore-forming toxins, 30
Porins
in antibiotic resistance, 262
in *Neisseria gonorrhoeae,* 2514-2515
Pork tapeworm, 3286t, 3288. *See also* Tapeworms.
Porphyria cutanea tarda, hepatitis C–related, 1962
Porphyromonas [spp.], 2811, 2812
in oral cavity, 787, 787t, 789
microbiology of, 2839, 2839t
Porphyromonas gingivalis
colonization by, 2839
odontogenic infections from, 788, 788f, 789
virulence factors of, 2814, 2814t, 2840
Porphyromonas intermedia, odontogenic infections from, 788, 788f, 789
Portal vein, in pyogenic liver abscess, 951, 952t
Posaconazole, 510
for aspergillosis, 2968t, 2969
for brain abscess, 1160-1161
for Chagas' disease, 3162
for dark-walled fungal infections, 3072
for endophthalmitis, 1411
for eumycetoma, 2995
for fusariosis, 3073
for mucormycosis, 2979
Positron emission tomography (PET), for brain abscess, 1158-1159
Postanginal sepsis/septicemia, 754, 754f, 756, 794, 794f
Postantibiotic effect, 278
of aminoglycosides, 334
Postcataract endophthalmitis, 1407-1411, 1407f, 1408f
Postgonococcal urethritis, 1351
Postherpetic neuralgia, 1783
Postinfectious bronchitis, 803-805, 804t
Postinfectious encephalomyelitis, 1143-1147
Post–kala-azar dermal leishmaniasis, 3145t, 3148-3149
Post-Lyme disease syndrome, 2806
Postoperative infections, 3533-3545. *See also* Nosocomial infections; Wound infections.
after gynecologic surgery, 1376-1378, 1377t
cardiopulmonary bypass and, 3538
causative factors in, 3533-3534
episiotomy, 1375
foreign material and, 3537
from streptococci, 1178
hematogenous seeding in, 3535-3536
historical perspective on, 3533
host factors in, 3536-3537
immunologic factors in, 3537-3538
in asplenia, 3528
in clean wounds, 3536
in contaminated wounds, 3536
in heart transplants, 3503
in renal transplants, 3503
investigational models of, 3537, 3539t
microbial load in, 3534, 3534f, 3534t
of head and neck, 800
oxygen administration and, 3537-3538
pathogenesis and pathophysiology of, 3534-3538, 3539t
pathogens in

Postoperative infections *(Continued)*
species and sources of, 3534-3536, 3535t
virulence factors in, 3536-3537
prevention of, 480-481
antibiotics in, 3538-3544, 3543t
cost-benefit analysis for, 3544
delivery methods for, 3542, 3543t
novel approaches to, 3542, 3543t
regimens of, 3542, 3543t
resistance to, 3539-3540
selection of, 3541
timing and duration of, 3541-3542
cytokines in, 3538
infection control measures in, 3540, 3540t
prophylaxis for, 480-481
rates of, by site, 3538t
risk factors for, 3534t, 3536-3537, 3537t
procedure-related, 3537-3538
skin flora and, 3535
surveillance for, 3454t, 3544-3545
tissue trauma and, 3537
transfusions and, 3538
wound microenvironment and, 3537
Postpartum fever, of unknown origin, 1374-1375
Postpoliomyelitis syndrome, 2144
Postsplenectomy sepsis, 734, 3526-3528, 3526f-3528f, 3526t, 3530
Poststreptococcal autoimmune neuropsychiatric disorders associated with streptococci, 2384
Poststreptococcal glomerulonephritis. *See* Glomerulonephritis, poststreptococcal.
Posttransplant lymphoproliferative disorder, 3510
Posttransplantation syndrome, viral infections in, specimen collection in, 233t
Posttraumatic endophthalmitis, 1407t, 1408
Postvaccination encephalomyelitis/encephalopathy, 1745, 2053
Potassium iodide, for sporotrichosis, 2987
Pott's disease, 1329, 2879
Pott's puffy tumor, 777
Pouch of Douglas, 927
Poultry, *Salmonella enteritidis* infections from, 2639-240, 2639f
Povidone-iodine
catheter infection prophylaxis with, 481, 482
disinfection with, 479, 3336
for mediastinitis, 1074
Powassan virus, 1929, 1941. *See also* Tick-borne encephalitis.
Poxviruses, 1742-1755
characteristics of, 1742-1744, 1743f
genera of, 1742
in HIV vaccine testing, 1712
interleukin-18 expression by, 122
molluscipoxviruses, 1338-1344, 1753-1754
orthopoxviruses, 1742-1749
parapoxviruses, 1753
pathogenesis of, 1744
treatment of, 1749
yatapoxviruses, 1754-1755
PPNP, in infection susceptibility, 46
Practice guidelines, Web sites for, 3659t
Practice tools, Web-based, 3660-3661, 3661t
Prayer, 604
Praziquantel
adverse effects of, 581t
for cysticercosis, 3290, 3496
for fluke infections, 572t
for helminthic disease, 570t
for intestinal flukes, 3277t
for lung flukes, 3277t
for platyhelminths, 595-596
for schistosomiasis, 3277t, 3280
for tapeworms, 575t, 3289, 3290

Prealbumin, nutritional status and, 140, 140t
Prednisolone, for meningitis, 1117
Prednisone. *See also* Corticosteroids.
  for allergic bronchopulmonary aspergillosis,
      2963t
  for aphthous esophageal ulceration, 1234
  for chronic obstructive pulmonary disease, 810t
  for cysticercosis, 580t
  for disseminated *Mycobacterium avium*
      complex disease, 2906
  for hepatitis, 1437
  for herpes zoster, 1784
  for infectious mononucleosis, 1814
  for leprosy reversal reactions, 2895
  for Marshall's (PFAPA) syndrome, 1208
  for ocular syphilis, 1418
  for pericarditis, 1062
  for *Pneumocystis,* 3089
      for prophylaxis, 3090
  for *Pneumocystis jirovecii,* 558, 1685t
  for pulmonary tuberculosis, 2870
  for rheumatic fever, 2385, 2385t
  for transplant immunosuppression, infections
      and, 3478
  in cytomegalovirus reactivation, 1794-1795
  metronidazole interactions with, 393t
Preemptive therapy, 620
Pregnancy
  acute fatty liver of, 1436
  American trypanosomiasis in, 3158
  anthrax in, post-exposure prophylaxis for,
      3622t
  antimicrobial therapy in, 244-245
  bacterial vaginosis in, 1366-1367
  bacteriuria in, 887
  BK virus in, 1858-1859, 1859t
  blastomycosis in, 3034
  Brucella in, 2671
  Campylobacter fetus in, 2553
  cephalosporins in, 304
  Chlamydia trachomatis in
      complications of, 2249, 2447t
      neonatal infections from, 1250-2251, 2447t
      treatment of, 1250
  cytomegalovirus in, 1789
  delivery in. *See* Delivery.
  dengue fever in, 1938
  donovanosis in, 2749
  ectopic, after pelvic inflammatory disease,
      2249
  enteroviruses in, 2137, 2153
  giardiasis in, 3202t, 3203
  hepatitis A in, 2173
  hepatitis B in, 1874, 1884, 1884t
      chronic, treatment of, 1449
  hepatitis C in, 1965-1966
  hepatitis E in, 2209-2210, 2210f
  herpes simplex virus in, 1771-1772
      peripartum care and, 3410, 3410t
  HIV infection in, 1622
      detection of, 1519
      prevention of, 1495-1496, 3403-3404
          antiretroviral therapy in, 1621, 1622-1626,
              1625t
          transmission of, 1470, 1490-1491
          treatment of, 1626-1627
  HTLV in, 2104-2105, 2104t, 2105f, 2111-2112,
      2113
  human papillomavirus in, 1843
  immunizations in, 3575, 3577, 3644
  intra-amniotic infection syndrome in, 1372-
      1373
  JC virus in, 1858-1859, 1859t
  labor and delivery in. *See* Delivery; Labor.
  Lassa fever in, 2095

Pregnancy *(Continued)*
  Listeria monocytogenes in, 2480
  lymphocytic choriomeningitis in, 2095
  malaria in, 579t, 3125, 3127
  measles in, 2034-2035
  mumps in, 2005-2006
  Neisseria gonorrhoeae in, 2522
  nitrofurantoin in, 475-476
  parvovirus B19 in, 1895, 1896
  poliomyelitis in, 2137, 2143
  Q fever in, 2297
  quinolones in, 467
  Rocky Mountain spotted fever in, 2291
  rubella in, 1921, 1922-1923
      from reinfections, 1922
      vaccination for, 1924
  South American hemorrhagic fevers in, 2095
  Streptococcus agalactiae (group B) in, 2425,
      2428
      chemoprophylaxis for, 2430-2431, 2431t
  syphilis in, 2781
  toxoplasmosis in, 3180
      diagnosis of, 3186-3187
      treatment of, 3190-3191
  travel in, 3644
  trichomoniasis in, 1362, 3206, 3208
  trimethoprim in, 447
  tuberculosis in, 2872
  urinary tract infections in, 892-893
  vancomycin in, 421
  varicella in, 1782-1783
      prevention of, 1785
Prematurity
  acute pyelonephritis and, 892-893
  Chlamydia trachomatis and, 2249
  respiratory syncytial virus and, 2017, 2017t
Preoptic area, in thermoregulation, 6f, 707-708
Preseptal cellulitis, 1421-1424, 1421f-1423f
Pressure ulcers
  in elderly, 3519-3520
  in spinal cord injury, 3515-3516
  infected, 1184
Presumed ocular histoplasmosis syndrome, 3021,
      3025
Preterm infants. *See* Prematurity.
Pretracheal space, 790, 790f
  infections of, 793. *See also* Odontogenic
      infections.
Prevention, 169-171, 620
  preemptive, 620
  primary, 170-171
  risk assessment in, 169-170
  secondary, 171, 620
  strategies for, 169
  tertiary, 171
Prevotella [spp.], 2811, 2812
  antibiotic resistance in, 2844-2845
  appendicitis from, 969
  empyema from, 846
  in oral cavity, 787, 787t, 789
  microbiology of, 2839, 2839t
  pericarditis from, 1059
  peritonitis from, 938
  treatment of, 2844, 2844t
      with metronidazole, 389t
      with tetracyclines, 360t
  virulence factors of, 2814, 2814t
Prevotella intermedia
  odontogenic infections from, 788, 788f, 789
  virulence factors of, 2840
Prevotella melaninogenica
  brain abscess from, 1157, 1158t
  carbapenems for, 313t
  endocarditis from, 992
  in gingival crevices, 2839

Prevotella melaninogenica (Continued)
  in oral cavity, 787, 787t, 789
  lung abscess from, 854
  secondary peritonitis from, 932, 936
  treatment of
      with chloramphenicol, 367t
      with penicillins, 284t, 287, 288t
  virulence factors of, 2840, 2840t
Priftin, 494
Primaquine, 585
  adverse effects of, 581t
  drug interactions with, 694t
  for malaria, 573t, 574t, 3134t, 3136
      for prophylaxis, in travelers, 3642
  for *Pneumocystis,* 3088
  for *Pneumocystis jirovecii,* 575t, 1685t
  indications for, 569t
  structure of, 585f
Primaquine-clindamycin, for *Pneumocystis
      jirovecii,* 569t
Primary amebic meningoencephalitis, 3111-3119
  clinical features of, 3116, 3116t
  diagnosis of, 3117
  epidemiology of, 3114
  etiology of, 3112, 3112f
  pathogenesis and pathophysiology of, 3114-
      3115
  prevention of, 3119
  treatment of, 3118
Primary effusion lymphoma, 1602, 1605, 1810,
      1830, 1830f
  from Epstein-Barr virus, 1810
  from human herpesvirus 8, 1830, 1830f
Primates, nonhuman
  as HIV reservoir, 2119
  hepatitis B virus in, 1832-1834, 1832f
  hepatitis E virus from, 2208
  hepatitis E virus in, 2208
  herpes B virus in. *See* Herpes B virus.
  HIV in, 2119
Prion(s), 2219-2221, 2219-2231, 2219t
  characteristics of, 2219-2221, 2219t
  discovery of, 2219
  laboratory diagnosis of, 2219
  molecular biology of, 2219-2221
Prion diseases
  chronic wasting disease, 2230
  clinical features of, 2222t
  course of, 2222t
  Creutzfeldt-Jakob disease, 2222-2228, 2222t,
      2230
  diagnosis of, 2222t
  epidemiology of, 2222t
  etiology of, 2222t
  fatal familial insomnia, 230, 2222t, 2229
  geographic distribution of, 2222t
  Gerstmann-Sträussler-Scheinker syndrome,
      222t, 2228-2229
  infection control measures for, 2230-2231,
      3341
  insomnia in, 2220, 2229
  kuru, 222t, 2221-2222, 2230
  prevention of, 2230
  treatment of, 2230
Prion protein, 2219-2221, 2219t
  assays for, 2225
  isoforms of, 2225
Prion protein gene, in infection susceptibility, 46,
      48
Prisons, tuberculosis spread in, 2858
Pristinamycin, 425
PRO 140, 20, 20t
PRO 542, 20, 20t
Proanthocyanidins, 605, 606f
  in urinary tract infections, 20t, 21

Probenecid
  drug interactions with, 525
  for gonococcal pelvic inflammatory disease, 2525, 2525t
  for syphilis, 2782
  oseltamivir interactions with, 536
  quinolones with, 459
  with cidofovir, for cytomegalovirus retinitis, 1792-1793
Probiotics, for gastrointestinal disease, 1218
Procaine penicillin. See Penicillin G.
Procalcitonin, in bacterial meningitis, 1103
Procoagulant response, 910, 910f
Proctitis/proctocolitis
  from Chlamydia trachomatis, 2246, 2247t, 2250
  from herpes simplex virus, 1766-1767, 1773t.
    See also Herpes simplex virus, genital.
  from Neisseria gonorrhoeae, 1267, 2520
  in HIV infection, 1580, 1580t
Proctoscopy, in gastrointestinal infections, 1224
Proglottids, 3285, 3287f
Progressive bacterial synergistic gangrene, 1181-1182, 1181f, 1183t
Progressive multifocal leukoencephalopathy, 1856-1861
  clinical features of,1858t, 1858
  diagnosis of, 1859-1861
  epidemiology of, 1857
  etiology of, 1857
  in HIV infection, 525, 1589-1591, 1590f, 1697-1698
  in transplant recipients, 3509
  pathogenesis of, 1857-1858
  prevention of, 1861
  treatment of, 1861
Proguanil
  adverse effects of, 581t
  for malaria, 3129, 3133, 3134t, 3135
    for prophylaxis, 3137-3138, 3137t
    resistance to, 3129. See also Malaria, drug-resistant.
  for Plasmodium falciparum prophylaxis, 587
Properdin, 69, 70t, 74t
  deficiency of, 81, 82t, 87, 151t
Prophylaxis. See Prevention.
Propionibacterium [spp.], 2851
  gram stain of, 2849, 2850f
  pericarditis from, 1059
  treatment of
    with macrolides, 397t
    with quinupristin-dalfopristin, 425
Propionibacterium acnes
  cardiovascular device infections from, 1023
  chloramphenicol for, 367t
  endophthalmitis from, 1408, 1411
  mupirocin for, 485t
  otitis externa from, 766
  prosthetic vascular graft infections from, 1037
  shunt infections from, 1035, 1127, 1127t
  topical antibacterials for, 483
  transient bacteremia from, 978
Propionibacterium propionicum, canaliculitis from, 2924
Prostadynia, 894
Prostaglandins, in neutrophil migration, 98
Prostatic abscess, 894, 894f, 1383t, 1384
  in melioidosis, 2625, 2628, 2628f
Prostatic antibacterial factor, 1382
Prostatitis, 893-895, 1382-1384
  acute bacterial (type I), 893-894, 894f, 895, 1382, 1383t
  asymptomatic inflammatory, 1383-1384, 1383t
  chronic bacterial (type II), 894, 895, 1382-1383, 1382t

Prostatitis (Continued)
  chronic, with chronic pelvic pain, 1382, 1383, 1383t
  classification of, 893, 893t, 1382, 1382t
  diagnosis of, 1382, 1382t
  from Blastomyces dermatitidis, 3033, 3033f
  from Chlamydia trachomatis, 1352, 2246, 2247t
  from herpes simplex virus, 1766. See also Herpes simplex virus, genital.
  from Ureaplasma urealyticum, 1352
  granulomatous, 1383t, 1384
  in HIV infection, 1384, 1385-1386
  nonbacterial (type III), 894, 1382, 1382t, 1383, 1383t
  treatment of, 894-895
    with quinolones, 460
  tuberculous, 1383t, 1384
Prostatosis, 894
Prostheses, Staphylococcus aureus infections of, 2346
Prosthetic joint infections, 1332-1336
  clinical presentation of, 1333, 1333t
  diagnosis of, 1333-1334, 1334f
  from Staphylococcus epidermidis, 2357
  laboratory culture in, 1334, 1334t
  microbiology of, 1332-1333, 1333t
  pathogenesis of, 1332-1333
  prevention of, 1335-1336
  treatment of, 1334-1335
Prosthetic valve infections, 1024-1032. See also
    Cardiovascular device infections;
    Endocarditis, prosthetic valve.
  from Coxiella burnetii, 2300
Prosthetic vascular grafts, infections of, 1036-1039
Prostitutes, HIV infection in, 1480, 1482
Protease inhibitors, 1663-1668, 1665t
  combination therapy with, 1672
  drug interactions with, 695t
    with antiepileptics, 1596-1597
    with rifamycin, 376t
  for AIDS dementia, 1586
  for perinatal HIV transmission prevention, 1625t
  pediatric, 1646t, 1648t
  resistance to, 1667-1668
  structures of, 1664f
Proteases, of Pseudomonas aeruginosa, 2595
Protein(s)
  acute-phase, 709-710, 710t
  in cerebrospinal fluid, 1081, 1081t
  viral, 1730-1731, 1731f
Protein binding, in antimicrobials, 246, 273
Protein C, activated, 910
  for sepsis, 921
Protein C receptor, 910
Proteinuria, in urinary tract infections, 884
Proteolytic fragmentation, of adhesins, 16, 16f, 16t
Proteus [spp.], 2580
  beta-lactamase production by, 257
  endocarditis from, 991
  in peritoneal dialysis, 941
  mycotic aneurysm from, 1008
  secondary peritonitis from, 937
  suppurative thrombophlebitis from, 1004
  treatment of, with penicillins, 288t
  urinary tract infections from, 881, 882, 2580
Proteus aeruginosa, peritonitis from, 942
Proteus mirabilis, 2580
  peritonitis from, 937, 938, 939
    secondary, 937
  prostatitis from, 894
  treatment of

Proteus mirabilis (Continued)
  with aminoglycosides, 334t-335t
  with carbapenems, 313t
  with cephalosporins, 298t
  with chloramphenicol, 367t
  with combination therapy, 249
  with mupirocin, 485t
  with penicillins, 284t, 288t
  with quinolones, 455t
  with rifamycin, 374t
  with sulfonamides, 441t
  with trimethoprim, 444t
  with trimethoprim-sulfamethoxazole, 444
  urinary tract infections from, 2580
  catheter-related, 3372
Proteus vulgaris, 2580
  treatment of
    with carbapenems, 313t
    with mupirocin, 485t
    with penicillins, 284t
    with quinolones, 455t
    with rifamycin, 374t
Prothionamide, for leprosy, 499
Proton motive force, 262
Proton pump inhibitors, for Helicobacter pylori infections, 2563
Prototheca [spp.]
  in immunocompromised host, 1184
  laboratory studies of, 229
Prototheca wickerhamii, 3076f, 3076t, 3077
  skin infections from, 1184
Prototheca zofii, 3076t, 3077
Protozoa
  classification of, 3095, 3095t, 3096t
  coccidian, 3228-3232
Protozoal infections, 568, 3095. See also specific infections.
  brain abscess in, 1152, 1155, 1157, 1158, 1158t
  clinical features of, 3096t
  complement resistance in, 77
  complement-dependent killing in, 77
  diagnosis of, 3096t
  epidemiology of, 3096t
  geographic distribution of, 3096t
  meningitis in, 1084t, 1088
    clinical features of, 1101
    diagnosis of, 1104-1105
    treatment of, 1106t
  syndrome of abdominal pain, diarrhea, and eosinophilia from, 1281t, 1283
  transmission of, 3096t
  treatment of, 582-583, 583f
Providencia [spp.], 2580
  endocarditis from, 991
  suppurative thrombophlebitis from, 1004
  treatment of
    with aminoglycosides, 334t-335t
    with penicillins, 284t, 288t
Providencia rettgeri, 2580
  quinolones for, 455t
  rifamycin for, 374t
Providencia stuartii, 2580
  quinolones for, 455t
  rifamycin for, 374t
Prp 27-30, 2219, 2220. See also Prion(s).
PRP, in infection susceptibility, 48
Pruritus. See Antipruritics.
Pseudallescheria boydii, 3068-3069, 3068f, 3076t
  brain abscess from, 1152, 1155, 1158t, 1160-1161, 3068-3069
  endocarditis from, 993
  mycetoma from, 299t, 2991-2995, 2992t, 2994f, 3068

Pseudallescheria boydii (Continued)
  pulmonary infections from
    in cystic fibrosis, 872
    in immunocompromised host, 3436
  skin lesions from, in immunocompromised
    host, 3439
Pseudoaneurysms
  infections of, 1007
  mycotic, in injection drug users, 3467-3468
Pseudoappendicitis, from *Campylobacter jejuni*,
  2552
Pseudohyphae, 229
Pseudoinfections, from *Bacillus,* 2493
Pseudolymphangitis, 1212
Pseudomembranous colitis, 1249-1259
  from *Candida,* 1250
  from clindamycin, 1265f
  from *Clostridium difficile,* 1223, 1249-1252,
    1251f
    agents inciting, 1252, 1252t
    clindamycin and, 410, 411
    clinical manifestations of, 1253-1254, 1254f
    diagnosis of, 1255-1257, 1256t
    endoscopy of, 1256
    epidemic strains in, 1253
    epidemiology of, 1252-1253, 1252t
    etiology of, 1250
    factors contributing to, 1252-1253
    incidence of, 1252
    lincomycin and, 410
    metronidazole and, 392
    microbiology of, 1251-1252
    normal flora and, 1218
    pathogenesis of, 1254-1255
    pathology of, 1255, 1255f
    prevention of, 1258
    recurrent, 1258
    reservoirs of, 1253
    surgery for, 1258
    treatment of, 1257-1258, 1257t, 1258t
      with teicoplanin, 424
      with vancomycin, 423
  from *Clostridium perfringens,* 1250
  from erythromycin, 400
  from penicillins, 287
  from *Staphylococcus aureus,* 1250, 1250f
  from trimethoprim-sulfamethoxazole, 445
  historical overview of, 1250-1251, 1250f,
    1251f
Pseudomonas [spp.], 2751t, 2759-2760
  beta-lactamase production by, 260
  cardiovascular device infections from, 1023
  endocarditis from, 991
    treatment of, 999-1000
  exotoxin A of, 27
  identification of, 220, 220t, 221t
  in peritoneal dialysis, 941
  keratitis from, 1397-1400
  quinolone-resistant, 465
  sinusitis from, 782, 782t
  treatment of
    with penicillins, 284t, 288t
    with rifamycin, 374t
  urinary tract infections from, 881, 882
Pseudomonas aeruginosa, 2587-2608
  adherence of, 2592-2594
  alginate antibodies in, 2598
  aminoglycoside susceptibility to, 332-333, 332t
  anatomic barriers to, 2589-2590
  antimicrobial kill curves for, 275, 275f
  arthritis from, 1312, 1312t, 2602-2603
  as opportunist, 3, 4
  bacteremia from, 736, 2599-26001, 2600f
  beta-lactamase production by, 257
  biofilm formation in, 2598

Pseudomonas aeruginosa (Continued)
  blood-stream dissemination of, 2598-2599
  bone infections from, 2602-2603
  brain abscess from, 1151, 1157, 1158t
  burn infections from, 2605-2606
  chronic respiratory tract infections from, 2602
  clinical manifestations of, 2599-2608
  colonization by, 2592-2594
  community-acquired, 2588
  conjunctivitis from, 1391
    in neonate, 1393
  COPD exacerbations from, 809
  cystic fibrosis transmembrane conductance
    regulator in, 2592, 2593f
  cytotoxin of, 2596
  ecthyma gangrenosum from, 733, 736, 1186
  endocarditis from, 2606
    in intravenous drug users, 992
    prosthetic valve, 1030
    treatment of, 999-1000
  endovascular infections from, 2606
  entry of, 2592-2594, 2593f
  epidemiology of, 2588-2589
  exoenzymes of, 2596
  exotoxin A of, 28, 2595-2596
  eye infections from, 2604
  falgella of, 2594
  febrile neutropenia from, 2606-2607
  folliculitis from, 733, 736, 1175
  gangrene from, 1181, 1182, 1183t, 1186
  genetic regulation of, 7
  history of, 2588
  immunotherapy for, 2599
  in coronary artery stents, 1040
  in cystic fibrosis, 870-871
  in HIV infection, 2607
  keratitis from, 1397-1400
  lipopolysaccharide of, 2588, 2588f, 2595
  lung abscess from, 854
  meningitis from, 1087, 1106t, 1114, 2604
  microbiology of, 2587-2588
  morphology of, 2587, 2587f
  multidrug resistant, 2607-2608
  mycotic aneurysms from, 1008
  necrotizing fasciitis from, 2341
  nosocomial, 2588-2589
  osteomyelitis from, 1324
    hyperbaric oxygen for, 566
  otitis from, 766, 2604-2605
  pancreatic infections from, 962
  pathogenesis of, 2589-2599
    bacterial factors in, 2592-2599
    host factors in, 2589-2592
  phospholipase of, 2596
  physiologic barriers to, 2589-2590
  pili of, 2593-2594
  pneumonia from, 2598, 2601-2602
    aspiration, 835
    chest film in, 829
    chronic, 2602
    community-acquired, 831-833
    in cystic fibrosis, 870, 872
    in HIV infection, 1570
    nosocomial, 835-836, 3367t
    treatment of, 836-839, 837t, 838t
  proteases of, 2595
  quinolone-resistant, 454
  quorum sensing by, 2597-2598
  resistance to, 2589-2595
  rhamnolipid of, 2596
  secondary peritonitis from, 932, 936
    treatment of, 938, 939
  sinusitis from, 776, 776t, 782, 782t
  skin infections from, 733, 736, 1186, 2605-
    2606

Pseudomonas aeruginosa (Continued)
  soft tissue infections from, 2605-2606
  structure of, 2587-2588, 2587f
  suppurative thrombophlebitis from, 1003, 1004
  tissue spread of, 2598
  toxin production by, 2595-2596
  transient bacteremia from, 978
  treatment of, 2607-2608
    antimicrobial selection in, 246
    with aminoglycosides, 334t-335t, 344, 344t
      combination therapy with, 336t, 337t
      postantibiotic effect in, 334
    with carbapenems, 313t
    with cephalosporins, 298t
    with chloramphenicol, 367t
    with combination therapy, 248, 336t, 337t
    with mupirocin, 485t
    with penicillins, 284t, 288t
    with quinolones, 455t, 463
    with rifamycin, 374t, 382
    with sulfonamides, 441t
    with tetracyclines, 359t
    with trimethoprim, 444t
    with vancomycin, 359t
  type III secretion factors of, 2596
  typhlitis from, 973
  urinary tract infections from, 2605
    catheter-related, 3372
  vaccines for, 2599, 2599t
  virulence of, 2592, 2594t, 2597-2598
    iron acquisition in, 2595
    pyocyanin in, 2596-2597
    reactive oxygen species in, 2597
Pseudomonas cepacia, endocarditis from, 991
Pseudomonas fluorescens, 2587, 2759-2760
  from red blood cell transfusion, 3388
Pseudomonas luteola, 220t, 2760
Pseudomonas oryzihabitans, 220t, 2760
Pseudomonas (Burkholderia) pseudomallei,
  chloramphenicol for, 367t
Pseudomonas putida, 2587, 2760
Pseudomonas quinolone system, 2597-2598
Pseudomonas stutzeri, 2760
Pseudomycetoma, 3057
Pseudo-nitzschia pungens, 3256, 3256t
Pseudophakic endophthalmitis, 1407t, 1408
Pseudopod, by enteropathogenic *Escherichia coli,*
  9, 9f
Psittacosis, 2251, 2256-2258
  endocarditis in, 993
  history in, 823t
  isolation precautions for, 3330t
  vs. enteric fever, 1278
Psoas abscess, 1200-1201
  in melioidosis, 2625, 2627f
Psoriasis, genital lesions in, 1344-1345
Psorophora spp.
  Rocio encephalitis from, 1945, 1945t
  Venezuelan equine encephalitis from, 1915
Psychotropic agents, rifamycin interaction with,
  376t
Pterygoid space, 790, 790f
  infections of, 791-792. *See also* Odontogenic
    infections.
Pubic lice, 3302-3304, 3302f, 3303f
Public Health Security and Bioterrorism and
  Response Act, 3600
Puerperal infections, 1373-1376, 1373f
  from streptococcus group C, 2444
  from streptococcus group G, 2444
Pulmonary abscess. *See* Lung abscess.
Pulmonary artery catheters, infections of, 3355
Pulmonary defense systems, impairment of, 821-
  822
Pulmonary edema, in malaria, 3125

Pulmonary embolism
  fever from, 726
  in airplane passengers, 3644
  in spinal cord injury, 3514-3515
  pleural effusion and, 847, 849
Pulmonary eosinophilia, 835
Pulmonary host defenses, 820-822
Pulmonary hypertension, in HIV infection, 1573
Pulmonary infections. *See also* Pneumonia;
    Respiratory tract infections; *and specific
    infections.*
  anaerobic, 2812
    from gram-negative bacilli, 2841
  from *Aspergillus,* 3035-3036
    chronic, 2963
    invasive, 2963-2964, 2964, 2966-2967
  from *Blastomyces dermatitidis,* 3029-3031,
      3029t, 3030f-3032f
    treatment of, 3036-3037, 3036t
  from *Clostridium,* 2830
  from *Coccidioides immitis,* 3042-3043, 3043f-
      3045f
  from *Cryptococcus neoformans,* 3002-3003,
      3003f, 3003t, 3007
  from *Fusarium,* in immunocompromised host,
      3436
  from mucormycosis, 2977, 2978f, 2979f
  from *Paracoccidioides brasiliensis,* 3064,
      3064f, 3065f
  from *Plasmodium falciparum,* 3125
  from *Pseudallescheria boydii,* 3068-3069, 3076t
  from *Pseudomonas aeruginosa,* 2592, 2598
  from *Rhodococcus equi,* 2472-2473
  from *Salmonella,* 2647t
  from *Scedosporium apiospermum*
    in cystic fibrosis, 872
    in immunocompromised host, 3436
  from *Schistosoma,* 3279
  from *Sporothrix schenckii,* 2985, 2986, 2986f,
      2987
  from *Streptococcus anginosus* group, 2455
  from *Toxoplasma gondii,* 3176, 3179
  in burn patients, 3550
  in cancer patients, 3434-3437, 3457
  in cystic fibrosis, 869-873
    microbiology of, 870-872
    treatment of, 892
  in immunocompromsed host, laboratory
      diagnosis of, 3428
  in stem cell transplant, 3488, 3493-3495
  in travelers, 3647t, 3648t, 3651
  risk factors for, 823t, 858-859
  treatment of, with clindamycin, 411
Pulmonary infiltrates
  in immunocompromised host, 3436
  with esoinophilia, 835
Pulmonary nodules
  differential diagnosis of, 861t
  in coccidioidomycosis, 3043, 3044f
  radiographic appearance of, 861t
Pulmonary sarcoidosis, chest film in, 862f
Pulmonary surfactant, 820
Pulpitis, 790-791
Pulsed-field gel electrophoresis, 222
  for foodborne disease, 1294
  of *Burkholderia cepacia,* 2617
Puncture wounds, osteomyelitis in, from
    Pseudomonas aeruginosa, 2603
Pure red cell aplasia, from parvovirus B19, 1894,
    1896
Purine nucleoside phosphorylase deficiency, 150t
Purpura, 730t, 731, 732, 734. *See also* Rash.
  in sepsis, 917
  thrombotic thrombocytopenic, in HIV
      infection, 1561

Purpura fulminans, 735
Purtilo's syndrome, 1435, 1807
Pustules, 731-732, 734. *See also* Rash.
  causes of, 734
Puumala virus, 2086-2089, 2086t
  as biological weapon, 3627-3629, 3628t
Pyelography, intravenous, of urinary tract
    infections, 897-898
Pyelonephritis
  acute, 875
    antimicrobial therapy for, 889-890, 890f
    papillary necrosis in, 876, 876f
    pathology of, 875
    prematurity and, 892-893
  catheter-related, 3373
  chronic, 875-876, 875f
  emphysematous, 890, 890f, 897
  from *Candida,* 2946
  hematogenous route in, 876
  in elderly, 3517-3518
  in spinal cord injury, 3514
  in transplant recipients, 3503, 3509
  nitrofurantoin for, 474
  xanthogranulomatous, 895
    imaging of, 899, 899f
Pyloric stenosis, infantile hypertrophic,
    erythromycin and, 400
Pyocyanin, in *Pseudomonas aeruginosa*
    infections, 2596-2597
Pyoderma
  from *Streptococcus pyogenes* (group A), 2368-
      2370, 2369f
  in poststreptoccocal acute glomerulonephritis,
      2387t
  quinolones for, 463-464
  topical antibacterial therapy for, 482
Pyoderma gangrenosum, 1184t
  in immunocompromised host, 3439
Pyodermas, 1172-1180
  subcutaneous abscess in, 1191
Pyogenic infections, liver abscess in, 951-955
Pyogenic orchitis, 1385
Pyomyositis, 1195-1197. *See also* Myositis.
  from *Staphylococcus aureus,* 2347-2348
  in injection drug users, 3464
Pyopneumothorax, from *Coccidioides immitis,*
    3043, 3045f
PYR test, 216t
  for *Enterococcus,* 217t, 218
Pyrantel pamoate
  adverse effects of, 582t
  drug interactions with, 695t
  for ascariasis, 571t, 3263
  for enterobiasis, 572t, 3266
  for helminthic disease, 570t
  for hookworms, 3264
  for intestinal nematodes, 593
  for *Moniliformis moniliformis,* 574t
  for *Trichostrongylus,* 576t
Pyrazinamide
  dosage of, 676t-677t
  for brain abscess, 1159t
  for tuberculosis, 492, 1681t, 2867, 2868, 2868t,
      2869
    in HIV infection, 1687t, 1699, 2870, 2871t
  formulations of, 649t
Pyrethrins
  adverse effects of, 582t
  for lice, 3303-3304
Pyridoxine, for *Mycobacterium tuberculosis*
  in HIV infection, 1687t, 1699
  in latent infections, 2874
Pyrimethamine
  adverse effects of, 582t
  for brain abscess, 1159t

Pyrimethamine *(Continued)*
  for *Isospora belli,* 1689t
  for malaria, 587-588, 3133, 3134-3135, 3134t
    mechanism of action of, 3129
    resistance to, 3129, 3133. *See also* Malaria,
        drug-resistant.
  for *Pneumocystis,* for prophylaxis, 3090
  for *Pneumocystis jirovecii,* 575t, 1681t, 1683t
  for *Toxoplasma gondii,* 576t, 580t, 3188
    in chorioretinitis, 3190
    in congenital infections, 3191
    in encephalitis, 1587
      for prophylaxis, 3190
    in HIV infection, 1682t, 1683t, 1685t, 1695
    in immunocompromised host, 3188-3190,
        3189t
      for prophylaxis, 3191, 3504
    in pregnancy, 3190-3191
  prophylactic, for transplant recipients, 3483,
      3504
  structure of, 588f
Pyrimethamine-sulfadiazine, 569t
  for toxoplasmic encephalitis, 443
Pyrimethamine-sulfadoxine, 573t, 574t, 578t
  for malaria, 573t, 574t, 578t
  for *Toxoplasma gondii,* 3190
    for encephalitis prophylaxis, 3190
Pyrogen(s)
  endogenous
    in acute-phase response, 709-710, 710t
    in febrile response, 708-709, 709f, 711
    in immune response, 712
  exogenous, 708
Pyrogenic cytokines, in sepsis syndrome, 712
Pyrrolidinyl, with quinolones, 451
L-Pyrrolidonyl-β-naphthylamide, 216t
  for *Enterococcus,* 217t, 218
Pythiosis, 2981
Pyuria
  in urethral syndrome, 886
  in urinary tract infections, 884

Q

Q fever *(Coxiella burnetii),* 2296-2301
  chronic, 2299-2300
  clinical manifestations of, 2297-2301
  endocarditis in, 993, 2299-2300, 2299f
    quinolones for, 465
    treatment of, 1001
  epidemiology of, 2297
  etiology of, 2296-2297, 2296f
  hepatitis in, 1436, 2300
  history in, 823t
  in immunocompromised host, 2300-2301
  isolation precautions for, 3330t
  meningoencephalitis in, 2300
  pathogenesis of, 2297
  pneumonia in, 2297-2299, 2298f
  prevention of, 2301, 3330t
  rifamycin for, 382
  self-limited febrile illness in, 2297
  vs. enteric fever, 1275t
Qinghaosu, 606f
QT interval, quinolone effects on, 466-467
Quantiferon-TB test, 227-228, 2861
Quaternary ammonium compounds, disinfection
    with, 3337-3338
Queensland tick typhus, 2285t, 2287t, 2292-2293
Quinacrine
  drug interactions with, 695t
  for giardiasis, 3202, 3202t
Quinidine, 569t
  cardiotoxicity of, 3135-3136
  for malaria, 574t, 586, 3133, 3134t, 3135-3136

Quinidine *(Continued)*
   mechanism of action of, 3129
   resistance to, 3129. *See also* Malaria, drug-
     resistant.
Quinine, 569t
   adverse effects of, 582t
   drug interactions with, 696t
   for babesiosis, 571t, 3213, 3214
   for malaria, 573t, 578t, 585-586, 585f, 3129,
     3134t, 3135
   resistance to, 3129. *See also* Malaria, drug-
     resistant.
Quinolones, 451-467. *See also specific agents.*
   absorption of, 457
   adverse effects of, 466-467
   age and, 244
   antimicrobial activity of, 454, 455t, 456-457, 456t
   distribution of, 457, 458t
   dosage of, 458, 458t, 672t-675t
   drug interactions with, 458-459, 691t
   elimination of, 457-458, 458t
   for acute pyelonephritis, 889
   for bacteremia, 464-465
   for brain abscess, 1159, 1159t
   for endocarditis, 465
   for enterccoccal infections, 997, 2416
   for enterococcal endocarditis, 997
   for gastrointestinal infections, 460-462
   for intra-abdominal infections, 461-462
   for keratitis, 1399
   for *Legionella,* 27278
   for leprosy, 2894
   for meningitis, 465, 1113, 1114
   for mycobacteria, 464
     nontuberculous, 497
   for *Mycoplasma pneumoniae,* 2278
   for *Neisseria gonorrhoeae,* 2524t, 2525
   for neutropenia, 464-465
   for prostatitis, 460, 895
   for *Pseudomonas* endocarditis, 1000
   for psittacosis, 2257
   for respiratory infections, 462-463
   for secondary peritonitis, 939
   for sepsis, 919
   for sexually transmitted disease, 460
   for staphylococcal endocarditis, 999
     prosthetic valve, 1027
   for traveler's diarrhea, 1243
   for tuberculosis, 494, 2867
   for typhoid fever, 2648-2649, 2649t
   for urethritis, 1207
   for urinary tract infections, 459-460, 890
   for urogenital chlamydial infections, 2247t,
     2249, 2250
   formulations of, 648t
   in preemptive pancreatic infection treatment,
     965t
   mechanism of action of, 451-453
   pharmacology of, 457-459, 457t
   pneumococci resistant to, 185
   postantibiotic effect of, 457
   prophylactic, in cancer-related febrile
     neutropenia, 3442-3446, 3444f, 3445f
   resistance to, 453-454, 465-466
     by *Neisseria gonorrhoeae,* 186, 2519
     by *Salmonella,* 2640
     by *Staphylococcus aureus,* 2334t
     efflux in, 263
     in elderly, 3522
     outer membrane permeability in, 262
     target enzyme alteration in, 265
   respiratory tract
     for pneumonia, 837-839, 837t, 838t
     in cystic fibrosis, 872
     pneumococcal resistance to, 837, 837t

Quinolones *(Continued)*
   structure of, 451, 452f
   uses of, 459-465
   with other antimicrobial agents, 457
Quinsy, 754, 756
Quinupristin
   for pneumonia, 837-839, 837t, 838t
   pneumococcal resistance to, 837, 837t
Quinupristin-dalfopristin, 425-427
   adverse effects of, 427
   antimicrobial activity of, 425-426
   distribution of, 426-427
   dosage of, 427, 668t-669t
   drug interactions with, 427
   elimination of, 426-427
   for *Enterococcus,* 2417
     multidrug-resistant, 1028, 1029t
   for penicillin-resistant enterococcal
     endocarditis, 997
   for shunt infections, 1129t, 1130
   for *Staphylococcus,* 424t, 2336-2337
   formulations of, 648t
   mechanism of action of, 425
   pharmacology of, 426
   resistance to, 426
     by *Staphylococcus aureus,* 2334t
   uses of, 427
Quorum sensing, 8

R

Rabies, 2047-2054
   clinical features of, 2050-2051
   course of, 2050, 2051t
   diagnosis of, 252f, 2051-252
   differential diagnosis of, 2052-2053
   epidemiology of, 2047t, 2048-2049, 2048f,
     2049f
   furious, 2050-2051, 2051t
   geographic distribution of, 3640f
   historical perspective on, 2047
   host susceptibility to, 2051t
   immune response to, 2050
   paralytic (dumb), 2051, 2051t
   pathogenesis of, 2049-2050
   pathology of, 2049-2050, 2050f
   prevention of, 2053-2054, 2054f. *See also*
     Rabies vaccine.
   transmission of, 2050
   treatment of, 2054
Rabies immune globulin, 2053, 3574
Rabies vaccine, 2053-2054, 3571
   acute disseminated encephalomyelitis from,
     2053
   for bites, 3554t
   for elderly, 3522
   for travelers, 3639f, 3640
Rabies virus
   genome of, 2047, 2048t
   receptors for, 1732t
   replication of, 2048, 2049
   structure of, 2047, 2048t
RAC, in oxidative burst, 101
Racecadotril, for rotavirus, 1909
Racemose cysticercosis, 3290
Radiation therapy
   for Kaposi's sarcoma, 1603
   for primary central nervous system lymphoma,
     1589, 1608
   in stem cell transplant, 3486-3487
   of head and neck, complications of, 800
Radiculitis, 1143
Radiculopathy
   cytomegalovirus, 1791
   progressive, in HIV infection, 1595, 1597t

Radioallergosorbent test, for beta-lactam
   antibiotic allergy, 323
Radiography
   chest, 3013-3025
     cavitary lesions on, 854t, 855, 860, 861t
     diffuse infiltrates and fibrosis on, 861t
     for acute pneumonia, 823, 828-830, 829f
     for anthrax, 3619, 3619f
     for aspergillosis, 2964, 2964f, 2966-2967
     for blastomycosis, 867f, 3030, 3030f-3032f,
       3031
     for bronchiolitis, 816
     for chronic pneumonia, 860, 860f-867f, 861t
     for coccidioidomycosis, 864f, 3042-3043,
       3043f-3045f
     for croup, 762, 762f
     for cryptococcosis, 3002, 3003, 3003f, 3004,
       3007
     for *Francisella tularensis* pneumonia, 2681,
       2681f
     for histoplasmosis, 863f, 3018-3109, 3018f
     for HIV-related pulmonary complications,
       1568, 1568t
     for *Legionella,* 2727f, 2728f
     for lung abscess, 855, 855f
     for lymphangioleiomyomatosis, 863f
     for mucormycosis, 2977, 2977f, 2978f
     for *Mycobacterium avium* complex
       infections, 864f, 2899f, 2900f
     for nocardiosis, 2918, 2918f
     for *Paracoccidioides brasiliensis,* 3064,
       3064f, 3065f
     for pleural effusion/empyema, 847, 848f,
       849
     for pneumococcal pneumonia, 2400
     for *Pneumocystis* pneumonia, 3085,3085f,
       3082-3084, 3084f
     for psittacosis, 2257
     for Q fever, 2298, 2298f
     for respiratory syncytial virus, 2014
     for *Rhodococcus equi* pneumonia, 865f
     for tropical pulmonary eosinophilia, 3274f,
       3275
     for tuberculoma, 2865, 2865f
     for tuberculosis, 864f, 865f, 2864, 2864f,
       2866
     lobar consolidation on, 861t
      differential diagnosis of, 861t
     patchy infiltrates on, 861t
      differential diagnosis of, 861t
   for brain abscess, 7f, 1155-1157, 1158-1159
   for central nervous system infections, 1082,
     1103, 1104f, 1135
   for Creutzfeldt-Jakob disease, 2224-2225,
     2226
   for epidural abscess, 1167, 1167f
   for hepatic fibrosis, 1963-1964
   for mediastinitis, 1072, 1072f
   for melioidosis, 2625f, 2626f
   for meningitis
     acute, 1082, 1103, 1104f
     chronic, 1082, 1135
   for miliary tuberculosis, 2876, 2876f
   for mucormycosis, 2977, 2977f, 2978, 2978f
   for odontogenic infections, 780, 796f, 1135
   for orbital infections, 1423, 1423f
   for prosthetic joint infections, 1333, 1334f
   for psoas abscess, 1200
   for pyomyositis, 1197
   for secondary peritonitis, 935
   for sinusitis, 778
   for subdural empyema, 1164-1165, 1166f
   for suppurative intracranial thrombosis, 1169,
     1169f
Radioimmunoassay, 58

Radioimmunoprecipitation, for HIV infection, 1516
Radionuclide cholescintigraphy, 956
Radionuclide scanning
    for intraperitoneal abscess, 943, 944f
    for pneumonia, 830
    for urinary tract infections, 898, 899f
RAG-1, 59
RAG-2, 59
Ralstonia [spp.], 2751t, 2760
Ralstonia pickettii, 221t, 2760
Ramichloridium mackenziei, brain abscess from, 3070
Ramoplanin, for vancomycin-resistant enterococcal endocarditis, 997
Ramsay Hunt syndrome, 1783
Ranitidine, for *Helicobacter pylori*, 2563
RANTES, in HIV susceptibility, 45, 45t
Rapamycin, for transplant immunosuppression, infections and, 3478
Rape, of children, HIV infection from, 1651
Rapid antigen detection tests
    for bronchiolitis, 816
    for croup, 763
    for pharyngitis, 755
    for streptococcal pharyngitis, 2366-2367
Rapid hepatitis B sAg/eAg test, 237, 237t
Rapid plasma reagin assay
    for endemic treponematoses, 2787
    for syphilis, 2778, 2779
Rash, 2149. *See also* Exanthem(s); Skin infections.
    approach to patient with, 729-731
    diaper, from *Candida*, 2944, 2944f, 2951
    differential diagnosis of, 731-734, 731t
    diffuse erythematous, 733
    distribution of, 730-731
    drug-related, 731
        in HIV infection, 742
        in infectious mononucleosis, 1806, 1806f, 1806t
    etiology of, 730t
    evaluation of, 729-731
    extent of, 730-731
    febrile, 729-742. *See also* Fever.
    from nitrofurantoin, 475
    from quinolones, 466
    from rifamycin, 377-378
    from teicoplanin, 424
    from vancomycin, 421
    histologic findings in, 731t
    history in, 729
    in alphavirus infections, 1916
    in bartonellosis, 739-740
    in borreliosis, 738-739
    in candidiasis, 739
    in *Capnocytophaga canimorsus* infections, 738
    in coccidiodomycosis, 3043
    in coxsackievirus infections, 2149-2150
    in cytomegalovirus infections, 1790
    in dengue fever, 739, 1938, 3653f
    in dermatophytosis, 3054-3058, 3055f-3057f
    in disseminated gonococcal infections, 2522, 2522f
    in Ebola fever, 739
    in echovirus infections, 2149-2150
    in ehrlichiosis, 740
    in encephalitis, 1145
    in endocarditis, 736
    in enterovirus infections, 2149-2150
    in epidemic typhus, 2304, 2304t
    in erythema infectiosum (fifth disease), 732, 1893-1894, 1893f
    in erythema multiforme, 732

Rash (*Continued*)
    in hand-foot-mouth disease, 2150
    in hepatitis B, 1877
    in herpes simplex virus infections, 732
    in herpes zoster, 1783, 1783f
    in HIV infection, 741-742, 741t
    in hookworm infections, 3264
    in HTLV, 2108f, 2111
    in human herpes 6 infections, 739
    in human parvovirus B19 infections, 732
    in immunocompromised host, 13t, 741-742
    in infectious mononucleosis, 1806, 1806f, 1806t
    in Kawasaki syndrome, 755, 3316
    in Lyme disease, 734, 738, 2798, 2801-2802, 2801f, 2802t, 3314f
    in malaria, 734
    in Marburg fever, 739
    in measles, 2033, 2033f
    in Menangle virus infections, 2043-2044
    in meningitis, 1100, 1186
    in meningococcal sepsis, 2503, 2505f
    in meningococcemia, 735-736, 1186
    in monkeypox, 740-741
    in murine typhus, 2307
    in mycoplasmal infections, 2274f, 2275
    in *Neisseria gonorrhoeae* infections, 736
    in orthopoxvirus infections, 740-741
    in orthoreovirus infections, 1899
    in *Pseudomonas* infections, 736
    in respiratory syncytial virus infections, 2015t
    in rheumatic fever, 733, 737
    in rickettsial infections, 730, 731t, 734, 738, 2286, 2290, 2290f, 2291f, 2296
    in rickettsialpox, 2295
    in Rocky Mountain spotted fever, 734, 738
    in rubella, 1922
    in salmonellosis, 730, 730t, 733
    in scarlet fever, 737-738
    in schistosomiasis, 3278
    in sepsis, 735
    in smallpox, 740, 1746-1747, 1746f, 1747f, 3614, 3614f, 3615f
    in spotted fevers, 730, 731t, 2287t, 2290, 2290f, 2291f, 2292-2293
    in staphylococcal infections, 736-737
    in staphylococcal scalded skin syndrome, 732, 733, 737
    in staphylococcal toxic shock syndrome, 737, 738t
    in stem cell transplant, 3488
    in Stevens-Johnson syndrome, 732, 733
    in streptococcal infections, 737-738
    in streptococcal toxic shock syndrome, 738, 738t
    in strongyloidiasis, 3265
    in Sweet syndrome, 734-735
    in syphilis, 733
    in tick-borne disease, 734
    in tinea, 3054-3058, 3055f-3057f
    in toxic epidermal necrolysis, 732, 733
    in toxic shock syndrome, 732, 733
    in travelers, 3652, 3653f
    in typhoid fever, 1186
    in vaccinia, 1745
    in varicella, 740, 1782
    in variola, 740, 1746-1747, 1746f, 1747f
    in West Nile virus infections, 732
    lesion characteristics in, 730-732, 730t. *See also* Skin lesions.
    maculopapular, 732-733
    nodular, 733, 733t
    noninfectious causes of, 731
    pathogenesis of, 731

Rash (*Continued*)
    pathogens causing, 731t
    pediatric, from viral infections, 234, 235t
    petechial, 734
    physical examination in, 729-730
    purpuric, 734
    terminology of, 731
    timing of, 731, 731t
    types of, 730-732, 730t
    vesicobullous, 733-734
    vesicular
        differential diagnosis of, 1784
        viral, 233t
Rat(s)
    Penicillium marneffei in, 3074
    plague from, 2691, 2692-2693
    Rickettsia typhi from, 2306-2308
    Seoul virus from, 2086t, 2087-2089
Rat-bite fever, 2708-2710
    clinical manifestations of, 2709
    diagnosis of, 2709
    epidemiology of, 2709
    from *Spirillum minus*, 2708, 2709t, 2810
    from *Streptobacillus moniliformis*, 2708, 2709t
    treatment of, 2710
    vs. enteric fever, 1274t, 1277
Ravuconazole, 510
    for aspergillosis, 2968t, 2969
Raynaud's phenomenon, from *Mycoplasma pneumoniae*, 2274-2275, 2274f, 2276
Reactive airway disease. *See also* Asthma.
    bronchiolitis and, 814-815, 816
Reactive arthritis, 1354-1355, 2247-2248
    from *Chlamydia trachomatis*, 1354-1355, 2247-2248
    urethritis and, 1354-1355, 1414, 2247-2248
    uveitis and, 1354-1355, 1414
Reactive oxygen species, in *Pseudomonas aeruginosa*, 2597
Reassortant rotavirus tetravalent vaccine, 1238
Receptor-mediated endocytosis, viral, 1733, 1733f
Receptors, viral, 1732-1733, 1732t
Recombinant immunoblot assay, for hepatitis virus, 237
Recombination activating genes, 59
Rectal biopsy, 1224
    for *Campylobacter jejuni*, 2551
Rectal infections. *See* Proctitis/proctocolitis.
Rectal lesions, in genital herpes, 1766-1767, 1767f
Rectal swabs, collection and transport of, 207t
Rectal temperature, 3, 703-704. *See also* Temperature.
Rectocolitis. *See* Colitis; Proctitis/proctocolitis.
Recurrent respiratory papillomatosis, 1843. *See also* Human papillomavirus(es).
    clinical features of, 1847
    treatment of, 1850
Red bugs, 3310-3311, 3311f
Red cell. *See under* Erythrocyte.
Red eye, differential diagnosis of, 1393-1394
Red man syndrome, from vancomycin, 421
Red mange, 3311
Red tides, 3255-3256, 3255f, 3256t
Reduction-modifiable protein, in *Neisseria gonorrhoeae*, 2516
Reflux
    gastroesophageal, in HIV infection, 1575
    vesicoureteral. *See* Vesicoureteral reflux.
Reflux nephropathy, 886
Regulon, in pathogenicity control, 7
Rehydration. *See* Fluid management.

Reiter's syndrome, 1354-1355, 2247-2248
  from *Campylobacter jejuni,* 2555
  from *Shigella,* 2659
  in HIV infection, 1555-1556
  urethritis in, 1354-1355, 1414, 2247-2248
  uveitis in, 1354-1355, 1414
  vs. bacterial arthritis, 1315
Relapsing fever, 2795-2797
  clinical manifestations of, 2796, 2796t
  diagnosis of, 2796-2797, 2797f
  epidemiology of, 2795-2796
  louse-borne, 2795, 2797
  pathophysiology of, 2796
  tick-borne, 2795, 2796, 2797f, 3312-3314,
    3313f, 3313t
  treatment of, 2797
  vs. enteric fever, 1274t, 1277
Renal actinomycosis, 2928
Renal calculi, in urinary tract infections, 881,
  881f
Renal candidiasis, 2946, 2947, 2947f, 2950
Renal clearance, 274
Renal failure
  drug dosages in, 635, 651t-685t
  in leptospirosis, 2792
  pulmonary tuberculosis in, treatment of, 2872
  rifamycin and, 377
Renal inflammation, chronic, catheter-related,
  3373
Renal insufficiency
  adefovir dipivoxil in, 521, 521t
  amantadine in, 522t
  antimicrobial therapy in, 888-889
  cephalosporin dosage in, 302t, 303
  chloramphenicol in, 368
  famciclovir in, 526t
  foscarnet in, 527, 528t
  ganciclovir in, 529t
  quinolone dosage in, 458, 458t
  sulfonamides in, 442
  valacyclovir dosage in, 518, 519t
  valganciclovir in, 529t
  vancomycin in, 420-421
Renal toxicity
  of aminoglycosides, 339-341, 339f, 340t, 341t
  of amphotericin B, 2967
  of penicillins, 286
Renal transplantation
  BK virus infections in, 1858-1861
  cytomegalovirus infections in, 1796
    from donor organ, 1794
    prevention of, 1793-1794
  infections in, 3502t, 3503. *See also*
    Transplantation, infections in.
  JK virus infections in, 1859-1861
  Kaposi's sarcoma in, 1829-1830
  mycotic aneurysms in, 1007
  pentoxifylline in, 560
  survival in, 3501, 3501t
  toxoplasmosis in, 3177t, 3178
  urinary tract infections in, 883
Reoviruses, 1899
  receptors for, 1732t
Reproductive tract. *See under* Genital;
  Genitourinary tract infections.
Respiratory burst
  abnormalities of, 106-108
  in chronic granulomatous disease, 155, 155f
  in neutrophils, 99-101, 100f
Respiratory dysfunction, in poliomyelitis, 2143
Respiratory syncytial virus, 2009-2021
  age distribution of, 2011-2012, 2012f
  airway hyperreactivity from, 2015t, 2016t,
    2019

Respiratory syncytial virus *(Continued)*
  antigenic variation in, 2010-2011
  apnea from, 2018-2019
  bronchiolitis from, 812-813, 813t, 2014-2016
  characteristics of, 2009-2010, 2009f
  classification of, 2009
  clinical manifestations of, 2014-2017, 2014f,
    2015t, 2016t
    nonrespiratory, 2017
  colds from, 747-750, 747t
  collection of, 233t
  complications of, 2017-2019
    acute, 2018-2019
    in immunocompromised host, 2017t, 2018
    long-term, 2019
    risk factors for, 2017-2018, 2017t
  croup from, 760t, 761
  culture of, 2010, 2010f, 2019
  diagnosis of, 2019-2020
  epidemiology of, 2011-2012, 2012f
  genome of, 2009-2010, 2010f
  historical perspective on, 2009
  hospitalization for, 2012, 2016-2017, 2016t,
    2017t
  human metapneumovirus and, 2028-2029
  hypoxemia from, 2014, 2018-2019
  immunization for, 2021
  in animals, 2011
  in chronic obstructive pulmonary disease, 808
  in hematologic malignancies, 3435
  in immunocompromised host, 2018, 2019t
  in stem cell transplant, 3494-3495
  in transplant recipients, 3509
  incidence and prevalence of, 2011-2012, 2011t
  laboratory tests for, 234
  myocarditis from, 1053, 1053t
  nosocomial, 2017
    prevention of, 2020-2021
  otitis media from, 2014-2015, 2015t, 2016,
    2016t
  pathogenesis of, 2012-2014
  pneumonia from, 2011-2012, 2014-2017
  prevention of, 2020-2021
  radiography in, 2014
  recurrent, 2012
  seasonal occurrence of, 2011
  sinusitis from, 772-780
  structure of, 2009-2010, 2009f
  tracheobronchitis from, 2014, 2015, 2015t
  treatment of, 2020
    in immunocompromised host, 2018
    with antiviral drugs, 515t
    with interferons, 534
    with palivizumab, 558
    with ribavirin, 538
  vaccine for, 2012
  wheezing from, 2015t, 2016t, 2019
  with bacterial coinfection, 2019
Respiratory syncytial virus immune globulin,
  2021, 3574
  for immunocompromised host, 2018
  for otitis media, 770
Respiratory syncytial virus vaccine, for otitis
  media, 770, 770t
Respiratory tract
  host defenses in, 36, 820-822, 820t
    impairment of, 821-822
  in peritonitis, 935, 940
  specimen collection and transport from, 206t
Respiratory tract infections, 2530. *See also*
  Pneumonia; Pulmonary infections; *and*
  specific types.
  acute, 174-176
  brain abscess from, 1151t, 1152

Respiratory tract infections *(Continued)*
  chronic, from *Pseudomonas aeruginosa,* 2602
  cough in, 803, 803t, 804t
  from *Acinetobacter,* 2634
  from adenoviruses, 1838
  from *Brucella,* 2671
  from *Candida,* 2945
  from *Chlamydia (Chlamydophila)*
    pneumoniae, 2258-2266
  from *Chlamydia psittaci,* 2251, 2256-2258
  from coronaviruses, 1990-1996
  from *Corynebacterium diphtheriae,* 2460,
    2460f, 2461-2462, 2461f
  from coxsackieviruses, 2150
  from *Enterococcus,* 2413
  from enteroviruses, 2150-2151
  from *Haemophilus influenzae,* 2661-2662
  from human metapneumovirus, 2028-2029,
    2028t, 2029t
  from influenza virus, 2070-2071, 2070t
  from *Kingella,* 2533
  from microsporidia, 3238t, 3244, 3245
  from *Moraxella (Branhamella) catarrhalis,*
    2530-2531, 2531f
  from *Mycobacterium avium* complex, 2897,
    2898, 2899-2901, 2900f, 2901f, 2901t,
    2902, 2903-2905, 2906
  from *Neisseria meningitidis,* 2506
  from *Nocardia,* 2917-2918, 2918f
  from orthoreoviruses, 1899
  from parainfluenza viruses, 1998-2001
  from *Pasteurella,* 2689
  from respiratory syncytial virus, 812-813,
    2009-2021
  from SARS virus, 1990-1996
  from *Staphylococcus aureus,* 2345
  from streptococcus group C, 2444
  from streptococcus group G, 2444
  hospitalization for, 2012, 2016-2017, 2016t,
    2017t
  in dialysis, 87
  in stem cell transplant, 3488, 3493-3495, 3494-
    3495
  in travelers, 3647t, 3648t, 3651
  laboratory tests for, 208, 209t
  nosocomial, 2531, 3362-3368
    definition of, 3362-3363, 3363t
    diagnosis of, 3366-3367
    epidemiology of, 3363
    etiology of, 3365-3366, 3365t
    pathogenesis of, 3364-3365
    prevention of, 3368, 3368t
    risk factors for, 3363-3364, 3364t
    treatment of, 3367-3368, 3367t
  outpatient parenteral antimicrobial therapy for,
    629t, 630
  pediatric, from nontypeable *Haemophilus*
    influenzae, 2663
  specimen collection and transport from, 206t
  treatment of
    with quinolones, 462-463
    with trimethoprim-sulfamethoxazole, 446
  upper tract, 747-750
    from adenoviruses, 1838
    from *Chlamydia (Chlamydophila)*
      pneumoniae, 2258-2266
    from enteroviruses, 2150
    from microsporidia, 3238t, 3244, 3245
    from respiratory syncytial virus, 2014-2016
    from rhinoviruses, 2185-2192, 2189
    laryngitis in, 758-759
    laryngotracheobronchitis in, 760-764
    otitis media and, 767
    pharyngitis in, 752-757

Respiratory tract infections (*Continued*)
  viral
    laboratory tests for, 234
    specimen collection in, 233t
Respiratory tract quinolones
  for pneumonia, 837-839, 837t, 838t
    in cystic fibrosis, 872
  pneumococcal resistance to, 837, 837t
Respiratory viruses
  interferons for, 534-535
  ribavirin for, 538
Respirovirus, 1998
Restriction fragment length polymorphism, 222
  of *Mycobacterium tuberculosis,* 2854t, 2855
Retina, in endocarditis, 982, 983f
Retinal necrosis, acute, 1416, 1417f, 1418
Retinitis. *See also* Chorioretinitis.
  from *Bartonella henselae,* 1417, 1417f
  from *Baylisascaris procyonis,* 3295
  from *Candida,* 1409, 1411, 1417, 2947-2948,
    2948f, 2951
  from *Cryptococcus neoformans,* 3005
  from cytomegalovirus, 1415-1416, 1559-1560,
    1790-1793, 1791f
    antiviral drugs for, 515t
    cidofovir for, 525
    fomivirsen for, 527
    foscarnet for, 528
    in HIV infection, 1684t-1686t, 1696-1697
    treatment of, 527-528, 1792-1793
  from herpes simplex virus, 1769
  from *Toxocara,* 3295
  from *Toxoplasma,* 1560
  from varicella-zoster virus, 1560
  in cat-scratch disease, 1417, 1417f
  in HIV infection, 1559-1560
Retinol, 141
Retinopathy, in HIV infection, 1559
Retroperitoneal space, 928
Retropharyngeal space, 790, 790f
  infections of, 793, 797, 797t. *See also*
    Odontogenic infections.
Retrotransposons, 2120-2121, 2120f
Retroviral syndrome
  acute, 1552-1553, 1552t, 1553f
  HIV testing in, 1520
Retroviridae, 2098
Retroviruses. *See also* Human immunodeficiency
    virus (HIV); Human T-cell lymphotropic
    virus (HTLV).
  animal, 2119-2120
  as agents of zoonoses, 2119
  classification of, 2119-2120
  cross-species transmission of, 1521
  discovery of, 2119
  genome of, 2120-2121, 2120f
  lenti, 2119-2120
  long terminal repeats in, 2127-2128, 2128f
  mobile DNA elements in, 2120-2121, 2120f
  oncogenic, 2119
  origin of, 2119
  replication of, 1734, 2103, 2119
  structure of, 2120, 2120f
  zoonotic, 1521
Reverse transcriptase, in HIV, 2119, 2123t, 2125,
    2130f
Reverse transcriptase inhibitors, prophylactic,
    after occupational exposure to HIV, 3402,
    3402t
Reverse transcriptase–polymerase chain reaction
    (RT-PCR) assay
  for hepatitis E virus, 2211
  for human metapneumovirus, 2030
  for rabies, 2052
  for respiratory syncytial virus, 2019

Reye's syndrome, 1144, 1783
  enteroviruses and, 2149
  in influenza, 2071
Rh immune globulin, 3574
Rhabdomyolysis, 1202
Rhabdoviruses, 2047-2054. *See also* Rabies.
  characteristics of, 2047-2048, 2047t, 2048f,
    2048t
  classification of, 2047, 2047t
Rhamnolipid, of *Pseudomonas aeruginosa,* 2596
Rheumatic fever, 737-738, 756, 757, 2380-2386
  clinical manifestations of, 2382-2384, 2383f
  diagnosis of, 2384-2385, 2384t
  epidemiology of, 2381-2382
  etiology of, 2380-2381, 2380t
  history of, 2380
  pathogenesis of, 2380-2381
  pathology of, 2381
  prevention of, 2385-2386, 2386t
    erythromycin in, 401t
    streptococcal pharyngitis treatment in, 2368
    sulfonamides in, 443
    vs. endocarditis prevention, 1049
  rash in, 733
  skin lesions in, 737
  treatment of, 2385, 2385t
Rheumatoid arthritis. *See also* Arthritis.
  juvenile, fever in, 727
  parvovirus B19 and, 1894
  pleural effusion and, 847, 849
Rheumatoid factor, 65
  in endocarditis, 980
Rheumatologic disease, complement in, 78, 87
Rhinitis
  from adenoviruses, 1838
  from microsporidia, 3244
  from respiratory syncytial virus, 2015t
Rhinocerebral mucormycosis, 2975-2977, 2976f,
    2977f
  orbital cellulitis in, 1423, 2975-2977, 2976f,
    2977f
Rhinocladiella aquaspersa, chromoblastomycosis
    from, 2988-2991
Rhinorrhea, from human metapneumovirus, 2028-
    2029, 2028t, 2029f
Rhinoscleroma, from *Klebsiella pneumoniae*
    subsp. *rhinoscleromatis,* 2578-2579
Rhinosporidium seeberi, 3075-3077, 3076f, 3076t
  laboratory studies of, 229
Rhinoviruses, 2185-2192
  adhesin-based therapies for, 20t, 21
  asthma from, 2190
  biology of, 2187
  bronchiolitis from, 813, 813t
  characteristics of, 2185-2187, 2186f
  classification of, 2185
  clinical manifestations of, 749, 2189-2190,
    2190f
  colds from, 747-750, 747t. *See also* Common
    cold.
  collection of, 233t
  course of, 2189, 2190f
  croup from, 761
  culture of, 2191
  diagnosis of, 749, 2191
  enteroviruses and, 2185
  epidemiology of, 2187
  genome of, 2187
  historical perspective on, 2185
  immune response to, 2189
  immunotypes of, 2187
  infections/illness rates for, 2187
  inflammatory pathways for, 2188t, 2189
  laryngitis from, 758, 759t
  lower respiratory infections from, 2189

Rhinoviruses (*Continued*)
  otitis media from, 2189-2190
  pathogenesis of, 2188-2189, 2188t
  prevention of, 2192
  receptor-binding group of, 21
  receptor for, 1732t
  replication of, 2187
  seasonal occurrence of, 747-748, 2187
  serotypes of, 2185
  sinusitis from, 776, 776t, 2189
  structure of, 2185-2186, 2186f
  transmission of, 2187-2188
  treatment of, 2192
  vaccines for, 2192
Rhipicephalus sanguineus, 2288
  as boutonneuse fever vector, 2292
  as canine ehrlichiosis vector, 2310
Rhizobium [spp.], 2751t, 2760-2761
Rhizobium radiobacter, 2760-2761
Rhizomucor spp., 229
  appearance of in tissue, 2936f, 2938t
  mucormycosis from, 2974, 2974f, 2977f
Rhizopus spp., 2974, 2974t
  characteristics of, 2974-2975, 2974f
  mucormycosis from, 2974-2980
  sclerosing mediastinitis from, 1075
Rhodnius prolixus, Chagas' disease from, 3157-
    3158, 3158f, 3159
Rhodococcus [spp.], 228-229, 2472, 2473
Rhodococcus equi, 2472-2473
  identification of, 229
  laboratory identification of, 219, 219t
  pneumonia from
    chest film in, 865f
    in HIV infection, 1570, 1570f
  splenic abscess from, 967, 967t
  treatment of
    with linezolid, 437, 437t
    with rifamycin, 382
    with vancomycin, 418
Rhodococcus erythropolis, 2473
Rhodococcus fasciens, 2473
Rhodococcus rhodochrous, 2473
Rhodotorula spp., 3074
*Rho*GDI, in oxidative burst, 101
Ribavirin, 515t, 536-538
  dosage of, 682t-683t
  drug interactions with, 696t
  for arenavirus infections, 2096
  for bronchiolitis, 817
  for Crimean-Congo hemorrhagic fever, 2089
  for hantavirus pulmonary syndrome, 2089
  for hemorrhagic fever with renal syndrome,
    2089
  for Hendra virus, 2041
  for hepatitis C, 538
    in acute infections, 1969
    in chronic infections, 1453-1455, 1454t,
      1967, 1967f
    in HIV infection, 1691t
    with HIV coinfection, 1971, 1971f
  for human metapneumovirus, 2030
  for Lassa fever, 2096
  for measles, 2036
  for Nipah virus, 2042
  for poxvirus infections, 1749
  for respiratory syncytial virus, 538, 2020
    in immunocompromised host, 2018, 3435
  for respiratory viruses, 538
  for Rift Valley fever, 2089
  for SARS, 1996
  for South American hemorrhagic fevers, 2096
  formulations of, 649t
  structure of, 536, 537f
  toxicity of, 1968

Ribosomal protection proteins, in tetracycline resistance, 358-359
Ribosomes, in *Staphylococcus aureus* resistance, 2335
Ricin toxin, isolation precautions for, 3330t
Rickettsia [spp.]
  bacteriology of, 2284
  classification of, 2284, 2284f
  clinical manifestations of, 2286, 2287t
  cytoplasmic replication of, 123
  diagnosis of, 2286
  encephalitis from, 1145, 1146, 2290
  epidemiology of, 2286
  genome of, 2286
  historical perspective on, 2284-2286, 2285t
  in myocarditis, 1055
  in travelers, 3647t, 3648t, 3649
  meningitis from, 1084t, 2290
  nonpathogenic, 2286
  of unknown pathogenicity, 2288
  pathophysiology of, 2286
  rash from, 730, 731t, 734, 738, 2290, 2290f, 2291f
  rash in, 730, 731t, 734, 738, 2290, 2290f, 2291f
  spotted fever group, 2287-2293
  target cells of, 2287t
  vectors of, 2285t
  vs. enteric fever, 1275t, 1278
Rickettsia aeschlimanii, 2287t
Rickettsia africae, 2285t, 2287t, 2292-2293
Rickettsia akari, 2284, 2295-2296
Rickettsia australis, 2285t, 2287t, 2292-2293
Rickettsia conorii, 2292-2293
Rickettsia felis, 2284, 2285t, 2287t, 2293, 2306
Rickettsia heilongjiang, 2287t
Rickettsia helvetica, 2285t, 2287t, 2293
Rickettsia honei, 2285t, 2287t, 2292-2293
Rickettsia japonica, 2285t, 2287t, 2292-2293
Rickettsia mongolotimonae, 2287t
Rickettsia prowazekii, 2285t, 2287t, 2303-2305
  isolation precautions for, 3330t
Rickettsia rickettsii, 2287-2292. *See also* Rocky Mountain spotted fever.
  as bioterrorism agent, 2288
  host cell defenses and, 10
Rickettsia sibirica, 2285t, 2287t, 2292
Rickettsia slovaca, 2285t, 2287t, 2292-2293
Rickettsia typhi, 2284
Rickettsiaceae, classification and taxonomy of, 2284, 2284f
Rickettsialpox, 2287t, 2295-2296, 2295f, 2295t
Rifabutin. *See also* Rifamycin.
  chloramphenicol interactions with, 369t
  dosage of, 676t-677t
  for *Mycobacterium avium* complex, 2903-2906, 2904t
    for prophylaxis, 2906
    in HIV infection, 1682t, 1683t, 1687t, 1700
  for nontuberculous mycobacterial infections, 496, 2910, 2911, 2913t
  for tuberculosis, 493-494
    in HIV infection, 1700, 2870-2871, 2871t
  formulations of, 649t
  structure of, 375f
Rifalazil, 383
Rifampin
  dosage of, 676t-677t
  drug interactions with, 491-492, 491t
  for brain abscess, 1159t
  for *Brucella*, 2672
  for chlamydial endocarditis, 1001
  for epiglottitis, 786
  for experimental endocarditis, 1048
  for *Haemophilus influenzae*, 2665

Rifampin *(Continued)*
  for leprosy, 498, 2893, 2894
  for meningitis, 1106t, 1107t, 1113, 1114, 1115, 1117
    for prevention, 1117, 1118
  for *Mycobacterium avium* complex, 2903-2906
  for *Neisseria meningitidis*, 2507, 2507t, 2509
  for nontuberculous mycobacterial infections, 496, 2910, 2911, 2913t
  for osteomyelitis, 1324t
  for prosthetic joint infections, 1335
  for Q fever endocarditis, 1001
  for Q fever pneumonia, 2299
  for scrub typhus, 2310
  for staphylococcal endocarditis, 999, 2344t
    prosthetic valve, 1026t, 1027
  for *Staphylococcus aureus* nasal carriage, 1176
  for *Streptococcus agalactiae* (group B), 2429
  for streptococcus group C, 2445
  for *Streptococcus pneumoniae* meningitis, 2405
  for tuberculosis, 491-492, 491t, 2867
    in children, 2872
    in HIV infection, 1681t, 1687t, 1699, 1700, 2870, 2871t, 2872
    latent, 2873
    regimens for, 2868, 2868t, 2869
  formulations of, 649t
  hepatic function and, 245
  in metabolic disorders, 244
  metronidazole interactions with, 393t
  resistance to, by *Staphylococcus aureus*, 2334t
Rifampin-ciprofloxacin, for *Staphylococcus aureus* osteomyelitis, 2346-2347
Rifamycin, 374-383
  adverse reactions to, 376-378
  antibacterial activity of, 374, 374t
  drug interactions with, 376, 376t, 696t
  for *Brucella*, 382
  for *Burkholderia cepacia*, 382
  for *Chlamydia*, 382
  for *Chlamydophila*, 382
  for *Clostridium difficile*, 382-383
  for *Cryptosporidium parvum*, 383
  for ehrlichiosis, 382
  for *Enterococcus*, 381
  for fungal infections, 383
  for *Helicobacter pylori*, 382
  for *Legionella*, 382
  for Mediterranean spotted fever, 382
  for nontuberculous mycobacterial infections, 379
  for orthopedic implant infections, 380-381
  for pruritus, 383
  for *Pseudomonas aeruginosa*, 382
  for Q fever, 382
  for *Rhodococcus equi*, 382
  for staphylococcal endocarditis, 379-380
  for staphylococcal osteomyelitis, 380-381
  for *Staphylococcus aureus*, 381
  for *Streptococcus*, 381
  for tuberculosis, 378
  in foreign body infection prevention, 381
  in meningitis chemoprophylaxis, 381-382
  mechanism of action of, 374
  pharmacology of, 374-376
  resistance to, 374
  structure of, 375f
Rifapentine. *See also* Rifamycin.
  for tuberculosis, 494
  formulations of, 649t
  structure of, 375f
Rifaximin, 383
  for cryptosporidiosis, 3222
  for *Shigella*, 2659t

Rift Valley fever, 2086-2089, 2086t
  as biological weapon, 3627-3629, 3627t
  clinical features of, 3629t
Rimantadine, 515t
  activity spectrum of, 521
  dosage of, 682t-683t
  drug interactions with, 522-523
  for hepatitis C, 523
  for influenza, 523, 805, 2072-2073, 2072t
    for prophylaxis, 2078
    in HIV infection, 1682t
  formulations of, 649t
  mechanism of action of, 522
  pharmacokinetics of, 522
  resistance to, 522, 2073
  side effects of, 2072t, 2073
  structure of, 521f
  toxicity of, 523
Ringworm. *See* Tinea.
Rio Bravo virus, 1945t
Risk
  assessment of, 169-170
  attributable, 162-163, 162f
  relative, 162-163, 162f
Risus sardonicus, from tetanus, 2818, 2818f
Ritonavir, 1664-1666, 1665t
  dosage of, 684t-685t
  drug interactions with, 696t-697t
  for perinatal HIV transmission prevention, 1625t, 1626
  for tuberculosis, in HIV infection, 2870
  formulations of, 649t
  pediatric, 1646t
  structure of, 1663f
Ritter's disease. *See* Staphylococcal scalded skin syndrome.
Rituximab, for HIV-related non-Hodgkin's lymphoma, 1607
River blindness, 1405, 3273-3274
RNA glycosidase toxins, 25t
RNA reverse-transcribing viruses, 2098. *See also* Human T-cell lymphotropic virus (HTLV).
RNAIII-activating protein, 2325
Rochalimaea (Bartonella) quintana, 2733
Rochalimaea (Bartonella) vinsonii, 2733
Rocio encephalitis, 1945
Rocky Mountain spotted fever, 2288-2292, 2290t, 3312, 3313t, 3314, 22827t
  prevention of, 3315
  rash in, 730, 731t, 732-733, 734, 738, 2290, 2290f, 2291f
  vs. ehrlichiosis, 2314, 2314t
  vs. enteric fever, 1275t, 1278
  vs. murine typhus, 2308
Rocky Mountain wood tick, 3312-3314, 3313f, 3313t
Rodent-borne infections
  arenavirus, 2090-2096, 2091t
  hantavirus, 2086-2089, 2086t
Romaña's sign, 3159, 3160f
Rosacea, topical antibacterial therapy for, 482-483
Rosai-Dorfman disease, 1210
Rose spots, 730, 733
  in typhoid fever, 1186
Roseola infantum, 1822, 1822f
Roseomonas [spp.], 2751t, 2761
Roseomonas gilardii, 2761
Ross River virus, 238, 1913-1919, 1914t. *See also* Alphaviruses.
Rotaviruses, 1902-1910
  classification of, 1905-1906
  clinical manifestations of, 1904
  collection of, 233t
  diagnosis of, 1908

Rotaviruses *(Continued)*
 diarrhea from, 178
  noninflammatory, 1239
 disinfection/sterilization and, 3341
 epidemiology of, 1906-1907, 1906f, 1907f
 gastrointestinal infections from, 235
 historical perspective on, 1902
 immune response to, 1907-1908
 pathogenesis of, 1904-1905
 prevention of, 1909-1910
 receptor for, 1732t
 replication of, 1903-1904
 serology of, 1905-1906
 structure of, 1902-1903, 1902f, 1903f
 transmission of, 1907
 treatment of, 1909
 vaccine for, 1226, 1238, 1909
 weanling diarrhea from, 1237, 1238
Roth spots, 736
 in endocarditis, 982, 983f, 984
Rothia dentocariosa, 2471
 endocarditis from, 992
Rothia mucilaginosa, 217t, 218
 endocarditis from, 992
Roundworms. *See* Nematodes.
Rous sarcoma virus, 2119
Roxithromycin, 408
 dosage of, 664t-665t
 drug interactions with, 697t
 for chlamydial pneumonia, atherosclerosis
   after, 2265
 for cryptosporidiosis, 3222
 for *Isospora belli,* in HIV infection, 1689t
 for *Toxoplasma gondii* encephalitis
   prophylaxis, 3190
 formulations of, 648t
Rubella, 1921-1924
 clinical features of, 1922-1923, 1923t
 complications of, 1922
 congenital, 1921, 1922-1923, 1923t
  diagnosis of, 1923-1924
  prevention of, 1924
 conjunctivitis in, 1390
 diagnosis of, 1923-1924
 epidemiology of, 1921
 from reinfections, 1921-1922
 immunity to, 1921-1922, 1924
 pathogenesis of, 1922
 prevention of, 1924
 transmission of, 1921
 treatment of, 1924
 vaccine for, 1921-1924, 3571. *See also*
   Measles, mumps, rubella (MMR) vaccine.
  complications of, 1924
  efficacy of, 1921-1923, 1924
  in pregnancy, 1924
Rubella virus
 collection of, 233t
 pancreatic infections from, 959t, 960
Rubeola. *See* Measles virus.
Rubulavirus, 1998
Russian spring-summer encephalitis, 1928, 1929.
   See also Tick-borne encephalitis.
Rusty sputum, 824, 824f

S

S protein, 70t, 74t
S6-14-03 virus, 1900
Sabethes spp., yellow fever from, 1929
Sabia virus, 2090-2096, 2092t
 as biological weapon, 3627-3629, 3627t
 Brazilian hemorrhagic fever from, 2090-2096,
   2091t. *See also* South American
   hemorrhagic fevers.

Sabin-Feldman dye test, for toxoplasmosis, 3182
Saccharomyces cerevisiae, 3074
 vulvovaginitis from, 1362
Sacral radiculopathy, from herpes simplex virus,
   1766-1767, 1767f, 1773t
Sacroiliac joint, osteomyelitis of, 1329
Sacroiliitis, in Reiter's syndrome, 1354-1355
Sae, 2325
Sagittal sinus thrombophlebitis, 1168-1170, 1169f
St. John's wort, 610
 for depression, 609
St. Louis encephalitis, 235t, 1146
 clinical features of, 1940-1944
 diagnosis of, 1942
 epidemiology of, 1932t, 1933, 1935f
 historical perspective on, 1928
 meningitis and, 1085
 pathogenesis of, 1937-1938
 prevention of, 1944
 treatment of, 1944
Saksenaea [spp.], mucormycosis from, 2974, 2978
Salicylates
 for fever, 713
 for Kawasaki disease, 3318
 for rheumatic fever, 2385, 2385t
Salicylazosulfapyridine, 441
Salicylic acid, for cutaneous warts, 1848
Saliva
 HIV transmission in, 1489, 1492
 in HIV testing, 1512
Salivaria [spp.], 3157
Salivary gland infections, 797t, 799
Salmeterol, for chronic obstructive pulmonary
   disease, 810t
Salmon River virus, 1899
Salmonella [spp.], 2636-2650
 antisera identification of, 221
 appendicitis from, 969
 bacteremia from, 2646
  in HIV infection, 2649-2650
  treatment of, 2649
 classification of, 2637, 2637t
 clinical manifestations of, 2644-2646
 clonal analysis of, 5
 culture of, 1224
 diarrhea from, 178
 DT104, 1295-1296
 endocytosis by, 2642, 2642f
 enteric fever from, 1273, 1274t, 2644-2646
 enteric fever–like syndrome from, 1276-1277
 enteritis from, 1266-1267
  quinolones for, 461
 epidemiology of, 2638-2641
 extraintestinal complications of, 2646, 2647t
 foodborne disease from, 1288, 1291-1292,
   2639-2640, 2639f, 2650
 gastric acid and, 1217
 genome of, 2637
 history of, 2636
 host cell invasion by, 9
 host response to, 2644
 in HIV infection, 2646, 2649-2650
  treatment of, 1683t, 1689t, 1701
 innate immunity in, 2644
 intestinal epithelium and, 2642-2643, 2642f
 invasiveness of, 1222
 macrophage response to, 2643-2644
 meningitis from, 1087, 1114
 microbiology of, 2637-2638
 mycotic aneurysm from, 1008
 Newport, 1296
 nitric oxide resistance of, 2643-2644
 nontyphoidal
  chronic carriage of, 2650
  DT104, 2640

Salmonella [spp.] *(Continued)*
 epidemiology of, 2638-2641, 2639f, 2641f
 gastroenteritis from, 2644
  in HIV infection, 1241
 multidrug-resistant, 2640, 2641f
 nosocomial, 2640-2641
 treatment of, 2649
 pathogenesis of, 2641-2644
 pathogenicity islands of, 2642-2644
 postsplenectomy sepsis from, 3528
 prevention of, 2650
 rash in, 730, 730t, 733
 resistance to
  by antimicrobials, 185-186
  cytokines in, 157f
 secretory system of, 2642
 serotypes of, 2637, 2637t
 splenic abscess from, 967, 967t
 subtyping of, 2638
 susceptibility to, 47, 123
 T3SS, 2644
 taxonomy of, 2637, 2637t
 transmission of, 177
 treatment of
  with aminoglycosides, 334t-335t
  with cephalosporins, 298t
  with chloramphenicol, 366, 370
  with penicillins, 284t, 288t
  with quinolones, 455t
  with sulfonamides, 441t
  with trimethoprim, 444t
  with trimethoprim-sulfamethoxazole, 446
 vascular infections from, 2646
 with schistosomiasis, 3279-3280
Salmonella choleraesuis, mycotic aneurysm from, 1008
Salmonella enterica
 enteric fever from, 1273
 quinolones for, 461
Salmonella enteritidis
 mycotic aneurysm from, 1008
 risk for, 163
Salmonella newport, 186
Salmonella paratyphi, 2645
 chloramphenicol for, 367t
 epidemiology of, 2638
Salmonella typhi
 antibiotic-resistant, 2638, 2638t
 enteric fever from, 2645
 epidemiology of, 2638
 gastrointestinal infections from, 1216
 multidrug resistance of, 366
 mycotic aneurysm from, 1008
 pancreatitis from, 959, 959t
 penicillins for, 288t
 skin lesions from, 1186
 treatment of, 2648-2649, 2649t
  with chloramphenicol, 367t
  with macrolides, 401t
  with mefloquine, 586
 vaccine for, 2646-2647
 Widal test for, 1275
Salmonella typhimurium
 cephalosporin resistance of, 262
 DT104, antimicrobial resistance of, 186
 evolution of, 6
 regulation of, 7t
 resistance of, 366
 survival by, 9
Salpingitis
 from *Chlamydia trachomatis,* 2247t, 2248-
   2249
 from herpes simplex virus, 1766. *See also*
   Herpes simplex virus, genital.
 from *Mycoplasma genitalium,* 2281, 2281t
 from *Neisseria gonorrhoeae,* 2514, 2515f

Salpingitis (Continued)
  in pelvic inflammatory disease, 1378-1380, 1378f, 1379t
San Joaquin Valley fever, 3040. See also Coccidioides immitis.
Sand fleas, 3310
Sand flies
  control measures for, 3154
  leishmaniasis from, 3146
SAP, 153
Saphenous venectomy, cellulitis after, 1178, 1180
SAPHO syndrome, 1328
Sapoviruses, 2196. See also Caliciviruses.
  gastrointestinal infections with, 235
Sappinia diploidea, 577t
  characteristics of, 3112, 3113f
  meningitis from, 3112, 3113f, 3114, 3117, 3118, 3119
Sapporo virus, 2196. See also Caliciviruses.
Saquinavir, 1663-1664, 1665t
  dosage of, 684t-685t
  for perinatal HIV transmission prevention, 1625t, 1626
  formulations of, 649t
  pediatric, 1646t
  resistance to, 1668
  structure of, 1663f
Sarcocystis spp., 3232
Sarcoidosis
  fever in, 726
  meningitis in, 1138-1139
  pulmonary, chest film in, 862f
Sarcophagidae, myiasis from, 3307-3310, 3308t
Sarcoptes scabiei, 575t, 1341, 1341f, 1343, 3304, 3304f. See also Scabies.
  in HIV infection, 1558, 1559f
Sarin nerve gas attack, 3591, 3624
SARS. See Severe acute respiratory syndrome (SARS).
Saturated solution of potassium iodide, for sporotrichosis, 2987
Saxitoxins, 3255
Scabies, 1341, 1341f, 3304f-3306f, 3304-3307
  clinical features of, 1338-1339, 1341, 1341f, 3304-3306, 3305f, 3306f
  diagnosis of, 1343
  epidemiology of, 3304
  in HIV infection, 1558, 1559f
  institutional outbreaks of, 3307
  ivermectin for, 595
  nodular, 3305, 3305f, 3306f
  Norwegian (crusted), 3305, 3306, 3306f, 3307
  in HIV infection, 1558, 1559f
  staphylococcal coinfection in, 3305
Scabies incognito, 3305
Scalp. See also Hair.
  candidiasis of, alopecia and, 2944. See also Alopecia.
  dermatophytosis of, 3051, 3053, 3056, 3057f. See also Tinea capitis.
  dissecting cellulitis of, 1179
  pediculosis of, 3302-3304, 3302f, 3303f
Scarlet fever, 737-738
  rash in, 737-738
  staphylococcal, 737, 1175
  streptococcal, 2365
Scavenger receptor, 124
  in phagocytosis, 37
Scedosporium spp., 229
Scedosporium apiospermum, 3068-3069, 3068f, 3076t
  brain abscess from, 1152, 1155, 1158t, 1160-1161, 3068-3069
  endocarditis from, 993

Scedosporium apiospermum (Continued)
  mycetoma from, 299t, 2991-2995, 2992t, 2994f, 3068
  pulmonary infections from
    in cystic fibrosis, 872
    in immunocompromised host, 3436
  skin lesions from, in immunocompromised host, 3439
Scedosporium prolificans, 3069, 3069f, 3070, 3076t
SCH-C, 20, 20t
Schistosoma [spp.]. See also Schistosomiasis.
  praziquantel for, 595
  susceptibility to, 47
Schistosoma haematobium
  collection and transport of, 207t
  pancreatic infections from, 959t, 960
  praziquantel for, 575t
Schistosoma japonicum, praziquantel for, 575t
Schistosoma mansoni
  oxamniquine for, 596
  treatment of, 575t
  vs. enteric fever, 1278
Schistosoma mekongi, praziquantel for, 575t
Schistosomiasis
  acute, 3278
    vs. malaria, 3133
  chronic, 3278-3280
  clinical syndromes of, 3278-3280
  coinfection in
    with hepatitis, 3280
    with salmonellosis, 3279-3280
  dermatitis in, 3278, 3294t, 3298
  diagnosis of, 3280
  egg types in, 3279f, 3281f
  epidemiology of, 3276-3277, 3277t
  etiology of, 3276, 3277t
  pathogenesis of, 3277-3278, 3277t
  prevention and control of, 3281
  syndrome of abdominal pain, diarrhea, and eosinophilia from, 1281t, 1282
  treatment of, 3277t, 3280
    with praziquantel, 595
  vs. malaria, 3133
  worm life cycle in, 3276, 3278f
Schlichter test, 223
Schools
  hepatitis A outbreaks in, 2171, 2171f, 2178
  rhinovirus outbreaks in, 2188
Schwann cells, Mycobacterium leprae in, 2889
Sclerosing cholangitis
  HIV-related, 956-957
  in cryptosporidiosis, 3220, 3221
Sclerotic bodies, in chromoblastomycosis, 2989, 2990f
Scopulariopsis spp., 3073
Scrapie, 2219, 2219t
Screening
  for cervical cancer, 1850-1851, 1851t
    in HIV infection, 1610, 1611t
  for Chlamydia trachomatis, 2251
Screwworms, myiasis from, 3308-3310, 3308t
Scrofula, 1206-1207
Scrotum
  elephantiasis of, 3271, 3271f
  Fournier's gangrene of, 1190, 1191
Scrub typhus, 2287t, 2309-2310, 2309f, 2310t, 3311
Scurvy, 141
Scytalidium infections, 3054, 3058, 3059
Seadornaviruses, 1900-1901
Seafood. See Fish; Shellfish.
Sealpox, 1753
Seborrheic blepharitis, 1420

Seborrheic dermatitis, from Malassezia, 3061
Secondary attack rate, 167
Secretion factors, of Pseudomonas aeruginosa, 2596
Secretions
  in host defense, 35-36
  of Enterobacteriaceae, 2571-2572
Secretory piece and protein, 35
Secretory vesicles, 94, 94t
Seizures
  febrile, 712-713
    prevention of, 714
  in central nervous system infections, 1083
  in HIV infection, 1596-1597, 1597f
Selectins, 132
  in neutrophil adhesion, 96
Selective gut decontamination, in pancreatic infections prevention, 962
Selenium, 142, 143f
Semen, as HIV vector, 1385-1386
Semilunar valves, in endocarditis, 981
Semliki Forest virus, 1913-1919, 1914t. See also Alphaviruses.
SEN virus, 1427
Sendai virus, 1998, 2001
Sennetsu neorickettsiosis, 2311, 2311t, 2312, 2315-2316
Sensitivity, in epidemiologic studies, 161
Seoul virus, 2086-2089, 2086t
  as biological weapon, 3627-3629, 3628t
Sepik virus, 1945t
Sepsis, 906-922. See also Septicemia.
  acute lung injury in, 917
  adrenal insufficiency in, 915-916
  catheter-related, without suppurative thrombophlebitis, 1002-1003
  cerebral function in, 915
  circulation in, 916-917
  clinical manifestations of, 915-918
  continuum of, 916
  corticosteroids for, 559
  cultures in, 918
  cutaneous manifestations of, 917-918
  cytokine levels in, 918
  definitions of, 906, 906t
  diagnosis of, 918
  differential diagnosis of, 918
  epidemiology of, 907
  etiology of, 3427-3428
  fluid management for, 919-920
  from Aeromonas, 2754
  from Capnocytophaga, 2731
  from Pseudomonas aeruginosa, 2598-2599
  gastrointestinal injury in, 917
  gram-negative, 86
  hepatic dysfunction in, 917
  host defenses in, 922
  hydrocortisone for, 920
  hyperglycemia in, prevention of, 921-922
  hypothalamic-pituitary-adrenal axis in, 915
  immune dysfunction in, 917
  in asplenia, 734
  in prosthetic valve endocarditis, 1030
  meningococcal, petechiae from, 2503, 2503f-2505f
  muscle proteolysis in, 1202
  neonatal
    from Enterococcus, 2413-2414
    from nontypeable Haemophilus influenzae, 2663
    from streptococcus group G, 2444
  nervous system in, 915-916
  neuroendocrine system in, 915-916
  nutritional support in, 921
  pathogenesis of, 907-915

Sepsis *(Continued)*
  pathology of, 910-911
  pentoxifylline for, 560
  postanginal, 754, 754f, 794, 794f
  postsplenectomy, 734, 3526-3528, 3526f-3528f, 3526t, 3530
  prognosis of, 922
  purpura fulminans in, 735
  rash in, 735
  renal dysfunction in, 917
  secondary infections in, prevention of, 921
  severe, 906, 906t
    microbial triggers for, 913-915, 913f
    pathologic responses to, 911-912
    sites of, 913, 913f, 914
  symmetric peripheral gangrene in, 735
  treatment of, 918-921, 919t
    surgical drainage in, 919
    with anti-inflammatory therapy, 559, 920-921
    with antimicrobial therapy, 918-919, 919t
    with vasopressin, 920
  vs. malaria, 3132
Sepsis syndrome
  bacterial lipopolysaccharide in, 712, 714
  etiology of, 3427-3428
  pyrogenic cytokines in, 712
Septata spp., 3237, 3238t. *See also* Microsporidia.
Septic abortion, 1375-1376, 1377t
  from *Campylobacter jejuni,* 2552
Septic arthritis. *See* Arthritis.
Septic cavernous sinus thrombosis, 794, 795f. *See also* Odontogenic infections.
Septic conditions. *See also* under Suppurative.
Septic pelvic thrombophlebitis, 1374-1375
Septic shock, 40, 906, 906t, 912-913
  adrenal insufficiency in, 918
  complement in, 86
  continuum of, 916
  from viridans streptococci, 2436-2437
Septic thrombophlebitis, 917. *See also* Thrombophlebitis, suppurative.
  from *Candida,* 2947
  in injection drug users, 3467-3468
  pelvic, 1374-1375
Septicemia. *See also* Bacteremia.
  from *Vibrio vulnificus,* 2546
  from *Yersinia enterocolitica,* 2699
  lipooligosaccharide levels in, 2504
  postanginal, 754, 754f, 756
Serine proteases, 75
Seroincidence surveys, 165
Seroprevalence survey, 165
Serratia [spp.], 2579-2580
  cardiovascular device infections from, 1023
  percutaneous intravascular device infections from, 3356
  peritonitis from, treatment of, 938, 939
  suppurative thrombophlebitis from, 1004
  treatment of
    with aminoglycosides, 334t-335t
    with cephalosporins, 298t
    with penicillins, 284t, 288t
Serratia liquefaciens, 2579
Serratia marcescens, 2579
  artificial heart infections from, 1035
  endocarditis from, 991
  in chronic granulomatous disease, 155, 156
  meningitis from, 1087
  mycotic aneurysm from, 1008
  pneumonia from, 836
  toxin secretion in, 26
  transient bacteremia from, 978

Serratia marcescens (Continued)
  treatment of
    with aminoglycoside combination therapy, 337t
    with aminoglycosides, 344t
    with carbapenems, 313t
    with chloramphenicol, 367t
    with mupirocin, 485t
    with quinolones, 455t
    with rifamycin, 374t
    with sulfonamides, 441t
    with trimethoprim, 444t
Serum amyloid A, in acute-phase response, 709
Serum antimicrobial dilution titer, 250
Serum bactericidal titer, 223, 250
  in endocarditis therapy monitoring, 995
Serum sickness, with penicillins, 286
Setaria labiatopapillosa, ocular infections from, 3273
Severe acute respiratory syndrome (SARS), 175-176, 176t, 3630
  characteristics of, 1991-1992, 1992f
  clinical features of, 176, 176t, 1995
  diagnosis of, 1995-1996
  disinfection/sterilization and, 3341
  emergence of, 1990, 1993
  emergency preparedness for, 192, 194-201
  epidemiology of, 161, 1993, 1993f
  from human metapneumovirus, 2029
  genome of, 1991-1992, 1991f
  history in, 823t
  isolation precautions for, 3330
  pathogenesis of, 1994
  prevention of, 1996, 3330, 3341
  reappearance of, 1993, 1996
  replication of, 1991-1992
  transmission of, 176, 177f, 1993
  treatment of, 1996
  virus of, 238
Severe inflammatory response syndrome, rash in, 735
Sex hormones, in female HIV infection, 1630
Sexual abuse/assault, of children, HIV infection from, 1651
Sexual behavior, in HIV infection transmission, 1470, 1488-1490
Sexually reactive arthritis, 1354-1355, 2247-2248
Sexually transmitted diseases. *See also specific diseases.*
  donovanosis in, 2749
  genital lesions in, 1338-1345, 1338-1445. *See also* Genital lesions.
  in HIV transmission, 1470, 1472, 1489, 1619
  in travelers, 3642
  inguinal lymphadenopathy in, 1207-1208, 1210
  laboratory studies for, 212-213
  public health control measures in, 2526-2527
  sex partner management in, 2526
  treatment of
    in HIV infection prevention, 1619
    with quinolones, 460
    with trimethoprim-sulfamethoxazole, 446
  urinary tract infections in, 876
Shaving, preoperative, 3540
Shell temperature, 704, 707-708. *See also* Temperature.
Shell vial spin amplification, of respiratory viruses, 234
Shellfish
  calicivirus infections from, 2197
  cognitive/memory impairment from, 3256, 3256t
  diarrhea from, 3256, 3256t
  hepatitis A from, 2166, 2171, 2171f
  hepatitis E from, 2208
  neurologic illness from, 3255-3256, 3255f, 3256t

Shellfish poisoning, 1289-1290, 1290t
  from *Vibrio parahaemolyticus,* 2545
  treatment of, 1296
Shewanella [spp.], 2751t, 2761
Shewanella algae, 2761
Shewanella putrefaciens, 2761
Shiga toxin, 29, 1220
  Escherichia coli, 2573t, 2576-2577, 2577f
    foodborne disease from, 1289
  Shigella dysenteriae, 2577
Shiga-like toxin, 29, 1220
Shigella [spp.], 178, 1264, 1265t, 2655-2660
  antisera identification of, 221
  control of, 2659-2660
  culture of, 1224
  diagnosis of, 2657-2658, 2658f
  diarrhea from, 178
  epidemiology of, 2656-2657
  foodborne disease from, 1288, 2657, 2659
  gastrointestinal infections from, 1216
  host cell invasion by, 9
  identification of, 2655
  immunity to, 2659-2660
  in HIV infection, 1689t, 1701
  invasiveness of, 1222, 2656
  isolation of, 2655
  microbiology of, 2655, 2655f
  organism numbers in, 1216
  pathogenesis of, 2656, 2656t
  plasmid-encoded, 6t
  regulation of, 7t
  reservoirs for, 2657
  sigmoidoscopy in, 1264
  spread of, 2657
  survival by, 9
  toxigenicity of, 2656
  transmission of, 177
  treatment of, 2658-2659, 2659t
    with antimicrobials, 1226
    with azithromycin, 401t
    with cephalosporins, 298t
    with chloramphenicol, 367t
    with erythromycin, 401t
    with penicillins, 284t
    with quinolones, 455t, 461
    with sulfonamides, 441t
    with tetracyclines, 359t
    with trimethoprim, 444t
    with vancomycin, 359t
  vaccines for, 2659-2660
  virulence of, 2656, 2656t
  weanling diarrhea from, 1237
  worldwide incidence of, 2657
Shigella dysenteriae, 1264, 1265f
  antimicrobial-resistant, 185
  diarrhea from, 178
  neuroenterotoxin of, 1220
  toxins of, 29, 2577. *See also* Shiga toxin.
Shigella flexneri, 1264
  cytoplasmic replication of, 123
  gastric acid and, 1217
Shigella sonnei, clones of, 5
Shingles. *See* Herpes zoster.
Shock
  endotoxic, complement in, 86
  in meningococcal disease, 2504
  septic, 906, 906t, 912-913
    adrenal insufficiency in, 918
    complement in, 86
    continuum of, 916
    from viridans streptococci, 2436-2437
  vasoconstrictive, 912-913
Shock liver, 1436
Short consensus repeats, 75

Shunt infections. *See* Cerebrospinal fluid shunt infections.
Sialadenitis, 797t, 799
  from mumps virus, 2004
Sialic acid, in complement activation, 74
Siberian tick typhus, 2285t, 2287t, 2292
Siberian tick-borne encephalitis virus, 1934
Sickle cell disease/trait
  bacteriuria and, 883
  malaria and, 35, 43, 44, 46, 3126
  Mycoplasma pneumoniae in, 2274f, 2275
  osteomyelitis in, 1329
Siderophores, 2572
  in *Burkholderia cepacia,* 2617
  in *Pseudomonas aeruginosa,* 2595
Sigmoidoscopy, in pseudomembranous enterocolitis, 1264
Signal transducer and activator of transcription 1, 151t, 157
Signaling lymphocyte-activation molecule–associated protein, 153
Silver nitrate
  conjunctivitis from, 1392
  for burns, 3548
Silver sulfadiazine, 441, 484t
  for burns, 3549
Simian herpes B virus. *See* Herpes B virus.
Simian immunodeficiency virus, 181-182, 1521, 1528, 2119
  in HIV vaccine testing, 1708, 1712
Sin Nombre virus, 739, 2086-2089, 2086t
  as biological weapon, 3627-3629, 3628t
Sindbis virus, 1913-1919, 1914t. *See also* Alphaviruses.
  ribavirin-resistant, 537
Single-photon emission computed tomography (SPECT)
  for brain abscess, 1158-1159
  for primary central nervous system lymphoma, 1608
Singlet oxygen, in neutrophil bactericidal activity, 102
Sinography, for prosthetic vascular graft infections, 1037-1038
Sinus histiocytosis, with lymphadenopathy, 1210
Sinus puncture and aspiration
  in acute sinusitis, 776, 776t
  in chronic sinusitis, 781, 782t
  specimen collection and transport for, 206t
Sinus puncture and lavage, 780, 781
Sinuses, anatomy and physiology of, 773, 773t
Sinusitis, 772-782
  acute, 772-780
  bacterial, 775-776, 776t
  brain abscess from, 1151t, 1152
  chronic, 780-782
    fungal, 778, 2962
    postsurgical, 782, 782t
    presurgical, 780-781, 781f
  classification of, 773t, 777-778, 778t
  clinical features of, 777
  complications of, 778-779
  diagnosis of, 777-778, 778t
  epidemiology of, 773-774
  etiology of, 776-777, 776t, 777t
  from *Actinomyces,* 2926
  from anaerobic gram-negative bacilli, 2841
  from *Aspergillus,* 2962, 2964-2965
  from *Chlamydia (Chlamydophila) pneumoniae,* 2262
  from *Haemophilus influenzae,* 775, 776, 776t, 2663
  from measles virus, 2035
  from microsporidia, 3238t, 3244, 3247-3249, 3248t

Sinusitis *(Continued)*
  from *Moraxella (Branhamella) catarrhalis,* 2531
  from *Pseudallescheria boydii,* 3068-3069
  from rhinoviruses, 2189
  from *Streptococcus pneumoniae,* 2399, 2404
  fungal, 777, 777t, 781, 2962
    allergic, 2962, 3070-3071, 3071f
      from *Aspergillus,* 2962
  in common cold, 772, 773-774, 774, 774f, 775f, 2189
  in immunocompromised host, 3437
  in rhinocerebral mucormycosis of, 2975-2977, 2977f
  maxillary, 794. *See also* Odontogenic infections.
  nosocomial, 776-777
  orbital/preseptal cellulitis in, 1421-1424, 2975-2977, 2976f, 2977f
  pathogenesis of, 774-775
  severity of, 777, 778t
  specimen collection in, 776, 776t
  subdural empyema from, 1164-1165
  suppurative intracranial thrombophlebitis from, 794, 795f, 797t, 799-800, 1168-1170, 1169f
  treatment of, 779-780
    with quinolones, 463
    with telithromycin, 407
  viral, 774-775, 776, 776t
  vs. common cold, 755
SipA, 2642
SipC, 2642
Sirolimus, for transplant immunosuppression, infections and, 3478
Sisomicin
  names and sources of, 329t
  structure of, 329f, 330
Sitafloxacin, for psittacosis, 2257
Six Gun City virus, 1899
Sixth disease, 1822, 1822f
Sjögren's syndrome
  meningitis in, 1139
  vs. chronic bacterial parotitis, 799
Skin
  acidity of, 35
  barrier functions of, 3423
  disinfection of, 479
  embolic lesions of, in *Staphylococcus aureus* endocarditis, 2342, 2342f
  in host defense, 35
  in sepsis, 917
  nitrofurantoin effects on, 475
  portals of entry in, 3423-3424
  preoperative preparation of, 3540
  rifamycin effects on, 377-378
  ulcers of. *See* Ulcer(s), cutaneous.
Skin flora, 3423-3424, 3423f
  postoperative infections and, 3535, 3544, 3544t
Skin infections
  anaerobic, 2813
  chronic, 1184
  classification of, 1173t
  clinical features of. *See* Skin lesions.
  etiology of, 1173t
  from anaerobic gram-negative bacilli, 2843
  from *Aspergillus,* 2966, 2966f
  from *Bacillus anthracis,* 2486, 2487f
  from *Blastomyces dermatitidis,* 3027, 3029t, 3030t, 3031-3032, 3032f, 3033f
  from *Candida,* 2942-2944
    in disseminated disease, 739, 1187, 2943, 2943f
  from *Coccidioides immitis,* 3043, 3044, 3045f
  from *Corynebacterium diphtheriae,* 2462

Skin infections *(Continued)*
  from *Cryptococcus neoformans,* 3003t, 3004-3005, 3004f
  from dermatophytes, 3051-3059
  from *Erysipelothrix rhusiopathiae,* 2497, 2497f
  from *Francisella tularensis,* 2681
  from human herpesvirus 6, 1823
  from *Lacazia loboi,* 3075, 3075f, 3076t
  from *Legionella micdadei,* 2726
  from *Malassezia,* 3060
  from microsporidia, 3244
  from mucormycosis agents, 2978, 2980
  from *Mycobacterium leprae,* 2890-2891, 2890f-2892f
  from nontuberculous mycobacteria, 2910t, 2911-2912, 2913t
  from *Paracoccidioides brasiliensis,* 3064-3065, 3065f
  from *Pasteurella,* 2688
  from *Pseudomonas aeruginosa,* 2589-2590, 2605-2606
  from schistosomes, 3278, 3294t, 3298
  from *Scytalidium,* 3058, 3059
  from *Sporothrix schenkii,* 2984-2985, 2984f
  from *Staphylococcus aureus,* 2339-2342, 2340f
  from *Streptococcus agalactiae* (group B), 2427-2428
  from streptococcus group C, 2443
  from streptococcus group G, 2443
  from *Streptococcus pyogenes* (group A), 2370-2374
  from *Vibrio vulnificus,* 2546
  in bacteremia, 1186
  in *Bartonella* bacillary angiomatosis, 2735, 2735f
  in cancer, 3438-3439
  in elderly, 3519-3520
  in endocarditis, 982, 983f, 1044
  in HIV infection, 742
  in immunocompromised host, 1184, 3438-3439
    laboratory diagnosis of, 3428
  in injection drug users, 3463
  in melioidosis, 2625, 2626f, 2627f
  in travelers, 3652, 3653f
  intravascular device-related, prevention of, 3356
  laboratory studies for, 213
  lymphadenitis in, 1209t, 1211
  metronidazole for, 394
  papillomatous, in yaws, 2786-2787, 2786f, 2787f
  prevention of, in travelers, 3643
  prophylaxis for, topical antibacterial therapy in, 480-481
  seborrheic, in HIV infection, 1557, 1558f
  secondary, 1184-1185
  self-induced, 1185
  specimen collection and transport for, 207t
  treatment of
    outpatient parenteral therapy in, 629t, 630
    with daptomycin, 428
    with quinolones, 463-464
Skin lesions. *See also* Rash *and specific types.*
  characteristics of, 730-732, 730t
  genital, 1344-1345. *See also* Genital lesions.
Skin tests. *See also specific tests.*
  for beta-lactam antibiotic sensitivity, 322-323
  for chronic pneumonia, 863
  for coccidioidomycosis, 3047
  for tuberculosis, 2860-2861, 2861t, 2872, 2872t
Skull fractures, cerebrospinal leak in
  chemoprophylaxis for, 1103
  radiography of, 1103
  surgery for, 1117

Sleep problems, in prion diseases, 2220, 2229
Sleeping sickness. See African trypanosomiasis.
Slim disease, 1554
Small intestine, 927, 927f. See also under
    Gastrointestinal; Intestinal.
  abnormal bacterial colonization in, 1243-1244
  disorders of, in HIV infection, 1579-1580,
    1580t
  epithelium of, T cells in, 122
  flora of, in secondary peritonitis, 932
  Giardia lamblia of, 1270
  in tropical sprue, 1304
  Isopora belli of, 1270
  transplantation of, infections in, 3505. See also
    Transplantation, infections in.
  ulcers of. See Peptic ulcers.
Smallpox, 237, 740-741, 1746-1747, 1746f,
    1747f, 1747t
  as biological weapon, 3592-3593, 3612-3617
    emergency preparedness for, 3616-3617
    epidemiology of, 3613
    historical perspective on, 3594, 3612-3613
    infection control measures for, 3616
    potential impact of, 3592-3593
  clinical features of, 740, 1746-1747, 1746f,
    1747f, 3614, 3614f, 3615f
  conjunctivitis from, 1389-1390
  diagnosis of, 3615-3616
  disinfection/sterilization and, 3342
  epidemic potential of, 3592-3593
  epidemiology of, 3613
  flat, 3614
  hemorrhagic, 3614
  isolation precautions for, 3329, 3330t
  laboratory studies for, 237
  modern outbreaks of, 3592
  ordinary, 3614
  pathogenesis of, 3613-3614
  public health impact of, 3616-3617
  rash in, 740
  specimen collection in, 233t
  transmission of, 3616
  treatment of, 1749
  vaccination for, 740-741, 1744, 3571-3572
    complications of, 740-741, 1743f, 1744-
      1746. See also Vaccinia.
  vaccine for, 740-741, 1744, 3571-3572, 3592,
    3616-3617
    complications of, 740-741, 1743f, 1744-
      1746. See also Vaccinia.
    for outbreaks, 3593, 3599, 3616-3617
    monkeypox prophylaxis and, 1747, 1748
    routine use of, 3592
  vs. varicella, 740
Snakebites, 3553-3554
  antivenin for, 66
SNARE complex, clostridial neurotoxin attack of,
    28
Snow Mountain virus, 2195, 2196. See also
    Caliciviruses.
Sodium bicarbonate, tetracycline with, 364t
Sodium dodecyl sulfate–polyacrylamide gel
    electrophoresis, of Moraxella (Branhamella)
    catarrhalis, 2530
Sodium hypochlorite, disinfection with, 3334,
    3341
Sodium stibogluconate, adverse effects of, 582t
Soft tissue infections. See also Abscess; Cellulitis.
  anaerobic, 2813
  from Acinetobacter, 2634
  from Aeromonas, 2754
  from anaerobic gram-negative bacilli, 2843
  from Arcanobacterium haemolyticum, 2470
  from Bacillus, 2495
  from Clostridium, 2830-2831

Soft tissue infections (Continued)
  from nontuberculous mycobacteria, 2910t,
    2911-2912, 2913t
  from Pasteurella, 2688
  from Pseudomonas aeruginosa, 2605-2606
  from Salmonella, 2647t
  from Staphylococcus aureus, 2339-2342
  from Streptococcus agalactiae (group B),
    2427-2428
  from streptococcus group C, 2443
  from streptococcus group G, 2443
  from Streptococcus pyogenes (group A), 2370-
    2374
  from Vibrio vulnificus, 2546
  in elderly, 3519-3520
  in injection drug users, 3463-3464
  laboratory studies for, 213
  prophylaxis for, topical antibacterial therapy in,
    480-481
  treatment of
    outpatient parenteral therapy in, 629t, 630
    with daptomycin, 428
    with quinolones, 463-464
Solid-phase immunosorbent assay, 57, 58f, 59
Sordarins, 511
Sore throat. See Pharyngitis.
Sortase, in Staphylococcus aureus, 2326, 2327f
South Africa, HIV infection in, 1466, 1467f
South American hemorrhagic fevers, 2090-2096
  as biological weapon, 3627-3629, 3627t
  clinical manifestations of, 2091t, 2095, 3629t
  diagnosis of, 2095
  disinfection/sterilization and, 3342
  epidemiology/epizootology of, 2091t, 2093
  in pregnancy, 2095
  pathogenesis of, 2091t, 2094
  prevention of, 2091t, 2095
  treatment of, 2091t, 2095
  vaccines for, 2096
  virus characteristics in, 2091t, 2092
Southeast Asian ovalocytosis, malaria and, 3127
Southern flying squirrels, as typhus reservoir,
    2304, 2305
Southern hybridization, 12
Southern tick-associated rash illness, 3314
Sowda, 3273
SP-40,40, 70t
Sparfloxacin
  dosage of, 674t-675t
  for leprosy, 499
  for pneumonia, 837-839, 837t, 838t
  for psittacosis, 2257
  for urinary tract infections, 460
  formulations of, 648t
  pneumococcal resistance to, 837, 837t
Sparganosis, 3286, 3286t, 3292
Spas, legionnaires' disease prevention in, 2720
Spasmodic croup, 760. See also
    Laryngotracheobronchitis.
Specific granules, deficiency of, 108
Specificity, in epidemiologic studies, 161
Specimens
  collection and transport of, 204, 205t-207t, 208
  microscopic observation of, 214, 214t
  selection of, 204
SPECT (single-photon emission computed
    tomography)
  for brain abscess, 1158-1159
  for primary central nervous system lymphoma,
    1608
Spectinomycin
  antimicrobial activity of, 333, 334t-335t
  chemical family of, 330t
  dosage of, 660t-661t
  drug interactions with, 697t

Spectinomycin (Continued)
  for Neisseria gonorrhoeae, 350, 2524t, 2525,
    2526
  names and sources of, 329t
  structure of, 329f
Sperm, production and transport of, 1381
Spermatogenesis, famciclovir effects on, 526
Spermicides
  in HIV infection, 1494
  in Neisseria gonorrheae prophylaxis, 2527
  in urinary tract infections, 876
SPH 16111–related viruses, 1945t
Sphenoid sinus
  anatomy and physiology of, 773, 773t
  infections of. See Sinusitis.
Sphingobacterium [spp.], 2751t, 2761-2762
Sphingobacterium multivorum, 2761-2762
Sphingobacterium spiritivorum, 2761-2762
Sphingomonas [spp.], 2751t, 2762
Sphingomonas paucimobilis, 220t, 2762
Spider bites, 3653f
Spider mites, 3311
Spinal abscess, 1165-1168. See also Myelitis.
  from Coccidioides immitis, 3044, 3046f
  in injection drug users, 3471-3472
  tuberculous, 2879
Spinal cord infections. See Myelitis.
Spinal cord injury, infections in, 3512-3516
Spinal osteomyelitis, 1326-1327, 1326f
  from Aspergillus, 2966, 2966f
  from Candida, 2946, 2947, 2947f
  from Coccidioides immitis, 3044, 3045f
  from Pseudomonas aeruginosa, 2602-2603
  in injection drug users, 3465
Spinal paralytic poliomyelitis, 2142-2143. See
    also Poliomyelitis.
Spinal subdural empyema, 1164-1165
Spinal tap. See Lumbar puncture.
Spiramycin
  adverse effects of, 582t
  dosage of, 664t-665t
  for cryptosporidiosis, 3222
  for isosporiasis, in HIV infection, 1689t
  for toxoplasmosis, 576t, 589
    in congenital infections, 3191
    in pregnancy, 3188, 3190-3191
  indications for, 569t
Spirillum minus, 2810
  endocarditis from, 993
  penicillins for, 288t
  rat-bite fever from, 2708, 2709t
  treatment of, 2710
Spirochetes
  laboratory tests for, 2778, 2778f
  meningitis from, 1084t, 1088
    diagnosis of, 1085, 1103-1104
    treatment of, 1106t, 1115
Spirometra mansonoides, 3286t, 3292. See also
    Tapeworms.
Spleen
  abscess of, 967-968, 967t
    in endocarditis, 982
    in injection drug users, 3470-3471
    in melioidosis, 2627f
  absence of. See Asplenia.
  anatomy of, 120-121, 121f
  candidiasis of, 2947, 2947f, 2950
  enlarged
    in endocarditis, 984
    in malaria, 3126, 3127
  evaluation of, 3525-3526
  immune functions of, 3423
    in Streptococcus pneumoniae infection, 2397
  in Bartonella bacillary angiomatosis, 2735,
    2736f

Spleen *(Continued)*
in salmonellosis, 2647t
in schistosomiasis, 3279
infarction of, in endocarditis, 982
red pulp of, 120-121, 121f
rupture of
in infectious mononucleosis, 1806-1807
in malaria, 3126
white pulp of, 120-121, 121f
Splendore-Hoeppli phenomenon, 2981
Splenectomy. *See also* Asplenia.
alternatives to, 3530
indications for, 3524, 3534t
infections after, 158, 3526-3530
Splenomegaly
in endocarditis, 984
in malaria, 3126, 3127
Split pleura sign, 848
Spondweni virus, 1945t
Spondylitis, tuberculous, 2879, 2879f
Spondylodiskitis, 1326-1327, 1326f
Sponge bath, for fever, 713, 714, 715
Spontaneous abortion
from *Brucella,* 2671
from *Chlamydia trachomatis,* 2249
from hepatitis E virus, 2210
from parvovirus B19, 1895, 1896
Spores, in gram-positive rods, 218
Sporothrix schenckii, 2984-2987
appearance of in tissue, 2938t, 2986-2987, 2987f
characteristics of, 2984
clinical manifestations of, 2984-2986
transmission of, 2984
Sporotrichosis, 2984-2987
arthritis in, 1318
clinical features of, 2984-2986
diagnosis of, 2986-2987
differential diagnosis of, 2984-2985, 2985t
epidemiology of, 2984
etiology of, 2984
extracutaneous, 2985-2986, 2985f, 2986f
multifocal, 2986, 2986f
in HIV infection, 2986, 2987
lymphocutaneous, 1211-1213, 2984-2985, 2985f
meningitis in, 1134, 1134f, 1135, 1138
prognosis of, 2987
treatment of, 2987
with amphotericin B, 504
with itraconazole, 508
with ketoconazole, 507
Spotted fevers, 2287-2293. *See also under Rickettsia.*
clinical findings in, 2287t
discovery of, 2285t
vectors of, 2285t
Sprue, 1301
tropical. *See* Tropical sprue.
Sputum
characteristics of, 824, 824f
collection and transport of, 206t, 826, 863
currant-jelly, 824, 824f
Nocardia colonization by, 2918
rusty, 824, 824f
Sputum examination, 854
antigen detection in, 826
culture in, 208, 825-826
in pneumococcal pneumonia, 2400, 2401, 2401t
direct fluorescent antibody tests in, 826
gram stain in, 823-825, 824f, 825f
in acute pneumonia, 823-826, 824f, 825f
in chronic pneumonia, 862-863
in lung abscess, 855

Sputum examination *(Continued)*
in *Pneumocystis* pneumonia, 3087
in tuberculosis, 825, 825f
polymerase chain reaction in, 826
sample collection for, 206t, 826, 863
transtracheal aspiration for, 826
Squamous intraepithelial neoplasia
anal, 1611
in HIV infection, 1609
cervical, 1610-1611
Squirrels, as typhus reservoir, 2304, 2305
SrrAB, 2325
Stains, 214, 214t
for yeast, 2937
Gram. *See* Gram stain.
Standard precautions, 3326-3327
HIV and, 3395-3396
Staphylococcal respiratory response, 2325
Staphylococcal scalded skin syndrome, 737, 1174, 1174f, 2321
clinical aspects of, 2330, 2330f
exfoliative toxins in, 2329-2330, 2330f
pathogenesis of, 2330
vs. toxic epidermal necrolysis, 737
Staphylococcal scarlet fever, 737, 1175
Staphylococcal secretory antigen, in endocarditis, 990
Staphylococcal toxic shock syndrome. *See* Toxic shock syndrome, staphylococcal.
Staphylococcus [spp.]
adherence of, 1022-1023
antibiotic resistance of, 263t
beta-lactamase production by, 256
brain abscess from, 1151, 1153, 1154
cardiovascular device infections from, 1023
catheter-related infections from, 3349
coagulase-negative, 2352-2358, 2352t
antibiotic susceptibility of, 2353
catheter infections from, 2354-2355
cerebrospinal fluid, 2355
ecology of, 2352-2353
endocarditis from, 2354
epidemiology of, 2353
genetics of, 2353
graft infections from, 1037
identification of, 2352, 2352t
nosocomial bacteremia from, 2353-2354
treatment of
with carbapenems, 313t
with linezolid, 437, 437t
with quinolones, 456t
urinary tract infections from, 2355-2356, 2356t
vancomycin-resistant, 419
virulence factors of, 2353
vs. coagulase-positive, 217, 217t
conjunctivitis from, 1391-1392
in neonate, 1393
endocarditis from, 990
prosthetic valve, 1026-1027, 1026t
treatment of, 998-999
enterotoxins of, 29-30
foodborne disease from, 1219, 2332
from platelet transfusion, 3388
habitat of, 2321-2322
in susceptibility testing, 224
keratitis from, 1397-1400
mycotic aneurysm from, 1008
pancreatic infections from, 961
prostatitis from, 894
quinolone-resistant, 465
quinupristin-dalfopristin–resistant, 426
rash from, 736-737
in HIV infection, 742
shunt infections from, 1035, 1127-1130, 1127t

Staphylococcus [spp.] *(Continued)*
species in, 2321, 2323t
splenic abscess from, 967, 967t
subdural empyema from, 1164-1165
toxins of, in severe sepsis, 914-915
transient bacteremia from, 978
treatment of
with clindamycin, 411
with daptomycin, 428
with fusidic acid, 326, 326t
with quinupristin-dalfopristin, 424t, 425
with rifamycin, 379
with teicoplanin, 424t, 425
with vancomycin, 418, 424t
urinary tract infections from, 878, 882
vancomycin-resistant, 264, 264t
Staphylococcus aureus, 3, 2321-2348
antibiotic resistance of, 184-185, 2333-2336, 2334t, 2338, 2353
drug efflux in, 2335-2336, 2336t
ribosome modification in, 2335
to beta-lactams, 2333, 2334t
to erythromycin, 398
to glycopeptides, 2334t, 2335
to macrolide-lincosamide-streptogramin B, 2334t, 2335-2336
to methicillin. *See Staphylococcus aureus,* methicillin-resistant.
to penicillins, 2333, 2334t
to quinolones, 2336
arthritis from, 1312, 1312t
Bacillus subtilis and, 2321, 2332
bacteremia from, 2342
beta-lactamase–producing, 281
biofilm of, 2325-2326, 2326f
brain abscess from, 1151, 1153, 1154, 1157, 1158t
bursitis from, 1319
capsular polysaccharides of, 2321, 2322t
capsule of, 2326, 2326f
carbuncles from, 1175, 2340
cardiac occlusion device infections from, 1036
carriage of, 2322, 2338-2339
decontamination for, 2339
mupirocin for, 480-481
nasal, 2322, 2338-2339
eradication of, 1176, 3540
topical antibacterial therapy for, 483-484
catheter-related infections from, 3349
cell surface determinants in, 2325-2328, 2326f, 2327f, 2327t, 2328f, 2329f
cellulitis from, 2341, 2341f
characteristics of, 2321, 2323f
clinical aspects of, 2337-2338
colonization from, rifamycin for, 381
conjunctivitis from, 1391
culture of, 2322-2324
cytotoxins of, 2321, 2322t
empyema from, 846
endocarditis from, 379-380, 978, 979, 980, 990, 1024, 1025, 1030, 1044, 2342-2345
clinical features of, 2343, 2344f
diagnosis of, 2344, 2344t
embolic skin lesions in, 2342, 2342f
epidemiology of, 2342-2343
host defense in, 2343
in injection drug users, 992, 2344-2345
methicillin-resistant, 998-999
mitral valve in, 2342, 2343f
neurologic complications of, 2344
pathogenesis of, 2343
platelets in, 2343
prosthetic valve, 1024, 1025, 1030
rifamycin for, 379-380

Staphylococcus aureus (Continued)
    treatment of, 998-999, 2344t
    vascular complications of, 2344
  endophthalmitis from, 1408
  enterotoxins of, 2321, 2330, 2332
  enzymes of, 2321, 2322t
  epidemiology of, 2325, 2337
  epidural abscess from, 1165-1167
  erysipelas from, 2341
  exoenzymes of, 2328-2329
  exoproteins of, 2325
  folliculitis from, 2340
  foodborne disease from, 1286-1288, 1294, 1294t, 2339
  furuncles from, 1175, 2340
  graft infections from, 1037, 1039, 1040, 1041, 2357
  hemolysins of, 2329
  hidradenitis suppurativa from, 2340
  identification of, 217, 217t, 2322-2324
  impetigo from, 1172
  in chronic granulomatous disease, 155, 156f
  in cystic fibrosis, 870
  in invasive nonsurgical cardiac procedures, 1040
  in neutrophil disorders, 154
  in peritoneal dialysis, 941
  infectious syndromes with, 2339-2348
  insertion sequences of, 2332
  keratitis from, 1397-1400
  lipoteichoic acids of, 2327
  liver abscess from, 952
  lung abscess from, 854
  mastitis from, 2340
  mastoiditis from, 771
  meningitis from, 1088, 1106t, 1114, 2345
  methicillin-resistant, 184-185
    carriage of, 2339
    cephalosporins for, 296, 298t
    community-acquired, 184, 2334
    contact precautions for, 3329
    coresistance patterns in, 2336, 2336t
    decontamination scheme for, 2338, 2338t
    hospital-acquired, 2333
    mechanism of, 2334-2335
    nasal carriage of, 2322
    Panton-Valentine toxin in, 2329, 2329f
    penicillin-binding protein in, 264
    postoperative infections from, 3539-3540, 3540
    quinupristin-dalfopristin for, 427
    SCC*mec* resistance island of, 2333
    skin infections from, 737
    vancomycin for, 422, 918-919
  molecular analysis of, 2321, 2322t, 2323-2324
  morphologic variants of, 2323
  mortality rates in, 2337, 2337t
  mycotic aneurysm from, 1006, 1007
  necrotizing fasciitis from, 2341-2342
  noninflammatory diarrhea from, 1239
  nutritionally variant streptococci around, 2440
  osteomyelitis from, 1324, 1324t, 2345-2347, 2345t, 2347f
    hyperbaric oxygen for, 566
    rifamycin for, 380-381
  otitis externa from, 766
  otitis media from, 767t
  Panton-Valentine toxin of, 2329, 2329f
  pathogenicity (genomic) islands of, 2332-2333
  peptidoglycans in, 2327-2328, 2328f
  pericarditis from, 1059, 2345
  plasmid-encoded, 6t
  pneumonia from
    aspiration, 835
    chest film in, 829, 830f

Staphylococcus aureus (Continued)
  community-acquired, 831-833
    in cystic fibrosis, 870, 872
    nosocomial, 836, 3364, 3365, 3365t, 3367t, 3368
    sputum in, 825, 825f
    treatment of, 836-839, 837t, 838t
  preseptal cellulitis from, 1422-1424
  prevention of, 2337
  primary peritonitis from, 929
  prostatitis from, 893
  prosthesis infections from, 1332, 1333, 1333t, 2346
  pseudomembranous colitis from, 1250, 1250f
  pulmonary infections from, 2345
  pyomyositis from, 1195, 1196, 2347-2348
  quinolone-resistant, 454
  regulation of, 7t
  regulatory systems of, 2324-2325, 2324f
  resistance by, 2321
  risk factors for, 2338, 2338t
  sepsis from, 907
  septic arthritis from, 2347
  septic bursitis from, 2347
  shunt infections from, 1127-1130, 1127t
  sinusitis from, 776, 776t, 777, 782, 782t
  skin infections from, 2339-2342
  skin lesions from, 737
  small colony variants of, 2323
  soft tissue infections from, 2339-2342
  staphylococcal scalded skin syndrome from, 737
  subdural empyema from, 1164-1165
  superantigens of, 2321, 2322t, 2330-2332
    toxins of, in Kawasaki disease, 3318
  suppurative thrombophlebitis from, 1004, 1168
  surface adhesins of, 2326-2327, 2326f, 2326t
  surface proteins of, 2321, 2322t
  teichoic acids of, 2327
  toxic shock syndrome from, 2321. *See* Toxic shock syndrome, staphylococcal.
  toxin-related disease from, 2339
  toxins of, 1221
    in Kawasaki disease, 3318
  transposons of, 2332
  treatment of, 2336-2337
    with aminoglycosides, 334t-335t, 344t
      in combination therapy, 336t
    with carbapenems, 313t
    with chloramphenicol, 367t
    with clindamycin, 409, 409t
    with daptomycin, 2337
    with lincomycin, 409
    with linezolid, 437, 437t, 438, 2336-2337
    with macrolides, 397t
    with mupirocin, 485t
    with penicillins, 284t, 287, 288t
    with quinolones, 456t
    with quinupristin-dalfopristin, 2336-2337
    with rifamycin, 374t
    with sulfonamides, 441t
    with tetracyclines, 359t
    with trimethoprim, 444t
    with trimethoprim-sulfamethoxazole, 444
    with vancomycin, 359t
  vancomycin-intermediate, 185
    nosocomial transmission of, prevention of, 3329
  vancomycin-resistant, 185, 419
    nosocomial transmission of, prevention of, 3329
  virulence factors in, 3536
  wound infections from, 2341
Staphylococcus capitis, endocarditis from, 990

Staphylococcus epidermidis, 2352-2358
  bacteremia from, in immunocompromise, 2356
  catheter infections from, 2354-2355
  endocarditis from, 990, 2354
    prosthetic valve, 1024, 1025, 1030
    treatment of, 380, 999
  graft infections from, 2357
  identification of, 217, 217t
  in blood culture, 210
  in peritoneal dialysis, 941
  infections from, 2352t
  keratitis from, 1397-1400
  meningitis from, 1088, 1106t
  nosocomial infections from, 2353
  ocular infections from, 2357
  osteomyelitis from, 2356-2357
    hyperbaric oxygen for, 566
  otitis externa from, 766
  pancreatic infections from, 962
  pediatric infections from, 2357
  prosthetic joint infections from, 2357
  resistance of, 2353
    plasmids in, 2353
  shunt infections from, 1127-1130, 1127t, 2355
  sinusitis from, 782, 782t
  suppurative thrombophlebitis from, 1004
  susceptibility of, 2353
  treatment of
    with aminoglycosides, 344t
      in combination therapy, 336t, 337t
    with cephalosporins, 298t
    with clindamycin, 409t
    with macrolides, 397t
    with mupirocin, 485t
    with penicillins, 284t, 288t
    with rifamycin, 374t
    with trimethoprim, 444t
  urinary tract infections from, catheter-related, 3372
Staphylococcus haemolyticus, 2353
Staphylococcus hominis, 2352
Staphylococcus intermedius, from animal bites, 3552
Staphylococcus lugdunensis, endocarditis from, 990, 2354
  prosthetic valve, 1030
Staphylococcus pneumoniae, pericarditis from, 1059
Staphylococcus saccharolyticus, 2352, 2848
Staphylococcus saprophyticus
  endocarditis from, 990
  laboratory identification of, 217
  nitrofurantoin for, 473
  urinary tract infections from, 2355-2356, 2356t
  virulence factors of, 2353
Statins, in sepsis prevention, 922
Stavudine, 1657t, 1658
  dosage of, 684t-685t
  drug interactions with, 697t
  formulations of, 649t
  neurotoxicity of, 1594t
  pediatric, 1646t
  prophylactic
    after occupational exposure to HIV, 3402, 3402t
    in pregnancy, 3404
    for perinatal HIV transmission, 1625t
  structure of, 1656f
Steam sterilization, 3337t, 3338
  flash method of, 3339
Steatosis, hepatic, in HIV-infected women, 1630-1631
Steeple sign, in croup, 762, 762f

Stegomeyia spp., alphavirus infections from, 1916
Stem cell transplantation. *See* Hematopoietic stem cell transplantation; Transplantation.
Stenotrophomonas [spp.]
  cardiovascular device infections from, 1023
  identification of, 220
Stenotrophomonas maltophilia, 2615-2620
  carbapenems for, 313t
  clinical manifestations of, 2618
  identification of, 221t
  meningitis from, 1114
  pathogenesis of, 2616-2617
  peritonitis from, treatment of, 938, 939
  pneumonia from, 2618
  prevention of, 2619-2620
  pulmonary infections from
    in cystic fibrosis, 871
    nosocomial, 3367t
  sinusitis from, 782
  taxonomy of, 2615
  treatment of, 2619
    with aminoglycosides, 334t-335t
    with penicillins, 288t
    with quinolones, 455t
    with trimethoprim, 444t
    with trimethoprim-sulfamethoxazole, 444
  virulence factors of, 2616-2617
Stent infections
  coronary artery, 1040
  peripheral vascular, 1036
Stercoraria spp., 3157
Sterilization. *See also* Disinfection.
  bioterrorism and, 3342
  definition of, 3331
  in hospitals, 3331-3333, 3332t
  methods of, 3337t, 3338-3340
  with ethylene oxide, 3337t, 3339
  with hydrogen peroxide gas plasma, 3337t, 3339-3340
  with peracetic acid, 3337t, 3340
  with steam, 3337t, 3338
    in flash method, 3339
Sternal wound infections, in heart transplants, 3503
Steroid hormones, anabolic, for weight loss, 145
Steroids. *See* Corticosteroids.
Stevens-Johnson syndrome, 732, 733
  from *Mycoplasma pneumoniae,* 2274, 2274f
Stibogluconate
  for leishmaniasis, 591
  for post–kala-azar dermal leishmaniasis, 3153
  for trypanosomiasis, 569t
  for visceral leishmaniasis, 3153
Stillbirth
  from *Chlamydia trachomatis,* 2249
  from hepatitis E virus, 2210
  from parvovirus B19, 1895, 1896
Still's disease, fever in, 727
Stomach. *See under* Gastric; Gastrointestinal.
Stomatitis
  aphthous, 798-799
    differential diagnosis of, 754, 756
    in immunocompromised host, 798-799
    in Marshall's syndrome, 756
    vs. herpetic pharyngitis, 756
  from herpes simplex virus, 1765-1766
  gangrenous, 798
  in immunocompromised host, 798-799, 3424-3425, 3437
  vesicular, 2150
Stomatococcus mucilaginosus, 2446. *See also Rothia mucilaginosa.*
  endocarditis from, 992
Stool examination
  culture in, 1224
  for *Campylobacter,* 2553, 2554f

Stool examination *(Continued)*
  for cestodes, 3288-3289
  for *Cryptosporidium,* 3220, 3221f
  for *Cyclospora,* 3229
  for *Entamoeba histolytica,* 3104
  for *Giardia lamblia,* 3202
  for microsporidia, 3246, 3246t
  for ova and parasites, 2207t, 3202
  for *Salmonella,* 2637
  for *Shigella,* 2658, 2658f
  in helminthic infections, 3293
  laboratory tests in, 212
  specimen collection and transport for, 207t
Strain typing, 222
Strategic National Stockpile, 3599
Strawberry tongue, 734
Streptidine, 329f
Streptobacillus moniliformis, 2708-2710
  bacteriology of, 2708-2709
  clinical manifestations of, 2709
  endocarditis from, 992
  epidemiology of, 2709
  laboratory detection of, 2709
  splenic abscess from, 967, 967t
  treatment of, 2710
    with penicillins, 288t
Streptococcal pyogenic exotoxin, Kawasaki disease and, 3318
Streptococcal toxic shock syndrome. *See* Toxic shock syndrome, streptococcal.
Streptococcus [spp.], 1182, 2360-2362
  animal isolated, 2362t
  appendicitis from, 969
  arthritis from, 1312, 1312t
  beta-hemolytic, 2441-2447. *See also* Streptococcus group C; Streptococcus group G
  brain abscess from, 1151, 1154, 1157, 1158t
  bursitis from, 1319
  classification of, 2360-2362, 2360f, 2361f, 2361t, 2362t
  diverticulitis from, 972
  endocarditis from, 988-990
    prosthetic valve, 1027, 1027t
    treatment of, 995-998
  enterococcal, 2361
  exotoxins of, 29
  gangrene from, 1181, 1183t, 1187, 1188t, 1189-1191
  hemolytic
    classification of, 2360-2361, 2360f, 2361f
    endocarditis from, 988
    identification of, 217t, 218
    linezolid for, 437, 437t
  human isolated, 2361t
  in oral cavity, 787, 787t
  in peritoneal dialysis, 941
  keratitis from, 1397-1400
  liver abscess from, 952
  myositis from, 1197-1198
  nonhemolytic, identification of, 217t, 218
  osteomyelitis from, 1324
  penicillin-sensitive, 995-996
  pharyngitis from. *See* Pharyngitis, streptococcal.
  preseptal cellulitis from, 1422-1424
  rash from, 737-738
    in HIV infection, 742
  resistance of, 263t
    to penicillin, 996-998
  sinusitis from, 782, 782t
  splenic abscess from, 967, 967t
  subdural empyema from, 1164-1165
  toxins of, in severe sepsis, 914-915
  treatment of

Streptococcus [spp.] *(Continued)*
  with daptomycin, 428
  with macrolides, 401t, 402-403
  with quinolones, 456t
  with quinupristin-dalfopristin, 425
  with rifamycin, 381
  with vancomycin, 418
  typhlitis from, 973
  viridans. *See Streptococcus viridans* group.
Streptococcus acidominimus, classification of, 2435, 2435t
Streptococcus adjacens (Granulicatella adiacens), 2440
  endocarditis from, 979
Streptococcus agalactiae (group B), 2361t, 2423-2431, 2427t
  adherence of, 2425
  arthritis from, 2427
  classification of, 2423-2424
  clinical manifestations of, 2426-2429, 2427t
  colonization of, 2424, 2424t
  diagnosis of, 2429
  endocarditis from, 989, 2427
    prosthetic valve, 1027
  epidemiology of, 2424-2425
  history of, 2423
  host defenses against, 2425-2426
  identification of, 2423
  in female genital tract, 2427
  in neonates, 2426-2427
  in pregnancy, 2425
  incidence of, 2425
  inflammatory mediators of, 2426
  intra-amniotic infection syndrome from, 1372-1373
  invasive, 2425, 2429
  meningitis from, 1087, 1106t, 1114, 1118, 2428
  morphology of, 2423
  osteomyelitis from, 2427
  pathogenetic mechanisms of, 2425-2426
  pneumonia from, 2427
  predisposing factors for, 2427, 2427t
  prevention of, 2430-2431, 2431t
  skin infections from, 2427-2428
  soft tissue infections from, 2427-2428
  transmission of, 2424-2425
  treatment of, 2429-2430, 2430t
    with carbapenems, 313t
    with cephalosporins, 298t
    with chloramphenicol, 367t
    with macrolides, 397t
    with mupirocin, 485t
    with nitrofurantoin, 473
    with penicillins, 284t, 287, 288t
    with quinolones, 456t
    with rifamycin, 374t
  typing of, 2423-2424
  vaccines for, 2431
  virulence factors of, 2426
Streptococcus anginosus group, 2435, 2435t, 2451-2455
  abdominal infections from, 2454-2455
  bacteremia from, 2454
  bacteriology of, 2451
  brain abscess from, 1151, 1157, 1158t
  central nervous system infections from, 2454
  classification of, 2361t, 2435, 2435t
  empyema from, 847
  endocarditis from, 988-990, 2454
  epidemiology of, 2436t
  habitat of, 2452-2453
  head and neck infections from, 2454
  identification of, 217t, 218
  pathogenicity of, 2453-2454
  sinusitis from, 776, 776t, 782t

Streptococcus anginosus group *(Continued)*
taxonomy of, 2451-2452, 2452f, 2452t
thoracic infections from, 2455
treatment of, 2455
Streptococcus anginosus-constellatus,
classification of, 2435, 2435t
Streptococcus aureus, toxic shock syndrome
from, 2331-2332, 2331t
Streptococcus bovis, 2417-2418
classification of, 2361t
endocarditis from, 988, 989
prosthetic valve, 1027
laboratory identification of, 217t, 218
penicillins for, 288t
Streptococcus canis, 2362t
*Streptococcus constellatus. See Streptococcus
anginosus* group.
Streptococcus cristatus, 2436t
Streptococcus defectivus (Abiotrophia defectiva), 2440
endocarditis from, 979
Streptococcus dysgalactiae, 2441, 2441t
Streptococcus dysgalactiae subsp. *dysgalactiae,*
2362t
Streptococcus dysgalactiaei subsp. *equisimilis,*
2361t
Streptococcus epidermidis, meningitis from,
vancomycin for, 423
Streptococcus equi, microbiology of, 2441t, 2442
Streptococcus equi subsp. *equi,* 2362t
Streptococcus equi subsp. *zooepidemicus,* 2362t
Streptococcus equinus, endocarditis from, 989
Streptococcus equisimilis, 2441-2442, 2441t
Streptococcus gordonii, 2436t
endocarditis from, 979
tolerance of, 2440
Streptococcus group A. *See Streptococcus
pyogenes* (group A).
Streptococcus group B. *See Streptococcus
agalactiae* (group B).
Streptococcus group C, 2445
arthritis from, 2443
bacteremia from, 2444-2445
clinical manifestations of, 2442-2445
endocarditis from, 2444
epidemiology of, 2442
meningitis from, 2444
microbiology of, 2441-2442, 2441t
osteomyelitis from, 2443
pharyngitis from, 754, 2442-2443. *See also*
Pharyngitis, streptococcal.
puerperal infections from, 2634
respiratory tract infections from, 2444
skin/soft tissue infections from, 2443
tolerance of, 2445
treatment of, 2445
Streptococcus group G, 2445
arthritis from, 2443
bacteremia from, 2445
clinical manifestations of, 2442-2445
endocarditis from, 2444
epidemiology of, 2442
meningitis from, 2444
microbiology of, 2442
neonatal sepsis from, 2444
osteomyelitis from, 2443
pharyngitis from, 754, 2442-2443. *See also*
Pharyngitis, streptococcal.
puerperal infections from, 2444
respiratory tract infections from, 2444
skin/soft tissue infections from, 2443
treatment of, 2445-2446
Streptococcus group M, pyoderma from, 2369
Streptococcus infantarius, endocarditis from, 989
Streptococcus iniae, 2362t, 2446
cellulitis from, 1184

*Streptococcus intermedius. See Streptococcus
anginosus* group.
Streptococcus macedonicus, endocarditis from,
989
*Streptococcus milleri. See Streptococcus
anginosus* group.
Streptococcus mitior
classification of, 2435, 2435t
endocarditis from, 988
epidemiology of, 2436t
Streptococcus mitis, 2435, 2435t
antibiotic resistance of, 2440
biochemical characteristics of, 2436t
classification of, 2361t
epidemiology of, 2436t
identification of, 217t, 218
in synthetic carotid patches, 1041
odontogenic infections from, 788, 788f, 789
tolerance of, 2440
Streptococcus morbillorum, 2435
biochemical characteristics of, 2436t
classification of, 2435, 2435t
Streptococcus mutans, 2435, 2435t
biochemical characteristics of, 2436t
classification of, 2361t, 2435, 2435t
dental caries from, 788, 788f, 2436
endocarditis from, 978, 988, 989
epidemiology of, 2436t
identification of, 217t, 218
Streptococcus nutritionally variant (deficient)
group, 2440-2441
Streptococcus oralis, 2436t
antibiotic resistance of, 2440
odontogenic infections from, 788, 788f
Streptococcus parasanguinis, 2436t
Streptococcus pneumoniae, 2361t, 2392-2407
adherence of, 2394
anatomy of, 2392-2393, 2393f
anticapsular antibody to, 2396-2397
antigen detection for, 828
antisera identification of, 221
bronchitis exacerbation from, 2400
capsule of, 2392-2393, 2393f
colonization by, 2394, 2397
complement activation by, 2396
conjunctivitis from, 1391
in neonate, 1393
culture of, 208
diagnosis of, 828, 829
empyema from, 846
endocarditis from, 988, 989
prosthetic valve, 1027
treatment of, 1000
epidemiology of, 2393-2394, 2394f, 2395f
factors predisposing to, 2397-2398, 2397t, 2398t
history of, 2392
identification of, 218
immunologic defenses against, 2396-2397
in chronic obstructive pulmonary disease
in exacerbations, 809
in stable disease, 808
in HIV infection, 1486, 2398
treatment of, 1682t, 1699
in susceptibility testing, 224
infections from, 2398-2402, 2399f
inflammatory response produced by, 2396
invasiveness of, 2394-2395
keratitis from, 1397-1400
mastoiditis from, 771
meningitis from, 1087, 1106t, 1112-1113,
1118, 1119, 2399-2400, 2437-2439
antibiotic susceptibility in, 2403t
prevention of, 1118, 1119
treatment of, 1106t, 1112-1113, 2405
vancomycin for, 422-423

Streptococcus pneumoniae (Continued)
microbiology of, 2392
mycotic aneurysm from, 993
otitis media from, 767, 767t, 2399
treatment of, 2404
pathogenetic mechanisms of, 2394-2396
peritonitis from, 929
phagocytosis of, 2395
physiology of, 2392-2393
pneumonia from. *See* Pneumococcal
pneumonia.
postsplenectomy sepsis from, 3527
preseptal cellulitis from, 1422-1424
prevention of, 2405-2407, 2406t
resistance of, 185, 2402-2404
to erythromycin, 397
to penicillin, 185, 836-837, 837t, 1112
to quinolones, 185, 466
to vancomycin, 419
serotypes of, 175, 2392-2393
sinusitis from, 775, 776, 776t, 779, 780, 781t,
2399, 2404
splenic defenses against, 2397
susceptibility of, 2402-2404, 2403t
to penicillin, 2402, 2403t
transformation in, 2393
treatment of, 2404-2405
with aminoglycosides, 334t-335t
postantibiotic effect in, 334
with carbapenems, 313t
with cephalosporins, 298t
with chloramphenicol, 367t
with clindamycin, 409, 409t
with lincomycin, 409
with linezolid, 437, 437t, 438
with macrolides, 397t, 401t, 407
with mupirocin, 485t
with penicillins, 284t, 287, 288t
with quinolones, 456t
with rifamycin, 374t
with sulfonamides, 441t
with tetracyclines, 358, 359t
with trimethoprim, 444t
with trimethoprim-sulfamethoxazole, 444
with vancomycin, 359t
vaccine for, 839, 1119, 2405-2407, 2406t. *See
also* Pneumococcal vaccine.
virulence of, 2395-2396, 2396t
Streptococcus porcinus, 2362t
Streptococcus pyogenes (group A), 2361t, 2362-
2375
antisera identification of, 221
bacteremia from, 2375
cellulitis from, 1178, 1180, 2370-2371,
2371f
perianal, 2375
conjunctivitis from, 1391
description of, 2362-2365, 2364f
empyema from, 846-847
endocarditis from, 978
erysipelas from, 1177, 2341, 2370, 2371f
exotoxins of, 29
extracellular products of, 2364
gangrene from, 1181, 1183t
glomerulonephritis from, 2386-2387. *See also*
Glomerulonephritis.
history of, 2362
impetigo from, 1172, 2339-2340
in sepsis, 907
keratitis from, 1397-1400
laboratory tests of, 208
lymphangitis from, 1211, 1212, 2375
meningitis from, 1087
myonecrosis from, 2372
myositis from, 2372, 2372f

Streptococcus pyogenes (group A) *(Continued)*
necrotizing fasciitis from, 2341, 2371-2372
vs. necrotizing myositis, 1197-1198
nephritogenic, 2386
nonsuppurative sequelae from, 2380t
otitis media from, 767, 767t
phage-encoded, 6t
pharyngitis from, 738, 753-754, 2364-2368.
See also Pharyngitis.
clinical manifestations of, 2365
diagnosis of, 2365-2367
epidemiology of, 2364-2365, 2364f
nonsuppurative complications for, 2365
rapid antigen detection tests for, 2366-2367
rheumatic fever after, 2382
suppurative complications for, 2365
throat culture for, 2366, 2368
treatment of, 2367-2368, 2367t
with clindamycin, 411
with telithromycin for, 407
vs. nonstreptococcal sore throat, 2366
pneumonia from, 2375
postpartum endometritis from, 1374
primary peritonitis from, 929
pyoderma from, 2368-2370, 2369f
resistance of, to erythromycin, 397
rheumatic fever from, 2380-2381, 2380t. *See also* Rheumatic fever.
rifamycin for, 374t
scarlet fever from, 737-738, 2365
sinusitis from, 776, 776t
skin infections from, 2369, 2369f, 2370-2374
skin lesions from, 737-738
soft tissue infections from, 2370-2374
somatic constituents of, 2363, 2363f
superantigen toxins of, in Kawasaki disease, 3318
toxic shock syndrome from, 738, 738t, 2372-2375. *See also* Toxic shock syndrome, streptococcal.
treatment of
with aminoglycoside combination therapy, 336t
with carbapenems, 313t
with cephalosporins, 298t
with chloramphenicol, 367t
with clindamycin, 409, 409t, 411
with lincomycin, 409
with linezolid, 437, 437t
with macrolides, 397t, 407
with mupirocin, 485t
with penicillins, 284t, 287, 288t
with quinolones, 456t
with sulfonamides, 441t
with trimethoprim, 444, 444t
with trimethoprim-sulfamethoxazole, 444
virulence factors of, 2363, 2363f
vs. infectious mononucleosis, 1813
vulvovaginitis from, 2375
Streptococcus salivarius, 2435, 2435t
biochemical characteristics of, 2436t
classification of, 2361t, 2435, 2435t
endocarditis from, 988
epidemiology of, 2436t
tolerance of, 2440
Streptococcus sanguis, 2436t
antibiotic resistance of, 2440
aphthous stomatitis from, 798
classification of, 2435, 2435t
endocarditis from, 978, 979-980, 988
mupirocin for, 485t
odontogenic infections from, 788, 788f, 789
tolerance of, 2440

Streptococcus suis, 2362t
endocarditis from, 989
Streptococcus uberis, 2435, 2435t
Streptococcus vestibularis, 2436t
Streptococcus viridans group, 2435-2440, 2439
bacteremia from, 2436, 2437, 2438
biochemical characteristics of, 2435, 2436t
classification of, 2361t, 2435, 2435t, 2436t
empyema from, 847
endocarditis from, 988, 989, 2436-2438, 2436t, 2437t
teicoplanin for, 425
epidemiology of, 13-14
identification of, 2435
in stem cell transplant, 3492
meningitis from, 2438-2439
microbiology of, 2435
pathogenicity of, 2436-2437
pneumonia from, 2439
resistance of, 2439-2440
septic shock from, 2436-2437
tolerance of, 2440
treatment of, 2439-2440
with aminoglycosides, 336t, 337t, 344t
with cephalosporins, 298t
with chloramphenicol, 367t
with clindamycin, 409t
with combination therapy, 248
with macrolides, 397t
with penicillins, 284t, 288t
with rifamycin, 374t
Streptococcus zooepidemicus, 2441t, 2442
pharyngitis from, 2443
Streptogramins, 425-427. *See also* Quinupristin-dalfopristin.
resistance to, 262-263, 263t
by *Staphylococcus aureus,* 2334t, 2335-2336
Streptokinase, 2364
for pleural effusion/empyema, 851
Streptolysin, 2364
Streptomyces [spp.], laboratory tests for, 228-229
Streptomyces avermitilis, ivermectin for, 594
Streptomyces somaliensis, mycetoma from, 2991-2995, 2992t
Streptomycin
antimicrobial activity of, 333, 334t-335t
chemical family of, 330t
dosage of, 660t-661t, 676t-677t
for actinomycetoma, 2995
for *Brucella,* 2672
for bubonic plague, 1211
for *Calymmatobacterium granulomatis,* 2750
for culture-negative endocarditis, 1001
for enterococcal endocarditis, 997, 998, 2416, 2416t
of prosthetic valve, 1027t, 1028, 1028t
with penicillin resistance, 996
for experimental endocarditis, 1048
for *Francisella tularensis,* 2682
for nontuberculous mycobacterial infections, 496
for plague, 3603
for rat-bite fever, 2710
for streptococcal endocarditis, 995-996
of prosthetic valve, 1027t
for tuberculosis, 493, 2867, 2868, 2868t
in HIV infection, 2870, 2871t, 2872
for tularemia, in bioterrorism attack, 3610t, 3611
for viridans streptococcal endocarditis, 2437t, 2438
for *Yersina pestis,* 2696
formulations of, 647t, 649t
names and sources of, 329t
once-daily dosage regimens for, 348t
structure of, 328, 329f, 330

Stress, immunologic effects of, 40
Stridor
differential diagnosis of, 763
in croup, 762, 763
in epiglottitis, 763
Stroke, fever of unknown origin in, 721
Strongyloides [spp.], pulmonary infiltrates with eosinophilia from, 835
Strongyloides stercoralis, 3261t, 3264-3266
adult T-cell leukemia/lymphoma and, 2109, 2111
culture of, 1224
diarrhea from, 1242
in immunocompromised host, 3438
pancreatic infections from, 959t, 960
pneumonia from, in HIV infection, 1572
syndrome of abdominal pain, diarrhea, and eosinophilia from, 1281, 1281t
treatment of, 575t
with ivermectin, 595
with thiabendzole, 593
Stye, 1419
Subacute sclerosing panencephalitis, 2032, 2034
Subaortic stenosis, idiopathic hypertrophic, endocarditis in, 976
Subconjunctival hemorrhage, in acute hemorrhagic conjunctivitis, 1389, 2136, 2137, 2156
Subcutaneous nodules, in blastomycosis, 3029t, 3033
Subcutaneous tissue infections, 1187-1191, 1188t
differential diagnosis of, 1188t
etiology of, 1188t
factitial, 1188t
injection site, 1188t
primary, 1187-1191, 1188t
secondary, 1187-1191
terminology of, 1187
Subdural empyema, 1164-1165
clinical features of, 1079-1080
in injection drug users, 3471
Subhepatic space, 927-928, 927f, 928f
abscess of, 928
Sublingual space, 790, 790f
infections of, 754, 756, 792-793, 793, 793f. *See also* Odontogenic infections.
Submandibular abscess, actinomycotic, 2925, 2925f
Submandibular space, 790, 790f
infections of, 754, 756, 792-793, 793, 793f. *See also* Odontogenic infections.
Submaxillary space, 790, 790f
infections of, 792-793
Submental space, 790, 790f
infections of, 792-793
Subpectoral lymphadenitis, 1205
Subperiosteal abscess, 1421-1424, 1421f, 1423f
in suppurative thrombophlebitis, 1003
Subphrenic space, 927, 927f, 928f
abscess of, 928, 943
Substance abuse. *See also* Injection drug users.
hepatitis A and, 2171, 2178
Sul1, 265
Sul2, 265
Sulbactam, 316-317, 316f
Sulfacetamide sodium, 441
Sulfadiazine, 440, 440f
dosage of, 670t-671t
for brain abscess, 1159t
for paracoccidioidomycosis, 3065
for rheumatic fever, 2385-2386, 2385t
for toxoplasmosis, 576t, 3188
in congenital infections, 3191
in encephalitis, 1587
in HIV infection, 1683t, 1685t, 1695

Sulfadiazine (Continued)
  in immunocompromised host, 3188-3190, 3189t
  in pregnancy, 3190-3191
    with chorioretinitis, 3190
  formulations of, 648t
Sulfadimethoxine, for paracoccidioidomycosis, 3065
Sulfadoxine, 441
  dosage of, 670t-671t
  formulations of, 648t
Sulfadoxine-pyrimethamine
  drug interactions with, 697t
  for malaria, 441, 3133, 3134-3135, 3134t
    mechanism of action of, 3129
    resistance to, 3129, 3133. See also Malaria, drug-resistant.
Sulfaguanidine, 441
Sulfameter, 441
Sulfamethizole
  dosage of, 670t-671t
  formulations of, 648t
Sulfamethoxazole, 440-441, 440f. See also Trimethoprim-sulfamethoxazole.
  dosage of, 670t-671t
  for actinomycetoma, 2995
  for nocardiosis, 2920, 2920t
  for paracoccidioidomycosis, 3065
  formulations of, 648t
  Staphylococcus aureus resistance to, 2334t
Sulfamethoxypyridazine, 441
  for paracoccidioidomycosis, 3065
Sulfanilamide, 440, 440f
Sulfasuxidine, 441
Sulfathalidine, 440, 440f, 441
Sulfisoxazole, 440, 440f
  dosage of, 670t-671t
  for otitis media prevention, 769
Sulfonamides, 440-443
  adverse reactions to, 442
  age and, 244
  antimicrobial activity of, 441, 441t
  classification of, 440
  derivation of, 440
  distribution of, 442, 442t
  drug interactions with, 443, 697t-698t
  for gastrointestinal infections, 441
  for gestational bacteriuria, 893
  for Neisseria meningitidis, 2509
  for nocardiosis, 2919-2920, 2920t
  for nontuberculous mycobacteria, 497
  for paracoccidioidomycosis, 3065
  for parasites, 588
  in renal insufficiency, 442
  long-acting, 441
  mechanism of action of, 441
  medium-acting, 440-441
  pharmacology of, 442, 442t
  resistance to, 265, 441-442
  short-acting, 440-441
  structure of, 440, 440f
  topical, 441
  uses of, 443
Sulfonamide-trimethoprim, 248
Sulfoxone, for leprosy, 499
Sulfur granules, in actinomycosis, 2930-2931, 2930f
Superantigens
  bacterial toxins of, in Kawasaki disease, 3317-3318
  in Staphylococcus aureus, 2330-2331
  in Streptococcus pyogenes, 2364
Superinfections
  erythromycin and, 400
  tetracyclines and, 363t, 365

Superior sagittal thrombophlebitis, 1168-1170, 1169f
Superoxide anion, in neutrophil bactericidal activity, 102
Superoxidized water, disinfection with, 3334
Suppurative conditions. See also Sepsis.
Suppurative lymphadenitis. See Lymphadenitis/lymphadenopathy.
Suppurative parotitis, 797t, 799
Suppurative thrombophlebitis
  in burn patients, 3550
  intracranial, 794, 795f, 1168-1170, 1169f
    cavernous sinus, 794, 795f, 797t, 1168-1170, 1169f
    lateral sinus, 1168-1170
    sagittal sinus, 1168-1170, 1169f
  jugular, 754, 754f, 794, 794f
    lung abscess and, 854
    treatment of, 797, 797t
Suppurative thyroiditis, 800
Supraglottitis, 784-786
  vs. croup, 763
Suprapubic catheterization, 3374
  infections from. See Urinary tract infections, catheter-related.
Sural nerve biopsy, in HIV-related neuropathy, 1593-1594
Suramin
  adverse effects of, 582t
  for African trypanosomiasis, 590, 3168, 3168t
  for American trypanosomiasis, 576t
  for Trypanosomatidae, 569t
Surfactant, 820
  in Pseudomonas aeruginosa resistance, 2590
Surgery
  infections after. See Postoperative infections.
  laser. See Laser surgery.
  skin preparation for, 3540
Surveillance
  active, 164
  community-based, 164
  for antimicrobial resistance, 164, 265, 266f
  syndromic, for bioterrorist attacks, 3598
  for nosocomial infections, 3323
Susceptibility, definition of, 223
Susceptibility testing, 222-224
  for Bartonella, 2742-2743
  for mycobacteria, 227
  for Mycobacterium tuberculosis, 2854t, 2855
  for viruses, 238-239
  issues in, 224
  minimal bactericidal concentration in, 223
  minimal inhibitory concentration in, 222, 223
  terminology in, 222-223
Sutterella spp., 2844t
Sutures, cardiac, infections of, 1035-1036
Sweat chloride test, for cystic fibrosis, 869
Sweet syndrome, 730, 730t, 1179, 3439
  skin lesions in, 734-735
  vs. cellulitis, 1179
Swimmer's ear, 766
  from Pseudomonas aeruginosa, 2604
Swimmer's itch, 3278, 3294t, 3298
Swimming pool granuloma, 1212, 1213
Swine, hepatitis E virus in, 2208-2209
Swyer-James syndrome, 817-818
Sycosis barbae, 1175, 2340
Sydenham's chorea, in rheumatic fever, 2383-2384
Sylvatic (epidemic) typhus, 2303-2305, 2308. See also Typhus.
Symmetric peripheral gangrene, 735
Sympathetic nervous system, in systemic response, 909

Synaptaxin, in botulism, 2823, 2824f
Synaptobrevin, in botulism, 2823, 2824f
Syndrome of abdominal pain, diarrhea, and eosinophilia, 1280-1283, 1281t
Synergism, 274
  in combination therapy, 248
Synergistic necrotizing cellulitis, 1188t, 1191, 1200
Synergy testing, 223
Synovial fluid, collection and transport of, 206t
Synovitis, acne, plantar pustulosis, hyperostosis, osteitis, 1328
Syphilids, pustular, 2773
Syphilis, 2768-2783. See also Treponema pallidum.
  atypical, 2777-2778
  cardiovascular, 2776
  central nervous system in, 2774-2776. See also Neurosyphilis.
  chancre in, 2771, 2772-2773, 2772f, 2773f
  clinical manifestations of, 2772-2778
  condylomata lata in, 1340, 1340f, 1341-1342
  congenital, 2777, 2777t
    tests for, 2780
  darkfield examination for, 2778, 2778f
  diagnosis of, 1342-1343, 2778-2780, 2778f, 2778t, 2780t
  endemic, 2787
  epidemiology of, 1342, 2770, 2770f
  etiology of, 2769-2770
  gastrointestinal, 1269, 2774
  genital lesions in, 733, 1339-1344, 1340f, 1342t
    characteristics of, 1339-1340, 1340f
    clinical features of, 1339, 1340, 1340f
    duration of, 1341-1342
    presentation of, 1338-1339
  gumma in, 2776-2777
  hepatitis in, 2774
  history of, 2768-2769
  immunity to, 2783
  in HIV infection, 742, 1342, 1690t, 1701-1702, 2782, 2783
  in injection drug users, 3473
  incubating, 2772
  late, 2774, 2782
  late benign, 2776-2777
  latent, 2774
  meningitis in, 1583-1584
  mucous patches in, 2773-2774, 2774f
  nontreponemal reaginic tests for, 2778-2779
    false-positive, 2780, 2780t
  obliterative endarteritis in, 2771, 2771f
  ocular, 1400, 1415, 1418, 2782
  otitis in, 2782
  papules in, 2773
  pathogenesis of, 2770-2771
  persistent, 2782
  polymerase chain reaction for, 2780
  primary, 2772-2773, 2772f, 2773f
  retreatment of, 2782
  secondary (disseminated), 2773-2774, 2773t, 2774f
  serologic tests for, 2778, 2778t
    false-positive, 2780, 2780t
  skin lesions in, 733
  stages of, 2770-2771
  transfusion-related, 3388
  treatment of, 1344, 2780-2783, 2781t
    Jarish-Herxheimer reaction in, 2782-2783
    penicillin allergy in, 2782
  treponemal tests for, 2779
  untreated, 2771-2772
Syphilitic meningitis, 1088

Systemic inflammatory response syndrome, 906t.
  See also Sepsis.
  etiology of, 3427-3428
Systemic lupus erythematosus
  autoantibodies in, 79
  complement deficiency in, 79-80, 87
  immune complex clearance in, 80-81
  meningitis in, 1139
  pleural effusion in, 847, 849, 862f

T

T cell(s), 3183-3185, 3184f. *See also* CD4; CD8;
    Lymphocyte(s).
  activation of, 61-62, 63f, 132
  antigen recognition by, 124
  antigen-specific memory of, 134
  assay of, 152, 153t
  B cell interactions with, 61, 62f
  congenital defects in, 152-153, 153t
  cytolytic, in myocarditis, 1054
  cytotoxic
    in HIV infection, 1530-1531, 1530t, 1708,
        1709
    in HIV nonprogression, 1532
    in HIV vaccines, 1712-1713
  defects in, 66
  hypersensitivity reactions, 152-153, 153t
  in autoimmunity, 65
  in hypersensitivity reactions, 319t, 320
  in immunodeficiency, 150t
  in intestinal mucosa, 122
  in primary immune response, 56
  lymph node entry of, 121
  memory, 134
  naive, 134
  peripheral, 132
  priming of, 132-133
  pulmonary, 821
  regulatory, 134-135
  signals for, 61, 62f
  suppressor, 134-135
T cell receptor, antigen presentation to, 37
T helper cells, CD4+, activated, 61, 62f
T84 cells, neutrophil migration across, 98
T-1249 peptide, 21
Tacaribe viruses, 2090, 2093-2094
Tache noire, 734
Tachipleistophora spp., in HIV infection, 1701
Tachycardia
  in myocarditis, 1056
  ventricular, erythromycin and, 400
Tacrolimus
  chloramphenicol interactions with, 369t
  for transplant immunosuppression, infections
      and, 3478
  in cytomegalovirus reactivation, 1795
  metronidazole interactions with, 393t
Taenia [spp.] *See also* Tapeworms.
  albendzole for, 592
Taenia crassiceps, 3292
Taenia multiceps, 3286t, 3292
Taenia saginata, 3286t, 3288
  syndrome of abdominal pain, diarrhea, and
      eosinophilia from, 1281t, 1283
  treatment of, 575t
Taenia serialis, 3292
Taenia solium, 1202, 3286t, 3288, 3289-3290. *See
    also* Cysticercosis; Tapeworms.
  syndrome of abdominal pain, diarrhea, and
      eosinophilia from, 1281t, 1283
  treatment of, 575t, 595
Tafenoquine, for malaria, 3136
Tamm-Horsfall protein, 36, 879, 879f
Tanapox, 1754-1755

Tapeworms
  anatomy of, 3285, 3287f
  beef, 3286t, 3288
  characteristics of, 3285-3286, 3286f
  diagnosis of, 3259t, 3288-3289
  dual infections with, 3286
  dwarf, 3286t, 3287-3288
  fish, 3286t, 3287
  host range of, 3286-3287
  immune response to, 3287
  invasive, 3289-3292
  life cycle of, 3285-3286, 3286f
  management of, 3289
  pathogenicity of, 3287
  pork, 3286t, 3288
  prevention of, 3292
  syndrome of abdominal pain, diarrhea, and
      eosinophilia from, 1281t, 1283
  treatment of, 570t, 575t, 595-596
Tat, 1602
Taunton virus, 2195. *See also* Caliciviruses.
Tazobactam, 317, 317f
  for febrile neutropenia, 3450-3454, 3451t
Tears, in host defense, 36
Teeth. *See also under* Dental.
  discoloration of, from tetracycline, 363-364
Teichoic acid
  in *Staphylococcus aureus,* 2327
  in *Streptococcus pneumoniae,* 2393, 2396
Teicoplanin, 423-425
  adverse effects of, 424-425
  antimicrobial activity of, 423-424
  dosage of, 668t-669t
  for *Clostridium difficile*–associated colitis,
      1258, 1258t
  for enterococcal endocarditis, 2417
    vancomycin-resistant, 997
  for febrile neutropenia, 3451t, 3452, 3453,
      3453t
  for shunt infections, 1129t, 1130
  for staphylococcal endocarditis, 999
  for *Staphylococcus,* 424t
  for *Streptococcus agalactiae* (group B), 2429
  pharmacokinetics of, 424
  resistance to, 423-424
    by *Enterococcus,* 264
    by *Leuconostoc,* 2418
  uses of, 425
Telbivudine, for chronic hepatitis B, 1448, 1448t,
    1881
Telithromycin
  adverse reactions to, 407
  antimicrobial activity of, 407
  chemistry of, 406, 407f
  dosage of, 664t-665t
  drug interactions with, 407, 698t
  for pneumonia, 837-839, 837t, 838t
  formulations of, 648t
  in vitro susceptibilities to, 397t
  mechanism of action of, 406
  pharmacology of, 407
  pneumococcal resistance to, 837, 837t
  resistance to, 406-407
  uses of, 407-408
Temafloxacin, 451
  adverse effects of, 467
  for streptococcal endocarditis, 995
Temperature
  age and, 705, 707
  axillary, 704-705
  core, 704, 705
  diurnal variability in, 705, 706-707, 706f
  elevated. *See* Fever.
  gender and, 705, 706, 707
  in elderly, 3521-3522

Temperature *(Continued)*
  in infections, 910
  in virulence gene expression, 7
  measurement of, 703-707
    anatomic variability in, 704-705
    observer variability in, 703-704
    physiologic variability in, 705
  normal values for, 703, 705-707, 706f
  oral, 703-704
  rectal, 703-704, 705
  regulation of, 707-708, 708f
  set-point, 707-708
  shell, 704
  skin, 705
  tympanic membrane, 704, 705
  upper limit of, 710
Temporal arteritis
  empirical corticosteroids for, 725
  fever in, 725, 726-727
Temporal space, 790, 790f
  infections of, 791-792, 792f. *See also*
      Odontogenic infections.
Tenofovir, 542, 1656f, 1657t, 1659
  dosage of, 684t-685t
  drug interactions with, 698t
  for chronic hepatitis B, 1448, 1448t,
      1881
  for hepatitis B virus, 1691t
  formulations of, 649t
  pediatric, 1646t
Tenosynovitis
  from nontuberculous mycobacteria, 2910t,
      2912
  from *Sporothrix schenckii,* 2985, 2985f,
      29862987
Terbinafine
  dosage of, 678t-679t
  for chromoblastomycosis, 2990, 2991
  for dermatophytosis, 3050t, 3058-3059
  formulations of, 649t
Terconazole
  for vulvovaginal candidiasis, 1364
  formulations of, 649t
Terrorism. *See* Bioterrorism.
Testis
  anatomy of, 1381, 1381f
  bacterial infections of, 1385
  infections of. *See* Orchitis.
Testosterone, for weight loss, 145
Tet, in tetracycline resistance, 358, 360t
Tetanolysin, 2817
Tetanospasmin, 2817, 2818
  in botulism, 2824
Tetanus, 1147-1148, 2817-2821. *See also*
    Clostridium tetani.
  cephalic, 2819, 2819f
  classification of, 2818
  clinical manifestations of, 2818-2819, 2818f,
      2819f
  diagnosis of, 2819
  epidemiology of, 2817, 2817f
  generalized, 2818, 2818f, 2819f
  history of, 2817
  in injection drug users, 3472
  localized, 2818-2819
  neonatal, 2819, 2819f
  pathogenesis of, 2818
  prophylaxis against, 2821. *See also* Diphtheria,
      tetanus, pertussis (DTP) vaccine; Tetanus
      immune globulin; Tetanus toxoid.
    for bites, 3554t
  spasm in, 2818, 2819-2820, 2819f
  stages of, 2818
  treatment of, 2819-2821, 2820t
  vs. rabies, 2052-2053

Tetanus and diphtheria toxoids, 3562-3564, 3564t. *See also* Diphtheria, tetanus, pertussis (DTP) vaccine.
Tetanus immune globulin, 66, 3574
  in pediatric HIV infection, 1650
Tetanus toxin, 26-28, 2817, 2818
Tetanus toxoid, 3572, 3572t
Tetanus toxoid vaccine, 66, 2821
  for adults, 346f, 347f
  with group B streptococcal polysaccharide, 2431
TetM, in tetracycline resistance, 265
Tetracycline(s), 356-366
  absorption of, 360, 362t
  activity spectrum of, 357-358, 359t, 360t
  age and, 244
  bone effects of, 363
  classification of, 356, 358t
  dosage of, 662t-663t
  drug interactions with, 364, 365, 698t
  elimination of, 362
  food interactions with, 364t, 365
  for actinomycosis, 2931, 2931t
  for amebiasis, 3106, 3106t
  for amebic meningitis, 1115
  for balantidiasis, 571t, 3233
  for *Brucella*, 2672
  for bubonic plague, 1211
  for *Calymmatobacterium granulomatis*, 2750
  for chlamydial endocarditis, 1001
  for chlamydial pneumonia, 2263
  for *Dientamoeba fragilis*, 572t
  for ehrlichiosis, 2315
  for epidemic typhus, 2305
  for *Francisella tularensis*, 2682, 3609-3610, 3609t
  for *Helicobacter pylori*, 2563
  for malaria, 573t, 578t
  for *Mycoplasma pneumoniae*, 2278
  for nontuberculous mycobacteria, 497
  for parasites, 589
  for periodontitis, 796, 796t
  for pneumonia, 837-839, 837t, 838t
  for psittacosis, 2257
  for rat-bite fever, 2710
  for relapsing fever, 2797
  for rickettsial diseases, 2293
  for Rocky Mountain spotted fever, 2091
  for secondary peritonitis, 938
  for trachoma, 1391
  for urethritis, 1207
  formulations of, 647t
  gastrointestinal effects of, 363t, 364
  half-life of, 360
  hepatic effects of, 245, 363t, 364
  history of, 356
  hypersensitivity reactions from, 362
  in breast milk, 361
  in liver disease, 362
  in noninfectious conditions, 366
  in pregnancy, 245
  in renal insufficiency, 362, 363t
  indications for, 365-366, 365t, 569t
  mechanism of action of, 356-358
  minimal inhibitory concentrations of, 359t
  neurotoxicity of, 363t, 364-365
  penicillin with, 365
  pharmacokinetics of, 360
  pharmacology of, 360-362, 362t
  photosensitivity from, 362
  pigmentation changes from, 362-363
  placenta crossing of, 361
  pneumococcal resistance to, 837, 837t
  prophylactic, for tularemia, 3609-3610, 3609t
  renal effects of, 245, 363t, 364
  resistance to, 358-359, 360t, 361t

Tetracycline(s) *(Continued)*
  by *Neisseria gonorrhoeae*, 2519
  by *Staphylococcus aureus*, 2334t
  by *Streptococcus agalactiae* (group B), 2426
  efflux in, 262, 263t
  enzymes in, 262
  ribosomal binding alteration in, 263
  tetM in, 265
  side effects of, 363t
  structure of, 356, 357f
  superinfections from, 363t, 365
  teeth discoloration from, 363-364
  tissue distribution of, 360-361
Tetranychus urticae, 3311
Textbooks, online, 3659t
Thailand, HIV infection in, 1468
Thalassemia, malaria protection from, 43
Thalidomide, 560
  for aphthous esophageal ulceration, 1234
  for aphthous stomatitis, 798
  for erythema nodosum leprosum, 499, 2895
  for meningitis, 1116
  for microsporidiosis, 3248
Thallium 201 single photon emission computed tomography (^{201}Tl-SPECT), for brain abscess, 1158-1159
Theophylline
  for chronic obstructive pulmonary disease, 810t
  quinolone effects on, 458-459
Therapeutic abortion, septic, 1375-1376, 1377t
Thermal injury, 158. *See also* Burn infections.
Thermogenesis, infection-related, 910
Thermometry, 703-707. *See also* Temperature, measurement of.
Thermoregulation, 707-708
Thiabendazole
  drug interactions with, 698t
  for *Angiostrongylus cantonensis* meningitis, 1115
  for capillariasis, 3298
  for chromoblastomycosis, 2990
  for cutaneous larva migrans, 571t, 3296
  for dracunculiasis, 3269-3270, 3270f
  for intestinal nematodes, 593
  for strongyloidiasis, 575t, 3265
Thiacetazone, for leprosy, 499
Thienamycin, 312, 312f
Thoracentesis, for pleural effusion/empyema, 850-851
Thoracic actinomycosis, 2926, 2927f
Throat culture
  in poststreptoccocal acute glomerulonephritis, 2388
  in streptococcal pharyngitis, 2366, 2368
  laboratory tests of, 208
  specimen collection and transport for, 206t
Throat, sore. *See* Pharyngitis.
Thrombocidins, in endocarditis, 980
Thrombocytopenia, 3427
  from cytomegalovirus, 1790
  from Epstein-Barr virus, 1806
  from rubella, 1922
  from teicoplanin, 425
  in endocarditis, 985
  in HIV infection, 1560-1561
  in sepsis, 916
  X-linked, Wiskott-Aldrich syndrome protein in, 153
Thromboembolic disease, fever in, 726
Thrombophlebitis
  septic, 917
    from *Candida*, 2947, 2951
    in injection drug users, 3467
    pelvic, 1374-1375
    suppurative, 1002-1005

Thrombophlebitis *(Continued)*
  clinical manifestations of, 1003-1004
  epidemiology of, 1002-1003
  etiology of, 1004
  in burn patients, 3550
  intracranial, 794, 795f, 1168-1170, 1169f
    cavernous sinus, 794, 795f, 797t, 1168-1170, 1169f, 1421-1424
    lateral sinus, 1168-1170
    sagittal sinus, 1168-1170, 1169f
  jugular, 754, 754f, 794, 794f
    lung abscess and, 854
    treatment of, 797, 797t
  laboratory findings in, 1004
  pathogenesis of, 1003
  pathology of, 1003
  prevention of, 1005
  superficial, 1003
  treatment of, 1004-1005
Thrombosis
  deep venous, in airplane passengers, 3644
  nonbacterial, in endocarditis, 977
Thrombotic thrombocytopenic purpura, in HIV infection, 1561
Thrush, 2940-2941, 2940f, 2941f
  chronic, 2944
  in immunocompromised host, 798-799, 2944, 3437, 3483
  prevention of, in transplant recipients, 3483
  treatment of, 2950-2951
Thymocytes
  double-positive, 131
  in HIV infection, 1535
Thymosin-alpha$_1$, 560
Thymus
  in CD4$^+$ T-cell selection, 131
  in CD8$^+$ T-cell selection, 131
Thyroglossal duct cysts, infected, 799-800
Thyroiditis, suppurative, 800
Thyrotoxicosis, diarrhea in, 1243
Tic douloureux, 1783
Ticarcillin, 291-292, 292f
  antimicrobial activity of, 333, 334t-335t
  dosage of, 652t-653t
  for anaerobes, 284t
  for bacilli, 284t
  for Enterobacteriaceae, 284t
  for peritonitis, 938
  for *Pseudomonas*, 284t
  for *Pseudomonas aeruginosa*, 275, 275f
  for secondary peritonitis, 937t
  formulations of, 646t
  minimal inhibitory concentration of, 284t
  uses of, 287, 288t
Ticarcillin-clavulanate, 316
  dosage of, 652t-653t
  for *Stenotrophomonas maltophilia*, 2619
  formulations of, 646t
Ticarcillin–clavulanic acid, for postoperative gynecologic infections, 1377t
Tick(s)
  biology and ecology of, 3312
  bites of, 3313
  eradication and control of, 3313-3314
  hard, 3312, 3313t
  in relapsing fever transmission, 2795-2796
  soft, 3312, 3313t
  species of, 3313t
Tick paralysis, 3314
Tick-borne encephalitis, 3311, 3312-3315
  clinical features of, 1941-1942
  diagnosis of, 1942
  epidemiology of, 1934-1935
  historical perspective on, 1928
  pathogenesis of, 1937-1938

Tick-borne encephalitis *(Continued)*
  prevention of, 1928, 1944
  treatment of, 1944
  vaccines for, 1944
    for travelers, 3639t, 3641
    vs. Lyme borreliosis, 1942
Tick-borne flavivirus hemorrhagic fever, clinical
    features of, 3629t
Tick-borne infections, 3312-3315. *See also*
    Zoonosis(es).
  babesiosis, 3209-3211
  boutonneuse fever, 2287-2293
  Colorado tick fever, 1900-1901, 1900f
  Crimean-Congo hemorrhagic fever, 2086t,
    2087-2089
  ehrlichioses, 235, 2311t, 2312, 3312, 3313t, 3314
  encephalitic. *See* Tick-borne encephalitis.
  epidemiology of, 2286, 3312, 3313t
  Eyach virus, 1901
  from coltiviruses, 1900-1901
  from orbiviruses, 1899
  from *Rickettsia slovaca,* 2285t, 2287t, 2293
  from seadornaviruses, 1900-1901
  geographic distribution of, 1927f, 2286, 3313t
  Lyme disease. *See* Lyme disease.
  Omsk hemorrhagic fever, 1945
  prevention of, 1901, 3314-3315
  rash in, 734
  relapsing fever, 3312-3314, 3313f, 3313t
  rickettsioses, 2287-2293
  Rocky Mountain spotted fever, 2287-2292,
    2288-2289, 2289f
  Southern tick-associated rash illness, 3314
  spotted fevers, 2287-2293
  tick behavior and, 2286
Tigecycline, 358, 358t
  for nontuberculous mycobacterial pulmonary
    disease, 2911
Tight junction apparatus cadherins, 9
Time above minimal inhibitory concentration,
    278
Tinea. *See also* Dermatophyte(s);
    Dermatophytoses.
  clinical features of, 3054-3057, 3055f-3057f
  diagnosis of, 3058
  epidemiology of, 3052-3053, 3052t, 3053t
  etiology of, 3051-3052, 3052t, 3053t
  pathogenesis of, 3053-3054
  terminology of, 3054
  treatment of, 3058-3059, 3059t
    with nitraconazole, 508-509
Tinea barbae, 3056
Tinea capitis, 3056-3057, 3057f
  age and, 3053
Tinea corporis, 3055, 3055f
Tinea cruris, 3054-3055
Tinea faciei, 3056, 3056f
Tinea imbricata, 3055-3056, 3055f
Tinea incognito, 3054
Tinea manum, 3056
Tinea nigra, 3061
Tinea pedis, 3054
Tinea versicolor, 3060
Tinidazole, 1362
  adverse effects of, 582t
  for amebiasis, 571t, 3106, 3106t
  for giardiasis, 3202t
  for luminal protozoa, 582-583
  for trichomoniasis, 576t, 3207-3208
  indications for, 568t
Tioconazole
  for onychomycosis, 3058
  for vulvovaginal candidiasis, 1364
Tioman virus, laboratory studies for, 238
Tissue tropism, 34-35

TLR2, in infection susceptibility, 48
TLR4
  in infection susceptibility, 48
  in mycobacterial disease susceptibility, 44t
Tobramycin, 329f, 330
  antimicrobial activity of, 333, 334t-335t
  dosage of, 660t-661t
  for bacterial arthritis, 1316t
  for brain abscess, 1159t
  for febrile neutropenia, 3450-3452, 3451t
  for meningitis, 1106t, 1107t
  for osteomyelitis of jaw, 797t
  for *Pseudomonas aeruginosa,* 275, 275f
  for *Pseudomonas aeruginosa* pneumonia, 2602
  for *Pseudomonas* endocarditis, 1000
  for pulmonary infections, in cystic fibrosis, 872
  for shunt infections, 1129t
  for staphylococcal endocarditis, 998
  for streptococcal endocarditis, 995
  formulations of, 647t
  names and sources of, 329t
  once-daily dosage regimens for, 347, 347t
Toenails. *See* Nails.
Togaviruses, 1913
Toll gene family, 34
Toll-like receptor(s), 37-38, 37t, 123-124
  cellular distribution of, 38, 39t
  in cytokine production, 38, 38f
  in leprosy, 2888
  signaling pathways of, 38-39, 38f
Toll-like receptor 4, 907, 907f
  gene polymorphisms in, 913
  in Enterobacteriaceae lipopolysaccharide, 2572
Toll-like receptor gene, 34
Toluidine red unheated syphilis test, 2778
TonB, in iron acquisition, 2572
Tongue, strawberry, 734
Tonsillectomy
  indications for, 757
  paralytic poliomyelitis and, 2143
Tonsillitis
  exudative, rheumatic fever after, 2381-2382
  from *Actinomyces,* 2926
  from adenoviruses, 1837-1839, 1837t
  from *Corynebacterium diphtheriae,* 2460,
    2460f
  from *Streptococcus pyogenes* (group A), 2365
Topical antibacterial therapy, 478-487. *See also*
    specific agent.
  advantages of, 478-479, 479t
  for acne vulgaris, 483
  for erythrasma, 482-483
  for pyoderma, 482
  for rosacea, 482-483
  for *Staphylococcus aureus* nasal carriage, 483-
    484
  prophylaxis with
    in burn wound infections, 482
    in catheter-related infections, 481
    in clean wound infections, 479-480
    in dialysis catheter infections, 481-482
    in operative wound infections, 480-481
    in recurrent skin/soft tissue infections, 480-481
  skin disinfection with, 479
Topoisomerase, quinolone inhibition of, 451-453
Toronto virus, 2195, 2196, 2197. *See also*
    Caliciviruses.
Toroviruses, 2203
  characteristics of, 1992
  discovery of, 1990-1991
  gastroenteritis from, 1239
  laboratory diagnosis of, 1996
Toscana virus, 2089
Tosufloxacin, 451
  for psittacosis, 2257

Total body clearance, 274
Total oral clearance, 274
Total parenteral nutrition, 144. *See also*
    Nutritional support.
  catheters for, infections of, 3352-3355, 3353t,
    3354t
Toxic epidermal necrolysis, 732, 733, 1174
  vs. staphylococcal scalded skin syndrome, 737
Toxic megacolon
  in amebic colitis, 3103
  in American trypanosomiasis, 3158, 3160, 3163
Toxic shock syndrome
  from influenza virus, 2071
  intravenous immune globulin for, 558
  nonmenstrual, 184, 2331
  skin lesions in, 1175
  staphylococcal, 737, 738t, 2321, 2331-2332,
    2331t
    diagnosis of, 2331-2332, 2331t
    menstrual, 2331
    nonmenstrual, 184, 2331
    predisposing factors to, 2331
    prevention of, 2332
    treatment of, 2332
  streptococcal, 737-738, 738t, 2331-2332,
    2331t, 2372, 2372f
    case definition for, 2372, 2373t
    clinical manifestations of, 2373-2374
    cytokine induction in, 2372-2373
    exotoxins in, 2364
    factors in, 2372, 2373t
    necrotizing fasciitis in, 1189
    pathogenesis of, 2372
    prophylaxis for, 2375
    secondary, 2375
    treatment of, 2374
  toxins of, 29-30, 2330
  in severe sepsis, 914-915
Toxic shock syndrome toxin-1, in Kawasaki
    disease, 3318
Toxic shock–like syndrome, streptococcal,
    necrotizing fasciitis in, 1189
Toxin(s), 24-31. *See also* Enterotoxins.
  adenylate cyclase, 25t
  attachment of, 26-27
  botulinum. *See* Botulinum toxin(s).
  classification of, 24, 25t
  deamidating, 25t
  entry of, 26-27
  exfoliative, 29
  glucosylating, 25t
  in gastrointestinal infections, 1219, 1220t
  mechanism of action of, 27-31
  membrane-damaging, 30
  metalloprotease, 25t
  of *Bacillus anthracis,* 27, 2485
  of *Bacteroides fragilis,* 1221
  of *Bordetella pertussis,* 27-28, 2702
  of *Clostridium botulinum,* 27, 30-31, 2822-
    2825, 2824f, 2825t
  of *Clostridium difficile,* 29, 207t, 1221, 1239
  of *Clostridium tetani,* 26-28, 2817, 2818
  of *Corynebacterium diphtheriae,* 26-28,
    1055
  of Enterobacteriaceae, 2571-2572
  of *Pseudomonas aeruginosa,* 2595-2596
  of *Staphylococcus aureus,* 2339
  pore-forming, 30
  regulation of, 24, 26, 26t
  RNA glycosidase, 25t
  secretion of, 24, 26, 26t
  Shiga, 29, 1220, 2573t, 2576-2577,
    2577f
  synthesis of, 24, 26
  therapeutic uses of, 30-31

Toxocara canis
  ocular infections from, 3294-3295
  syndrome of abdominal pain, diarrhea, and
      eosinophilia from, 1281t, 1282
  treatment of, 576t
  visceral infections from, 3293-3294, 3294t
Toxocara cati, 3293, 3294t
Toxocariasis, 1416, 3293-3294, 3294t
Toxoid, definition of, 3557
Toxoplasma [spp.]
  acute pancreatitis from, 959, 959t
  central nervous system lymphoma and, 1608
  in HIV infection
      encephalitis from, 1587, 1588f
      retinitis from, 1560
      treatment of, 580t
Toxoplasma gondii, 568, 584, 3170-3193
  brain abscess from, 1152, 1155, 1157, 1158,
      1158t
  characteristics of, 3170-3172
  chorioretinitis from, 3176, 3177, 3179-3180,
      3179f
      diagnosis of, 3186
      in pregnancy, 3191
      treatment of, 3186, 3190
  clinical manifestations of, 3176-3181
  congenital infections from, 3170, 3180-3181
      diagnosis of, 3187-3188
      incidence of, 3193t
      prevention of, 3191-3193
      treatment of, 3191
  course of, 3176-3177
  diagnosis of, 3181-3188
      antibody tests for, 3182-3183
      cerebrospinal fluid analysis in, 3185
      culture in, 3181-3182
      histologic, 3182
      in congenital infections, 3187-3188
      in encephalitis, 3183-3185, 3184f
      in immunocompetent host, 3185
      in immunocompromised host, 3185-3186
      in ocular infections, 3186
      in pregnancy, 3186-3187, 3192
      radiologic, 3183-3185, 3184f
      serologic, 3182-3183
  encephalitis from, 3175-3176, 3175f, 3179-
      3180
      diagnosis of, 3183-3186, 3184f, 3192f
      prevention of, 3190
      treatment of, 3188-3190, 3189t
  genetic susceptibility to, 3174
  histopathology of, 3182
  host cell entrance by, 8-9
  immune response to, 3173-3174
  in HIV infection, 1695, 3177, 3179-3180. *See
      also Toxoplasma gondii,* in
      immunocompromised host.
      encephalitis from, 1587, 1588f
      pneumonia from, 1572
      prophylaxis against, 1682t, 1683t, 1684t
      treatment of, 1685t, 1695-1696
  in immunocompromised host, 3177-3180
      diagnosis of, 3185-3186
      prevention of, 3188-3190, 3189t
      treatment of, 3188-3190, 3189t
  in oocysts, 3170, 3171f
  in pregnancy, 3180
      diagnosis of, 3186-3187
      treatment of, 3190-3191
  in tachyzoites, 3170-3171, 3171f
  in tissue cysts, 3171-3172, 3171f
  in transplant recipients, 3177-3179, 3496,
      3504, 3508. *See also Toxoplasma gondii,*
      in immunocompromised host.
  isolation of, 3181-3182

Toxoplasma gondii (Continued)
  lymphadenitis from, 1210, 3175f, 3176, 3177
  myalgias in, 1201
  myelitis from, 3179
  myocarditis from, 1053, 1055, 1055f, 3175f,
      3176, 3177
  myositis from, 3175f, 3176, 3177
  pathogenesis of, 3173-3174
  pathology of, 3174-3176, 3175f
  prevention of, 3177, 3191-3193
  pulmonary infections from, 3176, 3179
  strains of, 3170
  transmission of, 3172-3173, 3172f
  treatment of, 569t, 576t, 580t, 3188-3191
      for congenital infections, 3191
      for ocular infections, 3190
      immunologic, 3188
      in immunocompetent host, 3188
      in immunocompromised host, 3188-3190,
          3189t
      in pregnancy, 3190-3191
      pharmacologic, 3188
      with azithromycin, 403
      with clarithromycin, 403
      with clindamycin, 589
      with pyrimethamine, 588
      with spiramycin, 589
      with sulfonamides, 443
      with trimethoprim-sulfamethoxazole, 447
  vs. enteric fever, 1275t
  vs. infectious mononucleosis, 1812-1813
ToxR protein, 8
Trace metals, 142-143, 143t
  for elderly patient, 146, 146t
Tracheal aspirate, collection and transport of,
      206t
Tracheal cytotoxin, 27
  of *Bordetella pertussis,* 2702, 2703
Tracheitis, 758-759, 764. *See also* Laryngitis;
      Laryngotracheobronchitis.
  bacterial, 764
  from adenoviruses, 1838
Tracheobronchitis. *See also* Laryngo-
      tracheobronchitis.
  from *Aspergillus,* 2964
  from respiratory syncytial virus, 2014, 2015,
      2015t
Trachipleistophora spp., 574t, 3237, 3238t, 3245-
      3246. *See also* Microsporidia.
Trachoma, 1390-1391, 2244, 2244t. *See also
      Chlamydia trachomatis.*
  diagnosis of, 2242
  grading of, 2244, 2244t
  keratitis in, 1400
  pathogenesis of, 2241
  susceptibility to, tumor necrosis factor in, 47
  treatment of, 405, 2244, 2244t
Trade names, drug, tables of, 635t-646t
Transactivator protein, class II, in MHC class II
      molecule expression, 125
Transducers, infections of, in hemodynamic
      monitoring, 3355-3356, 3356t
Transferrin, nutritional status and, 140, 140t
Transformation, 5
  in *Streptococcus pneumoniae,* 2393
Transfusions
  Chagas' disease from, 3158, 3163
  cytomegalovirus infection from, 1789
  Epstein-Barr virus infection from, 1789
  erythrocyte
      for chronic granulomatous disease,
          109
      for sepsis, 920
  febrile neutropenia from, 3433
  for hydrops fetalis, 1896

Transfusions (Continued)
  granulocyte
      for cancer-related febrile neutropenia, 3458
      for granulocytopenia, 109
  hepatitis A from, 2166-2167, 2178
  hepatitis B from, 1430
  hepatitis C from, 1451, 1452, 1453, 1965, 1969
  hepatitis G from, 1984-1987
  hepatitis-associated aplastic anemia and, 1985
  HIV infection from, 1469, 1470, 1490
      prevention of, 1495
      screening for, 1520
  HTLV infection from, 2106
      prevention of, 2113
  in peritonitis, 940
  infections from
      in transplant recipients, 3480
      nosocomial, 3385-3388, 3385f, 3386t, 3387t
      postoperative, 3538
  intrauterine, for hydrops fetalis, 1896
  leukocyte
      for chronic granulomatous disease, 109
      for granulocytopenia, 109
  plasma
      complement replacement via, 88
      in peritonitis, 940
  TT virus infection from, 1987-1988
  West Nile virus from, 3387
Transient aplastic crisis, from parvovirus B19,
      1894, 1896
Transient erythroblastopenia of childhood, 1894,
      1896
Translocated intimin receptor, in *E. coli*
      adherence, 1221
Transmissible neurodegenerative diseases, 2219-
      2231. *See also* Prion diseases.
Transmission, routes of, 168-169
Transmission-based precautions, 3327-3330,
      3327t, 3328t, 3330t
Transplantation. *See also* Immunocompromised
      host *and specific tissue and organs.*
  adenovirus in, 1839
  aspergillosis in, 2960-2961
  Creutzfeldt-Jakob disease in, 2222, 2223
  cryptococcosis in, 3000, 3508
  cytomegalovirus in. *See* Cytomegalovirus, in
      transplant recipients.
  Epstein-Barr virus in, 3509-3510
  febrile neutropenia in, 3483-3484
  fever in, 721
  hepatitis B in, 1449-1450, 1877-1878, 1881-
      1882, 3507
  hepatitis C in, 3507
  hepatitis G in, 1986
  herpes simplex virus in, 3508
  HIV in, 3480
      screening for, 1520
  human herpesvirus 6 in, 1823, 3508
  human herpesvirus 8 in, 3509
  immunization and, 3481-3482
  immunosuppression in, infections and, 3477-
      3479
  infections in
      approach to fever in, 3483-3484
      bacteremic, 3506
      central nervous system, 3507-3508, 3507t
      characteristics of, 3502-3505, 3502t
      clinical features of, 3502-3505
      cutaneous, 3505-3506, 3505t
      epidemiology of, 3502t
      frequency of, 3502, 3502t
      gastrointestinal, 3506-3507
      graft vulnerability to, 3477, 3478t
      host factors in, 3477
      immunosuppression and, 3477-3479

Transplantation *(Continued)*
    in solid organ transplants, 3501-3510. *See also specific organs.*
    in stem cell transplants, 3486-3497. *See also* Hematopoietic stem cell transplantation.
    intra-abdominal, 3506-3507
    latent, 3479, 3502
    microbial agents of, 3479-3480, 3479t, 3480t, 3503t
    monitoring for, 3481
    mortality in, 3502t
    pretransplant evaluation for, 3480-3481, 3481t
    prevention of, 3481-3483, 3482t, 3483t
    pulmonary, 3506, 3509
    risk factors for, 3476-3484, 3476t
    sites of, 3502t
    sources of, 3479-3480
    surgical factors in, 3477, 3477f
    timing of, 3476, 3501-3502, 3501f, 3502f
    transfusion-related, 3480, 3480t
    transmission of, 3479-3480
    transplant type and, 3477, 3477f, 3502-3503, 3502t
    types of, 3502-3510, 3502t
    underlying disease and, 3477
    urinary tract, 3503, 3509
    wound, 3506
  Kaposi's sarcoma in, 1829-1830, 3509
  lymphoproliferative disease in, 3510
  mucormycosis in, 2975-2980
  nocardiosis in, 3508
  outcome in, 3501, 3501t
  polyomavirus in, 3509
  routine laboratory studies in, 3480-3481, 3481t
  skin lesions in, 741-742, 741t, 3505-3506
  survival in, 3501t
  toxoplasmosis in, 3177-3179, 3177t, 3496, 3504, 3508. *See also Toxoplasma gondii,* in immunocompromised host.
  tuberculosis in, 3480, 3481
  varicella-zoster virus in, 3439, 3494, 3508
  xenotransplantation, retrovirus transmission in, 1521
Transporter associated with antigen processing, 126
Transposable elements, 2120-2121, 2120f
Transposition, in antibiotic resistance, 255
Transposons
  conjugative, 255
  in antibiotic resistance, 253, 254-255, 254f
  in virulence gene identification, 10
Transtracheal aspiration
  for sputum collection, 826
  specimen collection and transport in, 206t
Transverse myelitis, 1147
  from enteroviruses, 2149
  from herpes simplex virus, 1766-1767, 1767f
  in schistosomiasis, 3279
Trauma
  gas gangrene from, 2832
  intraperitoneal abscess in, 943
  maxillofacial, 800
  pyogenic liver abscess in, 951, 952t
Travelers
  air travel–related problems in, 3644
  altitude sickness in, 3644
  amebiasis, in prevention of, 3107
  bloodborne diseases in, prevention of, 3642
  chronic pneumonia in, 858
  dengue in, 3647t, 3648t, 3649
  diarrhea in, 1241-1243, 1242t, 1243t, 3642, 3643, 3643f, 3652. *See also* Diarrhea, traveler's.
  eosinophilia in, 3652, 3654

Travelers *(Continued)*
  fever of unknown origin in, 720-721, 721t, 3646-3648, 3647t
  foodborne infections in, prevention of, 3642
  hepatitis in, 2171f, 2172, 2178, 3647t, 3648t, 3649
  HIV infection in, prevention of, 3642
  immunizations for, 3575, 3637-3641. *See also specific vaccines.*
    interactions among, 3641
    recommendations for, 3639t
    spacing of, 3641
  infections in
    asymptomatic, screening for, 3654
    clinical features of, 3647t
    examples of, 3647t
    exposure history for, 3648, 3647t
    history in, 3646-3648, 3647t
    incubation periods for, 3648t
  information sources for, 3638t
  jet lag in, 3644
  key preventive behaviors for, 3642-3644
  leptospirosis in, 3647t, 3648t, 3649
  malaria in, 3128, 3129, 3647t, 3649, 3648t, 3649t
    prevention of, 3642
  medical care for
    during travel, 3644
    pretravel, 3637-3641
  medical kit for, 3644
  mosquito-borne infections in. *See also* Travelers, malaria in.
    prevention of, 3642
  motion sickness in, 3644
  numbers and destinations of, 3638f
  parasitic infections in, 3652-3654
  paratyphoid fever in, 3647t, 3648t, 3649
  pretravel management of, 3637-3641
  respiratory infections in, 3647t, 3648t, 3649-3651
  rickettsial diseases in, 3647t, 3648t, 3649
  sexually transmitted diseases in, 3642
  skin disorders in, 3652, 3653f
    prevention of, 3643
  tuberculosis in, prevention of, 3644
  typhoid fever in, 3647t, 3648t, 3649
Trematodes, 3276-3284
  diagnosis of, 3259t
  intestinal, 3277t, 3279f, 3282-3283
  liver, 3277t, 3279f, 3281-3282, 3281f
  lung, 3277t, 3279f, 3283
  syndrome of abdominal pain, diarrhea, and eosinophilia from, 1281t, 1283
  treatment of, 570t, 572t, 595-596
Trench fever, 740
  from *Bartonella quintana,* 2734
Trench mouth, 754, 756, 791, 2841
Treponema [spp.], 2785
Treponema carateum, 2769, 2785, 2787
Treponema denticola, odontogenic infections from, 788, 788f
Treponema pallidum, 2768-2783. *See also* Syphilis.
  antibodies to, 59, 2778t, 2779, 2780
  characteristics of, 2769-2770
  darkfield examination for, 1342-1343
  diagnosis of, 1342-1343
  direct examination of, 2778, 2778f
  hemagglutination assay for, 58, 2778t, 2779, 2787
  in HIV infection, 1690t, 1701-1702, 2782, 2783
  isolation of, 2780
  keratitis from, 1400

Treponema pallidum (Continued)
  meningitis from, 1583-1584
    acute, 1088
      clinical features of, 1100
      diagnosis of, 1103-1104
      treatment of, 1106t, 1115
    chronic, 1138, 1140
  pathogenesis of, 2770-2771
  penicillins for, 288t
  syphilis from. *See* Syphilis.
  uveitis from, 1414-1415
Treponema pallidum subsp. *endemicum,* 2769, 2785, 2787
Treponema pallidum subsp. *pallidum,* 2769, 2785
Treponema pallidum subsp. *pertenue,* 2769, 2785, 2786-2787, 2786f, 2787f
Treponematoses, endemic, 2785-2788
  clinical manifestations of, 2786
  diagnosis of, 2787-2788
  epidemiology of, 2785-2786
  public health control of, 2788
  treatment of, 2788
Triamcinolone, for chronic obstructive pulmonary disease, 810t
Triatoma infestans, Chagas' disease from, 3159
Triazoles, 507
Tribec virus, 1899
Trichinella [spp.], 3268, 3268t, 3293
Trichinella nativa, syndrome of abdominal pain, diarrhea, and eosinophilia from, 1281t, 1282
Trichinella spiralis, 1266
  syndrome of abdominal pain, diarrhea, and eosinophilia from, 1281t, 1282
  treatment of, 576t
  vs. enteric fever, 1275t
Trichinosis, 1202, 3268-3269, 3268t, 3269f, 3269t
  myositis in, 1202
Trichloroacetic acid
  for genital warts, 1849
  for human papillomavirus, 1691t
Trichoderma spp., 3073
Trichomonas [spp.], 3207
  collection and transport of, 207t
  metronidazole-resistant, 390
Trichomonas tenax, 3205
Trichomonas vaginalis, 212, 1361-1362, 1362t, 1363f, 1363t, 1628, 3205-3208
  clinical manifestations of, 3206-3207
  diagnosis of, 1360, 1361f, 3207
  epidemiology of, 3205-3206
  in pregnancy, 1362, 3206, 3208
  metronidazole for, 393
    resistance to, 3208
  transmission of, 3206
  treatment of, 576t, 580t, 3207-3208
  urethral syndrome from, 1352
  urethritis from, 1348, 1351, 3207. *See also* Urethritis, nongonococcal.
Trichophyton [spp.], 3051-3059. *See also* Dermatophyte(s); Dermatophytoses.
Trichophyton concentricum, 3052t, 3053, 3054
  tinea imbricata from, 3055-3056, 3055f
Trichophyton erinacei, 3052, 3052t
  tinea corporis from, 3055, 3055f
Trichophyton gourvilii, 3052t, 3053, 3053t
Trichophyton interdigitale, 3052, 3052t, 3053, 3054
Trichophyton mentagrophytes, nail infections from, 3057
Trichophyton mentagrophytes complex
  classification of, 3051-3052, 3052t
  tinea pedis from, 3054
Trichophyton quinckeanum, 3052, 3052t, 3053-3054

Trichophyton rubrum, 3052-3053, 3052t
  deep infections from, 3057, 3057f
  nodular folliculitis from, 3055
  onychomycosis from, 3057
  tinea corporis from, 3055
  tinea cruris from, 3054-3055
  tinea faciei from, 3056, 3056f
  tinea manum from, 3056
  tinea pedis from, 3054
Trichophyton schoenleinii, 3052t, 3053, 3053t,
    3058
  favus from, 3051, 3053, 3056
Trichophyton simii, 3052, 3052t
Trichophyton soudanense, 3052t, 3053, 3053t
  nail infections from, 3057
Trichophyton tonsurans, 3052t, 3053, 3053t,
    3054, 3056
Trichophyton verrucosum, 2053t, 3052, 3052t,
    3054
  tinea corporis from, 3055
Trichophyton violaceum, 3052t, 3053, 3053t
Trichophyton yaoundei, 3052t, 3053, 3053t
Trichosporon asahii, 3073
Trichosporon [spp.], 3073, 3076t
  white piedra from, 3061
Trichosporon asteroides, 3073
Trichosporon beigelii, 3061
  endocarditis from, 993
Trichosporon capitatum, 3074
Trichosporon cutaneum, 3073
Trichosporon inkin, 3061, 3073
Trichosporon mucoides, 3061, 3073
Trichosporon ovoides, 3061, 3073
Trichostrongylus spp., treatment of, 576t
Trichuris trichiura, 3261t, 3263-3264, 3263f
  treatment of, 576t, 592
Triclabendazole, for flukes, 572t, 577t
  intestinal, 3277t
  liver, 3277t, 3282
Triclosan, skin disinfection with, 479
Tricuspid valve, in endocarditis, 984
Trifluorothymidine, 524f
Trifluridine, 515t, 538
  for herpes simplex virus, 1686t
  for ocular vaccinia, 1403
  for vaccinia conjunctivitis, 1390t
Trigeminal neuralgia, 1783
Trimethoprim, 440, 443-447
  adverse effects of, 445
  antimicrobial activity of, 444, 444t
  dosage of, 670t-671t
  drug interactions with, 445, 698t-699t
  for acute pyelonephritis, 889
  for lower urinary tract infections, 890
  for malaria, 587-588
  for *Pneumocystis jirovecii* pneumonia, 575t
  for relapsing urinary tract infections, 891
  formulations of, 648t
  in pregnancy, 447
  mechanism of action of, 443, 443f
  pharmacology of, 445
  resistance to, 265, 444-445
    by *Staphylococcus aureus,* 2334t
  structure of, 443, 443f
  uses of, 446-447
  with other antimicrobial agents, 445-446
Trimethoprim-dapsone, for *Pneumocystis,* 3088
Trimethoprim-sulfamethazole
  dosage of, 670t-671t
  for brain abscess, 1159t
  for cyclosporiasis, 3229
  for isosporiasis, 3232
  for *Pneumocystis,* 3088
    for prophylaxis, 3089-3090

Trimethoprim-sulfamethazole *(Continued)*
  for *Pneumocystis jirovecii,* for prophylaxis,
    3447, 3447t
  for pneumonia, 837-839, 837t, 838t
  for *Toxoplasma gondii*
    for encephalitis prophylaxis, 3190
    in immunocompromised host, 3189, 3189t
  for transplant-related toxoplasmosis
    prophylaxis, 3177
  formulations of, 648t
  prophylactic, for transplant recipients, 3177, 3482
Trimethoprim-sulfamethoxazole
  antimicrobial activity of, 444
  for actinomycetoma, 2995
  for acute pyelonephritis, 889
  for chronic granulomatous disease, 107
  for COPD exacerbations, 811t
  for *Cyclospora,* 572t
  for dialysis-related peritonitis, 942t
  for *Isospora belli,* 1689t-1690t
  for *Listeria monocytogenes,* 2483
  for lower urinary tract infections, 890
  for melioidosis, 2629t
  for meningitis, 1106t, 1107t
  for nocardiosis, 2920, 2920t, 2921
    for prophylaxis, 2921
  for paracoccidioidomycosis, 3065
  for parasites, 588
  for *Pneumocystis jirovecii,* 569t, 575t, 580t,
    1568, 1681t, 1683t, 1685t, 1692-1693,
    1694-1698
    pediatric, 1649
  for prostatitis, 895
  for Q fever endocarditis, 1001
  for relapsing urinary tract infections, 891
  for *Salmonella,* 2650
  for *Shigella,* 1689t
  for *Stenotrophomonas maltophilia,* 2619
  for *Toxoplasma gondii,* 1682t, 1685t
    for chorioretinitis prophylaxis, 3190
  for traveler's diarrhea, 1243
  for urinary tract infections, 446
    recurrent, 892
  for Whipple's disease, 1309, 1310t
  in HIV infection, 1567
  indications for, 569t
  resistance to, 444
    pneumococcal, 837, 837t
Trimetrexate
  for *Pneumocystis,* 3088, 3089
  for *Pneumocystis jirovecii,* 1685t, 1693-1694
  formulations of, 648t
Trioleandomycin, 408
Trismus, from tetanus, 2818, 2818f
Tropheryma [spp.], 228-229
Tropheryma whipplei, 1145, 1306, 1306f
  detection of, 1309
  encephalititis from, 1145
  endocarditis from, 993
  laboratory tests for, 228
  prosthetic valve endocarditis from, 1026
  uveitis from, 1417
  Whipple's disease from, 1145
Tropical eosinophilia, 835
Tropical polymyositis, 1194-1197. *See also*
    Myositis.
Tropical pulmonary eosinophilia, 3274-3275, 3274f
  diethylcarbamazine for, 572t
Tropical spastic paraparesis, 2108t, 2110-2111
  transfusion-related, 2106
  treatment of, 2112-2113
Tropical sprue, 1301-1305
  clinical manifestations of, 1303-1304
  diagnosis of, 1304

Tropical sprue *(Continued)*
  epidemiology of, 1301-1302
  etiology of, 1302-1303
  intestinal abnormalities in, 1304
  morphology of, 1304
  pathogenesis of, 1303f
  treatment of, 1305
Tropism, cellular (tissue), 34-35
Trovafloxacin, 451
  adverse effects of, 467
  dosage of, 674t-675t
  for gonococcal urethritis, 460
  for intra-abdominal infections, 461
  for meningitis, 465, 1113
  for penicillin-resistant enterococcal
    endocarditis, 997
  for peritonitis, 939
  for pneumonia, 837-839, 837t, 838t
  for respiratory infections, 462
  for secondary peritonitis, 937t
  formulations of, 648t
  pneumococcal resistance to, 837, 837t
Trypanosoma [spp.]
  characteristics of, 3156-3157
  classification of, 3157
  geographic distribution of, 3157, 3157f
  keratoconjunctivitis from, 1147-1148, 1393,
    1405
  life cycle of, 3157, 3158f
  neuritis from, 1147-1148
  transmission of, 3157-3158
Trypanosoma brucei complex, 3157. *See also*
    Trypanosomiasis, African.
Trypanosoma brucei subsp. *brucei,* 3157
Trypanosoma brucei subsp. *gambiense*
  myocarditis from, 1053
  treatment of, 576t, 590-592
Trypanosoma brucei subsp. *rhodesiense,* 3157
  myocarditis from, 1053
  treatment of, 576t, 590-592
Trypanosoma cruzi, 3157-3158, 3158f. *See also*
    Trypanosomiasis, American.
  complement-dependent killing of, 77
  life cycle of, 3157, 3158f
  myocarditis from, 1053
  neuritis from, 1147-1148
  transfusion-related, 3388
  transmission of, 3157-3158
  treatment of, 576t, 580t, 590-592
Trypanosoma gambiense, neuritis from, 1147-
    1148
Trypanosoma rhodesiense, neuritis from, 1147-
    1148
Trypanosomatidae infections, 568
  treatment of, 569t, 576t, 580t
Trypanosomes, specimen collection and transport
    in, 205t
Trypanosomiasis, 3156-3163
  African, 3165-3169
    clinical features of, 3166-3167
    course of, 3166-3167
    diagnosis of, 3167-3168, 3167f
    epidemiology of, 3166
    etiology of, 3165
    neuritis in, 1147-1148
    ocular involvement in, 1147-1148, 1393, 1405
    pathogenesis and pathophysiology of, 3165-
      3166
    prevention of, 3169
    treatment of, 569t, 576t, 590-592, 3168-3169
    vs. malaria, 3133
  American, 3156-3163
    clinical features of, 3159-3160, 3160f
    congenital, 3158

Trypanosomiasis *(Continued)*
course of, 3159-3160
diagnosis of, 3161-3162
epidemiology of, 3159
etiology of. *See also Trypanosoma cruzi.*
in immunocompromised host, 3160-3161
myocarditis in, 1053, 1055
pathology of, 3158, 3158f
prevention of, 3163
reactivation, 3160-3161
transfusion-related, 3158, 3163
treatment of, 569t, 576t, 590-592, 3162-3163
in HIV infection, 1692t
hypergammaglobulinemia in, 65
Trypanozoon spp., 3157
Tsukamurella [spp.], 228-229
Tsukamurella paurometabola, 2473
TT virus, 1987-1988
Tuberculin test, 2860-2861, 2861t
in HIV infection, 2861
positivity of
criteria for, 2872, 2872t
treatment for, 2874-2875
Tuberculoid leprosy, 1147-1148
Tuberculoma
intracranial, 2878
pulmonary, 2865, 2865f
Tuberculosis, 2852-2883
age influence on, 2862
aortic, 2882-2883
arthritis in, 1319
atypical, chest film in, 864f
case rate for, 2855-2856, 2856f, 2856t
caseous material in, 2859
central nervous system, 2877-2878, 2877f
cervical lymphadenitis in, 1206-1207
chest film in, 864f, 865f
complications of, corticosteroids for, 558-559
contact exposure to, treatment of, 2873-2874, 2873f
contact tracing in, 858
cutaneous, 2882
emergence of, 182-183
endobronchial, 2865
epidemiology of, 2855-2859
epididymitis in, 1384
erythema induratum in, 733
extrapulmonary, 1319, 2875-2883
in HIV infection, 2875
treatment of, 2875
fever in, 726
gastrointestinal, 1269, 2881
in HIV infection, 2881
vs. enteric fever, 1274t, 1277-1278
genetic factors in, 43, 44, 44t, 2858
genitourinary, 2880-2881, 2880t
hematologic abnormalities in, 2876-2877
hepatic, 2881
history of, 2852-2853
hypersensitivity in, 2861-2862
immunity in, 2859-2860
in adolescents, 2862, 2863f
in children, 2862
in elderly, 2863, 3519
in HIV infection, 182-183, 1472, 1481, 1486-
1487, 1561, 1568, 1570-1571, 1570f,
2863, 2865, 2865t
epidemiology of, 2857
extrapulmonary, 2875
gastrointestinal, 2881
genitourinary, 2880
in developing world, 1472
latent, 2874
miliary, 2877

Tuberculosis *(Continued)*
peripheral lymphadenitis in, 2882, 2882f
progression of, 2858
prophylaxis against, 1681t, 1700
spread of, 2858-2859
treatment of, 1687t, 1699-1700
multidrug resistance in, 489, 2869
in immigrants, 2855, 2856f, 2856t
in immunocompromised host, 3436-3437. *See
also* Tuberculosis, in HIV infection.
in infancy, 2862
in injection drug users, 3469
in lower lung field, 2865
in midadulthood, 2862-2863
in transplantation, 3480, 3481
in travelers, prevention of, 3644
incidence of, 2856, 2856t
keratitis in, 1400
laboratory findings in, 2866
laryngeal, 759
late generalized, 2876
late hematogenous, 2863
latent
in HIV infection, 2874
tests for, 227-228, 2861
treatment of, 2872-2874, 2872t
lymph node, 2881-2881
measles in, 2035
meningitis in, 1135, 1136, 2877-2878, 2877f
in immunocompromised host, 1140
microbiology of, 2853-2855, 2854t
miliary, 2875-2876, 2876f, 2876t
cryptic, 2876
effusion in, 2878
in HIV infection, 2877
morbidity in, 2855-2857
mortality in, 2855-2857
nonreactive, 2859, 2876
nosocomial
control of, 2858-2859
prevention of, 3327-3329
spread of, 2858
ocular, 1415-1416, 1416f, 1418
pancreatic, 2881
pathogenesis of, 2861-2863, 2863f
pericarditis in, 1059, 1060, 1060f, 1062
peripheral osteoarticular, 2880
physical examination in, 2866
pleural effusion in, 2878
pleurisy in, 847
diagnosis of, 849
postprimary (adult-type), 2864-2865, 2864f
primary (childhood), 2862, 2863-2864
primary hepatic, 2877
primary infections in, 2861-2862
progression of, 2858
proliferative response in, 2859
prostatitis in, 1383t, 1384
pulmonary, 2863-2875
after childhood, 2864
apical localization of, 2862
cancer in, 2867
chronic, 2862
diagnosis of, 2866
drug-resistant, 2867, 2867t
in HIV infection. *See* Tuberculosis, in HIV
infection.
radiography of, 2866
reinfections in, 2862
renal, 2880, 2880t
risk factors for, 2857, 2863
sclerosing mediastinitis in, 1075
skeletal, 2879-2880, 2879f
spread of, 2857, 2858-2859

Tuberculosis *(Continued)*
sputum in, 825, 825f, 826
susceptibility to, 48
symptoms of, 2865-2866
treatment of, 334t-335t, 344t, 403, 489-496,
490t-492t, 2867-2875. *See also*
Antituberculous drugs *and specific agents.*
collapse therapy in, 2878
interferon in, 555-556
paradoxical response in, 1700
resistance in, 48, 184, 2857, 2858, 2867
in HIV infection, 489, 2869
vaccination in, 2875
tuberculin converters in, 2874
tuberculin positivity in, 2856, 2856f, 2856t
tuberculin test for, 2860-2861, 2861t
tuberculin test in, 2860-2861, 2861t
in HIV infection, 2861
positivity of
criteria for, 2872, 2872t
treatment for, 2874-2875
worldwide distribution of, 2856-2857, 2857t
Tubo-ovarian abscess, 1378, 1379t, 1380
Tularemia, 2674-2683, 3607-3611. *See also
Francisella tularensis.*
as biological weapon, 3607-3611
clinical features of, 3607-3608, 3608t
diagnosis of, 3608-3609, 3608t
differential diagnosis of, 3608t
infection control measures for, 3610
postexposure prevention for, 3609-3610,
3609t, 3611t
treatment of, 3610t, 3611, 3611t
vaccine for, 3610
clinical manifestations of, 2678-2681
cutaneous, 2681
disinfection/sterilization and, 3342
epidemiology of, 2676-2677, 2676f, 2677f
glandular, 2679
history in, 823t
incidence of, 2676, 2676f
isolation precautions for, 3330t
oculoglandular, 2679-2680
pharyngeal, 2680
pneumonic, 2680-2681, 2681f
prevention of, 2683
treatment of, 2682-2683
with quinolones, 465
typhoidal, 2680
ulceroglandular, 2679, 2679f
Tumbu fly, myiasis from, 3307-3308, 3308t
Tumor necrosis factor
gene polymorphisms in, 913
in hepatitis B susceptibility, 45
in infections susceptibility, 47
in lesishmaniasis susceptibility, 44t
in malaria susceptibility, 44t
in severe sepsis, 912
in shock, 914
in systemic response, 908
Tumor necrosis factor-α, 38, 38t
as pyrogen, 708-709, 711-712
in acute-phase response, 39
in HIV infection, 1536, 1538, 1539, 1539f
in melioidosis, 2624
in meningococcal disease, 2508
in *Pseudomonas aeruginosa* resistance, 2590
in *Streptococcus agalactiae* (group B),
2426
Tumor necrosis factor-β, in HIV replication,
1539, 1539f
Tungiasis, 3310
Turicella otitidis, 2471
Turkey rhinotracheitis virus, 2026-2027, 2027f

24-hour area under serum concentration curve:minimal inhibitory concentration ratio, 277-278, 277f

Twins, disease susceptibility in, 43, 43t

Tympanic membrane temperature, 704, 705. *See also* Temperature.

Tympanocentesis, 768, 769

Tympanometry, 768

Tympanostomy tubes, 770-771

Typhlitis, 973, 3457
  chemotherapy-induced, 3438, 3457
  etiology of, 3421t
  from *Clostridium,* 2834, 2835t, 2836
  in stem cell transplant, 3421t, 3488

Typhoid fever, 1267. *See also* Enteric fever.
  chloramphenicol-resistant, 370
  cystic fibrosis and, 46
  diarrhea in, 1242
  epidemiology of, 2638
  fever in, 723, 723f
  from *Francisella tularensis,* 2680
  from *Salmonella typhi,* 2644-2645
  geographic distribution of, 3640f
  history of, 2636
  in travelers, 3647t, 3648t, 3649
  rash in, 730, 733, 1186
  rose spots in, 730, 1186
  skin lesions in, 1186
  treatment of, 2648-2649, 2649t

Typhoid vaccine, 1226, 2646-2647, 3572
  for travelers, 3639, 3639t

Typhus
  African tick, 2090t, 2285t, 2287t, 2292-2293, 3653f
    vs. malaria, 3133
  endemic, 1275t
  epidemic, 1275t, 2285t, 2286, 2287t, 2303-2305, 2308
  history of, 2636
  murine, 2287t, 2306-2308
  Queensland tick, 2287t
  scrub, 1275t, 2287t, 2309-2310, 2309f, 2310t, 3311
  Siberian tick, 2285t, 2287t, 2292
  vs. enteric fever, 1275t

Tyrosine kinase, in *Pseudomonas aeruginosa,* 2592

Tzanck smear, for herpes simplex virus, 1343

U

Uganda, HIV infection in, 1467, 1467f

Ukraine, HIV infection in, 1466, 1466f

Ulcer(s)
  aphthous
    esophageal, 1233, 1233t
    in acute retroviral syndrome, 1552, 1553f
    oral. See Ulcer(s), oral.
  Buruli, 2912
  Chiclero's, 3145t, 3149, 3150
  corneal, 1388. *See also* Keratitis.
    from microsporidia, 1405, 3238t, 3243-3245, 3248t, 3249
    vs. conjunctivitis, 1393
  cutaneous
    chronic, 1184
    diabetic, 1184
    from guinea worm, 3269-3270, 3270f
    from nontuberculous mycobacteria, 2910t, 2912, 2913t
    in aspergillosis, 2966, 2966f
    in blastomycosis, 3032, 3033f
    in chromoblastomycosis, 2989, 2989f
    in cryptococcosis, 3004-3005, 3004f

Ulcer(s) *(Continued)*
    in injection drug users, 3463-3464
    in leishmaniasis, 3149f
    in spinal cord injury, 3515-3516
    in syphilis, 733
  esophageal, 1233, 1233t
    from *Corynebacterium diphtheria,* 1180-1181
    from *Entamoeba histolytica,* 3100, 3100f
    from *Francisella tularensis,* 2679, 2679f
    genital, 1338-1344, 1339f-1341f, 1342t. *See also* Genital lesions.
      from *Haemophilus ducreyi,* 2667
      in HIV infection, 1489, 1630
    in donovanosis, 2748-2749, 2749f
    in histoplasmosis, 3019, 3020, 3021, 3021f
    laboratory studies for, 213
    membranous, 1180
    neurotrophic, in leprosy, 2895
    oral, 754, 798
      differential diagnosis of, 754, 756
      in acute retroviral syndrome, 1552, 1553f
      in hand-foot-mouth disease, 798-799, 2150
      in herpes simplex virus infection, 1765-1766, 1766f, 1773-1774, 1773t. *See also* Herpes simplex virus, orofacial.
      in histoplasmosis, 3021, 3021f
      in HIV infection, 1555
      in immunocompromised host, 798-799
      in Marshall's syndrome, 1208
      in paracoccidioidomycosis, 3064-3065, 3065f
      vs. herpetic pharyngitis, 756
    peptic
      blood group O–associated, 46
      clarithromycin for, 405
      from *Candida albicans,* 1269
      from *Helicobacter pylori,* 2560-2561, 2561, 2561f
      in HIV infection, 1576
    pressure
      in elderly, 3519-3520
      in spinal cord injury, 3515-3516
      infected, 1184

Ulcerative blepharitis, 1420

Ulcerative gingivitis, acute necrotizing, 754, 756, 791
  treatment of, 796, 796t

Ulcerative postdysenteric colitis, 3103

Ulceroglandular syndrome, 1208, 1209t

Ultrasonography
  for cholecystitis, 956f
  for intraperitoneal abscess, 943-944
  for perinephric abscess, 895, 896f
  for pleural effusion/empyema, 847-848
  for secondary peritonitis, 935
  for splenic abscess, 968
  for urinary tract infections, 897, 898f, 899f

Upper respiratory infections. See Respiratory tract infections.

Urea, for onychomycosis, 3058

Ureaplasma [spp.], 2270

Ureaplasma diversum, 2281t

Ureaplasma parvum, 2280-2282

Ureaplasma urealyticum, 2280-2282, 2281t
  diagnosis of, 1348
  in urinary tract infections, 882
  postpartum endometritis from, 1374
  treatment of
    with linezolid, 437, 437t
    with macrolides, 403
    with quinupristin-dalfopristin, 425
  urethritis from, 1347-1355. *See also* Urethritis, nongonococcal.

Urease breath tests, for *Helicobacter pylori,* 2562, 2562t

Ureidopenicillins, 287, 288t, 292-293, 292f
  in preemptive pancreatic infection treatment, 965t
  susceptibility to, 283-284

Uremia, in endocarditis, 984

Ureteral stenosis, from BK virus, 1858

Ureteritis, from microsporidia, 3243

Urethra
  female, in urinary tract infections, 880
  length of, in host defense, 36

Urethral syndrome, 886, 1352
  from *Chlamydia trachomatis,* 1352

Urethritis, 1347-1355
  as sexually transmitted disease, 1350
  asymptomatic, 1351-1352
  from *Candida,* 2946, 2950
  from *Chlamydia trachomatis,* 1347-1355, 2245f, 2246, 2247t
    treatment of, 1352-1354, 2247t, 2249-2250
  from herpes simplex virus, 1766. See also Herpes simplex virus, genital.
  gonococcal, 2519, 2520f
    clinical features of,1347, 1349-1350
    complications of, 1352
    diagnosis of, 1350
    etiology of, 1349
    in females, 1352
    quinolones for, 460
    treatment of, 1352-1354
  in HIV infection, 1349
  laboratory findings in, 1347-1349, 1348f
  meningococcal, 2506
  nongonococcal, 1347-1355, 2245f, 2246, 2247t
    clinical features of, 1347, 1349-1350, 2246
    complications of, 1350, 2246
    diagnosis of, 1350, 2246
    etiology of, 1349t, 1350-1351, 2246
    from *Chlamydia trachomatis,* 1347-1355, 2245f, 2246, 2247t, 2248
    from *Mycoplasma genitalium,* 2281, 2281t
    from *Trichomonas vaginalis,* 1348, 1351, 3207
    from *Ureaplasma urealyticum,* 2281, 2281t
    in females, 1352, 2248, 2250
    in Reiter's syndrome, 1354-1355, 2247-2248
    macrolides for, 401t
    recurrent, 1353-1354
    treatment of, 1352-1354, 2247t, 2249
  noninfectious, 1349
  physical examination in, 1347
  postgonococcal, 1351
  treatment of, for sexual partners, 1352, 1354
  urethral syndrome from, 1352

Urgency, 891

Urinalysis, 211
  in endocarditis, 985
  in HIV testing, 1512
  in pneumonia, 828
  microscopic examination of, 884, 884t
  pH of, in urinary tract infection treatment, 888
  specimen collection and transport for, 207t, 885, 3374
  specimen collection and transport in, 207t

Urinary antigen assay, pneumonia diagnosis by, 208

Urinary anti-infectives
  dosage of, 674t-675t
  formulations of, 648t

Urinary calculi
  catheter-related, 3373
  in urinary tract infections, 881, 881f

Urinary obstructions, catheter-related, 3373

Urinary tract catheterization. *See also* Urinary
   tract infections, catheter-related.
  intermittent, 3374
  prevention of, 3374
  suprapubic, 3374
Urinary tract infections, 875-901. *See also*
   Bacteriuria; Cystitis; Pyelonephritis.
  ascending route of, 876
  bacteria in, 881-882
  calculi in, 881, 881f
  catheter-related, 3370-3377
    from long-term catheterization, 3372t, 3373-
      3374
    from short-term catheterization, 3372-3373,
      3372t
    historical perspective on, 3370
    pathogenesis of, 3370-3371
    patient-patient transmission of, 3377
    prevention of, 3374-3376
    risk factors for, 3371
    treatment of complications of, 3376-3377
  chronic, 875
  clinical manifestations of, 884
  coagulase-negative staphylococcal, 2355-2356,
    2356t
  complementary and alternative medicine for,
    20, 21, 604t
  complicated, 875
  cranberry juice for, 20t, 21
  diagnosis of, 884-886
    culture in, 885-886
    microscopic examination in, 884, 884t
    presumptive, 884, 884t
    site localization in, 886
  epidemiology of, 881-883, 883t
  Escherichia coli P fimbriae in, 19-20, 19f
  from *Actinomyces,* 2928
  from *Blastomyces dermatitidis,* 2946, 2950
  from *Candida,* 2946, 2950
  from *Corynebacterium urealyticum,* 2469-2470
  from *Enterococcus,* 2412
  from *Escherichia coli,* 2574
  from *Klebsiella pneumoniae,* 2578
  from microsporidia, 3243
  from *Proteus,* 2580
  from *Proteus mirabilis,* 2580
  from *Pseudomonas aeruginosa,* 2605
  fungal, 892
  hematogenous route of, 876
  host response in, 879-881, 879f, 879t, 881f
  host-parasite interaction in, 876-881
  imaging of, 896-900, 897f-900f
  in cancer, 3438
  in children, 886-887
    imaging of, 899-900, 900f
  in elderly, 3517-3518
  in females, 886, 886f, 887
  in HIV infection, 1385-1386
  in immunocompromised host, 3438
    laboratory diagnosis of, 3429
  in males, 876, 887, 888
  in pregnancy, 892-893
  in spinal cord injury, 3513-3514
  in transplant recipients, 3487, 3503, 3509
  kidney function in, 884
  laboratory tests for, 211
  lower tract, 890-891
  lymphatic route of, 876
  microorganisms in, 876-878, 877t
  natural history of, 886-887
  nitrofurantoin for, 474
  nosocomial, 3370-3377. *See also* Urinary tract
    infections, catheter-related.
  pathogenesis of, 876-881

Urinary tract infections *(Continued)*
  pathology of, 875-876, 875f, 876f
  proteinuria in, 884
  pyuria in, 884
  recurrent
    methenamine for, 476-477
    nitrofurantoin for, 475
    periurethral colonization in, 880
  reinfections in, 875
    treatment of, 891-892
  relapsing, 875
    treatment of, 891
  remission in, 887
  resistance to, 36
  risk factors for, 883
  symptoms of, 884
  treatment of, 887-892, 901f
    considerations in, 887-888
    hydration in, 888
    surgery in, 900-901
    urinary pH in, 888
    with analgesics, 888
    with antimicrobial agents, 888-892
    with quinolones, 459-460
    with sulfonamides, 443
    with trimethoprim-sulfamethoxazole, 446
  uncomplicated, 875
  vesicoureteral reflux in, 881, 882f, 886
Urine
  acidification of, 888
    methenamine and, 476
  bactericidal properties of, 36, 879, 888
  collection of, 207t, 885
    external devices for, 3374
  culture of, 207t, 211, 885-886
  examination of. *See* Urinalysis.
  formaldehyde concentration in, methenamine
    and, 476
Urine antigen testing, for *Legionella
    pneumophila,* 2718, 2718t
Urogenital infections. *See under* Genital;
    Genitourinary tract infections.
Urokinase, for pleural effusion/empyema, 851
Uromucoid, 879, 879f
Uropathogens, 876-878, 877t
Uroplakin, *Escherichia coli* binding to, 878
Urosepsis, 875
Ursodeoxycholic acid, for hepatitis, 1437
US28, 98
Ushers, 8
Usutu virus, 1945t
Uta, 3145t, 3149, 3150
Uterine infections
  postpartum, 1373-1375
  prenatal, 1372-1373
Uterus, 927
  dysfunctional bleeding from, in HIV infection,
    1630
Uveitis, 1413-1418
  autoimmune, 1414
  classification of, 1413, 1413t
  clinical features of, 1414-1417
  diagnosis of, 1417-1418
  epidemiology of, 1414
  etiology of, 1413t, 1414, 1414f
  from *Bartonella henselae,* 1417, 1417f
  from *Brucellosis,* 1417
  from *Candida,* 1417, 1418, 2947-2948, 2948f,
    2951
  from cytomegalovirus, 1415-1416
  from herpes simplex virus, 1416, 1418,
    1773t
  from *Histoplasma capsulatum,* 3021
  from HTLV, 2111

Uveitis *(Continued)*
  from *Mycobacterium tuberculosis,* 1416, 1416f
  from rifabutin, 493
  from rifamycin, 377
  from *Toxocara,* 1416
  from *Toxoplasma gondii,* 3176, 3177, 3179-
    3180, 3179f
    diagnosis of, 3186
    treatment of, 3186, 3190
  from *Treponema pallidum,* 1414-1415
  granulomatous, 1413, 1413f
  in acute retinal necrosis, 1416, 1417f
  in leprosy, 1417
  in leptospirosis, 1416-1417
  in Lyme disease, 1417
  in Reiter's syndrome, 1354-1355, 1414
  in Whipple's disease, 1417
  pathophysiology of, 1414
  terminology for, 1413, 1413t
  treatment of, 1418
  vs. conjunctivitis, 1393

V

V factor, 216t
  in *Haemophilus influenzae* growth, 2661
VacA, 2558, 2559
Vaccine(s), 3557-3585. *See also specific diseases
    or vaccines.*
  adjuvants for, 3557, 3558
  administration route for, 3558
  adverse effects of, 3559, 3560-3561, 3560t,
    3580t-3581t
    compensation for, 3582
    reporting of, 3579, 3582
  age and, 3558
  assessment of need for, 3578-3579
  bacille Calmette-Guérin, 2320, 2875
    parenteral exposure through, 123
  combination, 3579
  complement deficiency and, 88
  conjugate, B cells in, 62, 63f
  constituents of, 3557
  contraindications to, 3583t-3584t
  currently available, 3561-3574, 3562t
  definition of, 3557
  determinants of immunogenicity from, 3557-
    3558
  development of, 3559-3561, 3560t, 3561t
  dosage for, 3558
  for health care workers, 3575
  for HIV-infected patients, 3577-3578, 3578t
  for immunocompromised hosts, 3577-3578,
    3578t
  for occupational exposures, 3575
  for pregnant patients, 3575, 3577
  for travel, 3575
  handling of, 3578
  immune response to
    measurement of, 3559
    mobilization of, 3558-3559
    temporal course of, 3559
    unanticipated, 3559
  immunization principles and, 3560-3561,
    3560t, 3561t
  immunologic basis for, 3557
  improving coverage with, 3582, 3584-3585
  information sources for, 3585
  interrupted schedules of, 3579
  intervals between, 3579
  live vs. killed or subunit, 3558
  major histocompatibility complex and, 3558
  P fimbriae in, 19
  parent and patient education on, 3579

Vaccine(s) (Continued)
  postexposure, 3578
  records of, 3579
  safety of, 3560-3561, 3561t
  schedules of
    for adults, 3575, 3576f, 3577f
    for children, 3563f, 3564t, 3574-3575
  simultaneous administration of, 3579
  standards for, 3582, 3582t-3584t
  storage of, 3578
  use of, 3574-3585
Vaccinia, 740-741, 1743f, 1744-1746
  as zoonosis, 1746
  generalized, 740-741, 1745
  in HIV vaccine testing, 1714
  keratoconjunctivitis in, 1390, 1390t, 1402,
    1403
  pancreatic infections in, 959t, 960
  progressive, 1744-1745
  treatment of, 1749
  vaccine for, 740-741
Vaccinia immune globulin, 1745, 3574
  for conjunctivitis, 1390t
  for eczema vaccinatum, 1745
  for poxvirus infections, 1749
  for progressive vaccinia, 1745
Vagina
  anaerobic colonization of, 2839
  aphthous ulcers of, 1345
  in host defense, 36
  in urinary tract infections, 880
  lesions of. See Genital lesions.
Vaginal cuff cellulitis, postoperative, 1376-1377,
    1377t
Vaginal flora
  assessment of, 1360-1361
  in secondary peritonitis, 932-933
  Mycoplasma spp. in, 2281
Vaginal secretions
  abnormal, 1358, 1358t
  examination of, 1360-1361, 1360f
  normal, 1357-1358, 1358f, 1358t
  sampling of, 1360
Vaginal warts. See Genital warts.
Vaginitis emphysematosa, 3206
Vaginitis/vulvovaginitis, 212, 1357-1370
  desquamative inflammatory, 1367-1368, 1367f,
    1367t, 1368f
  emphysematous, 3206
  estrogen deficiency, 1369
  examination in, 1359-1360, 1359t, 1360f
  from Candida, 1344, 1362-1365, 1363f, 1364f,
    1364t, 1369, 2942, 2942f, 2946, 2951
    genital herpes and, 1768
    in HIV infection, 1628
  from herpes simplex virus, 1768
  from Saccharomyces cerevisiae, 1362
  from Streptococcus agalactiae (group B),
    2424, 2431
  from Streptococcus pyogenes (group A), 2375
  from Trichomonas vaginalis, 1361-1362,
    1362t, 1363f, 1363t, 3205-3208
    in HIV infection, 1628
  gonococcal, 2523
  history in, 1358-1359, 1359t
  in neonate, 1359
Vaginosis, bacterial, 1365-1367, 1366f, 1366t
  anaerobic, 2813
  clue cells in, 1360
  from gram-negative bacilli, 2842
  in HIV infection, 1628
  laboratory studies for, 212
  pelvic inflammatory disease and, 1378
Vagococcus spp., 217t, 218

Valacyclovir, 515t. See also Acyclovir.
  activity spectrum of, 516
  dosage of, 682t-683t
    in renal insufficiency, 518, 519t
  drug interactions with, 686t
  for cytomegalovirus infection, in transplant
    recipients, 1795-1796
  for genital herpes, 1344, 1769
  for herpes B virus infection, 1834, 1834t
  for herpes simplex keratitis, 1402t
  for herpes simplex virus infection, 519, 519t,
    1773t-1774t, 1774
    in HIV infection, 1683t
  for herpes virus B infection, 520
  for herpes zoster, 1784
  for herpes zoster ophthalmicus, 1403t
  for herpesvirus infection, 1760t, 1761
  for human herpesvirus 6 infection, 1823
  for varicella-zoster virus infection, in HIV
    infection, 1686t
  formulations of, 649t
  pharmacokinetics of, 517-518, 519t
  toxicity of, 518
  uses of, 518-520
Valganciclovir, 515t, 528-530
  activity spectrum of, 528
  dosage of, 682t-683t
  drug interactions with, 692t
  for cytomegalovirus infection, 530, 1792
    in encephalitis, 1591
    in HIV infection, 1683t, 1685t-1686t, 1697
    in transplant recipients, 1793-1796, 3493
  for herpesvirus infection, 1760t, 1761
  formulations of, 649t
  in renal insufficiency, 529t
  pharmacokinetics of, 529
  prophylactic, for transplant-related
    cytomegalovirus infections, 3482
Valley fever, 3040. See also Coccidioides immitis.
Valtorcitabine, for chronic hepatitis B, 1448,
    1448t
Van C, in Enterococcus resistance, 264
Vancomycin, 417-423
  administration of, 420
  adverse reactions to, 421
  antimicrobial activity of, 418
  distribution of, 419-420
  dosage of, 668t-669t
    in renal insufficiency, 420-421
    monitoring of, 422
  drug interactions with, 421-422, 699t
  excretion of, 420
  for asplenia, 3529
  for bacillary infections, 418, 2495
  for bacterial arthritis, 1316t
  for brain abscess, 1157, 1159t
  for cavernous sinus thrombosis, 1424
  for cellulitis, 1180
  for Chryseobacterium meningosepticum, 2758
  for Clostridium difficile–associated colitis, 423,
    1257, 1258, 1258t
  for dialysis-related peritonitis, 942, 942t
  for endocarditis, 1050t
  for endophthalmitis, 1410-1411
  for enterococcal endocarditis, 998, 2416,
    2416t
    penicillin-resistant, 996, 997
    prosthetic valve, 1027-1028, 1027t, 1028t
  for enterococcal infections, 2416. See also
    Vancomycin, resistance to, by enterococci.
  for febrile neutropenia, 3451t, 3452, 3453f,
    3453t
  for listeriosis, 2483
  for meningitis, 1106t, 1107t, 1113, 1114

Vancomycin (Continued)
  for methicillin-resistant Staphylococcus aureus,
    184-185
  for orbital/preseptal cellulitis, 1423f, 1424
  for osteomyelitis, 1324t, 1325
  for pneumococcal pneumonia, 2405
  for primary peritonitis, 931
  for sepsis, 919t
  for shunt infections, 1129t, 1130
  for staphylococcal endocarditis, 998-999, 2344t
    prosthetic valve, 1026t, 1027
  for staphylococcal infections, 424t
  for streptococcal endocarditis, 995
    prosthetic valve, 1027t
  for Streptococcus agalactiae (group B), 2429,
    2430, 2430t
  for Streptococcus anginosus group, 2455
  for Streptococcus bovis, 2418
  for streptococcus group C, 2445
  for Streptococcus pneumoniae meningitis, 2405
  for viridians streptococcal meningitis, 2439
  formulations of, 648t
  mechanism of action of, 417-418
  minimal inhibitory concentrations of, 359t
  pharmacology of, 419-421
  prophylactic, perioperative, 3543t
  resistance to, 418-419
    by enterococci, 185, 264, 264t, 418-419,
      2335, 2415, 2417
      contact precautions and, 3329
      disinfection/sterilization and, 3341-3342
      in pseudomembranous colitis, 1252
      linezolid for, 438
      metronidazole for, 392-393
    by Erysipelothrix rhusiopathiae, 2498
    by Leuconostoc, 2418
    by Staphylococcus, 185, 264, 264t
    by Staphylococcus aureus, contact
      precautions and, 3329
  structure of, 417
  teicoplanin interaction with, 424
  tolerance to, by streptococcus group G, 2446
  uses of, 422-423
Varicella. See also Varicella-zoster virus.
  clinical manifestations of, 1783
  conjunctivitis from, 1389
  diagnosis of, 1784
  differential diagnosis of, 1784
  epidemiology of, 1781
  etiology of, 1781
  historical perspective on, 1781
  in immunocompromised host, 1782, 1783, 1785
  in neonate, 1782-1783
    prevention of, 1785
  in pregnancy, prevention of, 1785
  ocular involvement in, 1389, 1401, 1402
  pathogenesis of, 1782
  prevention of, 1785
  rash in, 740
  Reye's syndrome in, 1783
  treatment of, 1784-1785
  vs. enteroviral infections, 2150
  vs. smallpox, 1747f
  vs. variola, 740
Varicella vaccine, 1785, 3563f, 3564t, 3572-3573
  schedule for children, 3564t
Varicella-zoster immune globulin, 1785, 3574
  for adults, 346f, 347f
  for HIV infection, 1682t
  for pediatric HIV infection, 1650
Varicella-zoster immune plasma, 1785
Varicella-zoster virus, 1780-1785
  acute pancreatitis from, 959t, 959t
  acute retinal necrosis from, 1416, 1417f

Varicella-zoster virus (Continued)
  acyclovir-resistant, foscarnet for, 528
  antiretroviral therapy effect on, 1561
  Bell's palsy from, 1766
  cerebellar ataxia from, 1782
  characteristics of, 1781
  clinical features of, 1758, 1758t, 1760t, 1782-
    1784, 1783f
  collection of, 233t
  diagnosis of, 1761, 1784
  differential diagnosis of, 1784
  encephalitis from, 1782, 1783
  epidemiology of, 1759, 1759t, 1780, 1781-
    1782
  genome of, 1781
  historical perspective on, 1781
  immune response in, 1758
  in HIV infection, 1556, 1561
    retinitis from, 1560
    treatment of, 1682t, 1683t, 1686t-1687t,
      1696
  in immunocompromised host, 1782, 1783-
    1784, 1785, 3439, 3494
  in neonate, 1782-1783
  in pregnancy, 1782-1783
  in transplant recipients, 3439, 3494, 3508
  isolation of, 1781
  keratitis from, 1401-1403, 1402t, 1782, 1783
  laryngitis from, 759
  meningitis from, 1085, 1101, 1783
  occupational exposure to, management of,
    3413-3414
  ocular complications from, 1389, 1401-1403,
    1402t, 1416, 1417f, 1782, 1783
  pathogenesis of, 1782
  pediatric, 234
  pneumonitis from, 1782
  prevention of, 1760t, 1761, 1785
  reactivation of. See Herpes zoster.
  replication of, 1781
  structure of, 1743f, 1756-1757, 1756t, 1757f,
    1781
  susceptibility testing for, 238
  transmission of, 1759-1761, 1759t, 1782
    nosocomial, 3410-3414, 3412f, 3413f
      investigation of, 3411-3413, 3412f, 3413f
      mechanisms of, 3411
      prevention of, 3411
      risk of, 3410-3411
    treatment of, 1760t, 1761, 1784-1785
      with acyclovir, 519-520
      with antiviral drugs, 515t
      with brivudin, 540
  variants of, 1781
  varicella from. See Varicella.
Variola virus, 1743f. See also Smallpox.
Vascular candidiasis, 2947
Vascular closure devices, femoral artery,
  infections of, 1040
Vascular device-associated infections, 3347-3358.
  See also Intravascular devices, percutaneous,
  infections due to.
Vascular gangrene, 1188t
Vascular insufficiency, osteomyelitis in, 1327-
  1328, 1327t
Vascular prosthetic grafts, infections of, 1036-
  1039
Vasculitis. See also Arteritis; Endarteritis.
  factor H deficiency in, 82
  from Campylobacter fetus, 2553
  from Candida, 2947, 2951
  from Chlamydia (Chlamydophila) pneumoniae,
    atherosclerosis and, 2263-2266
  from parvovirus B19, 1895

Vasculitis (Continued)
  from Salmonella, 2646
  in chronic leptomeningeal infections, 1144
  in injection drug users, 3467-3468, 3468f
  syndrome of abdominal pain, diarrhea, and
    eosinophilia from, 1281t, 1283
Vasoconstriction, inflammation-induced, 912-913
Vasopressin, for sepsis, 920
VDRL test, 2778, 2779, 2780
  for endemic treponematoses, 2787
Vector-borne disease, 178-181, 179f-181f. See
  also Zoonoses.
Vegetables, Salmonella in, 2640
Veillonella spp., 2848, 2849
  chloramphenicol for, 367t
  in oral cavity, 787, 787t
Velocardiofacial syndrome, 150t
Vena cava filters, infections of, 1041
Veneral Disease Research Laboratory test, 2778,
  2779, 2780
  for endemic treponematoses, 2787
Venereal disease. See Sexually transmitted
  diseases.
Venereal warts. See Genital warts; Human
  papillomavirus(es).
Venezuelan equine encephalitis, 235t, 1913-1919,
  1914t. See also Alphaviruses.
  isolation precautions for, 3330t
Venezuelan hemorrhagic fever, 2090-2096, 2091t.
  See also South American hemorrhagic
  fevers.
  as biological weapon, 3627-3629, 3627t
Veno-occlusive disease, in stem cell transplant,
  3487
Venotomy, for suppurative thrombophlebitis,
  1005
Venous sinus thrombosis, 1168-1170, 1169f
  suppurative intracranial, 794, 795f, 1168-1170,
    1169f
    cavernous, 794, 795f, 797t, 1168-1170,
      1169f
    lateral, 1168-1170
    sagittal, 1168-1170, 1169f
Venous thrombosis. See also Suppurative
  thrombophlebitis.
  in airplane passengers, 3644
Ventilator-associated pneumonia, 835-836, 3362-
  3368. See also Pneumonia, nosocomial.
  diagnosis of, 827
  lung abscess from, 854
Ventriculitis
  shunt-related, 1128
  vancomycin for, 420, 422-423
Verrucae. See Human papillomavirus(es); Warts.
Verruga peruana, 739-740, 3653f
  from Bartonella bacilliformis, 2733-2734,
    2734f
Vertebral osteomyelitis, 1326-1327, 1326f
  from Aspergillus, 2966, 2966f
  from Candida, 2946, 2947f
  from Coccidioides immitis, 3044, 3045f
  from Pseudomonas aeruginosa, 2602-2603
  in injection drug users, 3465
Vertigo, minocycline and, 364
Vesicles, 730t, 731. See also Rash.
  causes of, 733-734
Vesicobullous eruptions, differential diagnosis of,
  733-734
Vesicoureteral reflux
  bacteriuria in, 887
  imaging of, 900, 900f
  in urinary tract infections, 881, 882f,
    886
  intrarenal, 886

Vesicular rash. See also Rash.
  differential diagnosis of, 1784
Vesicular stomatitis, 2150
Vesicular stomatitis virus, 2044-2046, 2045t
  adherence by, 14f
  receptor for, 1732t
Vesiculobullous eruptions, 733-734. See also
  Rash.
Vesiculoviruses, 2044-2046, 2045t, 2047
Vesiviruses, 2196
Vestibular toxicity, of aminoglycosides, 341, 343
Vestibulitis, 1369-1370, 1370f
Viannia spp., 3145t, 3146-3147
Vibrio [spp.], 2544, 2546
  bullous eruptions from, 734
  culture of, 1224
  endocarditis from, 992
  isolation precautions for, 3330t
  laboratory identification of, 220
  laboratory detection of, 212
  tetracyclines for, 358
Vibrio alginolyticus, 2546
  dysentery from, 1266
Vibrio carchariae, 2546
Vibrio cholerae, 2536-2542. See also Cholera.
  diarrhea from, electrolyte concentration in,
    2537, 2537t
  dysentery from, 1266
  enterotoxin of, 29, 2537
  environment of, 2537-2538, 2538f
  foodborne disease from, 1288, 1292, 2538
  gastric acid and, 1217
  genetic regulation of, 7, 8
  identification of, 2537
  isolation of, 2537
  microbiology of, 2536-2537
  non-O1, 2547
  O1, 2537, 2539
  O1 El Tor, 2537, 2540, 2541f
  O139, 177, 2537, 2539, 2540, 2541f
  O139 (Bengal), noninflammatory diarrhea
    from, 1239-1240
  phage-encoded, 6t
  regulation of, 7t
  serotypes of, 2536-2537
  transmission of, 2538-2539, 2539f
  vaccines for, 3562
Vibrio cincinnatiensis, 2546
Vibrio damsela, dysentery from, 1266
Vibrio fluvialis, 2546
  dysentery from, 1266
Vibrio furnissii, 2546
Vibrio hollisae, 2546
  dysentery from, 1266
Vibrio metschnikovii, 2546
Vibrio mimicus, 2547
Vibrio parahaemolyticus, 2544-2545
  cytotoxin of, 1221
  dysentery from, 1266
  enterotoxin of, 1220
  foodborne disease from, 1288, 2544,
    2545
Vibrio vulnificus, 2545-2546
  aminoglycosides for, 344t
  bullous eruptions from, 734, 3653f
  cellulitis from, 1179
  dysentery from, 1266
  in hepatic impairment, 908
Vidarabine, 515t, 524f, 538-539
  dosage of, 682t-683t
  drug interactions with, 699t
  for ocular vaccinia, 1390t, 1403
Video-assisted thorascopic surgery (VATS), for
  pleural effusion/empyema, 851

Vincent's angina, 754, 756, 791, 2841
Vincristine
  for HIV-related non-Hodgkin's lymphoma,
    1605
  neurotoxicity of, 1594t
Violacein, in *Chromobacterium violaceum,* 2755
Viral capsid, 1730-1731, 1731f
Viral hemorrhagic fevers, 237. *See also specific*
    fevers.
  arenavirus, 2090-2096, 2091t
  as biological weapons, 3626-3629,
    3626t-3629t
  clinical features of, 3629t
  isolation precautions for, 3329, 3330t
  rash in, 739
Viral infections. *See also* Virus(s) *and specific*
    infections and viruses.
  antiviral drugs for, 514-542, 515t
  cell-mediated immunity in, 122
  chronic, 1737
  defenses against, 126-127
  genetic susceptibility to, 43
  immunomodulators in, 514
  laboratory tests for, 232-239, 235t, 237t
  latent, 1737
  pathogenesis of, 1735
  pediatric, 234-235, 235t
  persistent, 1737-1738
  virulence of, in selenium deficiency, 142
  vitamin A for, 141
  vs. enteric fever, 1274t
Viral proteins, 1730-1731, 1731f
Viral rhinosinusitis, 772. *See also* Common cold.
Viral set point, 2121
Viramidine, 541
Viremia, 1736-1737, 1736f
Virginiamycin, 425
Viridans streptococci. *See Streptococcus viridans*
    group.
Virions, 1729, 1730f
Virulence, 167
  definition of, 3
  genetic regulation of, 6-8, 7t
  molecular perspective on, 3-12
Virulence factors
  definition of, 3
  phage-encoded, 5, 6t
  plasmid-encoded, 5, 6t
Virulence genes, 10-11
  horizontal exchange of, 5, 6t
Virus(es). *See also under* Viral.
  antibody neutralization of, 55
  assembly of, 1730-1731
  classification of, 1729, 1730t
  collection and transport of, 232, 233t, 234
  complement interactions with, 77
  enveloped, 1730-1731
  genome of, 1729-1730, 1730t
    replication of, 1733-1734
  historical perspective on, 1729
  host cell manipulation by, 10
  host entry by, 1735-1736
  interactions of
    with cell, 1731-1735
    with environment, 1738
    with host, 1735-1738
  oncogenic, 1738
  pathogenicity of, 1735
  persistence of, 1737-1738
  proteins of, 1730-1731, 1731f
  receptor-mediated endocytosis of, 1733, 1733f
  receptors for, 1732-1733, 1732t
  replication of, 1731-1735
    attachment in, 1731-1733, 1732f

Virus(es) *(Continued)*
  cell killing in, 1734, 1734f
  cell penetration in, 1733, 1733f
  disassembly in, 1733, 1733f
  drug targeting of, 1734-1735
  genomic, 1733-1734
  stages in, 1732
  routes of spread of, 1735-1737, 1735f, 1736f
  structure of, 1729-1731, 1730f, 1731f
  susceptibility testing for, 238-239
  symmetry of, 1730, 1730f
  tropism of, 1732, 1737
  virulence of, 1735
    determinants of, 1738
Virus particles, 1729, 1730f
Virus-associated hemophagocytic syndrome,
    1894-1895
Visceral larva migrans
  from *Baylisascaris procyonis,* 3294, 3295
  from *Toxocara,* 3293-3294, 3294t
  vs. enteric fever, 1275t, 1278
Visceral leishmaniasis, 3145t, 3147-3149, 3148.
    See also Leishmaniasis.
Viscerotropic leishmaniasis, 3145t, 3148
Vision loss
  from ethambutol, 493
  in cryptococcosis, 3005
  in endophthalmitis, 1411
  in mucormycosis, 2976
  in onchocerciasis, 3273-3274
Vitamin(s)
  fat-soluble, 141
  for elderly patient, 146, 146t
  water-soluble, 141-144
Vitamin A, 141
  deficiency of, 141, 606-607
    in acute respiratory infections, 175
    in elderly patient, 146, 146t
    in perinatal HIV transmission, 1621
  for measles, 2036
  for measles pneumonia, 604t, 606-607
Vitamin B_{12} deficiency, in elderly patient, 146,
    146t
Vitamin C, 141-142
  deficiency of, 141-142
  for colds, 604t, 608-609, 750
Vitamin D receptor
  in hepatitis B susceptibility, 45
  in infection susceptibility, 48
Vitamin E, 141
  deficiency of, in elderly patient, 146, 146t
  for elderly patient, 146-147, 146t
Vitrectomy
  for biopsy, 1409, 1410, 1410f
  for endophthalmitis, 1410, 1411
  for ocular candidiasis, 1418
Vitreous, aspiration of, 1409, 1410, 1410f
Vitronectin, 70t, 74t
Vittaforma corneae, 3237, 3238t. *See also*
    Microsporidia.
  treatment of, 574t
Vittaforma (Nosema) ocularum, keratitis from,
    1405
Vogt-Koyanagi-Harada syndrome, meningitis in,
    1139
Vomiting, 1238-1239, 1239t
Voriconazole, 503f, 510
  dosage of, 678t-679t
  drug interactions with, 699t
  for allergic fungal sinusitis, 3072
  for aspergillosis, 2968, 2968t
  for blastomycosis, 3037
  for brain abscess, 1159t, 1160, 1161
  for cancer-related febrile neutropenia, 3455

Voriconazole *(Continued)*
  for candidiasis, 2949-2951
  for coccidioidomycosis, 3048-3049
  for dark-walled fungal infections, 3072
  for endophthalmitis, 1411
  for eumycetoma, 2995
  for fusariosis, 3073
  for pseudallescheriasis, 3069
  for *Scedosporium prolificans,* 3069
  formulations of, 649t
  prophylactic, for transplant recipients, 3483
Vulva
  lichen sclerosus of, 1369
  verrucous lesions of, 1341, 1841-1850, 1846f.
    See also Genital lesions; Genital warts;
    Human papillomavirus(es).
Vulvar vestibulitis, 1369-1370, 1370f
Vulvitis, 1369
  focal, 1369-1370, 1370f
Vulvovaginitis. *See* Vaginitis/vulvovaginitis.

W

W-1 antigen, 3028, 3029
Walking pneumonia, 2273
Wangiella (Exophiala) dermatitidis, brain abscess
    from, 3070, 3076t
Warble, 3308
Warfarin
  metronidazole interactions with, 393t
  quinolone effects on, 459
Warts, 151t. *See also* Human papillomavirus(es).
  anogenital, 1341-1344, 1842-1850, 1846f. *See*
    also Genital warts.
  cutaneous, 1842, 1844f, 1845
    in epidermodysplasia verruciformis, 1842,
      1845, 1850
    treatment of, 1848
  oral, 1847, 1850
  plane, 1842, 1845
  plantar, 1842, 1845
Waste, infectious, 3342, 3343t
Wasting, 140
  in HIV infection, 145-146, 1554
Water intake. *See* Fluid management.
Water, superoxidized, disinfection with, 3334
Water systems
  in cholera prevention, 2541-2542
  in *Legionella* infection prevention, 2711, 2712,
    2713, 2720, 2728
Waterborne disease, 1291, 1291t
  bioterrorism-related, isolation precautions for,
    3330t
  cryptosporidiosis as, 3217
  gastrointestinal, 1215-1216, 1216t
  giardiasis as, 3200
  hepatitis A as, 2166, 2171, 2171f, 2172
  hepatitis E as, 2207, 2207f, 2208
  in travelers, 3643
  microsporidiosis as, 3249
  shigellosis as, 2657, 2659
  toxoplasmosis as, 3173
Wayson stain, for *Yersina pestis,* 2695-2696
Weanling diarrhea, 1237-1238
Weeksella [spp.], 2751t, 2762
Weeksella virosa, 2762
Weeksella zoohelcum, 2762
Wegener's granulomatosis
  chest film in, 866f
  meningitis in, 1139
Weight loss, in acquired immunodeficiency
    syndrome, 145-146
Weil-Felix test, 2307
Weil's disease, 2792

Well's syndrome, 1180
Wesselsbron virus, 1945t
West African trypanosomiasis. *See also*
    Trypanosomiasis, African.
    treatment of, 576t
West Nile encephalitis, 179-180, 180f, 235-236,
    235t, 1145, 1146
    clinical features of, 1940, 1940f
    course of, 1940, 1940f
    diagnosis of, 1942
    epidemiology of, 1932t, 1933-1934, 1933f-1935f
    geographic distribution of, 1927f
    historical perspective on, 1928
    in elderly, 3521
    pathogenesis of, 1937-1938
    prevention of, 1944
    rash from, 732
    transfusion-related, 3387
    treatment of, 1944
Western blot, 57-58
    for *Borrelia burgdorferi*, 2804, 2805f
    for HIV infection, 1508t, 1514-1516, 1514f,
        1515f, 1516t
Western equine encephalitis, 235t, 1913-1919,
    1914t. *See also* Alphaviruses.
    isolation precautions for, 3330t
Wet mounts, 214
Whataroa virus, 1913-1919, 1914t. *See also*
    Alphaviruses.
Wheezing
    differential diagnosis of, 816
    in bronchiolitis, 814-815
    in human metapneumovirus infection, 2028-
        2029, 2028t, 2029t
    in respiratory syncytial virus infection, 761,
        816, 2015t, 2016t, 2019
Whipple's disease, 1145, 1306-1310
    clinical features of, 1308-1309, 1308t
    endocarditis in, 993
    epidemiology of, 1307
    etiology of, 1306-1307, 1306f
    pathogenesis of, 1307
    pathology of, 1307-1308, 1308f
    treatment of, 1309-1310, 1310t
    uveitis in, 1417
Whipworm, 576t
White blood cell transfusion
    for chronic granulomatous disease, 109
    for granulocytopenia, 109
White blood cells, in cerebrospinal fluid, 1081,
    1081t
White piedra, 3061, 3073
Whitewater Arroyo virus, 2093-2094
Whitfield's ointment
    for dermatophytosis, 3058
    for tinea nigra, 3061
Whitlow, herpetic, 1769, 1769f, 1773t
Whooping cough. *See Bordetella* [spp.]; Pertussis.
Widal test, for *Salmonella typhi*, 1275
Wilson's disease, 1436
WIN compounds, 20t, 21
Winter vomiting disease, 1238-1239, 1239t
Wiskott-Aldrich syndrome, 150t
    laboratory studies in, 149
    severe combined immunodeficiency in, 66
    T-cell function in, 153
Wiskott-Aldrich syndrome protein, 153
Wohlfahrtia magnifica, myiasis from, 3308-3310,
    3308t
Wolbachia spp., 577t, 2311, 2312, 3272, 3273
    classification of, 2284
    in filariasis, 2286, 3271
    pathogenesis of, 2286
    vectors of, 2285t

Women
    genitourinary infections in, 876, 886, 886f, 887
        anaerobic, 2813
        from gram-negative bacilli, 2842
        from *Clostridium*, 2830
        from HIV, 1619. *See also* Women, HIV
            infection in.
        from *Mycobacterium tuberculosis*, 2880-
            2881
        from *Streptococcus agalactiae* (group B), 6
        sexually transmitted. *See* Sexually
            transmitted diseases.
    gynecologic surgery in, surgical site infections
        in, 1376-1378, 1377t
    HIV infection in, 1616-1632
        bacterial infections in, 1627
        bacterial vaginosis in, 1628
        cervicovaginal shedding in, 1628-1630
        clinical manifestations of, 1627-1631
        epidemiology of, 1617-1618
        genital ulcers in, 1630
        human papillomavirus infection in, 1629
        in United States, 1617
        Kaposi's sarcoma in, 1627-1628
        malignancy in, 1627-1628
        menstruation in, 1489, 1619, 1630
        metabolic complications of, 1630-1631
        mucopurulent cervicitis in, 1628
        opportunistic processes in, 1627-1630
        ovulation in, 1630
        pelvic inflammatory disease in, 1628-1629
        prognosis of, 1631
        sex hormones in, 1630
        treatment of, 1631-1632
        Trichomonas vaginitis in, 1628
        vulvovaginal candidiasis in, 1627, 1628
        worldwide prevalence of, 1617-1618
    temperature in, 705, 706, 707
    urinary tract infections in, 876, 886, 886f, 887
World Wide Web, 3658-3660. *See also* Digital
    resources.
Wound(s)
    clean, 3534, 3534t
    clean-contaminated, 3534, 3534t
    contaminated, 3534, 3534t
Wound botulism, 2823, 2824-2825
    in injection drug users, 3472
Wound diphtheria, 1180-1181
Wound infections
    bite, 3552-3555
    burn, 3547-3551
    Clostridium in, 2830-2831, 2837
    Enterococcus in, 2413
    laboratory studies for, 213
    postoperative. *See* Postoperative infections.
    Pseudomonas aeruginosa in, 2589-2590
        osteomyelitis from, 2603
    specimen collection and transport from, 207t
    staphylococcal, 2341
    topical antibacterial therapy for, 479-481
Wound myiasis, 3307-3310, 33108t
Wuchereria bancrofti, 3270-3272, 3270f-3272f
    diethylcarbamazine for, 594
    lymphangitis from, 1208, 1212
    sclerosing mediastinitis from, 1075
    treatment of, 572t, 577t
    tropical pulmonary eosinophilia and, 3274-3275

X

X factor, 216t
    in *Haemophilus influenzae* growth, 2661
Xenopsylla cheopis, as murine typhus vector,
    2306

Xenotransplantation. *See also* Transplantation.
    retrovirus transmission in, 1521
Xigris, for sepsis, 921
X-linked agammaglobulinemia, chronic
    meningoencephalitis in, 2154-2155
X-linked immunodeficiency with hyperIgG
    syndrome, cryptosporidiosis in, 3218
X-linked lymphoproliferative disease, 1435, 1807,
    2151
    treatment of, 1814-1815
X-linked neutropenia, Wiskott-Aldrich syndrome
    protein in, 153
Xylitol, for otitis media, 769-770
Xylohypha (Cladophialophora) bantiana, brain
    abscess from, 3070, 3070f

Y

Yatapoxviruses, poxvir
Yaws, 2786-2787, 2786f, 2787f
Yeast, 229, 230t. *See also* Fungi *and specific
    yeasts.*
    appearance of, in tissue, 2936f-2937f, 2938t
    forms of, 2935
    identification of, 230, 230t, 231, 232f
    spores of, 2935-2936
    vs. molds, 2935
Yeast infections, vaginal, 1344
Yellow fever
    as biological weapon, 3627-3629, 3628t
    clinical features of, 1938, 3629t, 3653f
    diagnosis of, 1942
    epidemiology of, 1929
    geographic distribution of, 1927, 1927f, 3640f
    hepatitis from, 1435
    immunization for, for elderly, 3522
    outbreaks of, 1932t
    pathogenesis of, 1935-1936
    prevention of, 1943
    treatment of, 1943
    vaccine for, 1943, 3573
        for travelers, 3639-3640, 3639t
    vs. malaria, 3133
Yersinia [spp.], 2691-2700
    appendicitis from, 969
    endocarditis from, 992
    invasiveness of, 1222
    laboratory detection of, 212
    plasmid-encoded, 6t
    regulation of, 7t
Yersinia enterocolitica, 2697-2700
    characteristics of, 2698
    culture of, 1224
    diagnosis of, 2699
    enteric fever from, 1274t
    enteric fever–like syndrome from, 1276-1277
    enteritis from, 1267
    enterocolitis from, 2699
    epidemiology of, 2698-2699, 2698f
    erythema nodosum from, 2699
    foodborne disease from, 1289, 1292
    from red blood cell transfusion, 3388
    history of, 2697-2698
    mesenteric adenitis from, 1279, 1279t, 1280
    pathogenesis of, 2699
    pharyngitis from, 755, 756, 2365, 2699
    pyogenic liver abscess from, 952
    reactive polyarthritis from, 2699
    septicemia from, 2699
    treatment of, 2699-2700
        with quinolones, 455t
        with trimethoprim-sulfamethoxazole, 444
Yersinia frederiksenii, 2700
Yersinia intermedia, 2700

Yersinia kristensenii, 2700
Yersinia pestis, 2691-2697. *See also* Plague.
  as biological weapon, 3601-3604, 6303t
  characteristics of, 2691
  culture of, 3603
  disinfection/sterilization and, 3342
  evolution of, 6
  isolation precautions for, 3329-3330, 3330t
  laboratory detection of, 213-214
  pathogenesis of, 2693
Yersinia pseudotuberculosis
  characteristics of, 2698
  diagnosis of, 2699
  enteric fever from, 1274t
  enteric fever–like syndrome from, 1276-1277
  epidemiology of, 2699
  history of, 2697-2698
  in plague bacillus study, 10
  mesenteric adenitis from, 1279, 2699
  pathogenesis of, 2699
  treatment of, 2700
Yogurt
  for rotavirus, 1909
  for vulvovaginal candidiasis, 1365

Z

Zalcitabine, 1657t, 1658
  dosage of, 684t-685t
  drug interactions with, 699t
  for perinatal HIV transmission prevention, 1625t
  formulations of, 649t
  neurotoxicity of, 1594t
  pancreatitis from, 1579
  pediatric, 1646t
  resistance to, 1660
  structure of, 1656f

Zanamivir, 515t, 539-540
  dosage of, 682t-683t
  for influenza, 805, 2072t, 2073-2074
    for prophylaxis, 2078
  formulations of, 649t
  side effects of, 2072t, 2074
  structure of, 536f
Zidovudine, 1655-1657, 1657t
  dosage of, 684t-685t
  drug interactions with, 700t
  for AIDS dementia, 1586
  for postexposure prophylaxis, 1672
  formulations of, 649t
  ganciclovir interactions with, 529
  in pregnancy, 1626-1627
  myopathy from, 1596
  neurotoxicity of, 1594t, 1597t
  pediatric, 1646t
  prophylactic
    adverse reactions to, 3403
    after occupational exposure to HIV, 3402, 3402t
    for perinatal HIV transmission, 1621-1624, 1625t, 1640t
    in pregnancy, 3403
  resistance to, 1660
  structure of, 1656f
Ziehl-Neelsen stain, for mycobacteria, 225
Zika virus, 1945t
Zinc
  deficiency of, 142
    in elderly patient, 146, 146t
    prostatitis and, 1382
  for colds, 604t, 608, 750
  for diarrhea, 604t, 607
  in inflammation, 39
ZO-1, 9

Zoonoses, 4, 178-181, 3630-3636. *See also specific infections and vectors.*
  animal reservoirs for, 3632t, 3633t, 3634-3635
  classification of, 3630, 3631t-3632t
  defining criteria for, 3630
  diagnosis of, 3635-3636
  distribution of
    geographic, 3632-3634
    in nature, 3634-3635
  epidemiology of, 3632-3635
  etiology of, 3631t-3632t
  examples of, 3631t-3632t
  from *Campylobacter,* 2549-2550
  from paramyxoviruses, 2038-2044
    classification of, 2038, 2039f
    Hendra virus, 2038-2041, 2039f, 2039t
    Menangle virus, 2038-2039, 2042-2044
    Nipah virus, 2038-2039, 2039t, 2040f, 2041-2042, 2043f
    structure of, 2039, 2040f
  from vesicular stomatitis virus, 2044-2046, 2045t
  from *Yersinia enterocolitica,* 2698
  public health impact of, 3630-3634
  relapsing fever as, 2795-2797
  retrovirus infections as, 2119
  risk factors for, 3631t-3632t, 3633t
  transmission of, 3631t-3632t
Zoster. *See* Varicella-zoster virus.
Zoster ophthalmicus, acyclovir for, 519, 520
Zoster sine herpes, 1085
Zygomycetes, 229, 2974, 2974t
  in stem cell transplant, 3496
Zygomycosis, 2973. *See also* Mucormycosis.